*Principles and Practice of*

# ENDOCRINOLOGY
## AND
# METABOLISM

# Principles and Practice of
# ENDOCRINOLOGY
# AND
# METABOLISM

## THIRD EDITION

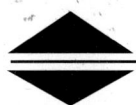

**EDITOR**

# Kenneth L. Becker

**ASSOCIATE EDITORS**
**John P. Bilezikian**
**William J. Bremner**
**Wellington Hung**
**C. Ronald Kahn**
**D. Lynn Loriaux**
**Eric S. Nylén**
**Robert W. Rebar**
**Gary L. Robertson**
**Richard H. Snider, Jr.**
**Leonard Wartofsky**

## With 330 Contributors

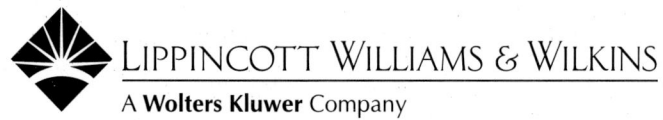

LIPPINCOTT WILLIAMS & WILKINS
A **Wolters Kluwer** Company
Philadelphia · Baltimore · New York · London
Buenos Aires · Hong Kong · Sydney · Tokyo

*Acquisitions Editor*: Lisa McAllister
*Developmental Editor*: Anne Snyder
*Supervising Editor*: Mary Ann McLaughlin
*Production Editor*: Shannon Garza, Silverchair Science + Communications
*Manufacturing Manager*: Colin Warnock
*Cover Designer*: Joan Greenfield
*Compositor*: Silverchair Science + Communications
*Printer*: World Color/Rand McNally

**Library of Congress Cataloging-in-Publication Data**

Principles and practice of endocrinology and metabolism / editor, Kenneth L. Becker ; associate editors, John P. Bilezikian ... [et al.].--3rd ed.
   p. ; cm.
  Includes bibliographical references and index.
  ISBN 0-7817-1750-7
   1. Endocrinology. 2. Endocrine glands--Diseases. 3. Metabolism--Disorders. I. Becker, Kenneth L.
  [DNLM: 1. Endocrine Diseases. 2. Metabolic Diseases. WK 100 P957 2000]
  RC648 .P67 2000
  616.4--dc21
                        00-022095

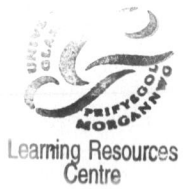
Care has been taken to confirm the accuracy of the information presented and to describe generally accepted practices. However, the authors, editors, and publisher are not responsible for errors or omissions or for any consequences from application of the information in this book and make no warranty, expressed or implied, with respect to the currency, completeness, or accuracy of the contents of the publication. Application of this information in a particular situation remains the professional responsibility of the practitioner.

The authors, editors, and publisher have exerted every effort to ensure that drug selection and dosage set forth in this text are in accordance with current recommendations and practice at the time of publication. However, in view of ongoing research, changes in government regulations, and the constant flow of information relating to drug therapy and drug reactions, the reader is urged to check the package insert for each drug for any change in indications and dosage and for added warnings and precautions. This is particularly important when the recommended agent is a new or infrequently employed drug.

Some drugs and medical devices presented in this publication have Food and Drug Administration (FDA) clearance for limited use in restricted research settings. It is the responsibility of health care providers to ascertain the FDA status of each drug or device planned for use in their clinical practice.

10 9 8 7 6 5 4 3 2 1

# EDITOR

**Kenneth L. Becker,** MD, PhD
Professor of Medicine
Professor of Physiology and
    Experimental Medicine
Director of Endocrinology and Metabolism
George Washington University School of Medicine
    and Health Sciences
Veterans Affairs Medical Center
Washington, DC

# ASSOCIATE EDITORS

**John P. Bilezikian,** MD
Professor of Medicine and Pharmacology
Department of Medicine
Columbia University College of Physicians and Surgeons
New York, New York

**William J. Bremner,** MD, PhD
Robert G. Petersdorf Professor and Chairman
Department of Medicine
University of Washington School of Medicine
Seattle, Washington

**Wellington Hung,** MD, PhD
Professor Emeritus of Pediatrics
Georgetown University School of Medicine
Professorial Lecturer in Pediatrics
George Washington University School of Medicine
    and Health Sciences
Washington, DC

**C. Ronald Kahn,** MD
Mary K. Iacocca Professor of Medicine
Harvard Medical School
President and Director, Research Division
Joslin Diabetes Center
Boston, Massachusetts

**D. Lynn Loriaux,** MD, PhD
Professor and Chair
Department of Medicine
Oregon Health Sciences University School of Medicine
Portland, Oregon

**Eric S. Nylén,** MD
Associate Professor of Medicine
Department of Endocrinology
George Washington University School of Medicine
    and Health Sciences
Veterans Affairs Medical Center
Washington, DC

**Robert W. Rebar,** MD
Professor
Department of Obstetrics and Gynecology
University of Cincinnati College of Medicine
Chief, Obstetrics and Gynecology
University Hospital
Cincinnati, Ohio
Associate Executive Director
American Society for Reproductive Medicine
Birmingham, Alabama

**Gary L. Robertson,** MD
Professor of Medicine and Neurology
Department of Endocrinology
Northwestern University Medical School
Chicago, Illinois

**Richard H. Snider, Jr.,** PhD
Chief Chemist
Endocrinology Research Laboratory
Veterans Affairs Medical Center
Washington, DC

**Leonard Wartofsky,** MD, MPH, MACP
Clinical Professor of Medicine
Georgetown University School
    of Medicine
Clinical Professor of Medicine
George Washington University School
    of Medicine and Health Sciences
Chair, Department of Medicine
Washington Hospital Center
Clinical Professor of Medicine
Howard University College
    of Medicine
Washington, DC
Professor of Medicine and Physiology
Uniformed Services University of the Health Sciences
    F. Edward Hébert School of Medicine
Bethesda, Maryland

**Alaa Abou-Saif,** MD
Gastroenterology Fellow
Department of Medicine
Division of Gastroenterology
Georgetown University School of Medicine
Washington, DC

**Gary M. Abrams,** MD
Associate Professor of Clinical Neurology
Department of Neurology
University of California, San Francisco,
    School of Medicine
San Francisco, California

**Thomas Aceto, Jr.,** MD
Professor of Pediatrics
Chairman Emeritus of Pediatrics
Saint Louis University School
    of Medicine
Cardinal Glennon Children's Hospital
St. Louis, Missouri

**Bharat B. Aggarwal,** PhD
Professor of Medicine and Biochemistry
Department of Bioimmunotherapy
Chief, Cytokine Research Section
University of Texas–Houston Medical
    School
M. D. Anderson Cancer Center
Houston, Texas

**Zalman S. Agus,** MD
Emeritus Professor of Medicine
University of Pennsylvania School
    of Medicine
Philadelphia, Pennsylvania

**Rexford S. Ahima,** MD, PhD
Assistant Professor of Medicine
Division of Endocrinology, Diabetes
    and Metabolism
University of Pennsylvania School
    of Medicine
Philadelphia, Pennsylvania

**Andrew J. Ahmann,** MD
Assistant Professor of Medicine
Director of Adult Diabetes Services
Oregon Health Sciences University
    School of Medicine
Portland, Oregon

**Abdullah A. Alarifi,** MD
Consultant Endocrinologist
Department of Medicine
King Faisal Specialist Hospital and
    Research Centre
Riyadh, Kingdom of Saudi Arabia

**K. George M. M. Alberti,** MD, DPhil,
    PRCP, FRCP
Professor of Medicine
Department of Diabetes and Metabolism
University of Newcastle upon Tyne
    Faculty of Medicine
Newcastle upon Tyne, England

**Melvin G. Alper,** MD
Private Practice, Ophthalmology
Chevy Chase, Maryland

**John K. Amory,** MD
Assistant Professor
Department of Medicine
University of Washington School
    of Medicine
Veterans Affairs Puget Sound Health
    Care System
Seattle, Washington

**Neil Aronin,** MD
Professor of Medicine and
    Cell Biology
Director, Division of Endocrinology
    and Metabolism
University of Massachusetts Medical
    School
Worcester, Massachusetts

**Louis J. Aronne,** MD
Clinical Associate Professor
    of Medicine
Weill Medical College of Cornell
    University
New York, New York

**Gilbert P. August,** MD
Professor of Pediatrics
Department of Endocrinology
George Washington University School
    of Medicine and Health Sciences
Children's National Medical Center
Washington, DC

**Lloyd Axelrod,** MD
Associate Professor of Medicine
Harvard Medical School
Physician and Chief of the James
    Howard Means Firm
Massachusetts General Hospital
Boston, Massachusetts

**Daiva R. Bajorunas,** MD
Senior Director, Clinical Research
Global Project Team Leader,
    Metabolism
Aventis Pharmaceuticals
Bridgewater, New Jersey

**H. W. Gordon Baker,** MD, PhD, FRACP
Associate Professor
Department of Obstetrics and Gynaecology
University of Melbourne School
    of Medicine
Royal Women's Hospital
Victoria, Australia

**James R. Baker, Jr.,** MD
Professor of Medicine
Department of Internal Medicine–
    Allergy and Immunology
Chief, Division of Allergy
University of Michigan Medical School
Ann Arbor, Michigan

**William A. Banks,** MD
Professor of Internal Medicine
Division of Geriatrics
Saint Louis University School of Medicine
St. Louis, Missouri

**Robert L. Barbieri,** MD
Kate Macy Ladd Professor of Obstetrics,
    Gynecology and Reproductive Biology
Harvard Medical School
Boston, Massachusetts

**Marcelo J. Barrionuevo,** MD
Assistant Professor
Department of Obstetrics and Gynecology
University of Miami School of Medicine
Margate, Florida

**David S. Baskin,** MD, FACS
Professor of Neurosurgery and
    Anesthesiology
Baylor College of Medicine
Houston, Texas

**Gerhard Baumann,** MD
Professor of Medicine
Northwestern University Medical Center
Chicago, Illinois

**Peter H. Baylis,** MD, FRCP, FAMS
Professor of Experimental Medicine
Dean, Department of Medicine
The Medical School
University of Newcastle upon Tyne
    Faculty of Medicine
Newcastle upon Tyne, England

**David V. Becker,** MD
Professor of Radiology and Medicine
Division of Nuclear Medicine
    and Endocrinology
Weill Medical College of Cornell University
New York Presbyterian Hospital
New York, New York

**Dorothy J. Becker,** MB, Bch
Professor of Pediatrics
University of Pittsburgh School
    of Medicine
Children's Hospital of Pittsburgh
Pittsburgh, Pennsylvania

**Kenneth L. Becker,** MD, PhD
Professor of Medicine
Professor of Physiology and
    Experimental Medicine
Director of Endocrinology and
    Metabolism
George Washington University School
    of Medicine and Health Sciences
Veterans Affairs Medical Center
Washington, DC

**Norman H. Bell,** MD
Distinguished University Professor
    of Medicine
Medical University of South Carolina
    College of Medicine
Charleston, South Carolina

**Bankim Bhatt,** MD
Medical Resident
Department of Medicine
Georgetown University School
    of Medicine
Washington Hospital Center
Washington, DC

**John P. Bilezikian,** MD
Professor of Medicine and
    Pharmacology
Department of Medicine
Columbia University College of
    Physicians and Surgeons
New York, New York

**Richard E. Blackwell,** MD, PhD
Professor of Obstetrics and
    Gynecology
University of Alabama School
    of Medicine
Birmingham, Alabama

**Vicky A. Blakesley,** MD, PhD
Director, Department of New Product
    Evaluation
International Division
Abbott Laboratories
Abbott Park, Illinois

**Stephen Bloom,** MA, MD, DSc, FRCPath,
    FRCP, FMedSci
Professor of Medicine
Department of Metabolic Medicine
Division of Investigative Science
University of London
Imperial College School of Medicine
London, England

**Manfred Blum,** MD
Professor of Clinical Medicine and
    Radiology
Director, Nuclear Endocrine Laboratory
New York University School
    of Medicine
New York, New York

**Nanci Bobrow,** PhD
Assistant Clinical Professor of Pediatrics
Cardinal Glennon Children's Hospital
Saint Louis University School of
    Medicine
St. Louis, Missouri

**Susan Bonner-Weir,** PhD
Associate Professor of Medicine
Harvard Medical School
Senior Investigator
Joslin Diabetes Center
Boston, Massachusetts

**Stefan R. Bornstein,** MD, PhD
Assistant Professor and Research Scholar
Pediatric and Reproductive
    Endocrinology Branch
National Institute of Child Health and
    Human Development
National Institutes of Health
Bethesda, Maryland

**Eric Bourekas,** MD
Assistant Professor of Radiology
Section of Diagnostic and Interventional
    Neuroradiology
Ohio State University College of
    Medicine and Public Health
Columbus, Ohio

**William J. Bremner,** MD, PhD
Robert G. Petersdorf Professor
    and Chairman
Department of Medicine
University of Washington School
    of Medicine
Seattle, Washington

**Edward M. Brown,** MD
Professor of Medicine
Endocrine–Hypertension Division
Harvard Medical School
Brigham and Women's Hospital
Boston, Massachusetts

**Henry B. Burch,** MD
Associate Professor of Medicine
Uniformed Services University of the
    Health Sciences F. Edward Hébert
    School of Medicine
Bethesda, Maryland
Department of Endocrine-Metabolic
    Service
Walter Reed Army Medical Center
Washington, DC

**Kenneth D. Burman,** MD
Professor of Medicine
Uniformed Services University of the
    Health Sciences F. Edward Hébert
    School of Medicine
Bethesda, Maryland
Clinical Professor
Department of Medicine
George Washington University School
    of Medicine and Health Sciences
Professor of Medicine
Georgetown University School
    of Medicine
Chief, Endocrine Section
Washington Hospital Center
Washington, DC

**Peter H. Byers,** MD
Professor of Pathology and Medicine
University of Washington School
    of Medicine
Seattle, Washington

**Enrico Carmina,** MD
Professor
Department of Endocrinology
University of Palermo
Palermo, Italy
Visiting Professor
Department of Obstetrics and
    Gynecology
Columbia University College of
    Physicians and Surgeons
New York, New York

**Thomas O. Carpenter,** MD
Professor of Pediatrics
Yale University School of Medicine
Yale–New Haven Hospital
New Haven, Connecticut

**Bruce R. Carr,** MD
Professor
Paul C. Macdonald Distinguished Chair
    in Obstetrics and Gynecology
Director, Division of Reproductive
    Endocrinology
University of Texas Southwestern
    Medical Center at Dallas
    Southwestern Medical School
Dallas, Texas

**Veronica M. Catanese,** MD
Assistant Professor
Department of Medicine and
    Cell Biology
New York University School
    of Medicine
New York, New York

**Donald Chakeres,** MD
Professor of Radiology
Ohio State University College of
    Medicine and Public Health
Columbus, Ohio

**John R. G. Challis,** PhD, Dsc, FIBiol,
FRCOG, FRSC
Department of Physiology
Medical Sciences Building
University of Toronto Faculty
of Medicine
Toronto, Ontario
Canada

**Philippe Chanson,** MD
Professor of Medicine
Department of Endocrinology
University Paris XI
Bicêtre University Hospital
Le Kremlin-Bicêtre
France

**William W. Chin,** MD
Professor of Medicine
Harvard Medical School
Boston, Massachusetts
Vice President, Lilly Research
Laboratories
Eli Lilly & Co.
Lilly Corporate Center
Indianapolis, Indiana

**George P. Chrousos,** MD
Chief, Pediatric and Reproductive
Endocrinology Branch
National Institutes of Health
Bethesda, Maryland

**Richard V. Clark,** MD, PhD
Principal Clinical Research Physician
Clinical Pharmacology–Exploratory
Department
Glaxo Wellcome Research and
Development
Research Triangle Park, North Carolina

**Thomas L. Clemens,** MD, PhD
Professor of Medicine and Molecular and
Cellular Physiology
Department of Internal Medicine/
Endocrinology
University of Cincinnati College
of Medicine
Cincinnati, Ohio

**Fredric L. Coe,** MD
Professor
Departments of Medicine and Physiology
University of Chicago Pritzker School
of Medicine
Chicago, Illinois

**Joshua L. Cohen,** MD
Associate Professor of Medicine
Department of Endocrinology
George Washington University School
of Medicine and Health Sciences
Washington, DC

**Régis Cohen,** MD, PhD
Praticien Hospitalier
Endocrine Staff Physician
Avicenne Hospital
Bobigny, France
University of Leonardo Da Vinci
Paris, France

**Warren E. Cohen,** MD
Associate Clinical Professor of Pediatrics
and Neurology
George Washington University School
of Medicine and Health Sciences
Washington, DC
Medical Director, United Cerebral Palsy
Nassau County, New York

**Alessandra Colantoni,** MD
Assistant Professor of Medicine
Department of Gastroenterology
and Hepatology
Loyola University of Chicago Stritch
School of Medicine
Loyola University Medical Center
Maywood, Illinois

**Richard J. Comi,** MD
Associate Professor of Medicine
Section of Endocrinology
and Metabolism
Dartmouth Medical School
Dartmouth–Hitchcock Medical Center
Hanover, New Hampshire

**Paul E. Cooper,** MD, FRCPC
Associate Professor of Neurology
Departments of Clinical Neurological
Sciences and Medicine
University of Western Ontario Faculty
of Medicine and Dentistry
Health Sciences Addition
London, Ontario
Canada

**Dalila B. Corry,** MD
Associate Clinical Professor
of Medicine
Department of Medicine
University of California, Los Angeles,
UCLA School of Medicine
Los Angeles, California
Chief, Nephrology
Olive View Medical Center
Sylmar, California

**Francesco Cosentino,** MD, PhD
Assistant Professor
Department of Experimental Medicine
and Pathology
University "La Sapienza"
Rome, Italy
Senior Research Associate
Cardiovascular Research
Department of Cardiology
University Hospital
Zurich, Switzerland

**Felicia Cosman,** MD
Associate Professor of Clinical
Medicine
Department of Medicine
Columbia University College of
Physicians and Surgeons
New York, New York
Helen Hayes Hospital
West Haverstraw, New York

**Brian M. Cox,** PhD
Professor of Pharmacology
and Neuroscience
Department of Pharmacology
Uniformed Services University of the
Health Sciences F. Edward Hébert
School of Medicine
Bethesda, Maryland

**Glenn R. Cunningham,** MD
Associate Chief of Staff
Department of Medicine
University of Texas–Houston Medical
School
Veterans Affairs Medical Center
Houston, Texas

**Mary F. Dallman,** PhD
Professor of Physiology
University of California, San Francisco,
School of Medicine
San Francisco, California

**Daniel N. Darlington,** PhD
Associate Professor of Surgery
Departments of Surgery
and Physiology
University of Maryland School
of Medicine
Baltimore, Maryland

**Philip Darney,** MD, MSc
Professor of Obstetrics, Gynecology,
and Reproductive Sciences
University of California, San Francisco,
School of Medicine
San Francisco General Hospital
San Francisco, California

**Harish P. G. Dave,** MB, ChB, MRCP(UK)
Associate Professor of Medicine
Department of Hematology
George Washington University School
of Medicine and Health Sciences
Veterans Affairs Medical Center
Washington, DC

**Faith B. Davis,** MD
Professor of Medicine and Cell Biology
and Cancer Research
Albany Medical College
Staff Physician
Stratton Veterans Affairs Medical
Center
Albany, New York

**Paul J. Davis,** MD
Professor of Medicine and Cell Biology
    and Cancer Research
Senior Associate Dean for
    Clinical Research
Albany Medical College
Research Physician
Wadsworth Center, New York State
    Department of Health
Staff Physician
Stratton Veterans Affairs Medical
    Center
Albany, New York

**Suzanne M. Jan De Beur,** MD
Assistant Professor of Medicine
Johns Hopkins University School
    of Medicine
Baltimore, Maryland

**Ralph A. DeFronzo,** MD
Professor of Medicine
Chief, Diabetic Division
Member, Nephrology Division
University of Texas Medical School at
    San Antonio
University Health Center
San Antonio, Texas

**David M. De Kretser,** MD, MBBS, FRACP
Professor and Director
Monash Institute of Reproduction
    and Development
Monash University
Monash Medical Centre, Clayton
Clayton, Victoria
Australia

**Nicola De Maria,** MD
Research Associate
Liver Transplant Program
Loyola University Medical Center
Maywood, Illinois

**David P. Dempsher,** MD, PhD
Associate Professor of Pediatrics
Cardinal Glennon Children's
    Hospital
Saint Louis University School of
    Medicine
St. Louis, Missouri

**David W. Dempster,** PhD
Professor of Clinical Pathology
Columbia University College of
    Physicians and Surgeons
New York, New York
Director, Regional Bone Center
Helen Hayes Hospital
West Haverstraw, New York

**Luca deSimone**
Nephrology Fellow
Beth Israel Medical Center
New York, New York

**Gerard M. Doherty,** MD
Associate Professor of Surgery
Section of Surgical Oncology
    and Endocrinology
Washington University School
    of Medicine
St. Louis, Missouri

**Allan L. Drash,** MD
Emeritus Professor of Pediatrics
University of Pittsburgh School of
    Medicine
Pittsburgh, Pennsylvania

**Marc K. Drezner,** MD
Professor of Medicine
Head, Section of Endocrinology,
    Diabetes, and Metabolism
University of Wisconsin Medical School
Madison, Wisconsin

**Alan Dubrow,** MD
Clinical Assistant Professor
    of Medicine
Department of Nephrology
Beth Israel Deaconess Medical Center
New York, New York

**D. Robert Dufour,** MD
Clinical Professor of Pathology
George Washington University School
    of Medicine and Health Sciences
Washington, DC
Uniformed Services University of the
    Health Sciences F. Edward Hébert
    School of Medicine
Bethesda, Maryland
Chief, Pathology and Laboratory
    Medicine Service
Veterans Affairs Medical Center
Washington, DC

**Roberta P. Durschlag,** PhD, RD
Clinical Assistant Professor
Department of Health Sciences
Boston University School of Medicine
Boston, Massachusetts

**Richard C. Eastman,** MD
Cygnus, Inc.
Redwood City, California

**George S. Eisenbarth,** MD, PhD
Professor of Pediatrics, Immunology,
    and Medicine
University of Colorado Health
    Sciences Center
Barbara Davis Center for
    Childhood Diabetes
Denver, Colorado

**George M. Eliopoulos,** MD
Associate Professor of Medicine
Harvard Medical School
Beth Israel Deaconess Medical Center
Boston, Massachusetts

**William J. Ellis,** MD
Associate Professor and Clinic Director
Department of Urology
University of Washington School of
    Medicine
Seattle, Washington

**Abby Erickson,** BA
Colorado Center for Bone Research
Lakewood, Colorado

**Gregory F. Erickson,** PhD
Professor
Department of Reproductive
    Medicine
University of California, San Diego,
    School of Medicine
La Jolla, California

**Eric A. Espiner,** MD, FRACP, FRS(NZ)
Professor
Department of Endocrinology
University of Otago
Christchurch School of Medicine
Christchurch Public Hospital
Christchurch, New Zealand

**Jan Fahrenkrug,** MD, DMSci
Professor
Department of Clinical Chemistry
University of Copenhagen Faculty
    of Health Sciences
Bispebjerg Hospital
Copenhagen, Denmark

**Kenneth R. Falchuk,** MD
Associate Professor of Medicine
Harvard Medical School
Beth Israel Deaconess Medical
    Center
Boston, Massachusetts

**Murray J. Favus,** MD
Professor of Medicine
University of Chicago Pritzker School
    of Medicine
Chicago, Illinois

**Eva L. Feldman,** MD, PhD
Professor of Neurology
University of Michigan Medical
    School
Ann Arbor, Michigan

**Jo-David Fine,** MD, MPH
Professor
Department of Dermatology
University of North Carolina
    at Chapel Hill School of Medicine
Chapel Hill, North Carolina

**James D. Finkelstein,** MD
Senior Clinician
Department of Medicine
Veterans Affairs Medical Center
Washington, DC

**Jeffrey S. Flier,** MD
George C. Reisman Professor
    of Medicine
Harvard Medical School
Beth Israel Deaconess Medical Center
Boston, Massachusetts

**Ruth C. Fretts,** MD, MPH
Assistant Professor
Department of Obstetrics and Gynecology
Harvard Medical School
Beth Israel Deaconess Medical Center
Boston, Massachusetts

**Om P. Ganda,** MD
Associate Clinical Professor
Department of Medicine
Harvard Medical School
Joslin Diabetes Center
Beth Israel Deaconess Medical Center
Boston, Massachusetts

**Luigi Garibaldi**
Beth Israel Medical Center
Newark, New Jersey

**Gary W. Gibbons,** MD
Associate Clinical Professor of Surgery
Harvard Medical School
Director, Quality Improvement
Department of Surgery
Beth Israel Deaconess Medical Center
Boston, Massachusetts

**John R. Gill, Jr.,** MD
Scientist, Emeritus
Hypertension-Endocrine Branch
National Heart, Lung, and Blood
    Institute
National Institutes of Health
Bethesda, Maryland

**Henry N. Ginsberg,** MD
Professor of Medicine
Columbia University College of
    Physicians and Surgeons
New York, New York

**Joel S. Glaser,** MD
Professor
Departments of Ophthalmology
    and Neurology
University of Miami School
    of Medicine
Bascom Palmer Eye Institute
Miami, Florida
Department of Ophthalmology
Cleveland Clinic of Florida
Coral Gables, Florida

**Allan R. Glass,** MD
Adjunct Professor of Medicine
Uniformed Services University of the
    Health Sciences F. Edward Hébert
    School of Medicine
Bethesda, Maryland

**Philip W. Gold,** MD
Branch Chief
Department of Intramural
    Research Programs
National Institute of Mental Health
National Institutes of Health
Bethesda, Maryland

**Alisa B. Goldberg,** MD
Assistant Adjunct Professor
Department of Obstetrics, Gynecology
    and Reproductive Sciences
University of California, San Francisco,
    School of Medicine
San Francisco General Hospital
San Francisco, California

**Ira J. Goldberg,** MD
Professor of Medicine
Columbia University College of
    Physicians and Surgeons
New York, New York

**Stuart L. Goldberg,** MD
Assistant Director, Bone Marrow
    Transplantation Program
Temple University School
    of Medicine
Philadelphia, Pennsylvania

**Allison B. Goldfine,** MD
Instructor of Medicine
Department of Cellular and
    Molecular Physiology
Harvard University
Joslin Diabetes Center
Boston, Massachusetts

**Allan L. Goldstein,** PhD
Chair, Department of Biochemistry
    and Molecular Biology
George Washington University School
    of Medicine and Health Sciences
Washington, DC

**David S. Goldstein,** MD, PhD
Chief, Clinical Neurocardiology
    Section
National Institutes of Health
Bethesda, Maryland

**David Goltzman,** MD
Professor of Medicine and Physiology
McGill University Faculty
    of Medicine
Royal Victoria Hospital
Montreal, Quebec
Canada

**Esther A. Gonzalez,** MD
Assistant Professor
Division of Nephrology
Saint Louis University School
    of Medicine
St. Louis, Missouri

**Michael N. Goodman,** PhD
Professor of Medicine
Department of Internal Medicine
University of California, Davis,
    School of Medicine
Sacramento, California

**Phillip Gorden,** MD
Director Emeritus
National Institute of Diabetes and
    Digestive and Kidney Diseases
National Institutes of Health
Bethesda, Maryland

**Frederic D. Gordon,** MD
Assistant Professor of Medicine
Department of Hepatobiliary Surgery
    and Liver Transplantation
Tufts University School of Medicine
Lahey Clinic Medical Center
Boston, Massachusetts

**Daryl K. Granner,** MD
Joe C. Davis Professor of
    Biomedical Science
Professor of Molecular Physiology,
    Biophysics, and Internal Medicine
Vanderbilt University School
    of Medicine
Director, Vanderbilt Diabetes Center
Staff Physician
Veterans Affairs Hospital
Nashville, Tennessee

**Søren Gräs,** MD
Senior Registrar
Department of Obstetrics and
    Gynaecology
Herlev University Hospital
Herlev, Denmark

**Douglas A. Greene,** MD
Executive Vice President
Department of Clinical Sciences
    and Product Development
Merck & Co., Inc.
Rahway, New Jersey

**David A. Gruenewald,** MD, FACP
Assistant Professor of Medicine
University of Washington School
    of Medicine
Veterans Affairs Puget Sound Health
    Care System
Seattle, Washington

**Joel F. Habener,** MD
Professor of Medicine
Laboratory of Molecular
    Endocrinology
Harvard Medical School
Massachusetts General Hospital
Boston, Massachusetts

**Philippe A. Halban,** PhD
Professor of Medicine
Louis-Jeantet Research Laboratories
Geneva University Medical Center
Geneva, Switzerland

**Nicholas R. S. Hall,** PhD
Health and Human Performance
Orlando, Florida

**Allan G. Halline,** MD
Assistant Professor of Medicine
Section of Digestive and
   Liver Diseases
University of Illinois at Chicago
   College of Medicine
Chicago, Illinois

**Stephen G. Harner,** MD
Professor of Otolaryngology
Department of Otolaryngology
Mayo Medical School
Rochester, Minnesota

**Marianne Hatle,** MD
Resident
University of Maryland School
   of Medicine
Baltimore, Maryland

**Michael J. Hausmann,** MD
Professor
Department of Nephrology
Faculty of Health Sciences
Ben Gurion University of the Negev
Scroka Medical Center
   of Kupat Holim
Beer Sheva, Israel

**Karin Hehenberger,** MD, PhD
Research Fellow
Joslin Diabetes Center
Harvard Medical School
Boston, Massachusetts

**J. Fielding Hejtmancik,** MD, PhD
Medical Officer
National Eye Institute
National Institutes of Health
Bethesda, Maryland

**Geoffrey N. Hendy,** PhD
Professor of Medicine
McGill University Faculty
   of Medicine
Royal Victoria Hospital
Montreal, Quebec
Canada

**James V. Hennessey,** MD
Associate Professor of Medicine
Division of Endocrinology
Brown University School of Medicine
Rhode Island Hospital
Providence, Rhode Island

**Jules Hirsch,** MD
Professor Emeritus and
   Physician-in-Chief Emeritus
Laboratory of Human Behavior and
   Metabolism
Rockefeller University
Rockefeller University Hospital
New York, New York

**Angelica Lindén Hirschberg,** MD, PhD
Associate Professor of Obstetrics
   and Gynecology
Karolinska Institute
Karolinska Hospital
Stockholm, Sweden

**Max Hirshkowitz,** MD
Associate Professor
Department of Psychiatry
Baylor College of Medicine
Director, Sleep Center
Houston Veterans Affairs
   Medical Center
Houston, Texas

**Gary D. Hodgen,** PhD
Professor
Department of Obstetrics and
   Gynecology
Eastern Virginia Medical School
Chair
The Howard and Georgeanna
   Jones Institute for Reproductive
   Medicine
Norfolk, Virginia

**Edward W. Holmes,** MD
Chairman, Department
   of Medicine
University of Pennsylvania School
   of Medicine
Philadelphia, Pennsylvania

**Jens J. Holst,** MD
Department of Medical Physiology
University of Copenhagen Faculty
   of Health Sciences
The Panum Institute
Copenhagen, Denmark

**Robert N. Hoover,** MD, ScD
Director, Epidemiology and
   Biostatistics Program
National Cancer Institute
National Institutes of Health
Bethesda, Maryland

**Gabriel N. Hortobagyi,** MD
Professor of Medicine, Chairman
Department of Breast and Gynecologic
   Medical Oncology
University of Texas–Houston
   Medical School
M. D. Anderson Cancer Center
Houston, Texas

**Eva Horvath,** PhD
Associate Professor of Pathology
Department of Laboratory Medicine
Division of Pathology
University of Toronto Faculty of Medicine
St. Michael's Hospital
Toronto, Ontario
Canada

**Barbara V. Howard,** PhD
President, MedStar Clinical Research
   Institute
Washington, DC

**William James Howard,** MD
Professor of Medicine
George Washington University School
   of Medicine
Senior Vice President and Medical
   Director
Washington Hospital Center
Washington, DC

**Ilpo Huhtaniemi,** MD, PhD
Professor of Physiology
University of Turku Faculty
   of Medicine
Turku, Finland

**Wellington Hung,** MD, PhD
Professor Emeritus of Pediatrics
Georgetown University School
   of Medicine
Professorial Lecturer in Pediatrics
George Washington University School
   of Medicine and Health Sciences
Washington, DC

**Mehboob A. Hussain,** MD
Department of Medicine
New York University School of Medicine
New York, New York

**Philip M. Iannaccone,** MD, PhD
George M. Eisenberg Professor
Department of Pediatrics
Northwestern University
   Medical School
Children's Memorial Institute of
   Education and Research
Chicago, Illinois

**Ivor M. D. Jackson,** MB, ChB
Professor of Medicine
Division of Endocrinology
Brown University School
   of Medicine
Rhode Island Hospital
Providence, Rhode Island

**Richard V. Jackson,** MBBS, FRACP
Associate Professor of Medicine
University of Queensland Faculty
   of Health Sciences
Greenslopes Private Hospital
Queensland, Australia

**Lois Jovanovic,** MD
Clinical Professor of Medicine
University of Southern California School
    of Medicine
Los Angeles, California
Director and Chief Scientific Officer
Sansum Medical Research Institute
Santa Barbara, California

**William A. Jubiz,** MD
Director
Endocrinology Center
Cali, Colombia

**C. Ronald Kahn,** MD
Mary K. Iacocca Professor of Medicine
Harvard Medical School
President and Director, Research
    Division
Joslin Diabetes Center
Boston, Massachusetts

**Cynthia G. Kaplan,** MD
Associate Professor of Pathology
SUNY at Stony Brook School of Medicine
    Health Sciences Center
Stony Brook, New York

**Edwin L. Kaplan,** MD, FACS
Professor of Surgery
University of Chicago Pritzker School
    of Medicine
Chicago, Illinois

**Abba J. Kastin,** MD
Chief of Endocrinology
Departments of Medicine
    and Neuroscience
Tulane University School of Medicine
Veterans Affairs Medical Center
New Orleans, Louisiana

**Laurence Katznelson,** MD
Assistant Professor of Medicine
Harvard Medical School
Massachusetts General Hospital
Boston, Massachusetts

**Harry R. Keiser,** MD
Scientist Emeritus
National Heart, Lung, and Blood Institute
    Clinical Center
National Institutes of Health
Bethesda, Maryland

**Ellie Kelepouris,** MD
Professor of Medicine
Temple University School of Medicine
Philadelphia, Pennsylvania

**Craig M. Kessler,** MD
Professor of Medicine and Pathology
Chief, Division of Hematology-Oncology
Georgetown University School of Medicine
Lombardy Cancer Center
Washington, DC

**Parvez Khatri,** MD
Fellow, Department of
    Medicine/Nephrology
George Washington University School
    of Medicine and Health Sciences
Washington, DC

**Paul L. Kimmel,** MD
Professor of Medicine
George Washington University School
    of Medicine and Health Sciences
Washington, DC
Director, Diabetic Nephropathy
    Program
Division of Kidney, Urologic, and
    Hematologic Diseases
National Institute of Diabetes and
    Digestive and Kidney Diseases
National Institutes of Health
Bethesda, Maryland

**George L. King,** MD
Professor of Medicine
Acting Director of Research
Joslin Diabetes Center
Harvard Medical School
Boston, Massachusetts

**Anne Klibanski,** MD
Professor of Medicine
Harvard Medical School
Chief, Neuroendocrine Unit
Massachusetts General Hospital
Boston, Massachusetts

**Mitchel A. Kling,** MD
Associate Professor of Psychiatry
    and Medicine
University of Maryland School
    of Medicine
Veterans Affairs Medical Center
Baltimore, Maryland

**Mark Korson,** MD
Associate Professor of Pediatrics
Division of Genetics
Tufts University School of Medicine
New England Medical Center
Boston, Massachusetts

**Kalman Kovacs,** MD, PhD
Professor of Pathology
Department of Laboratory Medicine
Division of Pathology
University of Toronto Faculty of Medicine
Saint Michael's Hospital
Toronto, Ontario
Canada

**Andrzej S. Krolewski,** MD, PhD
Associate Professor of Medicine
Chief, Section of Genetics and
    Epidemiology
Harvard Medical School
Research Division
Joslin Diabetes Center
Boston, Massachusetts

**Robert J. Kurman,** MD
Richard W. TeLinde Distinguished
    Professor of Gynecologic
    Pathology
Departments of Gynecology, Obstetrics,
    and Pathology
Johns Hopkins University School
    of Medicine
Baltimore, Maryland

**John C. LaRosa,** MD, FACP
President
SUNY Downstate Medical Center
    College of Medicine
University Hospital of Brooklyn
Brooklyn, New York

**Robert B. Layzer,** MD
Professor Emeritus of Neurology
University of California, San Francisco,
    School of Medicine
San Francisco, California

**Jacques LeBlanc,** MD
Professor Emeritus of Physiology
Université Laval Faculty
    of Medicine
Quebec City, Canada

**Peter A. Lee,** MD, PhD
Professor of Pediatrics
Pennsylvania State University
    College of Medicine
The Milton S. Hershey Medical
    Center
Hershey, Pennsylvania

**Z. M. Lei,** MD, PhD
Assistant Professor of Obstetrics
    and Gynecology
University of Louisville School
    of Medicine
Louisville, Kentucky

**Hoyle Leigh,** MD
Professor of Psychiatry
University of California, San Francisco,
    School of Medicine
San Francisco, California

**Derek LeRoith,** MD, PhD
Chief, Molecular and Cellular
    Endocrinology Branch
National Institute of Diabetes and
    Digestive and Kidney Diseases
National Institutes of Health
Bethesda, Maryland

**Michael A. Levine,** MD
Professor of Pediatrics, Medicine,
    and Pathology
Director, Pediatric Endocrinology
Johns Hopkins University School
    of Medicine
Baltimore, Maryland

**Jonathan J. Li,** PhD
Director, Division of Etiology and
  Prevention of Hormone-Associated
  Cancers
Professor of Pharmacology, Toxicology
  and Preventive Medicine
University of Kansas School of Medicine
Kansas Cancer Institute
Kansas City, Kansas

**Sara Antonia Li,** MD
Associate Director
Hormonal Carcinogenesis Laboratory
University of Kansas School of Medicine
Kansas Cancer Institute
Kansas City, Kansas

**Robert D. Lindeman,** MD
Professor Emeritus of Medicine
Department of Internal Medicine
University of New Mexico School
  of Medicine
University of New Mexico Hospital
Albuquerque, New Mexico

**Robert Lindsay,** MBChB, PhD, FRCP
Professor of Clinical Medicine
Columbia University College of
  Physicians and Surgeons
New York, New York
Chief of Internal Medicine
Helen Hayes Hospital
West Haverstraw, New York

**Timothy O. Lipman,** MD
Professor of Medicine
Georgetown University School of Medicine
Chief, Gastroenterology–Hepatology
Nutrition Section
Veterans Affairs Medical Center
Washington, DC

**Virginia A. Livolsi,** MD
Professor of Pathology
Department of Pathology and
  Laboratory Medicine
University of Pennsylvania School
  of Medicine
Philadelphia, Pennsylvania

**Rogerio A. Lobo,** MD
Willard C. Rappleye Professor
  of Obstetrics and Gynecology
Chairman, Department of Obstetrics
  and Gynecology
Columbia University College of
  Physicians and Surgeons
Columbia Presbyterian Medical Center
Director, Sloane Hospital for Women
New York, New York

**Rebecca J. Locke**
Research Assistant
Columbia University College of
  Physicians and Surgeons
New York, New York

**Christopher J. Logethetis,** MD
Chairman and Professor
Department of Genitourinary
  Medical Oncology
University of Texas–Houston
  Medical School
M. D. Anderson Cancer Center
Houston, Texas

**D. Lynn Loriaux,** MD, PhD
Professor and Chair
Department of Medicine
Oregon Health Sciences University
  School of Medicine
Portland, Oregon

**Harvey S. Luksenburg,** MD
Assistant Professor of Medicine
George Washington University School
  of Medicine and Health Sciences
Washington, DC

**Thomas F. Lüscher,** MD
Professor and Head of Cardiology
Hospital Universitaire de Zurich
Zurich, Switzerland

**Ruth S. MacDonald,** RD, PhD
Professor of Nutrition
Department of Food Science and
  Human Nutrition
University of Missouri–Columbia School
  of Medicine
Columbia, Missouri

**Michelle Fischmann Magee,** MD, MB, BCh, BAO
Medical Director, Diabetes Team
MedStar Clinical Research Institute
Washington Hospital Center
Washington, DC

**Robert W. Mahley,** MD, PhD
Professor of Pathology and Medicine
Director, Gladstone Institute of
  Cardiovascular Disease
University of California, San Francisco,
  School of Medicine
San Francisco, California

**Christos S. Mantzoros,** MD, Dsc
Assistant Professor of Medicine
Department of Internal Medicine
Harvard Medical School
Beth Israel Deaconess Medical Center
Boston, Massachusetts

**Eleftheria Maratos-Flier,** MD
Associate Professor of Medicine
Research Division
Harvard Medical School
Joslin Diabetes Center
Boston, Massachusetts

**Paul Marik,** MBBCh, FCP(SA), FRCP(C), FCCM, FCCP
Department of Critical Care
Mercy Hospital of Pittsburgh
Pittsburgh, Pennsylvania

**Kevin J. Martin,** MB, BCh, FACP
Professor of Internal Medicine
Department of Nephrology
Director, Division of Nephrology
Saint Louis University School
  of Medicine
St. Louis, Missouri

**William D. Mathers,** MD
Professor of Ophthalmology
Oregon Health Sciences University
  School of Medicine
Casey Eye Institute
Portland, Oregon

**Paul N. Maton,** MD, FRCP, FACP, FACG
Digestive Disease Specialists
  Incorporated
Digestive Disease Research Institute
Oklahoma City, Oklahoma

**Alvin M. Matsumoto,** MD
Professor
Department of Medicine
University of Washington School
  of Medicine
Chief of Gerontology
Veterans Affairs Puget Sound Health
  Care System
Seattle, Washington

**Ernest L. Mazzaferri,** MD, MACP
Professor Emeritus and Chairman
Department of Internal Medicine
Ohio State University College of
  Medicine and Public Health
Columbus, Ohio

**Alan M. McGregor,** MA, MD, FRCP
Professor of Medicine
King's College
Guy's, King's and St. Thomas' School
  of Medicine
London, England

**Karim Meeran,** MD, MRCP
Senior Lecturer
Division of Endocrinology
  and Metabolism
University of London Imperial College
  School of Medicine
Hammersmith Hospital
London, England

**Minesh P. Mehta,** MD, MB, ChB
Associate Professor and Chairman
Department of Human Oncology
University of Wisconsin Medical School
Madison, Wisconsin

**James C. Melby,** MD
Professor of Medicine and Physiology
Boston University School
  of Medicine
Boston Medical Center
Boston, Massachusetts

**Stephen A. Migueles,** MD
Fellow, Infectious Diseases
Laboratory of Immunoregulation
National Institute of Allergy and
    Infectious Diseases
National Institutes of Health
Bethesda, Maryland

**Donald L. Miller,** MD
Professor of Radiology and
    Nuclear Medicine
Uniformed Services University of the
    Health Sciences F. Edward Hébert
    School of Medicine
Bethesda, Maryland

**Elizabeth A. Miller**
Urology Resident
University of Washington School of
    Medicine
Seattle, Washington

**Paul D. Miller,** MD
Clinical Professor
Department of Medicine
University of Colorado Health
    Sciences Center
Denver, Colorado

**Dolly Misra,** MD
Assistant Clinical Professor of Medicine
Division of Endocrinology and Metabolism
George Washington University School
    of Medicine and Health Sciences
Washington, DC
Diabetes and Endocrine Consultants
Waldorf, Maryland

**Mark E. Molitch,** MD
Professor of Medicine
Center for Endocrinology, Metabolism,
    and Molecular Medicine
Northwestern University Medical School
Chicago, Illinois

**Chulso Moon,** MD, PhD
Clinical Fellow
Department of Medicine
University of Texas–Houston
    Medical School
M. D. Anderson Cancer Center
Houston, Texas

**Arshag D. Mooradian,** MD
Professor of Medicine
Director of Endocrinology, Diabetes
    and Metabolism
Saint Louis University School of Medicine
St. Louis, Missouri

**Gregory P. Mueller,** PhD
Professor of Physiology
Uniformed Services University of the
    Health Sciences F. Edward Hébert
    School of Medicine
Bethesda, Maryland

**Beat Müller,** MD
Department of Internal Medicine
Division of Endocrinology
University Hospitals
Basel, Switzerland

**Susan E. Myers,** MD
Assistant Professor of Pediatrics
Saint Louis University School of Medicine
Cardinal Glenn Children's Hospital
St. Louis, Missouri

**David J. Nashel,** MD
Professor of Medicine
Georgetown University School of Medicine
Chief of Medical Service
Veterans Affairs Medical Center
Washington, DC

**Adnan Nasir,** MD, PhD
Department of Dermatology
University of North Carolina
    at Chapel Hill School of Medicine
Chapel Hill, North Carolina

**Jeffrey A. Norton,** MD
Professor of Surgery
Vice Chairman, Department of Surgery
University of California, San Francisco,
    School of Medicine
San Francisco Veterans Affairs
    Medical Center
San Francisco, California

**Robert H. Noth,** MD
Associate Professor of Medicine
Department of Internal Medicine
University of California, Davis,
    School of Medicine
Davis, California
Veterans Affairs Outpatient Clinic
Martinez, California

**Jennifer A. Nuovo**
Endocrinologist
MedClinic of Sacramento
Sacramento, California

**Eric S. Nylén,** MD
Associate Professor of Medicine
Department of Endocrinology
George Washington University School
    of Medicine and Health Sciences
Veterans Affairs Medical Center
Washington, DC

**Donna M. Arab O'Brien,** MD
Department of Medicine
Division of Endocrinology
St. Joseph's Health Centre
Toronto, Ontario
Canada

**Mary Oehler,** MD
Staff Radiologist
Mount Carmel East Hospital
New Albany, Ohio

**Robert A. Oppenheim,** MD
Naperville Eye Associates
Naperville, Illinois

**Jeffrey L. H. O'Riordan**
Emeritus Professor of Metabolic Medicine
University College
London, United Kingdom

**Steven J. Ory,** MD
Clinical Associate Professor of Obstetrics
    and Gynecology
University of Miami School of Medicine
Miami, Florida

**Harry Ostrer,** MD
Associate Professor of Pediatrics
    and Pathology
Human Genetics Program
New York University School of Medicine
New York, New York

**Weihong Pan,** MD, PhD
Assistant Professor of Medicine
Tulane University School of Medicine
New Orleans, Louisiana

**Yogesh C. Patel,** MD, PhD, FACP, FRCP(C),
    FRACP, FRSC
Professor of Medicine
Director, Division of Endocrinology
    and Metabolism
McGill University Faculty of Medicine
Royal Victoria Hospital
Montreal, Quebec
Canada

**Gary R. Peplinski,** MD
Surgical Service
San Francisco Veterans Affairs
    Medical Center
San Francisco, California

**Ora Hirsch Pescovitz,** MD
Professor of Pediatrics, Physiology,
    and Biophysics
Department of Pediatric Endocrinology
Indiana University School of Medicine
James Whitcomb Riley Hospital
    for Children
Indianapolis, Indiana

**Kristina C. Pfendler,** MD
Postdoctoral Scholar
Department of Obstetrics and
    Gynecology
University of California, San Francisco,
    School of Medicine
San Francisco, California

**Joseph J. Pinzone,** MD
Assistant Professor of Medicine
Department of Internal Medicine
George Washington University School
    of Medicine and Health Sciences
Washington, DC

**Mark R. Pittelkow,** MD
Professor of Dermatology, Biochemistry,
and Molecular Biology
Mayo Medical School
Consultant, Department of Dermatology
Mayo Clinic
Rochester, Minnesota

**Stephen R. Plymate,** MD
Research Professor of Medicine
University of Washington School
of Medicine
Veterans Affairs Puget Sound Health
Care System
Seattle, Washington

**Ke-Nan Qin,** MD
Fellow of Pediatric Endocrinology
Department of Pediatrics
University of Chicago Pritzker School
of Medicine
University of Chicago Children's Hospital
Chicago, Illinois

**Ralph Rabkin,** MB, Bch, MD
Professor of Medicine and Nephrology
Department of Medicine
Stanford University School of Medicine
Stanford, California
Veterans Affairs Palo Alto Health
Care System
Palo Alto, California

**Miriam T. Rademaker,** PhD
Professor of Medicine
University of Otago
Christchurch School of Medicine
Christchurch, New Zealand

**Lawrence G. Raisz,** MD
Professor of Medicine
Department of Endocrinology
University of Connecticut School
of Medicine
University of Connecticut Health Center
Farmington, Connecticut

**Lawrence I. Rand,** MD
Clinical Assistant Professor
of Ophthalmology
Harvard Medical School
Boston, Massachusetts

**Ch. V. Rao,** PhD
Professor and Director
Department of Obstetrics and Gynecology
University of Louisville School of Medicine
Louisville, Kentucky

**Robert E. Ratner,** MD
Associate Clinical Professor of Medicine
George Washington University School
of Medicine and Health Sciences
Director, MedStar Clinical
Research Institute
Washington, DC

**Gerald M. Reaven,** MD
Professor of Medicine
Stanford University School
of Medicine
Stanford, California

**Robert W. Rebar,** MD
Professor
Department of Obstetrics
and Gynecology
University of Cincinnati College
of Medicine
Chief, Obstetrics and Gynecology
University Hospital
Cincinnati, Ohio
Associate Executive Director
American Society for
Reproductive Medicine
Birmingham, Alabama

**Robert S. Redman,** DDS, MSD, PhD
Chief, Oral Diagnosis Section,
Dental Service
Veterans Affairs Medical Center
Washington, DC
Clinical Associate Professor
Department of Oral and
Maxillofacial Pathology
University of Maryland School
of Medicine
Baltimore College of Dental Surgery
Baltimore, Maryland

**H. Lester Reed,** MD
Clinical Professor of Medicine
University of Auckland Faculty of
Medical and Health Sciences
Middlemore Hospital
Auckland, New Zealand

**Domenico C. Regoli,** MD
Professor Emeritus
Department of Pharmacology
Universite de Sherbrooke
Faculte de Medecine
Sherbrooke, Quebec
Canada

**Jens F. Rehfeld,** MD, DSc
Professor of Clinical Biochemistry
University of Copenhagen Faculty
of Health Sciences
Copenhagen University Hospital
Copenhagen, Denmark

**Robert L. Reid,** MD, FRCS(C)
Professor
Department of Obstetrics
and Gynaecology
Queen's University School
of Medicine
Faculty of Health Sciences
Kingston General Hospital
Kingston, Ontario
Canada

**Russel J. Reiter,** PhD
Professor of Neuroendocrinology
Department of Cellular and
Structural Biology
University of Texas Medical School
at San Antonio
University Health Center
San Antonio, Texas

**Matthew D. Ringel,** MD
Assistant Professor of Medicine
Uniformed Services University of the
Health Sciences F. Edward Hébert
School of Medicine
Bethesda, Maryland
Assistant Clinical Professor of Medicine
George Washington University School
of Medicine and Health Sciences
Section of Endocrinology
Washington Hospital Center
Washington, DC

**Antonio Rivera ,** MD
Fellow, Department of Medicine
Section of Renal Diseases and
Hypertension
George Washington University Medical
Center
Washington, DC

**Gary L. Robertson,** MD
Professor of Medicine and Neurology
Department of Endocrinology
Northwestern University Medical School
Chicago, Illinois

**R. Paul Robertson,** MD
Professor of Medicine
and Pharmacology
Scientific Director, Pacific Northwest
Research Institute
Seattle, Washington

**Simon P. Robins,** PhD, Dsc
Head, Skeletal Research Unit
Rowett Research Institute
Aberdeen, Scotland

**Alan D. Rogol,** MD, PhD
Professor of Clinical Pediatrics
Department of Pediatrics
University of Virginia School
of Medicine
University of Virginia Medical Center
Charlottesville, Virginia
Clinical Professor of Internal Medicine
Virginia Commonwealth University
School of Medicine
Richmond, Virginia

**Prashant K. Rohatgi,** MB, MD
Professor of Medicine
George Washington University School
of Medicine and Health Sciences
Veterans Affairs Medical Center
Washington, DC

**Mikael Rørth,** MD
Professor of Clinical Oncology
University of Copenhagen Faculty
  of Health Sciences
Rigshospitalet
Copenhagen, Denmark

**Robert L. Rosenfield,** MD
Professor of Pediatrics and Medicine
Department of Pediatric Endocrinology
University of Chicago Pritzker School
  of Medicine
Chicago, Illinois

**Robert K. Rude,** MD
Professor of Medicine
University of Southern California School
  of Medicine
Los Angeles, California

**Neil B. Ruderman,** MD, DPhil
Professor
Department of Medicine and Physiology
Boston University School of Medicine
Boston, Massachusetts

**James W. Russell,** MD
Assistant Professor
Department of Neurology
University of Michigan Medical School
Ann Arbor GRECC
Ann Arbor, Michigan

**Lester B. Salans,** MD
Adjunct Professor
The Rockefeller University
Clinical Professor of Medicine
Mt. Sinai School of Medicine
New York, New York

**Salil D. Sarkar**
Department of Radiology
SUNY Health Sciences Center at
  Brooklyn College of Medicine
Brooklyn, New York

**David H. Sarne,** MD
Associate Professor of Medicine
Department of Internal Medicine
University of Illinois at Chicago College
  of Medicine
Chicago, Illinois

**Ernst J. Schaefer,** MD
Professor of Medicine
Lipid Division
Tufts University School of Medicine
New England Medical Center
Boston, Massachusetts

**Isaac Schiff,** MD
Joe Vincent Meigs Professor of Gynecology
Department of Obstetrics and Gynecology
Harvard Medical School
Massachusetts General Hospital
Boston, Massachusetts

**R. Neil Schimke,** MD
Professor of Medicine and Pediatrics
Chief, Division of Endocrinology
  and Genetics
University of Kansas School of Medicine
Kansas City, Kansas

**James R. Schreiber,** MD
Elaine and Mitchell Yanow Professor
  and Head
Department of Obstetrics and
  Gynecology
Washington University School
  of Medicine
St. Louis, Missouri

**David E. Schteingart,** MD
Professor of Internal Medicine
Division of Endocrinology
  and Metabolism
University of Michigan Medical School
Ann Arbor, Michigan

**Ellen W. Seely,** MD
Assistant Professor of Medicine
Director of Clinical Research
Endocrine-Hypertension Division
Harvard Medical School
Brigham and Women's Hospital
Boston, Massachusetts

**Markus J. Seibel,** MD, PD
Associate Professor of Medicine
Division of Endocrinology and
  Metabolism
University of Heidelberg Medical School
Heidelberg, Germany

**Elizabeth Shane,** MD
Professor of Medicine
Columbia University College of
  Physicians and Surgeons
New York, New York

**Lawrence E. Shapiro,** MD
Clinical Professor of Medicine
SUNY at Stony Brook School of Medicine
  Health Sciences Center
Stony Brook, New York
Director, Division of Endocrinology
Winthrop University Hospital
Mineola, New York

**Meeta Sharma,** MBBS, MD
Assistant Director, Diabetes Team
Division of Endocrinology
Georgetown University School
  of Medicine
MedStar Diabetes Institute
Washington Hospital Center
Washington, DC

**R. Michael Siatkowski,** MD
Associate Professor of Ophthalmology
Dean A. McGee Eye Institute
Oklahoma City, Oklahoma

**Omega L. Silva,** MD
Professor Emeritus of Medicine
George Washington University
  School of Medicine and
  Health Sciences
Washington, DC

**Shonni J. Silverberg,** MD
Associate Professor of Medicine
Columbia University College of
  Physicians and Surgeons
New York, New York

**Joe Leigh Simpson,** MD
Ernst W. Bertner Chairman
  and Professor
Department of Obstetrics
  and Gynecology
Baylor College of Medicine
Houston, Texas

**Ethel S. Siris,** MD
Madeline C. Stabile Professor
  of Clinical Medicine
Department of Medicine
Columbia University College of
  Physicians and Surgeons
New York, New York

**Glen W. Sizemore,** MD
Professor of Medicine
Division of Endocrinology and
  Metabolism
Loyola University of Chicago Stritch
  School of Medicine
Maywood, Illinois

**Niels E. Skakkebaek,** MD
Professor of Growth
  and Reproduction
University of Copenhagen Faculty
  of Health Sciences
Rigshospitalet
Copenhagen, Denmark

**Celia D. Sladek,** PhD
Professor and Acting Chair
Department of Physiology
  and Biophysics
Finch University of Health Sciences
  Chicago Medical School
North Chicago, Illinois

**John R. Sladek, Jr.,** PhD
Professor and Chairman
Department of Neuroscience
Finch University of Health Sciences
  Chicago Medical School
North Chicago, Illinois

**Eduardo Slatopolsky,** MD
Renal Division
Washington University School
  of Medicine
St. Louis, Missouri

**Robert C. Smallridge,** MD
Professor of Medicine
Mayo Medical School
Chair, Endocrine Division
Mayo Clinic
Jacksonville, Florida

**Robert J. Smith,** MD
Professor of Medicine
Chief of Endocrinology
Brown University School of Medicine
Director, Hallett Diabetes Center
Rhode Island Hospital
Providence, Rhode Island

**Richard H. Snider, Jr.,** PhD
Chief Chemist
Endocrinology Research Laboratory
Veterans Affairs Medical Center
Washington, DC

**Phyllis W. Speiser,** MD
Professor of Clinical Pediatrics
Department of Pediatrics
New York University School of Medicine
New York, New York
North Shore University Hospital
Manhasset, New York

**Harvey J. Stern,** MD, PhD
Genetics and IVF Institute
Fairfax, Virginia

**Martin J. Stevens,** MD
Associate Professor of Internal Medicine
University of Michigan Medical School
Ann Arbor, Michigan

**Andrew F. Stewart,** MD
Professor of Medicine
Chief, Division of Endocrinology
University of Pittsburgh School of Medicine
Pittsburgh, Pennsylvania

**Elizabeth A. Streeten,** MD
Clinical Assistant Professor of Medicine
Department of Endocrinology, Diabetes,
    and Obesity
University of Maryland School of Medicine
Baltimore, Maryland

**Gordon J. Strewler,** MD
Professor of Medicine
Department of Medical Service
Harvard Medical School
Boston, Massachusetts
Veterans Affairs Boston Healthcare System
West Roxbury, Massachusetts

**Martin I. Surks,** MD
Professor of Medicine and Pathology
Department of Medicine
Albert Einstein College of Medicine
    of Yeshiva University
Montefiore Medical Center
Bronx, New York

**Arthur L. M. Swislocki,** MD
Associate Professor of Medicine
Department of Internal Medicine
University of California, Davis,
    School of Medicine
Davis, California
Veterans Affairs Outpatient Clinic
Martinez, California

**Shahrad Taheri,** MSc, MB, MRCP
Wellcome Trust Research Fellow
Division of Endocrinology
    and Metabolism
University of London Imperial College
    School of Medicine
Hammersmith Hospital
London, England

**Robert J. Tanenberg,** MD, FACP
Professor of Medicine
Section of Endocrinology
    and Metabolism
Brody School of Medicine
East Carolina University School
    of Medicine
Greenville, North Carolina

**Kamal Thapar,** MD
Assistant Professor of Neurosurgery
University of Toronto Faculty
    of Medicine
Toronto Western Hospital,
    University Health
Toronto, Ontario
Canada

**Ramesh K. Thapar,** MD
Senior Resident
Department of Psychiatry
University of Maryland School
    of Medicine
Baltimore, Maryland

**Michael A. Thomas,** MD
Associate Professor
Department of Clinical Obstetrics
    and Gynecology
University of Cincinnati College
    of Medicine
Cincinnati, Ohio

**Christopher J. Thompson,** MB, ChB,
    MD, FRCPI
Consultant Physician and
    Endocrinologist
Department of Endocrinology
Royal College of Surgeons
    in Ireland
Beaumont Hospital
Dublin, Ireland

**Keith Tornheim,** PhD
Associate Professor of Biochemistry
Boston University School
    of Medicine
Boston, Massachusetts

**David J. Torpy,** MBBS, PhD, FRACP
Senior Lecturer
Department of Medicine
University of Queensland
Faculty of Health Sciences
Brisbane, Australia

**Carmelita U. Tuazon,** MD, MPH
Professor of Medicine
George Washington University School
    of Medicine and Health Sciences
Washington, DC

**Catherine Tuck,** MD
Assistant Professor of Medicine
Columbia University College of
    Physicians and Surgeons
New York, New York

**Michael L. Tuck,** MD
Professor of Medicine
University of California, Los Angeles,
    UCLA School of Medicine
Los Angeles, California
Veterans Affairs Medical Center, Sepulveda
Sepulveda, California

**Stephen Jon Usala,** MD, PhD
Clinical Associate Professor
Department of Medicine
Texas Tech University Health Sciences
    Center School of Medicine
Amarillo, Texas

**Eve Van Cauter,** PhD
Professor of Medicine
University of Chicago Pritzker School
    of Medicine
Chicago, Illinois

**Greet H. Van Den Berghe,** MD, PhD
Associate Professor of Intensive
    Care Medicine
Catholic University of Leuven
Leuven, Belgium

**David H. Van Thiel,** MD
Director of Transplantation
Loyola University of Chicago Stritch
    School of Medicine
Loyola University Medical Center
Liver Transplant Office
Maywood, Illinois

**Joseph G. Verbalis,** MD
Professor of Medicine and Physiology
Georgetown University School of Medicine
Washington, DC

**Robert Volpé,** MD, FRCP(C), MACP, FRCP
    (Edin & Lord)
Professor Emeritus
Department of Medicine
University of Toronto Faculty of Medicine
Toronto, Ontario
Canada

**Steven G. Waguespack,** MD
Fellow, Adult and Pediatric
   Endocrinology
Departments of Medicine and Pediatrics
Division of Endocrinology
Indiana University School of Medicine
Riley Children's Hospital
Indianapolis, Indiana

**Brian Walsh,** MD
Director, Menopause Center
Department of Obstetrics
   and Gynecology
Harvard Medical School
Brigham and Women's Hospital
Boston, Massachusetts

**David O. Walterhouse,** MD
Assistant Professor of Pediatrics
Northwestern University Medical School
Children's Memorial Hospital
Chicago, Illinois

**Emily C. Walvoord,** MD
Senior Fellow
Department of Pediatric Endocrinology
   and Diabetology
Indiana University School of Medicine
Riley Hospital for Children
Indianapolis, Indiana

**James H. Warram,** MD, ScD
Senior Investigator
Section on Genetics and Epidemiology
Research Division
Harvard Medical School
Joslin Diabetes Center
Boston, Massachusetts

**Michelle P. Warren,** MD
Professor of Obstetrics and Gynecology
   and Medicine
Wyeth Ayerst Professor of
   Women's Health
Columbia University College of
   Physicians and Surgeons
New York, New York

**Leonard Wartofsky,** MD, MPH, MACP
Clinical Professor of Medicine
Georgetown University School
   of Medicine
Clinical Professor of Medicine
George Washington University School
   of Medicine and Health Sciences
Chair, Department of Medicine
Washington Hospital Center
Clinical Professor of Medicine
Howard University College
   of Medicine
Washington, DC
Professor of Medicine and Physiology
Uniformed Services University of the
   Health Sciences F. Edward Hébert
   School of Medicine
Bethesda, Maryland

**Stephen I. Wasserman,** MD
Helen M. Ranney Professor of Medicine
Chair, Department of Medicine
University of California, San Diego,
   School of Medicine
La Jolla, California

**Colleen Weber,** RN
Pediatric Endocrine Nurse
Cardinal Glennon Children's Hospital
St. Louis, Missouri

**Anthony Peter Weetman,** MD, FRCP, DSc
Professor of Medicine
University Department of Clinical Sciences
University of Sheffield School of Medicine
Northern General Hospital
Sheffield, England

**Gordon C. Weir,** MD
Professor of Medicine
Research Division
Harvard Medical School
Joslin Diabetes Center
Boston, Massachusetts

**Laura S. Welch,** MD
Director, Occupational and
   Environmental Medicine
Georgetown University School of Medicine
Washington Hospital Center
Washington, DC

**Samuel A. Wells, Jr.,** MD
Professor of Surgery
Washington University School
   of Medicine
St. Louis, Missouri

**Jon C. White,** MD, FACS
Director of Surgical Intensive Care
Department of Surgery
Veterans Affairs Medical Center
Associate Professor of Surgery
George Washington University School
   of Medicine and Health Sciences
Washington, DC

**Perrin C. White,** MD
Professor of Pediatrics
University of Texas Southwestern
   Medical Center at Dallas
Southwestern Medical School
Dallas, Texas

**Michael P. Whyte,** MD
Medical-Scientific Director
Department of Metabolic and
   Molecular Research
Professor of Medicine, Pediatrics,
   and Genetics
Division of Bone and Mineral Diseases
Washington University School
   of Medicine
Barnes–Jewish Hospital
St. Louis, Missouri

**Gordon H. Williams,** MD
Professor of Medicine
Harvard Medical School
Chair, Endocrine-Hypertension
   Division
Brigham and Women's Hospital
Boston, Massachusetts

**Stephen J. Winters,** MD
Professor of Medicine
Chief, Division of Endocrinology
   and Metabolism
University of Louisville School
   of Medicine
Louisville, Kentucky

**Joseph I. Wolfsdorf,** MB, BCh
Associate Professor of Pediatrics
Department of Medicine
Division of Endocrinology
Harvard Medical School
Children's Hospital National
   Medical Center
Boston, Massachusetts

**I-Tien Yeh,** MD
Associate Professor
Department of Pathology
University of Texas Medical School
   at San Antonio
University Health Center
San Antonio, Texas

**Paul M. Yen,** MD
Chief, Molecular Regulation and
   Neuroendocrinology
Clinical Endocrinology Branch
National Institute of Diabetes and
   Digestive and Kidney Disease
National Institutes of Health
Bethesda, Maryland

**James E. Zadina,** PhD
Professor of Medicine
Tulane University School
   of Medicine
Director, Neuroscience
   Laboratory
Department of Research
Veterans Affairs Medical Center
New Orleans, Louisiana

**Gary P. Zaloga,** MA, MD
Director of Critical Care Medicine
Department of Medicine
Georgetown University School
   of Medicine
Washington Hospital Center
Washington, DC

**Charles Zaloudek,** MD
Professor
Department of Pathology
University of California, San Francisco,
   School of Medicine
San Francisco, California

**Carol Zapalowski,** MD, PhD
Colorado Center for Bone Research
Lakewood, Colorado

**Thomas R. Ziegler,** MD
Associate Professor of Medicine
Division of Endocrinology/Metabolism
Emory University School of Medicine
Atlanta, Georgia

**Michael Zinger,** MD
Clinical Instructor
Department of Obstetrics
  and Gynecology
Division of Reproductive
  Endocrinology
University of Cincinnati College
  of Medicine
Cincinnati, Ohio

# PREFACE

This third edition of *Principles and Practice of Endocrinology and Metabolism* has been substantially and systematically revised. All of the chapters have been updated, many have been entirely rewritten, and many deal with completely new topics. Furthermore, additional important information and references have been added up until the very date of printing.

The new chapters covering topics that did not appear in depth in the prior edition include: Molecular Biology: Present and Future; Pituitary Tumors: Overview of Therapeutic Options; The Incidental Adrenal Mass; Appetite; Pancreas and Islet Transplantation; Syndrome X; Endocrine Effects on Lipids; Compendium of Growth Factors and Cytokines; The Endocrine Blood Cells; The Endocrine Adipocyte; and Endocrine Disorders in Human Immunodeficiency Virus Infection.

We would like to welcome the authors of these chapters, and also the new authors who have updated, extensively revised, or have entirely rewritten chapters on topics that appeared in the last edition.

A new section has been added to this textbook: Endocrinology of Critical Illness. The six chapters comprising this section address the multiple aspects of this condition in a manner that is unique. Critical illness, which to some extent afflicts the great bulk of humankind at some time in their lives, has enormous hormonal and metabolic dimensions that relate directly to the diagnosis of the illness, influence the response of the host and the consequent evolution of the condition, and play a role in its outcome. The specific chapters include Critical Illness and Systemic Inflammation, Endocrine Markers and Mediators in Critical Illness, The Hypothalamic–Pituitary–Adrenal Axis in Stress and Critical Illness, Neuroendocrine Response to Acute versus Prolonged Critical Illness, Fuel Metabolism and Nutrient Delivery in Critical Illness, and Endocrine Therapeutics in Critical Illness. These subjects are of great importance to every endocrine clinician as well as many who are involved in fundamental endocrine research.

Overall, the goal of this textbook is to continue to provide, in a readable, understandable, and well-illustrated format, the clinical and basic information on endocrinology and metabolism that will be useful to both clinicians and basic scientists. We also wish this book to be a useful source of information for internists, house staff, and medical students. We have attempted to cover the field thoroughly and broadly, to include most of the known endocrine and metabolic disorders and hormonal messenger molecules, to furnish appropriate and current references, and to be of practical benefit to our readers.

A complete CD version of this entire textbook is available. It contains approximately 4000 self-assessment questions that have been assembled and edited by Dr. Meeta Sharma.

I wish to acknowledge the very helpful library assistance of Joanne Bennett. I am very grateful for the indispensable editorial and pharmaceutical aid of my Editorial Assistant, Roberta L. Brown, Pharm. D.

Kenneth L. Becker, MD, PhD

# PREFACE TO THE FIRST EDITION

Although there are several excellent large textbooks of endocrinology, we have felt the need for a book which would aim at encompassing all aspects of the field, a book which would be disease-oriented, would have practical applicability to the care of the adult and pediatric patient, and could be consulted to obtain a broad range of pathophysiologic, diagnostic, and therapeutic information.

To fulfill this goal we called upon not only eminent specialists in endocrinology but also upon experts in many fields of medicine and science. The first part of the book surveys general aspects of endocrinology. The eight succeeding parts deal with specific fields of endocrinology: The Endocrine Brain and Pituitary Gland, The Thyroid Gland, Calcium and Bone Metabolism, The Adrenal Glands, Sex Determination and Development, Endocrinology of the Female, Endocrinology of the Male, and Disorders of Fuel Metabolism. Each of these parts contains relevant anatomic, physiologic, diagnostic, and therapeutic information and, when indicated, pediatric coverage of the topic.

Diffuse Hormonal Secretion expounds upon the fact that endocrine function is not confined to anatomically discrete endocrine glands but is also intrinsic to all tissues and organs. This part is divided in two; it first presents a discussion of hormones which have a diffuse distribution and are not reviewed elsewhere in the book, and subsequently it deals with body constituents which are important sites of hormonal secretion.

Heritable Abnormalities of Endocrinology and Metabolism underlines the importance of genetics in the causation of many endocrine and metabolic abnormalities. Endocrine and metabolic dysfunction in the young and in the aged is the subject of a separate part, because in both of these age groups hormonal function as well as endocrine disorders differ profoundly from those of individuals in their middle decades.

Interrelationships Between Hormones and the Body discusses the impact of hormones on the soma and addresses clinical aspects of the disorders they may engender. Hormones and Cancer examines the phenomenon of hormone-induced neoplasms, elaborating on the fact that all neoplasms secrete hormones, that several of these hormones can cause additional clinical disorders, and that some neoplasms respond therapeutically to hormonal manipulation.

The ensuing part, entitled Endocrine and Metabolic Effects of Toxic Agents deals with the sometimes subtle, sometimes profound influence of four nearly omnipresent agents: medication, alcohol, tobacco, and cannabis; it also addresses the consequences of environmental toxins on the endocrine system. The last part deals with the therapeutic use of drugs in endocrinology and the proper interpretation of laboratory values. It offers an extensive table on the clinical use of endocrine-related drugs, a table on reference values, and an outline of the dynamic procedures used in endocrinology. The goal of these tabular chapters is to facilitate the day-to-day evaluation and therapy of the endocrine patient.

As a rule, the emphasis of this textbook is on the endocrinology of the human being. Animal data are presented only when contributing to a better understanding of human physiology and pathology. To maximize current relevance, historical information is kept to a minimum. While efforts were made to avoid repetition, the coverage of certain topics may recur when viewed from different standpoints. It is hoped that this will provide a wider dimension of the understanding of endocrine and metabolic function and dysfunction.

In order not to interrupt continuity, bibliographic references are grouped at the end of each part. Finally, with the interest of the reader in mind, particular attention was given to composing an index as detailed as possible.

I wish to thank the associate editors of this text for their skill, their enthusiasm, and their hard work. We all are very grateful for the expertise of our many eminent contributors. During the preparation of the manuscripts, there was considerable intercommunication between these contributors and their respective editors concerning both content and presentation.

I wish to acknowledge the participation of Richard H. Snider, PhD, and Eric S. Nylén, MD, who have provided outstanding editorial assistance throughout the preparation of the textbook.

The field of endocrinology and metabolism is evolving rapidly. New data are being developed continuously, and with this in mind, all contributors were encouraged to add up-to-date information until nearly the date of publication.

There are numerous matters upon which there is no current common agreement, and logical arguments can be marshaled to buttress diametrically different viewpoints. This textbook is written by many authors; though most of the beliefs and conclusions of the contributors tend to reflect those of the editors, no attempt was made to impose a uniformity of pathophysiologic, diagnostic, or therapeutic viewpoints, and the book does not lack for differences of opinion.

We hope that the *Principles and Practice of Endocrinology and Metabolism* will be a relevant sourcebook for those interested in the science and the practice of this fascinating discipline, whether they be clinicians, basic scientists, allied health personnel, or students.

Kenneth L. Becker, MD, PhD

# CONTENTS

# PART III   THE THYROID GLAND

## *Leonard Wartofsky, Editor*

# PART IV   CALCIUM AND BONE METABOLISM

## *John P. Bilezikian, Editor*

## PART V THE ADRENAL GLANDS

### *D. Lynn Loriaux, Editor*

# PART VI  SEX DETERMINATION AND DEVELOPMENT
## Robert W. Rebar and William J. Bremner, Editors

# PART VII  ENDOCRINOLOGY OF THE FEMALE
## Robert W. Rebar, Editor

# PART VIII  ENDOCRINOLOGY OF THE MALE
## *William J. Bremner, Editor*

# PART IX  DISORDERS OF FUEL METABOLISM
## *C. Ronald Kahn, Editor*

# P A R T  X  DIFFUSE HORMONAL SECRETION

*Eric S. Nylén, Editor*

# PART XI  HERITABLE ABNORMALITIES OF ENDOCRINOLOGY AND METABOLISM

*Kenneth L. Becker, Editor*

# PART XII  IMMUNOLOGIC BASIS OF ENDOCRINE DISORDERS

*Leonard Wartofsky, Editor*

# PART XIII ENDOCRINE AND METABOLIC DYSFUNCTION IN THE GROWING CHILD AND IN THE AGED

## Wellington Hung, Editor

# PART XIV INTERRELATIONSHIPS BETWEEN HORMONES AND THE BODY

## Kenneth L. Becker, Editor

# PART XV HORMONES AND CANCER
## *Kenneth L. Becker, Editor*

# PART XVI ENDOCRINOLOGY OF CRITICAL ILLNESS
## *Eric S. Nylén, Editor*

# PART XVII ENDOCRINE AND METABOLIC EFFECTS OF TOXIC AGENTS
## *Kenneth L. Becker, Editor*

# PART XVIII   ENDOCRINE DRUGS AND VALUES
## *Kenneth L. Becker, Editor*

# PART I

# GENERAL PRINCIPLES OF ENDOCRINOLOGY

KENNETH L. BECKER, EDITOR

# CHAPTER 1

# ENDOCRINOLOGY AND THE ENDOCRINE PATIENT

KENNETH L. BECKER, ERIC S. NYLÉN, AND RICHARD H. SNIDER, JR.

## DEFINITIONS

*Endocrinology* is the study of communication and control within a living organism by means of chemical messengers that are synthesized in whole or in part by that organism.

*Metabolism*, which is an integral part of the science of endocrinology, is the study of the biochemical control mechanisms that occur within living organisms. The term includes such diverse activities as gene expression; biosynthetic pathways and their enzymatic catalysis; the modification, transformation, and degradation of biologic substances; the biochemical mediation of the actions and interactions of such substances; and the means for obtaining, storing, and mobilizing energy.

The chemical messengers of endocrinology are the *hormones*, endogenous informational molecules that are involved in both intracellular and extracellular communication.

## ROLE OF THE ENDOCRINE SYSTEM

The mammalian organism, including the human, is multicellular and highly specialized with regard to sustaining life and reproductive processes. Reproduction requires gametogenesis, fertilization, and implantation. Subsequently, the new intrauterine conception must undergo cell proliferation, organogenesis, and differentiation into a male or female. After parturition, the newborn must grow and mature sexually, so that the cycle may be repeated. To a considerable extent, the endocrine system influences or controls all of these processes. Hormones participate in all physiologic functions, such as muscular activity, respiration, digestion, hematopoiesis, sense organ function, thought, mood, and behavior. The overall purpose of the coordinating, regulating, integrating, stimulating, suppressing, and modulating effects of the many components of the endocrine system is *homeostasis*. The maintenance of a healthy optimal internal milieu in the presence of a continuously changing and sometimes threatening external environment is termed *allostasis*.

## HORMONES

### CHEMICAL CLASSIFICATION

Most hormones can be classified into one of several chemical categories: *amino-acid derivatives* (e.g., tryptophan → serotonin and melatonin; tyrosine → dopamine, norepinephrine, epinephrine, triiodothyronine, and thyroxine; L-glutamic acid → γ-aminobutyric acid; histidine → histamine), *peptides* or *polypeptides* (e.g., thyrotropin-releasing hormone, insulin, growth hormone, nerve growth factor), *steroids* (e.g., progesterone, androgens, estrogens, corticosteroids, vitamin D and its metabolites), and *fatty acid derivatives* (e.g., prostaglandins, leukotrienes, thromboxanes).

### SOURCES, CONTROLS, AND FUNCTIONS

Previously hormones were thought to be synthesized and secreted predominantly by anatomically discrete and circum-

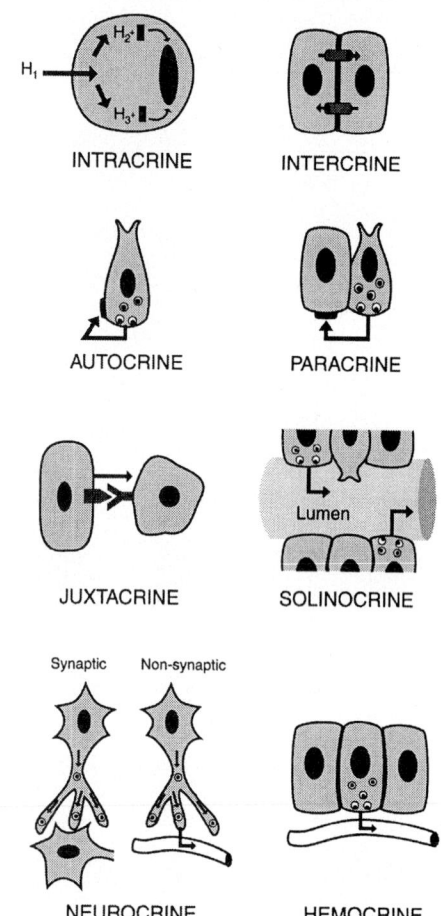

**FIGURE 1-1.** Different types of hormonal communication detailed in the chapter. The darkened areas on the cell membrane represent receptors. (*H*, hormone.) See text for explanations.

scribed glandular structures, called ductless glands (e.g., pituitary, thyroid, adrenals, gonads). However, many microscopic organoid-like groups of cells and innumerable other cells of the body contain and secrete hormones (see Chap. 175).

The classic "glands" of endocrinology have lost their exclusivity, and although they are important on physiologic and pathologic levels, the widespread secretion of hormones throughout the body by "*nonglandular*" *tissues* is of equal importance. Most hormones are known to have *multiple sources*. Moreover, the physiologic stimuli that release these hormones are often found to differ according to their locale. The response to a secreted hormone is not stereotyped but varies according to the nature and location of the target cells or tissues.

## TRANSPORT

### TYPES OF SECRETORY TRANSPORT

Hormones have various means of reaching target cells. In the early decades of the development of the field of endocrinology, hormones were conceived to be substances that traveled to distal sites through the blood. This is accomplished by release into the extracellular spaces and subsequent entrance into blood vessels by way of capillary fenestrations. The most appropriate term for such blood-bone communication is *hemocrine* (Fig. 1-1).

Several alternative means of hormonal communication exist, however. *Paracrine* communication involves the extrusion of hormonal contents into the surrounding interstitial spaces; the hormone then interacts with receptors on nearby cells (see Fig. 1-1 and Chaps. 4 and 175).[1] Direct paracrine transfer of cytoplasmic messenger molecules into adjacent cells may occur through specialized gap junctions (i.e., *intercrine* secretion).[2] Unlike hemocrine secretion, in which the hormonal secretion is diluted within the circulatory system, paracrine secretion delivers a very high concentration of hormone to its target site. *Juxtacrine* communication occurs when the messenger molecule does not traverse a fluid phase to reach another cell, but, instead, remains associated with the plasma membrane of the signaling cell while acting directly on an immediately adjacent receptor cell (e.g., intercellular signaling that is adhesion dependent and occurs between endothelial cells and leukocytes and transforming growth factor-α in human endometrium).[3,4]

Hormones may be secreted and subsequently interact with the same cell that released the substance; this process is *autocrine* secretion (see Fig. 1-1).[5] The secreted hormone stimulates, suppresses, or otherwise modulates the activity of the secreting cell. Autocrine secretion is a form of self-regulation of a cell by its own product.

When peptide hormones or other neurotransmitters or neuromodulators are produced by neurons, the term *neurocrine* secretion is used (see Fig. 1-1).[6] This specialized form of paracrine release may be *synaptic* (i.e., the messenger traverses a structured synaptic space) or *nonsynaptic* (i.e., the messenger is carried to its local or distal site of action by way of the extracellular fluid or the blood). Nonsynaptic neurocrine secretion has also been called *neurosecretion*. An example of neurosecretion is the release of vasopressin and oxytocin into the circulatory system by nervous tissue of the pituitary (see Chap. 25).

Several peptides and amines are secreted into the luminal aspect of the gut (e.g., gastrin, somatostatin, luteinizing hormone–releasing hormone, calcitonin, secretin, vasoactive intestinal peptide, serotonin, substance P).[7] This process may be called *solinocrine* secretion (see Fig. 1-1), from the Greek word for a hollow tube. Solinocrine secretion also occurs into the bronchi, the urogenital tract, and other ductal structures.[8]

Commonly, the same hormone can be transported by more than one of these means.[9]

Extracellular transportation may not always be necessary for hormones to exert their effects. For example, some known hormonal secretions that are transported by one or more of these mechanisms are also found in extremely low concentrations within the cytoplasm of many cells. In such circumstances, these hormones do not appear to be localized to identifiable secretion granules and probably act primarily within the cell. This phenomenon may be called *intracrine* secretion. As shown in Figure 1-1, the process comprising uptake of a hormone precursor $H_1$ and intracellular conversion into $H_2$ (e.g., estrogens) or $H_3$ (e.g., androgens) and subsequent binding and nuclear action is also a form of intracrine communication.

### OVERLAP OF EXOCRINE AND ENDOCRINE TYPES OF SECRETION

Classically, an *exocrine* gland is a specialized structure that secretes its products at an external or internal surface (e.g., sweat glands, sebaceous glands, salivary glands, oxyntic or gastric glands, pancreatic exocrine glandular system, prostate gland). An exocrine gland may be unicellular (e.g., mucous or goblet cells of the epithelium of mucous membranes) or multicellular (e.g., salivary glands). Many multicellular exocrine glands possess a structured histologic organization that is suited to the production and delivery of secretions that are produced in relatively large quantities. A specialized excretory duct or system of ducts usually constitutes an intrinsic part of the gland. Some exocrine glandular cells secrete their substances by means of destruction of the cells themselves (i.e., *holocrine* secretion); an example is the sebaceous glands. Other exocrine glandular cells secrete their substances by way of the loss of a portion of the apical cytoplasm along with the material being secreted (i.e., *apocrine* secretion); an example is the apocrine sweat glands. Alternatively, in many forms of exocrine secretion, the secretory cells release their products through the cell membrane, and the cell remains intact (i.e., *merocrine* secretion); an example is the salivary glands. The constituents of some exocrine glands, particularly those opening on the external surface of the body, sometimes function as *pheromones*, which are chemical substances that act on other members of the species.[10]

Many exocrine glands contain cells of the diffuse neuroendocrine system (see Chap. 175) and neurons; both cell types secrete *peptide hormones*. Peptide hormones, steroids, and prostaglandins are found in all exocrine secretions (e.g., sweat, saliva, milk, bile, seminal fluid; see Chap. 106).[11–14] Although they usually are not directly produced in such glands, thyroid and steroid hormones are found in exocrine secretions as well.[15–18]

The preferred approach is to view the term "exocrine" as a histologic-anatomic entity and not as a term that is meant to be antithetical to or to contrast with the term "endocrine." Endocrinologists are concerned clinically and experimentally with all means of hormonal communication. The word "endocrine" is best used in a global sense, indicating any and all means of communication by messenger molecules.

## TYRANNY OF HORMONE TERMINOLOGY

Hormones usually are named at the time of their discovery. Sometimes, the names are based on the locations where they were first found or on their presumed effects. However, with time, other locations and other effects are discovered, and these new locations or effects often are more physiologically relevant than the initial findings. *Hormonal names are often overly restrictive, confusing, or misleading.*

In many instances, such hormonal names have become inappropriate. For example, atrial natriuretic hormone is present in the brain, hypothalamus, pituitary, autonomic ganglia, and lungs as well as atrium, and it has effects other than natriuresis (see Chap. 178). Gastrin-releasing peptide is found in semen, far from the site of gastrin release. Somatostatin, which was found in the hypothalamus and named for its inhibitory effect on growth hormone, occurs in many other locations and has multiple other functions (see Chap. 169). Calcitonin, which initially was thought to play an important role in regulating serum calcium and was named accordingly, appears to exert many other effects, and its influence on serum calcium may be quite minor (see Chap. 53). Growth hormone–releasing hormone and arginine vasopressin are found in the testis, where effects on growth hormone release or on the renal tubular reabsorption of water are most unlikely. Vasoactive intestinal peptide is found in multiple tissues other than the intestines (see Chap. 182). Insulin, named for the pancreatic islets, is found in the brain and elsewhere.[19] Prostaglandins have effects that are far more widespread than those exerted in the secretions of the prostate, from which their name derives (see Chap. 172).

The endocrine lexicon also contains substances called hormones that are not hormones. In the human, melanocyte-stimulating hormone (MSH) is not a functional hormone, but it comprises amino-acid sequences within the proopiomelanocortin (POMC) molecule: α-MSH within the adrenocorticotropic hormone (ACTH) moiety, β-MSH within δ-lipotropin, and δ-MSH within the N-terminal fragment of POMC (see Chap. 14).

Numerous peptide hormones exist that, because of their effects on DNA synthesis, cell growth, and cell proliferation, have been called *growth factors* and *cytokines* (see Chaps. 173 and 174). These substances, which act locally and at a distance, often do not have the sharply delineated target cell selectivity that was attributed to them when they first were discovered. Their terminology also is confusing and often misleading.

Aside from occasional readjustments of hormonal nomenclature, no facile solution appears to exist to the quandary of terminology, other than an awareness of the pitfalls into which the terms may lead us.

## ENDOCRINE SYSTEM INTERACTION WITH ALL BODY SYSTEMS

Although speaking in terms of the cardiovascular, respiratory, gastrointestinal, and nervous systems is convenient, the endocrine system anatomically and functionally overlaps with all body systems (see Part X). Extensive overlap is found between the endocrine system and the nervous system (see Chaps. 175 and 176). Hormonal peptides are synthesized in the cell bodies of neurons, are transported along axons to nerve terminals, and are released at the nerve endings. Within these neurons, they coexist with classic neurotransmitters and often are coreleased with them. These substances play a role in *neuromodulation* or *neurosecretion* by means of the extracellular fluid. The nerves in which peptide hormones appear to play a role in the transmission of information are called *peptidergic* nerves.[20] It is the ample similarity of ultrastructure, histochemistry, and hormonal contents of nerve cells and of many peptide-secreting endocrine cells that has led to the concept of the diffuse neuroendocrine system.

## GENETICS AND ENDOCRINOLOGY

The rapid application of new discoveries and new techniques in genetics has revolutionized medicine, including the field of endocrinology. DNA probes have been targeted to selected genes, and the chromosomal locations of genes related to many hormones and their receptors have been determined. A complete map of the human genome is gradually emerging.[21] This approach has led to new knowledge about hormone biosynthesis and has provided important information concerning species differences and evolution. The elucidation of the chromosomal loci for genes controlling the biosynthesis of hormone receptors should provide insights into the physiologic effects of hormones. Clinically, these techniques have potential significance as a diagnostic aid in evaluating afflicted patients, a means of identifying asymptomatic heterozygotes, and a method for identification of unborn individuals at risk (i.e., prenatal diagnosis; see Chap. 240). Delineation of processes of genetic expression is revealing the mechanisms of hormonal disease (e.g., obesity[22]) and also may lead to gene therapy for some forms of endocrine illness or humoral-mediated conditions.[23]

## NORMAL AND ABNORMAL EXPRESSION OR MODULATION OF THE HORMONAL MESSAGE AND ITS METABOLIC EFFECT

A sophisticated and faultless machinery is required for appropriate hormonal expression. The hormonal messenger is subject to modifications that may occur anywhere from its initial synthesis to its final arrival at its target site. Subsequently, the expression of the message at this site (i.e., its action) may also be modified (see Chap. 4). The modulations or alterations of the hormonal message or its final action may be physiologic or pathologic. Table 1-1 summarizes some of the normal and abnormal modulations of a hormonal message and its subsequent metabolic effects.

On a physiologic level, the first steps in the genetic ordering of hormonal synthesis, the subsequent posttranslational processing of the hormone, the postsecretory extracellular transport, the receptor mediation of the hormone and subsequent transduction, and the inactivation and clearance of the hormone all contribute to *expressing, diversifying, focalizing, and specifying the hormonal message and its ultimate action.* On a pathologic level, all of these steps are subject to malfunction, causing disease.

Our increased knowledge of endocrine systems has forced us to rethink many traditional concepts. To dispel some common misconceptions, listing several "nots" of endocrinology may be worthwhile (Table 1-2).

## THE ENDOCRINE PATIENT

### FREQUENCY OF ENDOCRINE DISORDERS

In a survey of the subspecialty problems seen by endocrinologists, the six most common, in order of frequency, were found to be diabetes mellitus, thyrotoxicosis, hypothyroidism, nontoxic nodular goiter, diseases of the pituitary gland, and diseases of the adrenal gland. Some conditions seen by endocrinologists are infrequent or rare (e.g., congenital adrenal hyperplasia, pseudohypoparathyroidism), whereas others are relatively common (e.g., Graves disease, Hashimoto thyroiditis), and some are among the most prevalent diseases in general practice (e.g., diabetes mellitus, obesity, hyperlipoproteinemia, osteoporosis, Paget disease). The third most common medical problem encountered by general practitioners is diabetes mellitus, and the tenth most frequent problem is obesity.[66]

Of the total deaths in the United States (i.e., both sexes, all races, and all ages combined), diabetes mellitus is the seventh most common cause. The most common cause of death (heart disease) and the third most common (cerebrovascular accidents) are greatly influenced by metabolic conditions such as diabetes mellitus and hyperlipemia.[67]

### COST OF ENDOCRINE DISORDERS

The frequency and morbidity of endocrine diseases such as osteoporosis, obesity, hypothyroidism, and hyperthyroidism, and the grave consequences of other endocrine disorders such as Cushing syndrome and Addison disease demonstrate that the expense to society is considerable. In the case of diabetes, the health care expenditure is staggering. Approximately 10.3 million people have diabetes in the U.S., and an estimated 5.4 million have undiagnosed diabetes. Direct medical expenses attributed to diabetes total $44.1 billion. The total annual medical expenses of people with diabetes average $10,071 per capita, as compared to $2,669 for persons without diabetes.[68] Interestingly, these expenses may be less if the appropriate specialties are involved in the care.[69]

### FACTORS THAT INFLUENCE TEST RESULTS

In clinical medicine, hormonal concentrations usually are ascertained from two of the most easily obtained sources: blood and urine. The diagnosis of an endocrinopathy often depends on the demonstration of increased or decreased levels of these blood or urine constituents. However, several factors must be kept in mind when interpreting a result that appears to be abnormal. These may include age, gender, time of day, exercise, posture, emotional state, hepatic and renal status, presence of other illness, and concomitant drug therapy (see Chaps. 237 and 239).

### RELIABILITY OF THE LABORATORY DETERMINATION

The practice of clinical endocrinology far from a large medical center was previously hindered by the difficulty in obtaining blood and urine tests essential for appropriate diagnosis and follow-up care. However, accurate and rapid analyses now are provided by commercial laboratories. Nevertheless, wherever performed, some tests are unreliable because of methodologic difficulties. Other tests may be difficult to interpret because of a particular susceptibility to alteration by physiologic or pharmacologic factors (e.g., plasma catecholamines; see Chap. 86).

**TABLE 1-1.**

**Modulation of the Hormone Message and Its Subsequent Physiologic or Pathologic Metabolic Effects**

| Modulation | Explanation | Examples |
|---|---|---|
| Gene mutations | Alteration of one or more nucleotides within the DNA gene sequence may result in a missense gene, a nonsense gene, a gene deletion, or a gene conversion.[24,25] The mutation may affect hormone synthesis, enzymatic processing of the hormone, or synthesis of a receptor for a hormone. | Mutant proinsulin syndrome is characterized by a structurally abnormal proinsulin, which results in diminished bioactivity and diabetes.[26] A mutation involving the inwardly rectifying potassium (Kir) channels results in the syndrome of persistent hyperinsulinemic hypoglycemia of infancy, in which pancreatic B cells are dysfunctional.[27] Some nondiabetic Mexican Americans have mutation in the high-affinity sulfonyl urea receptor (*SUR1*) gene, which regulates insulin secretion. This may be an antecedent to the development of type 2 diabetes in some of these hyperinsulinemic persons.[28] Growth hormone resistance (i.e., Laron syndrome) is caused by point mutations in the gene coding for the human growth hormone receptor.[29,30] Mutations in the *NKCC2* gene (one of the $Na^+$-$K^+$-$Cl^-$ cotransporter isoforms) results in Bartter syndrome (hypokalemic metabolic acidosis, salt wasting, volume depletion, and hypercalciuria).[31] Pseudoaldosteronism type 1 (PAH1) is often due to a mutation of the amiloride-sensitive epithelial sodium channel.[32] |
| Chromosomal deletions | Loss of chromosomal material, with an associated loss of genes. | WAGR syndrome (Wilms tumor, aniridia, genitourinary malformations, mental retardation) may have an associated chromosomal deletion involving the gene coding for the β-subunit of follicle-stimulating hormone; its deficiency during embryonic development may cause the genitourinary abnormalities.[33] Ovarian dysgenesis (Turner syndrome) is the result of the loss of all or part of an X chromosome (see Chap. 90). CATCH 22 (cardiac defect, abnormal facies, thymic hypoplasia, cleft palate, hypocalcemia) is due to a deletion within chromosome 22.[34] |
| Alternative gene processing | Alternative splicing of the primary RNA transcript gives rise to multiple messenger RNAs, each encoding a different hormone (see Chap. 3). A similar phenomenon can occur during the synthesis of a hormonal receptor. | An alternative exon selection gives rise to the hormone calcitonin or the very differently structured[35] hormone calcitonin gene-related peptide (CGRP), a phenomenon that may be altered by a physiologic or pathologic change of the biosynthetic milieu (see Chap. 53).[35a] Many patients with medullary thyroid cancer have a greater CGRP-to-calcitonin secretion ratio than do normal persons. Alternative splicing can also produce different forms of receptors (e.g., thyroid receptors).[36,37] |
| Posttranslational processing | Most or all peptide hormones are synthesized in the form of large polypeptide precursors,[38] some of which contain more than one functionally distinct hormone (see Chap. 3). Subsequent proteolytic enzymatic processing releases these hormones in their bioactive state.[39] | In the paraneoplastic adrenocorticotropic hormone (ACTH) syndrome in which ACTH is biosynthesized by an extrapituitary tumor (see Chap. 219), much of the hormone that is detectable in the serum is of high-molecular-mass, incompletely processed bioinactive material (see Chaps. 14 and 75). |
| Alterations of transporting molecules | Many hormones are transported in the blood in association with protein carrier molecules. These substances facilitate transport and may provide a means of temporary storage of the hormone, protecting it from degradation or retarding its clearance. | Sex hormone–binding globulin (see Chap. 101) progressively decreases in concentration from infancy to prepuberty, gradually increasing the amount of unbound testosterone and estradiol; this augments the amount of free, tissue-available sex hormones before puberty.[40] In familial dysalbuminemic hyperthyroxinemia, a variant albumin possesses a high affinity for thyroxine; as a result, these euthyroid persons have a spuriously high total serum thyroxine.[41] |
| Endogenous antihormones | Circulating antihormones antagonize hormone action.[42] These substances, which differ slightly in structure from the hormones they antagonize, bind to the appropriate hormonal receptors but lack some or all bioactivity. | Some men with idiopathic azoospermia or oligospermia may have relatively inactive follicle-stimulating hormone isoforms.[43] |
| Antibodies to hormones or to their receptors | Although not present normally, antibodies to endogenous hormones may develop. Antibodies also may develop to a hormone receptor.[44] | Antiinsulin antibodies are found in the blood of patients with previously untreated type 1 diabetes.[45] In first-degree relatives of patients with type 1 diabetes, the presence of such antibodies may be a predictive marker for the disease.[46] Antiinsulin receptor antibodies may produce hypoglycemia through their continuous receptor stimulatory activity[47]; others can produce severe cellular resistance to both insulin and insulin-like growth factor-I.[48] Autoantibodies to the thyrotropin receptor of the thyroid follicular cell appear in Graves disease (see Chap. 42) and may cause the hyperthyroidism.[49] |
| Receptor or postreceptor mediation of hormone action | Hormones reversibly bind to specific high-affinity protein receptors, leading to intracellular events that culminate in the appropriate cellular response (see Chaps. 4, 32, and 72). Altered receptor function or altered *transduction* (i.e., the biochemical events beyond receptor binding) plays a role in the pathogenesis of several endocrine disorders. Some of these defects are the result of antibodies to receptors (as above) and others result from heritable or acquired (e.g., drug-induced) defects in the receptor or its subsequent transduction. These congenital or acquired conditions may be called *target cell resistance disorders.* | Steroid hormone resistance: vitamin D–dependent rickets type 2 (see Chaps. 63 and 70),[50] primary glucocorticoid resistance,[51] pseudohypoaldosteronism,[52] androgen resistance (see Chap. 96).[53] Thyroid hormone resistance: pituitary or generalized resistance to thyroid due to a receptor abnormality (see Chap. 32). Peptide hormone resistance: resistant ovary syndrome due to decreased responsivity to gonadotropins (see Chap. 96),[54,55] type A syndromes of insulin resistance and acanthosis nigricans (see Chap. 146),[56] congenital nephrogenic diabetes insipidus due to resistance to vasopressin.[57,58] Some cases of insulin resistance may be due to abnormalities of the GLUT4 insulin transporter system.[59] |
| Hormone inactivation and clearance | A hormone must be inactivated or removed from its target site so that its effect may terminate. Depending on the hormone, the mechanisms for such termination are hydrolysis by degradative enzymes, oxidation, reduction, deiodination, conjugation with glucuronide, and other methods.[60–64] Depending on the hormone, various tissues or organs are involved in their degradation or clearance from the circulation or from the body (e.g., liver, kidney, muscle, lung). | Ineffective hepatic degradation of endogenous estrogens may result in gynecomastia (see Chap. 120). Renal disease may result in poor degradation of the exogenous insulin administered to a type 1 diabetic, resulting in hypoglycemia. A deficiency of the 11β-hydroxysteroid dehydrogenase enzyme results in poor clearance of cortisol and a syndrome of mineralocorticoid excess[65] (see Chap. 80). The uridine diphospho-glucuronosyl-transferase (UGT) family of enzymes conjugate and inactivate steroid hormones in their target tissues, and modifications of their expression may influence hormonal responsivity.[65] |

**TABLE 1-2.**
**Several "Nots" of Modern Endocrinology**

1. Endocrinology is *not* only the study of internal secretions by ductless glands. It also deals with the secretions of groups of cells, of individual cells, and of the exocrine glands.

2. The secretion of a gland is *not* unihormonal. There is no gland and probably no hormone-secreting cell that secretes only one active substance.

3. Most hormones do *not* have a single source. With very few exceptions, hormones are produced in more than one location in the body and by more than one cell type.

4. In view of the extensive tissue distribution of most hormones, with some exceptions, the extirpation of any single gland or tissue that produces large amounts of a specific hormone usually does *not* remove that hormone from the body.

5. A hormone is *not* a substance that acts only at a distal site in the body. Its action often is within the immediate environs, and sometimes it acts on the very cell that secretes the hormone.

6. The term "endocrine" should *not* be used to connote a means of transport (i.e., the blood). A hormone is *not* only blood borne. It also may be borne by extracellular fluid, in lymph, across synapses, or in external secretions, and it may be carried in a functioning state within the confines of the cell itself.

7. A hormone does *not* in itself exert a specific action. It depends on arriving and interacting with an appropriate receptor that commences the transduction of the hormone message into an action.

8. The receptor-mediated actions of most hormones are *not* stereotyped. They often differ according to the site-specific characteristics of the receptors and their function at that time.

9. The name of a hormone does *not* necessarily indicate its exclusive site of production or its predominant physiologic action.

10. The endocrine system is *not* under the control of a separate and independent nervous system. Instead, the nervous and endocrine systems overlap on both a biochemical and a physiologic level.

11. The effects of hormones are *not* independent of their concentrations. They vary according to the quantity present at the site of action; an excess may cause effects entirely different from a physiologically sufficient amount.

12. The effects of hormones are *not* independent of the age of the individual. They vary with the developmental stage of an individual and with his or her age.

---

Although many tests are sensitive and specific, they all have innate interassay and intraassay variations that may be particularly misleading when a given value is close to the clinical "medical decision point" (see Chap. 237). Some laboratory differences are due to hormone heterogeneity (e.g., growth hormone has several isoforms, which bind differently to growth hormone–binding proteins).[70]

### DETERMINATION OF ABNORMAL TEST RESULTS

Not uncommonly, the intellectual or commercial enthusiasm engendered by a new diagnostic procedure of presumed importance is found to be unjustified, because the "test" was based on an invalid premise, because too few of ill patients were studied, because normative data to establish reference values were insufficient, or because subsequent studies were not confirmatory (see Chaps. 237 and 241).

The increased sophistication of medical testing has made the physician and the patient aware of the presence of "abnormalities" that may be harmless: physiologic deviations from that which is most common, or pathologic entities that commonly remain asymptomatic. Such findings may cause considerable worry, lead to the expense and risk of further diagnostic procedures, and even cause needless therapeutic intervention.

Some "abnormalities" are the result of methods of imaging. For example, sonography of the thyroid may demonstrate the presence of small nodules within the thyroid gland of a person without any palpable abnormality of that region of the gland; most such microlesions are benign or behave as if they were.

Another "abnormality" revealed by imaging is the occasional heterogeneous appearance of a normal pituitary gland on a computed tomography (CT) examination. Intermingled CT-lucent and CT-dense areas are seen on the scan, and such nonhomogeneous areas may be confused with a microadenoma.[71,72] The increasing use of magnetic resonance imaging (MRI) of the brain may reveal a bona fide asymptomatic microadenoma of the pituitary gland, but extensive endocrine workup often reveals many such lesions to be nonfunctional. They occur in as much as 10% of the normal population.[73]

Rathke cleft cysts of the anterior sella turcica or the anterior suprasellar cistern often are seen by MRI.[74] Although an occasional patient may have a large and symptomatic lesion,[75] most of these lesions are small and asymptomatic. During MRI or CT examination of the brain, the examiner often incidentally encounters a "primary empty sella," an extension of the subarachnoid space into the sella turcica with a resultant flattening of the pituitary gland in a patient without any pituitary lesion or any prior surgery of that region (see Chap. 11). Although some of these patients may be symptomatic, most have no associated symptoms or hormonal deficit. Another, albeit rare, lesion of the pituitary region seen on MRI is a sellar spine. This asymptomatic anatomic variant is an osseous spine arising in the midline from the dorsum sella that protrudes into the pituitary fossa; it may be an ossified remnant of the cephalic tip of the notochord.[76]

MRI or CT scanning of the abdomen may reveal the presence of harmless morphologic variations of the adrenal gland (i.e., incidentalomas) that sometimes leads to unnecessary surgery.[77] (See Chap. 84.)

### RISKS OF ENDOCRINE TESTING

Endocrine testing is not always benign. Many procedures can cause mild to marked side effects.[78–81] Other diagnostic maneuvers, particularly angiography, may result in severe illness.[82] The expected benefit of any procedure that is contemplated for a patient clearly should be greater than the risk.

### COST AND PRACTICABILITY OF ENDOCRINE TESTING

In addition to being aware of the many factors that influence hormonal values, the limitations of laboratory determinations, and the potential risks of some of these procedures, the endocrinologist must be aware of their expense, particularly because medical costs have increased at an annual rate that is almost twice the rate of overall inflation during the last several years.

A hypertensive patient with hypokalemia who is taking neither diuretics nor laxatives should undergo studies of the renin-angiotensin-aldosterone system, and appropriate pharmacologic or dietary manipulations of sodium balance should be instituted (see Chap. 90). But what should be done with the hypertensive patient who is normokalemic? Occasionally, such a person may have an aldosteronoma.[83] Should such normokalemic patients be studied? Similarly, should the approximately 25 million hypertensive patients in the United States undergo urinary collections for determinations of catecholamine metabolites to find the rare patient with pheochromocytoma? In the context of the individual physician-patient relationship, the answers to such questions may not be difficult, but they become more controversial when placed within the framework of fiscal guidelines.

## CONCLUSION

The complexity of the endocrine system presents a profound intellectual challenge. The macrosystem of endocrine glands secretes its hormones under the influence of other gland-based releasing factors or neural influences or both. The very act of secretion alters subsequent secretion by means of feedback controls (see Chap. 5). Superimposed on this already complex arrangement, the microsystem of dispersed, somewhat independent, but overlapping units throughout the body, as well as the continuous modulation of the receptors for the secreted hormones, allow general or focal actions that are coordinated with other body functions, tempered to the occasion, and appropriate to the needs of the individual. That such a complex system may go awry and that a dysfunction may have a considerable impact on the patient is not surprising.

Because endocrinology and metabolism are broad subjects that incorporate much, if not all, of normal body functions and disease states, they defy easy categorization. However, these enormous complexities, rather than deterring the clinician, researcher, or student, should provide a stimulus to probe deeper into areas difficult to understand and should hasten the eventual application of new developments to patient care.

# REFERENCES

1. Hofbauer LC, Khosla S, Dunstan CR, et al. The roles of osteoprotegerin and osteoprotegerin ligand in the paracrine regulation of bone resorption. J Bone Mineral Res 2000; 15:2.
2. Usadel H, Bornstein SR, Ehrhart-Bornstein M, et al. Gap junctions in the adrenal cortex. Horm Metab Res 1993; 25:653.
3. Zimmerman GA, Lorant DE, McIntyre TM, Prescott SM. Juxtacrine intercellular signaling: another way to do it. Am J Respir Cell Mol Biol 1993; 9:573.
4. Bush MR, Mele JM, Couchman GM, Walmer DK. Evidence of juxtacrine signaling for transforming growth factor alpha in human endometrium. Biol Reprod 1998; 59:1522.
5. Hashimoto K, Higashiyama S, Asada H, et al. Heparin-binding epidermal growth factor-like growth factor is an autocrine growth factor for human keratinocytes. J Biol Chem 1994; 269:20060.
6. Gouin FJ. Morphology, histology and evolution of Myriapoda and insects. 3. The nervous system and the neurocrine systems. Fortschr Zool 1965; 17:189.
7. Uvnas-Wallensten K. Luminal secretion of gut peptides. Clin Gastroenterol 1980; 9:545.
8. Van Minnen J. Production and exocrine secretion of LHRH-like material by the male rat reproductive tract. Peptides 1988; 9:515.
9. Becker KL. The coming of age of a bronchial epithelial cell. Am J Respir Crit Care Med 1994; 149:183.
10. Cohn BA. In search of human skin pheromones. Arch Dermatol 1994; 130:1048.
11. Corps AN, Brown KD, Rees LH, et al. The insulin-like growth factor I content in human milk increases between early and full lactation. J Clin Endocrinol Metab 1988; 67:25.
12. Hammami MM, Haq A, Al-Sedairy S. The level of endothelin-like immunoreactivity in seminal fluid correlates positively with semen volume and negatively with plasma gonadotropin levels. Clin Endocrinol 1994; 40:361.
13. Schmidt NA. Salivary cortisol testing in children. Issues Compr Pediatr Nurs 1998; 20:183.
14. Voss HF. Saliva as a fluid for measurement of estriol levels. Am J Obstet Gynecol 1999; 180:S226.
15. Nizankowska B, Abramowicz T, Korezowski R, Rusin J. Triiodothyronine and thyroxine in human, cow's and formula milk. Exp Clin Endocrinol 1988; 91:116.
16. Langer P, Moravec R, Ohradka B, Foldes O. Iodothyronines in human bile. Endocrinol Exp 1988; 22:35.
17. Shieh CC, Chang SC, Tzeng CR, et al. Measurement of testosterone in seminal plasma, saliva and serum by solid-phase enzyme immunoassay. Andrologia 1987; 19:614.
18. O'Rorke A, Kane MM, Gosling JP, et al. Development and validation of a monoclonal antibody enzyme assay for measuring progesterone in saliva. Clin Chem 1994; 40:454.
19. Hendricke SA, Roth J, Rishi S, Becker KL. Insulin in the nervous system. In: Krieger DT, Bronnstein MJ, Martin J, eds. Brain peptides. New York: John Wiley & Sons, 1983:403.
20. Bean AJ, Zhang X, Hokfelt T. Peptide secretion: what do we know? FASEB J 1994; 8:630.
21. Zabarovsky ER, Allikmets R, Kholodnyuk I, et al. Construction of representative NOTI linking libraries specific for the total human genome and chromosome 3. Genomics 1994; 20:312.
22. Perusse L, Chagnon YC, Weisnagel J, Bouchard C. The human obesity gene map: the 1998 update. Obes Res 1999; 7:111.
23. Moldawer LL, Edwards PD, Minter RM, et al. Application of gene therapy to acute inflammatory disease. Shock 1999; 12:83.
24. Atkinson J, Martin R. Mutations to nonsense codons in human genetic disease: implications for gene therapy by nonsense suppressor tRNAs. Nucleic Acids Res 1994; 22:1327.
25. Miller WL. Molecular biology of steroid hormone synthesis. Endocr Rev 1988; 9:295.
26. Oohoshi H, Ohgawara H, Nanjo K, et al. Familial hyperproinsulinemia associated with NIDDM. Diabetes Care 1993; 16:1340.
27. Abraham MR, Jahingir A, Alekseev AE, Terzic A. Channelopathies of inwardly rectifying potassium channels. FASEB J 1999; 13:1901.
28. Goksel DL, Fischbach K, Duggirala R, et al. Variant in sulfonylurea receptor-1 gene is associated with high insulin concentrations in nondiabetic Mexican Americans: SUR-1 gene variant and hyperinsulinemia. Hum Genet 1998; 103:280.
29. Duquesnoy P, Sobrier ML, Duriez B, et al. A single amino acid substitution in the exoplasmic domain of the human growth hormone GH receptor confers familial GH resistance (Laron syndrome) with positive GH-binding activity by abolishing receptor homodimerization. EMBO J 1994; 13:1386.
30. Rosenfeld RG, Rosenbloom AL, Guevara-Aguirre J. Growth hormone (GH) insensitivity due to primary GH receptor deficiency. Endocr Rev 1994; 15:369.
31. Haas M, Forbush B III. The $Na^+$-$K^+$-$Cl^-$ cotransporters. J Bioenerg Biomembr 1998; 30:161.
32. Torpy DJ, Chrousos GP. Hyper- and hypoaldosteronism. Vitam Horm 1999; 57:177.
33. Glaser T, Lewis WH, Brung GH, et al. The beta subunit of follicle stimulating hormone is deleted in patients with aniridia and Wilms' tumor allowing a further definition of the WAGR locus. Nature 1986; 321:882.
34. Sergi C, Serpi M, Müller-Navia J, et al. CATCH 22 syndrome: report of 7 infants with follow-up data and review of the recent advancements in the genetic knowledge of the locus 22q11. Pathologica 1999; 91:166.
35. Stojdl DF, Bell JC. SR protein kinases: the splice of life. Biochem Cell Biol 1999; 77:293.
35a. Franklyn JA, Sheppard MC. Hormonal control of gene expression. Clin Endocrinol (Oxf) 1988; 29:337.
36. Izumo S, Mahdavi V. Thyroid hormone receptor α isoforms generated by alternative splicing differentially activate myosin HC gene transcription. Nature 1988; 334:539.
37. Koenig RJ, Lazar MA, Hodin RA, et al. Inhibition of thyroid hormone action by a non-hormone binding c-erbA protein generated by alternative mRNA splicing. Nature 1989; 337:659.
38. Jung LJ, Kreiner T, Scheller RH. Prohormone structure governs proteolytic processing and sorting in the Golgi complex. Recent Prog Horm Res 1993; 48:415.
39. Seidah NG, Day R, Marcinkiewicz M, Chrétien M. Mammalian paired basic amino acid convertases of prohormones and proproteins. Annals N Y Acad Sci 1993; 680:135.
40. Belgorosky A, Rivarola MA. Progressive increase in non sex hormone-binding globulin-bound testosterone and estradiol from infancy to late puberty in girls. J Clin Endocrinol Metab 1988; 67:234.
41. Tang KT, Yang HJ, Choo KB, et al. A point mutation in the albumin gene in a Chinese patient with familial dysalbuminemic hyperthyroxinemia. Eur J Endocrinol 1999; 141:374.
42. Dahl KD, Bicsak TA, Hsueh AJW. Naturally occurring antihormones: secretion of FSH antagonists by women treated with a GnRH analog. Science 1988; 239:72.
43. Wang C, Dahl KD, Leung A, et al. Serum bioactive follicle-stimulating hormone in men with idiopathic azoospermia and oligospermia. J Clin Endocrinol Metab 1987; 65:629.
44. Bach JF. Antireceptor or antihormone autoimmunity and its relationship with the idiotype network. Adv Nephrol 1987; 16:251.
45. Palmer JP, Asplin CM, Clemons P, et al. Insulin antibodies in insulin-dependent diabetics before insulin treatment. Science 1983; 222:1337.
46. Yu L, Robles DT, Abiru N, et al. Early expression of antiinsulin autoantibodies of humans and the NOD mouse: evidence for early determination of subsequent diabetes. Proc Natl Acad Sci U S A 2000; 97:1701.
47. Di Paolo S, Georgino R. Insulin resistance and hypoglycemia in a patient with systemic lupus erythematosus: description of antiinsulin receptor antibodies that enhance insulin binding and inhibit insulin action. J Clin Endocrinol Metab 1991; 73:650.
48. Auclair M, Vigaroux C, Desbois-Mouthon C, et al. Antiinsulin receptor autoantibodies associate with insulin receptor substrate-1 and -2 and cause severe cell resistance to both insulin and insulin-like growth factor-I. J Clin Endocrinol Metab 1999; 84:3197.
49. Chiovato L, Santini F, Vitti P, et al. Appearance of thyroid stimulating antibody and Graves disease after radioiodine therapy for toxic nodular goitre. Clin Endocrinol 1994; 40:803.
50. Liberman UA, Eil C, Marx SJ. Clinical features of hereditary resistance to 1,25-dihydroxyvitamin D (hereditary hypocalcemic vitamin D resistant rickets type II). Adv Exp Med Biol 1986; 196:391.
51. Chrousos GP, Detera-Wadleigh SD, Karl M. Syndromes of glucocorticoid resistance. Ann Intern Med 1993; 119:1113.
52. Zennoro MC, Borensztein P, Seubrier F, et al. The enigma of pseudohypoaldosteronism. Steroids 1994; 59:96.
53. Zoppi S, Wilson CM, Harbison MD, et al. Complete testicular feminization caused by an amino-terminal truncation of the androgen receptor with downstream initiation. J Clin Invest 1993; 91:1105.
54. Talbert LM, Raj MH, Hammond MG, Greer T. Endocrine and immunologic ovary syndrome. Fertil Steril 1984; 42:7411.
55. Fraser IS, Russell P, Greco S, Robertson DM. Resistant ovary syndrome and premature ovarian failure in young women with galactosemia. Clin Reprod Fertil 1986; 4:133.

56. Suzuki Y, Hashimoto N, Shimada F, et al. Defects in insulin binding and receptor kinase in cells from a human with type A insulin resistance and from her family. Diabetologia 1991; 34:86.
57. Bichet DG, Razi M, Lonergan M, et al. Hemodynamic and coagulation responses to 1-desamino (8-D-arginine) vasopressin in patients with congenital nephrogenic diabetes insipidus. N Engl J Med 1988; 318:881.
58. Singer I, Forrest JN Jr. Drug-induced states of nephrogenic diabetes insipidus. Kidney Int 1976; 10:82.
59. Jung Cy, Lee W. Glucose transporters and insulin action: some insights into diabetes management. Arch Pharm Res 1999; 22:329.
60. Visser TJ, Kaptein E, Terpstra OT, Krenning EP. Deiodination of thyroid hormone by human liver. J Clin Endocrinol Metab 1988; 67:17.
61. Bunnett NW. Postsecretory metabolism of peptides. Am Rev Respir Dis 1987; 136:S27.
62. Roupas P, Herington AC. Receptor-mediated endocytosis and degradative processing of growth hormone by rat adipocytes in primary culture. Endocrinology 1987; 120:2158.
63. Benzi L, Ceechetti P, Ciccarone A, et al. Insulin degradation in vitro and in vivo: a comparative study in men. Evidence that immunoprecipitable, partially rebindable degradation products are released from cells and circulate in blood. Diabetes 1994; 43:297.
64. Yamaguchi T, Fukase M, Kido H, et al. Meprin is predominantly involved in parathyroid hormone degradation by the microvillar membranes of rat kidney. Life Sci 1994; 54:381.
65. Ferrari P, Lovati E, Frey FJ. The role of the II beta-hydroxysteroid dehydrogenase type 2 in human hypertension. J Hypertens 2000; 18:241.
66. Hum DW, Belanger A, Levesque E, et al. Characterization of UDP-glucuronyl-transferases active on steroid hormones. J Steroid Biochem Mol Biol 1999; 69:413.
67. National Center for Health Statistics. Monthly Vital Statistics Report 1999; 47(19):1.
68. American Diabetes Association. Economic consequences of diabetes mellitus in the U.S. in 1977. Diabetes Care 1998; 21:296.
69. Levetan CS, Passaro MD, Jablonski KA, Ratner RE. Effect of physician specialty on outcomes in diabetic ketoacidosis. Diabetes Care 1999; 22:1790.
70. Baumann G. Growth hormone heterogeneity in human pituitary and plasma. Horm Res 1999; 51(Suppl 1):2.
71. Roppolo HMN, Latchaw RE, Meyer JD, Curtin HD. Normal pituitary gland: 1. Macroscopic anatomy–CT correlation. Am J Neuroradiol 1983; 4:927.
72. Tihansky DP, Crossen J, Markowitz H. Pseudotumor artifact of the dorsum sella in CT scanning. Comput Radiol 1987; 11:241.
73. Hall WA, Luciano MG, Doppman JL, et al. Pituitary magnetic resonance imaging in normal human volunteers: occult adenomas in the general population. Ann Intern Med 1994; 120:817.
74. Kucharczyk W, Peck WW, Kelly WM, et al. Rathke cleft cysts: CT, MR imaging, and pathologic features. Radiology 1987; 165:491.
75. Hama S, Arita K, Tominago A. Symptomatic Rathke's cleft cyst coexisting with central diabetes insipidus and hypophysitis: case report. Endocr J 1999; 46:187.
76. Fujisawa I, Asato R, Togashi K, et al. MR imaging of the sellar spine. J Comput Assist Tomogr 1988; 12:644.
77. McGrath PC, Sloan DA, Schwartz RW, Kenady DE. Advances in the diagnosis and therapy of adrenal tumors. Curr Opin Oncol 1998; 10:52.
78. Ratzmann GW, Zollner H. Hypomagnesemia and hypokalemia in the insulin hypoglycemia test. Z Gesamte Inn Med 1985; 40:567.
79. Read RC, Doherty JE. Cardiovascular effects of induced insulin hypoglycemia in man during the Hollander test. Am J Surg 1972; 104:573.
80. Sobel RJ, Ariad S. Adverse cardiovascular responses to thyrotropin-releasing hormone (200 micrograms) in cardiac patients. Isr J Med Sci 1987; 23:1107.
81. Boice JD Jr. The danger of x-rays—real or apparent. N Engl J Med 1986; 315:828.
82. Hash RB. Intravascular radiographic contrast media: issues for family physicians. J Am Board Fam Pract 1999; 12(1):32.
83. Bravo EL, Tarazi RC, Dustan HP, et al. The changing clinical spectrum of primary aldosteronism. Am J Med 1983; 74:641.

# CHAPTER 2

# MOLECULAR BIOLOGY: PRESENT AND FUTURE

MEHBOOB A. HUSSAIN AND JOEL F. HABENER

The beginnings of molecular biology as a distinct discipline occurred in the late 1940s and early 1950s with the recognition that polynucleotides were the repository of *genetic information* in the form of *DNA* and the *transmitters of genetic information* in the form of *messenger RNA (mRNA)*, and that *transfer RNAs* are fundamental for the *assembly of amino acids into proteins*. Detailed descriptions of the historical developments of this modern era of molecular biology are provided in several books.[1–4] These were exciting times, as understanding progressed rapidly from the discovery by Avery and Brundage that *DNA was a genetic substance*; Chargaff established that *DNA is composed of four different deoxyribonucleotides (dATP, dGRP, dTTP, dCTP)*; Watson and Crick elucidated the *double-helical structure of DNA*; Jacob and Monod identified *mRNA as the intermediary in the transfer of information encoded in DNA to the assembly of amino acids into proteins*; Holly discovered *transfer RNAs*; and Nirenberg et al. discovered the genetic code (i.e., *each of the 21 amino acids is specified by a triplet of nucleotides, or codons, within the mRNA to be translated into a protein*).

In the 1960s, several major discoveries paved the way for the development of recombinant DNA technology and genetic engineering. Two of the major breakthroughs that made this possible were the discoveries of *reverse transcriptase*[5] and *restriction endonucleases*,[6–8] and techniques for determining the precise sequence of nucleotides in DNA.[9,10] Reverse transcriptase, which is found encoded in the RNA of certain tumor viruses, is the means by which the virus makes DNA copies of its RNA templates. It allows molecular biologists to copy mRNA into complementary DNA (cDNA), which is an essential step in the preparation of recombinant DNA for purposes of cloning.

Another fundamental discovery was that of restriction endonucleases, enzymes that cut DNA at specific sequences, typically of 4 to 10 base pairs. The application of specific restriction endonucleases allows for the cleavage of DNAs at precise locations, a property that is critical for the engineering of DNA segments.

A most critical and important discovery was the technologic methodology to *determine the sequential order of nucleotides in DNA*. Both chemical and enzymatic approaches were developed. Currently, the nucleotide sequences of DNAs are determined by sophisticated automated instruments using random enzymatic cleavages of DNAs labeled with fluorescent markers.

By fortunate coincidence, research into the mechanisms by which bacteria become resistant to certain antibiotics led to the discovery of bacterial *plasmids*, which are "viruses" that live within bacteria and lend genetic information to the bacteria to ensure their survival. Plasmids faithfully replicate within bacteria. Importantly, plasmid DNA is relatively simple in structure and is amenable to genetic engineering by excision of DNA sequences and insertion of *foreign DNA sequences*, which will replicate within bacteria without interference by the host bacterium. These plasmids have become useful vehicles in which to express and amplify foreign DNA sequences.

## CLONING OF GENES

**Complementary DNA Libraries.** The cloning of a particular expressed gene begins with the preparation and cloning of cDNAs from mRNAs of a particular cell (Fig. 2-1; Table 2-1) (for a more comprehensive description, see references 11 and 12). The cDNAs are prepared by *priming* the reverse transcription of mRNAs, using reverse transcriptase and short oligonucleotide fragments of oligodeoxyribothymidine, which preferentially bind to the 3'-polyadenylate, or poly(A), tract that is characteristic of cellular mRNAs. Alternatively, *random* oligonucleotides of different base compositions may be used. Double-stranded DNA is then prepared from the single-stranded cDNA by using DNA polymerase, and the cDNAs are inserted into bacterial plasmids that have been cleaved at a single site with a restriction endonuclease. To ensure a reasonably high efficiency of insertion of the foreign DNA into the plasmids, cohesive, or "sticky," ends are first prepared by adding short DNA

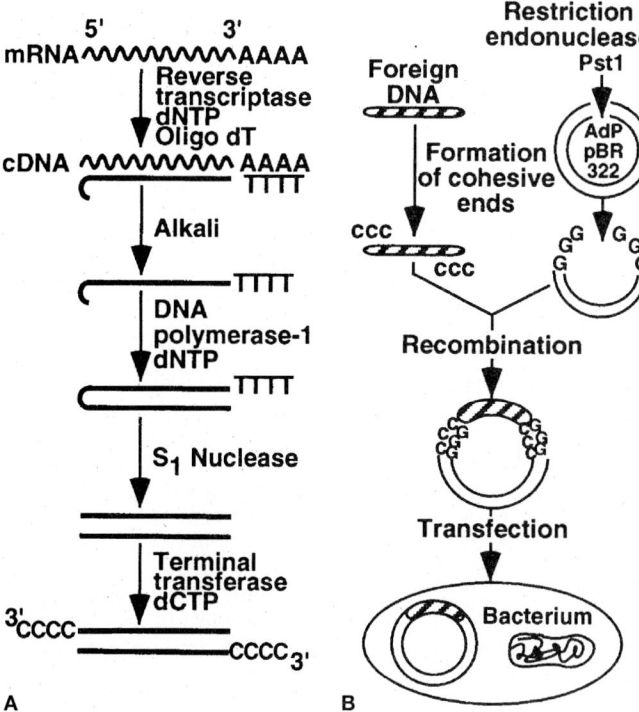

**FIGURE 2-1.** An approach used in construction and molecular cloning of recombinant DNA. **A,** Preparation of double-stranded DNA from an *mRNA* template. The enzyme reverse transcriptase is used to reverse-transcribe a single-stranded DNA copy complementary to the mRNA primed with an oligonucleotide of polydeoxythymidylic acid hybridized to the poly(A) tract at the 3' end of mRNA. A complementary copy of the DNA strand is then prepared with DNA polymerase. Ends of double-stranded DNA are made flush by cleavage with the enzyme S1 nuclease, and homopolymer extensions of deoxycytidine are synthesized on 3' ends of DNA with the enzyme terminal transferase. Oligo(dC) homopolymer extensions form sticky ends for purposes of insertion of DNA into a linearized bacterial plasmid on which complementary oligo(dG) homopolymer extensions have been synthesized. **B,** Insertion of foreign DNA into a bacterial plasmid for molecular cloning. A bacterial plasmid, typically pBR322, that has been specifically engineered for purposes of cloning DNA is linearized by cleavage with restriction endonuclease Pst I. Poly(dG) homopolymer extensions are synthesized onto 3' ends of plasmid DNA. Foreign DNA with complementary poly(dC) homopolymer extensions is hybridized to and inserted into the plasmid. Recombinant plasmid DNA is transfected into susceptible host strains of bacteria, in which plasmid replicates apart from bacterial chromosomal DNA. Bacteria are then grown on a plate containing tetracycline. Colonies that are resistant to tetracycline are tested for sensitivity to ampicillin. Because native plasmids contain genes encoding resistance to both tetracycline and ampicillin and the gene encoding resistance to ampicillin is inactivated by insertion of a foreign DNA at the Pst I site, bacterial colonies harboring plasmids with DNA inserts are resistant to tetracycline and sensitive to ampicillin. Subsequent screening of tetracycline-resistant, ampicillin-sensitive clones containing specific DNA-inserted sequences is carried out by either DNA hybridization with labeled DNA probes or by other techniques such as hybridization arrest and cell-free translation.

sequences to the ends of the foreign DNA and to the plasmids. Vectors that are commonly used are derivatives of the plasmid *pBR322*, which was engineered specifically for the purposes of cloning DNA fragments (see Fig. 2-1). Foreign DNA is inserted into a unique site that is prepared by endonuclease cleaving of a desired site within a polylinker, multiple cloning site engineered into the plasmid. This site is often located within the gene that codes for bacterial β-galactosidase. The backbone plasmid also carries a gene for resistance to ampicillin or tetracycline. Thus, bacteria containing the plasmids can be selected by their resistance to ampicillin or tetracycline; those specifically containing DNA inserts can be selected by their inability

**TABLE 2-1.**
**Approaches for the Selection of Cloned Complementary DNAs (cDNAs)**

NUCLEIC ACID HYBRIDIZATION
  *Hybridization selection and translation*
  *Hybridization arrest and translation*
  *Degenerate oligonucleotide probes*
    Direct hybridization to cDNA libraries
    Polymerase chain reaction (PCR)
PROTEIN EXPRESSION FROM CLONED cDNAs
  *Detection by antisera*
  *Detection by oligonucleotide containing protein-binding sites (transcription factors)*
SPECIALIZED APPROACHES
  *Rapid amplification of cDNA ends (RACE)*
  *Two-site interaction trap*

to express β-galactosidase and to cleave β-galactopyranoside (blue-white screening).

**Hybridization Screening.**    The recombinant plasmids containing DNA sequences that are complementary to the specific mRNAs of interest are identified by hybridizing recombinant plasmids to the initial mRNA preparations used in the cloning. The hybrid-selected mRNA is subsequently eluted and translated in a cell-free system appropriate for the protein under study. Alternatively, specific inhibition of the translation of an mRNA can be used to identify the DNA of interest: DNA that is complementary to the mRNA being translated will bind the RNA, thus precluding translation and reducing the amount of the protein being synthesized.

The initial techniques of hybridization selection and hybridization arrest, in which cell-free translation is used as the assay system, are now supplanted by hybridization of the bacterial colonies with synthetic oligonucleotide *probes* that are *labeled with phosphorus-32 ($^{32}P$)*. Mixtures of oligonucleotides in the range of 14 to 17 bases are prepared that are complementary to the nucleotide sequences predicted from the known amino-acid sequences of segments of the protein encoded by mRNA. Because of the degeneracy in the genetic code (there are 61 amino-acid codons and 20 amino acids), mixtures of from 24 to 48 oligonucleotides ordinarily represent all possible sequences complementary to a particular 14- to 17-base region of mRNA.

**Expression Screening.**    Later-generation cDNA libraries have been prepared in bacterial phages (λ gt-11) or hybrids between plasmids and phages (*phagemids*), which have been engineered to allow the bacteria infected with the recombinant phages to translate mRNAs expressed from the cDNAs, and thereby to produce the protein products encoded by the cDNAs. The desired sequence of interest can be selected at the protein level by screening the library of bacterial clones with an antiserum directed to the protein. When the desired product is a DNA-binding protein, the library can be screened with a labeled DNA duplex containing copies of the target sequence to which the protein binds.

**Yeast Two-Site Interaction Trap.**    The cloning of cDNAs encoding proteins that interact with other known proteins can be accomplished using the yeast two-site interaction trap, which functions much as a bait and fish system. The bait is a cDNA encoding a known protein that is engineered to bind to an enhancer in the promoter of a gene that encodes a factor essential for the survival of a yeast cell. The sequences (*fish*) in the cDNA library are engineered with a strong transcriptional transactivation domain, such as that from the herpes simplex virus and yeast transcription factors *VP16* or *Gal-4*, respectively. The occurrence of protein-protein interactions between the bait and one of the fish activates the expression of the yeast survival gene, which thereby allows for the selection and cloning of the yeast cell that harbors the described cDNA sequence from the cDNA library.

**Rapid Amplification of Complementary DNA Ends.** Most often cDNAs isolated by one or more of the approaches described above lack the complete sequence and are deficient in the 5' ends. The 5' sequences are determined by using the *rapid amplification of cDNA ends (RACE)* technique.

## GENOMIC LIBRARIES AND GENE ISOLATION

**Southern Blots and Hybridization Screening.** The techniques used in the cloning of genomic DNA are similar to those used for cloning cDNA, except that the genomic sequences are longer than the cDNA sequences and different cloning vectors are required. The common vectors are derivatives of the bacteriophage λ that can accommodate DNA fragments of 10 to 20 kilobases (kb). Certain hybrids of bacteriophages and plasmids, called *cosmids*, can accommodate inserts of DNA of up to 40 to 50 kb. Even larger segments of DNA up to 1 to 2 megabases (Mb) can be cloned and propagated in yeast and are called *yeast artificial chromosomes (YACs)*. In the cloning of genomic DNA, restriction fragments are prepared by partial digestion of unsheared DNA with a restriction endonuclease that cleaves the DNA into many fragments. DNA fragments of proper size are prepared by fractionation on agarose gels and are ligated to the bacteriophage DNA. The fragments of DNA containing the desired sequences can be detected by hybridization of a membrane blot prepared from the gel with a $^{32}$P-labeled cDNA, a *Southern blot*. The recombinant DNA is mixed with bacteriophage proteins, which results in the production of viable phage particles. The recombinant bacteriophages are grown on agar plates covered with growing bacteria. Then the bacteria are infected by a phage particle, which lyses the bacteria to form visible plaques. Specific phage colonies are transferred by nitrocellulose filters and are hybridized by cDNA probes labeled with $^{32}$P, similar to a Southern blot. Libraries of genomic DNA fragments and tissue-specific cDNAs from various animal species cloned in plasmids and bacteriophages are available from a number of commercial laboratories. The development of yeast chromosomal libraries that harbor large segments (several megabases) of chromosomal DNA has markedly accelerated the generation of gene linkage maps.

**Enhancer Traps.** One approach to identifying novel genes imbedded in the genome is to randomly insert a transcriptional reporter gene into chromosomal DNA that has been cleaved into 1- to 2-kb fragments by digestion with a restriction endonuclease. The family of ligated hybrid fragments is then cloned into plasmids that are individually introduced (transfected) into host cell lines (e.g., NIH or BHK fibroblasts). After the transfected cell lines are incubated with the cloned DNA fragments for 1 to 2 days, extracts are prepared from the cells and assayed for expression of the transcriptional reporter gene. Typical transcriptional reporter genes used are *firefly luciferase, bacterial chloramphenicol acetyl transferase*, or *bacterial alkaline phosphatase*. When, by chance, a transcriptional enhancer is encountered, as determined by the activation of the reporter gene, the particular cloned DNA fragment is sequenced and searched for transcribed exonic and/or intronic sequences of genes, many of which typically reside 100 to 1000 base pairs from the enhancer sequence. The transcribed sequences of genes usually, but not always, reside 3' (downstream) from enhancer sequences.

**Rapid Amplification of Genomic DNA Ends.** The principle of *rapid amplification of genomic DNA ends (RAGE)* is similar to that of RACE previously described and allows for the identification of unknown DNA sequences in genomic DNA. Oligonucleotide primers (*amplimers*) are annealed to the test genomic DNA sample and extended on the genomic DNA template with

DNA polymerase, and a second set of oligonucleotide primers is ligated to the extended ends. The extended DNA fragments are then amplified by polymerase chain reaction (see next section), isolated by electrophoresis on agarose gels, and sequenced.

## GENE AMPLIFICATION BY POLYMERASE CHAIN REACTION

The development of the *polymerase chain reaction PCR*, a technique for the rapid amplification of specific DNA sequences, constituted a major technological breakthrough.[13–16] This procedure relies on the unique properties of a thermally stable DNA polymerase (*Taq polymerase*) to allow for sequential annealing of small oligonucleotide primers that bracket a DNA sequence of interest; the result is successive synthesis of the DNA strands. Specific DNA sequences as short as 50 and as long as several thousand base pairs can be amplified over a million-fold in just a few hours by using an automated thermal cycler. The technique is so sensitive that DNA (genomic DNA or cDNA reverse-transcribed from RNA) from a single cell can be so amplified. Indeed, a sample containing only a single target DNA molecule can be amplified. The applications of this technique are diverse. Not only is it possible to amplify and to clone rare sequences for detailed studies, but also the technique has applications in the fields of medical diagnosis and forensics. Scarce viruses can be detected in a drop of serum or urine or a single white blood cell. Genotyping can be done from a blood or semen stain, saliva, or a single hair. Paradoxically, a major drawback of PCR is its exquisite sensitivity, which leaves open the possibility of false-positive results because of minute contaminations of the samples being tested. Thus, extreme precautions must be taken to avoid the introduction of contaminants.

PCR is carried out using DNA polymerase and oligonucleotide primers complementary to the two 3' borders of the duplex segment to be amplified. The objective of PCR is to *copy the sequence of each strand between the regions at which the oligonucleotide primers anneal*. Thus, after the primers are annealed to a denatured DNA containing the segment to be amplified, the primers are extended using DNA polymerase and the four deoxynucleotide triphosphates. Each primer is extended toward the other primer. The result is a double-stranded DNA (which itself is then denatured and annealed again with primer, and the DNA polymerase reaction is repeated). This cycle of steps (*denaturation, annealing, and synthesis*) may be repeated 60 times. At each cycle, the amount of duplex DNA segment doubles, because both new and old DNA molecules anneal to the primers and are copied. In principle (and virtually in practice), $2^n$ copies (where $n$ = number of cycles) of the duplex segment bordered by the primers are produced.

The heat-stable polymerase isolated from thermophilic bacteria (*Thermophilus aquaticus*), Taq polymerase, allows multiple cycles to be carried out after a single addition of enzyme. The DNA, an excess of primer molecules, the deoxynucleotide triphosphates, and the polymerase are mixed together at the start. Cycle 1 is initiated by heating to a temperature adequate to assure DNA denaturation, followed by cooling to a temperature appropriate for primer annealing to the now-single strands of the template DNA. Thereafter, the temperature is adjusted for DNA synthesis (*elongation*) to occur. The subsequent cycles are initiated by again heating to the denaturation temperature. Thus, cycling can be automated by using a computer-controlled variable-temperature heating block.

In addition to permitting automation, the use of the DNA polymerase of *T. aquaticus* has another advantage. The enzyme is most active between 70° and 75°C. Base pairing between the oligonucleotide primers and the DNA is more specific at this temperature than at 37°C, the optimal functioning temperature of *Escherichia coli* DNA polymerase. Consequently, the primers are less likely to anneal nonspecifically to unwanted DNA segments, especially when the entire genome is present in the target DNA.

## VARIATIONS OF POLYMERASE CHAIN REACTION

Simple modifications of the PCR conditions can expand the opportunities of the PCR. For example, synthesizing oligonucleotide primers that recognize domains (*motifs*) shared by cDNAs and their respective protein products, and choosing less stringent annealing conditions for the primers, permit new sequences of yet unknown DNAs to be generated with PCR, ultimately resulting in the discovery of new cDNAs belonging to the same family. For example, the pancreatic B-cell transcription factor *IDX-1* was identified by PCR using oligonucleotide primers that would anneal to sequences shared by the homeodomain transcription factor family.

PCR primers can be modified in their sequence and thus are not completely complementary to the template DNA. The amplified PCR product then carries the sequence of the primer and not the original DNA sequence. This strategy can be used to insert mutations site-specifically into known DNA sequences.

## APPROACHES TO THE QUANTITATIVE ASSESSMENT OF GENE EXPRESSION

### TRANSCRIPTION ASSAYS

**Nuclear Run-On Assays.**    Several assays are available that provide an *index of relative rates of gene transcription* (Fig. 2-2). A simple, straightforward assay is the *nuclear run-on assay* in which nuclei are isolated from tissue culture cells and nascent RNA chains are allowed to continue to polymerize in the presence of radiolabeled deoxyribonucleotides in vitro. This assay has the advantage that it surveys the density of nascent transcripts made from the endogenous genes of cells and, on average, is a good measure of gene transcription rates in response to the existing environmental conditions in which the cultured cells are maintained. Newly synthesized RNA is applied (hybridized) to a nylon membrane on which a cDNA target complementary to the desired RNA has been adsorbed. Radiolabeled RNA hybridized to the cDNA is determined in a radiation counter.

**Cell-Free In Vitro Systems.**    Rates of RNA synthesis can also be determined in broken cell or cell-free lysates to assess the relative strengths of different promoters. To restrict the newly synthesized radiolabeled RNA to a single size and, thus, to enable more ready detection by electrophoresis, a DNA template is used that does not contain guanine bases, called a *G-free cassette*. RNA synthesis is carried out in the absence of the guanine nucleotide. After synthesis of a specified length of RNA at the end of which guanine bases are encountered, RNA synthesis is terminated.

**Transfection of Promoter-Reporters in In Vivo Cell Culture.** Many of the currently used assays of gene transcription employ promoter sequences fused to genes encoding proteins that can be quantitated by bioassays (e.g., bacterial chloramphenicol acetyl transferase, firefly luciferase, alkaline phosphatase, or green fluorescent protein). The hybrid DNAs, so called *promoter-reporter DNAs*, are introduced into tissue culture cells by one of several *chemical methods* (i.e., DNA adsorbed to calcium phosphate precipitates, diethylaminoethyl (DEAE)-dextran incorporated into liposomes, or human artificial chromosomes [Table 2-2]); or *physical methods* (i.e., electroporation, direct microinjection of DNA, or ballistic injection using a gene gun [Table 2-3]). After introduction of the reporter DNA into the

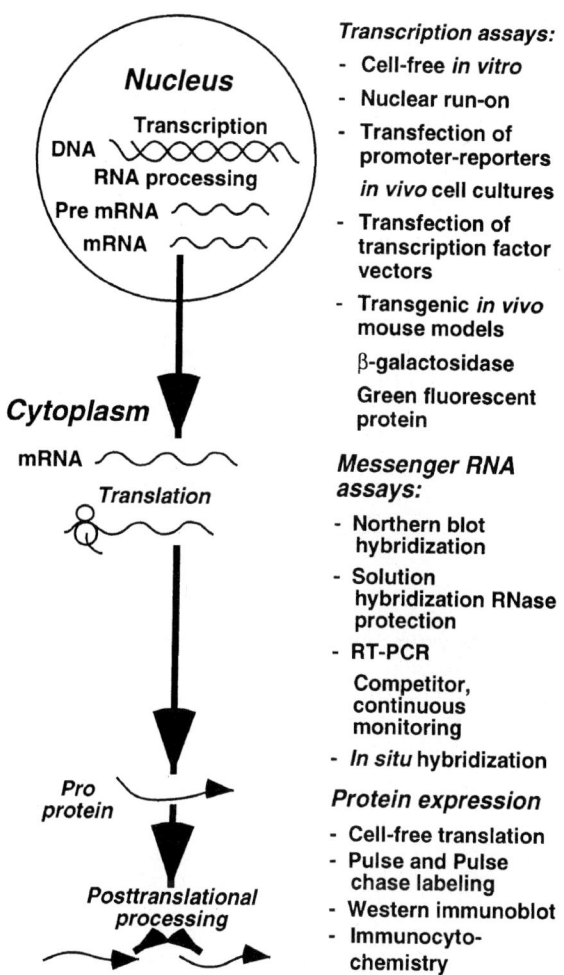

**FIGURE 2-2.** Approaches to the quantitative assessment of gene expression. Shown are the various types of assays that can be used to examine regulation of gene expression at various levels. (*mRNA*, messenger RNA; *RNase*, ribonuclease; *RT-PCR*, reverse transcription polymerase chain reaction.)

cells, the transfected cells are incubated for a specified time under the desired experimental conditions, the cells are harvested, and extracts are prepared for assays of the reporter-specific enzymatic activity. By these transfection methods, cell-type specificity for the expression of gene-promoter sequences can be determined by comparing promoter-reporter efficiencies in cells of different phenotypes. In addition, important transcriptional control sequences in the promoter can be mapped by DNA mutagenesis studies.

**Transfection of Transcription Factor Expression Vectors.** An extension of the promoter-reporter transfection approach is to cotransfect recombinant expression plasmids encoding transcription factors that bind to control sequences in the promoter DNA and activate transcription of the reporter. By this approach, critical functional components of transcription factors and critical bases in DNA control sequences can be examined experimentally.

**Transgenic In Vivo Mouse Models.**    A method developed for examining *specificity of tissue expression and efficiency of expression of promoter-reporter genes* is their introduction into mice in vivo, using transgenic technology (see the section Genetic Manipulations in Animals In Vivo). Recombinant promoter-reporter genes are injected into the pronucleus of fertilized mouse ova and implanted into surrogate females. The tissues of transgenic neonatal mice are examined for the tissue distribution and relative

**TABLE 2-2.**
**Chemical Methods for Introducing Genes into Mammalian Cells**

| Method | Advantages | Disadvantages |
|---|---|---|
| DNA–calcium phosphate | Cell death minimal | Good for ex vivo use only |
| | Important in the production of viral vectors | Low transfection efficiency |
| | Simple, inexpensive | Low transgene expression levels |
| | Expression transient or stable | Transient expression only |
| DNA-DEAE-dextran | More reproducible than DNA–calcium morphate | Good for ex vivo only |
| | Can carry large pieces of DNA (chromosomes) | Transient expression only |
| | Can be targeted | Works only in some cell types |
| | Nonimmunogenic | |
| | Preparations are pyrogen free | |
| DNA-lipid-protein (liposomes) | Can be targeted, transfection rates are better | |
| Human artificial chromosomes | Do not integrate into host chromosomes | Further development required |
| | Large inserts can be accommodated | |
| | Better transcription control | |

*DEAE*, diethylaminoethyl dextran.

strength of the expression of the reporter function. Commonly used reporter functions are the genes encoding either β-galactosidase or green fluorescent protein.

## MESSENGER RNA ASSAYS

**Northern Blot Hybridization.** RNA blotting (*Northern blotting*) is analogous to DNA blotting (*Southern blotting*). RNA is separated according to size by electrophoresis through agarose gels. Generally, the electrophoresis is performed under conditions that denature the RNA so that the effects of RNA secondary structure on the electrophoretic mobility of the RNAs can be minimized. Alkaline conditions are unsuitable; therefore, agents such as glyoxal, formaldehyde, or urea are used. The size-separated RNA is transferred by blotting to an immobilizing membrane without disturbing the RNA distribution along the gel. A labeled DNA is then used as a probe to find the position on the blot of RNA molecules corresponding to the probe. The immobilized RNA is incubated with DNA under conditions allowing annealing of the DNA to the RNA on the immobilized matrix. After washing away excess and unspecifically annealed DNA, the matrix is exposed to an x-ray film to detect the position of the probe. RNA blotting allows the estimation of the size of the RNA that is being detected. In addition, the intensity of the band on an x-ray film indicates the abundance of the RNA in the cell or tissue from which the RNA was extracted.

**Solution Hybridization Ribonuclease Protection.** To obtain more precise information on the amount of a specific RNA species in a certain cell or tissue, a single-stranded radioactive probe is generated that is complementary to a portion of the RNA being studied. An excess amount of this single-stranded probe is then mixed in solution with the total RNA of the cells or tissue being investigated. Digestion with ribonuclease of all single-stranded nucleic acids present after hybridization leaves the double-stranded species, consisting of the labeled probe annealed to its complementary RNA, in the solution. The contents of the solution are then size-separated on an electrophoretic gel, which is exposed to an x-ray film. Knowing the amount of input labeled single-stranded probe allows a quantification of the specific RNA present in the total RNA of the cells or tissue.

**In Situ Hybridization.** In situ hybridization with labeled single-stranded probes onto tissues is, in principle, similar to the ribonuclease protection assay. Detection and determination of the location of a certain species of RNA within a tissue is possible.

**Reverse Transcription Polymerase Chain Reaction.** *Reverse transcription polymerase chain reaction (RT-PCR)* can be used to quantitate the abundance of a specific RNA. This method is particularly practical when small amounts of tissue or cells are available to be analyzed. The RNA is reverse-transcribed to DNA with reverse transcriptase. The cDNA population is then subjected to PCR amplification with specific primers that recognize the cDNA in question. By choosing the number of PCR cycles within the linear range of product generated after each cycle (i.e., enough primers, nucleotides, and DNA polymerase in the reaction mixture for none of them to be the limiting factor of the reaction) and adding to the PCR reaction a defined amount of an artificial DNA template that is also recognized by the primer oligonucleotides but yields a different-sized product, one can detect differences in abundance of cDNA (and hence RNA in the original sample) among two or more samples. Newer methods allow for an on-line monitoring of each PCR reaction of the product generated. This is achieved by using primer oligonucleotides that can be monitored during the PCR reaction cycles by external optical devices. Such on-line continuous monitoring allows the performance of PCR reactions without prior determination of the number of cycles required to keep the PCR reaction within the linear range of amplification. Continuous PCR monitoring

**TABLE 2-3.**
**Physical Methods for Introducing Genes into Mammalian Cells**

| Method | Advantages | Disadvantages |
|---|---|---|
| Direct microinjection | High transfection rate | Good for ex vivo use only |
| Electroporation | High transfection rate | Good for ex vivo use only |
| | | Excessive cell death |
| Plasmid injection | Simple | Low transfection rate |
| | Up to 19 kb of DNA can be transferred to muscle | |
| | Good for use in DNA vaccines | |
| Ballistic injection | High transfection rate | Transient transfection |
| | Delivery of precise dosages of DNA | Considerable cell death |
| | Good for use in DNA vaccines | |

provides immediate information on abundance of a given cDNA species in PCR reactions. Knowledge of the absolute amount of labeled oligonucleotide primer added to the PCR reaction at the start can be used to determine the exact amount of the PCR product generated.

## PROTEIN EXPRESSION ASSAYS

**Cell-Free Translation.**    A commonly used method to analyze proteins encoded by mRNA is to translate the mRNA in cell-free translation systems in vitro. By this method, proteins can be radioactively labeled to a high specific activity. The cell-free translation also provides the primary protein product, such as a proprotein or prohormone, encoded by the mRNA.

**Pulse and Pulse-Chase Labeling.**    Studies of protein syntheses can also be carried out in vivo by incubation of cultured cells or tissues with radioactive amino acids (*pulse labeling*). Posttranslational processing (e.g., enzymatic cleavages of prohormones) can be assessed by first incubating the cells or tissues for a short time with radioactive amino acids and then incubating them for an additional period with unlabeled amino acids (*pulse-chase labeling*).

**Western Immunoblot.**    Another approach to the analyses of particular cellular proteins is the *Western immunoblot* technique. Proteins in cell extracts are separated by electrophoresis on polyacrylamide or agarose gels and transferred to a nylon or nitrocellulose membrane, which is then treated with a solution containing specific antibodies to the protein of interest. The antibodies that are bound to the protein fixed to the membrane are detected by any one of several methods, such as secondary antibodies tagged with radioisotopes, fluorophores, or enzymes.

**Immunocytochemistry.**    A refinement of the Western immunoblot technique is the detection of specific proteins within cells by *immunocytochemistry* (immunohistochemistry). Cultured cells or tissue sections are fixed on microscope slides and treated with solutions containing specific antibodies. The antibodies that are bound to the proteins within the cells are detected with fluorescently tagged secondary antibodies or by an avidin-biotin complex. Immunocytochemistry is a powerful technique when used for the simultaneous detection of two or even three different proteins with examination by confocal microscopy.

## DNA-PROTEIN INTERACTION ASSAYS

### ELECTROPHORETIC MOBILITY GEL SHIFT AND SOUTHWESTERN BLOTS

The binding of proteins such as transcription factors to DNA sequences is commonly done by two approaches: *electrophoretic mobility shift assay (EMSA)* and *Southwestern blotting*. Typically, EMSA consists of incubation of protein extracts with a radiolabeled DNA sequence or probe. The mixture is then analyzed by electrophoresis on a nondenaturing polyacrylamide gel, followed by autoradiography or autofluorography to evaluate the distribution of the radioactivity or fluorescence in the gel. Interactions of specific proteins with the DNA probe are manifested by a retardation of the electrophoretic migration of the labeled probe, or *band shift*. The EMSA technique can be extended to include antibodies to specific proteins in the incubation mixture. The interaction of a specific antibody with a protein bound to the DNA probe causes a further retardation of migration of the DNA-protein complex, leading to a *super shift*.

### PROTEIN-PROTEIN INTERACTION ASSAYS

A number of different assays are used to determine and evaluate protein-protein interactions. Two in vitro assays are *coimmunopre-*

*cipitation* and *polyhistidine-tagged glutathione sulfonyl transferase (GST) pull-down*. Two in vivo assays are the yeast and mammalian two-site interaction assays.

**Coimmunoprecipitation.**    The commonly used coimmunoprecipitation assay makes use of antisera to specific proteins. In circumstances in which two different proteins, A and B, associate with each other, an antiserum to protein A will immunoprecipitate not only protein A, but also protein B. Likewise, an antiserum to protein B will coimmunoprecipitate proteins B and A. In practice, the proteins under investigation are radiolabeled by synthesis in the presence of radioactive amino acids, either in cell-free transcription-translation systems in vitro, or in cell culture systems in vivo. Coimmunoprecipitated proteins are detected by gel electrophoresis and autoradiography. Alternatively, the proteins so immunoprecipitated or coimmunoprecipitated can be assayed by Western immunoblot techniques.

**Glutathione Sulfonyl Transferase Pull-Down.**    GST is an enzyme that has a high affinity for its substrate, glutathione. This property of high-affinity interactions has been exploited to develop a cloning vector plasmid encoding GST and containing a polylinker site that allows for the insertion of coding sequences for any protein of interest. Thus, if protein A is believed to interact with protein B, the coding sequence for either protein A or protein B can be inserted into the GST vector. The GST–protein A or B fusion protein is synthesized in large amounts by multiplication and expression of the plasmid vector in bacteria. The GST-fusion protein is then incubated with either labeled or unlabeled proteins in extracts of cells or nuclei. Proteins in the extracts bound to protein A or B in the GST-fusion protein are *pulled down* from the extracts by capturing the GST on glutathione-agarose beads. Proteins are released from the beads and analyzed by either gel electrophoresis and autoradiography (*labeled proteins*) or by Western immunoblot (*unlabeled proteins*). Similar methods using polyhistidine tag in place of GST are also used for pull-down experiments.

**Far Western Protein Blots.**    A variation on the Western blotting technique is the *Far Western blot*. In this technique, a radiolabeled or fluorescence-labeled known protein (instead of an antibody) is applied to a membrane to which proteins from an electrophoretic gel have been transferred. If the known protein binds to any one or more proteins on the membrane, it is detected as a labeled band by autoradiograph or autofluorography. Relatively strong protein-protein interactions are required for this approach to succeed.

**Yeast and Mammalian Cell Two-Site Interaction Traps.**    The two-site interaction traps are useful for demonstrating protein-protein interactions in vivo. The principle of the approach is that, when a specific protein-protein interaction occurs, it reconstitutes an active transcription factor which then activates the transcription of a reporter gene. The cells (yeast or mammalian) are programmed to constitutively express a strong DNA-binding domain, such as *Gal-4*, fused to the expression sequence of the selected protein, protein A (*the bait*). The cells are also programmed to express a transcriptional reporter (e.g., CAT or luciferase linked to a promoter) that has binding sites for Gal-4. Thus, protein A anchors to the DNA-binding site of the reporter promoter via the Gal-4 binding domain but does not activate transcription of the reporter gene, and no reporter function is expressed. Protein B, however, is expressed as a fusion protein with a strong transcriptional activator sequence (e.g., the transcriptional transactivation domain of Gal-4 or of VP16). This transcriptional activation domain–protein B fusion protein does not bind DNA, but when, or if, protein B physically interacts with (binds to) protein A, a fully active transcription factor is reconstituted, the promoter reporter gene is transcribed, and the reported function is expressed.

The yeast two-hybrid system can be used to clone proteins that interact with a bait protein such as protein A. In this instance, a cDNA protein expression library is prepared or obtained that has all of the cDNAs of a given tissue fused to a coding sequence for a transactivation domain (e.g., VP16). Further, the reporter consists of a survival factor essential for the growth of the yeast cell. Thus, when a cDNA encodes a protein B (fish) that interacts with the bait protein A, the yeast cell expresses the survival protein and survives, whereas the other yeast cells die.

## GENETIC MANIPULATIONS IN ANIMALS IN VIVO

### TRANSGENIC APPROACHES

To create transgenic mice, DNA is injected into the male pronucleus of one-cell mammalian embryos (fertilized ova) that are then allowed to develop by insertion into the reproductive tract of pseudopregnant foster mothers (Fig. 2-3A). The transgenic animals that develop from this procedure contain the foreign DNA integrated into one or more of the host chromosomes at an early stage of embryo development. As a consequence, the foreign DNA is generally transmitted to the germline, and, in a number of instances, the foreign genes are expressed. Because the foreign DNA is injected at the one-cell stage, a good chance exists that the DNA will be distributed among all the progeny cells as development proceeds. This situation provides an opportunity to analyze and compare the qualitative and quantitative efficiencies of expression of the genes among various organs. The technique is quite efficient; >50% of postinjection ova produce viable offspring, and, of these, ~10% efficiently carry the foreign genes. In the transgenic animals, the foreign genes can be passed on and expressed at high levels in subsequent generations of progeny.

Transgenic approaches can also be used to prevent the development of the lineage of a particular cell phenotype or to impair the expression of a selected gene. A cell lineage can be ablated by targeting a microinjected DNA containing a subunit of the diphtheria toxin to a particular cell type, using a promoter sequence specifically expressed in that cell type. The diphtheria toxin subunit inhibits protein synthesis when expressed in a cell, thereby killing the cell. The expression of a particular gene can be impaired by similar cell promoter–specific targeting of a DNA expression vector to a cell that produces an antisense mRNA to the mRNA expressed by the gene of interest. The antisense mRNA hybridizes to nuclear transcripts and processed mRNAs; this results in their degradation by double-stranded RNA–specific nucleases, thereby effectively attenuating the functional expression of the gene. The efficacy of the impairment of the mRNA can be enhanced by incorporating a ribozyme *hammerhead* sequence in the expressed antisense mRNA so as physically to cleave the mRNA to which it hybridizes. Another approach to producing a particular gene loss of function is to direct expression of a dominant negative protein (e.g., a receptor made deficient in intracellular signaling by an appropriate mutation, or a mutant transcription factor deficient in transactivation functions but sufficient for DNA binding). These dominant negative proteins compete for the essential functions of the wild-type proteins, resulting in a net loss of function.

Another approach, termed *targeted transgenesis*, combines targeted homologous recombination in embryonic stem (ES) cells with gain-of-function transgenic approaches.[11,12,17] This method allows for targeted integration of a single-copy transgene to a single desired locus in the genome and thereby avoids problems of random and multiple-copy integrations, which may compromise faithful expression of the transgene in the conventional approach.

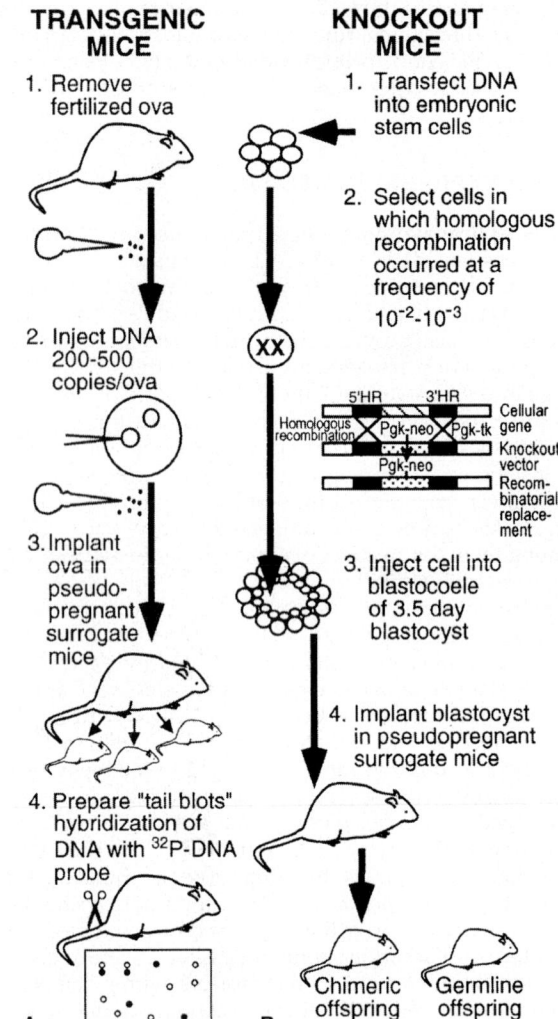

**FIGURE 2-3.** Approaches for (**A**) the integration of a foreign gene into the germline of mice, and (**B**) disruption or knock-out of a specific gene. **A,** DNA containing a specific foreign gene is microinjected into the male pronucleus of fertilized ova obtained from the oviduct of a mouse. Ova are then implanted into the uterus of pseudopregnant surrogate mothers. Progeny are analyzed for the presence of foreign genes by hybridization with $^{32}$P-labeled DNA probe and DNA prepared from a piece of tail from a mouse, which has been immobilized on a nitrocellulose filter (tail blots). **B,** To create a knock-out of a gene, pluripotential embryonic stem (*ES*) cells are used in vitro to introduce an engineered plasmid DNA sequence that will recombine with a homologous gene that is targeted. The recombination excises a portion of the gene in the ES cells, rendering it inactive (no longer expressible). ES cells in which the homologous recombination occurred successfully are selected by a combined positive-negative drug selection. The engineered ES cells are injected into the blastocoele of 3.5-day blastocysts that are then implanted into the uterus of pseudopregnant mice. The offspring are both chimeric and germline for expression of the knock-out gene and must be cross-bred to homozygosity for the genotype of a complete knock-out of the gene that is targeted for disruption.

### GENE ABLATION (KNOCK-OUTS)

A major advance beyond the *gain-of-function* transgenic mouse technique has been the development of methods for producing *loss of function* by targeted disruption or replacement of genes. This approach uses the techniques of homologous recombination in cultured pluripotential ES cells, which are then injected into mouse blastocysts and implanted into the uteri of pseudopregnant mice (Fig. 2-3B). The targeting vector contains a core *replacement* sequence consisting of an expressed-cell lethal-drug

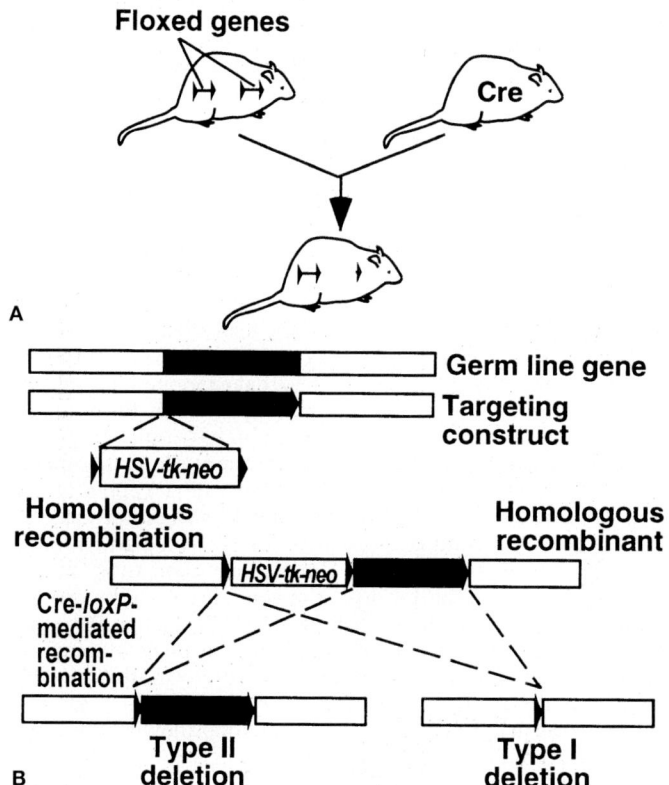

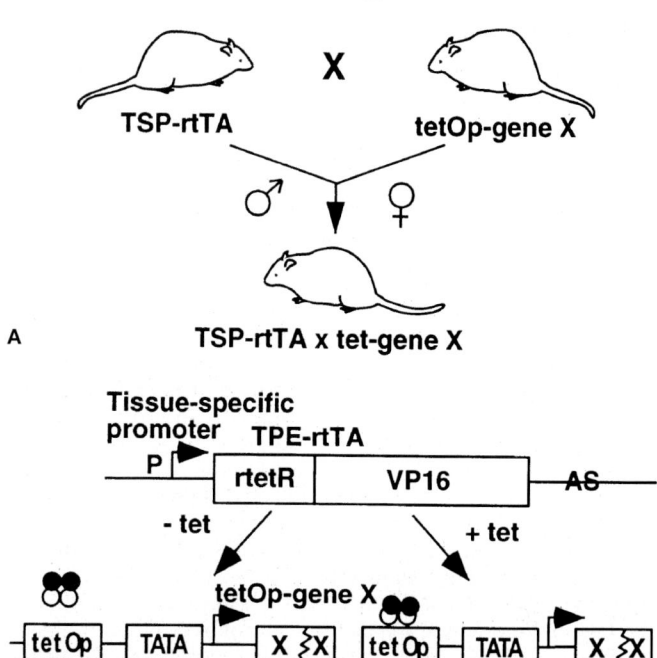

**FIGURE 2-4.** Schema of the Cre-loxP approach to conditionally knock out a specifically targeted gene in mice. **A,** The approach requires the creation of two separate strains of transgenic mice that are crossed to produce double transgenic mice to effect the conditional gene knockouts. One mouse strain is created so as to replace the gene of interest by one that has been flanked by loxP recombination sequences (*floxed*), using targeted recombinational gene replacement in embryonic stem cells as illustrated in Figure 2-3B. The other mouse strain is a transgenic mouse in which the Cre recombinase enzyme expression vector is targeted to the tissue of interest using a tissue-specific promoter, such as the proinsulin gene promoter, to target and restrict expression to pancreatic B cells. **B,** A more detailed depiction of the strategy for preparation of the gene replacement by homologous recombination to generate mice with a floxed gene. This approach is similar to that described in Figure 2-3B to create knock-out mice.[18]

**FIGURE 2-5.** Diagram showing the approach to reversible conditional expression of a gene in mice, using a tetracycline-inducible gene expression system. **A,** As in the Cre-loxP system (see Fig. 2-4A), the tetracycline-inducible gene system requires the creation of two independent strains of transgenic mice. One strain of mice targets the expression of a specially engineered transcription factor (*rtTA*) to the tissue of interest, using a tissue-specific promoter (*TSP*). **B,** the rtTA transcription factor consists of a modification of the bacterial tetracycline-responsive repressor that has been genetically engineered so as to convert it into a transcriptional transactivator when exposed to tetracycline or one of its analogs. The other mouse strain is one in which a gene of interest is introduced, usually driven by a ubiquitous promoter such as a viral promoter (CMV, RSV) or an actin promoter. The gene of interest could be one encoding an antisense RNA to a messenger RNA of a protein that is to be knocked out. The creation of double transgenic mice then allows for the expression of the gene of interest in a specific tissue under the control of the induced tetracycline. (See text for more detailed description.[57]) (*tet op,* tetracycline resistance operon; *P,* promoter; *AS,* antisense; *TPE,* tissue promoter element.)

resistance gene (*selectable marker*) (e.g., neomycin [*Pgk-neo*]) flanked by sequences homologous to the targeted cellular gene, and a second selectable marker gene (e.g., thymidine kinase [*pgk-tk*]). The ES cells are transfected with the gene-specific targeting vector. Cells that take up vector DNA and in which homologous recombination occurs are selected by their resistance to neomycin (*positive selection*). To select against random integration, a susceptibility to killing by thymidine kinase (*negative selection*) is used; only homologous recombination in which the thymidine kinase gene has been lost will confer survival benefit. Because the ES cells are injected into multicellular 3.5-day blastocysts, many of the offspring are mosaics, but some are germline heterozygous for the recombined gene. F1 generation mice are then bred to homozygosity so as to manifest the phenotype of the gene knock-out. Using this approach of targeted gene disruption, literally thousands of *knock-out* mice have been created. Many of these knock-out mice are models for human genetic disorders (e.g., those of endocrine systems such as pancreatic agenesis [homeodomain protein IDX-1], familial hypocalciuric hypercalcemia [calcium receptor], intrauterine growth retardation [insulin-like growth factor-II receptor], salt-sensitive hypertension [atrial natriuretic peptide], and obesity [$\alpha_3$-adrenergic receptor]).

## CONDITIONAL (DEVELOPMENTAL) INTERRUPTION OF GENE EXPRESSION

Although targeted transgenesis using chosen site integration and targeted disruption of genes has proven helpful in analyses of the functions of genes, conditionally to induce expression of transgenes or conditionally to inactivate a specific gene is useful. Early on, randomly integrated vectors for the expression of transgenes used the metallothionein promoter that is readily inducible by the administration of heavy metals to transgenic mice. Now techniques have been developed to conditionally inactivate targeted genes in a defined spatial and temporal pattern. Several approaches to achieve conditional gene inactivation have been developed. Two of these approaches are (a) the Cre recombinase–loxP system (Fig. 2-4)[18] and (b) the tetracycline-inducible transactivator vector (tTA) system (Fig. 2-5).[19] Occasionally, both of these systems have been used effectively to knock out (Cre-loxP) or to attenuate (reverse tTA) the expression of specific genes. Both the Cre-loxP and reverse tTA systems require the creation of two independent strains of transgenic mice, which are then crossed to produce *double transgenic mice.*

## CRE RECOMBINASE–LOXP SYSTEM

The Cre-loxP approach is based on the Cre-loxP recombination system of bacteriophage P1 (see Fig. 2-4). This system is capable of mediating loxP site-specific recombination in embryonal stem cells and in transgenic mice. Conditional targeting requires the generation of two mouse strains. One transgenic strain expresses the Cre recombinase under control of a promoter that is cell-type specific or developmental stage specific. The other strain is prepared by using ES cells to effect a replacement of the targeted gene with an exact copy that is flanked by loxP sequences required for recombination by the Cre recombinase. The recombined gene is said to be *floxed*. The presence of the loxP sites does not interfere with the functional expression of the gene and will be normally expressed in all of its usual tissues not coexpressing the Cre recombinase. In those tissues in which the Cre is expressed by virtue of its tissue-specific promoter, the target gene will be deleted by homologous recombination. Thus, the Cre-loxP system acts like a timer in which the events that are to take place are predetermined by the prior reprogramming of the genes: the target gene will be ablated during development where and when the promoter chosen to drive the expression of Cre is activated. Thus, a disadvantage of the Cre-loxP system is the lack of control over when the gene knock-out will take place, because it is preprogrammed in the system. Newer genetically engineered Cre derivatives allow for pharmacologic activation of the recombinant event. A potential advantage of the Cre-loxP system is that one can theoretically generate extensive collections of mice expressing the Cre recombinase specifically and individually in many different tissues so that these mice could be made commercially available to investigators.

## CONDITIONAL TETRACYCLINE-INDUCIBLE FORWARD AND REVERSE TRANSACTIVATOR VECTOR SYSTEMS

The Cre-loxP system leads to the irreversible targeted disruption of a particular gene at the time that the promoter encoding the Cre recombinase is activated during development. Having available a system that can be reversibly activated at any time would be desirable. A system that holds promise in this regard is the tetracycline-inducible transactivator vector (forward or reverse tTA), which, in response to tetracycline, switches on a specific gene bearing a promoter containing the tetracycline-responsive operon (see Fig. 2-5). This system allows any recombinant gene marked by the presence of the tet operon to be turned on or off at will simply by the administration of a potent tetracycline analog to the transgenic mice. The vectors were engineered from the sequences of the *E. coli* bacterial tetracycline resistance operon (tet op), in which a repressor sits on the operon, keeping the resistance gene off. When tetracycline binds to the repressor, it is deactivated, falls off of the operon, and turns on the gene. First, the repressor was converted into an activator by fusing the DNA-binding domain to the potent activator sequence (VP16) of the herpes simplex virus. In this system, tetracycline turned off the activator (tet-off) and thereby caused failure of expression of target genes containing the tet operon binding sites for the repressor turned into an activator. This tTA system required the continued presence of tetracycline to keep the gene off and withdrawal of the tetracycline to turn on the gene, raising problems of long and variable clearance times for the drugs. Turning the gene on by administration of tetracycline (tet-on) would be preferable. Therefore, the tTA vector was reengineered to reverse the action of tetracycline: in the current vector system, the binding of tetracycline to the reverse tTA enhances its binding to the tet operon. Theoretically, as the reverse tTA system now works, any gene can be reversibly turned on by the administration of tetracycline or one if its more potent analogs in the double transgenic mouse, which consists of a cross between a mouse that has the reverse tTA targeted to express in a specific tissue and a mouse that has a ubiquitously expressed transgene for any gene X under the control of the tet operon. The equivalent of gene knock-outs can be accomplished by constructing gene X in a context to express an antisense RNA containing a ribozyme sequence. When induced by tetracycline, antisense-ribozyme RNA binds to the mRNA expressed by gene X, cleaves it, and thereby functionally inactivates the gene.

## PROSPECTS FOR THE FUTURE FOR CONDITIONAL TRANSGENE EXPRESSION

The availability of the Cre-loxP and the forward and reverse tTA systems now makes it feasible to combine their key features in the creation of *triple transgenic mice* so that a targeted recombinational disruption of a gene can be accomplished by the administration of tetracycline. The Cre recombinase could be placed under the control of a tissue-specific promoter containing the tet operon uniquely responsive to the presence of tTA and targeted to a specific tissue by standard pronuclear injection targeted transgenesis. A second transgenic mouse is created with a ubiquitously expressed promoter during the expression of the reverse tTA. In the third mouse, the gene desired to be deleted would be replaced with an appropriately floxed gene. The latter mouse would be prepared by implantation of recombinantly engineered ES cells into blastocysts. The administration of tetracycline to the triple transgenic mouse would induce the Cre recombinase in a tissue-specific manner, thus allowing temporal and spatial control of gene knock-outs.

## EXPRESSED SEQUENCE TAGS

A very informative database of *expressed sequence tags (ESTs)* is being generated and placed in GenBank. Expressed sequence tags are prepared by random, single-pass sequencing of mRNAs from a repertoire of different tissues, mostly embryonic tissues (e.g., brain, eye, placenta, liver). Currently, the EST database contains ~50% of the estimated expressed genes in humans and mammals (70,000–80,000). The EST database will become extremely valuable when the sequences of the human, rat, and mouse genomes are completed.

# DNA ARRAYS FOR THE PROFILING OF GENE EXPRESSION

Two variants of DNA-array chip design exist.[20,21] The first consists of cDNA (sequences unknown) immobilized to a solid surface such as glass and exposed to a set of labeled probes of known sequences, either separately or in a mixture of the probes. The second is an array of oligonucleotide probes (sequences known, based on either known genes in GenBank or ESTs) that are synthesized either in situ or by conventional synthesis followed by on-chip immobilization (Fig. 2-6). The array is exposed to labeled sample DNA (unknown sequence) and hybridized, and complementary sequences are determined.

In cDNA chips, immobilized targets of single-stranded cDNAs prepared from a specific tissue are hybridized to single-stranded DNA fluorescent probes produced from total mRNAs to evaluate the expression levels of target genes.

## OLIGONUCLEOTIDE ARRAYS (GENOMIC AND EXPRESSED SEQUENCE TAGS)

The oligonucleotide gene chip ($1.28 \times 1.28$ cm$^2$) consists of a solid-phase template (glass wafer) to which high-density arrays of oligonucleotides (distance between oligonucleotides of 100 Å) are attached, with each probe in a predefined position in the array. Each gene EST is represented by 20 pairs of

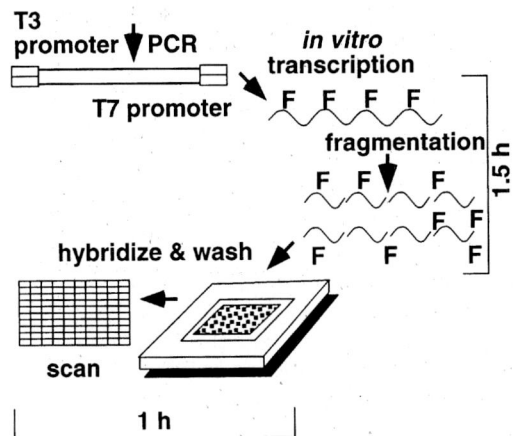

**FIGURE 2-6.** Sample preparation and hybridization for oligonucleotide assay. A complementary DNA (*cDNA*) is transcribed in vitro to RNA, and then reverse-transcribed to cRNA. This material is fragmented and tagged with a fluorescent tag molecule (*F*). The fragments are hybridized to an array of oligonucleotides representing portions of DNA sequences of interest. After washing, hybridization of the cRNA probe is detected by localization of the fluorescent signals. (*PCR*, polymerase chain reaction.)

25 base oligonucleotides from different parts of the gene (5' end, middle, and 3' end).

The specificity of the detection method is controlled by the presence of single-base mismatch probes. Pairs of perfect and single-base mismatch probes corresponding to each target gene are synthesized on adjacent areas on the arrays. This is done to identify and subtract nonspecific background signals. The gene chip is sensitive enough to detect one to five transcripts per cell and is much more sensitive than the Northern blot technique.

## COMPLEMENTARY DNA ARRAYS (SPECIFIC TISSUES)

Poly (A) mRNA is isolated from cells or tissue of interest, and synthesis of double-stranded cDNA is accomplished by reverse transcription of cDNA, followed by synthesis of double-stranded cDNA using DNA polymerase I. In vitro transcription of double-stranded cDNA to cRNA is accomplished using biotin-16-UTP and biotin-11-CTP for labeling and a T7 RNA polymerase as enzyme. This cRNA is used for hybridization with the *gene chip*. The gene chip is stained with R-physoerythrin streptavidin to detect biotin-labeled nucleotides, and different wash cycles are performed. Thereafter the gene chip is scanned digitally and analyzed by special software. (A grid is automatically placed over the scanned image of the probe array chip to demarcate the probe cells.) After grid alignment, the average intensity of each probe cell is calculated by the software, which then analyzes the patterns and generates a report.

The applications of the gene chip include:

1. Simultaneous analysis of temporal changes in gene expression of all known genes and ESTs.
2. Sequencing of DNA.
3. Large-scale detection of mutations and polymorphisms in specific genes (i.e., *BRCA1*, *HIV-1*, cystic fibrosis *CFTR*, β-thalassemia).
4. Gene mapping by determining the order of overlapping clones.

Expensive equipment for generating and analyzing the data using genechips is required. When the cloning of all genes is completed (Human Genome Project), the gene chip will allow monitoring of the expression of all known genes in various situations.

# STRATEGIES FOR MAPPING GENES ON CHROMOSOMES

## GENETIC LINKAGE MAPS AND QUANTITATIVE TRAIT LOCI

A *genetic linkage map* shows the relative locations of specific DNA markers along the chromosome.[22–27] Any inherited physical or molecular characteristic that differs among individuals and is easily detectable in the laboratory is a potential genetic marker. Markers can be expressed DNA regions or DNA segments that have no known coding function, but whose inheritance pattern can be followed. DNA sequence differences (polymorphisms; i.e., nucleotide differences) are especially useful markers because they are plentiful and easy to characterize precisely. Markers must be polymorphic to be useful in mapping. Alternative DNA polymorphisms exist among individuals, even among members of a single family, so that they are detectable among different families. Polymorphisms are variations in DNA sequence in the genome that occur every 300 to 500 base pairs. Variations within protein-encoding exon sequences can lead to observable phenotypic changes (e.g., differences in eye color, blood type, and disease susceptibility). Most variations occur within introns and have little or no effect on the phenotype (unless they alter exonic splicing patterns), yet these polymorphisms in DNA sequence are detectable and can be used as markers. Examples of these types of markers are: (a) *restriction fragment length polymorphisms* (RFLPs), which reflect sequence variations in DNA sites that are cleaved by specific DNA restriction enzymes; and (b) variable number of tandem repeat sequences (VNTRs), which are short repeated sequences that vary in the number of repeated units and, therefore, in length. The human genetic linkage map is constructed by observing how frequently any two polymorphic markers are inherited together.

Two genetic markers that are in close proximity tend to be passed together from mother to child. During gametogenesis, homologous recombination events take place in the metaphase of the first meiotic step (*meiotic recombination crossing-over*). This may result in the separation of two markers that originally resided on the same chromosome. The closer the markers are to each other, the more tightly linked they are and the less likely that a recombination event will fall between and separate them. *Recombination frequency* provides an estimate of the distance between two markers.

On the genetic map, distances between markers are measured in terms of *centimorgans* (cM), named after the American geneticist Thomas Hunt Morgan. Two markers are said to be 1 cM apart if they are separated by recombination 1% of the time. A genetic distance of 1 cM is roughly equal to a physical distance of 1 million base pairs of DNA (1 Mb). The current resolution of most human genetic map regions is approximately 10 Mb.

An inherited disease can be located on the map by following the inheritance of a DNA marker present in affected individuals but absent in unaffected individuals, although the molecular basis of a disease or a trait may be unknown. Linkage studies have been used to identify the exact chromosomal location of several important genes associated with diseases, including cystic fibrosis, sickle cell disease, Tay-Sachs disease, fragile X syndrome, and myotonic dystrophy.

## RESTRICTION ENZYMES AND CHROMOSOMAL MAPPING

The restriction endonucleases, which have been isolated from various bacteria, recognize short DNA sequences and cut DNA molecules at those specific sites. A natural biofunction of restriction endonucleases is to protect bacteria from viral infection or foreign DNA by destroying the alien DNA. Some restriction enzymes cut DNA very infrequently, generating a small number of very large fragments, whereas other restriction enzymes cut DNA more frequently, yielding many smaller fragments. Because hundreds of different restriction enzymes have been characterized, DNA can be cut into many different-sized fragments.

## PHYSICAL MAPS

Different types of physical maps vary in their degree of resolution. The lowest resolution physical map is the chromosomal (cytogenetic) map, which is based on the distinctive banding pattern observed by light microscopy of stained chromosomes. A cDNA map shows the locations of expressed DNA (exons) on the chromosomal map. The more detailed *cosmid contiguous DNA block (contig) map* depicts the order of overlapping DNA fragments spanning the genome (see the section High-Resolution Physical Mapping). A *macrorestriction map* describes the order and distance between restriction enzyme cleavage sites. The *highest resolution physical map* will be the complete elucidation of the DNA base-pair sequence of each chromosome in the human genome.

### LOW-RESOLUTION PHYSICAL MAPPING

**Chromosomal Map.**    In a chromosomal map, genes or other identifiable DNA fragments are assigned to their respective chromosomes, with distances measured in base pairs. These markers can be physically associated with particular bands (identified by cytogenetic staining) primarily by *in situ hybridization*, a technique that involves tagging the DNA marker with an observable label. The location of the labeled probe can be detected after it binds to its complementary DNA strand in an intact chromosome.

As with genetic linkage mapping, chromosomal mapping can be used to locate genetic markers defined by traits observable only in whole organisms. Because chromosomal maps are based on estimates of physical distance, they are considered to be physical maps. The number of base pairs within a band can only be estimated.

**Fluorescence In Situ Hybridization.**[28,29]    A fluorescently labeled DNA probe locates a DNA sequence detected on a specific chromosome. The fluorescence in situ hybridization (FISH) method allows for the orientation of DNA sequences that lie as close as 2 to 5 Mb. Modifications to the in situ hybridization methods, using chromosomes at a stage in cell division (interphase) when they are less compact, increase map resolution by an additional 100,000 base pairs.

A cDNA map shows the positions of expressed DNA regions (exons) relative to particular chromosomal regions or bands. (Expressed DNA regions are those transcribed into mRNA.) The cDNA is synthesized in the laboratory using the mRNA molecule as the template. This cDNA can be used to map the genomic region of the respective molecule. A cDNA map can provide the chromosomal location for genes whose functions are currently unknown (ESTs). For hunters of disease genes, the map can also suggest a set of candidate genes to test when the approximate location of a disease gene has been mapped by genetic linkage analysis.

### HIGH-RESOLUTION PHYSICAL MAPPING

Two current approaches to high-resolution mapping are termed *top-down* (producing a macrorestriction map) and *bottom-up* (resulting in a contig map). With either strategy, the maps represent ordered sets of DNA fragments that are generated by cutting genomic DNA with restriction enzymes. The fragments are then amplified by cloning or by PCR methods. Electrophoretic techniques are used to separate the fragments (according to size) into different bands, which are visualized by staining or by hybridization with DNA probes of interest. The

use of purified chromosomes, separated either by fluorescence-activated flow sorting from human cell lines or in hybrid cell lines, allows a single chromosome to be mapped.

A number of strategies can be used to reconstruct the original order of the DNA fragments in the genome. Many approaches make use of the ability of single strands of DNA and/or RNA to hybridize to form double-stranded segments. The extent of sequence homology between the two strands can be inferred from the length of the double-stranded segment. *Fingerprinting* uses restriction enzyme cleavage map data to determine which fragments have a specific sequence (*fingerprint*) in common and, therefore, overlap. Another approach uses linking clones as probes for hybridization to chromosomal DNA cut with the same restriction enzyme.

In top-down mapping, a single chromosome is cut (using *rare-cutter restriction enzymes*) into large pieces, which are ordered and subdivided; the smaller pieces are then mapped further. The resulting macrorestriction maps depict the order of and distance between locations at which rare-cutter restriction sites are found in the chromosome. This approach yields maps with more continuity and fewer gaps between fragments than contig maps, but map resolution is lower and the map may not be useful in finding particular genes. In addition, this strategy generally does not produce long stretches of mapped sites. Currently, this approach allows DNA pieces to be located in regions measuring ~100 kb to 1 Mb.

The development of *pulsed-field gel (PFG)* electrophoretic methods has improved the mapping and cloning of large DNA molecules. Whereas conventional gel electrophoretic methods separate pieces of DNA <40 kb in size, PFG separates molecules up to 10 Mb, allowing application of both conventional and new mapping methods to large genomic regions.

The bottom-up (contig) approach involves cutting the chromosome into small pieces, each of which is cloned and ordered. The ordered fragments form contigs, or contiguous DNA blocks. Currently, the resulting library of clones varies in size from 10 kb to 1 Mb. An advantage of this approach is the accessibility of these stable clones to other researchers. Contig construction can be verified by FISH, which localizes cosmids to specific regions within chromosomal bands.

*Contig maps* consist of a linked library of small overlapping clones of DNA representing a complete chromosomal segment. Although useful for finding genes localized in a small area, contig maps are difficult to extend over large stretches of a chromosome because all regions are not clonable. DNA probe techniques can be used to fill in the gaps, but they are time consuming.

Technological improvements now make possible the cloning of large DNA pieces using artificially constructed chromosome vectors that carry human DNA fragments as large as 1 Mb. These vectors are maintained in yeast cells (i.e., YACs).[30,31] Before YACs were developed, the largest cosmids carried inserts of only 20 to 40 kb. YAC methodology drastically reduces the number of clones to be ordered; many YACs span entire human genes. A more detailed map of a large YAC insert can be produced by *subcloning* (a process in which fragments of the original insert are cloned into smaller insert vectors). Because some YAC regions are unstable, large-capacity bacterial vectors have also been developed (*bacterial artificial chromosome, BAC*).

## SEPARATING CHROMOSOMES

*Flow-sorting* uses flow cytometry to separate, according to size, chromosomes isolated from cells during cell division, when they are condensed and stable.[32,33] As the chromosomes flow singly past a laser beam, they are differentiated by analyzing the amount of DNA present, and individual chromosomes are directed to specific collection tubes.

## SOMATIC CELL HYBRIDIZATION

In somatic cell hybridization, human cells and rodent tumor cells are fused (hybridized); over time, after the chromosomes mix, human chromosomes are preferentially lost from the hybrid cell until only one or a few remain. Those individual hybrid cells are then propagated and maintained as cell lines containing specific human chromosomes. Improvements to this technique have generated a number of hybrid cell lines, each with a specific single human chromosome.

Starting maps and sequences is relatively simple. Finishing them requires either development of new strategies or use of a combination of existing methods. After a sequence is determined, the task that remains is to fill in the many large gaps left by current mapping methods. One approach is a single chromosome microdissection, in which a piece of DNA is physically cut from a chromosomal region of particular interest and then broken up into smaller pieces and amplified by PCR or cloning. These fragments of DNA can then be mapped and sequenced by conventional methods.

## CHROMOSOME WALKING (POSITIONAL CLONING)

Chromosome walking, one strategy for cloning genes and filling gaps, involves hybridizing a primer of known sequence to a clone from an unordered genomic library and synthesizing a short complementary strand (called *walking on the chromosome*). The complementary strand is then sequenced and its end used as the next primer for further walking. In this way, the adjacent (previously unknown) region is identified and sequenced. The chromosome is thus systematically sequenced from one end to the other. Because primers must be synthesized chemically, a disadvantage of this technique is the need to construct a large number of different primers for walking large distances. Chromosome walking is also used to locate specific genes by sequencing the chromosomal segments between markers that flank the gene of interest (i.e., positional cloning).

The degree of difficulty encountered in finding a disease gene of interest depends largely on what information is already known about the gene and especially on what kind of DNA alterations cause the disease. Spotting the disease gene is difficult when disease results from a single altered DNA base; sickle cell anemia is an example of such a case, as are probably most major human inherited diseases. When disease results from a large DNA rearrangement, the anomaly can be detected as alterations in the physical map of the region or even by direct microscopic examination of the chromosome. The location of these alterations pinpoints the site of the gene.

## CANDIDATE GENE APPROACH

Another approach to identifying a disease-causing or disease-related gene is the *candidate gene approach*. Here, a gene known to be important in the development or function of a certain organ or organ system is analyzed for mutations in a cohort with the disease and compared with the gene in a healthy control group. This approach has been valuable in identifying single gene mutations in well-defined, relatively small pedigrees. With the possibility for large-scale genome-wide screening using DNA-array technology, this approach may be applied to large cohorts in a widespread manner in the future.

# FUTURE PROSPECTS

## HUMAN GENOME PROJECT

The Human Genome Project was begun in 1990 by the U.S. government and is coordinated by the U.S. Department of Energy and the National Institutes of Health. Although it was originally conceived as a 15-year program, rapid technological advances as well as collaboration between genome projects of several countries (United Kingdom, Germany, Japan, France) and privately funded endeavors to sequence the human genome have accelerated the project to an expected completion date of 2001, with 90% of the genome available in the spring of 2000.[34] The Human Genome Project initiated by the U.S. government has set out to sequence the entire genome of one human individual (identity strictly secret), whereas the privately initiated effort is sequencing the entire genome of five different individuals. The latter approach is addressing the issue of some, although limited, variability in the genome of humans.

The goals of the Human Genome Project are to identify the estimated 80,000 expressed genes in human DNA; to determine the sequences of the ~3 billion chemical bases that make up the human DNA; to store the information in databases that will be made accessible to the public; to develop tools for data analysis; and to address the ethical, legal, and societal issues that may arise from the project. Furthermore, to allow comparison of genetic information among species and to address questions related to the interaction of humans with infectious pathogens, researchers are studying the genetic makeup of several nonhuman organisms, including *Drosophila melanogaster*, *Plasmodium falciparum*, and the laboratory mouse. The genomes of several organisms such as *E. coli*, *Saccharomyces cerevisiae*, *Caenorhabditis elegans*, *Bacillus subtilis*, *Synechtosis species*, *A. fulgidus*, *P. aerophilum*, *Haemophilus influenzae*, *M. thermoautrophicum*, *M. jannaschii*, *A. aolicolus*, *Borrelia burgdorferi*, *Treponema pallidum*, *Mycoplasma pneumoniae*, *M. genitalum*, *Chlamydia trachomatis*, *Rickettsia prowazekii*, *Helicobacter pylori*, and *Mycobacterium tuberculosis* are already known and accessible.

During progress of the Human Genome Project, several new goals have been formulated. For example, one goal is to identify regions of the human genome that differ from person to person. Although the majority of individuals' DNA sequences are the same, estimates are that humans are only ~99% identical genetically. These DNA sequence variations can have a major impact on how people's bodies respond to disease (i.e., to environmental insults, such as bacteria, viruses, and toxins; and to drugs and other therapies). Methods have been developed to rapidly detect different types of variation, particularly the most common type, called *single-nucleotide polymorphisms (SNPs)*, which occur approximately once every 100 to 300 bases. SNP maps will ultimately help identify multiple genes associated with complex diseases such as cancer, diabetes, vascular disease, and some forms of mental illness. These associations are difficult to establish with conventional gene-hunting methods because a single altered gene may make only a small contribution to disease risk.

The atlas of the human genome will revolutionize medical practice and biologic research into the twenty-first century and beyond. All human genes will be found, and accurate diagnostics will be developed for most inherited diseases. In addition, animal models for human disease research will be more easily developed, facilitating the understanding of gene function in health and disease.

Single genes associated with a number of diseases (e.g., cystic fibrosis, Duchenne muscular dystrophy, myotonic dystrophy, neurofibromatosis, diabetes mellitus, and retinoblastoma) have already been identified. Diseases caused by several genes or by a gene interacting with environmental factors can be studied more efficiently. Genetic susceptibilities have been implicated in many major disabling and fatal diseases, including heart disease, stroke, diabetes, and several kinds of cancer. The identification of these genes and their proteins will pave the way to more effective therapies and preventive measures.

The potential benefits of the Human Genome Project are manifold. Only some of the important potential applications

**TABLE 2-4.**
**Implications and Issues Arising from the Human Genome Project**

Fairness in the use of genetic information by insurers, employers, courts, schools, adoption, agencies, the military, etc.; that is, who should have access to information and how will it be used?

Privacy and confidentiality of genetic information; that is, who owns and controls information?

Psychological impact and stigmatization due to individual genetic differences. How does the genetic information affect the individual and impact on society's perception of the individual?

Genetic testing of an individual for a specific condition due to a family history of prenatal, carrier, presymptomatic testing, population screening.

Reproductive issues involving informed consent for procedures, use of genetic information in decision making, reproductive rights.

Clinical uses, education of health service providers, patients, and the general public. Implementation of standards and quality control measures in testing procedures.

Commercialization of products: issues include intellectual property rights, patents, copyrights, trade secrets, and accessibility of data and materials.

Unanticipated consequences of manipulations of the genome. Continued control through legislation, and its implications.

---

are discussed here. *Molecular medicine* (a term lending more significance to medicine and the understanding of human disease and its potential cure at the molecular level) will gain increasing importance in medical practice. Improved diagnosis and earlier detection of genetic predisposition to disease are already commonplace for certain conditions (cystic fibrosis, trisomy, fragile X syndrome, myotonic dystrophy, and neurofibromatosis). The design of drugs that are tailored to the demands imposed by genetic predisposition and the choice of treatment based on genetic information will allow a more rational approach to treatment.

*Microbial genomics,* which yields the sequence and function of microbial genes, can potentially identify new energy sources (biofuels) and identify bacteria useful in environmental remediation, toxic waste reduction, and industrial processing. New tools for risk assessment for exposure to radiation and toxic agents can be made more reliably at the genetic level with information on the human genome. Furthermore, comparison of genomic sequences can increase the capabilities to study evolution through germline mutations in lineages; examine migration of different population groups based on female genetic inheritance; investigate mutations on the Y chromosome to trace lineage and migration of males; and compare breakpoints in the evolution of mutations with ages of populations and historical events.

DNA forensic analysis aimed at proper identification of individuals involved in crimes and catastrophic events, establishment of paternity and family relationships, and matching of organ donors is already commonplace with the limited possibilities available today. The expansion of genetic information with the Human Genome Project should allow for improving the reliability of such tests.

Agriculture, livestock breeding, and bioprocessing are additional areas affected directly by the genome project. Understanding plant and animal genomes can potentially allow the creation of stronger, more resistant plants and animals. Bioengineered seeds are already being used to grow disease-resistant crops, thereby reducing costs in agriculture. Some additional applications that are already being tested experimentally are the design of pesticides, development of edible vaccines incorporated into food products, development of new environmental cleanup uses for plants like tobacco, and generation of animals and plants producing molecules to be used for the treatment of human conditions (i.e., clotting factors, hemoglobin).

Although human genome research itself does not pose any new ethical dilemma, the use of data arising from these studies presents challenges that need to be addressed before the data accumulate significantly. Some of the issues pertinent to the question are summarized in Table 2-4. To assist in policy development, the ethics component of the Human Genome Project is funding conferences and research projects to identify and consider relevant societal issues, as well as activities to promote public awareness of these topics.

## STEM CELLS

### EMBRYONIC STEM CELLS

ES cells are pluripotent cells that give rise to all adult cell types.[35] They can be derived from the *blastocyst*, a preimplantation-stage embryo,[36] or from *primordial germ cells*, cells of the early embryo that eventually differentiate into sperm and oocytes.[37] Mouse ES cells have been used for approximately a decade to generate genetically altered mice (*knock-out, knock-in, Cre recombinants*). Mouse ES cells are *pluripotent* in that they can differentiate into many cell types. ES cells, unlike fertilized eggs, cannot develop completely into individual organisms. ES cells that are placed into a uterus will never develop into an embryo. After desired manipulations, ES cells are injected into the cavity of a developing blastocyst, which ultimately develops into a *chimera* harboring all tissue cells from the original embryo as well as filiae of the artificially introduced ES cells. ES cells cannot develop into an embryo on their own; they must be placed into an artificial environment, one in which the host cells provide the placental tissues of the conceptus. The derivation of human ES cells from developing fetuses has opened exciting new possibilities for therapy as well as raising legal and ethical issues.[36,38]

To be able to generate tissue for potential transplantation or organ replacement, ES cells that are immunologically identical to the prospective host would need to be generated. This could possibly be achieved by *somatic nuclear transfer,* with a nucleus of a prospective host inserted into a *recipient enucleated oocyte* of either the same or a different species. From the embryo that developed, the inner cell mass of the blastocyst would need to be isolated and grown in vitro to yield ES cells, which then would need to be differentiated into the desired tissue. To date, not all of these steps have been mastered.

The *use of ES cells therapeutically has dangers, however.* Mouse ES cells are tumorigenic, growing into teratomas or teratocarcinomas when injected anywhere in the adult mouse. Human ES cells might behave similarly.

### PLURIPOTENT STEM CELLS IN ADULT ORGANS

Renewable tissues (blood, intestinal epithelium, epidermis) are considered to harbor stem cells that can, by multiplication, yield cells which can then further differentiate into cells of the respective host tissue.

Cells in the nervous system have been found to have the capacity to generate new neurons and glial cells (astrocytes and oligodendrocytes), and, because of this, they are considered to be neuronal stem cells.[39–41] These cells can be isolated from the wall of the lateral ventricle of the brain.[42] These cells, which constitute ~0.1% to 1% of the cells in the ependymal lining, express immature neural markers consistent with a stem-cell function.

In vitro, these stem cells divide in response to epidermal growth factor and fibroblast growth factor-2.[43] On dividing, they are thought to give rise to both neural and glial progeny. If these cells are transplanted into the intact brain, they integrate and differentiate into a range of neuronal and glial cells.[44,45] Moreover, these cells can regenerate blood cells when transplanted into lethally radiated host mice.

Human embryonic stem cells, which can be cloned[46] and grown for extended periods,[47] reside in the adult brain (Table 2-5).[48]

Another example of pluripotent stem cells is mesenchymal stem cells (MSCs), which can be isolated from bone marrow.[49] These cells can be expanded in culture and still differentiate into osteoblasts, osteocytes, chondrocytes, adipocytes, tendon-

**TABLE 2-5.**
**Human Stem Cells Isolated**

| Stem Cell Type | Source | Daughter Tissues |
|---|---|---|
| Embryonic (ES) | Embryo or fetal tissue | All types |
| Hematopoietic | Adult bone marrow | Blood cells (brain?) |
| Neuronal | Fetal brain | Neurons, glia (blood?) |
| Mesenchymal | Adult bone marrow | Muscle, bone, cartilage, tendon |

**TABLE 2-7.**
**Animals Cloned by Somatic Nuclear Transfer**

| Name of Animals | Property | Reference |
|---|---|---|
| Megan and Morag | Lambs from cultivated embryonic cells | Campbel, et al. Nature 1996; 380:64. |
| Dolly and Bonnie | Lambs from nucleus of cell from udder of an adult sheep | Wilmut, et al. Nature 1997; 385:810. |
| Polly and Molly | Lambs from transgenic fibroblasts expressing human factor IX | Schnieke, et al. Science 1997; 278:2130. |
| ACT3, ACT4, ACT5 | Calves from genetically modified fetal fibroblasts | Cibelli, et al. Science 1998; 280:1256. |
| Cumulina and clones | Mice from cumulus cells from mouse ovary | Wayakama, et al. Nature 1998; 394:369. |

associated cells, and myotubules[50]; they have been transplanted into children with osteogenesis imperfecta and into women who have undergone high-dose myelotoxic chemotherapy,[51,52] and used for Achilles tendon repair.[53]

Several ethical and biologic questions need to be addressed before ES cells can be used widely for human applications (Table 2-6).

## SOMATIC CELL CLONING IN VIVO

### BLASTOMERE SEPARATION

Cloning by blastomere separation (called "twinning") (Table 2-7) involves splitting a developing embryo soon after fertilization of the egg by a sperm to give rise to two or more embryos. The resulting organisms are identical twins (clones) containing DNA from both the mother and the father. This technique has been used for approximately one decade for generating transgenic or knock-out embryos and animals. Twinning in the sense of generating two or more genetically identical organisms has been practiced for thousands of years with plants.

### SOMATIC NUCLEUS TRANSFER

Cloning by somatic nucleus transfer involves the insertion of a nucleus of a cell from one single adult into an egg from which the original nucleus has been removed. This allows for the generation of an animal with the genetic information coming from one single adult (as opposed to cloning by blastomere separation). The technique of somatic nucleus transfer was attempted in the 1950s in frogs, and early attempts were conducted in mammals in the 1980s. In 1996, lambs were successfully cloned via somatic nucleus transfer from embryonic cells that had been cultured in vitro for several months. Dolly, the lamb that was cloned by transferring the nucleus of a cell from the udder of a 6-year-old sheep, gained broad attention. The theoretical possibility was created of generating an unlimited number of genetically identical individuals from one single parent. However, the clones generated through somatic nucleus transfer are not completely genetically identical to the donor animal. The mitochondrial DNA in the host oocyte originates from the mother. Dolly appears to be a healthy sheep and has reportedly given birth to a lamb named Bonnie per vias naturalis.

In 1997, a second lamb named Polly was generated by an additional cellular manipulation. Nuclei from fetal fibroblasts were modified in vitro to incorporate the cDNA for human factor IX under control of the β-lactoglobin promoter. These

**TABLE 2-6.**
**Biologic and Ethical Questions Pertinent to Use of Embryonic Stem (ES) Cells**

Are ES cells tumorigenic?

Can ES cells be forced to differentiate along a defined pathway?

Can all ES cells in vitro be made to differentiate simultaneously along the same pathway?

Can ES cell lines be derived from the patient's own tissue for ultimate tissue replacement?

Should ES cells be considered embryos?

"transgenic" fibroblasts were used as donor nuclei for somatic transfer. Polly, the lamb generated by this method, produces up to 40 g/L of human factor IX in its milk. Factor IX can now be isolated without much effort and used in therapeutic applications. Since these advances were reported, successful cloning of calves and mice has also been accomplished.

The majority of clones fail sometime during development, and some fail after birth. One report suggests that the immune defense system of animals cloned by somatic nucleus transfer may be impaired. Further, telomeres of cloned animals appear to be shorter, suggesting that the cells may have a reduced life span and the animals may manifest symptoms of premature aging. However, the offspring of Dolly appears to have telomeres of normal length. Some accomplishments of somatic nuclear transfer are summarized in Table 2-7.

## GENE KNOCK-OUT LIBRARIES

A main area of investigation when the entire genome of humans as well as that of laboratory animals (i.e., mice and rats) is known and large-scale mutation screening of the entire genome can be performed rapidly will be the study of the function of genes identified in the context of diseases and the consequences of mutations in these genes.

For this purpose, collections of knock-out mice strains are made available to researchers for analysis in various assay systems. Furthermore, tissue-specific ablation of certain genes with the Cre-loxP methodology are being provided to researchers. The effects of gene ablation in defined physiologic situations and the effects of drugs in an animal lacking the function of a defined gene can then be studied more efficiently.

## GENE THERAPY: VECTORS AND PROBLEMS[54]

The concept of gene therapy is the transfer of genetic information to a host organism or a specific tissue within an organism. The product of the delivered gene either may be missing or of insufficient quantity in the host (*replacement therapy*) or may be of pharmacologic/therapeutic value (e.g., immune modulation, vaccination). Agents carrying the DNA to target cells are called *vectors*. The requirements for an ideal vector are that it should accommodate an unlimited amount of inserted DNA, lack the ability of autonomous replication of its own DNA, be easily manufactured, and be available in a concentrated form. For most applications, it should have the ability to target specific cell types or limit its gene expression in the long term or in a controlled fashion. It should not be toxic or immunogenic. Such vectors do not exist, and none of the DNA delivery systems so far available for in vivo gene transfer is perfect. Thus, the advancement of gene therapy lies in the development and improvement of new gene vector systems.

Different ways of introducing genes into mammalian cells and tissues have been devised, the simplest being the inoculation of naked DNA by means of microinjection, electroporation, or bioballistics (known as the *gene gun* technique[55]). More elaborate and efficient ways include the use of self-assembling complexes of lipid-DNA (e.g., liposomes) protein-DNA, or lipid-protein-DNA, and viral vectors. The physicochemical methods of gene delivery are summarized in Tables 2-2 and 2-3.

Viral vectors can be fragments of viral DNA containing the DNA to be transferred or the viral particle itself.[56] The viral particle is rendered replication defective through the manipulation of the viral DNA, and the end product is a nonpathogenic viral vector carrying the genetic information of therapeutic interest. Many different types of virus have been used for gene-transfer purposes. The viruses holding most promise for future application in biomedicine (*retroviruses, adenoviruses,* and *adenoassociated viruses*) are discussed in the following sections.

**Retroviral Vectors.** The Moloney murine leukemia virus (MoMuLV) was the first virus used in developing a vector system for gene transfer. Parts of the retroviral genome that are involved in the replication of the MoMuLV—gag, pol, and env—are removed and replaced by a gene of interest. What remains of the retrovirus are the long terminal repeats harboring regulatory elements, integration signals, and transcription promoters, and a packaging signal. To produce retroviral vectors carrying the gene of interest, one must use a packaging cell line harboring the gag, pol, and env genes, which have previously been incorporated into the genome of such packaging cells. The vectors are produced in high titers in the packaging cells, purified, and injected into the organism (*in vivo gene therapy*) or put in contact with cells collected from the patient and maintained in cell culture (*ex vivo gene therapy*). Retroviral vectors have the ability to integrate their genomic material into the host genome as a result of the presence of the remaining retroviral regulatory sequences in the form of the long terminal repeats. Once integrated, the inserted gene can be expressed to produce the desired protein.

Advantages of retroviral vectors are that they are well characterized, they can be produced in high titers, and they have a high efficiency of infection. Disadvantages are the limited size of DNA (7–8 kb) that retrovirus vectors can accommodate, the requirement that the target cells be in cell division to allow for the integration of the vectors, and the potential for insertional mutagenesis due to retroviral vector integration at random in the genome. The latter feature has the potential to interrupt important genes in the cell, with serious consequences that include oncogenesis through the activation of protooncogenes or inactivation of tumor-suppressor genes.

*Lentiviruses* are a group of retroviruses that have the ability to infect and integrate their genome even in cells that are not dividing. Thus, the use of lentiviruses as gene therapy vectors is broader than that of other retroviruses and is under investigation.

**Adenoviral Vectors.** The human adenoviruses are nonenveloped DNA viruses with a linear double-stranded DNA of ~36 kb, encapsulated in an icosahedral capsoid measuring 70 to 100 nm in diameter. Adenoviruses are known pathogens in humans, and most, if not all, adult humans have been exposed to adenoviruses and have antibodies against adenovirus antigens.

An adenovirus does not depend on host-cell division for its replication, and the chromosome rarely integrates into the genome, remaining episomal in most cases. Integration seems to occur mainly in the presence of high levels of infection in dividing cells, but this event does not contribute significantly to the utility of these viruses as vectors. Adenoviral vectors have a broad spectrum of cell infectivity that includes virtually all postmitotic and mitotic cells; they also can be produced in high titers.

The genome of the adenovirus encodes ~15 proteins. Viral gene expression occurs in a coordinated fashion and is mainly directed by the E1A and E1B genes, localized within the 5' region of the adenoviral genome. These genes have transactivation functions for the transcription of various viral and host-cell genes. Because E1 genes are involved in adenoviral replication, their removal renders the virus replication incompetent. The removal also creates room for insertion of a foreign gene of therapeutic interest. An exogenous DNA can also replace the E3 region, which produces a product enabling the virus to evade the immune system. *Packaging cells* carrying adenoviral genes that provide transcomplementation functions are required to produce defective adenoviral vectors. Packaging cells of the NIH-293 cell lineage are human embryo kidney (HEK) cells that have been previously transformed with type 5 adenovirus. These cells retain the E1A and E1B regions of the viral genome covalently linked to their genomic DNA.

Disadvantages of the adenoviral vectors include the short duration of transgene expression, because the vector usually does not integrate stably into the host-cell genome. Further, the size of the inserted foreign DNA sequence is limited, and cellular and humoral immune responses are typically triggered against the adenoviral particles or against the host cell that eventually expresses adenoviral proteins, thus limiting the longevity of the adenovirus vector.

**Adenoassociated Viral Vectors.** Adenoassociated virus (AAV) is a small nonenveloped, nonpathogenic DNA virus belonging to the Parvoviridae family. The AAV genome is a single-strand DNA molecule of 4681 bases, including two inverted long terminal repeats (ITRs). ITRs are 145-base-long palindromic sequences involved in the regulation of the AAV cell cycle. They are located in the 5' and 3' terminal portions of the viral genome and serve as origins and initiators for DNA replication. Flanked by the ITRs, two large open-reading frames code for a regulatory protein and a structural protein, called *rep* and *cap*, respectively. The protein coding sequence located in the 5' region (rep gene) encodes four nonstructural proteins involved in the genomic replication. The 3' region contains the cap gene, which encodes three structural proteins required for the formation of the viral capsid. AAV is capable of replication in a cell only in the presence of a helper virus (adenovirus or herpes virus) that provides by transcomplementation the helper factors that are essential for its replication. In the absence of a helper virus, the AAV genome preferentially integrates into a specific site on the short arm of chromosome 19, between q13.3 and qter, called AAVS1. The ITRs as well as a rep transcript play an important role in this process, which results in a latent infection in mitotic as well as in postmitotic cells. Episomal virus and insertion in nonspecific sites has been documented.

Among the advantages of AAV as a potential gene vector in human gene therapy are the lack of relation to human diseases, broad infectivity spectrum, and ability to stably integrate into the host genome. This integration can occur in cells that are not dividing, although at a lower frequency than in dividing cells. The site-directed integration is also a most favorable property of AAV.

## DNA-BASED VACCINATION

Immunization with transfer of genetic material represents a novel approach to vaccination.[57,58] The technology involves transferal of a gene (encoding an antigenic protein cloned in an expression vector) to a host, leading to the induction of an immune response. Direct gene transfer may be undertaken using either viral vectors or recombinant plasmid DNA. Viral vectors have the disadvantages of being derived from pathogens (like traditional vaccines based on attenuated virus), and, therefore, are of limited interest for the purpose of immunization. In contrast, DNA plasmids encoding antigens are more frequently used because they do not have the inconvenience of classic vaccines: they are safe, inexpensive, easy to produce, heat stable, and amenable to genetic manipulation.

Currently, two main delivery systems are available for gene vaccination. Plasmid DNA is injected intramuscularly, or DNA is coated onto gold beads and transferred into the epidermis or dermis by a *bioballistic process (gene gun)*. The intramuscular injection is the most widely used method for immunization, and it consists of direct injection of naked DNA into skeletal muscle. Plasmid DNA in some instances is injected into muscle directly in saline solution or after injection of toxins or a local anesthetic to cause necrosis and regeneration of the injected muscle, thereby increasing the expression of the encoded antigen and amplifying the immunologic response. It is unclear whether the elevated antigen in regenerating muscle cells is due to an increased expression of the antigen gene or to the antigen contained within antigen-presenting cells that are recruited to the site of tissue damage. Humoral and cell-mediated immune responses have been induced by the direct intramuscular injection of plasmid DNA endocrine immunogens. An antibody response was first reported against an influenza virus protein in mice, and specific cytotoxic T-cell responses were also detected in different systems (i.e., human immunodeficiency virus infection and hepatitis B) after genetic immunization. Protective immunity was first demonstrated in mice injected intramuscularly with nucleoprotein DNA of influenza virus. In this model, researchers have indicated that both CD4+ and CD8+ T cells contributed to the protection. Protective immune responses have also been demonstrated in mice against *Leishmania major, Plasmodium yoelii, Mycobacterium tuberculosis*, dengue virus, and herpes simplex virus.

The bioballistic (gene gun) method uses a helium gas pressure-driven device to deliver gold particles coated with plasmid directly into the skin. When gene vaccines are administered by gene gun technology, most of the plasmid DNA is taken up by keratinocytes and some dermal fibroblasts; they become transfected and produce the encoded antigen. Humoral responses using bioballistic approaches were demonstrated using plasmids encoding human growth hormone and human α-antitrypsin.

The nature of the immune response elicited by these DNA vaccination approaches is not clearly understood. In an initial study, the suggestion was made that DNA vaccination elicits a cell-mediated immune response, because passive transfer of serum from immune mice did not engender protective immunity. Depletion experiments demonstrated that both CD4+ and CD8+ cell populations were involved in host protection against infection. However, some investigators have also reported an induction of immunoglobulins after gene gun–mediated immunization.

# REFERENCES

1. Angier N. Natural obsessions: the search for the oncogene. Boston: Houghton Mifflin, 1988.
2. Judson HF. The eighth day of creation: makers of the revolution in biology. Cold Spring Harbor: Cold Spring Harbor Press, 1996.
3. Hall SS. Invisible frontier: the race to synthesize a human gene. New York: Atlantic Monthly Press, 1987.
4. Morange MA. History of molecular biology. Cambridge, MA: Harvard University Press, 1998.
5. Baltimore D. RNA-dependent DNA polymerase in virions of RNA tumour viruses. Nature 1970; 226:1209.
6. Kelly TJ Jr, Smith HO. A restriction enzyme from *Hemophilus influenzae*. II. J Mol Biol 1970; 51:393.
7. Smith HO, Wilcox KW. A restriction enzyme from *Hemophilus influenzae*. I. Purification and general properties. J Mol Biol 1970; 51:379.
8. Danna K, Nathans D. Specific cleavage of simian virus 40 DNA by restriction endonuclease of *Hemophilus influenzae*. Proc Natl Acad Sci U S A 1971; 68:2913.
9. Maxam AM, Gilbert W. A new method for sequencing DNA. Proc Natl Acad Sci U S A 1977; 74:560.
10. Sanger F, Nicklen S, Coulson AR. DNA sequencing with chain-terminating inhibitors. Proc Natl Acad Sci U S A 1977; 74:5463.
11. Sambrook J, Fritsch EF, Maniatis T. Molecular cloning: a laboratory manual, 2nd ed. Cold Spring Harbor: Cold Spring Harbor Press, 1989.
12. Ausubel FM, Brend R, Kingston RE, et al. Current protocols in molecular biology. New York: John Wiley and Sons, 1993.
13. Saiki RK, Scharf S, Faloona F, et al. Enzymatic amplification of beta-globin genomic sequences and restriction site analysis for diagnosis of sickle cell anemia. Science 1985; 230:1350.
14. Freeman WM, Walker SJ, Vrana KE. Quantitative RT-PCR: pitfalls and potential. Biotechniques 1999; 26:112.
15. Wright PA, Wynford-Thomas D. The polymerase chain reaction: miracle or mirage: a critical review of its uses and limitations in diagnosis and research. J Pathol 1990; 162:99.
16. Mullis KB, Ferre F, Gibbs RA. The polymerase chain reaction. New York: Springer-Verlag, 1994.
17. Bronson SK, Smithies O. Altering mice by homologous recombination using embryonic stem cells. J Biol Chem 1994; 269:27155.
18. Rajewsky K, Gu H, Kuhn R, et al. Conditional gene targeting. J Clin Invest 1996; 98:600.
19. Gossen M, Freundlieb S, Bender G, et al. Transcriptional activation by tetracyclines in mammalian cells. Science 1995; 268:1766.
20. Ramsay G. DNA chips: state-of-the art. Nat Biotechnol 1998; 16:40.
21. Kurian KM, Watson CJ, Wyllie AH. DNA chip technology. J Pathol 1999; 187:267.
22. Donis-Keller H, Green P, Helms C, et al. A genetic linkage map of the human genome. Cell 1987; 51:319.
23. Grompe M, Gibbs RA, Chamberlain JS, Caskey CT. Detection of new mutation disease in man and mouse. Mol Biol Med 1989; 6:511.
24. Rikke BA, Johnson TE. Towards the cloning of genes underlying murine QTLs. Mamm Genome 1998; 9:963.
25. Leach RJ, O'Connell P. Mapping of mammalian genomes with radiation (Goss and Harris) hybrids. Adv Genet 1995; 33:63.
26. Martin N, Boomsma D, Machin G. A twin-pronged attack on complex traits. Nat Genet 1997; 17:387.
27. Farral M. Affected sibpair linkage tests for multiple linked susceptibility genes. Genet Epidemiol 1997; 14:103.
28. Chang SS, Mark HF. Emerging molecular cytogenetic technologies. Cytobios 1997; 90:7.
29. Luke S, Shepelsky M. FISH: recent advances and diagnostic aspects. Cell Vis 1998; 5:49.
30. Coulson A, Waterston R, Kiff J, et al. Genome linking with yeast artificial chromosomes. Nature 1988; 335:184.
31. Vollrath D, Davis RW, Connelly C, Hieter P. Physical mapping of large DNA by chromosome fragmentation. Proc Natl Acad Sci U S A 1988; 85:6027.
32. Roslaniec MC, Bell-Prince CS, Crissman HA, et al. New flow cytometric technologies for the 21st century. Hum Cell 1997; 10:3.
33. Ferguson-Smith MA. Genetic analysis by chromosome sorting and painting: phylogenetic and diagnostic applications. Eur J Hum Genet 1997; 5:253.
34. Collins FS. Shattuck lecture—medical and societal consequences of the Human Genome Project. N Engl J Med 1999; 341:28.
35. Vogel G. Harnessing the power of stem cells. Science 1999; 283:1432.
36. Thomson JA, Itskovitz-Eldor J, Shapiro SS, et al. Embryonic stem cell lines derived from human blastocysts [see comments] [published erratum appears in Science 1998; 282(5395):1827]. Science 1998; 282:1145.
37. Shamblott MJ, Axelman J, Wang S, et al. Derivation of pluripotent stem cells from cultured human primordial germ cells. Proc Natl Acad Sci U S A 1998; 95:13726.
38. Marshall E. A versatile cell line raises scientific hopes, legal questions. (News; comment). Science 1998; 282:1014.
39. McKay R. Stem cells in the central nervous system. Science 1997; 276:66.
40. Weiss S, van der Kooy D. CNS stem cells: where's the biology (a.k.a. beef)? J Neurobiol 1998; 36:307.
41. Alvarez-Buylla A, Temple S. Stem cells in the developing and adult nervous system. J Neurobiol 1998; 36:105.
42. Johansson CB, Momma S, Clarke DL, et al. Identification of a neural stem cell in the adult mammalian central nervous system. Cell 1999; 96:25.
43. Cattaneo E, McKay R. Proliferation and differentiation of neuronal stem cells regulated by nerve growth factor. Nature 1990; 347:762.
44. Gage FH, Kempermann G, Palmer TD, et al. Multipotent progenitor cells in the adult dentate gyrus. J Neurobiol 1998; 36:249.
45. Takahashi M, Palmer TD, Takahashi J, Gage FH. Widespread integration and survival of adult-derived neural progenitor cells in the developing optic retina. Mol Cell Neurosci 1998; 12:340.
46. Flax JD, Aurora S, Yang C, et al. Engraftable human neural stem cells respond to developmental cues, replace neurons, and express foreign genes. Nat Biotechnol 1998; 16:1033.
47. Svendsen CN, ter Borg MG, Armstrong RJ, et al. A new method for the rapid and long term growth of human neural precursor cells. J Neurosci Methods 1998; 85:141.
48. Eriksson PS, Perfilieva E, Bjork-Eriksson T, et al. Neurogenesis in the adult human hippocampus [see comments]. Nat Med 1998; 4:1313.
49. Prockop DJ. Marrow stromal cells as stem cells for nonhematopoietic tissues. Science 1997; 276:71.
50. Horwitz EM, Prockop DJ, Fitzpatrick LA, et al. Transplantability and therapeutic effects of bone marrow-derived mesenchymal cells in children with osteogenesis imperfecta [see comments]. Nat Med 1999; 5:309.
51. Koc H, Gurman G, Arslan O, et al. Is there an increased risk of graft-versus-host disease after allogeneic peripheral blood stem cell transplantation? Blood 1996; 15:2362.
52. Lazarus HM, Haynesworth SE, Gerson SL, et al. Ex vivo expansion and subsequent infusion of human bone marrow–derived stromal progenitor cells (mesenchymal progenitor cells): implications for therapeutic use. Bone Marrow Transplant 1995; 16:557.
53. Young RG, Butler DL, Weber W, et al. Use of mesenchymal stem cells in a collagen matrix for Achilles tendon repair. J Orthop Res 1998; 16:406.
54. Dani SU. The challenge of vector development in gene therapy. (In Process Citation). Braz J Med Biol Res 1999; 32:133.

55. Robinson HL. DNA vaccines: basic mechanisms and immune responses. Int J Mol Med 1999; 4:549.
56. Stone D, David A, Bolognani F, et al. Viral vectors for gene delivery and gene therapy within the endocrine system. J Endocrinol 2000; 164:103.
57. Davis HL. Plasmid DNA expression systems for the purpose of immunization. Curr Opin Biotechnol 1997; 8:635.
58. Seder RA, Gurunathan S. DNA vaccines: designer vaccines for the 21st century. N Engl J Med 1999; 341:277.

# CHAPTER 3

# BIOSYNTHESIS AND SECRETION OF PEPTIDE HORMONES

WILLIAM W. CHIN

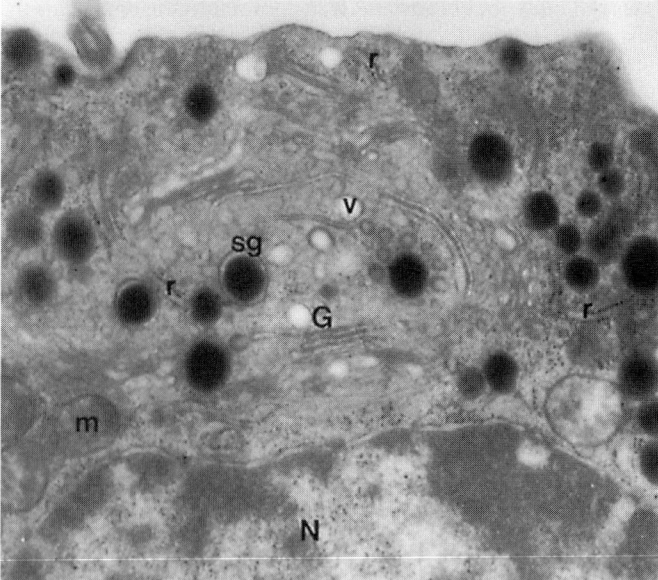

**FIGURE 3-1.** Electron micrograph of a rat lactotrope. The rat lactotrope in the anterior pituitary gland synthesizes and secretes prolactin. This electron micrograph reveals a portion of a lactotrope, including the two major compartments, nucleus (*N*) and cytoplasm. The nucleus is delineated by a double membrane, the nuclear envelope. The key organelles in the synthesis and processing of polypeptide hormones include the rough endoplasmic reticulum (*r*), Golgi stack (*G*), secretory vesicle (*v*), and secretory granule (*sg*). Mitochondria (*m*), the major source of cellular energy, are shown. The secretory granules are characterized by an electron-dense material representing condensed polypeptide hormone. (Courtesy of Gwen V. Childs, University of Texas at Galveston.)

In the endocrine system, hormones are factors produced by groups of cells clustered in specific tissues, commonly known as *glands,* and released into the general circulation to affect the function of distant target cells. Because hormones are responsible for the control of a complex metabolic milieu, they, along with the hormone-producing and target cells, participate in intricate regulatory networks (see Chaps. 4 and 5).

An important feature is *positive* regulation of hormone synthesis and secretion. For example, gonadotropin-releasing hormone (GnRH) from the hypothalamus stimulates production and release of the pituitary gonadotropins. Another common theme is regulation by *negative* feedback, by which a trophic hormone stimulates the production and secretion of a second hormone in a target cell that acts on the original gland to decrease secretion of the trophic hormone. For example, thyroid-stimulating hormone (TSH) is produced and secreted from the thyrotrope in the anterior pituitary gland. It stimulates the thyroid gland to synthesize and secrete thyroid hormones, which act on the thyrotrope to decrease further production and release of TSH. Thus, hormones may regulate the biosynthesis and release of other hormones. Moreover, hormones may control other cellular activities by determining the amount and activity of other proteins. This regulation occurs largely at the gene transcriptional level, although some regulation occurs at posttranscriptional, translational, and posttranslational levels.

In addition to operating at the broader level of the endocrine system, factors secreted from a given cell can influence cellular activities in adjacent or neighboring cells (i.e., paracrine effects) or within itself (i.e., autocrine effects; see Chap. 1). Intracellular communication effected by hormonal factors is critical for the integrated function of an organism. The pivotal and ubiquitous nature of hormones in these tasks makes understanding their synthesis and release essential.

This chapter describes the events that occur in the biosynthesis of polypeptide hormones in hormone-secretory cells, from the gene to the final, bioactive protein hormone, including the intracellular structures involved in this process. Insights about the regulation of the hormone-producing cell derived from studies involving recombinant DNA technology and molecular and cellular biology are highlighted.

## OVERVIEW OF PEPTIDE HORMONE SYNTHESIS AND SECRETION

Proteins are important as the backbones of polypeptide hormones and as integral components of enzymes that participate in the biosynthetic pathways of steroid and thyroid hormones as well as enzymes that participate in intracellular synthetic and degradative actions and in energy generation. They are critical membrane, receptor, and cytoskeletal molecules, and an appreciation of the pathways for polypeptide synthesis and their associated cellular structures is important. This section describes the general pathways of polypeptide synthesis, with an emphasis on the informational flow from the gene to the final functional protein and the cell structures involved in each of the steps in this highway of biochemical events.[1-3] The production of a functional protein hormone requires numerous steps, each one involving modifications or processing of precursor molecules.

The eukaryotic cell consists of two major compartments, the nucleus and cytoplasm (Figs. 3-1 and 3-2), which are delimited by plasma membranes that are topologically contiguous with one another (see Fig. 3-2). The nucleus is surrounded by a nuclear envelope consisting of an outer and inner membrane encompassing a cisternal space.[4] The nuclear envelope is perforated by nuclear pore complexes that permit communication of the nucleoplasm with the cytoplasm.

The nucleus contains much of the cellular nucleic acid or genetic material in the form of *genes,* which harbor the information necessary for the initial production of precursor RNAs and hence functional proteins. The cytoplasm contains multiple organelles that are involved in the synthesis of proteins and their processing. These events occur through an assembly-line arrangement, by which the initial protein precursors are altered by changes in their primary structures and by glycosylation and other chemical modifications. These organelles include the *endoplasmic reticulum* (ER), where initial protein synthesis occurs, and a complex membranous structure known as the *Golgi stack,* where further protein processing and posttranslational modifications, sorting, and translocation take place.

The secretory cell is differentiated from other cell types by the presence of *secretory granules* that emerge from the Golgi stack. These granules are specialized, membrane-bound organelles that

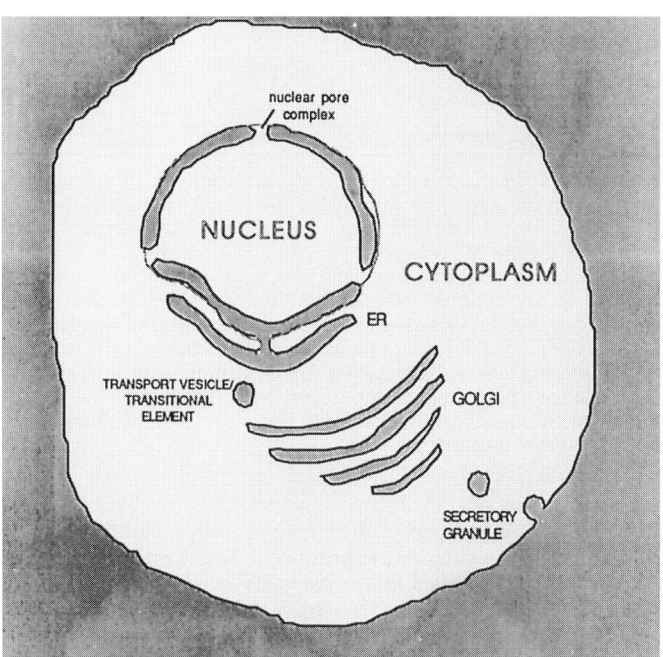

**FIGURE 3-2.** Diagram of the secretory cell. The secretory cell contains two major compartments: nucleus and cytoplasm. The nucleus is delimited by a nucleoplasmic membrane that is perforated by nuclear pore complexes. The nuclear membrane is contiguous with the endoplasmic reticulum (*ER*). Transport of polypeptides from the ER to the next organelle, the Golgi stack, is accomplished by way of transport vesicles or transitional elements. Polypeptide hormones exit from the Golgi stack by formation of secretory vesicles and granules. The stored polypeptide hormone in the secretory granule is released in the process of emiocytosis or exocytosis on receipt of the appropriate extracellular stimuli. The shaded areas represent topologically extracellular spaces. The lumen of the ER and Golgi are contiguous with the extracellular space.

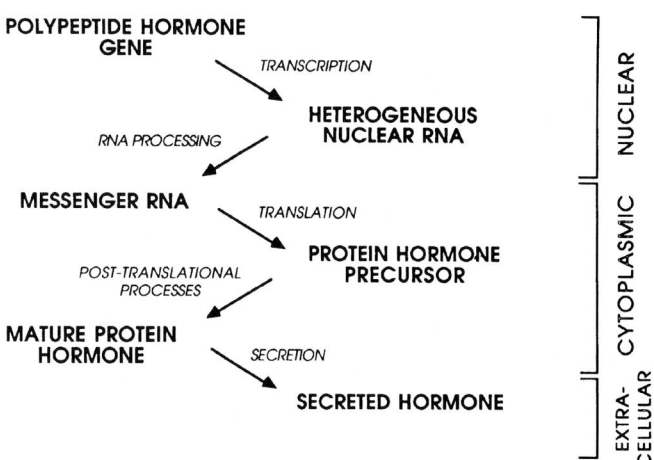

**FIGURE 3-3.** Informational flow from the polypeptide hormone gene to the bioactive secreted hormone. The *gene,* containing information in the form of DNA, is transcribed into heterogeneous nuclear RNA. This *heterogeneous nuclear RNA* is rapidly processed to form mature messenger RNA (mRNA). These events occur in the nucleus. The mRNA enters the cytoplasm, where it interacts with the protein synthetic machinery and undergoes translation, by which the *protein hormone precursor* is synthesized. Then numerous cotranslational and posttranslational processes occur in the rough endoplasmic reticulum and Golgi stack to yield the *mature protein hormone.* Secretory vesicles bud and emerge from the *trans*-Golgi to produce the secretory granule. In this state, the polypeptide hormone is stored and released on stimulation by the appropriate extracellular signals, whereupon the hormone enters the extracellular space. The *secreted hormone* may be acted on further by extracellular processes to yield other active hormone species and may be subjected to peripheral degradation.

contain polypeptide hormones in high concentration that may be stored for long periods. Stimulus-secretion coupling allows release of the hormone from the granule on physiologic demand.

The informational flow from the gene to the final protein is shown in Figure 3-3. Each protein produced by a cell is encoded by a gene. In a typical mammalian haploid genome, ~100,000 genes are grouped together into clusters called chromosomes. However, only a subset of these genes is expressed in a given cell. The genes in chromosomes are organized as chromatin with its DNA bound to basic histone and acidic nonhistone proteins. Specifically, the DNA is wrapped nearly twice around an histone-octamer core at regular intervals (i.e., every 140 nucleotides) to yield nucleosomes and a structure resembling beads on a string. These protein-DNA interactions provide the gene with vital secondary and tertiary structures. The DNA in this condensed form probably is transcriptionally inactive. However, modifications in this structure, dictated by developmental or regulated patterns, may determine whether a particular gene may be transcribed at all and, if so, at what rate. The role of chromatin structure in determining the breadth of cell-specific gene transcription remains to be clarified.

The information in a gene appears in the form of a double-stranded polymer of deoxyribonucleotides (DNA). The protein sequence is embedded in triplets of nucleotides in a tandem array dictated by the genetic code. The information present as DNA in a gene must be transferred to another molecule, RNA, which transfers the original information from the nucleus to the cytoplasm. The informational transfer from the gene to RNA is known as *transcription.* Initially, a precursor RNA, called heterogeneous nuclear RNA (hnRNA), is synthesized

using the original DNA in the gene as a template. This precursor molecule is then rapidly processed into the mature messenger RNA (mRNA).

The mRNA exits the nucleus to enter the cytoplasm. The mRNA molecule is a version of the gene with its data represented as a linear sequence of ribonucleic acids. The mRNA quickly interacts with the protein synthetic machinery, the ribosomes of the cytoplasm. The ribosome is a complex structure that contains ribosomal RNAs and its associated proteins. Within this structure, the information present in the mRNA is eventually transferred to protein information. The availability of several adapter molecules known as transfer RNA (tRNA) allows the information in the triplets of nucleotides (i.e., codons) in the mRNA to be converted to amino acids. Because one of four different nucleotides can occupy each position in a triplet codon, $4^3$ or 64 sequence possibilities exist. More codons are available than are necessary to encode the 20 essential amino acids. The genetic code contains redundancy or degeneracy so that a single amino acid may be represented by more than one codon. Because a protein molecule has a beginning and an end, the mRNA must contain information for the start and stop of translation. Important codons include AUG, or initiator methionine, which is the first amino acid of all newly synthesized polypeptides, and UAG, UAA, and UGA, which are termination codons.

Proteins destined for secretion are produced on ribosomes and possess a $NH_2$-terminal signal or leader peptide that interacts with cytoplasmic and ER receptors to mediate rapid ribosome–ER membrane association. This new complex allows newly synthesized proteins destined for secretion to enter the lumen of the ER, which is topologically located outside the cell. Soon after this occurs, cotranslational events take place, and the newly synthesized polypeptide is then sequestered within the cisternal space of the ER. The polypeptide then migrates from the ER through the Golgi stack, where further processing occurs. After the transfer from the *cis* to the medial to the *trans*

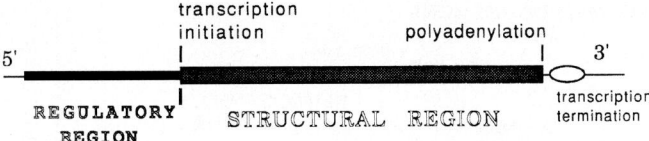

**FIGURE 3-4.** The transcriptional unit. Each polypeptide hormone or subunit is encoded by a transcriptional unit. This diagram shows the transcriptional unit that contains structural and regulatory regions. The regulatory region is shown at the 5'-flanking portion of the transcriptional unit. However, such regulatory elements may occur in other parts of the gene, including introns or 3'-flanking regions. The structural region is bounded by the transcriptional initiation or cap site at the 5' end and the polyadenylation site at the 3' end. The signals for transcription termination are more than 50 to 200 nucleotides downstream of the polyadenylation site.

regions of the Golgi complex, the maturing polypeptide hormone is sorted and transferred to the secretory granule. Polypeptides in secretory vesicles and granules are released into the extracellular space by fusion of the vesicle with the plasma membrane and by exocytosis of the contained material. Hormones in secretory granules are stored until the appropriate extracellular signal, generally a calcium flux, is received to prompt the release of the contents of the secretory granule. In response to the chemical signal, the membranes of the secretory granule fuse with the plasma membrane, and emiocytosis (i.e., regulated exocytosis) occurs.

In a series of alterations in precursor RNA and protein molecules, the eventually mature and bioactive polypeptide hormone is synthesized and secreted.

## GENE STRUCTURE

Polypeptide hormones may be encoded by single or multiple genes. Frequently, a hormone requires only intramolecular folding and formation of disulfide linkages in a single protein backbone to form the bioactive molecule. Sometimes, the bioactive hormone is formed by the covalent or noncovalent association of two or more subunits derived from a single gene or multiple genes. An example of the former is insulin, which is initially synthesized as a precursor with polypeptide subunits A and B interrupted by peptide C. However, during its intracellular processing, disulfide linkages are formed between subunits A and B, with the proteolytic cleavage and removal of peptide C. Two subunits are associated in a covalent manner to yield the bioactive insulin molecule. Major examples of the latter case are glycoprotein hormones (i.e., TSH and gonadotropins) (see Chaps. 15 and 16). In this family of hormones, each member consists of two subunits encoded by separate genes located on separate chromosomes. The subunits become associated in a noncovalent manner to form the bioactive dimer.[5]

Several hormones require proteolytic cleavage of the precursor molecule before the formation of the bioactive product. The major example is adrenocorticotropic hormone (ACTH) and β-lipotropin produced from the precursor preproopiomelanocortin by trypsin-like proteolytic cleavage at dibasic residues. Each polypeptide may require covalent modifications of its polypeptide backbone. In the glycoprotein hormones, each subunit contains several *N*-linked carbohydrate moieties, and the β subunit of human chorionic gonadotropin contains additional *O*-linked oligosaccharides. In yet other molecules, the addition of sulfate, phosphate, acetyl, and COOH-amide groups is necessary for full bioactivity. Bioactive peptides found in the brain-gut axis require a COOH-terminal amide group for full activity. This conversion is catalyzed by an α-amidation enzyme on substrate hormones that possess COOH-terminal sequences: X-Y-Gly → X-Y-NH$_2$.[6,7]

The gene that encodes the polypeptide hormone is part of a simple or complex transcriptional unit. A simple transcriptional

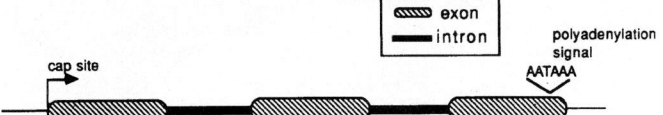

**FIGURE 3-5.** The structural region of the transcriptional unit. The structural region contains DNA information that is completely copied and transcribed into the heterogeneous nuclear RNA or RNA precursor. The important feature of eukaryotic structural regions of the gene is the presence of *exons* and *introns*. The exon contains sequences that are retained in the mature messenger RNA; the intron sequences are removed during RNA splicing in the nucleus. The first nucleotide of the structural region is known as the *cap site*, which is the point at which transcription begins in the first exon. The structural region terminates at the polyadenylation site, which is determined in part by the presence of a polyadenylation signal, AATAAA, located 15 to 20 nucleotides upstream of the polyadenylation site.

unit (Fig. 3-4) is composed of two major components: structural and regulatory. A simple unit produces a single mRNA, whereas a complex unit may yield multiple mRNAs, some of which may encode different proteins. The structural region encodes information that is ultimately found in mRNA (Fig. 3-5). However, in most eukaryotic genes, the coding region is not contiguous with that in the mRNA. Intervening or extraneous segments of DNA are placed between regions that eventually are found in mature mRNA. The coding regions in genes that are ultimately found in mRNA are known as *exons,* and the intervening sequences are known as *introns.* The role and function of introns are unknown, although introns separate functional domains in many polypeptides.[8] A similar exon encoding an epidermal growth factor (EGF)–like domain has been detected in genes encoding the low-density lipoprotein receptor, the precursor of EGF, and clotting factors IX and X.[9] These and other data suggest that introns may play important roles in the evolution of protein families. Moreover, introns may participate in alternate splicing of exons, leading to increased mRNA and polypeptide diversity.

The regulatory region contains elements that determine whether a gene is transcribed and, if so, in what quantity (Fig. 3-6). A structural region alone is ineffective in this informational flow. The presence of a regulatory region is obligatory for

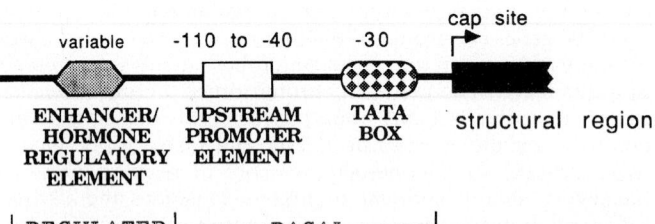

**FIGURE 3-6.** The regulatory region of the transcriptional unit. This diagram shows the important elements of the regulatory region. Only part of the structural region, including its cap site, is shown. The *TATA box* is located ~25 to 30 nucleotides upstream of the cap site. It is fixed in position and orientation and binds important binding proteins that allow interaction with RNA polymerase II. The *upstream promoter element* is located 40 to 110 nucleotides upstream of the cap site and binds critical proteins that also interact with the RNA polymerase II. The interplay of the upstream promoter element and TATA box are crucial for basal expression of a given structural region. Another element is the enhancer, which is located a variable distance from the cap site, including locations downstream of the cap site, and is independent of orientation. The enhancer element also binds to DNA-binding proteins that further augment or decrease transcription. Enhancer interactions determine regulation of gene expression above or below basal levels. A special subset of enhancers includes the hormone regulatory element, which mediates the effects of steroid and thyroid hormones and second messengers induced by polypeptide hormones.

the expression of its associated gene. The DNA in a gene is not found devoid of associated proteins in nature. Marked secondary, tertiary, and quaternary structure is found in genes located in chromatin, and covalent modifications of nucleotide residues are found within genes. In particular, methylation of cytosine residues may play an essential part in determining whether regulatory regions are "open" for transcription. The regulatory region plays an important role in moment-to-moment regulation of gene expression and in the tissue-specific and developmental programs of gene expression.

The process of transcription, whereby information in the gene as DNA is transformed into information as RNA, produces a large RNA precursor molecule (see Fig. 3-3).[10] The initial RNA transcript commences at the 5' end of the first exon, continues through the other exons and introns in the structural region, and terminates at the 3' end of the last exon. This hnRNA contains more information than in the mature mRNA because of the inclusion of intron sequences. The enzyme RNA polymerase II performs the transcription reaction using the DNA in the gene as the template. The first nucleotide in the RNA precursor transcript, generally a purine (A or G), is defined as the transcriptional start, also called the *cap site*. Subsequent ribonucleotides are polymerized during RNA elongation until the transcript is completed in the process of termination.

The initiation of transcription by RNA polymerase II often is the rate-limiting step in gene expression and is determined by the interaction of the enzyme with a number of nuclear factors and DNA elements in the regulatory region of the transcription unit.[11,12] Two types of elements participate in regulation of transcription of the typical eukaryotic gene. The first component is the *cis*-acting element, which is a DNA segment located in the regulatory region of a transcriptional unit. These *cis* elements are located near the structural region of a gene. Another component is the *trans*-acting element or factor, which usually consists of a DNA-binding protein present in the nucleus that is encoded by a gene separate from the transcriptional unit that is being regulated and interacts with a *cis*-regulatory element. These nuclear factors are said to "act in *trans*" to regulate gene expression. Mutations that affect *trans*-activation occur in distant genes but not in the gene that is being regulated. Interactions of *trans*-acting factors with *cis*-DNA elements determine tissue-specific, developmental, and regulated expression of genes.

Three important DNA elements—the TATA box, the upstream promoter element, and enhancers—occur in the regulatory region, which is commonly located at the 5'-flanking region of the transcriptional unit (see Fig. 3-6).[12,13] However, regulatory regions or elements thereof may occur in other sections of the transcriptional unit, including introns and 3'-flanking regions. The key elements include the *TATA box*, an AT-rich region located in a fixed position and orientation 25 to 30 nucleotides upstream from the cap site. This DNA element binds several TATA-binding proteins and associated factors found in the nucleus that allow for efficient interaction of RNA polymerase II with the transcriptional unit. The TATA box interactions, although not strictly required, are important for accurate and efficient initiation of transcription. The nature of the transcription initiation complex has been clarified. The components include at least seven transcription factors (i.e., TFIIA, TFIIB, TFIID, TFIIE, TFIIF, TFIIH, TFIIJ) and RNA polymerase II. A major constituent is TFIID, which is also a large multisubunit (>700-kDa) complex with at least eight proteins. One of these, the TATA-binding protein (TBP), allows the binding of TFIID to the TATA box or related Inr (initiator) sequences. The other components of TFIID have also been partially characterized and are known as coactivators or TBP-associated proteins (TAFs). They are essential for the communication of enhancer-binding protein signals to the basal transcriptional machinery and the subsequent regulation of gene expression. Basal transcription depends on the formation of a preinitiation complex involving TFIID-TFIIA-TFIIB, followed by the rapid entry of RNA polymerase II to facilitate the establishment of the transcriptional machinery.[14–16]

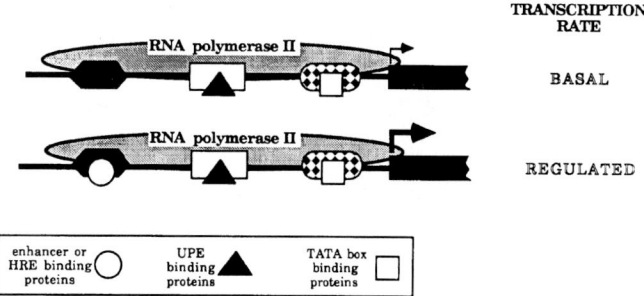

**FIGURE 3-7.** Regulation of transcriptional rates by interactions of *trans*-acting factors. Various permutations of interactions of nuclear binding proteins with various DNA elements within regulatory regions determine rates of transcription at the basal and regulated levels. Such proteins include the TATA box, the upstream promoter element (*UPE*), and enhancer or hormone regulatory element (*HRE*)–binding proteins.

The second DNA element is the *upstream promoter element* (UPE), which is located 60 to 110 nucleotides upstream from the cap site.[17] It includes elements such as the CCAAT and GC-rich (GGGCGG) boxes that bind to CAAT-binding proteins and SP1 (a cellular DNA-binding protein that interacts with the SV40 genome), respectively. These elements also associate with DNA-binding proteins that augment the efficiency of transcription by RNA polymerase II. These UPEs may or may not require specific TATA boxes to perform their function most efficiently. Together, the TATA box and UPEs are components close to the structural region and are essential for maintenance of basal levels of gene transcription (Fig. 3-7).

*Enhancers* are located in variable positions and may act independently of orientation. They may be located more distal than the promoter elements and are found up to several thousand nucleotides upstream or downstream of the transcriptional unit. These elements also bind proteins that enhance transcriptional rates or diminish them (i.e., silencers) in an ill-defined manner and constitute the foci of regulated transcription (see Fig. 3-7). Several proposed mechanisms include the cooperative interaction of a number of DNA-binding proteins to effect efficient formation of the transcription-initiation complex of RNA polymerase II with the regulatory or promoter region.[18] Another hypothesis suggests that the interaction of proteins with these elements opens up the configuration of DNA, perhaps by "bending" to allow access of the gene to the transcription machinery.

With recombinant DNA techniques, a reporter gene construct can be produced that may be transfected into foreign cells by gene transfer.[19,20] This allows the expression of the reporter gene with enhanced production of an enzyme or polypeptide product that is not normally produced in eukaryotic cells. The synthesis of such products may be detected by sensitive enzyme assays or radioimmunoassays. DNA constructs in which a structural region corresponding to the enzyme alone is transfected into cells are not expressed in the absence of regulatory regions. However, if a promoter element is placed 5' to the reporter gene, then expression may occur. Using such approaches, structural analysis of various portions of the 5'-regulatory regions of genes, including enhancer and upstream regulatory elements, may be performed.

After the RNA transcript is initiated, the RNA polymerase II continues the process of template reading by elongation of the transcript until termination occurs. The actual site of transcription termination is variable, located 50 to 200 or more nucleotides downstream from the 3' end of the last exon or polyadenylation site.[21] Although potential weak consensus sequences have been discerned that may determine the site at which the initial RNA transcript is terminated, the polyadenylation site appears to be obtained only by virtue of endonucleolytic cleavage of longer heterogeneous 3' ends of the hnRNA.

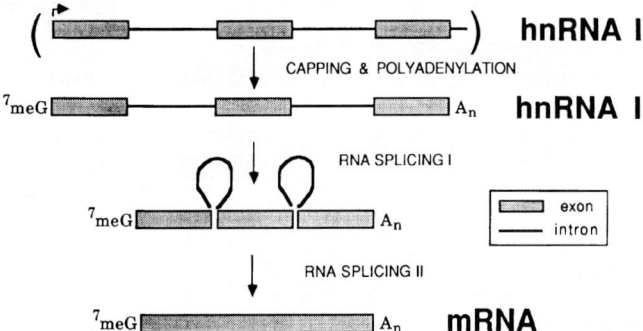

**FIGURE 3-8.** Gene transcription and RNA processing. The initial RNA transcript is known as heterogeneous nuclear RNA (*hnRNA I*). It contains exons and introns of the structural region and rapidly undergoes 5' capping with $^7$methylguanosine ($^7meG$) and 3' polyadenylation ($A_n$) (*hnRNA II*). Little heterogeneous nuclear RNA has been detected without 5' cap or 3' polyadenylated (*poly[A]*) tails. In a slower process, introns are removed by RNA splicing followed by religation of exon sequences. The mature messenger RNA (*mRNA*) is composed of fused exon sequences and contains a 5' cap and a 3' poly(A) tail.

The well-conserved consensus polyadenylation site sequence AAUAAA, which is located 15 to 20 nucleotides upstream from the polyadenylation site, and other proximal downstream sequences 10 to 12 nucleotides from the polyadenylation site, may serve as points of recognition for this processing event. Although the mechanisms of polyadenylation are not well known, the presence of the consensus sequences suggests a requirement for stem-loop formation and involvement of small nuclear ribonucleoproteins (snRNPs).

## MESSENGER RNA PROCESSING

The hnRNA product of gene transcription is rapidly processed in the nucleus with a half-time ($t_{1/2}$) of 5 to 20 minutes (Fig. 3–8).[22] Three major events transform the large heterogeneous RNA precursors into the mature RNA. First, at the 5' end of hnRNA, a $^7$methylguanosine residue is added to the first nucleotide of the transcript by means of a 5'-5' triphosphate bond after 20 to 30 nucleotides have been polymerized. This reaction is rapid ($t_{1/2}$ < 1 minute) and is catalyzed by the 5'-capping enzyme, including guanylyl and methyl transferases. The 5'-methyl cap associates with 5'-cap binding proteins, which favors the formation of a stable 40S translation-initiation complex and increases the stability and efficiency of translation of the eventual mature mRNA.[23]

The second modification occurs at the 3' end and involves the addition of a polyadenylate, or poly(A), tail. Polyadenylation includes the addition of 250 to 300 adenylate (A) residues at the polyadenylation site located at the 3' end of the RNA. This poly(A) tail, which is reduced to 30 to 250 residues during nuclear processing and export, may also be important for increased RNA stability. These two additions, capping and polyadenylation, occur within minutes after the synthesis of hnRNA and generally before RNA splicing; almost all isolated hnRNA contains both modifications.

The third major processing step involved in mRNA maturation is the removal of introns during RNA splicing.[24–26] This process includes endonucleolytic cleavage of introns and religation of exons. The 5' and 3' ends of introns have consensus sequences, as shown in Figure 3-9.

These consensus sequences may be necessary for the appropriate interaction of U1 snRNP species present in the nucleus to serve as a "splicing adapter" for the splicing process. Moreover, a polypyrimidine tract is located adjacent to the 3' AG residues and a critical adenylate residue in a branch sequence, 30 nucleotides upstream of the 3' end of the intron. The first step in the

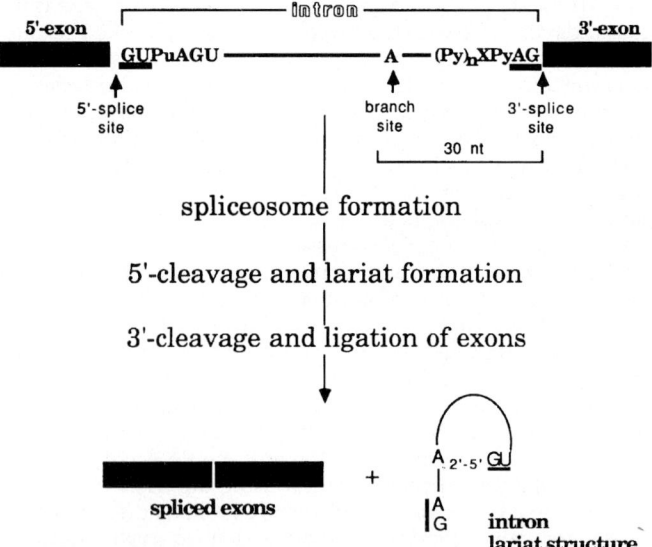

**FIGURE 3-9.** RNA splicing: consensus intron sequences and mechanisms for intron removal. A consensus sequence has been determined for the 5' and 3' ends of intron sequences. Data suggest the potential mechanism of intron removal by means of lariat formation preceded by interaction with nuclear RNAs. (*nt*, nucleotides.)

splicing process involves the formation of the *spliceosome*, which includes the hnRNA, U1 snRNP, and other factors. The initial event is endonucleolytic cleavage at the 5' splice site, followed by the formation of a 5'-2' phosphodiester bond between the 5' G and the downstream A located in a branch sequence. This "lariat" intermediate is then cleaved at the 3' end and degraded, and the exons are ligated.

The removal of introns from hnRNA must be precise; errors can change the exon or mRNA-coding regions. The sequence of removal of multiple introns within a gene is generally nonrandom, although the mechanism is unknown. Variations in the splicing pattern in a given hnRNA transcript can occur, and tissue-specific interactions of RNA splicing-modification proteins may dictate alternate patterns of intron-RNA splicing, causing altered mRNA forms.[27] In a complex transcriptional unit, an alternate exon choice, including alternative internal acceptor and donor site use, may yield different mRNA products. A complex transcriptional unit may also possess alternate transcriptional start sites in the same contiguous segment of DNA (i.e., in the same exon) or in multiple transcriptional start sites in different exons contributed by alternate exon choice. Another possible mechanism for diversity in the complex transcriptional unit is alternative final exon choice (i.e., differences in polyadenylation sites).

The splicing process is another rate-limiting step and takes place over 5 to 30 minutes; it is much slower than the capping and polyadenylation reactions. What role RNA splicing plays in the informational flow is unclear. However, the potential contribution of RNA diversity by RNA splicing has been discussed. There are mRNAs that lack poly(A) tails (e.g., histone mRNAs), mRNAs that lack a 5' cap (e.g., poliovirus mRNAs), and eukaryotic genes that lack introns. Such modifications are not essential for RNA maturation.

## RNA TRANSPORT

The newly synthesized mature mRNA is actively transferred from the nuclear to the cytoplasmic compartments by way of the nuclear pore complex (NPC). The NPC is a large multiple-component structure that is located in the nuclear envelope and serves as a channel for the movement of macromolecules such

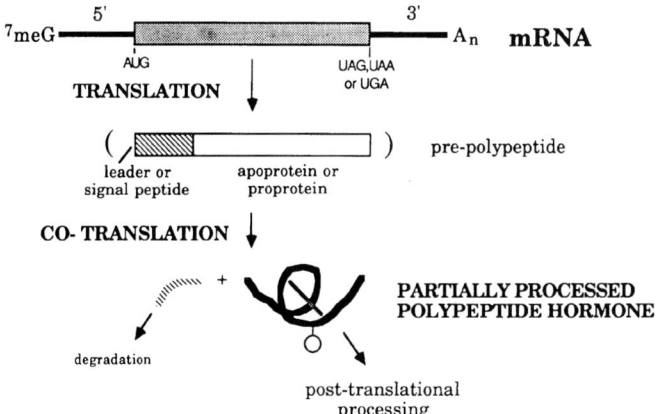

**FIGURE 3-10.** Structure and translation of messenger RNA (*mRNA*). In most cases, the mature mRNA represents the fusion of multiple exons. These sequences encode two major regions: translated and untranslated. The translated or coding region is delimited by the translation initiator codon, AUG, at its 5' end and the termination codon, UGA, UAA, UAG, at its 3' end. This coding region represents a series of codons in an open-reading frame that determines the amino-acid sequence of its encoded polypeptide. The 5' and 3' untranslated regions are shown. The mRNA enters the cytoplasm to interact with the ribosome. There, protein synthesis is initiated, and by way of a series of several cotranslational events, secretory polypeptide hormone precursors are processed. The steps involve cleavage of the signal or leader peptide, followed by addition of asparagine-linked carbohydrate moieties in glycoprotein subunits or hormones, and intramolecular folding with the formation of disulfide linkages. These events occur within the lumen of the rough endoplasmic reticulum. These partially processed polypeptide hormones are then shuttled to the Golgi stack, where these molecules are transported, sorted, and further processed posttranslationally to yield the bioactive hormone located in secretory granules or vesicles.

as RNAs. The mRNA and other RNAs subject to transport are closely associated with proteins and exist as ribonucleoproteins. Each RNA likely possesses distinct protein-targeting sequences that permit its export and import. This shuttling of mRNA from the nucleus to the cytoplasm is mediated by a large family of transport factors known collectively as *exportins* and *importins*. However, the precise nature of the interactions of these shuttling proteins, mRNAs, and the NPC is not well understood.[28]

## TRANSLATION

The structure of mRNA is shown in Figure 3-10. The exons encode two major regions of the mRNA: translated and untranslated. The translated or coding region contains the open reading frame, beginning from the initiation methionine codon to the termination codon. The untranslated regions flank the coding region and are known as 5' or 3' untranslated regions. The functions of the untranslated regions are not well established, but data indicate that the 5' untranslated region may be important in determining the efficiency of translation of the mRNA.[29,30] The 3' untranslated region may contain important RNA elements, especially several AU-rich sequences that determine the stability of mRNA in the cytoplasm.[31] Each of these regions may mediate its effects by binding to specific RNA-binding proteins.[32,33]

The mRNA in the cytoplasm rapidly interacts with the ribosome (see Fig. 3-10). The ribosome is a complex ribonuclear particle that contains 28S, 18S, and 5S RNAs, along with a group of ribosomal proteins. Among these proteins are factors responsible for the initiation, elongation, and termination of mRNA translation. For the typical mRNA, 3 to 15 ribosomes may be attached at any given time. As the ribosome reads the mRNA in the process of translation, amino acids are brought to the translation complex by way of adapter tRNA molecules.

These molecules are differentiated by the presence of anticodon structures (i.e., RNA sequences complementary to a particular codon) at one end and attachment sites for specific amino-acid residues at the other end of the L-shaped molecule. The reading of successive codons causes the alignment of the appropriate amino acids and polymerization to yield the polypeptide chain.

Translation initiation occurs at the initiator codon or AUG, which represents the amino residue methionine. Translation generally begins at the first AUG codon located at the 5' end of the mRNA. This initiation methionine codon is normally followed by an open reading frame of codons encoding amino acids until a termination codon is reached. When a UAG, UAA, or UGA is encountered, protein synthesis stops, and the nascent polypeptide chain is released from the ribosome complex. The context of the methionine codon that is used for translation initiation has been characterized further to include a consensus sequence: 5'-CCACCAUGG-3'.

This sequence nest presents the AUG as the most favorable initiation codon.[34] However, examples have been found in which the AUG is located 5' of the authentic start site. In these instances, the context may not be ideal or may be quickly followed by a termination codon in frame. Whether peptides encoded by these short-reading frames are eventually expressed is unknown.[35,36]

All polypeptide hormones and almost all other proteins destined for membrane, lysosome, ER, and Golgi stack locations or for secretion are encoded by a larger polypeptide precursor. All polypeptide hormones possess a signal or leader peptide that is a characteristic segment of protein located at the N-terminal end[37,38] (Table 3-1). Although no consensus primary sequence has been obtained for this signal peptide, it generally possesses a hydrophobic core preceded by basic amino-acid residues in its 16- to 30-amino-acid residue extent.

Several events occur before the entire polypeptide chain is synthesized (Fig. 3-11). After the synthesis of ~70 amino acids, the *signal recognition particle* (SRP), a group of six proteins and a small RNA (7S), interacts with the signal peptide to momentarily halt translation elongation in the RNA–ribosome-nascent protein complex.[39,40] The 7S RNA contains a signal peptide recognition and an elongation arrest domain. This complex then interacts with the SRP receptor, an integral membrane protein located on the cytoplasmic face of the ER. In this process, polyribosomes are attached to membranous structures associated with the endoplasmic reticulum to form the *rough ER* (RER). After this interaction occurs, translational arrest is relieved, and translation proceeds as usual. At this point, the signal peptide is vectorially transported through the membrane into the cisternal aspect of the ER. The newly synthesized protein has been translocated from the inside to the outside of the cell in a topologic sense.

As protein synthesis continues, the signal peptide is transiently immobilized in the membrane by virtue of its hydrophobic nature or its binding to a putative signal peptide receptor.[41,42] Although the nascent protein chain is transferred to the cisterna by way of an unknown, energy-dependent translocation process, a luminal surface enzyme, signal peptidase, rapidly performs proteolytic cleavage to remove the signal peptide. The transmembrane transport of the protein does not require signal peptide cleavage and may take place by way of a protein channel or, less likely, through lipid. If the protein is to be *N*-glycosylated (i.e., to contain asparagine-linked carbohydrate moieties), other enzymes and the dolichol-lipid oligosaccharide carrier provide core glycosylation in this cotranslational process. Moreover, protein folding and oxidation of cysteine residues in disulfide formation occur. At the completion of protein synthesis and complete transfer of the protein to the luminal space, the SRP complex dissociates from its receptor and is recycled into the cytoplasm. Polyribosomes also are disaggregated to form free ribosomes and RNA. The translation of the polypeptide hormone causes the synthesis of a polypeptide core derived from

**TABLE 3-1.**
**Polypeptide Hormones: Some of Their Precursor Proteins***

| Hormone[†] | Hormone Size (aa)[‡] | Precursor Size (aa)[§] | H/P (%)[¶] | Location in Precursor[#] | Copies[**] | Modifications[††] | Species[‡‡] | Comments[§§] |
|---|---|---|---|---|---|---|---|---|
| Prolactin | 198 | 198 | 100 | — | 1 | — | h | — |
| Growth hormone | 191 | 191 | 100 | — | 1 | — | h | — |
| Adrenocorticotropic hormone (ACTH) | 39 | 235 | 17 | M | 1 | P, CHO | m | Other peptides |
| Thyroid-stimulating hormone β (TSHβ) | 118 | 118 | 100 | — | 1 | CHO | h | — |
| Luteinizing hormone β (LHβ) | 121 | 121 | 100 | — | 1 | CHO | h | — |
| Follicle-stimulating hormone β (FSHβ) | 111 | 111 | 100 | — | 1 | CHO | h | — |
| α subunit | 92 | 92 | 100 | — | 1 | CHO | h | — |
| Vasopressin | 9 | 145 | 6 | N | 1 | Am | r | C neurophysin |
| Oxytocin | 9 | 106 | 8 | N | 1 | Am | r | C neurophysin |
| Corticotropin-releasing hormone (CRH) | 41 | 166 | 25 | C | 1 | Am | o | — |
| Growth hormone–releasing hormone (GHRH) | 44 | 107/108 | 41 | M | 1 | Am | h | — |
| Gonadotropin-releasing hormone (GnRH) | 10 | 69 | 15 | N | 1 | Am | h | C-GnRH–associated peptide (GAP) |
| Thyrotropin-releasing hormone (TRH) | 3 | 231 | 1 | D | 5I | Am | r | — |
| Parathyroid hormone (PTH) | 84 | 90 | 31 | C | 1 | — | h | — |
| Calcitonin | 32 | 116 | 28 | M(C) | 1 | Am | r | 21-aa katacalcin |
| Thyroxine (T₄) | 2 | ~2500 | <0.1 | D | 2I | — | | Thyroglobulin precursor |
| Somatostatin | <u>14</u>/28 | 92 | 15 | C | 1 | — | r | |
| Insulin | 51 | 86 | 59 | N & C | 1 | — | h | Subunits; C peptide |
| Glucagon | 29 | 160 | 18 | M | 3R | — | r | GLP-I and GLP-II |
| Pancreatic polypeptide (PP) | 36 | 66 | 55 | N | 1 | — | h | |
| Vasoactive intestinal polypeptide (VIP) | 28 | 149 | 19 | M | 2R | Am | h | PHM-27 |
| Gastrin | 34/<u>17</u>/14 | 85 | 20 | M(C) | 1 | Am | p | — |
| Gastrin-releasing peptide (GRP) | 27 | 125 | 22 | N | 1 | Am | h | — |
| Cholecystokinin (CCK) | 58/<u>39</u>/33/12/8 | 95 | 41 | M(C) | 1 | Am | r | — |
| Renin | 334 | 401 | 83 | C | 1 | — | m | — |
| Angiotensin | <u>8</u>/10 | 453 | 2 | N | 1 | — | r | — |
| Atriopeptin (ANH) | 24 | 127/128 | 19 | C | 1 | — | h | — |
| | | | | | | | r | — |
| Inhibin-α | 134 | 344 | 39 | C | 1 | CHO? | p | — |
| Inhibin-β_A | 116 | 424 | 27 | C | 1 | CHO? | p | — |
| Inhibin-β_B | 115 | ? | — | C | 1 | CHO? | p | — |
| Enkephalin | 5 | 239 | 2 | D | 7R | — | b | 6-met |
| Substance P | 11 | 93 | 12 | M | 1 | — | b | — |
| Substance K | 10 | 111 | 9 | M | 1 | — | b | — |
| Dynorphin A/B | <u>17</u>/13/32 | 236 | 7 | D | 6R | — | p | α- and β-neoendorphin Dynorphins A and B Leumorphin Dynorphin-32 |

GLP, glucagon-like peptide; PHM, peptide histidine methionine.
*Most polypeptide hormones are encoded in precursor proteins known as *proproteins* or *polyproteins*.
[†]Well-characterized polypeptide hormones are listed; one exception is thyroxine, which is a modified amino acid derived from a protein precursor.
[‡]Hormone sizes in amino-acid residues (aa) are given. In some instances several different-sized peptides possess biologic activities. The size of the major form is underlined.
[§]Hormone proprotein sizes in amino-acid residues (aa) are given and are, in general, deduced from complementary DNAs. The proprotein represents the translation product minus the signal peptide. *All* proproteins are initially synthesized with signal peptides (16–30 aa) attached at the N terminus. Some values are estimated due to uncertainty of signal peptide cleavage site.
[¶]Fraction of hormone to proprotein in percent.
[#]Location of hormone within proprotein: N, NH₂ terminal; C, COOH terminal; M, midregion; M(C), midregion toward C; D, dispersed.
[**]Copies of hormone within proprotein: I, identical; R, related.
[††]Modifications of the hormone: P, phosphorylation; CHO, glycosylation; Am, COOH-terminal α-amidation.
[‡‡]Species: h, human; o, sheep; b, cow; p, pig; r, rat; m, mouse.
[§§]Known peptides present in remainder of proprotein are noted.

the initial protein precursor, which is already modified, in some instances, by the addition of carbohydrate moieties and by folding and formation of intramolecular disulfide linkages. The precursor polypeptide encoded by mRNA is not found in vivo, because the signal peptide is removed before the completion of the polypeptide chain. The exit from the ER probably depends on appropriate protein assembly or conformation, but glycosylation is not required.

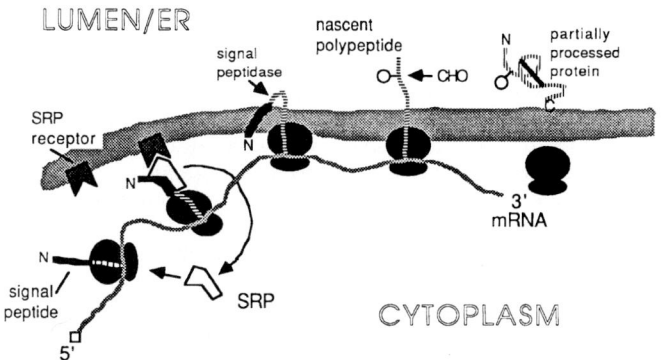

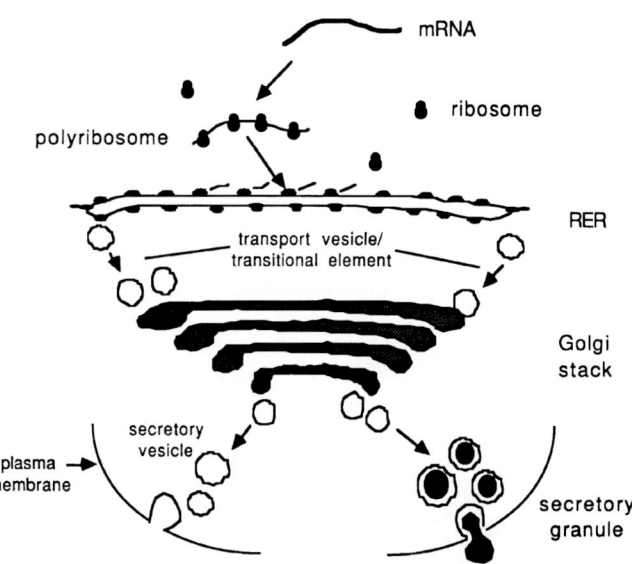

**FIGURE 3-11.** Details of translational and cotranslational processes. The messenger RNA (*mRNA*) interacts with the ribosome where protein synthesis is initiated. In the case of polypeptide hormones, the first segment of protein synthesized is the N-terminal signal or leader peptide. As soon as the signal peptide emerges from the ribosomal complex, a protein-RNA particle known as the signal recognition particle (*SRP*) associates with the signal peptide. This interaction allows the ribosomal-mRNA–nascent polypeptide complex to interact with the SRP receptor located on the cytoplasmic face of the endoplasmic reticulum (*ER*) membrane and brings the ribosome in close apposition to the ER to form the rough ER. The momentary translational arrest that occurs on interaction of the complex with SRP is released to allow further protein synthesis. Cleavage of the signal peptide from the apoprotein by signal peptidase and other modifications, including addition of asparagine-linked carbohydrates (*CHO*), intramolecular folding, and disulfide linkage formation, occurs coincidentally with release of ribosomes from the ER. In this manner, the partially processed protein, although initially synthesized in the cytoplasmic space, enters the luminal space.

**FIGURE 3-12.** The polypeptide hormone highway. Protein hormone synthesis is initiated in the cytoplasm on polyribosomes. The partially processed hormone, with the signal peptide removed and *N*-linked carbohydrate moieties attached and with appropriate folding, enters the lumen of the rough endoplasmic reticulum (*RER*). By way of transport vesicle–transitional elements, these partially processed products are transferred to the Golgi stack on fusion and release. In a serial process of budding formation of secretory vesicles and fusion, processed products are transferred through the Golgi stack, from which they exit as secretory vesicles or granules after sorting in the *trans* and *trans*-Golgi network compartments of the Golgi. Materials are then released from granules by the fusion of vesicles or granules with the plasma membrane.

## POSTTRANSLATION

Up to the translational and cotranslational steps in the ER, all secretory, membrane, lysosome, endogenous ER, and Golgi proteins have traversed the same biosynthetic path. After this point, the major task of sorting and transferring the proteins to the correct intracellular destinations must be completed. This complex process occurs in the Golgi stack and requires sorting signals among the proteins and sorting mechanisms in this organelle. A polypeptide hormone destined for regulated secretion must exit the ER, traverse the Golgi stack, and arrive properly in the secretory granule (Fig. 3-12).

The Golgi stack comprises a series of flattened, saccular membranous compartments that encompass four histologically and functionally distinct regions: the *cis*, *medial*, and *trans* regions of the Golgi complex and the *trans*-Golgi network (TGN)[43,44] (Fig. 3-13). The *cis*-Golgi region is most proximal to the transitional elements of the RER, and the TGN is most distal. The maintenance of distinct Golgi-specific antigens, unique enzyme markers, and different lectin-binding characteristics suggest that the compartments are not contiguous.

A *vesicle transfer model* has been proposed to account for transport of materials from the RER to the TGN. In this model, membrane vesicles form from the upstream compartment by budding at the rims of the Golgi plates and rejoin the adjacent downstream compartment by vesicle fusion and the interaction of microfilaments. The reiterative process of budding and fusion of secretory or transport vesicles causes vectorial transfer of proteins from the RER to the TGN in a unidirectional and energy-dependent process.

The newly synthesized polypeptide in the lumen of the RER is first translocated to the *cis*-Golgi region (see Fig. 3-12). From this point, the protein is transported and processed in the Golgi stack. This organelle may be appropriately considered an assembly line for posttranslational processing. It is here that *N*-linked carbohydrate cores are further modified among glycoproteins[45] (Fig. 3-14). This process involves digestion of

the high-mannose peripheral sugars in the *N*-linked carbohydrate cores by multiple glycosidases and subsequent addition of distal or terminal sugars by way of numerous glucosyltransferases. The steps in this process of carbohydrate maturation occur in different Golgi compartments. Other processes also

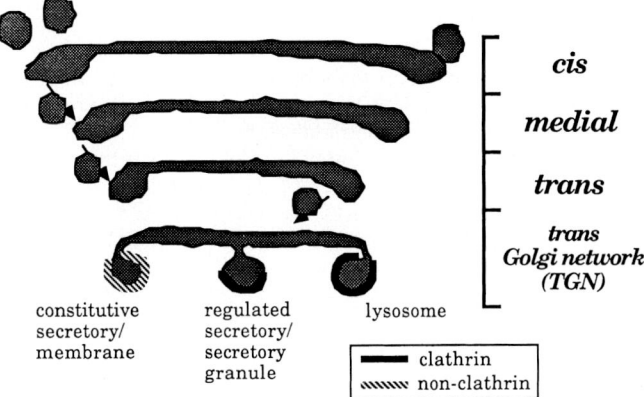

**FIGURE 3-13.** The Golgi stack. The Golgi stack consists of numerous membranous compartments, including *cis*, *medial*, and *trans*-Golgi elements. These compartments may be differentiated by the presence of specific enzymes. Partially processed protein hormones traverse this system by way of intermediate secretory vesicles in a budding-fusion reiterative process. In addition to transport, protein processing occurs. Sorting with routing to ultimate destinations in cellular sites is accomplished in the *trans*-Golgi network (*TGN*). Secretory peptides may be sorted to constitutive or regulated secretory pathways. Constitutive secretory pathways are equivalent to the pathways taken by membrane proteins, whereby non-clathrin-coated membrane segments are used. The regulated secretory-secretory granule pathway involves a clathrin-coated pit among membrane segments. This is similar to the pathway taken by lysosomal components. (Adapted from Griffiths G, Simons K. The trans Golgi network: sorting at the exit site of the Golgi complex. Science 1986; 234:438.)

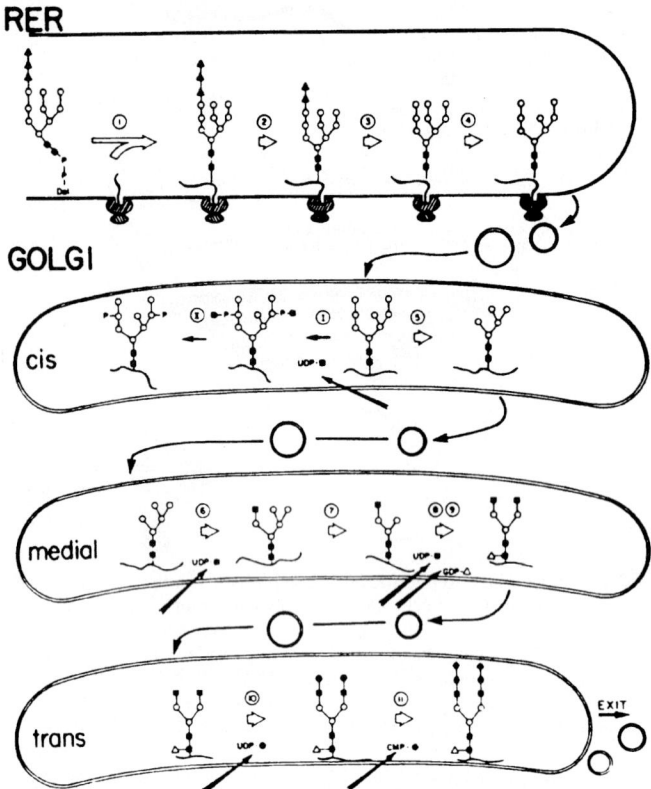

**FIGURE 3-14.** Proximal and distal glycosylation. The pathway of glycosylation in the rough endoplasmic reticulum (*RER*) and Golgi is shown. Core carbohydrate moieties are added cotranslationally by way of a dolichol-sugar intermediate (*Dol-*) to Asn residues in the protein backbone in the RER. Several glycosidases (steps 1–4) remove distal sugars in this compartment. Distal glycosylation occurs by the actions of mannosidases (steps 5–7) and glycosyl transferases (steps 6, 8–1) in the Golgi. Phosphorylation (I, II) of *N*-acetyl glucosamines in carbohydrate moieties in the *cis* Golgi occurs in proteins destined for lysosome localization. (From Kornfeld R, Kornfeld S. Assembly of asparagine-linked oligosaccharides. Annu Rev Biochem 1985; 54:631.)

occur, including phosphorylation, acetylation, sulfation, acylation, α-amidation of COOH termini, addition of ubiquitin, other modifications, and degradation.[46]

Another important function of the Golgi stack is the delivery of nascent polypeptides to the appropriate targets within the cell, which occurs in the *trans*-Golgi region or TGN.[47] The proteins destined for lysosomal sites are targeted to those organelles by way of the mannose-6-phosphate receptor.[48] In a similar manner, receptor and secretory proteins are targeted to membrane and secretory granule sites, respectively.[49–53] The nearly mature polypeptide emerges from the Golgi stack in the TGN, where transport organelles, known as secretory vesicles or granules, are formed. These vesicles allow the exit of the nearly mature protein hormone from the Golgi stack.

Secretory proteins are released from a cell by way of two pathways: the *constitutive pathway* and the *regulated pathway*.[54,55] The constitutive pathway is thought to be mediated by a passive aggregation sorting mechanism whereby peptide hormones form aggregates in the TGN, an action that is facilitated by acidic pH and high calcium concentrations in this compartment. The polarity of the secretory faces of epithelial cells enables proteins that are released in a nonregulated or constitutive manner to be released on the apical surface and regulated release to be performed at the basolateral surface. Whether such polarity of secretion exists in endocrine cells is unknown. Constitutive release generally involves the rapid exocytosis of newly synthesized peptides, but regulated secretion involves the classic secretory

granule and signaled degranulation, causing hormone- or factor-regulated release of hormones. Secretory peptides must be segregated into one pathway or the other. Regulated secretion involves the formation of secretory residues and granules composed of clathrin-containing membrane segments, as found in lysosomes. Proteins destined for regulated secretion must end up in a reservoir known as the secretory granule, where the polypeptide hormones are concentrated and stored. This pathway is now considered to operate by active sorting via a signal ligand receptor. Proteins destined for secretion in this manner clearly contain sorting signals in their precursor molecules. For instance, the precursors to proopiomelanocortin (POMC) and proenkephalin have a stretch of aliphatic hydrophobic and acidic amino-acid residues at the N termini that are necessary and sufficient for efficient sorting into secretory granules. Further, carboxypeptidase E (Cpe) appears to serve as a sorting receptor for these peptide signals as determined by biochemical and genetic approaches. In particular, the *Cpe*[fat], which harbors a mutant and ineffective Cpe, is obese, diabetic, and infertile. It has elevated levels of proinsulin in pancreatic B cells and of POMC in the anterior pituitary, and decreased insulin and ACTH release.[56]

Three types of vesicles are formed in the TGN. One is the secretory vesicle, which is not clathrin coated and mediates non–receptor-dependent transport of membrane proteins and protein to be secreted in the constitutive pathway. The other two are the secretory granule, which is partially clathrin coated and mediates the receptor-dependent transfer of regulated secretory peptides, and the lysosome, which is predominantly clathrin coated and mediates transport of lysosomal enzymes and proteins.[57] The secretory vesicle participates in the default, bulk-flow sorting system, but the others require the presence of "sorting patches" or sorting signals based on secondary and tertiary, but not primary, structures.[55] Although the secretory granules are derived from immature granules with clathrin-coated pits, the precise nature of the receptor-mediated sorting of peptide hormones is unknown.

Evidence exists for pH-regulated, receptor-dependent sorting in the *trans*-Golgi and TGN. The pH of the compartments decreases as the Golgi stack is traversed from *cis* to *trans* regions. Such gradients in pH may participate in the *molecular aggregation* of polypeptide hormones. Possibly, these aggregates formed in the process of hormone concentration may initiate the budding of secretory granules. Chloroquine, which prevents Golgi acidification, may inhibit granule formation by preventing aggregation in neutralized Golgi stacks.

Proteolytic processing of protein precursors (i.e., proproteins or polyproteins) to yield smaller bioactive peptides (see Table 3-1) also occurs in acidic Golgi and secretory vesicles.[58] Such proteolysis, however, is not required for packaging.

## SECRETORY GRANULE

Much has been learned about the nature of polypeptide hormones and secretory granules.[55,59,60] The hormones in this organelle are highly concentrated. In particular, a number of polypeptide hormones are condensed in a crystal lattice formation to increase the amount of hormone (up to 200-fold) in this organelle. Secretory granules allow cells to store enough hormone to be released on demand by extracellular signals at a level not possible by de novo synthesis. The $t_{1/2}$ of stored hormones may be days, whereas the $t_{1/2}$ of similar proteins in secretory vesicles may be minutes.

The size of secretory granules varies greatly, depending on the nature of the stored hormone. The condensation of hormone is demonstrated by the presence of electron-opaque or "dense" cores. The granule core is quite stable and is often visible even after exocytosis or in vitro enzymatic digestion of the granule membrane. It is osmotically inert yet sensitive to pH levels higher than 7.0.[55]

The formation of the secretory granule proceeds in stages, beginning in the *trans*-Golgi, where the initial hormone concentration may be observed. This aggregation process[60a] is facilitated by changes in pH, calcium concentration, and possible presence of other proteins such as secretogranins, chromogranins, and sulfated proteoglycans. Aggregates may form in different regions of the secretory granule. The colocalization of two or more polypeptide hormones in a granule may be observed. Within a cell, the relative distribution of two hormones is constant from granule to granule; however, variability in overall distribution is achieved from cell to cell. The mechanism by which the gonadotrope, a cell that generally produces luteinizing hormone (LH) and follicle-stimulating hormone (FSH), may be regulated to release LH and FSH differentially remains unclear.[61]

## SECRETION

Secretory granules release their contents by cytoskeletal protein-mediated movement of the granule toward the cellular surface.[61a] There, secretory granule membranes fuse with the plasma membrane and allow eversion or exocytosis of stored hormone.[62] This process of *emiocytosis* causes secretion of hormone. The mechanisms involved in stimulus-secretion coupling are not well known, although responses to cellular signals causing changes in intracellular calcium, ion currents, or intracellular pH may lead to these events.

In the unstimulated cell, a web of actin-associated microfilaments on the cytoplasmic face of the plasma membrane may act as a physical barrier to secretory granule fusion. However, changes in intracellular calcium, ion currents, or intracellular pH may cause differences in actin-binding protein interactions and alterations in the "secretory barrier" and permit exocytosis to occur.

Secretion and rapid membrane fusion of multiple secretory granules require an endocytotic pathway to retrieve the extra membranes resulting from exocytosis in the plasma membrane and to return them to the Golgi stack and lysosome.

## REGULATION OF POLYPEPTIDE HORMONE SYNTHESIS

Regulation of the biosynthesis of polypeptides may occur at any of the biosynthetic levels in the pathway (Table 3-2 and Fig. 3-4). Of major interest is the regulation of peptide hormone synthesis at the transcriptional level.

Studies using gene transfer and structure-function analysis have established that specific DNA elements in the regulatory region of the transcriptional unit are critical for determining transcriptional rates of various structural regions.[63,64] In particular, hormone-regulatory elements (HREs) have been characterized for glucocorticoid, estrogen, androgen progesterone, vitamin D, mineralocorticoid, retinoic acid, and thyroid hormone receptors. In each case, a DNA element 8 to 20 nucleotides long may be necessary and sufficient for conferring hormonal regulation to its associated structural region. Several factors, including the steroid and thyroid hormones, interact with nuclear receptor proteins, which interact with DNA elements directly to modulate gene transcription.[65–68] For the glucocorticoid receptor, the glucocorticoid ligand binds to the inactive glucocorticoid receptor in the cytoplasm, present in a complex with heat shock proteins, hsp 90 and hsp 70, and others.

The activated receptor-ligand complex interacts as a *trans*-acting factor to bind the DNA element corresponding to the glucocorticoid regulatory element (GRE). Studies have been performed on GREs in genes for mouse mammary tumor virus (*MMTV*) and murine sarcoma viruses, human metallothionein IIa, tyrosine aminotransferase, tryptophan oxygenase, and growth hormone, and in other genes. The long terminal repeat region of *MMTV* contains five GREs.[64,69] A consensus sequence

### TABLE 3-2.
### Loci of Genetic Regulation of Polypeptide Hormone Synthesis*

| TRANSCRIPTION | TRANSLATION |
|---|---|
| Initiation | Protein synthesis |
| Elongation | |
| Termination | POSTTRANSLATION |
| | Protein modification |
| POSTTRANSCRIPTION | Protein maturation |
| hnRNA processing | Peptide maturation |
| hnRNA stability | Peptide stability |
| | |
| mRNA | STORAGE |
| Stability | |
| | SECRETION |
| | |
| | POSTSECRETION |

*At each step in the pathway of biosynthesis of polypeptide hormones is potential regulation by factors and other hormones. At the transcriptional level, the major focus of regulation is at *transcription initiation*. However, regulation at elongation and termination steps is also possible. The various steps in heterogeneous nuclear RNA (*hnRNA*) processing, including splicing and hnRNA stability, may be regulated events. Messenger RNA (*mRNA*) stability is a major regulated step in determining the steady-state amounts of mRNA that will be translated into protein. Regulation at the translational level has been described and is a possible locus of regulation. Any of the posttranslational steps, including release of secretory granules, may also be focus of regulation. Extracellular processes (postsecretion), including serum protein binding of hormones, activation, and degradation, may also converge to determine the steady-state level of bioactive polypeptide hormone.

for the putative GRE is shown by the sequence 5'-GGTA-CANNNTGTTCT-3', in which N = A, C, G, or T.

The structures of the steroid and thyroid hormone receptors are better known. These hormone receptors are encoded by genes related to a viral oncogene, v-*erbA*.[70,71] The thyroid hormone receptor is encoded by the protooncogene c-*erbA*. Each receptor contains a stereotypic structure, including a protein that is ~45 to 60 kDa, with a central DNA-binding domain and a carboxyl-terminal ligand-binding domain. These and other regions mediate *trans*-activation, dimerization, and nuclear localization. The DNA-binding region consists of multiple cysteine and histidine residues that are critical for the formation of $Zn^{2+}$ fingers first described in the DNA-binding protein TFIIIa, a transcription regulatory factor for the 5S ribosomal gene in *Xenopus*.[72] This $Zn^{2+}$ finger interaction is a common motif for the binding of many eukaryotic proteins to DNA.[73–75]

The steroid–thyroid hormone receptors represent the first major examples of *trans*-acting factors well described in mammalian systems. The motif found in prokaryotic systems, particularly the interactions of cro and lambda repressor proteins with their target DNA elements in bacteriophage lambda, occurs with a homopolymeric dimer of subunits containing alpha helix–turn–alpha helix structure. The binding generally involves protein dimers; it requires a twofold axis of symmetry in the DNA sequence and involves the major groove of the target DNA over several helical turns. Data indicate that the thyroid hormone, retinoic acid, and vitamin D receptors are active only in the heterodimeric state, with other nuclear factors such as retinoid X receptors as their partners.

Hormones that act by way of surface membrane receptors may induce the production of second messengers that may directly or indirectly interact with DNA elements within the gene.[76–79] HREs may not be restricted to interactions observed with steroid–thyroid hormone receptor complexes, but they may involve other protein-DNA interactions. Advances in the isolation of such *trans*-acting factors and the identification of *cis*-acting HREs will probably speed an understanding of the molecular mechanisms of the hormonal regulation of gene expression at the transcriptional level.[80]

The presence of multiple enhancer elements or HREs in the regulatory regions of genes allows fine tuning of transcriptional

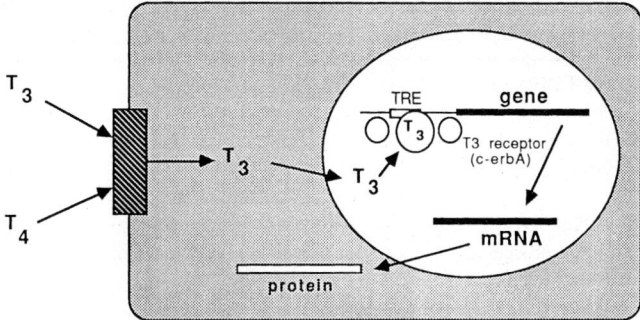

**FIGURE 3-15.** Thyroid hormone action. This diagram depicts the mechanism of action of thyroid hormones in the regulation of a thyroid hormone–responsive gene. Thyroxine ($T_4$) or triiodothyronine ($T_3$) enters the cell. $T_4$ is converted to $T_3$ intracellularly in many cells by means of 5'-deiodinase activity. $T_3$ then enters the nucleus, where it binds to the nuclear thyroid hormone receptor, which is encoded by c-*erbA*. This hormone nuclear receptor complex then serves as a *trans*-acting factor for binding to a thyroid hormone regulatory element (*TRE*), which may then positively or negatively regulate gene expression, with resultant production of RNA and protein derived from the thyroid hormone–regulated gene. (*mRNA*, messenger RNA.)

efficiency and influences the rate of production of the initial RNA transcript[81–85] (Fig. 3-15).

Other loci for regulation in this biosynthetic pathway include elongation and termination of transcription[86] (see Fig. 3-9). The various steps of RNA maturation, most notably RNA splicing, may also change mRNA levels encoding a particular polypeptide hormone, which ultimately determines the amount of polypeptide produced. The nuclear stability of the hnRNA and transport of the RNA from the nucleus to the cytoplasm also may be regulated. A major determinant of the steady-state levels of mRNA is cytoplasmic mRNA stability. Examples include the estrogen regulation of chicken liver vitellogenin mRNA, prolactin regulation of breast casein mRNA stabilities, and thyroid hormone control of the TSH β subunit.[87–89]

The interaction of mRNA with the protein synthetic machinery in the process of translation may be regulated. Several examples of translational control have been observed, including glucose regulation of the translational efficiency of insulin mRNA. Moreover, a number of the posttranslational processing events that occur in the RER and Golgi stack and the control of secretory granule formation and release may also be loci for regulation.

Even after proteins are released from the secretory cell, the bioactive peptide may be further acted on by degradative processes and proteolytic events that may activate proteins in extracellular steps to determine the bioactivity of a particular polypeptide hormone. A major example involves the cascade of the extracellular enzymatic conversion of the precursors of angiotensin II (see Chap. 79). Another example of postsecretion proteolytic processing of precursor polypeptides involves the conversion of iodinated thyroglobulin to the iodinated thyronines, thyroxine and triiodothyronine, in the follicular cell of the thyroid. Plasma stability of a polypeptide is a major determinant of the activity of the hormone in its eventual interaction with target cells.

## GENERATION OF DIVERSITY

A major example of the generation of diversity is the calcitonin and calcitonin gene–related peptide (CGRP) system. In this system, the C cell of the thyroid expresses a calcitonin-CGRP transcript that initially contains six exons. In the C cell, tissue-specific factors determine the use of the polyadenylation site in the fourth exon, but in the brain, transcription through the sixth exon, which encodes CGRP and the alternative polyadenylation site present in that exon, provides the alternative splicing

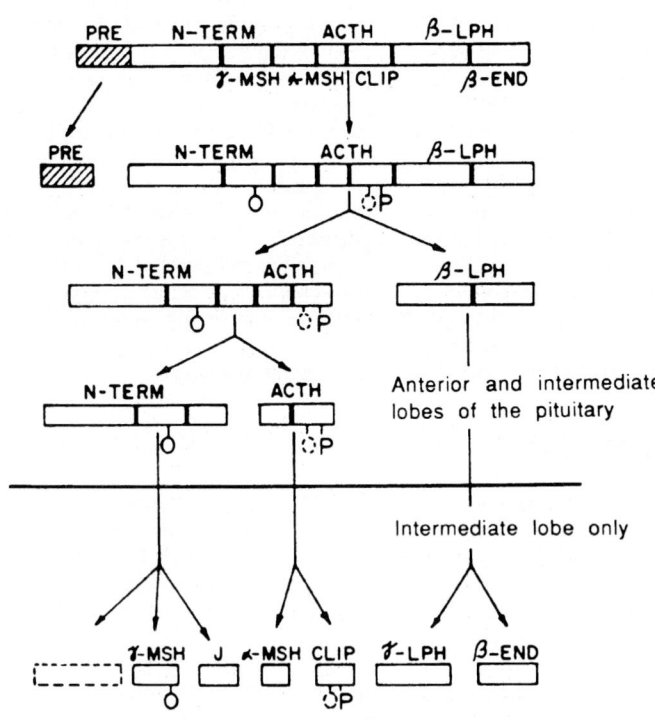

○ Glycosylation
⟡ Partial glycosylation
P Phosphorylation

▮ Dibasic amino acids
▨ Presequence

**FIGURE 3-16.** Alternative protein processing of the preproopiomelanocortin (*POMC*) precursor. In the anterior pituitary gland, the single POMC precursor is processed posttranslationally to produce adrenocorticotropic hormone (*ACTH*) and β-lipotropin (β-*LPH*). However, the intermediate lobe further processes these peptides to α-melanocyte-stimulating hormone (α-*MSH*), corticotropin-like intermediate lobe peptide (*CLIP*), γ-lipotropin (γ-*LPH*), and β-endorphin. (From Douglass J, Civielli O, Herbert E. Polyprotein gene expression: generation of diversity of neuroendocrine peptides. Annu Rev Biochem 1984; 53:665.)

and deletion of the fourth exon, which encodes calcitonin. The C cells express mostly calcitonin and not much CGRP; conversely, the hypothalamus produces mostly CGRP but not much calcitonin (see Chap. 53 and Fig. 53-1). Other examples of alternative splicing yielding different polypeptides include the synthesis of the alternate human growth hormone form, substance P, substance K, and protooncogenes.[90,91]

Alternative processing of polypeptides in a posttranslational process is important for the generation of polypeptide diversity.[92,93] A major example of this is the production of ACTH and β-lipotropin from the POMC precursor (Fig. 3-16). Using the same mRNA transcript, the anterior pituitary gland produces ACTH and β-lipotropin, and the intermediate lobe of the pituitary gland performs further alternate proteolytic processing and produces β-endorphin, corticotropin-like intermediate lobe peptide (CLIP), α-melanocyte-stimulating hormone, and other products (see Chap. 16).

## REFERENCES

1. Alberts B, Watson JD, Bray D, et al. Molecular biology of the cell. New York: Garland Publishing, 1994.
2. Matsudaira P, Berk A, Zipursky L, et al. Molecular cell biology. New York: WH Freeman Co, 1999.
3. Lewin BM. Genes VII. New York: Oxford University Press, 1999.
4. Newport JW, Douglass JF. The nucleus: structure, function, and dynamics. Annu Rev Biochem 1987; 56:535.
5. Chin WW. Organization and expression of glycoprotein hormone genes. In: Imura H, ed. The pituitary gland. New York: Raven Press, 1985:164.

6. Eipper BA, Mains RE, Glembotski CC. Identification in pituitary tissue of a peptide alpha-amidation activity that acts on glycine-extended peptides and requires molecular oxygen, copper, and ascorbic acid. Proc Natl Acad Sci U S A 1983; 80:5144.
7. Bradbury AF, Finnie MDA, Smyth DG. Mechanism of C-terminal amide formation by pituitary enzymes. Nature 1982; 298:686.
8. Gilbert W. Why genes in pieces? Nature 1978; 271:501.
9. Sudhoff TC, Russell DW, Goldstein JL, et al. Cassette of eight exons shared by genes for LDL receptor and EGF receptor. Science 1985; 228:893.
10. Nevins JR. The pathway of eukaryotic mRNA formation. Annu Rev Biochem 1983; 52:441.
11. Darnell JE Jr. Variety in the level of gene control in eukaryotic cells. Nature 1982; 297:365.
12. Rowley A, Dowell SJ, Diffley FX. Recent developments in the initiation of chromosomal DNA replication: a complex picture emerges. Biochim Biophys Acta 1994; 1217:239.
13. Albright SR, Tjian R. TAFs revisited: more data reveal new twists and confirm old ideas. Gene 2000; 242:1.
14. Zawel L, Reinberg D. Advances in RNA polymerase II transcription. Curr Opin Cell Biol 1992; 4:488.
15. Pugh BF, Tjian R. Diverse transcriptional functions of the multisubunit eukaryotic TFIID complex. J Biol Chem 1992; 267:679.
16. Conaway RC, Conaway JW. General initiation factors for RNA polymerase II. Annu Rev Biochem 1993; 62:161.
17. Busby S, Ebright RH. Promotor structure, promotor recognition, and transcription activation in prokaryocytes. Cell 1994; 79:743.
18. Ptashne M. Gene regulation by proteins acting nearby and at a distance. Nature 1986; 322:697.
19. Walker MD, Edlund T, Boulet AM, Rutter WJ. Cell-specific expression controlled by the 5'-flanking region of insulin and chymotrypsin genes. Nature 1983; 306:557.
20. Edlund T, Walker MD, Barr PJ, Rutter WJ. Cell-specific expression of the rat insulin gene: evidence for role of two distinct 5'-flanking elements. Science 1985; 230:912.
21. Platt T. Transcription termination and the regulation of gene expression. Annu Rev Biochem 1986; 55:339.
22. Brawerman G. Determinants of messenger RNA stability. Cell 1987; 48:5.
23. Shatkin AJ. mRNA cap binding proteins: essential factors for initiating translocation. Cell 1985; 40:223.
24. Padgett RA, Grabowski PJ, Konarska MM, et al. Splicing of messenger RNA precursors. Annu Rev Biochem 1986; 55:1119.
25. Sharp PA. Splicing of messenger RNA precursors. Science 1987; 253:766.
26. Keller W. The RNA lariat: a new ring to the splicing of mRNA precursors. Cell 1984; 39:423.
27. Andreadis A, Gallego ME, Nadal-Ginard B. Generation of protein isoform diversity by alternative splicing: mechanistic and biological implications. Annu Rev Cell Biol 1987; 3:207.
28. Weis K. Importins and exportins: how to get in and out of the nucleus. Trends Biol Sci 1998; 23:185.
29. Pelletier J, Sonenberg N. Insertion mutagenesis to increase secondary structure within the 5'-noncoding region of a eucaryotic mRNA reduces translational efficiency. Cell 1985; 40:515.
30. Darveau A, Pelletier J, Sonenberg A. Differential efficiencies of in vitro translation of mouse c-myc transcript differing in the 5'-untranslated region. Proc Natl Acad Sci U S A 1985; 82:2315.
31. Shaw G, Kamen R. A conserved AU sequence from the 3'-untranslated region of GM-CSF mRNA mediates selective mRNA degradation. Cell 1986; 46:659.
32. Nielsen DA, Shapiro DJ. Insights into hormonal control of messenger RNA stability. Mol Endocrinol 1990; 4:953.
33. Atwater JA, Wisdom R, Verma IM. Regulated mRNA stability. Annu Rev Genet 1990; 24:519.
34. Kozak M. Compilation and analysis of sequences upstream from the translational start site in eukaryotic mRNAs. Nucleic Acids Res 1984; 12:857.
35. Kozak M. Selection of initiation sites by eucaryotic ribosomes: effect of inserting AUG triplets upstream from the coding sequence for preproinsulin. Nucleic Acids Res 1984; 12:3873.
36. Kozak M. Bifunctional messenger RNAs in eukaryotes. Cell 1986; 47:481.
37. Von Heijne G. A new method for predicting signal sequence cleavage sites. Nucleic Acids Res 1986; 14:4683.
38. Gierasch LM. Signal sequences. Biochemistry 1989; 28:1.
39. Walter P, Gilmore R, Blobel G. Protein translocation across the endoplasmic reticulum. Cell 1984; 38:5.
40. Wickner WT, Lodish HF. Multiple mechanisms of protein insertion into and across membranes. Science 1985; 230:400.
41. Wiedmann M, Kurzchalia TV, Hartmann E, Rapoport TA. A signal sequence receptor in the endoplasmic reticulum membrane. Nature 1987; 328:830.
42. Dunphy WG, Rothman JE. Compartmental organization of the Golgi stack. Cell 1985; 42:13.
43. Mellman I, Warren G. The road taken: past and future foundations of membrane traffic. Cell 2000; 100:99.
44. Griffiths G, Simons K. The *trans* Golgi network: sorting at the exit site of the Golgi complex. Science 1986; 234:438.
45. Kornfeld R, Kornfeld S. Assembly of asparagine-linked oligosaccharides. Annu Rev Biochem 1985; 54:631.
46. Dice JF. Molecular determinants of protein half-lives in eukaryotic cells. FASEB J 1987; 1:349.
47. Sanders SL, Schekman R. Polypeptide translocation across the endoplasmic reticulum membrane. J Biol Chem 1992; 267:13791.
48. Kornfeld S. Trafficking of lysosomal enzymes in normal and disease states. J Clin Invest 1986; 77:1.
49. Munro S. Pelham HRB. A C-terminal signal prevents secretion of lumenal ER proteins. Cell 1987; 48:899.
50. Munro S, Pelham HRB. An HSP70-like protein in the ER: identity with the 78 kd glucose-regulated protein and immunoglobulin heavy chain binding protein. Cell 1986; 46:291.
51. Johnson LM, Bankaitis VA, Emr SD. Distinct sequence determinants direct intracellular sorting and modification for a yeast vacuolar protease. Cell 1987; 48:875.
52. Valls LA, Hunter CP, Rothman JH, Stevens TH. Protein sorting in yeast: the localization determinant of yeast vacuolar carboxypeptide Y residues in the propeptide. Cell 1987; 48:887.
53. Moore HH, Kelly RB. Re-routing of a secretory protein by fusion with human growth hormone sequences. Nature 1986; 321:443.
54. Kelly RB, Grote E. Protein targeting in the neuron. Annu Rev Neurosci 1993; 16:95.
55. Burgess TL, Kelly RB. Constitutive and regulated secretion of proteins. Annu Rev Cell Biol 1987; 3:243.
56. Loh YP, Snell CR, Cool DR. Receptor-mediated targeting of hormones to secretory granules. Role of carboxypeptidase E. Trends Endocrinol Metab 1997; 8:130.
57. Tooze J, Tooze SA. Clathrin-coated vesicular transport of secretory proteins during the formation of ACTH-containing secretory granules in AtT-20 cells. J Cell Biol 1986; 103:839.
58. Orci L, Ravazzola M, Storch M-J, et al. Proteolytic maturation of insulin is a post-Golgi event which occurs in acidifying clathrin-coated secretory vesicles. Cell 1987; 49:865.
59. Mellman I, Fuchs R, Helenius A. Acidification of the endocytic and exocytic pathways. Annu Rev Biochem 1986; 55:663.
60. Hong W, Tang BL. Protein trafficking along the exocytotic pathway. Bioassays 1993; 15:231.
60a. Gerdes HH, Glombik MM. Signal-mediated sorting to the regulated pathway of protein secretion. Anat Anz 1999; 181:447.
61. Inoue K, Kurosumi K. Ultrastructural immunocytochemical localization of LH and FSH in the pituitary of the untreated male rat. Cell Tissue Res 1984; 235:77.
61a. Gullberg U, Bengtsson N, Bulow E, et al. Processing and targeting of granule proteins in human neutrophils. J Immunol Methods 1999; 232:201.
62. DeLisle RC, Williams IA. Regulation of membrane fusion in secretory exocytosis. Annu Rev Physiol 1986; 48:225.
63. Thomas G, Thorne BA, Hruby DE. Gene transfer technique to study neuropeptide processing. Annu Rev Physiol 1988; 50:323.
64. Yamamoto KR. Steroid receptor regulated transcription of specific genes and gene networks. Annu Rev Genet 1985; 19:209.
65. Shupnik MA, Chin WW, Habener JF, Ridgway EC. Transcriptional regulation of the thyrotropin subunit genes by thyroid hormone. J Biol Chem 1985; 260:2900.
66. Larsen PR, Harney JW, Moore DD. Sequences required for cell type specific thyroid hormone regulation of rat growth hormone promoter activity. J Biol Chem 1986; 261:14373.
67. Wright PA, Crew MD, Spindler SR. Discrete positive and negative thyroid hormone-responsive transcription regulatory elements of the rat growth hormone gene. J Biol Chem 1987; 262:5659.
68. Flug F, Copp RP, Casanova J, et al. *Cis*-acting elements of the rat growth hormone gene which mediate basal and regulated expression by thyroid hormone. J Biol Chem 1987; 262:6373.
69. Jantzen HM, Strahle U, Gloss B, et al. Cooperativity of glucocorticoid response elements located far upstream of the tyrosine aminotransferase gene. Nature 1987; 49:29.
70. Weinberger C, Thompson CC, Ong ES, et al. The c-erb-A gene encodes a thyroid hormone receptor. Nature 1986; 324:64 1.
71. Green S, Chambon P. A super family of potentially oncogenic hormone receptors. Nature 1986; 324:615.
72. Brown DD. The role of stable complexes that repress and activate eucaryotic genes. Cell 1984; 37:359.
73. von Hippel PH, Bear DG, Morgan WD, McSwiggen JA. Protein-nucleic acid interactions in transcription: a molecular analysis. Annu Rev Biochem 1984; 53:389.
74. Harrison SC. A structural taxonomy of DNA-binding domains. Nature 1991; 353:715.
75. Pabo CO. Transcription factors: structural families and principles of DNA recognition. Annu Rev Biochem 1992; 61:1053.
76. Murdoch GH, Franco R, Evans RM, Rosenfeld RG. Polypeptide hormone regulation of gene expression. Thyrotropin-releasing hormone rapidly stimulates both transcription of the prolactin and the phosphorylation of a specific nuclear protein. J Biol Chem 1983; 258:15329.
77. Montminy MR, Sevarino KA, Wagner JA, et al. Identification of a cyclic AMP responsive element within the rat somatostatin gene. Proc Natl Acad Sci U S A 1986; 83:6682.
78. Hunter T, Karin M. The regulation of transcription by phosphorylation. Cell 1992; 70:375.
79. Habener JF. Cyclic AMP response element binding proteins: a cornucopia of transcription factors. Mol Endocrinol 1990; 4:1087.
80. Kadonaga JT, Tjian R. Affinity purification of sequence-specific DNA-binding proteins. Proc Natl Acad Sci U S A 1986; 83:5889.
81. Brent R. Repression of transcription in yeast. Cell 1985; 42:3.

82. Diamond MI, Miner JN, Yoshinaga SK, Yamamoto KR. Transcriptional factor interactions: selectors of positive and negative regulation from a single DNA element. Science 1990; 249:1266.

83. Guarente L. Yeast promoters: positive and negative elements. Cell 1984; 36:799.

84. Jones NC. Negative regulation of enhancers. Nature 1986; 321:202.

85. Maniatis T, Goodbourn S, Fischer JA. Regulation of inducible and tissue-specific gene expression. Science 1987; 236:1237.

86. Yanofsky C. Transcription attenuation. J Biol Chem 1988; 263:609.

87. Brock ML, Shapiro DJ. Estrogen stabilizes vitellogenin mRNA against cytoplasmic degradation. Cell 1983; 34:207.

88. Guyette WA, Matusik RJ, Rosen JM. Prolactin-mediated transcriptional and post-transcriptional control of casein gene expression. Cell 1979; 17:1013.

89. Krane IM, Spindel ER, Chin WW. Thyroid hormone decreases the stability and the poly(A) tract length of rat thyrotropin β-subunit messenger RNA. Mol Endocrinol 1991; 5:469.

90. Koenig RJ, Lazar MA, Hodin RA, et al. Inhibition of thyroid hormone action by a non-hormone binding c-erbA protein generated by alternative mRNA splicing. Nature 1989; 337:659.

91. Chew SL. Alternative splicing of mRNA as a mode of endocrine regulation. Trends Endocrinol Metab 1997; 8:405.

92. Douglass J, Civelli O, Herbert E. Polyprotein gene expression: generation of diversity of neuroendocrine peptides. Annu Rev Biochem 1984; 53:665.

93. Wilson HE, White A. Prohormones: their clinical relevance. Trends Endocrinol Metab 1998; 9:396.

# CHAPTER 4

# HORMONAL ACTION

DARYL K. GRANNER

## GENERAL FEATURES OF HORMONE SYSTEMS AND HISTORICAL PERSPECTIVE

Multicellular organisms use intercellular communication mechanisms to ensure their survival by coordinating the responses necessary for adjusting to constantly changing external and internal environments. Two systems comprising several highly differentiated tissues have evolved to serve these functions. One is the nervous system, and the other is the endocrine system, which classically has been viewed as using mobile hormonal messages that are secreted from one gland or tissue to act on a distant tissue. There is an exquisite convergence of these regulatory systems. For example, neural regulation of the endocrine system is important; many neurotransmitters resemble hormones in their synthesis, release, transport, and mechanism of action; and many hormones are synthesized in the nervous system (see Chap. 175). The focus of this chapter is the endocrine system and how hormones work.

The word *hormone* is derived from a Greek term that means to arouse to activity. Classically defined, a hormone is a substance that is synthesized in one organ and transported by the circulatory system to act on another tissue. However, this original description is too restrictive, because hormones can act on adjacent cells (i.e., paracrine action) and on the cell in which they were synthesized (i.e., autocrine action) without entering the circulation.

Early studies concentrated on defining the endocrine action of hormones by removing or ablating an organ to localize the site of production. An extract of the tissue was then used to restore the function, and this served as a bioassay for subsequent purification of the hormone and the elucidation of physiologic and biochemical actions. This classic era of the study of hormonal action was descriptive. During this period, many hormones were discovered, and their major effects were defined. Because it was assumed that hormones had a unique source and a single or predominant action, they were named for the tissue of origin (e.g., thyroid hormone) or for the action (e.g., growth hormone).

The next era of investigation of hormonal action was characterized by the discovery of many more hormones and by a more detailed analysis of how hormones work. The investigation of their functions was aided by methods and ideas previously exploited by endocrinologists, including the use of radioisotopes, the concept of turnover, improved means of purifying molecules, and the availability of sophisticated analytic machinery. Such studies changed the direction of research in hormonal action from a descriptive (i.e., organ or tissue) to a mechanistic (i.e., molecule or function) approach. *Where* a molecule worked was no longer as important as *how* it acted. A single hormone could have hemocrine (i.e., transportation through the blood), paracrine, or autocrine actions but affect the different target cells in a similar way, and some effects could be produced by a variety of hormones. For example, naming a single molecule the "growth hormone" was incorrect, because this hormone is but one of several—including the thyroid hormones, sex hormones, glucocorticoids, insulin, and various growth-promoting polypeptides—that are involved in growth, and growth promotion is only one of the actions of the so-called growth hormone.

The principles of hormone synthesis, storage, secretion, transport, metabolism, and feedback control were established during this period. A major contribution was the elaboration of the concept of hormone receptors, and of the properties of specificity and selectivity of response, how target cells are defined, how responses are modulated, how signals are transduced from the outside of a cell to its interior, and how hormones can be classified according to their mechanism of action.

The techniques of molecular biology and recombinant DNA have been applied to hormonal action with remarkable success. It is now possible to analyze hormonal effects on gene expression and to study which few nucleotides of the $3 \times 10^9$ in each haploid genome confer the response. Another exciting area is the overlapping spectrum of activity of components of hormonal action systems with nonhormonal proteins. Consider the similar features of the guanosine triphosphate (GTP)–binding proteins involved in the hormone-sensitive adenylate cyclase system with the transforming *RAS* oncogene family of proteins or with transducin, which is the protein that couples photoactivation to the visual response.[1,2] The homology of platelet-derived growth factor (*PDGF*) gene and the v-*sis* transforming gene is remarkable, as is the similarity between the insulin and epidermal growth factor receptors, both of which have intrinsic tyrosine kinase activity.[3–6] Researchers are exploring the molecular bases of endocrine diseases, such as pseudohypoparathyroidism, several types of dwarfism, Graves disease, certain types of extreme insulin resistance, testicular feminization, acromegaly, vitamin D resistance, and hereditary nephrogenic diabetes insipidus, to name a few.[7–14] This knowledge has challenged many of the earlier concepts of hormonal action and endocrine disease.

## TARGET CELL CONCEPT

There are ~200 types of differentiated cells in humans. Only a few produce hormones, but virtually all of the 75 trillion cells in a human body are targets of one or more of the ~50 known hormones. The concept of target cells is undergoing redefinition. It was thought that hormones affected a single cell type, or only a few kinds of cells, and that a hormone elicited a unique biochemical or physiologic action. For example, it was presumed that thyroid-stimulating hormone (TSH) stimulated thyroid growth and thyroid hormonogenesis; adrenocorticotropic hormone (ACTH, also called corticotropin) enhanced growth and function of the adrenal cortex; glucagon increased hepatic glucose production; and luteinizing hormone (LH) stimulated gonadal steroidogenesis. However, these same hormones also stimulate lipolysis in adipose cells.[15] Although the physiologic importance of this effect is unclear, the concept of unique sites of actions of these hormones is untenable. A more relevant example is that of insulin, which effects various responses in different cells and occasionally influences different processes within the same cell. It enhances glucose uptake and oxidation in muscle, lipogenesis in fat, amino acid transport in liver and lymphocytes, and protein synthesis in liver and muscle. These and other examples necessitated a reevaluation of the target cell concept.

With the delineation of specific cell-surface and intracellular hormone receptors, the definition of a target has been expanded to include any cell in which the hormone binds to its receptor, whether or not a biochemical or physiologic response has been determined. This definition also is imperfect, but it has heuristic merit, because it presumes that not all actions of hormones have been elucidated.

The response of a target cell is determined by the differentiated state of the cell, and a cell can have several responses to a single hormone. Cells can respond to a hormone in a hemocrine, paracrine, or autocrine manner. An example is the hormone gastrin-releasing peptide (also called mammalian bombesin). Gastrin-releasing peptide has hemocrine and paracrine actions in the gut but is produced by and stimulates the growth of small cell carcinoma cells of the lung.[16]

Several factors determine the overall response of a target cell to a hormone. The concentration of a hormone around the target cell depends on the rate of synthesis and secretion of the hormone, the proximity of target and source, the association-dissociation constants of the hormone with specific plasma carrier proteins, the rate of conversion of an inactive or suboptimally active form of the hormone into the active form, and the rate of clearance of the hormone from blood by other tissues or by degradation or excretion. The actual response to the hormone depends on the relative activity and state of occupancy, or both, of the specific hormone receptors on the plasma membrane or within the cytoplasm or nucleus; the metabolism of the hormone within the target cell; the presence of other factors within the target cell that are necessary for the hormone response; and postreceptor desensitization of the cell. Alterations of any of these processes can change the hormonal effect on a given target cell and must be considered in addition to the classic feedback loops.

# HORMONE RECEPTORS

## GENERAL FEATURES

One of the major challenges in making the hormone-based communication system work is depicted in Figure 4-1. Hormone concentrations are very low in the extracellular fluid, generally in the range of $10^{-15}$ to $10^{-9}$ M. This is much lower than that of the many structurally similar molecules (e.g., sterols, amino acids, peptides) and other molecules that circulate at concentrations in the $10^{-5}$ to $10^{-3}$ M range. Target cells must identify the various hormones present in small amounts and differentiate a given hormone from the 106- to 109-fold excess of other, often closely related, molecules. This high degree of discrimination is provided by cell-associated recognition molecules called *receptors*. Hormones initiate their bioeffects by binding to specific receptors, and because any effective control system must provide a means of stopping a response, hormone-induced actions usually terminate after the effector dissociates from the receptor.

A target cell is defined by its ability to bind a given hormone selectively by means of a receptor, an interaction that is often quantitated using radioactive ligands that mimic hormone binding. Several features of this interaction are important. The

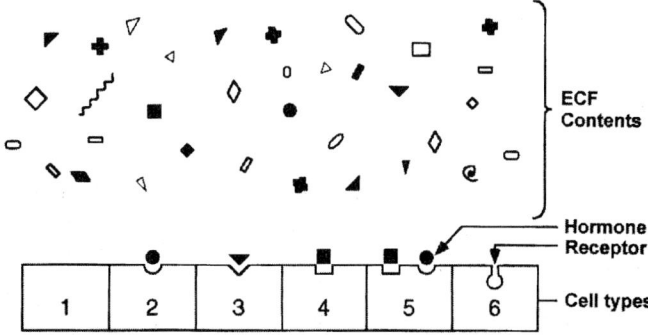

**FIGURE 4-1.** Specificity and selectivity of hormone receptors. Many different molecules circulate in the extracellular fluid (*ECF*), but only a few are recognized by hormone receptors. Receptors must select these molecules from among high concentrations of the other molecules. This simplified drawing shows that a cell may have no hormone receptors, have one receptor, have a receptor but no hormone in the vicinity, or have receptors for several hormones.

radioactivity must not alter the bioactivity of the ligand. The binding should be specific, in which case the ligand is displaceable by unlabeled agonist or antagonist. Binding should be saturable. Binding should occur within the concentration range of the expected biologic response.

## RECOGNITION AND COUPLING DOMAINS OF RECEPTORS

All receptors, whether for polypeptides or steroids, have at least two functional domains, and most have several more. A *recognition domain* binds the hormone, and a second region, the *coupling domain*, generates a signal that links hormone recognition to some intracellular function. The binding of hormone by receptor implies that some region of the hormone molecule has a conformation that is complementary to a region of the receptor molecule. The degree of similarity, or fit, determines the tightness of the association; this is measured as the affinity of binding. If the native hormone has a relative affinity of 1, other natural molecules range between 0 and 1. In absolute terms, this actually spans a binding affinity range of more than a trillion. Ligands with a relative affinity of more than 1 for some receptors have been synthesized and are used to study receptor biology.

*Coupling* (i.e., signal transduction) occurs in two ways. Polypeptide and protein hormones, and the catecholamines, bind to receptors located in the plasma membrane, and thereby generate signals that regulate various intracellular functions. Steroids, thyroid hormones, retinoids, and other hormones of this class interact with intracellular receptors, and this complex provides the initial signal.

The amino acid sequences of the recognition and coupling domains have been identified in many polypeptide hormone receptors. Hormone analogues with specific amino acid substitutions were used to change binding and alter the bioactivity of the hormone. Steroid hormone receptors also have these two functional domains; one site binds the hormone and the other binds to specific DNA regions. They also have other domains important for their function, which are described later. Several receptors have been characterized by recombinant DNA techniques, and structural analysis shows that these domains are highly homologous. This homology has been used to isolate cDNAs encoding several receptors that had not been obtained through classic protein purification procedures. The investigations have shown that these nuclear receptors are part of a large family of related proteins.[17] This family of proteins is thought to regulate gene transcription, often in association with other transcription factors and coregulatory molecules. The ligands for many of the proteins in this family have not been identified; these are called *orphan receptors*.

**TABLE 4-1.**
**A Comparison of Hormone Receptors with Transport Proteins**

| Feature | Receptors* | Plasma Transport Proteins |
| --- | --- | --- |
| Concentration | Very low | Very high |
| Binding affinity | Very high | Low |
| Binding specificity | High | Low |
| Saturability at physiologic concentrations | Yes | No |
| Reversibility of binding | Yes | Yes |
| Signal transduction | Yes | No |

*Hormone receptors are present at a concentration of a few thousand per cell and have a binding affinity (generally measured as the dissociation constant or $k_d$) in the $10^{-11}$ to $10^{-9}$ M range. Plasma transport proteins are more abundant (billions of molecules/µL) and have a binding affinity of $10^{-7}$ to $10^{-5}$ M.

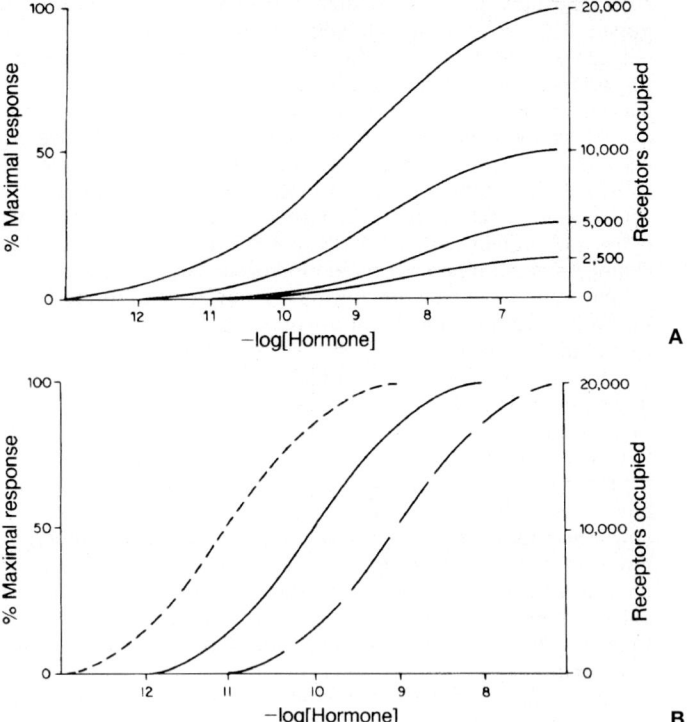

**A**

**B**

**FIGURE 4-3.** Changes of receptor occupancy have large effects on the biologic response when effector and receptor occupancy are tightly coupled. This can occur when the receptor number changes (**A**) or when the affinity of the receptor for the hormone changes (**B**). In the hypothetical case shown in (**A**), a decrease from 20,000 receptors per cell to 10,000 results in a 50% decrease of the maximal response, a $V_{max}$ effect. A decrease in affinity (i.e., *solid to interrupted line in* [**B**], *or rightward shift*) means that more hormone is required for a given effect, but the same maximal response can be obtained. This is a $K_m$ effect. (From Granner DK. Characteristics of hormone systems. In: Murray RK, Granner DK, Mayer PA, Rodwell VW, eds. Harper's biochemistry, 21st ed. Norwalk, CT: Appleton & Lange, 1988.)

The dual functions of binding and coupling ultimately define a receptor, and it is the coupling of hormone binding to signal transduction, called *receptor-effector coupling*, that provides the first step in the amplification of the hormonal response. This dual purpose also differentiates the target cell receptor from the plasma carrier proteins that bind hormone without generating a signal. It is important to differentiate the binding of hormones to receptors from the association that hormones have with various transport or carrier proteins. Table 4-1 lists several features of these functionally different classes of proteins.

## RECEPTOR OCCUPANCY AND BIOEFFECT

The concentrations of hormone required for occupancy of the receptor and for elicitation of a specific biologic response often are similar (Fig. 4-2A). This is especially true for steroid hormones, but some polypeptide hormones also exhibit this characteristic. This tight coupling is remarkable, considering the many steps that must occur between hormone binding and complex responses, such as transport, enzyme induction, cell lysis, or cell replication. When receptor occupancy and bioeffect are tightly coupled, significant changes in the latter occur when receptor occupancy changes. This happens when fewer receptors are available (Fig. 4-3A) or the affinity of the receptor changes but hormone concentration remains constant (see Fig. 4-3B). Otherwise, there is a marked dissociation of binding and effect, and a maximal bioeffect occurs when only a small percentage of the receptors are occupied (see effect 2 in Fig. 4-2B).

Receptors not involved in the elicitation of the response are called *spare receptors*. They are observed in the response of several polypeptide hormones and are thought to provide a means of increasing the sensitivity of a target cell to activation by low concentrations of hormone and to provide a reservoir of recep-

tors. The concept of spare receptors is operational and may depend on which aspect of the response is examined and which tissue is involved. For example, there is excellent agreement between LH binding and cyclic adenosine monophosphate (cAMP) production in rat testis and ovarian granulosa cells (there generally are no spare receptors when any hormone activates adenylate cyclase), but steroidogenesis in these tissues, which is cAMP dependent, occurs when fewer than 1% of the receptors are occupied (see effects 1 and 2 in Fig. 4-2).[18] Transcription of the phosphoenolpyruvate carboxykinase gene is

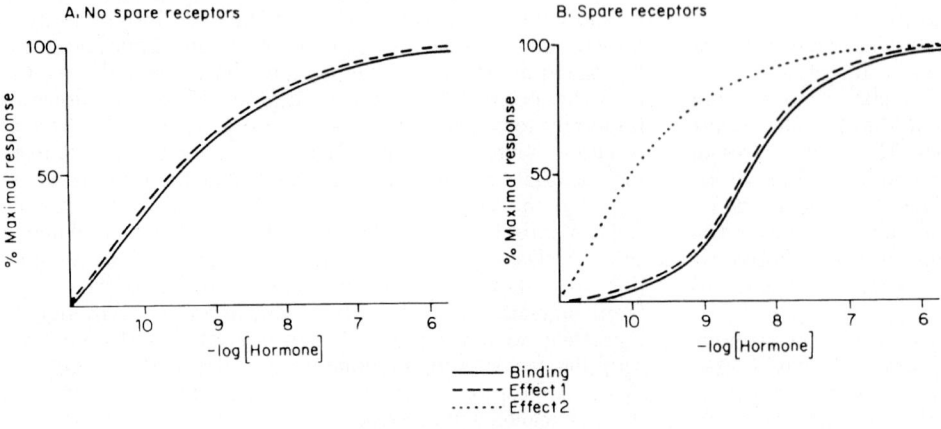

**FIGURE 4-2.** Hormone binding and biologic effect are compared in the absence (**A**) and presence (**B**, *effect 2*) of spare receptors. Some biologic effects in a tissue may be tightly coupled to binding, but others demonstrate the spare receptor phenomenon (e.g., compare effects 1 and 2 in **B**). (From Granner DK. Characteristics of hormone systems. In: Martin DW Jr, Mayer PA, Rodwell VW, Granner DK, eds. Harper's review of biochemistry, 20th ed. Los Altos, CA: Lange Medical Publications, 1985:501.)

**TABLE 4-2.**
**Classification of Steroids According to Their Action
as Glucocorticoids**

**AGONISTS**
  Dexamethasone
  Cortisol
  Corticosterone
  Aldosterone
**PARTIAL AGONISTS**
  11 β-Hydroxyprogesterone
  21-Deoxycortisol
  17 α-Hydroxyprogesterone
  Progesterone
**ANTAGONISTS**
  Testosterone
  17β-Estradiol
  19-Nortestosterone
  Cortisone
**INACTIVE STEROIDS**
  11 α-Hydroxyprogesterone
  Androstenedione
  11α,17α-Methyltestosterone
  Tetrahydrocortisol

  (From Granner D. Hormones of the adrenal cortex. In: Murray RK, Granner DK, Mayer PA, Rodwell VW, eds. Harper's biochemistry, 21st ed. Norwalk, CT: Appleton & Lange, 1988.)

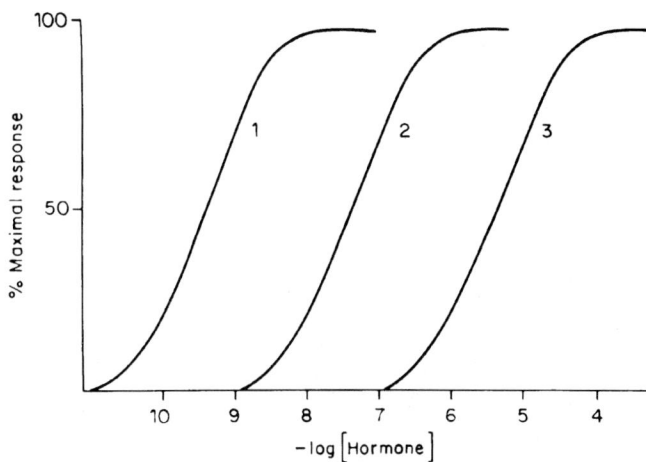

**FIGURE 4-4.** Within a class of hormones—glucocorticoids, for example—different molecules may have different potencies. In this case, hormones 1, 2, and 3 are all agonists, but very different concentrations are required to achieve a given biologic response. The binding of steroid to receptor would parallel each of these curves. (From Granner DK. Characteristics of hormone systems. In: Murray RK, Granner DK, Mayer PA, Rodwell VW, eds. Harper's biochemistry, 21st ed. Norwalk, CT: Appleton & Lange, 1988.)

repressed when far fewer than 1% of hepatoma cell insulin receptors are occupied, but there is a high correlation between insulin binding and amino acid transport in thymocytes.[19] Other examples of the dissociation of receptor binding and biologic effects include the effects of catecholamines on muscle contraction, lipolysis, and ion transport.[20] These end-responses presumably reflect a cascade or multiplier effect of the hormone.

Different responses within the same cell can require various degrees of receptor occupancy. For example, successively greater degrees of occupancy of the adipose cell insulin receptor increase, in sequence, lipolysis, glucose oxidation, amino acid transport, and protein synthesis.[21]

## AGONIST-ANTAGONIST CONCEPT

Molecules can be divided into four groups according to their ability to elicit a hormone receptor–mediated response. These classes are *agonists, partial agonists, antagonists,* and *inactive agents* (Table 4-2).

Agonists elicit the maximal response, although different concentrations may be required. In the example of Figure 4-4, 1, 2, and 3 could be porcine insulin, porcine proinsulin, and guinea pig insulin, respectively. In all systems tested, these insulins have the same rank order of potency, but each elicits a maximal response if present in sufficient concentration. Likewise, 1, 2, and 3 could be dexamethasone, cortisol, and corticosterone (see Table 4-2). Partial agonists evoke an incomplete response even when very large concentrations of the hormone are used, as shown by line B of Figure 4-5. Antagonists generally have no effects themselves, but they competitively inhibit the action of agonists or partial agonists (see lines A through C in Fig. 4-5). Many structurally similar compounds elicit no effect and have no effect on the action of the agonists or antagonists. These are classified as inactive agents and are represented as line D in Figure 4-5.

Partial agonists also compete with agonists for binding to and activation of the receptor, when they become partial antagonists. The extent of the inhibition of agonist activity caused by partial or complete antagonists depends on the relative concentration of the various steroids. Generally, much higher concentrations of the antagonist are required to inhibit an agonist than are necessary for the latter to exert its maximal effect. Because these con-

centrations are rarely achieved in vivo, this phenomenon is used for studies of the mechanism of action of hormones in vitro.

The binding of a ligand to the receptor must facilitate a change in this molecule so that it can bind to DNA. This phenomenon was first suggested in studies that used the steroids in Table 4-2.[22] The hypothesis assumes that agonists bind to and fully activate the receptor and elicit the maximal biologic response; that partial agonists fully occupy the receptor but afford incomplete activation and therefore a partial response; and that antagonists fully occupy the receptor, but because this complex is unable to bind to DNA, it elicits no intrinsic response but does inhibit the action of agonists.

## REGULATION OF RECEPTORS

The number of hormone receptors on or in a cell is in a dynamic state and can be regulated physiologically or be influenced by

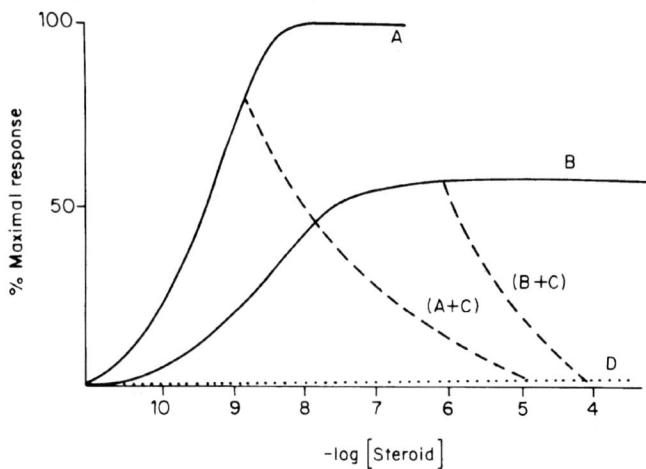

**FIGURE 4-5.** Classification of hormones according to their biologic activity. Steroids, for example, can be classified as agonists (*line A*), partial agonists (*line B*), antagonists (*C in A+C or B+C*), or inactive agents (*dotted line D*). This drawing represents induction of the enzyme tyrosine aminotransferase. (From Granner DK. Characteristics of hormone systems. In: Murray RK, Granner DK, Mayer PA, Rodwell VW, eds. Harper's biochemistry, 21st ed. Norwalk, CT: Appleton & Lange, 1988.)

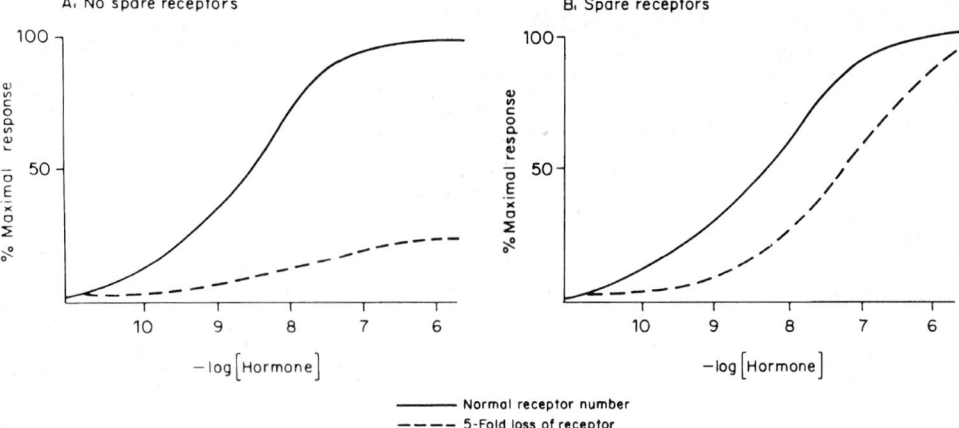

**FIGURE 4-6.** The effect a five-fold loss of receptors has on a biologic system that lacks (**A**) or has (**B**) spare receptors. (From Granner DK. Characteristics of hormone systems. In: Martin DW Jr, Mayer PA, Rodwell VW, Granner DK, eds. Harper's review of biochemistry, 20th ed. Los Altos, CA: Lange Medical Publications, 1985:502.)

diseases or therapeutic measures. The receptor concentration and affinity of hormone binding can be regulated.

Some changes can be acute and can significantly affect hormone responsiveness of the cell. For instance, cells exposed to β-adrenergic agonists for minutes to hours no longer activate adenylate cyclase in response to more agonist, and the biologic response is lost. This *desensitization* occurs by two mechanisms.[23] The loss of receptors, called *down-regulation*, involves the internal sequestration of receptors, segregating them from the other components of the response system, including the regulatory and catalytic subunits of adenylate cyclase. Removal of the agonist results in the return of receptors to the cell surface and restoration of hormonal sensitivity.[23] An example of a second form of desensitization of the β-adrenergic system involves the covalent modification of receptor by phosphorylation.[24] This cAMP-dependent process entails no change in receptor number and no translocation. Reconstitution experiments show that because the phosphorylated receptor is unable to activate adenylate cyclase, the activation and hormone binding domains are uncoupled.[23] Other examples of physiologic adaptation that is accomplished through down-regulation of receptor number by the homologous hormone include insulin, glucagon, thyrotropin-releasing hormone, growth hormone, LH, follicle-stimulating hormone, and catecholamines. A few hormones, such as angiotensin II and prolactin, *up-regulate* their receptors. The changes in receptor number can occur over a period of minutes to hours and are probably an important means of regulating biologic responses.

How the loss of receptor affects the biologic response elicited at a given hormone concentration depends on whether there are spare receptors (Fig. 4-6). Suppose there is a fivefold reduction in receptor number in a cell. With no spare receptors (see Fig. 4-6*A*), the maximal response obtained is 20% that of control, hence, the effect is on the $V_{max}$. With spare receptors (see Fig. 4-6*B*), the maximal response is obtained, but at five times the originally effective hormone concentration, analogous to a $K_m$ effect.

## STRUCTURE OF RECEPTORS

The acetylcholine receptor (AChR), which exists in relatively large amounts in the electric organ of *Torpedo californica*, was the first plasma membrane–associated receptor to be studied in detail. The AChR consists of four subunits: $\alpha_2$, β, γ, and δ.[25] The two α subunits bind acetylcholine.[26] The technique of site-directed mutagenesis has been used to show which regions of this subunit participate in the formation of the transmembrane ion channel, which is the major function of the AChR.[25]

Other receptors occur in very small amounts, and recombinant DNA techniques have been used to deduce many of the structures and to find and characterize new receptors. The insu-

lin receptor is a heterotetramer ($\alpha_2\beta_2$) linked by multiple disulfide bonds, in which the extramembrane α subunit binds insulin and the membrane-spanning β subunit transduces the signal through the tyrosine kinase component of the cytoplasmic portion of this polypeptide[27] (Fig. 4-7). The insulin-like growth factor-I (IGF-I) receptor has a similar structure, and the epidermal growth factor (EGF) and low-density lipoprotein receptors are similar in many respects[28–30] (see Fig. 4-7). Receptors that couple ligand binding to signal transduction through G-protein intermediaries characteristically have seven membrane-spanning domains.[31]

Members of the nuclear receptor superfamily have several functional domains: a *ligand-binding domain* in the carboxyl-terminal region, an adjacent *DNA-binding domain*, and one or more *trans*-activation domains. There may also be dimerization, nuclear translocation, and heat shock protein domains, and regions that allow for interactions with a number of other accessory factor and coregulatory proteins[17,32] (Fig. 4-8). The amino acid sequence homology is particularly strong in the various DNA-binding domains, and it was this feature that led to the elucidation of the nuclear receptor superfamily.[17]

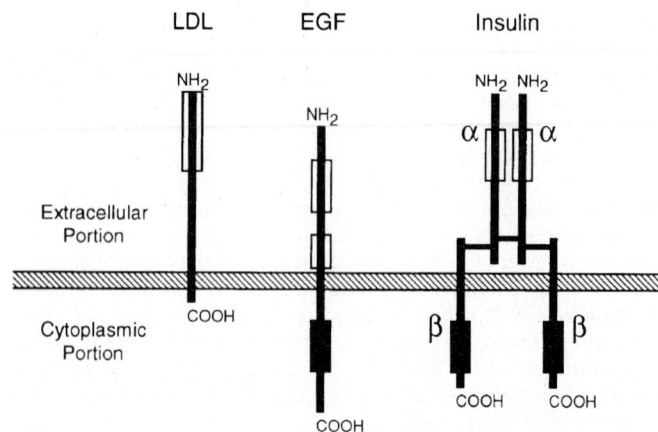

**FIGURE 4-7.** Schematic representation of the structures of the low-density lipoprotein (*LDL*), epidermal growth factor (*EGF*), and insulin receptors. The amino terminus (NH₂) of each is in the extracellular portion of the molecule. The carboxyterminus (*COOH*) is in the cytoplasm. The open boxes represent cysteine-rich regions that are thought to be involved in ligand binding. Each receptor has a short domain (~25 amino acids) that traverses the plasma membrane (*hatched line*) and an intracellular domain of variable length. The EGF and insulin receptors have tyrosine kinase activity associated with the cytoplasmic domain (■) and have autophosphorylation sites in this region. The insulin receptor is a heterotetramer connected by disulfide bridges (*vertical bars*).

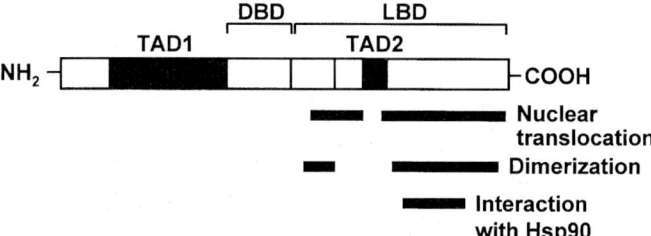

**FIGURE 4-8.** Nuclear receptor family members have several general domains. The amino-terminal region is most variable and often contains a *trans*-activating domain (*TAD1*). The DNA-binding domain (*DBD*) is most conserved, and this feature led to the discovery that these receptors are part of a large family of DNA-binding proteins. The hormone- or ligand-binding domain (*LBD*), which affords specificity, is located in the carboxy-terminal (*COOH*) region of the molecule and contains a second *trans*-activating domain (*TAD2*). Also shown are regions that allow for nuclear translocation, dimerization, and interaction with heat shock protein (*Hsp90*). Members of this family that have no known ligand are called *orphan receptors*.

## CLASSIFICATION OF HORMONES

A classification based on the location of receptors and the nature of the signal used to mediate hormonal action within the cell appears in Table 4-3, and general features of each group are listed in Table 4-4.

The hormones in group I are lipophilic. After secretion, these hormones associate with transport proteins, a process that circumvents the solubility problem while prolonging the plasma half-life by preventing the hormone from being metabolized and excreted. These hormones readily traverse the plasma membrane of all cells and encounter receptors in the cytosol or the nucleus of target cells. The ligand-receptor complex is assumed to be the intracellular messenger in this group.

The second major group consists of water-soluble hormones that bind to the plasma membrane of the target cell. These hormones regulate intracellular metabolic processes through intermediary molecules, called *second messengers* (the hormone itself is the first messenger), which are generated because of the ligand-receptor interaction. The second-messenger concept arose from the observation of Sutherland[33] that epinephrine binds to the plasma membrane of pigeon erythrocytes and increases intracellular cAMP. This was followed by a series of experiments in which cAMP was found to mediate the metabolic effects of many hormones. Hormones that use this mechanism are shown in group IIA. Several hormones, some of which were previously thought to affect cAMP, appear to use cyclic guanosine monophosphate (cGMP) (group IIB) or calcium or phosphatidylinositide metabolites (or both) as the intracellular signal (group IIC). The intracellular messenger has been identified as a protein kinase/phosphatase cascade for the hormones listed in group D.

A few hormones fit in more than one category (i.e., some hormones act through cAMP and $Ca^{2+}$), and assignments change with new information.

### MECHANISM OF ACTION OF GROUP I HORMONES

A schematic representation of the mechanism of action of group I hormones (see Table 4-3) is shown in Figure 4-9. These lipophilic molecules probably diffuse through the plasma membrane of all cells but encounter their specific, high-affinity receptor only within target cells. The hormone-receptor complex then undergoes an "activation" reaction that causes size, conformation, and surface charge changes that render it able to bind to chromatin. In some cases—with the glucocorticoid receptor, for example—this process involves the disruption of a receptor–heat shock protein complex. Whether the association

**TABLE 4-3.**
**Hormones and Their Actions: Classification According to Mechanism of Action**

**GROUP I. HORMONES THAT BIND TO INTRACELLULAR RECEPTORS**
Androgens
Calcitriol [1,25(OH)$_2$D$_3$]
Estrogens
Glucocorticoids
Mineralocorticoids
Progestins
Retinoic acid
Thyroid hormones (triiodothyronine and thyroxine)

**GROUP II. HORMONES THAT BIND TO CELL SURFACE RECEPTORS**
*A. The second messenger is cyclic adenosine monophosphate*
$\alpha_2$-Adrenergic catecholamines
$\beta_2$-Adrenergic catecholamines
Adrenocorticotropic hormone (ACTH)
Angiotensin II
Antidiuretic hormone (ADH)
Calcitonin
Chorionic gonadotropin
Corticotropin-releasing hormone (CRH)
Follicle-stimulating hormone (FSH)
Glucagon
Lipotropin (LPH)
Luteinizing hormone (LH)
Melanocyte-stimulating hormone (MSH)
Parathyroid hormone (PTH)
Somatostatin (SRIH)
Thyroid-stimulating hormone (TSH)

*B. The second messenger is cyclic guanosine monophosphate*
Atriopeptides
Nitric oxide

*C. The second messenger is calcium or phosphatidylinositides (or both)*
$\alpha_1$-Adrenergic catecholamines
Acetylcholine (muscarinic)
Angiotensin II
ADH
Epidermal growth factor (EGF)
Gonadotropin-releasing hormone
Platelet-derived growth factor
Thryotropin-releasing hormone

*D. The second messenger is a kinase/phosphatase cascade*
Chorionic somatomammotropin
Erythropoietin
Fibroblast growth factor
Growth hormone
Insulin
Insulin-like growth peptides (IGF-I, IGF-II)
Nerve growth factor
Oxytocin
Prolactin

**SUBCLASSIFICATION OF GROUP IIA HORMONES**
*Hormones that stimulate adenylate cyclase ($H_s$)*
ACTH
ADH
$\beta$-Adrenergics
Calcitonin
CRH
FSH
Glucagon
Human chorionic gonadotropin
LH
LPH
MSH
PTH
TSH

*Hormones that inhibit adenylate cyclase ($H_i$)*
$\alpha_2$-Adrenergics
Acetylcholine (muscarinic: M$_2$)
Angiotensin II
Opioids
SRIH

(Modified from Granner D. Hormones of the adrenal cortex. In: Murray RK, Granner DK, Mayer PA, Rodwell VW, eds. Harper's biochemistry, 21st ed. Norwalk, CT: Appleton & Lange, 1988.)

**TABLE 4-4.**
**General Features of Hormone Groups**

| Feature | Group I | Group II |
|---|---|---|
| Types | Steroids | Polypeptides |
| | Iodothyronines | Proteins |
| | Calcitriol | Glycoproteins |
| | | Catecholamines |
| Solubility | Lipophilic | Hydrophilic |
| Transport proteins | Yes | No |
| Plasma half-life | Long (hours, days) | Short (minutes) |
| Receptor | Intracellular | Plasma membrane |
| Mediators | Receptor-hormone complex | Cyclic adenosine monophosphate, cyclic guanosine monophosphate, $Ca^{2+}$, diacylglycerol, kinase cascades, phosphatidyl inositides, others |

and activation processes occur in the cytoplasm or nucleus appears to depend on the specific hormone. The hormone-receptor complex binds to specific regions of DNA and activates or inactivates specific genes.[34,35] By selectively affecting gene transcription and the production of the respective messenger RNAs (mRNAs), the amounts of specific proteins are changed, and metabolic processes are influenced. The effect of each of these hormones is specific; generally, the hormone affects <1% of the proteins or mRNAs in a target cell.

The nuclear actions of steroid hormones predominate and are well defined, but direct actions of these hormones in the cytoplasm and on various organelles and membranes also have been described.[36] An effect of estrogens, cAMP, and glucocorticoids on mRNA degradation rates has been demonstrated.[37–40] Glucocorticoids also affect posttranslational processing of some proteins.[41]

Although the biochemistry of gene transcription in mammalian cells is not completely understood, a general model of the structural requirements of steroid regulation of gene transcription can be drawn (Fig. 4-10). Steroid-regulated genes must be in regions of "open" or transcriptionally active chromatin (depicted as the bubble in Fig. 4-9), as defined by their susceptibility to digestion by the enzyme DNase I.[42] The open or closed conformation of chromatin may be regulated by the extent of acetylation of the histones that combine with DNA to form chromatin (discussed later this section). Genes have at least two separate regulatory regions in the DNA sequence immediately 5' of the transcription initiation site. The first of these, the basal promoter element (BPE), is generic, because it is present in some form in all genes.[43] This is depicted as containing the consensus sequence GTATA (A/T)A(A/T), called the TATA box (see Chap. 3), because this is the structure found most frequently. Another common component of the BPE is the CAAT box; this sequence or some equivalent structure usually is present. The BPE appears to specify the site of RNA polymerase II attachment to DNA and therefore the accuracy of transcript initiation.[44]

A second regulatory region is located slightly farther upstream than the BPE, and this may also consist of several discrete elements. This region modulates the frequency of transcript initiation and is less dependent on position and orientation. In these respects, it resembles the transcription enhancer elements found in other genes.[45,46] The regulatory region consists of two types of DNA elements in genes that respond to hormones. *Hormone response elements (HREs)* are short segments of DNA that bind a specific *hormone receptor/ligand complex.*[32,34,35] HREs are often capable of regulating transcription from test promoter/reporter gene constructs, but in most physiologic circumstances, other DNA element/protein complexes are required. The HRE usually is found within 250 nucleotides of the transcription initiation site, but the precise location of the HRE varies from gene to gene.

Identification of an HRE requires that it bind the hormone-receptor complex more avidly than does surrounding DNA or DNA from another source. The HRE also must confer hormone responsiveness. Putative regulatory sequence DNA can be ligated to reporter genes to assess this point. Usually, these fusion genes contain reporter genes not ordinarily influenced by the hormone, and these genes often are not expressed in the tissue being tested. Commonly used reporter genes are firefly luciferase or bacterial chloramphenicol acetyltransferase. The fusion gene is transfected into a target cell, and if the hormone

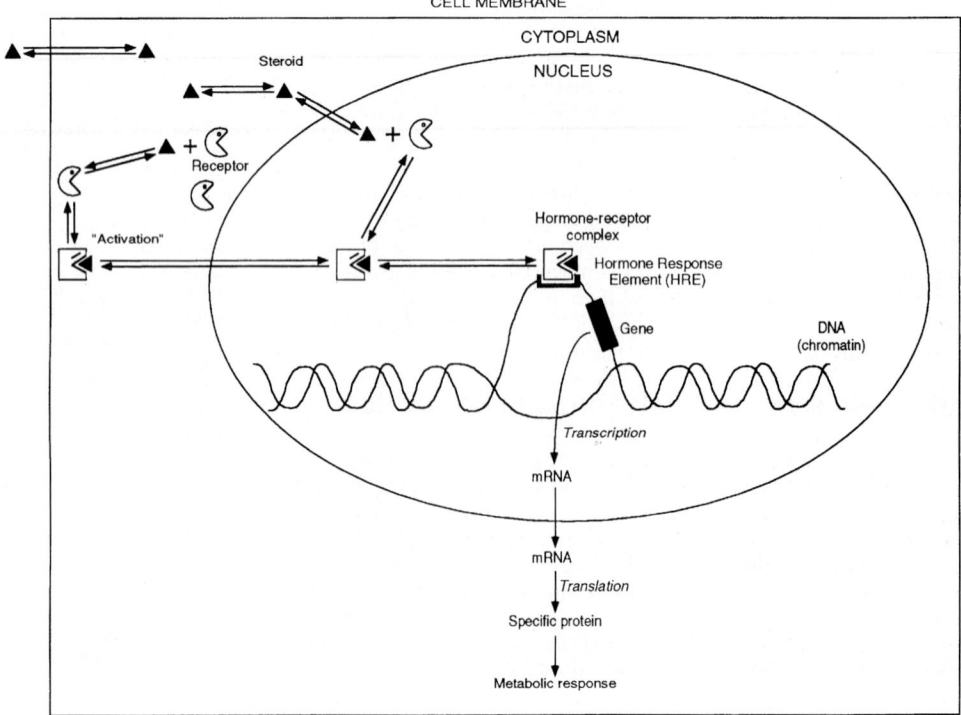

**FIGURE 4-9.** A general model of group I hormone action. The hormone binds to intracellular receptors in the cytoplasm or the nucleus and causes a conformational change. The hormone-receptor complex then binds to a specific region on DNA called the *hormone response element.* This interaction, with the help of various accessory factors and coregulators, results in the activation or repression of a restricted number of genes. The hormone response elements and associated factor elements are called *hormone response units.* The "bubble" indicates that this region of DNA is open or accessible to the transcription complex. These regions of DNA are often found to be sensitive to digestion by the enzyme DNase I.

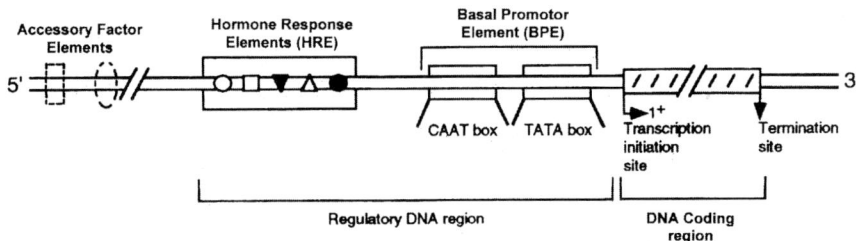

**FIGURE 4-10.** Structural requirements for hormonal regulation of gene transcription. Transcription starts at the arrow, where 1+ signifies the first nucleotide of the gene that is transcribed or copied. Immediately adjacent, on the 5' upstream side, is the basal promoter element, which generally consists of a TATA box and other components, such as a CAAT box. Hormone response elements (which bind the liganded receptor) can be anywhere in the 5' region or in the gene itself. Other DNA elements (accessory factor elements) that cooperate with the hormone response elements to regulate transcription can also be located at various sites. Together these form a hormone response unit.

now regulates the transcription of the reporter gene, an HRE is functionally defined. Position, orientation, and base-substitution effects can be precisely described using this technique.

Although HREs do transmit a hormone response in simple promoter test conditions, the situation is much more complex in most naturally occurring genes. The HRE must interact with other elements (and associated binding proteins) to function optimally. Such assemblies of *cis*-acting DNA elements and *trans*-acting factors are called *hormone response units (HRUs)*.[45] An HRU, therefore, consists of one or more HREs and one or more DNA elements with associated accessory factors (Fig. 4-11). In complex promoters—regulated by a variety of hormones—certain accessory factor components of one HRU (glucocorticoid) may be part of that for another (retinoic acid). This arrangement may provide for the hormonal integration of complex metabolic responses.

The communication between an HRU and the basal transcription apparatus is accomplished by one or more of a class of coregulator molecules (see Fig. 4-11). The first of these described was the cAMP response element binding (CREB) protein, so-called CBP. CBP, through an amino terminal domain, binds to phosphorylated serine 137 of CREB and facilitates transactivation in response to cAMP. It thus is described as a coactivator. CBP and its close relative, p300, interact with a number of signaling molecules, including activator protein-1, signal transducers and activators of transcription, nuclear receptors, and CREB.[46]

CBP/p300 also binds to the p160 family of coactivators—described in the next paragraph—and to a number of other proteins. It is important to note that CBP/p300 also has intrinsic histone acetyltransferase (HAT) activity. The importance of this is described later in this section. Some of the many actions of CBP/p300 appear to depend on intrinsic enzyme activities and the ability of this protein to serve as a scaffold for the binding of other proteins.

Three other families of coactivator molecules, all of ~160 kDa, have been described. These members of the p160 family of coactivators include (a) SRC-1 and NCoA-1; (b) GRIP 1, TIF2, and NCoA-2; and (c) p/CIP, ACTR, AIB1, RAC3, and TRAM-1.[47] The different names for members within a subfamily often represent species variations or minor splice variants. There is ~35% amino acid identity between members of the different subfamilies.

The role of these many coactivators is still evolving. It appears that certain combinations are responsible for specific ligand-induced actions through various receptors. The role of HAT is particularly interesting. Mutations of the HAT domain disable many of these transcription factors. Current thinking holds that these HAT activities acetylate histones and result in the remodeling of chromatin into a transcription-efficient environment.[48] In keeping with this hypothesis, histone deacetylation is associated with the inactivation of transcription.

In certain instances, the removal of a corepressor complex through a ligand-receptor interaction results in the activation of transcription. For example, in the absence of hormone, the thyroid or retinoic acid receptors are bound to a corepressor complex containing N-CoR or SMRT and associated proteins, some of which have histone deacetylase activity.[47] The target gene is repressed until the binding of hormone to the thyroid receptor results in the dissociation of this complex, and gene activation then ensues.

## MECHANISM OF ACTION OF GROUP II HORMONES

Most group II hormones are water soluble, have a short plasma half-life and no transport proteins, and initiate a response by binding to a receptor located in the plasma membrane (see Tables 4-3 and 4-4).

### CYCLIC ADENOSINE MONOPHOSPHATE AS THE SECOND MESSENGER

Cyclic AMP (3',5' adenylic acid), a ubiquitous nucleotide derived from adenosine triphosphate (ATP) through the action of the enzyme adenylate cyclase (Fig. 4-12), plays a crucial role in the action of several hormones. The intracellular level of cAMP is increased or decreased by various hormones (see Table 4-3). This effect varies from tissue to tissue and sometimes within a given tissue, depending on which specific hormone-receptor interactions occur. For example, epinephrine causes large increases of cAMP in muscle and relatively small changes in liver; the opposite is true of glucagon.

Tissues that respond to several hormones of this group do so through unique receptors converging on a single class of adenylate cyclase molecules. The best example of this is the adipose cell in which epinephrine, ACTH, TSH, glucagon, LH, melanocyte-

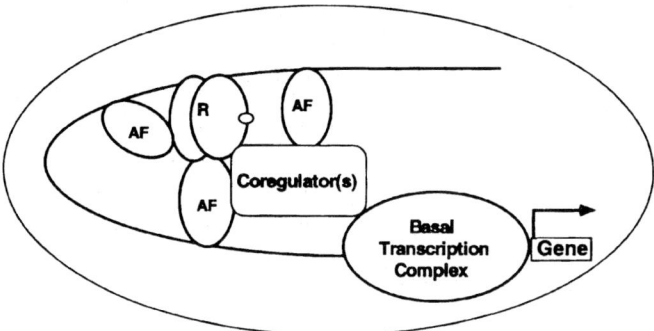

**FIGURE 4-11.** The hormone response unit (*HRU*). The HRU is an assembly of DNA elements and bound proteins. An essential component is the hormone response element with ligand-bound receptor (*R*). Also important are the accessory factor (*AF*) elements with bound transcription factors. More than two dozen of these accessory factors have been linked to hormone effects on transcription. The AFs can interact with each other or with the nuclear receptors. The components of the HRU communicate with the basal transcription machinery through a coregulator complex. The components of the coregulator complex, some of which are described in the text, provide for the direction and specificity of the hormone response. (From Granner DK. Hormone action. In: Murray RK, Granner DK, Mayes PA, Rodwell VW, eds. Harper's biochemistry, 25th ed. Norwalk, CT: Appleton & Lange, 1999.)

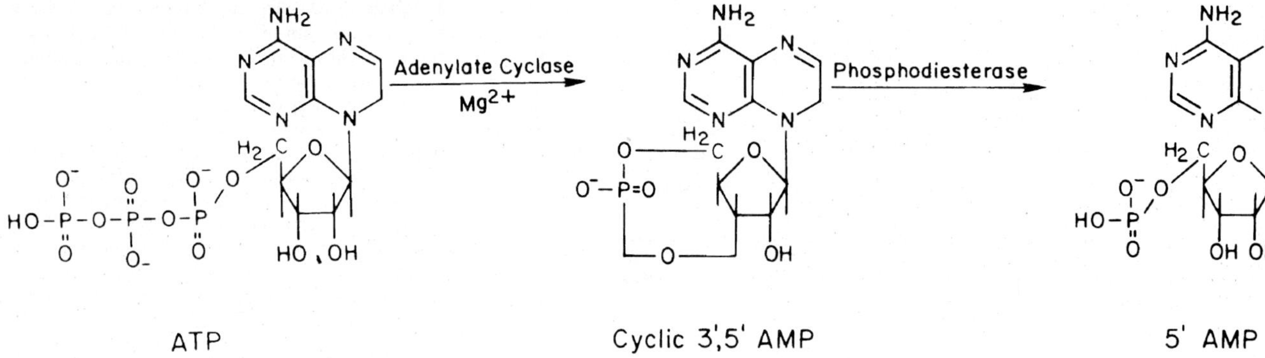

**FIGURE 4-12.** The formation and metabolism of cyclic adenosine monophosphate (*AMP*). (*ATP*, adenosine triphosphate.)

stimulating hormone, and vasopressin stimulate adenylate cyclase and increase cAMP.[15] Combinations of maximally effective concentrations are not additive, and treatments that destroy one receptor response have no effect on the response of other hormones. Some actions of cAMP occur outside the nucleus, presumably by mediating changes in the degree of phosphorylation of critical enzymes involved in metabolic processes, such as glycogenolysis, gluconeogenesis, and lipolysis.[49] Effects of cAMP on the transcription of many genes have been described, and this clearly is a major action of this molecule.[50]

### ADENYLATE CYCLASE SYSTEM

The components of this system in mammalian cells are shown in Figure 4-13. The interaction of the hormone with its receptor causes the activation or inactivation of adenylate cyclase. This process is mediated by two GTP-dependent regulatory protein complexes, designated $G_s$ (stimulatory) and $G_i$ (inhibitory), each of which is composed of three subunits: $\alpha$, $\beta$, and $\gamma$ (see Fig. 4-13). These G proteins are part of a large family with more than 20 members that mediate many biologic processes in addition to hormone responses[51] (Table 4-5). Adenylate cyclase, located on the inner surface of the plasma membrane, catalyzes the formation of cAMP from ATP in the presence of magnesium (see Fig. 4-12).

What was originally considered a single protein with hormone binding and catalytic domains was found to be a system of extraordinary complexity. Biochemical and genetic studies have established the biochemical uniqueness of the hormone-receptor, GTP-regulatory, and catalytic domains of the adenylate cyclase complex.

Two parallel systems, stimulatory (s) and inhibitory (i), converge on the catalytic molecule (C). Each system consists of a receptor, $R_s$ or $R_i$, and a regulatory complex, $G_s$ or $G_i$. $G_s$ and $G_i$ are trimers composed of $\alpha$, $\beta$, and $\gamma$ subunits (see Fig. 4-13) and are so called because they bind and hydrolyze GTP. The $\alpha_s$ and $\alpha_i$ are unique proteins of 39 to 46 kDa; the $\beta$ subunits are 37-kDa proteins, and the $\gamma$ subunits are 8-kDa proteins.[51] The binding of a hormone to $R_s$ or $R_i$ yields a receptor-mediated activation of G, which requires $Mg^{2+}$-dependent guanosine diphosphate (GDP)/GTP exchange by $\alpha$ and the subsequent dissociation of $\beta$ and $\gamma$ from $\alpha$.

The $\alpha_s$ subunit has GTPase activity; the active form, $\alpha_s \times$ GTP, is inactivated on hydrolysis of the GTP to GDP, and the trimeric $G_s$ complex is reformed.[52] Cholera toxin, an irreversible activator of cyclase, causes adenosine diphosphate (ADP) ribosylation of $\alpha_s$ on arginine at position 201 in the protein, and in so doing, inactivates the GTPase; $\alpha_s$ remains in the active form.[53,54] The $\alpha_i$ also has GTPase activity; however, because GDP does not freely dissociate from $\alpha_i$, the latter is reactivated by an exchange of GTP for GDP. Pertussis toxin irreversibly activates adenylate cyclase by promoting the ADP ribosylation of $\alpha_i$ on a cysteine residue, which prevents this subunit from being activated by ligand-bound receptor.[55]

The exact mechanism of activation and inactivation of the adenylate cyclase moiety has not been established.[55a] The $\alpha_s$ form

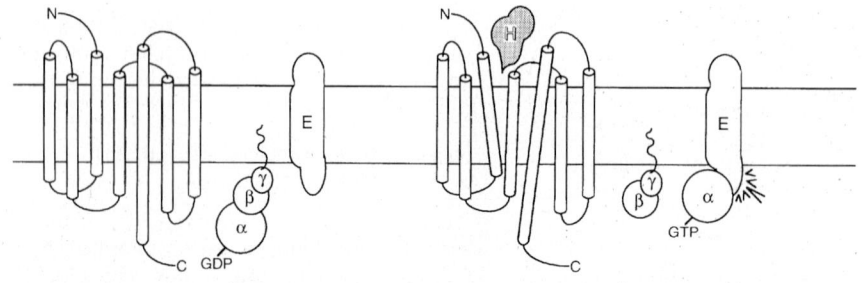

No Hormone: inactive effector          Bound Hormone: active effector

**FIGURE 4-13.** Components of the hormone receptor–G-protein effector system. Receptors that couple to effectors through G proteins typically have seven membrane-spanning domains. The amino (*N*) and carboxy (*C*) termini are shown. In the absence of hormone (*left*), the heterotrimeric G-protein complex (i.e., $\alpha$, $\beta$, $\gamma$) is in an inactive, guanosine diphosphate (*GDP*)–bound form and is probably not associated with the receptor. This complex is anchored to the plasma membrane through prenylated groups on the $\beta\gamma$ subunits (*wavy lines*) and perhaps by myristoylated groups on $\alpha$ subunits. On binding of hormone to the receptor, there is a presumed conformational change of the receptor and activation of the G-protein complex. This results from the exchange of GDP and guanosine triphosphate (*GTP*) on the $\alpha$ subunit, after which $\alpha$ and $\beta\gamma$ dissociate. The $\alpha$ subunit binds to and activates the effector (*E*). E can be adenylate cyclase ($\alpha_s$), a $K^+$ channel ($\alpha_i$, $\alpha_o$), phospholipase C-$\beta$ ($\alpha_q$), or other molecule. The $\beta\gamma$ subunit can also have direct actions on E.

**TABLE 4-5.**
**Classes and Functions of G Proteins**

| Class and Type* | Stimulus | Effector | Effect |
|---|---|---|---|
| $G_s$ | | | |
| $\alpha_s$ | Glucagon, β adrenergics | ↑ Adenylate cyclase | Gluconeogenesis<br>Lipolysis<br>Glycogenolysis |
| $\alpha_{olf}$ | Odorant | ↑ Adenylate cyclase | Olfaction |
| $G_i$ | | | |
| $\alpha_{i1}$ | Acetylcholine | ↓ Adenylate cyclase<br>↑ Potassium channels | Slowed heart rate |
| $\alpha_{i2}$ | $\alpha_2$ Adrenergics<br>$M_2$ Cholinergics | | |
| $\alpha_0$ | Opioids, endorphins | ↑ Potassium channels<br>↓ Calcium channels | Neuronal electrical activity |
| $\alpha_t$ | Light | ↑ Cyclic guanosine monophosphate phosphodiesterase | Vision |
| $G_q$ | | | |
| $\alpha_q$ | $M_1$ Cholinergics<br>$\alpha_1$ Adrenergics | ↑ Phospholipase C-$\beta_1$ | ↑ Muscle contraction and<br>↑ blood pressure |
| $\alpha_{q1}$ | $\alpha_1$ Adrenergics | ↑ Phospholipase C-$\beta_2$ | |
| $G_{12}$ | | | |
| $\alpha_{12}$ | ? | ? | ? |

*The four major classes of mammalian G proteins ($G_s$, $G_i$, $G_q$, $G_{12}$) are based on protein sequence homology. Representative members of each are shown, along with known stimuli, effectors, and well-defined biologic effects. More than 20 different α subunits have been identified.

can stimulate adenylate cyclase directly, and in some instances, the βγ complex, which is tightly associated and always acts as a unit, augments this action.

Less is known about how hormones inhibit adenylate cyclase activity. Direct inhibitory effects of $G_i$ protein on adenylate cyclase have been difficult to detect. One hypothesis is that the βγ complex that is liberated from $G_i$, which exists in most cells in great abundance over $G_s$, could bind to and inactivate $\alpha_s$. This would effectively shut off the stimulatory signals. Alternatively, βγ may directly inhibit some forms of adenylate cyclase. The α subunits and the βγ complex have actions independent of those on adenylate cyclase. Some forms of $\alpha_s$ stimulate $Ca^{2+}$ channels and inhibit $K^+$ channels. Similarly, some forms of $\alpha_i$ stimulate $K^+$ channels and inhibit $Ca^{2+}$ channels. Other subunits, particularly those of the $G_q$ family (see Table 4-5), are involved in the activation of members of the phospholipase C group of enzymes. This is important in the generation of the intracellular signals of inositol triphosphate and diacylglycerol. The βγ complex also can stimulate $K^+$ channels and activate certain isoforms of phospholipase C.[51]

Members of the family of G proteins mediate a variety of important processes (see Table 4-5). Transducin, the protein that is important in coupling light to photoactivation in the retina, is a member of the G-protein family, as are the proteins involved in smell and taste.[56] The products of the RAS oncogenes, which are involved in regulating cell growth, are members of the larger superfamily.[57] The G proteins are themselves a family within the large superfamily of GTPases and can be classified according to sequence homology into at least four subfamilies, as illustrated in Table 4-5. There are more than 20 α subunits, and there are at least four β subunits and six γ subunits. There are at least five adenylate cyclase molecules.[58] There may well be more members of each group.

Pseudohypoparathyroidism, an "experiment of nature," is a syndrome characterized by hypocalcemia and hyperphosphatemia, the biochemical hallmarks of hypoparathyroidism, and by several congenital defects (see Chap. 60). Individuals with pseudohypoparathyroidism do not have defective parathyroid function; they secrete large amounts of bioactive parathyroid hormone. Some have target organ resistance on the basis of a postreceptor defect. They are partially deficient in G protein (probably only the $\alpha_s$ subunit) and fail to couple binding to adenylate cyclase stimulation.[58,59] The observation that patients with pseudohypoparathyroidism often have defective responses to other hormones, including TSH, glucagon, and β-adrenergic agents, is not surprising.[60] Many G-protein–linked endocrinopathies have now been described (see Chap. 60). (See ref 60a.)

Approximately 40% of persons with acromegaly have a G-protein–linked disease. These individuals have one of two mutations in the $\alpha_s$ subunit that affects the intrinsic GTPase activity of this protein. One mutation, at arginine position 201, affects the same site that is ADP ribosylated by cholera toxin.[12] The constitutive overproduction of cAMP results in excessive release of growth hormone and somatotropic cell adenomas. In this way, $\alpha_s$ functions as an oncogene. Other α-subunit mutations that affect the GTPase domain result in tumors of the adrenal cortex and ovary.[61]

## CYCLIC ADENOSINE MONOPHOSPHATE–DEPENDENT PROTEIN KINASE

In prokaryotic cells, cAMP binds to a specific protein, catabolite regulatory protein, which binds directly to DNA and influences gene expression.[62] The analogy of this to steroid hormone action is apparent. In eukaryotic cells, cAMP binds to protein kinase A (PKA), which is a heterotetrameric molecule consisting of two regulatory subunits (R) and two catalytic subunits (C).[63] Cyclic AMP binds to the regulatory subunits and yields the following reaction:

$$4\,cAMP + R_2C_2 \rightleftharpoons R_2 \times (4\,cAMP) + 2C.$$

The $R_2C_2$ complex has no enzymatic activity, but the binding of cAMP by R dissociates R from C, thereby activating the latter. The active C subunit catalyzes the transfer of the γ-phosphate of ATP ($Mg^{2+}$) to a serine or threonine residue in various proteins. The consensus phosphorylation sites of PKA are -Arg-Arg-X-Ser- and -Lys-Arg-X-X-Ser-, in which X can be any amino acid.[64]

Protein kinase activities originally were described as cAMP dependent or cAMP independent. This area has also become considerably more complex, because protein phosphorylation is recognized as a general regulatory mechanism. Dozens of protein kinases have been described. All are unique molecules and show considerable variability with respect to subunit composition, molecular weight, autophosphorylation, $K_m$ for ATP, and substrate specificity.[65]

## PHOSPHOPROTEINS

The effects of cAMP in eukaryotic cells are thought to be mediated by protein phosphorylation and dephosphorylation.[66] The effect of cAMP, including such diverse processes as steroidogenesis, secretion, ion transport, carbohydrate and fat metabolism, enzyme induction, gene regulation, and cell growth and replication, could be conferred by a specific protein kinase, a specific phosphatase, or by specific substrates for phosphorylation. Many substrates have been identified. For example, the transcription factor, CREB, mediates many of the effects of cAMP on gene transcription.[67,68] CREB binds to the cAMP response element in the unphosphorylated state but is much more active in stimulating transcription after it has been phosphorylated by PKA.[69] Phosphorylation on serine 133 allows CREB to bind to the coactivator CBP.[46] This complex is associated with enhanced rates of transcription of target genes.

## PHOSPHODIESTERASES AND PHOSPHOPROTEIN PHOSPHATASES

Reactions caused by hormones in class IIA can be terminated in several ways, including the hydrolysis of cAMP by phosphodiesterases.[70] The presence of these hydrolytic enzymes ensures a rapid turnover of the signal (i.e., cAMP), and there is a rapid termination of the biologic process after the hormonal stimulus is removed. The cAMP phosphodiesterases exist in low- and high-$K_m$ forms and are themselves subject to regulation by hormones and by intracellular messengers such as calcium, probably acting through calmodulin.[71–73] Inhibitors of phosphodiesterase, most notably xanthine derivatives, increase intracellular cAMP and mimic or prolong the actions of hormones.

Another means of controlling hormonal action is the regulation of the protein dephosphorylation reaction. There are two classes of phosphoprotein phosphatases. One group attacks phosphate on threonine or serine residues, another attacks phosphotyrosine. The threonine or serine protein phosphatases have been divided into two groups. Type 1 enzymes dephosphorylate the β subunit of phosphorylase kinase and are inhibited by small heat- and acid-stable proteins (i.e., inhibitors 1 and 2). The type 2 enzymes dephosphorylate the α subunit of phosphorylase kinase preferentially and are insensitive to the inhibitor proteins.[74] There are a few members of each group, but there are many more protein kinases than there are phosphatases.

The regulatory role of phosphatases has been best worked out in the case of glycogen metabolism.[75] Certain phosphatases may attack specific residues; for example, some phosphatases remove phosphate from tyrosine residues.[76]

## EXTRACELLULAR CYCLIC ADENOSINE MONOPHOSPHATE

Some cAMP leaves cells and can be readily detected in extracellular fluids. The actions of glucagon on liver and of vasopressin or parathyroid hormone on the kidney are reflected in elevated levels of cAMP in plasma and urine, respectively.[77] This led to diagnostic tests of target organ responsiveness. Extracellular cAMP has little or no bioactivity in mammals, but it is an extremely important intercellular messenger in lower eukaryotes and prokaryotes.

## HORMONES THAT ACT THROUGH CYCLIC GUANOSINE MONOPHOSPHATE

Cyclic GMP is made from GTP by the enzyme guanylate cyclase, which exists in soluble and membrane-bound forms.[78–80] Each of these isozymes has unique kinetic, physiochemical, and antigenic properties. For some time, cGMP was thought to be the functional counterpart of cAMP, but it became apparent that cGMP had a unique place in hormonal action. The atriopeptins, a family of peptides produced in cardiac atrial tissues, cause natriuresis, diuresis, vasodilation, and inhibition of aldosterone secretion (see Chap. 178). These peptides, such as atrial natriuretic factor, bind to and activate the membrane-bound form of guanylate cyclase. This causes an increase of cGMP, as much as 50-fold in some cases, which is thought to mediate these effects. Other evidence links cGMP to vasodilation. A series of compounds, including nitric oxide, nitroprusside, nitroglycerin, sodium nitrite, and sodium azide, cause smooth muscle relaxation and are potent vasodilators. These agents increase cGMP by activating nitric oxide synthase, which in turn produces nitric oxide. Nitric oxide activates the soluble form of guanylate cyclase. Inhibitors of cGMP phosphodiesterase enhance and prolong these responses. The increased cGMP activates cGMP-dependent protein kinase, which phosphorylates several smooth muscle proteins, including the myosin light chain. Presumably, this is involved in relaxation of smooth muscle and vasodilation. A cGMP phosphodiesterase attenuates these responses. Sildenafil (Viagra) is a potent phosphodiesterase inhibitor. The use of this compound in erectile dysfunction is based on the fact that it prolongs the accumulation and action of cGMP on penile smooth musculature.

## HORMONES THAT ACT THROUGH CALCIUM AND PHOSPHATIDYLINOSITIDES

Ionized calcium is an important regulator of various cellular processes, including muscle contraction, stimulus-secretion coupling, the blood clotting cascade, enzyme activity, and membrane excitability. It also is an intracellular messenger of hormonal action.[81,82]

**Calcium Metabolism.** The extracellular calcium concentration is ~1.2 mM and is rigidly controlled. The intracellular free concentration of this ion ($Ca^{2+}$) is much lower, ~100 to 200 nM, and the concentration associated with intracellular organelles is in the range of 1 to 20 μM. Despite this 5000- to 10,000-fold concentration gradient and a favorable transmembrane electrical gradient, $Ca^{2+}$ is restrained from entering the cell. Resting (basal) $Ca^{2+}$ concentrations are determined by the activities of several $Ca^{2+}$ exchangers and/or $Ca^{2+}$ pumps located in the plasma membrane and endoplasmic reticulum membrane. Hormones can raise cytosolic $Ca^{2+}$ via three mechanisms: (a) activation of ligand-gated $Ca^{2+}$ channels in plasma membrane; (b) depolarization of the plasma membrane that activates inward-directed voltage-gated $Ca^{2+}$ channels in the plasma membrane; and (c) activation of phospholipase c (PLC) through a $G_q$ (G protein) mechanism, or by tyrosine phosphorylation, to generate inositol trisphosphate ($IP_3$), which stimulates release from intracellular $Ca^{2+}$ reservoirs. $Ca^{2+}$ concentrations are rapidly returned to the basal concentrations by a reversal of one or more of these mechanisms, as a sustained elevation of $Ca^{2+}$ is toxic to cells.

Two observations led to the current understanding of how $Ca^{2+}$ serves as an intracellular messenger of hormonal action. The first was the ability to quantitate the rapid changes of intracellular $Ca^{2+}$ concentration that are implicit in a role for $Ca^{2+}$ as an intracellular messenger. Such evidence was provided by various techniques, including the use of quin-2 or fura-2, fluorescent $Ca^{2+}$ chelators.[83] Rapid changes of $Ca^{2+}$ in the submicromolar range can be quantitated using these compounds. The second important observation linking $Ca^{2+}$ to hormonal action involved the definition of the intracellular targets of $Ca^{2+}$ action. The discovery of a $Ca^{2+}$-dependent regulator of phosphodiesterase activity provided the basis for understanding how $Ca^{2+}$ and cAMP interact within cells.[73]

**Calmodulin.** The major calcium-dependent regulatory protein is calmodulin, a 17-kDa protein that is homologous to

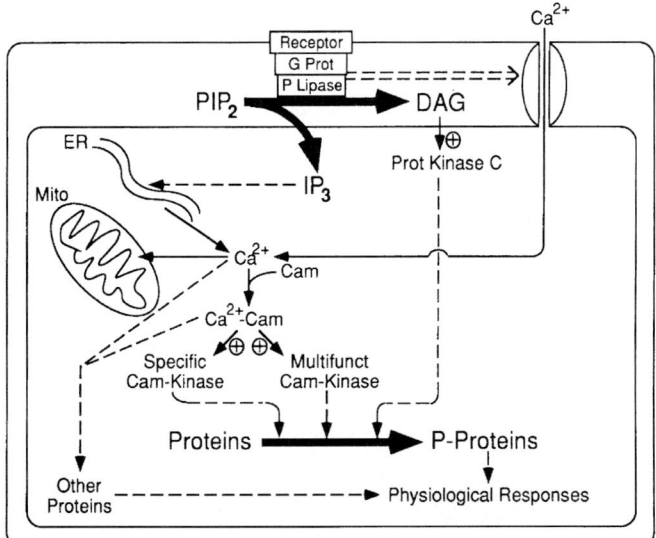

**FIGURE 4-14.** Many hormone effects are mediated by phosphatidylinositide metabolites and by ionic calcium ($Ca^{2+}$). Certain hormone-receptor interactions are coupled through a G-protein complex to a membrane-associated enzyme, phospholipase C. This enzyme catalyzes the hydrolysis of phosphatidylinositol bisphosphate ($PIP_2$) into diacylglyceride ($DAG$) and inositol triphosphate ($IP_3$). These intracellular messengers activate specific enzymes. DAG directly activates protein kinase C. $IP_3$ combines with a specific receptor on $Ca^{2+}$-containing intracellular organelles (e.g., the endoplasmic reticulum [$ER$]), releasing $Ca^{2+}$ into the cytoplasm. $Ca^{2+}$, in combination with calmodulin ($Cam$), activates enzymes such as the specific Cam-kinase and a multifunctional Cam-kinase. $Ca^{2+}$-Cam also binds to and changes the activity of a number of other proteins. (*Prot*, protein.) (Courtesy of John Exton.)

the muscle protein troponin C in structure and function.[84,85] Calmodulin has four $Ca^{2+}$-binding sites, and full occupancy of these leads to a marked conformational change of the protein. This conformational change is linked to the ability of calmodulin to activate enzymes. Calmodulin can be a constituent subunit of complex proteins. For example, it is the δ subunit of phosphorylase b kinase.[86] The interaction of $Ca^{2+}$ with calmodulin and the resultant change of activity of the latter are similar conceptually to the binding of cAMP to protein kinase and the subsequent activation of this molecule.

Calmodulin participates in regulating various protein kinases and enzymes of cyclic nucleotide generation and degradation.[86a] As shown in Figure 4-14, the $Ca^{2+}$-calmodulin complex activates specific calmodulin-dependent protein kinases and a multifunctional calmodulin-dependent protein kinase. Other enzymes are regulated directly (adenylate cyclase, cyclic nucleotide phosphodiesterase, phosphorylase kinase) or indirectly ($Ca^{2+}$/$Mg^{2+}$-ATPase, glycerol-3-phosphate dehydrogenase, glycogen synthase, guanylate cyclase, myosin kinase, nicotinamide-adenine dinucleotide (NAD) kinase, phospholipase $A_2$, pyruvate carboxylase, pyruvate dehydrogenase, and pyruvate kinase) by $Ca^{2+}$, probably through calmodulin.

Along with its effects on enzymes and ion transport, $Ca^{2+}$-calmodulin regulates the activity of many structural elements in cells. These include the actin-myosin complex of smooth muscle, which is under β-adrenergic control, and various microfilament-mediated processes in noncontractile cells, including cell motility, conformation changes, the mitotic apparatus, granule release, and endocytosis. Calcium regulates the transcription of the *FOS* gene by phosphorylating CREB, probably through the mechanism described in Figure 4-14. This is an interesting example of the convergence of two different signal transduction pathways: the cAMP system and the $Ca^{2+}$ system.[87]

**Calcium as a Mediator of Hormonal Action.** A role for ionized calcium in hormonal action is suggested by observa-

tions that the effect of many hormones is blunted in $Ca^{2+}$-free media or when intracellular calcium is depleted; can be mimicked by agents that increase cytosolic $Ca^{2+}$, such as the $Ca^{2+}$ ionophore A23187; and involves changes of cellular calcium flux. These processes have been studied in some detail in the pituitary, smooth muscle, platelets, and salivary gland, but most is known about how vasopressin and α-adrenergic catecholamines regulate glycogen metabolism in the liver.

Phosphorylase activation results from the conversion of phosphorylase b to phosphorylase a through the action of the enzyme phosphorylase b kinase. This enzyme contains calmodulin as its δ subunit, and its activity is increased through $Ca^{2+}$ concentration ranges of 0.1 to 1.0 μM. Addition of $\alpha_1$-agonists or vasopressin to isolated hepatocytes causes a threefold increase of cytosolic $Ca^{2+}$ (from 0.2 to 0.6 μM) within a few seconds. This change precedes and equals the increase in phosphorylase a activity, and the hormone concentrations required for both processes are comparable.[88,89] This effect on $Ca^{2+}$ is inhibited by $\alpha_1$-antagonists, and removal of the hormone causes a prompt decline of cytosolic $Ca^{2+}$ and phosphorylase a. The initial source of the $Ca^{2+}$ appears to be intracellular organelle reservoirs, which seem to be sufficient for the early effects of the hormones. More prolonged action appears to require enhanced influx, inhibition of $Ca^{2+}$ efflux, or both through the $Ca^{2+}$ pump. The latter may depend on concomitant increases of cAMP.

**Role of Phosphatidylinositide Metabolism in $Ca^{2+}$-Dependent Hormonal Action.** Some signal must provide communication between the hormone receptor on the plasma membrane and the intracellular $Ca^{2+}$ reservoirs. This is accomplished by the products of phosphatidylinositide metabolism.[82] Phosphatidylinositol 4,5-bisphosphate is hydrolyzed to 1,4,5-triphosphate ($IP_3$) and diacylglycerol through the action of phospholipase C (see Fig. 4-14). These two signals activate different pathways. $IP_3$ binds to a receptor on the surface of intracellular organelles that serve as $Ca^{2+}$ repositories. The binding of $IP_3$ to this receptor (which is similar to the ryanodine receptor) opens these $Ca^{2+}$ channels, and cytosolic free $Ca^{2+}$ increases.[82] $Ca^{2+}$ enters into cells from the extracellular fluid. Diacylglycerol activates protein kinase C, and this enzyme alters metabolic processes by phosphorylating various substrate proteins.

Steroidogenic agents, including ACTH and cAMP in the adrenal cortex; angiotensin II, $K^+$, serotonin, ACTH, and dibutyryl cAMP in the zona glomerulosa of the adrenal; LH in the ovary; and LH and cAMP in the Leydig cells of the testes have been associated with increased amounts of phosphatidic acid, phosphatidylinositol, and polyphosphatidylinositides in the respective target tissues.[90]

Other examples include the addition of thyrotropin-releasing hormone to pituitary cells, which is followed within 15 seconds by a marked increase of inositol degradation by phospholipase C. The intracellular levels of inositol diphosphate and triphosphate increase markedly, mobilizing intracellular calcium. This activates calcium-dependent protein kinase, which phosphorylates several proteins, one of which appears to be involved in TSH release.[91] Calcium also appears to be the intracellular mediator of gonadotropin-releasing hormone action on LH release, which probably involves calmodulin.[92]

The roles that $Ca^{2+}$ and phosphoinositide breakdown products may play in hormonal action are shown in Figure 4-14. In this scheme, the phosphoinositide products are the second messengers, and $Ca^{2+}$ is a tertiary messenger. Hormones that couple through G proteins generate signals by this mechanism, as do some hormones that initiate signal transduction by the activation of an intrinsic tyrosine kinase activity in the receptor. It is likely that several examples of the complex networking of intracellular messengers will be discovered.

## HORMONES THAT USE A KINASE OR PHOSPHATASE CASCADE AS THE INTRACELLULAR MESSENGER

This important group of hormones had been listed under the category of "intracellular mediator unknown." A major breakthrough came with the discovery that the EGF receptor contained an intrinsic tyrosine kinase activity that was activated on the binding of the ligand, EGF.[93] Shortly thereafter, the insulin and IGF-I receptors were also found to contain intrinsic, ligand-activated tyrosine kinase activity.[27,94] Several receptors, generally those involved in binding ligands involved in growth control, have intrinsic tyrosine kinase activity or associate with proteins that are tyrosine kinases.[95] Another distinguishing feature of this class of hormone action is that these kinases preferentially phosphorylate tyrosine residues, and tyrosine phosphorylation is infrequent (<0.03% of total amino acid phosphorylation) in mammalian cells.[4]

Some of the hormones, such as EGF, that activate tyrosine kinases activate phospholipase C and exert effects through $Ca^{2+}$ and $IP_3$ or diacylglycerol. Investigators have considered that tyrosine kinase activation could also initiate a phosphorylation and dephosphorylation cascade that involved the action of one or several other protein kinases and the counterbalancing actions of phosphatases. Considerable evidence supports this hypothesis. Two mechanisms are used to initiate this cascade. Some hormones—such as growth hormone, prolactin, erythropoietin, and the cytokines—initiate their action by activating tyrosine kinase, but this activity is not an integral part of the hormone receptor. The hormone-receptor interaction somehow activates cytoplasmic protein tyrosine kinases (PTKs), such as Tyk-2, Jak-1, or Jak-2.[96] These PTKs phosphorylate one or more cytoplasmic proteins, which then associate with other docking proteins through binding to Src homology 2 domains, ~100 amino acid–long segments that are referred to as SH2 domains. Further steps must be elucidated, but it is presumed that hormones of this class mediate their effects, at least in part, through a kinase cascade that is initially activated by PTK.

Activation of the intrinsic tyrosine kinase activity of the insulin receptor results in the phosphorylation of a substrate, called the *insulin receptor substrate (IRS)*, on tyrosine residues. At least four IRS proteins have been identified. Phosphorylated IRS proteins bind to the SH2-domains of a variety of proteins that presumably are directly or indirectly involved in mediating different effects of insulin. For example, the binding of IRS-2 to PI-3 kinase results in the activation of the latter, and this links insulin action to phosphoinositide metabolism and thereby to many physiologic processes, including translocation of the glucose transporter and the regulation of genes involved in metabolism. The growth-promoting effects of insulin, and of IGF-I, appear to result from the phosphorylation of IRS-1 by the insulin receptor. Phosphorylated IRS-1 binds to another SH2 domain–containing protein, GRB-2, which, in turn, activates the MAP kinase pathway. The result of this interaction is the activation of a cascade of threonine or serine kinases.[97] The exact role of the many docking proteins, kinases, and phosphatases in insulin action remains to be established. It is particularly important to link these various pathways to the well-established physiologic and biochemical actions of this hormone, and to decipher how the specificity of hormone action is achieved by the many hormones that use one or more of the components of this complex array of signaling proteins.

## REFERENCES

1. Robishaw JD, Russell DW, Harris BA, et al. Deduced primary structure of the α-subunit of the GTP-binding stimulatory protein of adenylate cyclase. Proc Natl Acad Sci U S A 1986; 83:1251.
2. Obin M, Nowell T, Taylor A. The photoreceptor G-protein transducin (Gt) is a substrate for ubiquitin-dependent proteolysis. Biochem Biophys Res Commun 1994; 200:1169.
3. Waterfield MD, Scrace GT, Whittle N, et al. Platelet-derived growth factor is structurally related to the putative transforming protein p28$^{sis}$ of simian sarcoma virus. Nature 1983; 304:35.
4. Goldstein J, Brown M, Anderson RGW, et al. Receptor-mediated endocytosis. Annu Rev Cell Biol 1985; 1:1.
5. Hunter GK, Cooper JA. Protein-tyrosine kinases. Annu Rev Biochem 1985; 54:897.
6. Sahal D, Ramachandvan J, Fujita-Yamaguchi Y. Specificity of tyrosine protein kinases of the structurally related receptors for insulin and insulin-like growth factor I: Tyr-containing synthetic polymers as specific inhibitors or substrates. Arch Biochem Biophys 1988; 260:416.
7. Spiegel AM, Levine MA, Aurbach GD. Deficiency of hormone receptor-adenylate cyclase coupling protein: basis for hormone resistance in pseudo-hypoparathyroidism. Am J Physiol 1982; 243:E37.
8. Laron Z, Kowadlo-Silbergeld A, Eshet R, Pertzelan A. Growth hormone resistance. Ann Clin Res 1980; 12:269.
9. Davies TF. Diseases of the TSH receptor. Clin Endocrinol Metab 1983; 12:79.
10. Kahn CR, Flier JS, Bar RS, et al. The syndromes of insulin resistance and acanthosis nigricans. N Engl J Med 1976; 294:739.
11. Griffin JE, Wilson JD. The syndromes of androgen resistance. N Engl J Med 1980; 302:198.
12. Landis CA, Masters SB, Spada A, et al. GTPase inhibiting mutations activate the alpha chain of $G_s$ and stimulate adenyl cyclase in human pituitary tumors. Nature 1989; 340:692.
13. Kristjansson K, Rut AR, Hewison M, et al. Two mutations in the hormone binding domain of the vitamin D receptor cause tissue resistance to 1,25-dihydroxyvitamin D. J Clin Invest 1993; 92:12.
14. Rosenthal W, Antaramian A, Gilbert S, Birnbaumer M. Nephrogenic diabetes insipidus: a $V_2$ vasopressin receptor unable to stimulate adenylyl cyclase. J Biol Chem 1993; 268:13030.
15. Butcher RW, Baird CE. Effects of prostaglandins on adenosine 3,5 monophosphate levels in fat and other tissues. J Biol Chem 1968; 243:1713.
16. Cuttitta F, Carney DN, Mulshine J, et al. Bombesin-like peptides can function as autocrine growth factors in human small cell lung cancer. Nature 1985; 316:823.
17. Evans R. The steroid and thyroid hormone receptor superfamily. Science 1988; 240:889.
18. Dufau ML, Catt KJ. Gonadotropin receptors and regulation of steroidogenesis in the testes and ovary. Vitam Horm 1978; 36:461.
19. Andreone TL, Beale EG, Bar R, Granner DK. Insulin decreases phosphoenolpyruvate carboxykinase (GTP) mRNA activity by a receptor mediated process. J Biol Chem 1982; 257:35.
20. Macquire MD, Ross EM, Gilman AG. β-Adrenergic receptor: ligand binding properties and the interaction with adenylyl cyclase. Adv Cyclic Nucleotide Res 1977; 8:1.
21. Kono T, Barham FW. The relationship between the insulin-binding capacity of fat cells and the cellular response to insulin: studies with intact and trypsin-treated cells. J Biol Chem 1971; 246:6210.
22. Samuels HH, Tomkins GM. Relation of steroid structure to enzyme induction in hepatoma tissue culture cells. J Mol Biol 1970; 52:57.
23. Benovic JL, Pike LJ, Cerione RA, et al. Phosphorylation of the mammalian β-adrenergic receptor by cyclic AMP-dependent protein kinase. J Biol Chem 1985; 260:7094.
24. Sibley DR, Benovic JL, Caron MG, Lefkowitz RJ. Phosphorylation of cell surface receptors: a mechanism for regulating signal transduction pathways. Endocr Rev 1988; 9:38.
25. Mishina M, Tobimatsu T, Imoto K, et al. Location of functional regions of acetylcholine receptor α-subunit by site-directed mutagenesis. Nature 1985; 313:364.
26. Gotti C, Frigerio F, Bolognesi M, et al. Nicotinic acetylcholine receptor: a structural model for alpha-subunit peptide 188–20, the putative binding site for cholinergic agents. FEBS Lett 1988; 228:118.
27. Kasuga M, Karlsson FA, Kahn CR. Insulin stimulates phosphorylation of the 95,000 dalton subunit of its own receptor. Science 1982; 215:185.
28. Massague J, Czech MP. The subunit structures of two distinct receptors for insulin-like growth factors I and II and their relationship to the insulin receptor. J Biol Chem 1982; 257:5038.
29. Ullrich A, Coussens L, Hayflick JS, et al. Human epidermal growth factor cDNA sequence and aberrant expression of the amplified gene in A431 epidermoid carcinoma cells. Nature 1984; 309:418.
30. Russell DW, Schneider W, Yamamoto T, et al. Domain map of the LDL receptor: sequence homology with the epidermal growth factor precursor. Cell 1984; 37:577.
31. Dohlman HG, Thorner J, Caron MG, Lefkowitz RJ. Model systems for the study of seven-transmembrane-segment receptors. Annu Rev Biochem 1991; 60:653.
32. Yamamoto KR. Steroid receptor regulated transcription of specific genes and gene networks. Annu Rev Genet 1985; 19:209.
33. Sutherland EW. An introduction. In: Robison GA, Butcher RW, Sutherland EW, eds. Cyclic AMP. New York: Academic Press, 1971:1.
34. Beato M. Gene regulation by steroid hormones. Cell 1989; 56:335.
35. Lucas PC, Granner DK. Hormone response domains in gene transcription. Annu Rev Biochem 1992; 61:1131.
36. Reynhout JK, Smith LD. Studies on the appearance and nature of a maturation-inducing factor in the cytoplasm of amphibian oocytes exposed to progesterone. Dev Biol 1974; 38:394.

37. Brock ML, Shapiro DJ. Estrogen stabilizes vitellogenin mRNA against cyto-plasmic degradation. Cell 1983; 34:207.
38. Diamond DJ, Goodman HM. Regulation of growth hormone mRNA synthesis by dexamethasone and triiodothyronine. J Mol Biol 1985; 181:41.
39. Petersen DD, Koch SR, Granner DK. 3' noncoding region of phosphoenolpyruvate carboxykinase mRNA contains a glucocorticoid-responsive mRNA stabilizing element. Proc Natl Acad Sci U S A 1989; 86:7800.
40. Hod Y, Hanson R. Cyclic AMP stabilizes the messenger RNA for phosphoenolpyruvate carboxykinase (GTP) against degradation. J Biol Chem 1988; 263:7747.
41. Firestone GL, Payvar F, Yamamoto KR. Glucocorticoid regulation of protein processing and compartmentalization. Nature 1982; 300:221.
42. Weintraub H, Groudine M. Chromosomal subunits in active genes have an altered conformation. Science 1976; 93:848.
43. Baker C, Ziff E. Promoters and heterogeneous 5' termini of the mRNAs of adenovirus serotype 2. J Mol Biol 1981; 149:189.
44. McKnight SL, Kingsbury R. Transcriptional control signals of a eucaryotic protein coding gene. Science 1982; 217:316.
45. Wang J-Ch, Stromstedt P-E, Sugiyama T, Granner DK. The phosphoenolpyruvate carboxykinase gene glucocorticoid response unit. Identification of the functional domains of accessory factors HNF3 and HNF4 and the necessity of proper alignment of their cognate binding sites. Mol Endocrinol 1999; in press. 13:604.
46. Montminy M. Transcriptional regulation by cyclic AMP. Annu Rev Biochem 1997; 66:807.
47. Torchia J, Glass C, Rosenfeld MG. Co-activators and co-repressors in the investigation of transcriptional responses. Curr Opin Cell Biol 1998; 10:373.
48. Grunstein M. Histone acetylation in chromatin structure and transcription. Nature 1997; 389:349.
49. Denton RM. Early events in insulin actions. Adv Cyclic Nucleotide Protein Phosphorylation Res 1986; 20:293.
50. Lee KAW, Masson N. Transcriptional regulation by CREB and its relatives. Biochim Biophys Acta 1993; 1174:221.
51. Hepler JR, Gilman AG. G proteins. Trends Biochem Sci 1992; 17:383.
52. Brandt DR, Ross EM. GTPase activity of the stimulatory GTP-binding regulatory protein of adenylate cyclase, G$_s$: accumulation and turnover of enzyme-nucleotide intermediates. J Biol Chem 1985; 260:266.
53. Gill DM, Meren R. ADP-ribosylation of membrane proteins catalyzed by cholera toxin: basis of the activation of adenylate cyclase. Proc Natl Acad Sci U S A 1978; 15:3050.
54. Vaughan M. Choleragen, adenylate cyclase, and ADP-ribosylation. Harvey Lect 1983; 77:43.
55. Katada T, Ui M. Direct modification of the membrane adenylate cyclase system by islet-activating protein due to ADP-ribosylation of a membrane protein. Proc Natl Acad Sci U S A 1982; 79:3129.
55a. Gether U. Uncovering molecular mechanisms involved in activation of G protein-coupled receptors. Endocr Rev 2000; 21:90.
56. Nukada T, Tanabe T, Takahashi H, et al. Primary structure of the α-subunit of bovine adenylate cyclase-inhibiting G-protein deduced from the cDNA sequence. FEBS Lett 1986; 197:305.
57. Hurley JB, Simon MI, Teplow DB, et al. Homologies between signal transducing G proteins and *RAS* gene products. Science 1984; 226:860.
58. Farfel Z, Brickman AS, Kaslow HR, et al. Defect of receptor-cyclase coupling protein in pseudohypoparathyroidism. N Engl J Med 1980; 303:237.
59. Spiegel AM, Weinstein LS, Shenker A. Abnormalities in G protein-coupled signal transduction pathways in human disease. J Clin Invest 1993; 92:1119.
60. Levine MA, Downs RW Jr, Moses AM, et al. Resistance to multiple hormones in patients with Aurbach pseudohypoparathyroidism. Am J Med 1983; 74:545.
60a. Farfel Z, Bourne HR, Iiri T. The expanding spectrum of G protein diseases. N Engl J Med 1999; 340:1012.
61. Lyons J, Landis CA, Harsh G, et al. Two G protein oncogenes in human endocrine tumors. Science 1990; 249:655.
62. De Crombrugghe B, Busby S, Buc H. Cyclic AMP receptor protein: role in transcriptional activation. Science 1984; 224:831.
63. Beavo JA, Bechtel PJ, Krebs EG. Mechanisms of control for cAMP-dependent protein kinase from skeletal muscle. Adv Cyclic Nucleotide Res 1975; 5:241.
64. Kemp BE, Graves DJ, Benjamin E, Krebs EG. Role of multiple basic residues in determining the substrate specificity of cyclic AMP-dependent protein kinase. J Biol Chem 1977; 252:4888.
65. Hunter T. A thousand and one protein kinases. Cell 1987; 50:823.
66. Kuo JF, Greengard P. Cyclic nucleotide-dependent protein kinase: IV. Widespread occurrence of adenosine 3',5'-monophosphate-dependent protein kinase in various tissues and phyla of the animal kingdom. Proc Natl Acad Sci U S A 1969; 64:1349.
67. Montminy MR, Bilezikjian ML. Binding of a nuclear protein to the cyclic-AMP response element of the somatostatin gene. Nature 1987; 328:175.
68. Hoeffler JP, Meyer TE, Yun Y, et al. Cyclic AMP-responsive DNA-binding protein: structure based on a cloned placental cDNA. Science 1988; 242:1430.
69. Quinn PG, Granner DK. Cyclic AMP-dependent protein kinase regulates transcription of the phosphoenolpyruvate carboxykinase gene but not binding of nuclear factors to the cyclic AMP regulatory element. Mol Cell Biol 1990; 10:3357.
70. Wells JN, Hardman JG. Cyclic nucleotide phosphodiesterases. Adv Cyclic Nucleotide Res 1977; 8:119.
71. Strada SJ, Thompson JW. Multiple forms of cyclic nucleotide phosphodiesterases: anomalies or biologic regulators. Adv Cyclic Nucleotide Res 1977; 9:265.
72. Francis SH, Kono T. Hormone-sensitive cAMP phosphodiesterase in liver and fat cells. Mol Cell Biol 1982; 42:109.
73. Cheung WY, Lynch TJ, Wallace RW. An endogenous Ca$^{2+}$-dependent activator protein of brain adenylate cyclase and cyclic nucleotide phosphodiesterase. Adv Cyclic Nucleotide Res 1977; 9:233.
74. Cohen P. The structure and regulation of protein phosphatases. Annu Rev Biochem 1989; 58:453.
75. Dent P, Lavoinne A, Nakielny S, et al. The molecular mechanism by which insulin stimulates glycogen synthesis in mammalian skeletal muscle. Nature 1990; 348:302.
76. Walton KM, Dixon JE. Protein tyrosine phosphatases. Annu Rev Biochem 1993; 62:101.
77. Chase LR, Aurbach GD. Parathyroid function and the renal excretion of 3' adenylic acid. Proc Natl Acad Sci U S A 1967; 58:518.
78. Murad F, Mittal CK, Arnold WP, et al. Guanylate cyclase: activation by azide, nitro compounds, nitric oxide, hydroxyl radical and inhibition by hemoglobin and myoglobin. Adv Cyclic Nucleotide Res 1978; 9:145.
79. Takio K, Wade RD, Smith SF, et al. Guanosine cyclic 3,5 phosphate dependent protein kinase: a chimeric protein homologous with two separate protein families. Biochemistry 1984; 23:4207.
80. Chinkers M, Garbers DL. Signal transduction by guanylyl cyclases. Annu Rev Biochem 1991; 60:553.
81. Rasmussen H. The calcium messenger system. N Engl J Med 1986; 314:1094.
82. Berridge M. Inositol triphosphate and calcium signaling. Nature 1993; 361:315.
83. Tsien RY, Rink TJ, Poenie M. Measurement of cytosolic free Ca$^{2+}$ in individual cells using fluorescence microscopy with dual excitation wavelengths. Cell Calcium 1985; 6:145.
84. Watterson DM, Sharief F, Vanaman TC. The complete amino acid sequence of the Ca$^{2+}$-dependent modulator protein (calmodulin) of bovine brain. J Biol Chem 1980; 255:962.
85. Means AR, Chafouleas JG. Calmodulin in endocrine cells. Annu Rev Physiol 1982; 44:667.
86. Cohen P, Burchell A, Foulkes JG, et al. Identification of the Ca$^{2+}$-dependent modulatory protein as the fourth subunit of rabbit skeletal muscle phosphorylase kinase. FEBS Lett 1978; 92:287.
86a. Means AR. Regulatory cascades involving calmodulin-dependent protein kinases. Mol Endocrinol 2000; 14:4.
87. Sheng M, Thompson MA, Greenberg ME. CREB: a Ca(2+)-regulated transcription factor phosphorylated by calmodulin-dependent kinases. Science 1991; 252:1427.
88. Williamson JR, Cooper RH, Hoek JB. Role of calcium in the hormonal regulation of liver metabolism. Biochim Biophys Acta 1981; 639:243.
89. Blackmore PF, Hughes BP, Charest R, et al. Time course of α$_1$-adrenergic and vasopressin actions on phosphorylase activation: calcium efflux, pyridine nucleotide reduction, and respiration in hepatocytes. J Biol Chem 1982; 258:10488.
90. Farese RV. The role of the phosphatidate-phosphoinositide cycle in the action of steroidogenic hormones. Endocr Res 1985; 10:515.
91. Kolesnick RN, Musacchio I, Thaw C, Gershengorn MD. Thyrotropin (TSH)-releasing hormone decreases phosphatidylinositol and increases unesterified arachidonic acid in thyrotropic cells: possible early events in stimulation of TSH secretion. Endocrinology 1984; 114:671.
92. Conn PM, Staley D, Jinnah H, Bates M. Molecular mechanism of gonadotropin releasing hormone action. J Steroid Biochem 1985; 23:703.
93. Staros JV, Cohen S, Russo MW. Epidermal growth factor receptor: characterization of its protein kinase activity. In: Cohen P, Housley MD, eds. Molecular mechanism of transmembrane signaling. New York: Elsevier Science Publishing, 1985:253.
94. Ullrich A, Bell JA, Chen EY, et al. Human insulin receptor and its relationship to the tyrosine kinase family of oncogenes. Nature 1985; 313:756.
95. Fantl WJ, Johnson DE, Williams LT. Signaling by receptor tyrosine kinases. Annu Rev Biochem 1993; 62:453.
96. Argetsinger LS, Campbell GS, Yang X, et al. Identification of JAK2 as a growth hormone receptor-associated tyrosine kinase. Cell 1993; 74:237.
97. Cheatum B, Kahn CR. Insulin action and the insulin signaling network. Endocr Rev 1995; 16:117.

# CHAPTER 5

# FEEDBACK CONTROL IN ENDOCRINE SYSTEMS

DANIEL N. DARLINGTON AND MARY F. DALLMAN

The function of endocrine systems is *to maintain homeostasis of the organism and to perpetuate the species.* Homeostasis is maintained by the continual adjustment of nervous and endocrine systems in response to a changing environment. Because most endocrine systems are intimately related to the central nervous system and the autonomic nervous system (see Chaps. 8, 9, and 85), a *continual bidirectional flow of information*—one relaying the conditions in the organism, and the other directing neural and endocrine responses—is present and functions to maintain appropriate operating conditions.

To produce stable systems, it has been useful to apply the knowledge gained from the engineering discipline to physiologic control systems. The quantitative relations among system components in engineering and the mathematical description of these have been useful in describing biologic control systems.[1] The notion of a setpoint reference signal, which can be explicitly delineated in an engineered system, is, in most biologic systems, an apparent setpoint, deduced by the behavior of the system, and probably normally arises from the interaction of a hormone or metabolite with receptors and cellular function.

## FEEDBACK

### DEFINITION

*Feedback* is a process within a system that occurs when *the product or result of activity in the system modifies the factors that produce that product or result.* The result can modify these factors in either of two ways: (a) by stimulating the factors to generate more product (*positive feedback*), or (b) by inhibiting the factors so that fewer products are generated (*negative feedback*).

Mammalian organisms are composed of many feedback systems. Each system has its own specific function and is self-regulating. However, all of the systems are interconnected, making the overall system extremely complex. Usually, negative feedback is used to maintain a variable within a range that is advantageous for optimal cellular function. When an internal or external stimulus perturbs a regulated variable, neural or endocrine responses (or both) occur that counteract the disturbance and return the variable to within its normal range. Such performance requires a means to determine the level of activity or the concentration of the variable that is regulated.

### COMPONENTS

The components of a simple endocrine feedback system are shown in Figure 5-1. A *variable* is monitored by a *receptor* that is sensitive to changes in that variable. The receptor is connected to a structure or structures that process and integrate the signal generated by alterations in the variable. The *signal processor* includes a reference setpoint and a comparator element that compares the receptor input with the reference signal. The difference between input from the receptor and the setpoint is generated by the comparator, and the resulting error signal then modifies the existing activity of the effector endocrine gland. If the error signal is positive, the effector gland is stimulated to secrete, and the concentration of hormone in the circulation increases to levels that are adequate to effect the

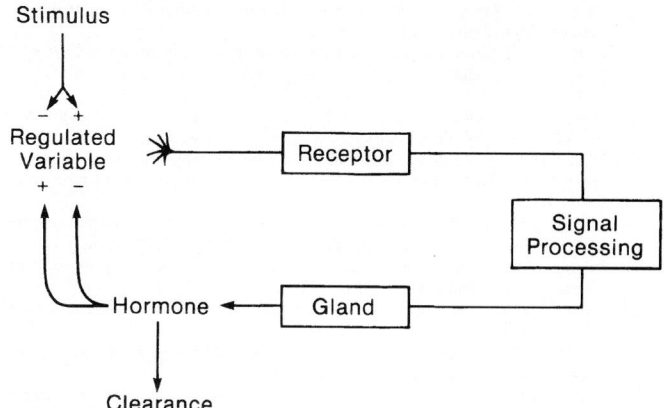

**FIGURE 5-1.** Model for a simple endocrine feedback system consisting of a variable being monitored by a receptor, a signal processor that analyzes the signal, and an endocrine gland with a secretion rate that is regulated by the processor. The concentration of free hormone in the circulation depends on the clearance of the hormone and the presence and concentration of specific binding protein in the circulation. Any change in the variable is sensed, and a response (hormone) is elicited to bring the variable back within its "normal" range.

normalization of the perturbed regulated variable. Because many hormones are secreted into the circulation, the concentration of hormone achieved is affected by the rate of clearance and by the amount of hormone that is bound in the plasma compartment by a specific carrier protein (i.e., only the free, unbound hormone is available to cellular receptors).

## LOCALIZATION OF COMPONENTS

The receptor, processing unit, and endocrine gland may all reside within a single cell or in a group of similar cells functioning in concert, or they may involve entirely separate and widely dispersed units. For example, the B cell (β cell, insulin-producing) of the pancreas is directly sensitive to changes in extracellular glucose concentration (see Chap. 134). An increase in blood glucose is thus sensed by the B cell and increases the rate of insulin synthesis and secretion. The increased concentration of insulin causes increased glucose transport into those cells that contain insulin receptors and a reduction in blood glucose concentration. The normalization of glucose concentration eliminates the stimulus to the B cell.

Arterial blood pressure is monitored by mechanoreceptors in the carotid artery and aortic arch. The central nervous system processes and integrates afferent information from the mechanoreceptors. The autonomic nervous and various endocrine systems represent the "gland" that secretes norepinephrine and various hormones; when there is a marked decrease in arterial pressure, the release of these hormones effectively restores arterial blood pressure to normal.

## AMPLIFICATION OF OUTPUT

All feedback systems amplify their outputs (glandular secretions) to correct for the effects of perturbations. The effectiveness of this amplification in maintaining a regulated variable within the normal range is termed the *gain* of the system. The gain of a system is determined by comparing the magnitude of excursion of a regulated variable under conditions in which the feedback loop is abolished with the magnitude of excursion under conditions in which the feedback loop is intact.

Figure 5-2 shows a theoretical situation in which the control of glucose is examined. At the moment of onset of the glucose infusion, the pancreatic B cells are either removed from the system or left intact. In the absence of the B cells, insulin secretion would not occur, and the blood glucose concentration would

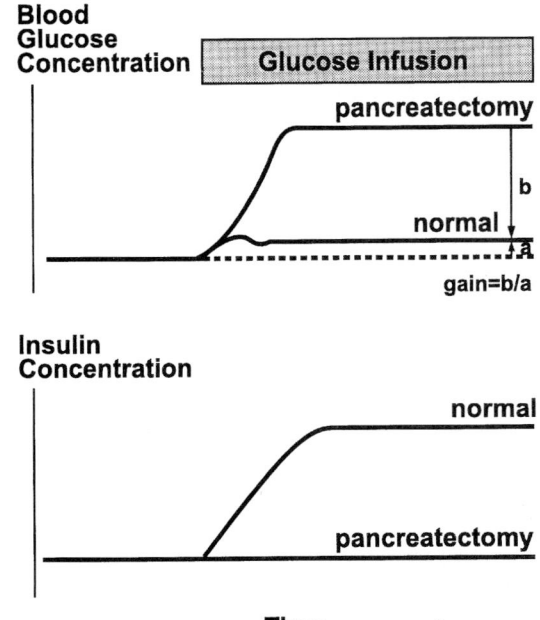

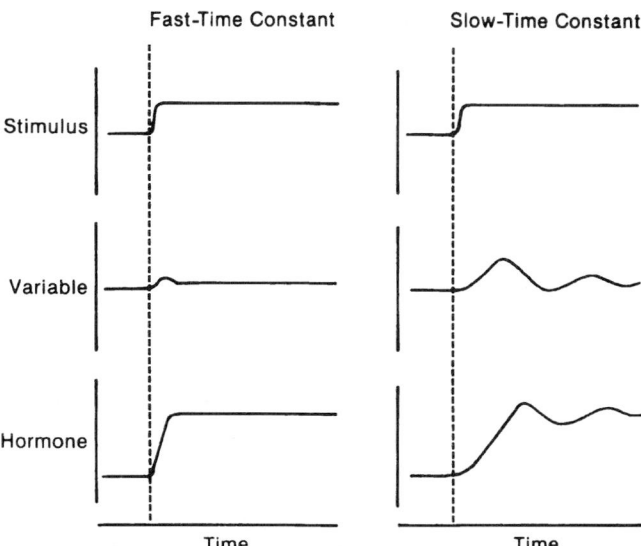

**FIGURE 5-3.** Comparison of the effectiveness of feedback systems (hypothetical) with fast- and slow-time constants. Notice that for the same stimulus, the feedback system with the fast-time constant regulates the variable near normal levels and does not overshoot or undershoot as does the feedback system with the slow-time constant.

**FIGURE 5-2.** Gain in an endocrine feedback system. The diagram shows the (hypothetical) blood glucose (*top*) and insulin (*bottom*) concentrations before and during infusion of glucose. The gain is defined as the ratio of the difference between the responses (perturbed glucose levels) of the open-loop and closed-loop conditions (*arrow b*) and the difference between the response of the closed-loop glucose and the pre-infusion levels (*arrow a*). The gain is an index of feedback loop effectiveness. (Redrawn from Guyton AC. Textbook of medical physiology, 5th ed. Philadelphia: WB Saunders, 1976.)

increase because of the glucose infusion in proportion to the infusion rate. The steady-state glucose concentration would be determined by the volume into which glucose is distributed and the rate at which glucose is lost from that volume of distribution in the absence of insulin. With the B cells of the pancreas in the system (i.e., under closed-loop conditions), the infusion-induced increase in blood glucose concentration would increase the concentration of glucose bathing the pancreatic B cell and cause secretion of insulin. The elevated insulin concentration activates increased target cell uptake of glucose, lowering the circulating glucose levels. Glucose concentration in the open-loop condition increases well above the normal range; whereas under closed-loop control, glucose concentration is maintained close to the normal range.

The error in the regulation of blood glucose is the difference between the preinfusion value (see Fig. 5-2, dotted line) and the new level (see Fig. 5-2, arrow a). The degree by which the variable (glucose) is controlled is the difference between the open-loop glucose concentration and the closed-loop glucose concentration (see Fig. 5-2, arrow b). The gain of the system can then be calculated as the ratio between arrow b and arrow a.[2] In this example, the difference between the open-loop and closed-loop response is 10 units, and the difference between the closed-loop response and preinfusion levels is 2 units. The gain of this system is, therefore, 10/2, or 5 (usually denoted as a negative number to show normalization). Thus, for each unit increase of the controlled variable under closed-loop conditions, there would be a five-fold change if the feedback loop were open.

## TIME CONSTANTS

The effectiveness of feedback can also be described in terms of the time elapsed between the onset of the stimulus (the change in the regulated variable) and the effect of the system response. This is a function of the time constant of each component of the feedback loop. In a multicomponent feedback system, the component with the slowest time constant determines the delay time between stimulus and response (time constant of the system). Figure 5-3 compares the imagined performance of two systems, one with a fast-time constant (left) and the other with a slow-time constant (right). Time constants may clarify the requirement for the hierarchical feedback loops that are so commonly encountered in biologic systems.

The time constants for transmission of neural information are in the milliseconds to seconds range. Peptide and protein hormones, acting on receptors in the plasma membrane to alter intracellular concentrations of a second messenger, exert many of their primary effects on cellular function over the range of seconds to minutes. Still slower, in hours, are the effects of steroid and thyroid hormones, which are mediated by alterations in the rate of gene transcription and translation, and of protein synthesis. Interestingly, those hormones with the longest time constants (adrenal and gonadal steroids, hepatic somatomedins) are secreted by glands controlled by other hormones with faster time constants, and these systems exhibit high-gain feedback control. Moreover, the feedback inhibition exerted by these hormones with characteristically slow target effects may be mediated by mechanisms with faster time constants than those of their target effects. Thus, the overall performance of a relatively slow system may appear tighter than anticipated and more like that of a system with an overall fast-time constant.

For instance, the secretion of glucocorticoids is regulated by a cascade system in which corticotropin-releasing hormone (CRH), secreted from the median eminence of the hypothalamus in response to appropriate stimulation, acts on corticotropes in the anterior pituitary to cause synthesis and secretion of adrenocorticotropic hormone (ACTH). ACTH, likewise, acts on the zona fasciculata cells of the adrenal cortex to stimulate the synthesis and secretion of cortisol and corticosterone (see Chap. 14). The initiation of a stimulus to CRH until a rise in circulating concentration of cortisol or corticosterone occurs requires <5 minutes. The minimum time required for cortisol to increase gluconeogenesis, enabling increased hepatic glucose secretion, may be ~2 hours. If insulin-induced hypoglycemia were the stimulus that provoked CRH secretion, return of the extracellular glucose concentration to normal would relieve the stimulus to CRH. However, in the absence of a more rapid cortisol feedback effect on the hypothalamic CRH-secreting cells and on the corticotrope cells that secrete ACTH, there would clearly be an overshoot in the amount of cortisol secreted in response to the stimulus of hypoglycemia because of the lag time between the elevated concentrations of cortisol in the circulation and the effect of these elevated levels on peripheral target cells. The direct feedback effects of cortisol, the other steroid hormones, and thyroid hormones on their trophic hormonal controllers allow tighter control of these systems.

## LOADS ON ENDOCRINE SYSTEMS

Endocrine systems have the ability to restore homeostasis in response to varying degrees of perturbation. The load on the system is the degree or strength of the perturbation. In response to the perturbation, the endocrine system adjusts the amount of "free" circulating hormone in an attempt to regain homeostasis. The amount of free circulating hormone (or hormonal load) is dependent on the secretion and clearance rates of the hormone, and the production and clearance rates of the specific hormone-binding proteins. Newly secreted free hormone is immediately accessible to clearance from the circulation by metabolism in liver, kidney, and other tissues, and by filtration and excretion by the kidney. Moreover, many hormones are bound in the circulation by high-affinity specific binding globulins. The "bound" hormone is unavailable for diffusion into the interstitial fluid and cannot affect the target organ or tissue. However, the bound and free hormone exists in an equilibrium in plasma such that as free hormone is cleared, bound hormone becomes free. Bound hormone acts as a storage of free hormone. If, for any reason, the rate of metabolism or clearance changes, or if the production or clearance rates of its specific binding hormone changes, then the input signal to the endocrine gland that is producing the hormone must change to accommodate the change in load of free hormone.

## EXAMPLES OF FEEDBACK IN ENDOCRINE SYSTEMS

Importantly, our current state of knowledge does not allow us to apply all these principles to most endocrine systems. Nonetheless, there is plentiful evidence for the existence of feedback regulation in all endocrine systems. Knowledge of this feedback has been used in the design and interpretation of many clinical tests for the determination of endocrine disorders.

### HYPOTHALAMIC–PITUITARY–TARGET ENDOCRINE FEEDBACK

#### LONG-LOOP FEEDBACK

One of the most clinically obvious and simplest forms of negative feedback control in endocrine systems involves suppression of the secretion of a trophic factor (or hormone) by the hormone it stimulates. For example, hormone A stimulates the secretion of hormone B, which in turn suppresses the secretion of hormone A. Hormone B may suppress the secretion of hormone A by acting directly on the cells that secrete A, or indirectly, by acting on the cells (or neurons) that stimulate the secretion of A. This type of control is exemplified in the relations between the hypothalamus, anterior pituitary gland, and peripheral endocrine glands controlled by pituitary hormones. The hypothalamus secretes neurohormones that stimulate (or inhibit) the secretion of specific anterior pituitary hormones, which in turn stimulate a peripheral target gland to secrete hormone and, with sufficient stimulation, to grow (see Chaps. 8 and 9).

In Figure 5-4, CRH-containing neurons in the hypothalamus release CRH into the hypophysial portal system.[3] ACTH released from corticotropes in response to CRH stimulates cor-

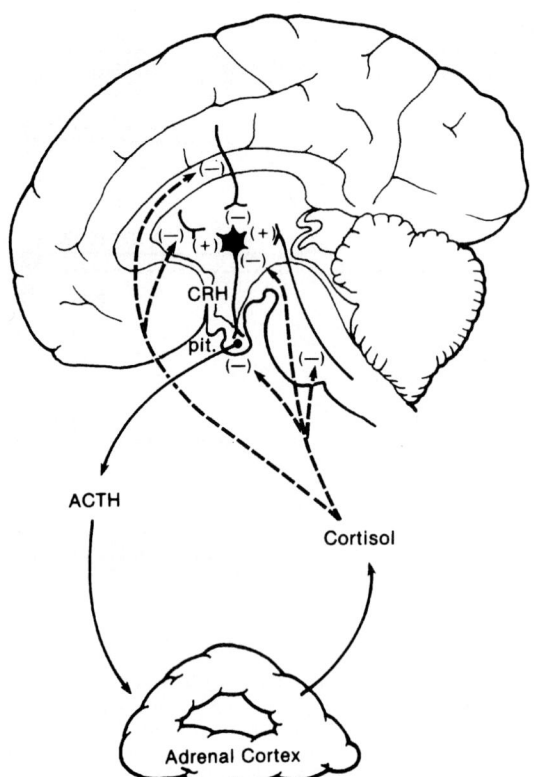

**FIGURE 5-4.** Simplified feedback loop in the hypothalamic–pituitary–adrenal cortical system. (*ACTH*, adrenocorticotropin hormone; *CRH*, corticotropin-releasing hormone; *pit.*, pituitary.) The *dotted arrows* show the sites of feedback by cortisol.

tisol synthesis and secretion from the adrenal cortex. Cortisol acts to inhibit the secretion of ACTH from the corticotrope and to inhibit CRH secretion from the hypothalamic neuron, and it may also act on extrahypothalamic sites that regulate CRH synthesis and secretion.[4,5] Clinically, the feedback effects of cortisol are important. Long-term therapy with pharmacologic amounts of glucocorticoids suppresses ACTH secretion to the extent that the adrenal cortices atrophy and become unresponsive to ACTH. The atrophic adrenal cortex does not secrete normal quantities of cortisol, and the abrupt discontinuation of exogenous glucocorticoids may lead to a patient who displays all the signs of cortisol deficiency (see Chaps. 76 and 78).

The feedback effects of cortisol on ACTH release is an example of long-loop feedback: secretion of the peripheral gland affecting the secretion of the pituitary trophic hormone. Long-loop feedback occurs in most of the anterior pituitary hormone systems and is most apparent when the capacity for hormone synthesis or secretion in the peripheral target gland is compromised or abolished. The magnitude of the effects of inhibiting or removing the long-loop feedback signal on circulating concentrations of the appropriate pituitary trophic hormone (i.e., the effects of opening the feedback loop) is large. The dramatic increases in the circulating concentrations of the pituitary trophic hormone that occur under conditions in which there is an abnormally low feedback signal from the target endocrine gland are useful clinically in *distinguishing between a primary and a secondary disturbance* in an endocrine system. For instance, hypothyroidism could arise from a primary disturbance in the synthesis of thyroxine in the thyroid gland, or it could result from lack of stimulation of the thyroid gland by thyrotropin (thyroid-stimulating hormone [TSH]). In both cases, circulating thyroxine concentrations would be low; if the defect were due to a primary thyroidal disturbance, TSH concentrations would be high, whereas if the defect were due to lack of TSH secretion, circulating concentrations would be low.

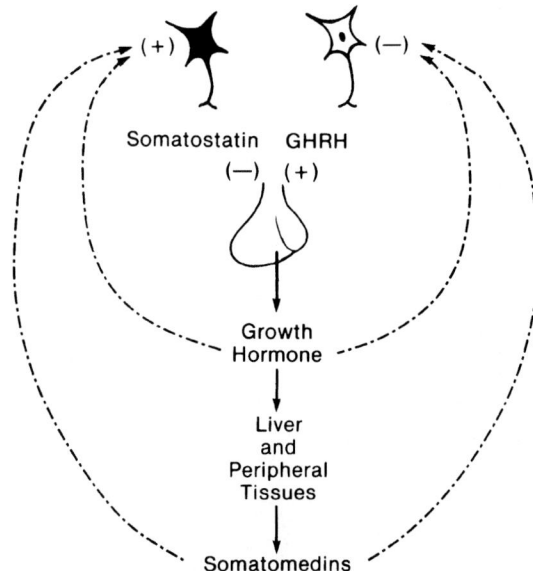

**FIGURE 5-5.** Long- and short-loop feedback. Neurons in the hypothalamus release somatostatin and growth hormone–releasing hormone (*GHRH*) into the circulation that bathe the growth hormone–secreting cell (somatotrope). Growth hormone stimulates somatomedin C formation in peripheral tissues. Both growth hormone and somatomedins act at the level of the hypothalamus to inhibit growth hormone release.

## SHORT-LOOP FEEDBACK

Evidence also exists for short-loop inhibition of secretion of hypothalamic-releasing hormones by the trophic hormones of the anterior pituitary. For example, growth hormone secreted by somatotropes in the anterior pituitary stimulates secretion of insulin-like growth factors from the liver and other peripheral tissues (see Chaps. 12 and 173). The somatomedins exhibit long-loop feedback on growth hormone secretion. However, growth hormone has an effect on the hypothalamic-releasing and release-inhibiting hormones that regulate its secretion (Fig. 5-5). There is evidence suggesting that this feedback can occur either by inhibiting the secretion of growth hormone–releasing hormone or by stimulating the secretion of growth hormone–inhibiting hormone (somatostatin) into the hypophysial portal circulation.[6,7] There is growing evidence that similar short-loop feedback circuits exist for the other hypophysial hormones. Quantitatively, these appear to be less important than the long-loop feedback, and they may serve as a fine-tuning system within the central nervous system.

## ULTRASHORT-LOOP FEEDBACK

Ultrashort-loop feedback is suspected to occur when a hormone acts on its own cell type to inhibit further secretion of itself. There is little evidence for this phenomenon; however, it could be of considerable importance in the regulation of secretion of posterior pituitary hormones. In the hypothalamus, collateral axons of oxytocin and vasopressin neurons make contact with other oxytocin and vasopressin neurons.[8,9] These cell–cell interactions could help to sharpen and synchronize the secretion of hormone in a given cell type. In the anterior pituitary, vasoactive intestinal peptide (VIP) stimulates secretion of prolactin from lactotropes. However, this effect may be autocrine/paracrine in nature, because lactotropes express and secrete both VIP and prolactin into the extracellular fluid (Fig. 5-6). Thus, VIP can then stimulate secretion of VIP/prolactin from its own or neighboring lactotropes.[10–12]

## FEEDBACK EFFECTS ON AMPLITUDE AND PULSE FREQUENCY: THE GONADOTROPIN SYSTEM

Many, and perhaps most, anterior pituitary hormones are secreted in a pulsatile manner (i.e., surges in secretion occur at

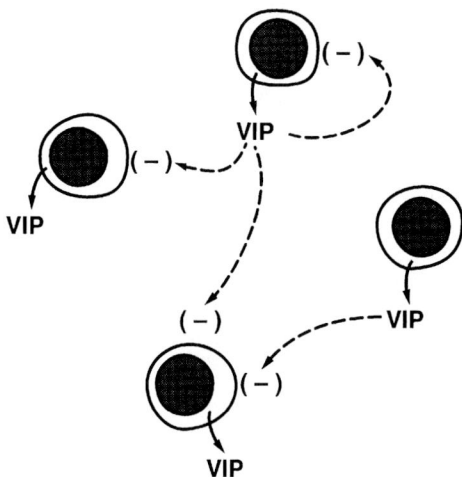

**FIGURE 5-6.** Ultrashort-loop feedback. Vasoactive intestinal peptide (*VIP*) is secreted from lactotropes with prolactin in the anterior pituitary. VIP can stimulate further secretion of VIP/prolactin from the same cell or from neighboring lactotropes (autocrine and paracrine).

regular intervals). Evidence suggests that this arises from synchronous bursts of activity in hypothalamic neurons that secrete the appropriate releasing factors. The gonadal endocrine system has been best studied from this point of view. The gonadotropin-releasing hormone (GnRH) is released in bursts that appear to drive secretion of luteinizing hormone (LH) in episodes (see Chap. 16). In humans and in subhuman primates, GnRH and LH concentrations in hypophysial and systemic blood demonstrate cycles with periods of 2 to 4 hours. LH stimulates testosterone secretion in men and ovulation, luteal formation, and estrogen and progesterone secretion in women.

## NEGATIVE FEEDBACK BY SEX STEROIDS

Testosterone, estrogen, and progesterone exert long-loop feedback on the cycle amplitude and frequency of GnRH and LH. Testosterone and progesterone decrease the frequency and amplitude of the GnRH cycles and thus lower the mean concentration of LH in the circulation. The absence of both hormones leads to acceleration of the cycle frequency and amplitude. The effects of estradiol are complex. Low concentrations of estradiol or high concentrations of estradiol in the presence of progesterone inhibit both the frequency and amplitude of LH secretory pulses, thus decreasing both minimum and maximum concentrations of LH in the circulation.[13,13a,14]

## POSITIVE FEEDBACK BY SEX STEROIDS

Conversely, during the late follicular phase of the menstrual cycle, high concentrations of unopposed estradiol increase pulse frequency and pulse amplitude of LH.[13] Thus, a single hormone (estradiol) exerts either negative or positive effects on its trophic hormone, depending on the duration, concentration, and conditions of exposure. The unstable behavior of the gonadal system in this example of positive feedback is characteristic of positive feedback systems. The positive effect of estradiol leads to increasingly frequent and large pulses of LH that in turn lead to increasing secretion of estradiol until the system becomes too unstable to exist, and ovulation occurs. Because the ovum-containing follicle was the primary source of estradiol-secreting granulosa cells, ovulation disrupts the system, and the whole process can begin again (see Chaps. 94 and 95).

## PARTURITION AND SUCKLING

The female reproductive system provides two other good examples of positive feedback: parturition- and suckling-induced oxytocin secretion. In both of these examples, there is a neuroendocrine control loop. In the former, stretch receptors in the uterine cervix are stimulated by presentation of the infant's head; the receptors, in turn, activate neural pathways in the spinal cord and the brainstem that cause secretion of oxytocin from the posterior pituitary. Oxytocin interacts with receptors on the uterine myometrium to cause uterine contraction and further stretch of the uterine cervix. The positive feedback cycle is ended with delivery of the baby and cessation of uterine stretch (see Chaps. 25 and 109). With suckling, stimulation of the nipple activates stretch receptors in the nipples that stimulate spinal cord and brainstem pathways to oxytocin secretion. Oxytocin then causes myoepithelial cell contraction in milk ducts of the breast and milk letdown. The cycle is interrupted when suckling stops (see Chaps. 25 and 106).

## REGULATED VARIABLES

All controlled variables of an organism are *monitored* by receptors and processors that ensure that the variables are maintained within a relatively narrow normal range. When an internal or external stimulus changes or perturbs a regulated variable, the change is sensed and corrected by the nervous and endocrine systems. Some examples of variables that are regulated largely by activity in the autonomic nervous system and by hormones include blood pressure, blood oxygen and carbon dioxide tension, extracellular fluid volume, tissue substrates, metabolites and ions, the composition of filtrate in the kidney tubules, blood flow to different vascular beds, and enzyme production by exocrine glands. All of these variables are regulated by the feedback arrangement described earlier (see Fig. 5-1). Each variable is monitored by a sense organ that is connected to an information processor that controls neural or glandular secretion. The sense organ can be a modified structure that is (a) connected to the central nervous system, (b) connected to the gland, or (c) an integral part of the endocrine effector cell. The effector organ can be an endocrine gland (adrenal cortex, pancreas) or an autonomic postganglionic nerve terminal. When the concentration or level of function of a regulated variable is perturbed, a neural or hormonal response occurs that rectifies the perturbation.

## ENDOCRINE CELLS AS RECEPTORS AND EFFECTORS

Some blood-borne agents (nonhormonal) have profound effects on the secretion of certain endocrine gland cells. The action of glucose on the pancreatic B cell was mentioned earlier. The overall effect of glucose-stimulated insulin secretion is to reduce elevated blood glucose levels to the normal range by removing glucose from the blood and facilitating storage in other tissues. Clearly, the action of insulin reduces the stimulus to its secretion. Another example of this kind is the direct effect of potassium on aldosterone secretion from cells of the adrenal zona glomerulosa (see Chap. 79). Small increases in the extracellular fluid concentration of potassium increase aldosterone synthesis and secretion. Aldosterone facilitates secretion of potassium by cells of the distal tubule of the kidney, thus reducing the extracellular fluid concentration of this cation.[15] This type of feedback regulation also exists for gastrointestinal secretions. The gut hormones are secreted from polarized cells in the intestine that are stimulated by gut contents on the luminal surface and that secrete hormones from the basal surface.

Examples also can be given of direct stimulation of one endocrine gland that causes recruitment of another hormonal system. The chief cells of the parathyroid glands are directly sensitive to the concentration of ionized calcium in the extracellular fluid (Fig. 5-7; see Chap. 51). If the plasma concentration of ionized calcium decreases, the chief cells respond to the decrease in calcium with an increased rate of secretion of parathyroid hormone. Parathyroid hormone facilitates calcium

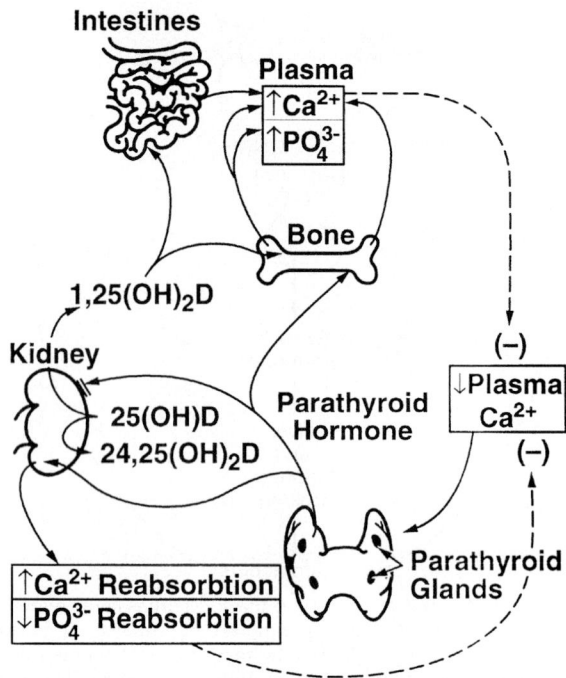

**FIGURE 5-7.** Feedback regulation of plasma calcium levels. A decrease in extracellular fluid ionized calcium concentration ($Ca^{2+}$) stimulates the release of parathyroid hormone phosphate acts to increase plasma calcium by facilitating calcium reabsorption from kidney, calcium release from bone, and formation of 1,25-dihydroxycholecalciferol (*1,25[OH]$_2$D*) from 25-hydroxycholecalciferol (*25[OH]D*). (It also attenuates formation of the inactive form of the hormone, 24,25-dihydroxycholecalciferol [*24,25(OH)$_2$D*].) 1,25(OH)$_2$D increases calcium release from bone and the intestinal absorption of calcium. The dotted lines show the restitution of plasma calcium concentration.

reabsorption by the renal tubules and increases the release of calcium from bone. This hormone also facilitates the formation of 1,25-dihydroxycholecalciferol.[16] This vitamin D metabolite further facilitates calcium release from bone and increases intestinal absorption of calcium (see Chap. 54). Although the regulation of the ionized calcium concentration in plasma is more complex than described here (see Chap. 49), this exemplifies how hormonal systems can be recruited for regulation of a variable.

## RECEPTORS IN PROXIMITY TO THE ENDOCRINE GLAND

Endocrine tissue may modify its hormonal secretory rate as a regulated variable changes but may not actually sense the change itself. For example, the macula densa comprises a specialized cell type that senses sodium or chloride transport from the distal tubular filtrate of the kidney (Fig. 5-8). The macula densa is adjacent to the juxtaglomerular cells in the afferent arterioles entering the Bowman capsule. A fall in plasma sodium concentration is reflected in the sodium concentration in the tubular ultrafiltrate. A decrease in sodium delivery to the distal tubule is sensed by the macula densa cells. The macula densa stimulates the juxtaglomerular cells to secrete renin.[17] Renin, released into the general circulation, cleaves the terminal 10 amino acids from angiotensinogen, producing angiotensin I. Angiotensin I is converted in the circulation (particularly as it passes through the pulmonary vascular bed) to angiotensin II. Angiotensin II stimulates the secretion of aldosterone from the cells of the adrenal zona glomerulosa, and the effect is the stimulation of sodium reabsorption and potassium and hydrogen excretion in the renal distal tubule.[15] The net movement of sodium into the extracellular fluid compartment increases the

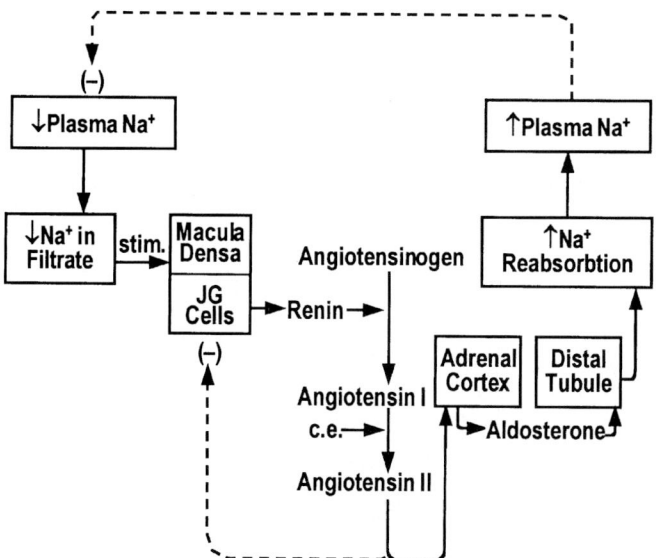

**FIGURE 5-8.** Feedback regulation of plasma sodium levels and the existence of two feedback loops in the system (*dotted lines*). As plasma sodium [*Na⁺*] falls, the macula densa in the renal distal tubule senses the sodium fall in the filtrate and stimulates renin release from the juxtaglomerular (*JG*) cells. Renin enzymatically converts angiotensinogen (in the blood) into angiotensin I. Angiotensin I is enzymatically converted to angiotensin II, which stimulates aldosterone release. Aldosterone facilitates sodium reabsorption from the distal tubules, which leads to an increase in plasma sodium. (*c.e.,* converting enzyme; *stim.,* stimulates.)

plasma sodium concentration and relieves the stimulus to renin secretion.

The regulation of renin secretion, however, involves two feedback loops. Aldosterone facilitates sodium reabsorption and thus removes the initial stimulus to renin secretion; however, angiotensin II also directly inhibits renin secretion from the juxtaglomerular cells (see Fig. 5-8). Again, as with the hypothalamic–pituitary target gland cascades, the hormonal feedback may serve to inhibit the system more rapidly than would occur with the full restitution of plasma sodium concentration, thus preventing excessive secretion of aldosterone and gaining greater efficiency of the system (see Chaps. 79 and 183).

## RECEPTORS THAT CAN INITIATE MULTISYSTEM RESPONSES

Multisystem control involves specialized receptor organs that are directly connected to or embedded in central components of the autonomic nervous system. Organizationally, the autonomic pathways in the medulla, pons, midbrain, and hypothalamus constitute this central system. Afferent input is provided from chemoreceptors, high- and low-pressure baroreceptors, and other peripheral receptors by way of the spinal cord and cranial nerves. Chemosensitive structures exist in the brain and include the circumventricular organs, glucose receptors and osmoreceptors in the hypothalamus, medullary cells that are sensitive to pH, and cells throughout this region of the brain that contain receptors for steroid hormones[4,18,19] and insulin.[20] The types of response generated by alterations in input from these receptors tend to involve multiple systems (see Chaps. 8 and 9).

The efferent sympathetic and parasympathetic components of the autonomic nervous system innervate all endocrine tissue and can modify the secretion of glands. For example, the well-known cephalic phase of digestion includes vagal stimulation of insulin secretion, which occurs well in advance of substrate (glucose) stimulation of the pancreatic B cell. Insulin secretion, however, is just one of a set of autonomically mediated responses that occurs to the sight, smell, or taste of food. Also included in this phase of digestion is increased salivation,

increased gastric motility and acid secretion, and increased gastrin secretion.

Stimulation of both central and peripheral receptors occurs with signals that regulate energy balance. In addition to the neural and hormonal feedback information from the alimentary system that occurs with ingestion of food, occupancy of central receptors for glucocorticoids and insulin appears to be critical for overall regulation of energy balance.[20,21] Glucocorticoids and insulin, apparently through their actions on the central nervous system,[20,21] are, respectively, stimulatory and inhibitory to food intake; by contrast, their peripheral effects are, respectively, inhibitory and stimulatory to energy storage.

It appears likely that the reciprocal effects of glucocorticoids and insulin on food intake are mediated, in part, through their opposing actions on the orexigenic peptide that is synthesized in the arcuate nuclei of the hypothalamus, neuropeptide Y.[20,21] Insulin inhibits[20] and glucocorticoids stimulate[21] neuropeptide Y synthesis and secretion. Neuropeptide Y stimulates food intake in satiated animals and, over the long term, causes obesity. Axons containing neuropeptide Y, in turn, innervate nearby hypothalamic cell groups that are known to constitute a neural network that determines food intake.

The metabolic effects of glucocorticoids and insulin on energy balance (see Chaps. 72 and 135) are antagonistic to each other and are opposite in direction to their central, antagonistic effects on energy acquisition. Thus, this bihormonal effector and signaling system serves as a relatively simple overall regulator of energy stores.

Stimulation of peripheral receptors occurs with severe hemorrhage (Fig. 5-9). A sudden decrease in arterial blood pressure and venous return occasioned by a rapid hemorrhage of 20% of the blood volume is registered by the peripheral stretch receptors in the great veins and atria and in the aortic arch and carotid arteries. The information leads to increased autonomic sympathetic activity and the secretion of epinephrine from the adrenal medulla. Secreted catecholamines act to increase heart rate and stroke volume (by way of chronotropic and inotropic actions on cardiac muscle) and to increase peripheral vascular resistance by constriction of vascular smooth muscle[22,23] (see Chap. 85).

Increased sympathetic outflow to the juxtaglomerular cells of the kidney and decreased renal perfusion pressure or flow cause renin secretion[24,25] and, thus, an increase in circulating angiotensin II concentration. Angiotensin II acts directly on arterial smooth muscle to cause vasoconstriction and, therefore, increased arterial blood pressure. Angiotensin II, by way of an action on the subfornical organ, also stimulates the conscious desire to drink fluids and further augment sympathetic activity.[19,26] Moreover, angiotensin II acts on the adrenal glomerulosal cells to stimulate the secretion of aldosterone,[27] which causes increased reabsorption of sodium by the kidney and aids in the restoration of the extracellular fluid volume.

The hemorrhage-induced alteration in atrial baroreceptor input to the brain also causes stimulation of vasopressin secretion, which causes direct constriction of the vascular smooth muscle and, through its action on kidney, antidiuresis (see Chaps. 25 and 206). All of these hormonal actions contribute to the maintenance of cardiac function and adequate perfusion pressure.[28,29] In addition, the behavioral and renal actions of the hormones tend to restore extracellular fluid volume to normal. Clearly, in some situations, if one hormonal system is removed, the other systems "take over" to maintain arterial blood pressure within its normal range. However, all the systems are necessary to combat severe changes in the system. For example, resting arterial pressure is not affected by pharmacologic blockade of the receptors for vasopressin or angiotensin II. However, the administration of these same blocking agents or blockade of the sympathetic nervous system seriously impairs the restitution of arterial pressure after hemorrhage.[30]

The endocrine responses to hemorrhage enumerated earlier and in Figure 5-9 do not represent a complete list of the hor-

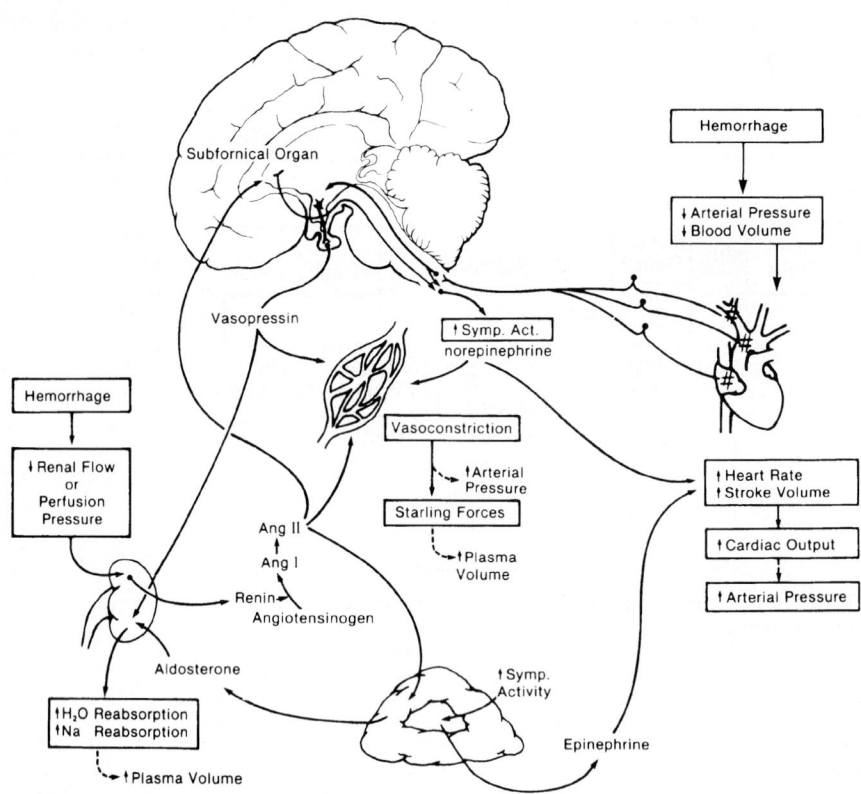

**FIGURE 5-9.** Example of complex feedback regulation of blood pressure and blood volume after hemorrhage. (*Ang*, angiotensin; *Symp. Act.*, sympathetic activity.)

monal changes elicited by hemorrhage-induced changes in baroreceptor input to hypothalamic control systems. Increased secretion of ACTH, growth hormone, and pancreatic glucagon occurs, and pancreatic insulin secretion decreases. After the surgical removal of baroreceptor input to the central autonomic pathways, hemorrhage no longer elicits either vasopressin or ACTH secretion, strongly suggesting that it is this information that drives the responses.

## CONCLUSION

Feedback information allows the control systems to adjust appropriately to the internal conditions and to diminish overshoots in endocrine responses that are occasioned by long delays between hormonal secretion and target tissue response.

## REFERENCES

1. Houk JC. Control strategies in physiological systems. FASEB J 1988; 2:97.
2. Guyton AC. Textbook of medical physiology, 9th ed. Philadelphia: WB Saunders, 1996:7.
3. Engler D, Redei E, Kola I. The corticotropin-release inhibitory factor hypothesis: a review of the evidence for the existence of inhibitory as well as stimulatory hypophysiotropic regulation of adrenocorticotropin secretion and biosynthesis. Endocrine Rev 1999; 20:460.
4. Keller-Wood ME, Dallman MF. Corticosterone inhibition of ACTH secretion. Endocr Rev 1984; 5:1.
5. Dallman MF, Akana SF, Levin N, et al. Corticosteroids and the control of function in the hypothalamic-pituitary-adrenal (HPA) axis. Ann NY Acad Sci 1994; 746:22.
6. Frohman LA, Jansson J. Growth-hormone releasing hormone. Endocr Rev 1986; 7:223.
7. Muller EE. Neural control of somatotropic function. Physiol Rev 1987; 67:962.
8. Dreifuss JJ, Kelly JS. Recurrent inhibition of antidromically identified rat supraoptic neurons. J Physiol (Lond) 1972; 200:87.
9. Moos F, Freund-Merier MJ, Guerne Y, et al. Release of oxytocin and vasopressin by magnocellular nuclei in vitro: specific facilitatory effects of oxytocin on its own release. J Endocrinol 1984; 102:63.
10. Denef C. Paracrine interactions in the anterior pituitary. Clin Endocrinol Metab 1986; 15:1.
11. Schwartz J, Cherny R. Intercellular communication within the anterior pituitary influencing the secretion of hypophysial hormones. Endocr Rev 1992; 13:453.
12. Lambertz SW, Macleod RM. Regulation of prolactin secretion at the level of the lactotroph. Physiol Rev 1990; 70:279.
13. Plant TM. Gonadal regulation of hypothalamic gonadotropin-releasing hormone release in primates. Endocr Rev 1986; 7:75.
13a. Evans JJ. Modulation of gonadotropin levels by peptides acting at the anterior pituitary gland. Endocr Rev 1999; 20:46.
14. Vitale ML, Chiocchio SR. Serotonin, a neurotransmitter involved in the regulation of luteinizing hormone release. Endocr Rev 1993; 14:480.
15. Carey RM, Sen S. Recent progress in the control of aldosterone secretion. Recent Prog Horm Res 1986; 42:251.
16. MacDonald BR. Parathyroid hormone, prostaglandins and bone resorption. World Rev Nutr Diet 1986; 47:163.
17. Schnermann J. Juxtaglomerular cell complex and the regulation of renal salt. Am J Physiol 1998; 274:2263.
18. Dallman MF. Viewing the ventromedial hypothalamus from the adrenal gland. Am J Physiol 1984; 246:R1.
19. Reid IA. Actions of angiotensin II on the brain: mechanisms and physiologic role. Am J Physiol 1984; 246:F533.
20. Schwartz MW, Figlewicz DP, Baskin DG, et al. Insulin in the brain: a hormonal regulator of energy balance. Endocr Rev 1992; 13:387.
21. Dallman MF, Strack AM, Akana SF, et al. Feast and famine: critical role of glucocorticoids with insulin in daily energy flow. Front Neuroendocrinol 1993; 14:303.
22. Darlington DN, Tehrani MJ. Blood flow, vascular resistance, and blood volume after hemorrhage in conscious adrenalectomized rat. J Appl Physiol 1997; 83:1648.
23. Darlington DN, Jones RO, Marzella L, Gann DS. Changes in regional vascular resistance and blood volume after hemorrhage in fed and fasted awake rats. J Appl Physiol 1995; 78:2025.
24. Darlington DN, Keil LC, Dallman MF. Potentiation of hormonal responses to hemorrhage and fasting, but not hypoglycemia in conscious adrenalectomized rats. Endocrinology 1989; 125:1398.
25. Darlington DN, Chew G, Ha T, et al. Corticosterone, but not glucose, treatment enables fasted adrenalectomized rats to survive moderate hemorrhage. Endocrinology 1990; 127:766.
26. Thrasher TN, Keenan CR, Ramsay DJ. Cardiovascular afferent signals and drinking in response to hypotension in dogs. Am J Physiol 1999; 277:R795.
27. Burnay MM, Python CP, Vallotton MB, et al. Role of the capacitative calcium influx in the activation of steroidogenesis by angiotensin-II in adrenal glomerulosa cells. Endocrinology 1994; 135:751.
28. Dampney RA. Functional organization of central pathways regulating the cardiovascular system. Physiol Rev 1994; 74:323.
29. Herd JA. Cardiovascular response to stress. Physiol Rev 1991; 71:305.
30. Rossi NF, Shrier RW. Role of arginine vasopressin in regulation of systemic arterial blood pressure. Annu Rev Med 1986; 37:13.

# CHAPTER 6

# ENDOCRINE RHYTHMS

EVE VAN CAUTER

Pronounced temporal oscillations ranging in period from a few minutes to a year occur throughout the endocrine system. These oscillations are part of the wide variety of rhythms that exist in all living organisms. Rhythms with a period of ~24 hours have been called *circadian,* from the Latin *circa diem,* meaning "around a day." According to the terminology of circadian biology, 24-hour rhythms should only be referred to as circadian if they are primarily driven by an endogenous clock system. However, it has become increasingly apparent that nearly all 24-hour rhythms partly reflect the influence of an *endogenous circadian pacemaker located in the hypothalamus* and partly the *influence of other events occurring with a 24-hour periodicity,* such as the alternation of waking and sleeping, light and dark, food intake, and postural changes. Thus, the use of the term *circadian* is often extended to *all diurnal variations recurring regularly at a time interval of ~24 hours.*

Circadian rhythms have been used to separate two further classes of biologic rhythms: *ultradian* rhythms, with periods shorter than 24 hours, and *infradian* rhythms, with periods longer than 24 hours. The pulsatile release of pituitary hormones belongs to the ultradian range. The menstrual cycle and the seasonal variations in the reproductive system are infradian rhythms. Reproducible circadian changes occur in the secretory pattern of the *vast majority* of hormones.

## CIRCADIAN RHYTHMS

### BASIC MECHANISMS

There is virtually neither a tissue nor a function in the human organism that does not exhibit regular changes from day to night. Distinct patterns of secretion recur at 24-hour intervals for essentially all hormones. Much of the temporal variability and organization of endocrine release ultimately results from the activity of two interacting time-keeping mechanisms in the central nervous system: endogenous circadian rhythmicity and sleep-wake homeostasis (Fig. 6-1). In mammals, endogenous circadian rhythmicity is generated by a pacemaker or group of oscillators located in the paired suprachiasmatic nucleus (SCN) of the hypothalamus.[1] Sleep-wake homeostasis is an hourglass-like mechanism relating the amount and quality of sleep to the duration of prior wakefulness.[2]

The endogenous nature of human circadian rhythms has been established by experiments in which subjects were isolated in a soundproof chamber with no time cues available. Under those conditions, the subjects show *free-running rhythms* with periods, which deviate slightly from 24 hours and vary from one individual to another. In humans, the endogenous "free-running" period is usually slightly longer than 24 hours. In the past few years, enormous progress has been made in elucidating the molecular and genetic mechanisms underlying the generation of circadian rhythms in mammals. After the discovery of the first mammalian circadian clock gene, called *Clock,*[3,4] a number of other mammalian clock genes were rapidly identified and sequenced.[5] Intense efforts are now under way to understand how these genes and their protein products interact with each other through a series of activational and inhibitory pathways to produce the precise periodicity of the circadian signal generated in the SCN.

Environmental agents, primarily the *light-dark cycle* (i.e., *photic cues*), affect the expression and properties of the circadian

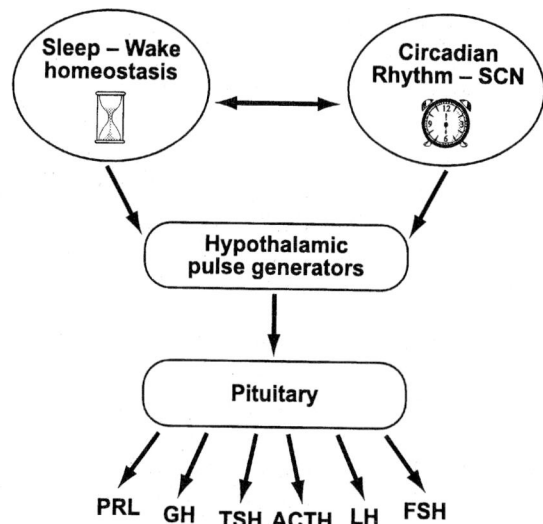

**FIGURE 6-1.** Schematic representation of the central mechanisms involved in the control of temporal variations in pituitary hormone secretions over the 24-hour cycle. Sleep-wake homeostasis is in an hourglass-like mechanism, which relates the propensity for deep non-rapid eye movement (non-REM) sleep to the amount of prior wakefulness. Circadian rhythmicity is an endogenous near-24-hour oscillation generated in the suprachiasmatic nuclei (*SCN*) of the hypothalamus and transmitted via neural as well as humoral mechanisms. (*ACTH,* adrenocorticotropic hormone; *FSH,* follicle-stimulating hormone; *GH,* growth hormone; *LH,* luteinizing hormone; *PRL,* prolactin; *TSH,* thyrotropin-stimulating hormone.)

signal. Light exposure in the later part of the subjective night and in the early part of the subjective day (e.g., around dawn) generally advances the phase of the circadian oscillation. In contrast, light exposure in the later part of the subjective day and during the early part of the subjective night (e.g., around dusk) delays circadian phase. Light-dark information reaches the SCN via a direct afferent pathway from the retina as well as an indirect projection via the intergeniculate leaflet of the thalamus.[1] There also is good evidence to indicate that *nonphotic cues* are also capable of altering circadian function. Many of the nonphotic stimuli that induce phase shifts in the circadian clock appear to do so by either stimulating physical activity or activating the pathways by which information about the activity-rest state of the organism reaches the clock.[1] Phase-shifts may occur when activity pathways are stimulated during the normal rest period or, vice-versa, when rest is enforced during the normal active period. As is the case for light, the magnitude and direction of the phase-shifts depend on their timing relative to the internal circadian clock. There is now substantial evidence to indicate that the Raphe nuclei of the brainstem are involved in mediating the effects of activity on the circadian clock.

Sleep-wake homeostasis is thought to involve a putative *neural sleep factor (factor "S")* that rises during waking and decays exponentially during sleep,[2] and regulates the timing, amount, and intensity of the deeper stages of sleep. These stages of deep sleep correspond to stages III and IV of *non–rapid-eye-movement (REM)* sleep, usually referred to as *slow-wave (SW) sleep* because of the appearance of well-defined waves in the frequency range 0.5 to 4.0 Hz in the electroencephalogram. The neuroanatomical and neurochemical basis of sleep-wake homeostasis has not been entirely elucidated but appears to involve the basal forebrain cholinergic region and *adenosine,* a neuromodulator of which the extracellular concentrations in this region increase during sustained wakefulness and decrease during sleep.[6] The mechanisms controlling sleep propensity and maintenance in the human appear to be somewhat different from those occurring in most other mammalian species. Indeed, *human sleep is generally consolidated* in a single 7-

to 9-hour period, whereas *fragmentation* of the sleep period in several bouts is the rule in most other mammals. Possibly as a result of this consolidation of the sleep period, the wake-sleep and sleep-wake transitions in the human are associated with physiologic changes—and, in particular, endocrine changes—that are *more marked than those observed in animals*. Humans are also unique in their *capacity to maintain wakefulness* despite an increased pressure to sleep. While decrements in mood and cognitive function associated with such behaviors have long been recognized, these behaviors have been found to be associated with endocrine and metabolic alterations that may result in long-term adverse health consequences.[6a]

The pathways by which circadian rhythmicity, sleep-wake homeostasis, and their interactions modulate hormonal release are largely unknown. At the level of the central nervous system (see Fig. 6-1), humoral and/or neural signals originating from the hypothalamic circadian pacemaker and from brain regions involved in sleep regulation affect the activity of the hypothalamic structures responsible for the pulsatile release of neuroendocrine factors (e.g., corticotropin-releasing hormone [CRH], growth hormone–releasing hormone [GHRH], etc.), which stimulate or inhibit intermittent secretion of pituitary hormones. It appears that stimulatory or inhibitory effects of sleep on endocrine release are primarily associated with SW sleep, rather than REM sleep. Theoretically, the modulation of neuroendocrine release by sleep and circadian rhythmicity could be achieved by modulation of pulse amplitude, modulation of pulse frequency, or a combination of both. The data available so far seem to indicate that circadian rhythmicity of pituitary hormonal release is achieved primarily by modulation of pulse amplitude without changes in pulse frequency, whereas sleep-wake and REM/non-REM transitions affect pulse frequency. Pituitary hormones that influence endocrine systems not directly controlled by hypothalamic factors probably mediate, at least partially, the modulatory effects of sleep and circadian rhythmicity on these systems (e.g., counterregulatory effects of growth hormone [GH] and cortisol on glucose regulation).

Figure 6-2 shows examples of 24-hour patterns of plasma cortisol, thyrotropin (thyroid-stimulating hormone [TSH]), prolactin (PRL), and GH levels observed in normal young men in the presence (left) and in the absence (right) of sleep. To eliminate the effects of feeding, fasting, and postural changes, the subjects remained recumbent throughout the study, and the normal meal schedule was replaced by intravenous glucose infusion at a constant rate. These profiles exemplify the high degree of temporal organization provided by circadian rhythms in the endocrine system. As is the case for the majority of hormones, the plasma levels of these four pituitary-dependent hormones follow a pattern that repeats itself day after day. The nocturnal rise of TSH starts in the evening, at a time when cortisol secretion is quiescent, and ends at the beginning of the sleep period, when GH and PRL concentrations surge. The early morning period is associated with low TSH, low PRL, and low GH concentrations but high cortisol levels. Thus, the release of these four hormones follows a highly coordinated temporal program that results from interactions between circadian rhythmicity, sleep, and pulsatile release. It is apparent that the presence or absence of sleep had only modest effects on the wave shape of the cortisol profile but markedly affected the profilers of TSH, PRL, and GH. Thus, the relative contributions of circadian rhythmicity and sleep-wake homeostasis vary from one endocrine axis to the other, but, as will be shown in subsequent sections, inputs from both central nervous system processes can be recognized in the majority of 24-hour hormonal patterns.

## MEDICAL IMPLICATIONS

Among the medical implications of circadian rhythms, those relating to clinical diagnosis are the most obvious. Indeed, because of the wide amplitude of certain rhythms, the estimation

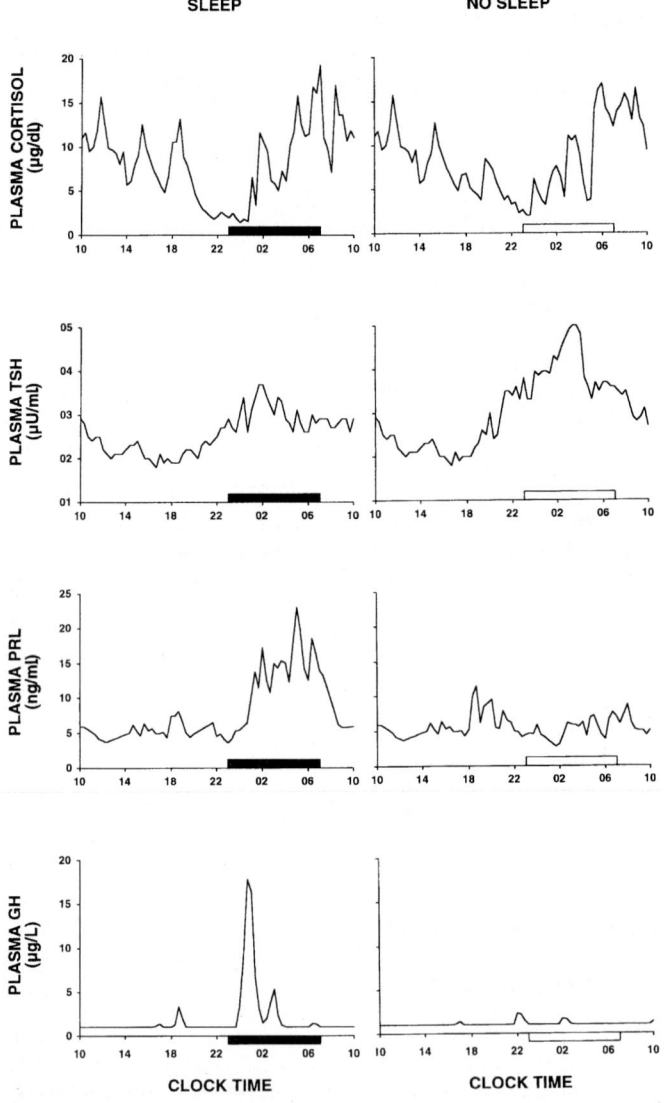

**FIGURE 6-2.** From top to bottom: Temporal profiles of plasma cortisol (*COR*), thyrotropin (thyroid-stimulating hormone [*TSH*]), prolactin (*PRL*), and growth hormone (*GH*) in a healthy male adult studied over a 24-hour cycle with a normal sleep period (*left*) or continuously awake (*right*). The black bars denote the sleep periods; the open bars the periods of nocturnal sleep deprivation.

of the mean level of a parameter from a single measurement may involve an error exceeding 100%. For example, a plasma cortisol level of 15 µg/dL (i.e., 414 nmol/L) at 8:00 a.m. is perfectly normal, whereas the same value obtained at 8:00 p.m. is suggestive of some form of hypercortisolism. Differentiation between normal and pathologic levels may be greatly improved by adequately selecting the time of sample collection. To illustrate this concept, Figure 6-3 shows the mean of 56 profiles of plasma cortisol from patients with Cushing syndrome as compared with the mean of 60 profiles obtained in normal subjects. Overlap between individual values from the two groups of subjects should be expected at all times except between 10:00 p.m. and 2:00 a.m., when the mean cortisol level allows for the discrimination between healthy controls and patients with hypercortisolism in 114 out of 116 cases. As discussed later in this section, it is also important to find out whether the patient has been recently involved in night work or has just returned from transmeridian travel when interpreting certain hormonal data for diagnostic purposes.

Another medical implication of circadian rhythms is based on the fact that the response of the organism to many stimuli depends on the time at which that stimuli is applied. This find-

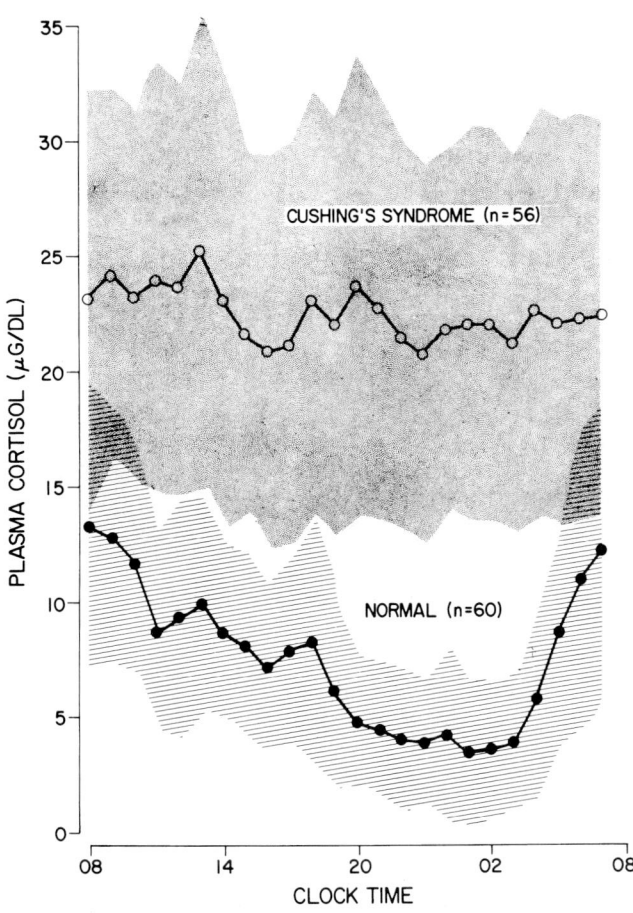

**FIGURE 6-3.** Mean, across individuals, of the 24-hour profile of plasma cortisol in 60 normal subjects (*closed circles*) and 56 patients with Cushing syndrome (*open circles*). The hatched and shaded areas represent one standard error of the mean above and below the mean for normal subjects or patients with Cushing syndrome, respectively.

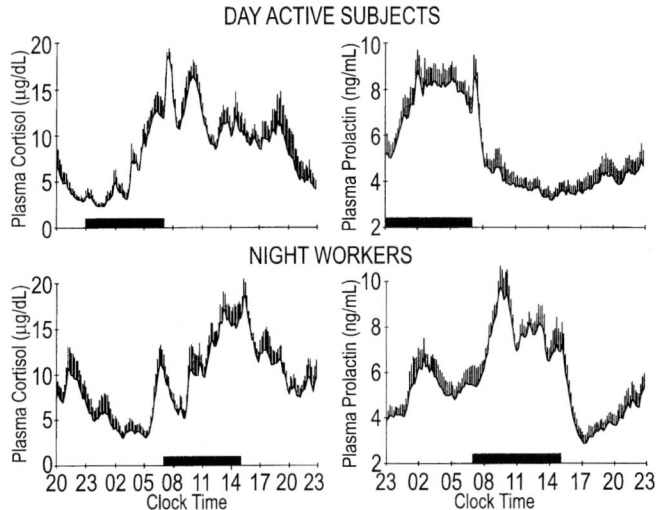

**FIGURE 6-4.** Mean 24-hour profiles of plasma cortisol (*left*) and prolactin (*right*), either in healthy subjects who work during the daytime or in healthy subjects who have been working during the night for at least 2 years. The vertical lines at each time point represent the standard error of the mean. The black bars represent the sleep periods. (Data from Weibel L, Follenius M, Spiegel K, et al. Comparative effect of night and daytime sleep on the 24-hour cortisol secretory profile. Sleep 1995; 18:549; Weibel L, Spiegel K, Follenius M, et al. Internal dissociation of the circadian markers of the cortisol rhythm in night workers. Am J Physiol 1996; 270:E608; Spiegel K, Weibel L, Gronfier C, et al. Twenty-four hour prolactin profiles in night workers. Chronobiol Int 1996; 13:283.)

ing forms the theoretical basis of *chronopharmacology* (i.e., the investigation of drug effects as a function of their time of administration) and of *chronotherapy* (i.e., the design of better protocols of treatment that take into account the chronobiologic characteristics of the system).[7]

Abnormal 24-hour regulation of endocrine and other physiologic functions occur in a variety of highly prevalent conditions, including *shift work, "jet lag"* (see Chap. 10), *blindness, major depressive illness* (see Chap. 201), and *sleep disorders*. The health symptoms of shift workers and the general feeling of discomfort experienced after a transmeridian flight are well-known consequences of the *desynchronization between internal and external time*. Both are associated with a variety of physical and performance deficits. The *jet lag syndrome* usually includes symptoms of fatigue, subjective discomfort, sleep disturbances, reduced mental and psychomotor performance, and gastrointestinal tract disorders. The malaise partly reflects a state of internal desynchrony, because different physiologic systems adapt to abrupt shifts of environmental time at different rates. The syndrome subsides as adaptation to local time is achieved. Unless the condition of jet lag is repeated at frequent time intervals for prolonged periods of time (as in the case of air transportation professionals), this transient syndrome is not thought to be associated with long-term adverse effects on physical and mental health. In contrast, *shift work*, which is voluntarily accepted by millions of workers, is a *major health hazard*, involving an increased risk of cardiovascular illness, gastrointestinal disorders, psychosocial symptoms, sleep disturbances, substance abuse, reduced immune function, and infertility.[8–10] Shift workers are generally in a condition of chronic

sleep debt,[9] which could in itself result in endocrine and metabolic disturbances. Workers on permanent or rotating night shifts do not fully adapt to these schedules, even after several years,[11,12] and live in a chronic state of internal desynchrony of the endocrine system. An example is shown in Figure 6-4, which compares mean 24-hour profiles of plasma cortisol and PRL in permanent night workers as compared with day workers.[13–15] The components of these endocrine rhythms, which are primarily controlled by sleep-wake homeostasis (e.g., sleep-related PRL secretion), partly adapted to the night schedule, whereas components reflecting circadian timing (i.e., onset of the early morning elevation of cortisol secretion) showed little, if any, adaptation. As a result, the night workers had to initiate sleep when cortisol levels were already high and maintain wakefulness despite elevated concentrations of PRL, a hormone thought to be involved in sleep regulation.

Abnormal synchronization of circadian rhythms, including hormonal rhythms, have also been observed in totally blind subjects. These disturbances are thought to reflect a lack of entrainment to the 24-hour environmental periodicity that is due to the absence of photic synchronization.

In severely depressed subjects, early timing of a number of circadian rhythms, including hormonal rhythms, has been observed. These findings provide the basis for the *phase-advance hypothesis for affective illness*, which proposes that abnormalities in circadian time-keeping are involved in the pathophysiology of depression.[16] Patients experiencing *sleep apnea*, a condition in which frequent awakenings interrupt sleep, have abnormalities of sleep-related endocrine release. When the condition is untreated, nocturnal PRL and GH levels do not increase to the same extent as in healthy subjects with normal sleep. Studies that have examined the impact of treatment with continuous positive airway pressure have demonstrated that treatment of the sleep disorder partly normalizes the endocrine alteration.[17,17a] This is illustrated in the profiles shown in Figure 6-5 in the case of GH. After 3 months of treatment, nasal continuous positive airway pressure therapy increases plasma insulin-like growth factor-I levels in men with severe obstructive sleep

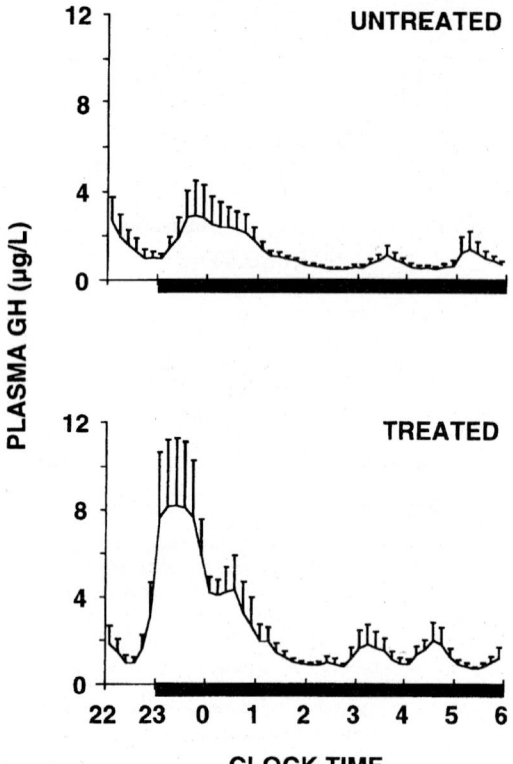

**FIGURE 6-5.** Mean profiles of plasma growth hormone (*GH*) in patients with sleep apnea studied before (*top*) and after (*bottom*) treatment with continuous positive airway pressure. The vertical line at each time point represents the standard error of the mean. (Data from Saini J, Krieger J, Brandenberger G, et al. Continuous positive airway pressure treatment: effects on growth hormone, insulin and glucose profiles in obstructive sleep apnea patients. Horm Metab Res 1993; 25:375. Reproduced from Van Cauter E, Spiegel K. Circadian and sleep control of hormonal secretions. In: Turek FW, Zee PC, eds. Regulation of sleep and circadian rhythms. New York: Marcel Dekker, Inc., 1999:397.)

apnea.[18] In children, surgical correction of obstructive sleep apnea may restore GH secretion and a normal growth rate.[19]

Age-related changes in endocrine, metabolic, and behavioral circadian rhythms have been well described.[20,21] One of the most prominent changes is a reduction in rhythm amplitude. The overall findings of a study that examined age-related differences in 24-hour endocrine rhythms and sleep in healthy subjects are shown in Figure 6-6. The cortisol and TSH rhythms were dampened in the older group. A decrease by at least 50% in the nocturnal release of both GH and melatonin was observed in the older volunteers, and SW sleep was drastically diminished. Deficits in the maintenance and depth of nocturnal sleep are generally paralleled by decreased alertness during the daytime. Many circadian rhythms are also phase advanced in older subjects such that specific phase points of the rhythms occur earlier than in young subjects.[21] The alterations in circadian regulation are closely associated with changes in sleep-wake habits (i.e., earlier bedtimes and waketimes).

## ULTRADIAN RHYTHMS

### PERIOD RANGE AND ORIGIN

The term *ultradian* is primarily used to designate rhythmicities with periods ranging from fractions of hours to several hours. In the hourly range, the most prominent ultradian rhythms are the alteration of REM and non-REM stages in sleep and the pulsatility of hormonal secretions. Oscillations in the 80- to 120-minute

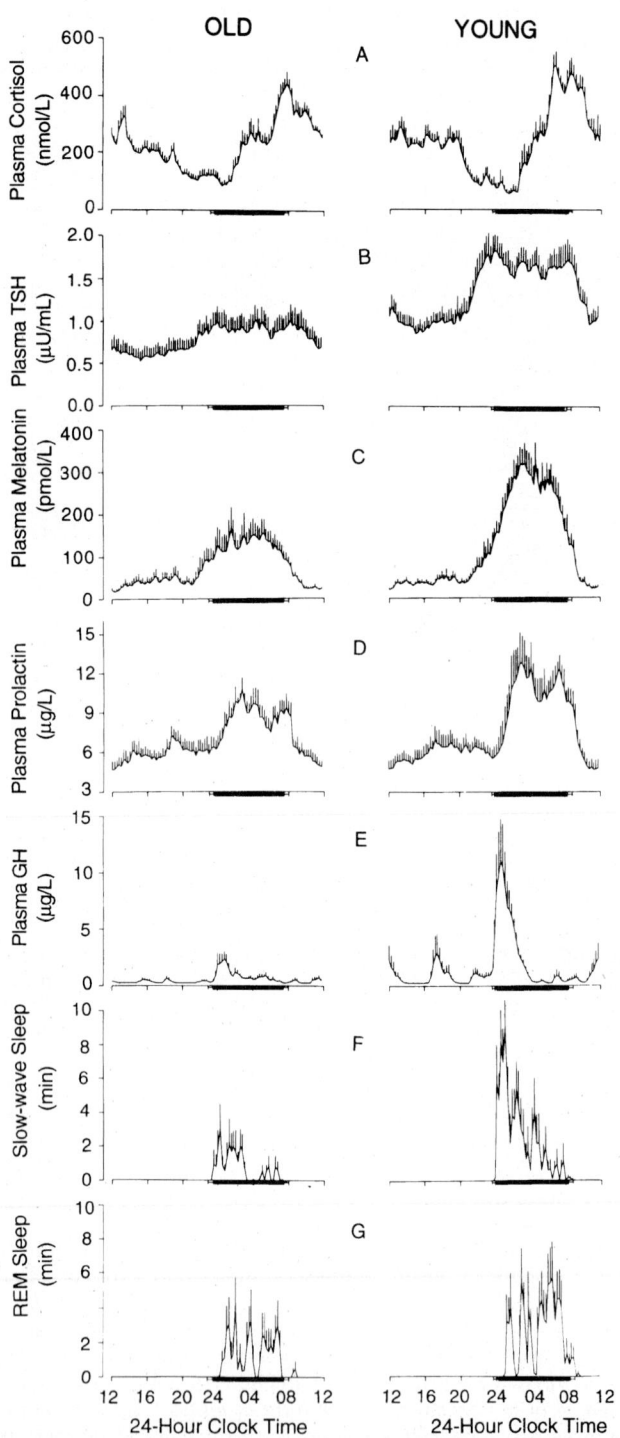

**FIGURE 6-6.** From top to bottom, mean 24-hour profiles of plasma cortisol, thyrotropin (thyroid-stimulating hormone [*TSH*]), melatonin, prolactin, and growth hormone (*GH*) levels, and distribution of slow-wave (*SW*) and rapid-eye-movement (*REM*) stages in sleep in old and young subjects. The distribution of SW and REM is expressed in minutes of each 15-minute sampling interval spent in the corresponding stage. Vertical lines at each time point represent the standard error of the mean. The black bars correspond to the mean sleep period. (From van Coevorden A, Mockel J, Laurent E, et al. Neuroendocrine rhythms and sleep in aging. Am J Physiol 1991; 260:E651.)

range also occur at the rate of urine flow and gastric motility. Pulsatile hormonal release is ubiquitous in the endocrine system. Indeed, the plasma levels of most hormones undergo episodic fluctuations of variable duration and magnitude, referred to as secretory *"episodes"* or *"pulses."* These pulses recur at 1- to 4-

hour intervals (see Fig. 6-2). Pulsatility has been observed for anterior and posterior pituitary hormones; for hormones directly under their control; and for other endocrine variables, such as insulin, glucagon, and renin. The long-disputed theory that ultradian variations of brain activity—similar to those occurring during sleep—were also present during wake (constituting a *basic rest-activity cycle*) has received some experimental support. One study demonstrated the existence of an ultradian rhythm of brain electrical activity in the frequency range of 13 to 35 Hz, an index of central alertness, during waking.[22] Furthermore, it appeared that pulses of cortisol release were significantly associated with increases in this marker of alertness.

In discussing the origin of ultradian hormonal fluctuations, one must distinguish two general cases: that of the hormones under direct hypothalamic control and that of hormones that are part of more peripheral endocrine systems. In the first case, periodic release ultimately reflects phasic neural activation, whereas in the second case, oscillatory behavior is a property of the dynamics of local regulatory networks. The episodic pulses of anterior pituitary hormones, which are representative of the first case, result from secretion in discrete bursts in response to pulsatile stimulation and/or inhibition by hypothalamic factors. The specific hypothalamic mechanism controlling pulsatile release appears to be different for each pituitary axis, but common stimuli may operate in different axes. The state of knowledge is most advanced in the case of the gonadotropins, for which pulsatile release is caused by intermittent discharges of gonadotropin-releasing hormone (GnRH) into the pituitary portal circulation. The GnRH pulses are obtained by synchronous discharges of GnRH-containing neurons in the arcuate of the mediobasal hypothalamus.[23] Sharp increases in the frequency of hypothalamic multiunit electrical activity are associated with each pulse of peripheral luteinizing hormone (LH) level.[23] The pulsatile behavior is intrinsic to the GnRH neurons, as attested by their coordinate secretion in tissue cultures.[24] Intermittent stimulation by pituitary hormones is then in turn responsible for the episodic release of hormones under their control (see Chap. 16).

For hormones other than those controlled by the hypothalamo-pituitary axis, the mechanisms causing episodic variations in plasma levels are generally less well understood. Notable exceptions are the ultradian 1- to 2-hour oscillations of insulin secretion that occur after meal ingestion, as well as during constant glucose infusion or continuous enteral nutrition.[25,26] Theoretical and experimental evidence suggests that in conditions of normal glucose tolerance, these oscillations arise from the negative feedback interactions linking insulin and glucose.[26]

## PHYSIOLOGIC SIGNIFICANCE

The physiologic significance of hormonal pulsatility has been first demonstrated by experiments showing that normal LH and follicle-stimulating hormone (FSH) levels may be restored by pulsatile, but not continuous, administration of exogenous GnRH to primates with lesions in the hypothalamus that had abolished endogenous GnRH production.[23] These findings were rapidly applied to the treatment of a variety of disorders of the pituitary-gonadal axis, using either pulsatile GnRH administration to correct a deficient production of endogenous GnRH or long-acting GnRH analogs to induce pituitary desensitization.[27] Similar approaches have been investigated for other hypothalamo-pituitary axes.

## METHODOLOGIC ASPECTS OF THE STUDY OF ENDOCRINE RHYTHMS

### DIURNAL VARIATIONS

To investigate circadian hormonal rhythms, a group of individuals is usually studied for a minimum of 24 hours each, following the same experimental protocol. The demonstration of

circadian rhythmicity is then based on the observation of consistently reproducible characteristics in the set of 24-hour profiles obtained. To validate such an approach, the group of subjects should be as homogeneous as possible, not only in terms of physical parameters, such as age and gender, but also in terms of living habits, such as bedtimes and meal schedules. To maximize interindividual synchronization, the volunteers should comply with a standardized schedule of meals and bedtimes for several days before the investigation. Blood sampling is usually done at regular intervals through a catheter inserted into a forearm vein. During bedtime hours, the catheter is connected to plastic tubing extending to an adjacent room to collect blood samples without disturbing the subject. Because of the major modulatory effects exerted by sleep stages on hormonal release, it is important to obtain *polygraphic sleep recordings* using standardized methods for recording and scoring. If polygraphic monitoring is not possible, estimates of sleep onset and awakenings should be carefully recorded. Daytime naps should be avoided. To obtain valid estimations of the circadian parameters, it is necessary to sample at intervals not exceeding 1 hour. Indeed, the pulsatile variations may bias the estimation of the characteristics of the circadian rhythm if sampling is less frequent. Procedures to analyze 24-hour hormonal profiles usually involve the fitting of a smooth curve to the data. The times of occurrence of the maximum and the minimum of the best-fit curve are often referred to as, respectively, the acrophase and the nadir. The amplitude of the circadian rhythm may be estimated as 50% of the difference between the maximum and the minimum of the best-fit curve.

## PULSATILE VARIATIONS

The definition of an optimal sampling protocol to study pulsatile hormonal fluctuations depends on the type of phenomenon under study. Presently, sampling at 1-minute intervals represents probably the fastest rate technically achievable with reasonable precision. Sampling every few minutes uncovers high-frequency, low-amplitude variations superimposed on the slower pulsatile release occurring at hourly intervals. These intensified rates of venous sampling may not allow for the estimation of the characteristics of major secretory bursts, because the total duration of sampling compatible with this rate of blood withdrawal limits the observed number of large peaks. Sampling rates of 20 and 30 minutes only detect major pulses lasting >1 hour.

The analysis of pulsatile variations may be considered at two levels. The researcher may wish to define and characterize significant variations in peripheral levels based on estimations on the size of measurement error (i.e., primarily assay error). However, under certain circumstances, it is possible to mathematically derive secretory rates from the peripheral concentrations. This procedure, often referred to as *deconvolution*, often reveals more pulses of secretion than the analysis of peripheral concentrations. It also more accurately defines the temporal limits of each pulse.

The association between pulsatile GH secretion and sleep stages in a single individual is shown in Figure 6-7.[28] The profile shown on the top represents the plasma levels of GH measured at 15-minute intervals. Three pulses were found significant using a pulse detection algorithm (i.e., ULTRA[28]). The corresponding profile of GH secretory rates calculated by deconvolution is shown in the second profile from the top. A single compartment model for GH disappearance with a half-life of 19 minutes and a volume of distribution of 7% of the body weight was used in this calculation. Pulse analysis of the secretory rates now reveals the occurrence of three additional pulses of GH secretion. The three lower profiles show the percentages of each 15-minute sampling interval spent in stages of wake, SW, and REM, respectively. When the profile of plasma concentrations is compared with the SW profile, it appears that

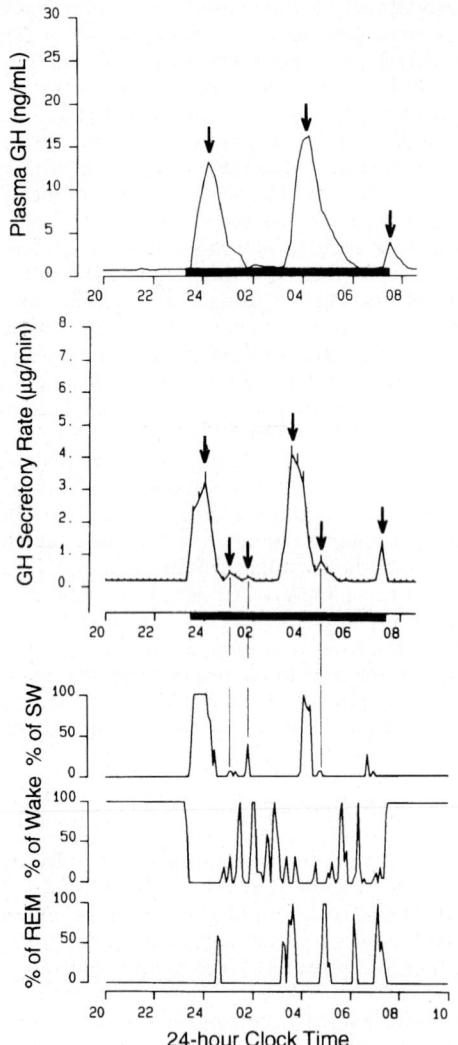

**FIGURE 6-7.** 24-hour profile of plasma growth hormone (*GH; top*) sampled at 15-minute intervals in a normal man. The black bar indicates the sleep period. The second panel from the top shows the profile of GH secretory rates derived by deconvolution from the profile of plasma concentrations. Significant pulses of plasma levels and secretory rates are indicated by arrows. The three lower panels represent the temporal distribution of slow-wave (*SW*) stages (*III + IV*), wake, and rapid eye movement (*REM*) during sleep. Vertical lines indicate the temporal association between pulses of GH secretion and SW stages. (From Van Cauter E. Computer-assisted analysis of endocrine rhythms. In: Rodbard D, Forti G, eds. Computers in endocrinology. New York: Raven Press, 1990:59.)

subsequent to its initiation in concomitance with the beginning of the first SW period, the sleep-onset GH pulse spanned the first 3 hours of sleep, without apparent modulation by non-REM and REM stages. However, the profile of secretory rates clearly reveals that GH was preferentially secreted during the SW stage, with interruptions of secretory activity coinciding with the intervening REM or wake stages. Deconvolution demonstrated a closer association between SW stages and active GH secretion than the analysis of plasma levels, because the temporal limits of each pulse were more accurately defined and additional pulses were revealed. The validity of the deconvolution procedure is critically dependent on the knowledge of the clearance kinetics of the hormone under study; extra caution in interpreting the data must be exerted, because this procedure involves an amplification of measurement error, with increased risk of false-positive error.

Whether examining peripheral concentrations or secretory rates, there are two major approaches to analyzing the episodic

fluctuations. The first, and most commonly used, is the time domain analysis in which the data are plotted against time and pulses are detected and identified. The second is the analysis in the frequency domain in which amplitude is plotted against frequency or period. These two approaches differ fundamentally both in the mathematical treatment of the data and in the questions they may help to resolve; therefore, they should be viewed as being complementary. The regularity of pulsatile behavior may be quantified by both approaches (i.e., by examining the distribution of interpulse intervals derived from a time domain analysis or by examining the distribution of spectral power in a frequency domain analysis). Additionally, another analytical tool, the *approximate entropy*, has been introduced to quantify regularity of oscillatory behavior in endocrine and other physiologic time series.[29,30]

## RHYTHMS IN THE SOMATOTROPIC AXIS

In normal subjects, the 24-hour profile of plasma GH consists of stable low levels abruptly interrupted by bursts of secretion (see Figs. 6-2, 6-5, 6-6, and 6-7). The most reproducible secretory pulse occurs shortly after sleep onset, in association with the first phase of SW sleep.[31] Other secretory pulses may occur in later sleep and during wakefulness in the absence of any identifiable stimulus. In women, daytime GH pulses are more frequent than in men, and the sleep-associated pulse, although still present, does not generally account for most of the 24-hour GH release. The secretory profile is less regular in women than in men.[32] Circulating estradiol concentrations play an important role in determining overall levels of spontaneous GH secretion.[33] Sleep onset elicits a pulse in GH secretion whether sleep is advanced, delayed, interrupted, or fragmented. Delta wave electroencephalographic activity consistently precedes the elevation in plasma GH levels. While SW sleep is clearly a major determinant of the 24-hour profile of GH secretion in humans, there is also evidence for the existence of a circadian modulation of the occurrence and height of GH pulses, reflecting decreased somatostatin inhibition in the evening and nocturnal hours.[34] Administration of a specific GHRH antagonist results in a near total suppression of sleep-related GH release, indicating an important role for GHRH in the control of nocturnal GH secretion.[35]

Two studies involving pharmacologic stimulation of SW sleep have provided evidence for a common mechanism in the control of SW sleep and GH secretion and have indicated that compounds, which increase SW sleep, could represent a novel class of GH secretagogues. Indeed, enhancement of SW sleep by oral administration of low γ-hydroxybutyrate (a naturally occurring metabolite of γ-aminobutyric acid used in the treatment of narcolepsy) or ritanserin (a selective 5HT$_2$ receptor antagonist) results in simultaneous and highly correlated increases of nocturnal GH release.[36,37]

The total amount and the temporal distribution of GH release are strongly dependent on age.[31] A pulsatile pattern of GH release, with increased pulse amplitude during sleep, is present in prepubertal boys and girls. During puberty, the amplitude of the pulses, but not the frequency, is increased, particularly at night. Maximal overall GH concentrations are reached in early puberty in girls and in late puberty in boys. Age-related decreases in GH secretion have been well documented in both men and women and are illustrated in Figure 6-6.

There is a marked suppression of GH levels throughout the 24-hour span in obese subjects. In normal-weight subjects, fasting, even for only 1 day, enhances GH secretion via an increase in both pulse amplitude and pulse frequency.[38] Nonobese juvenile or maturity-onset diabetic patients hypersecrete GH during wakefulness as well as during sleep, primarily because of an increase in the amplitude of pulses.[39] This abnormality may disappear when blood sugar levels are strictly controlled. In acromegaly, GH is hypersecreted throughout the 24-hour span, with a pulsatile pattern superimposed on elevated basal levels, indicative of the presence of tonic secretion.[40,41] After trans-sphenoidal surgery, a normal circadian pattern of GH release can be restored.[41] In contrast, bromocriptine therapy lowers the overall GH secretion but does not lead to the resumption of normal 24-hour profiles.

## RHYTHMS IN THE PITUITARY-ADRENAL AXIS

Twenty-four-hour profiles of cortisol typical of normal subjects are shown in Figures 6-2, 6-3, 6-4, and 6-6. The patterns of plasma adrenocorticotropic hormone (ACTH) and cortisol variations show an early morning maximum, declining levels throughout daytime, a quiescent period of minimal secretory activity, and an abrupt elevation during late sleep. With a 15-minute sampling rate, ~15 pulses of ACTH and cortisol can be detected in a 24-hour span. The cortisol profiles shown in the upper panels of Figure 6-2 illustrate the remarkable persistence of the wave shape of the rhythm in the absence of sleep and support the notion that the 24-hour periodicity of corticotropic activity is primarily controlled by circadian rhythmicity. Nevertheless, modulatory effects of the sleep or wake condition have been clearly demonstrated. Sleep onset is reliably associated with a short-term inhibition of cortisol secretion,[42–44] although this effect (which appears to be related to slow-wave stages[45]) may not be detectable when sleep is initiated at the peak of corticotropic activity (i.e., in the morning[13]). Conversely, awakening at the end of the sleep period is consistently followed by a pulse of cortisol secretion.[46,47] During sleep deprivation, these rapid effects of sleep onset and sleep offset on corticotropic activity are obviously absent, and the amplitude of the rhythm is reduced as compared with normal conditions (see Fig. 6-2).

In addition to the immediate modulatory effects of sleep-wake transitions on cortisol levels, nocturnal sleep deprivation—even partial—results in higher-than-normal cortisol concentrations on the following evening.[48] Sleep loss, thus, appears to delay the normal return to evening quiescence of the corticotropic axis. This suggests that sleep loss may slow down the rate of recovery of the hypothalamic–pituitary–adrenal axis response after a challenge.

A circadian variation parallel to that of cortisol occurs for the plasma levels of adrenal steroids.[49] Figure 6-8 shows the mean 24-hour profiles of cortisol, 11-hydroxyandrostenedione, dehydroepiandrosterone, and androstenedione (AD) for 10 normal young men. The amplitude of the circadian variation in 11-hydroxyandrostenedione levels, a steroid derived from adrenal AD, is essentially similar to that of cortisol, whereas the amplitude of the variations in dehydroepiandrosterone and AD levels, two steroids of partially gonadal origin, is much lower.[49] Pulses of the plasma concentrations of adrenal steroids occur in remarkable synchrony with bursts of cortisol secretion, indicating that pulsatile ACTH release is reflected in the temporal organization of all adrenal secretions.

A distinct circadian rhythm of serum cortisol levels emerges at ~6 months of age. Once this periodicity has been established, it persists throughout adulthood and has been observed through the ninth decade.[21] The overall pattern of the rhythm remains unchanged (see Fig. 6-6), but in older subjects, the nadir is advanced by 1 to 2 hours and the amplitude is decreased.[21] In women, oral contraceptive therapy results in a large increase of the mean cortisol level and of the amplitude of the rhythm resulting from an estrogen-induced elevation of transcortin-binding capacity. Thus, when hypercortisolism is suspected in a female patient, it is essential to know whether the patient is receiving estrogen treatment.

The 24-hour profile of pituitary-adrenal secretion remains unaltered in a wide variety of pathologic states. Disease states in which alterations of the cortisol rhythm have been

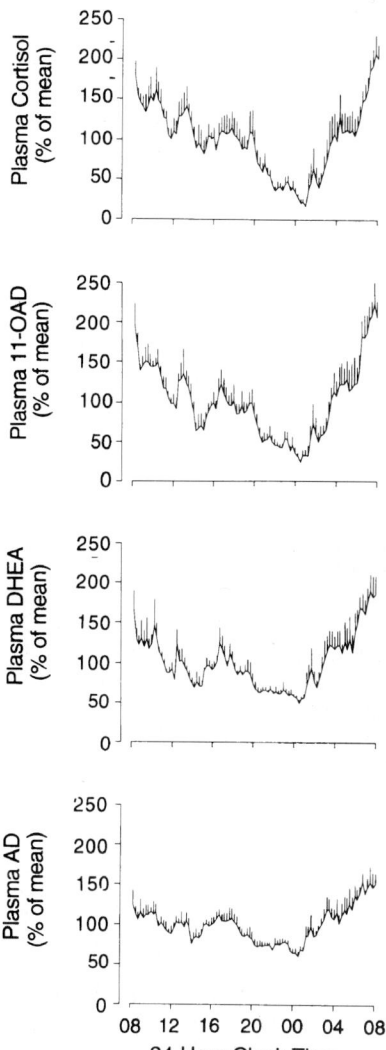

**FIGURE 6-8.** Mean 24-hour profiles of plasma cortisol, 11-hydroxyandrostenedione (*11-OAD*), dehydroepiandrosterone (*DHEA*), and androstenedione (*AD*) obtained at 15-minute intervals in 10 normal young men. For each subject and each hormone, the data were expressed as a percentage of the individual 24-hour mean before calculating group values. The vertical bars at each time point represent the standard error of the mean. (Data from Lejeune-Lenain C, Van Cauter E, Desir D, et al. Control of circadian and episodic variations of adrenal androgens secretion in man. J Endocrinol Invest 1987; 10:267.)

observed[50] include primarily (a) disorders involving abnormalities in binding and/or metabolism of cortisol, (b) the various forms of Cushing syndrome, and (c) severe depression.

The relative amplitude of the circadian rhythm and of the episodic fluctuations of cortisol is blunted in patients with liver disease and in patients with anorexia nervosa, primarily because of the decreased metabolic clearance of cortisol. In contrast, in hyperthyroidism, for which cortisol production and peripheral metabolism are increased, episodic pulses are enhanced. In hypothyroid patients, there is diminished cortisol clearance, the mean level is markedly elevated, and the relative amplitude of the rhythm is, therefore, dampened. Figure 6-9 illustrates typical 24-hour cortisol patterns of plasma cortisol and cortisol secretory rates in a patient with pituitary Cushing disease and a patient with major endogenous depression as compared with a normal subject. In patients with Cushing syndrome secondary to adrenal adenoma or ectopic ACTH secretion, the circadian variation of plasma cortisol is invariably absent. However, in pituitary-dependent Cushing disease, a low-amplitude circadian variation may persist, suggesting that

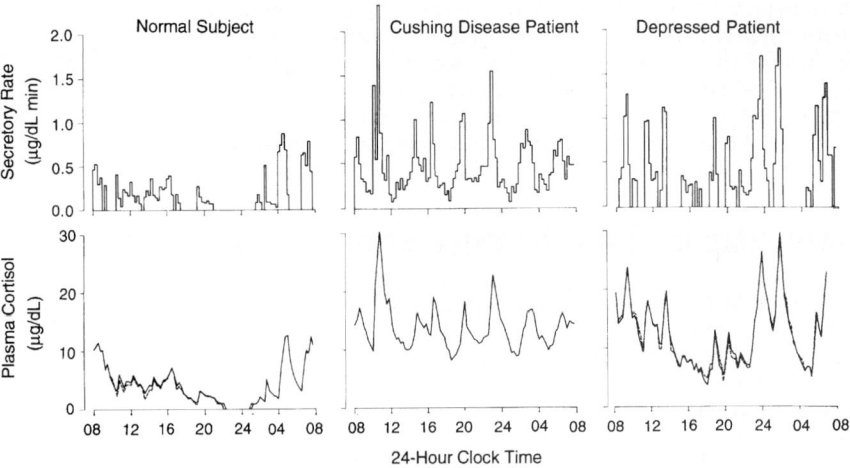

**FIGURE 6-9.** Twenty-four-hour profiles of cortisol secretory rate (*top*) and plasma cortisol (*bottom*) in a normal subject (*left*), a patient with pituitary Cushing disease (*middle*), and a patient with major endogenous depression of the unipolar subtype (*right*). Cortisol secretory rates were derived from plasma levels using a two-compartment model for cortisol distribution and metabolism. Note that circadian rhythmicity is markedly attenuated in the subject with Cushing disease, but it is preserved in the depressed patient. Cortisol secretion is entirely intermittent in the normal subject and the depressed patient, but the secretory pattern of the patient with Cushing disease shows evidence of tonic cortisol release.

there is no defect in the neural clock generating the periodicity. Cortisol pulsatility is blunted in ~70% of patients with Cushing disease, suggesting autonomous tonic secretion of ACTH by a pituitary tumor. However, in ~30% of these patients, the magnitude of the pulses is instead enhanced. These "hyperpulsatile" patterns could be caused by enhanced hypothalamic release of CRH or persistent pituitary responsiveness to CRH. Hypercortisolism with persistent circadian rhythmicity and increased pulsatility is found in a majority of acutely depressed patients. In these patients, who do not develop the clinical signs of Cushing syndrome despite the high cortisol levels, the quiescent period often occurs earlier than in normal subjects of comparable age. This *phase-advance* could reflect an alteration in the regulation of the circadian pacemaker system. When a clinical remission is obtained, the hypercortisolism and the abnormal timing of the quiescent period disappear, indicating that these disturbances are "state" rather than "trait" dependent. Contrasting with the increased cortisol pulsatility that characterizes many patients with major depression, a few studies have suggested that pulsatile variations are of lower amplitude in post-traumatic stress disorder and chronic fatigue syndrome.[51,52]

## RHYTHMS IN PROLACTIN SECRETION

Under normal conditions, the 24-hour profile of plasma PRL levels (see Chap. 13) follows a bimodal pattern, with minimal concentrations around noon, an afternoon phase of augmented secretion, and a major nocturnal elevation starting shortly after sleep onset and culminating around midsleep. Episodic pulses occur throughout the 24-hour span. Morning awakening is consistently associated with a brief PRL pulse.[53,54] Studies on PRL during daytime naps or after shifts of the sleep period have demonstrated that sleep onset is invariably associated with an increase in PRL secretion. This is well illustrated by the profiles shown in Figure 6-2 in the presence and in the absence of sleep and in Figure 6-4, which compares the profiles of day and night workers. However, a sleep-independent circadian component of PRL secretion may be observed in some individuals, particularly in women.[54] An example may be seen in the PRL profiles of night workers (see Fig. 6-4) in whom a nocturnal elevation occurred despite nocturnal activity.[15]

When sleep structure is characterized by power spectral analysis of the electroencephalogram, a close temporal association between increased PRL secretion and SW activity is clearly apparent.[55] Conversely, prolonged awakenings, which interrupt sleep, are consistently associated with decreasing PRL concentrations. Thus, shallow and fragmented sleep is generally associated with lower nocturnal PRL levels. This is

indeed what is observed in elderly subjects (see Fig. 6-6),[21] who have an increased number of awakenings and markedly decreased amounts of SW sleep, and in whom a dampening of the nocturnal PRL rise is evident. Benzodiazepine hypnotics taken at bedtime often cause an increase in the nocturnal PRL rise, resulting in concentrations in the pathologic range for part of the night.[56]

Absence or blunting of the nocturnal increase of plasma PRL has been reported in a variety of pathologic states, including uremia, breast cancer in postmenopausal women, and Cushing disease. In subjects with insulin-dependent diabetes, the circadian and sleep modulation of PRL secretion is preserved, but overall levels are markedly diminished.[57] In hyperprolactinemia associated with prolactinomas, the nocturnal elevation of PRL is preserved in patients with microadenomas but altered in patients with macroadenomas.[58] Selective removal of PRL-secreting microadenomas can result in the normalization of the PRL pattern.

## RHYTHMS IN THE GONADOTROPIC AXIS

Rhythms in the gonadotropic axis cover a wide range of frequencies, from episodic release in the ultradian range to diurnal rhythmicity and monthly and seasonal cycles. These various rhythms interact to provide a coordinated temporal program governing the development of the reproductive axis and its operation at every stage of maturation. The following summary is centered on 24-hour rhythms and their interaction with pulsatile release at the various stages of maturation of the human reproductive system. More detailed reviews may be found elsewhere.[50,59,60]

Before puberty, LH levels are very low. Both LH and FSH appear to be secreted in a pulsatile pattern but with a very low amplitude, which is insufficient to activate the gonad. The onset of puberty is associated with an augmentation of pulsatile activity in a majority of both girls and boys. In pubertal children, the magnitude of the nocturnal pulses of LH and FSH is consistently increased during sleep. As the pubescent child enters adulthood, the daytime pulse amplitude increases as well, eliminating or diminishing the diurnal rhythm. In pubertal girls, there is a diurnal variation of circulating estradiol levels, with higher concentrations during the daytime than during the nighttime. The lack of parallelism between gonadotropin and estradiol levels reflects a 6- to 8-hour delay between gonadotropin stimulation and the subsequent ovarian response. In pubertal boys, the nocturnal rise of testosterone coincides with the elevation of gonadotropins.

Patterns of LH release in adult men exhibit large interindividual variability. The diurnal variation is dampened and may become undetectable. A marked diurnal rhythm in circulating testosterone levels in young adults, with minimal levels in the late evening and maximal levels in the early morning, has been well demonstrated. In young male adults, the amplitude of the circadian variation averages 25% of the 24-hour mean.[49] In older men, the amplitude of LH pulses is decreased, and no significant diurnal pattern can be detected. However, the circadian rhythm in testosterone remains apparent, although markedly dampened.

In adult women, the 24-hour variation in plasma LH is modulated by the menstrual cycle. In the early follicular phase, LH pulses are large and infrequent, and a slowing of the frequency of secretory pulses occurs during sleep. In the midfollicular phase, pulse amplitude is decreased, pulse frequency is increased, and frequency modulation of LH pulsatility by sleep is less apparent. Pulse amplitude increases again by the late follicular phase. No modulation by sleep is apparent until the early luteal phase, when nocturnal slowing of pulsatility is again evident. During the luteal-follicular transition, there is a four- to five-fold increase in LH pulse frequency, which accompanies the selective FSH rise necessary for normal folliculogenesis. Toward menopause, gonadotropin levels are elevated but show no consistent circadian pattern.

Abnormal ultradian and/or circadian hormonal profiles have been found in a wide variety of reproductive disorders. The findings pertaining to disorders of female and male reproduction for which an abnormal function of the hypothalamic pulse generator and/or its modulation by diurnal rhythmicity seem to be primarily involved have been reviewed elsewhere.[50,59,60]

## RHYTHMS IN THE THYROTROPIC AXIS

In normal adult men and women, TSH levels are low throughout the daytime and begin to increase in the late afternoon or early evening.[61] Maximal levels occur shortly before sleep. During sleep, TSH levels generally decline slowly. A further decrease occurs in the morning hours (see Figs. 6-2 and 6-6). Studies involving sleep deprivation and shifts of the sleep-wake cycle have consistently indicated that an inhibitory influence is exerted on TSH secretion during sleep. Interestingly, when sleep occurs during daytime hours, TSH secretion is not suppressed significantly below normal daytime levels. When the depth of sleep is increased by prior sleep deprivation, the nocturnal TSH rise is even further blunted. There is a consistent association between descending slopes of TSH concentrations and SW stages.[62] The pronounced enhancing effect of sleep deprivation on the nighttime TSH rise is illustrated in Figure 6-2. The timing of the evening rise seems to be controlled by circadian rhythmicity. The temporal pattern of TSH secretion seems to reflect both tonic and pulsatile release, with both the frequency and the amplitude of the pulses increasing during the nighttime. Pulses of TSH secretion persist during somatostatin or dopamine treatment, suggesting that the control of pulsatility is largely thyrotropin-releasing hormone dependent.[61]

Because triiodothyronine and thyroxine are largely bound to serum protein, the existence of a circadian rhythm independent of postural changes has been difficult to establish. However, under conditions of sleep deprivation, the increased amplitude of the TSH rhythm results in an increased amplitude of the triiodothyronine rhythm, which becomes detectable in a majority of subjects.

The fact that the inhibitory effects of sleep on TSH secretion are time dependent may cause, under certain circumstances, elevations of plasma TSH levels, which reflect the misalignment of sleep and circadian timing. Figure 6-10 shows the mean profiles of plasma TSH levels observed in a group of normal young men in the course of adaptation to simulated jet

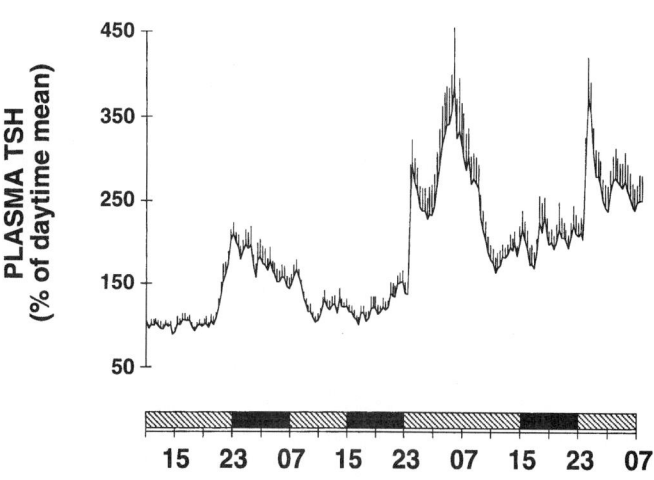

**FIGURE 6-10.** Mean (and standard error of the mean) profiles of plasma thyrotropin (thyroid-stimulating hormone [*TSH*]) from eight normal young men who were subjected to an 8-hour advance of the sleep-wake and dark-light cycles. Black bars indicate bedtime periods. (Data from Hirschfeld U, Moreno-Reyes R, Akseki E, et al. Progressive elevation of plasma thyrotropin during adaptation to simulated jet lag: effects of treatment with bright light or zolpidem. J Clin Endocrinol Metab 1996; 81:3270.)

lag.[63] After a 24-hour baseline period, the sleep-wake cycle and the dark period were abruptly advanced by 8 hours. In the course of adaptation, TSH levels increased progressively, because daytime sleep failed to inhibit TSH, and nighttime wakefulness was associated with large circadian-dependent TSH elevations. As a result, mean TSH levels after awakening from the second shifted sleep period were more than two-fold higher than during the same time interval after normal nocturnal sleep. This study demonstrates that the subjective discomfort and fatigue associated with jet lag may involve a prolonged elevation of a hormonal concentration in the peripheral circulation.

In older adults, there is an overall decrease of TSH levels (see Fig. 6-6), but the rhythm persists, albeit slightly dampened and with an earlier evening rise than in younger adults.[64] Fasting decreases overall TSH levels by decreasing pulse amplitude, resulting in a dampening of the nocturnal surge.[65]

A decreased or absent nocturnal rise of TSH has been observed in a wide variety of nonthyroidal illnesses, suggesting that hypothalamic dysregulation generally affects the circadian TSH surge. The nocturnal TSH surge is diminished or absent in hyperthyroidism, central hypothyroidism, and in various conditions of hypercortisolism. The lack of normal nocturnal elevation of TSH levels also appears to be a sensitive index of preclinical hyperthyroidism. In poorly controlled diabetic states, whether type 1 or type 2, the surge also disappears.[66] Correction of hyperglycemia is associated with a reappearance of the nocturnal elevation.[66]

## RHYTHMS IN GLUCOSE REGULATION

In normal humans, glucose tolerance varies with the time of day.[67] Figure 6-11 illustrates circadian variations in glucose tolerance to oral glucose, identical meals, constant glucose infusion, and enteral nutrition in normal subjects. Plasma glucose responses to oral glucose, intravenous glucose, or meals are markedly higher in the evening than in the morning. Overnight studies of subjects sleeping in the laboratory have consistently observed that despite the prolonged fasting condition,

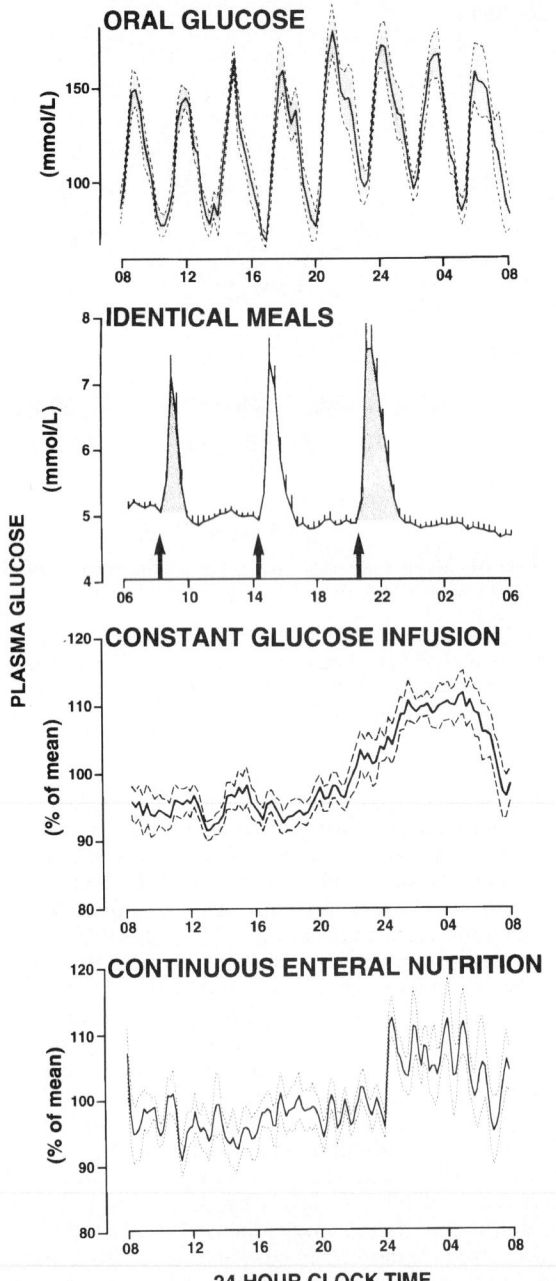

**FIGURE 6-11.** Twenty-four-hour pattern of blood glucose changes in response to oral glucose (*top panel;* 50 g glucose every 3 hours), identical meals, constant glucose, and continuous enteral nutrition in normal young adults. At each time point, the mean glucose level is shown with the standard error of the mean. (Reproduced from Van Cauter E, Polonsky KS, Scheen AJ. Roles of circadian rhythmicity and sleep in human glucose regulation. Endocr Rev 1997; 18:716.)

ation in glucose tolerance is partly driven by the wide and highly reproducible 24-hour rhythm of circulating levels of cortisol, an important counterregulatory hormone.[68] Diminished insulin sensitivity and decreased insulin secretion in relation to elevated glucose levels are both involved in causing reduced glucose tolerance later in the day. During the first part of the night, decreased glucose tolerance is due to decreased glucose utilization both by peripheral tissues (relaxed muscles and rapid insulin-like effects of sleep-onset GH secretion) and by the brain (imaging studies have demonstrated a reduction in glucose uptake during SW sleep). During the second part of the night, these effects subside, as sleep becomes more shallow and fragmented. Thus, complex interactions of circadian and sleep effects result in a consistent and predictable pattern of changes of the setpoint of glucose regulation over the 24-hour cycle.

Human insulin secretion is a complex oscillatory process including rapid pulses recurring every 10 to 15 minutes superimposed on slower, ultradian oscillations with periods in the 90- to 120-minute range.[26] The ultradian oscillations are tightly coupled to glucose, and the periodicity of the insulin secretory oscillations can be entrained to the period of an oscillatory glucose infusion, supporting the concept that these ultradian oscillations are generated by the glucose-insulin feedback mechanism.[69] Stimulatory effects of sleep on insulin secretion are mediated by an increase in the amplitude of the oscillation.[70] The rapid 10- to 15-minute pulsations seem to have a different origin from that of the ultradian oscillations.[26] Indeed, they may appear independently of glucose, because they have been observed in the isolated perfused pancreas and in isolated islets. Thus, the existence of an intrapancreatic pacemaker generating rapid oscillations has been postulated.

In obese and diabetic subjects, the diurnal and ultradian variations in glucose regulation are abnormal. In obesity, the morning versus evening difference in glucose tolerance observed in normal subjects is abolished. In type 1 diabetic patients, the increase in glucose levels and/or insulin requirements, which occurs in a prebreakfast period ranging from 5:00 a.m. to 9:00 a.m., has been called the *dawn phenomenon.*[71] A role for nocturnal GH secretion in the pathogenesis of the dawn phenomenon has been demonstrated in some, but not all, studies. The observation of a dawn phenomenon in type 2 diabetes patients under normal dietary conditions has been less consistent. Prominent diurnal variations in glucose levels and insulin secretion in both normal subjects and diabetic patients become apparent during prolonged fasting.[72] Figure 6-12 illustrates these variations in diabetic patients and age-, sex-, and weight-matched controls studied during a 24-hour fast following an overnight fast.[72] As expected, glucose levels initially declined as a result of the fasting condition, but started rising again in the late evening to reach a morning maximum. The nocturnal rise of glucose during prolonged fasting could represent a normal diurnal variation in the setpoint of glucose regulation amplified by counterregulatory mechanisms activated by the fasting condition.

The rapid and ultradian oscillations of insulin secretion are perturbed in type 2 diabetes and in impaired glucose tolerance without hyperglycemia. The rapid pulses appear to be less regular and of shorter duration than in normal subjects.[73,74] A less regular oscillatory pattern may already be detected in relatives of patients with type 2 diabetes. The ultradian oscillations, which have an exaggerated amplitude in obese subjects without apparent changes in frequency or pattern of recurrence, are irregular and of lower amplitude in subjects with established type 2 diabetes.[75–77] Disturbances in the pattern of entrainment of insulin secretion to oscillatory glucose infusions are evident in type 2 diabetes patients, in nondiabetic subjects with impaired glucose tolerance,[77] and in nondiabetic first-degree relatives of subjects with type 2 diabetes.[26]

glucose levels remain stable or fall only minimally across the night, contrasting with the clear decrease that is associated with daytime fasting. Thus, a number of mechanisms operative during nocturnal sleep must intervene to maintain stable glucose levels during the overnight fast. Experimental protocols using intravenous glucose infusion or enteral nutrition (the two experimental conditions allowing for the study of nighttime glucose tolerance during sleep without awakening the subjects) have shown that glucose tolerance deteriorates further as the evening progresses, reaches a minimum around midsleep, and then improves to return to morning levels (see Fig. 6-11).[67] There is evidence to indicate that this diurnal vari-

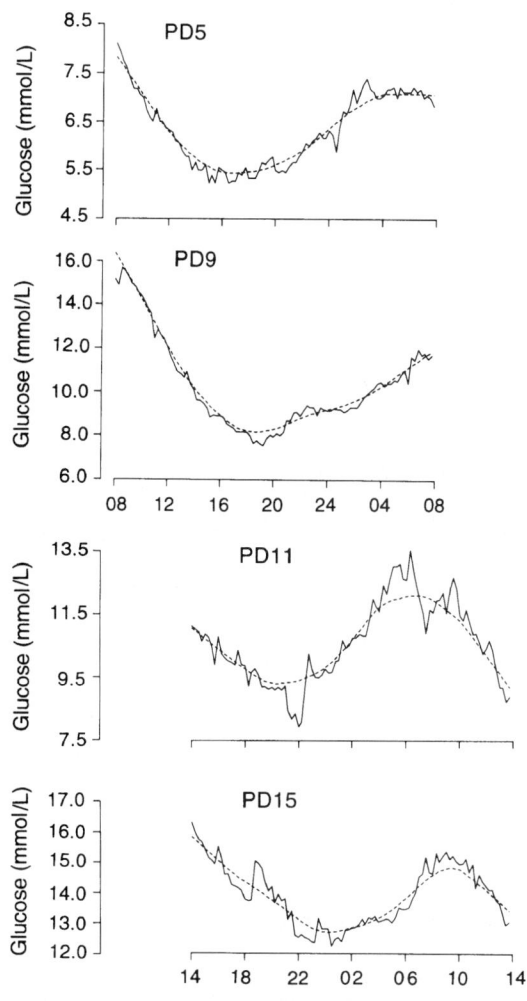

**FIGURE 6-12.** Individual 24-hour glucose profiles from four subjects with type 2 diabetes who remained fasted throughout the study period. The two upper profiles were obtained from 8 a.m. the first day until 8 a.m. the next day. The two lower profiles were obtained from 2 p.m. the first day until 2 p.m. the next day. Irrespective of the timing of the beginning of the fasting period, glucose concentrations started increasing in the evening and peaked in the morning. The dashed lines represent the best-fit curve. (From Shapiro ET, Polonsky KS, Copinschi G, et al. Nocturnal elevation of glucose levels during fasting in noninsulin-dependent diabetes. J Clin Endocrinol Metab 1991; 72:444.)

# REFERENCES

1. Turek FW. Circadian rhythms. Horm Res 1998; 49:109.
2. Borbely AA. Processes underlying sleep regulation. Horm Res 1998; 49:114.
3. Vitaterna MH, King DP, Chang AM, et al. Mutagenesis and mapping of a mouse gene, Clock, essential for circadian behavior. Science 1994; 264:719.
4. King DP, Zhao Y, Sangoram AM, et al. Positional cloning of the mouse circadian Clock gene. Cell 1997; 89:641.
5. Dunlap JC. Molecular bases for circadian clocks. Cell 1999; 96:271.
6. Porkka-Heiskanen T, Strecker RE, Thakkar M, et al. Adenosine: a mediator of the sleep-inducing effects of prolonged wakefulness. Science 1997; 276:1255.
6a. Spiegel K, Leproult R, Van Cauter E. Impact of sleep debt on metabolic and endocrine function. Lancet 1999; 9:1435.
7. Reinberg AE. Concepts in chronopharmacology. Annu Rev Pharmacol Toxicol 1992; 32:51.
8. Czeisler CA, Johnson MP, Duffy JF, et al. Exposure to bright light and darkness to treat physiologic maladaptation to night work. N Engl J Med 1990; 322:1253.
9. Tepas DI, Carvalhais AB. Sleep patterns of shiftworkers. Occup Med 1990; 5:199.
10. Van Reeth O. Sleep and circadian disturbances in shift work: strategies for their management. Horm Res 1998; 49:158.
11. Roden M, Koller M, Pirich K, et al. The circadian melatonin and cortisol secretion pattern in permanent night shift workers. Am J Physiol 1993; 265:R261.
12. Folkard S, Minors DS, Waterhouse JM. Chronobiology and shift work: current issues and trends. Chronobiologia 1985; 12:31.
13. Weibel L, Follenius M, Spiegel K, et al. Comparative effect of night and daytime sleep on the 24-hour cortisol secretory profile. Sleep 1995; 18:549.
14. Weibel L, Spiegel K, Follenius M, et al. Internal dissociation of the circadian markers of the cortisol rhythm in night workers. Am J Physiol 1996; 270:E608.
15. Spiegel K, Weibel L, Gronfier C, et al. Twenty-four hour prolactin profiles in night workers. Chronobiol Int 1996; 13:283.
16. Wehr TA, Goodwin FK. Biological rhythms in manic-depressive illness. In: Wehr TA, Goodwin FK, eds. Circadian rhythms in psychiatry. Pacific Grove, CA: Boxwood Press, 1983;129.
17. Van Cauter E, Spiegel K. Circadian and sleep control of hormonal secretions. In: Turek FW, Zee PC, eds. Regulation of sleep and circadian rhythms. New York: Marcel Dekker, Inc., 1999:397.
17a. Saini J, Krieger J, Brandenberger G, et al. Continuous positive airway pressure treatment: effects on growth hormone, insulin and glucose profiles in obstructive sleep apnea patients. Horm Metab Res 1993; 25:375.
18. Grunstein RR, Handelsman DJ, Lawrence SJ, et al. Neuroendocrine dysfunction in sleep apnea: reversal by continuous positive airways pressure therapy. J Clin Endocrinol Metab 1989; 68:352.
19. Goldstein SJ, Wu RHK, Thorpy MJ, et al. Reversibility of deficient sleep entrained growth hormone secretion in a boy with achondroplasia and obstructive sleep apnea. Acta Endocrinol 1987; 116:95.
20. Czeisler CA, Chiasera AJ, Duffy JF. Research on sleep, circadian rhythms and aging: applications to manned spaceflight. Exp Gerontol 1991; 26:217.
21. van Coevorden A, Mockel J, Laurent E, et al. Neuroendocrine rhythms and sleep in aging. Am J Physiol 1991; 260:E651.
22. Chapotot F, Gronfier C, Jouny C, et al. Cortisol secretion is related to electroencephalographic alertness in human subjects during daytime wakefulness. J Clin Endocrinol Metab 1998; 83:4263.
23. Hotchkiss J, Knobil E. The menstrual cycle and its neuroendocrine control. In: Knobil E, Neil JD, eds. The physiology of reproduction, 2nd ed. New York: Raven Press, 1994:711.
24. Wetsel WC, Valenca MM, Merchenthaler I, et al. Intrinsic pulsatile secretory activity of immortalized luteinizing hormone-releasing hormone-secreting neurons. Proc Natl Acad Sci U S A 1992; 89:4149.
25. Simon C, Brandenberger G, Follenius M. Ultradian oscillations of plasma glucose, insulin, and C-peptide in man during continuous enteral nutrition. J Clin Endocrinol Metab 1987; 64:669.
26. Polonsky KS, Sturis J, Van Cauter E. Temporal profiles and clinical significance of pulsatile insulin secretion. Horm Res 1998; 49:178.
27. Conn PM, Crowley WF. Gonadotropin-releasing hormone and its analogues. N Engl J Med 1991; 324:93.
28. Van Cauter E. Computer-assisted analysis of endocrine rhythms. In: Rodbard D, Forti G, eds. Computers in endocrinology. New York: Raven Press, 1990:59.
29. Pincus SM, Keefe DL. Quantification of hormone pulsatility via an approximate entropy algorithm. Am J Physiol 1992; 262:E741.
30. Pincus SM, Goldberger AL. Physiologic time-series analysis: what does regularity quantify? Am J Physiol 1994; 266:H1643.
31. Van Cauter E, Plat L, Copinschi G. Interrelations between sleep and the somatotropic axis. Sleep 1998; 21:553.
32. Pincus SM, Gevers EF, Robinson IC, et al. Females secrete growth hormone with more process irregularity than males in both humans and rats. Am J Physiol 1996; 270:E107.
33. Ho KY, Evans WS, Blizzard RM, et al. Effects of sex and age on the 24-hour profile of growth hormone secretion in man: importance of endogenous estradiol concentrations. J Clin Endocrinol Metab 1987; 64:51.
34. Jaffe C, Turgeon D, DeMott Friberg R, et al. Nocturnal augmentation of growth hormone (GH) secretion is preserved during repetitive bolus administration of GH-releasing hormone: potential involvement of endogenous somatostatin: a clinical research center study. J Clin Endocrinol Metab 1995; 80:3321.
35. Ocampo-Lim B, Guo W, DeMott Friberg R, et al. Nocturnal growth hormone (GH) secretion is eliminated by infusion of GH-releasing hormone antagonist. J Clin Endocrinol Metab 1996; 81:4396.
36. Gronfier C, Luthringer R, Follenius M, et al. A quantitative evaluation of the relationships between growth hormone secretion and delta wave electroencephalographic activity during normal sleep and after enrichment in delta waves. Sleep 1996; 19:817.
37. Van Cauter E, Plat L, Scharf M, et al. Simultaneous stimulation of slow-wave sleep and growth hormone secretion by γ-hydroxybutyrate in normal young men. J Clin Invest 1997; 100:745.
38. Hartman ML, Veldhuis JD, Johnson ML, et al. Augmented growth hormone (GH) secretory burst frequency and amplitude mediate enhanced GH secretion during a two-day fast in normal men. J Clin Endocrinol Metab 1992; 74:757.
39. Edge JA, Dunger DB, Matthews DR, et al. Increased overnight growth hormone concentrations in diabetic compared with normal adolescents. J Clin Endocrinol Metab 1990; 71:1356.
40. Gelato MC, Oldfield E, Loriaux DL, Merriam GR. Pulsatile growth hormone secretion in patients with acromegaly and normal men: the effects of growth hormone-releasing hormone infusion. J Clin Endocrinol Metab 1990; 71:585.
41. Hartman ML, Veldhuis JD, Vance ML, et al. Somatotropin pulse frequency and basal concentrations are increased in acromegaly and are reduced by successful therapy. J Clin Endocrinol Metab 1990; 70:1375.

42. Weitzman ED, Zimmerman JC, Czeisler CA, Ronda JM. Cortisol secretion is inhibited during sleep in normal man. J Clin Endocrinol Metab 1983; 56:352.

43. Born J, Muth S, Fehm HL. The significance of sleep onset and slow wave sleep for nocturnal release of growth hormone (GH) and cortisol. Psychoneuroendocrinology 1988; 13:233.

44. Van Cauter E, Blackman JD, Roland D, et al. Modulation of glucose regulation and insulin secretion by circadian rhythmicity and sleep. J Clin Invest 1991; 88:934.

45. Follenius M, Brandenberger G, Bardasept J, et al. Nocturnal cortisol release in relation to sleep structure. Sleep 1992; 15:21.

46. Spath-Schwalbe E, Gofferje M, Kern W, et al. Sleep disruption alters nocturnal ACTH and cortisol secretory patterns. Biol Psychiatry 1991; 29:575.

47. Pruessner JC, Wolf OT, Hellhammer DH, et al. Free cortisol levels after awakening: a reliable biological marker for the assessment of adrenocortical activity. Life Sci 1997; 61:2539.

48. Leproult R, Copinschi G, Buxton O, Van Cauter E. Sleep loss results in an elevation of cortisol levels the next evening. Sleep 1997; 20:865.

49. Lejeune-Lenain C, Van Cauter E, Desir D, et al. Control of circadian and episodic variations of adrenal androgens secretion in man. J Endocrinol Invest 1987; 10:267.

50. Van Cauter E, Turek FW. Endocrine and other biological rhythms. In: DeGroot LJ, ed. Endocrinology. Philadelphia: WB Saunders, 1995:2487.

51. Yehuda R, Teicher MH, Trestman RL, et al. Cortisol regulation in posttraumatic stress disorder and major depression: a chronobiological analysis. Biol Psychiatry 1996; 40:79.

52. MacHale SM, Cavanaugh JTO, Bennie J, et al. Diurnal variation of adrenocortical activity in chronic fatigue syndrome. Neuropsychobiology 1998; 38:213.

53. Spiegel K, Follenius M, Simon C, et al. Prolactin secretion and sleep. Sleep 1994; 17:20.

54. Waldstreicher J, Duffy JF, Brown EN, et al. Gender differences in the temporal organization of prolactin (PRL) secretion: evidence for a sleep-independent circadian rhythm of circulating PRL levels: a clinical research center study. J Clin Endocrinol Metab 1996; 81:1483.

55. Spiegel K, Luthringer R, Follenius M, et al. Temporal relationship between prolactin secretion and slow-wave electroencephalographic activity during sleep. Sleep 1995; 18:543.

56. Copinschi G, Van Onderbergen A, L'Hermite-Balériaux M, et al. Effects of the short-acting benzodiazepine triazolam, taken at bedtime, on circadian and sleep-related hormonal profiles in normal men. Sleep 1990; 13:232.

57. Iranmanesh A, Veldhuis JD, Carlsen EC, et al. Attenuated pulsatile release of prolactin in men with insulin-dependent diabetes mellitus. J Clin Endocrinol Metab 1990; 71:73.

58. Seki K, Uesato T, Kato K, Shima K. Twenty-four hour secretory pattern of prolactin in hyperprolactinaemic patients with pituitary micro- and macroadenomas. Acta Endocrinol 1984; 106:433.

59. Hayes FJ, Crowley WFJ. Gonadotropin pulsations across development. Horm Res 1998; 49:163.

60. Filicori M, Tabarelli C, Casadio P, et al. Interaction between menstrual cyclicity and gonadotropin pulsatility. Horm Res 1998; 49:169.

61. Behrends J, Prank K, Dogu E, Brabant G. Central nervous system control of thyrotropin secretion during sleep and wakefulness. Horm Res 1998; 49:173.

62. Goichot B, Brandenberger G, Saini J, et al. Nocturnal plasma thyrotropin variations are related to slow-wave sleep. J Sleep Res 1992; 1:186.

63. Hirschfeld U, Moreno-Reyes R, Akseki E, et al. Progressive elevation of plasma thyrotropin during adaptation to simulated jet lag: effects of treatment with bright light or zolpidem. J Clin Endocrinol Metab 1996; 81:3270.

64. van Coevorden A, Laurent E, Decoster C, et al. Decreased basal and stimulated thyrotropin secretion in healthy elderly men. J Clin Endocrinol Metab 1989; 69:177.

65. Romijn JA, Adriaanse R, Brabant G, et al. Pulsatile secretion of thyrotropin during fasting: a decrease of thyrotropin pulse amplitude. J Clin Endocrinol Metab 1990; 70:1631.

66. Bartalena L, Cossu E, Grasso L, et al. Relationship between nocturnal serum thyrotropin peak and metabolic control in diabetic patients. J Clin Endocrinol Metab 1993; 76:983.

67. Van Cauter E, Polonsky KS, Scheen AJ. Roles of circadian rhythmicity and sleep in human glucose regulation. Endocr Rev 1997; 18:716.

68. Plat L, Byrne MM, Sturis J, et al. Effects of morning cortisol elevation on insulin secretion and glucose regulation in humans. Am J Physiol 1996; 270:E36.

69. Sturis J, Polonsky KS, Mosekilde E, Van Cauter E. Computer model for mechanisms underlying ultradian oscillations of insulin and glucose. Am J Physiol 1991; 260:E801.

70. Simon C. Ultradian pulsatility of plasma glucose and insulin secretion rates: circadian and sleep modulation. Horm Res 1998; 49:185.

71. Bolli GB, Gerich JE. The "dawn phenomenon": a common occurrence in both non-insulin-dependent and insulin-dependent diabetes mellitus. N Engl J Med 1984; 310:746.

72. Shapiro ET, Polonsky KS, Copinschi G, et al. Nocturnal elevation of glucose levels during fasting in noninsulin-dependent diabetes. J Clin Endocrinol Metab 1991; 72:444.

73. Lang DA, Matthews DR, Burnett M, Turner RC. Brief, irregular oscillations of basal plasma insulin and glucose concentrations in diabetic man. Diabetes 1981; 30:435.

74. O'Rahilly S, Turner R, Matthews D. Impaired pulsatile secretion of insulin in relatives of patients with non-insulin-dependent diabetes. N Engl J Med 1988; 318:1225.

75. Polonsky KS, Given BD, Hirsch LJ, et al. Abnormal patterns of insulin secretion in non-insulin-dependent diabetes mellitus. N Engl J Med 1988; 318:1231.

76. Simon C, Brandenberger G, Follenius M, Schlienger JL. Alteration in the temporal organisation of insulin secretion in Type 2 (non-insulin-dependent) diabetic patients under continuous enteral nutrition. Diabetologia 1991; 34:435.

77. O'Meara NM, Sturis J, Van Cauter E, Polonsky KS. Lack of control by glucose of ultradian insulin secretory oscillations in impaired glucose tolerance and in non-insulin-dependent diabetes mellitus. J Clin Invest 1993; 92:262.

# CHAPTER 7

# GROWTH AND DEVELOPMENT IN THE NORMAL INFANT AND CHILD

GILBERT P. AUGUST

The pediatric population is composed of *continually changing individuals.* Thus, a knowledge of normal developmental changes is required for the clinician to recognize deviant growth and development and abnormalities in the hormonal milieu.

## HEIGHT AND WEIGHT

Height and weight standards derived from one ethnic group cannot always be applied to other ethnic groups. Furthermore, use of current standards is important, because growth data obtained from a previous generation may not apply to the present generation. The National Health Survey collected growth and anthropometric data on American children from 1963 to 1974 (Table 7-1).[1–9] These data provide standards that can be correlated with sex, race, and socioeconomic status. The growth charts distributed by pharmaceutical companies are derived from these National Health Survey data. Because the growth standards of American white and black children do not differ significantly, a single growth standard can be used. Significant differences do exist, however, in the growth standards of American children of Asian descent.[7]

Figures 7-1 through 7-4 show the current growth data from the National Health Survey. In Table 7-1, the mean heights, mean weights, and standard deviations (SDs) for children 2 to 18 years of age are detailed. The standard deviation is useful in evaluating extreme deviations in growth (e.g., heights and weights below the standard curves).[10] Children whose heights or weights are below the standard curves constitute a significant proportion of the population, because the commonly used growth charts provide data from only the 5th through the 95th percentiles.

For children aged 2 to 18 years, growth curves for as low as 2 SD below the mean are available. These curves are more in keeping with the usual definition of "normal" as comprising 95% of the population. Only 2.5% of children would be considered as "short" by these standards (Figs. 7-1 through 7-4).

The National Center for Health Statistics has revised the current growth charts to reflect a more contemporaneous standard. The new charts contain data from the 3rd to 97th percentiles. The new growth charts are available on the internet at http://www.cdc.gov/growthcharts.

**TABLE 7-1.**
**Height and Weight of Children, Body Proportions, and Error of Prediction of Adult Height (United States)**

| | Height and Weight (Mean and Standard Deviation [SD]; Ages 2–18 yr)[3] | | | | | | | | Body Proportions (Sitting Height/Stature Ratio [× 100])[4,5] | | | | | | | | Error of Height Prediction (±90% Confidence Range in cm)*[33,39] | | | |
|---|---|---|---|---|---|---|---|---|---|---|---|---|---|---|---|---|---|---|---|---|
| | Males | | | | Females | | | | Males | | | | Females | | | | RWT | | TW2 Mark 2 | |
| Age (yr) | Height (cm) | SD | Weight (kg) | SD | Height (cm) | SD | Weight (kg) | SD | White | SD | Black | SD | White | SD | Black | SD | Boys | Girls | Boys† | Girls‡ |
| 2 | 88.3 | 3.8 | 12.74 | 1.60 | 87.2 | 4.6 | 12.19 | 1.46 | — | — | — | — | — | — | — | — | 6.4 | 6.4 | — | — |
| 3 | 95.0 | 3.7 | 14.61 | 1.54 | 95.0 | 3.1 | 14.48 | 1.78 | — | — | — | — | — | — | — | — | 6.1 | 6.1 | — | — |
| 4 | 102.7 | 4.3 | 16.85 | 2.24 | 100.8 | 4.0 | 15.88 | 1.84 | — | — | — | — | — | — | — | — | 5.7 | 5.7 | — | — |
| 5 | 108.9 | 5.0 | 18.55 | 2.50 | 107.9 | 4.9 | 18.07 | 2.39 | — | — | — | — | — | — | — | — | 5.4 | 5.4 | — | 6.1 |
| 6 | 116.1 | 4.7 | 21.31 | 2.65 | 115.4 | 5.4 | 20.99 | 4.04 | 54.8 | 1.33 | 53.0 | 1.39 | 54.6 | 1.54 | 52.6 | 1.23 | 5.0 | 5.1 | 7.7 | 5.8 |
| 7 | 122.6 | 4.7 | 24.00 | 3.71 | 120.6 | 5.0 | 22.24 | 2.91 | 54.0 | 1.34 | 52.4 | 1.19 | 53.8 | 1.51 | 52.1 | 1.18 | 4.8 | 5.1 | 7.6 | 5.8 |
| 8 | 128.1 | 5.7 | 26.37 | 4.52 | 127.4 | 5.0 | 26.32 | 4.98 | 53.6 | 1.20 | 51.6 | 1.24 | 53.2 | 1.79 | 51.6 | 1.52 | 4.8 | 5.1 | 6.7 | 5.6 |
| 9 | 131.6 | 6.2 | 28.83 | 5.57 | 133.2 | 6.5 | 30.84 | 7.02 | 52.9 | 1.66 | 51.4 | 1.51 | 52.7 | 1.45 | 50.7 | 1.49 | 5.0 | 5.2 | 6.7 | 5.9 |
| 10 | 138.8 | 6.3 | 33.57 | 7.47 | 138.5 | 6.7 | 32.62 | 6.41 | 52.3 | 1.41 | 50.8 | 2.26 | 52.2 | 1.28 | 50.8 | 2.77 | 5.3 | 5.2 | 6.6 | 5.4 |
| 11 | 143.4 | 6.2 | 36.87 | 7.44 | 144.0 | 7.9 | 37.56 | 7.97 | 51.9 | 1.36 | 50.5 | 2.35 | 52.0 | 1.92 | 50.4 | 1.23 | 5.7 | 5.2 | 6.3 | 4.9 |
| 12 | 149.9 | 7.6 | 41.85 | 11.40 | 151.9 | 8.0 | 44.89 | 11.01 | 51.4 | 1.17 | 49.7 | 1.41 | 52.1 | 1.28 | 50.4 | 1.44 | 6.0 | 5.1 | 6.3 | 4.9 |
| 13 | 154.2 | 7.2 | 45.61 | 10.90 | 157.1 | 6.8 | 48.88 | 10.77 | 51.3 | 1.16 | 50.3 | 2.01 | 52.3 | 1.31 | 50.6 | 1.28 | 6.2 | 4.8 | 6.1 | 4.8 |
| 14 | 164.2 | 8.9 | 54.71 | 12.28 | 159.1 | 5.6 | 51.76 | 11.91 | 51.4 | 1.24 | 49.9 | 1.39 | 52.5 | 1.27 | 51.0 | 1.65 | 5.9 | 3.9 | 5.6 | 3.9 |
| 15 | 167.8 | 8.4 | 56.89 | 13.13 | 161.5 | 7.2 | 55.20 | 10.90 | 51.7 | 1.30 | 49.8 | 1.28 | 52.6 | 1.33 | 51.2 | 1.52 | 5.0 | — | 5.3 | — |
| 16 | 173.2 | 7.8 | 63.41 | 11.39 | 163.8 | 6.0 | 56.73 | 11.91 | 51.9 | 1.31 | 50.0 | 1.51 | 53.0 | 1.32 | 51.0 | 1.38 | 3.1 | — | 4.8 | — |
| 17 | 176.8 | 7.2 | 69.88 | 13.07 | 161.4 | 6.8 | 57.95 | 11.49 | 52.0 | 1.25 | 50.6 | 1.46 | 53.0 | 1.27 | 51.5 | 1.37 | — | — | — | — |
| 18 | 177.0 | 5.5 | 72.27 | 16.37 | 163.9 | 5.6 | 59.52 | 10.10 | — | — | — | — | — | — | — | — | — | — | — | — |

*RWT*, Roche-Wainer-Thissen method; *TW2 Mark 2*, Tanner-Whitehouse system.
*Uses midrange parental stature in the regression equations for height prediction.
†Applies to boys for whom previous growth data were not obtained.
‡Applies to premenarcheal girls for whom previous growth data and previous bone age data were not obtained.

Socioeconomic status was found to play a small but significant adverse role in the growth of children with very low family incomes.[6]

Beyond age 2 to 3 years, children grow throughout childhood until puberty along a particular height percentile channel that is determined by genetic factors. The normal pubertal growth spurt is reflected by an upward shift in height percentile. As growth decelerates later in puberty with impending epiphyseal closure, a shift downward in height percentile occurs, so that adult height more closely approximates the prepubertal percentile ranking. The reason for these shifts lies in the cross-sectional character of the standard growth charts. Cross-sectional data mask normal longitudinal growth patterns. The growth charts derived from studies in Britain have superimposed longitudinal growth lines that represent temporal variations in the onset of puberty.[11] Similar data are available for North American children.[12]

A shift in height percentile can also occur during infancy when growth velocities are adjusted in children whose birth lengths are either "too long" or "too short" in comparison with their parents' heights. The shift upward in percentile generally takes place within the first 6 months of life and is usually completed by 12 months of age. The shift downward in percentile begins later, generally after 3 months of age, and is completed by 18 months of age.[13]

The influence of midparental stature on the interpretation of a child's growth status is considered to be of such importance by some workers that conversion graphs and adjustment formulas have been developed. Tanner and coworkers[14] developed such curves for British children, and adjustment tables are now available for American children.[15] Parental heights can also be used to predict target adult height.[16] This can be valuable when the effects of a treatment are analyzed.

The standard growth charts derived from the National Health Survey data are not as applicable for tracking the growth of premature infants or children small for gestational age. However, growth standards are available for such children through 4 years of age.[17,18] These growth charts must be adjusted for the degree of low birth weight.[19] Further, infants small for gestational age may not truly "catch up" when their heights are compared with those of their siblings.[20,21]

Whenever sufficient data exist to construct growth charts for children with constitutional diseases, those standards should be used for comparison of current growth status and for expected adult height. Such growth standards are available for children with achondroplasia, Down syndrome, diastrophic dysplasia, Duchenne muscular dystrophy, Klinefelter syndrome, Noonan syndrome, pseudoachondroplasia, Russell-Silver syndrome, spondyloepiphyseal dysplasia, and William syndrome.[22] Similar information is available for children with gonadal dysgenesis.[23,24]

Careful attention to detail is important to produce accurate height measurements that can be used to track a child's growth (Fig. 7-5). Length should be measured on a horizontal board with the head held firmly against the upright at one end and the length determined by sliding the movable upright against the child's heels. Length should be determined until 3 years of age. The growth curve from birth until 3 years of age is standardized on length. Height must be measured using a wall-mounted instrument or tape. This permits the child to stand fully upright. The feet should be together, the back and heels should be pressed against the wall or vertical part of the measuring instrument, and the head should be held in the Frankfort horizontal plane with upward pressure exerted under the child's mastoid process to hold the correct position and to measure maximal height. The measurement of height is taken by sliding a right-angle block downward until it touches the child's head; the height can then be read from the vertically mounted rule. Accurate, reproducible height measurements cannot be obtained from the commonly used height-measuring devices attached to weighing scales. The importance of adhering to the correct technique is documented in the National Health Survey data.[1–6]

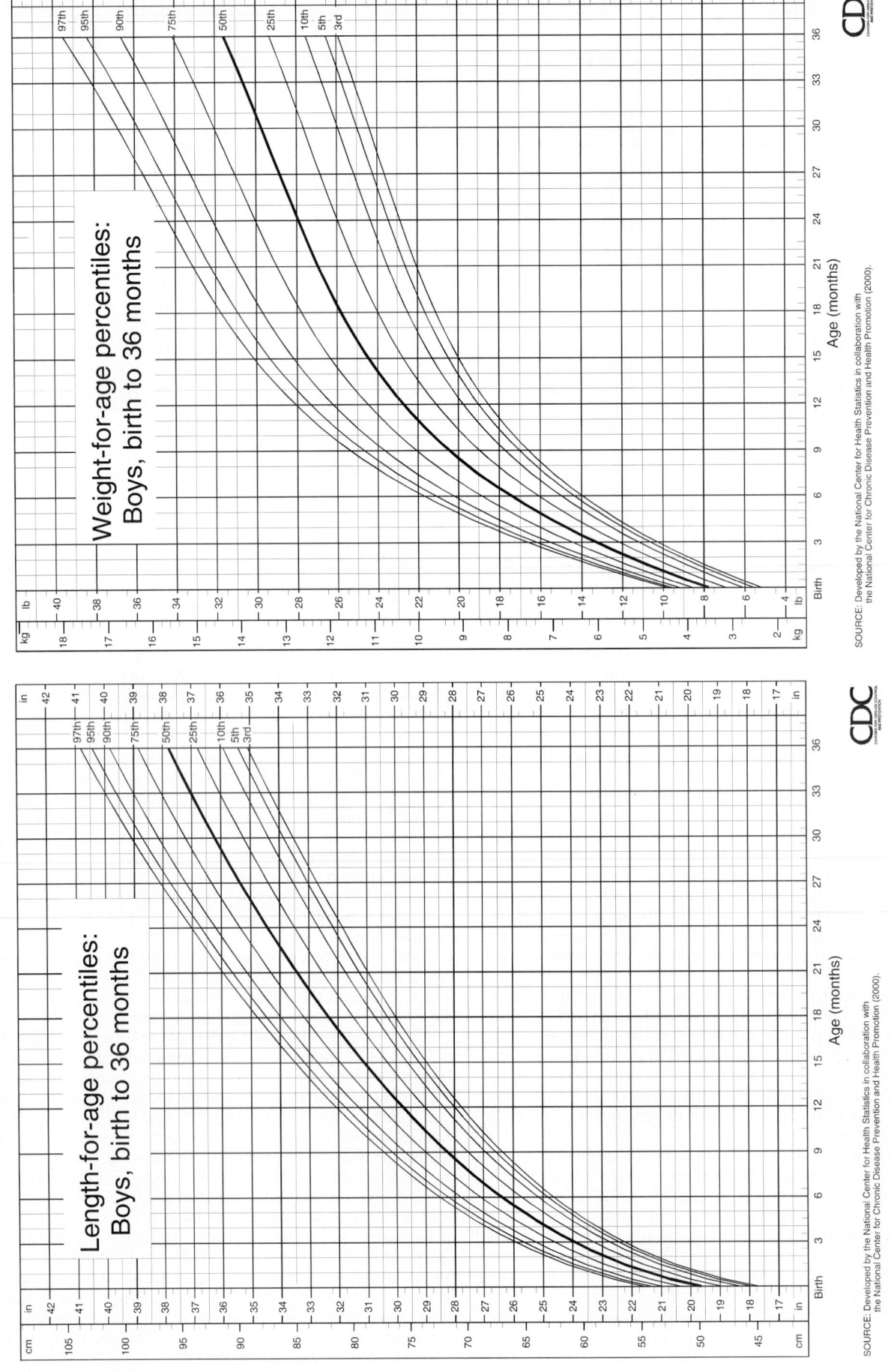

**FIGURE 7-1.** Length and weight of boys. Birth to 36 months of age. Centers for Disease Control and Prevention, National Center for Health Statistics. CDC growth charts: United States. Full size charts are available on the internet at http://www.cdc.gov/nchs/about/major/nhanes/growthcharts/charts.htm May 30, 2000.

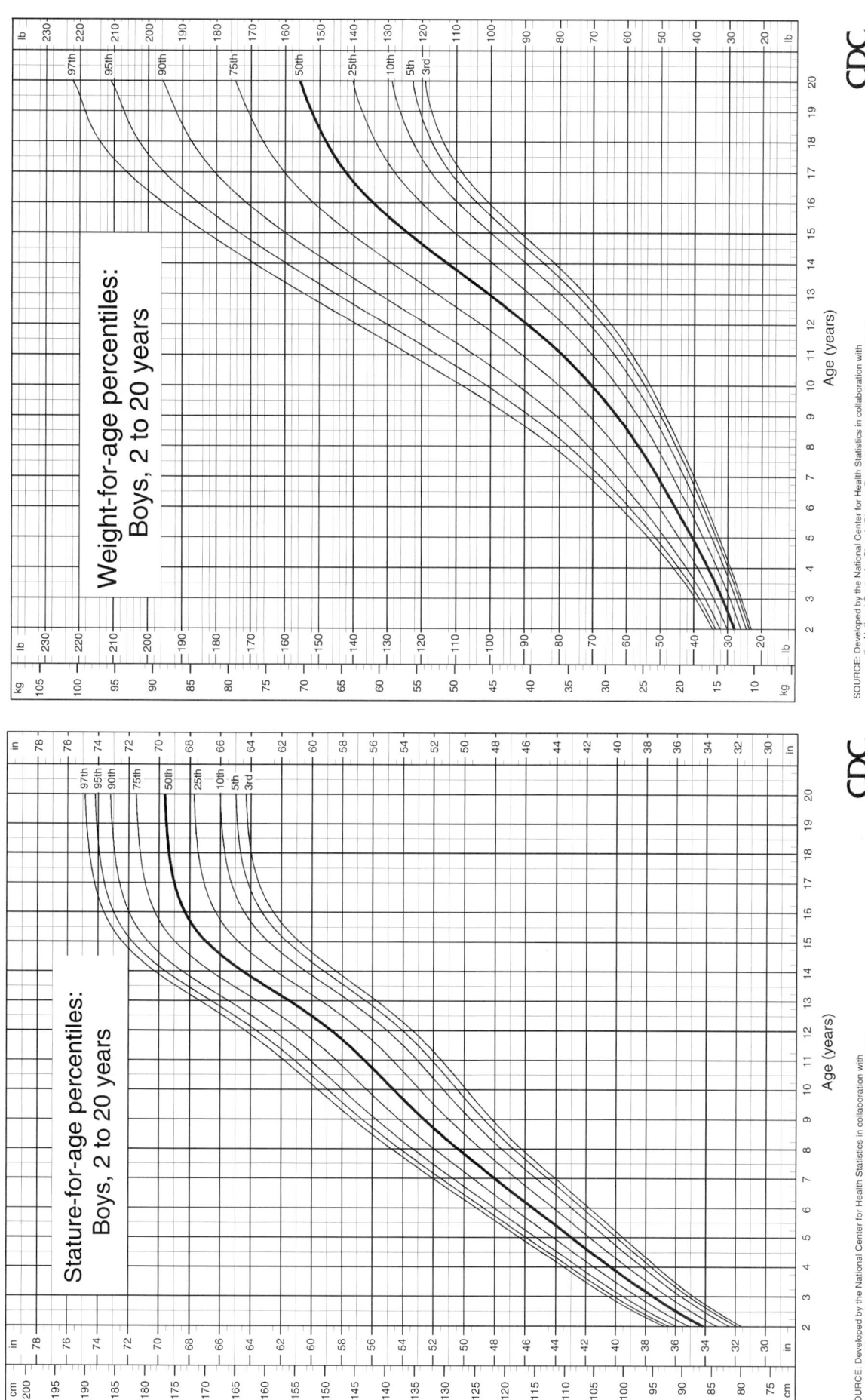

**FIGURE 7-2.** Height and weight of boys, 2 to 20 years of age. Centers for Disease Control and Prevention, National Center for Health Statistics. CDC growth charts: United States. Full size charts are available on the internet at http://www.cdc.gov/nchs/about/major/nhanes/growthcharts/charts.htm May 30, 2000.

CDC Growth Charts: United States

CDC Growth Charts: United States

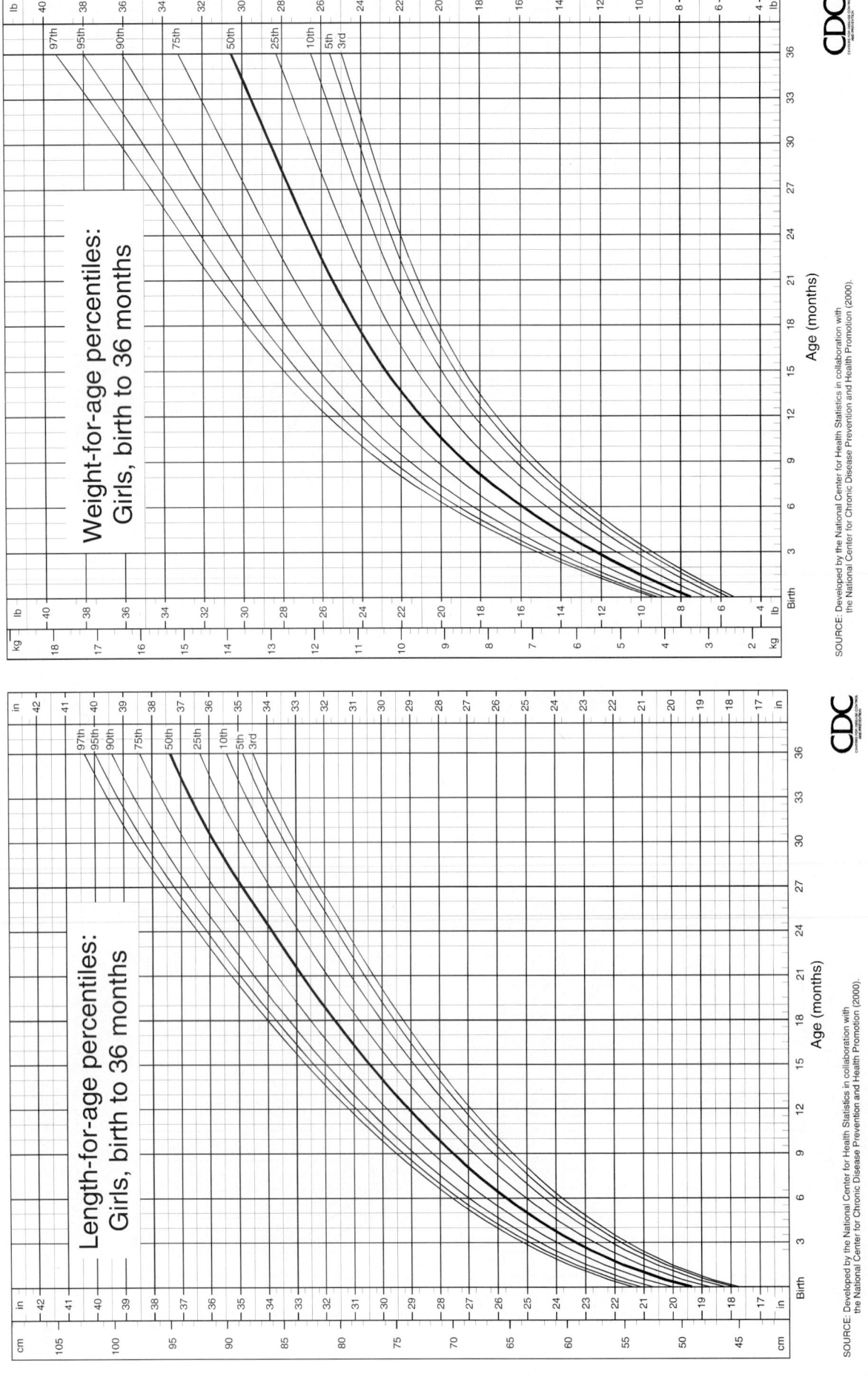

Weight-for-age percentiles:
Girls, birth to 36 months

Length-for-age percentiles:
Girls, birth to 36 months

SOURCE: Developed by the National Center for Health Statistics in collaboration with
the National Center for Chronic Disease Prevention and Health Promotion (2000).

SOURCE: Developed by the National Center for Health Statistics in collaboration with
the National Center for Chronic Disease Prevention and Health Promotion (2000).

**FIGURE 7-3.** Length and weight of girls. Birth to 36 months of age. Centers for Disease Control and Prevention, National Center for Health Statistics. CDC growth charts: United States. Full size charts are available on the internet at http://www.cdc.gov/nchs/about/major/nhanes/growthcharts/charts.htm May
30, 2000.

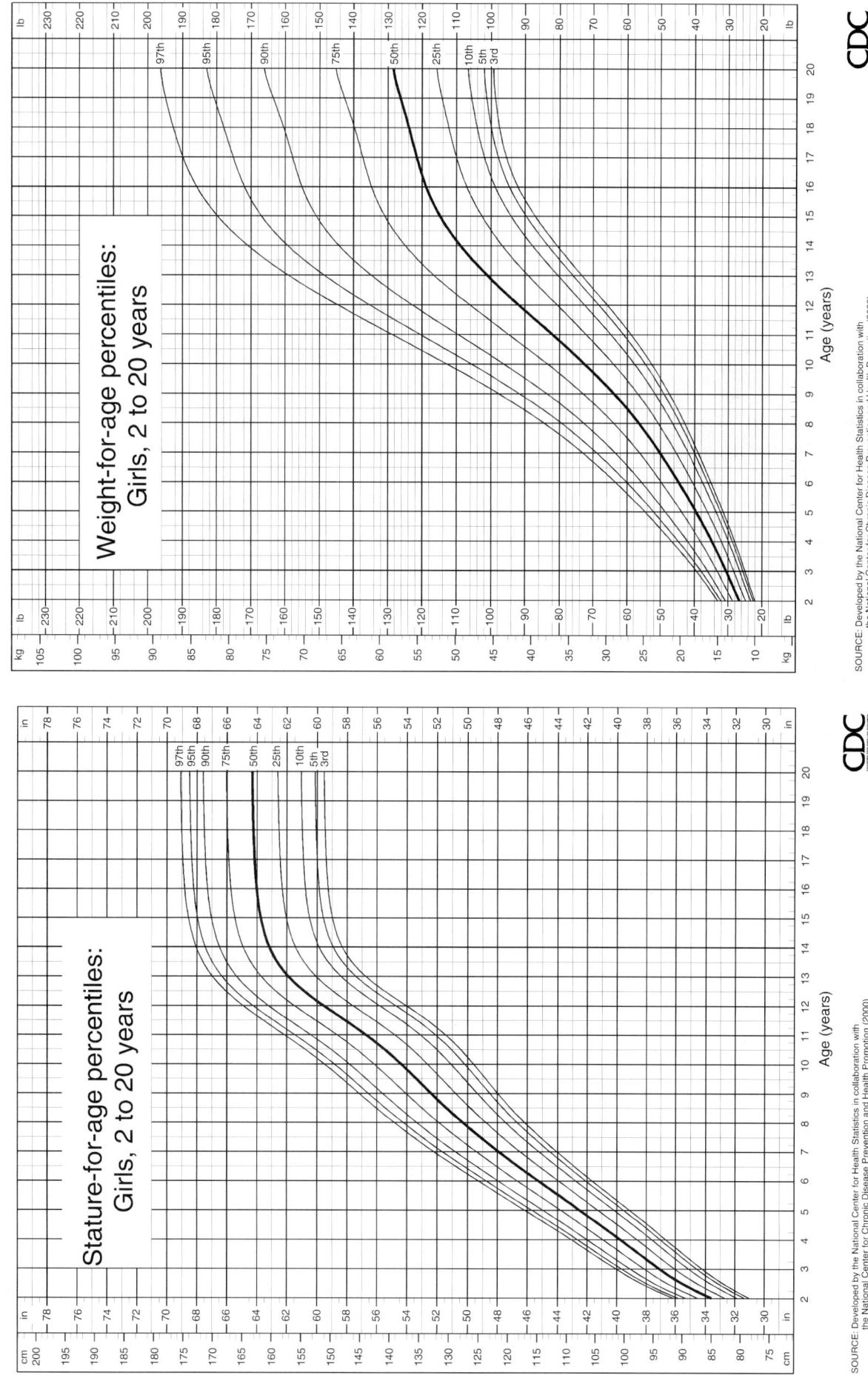

**FIGURE 7-4.** Height and weight of girls, 2 to 20 years of age. Centers for Disease Control and Prevention, National Center for Health Statistics. CDC growth charts: United States. Full size charts are available on the internet at http://www.cdc.gov/nchs/about/major/nhanes/growthcharts/charts.htm May 30, 2000.

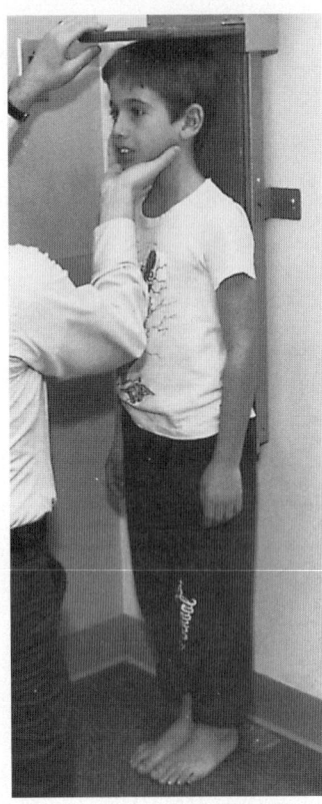

**FIGURE 7-5.** Technique of accurate measurement of standing height.

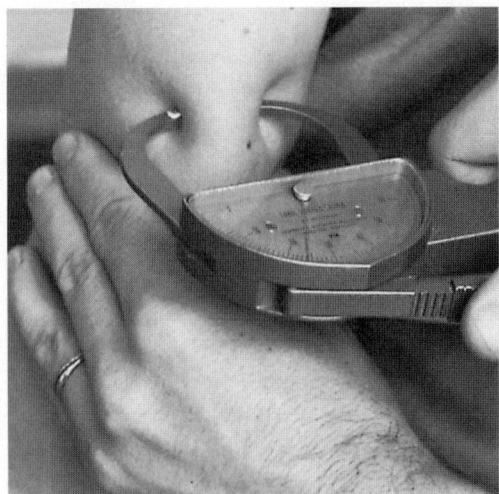

**FIGURE 7-6.** Measurement of skinfold thickness with the Lange caliper.

## GROWTH VELOCITY

The standard growth charts with their height percentiles are *growth attainment* charts, which represent how much height the child has attained by a particular age. A concept that is often more useful, especially when evaluating the longitudinal growth of an individual child, is *growth velocity*, which depicts growth during a given period. The difference in height at the beginning and end of a given period of time is annualized and then expressed as centimeters per year.[11,12] The X-axis on a growth velocity chart is the chronologic age; the Y-axis is the growth velocity in centimeters per year. These charts take into consideration the variability in height velocity caused by the normal variability in age of onset of puberty.

An advantage of height velocity charts is their ability to demonstrate more quickly an aberration of growth or the effects of treatment. Short-term growth velocity data, however, may be subject to error because of marked seasonal variation; children generally grow faster in the spring through early summer.[24]

The growth velocity charts clearly demonstrate that a child's growth rate is most rapid during infancy and puberty and is relatively stable during the elementary school years.

Although these charts present height velocity percentiles ranging from the 3rd to 97th percentiles, these may not represent the biologic normal range. Longitudinal growth that is consistently below the 10th percentile may not be sufficient to maintain a child in a single height attainment percentile; instead, that child may demonstrate a downward shift in height percentile.[25]

## SKINFOLD THICKNESS

Skinfold thickness is used as a measure of total body fat.[26] In research studies, more than one site needs to be measured, but for clinical use, the more readily accessible triceps skinfold is commonly used. The National Health Survey used a carefully standardized technique to measure the triceps skinfold. The Lange caliper (Fig. 7-6) was used on a skinfold parallel to the long axis of the arm over the triceps muscle halfway between the elbow and acromial process of the scapula; care was taken to apply the caliper so that the pressure plates remained parallel to each other. Table 7-2 presents the normal values.[27–29]

## BODY MASS INDEX

Body mass index (BMI) is another convenient measure of body fat. It is derived by calculating the weight in kilograms divided by the the height in meters squared. Population ranges for American children are now available according to ethnic group for ages 5 to 17 years.[30] The 15th, 50th, and 85th percentiles for each ethnic group appear in Table 7-3. The BMI will assume greater applicability once the new BMI curves are available from the National Center for Health Statistics. For adults, grade 1 obesity is defined as a BMI of over 25 and grade 2 obesity as a BMI over 30. Similar cutoff levels have been suggested for late adolescence. These BMI values are close to the 80th and 95th percentiles, respectively, on the National Center for Health Statistics charts.[31]

## BONE AGE

The concept of bone age is based on the skeletal changes that occur with the physical growth and maturation of the child. These skeletal changes include the calcification, growth, and shaping of the epiphyseal centers of the bones and their eventual fusion with the diaphyses. The fact that these changes occur in a regular sequence in the different bones as determined by the radiographic examination of normally developing children permits one to estimate a bone age for a particular child. Any of a number of techniques can be used, as well as any part of the skeleton. The most popular method in the United States compares a single anteroposterior radiograph of the left hand and wrist with the series of standard films in the atlas compiled by Greulich and Pyle.[32] In Europe, the Tanner method is used to calculate the bone age of the left hand and wrist by using maturity indicators for each bone, so that a composite score is derived.[33] The Tanner-Whitehouse method has been standardized for American children aged 8 to 16 years.[34]

As with any other laboratory test, there is a mean population bone age that corresponds to the particular best fit in the Greulich and Pyle atlas and a standard deviation or range of

**TABLE 7-2.**
Percentiles for Triceps Skinfold Thickness (in Millimeters) by Year of Age[27,28]

| Age (yr) | Males | | | | | | | Age | Females | | | | | | |
|---|---|---|---|---|---|---|---|---|---|---|---|---|---|---|---|
| | 5th | 10th | 25th | 50th | 75th | 90th | 95th | | 5th | 10th | 25th | 50th | 75th | 90th | 95th |
| **WHITES** | | | | | | | | | | | | | | | |
| 6 | 5.0 | 6.0 | 6.5 | 8.0 | 9.5 | 12.0 | 13.0 | 6 | 6.0 | 6.5 | 8.0 | 10.0 | 11.0 | 14.0 | 16.0 |
| 7 | 5.0 | 6.0 | 7.0 | 8.0 | 10.0 | 12.0 | 14.5 | 7 | 6.5 | 7.0 | 8.0 | 10.0 | 12.5 | 16.0 | 18.0 |
| 8 | 5.0 | 6.0 | 7.0 | 8.0 | 11.0 | 14.0 | 17.0 | 8 | 6.0 | 7.0 | 9.0 | 11.0 | 14.0 | 18.0 | 20.0 |
| 9 | 5.0 | 6.0 | 7.0 | 9.0 | 12.0 | 17.0 | 21.0 | 9 | 7.0 | 8.0 | 9.0 | 11.5 | 15.0 | 20.0 | 22.5 |
| 10 | 5.5 | 6.0 | 7.5 | 9.5 | 13.0 | 16.0 | 20.0 | 10 | 6.0 | 7.0 | 9.0 | 12.0 | 16.0 | 20.0 | 23.0 |
| 11 | 5.5 | 6.0 | 8.0 | 10.0 | 14.0 | 19.0 | 22.0 | 11 | 7.0 | 7.5 | 9.0 | 12.0 | 16.0 | 20.1 | 22.0 |
| 12 | 5.2 | 5.7 | 7.2 | 9.7 | 13.6 | 19.8 | 23.2 | 12 | 6.1 | 7.1 | 9.2 | 12.0 | 16.0 | 22.1 | 25.1 |
| 13 | 4.8 | 5.4 | 7.1 | 9.4 | 13.4 | 19.7 | 22.6 | 13 | 6.6 | 7.6 | 9.6 | 12.7 | 17.2 | 22.7 | 25.4 |
| 14 | 4.3 | 5.0 | 6.3 | 8.2 | 12.5 | 17.4 | 21.2 | 14 | 7.3 | 8.5 | 11.0 | 14.2 | 18.7 | 23.5 | 26.8 |
| 15 | 4.3 | 4.8 | 6.0 | 7.8 | 11.2 | 16.4 | 21.3 | 15 | 7.5 | 8.8 | 12.0 | 15.1 | 20.0 | 25.4 | 29.9 |
| 16 | 4.2 | 5.0 | 5.9 | 7.6 | 11.6 | 16.5 | 20.5 | 16 | 8.1 | 9.7 | 12.3 | 16.0 | 21.1 | 25.5 | 29.1 |
| 17 | 4.1 | 4.5 | 5.6 | 7.7 | 11.6 | 15.8 | 20.7 | 17 | 8.5 | 10.1 | 12.4 | 16.3 | 20.8 | 25.3 | 29.5 |
| **BLACKS** | | | | | | | | | | | | | | | |
| 6 | 4.0 | 5.0 | 5.5 | 7.0 | 8.0 | 10.0 | 11.0 | 6 | 5.0 | 5.0 | 6.0 | 7.0 | 9.0 | 11.0 | 14.0 |
| 7 | 4.0 | 4.0 | 5.0 | 6.0 | 7.0 | 9.0 | 10.0 | 7 | 5.0 | 5.0 | 6.0 | 7.5 | 9.0 | 12.0 | 16.0 |
| 8 | 4.0 | 4.0 | 5.0 | 6.5 | 8.0 | 12.0 | 13.0 | 8 | 5.0 | 5.0 | 6.5 | 8.0 | 11.0 | 14.0 | 20.0 |
| 9 | 4.0 | 4.0 | 5.0 | 6.5 | 8.0 | 11.0 | 14.0 | 9 | 5.0 | 6.0 | 7.0 | 9.0 | 12.5 | 15.5 | 19.0 |
| 10 | 4.0 | 4.0 | 5.5 | 7.0 | 9.0 | 11.0 | 13.0 | 10 | 5.0 | 6.0 | 7.0 | 9.0 | 12.0 | 20.0 | 20.2 |
| 11 | 4.0 | 4.0 | 6.0 | 7.0 | 9.0 | 12.0 | 18.0 | 11 | 4.0 | 6.0 | 7.0 | 10.0 | 12.0 | 20.0 | 25.0 |
| 12 | 3.8 | 4.7 | 5.6 | 7.4 | 10.3 | 15.3 | 23.2 | 12 | 6.0 | 6.5 | 7.7 | 10.6 | 16.2 | 22.5 | 25.6 |
| 13 | 3.6 | 4.2 | 5.2 | 7.2 | 10.3 | 15.6 | 25.2 | 13 | 6.0 | 6.3 | 7.7 | 9.8 | 13.6 | 23.9 | 27.2 |
| 14 | 3.6 | 4.1 | 4.8 | 6.4 | 8.4 | 14.2 | 19.2 | 14 | 5.5 | 6.7 | 10.0 | 12.5 | 17.3 | 22.1 | 24.6 |
| 15 | 3.9 | 4.2 | 5.1 | 6.4 | 7.7 | 10.6 | 14.7 | 15 | 7.2 | 8.2 | 10.2 | 12.8 | 17.9 | 22.7 | 25.8 |
| 16 | 4.0 | 4.3 | 4.9 | 6.7 | 8.9 | 11.7 | 12.8 | 16 | 7.0 | 7.6 | 9.6 | 13.1 | 17.8 | 26.4 | 31.5 |
| 17 | 4.2 | 4.6 | 5.3 | 6.1 | 8.5 | 14.0 | 15.8 | 17 | 7.1 | 7.6 | 10.7 | 13.4 | 18.2 | 23.3 | 25.8 |

expected values. The normal range of expected bone ages for a child younger than 1 year of age is ±3 to 6 months; for a child of 6 to 11 years of age, the range is ±2 years; and for a child of 12 to 14 years of age, the range is ±2 years.[35]

The National Health Survey compared the bone ages of contemporary children with those derived from the original study of Greulich and Pyle between 1917 and 1942. The original study population was composed of upper-middle-class children in Cleveland. In children aged 6 to 11 years, good congruence was seen except that contemporary 10- and 11-year-old children showed a significant retardation in bone age of 0.2 to 0.65 years.[36]

The assumption that bone age advances 1 year for each calendar year may not be correct; bone age advances more rapidly than chronologic age during the onset of puberty and during peak height velocity of puberty. At these times, the average advancement in bone age over chronologic age is 1.73 years, with a range of 0.8 to 2.8 years.[37] Bone age advancement should not be attributed falsely to therapeutic intervention. These results serve as another example of the difference between normal longitudinal growth of a single child and the cross-sectional standards that are usually available for tracking a child's growth and development.[37]

The determination of bone age can be useful if one remains aware of its limitations. The particular standard used must be verified for the population being studied. The person interpreting the bone age radiograph must be consistent. Separate male and female standards exist, and there is a range of normal (see Chaps. 18 and 217).

## HEIGHT PREDICTION

One of the most common applications of a bone age determination is the prediction of eventual adult height. Bayley and Pinneau[38] published prediction tables based on the percentage

of adult height attained at various bone ages. The tables were further refined by separating the children whose bone ages were >1 year advanced or retarded compared with chronologic age. Separate prediction tables are provided for these children as well as for males and females.

More mathematically refined systems have been proposed that use regression formulas with the addition of variables such as weight, midparental stature, growth velocity, and menarcheal status. The Roche-Wainer-Thissen (RWT) method uses the child's recumbent length rather than standing height and is standardized for American children.[39] The Tanner-Whitehouse system (TW2 Mark 2) is standardized for British children.[33] It includes a larger number of children at the extremes of the standardizing group and thus tries to counter one criticism of height prediction methods—that they are most accurate for the prediction of the final adult height of normal children whose bone ages are not significantly retarded. In addition, the TW2 Mark 2 system no longer takes into account midparental stature in the prediction regression formulas, as did the previous formulas.

Regardless of which system is used for the prediction of adult height, the prediction always has an error. For the RWT method, the ±90% confidence range for a prediction is given in Table 7-1. For the TW2 Mark 2 system, the error is stated as a residual standard deviation. For comparison purposes, in Table 7-1, the residual standard deviation has been multiplied by 1.645 to provide the 90% confidence range for a predicted adult height. To obtain a 95% confidence range, the residual standard deviation is multiplied by ±1.96. For normal children, these two methods are comparable and appear more accurate than the older Bailey and Pinneau tables[39]; the stated error in the latter method is 5.1 cm for ±2 SD. In a comparative study of the three methods that examined Finnish children, the RWT method was slightly more accurate.[40,41]

**TABLE 7-3.**
**Body Mass Index Centiles for Children 5–17 Years of Age**

| | Age (yr) | | | | | | | | | | | | |
|---|---|---|---|---|---|---|---|---|---|---|---|---|---|
| Centile | 5 | 6 | 7 | 8 | 9 | 10 | 11 | 12 | 13 | 14 | 15 | 16 | 17 |
| MALES | | | | | | | | | | | | | |
| **Asian** | | | | | | | | | | | | | |
| 15th | 14.0 | 14.1 | 14.3 | 14.5 | 14.7 | 15.0 | 15.4 | 16.0 | 16.6 | 17.3 | 18.0 | 18.6 | 19.2 |
| 50th | 15.0 | 15.0 | 15.2 | 15.6 | 16.0 | 16.6 | 17.1 | 17.8 | 18.4 | 19.2 | 19.9 | 20.6 | 21.2 |
| 85th | 15.5 | 15.7 | 16.1 | 16.9 | 17.9 | 19.1 | 20.0 | 20.7 | 21.2 | 21.8 | 22.5 | 23.4 | 23.8 |
| **Black** | | | | | | | | | | | | | |
| 15th | 14.4 | 14.4 | 14.6 | 14.8 | 15.1 | 15.4 | 15.8 | 16.3 | 17.0 | 17.7 | 18.3 | 18.9 | 19.6 |
| 50th | 15.5 | 15.5 | 15.8 | 16.1 | 16.5 | 17.1 | 17.7 | 18.3 | 19.0 | 19.7 | 20.5 | 21.2 | 21.7 |
| 85th | 16.8 | 17.0 | 17.4 | 18.3 | 19.4 | 20.6 | 21.6 | 22.3 | 22.8 | 23.4 | 24.1 | 25.1 | 25.5 |
| **Latino** | | | | | | | | | | | | | |
| 15th | 14.6 | 14.7 | 14.9 | 15.1 | 15.4 | 15.6 | 16.1 | 16.6 | 17.3 | 18.0 | 18.6 | 19.2 | 19.9 |
| 50th | 15.9 | 16.0 | 16.2 | 16.6 | 17.0 | 17.6 | 18.1 | 18.8 | 19.5 | 20.2 | 21.0 | 21.7 | 22.3 |
| 85th | 18.0 | 18.2 | 18.6 | 19.5 | 20.7 | 21.9 | 22.9 | 23.6 | 24.2 | 24.8 | 25.6 | 26.5 | 27.0 |
| **White** | | | | | | | | | | | | | |
| 15th | 14.4 | 14.4 | 14.6 | 14.9 | 15.1 | 15.4 | 15.8 | 16.3 | 17.0 | 17.7 | 18.3 | 18.9 | 19.6 |
| 50th | 15.5 | 15.6 | 15.8 | 16.2 | 16.6 | 17.1 | 17.7 | 18.4 | 19.1 | 19.8 | 20.5 | 21.3 | 21.8 |
| 85th | 17.1 | 17.3 | 17.7 | 18.6 | 19.7 | 20.9 | 21.9 | 22.6 | 27.0 | 23.7 | 24.5 | 25.4 | 25.9 |
| FEMALES | | | | | | | | | | | | | |
| **Asian** | | | | | | | | | | | | | |
| 15th | 13.6 | 13.8 | 14.0 | 14.2 | 14.4 | 14.8 | 15.4 | 16.1 | 16.9 | 17.7 | 18.1 | 18.4 | 18.6 |
| 50th | 14.5 | 14.6 | 14.9 | 15.3 | 15.8 | 16.5 | 17.3 | 18.2 | 19.0 | 19.6 | 20.0 | 20.2 | 20.6 |
| 85th | 15.7 | 16.1 | 16.7 | 17.7 | 18.8 | 20.0 | 21.2 | 22.2 | 23.0 | 23.5 | 23.8 | 24.0 | 24.5 |
| **Black** | | | | | | | | | | | | | |
| 15th | 14.0 | 14.2 | 14.4 | 14.6 | 14.8 | 15.2 | 15.8 | 16.6 | 17.4 | 18.1 | 18.6 | 18.9 | 19.1 |
| 50th | 15.4 | 15.5 | 15.8 | 16.2 | 16.7 | 17.4 | 18.3 | 19.2 | 20.0 | 20.7 | 21.1 | 21.3 | 21.6 |
| 85th | 17.7 | 18.1 | 18.8 | 19.8 | 21.0 | 22.3 | 23.5 | 24.6 | 25.4 | 25.9 | 26.2 | 26.5 | 26.9 |
| **Latina** | | | | | | | | | | | | | |
| 15th | 14.3 | 14.5 | 14.7 | 14.9 | 15.1 | 15.5 | 16.1 | 16.9 | 17.7 | 18.5 | 19.0 | 19.2 | 19.5 |
| 50th | 15.5 | 15.6 | 15.9 | 16.3 | 16.9 | 17.6 | 18.4 | 19.3 | 20.2 | 20.8 | 21.2 | 21.4 | 21.8 |
| 85th | 18.1 | 18.5 | 19.2 | 20.2 | 21.4 | 22.7 | 24.0 | 25.1 | 25.9 | 26.4 | 26.7 | 27.0 | 27.5 |
| **White** | | | | | | | | | | | | | |
| 15th | 13.7 | 14.0 | 14.1 | 14.3 | 14.5 | 14.9 | 15.5 | 16.3 | 17.1 | 17.8 | 18.3 | 18.5 | 18.8 |
| 50th | 14.9 | 15.0 | 15.3 | 15.7 | 16.2 | 16.9 | 17.7 | 18.6 | 19.4 | 20.1 | 20.5 | 20.7 | 21.0 |
| 85th | 16.5 | 16.9 | 17.6 | 18.6 | 19.7 | 21.0 | 22.2 | 23.2 | 24.0 | 24.5 | 24.8 | 25.1 | 25.5 |

(Data modified from Rosner B, Prineas R, Loggie J, Daniels SR. Percentiles for body mass index in US children 5 to 17 years of age. J Pediatrics 1998; 132:211.)

The important issue is not how well the various height prediction systems work in normal children but rather how well they work in children with abnormal growth patterns. In children with familial tall stature, the Tanner method was slightly more accurate than the other two methods.[41] Both the RWT and Tanner methods, however, overestimated adult height in children with precocious puberty or gonadal dysgenesis; the Bailey and Pinneau tables were more accurate in these conditions. The overestimation for children with precocious puberty ranged from 30 cm at 5 years of age to just 5 cm at 13 years of age. The overestimation of adult height was 10 cm at the earlier ages in children with gonadal dysgenesis. The greater accuracy of height prediction with increasing age of the patient also holds true for children with constitutional tall stature.[42] In addition, the RWT and Tanner methods both overestimated the adult heights of children with primordial short stature.[41]

These studies used the older Tanner methods. Tanner and coworkers[33] point out several limitations to the accuracy of their new formulas that should apply to other height prediction systems. Although the formulas take into account several variables, some unpredictability still exists, as reflected in the residual standard deviation. Tanner and co-workers[33] point out that no particular reason exists that the equations should be valid in cases of precocious puberty or achondroplasia.

In part, the error in height prediction, measured by whatever means, may be due to the variability in total height gained during puberty. In a review[43] of four studies of American children, from the onset of puberty, girls had an average gain in height of 25.4 to 31 cm, and boys had an average gain in height of 28.2 to 31 cm. The standard deviations ranged from 4 to 6.8 cm for girls and 4.3 to 5.5 cm for boys. Thus, although considerable height was gained during puberty, considerable variability was seen as well. Similar results were reported in European studies.[43] Confounding this further is the inverse relationship between height obtained during puberty and the age of onset of puberty.[44] This phenomenon may be related to the shortened duration of puberty, at least in girls, with the later onset of puberty.[45]

Finally, an additional caution arises from a study that compared the final adult height achieved by short children with normal bone ages and by short children with significantly retarded bone ages with predictions of the children's height using the Bailey and Pinneau tables.[46] Although only 1 of 17 children with normal bone age had an overpredicted adult height, 5 of 10 children with a retarded bone age had an overprediction of their adult height—they failed to reach an adult height within 5.1 cm of the predicted height.[46] This is the group of children for whom the physician is most often called on to

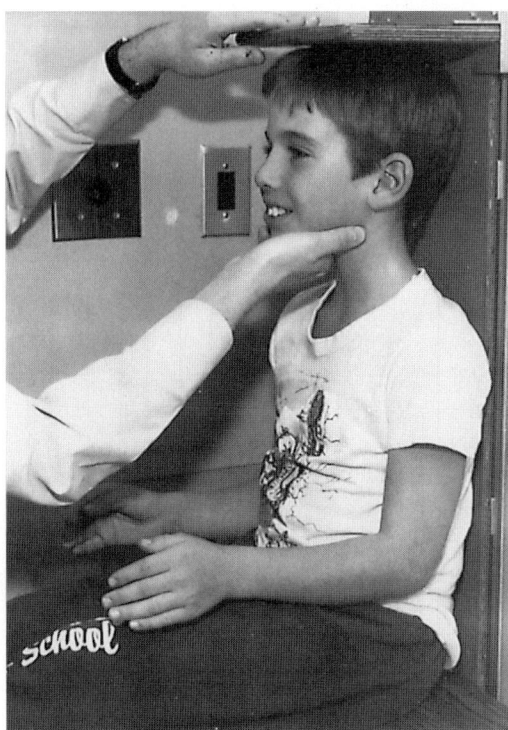

**FIGURE 7-7.** Technique of accurate measurement of sitting height.

use height prediction tables and provide reassurance to the patient and family.

A comparison of predicted adult height, based on bone age and current height, with the predicted genetic target adult height based on parental heights is often useful.[16] This is of importance when determining if the child's current height is inconsistent with genetic potential or when one is evaluating the effects of a therapeutic intervention.

### BODY PROPORTIONS

Significant racial differences exist in regard to body proportions. The sitting/standing height ratio was determined during the National Health Survey.[4,5] These data are presented in Table 7-1. Careful attention to detail is required. Height measurement using a wall-mounted instrument is required. Sitting height is measured on a sitting height table, with the child sitting erect in a standardized manner and with the head held in the Frankfort plane[4,5] (Fig. 7-7).

### GENITAL DEVELOPMENT

Table 7-4 presents the normal standards for penile and testicular size.[47–49] Penile length is a stretched length; traction is applied to the penis and the rule is applied firmly to the root of the penis. Too often, the suprapubic fat pad is not compressed enough so that one obtains a penile length that is artifactually too short (see Chap. 93).

## DEVELOPMENTAL ENDOCRINOLOGY

The pediatric patient undergoes continuous change that is reflected not only in growth rates but also in the secretory activity of the endocrine system. The perinatal period is one of rapid change in the endocrine system when the child is adjusting to extrauterine life (Table 7-6). This is further complicated by the differences that may exist in hormonal levels in the full-term

**TABLE 7-4.**
**Penile and Testicular Size During Childhood**

| Age (yr) | Penis Length* | | Testis Length | |
|---|---|---|---|---|
| | cm | SD | cm† | SD |
| 0.2–2.0 | 2.7 | 0.5 | 1.4 | 0.4 |
| 2.1–4.0 | 3.3 | 0.4 | 1.2 | 0.4 |
| 4.1–6.0 | 3.9 | 0.9 | 1.5 | 0.6 |
| 6.1–8.0 | 4.2 | 0.8 | 1.8 | 0.3 |
| 8.1–10.0 | 4.9 | 1.0 | 2.0 | 0.5 |
| 10.1–12.0 | 5.2 | 1.3 | 2.7 | 0.7 |
| 12.1–14.0 | 6.2 | 2.0 | 3.4 | 0.8 |
| 14.1–16.0 | 8.6 | 2.4 | 4.1 | 1.0 |
| 16.1–18.0 | 9.9 | 1.7 | 5.0 | 0.5 |
| 18.1–20.0 | 11.0 | 1.1 | 5.0 | 0.3 |

SD, standard deviation.
At age 10 years, the mean testicular volume, using the Prader orchidometer, is 1.8 cm, with the 10th to 90th range being 1.0 to 2.0.
*The penile lengths in this table are shorter than those found by Schonfeld.[49] This may be related to the degree of stretching of the penis (see Chap. 90).
†See Chapter 93 for testicular size in terms of volume.
(Data from Winter JSD, Faiman C. Pituitary-gonadal relations in male children and adolescents. Pediatr Res 1972; 6:126; and from Zachmann M, Prader A, Kind HP, et al. Testicular volume during adolescence: cross sectional and longitudinal studies. Helv Paediatr Acta 1974; 29:61.)

versus preterm infant. This section outlines some of these hormonal variations. As a general rule, one can divide the analysis of hormonal secretory activity into the following developmental periods: fetal, perinatal, childhood, and pubertal.[50,51]

### GROWTH HORMONE AND INSULIN-LIKE GROWTH FACTORS

Immunoreactive growth hormone is found in human anterior pituitary glands as early as the seventh week of gestation.[49] Pituitary growth hormone increases from 0.44 μg per gland at 10 to 14 weeks of gestation to a mean of 675 μg per gland at term. However, pituitary growth hormone level is fairly constant after 25 weeks of gestation. Growth hormone is also detectable in fetal serum in high concentration. These high concentrations of growth hormone may be a reflection of hypothalamic-pituitary neuroendocrine immaturity. At 10 to 14 weeks of gestation, the mean growth hormone level in fetal serum is 65 ng/mL, and it rises rapidly to a peak fetal concentration of 132 ng/mL at 20 to 25 weeks of gestation. Thereafter, serum growth hormone declines to 35 ng/mL at 35 to 40 weeks of gestation.

The postulated immature neuroendocrine control of growth hormone secretion persists into the neonatal period. Growth hormone is not suppressed by glucose until 1 month of age, and the normal sleep-induced rise in serum growth hormone levels does not appear until 3 months of age.[51]

**TABLE 7-5.**
**Normal Values for Insulin-Like Binding Protein-2 (IGFBP-2)**

| Age (yr) | ng/mL |
|---|---|
| 0–1 | 348–922 |
| 1–2 | 280–750 |
| 2–6 | 275–700 |
| 6–10 | 200–540 |
| 10–15 | 200–470 |
| 15–25 | 215–518 |
| 25–45 | 220–570 |
| 45–65 | 225–710 |
| 65–75 | 225–850 |

(Data from Endocrine Sciences, Calabasas Hills, CA.)

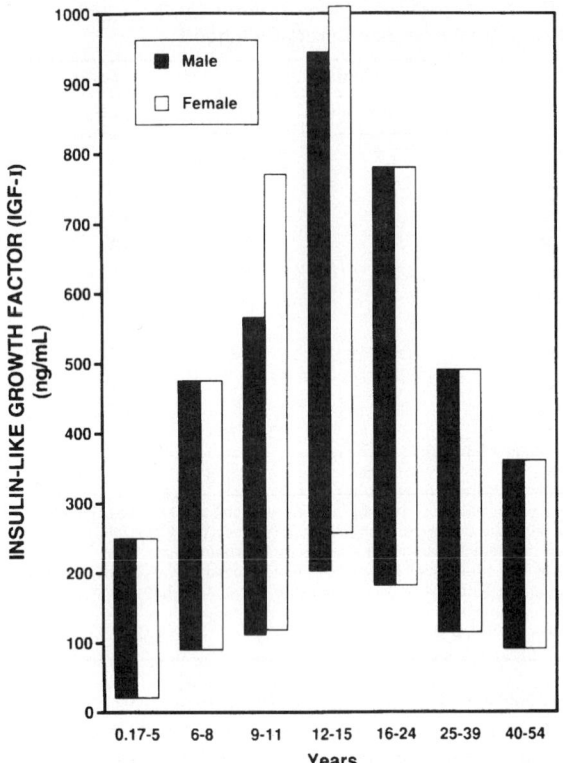

**FIGURE 7-8.** Variation of insulin-like growth factor-I with age and sex. (Data derived from the normal values provided by Quest Diagnostic Nichols Institute, San Juan Capistrano, California.)

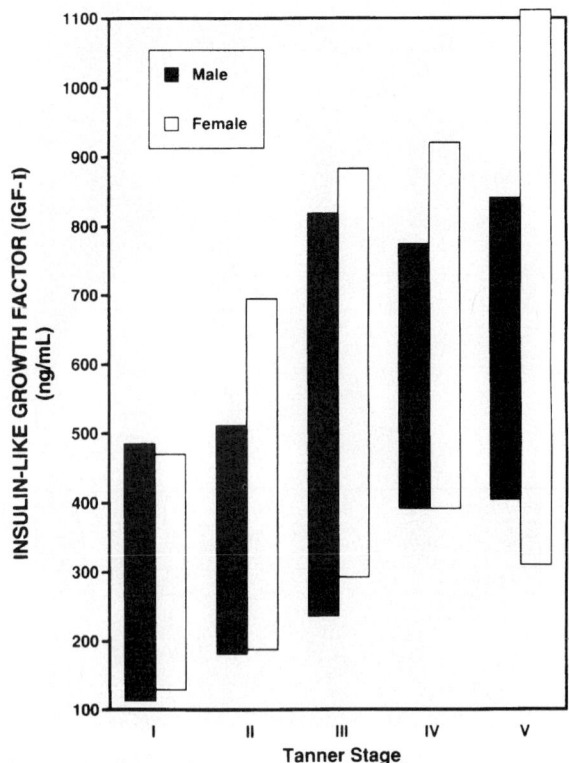

**FIGURE 7-9.** Variation of insulin-like growth factor-I with stage of puberty and sex. (Data derived from the normal values provided by Quest Diagnostic Nichols Institute, San Juan Capistrano, California.)

Insulin-like growth factor-I (IGF-I) plasma concentrations show a marked age-related pattern. The normal ranges, as reported by the Quest Diagnostic Nichols Institute, are shown in Figures 7-8 and 7-9. The range is large, and a marked overlap of values is seen when one compares the lower range of normal with values typically associated with growth hormone deficiency. Plasma IGF-I levels increase with age; during puberty concentrations are reached that would be associated with acromegaly if encountered in an adult. After puberty, the levels decline to the normal adult range. Females generally have IGF-I levels ~20% higher than those of males. The normal level of IGF-I may correlate better with the child's physiologic development. Such a relation is seen during puberty (see Fig. 7-9). For prepubertal boys, a similar relation with bone age may be valid as well.[52,53] Insulin-like growth factor–binding protein-3 (IGFBP-3) has been suggested as another serum protein reflective of growth hormone secretion and function.[54] In a manner similar to IGF-I, normal values for IGFBP-3 vary according to age and stage of puberty (Fig. 7-10).

Measurement of insulin-like growth factor–binding protein-2 (IGFBP-2) has been proposed as another aid in the diagnosis of growth hormone deficiency[55] (see Table 7-5). Interestingly, IGFBP-2 is increased in growth hormone deficiency, rather than being decreased as is the case with both IGF-I and IGFBP-3.

## ADRENOCORTICOTROPIC HORMONE AND ADRENOCORTICAL STEROIDS

Adrenocorticotropic hormone (ACTH) is detectable in fetal serum as early as 10 to 14 weeks of gestation. The concentration of ACTH declines toward term, falling from 249 pg/mL ± 65 SE (standard error) to 143 pg/mL ± 9 SE at term. By 1 week of age, the serum ACTH levels are similar to those found in older children. The pattern of adrenal corticosteroids secreted varies from those found in older children. This is due to the presence of a fetal zone in the adrenal gland that constitutes 70% to 85% of the total weight of the adrenal gland at term. In both full-

term and premature infants, the fetal zone undergoes rapid involution after birth, so that it constitutes just 10% of the adrenal gland by 4 to 5 months of age.[56] Plasma concentrations of adrenal steroids are shown in Figure 7-11.

## THYROID-STIMULATING HORMONE AND THYROID HORMONES

As with the previously discussed hormone systems, thyroid function varies greatly depending on gestational age and perinatal circumstances (see Chap. 47). Thyroid-stimulating hormone (TSH) is detected in fetal serum as early as 10 weeks of gestation; however, the levels are low—only 2.4 µU/mL ± 0.14 SE at 10 to 20 weeks of gestation. This increases to 9.6 µU/mL ± 0.93 SE at 25 to 30 weeks of gestation. The increase in TSH is accompanied by increases in mean free thyroxine ($T_4$) and total

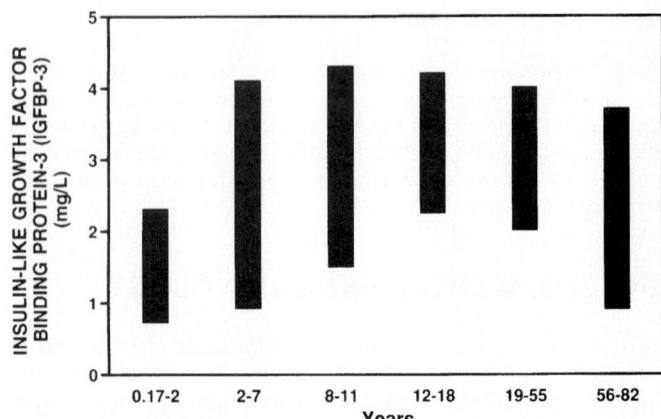

**FIGURE 7-10.** Variation of insulin-like growth factor–binding protein-3 with age. (Data derived from the normal values provided by Quest Diagnostic Nichols Institute, San Juan Capistrano, California.)

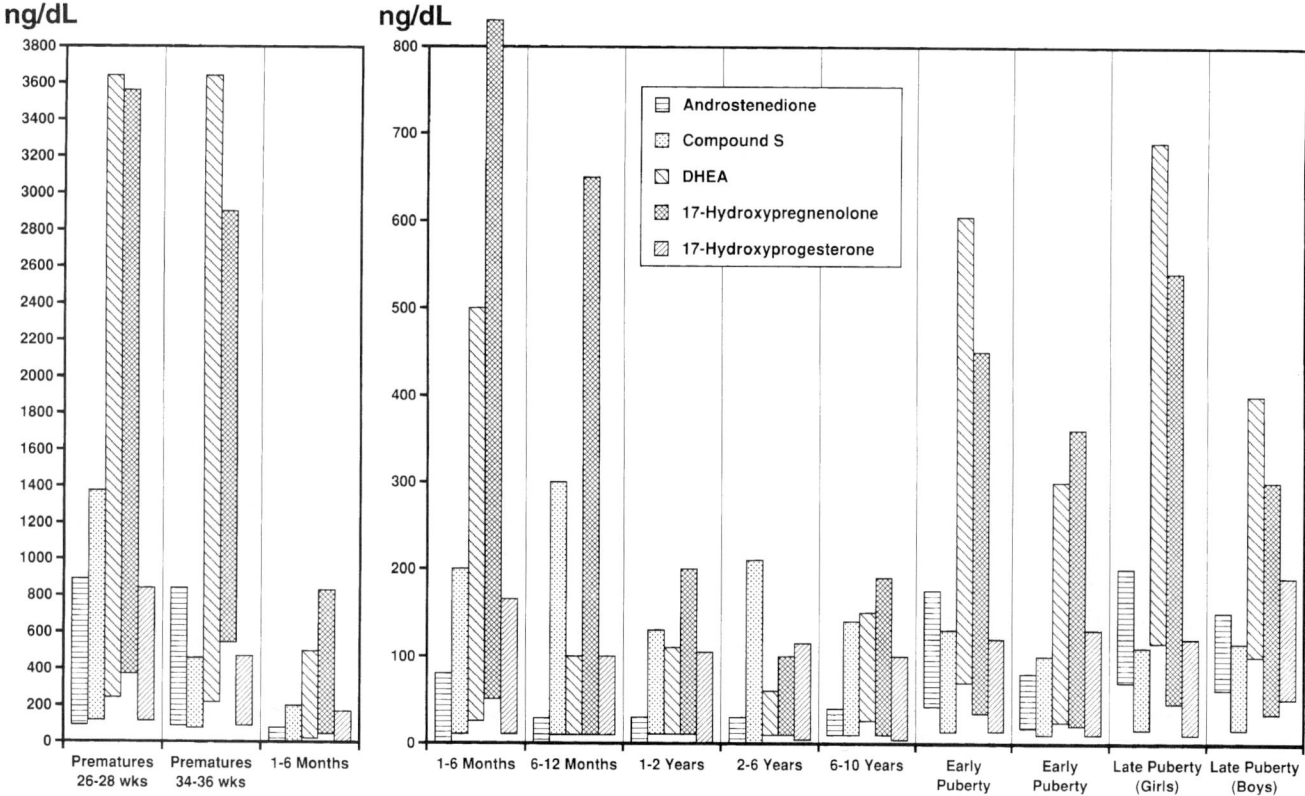

**FIGURE 7-11.** Variation of selected adrenal steroids with age and onset of puberty. (*DHEA*, dehydroepiandrosterone.) (Data derived from the normal values provided by Endocrine Sciences, Calabasas Hills, California.)

$T_4$ serum concentrations. Free $T_4$ increases from 1.8 ng/dL at 10 to 20 weeks of gestation, to 2.6 ng/dL at 22 weeks, to 3 ng/dL at 30 weeks, and to 4 ng/dL at term. The rise in mean $T_4$-binding globulin during this period helps to produce an increase in serum $T_4$ levels, which rise from 3 µg/dL at 20 weeks of gestation to 9.4 µg/dL (range, 5.7–15.6) at 30 weeks of gestation. Without any further rise in $T_4$-binding globulin, the fetal $T_4$ rises to 10.1 µg/mL at 35 weeks of gestation (range, 6.1–16.8) and to 10.9 µg/dL by term (range, 6.6–18.1).[57,58] Between 30 and 40 weeks of gestation, some further maturation seems to take place of the hypothalamic systems responsible for the feedback inhibition of TSH by circulating thyroid hormones. This is suggested by the fall in serum TSH concentration to 8.9 µU/mL ± 0.93 SE at term as the serum free $T_4$ rises.[59] New second- and third-generation TSH assays have been introduced, and the absolute values listed should be viewed relative to the newer assays.

The perinatal period is associated with marked changes in thyroid hormone levels. Within a half hour of birth, the serum TSH level rises to a mean of slightly over 18 µU/mL and then rapidly returns to normal within a day. The rise in serum TSH is paralleled within 24 hours by rises in serum $T_4$ and triiodothyronine ($T_3$) levels; $T_3$ levels then decline in a few days, and $T_4$ levels decline in a few weeks. Similar but less marked changes are seen in premature infants.[59] The rise in serum $T_3$ is not completely dependent on the rise in TSH but rather is also due to a change in the peripheral conversion of $T_4$ to $T_3$, as opposed to reverse $T_3$, which occurs in the prenatal period[59] (see Chaps. 15, 33, and 47). The changes in thyroid hormone levels during the neonatal period in premature infants is also dependent on the degree of prematurity and the infant's health status.[60]

## LUTEINIZING HORMONE, FOLLICLE-STIMULATING HORMONE, AND THE SEX STEROIDS

As early as the 10th week of gestation, luteinizing hormone (LH) and follicle-stimulating hormone (FSH) are found in fetal pituitary glands. Serum LH and FSH levels in the fetus are high, well within the adult castrate range. Higher fetal serum FSH levels are found in females. Toward term, serum LH and FSH levels decline to the low levels typically found at term, but shortly after birth, serum levels of LH and FSH rise again, with LH levels higher in the male and FSH levels higher in the female. Serum LH and FSH levels may not decline to the concentrations deemed typical of childhood for 6 to 12 months (Table 7-6; see also Chaps. 16 and 91). Marked differences appear to exist in the patterns of immunoreactive LH and FSH as compared with bioactive LH and FSH. The ratios also appear to vary with age and stage of development.[61–63]

The fetal serum estradiol level does not differ in males and females, but males have higher serum levels of testosterone before the 20th week of gestation, corresponding to the period of development of the male external genitalia. The serum testosterone level ranges from 100 to 600 ng/dL.[64] The fetal serum testosterone level declines toward term, but in cord blood, it remains higher in males than in females. Coincident with the postnatal surge of LH, serum testosterone levels in males rise again to midpubertal levels, remaining higher than concentrations thought appropriate for childhood until 4 to 9 months of age.[65–68] The normal concentrations of these hormones and some other adrenal hormones are presented in Table 7-6 and Figure 7-11.

Although the serum androstenedione level is in the typical prepubertal range by 1 year of age, it begins to rise again before any manifestations of puberty. Androstenedione begins to rise at 8 years of age in boys and at 7 years of age in girls.

A similar pattern can be seen for dehydroepiandrosterone and for dehydroepiandrosterone sulfate. The rise in these hormones starts at 7 years of age in boys and at 6 years of age in girls. Similar to other adrenal androgens, dehydroepiandrosterone sulfate also manifests serum concentrations that vary with the child's age. In premature infants, the mean serum concentration is 263 µg/dL ± 40.1 SD; in full-term infants, 58.9 µg/dL ± 4.5 SD; in male children 1 to 6 years of age, 15.4 µg/dL ± 6.8 SD; in female children 1 to 6 years of age, 24.7 µg/dL ± 11.1 SD; in male children 6 to 8 years of age, 18.8 µg/dL ± 4.1 SD; in female chil-

**TABLE 7-6.**
**Blood Concentrations of Gonadotropins, Gonadal Steroids, Renin, and Aldosterone in Infancy and Childhood**

| | LH and FSH (Serum, Median and Range)*[62,64] | | | | | Gonadal Steroids (Serum, Median and Range or SD)[64–69] | | | | | Plasma Renin Activity, Plasma Aldosterone, and Urinary Aldosterone (Geometric Mean and Range)[70] | | | |
|---|---|---|---|---|---|---|---|---|---|---|---|---|---|---|
| | *LH, mIU/mL* | | *FSH, mIU/mL* | | | Testosterone, ng/dL | | Estradiol, ng/dL | | | Plasma Renin Activity ng/mL/hr | Plasma Aldo-sterone ng/dL | | Urinary Aldosterone g/24 hr/ 1.73 M² |
| Age | *Male* | *Female* | *Male* | *Female* | Age | *Male* | *Female* | *Male* | *Female* | Age | | | Age | |
| 1–8 d | 18.9† (14–23.4) | 10.4 (5.9–15.8) | 1.6 (0–10.8) | 2.7 (0–35) | Cord | 33.8 (9.5†) | 26.4 (7.4†) | 550 (266–1569) | 810 (500–1475) | 0.25–3 mo | 9.8 (4.0–23.8) | 66 (25–213) | 0.5–3 mo | 14.3 (6.1–46.3) |
| 1–2 mo | 23.4† (9.9–70.2) | 14.9 (5.9–38.3) | 4.3 (0–27.5) | 9 (1.3–44.2) | 1–8 d | 20 (15–45) | 15 (10–30) | 1.9 (0–2.4) | 1 (0–3.1) | | | | 3–6 mo | 10.4 (4.0–23.6) |
| 2–4 mo | 11.3 (5.4–18) | 17.6 (4.5–32.9) | 3.8† (0–17.5) | 6.4 (0–80) | 9–30 d | 160 (80–330) | 15 (10–25) | 2 (0–3.6) | 2 (0–3.5) | 3–12 mo | 4.5 (1.5–10.2) | 24 (7–108) | 6–12 mo | 13.4 (4.3–30.5) |
| 4–12 mo | 7.7 (0–14.9) | 8.1 (0–14.4) | 1.3† (0–4.6) | 6.8 (0–35.3) | 1–2 mo | 190 (55–385) | 7 (0–40) | 1 (0–3.1) | 1 (0–5.1) | 1–4 yr | 4.4 (1.7–11.8) | 16 (3–77) | 1–4 yr | 11.5 (4.1–26.1) |
| 1–2 yr | 8.6 (0–14.9) | 9 (7.2–15.8) | 2† (0–8) | 4.7 (1.7–12.3) | 2–4 mo | 115 (5–330) | 5 (0–15) | 1.1 (0–3.4) | 1.3 (0–7.3) | 4–8 yr | 2.9 (0.9–9.2) | 14 (5–44) | 4–8 yr | 5.3 (1.7–10.6) |
| 2–4 yr | 6.8 (0–9.5) | 6.8 (0–9.5) | 3.1 (0–4.5) | 4.6 (0–8.3) | 4–12 mo | 7.5 (0–120) | 5 | 1.2 (0–2.9) | 1 (0–1.9) | 8–16 yr | 2 (0.9–7.6) | 10 (4–22) | 8–16 yr | 2.9 (1.0–7.9) |
| | | | | | 1–2 yr | 5 (0–10) | 5 (0–10) | 1 (0–2.7) | 1.1 (0–1.8) | | | | | |

LH, luteinizing hormone; FSH, follicle-stimulating hormone; SD, standard deviation.
*Several different LH and FSH assays are being used. The data here should be viewed as relative levels of gonadotropins.
†A significant male versus female difference.

dren 6 to 8 years of age, 30.4 µg/dL ± 7.6 SD; in male children 8 to 10 years of age, 58.6 µg/dL ± 10.1 SD; and in female children 8 to 10 years of age, 117.3 µg/dL ± 41.7 SD[69] (see Chaps. 91 and 92).

## RENIN AND ALDOSTERONE

The plasma concentrations of renin and aldosterone are markedly elevated in the newborn and decline slowly to accepted normal levels[70] (see Table 7-6).

## REFERENCES

1. National Center for Health Statistics. Height and weight of children, United States. Vital and Health Statistics, PHS Pub. No. 1000—series 11, No. 104. Public Health Service. Washington: Government Printing Office, September 1970.
2. National Center for Health Statistics. Height and weight of youths 12–17 years, United States. Vital and Health Statistics, PHS Pub. No. 1000—series 11, No. 124. Public Health Service. Washington: Government Printing Office, January 1973.
3. National Center for Health Statistics. NCHS growth curves for children birth–18 years, United States. Vital and Health Statistics, PHS Pub. No. 1000—series 11, No. 165. Public Health Service. Washington: Government Printing Office, November 1977.
4. National Center for Health Statistics. Body dimensions and proportions, white and Negro children 6–11 years, United States. Vital and Health Statistics, PHS Pub. No. 1000—series 11, No. 143. Public Health Service. Washington: Government Printing Office, December 1974.
5. National Center for Health Statistics. Body weight, stature, and sitting height, white and Negro youths 12–17 years, United States. Vital and Health Statistics, PHS Pub. No. 1000—series 11, No. 126. Public Health Service. Washington: Government Printing Office, August 1973.
6. National Center for Health Statistics: Height and weight of children: socio-economic status. Vital and Health Statistics, PHS Pub. No. 1000—series 11, No. 119. Public Health Service. Washington: Government Printing Office, October 1972.
7. Barr GD, Allen CM, Shinefield HR. Height and weight of 7500 children of three skin colors. Am J Dis Child 1972; 124:866.
8. Wingerd J, Schoen EJ, Solomon IL. Growth standards in the first two years of life based on measurements of white and black children in a prepaid healthcare program. Pediatrics 1971; 47:818.
9. Wingerd J, Solomon IL. Parent-specific height standards for pre-adolescent children of three racial groups, with method for rapid determination. Pediatrics 1973; 52:555.
10. Lippe BM. Short stature in children: evaluation and management. J Pediatr Health Care 1987; 1:313.
11. Tanner JM, Whitehouse RM. Clinical longitudinal standards for height, weight, height velocity, weight velocity, and stages of puberty. Arch Dis Child 1976; 51:170.
12. Tanner JM, Davies PSW. Clinical longitudinal standards for height and weight velocity for North American children. J Pediatr 1985; 107:317.
13. Smith DW, Truog W, Rogers JE, et al. Shifting linear growth during infancy: illustration of genetic factors in growth from fetal life through infancy. J Pediatr 1976; 89:225.
14. Tanner JM, Goldstein H, Whitehouse RH. Standards for children's heights at ages 2–9 years allowing for heights of parents. Arch Dis Child 1970; 45:755.
15. Himes JH, Roche AF, Thissen D, Moore WM. Parent-specific adjustments for evaluation of recumbent length and stature of children. Pediatrics 1985; 75:304.
16. Luo ZC, Albertson-Wikland K, Karlberg J. Target height predicted by parental heights in a population-based study. Pediatr Res 1998; 44:563.
17. Cruise MO. A longitudinal study of the growth of low birth weight infants. I. Velocity and distance growth, birth to 3 years. Pediatrics 1973; 51:620.
18. Fritzhardinge PM, Steven EM. The small-for-date infant. I. Later growth patterns. Pediatrics 1972; 49:671.
19. Guo SS, Roche AE, Chumlea W, et al. Adjustments to the observed growth of preterm low birth weight infants for application to infants who are small for gestational age at birth. Acta Med Auxol 1998; 30:71.
20. Strauss RS, Dietz WH. Growth and development of term infants born with low birth weight: effects of genetic and environmental factors. J Pediatr 1998; 133:67.
21. Leger J, Limoni C, Collin D, Czernichow P. Prediction factors in the determination of final height in subjects born small for gestational age. Pediatr Res 1998; 43:808.

22. Ranke MB. Disease-specific growth charts: do we need them? Acta Paediatr Scand 1989; 356(Suppl):17.

23. Park E, Bailey JD, Cowell CA. Growth and maturation of patients with Turner's syndrome. Pediatr Res 1983; 17:1.

24. Lyon AJ, Preece MA, Grant DB. Growth curves for girls with Turner syndrome. Arch Dis Child 1985; 60:932.

25. Marshall WA. Evaluation of growth rate in height over periods of less than one year. Arch Dis Child 1971; 46:414.

26. Cureton KJ, Boileau RA, Lohman TG. A comparison of densitometric, potassium-40 and skinfold estimates of body composition in prepubescent boys. Hum Biol 1975; 47:321.

27. National Center for Health Statistics. Skinfold thickness of children 6–11 years. Vital and Health Statistics, PHS Pub. No. 1000—series 11, No. 120. Public Health Service, Washington: Government Printing Office, October 1972.

28. National Center for Health Statistics. Skinfold thickness of youths 12–17 years, United States. Vital and Health Statistics. PHS Pub. No. 1000—series 11, No. 132. Public Health Service, Washington: Government Printing Office, January 1974.

29. Sann L, Durand M, Picard J, et al. Arm fat and muscle areas in infancy. Arch Dis Child 1988; 63:256.

30. Rosner B, Prineas R, Loggie J, Daniels SR. Percentiles for body mass index in U.S. children 5 to 17 years of age. J Pediatr 1998; 132:211.

31. Dietz WH, Robinson TN. Use of the body mass index (BMI) as a measure of overweight in children and adolescents. J Pediatr 1998; 132:191.

32. Greulich W, Pyle SL. A radiographic standard of reference for the growing hand and wrist. Chicago: Year Book Medical Publishers, 1971.

33. Tanner JM, Whitehouse RH, Cameron N, et al. Assessment of skeletal maturity and prediction of adult height (TW2 method), 2nd ed. London: Academic Press, 1983.

34. Tanner J, Oshman D, Bahhage F, Healy M. Tanner-Whitehouse bone age reference values for North American children. J Pediatr 1997; 131:34.

35. Graham CB. Assessment of bone maturation: methods and pitfalls. Radiol Clin North Am 1972; 10:185.

36. National Center for Health Statistics. Skeletal maturity of children 6–11 years. Vital and Health Statistics, PHS Pub. No. 1000—series 11, No. 140. Public Health Service. Washington: Government Printing Office, November 1974.

37. Buckler JMH. Skeletal age changes in puberty. Arch Dis Child 1984; 59:115.

38. Bailey N, Pinneau SR. Tables for predicting adult height from skeletal age: revised for use with the Greulich-Pyle hand standards. J Pediatr 1952; 14:423.

39. Roche AF, Wainer H, Thissen D. The RWT method for the prediction of adult stature. Pediatrics 1975; 56:1026.

40. Lenko HL. Prediction of adult height with various methods in Finnish children. Acta Paediatr Scand 1979; 68:85.

41. Zachmann M, Sobradillo B, Frank H, Prader A. Bayley-Pinneau, Roche-Wainer-Thissen and Tanner height predictions in normal children and in patients with various pathologic conditions. J Pediatr 1978; 93:749.

42. de Waal WJ, Greyn-Fokker MH, Stijnen TH, et al. Accuracy of final height prediction and effect of growth-reductive therapy in 362 constitutionally tall children. J Clin Endocrinol Metab 1996; 81:1206.

43. Abbassi V. Growth and normal puberty. Pediatrics 1998; 102:507.

44. August GP, Julius JR, Blethen SL. Adult height in children with growth hormone deficiency who are treated with biosynthetic growth hormone: the National Cooperative Growth Study experience. Pediatrics 1998; 102:512.

45. Marti-Henneberg C, Vizmanos B. The duration of puberty in girls is related to the timing of its onset. J Pediatr 1997; 131:618.

46. Blethen SL, Gaines S, Weldon V. Comparison of predicted and adult heights in short boys: effect of androgen therapy. Pediatr Res 1984; 18:467.

47. Winter JSD, Faiman C. Pituitary-gonadal relations in male children and adolescents. Pediatr Res 1972; 6:126.

48. Zachmann M, Prader A, Kind HP, et al. Testicular volume during adolescence: cross sectional and longitudinal studies. Helv Paediatr Acta 1974; 29:61.

49. Schonfeld WA. Primary and secondary sexual characteristics: study of their development in males from birth through maturity, with biometric study of penis and testes. Am J Dis Child 1943; 65:535.

50. Belisle S, Tulchinsky D. Amniotic fluid hormones. In: Tulchinsky D, Ryan KJ, eds. Maternal-fetal endocrinology. Philadelphia: WB Saunders, 1980:169.

51. Gluckman PD, Grumbach MM, Kaplan SL. The human fetal hypothalamus and pituitary gland: the maturation of neuroendocrine mechanisms controlling the secretion of fetal pituitary growth hormone, prolactin, gonadotropin, and adrenocorticotropin-related peptides. In: Tulchinsky D, Ryan KJ, eds. Maternal-fetal endocrinology. Philadelphia: WB Saunders, 1980:196.

52. Cacciari E, Cicognani A, Pirazzoli P, et al. Differences in somatomedin-C between short-normal subjects and those of normal height. J Pediatr 1985; 106:891.

53. Juul A, Bang P, Hertel NT, et al. Serum insulin-like growth factor-I in 1030 healthy children, adolescents, and adults: relation to age, sex, stage of puberty, testicular size, and body mass index. J Clin Endocrinol Metab 1994; 78:744.

54. Blum WF, Albertsson-Wikland K, Rosberg S, Ranke MB. Serum levels of insulin-like growth factor I (IGF-I) and IGF binding protein 3 reflect spontaneous growth hormone secretion. J Clin Endocrinol Metab 1993; 76:1610.

55. Smith WJ, Nam TJ, Underwood LE, et al. Use of Insulin-like growth factor-binding protein-2 (IGFBP-2), IGFBP-3, and IGF-I for assessing growth hormone status in short children. J Clin Endocrinol Metab 1993; 77:1294.

56. Sperling MA. Newborn adaptation: adrenocortical hormones and ACTH. In: Tulchinsky D, Ryan KJ, eds. Maternal-fetal endocrinology. Philadelphia: WB Saunders, 1980:387.

57. Oddie TH, Fisher DA, Bernard B, Lam RW. Thyroid function at birth in infants of 30 to 45 weeks gestation. J Pediatr 1977; 90:803.

58. Burrow GN, Fisher DA, Larsen PR. Maternal and fetal thyroid function. N Engl J Med 1994; 331:1072.

59. Fisher DA, Klein AH. The ontogenesis of thyroid function and its relationship to neonatal thermogenesis. In: Tulchinsky D, Ryan KJ, eds. Maternal-fetal endocrinology. Philadelphia: WB Saunders, 1980:281.

60. Van Wassenaer AG, Kok JH, Dekker FW, De Vulder JJM. Thyroid function in very preterm infants: influences of gestational age and disease. Pediatr Res 1997; 42:604.

61. Beitins IZ, Padmanabhan V. Bioactivity of gonadotropins. Endocrinol Metab Clin North Am 1991; 20:85.

62. Beck-Peccoz P, Padman V, Baggiani AM, et al. Maturation of hypothalamic-pituitary-gonadal function in normal human fetuses: circulating levels of gonadotropins, their common α-subunits and free testosterone, and discrepancy between immunological and biological activities of circulating follicle-stimulating hormone. J Clin Endocrinol Metab 1991; 73:525.

63. Kletter GB, Padmanabhan V, Brown MB, et al. Serum bioactive gonadotropin during male puberty: a longitudinal study. J Clin Endocrinol Metab 1993; 76:432.

64. Reyes FI, Boroditsky RS, Winter JSD, Faiman C. Studies on human sexual development. II. Fetal and maternal serum gonadotropin and sex steroid concentrations. J Clin Endocrinol Metab 1974; 38:612.

65. Forest MC, Cathiard AM, Bertrand JA. Evidence of testicular activity in early infancy. J Clin Endocrinol Metab 1973; 37:148.

66. Forest M, Cathiard AM. Pattern of plasma testosterone and Δ-4-androstenedione in normal newborns: evidence for testicular activity at birth. J Clin Endocrinol Metab 1975; 41:977.

67. Winter JSD, Faiman C, Hobson WC, et al. Patterns of serum gonadotropin concentrations from birth to four years of age in man and chimpanzee. J Clin Endocrinol Metab 1975; 40:545.

68. Winter JSD, Hughes IA, Reyes FI, et al. Pituitary-gonadal relations in infancy. II. Patterns of serum gonadal steroid concentration in man from birth to two years of age. J Clin Endocrinol Metab 1976; 42:679.

69. Reiter ED, Fuldaurer VG, Root AW. Secretion of the adrenal androgen, dehydroepiandrosterone sulfate, during normal infancy, childhood, in sick infants and in children with endocrinologic abnormalities. J Pediatr 1977; 90:766.

70. Fiselier T, Monnens L, van Munster P, et al. The renin-angiotensin-aldosterone system in infancy and childhood in basal conditions and after stimulation. Eur J Pediatr 1984; 143:18.

# PART II

# THE ENDOCRINE BRAIN AND PITUITARY GLAND

GARY L. ROBERTSON, EDITOR

# CHAPTER 8

# MORPHOLOGY OF THE ENDOCRINE BRAIN, HYPOTHALAMUS, AND NEUROHYPOPHYSIS

JOHN R. SLADEK, JR., AND CELIA D. SLADEK

## OVERVIEW OF THE HYPOTHALAMUS

The human hypothalamus is a tiny wedged-shaped mass of tissue, composed primarily of gray matter, that subserves widespread functions, ranging from those considered somewhat automatic (i.e., autonomic) to more complex behaviors requiring a high level of integration. The hypothalamus is situated in the ventralmost diencephalon (Fig. 8-1). It is bounded laterally by portions of the subthalamus; medially by the vertically oriented, slitlike third ventricle; rostrally by the lamina terminalis; caudally by the mesencephalon; and dorsally by the thalamus. Ventrally, the hypothalamus is contiguous with the infundibulum and pituitary stalk; the latter serves to transmit axons en route to the neurohypophysis. On the ventral surface of the brain, the hypothalamus appears as a prominent set of protuberances, the paired mammillary bodies caudally, and the midline infundibular eminence. The boundaries of the hypothalamus are easily identified by the optic chiasm rostrally and by the caudal edge of the mammillary bodies as they are situated at the rostral limit of the interpeduncular fossa. Here, the caudal limits of the hypothalamus merge with the midbrain.

Classic neuroanatomic techniques have been used to identify hypothalamic nuclei cytoarchitectonically. Some nuclei are relatively easy to identify microscopically, based on size or packing density of neurons; others benefit from placement close to readily identified landmarks such as the third ventricle or the optic chiasm. Prominent myelinated fiber bundles punctuate the relatively nondescript nuclear divisions of the hypothalamus, indicating the diverse reciprocal connections that exist between the hypothalamus and numerous brain regions. The fornix and mammillary fasciculus interconnect the hypothalamus with, for example, the hippocampus, the thalamus, and the brainstem. Other brain regions influence hypothalamic function through pathways that are seen to advantage with current histochemical methods. These systems, which include the medial forebrain bundle and the dorsal longitudinal fasciculus, interconnect the hypothalamus with olfactory areas rostrally and with autonomic centers of the brainstem and spinal cord caudally. Thus, the hypothalamus is an important link between the forebrain and brainstem, integrating visceral, endocrine, and behavioral functions through a highly ordered set of reciprocating circuits.

## NUCLEAR TOPOGRAPHY

### HYPOTHALAMIC ZONES

Because the hypothalamus is so rich in perikaryal groups and so poor in landmarks (e.g., myelinated fiber bundles), the prudent approach is to consider easily identified *hypothalamic zones* as geographic points with respect to the more than two dozen classically identified hypothalamic nuclei, as detailed by Nauta and Haymaker.[1] Zones in both longitudinal and coronal planes are illustrated in Figure 8-2.

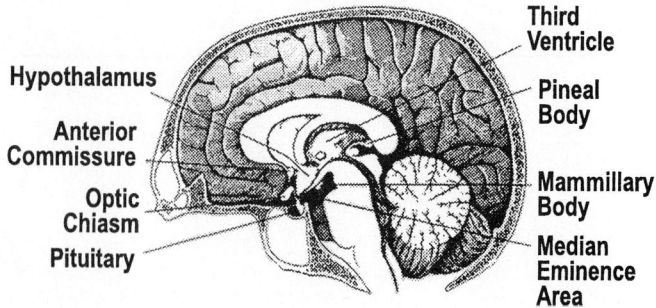

**FIGURE 8-1.** Human hypothalamus in sagittal section. The hypothalamus is bounded anteriorly by the lamina terminalis, the tissue that bridges the anterior commissure and optic chiasm; posteriorly by the brainstem; and dorsally by the overlying thalamus (adjacent to the label for the third ventricle). The hypothalamus is relatively small in comparison to other brain regions, yet is intimately involved in mediating or moderating many brain and endocrine functions. (From Krieger DT, Hughes JC, eds. Neuroendocrinology. Sunderland, MA: Sinauer Associates, 1980:3.)

**Longitudinal Plane.**   The longitudinal zones are based on the phylogenetically primitive organization of lower vertebrates, in which the hypothalamus is characterized by a relatively cell-rich *medial zone*. A somewhat acellular *lateral zone* is separated from the medial zone by a prominent fiber bundle, the fornix. The medial zone can be subdivided further into a *midline zone* that is immediately adjacent to the third ventricle and contains a relatively homogeneous nuclear mass called the *periventricular stratum*. The more laterally placed portions of the medial hypothalamic zone contain reasonably differentiated cell clusters, including the medial preoptic, anterior hypothalamic, ventromedial, dorsomedial, paraventricular, posterior, and premammillary nuclei.

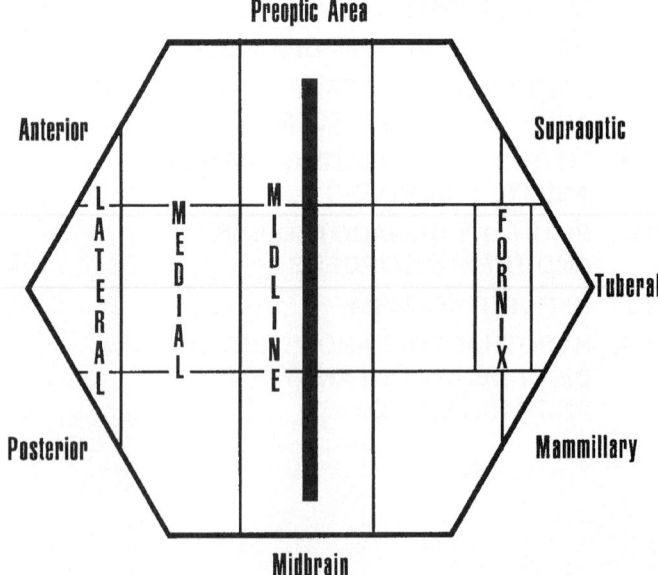

**FIGURE 8-2.** Diagram showing anatomic relationship of hypothalamic nuclei, by zones. Here, the hypothalamus is considered as a hexagon, bordered anteriorly by the preoptic area and posteriorly by the midbrain. The third ventricle (*wide black line*) forms its midline. Most hypothalamic nuclei can be found within three longitudinal zones, designated as midline, medial, and lateral in relation to the third ventricle and fornix. These zones can be further subdivided into three anteroposterior regions or levels (supraoptic, tuberal, and mammillary), allowing identification of hypothalamic nuclei by position, an approach that is much simpler than distinguishing the nuclei by the classic cytoarchitectonic method. The three levels, shown in the coronal plane in Figure 8-3, depict the essential hypothalamic nuclei.

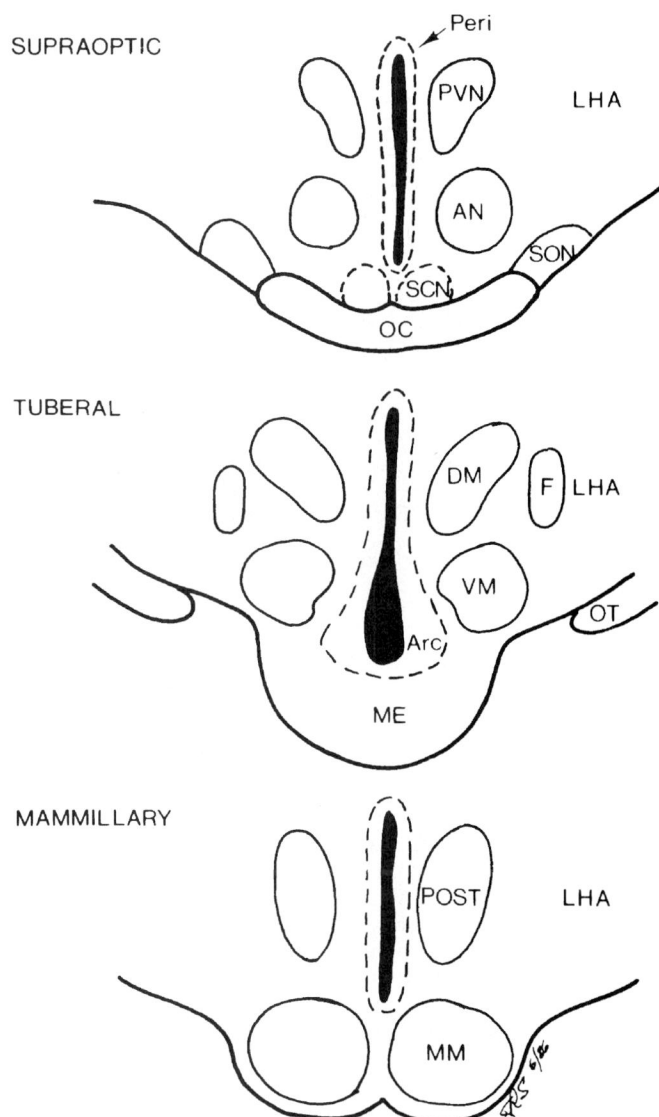

**FIGURE 8-3.** The hypothalamus in the coronal plane, demonstrating the relative positions of hypothalamic nuclei. At the supraoptic level, the midline zone (*dashed line*) consists of the periventricular nucleus (*Peri*) and its ventral expansion, the suprachiasmatic nucleus (*SCN*). The periventricular nucleus continues through the more caudal levels. At tuberal levels, the SCN is replaced by the arcuate nucleus (*Arc*). The medial zone, defined as all the tissue between the fornix laterally and the periventricular nucleus medially, contains five major hypothalamic nuclei that essentially replace each other positionally at each level. Thus, the paraventricular (*PVN*) and anterior (*AN*) nuclei, which occupy the supraoptic level, are replaced by the dorsomedial (*DM*) and ventromedial (*VM*) nuclei at tuberal levels; these nuclei in turn are replaced by the posterior nucleus (*POST*) at the most caudal, mammillary level. The lateral zone consists almost exclusively of the lateral hypothalamic area (*LHA*), with the exception of the supraoptic nucleus (*SON*), which is seen at supraoptic levels. The third ventricle appears as the dark structure in the midline. (*F*, fornix; *ME*, median eminence; *MM*, mammillary body; *OC*, optic chiasm; *OT*, optic tract.)

**Coronal Plane.**    For convenience, the hypothalamus in the coronal plane can be further subdivided anteroposteriorly into three regions: the *supraoptic, tuberal,* and *mammillary* regions (Figs. 8-3 and 8-4). The supraoptic region includes that portion of the hypothalamus situated between the optic chiasm and tuber cinereum. The tuberal zone extends caudally to the most anterior portion of the mammillary bodies. The mammillary region includes the most caudal hypothalamus to the mesodiencephalic junction.

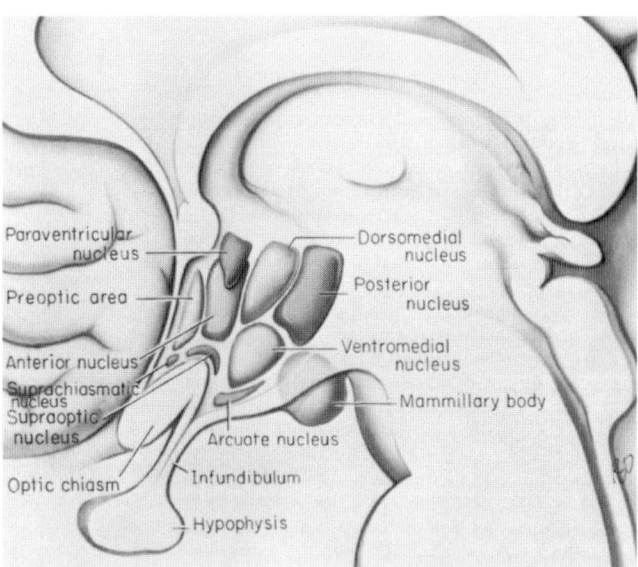

**FIGURE 8-4.** The hypothalamus in a parasagittal plane, showing the relative positions of major nuclei. These relationships can be better appreciated by comparing this figure with Figures 8-1 and 8-3. For example, three nuclear groups, the paraventricular, dorsomedial, and posterior, appear to replace one another as one proceeds anatomically, rostrally to caudally, through the three major coronal levels—supraoptic, tuberal, and mammillary (see Fig. 8-3). (From Carpenter MB, Sutin J, eds. Human neuroanatomy. Baltimore: Williams & Wilkins, 1983:553.)

The midline zone accordingly contains the periventricular stratum throughout most of its rostrocaudal extent. At tuberal regions, the ventral periventricular stratum expands laterally to accommodate the arcuate (infundibular) nucleus. At supraoptic levels, a ventral region of the periventricular stratum is identified as the suprachiasmatic nucleus. Although numerous other fine points of periventricular zone anatomy exist, one could consider the two subcomponents of this region as the suprachiasmatic and arcuate nuclei. The medial hypothalamic zone, defined as all remaining tissue lateral to the periventricular stratum and medial to the descending limb of the fornix, contains the paraventricular and anterior hypothalamic nuclei at supraoptic levels, the dorsomedial and ventromedial nuclei at tuberal levels, and the posterior hypothalamic nucleus at mammillary levels (see Fig. 8-3). Thus, as one proceeds rostrally to caudally through the three hypothalamic regions, a gradual replacement of these well-differentiated nuclei is seen. The lateral hypothalamic zone is relatively undistinguished, with the lateral hypothalamic area occupying most of this zone in all three regions. The lone exception is the supraoptic nucleus, which is seen at the supraoptic level. Because of the complex nature of the paraventricular nucleus, it is sometimes considered as part of the periventricular zone, but the alarlike lateral extensions of this nucleus clearly place a large part of it within the medial zone.

## PREOPTIC AREA

The preoptic area, located rostral to the strict limits of the hypothalamus, contains nuclei in all three (medial to lateral) zones, including the preoptic periventricular, medial preoptic, and lateral preoptic nuclei (see Fig. 8-4). Functionally, the preoptic region is integrated with the remainder of the hypothalamus because it includes neurons that regulate anterior pituitary function as well as structures that are essential for fluid and electrolyte balance. A full description of these hypothalamic regions and nuclei may be found in two classic accounts.[1,2]

**FIGURE 8-5.** Major hypothalamic pathways. Pathways to the hypothalamus arise from several areas, including olfactory, limbic, and brainstem regions; reciprocal circuits exist, particularly to autonomic centers of the caudal medulla and spinal cord. The dorsal longitudinal fasciculus conveys most of the descending information to brainstem nuclei and is identified by the parallel, opposite arrows in this drawing. Another major pathway, the fornix, carries higher cortical information from the hippocampus (*Hipp.*) to the mammillary nucleus. (*AV,* nucleus ventralis anterior of thalamus; *BL, Ce.,* and *Co.,* basolateral, central, and cortical amygdaloid nuclei; *Bulb. olf.,* olfactory bulb; *Coll. sup.,* superior colliculus; *H,* hypothalamus; *M,* mammillary body; *MD,* dorsomedial thalamic nucleus; *N. Dors. n. X,* dorsal motor vagal nucleus; *N. loc. coer.,* locus coeruleus; *N. raphe,* nuclei of the raphe; *N. tr. solit.,* nucleus tractus solitarius; *Olf. Cort.,* olfactory cortex; *Optic ch.,* optic chiasma; *Periaq. gr.,* periaqueductal gray; *Prefr. cort.,* prefrontal cortex; *RF,* reticular formation; *S,* septum; *VM,* ventromedial hypothalamic nucleus.) (From Brodal A, ed. Neurological anatomy in relation to clinical medicine, 3rd ed. New York: Oxford University Press, 1981:698.)

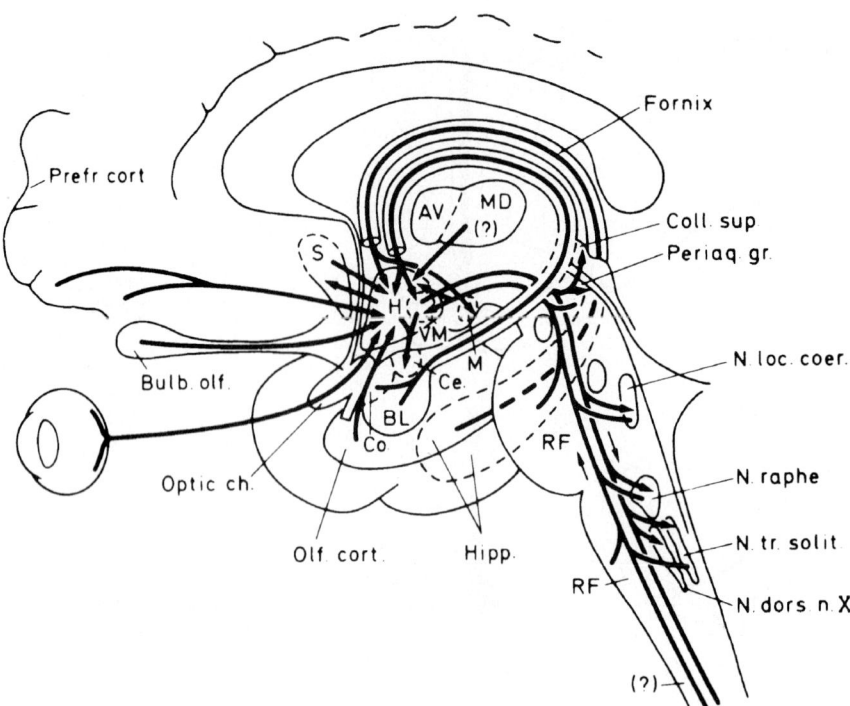

## CLASSIC PATHWAYS

### AFFERENT PATHWAYS

Afferent pathways to hypothalamic nuclei arise primarily from the brainstem, thalamus, basal ganglia, cerebral cortex, and olfactory areas. The detailed anatomy of these connections and hypothalamic interconnections is described in several fine reviews.[1,3,4] Briefly, the reticular formation and visceral centers of the brainstem connect with the hypothalamus through two prominent pathways, the mammillary peduncle and the dorsal longitudinal fasciculus. Visceral and somatic information also reaches the hypothalamus from the locus ceruleus, vagal nuclei, periaqueductal gray area, and nuclei of the solitary tract (Fig. 8-5). The fornix transmits fibers from the hippocampus by direct projections to the mammillary bodies. Additional afferents from the piriform cortex and the amygdala also reach the hypothalamus, probably by other routes. Olfactory information through the medial forebrain bundle and stria terminalis reaches the hypothalamus either directly or indirectly through the previously mentioned cortical regions, the stria terminalis being the primary pathway from the amygdala. Most of the afferent pathways are reciprocal; thus, the hypothalamic efferent connections are extensive.

### EFFERENT PATHWAYS

The dorsal longitudinal fasciculus transmits information to brainstem reticular centers as well as to visceral and somatic efferent nuclei. This system descends caudally to innervate preganglionic autonomic centers of the spinal cord, particularly the intermediolateral gray column.[5,6] Although the hypothalamus was once thought to interconnect with autonomic centers by multisynaptic pathways, it is now clear that the dorsal motor nucleus of the vagus, the nuclei of the solitary tract, and the nucleus ambiguus receive direct projections from the paraventricular nucleus of the hypothalamus. Thus, reciprocal connections between these regions form an integrated autonomic circuit. Other fibers reach the brainstem through the medial forebrain bundle.

Hypothalamic efferents projecting to the thalamus traverse the mammillothalamic tract to the anterior nucleus of the thalamus, where they are relayed to the cerebral cortex. Other efferent fibers ascend over the more diffuse periventricular system. The hypothalamus is connected with the neurohypophysis by the hypothalamo-neurohypophysial tract, a system of unmyelinated fibers that terminates in the neurohypophysis for the purpose of storing and then delivering vasopressin, oxytocin, and possibly other endogenous peptides such as dynorphin to the pituitary blood.

### HYPOTHALAMO-NEUROHYPOPHYSIAL SYSTEM

In contrast to other hypothalamic nuclei, the paraventricular and supraoptic nuclei are easy to identify (Fig. 8-6). Each nucleus contains the largest nerve cells in the hypothalamus (Fig. 8-7). The cells stain densely with common dyes that reveal the abundant ribonucleoprotein (i.e., Nissl substance) in their perikaryal cytoplasm. Ultrastructurally, the protein-synthesizing machinery of these neurons also is evident and reflects their high level of activity with respect to the manufacture of vasopressin, oxytocin, and coexistent peptides. The neurons are revealed in excellent detail when stained immunohistochemically with antibodies directed against specific hypothalamic peptides (see Fig. 8-7).[7,8] Such analysis has revealed that oxytocin neurons also contain cholecystokinin[9] and that vasopressin neurons also contain dynorphin.[10] Axons from the supraoptic and paraventricular nuclei as well as associated accessory nuclei of the hypothalamus project ventrally and caudally (see Fig. 8-6) to the underlying neurohypophysis, where they release oxytocin, vasopressin, and associated peptides into the peripheral circulation to regulate fluid and electrolyte balance and to initiate the smooth muscle contraction that is associated with lactation and parturition.

Other neurons of the paraventricular nucleus are global, with widespread connections to autonomic centers of the brainstem and spinal cord, and to the forebrain and cortical areas, including the septum, cingulum, and hippocampus.[11a] These far-reaching interconnections focus attention on oxytocin and vasopressin as more than simply neurohypophysial hormones. The demonstration of these peptides in presynaptic nerve terminals suggests that they may function as neurotransmitters.

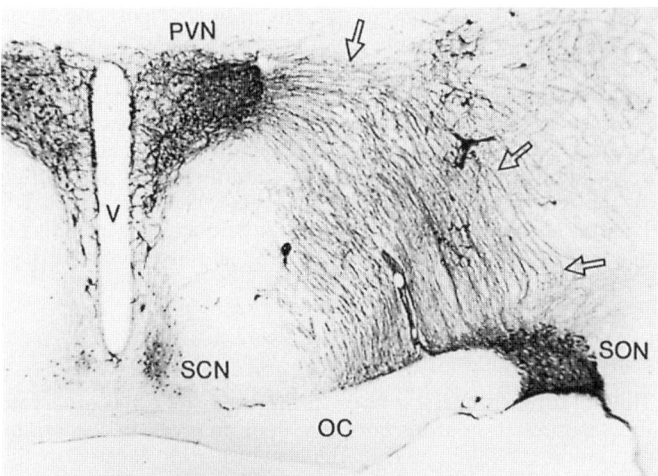

**FIGURE 8-6.** Immunohistochemical staining for neurophysins associated with vasopressin and oxytocin reveals the extent of the neurohypophysial system at the supraoptic level of the rat hypothalamus. Dense staining is seen within neurons of the paraventricular (*PVN*) and supraoptic (*SON*) nuclei. A ventral flow of axons from each nucleus (*arrows*) represents the origin of the hypothalamo-neurohypophysial tract as it courses to the posterior pituitary. Stained neurons also are seen within the suprachiasmatic nucleus (*SCN*); however, this nucleus does not contribute fibers to the neural lobe. (*OC*, optic chiasm; *V*, third ventricle.) Original magnification ×30

## CHEMICAL NEUROANATOMY

### HORMONES AS CHEMICAL NEUROTRANSMITTERS

The hypothalamus is one of the most complicated areas of the brain with respect to chemical neurotransmitters because of the small amount of tissue occupied by the hypothalamus and the great number of transmitter substances located within hypothalamic nerve cells and associated fiber systems.[12] The classic studies of Bargmann[13] and of Scharrer and Scharrer,[14] who are credited with describing the principles of neurosecre-

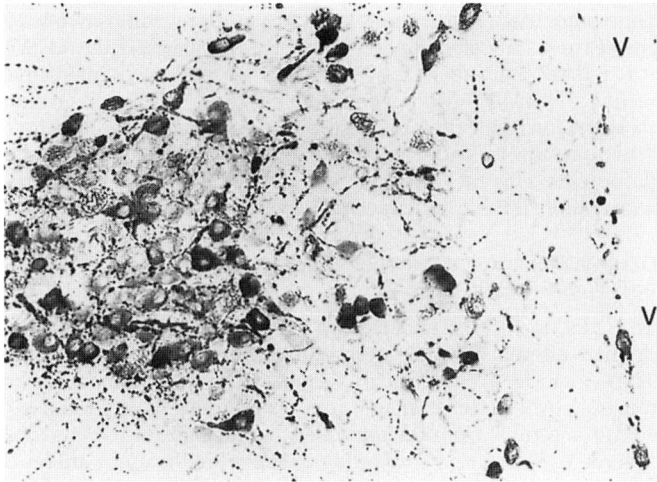

**FIGURE 8-7.** Appearance of neurons of the paraventricular nucleus after immunohistochemical staining for vasopressin. This set of magnocellular neurons occupies a subnucleus of the paraventricular nucleus that contains primarily vasopressin neurons that project to the neural lobe.[30] The neurons are large, multipolar, and possess beaded processes. The position of the third ventricle is indicated (*V*). Original magnification ×350

tion, brought to light the unique chemical characteristics of neurons of the supraoptic and paraventricular nuclei. The introduction in the early 1960s of the Falck-Hillarp histofluorescence method[15] allowed identification of the catecholamines dopamine and norepinephrine within the hypothalamus. Most notable were the dopaminergic neurons of the tuberoinfundibular system, which are involved in regulating the release of anterior pituitary substances.[16] A decade later, immunohistochemical methods[17] increased the list of known hypothalamic chemical neurotransmitters and modulators to include substances such as luteinizing hormone–releasing hormone, corticotropin-releasing hormone, vasoactive intestinal peptide, neurotensin, somatostatin, enkephalin, endorphin, cholecystokinin, galanin, and several others.[18,19] Although the discovery of luteinizing hormone–releasing hormone[20] and somatostatin within hypothalamic, preoptic, and adjacent regions of the endocrine hypothalamus was not surprising, the finding of "gut peptides" and the discovery of a complex system of opioid neurons[21] have redefined the hypothalamus, based on the chemical cytoarchitecture of transmitters and hormones.[18,21a]

The application of in situ hybridization techniques to localize messenger RNA for these peptides indicates that this wide array of peptides is synthesized in the hypothalamus and that neurons have the capacity to synthesize multiple regulatory peptides simultaneously.[22] The specific peptides produced by a given neuron are not static but depend on the stimuli received by that cell.[22,23] For example, hypophysectomy dramatically increases the expression of galanin in the vasopressin neurons of the supraoptic nucleus and of cholecystokinin in the oxytocin neurons, but salt loading induces the expression of tyrosine hydroxylase in the vasopressin neurons and of corticotropin-releasing hormone in the oxytocin neurons.[24] The role of these simultaneously released peptides is not completely defined, but in at least some instances, they interact to regulate hormone release from the anterior pituitary or to modulate hormone release from the posterior pituitary.

### VASOPRESSIN RELEASE AS A MODEL OF INTERACTIVE CHEMICAL CIRCUITRY

#### NOREPINEPHRINE REGULATION OF VASOPRESSIN AND OXYTOCIN

The role of afferents to the paraventricular and supraoptic nuclei is considered relative to the regulation of vasopressin release as exemplary of the kind of functionally interactive chemical circuitry that is being revealed with respect to hypothalamic neuroanatomy. The supraoptic and paraventricular nuclei receive dense, diverse afferent inputs, many arising from the brainstem reticular formation. One of these is a well-defined system of noradrenergic afferents to vasopressin neurons of the supraoptic and paraventricular nuclei (Fig. 8-8). The paraventricular nuclei in turn send reciprocal peptidergic fibers to the reticular core of the brainstem. Norepinephrine-containing perikaryal groups in the brainstem have been designated A1 to A7.[25] These noradrenergic neurons originally were seen primarily within the reticular formation of the pons and medulla. Later, attention focused on groups A1, A2, A5, and A7 as projecting to the hypothalamus through a ventral pathway that ascends within the dorsal portion of the reticular formation of the brainstem, entering the medial forebrain bundle at hypothalamic levels in association with serotonergic and dopaminergic systems from the brainstem.[26] On reaching the hypothalamus, these fibers exit the medial forebrain bundle to supply the supraoptic and paraventricular nuclei. The densest patterns of noradrenergic fibers—perhaps the densest patterns in the entire brain—are seen in the mammalian hypothalamus[27,28] (Fig. 8-9). These fibers appear in contact with the cell bodies of the magnocellular neurons, lending further support to the concept that norepinephrine plays a role in the regulation of neurohypophysial peptides.[29]

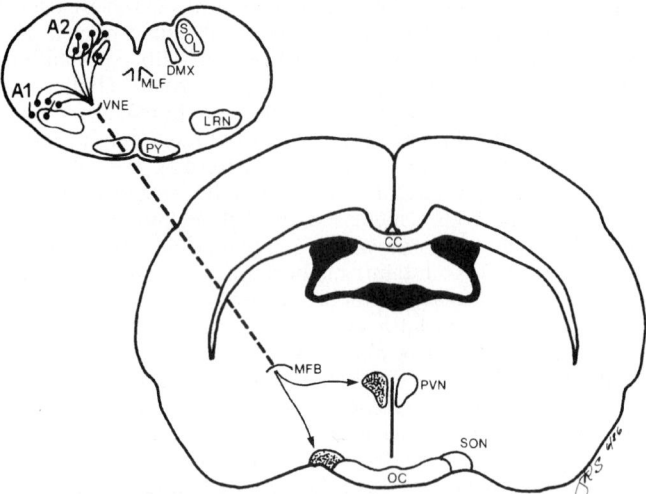

**FIGURE 8-8.** Ascending noradrenergic axons reach the magnocellular nuclei of the hypothalamus through the ventral norepinephrine pathway (*VNE*) of the brainstem, which continues rostrally in the medial forebrain bundle (*MFB*) of the diencephalon. The neurons of origin of this system (*A1, A2*) are located in the lateral reticular formation of the medulla near the lateral reticular nucleus (*LRN*) and in an area of the dorsomedial medulla that is important in cardiovascular regulation—the nucleus solitarius (*SOL*) and the dorsal motor vagal nucleus (*DMX*), respectively. This pathway, which is probably reciprocal from the paraventricular nucleus (*PVN*), supplies a dense noradrenergic innervation to the magnocellular nuclei, as shown for the monkey (also see Fig. 8-9). (*CC*, corpus callosum; *MLF*, medial longitudinal fasciculus; *OC*, optic chiasm; *PY*, pyramidal tract; *SON*, supraoptic nucleus.)

In subsequent studies, the simultaneous demonstration of catecholamine fluorescence and peptide immunohistochemistry[30] revealed a consistent juxtaposition between catecholamine varicosities and magnocellular perikarya in the supraoptic and paraventricular nuclei in both rodents[31] and primates.[32] Specifi-

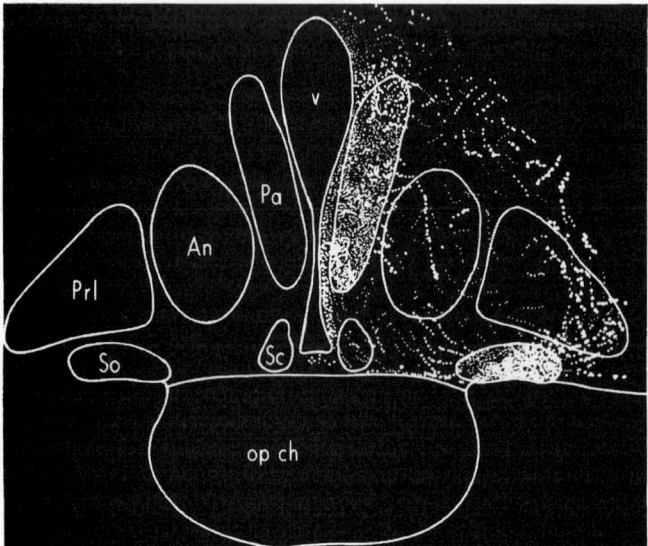

**FIGURE 8-9.** Patterns of catecholamine innervation of hypothalamic nuclei at a supraoptic level in the rhesus monkey. Exceptionally dense patterns exist in the paraventricular (*Pa*) and supraoptic (*So*) nuclei; less impressive patterns are seen in other nuclei at this level. Depictions such as this led to intense examination of the role of catecholamines in the release of neurohypophysial peptides. (*An*, anterior nucleus; *op ch*, optic chiasma; *Prl*, lateral preoptic nucleus; *Sc*, suprachiasmatic nucleus; *v*, third ventricle.) (From Hoffman GE, Felten DL, Sladek JR Jr. Monoamine distribution in primate brain. III. Catecholamine-containing varicosities in the hypothalamus of *Macaca mulatta*. Am J Anat 1976; 147:501.)

cally, vasopressin-containing neurons in ventral portions of the supraoptic nucleus and the major vasopressin subcomponent of the paraventricular nucleus were seen to be studded with brightly fluorescent catecholamine-containing varicosities. In contrast, oxytocin neurons received far fewer fluorescent fibers on their cell bodies and proximal dendrites. The preferential innervation of vasopressin neurons primarily reflects innervation by the A1 noradrenergic cells of the ventrolateral medulla.[33–35] The sparse innervation of the oxytocin neurons reflects innervation of the nuclei by the A2 noradrenergic cell group that does not differentiate between oxytocin and vasopressin neurons.[35]

## CATECHOLAMINES, VASOPRESSIN, AND AUTONOMIC REGULATION

The noradrenergic cell groups in the brainstem that innervate the vasopressin neurons are intimately involved in autonomic regulation. The A2 catecholamine neurons are located in the nucleus of the tractus solitarius, which receives baroreceptor information from the carotid sinus and aortic arch. This information is also transmitted to the A1 cells in the ventrolateral medulla that project to the vasopressin neurons.[36] The paraventricular nucleus is also innervated by the locus ceruleus (A6), an important autonomic relay center.[37] Thus, the catecholamine input to the supraoptic and paraventricular nuclei represents a source of autonomic regulation of neurohypophysial function. These pathways are important because blood pressure, blood volume, and the partial pressure of oxygen are potent regulators of vasopressin release from the neural lobe.

Stimulation of the A1 region results in an increase in blood pressure and enhanced vasopressin release, and inhibition of this region prevents baroreceptor-initiated secretion of vasopressin.[38] This response is prevented by destruction of the catecholamine terminals in the supraoptic and paraventricular nuclei[39] but is not prevented by administration of adrenergic antagonists.[40] This can be explained by the finding that, in addition to norepinephrine, the A1 neurons produce neuropeptide Y, adenosine triphosphate (ATP), and substance P.[41,42] Pharmacologic evidence indicates that these neuroactive substances participate in the excitation of vasopressin neurons by the A1 pathway.[43,44]

The central role of the paraventricular nucleus and vasopressin in blood pressure regulation and other autonomic functions was underscored by the finding of reciprocal pathways containing vasopressin and oxytocin in the same brainstem regions that give origin to the ascending noradrenergic fibers to the supraoptic and paraventricular nuclei. The finding of neurophysin-positive varicosities in juxtaposition to norepinephrine perikarya in the A1, A2, A5, and A7 brainstem groups suggests a functionally interactive reciprocal circuit.[45] Moreover, microinjection of vasopressin into these regions has profound effects on cardiovascular function. Thus, a reciprocal pathway involving catecholamine afferents and vasopressin efferents is one mechanism involved in hypothalamic modulation of the autonomic nervous system.

## OTHER CHEMICALLY DEFINED AFFERENTS AND VASOPRESSIN RELEASE

The paraventricular and supraoptic nuclei receive chemically defined afferents from other central nervous system sites.[46,47] These include serotonergic projections from the midbrain raphe nuclei, GABAergic (transmitting or secreting γ-aminobutyric acid) projections from the region of the nucleus accumbens, and several hypothalamic projections. The hypothalamic afferents include cholinergic[48] and GABAergic projections arising from cells near the paraventricular and supraoptic nuclei, β-endorphinergic afferents from the arcuate nucleus, histaminergic afferents from the tuberomammillary nuclei,[49,50] dopaminergic afferents from neurons in the A11, A12, and A13 groups,[51] and numerous projections from the preoptic region, including projections from the subfornical organ and the organum vasculosum of the lamina terminalis. The chemical nature of these last projections includes glutamatergic, GABAergic, angiotensinergic, and atriopeptidergic fibers. The functional role of many of these afferents is unknown, but the afferents from the preoptic region and the circumventricular organs clearly are intimately involved in the osmotic regulation of vasopressin release as part of their role in fluid and electrolyte balance. A particularly important role for the classic excitatory amino acid neurotransmitter glutamate in regulating hypothalamic activity has been suggested by the presence of numerous immunocytochemically identified glutamatergic synapses in the hypothalamus and the finding that glutamate antagonists virtually eliminate excitatory postsynaptic potentials in the paraventricular, supraoptic, and arcuate nuclei. Thus, the hypothalamus continues to emerge as a complex brain region in which a wide variety of classic and more recently discovered transmitters serve numerous endocrine and other functions related to autonomic, limbic, and pituitary activity.[52]

# REFERENCES

1. Nauta WJH, Haymaker W. Hypothalamic nuclei and fiber connections. In: Haymaker W, Anderson E, Nauta WJH, eds. The hypothalamus. Springfield, IL: Charles C Thomas, 1969:136.
2. Crosby EC, Woodburne RT. The comparative anatomy of the preoptic area and the hypothalamus. Research Publications—Association for Research in Nervous and Mental Disease. New York: Raven Press, 1939; 20:52.
3. Brodal A. The autonomic nervous system: the hypothalamus. In: Brodal A, ed. Neurological anatomy in relation to clinical medicine. New York: Oxford University Press, 1981:698.
4. Palkovits M, Zaborszky L. Neural connections of the hypothalamus. In: Morgane PJ, Panksepp J, eds. Handbook of the hypothalamus, vol 1. Anatomy of the hypothalamus. New York: Marcel Dekker, 1979:379.
5. Swanson LW, Kuypers HBJM. The paraventricular nucleus of the hypothalamus: cytoarchitectonic subdivision and organization of projections to the pituitary, dorsal vagal complex, and spinal cord as demonstrated by retrograde fluorescence double-labeling methods. J Comp Neurol 1980; 194:555.
6. Nilaver G, Zimmerman EA, Wilkins J, et al. Magnocellular hypothalamic projections to the lower brainstem and spinal cord of the rat. Neuroendocrinology 1980; 30:150.
7. Swaab D, Pool C, Nijveldt F. Immunofluorescence of vasopressin and oxytocin in the rat hypothalamo-neurohypophyseal system. J Neural Transm 1975; 36:195.
8. Silverman AJ, Zimmerman EA. Magnocellular neurosecretory system. Annu Rev Neurosci 1983; 6:357.
9. Vanderhagen JJ, Lotstra F, Vandesand F, Dierickx K. Coexistence of cholecystokinin and oxytocin-neurophysin in some magnocellular hypothalamo-hypophyseal neurons. Cell Tissue Res 1981; 221:227.
10. Watson SJ, Akil H, Fischli W, et al. Dynorphin and vasopressin: common localization in magnocellular neurons. Science 1982; 216:85.
11. Buijs RA. Intra- and extrahypothalamic vasopressin and oxytocin pathways in the rat: pathways to the limbic system, medulla oblongata and spinal cord. Cell Tissue Res 1978; 192:423.
11a. Jordan J, Shannon JR, Black BK, et al. The pressor response to water drinking in humans: a sympathetic reflex? Circulation 2000; 101:504.
12. Hoffman GH, Phelps CJ, Khachaturian H, Sladek JR Jr. Neuroendocrine projections to the median eminence. In: Pfaff DW, Ganten D, eds. Current topics in neuroendocrinology, vol 7. Morphology of hypothalamus and its connections. New York: Springer-Verlag, 1986:161.
13. Bargmann W. über der neurosekretorische Vernupfung von Hypothalamus und Neurohypophyse. Z Zellforsch 1949; 34:610.
14. Scharrer E, Scharrer B. Hormones produced by neurosecretory cell. Recent Prog Horm Res 1954; 10:183.
15. Falck B, Hillarp N-A, Thieme G, Torp A. Fluorescence of catecholamines and related compounds condensed with formaldehyde. J Histochem Cytochem 1962; 10:348.
16. Fuxe K, Hökfelt T. The influence of central catecholamine neurons on the hormone secretion from the anterior and posterior pituitary. In: Stutinsky F, ed. Neurosecretion. Berlin: Springer-Verlag, 1967:166.
17. Sternberger L, Hardy P, Cuculis J, Meyer H. The unlabeled antibody enzyme method in immunohistochemistry: preparation and properties of soluble antigen-antibody complex (horseradish peroxidase-antihorseradish peroxidase) and its use in identification of spirochetes. J Histochem Cytochem 1969; 18:315.
18. Hökfelt T, Elde R, Fuxe K, et al. Aminergic and peptidergic pathways in the nervous system with special reference to the hypothalamus. In: Reichlin S, Baldessarini RJ, Martin BJ, eds. The hypothalamus. Research Publications—Association for Research in Nervous and Mental Disease. New York: Raven Press, 1978:69.
19. Gai WP, Geffen LB, Blessing WW. Galanin immunoreactive neurons in the human hypothalamus: colocalization with vasopressin-containing neurons. J Comp Neurol 1990; 298:265.
20. Hoffman GE, Melnyk V, Hayes T, et al. Immunocytology of LHRH neurons. In: Scott DE, Kizlowski GP, Weindl A, eds. Brain-endocrine interactions, vol III. Neural hormones and reproduction. Basel: S Karger, 1978:67.
21. Watson SJ, Khachaturian H, Akil H, et al. Comparison of the distribution of dynorphin systems and enkephalin systems in brain. Science 1982; 218:1134.
21a. Patrick RL. Synaptic clefts are made to be crossed: neurotransmitter signaling in the central nervous system. Toxicol Pathol 2000; 28:31.
22. Lightman SL, Young WS III. Vasopressin, oxytocin, dynorphin, enkephalin and corticotrophin releasing factor mRNA stimulation in the rat. J Physiol (Lond) 1987; 394:23.
23. Meister B, Villar MJ, Ceccatelli S, Hökfelt T. Localization of chemical messengers in magnocellular neurons of the hypothalamic supraoptic and paraventricular nuclei: an immunohistochemical study using experimental manipulations. Neuroscience 1990; 37:603.
24. Meister B. Gene expression and chemical diversity in hypothalamic neurosecretory neurons. Mol Neurobiol 1993; 7:87.
25. Dahlström A, Fuxe E. Evidence for the existence of monoamine-containing neurons in the central nervous system. I. Demonstration of monoamines in the cell bodies of brainstem neurons. Acta Physiol Scand 1965; 62:1.
26. Ungerstedt U. Stereotaxic mapping of the monoamine pathways in the rat brain. Acta Physiol Scand 1971; 367:1.
27. Cheung Y, Sladek JR Jr. Catecholamine distribution in feline hypothalamus. J Comp Neurol 1975; 164:339.
28. Hoffman GE, Felten DL, Sladek JR Jr. Monoamine distribution in primate brain. III. Catecholamine-containing varicosities in the hypothalamus of *Macaca mulatta.* Am J Anat 1976; 147:501.
29. Sladek JR, Sladek CD. Neurological control of vasopressin release. Fed Proc 1985; 44:66.
30. Sladek JR Jr, McNeill TH. Simultaneous monoamine histofluorescence and neuropeptide immunocytochemistry. IV. Verification of catecholamine-neurophysin interactions through single section analysis. Cell Tissue Res 1980; 210:181.
31. McNeill TH, Sladek JR Jr. Simultaneous monoamine histofluorescence and neuropeptide immunocytochemistry. II. Correlative distribution of catecholamine varicosities and magnocellular neurosecretory neurons in the rat hypothalamic paraventricular and paraventricular nuclei. J Comp Neurol 1980; 193:1023.
32. Sladek JR Jr, Zimmerman EA. Simultaneous monoamine histofluorescence and neuropeptide immunocytochemistry. VI. Catecholamine innervation of vasopressin and oxytocin neurons in the rhesus monkey hypothalamus. Brain Res Bull 1983; 9:431.
33. Sawchenko PE, Swanson LW. The organization of noradrenergic pathways from the brainstem to the paraventricular and supraoptic nuclei in the rat. Brain Res Rev 1982; 4:275.
34. McKellar S, Loewy AD. Organization of some brainstem afferents to the paraventricular nucleus of the hypothalamus in the rat. Brain Res 1981; 217:351.
35. Cunningham ET Jr, Sawchenko PE. Reflex control of magnocellular vasopressin and oxytocin secretion. Trends Neurosci 1991; 14:406.
36. Day TA, Sibbald JR. A1 cell group mediates solitary nucleus excitation of supraoptic vasopressin cells. Am J Physiol 1989; 257:R1020.
37. Sladek JR Jr. Central catecholamine pathways to vasopressin neurons. In: Schrier RW, ed. Vasopressin. New York: Raven Press, 1985:343.
38. Blessing WW, Willoughby JO. Inhibiting the rabbit caudal ventrolateral medulla prevents baroreceptor-initiated secretion of vasopressin. J Physiol (Lond) 1985; 367:253.
39. Lightman SL, Todd K, Everitt BJ. Ascending noradrenergic projections from the brainstem: evidence for a major role in the regulation of blood pressure and vasopressin secretion. Exp Brain Res 1984; 55: 145.
40. Day TA, Renaud LP, Sibbald JR. Excitation of supraoptic vasopressin cells by stimulation of the A1 noradrenaline cell group: failure to demonstrate role for established adrenergic or amino acid receptors. Brain Res 1990; 516:91.
41. Bittencourt JC, Benoit R, Sawchenko PE. Distribution and origins of substance P-immunoreactive projections to the paraventricular and supraoptic nuclei: partial overlap with ascending catecholaminergic projections. J Chem Neuroanat 1991; 4:63.
42. Lundberg JM, Pernow J, Lacroix JS. Neuropeptide Y: sympathetic cotransmitter and modulator? News Physiol Sci 1989; 4:13.
43. Day TA, Sibbald JR, Khanna S. ATP mediates an excitatory noradrenergic neuron input to supraoptic vasopressin cells. Brain Res 1993; 607:341.
44. Sibbald JR, Wilson BKJ, Day TA. Neuropeptide Y potentiates excitation of supraoptic neurosecretory cells by noradrenaline. Brain Res 1989;499: 164.
45. Sladek JR Jr, Sladek CD. Anatomical reciprocity between magnocellular peptides and noradrenaline in putative cardiovascular pathways. Prog Brain Res 1983; 60:437.
46. Sladek CD, Armstrong WE. Effect of neurotransmitters and neuropeptides on vasopressin release. In: Gash DM, Boer GJ, eds. Vasopressin. New York: Plenum Publishing, 1987:275.
47. Renaud LP, Bourque CW. Neurophysiology and neuropharmacology of hypothalamic magnocellular neurons secreting vasopressin and oxytocin. Prog Neurobiol 1991; 36:131.
48. Mason WT, Ho YW, Eckenstein F, Hatton GI. Mapping of cholinergic neurons associated with rat supraoptic nucleus: combined immunocytochemical and histochemical identification. Brain Res Bull 1983; 11:617.
49. Kjaer A, Larsen PJ, Knigge U, et al. Histamine stimulates c-fos expression in hypothalamic vasopressin, oxytocin, and corticotropin releasing hormone-containing neurons. Endocrinology 1994; 134:482.

50. Atkins VJ, Bealer SL. Hypothalamic histamine release, neuroendocrine and cardiovascular responses during tuberomammillary nucleus stimulation in the conscious rat. Neuroendocrinology 1993; 57:849.
51. Lindvall O, Bjorklund A, Skagerberg G. Selective histochemical demonstration of dopamine terminal systems in rat di- and telencephalon: new evidence for dopaminergic innervation of hypothalamic neurosecretory nuclei. Brain Res 1984; 306:19.
52. Levey AI. Molecules of the brain. Hosp Pract (Off Ed) 2000; 35(2):41 and 51.

# CHAPTER 9

# PHYSIOLOGY AND PATHOPHYSIOLOGY OF THE ENDOCRINE BRAIN AND HYPOTHALAMUS

PAUL E. COOPER

The brain and endocrine system have been linked since the 1940s, when the hypothalamus was first assigned a central role in the control of anterior pituitary secretion.[1,2]

This chapter discusses the functional neuroanatomy of the hypothalamic-pituitary unit, as well as the important nonendocrine functions of the hypothalamus.

## HYPOTHALAMIC-PITUITARY UNIT

### EMBRYOLOGY

Between the third and fourth weeks of embryonic development, a longitudinal groove, the *sulcus limitans,* appears in the lumen of the neural tube. This sulcus divides the alar (dorsal) plate from the basal (ventral) plate. The basal plate plays no part in the development of the hypothalamus or pituitary, participating only in the formation of nervous tissue caudal to the diencephalon. At ~5.5 weeks, the alar plate, in the region that gives rise to the diencephalon, develops a longitudinal groove contiguous with the sulcus limitans. This groove, the *hypothalamic sulcus,* divides the alar plate into a dorsal portion, which gives rise to the thalamus, and a ventral portion, which gives rise to the hypothalamus[3] (Fig. 9-1*A* and *B*).

During the fifth week of embryonic life, the anterior pituitary begins to form as a diverticulum (*Rathke pouch*) of the buccal cavity. It expands dorsally to join the basal portion of the forebrain (see Fig. 9-1*C*) so that by the eighth week, the posterior pituitary, which begins as a diverticulum of the floor of the third ventricle, has contacted the Rathke pouch and been invested by it. By the 11th week, the cavity of the Rathke pouch becomes flattened and loses its connection with the buccal cavity.[3] Remnants of its attachment to the buccal cavity form the craniopharyngeal duct, residual cells of which persist in the posterior lobe of the pituitary, the hypophysial stalk, and the basisphenoid. Traditionally, these residual cells are thought to be the origin of craniopharyngioma; however, because craniopharyngiomas occasionally develop in the sella or along the craniopharyngeal duct itself, this idea on the origin of these tumors has been questioned. Careful examination of the superior pharynx in infants and adults almost always reveals a *pharyngeal hypophysis* at the buccal end of the craniopharyngeal duct. It is composed mainly of undifferentiated epithelial cells with a few chromophobes and chromophils, although rarely this residual pharyngeal hypophysial tissue has been reported to produce excessive pituitary hormone secretion.

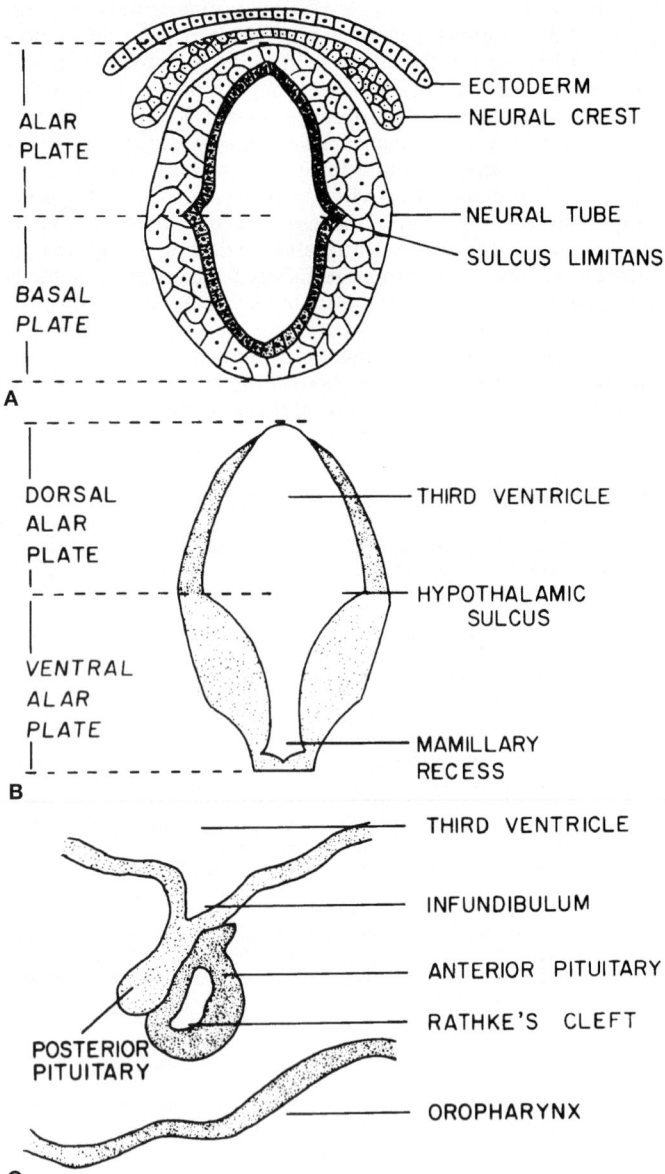

**FIGURE 9-1. A,** Cross section of a human embryo (3.5 weeks) through the first cervical somite. **B,** Cross section of a human embryo (5.5 weeks) in the region of the diencephalon. **C,** Midsagittal section of the hypothalamus of a human embryo (11 weeks).

## FUNCTIONAL NEUROANATOMY

Neuroanatomically, the traditional borders of the hypothalamus are the lamina terminalis (rostrally); the posterior edge of the mammillary body (caudally); the hypothalamic sulcus (dorsally); the floor of the third ventricle (ventrally); and the internal capsule, basis pedunculi, and subthalamus (laterally). The hypothalamus usually is divided into three regions: the chiasmatic (preoptic region), the tuberal region, and the mammillary complex. Of these three, the first two contain the neuronal groups and tracts that are of most significance in neuroendocrine regulation (Table 9-1).

Histologically, the hypothalamus contains two types of neurons: large (magnocellular) and small (parvicellular). Magnocellular neurons are of two classes: those that secrete arginine vasopressin (AVP) and neurophysin II, and those that secrete oxytocin and neurophysin I. AVP often is colocalized with dynorphin or angiotensin II, whereas oxytocin frequently is colocalized with cholecystokinin (CCK), corticotropin-releasing

**TABLE 9-1.**
**Hypothalamic Regions and Nuclei of Neuroendocrine Interest**

| Region | Nucleus | Functional Significance |
|---|---|---|
| **Chiasmatic (preoptic) region** | Suprachiasmatic | Major circadian pacemaker |
| | Sexually dimorphic | Unknown; ? male sexual behavior |
| | Supraoptic | Oxytocin and vasopressin secretion |
| | Paraventricular | Oxytocin and vasopressin secretion |
| **Tuberal** | Ventromedial | Feeding, aggression, sexual behavior, gonadotropin secretion; ? influence on higher cortical function and behavior |
| | Dorsomedial | Uncertain |
| | Infundibular (arcuate) | Pituitary secretion, particularly gonadotropins |
| | Lateral tuberal | Feeding and metabolism |
| | Tuberomammillary | Uncertain |

hormone (CRH), metenkephalin, or proenkephalin. Parvicellular neurons contain a variety of neuropeptides or biogenic amines, many of which are colocalized.

The parvicellular neurons of the hypothalamus that are found in the immediate periventricular region of the third ventricle, from the preoptic area to the mammillary bodies, project to the median eminence, where their neurosecretory products are released to influence anterior pituitary function. Functionally discrete groups of parvicellular neurons have been located in the anterior preoptic region, the paraventricular nucleus, and the arcuate nucleus.

The more medial area of the hypothalamus has collections of neurons that receive inputs from the brainstem and the limbic system. They, in turn, project to the periventricular zone, the limbic system, the brainstem, and the spinal cord in a circuit that is suited to the coordination of endocrine, autonomic nervous, and more complex behavioral responses to ensure homeostasis.

In the lateral hypothalamic area is found the medial forebrain bundle, a neural pathway that connects the brainstem reticular formation with the septum and the limbic system and also has input into the periventricular secretory neurons.

## HYPOPHYSIOTROPIC HORMONES

The anterior pituitary is known to produce six peptide hormones (Table 9-2). The secretion of each of these is under the control of one or more hypothalamic neuropeptides and several other classic neurotransmitters. A comprehensive review of these intricate interactions has been published elsewhere.[4]

In primates, a few neurons containing *gonadotropin-releasing hormone* (GnRH) are found in clusters above the optic chiasm, medial to the supraoptic nuclei, but most are found in the medial basal hypothalamus.[5] Their axons project to the median eminence, where GnRH is released in a pulsatile fashion. In humans, GnRH-positive neurons are found in the arcuate nucleus.[4] The GnRH-containing neurons of the medial basal hypothalamus have an intrinsic firing pattern that results in the pulsatile release of GnRH. Norepinephrine, epinephrine, serotonin, acetylcholine, and N-methyl D-aspartic acid all stimulate GnRH release, as do angiotensin II (probably through its action on norepinephrine) and neuropeptide Y.[4] Opioid peptides and γ-aminobutyric acid (GABA) inhibit GnRH release.[4]

CRH-containing neurons are found in the medial portion of the paraventricular nucleus. From there, they project to the median eminence, where they release CRH in a pulsatile fashion (see Chap. 8). CRH release is stimulated by norepinephrine, epinephrine, serotonin, glutamine, aspartamine, acetylcholine, angiotensin II, and neuropeptide Y, and is inhibited by GABA, AVP, opioid peptides, and substance P.[4]

Neurons containing *thyrotropin-releasing hormone* (TRH) are found in the periventricular portion of the paraventricular nucleus and in a similar location in the anterior hypothalamus. They project to the median eminence through the lateral retrochiasmatic area.[5] TRH release is responsive to triiodothyronine ($T_3$) and thyroxine ($T_4$) levels. It also is stimulated by norepinephrine, dopamine, and serotonin, and is inhibited by GABA and opioid peptides.[4]

Prolactin release is inhibited by dopamine and stimulated by TRH and vasoactive intestinal peptide (VIP). Dopamine-containing neurons are found in the arcuate nucleus and the preoptic ventricular nucleus.[6] They project into hypothalamic regions rich in TRH and somatostatin. VIP-containing neurons are found in the paraventricular nucleus and project to the median eminence. They also are found in the suprachiasmatic nucleus.

Neurons containing *growth hormone–releasing hormone* are found in the arcuate nucleus, just lateral to the median eminence. Their nerve terminals project to the median eminence and pituitary stalk.[7,8] The release of growth hormone–releasing hormone is stimulated by norepinephrine and serotonin.[4]

Neurons containing somatostatin (*growth hormone release–inhibiting hormone*) are distributed widely in the central nervous system (see Chap. 169). In the hypothalamus, they are localized to neurons in the paraventricular nucleus. Their axons travel laterally and ventrally toward the optic chiasm and then caudally to the median eminence. The arcuate and ventromedial nuclei receive somatostatinergic innervation from other sources. Many somatostatin-containing nerve terminals are found in the ventromedial arcuate complex, the suprachiasmatic nucleus, the ventral premammillary nuclei, and the organum vasculosum of the lamina terminalis.[5,9]

## HYPOTHALAMIC NEURAL CONNECTIONS

Hypothalamic afferent pathways carry important information on emotion and visceral function. Ascending visceral afferents convey data to the hypothalamus from baroreceptors, volume

**TABLE 9-2.**
**Anterior Pituitary and Hypophysiotropic Hormones**

| Pituitary Hormones | Hypophysiotropic Hormones | |
| | *Name* | *Structure* |
|---|---|---|
| Luteinizing hormone (*LH*) and follicle-stimulating hormone (*FSH*) | Gonadotropin-releasing hormone (*GnRH*) | 10 amino acids |
| Pro-opiomelanocortin (contains corticotropin and β-endorphin) | Corticotropin-releasing hormone (*CRH*) | 41 amino acids |
| Thyrotropin (*TSH*) | Thyrotropin-releasing hormone (*TRH*) | 3 amino acids |
| Prolactin (*PRL*) | Prolactin-releasing factor (*PRF*) | Unknown (TRH and VIP)* |
| | Prolactin release–inhibiting hormone (*PIH*) | Dopamine |
| Growth hormone | Growth hormone–releasing hormone (*GHRH*) | 44 amino acids |
| | Growth hormone release–inhibiting hormone (somatostatin) | 14 amino acids |

*Both TRH and vasoactive intestinal peptide (*VIP*) release prolactin in vivo and in vitro. Whether either is a physiologically important PRF is uncertain.

receptors, and taste receptors. These inputs reach the hypothalamus over poorly defined pathways that relay in the reticular formation and midline thalamic nuclei. Somatosensory information also reaches the hypothalamus. The limbic system has rich afferent connections to the hypothalamus. The medial forebrain bundle serves as an important integrative pathway between the brainstem and the limbic system. The amygdala sends fibers to the hypothalamus through the stria terminalis, and the fornices relay information from the hippocampal formation to the mammillary bodies of the hypothalamus. The mammillary bodies also receive input from and provide input to the anterior thalamic nuclei through the mammillothalamic tract and, therefore, are indirectly connected to the cingulate cortex. Finally, afferent hypothalamic connections from the dorsomedial thalamic nucleus and direct corticohypothalamic connections from the orbital surface of the frontal lobe are found.[10]

Two major hypothalamic efferent pathways are the dorsal longitudinal fasciculus and the mammillotegmental fasciculus. The fibers of the dorsal longitudinal fasciculus terminate in the dorsal motor nucleus of the vagus, the salivatory and lacrimal nuclei, the intermediolateral cell column of the thoracolumbar cord, and the sacral autonomic area. In addition, efferents from this tract go to various brainstem motor nuclei connected with eating and drinking, and to spinal cord motor neurons that participate in the shivering that raises body temperature. The fibers of the mammillotegmental fasciculus end in the raphe nuclei of the midbrain and pons. Finally, the mammillothalamic fasciculus contains two-way connections with the anterior nuclei of the thalamus.[10]

Through these rich connections, the hypothalamus monitors and influences body functions, preserving the constancy of the internal milieu.

## SUPRACHIASMATIC NUCLEUS

The suprachiasmatic nucleus is responsible for generating circadian rhythms in all mammals, including humans. It is composed of neurons that contain AVP, VIP, neuropeptide Y, and neurotensin. A marked seasonal variation exists in suprachiasmatic nucleus cell numbers and volumes in humans, with summer values being approximately half those found in the fall. Hypothalamic tumors that involve the anterior hypothalamus disturb circadian rhythms in humans.[11,12]

The volume of the suprachiasmatic nucleus and the number of cells is similar in men and women, although the shape of the nucleus is different.[13] Homosexual males have been reported to have a suprachiasmatic nucleus that is 1.7 times larger than that in heterosexual males and contains 2.1 times as many cells.[14] The functional implication of this finding, if confirmed, remains to be determined.

## SEXUALLY DIMORPHIC NUCLEUS

The sexually dimorphic nucleus, or intermediate nucleus, is found in the preoptic area. It contains twice as many cells in young adult males as in comparable adult females.[15] Cell numbers in the nucleus are similar in males and females at birth and not until ~4 years of age can any difference be detected. No difference in cell number in this nucleus is observed when the brains of homosexual and heterosexual males are compared.[14,16]

The third nucleus of the interstitial nuclei of the anterior hypothalamus has been found to be larger in males than in females, and is approximately half as large in homosexual males as in heterosexual males.[17] This finding, which has not been confirmed, suggests yet another hypothalamic area that is dimorphic with respect to gender as well as sexual orientation.

## BLOOD SUPPLY OF THE HYPOTHALAMIC-PITUITARY UNIT

The hypothalamus receives its arterial blood supply from the circle of Willis, the internal carotid and posterior cerebral arter-

ies. Apart from blood that drains into the pituitary gland, most blood from the hypothalamus enters the basal vein of Rosenthal through numerous small venous plexuses in and around the hypothalamus.

The blood supply of the pituitary gland is more complex (see Chap. 11). The posterior pituitary (neurohypophysis) is supplied by blood directly from the inferior hypophysial artery and drains into the inferior hypophysial veins. At its most rostral portion, in the median eminence, the neurohypophysis is supplied by the superior hypophysial arteries; free communication exists between the blood supply of the median eminence and that of the posterior pituitary. Apart from the most superficial layers of the gland, which are supplied by small capsular arteries, the anterior pituitary gland lacks a direct arterial blood supply. Blood is supplied to the median eminence by the superior hypophysial arteries, and the major venous drainage of the median eminence is through the portal veins to the anterior pituitary. Blood then drains from the anterior pituitary into the posterior pituitary, from which it enters the cavernous sinus or returns to the median eminence. This anatomic configuration means that blood from the median eminence, rich in hypothalamic factors and neurotransmitters, is directed toward the anterior pituitary, where it influences the secretion of pituitary hormones. Whether blood from the anterior pituitary, rich in pituitary hormones, returns to the median eminence to participate in feedback control and other possible effects on the brain is debated.[18,19]

## ANATOMY OF THE PARAPITUITARY AREA

Disorders of the hypothalamic-pituitary unit may be seen clinically because of neuroendocrine dysfunction or because of symptoms caused by compression of local structures. To fully understand the symptoms produced by compression, one must understand the anatomy of the parapituitary area (Fig. 9-2).

The *pituitary gland* rests in the sella turcica. Inferiorly, it is bounded by the sphenoid sinus. Superiorly, it is separated from the cranial cavity by a double layer of dura mater, the *diaphragma sellae*; through this passes the *pituitary stalk.* Normally, the dura tightly surrounds the stalk. If the opening is larger or if the intracranial pressure is increased, however, the arachnoid membrane may herniate into the sella, displacing the pituitary gland peripherally and enlarging the sella—the *empty sella syndrome* (see Chaps. 11 and 17). The diaphragma sellae is pain sensitive; stretching of this tissue by pituitary enlargement may give rise to frontotemporal headaches.

The *optic chiasm* lies 3 to 10 mm above the pituitary fossa. In 90% of persons, the chiasm is partly or completely above the diaphragma. Of the remaining 10% of persons, approximately half have an anteriorly placed chiasm ("prefixed") and half have a posteriorly placed chiasm ("postfixed").[20] This anatomic variability accounts for the lack of visual field abnormalities in some patients with a large suprasellar extension of a pituitary tumor. Compression of the optic chiasm by a pituitary tumor usually affects the crossing fibers in the chiasm. These come from the nasal portions of the retina, which serve the temporal fields. Thus, the typical visual field abnormality that occurs in chiasmatic compression is a bitemporal hemianopsia. Because the most inferiorly placed fibers in the optic chiasm carry information from the superior visual fields, tumors pushing on the chiasm from below tend to cause superior quadrantanopsias of the bitemporal variety, whereas lesions pushing on the chiasm from above cause inferior bitemporal quadrantanopsias. Unfortunately, several exceptions to these rules do occur. Lesions in and around the optic chiasm tend to produce incongruous visual field defects (i.e., of a different configuration in each eye; see Chap. 19).

Immediately lateral to the pituitary gland are the *cavernous sinuses*. Within each is found the carotid artery and its sympathetic plexus; cranial nerves III, IV, and VI; and the ophthalmic

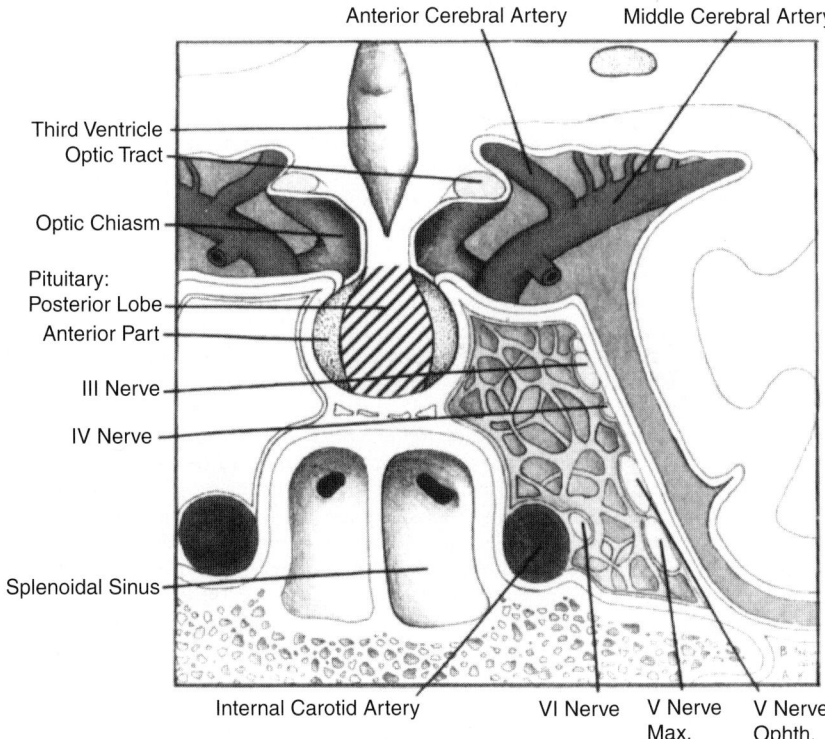

Anterior Cerebral Artery    Middle Cerebral Artery

Third Ventricle
Optic Tract

Optic Chiasm

Pituitary:
Posterior Lobe
Anterior Part

III Nerve

IV Nerve

Splenoidal Sinus

Internal Carotid Artery    VI Nerve    V Nerve    V Nerve
Max.    Ophth.

**FIGURE 9-2.** Anatomic relationships of the pituitary fossa and cavernous sinus. The lateral wall of the sella turcica is formed by the cavernous sinus. The sinus contains the carotid artery, two branches of the fifth cranial nerve (ophthalmic [*Ophth.*] and maxillary [*Max.*]), the third nerve (oculomotor), the fourth nerve (trochlear), and the sixth nerve (abducens). The optic chiasm and optic tract are located superior and lateral, respectively, to the pituitary. (*A*, artery; *N*, nerve.) (From Martin JB, Reichlin S, Brown GM, eds. Clinical neuroendocrinology. Philadelphia: FA Davis, 1987:447.)

and maxillary divisions of the trigeminal nerve. Sudden expansion of a pituitary tumor into the cavernous sinus may produce cranial nerve palsy. Conversely, an aneurysm of the cavernous portion of the carotid artery can erode laterally and mimic the plain skull radiographic appearance of a pituitary tumor and even lead to mild hypopituitarism.

## FUNCTIONS OF THE NONENDOCRINE HYPOTHALAMUS

### TEMPERATURE REGULATION

For the body to function efficiently, its temperature must be maintained within narrow limits. Wide variations beyond this range can result in serious metabolic derangement and death. The hypothalamus ensures that the heat gained by the body from metabolic activity, and in some circumstances from the environment, is balanced by the heat lost.[21,22]

The preoptic anterior hypothalamus contains thermosensitive neurons that monitor the temperature of blood (Fig. 9-3). Experiments have shown that serotonin (5-hydroxytryptamine) released in this area stimulates hypothalamic heat production centers. This effect is blocked by norepinephrine or epinephrine.

The caudolateral portion of the hypothalamus is insensitive to changes in body temperature, but the regulatory center that determines the normal setpoint of 37°C is located here. The injection of acetylcholine-like substances into this region causes profound and long-lasting hypothermia. It also is through this area that the main pathways controlling heat loss and heat conservation travel to the midbrain, pons, medulla, and spinal cord.

Intraventricular injection of the neuropeptides mammalian bombesin, neurotensin, TRH, somatostatin, and β-endorphin decreases body temperature and thus implicates these substances in thermoregulation. CRH appears to be an important mediator of thermogenesis in response to serotonin and its agonists and to cytokines. No peptide or group of peptides, however, has been singled out as the physiologic regulator of body temperature.[20] In some experiments, prostaglandin $E_2$ has increased body temperature.

Hypothalamic injury after head trauma or cerebral infarction can produce prolonged hypothermia resulting either from a change in the setpoint or from an impairment of heat production mechanisms. *Paroxysmal hypothermia* has been described in a few patients. These persons appear to have a temporary alteration in setpoint, with the body temperature falling to 32°C or lower. The hypothermia may last for minutes to days and is associated with fatigue, decreased alertness, hypoventilation, and even cardiac arrhythmia. The loss of body heat is caused by increased sweating and vasodilation. Although the paroxysmal nature of these episodes has suggested an epileptic etiology, the attacks are not prevented by use of anticonvulsants.[21]

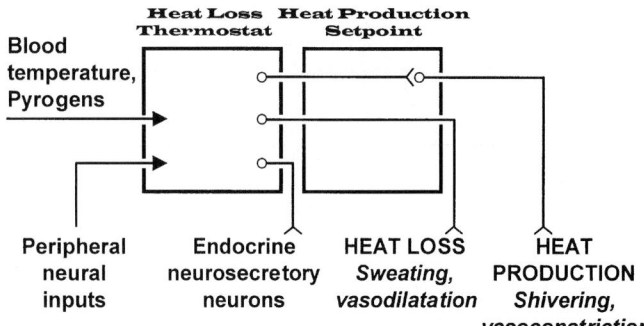

PREOPTIC ANTERIOR    POSTERIOR
HYPOTHALAMUS    HYPOTHALAMUS

**Heat Loss    Heat Production**
**Thermostat    Setpoint**

Blood
temperature,
Pyrogens

Peripheral    Endocrine    HEAT LOSS    HEAT
neural    neurosecretory    *Sweating,*    PRODUCTION
inputs    neurons    *vasodilatation*    *Shivering,*
*vasoconstriction*

**FIGURE 9-3.** Hypothalamic temperature regulation mechanisms. The preoptic anterior hypothalamic area functions as a thermostat and contains mechanisms for regulation of heat loss. The posterior hypothalamus integrates heat production mechanisms. Lesions of the preoptic anterior hypothalamic area cause hyperthermia; lesions of the posterior hypothalamus cause hypothermia or poikilothermia. (Modified from Myers RD. Ionic concepts of the set-point for body temperature. In: Lederis K, Cooper KE, eds. International symposium on recent studies of hypothalamic function, Calgary, 1973. Basel: S Karger, 1974:371; and from Cooper PE, Martin JB. Neuroendocrinologic diseases. In: Rosenberg R, ed. Comprehensive neurology. New York: Raven Press, 1991:608.)

*Paroxysmal hyperthermia* can occur in some conditions. Acute damage to the preoptic anterior hypothalamus from surgery, subarachnoid hemorrhage, or cerebral infarction can lead to profound impairment of heat loss mechanisms, and the resulting hyperthermia can be lethal. *Cyclic hyperthermia* has been seen in some patients, but the neuropathologic substrate for this condition is unknown. Some have responded to therapy with phenytoin. Sustained hyperthermia probably is not seen in hypothalamic dysfunction. Reported case studies of prolonged hyperthermia attributed to hypothalamic dysfunction have not excluded an underlying malignancy or unrecognized infection. *Cyclic hypothermia*, responsive to treatment with anticonvulsant agents, such as clonidine or cyproheptadine, has been described.[23]

Large lesions in the posterior hypothalamus or lesions in the brainstem that damage the hypothalamic outflow tracts may result in *poikilothermia*, a condition in which the body temperature varies with environmental temperature. Most affected patients have hypothermia, although in hot, humid conditions, hyperthermia may be a problem.[21]

During *fever*, the body's temperature setpoint is elevated, although the ability to regulate temperature around the new setpoint is normal.[24] In response to an infection or other cause of inflammation, the body's inflammatory cells—primarily monocytes—release cytokines,[25] which act at the hypothalamus to cause fever.[24] Interleukin-1 (IL-1) releases phospholipases in the hypothalamus that, in turn, release arachidonic acid from plasma membranes. Arachidonic acid causes a rise in prostaglandin E, which raises the body temperature setpoint. Treatment with acetylsalicylic acid or acetaminophen to reduce fever probably affects this process. Animal studies suggest that the action of IL-1 occurs in the preoptic anterior hypothalamus through the reduction of the sensitivity of "warm-sensitive" neurons, allowing the body to tolerate a higher temperature. Once this new setpoint has been established, the hypothalamus uses normal physiologic mechanisms to maintain body temperature by peripheral vasoconstriction, reduced sweating, and, if necessary, increases in heat production through shivering.

Tumor necrosis factor (TNF) is another cytokine that alters the setpoint in the hypothalamus and increases the production of IL-1 locally, in the hypothalamus. Most TNF seems to be produced in macrophages stimulated by bacterial endotoxin. Interleukin-6 (IL-6) and interferon-γ also act directly at the hypothalamus to raise the setpoint.

The exact role of the cytokines in regulating body temperature and in causing fever is unclear because complex interactions exist among these compounds. IL-1, for example, stimulates its own production and interferon-γ stimulates IL-1 production, whereas interleukin-4 suppresses the production of IL-1, TNF, and IL-6. IL-1 production also is inhibited by glucocorticoids and prostaglandin E.

The *fulminant hyperthermia* (malignant hyperthermia) that can occur during anesthesia is not hypothalamic in origin. Rather it results from excessive muscle contraction caused by an abnormality of the muscle membrane. Another syndrome of hyperthermia is the neuroleptic malignant syndrome. This condition, characterized clinically by hyperthermia, rigidity of skeletal muscles, autonomic instability, and fluctuating levels of consciousness, has been associated with the use of major tranquilizers, rapid withdrawal from treatment with dopaminergic agents (e.g., L-dopa or bromocriptine), and, less commonly, the use of tricyclic antidepressants. The common denominator in the syndrome seems to be an alteration in dopamine function in the hypothalamus. Treatment consists of discontinuing the use of neuroleptics, providing general support, and administering anticholinergics for mild cases, bromocriptine (5 mg orally or nasogastrically four times daily) for more severe cases, and benzodiazepines or dantrolene (2–3 mg/kg per day intravenously to a maximum of 10 mg/kg per day) for resistant cases.[26,27]

## APPETITE REGULATION

In most animals, the body is able to balance its intake of food and output of energy to maintain body weight. It is the hypothalamus that receives inputs from the periphery that either stimulate or inhibit the intake of food, and it is the hypothalamus that, likewise, sends signals to other parts of the brain to influence endocrine, autonomic, and motor nervous system function.[28] The interaction between the limbic system and the hypothalamus is critical in translating the need for food into behaviors such as hunting and stalking.

The destruction of both ventromedial nuclei in the rat or the cat markedly increases food intake for a few days. As the animal becomes obese, the overeating decreases; if it is then fasted back to ideal weight and given free access to food, the animal again increases its food intake until it becomes obese. Lesions of the ventromedial nuclei, however, do not produce a pure syndrome of obesity. During the phase of overeating, the animals often are irritable and aggressive, becoming lethargic and passive when the increased weight is achieved. The pituitary gland is not necessary for the weight gain because hypophysectomized animals also become obese. If hyperphagia is prevented by tube feeding, the animals still become obese. Hyperinsulinemia has been observed in lesioned animals within minutes of surgery; if this is prevented by lesioning the pancreatic B cells with streptozocin, the obesity and hyperphagia are prevented.

Classic neurophysiology explained the hyperphagia in animals with a lesion of the ventromedial nuclei on the basis of unopposed activity of a hypothalamic "feeding center" in the lateral hypothalamus. Implantation of electrodes in this lateral area causes, after stimulation, marked increases in food intake, whereas destruction of this area causes aphagia, even in animals with concomitant ventromedial nuclei lesions.

The limbic system plays an important role in appetite. One suggested interaction is that the urge to eat arises in the hypothalamus and the limbic structures modify food intake through a discriminative function. Bilateral lesions in the amygdala cause prolonged aphagia and adipsia. Stimulation of this same area in the fed animal does not cause increased eating, but intake increases if the stimulation is performed while the animal is eating.

Cells in the ventromedial hypothalamus also monitor blood glucose levels and coordinate the hypothalamic response to hypoglycemia. Although hypothalamic lesion studies have shown that blood glucose is decreased on stimulation of the anterior and tuberal regions medially, acute hypothalamic damage tends to produce hyperglycemia by activation of the sympathetic nervous system and a resulting glycogenolysis in the liver. Another important effect is the elevation of growth hormone, a contrainsulin hormone, which causes glucose levels to rise. In patients deficient in growth hormone, on either a hypothalamic or a pituitary basis, profound hypoglycemia can occur and may even be a presenting symptom, especially in children.

Many of the features of lateral hypothalamic lesions in animals have been thought to result from damage to the nigrostriatal bundle, a dopamine-containing tract connecting the substantia nigra to the basal ganglia. Lesions in this tract cause anorexia and weight loss, whereas lesions in the ventral adrenergic bundle, a norepinephrine-containing tract originating in the locus coeruleus, cause hyperphagia and obesity. Serotonin is thought to inhibit eating, whereas GABA agonists have the opposite effect.

Of interest has been the putative role of neuropeptides in the regulation of appetite. The gastrointestinal peptides CCK, bombesin, and glucagon can inhibit feeding behavior through an action on the vagal nucleus. Neuropeptide Y can cause hypothalamic obesity by inhibiting sympathetic drive and stimulating insulin release.[29]

An important putative stimulator of appetite is β-endorphin. One potential mechanism for this action is its ability to stimulate the release of insulin. Other neurotransmitters have been assumed to play a role in the control of appetite. Experimentally, the following substances *decrease appetite*: norepinephrine, serotonin, CCK, neurotensin, bombesin, TRH, naloxone, somatostatin, and VIP. The following substances *increase appetite*: dopamine, GABA, β-endorphin, enkephalin, and neuropeptide Y.[30] (Also see Chap. 125.)

Increased oxidation of fatty acids raises levels of 3-hydroxybutyrate, which can reduce food intake through an action at the level of the hypothalamus. The *ob*, *db*, and *fa* genes have all been implicated in the regulation of feeding in animals through production of a circulating factor. In the case of the *ob* gene, this circulating factor is leptin. Genetically obese mice have a leptin deficiency that, when corrected, leads to a reduction in food intake with a resulting fall in body weight. Leptin levels have been found to be high in obese humans. This suggests an insensitivity to endogenous leptin in these individuals.[31] A discussion of the role of other peptides such as uncoupling proteins, agouti protein, melanocortin receptor isoforms, melanin-concentrating hormone, and the proteins responsible for the tub and fat monogenic mouse models of obesity is beyond the scope of this chapter but has been reviewed.[32]

Hypothalamic tumors that cause hyperphagia, aggressive behavior, and the development of marked obesity have been described. Similar clinical syndromes can be seen in patients with hypothalamic damage caused by radiation therapy or encephalitis. For many years, the syndromes of anorexia nervosa and bulimia nervosa have been considered by many to be purely psychiatric; however, the finding of reduced serotonin levels in the cerebrospinal fluid of patients with bulimia nervosa, the low cerebrospinal fluid levels of norepinephrine in patients with anorexia nervosa, and the enhanced secretion of CCK-8-S in patients with anorexia nervosa suggest that neurotransmitter or neuropeptide abnormalities could be responsible for at least some of the clinical features of these syndromes.[33] The question remains whether these changes are a result of the condition or its cause (see Chap. 128).

## EMOTION AND LIBIDO

The anatomic substrate for emotion is widespread and not confined to any single area of the brain; the frontal and temporal lobes, the limbic system, and the hypothalamus all participate in emotion. The hypothalamus is thought to play an important role in the integration and expression of emotion, especially sexual and aggressive behaviors.[34]

The hypothalamus is necessary for angry behavior in cats. If all cerebral tissue rostral to the tuberal region is removed, angry behavior still can be induced by minor stimuli, but if the remaining hypothalamus then is removed, this activity no longer can be provoked. Electrical stimulation of the caudal hypothalamus in the cat can elicit rage reactions.

Bilateral anteromedial hypothalamic lesions cause normally friendly cats to become aggressive, as do bilateral lesions in the ventromedial nuclei, or electrical stimulation in the perifornical region or the periaqueductal gray area between the third and fourth ventricles.

The limbic system appears to exert a tonic inhibition on the perifornical region of the hypothalamus. Damage to these inhibitory pathways or stimulation in this area results in angry behavior.

Ablation of certain areas in the hypothalamus produces fearful behavior, and stimulation of certain hypothalamic areas in the dorsal hippocampal formation and the septal region produces pleasure reactions. For such reactions to occur, the basal telencephalon and thalamus must be intact.

Some humans report a pleasurable or glowing feeling with electrical stimulation in the septal area; others report a feeling of sexual gratification.

Primates from which the amygdala, piriform cortex, and part of the hippocampal formation have been removed bilaterally exhibit several behavioral disturbances, including hypersexuality, loss of discrimination of taste for thirst-quenching liquids, hyperoral behavior, and loss of awareness of harmful or painful objects (*Klüver-Bucy syndrome*).

Rage attacks have occurred in patients with lesions in the caudal hypothalamus, the subthalamus, and even the midbrain. They also have been induced by manipulation of the hypothalamus during surgery. Fear and rage in patients with hypothalamic disorders usually occur in situations that normally would be associated with these same emotions, but in lesser degrees. In those cases examined pathologically, lesions of the basal portion of the brain, especially the descending pathways to the hypothalamus from the cerebral cortex, or the ventromedial nuclei, usually are found.

Stimulation of the posterior portion of the hypothalamus in humans can arouse feelings of fear and horror. Lesions of the mammillary bodies and vicinity are associated with drowsiness, somnolence, apathy, and indifference. Psychosurgery directed at the medial posterior hypothalamus or the caudolateral region has caused apathy in previously aggressive persons. Euphoria rarely is seen in adults with hypothalamic disease but is seen in children as part of the *diencephalic syndrome.* This syndrome most commonly manifests in infancy as failure to thrive; a glioma of the anterior hypothalamus usually is found. Children with this condition are emaciated despite normal or excessive food intake, and are described as jovial and as having excessive energy. Approximately 50% of affected children have nystagmus. A tendency to hypoglycemia also may bring these children to medical attention. Despite growth failure, growth hormone levels usually are elevated. Computed tomography demonstrates abnormalities in most cases (see Chap. 18).

Normal libido is the product of an interaction between hypothalamic and extrahypothalamic sites. Usually, hypothalamic damage leads to decreased GnRH levels and reduced libido. Hypersexuality is a rare accompaniment of hypothalamic disease and may be seen with or without increased libido.[35] Paroxysmal hypersexuality consisting of sexual urges, genital sensations, and orgasm has been observed in association with temporal lobe tumors or epilepsy but not with primary hypothalamic disease. Altered sexual preference has been described in association with hypothalamic lesions.[36]

Epileptiform activity in the temporal lobe has been linked to violent behavior. This is extremely rare, however. In a review of 5400 patients with epilepsy, violent behavior during a seizure was found in only 19 cases.[37]

Evidence is accumulating to suggest that the hypothalamus plays a role in the symptoms of fibromyalgia and chronic fatigue syndrome.[38]

## AUTONOMIC FUNCTIONS

The hypothalamus plays an important role in the integration of the functions of the autonomic nervous system.[39]

### CARDIOVASCULAR FUNCTIONS

Signals of cardiovascular status are sent to the brain from baroreceptors and chemoreceptors at the carotid sinus and aortic arch, and from pressure/volume receptors in the atrium. This information is fed into the nucleus of the tractus solitarius, as well as into cells of the paramedian reticular nuclei in the medulla. In the medulla, these afferent signals are modulated by inputs from higher centers, particularly the hypothalamus.

The main sympathetic outflow to the heart begins in the paraventricular nucleus of the hypothalamus. Some of the paraventricular neurons project to the intermediolateral cell column of the spinal cord (the site of origin of preganglionic sympathetic neurons), whereas others project to the dorsal motor nucleus of the vagus where they can influence parasympathetic output to the heart.[40]

Stimulation of the anterior hypothalamus, particularly the preoptic area, causes bradycardia, hypotension, and decreased baroreflex activity. Such stimulation also can lower the threshold for ventricular fibrillation and cause a variety of electrocardiographic changes. Such changes are common in patients with subarachnoid hemorrhage.

Hypothalamic disease also may cause hypertension, and the disrupted autonomic function that occurs in subarachnoid hemorrhage can cause myocardial necrosis, an effect blocked by sympathetic blockade.

The hypothalamus receives input from the nucleus of the tractus solitarius and relays information from higher cortical centers to brainstem vasomotor centers. The many and varied cardiovascular phenomena that occur in response to emotion, especially hypertension and cardiac arrhythmias, probably are mediated by the hypothalamus.[40]

The anterior portion of the ventral third ventricle has been shown, by lesion studies, to be a site at which body fluid homeostasis and arterial blood pressure are regulated. Angiotensin II levels reflect changes in serum osmolality or sodium concentration. In addition, the area receives sensory neural input from the kidney, carotid sinus, and other baroreceptors. Output from this area can induce vasoconstriction (through the sympathetic nervous system), and abnormal function of this region has been implicated in the pathogenesis of hypertension.[41]

## RESPIRATION

Acute pulmonary edema has been described in association with numerous injuries to the central nervous system, such as increased intracranial pressure, epilepsy, and hypothalamic injury.[41a] Classically, *neurogenic pulmonary edema* was defined as normal pulmonary capillary wedge pressures with increased protein content of edema fluid in the lung. One hypothesis has been that noncardiac pulmonary edema can be caused by excessive sympathetic outflow from the hypothalamus. Virtually all cases of this type of pulmonary edema, however, are accompanied by system hypertension; therefore, when the experimental physiologic data are reviewed, separation of cardiac from noncardiac causes of edema is impossible. Most of the data support centrally induced systemic hypertension as the cause of the syndrome.[42]

## GASTROINTESTINAL FUNCTIONS

Under normal resting conditions, gastric motility is relatively autonomous. Higher cortical centers, including the neocortex and limbic lobe, may influence gastric activity through their connections with the hypothalamus. Afferent signals go to the gut through the vagus nerves.

Electrical stimulation of areas of the rostral hypothalamus causes a prompt fall in gastric pH, an effect that is prevented by vagotomy. Stimulation of the tuberal and caudolateral areas of the hypothalamus causes reduced secretion of gastric acid that is of slower onset. This is unaffected by vagotomy but is prevented by bilateral adrenalectomy.

Stimulation and ablation studies in the monkey have shown that cortical areas affect peristalsis, the volume of gastric secretion, and its enzyme and acid content. Similar effects can be seen with stimulation or lesioning of the amygdala.

Bilateral lesions in the anterolateral hypothalamus increase basal gastric acid secretion, an effect that is abolished by interruption of the fibers of the fornix and medial forebrain bundle. This observation suggests that the limbic lobe and frontal neocortex normally exert a tonic, inhibitory effect on basal gastric secretion.

Prolonged hypothalamic stimulation often results in hemorrhage and ulceration in the gastric mucosa of monkeys and dogs, whereas sympathectomy prevents the hemorrhage but not the ulceration.

Lesions anywhere from the rostral hypothalamus to the region of the vagal nuclei in the medulla oblongata may cause acute hemorrhagic erosions of the gastric mucosa; extensive ulceration of the lower esophagus and stomach; and acute perforation of the esophagus, stomach, and duodenum. Such lesions are most likely to occur after damage to or pressure on the hypothalamus, particularly its tuberal region.

## BIOLOGIC RHYTHMS

Biologic rhythms are ubiquitous in the animal and plant kingdoms, occurring in single cells, tissues, organs, individual animals, and populations (see Chap. 6). Their periods range from milliseconds to years. Many endocrine rhythms are *circadian*, having a period ~24 hours long.[43] *Ultradian* rhythms, with periods shorter than 24 hours, and *infradian* rhythms, with periods longer than 24 hours, certainly exist, but the neural mechanisms responsible for these rhythms are debated. Circadian rhythms have been studied extensively. Integrity of the retinohypothalamic projection, which terminates in the suprachiasmatic nucleus, appears to be essential for the light entrainment of circadian rhythms, and the suprachiasmatic nucleus appears essential for circadian rhythmicity. Ablation of the suprachiasmatic nucleus is associated with the loss of all circadian rhythms. The exact functioning of the suprachiasmatic nucleus in the generation of circadian rhythms is unknown, but at least two coupled oscillators appear to exist. These oscillators cause the circadian variations seen in brain monoamines, plasma amino acids, corticotropin and cortisol, growth hormone, prolactin, vasopressin, aldosterone, insulin, glucose, and sex steroids, as well as pineal activity, body temperature, and autonomic function.[44]

## MEMORY

The hypothalamus is closely linked to nervous structures associated with memory function: the reticular formation, hippocampal formation, and other limbic structures.[45,46] Although lesions in the mammillary bodies are found in virtually all cases of *Wernicke-Korsakoff syndrome* (retrograde amnesia, confabulation, apathy),[47] the memory deficit in this condition has been thought to correlate best with lesions in the dorsomedial nucleus of the thalamus. Nonetheless, a case report of a brain-injured patient who was studied using magnetic resonance imaging suggests that, at least in trauma, hypothalamic injury alone, without accompanying thalamic injury, can cause marked, relatively focal, memory deficits.[48] Many patients with hypothalamic lesions exhibit disturbances of short-term memory, with sparing of immediate recall and long-term memory. Bilateral hippocampal lesions are associated with severe memory disturbance, although some controversy exists about whether involvement of the fornices, the major outflow tract of the hippocampal formation, produces permanent memory loss. Evidence suggests that fornix transection can cause wide-ranging memory disturbance in humans (see Chap. 176).[49]

## SLEEP

The region of the hypothalamic-midbrain junction appears to play an important role in sleep and wakefulness. Two types of patients were seen in the encephalitis pandemics[50] of 1917 and 1920: those with prolonged somnolence and ophthalmoplegia, and those with agitation and hyperkinesia. Pathologically, somnolence correlated with damage to the tegmentum of the midbrain, and agitation was seen in patients with anterior hypothalamic lesions. Damage to the hypothalamic-midbrain junction by multiple sclerosis, abscess, or infarction has been described as causing hypersomnia or inversion of the sleep-waking cycles. Some studies support the concept of a "sleep center" in the anterior hypothalamus that, if damaged, causes hyperactivity and sleeplessness, whereas the posterior hypothalamus appears to be involved in the production of rapid eye movement sleep.

The ascending reticular formation participates in normal wakefulness. Damage to it results in coma (complete unresponsiveness). Alternatively, the hypothalamus seems to be the generator of normal sleep-wake cycles. Damage to the hypothalamus causes either excessive wakefulness or somnolence (i.e., an unresponsive state from which the patient can be aroused, at least temporarily).

## HYPOTHALAMIC SYNDROMES

Several clinical syndromes have been attributed to hypothalamic dysfunction.[51] Previously, patients have been described who had autonomic overactivity associated with tumors in the region of the hypothalamus and third ventricle. This was termed *diencephalic epilepsy,* although its epileptic nature is in doubt because electroencephalograms do not show seizure activity during spells and the condition does not respond to administration of anticonvulsants.

Glioma of the anterior hypothalamus in early childhood produces a clinical syndrome characterized by profound emaciation despite normal or excessive food intake, excess energy, and euphoria—the *diencephalic syndrome of infancy* (see Chap. 18).

*Kleine-Levin syndrome* is characterized by episodes of somnolence followed by hyperactivity, irritability, and increased appetite. Adolescent boys are most commonly affected. The attacks occur every 3 to 6 months and last days to weeks. The cause is unknown, and the specific hypothalamic pathology has not been determined.[52]

## REFERENCES

1. Fortier C. Obituary: Geoffrey Wingfield Harris. Endocrinology 1972; 90:851.
2. Bajusz E, Ernst A. Scharrer. Editorial. Neuroendocrinology 1965; 1:65.
3. Hamilton WJ, Boyd JD, Mossman HW. Human embryology: prenatal development of form and function, 3rd ed. Cambridge: W Heffer & Sons, 1962:315.
4. Palkovits M. Neuropeptides in the brain. In: Martini L, Ganong WF, eds. Frontiers in neuroendocrinology, vol 10. New York: Raven, 1988:1.
5. Page RB. Neuropharmacology of anterior pituitary control. In: Barrow DL, Selman WR, eds. Neuroendocrinology, vol 5. Concepts in neurosurgery. Baltimore: Williams & Wilkins, 1992:31.
6. Müller EE, Nisticò G. Brain messengers and the pituitary. San Diego, CA: Academic Press, 1989:1.
7. Jacobowitz DM, Schulte H, Chrousos GP, Loriaux DL. Localization of GRF-like immunoreactive neurons in rat brain. Peptides 1984; 4:521.
8. Merchenthaler I, Thomas CR, Arimura A. Immunocytochemical localization of growth hormone releasing factor (GHRF)-containing structures in the rat brain using anti-rat GHRF serum. Peptides 1984; 5:1071.
9. Beal MF, Mazurek MF, Martin JB. A comparison of somatostatin and neuropeptide Y distribution in monkey brain. Brain Res 1987; 10:405.
10. Barr M, Kiernan JA. The human nervous system: an anatomical viewpoint, 6th ed. Philadelphia: JB Lippincott, 1993:181.
11. Schwartz WJ, Bosis NA, Hedley-Whyte ET. A discrete lesion of ventral hypothalamus and optic chiasm that disturbed the daily temperature rhythm. J Neurol 1986; 233:1.
12. Cohen RA, Albers HE. Disruption of human circadian and cognitive regulation following a discrete hypothalamic lesion: a case study. Neurology 1991; 41:726.
13. Swaab DF, Hofman MA, Lucassen PJ, et al. Functional neuroanatomy and neuropathology of the human hypothalamus. Anat Embryol (Berl) 1993; 187:317.
14. Swaab DF, Fliers E, Partiman TS. The suprachiasmatic nucleus of the human brain in relation to sex, age and senile dementia. Brain Res 1985; 342:37.
15. Swaab DF, Hofman MA. An enlarged suprachiasmatic nucleus of the human brain in homosexual men. Brain Res 1990; 537:141.
16. Swaab DF, Hofman MA. Sexual differentiation of the human hypothalamus: ontogeny of the sexually dimorphic nucleus of the preoptic area. Dev Brain Res 1988; 44:314.
17. LeVay S. A difference in hypothalamic structure between heterosexual and homosexual men. Science 1991; 253:1034.
18. Bergland RM, Page RB. Can the pituitary secrete directly to the brain? (Affirmative anatomical evidence.) Endocrinology 1978; 102:1325.
19. Page RB. Pituitary blood flow. Am J Physiol 1982; 243:E427.
20. Banna M. Terminology, embryology and anatomy. In: Hankinson J, Banna M, eds. Major problems in neurology, vol 6. Pituitary and parapituitary tumors. London: WB Saunders, 1976:1.
21. Cooper PE. Disorders of the hypothalamus and pituitary gland. In: Joynt RJ, ed. Clinical neurology, vol 3. Philadelphia: JB Lippincott, 1993:1.
22. Rothwell NJ. CNS regulation of thermogenesis. Crit Rev Neurobiol 1994; 8:1.
23. Kloos RT. Spontaneous periodic hypothermia. Medicine 1995; 74:268.
24. Cooper KE. The neurobiology of fever: thoughts on recent developments. Annu Rev Neurosci 1987; 10:297.
25. Reichlin S. Neuroendocrine-immune interactions. N Engl J Med 1993; 329:1246.
26. Rosenberg MR, Green M. Neuroleptic malignant syndrome—review of response to therapy. Arch Intern Med 1989; 149:1927.
27. Gratz SS, Levinson DF, Simpson GM. The treatment and management of neuroleptic malignant syndrome. Prog Neuropsychopharmacol Biol Psychiatry 1992; 16:425.
28. Bray GA, Fisler J, York DA. Neuroendocrine control of the development of obesity: understanding gained from studies of experimental animal models. Front Neuroendocrinol 1990; 11:128.
29. York DA. Lessons from animal models of obesity. Endocrinol Metab Clin North Am 1996; 25:781.
30. Cezayirli RC, Robertson JT. Pharmacologic modulation of hypothalamic control of appetite. In: Givens JR, ed. The hypothalamus. Chicago: Year Book Medical Publishers, 1984:115.
31. Considine RV, Sinha MK, Heiman ML, et al. Serum immunoreactive-leptin concentrations in normal-weight and obese humans. New Engl J Med 1996; 334:292.
32. Bessesen DH, Faggioni R. Recently identified peptides involved in the regulation of body weight. Semin Oncol 1998; 25(Suppl 6):28.
33. Leibowitz SF. Brain monoamine projections and receptor systems in relation to food intake, diet preference, meal patterns, and body weight. In: Brown GM, Koslow SH, Reichlin S, eds. Neuroendocrinology and psychiatric disorders. New York: Raven Press, 1983:383.
34. Van de Poll NE, Van Goozen SH. Hypothalamic involvement in sexuality and hostility: comparative psychological aspects. Prog Brain Res 1992; 93:343.
35. Plum F, VanUitert R. Nonendocrine diseases and disorders of the hypothalamus. In: Reichlin S, Baldessarini RJ, Martin JB, eds. The hypothalamus. New York: Raven Press, 1978:415.
36. Miller BL, Cummings JL, McIntyre H, et al. Hypersexuality or altered sexual preference following brain injury. J Neurol Neurosurg Psychiatry 1986; 49:867.
37. Delgado-Escueta AV, Mattson RH, King L, et al. The nature of aggression during epileptic seizures. N Engl J Med 1981; 305:711.
38. Crofford LJ, Demitrack MA. Evidence that abnormalities of central neurohormonal systems are key to understanding fibromyalgia and chronic fatigue syndrome. Rheum Dis Clin North Am 1996; 22:267.
39. Grossman A, ed. Neuroendocrinology of stress. Baillieres' clinical endocrinology and metabolism, vol 1. London: Baillieres Tindall, 1987:247.
40. Valeriano J, Elson J. Electrocardiographic changes in central nervous system disease. Neurol Clin 1993; 11:257.
41. Samuels MA. Neurally induced cardiac damage. Neurol Clin 1993; 11:273.
41a. Keegan MT, Lanier WL. Pulmonary edema after resection of a fourth ventricle tumor: possible evidence for a medulla-mediated mechanism. Mayo Clin Proc 1999; 74:264.
42. Simon RP. Neurogenic pulmonary edema. Neurol Clin 1993; 11:309.
43. Aschoff J. Circadian rhythms: general features and endocrinological aspects. In: Kreiger DT, ed. Endocrine rhythms. New York: Raven Press, 1979:1.
44. Moore RY. The anatomy of central neural mechanisms regulating endocrine rhythms. In: Kreiger DT, ed. Endocrine rhythms. New York: Raven Press, 1979:63.
45. Zola-Morgan S, Squire LR. Neuroanatomy of memory. Annu Rev Neurosci 1993; 16:547.
46. Wilson MA, McNaughton BL. Reactivation of hippocampal ensemble memories during sleep. Science 1994; 265:676.
47. Pitella JE, Giannetti AV. Morphometric study of the neurons in the medial mammillary nucleus in acute and chronic Wernicke's encephalopathy. Clin Neuropathol 1994; 13:26.
48. Dusoir H, Kapur N, Byrnes DP, et al. The role of diencephalic pathology in human memory disorder: evidence from a penetrating paranasal brain injury. Brain 1990; 113:1695.
49. Gaffan EA, Gaffan D, Hodges JR. Amnesia following damage to the left fornix and to other sites: a comparative study. Brain 1991; 114:1297.
50. Creisler CA, Klerman EB. Circadian and sleep-dependent regulation of hormone release in humans. Recent Prog Horm Res 1999; 54:97.
51. Martin JB. Neurologic manifestations of hypothalamic disease. Prog Brain Res 1992; 93:31.
52. Mukaddes NM, Alyanak B, Kora ME, Polvan O. The psychiatric symptomatology in Kleine-Levin syndrome. Child Psychiatry Hum Dev 1999; 29:253.

# CHAPTER 10

# PINEAL GLAND

RUSSEL J. REITER

## MORPHOLOGY AND INNERVATION

### GROSS ANATOMY

The pineal gland, so called because of its resemblance to a pine cone (Latin *pineas*), is a multifaceted endocrine organ whose secretory products directly or indirectly affect every organ and cell in the body. Embryologically, it is derived from neuroectoderm as an outgrowth of the diencephalon. In adults, it is attached to the posterodorsal aspect of the diencephalon, and its proximal portion is invaginated by the pineal recess of the third ventricle (Fig. 10-1). The gland weighs ~130 mg, with great individual variation seen, and is ~1 cm long. The blood supply to the gland is derived from the posterior choroidal branches of the posterior cerebral arteries. The pineal gland has a copious blood supply. In advanced age, it may acquire calcium deposits (corpora arenacea, acervuli), which are visible on skull radiographs.

### INNERVATION

The pineal gland is innervated by sympathetic axons and by axons coming directly from the brain.[1] Postganglionic sympathetic axons arrive in the pineal from perikarya located in the superior cervical ganglia. The cell bodies of the preganglionic fibers that end in the ganglia are located in the intermediolateral cell column of the upper thoracic cord. The neurons in the intermediolateral cell columns receive terminals from, among other sources, perikarya in the hypothalamus, possibly in the paraventricular nuclei; these nuclei are connected to the suprachiasmatic nuclei, which receive a prominent input from the ganglion cells of the retinas through the retinohypothalamic tract. Through this complex series of neurons, the *retinas are*

*functionally related to the pineal gland.* Sympathetic innervation of the pineal is essential for the rhythmic metabolism of indoleamines and for the pineal's endocrine functions. The sympathetic neurotransmitter mediating the cyclic production of pineal indoleamines is norepinephrine.

Besides sympathetic innervation, the pineal gland receives axons directly from the brain that enter through the stalk. The function of these fibers relative to the physiology of the pineal is unknown.

## HISTOLOGY

The major cellular elements within the pineal gland are the *pinealocytes*, which are arranged into cords or follicles separated by connective tissue septa. With advancing age, the septa become more prominent. Ultrastructurally, the pinealocytes have one to several cytoplasmic processes that typically terminate near the many capillaries perfusing the gland. The nerve endings in the pineal gland usually lie close to the pinealocyte processes in the perivascular spaces, but true morphologic synapses are not obvious.

## INDOLEAMINE METABOLISM

### MELATONIN

Within the pinealocyte, tryptophan, an amino acid taken up from the blood, is metabolized to a variety of potential hormones (Fig. 10-2).[2] The compound that has been most thoroughly investigated is *N*-acetyl-5-methoxytryptamine, or melatonin. Tryptophan is initially metabolized to serotonin (5-hydroxytryptamine); the concentration of this monoamine in the pineal gland exceeds that in any other organ. Especially

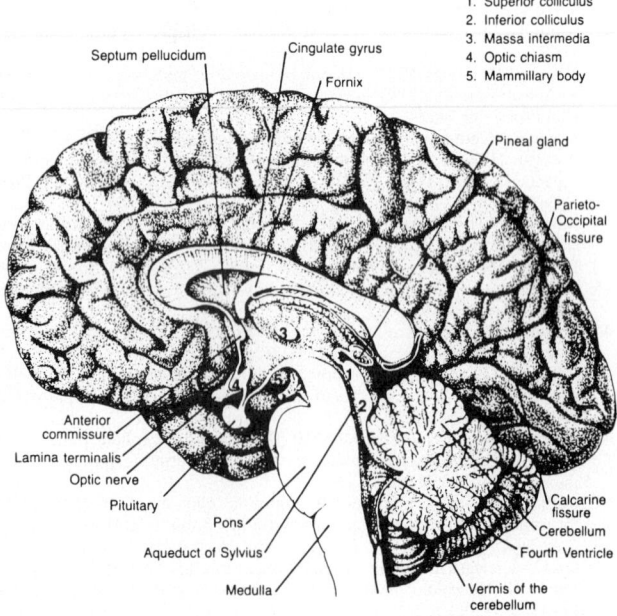

1. Superior colliculus
2. Inferior colliculus
3. Massa intermedia
4. Optic chiasm
5. Mammillary body

**FIGURE 10-1.** Midsagittal view of the human brain showing the relationship of the pineal gland to other neural structures.

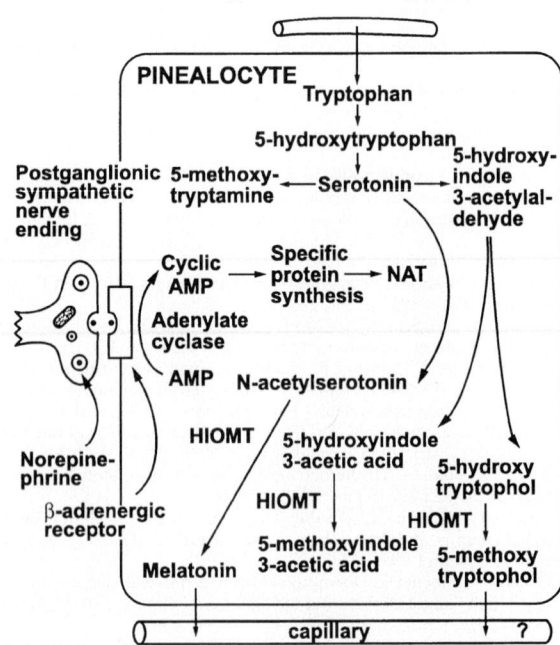

**FIGURE 10-2.** Interactions of postganglionic sympathetic neurons with the endocrine unit of the pineal gland, the pinealocyte, and the conversion of tryptophan to a variety of indole products. Within the pinealocyte, cyclic adenosine monophosphate (*AMP*) acts as a second messenger to stimulate the activity of serotonin *N*-acetyltransferase (*NAT*), primarily during darkness. Serotonin also is acted on by hydroxyindole-*O*-methyltransferase (*HIOMT*) to form 5-methoxytryptamine, and by monoamine oxidase to form 5-hydroxyindole-3-acetylaldehyde. Melatonin is a major secretory product of the pineal gland. (Modified from Reiter RJ, MacLeod RM, Müller EE, eds. Neuroendocrine perspectives, vol 3. New York: Elsevier, 1984:350.)

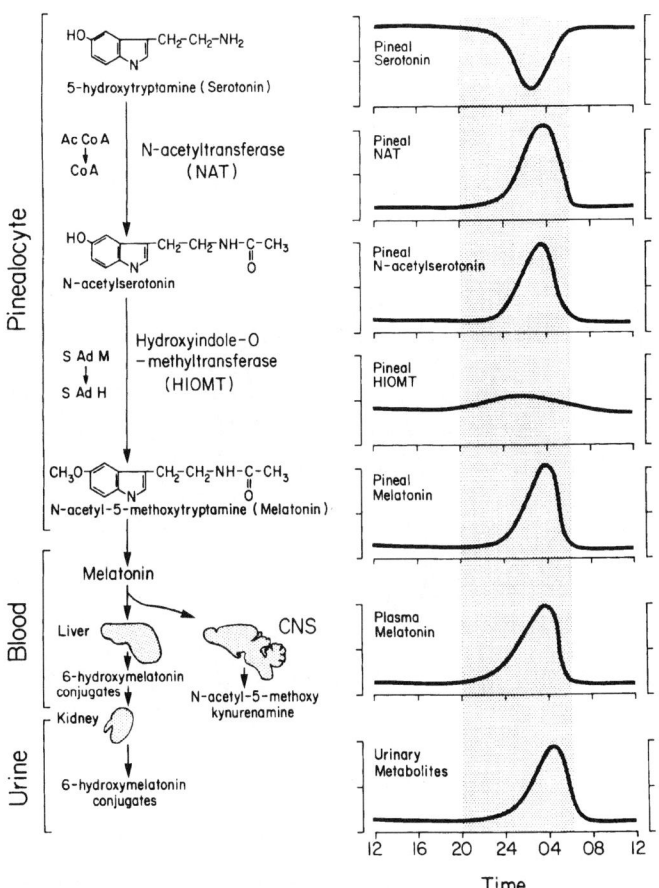

**FIGURE 10-3.** Pineal, blood, and urinary rhythms of various constituents. Methods are available for estimating blood and urinary levels of melatonin and its metabolites. The shaded area in the right half of the figure represents the daily dark period. (*Ac Co A*, Acetyl coenzyme A; *CoA*, coenzyme A; *S Ad M*, S-adenosyl methionine; *S Ad H*, S-adenosyl homocysteine; *CNS*, central nervous system.) (From Reiter RJ. Pineal indoles: production, secretion and actions. In: Muller CE, MacLeod RM, eds. Neuroendocrine perspectives, vol 13. Amsterdam: Elsevier, 1984:358.)

during the daily dark period, serotonin is *N*-acetylated by the enzyme serotonin *N*-acetyltransferase to form *N*-acetylserotonin.[3] The activity of *N*-acetyltransferase increases many-fold during darkness (Fig. 10-3). *N*-acetylserotonin is converted to melatonin by the action of hydroxyindole-*O*-methyltransferase. Once formed, melatonin is rapidly secreted into the blood vascular system and, as a consequence, plasma melatonin levels typically are highest at night, when pineal melatonin production is greatest.

### SEROTONIN

Hydroxyindole-*O*-methyltransferase also acts directly on serotonin, converting it to 5-methoxytryptamine (see Fig. 10-2), a compound that has been proposed as a pineal hormone. Serotonin also is metabolized by monoamine oxidase; the product is eventually converted to 5-methoxytryptophol and 5-methoxyindoleacetic acid, the former of which possibly is released from the pineal.

### INFLUENCE OF HORMONES AND DRUGS ON MELATONIN SECRETION

Most of what is known about the interactions of the postganglionic neurotransmitter norepinephrine with the pinealocyte comes from observations in animals, although the relationships probably are similar in humans. Norepinephrine is released

into the synaptic cleft, primarily during the daily dark period, after which it acts primarily on β-adrenergic receptors on the pinealocyte membrane, where it stimulates cyclic adenosine monophosphate production and, eventually, *N*-acetyltransferase activity and melatonin synthesis (see Fig. 10-2).[4] Alpha receptors on the pinealocyte membrane also may be involved in mediating the nocturnal rise in melatonin. In humans, the peripheral infusion of isoproterenol, a β-receptor agonist, does not increase blood levels of melatonin as readily as it does in some animals. In addition, orciprenaline and L-dopa are ineffective in altering circulating melatonin in humans. The inability of isoproterenol to stimulate human pineal melatonin production may relate to the relative insensitivity of the pinealocyte β-receptors to the agonist throughout most of the day; animal studies have shown that either the number of receptors or their affinity for the ligand is greatly increased at night.[5] Circulating norepinephrine may be relatively ineffective in promoting pineal melatonin production because the sympathetic nerve endings in the pineal gland have an active uptake mechanism for the catecholamine, thereby protecting the pinealocytes from circulating norepinephrine.

Other drugs that seem incapable of altering blood melatonin levels in humans include scopolamine, amphetamine, thyrotropin-releasing hormone, luteinizing hormone–releasing hormone, and desaminocys-D-arg-vasopressin.[5] Both clonidine and dexamethasone have been reported to lower plasma levels of melatonin. In general, pineal melatonin production seems to be out of the usual endocrine feedback loop.

### PLASMA LEVELS OF MELATONIN AND ITS METABOLISM

Plasma levels of melatonin seem to reflect closely the amount being synthesized and secreted by the pineal gland (see Fig. 10-3).[6] When pineal melatonin production increases at night, plasma levels rise accordingly. In the few individuals in whom the pineal has been surgically removed because of tumors in the epithalamic region, plasma levels of melatonin either are severely depressed or are undetectable.[7] In animals, pinealectomy is associated with very low or nonmeasurable amounts of melatonin in plasma.

The nocturnal rise in plasma melatonin levels has been measured by bioassay, radioimmunoassay, and gas chromatography–mass spectrometry.[7a] Depending on the technique used, daytime levels of plasma melatonin range from undetectable to 20 pg/mL. At night, values may increase to 300 pg/mL; however, with the most specific methods, nighttime levels typically are <50 pg/mL. Short-term rises may be superimposed on the 24-hour cycle of melatonin production because of the episodic secretion of melatonin by the pineal gland. Although the amplitude of the circadian melatonin varies widely between individuals, the rhythm is highly reproducible within each person.

Most melatonin in the plasma may be bound to proteins, especially albumin. Melatonin readily penetrates cell membranes and tissue barriers (e.g., the blood–brain barrier). Some of its primary sites of action are undoubtedly in the central nervous system (see ref. 7b). Because of its rapid metabolism, usually <1% of exogenously administered melatonin escapes into the urine in unmetabolized form.

Melatonin is enzymatically degraded in at least two sites, the liver and the brain (see Fig. 10-3).[2] In animals, melatonin is rapidly metabolized in the liver. Humans with hepatic cirrhosis reportedly have higher than normal daytime levels of plasma melatonin, which implicates the liver as the primary site of its metabolism. In addition, the half-life of plasma melatonin is longer in humans with impaired liver function than in those with normal liver function.

In the liver, melatonin is chiefly metabolized to 6-hydroxymelatonin; this is conjugated to sulfuric acid and, to a much lesser extent, to glucuronic acid. A small amount of melatonin is converted to *N*-acetylserotonin in the liver and appears in the blood as a sulfate or glucuronide conjugate. Melatonin taken up by the central nervous system is converted in part to *N*-acetyl-5-methoxykynurenamine, which, along with the hepatic metabolites of melatonin, is excreted in the urine.

Besides its enzymatic degradation, melatonin is nonenzymatically metabolized when it scavenges free radicals. Melatonin's ability to scavenge the highly toxic hydroxyl radical is one of the newly discovered functions of this widely acting hormone.

## FACTORS INFLUENCING PLASMA MELATONIN RHYTHM

### LIGHT–DARK CYCLE

The primary factor determining plasma melatonin levels is the prevailing light–dark environment.[8] The rhythmic production and secretion of melatonin is synchronized by the light–dark cycle. Typically, daytime is associated with low plasma melatonin levels and nighttime is associated with high levels (see Fig. 10-3).[6] Blind humans with no retinal light perception exhibit *free-running melatonin cycles,* with periods of ~24.7 hours. In these persons, the highest plasma melatonin values can occur either at night or during the day.[9]

The rise in plasma melatonin levels in sighted humans may actually precede the removal of artificial light at bedtime.[5] Short-term dark exposure during the day typically is not associated with increased circulating melatonin levels. When persons are exposed to light during the normal dark period, however, plasma melatonin levels drop rapidly if the light has a brightness of 2500 lux or more (2500 lux is roughly four to five times the intensity of normal room light but considerably less than the intensity of sunlight).[10] Individuals awakened at night and exposed to darkness or low light intensities (<300 lux) typically do not exhibit a marked alteration in the rhythmic production of melatonin.

When the light–dark cycle is shifted, such as in transmeridian travel or with a new rest–activity schedule, the melatonin rhythm also is shifted; however, the change is not immediate.[11] Thus, if humans are phase-shifted by 12 hours, elevated levels of blood melatonin and its urinary metabolites may not occur for several days. Within 7 to 12 days, depending somewhat on age (see later), the melatonin cycle readjusts to the prevailing light–dark environment so that elevated levels coincide with the period of darkness. The interval required for reentrainment of the melatonin cycle also depends on the magnitude of the phase shift: the greater the phase shift, the greater the interval required for the melatonin rhythm to reentrain.

Nocturnal secretion of melatonin seems unrelated to sleep stage.[12] Maximal plasma melatonin levels usually appear before the maximal rapid eye movement sleep peak.

In animals that experience natural photoperiodic and temperature conditions throughout the year, season has a significant influence on the plasma melatonin rhythm, affecting both the duration and the magnitude of the nocturnal rise.[2] In humans, who live under more controlled environmental conditions, the influence of season is less obvious but may be measurable.[13]

### AGE AND SEXUAL MATURATION

Age substantially influences the pattern of melatonin production (Fig. 10-4). Whereas the day–night periodicity in plasma melatonin levels probably is not present at birth, by the end of the first year of life children exhibit a robust rhythm.[14] The highest nighttime levels of melatonin occur in children 1 to 5 years of age. Several reports document a significant attenuation of the nocturnal rise in plasma melatonin levels between 5 and 15 years of age (Fig. 10-5).[15] This decrease is of particular interest because of its possible relationship to pubertal develop-

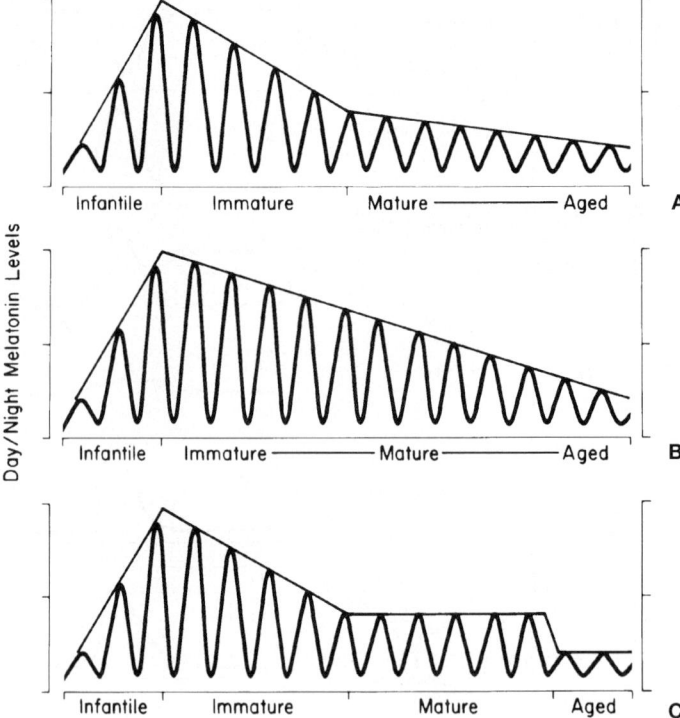

**FIGURE 10-4.** Changes in blood melatonin levels as a function of age. During the infantile period (age 0 to 1 year), the melatonin rhythm matures; after the first year of age, a decrease is seen in nocturnal melatonin levels. The drop in nighttime melatonin may be rapid (**A** and **C**) or gradual (**B**) from 5 to 15 years of age (immature period). Low nocturnal melatonin titers in advanced age may be a consequence of a gradual reduction (**A** and **B**) or associated with some critical event late in life (**C**).

ment. In animals, the activated pineal gland, or exogenous melatonin administration, can retard sexual maturation.[16] Hence, the gradual decrease in nocturnal plasma melatonin levels as humans mature sexually may permit the establishment of adult neuroendocrine-gonadal relationships.[17]

The decrease in nighttime melatonin levels in the decade beginning at 5 years of age has not been universally demonstrated. Even

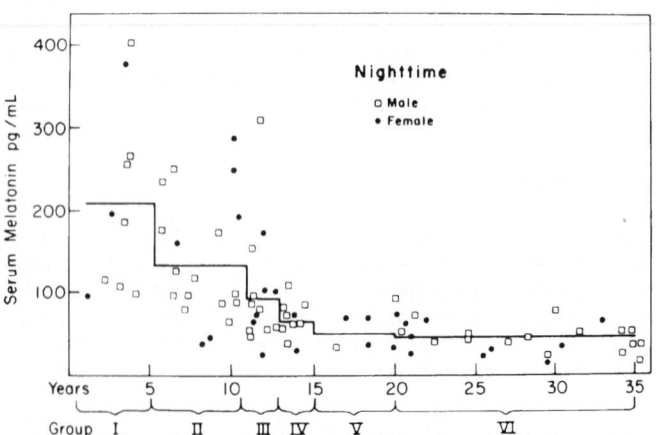

**FIGURE 10-5.** Nocturnal serum melatonin values in male and female subjects aged 1 to 35 years. Values are plotted against chronologic age and state of sexual development (Tanner stages I to VI). Between 5 and 15 years of age, as individuals pass through puberty, nocturnal melatonin levels decrease by roughly 75%. (From Waldhauser F, Dietzel M. Daily and annual rhythms in human melatonin secretion: role in puberty control. Ann N Y Acad Sci 1985; 435:205.)

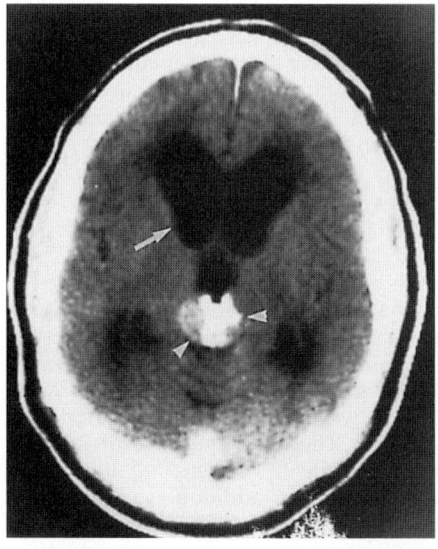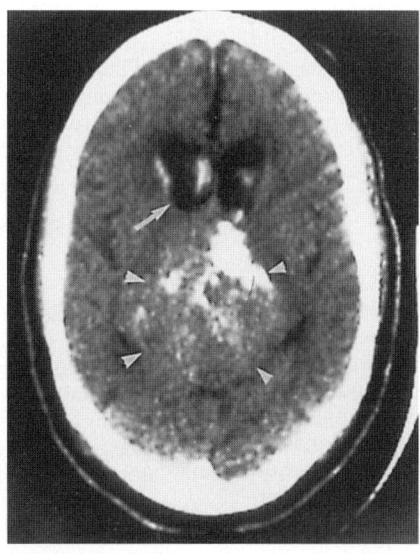

A,B

**FIGURE 10-6.** Computed tomographs (*CTs*) of a 67-year-old man with Parinaud syndrome and deteriorating mental status. Four years previously, the CT scan shown in **A** was obtained because of disorientation and dementia thought to be secondary to increased intracranial pressure. A 2-cm mass was seen in the pineal region (*arrowheads*) with triventricular dilation (*arrow*) (third and lateral ventricles). The fourth ventricle was not involved. The patient refused definitive surgery, and a ventriculoperitoneal shunt was performed. In the CT scan shown in **B**, the lesion has grown to 7 cm; the ventricles decreased in size considerably after shunt placement. (Courtesy of Dr. Frederick T. Borts.)

if a reduction in the ability of the pineal to secrete melatonin is correlated with pubertal onset, this does not mean that the indoleamine normally limits the maturation of the reproductive system. The case could be that gonadotropins or sex steroids secreted by the pituitary and gonads, respectively, inhibit the conversion of serotonin to melatonin in the pineal gland. Finally, the decrease in plasma melatonin may be merely a function of age and not causally related to the status of the reproductive organs. In one case report, however, a strong correlation was found between the decrease in circulating melatonin and pubertal onset.

After adolescence, most individuals continue to exhibit a 24-hour rhythm in plasma melatonin production and the urinary excretion of metabolites. In advanced age, however, the ability of the pineal to produce melatonin is severely limited, especially at night. In elderly persons, a nocturnal rise in melatonin is barely detectable.

### AVERSIVE STIMULI

Aversive stimuli, which cause the release of large amounts of catecholamines into the systemic circulation, have been investigated for their effects on the discharge of melatonin from the pineal gland. In general, procedures such as electroconvulsive therapy, pneumoencephalography, and lumbar puncture, and conditions such as excessive short-term exercise, insulin-induced hypoglycemia, and psychologic conflict have a minor influence on daytime plasma melatonin levels.[5] In one study, however, strenuous exercise in women significantly increased daytime circulating melatonin levels.[18] The consequences of short-term rises in plasma melatonin during the day are unknown.

### POSSIBLE SEX STEROID FEEDBACK

Several studies have described plasma melatonin levels as a function of the human menstrual cycle. The rationale for these studies was that, if melatonin has an antigonadotropic action in humans, as it has in some other mammalian species, then perhaps ovarian secretory products may limit pineal melatonin secretion at the time of ovulation. In some studies, nocturnal plasma melatonin levels were found to be lower during the midmenstrual cycle (ovulation) than during the postmenstrual or premenstrual periods.[19] These results suggest that the midcycle lessening of the nocturnal melatonin increase may permit the release of pituitary gonadotropins required for ovulation. Not all investigators have reported menstrual cycle variations in the 24-hour melatonin rhythms, however. In acyclic athletic women, higher than normal circulating melatonin values have been reported.

Melatonin secretion has not been found to be linked to prolactin, growth hormone, adrenocorticotropin, testosterone, or luteinizing hormone.[5]

## CLINICAL IMPLICATIONS

### SEXUAL MATURATION

The pineal gland and melatonin have been implicated in several clinical entities.[5] Besides the possible link between gradually decreasing nocturnal melatonin levels and pubertal development (see Fig. 10-5), pineal tumors may alter sexual maturation (also see Chap. 92).[20,21] Tumors of the pineal gland are more prevalent in men than in women and may either retard or advance sexual development.[20] The opposite responses to space-occupying lesions of the pineal region are explained on the basis of cellular origin (i.e., parenchymal or nonparenchymal) and the consequential endocrine capabilities of the tumorous mass. In addition, these tumors can cause increased intracranial pressure and, because of associated hydrocephalic dilation of the third ventricle, *Parinaud syndrome* (paralysis of upward gaze and slightly dilated pupils that react normally on accommodation but not to light) (Fig. 10-6). Hypermelatoninism with an enlarged pineal gland has been shown to be associated with delayed sexual development.

### OVULATORY RELATIONSHIPS

The observation that nocturnal melatonin levels may be lowest at the time of ovulation in women suggests that a decrease in the indoleamine concentration may permit ovulation.[19] In animals, exogenously injected melatonin can inhibit both the release of ova and the surge of ovulatory hormones associated with this process. Melatonin may have a similar antiovulatory capability in humans when given in pharmacologic doses.[22] Higher than normal nocturnal melatonin secretion is associated with hypothalamic amenorrhea in women, and with delayed puberty.[23]

### PSYCHOLOGICAL INTERRELATIONSHIPS

A possible link between various types of depression and pineal function has been proposed. Several psychiatric diseases have a strong seasonal component; one of these is seasonal affective disorder.[24] This condition is characterized by recurring periods of depression during the winter months, when the natural day length is shortest. Typical symptoms are hypersomnia, excessive eating, a craving for carbohydrates, and sadness. Phototherapy for this disorder entails exposing the patient to bright (2500 lux), full-spectrum artificial light, usually early in the morning. The symptoms normally associated with seasonal depression are greatly reduced by phototherapy but are partially reinstated if melatonin is given orally during the period of phototherapy. Bright light early in the morning prevents the phase delay in the melatonin rhythm that may be typical of patients with seasonal affective disorder.

## SLEEP

Persons given exogenous melatonin report feeling sleepy. Under usual conditions, high plasma melatonin levels are associated with the nightly sleep interval.[25] Melatonin has been reported to affect brain levels of serotonin, a compound that may be important in the initiation or maintenance of sleep. In various studies, melatonin given orally or sprayed intranasally facilitated the onset of sleep or led to tiredness, and generally had a sedative effect. Melatonin is being touted as a sleep-enhancing agent, although the data is contradictory.[25a]

## JET LAG AND OTHER BIOLOGIC RHYTHM DISORDERS

Jet lag has been related to elevated melatonin levels during times that the concentration of this indoleamine should be low.[11] Flight across time zones is associated with a phase shift in the sleep–activity cycle. The circulating melatonin rhythm requires time to readjust, and during this interval melatonin levels are elevated or depressed at unusual times. This lack of synchrony is believed to be related to the fatigue associated with jet lag.[26] Melatonin administration is being tested as a therapy for jet lag. The ability of melatonin to influence jet lag relates to its influence on the biologic clock (i.e., the suprachiasmatic nuclei). The neurons in these nuclei contain numerous receptors for melatonin.[27] The membrane receptors on which melatonin acts are part of the superfamily of receptors that possess seven transmembrane domains. The receptors are pertussis toxin sensitive and G-protein linked. Cyclic adenosine monophosphate (cAMP) functions as the intracellular messenger.[28]

## TUMOR GROWTH

The possibility that the pineal gland and melatonin may be related to tumor growth has received much attention.[29] The interactions of the pineal gland with tumor promotion are most obvious in the case of malignant growths that are dependent on sex steroids or prolactin. In addition, because of its free radical scavenging ability (see later), melatonin may prevent DNA damage that precedes tumor initiation.

Depressed nocturnal plasma melatonin levels in patients with mammary cancer may contribute to tumor growth. In premenopausal and postmenopausal women with clinical stage I and II mammary carcinogenesis, the nocturnal melatonin rise was attenuated in those with estrogen receptor–positive tumors, compared to those with estrogen receptor–negative mammary growths.[30] In the patients with estrogen receptor–positive tumors, a strong negative correlation was seen between plasma melatonin concentrations and estrogen receptors in the tumor. Whether the lower levels of melatonin in these women were a cause or an effect of the tumor, or an unrelated temporal association, was impossible to determine. Melatonin is known to suppress cellular proliferation and tissue growth.[29]

## FREE RADICAL SCAVENGING

Melatonin has been shown to be a highly effective scavenger of the hydroxyl radical, singlet oxygen, and the peroxynitrite anion, and it stimulates the activity of several antioxidative enzymes.[31] Because of its multiple antioxidative actions, melatonin has been tested for its ability to reduce oxidative damage due to ionizing radiation and a variety of xenobiotics; in these

tests pharmacologic levels of melatonin have been shown to efficiently abate oxidative damage.[32] These findings have generated interest in the potential use of melatonin in the treatment of neurodegenerative diseases of the aged that may involve free radical damage to neurons.[31,33] Examples of such conditions include Alzheimer, Parkinson, and Huntington diseases.

## CONCLUSION

The human pineal gland is a highly active organ that secretes at least one indole hormone, melatonin, and possibly several other active substances, either indoleamines or peptides. Assays are available to measure melatonin in bodily fluids[34] and its metabolites in the urine. The cyclic production of melatonin is highly characteristic, with highest levels occurring during the dark/sleep phase. The consequences of altered melatonin rhythms are incompletely understood but likely relate to several clinical entities. In addition, some persons probably have an excess (hypermelatoninism)[17] or deficiency (hypomelatoninism)[35] in melatonin production and secretion.

## REFERENCES

1. Vollrath L. Functional anatomy of the human pineal gland. In: Reiter RJ, ed. The pineal gland. New York: Raven Press, 1984:285.
2. Reiter RJ. Pineal melatonin: cell biology of its synthesis and of its physiological interactions. Endocr Rev 1991; 12:151.
3. Reiter RJ. Pineal gland: interface between the photoperiodic environment and the endocrine system. Trends Endocrinol Metab 1991; 2:13.
4. Pangerl B, Pangerl A, Reiter RJ. Circadian variations of adrenergic receptors in the mammalian pineal gland: a review. J Neural Transm 1990; 81:17.
5. Vaughan GM. Melatonin in humans. Pineal Res Rev 1984; 2:141.
6. Arendt J. Mammalian pineal rhythms. Pineal Res Rev 1985; 3:161.
7. Neuwelt EA, Lewy AJ. Disappearance of plasma melatonin after removal of neoplastic pineal gland. N Engl J Med 1983; 308:1132.
7a. Cook MR, Graham C, Kavet R, et al. Morning assessment of nocturnal melatonin secretion in older women. J Pineal Res 2000; 28:41.
7b. Witt-Enderby PA, Li PK. Melatonin receptors and ligands. Vitamin Horm 2000; 58:321.
8. Reiter RJ. The mammalian pineal gland as an end organ of the visual system. In: Wetterberg L, ed. Light and biological rhythms in man. Oxford: Pergamon, 1993:145.
9. Lewy AJ, Newsome DA. Different types of melatonin circadian secretory rhythms in some blind subjects. J Clin Endocrinol Metab 1983; 56:1103.
10. Lewy AJ, Wehr TA, Goodwin FK, et al. Light suppresses melatonin secretion in humans. Science 1980; 210:1267.
11. Fevre-Montange M, Van Cauter E, Retetoff S, et al. Effects of "jet lag" on hormonal pattern. II. Adaptation of melatonin circadian periodicity. J Clin Endocrinol Metab 1978; 52:642.
12. Vaughan GM, Allen JP, de la Pena A. Rapid melatonin transients. Waking Sleeping 1979; 3:169.
13. Stokkan KA, Reiter RJ. Melatonin rhythms in Arctic urban residents. J Pineal Res 1994; 16:33.
14. Attanasio A, Borelli P, di Rocco E, et al. Clinical significance of melatonin in children. In: Gupta D, Borelli P, Attanasio A, eds. Pediatric neuroendocrinology. London: Croom Helm, 1985:203.
15. Waldhauser F, Dietzel M. Daily and annual rhythms in human melatonin secretion: role in puberty control. Ann N Y Acad Sci 1985; 453:205.
16. Reiter RJ. The pineal and its hormones in the control of reproduction. Endocr Rev 1980; 1:109.
17. Puig-Domingo M, Webb SM, Serrano J, et al. Melatonin-related hypogonadotropic hypogonadism. N Engl J Med 1992; 17:81.
18. Carr DB, Reppert SM, Mullen B, et al. Plasma melatonin increases during exercise in women. J Clin Endocrinol Metab 1981; 53:224.
19. Hariharasubramanian N, Nair NPV, Pilapel C, et al. Plasma melatonin levels during menstrual cycle: changes with age. In: Gupta D, Reiter RJ, eds. The pineal gland and puberty. London: Croom Helm, 1986:166.
20. Vaughan GM, Meyer GG, Reiter RJ. Evidence for a pineal-gonadal relationship in the human. In: Reiter RJ, ed. The pineal and reproduction. Basel: Karger, 1978:191.
21. Herrick MK. Pathology of pineal tumors. In: Neuwelt EA, ed. Diagnosis and treatment of pineal region tumors. Baltimore: Williams & Wilkins, 1984:31.
22. Voordouw BCG, Euser R, Verdonk RER, et al. Melatonin and melatonin-progestin combinations alter pituitary-ovarian function in women and can inhibit ovulation. J Clin Endocrinol Metab 1992; 74:108.
23. Berga SL, Mortola JF, Yen SSC. Amplification of nocturnal melatonin secretion in women with functional hypothalamic amenorrhea. J Clin Endocrinol Metab 1988; 66:242.

24. Rosenthal NE, Sack DA, James SP, et al. Seasonal affective disorder and phototherapy. Ann N Y Acad Sci 1985; 453:260.
25. Wurtman RJ, Lieberman HR. Melatonin secretion as a mediator of circadian variations in sleep and sleepiness. J Pineal Res 1985; 2:301.
25a. Spitzer RL, Terman M, Williams JB, et al. Jetlag: clinical features, validation of a new syndrome-specific scale, and lack of response to melatonin in a randomized, double-blind trial. Am J Psychiatry 1999; 156:1392.
26. Daan S, Lewy AJ. Scheduled exposure to daylight: a potential strategy to reduce "jet lag" following transmeridian flight. Psychopharmacol Bull 1984; 20:566.
27. Liu C, Weaver DR, Jin X, et al. Molecular dissection of two distinct actions of melatonin on the suprachiasmatic circadian clock. Neuron 1997; 19:91.
28. Delagrange P, Guardiola-Lemaitre B. Melatonin, its receptors, and its relationships with biological rhythm disorders. Clin Neuropharmacol 1997; 20:482.
29. Blask DE. Melatonin in oncology. In: Yu HS, Reiter RJ, eds. Melatonin. Boca Raton: CRC Press, 1993:447.
30. Tamarkin L, Danforth D, Lichter A, et al. Decreased nocturnal plasma melatonin peak in patients with estrogen positive breast cancer. Science 1982; 216:1003.
31. Reiter RJ. Oxidative damage in the central nervous system: protection by melatonin. Prog Neurobiol 1998; 56:1.
32. Reiter RJ, Tang L, Garcia JJ, Muñoz-Hoyos A. Pharmacological actions of melatonin in oxygen radical pathophysiology. Life Sci 1997; 60:2255.
33. Brusco LI, Marquez M, Cardinali DP. Monozygotic twins with Alzheimer's disease treated with melatonin: case report. J Pineal Res 1998; 25:260.
34. Miles A. Melatonin: perspectives in the life sciences. Life Sci 1989; 44:375.
35. Li Y, Jiang H, Wang ML, et al. Rhythms of serum melatonin in patients with spinal lesions at the cervical, thoracic, or lumbar region. Clin Endocrinol (Oxf) 1989; 30:47.

# CHAPTER 11

# MORPHOLOGY OF THE PITUITARY IN HEALTH AND DISEASE

KAMAL THAPAR, KALMAN KOVACS, AND EVA HORVATH

In 1886, the French neurologist Pierre Marie proposed that the pituitary gland plays a fundamental role in the development of acromegaly. Since then, remarkable progress has been made in understanding hypophysial structure and function, the biochemistry of pituitary hormones, the regulation of pituitary hormone synthesis and release, and the morphologic and clinical manifestations of pituitary abnormalities. This chapter focuses on pituitary morphology in health and disease. Because the hypothalamus is closely related to the pituitary, diseases of the hypothalamus also are summarized.

## THE NORMAL PITUITARY[1,2]

### EMBRYOLOGY

The pituitary gland is derived from two sources. The *epithelial* part, which includes the pars distalis, pars intermedia, and pars tuberalis, originates from an evagination of the stomodeal ectoderm called the *Rathke pouch*. The *neural* portion, which includes the pars infundibularis or infundibulum, the neural stalk, and the pars posterior or pars nervosa, arises from the floor of the diencephalon.

The Rathke pouch is detectable at approximately the third week of gestation as a small, thin-walled vesicle in the roof of the stomodeum, which is the primitive buccal cavity. After increasing in size, it adheres to the infundibulum. Its distal end becomes narrower and forms the craniopharyngeal canal, which subsequently is obliterated, although in some cases it may remain patent until the end of intrauterine life or even

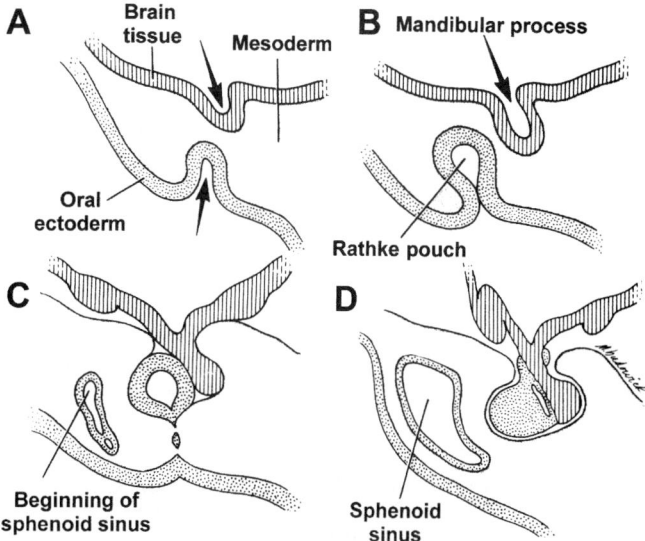

**FIGURE 11-1.** Embryogenesis of pituitary gland. **A,** Early invagination of primitive stomodeum and infundibular process. **B,** Growth of mesoderm constricts Rathke pouch. **C,** Further development pinches off Rathke pouch from oral cavity. **D,** Rathke cleft components develop into the pars distalis, pars tuberalis, and possibly the pars intermedia. Infundibular process develops into infundibular stalk and pars nervosa. (From Tindall GT, Barrow DL. Disorders of the Pituitary. St Louis: Mosby, 1986:10, with permission.)

after birth. The anterior wall of its proximal portion, where cell replication is faster, gives rise to the pars distalis; the posterior wall develops to become the pars intermedia. The anterolateral part of the Rathke pouch grows upward on both sides, in front of the infundibulum, forming the pars tuberalis (Fig. 11-1).

By the end of the third month of intrauterine life, the gross features of the pituitary gland are clearly recognizable. The infundibulum becomes elongated, and the pituitary is embedded deeper in the sella turcica. The neurohypophysis differentiates into the proximal median eminence and the distal posterior lobe, which are connected by the hypophysial stalk.

Pituitary hormones are synthesized early in embryonic life. In humans, growth hormone (GH) and adrenocorticotropic hormone (ACTH) can be demonstrated by immunocytology and radioimmunoassay at approximately the ninth week of gestation. These two hormones are soon followed by the appearance of the α and then the β subunits of glycoprotein hormones: thyroid-stimulating hormone (TSH), follicle-stimulating hormone (FSH), and luteinizing hormone (LH). Prolactin is the last adenohypophysial hormone to be produced; it can be detected at approximately the 20th week of intrauterine life. Vasopressin and oxytocin are found at ~10 weeks of gestation.

Histologic differentiation also takes place early. Acidophilic cells are noticeable at approximately the third month of gestation; basophilic cells appear a little later. In approximately the eighth week of embryonic life, a large connective tissue mass carrying blood vessels to the developing anterior lobe becomes visible. The neurosecretory material in the posterior lobe can be recognized at approximately the fifth month of gestation.

### ANATOMY

The pituitary lies in the sella turcica, or hypophysial fossa, at the base of the brain; it is surrounded by the sphenoid bone. The pituitary gland is an oval, bean-shaped, bilaterally symmetric organ measuring ~13 mm transversely, 9 mm anteroposteriorly, and 6 mm vertically.

The average weight of the pituitary is 0.6 g; it ranges from 0.4 g to 0.8 g in adults, and averages 0.1 g at birth. A reduction in weight is evident in old age, and an increase occurs during pregnancy and lactation. The pituitary gland weighs somewhat

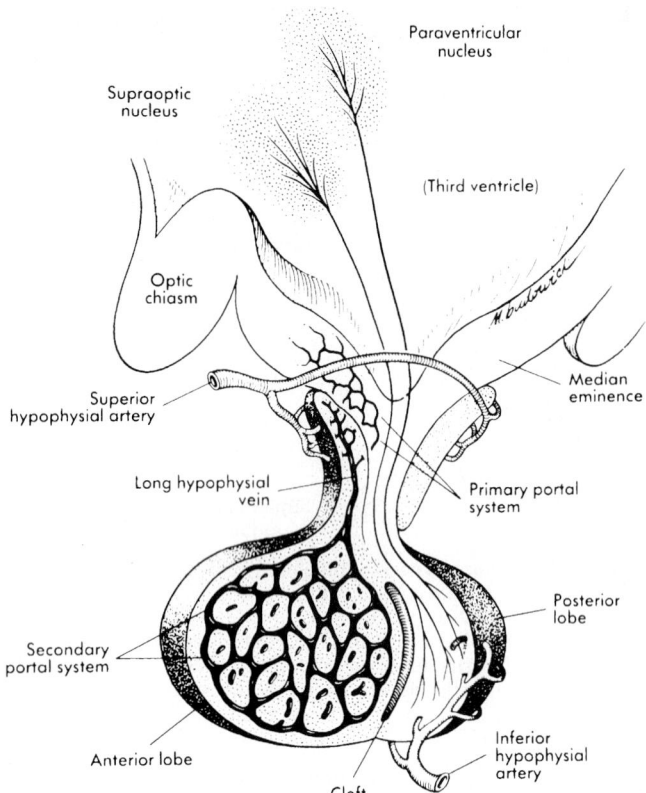

**FIGURE 11-2.** Sagittal diagram of the pituitary and its important anatomic features, including blood supply. (From Tindall GT, Barrow DL. Disorders of the Pituitary. St Louis: Mosby, 1986:11, with permission.)

more in multiparous women than in nulliparous women or in men. The anterior lobe is larger than the posterior lobe, constituting ~80% of the organ. The cut surface of the adenohypophysis is brownish red and can be distinguished from the sharply demarcated grayish neurohypophysis.

The pituitary is covered by the dura, a dense layer of connective tissue that lines the sella. The sella diaphragm, the connective tissue dura covering the superior surface of the sella, has a small central opening that is penetrated by the hypophysial stalk. The diameter of the opening is ~5 mm.

Well protected in the bony sella, the pituitary is located in the vicinity of several structures. The lateral walls of the sella on both sides are close to the cavernous sinuses, the internal carotid arteries, and the oculomotor, trochlear, and abducent nerves. Below and in front of the sella lies the sphenoid sinus, which is separated from the sella by a thin layer of bone. Above the sellar diaphragm and in front of the hypophysial stalk is the optic chiasm. Above the roof of the sella is the median eminence, the hypothalamus, and the third ventricle of the brain.

Anatomically, the pituitary is divided into two different structures: the adenohypophysis, which consists of the pars distalis, the pars intermedia, and the pars tuberalis; and the neurohypophysis, which consists of the median eminence, the hypophysial stalk, and the pars posterior or pars nervosa. The pars distalis, the largest part of the adenohypophysis, is the main site of adenohypophysial hormone synthesis and discharge. In humans, the pars intermedia is rudimentary, and its functional significance is unknown. The pars tuberalis, the upward extension of the adenohypophysis, surrounds two sides of the hypophysial stalk and consists of adenohypophysial cells, primarily gonadotropes and thyrotropes. The pars nervosa, the downward extension of the brain, is connected to the hypothalamus by the hypophysial stalk (Fig. 11-2).

## BLOOD SUPPLY

Blood is supplied to the pituitary by the superior and inferior hypophysial arteries, which arise from the internal carotid arteries. The superior hypophysial arteries penetrate the infundibulum and terminate in the surrounding capillary network. The hypothalamic hormones are synthesized in different structural parts and are transported along the nerve fibers to the infundibulum, where they permeate through the capillary walls into the blood. The larger parallel veins deriving from these capillaries are the long portal vessels. They extend downward in the hypophysial stalk and terminate in adenohypophysial capillaries, which carry high concentrations of hypothalamic hormones. The short portal vessels, originating in the distal part of the hypophysial stalk and posterior lobe, also run to the adenohypophysis. Approximately 70% to 90% of the adenohypophysial blood supply is carried by long portal vessels and 10% to 30% is carried by short portal vessels. A descending branch of the superior hypophysial artery known as the *loral artery* provides some direct arterial blood supply to the anterior lobe without passing through the infundibulum. The capsular arteries, arising from the inferior hypophysial arteries, transport additional arterial blood to the pituitary capsule and a few rows of adenohypophysial cells under the capsule. The inferior hypophysial arteries carry blood to the neurohypophysis. Venous blood is transported from the pituitary by neighboring venous sinuses to the jugular veins. It appears that blood flow may be reversed, and some blood may flow from the adenohypophysis to the brain. The neurohypophysis has an important role in directing blood either to the adenohypophysis or to the hypothalamus. Electron microscopic studies show that the adenohypophysial capillaries are lined by fenestrated endothelium. A subendothelial space and a distinct basement membrane can be seen under the endothelial layer.

## INNERVATION

Despite its close proximity to the nervous system, the adenohypophysis has no direct nerve supply, except for a few sympathetic nerve fibers that penetrate the anterior lobe along the vessels. The nerve fibers may affect adenohypophysial blood flow but play no direct role in the regulation of adenohypophysial hormone secretion. The regulatory role of the hypothalamus is neurohumoral; it is manifested by stimulating and inhibiting hormones produced in the hypothalamus and transported by the portal vessels to the adenohypophysis.

The posterior lobe is richly innervated through the hypophysial stalk by the supraopticohypophysial and tuberohypophysial tracts. The former originates in the supraoptic and paraventricular nuclei, the two magnocellular nuclei of the anterior hypothalamus, and transports the neurosecretory material along the unmyelinated nerve fibers from the hypothalamus to the posterior lobe. The latter arises in the central and posterior hypothalamus.

## CYTOLOGIC FEATURES

### ADENOHYPOPHYSIS

Although cytologic details have been studied extensively, many questions remain unanswered. Immunocytologic and electron microscopic studies have helped investigators to define various cell types and to develop a functional cell classification that allows correlation of structural features with hormone production and endocrine activity.

The long-accepted notion that the adenohypophysis consists of three cell categories—acidophilic, basophilic, and chromophobic—no longer is tenable. However, because of its convenience and simplicity, and the weight of tradition, this concept continues to influence terminology, especially that related to pathology. An alternative *functional nomenclature* based on immunocytologic and ultrastructural findings has been developed and is gaining widespread acceptance. This nomenclature recognizes five different cell types that produce the six known adenohypophysial hormones. Of the five cell types, two—GH cells and prolactin cells—belong to the acidophilic series. The three other cell types belong to the basophilic series: corticotropes produce ACTH and other fractions of the pro-opiomelanocortin molecule, thyrotropes synthesize TSH, and gonadotropes make FSH and LH. Chromophobic cells are insufficiently granulated to be stained with acidic or basic dyes. Ultrastructurally, however, cells classed as chromophobes on the basis of light microscopic findings contain enough secretory granules and other characteristic fine structural features to be identified as distinct cell types.

The cellular composition of the human adenohypophysis probably results from competition among various inducers acting on pluripotential precursor cells. Although the cell population in the glandular acini is not homogeneous, a general pattern of distribution of various cell types usually can be discerned in the normal adenohypophysis. This pattern may be altered in various diseases, especially diseases of the target glands—the adrenal cortex, thyroid, and gonads.

**Somatotropes.** Growth hormone cells, or somatotropes, are stained by acid dyes. They usually are abundant, accounting for ~50% of the adenohypophysial cells, and are located mainly in the lateral wings. The association of gigantism and acromegaly with acidophilic tumors first suggested that GH is produced in acidophilic cells. On electron microscopic examination, GH cells are seen to contain well-developed rough-surfaced endoplasmic reticulum, prominent Golgi complexes, and numerous secretory granules measuring 300 to 600 nm. The relative numeric proportions, distribution, and morphologic features of GH cells are remarkably constant in the human adenohypophysis and are not noticeably affected by age, sex, or various diseases. Pituitaries of cretins may show a reduced number of GH cells, but this is not a common finding in adult primary hypothyroidism. Prepubertal GH deficiency is associated with dwarfism, but the number, size, and morphologic appearance of GH cells often are normal. This finding is consistent with the fact that growth hormone–releasing hormone (GHRH) administration increases blood GH levels in these dwarfs and accelerates growth. As might be expected, in the adenohypophyses of patients with tumors that produce GHRH, GH-cell hyperplasia, and, less frequently, adenoma formation may be evident.

**Lactotropes.** Prolactin cells, or lactotropes (or mammotropes), constitute ~15% to 20% of adenohypophysial cells. They are acidophilic or chromophobic and stain with erythrosin and carmoisin. However, these stains are not reliable and should be replaced by immunocytologic techniques, which demonstrate prolactin in the Golgi apparatus and secretory granules. Prolactin cells are randomly scattered throughout the adenohypophysis, showing a concentration at the posterolateral edges, close to the neural lobe. On electron microscopic examination, prolactin cells appear either densely granulated, containing large secretory granules measuring up to 700 nm, or sparsely granulated, possessing prominent rough-surfaced endoplasmic reticulum, conspicuous Golgi complexes, and sparse, spherical, oval, or irregular secretory granules measuring 150 to 300 nm. The densely granulated cells are thought to be resting cells; sparsely granulated cells are assumed to be engaged in hormone secretion. Granule extrusion, regarded as a morphologic sign of hormone secretion, occurs on the capillary side of prolactin cells. A characteristic ultrastructural feature of prolactin cells is *misplaced exocytosis*, or extrusion of secretory granules from the cell on the lateral cell surface distant from capillaries, and intracellular extensions of the basement membranes.

The number of prolactin cells varies considerably under certain conditions. Prolactin cells are the last to appear in the fetal pituitary. Because of the effect of maternal estrogen, they are numerous in the adenohypophyses of newborns. With the cessation of the estrogen effect, their numbers soon decrease and remain low during childhood. The number of prolactin cells increases spectacularly during pregnancy and lactation. This is a true hyperplasia and may explain the greater weight of the pituitary found in multiparous women. Nonetheless, there are no significant differences in the number of prolactin cells between men and nulliparous women, and no regression of prolactin cells is found in old age. Estrogen treatment and primary hypothyroidism of long duration may result in hyperplasia of prolactin cells.

**Corticotropes.** Corticotropes are ACTH-producing cells that make up ~15% to 20% of adenohypophysial cells. They stain positively with periodic acid–Schiff (PAS) stain and lead hematoxylin, stain with basic dyes, and are located mainly in the central mucoid wedge, where they are the predominant cell type. Corticotropes produce ACTH and other fragments of the pro-opiomelanocortin molecule, such as β-lipotropin (β-LPH) and endorphins. Positivity to PAS stain is explained by the carbohydrate moiety of the prohormone. Corticotropes are also seen lining the cystic cavities of the pars intermedia. Cells containing immunoreactive ACTH frequently spread into the posterior lobe. The endocrinologic significance of this change, called *basophilic cell invasion*, is unknown. On electron microscopic examination, corticotropes contain a widely dispersed, moderately developed, rough-surfaced endoplasmic reticulum, a prominent Golgi apparatus, a few bundles of microfilaments, and numerous spherical or irregular secretory granules that vary in electron density, often line up along the cell membrane, and measure 300 to 600 nm. In anencephaly, corticotropes fail to show a normal development and are nearly absent from the adenohypophysis. In long-standing hypocortisolism, corticotropes may increase in number and size and become vacuolated. In patients with tumors that produce corticotropin-releasing hormone (CRH), corticotropes may undergo hyperplasia, indicating that CRH induces their proliferation.

The best-known morphologic abnormality of corticotropes in postnatal life is *Crooke hyaline change,*[1] the deposition of a homogeneous, glassy, PAS-negative material in the cytoplasm that contains no ACTH. It corresponds to an accumulation of microfilaments seen in electron microscopic studies (Fig. 11-3).

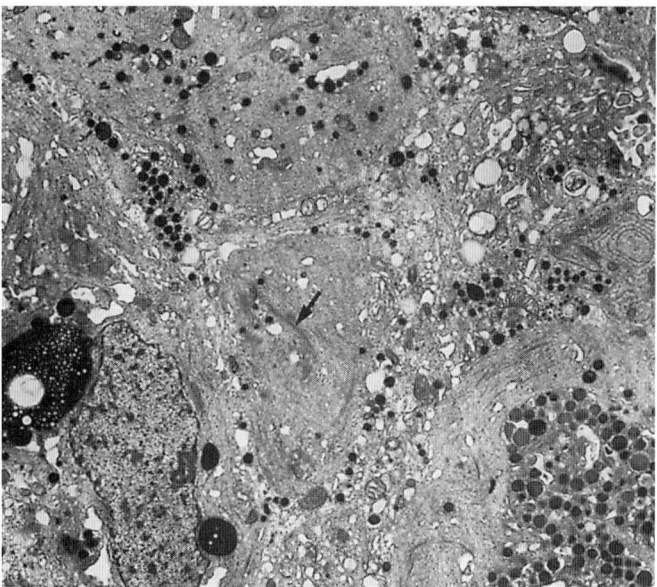

**FIGURE 11-3.** Crooke cells. Note accumulation of microfilaments (*arrow*) in the nontumorous portion of the adenohypophysis harboring an adrenocorticotropic hormone–secreting adenoma. ×7800

Crooke hyalinization, which is caused by cortisol excess, occurs in patients with Cushing disease, glucocorticoid hormone–producing adrenal tumors, and paraneoplastic ("ectopic") ACTH syndrome, and after protracted treatment with pharmacologic doses of cortisol or its derivatives. The changes are reversible: the hyaline material disappears with the removal of cortisol- or ACTH-producing tumors, or with the discontinuation of glucocorticoid therapy.

**Thyrotropes.**   Thyrotropes are TSH-producing cells that constitute ~5% of adenohypophysial cells, making them the least numerous in this structure. They are basophilic, stain positively with PAS, aldehyde fuchsin, and aldehyde thionin, and are located mainly in the anteromedial portion of the pars distalis in the mucoid wedge. On electron microscopic examination, they usually have large cytoplasmic processes and contain short, rough-surfaced endoplasmic reticulum membranes, well-developed Golgi complexes, numerous microtubules, and spherical secretory granules that often line up along the cell membrane and measure 100 to 250 nm.

Thyrotropes often increase in number and size in patients with long-standing primary hypothyroidism and transform into so-called thyroidectomy cells. These cells are large thyrotropes with a vacuolated cytoplasm, dilated endoplasmic reticulum cisternae, and large PAS-positive lysosomal globules. Diffuse or nodular thyrotrope hyperplasia may be marked in untreated long-standing primary hypothyroidism; adenomas composed of thyrotropes may be noted. In patients with hyperthyroidism, thyrotropes are sparse, small, and dense.

**Gonadotropes.**   Gonadotropes are FSH/LH-producing cells that constitute about 10% of adenohypophysial cells. Many gonadotropes are found in the central mucoid wedge, but they are also randomly distributed in the lateral wings, often close to prolactin cells. Gonadotropes are basophilic, PAS-positive cells. Most produce both FSH and LH, which can be demonstrated immunocytologically in the cytoplasm. Some gonadotropes, however, contain only FSH or LH. On electron microscopic examination, gonadotropes are characterized by a spherical nucleus and an abundant cytoplasm with a well-developed rough-surfaced endoplasmic reticulum, a conspicuous Golgi complex, and two populations of secretory granules, one with a mean diameter of 250 nm and the other with a diameter of 400 nm or more. Other gonadotropes contain only secretory granules averaging 250 nm in diameter. There are several transitional forms, indicating that gonadotropes derive from the same precursor with the ability to produce both FSH and LH.

After removal of the gonads, castration cells (gonadectomy cells) are apparent in the pituitary. These cells are large gonadotropes with pale vacuolated cytoplasm and a peripherally located nucleus. In some castration cells, the entire cytoplasm appears to be transformed into one large vacuole, endowing the cell with a signet-ring appearance. On electron microscopic examination, the most prominent finding is marked dilation of the endoplasmic reticulum membrane network and a reduced number of secretory granules. The effect of gonadal steroids on the morphology of human gonadotropes has not been sufficiently documented.

### POSTERIOR LOBE AND PITUITARY STALK

The posterior lobe, the downward extension of the central nervous system, is composed of nerve fibers, axon terminals, glial cells called *pituicytes,* and neurosecretory material stored in nerve endings in the form of granules that stain with Gomori chromalum-hematoxylin, aldehyde fuchsin, and aldehyde thionin. Immunocytologic techniques conclusively reveal the presence of vasopressin, oxytocin, and their carrier protein, neurophysin, in the neurosecretory material.

The pituitary stalk, which connects the hypothalamus and median eminence with the pituitary, contains unmyelinated nerve fibers that terminate in the posterior lobe and portal vessels, and transport releasing and inhibiting hormones to the anterior lobe.

## THE ABNORMAL ADENOHYPOPHYSIS[1a,2]

Diseases of the adenohypophysis can be broadly divided into (a) developmental abnormalities; (b) vascular disorders; (c) inflammatory conditions; (d) miscellaneous alterations, including deposition of various substances; (e) hyperplasias; and (f) neoplasms.

### DEVELOPMENTAL ABNORMALITIES

**Pituitary Aplasia.**   Pituitary aplasia, the congenital absence of the hypophysis, is a rare abnormality that is often accompanied by other malformations. The agenesis may involve the entire pituitary gland or the adenohypophysis and is caused by defective formation of the Rathke pouch. If the affected newborn survives, severe hypopituitarism develops. Pituitary hypoplasia is the milder form of the same defect.

**Anencephaly.**   In anencephaly, the brain, including the hypothalamus, is missing; thus, no neurohumoral regulation is exerted on the pituitary. The posterior lobe is present in some cases and absent in others. The anterior lobe is reduced in size and contains decreased numbers of corticotropes. The other adenohypophysial cell types are well developed and show no major abnormalities.

**Persistent Remnants of the Rathke Pouch.**   Remnants of the Rathke pouch persist in 20% to 50% of human pituitaries in the form of squamous cell nests. The nests vary in size and are located at the distal end of the stalk close to the anterior lobe.

**Persistent Cleft of the Rathke Pouch.**   Persistence of the cleft of the Rathke pouch is a harmless congenital defect and a common autopsy finding. The cleft fails to close and a distended, colloid-filled space is seen between the anterior and posterior lobes. Although this cleft is generally microscopic in proportion, it rarely may accumulate sufficient colloidal material to become an expansile and clinically significant intrasellar and suprasellar mass. These are known as *Rathke cleft cysts,* as discussed later (see the section on neoplasms). Although these lesions are most certainly not neoplastic in nature, they are discussed under the heading of neoplasms both for convenience and because they frequently mimic clinically and radiologically true cystic neoplasms of the sellar region.

**Pituitary Dystopia.**   Pituitary dystopia is a rare condition characterized by a failure of union of the neurohypophysis and adenohypophysis during early development. The pituitary stalk is foreshortened, resulting in an extrasellar location of the neural lobe and a failure of the latter to descend into the sella. Usually, there is no physical attachment between the neurohypophyses and the adenohypophyses, although, occasionally, the two may be tenuously attached by strands of tissue. The anomaly is generally inconsequential, most cases being incidental autopsy findings. Rarely, it may be accompanied by other abnormalities such as hypogonadism, growth retardation, or other congenital anomalies.

**Septo-Optic Dysplasia.**   Septo-optic dysplasia is a complex developmental disorder characterized by variable and often partial expression of midline structural abnormalities of the brain, hypoplasia of the optic nerves, and hypothalamic dysfunction. The last may manifest as anterior and posterior pituitary failure on a hypothalamic basis. Additional features of hypothalamic dysfunction may also be present, including alterations of temperature regulation, hyperphagia, and precocious puberty. The full syndrome is expressed in only a few cases; most patients come to medical attention during early childhood with pituitary insufficiency and visual dysfunction. Septo-optic dysplasia is a medically treatable condition that is wholly compatible with life.

**Anatomic Variations.**   Anatomic variations in the shape and position of the pituitary and its relationships to neighboring tissues are common. Although these differences have no major clinical significance, they may be important to radiologists and neurosurgeons.

**Pharyngeal Pituitary.** In virtually all persons, a small ectopic focus of anterior pituitary tissue persists throughout life, and can usually be identified as a minute, oval, midline nodule embedded within the sphenoid bone. Known as the *pharyngeal pituitary,* this remnant of the Rathke pouch is usually <5 mm in size and is most frequently located deep within the mucosa or periosteum, beneath or near the vomerosphenoidal articulation; less often, it may be found in the nasopharynx or even within the nasal cavity. It is surrounded by a thin connective tissue capsule and consists of small clusters of chromophobic cells mixed with a few acidophilic and basophilic cells. In contrast to the pars distalis, the pharyngeal pituitary is richly innervated but has no portal blood supply; thus, it receives no hypothalamic hormones directly that might otherwise affect its secretory activity. Although immunocytologic techniques have disclosed various adenohypophysial hormones in the pharyngeal pituitary, this structure has no major endocrinologic significance and shows no marked histologic changes in patients with endocrine disorders. It cannot take over the function of the adenohypophysis after hypophysectomy or destructive adenohypophysial disease. The only clinically relevant feature of the pharyngeal pituitary is that it rarely may be the site for pituitary adenoma development.[1–3] Most such tumors have been situated within the sphenoid sinus, and both nonfunctioning and hormonally active tumors have been reported. With respect to the latter, GH-producing tumors have been reported most commonly, followed in frequency by prolactin-producing and ACTH-producing adenomas. In the true "ectopic" pituitary adenoma, the intrasellar pituitary should be normal, although rarely, simultaneous development of an intrasellar and noncontiguous ectopic pituitary tumor has been reported. Another rare site for ectopic pituitary adenomas is the suprasellar region. Such "ectopic" tumors presumably arise from adenohypophysial cells of the pars tuberalis situated on the supradiaphragmatic portion of the pituitary stalk.

**Empty Sella Syndrome.** The term *empty sella* refers to the anatomic state resulting from the intrasellar herniation of the subarachnoid space through a defective and enlarged diaphragmatic aperture. The result is compression and posterior displacement of the pituitary gland, enlargement of the sella, and a seemingly "empty" appearance of the sella on both gross and radiologic examination. It is of clinical and pathophysiologic importance to distinguish those cases of empty sella occurring without identifiable cause (i.e., primary empty sella) from those resulting from a loss of intrasellar volume, such as would occur after an infarction, surgery, or the radionecrosis of an intrasellar neoplasm (i.e., secondary empty sella).

PRIMARY EMPTY SELLA SYNDROME.[4] Anatomic defects in the diaphragma sellae of 5 mm or more have been demonstrated in ~40% of consecutive autopsies, with >20% exhibiting intrasellar extension of the subarachnoid space[5] and 5% showing a fully developed empty sella.[6] Whether such abnormalities *alone* are the cause of primary empty sella syndrome, a predisposing factor to it, or simply the result of some other process remains uncertain. Because most of these features have been incidental autopsy findings in persons without neurologic or endocrine symptoms, it is likely that additional factors contribute to the clinical syndrome. Elevated intracranial pressure is a potentially important contributing factor because it has been documented in patients with primary empty sella syndrome. Ten percent of patients with *benign intracranial hypertension* have a coexisting empty sella. This latter relationship is especially intriguing because both conditions share overlapping clinical profiles.[7]

Most cases of primary empty sella are discovered incidentally in patients who do not have symptoms. In the few patients who do have symptoms, the clinical profile is characteristic. Eighty percent of cases occur in middle-aged women, many of

whom are obese and hypertensive. Spontaneous cerebrospinal fluid rhinorrhea, usually through a markedly thinned and eroded sellar floor, may complicate the primary empty sella in up to 10% of cases involving symptoms. Clinically evident pituitary dysfunction is unusual. Subtle abnormalities of the GH axis, appreciable only on dynamic endocrine testing, have been reported, as have rare accounts of panhypopituitarism.[8] A modest hyperprolactinemia on the basis of stalk distortion occurs in fewer than 10% of patients. (The occasional occurrence of a pituitary microadenoma, most often a prolactin-producing adenoma, in association with primary empty sellar syndrome is purely coincidental.) In the most exceptional instances, intrasellar prolapse of the optic chiasm may be a source of visual dysfunction. In most cases, objective ophthalmologic findings, although rarely present, are the result of coexisting benign intracranial hypertension and not of the empty sella per se.

The gross pathologic features of the condition include an enlarged and thin-walled, thinned-floor sella, the diaphragm of which consists of a narrow rim. A markedly flattened pituitary gland can be seen displaced against the posterior sellar wall. Despite marked distortion of the gland, its histologic appearance and immunochemical integrity remain largely intact.

SECONDARY EMPTY SELLA SYNDROME. A secondary empty sella most commonly occurs after surgical extirpation or radiotherapy of a pituitary adenoma. The diaphragm may be developmentally deficient, eroded by the primary tumor, or affected by its treatment, permitting the descent of both the chiasm and the chiasmatic cistern into the sella. Because the latter may become entrapped and kinked by arachnoid adhesions and scar tissue, visual dysfunction is a common mode of presentation in patients with secondary empty sella syndrome. Secondary empty sella syndrome also may occur in the setting of atrophy of a nontumorous pituitary or of pituitary adenomas that have previously undergone massive hemorrhage or infarction, as in Sheehan syndrome and pituitary apoplexy, respectively.

## CIRCULATORY DISTURBANCES

**Pituitary Hemorrhage.** Hemorrhages of the pituitary are rare. They may develop in patients with head trauma, various hematologic abnormalities, or increased intracranial tension. In rapidly growing pituitary adenomas, intrahypophysial pressure may increase, leading to compression of intrahypophysial or extrahypophysial portal vessels and the arrest of portal circulation. Vessels may undergo a subtle, hypoxic injury noticeable on electron microscopic examination. If the damage is severe, the vascular walls cannot withstand the elevations in blood pressure and they rupture, resulting in hemorrhage. Pituitary apoplexy is the extreme variant of this process (see later in this chapter).

**Pituitary Infarction.** Pituitary infarction is a noninflammatory, coagulative necrosis caused by ischemia secondary to interruption of the blood supply. Small adenohypophysial infarcts are common, being found in ~1% to 6% of autopsies of unselected adult subjects. The lesions remain unrecognized clinically and can be detected only by histologic examination. A loss of 75% of adenohypophysial tissue produces no clinical symptoms of hypopituitarism and no biochemical abnormalities.

Pituitary necrosis can be associated with several diseases. Postpartum pituitary necrosis (*Sheehan syndrome*) occurs in women who experienced severe blood loss and were in hypovolemic shock about the time of delivery. During shock, the pituitary circulation may be interrupted and the anterior lobe undergoes ischemic infarction. Adenohypophysial necrosis also may occur in nonobstetric shock, but less frequently than in women with severe circulatory failure secondary to obstetric hemorrhage. This suggests that pregnancy predisposes women to pituitary necrosis, but neither the site of sensitization nor the mechanism leading to necrosis is known (see Chap. 17).

Necrotic foci of varying sizes can be found in the pituitaries of patients with diabetes mellitus, head trauma, cerebrovascular accidents, increased intracranial pressure, and epidemic hemorrhagic fever. Pituitary infarction develops after disruption of the pituitary stalk, which causes an arrest of the adenohypophysial circulation. Adenohypophysial infarcts often can be seen in patients who were maintained on mechanical respirators before they died. The lesions represent coagulative infarcts and often are accompanied by severe hypoxic lesions of the brain.

The pathogenesis of pituitary infarction is unclear, and the mechanism of arrest of the adenohypophysial circulation is not known. Proposed causes include embolism, thrombosis, disseminated intravascular coagulation, vascular compression, vasospasm, and primary capillary damage.

In postpartum pituitary necrosis, Sheehan postulated that severe spasm develops in those arterioles from which portal vessels arise.[2] Vasospasm is followed by hypophysial ischemia and secondary thrombosis, resulting in coagulative infarcts that usually spare the posterior lobe and hypophysial stalk because these areas have a rich arterial blood supply.

In cases of postpartum pituitary necrosis, infarcted areas may be large, involving more than 90% of the anterior lobe. Adenohypophysial cells are not capable of sufficient regeneration. Thus, when there is extensive infarction, permanent hypopituitarism develops. Because modern obstetric care usually prevents blood loss and obstetric shock in pregnant women, Sheehan syndrome has become rarer.

*Fibrous atrophy* is the final phase of ischemic necrosis of the anterior lobe. The necrotic areas are replaced by fibrous tissue. The sequence of events is identical to that occurring in infarcts of other organs.

Necrotic foci may occur in the posterior lobe and hypophysial stalk in association with head injuries, increased intracranial pressure, and obstetric and nonobstetric shock. These patients may develop diabetes insipidus.

**Pituitary Apoplexy.**   Classically defined, pituitary apoplexy[9,10] refers to the abrupt and occasionally catastrophic occurrence of acute hemorrhagic infarction of a pituitary adenoma. The clinical syndrome is easily recognized, consisting of acute headache, meningismus, visual impairment, ophthalmoplegia, and alterations in consciousness. Without timely intervention, patients may die of subarachnoid hemorrhage or acute, life-threatening hypopituitarism. As defined herein, pituitary apoplexy is a complication in 1% to 2% of all pituitary adenomas. "Silent," or subclinical, hemorrhage into a pituitary adenoma is considerably more common, as evidenced by the finding of hemorrhage, necrosis, or cystic change in up to 10% of all surgical specimens. There is little consensus as to which tumor types, if any, are most susceptible to apoplectic hemorrhage. Some have suggested that hormonally active tumors associated with acromegaly and Cushing disease are especially prone to apoplexy, whereas others have found large nonfunctioning tumors to bear the greatest risk. In the experience of the authors, large nonfunctioning pituitary tumors, particularly silent corticotrope adenomas, appear to have the highest inherent tendency to undergo apoplectic hemorrhage.

The pathophysiologic basis of pituitary apoplexy remains speculative. Ischemic necrosis of a rapidly growing tumor, intrinsic vascular abnormalities peculiar to pituitary tumors, and compression of the superior hypophysial artery against the sellar diaphragm have all been suggested as mechanisms contributing to apoplectic hemorrhage.[11] Predisposing factors loosely associated with apoplexy include bromocriptine therapy, anticoagulation, diabetic ketoacidosis, head trauma, estrogen therapy, and pituitary irradiation. Most cases, however, occur in the absence of any known predisposing condition.

Chronologically, apoplexy begins with infarction of the tumor and the surrounding gland and is followed by hemorrhage and edema. This sudden increase in both pressure and volume within the tumor causes precipitous expansion of the tumor followed by mechanical compression of the optic apparatus and of structures within the cavernous sinus. The bulk of the hemorrhage is generally contained within a tense tumor "capsule," although an extravasation of blood into the subarachnoid space frequently occurs. Obstructive hydrocephalus may further complicate apoplexy in large macroadenomas, particularly those having a significant suprasellar component. Glandular destruction of varying degree is a regular pathologic feature of apoplexy; this results in partial or total and transient or permanent hypopituitarism. Fortunately, the anterior pituitary has an astonishing reserve capacity; at least 75% to 90% of the gland must be destroyed before permanent endocrine deficits develop. The posterior pituitary, which has its own blood supply, generally escapes injury. Accordingly, diabetes insipidus only rarely is a complication of pituitary apoplexy (see Chap. 26).

Histologically, most pituitary apoplexy specimens have a fairly uniform appearance, consisting primarily of blood and necrotic tumor. Often, only "ghosts" of neoplastic cells remain. A typical adenoma pattern still may be demonstrated with reticulin stains, thus confirming the presence of an underlying adenoma.

Rare instances of pituitary apoplexy causing *complete autoinfarction* of a pituitary adenoma and resulting in spontaneous endocrinologic cure have been known to occur. In addition to the acute and subacute complications noted previously, a late manifestation of pituitary apoplexy is the secondary empty sella syndrome.

## INFLAMMATORY DISORDERS OF THE PITUITARY

**Inflammation.**   The pituitary gland rarely may be subject to a variety of inflammatory disorders, the pathogenesis of which ranges from acute suppuration to chronic granulomatous conditions to autoimmune processes. Despite the diversity of pathologic processes represented, their somewhat generic clinical presentation as nonfunctioning sellar masses frequently prompts a preoperative diagnosis of pituitary adenoma; their inflammatory nature is revealed only after pathologic examination of the surgical specimen.

**Infectious Diseases of the Pituitary Gland.**[4,12]   With the availability of effective antimicrobial therapy, acute bacterial infection of the pituitary gland has become an exceedingly rare event that periodically surfaces in the form of isolated case reports. In many cases, neither a cause nor a predisposing condition can be found. Those of known etiology, however, appear to arise in one of two clinical settings. The first, and perhaps most important, mechanism involves secondary extension from a preexisting, anatomically contiguous purulent focus. An acute sphenoid sinusitis is most often implicated; less commonly, osteomyelitis of the sphenoid bone, cavernous sinus thrombophlebitis, peritonsillar abscess, mastoiditis, purulent otitis media, or bacterial meningitis serves as the inciting focus. The second mechanism underlying purulent hypophysitis is septicemia, with pituitary infection being a complication of hematogenous dissemination from any of numerous distant septic foci (pneumonia, osteomyelitis, endocarditis, septic abortion, retroperitoneal abscess). Microabscesses, particularly of the posterior lobe, are occasional autopsy findings in patients succumbing to overwhelming sepsis. In this context, they likely represent a clinically insignificant preterminal complication. Of note, postoperative pituitary abscess complicating transsphenoidal surgery is exceedingly rare.

The symptoms of pituitary abscess often are indistinguishable from those of other sellar masses (headache, chiasmatic syndrome, hypopituitarism). When they are accompanied by symptoms of meningitis, however, the possibility of pituitary abscess should always be strongly considered.[13] The bacteriology of pituitary abscess is diverse. When an organism can be isolated, *Staphylococcus aureus*, *Diplococcus pneumoniae*, group A

*Streptococcus, Klebsiella* sp., and *Citrobacter diversus* have been reported most often.[12] A surprising number of pituitary abscesses has developed in the setting of a preexisting sellar lesion, such as pituitary adenoma, craniopharyngioma, or Rathke cleft cyst.[12,13] Why such lesions should be especially vulnerable to abscess formation remains speculative, but it may be related to poor circulation or areas of necrosis present in some such lesions. The histologic picture of pituitary abscess is remarkable for extensive tissue destruction, as evidenced by necrosis and a dense polymorphonuclear inflammatory infiltrate. The mortality associated with pituitary abscess is high, approaching 28% in the absence of meningitis, and 45% when associated with meningitis.[13]

Pituitary infections also may be caused by a variety of other agents. *Tuberculosis,* still endemic in certain areas, was historically an important cause of hypopituitarism.[12] In most instances, parapituitary involvement has been secondary to dense, plaque-like basilar meningitis. Secondary arteritis, a frequent accompaniment, can result in infarction of the pituitary stalk. Intrasellar "tuberculomas" usually are associated with widespread destruction of the pituitary, frequently are calcified, and almost always are associated with active tuberculosis elsewhere. When it causes symptoms, tuberculous involvement of the pituitary or its stalk manifests as anterior pituitary failure or diabetes insipidus. *Syphilis,* now uncommon in its consummate forms, was historically an important cause of destructive granulomatous inflammation of the pituitary. Manifesting as a discrete gummatous lesion or as diffuse scarring, the eventual result of syphilitic infection is massive destruction of the gland and, in some cases, hypopituitarism.[8]

Mycotic infection, notably aspergillosis, also has been reported to involve the sellar, parasellar, and orbital regions, presenting as an inflammatory mass. Parasitic infiltration of the sellar and parapituitary regions by *Cysticercus* and *Echinococcus* organisms has been known to produce a mass in this region. Finally, in the context of the acquired immunodeficiency syndrome and other immunosuppressed states, an additional spectrum of pituitary infection has emerged, including agents such as *Pneumocystis carinii, Toxoplasma gondii,* and cytomegalovirus.[14] The clinical significance of pituitary involvement by these agents is still poorly understood.

**Lymphocytic Hypophysitis.**    Lymphocytic hypophysitis is a destructive, inflammatory disorder of the anterior pituitary; it is presumed to be autoimmune in nature.[1,2,15–17] Occurring almost exclusively in women, the disease is often temporally related to pregnancy. Almost 70% of reported cases have occurred either during pregnancy or within the first postpartum year; only occasionally are women beyond reproductive age affected. Rarely, lymphocytic hypophysitis may occur in men.[17] Aside from the fact that women are generally more prone to autoimmune conditions, no explanations exist for the strong female preponderance in lymphocytic hypophysitis. Frequently, concurrent or prior autoimmune disease of other endocrine glands (i.e., Hashimoto thyroiditis, adrenalitis) can be demonstrated, suggesting that lymphocytic hypophysitis is but one component of a generalized polyglandular autoimmune syndrome. That antipituitary antibodies, most often directed against the prolactin cell, have been detected in the serum of some affected patients strongly supports an autoimmune etiology. Whether the process is generated by humoral as well as cell-mediated mechanisms remains uncertain. The clinical presentation includes headache and visual defects caused by an expanding sellar mass, amenorrhea and galactorrhea as the result of moderate hyperprolactinemia, and varying degrees of hypopituitarism.

Grossly, the inflammatory response underlying lymphocytic hypophysitis produces an enlarged, firm pituitary gland, which often extends into the suprasellar space and may be accompanied by enlargement of the sella. Microscopically, the process is restricted to the anterior pituitary, where normal glandular

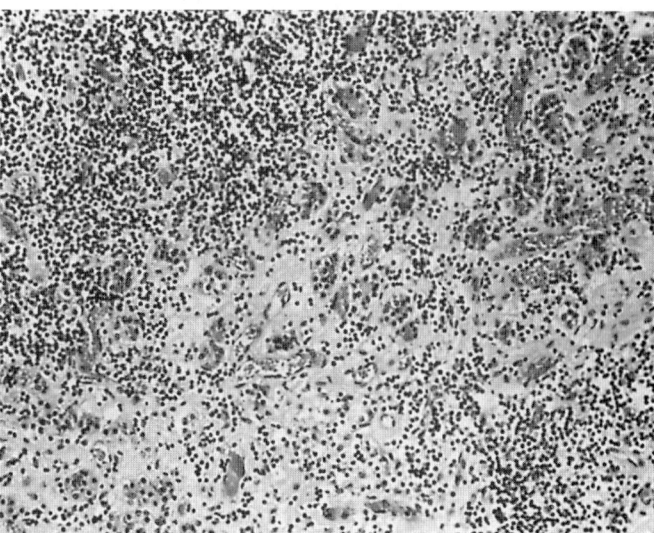

**FIGURE 11-4.** Lymphocytic hypophysitis. Note massive mononuclear cell infiltration and extensive destruction of adenohypophysial parenchyma. Hematoxylin-eosin stain; ×100

architecture is disrupted by an extensive infiltration of lymphocytes, plasma cells, eosinophils, and macrophages[15] (Fig. 11-4). Both the structural and the immunohistochemical integrity of involved cells are lost. In especially extensive cases, loosely organized lymphoid follicles and germinal centers may be present. The chronicity of the process is evidenced by varying degrees of fibrotic change. At the microscopic level, tuberculosis, syphilis, sarcoidosis, giant-cell granuloma, and postpartum pituitary infarction all may be considered in the differential diagnosis. Because the posterior lobe escapes injury, diabetes insipidus is not a feature of this condition.

The potentially lethal nature of lymphocytic hypophysitis is illustrated by the fact that many early descriptions of the condition stemmed from necropsy studies. Improved recognition of this condition coupled with hormone replacement therapy has rendered lymphocytic hypophysitis a curable disease.

**Granulomas.**    In addition to tuberculosis and syphilis, which are the two principal granulomatous infections affecting the pituitary, two additional noninfectious granulomatous processes may present as pituitary granulomas: sarcoidosis and giant-cell granuloma.

SARCOIDOSIS.    Considered one of the "great imitators," sarcoidosis is known for its tendency to involve pituitary-hypothalamic structures.[1,2,4,18,19] Therefore, it serves as a diagnosis of exclusion for masses and other destructive inflammatory processes occurring in this region. Sarcoidosis is a relatively common, multisystem inflammatory disorder of unknown origin. It most commonly affects the lungs, lymph nodes, skin, and eyes, but virtually no organ system is spared. Clinically apparent nervous system involvement occurs in ~5% of cases and may involve the cranial, spinal, or peripheral compartments.

Within the cranium, sarcoidosis has a predilection for the base of the brain, where it entraps cranial nerves and hypothalamic-pituitary structures in an adhesive and infiltrative arachnoiditis. Discrete parenchymal masses occur much less frequently. Involvement of the pituitary, infundibulum, and hypothalamic structures occurs in ~1% of patients with established systemic disease. Rarely, isolated involvement of these structures may be the initial or sole feature of sarcoidosis.

The clinical manifestations of sellar region sarcoidosis are variable and generally reflect hypothalamic or infundibular damage. Diabetes insipidus, somnolence, obesity, abnormal temperature regulation, hyperprolactinemia, and hypopituitarism have all been reported. With respect to the last of these, gonadotropic, thyrotropic, and adrenocorticotropic function is most commonly impaired. Although pathologic involvement of the adenohypophysis may be demonstrated, hypopituitarism in the setting of sarcoidosis is generally considered to be the result of injury to the hypophysiotropic areas of the hypothalamus or to the pituitary stalk. That many patients with diminished pituitary function retain responsiveness to exogenously administered hypothalamic releasing factors argues against excessive functional damage to hormone-producing cells of the anterior pituitary.

The histologic appearance of sarcoidosis in the pituitary-hypothalamic region is similar to that of sarcoidosis in other organs. Noncaseating granulomas, consisting of giant cells, lymphocytes, and macrophages, can be seen in the anterior and posterior pituitary, the infundibulum, and the hypothalamus. Blood vessels often are involved by the inflammatory process. Depending on the stage of the disease, scar formation of varying degrees may be evident. Although necrosis—the histologic hallmark of tuberculosis and other infectious processes—is absent in sarcoidosis, noncaseating granulomas may be a feature of numerous infectious processes. Thus, special stains and cultures for fungi and tubercle bacilli must be performed to exclude an infectious cause, particularly in the absence of known systemic sarcoidosis.

GIANT-CELL GRANULOMA.   Giant-cell granuloma of the pituitary[1,2,19] is a rare condition, the earliest description of which stemmed from autopsy studies. Although historically the disease was seldom diagnosed during life, increasing awareness of giant-cell granuloma as a distinct clinicopathologic entity has led to its periodic detection among surgical specimens from patients harboring mass lesions of the sella. Like that of sarcoidosis, the etiology of giant-cell granuloma remains obscure. Because some histopathologic features are common to both conditions, immune-mediated mechanisms, perhaps similar to those postulated for sarcoidosis, have been invoked as underlying the development of giant-cell granuloma as well. In contrast to sarcoidosis, however, giant-cell granuloma is a disease virtually exclusive to the pituitary gland; exceptional accounts of histologically similar granulomas have been reported in the adrenals.

Topologically, the anterior lobe of the pituitary is hardest hit by giant-cell granuloma; neurohypophysial involvement occurs less frequently, and hypothalamic involvement is distinctly unusual. Histologically, the appearance is that of a noncaseating granulomatous inflammation, with giant cells bearing Schumann bodies, abundant histiocytes, and occasional lymphocytes. Extensive parenchymal destruction is the rule, eventually accompanied by fibrosis and scar formation. The clinical picture generally is dominated by hypopituitarism, which also may be accompanied by diabetes insipidus and moderate hyperprolactinemia, depending on the degree of damage to the pituitary stalk. The inflammatory process often is a source of considerable glandular enlargement, so much so that most surgically treated cases have masqueraded preoperatively as nonfunctioning pituitary macroadenomas.

## MISCELLANEOUS CONDITIONS

**Langerhans Cell Histiocytosis (Histiocytosis X).**   Classified under the rubric *Langerhans cell histiocytosis*[1,2,4,19,20] are several related but poorly understood nonneoplastic processes that are unified pathologically by their content of highly characteristic histiocyte-like cells. The extent and nature of organ involvement as well as the clinical course in Langerhans cell histiocytosis is variable. Ranging from the fulminant, generalized, and frequently lethal Letterer-Siwe disease, to the multifocal eosinophilic granulomas of Hand-Schüller-Christian disease, to the relatively innocent solitary eosinophilic granuloma of bone, hypothalamic-pituitary involvement may be a feature of each.

Central nervous system involvement is a common feature of Langerhans cell histiocytosis, although only rarely do central nervous system lesions occur in the absence of disease elsewhere.[20] There is an apparent predilection for involvement of the hypothalamus, infundibulum, and posterior pituitary.[19,20] The anterior lobe is affected far less often. In most cases, involvement of these structures represents extension from an adjacent bony lesion, although occasionally, in the context of disseminated disease, parapituitary and meningeal involvement occurs in the absence of bony disease. Diabetes insipidus generally is the earliest and most prominent feature of pituitary involvement, reflecting posterior pituitary, infundibular, or hypothalamic infiltration. Perturbations of anterior pituitary function (typically GH deficiency) may occur; less often there may be a deficiency of other hormones. These are considered to be secondary to disease of the hypothalamus or pituitary stalk. Sometimes, damage to the stalk may be so extreme as to render the anterior lobe functionally, if not physically, disconnected from the hypothalamus. Moderate degrees of hyperprolactinemia also may be a feature of the condition, again reflecting hypothalamic or stalk injury.

The histologic picture of Langerhans cell histiocytosis is typical of disease elsewhere and is characterized by infiltrates of histiocytes (often foamy in appearance), eosinophils, and lymphocytes. The essential component of the infiltrate is the Langerhans cell, a large mononuclear cell resembling a histiocyte and expressing S-100 protein as well as HLA-DR and CD1 antigens. The ultrastructural presence of Birbeck granules, which are pentalaminar tubular structures found in the cytoplasm of the Langerhans cell, is pathognomonic. A definitive diagnosis of Langerhans cell histiocytosis rests on the characteristic cytologic features of the Langerhans cell and the accompanying infiltrate. The identification of Birbeck granules and the antigenic determinant CD1 is confirmatory.

**Idiopathic Medical Conditions.**   Dysfunction of the hypothalamic-pituitary axis remains a poorly characterized component of many idiopathic medical conditions.[1,2,9] These include the Laurence-Moon-Biedl syndrome, cerebral gigantism or Sotos syndrome, the Prader-Willi syndrome, and anorexia nervosa. Even at a purely clinical level, the endocrinologic aberrations accompanying these disorders are, at best, incompletely understood. Correspondingly, pathologic studies of hypothalamic and pituitary tissues in each of these conditions have been few and the findings inconsistent. In all cases, if pathologic correlates of hypothalamic-pituitary dysfunction can be identified, it is usually the hypothalamus that shows a more consistent pattern of pathologic change; primary pathologic features in the pituitary are inconspicuous or absent in these disorders.[19]

**Deposits.**   Deposits of various substances may be accompanied by anterior hypopituitarism. *Amyloid* deposits in the pituitary occur outside the cell in the walls of blood vessels and the interstitium and are part of the amyloidosis of other organs, mainly the kidneys, liver, spleen, and intestines. Pituitary amyloid is regarded as immune amyloid and has the same staining characteristics and ultrastructural appearance as amyloid in other organs. In some pituitary adenomas, especially prolactin-producing adenomas, the adenoma cells may produce amyloid that is different ultrastructurally from immune amyloid. In cells with massive amyloid accumulation, the plasmalemma becomes disrupted, and amyloid can be identified in the extracellular space. In hemochromatosis and hemosiderosis, *iron* pigment may be deposited in the cytoplasm of adenohypophysial cells (see Chap. 131). Iron storage is uneven, it occurs most extensively in the cytoplasm of gonadotropes compared with other cell types. Preferential iron deposits in gonadotropes may explain the occurrence of hypogonadism with iron overload. Electron microscopic examination demonstrates hemosiderin and ferritin particles in the cytoplasm of the adenohypophysial cells; this is incorporated into lysosomal dense bodies. Prussian blue staining combined with an immunoperoxidase technique discloses iron and adenohypophysial hormones in the cytoplasm of the same cells, which is consistent with the assumption that iron uptake does not block hormone production. Iron accumulation may be accompanied by fibrosis, which accounts for the development of adenohypophysial insufficiency. In some pituitary tumors, transferrin has been shown to exhibit stimulatory growth factor-like properties.[21]

*Calcium* deposits can be demonstrated at the site of necrosis or in pituitary tumors, especially craniopharyngiomas and prolactin-producing adenomas. Calcification is not so marked as to cause hypopituitarism.

In Hurler syndrome, or gargoylism, *mucopolysaccharides* accumulate in the pituitary. The adenohypophysial cells, mainly acidophilic cells, exhibit marked cytoplasmic vacuolization. Electron microscopic studies show granular membranous bodies and prominent lipid-laden lysosomes in some basophilic cells.

## ADENOHYPOPHYSIAL CELL HYPERPLASIA[1,2,10,22]

By definition, hyperplasia refers to a nonneoplastic increase in cell number. Although it is generally accepted that *physiologic* hyperplasia regularly affects the pituitary gland (e.g., prolactin cell hyperplasia of pregnancy), the occurrence of pathologic forms of pituitary cell hyperplasia has long been questioned. It is now certain that *pathologic* forms of hyperplasia, although rare, do occur, and occasionally can be the source of both pituitary enlargement and a hypersecretory state in the absence of pituitary adenoma formation.[22] Although a small increase in prolactin, ACTH, and TSH adenomas or "tumorlets" occurs in the setting of protracted estrogen administration, Addison disease, and hypothyroidism, respectively, there is little evidence to suggest that pituitary cell hyperplasia is a common precursor of adenoma formation in humans.[10,23] Moreover, pituitary adenomas are rarely surrounded by a zone of hyperplastic cells of similar type.

Beyond the conceptual uncertainties surrounding adenohypophysial cell hyperplasia are the real practical difficulties confounding its detection. Even when present, pituitary hyperplasia is difficult to diagnose, even by experienced pituitary pathologists. The small and frequently fragmented nature of surgical specimens coupled with the normal acinar, and sometimes nodular, histologic pattern of normal pituitary cells significantly complicates the identification of hyperplastic foci. Hyperplasia is best recognized on reticulin-stained specimens and by immunohistochemical techniques. The essential pathologic feature is expansion of acini with retention of the overall acinar morphology. Morphologically, pituitary cell hyperplasia can be focal, nodular, or diffuse, and generally involves cells of a single type; rarely, several cell types may be affected simultaneously.

**Prolactin Cell Hyperplasia.** The most common form of prolactin cell hyperplasia is physiologic and occurs during pregnancy and lactation. In this context, proliferation of prolactin cells results in a doubling of the size of the gland. Another common form of prolactin cell hyperplasia is that which occurs as the result of the *stalk section effect* (i.e., interruption of dopamine delivery to the anterior lobe caused by any of several sellar and suprasellar lesions). The presence of prolactin hyperplasia adjacent to some corticotrope adenomas remains unexplained. In cases of long-standing primary hypothyroidism, prolactin cell hyperplasia is an occasional accompaniment, one that presumably reflects the trophic effects of thyrotropin-releasing hormone (TRH) on pituitary lactotropes. Furthermore, stores of hypothalamic dopamine are known to be diminished in untreated hypothyroidism. Accordingly, loss of tonic dopaminergic inhibition provides an additional neuroendocrine mechanism for lactotrope hyperplasia in this circumstance. Isolated lactotrope hyperplasia as the primary cause of hyperprolactinemia is exquisitely rare, as is the coexistence of prolactin cell hyperplasia with a prolactinoma.

**Growth Hormone Cell Hyperplasia.** Growth hormone cell hyperplasia is a rare phenomenon. In virtually all instances, somatotrope hyperplasia occurs as the result of an extrapituitary GHRH-producing tumor (e.g., pancreatic islet cell tumor, pheochromocytoma, bronchial and intestinal carcinoids, small-cell carcinoma of the lung).[24] In response to the stimulatory effect of GHRH, pituitary somatotropes enlarge, proliferate, and produce excess GH; acromegaly is the clinical result. Despite persistent stimulation by GHRH and the development of somatotrope hyperplasia, adenomatous transformation rarely occurs in this setting, even after protracted periods of stimulation. Although GHRH-producing tumors are rare causes of acromegaly, they should always be considered in the differential diagnosis. Idiopathic GH cell hyperplasia has yet to be conclusively demonstrated as a cause of acromegaly (see Chap. 219).

**Corticotrope Cell Hyperplasia.** Considerable debate surrounds the role of idiopathic corticotrope hyperplasia as a cause of Cushing disease. In the experience of the authors, corticotrope hyperplasia alone, or in combination with a corticotrope adenoma, is responsible for up to 10% of all cases of pituitary-dependent Cushing disease.[22] Theoretically, such cases of Cushing disease should be more refractory to cure by all but total hypophysectomy because hyperplastic foci either remain or are newly induced from the ongoing hyperplastic stimulus. Less controversial, and generally acknowledged, is the occurrence of corticotrope hyperplasia in response to a variety of extrapituitary CRH-producing tumors (e.g., neuroendocrine neoplasms, hypothalamic or adenohypophysial gangliocytomas; see Chaps. 75 and 219). In this setting, hyperplasia may result in considerable glandular enlargement, at times sufficient to mimic a pituitary adenoma. Not surprisingly, nodular hyperplasia of pituitary corticotropes is regularly seen in untreated Addison disease.[25]

**Thyrotrope Hyperplasia.** Hyperplasia of TSH-producing cells occurs exclusively in the context of long-standing primary hypothyroidism.[26] Frequently, such hyperplasia can be so pronounced as to enlarge the pituitary and simulate an adenoma. Pituitary surgeons should be aware of this lesion because numerous cases of thyrotrope hyperplasia have inadvertently been treated with surgical resection without the benefit of medical therapy. Thyroid hormone replacement alone is curative in many cases. Given the trophic effect of TRH on lactotropes, prolactin cell hyperplasia may be found to coexist with thyrotrope hyperplasia.

**Gonadotrope Hyperplasia.** Hyperplasia of gonadotropes is a rare occurrence that often is difficult to recognize, even in pronounced cases. It has been found in the pituitaries of patients in whom primary hypogonadism commenced at a young age, although it is not encountered among autopsied pituitaries of postmenopausal women. Gonadotrope hyperplasia is not a cause of pituitary enlargement, nor is it an accompanying feature or a likely predecessor to gonadotrope adenoma formation.

## PITUITARY NEOPLASMS

Numerous tumor types occur in the sellar region; they can be epithelial or mesenchymal and benign or malignant[4,10] (Table 11-1). Some tumors also occur elsewhere; their histologic appearance is the same in the pituitary as in other organs. Some small tumors cause no clinical or biochemical abnormalities, whereas others destroy large areas of the pituitary, resulting in anterior hypopituitarism, diabetes insipidus, and hyperprolactinemia. Other tumors cause syndromes of hormonal hyperfunction (see Chaps. 12 to 16).

### PITUITARY ADENOMAS

#### EPIDEMIOLOGY

Pituitary adenomas are benign epithelial neoplasms derived from and composed of adenohypophysial cells. They account for ~10% to 15% of all intracranial neoplasms. Depending on the population surveyed, their reported annual incidence var-

**TABLE 11-1.**
**Tumors and Nontumorous Lesions of the Sellar Region**

| | |
|---|---|
| Abscess | Granular cell tumor |
| Adenoma (pituitary) | Granulomas |
| Angioma | Hamartoma |
| Carcinoma (pituitary) | Histiocytosis X |
| Carcinoma (sphenoid sinus, nasopharynx) | Leukemia |
| Cholesteatoma | Lymphocytic hypophysitis |
| Chordoma | Lymphoma |
| Choristoma | Melanoma |
| Craniopharyngioma | Meningioma |
| Dermoid cyst | Metastasis (carcinoma, sarcoma) |
| Epidermoid cyst | Paraganglioma |
| Fibroma | Plasmacytoma |
| Gangliocytoma | Rathke cleft cyst |
| Ganglioneuroma | Sarcoidosis |
| Germinoma | Sarcoma |
| Glioma (optic nerve, neurohypophysis, hypothalamus) | Syphilis |
| | Teratoma |
| Glomangioma | Tuberculosis |

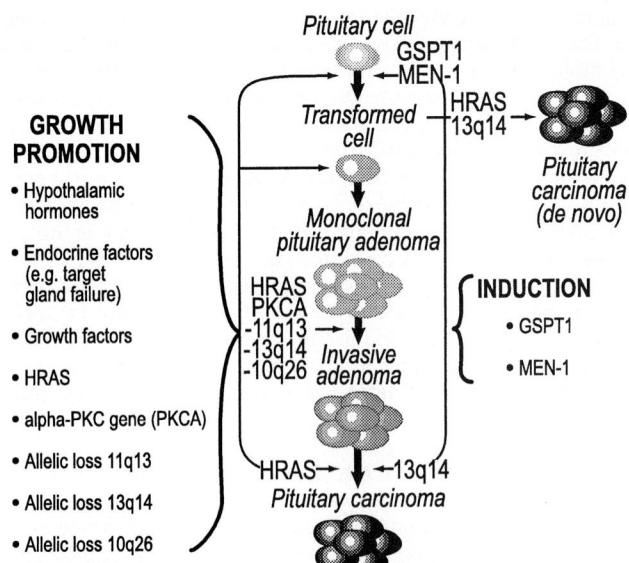

**FIGURE 11-5.** Molecular events that are considered important in the development and progression of pituitary adenomas. Conceptually, the events contributing to pituitary tumor development can be distinguished as tumor induction events (*right panel*) and tumor promotion events (*left panel*). Tumor induction events represent specific genomic mutations that may be early transforming events (gsp, multiple endocrine neoplasia type 1 [*MEN1*]). Tumor promotion events represent growth-promoting events, which include additional mutations (PKC-α, H-ras), stimulation by hypothalamic hormones, or modulation by the endocrine status of the patient (i.e., Nelson syndrome).

ies from 1.0 to 7.6 per 100,000 population.[1,10] By this measure, pituitary tumors not only are the dominant form of neoplasia arising in the sellar region, but also are among the most frequent primary intracranial tumors encountered in clinical practice. These figures, derived primarily from neurosurgical series, may even underestimate the true incidence of pituitary adenomas, because their frequency in unselected autopsy cases approaches 25%.[10] Thus, neoplastic transformation in the pituitary can be considered an exceedingly common event, albeit one that may not always manifest itself clinically.

Although no age group is exempt from the development of pituitary tumors, there is a clear tendency for these lesions to become more common with age, with the highest incidence occurring between the third and sixth decades of life. Only rarely are they diagnosed in prepubertal patients. Based on surgical series, a female preponderance appears to exist, with women of child-bearing age being at greatest risk for tumor development. The basis of this increased susceptibility in women is uncertain. It may be that the susceptibility is more apparent than real, because manifestations of pituitary dysfunction are generally more conspicuous in premenopausal women, prompting earlier diagnosis by both patients and physicians. Moreover, the incidence of pituitary adenomas in autopsy series is equally distributed between the sexes.[10]

### PATHOGENESIS AND MOLECULAR BIOLOGY[2,10,23]

Accumulating evidence indicates the development of pituitary adenomas to be a multistep and multicausal process that, in its most abbreviated form, consists of an irreversible tumor initiation phase followed by a tumor promotion phase (Fig. 11-5). The events necessary to accomplish the process are only superficially understood. Nonetheless, it is known that hereditary predisposition, endocrine and hypothalamic factors, and specific genomic mutations all appear to have some pathophysiologic role in the initiation or progression of pituitary adenomas. Before considering the relative contribution of each of these to pituitary tumor development, it is important to acknowledge that tumor development in the pituitary is a monoclonal process. This observation is of considerable conceptual relevance and provides the background on which other pathophysiologic events must be integrated.

### CLONAL ORIGINS[10,23]

One of the most fundamental and historically contentious issues surrounding pituitary tumorigenesis relates to whether

transformation in the pituitary is primarily the product of hypothalamic dysfunction or simply the result of an acquired transforming mutation intrinsic to an isolated adenohypophysial cell. The *hypothalamic hypothesis* suggests that pituitary adenomas arise as the eventual, downstream, and seemingly passive consequence of excessive trophic influences, emanating from a dysfunctional hypothalamus. Alternatively, the *pituitary hypothesis* suggests that pituitary adenomas arise as the direct result of an intrinsic pituitary defect, with neoplastic transformation occurring in relative autonomy of hypothalamic trophic influence. Whereas substantial evidence exists in support of both possibilities, the latter concept has been especially favored in view of the lack of peritumoral hyperplasia in association with pituitary adenomas and because many pituitary tumors can be definitively "cured" when completely removed. Neither of these would be expected were hypothalamic overstimulation the dominant tumorigenic mechanism.

Further strengthening the idea that pituitary adenomas result from somatic mutations that occur at the level of a single, susceptible, adenohypophysial cell have been reports concerning their clonal composition. Using the strategy of allelic X-chromosome inactivation analysis, which assesses restriction fragment length polymorphisms and differential methylation patterns in various X-linked genes, several independent laboratories have confirmed a monoclonal composition for virtually all pituitary adenomas.[27,28] Validation of the monoclonal nature of pituitary adenomas has been an important conceptual advance because it has established pituitary adenomas as monoclonal expansions of a single, somatically mutated, and transformed adenohypophysial cell. Were hypothalamic overstimulation the dominant initiating event, then a population of anterior pituitary cells should simultaneously be affected and a polyclonal tumor would be the expected result; this has not been the case.

### HYPOTHALAMIC FACTORS AND PITUITARY TUMORIGENESIS

Whereas the demonstration that pituitary adenomas are monoclonal derivatives of a single transformed adenohypophysial cell does conform well to existing paradigms of human tumorigenesis, it should not be interpreted as somehow exonerating hypothalamic influences of a role in pituitary tumor development. On the contrary, the culpability of hypothalamic hormones in pituitary tumorigenesis continues to gain strength, and there has been renewed interest in integrating a role for these hormones in the current multistep monoclonal model.[29] The class of hypothalamic hormones at issue are the hypothalamic hypophysiotropic hormones, which primarily include GHRH, somatostatin (SRIF), CRH, TRH, gonadotropin-releasing hormone (GnRH), and dopamine. Produced in hypothalamic nuclei, descending via the portal circulation, and binding to specific membrane receptors on their respective adenohypophysial target cells, these hormones govern the secretory and proliferative activity of each of the principal pituitary cell types. In logical extension of their physiologic trophic activities has been the implication that aberrant activity of these regulatory hormones in the form of excess stimulation or deficient inhibition may contribute to the genesis and/or progression of pituitary adenomas. For example, in states of pathologic GHRH excess, as occurs with rare GHRH-producing tumors (pancreatic endocrine tumors, carcinoids, pheochromocytomas, and hypothalamic hamartomas/gangliocytomas), chronic GHRH stimulation leads to hyperplasia of pituitary somatotropes, GH hypersecretion, and clinical acromegaly. Depending on the duration of exposure to the excess GHRH, progression from somatotrope hyperplasia to adenomatous transformation has been documented in some, but not all instances.[24] A parallel phenomenon has been demonstrated in transgenic mice bearing the human GHRH transgene. That these animals develop gigantism, elevated GH levels, somatotrope hyperplasia, and, eventually, GH-producing pituitary adenomas, provides compelling and conclusive evidence of the tumor-promoting properties of GHRH.[30] To date, analogous data implicating other hypophysiotropic hormones have been comparatively few; however, the convincing precedence provided by these GHRH data lends, at the very least, some plausibility to the idea that other hypophysiotropic hormones may also share similar tumorigenic potential. Whereas a specific somatic mutation of an adenohypophysial cell is requisite to adenomatous transformation, hypophysiotropic hormones may modify the cell's susceptibility for such a mutation to occur. Some hypophysiotropic hormones (GHRH, CRH, TRH) are known to induce early-response genes in their respective adenohypophysial target cells, mustering a potent, yet physiologic mitogenic response. Were it to occur, not only would the aberrant overactivity of these regulatory hormones be accompanied by increased proliferative activity of relevant adenohypophysial cells, but the possibility for a transforming mutation also would be correspondingly increased. The extent to which this actually does occur among pituitary adenomas is unknown, although abnormal hypothalamic and other neuroendocrine responses have been demonstrated in patients with pituitary adenomas, including those having undergone "successful" tumor removal.[31]

Tumor initiation aside, a more persuasive role for hypothalamic hormones can be envisaged during the tumor progression phase of pituitary tumorigenesis. Given that pituitary adenomas frequently express and retain responsiveness to hypothalamic hormones, the latter have been implicated in facilitating proliferation of the transformed clone. Of particular interest have been a number of reports wherein pituitary tumors themselves were shown to express at the protein and/or mRNA level various hypophysiotropic hormones together with their corresponding receptors. Somatotrope adenomas have been shown to express both GHRH-mRNA transcripts and protein,[32,33] experimental corticotrope adenomas have been shown to express CRH-mRNA transcripts,[34] thyrotrope adenomas have been shown to express TRH mRNA,[35] and gonadotrope adenomas have been shown to express GnRH mRNA and protein.[36] These data strongly suggest the possibility that pituitary adenomas may be subject to autocrine and/or paracrine regulation by endogenously produced hypophysiotropic hormones. In the case of GH-secreting pituitary adenomas, tumoral expression of GHRH mRNA was shown to be an adverse event—one associated with higher proliferative activity, invasiveness, increased secretory activity, and a reduced likelihood of postoperative remission.[37]

In view of the foregoing, it should be clear that despite the monoclonal constitution of pituitary adenomas, a potential role of hypothalamic hormones in their genesis and/or progression is not easily dismissed (see Fig. 11-5).

## ENDOCRINE FACTORS

A recurring theme, one borne from both experimental study and clinical observation, relates to the possible predisposing, promoting, or perhaps even the inductive effect of certain altered endocrine states to the development of pituitary adenomas. Of particular relevance are those states of target-gland failure wherein the pituitary is no longer subject to negative feedback effects imposed by target-gland hormones. For example, within the pituitary glands of patients with Addison disease and primary hypothyroidism of long duration, the respective frequencies of corticotrope and thyrotrope "tumorlets" was higher than that observed in control individuals.[25,26] Admittedly, only a loose correlation, but stronger still, and of greater clinical concern is the behavior of corticotrope adenomas and thyrotrope adenomas in the setting of bilateral adrenalectomy (Nelson syndrome) and prior thyroidectomy, respectively.[38] That such tumors tend to be notoriously more aggressive than those having an intact pituitary-target gland axis emphasizes the potential importance of negative-feedback inhibition in modulating the behavior and progression of these neoplasms.

A final endocrine issue, one having been repeatedly implicated in pituitary adenoma development, particularly PRL-producing adenomas, concerns the role of estrogen as a contributor to transformation and/or neoplastic progression in the pituitary. The tumor-promoting properties of this sex steroid are mediated by specific estrogen receptors which, when ligand activated, dimerize and bind to specific DNA-addressing sites to induce transcription of various target genes governing cell proliferation. Whereas chronic estrogen administration routinely induces prolactinomas in rodents, evidence in favor of a similar relationship in humans has been less convincing. The increasing frequency with which prolactinomas were being diagnosed in the 1970s paralleled the use of oral contraceptives in women, a phenomenon that once invited speculation about a possible causal or predisposing effect of the latter in the development of the former. Several case-controlled studies, however, have failed to substantiate such a relationship.[39] Still, estrogens are known to alter the morphology and secretory activity of human adenohypophysial cells, indicating that the anterior pituitary is an important target tissue for estrogen action.[40] The observation that the hormonal milieu of pregnancy can, in some instances, stimulate prolactinoma growth indicates a potential responsiveness of these tumors to estrogenic stimulation. That human pituitary adenomas express estrogen receptors has been recognized for some time. In addition, estrogen receptor mRNA transcripts are present in all types of pituitary adenomas and in all cell types of the normal anterior pituitary gland.[41] In at least a single but noteworthy instance, one involving a transsexual patient, high-dose estrogen therapy correlated with the development of a human PRL-producing pituitary adenoma.[42] Thus, the link between estrogens and human pituitary tumor formation remains somewhat circumstantial, but sufficiently so, that it cannot be entirely dismissed.

**Genomic Alterations: Oncogene Activation.**    Accompanying the realization that the somatic mutation of an isolated adenohypophysial cell is an event requisite to pituitary tumorigenesis has been a vigorous attempt to identify and characterize the responsible mutation. Of the genomic and cellular alterations known to occur in pituitary adenomas, relatively few appear to involve activating mutations of known oncogenes. To date, activating mutations of only two oncogenes have been reported in pituitary adenomas: gsp and H-ras. Whereas the former is encountered with some regularity in somatotrope adenomas and periodically in other pituitary adenoma types, the latter has been identified in only isolated instances.

The only consistent evidence favoring oncogene activation as a transforming mechanism in the pituitary stems from the discovery and characterization of the gsp oncogene, an oncogene first identified in GH-producing pituitary adenomas.[43,44] The signal transduction cascades governing the secretory and proliferative functions of pituitary somatotropes converge on the adenylate cyclase second messenger system. In the normal state, the hypothalamic hypophysiotropic hormone (GHRH) is the principal positive regulator of somatotrope function. After binding to its membrane receptor on the somatotrope cell surface, the GHRH-proliferative signal is coupled to a stimulatory, heterotrimeric G-protein, termed Gs, which binds GTP and activates adenylate cyclase. This results in elevations of cAMP levels that, through a series of poorly characterized downstream events, ultimately lead to GH secretion and somatotrope proliferation. Adenylate cyclase activation is normally a self-limiting, transient, and tightly regulated event. This is because one structural component of Gs, known as the α chain, maintains intrinsic GTPase activity that, after transducing the signal, hydrolyzes GTP and returns Gs to its inactive state, thus terminating the trophic signal. Activating mutations of gsp are the result of point mutations in the α chain gene of Gs. The mutant alpha chain has deficient GTPase activity and is therefore incapable of hydrolyzing GTP and "turning off" the proliferative signal. Therefore, such mutant forms of the α chain stabilize Gs in its active configuration, thus mimicking the trophic effects of persistent GHRH action. Bypassing the tight regulatory control normally provided by GHRH, somatotropes bearing the mutant α chain of Gs constitutively activate adenylate cyclase, providing an autonomous and unrestrained capacity for cell proliferation and GH secretion.

Whereas in North American and European studies, activating mutations of gsp have been reported in ~40% of somatotrope adenomas,[44] in Japan, such mutations are rare events.[45] In neither geographic setting, however, does their presence confer any significantly distinctive clinical, behavioral, biochemical, or radiologic characteristics to the tumor. In one report, tumors exhibiting gsp mutations occurred in older patients, were smaller, and had lower basal GH levels than wild-type tumors, although this has not been uniformly observed.[31,44]

Activating mutations of the Gs α chain have also been identified in 10% of clinically nonfunctioning pituitary adenomas and very recently, in 5% of corticotrope adenomas.[46–48] That such mutations should occur in tumors not somatotropic in nature suggests that stimulatory G proteins may underlie intracellular signaling in other cell types as well. As in the case of somatotrope adenomas, nonfunctioning and corticotrope adenomas bearing mutations of gsp do not appear to differ clinically from those tumors lacking this mutation.

Aside from gsp mutations that have been identified with some regularity, the search for additional activating mutations involving other candidate oncogenes has not proved particularly informative. The only relevant finding concerns the very occasional demonstration of mutations involving the H-ras oncogene among isolated pituitary tumors. The first dedicated study of ras mutations in the pituitary involved the screening of 19 pituitary adenomas wherein an activating mutation of ras was identified in only a single instance.[49] The noteworthy feature of this case, a prolactinoma, pertained to the unusual aggressiveness of the tumor; the tumor was remarkable for a rather early age of onset, multiple recurrences, very high prolactin levels, resistance to dopamine agonist therapy, and unrelenting invasiveness that ultimately proved fatal. In a subsequent genomic screening of 44 pituitary adenomas, none were found to have mutations of ras.[50] In a third study, one focusing on pituitary carcinomas, mutations of H-ras were demonstrated in three of five distant metastases but in none of the primary pituitary lesions, nor in any invasive pituitary adenoma.[51] Of these, two were corticotrope carcinomas and the third was a lactotrope carcinoma. Collectively, these data suggest that mutations of ras, while uncommon events in pituitary tumorigenesis, do appear to be associated with an unusually aggressive phenotype and are likely late events in pituitary tumor progression. Furthermore, the presence of H-ras mutations in secondary deposits but not in the primary lesion of pituitary carcinomas is especially intriguing for it suggests that this mutation may play a role in initiating and/or sustaining distant pituitary metastases (see Fig. 11-5).

## GENOMIC ALTERATIONS: TUMOR-SUPPRESSOR GENE INACTIVATION

**MEN1 Tumor-Suppressor Gene.**    Genetic predisposition to pituitary tumor development is restricted to a single and uncommon condition, the MEN1 syndrome. This autosomal-dominant condition is characterized by the simultaneous development of tumors involving the parathyroid glands, pancreatic islet cells, and the pituitary. A variably penetrant condition, only 25% of patients develop pituitary tumors, the majority of which are macroadenomas associated primarily with GH and/or PRL hypersecretion.[1,10] Approximately 3% of all pituitary adenomas occur in the context of MEN1. The nature of the genetic defect in MEN1 has recently been identified and involves allelic loss of a putative tumor-suppressor gene at the 11q13 locus.[52,53] In its recessive behavior, the MEN1 gene is typical of a tumor-suppressor gene, with susceptible individuals inheriting a germline mutation of one of the two 11q13 alleles. Subsequent spontaneous mutation, inactivation, or deletion of the remaining normal 11q13 locus in susceptible endocrine tissues ultimately leads to tumor formation in the involved tissue.

Once believed to be a genetic defect that accounted for pituitary adenomas occurring exclusively in the context of MEN1, several studies have also demonstrated loss of the 11q13 locus in seemingly sporadic pituitary adenomas. In the earliest of these, allelic deletions of 11q13 were found in two of three sporadic prolactinomas.[52] Subsequently, 4 of 12 sporadic GH cell adenomas were found to have deletions involving the 11q13 locus.[54] More recently, allelic deletions of chromosome 11 were found in 18% of pituitary adenomas of all major types.[55] Collectively, these data suggest that the 11q13 locus is the site of an important tumor-suppressor gene, the inactivation of which may be of pathogenic relevance to the development of both sporadic and MEN1–related pituitary adenomas.

**p53 Tumor-Suppressor Gene.**    Mutations of the p53 gene represent the single most common nonrandom genomic alteration encountered in human cancer.[56] The contribution of p53 gene mutations to pituitary tumorigenesis remains unsettled. Much of the difficulty in implicating or excluding a role for p53 mutations in these tumors has centered on the apparent incongruity between data obtained by conventional genomic screening from that provided by p53 immunohistochemistry studies.[57] On the one hand, in all of three studies wherein the p53 gene was screened at the usual mutational "hot spots," not a single pituitary tumor was identified as having a p53 mutation.[50,58] Alternatively, in several reports wherein pituitary tumors were studied immunohistochemically, conclusive nuclear accumulation of p53 protein was demonstrated in some pituitary tumors.[57,59] In one report, nuclear accumulation of p53 was selectively present in none, 15%, and 100% of noninvasive adenomas, invasive adenomas, and pituitary carcinomas, respectively. Moreover, the growth fractions of p53 immunopositive tumors were significantly higher than those immunonegative for p53.[59] In reconciling the genomic screening and immunohistochemical data, it is important to acknowledge the different inferences permissible by each methodology. Whereas p53 immunohistochemistry analysis was once regarded as a surrogate means of detecting underlying gene mutations, the concordance between these two methods has not proved as strong as previously believed, and the former cannot be regarded as unequivocal proof of the latter. Therefore, the weight of existing evidence argues against p53 gene mutations as events that contribute to pituitary tumor development and/or their progression. Still, the inability to invoke an underlying gene mutation as the basis for the observed accumulation of p53 protein among aggressive pituitary tumors should not diminish the practical utility of this protein as an immunohistochemical marker of aggressive behavior in this tumor system. Moreover, alternative and equally relevant pathophysiologic mechanisms other than p53 gene mutations may account for p53 immunopositivity. Precedence in support of this has been provided by other human tumors, such as sarcomas and cervical carcinomas, wherein immunohistochemically apparent p53 accumulation reflects complex formation, sequestration, and resultant inactivation of wild-type p53 by other proteins, producing a state functionally equivalent to that occurring with a gene mutation; similar mechanisms may be operative in pituitary tumors.[56]

**13q14.**    The first of the tumor-suppressor genes to be identified, the retinoblastoma gene (Rb) remains the prototypical example of this class of genes. Beyond its role in the development of familial retinoblastoma and various other malignancies and its overall contribution to cell-cycle regulatory control, studies of the Rb gene added a new dimension to the very concept of human cancer, illuminating recessive aspects of the process and the oncogenic consequences that accompany loss of protective genomic elements. The implication that the Rb gene might be involved in pituitary tumorigenesis had a somewhat serendipitous beginning. Transgenic mice in which one of the two germline Rb alleles had been deactivated failed to develop retinoblastomas as anticipated; instead they developed large, high-grade, invasive pituitary tumors.[60] On further analysis, these tumors were shown to have lost the remaining normal Rb allele, convincingly implicating a second Rb "hit" as the basis for pituitary tumor development in this model. All of these tumors were found to be corticotropic in nature, immunoreactive for ACTH, and of pars intermedia origin (unpublished observations).

Prompted by the provocative nature of these findings, a number of recent studies have sought to determine the relevance of Rb mutations in human pituitary tumors. In the first report, none of 18 informative pituitary tumors exhibited allelic Rb loss.[61] This was further confirmed in a study of 30 informative pituitary adenomas wherein none was found to exhibit loss of heterozygosity (LOH) at the Rb gene locus.[62] In another study, however, LOH was found at the Rb locus in all of seven pituitary carcinomas, including their metastatic deposits, and in all of six highly invasive pituitary adenomas.[63] The significance of these latter observations vis-à-vis Rb gene mutations, however, was undermined by the finding of Rb protein in tumors exhibiting LOH at the Rb locus. In reconciling the apparent discordance between Rb gene and protein status, together with the two previous studies that excluded Rb mutations within pituitary tumors, the conclusion was made that another putative tumor-suppressor gene, one present on 13q14 but distinct from Rb, must be involved in pituitary tumor progression (see Fig. 11-5).[63]

### OTHER GENOMIC ALTERATIONS

**Protein Kinase C Gene.**    Another genomic alteration identified in pituitary adenomas, specifically invasive ones, relates to the protein kinase C (PKC) family of second messengers. PKC family members are ubiquitous, membrane-bound, intracellular kinases whose function is to phosphorylate serine or threonine residues on important substrate proteins. Such kinase activity is thought to govern several important cellular pro-

cesses, including the transmembrane signaling underlying cell proliferation and differentiation. Altered or aberrant PKC activity has been demonstrated in several human tumors, including pituitary adenomas. In comparison with normal pituitary tissue, increased PKC protein expression was identified in pituitary adenomas. More recently, it has been demonstrated that the specific PKC isoform that is overexpressed in pituitary tumors is PKC-α. Interestingly, this particular PKC isoform has been favored as the isoform that mediates the mitogenic functions of PKC. Not only was PKC-α found to be overexpressed in pituitary adenomas, but invasive adenomas also exhibited a conserved point mutation of the PKC-α gene.[64]

**Cytogenetic Changes.**    Perhaps the most graphic evidence in support of the concept that neoplasia represents the successive accumulation of genetic alterations is derived from cytogenetic studies of tumor cells. In the case of pituitary adenomas, given their low intrinsic mitotic activity and overall benign constitution, metaphase preparations are not easily procured, and few direct cytogenetic analyses have been successfully performed. Of those that have, cytogenetic aberrations appeared more commonly among functioning pituitary adenomas than in endocrine-inactive ones.[65,66] Overall, rearrangements involving chromosomes 17 and 19 were most commonly observed; trisomy of chromosome 7 as well as structural abnormalities of chromosomes 18p, 1, and 4 were observed less often. Given the limited number of cytogenetic analyses performed on pituitary adenomas to date, it is impossible to determine the pathophysiologic significance of the chromosomal aberrations so far cataloged. Whether such alterations are nonrandom events that contribute to tumor initiation and/or progression remains uncertain. Alternatively, such alterations may simply represent genetic instability inherent to neoplastic cells, being neither important nor informative to the evolution or progression of pituitary adenomas.

### GENERAL FEATURES OF PITUITARY ADENOMAS[1,10]

From clinical, pathologic, and biologic standpoints, tumors of the pituitary gland are a heterogeneous group. Underlying much of this heterogeneity is the fact that the normal adenohypophysis is composed of five principal cell types, each of which is susceptible to neoplastic transformation. The resulting adenoma tends to maintain the secretory activity nomenclature and some of the morphologic features of the cell of origin. Up to 70% of pituitary adenomas are hormonally active lesions that produce distinctive alterations in the endocrine equilibrium. The remainder are incapable of secreting a biologically active hormonal product and are referred to as *nonfunctional*. Further contributing to their overall heterogeneity are their variable and often unpredictable growth characteristics. Whereas some tumors exist largely as microadenomas, maintain a well-defined margin, and show little appreciable growth over time, others exhibit rapid proliferation rates and are markedly invasive or compressive of adjacent bony, neural, or vascular structures. This tremendous variation in biologic behavior cannot be predicted on morphologic grounds alone. Even the exceptional pituitary carcinoma, so defined on the basis of its metastatic capability, may appear entirely benign histologically.

The clinical presentation of pituitary adenomas also is variable, although three principal patterns are recognized. The first involves pituitary hyperfunction, in the form of several characteristic hypersecretory states. Hypersecretion of prolactin, GH, ACTH, and, rarely, TSH, produces their corresponding clinical phenotypes: amenorrhea-galactorrhea syndrome, acromegaly or gigantism, Cushing disease, and secondary hyperthyroidism, respectively.[1,4,67] By contrast, some pituitary adenomas produce symptoms of anterior pituitary deficiency, resulting from compression of the nontumorous pituitary or damage to the pituitary stalk or hypophysiotropic areas of the hypothalamus. This usually occurs insidiously in the context of large, nonfunctioning pituitary adenomas, but occasionally it may occur acutely in the setting of pituitary apoplexy. In the face of chronic compression, the various secretory cells of the pituitary differ in their functional reserve. Because gonadotropes are the most vulnerable, they usually are affected first, followed sequentially by thyrotropes and somatotropes. Corticotropes demonstrate the greatest functional resilience and generally are the last to be affected. Finally, the clinical presentation of a pituitary adenoma may be a neurologic one, with or without coexisting endocrinopathy. Given its strategic location at the skull base, a growing adenoma produces a predictable array of neurologic signs and symptoms. Suprasellar extension with compression of the optic chiasm results in a characteristic bitemporal hemianopic pattern of vision loss (see Chap. 20). Encroachment on the hypothalamus causes alterations of sleep alertness and behavior (see Chap. 9). Transgression of the lamina terminalis can bring these tumors into the region of the third ventricle, where obstruction to the flow of cerebrospinal fluid results in obstructive hydrocephalus. Lateral penetration of the tumor into the cavernous sinus occurs commonly, occasionally ensheathing the cavernous segment of the carotid artery and functionally compromising cranial nerves transiting the sinus. Some tumors extend in other directions and, if sufficiently large, can involve the anterior, middle, and, occasionally, posterior cranial fossae to produce a full spectrum of neurologic deficits.

A final endocrinologic feature of pituitary adenomas, one that is common to many neoplastic, compressive, or infiltrative lesions affecting the sellar region, is moderate hyperprolactinemia. The blood prolactin levels are not extremely high, usually below 200 ng/mL. In addition, TRH stimulation, although not reliable as a test, may further increase the blood prolactin levels, whereas patients with prolactin-producing pituitary adenomas may exhibit no response or a blunted response to TRH. In patients with non–prolactin-producing tumors, the mechanism of hyperprolactinemia is explained by the so-called "stalk section effect." Because prolactin secretion is suppressed by hypothalamic dopamine, interference with the synthesis, discharge, or adenohypophysial transport of dopamine may relieve pituitary prolactin cells from dopaminergic inhibition, resulting in increased prolactin release and hyperprolactinemia (see Chap. 13).

As a rule, prolactin elevations in excess of 200 ng/mL are virtually always indicative of autonomous prolactin secretion from a neoplasm, either a prolactinoma or a plurihormonal pituitary tumor with a lactotropic component.

## MEANS OF CLASSIFICATION

Since pituitary adenomas were first recognized, substantial effort has been devoted to classifying them into distinct groups. Endocrinologic classifications emphasize clinical manifestations of the disease or the dominant endocrine abnormality as assessed biochemically, most often with radioimmunoassay of blood hormone levels. Pathologic classifications hinge on structural features of adenoma cells and emphasize morphologic tumor markers. Modern pathologic classifications are based on sophisticated morphologic methods, such as immunocytochemistry analysis, ultrastructural analysis, immunoelectron microscopy, and morphometry. The conventional pathologic methods have been integrated with the powerful applications of molecular science. Methodologies such as in situ hybridization and Northern blot analysis permit the classification of pituitary adenomas on the basis of specific gene expression patterns (Fig. 11-6). Although these methods as well as those that catalog pituitary adenomas on the basis of specific genomic alterations are currently of research interest only, they will assume increasing importance in both the classification of pituitary adenomas and the prediction of their biologic behavior.

Useful classifications are those that permit conclusions based on biologic behavior, prognosis, and response to various treatment modalities. Thus, pituitary adenomas are classified accord-

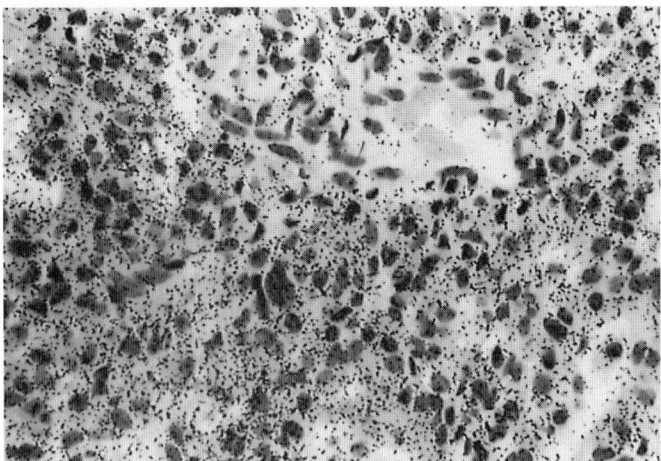

**FIGURE 11-6.** Cellular distribution of pro-opiomelanocortin (*POMC*) mRNA in a corticotrope adenoma from a patient with Nelson syndrome as demonstrated by the method of in situ hybridization. The distribution of the black silver grains corresponds to the distribution of POMC mRNA. Original magnification ×400

ing to the staining affinities of the cell cytoplasm, size, growth pattern, endocrine activity, histologic features, hormone synthesis and content, granularity of cell cytoplasm, cellular composition and cytogenesis, or electron microscopic characteristics.

On the basis of tinctorial features of the cell cytoplasm, acidophilic, basophilic, and chromophobic adenomas can be distinguished. Acidophilic adenomas were assumed to cause GH overproduction and, consequently, gigantism and acromegaly. Basophilic adenomas were thought to secrete ACTH and were linked to Cushing disease. Chromophobic adenomas were considered endocrinologically inactive tumors not associated with hormone excess. However, it has been clearly shown that acidophilic adenomas can synthesize hormones other than GH, such as prolactin, or can be endocrinologically inactive. Some basophilic adenomas represent silent corticotrope cell adenomas unaccompanied by ACTH excess or they produce hormones other than ACTH. Chromophobic adenomas may not be associated with hormone overproduction; however, this is not a general rule because more than half of all chromophobic adenomas are endocrinologically active tumors, secreting GH, prolactin, ACTH, TSH, FSH, LH, or the α subunit. The classification of pituitary adenomas on the grounds of the staining affinities of the cell cytoplasm has limited value because it does not consider hormone production, cellular composition, or cytogenesis, and because it fails to correlate structural features with secretory activity.

## GROWTH PATTERNS

Based on size, pituitary adenomas can be divided into microadenomas and macroadenomas. Microadenomas measure <10 mm in greatest diameter and macroadenomas measure >10 mm. This classification is useful because a prognosis can be based on tumor size. Large tumors usually are difficult to remove completely, and recurrences are more frequent than with small, well-demarcated tumors confined to the sella. There are no light or electron microscopic differences between microadenomas and macroadenomas.

Pituitary tumors grow either by expansion or by invasion and can be divided on the basis of growth patterns as follows:

Grade 0: Intrapituitary microadenoma; normal sellar appearance.
Grade 1: Intrapituitary microadenoma; focal bulging of sellar wall.
Grade 2: Intrasellar macroadenoma; diffusely enlarged sella; no invasion.

**TABLE 11-2.**
**Size and Frequency of Gross Local Invasion among the Major Pituitary Tumor Types**

| Pituitary Tumor Type | % Microadenoma | % Invasion | % Macroadenoma | % Invasion | Overall Incidence of Invasion (%) |
|---|---|---|---|---|---|
| GH cell adenoma | 14 | 0 | 86 | 50 | 50 |
| PRL cell adenoma | 33 | — | 67 | — | 52 |
| Mixed GH-PRL cell adenoma | 26 | 0 | 74 | 31 | 31 |
| ACTH cell adenoma (Cushing disease) | 87 | 8 | 13 | 62 | 15 |
| ACTH cell adenoma (Nelson syndrome) | 30 | 17 | 70 | 64 | 50 |
| Silent ACTH adenoma | 0 | 0 | 100 | 82 | 82 |
| Gonadotrope adenoma | 0 | 0 | 100 | 21 | 21 |
| Thyrotrope adenoma | 0 | 0 | 100 | 75 | 75 |
| Null cell adenoma | 2 | — | 98 | — | 42 |
| Plurihormonal adenoma | 25 | 31 | 75 | 59 | 52 |

*ACTH*, adrenocorticotropic hormone; *GH*, growth hormone; *PRL*, prolactin.
(Modified from Scheithauer BW, Kovacs K, Laws ER Jr, Randall RV. Pathology of invasive pituitary adenomas with special reference to functional classification. J Neurosurg 1986; 65:733.)

Grade 3: Macroadenoma; localized sellar invasion and/or destruction.

Grade 4: Macroadenoma; extensive sellar invasion and/or destruction.

Tumors are further subclassified on the basis of their extrasellar extensions, whether suprasellar or parasellar. Pituitary carcinomas (i.e., pituitary tumors with demonstrated metastatic spread) are sometimes designated as Grade 5.

**Intrapituitary and Intrasellar Adenomas.** Intrapituitary adenomas are confined to the substance of the pituitary; intrasellar adenomas are located in the sella. These adenomas neither erode the sella nor invade parasellar tissue. They grow slowly, are well circumscribed, and are surrounded by a pseudocapsule consisting of condensed reticulin fibers and compressed rows of adenohypophysial cells; they have no fibrous capsule such as benign tumors may have elsewhere.

**Diffuse Adenomas.** Diffuse adenomas are large and expansive; they may fill the entire sella and cause focal erosion of the sellar wall.

**Invasive Adenomas.** Invasive adenomas grow more rapidly than do expansive adenomas. They have no sharp borders, they erode the sella and spread into neighboring tissue, they may infiltrate the sphenoid bone and invade the posterior lobe and cavernous sinus, and they may compress the optic nerve and other cranial nerves in the vicinity. Invasive adenomas may spread into the brain, penetrate into the third ventricle, and compress or destroy the hypothalamus and pituitary stalk. The aggressive behavior of invasive adenomas, although frequently translated into diminished surgical cure rates, is generally not reflected in their histologic features. Invasive adenomas exhibiting extreme local aggressiveness frequently maintain a deceptively innocent histologic appearance. In general, the usual morphologic markers of tumor aggressiveness (i.e., pleomorphism, nuclear atypia, increased cellularity, mitotic activity) correlate poorly with the invasive tendency, proliferative capacity, potential for recurrence, or overall biologic behavior of an adenoma.

The incidence of local invasion depends not only on the different pituitary tumor types, but also on how the phenomenon is defined. Depending on the criteria used, invasion can be demonstrated radiologically, intraoperatively, and microscopically in 10%, 35%, and 90% of all pituitary adenomas, respectively.[68] Not surprisingly, microscopic evidence of dural invasion increases with tumor size, being evident in 66% of microadenomas, 87% of macroadenomas, and 94% of macroadenomas with suprasellar extension. Because microscopic evidence of dural invasion is so ubiquitous a finding, it is a poor index of tumor aggressiveness. Therefore, it has become common practice to designate adenomas as "invasive" on the basis of radiologic or intraoperative evidence of gross invasion. The frequency of invasion among the various tumor types is presented in Table 11-2.

Because the histopathologic features of pituitary adenomas correlate poorly with their clinical aggressiveness, the development of a reliable and informative strategy to predict their biologic behavior has remained one of the most inscrutable aspects of pituitary tumor biology. During the past decade, numerous strategies have been applied to the problem of predicting the proliferative potential of pituitary adenomas.[10] Previously considered to be of research interest only, some of these methods are beginning to reach levels of clinical applicability.

In attempting to distinguish mitotically active pituitary adenomas, which are prone to recurrence, from the more indolent ones, which are amenable to surgical cure, the presence of several cell-cycle–specific proliferation markers has been studied in pituitary adenomas. Two of these, Ki67 and proliferating cell nuclear antigen (PCNA), have been particularly informative from a clinical standpoint. The former is a cell-cycle–specific, nuclear-associated antigen of uncertain function whose expression is restricted to proliferating cells in the G1-to-M phase of the cell cycle. Thus, its immunochemical presence and relative abundance in tumor tissue provides some measure of the proliferative activity of a tumor. In one study, invasive adenomas expressed twice the amount of Ki67 protein as did noninvasive adenomas.[69] Subsequent studies of Ki67 expression using MIB-1, an antibody that recognizes the Ki67 on better preserved and formalin-fixed preparations, have expanded our understanding of the cell kinetics of pituitary tumors.[70] Specifically, (a) the growth fractions of pituitary tumors are low, most indices being <5%; (b) mean growth fractions are significantly higher among invasive adenomas and highest among pituitary carcinomas when compared with noninvasive adenomas (4.7%, 11.9%, and 1.4%, respectively); (c) virtually all noninvasive adenomas had growth fractions <3%, whereas those of most invasive adenomas and pituitary carcinomas were higher; and (d) the growth fraction of hormonally active pituitary tumors was significantly higher than that of endocrinologically inactive pituitary adenomas. Although these data suggest that a significant correlation does exist between Ki67 expression and pituitary tumor behavior, all reports to date have been retrospective in nature. Accordingly, prospective studies will be required to determine the long-term prognostic significance of this marker.

PCNA is a critical accessory protein of the enzyme DNA polymerase-δ. The former is an essential component of the replicon, the multimeric complex that polymerizes DNA nucleotides during leading-strand DNA replication just before cell division. Therefore, the nuclear expression of PCNA is a requirement for all replicating cells. PCNA expression has been studied in a large group of pituitary adenomas of all sizes and various immunotypes, including nonrecurrent and recurrent tumors.[71] The expression of PCNA was significantly higher among recurrent pituitary adenomas than among nonrecurrent ones. Furthermore, the PCNA index was higher in larger tumors, particularly those exhibiting extrasellar extension. Among recurrent tumors, a higher PCNA index tended to be accompanied by a shorter disease-free interval.

Flow cytometric analysis, although prognostically informative for many human epithelial malignancies, has been less than enlightening when applied to pituitary adenomas.[23] Although ploidy analyses have shown many pituitary adenomas to have either diploid or aneuploid complements, neither have been reliably correlated with the invasiveness or potential for recurrence of an adenoma. Similarly, S-phase fractions of pituitary adenomas, as determined by flow cytometry, do not appear to be prognostically informative. The S-phase fraction of cycling cells also has been determined in situ after the in vivo administration of bromodeoxyuridine (BrDU), a thymidine analog. The incorporated BrDU in cycling cells is revealed by immunohistochemistry analysis using an anti-BrDU antibody. Because pituitary adenomas have relatively low proliferation rates overall, the S-phase fractions usually are small, generally <0.5%. The consistent finding that tumors associated with Nelson syndrome have the highest S-phase fractions validates the aggressiveness observed clinically in this group of tumors. The narrow range of observed S-phase fractions in pituitary adenomas overall, however, limits the sensitivity of this technique in distinguishing subtle differences in S-phase fractions between aggressive and nonaggressive pituitary adenoma variants.

**Carcinoma of the Pituitary Gland.**   Despite their epithelial nature and the regularity with which many pituitary adenomas exhibit aggressive local behavior, it remains a mystery why so few are capable of metastatic dissemination. Metastasizing pituitary tumors of adenohypophysial origin (i.e., pituitary carcinomas) are rare. A recent review identified 52 cases of pituitary carcinoma to which 12 new cases were added.[72] Pituitary carcinoma is a precisely defined entity that includes only those tumors of adenohypophysial type with demonstrated craniospinal or systemic metastases.[1,10] In contrast to most human carcinomas, the usual histologic markers of malignancy (nuclear atypia and pleomorphism, mitotic activity, necrosis, hemorrhage, invasiveness) are insufficient to permit an unqualified diagnosis of pituitary carcinoma; these features are commonly seen in ordinary pituitary adenomas. Instead, the diagnosis is predicated on tumor behavior, being relatively independent of histologic features. Among reported cases of pituitary carcinoma, metastatic dissemination most often involved the cerebrospinal fluid axis. Numerous extraneural metastatic sites have also been reported, including bone, liver, lymph nodes, lung, kidney, and heart.

Pituitary carcinomas primarily affect adults, although their clinical presentation is variable. In some patients, the initial course is indistinguishable from that of a benign pituitary adenoma. Local invasion is variably present, and the histologic characteristics of the tumor may be entirely benign. A protracted course, often punctuated by multiple local recurrences, is then followed by metastatic dissemination. In many such cases, a clear escalation in histologic abnormalities is observed when primary tumors are compared with metastatic deposits. In this setting, the process appears to be one of malignant transformation in a preexisting benign adenoma. Alternatively, the behavior of other pituitary carcinomas is indicative of de novo malignancy. Such tumors are biologically malignant from the onset, beginning as rapidly growing, relentlessly invasive, cytologically atypical tumors that promptly give way to metastatic dissemination.

Although both hormonally active and nonfunctioning pituitary carcinomas have been described, the former appear to predominate. Pituitary carcinomas composed of ACTH cells (particularly in the context of Nelson syndrome), prolactin cells, and GH cells are most frequently represented. As a rule, metastatic deposits should retain the immunotype of the primary tumor. Because the pituitary is often the recipient of metastatic carcinomas originating systemically, the far more common occurrence of metastatic deposits to the pituitary must be excluded by careful clinical and pathologic examination before arriving at a diagnosis of primary pituitary carcinoma.

The factors that underlie the capacity for metastatic dissemination in pituitary carcinomas remain obscure. Their mode of spread, however, is more fully understood. Craniospinal involvement appears to begin with invasion of the subarachnoid space and eventual dissemination by cerebrospinal fluid flow. Intracranial deposits involving brain parenchyma likely develop as the result of tumor permeation into perivascular (Virchow-Robin) spaces or by venous sinus invasion. Extracranial spread of pituitary carcinomas involves both hematogenous and lymphatic routes. Invasion of the cavernous sinus provides the necessary venous access for transport of tumor cells to the internal jugular vein through the petrosal system. Whereas the pituitary lacks lymphatic drainage, invasion of the tumor into the skull base provides access to the rich lymphatic network, permitting systemic dissemination. Death from pituitary carcinoma usually is the consequence of extensive intracranial disease and not the result of extraneural deposits per se. Because neither the presence nor the treatment of systemic metastases appears to alter the prognosis of pituitary carcinomas, the frequency of metastases, particularly nonfunctioning ones, is likely underreported.

## CLASSIFICATION OF PITUITARY ADENOMAS BY HORMONE PRODUCTION[1,2,10]

Pituitary adenomas can be classified according to hormone production, on the basis of clinical presentation and blood hormone levels as assessed by radioimmunoassay. Thus, functioning adenomas, which produce GH, prolactin, ACTH, TSH, FSH, LH, or the α subunit, can be distinguished clinically from nonfunctioning adenomas, which are not associated with hormone excess. It is evident that all known adenohypophysial hormones can be secreted by pituitary adenoma cells.

A unifying pituitary adenoma classification encompasses histologic, immunocytochemical, and ultrastructural features of tumor cells and emphasizes the importance of hormone production, cellular composition, and cytogenesis. Such a classification stresses structure–function relationships and correlates the morphologic appearance of adenoma cells with their secretory activity.

All known adenohypophysial cell types can give rise to adenoma. The prevalence of each type is as follows: prolactin cell adenoma, 26%; null cell adenoma, 17%; GH cell adenoma, 14%; corticotrope cell adenoma, 15%; plurihormonal adenoma, 13%; oncocytoma, 6%; gonadotrope cell adenoma, 8%; and thyrotrope cell adenoma, 1%. The morphologic features of pituitary adenomas can reveal their cellular composition, hormone production, and, in some cases, cytogenesis.

**Growth Hormone Cell Adenomas.**   Growth hormone cell adenomas are associated with elevated blood GH concentrations and acromegaly or gigantism (see Chap. 12). On light microscopic examination they appear either acidophilic or chromophobic. On electron microscopic examination, acidophilic adenomas are *densely granulated*, and chromophobic adenomas are *sparsely granulated*. Separating these two subtypes has practical importance. Densely granulated tumors have a better prognosis; they have a slower growth rate, tend to be easier to remove surgically, and recur less frequently after surgery. The densely granulated adenoma cells resemble GH cells seen in the nontumorous pituitary and are characterized by well-developed, rough-surfaced endoplasmic reticulum, a conspicuous Golgi apparatus, and numerous spherical, evenly

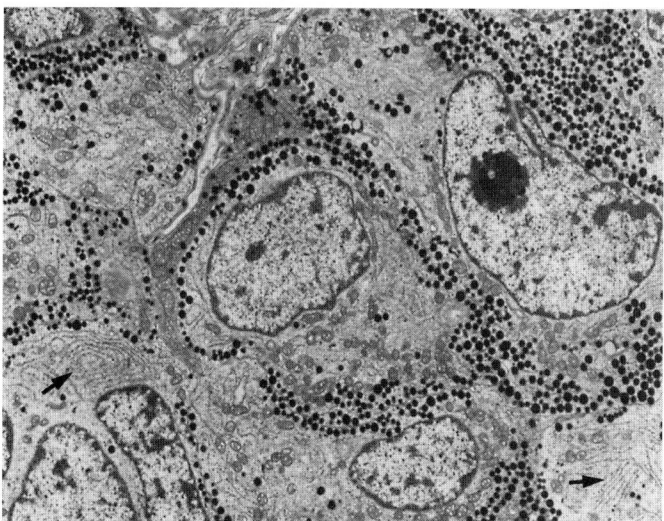

**FIGURE 11-7.** Ultrastructural features of densely granulated growth hormone cell adenoma. Note well-developed, rough-surfaced endoplasmic reticulum (*arrows*) and numerous large secretory granules. ×5600

electron-dense secretory granules measuring 250 to 650 nm (Fig. 11-7). The cells constituting sparsely granulated adenomas differ from GH cells of the nontumorous adenohypophysis. They possess irregular indented nuclei, rough-surfaced and smooth-surfaced endoplasmic reticulum, a conspicuous Golgi apparatus, several centrioles and cilia, fibrous bodies composed of microfilaments and smooth-walled tubules, and a few spherical, evenly electron-dense secretory granules measuring 100 to 300 nm (Fig. 11-8). No correlation has been noted between serum GH levels and granularity of the cell cytoplasm; both densely and sparsely granulated GH cell adenomas can be associated with markedly or slightly elevated GH levels as well as with severe and rapidly progressing or mild and slowly advancing acromegaly.

**Prolactin Cell Adenomas.**   Prolactin cell adenomas are associated with hyperprolactinemia, amenorrhea, galactorrhea, and infertility (see Chap. 13). In men, symptoms include decreased libido and impotence. In some cases, endocrine manifestations are subtle or absent, and only local symptoms call attention to a pituitary tumor. Markedly elevated serum prolactin levels (i.e., >150–200 ng/mL) confirm the clinical diagnosis of a prolactin-producing pituitary adenoma.

Prolactin-producing adenomas can occur at any age but most often are diagnosed in young women. Based on surgical material, women are more frequently affected than men, but in unselected adult autopsies, no sex difference can be demonstrated. Since the introduction of bromocriptine therapy, the number of prolactin-producing tumors treated surgically has declined.

Patients with prolactin cell adenomas can be effectively treated with various dopaminergic agonists. Depending on the sex of the patient, the treatment abolishes the amenorrhea, stops the galactorrhea, increases the libido, and cures the infertility (see Chap. 13); serum prolactin levels show a marked decline. The tumor regresses, as assessed by various imaging techniques. Local symptoms, such as visual disturbances, often disappear. The effects of treatment are reversible; if drug administration is discontinued, the tumor regrows, serum prolactin levels rise, and clinical symptoms reappear. As a result of bromocriptine medication, the tumor cells themselves decrease in size, indicating that tumor regression is mainly a result of a reduction in cell volume. In addition to an overall reduction in cytoplasmic volume, there also is a significant reduction in the volume density of the hormone's synthetic and secretory apparatus (rough endoplasmic reticulum and Golgi complex). Overall, this gives a hypercellular appearance to the tumor. The tumoristatic effects of bromocriptine are especially well visualized by electron microscopic examination, in which cells become irregularly shaped, contain heterochromatic nuclei, and maintain a scant cytoplasm with markedly involuted Golgi complexes. The size and volume density of secretory granules remain unaffected. All these ultrastructural changes are fully reversible on discontinuation of the drug. Prolonged exposure to bromocriptine also may result in fibrotic change within the tumor, an alteration that may adversely complicate surgical extirpation. The presence of cell necrosis after bromocriptine administration also has been reported. Whether bromocriptine is cytotoxic is difficult to assess because foci of necrosis, hemorrhage, and fibrosis may occur in prolactin-producing adenomas without dopaminergic agonist treatment.

HISTOPATHOLOGY.   Histologically, prolactin cell adenomas most often are chromophobic or slightly acidophilic, exhibiting distinct prolactin immunostaining in the Golgi complex and secretory granules. On electron microscopic examination, prolactin cell adenomas can be separated into densely granulated and sparsely granulated variants. Densely granulated prolactin cell adenomas are rare. The adenoma cells resemble nontumorous resting prolactin cells and are characterized by prominent rough-surfaced endoplasmic reticulum, conspicuous Golgi complexes, and numerous spherical, oval, or irregularly shaped secretory granules measuring up to 700 nm. Sparsely granulated prolactin cell adenomas are the most frequent tumor type in the human pituitary. The adenoma cells possess a prominent rough-surfaced endoplasmic reticulum, a conspicuous Golgi apparatus, and sparse, spherical, and oval, or irregularly shaped, evenly electron-dense secretory granules measuring 150 to 300 nm (Fig. 11-9). The rough-surfaced endoplasmic reticulum membranes form concentric cytoplasmic whorls, called *nebenkerns*. Another characteristic ultrastructural feature of prolactin cell adenomas is the presence of *misplaced exocytosis*—extrusion of secretory granules on the lateral side of the cell, distant from capillaries and intercellular extensions of the basement membrane. Granule extrusion also occurs on the capillary side of prolactin cells.

Prolactin cell adenomas may produce an amyloid-like substance and exhibit various degrees of calcification, sometimes so extensive as to be visible with imaging techniques. Amyloid deposition and calcification are characteristic but not pathognomonic; they most frequently occur in prolactin cell adenomas but occasionally may be present in other adenoma types.

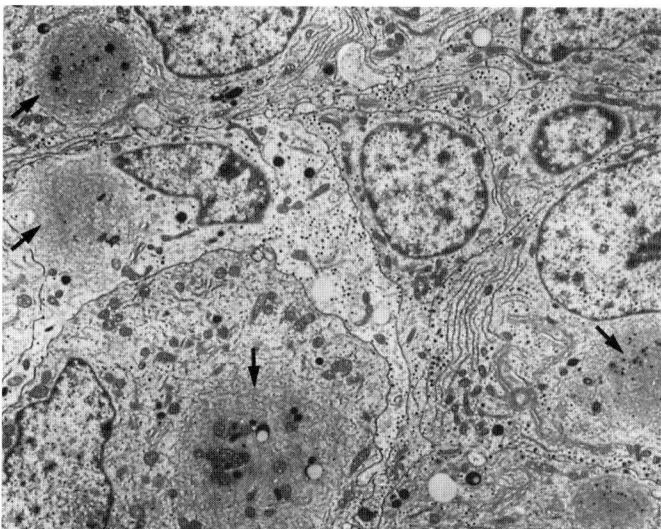

**FIGURE 11-8.** Sparsely granulated growth hormone–producing adenoma with fibrous bodies (*arrows*). The secretory granules are sparse and small. ×5600

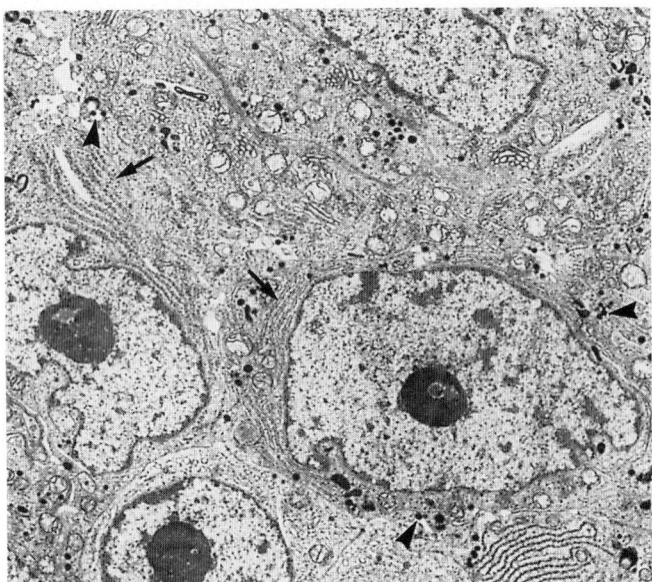

**FIGURE 11-9.** Sparsely granulated prolactin cell adenoma with prominent rough-surfaced endoplasmic reticulum membranes (*arrows*) and misplaced exocytosis (extrusion of secretory granules into the extracellular space, distant from the basement membrane; *arrowheads*). ×7800

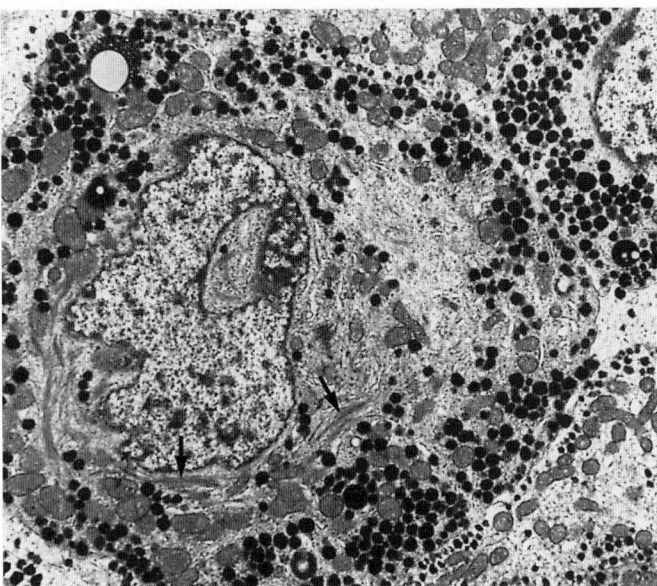

**FIGURE 11-10.** Electron microscopic appearance of densely granulated corticotrope cell adenoma. Note the irregular or dented shape of secretory granules and bundles of type I filaments (*arrows*). ×9800

**Corticotrope Adenomas.** Corticotrope adenomas produce ACTH and other peptides of the pro-opiomelanocortin molecule, such as β-LPH and endorphins. They may secrete hormones excessively and may be associated with Cushing disease or Nelson syndrome (see Chap. 75). In Cushing disease, the excess ACTH stimulates the adrenal cortex and causes various degrees of hypercortisolism. Historically, bilateral adrenalectomy was undertaken because the ACTH-producing pituitary adenoma either was unrecognized or was unsuccessfully treated. With the development of increasingly precise imaging technology and superior microsurgical techniques, bilateral adrenalectomy is now a procedure of last resort that is rarely required in the management of Cushing disease. Accordingly, new cases of Nelson syndrome are becoming increasingly uncommon. When bilateral adrenalectomy is necessary to control refractory Cushing disease, the clinical picture is characteristic. As hypercortisolism regresses, the tumor frequently behaves in a "disinhibited" fashion, tending to grow more rapidly and to produce large amounts of ACTH and other pro-opiomelanocortin–derived peptides. Patients become hyperpigmented, and the tumor tends to be far more aggressive and invasive than are those corticotropic adenomas that have an intact pituitary-adrenal axis. Furthermore, only a few patients with Nelson syndrome are cured by surgery and radiotherapy; up to 20% of these patients succumb to uncontrolled local tumor growth. Such aggressive behavior has been ascribed to the loss of negative glucocorticoid feedback resulting from the adrenalectomy; this suggests that corticotrope adenomas, as a whole, are not entirely autonomous, but are subject to feedback and modulation of their secretory activity and growth rate by glucocorticoid hormones.

Importantly, more than 80% of the adenomas responsible for Cushing disease are microadenomas. Because many are only a few millimeters in diameter, they frequently evade detection, even with the most sophisticated imaging techniques. Given their small size, these tumors present technical difficulties, both to surgeons and to pathologists. From a surgical standpoint, corticotrope microadenomas rarely are situated on the surface of the gland and are exposed only after a thorough dissection of a seemingly normal gland. Most arise in the midline of the pituitary, within the so-called *mucoid wedge*, an area in which corticotropes are most numerous. The surgical specimen provided to the pathologist frequently is small and fragmented; as a

result, considerable patience and skill are required to differentiate adenomatous elements from the normal glandular tissue. Whereas 10% to 15% of microadenomas demonstrate local invasion, fully 60% of macroadenomas are grossly invasive.

HISTOPATHOLOGY. Histologically, corticotrope adenomas usually are basophilic and exhibit various degrees of PAS and lead-hematoxylin positivity. Immunoperoxidase staining reveals ACTH and other fragments of the pro-opiomelanocortin molecule in the cytoplasm of adenoma cells. On electron microscopic examination, adenomatous corticotropes often resemble nonadenomatous corticotropes; they possess well-developed, rough-surfaced endoplasmic reticulum, prominent Golgi apparatuses, and numerous spherical secretory granules that vary in electron density, often line up along the cell membrane, and measure 250 to 700 nm (Fig. 11-10). In corticotrope adenomas removed from patients with Cushing disease, bundles of microfilaments usually are present, whereas in adenomas removed from patients with Nelson syndrome, microfilaments are inconspicuous or absent. Otherwise, no ultrastructural differences exist between the corticotrope adenomas of patients with Cushing disease and Nelson syndrome.

A few actively secreting corticotrope adenomas are chromophobic and possess only sparse, fine, PAS-positive cytoplasmic granules. These tumors immunostain for ACTH and related peptides, indicating that they arise in and consist of corticotropes. On electron microscopic examination, chromophobic corticotrope adenoma cells are sparsely granulated and appear less differentiated than their basophilic, densely granulated counterparts. Chromophobic tumors usually are larger, grow faster, tend to be invasive, and recur more frequently than basophilic adenomas, which generally are small, measuring only a few millimeters in diameter.

**Silent Corticotrope Adenomas.**[1,2,10,22] Silent corticotrope adenomas immunostain for ACTH and related peptides but are not associated with clinical or biochemical evidence of ACTH excess. On light microscopic examination, these tumors are basophilic or chromophobic, show various degrees of PAS positivity, and immunostain for ACTH, β-LPH, and endorphins. On electron microscopic examination, silent corticotrope cell adenomas are a heterogeneous group. In some cases, the ultrastructural features of tumor cells are indistinguishable from those of actively secreting tumors, such as are associated with Cushing disease or Nelson syndrome. In other cases, an increase in the size and number of lysosomes, *crinophagy* (uptake of secretory granules by lysosomes), and marked underdevelopment or involution of the Golgi apparatus suggest a defect in various steps involving hormone synthesis, packaging, or discharge. Two distinct silent corticotrope adenomas, designated *silent corticotrope adenomas subtypes I and II*, have been identified as specific clinicopathologic entities. A third, no longer considered corticotropic in nature, is designated *silent subtype III*. For the most part, silent subtypes I through III present clinically as large and invasive nonfunctioning sellar masses.[1,17] In some instances, hyperprolactinemia is present, sometimes at a level higher than that attributable to the stalk section effect. Accordingly, it has been suggested that some silent subtypes may facilitate prolactin release from nontumorous lactotropes or are themselves capable of prolactin secretion. These findings are particularly applicable to silent subtype III, a tumor frequently seen in women, and therefore often is diagnosed before operation as a prolactinoma. The reason that some silent subtype III tumors have been responsible for acromegaly remains a total mystery. A peculiarity of silent subtype tumors relates to their propensity to undergo apoplectic hemorrhage. In the experience of the authors, more than 40% of silent subtype adenomas presented in this fashion.[22] In all, the silent subtype tumors are enigmatic entities, whose cytogenesis and overall biology warrants further study.

**Thyrotrope Adenomas.** With fewer than 100 cases reported, TSH-secreting adenomas are the least common pituitary tumor phenotype, accounting for only 1% of all pituitary adenomas. Of reported cases, most thyrotrope adenomas have been large, aggressive macroadenomas, both compressive and invasive of surrounding structures.[73] Usually, the accompanying clinical history is remarkable for some form of thyroid dysfunction. It once was believed that most arose in the context of long-standing primary hypothyroidism, presumably by way of feedback inhibitory loss, induction of thyrotrope hyperplasia, and, later, adenoma formation. Although such a perspective was compatible with earlier experimental studies in which thyroidectomy induced pituitary thyrotrope adenomas in rodents, careful clinicopathologic correlations of human thyrotrope adenomas indicate an alternate sequence of likely events.[10,23] In many patients, the initial manifestations appear to be those of hyperthyroidism and goiter, events wholly compatible with TSH hypersecretion by the tumor. Because secondary (i.e., pituitary-dependent) hyperthyroidism previously was not a well-recognized condition, many such patients were incorrectly thought to have primary hyperthyroidism and were subjected to some form of thyroid ablation. This served to ameliorate symptoms, but sometimes was followed later by accelerated tumor growth, optic nerve compression, or recurrence of the hyperthyroid state. Only then was the pituitary correctly identified as the site of pathologic involvement. The invasive nature of these tumors appears to be related to two factors, the first of which is the typical diagnostic delay. A more cogent factor, however, is the loss of feedback inhibition. In the same way that end-organ ablation contributes to tumor aggressiveness in the context of Nelson syndrome, similar disinhibiting influences may be operative in the progression of TSH adenomas in the setting of prior thyroidectomy. The routine availability of sensitive TSH assays coupled with general awareness of the thyrotrope adenoma as a potential, though rare, cause of hyperthyroidism should permit more expeditious diagnosis of this tumor type, perhaps while it is still in the microadenoma stage.[67] Furthermore, thyrotrope adenomas commonly cosecrete in excess a free $\alpha$ subunit that, if present, may be a helpful diagnostic clue suggesting a pituitary source over a primary thyroid cause of hyperthyroidism (see Chaps. 15 and 42).

HISTOPATHOLOGY. On light microscopic examination, thyrotrope adenomas are chromophobic, containing a few small cytoplasmic granules mainly at the cell periphery that stain for PAS, aldehyde fuchsin, and aldehyde thionin. TSH can be demonstrated immunocytologically in the cytoplasm of the adenoma cells. Occasionally, immunostaining shows only slight or no TSH immunopositivity, suggesting that little hormone is stored in the cytoplasm or that abnormal TSH is produced that is not immunoreactive but may have bioactivity. On electron microscopic examination, thyrotrope adenomas consist of elongated, angular, or irregular cells with long cytoplasmic processes, scanty rough-surfaced endoplasmic reticulum, an inconspicuous Golgi apparatus, and numerous microtubules. Secretory granules are sparse and spherical, vary slightly in electron density, line up along the cell membrane, and measure 50 to 200 nm. Thyrotrope adenomas often differ in their ultrastructural appearance from nontumorous thyrotropes. In some cases, they consist of highly differentiated thyrotropes with an abundant, slightly dilated, rough-surfaced endoplasmic reticulum, a conspicuous Golgi apparatus, and varying numbers of secretory granules in the range of 50 to 250 nm.

**Gonadotrope Adenomas.** Gonadotrope adenomas produce FSH, FSH and LH, or, rarely, LH alone. They are identified more frequently in older patients. The clinical manifestations of gonadotrope cell adenomas are not clearly defined; patients may show varying degrees of hypogonadism, decreased libido, impotence, and elevated serum FSH/LH concentrations.

HISTOPATHOLOGY. On light microscopic examination, gonadotrope adenomas appear chromophobic and may contain sparse PAS-positive cytoplasmic granules. Immunostaining reveals FSH, LH, or both in the cytoplasm of adenoma cells. On electron microscopic examination, sexual dichotomy is evident. In men, adenomatous gonadotropes usually are less differentiated and have a few rough-surfaced endoplasmic reticulum membranes, a moderately developed Golgi apparatus, several microtubules, and sparse, spherical secretory granules that vary slightly in electron density, line up along the cell membrane, and measure 100 to 300 nm. In women, adenomatous gonadotropes are more differentiated and resemble their nontumorous counterparts. The prominent honeycomb-like Golgi complex consists of several dilated sacculi and vesicles containing a few immature secretory granules. Secretory granules are sparse and randomly distributed, vary slightly in electron density, and measure 50 to 150 nm.

**Null Cell Adenomas.** Null cell adenomas have no histologic, immunocytologic, or electron microscopic markers and are not associated clinically and biochemically with any known hormone excess. Although these tumors are endocrinologically inactive and contain no known hormones, they possess the organelles necessary for hormone secretion and have secretory granules.[1] It may be that these tumors produce biologically inactive hormone fragments, precursor molecules, or hormones unidentified at present.

Together, null cell adenomas and their oncocytic variants (discussed later) account for almost one-fourth of all pituitary adenomas. Both are nonfunctioning sellar masses and are typically seen during middle or old age. They tend to be slow-growing lesions, with some likely growing for years subclinically before manifesting themselves clinically. Despite the regularity with which these tumors are encountered in clinical practice, and the fact that their existence has been known for almost two decades, fundamental questions concerning their causation, cytogenesis, and biology remain unanswered.[2,10,74] That these tumors frequently share morphologic similarities with undifferentiated gonadotrope adenomas has fueled speculation that null cell adenomas may be neoplastic offshoots of gonadotropic lineage. Compelling support for such a notion was provided by the finding that 80% of null cell adenomas and oncocytomas express glycoprotein hormone genes.[10] Furthermore, both gonadotropin release and gonadotropin-releasing hormone responsiveness have been demonstrated in null cell adenomas maintained in tissue culture. Alternatively, there is preliminary evidence favoring the existence of nonneoplastic null cells scat-

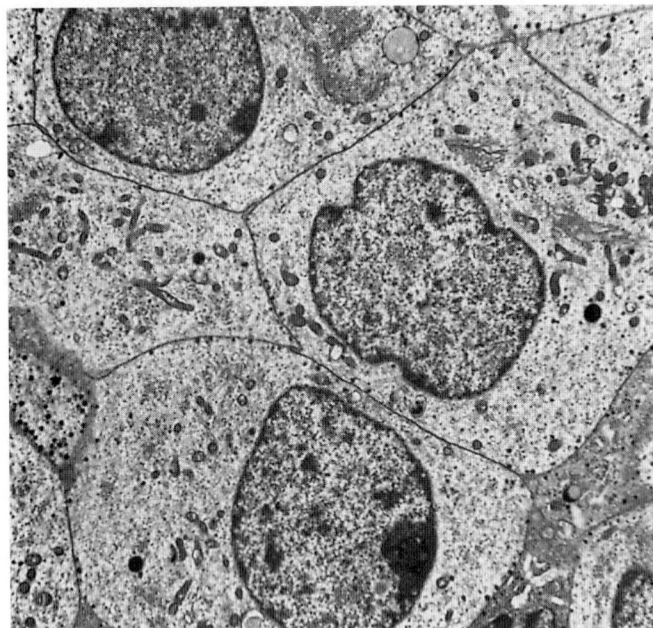

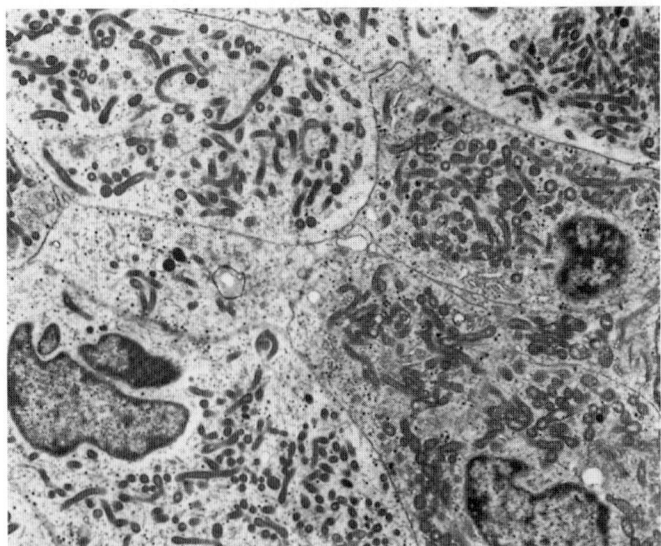

**FIGURE 11-12.** Pituitary oncocytoma showing abundance of mitochondria. ×7000

**FIGURE 11-11.** Null cell adenoma. The small adenoma cells contain poorly developed cytoplasmic organelles and sparse, small secretory granules. ×9800

tered throughout the normal pituitary.[75] It is speculated that such "normal" null cells may be transitional, undifferentiated, or precursor cells that are capable of shifting from hormonally inactive to hormonally active states. Should null cells be validated as cellular constituents of the normal pituitary, null cell adenomas could be envisioned as their neoplastic derivatives.

**HISTOPATHOLOGIC CHARACTERISTICS.** On light microscopic examination, null cell adenomas are chromophobic; immunocytologically, they contain no adenohypophysial hormones. In many tumors, however, small groups of adenoma cells or randomly scattered individual cells immunostain for one or more pituitary hormones, most frequently FSH or the α subunit, less frequently TSH, LH, and prolactin, and occasionally GH or ACTH. Consistent with these findings, in vitro studies reveal that most null cell adenomas produce FSH, TSH, LH, or the α subunit; these hormones can be demonstrated by radioimmunoassay in tumor culture. It is not clear whether this means multidirectional differentiation from an uncommitted precursor, tumor cell heterogeneity, or gradual dedifferentiation. On electron microscopic examination, null cell adenomas are characterized by closely apposed, polyhedral or irregularly shaped cells with pleomorphic or indented nuclei and poorly developed cytoplasm possessing a few rough endoplasmic reticulum profiles, a moderately developed Golgi apparatus, and microtubules, which may be abundant in some cells. The secretory granules are sparse and spherical, vary slightly in electron density, line up along the cell membrane, and measure 100 to 200 nm (Fig. 11-11). Oncocytic transformation (i.e., the increase of cytoplasmic volume occupied by mitochondria) is common in null cell adenomas.

Because of the lack of endocrine symptoms, some null cell adenomas are recognized only when they enlarge and spread outside the sella, causing local symptoms such as visual disturbances, headache, or injury of cranial nerves.

**Oncocytomas.** Oncocytomas represent the oncocytic variant of null cell adenomas. The term *oncocytosis* is used to describe tumor cells that exhibit intracellular mitochondrial accumulation. Thus, oncocytomas differ from null cell adenomas only insofar as the cells of the former contain massive numbers of large mitochondria. Both tumors share a similar clinical profile that is dominated by the neurologic and endocrinologic sequelae of an expansile, nonfunctioning sellar mass.

Like null cell adenomas, oncocytomas are unaccompanied by clinical or biochemical evidence of oversecretion of adenohypophysial hormones, have no morphologic markers that would reveal their cytogenesis, occur most frequently in older men and women, and are rarely diagnosed in patients younger than 40 years.

**HISTOPATHOLOGY.** On light microscopic examination, oncocytomas are chromophobic or acidophilic. The acidophilia is not the result of staining of secretory granules but of the uptake of acid dyes by accumulating mitochondria. Immunostaining of oncocytoma cells fails to demonstrate pituitary hormones. In many cases, however, small groups of adenoma cells or randomly scattered individual cells immunostain for FSH, the alpha subunit, LH, or TSH, indicating that oncocytoma cells do not lose their potential to produce hormones or that they can differentiate to a hormone-producing cell line. Electron microscopic examination reveals abundant cytoplasmic mitochondria (Fig. 11-12), which may be extensive, filling as much as 50% of the cytoplasm (compared with ~8% normally). In some tumors, a transition can be seen between null cell adenoma and oncocytoma. The authors use the term *oncocytoma* only when abundant mitochondria are evident in practically every adenoma cell.

**Plurihormonal Adenomas.** Plurihormonal adenomas produce more than one hormone and can be divided into *monomorphous* and *plurimorphous* types. Monomorphous plurihormonal adenomas consist of one morphologically distinct cell type that produces two or more hormones; the cell may differ morphologically from known adenohypophysial cells. Plurimorphous plurihormonal adenomas are composed of two or more morphologically distinct cell types, each producing different hormones; they are similar in ultrastructural appearance to their nontumorous counterparts. Immunocytologic techniques are required to establish the diagnosis. Electron microscopic examination may fail to reveal the cellular origin of the adenoma because ultrastructural features may not be distinct or the tumor may consist of cells not recognized in nontumorous adenohypophyses.

In the experience of the authors, 12% of surgically removed pituitary adenomas are plurihormonal. The most frequent hormonal combination produced is GH and prolactin. Three morphologically distinct adenoma types produce GH and prolactin simultaneously: acidophil stem cell adenoma, mammosomatotrope adenoma, and mixed GH cell–prolactin adenoma.

**ACIDOPHIL STEM CELL ADENOMAS.** Acidophil stem cell adenomas grow rapidly, often spreading into neighboring tissues.

They are associated with various degrees of hyperprolactinemia. In some patients, clinical features of acromegaly may be apparent despite normal serum GH levels. Acidophil stem cell adenomas are monomorphous, bihormonal tumors that consist of one cell type, which is assumed to represent the common progenitor of GH cells and prolactin cells. Immunocytologic techniques demonstrate both prolactin and GH in the cytoplasm of the same adenoma cells. Immunostaining for GH often is weak or absent. On electron microscopic examination, acidophil stem cell adenomas are composed of closely apposed elongated cells with irregular nuclei and well-developed cytoplasm containing dispersed, short profiles of rough-surfaced endoplasmic reticulum, an inconspicuous Golgi apparatus, fibrous bodies containing microfilaments and smooth-walled tubules, multiple centrioles and cilia, and sparse, irregular secretory granules measuring 100 to 300 nm. Some exocytosis may be evident. Oncocytic change and mitochondrial gigantism occur in most tumors. The correlation between tumor size and blood prolactin concentrations, which is apparent in patients with sparsely granulated prolactin cell adenomas, is often absent in patients with acidophil stem cell adenomas; relatively large tumors may be accompanied by only slight or moderate hyperprolactinemia.

MAMMOSOMATOTROPE CELL ADENOMAS.   Mammosomatotrope cell adenomas are slowly growing tumors accompanied by elevated serum GH concentrations, acromegaly, and, in some cases, mild hyperprolactinemia. These monomorphous, bihormonal tumors consist of acidophilic cells. Immunocytologic methods demonstrate GH and prolactin in the cytoplasm of the same adenoma cells. On electron microscopic examination, the adenoma cells appear to be well differentiated and resemble densely granulated GH cells. The secretory granules are often irregular; they may be evenly electron dense or have a mottled appearance, and they measure 200 to 2000 nm. Exocytosis and large extracellular deposits of secretory material are characteristic features.

MIXED GROWTH HORMONE CELL–PROLACTIN CELL ADENOMAS.   Mixed GH cell–prolactin cell adenomas are associated with elevated serum GH levels, acromegaly, hyperprolactinemia, and, occasionally, galactorrhea, amenorrhea, decreased libido, and impotence. These bimorphous, bihormonal tumors are composed of two morphologically distinct cell types: densely or sparsely granulated GH cells and prolactin cells. The two cell types form small groups; in several areas, individual cells are interspersed. Immunostaining demonstrates GH and prolactin in the two different cell populations. Electron microscopic examination shows two morphologically distinct cell types. Every combination may occur; most frequently, densely granulated GH cells and sparsely granulated prolactin cells are identified.

UNUSUAL PLURIHORMONAL ADENOMAS.   Occasional, unusual plurihormonal pituitary adenomas produce bizarre combinations of two or more hormones, such as GH and TSH; prolactin and TSH; GH, prolactin, and TSH; and, less frequently, GH, prolactin, and ACTH, or GH, prolactin, FSH/LH, and the α subunit. Such tumors may be monomorphous or plurimorphous. The cell type or types constituting the tumors often cannot be identified, even with detailed electron microscopic investigation. In a few cases, however, two or more ultrastructurally distinct cell types resembling their nontumorous counterparts can be recognized. The hormone content and ultrastructural features of adenomas cannot always be correlated.

On light microscopic examination, the unusual plurihormonal adenomas consist of chromophobic, acidophilic, or basophilic cells, or a mixture of cells that stain differently with different histologic techniques. Clinically and biochemically, the secretion of several hormones may be apparent; acromegaly may be accompanied by hyperthyroidism, hypercorticism, or hyperprolactinemia. Some components may be silent. Immunostaining demonstrates hormones in the cell cytoplasm, but hormone production is not always reflected in hypersecretory symptoms clinically, or in increased serum hormone levels.

Plurihormonal adenomas, which are difficult to classify, clearly show that the one cell–one hormone theory, which has dominated pituitary cytophysiology and cytopathology for many years, is oversimplified and requires revision.

Beyond the conceptual importance underlying the phenomenon of plurihormonality is a potentially important clinical issue. Although unproven, there is some suggestion that some plurihormonal tumors behave more aggressively than do their monohormonal counterparts.[10,75,76] In the case of other endocrine tumors (e.g., pancreatic tumors, medullary carcinoma of the thyroid), plurihormonal tumors are thought to portend a more malignant course than that of monohormonal tumors. Evidence in support of a similar occurrence in the pituitary remains inconclusive. It is known, however, that most plurihormonal pituitary adenomas are macroadenomas at presentation, even in the presence of a hypersecretory syndrome. Furthermore, ~50% of all plurihormonal pituitary adenomas are grossly invasive at the time of diagnosis.[76]

## MALIGNANT PITUITARY LESIONS

### PRIMARY MALIGNANT NEOPLASMS

Primary malignant neoplasms of the hypophysis include carcinomas and sarcomas; they are extremely rare.

**Primary Adenohypophysial Carcinomas.**   Primary adenohypophysial carcinomas, which are derived from anterior pituitary cells, may secrete GH, prolactin, or ACTH or may not be associated with hormone production. They are rare and were discussed earlier. Electron microscopic and immunocytologic studies fail to distinguish between benign and malignant tumors.

**Sarcomas.**   Sarcomas of the adenohypophysis include fibrosarcoma, osteosarcoma, and undifferentiated sarcoma. With few exceptions, virtually all have occurred after radiotherapy for either pituitary adenoma, craniopharyngioma, or retinoblastoma. Fibrosarcomas, in particular, are most commonly the consequence of radiotherapy to a pituitary adenoma. Histologically, these tumors exhibit marked cellular and nuclear pleomorphism, replete with mitotic figures, areas of necrosis, and hemorrhage. In many instances, the sarcomatous component can be seen to be intimately admixed within the substance of a persistent pituitary adenoma. Thus, it has been suggested that radiotherapy induces fibrosarcoma formation by transforming fibroblastic elements within the original adenoma. The latency period for sarcomatous transformation is variable; an average period of 11 years has been reported.[10,19] Postirradiation sarcomas are virtually always high-grade malignancies typified by rapid growth, relentless local invasion, and a survival period rarely exceeding a few months.

### SECONDARY NEOPLASMS

Secondary neoplasms of the pituitary most often are found incidentally at autopsy and are not associated with clinical symptoms or biochemical abnormalities. They occur in 1% to 5% of patients with cancer. The most commonly observed endocrine abnormality is diabetes insipidus (see Chap. 26), which occurs in patients with metastatic carcinoma of the posterior lobe, hypophysial stalk, or hypothalamus. Compression or destruction of the production site of hypothalamic releasing and suppressing hormones or interference with adenohypophysial blood flow (either by blocking transport of hypothalamic hormones to the adenohypophysis or by inducing ischemia) also may account for the development of endocrine symptoms. Local symptoms may be apparent; however, anterior hypopituitarism is rare because a substantial part of the adenohypophysis must be destroyed before a decrease in adenohypophysial hormone secretion becomes manifest clinically and biochemically. Hypophysial metastases usually occur at an advanced stage of neoplastic disease, when the malignant process involves several organs. Affected patients rarely live long enough to develop anterior hypopituitarism. Only rarely are symptoms of pituitary metastases the first manifestation of a systemic malignancy.[77]

Hypophysial metastases may come from different primary sources, such as carcinomas of the bronchus, colon, prostate, larynx, or kidney; malignant melanoma; sarcomas; and hematologic malignancies. In the last of these categories, plasmacytoma is notorious for its periodic presentation in the sellar region. Many plasmacytomas of the sellar region have occurred in the absence of known systemic disease, presenting as seemingly ordinary pituitary adenomas. Regardless of therapy, most eventually evolve into full-blown multiple myeloma. For women, carcinoma of the breast is the most common primary lesion that metastasizes to the pituitary. In men, carcinoma of the lung is the most culpable primary tumor.

Metastases to the posterior lobe are more frequent than to the anterior lobe, presumably because the posterior lobe has a rich direct arterial blood supply. Metastatic tumor deposits usually occur first in the pituitary stalk or posterior lobe and permeate the anterior lobe, either by direct extension from the hypophysial stalk or posterior lobe, or through the portal circulation, by long or short portal vessels. However, isolated metastases may occur in the anterior lobe, indicating that the secondary tumor in the adenohypophysis is not invariably the result of prior involvement of the posterior lobe and hypophysial stalk; in the genesis of adenohypophysial metastases, routes other than the portal circulation must be considered. Tumor cells may also spread from perihypophysial tissues to the pituitary.

In patients with disseminated carcinomatosis, infiltration of long portal vessels by carcinoma cells leads to vascular occlusion and subsequent ischemia, causing adenohypophysial infarcts. The necrotic foci are not large enough to cause hypopituitarism.

## CRANIOPHARYNGIOMAS

Craniopharyngiomas are histologically benign tumors that are thought to arise from remnants of the Rathke pouch. Such embryonic squamous cell "nests" extend from the tuber cinereum to the pituitary gland, presumably along the track of an incompletely involuted hypophysial-pharyngeal duct. By virtue of their location, craniopharyngiomas simultaneously compromise the function of several intracranial structures and produce numerous clinical effects, including vision loss, anterior and posterior pituitary dysfunction, and increased intracranial pressure. Despite their "benign" nature, craniopharyngiomas can offer considerable resistance to successful treatment.

Craniopharyngiomas account for ~3% of intracranial tumors. They primarily affect children, for whom they represent the most common nonglial brain tumor and 10% of all intracranial neoplasms. The age-related incidence of craniopharyngiomas is bimodal, with a major, early peak between 5 and 10 years of age, and a second, smaller peak between 50 and 60 years of age. A slight male preponderance has generally been noted.

Topologically, most craniopharyngiomas are suprasellar in location. Those so situated can compress the optic apparatus, cause hydrocephalus by indenting the third ventricle, encroach on hypothalamic structures, distort the infundibulum and pituitary, and penetrate cerebrospinal fluid spaces to gain access to the middle and posterior cranial fossae. Twenty percent of craniopharyngiomas originate within the sella, producing sellar enlargement in a fashion similar to that produced by pituitary adenomas. Almost half of all craniopharyngiomas are cystic, 15% are solid, and the remainder are made up of both solid and cystic elements. Although generally well circumscribed, craniopharyngiomas are not encapsulated lesions and therefore are often tenaciously adherent to basal neural and vascular structures. It is this feature of craniopharyngiomas that frequently undermines successful attempts at a safe and curative resection.

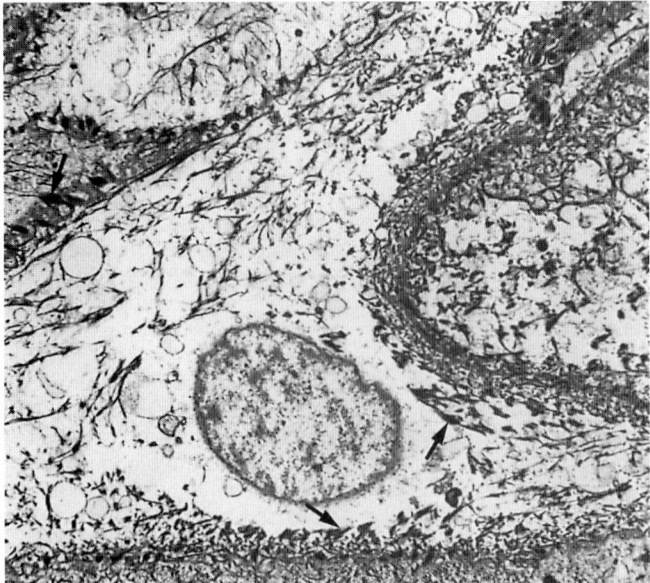

**FIGURE 11-13.** Epithelial component of craniopharyngioma showing tonofilaments (*arrows*) and absence of secretory granules. ×8000

There has been an increasing tendency to view craniopharyngiomas as being either classically *adamantinomatous* or *papillary* in nature, which is a distinction that some believe to be of clinical, pathologic, and prognostic significance.[78,79]

**Adamantinomatous Craniopharyngioma.** Adamantinomatous craniopharyngioma represents the classic cystic craniopharyngioma of childhood. It frequently is a bulky, partially calcified tumor that tenaciously insinuates itself around basal brain structures. On gross sectioning, it oozes a viscid admixture of shimmering cholesterol crystals and calcific desquamated debris that, in appearance and consistency, often is described as "machinery oil." On light microscopic examination, this variant exhibits an intricate pattern of epithelial growth, including intermixed islands of solid and cystic epithelium within a matrix of variably cellular connective tissue. Nests or cords of columnar and squamous epithelial cells can be demonstrated. Lymphocytes, macrophages, clusters of foamy cells, cholesterol crystals, keratin deposits, necrotic debris, and polymorphonuclear leukocytes often are present. Calcification, ranging from areas visible only with a microscope to palpable concretions, is common. Rarely, frank bone formation may be present. Cyst formation is presumably the result of degeneration of squamous cells, accumulation of keratinous debris, and perivascular stromal degeneration. The results of immunohistochemical studies are conclusively negative for adenohypophysial hormones, indicating that craniopharyngiomas do not originate in adenohypophysial cells and are not capable of hormone production. The results of immunostaining for keratin are positive. Electron microscopic examination shows bundles of tonofilaments, prominent desmosomal attachments, and an absence of secretory granules (Fig. 11-13).

**Papillary Craniopharyngioma.** The clinical, radiologic, and pathologic profile of papillary craniopharyngioma deviates considerably from that of the conventional adamantinomatous variant.[78,79] Accounting for ~10% of all craniopharyngiomas, the papillary variant occurs almost exclusively in adults. It usually is suprasellar in location and frequently involves, or arises within, the third ventricle. Most papillary variants are solid or have only a relatively minor cystic component. Papillary craniopharyngiomas are more discretely circumscribed than classic craniopharyngiomas and lack the calcification and "machinery oil" content so typical of adamantinomatous tumors. Liquid contents, although rarely present, generally are clear. Lacking tenacious adhesions to basal brain structures, the papillary craniopharyngioma is reputed to be more readily separable from surrounding structures. Histologically, it consists of a well-differentiated, albeit less complex, epithelial pattern than that of the adamantinomatous variant. Prominent, stratified, squamous-lined papillae, devoid of columnar palisading, microcystic degeneration, calcification, keratinous nodules, and cholesterol clefts, are characteristic. Whereas the papillary variant is regarded by some as being more amenable to complete and curative resection, not all are in agreement with this view.[78–81]

Both forms of craniopharyngioma are histologically benign. Mitotic figures and other features of histologic aggressiveness generally are not seen. Despite their histologic benignity, craniopharyngiomas, particularly the adamantinomatous type, are notorious for their high rate of postoperative recurrence. Even among tumors resected radically, a procedure sometimes accompanied by considerable functional deficit, recurrence rates as high as 25% have been reported. For lesser degrees of resection, recurrence of symptoms is virtually guaranteed, often within 3 years of surgery. Radiotherapy for incompletely excised lesions has proved effective in forestalling recurrence (see Chap. 22). Malignant transformation is exquisitely rare; only a single case of malignant craniopharyngioma has been described.

Craniopharyngiomas, both adamantinomatous and papillary, have been shown to express estrogen receptor mRNA and protein. The significance of this finding remains to be determined.[82]

**Rathke Cleft Cysts.** Rathke cleft cysts are epithelial cysts apparently derived from remnants of the Rathke pouch. At autopsy, roughly one-fifth of pituitaries contain macroscopic remnants of the Rathke pouch in the form of discontinuous cystic remnants or microscopic clefts at the interface of the anterior and posterior lobes. Occasionally, these Rathke cleft remnants, as the result of progressive accumulation of colloidal secretions, become sufficiently large and compress surrounding structures. Most cases involving symptoms present as expansile intrasellar masses, occasionally having a suprasellar component. Only exceptionally are they entirely suprasellar in location. Local compressive effects are the basis for presentation in most cases involving symptoms, with headache, hypopituitarism, hyperprolactinemia, visual disturbance, and, rarely, diabetes insipidus being the principal clinical features.[83]

Rathke cleft cysts are thin-walled, uniloculate, and filled with fluid, the composition of which ranges from watery to mucinous. The cyst wall frequently is composed of a single layer of cuboidal or columnar, ciliated, or mucin-producing epithelium. Small numbers of adenohypophysial cells also may be evident. Calcification is rare, as is amyloid deposition. Although the epithelial pattern is considerably less complex than that of craniopharyngioma, the distinction between these two entities occasionally can be troublesome, emphasizing the importance of generous tissue sampling. Rarely, pituitary adenomas can be found to be admixed with elements of a Rathke cleft cyst. Such biopsy results usually represent the simultaneous sampling of two distinct lesions. Even rarer are more complex lesions, in which Rathke cyst components are intimately associated with adenoma and even squamous metaplasia; such lesions have been termed *transitional cell tumors of the pituitary*. Whether these are distinct clinicopathologic entities or simply the collision of two distinct lesions remains to be determined.

Rathke cleft cysts are definitively treated by drainage and marsupialization of the cyst wall, a procedure that usually results in cure. Recurrences are unusual.

# PATHOLOGY OF THE NEUROHYPOPHYSIS AND HYPOTHALAMUS[2,4,10,19]

Clinically significant diseases of the posterior lobe are rare. Endocrinologically, they can be divided into conditions associated with increased or decreased vasopressin secretion. Several abnormalities are unaccompanied by endocrine alterations.

## INAPPROPRIATE SECRETION OF VASOPRESSIN

Inappropriate secretion of vasopressin, or the Schwartz-Bartter syndrome, is the result of vasopressin hypersecretion, either from the posterior pituitary or from extrahypophysial neoplasms (see Chaps. 27 and 219). Renal sodium loss and hyponatremia are characteristic features. Several diseases, including meningitis, myxedema, and cerebral lesions, may be associated with increased vasopressin discharge. Paraneoplastic ("ectopic") vasopressin secretion may occur in various neoplasms, but is seen mainly in carcinoma of the bronchus. Vasopressin can be extracted from the extrapituitary tumors of patients with vasopressin excess, providing evidence for paraneoplastic ("ectopic") production of the hormone.

## DIABETES INSIPIDUS

Diabetes insipidus is characterized clinically by polyuria and polydipsia (see Chap. 26). In most cases it is caused by vasopressin deficiency resulting from the destruction of supraoptic and paraventricular nuclei, which is where vasopressin is synthesized, or by organic damage to the hypophysial stalk or posterior lobe, which is the site of vasopressin discharge. Morphologically, various lesions can be seen in the hypothalamus, especially in the nucleus supraopticus or along the supraopticohypophysial tract. Selective destruction of the posterior lobe results in only moderate and temporary polyuria and polydipsia. Causes include lesions resulting from head trauma, transection of the hypophysial stalk, meningoencephalitis, sarcoidosis, granulomas, Langerhans histiocytosis, primary tumors, metastatic carcinomas, lymphomas, and leukemias. Of note, pituitary adenomas, including large and invasive ones, are virtually never accompanied by diabetes insipidus as an initial feature of the tumor. The preoperative presence of diabetes insipidus in association with a sellar region mass argues strongly against a diagnosis of pituitary adenoma, however suggestive the imaging studies may be. In *idiopathic diabetes insipidus*, no destructive lesions can be recognized grossly in the hypothalamus, hypophysial stalk, or posterior pituitary. Histologically, nerve cells of the supraoptic and paraventricular nuclei may show a marked reduction in number and size and loss of stainable neurosecretory material. Immunostaining demonstrates an absence of vasopressin in the hypothalamus, hypophysial stalk, and posterior lobe.

The *renal form of diabetes insipidus* (nephrogenic diabetes insipidus) is caused by end-organ failure. Renal tubular cells fail to respond to the antidiuretic effect of vasopressin, resulting in polyuria and polydipsia. No lesions are evident in the hypothalamus, hypophysial stalk, or posterior lobe. Vasopressin synthesis and release are not impaired.

## BASOPHILIC CELL INVASION

Basophilic cell invasion of the pituitary is a frequent autopsy finding in older men. It causes no clinical symptoms and cannot be detected by gross examination of the pituitary. Histologically, single or small groups of basophilic cells are seen to creep into the posterior lobe. In some cases, large groups of basophilic cells deeply invade the posterior lobe. The cytoplasm of basophilic cells is PAS-positive and contains ACTH and other fragments of the pro-opiomelanocortin molecule, indicating that these cells are related to corticotropes. However, they differ from the corticotropes located in the anterior lobe: they are smaller and denser, and, except for occasional cases, do not show Crooke hyalinization as a result of cortisol excess. Basophilic cell invasion is not apparent before puberty and cannot be correlated with any clinical endocrine abnormality. From a practical standpoint, the phenomenon of basophil invasion is important only insofar as its presence in a surgical specimen should not be mistaken for a corticotrope adenoma invading the neural lobe of the gland.

## MISCELLANEOUS FINDINGS

*Squamous cell nests*, which are *glandular structures* resembling salivary glands, and focal *mononuclear cell infiltration* are common incidental findings at autopsy in the posterior lobe and distal end of the hypophysial stalk. *Hemorrhages, necroses,* and *granulomas* were reviewed in the discussion on diseases of the anterior lobe.

## INTERRUPTION OF THE HYPOPHYSIAL STALK

Interruption of the hypophysial stalk causes distinct changes along the entire supraopticohypophysial tract. Surgical transection or disruption of the hypophysial stalk secondary to head trauma or organic diseases leads to atrophy of the supraoptic and, to a lesser extent, the paraventricular nuclei, as well as the posterior lobe. Various diseases, such as infections, granulomas, sarcoidosis, and neoplasms, can destroy the supraoptic and paraventricular nuclei and disrupt the hypophysial stalk, thereby impairing the innervation of the posterior lobe. Because the normal functional activity of the posterior lobe depends on the integrity of its nerve supply, diabetes insipidus develops in the absence of innervation. Morphologically, the posterior lobe undergoes marked involution; loss of stainable neurosecretory material and hormone content can be demonstrated. On radioimmunoassay, vasopressin concentrations become undetectable; histologically, neurohypophysial tissue is replaced by a fibrous scar. Atrophy of the posterior lobe is noticeable in some cases of anterior hypopituitarism. In postpartum hypopituitarism, atrophy of the supraoptic and paraventricular nuclei and of the hypophysial stalk and posterior lobe may occur.

## NEOPLASMS

Neoplasms in the posterior lobe, hypophysial stalk, and hypothalamus are uncommon. *Secondary carcinomas* were discussed earlier in relation to the anterior lobe.

### GRANULAR CELL TUMORS

Granular cell tumors (choristomas, or tumorlets) are the most common primary tumors in the posterior lobe and distal part of the hypophysial stalk. They are found in 1% to 8% of unselected adult autopsies, mainly in the elderly. Usually small (1–2 mm or less), they can be detected histologically. Granular cell tumors are slow-growing, histologically benign, sharply demarcated but unencapsulated nodules that usually are not associated with clinical symptoms or biochemical abnormalities and are recognized incidentally at autopsy. Rare granular cell tumors grow rapidly and become large, causing headaches, vision disturbances, diabetes insipidus, and anterior hypopituitarism.[10] Because of increased intracranial pressure or cranial nerve compression, surgical removal of the tumor may be necessary.

Histologically, granular cell tumors consist of loosely apposed, large, spherical, oval, or polygonal cells with eccentric nuclei and abundant, coarsely granular cytoplasm. Numerous large granules that stain strongly with PAS, luxol fast blue, and alcian blue almost fill the entire cytoplasm. On electron microscopic examination, the granules correspond to large, membrane-bound, unevenly electron-dense lysosomes. Immunostains reveal an absence of adenohypophysial or neurohypophysial hormones, but may show S-100 protein in the cytoplasm. Granular cell tumors appear to originate in pituicytes, the special glial cells of the posterior lobe.

### GLIOMAS

Other neoplasms are rare in the posterior lobe. Gliomas may originate in pituicytes of the posterior lobe; their histologic features are identical to those of glial tumors deriving from the central nervous system. Most gliomas involving the posterior lobe originate in the hypothalamus or median eminence and spread downward to the posterior lobe. Diabetes insipidus may develop as a result of massive destruction of the hypothalamus, the hypophysial stalk, or the posterior lobe.

Most gliomas that involve the hypothalamus, stalk, and posterior lobe are low-grade astrocytomas of pilocytic type. Malignant gliomas arising in these structures are extremely rare, most being a long-term complication of radiotherapy for a sellar region tumor. Postirradiation gliomas occurring in the region generally have been either anaplastic astrocytomas or glioblastomas. The mean latency period is ~10 years.[19] They invariably are aggressive lesions, with most patients dying within months of the diagnosis.

### GANGLIOCYTOMAS (HAMARTOMAS) OF THE SELLAR REGION

Lesions composed of neurons can occasionally form symptomatic masses in the sellar region. In fact, constituting this group are a collection of entities, ranging from simple hypothalamic hamartomatous growths on the one hand, to intriguing intrasellar neoplasms composed of both neuronal and adenohypophysial elements. As a group, however, they remain unified by their content of fully differentiated ganglion cells that appear mature and are accompanied by neuropil.

The nomenclature surrounding these lesions has been as diverse as it has been confusing, wherein designations such as ganglioneuroma, neuronal hamartoma, gangliocytoma, choristoma, gangliocytoma-pituitary adenoma, pituitary adenoma–adenohypophysial choristoma, and a medley of neologisms of one form or another have been inconsistently, interchangeably, and, at times, arbitrarily applied. Understandably, some of this variation in terminology reflects differing views on the presumed histogenetic origins of these lesions, an issue that currently is far from settled. It is important to recognize that two topologically distinct variants exist: one arising in the hypothalamus and the second within the sella. Of the former entities that arise in or remain physically attached to the hypothalamus, the term *hypothalamic neuronal hamartoma* is applied. Of the intrasellar variants, the majority of which are intimately admixed within the substance of a pituitary adenoma, the terms *pituitary adenoma-adenohypophysial neuronal choristoma* (PANCH)[84] or *mixed pituitary adenoma-gangliocytoma* are applied.[85] Both hypothalamic and intrasellar variants are discussed separately.

**Hypothalamic Neuronal Hamartoma.**    Not uncommonly, a well-defined mass composed of mature central ganglionic tissue projecting in the leptomeninges from the base of the brain will be encountered. In fact, when carefully sought, minute, macroscopic and nodular foci of ectopic hypothalamic tissue may be found incidentally in ~20% of random autopsies. This is usually attached to the ventral hypothalamus, the adjacent pia, or on the surface of the proximal posterior cerebral arteries. Although such hamartomatous nodules are clinically insignificant, rarely they may grow to several centimeters in size and compress surrounding structures. Some retain a thick pedicular attachment to the hypothalamus, tuber cinereum, or mammillary bodies, whereas others form a sessile solitary mass.

Most symptomatic examples occur in young males, in whom precocious puberty is the best known manifestation. In some instances, GnRH can be detected immunohistochemically within the neurons of such hamartomas, providing a neuroendocrinologic basis for accelerated sexual maturation. This is not, however, a universal nor a necessary finding. Precocious puberty in immunonegative cases is presumably the result of hypothalamic compression. Rarely, hypothalamic neuronal hamartomas may produce GHRH and clinical acromegaly on a hypothalamic basis, a condition dubbed *hypothalamic acromegaly*. In such cases, the pituitary may show either hyperplasia or adenomas of GH-producing cells. In addition to other features of hypothalamic dysfunction (somnolence, hyperphagia, autonomic disturbances, and diabetes insipidus), these tumors are associated with a peculiar form of epilepsy, one characterized by laughing (*gelastic seizures*).

Grossly, the mass in most symptomatic examples will be only 1 to 2 cm in size and often lies behind the pituitary stalk. It is pale, of firm consistency, and has homogeneous cut surfaces. Microscopically, the composition of the tissue resembles that of cerebral gray matter, both qualitatively and quantitatively. The neurons can vary in size, shape, and number, and both unipolar and multipolar forms are represented. Overall, these elements fully resemble mature hypothalamic neurons, although they are often disposed in clusters. Both myelinated and unmyelinated fibers course among them, forming compact bundles in some areas. Axonal processes may also appear to form ill-defined tracts, particularly among examples having pedicular attachment to the hypothalamus. In all examples, the neuronal elements are supported by a normal complement of glial cells of different kinds, although a variable amount of fibrillary gliosis may be found.

Immunohistochemical stains reveal a variety of hypothalamic-releasing peptides that normally reside within the cytoplasm of hypothalamic neurons: immunopositivity for GnRH, somatostatin, GHRH, and CRH may be detectable. In most cases, the immunohistochemical presence of these factors is regarded as a physiologic finding, and should not necessarily imply that these lesions are engaged in pathologic hormone hypersecretion. However, in the appropriate clinical context, such as with precocious puberty or the rare instance of acromegaly, the trophic effects of these hormones and their pathologic contribution to the endocrinopathy cannot be dismissed.

If they are symptomatic and surgically accessible, therapy for hypothalamic neuronal hamartomas is directed primarily at relief of the mass effect. When technically feasible, surgical resection has been successful not only in ameliorating mass effects, but also in regressing secondary sexual characteristics in those experiencing precocious puberty and in improving seizure control. For lesions less amenable to total resection by virtue of their deep intrahypothalamic location or other factors limiting surgical accessibility, partial resection may also be of some symptomatic benefit; residual hamartomatous tissue should grow slowly, if at all.

**Hypothalamic Hamartoblastoma.** A special variant of hypothalamic hamartoma is the hypothalamic hamartoblastoma, which occurs in infants and neonates and is associated with other multiple congenital abnormalities. The most frequent of the co-existing anomalies have included pituitary agenesis; dwarfism; dysmorphic facies; short, broad, or absent olfactory bulbs; hypoplastic thyroid and adrenals; cryptorchidism; various renal and cardiac malformations; anorectal atresia; syndactyly; and short metacarpals. This lethal syndrome is sometimes referred to as the Pallister-Hall syndrome. The hamartomatous lesion in this condition differs in several subtle respects from the more common hypothalamic hamartoma described earlier. As might be expected from the young age of affected patients, the lesion tends to be more cellular and less differentiated than the typical hypothalamic hamartoma found in older patients, hence the designation hamartoblastoma. A process morphologically intermediate between neoplasm and malformation, the hamartoblastoma is composed of ill-defined clusters of uniform, primitive-appearing, immature neurons unassociated with atypia or mitoses; neuronal differentiation appears incomplete.

**Intrasellar Adenohypophysial Neuronal Choristoma.** The intriguing neoplasm of the sellar region known as an *intrasellar adenohypophysial neuronal choristoma*, which, for lack of better designations, has previously been known under the terms *intrasellar adenohypophysial neuronal choristoma* or the *intrasellar gangliocytoma*. It is a composite neoplasm composed of adenohypophysial cells and ganglion-like cells to which the appellation *pituitary adenoma-neuronal choristoma* (PANCH) has been applied in an attempt to highlight the duality of its composition.[84] In a comprehensive review reiterating the composite neuronal and adenohypophysial nature of this

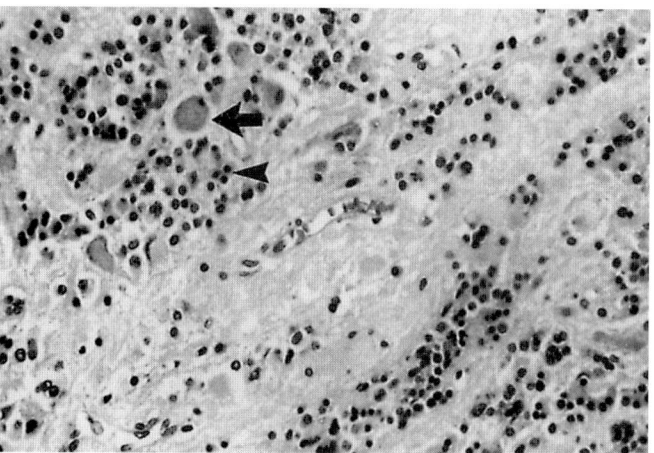

**FIGURE 11-14.** Adenohypophysial neuronal choristoma. The specimen is from a patient with acromegaly and a large intrasellar and suprasellar mass that was presumed to be an ordinary growth hormone–secreting adenoma. After transsphenoidal resection, the surgical specimen revealed an adenohypophysial neuronal choristoma intermixed within the substance of a growth hormone–secreting pituitary adenoma. Adenoma cells (*arrowhead*) intermixed with fully differentiated neurons (*arrow*) are evident in the specimen. These neurons were shown to contain growth hormone–releasing hormone. Original magnification ×400

neoplasm, the authors indicated a preference for the appellation "mixed adenoma-gangliocytoma."[85]

This lesion, although sharing some histologic similarities with the hypothalamic hamartoma, differs in several topologic and biologic respects. First and foremost, adenohypophysial neuronal choristomas are intrasellar lesions that have no physical attachment to the hypothalamus. Second, they are generally associated with—or more precisely—are intimately admixed with an endocrinologically functioning pituitary adenoma. Accordingly, they are virtually always symptomatic lesions of which the presence is heralded by a hypersecretory state. Finally, the neuronal component of this lesion, like the adenohypophysial component, are both genuinely neoplastic in nature.

The basic lesion consists of islands of ganglion-like cells and accompanying neuropil interspersed within the substance of a pituitary adenoma (Fig. 11-14). The ratio of adenohypophysial cells to neuronal elements can vary considerably, but as a rule, both will be strongly represented. The adenohypophysial cells in virtually all instances are chromophobic and sparsely granulated in nature. They may be disposed in nests, sheets, or otherwise scattered among the neuronal elements. With respect to the latter, the ganglion-like cells are of varying size and number, contain an abundant cytoplasm, complete with peripheral Nissl substance and neuronal processes containing Herring bodies. The ganglion cells fully resemble normal hypothalamic neurons.

Of reported cases, most have occurred in the setting of acromegaly, wherein patients have had the clinical, radiologic, and endocrinologic features of a typical GH-producing pituitary adenoma. On examination of the surgical specimen, a somatotrope adenoma is encountered, invariably of the sparsely granulated type, in which are interspersed varying numbers of neuronal elements, the morphology of which resembles well-differentiated ganglionic cells. Some of these ganglion cells have been found to be immunoreactive for GHRH, whereas others are immunoreactive for somatostatin. Less frequently, the lesion occurs in the setting of Cushing disease, wherein the adenoma is of the corticotropic type accompanied by ganglion cells immunoreactive for CRH. Only rarely is the adenohypophysial tumor a prolactinoma or a clinically nonfunctioning-pituitary adenoma.

Previously, hypotheses concerning the origin of these lesions centered on the seemingly displaced hypothalamic neurons in the pituitary fossa that, as a result of their secretion of trophic factors, might have a paracrine inductive effect on adjacent adenohypophysial cells, stimulating their growth and eventual neoplastic transformation. According to this view, pituitary adenoma formation is regarded as a secondary, downstream event. Subsequently, however, an alternative hypothesis has been proposed that features adenohypophysial cells as the instigators of the process, rather than seemingly passive targets of paracrine effect.[84] Supported by compelling morphologic evidence, this hypothesis suggests that pituitary adenoma formation is the primary event, and the ganglionic component of the lesion arises as the consequence of neuronal metaplasia of neoplastic adenohypophysial cells. When subjected to careful ultrastructural study, morphologic changes that are indicative of a metaplastic process beginning in adenohypophysial cells that gradually gives way to cells having intermediate and, eventually, fully neuronal features can be seen. Whereas metaplastic change is a well-known phenomenon in both normal and neoplastic adenohypophysial cells, as it is in other neuroendocrine neoplasms, actual induction of such metaplastic change has yet to be demonstrated experimentally. A third hypothesis is that both adenohypophysial and neuronal components of this tumor arise from a common, but as yet hypothetical, progenitor cell sequestrated in the sella as an embryonal tissue nest.

Because this entity is relatively new, with only small numbers of cases having been collected, and virtually no long-term follow-up data available, it is unclear whether the behavior of these mixed lesions differs significantly from that of the corresponding pituitary adenoma.

The isolated intrasellar gangliocytoma is a lesion unassociated with a pituitary adenoma and anatomically distinct from the hypothalamus.[85] Although an adenoma was not found in any of seven cases, three examples were associated either with Cushing disease or with acromegaly, a situation not readily explained by a purely gangliocytic tumor. The authors have not encountered such a pure gangliocytic lesion in the sella, particularly in the setting of a hypersecretory state—when an accompanying pituitary adenoma or hyperplasia has always been present.

# REFERENCES

1. Hague K, Post KD, Morgello S. Absence of peritumoral Crooke's change is associated with recurrence in surgically treated Cushing's disease. Surg Neurol 2000; 53:77.

1a. Kovacs K, Horvath E. Tumors of the pituitary gland. In: Hartmann WH, Sobin LH, eds. Atlas of tumor pathology, fascicle 21, series 2. Washington, DC: Armed Forces Institute of Pathology, 1986:1.

2. Horvath E, Scheithauer B, Kovacs K, et al. Regional neuropathology: hypothalamus and pituitary. In: Graham D, Lantos P, eds. Greenfield's Neuropathology. London: Arnold, 1997:1007.

3. Lloyd RV, Chander WF, Kovacs K, Ryan N. Ectopic pituitary adenomas with normal anterior pituitary glands. Am J Surg Pathol 1986; 10:546.

4. Thapar K, Kovacs K, Scheithauer B, et al. Classification and pathology of sellar and parasellar tumors. In: Tindall G, Cooper P, Barrow D, eds. The Practice of Neurosurgery. Baltimore: Williams & Wilkins, 1996:1021.

5. Bergland RM, Ray BS, Torack RM. Anatomical variations in the pituitary gland and adjacent structures in 225 human autopsy cases. J Neurosurg 1968; 28:93.

6. Kaufman B, Chamberlin WB Jr. The ubiquitous "empty" sellar turcica. Acta Radiol Diagn (Stockh) 1972; 13:413.

7. Weisberg LA, Housepian EM, Saur DP. Empty sella syndrome as a complication of benign intracranial hypertension. J Neurosurg 1975; 43:177.

8. Brismar K, Efendic S. Pituitary function in the empty sella syndrome. Neuroendocrinology 1981; 32:70.

9. McFadzean R, Teasdale G. Pituitary apoplexy. In: Landolt A, Vance M, Reilly P, eds. Pituitary Adenomas. Edinburgh: Churchill Livingstone, 1996:485.

10. Thapar K, Kovacs K. Tumors of the sellar region. In: Bigner DD, McLendon RE, Bruner JM, eds. Russel and Rubinstein's pathology of tumors of the nervous system, 6th ed. Baltimore: Williams & Wilkins, 1998:561.

11. Cardosa ER, Peterson EW. Pituitary apoplexy: a review. Neurosurgery 1984; 14:363.

12. Berger SA, Edberg SC, David G. Infectious disease in the sella turcica. Rev Infect Dis 1986; 8:747.

13. Domingue JN, Wilson CB. Pituitary abscesses: report of seven cases and review of the literature. J Neurosurg 1977; 46:601.

14. Sano T, Kovacs K, Scheithauer BW, et al. Pituitary pathology in acquired immunodeficiency syndrome. Arch Pathol Lab Med 1989; 113:1066.

15. Beressi N, Beressi JP, Cohen R, Modigliani E. Lymphocytic hypophysitis: a review of 145 cases. Ann Med Interne (Paris) 1999; 150:327.

16. Feigenbaum SL, Martin MC, Wilson CB, Jaffe RB. Lymphocytic adenohypophysitis: a pituitary mass lesion occurring in pregnancy. Proposal for medical treatment. Am J Obstet Gynecol 1991; 164:1549.

17. Lee JH, Laws ER Jr, Guthrie BL, et al. Lymphocytic hypophysitis: occurrence in two men. Neurosurgery 1994; 34:159.

18. Capellan JIL, Olmedo C, Martin JM, et al. Intrasellar mass with hypopituitarism as a manifestation of sarcoidosis. J Neurosurg 1990; 73:283.

19. Scheithauer BW. The neurohypophysis. In: Kovacs K, Asa SL, eds. Functional endocrine pathology. Boston: Blackwell, 1991:170.

20. Nishio S, Mizuno J, Barrow DL, et al. Isolated histiocytosis X of the pituitary gland: case report. Neurosurgery 1987; 21:718.

21. Tampanaru-Sarmesiu A, Stefaneanu L, Thapar K, et al. Transferrin and transferrin receptor in human hypophysis and pituitary adenomas. Am J Pathol 1998; 152:413.

22. Horvath E, Kovacs K. The adenohypophysis. In: Kovacs K, Asa SL, eds. Functional endocrine pathology. Boston: Blackwell, 1991:245.

23. Thapar K, Kovacs K, Laws ER Jr. The pathology and molecular biology of pituitary adenomas. Adv Tech Stand Neurosurg 1995; 22:4.

24. Sano T, Asa SL, Kovacs K. Growth hormone-releasing hormone–producing tumors: clinical, biochemical, and morphological manifestations. Endocr Rev 1988; 9:357.

25. Scheithauer BW, Kovacs K, Randall RV. The pituitary in untreated Addison's disease: a histologic and immunocytologic study of 18 adenohypophyses. Arch Pathol Lab Med 1983; 107:484.

26. Scheithauer BW, Kovacs K, Randall RV, Ryan N. Pituitary gland in hypothyroidism. Histologic and immunocytologic study. Arch Pathol Lab Med 1985; 109:499.

27. Herman V, Fagan J, Gonsky R, et al. Clonal origin of pituitary adenomas. J Clin Endocrinol Metab 1990; 71:1427.

28. Schulte HM, Oldfield EH, Allolio B, et al. Clonal composition of pituitary adenomas in patients with Cushing's disease: determination by X chromosome inactivation analysis. J Clin Endocrinol Metab 1991; 73:1302.

29. Faglia G, Spada A. The role of the hypothalamus in pituitary neoplasia. Baillieres Clin Endocrinol Metab 1995; 9:225.

30. Asa S, Kovacs K, Stefaneanu L, et al. Pituitary adenomas in mice transgenic for growth hormone-releasing hormone. Endocrinology 1992; 131:2083.

31. Melmed S. Acromegaly. In: Melmed S, ed. The Pituitary. Cambridge: Blackwell Science, 1995:413.

32. Levy A, Lightman S. Growth hormone-releasing hormone transcripts in human pituitary adenomas. J Clin Endocrinol Metab 1992; 74:1474.

33. Rauch C, Li J, Croissandeau G, et al. Characterization and localization of an immunoreactive growth hormone-releasing hormone precursor form in normal and tumoral human anterior pituitaries. Endocrinology 1995; 136:2594.

34. Castro M, Brooke J, Bullman A, et al. Synthesis of corticotropin-releasing hormone (CRH) in mouse corticotropic tumour cells expressing the human proCRH gene, intracellular storage and regulated secretion. J Mol Endocrinol 1991; 7:97.

35. Pagesy P, Li JY, Rentier-Delrue F, et al. Growth hormone and somatostatin gene expression in pituitary adenomas with active acromegaly and minimal plasma growth hormone elevation. Acta Endocrinol 1990; 122:745.

36. Miller G, Alexander J, Klibanski A. Gonadotropin-releasing hormone messenger RNA expression in gonadotroph tumors and normal human pituitary. J Clin Endocrinol Metab 1996; 81:80.

37. Thapar K, Kovacs K, Stefaneanu L, et al. Overexpression of the growth hormone-releasing hormone gene in acromegaly associated pituitary tumor: an event associated with neoplastic progression and aggressive behavior. Am J Pathol 1997; 151:769.

38. Thapar K, Kovacs K, Muller P. Clinical-pathologic correlations of pituitary tumors. Baillieres Clin Endocrinol Metab 1995; 9:243.

39. Molitch ME. Pathologic hyperprolactinemia. Endocrinol Metab Clin North Am 1992; 21:877.

40. Scheithauer BW, Kovacs K, Randall RV, Ryan N. Effects of estrogen on the human pituitary: a clinicopathologic study. Mayo Clin Proc 1989; 64:1077.

41. Stefaneanu L, Kovacs K, Horvath E, et al. In situ hybridization of estrogen receptor mRNA in human adenohypophysial cells and pituitary adenomas. J Clin Endocrinol Metab 1994; 78:83.

42. Kovacs K, Stefaneanu L, Ezzat S, et al. Prolactin producing pituitary adenoma in a male to female transsexual patient following protracted estrogen administration: a morphologic study. Arch Pathol Lab Med 1994; 118:562.

43. Vallar L, Spada A, Giannattasio G. Altered Gs and adenylate cyclase activity in human GH secreting pituitary tumors. Nature 1987; 330:566.

44. Landis CA, Harsh G, Lyons J, et al. Clinical characteristics of acromegalic patients whose pituitary tumors contain mutant Gs protein. J Clin Endocrinol Metab 1990; 71:1416.

45. Yoshimoto K, Iwahana H, Fukuda A, et al. Rare mutations of the Gs alpha subunit in human endocrine tumors. Mutation detection by polymerase chain reaction-primer introduced restriction analysis. Cancer 1993; 72:1286.

46. Tjordman K, Stern N, Ouaknine G, et al. Activating mutations of the Gs alpha gene in nonfunctioning pituitary tumors. J Clin Endocrinol Metab 1993; 77:765.

47. Williamson E, Daniels M, Foster S, et al. Gs alpha and gi2 alpha mutations in clinically non-functioning pituitary tumors. Clin Endocrinol 1994; 41:815.

48. Williamson E, Ince P, Harrison D, et al. G-protein mutations in human pituitary adrenocorticotrophic hormone-secreting adenomas. Eur J Clin Invest 1995; 25:128.
49. Karga HJ, Alexander JM, Hedley-White ET, et al. Ras mutations in human pituitary tumors. J Clin Endocrinol Metab 1992; 74:914.
50. Herman V, Drazin NZ, Gonsky R, et al. Molecular screening of pituitary adenomas for gene mutations and rearrangements. J Clin Endocrinol Metab 1993; 77:50.
51. Pei L, Melmed S, Scheithauer BW, et al. H-ras mutations in human pituitary carcinoma metastases. J Clin Endocrinol Metab l994; 78:842.
52. Bystrom C, Larsson C, Blomberg C, et al. Localization of the MEN1 gene to a small region within chromosome 11q13 by deletion mapping tumors. Proc Natl Acad Sci U S A 1990; 87:1968.
53. Chandrasekharappa S, Guru C, Manickam P, et al. Positional cloning of the gene for multiple endocrine neoplasia—type 1. Science 1997; 276:404.
54. Thakkar R, Pook M, Wooding C, et al. Association of somatotrophinomas with loss of alleles on chromosome 11 and with Gsp mutations. J Clin Invest 1993; 91:2815.
55. Boggild M, Jenkinson S, Pistorello M, et al. Molecular genetic studies of sporadic pituitary tumors. J Clin Endocrinol Metab l994; 78:387.
56. Harris C, Hollstein M. Clinical implications of the p53 tumor-suppressor gene. N Engl J Med 1993; 329:1318.
57. Thapar K, Scheithauer BW, Kovacs K, et al. p53 expression in pituitary adenomas and carcinomas: correlation with invasiveness and tumor growth fractions. Neurosurgery 1996; 38:765.
58. Levy A, Hall L, Yeudall WA, et al. p53 gene mutations in pituitary adenomas: rare events. Clin Endocrinol 1994; 41:809.
59. Buckley N, Bates AS, Broome J, et al. p53 protein accumulates in Cushings adenomas and invasive non-functional adenomas. J Clin Endocrinol Metab 1994; 79:1513.
60. Jacks T, Fazeli A, Schmitt EM, et al. Effects of an Rb mutation in the mouse. Nature 1992; 359:295.
61. Cryns VL, Alexander JP, Klibanski A, Arnold A. The retinoblastoma gene in human pituitary tumors. J Clin Endocrinol Metab 1993; 77:644.
62. Zhu J, Leon S, Beggs A, et al. Human pituitary adenomas show no loss of heterozygosity at the retinoblastoma gene locus. J Clin Endocrinol Metab 1994; 78:922.
63. Pei L, Melmed S, Scheithauer B, et al. Frequent loss of heterozygosity at the retinoblastoma susceptibility gene (RB) locus in aggressive pituitary tumors: evidence for a chromosome 13 tumor suppressor gene other than RB. Cancer Res 1995; 55:1613.
64. Capra E, Rindi G, Pompei-Spina M, et al. Chromosomal abnormalities in a case of pituitary adenoma. Cancer Genet Cytogenet 1993; 681:40.
65. Rock J, Babu V, Drumheller T, et al. Cytogenetic findings in pituitary adenomas: results of a pilot study. Surg Neurol 1993; 40:224.
66. Alvaro V, Levy L, Deburay C, et al. Invasive human pituitary tumors express a point mutated alpha-protein kinase-C. J Clin Endocrinol Metab 1993; 77:1125.
67. Klibanski A, Zervas N. Diagnosis and management of hormone-secreting pituitary adenomas. N Engl J Med 1991; 324:822.
68. Scheithauer BW, Kovacs K, Laws ER Jr, Randall RV. Pathology of invasive pituitary adenomas with special reference to functional classification. J Neurosurg 1986; 65:733.
69. Knosp E, Kitz K, Perneczky A. Proliferation activity in pituitary adenomas. Measurement by monoclonal antibody Ki. Neurosurgery 1989; 25:927.
70. Thapar K, Kovacs K, Scheithauer B, et al. Proliferative activity and invasiveness among pituitary adenomas and carcinomas: an analysis using the MIB-1 antibody. Neurosurgery 1996; 38:99.
71. Hsu DW, Hakim F, Biller BMK, et al. Significance of proliferating cell nuclear antigen index in predicting pituitary adenoma recurrence. J Neurosurg 1993; 78:753.
72. Pemicone PJ, Scheithauer BW, Sebo TJ, et al. Pituitary carcinoma. A clinicopathologic study of 15 cases. Cancer 1997; 79:804.
73. Gesundheit N, Petrick PA, Nissim M, et al. Thyrotropin-secreting pituitary adenomas. Clinical and biochemical heterogeneity. Case reports and follow-up of nine patients. Ann Intern Med 1989; 111:827.
74. Kovacs K, Asa SL, Horvath E, et al. Null cell adenomas of the pituitary: attempts to resolve their cytogenesis. In: Leschago J, Kameya T, eds. Endocrine pathology update. New York: Field & Wood, 1990:17.
75. Kovacs K, Horvath E, Asa SL, et al. Pituitary cells producing more than one hormone. Human pituitary adenomas. Trends Endocr Metab 1989; 1:104.
76. Thapar K, Stefaneanu L, Kovacs K, et al. Plurihormonal pituitary tumors: beyond the one cell-one hormone theory. Endocr Pathol 1993; 4:1.
77. Branch CL, Laws ER Jr. Metastatic tumors of the sella turcica masquerading as primary pituitary tumors. J Clin Endocrinol Metab 1987; 65:649.
78. Burger P, Scheithauer B. Tumors of the central nervous system. Third series, fascicle 10. Washington, DC: Armed Forces Institute of Pathology, 1994.
79. Crotty R, Scheithauer B, Young W, et al. Papillary craniopharyngioma: a clinicopathological study of 48 cases. J Neurosurg 1995; 83:206.
80. Crotty T, Scheithauer BW, Young WF, Davis D. Papillary craniopharyngiomas: a morphological and clinical study of 46 cases. Endocr Pathol 1992; 3(Suppl):S6(abst).
81. Weiner H, Wishoff J, Rosenberg M, et al. Craniopharyngiomas: a clinicopathologic analysis of factors predictive of recurrence and functional outcome. Neurosurgery 1994; 35:1001.
82. Thapar K, Stefaneanu L, Kovacs K, et al. Estrogen receptor gene expression in craniopharyngioma: an in situ hybridization study. Neurosurgery 1994; 35:1012.
83. Brassier G, Morandi X, Tayiar E, et al. Rathke's cleft cysts: surgical-MRI correlation in 16 symptomatic cases. J Neuroradiol 1999; 26:162.
84. Horvath E, Kovacs K, Scheithauer BW, et al. Pituitary adenoma with neuronal choristoma (PANCH): composite lesion or lineage infidelity? Ultrastruct Pathol 1994; 18:565.

# SECTION A

# ADENOHYPOPHYSIS

# CHAPTER 12

# GROWTH HORMONE AND ITS DISORDERS

GERHARD BAUMANN

Growth hormone (GH) is a polypeptide hormone produced by the somatotrope cells in the pituitary gland. It is the master anabolic hormone and possesses numerous bioactivities related to somatic growth, body composition, and intermediary metabolism. Many of the biologic actions of GH are mediated through insulin-like growth factor-I (IGF-I), but GH also has direct effects independent of IGF-I. Unlike most other hormones, GH is species specific, not only in its structure but also partially in its function. Its "one-way species specificity" refers to the fact that primate GHs are active in lower (evolutionarily earlier) species, but GHs of lower species are inactive in primates, including humans. GH regulation and, in part, GH action also differ among species. This chapter focuses primarily on human GH and its biology.

## GROWTH HORMONE GENES

In humans, GH is encoded by two genes on the long arm of chromosome 17.[1] They are part of a gene-duplication cluster that also includes the genes for chorionic somatomammotropin (placental lactogen), a protein highly homologous with GH (Fig. 12-1). The GH genes are named *GH-N* (or GH-1) and *GH-V* (or GH-2); the former is expressed in the pituitary, the latter in the placenta. GH-V is also called *placental GH*. The two GH genes are similar in structure; both are composed of five exons and four introns; each spans ~1.6 kb.

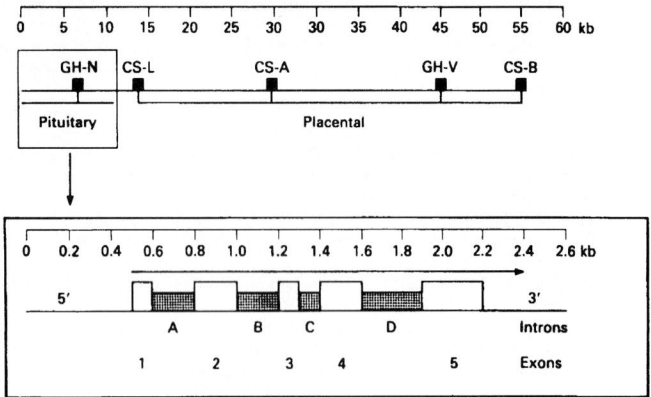

**FIGURE 12-1.** Human growth hormone locus on chromosome 17q22-24. The top panel shows the organization of the locus with the two GH genes (GH-N and GH-V) and the three chorionic somatomammotropin genes (CS-L, CS-A, CS-B). CS-L is probably a pseudogene. The bottom panel shows the GH-N gene in more detail, with five exons and four introns. GH-N is expressed in the pituitary, the other genes in the locus exclusively in the placenta. (From Parks JS. Molecular biology of growth hormone. Acta Paediatr Scand 1989; 349[Suppl]:127.)

## GROWTH HORMONE STRUCTURE

Human GH is heterogeneous and consists of several molecular variants (Fig. 12-2).[2] The principal form is a 191-amino-acid, single-chain protein with a molecular weight of ~22,000. It is the most abundant form (~90%–95% of pituitary GH), generally referred to as "GH" or "22K GH." Two disulfide loops are present, and the three-dimensional structure is a twisted bundle of four α-helices (Fig. 12-3).[3] Two independent receptor-binding sites are located on opposite surfaces of GH, allowing for ligand-induced receptor dimerization (see later). GH-V (placental GH) has a similar primary structure; it differs from GH-N (22K GH) in 13 of the 191 amino-acid positions (see Fig. 12-2). One important difference is the glycosylation consensus site at asparagine 140; GH-V exists as a glycosylated as well as nonglycosylated protein. The second most abundant GH form after 22K GH is an mRNA splice variant that lacks an internal sequence of 15 amino acids. Its molecular weight is ~20,000, and hence it is known as "20K GH." It accounts for 5% to 7% of pituitary GH. Other minor variants include an $N_\alpha$-acylated and two deamidated variants (see Fig. 12-2). Little is known about the bioactivities or significance of these minor GH forms. In addition to the monomeric forms of

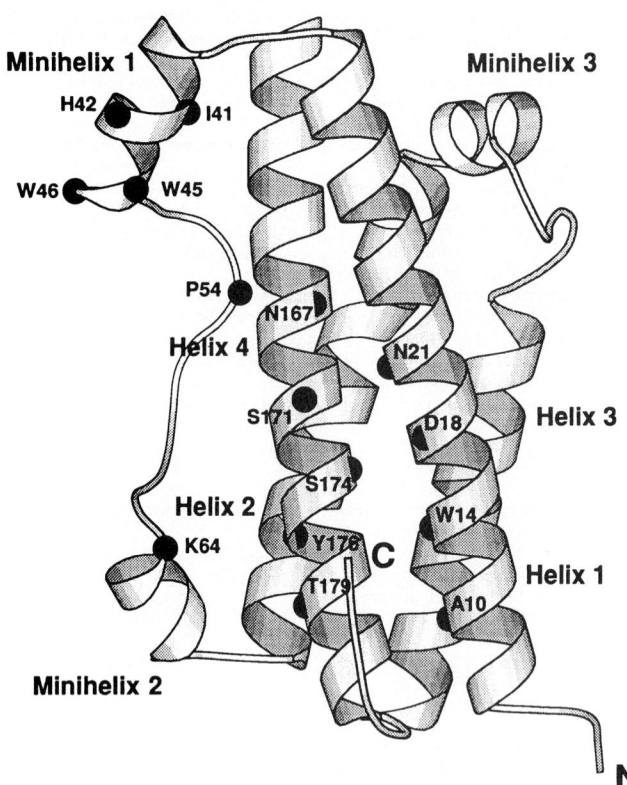

**FIGURE 12-3.** Three-dimensional structure of human growth hormone (22K), depicted as a ribbon diagram. The four main α-helices are shown together with three minihelices within the connecting loops. Some residues mutated for technical purposes are indicated; they are not relevant in this context. (N, amino terminus; C, carboxy terminus.) (From Ultsch MH, Somers W, Kossiakoff AA, de Vos AM. The crystal structure of affinity-matured human growth hormone at 2 Å resolution. J Mol Biol 1994; 236:286.)

GH just described, GH also exists as an oligomeric series of up to at least pentameric GH.[4] Both noncovalent and disulfide-linked oligomers occur, and homo- as well as heterooligomers composed of the various monomeric forms exist in the pituitary and plasma. The biologic significance of GH oligomers is unclear, but they likely act as modulators of overall GH activity because of their different affinities for the GH receptor. The existence of so many molecular forms of GH is one reason for the difficulty with GH measurements and the discrepant results obtained by different assays (see later).

**FIGURE 12-2.** Primary structure of human growth hormone and its variants. The polypeptide shown is GH-N (22K). Amino-acid substitutions in GH-V are indicated next to the involved residues. The sequence connected by the heavy line (residues 32–46) is deleted in 20K GH. The tree structure at Asn-140 denotes glycosylation in GH-V. The *asterisks* indicate sites of deamidation, the dot at the amino terminus acylation. (From Baumann G. Growth hormone heterogeneity: genes, iso-hormones, variants and binding proteins. Endocr Rev 1991; 12:424.)

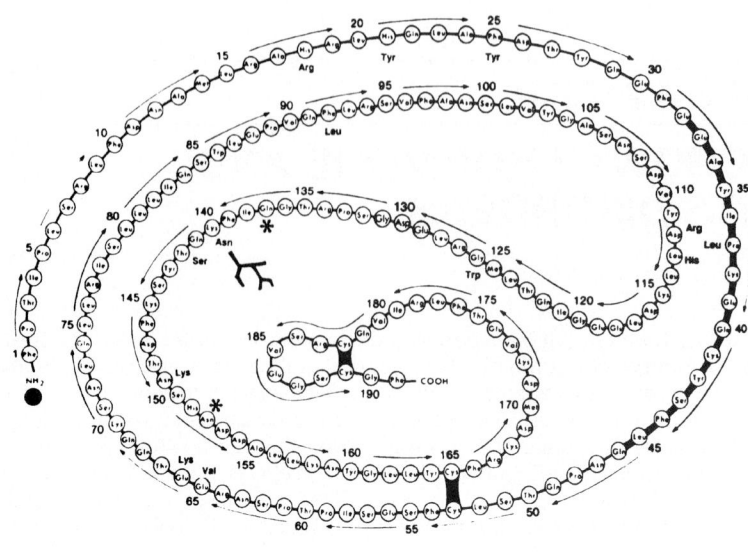

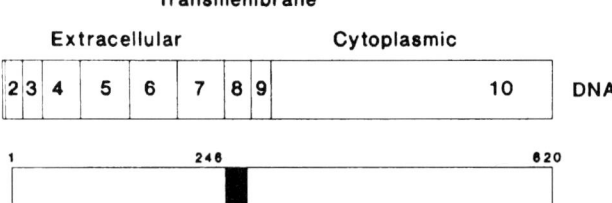

**FIGURE 12-4.** Schematic representation of the growth hormone receptor (*GHR*) complementary DNA (*top*) and protein (*bottom*). The GHR is encoded by 10 exons; exons 2–7 encode the extracellular domain, exon 8 the transmembrane domain, and exons 9 and 10 the cytoplasmic domain. The numbers in the upper panel denote the exons; those in the lower panel the amino acids. The transmembrane domain is shaded in black. (Adapted from Kelly PA, Djiane J, Postel-Vinay M-C, Edery M. The prolactin/growth hormone receptor family. Endocr Rev 1991; 12:235.)

## GROWTH HORMONE RECEPTOR

The GH receptor (GHR) is a 620-amino-acid, ~130 kDa, single-chain glycoprotein with a single transmembrane domain, a large extracellular domain containing the GH-binding site, and an intracellular domain involved in GH signaling (Fig. 12-4).[5] The extracellular domain also occurs separately as a soluble GH-binding protein (GHBP, see later). The GHR is a member of the cytokine receptor family that also includes the receptors for prolactin, erythropoietin and other hematopoietic growth factors, many of the interleukins, and others.[6] The GHR is encoded by a single gene located on the short arm of chromosome 5. The gene spans at least 87 kb and is divided into 10 exons and 9 introns.[7] Exons 2–7 encode the extracellular domain, exon 8 the transmembrane domain, and exons 9 and 10 the intracellular domain. The GHR is expressed ubiquitously, with the liver being the organ most enriched in GHRs. In addition to the full-length GHR, two variants of the GHR are found in humans. A version lacking the 22 amino acids encoded by exon 3 is differentially expressed among tissues[8] and/or in different individuals.[9] This internal deletion near the amino terminus has no known functional consequence. The second variant is a GHR truncated at nine amino acids beyond the transmembrane domain, so that it lacks most of the intracellular domain.[10] This variant is also expressed ubiquitously. The absence of an intracellular domain renders this variant incapable of signaling and favors prolonged persistence on the cell membrane. The latter may be the reason why this receptor variant contributes substantially to GHBP generation (see later). This truncated GHR variant modulates GH action by forming heterodimers with full-length GHRs, thereby sequestering some of the GHRs in a nonfunctional state.

GH initiates its action first by binding to the GHR through site 1 on one of its surfaces; this is then followed by binding of a second GHR to site 2 on the other surface of GH.[11] This results in a complex containing two GHRs in association with GH (Fig. 12-5). This GH-induced dimerization of the GHR is critical for GHR signaling and GH action. The functional domains of the GHR are depicted in Figure 12-6. Intracellular signaling is initiated by binding of JAK2 (Janus kinase 2) to a proline-rich region (Box 1) in the proximal intracellular part of the GHR, followed by a JAK2-mediated tyrosine phosphorylation cascade involving JAK2 itself, the GHR, signal transducers and activators of transcription (Stats) 1, 3, and 5, insulin-receptor substrates (IRS) 1 and 2, components of the mitogen-activated protein kinase (MAPK), the protein kinase C, and phosphatidyl inositol-3 kinase pathways, and several other intracellular signaling and adapter proteins, not all of which are known (Fig. 12-7).[12] Gene transcription is then activated through these pathways. Interestingly, as of this writing, the precise pathway responsible for activation of IGF-I gene transcription is not known.

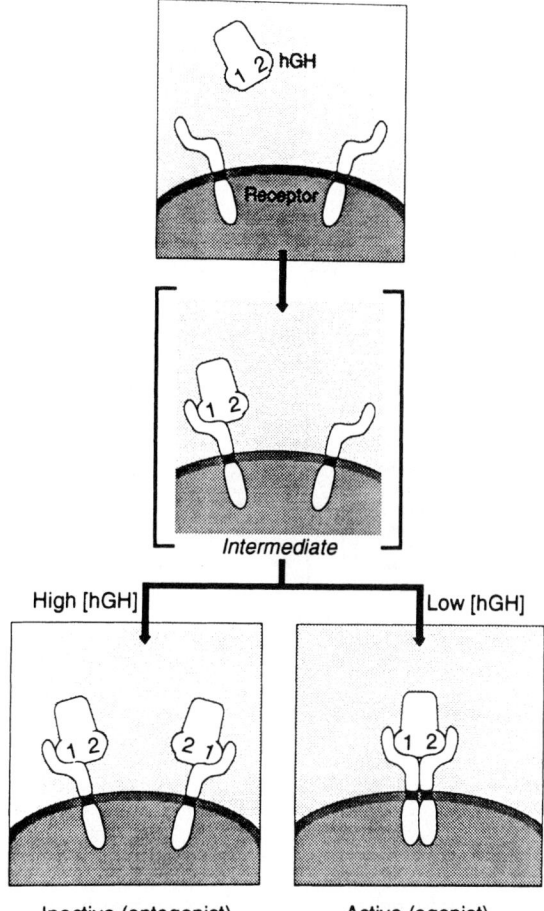

**FIGURE 12-5.** Schematic representation of growth hormone (*GH*)–induced dimerization of two growth hormone receptors (*GHRs*). Binding occurs first through site 1 on GH, followed by binding of a second GHR to site 2 on GH. The dimerized GHR (2:1) complex (*lower right*) is active in transducing the GH signal. At very high (pharmacologic) GH concentrations (*lower left*), the ratio of GH to GHR is high enough to saturate GHRs through site 1 binding, with the GHR trapped in an inactive 1:1 complex. This occurs at GH levels that are not seen in vivo. However, recognition of the potential existence of an inactive 1:1 complex was important in developing a GH antagonist (see text on treatment for acromegaly). (*hGH*, human growth hormone.) (From Fuh G, Cunningham BC, Fukunaga R, et al. Rational design of potent antagonists to the growth hormone receptor. Science 1992; 256:1677.)

The GHR binds GH variants with different affinities. The 20K variant as well as the oligomeric GH forms have lower affinity than monomeric 22K GH, but GH-V is equipotent to 22K GH. Little is known about the binding of the other GH variants.

## GROWTH HORMONE–BINDING PROTEIN

The GHBP is the soluble, extracellular domain of the GHR. In humans and many other species, the GHBP is generated from the GHR by proteolysis; in rodents it is derived from the GHR gene via alternative splicing.[13] The GHBP circulates in plasma in nanomolar concentrations, sufficient to complex a substantial part (~50%) of plasma GH. The serum GHBP level appears to reflect the GHR abundance of the organism, especially in the liver. The biologic significance or importance of the GHBP is not known; it is evolutionarily conserved throughout the vertebrates and is generated by different mechanisms in different species, suggesting an important role. The GHBP modulates GH action through a variety of mechanisms. It inhibits GH

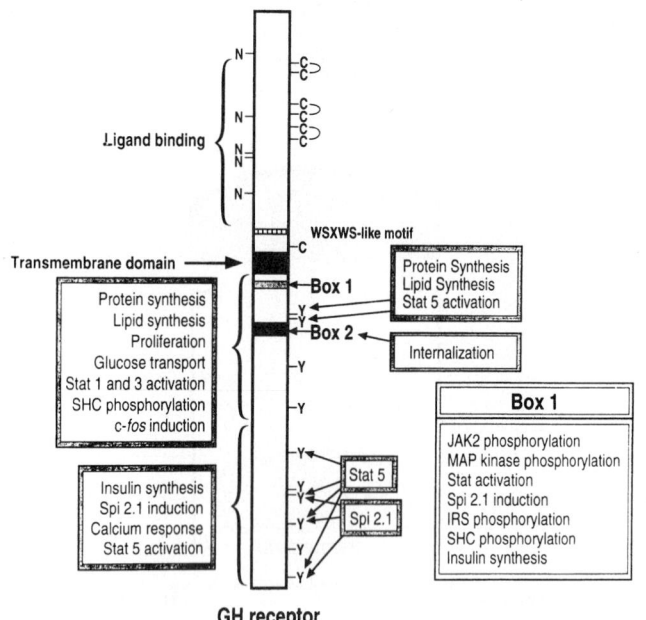

**FIGURE 12-6.** Functional domains of the growth hormone receptor (extracellular domain is on top). The proline-rich Box 1 is crucial for JAK2 (Janus kinase 2) binding and initiation of most of the signaling events. (*C*, extracellular cysteines, only one of which is free [*not disulfide linked*]; *N*, potential N-linked glycosylation sites; *Y*, intracellular tyrosines, important for phosphorylation and docking of signaling molecules; *WSXWS*, tryptophan-serine motif; *Stat*, signal transducer and activator of transcription; *SHC*, Src homology containing protein; *MAPK*, mitogen-activated protein kinase; *Spi 2.1*, serine protease inhibitor 2.1; *IRS*, insulin receptor substrate.) (From Argetsinger LS, Carter-Su C. Mechanisms of signaling by growth hormone receptor. Physiol Rev 1996; 76:1089.)

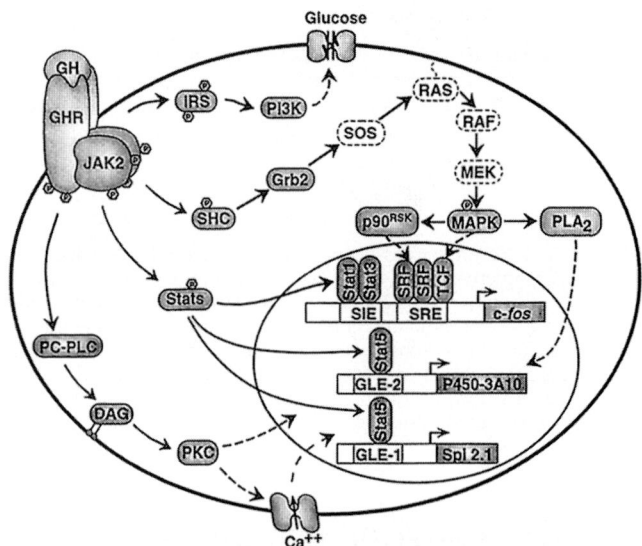

**FIGURE 12-7.** Intracellular signaling pathways of the growth hormone receptor (*GHR*) (partial rendition). Principal pathways are the signal transducer and activator of transcription (*Stat*), protein kinase C (*PKC*), mitogen-activated protein kinase (*MAPK*), and insulin receptor substrate (*IRS*) pathways. The inner ellipse represents the nucleus. Transcriptional elements, their cognate transcription factors, and transactivated genes are shown. (*GH*, growth hormone; *P*, phosphorylated sites; *JAK2*, Janus kinase 2; *PC*, phosphatidyl choline; *PLC*, phospholipase C; *DAG*, diacylglycerol; *PI3K*, phosphatidyl-inositol-3 kinase.) (From Argetsinger LS, Carter-Su C. Mechanisms of signaling by growth hormone receptor. Physiol Rev 1996; 76:1089.)

action by competing with the GHR for ligand and by generating "unproductive" heterodimers with the GHR at the cell surface, as opposed to the GHR homodimers necessary for signaling. The GHBP also prolongs the half-life of GH in the circulation by complexing GH, thereby delaying its elimination. The net effect of these modulatory activities in the intact organism is not well understood.

In the circulation, GH also binds (with low affinity) to one or more proteins related to $\alpha_2$-macroglobulin.[14] This complex accounts for no more than 5% of total GH in serum.

## SOMATOTROPE DEVELOPMENT AND GROWTH HORMONE

Several pituitary transcription factors are involved in pituitary somatotrope development. Their consideration is important here because mutations in their respective genes lead to abnormalities in the GH axis. The reader is referred to Chapters 8 and 11 for a full discussion of pituitary ontogeny. Developmental genes relevant to GH include the Prop-1, Pit-1 (also known as Pou1f1), and GH-releasing hormone receptor (GHRH-R) genes. These genes are expressed sequentially during anterior pituitary development; each is more restrictive in its impact on different cell types; and each is dependent on the activity of the preceding one.[15] Prop-1 and Pit-1 are POU-homeodomain transcription factors, the GHRH-R is a seven transmembrane domain receptor signaling through the cyclic adenosine monophosphate (cAMP) pathway. Prop-1 is important for development of the gonadotrope, somatotrope, lactotrope, and thyroptrope lineages. Pit-1, under the direction of Prop-1, is involved in differentiation of somatotropes, lactotropes, and thyrotropes. The GHRH-R, which is exclusively expressed in

somatotropes under the direction of Pit-1, is critical for the normal expansion of the somatotrope population. The GHRH-R is also necessary for GH synthesis and secretion (see later).

## SECRETION

### NEURAL CONTROL

GH secretion is under neural control from the hypothalamus through at least two and possibly three hypophysiotropic factors: GH-releasing hormone (GHRH), somatostatin, and probably ghrelin (see following section). The GHRH neurons are located primarily in the arcuate and ventromedial nuclei, and somatostatin neurons are located primarily in the anterior periventricular area of the hypothalamus. GHRH and somatostatin release are controlled by a complex and incompletely understood neural network, involving α-adrenergic, dopaminergic, serotoninergic, cholinergic, and histaminergic inputs. In general, α-adrenergic, dopaminergic, serotoninergic, and cholinergic signals stimulate GH secretion. The limbic system plays an important role in GH secretion. A full discussion of the neural pathways regulating GH secretion is beyond the scope of this chapter. From a practical standpoint, it is important to know the physiologic stimuli leading to GH secretion, the principal pharmacologic agents used to test GH secretory capacity, and the peripheral feedback control of GH secretion.

### GROWTH HORMONE–RELEASING HORMONE AND THE GROWTH HORMONE–RELEASING HORMONE RECEPTOR

GHRH is a 40- to 44-amino-acid peptide isolated first from pancreatic tumors that produced it ectopically,[16,17] and subsequently from the hypothalamus (Fig. 12-8). Its gene, located on chromosome 20q, encodes a 108-amino-acid precursor from which GHRH is derived by proteolytic cleavage. It is expressed

```
                5            10            15            20
GHRH 1-40:  Tyr—Ala—Asp—Ala—Ile—Phe—Thr—Asn—Ser—Tyr—Arg—Lys—Val—Leu—Gly—Gln—Leu—Ser—Ala—Arg—
                25            30            35            40
            Lys—Leu—Leu—Gln—Asp—Ile—Met—Ser—Arg—Gln—Gln—Gly—Glu—Ser— Asn—Gln—Glu—Arg—Gly—Ala
------------------------------------------------------------------------------------------
                5            10            15            20
GHRH 1-44:  Tyr—Ala—Asp—Ala—Ile—Phe—Thr—Asn—Ser—Tyr—Arg—Lys—Val—Leu—Gly—Gln—Leu—Ser—Ala—Arg—
                25            30            35            40      44
            Lys—Leu—Leu—Gln—Asp—Ile—Met—Ser—Arg—Gln—Gln—Gly—Glu—Ser— Asn—Gln—Glu—Arg—Gly—Ala—Arg—Ala—Arg—Leu—NH₂
```

**FIGURE 12-8.** Amino-acid sequence of growth hormone–releasing hormone (*GHRH*) 1-40 (*top*) and 1-44 (*bottom*). GHRH 1-44 has four additional amino acids at the C-terminal end of the molecule and is amidated.

in highest concentration in the hypothalamus, but also in other parts of the brain, in the gut, and in other tissues. The extrahypothalamic role of GHRH is largely unknown; it may act as a sleep inducer. GHRH is released from the median eminence into the pituitary portal system and is the principal stimulatory hypophysiotropic factor promoting GH secretion. (As mentioned earlier, GHRH is also important for the development of somatotrope cells[15] and for GH synthesis.[18]) GHRH, on reaching the somatotropes, interacts with the GHRH-R, which is a seven transmembrane, $G_s\alpha$-coupled receptor that signals through the cAMP and $Ca^{2+}$-channel pathways (Fig. 12-9). Activation of these pathways effects GH release from secretory granules as well as GH gene transcription. The GHRH-R is expressed in a variety of tissues, but its biologic role in extrapituitary sites is unknown. GHRH is rapidly inactivated in plasma by an amino peptidase that cleaves the N-terminal dipeptide. Ectopic production of GHRH can occur in carcinoid and pancreatic islet tumors.

## SOMATOSTATIN AND SOMATOSTATIN RECEPTORS

Somatostatin is a cyclical peptide that exists in two forms: somatostatin-14 and somatostatin-28, the latter being extended at the amino terminus (Fig. 12-10; see Chap. 169). In humans, both somatostatins are encoded by a single gene on the long arm of chromosome 3, and a 92-amino-acid precursor is differentially processed to the two somatostatin forms, in part in a tissue-specific manner. In the hypothalamus, somatostatin-14 is the predominant form. Somatostatin is widely expressed throughout the central nervous system, the gut, and the pan-

creas. In extrahypothalamic sites, somatostatin has inhibitory effects on insulin secretion, gut hormone secretion, gut motility, and pancreatic and gastrointestinal exocrine secretions. In the hypothalamic-pituitary system, somatostatin inhibits GH and thyroid-stimulating hormone (TSH) secretion. Five somatostatin receptor subtypes are known; normal human pituitary expresses subtypes 1, 2, and 5.[19] These receptors are members of the seven transmembrane domain, G protein–coupled class. Interaction of somatostatin with its receptors induces coupling to $G_i$ and $G_o$ proteins, which in turn inhibits cAMP production and $Ca^{2+}$-channel fluxes, thereby blocking release of GH (and other hormones).[19]

## GROWTH HORMONE–RELEASING PEPTIDES AND THE GROWTH HORMONE–RELEASING PEPTIDE RECEPTOR

GHRPs are a class of short peptides (5–6 amino acids) that are extremely potent as pharmacologic GH secretagogues. The first prototypes (GHRP-5 and GHRP-6) were described in the early 1980s,[20] and many peptide and nonpeptide analogs have since been synthesized. GHRPs are not entirely specific for GH; they also act to release adrenocorticotropic hormone (ACTH) and prolactin, although the effect on these hormones is relatively modest. The cloning of a specific GHRP receptor in 1996 moved this field from the pharmacologic to the physiologic realm,[21] and a natural ligand, ghrelin, has been identified.[21a] The GHRP receptor is also a seven transmembrane domain, G protein–coupled receptor that interacts with $G\alpha_{11}$. It is expressed in the hypothalamus and

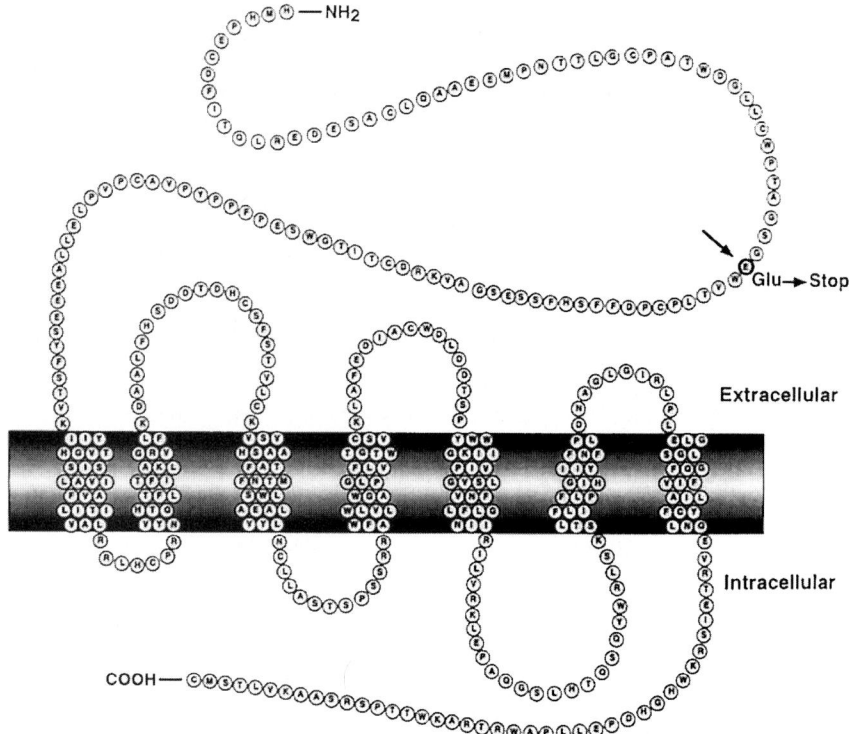

**FIGURE 12-9.** Primary structure of the growth hormone–releasing hormone (*GHRH*) receptor, showing the seven transmembrane helices. The location of a nonsense mutation responsible for familial GHRH-resistant dwarfism is also shown (see text on congenital growth hormone deficiency). (From Maheshwari HG, Silverman BL, Dupuis J, Baumann G. Phenotype and genetic analysis of a syndrome caused by an inactivating mutation in the growth hormone releasing hormone receptor: dwarfism of Sindh. J Clin Endocrinol Metab 1998; 83:4065.)

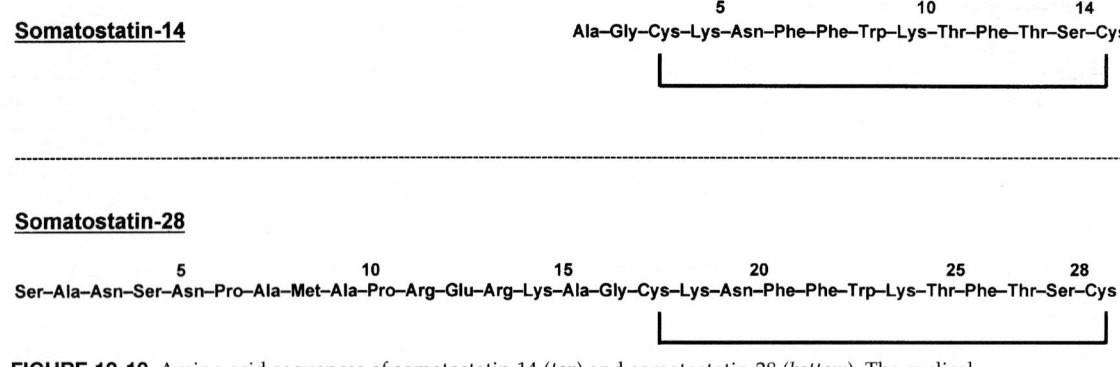

**FIGURE 12-10.** Amino-acid sequences of somatostatin-14 (*top*) and somatostatin-28 (*bottom*). The cyclical nature is indicated by the Cys-Cys bond.

to a lesser degree in the pituitary. Ghrelin is expressed in the stomach and hypothalamus; it must be considered as a potential candidate for the regulation of GH secretion. Of interest is that its action on GH secretion is dependent on a functional GHRH system, and that GHRH and GHRP have synergistic actions in vivo. In contrast, the effect of GHRP on ACTH and prolactin release is independent of GHRH. The principal site of action of GHRP on the release of GH, ACTH, and prolactin is the hypothalamus, although for GH a direct, minor effect is also present at the pituitary level. The precise role of the GHRP system in the regulation of GH secretion remains to be determined.

## FEEDBACK CONTROL

Negative feedback on GH secretion is exerted by IGF-I (a long feedback loop) and by GH itself (a short feedback loop). IGF-I inhibits GH secretion at both the hypothalamic and pituitary levels by influencing GHRH and somatostatin production (hypothalamus) and by interfering with GHRH action (pituitary). GH inhibits its own secretion by modulating GHRH and somatostatin secretion in the hypothalamus. These feedback effects are superimposed on the neural control mentioned earlier.

## OTHER CONTROL MECHANISMS

Other important control mechanisms for GH secretion are estrogen- and age-dependent changes. Estrogen has a generally stimulating effect on GH secretion, which results in a distinct sexual dimorphism of GH secretion during the reproductive years. Estrogen can also be used to "prime" a patient to maximize response to pharmacologic stimuli. The estrogen effect may in part be mediated by induction of a peripheral GH-resistant state, with lowering of serum IGF-I levels.

Pronounced developmental changes occur in GH secretion over the life span. In late fetal and neonatal life, GH secretion is very high and partly unregulated, perhaps in part because of the immaturity of the GHR system and low IGF-I levels. After birth, GH secretion rapidly falls to childhood levels, to be up-regulated again during puberty in response to sex steroids. Thereafter, GH secretion declines progressively by ~15% per decade, reaching very low levels in old age. This process has been termed "somatopause" and is in part responsible for the body compositional changes associated with aging. Both genders are affected by this age-dependent decline.

The principal *physiologic short-term* regulators of GH secretion are (a) neural endogenous rhythm, (b) sleep, (c) stress, including exercise, and (d) nutritional and metabolic signals.

The integrated result of the multiple inputs into the control of GH secretion is a diurnal rhythm of pulsatile secretion that is fairly constant in periodicity but varies widely in amplitude. The highest peaks in serum GH are seen during phase IV (slow wave) sleep, typically 1 to 2 hours after falling asleep. Pulses of smaller amplitude occur throughout the day, on average approximately every 2 hours.[22] Many of these pulses are too small to be measured in conventional assays, and perhaps too small to have much biologic activity. Women of reproductive age generally have higher amplitudes as well as higher interpeak GH levels—an effect that has been attributed to estrogen (Fig. 12-11). The extent to which metabolic changes due to intermittent meals influence GH secretion is unclear; available data suggest that under physiologic circumstances, such effects are minor at best. However, fasting, malnutrition, and obesity have profound effects on GH production (see later). The variability of serum GH levels makes it clear that sampling at single, random time points cannot be used for diagnostic purposes, and that dynamic testing under standardized conditions or diurnal sampling is necessary to arrive at a diagnosis of GH under- or overproduction.

There is no known differential secretion or specific stimulus for any of the GH variants. Indeed, they appear to be cosecreted in response to a variety of physiologic or pharmacologic stimuli. However, they have different plasma half-lives, and hence their relative proportions in plasma may differ from that in the pituitary. The average plasma half-life of GH (representing mostly monomeric 22K GH) is ~17 minutes.[23] The 20K variant and oligomeric forms have longer half-lives.

After secretion, GH binds to GHBP in the circulation. This occurs very rapidly, with maximal binding achieved within a few minutes. The amount of GH bound to GHBP varies, depending on the GHBP level in a given person, the GH concentration (which may partially saturate the GHBP), and the time after a secretory pulse. On the average, 40% to 50% of plasma GH is bound to the GHBP.[24] The bound fraction has delayed clearance, dampens the oscillations of serum GH, and serves as a circulating GH reservoir. The GHBP level in serum is not influenced by GH pulses; it exhibits no or minimal diurnal variation.

## REGULATION OF PLACENTAL GROWTH HORMONE SECRETION

GH-V or placental GH is secreted during pregnancy into the maternal (but not fetal) circulation. This process is not regulated by the factors just described for pituitary GH regulation. The principles regulating GH-V secretion are unknown; it may simply be released constitutively as a function of syncytiotrophoblast mass. Plasma GH-V levels increase progressively during the second trimester to reach a plateau in the third trimester (Fig. 12-12). Concomitantly, pituitary GH-N levels are suppressed, presumably via negative feedback by GH-V and IGF-I. GH-V binds to GHR with the same affinity as GH-N; its high plasma levels may be responsible for some of the fluid retention and changes in physical features seen in late pregnancy.

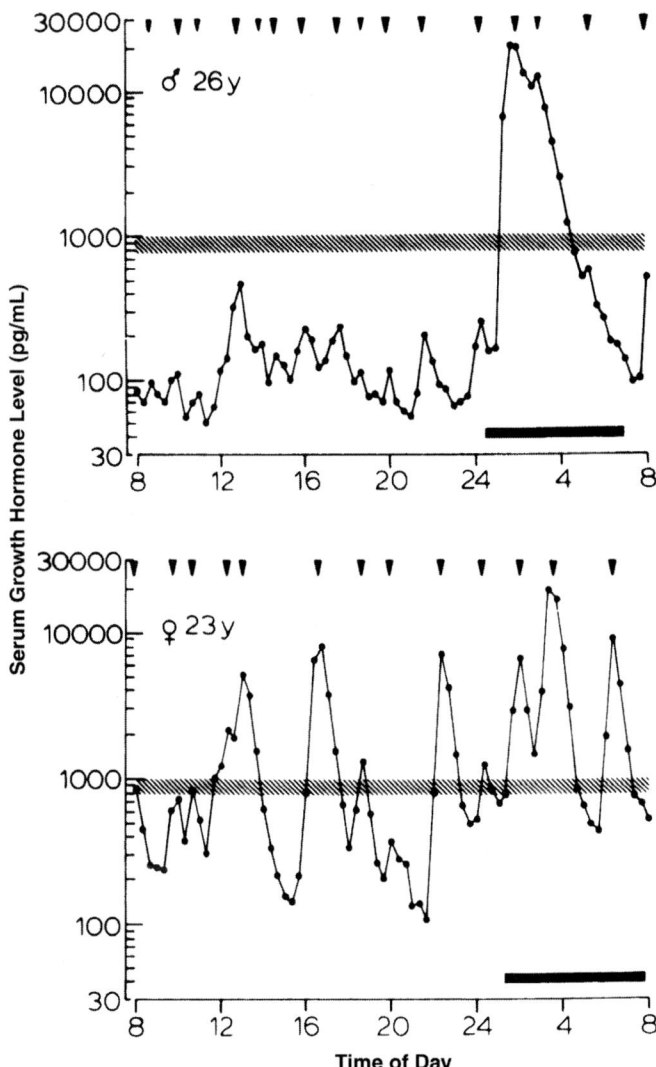

FIGURE 12-11. Characteristic diurnal profiles of serum growth hormone (*GH*) levels in a young man (*top*) and a young woman (*bottom*). Women of reproductive age have a higher baseline and a greater average pulse amplitude than men. The ordinate is logarithmic to emphasize the presence of small secretory peaks throughout the day; note that the units for GH are pg/mL. The black bar indicates the period of sleep; the shaded bar shows the 1 ng/mL level that represents the detection limit in many conventional assays; the triangles on top indicate the secretory events as defined by a pulse-detection program. (Adapted from Winer LM, Shaw MA, Baumann G. Basal plasma growth hormone levels in man: new evidence for rhythmicity of growth hormone secretion. J Clin Endocrinol Metab 1990; 70:1678.)

# REGULATION OF THE GROWTH HORMONE RECEPTOR AND BINDING PROTEIN

For reasons of accessibility, little is known about the regulation of GHRs in human tissues. Therefore, much of the information about GHR regulation is based on (a) animal studies and (b) GHBP measurements in humans, using the GHBP as a surrogate for the GHR. Based on the comparison between direct GHR data in animals and GHBP data in humans, the GHBP level in serum appears to be a reasonable index of GHR abundance in tissues, primarily the liver.

The main regulator of GHR/GHBP abundance is ontogeny. In fetal and neonatal life, GHR expression is very low, and serum GHBP levels are correspondingly low. This is a physio-

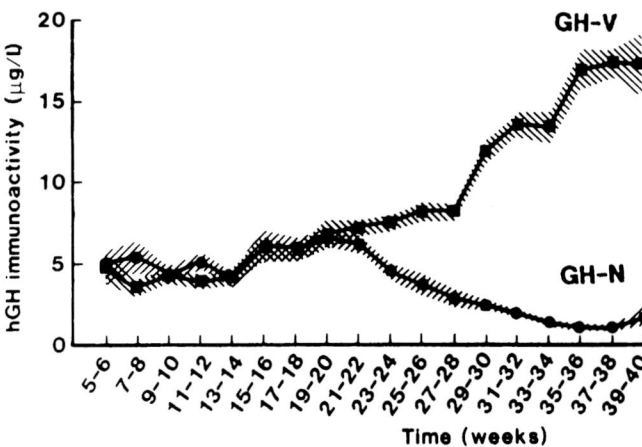

FIGURE 12-12. Plasma levels of the growth hormones GH-N and GH-V during pregnancy. Pituitary GH-N is gradually supplanted by placental GH-V. (*hGH*, human growth hormone.) (From Baumann G. Growth hormone heterogeneity: genes, isohormones, variants and binding proteins. Endocr Rev 1991; 12:424; as adapted from Frankenne F, Closset J, Gomez F, et al. The physiology of growth hormones [GHs] in pregnant women and partial characterization of the placental GH variant. J Clin Endocrinol Metab 1988; 66:1171.)

logic GH-resistant condition, with high GH and low IGF-I levels. Postnatally a rapid up-regulation of the GHR and GHBP occurs, coincident with the emergence of GH responsivity.[25] This process continues throughout childhood, until in the late teens GHBP levels (and presumably GHR levels) reach adult levels. GHBP levels remain constant through adult life until approximately age 60, when a progressive decline ensues that continues until the tenth decade.[26] This decline is accompanied by a decline in IGF-I levels and constitutes part of the somatopause. Thus, in old age the changes caused by the decreasing GH secretion are further amplified by the development of GH resistance. Similar changes in GHR expression have been shown in aging animals. Women of reproductive age have slightly higher GHBP levels than men.

Estrogens, particularly if given orally, up-regulate serum GHBP, whereas androgens tend to lower GHBP. Interestingly, no discernible change is seen in GHBP level during puberty in either sex. The effect of GH itself on the GHBP in humans is controversial. The majority of studies find no significant change in GHBP levels in GH deficiency or in response to GH treatment. However, some reports show an up-regulation, and others a down-regulation of GHBP by GH. On balance, the effect of GH on serum GHBP (and probably, hence, on GHR) in humans is neutral or at least inconsistent. This differs from the case in rodents, in which the GHR (and the GHBP) expression is up-regulated by GH. Another important regulator of GHR/GHBP expression is nutritional status, probably, at least in part, mediated by insulin. A strong positive correlation exists between body mass index and serum GHBP, and IGF-I levels and GH responsivity vary in parallel as a function of adiposity and nutritional status.[13]

# ACTIONS OF GROWTH HORMONE

Growth hormone has numerous biologic actions, many occurring in concert to enhance protein anabolism and tissue accretion. GH can act directly as well as indirectly through IGF-I, also known as somatomedin C. The mitogenic and proliferative actions of GH are mediated through IGF-I, whereas some of the metabolic actions are direct GH effects. GH has no specific target organ; it acts on most if not all tissues through the ubiquitously expressed GHR.

## INSULIN-LIKE GROWTH FACTORS AND THEIR BINDING PROTEINS

The existence of GH-dependent factors that might mediate the action of GH was first suggested by the report that $SO_4$ incorporation into growth cartilage chondroitin sulfate was reduced by hypophysectomy, but that exposure of cartilage to GH in vitro could not correct the abnormality. In contrast, serum from animals treated with GH was highly effective in restoring $SO_4$ uptake, implicating a GH-dependent "sulfation factor."[27] Sulfation factor was later renamed somatomedin, and the "somatomedin hypothesis" was born. It soon became clear that somatomedin was identical to "nonsuppressible insulin-like activity," which led to the characterization of IGF-I and IGF-II. The IGFs are proinsulin-like molecules that are produced in many tissues in response to GH and other regulators. IGF-I production is highly GH-dependent, whereas IGF-II production is less dependent on GH. IGFs act both locally in a paracrine/autocrine fashion and distantly in a hormone-like mode. They have mitogenic and metabolic activities and act through the type I IGF receptor, which is structurally similar to the insulin receptor. Six binding proteins for IGF (IGFBP) are present in serum and interstitial fluid; they may either enhance or decrease IGF activity.[28] In addition, three IGFBP-related proteins bind IGFs with low affinity,[29] for a total of nine proteins in the IGFBP family. IGFBP-1 is insulin dependent and has primarily inhibitory activity in vivo. IGFBP-2 is inversely GH dependent; its biologic role is incompletely understood. IGFBP-3 is the major IGFBP in serum; it is highly GH dependent, and it serves primarily to retain IGFs in the circulation by forming a 150-kDa ternary complex involving IGF, IGFBP-3, and another GH-dependent protein called acid-labile subunit (ALS). This complex is responsible for the high IGF concentrations in serum and serves as a circulating IGF reservoir. Most of the circulating IGF is bound in this complex. IGFBP-4, IGFBP-5, and IGFBP-6 are in part associated with the extracellular matrix and modulate IGF action through restricting or enhancing IGF access to the IGF receptor. IGFBP structure and activity is modulated by proteases that cleave the IGFBPs, thereby decreasing IGF-binding affinity. Protease activity is regulated by a variety of physiologic and pathologic conditions. IGFBPs and their fragments may have activities of their own (such as antianabolic activity) that are independent of their IGF-binding properties. A full description of the complex IGF-IGFBP system is beyond the scope of this chapter; from a clinical standpoint, an understanding of IGFBP-3 and IGFBP-2 is most important because they can be used diagnostically.

## INSULIN-LIKE GROWTH FACTOR RECEPTOR

IGF-I and IGF-II bind to and signal through the IGF receptor (also known as type I IGF receptor). IGF-II also binds to the mannose-6-phosphate/type II IGF receptor, but to date no convincing evidence exists that the lysosomal pathway connected to this receptor is relevant to GH action. The type I IGF receptor is structurally homologous to the insulin receptor; it has a tetrameric structure with two extracellular α-subunits covalently connected to two β-subunits through disulfide bonds. The β-subunits have intrinsic tyrosine kinase activity and signal through a phosphorylation cascade involving IRS-1 and IRS-2, PI3-kinase, MAPK, and other pathways. The IGF receptor differs functionally from the insulin receptor in that it promotes primarily mitogenic/proliferative rather than metabolic activities. Because both receptors share intracellular pathways, it is presently not clear how this relative specificity of actions is conferred. Nevertheless, some crosstalk occurs between the IGF and the insulin systems at high ligand concentrations. The IGF receptor is widely expressed in tissues, with the exception

**TABLE 12-1.**
**Bioactivities of Growth Hormone (GH)**

| Direct GH Effects | IGF-mediated Effects | Both (or Unknown) |
|---|---|---|
| Lipolysis | Chondrocyte clonal expansion | Insulin antagonism |
| Amino-acid transport in muscle | Sulfate incorporation into cartilage | Islet cell hyperplasia |
| Acute hypoglycemic action | DNA and RNA synthesis | Erythropoiesis |
| IGF-I production | Phosphorus and Na$^+$ retention in kidney | Nitrogen retention |
| IGFBP-3 and ALS production | Linear growth in bones | Somatic growth* |
| Prechondrocyte differentiation | | Enhancement of immune function? |
| Lactogenesis | | |
| Somatostatin secretion in hypothalamus | | |

*IGF-I*, insulin-like growth factor-I; *IGFBP-3*, insulin-like growth factor binding protein-3; *ALS*, acid-labile subunit.
*Somatic growth is possible but suboptimal with IGF-I alone. GH assists IGF action through several ancillary effects, such as changing in vivo IGF kinetics through IGFBP-3 and ALS production, synthesizing protein in muscle, differentiating prechondrocytes, etc.

of liver, where it is expressed at very low levels. The IGF system is described in detail in Chapter 173.

Because of the widespread expression of the GHR, the IGFs, and the IGF receptor, discerning which of the ultimate biologic actions of GH are direct and which are IGF-mediated has been difficult. Table 12-1 lists the principal GH actions and attempts to assign them to direct and IGF-mediated pathways. In many cases, this assignment is tentative, and both direct and indirect mediation may occur.

The principal bioactivities of the GH/IGF system relevant to the intact organism and to clinical medicine are nitrogen retention, protein anabolism, linear growth, lipolysis, insulin antagonism (diabetogenesis), Na$^+$ retention, and negative feedback on GH secretion (short- and long-loop feedback). GH is best viewed as the master postnatal anabolic hormone orchestrating a cascade of activities leading to lean body mass accretion. The exception is adipose tissue, in which GH is largely catabolic. Human GH has lactogenic properties because it can bind to prolactin receptors. This is not a property of animal GHs, and its biologic importance in humans is uncertain. Also unclear is the importance of GH for the immune system; no overt abnormality in immune function is seen in cases of GH deficiency or in GH resistance.

## MEASUREMENT OF PLASMA GROWTH HORMONE

The measurement of GH in blood is problematic because of the heterogeneous nature of GH. This heterogeneity is one reason for the observation that different assay designs can yield different results for the same blood sample.[30] Plasma GH is measured either by conventional polyclonal radioimmunoassay or by a variety of monoclonal immunoradiometric or immunoenzymatic assays. Monoclonal assays frequently yield lower readings than polyclonal assays. This is in part due to the fact that some of the GH variants are not fully reactive in monoclonal assays, but other, poorly understood matrix effects are also involved. The problem of nonreproducibility of results among assays and laboratories can present a diagnostic dilemma in the classification of a patient as GH deficient or normal. Discrepancies are particularly notable among monoclonal assays. The need exists for a universal standard and assay design that permits comparison of GH determinations among different laboratories.

**TABLE 12-2.**
**Dynamic Tests for Growth Hormone Secretion**

| Stimulatory | Dose/Administration |
|---|---|
| Insulin hypoglycemia | 0.05–0.10 U/kg iv |
| L-dopa | Adults: 500 mg po |
| | Children: 250 mg po |
| Arginine infusion | 0.5 g/kg iv over 30 min (30 g maximum) |
| GHRH | 1 µg/kg iv |
| Clonidine | Adults: 250 µg po |
| | Children: 125 µg po |
| Glucagon | 1 mg sc or im |
| GHRP* | Dose depends on type of GHRP (1 µg/kg iv for GHRP-2 or hexarelin) |
| GHRH-arginine combined | |
| GHRH-GHRP combined* | |
| **Inhibitory** | |
| Glucose-tolerance test | 75 or 100 g po |

*iv*, intravenous; *po*, by mouth; *sc*, subcutaneous; *im*, intramuscular; *GHRH*, growth hormone–releasing hormone; *GHRP*, growth hormone–releasing peptide.
*Not yet in standard use.
Stimulatory tests can be enhanced by pretreatment with estrogen, pyridostigmine, or propranolol.

## DYNAMIC TESTS OF GROWTH HORMONE SECRETION

Because of the pulsatile nature of GH secretion, plasma GH levels vary widely in normal subjects. It follows that a single GH measurement is not diagnostic for an abnormality in the GH axis. Therefore, dynamic testing of the response of plasma GH to standardized provocative or inhibitory tests is mandatory for the evaluation of GH disorders. Table 12-2 lists the dynamic tests in clinical use. This topic has been comprehensively reviewed.[31] Among the provocative tests, the insulin-tolerance test is considered the "gold standard," as it is a potent and reliable stimulus for GH release. Its disadvantage is that induction of hypoglycemia can be risky, and, therefore, the test must be closely supervised. For the test to be valid, a drop in blood glucose by at least 50% from the starting level must be achieved. GHRH testing has not proven to be as useful as anticipated because the GH response is highly variable, presumably because of differences in prevailing somatostatin tone. Clonidine is used successfully in children, but in adults it is a relatively weak stimulus for GH release. In normal subjects, the highest serum GH levels are seen after combined GHRH-GHRP stimulation. However, the clinical utility of this potent test in the diagnosis of GH deficiency is not yet known.

For research purposes, circadian sampling of blood for GH measurements is probably the best procedure to assess spontaneous GH secretion. The frequency of sampling should be at least every 20 minutes for accurate estimation of secretion rate. This can be done over a 24-hour period or overnight, when most of the GH secretion occurs. A variant of circadian sampling is continuous blood withdrawal by a pump. This yields a pooled "average" GH level but does not permit detection of secretory pulses. These maneuvers are cumbersome and impractical for general diagnostic purposes; they are largely reserved for investigational use. An additional limitation is that the GH secretion rate is quite variable among normal subjects, and the boundary between normal and deficient GH secretion rates is ill defined.

Measurement of urinary GH excretion has been advocated as a possible estimate of GH secretion rate. This method is technically feasible, but only a small fraction (≤0.01%) of the daily GH production is excreted in the urine. This, combined with substantial day-to-day variability and dependence on renal function, has made it difficult to establish urine GH determination as a reliable index of GH production rate. Measurement of urine GH as a clinical test has therefore been largely abandoned.

The GHRH-stimulation test cannot be used to distinguish reliably between hypothalamic and pituitary GH deficiency. This is similar to the failure of testing with other hypothalamic releasing hormones (gonadotropin-releasing hormone [GnRH], thyrotropin-releasing hormone [TRH], corticotropin-releasing hormone [CRH]) to clearly differentiate hypothalamic from pituitary disease.

Pituitary function tests must be interpreted in the context of other clinical assessments. They can yield misleading results in some conditions not associated with hypothalamic-pituitary disease. Examples are obesity, hypothyroidism, or hypercorticism, in which the GH response to all stimuli tends to be blunted. Conversely, malnutrition, catabolic conditions, or stress may be associated with elevated GH levels that are not normally suppressible.

## CLINICAL USE OF INSULIN-LIKE GROWTH FACTOR-I AND INSULIN-LIKE GROWTH FACTOR–BINDING PROTEIN MEASUREMENTS

Plasma IGF-I can be used as a surrogate measurement for GH. Unlike GH, its plasma level fluctuates very little throughout the day. Because IGF-I is highly GH dependent, its serum level reflects GH secretory status and can be used as an index for "integrated GH secretion." The same is true for IGFBP-3, another GH-dependent factor. However, such measurements must be interpreted in the context of other clinical information. IGF-I is also highly dependent on nutritional status and is influenced by age, catabolic disease, etc. IGF-I and IGFBP-3 levels are best used in conjunction with dynamic GH measurements or for longitudinal follow-up in conditions that are already diagnosed as primary GH disorders. IGFBP-2 is inversely GH dependent and may be used as an ancillary measurement. IGF-II, although GH dependent to some degree, has not proven to be of clinical use in the diagnosis of GH disorders. In the measurement of IGFs, separation of IGF from the IGFBPs before measurements is imperative to avoid spurious results due to interference of IGFBPs in the assay. Several strategies can be used to accomplish this, such as acid ethanol extraction, $C_{18}$ column separation, and acid gel filtration.

## ABNORMAL SECRETION OF GROWTH HORMONE

### DEFICIENCY OF GROWTH HORMONE

GH deficiency results from various causes, and the clinical manifestations depend on the age of the patient when the disease first occurs. The condition may be hereditary or acquired, and GH deficiency may be isolated or combined with other pituitary hormone deficiencies. Subdividing GH deficiency into childhood onset and adult onset categories is useful, because some of the clinical manifestations are different.

#### ETIOLOGY

**Congenital Growth Hormone Deficiency.** Table 12-3 lists the causes of GH deficiency. Among the congenital causes, between 5% and 30% have a familial pattern, which suggests a genetic basis. Known genetic causes of *combined* pituitary hormone deficiency involve the transcription factors Prop-1 and Pit-1, both members of the POU-homeodomain family of proteins critical for tissue differentiation. These genes are sequentially expressed during pituitary ontogeny, and Pit-1 is dependent on the expression of Prop-1 (of which the full name is "Prophet of Pit-1"). Inactivating mutations in the PROP1 gene lead to defective pituitary development, with TSH, luteinizing hormone, follicle-stimulating hormone, GH, and prolactin deficiency.[32] A two-base deletion in a hot spot in the

**TABLE 12-3.**
**Causes of Growth Hormone (GH) Deficiency**

**CONGENITAL**

| *Genetic* | *Mutant Gene* | *Inheritance* |
|---|---|---|
| 1. Isolated GH deficiency | GHN | AR; AD |
| | GHRHR | AR |
| | Locus near *btk* | X-linked |
| 2. Combined pituitary hormone deficiency | PROP1 | AR |
| | PIT1 | AR |
| 3. Pituitary developmental defect | HESX1(– Rpx) | AR |

*Other*
   Birth trauma (breech delivery, asphyxia, etc.)
   Midline defects
   Pituitary agenesis
   Anencephaly

**ACQUIRED POSTNATALLY**

*Tumors*
   Pituitary adenoma
   Craniopharyngioma
   Glioma, meningioma, pinealoma, etc.
   Metastatic tumor (rare)

*Trauma*

*Cranial radiation therapy*

*Bleeding/infarction*
   Sheehan syndrome
   Pituitary apoplexy

*Granulomatous disease*
   Sarcoid, tuberculosis, syphilis, histiocytosis X

*Infiltrative disease*
   Hemochromatosis, amyloidosis

*Infections*
   Meningitis, abscess

*Autoimmune hypophysitis*

*Functional*
   Emotional deprivation syndrome

*Idiopathic*
   Presumed GHRH deficiency or insufficiency

*AR*, autosomal recessive; *AD*, autosomal dominant; *btk*, Bruton's tyrosine kinase; *GHRHR*, growth hormone–releasing hormone receptor.

PROP1 gene, with resulting frameshift, is the most common cause.[33] The clinical phenotype is one of familial dwarfism, with hypothyroidism and hypogonadism. Of interest, pituitary enlargement frequently occurs in affected patients—a finding whose pathogenesis is not clear. Mutations in the PIT1 gene are another cause of combined pituitary hormone deficiency.[34] At least eight different mutations have been described; most are recessively inherited, but some are dominant negative (i.e., the abnormal gene product interferes with that derived from the normal allele). Pit-1 is important for development of somatotropes, lactotropes, and thyrotropes; affected patients suffer from GH, prolactin, and TSH deficiency. They do not develop pituitary enlargement as is seen in patients with PROP1 mutations. Known genetic causes of *isolated* GH deficiency include inactivating mutations in the GHRHR gene and in the GHN gene. GHRH action is required for somatotrope proliferation (late in pituitary development) and for GH synthesis and secretion. A defective GHRHR impacts all these mechanisms, and affected patients have pituitary hypoplasia and severe isolated GH deficiency.[35,36] The clinical phenotype is one of proportionate dwarfism with relative microcephaly, normal fertility, and normal lactation.[36] Mutations in the GHN gene affect GH production directly.[37] The GH locus is prone to deletions because of gene duplication, which includes homologous sequences in the regions flanking the duplicated genes. Deletions of 6.7, 7.0, and 7.6 kb are typical; affected homozygous patients have severe GH deficiency (termed type IA). A similar phenotype occurs with other severely inactivating mutations, such as nonsense and frameshift mutations. A milder form (termed type IB) is seen with less disabling mutations, such as missense mutations in which some, albeit abnormal, GH is produced. In type IA, secondary resistance to exogenous GH administration is seen frequently, but not always, because of the formation of high-titer anti-GH antibodies to the "foreign" GH protein. Patients with type IB, on the other hand, respond well to exogenous GH because they are immune tolerant to GH. A special case in this category is a bioinactive GH.[38] Dominantly inherited GHN gene mutations (termed type II) are caused by splice-site mutations in one allele that result in skipping of exon 3, with the resultant abnormal GH protein exerting a deleterious (dominant negative) influence on the normal GH produced by the intact allele. Improper disulfide pairing/aggregation or deranged transport to secretory granules are postulated mechanisms. In one case, a mutant GH was shown to act as an antagonist at the level of the GHR.[39] Yet another type of isolated GH deficiency is inherited in an X-linked manner (termed type III). The gene involved is unknown but resides close to the gene for "Bruton tyrosine kinase," an enzyme that is crucial for B-lymphocyte function. Hence, this type of GH deficiency is usually associated with hypo- or agammaglobulinemia. Interestingly, defects in the GHRH gene have not been identified to date, despite the fact that many cases of idiopathic GH deficiency are thought to be due to GHRH deficiency.

The majority of cases of congenital GH deficiency (isolated or combined) are sporadic; they are thought to be caused by birth trauma, cerebral insults, and congenital malformations or tumors affecting hypothalamic-pituitary development or function. Approximately 10% of such patients have abnormal magnetic resonance imaging (MRI) scans. In one family affected with two cases of septo-optic dysplasia, an inactivating mutation has been found in the gene encoding the early developmental transcription factor Hesx1, also known as Rpx (Rathke Pouch Homeobox).[40] The incidence of GH deficiency is estimated as 1 per 4000 to 10,000 births.

**Acquired Growth Hormone Deficiency.** GH deficiency can be acquired at any time during the life span, depending on when a hypothalamic-pituitary lesion or insult occurs. As already indicated, normal aging is associated with declining GH secretion during adulthood, and senescence resembles progressive GH insufficiency. During the growing years, the hallmark of GH deficiency is growth retardation; in adult life, the signs are more subtle changes in body composition and metabolism. Because of the lack of obvious manifestations, GH deficiency in adults is often not recognized, being diagnosed only after a long delay, or not considered clinically important. Moreover, only recently has GH deficiency in adults become amenable to therapy.

With pituitary lesions, the pattern of loss of pituitary hormones tends to follow a certain order: GH, gonadotropins, and prolactin tend to be lost early, whereas TSH and ACTH are affected later. This may be related to the abundance and/or spatial distribution of the respective cell types, with somatotropes being the most prevalent (accounting for ~50% of the anterior pituitary mass).

**CLINICAL PRESENTATION AND DIAGNOSIS**

In childhood, GH deficiency soon declares itself because of growth retardation. The GH dependence of somatic growth begins at or shortly after birth. If coexistent TSH deficiency is present, the resulting hypothyroidism contributes to and aggravates growth retardation. Organic causes for GH deficiency should be sought, but frequently no lesion is found, leading to the diagnosis of idiopathic GH deficiency. This entity is attributed to partial GHRH deficiency, although direct proof is

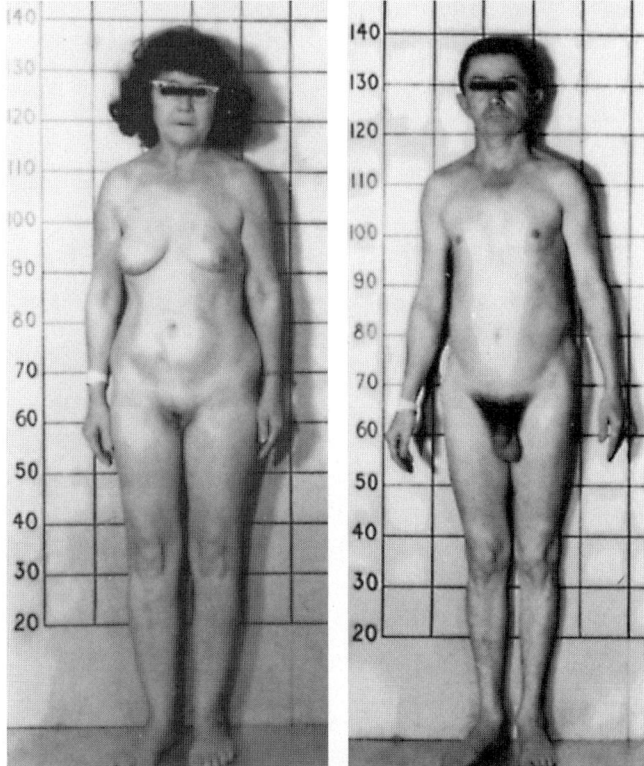

A

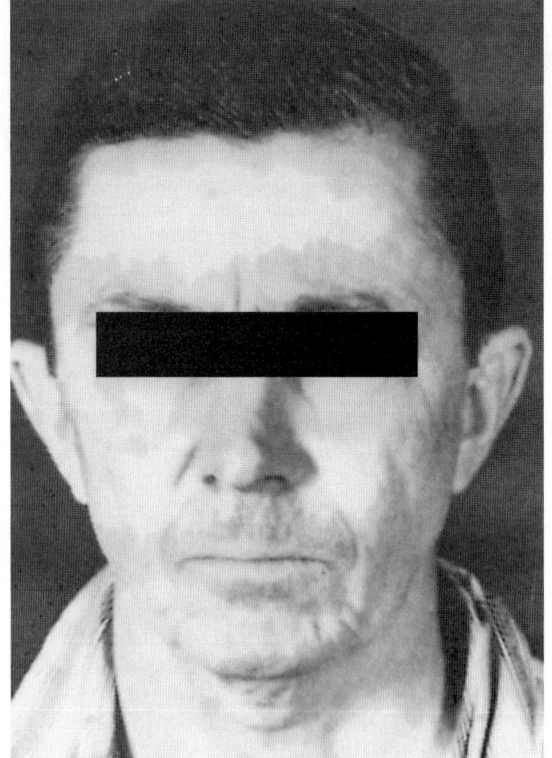

B

**FIGURE 12-13. A,** Two siblings with familial isolated growth hormone (*GH*) deficiency. Note the proportionate short stature and normal sexual development. **B,** The "child-like," finely wrinkled face of a 41-year-old man with isolated GH deficiency.

difficult. Growth retardation due to GH deficiency results in proportionate dwarfism and a progressive deviation from the normal growth curve. Untreated severe isolated GH deficiency results in adult heights of 120–140 cm in males and 110–130 cm in females. Other manifestations of GH deficiency during childhood are hypoglycemia, micropenis, and craniofacial abnormalities with saddle nose and facial hypoplasia. Patients tend to be "chubby" because of increased adipose tissue, particularly in the truncal area. Bone maturation is delayed by several years, and puberty is delayed by 2 to 3 years. Postpubertal men have a characteristic, high-pitched voice. The impact of GH deficiency on somatic growth and development is described in detail in Chapters 18, 92, and 198; Figure 12-13 shows the phenotype of adult patients with isolated GH deficiency. GH deficiency must be differentiated from other forms of short stature (constitutional, idiopathic, familial, etc.) that are much more common.

In adults, GH deficiency should be suspected when a pituitary or hypothalamic lesion is found, or when a history of childhood GH deficiency is present. Patients who had idiopathic GH deficiency during childhood may or may not be GH deficient as adults, so that retesting of GH secretion in adulthood is required. Approximately two-thirds of such patients are found to have normal GH secretion as adults.[41] One explanation for this phenomenon is that GH secretion rates during childhood and particularly during puberty are higher than in adult life, and that a partial limitation in GH production may yield levels that are inadequate during the growth years but sufficient in adulthood. Patients with pituitary lesions should be tested for GH deficiency even in the absence of other pituitary hormone deficiencies because somatotrope dysfunction may be an early manifestation of pituitary failure. This has therapeutic consequences, because such patients may benefit from GH treatment. The clinical manifestations of the adult GH deficiency syndrome are listed in Table 12-4.

Diagnosis relies on the demonstration of an underlying cause (a pituitary or hypothalamic lesion, a genetic defect, or a history of radiation), on provocative tests of GH secretion, and on IGF-I measurement. A low serum IGFBP-3 and a high IGFBP-2 level can be used as corroborative indicators. The typical, but arbitrary, cutoff for a normal peak GH level in response to provocative tests is 5 to 7 ng/mL in a polyclonal assay, and 2.5 to 3.5 ng/mL in a monoclonal assay. The Growth Hormone Research Society Consensus Guidelines for adult GH deficiency define a cutoff of 3 ng/mL in response to an insulin-tolerance test as "severe GH deficiency," with a gray zone between 3 and 5 ng/mL, using a polyclonal assay.[42] These cutoffs cannot be absolute because of the problems inherent in the assays mentioned above, and because of interindividual variations in GH response. Furthermore, tests that are less potent than the insulin-tolerance test may yield a lower GH response. Therefore, provocative tests must be interpreted in the clinical context. A finding of a low

**TABLE 12-4.**
**Clinical Manifestations of Growth Hormone Deficiency in Adults**

Increased adiposity, especially truncal/visceral
Decreased lean body mass
Decreased body fluid
Osteopenia
Thin, dry skin, with fine wrinkles
Poor sweating and impaired temperature regulation
Decreased muscular strength
Decreased exercise performance
Decreased energy and vitality
Decreased psychosocial well-being: depression, social isolation, anxiety
Elevated cholesterol, particularly low-density lipoprotein cholesterol
Hyperinsulinemia (obesity related)

difficult to obtain. Patients with idiopathic GH deficiency usually have blunted, but not absent, GH responses to secretagogues. As already mentioned, the boundaries between normal, insufficient, and deficient GH secretion are ill defined because GH secretion rates are highly variable in normal people. This may render the diagnosis of idiopathic GH deficiency

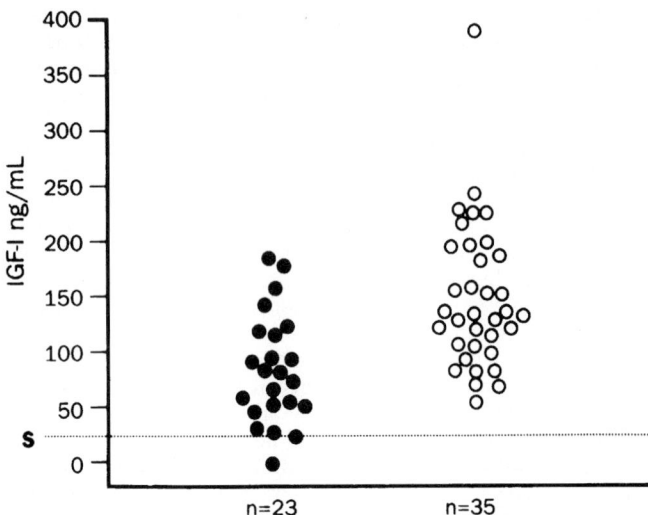

**FIGURE 12-14.** Serum insulin-like growth factor-I (*IGF-I*) levels in adult hypopituitary patients, aged 17 to 77 years (*closed circles*), compared to those in age-matched normal controls (*open circles*). All patients had growth hormone deficiency, as assessed by the insulin-tolerance test, and deficiency of other pituitary hormones. Note the overlap between normal and hypopituitary IGF-I levels. (*S*, assay sensitivity for IGF-I [25 ng/mL]; *n*, number of subjects tested.) (Adapted from Hoffman DM, O'Sullivan AJ, Baxter RC, Ho KKY. Diagnosis of growth-hormone deficiency in adults. Lancet 1994; 343:1064.)

serum IGF-I level is helpful in the absence of other causes for decreased IGF production, such as nutritional deprivation. However, difficulty arises because of the wide normal range for IGF-I levels. IGF-I levels are highly age dependent and must be judged against age-appropriate normative values. In very young children, in whom IGF-I levels are naturally low, differentiation of GH deficiency from normal production may be difficult based on the IGF-I level. In adults, particularly older adults, considerable overlap also exists between the normal IGF-I range and that seen in GH deficiency (Fig. 12-14).

## TREATMENT

GH deficiency can be treated successfully with recombinant human GH, given subcutaneously once daily at bedtime. The bedtime dosing is designed to at least partially mimic the normal GH secretory pulse occurring after sleep onset. The dose for children is 25 to 50 μg/kg per day; for adults it is 3 to 12 μg/kg per day. Studies have suggested that in adults administration of an absolute daily dose (e.g., 200–400 μg per day) may be more appropriate than dosing based on kilograms of body weight. This regimen is more physiologic because normal GH secretion is inversely related to adiposity, and weight-based dosing does not consider this. Women of reproductive age or those on estrogen treatment need higher GH doses to maintain normal IGF-I levels, as would be expected from the higher GH-secretion rates in normal women.

GH therapy is highly effective in reversing the manifestations of GH deficiency. The effect on children is growth acceleration to normal or even "catch-up" growth velocity, and normal adult height can be achieved provided that treatment starts early and is maintained until epiphyseal fusion occurs. Pediatric use of GH is described in detail in Chapters 18, 92, and 198. In adults, the principal effects are normalization of body composition (i.e., a decrease in adipose tissue, particularly visceral fat; Fig. 12-15), an increase in lean body mass and body fluid, an increase in bone mineral density, and a decrease in low-density lipoprotein cholesterol.[43] Other effects, such as improved muscular strength, endurance, energy, and psychosocial well-being, have also been reported in many, but not all, studies. Several years are probably required to realize the full benefit of GH therapy in adults. GH therapy for adults has begun only in the past decade, and its

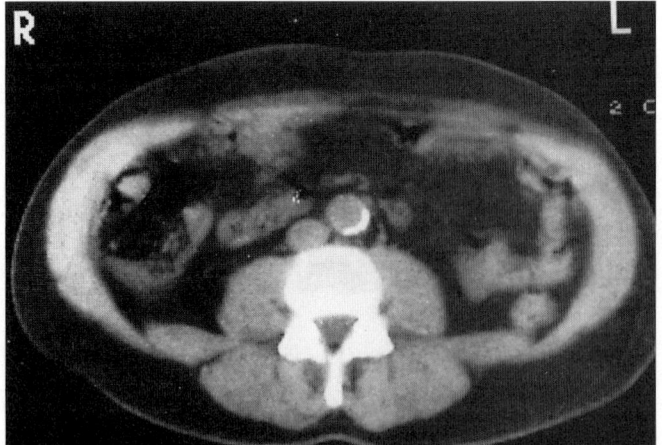

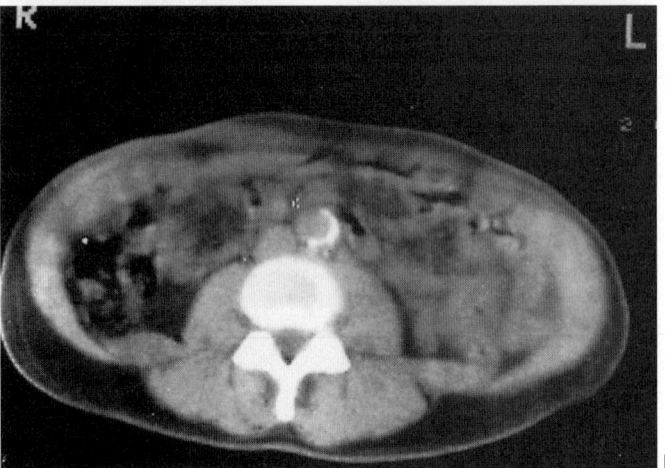

**FIGURE 12-15.** Transverse computed tomographic scan at the L3–L4 level before (**A**) and after 6 months of growth hormone therapy (**B**). Note the reduction of both visceral and subcutaneous adipose tissue (*dark areas*). (*R*, right; *L*, left.) (From Bengtsson B-A, Edén S, Lönn L, et al. Treatment of adults with growth hormone [GH] deficiency with recombinant human GH. J Clin Endocrinol Metab 1993; 76:309.)

ultimate outcome is still not fully known. One important unanswered question is whether the shortened life span of hypopituitary patients[44] can be prolonged with GH therapy.[44a]

GH dosing is monitored in children by observation of growth velocity and serum IGF-I, and in adults by serum IGF-I levels, which should be maintained in the age-appropriate normal range. Side effects are rare in children; adults, particularly the elderly, are more prone to side effects, such as transient edema, carpal tunnel syndrome, arthralgia, and myalgia, but these symptoms can be minimized or largely avoided by proper dosing. GH secretion naturally declines with age, and dosing accordingly should be adjusted based on age. Carbohydrate intolerance has not proved to be a major problem in GH-replacement therapy. Typically, insulin levels increase initially, but glucose levels remain normal. This is physiologically appropriate and inherent in the correction of the GH-deficient state. Nevertheless, glycemia should be monitored after institution of GH therapy, which may unmask a latent diabetic propensity. As adiposity diminishes over time, insulin levels tend to fall back to baseline values.

## GROWTH HORMONE INSENSITIVITY

A condition that clinically resembles GH deficiency is GH insensitivity, which can range from absolute GH resistance to varying degrees of mild GH insensitivity. It may be congenital/genetic or acquired.

## GENETIC CAUSES

Genetic GH resistance, also known as Laron syndrome, is due to inactivating mutations in the *GHR* gene.[45] Inheritance is autosomal recessive. Over 250 patients have been reported worldwide; significant consanguineous clusters have been described in Israel, Ecuador, and the Bahamas. Over 35 different mutations (deletions and nonsense, splice-site, and missense mutations) have been identified to date. Most are found in the extracellular domain of the receptor and inactivate the GH binding site. Other mutations include one that interferes with receptor dimerization, some that result in skipping of exon 8 (which encodes the transmembrane domain), and some that severely truncate the intracellular domain. Of interest is a mutation that has a dominant negative effect because the abnormal, truncated receptor interferes with normal receptor signaling owing to heterodimer formation between normal and mutant receptor.[46] The type of mutation determines whether the GHBP activity in plasma is absent or low (the majority of cases), normal, or even high (e.g., when the mutant receptor lacks a transmembrane domain).[47]

The phenotype is similar to that of severe GH deficiency. Children are near-normal at birth but show all the signs and symptoms associated with GH deficiency described earlier. Facial dysplasia may be even more pronounced than in GH deficiency. Heterozygotes are physically normal. IGF-I and IGFBP-3 levels are very low, but in contrast to GH deficiency, GH levels are elevated, both in the basal state and after stimulation. This is due to lack of negative feedback on GH production by IGF-I and by GH. Treatment with GH is ineffective, but therapy with IGF-I has resulted in growth rates that approach, but do not quite reach, those seen with GH therapy in GH-deficient children. Numerous problems exist with IGF-I therapy, such as abnormal pharmacokinetics because of low IGFBP-3 levels, limited availability of IGF-I, and absence of direct GH effects, that render therapy for this rare condition difficult.

Milder *heterozygous* mutations or polymorphisms in the GH receptor have been suggested as a possible explanation of idiopathic short stature.[48] However, in view of the fact that heterozygous relatives of Laron syndrome patients are of normal height, it is difficult to explain how milder heterozygous mutations would cause short stature.

Pygmies have a primary, possibly genetic, form of partial GH resistance. This has been attributed to low GHR expression, based on low serum GHBP levels.[49] Pygmies may also have partial IGF-I insensitivity, as postulated from the lack of an IGF-mediated proliferative response of lymphocytes derived from pygmies.[50] The exact reasons for pygmies' short stature remain to be elucidated.

## ACQUIRED CAUSES

Many medical conditions are associated with GH insensitivity of varying degrees (Table 12-5). These conditions are characterized by low IGF-I levels, elevated GH levels, and low GHBP levels. Decreased hepatic GHR expression has been demonstrated in corresponding animal models. GH insensitivity contributes to and aggravates catabolism in those disorders that are already prone to catabolism because of oversecretion of stress hormones such as glucocorticoids, catecholamines, and glucagon. To date, influencing the GH-resistant state has not been possible, except by treating the underlying cause. Attempts to overcome the resistance with large doses of exogenous GH have had mixed results, depending on the type of catabolic condition being treated. A study of GH treatment in critically ill patients resulted in a higher mortality. Therefore such therapy cannot be recommended at present except in the context of carefully controlled studies.

## HYPERSECRETION OF GROWTH HORMONE (ACROMEGALY)

Overproduction of GH, usually by a pituitary tumor, causes acromegaly in adults and pituitary gigantism in prepubertal

**TABLE 12-5.**
**Conditions Associated with Growth Hormone (GH) Resistance**

*Genetic*
  Laron syndrome (primary GHR deficiency)
  Pygmies*
*Physiologic*
  Fetal and neonatal life
  Senescence
*Acquired*
  Malnutrition
  Acute fasting
  Uncontrolled diabetes mellitus (particularly type 1)
  Critical illness
  Liver cirrhosis
  Chronic renal failure
  Hypothyroidism

*GHR*, growth hormone receptor.
*Pygmies may have a combination of GH and insulin-like growth factor-I resistance (see text).

children. Acromegaly is a disease of insidious onset that usually is not recognized until the progressive overgrowth of connective tissue and bone has caused striking changes of appearance. The prevalence of acromegaly is estimated to be ~1 in 20,000.[51] Its peak incidence is between the fourth and sixth decades.

### ETIOLOGY AND PATHOGENESIS

The great majority (>99%) of cases of acromegaly are caused by a pituitary adenoma, either pure somatotrope or occasionally somatomammotrope in origin. The adenoma is usually sporadic but may occur as part of the multiple endocrine neoplasia type 1 (MEN1) syndrome. Rarely, acromegaly may result from somatotrope hyperplasia, induced by excess production of GHRH from an ectopic source (carcinoids, islet cell tumors, small cell carcinoma) or by hamartomas or gangliocytomas in the hypothalamic or pituitary area. GHRH was first isolated from such an ectopic source in the pancreas,[16,17] but only ~50 cases of ectopic GHRH-induced acromegaly have been described.[52] Only one clearly documented case exists of acromegaly due to ectopic production of GH (by an islet cell tumor).[53] McCune-Albright syndrome is another disorder that can be associated with acromegaly and gigantism.

Although the role of a primary pituitary or hypothalamic disorder as the initiating cause of acromegaly was disputed for years, it is now clear that many GH-secreting tumors are monoclonal and harbor an activating mutation of the $G_s\alpha$ protein subunit. As indicated above, the GHRH-R signals through the $G_s$-cAMP pathway, and constitutive activation of $G_s\alpha$ essentially bypasses GHRH-regulated somatotrope growth, GH synthesis, and GH secretion. Thus, in a substantial proportion of tumors, a somatic mutation seems to be responsible for the disease.[54] McCune-Albright syndrome, a disorder with widespread constitutive activation of $G_s\alpha$, probably causes GH overproduction through the same mechanism.[55] In MEN1, tumorigenesis is a function of the loss of both alleles of a tumor-suppressor gene, the menin gene.[56] Thus, except in rare cases of ectopic (or eutopic) GHRH overproduction, acromegaly appears to be a primary pituitary disorder.

### CLINICAL AND LABORATORY MANIFESTATIONS

The clinical manifestations of acromegaly relate to the hormonal effects of GH and IGF-I on the one hand, and to local tumor-mass effects on the other. Table 12-6 lists the principal clinical and laboratory findings recorded in a large series of patients with acromegaly; Figures 12-16 to 12-18 illustrate typi-

**TABLE 12-6.**
**Clinical and Laboratory Findings in 57 Patients with Acromegaly**

| Finding | % |
| --- | --- |
| Recent acral growth | 100 |
| Sella volume >1300 mm³ | 96 |
| Excessive sweating | 91 |
| Heel-pad thickness >22 mm | 91 |
| Weakness | 88 |
| Arthralgias | 72 |
| Abnormal glucose tolerance test | 68 |
| Malocclusion of teeth | 68 |
| New skin tags | 58 |
| Serum phosphorus >4.5 mg/dL | 48 |
| Carpal tunnel syndrome | 44 |
| Hypertension (blood pressure >150/95 mm Hg) | 37 |
| Fasting plasma glucose >110 mg/dL | 30 |
| Serum testosterone (males) <300 ng/mL | 23 |
| Serum prolactin >25 ng/mL | 16 |
| 8 a.m. serum cortisol <8.0 μg/dL | 0.4 |

(From Clemmons DR, Van Wyk JJ, Ridgway EC, et al. Evaluation of acromegaly by radioimmunoassay of somatomedin-C. N Engl J Med 1979; 301:1138.)

cal features. The symptoms and signs of acromegaly can be divided into three categories: (a) *physical changes* related to excessive amounts of GH and IGF-I, (b) *metabolic effects* of excessive amounts of GH, and (c) *local effects* of the pituitary tumor.

Identifying acromegaly on the basis of appearance alone can be difficult. Because these changes occur slowly, often only the examination of old photographs can confirm the suspicion and help determine the time of onset (see Fig. 12-17). A delay in diagnosis is unfortunate because a surgical cure is much more likely when the tumor is small, and the more prominent bony changes are only partially reversible. In experienced surgical hands, transsphenoidal adenomectomy is curative for the majority of microadenomas (<1 cm in diameter), but cures are more difficult to achieve for macroadenomas (see later). Somatotrope tumors have a propensity for local invasion, including of bone, which makes eradication of all cells extraordinarily difficult once the tumor has progressed beyond the boundaries of the pituitary gland.

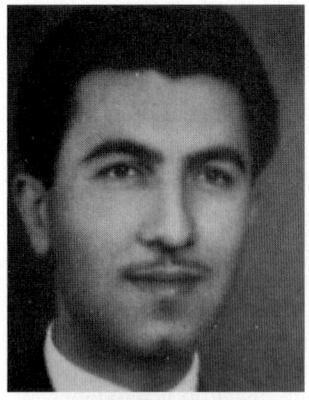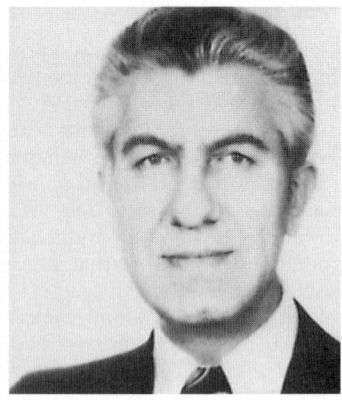

A,B

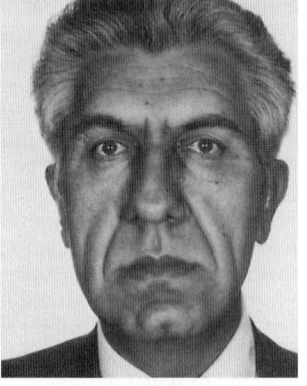

C

**FIGURE 12-17. A–C,** Progressive acromegalic changes in a 58-year-old man. Old photographs are useful to evaluate whether a diagnosis of acromegaly should be considered or to document progression of the disease.

The physical changes (see Figs. 12-16 to 12-18) include a general coarsening of features. Acral growth of bone and soft tissues is seen (a finding that gave the disease its name). Patients typically have large, spadelike hands, with a characteristic swelling of subcutaneous tissues that is more doughy than edematous (see Fig. 12-18). This results in a change in ring, glove, and shoe size—key anamnestic elements that should be actively sought. Bony overgrowth in the skull leads to frontal bossing, mandibular growth, prognathism, and dental malocclusion. Bony overgrowth leads to bone spurs in the spine and around the large joints, sometimes giving rise to spinal stenosis or other nerve compression syndromes. Carpal tunnel syndrome is a classic

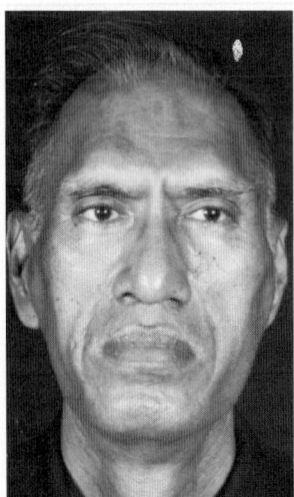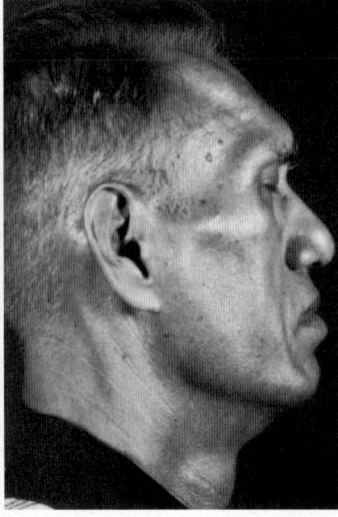

**FIGURE 12-16.** A 64-year-old man with acromegaly. Note the prominent jaw, the large zygomatic arches and supraorbital ridges. The bony overgrowth results in a comparative hollowing of the temporal region. The nose and ears are enlarged. The skin folds are exaggerated, the skin is tough and oily, and the sebaceous glands and pores are enlarged.

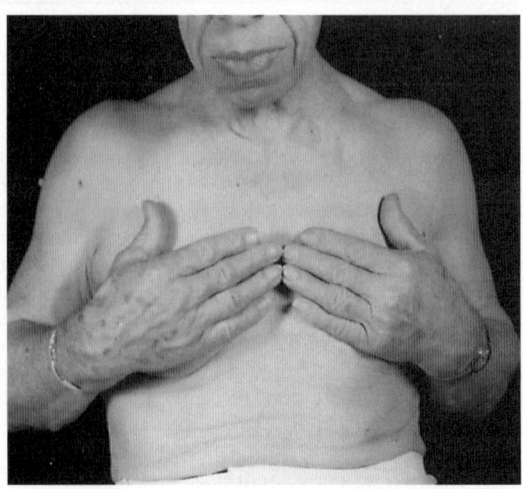

**FIGURE 12-18.** Enlarged hands of a man with acromegaly. Both bony enlargement and soft tissue swelling are present. The skin is thickened. A large skin tag is located in the right deltoid region and skeletal deformity is present.

early sign of acromegaly; it is also seen with exogenous GH treatment for GH deficiency (see earlier). A barrel deformity of the chest may occur as a result of rib elongation and kyphosis. Laryngeal overgrowth and thickened vocal cords, together with cranial hyperpneumatization, causes a characteristic deep, sonorous voice. The tongue is large and hypertrophic, sometimes with dental impressions at its borders. Sleep apnea is a common finding, at least in part because of pharyngeal obstruction. The skin is coarse and oily, and skin tags are common. Patients complain of excessive sweating and body odor. Galactorrhea may be present in women. The large joints may show deformities, and the calvarium is thickened. Arthralgias and osteoarthritis-like arthropathies are common. General visceromegaly is present.

Cardiac enlargement commonly occurs, and abnormalities invariably are seen on tests of dynamic cardiac function.[57] This probably results from a combination of direct effects of GH and IGF-I on myocardial growth and the sequelae of hypertension, hyperlipidemia, and diabetes, all of which are associated with acromegaly. Before effective means of treating acromegaly were available, premature cardiovascular death was responsible for a significantly shortened life span.

Acromegaly predisposes to colonic polyp formation,[58] and the incidence of colon cancer is probably also increased.[59]

The metabolic effects of excess GH and IGF-I relate to sodium retention, insulin antagonism, phosphate retention, abnormal calcium metabolism, and heightened bone turnover. One-third of acromegalic patients have hypertension.[60] Carbohydrate intolerance is common, and frank diabetes mellitus is seen in 10% to 20% of patients. Hyperlipidemias of various types occur in the presence and even absence of diabetes. Serum phosphorus levels are elevated, as are levels of 1,25-hydroxyvitamin D. There is increased calcium absorption and excretion, as well as hydroxyproline excretion as a manifestation of increased bone turnover.

Local tumor effects include headaches, visual field abnormalities due to optic chiasm compression, oculomotor paresis due to cavernous sinus invasion, galactorrhea due to stalk compression, and panhypopituitarism (uncommon). Headaches are characteristic for acromegaly, may be severe, and often exceed those seen with other pituitary tumors of similar or larger size. A cephalgic property may be inherent in excess GH or some other substance cosecreted from somatotrope tumors, as is also suggested by the sudden and dramatic relief of headaches by administration of somatostatin or its analogs (see later).

### DIAGNOSTIC TESTING

In acromegaly, GH secretion remains pulsatile, with increased amplitude and failure to completely cease between pulses. Pulse frequency may also be increased. GH levels vary widely, both within and outside the normal range. Therefore, a random GH level is not diagnostic of acromegaly, just as it cannot be diagnostic of hypopituitarism. The mixture of GH molecular variants secreted in acromegaly does not differ from the mixture secreted normally. Dynamic testing of GH *suppressibility* is required for diagnosis.

The diagnosis of acromegaly has been facilitated by IGF-I measurement. An elevated serum IGF-I level is almost pathognomonic for acromegaly, as few other conditions cause high IGF-I levels. Furthermore, IGF-I is highly sensitive to even mild elevation of GH secretion. When acromegaly is suspected, serum IGF-I measurement should be performed as a screening test. This should then be followed by a standard oral glucose-tolerance test (75 or 100 g glucose). Glucose normally suppresses GH secretion, with plasma levels of <1 ng/mL within an hour or two of glucose administration. In acromegaly, GH levels are not normally suppressible and may even increase in response to glucose. Lack of suppression by glucose to <1 ng/mL is the definitive diagnostic test in the proper clinical setting suggesting acromegaly.

The severity of clinical manifestations is notoriously poorly correlated with serum GH levels; correlation with IGF-I levels may be better. IGF-I may be elevated, and clinical disease

present, even at a mean GH level of 5 ng/mL.[61] The hallmark of acromegaly, even in such mild cases, is the absence of cessation of GH secretion, which results in higher than normal interpulse nadirs and a lack of glucose-induced suppressibility of GH to <1 ng/mL. Frequently, patients with acromegaly have a paradoxical GH response to TRH or GnRH—findings that support the diagnosis but are not entirely specific. Measurements of IGFBPs or GHBP are not useful in the diagnosis of acromegaly. In the ectopic GHRH syndrome, peripheral serum GHRH levels are substantially elevated.[52] However, this syndrome is so rare that routine screening is not recommended.

Pituitary imaging (MRI or computed tomographic scanning) frequently reveals a macroadenoma that may extend in any direction. Conventional radiography may show a ballooned sella turcica, the bony skull deformities described earlier, and enlarged sinuses.

### TREATMENT

The goal of treatment is two-fold: complete eradication of the tumor and normalization of GH and IGF-I secretion. The criteria for cure have changed over the years, with progressive lowering of the GH threshold from 10 to 5 to 2 ng/mL. Cure rates quoted in the literature are correspondingly variable. Criteria for a true cure should be very stringent, with normal suppressibility of GH and serum IGF-I in the normal range. Many patients, although substantially improved with respect to clinical disease, do not achieve this criterion, but rather have low-grade, residual acromegaly.

The primary form of therapy is transsphenoidal adenomectomy. For microadenomas (<1 cm), the surgical cure rate in experienced hands ranges from 60% to 90%; for larger tumors it is from 35% to 71%.[62–64] These numbers partly depend on the stringency of the criteria used to determine a cure. Early diagnosis is the key to a successful eradication of a small tumor. Selective removal of the adenoma should leave the rest of the pituitary intact, and postoperative hypopituitarism is uncommon. It cannot be emphasized enough that surgical outcomes depend on the experience and skill of the neurosurgeon; this procedure should be performed only in specialized centers.

Radiation therapy is used for patients who are not cured by surgery alone. It can be delivered as conventional x-ray therapy, as proton beam therapy, or in the form of the gamma knife (multiport, collimated cobalt-60 therapy). Radioactive pituitary implants have largely been abandoned. All three radiation modalities are attended by development of hypopituitarism. Moreover, they are slow in their onset of action, with conventional x-ray therapy requiring 5 to 10 years or more to lower GH levels to an acceptable range. Proton beam therapy acts faster but has been complicated by optic and oculomotor nerve damage and seizure disorders; its availability is limited to institutions that possess a cyclotron. Experience with gamma knife therapy is still limited; it is reserved for small tumors and, thus, is not well suited for those patients with macroadenomas who are most in need of radiation therapy.

Medical therapy is available in the form of dopamine agonists (bromocriptine, cabergoline) and somatostatin analogs (octreotide). These agents are largely reserved for patients with residual disease after surgery; they have generally not been used as primary therapy, although one study suggested that octreotide monotherapy may be considered for patients for whom a surgical cure is not anticipated.[65] In contrast to their great efficacy in the treatment of prolactinomas, dopamine agonists are not very effective in acromegaly, either in lowering GH levels or in shrinking tumor size. High doses are needed, and patient acceptance is poor because of side effects. Octreotide, on the other hand, is quite effective; its main drawback is that it has to be given by injection three times a day. However, long-acting analogs (lanreotide) or formulations (octreotide LAR) have been developed and are effective when injected in 20- to 40-mg doses at biweekly or monthly intervals. Octreotide can have a marked, immediate effect in relieving headaches—a phenomenon that is poorly understood. Future medical therapy may include use of a GH antagonist that is presently in clinical trials. Antagonism at the GHR level is based on the disabling of binding site 2 in the GH molecule, thereby preventing productive GHR dimerization. Preliminary results show that this antagonist is very effective in blocking GH action in patients with residual acromegaly. The hope is that the combination of agents that decrease GH secretion with one that blocks GH action will finally meet the difficult challenge of treating patients who suffer from residual acromegaly despite the best efforts at optimizing surgical and radiologic therapy.

## HYPERSENSITIVITY TO GROWTH HORMONE

GH hypersensitivity states have not been widely appreciated, but at least one such condition is very common: obesity. In obesity, IGF-I levels tend to be high or normal despite decreased GH secretion. GHBP levels are high, likely indicating increased GHR expression.[13] This constellation is the opposite of that in malnutrition, which is associated with GH insensitivity. Obese children grow faster than lean children[66]—an old observation that was not understood until recently. Hyperinsulinemia was proposed as an explanation, but insulin does not promote linear growth. Other than enhanced growth, the pathophysiologic consequences of the GH hypersensitivity associated with obesity are not clear; further studies are required to determine whether it contributes to increased morbidity.

Considerable advances have been made in our understanding of the GHRH–GH–IGF axis during the past few years. The genetic control of pituitary development and somatotrope function has been partially elucidated, with human disease linked to several control factors, such as Rpx, Prop-1, Pit-1, GHRH-R, and $G_s\alpha$. GH action has become far better understood through detailed molecular modeling of the GH-GHR interaction, the study of GHR mutations and their functional consequences, the partial elucidation of the GHR signaling cascade, and the assessment of GHR regulation through GHBP measurements in various physiopathologic conditions. GH therapy for adults with hypopituitarism has come of age, with several new insights gained about the importance of GH in maintaining normal body composition and metabolism during adult life.

## REFERENCES

1. Chen EY, Liao YC, Smith DH, et al. The growth hormone locus: nucleotide sequence, biology and evolution. Genomics 1989; 4:479.
2. Baumann G. Growth hormone heterogeneity: genes, isohormones, variants and binding proteins. Endocr Rev 1991; 12:424.
3. Ultsch MH, Somers W, Kossiakoff AA, de Vos AM. The crystal structure of affinity-matured human growth hormone at 2 Å resolution. J Mol Biol 1994; 236:286.
4. Stolar MW, Amburn K, Baumann G. Plasma "big" and "big-big" growth hormone (GH) in man: an oligomeric series composed of structurally diverse GH monomers. J Clin Endocrinol Metab 1984; 59:212.
5. Leung DW, Spencer SA, Cachianes G, et al. Growth hormone receptor and serum binding protein: purification, cloning and expression. Nature 1987; 330:537.
6. Kelly PA, Djiane J, Postel-Vinay M-C, Edery M. The prolactin/growth hormone receptor family. Endocr Rev 1991; 12:235.
7. Godowski PJ, Leung DW, Meacham LR, et al. Characterization of the human growth hormone receptor gene and demonstration of a partial gene deletion in two patients with Laron-type dwarfism. Proc Natl Acad Sci U S A 1989; 86:8083.
8. Mercado M, Davila N, McLeod JF, Baumann G. Distribution of growth hormone receptor messenger ribonucleic acid containing and lacking exon 3 in human tissues. J Clin Endocrinol Metab 1994; 78:731.
9. Wickelgren RB, Landin KL, Ohlsson C, Carlsson LM. Expression of exon 3-retaining and exon 3-excluding isoforms of the human growth hormone-receptor is regulated in an interindividual, rather than a tissue-specific manner. J Clin Endocrinol Metab 1995; 80:2154.
10. Dastot F, Sobrier M-L, Duquesnoy P, et al. Alternatively spliced forms in the cytoplasmic domain of the human growth hormone (GH) receptor regulate its ability to generate soluble GH-binding protein. Proc Natl Acad Sci U S A 1996; 93:10723.
11. Cunningham BC, Ultsch M, De Vos AM, et al. Dimerization of the extracellular domain of the human growth hormone receptor by a single hormone molecule. Science 1991; 254:821.
12. Carter-Su C, Smit LS. Signaling via JAK kinases: growth hormone receptor as a model system. Recent Prog Horm Res 1998; 53:61.
13. Baumann G. Growth hormone binding proteins: state of the art. J Endocrinol 1994; 141:1.
14. Kratzsch J, Selisko T, Birkenmeier G. Identification of transformed alpha 2-macroglobulin as a growth hormone-binding protein in human blood. J Clin Endocrinol Metab 1995; 80:585.
15. Sornson MW, Wu W, Dasen JS, et al. Pituitary lineage determination by the Prophet of Pit-1 homeodomain factor defective in Ames dwarfism. Nature 1996; 384: 327.
16. Rivier J, Spiess J, Thorner M, Vale W. Characterization of a growth hormone-releasing factor from a human pancreatic islet tumour. Nature 1982; 300:276.
17. Guillemin R, Brazeau P, Bohlen P, et al. Growth hormone–releasing factor from a human pancreatic tumor that caused acromegaly. Science 1982; 218:585.
18. Barinaga M, Yamamoto G, Rivier C, et al. Transcriptional regulation of growth hormone gene expression by growth hormone releasing factor. Nature 1983; 306:84.
19. Reisine T, Bell GI. Molecular biology of somatostatin receptors. Endocr Rev 1995; 16:427.
20. Bowers CY, Momany FA, Reynolds GA, Hong A. On the in vitro and in vivo activity of a new synthetic hexapeptide that acts on the pituitary to specifically release growth hormone. Endocrinology 1984; 114:1537.
21. Smith RG, Van der Ploeg LH, Howard AD, et al. Peptidomimetic regulation of growth hormone secretion. Endocr Rev 1997; 18:621.
21a. Kojima M, Hosada H, Date Y, et al. Ghrelin is a growth-hormone-releasing acylated peptide from stomach. Nature 1999; 402:656.
22. Winer LM, Shaw MA, Baumann G. Basal plasma growth hormone levels in man: new evidence for rhythmicity of growth hormone secretion. J Clin Endocrinol Metab 1990; 70:1678.
23. Faria ACS, Veldhuis JD, Thorner MO, Vance ML. Half-time of endogenous growth hormone (GH) disappearance in normal man after stimulation of GH secretion by GH-releasing hormone and suppression with somatostatin. J Clin Endocrinol Metab 1989; 68:535.
24. Baumann G, Amburn K, Shaw M. The circulating growth hormone–binding protein complex: a major constituent of plasma growth hormone in man. Endocrinology 1988; 122:976.
25. Daughaday WH, Trivedi B, Andrews BA. The ontogeny of serum GH binding protein in man: a possible indicator of hepatic GH receptor development. J Clin Endocrinol Metab 1987; 65:1072.
26. Maheshwari H, Sharma L, Baumann G. Decline of plasma growth hormone binding protein in old age. J Clin Endocrinol Metab 1996; 81:995.
27. Salmon WD Jr, Daughaday WH. A hormonally controlled serum factor which stimulates sulfate incorporation by cartilage in vitro. J Lab Clin Med 1957; 49:825.
28. Clemmons DR. Insulin-like growth factor binding proteins and their role in controlling IGF actions. Cytokine Growth Factor Rev 1997; 8:45.
29. Burren CP, Wilson EM, Hwa V, et al. Binding properties and distribution of insulin-like growth factor binding protein–related protein 3 (IGFBP-rP3/NovH), an additional member of the IGFBP superfamily. J Clin Endocrinol Metab 1999; 84:1096.
30. Châtelain P, Bouillat B, Cohen R, et al. Assay of growth hormone levels in human plasma using commercial kits: analysis of some factors influencing the results. Acta Paediatr Scand 1990; 370(Suppl):56.
31. Shalet SM, Toogood A, Rahim A, Brennan BMD. The diagnosis of growth hormone deficiency in children and adults. Endocr Rev 1998; 19:203.
32. Wu W, Cogan JD, Pfäffle RW, et al. Mutations in PROP1 cause familial combined pituitary hormone deficiency. Nature Genet 1998; 18:147.
33. Cogan JD, Wu W, Phillips JA 3rd, et al. The PROP1 2-base pair deletion is a common cause of combined pituitary hormone deficiency. J Clin Endocrinol Metab 1998; 83:3346.
34. Tatsumi K, Miyai K, Notomi T, et al. Cretinism with combined hormone deficiency caused by a mutation in the PIT1 gene. Nat Genet 1992; 1:56.
35. Wajnrajch MP, Gertner JM, Harbison MD, et al. Nonsense mutation in the human growth hormone-releasing hormone receptor causes growth failure analogous to the little (lit) mouse. Nat Genet 1996; 12:88.
36. Maheshwari HG, Silverman BL, Dupuis J, Baumann G. Phenotype and genetic analysis of a syndrome caused by an inactivating mutation in the growth hormone releasing hormone receptor: dwarfism of Sindh. J Clin Endocrinol Metab 1998; 83:4065.
37. Phillips JA III, Cogan JD. Genetic basis of endocrine disease 6: molecular basis of familial human growth hormone deficiency. J Clin Endocrinol Metab 1994; 78:11.
38. Takahashi Y, Shirono H, Arisaka O, et al. Biologically inactive growth hormone caused by an amino acid substitution. J Clin Invest 1997; 100:1159.
39. Takahashi Y, Kaji H, Okimura Y, et al. Short stature caused by a mutant growth hormone. N Engl J Med 1996; 334:432.
40. Dattani MT, Martinez-Barbera JP, Thomas PQ, et al. Mutations in the homeobox gene HESX1/Hesx1 associated with septo-optic dysplasia in human and mouse. Nat Genet 1998; 19:125.
41. Tauber M, Moulin P, Pienkowski C, et al. Growth hormone (GH) retesting and auxological data in 131 GH-deficient patients after completion of treatment. J Clin Endocrinol Metab 1997; 82:352.
42. Consensus guidelines for the diagnosis and treatment of adults with growth hormone deficiency: summary statement of the Growth Hormone Research Society Workshop on Adult Growth Hormone Deficiency. J Clin Endocrinol Metab 1998; 83:379.
43. Carroll PV, Christ ER, Bengtsson BA, et al. Growth hormone deficiency in adulthood and the effects of growth hormone replacement: a review. J Clin Endocrinol Metab 1998; 83:382.

44. Rosén T, Bengtsson BA. Premature mortality due to cardiovascular disease in hypopituitarism. Lancet 1990; 336:285.

44a. Bulow B, Hagmar L, Eskilsson J, Erfurth EM. Hypopituitary females have a high incidence of cardiovascular morbidity and an increased prevalence of cardio-vascular risk factors. J Clin Endocrinal Metab 2000; 85:574.

45. Rosenfeld RG, Rosenbloom AL, Guevara-Aguirre J. Growth hormone (GH) insensitivity due to primary GH receptor deficiency. Endocr Rev 1994; 15:369.

46. Ayling RM, Ross R, Towner P, et al. A dominant-negative mutation of the growth hormone receptor causes familial short stature. Nat Genet 1997; 16:13.

47. Parks JS, Brown MR, Faase ME. The spectrum of growth-hormone insensitivity. J Pediatr 1997; 131:S45.

48. Goddard AD, Dowd P, Chernausek S, et al. Partial growth-hormone insensitivity: the role of growth-hormone receptor mutations in idiopathic short stature. J Pediatr 1997; 131:S51.

49. Baumann G, Shaw MA, Merimee TJ. Low levels of high-affinity growth hormone–binding protein in African pygmies. N Engl J Med 1989; 320:1705.

50. Geffner ME, Bersch N, Bailey RC, Golde DW. Insulin-like growth factor I resistance in immortalized T cell lines from African Efe Pygmies. J Clin Endocrinol Metab 1995; 80:3732.

51. Alexander L, Appleton D, Hall R, et al. Epidemiology of acromegaly in the Newcastle region. Clin Endocrinol (Oxf) 1980; 12:71.

52. Faglia G, Arosio M, Bazzoni N. Ectopic acromegaly. Endocrinol Metab Clin North Am 1992; 21:575.

53. Melmed S, Ezrin C, Kovacs K, et al. Acromegaly due to secretion of growth hormone by an ectopic pancreatic islet-cell tumor. N Engl J Med 1985; 312:9.

54. Landis CA, Harsh G, Lyons J, et al. Clinical characteristics of acromegalic patients whose pituitary tumors contain mutant $G_s$ protein. J Clin Endocrinol Metab 1990; 71:1416.

55. Weinstein LS, Shenker A, Gejman PV, et al. Activating mutations of the stimulatory G protein in the McCune-Albright syndrome. N Engl J Med 1991; 325:1688.

56. Chandrasekharappa SC, Guru SC, Manickam P, et al. Positional cloning of the gene for multiple endocrine neoplasia-type 1. Science 1997; 276:404.

57. Martin JB, Kerber RE, Sherman MB, et al. Cardiac size and function in acromegaly. Circulation 1977; 56:863.

58. Delhougne B, Deneux C, Abs R, et al. The prevalence of colonic polyps in acromegaly: a colonoscopic and pathological study in 103 patients. J Clin Endocrinol Metab 1995; 80:3223.

59. Orme SM, McNally RJ, Cartwright RA, Belchetz PE. Mortality and cancer incidence in acromegaly: a retrospective cohort study. United Kingdom Acromegaly Study Group. J Clin Endocrinol Metab 1998; 83:2730.

60. Minniti G, Moroni C, Jaffrain-Rea ML, et al. Prevalence of hypertension in acromegalic patients: clinical measurement versus 24-hour ambulatory blood pressure monitoring. Clin Endocrinol (Oxf) 1998; 48:149.

61. Daughaday WH, Starkey RH, Saltman S, et al. Characterization of serum growth hormone (GH) and insulin-like growth factor I in active acromegaly with minimal elevation of serum GH. J Clin Endocrinol Metab 1987; 65:617.

62. Davis DH, Laws ER, Ilstrup DM, et al. Results of surgical treatment for growth hormone–secreting pituitary adenomas. J Neurosurg 1993; 79:70.

63. Abosch A, Tyrell JB, Lamborn KR, et al. Transsphenoidal microsurgery for growth hormone-secreting pituitary adenomas: initial outcome and long-term results. J Clin Endocrinol Metab 1998; 83:3411.

64. Swearingen B, Barker FG II, Katznelson L, et al. Long-term mortality after transsphenoidal surgery and adjunctive therapy for acromegaly. J Clin Endocrinol Metab 1998; 83:3419.

65. Newman CB, Melmed S, George A, et al. Octreotide as primary therapy for acromegaly. J Clin Endocrinol Metab 1998; 83:3034.

66. Forbes GB. Nutrition and growth. J Pediatr 1977; 91:40.

# CHAPTER 13

# PROLACTIN AND ITS DISORDERS

LAURENCE KATZNELSON AND ANNE KLIBANSKI

## NORMAL CONTROL OF PROLACTIN SECRETION

Prolactin secretion is controlled by dual inhibitory and stimulatory factors (Fig. 13-1). This hormone is unique among anterior pituitary hormones, because it is primarily regulated through tonic inhibition. Two decades of investigation have demonstrated the presence of one or more prolactin-inhibiting factors (PIFs).[1]

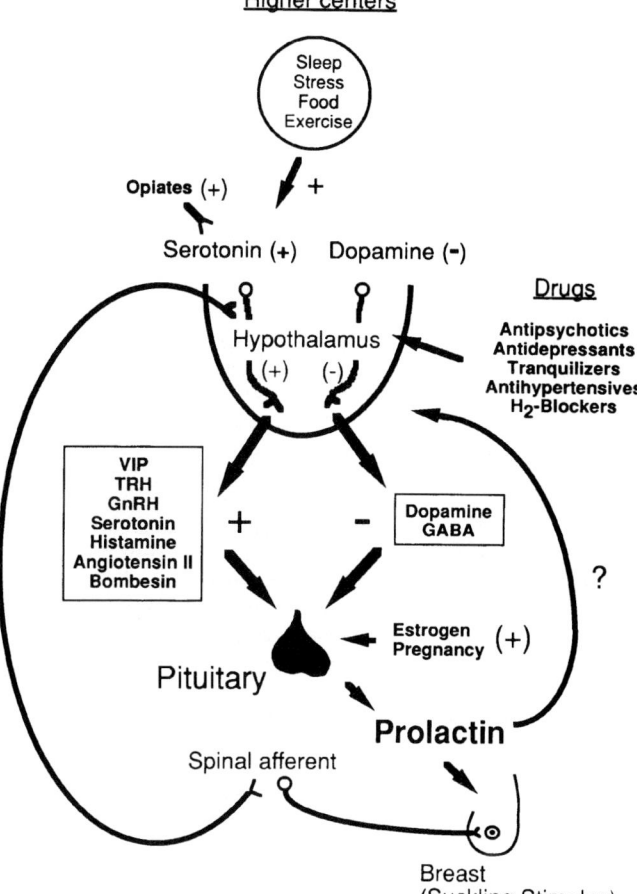

**FIGURE 13-1.** Regulation of prolactin secretion. Prolactin release is under tonic inhibition by prolactin inhibiting factors, predominantly dopamine. Prolactin release is stimulated by a number of factors, including vasoactive intestinal peptide (*VIP*), thyroid-releasing hormone (*TRH*), and gonadotropin-releasing hormone (*GnRH*). Estrogens, pregnancy, and breast suckling stimulate prolactin release. Within the hypothalamus, serotinergic and dopaminergic pathways are stimulatory and inhibitory, respectively, to prolactin release. (*GABA*, γ-aminobutyric acid.) (Modified from Molitch ME. Pathologic hyperprolactinemia. Endocrinol Metab Clin North Am 1992; 21:877.)

*Dopamine* is the most important PIF described. Multiple studies support the hypothesis that dopamine acts as an inhibiting factor. In vitro studies reveal that high-affinity dopamine receptors ($D_2$) are present on lactotrope membranes, and after binding occurs, inhibition of adenylate cyclase is demonstrated.[2,3] This results in a decrease in cyclic adenosine monophosphate (cAMP) production and the release of prolactin. Dopamine also directly inhibits prolactin biosynthesis at the level of RNA transcription. Dopamine is produced in higher nuclei in the brain and is secreted into the portal circulation to reach the pituitary. Infusion of dopamine in humans, resulting in serum dopamine concentrations similar to those found in portal blood, causes a reduction in prolactin secretion.[4] Dopamine receptor blockade results in prolactin elevation.[5] After dopamine is removed, as during pituitary stalk section, prolactin is rapidly released. These studies all point to a direct inhibitory effect of dopamine on pituitary lactotrope secretion. Most pharmacologic agents that cause prolactin release act either by blockade of dopamine receptors (e.g., haloperidol, phenothiazines) or by dopamine depletion in the tuberoinfundibular neurons (e.g., reserpine, α-methyldopa).

Another potential PIF includes a 56-amino-acid PIF identified within the precursor for gonadotropin-releasing hormone (GnRH). This *GnRH-associated peptide* (GAP) inhibits prolactin secretion and reduces prolactin secretion in rats, but the role of GAP in modulating prolactin secretion in humans remains unconfirmed.[6] Data also support the role of γ-*aminobutyric acid* (GABA) as a PIF. GABA is secreted into the portal circulation, with a resulting inhibitory effect on prolactin secretion, and GABA receptors have been detected on lactotropes.[7] However, the physiologic importance of GABA in prolactin regulation is unclear.

Stimulatory factors also regulate prolactin secretion. These substances may act directly on the pituitary or may act indirectly by means of dopaminergic blockade or depletion at the level of the hypothalamus. *Estrogens* are important physiologic stimulators of prolactin release.[8] In vitro studies show that estradiol increases prolactin biosynthesis, consistent with a direct stimulatory effect of estrogen on lactotrope function.[9] Chronic exposure to estrogens increases lactotrope number and size (i.e., "pregnancy cells"), and acute administration increases prolactin secretion within hours.[10] Estrogens may also indirectly increase prolactin levels by altering dopaminergic tone and by increasing responsiveness to other neuromodulators.

*Thyrotropin-releasing hormone* (TRH) stimulates the synthesis and release of prolactin in vivo and in vitro from normal and neoplastic lactotropes. Although pharmacologic doses of TRH result in a rapid release in prolactin after intravenous administration in humans, the physiologic role of TRH in modulating prolactin secretion is not established.[11] For example, suckling leads to release of prolactin without an accompanying heightened release of TRH. Hypothyroidism results in an increase in TSH and the prolactin response to TRH, and elevations in basal prolactin levels may be seen in primary hypothyroidism. The suggestion has been made that decreased hypothalamic dopamine may play a role in the hyperprolactinemia associated with hypothyroidism.

*Vasoactive intestinal peptide* (VIP) may selectively stimulate or potentiate the TRH effect on prolactin release.[12] Evidence exists for VIP receptors on lactotropes and VIP may stimulate prolactin release in vitro. Immunoneutralization of VIP effects through administration of anti-VIP antisera diminishes the prolactin response to stimuli, including suckling, a finding that again suggests a role of VIP as a stimulatory factor.[13] Data suggest that VIP may be produced in the pituitary and may stimulate prolactin release through a paracrine or autocrine mechanism.[14] The clinical significance of VIP in prolactin regulation in humans is unknown.

*GnRH* may also have stimulatory properties. The administration of GnRH induces the acute release of prolactin in normally cycling women and hypogonadal patients.[15] Moreover, incubation of human lactotropes with GnRH in vitro results in prolactin secretion.[16] These investigations suggest that GnRH, directly or through a paracrine mechanism involving gonadotropes, may be important in evoking prolactin release.

Investigations have suggested a role for *galanin* as a potent stimulator of prolactin release. Galanin is a 29-amino-acid peptide widely distributed in the central and peripheral nervous system. In the rat, intracerebroventricular injections of galanin may increase prolactin levels.[17] However, intravenous administration of galanin in humans does not raise serum prolactin levels.[18] The physiologic role of galanin in human prolactin regulation remains controversial.

*Serotonin* is another factor that may stimulate prolactin secretion.[19] Administration of serotonin antagonists decreases prolactin levels. Serotonin agonists appear to enhance prolactin secretion through specific serotonin receptors, perhaps explaining why only specific serotonin antagonists are capable of lowering prolactin secretion.[20]

Other factors that may have stimulatory roles include *bombesin, angiotensin II, histamine (H₂) antagonists*, and *opiates*.

Human prolactin structure has partial homology with growth hormone, perhaps accounting for the lactotropic activity of growth hormone. Heterogeneous forms of prolactin are found in the circulation. Eighty-five percent of prolactin (23 kDa) detected in the pituitary and secreted into serum is nonglycosylated, but glycosylated forms have been detected.[21] Approximately 8% of prolactin extractable from the pituitary is dimeric, and an additional 1% to 5% is polymeric, linked by disulfide bonds.[22] These forms include "big," "big-big," and "little" or "native" prolactins. The significance of these forms is unknown. The larger forms of prolactin may have decreased rates of binding to the prolactin receptor and possess diminished bioactivity relative to monomeric, nonglycosylated prolactin. These forms may represent nonspecific hormonal aggregates or binding of prolactin to serum proteins. Some patients have normal reproductive function but elevated serum prolactin values; the prolactin in these patients is composed of a relatively increased component of polymeric prolactin.[23] In such patients, the elevated prolactin levels may reflect increased levels of polymeric prolactin with decreased bioactivity. The suggestion has been made that certain isotypes of prolactin, specifically iso-B prolactin, may be elevated in the sera of patients with infertility and pregnancy wastage.[24] This isotype may be more resistant to bromocriptine therapy than native prolactin. However, these reports need to be confirmed. The significance of the remaining fraction of glycosylated prolactin is unknown.

## CLINICAL ASPECTS OF PROLACTIN PHYSIOLOGY

The physiologic causes of hyperprolactinemia are summarized in Table 13-1. The following sections describe clinical aspects of prolactin physiology.

### DIURNAL AND MENSTRUAL CYCLE VARIATION

Prolactin is secreted in a pulsatile fashion with 4 to 14 pulses per day (60% occur during sleep).[25] Prolactin secretory pulses begin 60 to 90 minutes after the onset of sleep.[26] The amplitude of pulses varies greatly among individuals, with peak levels occurring during the late hours of sleep. Such rises are not clearly associated with any specific stage of sleep. Although some studies have suggested that prolactin varies during the menstrual cycle, the precise nature of this relationship remains unclear. Several investigators have shown that prolactin levels are significantly higher during the ovulatory and luteal phases, particularly at midcycle.[27] This midcycle rise may be the result of increased circulating periovulatory estradiol levels. However, other studies have not confirmed this finding. Prolactin is probably not necessary for ovulation, because ovulatory periods may occur in women taking bromocriptine, a medication that suppresses prolactin.

**TABLE 13-1.**
**Physiologic Causes of Hyperprolactinemia**

Pregnancy
Postpartum state
    Nonnursing: days 1–7
    Nursing: with suckling
Neonatality
Estrogen therapy
Stress
Sleep
Hypoglycemia
Intercourse
Nipple stimulation
Exercise

## EATING

Abrupt rises in serum prolactin levels occur within an hour of eating in normal and pregnant hyperprolactinemic individuals, but they do not rise in those with prolactinomas. Amino acids metabolized from protein components of meals appear to be the main stimulants to prolactin secretion.[28]

## STRESS

Prolactin rises during stress, including physical exertion, surgery, sexual intercourse, insulin hypoglycemia, and seizures. The nature and teleologic significance of these changes is unknown. In women, nipple stimulation, chest wall trauma or surgery, and herpes zoster infection of the breast may result in increases in prolactin levels, in part through afferent neural pathways.[29] In contrast, nipple stimulation in men does not cause increased prolactin levels.

## AGE

Mean levels of prolactin are slightly higher in premenopausal women than in men, probably because of a direct effect of estrogen on pituitary prolactin secretion or estrogen-induced alterations in dopaminergic tone.[30] Some studies suggest that prolactin levels progressively decline in women with age, particularly after the menopause.[31] The responsiveness of prolactin to various pharmacologic agents (e.g., TRH) declines with age in women, probably because of postmenopausal estrogen deficiency.

## NORMAL STATES

The only established role of prolactin is to initiate and maintain lactation. Prolactin levels increase progressively with pregnancy. Estrogens play a major role in stimulation of prolactin levels, which peak at term (at 100–300 ng/mL).[32] Lactation begins when estradiol levels fall at parturition. During the first 4 to 6 weeks after delivery, prolactin levels increase in the circulation to 60 times higher than baseline levels within 20 to 30 minutes of nursing.[33] This elevation is associated with enhanced prolactin pulse amplitude without alteration of pulse frequency.[34] The nursing stimulus effectively promotes acute prolactin release through afferent spinal neural pathways. With continued nursing, the nipple stimulation itself elicits progressively less prolactin release, and in the weeks after initiation of lactation, basal and nursing-induced prolactin pulses decrease, although lactation continues.[33] Within 4 to 6 months after delivery, basal prolactin levels are normal, without a nursing-induced rise. The full explanation for the attenuation in basal and nursing-induced prolactin levels with continued nursing is unknown.

## CLINICAL MANIFESTATIONS OF HYPERPROLACTINEMIA

The amenorrhea-galactorrhea syndrome is the classic description of the clinical manifestation of hyperprolactinemia. However, a spectrum of reproductive disorders may be seen. Prolactin elevations are found in approximately 20% of patients with secondary amenorrhea.[35] Women with hyperprolactinemia may have more subtle abnormalities in gonadal function, including oligomenorrhea or alterations in luteal phase function. A subset of infertile women has been described with mild hyperprolactinemia in whom fertility was restored with bromocriptine therapy. Galactorrhea affects only ~30% of female patients with hyperprolactinemia, but the presence of galactorrhea in a woman with an ovulatory disorder greatly increases the chance that hyperprolactinemia is the underlying cause of the amenorrhea.[36] Patients with primary amenorrhea and delayed puberty may have hyperprolactinemia.[37]

Galactorrhea occurs in as many as 25% of women with normal serum prolactin levels. However, patients with idiopathic galactorrhea may demonstrate intermittent hyperprolactinemia. In a study of nine normoprolactinemic women with galactorrhea, eight patients had elevated levels of prolactin during sleep.[38] Several studies have shown that infertile, normoprolactinemic women with luteal phase defects may show improved luteal function or fertility after administration of bromocriptine therapy.[38] Unrecognized hyperprolactinemia may occur in a subset of patients with presumed normoprolactinemic galactorrhea and luteal phase defects.

Hypogonadism is frequently found in patients with hyperprolactinemia. In women, hypogonadism includes abnormal menstrual function, dry vaginal mucosa, and dyspareunia, and in men and women, the features include fatigue and diminished libido. Multiple potential mechanisms have been hypothesized for the induction of hypogonadism by prolactin, and the antigonadotropic actions of prolactin may occur at multiple levels. Frequently, the hypogonadism is associated with decreased or inappropriately normal levels of luteinizing hormone (LH) and follicle-stimulating hormone (FSH) relative to the state of estrogen deficiency. Multiple investigations suggest that prolactin may suppress spontaneous LH release through decreases in endogenous GnRH levels. In castrated rats, administration of graded doses of prolactin suppress LH levels, and prolactin appears to exert a negative feedback effect on its own secretion by means of a short-loop negative feedback at the level of the hypothalamus.[39,40] This feedback may be mediated through an increase in dopamine inhibitory tone. This increased hypothalamic dopamine tone, along with opiates and other factors, may suppress GnRH with a resultant decrease in LH pulses. The restoration of ovulatory menstrual periods in hyperprolactinemic women by pulsatile exogenous GnRH administration confirms the importance of endogenous GnRH abnormalities as the key mechanism of hypogonadism in these women.[41] Prolactin may modulate androgen secretion at the level of the adrenal gland and ovary, resulting in increased secretion of dehydroepiandrosterone sulfate and testosterone.[42] Altered ratios of estrogens and androgens may result in further abnormal gonadal function, with evidence of clinical hyperandrogenism.

If the underlying cause of the increased prolactin is a pituitary macroadenoma, the adenoma could cause compression of the normal, adjacent pituitary gland with a resultant decrease in gonadotrope function.

Men with hyperprolactinemia may have clinical manifestations of hypogonadism, such as decreased libido, impotence, infertility due to oligospermia, and gynecomastia. Galactorrhea is rare in hyperprolactinemic men because of a lack of estrogen priming of the breast.

## DIFFERENTIAL DIAGNOSIS AND CLINICAL APPROACH TO HYPERPROLACTINEMIA

As shown in Tables 13-1 and 13-2, hyperprolactinemia has multiple causes. The measurement of prolactin level should be repeated with the patient in a nonstimulated state, and, if possible, after an overnight fast in a nonstressed state. Because prolactin may be secreted to a modest degree after a breast examination, a subsequent mild increase in prolactin levels would warrant a repeat determination. Although Table 13-2 demonstrates the existence of several pathologic causes of prolactin elevation, pituitary tumors are clinically the most important. Prolactin-secreting pituitary adenomas are the most common type of pituitary tumors and may account for as many as 40% to 50% of all pituitary tumors.[43] Hyperprolactinemia may be detected in as many as 40% of patients with acromegaly and has been reported in patients with Cushing disease. Hyperprolactinemic patients with suggestive clinical manifestations should be evaluated for acromegaly and Cushing disease.

TABLE 13-2.
**Pathologic and Pharmacologic Causes of Hyperprolactinemia**

| PITUITARY DISEASE | NEUROGENIC CAUSES |
|---|---|
| Prolactin-secreting tumors | Chest wall trauma |
| Acromegaly | Chest wall lesions |
| Cushing disease | Herpes zoster |
| Empty sella syndrome | Breast stimulation |
| **PITUITARY STALK SECTION** | **MEDICATIONS** |
| Clinically nonfunctioning pitu- itary tumors | Phenothiazines |
| | Tricyclic antidepressants |
| Trauma | Metoclopramide |
| | Cimetidine |
| **HYPOTHALAMIC INFILTRATIVE OR DEGENERATIVE DISEASE** | Methyldopa |
| | Reserpine |
| | Calcium-channel blockers |
| Craniopharyngiomas | Cocaine |
| Meningiomas | |
| Dysgerminomas | **OTHER** |
| Gliomas | Renal failure |
| Lymphoma | Liver disease |
| Metastatic disease | Primary hypothyroidism |
| Tuberculosis | Ectopic hormone production |
| Sarcoidosis | Seizures |
| Eosinophilic granuloma | |
| Irradiation | |

(Adapted from Molitch ME. Pathologic hyperprolactinemia. Endocrinol Metab Clin North Am 1992; 21:877)

Substantial elevation in prolactin (>150 ng/mL) in a nonpuerperal state usually indicates a pituitary tumor. Good correlation exists between radiographic estimates of tumor size and prolactin levels, and very high levels of prolactin are associated with larger tumors. Prolactinomas are classified as microadenomas (<10 mm) and macroadenomas (>10 mm). The finding of a substantial elevation in serum prolactin in association with a pituitary lesion larger than 10 mm by radiographic analysis supports the diagnosis of a macroprolactinoma.

Modest levels of prolactin elevation (25–100 ng/mL) may be associated with several diagnoses. All other causes of hyperprolactinemia should be excluded before a tumor is considered. Primary hypothyroidism and pregnancy should be excluded. Chronic renal disease is associated with elevations in prolactin, probably because of altered metabolism or clearance of prolactin or decreases in dopaminergic tone.[44] Hemodialysis does not usually reverse the hyperprolactinemia.

Multiple pharmacologic causes of hyperprolactinemia are found. Ingestion of phenothiazines and other neuroleptics is a common cause for elevations in serum prolactin.[44a] One diagnostic problem is the evaluation of patients with psychiatric disease who are receiving phenothiazines and are found to have an elevated prolactin level. A magnetic resonance image (MRI) should be obtained for patients whose prolactin levels are above 100 ng/mL. Levels lower than 100 ng/mL are consistent with neuroleptic administration, and a scan is unnecessary unless other symptoms suggest a pituitary tumor. This strategy is based on the finding that most patients receiving neuroleptics with modest prolactin elevations have no evidence of a pituitary abnormality on MRI. Other pharmacologic agents associated with hyperprolactinemia include reserpine, α-methyldopa, cimetidine, and opiates.

Estrogen may increase prolactin levels, as is seen in pregnancy. However, the estrogen concentrations in typical oral contraceptives (e.g., 35 μg of ethinyl estradiol) are not associated with hyperprolactinemia, and no evidence exists that postmenopausal replacement estrogen causes elevations in serum prolactin. Any intrasuprasellar mass may lead to modest prolactin elevations through stalk compression, and the evaluation should include an MRI. These masses include primary pituitary tumors or meningiomas and craniopharyngiomas. Hypothalamic disorders, including destructive lesions such as tumors and granulomatous diseases, may lead to hyperprolactinemia by interfering with normal dopaminergic tone.

If an elevated serum prolactin level is not associated with primary hypothyroidism, pregnancy, or pharmacologic agents, a pituitary radiographic scan should be performed to rule out the presence of a prolactin-secreting pituitary tumor or other lesions. Microprolactinomas should be differentiated from macroprolactinomas. An MRI is the most sensitive tool for evaluating the sellar and suprasellar areas. If the scan shows normal sellar and extrasellar contents and no clear secondary cause of the elevated prolactin is present, the diagnosis of idiopathic hyperprolactinemia is made. This syndrome may be the result of a small tumor that is beyond the sensitivity of the scanning technique.

The evaluation should include assessment of gonadal status, such as the presence of oligomenorrhea or amenorrhea in women and of sexual dysfunction in men. This impacts therapy, as is described later. No stimulatory or suppressive endocrine tests are available that aid in the evaluation of elevated prolactin levels. For example, a TRH test cannot be used to diagnose a pituitary tumor; although tumors typically have blunted responses after TRH stimulation, this response can be seen with other disorders.

## TREATMENT FOR PROLACTINOMAS

Treatment depends on whether the patient has hyperprolactinemia due to an underlying cause such as drugs or hypothyroidism, or due to a prolactinoma. If the evaluation suggests the presence of a microprolactinoma, three treatment options are available: medical therapy with a dopamine agonist, careful follow-up without treatment, and, rarely, surgery. All patients with macroadenomas should be treated.

### MEDICAL THERAPY

Almost all patients with hyperprolactinemia due to pituitary disease can be effectively treated medically with the dopamine agonist bromocriptine (see Chap. 21). Bromocriptine lowers serum prolactin in patients with pituitary tumors and all other causes of hyperprolactinemia. A review of early studies of bromocriptine therapy for more than 400 hyperprolactinemic patients showed that normoprolactinemia or return of ovulatory menses occurred in 80% to 90% of patients.[45] Bromocriptine effectively decreases prolactin levels, normalizes reproductive function, and reverses galactorrhea. In this series, return of menstrual function was accompanied in some patients by prolactin levels that were significantly reduced but not normal. This suggests that the reduction of prolactin levels in some patients to slightly elevated levels may be sufficient for return of gonadal function. Bromocriptine is also useful in treating galactorrhea in patients with normoprolactinemic galactorrhea.

The onset of the effects of bromocriptine is rapid, usually occurring within 1 to 2 hours. The greatest decrease in prolactin levels occurs at the initiation of therapy; however, normalization may take weeks. The biologic half-life of bromocriptine is similar to its plasma half-life. Discontinuation of the drug is typically followed by a return of prolactin to elevated values. Bromocriptine decreases prolactin production and secretion, with a resultant reduction in lactotrope size and a subsequent decrease in tumor size.[46]

Therapy should be initiated slowly because side effects, including nausea, headache, dizziness, nasal congestion, and constipation, may occur. Gastrointestinal side effects may be minimized by starting with a very low dose (e.g., 1.25 mg, or one-half tablet) taken at night with a snack, and increasing the dose by 1.25 mg over 4- to 5-day intervals, as tolerated. This progression is continued until a dosage that normalizes prolactin levels is reached. The rate of dosage escalation is dictated by the clinical situation, such as the presence of mass effects. Side effects can usually be improved by continuing the medication at the same dosage or by temporarily reducing the dosage. If patients stop taking the medication for a few days, therapy should be reinstituted at a lower dosage, because side effects may return. Rarely, long-term therapy may result in side effects, including painless cold-induced digital vasospasm, alcohol intolerance, dyskinesia, and psychiatric reactions, including fatigue, depression, and anxiety.

To reduce the gastrointestinal side effects, bromocriptine has been administered intravaginally. Reductions in prolactin similar to that attained by oral bromocriptine have been achieved with the intravaginal route.[47] Gastrointestinal side effects are less common, and therapy may be more effective with vaginally administered bromocriptine.[48]

Cabergoline is an ergoline derivative with selective, potent, and long-lasting dopaminergic properties and is highly effective in the management of hyperprolactinemia. Because of the ease of administration of cabergoline (i.e., once or twice weekly) and its improved side-effect profile relative to bromocriptine, patients show a high rate of compliance. Administration of cabergoline at doses as high as 1.0 mg twice weekly to 113 patients with microprolactinomas resulted in normalization of prolactin levels in 95%.[49] In another study, administration of cabergoline resulted in normalization of prolactin levels in 25 of 26 patients with microprolactinomas.[50] Cabergoline appears to be better tolerated than bromocriptine and may play an important role in the management of patients intolerant of or resistant to bromocriptine. In a multicenter, randomized, 24-week trial involving 459 women, cabergoline was more effective and better tolerated than bromocriptine.[51] In a study of 27 patients with prolactinomas resistant to bromocriptine or the investigational dopamine agonist CV 205-502, including 19 subjects with macroadenomas, cabergoline administration resulted in normalization of prolactin values in 47% of patients with macroadenomas and in all patients with microadenomas.[52] Therefore, use of cabergoline may be considered in all subjects with hyperprolactinemia, including those who are poorly tolerant of or resistant to bromocriptine.[52a]

Other dopamine agonists are available, but not in the United States; these include CV 205-502 and a long-acting preparation of bromocriptine mesylate, Parlodel LAR. CV 205-502 is a nonergot, long-acting dopamine agonist that appears to have increased $D_2$-receptor binding compared with bromocriptine. Either CV 205-502 or bromocriptine was administered in a randomized double-blind fashion to 22 patients with microprolactinomas.[53] In this study, 91% of the patients who received CV 205-502 and 56% of those who received bromocriptine had normalization of prolactin levels. Side effects were less common in the group receiving CV 205-502, and the drug may be useful in those patients intolerant to bromocriptine.[54] CV 205-502 also is effective in the management of macroprolactinomas.[55]

Pergolide is a dopamine agonist approved by the U.S. Food and Drug Administration for the treatment of Parkinson disease. Although not approved for use in the management of hyperprolactinemia, studies have shown that pergolide has a comparable side-effect profile to bromocriptine and may reduce prolactin levels in patients unresponsive to bromocriptine.[56,56b] With the availability of cabergoline, pergolide is rarely used as an alternative to bromocriptine.

### SURGERY

Although surgery is not a primary mode of management for patients with prolactinomas, it may be indicated in several settings. These include patients with large tumors causing visual field deficits unresponsive to bromocriptine, those unable to tolerate dopamine agonist therapy because of its side effects, those with cystic tumors that do not respond to medical therapy, and those with tumor apoplexy. A transsphenoidal approach is used almost exclusively. When the procedure is performed by experienced surgeons, the morbidity rate is negligible. The mortality rate is less than 0.27%, and the major morbidity rate is 3%.[57]

A theoretic advantage of curative surgery is avoidance of long-term medication. However, clinical evidence is lacking. Among 28 patients with microprolactinomas, 24 were cured with transsphenoidal surgery based on normalization of serum prolactin levels. After approximately 4 years, 50% of these initially "cured" patients had recurrence of hyperprolactinemia, although none had radiographic evidence of tumor growth.[58] Another study found a recurrence rate of 39% after approximately 5 years.[59] In one study of patients with normal prolactin values after surgery, the overall recurrence rate was 26% at a mean follow-up of 9.2 years.[60] An immediately postoperative serum prolactin value of <5 ng/mL was associated with a recurrence rate of approximately 20%. These data suggest that, although surgery may result in normalization of prolactin levels initially in patients with microprolactinomas, risk of recurrence is relatively high. In addition, achievement of a low-normal serum prolactin level is an important predictive factor for long-term cure.

Surgical cure rates for macroprolactinomas are approximately 32%, with cure defined as normal prolactin levels after surgery.[45] Surgical cure is inversely proportional to serum prolactin levels and tumor size. Unfortunately, the recurrence rate in macroprolactinomas has been reported to be as high as 80% after curative surgery,[58] although another report indicates that recurrence rates as low as 26% can be achieved.[60]

### RADIATION THERAPY

Conventional radiotherapy (4500–5000 rad) or, rarely, proton beam therapy may be indicated in patients who are not able to tolerate medical therapy.

## MANAGEMENT OF MICROPROLACTINOMAS

The decision to institute medical therapy in patients with microprolactinomas is based on the metabolic consequences of hyperprolactinemia and tumor size. Patients with hyperprolactinemia are usually hypogonadotropic and have accompanying menstrual irregularities. Dopamine agonist therapy can restore menstrual function in most patients with amenorrhea. Luteal phase defects associated with hyperprolactinemia can also be reversed with bromocriptine therapy. Ovulation rates greater than 90% have been reported, with induction of pregnancy in more than 80% of patients.[61] Galactorrhea is not an absolute indication for dopamine agonist therapy, unless the degree of galactorrhea is significantly bothersome to the patient. The presence of amenorrhea is an indication for medical therapy because of the risk of osteoporosis associated with hyperprolactinemic amenorrhea. Some women with microprolactinomas may choose not to have therapy if they show no evidence of hypogonadism or amenorrhea and if they do not desire fertility. Reduction of prolactin levels frequently restores libido and increases sperm counts in hyperprolactinemic men.

Patients with microprolactinomas and those without radiographic evidence of pituitary tumors can sometimes be followed without therapy. Studies investigating the natural history of such tumors have shown that prolactin elevations usually remain stable and, in some cases, spontaneously normalize.[62] In a study of 41 patients with idiopathic hyperprolactinemia, based on normal computed tomographic scans for 5.5 years, 67% of patients whose initial prolactin values were less than 57 ng/mL had normalization of prolactin levels.[63] None of the patients with initial prolactin values above 60 ng/mL showed normalization.

These and other data suggest that the degree of prolactin elevation is a prognostic factor for spontaneous resolution. When 38 untreated patients with microprolactinomas were followed for an average of 50.5 months, 36.6% had an increase, 55.3% had a spontaneous decrease, and 13.1% had no change in prolactin levels.[64] A prospective study of untreated hyperprolactinemic women showed that basal menstrual function is an important variable in predicting progression of the prolactin level.[65] In this study, patients with normal initial menstrual function were more likely to have normalization of prolactin levels, and patients with oligomenorrhea or amenorrhea were more likely to have no change or increases in prolactin levels. Most microprolactinomas do not exhibit evidence of further growth, and prolactin levels may spontaneously normalize.

An important aspect of the natural history of microprolactinomas is that most tumors do not significantly increase in size. Although many of these studies used insensitive radiographic techniques, such as skull films and tomograms, they demonstrated that in patients with microprolactinomas and no radiographic evidence of a tumor, tumor size increased in 0% to 22% of patients.[61,63–66] In a study of 43 patients with presumed microadenomas with a mean follow-up period of 5.4 years, only 2 patients showed evidence of tumor progression.[66] In a prospective study, 27 women were followed for an average of 5.2 years.[65] Of 14 women with normal baseline radiographic studies, 4 developed evidence of an adenoma, although none developed a macroadenoma. Of the 13 women with evidence of a tumor at baseline, only 2 showed worsening of radiographic findings. This study suggests that, although tumor growth may occur in as many as 22% of cases, it is rarely accompanied by clinical symptoms from mass effects. Follow-up of untreated patients should include serial measurement of prolactin levels and periodic MRI scans, because tumor progression may not be accompanied by an increase in prolactin levels.

The presence of osteoporosis is a key factor in the decision to institute therapy. Hyperprolactinemia is associated with trabecular and cortical osteopenia. Fourteen young hyperprolactinemic women with prolactin levels ranging from 22 to 99 ng/mL and amenorrhea for 1 to 18 years had significantly decreased cortical bone density compared with normal women.[67] Additional studies have shown that hyperprolactinemic women may have trabecular osteopenia with spinal bone density 10% to 25% below normal.[68–70] Spinal bone density in hyperprolactinemic women correlates with serum androgen levels and relative percentage of ideal body weight.[68,71,72] Decreased bone density is thought to be due to hypogonadism and not a direct effect of prolactin, because hyperprolactinemic women with normal menstrual function do not have associated bone loss.[68] Figure 13-2 shows that hyperprolactinemic patients with hypogonadism have lower bone density than eugonadal hyperprolactinemic women. The decreased bone density in the hyperprolactinemic women with amenorrhea also correlates with the duration of amenorrhea.[70]

An important question is whether treatment of hyperprolactinemic amenorrhea may result in improvement in bone density. A prospective series in which 32 women with hyperprolactinemic amenorrhea were randomized to medical therapy or no therapy showed that resumption of menses with medical therapy was associated with a significant increase in cortical bone density, mostly during the first 12 months of therapy.[70] However, the cortical bone density achieved in this series remained below that of normal women. Of 38 women with prolactinomas examined 2 to 5 years after surgery, cortical bone mass was below normal in both cured and uncured patients, a finding which suggests that remission of hyperprolactinemia may not lead to normalization of bone density.[73] Therapy for hyperprolactinemic amenorrhea with resumption of menses may lead to improvement in but not normalization of bone density.

Another important question is whether hyperprolactinemic amenorrhea is associated with progressive, accelerated bone loss. In a study of 52 hyperprolactinemic women and 41 controls over a mean period of 1.8 years, trabecular osteoporosis was marked in women with hyperprolactinemic amenorrhea, and bone loss progressed in untreated women by an average of 3.8% per year.[71] Conversely, in another study of 56 hyperpro-

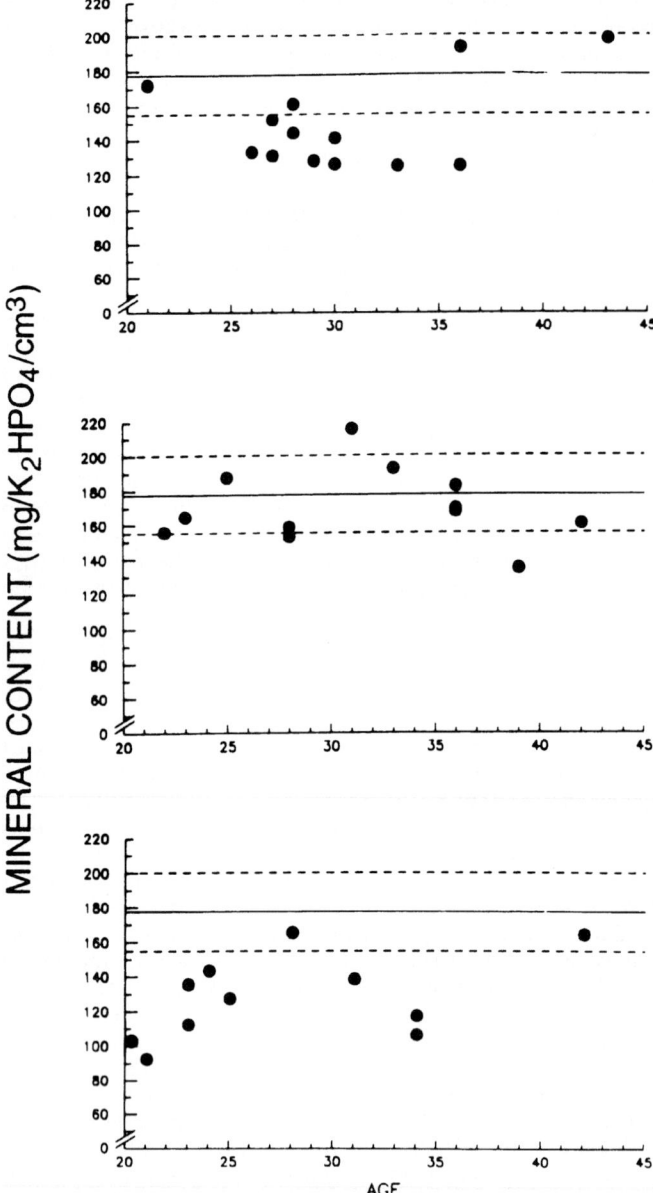

**FIGURE 13-2.** Spinal bone density in 13 women with hyperprolactinemic amenorrhea (*top*), 12 eumenorrheic hyperprolactinemic women (*middle*), and 11 women with hypothalamic amenorrhea (*bottom*). The mean ± 1 standard deviation for 19 normal women is shown by the solid and dashed horizontal lines, respectively. (Reprinted from Klibanski A, Biller BM, Rosenthal DI, et al. Effects of prolactin and estrogen deficiency in amenorrheic bone loss. J Clin Endocrinol Metab 1988; 67:124.)

lactinemic women, spinal bone density in women with amenorrhea did not decrease significantly over an average of 4.7 years.[72] These studies suggest that a subgroup of women with hyperprolactinemic amenorrhea may be at risk for progressive osteoporosis, including those women with decreased percentages of ideal body weight and lower serum androgen levels. Because osteoporosis is common in women with hyperprolactinemic amenorrhea, the authors recommend treatment of amenorrheic women to improve bone density or at least prevent further deterioration.

## MANAGEMENT OF MACROPROLACTINOMAS

Unlike patients with microprolactinomas, those with macroprolactinomas always require therapy. Patients with macroade-

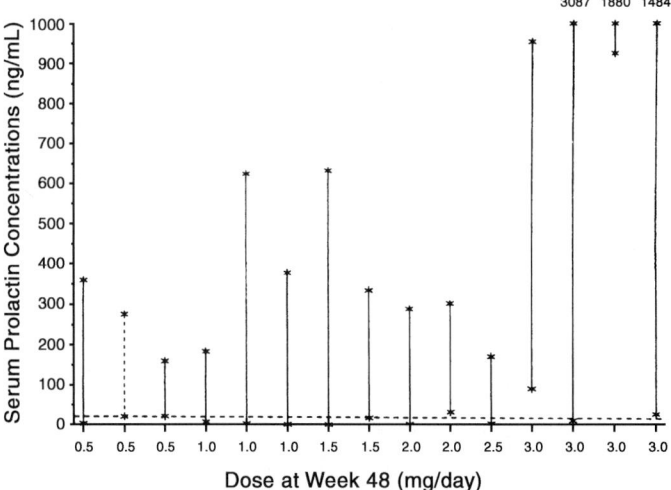

**FIGURE 13-3.** Individual serum prolactin levels at baseline and 48 weeks according to final dose in macroprolactinoma patients treated with cabergoline. The *dotted horizontal line* indicates normal serum prolactin (<20ng/mL). The *dotted vertical line* refers to a patient who normalized PRL at week 6 but did not complete 48 weeks because of a complication (pituitary hemorrhage). (From Biller BM, Molitch ME, Vance ML, et al. Treatment of prolactin-secreting macroadenomas with the once-weekly dopamine agonist cabergoline. J Clin Endocrinol Metab 1996; 81:2338, with permission.)

nomas may have evidence of local mass effects due to the tumor mass, with resultant visual field abnormalities, and hypopituitarism due to compression of the normal pituitary gland. Aggressive management is required to prevent or reverse these complications. Bromocriptine therapy results in significant tumor shrinkage in as many as 75% of patients. Tumor size reduction may occur in weeks or over many months, and this reduction is frequently accompanied by an improvement in visual field abnormalities and pituitary function. Visual field deficits have been reported to improve within hours of institution of medical therapy. Of 27 patients treated with bromocriptine, 64% experienced a reduction in tumor size of at least 50%.[74] Tumor shrinkage often occurred within 6 weeks. Sixty-six percent of patients had normalization of prolactin levels, but the fall in prolactin levels did not always correlate with reductions in tumor size.

Administration of cabergoline may lead to reduction in prolactin levels, tumor shrinkage, and restoration of gonadal function in patients with macroprolactinomas. When cabergoline was administered to 14 patients with macroprolactinomas, tumor shrinkage was observed in 13 (93%), and complete disappearance was documented in 2 patients.[75] In one such study, cabergoline was administered to 15 patients with macroprolactinomas in a multicenter, 48-week trial (see Fig. 13-3).[76] Normalization of prolactin levels was achieved in 73% of subjects, and mean reduction in tumor size was 31%. In this study, tumor shrinkage often occurred during the first 8 weeks; however, in some subjects, reductions in tumor volume were not seen until 24 weeks. Therefore, cabergoline may have an important role in the management of patients with macroprolactinomas.[77] Dosages of 0.5 to 3.0 mg cabergoline per week are often sufficient for maximal effects. The drug may be useful as first line therapy in patients with macroprolactinomas or in those who are intolerant of or resistant to bromocriptine.[52]

The heterogeneity of prolactinoma responses to bromocriptine may be the result of variable density of the $D_2$ receptor on tumor membranes. Good correlation exists between the density of dopaminergic binding sites and maximal inhibition of adenylate cyclase activation in bromocriptine-responsive and bromocriptine-resistant prolactinomas.[78] This suggests that bromocriptine response depends on the

density of the $D_2$ receptor. A study of 46 prolactinomas in patients undergoing surgery because of failure to respond to bromocriptine or local compression showed no evidence of mutations in the $D_2$ coding sequence.[79] Alterations in receptor density or function probably explain the lack of dopamine agonist effect in these patients.

Medical therapy represents the initial option for patients with macroprolactinomas with no or stable visual field deficits because of the low cure rates associated with surgery in such patients. Although transsphenoidal surgery is not used as a primary therapy for patients with macroprolactinomas, no data are available directly comparing the use of dopamine agonists with surgery as primary therapy for macroadenomas. Specific circumstances, such as the presence of a cystic prolactinoma (which often does not respond fully to dopamine agonist therapy), may predict a poor initial response to bromocriptine therapy in these patients. Cabergoline or bromocriptine is a useful adjunctive therapy in patients with large tumors, for which complete resection has not been possible.

Most men with diagnosed prolactinomas have macroadenomas. In women, most tumors are microadenomas. In part, this difference may reflect the fact that women present earlier than men for evaluation because of complaints of menstrual disturbances. In men with hyperprolactinemia-induced hypogonadism and normal residual pituitary function, 3 to 6 months may be required for testosterone levels to increase, normal sexual function to be restored, and sperm counts and motility to increase after prolactin levels normalize.[80]

## PREGNANCY AND PROLACTINOMAS

Many women with hyperprolactinemia present with infertility; bromocriptine is typically used to normalize prolactin levels and allow normal ovulation to occur. After pregnancy is established, bromocriptine should be discontinued if no evidence of local tumor compression is seen. Pregnancy in normal women leads to increased pituitary size through estrogen-stimulated lactotrope hyperplasia. For patients with prolactinomas, the concern is that the high estrogen levels associated with pregnancy may lead to lactotrope stimulation and tumor growth, with resulting local complications, including visual field deficits, headaches, and diabetes insipidus. In a review of the data on pregnancy outcomes in hyperprolactinemic patients, clinically significant tumor enlargement (e.g., causing headaches, visual deficits) were found in as many as 5.5% of patients with microprolactinomas.[81] Patients with microprolactinomas should be followed carefully during pregnancy, with visual field monitoring at monthly intervals.

In contrast to patients with microprolactinomas, 15.5% to 35.7% of patients with macroadenomas are at risk for clinically significant tumor enlargement during any trimester of pregnancy. Although some centers recommend transsphenoidal resection of the macroadenomas before conception, surgical resection does not prevent symptomatic enlargement during pregnancy. Monitoring of serum prolactin levels throughout pregnancy is not clinically useful, because prolactin levels increase markedly during pregnancy. The decision to reinstitute therapy depends on the development of clinical symptoms, not the serum prolactin level. If a complication due to tumor growth does occur, it is rapidly reversible with the reinstitution of bromocriptine therapy, which is then continued through term.

The outcome of bromocriptine-induced pregnancies is comparable to that of normal pregnancies. A large, international experience with bromocriptine and pregnancy suggests that bromocriptine therapy does not result in complications for the fetus[82] (see Chap. 110).

Experience with cabergoline and pregnancy is much more limited. In the largest such study (226 pregnancies induced by cabergoline) no evidence was found of increased pregnancy-associated complications or birth defects in these women compared to women who did not receive cabergoline.[83] However, until the experience with cabergoline is more widespread, bromocriptine is recommended as a first-choice therapy for hyperprolactinemic women seeking pregnancy.

After delivery, breast-feeding appears to be safe in patients not receiving bromocriptine. Patients with macroadenomas should continue to be followed closely, and the decision to institute therapy should depend on tumor size and clinical symptoms.

Patients with hyperprolactinemia should undergo a complete evaluation to determine the underlying cause of the elevated prolactin level. If idiopathic hyperprolactinemia or a prolactinoma is the cause, dopamine agonist therapy is highly efficacious in lowering prolactin levels, restoring gonadal function, and reversing local tumor complications.

# REFERENCES

1. Blackwell RE. Hyperprolactinemia. Evaluation and management. Endocrinol Metab Clin North Am 1992; 21:105.
2. Foord SM, Peters JR, Dieguez C, et al. Dopamine receptors on intact anterior pituitary cells in culture: functional association with the inhibition of prolactin and thyrotropin. Endocrinology 1983; 112:1567.
3. Schettini G, Cronin MJ, MacLeod RM. Adenosine 3',5'-monophosphate (cAMP) and calcium-calmodulin interrelation in the control of prolactin secretion: evidence for dopamine inhibition of cAMP accumulation and prolactin release after calcium mobilization. Endocrinology 1983; 112:1801.
4. Leblanc H, Lachelin GC, Abu-Fadil S, Yen SS. Effects of dopamine infusion on pituitary hormone secretion in humans. J Clin Endocrinol Metab 1976; 43:668.
5. Rivera JL, Lal S, Ettigi P, et al. Effect of acute and chronic neuroleptic therapy on serum prolactin levels in men and women of different age groups. Clin Endocrinol 1976; 5:273.
6. Nikolics K, Mason AJ, Szonyi E, et al. A prolactin-inhibiting factor within the precursor for human gonadotropin-releasing hormone. Nature 1985; 316:511.
7. Grossman A, Delitala G, Yeo T, Besser GM. GABA and muscimol inhibit the release of prolactin from dispersed rat anterior pituitary cells. Neuroendocrinology 1981; 32:145.
8. Raymond V, Beaulieu M, Labrie F, Boissier J. Potent antidopaminergic activity of estradiol at the pituitary level on prolactin release. Science 1978; 200:1173.
9. Maurer RA. Estradiol regulates the transcription of the prolactin gene. J Biol Chem 1982; 257:2133.
10. Scheithauer BW, Sano T, Kovacs KT, et al. The pituitary gland in pregnancy: a clinicopathologic and immunohistochemical study of 69 cases. Mayo Clin Proc 1990; 65:461.
11. Bowers CY, Friesen HG, Hwang P, et al. Prolactin and thyrotropin release in man by synthetic pyroglutamyl-histidyl-prolinamide. Biochem Biophys Res Commun 1971; 45:1033.
12. Kato Y, Iwasaki Y, Iwasaki J, et al. Prolactin release by vasoactive intestinal polypeptide in rats. Endocrinology 1978; 103:554.
13. Abe H, Engler D, Molitch ME, et al. Vasoactive intestinal peptide is a physiological mediator of prolactin release in the rat. Endocrinology 1985; 116:1383.
14. Hagen TC, Arnaout MA, Scherzer WJ, et al. Antisera to vasoactive intestinal polypeptide inhibit basal prolactin release from dispersed anterior pituitary cells. Neuroendocrinology 1986; 43:641.
15. Casper RF, Yen SS. Simultaneous pulsatile release of prolactin and luteinizing hormone induced by luteinizing hormone–releasing factor agonist. J Clin Endocrinol Metab 1981; 52:934.
16. Denef C, Andries M. Evidence for paracrine interaction between gonadotrophs and lactotrophs in pituitary cell aggregates. Endocrinology 1983; 112:813.
17. Koshiyama H, Kato Y, Inoue T, et al. Central galanin stimulates pituitary prolactin secretion in rats: possible involvement of hypothalamic vasoactive intestinal polypeptide. Neurosci Lett 1987; 75:49.
18. Giustina A, Licini M, Schettino M, et al. Physiological role of galanin in the regulation of anterior pituitary function in humans. Am J Physiol 1994; 266:E57.
19. Wehrenberg WB, McNicol D, Frantz AG, Ferin M. The effects of serotonin on prolactin and growth hormone concentrations in normal and pituitary stalk-sectioned monkeys. Endocrinology 1980; 107:1747.
20. Falaschi P, Rosa M, Rocco A, et al. Effect of ritanserin, specific 5HT-2 antagonist, on PRL secretion in normal subjects and in different hyperprolactinaemic conditions. Clin Endocrinol 1991; 34:449.
21. Lewis UJ, Singh RN, Sinha YN, Vanderlaan WP. Glycosylated human prolactin. Endocrinology 1985; 116:359.
22. Whitaker MD, Klee GG, Kao PC, et al. Demonstration of biological activity of prolactin molecular weight variants in human sera. J Clin Endocrinol Metab 1984; 58:826.
23. Corenblum B. Asymptomatic hyperprolactinemia resulting from macroprolactinemia. Fertil Steril 1990; 53:165.
24. Ben-David M, Schenker JG. Transient hyperprolactinemia: a correctable cause of idiopathic female infertility. J Clin Endocrinol Metab 1983; 57:442.
25. Veldhuis JD, Johnson ML. Operating characteristics of the hypothalamo-pituitary-gonadal axis in men: circadian, ultradian, and pulsatile release of prolactin and its temporal coupling with luteinizing hormone. J Clin Endocrinol Metab 1988; 67:116.
26. Sassin JF, Frantz AG, Weitzman ED, Kapen S. Human prolactin: 24-hour pattern with increased release during sleep. Science 1972; 177:1205.
27. Franchimont P, Dourcy C, Legros JJ, et al. Prolactin levels during the menstrual cycle. Clin Endocrinol 1976; 5:643.
28. Carlson HE. Prolactin stimulation by protein is mediated by amino acids in humans. J Clin Endocrinol Metab 1989; 69:7.
29. Boyd AED, Spare S, Bower B, Reichlin S. Neurogenic galactorrhea-amenorrhea. J Clin Endocrinol Metab 1978; 47:1374.
30. Katznelson L, Riskind PN, Saxe VC, Klibanski A. Prolactin pulsatile characteristics in postmenopausal women. J Clin Endocrinol Metab 1998; 83:761.
31. Vekemans M, Robyn C. Influence of age on serum prolactin levels in women and men. BMJ 1975; 4:738.
32. Rigg LA, Lein A, Yen SS. Pattern of increase in circulating prolactin levels during human gestation. Am J Obstet Gynecol 1977; 129:454.
33. Noel GL, Suh HK, Frantz AG. Prolactin release during nursing and breast stimulation in postpartum and nonpostpartum subjects. J Clin Endocrinol Metab 1974; 38:413.
34. Nunley WC, Urban RJ, Kitchin JD, et al. Dynamics of pulsatile prolactin release during the postpartum lactational period. J Clin Endocrinol Metab 1991; 72:287.
35. Franks S, Murray MA, Jequier AM, et al. Incidence and significance of hyperprolactinaemia in women with amenorrhoea. Clin Endocrinol 1975; 4:597.
36. Jacobs HS, Franks S, Murray MA, et al. Clinical and endocrine features of hyperprolactinaemic amenorrhoea. Clin Endocrinol 1976; 5:439.
37. Patton ML, Woolf PD. Hyperprolactinemia and delayed puberty: a report of three cases and their response to therapy. Pediatrics 1983; 71:572.
38. Asukai K, Uemura T, Minaguchi H. Occult hyperprolactinemia in infertile women. Fertil Steril 1993; 60:423.
39. Bergland RM, Page RB. Can the pituitary secrete directly to the brain? (Affirmative anatomical evidence). Endocrinology 1978; 102:1325.
40. Park SK, Selmanoff M. Hyperprolactinemia suppresses the luteinizing hormone responses to N-methyl-D-aspartate, epinephrine, and neuropeptide-Y in male rats. Endocrinology 1993; 133:2091.
41. Polson DW, Sagle M, Mason HD, et al. Ovulation and normal luteal function during GnRH treatment of women with hyperprolactinaemic amenorrhoea. Clin Endocrinol 1986; 24:531.
42. Lobo RA, Kletzky OA, Kaptein EM, Goebelsmann U. Prolactin modulation of dehydroepiandrosterone sulfate secretion. Am J Obstet Gynecol 1980; 138:632.
43. Klibanski A, Zervas NT. Diagnosis and management of hormone-secreting pituitary adenomas. N Engl J Med 1991; 324:822.
44. Cowden EA, Ratcliffe WA, Ratcliffe JG, et al. Hyperprolactinaemia in renal disease. Clin Endocrinol 1978; 9:241.
44a. Kleinberg DL, Davis JM, de Coster R, et al. Prolactin levels and adverse events in patients treated with risperidone. J Clin Psychopharm 1999; 19:57.
45. Molitch ME. Pathologic hyperprolactinemia. Endocrinol Metab Clin North Am 1992; 21:877.
46. Bassetti M, Spada A, Pezzo G, Giannattasio G. Bromocriptine treatment reduces the cell size in human macroprolactinomas: a morphometric study. J Clin Endocrinol Metab 1984; 58:268.
47. Vermesh M, Fossum GT, Kletzky OA. Vaginal bromocriptine: pharmacology and effect on serum prolactin in normal women. Obstet Gynecol 1988; 72:693.
48. Kletzky OA, Vermesh M. Effectiveness of vaginal bromocriptine in treating women with hyperprolactinemia. Fertil Steril 1989; 51:269.
49. Webster J, Piscitelli G, Polli A, et al. Dose-dependent suppression of serum prolactin by cabergoline in hyperprolactinaemia: a placebo controlled, double blind, multicentre study. European Multicentre Cabergoline Dose-Finding Study Group. Clin Endocrinol 1992; 37:534.
50. Muratori M, Arosio M, Gambino G, et al. Use of cabergoline in the long-term treatment of hyperprolactinemic and acromegalic patients. J Endocrinol Invest 1997; 20:537.
51. Webster J, Piscitelli G, Polli A, et al. A comparison of cabergoline and bromocriptine in the treatment of hyperprolactinemic amenorrhea. N Engl J Med 1994; 331:904.
52. Colao A, Di Sarno A, Sarnacchiaro F, et al. Prolactinomas resistant to standard dopamine agonists respond to chronic cabergoline treatment [see comments]. J Clin Endocrinol Metab 1997; 82:876.
52a. Cabergoline in the treatment of hyperprolactinemia: a study in 455 patients. J Clin Endocrinol Metab 1999; 84:2518.

53. Homburg R, West C, Brownell J, Jacobs HS. A double-blind study comparing a new non-ergot, long-acting dopamine agonist, CV 205-502, with bromocriptine in women with hyperprolactinaemia. Clin Endocrinol 1990; 32:565.
54. van-der-Lely AJ, Brownell J, Lamberts SW. The efficacy and tolerability of CV 205-502 (a nonergot dopaminergic drug) in macroprolactinoma patients and in prolactinoma patients intolerant to bromocriptine. J Clin Endocrinol Metab 1991; 72:1136.
55. Vance ML, Lipper M, Klibanski A, et al. Treatment of prolactin-secreting pituitary macroadenomas with the long-acting non-ergot dopamine agonist CV 205-502. Ann Intern Med 1990; 112:668.
56. Kletzky OA, Borenstein R, Mileikowsky GN. Pergolide and bromocriptine for the treatment of patients with hyperprolactinemia. Am J Obstet Gynecol 1986; 154:431.
56a. Freda PU, Andreadis CI, Khandji AG, et al. Long-term treatment of prolactin-secreting macroadenomas with pergolide. J Clin Endocrinol Metab 2000; 85:8.
57. Zervas NT. Surgical results in pituitary adenomas: results of an international study. In: Black PM, Zervas NT, Ridgway EC, Martin JB, eds. Secretory tumors of the pituitary gland. New York: Raven Press, 1984:377.
58. Serri O, Rasio E, Beauregard H, et al. Recurrence of hyperprolactinemia after selective transsphenoidal adenomectomy in women with prolactinoma. N Engl J Med 1983; 309:280.
59. Schlechte JA, Sherman BM, Chapler FK, VanGilder J. Long term follow-up of women with surgically treated prolactin-secreting pituitary tumors. J Clin Endocrinol Metab 1986; 62:1296.
60. Feigenbaum SL, Downey DE, Wilson CB, Jaffe RB. Transsphenoidal pituitary resection for preoperative diagnosis of prolactin-secreting pituitary adenoma in women: long term follow-up. J Clin Endocrinol Metab 1996; 81:1711.
61. Bergh T, Nillius SJ, Wide L. Bromocriptine treatment of 42 hyperprolactinaemic women with secondary amenorrhoea. Acta Endocrinol 1978; 88:435.
62. Weiss MH, Teal J, Gott P, et al. Natural history of microprolactinomas: six-year follow-up. Neurosurgery 1983; 12:180.
63. Martin TL, Kim M, Malarkey WB. The natural history of idiopathic hyperprolactinemia. J Clin Endocrinol Metab 1985; 60:855.
64. Sisam DA, Sheehan JP, Sheeler LR. The natural history of untreated microprolactinomas. Fertil Steril 1987; 48:67.
65. Schlechte J, Dolan K, Sherman B, et al. The natural history of untreated hyperprolactinemia: a prospective analysis. J Clin Endocrinol Metab 1989; 68:412.
66. March CM, Kletzky OA, Davajan V, et al. Longitudinal evaluation of patients with untreated prolactin-secreting pituitary adenomas. Am J Obstet Gynecol 1981; 139:835.
67. Klibanski A, Neer RM, Beitins IZ, et al. Decreased bone density in hyperprolactinemic women. N Engl J Med 1980; 303:1511.
68. Klibanski A, Biller BM, Rosenthal DI, et al. Effects of prolactin and estrogen deficiency in amenorrheic bone loss. J Clin Endocrinol Metab 1988; 67:124.
69. Koppelman MC, Kurtz DW, Morrish KA, et al. Vertebral body bone mineral content in hyperprolactinemic women. J Clin Endocrinol Metab 1984; 59:1050.
70. Klibanski A, Greenspan SL. Increase in bone mass after treatment of hyperprolactinemic amenorrhea. N Engl J Med 1986; 315:542.
71. Biller BM, Baum HB, Rosenthal DI, et al. Progressive trabecular osteopenia in women with hyperprolactinemic amenorrhea [see comments]. J Clin Endocrinol Metab 1992; 75:692.
72. Schlechte J, Walkner L, Kathol M. A longitudinal analysis of premenopausal bone loss in healthy women and women with hyperprolactinemia. J Clin Endocrinal Metab 1992; 75:698.
73. Schlechte JA, Sherman B, Martin R. Bone density in amenorrheic women with and without hyperprolactinemia. J Clin Endocrinol Metab 1983; 56:1120.
74. Molitch ME, Elton RL, Blackwell RE, et al. Bromocriptine as primary therapy for prolactin-secreting macroadenomas: results of a prospective multicenter study. J Clin Endocrinol Metab 1985; 60:698.
75. Ferrari C, Paracchi A, Mattei AM, et al. Cabergoline in the long-term therapy of hyperprolactinemic disorders. Acta Endocrinol 1992; 126:489.
76. Biller BM, Molitch ME, Vance ML, et al. Treatment of prolactin-secreting macroadenomas with the once-weekly dopamine agonist cabergoline. J Clin Endocrinol Metab 1996; 81:2338.
77. Ferrari CI, Abs R, Bevan JS, et al. Treatment of macroprolactinoma with cabergoline: a study of 85 patients. Clin Endocrinol 1997; 46:409.
78. Pellegrini I, Rasolonjanahary R, Gunz G, et al. Resistance to bromocriptine in prolactinomas. J Clin Endocrinol Metab 1989; 69:500.
79. Friedman E, Adams EF, Hoog A, et al. Normal structural dopamine type 2 receptor gene in prolactin-secreting and other pituitary tumors. J Clin Endocrinol Metab 1994; 78:568.
80. De Rosa M, Colao A, Di Sarno A, et al. Cabergoline treatment rapidly improves gonadal function in hyperprolactinemic males: a comparison with bromocriptine. Eur J Endocrinol 1998; 138:286.
81. Molitch ME. Pregnancy and the hyperprolactinemic woman. N Engl J Med 1985; 312:1364.
82. Turkalj I, Braun P, Krupp P. Surveillance of bromocriptine in pregnancy. JAMA 1982; 247:1589.
83. Robert E, Musatti L, Piscitelli G, Ferrari CI. Pregnancy outcome after treatment with the ergot derivative, cabergoline. Reprod Toxicol 1996; 10:333.

# CHAPTER 14

# ADRENOCORTICOTROPIN: PHYSIOLOGY AND CLINICAL ASPECTS

DAVID J. TORPY AND RICHARD V. JACKSON

The existence of an adrenocorticotropic factor was predicted by classic pituitary ablation/pituitary extract replacement experiments.[1,2] Ovine and human adrenocorticotropin hormone (ACTH) were later isolated and sequenced.[3,4] ACTH, a 39 amino acid peptide secreted by the corticotropes (located centrally in the anterior pituitary gland), stimulates adrenocortical steroid synthesis. Measurement of this peptide, formerly difficult, is now reliable and practical, although ACTH measurements are most useful when autonomous secretion or pathologic suppression of ACTH release is suspected. ACTH release is stimulated by the hypothalamic secretion of corticotropin-releasing hormone (CRH) and arginine vasopressin (AVP)—in response to stress and the circadian rhythm—and inhibited by negative feedback from circulating cortisol. A number of acquired or inherited disorders of ACTH secretion may be manifested by hypercortisolism, adrenal insufficiency, or hyperpigmentation.

## SYNTHESIS AND PROCESSING OF PROOPIOMELANOCORTIN

When ACTH is synthesized in the anterior pituitary gland by the corticotropes, it is derived from a much larger precursor, a 241 amino acid peptide, proopiomelanocortin (POMC)[5] (Fig. 14-1). The human POMC 8-Kb gene is located on chromosome 2p23.3, consisting of a 400 to 700 bp promoter, three exons, and two introns.[6,7] The main regulators of POMC transcription are CRH and glucocorticoids. CRH increases POMC transcription through a cyclic adenosine monophosphate–mediated mechanism, whereas glucocorticoids inhibit transcription. In the pituitary, prohormone convertase 1 (PC1) cleaves POMC into ACTH and two other large polypeptides, N-terminal peptide and β-lipotropin.[8] The roles of these large peptides, which are cosecreted in equimolar amounts to ACTH, are unknown. β-lipotropin was so named because of a mild lipolytic activity[9] that has doubtful relevance in humans. Formerly, β-lipotropin was measured by some investigators as a substitute for ACTH. In the brain, ACTH is cleaved by prohormone convertase 2 (PC2), yielding α-melanocyte-stimulating hormone (α-MSH) and corticotropin-like intermediate lobe peptide (CLIP), which are also produced in the human fetal pituitary intermediate lobe. These peptides are not produced in the adult, where the intermediate lobe is no longer present. Although MSH sequences (α-MSH, β-MSH, γ-MSH) are contained within POMC fragments, ACTH itself has melanotropic action, increasing melanin synthesis, and may itself lead to pigmentation in hypersecretory states. No MSH peptides are released from the anterior pituitary in humans, nor are these peptides found in human blood. MSH activity in human blood results from MSH sequences contained within ACTH and possibly within β-lipotropin and the N-terminal fragment of POMC.

Animal studies have revealed a role for α-MSH in the regulation of food intake, acting through the brain melanocortin-4 receptor. Studies in Mexican-Americans have shown an association between inheritance of the POMC region of chromosome 2, serum leptin concentration, and obesity.[10] POMC gene mutations can result in a monogenic disorder of early-onset obesity, adrenal insufficiency, and red hair.[11]

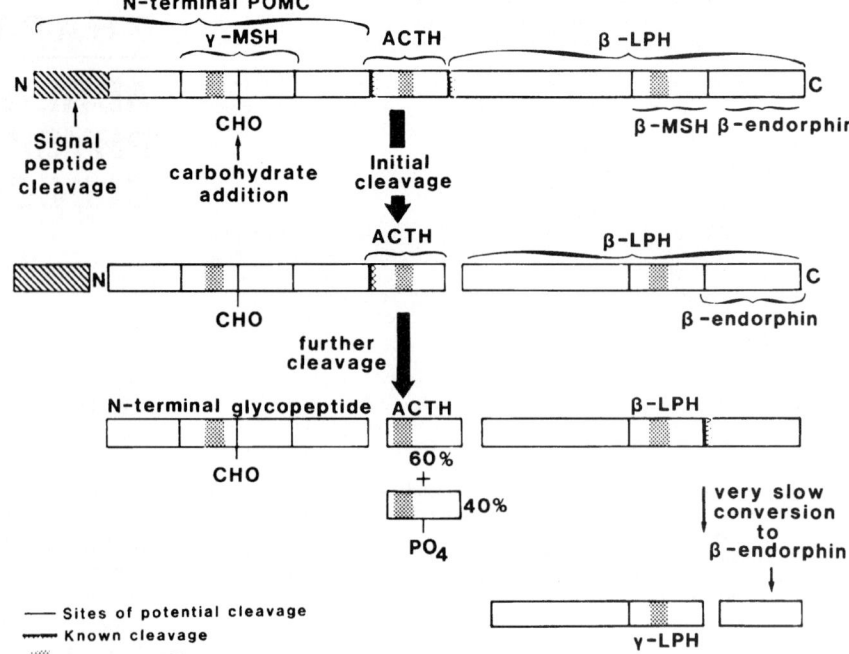

**FIGURE 14-1.** Processing of human proopiomelanocortin (*POMC*). The processing proceeds in stages, yielding a variety of forms of secreted peptides; N-terminal peptide, adrenocorticotropic hormone (*ACTH*), and β-lipotropin are the principal circulating forms. Approximately 40% of ACTH has a posttranslational addition of a phosphate moiety. (*γMSH*, gamma-melanocyte-stimulating-hormone; *LPH*, lipotropin; *CHO*, carbohydrate; *PO₄*, phosphate.)

## FUNCTIONS OF ADRENOCORTICOTROPIN

The primary action of ACTH is to promote steroidogenesis—that is, to enhance the synthesis and secretion of glucocorticoids, mineralocorticoids, and weak androgenic steroids of the adrenal cortex. However, the main physiologic controller of aldosterone release is the renin-angiotensin system (see Chap. 17). The N-terminal 18 amino acids are capable of cortisol release but are subject to rapid degradation; hence, the N-terminal 24 amino acids are used clinically to stimulate ACTH release (cosyntropin). ACTH acts on a specific 297-amino acid cell surface receptor that belongs to the $G_s$-protein–coupled 7-transmembrane superfamily of receptors. The ACTH receptor (also known as the melanocortin-2 receptor) gene is located at chromosome 18p11.1.[12,13] The ACTH receptor acts via a cyclic adenosine monophosphate–dependent second messenger pathway to increase adrenal lipoprotein uptake from plasma and increase the transcription rates of genes for enzymes involved in steroidogenesis. Increased low-density lipoprotein uptake is facilitated by an increase in cell-surface low-density lipoprotein receptors. In contrast, ACTH has a smaller effect on zona fasciculata hydroxymethylglutaryl-coenzyme A reductase levels and hence cholesterol synthesis.[14,15] Acutely, ACTH increases the activity of the rate-limiting enzyme of adrenal steroidogenesis, the $P450_{SCC}$ enzyme that catalyzes the conversion of cholesterol to Δ⁵-pregnenolone. Chronically, ACTH increases the activity of other adrenal enzymes involved in steroidogenesis. ACTH also stimulates protein synthesis, resulting in adrenal hypertrophy and hyperplasia. The activity of phenylethanolamine-*N*-methyltransferase, the enzyme that catalyzes epinephrine production (see Chap. 85), is dependent on cortisol, and hence ACTH levels. ACTH has a trophic effect on tyrosine hydroxylase activity, the enzyme responsible for catalyzing the rate-limiting step in catecholamine biosynthesis, and increases the rate of melanin synthesis in melanocytes, which leads to skin pigmentation.

## REGULATION OF ADRENOCORTICOTROPIN SECRETION

The anterior pituitary contains ~600 μg of ACTH.[16] ACTH, which is released on a pulsatile basis with peaks at ~30-minute intervals,[17] is subject to intravascular enzymatic degradation with a plasma disappearance half-life of 7 to 12 minutes.[18] Cortisol pulses follow those of ACTH by ~30 minutes, although not all cortisol peaks follow those of ACTH.[19] The relationship between increasing levels of ACTH and consequent cortisol secretion is defined by a sigmoidal curve.[20] Very high levels of ACTH do not further increase plasma cortisol concentrations, although the duration of a cortisol secretory burst continues to increase.[21]

Under some circumstances, the relation between ACTH and cortisol secretion is disturbed. In chronic stress, such as critical illness, a greater cortisol release occurs for an additional given ACTH stimulus because of adrenal hypertrophy and altered adrenal enzyme activities, which favor production of cortisol over that of adrenal androgens.[22] Elevated ACTH levels after appropriate stimuli, with blunted or normal cortisol responses, are seen in myotonic dystrophy,[23] a multisystem genetic disorder, and fibromyalgia,[24] an idiopathic pain syndrome. In these cases, the primary defect is thought to lie in ACTH regulation rather than an altered ACTH bioactivity or adrenal hyporesponsiveness.

Regulation of ACTH release is subject to three themes: stress, the circadian rhythm, and glucocorticoid negative feedback. Stress, defined as a threat to homeostasis, derives from such factors as sepsis, trauma, or emotion. In response to stress, ACTH release is greatly increased; consequently, the secretion of cortisol, the principal glucocorticoid in humans, can increase five-fold. The principal functions of cortisol during stress are to restrain the immune system, by reducing production of potentially damaging cytokines[25]; augment the effects of catecholamines on the vascular system; mobilize glucose and fatty acids for metabolic use; and sharpen cognition to allow appropriate behavioral responses. During starvation, cortisol acts to increase hepatic glucose production for use as energy.

ACTH secretion follows a light-entrained circadian rhythm with peak cortisol blood levels attained at ~6:00 a.m. to 8:00 a.m. and the lowest concentrations at approximately midnight.[26,27,27a] In animals, the circadian rhythm is based on serotonergic pathways arising from the suprachiasmatic nucleus,[28] although the mechanism—or indeed the function—of circadian ACTH release in humans is unknown. In humans, severe disturbances of circadian ACTH release following transmeridian travel require several days to be reentrained[29] (see Chap. 6).

Normally, glucocorticoid negative feedback controls ACTH release; however, stress and circadian factors make ACTH release less susceptible to feedback inhibition. At physiologic levels of cortisol, the brain, rather than the pituitary, is the main site of feedback inhibition.[30] Cortisol acts at two types of receptors in the hypothalamus and hippocampus to inhibit CRH release; these are type-1 (mineralocorticoid) and type-2 (classic glucocorticoid) receptors. The high affinity type-1 receptors are thought to mediate suppression of CRH release in response to basal conditions, whereas type-2 receptors mediate stress-level cortisol inhibition.[31,32] Both rapid and delayed feedback of glucocorticoids on ACTH secretion are observed. Rapid feedback is responsive to the rate of change in glucocorticoid concentrations; delayed feedback responds to absolute circulating glucocorticoid levels.[33]

The progressive rise in plasma ACTH, which occurs during pregnancy, is associated with increased total and free cortisol (two- to three-fold). This may be due to stimulation of the maternal pituitary corticotropes by placental CRH.[34] Transiently reduced central CRH secretion and relative hypocortisolism in the postpartum period may contribute to the mood and autoimmune phenomena observed at this time.

Leptin is a peptide hormone produced by adipocytes. It was isolated after studies of the leptin-deficient *ob/ob* (obese) mouse.[35] Leptin acts on specific neuropeptide/neurotransmitter pathways of the central nervous system and through these modulatory effects inhibits appetite. Starvation is associated with low leptin levels and hypercortisolism. Moreover, plasma leptin and cortisol have an inversely related circadian rhythm.[36] These findings suggest a close relationship between the hypothalamic–pituitary–adrenal (HPA) axis and leptin. Leptin inhibits ACTH secretion by inhibiting CRH synthesis.[37] Leptin also inhibits adrenocortical enzyme activity.[38] Hence, low leptin levels may account for the physiologic hypercortisolism of starvation, allowing stimulation of fuel catabolism and liberating amino acids and glucose[39] (see Chap. 186).

## MECHANISM OF CONTROL OF ACTH SECRETION

As previously stated, pituitary ACTH secretion is subject to regulation by the hypothalamic hormones, principally CRH and AVP (Fig. 14-2).[40] These hypophysiotropic factors are secreted into the hypothalamic-pituitary portal circulation at the median eminence from neurons arising in the parvicellular portion of the hypothalamic paraventricular nucleus. CRH, a 41 amino acid peptide discovered in 1981,[41] is regarded as the main proximate regulator of ACTH secretion, acting via the CRH-R1 receptor.[42,43] The effects of CRH and AVP are synergistic with respect to ACTH release.[44] Both CRH and AVP have been used to stimulate ACTH release in clinical studies.

The hypophysiotropic peptides are themselves regulated by a host of neurotransmitter pathways. Research into the role and importance of these pathways in humans has relied on indirect studies of pharmacologic agents through measurement of ACTH and cortisol release. In vitro studies of hypothalamic organ systems and animal preparations have allowed further insights. Importantly, CRH secretion is stimulated by noradrenergic neurons arising in the brainstem.[45] These are themselves innervated by CRH neurons, which provide a reverberating feedback loop to link the two great effectors of the stress response (the HPA axis and the sympathetic nervous system)[46] and are under tonic inhibition by central opioid pathways.[47] Other neurotransmitter systems that stimulate the CRH neuron include acetylcholine, serotonin, and neuropeptide Y. CRH secretion and central noradrenergic nuclei are inhibited by the gamma amino butyric acid/benzodiazepine system.[48] Other neurotransmitter systems with inhibitory effects on the CRH neuron include substance P and arcuate nucleus-derived POMC.

A major regulator of ACTH release is the immune system. Cytokines—produced in inflammatory sites with a time course favoring consecutive release of TNF-α, interleukin-1, and interleukin-6 (IL-6)—are potent releasers of ACTH and cortisol. Acutely, IL-6 may act principally at the brain and hypothalamus to indirectly cause release of ACTH, although the pituitary

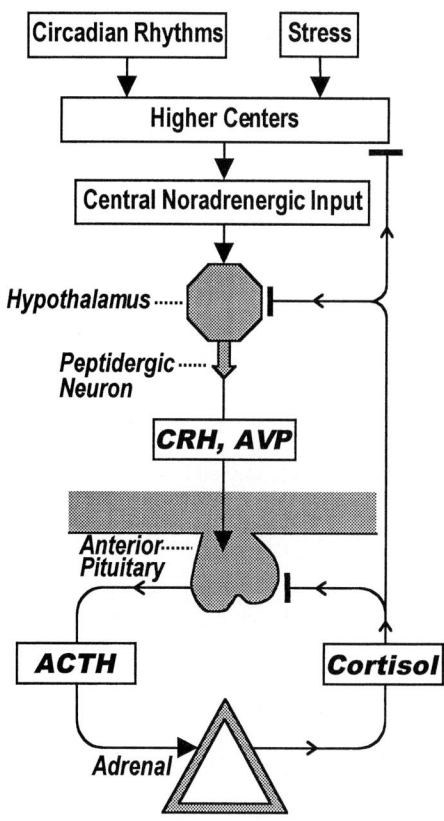

**FIGURE 14-2.** Neuroendocrine regulation of the hypothalamic–pituitary–adrenal (*HPA*) axis in humans. The circadian rhythm, stress, and feedback inhibition from circulating cortisol are the major regulators of HPA axis function. The two major secretagogues controlling adrenocorticotropin hormone (*ACTH*) release are corticotropin-releasing hormone (*CRH*) and arginine vasopressin (*AVP*). Noradrenergic input from the brainstem comprises a major stimulatory path to CRH release and links the HPA axis and the sympathetic nervous system.

and adrenal can also be stimulated directly.[49] In this regard, IL-6 in particular may be considered a hormone that is the major link between the immune system and the HPA axis. The result is a classic feedback loop between IL-6 and the HPA axis, in which cytokines stimulate the axis and cortisol suppresses the immune system and release of cytokines.[50]

## MEASUREMENT OF ADRENOCORTICOTROPIN

Traditional radioimmunoassays rely on a single-site antibody that measures both intact ACTH and abnormal ACTH, or POMC fragments, such as may be secreted from ectopic ACTH-secreting tumors. The highest correlation between the radioimmunoassay and bioassay of ACTH is found with "midportion" assays (i.e., assays using antisera that cross-react with the midportion of the ACTH molecule). These antisera bridge the sites of proteolytic cleavage of ACTH in the 15-amino acid to 18-amino acid portion, thus binding to the portion of the molecule responsible for the steroidogenic activity.[51]

Greater sensitivity and specificity have been reported for the two-site immunoradiometric assay. Two different antibodies are used, each directed to a different portion of the ACTH molecule. For ACTH to be detected in this assay, each site must be bound to its respective antibody. The detection limit is as low as 2 to 3 pg/mL of plasma, making it possible to measure ACTH without extraction, even in samples with suppressed ACTH levels. Nonetheless, these immunoradiometric assays may fail to detect aberrant large molecular mass forms of ACTH, resulting in misleadingly low levels.[52] Detection of large molecular

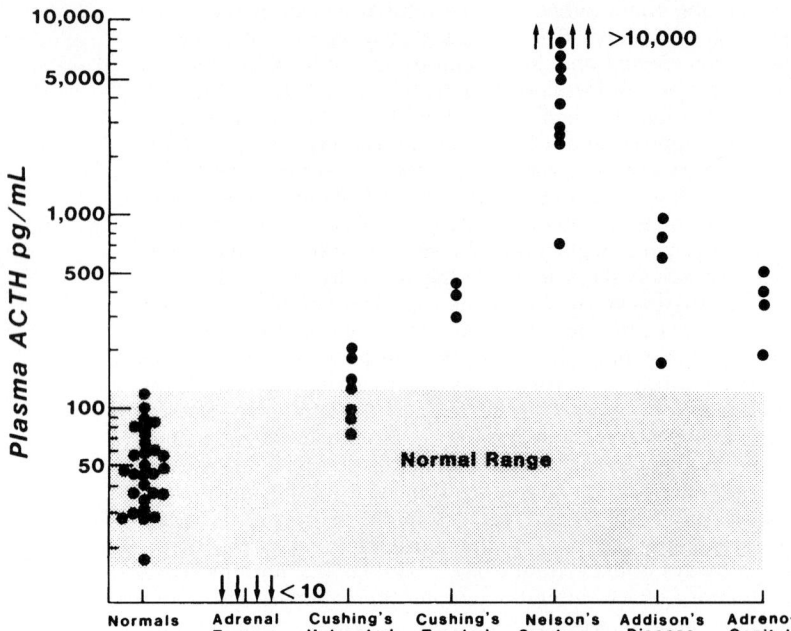

**FIGURE 14-3.** Plasma adrenocorticotropic hormone (*ACTH*) concentrations in pituitary-adrenal disorders, as determined with an assay using an N-terminal ACTH antiserum. Patients with treated Cushing disease had previous bilateral adrenalectomy, no history of pituitary irradiation, and were taking replacement doses of corticosteroids. Patients with Nelson syndrome had the classic features, except visual field defects were not present in all cases.

mass forms of ACTH is usually indicative of ectopic (extrapituitary) ACTH production.

Samples for the measurement of ACTH must be collected and immediately placed on ice for plasma separation within a short period. Plasma must be stored frozen until assay. This is necessary to prevent catabolism of ACTH by circulating peptidases. Mishandling of samples for clinical ACTH measurement leads to falsely low ACTH levels.

## BASAL PLASMA ACTH CONCENTRATIONS: CLINICAL APPLICATIONS

In many circumstances, because the levels of plasma or urinary cortisol are directly related to those of ACTH and can be measured more economically, cortisol levels can be used as an indirect index of ACTH activity. However, there are several circumstances in which the measurement of ACTH is invaluable. These include the differential diagnosis of ACTH-dependent or independent Cushing syndrome (see Chap. 75); measurement of ACTH in the inferior petrosal sinuses for definitive diagnosis of pituitary Cushing syndrome; the differential diagnosis of adrenal insufficiency; and the monitoring of Nelson syndrome. Typical plasma ACTH concentrations found in pituitary-adrenal disorders are shown in Figure 14-3. Substantial overlap exists between the ACTH values in ectopic Cushing and pituitary-dependent Cushing syndrome; hence, ACTH can not be used to differentiate these disorders, although ACTH levels >2000 pg/mL, in the setting of hypercortisolism, are virtually pathognomic of ectopic Cushing syndrome. Very high ACTH values are also seen in Nelson syndrome. Even in severe, untreated primary adrenal insufficiency, plasma ACTH rarely exceeds 2000 pg/mL. Low or undetectable plasma ACTH values occur in patients with hypopituitarism during or after exogenous corticosteroid administration and in patients with cortisol-secreting tumors (e.g., adrenal adenoma).

Measurement of plasma ACTH in samples obtained simultaneously from the inferior petrosal sinuses and peripheral plasma forms the basis of the currently most definitive test for differentiation of pituitary and ectopic sources of ACTH in ACTH-dependent Cushing syndrome. Ratios of >2:1 before CRH injection and >3:1 after CRH injection indicate pituitary Cushing syndrome.[53] The test is generally only necessary in selected cases of ACTH-dependent Cushing syndrome that have eluded diagnosis through less invasive testing.

In adrenal insufficiency, ACTH concentrations can be used to distinguish pituitary from adrenal causes. Inappropriately low or low-normal ACTH levels in the setting of adrenocortical deficiency are indicative of ACTH deficiency that is due to pituitary or hypothalamic disease. High ACTH levels in this setting are seen in primary adrenal insufficiency.

## DYNAMIC TESTING OF ADRENOCORTICOTROPIN SECRETORY FUNCTION

In states of possible autonomous ACTH hypersecretion, dexamethasone is used to inhibit ACTH secretion, and the plasma cortisol concentration or urinary cortisol excretion can be used to estimate ACTH secretory function (see Chap. 74). This technique is used in the diagnosis and differential diagnosis of Cushing syndrome and has been used to demonstrate hypercortisolism in melancholic depression.

Many stimuli have been used to stimulate ACTH secretion for clinical diagnostic purposes. Indications include Cushing syndrome and hypoadrenalism. The most frequently used test of HPA reserve is the cosyntropin stimulation test. This test is based on the rationale that if adrenal cortisol reserves are normal, the hypothalamic CRH and pituitary ACTH reserves must also be normal. Typically 250-μg ACTH (1–24) is administered intravenously and cortisol levels measured at baseline, 30 minutes, and 60 minutes. If plasma cortisol levels rise above 19 μg/dL at 30 (or 60) minutes, this is interpreted as a normal adrenal response. Peak cortisol levels of 16 μg/dL at 60 minutes occur after intramuscular cosyntropin.[54] In general, this is used to demonstrate both pituitary ACTH-secretory integrity and normal adrenal-cortisol secretory function, because adrenal atrophy develops rapidly in states of ACTH deficiency. An abnormal cosyntropin test is highly specific for adrenal insufficiency. In cases of pituitary or hypothalamic damage, in which sufficient time may not have passed to allow adrenal atrophy from ACTH deprivation, the cosyntropin test is normal.

However, glucocorticoid deficiency crises have occurred in individuals with a normal cosyntropin test, especially in patients with central hypoadrenalism (pituitary or hypothalamic causes) who may be mistakenly diagnosed as normal in as many as 40% of cases.[55] Low sensitivity of the 250-μg cosyntropin test has led to studies using a lower, more physiologic,

1-μg dose, which produces cortisol responses in normal subjects comparable to those obtained with 250-μg cosyntropin and appears more reliable in the diagnosis of central adrenal insufficiency.[56] A safe, reliable single test for assessing the functional reserve of the HPA axis[57] is still not available. Therefore, good clinical judgment is needed to select the correct test, or combination of tests, to determine whether there is an abnormality of HPA axis function.

Insulin-induced hypoglycemia involves the intravenous injection of 0.15 IU/kg insulin into a fasting subject. Hypoglycemia induces a profound and sustained hypercortisolism (cortisol >19 μg/dL). Careful medical supervision is essential, and the test is contraindicated in patients older than age 60 or in those who have had myocardial ischemia or epilepsy. This test, because of vast accumulated experience, is often regarded as the gold standard against which other tests of HPA axis reserve are compared.

The CRH test (see Chaps. 74, 75, and 76) involves the intravenous injection of CRH (1 μg/kg) with measurement of ACTH and cortisol at –1, 15, 30, 45, and 60 minutes. The test directly measures corticotrope function and offers the potential to separate pituitary from hypothalamic causes of ACTH deficiency, because pituitary lesions produce an attenuated ACTH/cortisol response to CRH.[58] Peak cortisol levels are similar to those observed in the ACTH stimulation test. Metyrapone inhibits the 11-hydroxylase enzyme, thereby inhibiting cortisol synthesis and leading to high levels of its immediate precursor, 11-deoxycortisol, which is stimulated by a lack of cortisol feedback and consequent ACTH hypersecretion (see Chap. 74). This test is used in the differential diagnosis of ACTH-dependent Cushing syndrome; patients with ectopic Cushing syndrome are less sensitive to glucocorticoid feedback, so the 11-deoxycortisol response is lower than in pituitary Cushing syndrome[59] (see Chaps. 74, 75, and 219).

## CLINICAL MANIFESTATIONS OF DISORDERS OF ADRENOCORTICOTROPIN EXCESS

Hyperpigmentation is common when ACTH levels exceed 300 pg/mL (Fig. 14-4). The highest ACTH levels are seen in Addison disease, Nelson syndrome, and ectopic ACTH secretion. Clinically, the hyperpigmentation is found particularly in areas of increased pressure (elbows, knuckles, knees) and is accentuated in areas of normal pigmentation (areolae, genitalia, palmar creases). Surfaces (such as the mucosal) that are not normally pigmented may exhibit hyperpigmentation. Scars acquired after the onset of ACTH excess also may exhibit hyperpigmentation (see Chap. 76).

Most cases of primary adrenal insufficiency are due to autoimmunity; infiltration or infection of the adrenal gland; or, rarely, X-linked adrenoleukodystrophy. Each of these may be associated with specific clinical features such as other immune disorders (type II autoimmune polyglandular syndrome), infectious manifestations, or neurologic disease, respectively.

Congenital resistance to ACTH may occur in isolated familial glucocorticoid deficiency, an autosomal recessive disorder that is due to a mutation of the ACTH receptor.[60] Affected children have hypoglycemic episodes, hyperpigmentation, and failure to thrive. Mineralocorticoid production is normal, and there is no cortisol response to exogenous ACTH. Patients with the Allgrove syndrome (ACTH resistance, achalasia, and alacrima) have ACTH resistance but lack mutations in the gene for the ACTH receptor.[61]

Nelson syndrome entails the development of an invasive ACTH-secreting macroadenoma after bilateral adrenalectomy to alleviate the hypercortisolism of pituitary ACTH-dependent Cushing syndrome.[62] Severe pigmentation occurs, and ACTH levels may be used as a tumor marker, particularly after pituitary surgery has made the identification of a pituitary tumor on magnetic resonance imaging unreliable. The development of Nelson syndrome could be prevented in children by presurgical pituitary irradiation.[63] Nelson syndrome is not a universal concomitant of bilateral adrenalectomy; an association between the development of Nelson syndrome and the presence of a glucocorticoid receptor mutation has been found.[64] Because bilateral adrenalectomy is now rarely performed in pituitary corticotropinoma cases, Nelson syndrome is correspondingly rare.

Autonomous excess secretion of ACTH produces hypercortisolism and Cushing syndrome.[65,66] The source of ACTH is generally a pituitary adenoma, although 10% to 20% of cases are due to an ectopic neuroendocrine tumor, most commonly a bronchial carcinoid. Clinical features of Cushing syndrome include centripetal obesity, muscle weakness, osteoporosis, skin thinning with bruising and striae, glucose intolerance, hirsutism, and hypertension. The presence of hyperpigmentation in the context of Cushing syndrome tends to suggest ectopic paraneoplastic ACTH production, in which the ACTH levels are often very high (see Chap. 219).

## CLINICAL MANIFESTATIONS OF ADRENOCORTICOTROPIN DEFICIENCY

A number of pituitary pathologies can lead to ACTH deficiency, including pituitary tumor, autoimmune lymphocytic hypophysitis (often postpartum), and granulomatous infiltration. Pituitary hormone deficiencies occasionally develop without apparent cause, although the most common cause in adults is a pituitary tumor, or treatment with surgery or irradiation.

ACTH deficiency is generally a late manifestation of pituitary disease, following growth hormone deficiency (poor growth in children), gonadotropin deficiency (loss of menses in women, loss of libido in men), and hypothyroidism (see Chap. 45) that is generally mild in pituitary disease but may be symptomatic with fatigue and cold intolerance.

ACTH deficiency produces hypoadrenalism. Loss of pigmentation may be apparent, particularly in children. Hypoadrenalism commonly causes fatigue and hypotension, which is often postural. Hyponatremia may be evident because glucocorticoids contribute to the maintenance of renal free water excretion; symptomatic hypoglycemia can occur. Mineralocorti-

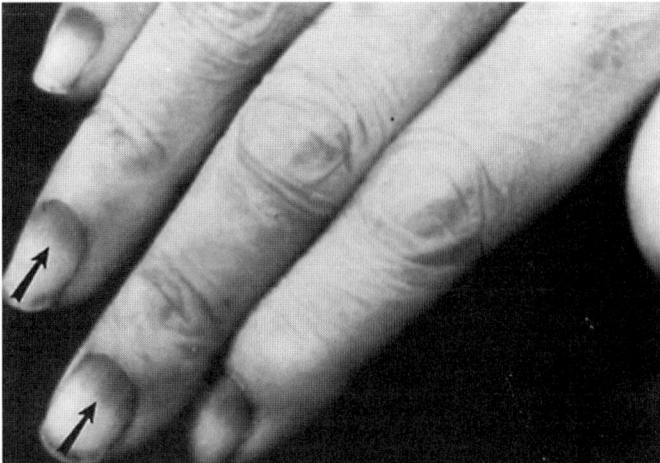

**FIGURE 14-4.** Pigmented lunulae in a patient with the paraneoplastic adrenocorticotropic hormone (*ACTH*) syndrome who developed severe hyperpigmentation of rapid onset 3 months previously. More commonly, pigmentation of the nails related to excess ACTH is longitudinal rather than transverse, as in this patient. (For other examples of hyperpigmentation related to excess ACTH, see Chaps. 76 and 219.)

coid production is regulated chiefly by angiotensin II and the potassium ion, thus mineralocorticoid deficiency does not develop in states of ACTH deficiency.

Isolated ACTH deficiency is rare, because pituitary pathologies such as tumor, radiation, or autoimmune disease typically spare the corticotropes until deficiencies of growth hormone, gonadotropins, and, finally, thyroid-stimulating hormone emerge. However, most cases of isolated ACTH deficiencies are likely to be autoimmune because of an association with other autoimmune disorders[67] or antipituitary antibodies.[68] Congenital ACTH deficiency that is due to a defect in POMC cleavage has been described.[69] Undetectable ACTH levels, normal cortisol levels, and increased cortisol secretory sensitivity to ACTH have been reported in a single patient. Two point mutations of the ACTH receptor gene were detected, suggesting the existence of an ACTH hypersensitivity syndrome.[70] Acquired isolated CRH deficiency has also been suggested, based on a lack of ACTH response to insulin hypoglycemia but a normal response to exogenous CRH.[71] The CRH stimulation test will probably not allow sufficiently accurate separation of pituitary or hypothalamic causes of ACTH deficiency[58] to be used as a gold standard test, but it may be useful along with other tests to assist clinical decision making.

A transient functional deficiency of ACTH release occurs after prolonged supraphysiologic glucocorticoid exposure, such as occurs in response to treatment with antiinflammatory doses of glucocorticoids or to correction of Cushing syndrome. Rapid restoration of ACTH release with CRH infusion suggests that the defect may be due predominantly to reduced CRH secretion.[72] This functional deficiency may last for as many as 2 years before normal HPA axis dynamics are restored, although a 6- to 9-month recovery course is often observed.[73]

# REFERENCES

1. Smith PE. Hypophysectomy and a replacement therapy in the rat. Am J Anat 1930; 45:205.
2. Collip JB, Anderson EM, Thomson DL. The adrenocorticotropic hormone of the anterior lobe. Lancet 1933; 2:347.
3. Li CH, Beschwind II, Cole RD, et al. Amino acid sequence of α corticotropin. Nature 1955; 176:687.
4. Lee TH, Lerner AB, Buettner-Janusch U. Isolation and structure of human corticotropin (ACTH). J Am Chem Soc 1959; 81:6084.
5. Eipper BA, Mains RE. Structure and biosynthesis of pro-adrenocorticotropin/endorphin and related peptides. Endocr Rev 1980; 1:1.
6. Satoh H, Mori S. Subregional assignment of the proopiomelanocortin gene (POMC) to human chromosome band 2p23.3 by fluorescence in situ hybridization. Cytogenet Cell Genet 1997; 76:221.
7. Chang AC, Cochet M, Cohen SN. Structural organization of human genomic DNA encoding the proopiomelanocortin peptide. Proc Natl Acad Sci U S A 1980; 77:4890.
8. Marcinkiewicz M, Day R, Seidah NG, Chretien M. Ontogeny of the prohormone convertases PC1 and PC2 in the mouse hypophysis and their colocalization with corticotropin and α-melanotropin. Proc Natl Acad Sci U S A 1993; 90:4922.
9. Li CH, Barafi L, Chretien M, Chung D. Isolation and structure of β-LPH from sheep pituitary glands. Nature 1965; 208:1093.
10. Comuzzie AG, Hixson JE, Almasy L, et al. A major quantitative trait locus determining serum leptin levels and fat mass is located on human chromosome 2. Nat Genet 1997; 15:273.
11. Krude H, Biebermann H, Luck W, et al. Severe early-onset obesity, adrenal insufficiency and red hair pigmentation caused by POMC mutations in humans. Nat Genet 1998; 19:155.
12. Mountjoy KG, Robbins LS, Mortrud MT, Cone RD. The cloning of a family of genes that encode the melanocortin receptors. Science 1992; 257:1248.
13. Magenis RE, Smith, L, Nadeau JH, et al. Mapping of the ACTH, MSH, and neural (MC3 and MC4) melanocortin receptors in the mouse and human. Mammalian Genome 1994; 5:503.
14. Shima S, Mitsunaga M, Nakao T, et al. Effect of ACTH on cholesterol dynamics in rat adrenal tissue. Endocrinology 1972; 98:808.
15. Brody RI, Black VH. Differential ACTH response of immunodetectable HMG CoA reductase and cytochromes P450 (17 alpha) and P450 (21) in guinea pig adrenal outer zone cell types, zona glomerulosa and zona fasciculata. Endocr Res 1991; 17:195.
16. Frohman LA. Diseases of the anterior pituitary. In: Felig P, Baxter JD, Broadu AE, Frohman LA, eds. Endocrinology and Metabolism, 2nd ed. New York: McGraw-Hill 1987:247.
17. Gallagher TF, Yoshida K, Roffwarg HD, et al. ACTH and cortisol secretory patterns in man. J Clin Endocrinol Metab 1973; 36:1058.
18. Krieger DT, Allen W. Relationship of bioassayable and immunoassayable plasma ACTH and cortisol concentration in animal subjects and in patients with Cushing's disease. J Clin Endocrinol Metab 1975; 10:675.
19. Horrocks PM, Jones AF, Ratcliffe WA, et al. Patterns of ACTH and cortisol pulsatility over twenty-four hours in normal males and females. Clin Endocrinol (Oxf) 1990; 32:127.
20. Schurmeyer TH. On the relationship between ACTH and cortisol secretion. Horm Metab Res Suppl 1987; 16:6.
21. Keller-Wood ME, Dallman MF. Corticosteroid inhibition of ACTH secretion. Endocr Rev 1984; 5:1.
22. Reincke M, Lehmann R, Karl M, et al. Severe illness. Neuroendocrinology. Ann NY Acad Sci 1995; 771:556.
23. Grice JE, Jackson RV, Hockings GI, et al. Adrenocorticotropin hyperresponse to the corticotropin-releasing hormone-mediated stimulus of naloxone in patients with myotonic dystrophy. J Clin Endocrinol Metab 1995; 80:179.
24. Crofford LJ, Engleberg NC, Demitrack MA. Neurohormonal perturbations in fibromyalgia. Baillieres Clin Rheumatol 1996; 10:365.
25. Munck A, Guyre PM, Holbrook, NJ. Physiological functions of glucocorticoids in stress and their relation to pharmacological actions. Endocr Rev 1984; 5:25.
26. Sack RL, Lewy AJ, Blood ML, et al. Circadian rhythm abnormalities in totally blind people: incidence and clinical significance. J Clin Endocrinol Metab 1992; 75:127.
27. Krieger DT. Rhythms of ACTH and corticosteroid secretion in health and disease and their experimental modification. J Steroid Biochem 1975; 6:785.
27a. Luboshitzky R. Endocrine activity during sleep. J Pediatr Endocrinol Metab 2000; 13:13.
28. Banky Z, Molnar J, Csernus V, Halasz B. Further studies on circadian rhythms after local pharmacological destruction of the serotoninergic innervation of the rat suprachiasmatic region before the onset of the corticosterone rhythm. Brain Res 1988; 445:222.
29. Desir D, Van Cauter E, Fang VS, et al. Effects of "jetlag" on hormonal patterns. I. Procedures, variations in total plasma proteins, and disruption of adrenocorticotropin cortisol periodicity. J Clin Endocrinol Metab 1981; 52:628.
30. Levin N, Shinsako J, Dallman M. Corticosterone acts on the brain to inhibit adrenalectomy-induced adrenocorticotropin secretion. Endocrinology 1988; 122:694.
31. Reul JHM, de Kloet ER. Two receptor systems for corticosterone in rat brain: microdistribution and differential occupation. Endocrinology 1985; 117:2505.
32. Ratka A, Sutanta W, Bloemers M, de Kloet ER. On the role of brain mineralocorticoid (Type I) and glucocorticoid (Type II) receptors in neuroendocrine regulation. Neuroendocrinology 1989; 50:117.
33. Dallman MF, Akana SF, Levin N, et al. Corticosteroids and the control of function in the hypothalamo–pituitary–adrenal (HPA) axis. Ann NY Acad Sci 1994; 746:22.
34. Magiakou MA, Mastorakos G, Rabin D, et al. Hypothalamic corticotropin-releasing hormone suppression during the postpartum period: implications for the increase in psychiatric manifestations at this time. J Clin Endocrinol Metab 1996; 81:1912.
35. Zhang Y, Proneca R, Maffei M, et al. Positional cloning of the mouse obese gene and its human homologue. Nature 1994; 372:425.
36. Licinio J, Mantzoros C, Negrao AB, et al. Human leptin levels are pulsatile and inversely related to pituitary-adrenal function. Nat Med 1997; 3:575.
37. Heiman ML, Ahima RS, Craft LS, et al. Leptin inhibition of the hypothalamic–pituitary–adrenal axis in response to stress. Endocrinology 1997; 138:3859.
38. Bornstein SR, Uhlmann K, Haidan A, et al. Evidence for a novel peripheral action of leptin as a metabolic signal to the adrenal gland: leptin inhibits cortisol release directly. Diabetes 1997; 46:1235.
39. Flier JS. Clinical review 94: What's in a name? In search of leptin's physiologic role. J Clin Endocrinol Metab 1998; 83:1407.
40. Orth DN, Jackson RV, DeCherney GS, et al. Effect of synthetic ovine corticotropin releasing factor: dose response of plasma ACTH and cortisol. J Clin Invest 1983; 71:587.
41. Vale W, Spiess J, Rivier C, Rivier J. Characterization of a 41-residue ovine hypothalamic peptide that stimulates secretion of corticotropin and β-endorphin. Science 1981; 213:1394.
42. Castro MG, Morrison E, Perone MJ, et al. Corticotrophin-releasing hormone receptor type 1: generation and characterization of polyclonal anti-peptide antibodies and their localization in pituitary cells and cortical neurones in vitro. J Neuroendocrinol 1996; 8:521.
43. Webster EL, Lewis DB, Torpy DJ, et al. In vivo and in vitro characterization of antalarmin, a nonpeptide corticotropin-releasing hormone (CRH) receptor antagonist: suppression of pituitary ACTH release and peripheral inflammation. Endocrinology 1996; 137:5747.
44. DeBold CR, Sheldon WR, DeCherney GS, et al. Arginine vasopressin potentiates adrenocorticotropin release induced by ovine corticotropin-releasing factor. J Clin Invest 1984; 73:533.
45. Al-Damluji S, Perry L, Tolin S, et al. Alpha-adrenergic stimulation of corticotropin secretion by a specific central mechanism in man. Neuroendocrinology 1987; 45:68.
46. Chrousos GP, Gold PW. The concepts of stress and stress system disorders. Overview of physical and behavioral homeostasis. JAMA 1992; 267:1244.
47. Jackson RV, Grice JE, Hockings GI, Torpy DJ. Naloxone-induced ACTH release: mechanism of action in humans. Clin Endocrinol (Oxf) 1995; 43:423.

48. Torpy DJ, Grice JE, Hockings GI, et al. Alprazolam blocks the naloxone-stimulated hypothalamo–pituitary–adrenal axis in man. J Clin Endocrinol Metab 1993; 76:388.
49. Papanicolaou DA, Wilder RL, Manolagas SC, Chrousos GP. The pathophysiologic roles of interleukin-6 in human disease. Ann Intern Med 1998; 128:127.
50. Chrousos GP. The hypothalamic–pituitary–adrenal axis and immune-mediated inflammation. N Engl J Med 1995; 332:1351.
51. Nicholson WE, Davis DR, Sherrell BJ, Orth DN. Rapid radioimmunoassay for corticotropin in unextracted human plasma. Clin Chem 1984; 30:259.
52. Findling JW, Engeland WC, Raff H. The use of immunoradiometric assay for the measurement of ACTH in human plasma. Trends Endocrinol Metab 1990; 1:283.
53. Oldfield EH, Doppman JL, Nieman LK, et al. Petrosal sinus sampling with and without corticotropin releasing hormone for the differential diagnosis of Cushing's syndrome. N Engl J Med 1991; 325:897.
54. Longui CA, Vottero A, Harris AG, Chrousos GP. Plasma cortisol responses after intramuscular corticotropin 1-24 in healthy men. Metabolism 1998; 47:1419.
55. Hockings GI, Strakosch CR, Jackson RV. Secondary adrenocortical deficiency: avoiding potentially fatal pitfalls in diagnosis and treatment. Med J Aust 1997; 166:400.
56. Thaler LM, Blevins L Jr. The low dose (1 μg) adrenocorticotropin stimulation test in the evaluation of patients with suspected central adrenal insufficiency. J Clin Endocrinol Metab 1998; 83:2726.
57. Streeten DH, Anderson GH Jr, Bonaventura MM. The potential for serious consequences from misinterpreting normal responses to the rapid adrenocorticotropin test. J Clin Endocrinol Metab 1996; 81:285.
58. Schulte HM, Chrousos GP, Avgerinos P, et al. The corticotropin releasing hormone test: a possible aid in the evaluation of patients with adrenal insufficiency. J Clin Endocrinol Metab 1984; 58:1064.
59. Avgerinos PC, Nieman LK, Oldfield EH, Cutler GB Jr. A comparison of the overnight and the standard metyrapone test for the differential diagnosis of adrenocorticotrophin-dependent Cushing's syndrome. Clin Endocrinol (Oxf) 1996; 45:483.
60. Weber A, Topperi J, Harvey RD, et al. Adrenocorticotropin receptor gene mutations in familial glucocorticoid deficiency: relationships with clinical features in four families. J Clin Endocrinol Metab 1995; 80:65.
61. Heinrichs C, Tsigos C, Deschepper J, et al. Familial adrenocorticotropin unresponsiveness associated with alacrima and achalasia: biochemical and molecular studies in two siblings with clinical heterogeneity. Eur J Pediatr 1995; 154:191.
62. Negesser SK, van Seters AP, Kievit J, et al. Long-term results of total adrenalectomy for Cushing's disease. World J Surg 2000; 24:108.
63. Jennings AS, Liddle GW, Orth DN. Results of treating childhood Cushing's disease with pituitary irradiation. N Engl J Med 1977; 297:957.
64. Karl M, von Wichert G, Kempter E, et al. Nelson's syndrome associated with a somatic frame mutation in the glucocorticoid receptor gene. J Clin Endocrinol Metab 1996; 81:124.
65. Newell-Price J, Trainer P, Besser M, Grossman A. The diagnosis and differential diagnosis of Cushing's syndrome and pseudo-Cushing's states. Endocr Rev 1998; 19:647.
66. Orth DN. Cushing's syndrome. N Engl J Med 1995; 332:791.
67. Shigemasa C, Kouchi T, Veta Y, et al. Evaluation of thyroid function in patients with isolated ACTH deficiency. Am J Med Sci 1992; 304:279.
68. Sugiura M, Hashimoto A, Shizawa M, et al. Heterogeneity of anterior pituitary cell antibodies detected in insulin dependent diabetes mellitus and ACTH deficiency. Diabetes Res 1980; 3:11.
69. Nussey SS, Soo SC, Gibson S, et al. Isolated congenital ACTH deficiency. A cleavage enzyme defect? Clin Endocrinol (Oxf) 1993; 39:381.
70. Hiroi N, Yakushiji F, Shimojo M, et al. Human ACTH hypersensitivity syndrome associated with abnormalities of the ACTH receptor gene. Clin Endocrinol (Oxf) 1998; 48:129.
71. Nishihara E, Kimura H, Ishimaru T, et al. A case of adrenal insufficiency due to acquired hypothalamic CRH deficiency. Endocr J 1997; 44:121.
72. Gomez MT, Magiakou MA, Mastorakos G, Chrousos GP. The pituitary corticotroph is not the rate limiting step in the postoperative recovery of the hypothalamic–pituitary–adrenal axis in patients with Cushing syndrome. J Clin Endocrinol Metab 1993; 77:173.
73. Graber RL, Ney RL, Nicholson WE, et al. Natural history of pituitary-adrenal recovery following long-term suppression with corticosteroids. J Clin Endocrinol Metab 1965; 25:11.

# CHAPTER 15

# THYROID-STIMULATING HORMONE AND ITS DISORDERS

JOSHUA L. COHEN

## THYROID-STIMULATING HORMONE STRUCTURE, BIOSYNTHESIS, AND FUNCTION

### GLYCOPROTEIN HORMONE STRUCTURE

Thyroid-stimulating hormone (TSH, thyrotropin) is one of a family of glycoprotein hormones that also includes follicle-stimulating hormone (FSH), luteinizing hormone (LH), and human chorionic gonadotropin (hCG, Table 15-1). These hormones each consist of two dissimilar subunits, α and β, held together by strong noncovalent bonds.[1] Each subunit consists of a polypeptide core that is stabilized by internal disulfide bonds and glycosylated at specific residues. The α subunits of all the glycoprotein hormones are identical and are highly conserved among different species. The β subunits of different hormones have extensive sequence homologies.

The glycoprotein hormones bind to membrane receptors in their target tissues. Hormonal specificities are determined by the respective β subunits. However, hCG and LH have weak intrinsic TSH bioactivity. The isolated α and β subunits are not bioactive. However, both α-TSH and β-TSH subunits contain receptor-binding domains. Modifications of amino-acid residues or of the carbohydrate side chains can result in TSH analogs with enhanced bioactivity or altered metabolic clearance.[2]

TSH has a molecular mass of ~28 kDa. It is glycosylated at two sites on the α subunit and at one site on the β subunit. Glycosylation is required for subunit association, intracellular processing of the precursors to the secretory form of the hormone, and metabolic clearance of secreted hormone. Chemically deglycosylated TSH binds to its receptor but does not elicit a biologic response, suggesting that the glycosyl residues may have a role in receptor activation.[3]

The x-ray crystallographic structure of hCG is known,[4] and a homologous structure for TSH has been proposed.[5] The α and β subunits of the glycoprotein hormones share a common structural motif consisting of a central "cystine knot" formed by disulfide bonds, with two hairpin loops on one side of the knot and a single loop on the other. This cystine knot structure is found in growth factors and hormones, including platelet-derived growth factor, nerve growth factor, inhibins, and others.[5] Another structural element presumed common to hCG, TSH, and the other glycoprotein hormones is a "seat-belt" region near the carboxyl terminus of the β subunit that wraps around the α subunit to maintain the heterodimeric structure.

### BIOSYNTHESIS OF THYROID-STIMULATING HORMONE

Separate genes encode the α-TSH and β-TSH subunits.[6] The human α gene is present in a single copy on chromosome 6 and is transcribed in all pituitary and placental cells synthesizing glycoprotein hormones. The human β-TSH gene is on chromosome 1. Hence, regulation of TSH gene transcription requires control of separate DNA regulatory elements for each subunit gene. Although all of the β subunits probably evolved from a common ancestor, β subunit genes are on separate chromosomes and do not form a single linkage group (see Table 15-1).

**TABLE 15-1.**
**Characteristics of Human Glycoprotein Hormones**

| Hormone | Subunit Structure | Molecular Mass (daltons) | Carbohydrate | β-Subunit Amino Acids | Number of β-Subunit Oligosaccharide Chains | β-Subunit Gene, Chromosome Number |
|---|---|---|---|---|---|---|
| Thyroid-stimulating hormone (TSH) | α-, β-TSH | 28,000 | 16% | 112 | 1 | 1 |
| Follicle-stimulating hormone (FSH) | α-, β-FSH | 29,000 | 32% | 118 | 2 | 11 |
| Luteinizing hormone (LH) | α-, β-LH | 29,000 | 16% | 112 | 1 | 19 |
| Human chorionic gonadotropin (hCG) | α-, β-hCG | 46,000 | 31% | 145 | 6 | 19 |

The α-TSH and β-TSH apoprotein cores are transcribed as prehormones, starting with leader sequences of hydrophobic amino acids that direct the nascent chains through the rough endoplasmic reticulum membrane (see Chap. 3). Pituitary glands contain excess α subunit relative to their β subunit content, and free subunits as well as intact hormone are secreted by the thyrotrope. Free α subunit generally can be detected in serum from euthyroid persons. It is increased in persons with primary hypothyroidism; free β-TSH also can be detected. Free α subunit (secreted by gonadotropes) also is increased in postmenopausal women. Free α subunit contains an additional oligosaccharide group that prevents it from combining with β-TSH.[5]

*Thyrotropin-releasing hormone* (TRH) stimulates α-TSH and β-TSH subunit gene transcription by inducing or activating specific transcriptional regulatory factors.[7,8] Triiodothyronine ($T_3$) causes a rapid fall in transcription of the α-TSH and β-TSH genes.[9] The synthesis of β-TSH appears to be the rate-limiting step and a major regulatory point in the control of TSH. Regulatory regions involved in $T_3$ suppression of subunit gene transcription (*negative $T_3$ response elements, TREs*) have been identified for both the α-TSH and β-TSH genes.[6] These negative TREs contain nucleotide sequences for interaction with the β receptor.[10]

Glycosylation of the subunits begins cotranslationally, with the transfer of preassembled oligosaccharides to specific asparagine residues.[3] Initial core glycosylation is required for the polypeptide chains to assume their tertiary structures and associate into heterodimers of α-TSH and β-TSH. Glycosylation of TSH also is under hormonal control by TRH and thyroid hormone.[3] TSH from patients with severe primary hypothyroidism and TSH released acutely by TRH stimulation differ in glycosylation compared to basal TSH.[11] TSH extracted from sera of patients with nonthyroid illnesses also has alterations in glycosylation. Because alterations in glycosylation affect its biologic properties, control of TSH glycosylation may be of physiologic significance.

### THYROID-STIMULATING HORMONE RECEPTOR

The TSH receptor is a member of the superfamily of *guanine nucleotide regulatory protein (G protein)–coupled receptors*.[12,13] Binding of TSH stimulates receptor interaction with the α subunit of the $G_s$ protein. This leads to the release of guanosine diphosphate (GDP) from the α subunit and its replacement with guanosine triphosphate (GTP) as well as dissociation of the G protein into α and βγ subunits that stimulate adenylate cyclase, increasing intracellular cyclic adenosine monophosphate (cAMP) and activating protein kinase A. At higher TSH concentrations, the receptor may interact with other G proteins, leading to modulation of other intracellular signaling pathways such as the $Ca^{2+}$, phosphatidylinositol phosphate, protein kinase C cascade.[14]

The TSH receptor gene was cloned by probing thyroid complementary DNA (cDNA) libraries with oligonucleotide probes complementary to cDNA sequences coding for segments of the LH/hCG and FSH hormone receptors thought likely to be conserved in the TSH receptor.[15] The TSH receptor gene, located on chromosome 14, contains 10 exons coding for a 764-amino-acid polypeptide (including a 21-amino-acid leader sequence). The apoprotein core of the TSH receptor has a molecular mass of 84.5 kDa.[16] Functional recombinant receptor has been expressed in stably trans-

fected Chinese hamster ovary cells and has been used for bioassay of TSH and of thyroid-stimulating immunoglobulin (TSI) activity.

The TSH receptor and other G protein–coupled receptors contain three major structural and functional domains (Fig. 15-1). The extracellular region is the site of receptor-ligand interaction and also is involved in signal transduction. The membrane-spanning region contains seven hydrophobic transmembrane segments joined by short extracellular and cytoplasmic connecting loops. The transmembrane segments and connecting loops interact with the G-protein α subunit. The cytoplasmic tail contains phosphorylation sites that may be targets for protein kinases to regulate receptor activity. Binding of TSH to the extracellular domain results in a conformational change that alters the interaction of the membrane-spanning domain with the $G_s\alpha$ subunit, leading to activation of the GDP/GTP cycle.

The extracellular region of the TSH receptor contains 398 amino acids, including six potential glycosylation sites. A major structural feature of the extracellular domain of the glycoprotein receptors is the presence of "leucine-rich repeats" (LRRs). Proteins containing LRRs generally have functions involving interaction with polypeptide ligands.[17] Based on the crystallographic structure of ribonuclease inhibitor, an LRR-containing protein, a model of the extracellular domain of the TSH receptor has been proposed.[18] The LRRs form a concave surface in the extracellular domain that can provide an extensive area for interaction with the hormone. This model is compatible with studies that have identified multiple regions in the TSH α and β subunits involved in hormone binding.

### BIOLOGIC ACTIONS OF THYROID-STIMULATING HORMONE

Within the thyroid, TSH stimulates virtually all metabolic and cellular processes involved in the synthesis and secretion of thyroid hormones, including iodine uptake and organification, thyroglobulin synthesis, iodotyrosine coupling, colloid droplet formation, and iodothyronine secretion.[19] TSH also stimulates intermediary metabolism as well as protein and nucleic acid synthesis and thyroid growth. Clinically observable effects of TSH on the normal thyroid gland include thyroid gland enlargement, increased radioactive iodine uptake, and increased secretion of thyroxine ($T_4$) and $T_3$.

### CONTROL OF THYROID-STIMULATING HORMONE SECRETION: NEURAL AND HUMORAL MODULATORS

#### NEURAL CONTROL OF THYROID-STIMULATING HORMONE SECRETION

The thyrotrope secretes TSH in response to humoral signals (Fig. 15-2). The hypothalamic neurohormones TRH, somatostatin, and dopamine are released under control of the central nervous system. Thyroid hormones feed back to suppress TSH release. Other hormones, including corticosteroids and cytokines, also can modulate TSH secretion.

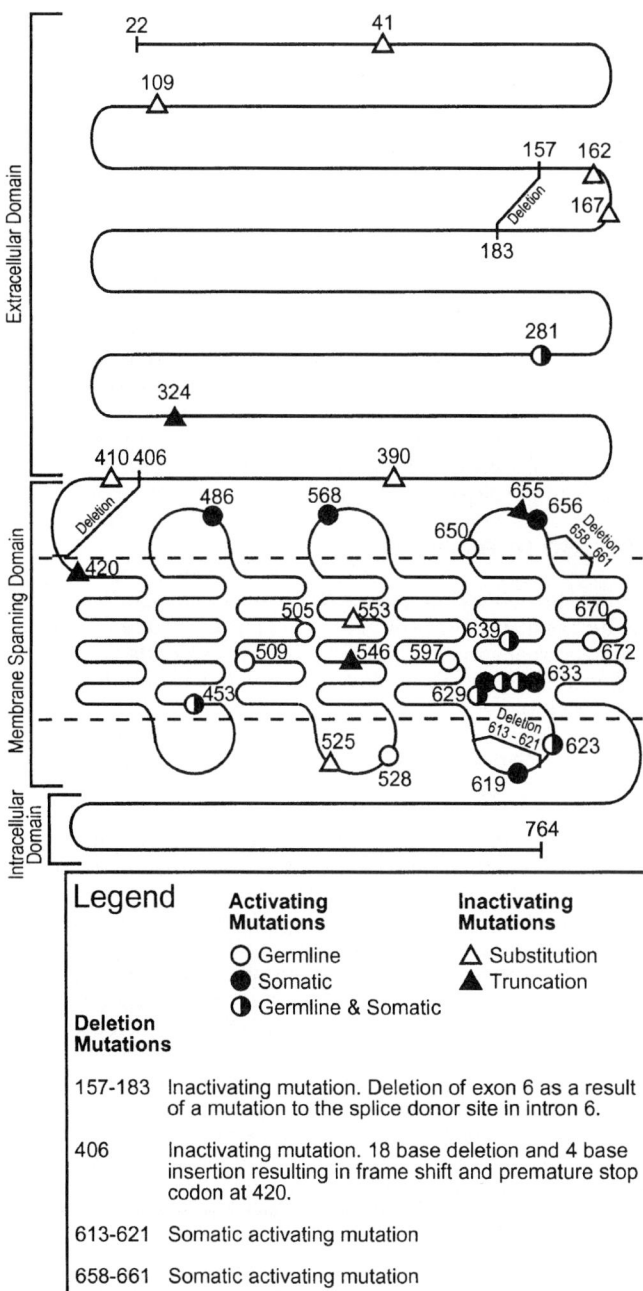

FIGURE 15-1. Schematic illustration of the human thyrotropin receptor with the sites of mutations resulting in constitutive activation or loss of function.[82–100] The initial 21 amino acids form the leader sequence and are cleaved during intracellular processing of the receptor. Germline activating mutations have been found in families with hereditary thyrotoxicosis and in neonates with nonautoimmune thyrotoxicosis. Somatic activating mutations have been found in solitary toxic nodules and toxic multinodular glands. (A database of thyroid-stimulating hormone receptor mutations is accessible through the internet at http://www.uni-leipzig.de/innere/TSH.)

Physiologic alterations in TSH secretion in response to factors such as circadian rhythm, cold exposure (in neonates and lower animals), and stress are controlled by the central nervous system through pathways that project to hypothalamic nuclei to modulate hypothalamic releasing hormone secretion. Numerous neurotransmitters, including biogenic amines, amino acids, endogenous opioids, and neuropeptides, have been found to modulate TSH secretion in animals.[20,21] For example, in rats, the TSH response to cold exposure appears to be mediated by α-adrenergic pathways.

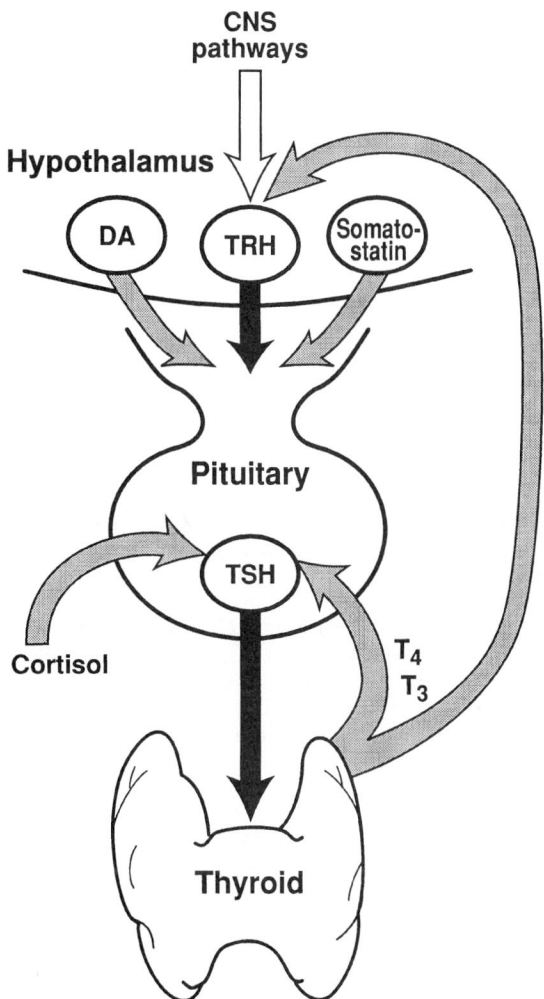

FIGURE 15-2. Interactions of the major humoral mediators of thyroid-stimulating hormone (*TSH*) secretion. Solid arrows denote stimulatory effect; shaded arrows denote inhibitory effect. (*DA*, dopamine; *TRH*, thyrotropin-releasing hormone; $T_4$, thyroxine; $T_3$, triiodothyronine.)

## THYROTROPIN-RELEASING HORMONE

TRH, a tripeptide (pyroglutamyl-histidyl-proline amide), was one of the first hypothalamic releasing hormones to be isolated and characterized (Fig. 15-3). The mammalian TRH prohormone contains multiple copies of the sequence Gln-His-Pro-Gly, suggesting that several TRH molecules could be derived from each precursor.[22] The highest density of TRH-containing cells in the central nervous system is found in the hypothalamic paraventricular nucleus.[23] TRH also is distributed extensively in the extrahypothalamic brain and in nonneuronal tissue, including the heart and testis.[24] High-affinity TRH receptors are widely distributed; many behavioral, pharmacologic, and neurophysiologic effects have been reported after TRH administration. Hence, TRH may function as a neurotransmitter.[21] However, probably only TRH released into the hypothalamic-pituitary portal circulation is involved in control of TSH secretion. Transcription of TRH is also under negative feedback regulation by $T_3$. TREs have been identified in the regulatory region of the TRH gene.[24]

The binding of TRH to its G-protein–coupled receptor on the thyrotrope stimulates hydrolysis of the membrane lipid phosphatidylinositol 4,5-bisphosphate to yield inositol 1,4,5-triphosphate and diacylglycerol[25]; each of these may function as an intracellular second messenger (see Chap. 4). Inositol triphosphate stimulates the mobilization of calcium from intracellular stores. Free calcium is bound rapidly by the calcium-binding protein calmodulin. The resulting complex activates kinases that phosphor-

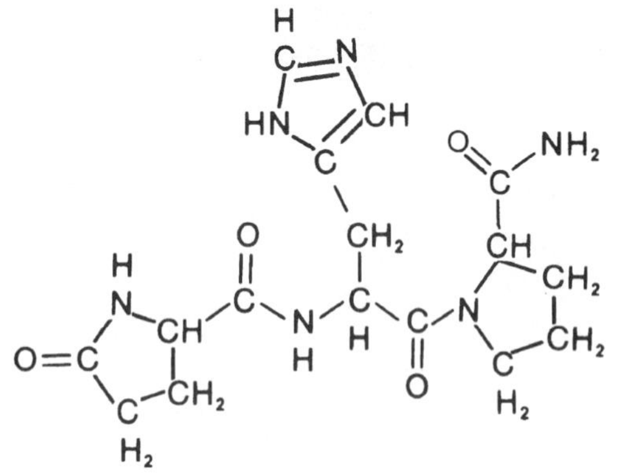

$$(pyro)Glu \quad - \quad His \quad - \quad Pro(NH_2)$$

**FIGURE 15-3.** Chemical structure of thyrotropin-releasing hormone (*TRH*). TRH is the smallest identified hypophysiotropic hormone. Cyclization of the glutamate and amidation of the proline are required for full bioactivity.

ylate proteins involved in the exocytosis of secretory granules. Diacylglycerol activates protein kinase C, leading to phosphorylation of other proteins that also may be needed for TSH secretion. TRH also stimulates adenylate cyclase in the pituitary.

Experimental evidence for the role of TRH in the control of TSH includes the observation that hypothalamic lesions that reduce TRH content cause a decrease in TSH secretion and hypothyroidism. In addition, the administration of anti-TRH antiserum to neutralize endogenous TRH causes a decrease in basal and cold-stimulated TSH levels in normal and hypothyroid rats.[21]

TRH administration also stimulates prolactin release. The physiologic role of TRH in the normal control of prolactin secretion is unclear, however (see Chap. 13). Prolactin, but not TSH, is elevated in nursing women. The administration of anti-TRH antibody does not block the physiologic prolactin rise during pregnancy or suckling. Hyperprolactinemia and galactorrhea have been observed in primary hypothyroidism.

Normally, TRH does not stimulate the secretion of other pituitary hormones. However, growth hormone release is stimulated by TRH administration in many patients with acromegaly and in some patients with renal failure, liver disease, anorexia nervosa, and depression. TRH stimulates the release of adrenocorticotropin in some patients with Cushing disease or Nelson syndrome, and the release of intact gonadotropin, α subunit, or free β subunit in patients with pituitary adenoma of gonadotrope origin.[26]

## THYROID HORMONES

Serum TSH levels are extremely sensitive to changes in circulating thyroid hormone concentrations. The administration of small doses of $T_4$ or $T_3$ to euthyroid persons suppresses basal TSH levels and blunts the TSH response to TRH. Conversely, the administration of iodide, which slightly decreases thyroid secretion of $T_4$ and $T_3$, causes increased basal TSH concentrations and enhanced TSH responses to TRH.[27] An inverse log-linear relationship is seen between changes in TSH and alterations in free $T_4$ or free $T_3$ levels.[28]

Thyroid hormone suppression of TSH secretion is initiated by $T_3$ binding to a nuclear receptor. $T_4$-induced suppression of TSH is mediated by its intrapituitary deiodination to $T_3$.[29] Monodeiodinase activity is high in the pituitary, and 50% to 60% of intrapituitary $T_3$ comes from local conversion of $T_4$ to $T_3$. Hence, the serum TSH concentration may be more dependent on serum $T_4$ than on serum $T_3$.

In addition to inhibiting TSH biosynthesis, $T_3$ administration also reduces the number of TRH receptors on thyrotropes and might thereby reduce their sensitivity to TRH.[30]

## DOPAMINE AND SOMATOSTATIN

The administration of dopamine, L-dopa, or bromocriptine to normal or hypothyroid individuals decreases their basal TSH concentrations and maximum TSH responses to TRH.[21] In addition, the dopamine-receptor blocking agents, metoclopramide and domperidone, increase TSH concentrations in both euthyroid and hypothyroid persons, a finding that supports a physiologic role for endogenous dopamine secretion in suppressing TSH release. Because neither dopamine nor domperidone crosses the blood–brain barrier, the effects of dopamine most likely are mediated directly at the thyrotrope.

Somatostatin may be a physiologic inhibitor of TSH secretion. The infusion of somatostatin lowers TSH levels in hypothyroid patients and suppresses the normal nocturnal rise in TSH.[21] In addition, the release of somatostatin from the hypothalamus is stimulated by $T_3$.[31] Finally, the administration of anti-somatostatin antiserum to rats causes an increase in basal serum TSH levels, and in cold- or TRH-stimulated TSH release.

## STEROID HORMONES

Steroid hormones modulate TSH secretion. Corticosteroids inhibit basal and TRH-stimulated TSH levels and block the normal nocturnal surge in TSH. The effects of steroids on pituitary responsiveness to TRH may be mediated by modulation of TRH receptors on thyrotropes.

## INTEGRATED CONTROL OF THYROID-STIMULATING HORMONE SECRETION

The secretion of TSH is controlled by the integrated thyrotrope response to humoral signals. The inhibitory effect of thyroid hormones on TSH secretion results in a closed-loop negative-feedback control system for the tight regulation of the concentration of thyroid hormone, which is sensed by the thyrotrope. A deviation of the thyroid hormone concentration from the setpoint of the control system alters TSH release, thereby causing a change in the secretion of thyroid hormones that returns their concentrations toward the setpoint. The setpoint of this "thyrostat" is established by stimulatory and inhibitory hypothalamic releasing hormones (TRH, somatostatin, dopamine) and other mediators that determine the sensitivity of the thyrotrope to inhibition by $T_3$. Thus, differences in thyroid hormone levels among individuals, or differences in responsiveness to environmental or physiologic conditions, reflect differences in the thyrotrope setpoints.

Support for this model is provided by the observation that hypothalamic lesions to thyroidectomized rats blunt the expected increase in TSH and enhance the suppressive effects of low doses of thyroid hormones. Chronic intrathecal infusion of TRH in patients with amyotrophic lateral sclerosis produces a sustained rise in serum thyroid hormone and TSH levels, suggesting that the infusion raises the pituitary setpoint.[32] In children with hypothyroidism resulting from idiopathic TRH deficiency, TSH release is more sensitive to inhibition by $T_4$, suggesting that thyrotrope sensitivity to thyroid hormone suppression is increased in the absence of TRH.[33]

## CONTROL OF THYROID-STIMULATING HORMONE SECRETION: PHYSIOLOGIC MODULATION

### EFFECTS OF AGE AND SEX

TSH is first detectable in fetal serum at ~13 weeks' gestational age, approximately the same time as the onset of fetal thyroid iodine uptake. The TSH level remains low until the 18th to 20th week of gestation, when it rises abruptly. At birth, the serum TSH concentration is ~10 µU/mL. It then rises rapidly, reaching levels of 75 to 150 µU/mL by 30 minutes after birth.[34] Levels then decline and are within the usual childhood range by 2 to 3 days after birth. The serum TSH concentration declines slightly during childhood and adolescence.[35]

The mean TSH concentration in euthyroid adults is 1.4 to 2.0 µU/mL. Levels do not differ significantly between men and women. Serum TSH levels do not change between adolescence and the age of 60 years. A study of the 24-hour profile of TSH secretion using a sensitive TSH assay found that mean TSH levels were decreased in healthy older men compared to younger control subjects.[36] The normal diurnal rhythm was preserved (see Chap. 199).

## DAILY RHYTHM

TSH levels rise to a peak between midnight and the early morning hours; a nadir in TSH concentration occurs in late afternoon.[21] TSH secretion is pulsatile, most likely in response to pulsatile release of TRH.[37] Six to 10 major pulses per 24 hours are noted. The nocturnal rise in TSH levels is associated with increased TSH pulse amplitude. Alterations in dopaminergic and somatostatinergic tone may modulate the TSH pulse size.

## EFFECTS OF STRESS

The serum TSH concentration is transiently depressed after stressful medical procedures such as treadmill exercise or gastroscopy, and for 1 to 2 days after elective surgery. These transient decreases may result from the inhibitory effects of increased serum cortisol.

Although exposure to cold is an important stimulus for TSH release in some animals, temperature effects in humans are more limited. Exposure of neonates 3 hours after birth to a decreased ambient temperature causes an increase in serum TSH levels compared to those in age-matched control subjects.[34] Elevated serum TSH levels also are noted during hypothermic cardiac surgery in infants.[38] In adults, small and inconsistent effects on serum TSH values have been reported as a result of acute or chronic cold exposure.[21]

## EFFECTS OF FASTING AND SEVERE ILLNESS

Fasting is associated with decreased 5'-monodeiodinase activity, which causes a fall in extrathyroidal conversion of $T_4$ to $T_3$ and an increase in reverse $T_3$ (see Chap. 36). Because similar changes have been observed in patients with numerous acute or chronic illnesses, fasting has been used as a model for the effects of illness on thyroid function. Despite the low $T_3$ concentration, basal TSH levels are either unchanged or decreased, and the TSH response to TRH generally is impaired. Thyrotrope responsiveness to thyroid hormones is intact because the administration of $T_3$ during a fast results in further suppression of TSH, whereas the administration of iodide (to reduce circulating thyroid hormone concentrations) restores normal TSH responsiveness to TRH.[39]

Basal TSH levels generally have been reported to be normal in euthyroid persons during mild or moderate illness. However, the pituitary-hypothalamic regulation of TSH may be impaired in some severely ill patients. In a study of patients who became severely ill while undergoing bone marrow transplantation, serum TSH decreased to subnormal or undetectable levels in most patients in whom serum $T_4$ values declined.[40] The decrease in TSH generally preceded the decline in $T_4$. With recovery, serum $T_4$ and TSH levels returned to normal.

These findings suggest that the setpoint of circulating thyroid hormone is decreased during fasting and severe illness. This could be the result of altered secretion of hypothalamic-releasing hormones, such as TRH or somatostatin. The post-

mortem hypothalamic content of TRH mRNA, measured by in situ hybridization, has been reported to be reduced in severely ill individuals.[23] Infusion of the cytokines interleukin-1 (IL-1) or tumor necrosis factor-α in rats alters TSH levels and thyroid cell function.[41] Also, administration of IL-1β to rats causes a decrease in the hypothalamic content of TRH mRNA.[42] These immunomodulators may play a role in the hypothalamic and pituitary responses to stress and illness. During recovery from severe illness, TSH levels may be transiently elevated.[43]

## CLINICAL APPLICATIONS OF THYROID-STIMULATING HORMONE MEASUREMENT

### THYROID-STIMULATING HORMONE ASSAY

The radioimmunoassays initially used for routine clinical measurement of TSH have been replaced by more sensitive two-site noncompetitive immunometric assays (IMAs). These assays use two antibodies with specificity toward separate epitopes on TSH. One antibody is attached to a solid-phase support and the other antibody is labeled. Enzymes, luminescent or fluorescent compounds, and iodine-125 have been used as antibody labels.[28,44] Luminescent labels now are used most commonly. Binding of the two antibodies to TSH results in the formation of a labeled "sandwich" that is separated from the noncomplexed reagents and measured. IMAs are specific for the measurement of TSH and generally free from interference. Rarely, falsely elevated serum TSH levels have been reported because of the presence in serum of heterophilic antibodies that neutralize the reagent anti-TSH antibody.[45]

With the introduction of the IMAs, a confusing nomenclature has developed based on the claimed sensitivity (e.g., "highly sensitive," "ultrasensitive," "supersensitive"). The American Thyroid Association has proposed that assays should be characterized by a functional criterion and that a TSH assay should be designated as "sensitive" only if sera from thyrotoxic persons yield results >3 log standard deviations below the mean of normal euthyroid persons.[46] More than 95% of sera from thyrotoxic persons would be expected to have TSH levels below the lower limit of normal in an assay meeting this criterion. Most commercial IMAs appear capable of meeting that standard.[47]

Clinical chemists have traditionally reported as the *analytic sensitivity* or detection limit of an assay the lowest TSH level statistically distinguishable from zero concentration by measurement of replicate samples in the same assay run. Such a definition of sensitivity may be clinically misleading, because a single measurement of a specimen containing TSH at the analytic threshold concentration would yield a result of zero 50% of the time. Furthermore, analytic sensitivity is a function of *within-assay* variance and does not assess the reliability of *between-assay* comparisons, which are more likely to be clinically useful in the diagnosis and treatment of an individual patient. As an alternative to analytic sensitivity, the proposal has been made that assay sensitivity be characterized by a criterion based on interassay variability. Specifically, the "lower limit of interassay quantitative measurement,"[48] or *functional sensitivity*, of an assay is the TSH concentration for which the interassay coefficient of variation is less than some preestablished threshold (generally 20%) to permit reliable quantitative comparisons between specimens measured in different assay runs.

A "generational" classification of TSH assays has been proposed[49] (Table 15-2). Each generation is approximately an order of magnitude more sensitive than the previous one. Both second- and third-generation assays distinguish suppressed TSH levels in hyperthyroidism from normal values. However, the third-generation assay further differentiates partial suppression of basal TSH concentrations in some patients with

**TABLE 15-2.**
**Properties of Thyroid-Stimulating Hormone (TSH) Assays**

| Generation | Method | Label | Functional Sensitivity (μU/mL) | Clinical Characteristics |
|---|---|---|---|---|
| First | RIA | $^{125}$I | 1–2 | Distinguishes hypothyroid from euthyroid sera |
| Second | IMA | $^{125}$I, enzyme, fluorescent, luminescent | 0.1–0.2 | Distinguishes suppressed TSH in clinically thyrotoxic individuals from healthy euthyroid controls |
| Third | IMA | Luminescent | 0.01–0.02 | Distinguishes complete suppression in hyperthyroidism from other causes of partial TSH suppression |

*RIA*, radioimmunoassay; *$^{125}$I*, iodine-125; *IMA*, immunometric assay.

subclinical hyperthyroidism, nonthyroid illness, glucocorticoid therapy, and other clinical states (Table 15-3) from the more complete suppression of basal TSH concentrations in overt hyperthyroidism.[50]

Measurement of TSH is frequently used as the initial, and sometimes sole, thyroid function test.[51] This approach is generally sensitive and specific in the ambulatory population, in which the finding of a normal TSH level is strong evidence that a patient is euthyroid, and an abnormal TSH has a high likelihood of being due to thyroid dysfunction. However, abnormally high or low TSH values (compared to those of an ambulatory euthyroid control population) are frequently noted in hospitalized patients as a result of the effects of nonthyroid illness, acute psychiatric illness, or glucocorticoid therapy.[52,53] Therefore, diagnoses of hypothyroidism or hyperthyroidism in hospitalized patients should be based on clinical evaluation, measurement of free thyroid hormone levels, and other indices of thyroid function, rather than on TSH measurement alone.

The TRH stimulation test has been used in the assessment of mild thyroid dysfunction and in the functional evaluation of the hypothalamic–pituitary–thyroid axis.[54] The test entails measuring serum TSH levels at baseline and after the bolus intravenous administration of TRH. A dose-response relation between administered TRH and peak TSH levels is observed for TRH doses of 6.25 to 400 μg. In clinical practice, a TRH dose sufficient to produce a maximal TSH response is used. The peak TSH response occurs 20 to 40 minutes after TRH administration. If a primary thyroid disorder is suspected, measurement

of TSH levels at baseline and at 20 or 30 minutes after TRH administration is sufficient (Fig. 15-4). If pituitary or hypothalamic dysfunction is suspected, TSH measurements should be continued for 2 to 3 hours at 30- to 60-minute intervals. During the first 5 minutes after TRH administration, side effects may include mild nausea, headache, a transient rise in blood pressure, light-headedness, a peculiar taste sensation, a flushed feeling, and urinary urgency.[54]

TRH testing may be viewed as a means of amplifying and detecting small differences in TSH secretion due, most importantly, to alterations in serum $T_4$ or $T_3$ concentrations. A slight excess of $T_4$ or $T_3$ blunts or completely blocks the TSH response to TRH, whereas small decrements in thyroid hormone levels enhance the response. The peak TSH response to TRH is proportional to the basal serum TSH level.[55] Expressed as a multiple of the basal TSH, the peak TSH is a mean 8 to 9.5 times higher. However, considerable variability is seen in individual responses (range: 3- to 23-fold increment in euthyroid persons).

In addition to thyroid hormone concentrations, other factors can alter the TSH response to TRH (see Table 15-3). In patients with severe illnesses, the TSH response to TRH is likely to be diminished. Cortisol and other neurohumoral factors secreted in response to stress, malnutrition, and the administration of glucocorticoids or dopamine all may contribute to the blunted TSH response. In patients with a subnormal basal TSH level, however, the magnitude of the TSH response to TRH does not distinguish those in whom TSH is suppressed as a result of intercurrent illness from those in whom it is suppressed as a result of partial suppression of the pituitary by slight excess of free thyroid hormone (i.e., patients with autonomous thyroid nodules or exogenous thyroid hormone suppression).[55]

**TABLE 15-3.**
**Clinical Influence on Basal Thyroid-Stimulating Hormone (TSH) and TSH Response to Thyrotropin-Releasing Hormone**

**INCREASED TSH AND ENHANCED RESPONSE**
  Hypothyroidism
  Drugs
    Iodine
    Oral cholecystographic agents
    Amiodarone
    Dopamine receptor-blocking agents
**DECREASED TSH AND BLUNTED RESPONSE**
  Hyperthyroidism
  Severe illnesses
  Chronic renal failure
  Starvation
  Depression
  Anorexia nervosa
  Growth hormone therapy or acromegaly
  Drugs
    Somatostatin agonists
    Glucocorticoids
    Oral contraceptives
    Dopamine agonists
    Bexarotene (retinoid X receptor agonist)

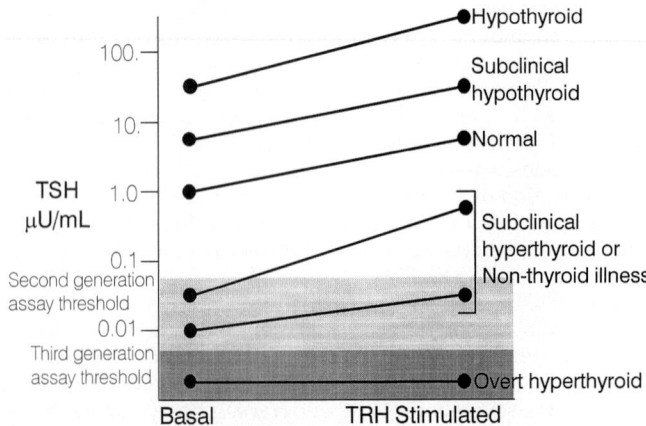

**FIGURE 15-4.** Typical thyroid-stimulating hormone (*TSH*) responses to the administration of thyrotropin-releasing hormone (*TRH*) under different conditions. Basal TSH is suppressed in overt thyrotoxicosis and does not respond to TRH. The blunted TSH response in patients with nonthyroid illness may be similar to the response in patients with subclinical hyperthyroidism. Patients with subclinical hyperthyroidism or nonthyroid illness may have a basal TSH below the detection threshold for second-generation TSH assays.

In general, if the basal TSH level exceeds the functional sensitivity threshold of the assay system and, therefore, can be accurately measured, then measurement of the TRH-stimulated TSH level does not provide additional information regarding the cause of the suppressed TSH. With the improvement in sensitivity of TSH assays, the TRH-stimulation test is not generally required in the evaluation of primary hypothyroidism or hyperthyroidism with suppressed TSH. However, the TRH-stimulation test may be useful in the evaluation of central hypothyroidism, in the rare patient with TSH-dependent hyperthyroidism, and in some patients with functioning pituitary tumors that respond to TRH stimulation (e.g., acromegaly).

## THYROID-STIMULATING HORMONE IN PRIMARY HYPOTHYROIDISM

The basal serum TSH concentration is increased in patients with intrinsic failure of the thyroid gland (primary hypothyroidism) of all causes. The magnitude of the increase is roughly proportional to the severity of disease.[56] In general, basal TSH levels show a better inverse correlation with serum $T_4$ levels than with serum $T_3$ levels; this is because of the importance of the uptake of serum $T_4$ and its intracellular deiodination as a source of $T_3$ in the thyrotrope.[29] In some persons, elevated TSH levels may be found with normal serum $T_3$ concentrations but decreased serum $T_4$ values. Such findings are common in patients with early thyroid gland failure, patients with mild iodine deficiency, and some patients with Graves disease who have been given long-term antithyroid drug treatment.

The isolated elevation of serum TSH levels with normal serum $T_4$ and $T_3$ concentrations in the absence of clinical signs or symptoms of hypothyroidism has been termed *subclinical hypothyroidism*. This condition has an overall prevalence of 2% to 7% and is particularly common in older women. Overt hypothyroidism develops at a rate of 5% to 10% per year in persons with elevated TSH levels and positive antithyroid antibodies.[57]

Measurement of the serum TSH level remains a sensitive test for the diagnosis of primary hypothyroidism in severely ill patients because basal TSH levels, although sometimes partially attenuated, remain higher than normal during intercurrent illness in patients with moderate or severe hypothyroidism. The diagnosis of hypothyroidism should be confirmed by measurement of the free $T_4$ value, however. Patients with mildly elevated TSH and normal free $T_4$ concentrations generally should undergo repeated thyroid function testing after discharge from the hospital to confirm the diagnosis of hypothyroidism.

The TSH response to TRH is exaggerated in patients with primary hypothyroidism. However, TRH testing should not be needed in the evaluation of suspected hypothyroidism if the basal serum TSH level is elevated.

## THYROID-STIMULATING HORMONE IN HYPERTHYROIDISM

Circulating TSH is suppressed in hyperthyroidism of all causes except in the rare patients with TSH-dependent thyrotoxicosis. In clinically hyperthyroid patients, the basal TSH level measured with a third-generation assay (functional sensitivity of <0.01 µU/mL) is <0.01 µU/mL; in most patients, TSH is undetectable.[28,58] Serum TSH generally remains undetectable after TRH stimulation in these patients.

Slight overproduction of $T_4$ and $T_3$ in patients with autonomous nodular goiter or mild Graves disease may suppress TSH values without raising free $T_4$ or free $T_3$ levels above the normal range (subclinical hyperthyroidism). Suppression of the hypothalamic-pituitary axis may be less complete in patients with subclinical hyperthyroidism. In some, the basal TSH level is undetectable, whereas in others, it is detectable but suppressed below the normal range for ambulatory persons. If the basal TSH value is detectable, a TSH increment in response to TRH

also is measurable. If the basal TSH level is undetectable, a slight increment after TRH stimulation sometimes may be noted.[28,58]

A second-generation TSH assay distinguishes suppressed TSH in hyperthyroidism from euthyroid levels. However, patients with partial TSH suppression also may have undetectably low TSH levels with this assay (see Fig. 15-4). If more precise measurement of thyrotrope suppression is required (i.e., to distinguish partial TSH suppression due to nonthyroid illness from thyrotoxicosis in hospitalized patients), measurement with a more sensitive assay or TRH-stimulation testing may be helpful.

## EVALUATION OF THERAPY FOR THYROID DISEASES

The adequacy of thyroid hormone replacement therapy in primary hypothyroidism can be evaluated by measuring the serum TSH concentration. Normalization of serum TSH levels should be sought as a therapeutic end point in adults.[59] The threshold for suppression of TSH has been reported to be elevated in infants with congenital hypothyroidism, who may show a persistently elevated TSH level in spite of the administration of adequate doses of replacement $T_4$.[60]

After the return of free $T_4$ from elevated to normal levels, the thyrotrope may remain suppressed for 4 to 6 weeks.[61] Therefore, TSH is not an accurate indicator of thyroid status in thyrotoxic patients whose thyroid hormone levels are changing. Free $T_4$ (and free $T_3$) should be measured in the short-term follow-up of hyperthyroid patients being treated with antithyroid drugs or during the immediate period after treatment with radioactive iodine.

TSH should be measured by a third-generation assay to confirm complete suppression by exogenous thyroid hormone in patients with thyroid cancer. If a second-generation assay is used, then TSH should be measured after TRH stimulation to determine the degree of suppression.[28,58]

## DISORDERS OF THYROID-STIMULATING HORMONE CONTROL

### DISORDERS CAUSING HYPOTHYROIDISM

#### CENTRAL HYPOTHYROIDISM

Central hypothyroidism results from failure of the pituitary to secrete biologically active TSH. Central hypothyroidism should be considered in patients who have clinical features of hypothyroidism or hypothalamic-pituitary dysfunction, low serum $T_4$ concentrations, and serum TSH levels that are not elevated. In patients with no clinical manifestations of myxedema and no other evidence of hypopituitarism, other causes of low serum $T_4$ without elevated serum TSH also should be considered, such as decreased thyroid hormone–binding proteins or severe illness. Patients with central hypothyroidism constitute several groups (Table 15-4), as described below.

**Combined Pituitary Hormone Deficiency (Idiopathic Hypopituitarism).** Patients with combined pituitary hormone deficiency (CPHD) have no antecedent histories of disease or injury that could cause hypopituitarism. Clinical features vary. Cases may be sporadic or familial in occurrence. Hypothyroidism alone is rare; patients generally present in childhood with growth hormone deficiency. Patients then go on to develop varying degrees of TSH, prolactin, and gonadotropin deficiencies. However, the patients do not have diabetes insipidus or neurologic deficits. In some families with CPHD, mutations in *pituitary-specific transcriptional factors (Pit-1, Prop-1)* have been identified (Table 15-5).[62-64]

**Isolated Thyroid-Stimulating Hormone Deficiency.** In patients with isolated thyroid-stimulating hormone deficiency, basal serum TSH values may be low, normal, or slightly elevated; TRH stimulation generally causes a rise in serum TSH levels. The chronic administration of TRH can restore thyroid

**TABLE 15-4.**
**Causes of Central Hypothyroidism**

**Congenital Hypopituitarism**
  Combined pituitary hormone deficiency
  Isolated thyrotropin-releasing hormone deficiency
  Isolated thyroid-stimulating hormone deficiency
**Hypothalamic Lesions**
  Congenital (cysts, midline defects, familial syndromes)
  Neoplastic (craniopharyngioma, dysgerminoma, meningioma, glioma)
  Infectious (encephalitis, fungal diseases, tuberculosis)
  Infiltrative (sarcoidosis, eosinophilic granulomatosis, lipid storage diseases)
  Traumatic (closed head injury, radiation necrosis, postsurgical)
**Pituitary Lesions**
  Neoplastic (adenoma, craniopharyngioma, metastases)
  Ischemic or hemorrhagic necrosis (postpartum, diabetes mellitus, arteritis, sickle cell anemia, pituitary apoplexy)
  Infiltrative (hemochromatosis, sarcoidosis)
  Cavernous sinus thrombosis
  Autoimmune hypophysitis

hormones to normal levels. Hence, the hypothyroidism is thought to result from impaired release of TRH from the hypothalamus. Rarely, familial cases with mutations in the β-TSH gene (see Table 15-5) have been described. Mutations have included a truncated β-TSH transcript as a result of a premature stop codon; a single amino-acid substitution resulted in a β-TSH that was unable to heterodimerize, and a frame-shift mutation resulted in reduced amounts of TSH with decreased bioactivity.[65,66] In another patient, loss-of-function mutations of the TRH receptor were reported (see Table 15-5).[67]

**Hypothalamic Lesions.**    Destructive lesions of the hypothalamus may result in central hypothyroidism. Generally, multiple pituitary hormones are involved, and patients often have diabetes insipidus. Serum prolactin levels may be mildly elevated because of interruption of the tonic dopaminergic lactotrope inhibitory pathway. In addition to hormone deficiencies, patients may have neurologic abnormalities and other manifestations of hypothalamic disease, such as disturbances of autonomic function, temperature regulation, food and water intake, and sleep cycle, as well as emotional lability.

TSH with reduced bioactivity has been found in the serum of patients with hypothalamic hypothyroidism; long-term treatment with TRH increases the bioactivity of their TSH.[68]

These findings might explain why some patients with hypothalamic disorders have hypothyroidism despite showing normal or slightly increased levels of immunoreactive TSH.

**Pituitary Lesions.**    Pituitary lesions also cause hypothyroidism. Hypothalamic disturbances, visual field cuts, and parasellar abnormalities may be observed if an extrasellar extension of the lesion is present. Pituitary adenomas rarely cause hypothyroidism if they have not grown large enough to cause distortion and enlargement of the margins of the sella turcica.[69]

## THYROID-STIMULATING HORMONE AND THYROTROPIN-RELEASING HORMONE TESTING IN HYPOTHALAMIC-PITUITARY DISEASE

Basal TSH levels may be normal, low, or slightly elevated in patients with central hypothyroidism. Basal TSH values do not correlate with free $T_4$ levels, and TRH-stimulated TSH values are not proportional to basal TSH values.[55] Therefore, clinical evaluation and measurement of free $T_4$ should be used in confirming the diagnosis of suspected central hypothyroidism and in titrating thyroid hormone replacement therapy in patients with central hypothyroidism.

Initially, the proposal was made that TRH testing should differentiate pituitary from hypothalamic causes of central hypothyroidism, with pituitary dysfunction causing a blunted or absent TSH response and hypothalamic disease resulting in a normal or exaggerated TSH rise that is delayed or prolonged. Although such classic patterns are found in many patients, the responses often overlap. Normal or "hypothalamic" patterns have been observed in patients with pituitary lesions, and the serum TSH response has been flat in some patients with suprasellar disease.[70] Thus, the anatomic site of the central lesion may not always correlate with the expected functional consequences on TRH responsiveness. Abnormal serum TSH responses to TRH (i.e., blunted or delayed peaks) also are noted frequently in patients with pituitary or hypothalamic diseases even when the patients appear clinically euthyroid and their serum thyroid hormone levels are normal.[71]

## DISORDERS CAUSING HYPERTHYROIDISM

### THYROID-STIMULATING HORMONE–INDUCED HYPERTHYROIDISM

Hyperthyroidism induced by TSH has been described in a small group of thyrotoxic patients in whom serum TSH levels are normal or increased (see Chap. 42). If signs and symptoms of thyrotoxicosis are absent in a patient with elevated thyroid

**TABLE 15-5.**
**Identified Molecular Defects in Thyroid-Stimulating Hormone (TSH) and TSH Receptor Function**

| Defect | Genetics | Clinical Syndrome | References |
|---|---|---|---|
| **Pit1/PROP1 deficiency** | Heterozygous, dominant | Combined pituitary hormone deficiency | 63, 64 |
|  | Homozygous, recessive |  |  |
|  | Compound heterozygous, recessive |  |  |
| **TRH receptor loss of function** | Compound heterozygous, recessive | Central hypothyroidism | 67 |
| **Hereditary TSH deficiency** | Homozygous, recessive | Central hypothyroidism | 65, 66 |
| **TSH receptor constitutive activation** | Germline: autosomal dominant | Nonautoimmune familial hyperthyroidism | 93–97 |
| **TSH receptor constitutive activation** | Acquired: somatic mutation | Autonomously functioning thyroid nodules, toxic nodular goiter | 86–91 |
| **TSH receptor loss of function** | Homozygous, recessive | Congenital hypothyroidism, TSH resistance | 98–100 |
|  | Compound heterozygous, recessive |  |  |
| **$G_s\alpha$ constitutive activation** | Acquired during embryogenesis | McCune-Albright syndrome; hyperthyroidism | 105 |
| **$G_s\alpha$ constitutive activation** | Acquired somatic mutation | Toxic nodular goiter | 87, 88 |
| **$G_s\alpha$ loss of function** | Heterozygous, dominant | Albright's hereditary osteodystrophy; TSH resistance | 105 |

*TRH*, thyrotropin-releasing hormone.
A database of TSH receptor mutations is accessible through the internet at http://www.uni-leipzig.de/innere/TSH.

**TABLE 15-6.**

**Causes of Hyperthyroxinemia with Nonsuppressed Thyroid-Stimulating Hormone (TSH)**

**INCREASED THYROXINE (T₄)-BINDING PROTEINS (FREE T₄ NORMAL)**

Increased thyroxine-binding globulin (TBG)

Inherited

Acquired

Increased thyroxine-binding prealbumin (TBPA)

Increased albumin binding

**IMPAIRED T₄ TO TRIIODOTHYRONINE (T₃) CONVERSION**

Drugs

Amiodarone

Oral cholecystographic agents

Propranolol

**DISORDERS CAUSING HYPERTHYROIDISM**

TSH-secreting pituitary tumor

Secreting TSH only

Cosecreting growth hormone or prolactin

Selective pituitary resistance to thyroid hormone

Nonpituitary tumor secreting factor with thyrotropin-releasing hormone (TRH)-like bioactivity

**ACUTE MEDICAL ILLNESS**

**ACUTE PSYCHIATRIC ILLNESS**

**AMPHETAMINE OVERDOSAGE**

**INTERMITTENT T₄ REPLACEMENT THERAPY**

**GENERALIZED RESISTANCE TO THYROID HORMONES**

---

hormone concentrations and normal serum TSH levels, other causes of hyperthyroxinemia with nonsuppressed TSH also should be considered (Table 15-6). Patients with TSH-induced hyperthyroidism have clinical evidence of a stimulated thyroid gland, including diffuse goiter and elevated radioactive iodine uptake. Extrathyroidal manifestations of Graves disease are lacking, and the assay of TSI is negative.[72] Two groups of abnormalities have been described.

**Thyroid-Stimulating Hormone–Producing Pituitary Tumors.** In patients with TSH-producing pituitary tumors, basal intact TSH levels are elevated but are not stimulated by TRH or suppressed by exogenous thyroid hormone. Free β-TSH is undetectable; however, free α subunit levels are elevated and the molar ratio of free α subunit to intact TSH is >1.[73,74] Computed tomography or magnetic resonance imaging generally reveals a pituitary lesion. However, these patients are best distinguished from those with nonneoplastic hypersecretion of TSH by measurement of the ratio of free α subunit to intact TSH and the response of TSH to TRH. TSH-producing pituitary tumors may cosecrete growth hormone or prolactin. The initial treatment of TSH-producing pituitary tumors is surgical resection, sometimes followed by postoperative irradiation. If hyperthyroidism persists, the long-acting somatostatin analog octreotide acetate has been shown to decrease serum TSH levels and cause reduction in tumor size.[73,75] Finally, thyroid ablation can be used for persistent thyrotoxicosis.

**Nonneoplastic Hypersecretion of Thyroid-Stimulating Hormone.** TSH-dependent hyperthyroidism has been described in the absence of a TSH-secreting pituitary tumor. These patients have *selective pituitary resistance to thyroid hormone (PRTH)*, a variant of the syndrome of *generalized resistance to thyroid hormone (GRTH)*.[76,77] The thyroid hormone resistance syndromes are inherited in an autosomal dominant fashion. Considerable clinical overlap is found between GRTH and PRTH. The free thyroid hormone levels are elevated in both. Clinical manifestations of hyperthyroidism in PRTH are variable. Laboratory findings in PRTH and GRTH are similar and are distinguished from the findings in subjects with TSH-secreting pituitary tumors.

Basal serum TSH levels are normal or slightly elevated and are stimulated by TRH. The administration of T₃ suppresses basal TSH levels and blunts the TSH response to TRH. Serum free α subunit levels are normal, and the molar ratio of free α subunit to intact TSH is <1. Thus, TSH secretory dynamics are qualitatively normal.

The thyroid hormone resistance syndromes are the result of *mutations in the T₃ nuclear receptor (TR)*. Similar mutations in the TRβ gene have been described in both GRTH and PRTH.[74] Hence GRTH and PRTH are alternate phenotypic expressions of a common underlying genotype. The mechanism responsible for this phenotypic variation has not yet been established. Because both the normal and mutant receptor genes may be expressed, the dominant receptor isoform (normal or mutant) may vary in different organs and in different individuals.

The treatment of nonneoplastic TSH-dependent hyperthyroidism is difficult. Antithyroid drug therapy may increase TSH levels further, causing enlargement of the goiter and possibly enhancing abnormal thyrotrope growth. Thyroxine administration may suppress the TSH but worsens symptoms of thyrotoxicosis. The pharmacologic suppression of TSH secretion has been attempted. Some patients have responded to bromocriptine or octreotide. Other patients have been treated successfully with 3,5,3'-triiodothyroacetic acid (TRIAC) or with D-thyroxine.[74]

### PARANEOPLASTIC THYROID-STIMULATING HORMONE PRODUCTION

A convincing case of ectopic production of TSH by a nonpituitary tumor has not been reported. A patient with hepatocellular carcinoma, thyrotoxicosis, and nonsuppressed TSH has been described.[78] Neither TSH nor TRH immunoreactivity could be detected in the tumor, and the hypothesis was made that the tumor was producing a factor with TRH bioactivity.

### HYPERTHYROIDISM IN TROPHOBLASTIC DISEASE

Hyperthyroidism has been observed in patients with trophoblastic neoplasms such as hydatidiform mole and choriocarcinoma.[79] Research has found that the thyrotropic activity isolated from hydatidiform moles copurifies with hCG and that highly purified hCG has weak intrinsic thyrotropic bioactivity[75] (see Chaps. 42, 112, and 219). Because hCG concentration may be high in patients with trophoblastic tumors, even weak intrinsic thyrotropic activity could stimulate the thyroid enough to cause thyrotoxicosis. The TSH bioactivity of hCG is enhanced by the removal of amino acids from its carboxyl terminus and by the removal of sialic acid residues from its carbohydrate side chains.[80] Hence, the proposal has been made that the thyroid stimulator in hyperthyroidism resulting from trophoblastic disease may be a structurally variant hCG, either transcribed from an abnormal hCG gene or altered by post-translational modifications.

### DEFECTS IN THYROID-STIMULATING HORMONE RECEPTOR FUNCTION

Since the cloning of the human TSH receptor, a number of mutations and polymorphisms have been reported (see Table 15-5).[81–84] Several groups of patients have been described.

### AUTONOMOUSLY FUNCTIONING THYROID NODULES

Mutations to the TSH receptor or to the G_s protein that result in constitutive activation of the cAMP cascade occur in some *autonomously functioning thyroid nodules (AFTNs)*.[85–91] TSH receptor–activating mutations have been reported in 8% to 82% of solitary AFTNs as well as in autonomous nodules within multinodular thyroid glands. These mutations are found only in the autonomous nodule and not in adjacent normal thyroid tissue or in peripheral cells; hence, they are nongermline somatic mutations. Activating somatic mutations to G$_s$α also have been reported in 0% to 38% of AFTNs. In addition, hyperthyroidism is frequently noted in patients with *McCune-Albright syndrome* who are mosaics for somatic G$_s$α-activating mutations acquired during embryogenesis. Not all AFTNs are the result of mutations to these components of the cAMP cascade, however, because autonomous nodules *without* mutations to either protein are also encountered frequently.

Transfected cells expressing the mutant receptor or G$_s$ protein have elevated basal levels of cAMP compared to cells transfected with the wild-type receptor or G$_s$. Stimulation by TSH generally causes a further increment in cAMP levels. The receptor-activating mutations are predominantly localized to the membrane-spanning region of the receptor within the transmembrane segments and connecting loops that interact with G$_s$α (see Fig. 15-1). Presumably, as a result of the conformational change in the receptor caused by the mutation, it is more effective in constitutively activating G$_s$α.

### FAMILIAL NONAUTOIMMUNE HYPERTHYROIDISM

*Hereditary thyrotoxicosis with diffuse hyperplasia of the thyroid* has been described in several families.[92–97] Inheritance of the syndrome is autosomal dominant. It is distinct from Graves disease because *no markers of autoimmunity* such as TSI, lymphocytic infiltrates, or ophthalmopathy are found. Clinical characteristics vary. Individuals generally present during infancy or early childhood, but some have been young adults at the time of diagnosis; hyperthyroidism ranges from mild to severe. Goiter may not be present initially but tends to grow over time. Hyperthyroidism generally recurs if the patient is treated with subtotal thyroidectomy or with less than complete radioiodine ablation. TSH receptor–activating mutations have been identified and characterized in these patients. The mutations are located in the same regions of the TSH receptor as the activating mutations in AFTNs (see Fig. 15-1); in some cases they are identical. However, the constitutive activity of the TSH receptor in this familial syndrome is generally less than the constitutive activity of the mutated receptors in AFTNs. Severe congenital activating mutations may have a high likelihood of being lethal in utero. In addition to the familial cases, several sporadic cases of congenital hyperthyroidism with activating mutations to the TSH receptor have been reported. These apparently are de novo germline mutations, because neither parent carried the mutated gene.

Constitutive activating mutations of G protein–coupled receptors also have been described in other clinical syndromes, including *familial male precocious puberty* (LH receptor), *continued spermatogenesis after hypophysectomy* (FSH receptor), *autosomal dominant hypoparathyroidism* (calcium receptor), and in a rare form of *dwarfism associated with PTH-independent hypercalcemia* (PTH receptor).[81]

### RESISTANCE TO THYROID-STIMULATING HORMONE

Several cases of TSH resistance as a result of TSH receptor loss-of-function mutations have been reported (see Table 15-5).[98–100] All patients have *elevated TSH levels*; in most, the radioactive iodine uptake and the free T$_4$ are normal or only slightly low, consistent with partial TSH unresponsiveness compensated by the elevated TSH. Cases of severe congenital hypothyroidism with hypoplasia of the thyroid also occur, however. Inheritance is autosomal recessive; affected individuals are compound heterozygous or homozygous for TSH receptor mutations. Heterozygotes are unaffected.

TSH-stimulated cAMP production is reduced or absent in cells transfected with the mutant receptor. Several mechanisms may cause the loss-of-function mutation. Some mutant TSH receptors cannot be detected in the plasma membrane. In some of these mutants, a premature stop codon results in production of a truncated polypeptide; in others an amino acid substitution

or deletion may lead to abnormal intracellular processing of the mutant TSH receptor and its consequent failure to appear on the cell surface. A second group of loss-of-function mutations exhibits decreased TSH binding as a result of mutations in the extracellular TSH-binding domain. Finally, in a third group of mutations, TSH binding is normal or near normal, but the cAMP response is impaired. These mutations, which have been localized within the extracellular and membrane-spanning domains (see Fig. 15-1), presumably result in defective coupling to G$_s$α.

TSH resistance occurs in patients with *pseudohypoparathyroidism type 1a*, who have *Albright hereditary osteodystrophy* (brachydactyly, subcutaneous ossifications, short stature, round face; see Chap. 60). These patients are heterozygous for loss-of-function mutations in the G$_s$α gene that result in partial loss of G$_s$α activity. They have variable patterns of hormone dysfunction involving end-organ responses to PTH, TSH, and gonadotropins in addition to the skeletal deformities.[101]

## CLINICAL USE OF RECOMBINANT HUMAN THYROID-STIMULATING HORMONE

Recombinant human TSH has been produced by cotransfecting Chinese hamster ovary cells with cDNA coding for α and β-TSH.[102] Glycosylation of recombinant human TSH is not identical to that of native human TSH. It is bioactive, however, and has undergone initial clinical trials in patients with thyroid cancer.[103] Results of whole body radioiodine scans in patients who had undergone thyroidectomy were evaluated after patients were treated with recombinant human TSH to stimulate radioiodine uptake, and were compared to scans obtained in the same patients after withdrawal of T$_3$ suppression and stimulation by endogenous TSH. In most patients, visualization of residual thyroid activity and metastatic uptake was comparable after both stimulation procedures.[104]

## REFERENCES

1. Pierce JG, Parsons TF. Glycoprotein hormones: structure and function. Annu Rev Biochem 1981; 50:465.
2. Szkudlinski MW, The NG, Grossmann M, et al. Engineering human glycoprotein hormone superactive analogues. Nature Biotech 1996; 14:1257.
3. Magner JA. Thyroid-stimulating hormone: biosynthesis, cell biology and bioactivity. Endocr Rev 1990; 11:354.
4. Lapthorn AJ, Harris DC, Littlejohn A, et al. Crystal structure of human chorionic gonadotropin. Nature 1994; 369:455.
5. Grossmann M, Weintraub BD, Szkudlinski MW. Novel insights into the molecular mechanisms of human thyrotropin action: structural, physiological, and therapeutic implications for the glycoprotein hormone family. Endocr Rev 1997; 18:476.
6. Chin WW, Can FE, Burnside J, Darling DS. Thyroid hormone regulation of thyrotropin gene expression. Recent Prog Horm Res 1993; 48:393.
7. Kim MK, McClaskey JH, Bodenner DL, Weintraub BD. An AP-1-like factor and the pituitary-specific factor Pit-1 are both necessary to mediate hormonal induction of human thyrotropin β gene expression. J Biol Chem 1993; 268:23366.
8. Steinfelder HJ, Wondisford FE. Thyrotropin (TSH) β-subunit gene expression—an example for the complex regulation of pituitary hormone genes. Exp Clin Endocrinol Diabetes 1997; 105:196.
9. Shupnik MA, Ridgway EC. Triiodothyronine rapidly decreases transcription of the thyrotropin subunit genes in thyrotropic tumor explants. Endocrinology 1985; 117:1940.
10. Can FE, Wong NCW. Characteristics of a negative thyroid hormone response element. J Biol Chem 1994; 269:4175.
11. Magner JA, Kane J, Chou ET. Intravenous thyrotropin (TSH)-releasing hormone releases human TSH that is structurally different from basal TSH. J Clin Endocrinol Metab 1992; 74:1306.
12. Boume HR, Sanders DA, McCormick F. The GTPase superfamily: a conserved switch for diverse cell functions. Nature 1990; 348:125.
13. Ji TH, Grossmann M, Ji I. G protein-coupled receptors. I. Diversity of receptor-ligand interactions. J Biol Chem 1998; 273:17299.
14. Laugwitz KL, Allgeier A, Offermanns S, et al. The human thyrotropin receptor: a heptahelical receptor capable of stimulating members of all four G protein families. Proc Natl Acad Sci U S A 1996; 93:116.

15. Parmentier M, Libert F, Maenhaut C, et al. Molecular cloning of the thyrotropin receptor. Science 1989; 246:1620.
16. Vassart G, Dumont JE. The thyrotropin receptor and the regulation of thyrocyte function and growth. Endocr Rev 1992; 13:596.
17. Kobe B, Deisenhofer J. A structural basis of the interactions between leucine-rich repeats and protein ligands. Nature 1995; 374:183.
18. Jiang X, Dreano M, Buckler DR, et al. Structural predictions for the ligand-binding region of glycoprotein hormone receptors and the nature of hormone-receptor interactions. Structure 1995; 3:1341.
19. Tong W. Actions of thyroid-stimulating hormone. In: Greep RO, Astwood EB, eds. Handbook of physiology, section 7, Endocrinology; vol III, Thyroid. Baltimore: Williams & Wilkins, 1974:255.
20. Toni R, Lechan RM. Neuroendocrine regulation of thyrotropin-releasing hormone (TRH) in the tuberoinfundibular system. J Endocrinol Invest 1993; 16:715.
21. Morley JE. Neuroendocrine control of thyrotropin secretion. Endocr Rev 1981; 2:396.
22. Lechan RM, Wu P, Jackson IMD, et al. Thyrotropin-releasing hormone precursor: characterization in rat brain. Science 1986; 231:159.
23. Fliers E, Wiersinga WM, Swaab DF. Physiological and pathophysiological aspects of thyrotropin-releasing hormone gene expression in the human hypothalamus. Thyroid 1998; 8:921.
24. Wilber JF, Xu AH. The thyrotropin-releasing hormone gene cloning, characterization, and transcriptional regulation in the central nervous system, heart and testis. Thyroid 1998; 8:897.
25. Gershengorn MC. Mechanism of thyrotropin releasing hormone stimulation of pituitary hormone secretion. Annu Rev Physiol 1986; 48:515.
26. Daneshdoost L, Gennarelli TA, Bashey HM, et al. Recognition of gonadotroph adenomas in women. N Engl J Med 1991; 324:589.
27. Vagenakis AG, Rapoport B, Azizi F, et al. Hyperresponse to thyrotropin-releasing hormone accompanying small decreases in serum thyroid hormone concentrations. J Clin Invest 1974; 54:913.
28. Spencer CA, LoPresti JS, Patel A, et al. Applications of a new chemiluminometric thyrotropin assay to subnormal measurement. J Clin Endocrinol Metab 1990; 70:453.
29. Larsen PR. Thyroid-pituitary interaction. N Engl J Med 1982; 306:23.
30. Gershengorn MC. Thyrotropin-releasing hormone receptor: cloning and regulation of its expression. Recent Prog Horm Res 1993; 48:341.
31. Berelowitz M, Maeda K, Harris S, Frohman LA. The effect of alterations in the pituitary-thyroid axis on hypothalamic content and in vitro release of somatostatin-like immunoreactivity. Endocrinology 1980; 107:24.
32. Kaplan MM, Taft JA, Reichlin S. Munsat TL. Sustained rises in serum thyrotropin, thyroxine, and triiodothyronine during long term, continuous thyrotropin-releasing hormone treatment in patients with amyotrophic lateral sclerosis. J Clin Endocrinol Metab 1986; 63:808.
33. Sato T, Ishiguro K, Suzuki Y, et al. Low setting of feedback regulation of TSH secretion by thyroxine in pituitary dwarfism with TSH-releasing hormone deficiency. J Clin Endocrinol Metab 1976; 42:385.
34. Fisher DA, Odell WD. Acute release of thyrotropin in the newborn. J Clin Invest 1969; 48:1670.
35. Penny R, Spencer CA, Frasier SD, Nicoloff JT. Thyroid-stimulating hormone and thyroglobulin levels decrease with chronological age in children and adolescents. J Clin Endocrinol Metab 1983; 56:177.
36. Van Coevorden A, Laurent E, Decoster C, et al. Decreased basal and stimulated thyrotropin secretion in healthy elderly men. J Clin Endocrinol Metab 1989; 69:177.
37. Brabant G, Prank K, Ranft U, et al. Physiological regulation of circadian and pulsatile thyrotropin secretion in normal men and women. J Clin Endocrinol Metab 1990; 70:403.
38. Wilber JF, Baum D. Elevation of plasma TSH during surgical hypothermia. J Clin Endocrinol Metab 1970; 31:372.
39. Gardner DF, Kaplan MM, Stanley CA, Utiger RD. Effect of tri-iodothyronine replacement on the metabolic and pituitary response to starvation. N Engl J Med 1979; 300:579.
40. Wehmann RE, Gregerman RI, Burns WH, et al. Suppression of thyrotropin in the low-thyroxine state of severe nonthyroidal illness. N Engl J Med 1985; 312:546.
41. Pang X-P, Hershman JM, Mirrel CJ, Pekary AE. Impairment of hypothalamic-pituitary-thyroid function in rats treated with human recombinant tumor necrosis factor-α (cachectin). Endocrinology 1989; 125:76.
42. Kakucska I, Romero LI, Clark BD, et al. Suppression of thyrotropin releasing hormone gene expression by interleukin 1-beta in the rat: implications for nonthyroid illness. Neuroendocrinology 1994; 59:129.
43. Bacci V, Schussler GC, Kaplan TB. The relationship between serum triiodothyronine and thyrotropin during systemic illness. J Clin Endocrinol Metab 1982; 54:1229.
44. van Heyningen V, Abbott SR, Daniel SG, et al. Development and utility of a monoclonal-antibody-based, highly sensitive immunoradiometric assay of thyrotropin. Clin Chem 1987; 33:1387.
45. Brennan MD, Klee GO, Preissner CM, Hay ID. Heterophilic serum antibodies: a cause for falsely elevated serum thyrotropin levels. Mayo Clin Proc 1987; 62:894.
46. Hay ID, Bayer MF, Kaplan MM, et al. American Thyroid Association assessment of current free thyroid hormone and thyrotropin measurements and guidelines for future clinical assays. Clin Chem 1991; 37:2002.
47. Spencer CA, Takeuchi M, Kazarosyan M. Current status and performance goals for serum thyrotropin (TSH) assays. Clin Chem 1996; 42:140.
48. Bayer MF. Performance criteria for appropriate characterization of "(highly) sensitive" thyrotropin assays. Clin Chem 1987; 33:630.
49. Nicoloff JT, Spencer CA. The use and misuse of the sensitive thyrotropin assays. J Clin Endocrinol Metab 1990; 71:553.
50. Saller B, Brod'a N, Heydarian R, et al. Utility of third generation thyrotropin assays in thyroid function testing. Exp Clin Endocrinol Diabetes 1998; 106:S29.
51. Ross DS, Daniels GH, Gouveia D. The use and limitations of a chemiluminescent thyrotropin assay as a single thyroid function test in an outpatient endocrine clinic. J Clin Endocrinol Metab 1990; 71:764.
52. Attia J, Margetts P, Guyatt G. Diagnosis of thyroid disease in hospitalized patients: a systematic review. Arch Intern Med 1999; 159:658.
53. Spencer C, Eigen A, Shen D, et al. Specificity of sensitive assays of thyrotropin (TSH) used as a screen for thyroid disease in hospitalized patients. Clin Chem 1987; 33:1391.
54. Hershman JM. Clinical application of thyrotropin-releasing hormone. N Engl J Med 1974; 290:886.
55. Spencer CA, Schwarzbein D, Guttler RB, et al. Thyrotropin (TSH)-releasing hormone stimulation test responses employing third and fourth generation TSH assays. J Clin Endocrinol Metab 1993; 76:494.
56. Bigos ST, Ridgway EC, Kourides IA, Maloof F. Spectrum of pituitary alterations with mild and severe thyroid impairment. J Clin Endocrinol Metab 1978; 46:317.
57. Tunbridge WMG, Brewis M, French JM, et al. Natural history of autoimmune thyroiditis. BMJ 1981; 282:258.
58. Ross DS, Ardisson U, Meskell MJ. Measurement of thyrotropin in clinical and subclinical hyperthyroidism using a new chemiluminescent assay. J Clin Endocrinol Metab 1989; 69:684.
59. Helfand M, Crapo LM. Monitoring therapy in patients taking levothyroxine. Ann Intern Med 1990; 113:450.
60. Schultz RM, Glassman MS, MacGillivray MH. Elevated threshold for thyrotropin suppression in congenital hypothyroidism. Am J Dis Child 1980; 134:19.
61. Vagenakis AG, Braverman LE, Azizi F, et al. Recovery of pituitary thyrotropic function after withdrawal of prolonged thyroid-suppression therapy. N Engl J Med 1975; 293:681.
62. Cohen LE, Wondisford FE, Radovick S. Role of Pit-1 in the gene expression of growth hormone, prolactin, and thyrotropin. Endocrinol Metab Clin North Am 1996; 25:523.
63. Pellegrini-Bouiller I, Bélicar P, Barlier A, et al. A new mutation of the gene encoding transcription factor Pit-1 is responsible for combined pituitary hormone deficiency. J Clin Endocrinol Metab 1996; 81:2790.
64. Deladoëy J, Flück C, Büyükgebiz A, et al. "Hot spot" in the PROP1 gene responsible for combined pituitary hormone deficiency. J Clin Endocrinol Metab 1999; 84:1645.
65. Doeker BM, Pfäffle RW, Pohlenz J, Andler W. Congenital central hypothyroidism due to a homozygous mutation in the thyrotropin β–subunit gene follows an autosomal recessive inheritance. J Clin Endocrinol Metab 1998; 83: 1762.
66. Hayashizaki Y, Hiraoka Y, Endo Y, Matsubara K. Thyroid stimulating hormone (TSH) deficiency caused by a single base substitution in the CAGYC region of the β-subunit. EMBO J 1989; 8:2291.
67. Collu R, Tang J, Castagné J, et al. A novel mechanism for isolated central hypothyroidism: inactivating mutations in the thyrotropin-releasing hormone receptor gene. J Clin Endocrinol Metab 1997; 82:1561.
68. Beck-Peccoz P, Amr S, Menzezes-Ferreira MM, et al. Decreased receptor binding of biologically inactive thyrotropin in central hypothyroidism. N Engl J Med 1985; 312:1085.
69. Klijn JGM, Lamberts SWJ, De Jong FH, et al. The importance of pituitary tumour size in patients with hyperprolactinaemia in relation to hormonal variables and extrasellar extension of tumour. Clin Endocrinol (Oxf) 1980; 12:341.
70. Patel YC, Burger HG. Serum thyrotropin (TSH) in pituitary and/or hypothalamic hypothyroidism: normal or elevated basal levels and paradoxical responses to thyrotropin-releasing hormone. J Clin Endocrinol Metab 1973; 37:190.
71. Snyder PJ, Jacobs LS, Rabello MM, et al. Diagnostic value of thyrotrophin-releasing hormone in pituitary and hypothalamic diseases. Ann Intern Med 1974; 81:751.
72. Weintraub BD, Gershengorn MC, Kourides IA, Fein H. Inappropriate secretion of thyroid stimulating hormone. Ann Intern Med 1981; 95:339.
73. Brucker-Davis F, Oldfield EH, Skarulis MC, et al. Thyrotropin-secreting pituitary tumors: diagnostic criteria, thyroid hormone sensitivity, and treatment outcome in 25 patients followed at the National Institutes of Health. J Clin Endocrinol Metab 1999; 84:476.
74. McDermott MT, Ridgway EC. Central hyperthyroidism. Endocrinol Metab Clin North Am 1998; 27:187
75. Gesundheit N, Petrick PA, Nissim M, et al. Thyrotropin-secreting pituitary adenomas: clinical and biochemical heterogeneity. Ann Intern Med 1989; 111:827.
76. Refetoff S, Weiss RE, Usala SJ. The syndromes of resistance to thyroid hormone. Endocr Rev 1993; 14:348.
77. Beck-Pecoz P, Forloni F, Cortelazz D, et al. Pituitary resistance to thyroid hormones. Horm Res 1992; 38:66.
78. Helzberg JH, McPhee MS, Zarling EJ, Lukert BP. Hepatocellular carcinoma: an unusual course with hyperthyroidism and inappropriate thyroid-stimulating hormone production. Gastroenterology 1985; 88:181.

79. Higgins HP, Hershman JM, Kenimer JG, et al. The thyrotoxicosis of hydatidiform mole. Ann Intern Med 1975; 83:307.

80. Hoermann R, Broecker M, Grossmann M, et al. Interaction of human chorionic gonadotropin (hCG) and asialo-hCG with recombinant human thyrotropin receptor. J Clin Endocrinol Metab 1994; 77: 1009.

81. Spiegel AM. Mutations in G proteins and G protein–coupled receptors in endocrine disease. J Clin Endocrinol Metab 1996; 81:2434.

82. Van Sande J, Parma J, Tonacchera M, et al. Somatic and germline mutations of the TSH receptor gene in thyroid diseases. J Clin Endocrinol Metab 1995; 80:2577.

83. Bodenner DL, Lash RW. Thyroid disease mediated by molecular defects in cell surface and nuclear receptors. Am J Med 1998; 105:524.

84. Morris JC. The clinical expression of thyrotropin receptor mutations. Endocrinologist 1998; 8:195.

85. Parma J, Duprez L, Van Sande J, et al. Somatic mutations in the thyrotropin receptor gene cause hyperfunctioning thyroid adenomas. Nature 1993; 365:649.

86. Holzapfel HP, Führer D, Wonerow P, et al. Identification of constitutively activating somatic thyrotropin receptor mutations in a subset of toxic multinodular goiters. J Clin Endocrinol Metab 1997; 82:4229.

87. Parma J, Duprez L, Van Sande J, et al. Diversity and prevalence of somatic mutations in the thyrotropin receptor and $G_s\alpha$ genes as a cause of toxic thyroid adenomas. J Clin Endocrinol Metab 1997; 82:2695.

88. Russo D, Arturi F, Wicker R, et al. Genetic alterations in thyroid hyperfunctioning adenomas. J Clin Endocrinol Metab 1995; 80:1347.

89. Duprez L, Parma J, Costagliola S, et al. Constitutive activation of the TSH receptor by spontaneous mutations affecting the N-terminal extracellular domain. FEBS Lett 1997; 409:469.

90. Tonacchera M, Chiovato L, Pinchera A, et al. Hyperfunctioning thyroid nodules in toxic multinodular goiter share activating thyrotropin receptor mutations with solitary toxic adenoma. J Clin Endocrinol Metab 1998; 83:492.

91. Führer D, Holzapfel HP, Wonerow P, et al. Somatic mutations in the thyrotropin receptor gene and not in the $G_s\alpha$ protein gene in 31 toxic thyroid nodules. J Clin Endocrinol Metab 1997; 82:3885.

92. Leclère J, Béné MC, Aubert V. Clinical consequences of activating germline mutations of TSH receptor, the concept of toxic hyperplasia. Horm Res 1997; 47:158.

93. Duprez L, Parma J, Van Sande J, et al. Germline mutations in the thyrotropin receptor gene cause non-autoimmune autosomal dominant hyperthyroidism. Nat Genet 1994; 7:396.

94. Führer D, Wonerow P, Willgerodt H, Paschke R. Identification of a new thyrotropin receptor germline mutation (Leu$^{629}$Phe) in a family with neonatal onset of autosomal dominant nonautoimmune hyperthyroidism. J Clin Endocrinol Metab 1997; 82:4234.

95. Schwab KO, Gerlich M, Broecker M, et al. Constitutively active germline mutation of the thyrotropin receptor gene as a cause of congenital hyperthyroidism. J Pediatr 1997; 131:899.

96. Grüters A, Schöneberg T, Biebermann H, et al. Severe congenital hyperthyroidism caused by a germ-line *neo* mutation in the extracellular portion of the thyrotropin receptor. J Clin Endocrinol Metab 1998; 83:1431.

97. Khoo DHC, Parma J, Rajasoorya C, et al. A germline mutation of the thyrotropin receptor gene associated with thyrotoxicosis and mitral valve prolapse in a Chinese family. J Clin Endocrinol Metab 1999; 84:1459.

98. Sunthoruthepvarakui T, Gottschalk ME, Hayashi Y, Refetoff S. Resistance to thyrotropin caused by mutations in the thyrotropin-receptor gene. N Engl J Med 1995; 332:155.

99. de Roux N, Misrahi M, Brauner R, et al. Four families with loss of function mutations of the thyrotropin receptor. J Clin Endocrinol Metab 1996; 81:4229.

100. Gagné N, Parma J, Deal C, et al. Apparent congenital athyreosis contrasting with normal plasma thyroglobulin levels and associated with inactivating mutations in the thyrotropin receptor gene: are athyreosis and ectopic thyroid distinct entities? J Clin Endocrinol Metab 1998; 83:1771.

101. Levine MA, Downs RW Jr, Moses AM, et al. Resistance to multiple hormones in patients with pseudohypoparathyroidism. Am J Med 1983; 74:545.

102. Thotakura NR, Desai BK, Bates LG, et al. Biological activity and metabolic clearance of a recombinant human thyrotropin produced in Chinese hamster ovary cells. Endocrinology 1991; 128:341.

103. Meier CA, Braverman LE, Ebner SA, et al. Diagnostic use of recombinant human thyrotropin in patients with thyroid carcinoma (phase I/II study). J Clin Endocrinol Metab 1994; 78:188.

104. Haugen BR, Pacini F, Reiners C, et al. A comparison of recombinant human thyrotropin and thyroid hormone withdrawal for the detection of thyroid remnant or cancer. J Clin Endocrinol Metab 1999; 84:3877.

105. Spiegel AM, Weinstein LS, Shenker A. Abnormalities in G protein coupled signal transduction pathways in human disease. J Clin Invest 1993; 92:1119.

# CHAPTER 16

# PITUITARY GONADOTROPINS AND THEIR DISORDERS

WILLIAM J. BREMNER, ILPO HUHTANIEMI, AND JOHN K. AMORY

The gonadotropins, luteinizing hormone (LH) and follicle-stimulating hormone (FSH), are large glycoproteins secreted from the anterior pituitary gland in response to hormonal signals from the brain and the gonads (Fig. 16-1). LH and FSH serve as intermediary messengers in the neuroendocrine system, which transmits environmental and central nervous system (CNS) information to the reproductive system. By transmitting the effects of exercise, diet, stress, and, in some species, of photoperiod and olfactory impulses, LH and FSH can stimulate ovarian and testicular function and therefore alter the physiology, fertility, and behavior of the host organism. In addition, pituitary gonadotropin secretion responds to hormonal signals returning from the gonads to allow integration of the function of the reproductive system, for example, during the menstrual cycle.

## STRUCTURE, SYNTHESIS, AND STORAGE OF GONADOTROPINS

### SUBUNIT COMPOSITION

The $\alpha$ and $\beta$ subunit structure of LH and FSH[1,2] is similar to that of thyroid-stimulating hormone and human chorionic gonadotropin (hCG; see Chaps. 15 and 112). Within each species, the $\alpha$ subunit is essentially identical in structure among the four hormones, whereas the $\beta$ subunit differs among the four hormones and determines the biologic function of the dimeric molecule. The two subunits must be bound together through noncovalent interactions to be bioactive; neither has significant activity alone.

### CARBOHYDRATE CONTENT

The approximate molecular mass of LH is 28 kDa and of FSH is 33 kDa; the $\alpha$ subunit common to both has a molecular mass of 14 kDa. These weights are approximate because of heterogeneity in the oligosaccharide (carbohydrate) moieties. The common $\alpha$ subunit has two N-linked carbohydrate side chains, LH-$\beta$ has one, and FSH-$\beta$ has two. Human chorionic gonadotropin-$\beta$ has, in addition to two N-linked carbohydrate moieties, four O-linked moieties in its C-terminal 32-amino-acid extension. The exact structure of these carbohydrate side chains is unknown and variable, but they contribute ~16% of the weight of the LH molecule. The composition of the carbohydrate side chains of a given hormone shows a certain degree of microheterogeneity.[3] The composition of these gonadotropin isoforms apparently varies according to the physiologic state and may, thus, determine the intrinsic bioactivity of the circulating gonadotropin at a given moment. However, the physiologic and pathophysiologic significance of this variability still remains unclear.

The sialic acid component of the carbohydrate side chain varies markedly in amount among the gonadotropins: 20 residues per molecule in hCG, 5 in FSH, and 1 or 2 in LH. The sialic acid content is directly related to the half-life of the hormone circulating in blood; hCG is cleared slowly, LH relatively rapidly, and FSH at an intermediate rate. In addition, the high degree of ter-

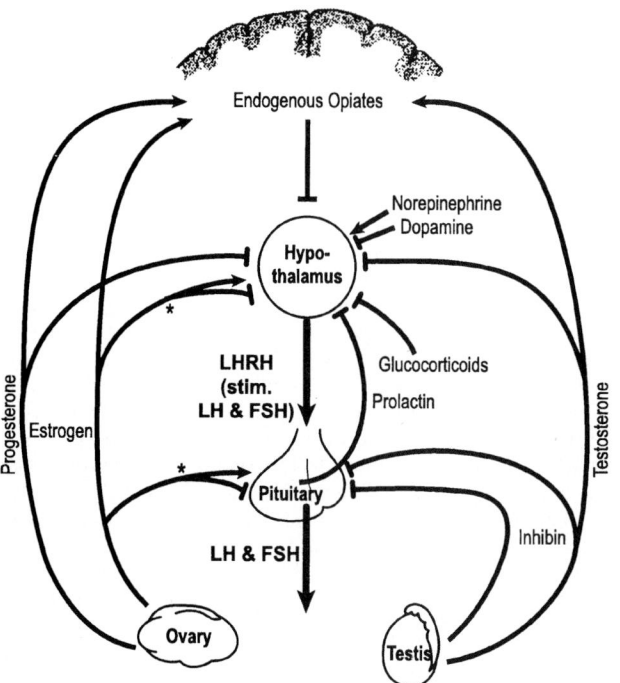

**FIGURE 16-1.** Schema for the control of gonadotropin secretion. (*Estrogen can be inhibitory or stimulatory to luteinizing hormone–releasing hormone [*GnRH*], depending on the level and duration of exposure, and perhaps other factors.) (←, stimulatory; ⊢, inhibitory; *stim.*, stimulates; *LH*, luteinizing hormone; *FSH*, follicle-stimulating hormone.)

minal sulfation of the carbohydrate termini in LH, as well as the rapid elimination of this type of glycoprotein through action of a specific liver receptor, contribute to the faster elimination rate of LH in comparison to FSH.[4] Progressive desialylation of the gonadotropins shortens their half-lives and, therefore, decreases their bioactivity in vivo, whereas their in vitro bioactivity may be retained.[5,6] Some of the deglycosylated hormones bind to receptors in vitro but do not stimulate adenylate cyclase, thereby functioning as competitive antagonists for the native hormone.[7]

The α and β subunits are products of separate genes for which the structures have been determined.[8,9] A single gene encodes the α subunit for the four glycoprotein hormones. The amino acid sequence contains a leader or signal peptide that is removed before addition of the carbohydrate moieties (see Chap. 3).

An important advance has been the expression in cultured mammalian cells of complementary DNA (cDNA) for the gonadotropins.[2] In mammalian cells, processing and glycosylation of the subunits, as well as combination and secretion, occurred in large quantities. In previously used bacterial cell systems, this had not been possible. The hormones produced by this recombinant technology are much purer than those obtained from human pituitaries or urine and can be produced in large quantities with constant quality. Significantly, they lack the postulated capability to transmit Creutzfeldt-Jakob disease, something which has halted the use of hormones prepared from human pituitaries[10] (see Chaps. 12 and 18). With this technology, one can also prepare gonadotropin analogs of different conformation and amino-acid or carbohydrate content, and test the structure and function relationships of these molecules, including possible antagonist compounds. Recombinant gonadotropins are now available for human LH, human FSH, and hCG.[11] The availability of these agents facilitates greatly the care of patients with gonadotropin deficiencies and aids ovarian priming procedures involved in artificial reproductive techniques such as in vitro fertilization (IVF) and intracytoplasmic sperm injection (ICSI).

The cells that synthesize and store gonadotropins in the anterior pituitary, the gonadotropes, are distributed singly in acini

made up largely of other cell types. Most gonadotropes stain with antibodies to both LH and FSH (or their β subunits), a finding that implies that the same cell produces both gonadotropins.[12] A few cells stain for either LH or FSH, but not for both (see Chap. 11).

Because of its better supply and similarity in action to LH, hCG has generally been used in diagnostic testing and in therapy (see Chaps. 93 and 97). Human menopausal gonadotropin (or menotropin), which is obtained from the urine of postmenopausal women, has an FSH-like and LH-like action; one preparation (Pergonal) has been used extensively to induce ovulation or spermatogenesis (see Chap. 97). Purified FSH and LH from urinary sources, as well as the recombinant form of FSH, are now available for clinical use.

## CONTROL OF SECRETION OF GONADOTROPINS

The synthesis and secretion of LH and FSH are under the control of luteinizing hormone–releasing hormone (LHRH, also called gonadotropin-releasing hormone, GnRH), and gonadal steroids and peptides, including inhibin and activin (see Fig. 16-1). GnRH is a decapeptide that is a product of hypothalamic neurosecretion and is carried by the hypothalamico-hypophysial portal system to the gonadotropic cells of the anterior pituitary (Fig. 16-2). Binding of GnRH to receptors on the pituitary gonadotropes causes the release of both FSH and LH.

During embryonic life, the cell bodies of GnRH-secreting neurons are detected in the olfactory placode, from where they gradually migrate to their final locations in the hypothalamus. This migration of GnRH neurons is disturbed in the most common X-linked form of Kallmann syndrome (hypogonadotropic hypogonadism and anosmia), due to mutation in an extracellular matrix protein, *anosmin*, and disturbance in development of the olfactory bulbs and tracts.[13] Other forms of hypogonadotropic hypogonadism have been found to be due to inactivating mutations in the GnRH-receptor gene.[14]

After the embryonic migration period, cell bodies of GnRH neurons are found predominantly in two regions of the primate hypothalamus: (a) anteriorly, especially in the medial preoptic area and the interstitial nucleus of the stria terminalis, and (b) in the tuberal regions, particularly the arcuate nucleus and adjacent paraventricular nucleus (see Chap. 8).[15,16] Physiologically important projections from these neurons go to the median eminence, where they terminate near the capillary bed of the portal system. Projections also are found to other CNS areas, such as the amygdala, hippocampus, and periaqueductal gray area, and to the posterior pituitary. The function of these projections is unknown, but the CNS projections could be important in the behavioral effects reported for GnRH. Stimulatory effects of GnRH on sexual behavior due to a direct CNS site of action have been reported in rodents.

## PULSATILE ACTIVITY

GnRH is secreted in pulses that vary in frequency from approximately one per hour to as few as one or two per 24 hours. In sheep, direct measurement of GnRH in portal blood simulta-

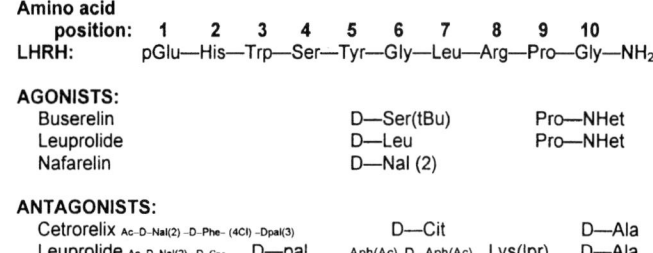

**FIGURE 16-2.** Amino-acid composition of luteinizing hormone–releasing hormone (*GnRH*) and some GnRH agonist analogs.

neously with the measurement of LH in peripheral blood demonstrated that each LH pulse is preceded by a GnRH pulse.[17]

To generate pulsatile secretory activity, many GnRH neurons must be synchronized to secrete almost simultaneously. This synchronized neural activity can be recorded by electrodes placed in the hypothalamus and correlates with pulsatile increases of LH into the circulation.[18] The neural mechanisms underlying this synchronous activity are not well understood (see Chap. 6).

## CONTROLLING FACTORS

GnRH secretory activity is affected by many CNS neurotransmitters and by gonadal steroids as well as other hormones. Opiates suppress gonadotropin secretion.[19] This effect is almost certainly mediated through an effect on GnRH secretion, because little evidence exists that opiates exert a direct effect on pituitary responsiveness to GnRH in vitro. Opiate antagonists, such as naloxone, can stimulate LH secretion in humans, suggesting a significant tonic inhibitory effect of endogenous opiates on GnRH secretion.[20] An important interaction occurs between the opiate effect and the prevailing steroid milieu, because naloxone administration increases LH levels in women in the late follicular and luteal phases but not in those in the early follicular phase or in postmenopausal women.[20,21] In monkeys, little β-endorphin enters the portal blood during the early follicular phase or in ovariectomized animals.[22] Levels of β-endorphin are markedly increased by estrogen and progesterone administration, a result that implies that these steroids may exert their inhibitory feedback effects partly through endogenous opiates.[23] In men, similar mechanisms may occur, because testosterone markedly slows the frequency of pulsatile LH secretions, and opiate blockade inhibits this effect.[24,25]

Catecholamines that arise in central neurons probably are important in the control of GnRH, although relatively few data supporting this concept are available for humans. Available evidence suggests that, in general, norepinephrine is stimulatory to GnRH secretion, and dopamine may be inhibitory, but further work is necessary, particularly studies on the effects of different steroidal milieux.[26] The roles of other neurotransmitters, including serotonin, γ-aminobutyric acid, and epinephrine, in the physiology of GnRH secretion are even less clear. Prolactin and glucocorticoids may exert inhibitory effects.

Gonadal steroids exert profound effects on gonadotropin secretion; in many situations, whether these effects are exerted at a hypothalamic or a pituitary level is difficult to ascertain. However, a change in the frequency of pulsatile LH secretion is generally assumed to reflect an effect on the hypothalamus, because the frequency of LH pulses closely mimics that of GnRH pulses. In studies based on this assumption, progesterone has been demonstrated to have an inhibitory effect on GnRH, converting the normally rapid LH pulses of the follicular phase to the much slower frequency characteristic of the luteal phase.[23] Similarly, testosterone administration leads to markedly slower LH pulse frequency in men, presumably through a hypothalamic effect.[24] Estradiol exerts both inhibitory and stimulatory effects, depending on the level and duration of exposure.

### EFFECTS OF LUTEINIZING HORMONE–RELEASING HORMONE ON GONADOTROPES

GnRH plays a central role in the biology of reproduction. GnRH interacts with high-affinity receptors on gonadotrope cells of the anterior pituitary. The GnRH receptor belongs to the family of seven transmembrane domain receptors, interacting on ligand binding with Gq.[27] This leads sequentially to activation of different phospholipases and release of free $Ca^{2+}$ and lipid-derived molecules as second messengers.[28] Activation of plasma membrane

$Ca^{2+}$ channels, mobilization of $Ca^{2+}$ from intracellular stores, and activation of calmodulin-stimulated cell responses play an important role in GnRH action.[29] In addition, the activation of phospholipase C (PL-C) is an early response, followed by those of phospholipase A-2 (PLA-2) and phospholipase D (PLD). Generation of second messengers inositol-1,4,5-triphosphate and diacylglycerol (DAG) mobilize intracellular pools of $Ca^{2+}$ and activate protein kinase C (PKC). Both $Ca^{2+}$-dependent conventional and $CA^{2+}$ independent novel PK isoforms are activated during this process. Arachidonic acid (AA), liberated by activated PLA-2, also participates in PKC activation. Crosstalk between $Ca^{2+}$, AA, and selected lipoxygenase products (e.g., leukotriene $C_4$), and the different PKC isoforms might generate compartmentalized signal transduction cascades on GnRH stimulation of the gonadotrope-producing cells. These include the mitogen-activated protein kinase (MAPK) cascade. Activation of c-jun and c-fos by GnRH stimulation can participate in transcriptional regulation through formation of the transcription factor AP-1. At least partly dissimilar signal transduction systems mediate the GnRH-stimulated acute secretion of gonadotropins and the more prolonged stimulation of new gonadotropin synthesis.

The events previously described lead to changes in intracellular protein kinase levels that are thought to be important in stimulating gonadotropin secretion and synthesis, although the detailed mechanisms of these stimulatory effects are unknown (see Chap. 4). Gonadotropin synthesis occurs through the classic process of ribosomal formation of peptide chains, followed by posttranslational modifications in the endoplasmic reticulum and Golgi apparatus (see Chap. 3). These modifications include cleavage of segments off the amino terminus of both the α and β subunits and the subsequent addition of carbohydrate moieties to form the mature gonadotropin molecules in the secretory granules. After synthesis and storage in granules, gonadotropins are available for release almost immediately after GnRH stimulation. After exocytosis, the gonadotropins diffuse rapidly into the nearby capillaries and appear in the venous effluent of the pituitary.

## THERAPEUTIC USEFULNESS OF LUTEINIZING HORMONE–RELEASING HORMONE

GnRH and its agonist analogs are important in the treatment of GnRH deficiency states, including menstrual and fertility disorders in women (see Chaps. 96 and 97) and hypothalamic causes of hypogonadism in men, such as Kallmann syndrome (see Chap. 115). However, GnRH infusion tests rarely give diagnostic information beyond that obtainable by measuring basal gonadotropin and gonadal steroid levels.

### PULSATILE VERSUS CONTINUOUS ADMINISTRATION[30]

Gonadotropin secretion does not follow the GnRH input signal exactly, particularly when GnRH is administered in a nonphysiologic pattern. Soon after GnRH became available for experimental use, researchers noted that continuous administration of this hormone (e.g., by constant intravenous infusion) did not lead to constant LH output but rather to a biphasic pattern of increase, implying that two pools of releasable hormone existed.[31] After the maximal response, a decline was seen in LH responsiveness that could not be explained by gonadal inhibitory feedback.[32] Pulsatile administration of GnRH was observed to cause persistent pulsatile secretion of LH, whereas continuous GnRH infusion caused a desensitization of pituitary responsiveness.[33] Continuous high-dose administration of GnRH over several days leads to almost complete failure of the ability of the pituitary to respond to GnRH secreted endogenously, yielding an experimentally induced hypogonadotropic hypogonadal state.[34]

## LUTEINIZING HORMONE–RELEASING HORMONE AGONISTS

The ability of continuous GnRH administration to inhibit pituitary gonadotropin production has been expanded greatly with the use of GnRH agonists (see Fig. 16-2).[35] Once-daily administration of the agonist analogs results in several days of increased gonadotropin secretion, followed by desensitization and a hypogonadotropic state with very low levels of gonadotropin and gonadal steroid production, or "medical castration." Such agonists have proved useful[36] in the treatment of many conditions, such as prostate cancer (Chap. 225), endometriosis (Chap. 98), precocious puberty (Chap. 92), uterine leiomyomas,[37] breast cancer, polycystic ovarian disease, cyclic porphyria, and acne, and for ovulation suppression and in vitro fertilization. Potentially useful applications include male contraception and the treatment of benign prostatic hypertrophy.

## LUTEINIZING HORMONE–RELEASING HORMONE ANTAGONISTS

Antagonist analogs of GnRH are undergoing active development.[35] These substances bind to GnRH receptors in the pituitary without stimulating gonadotropin secretion and block the effect of endogenous GnRH. Unlike GnRH agonists, they are immediately inhibitory, a potential advantage in the treatment of hormonally dependent conditions, such as prostate cancer. Antagonists may also prove superior to agonists in situations in which total gonadotropin inhibition is required, such as male contraceptive development, because even low levels of LH and FSH can partially support spermatogenesis.[38,39] In nonhuman primate studies, the administration of an GnRH antagonist, together with physiologic replacement dosages of testosterone (because the animals would otherwise be androgen deficient), reliably eliminates spermatogenesis.[40] Because the suppressive effect of the antagonist appears fully reversible, this combination shows promise for male contraceptive development (see Chap. 123).

## GONADOTROPIN-RELEASING HORMONE–ASSOCIATED PEPTIDE

GnRH (i.e., gonadotropin-releasing hormone) is synthesized in the hypothalamus as a part of a larger peptide, which is cleaved to yield GnRH and a larger fragment called gonadotropin-releasing hormone–associated peptide.[41] Some reports have demonstrated that this peptide stimulates secretion of gonadotropin, particularly FSH, from pituitary cells in vitro and inhibits prolactin secretion. The physiologic role of this peptide remains to be explored, however.

## EFFECTS OF GONADAL HORMONES ON GONADOTROPINS

### GONADAL STEROIDS

Gonadal steroids and proteins exert direct pituitary effects on gonadotropin secretion along with their effects on GnRH secretion. Estradiol, for example, exerts both negative and positive feedback effects directly on the pituitary. Testosterone administration inhibits LH and FSH secretion by a direct pituitary effect in men.[42] This effect is mediated in part by aromatization of testosterone to estradiol in vivo. Progesterone and testosterone also exert direct pituitary effects when studied in vitro, although these steroids have not been studied as definitively in vivo as has estradiol.

### INHIBIN

The major protein hormone product of the gonads is inhibin, a substance that has been studied for over 50 years,[43] and now has been characterized structurally.[44,45] Two 32-kDa forms of the glycoprotein, termed *inhibin A* and *inhibin B* and containing α and β subunits, have been described. Inhibin inhibits pituitary FSH secretion selectively, although at high levels it may also inhibit LH. Inhibin is produced in the Sertoli cells of the testis and in granulosa cells of the ovary, mainly under the stimulatory influence of FSH.[46,54]

The structure of inhibin bears an interesting homology to that of other substances such as transforming growth factor and *antimüllerian hormone*.[44,47] Antimüllerian hormone, also a product of Sertoli cells, leads to regression of the müllerian duct in the male embryo. Interestingly, alternative combinations of the subunits of inhibin (β-β instead of α-β) exert stimulatory effects on FSH secretion in vitro rather than the inhibitory effect of the inhibin molecule.[48,49] These β-β combinations are called *activins*. Whether or not activins are secreted from the gonads, and what their effects might be in vivo, are areas of current research activity. Surprisingly, one of the activins stimulates hemoglobin production in human bone marrow in vitro.[50] Many other effects of this family of substances have been described, including stimulation of early embryonic development and immunologic alterations. Follistatin, another protein produced by the gonads, also inhibits FSH secretion in primates.[51] The precise roles of inhibins, activins, and follistatin in the control of gonadotropin secretion are active areas of investigation.

In women, inhibin A is elevated in the luteal phase of the menstrual cycle, whereas inhibin B is elevated in the follicular phase.[52] Levels of both decline with age, implying a decrease in the quality of the remaining ovarian follicles. Inhibin B provides feedback inhibition of FSH, and a fall in inhibin B predates the oligomenorrhea and increases in FSH that signal menopause. In men, inhibin B is the physiologically important form of inhibin.[53] It exhibits a reciprocal relationship with FSH and a diurnal rhythm that appears to be independent of FSH or testosterone feedback.[54]

## LUTEINIZING HORMONE AND FOLLICLE-STIMULATING HORMONE IN PERIPHERAL BLOOD

LH and FSH circulate in blood predominantly in the monomeric form found in the pituitary gland; little evidence exists for prehormones or smaller active fragments. However, changes in properties, such as the ratio of bioactivity to immunoactivity, have been reported in various states of aging, steroid environments, and GnRH analog administration. Some of these changes are apparently due to inaccuracies in determination of gonadotropin immunoreactivity.[55] In monkeys, ovariectomy leads to a slight increase in molecular size and a decrease in the clearance rate of LH and FSH, which can be reversed by estrogen treatment. In aging men, the ratios of bioactivity to immunoactivity for both LH and FSH decrease.[56,57] During GnRH antagonist administration, FSH bioactivity decreases much more quickly than does immunoactivity. This phenomenon has been explained by the demonstration of FSH isoforms in human serum that block the bioeffect of FSH on the gonads.[58] Apparently, the secretion of these isoforms is stimulated by the GnRH antagonist. In all these situations, the conventional radioimmunoassays yield inaccurate assessments of the level of bioactive gonadotropins in blood. This error can be usually eliminated by use of two-site immunoassays.

### CLEARANCE

The gonadotropins are cleared from the blood by both the kidney and the liver. Small amounts are also bound to the gonads, but this accounts for little of the hormone clearance. Some 10%

to 20% of the hormone appears in a bioactive form in urine; most is metabolized in the hepatic and renal parenchyma. The half-life of FSH (4 to 5 hours) is much longer than that of LH (30 to 60 minutes); this is due partly to the higher sialic acid content of FSH, which impairs clearance, particularly by the liver, and partly to the high proportion of sulfated carbohydrate termini in LH, which accelerates its hepatic clearance.[4]

## MEASUREMENT

After the classical in vivo bioassays, the preferred method of gonadotropin measurements used to be radioimmunoassay using polyclonal antiserum. These assays now appear suboptimal due to their low sensitivity and poor specificity; in particular, they are unable to distinguish between low-normal and low levels. The second generation of immunoassays, using the noncompetitive immunometric principle and nonradioactive signaling systems (enzyme, fluorescence, chemiluminescence) are superior in terms of sensitivity and specificity. Gonadotropin concentrations are expressed in terms of partially purified preparations of pituitary or urinary hormones. The use of standards of different purity, and various antisera, leads to different reference ranges reported by individual laboratories and makes their comparisons difficult. This problem will be partly overcome when recombinant gonadotropins are adopted as standards. However, the gonadotropin patterns during physiologic changes, such as aging (see Chap. 199), puberty (see Chap. 91), pregnancy (see Chap. 112), and the menstrual cycle (see Chap. 95), as well as in pathologic conditions, are similar in reports from various laboratories. Most of the antibodies used in LH assays cross-react with hCG, so that LH measurements are artifactually elevated when hCG levels in serum are high, as in pregnancy and choriocarcinoma (see Chaps. 111 and 112). The possible presence of a common genetic variant of LH[59] should be kept in mind, because some commonly used immunoassay methods do not detect this structurally aberrant form of LH.

Sensitive, specific bioassays are now available for the measurement of both LH and FSH in human serum. More time-consuming and difficult to perform than immunoassays, these bioassays are not in common clinical use. In general, bioassays have confirmed the conclusions obtained with immunoassays. Some discrepancies are found, however (see above), and bioassay analysis is indicated when the immunoassay result does not fit the clinical picture.

## GONADAL EFFECTS OF GONADOTROPINS

The only known bioeffects of LH and FSH are in the gonads. LH and FSH stimulate cell growth and maintenance in both the testis and ovary (see Chaps. 94 and 113). As classically defined, LH stimulates steroidogenesis in both sexes, particularly testosterone synthesis, from Leydig cells in the male and from theca cells in the female. FSH stimulates spermatogenesis in the male and follicular development and estradiol secretion in the female. LH also induces ovulation from the mature follicle in the female and exerts a partial stimulatory effect on spermatogenesis in the male, probably mediated through increases in intratesticular levels of testosterone. LH and FSH were named for their initially described roles in females.

Both gonadotropins act through classic protein hormone–receptor mechanisms, involving a G protein–associated seven-transmembrane domain receptor.[60,61,62] After ligand binding, adenylate cyclase is activated, leading to increases in intracellular cyclic adenosine monophosphate (cAMP), which is the main second messenger involved in gonadotropin action. The cAMP activates protein kinase, and the resulting protein phosphorylation is thought to be important in the cellular effects of the gonadotropins.

In the testis, LH directly stimulates the synthesis of a *steroidogenic acute regulatory (StAR) protein*, which plays a key role in the transfer of cholesterol from the outer to the inner mitochondrial membrane. This is the site of the first step in steroid hormone biosynthesis from cholesterol to pregnenolone. Thereafter, the metabolic steps in the steroidogenic pathway leading to testosterone take place in the smooth endoplasmic reticulum. Testosterone exerts stimulatory effects on Sertoli cells and on spermatogenesis[39] (see Chap. 113). In men, this effect is probably mediated through the stimulatory effect of LH on intratesticular testosterone levels, because LH has no known direct effect on the seminiferous epithelium.

FSH binds to Sertoli cell and spermatogonial membranes in the testis. FSH is the major stimulator of seminiferous tubule growth during development. Because the tubules account for ~80% of the volume of the testis, FSH is of major importance in determining testicular size. FSH is important in the initial maturation of spermatogenesis during puberty; however, adult men can maintain sperm production despite very low blood levels of FSH if LH levels are normal.[39] The total numbers of sperm produced in the absence of FSH are low. Normalization of FSH levels leads to quantitatively normal sperm production.[63] These findings imply that the major physiologic role of FSH in men is to stimulate quantitatively normal levels of spermatogenesis.

Additional descriptions of ovarian and testicular effects of gonadotropins are presented in Chapters 90, 91, 94, 95, and 113.

## ABNORMALITIES OF GONADOTROPIN SECRETION AND ACTION

An outline of the causes of gonadotropin abnormalities is presented in Table 16-1. Other aspects of the pathophysiology of gonadotropins, as well as detailed discussions of the etiologies, diagnosis, and treatment of gonadotropin abnormalities, are included in Chapters 17, 92, 96, 97, 103, 114, 115. Pituitary tumors that produce gonadotropins are discussed below.

Genetic studies have detected several mutations in the gonadotropin and gonadotropin-receptor genes. The ligand mutations are exclusively of the loss-of-function type, whereas both loss- and gain-of-function mutations have been discovered in the receptor

**TABLE 16-1.**
**Abnormalities of Gonadotropins**

**DECREASED LEVELS**

*Hypothalamic Disease*

Craniopharyngioma

Other tumors (e.g., meningioma, gliomas, hamartoma, pinealoma, germinoma, metastatic)

Infiltrative disease (e.g., sarcoidosis, eosinophilic granuloma, tuberculosis, fungus infection, syphilis, hematologic malignancy)

Trauma

Vascular disease

Radiation therapy

Hypogonadotropic hypogonadism (e.g., Kallmann syndrome)

*Pituitary Disease*

Adenoma, including hemorrhage (pituitary apoplexy)

Infarction: postpartum (Sheehan syndrome), diabetes, arteritis, sickle cell crisis, shock

Metabolic: hemochromatosis, lymphocytic hypophysitis

*Other*

Stress

Anorexia nervosa

Athletic women with low body fat

Steroid abuse

**INCREASED LEVELS**

Paraneoplastic gonadotropin secretion

Precocious puberty

Primary gonadal failure

genes. In the latter, the signal transduction system of the receptor is partially activated in the absence of ligand hormone, resulting in constitutive activation of the hormonal effects. These mutations have been very educational in terms of unraveling certain details of the physiology of gonadotropin action as well as the pathogenesis of certain disorders of reproductive function.

Mutations in the FSH and LH β-subunit genes are extremely rare, probably due to the key role of these hormones in regulation of reproduction; no α-subunit mutations have so far been described. An inactivating LH-β mutation was found to cause absence of Leydig cells, lack of spontaneous puberty, and infertility in a male with normal early sexual differentiation.[64] Two females with homozygous mutations of the FSH-β gene have been described in the literature.[65,66] They both had primary amenorrhea with poor development of secondary sexual characteristics. One azoospermic male with similar mutations in the FSH-β gene has been described.[67] However, he may have suffered from an additional unrelated disturbance of Leydig cell function, because his testosterone level was low, and his LH level was high.

Inactivating LH-receptor mutations[67–69] in genetic males cause pseudohermaphroditism with severe Leydig cell hypoplasia, a finding that indicates a crucial role for the LH receptor in the stimulation of fetal testicular testosterone production and male sexual differentiation. In females, the phenotype of these mutations is anovulatory infertility and hypoestrogenism.[69,70]

An inactivating mutation in the FSH-receptor gene, an Ala→Val point mutation at position 198, has been detected in the extracellular domain of the receptor.[71] The homozygous females have hypergonadotropic primary or early-onset secondary amenorrhea with arrest of follicular development, a diagnosis often termed *resistant ovary syndrome*. The male phenotype was surprising, because only variable oligo-asthenozoospermia was found in these normally masculinized men, but no azoospermia or complete infertility.[72] This indicates that FSH action is not an absolute requirement for the pubertal initiation and maintenance of spermatogenesis or fertility. However, qualitatively and quantitatively normal spermatogenesis appears to be dependent on FSH action. Partially inactivating mutations of the FSH-receptor gene have been described; the phenotype of these individuals includes secondary amenorrhea, high circulating gonadotropin levels, and arrest of follicular growth at the early antral stage,[73] similar to that of patients with completely inactivating mutations. The role of FSH in ovarian and testicular function as indicated by the inactivating FSH ligand and receptor mutations is corroborated by very similar phenotypes observed in FSH-β[74] and FSH-receptor[75] knock-out mice.

Also, constitutively activating mutations are known for the LH and FSH-receptor genes. The former results in the familial male-limited, gonadotropin-independent, precocious puberty, "testotoxicosis."[76,77] The constitutive activity of the LH-receptor results in onset of testicular testosterone synthesis without LH action. No phenotype has been described in women affected with activation of LH-receptor mutations, apparently because premature LH activation has no effects on ovarian function without previous FSH priming, or because the prepubertal ovary does not express the LH receptor.

One case of a possible activating FSH-receptor mutation has been described in a male.[78] The subject was a male who had been hypophysectomized due to pituitary adenoma. Despite unmeasurable gonadotropin levels, he had persistently normal spermatogenesis. A mutation was found in his FSH-receptor gene, resulting in marginal constitutive activation of the FSH-receptor and probably in maintenance of spermatogenesis in the absence of FSH.

## GONADOTROPE ADENOMAS OF THE PITUITARY

Many pituitary adenomas, previously classified as nonfunctional, produce gonadotropins or their subunits.[79] Indeed, as many as

**TABLE 16-2.**
**Gonadotrope Adenomas of the Pituitary**

**PRESENTATION**

  **Mass effects:** Visual impairment, headache, radiologic evidence of a mass

  **Hormonal effects:** Oligomenorrhea or amenorrhea, male hypogonadism, rarely precocious puberty

**DIAGNOSTIC EVALUATION**

  **Mass effects:** Visual fields and acuity, magnetic resonance imaging of sella turcica and surrounding areas

  **Hormonal studies:** In a man with a macroadenoma, basal follicle-stimulating hormone (FSH), luteinizing hormone (LH), α subunit (LH-β and FSH-β if available); consider thyrotropin-releasing hormone stimulation test with measurement of same hormones. In a woman, measurement of FSH levels is not useful after menopause.

**THERAPY**

  Transsphenoidal surgery

  Radiation may be helpful to prevent recurrence

40% to 50% of all macroadenomas may originate in gonadotropes.[80] These tumors (Table 16-2) are generally recognized because of mass effects, such as visual impairment, headache, or the findings of sellar enlargement and pituitary mass on radiologic examination. The gonadotropins and their subunits that are produced only uncommonly lead to a clinical syndrome, partly explaining why these tumors were previously thought to be nonfunctional. Gonadotropin subunits have no known bioeffects, and the intact hormones are rarely produced in sufficient amount to cause a clinical syndrome. In fact, paradoxically, deficiencies of pituitary hormone secretion, especially of LH, are more commonly found, because the tumor mass compresses the normal pituitary, thereby impairing normal hormone production.

The hormones produced by gonadotrope adenomas are, in decreasing order of frequency, FSH, LH, α subunit, and LH-β subunit. The elevations may be small, however, and could easily be mistaken for the elevations seen in mild primary hypogonadism. The administration of thyrotropin-releasing hormone can sometimes be useful because, in normal subjects, this hormone only rarely increases the secretion of gonadotropins or their subunits, whereas it may stimulate the secretion of these substances in patients with gonadotrope adenomas.[81]

Magnetic resonance imaging evaluation is important in assessing the existence and extent of a gonadotrope adenoma. In addition, magnetic resonance imaging is helpful in determining the position of the optic chiasm, the possibility of hemorrhage in the pituitary, and the differentiation of an adenoma from an aneurysm. Management also should include a thorough evaluation of pituitary function, including thyroid and glucocorticoid axes, as well as the exclusion of a prolactinoma, because these tumors may be treated medically.

Therapy for gonadotrope adenomas has been reviewed.[82] Gonadotrope adenomas are principally treated with resection via the transsphenoidal approach. Indications for surgery include visual field and other neurologic deficits. Improvements are seen in as many as 90% of cases.[83] Irradiation can be used in patients with residual tumor after initial surgery to prevent recurrence, in patients who are poor surgical candidates, or in those whose tumors are surgically inaccessible; however, the incidence of pituitary dysfunction afterward is significant.[84] Medical therapies, such as administration of GnRH antagonists and somatostatin analogs, have been reported to decrease hormone levels; however, they do not cause regression of tumor size. Their role is probably limited to treating patients with aggressive tumors for whom other therapies have failed.

## REFERENCES

1. Bousfield GR, Perry WM, Ward DN. Gonadotropins: chemistry and biosynthesis. In: Knobil E, Neill JD, eds. The physiology of reproduction. New York: Raven Press, 1994:1749.

2. Gharib SD, Wierman ME, Shupnik MW, et al. Molecular biology of the pituitary gonadotropins. Endocr Rev 1990; 11:177.
3. Ulloa-Aguirre A, Midgley AR Jr, Beitins IZ, Padmanabhan V. Follicle-stimulating isohormones: characterization and physiological relevance. Endocr Rev 1995; 16:765.
4. Fiete D, Srivastava V, Hindsgaul O, Baenziger JU. A hepatic reticuloendothelial cell receptor specific for SO4-4GalNAc beta 1, 4GLcNAc beta 1,2Man alpha that mediates rapid clearance of lutropin. Cell 1991; 67:1103.
5. Van Hall EW, Vaitukaitis GT, Ross GT, et al. Effects of progressive desialylation on the rate of disappearance of immunoreactive hCG from plasma in rats. Endocrinology 1971; 89:11.
6. Dufau ML, Catt KJ, Tsuruhara T. Retention of in vitro biological activities by desialylated human luteinizing hormone and chorionic gonadotropin. Biochem Biophys Res Commun 1971; 44:1022.
7. Manjunath P, Sairam MR. Biochemical, biological and immunological properties of chemically deglycosylated human choriogonadotropin. J Biol Chem 1982; 257:7109.
8. Fiddes JC, Goodman HM. The gene encoding the common alpha subunit of the four human glycoprotein hormones. J Mol Appl Genet 1981; 1:3.
9. Talmadge K, Vamvakopoulos NC, Fiddes JC. Evolution of the genes for the beta subunits of human chorionic gonadotropin and luteinizing hormone. Nature 1984; 307:37.
10. Powell-Jackson J, Weller RO, Kennedy P, et al. Creutzfeldt-Jakob disease after administration of human growth hormone. Lancet 1985; 2:244.
11. LeCotonnec J-Y, Porchet HC, Beltrami V, et al. Clinical pharmacology of recombinant human follicle-stimulating hormone (FSH). 1. Comparative pharmacokinetics with urinary FSH. Fertil Steril 1994; 61:669.
12. Pelletier G, Robert F, Hardy J. Identification of human anterior pituitary cells by immunoelectron microscopy. J Clin Endocrinol Metab 1978; 46:534.
13. Seminara SB, Hayes FJ, Crowley WF Jr. Gonadotropin-releasing hormone deficiency in the human (idiopathic hypogonadotropic hypogonadism and Kallmann's syndrome): pathophysiological and genetic considerations. Endocr Rev 1998; 19:521.
14. De Roux N, Young J, Misrahi M, et al. A family with hypogonadotropic hypogonadism and mutations in the gonadotropin-releasing hormone receptor. N Engl J Med 1997; 337:1597.
15. Barry J. Immunofluorescence study for LRF neurons in man. Cell Tissue Res 1977; 181:1.
16. King JC, Anthony ELP. GnRH neurons and their projections in humans and other mammals. Peptides 1984; 5(Suppl 1):195.
17. Clarke IJ, Cummins JT. The temporal relationship between gonadotropin releasing hormone (GnRH) and luteinizing hormone (LH) secretion in ovariectomized ewes. Endocrinology 1982; 111:1737.
18. Wilson RC, Kesner JS, Kaufman J-M, et al. Central electrophysiologic correlates of pulsatile luteinizing hormone secretion in the rhesus monkey. Neuroendocrinology 1984; 39:256.
19. Reid RL, Hoff JD, Yen SSC, Li CH. Effects on pituitary hormone secretion and disappearance rates of exogenous β-endorphin in normal human subjects. J Clin Endocrinol Metab 1981; 51:1179.
20. Ropert JR, Quigley ME, Yen SSC. Endogenous opiates modulate pulsatile LH release in humans. J Clin Endocrinol Metab 1981; 52:583.
21. Reid RL, Quigley ME, Yen SSC. The disappearance of opioidergic regulation of gonadotropin secretion in postmenopausal women. J Clin Endocrinol Metab 1983; 57:1107.
22. Wehrenberg WB, Wardlaw SL, Frantz AG, Ferin M. β-Endorphin in hypophyseal portal blood: variations throughout the menstrual cycle. Endocrinology 1982; 111:879.
23. Soules MR, Steiner RA, Clifton DK, et al. Progesterone modulation of pulsatile luteinizing hormone secretion in normal women. J Clin Endocrinol Metab 1984; 58:378.
24. Matsumoto AM, Bremner WJ. Modulation of pulsatile gonadotropin secretion by testosterone in men. J Clin Endocrinol Metab 1984; 58:378.
25. Veldhuis JD, Rogol AD, Samojlik E, Ertel NH. Role of endogenous opiates in the expression of negative feedback actions of androgens and estrogens on pulsatile properties of luteinizing hormone secretion in man. J Clin Invest 1984; 74:47.
26. Barraclough CA, Wise PM. The role of catecholamines in the regulation of pituitary luteinizing hormone and follicle-stimulating hormone secretion. Endocr Rev 1982; 3:91.
27. Sealfon SC, Weinstein H, Millar RP. Molecular mechanisms of ligand interaction with the gonadotropin-releasing hormone receptor. Endocr Rev 1997; 18:180.
28. Conn PM. Gonadotropin-releasing hormone action. In: Adashi EY, Rock JA, Rosenwaks Z, eds. Reproductive endocrinology, surgery and technology. Philadelphia: Lippincott–Raven, 1996:163.
29. Naor Z, Harris D, Shacham S. Mechanism of GnRH receptor signaling: combinatorial cross-talk of Ca²⁺ and protein kinase C. Front Neuroendocrinol 1998; 19:1.
30. Urban RJ, Evans WS, Rogol AO, et al. Contemporary aspects of discrete peak-detection algorithms. 1. The paradigm of the luteinizing hormone pulse signal in men. Endocr Rev 1988; 9:3.
31. Bremner WJ, Paulsen CA. Two pools of luteinizing hormone in the human pituitary: evidence from constant administration of luteinizing hormone-releasing hormone. J Clin Endocrinol Metab 1974; 39:811.
32. Bremner WJ, Findlay JK, Lee VWK, et al. Feedback effects of the testis on pituitary responsiveness to GnRH infusions in the ram. Endocrinology 1980; 106:329.
33. Belchetz PE, Plant TM, Nakai Y, et al. Hypophysial responses to continuous and intermittent delivery of hypothalamic gonadotropin-releasing hormone. Science 1978; 202:631.
34. Veldhuis JD. Pathophysiologic features of episodic gonadotropin secretion in man. Clin Res 1988; 35:11.
35. Pechstein B, Nagaraja NV, Hermann R, et al. Pharmacokinetic-pharmacodynamic modeling of testosterone and luteinizing hormone suppression by cetrorelix in healthy volunteers. J Clin Pharmacol 2000; 40:266.
36. Vickery BH. Comparison of the potential for therapeutic utilities with gonadotropin-releasing hormone agonists and antagonists. Endocr Rev 1986; 7:115.
37. Friedman AF, Harrison-Atlas D, Barbieri RL. A randomized, placebo-controlled, double-blind study evaluating the efficacy of leuprolide acetate depot in the treatment of uterine leiomyomata. Fertil Steril 1989; 51:251.
38. Matsumoto AM, Karpas AE, Paulsen CA, et al. Reinitiation of sperm production in gonadotropin-suppressed normal men by administration of follicle stimulating hormone. J Clin Invest 1983; 72:1005.
39. Matsumoto AM, Paulsen CA, Bremner WJ. Stimulation of sperm production in gonadotropin-suppressed normal men by physiological dosages of human luteinizing hormone. J Clin Endocrinol Metab 1984; 59:882.
40. Bremner WJ, Bagatell CJ, Steiner RA. Gonadotropin-releasing hormone antagonist plus testosterone: a potential male contraceptive. J Clin Endocrinol Metab 1991; 73:465.
41. Nikolics K, Mason AJ, Szonyi E, et al. A prolactin-inhibiting factor within the precursor for human gonadotropin-releasing hormone. Nature 1985; 316:512.
42. Sheckter CB, Matsumoto AM, Bremner WJ. Testosterone administration inhibits gonadotropin secretion by an effect on the human pituitary. J Clin Endocrinol Metab 1989; 68:397.
43. Baker HWG, Bremner WJ, Burger HG, et al. Testicular control of FSH secretion. Recent Prog Horm Res 1977; 32:429.
44. Mason AJ, Hayflick JS, Ling N, et al. Complementary DNA sequences of ovarian follicular fluid inhibin show precursor structure and homology with transforming growth factor B. Nature 1985; 318:659.
45. Forage RG, Ring JM, Brown RW, et al. Cloning and sequence analysis of cDNA species encoding for the two subunits of inhibin from bovine follicular fluid. Proc Natl Acad Sci U S A 1986; 83:3091.
46. McLachlan RI, Matsumoto AM, Burger HG, et al. The relative roles of follicle-stimulating hormone and luteinizing hormone in the control of inhibin secretion in normal men. J Clin Invest 1988; 82:880.
47. Cate RL, Mattaliano RJ, Hession C, et al. Isolation of the bovine and human genes for müllerian inhibiting substance and expression of the human gene in animal cells. Cell 1986; 45:685.
48. Vale W, Rivier J, Vaughan J, et al. Purification and characterization of an FSH releasing protein from ovarian follicular fluid. Nature 1986; 321:776.
49. Ling N, Ying S-Y, Ueno N, et al. Pituitary FSH is released by a heterodimer of the β-subunits from the two forms of inhibin. Nature 1986; 321:779.
50. Yu J, Shao L, Lemas V, et al. Importance of FSH-releasing protein and inhibin in erythrodifferentiation. Nature 1987; 330:765.
51. Meriggiola MC, Dahl KD, Mather JP, Bremner WJ. Follistatin decreases activin-stimulated FSH secretion with no effect on GnRH-stimulated FSH secretion in prepubertal male monkeys. Endocrinology 1994; 134:1967.
52. Klein N, Illingworth P, Groome NP, et al. Decreased inhibin-B secretion is associated with the monotropic rise in older ovulatory women: a study of serum and follicular fluid inhibin-A and B levels in spontaneous menstrual cycles. J Clin Endocrinol Metab 1996; 81:2742.
53. Anawalt BD, Bebb RA, Matsumoto AM, et al. Serum inhibin B levels reflect Sertoli cell function in normal men with testicular dysfunction. J Clin Endocrinol Metab 1996; 81:3341.
54. Carlsen E, Olsson C, Petersen JH, et al. Diurnal rhythm in serum levels of inhibin B in normal men: relation to testicular steroids and gonadotropins. J Clin Endocrinol Metab 1999; 84:1664.
55. Jaakkola T, Ding Y-Q, Kellokumpu-Lehtinen P, et al. The ratios of serum bioactive/immunoreactive LH and FSH in various conditions with increased and decreased gonadotropin secretion: re-evaluation by ultrasensitive immunometric assay. J Clin Endocrinol Metab 1990:1496.
56. Warner BA, Dufau M, Santen RJ. Effects of aging and illness on the pituitary testicular axis in men: qualitative as well as quantitative changes in luteinizing hormone. J Clin Endocrinol Metab 1985; 60:263.
57. Tenover JS, Dahl KD, Hsueh AJW, et al. Serum bioactive and immunoreactive follicle-stimulating hormone levels and the response to clomiphene in healthy young and elderly men. J Clin Endocrinol Metab 1987; 64:1103.
58. Dahl KD, Bicsak TA, Hsueh AJW. Naturally occurring antihormones: secretion of FSH antagonists by women treated with a GnRH analog. Science 1988; 239:72.
59. Huhtaniemi I, Pettersson K. Mutations and polymorphisms in gonadotropin subunit genes: clinical relevance. Clin Endocr (Oxf) 1998; 48:675.
60. Catt KJ, Harwood JP, Clayton RN, et al. Regulation of peptide hormone receptors and gonadal steroidogenesis. Recent Prog Horm Res 1980; 36:557.
61. Segaloff DL, Ascoli M. The lutropin/choriogonadotropin receptor 4 years later. Endocr Rev 1993; 14:1496.
62. Simoni M, Gromoll J, Nieschlag E. The follicle-stimulating hormone receptor: biochemistry, molecular biology, physiology and pathophysiology. Endocr Rev 1997; 18:739.
63. Matsumoto AM, Karpas AE, Bremner WJ. Chronic human chorionic gonadotropin administration in normal men: evidence that follicle-stimulating hormone is necessary for the maintenance of quantitatively normal spermatogenesis in man. J Clin Endocrinol Metab 1986; 62:1184.

64. Weiss J, Axelrod L, Whitcomb RW, et al. Hypogonadism caused by a single amino acid substitution in the β subunit of luteinizing hormone. N Engl J Med 1992; 326:179.
65. Matthews CH, Borgato S, Beck-Peccoz P, et al. Primary amenorrhea and infertility due to a mutation in the β-subunit of follicle stimulating hormone. Nat Genet 1993; 5:83.
66. Layman LC, Lee E-J, Peak DB, et al. Delayed puberty and hypogonadism caused by mutations in the follicle-stimulating hormone β-subunit gene. N Engl J Med 1997; 337:607.
67. Phillip M, Arbelle JE, Segev Y, Parvari R. Male hypogonadism due to a mutation in the gene for the β-subunit of follicle-stimulating hormone. N Engl J Med 1998; 338:1729.
68. Kremer H, Kraaij R, Toledo SPA, et al. Male pseudohermaphroditism due to a homozygous missense mutation of the luteinizing hormone receptor gene. Nat Genet 1995; 9:10.
69. Latronico AC, Anasti J, Amhold I, et al. Testicular and ovarian resistance to luteinizing hormone caused by inactivating mutations of the luteinizing hormone-receptor gene. N Engl J Med 1996; 334:507.
70. Toledo SP, Brunner HG, Kraaij R, et al. An inactivating mutation of the luteinizing hormone receptor causes amenorrhea in a 46,XX female. J Clin Endocrinol Metab 1996; 81:3850.
71. Aittomäki K, Dieguez-Lucena JL, Pakarinen P, et al. Mutation in the follicle-stimulating hormone receptor gene causes hereditary hypergonadotropic ovarian failure. Cell 1995; 82:959.
72. Tapanainen JS, Aittomäki K, Jiang M, et al. Men homozygous for an inactivating mutation of the follicle-stimulating hormone (FSH) receptor gene present variable suppression of spermatogenesis and fertility. Nat Genet 1997; 15:205.
73. Beau I, Touraine P, Meduri G, et al. A novel phenotype related to partial loss of function mutations of the FSH receptor. J Clin Invest 1998; 102:1352.
74. Kumar TR, Wang L, Lu N, Matzuk MM. Follicle-stimulating hormone is required for ovarian follicle maturation but not male fertility. Nat Genet 1997; 15:201.
75. Dierich A, Sairam MR, Monaco L, et al. Impairing follicle-stimulating hormone (FSH) signaling in vivo: targeted disruption of the FSH receptor leads to aberrant gametogenesis and hormonal imbalance. Proc Natl Acad Sci U S A 1998; 95:13612.
76. Kremer H, Mariman E, Otten BJ, et al. Co-segregation of missense mutations of the luteinizing hormone receptor gene with familial male-limited precocious puberty. Hum Mol Genet 1993; 2:1779.
77. Shenker A, Laue L, Kosusgi S, et al. A constitutively activating mutation of the luteinizing hormone receptor in familial male precocious puberty. Nature 1993; 365:652.
78. Gromoll J, Simoni M, Neischlag E. An activating mutation of the follicle-stimulating hormone receptor autonomously sustains spermatogenesis in a hypophysectomized man. J Clin Endocrinol Metab 1996; 81:1367.
79. Snyder PJ. Gonadotroph cell adenomas of the pituitary. Endocr Rev 1985; 6:552.
80. Daneshdoost L, Gennarelli TA, Bashey HM, et al. Identification of gonadotroph adenomas in men with clinically nonfunctioning adenomas by the luteinizing hormone beta-subunit response to thyrotropin-releasing hormone. J Clin Endocrinol Metab 1993; 77:1352.
81. Daneshdoost L, Gennarelli TA, Bashey HM, et al. Recognition of gonadotroph adenomas in women. N Engl J Med 1991; 324:589.
82. Shomali ME, Katznelson L. Medical therapy for gonadotroph and thyrotroph tumors. Endocrinol Metab Clin North Am 1999; 28:223.
83. Black PM, Zervas NT, Candia G. Management of large pituitary adenomas by transsphenoidal surgery. Surg Neurol 1998; 29:443.
84. Snyder PJ, Fowble BF, Schatz NJ, et al. Hypopituitarism following radiation therapy of pituitary adenomas. Am J Med 1986; 81:457.

# CHAPTER 17

# HYPOPITUITARISM

JOSEPH J. PINZONE

The pituitary gland comprises anterior and posterior divisions. The anterior pituitary gland secretes adrenocorticotropic hormone (ACTH), thyroid-stimulating hormone (TSH), follicle-stimulating hormone (FSH), luteinizing hormone (LH), growth hormone (GH), and prolactin. The posterior pituitary gland secretes antidiuretic hormone (ADH) and oxytocin. Signs and symptoms of *hypopituitarism* result from reduced secretion of one or more of these hormones. Although some patients have total failure of pituitary function (i.e., *panhypopituitarism*), more commonly, only one or several hormones are deficient (i.e., *partial hypopituitarism*). Deficiency of only one pituitary hormone is

called *selective* or *isolated hypopituitarism*. This chapter will deal primarily with deficiencies of anterior pituitary hormones of adults (see Chaps. 25 and 26 for a more complete discussion of deficiencies of ADH and oxytocin and Chaps. 18 and 198 for pediatric neuroendocrine and GH dysregulation).

The most common selective deficiencies are those of GH or the gonadotropins. In progressive loss of pituitary function, as with a slowly growing pituitary adenoma, TSH, ACTH, and ADH are often the last to be diminished, not uncommonly in that order. Because the causes and manifestations of hypopituitarism are protean, the prevalence of hypopituitarism is difficult to estimate accurately. However, the major cause of hypopituitarism is pituitary tumors. Prevalence of pituitary tumors in the United States was reported to be 22,517, although this is probably an underestimate.[1]

Anterior pituitary hormone deficiencies lead to end-organ failure (e.g., diminished ACTH leads to decreased adrenal cortisol production). Syndromes associated with pituitary hormone insufficiency are termed *secondary* or *central* (e.g., decreased adrenal cortisol production that is due to diminished ACTH secretion is termed *secondary* or *central hypoadrenalism*). Technically, hormone deficiency syndromes resulting from hypothalamic failure should be called *tertiary*, but hypothalamic hormones are not measured in clinical practice. Consequently, conditions resulting from inadequate levels of either hypothalamic or pituitary hormones are referred to as secondary hormone deficiencies.

In general, pituitary hormone levels vary widely throughout the day and are dependent on feedback inhibition by target organ hormones. An exception to this is the maintenance of normal prolactin levels via tonic inhibition of prolactin secretion by dopamine.[2,3] An essential concept in the evaluation of pituitary dysfunction is that except for prolactin, measurement of pituitary hormone levels alone has no role in the diagnosis of pituitary hormone insufficiency. For example, a normal level of TSH does not rule out secondary hypothyroidism. It is important to remember that low thyroid hormone levels should lead to increased levels of TSH. Therefore, a "normal" or frankly low level of TSH in the presence of low thyroid hormone levels may be evidence of secondary hypothyroidism.

A variety of symptoms and signs—resulting from mass lesions (e.g., tumors) affecting the pituitary gland and from pituitary hormone deficiencies—may suggest hypopituitarism. Moreover, manifestations of hypopituitarism are often nonspecific and subtle; recognition is frequently delayed and misdiagnosis is common. The signs and symptoms of hormonal deficiency are inadequately relieved by symptomatic measures but respond well to specific hormone replacement therapy.

## PATHOGENESIS OF HYPOPITUITARISM

Table 17-1 lists many of the causes of hypopituitarism. There are no reliable statistics for the percentage of patients in each subgroup, but pituitary tumors represent the largest single category, and a *pituitary adenoma* (see Chap. 11) is the most common single cause of hypopituitarism in adults.

### TUMORS

Pituitary adenomas originate within the sella from one of the cell types found in the anterior pituitary. They may be secretory, with a resultant increase in the serum concentration of one of the pituitary hormones and evidence of, for example, Cushing syndrome or acromegaly. Alternatively, the adenoma may be *clinically nonfunctioning*, without evidence of hormonal hypersecretion; however, some clinically nonfunctioning tumors secrete hormonal precursors with diminished or absent biologic activity.[4] Even when an adenoma is hypersecretory, concomitant evidence of hypopituitarism is common because of the tumor effects on adjacent nontumorous pituitary tissue. Patients with microadenomas

**TABLE 17-1.**
**Pathogenesis of Hypopituitarism**

**TUMORS**
  Pituitary adenoma
  Craniopharyngioma
  Parasellar tumor (e.g., meningioma, glioma, pinealoma)
  Metastatic (especially lung and breast)
**OTHER MECHANICAL OR COMPRESSIVE LESIONS**
  Empty sella syndrome
  Neurosurgical procedure affecting the hypothalamic or pituitary region
  Head trauma (especially with a basal skull fracture)
  Carotid artery aneurysm impinging on the pituitary
**INFARCTION**
  Sheehan syndrome
  Pituitary apoplexy (bleeding into a preexisting pituitary tumor)
**RADIATION**
  Previous radiotherapy to the pituitary, hypothalamus, or head and neck region
**AUTOIMMUNE**
  Lymphocytic hypophysitis
**INFILTRATIONS AND INFECTIONS**
  Amyloidosis
  Histiocytosis X
  Hemochromatosis
  Idiopathic granulomatous hypophysitis
  Meningitis
  Pyogenic abscess
  Sarcoidosis
  Septic cavernous sinus
  Syphilis
  Tay-Sachs disease
  Tuberculosis
  Viral encephalitis
**MISCELLANEOUS**
  Recent discontinuation of glucocorticoid therapy
  Isolated gonadotropin deficiency (including Kallmann syndrome)
  Isolated growth hormone deficiency
  Idiopathic

(<10 mm) may or may not have hormone deficiencies; they most commonly have diminished gonadotropin secretion.[5,6] At least 30% of patients with macroadenomas (>10 mm) have a deficiency of one or more pituitary hormones, most commonly GH.[1]

*Craniopharyngiomas* (see Chap. 11) may be sellar—or more often, suprasellar—and frequently contain calcifications. These tumors are congenital and may cause growth retardation, diabetes insipidus (DI), or mass-related symptoms. They commonly cause hypopituitarism in children, but symptoms may not appear until adulthood.[7]

Other tumors can occur in the pituitary or hypothalamic area and cause compression and hypopituitarism. Among the many possibilities are meningiomas, gliomas, and metastases, especially from breast and lung cancer. *Pinealomas* (see Chap. 10) are worthy of special mention because they often respond well to radiotherapy. If the computed tomography (CT) or magnetic resonance imaging (MRI) scan shows a tumor in the pineal area, the serum and cerebrospinal fluid should be tested for α-fetoprotein and β-human chorionic gonadotropin, and the cerebrospinal fluid cytology should be checked. In the past, when biopsy of the pineal area was associated with a much greater risk, treatment was customarily initiated based on the previously described tests alone if the results were compatible with the diagnosis of pinealoma. However, these results were sometimes misleading. Biopsies in the pineal area can be done more safely now, and some physicians recommend that the diagnosis be confirmed by biopsy before treatment is initiated.[8]

The mechanisms by which pituitary tumors cause hypopituitarism include mechanical compression of normal pituitary tissue and interference with delivery of hypothalamic hormones to the pituitary via the hypothalamic-hypophysial portal system. In addition, supraphysiologic prolactin levels may diminish hypothalamic gonadotropin-releasing hormone (GnRH) secretion, resulting in decreased gonadotropin secretion and hypogonadism. A patient with a pituitary tumor of any size may have a deficiency of one or any combination of hormones. Therefore, upon diagnosis of a pituitary tumor, before therapy, the hypothalamic–pituitary–adrenal (HPA) axis and hypothalamic–pituitary–thyroid (HPT) axis should be evaluated, and prolactin should be measured. Evaluation of other axes may be undertaken, depending on individual circumstances. Hypopituitarism caused by a pituitary tumor may be reversible; surgical removal of the tumor or shrinkage via medical therapy is often accompanied by return of normal pituitary function. However, treatment of pituitary tumors with surgery or radiotherapy may worsen or cause hypopituitarism.

## OTHER MECHANICAL OR COMPRESSIVE LESIONS

The discovery of an enlarged sella turcica on a skull radiographic film suggests a pituitary tumor. However, the *empty sella syndrome* (see Chaps. 11 and 20) is another common cause of an enlarged sella.[9] The sella may be enlarged and the pituitary gland compressed by pressure from meningeal tissue that has herniated into the sella. Although the pituitary is atrophic and the sella cavity appears empty on radiologic studies, because there is sufficient residual functioning pituitary tissue, the patient is typically endocrinologically normal; nevertheless, hormonal deficiencies occasionally occur. A CT or MRI scan of the head can usually differentiate a pituitary tumor from the empty sella syndrome. Usually no pituitary tumor is present, but there occasionally may be a microadenoma in the residual pituitary tissue.

A *neurosurgical procedure* in the pituitary-hypothalamic region may lead to pituitary tissue destruction and hypopituitarism.[10] Severe *head trauma*, particularly if complicated by a basal skull fracture, may result in interruption of the pituitary stalk and consequent hypopituitarism.[11] Rarely, an intrasellar *carotid artery aneurysm* can cause compression and destruction of pituitary tissue and hypopituitarism.[12]

## INFARCTION

The pituitary gland enlarges during pregnancy, making it more vulnerable to a reduction in blood flow. *Sheehan syndrome* results from ischemic pituitary necrosis, which typically follows an episode of severe hypotension during pregnancy, usually a result of major blood loss at the time of delivery or shortly thereafter.[13] Symptoms are often obvious soon after delivery, but they may be delayed. The patient typically is unable to lactate postpartum and experiences amenorrhea or hypomenorrhea. Hypothyroidism usually occurs, and there may be concomitant hypoadrenalism. Sheehan syndrome has become much less common as obstetric techniques have improved. Rarely, the physician may see similar pituitary necrosis in a male or nonpregnant female patient who presumably has severely compromised pituitary blood flow from, for example, diabetes mellitus or sickle cell disease.

The acute and often dramatic symptoms of *pituitary apoplexy* (see Chap. 11) result from hemorrhagic infarction of a pituitary adenoma; hypopituitarism may result.[14] A pituitary tumor may have been diagnosed previously, or apoplexy may be its first recognized clinical manifestation. The patient may report severe headache and then become comatose; there may be an accompanying loss of vision and ophthalmoplegia from pressure on adjacent neural structures. A head CT scan shows hemorrhage in the pituitary area, and decompressive surgery may be needed on an emergency basis. Occasionally, a pituitary tumor may be totally destroyed by pituitary apoplexy, resulting in remission of hormonal and mechanical effects and cure of hormonal hypersecretion.[14a] An imaging study of a patient with a pituitary tumor may show evidence of old hemorrhage into the tumor, but the patient typically cannot recall any symptoms that might have been associated or may remember a severe headache without other complications. Such limited hemorrhages are much more common than the larger hemorrhages that cause the clinical syndrome of pituitary apoplexy.

Pituitary infarction from any cause may be life threatening; hormone replacement therapy with glucocorticoids and thyroid hormone should not be delayed and should be initiated before diagnosis. Pituitary imaging and neurosurgical consultation should be obtained immediately. With expedient, proper management, most patients do well.

## RADIATION

*Radiotherapy* (see Chap. 22), specifically to the pituitary area or as part of broader treatment of a head or neck tumor, may cause hypopituitarism.[15,16] Radiotherapy-induced hypopituitarism is dose dependent and often delayed. Most patients who receive radiotherapy will go on to develop partial or complete hypopituitarism. However, the length of time from the administration of radiotherapy to the onset of pituitary hormone deficiencies is highly variable. Therefore, patients who have received any form of pituitary or head and neck radiotherapy should undergo evaluation of pituitary function at regular intervals for life. Patients should be educated about symptoms of pituitary hormone deficiency and should be instructed to contact a physician if any of these symptoms develop. Some practitioners recommend evaluation of pituitary hormone axes every 3 months for the first year after radiotherapy and then yearly thereafter.[1] The regular interim visits should include evaluation of the HPA and HPT axes and measurement of prolactin. Axes that are failing but not yet in the abnormal range should be evaluated more frequently, or hormone replacement therapy should be initiated, depending on the clinical situation. In general, practitioners should have a low threshold for initiating hormone replacement therapy.

## AUTOIMMUNE

*Lymphocytic hypophysitis* refers to an autoimmune process that involves the anterior pituitary gland; it is most commonly seen in women in late pregnancy or postpartum, although it may occur in nonpregnant women or in men. There may be clinical signs of a pituitary mass or hypopituitarism, and there may be accompanying evidence of autoimmune disease elsewhere in the endocrine system.[17]

## INFILTRATIONS AND INFECTIONS

Many *infiltrative* or *infectious* processes can occasionally cause anterior or posterior pituitary dysregulation (see Table 17-1 and Chaps. 11 and 213). These diseases usually present with their respective classic signs and symptoms. Occasionally, hypopituitarism is the first, only, or most severe manifestation.

## MISCELLANEOUS

There are several miscellaneous causes of hypopituitarism, including the inevitable *idiopathic* classification.[18] One unfortunately common—although potentially preventable—cause is the *discontinuation of hormone therapy* in someone who has been receiving replacement for a known endocrine deficiency or who has been receiving pharmacologic doses for a nonendocrine disease. Patients taking glucocorticoid replacement therapy for primary or secondary hypoadrenalism have limited or no endogenous glucocorticoid production and should receive larger doses when significant physiologic stress occurs. In particular, pharmacologic (supraphysiologic) doses of glucocorticoids given as therapy for nonendocrine diseases, such as rheumatoid arthritis, may lead to adrenal atrophy and impair one's ability to produce endogenous glucocorticoids. Importantly, patients who

have received pharmacologic doses of glucocorticoids for 2 weeks or more may be at risk for hypoadrenalism, even after the glucocorticoids have been discontinued. After discontinuation, these patients may have the capacity to produce sufficient amounts of endogenous glucocorticoids during normal day-to-day functioning, but have a diminished capacity to produce sufficient glucocorticoids during times of significant physiologic stress for as long as 1 year afterward (see also Chap. 78).

Another category worthy of comment is *Kallmann syndrome* (see Chaps. 16 and 115), a form of isolated gonadotropin deficiency that sometimes can be diagnosed by history alone.[19] Usually, the patient consults a physician because he failed to go through puberty. If a very poor or absent sense of smell has been present since birth, it is likely that the patient has Kallmann syndrome, a congenital and sometimes familial form of hypogonadotropic hypogonadism, which is caused by a developmental failure of neuronal migration of the olfactory neurons and of the neurons responsible for GnRH secretion. Aplasia of the olfactory gyri and absence of the olfactory bulbs and tracts may be detected by MRI scan. This syndrome is not accompanied by a pituitary tumor or by clinical failure of the other pituitary functions. The physician must specifically inquire about the sense of smell, because the patient usually does not volunteer this seemingly insignificant detail. (Because the anosmia or hyposmia is congenital in Kallmann syndrome, a later onset might indicate a tumor, trauma, or sinusitis.) *Selective deficiency of GH* may occur as a familial or sporadic phenomenon (see Chaps. 12 and 198).

## DIAGNOSIS

### GENERAL PRINCIPLES

The history and physical examination (Fig. 17-1; see Tables 17-1 and 17-2) will usually help in the selection of subsequent laboratory studies. Some hormonal deficiencies or even a mass lesion may be inapparent from the history and physical examination alone and can be detected only by an appropriate laboratory and radiologic survey. The laboratory evaluation for

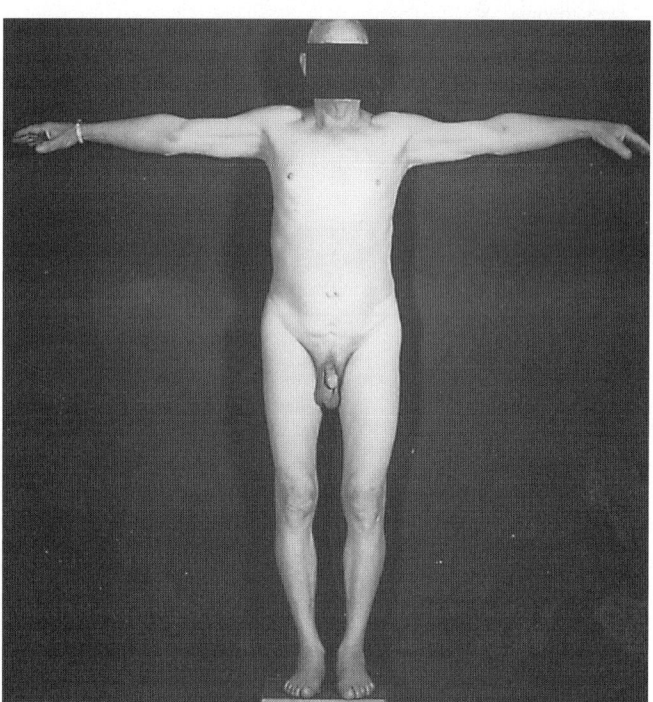

**FIGURE 17-1.** Hypopituitarism. A 55-year-old man with recent-onset hypopituitarism caused by a clinically nonfunctioning pituitary tumor. The skin is pale, and there is an almost total lack of body hair. Test results revealed a deficiency of gonadotropins and thyroid-stimulating hormone.

**TABLE 17-2.**
**Symptoms and Signs of Hypopituitarism**

**SPACE-OCCUPYING LESION OF THE SELLAR OR PARASELLAR REGION**

*SYMPTOMS*
Headache
Visual field defect or diminished visual acuity
Cranial nerve dysfunction
Anosmia
Seizure disorder

*SIGNS*
Visual field abnormalities detected on physical examination or formal testing
Retinal pallor on funduscopy
Cranial nerve palsy

**ADRENOCORTICOTROPIN DEFICIENCY**

*SYMPTOMS*
Weakness
Fatigue
Weight loss
Diminished sense of well-being
Neuroglycopenic symptoms

*SIGNS*
Pale skin, including nipples and areolae, with an inability to tan
Diminished axillary and pubic hair
Postural hypotension with inappropriately slow or normal pulse rate
Shock

**THYROID-STIMULATING HORMONE DEFICIENCY**

*SYMPTOMS*
Cold intolerance
Constipation
Fatigue
Lethargy
Weight gain
Diminished appetite
Slowing of cognitive and motor function
Deepening and hoarseness of the voice
Muscle cramping with symptoms of carpal tunnel syndrome
Menorrhagia

*SIGNS*
Myxedematous appearance
Skin is pale, cool, dry, and doughy
Slow pulse rate with narrowed pulse pressure
Dry coarse hair
Prolonged relaxation phase of deep tendon reflexes
Hypothermia
Hypoglycemia
Stupor
Respiratory depression
Short stature
Cretinism

**GONADOTROPIN DEFICIENCY IN MALES**

*SYMPTOMS*
Decreased libido
Impotence
Infertility
Shaving beard less and decline in the rate of progression of male pattern baldness
Fatigue
Muscle atrophy
Gynecomastia occasionally with galactorrhea
Hyposmia or anosmia
Delayed or interrupted puberty with delayed secondary sexual characteristic development, lack of deepening of voice, no need for deodorant, and concern about social acceptance
History of osteopenia or osteoporosis

*SIGNS*
Pale skin
Decreased axillary, facial, and pubic hair
Gynecomastia, occasionally with expressible galactorrhea
Small, soft testes
Small prostate gland
Persistence of a prepubertal or eunuchoid body habitus, including a small penis and testes

**GONADOTROPIN DEFICIENCY IN FEMALES**

*SYMPTOMS*
Menstrual disturbance, including dysfunctional uterine bleeding, oligomenorrhea, amenorrhea, and infertility
Hot flushes
Diminished libido
Atrophy of breast, vagina, and labia with dyspareunia
Galactorrhea
Failure to lactate postpartum
Delayed or interrupted puberty with delayed secondary sexual characteristics and menstruation, no need for deodorant, and concern about social acceptance
History of osteopenia or osteoporosis

*SIGNS*
Decreased axillary and pubic hair
Breast and genital atrophy
Expressible galactorrhea
Persistence of prepubertal body habitus

**GROWTH HORMONE DEFICIENCY**

*SYMPTOMS*
Increased abdominal adiposity
Reduced muscle mass and strength
Reduced vitality and energy
Depressed or labile mood
Social isolation
History of childhood growth hormone deficiency or short stature
History of osteopenia or osteoporosis

*SIGNS*
Obese with central fat distribution
Thin dry skin
Cool extremities
Short stature

**PROLACTIN DYSREGULATION**

*SYMPTOMS*
Symptoms of hypogonadism (see above), but with more galactorrhea in men and women and more gynecomastia in men
History of premature osteopenia or osteoporosis

*SIGNS*
Signs of hypogonadism (see above), but with more galactorrhea in men and women and more gynecomastia in men

**ANTERIOR PITUITARY HORMONE HYPERSECRETION**

*SYMPTOMS AND SIGNS OF HYPERPROLACTINEMIA*
See above and Chap. 13
*SYMPTOMS AND SIGNS OF CUSHING SYNDROME*
See Chaps. 14 and 75
*SYMPTOMS AND SIGNS OF ACROMEGALY*
See Chap. 12

**VASOPRESSIN DYSREGULATION**

*SYMPTOMS*
Polyuria
Polydipsia if thirst-sensing mechanism is intact

*SIGNS*
Dehydration

hypopituitarism can be divided into initial screening tests and supplemental tests that should be considered if the initial results are abnormal (Table 17-3).

The most effective initial approach to detecting adrenal or gonadal hypofunction is to assay the target gland hormones, even if the underlying defect is thought to be at the pituitary level. The serum concentrations of the target gland hormones are less variable than pituitary hormone levels and are generally more useful for differentiating subnormal from normal target gland function. If any of these target hormone values are diminished, the serum levels of the corresponding pituitary hormones should be measured. Because primary hypothyroidism is commonly seen in clinical practice, and because serum TSH is a very sensitive test used to diagnose primary hypothyroidism, many clinicians are in the habit of measuring TSH to diagnose hypothyroidism. However, if secondary hypothyroidism is suspected, the target gland hormone (free thyroxine [$FT_4$]) should be measured. Evaluation of GH deficiency in adults is typically not

**TABLE 17-3**
Laboratory Evaluation of Hypopituitarism

| Entity Being Evaluated | Initial Screening | Additional Tests |
|---|---|---|
| Thyroid-stimulating hormone (TSH) | Free thyroxine or free thyroxine index | TSH thyrotropin-releasing hormone stimulation |
| Luteinizing hormone (LH), follicle-stimulating hormone (FSH) | Male: total testosterone | Free testosterone |
| | | LH, FSH |
| | | Prolactin |
| | | Semen analysis |
| | Female: estradiol (omit if normal menses by history) | LH, FSH |
| | | Prolactin |
| | | Vaginal cytology |
| Corticotropin (ACTH) | Morning cortisol | Cosyntropin stimulation |
| | | Metyrapone stimulation |
| | | Insulin hypoglycemia |
| Prolactin | Prolactin | |
| Growth hormone | Insulin-like growth factor-I if excess is suspected | |
| Antidiuretic hormone (ADH) | If polyuria, 24-h urine volume and serum sodium | Water restriction test |
| | | ADH assay after dehydration |
| Mass lesion | MRI or CT head scan | Formal visual field examination |
| | | α-subunit measurement |

undertaken unless definite pituitary pathology is documented. Serum prolactin is usually measured as part of any evaluation for hypogonadism or hypopituitarism.

If a target gland hormone is definitely deficient, and the corresponding pituitary hormone concentration is clearly elevated, the diagnosis is primary target-gland failure. If, however, the pituitary hormone value is subnormal, this is consistent with deficiency at the level of the pituitary or hypothalamus. In the presence of frank target gland failure, a normal pituitary hormone concentration in the serum may represent biologically hypoactive hormone.[20]

The tests recommended in Table 17-3 usually provide good discrimination between normal and abnormal endocrine states, but false-positive and false-negative results are seen, often in conjunction with certain medications and diseases. Table 17-4 lists the fac-

**TABLE 17-4.**
Some Causes for Decreased or Increased Hormone Values Other Than Intrinsic Disease of the Respective Endocrine Gland

| Decreased Concentrations | Increased Concentrations* |
|---|---|
| **DECREASED THYROXINE** | **INCREASED THYROXINE** |
| Acromegaly | Amphetamines |
| Anabolic steroids | Clofibrate |
| Androgens | Congenital increased thyroxine-binding globulin |
| Anorexia nervosa | Estrogens (including pregnancy) |
| L-Asparaginase | Euthyroid hyperthyroxinemia |
| Congenital thyroxine-binding globulin deficiency | Liver disease |
| Danazol | Narcotic addiction |
| Dopamine | Perphenazine |
| Euthyroid sick (severe illness) | Porphyria |
| 5-Fluorouracil | **INCREASED CORTISOL** |
| Furosemide (acutely) | Congenital increased cortisol-binding globulin |
| Glucocorticoids | Estrogens (including pregnancy) |
| Halofenate | Hyperthyroidism |
| Liver disease | **INCREASED ESTRADIOL OR TESTOSTERONE** |
| Malnutrition | Estrogens (including pregnancy) |
| Mitotane | Hyperthyroidism |
| Nephrotic syndrome | **INCREASED PROLACTIN** |
| Phenylbutazone | Butyrophenones |
| Phenytoin | Estrogens (including pregnancy) |
| Salicylates (high doses) | Hypocortisolism |
| **DECREASED CORTISOL** | Hypothyroidism |
| Congenital cortisol-binding globulin deficiency | Liver disease |
| Liver disease | Methyldopa |
| Malnutrition | Metoclopramide |
| Nephrotic syndrome | Phenothiazines |
| Renal failure | Renal failure |
| **DECREASED ESTRADIOL OR TESTOSTERONE** | Reserpine |
| Acromegaly | Thioxanthenes |
| Androgens | |
| Hyperprolactinemia | |
| Hypothyroidism | |
| Obesity (massive) | |

*Also possible causes for falsely normal values in the presence of true endocrine hypofunction.

tors that can lower hormone values and cause false-positive diagnoses, and those that raise the hormone values and could obscure a true-positive result. Four general mechanisms account for most of this interference. First, the target gland hormones of the thyroid, adrenal gland, and gonads circulate partially bound to specific carrier proteins; any medication or disease that changes the hepatic synthesis of a carrier protein also changes the concentration of total hormone, even if the hormonally active free fraction remains constant throughout. Second, hypersecretion or hyposecretion of one pituitary hormone may cause a change in the concentration of another pituitary hormone. The latter abnormality disappears when the former is corrected by appropriate therapy. The suppression of gonadotropins by hyperprolactinemia is one example. Another is the increase of serum TSH concentration that occasionally can be seen in untreated primary or secondary hypoadrenalism.[21] Third, diseases that affect urinary excretion (e.g., uremia, nephrotic syndrome) or alter hepatic degradation (e.g., various liver diseases, hypothyroidism)—as well as severe, stressful illness—may alter hormone concentrations. The euthyroid sick syndrome, common in intensive care units or among other similarly stressed patients, mimics the laboratory findings of secondary hypothyroidism.[22] Fourth, some medications are a potential source of error. Phenytoin and high doses of salicylates can bind to the hormonal binding sites on thyroxine ($T_4$) binding proteins; this results in a decrease in total $T_4$ concentration, but the $FT_4$ determination remains unaltered. The information summarized in Table 17-4 can alert the physician to most cases of potential misinterpretation. However, if the clinical picture and the test results do not initially seem to agree, the prudent course is to review both carefully before rejecting either.

All patients with hypopituitarism should have an MRI or CT scan (see Chap. 20). In many cases, an MRI study is preferable, because it provides better anatomic detail, may detect a microadenoma that is not visible on a CT scan, is better able to demonstrate whether a mass lesion is impinging on the chiasm, and can better differentiate an aneurysm from other mass lesions. However, an MRI is more expensive than a CT scan, and in some clinical situations a CT scan is sufficient (e.g., if the only purpose is to rule out a large tumor that would be easily seen with either technique). With current methods, some small pituitary tumors cannot be detected by either imaging method. Absence of a visible mass does not definitively rule out a tumor, and periodic follow-up examinations may be indicated. When MRI or CT is performed, it should be a "dedicated" study with thin sections through the sellar and suprasellar area, performed with and without contrast.[1,23]

If a pituitary mass is found, neuroophthalmologic examination should be conducted by an ophthalmologist, including the determination of visual fields by computerized threshold or Goldmann perimetry (see Chap. 19). Periodic follow-up examinations also may be indicated, as after surgical removal of a pituitary tumor to determine whether there has been a change from the preoperative examination or as one of several ways to monitor a pituitary mass lesion for possible progression.

Additional tests may be indicated when certain specific diagnoses are being considered. In a patient with DI and a negative MRI result with no obvious underlying cause, sarcoidosis should be considered, and a cerebrospinal fluid examination for protein; a chest radiograph; and hepatic, bone marrow, or lymph node biopsy should be performed. Rarely, hemochromatosis (see Chap. 131) or other infiltrative or infectious disease may manifest as hypopituitarism (see Table 17-1). The physician should consider such a possibility and carry out appropriate screening tests if there are clues suggesting one of these conditions.

In a patient with a known pituitary or hypothalamic tumor, some preoperative endocrine testing is indicated, although the neurosurgery may result in further changes in endocrine status (Table 17-5). Hypothyroidism and hypoadrenalism should be sought. Untreated hypothyroidism increases the risk of an operative procedure; it is prudent to consider delaying pituitary exploration until the hypothyroidism is safely corrected.[24]

If hypoadrenalism and hypothyroidism coexist, the hypoadrenalism should be treated before, or along with, any hypothyroidism; restoration to a euthyroid state without correction of concomitant hypoadrenalism sometimes precipitates acute hypoadrenalism with adrenal crisis. If a pituitary tumor is clinically nonfunctioning, the physician may wish to obtain additional tests preoperatively to determine if the tumor is secreting one or more hormonal products that may be clinically silent. Prolactin, FSH, LH, and the α-subunit are all substances that under certain circumstances may fail to produce associated signs or symptoms. The α-subunit is a polypeptide chain that is part of the structures of FSH, LH, and TSH; the serum concentration of free α-subunit is increased above normal if a pituitary tumor secretes this peptide. If hypersecretion of any of these products is found, another measurement later in the course can serve as an additional criterion of the completeness of surgical resection or tumor recurrence. It is especially important to measure prolactin because the first-line therapy of a prolactin-secreting adenoma is usually dopamine agonist therapy and not surgery (see Chap. 13).

After pituitary surgery, close endocrinologic and neurosurgical evaluation is required (see Chap. 23 and Table 17-5). The immediate postoperative period should include measurement of serum sodium and urine-specific gravity at regular intervals, at first several times per day and then less frequently, for as long as 2 weeks after surgery. This regimen should diagnose immediate or delayed onset of DI or the syndrome of inappropriate ADH (SIADH); these conditions may occur with any manipulation of the pituitary or hypothalamus (see Chaps. 25 and 208). Stress doses of glucocorticoid supplementation should have been initiated preoperatively and may be tapered as the patient improves postoperatively. However, maintenance doses of glucocorticoids should continue until adequate functioning of the HPA axis is confirmed. Obviously, replacement of any target gland deficiencies should continue postoperatively. The first follow-up appointment should occur as early as needed, but definitely within the first month after discharge from the hospital. Intervals between subsequent visits during the first year after surgery can be individualized. Each postoperative visit should include a history and physical examination designed to determine the presence of hypopituitarism. Evaluation of HPA and HPT axis function and serum sodium should occur multiple times during the first postoperative year. Evaluation of HPA axis function and management of glucocorticoid therapy after surgery for Cushing disease or Cushing syndrome may be quite complex (see Chaps. 14, 23, and 75). Patients cured of Cushing disease or Cushing syndrome may require a protracted course of glucocorticoid supplementation. Medical therapy of Cushing syndrome may render the patient hypoadrenal, and replacement glucocorticoids and/or mineralocorticoids may be necessary.

The initial evaluation of hypopituitarism (including stimulation and suppression tests, 24-hour urine collections, visual field testing, and head CT or MRI scan) often can be conducted on an outpatient basis, unless the patient is acutely ill at the time of presentation. It is best to start with simple tests of baseline target-organ secretion and then to be selective in applying the many available additional tests. If a pituitary tumor is discovered and surgery is planned, the initial hormonal survey can be limited, and more extensive evaluation can be deferred until after surgery, at which time the need for long-term replacement therapy is determined.

Patients with hypopituitarism should have laboratory tests repeated annually or more often, depending on the clinical situation. In progressive forms of hypopituitarism, testing enables the detection of new deficits before they become symptomatic, and testing also can be used to monitor the adequacy of established hormonal regimens. The evaluation of pituitary and end-organ function is more completely discussed elsewhere (see Chaps. 33, 74, and 114). For long-term surveillance, if hypopituitarism has been caused by a definite or suspected mass lesion, annual visual field testing is usually indicated. The frequency

**TABLE 17-5.**
**Management of Hypopituitarism: Intercurrent Illnesses, Long-Term Follow-Up, and Perioperative Care at the Time of Pituitary Surgery**

**INTERCURRENT ILLNESSES AND LONG-TERM FOLLOW-UP**

Patient should wear medical alert bracelet or necklace and carry card in purse or billfold with diagnosis, endocrine medications, and physicians' names.

Instruct patient to double usual glucocorticoid dose for any vomiting, severe diarrhea, fever of 100°F (37.9°C) or higher, or severe respiratory infection. Divide into three or more doses daily. Continue usual doses of fludrocortisone and other endocrine medications. Do not increase glucocorticoids for headache, mental stress, or mild upper respiratory infection.

Assume that glucocorticoid taken within 1 hour before vomiting is not absorbed, and repeat dose. If repetitive vomiting over several hours interferes with absorption of oral glucocorticoids, seek prompt medical attention for therapy with intravenous glucocorticoids and saline.

If illness causes vomiting or diarrhea, encourage salty liquids.

When illness subsides, promptly decrease to maintenance glucocorticoid doses without tapering. Patient should be allowed to double glucocorticoid dose for illness without telephoning physician, but should contact physician if taking an increased dose for 7 days, or sooner if the patient is concerned.

Schedule routine office visits every 6 to 12 months. Review information concerning management of illness at each visit. Maintain good rapport so that patient will feel free to ask for advice. If patient misses an appointment, attempt to reestablish regular contact or check that the patient is receiving adequate alternative follow-up.

**PERIOPERATIVE CARE FOR SURGERY AFFECTING THE PITUITARY**

*Preoperatively*

Correct hypothyroidism before nonemergency surgery; first correct any concomitant hypoadrenalism. Glucocorticoid deficiency alone can be corrected immediately with treatment, but correction of major thyroid deficiency may take several weeks.

Minimum preoperative laboratory assessment: morning serum cortisol with further testing if value is subnormal, free thyroxine or free thyroxine index, and prolactin. First-line treatment for prolactin-secreting pituitary adenomas is usually dopamine agonist therapy (see Chap. 13).

Obtain formal visual field testing and ophthalmologic evaluation.

Administer hydrocortisone sodium succinate (Solu-Cortef) 100 mg by intravenous bolus or intramuscularly on call to the operating room, plus 100 mg intravenously during the procedure. Do not use cortisone acetate for this purpose because of its delayed onset of action.

*Postoperatively*

Administer hydrocortisone sodium succinate (Solu-Cortef) 25 to 50 mg intravenously every 6 hours initially. Then taper to normal replacement doses over several days to parallel clinical improvement (e.g., for uncomplicated recovery, halve total dose each 24 hours until at replacement levels). When patient can take oral medication without vomiting, give same doses orally. If the surgeon gives large doses of dexamethasone initially to minimize brain edema, this may be tapered to replacement dose.

Residual endogenous hypothalamic–pituitary–adrenal axis functioning may be evaluated by obtaining a serum cortisol measurement at 8:00 a.m., before the morning glucocorticoid dose. This is best done after glucocorticoids have been tapered to replacement doses. (If the patient is on dexamethasone, the serum cortisol will be truly reflective of endogenous cortisol production, because dexamethasone is not detected in the cortisol assay.) Therefore, if the patient has received a large dose of any glucocorticoid (except dexamethasone) within 24 hours before the serum cortisol measurement at 8:00 a.m., there is a risk that some of the exogenous glucocorticoid will be measured in the cortisol assay, invalidating this test. If preoperative adrenal function is normal, the postoperative course uncomplicated, and the residual anterior pituitary tissue thought to be sufficient for normal endocrine function, discontinuation of glucocorticoids for 24 hours, while under observation in the hospital, may allow a morning cortisol to be obtained without interference from exogenous glucocorticoids. In this situation, proper patient selection and close monitoring are of paramount importance. Evaluation of hypothalamic–pituitary–adrenal axis function and management of glucocorticoid therapy after surgery for Cushing disease or Cushing syndrome may be quite complex (see Chaps. 14, 23, and 75). Patients cured of Cushing disease or Cushing syndrome may require a protracted course of glucocorticoid supplementation.

Immediately following surgery, measure serum sodium and urine-specific gravity at regular intervals, at first several times per day and then less frequently, for as long as 2 weeks after surgery. This regimen should diagnose the immediate or delayed onset of diabetes insipidus or the syndrome of inappropriate antidiuretic hormone. For treatment options, see Chaps. 25 and 208.

Replacement of any target gland deficiencies should continue postoperatively. Laboratory assessment should evaluate for any new deficiencies, and elevated hormone levels should be remeasured to determine if cure has been effected.

Obtain postoperative visual field examination, whether or not the preoperative examination was abnormal. Determine timing of postoperative magnetic resonance imaging or computed tomography scanning in cooperation with the neurosurgeon, who should also be following the patient closely.

---

of head CT scanning or MRI is individualized, because both tests are expensive and the former involves radiation and iodide-contrast exposure. During the year immediately after removal of a mass lesion, the neurosurgeon or endocrinologist may wish to obtain more than one scan. If the lesion remains stable, the frequency of MRI or CT scans may revert to annual examinations for 1 or 2 years and then less fequently, unless there is some clinical suggestion of a recurrence. If a secretory tumor has been resected, a later rise in the serum concentration of the relevant hormone is one reason to suspect a recurrence and to repeat the CT or MRI scan.

It is important to recognize when symptoms are not caused by hypopituitarism. Patients with proven hypopituitarism may also develop other, more common conditions with symptoms that may be confused with the nonspecific symptoms of endocrine disease. For instance, anxiety and depression are common, and patients with hypopituitarism are not immune to such problems. In the presence of a new symptom, it should not be automatically assumed that the hormonal regimen should be changed. If endogenous serum hormone concentrations are normal, if the patient is already at the conventional upper limit of hormonal drug dosage, or if the patient has previously been stable on that dosage for many months, another diagnosis should be sought. A careful his-

tory and physical examination should be obtained, and hormone measurements should be repeated and other pertinent tests performed before making any medication changes.

## CLINICAL PRESENTATION AND DIAGNOSTIC TESTS

Patients with hypopituitarism first seek medical attention for relief of symptoms and signs related to (a) a space-occupying lesion in the sella turcica or parasellar region, and/or (b) pituitary hormone dysregulation (see Table 17-2).

### SPACE-OCCUPYING LESION OF THE SELLA TURCICA OR PARASELLAR REGION

In general, the larger the lesion in the sella turcica or parasellar region, the more likely is the lesion to compress surrounding structures, leading to pressure-related phenomena. A patient with a functioning pituitary tumor may present to a clinician with symptoms or signs of hormone excess (see Chaps. 12–16), pressure symptoms, and/or symptoms of diminished pituitary hormone secretion. Most commonly, a patient with a nonfunctioning pituitary tumor or other space-occupying lesion first seeks medical attention for pressure symptoms, even when hormonal deficiencies antedate these phenomena.

Headache, caused by traction on the meningeal membranes, is a common manifestation of a space-occupying sellar lesion. Often, such headaches are nonpulsatile, dull and poorly localized, and difficult or impossible to differentiate from many other forms of headache. Routine radiologic studies cannot be recommended to look for the small percentage of headache patients with pituitary tumors, unless there are additional clues such as new onset, progressive worsening, or incapacitating headaches; or an accompanying hormonal, ophthalmologic, or neurologic abnormality. Space-occupying lesions may compress the optic chiasm and lead to reports of diminished visual acuity or decreased peripheral vision. Further evaluation during the physical examination or by more formal methods of visual field testing may reveal deficits suggesting chiasmal compression (e.g., bitemporal hemianopia, superior lateral quadrantanopia; see Chap. 19).[25] Extraocular muscle paresis caused by pressure on the cranial nerves or nuclei lateral to the sella is seen occasionally. A large lesion can cause hypothalamic symptoms (see Chap. 9) or result in anosmia, seizures, or even symptoms of frontal or temporal lobe dysfunction. Stroke and subarachnoid bleeding are rare but more acute manifestations associated with very large sellar lesions and pituitary apoplexy, both of which may interrupt the sellar or parasellar vasculature.

### PITUITARY HORMONE DYSREGULATION

When a patient is suspected of having definite hypoadrenalism, hypothyroidism, or hypogonadism, the corresponding pituitary hormone should be assayed to determine whether the deficiency is *primary* (i.e., disease of the target gland itself) or *secondary* (i.e., insufficient stimulation of the target gland by the corresponding pituitary hormone). If the relevant pituitary hormone concentration is not clearly elevated, as it should be in the absence of feedback control, but instead is in the normal or subnormal range, a pituitary or hypothalamic cause must be suspected. To more accurately diagnose hypopituitarism, the pituitary hormone value should be checked before hormonal replacement is begun, because the exogenous target gland hormone would suppress the corresponding pituitary hormone. However, treatment, if urgent, need not always wait for the result.

Each anterior pituitary hormone is part of a tightly regulated axis composed of hypothalamic factors and target organ factors. Each component of the axis is involved in feedback regulation of the other components (see Chaps. 12–16). Pituitary hormones can be diminished alone or in combination; therefore, consideration of hypothalamic-pituitary target organ axes individually will provide a logical framework for diagnosing the complex and overlapping manifestations of hypopituitarism.

# ADRENOCORTICOTROPIN DEFICIENCY

The HPA axis is the most crucial and may be the most challenging pituitary axis to evaluate, because symptoms and signs of ACTH and cortisol deficiency are often nonspecific. Selective ACTH deficiency is rare; usually, other pituitary hormones are deficient as well.[26]

### SYMPTOMS

Physiologic effects of cortisol are protean. Consequently, cortisol deficiency often leads to subtle, nonspecific manifestations, but may be life threatening. Symptoms include weakness, fatigue, weight loss, and diminished sense of well-being. If a patient has neuroglycopenic symptoms and documented fasting hypoglycemia, evaluation for ACTH deficiency is indicated, along with a search for other causes (see Chaps. 158 and 161). Abdominal distress, including nausea and vomiting, is often noted. A history of recently discontinued glucocorticoids should be sought.

### SIGNS

Protracted secondary ACTH deficiency may lead to pale skin—including nipples and areolae—with decreased ability to tan. Diminished axillary and pubic hair may occur, especially in women. Postural hypotension is often seen; the pulse rate may be inappropriately normal or slow if concomitant hypothyroidism is present. With more acute hypoadrenalism, or during time of significant physiologic stress, patients may present with shock, which can be resistant to therapy.

### LABORATORY ASSESSMENT

The HPA axis comprises a tightly regulated feedback loop. The hypothalamus secretes corticotropin-releasing hormone (CRH) into the portal circulation, which is transported to the pituitary. There it acts to stimulate ACTH secretion into the peripheral circulation. ACTH stimulates cortisol secretion from the adrenal glands. Cortisol feeds back to inhibit CRH and ACTH secretion. Most cortisol is bound to cortisol-binding globulin (CBG), although the much smaller free or unbound component is the bioactive fraction. Factors that alter CBG production may affect total serum cortisol levels, which may not accurately reflect the free cortisol fraction. Estrogen stimulates hepatic production of CBG, whereas cirrhosis, nephrotic syndrome, and hyperthyroidism may lower CBG. However, in most clinical contexts, the total serum cortisol level is used to determine whether the adrenal glands are functioning properly. Many glucocorticoid preparations cross-react with the cortisol assay and should be avoided within 24 hours of testing.

In secondary hypoadrenalism, ACTH deficiency leads to decreased cortisol production by the adrenals; however, mineralocorticoid production typically remains adequate. Importantly, with most causes of *primary hypoadrenalism*, mineralocorticoid insufficiency is also present. Serum cortisol levels in normal persons and patients with hypoadrenalism often overlap considerably. Normally, serum cortisol levels demonstrate a diurnal variation. Peak cortisol levels usually occur between 6:00 and 8:00 a.m. and nadir at around 10:00 p.m. to midnight. With secondary hypoadrenalism, this diurnal variation may be maintained, but cortisol levels will be lower at any given time throughout the day. If CRH or ACTH secretion is abruptly interrupted, serum cortisol will drop to very low levels, often within hours. Therefore, pituitary apoplexy, Sheehan syndrome, and postoperative ACTH deficiency should be treated as emergent, potentially life-threatening situations. If hypoadrenalism is suspected and the patient is hypotensive, therapy with hydrocortisone, 100 mg intravenously every 8 hours, should not be delayed for diagnostic purposes. However, in this situation, measurement of the serum cortisol and ACTH level just before administration of glucocorticoids will be helpful diagnostically. Although the literature is often conflicting on this subject, one review provided the following guidelines: While a patient is hypotensive, a serum cortisol level ≥18 µg/dL is evidence of adequate HPA axis function. A level of 13 to 18 µg/dL is indeterminate, and hydrocortisone administration should be continued until further testing can be carried out. A serum cortisol level of 5 to 13 µg/dL is presumptive evidence of hypoadrenalism, and a level <5 µg/dL is regarded as definite evidence of hypoadrenalism.[27] If hypoadrenalism is diagnosed, a high ACTH level suggests primary hypoadrenalism, whereas a low or "normal" ACTH level suggests secondary hypoadrenalism.

With patients who are more stable, a variety of diagnostic tests can be utilized to determine whether hypoadrenalism exists. With each of these tests, an ACTH level may be drawn depending on the clinical context. Here, too, a frankly high ACTH level in a hypoadrenal patient would argue for primary hypoadrenalism, whereas a "normal" or low level would argue for secondary hypoadrenalism. The simplest test of the HPA axis is a cortisol level drawn between 6:00 and 8:00 a.m. A value of ≥19 µg/dL indicates an intact HPA axis, whereas a level <3 µg/dL is definite evidence of hypoadrenalism.[27] A value of 3 to 19 µg/dL is indeterminate and requires further testing. Because most patients *with or without hypoadrenalism* will have values in the indeterminate range, this test is of limited value.

The cosyntropin stimulation test is a convenient, safe, and generally reliable dynamic test of the HPA axis. Cosyntropin, the synthetic bioactive portion of ACTH, is injected intravenously at a dose of 250 µg, and serum cortisol is measured at 0, 30, and 60 minutes. A cortisol level ≥18 µg/dL at any point indicates that the adrenal glands can be stimulated adequately.[27] In most situations, this means that the HPA axis is intact. A lower value *might* indicate secondary hypoadrenalism. (See Chaps. 76 and 241 for the use of the ACTH test in primary hypoadrenalism [Addison disease].)

It should be noted that if secondary hypoadrenalism has occurred within the recent past (usually taken to mean the preceding few weeks), atrophy of the adrenal gland, normally seen with ACTH deficiency, may not have had sufficient time to occur. Consequently, endogenous adrenal production of cortisol may be insufficient because of lack of endogenous ACTH, whereas pharmacologically augmented cortisol production using intravenously administered cosyntropin *may still be possible*. Cosyntropin, 250 µg intravenously, is a supraphysiologic stimulus of cortisol production. This has led to interest in the use of ACTH 1 µg intravenously in place of a 250-µg dose as being possibly a more discriminating test of HPA axis integrity.[28]

The most reliable dynamic test of HPA axis function is the insulin tolerance test (ITT). The rationale is that severe hypoglycemia produces maximal physiologic stress and should stimulate the entire HPA axis leading to augmented cortisol production. The test is carried out by administering regular insulin 0.1 to 0.15 U/kg intravenously and measuring serum cortisol and blood glucose levels at 0, 30, and 60 minutes. Blood glucose at 30 and/or 60 minutes must be <40 mg/dL for the test to be valid. A cortisol level ≥18 µg/dL indicates an intact HPA axis, whereas a value <18 µg/dL *may* indicate secondary hypoadrenalism. This test is contraindicated in elderly patients and with patients who have seizures or those with cardiovascular or psychiatric disease. A physician must be present and the intravenous catheter must remain in place with a 50% dextrose solution available in case of hypoglycemia.

The metyrapone test, like the ITT, is a test of the entire HPA axis. Metyrapone blocks 11β-hydroxylase activity in the adrenal gland; 11β-hydroxylase catalyzes the conversion of 11-desoxycortisol (11-S) to cortisol in the final step of the cortisol biosynthetic pathway. Therefore, if metyrapone is given to a normal individual, cortisol production decreases; this stimulates the pituitary to secrete ACTH. ACTH then stimulates the cortisol biosynthetic pathway in the adrenal gland. However, because metyrapone is blocking the final step, 11-S accumulates. Proper functioning of the HPA axis is confirmed by an 11-S value >7.0 µg/dL. In a patient with secondary hypoadrenalism, diminished cortisol does not lead to a rise in ACTH, and the 11-S level remains ≤7 µg/dL. The metyrapone test requires an inpatient stay and may precipitate symptomatic adrenal insufficiency.

A less reliable test of hypoadrenalism, the urine free cortisol (UFC), measures free cortisol in a 24-hour urine collection. This test measures only the amount of cortisol that exceeds the binding capacity of CBG and is excreted in the urine; UFC levels are within the reference range in 20% of patients with hypoadrenalism.[29] In contrast, UFC is a good screening test for cortisol excess (see Chap. 14).

# THYROID-STIMULATING HORMONE DEFICIENCY

Symptoms and signs of secondary hypothyroidism are similar to those seen with primary hypothyroidism, although they often are milder. The essential diagnostic differences relate to interpretation of the results of the laboratory assessment.

## SYMPTOMS

Cold intolerance, constipation, fatigue, and lethargy are common symptoms. Weight gain despite diminished appetite may occur. Patients or family members may note a slowing of cognitive and motor function as well as a deepening and hoarseness of the voice. Muscle cramping, including symptoms of carpal tunnel syndrome, is sometimes present. Women of childbearing years may report menorrhagia.

## SIGNS

On physical examination, a myxedematous appearance with pale, cool skin that appears dry and doughy, and a large protruding tongue may be noted. Pulse rate is often slow and pulse pressure narrowed. Hair may be dry and sparse. Relaxation phase of the reflexes is prolonged. With more advanced hypothyroidism, hypothermia, hypoglycemia, stupor, and respiratory depression may, if left untreated, lead to death. In addition, children may demonstrate other age-dependent manifestations. Congenital hypothyroidism, although rarely of pituitary origin, may lead to cretinism (see Chap. 47). Linear growth may be inhibited in children and adolescents, leading to short stature.

## LABORATORY ASSESSMENT

The hypothalamus releases thyrotropin-releasing hormone (TRH) into the portal circulation. TRH is transported to the pituitary gland, where it causes release of TSH into the peripheral circulation. TSH binds to the thyroid, leading to release of $T_4$ and, to a lesser extent, the bioactive thyroid hormone, triiodothyronine ($T_3$). $T_4$ is converted to $T_3$ in peripheral tissues, including the pituitary. Both $T_4$ and $T_3$ exist primarily bound to thyroid-binding globulin and other blood proteins. The free fractions of $T_4$ and $T_3$ are the clinically important components. Many laboratories now utilize direct measurement of $FT_4$, which is the preferable way to measure serum $T_4$. However, sometimes the total $T_4$ and T uptake are used to calculate a $FT_4$ index ($FT_4I$), which estimates the $FT_4$ by taking into account variations in binding protein levels.

In secondary hypothyroidism, TSH deficiency leads to low levels of $FT_4$. Therefore, an $FT_4$ (or $FT_4I$), as well as a sensitive TSH assay, must be obtained. The $FT_4$ will be low, whereas TSH will be normal or subnormal. In contrast, with primary hypothyroidism, $FT_4$ is diminished but TSH is elevated as a compensatory response. The $T_3$ level can be normal or near normal in early hypothyroidism and is not usually measured as part of the initial workup. The $FT_4$ can differentiate hypothyroidism from most nonthyroidal laboratory abnormalities.[20] However, if the clinical setting suggests the possibility of the euthyroid sick syndrome (see Chap. 36), the $FT_4$ may be low, with a normal or subnormal TSH. This is thought to be a compensatory response that downregulates metabolism during physiologic stress, thereby preventing excessive catabolism. The underlying illness that is causing euthyroid sick syndrome should be treated; therapy with thyroid hormone is not recommended and may be harmful. In this situation, additional tests may be helpful; nevertheless, the clinician should be cautious in diagnosing hypothyroidism secondary to pituitary disease when a patient is experiencing a physically stressful illness or a period of caloric deprivation.

Rarely, a patient with long-standing primary hypothyroidism may develop significant pituitary enlargement and even chiasmal symptoms. Presumably, this occurs from chronic stimulation of the pituitary gland by the negative-feedback mechanism.[30] Furthermore, a patient rarely may have a pituitary tumor that secretes bioactive TSH or may have resistance to thyroid hormone. Both of these conditions can result in elevated or normal serum concentrations of TSH with concomitantly elevated thyroid hormone levels (see Chaps. 21 and 32).

A stimulation test with TRH is sometimes proposed to help differentiate secondary from tertiary (hypothalamic) hypothyroidism, but normal and abnormal results overlap considerably. Hence, this test result is often equivocal and should not be relied on as the sole criterion (see Chap. 33).

## GONADOTROPIN DEFICIENCY IN MEN

Most manifestations of decreased gonadotropin secretion in men are attributable to the resultant low testosterone levels. However, testosterone is converted to estrogens, and some manifestations of low LH and FSH may be due to low estrogen levels. Symptoms and signs of hypogonadism in men may be present for years before being appreciated and often are mistakenly attributed to normal aging. The patient's sexual partner may be the first to notice and, when appropriate, should also be queried about symptoms and signs.

### SYMPTOMS

In men with secondary hypogonadism, decreased libido, impotence, and infertility are common. The patient may note that he shaves less frequently and that there is a decline in the rate of progression of male pattern hair loss. With long-standing hypogonadism, fatigue and a loss of muscularity may be noted. A history of hyposmia or anosmia may be elicited from patients with Kallmann syndrome. If symptoms begin before or during puberty, the patient may demonstrate lack of deepening of the voice, no need for deodorant, and concerns about social acceptance. In some cases, it may be difficult to differentiate hypogonadotropic hypogonadism from delayed puberty (see Chaps. 7, 91, and 92).[31]

### SIGNS

Evidence on physical examination includes pale skin with decreased axillary, facial, and pubic hair. Small, soft testes and a small prostate gland may be noted. In cases where onset was before or during puberty, a small penis and eunuchoid body habitus may be appreciated. Osteopenia and osteoporosis may be associated with hypogonadism from any cause (see Chap. 64).

### LABORATORY ASSESSMENT

GnRH is secreted in a pulsatile fashion into the pituitary portal circulation and is the major regulator of LH secretion. For every pulse of GnRH secreted into the portal circulation, a resultant pulse of LH is secreted into the peripheral circulation. Peripheral LH stimulates testosterone production by the testes. Along with other factors, GnRH also regulates FSH secretion. Spermatogenesis is dependent on testosterone and FSH.

The initial test of this axis should be a serum total testosterone or a serum free testosterone. Testosterone, like $T_4$, is partially bound to serum proteins, and any alteration in the binding proteins also changes the total testosterone level. If a total serum testosterone is obtained initially and is found to be abnormal, this finding should be confirmed with a serum free testosterone measurement (see Chap. 114 for a discussion of free testosterone measurements).[32] Moreover, a low serum testosterone measurement should be followed up with a serum LH and FSH determination. In secondary hypogonadism, LH and FSH levels will be in the normal or subnormal range despite a low total or free testosterone level. In primary hypogonadism, total testosterone and free testosterone levels are low, but LH and FSH levels are elevated as a compensatory response. When viewed by adult norms, normal children have hypogonadotropic values of LH and FSH, and these assays are usually omitted prepubertally. (Hyperprolactinemia is a possible cause of hypogonadotropic hypogonadism, and a determination of prolactin should be part of any laboratory assessment of hypogonadism.) Because a stimulation test with GnRH rarely provides clinically useful information for the individual patient, the author does not currently recommend it as part of routine management (see Chap. 16). If

desired, in adults, testicular function can be evaluated with a semen analysis. Moreover, routine blood work in hypogonadal men may demonstrate a normocytic anemia.

## GONADOTROPIN DEFICIENCY IN WOMEN

Disrupted menstrual function, a very early manifestation of gonadotropin deficiency, often prompts premenopausal women to seek medical attention earlier in the course of hypogonadism than do men.

### SYMPTOMS

In women with secondary hypogonadism, menstrual dysfunction that manifests as dysfunctional uterine bleeding, oligomenorrhea, amenorrhea, or infertility is common. Diminished libido may occur. With persistence of hypogonadism, atrophy of breast tissue and of the vagina and labia may be noted. The latter may lead to dyspareunia. If prolactin is increased, galactorrhea may result. With Sheehan syndrome, failure to lactate postpartum may be noted. Hypogonadism with onset before or during puberty may result in delayed puberty; reports of lack of development of secondary sexual characteristics, including delayed menarche, and concerns about social acceptance may be present.

### SIGNS

Physical examination may reveal decreased axillary and pubic hair, and breast and genital atrophy (as well as expressible galactorrhea, if hyperprolactinemia is present). Osteopenia and osteoporosis are associated with hypogonadism from any cause (see Chap. 64). Signs of hypogonadism in adolescent girls include persistence of prepubertal body habitus with delayed breast, genital, and pubic hair development.

### LABORATORY ASSESSMENT

Peripheral LH stimulates estradiol and to a lesser extent testosterone production by the ovary. Along with other factors, GnRH also regulates FSH secretion. Ovulation is dependent on estradiol and FSH.

In general, no laboratory assessment is necessary if the patient reliably describes entirely normal menstrual cycles; the hormone assays usually are normal if the menses are normal. One exception to this is that hyperprolactinemia may be present even if menses are normal. If the menses are not perfectly normal, a serum estradiol value should be obtained, and if it is low, the physician also should obtain serum FSH, LH, and prolactin concentrations. Postmenopausal women suspected of having hypogonadism should have serum FSH, LH, and prolactin measured. Postmenopausal women typically have increased FSH and LH levels; thus, "normal" or subnormal values are consistent with secondary hypogonadism. Increased prolactin is associated with many causes of hypopituitarism.

## GROWTH HORMONE DEFICIENCY

Extensive research has led to improved characterization of the consequences of GH deficiency in adults and to a better understanding of the risks and benefits of treatment. Patient subgroups include those who have childhood-onset GH deficiency that persists into adulthood and those who have adult-onset GH deficiency. Although the presentation and response to therapy overlap considerably, variation between the subgroups has been noted.[33] The adult-onset subgroup frequently has other concomitant pituitary hormone deficiencies. Both subgroups may exhibit a varied constellation of symptoms and signs, and often have difficult diagnostic and management issues. GH replacement is expensive, requires many resources, and provides variable—

although often profound—benefit to adult patients. Therefore, it is important to identify patients at risk for GH deficiency and prudently utilize confirmatory diagnostic tests on the patients who might be appropriate candidates for GH replacement. Because of the complexity of the diagnostic and management issues surrounding GH deficiency in adults, it is advisable to have an endocrinologist involved throughout the care of these patients.

## SYMPTOMS

Adult patients with GH deficiency may report increased abdominal adiposity and reduced muscle mass that leads to decreased strength, reduced vitality and energy, and a diminished exercise capacity. Impaired psychological well-being is a major component of the GH deficiency syndrome in adults. A depressed and sometimes labile mood, anxiety, and social isolation are common symptoms.[34] Children with GH deficiency may report short stature compared with peers. A history of childhood GH deficiency should be sought in all patients with suspected hypopituitarism.

## SIGNS

Signs are often very subtle and nonspecific. Affect may be depressed or labile. Patients may be obese with centrally distributed fat. Skin may be thin and dry, and extremities may be cool because of poor venous circulation.[34] Parental heights may be used to calculate the predicted height of the patient; this may afford an objective criterion on which to base a diagnosis of short stature in cases of childhood-onset GH deficiency (see Chap. 7).

## LABORATORY ASSESSMENT

The hypothalamus secretes GH-releasing hormone into the pituitary portal circulation. GH-releasing hormone is transported to the pituitary, where it stimulates pulsatile GH secretion into the peripheral circulation. GH acts at liver and other tissues to induce insulin-like growth factor-I (IGF-I) synthesis and secretion. IGF-I is thought to mediate most of the metabolic and growth-enhancing effects of GH (see Chap. 12).

GH levels vary significantly throughout the day, and considerable disagreement exists about what constitutes laboratory confirmation of GH deficiency in adults. One definition of GH deficiency, in a patient with a compatible history, is a negative response to a standard GH stimulation test. A negative response may be taken to mean a peak serum GH of <5 ng/mL when measured by radioimmunoassay using a polyclonal antibody or <2.5 ng/mL when measured by immunoradiometric assay using monoclonal antibodies.[35] Because hypoglycemia stimulates GH secretion, the ITT is a reliable way to detect GH deficiency in adults. Serum samples for GH and glucose are collected every 15 to 30 minutes for 90 minutes after administration of insulin. The same prior-mentioned caveats and patient contraindications apply to the ITT when it is utilized to evaluate for GH deficiency. Other provocative testing agents have been used, including clonidine and arginine. For an outline of GH stimulation tests and a discussion of diagnostic criteria for GH deficiency in children, see Chapters 12, 18, and 198. A serum IGF-I level is not a sensitive and specific test on which, alone, to base the diagnosis of GH deficiency. There are many factors—including a complex set of binding proteins, age, and gender—that determine serum IGF-I levels. A low serum IGF-I value is helpful but not diagnostic, and a normal value does not rule out GH deficiency.

Osteopenia and osteoporosis are more prevalent in adults with GH deficiency; bone densitometry may be helpful as corroborative diagnostic information and to guide therapy. Measurement of plasma lipid and lipoprotein levels often reveals a profile consistent with an increased risk of coronary artery disease.[34] Formal muscle strength, exercise testing, and body composition testing is individualized.

# PROLACTIN DYSREGULATION

Prolactin elevation may occur because of oversecretion by a pituitary adenoma that may or may not be detectable on pituitary imaging. Moreover, several medications and certain physiologic processes may increase prolactin (see Table 17-4); a slightly elevated value should be repeated (see Chap. 13).[36] Rarely, serum prolactin may be elevated because of macroprolactinemia.[37] In this condition, the serum contains a large-molecular-mass form of prolactin that is immunoreactive but without significant bioactivity. If the serum prolactin level is >200 ng/mL but no pituitary tumor is visible by appropriate MRI, this possibility should be considered.

## SYMPTOMS

Hyperprolactinemia may be asymptomatic; an elevated serum value may be a clue to the presence of a pituitary tumor or pituitary stalk impingement.[36] However, prolactin elevation from any cause may result in signs and symptoms of hypogonadism in men or women.[38,39] A history of osteopenia or osteoporosis may be present.

## SIGNS

If hyperprolactinemia results in hypogonadism, the usual signs in men and women may occur (see respective sections of this chapter). Gynecomastia may occur in men. Galactorrhea occurs more commonly in women because estrogen priming of breast tissue facilitates this process.

## LABORATORY ASSESSMENT

Serum prolactin should be measured as part of any general screening for pituitary dysfunction (see Chap. 13). A persistently elevated prolactin value, without a pharmacologic, physiologic, or nonpituitary pathologic explanation (see Table 17-4) should be considered abnormal and likely due to a prolactin-secreting pituitary adenoma, even if pituitary imaging studies fail to demonstrate an abnormality. A moderately elevated serum prolactin may occur in disease or injury involving the hypothalamus. For serum prolactin, the upper limit of the normal range depends on which assay is used, but is typically 15 ng/mL for men and 20 ng/mL for women. Pituitary microadenomas that secrete prolactin (microprolactinomas) and macroadenomas that do not secrete prolactin but impinge on the pituitary stalk are typically associated with serum prolactin levels <250 ng/mL.[36] In contrast, macroadenomas that secrete prolactin (macroprolactinomas) are typically associated with prolactin levels >250 ng/mL.[36] Low prolactin levels are rare but may lead to failure of postpartum lactation.

# ANTERIOR PITUITARY HORMONE HYPERSECRETION

If the serum concentration of a pituitary hormone is shown to be inappropriately elevated (not just appropriately increased in response to a target gland deficiency), there may be a pituitary tumor present and concomitant hyposecretion of other pituitary hormones. Patients with symptoms of the amenorrhea-galactorrhea syndrome (see Chap. 13), acromegaly (see Chap. 12), or Cushing disease (see Chaps. 14 and 75) must be strongly suspected of harboring a hypersecretory pituitary tumor. The mechanism of *any associated hyposecretion* could be the compression of normal surrounding pituitary tissue by the tumor. However, in the case of a prolactin-secreting adenoma, concomitant hypogonadism may be caused by the hormonal effect of a high serum level of prolactin, suppressing gonadotropin production and decreasing the gonadal response to the gonadotropins.[39] Almost always, first-line treatment of a prolactinoma is dopamine agonist therapy; hence, measurement of serum prolactin should be part of the preoperative evaluation.

## VASOPRESSIN DYSREGULATION

Vasopressin (i.e., ADH) is synthesized in the magnocellular neurons of the anterior hypothalamus and transported and stored in the posterior pituitary gland. Vasopressin is secreted into the peripheral circulation and acts on the renal tubular cells to prevent free water loss. Serum osmolarity—and, to a lesser extent, volume status—regulate posterior pituitary vasopressin secretion. Deficiency of vasopressin may lead to polyuria, polydipsia, and free water loss with resultant hypernatremia. This condition is known as *central diabetes insipidus* (central DI) and can be temporary or permanent. It is common to lose several liters of water daily. Central DI usually indicates damage to the hypothalamus, either via suprasellar extension of a sellar or brain mass, trauma, or after extensive surgical resection. Appropriate secretion of vasopressin can often be seen with posterior pituitary damage if the hypothalamus remains intact. A patient who is alert, able to sense thirst, and can get to unlimited free water usually can drink enough to keep pace with free water losses. Of course, these patients need exogenous vasopressin treatment. However, a patient with DI and an altered sensorium or who is not able to free water is in a life-threatening situation; free water replacement and exogenous vasopressin treatment are urgently required. DI has other nonpituitary causes (see Chaps. 25 and 206).

Vasopressin excess causes SIADH and may result in free water retention and resultant hyponatremia. Among other causes, hypothalamic and/or pituitary pathology may lead to SIADH. This condition, too, may be temporary or permanent. SIADH may be asymptomatic initially, and when more advanced, severe hyponatremia can result in stupor, seizure, coma, or death. Treatment is primarily with free water restriction. SIADH also has nonpituitary causes (see Chaps. 25 and 206).

Diagnosis of central DI or SIADH is typically made by a history of polyuria or polydipsia, or by detecting serum sodium abnormalities in patients with known hypothalamic/pituitary pathology. Serum sodium and urine-specific gravity should be measured on all patients suspected of hypopituitarism. Patients who have undergone pituitary manipulation should have serum sodium measured routinely in the immediate postoperative period and at regular intervals for 2 weeks after surgery, because onset of SIADH or DI can be delayed (see Table 17-5). More extensive testing may be necessary (see Chaps. 25 and 206).

## OXYTOCIN DYSREGULATION

Oxytocin deficiency is rare and may result in problems during parturition (see Chap. 25). Oxytocin is not routinely measured.

## CONDITIONS THAT MIMIC HYPOPITUITARISM

The syndrome of hypopituitarism frequently includes nonspecific symptoms, such as weakness and fatigue. Because such symptoms are frequently psychogenic or, if organic, may be secondary to a variety of diseases, it is not cost-effective to screen specifically for hypopituitarism unless there are additional clues.

Two specific syndromes may superficially mimic hypopituitarism. *Anorexia nervosa* (see Chap. 128) is a form of deliberate chronic starvation, most commonly seen in young women and likely to have a psychiatric cause.[40] The presence of amenorrhea with low gonadotropin levels and borderline low thyroid function test results suggests pituitary disease, but these are compensatory hormonal changes seen in any form of starvation. A patient with anorexia nervosa appears obviously emaciated, an unexpected component of hypopituitarism.

In the syndrome of *autoimmune polyglandular hypofunction* (see Chap. 197), hormonal deficiencies of two or more endocrine glands are common, and if these are target glands of the pituitary, a pituitary cause naturally is considered.[41] However, measurement of the relevant pituitary hormones in this syndrome indicates that these are primary rather than secondary deficiencies. Furthermore, there may be other endocrine deficiencies that cannot be explained by hypopituitarism, such as diabetes mellitus or hypoparathyroidism. Circulating serum antibodies directed against endocrine tissues are often present. Lymphocytic hypophysitis also may be a component of this syndrome, but this represents a true cause of hypopituitarism.

## ENDOCRINE REPLACEMENT THERAPY

### GENERAL PRINCIPLES

Hypopituitarism can be an exceptionally satisfying condition to treat; most of its endocrine signs and symptoms can be completely relieved by suitable hormone replacement therapy. There are two general principles for prescribing a replacement regimen. First, the physician should perform suitable testing and treat only patients who are demonstrably borderline or deficient. Second, when there is failure of an endocrine target gland (e.g., thyroid, adrenal, gonad), regardless of whether the deficiency is primary or secondary, the physician should replace the target-gland hormone (e.g., cortisol) rather than the corresponding pituitary hormone (e.g., ACTH). Table 17-6 lists some commonly used endocrine replacement medications and typical adult doses.

When testing demonstrates borderline-low secretion of a hormone, particularly cortisol, in an asymptomatic patient, it is unclear whether the patient should be treated. Many patients with lower-than-normal glucocorticoid secretion can tolerate even a major stress adequately but, if possible, it is prudent not to take this risk. If the baseline serum cortisol concentration is borderline deficient, some physicians believe that extended treatment is better because the patient acquires the habit of taking glucocorticoid and may be more likely to think of increasing the dose appropriately at the time of an intercurrent illness. Others prefer to have the patient keep a supply of cortisol at home and take it only for intercurrent illness. The choice of treatment plan should be individualized.

More informed choices can be made if the physician becomes familiar with local costs of the various relevant diagnostic tests and of medications. In general, the costs of maintenance endocrine medications are low and are not of significant economic concern,

**TABLE 17-6.**
**Maintenance Medications for Hypopituitarism**

| Deficient Hormone | Medication (Typical Dose) |
|---|---|
| Thyroid-stimulating hormone | L-Thyroxine (75–150 µg, once daily) |
| Corticotropin | Cortisol (hydrocortisone) (20–30 mg daily, in two divided doses) |
| Luteinizing hormone, follicle-stimulating hormone* | Male: testosterone cypionate or enanthate (200–300 mg intramuscularly, every 3 wks), or daily skin patch<br>Female: conjugated estrogens (0.9–1.25 mg), days 1–25 each month, plus medroxyprogesterone acetate (5–10 mg) for days 12–25 |
| Growth hormone | 0.006 mg/kg per day (0.018 IU/kg/day) with incremental increases to keep IGF-I in the middle of the age adjusted reference range. Maximum 0.0125 mg/kg/day (0.0375 IU/kg/day) |
| Prolactin | None |
| Antidiuretic hormone | See Chaps. 25, 26, and 27 |

*For treatment of infertility, see Chaps. 97 and 118.

with the exceptions of GH therapy and gonadotropin treatment to promote fertility. For long-term follow-up, the most cost-effective strategy is to minimize hospitalizations. A central part of this strategy is to schedule follow-up office visits every 6 to 12 months after the patient is clinically stable. At these visits, the physician can answer questions and continue to educate the patient about his or her disease, as well as maintain a good rapport with the patient. This will increase the likelihood that the patient will phone for advice at a time when prompt treatment of an intercurrent illness can help prevent complications and hospitalization.

## GLUCOCORTICOID REPLACEMENT

Cortisol (i.e., hydrocortisone) or cortisone can be used for replacement therapy. Cortisone is converted to cortisol after ingestion. Cortisol is the predominant glucocorticoid secreted by the human adrenal gland, and an adult produces ~10 mg daily in the unstressed state.[42] There is a diurnal rhythm, with greater secretion in the morning and less in the evening. The serum half-life is ~1 hour.

When cortisol is used for adrenal replacement in the adult, it is commonly given in dosages of 30 mg daily; for example, 20 mg each morning and 10 mg each afternoon or evening. For smaller individuals, 20 mg daily is sufficient (e.g., 10 mg twice daily). This cortisol dosage exceeds normal daily adrenal secretion, but there are losses in absorption; also, undoubtedly, one to three doses daily is a less efficient mode of administration than the more continuous natural secretion. In the occasional patient who cannot reliably remember to take more than one dose daily, it may be best to give the entire dose in the morning (rather than risk undertreatment), or to use a glucocorticoid with a longer pharmacologic half-life. Some authors suggest every other day therapy. Cortisone is used interchangeably with cortisol, with 25 mg of cortisone considered equivalent to 20 mg of cortisol. Usually, there is little to favor one compound over the other, except habit or price. However, in severe liver disease, cortisol is preferable because the conversion of cortisone to cortisol occurs in that organ. Prednisone also can be substituted for cortisol, using the assumption that 5 mg of prednisone is equivalent to 20 mg of cortisol. Replacement doses of dexamethasone are not well defined, and there is considerable individual variation; the plasma disappearance half-life is longer than 4 hours, and once-daily dosing is often adequate. A typical dose would be 0.5 mg given at bedtime, with a range of 0.25 to 0.75 mg.

Although cortisol can be assayed in blood and urine, such determinations are not particularly useful in determining a replacement dose of cortisol for an individual patient. The serum half-life is short, so that the serum concentration can be above or below the normal range much of the time, even when a patient is responding well to the dose. The free cortisol in a 24-hour urine sample is often elevated on conventional cortisol dosage regimens.

Most patients do well on any of the aforementioned dosage regimens, manifesting no overt evidence of hypoadrenalism or Cushing syndrome. (However, one report suggests that in men with Addison disease, commonly used replacement doses of glucocorticoids may be associated with a low bone mineral density.[43]) Even allowing for the lesser efficiency of intermittent oral administration, it seems likely that the customarily used replacement doses are appropriate for most individuals. If, while using one of these regimens, a patient still has chronic symptoms that suggest hypoadrenalism, the physician should check for medication error or noncompliance. If neither is found, the symptoms are likely to be due to a cause other than hypoadrenalism. Some individuals experience a pleasant "high" with supraphysiologic doses of glucocorticoid, leading them to complain when they are returned to true replacement doses.[44] A patient's desire for euphoria is not a reason to continue higher-than-replacement doses indefinitely.

A patient with untreated or undertreated hypopituitarism potentially may be more vulnerable at the time of an intercurrent illness because of a lack of hormonal homeostatic mechanisms.

Before therapy, or if therapy is insufficient, such patients are very sensitive to infections, surgical procedures, or drugs such as sedatives or narcotics. Glucocorticoid doses conventionally are increased for significant physical illness or for operative procedures in an attempt to mimic the normal physiologic response to such situations. Interestingly, studies of patients undergoing operative procedures suggest that conventionally prescribed "stress doses" of glucocorticoid are larger and are maintained for a longer period than usually would be needed to mimic normal cortisol production.[45,46] A renal transplantation group reports that they no longer increase baseline immunosuppressive doses of glucocorticoid (5 to 10 mg of prednisone daily), even when patients are stressed by sepsis or surgery, and they believe such doses have been sufficient.[47] It is likely that the same would be true for intercurrent illnesses. However, until further data are available, the recommendation is to give conventional stress doses during times of intercurrent illness and perioperatively when there is no known contraindication to that approach. For some situations, however—such as surgery of a diabetic patient whose disease becomes difficult to control on higher glucocorticoid doses, or for a patient who becomes psychotic with high glucocorticoid doses—there are reasons to minimize the dosage. In such a situation, the author gives only the equivalent of two or three times the usual replacement doses on the day of surgery and taper to replacement doses within 3 days in the absence of postoperative complications. The patient should be monitored carefully for possible signs of hypoadrenalism and given supplemental glucocorticoid if indicated. Hypoadrenal symptoms are readily reversed if recognized and treated promptly. Table 17-5 summarizes current recommendations concerning glucocorticoid administration in the presence of intercurrent illness or perioperatively.

Patients whose hypoadrenalism is secondary to ACTH deficiency usually secrete normal or near-normal quantities of aldosterone in response to the still intact renin-angiotensin system, although their responses to salt restriction are not completely normal.[48] Hyponatremia in a patient with untreated hypopituitarism is most likely due to hypersecretion of ADH, rather than to mineralocorticoid deficiency; there usually is no evidence of salt or volume depletion, and the hyponatremia is rapidly corrected by glucocorticoid.[49] In contrast to patients with Addison disease, patients with secondary hypoadrenalism *rarely* need replacement therapy with the mineralocorticoid fludrocortisone. Moreover, cortisol has some intrinsic mineralocorticoid activity; occasionally it may be necessary to provide a small dose of fludrocortisone for a patient taking a synthetic glucocorticoid, such as dexamethasone, that has less mineralocorticoid activity.

Perioperative management of patients undergoing surgery that will affect the pituitary gland presents special challenges (see Chap. 23 and Table 17-5). Evaluation of HPA axis function and management of glucocorticoid therapy after surgery for Cushing disease or Cushing syndrome may be quite complex (see Chaps. 14 and 75). Patients cured of Cushing disease may require a protracted course of glucocorticoid supplementation. Medical therapy of Cushing syndrome may render the patient hypoadrenal, and replacement glucocorticoids and/or mineralocorticoids may be necessary.

## THYROID HORMONE REPLACEMENT

L-thyroxine (L-$T_4$) is the preferred replacement medication for patients with hypothyroidism (see Chap. 45). A typical replacement dosage of L-$T_4$ is 75 to 150 μg daily, with some patients requiring as little as 50 μg and others as much as 200 μg daily; the total replacement dose is usually ~1.6 μg/kg per day. Elderly patients may need ~25 to 50 μg less than younger individuals.[50–52] One dose daily is sufficient, because the half-life of L-$T_4$ is ~1 week. The serum level of $FT_4$ is used to judge the adequacy of the L-$T_4$ dose. The aim for most patients is to keep the $FT_4$ in the mid-normal range. If this goal is achieved, it is assumed that the body will convert $T_4$ to $T_3$ at a physiologically appropriate rate, and monitoring of the serum $T_3$ level is not required. The serum TSH, which is most helpful in choosing the correct replacement dosage in primary hypothyroidism, cannot serve this purpose in secondary hypothyroidism, a condition caused by a deficiency of TSH. If an individual is elderly, has cardiovascular disease, or is severely hypothyroid, it is prudent to start with 25 µg per day and gradually increase the dose by 25 µg per month until the $FT_4$ or $FT_4I$ normalizes. If the patient has none of these risk factors, the initial dose of 50 µg per day may be increased more rapidly in 25- to 50-µg increments. The correction of hypothyroidism in a patient with unrecognized hypoadrenalism can precipitate overt hypoadrenal crisis; the physician should begin glucocorticoid therapy before or along with the L-$T_4$ if there is concomitant hypoadrenalism. Severe hypothyroidism, resulting in myxedema coma, may initially require large doses of L-$T_4$.

## GONADAL STEROID REPLACEMENT

A hypogonadal state is not life threatening, and emergency therapy is not needed. Adults with a deficiency are treated with estrogens or androgens to improve sexual functioning and for a general feeling of enhanced vigor and well-being (Fig. 17-2). In the premenopausal woman, estrogen helps to protect against osteopenia and osteoporosis. However, if hyperprolactinemia is present, therapy with bromocriptine should be tried first, because the resultant suppression of prolactin may return the gonadotropins and the target gland hormones to normal. There also is concern that if a prolactinoma is present, its growth may be stimulated by estrogens. The same phenomenon may be seen with the administration of testosterone, presumably because of partial conversion of testosterone to estradiol.[53] Moreover, replacement of the gonadal hormones is relatively ineffective in the presence of hyperprolactinemia.[38] Testosterone therapy in hypogonadal men may avert or improve osteoporosis, restores skin and body hair to normal, and is beneficial to muscle function. Gonadal hormone replacement may be contraindicated in patients with a history of certain medical conditions (e.g., breast cancer, phlebitis, and pulmonary embolism in women, and cancer of the prostate or breast in men). Consequently, patients receiving long-term gonadal replacement therapy should be monitored for the possible development of breast or prostate cancer to allow prompt discontinuation of the hormone.

## TESTOSTERONE REPLACEMENT

Men may be treated with parenteral, transdermal, or oral androgens (see Fig. 17-2; see Chap. 119). The parenterally and transdermally administered androgen preparations are potent and have fewer important side effects than oral androgens. A testosterone transdermal system consists of a patch that is applied directly to the skin surface at 10:00 p.m. and delivers testosterone continuously; this regimen results in a serum testosterone concentration profile that mimics the normal circadian variation observed in healthy young men. A typical starting dose is one 5-mg patch. The dose can be increased or decreased to keep the morning testosterone level in the normal range. The most common adverse effect is irritation at the site of application of the patch. This can be treated with over-the-counter topical hydrocortisone cream applied after patch removal.

A traditional, reliable method of androgen replacement in men uses long-acting testosterone esters given intramuscularly, with effects lasting as long as 3 weeks. Typical dosages are 200 mg of testosterone cypionate or testosterone enanthate every 2 to 3 weeks or 300 mg every 3 weeks. Because the active androgen is testosterone itself, allergic or idiosyncratic reactions are not expected, unless there is a reaction to one of the other ingredients (e.g., cottonseed oil, sesame oil). Dose and schedule of administration should be adjusted to keep maximum and minimum levels in the normal range.

Oral androgens are often ineffective and may be associated with side effects such as cholestatic hepatitis, hepatic tumors, and peliosis hepatis. Their use is rapidly falling out of favor.

Elderly men with benign prostatic hypertrophy may develop urinary retention with the initiation of testosterone therapy; therefore, smaller doses may be appropriate. Moreover, the initiation of androgen therapy in a man who has not previously attained puberty results in physical changes and changes in libido, degree of aggression, and general outlook. Some male patients who have been hypogonadal for long periods may abandon androgens because these mental and behavioral changes are psychologically threatening. Therefore, starting doses should be smaller and should be increased very gradually (see Chaps. 92 and 119).

**A–C**

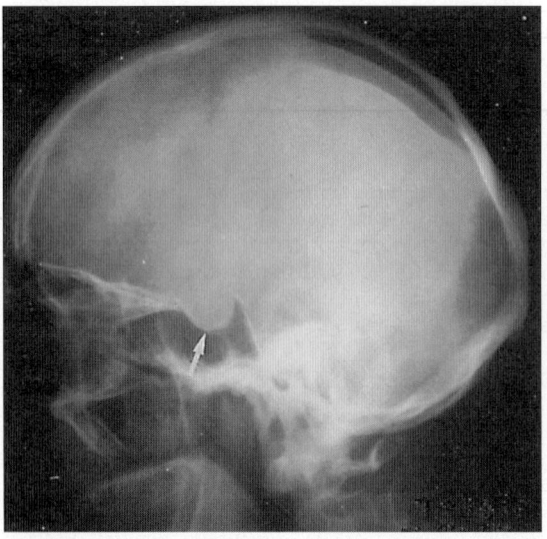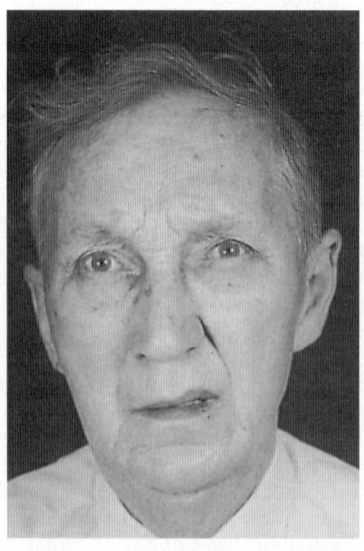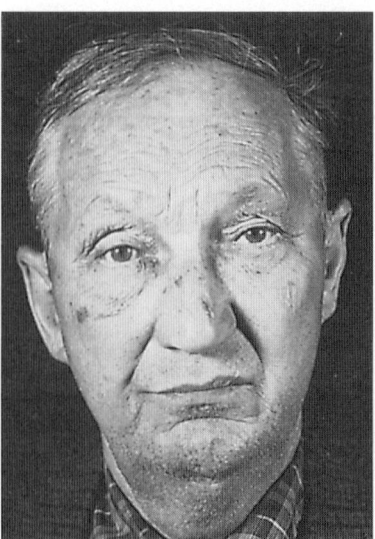

**FIGURE 17-2.** Clinically nonfunctioning pituitary tumor in a 53-year-old man. **A,** Skull radiograph film shows an enlarged, ballooned sella turcica (*arrow*) with eroded anterior and posterior clinoid processes. **B,** The patient has pale, "pasty" facies with no beard and fine wrinkling of the skin. Testing revealed gonadotropin deficiency. **C,** One year after having received testosterone injections every 3 weeks, the patient has responded to therapy.

## ESTROGEN REPLACEMENT

Premenopausal women are usually given cyclic oral estrogens, along with a progestogen for the final portion of the cycle (see Chap. 100). A typical regimen is 1 to 2 mg of micronized estradiol or 0.9 to 1.25 mg of conjugated estrogens daily for 25 consecutive days each month, taken orally (or estradiol, 0.05 to 0.1 mg per day, transdermally), with the addition of a progestogen, such as 5 to 10 mg of medroxyprogesterone acetate or 0.35 mg of norethindrone daily for the last 12 to 14 days of estrogen administration. Monthly withdrawal bleeding is expected. Standard oral contraceptive preparations containing a cyclic estrogen and progestogen are another option (see Chap. 104). Postmenopausal estrogen replacement regimens are discussed in Chapter 100.

In secondary hypogonadism, the gonads are usually intrinsically normal; they are lacking gonadotropin stimulation. Female patients with hypopituitarism are potentially capable of having fertility temporarily restored.[54] The use of gonadotropins and other drugs to restore fertility in such patients is discussed in Chapters 97 and 103.

## GROWTH HORMONE REPLACEMENT

Adults with GH deficiency may start therapy with 0.006 mg/kg per day (0.018 IU/kg per day) given as a daily subcutaneous injection. The dose may be increased based on relief of symptoms and signs, and should be limited by adverse effects. The aim is to keep the IGF-I level in the age- and sex-matched normal range. The maximum dose is 0.0125 mg/kg per day (0.0375 IU/kg per day).[35] Adverse effects include peripheral edema, arthralgias and myalgias, headache, paresthesias, and carpal tunnel syndrome.

A child with short stature resulting from GH deficiency should be evaluated for possible treatment if the epiphyses remain open (see Chaps. 12, 18, and 198).[55]

## VASOPRESSIN REPLACEMENT

ADH deficiency may lead to partial or total DI and has several forms of treatment (see Chap. 26). DI may be masked in the presence of hypoadrenalism and may come to clinical attention only after glucocorticoid therapy is initiated.

## PROLACTIN AND OXYTOCIN

Prolactin and oxytocin deficiency are not treated in clinical practice.

## REFERENCES

1. Vance ML. Hypopituitarism. N Engl J Med 1994; 330:1651.
2. LeBlanc H, Lachelin CL, Abu-Fadil S, et al. Effects of dopamine infusion on pituitary hormone secretion in humans. J Clin Endocrinol Metab 1976; 43:668.
3. DeRivera JL, Lal S, Ettigi P, et al. Effects of acute and chronic neuroleptic therapy on serum prolactin levels in men and women of different age groups. Clin Endocrinal (Oxf) 1976; 5:273.
4. Snyder P. Clinically nonfunctioning pituitary adenomas. Endocrinol Metab Clin North Am 1993; 22:163.
5. Stevenaert A, Beckers A, Vandalem JL, Hennen G. Early normalization of luteinizing hormone pulsatility after successful transsphenoidal surgery in women with microprolactinomas. J Clin Endocrinol Metab 1986; 62:1044.
6. Sauder SE, Frager M, Case GD, et al. Abnormal patterns of pulsatile luteinizing hormone secretion in women with hyperprolactinemia and amenorrhea: response to bromocriptine. J Clin Endocrinol Metab 1984; 59:941.
7. Styne DM. The therapy for hypothalamic-pituitary tumors. Endocrinol Metab Clin North Am 1993; 22:631.
8. Dempsey PK, Kondziolka D, Lunsford LD. Stereotactic diagnosis and treatment of pineal region tumours and vascular malformations. Acta Neurochir (Wien) 1992; 116:14.
9. Buchfelder M, Brockmeister S, Pichl J, et al. Results of dynamic endocrine testing of hypothalamic pituitary function in patients with a primary "empty" sella syndrome. Horm Metabol Res 1989; 21:57.
10. Nelson AT Jr, Tucker HSG Jr, Becker DP. Residual anterior pituitary function following transsphenoidal resection of pituitary macroadenomas. J Neurosurg 1984; 61:577.
11. Edwards OM, Clark JDA. Post-traumatic hypopituitarism. Medicine (Baltimore) 1986; 65:281.
12. Ooi TC, Russell NA. Hypopituitarism resulting from an intrasellar carotid aneurysm. Can J Neurol Sci 1986; 13:70.
13. Barkan AL. Case report: pituitary atrophy in patients with Sheehan's syndrome. Am J Med Sci 1989; 298:38.
14. Rolih CA, Ober KP. Pituitary apoplexy. Endocrinol Metab Clin North Am 1993; 22:291.
14a. Imaki T, Yamada S, Horada S, et al. Amelioration of acromegaly after pituitary infarction due to gastrointestinal hemorrhage from gastric ulcer. Endocr J 1999; 46:147.
15. Littley MD, Shalet SM, Beardwell CG, et al. Radiation-induced hypopituitarism is dose-dependent. Clin Endocrinol (Oxf) 1989; 31:363.
16. Constine LS, Woolf PD, Cann D, et al. Hypothalamic-pituitary dysfunction after radiation for brain tumors. N Engl J Med 1993; 328:87.
17. Cosman F, Post KD, Holub DA, Wardlaw SL. Lymphocytic hypophysitis: report of 3 new cases and review of the literature. Medicine (Baltimore) 1989; 68:240.
18. Van der Werff ten Bosch JJ, Bot A. Growth of males with idiopathic hypopituitarism without growth hormone treatment. Clin Endocrinol (Oxf) 1990; 32:707.
19. Rugarli EI, Ballabio A. Kallmann syndrome: from genetics to neurobiology. JAMA 1993; 270:2713.
20. Beck-Peccoz P, Amr S, Menezes-Ferreira MM, et al. Decreased receptor binding of biologically inactive thyrotropin in central hypothyroidism. N Engl J Med 1985; 312:1085.
21. Topliss DJ, White EL, Stockigt JR. Significance of thyrotropin excess in untreated primary adrenal insufficiency. J Clin Endocrinol Metab 1980; 50:52.
22. Surks MI, Chopra IJ, Mariash CN, et al. American Thyroid Association guidelines for use of laboratory tests in thyroid disorders. JAMA 1990; 263:1529.
23. Elster AD. Modern imaging of the pituitary. Radiology 1993; 187:1.
24. Ladenson PW, Levin AA, Ridgway EC, Daniels GH. Complications of surgery in hypothyroid patients. Am J Med 1984; 77:261.
25. Melen O. Neuro-ophthalmologic features of pituitary tumors. Endocrinol Metab Clin North Am 1987; 16:585.
26. Orme SM, Belchetz PE. Isolated ACTH deficiency. Clin Endocrinol (Oxf) 1991; 35:213.
27. Grinspoon SK, Biller BMK. Laboratory assessment of adrenal insufficiency. J Clin Endocrinol Metab 1994; 79:923.
28. Talwar V, Lodha S, Dash RJ. Assessing the hypothalamo-pituitary-adrenocortical axis using physiological doses of adrenocorticotropic hormone. QJM 1998; 91:285.
29. Snow K, Jiang NS, Kao PC, Scheithauer BW. Biochemical evaluation of adrenal dysfunction: the laboratory perspective. Mayo Clin Proc 1992; 67:1055.
30. Yamamoto K, Saito K, Takai T, et al. Visual field defects and pituitary enlargement in primary hypothyroidism. J Clin Endocrinol Metab 1983; 57:283.
31. Whitcomb RW, Crowley WF Jr. Male hypogonadotropic hypogonadism. Endocrinol Metab Clin North Am 1993; 22:125.
32. Rosenfield RL. Plasma testosterone binding globulin and indexes of the concentration of unbound androgens in normal and hirsute subjects. J Clin Endocrinol Metab 1971; 32:717.
33. Attanasio AF, Lamberts SWJ, Matranga AMC, et al. Adult growth hormone (GH)-deficient patients demonstrate heterogeneity between childhood onset and adult onset before and during human GH treatment. J Clin Endocrinol Metab 1997; 82:82.
34. Carroll PV, Christ ER, Bengtsson BA, et al. Growth hormone deficiency in adulthood and the effects of growth hormone replacement: a review. J Clin Endocrinol Metab 1998; 83:382.
35. Physicians' Desk Reference. 53rd ed. Montvale, NJ: Medical Economics Company, 1999.
36. Molitch ME. Pathologic hyperprolactinemia. Endocrinol Metab Clin North Am 1992; 21:877.
37. Jackson RD, Wortsman J, Malarkey WB. Macroprolactinemia presenting like a pituitary tumor. Am J Med 1985; 78:346.
38. Carter JN, Tyson JE, Tolis G, et al. Prolactin-secreting tumors and hypogonadism in 22 men. N Engl J Med 1978; 299:847.
39. Murray FT, Cameron DF, Ketchum C. Return of gonadal function in men with prolactin-secreting pituitary tumors. J Clin Endocrinol Metab 1984; 59:79.
40. Wade TD, Bulik CM, Neale M, Kendler KS, Anorexia nervosa and major depression: shared genetic and environmental risk factors. Am J Psychiatry 2000; 157:469.
41. Neufeld M, Maclaren NK, Blizzard RM. Two types of autoimmune Addison's disease associated with different polyglandular autoimmune syndromes. Medicine (Baltimore) 1981; 60:355.
42. Esteban NV, Loughlin T, Yergey AL, et al. Daily cortisol production rate in man determined by stable isotope dilution/mass spectrometry. J Clin Endocrinol Metab 1991; 72:39.
43. Zelissen PMJ, Croughs RJM, van Rijk PP, et al. Effect of glucocorticoid replacement therapy on bone mineral density in patients with Addison disease. Ann Intern Med 1994; 120:207.
44. Flavin DK, Fredrickson PA, Richardson JW, Merritt TC. Corticosteroid abuse: an unusual manifestation of drug dependence. Mayo Clin Proc 1983; 58:764.

45. Udelsman R, Norton JA, Jelenich SE, et al. Responses of the hypothalamic-pituitary-adrenal and renin-angiotensin axes and the sympathetic system during controlled surgical and anesthetic stress. J Clin Endocrinol Metab 1987; 64:986.
46. Chernow B, Alexander HR, Smallridge RC, et al. Hormonal responses to graded surgical stress. Arch Intern Med 1987; 147:1273.
47. Bromberg JS, Alfrey EJ, Barker CF, et al. Adrenal suppression and steroid supplementation in renal transplant recipients. Transplantation 1991; 51:385.
48. Williams GH, Rose LI, Dluhy RG, et al. Aldosterone response to sodium restriction and ACTH stimulation in panhypopituitarism. J Clin Endocrinol Metab 1971; 32:27.
49. Oelkers W. Hyponatremia and inappropriate secretion of vasopressin (antidiuretic hormone) in patients with hypopituitarism. N Engl J Med 1989; 321:492.
50. Davis FB, LaMantia RS, Spaulding SW, et al. Estimation of a physiologic replacement dose of levothyroxine in elderly patients with hypothyroidism. Arch Intern Med 1984; 144:1752.
51. Helfand M, Crapo LM. Monitoring therapy in patients taking levothyroxine. Ann Intern Med 1990; 113:450.
52. Toft AD. Thyroxine therapy. N Engl J Med 1994; 331:174.
53. Prior JC, Cox TA, Fairholm D, et al. Testosterone-related exacerbation of a prolactin-producing macroadenoma: possible role for estrogen. J Clin Endocrinol Metab 1987; 64:391.
54. Yen SSC. Female hypogonadotropic hypogonadism. Endocrinol Metab Clin North Am 1993; 22:29.
55. Saggese G, Federico G, Barsant S. Management of puberty in growth hormone deficient children. J Pediatr Endocrinol Metab 1999; 12(Suppl 1):329.

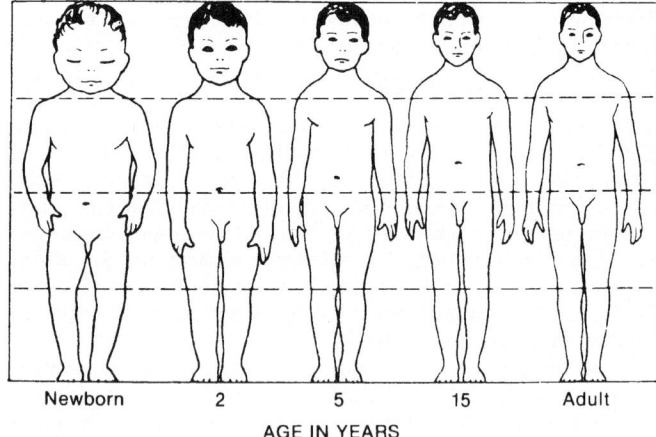

STATURE DIVIDED INTO QUARTERS

Newborn    2    5    15    Adult

AGE IN YEARS

**FIGURE 18-1.** Changes in body proportions with growth. The horizontal lines divide the figures into quarters. Note the following normal phenomena: progressive decrease in the relative size of the head, increase in the relative size of the lower extremities, and the progressive anatomic descent of the midpoint of the body. (From Sinclair D. Human growth after birth. Oxford: Oxford University Press, 1985:128.)

# CHAPTER 18

# HYPOTHALAMIC AND PITUITARY DISORDERS IN INFANCY AND CHILDHOOD

ALAN D. ROGOL

Disorders of the hypothalamus and pituitary gland in infants and children often manifest as abnormalities of growth. Pediatric manifestations may involve secondarily the thyroid gland, sexual development, or glucose homeostasis (see Chaps. 47 and 161).

## GROWTH PATTERN CONCEPTS

A child's growth pattern arises from a complex mixture of genetic potential, nutrition, psychological factors, and the secretion and interaction of many hormones (see Chaps. 7, 91, and 198).

### GROWTH VELOCITY

The patterns of growth and adolescent development can provide useful data that signal specific problems or simplify differential diagnoses. The rate of stature change, the growth velocity, may be derived from the growth chart (see Chap. 7). The growth chart also has a graph that depicts percentiles of weight for attained linear stature. This information may prove useful in evaluating problems such as malabsorption syndromes or chronic illness, in which most children are relatively

**FIGURE 18-2.** Normal standards for upper segment/lower segment (*US:LS*) body ratio during growth. (Measurements were obtained from 2100 Baltimore school children.) There is a significantly lower US:LS ratio for blacks (**B**) than for whites (**A**) at all ages because of a shorter upper segment and longer lower segment in blacks. There were no sex differences within either racial group up until approximately age 15 years. (Modified from McKusick VA. Heritable disorders of connective tissue, 3rd ed. St. Louis: Mosby, 1966:50.)

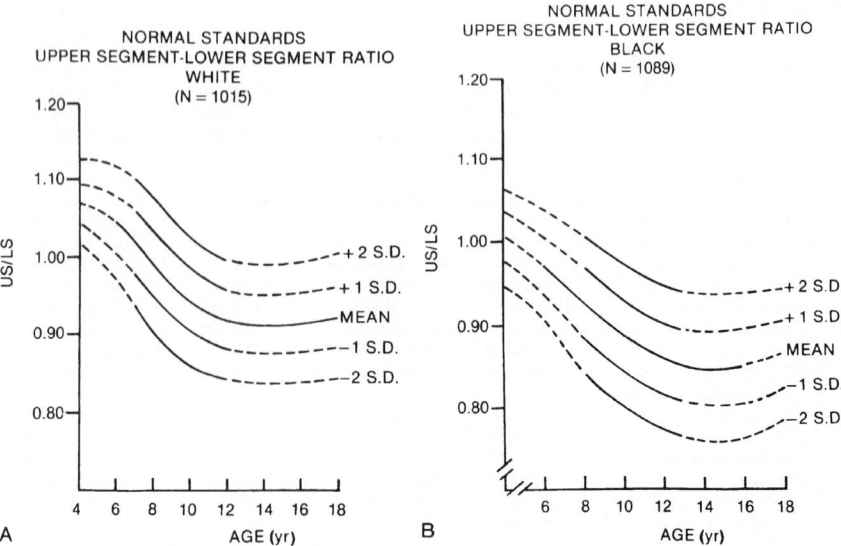

NORMAL STANDARDS
UPPER SEGMENT-LOWER SEGMENT RATIO
WHITE
(N = 1015)

US/LS

1.20
1.10
1.00
0.90
0.80

+2 S.D.
+1 S.D.
MEAN
-1 S.D.
-2 S.D.

4  6  8  10  12  14  16  18
AGE (yr)
A

NORMAL STANDARDS
UPPER SEGMENT-LOWER SEGMENT RATIO
BLACK
(N = 1089)

US/LS

1.20
1.10
1.00
0.90
0.80

+2 S.D.
+1 S.D.
MEAN
-1 S.D.
-2 S.D.

6  8  10  12  14  16  18
AGE (yr)
B

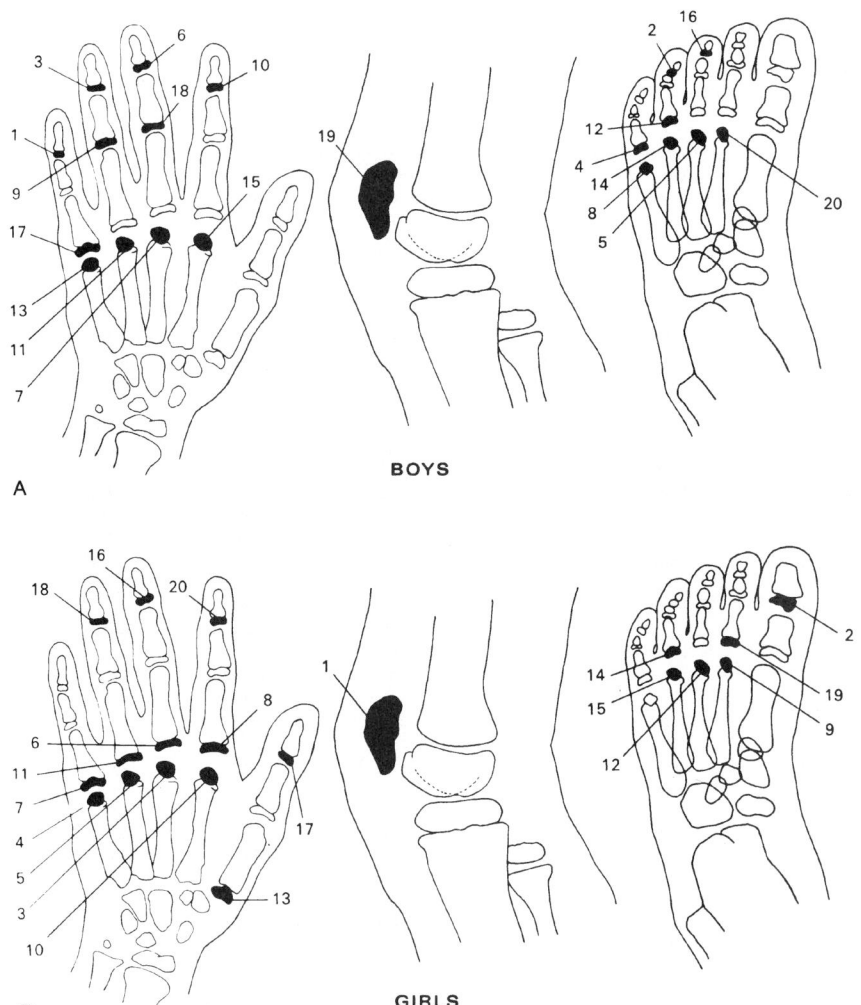

**FIGURE 18-3.** The 20 ossification centers of maximum predictive value in boys (**A**) and girls (**B**). The postnatal centers that have the greatest utility in skeletal assessment are in the hand, the knee, and the foot. The numbers indicate the relative predictive value of these postnatal ossification centers, number 1 being the most predictive. (From Garn SM, Rohman CG, Silverman FN, et al. Med Radiogr Photogr 1967; 43:45. Reprinted courtesy of Eastman Kodak Company.)

underweight for height, or hypopituitarism, in which children are relatively overweight for height.

## BODY SEGMENT RATIO

The body segment ratio (upper segment/lower segment ratio) is determined by measuring the lower segment (pubis to soles), subtracting that value from the height to calculate the upper segment (crown to pubis), and dividing the upper by the lower. These proportions change throughout development. At birth, the trunk is relatively long compared with the extremities, but by the end of puberty, the extremities are relatively longer than the trunk (Fig. 18-1). The body segment ratio at birth is ~1.7:1; it becomes ~1:1 by 8 to 10 years of age, reflecting the growth of long bones. Blacks are relatively long-limbed compared with whites and have upper/lower segment ratios of ~0.90 after puberty (Fig. 18-2). Tables of normal body segment ratios and arm span measurements have been published.[1]

The body segment ratio is affected in certain growth disorders. For example, many patients with chondrodystrophy have relatively short limbs compared with their upper segment; hypogonadal patients have increased limb length compared with their upper segment (eunuchoid proportions); and children with hypothyroidism may have a more infantile upper/lower segment ratio. Others have used the *span* (fingertip-to-fingertip) to delineate altered body proportions. The height and the span normally are within 5 cm of each other.

## SKELETAL AND DENTAL MATURATION

Skeletal and dental maturation may be used to assess a child's developmental (physiologic) status. A number of methods for obtaining the bone age have been developed, but the method of Greulich and Pyle[2] has proved to be the most practical screening procedure. A single radiograph of the left hand and wrist is obtained, and the epiphyseal development is compared with that of children of normal stature using an atlas. Other systems evaluate ossification centers in the hand, knee, and foot (Fig. 18-3). Together, these criteria allow a child's growth and developmental pattern to be determined (Fig. 18-3; Table 18-1). These data should help to determine whether a child's growth is within the range of normal (see Chaps. 7 and 217) or should be further evaluated.

## OTHER GROWTH CONCEPTS

*Height age* is the age for which a person's present height would be at the 50th percentile on the growth chart. *Short stature* usually is given a statistical definition, that is, a specific number of standard deviations (SD) below the expected mean for children of a certain chronologic age. A common definition is 2–3 SD below the mean for age; 2.5 SD, equivalent to the third percentile, often is used. *Tall stature* may be defined as 2–3 SD above the mean height for age; 2.5 SD, equivalent to the 97th percentile, often is used.

Growth velocity, or rate of incremental change, also has a normal range. *Growth failure* is often defined below the 10th to 25th percentile of the mean height velocity for age. The lowest values for both boys and girls between the ages of 2 and 12 years

**TABLE 18-1.**
**Age-at-Appearance Percentiles for Major Postnatal Ossification Centers**

| | PERCENTILES | | | | | |
|---|---|---|---|---|---|---|
| | Boys | | | Girls | | |
| OSSIFICATION CENTER | 5th | 50th | 95th | 5th | 50th | 95th |
| Head of humerus | 37g | 2w | 4m | 37g | 2w | 3m3 |
| Proximal epiphysis of tibia | 34g | 2w | 5w | 34g | 1w | 2w |
| Coracoid process of scapula | 37g | 2w | 4m2 | 37g | 2w | 5m |
| Cuboid of tarsus | 37g | 3w | 3m3 | 37g | 3w | 2m |
| Capitate of carpus | — | 3m | 7m | — | 2m | 7m |
| Hamate of carpus | 2w | 3m3 | 10m | 2w | 2m1 | 7m |
| Capitulum of humerus | 3w | 4m | 13m | 3w | 3m | 9m1 |
| Head of femur | 3w | 4m1 | 7m3 | 2w | 4m | 7m2 |
| Third cuneiform of tarsus | 3w | 5m2 | 19m | — | 2m3 | 14m3 |
| Greater tubercle of humerus | 3m | 10m | 2y4 | 2m2 | 6m1 | 13m3 |
| Primary center, middle segment of 5th toe | — | 12m2 | 3y10 | — | 9m | 2y1 |
| Distal epiphysis of radius | 6m2 | 12m1 | 2y4 | 4m3 | 10m | 2m2 |
| Epiphysis, distal segment of 1st toe | 8m2 | 12m3 | 2y1 | 4m3 | 9m2 | 20m1 |
| Epiphysis, middle segment of 4th toe | 5m | 14m3 | 2y11 | 5m | 11m | 3y |
| Epiphysis, proximal segment of 3rd finger | 9m1 | 16m2 | 2y5 | 5m | 10m1 | 19m2 |
| Epiphysis, middle segment of 3rd toe | 5m | 17m | 4y3 | 2m3 | 12m1 | 2y6 |
| Epiphysis, proximal segment of 2nd finger | 9m2 | 17m | 2y2 | 5m | 10m2 | 19m3 |
| Epiphysis, proximal segment of 4th finger | 9m3 | 18m | 2y5 | 5m | 11m | 20m |
| Epiphysis, distal segment of 1st finger | 9m | 17m1 | 2y8 | 5m | 12m | 20m3 |
| Epiphysis, proximal segment of 3rd toe | 11m | 19m | 2y6 | 6m1 | 12m3 | 22m3 |
| Epiphysis of 2nd metacarpal | 11m1 | 19m2 | 2y10 | 7m3 | 13m | 20m1 |
| Epiphysis, proximal segment of 4th toe | 11m2 | 19m3 | 2y8 | 7m2 | 15m | 2y1 |
| Epiphysis, proximal segment of 2nd toe | 11m3 | 21m | 2y8 | 7m3 | 14m2 | 2y1 |
| Epiphysis of 3rd metacarpal | 11m2 | 21m2 | 3y | 8m | 13m2 | 23m1 |
| Epiphysis, proximal segment of 5th finger | 12m | 22m1 | 2y10 | 8m | 14m2 | 2y1 |
| Epiphysis, middle segment of 3rd finger | 12m1 | 2y | 3y4 | 7m3 | 15m | 2y4 |
| Epiphysis of 4th metacarpal | 13m | 2y | 3y7 | 9m | 15m2 | 2y2 |
| Epiphysis, middle segment of 2nd toe | 10m3 | 2y1 | 4y1 | 6m | 14m1 | 2y3 |
| Epiphysis, middle segment of 4th finger | 12m | 2y1 | 3y3 | 7m3 | 15m | 2y5 |
| Epiphysis of 5th metacarpal | 15m1 | 2y2 | 3y10 | 10m2 | 16m2 | 2y4 |
| First cuneiform of tarsus | 10m3 | 2y2 | 3y9 | 6m | 17m1 | 2y10 |
| Epiphysis of 1st metatarsal | 16m3 | 2y2 | 3y1 | 11m3 | 19m | 2y3 |
| Epiphysis, middle segment of 2nd finger | 15m3 | 2y2 | 3y4 | 8m | 17m2 | 2y7 |
| Epiphysis, proximal segment of 1st toe | 17m2 | 2y4 | 3y4 | 10m3 | 18m3 | 2y5 |
| Epiphysis, distal segment of 3rd finger | 15m3 | 2y5 | 3y9 | 8m3 | 17m3 | 2y8 |
| Triquetrum of carpus | 6m | 2y5 | 5y6 | 3m2 | 20m2 | 3y9 |
| Epiphysis, distal segment of 4th finger | 16m2 | 2y5 | 3y9 | 8m3 | 18m1 | 2y10 |
| Epiphysis, proximal segment of 5th toe | 18m2 | 2y6 | 3y8 | 11m3 | 20m3 | 2y8 |
| Epiphysis of 1st metacarpal | 17m2 | 2y7 | 4y4 | 11m | 19m1 | 2y8 |
| Second cuneiform of tarsus | 14m2 | 2y8 | 4y3 | 9m3 | 21m3 | 3y |
| Epiphysis of 2nd metatarsal | 23m1 | 2y10 | 4y4 | 14m3 | 2y2 | 3y5 |
| Greater trochanter of femur | 23m | 3y | 4y4 | 11m2 | 22m1 | 3y |
| Epiphysis, proximal segment of 1st finger | 22m1 | 3y | 4y7 | 11m1 | 20m2 | 2y10 |
| Navicular of tarsus | 13m2 | 3y | 5y5 | 9m1 | 23m1 | 3y7 |
| Epiphysis, distal segment of 2nd finger | 21m3 | 3y2 | 5y | 12m3 | 2y6 | 3y4 |
| Epiphysis, distal segment of 5th finger | 2y1 | 3y4 | 5y | 12m | 23m2 | 3y6 |
| Epiphysis, middle segment of 5th finger | 23m1 | 3y5 | 5y10 | 10m3 | 23m3 | 3y7 |
| Proximal epiphysis of fibula | 22m2 | 3y6 | 5y3 | 16m | 2y7 | 3y11 |
| Epiphysis of 3rd metatarsal | 2y4 | 3y6 | 5y | 17m1 | 2y6 | 3y8 |
| Epiphysis, distal segment of 5th toe | 2y4 | 3y11 | 6y4 | 14m1 | 2y4 | 4y1 |
| Patella of knee | 2y6 | 4y | 6y | 17m3 | 2y6 | 4y |
| Epiphysis of 4th metatarsal | 2y11 | 4y | 5y9 | 21m1 | 2y10 | 4y1 |
| Lunate of carpus | 18m2 | 4y1 | 6y9 | 13m | 2y8 | 5y8 |
| Epiphysis, distal segment of 3rd toe | 3y | 4y4 | 6y2 | 16m2 | 2y9 | 4y1 |
| Epiphysis of 5th metatarsal | 3y1 | 4y5 | 6y4 | 2y1 | 3y3 | 4y11 |
| Epiphysis, distal segment of 4th toe | 2y11 | 4y5 | 6y5 | 16m2 | 2y7 | 4y1 |
| Epiphysis, distal segment of 2nd toe | 3y3 | 4y8 | 6y9 | 18m | 2y11 | 4y6 |
| Capitulum of radius | 3y | 5y3 | 8y | 2y3 | 3y11 | 6y3 |
| Scaphoid of carpus | 3y7 | 5y8 | 7y10 | 2y4 | 4y1 | 6y |
| Greater multangular of carpus | 3y7 | 5y11 | 9y | 23m1 | 4y1 | 6y4 |
| Lesser multangular of carpus | 3y1 | 6y3 | 8y6 | 2y5 | 4y2 | 6y |
| Medial epicondyle of humerus | 4y3 | 6y3 | 8y5 | 2y1 | 3y5 | 5y1 |
| Distal epiphysis of ulna | 5y3 | 7y1 | 9y1 | 3y4 | 5y5 | 7y8 |
| Epiphysis of calcaneus | 5y2 | 7y7 | 9y7 | 3y7 | 5y5 | 7y4 |
| Olecranon of ulna | 7y9 | 9y8 | 11y11 | 5y8 | 8y | 9y11 |
| Lateral epicondyle of humerus | 9y3 | 11y3 | 13y8 | 7y2 | 9y3 | 11y3 |
| Tubercle of tibia | 9y11 | 11y10 | 13y5 | 7y11 | 10y3 | 11y10 |
| Adductor sesamoid of 1st finger | 11y | 12y9 | 14y8 | 8y8 | 10y9 | 12y8 |
| Acetabulum | 11y11 | 13y7 | 15y4 | 9y7 | 11y6 | 13y5 |
| Acromion | 12y2 | 13y9 | 15y6 | 10y4 | 11y11 | 13y10 |
| Epiphysis, iliac crest of hip | 12y | 14y | 15y11 | 10y10 | 12y10 | 15y4 |
| Accessory epiphysis, coracoid process of scapula | 12y9 | 14y4 | 16y4 | 10y5 | 12y3 | 14y5 |
| Ischial tuberosity | 13y7 | 15y3 | 17y1 | 11y9 | 13y11 | 16y |

*g*, gestational age; *w*, week; *m*, month; *y*, year. Number following m or y refers to next smaller time unit (e.g., 9y4, 9 years, 4 months).
(From Garn SM, Rohmann CG, Silverman F. Radiographic standards for postnatal ossification and tooth calcification. N Med Radiogr Photogr 1967; 43:45, as modified by Silverman FN. Caffey's pediatric x-ray diagnosis: an integrated imaging approach. Chicago: Year Book Medical Publishers, 1985.)

approximate 1.75 inches (4.5 cm) per year. The average height increment during these years is ~2.5 inches (6.3 cm).

These principles and their use in the diagnosis, differential diagnosis, and therapy for growth-retarded children are described in Chapters 92 and 198. Dental maturation is discussed in Chapter 217.

# GROWTH FAILURE

Growth failure may be classified as follows: *hypopituitarism; emotional deprivation; chromosomal defects; systemic illness* (moderate to severe); *metabolic diseases*; and *chondrodystrophies.*

This classification is not all-inclusive but rather serves as a framework for discussing the approach to children with a failure to grow adequately. The major emphasis of this chapter is on hypopituitarism and emotional deprivation.

## HYPOPITUITARISM

Hypothalamic and pituitary dysfunction (partial or complete) may be classified using a number of systems: congenital versus acquired; isolated, partial, or panhypopituitarism; transient versus permanent; idiopathic versus organic; and primary (pituitary) versus secondary (affecting releasing factors).

The outline shown in Table 18-2 is a convenient list with which to organize a differential diagnosis of hypopituitarism in infants and children. It is not all-inclusive but highlights major categories of pituitary insufficiency. The criteria for the diagnosis of the growth hormone (GH) deficiency of hypopituitarism are as follows: *short stature; growth failure; no significant underlying illness; no evidence for emotional deprivation; delayed bone age; normal body proportions; low circulating levels of insulin-like growth factor-I* (IGF-I); and *subnormal responses to at least two stimuli for GH release.*

### CONGENITAL HYPOPITUITARISM

**Developmental Pituitary Disorders.** Developmental pituitary disorders may be so severe that they are incompatible with life. In some children, there is hypoplasia or absence of the pituitary gland, but in others, developmental anomalies of the hypothalamus appear to be responsible for the lack of pituitary development.[3,4] Anencephaly and holoprosencephaly (including arrhinencephaly, holotelencephaly, cyclopia, and cebocephaly) usually are incompatible with life. This group of anomalies compose a spectrum of developmental anomalies associated with failure of complete midline cleavage of the embryonic forebrain. The children either have no pituitary or a hypoplastic gland and have maldevelopment of the target organs. Atrophy of the adrenal glands always is present, and death usually occurs from adrenal insufficiency. A partial form of holoprosencephaly exists (Kallmann syndrome) in which patients have anosmia caused by the agenesis of the olfactory lobes, and hypogonadotropic hypogonadism secondary to failure of hypothalamic gonadotropin-releasing hormone secretion[5] (see Chaps. 16 and 115).

Absence or hypoplasia of the anterior pituitary is also an uncommon cause of hypopituitarism. The former usually is incompatible with life, but the latter has a spectrum ranging from severe to mild deficiency. The clinical presentation depends on the amount of functioning hypothalamic and pituitary tissue. The main features are severe hypoglycemia and shock because of adrenal failure.

The anterior pituitary lobe develops from an upward diverticulum of the primitive buccal cavity (Rathke pouch) in the nasopharynx and must migrate to its usual location within the sella turcica. There are a number of ectopic sites in which the gland may lodge, from the submucosa of the nasopharynx (pharyngeal pituitary) to the base of the brain. The pituitary stalk is the main neural connection between the hypothalamus (median eminence) and the posterior lobe of the pituitary. In addition to these neurons, there are the capillary loops of the hypothalamic-pituitary portal system providing the principal blood supply to the various portions of the anterior lobe.

Pituitary stalk interruption syndrome (hypoplasia of the anterior lobe, ectopic position of the posterior lobe, and interruption of the stalk) is strongly correlated with multiple anterior pituitary hormone deficiencies.[6] Injury may be developmental or secondary to transection of the stalk.

A number of other anomalies of the craniofacial area may coexist with hypopituitarism. The syndrome of basal encephalocele and hypothalamic–pituitary dysfunction should be mentioned because these patients all have a nasoepipharyngeal mass or unexplained "nasal polyp."[7] The diagnosis should be considered when evaluating a nasal mass, especially in conjunction with the associated findings of hypertelorism, broad nasal root, midline facial defects, optic atrophy, or optic coloboma.

**Inherited Pituitary Disorders**
GENETIC DISORDERS OF GROWTH HORMONE DEFICIENCY. Five to 30 percent of children with growth hormone deficiency have an affected first-degree relative, which is consistent with a genetic cause. These genetic anomalies may result in isolated or combined pituitary hormone deficiencies. The more common are POU1F1, homolog of the mouse Pit-1, and PROP-1 deficiencies, which lack not only GH, prolactin (Prl), and thyroid-stimulating hormone (TSH), but also the gonadotropins. The specific genes

to determine the level of plasma glucose frequently and to use GH and cortisol to treat refractory hypoglycemia.[12]

**Congenital Tumors**

CRANIOPHARYNGIOMA.   The most common tumor in the area of the pituitary of children is the craniopharyngioma[13] (see Chap. 11). It arises from the embryonic remains of the craniopharyngeal duct (Rathke pouch) and is of epithelial origin. This neoplasm commonly is cystic and often contains dark, thick, viscous fluid ("machinery oil"). Although congenital, it is so slow-growing that signs and symptoms often are not manifested until late in the first decade or in the second decade of life or even into adulthood. In addition to the signs of hypopituitarism, children and adolescents may have neurologic symptoms, including prolonged frontal headache, vomiting, or vision deficits—decreased acuity, diplopia, or photophobia. On examination, papilledema, optic nerve atrophy, and impaired visual fields are found in most; they indicate raised intracranial pressure. Older children and adolescents may have obesity or amenorrhea. In the asymptomatic patient, the diagnosis may be made by noting flecks of calcium in the suprasellar region or changes within the suprasellar area as evaluated on computed tomographic (CT) or magnetic resonance imaging (MRI; Fig. 18-4) studies. In a symptomatic patient, CT or MRI scanning is extremely helpful in confirming the diagnosis and determining the extent of the neoplasm.

Although craniopharyngioma is most commonly found in children, optic and third ventricle gliomas and arteriovenous malformations must be considered. The treatment is surgical

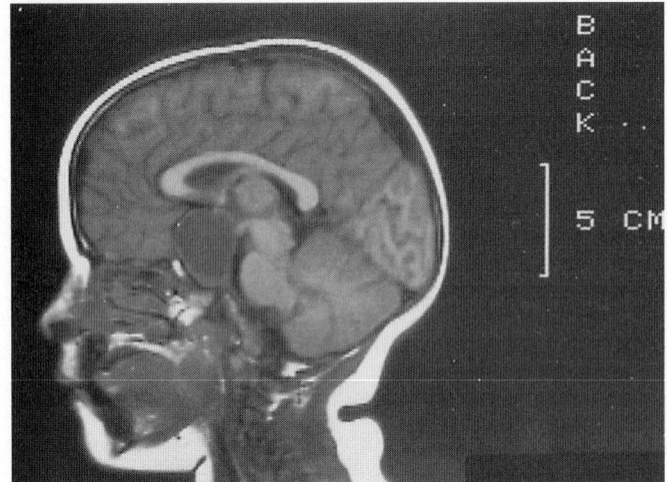
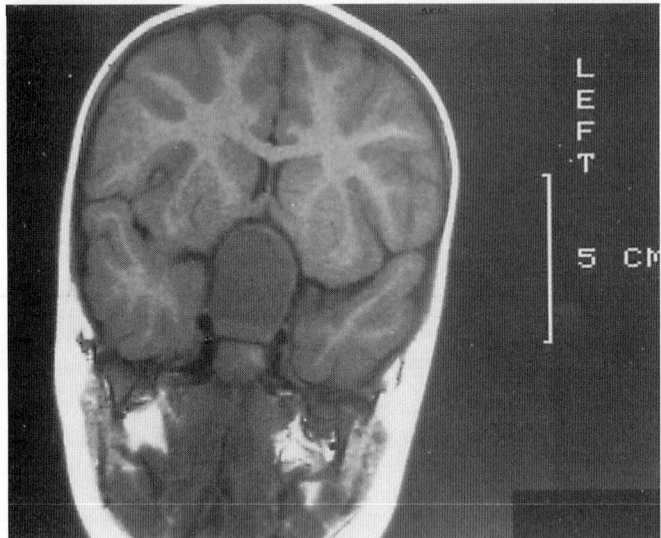

**FIGURE 18-4.** Computed tomographic (*CT*) scans of the brain of a 3-year-old girl with a craniopharyngioma. **A,** Sagittal view showing large suprasellar mass. **B,** Coronal view showing compression of pituitary gland and large suprasellar mass. (Courtesy of Dr. W. Cail, University of Virginia.)

encode members of the homeodomain family of transcription factors, which play an important role in the development of the human pituitary gland.[8] Other deficiencies are caused by growth hormone-releasing hormone receptor mutations.

ISOLATED GROWTH HORMONE DEFICIENCY AND PITUITARY DWARFISM.   The classification of familial GH deficiency primarily is descriptive and is based on the inheritance of the appropriate phenotype and lack of response to pharmacologic stimuli for GH secretion.[9] Six distinct groups based on the mode of inheritance and other hormone deficiencies have been defined (see Table 18-2). In only one, isolated GH deficiency type IA, have the pathophysiologic characteristics been defined: absence of the structural gene for GH (hGH-N).[10] The others apparently are a result of the lack of synthesis or secretion of the hypothalamic-releasing hormone, growth hormone–releasing hormone (GHRH), or to an excessive secretion of the inhibitory hormone, somatostatin. However, heterogeneity of structure and function exists within and among families with isolated GH deficiency and within and among families with pituitary deficiency, making the determination of the precise location of the defect difficult—hypothalamus or pituitary.[11]

Boys with severe GH deficiency and other anterior pituitary deficits may present with microphallus and hypoglycemia. The physical examination of the genitalia should alert the physician

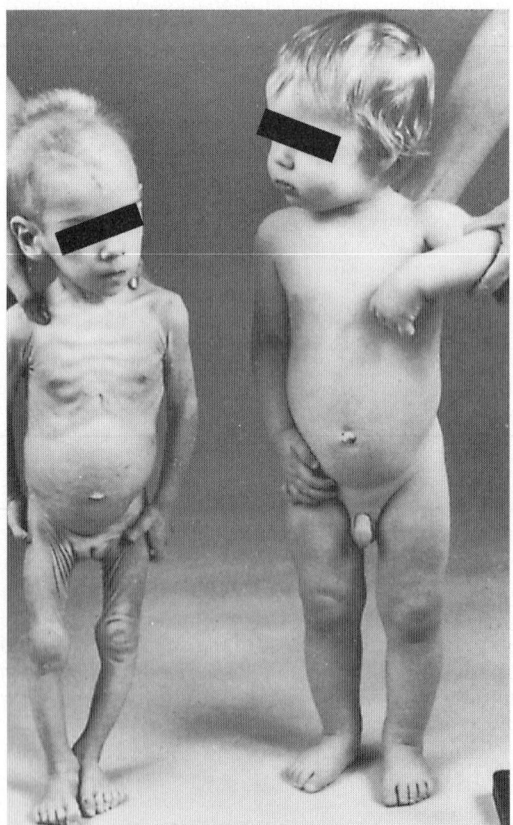

**FIGURE 18-5.** A 10-month-old child with diencephalic syndrome (*left*) next to a normal child of the same age (*right*). Despite striking emaciation, the infant appeared happy and alert and was extremely hyperactive. There was nystagmus. The feet and hands appeared large in comparison with the body. Basal growth hormone levels were high and were not suppressed adequately with glucose administration. At craniotomy, there was an optic glioma involving the optic nerves and chiasma that extended into the anterior hypothalamus and the posterior portion of the third ventricle. (From Häger A, Thorell JI. Studies on growth hormone secretion in a patient with the diencephalic syndrome of emaciation. Acta Paediatr Scand 1973; 62:231.)

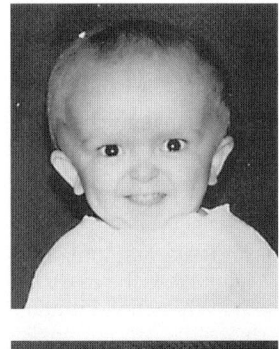
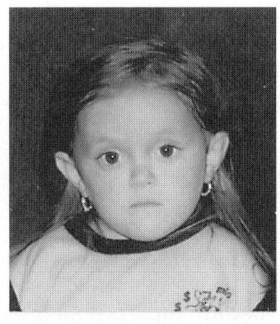
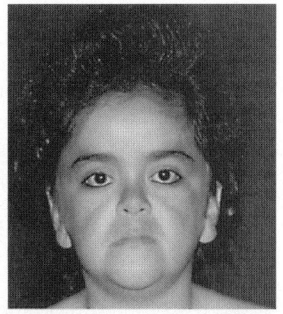
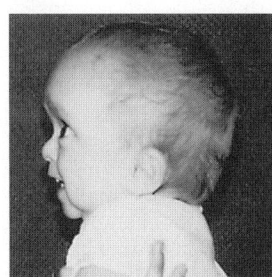
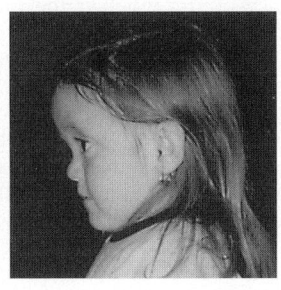
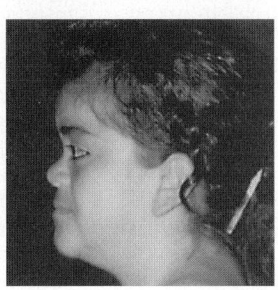

**FIGURE 18-6.** Three Ecuadorian patients with growth hormone receptor deficiency resulting from a point mutation at codon 180 of exon 6 of the growth hormone receptor: a boy aged 26 months (height, –8.2 SD), a girl aged 4.8 years (height –7.4 SD), and a woman aged 19 years (height, –6.5 SD). The vertical dimension of the face is decreased, the nasal bridge is hypoplastic, and the forehead is of normal dimension, giving the impression of craniomegaly, especially in the children. (Courtesy of J. Guevara-Aguirre, Institute for Endocrinology, Metabolism, and Reproduction, Quito, Ecuador; and A.L. Rosenbloom, University of Florida College of Medicine.)

and may be possible through the transsphenoidal approach. Aspiration of the cyst can decompress the mass and relieve symptoms but rarely is curative. Radiation therapy including intracystic application of radioactive pellets, although controversial, may be effective as adjuvant therapy to surgery. Tumor recurrence, even after "total" removal, is common. Hypopituitarism, especially GH deficiency, may be found preoperatively. Postoperatively, it is present in most patients, often in association with other defects in anterior pituitary function and central diabetes insipidus. Meticulous follow-up of growth velocity and pituitary target-organ function, and early replacement therapy greatly decrease the morbidity and mortality after surgery.

DIENCEPHALIC SYNDROME.    The diencephalic syndrome usually comprises a tumor in the diencephalon and the clinical picture of severe emaciation with relative conservation of growth rate, alert appearance, and relatively few neurologic signs. It is nearly always, but not exclusively, found in infancy.[14,15] There is a striking lack of subcutaneous fat. Often, the child seems inappropriately happy (Fig. 18-5). Some clinicians believe that it is related to the age of onset of compression of the hypothalamus because it is not seen in patients with craniopharyngiomas or other tumors within the same anatomic area that present later in childhood, although such tumors displace the third ventricle in a manner similar to that of opticochiasmatic gliomas. Although endocrinologic deficits may be present, they are inconstant and do not help in the diagnostic process. Most tumors are gliomas located in the anterior hypothalamus or in the opticochiasmatic system. The syndrome in infants with tumors placed more posteriorly is characterized by the early onset of vomiting and the absence or late onset of nystagmus, tremor, pallor, polyuria, papilledema, or optic atrophy. These patients are more likely to have malignant cells and raised protein concentrations in the cerebrospinal fluid than are children with more anteriorly placed tumors. These latter patients more often have nystagmus and optic atrophy. Vomiting appears later.[16]

Radiographic studies in patients with anteriorly placed tumors may show enlarged optic foramina and, less commonly, sellar alterations, evidence of increased intracranial pressure, and, rarely, calcification. Computed tomographic and MRI scans may be the best tools for defining the exact nature and extent of disease because the optic nerves, chiasm, and sellar and suprasellar regions can be visualized precisely.

The prognosis is poor, and the treatment remains controversial. Surgery is rarely curative, but it is important to obtain a pathologic diagnosis. Radiation therapy can dramatically reduce the mass of the tumor. However, the natural history is uncertain and variable. Thus, treatment for these often slow-growing tumors varies from no therapy, to surgical excision, to radiation therapy; however, one must be concerned with ultimate brain growth if a child younger than 2 to 3 years old undergoes radiation therapy. Because most series have been small and their data were collected over several decades when the approach to diagnosis, therapy, intensive postoperative care, and endocrinologic replacement therapy was in great flux, it is not surprising that no single therapeutic protocol has proved to be clearly superior.

**Defects in the Structure, Metabolism, or Secretion of Growth Hormone or Insulin-Like Growth Factor I**

BIOLOGICALLY INACTIVE GROWTH HORMONE.    Children with growth failure who have normal or elevated basal GH concentrations or a normal or increased response to pharmacologic stimuli, but diminished IGF-I concentrations that cannot be attributed to malnutrition, chronic illness, or other causes, may secrete a bioinactive (subactive) GH molecule. Bone and dental development are significantly delayed, and the body proportions are more appropriate for chronologic than height age. Although some investigators have proposed this hypothesis for short stature in the few children who fit into the diagnostic category, there is sparse evidence. Clearly, it is not the public health problem it was originally considered.[17] Findings in a single patient indicate that aggregation of serum GH may be responsible.[18] However, a mutation in the GH gene itself can produce a mutated form of GH (found to be expressed in *Escherichia coli*), which is clinically associated with short stature in the affected child.[19] The mutated GH binds avidly to the GHG receptor in the IM-9 cell line, but does not stimulate intracellular signaling pathways. Thus, it inhibits the bioeffects of native GH.

The growth hormone insensitive syndrome (GHIS) represents another defect in the mechanism of GH action[3,20] (Fig.18-6). These patients with familial dwarfism and clinical features of GH deficiency tend to be of normal birth weight, but growth velocity is retarded soon after birth. Motor development, bone maturation, and dental eruption are slow, and the anterior fontanelle may close later than average. The facial bones grow more slowly than the cranial vault. When the child has a small mid-face and mandible and a bulging forehead, macrocephaly should be considered.

The children tend to be obese and have a high-pitched voice. Although many of the original patients were of Semitic origin, subsequent patients have come from many ethnic backgrounds.

GH values are high basally and are elevated in response to pharmacologic stimuli, but IGF-I levels are low. The circulating GH molecules are biologically active. The pathogenesis of the defect is failure of the liver to respond to GH by generating IGF-I. Because the extracellular domain of the GH receptor is a growth hormone–binding protein (GHBP), this protein might be expected to be absent or defective in GHIS.[21] The initial direct evidence for a GH receptor defect in GHIS was that hepatocytes obtained at biopsy from a patient with this disorder did not bind tracer quantities of radiolabeled GH, although samples from control subjects undergoing abdominal surgery did.[22] Subsequently, the similarity of the circulating GHBP to the GH receptor (the former is the extracellular domain of the latter) led to the finding that GHBP was absent in patients with GHIS. The clinical and biochemical characteristics of GHIS have been reviewed.[23] Prominent biochemical abnormalities include low circulating levels of IGF-I, IGF-II, insulin-like growth factor–binding protein-3 (IGFBP-3), and GHBP; and levels of IGF-I, IGF-II, and IGFBP-3 that are higher in adults than in children without a change in the level of GHBP.[22] A number of treatment trials with recombinant human IGF-I are under way. In all the young patients, the growth rate is accelerated. Many patients had growth rates during therapy in the range of 8 to 10 cm per year. Because of the low IGFBP-3 levels at the onset of treatment and the lack of a buffer for the injected IGF-I, some patients experienced hypoglycemia.

GROWTH HORMONE NEUROSECRETORY DYSFUNCTION. Children with dysregulation of GH secretion meet the following criteria: *short stature; growth failure; bone age 2 or more years behind chronologic age; IGF-I levels low for age;* and *results for provocative tests for GH within normal limits.*[24] The children with GH deficiency meet these same criteria except that they have subnormal peak responses to provocative stimuli. Results of functional tests for other pituitary and target-gland hormones are normal. Malnutrition, systemic disease, and psychosocial dwarfism must be considered.

The normal child usually has more than six secretory episodes of GH per day, but children within this category usually have fewer than four. The number of secretory episodes, the amount of GH secreted, and the peak GH concentrations all are intermediate between values found for GH-deficient and normal children.

As greater numbers of slowly growing children are tested for GH neurosecretory dysfunction, the boundaries between normal and subnormal become more indistinct. It is not possible to determine with certitude from the 24-hour GH secretory pattern which children will respond favorably to therapy with GH. Given the expense and difficulty in determining a 24-hour secretory pattern, it may be prudent in selected children with growth failure to administer a 6-month therapeutic trial with GH. Marked acceleration in growth rate is the criterion for continued therapy. However, a number of such children respond to gonadal steroid hormone therapy with marked increases in endogenous GH secretion and growth rate.[25–28] In fact, for boys, if the child is within the pubertal age range, treatment with low doses of testosterone (50–100 mg intramuscularly each month) would be more appropriate than GH. The question of whether low-dose estradiol will augment GH secretion and ultimate growth in girls has been insufficiently explored.

### ACQUIRED HYPOPITUITARISM

**During Birth.** Perinatal complications, including breech or face presentation, can lead to pituitary insufficiency because of vascular compromise to the anterior hypophysis or to the hypothalamic area. Review of the birth records of patients with nonfamilial hypopituitarism indicates that more than half of all hypopituitary patients have an abnormal perinatal history—an incidence much higher than in the normal population. Magnetic resonance imaging studies may show an ectopic posterior pituitary gland ("bright spot") or interruption of the pituitary stalk.

**After Birth.** Trauma continues to be an important cause for hypopituitarism beyond the neonatal period. A blow to the head or face can cause bleeding in the hypothalamic area or may shear the pituitary stalk. Varying degrees of hypopituitarism result, but when the pituitary remains relatively intact, all the anterior pituitary hormones circulate in low concentrations except for high levels of prolactin.

The infiltrative diseases, whether infectious or granulomatous, may invade the hypothalamic areas that synthesize the releasing hormones or carry these factors to the median eminence. Pituitary insufficiency occurs whether the underlying disease is Langerhans cell histiocytosis (relatively commonly associated with hypopituitarism), meningitis or encephalitis caused by a number of organisms (e.g., tuberculosis), or is a result of autoimmune phenomena from primary or metastatic deposits in the hypothalamic area (see Chaps. 11 and 17). These latter causes are uncommon in adults and rare in children and adolescents.

All forms of hypothalamic–pituitary dysfunction may occur after intracranial surgery, irradiation therapy, or chemotherapy for neoplastic diseases. Data indicate growth failure and an abnormal GH secretory pattern among children who have survived acute lymphoblastic leukemia but who had received irradiation to the craniospinal axis or intrathecal therapy with antineoplastic agents.[29] The growth rate of such children should be followed carefully to determine which of the children might benefit from GH therapy (see Chap. 198).

Aneurysms of the internal carotid area and arteriovenous malformations in the hypothalamic area are uncommon. How-

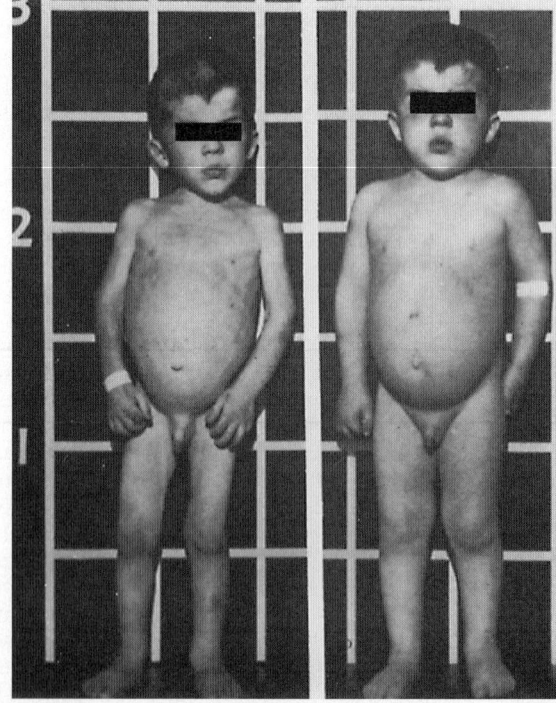

**FIGURE 18-7. Left,** A 5-year, 4-month-old child with deprivational dwarfism related to parental neglect, abuse, and malnutrition. The child is 84.5 cm (33.5 in.) in height, corresponding to a height age of 22 months; there is moderate mental retardation. There was patchy alopecia of the scalp, moderate hirsutism of the body, and a paucity of sweating. Note the sparse abdominal fat and the prominent abdomen; hepatomegaly was present. **Right,** the child was hospitalized, attended to, and provided unlimited food intake. Four months later, he had gained 5.2 kg (11.5 lb) and had grown 3.8 cm (1.5 in.). He became more active and playful, the body hair diminished, and he perspired normally. (From Copps SC, Gerritsen T, Smith DW, Waisman HA. Urinary excretion of 3,4-dihydroxyphenylalanine [DOPA] in two children of short stature and malnutrition. J Pediatr 1963;62:208.)

**TABLE 18-3.**
**Replacement Therapy for Pituitary Hormonal Deficiencies**

| Hormonal Deficiency | Pharmacologic Agent and Dose |
|---|---|
| Growth hormone | hGH, 0.3 mg/kg/wk subcutaneously (e.g., in divided daily doses). |
| Thyroid-stimulating hormone | L-Thyroxine, 2.5–5 µg/kg/d orally, ages 3 to 12; younger children may require up to 10 µg/kg/d. |
| Adrenocorticotropic hormone | Hydrocortisone, 12–18 mg/m²/d orally or its equivalent with other available glucocorticoid preparations. |
| Luteinizing hormone, follicle-stimulating hormone | *Men*[a]: Testosterone enanthate 200–300 mg IM every 2–3 weeks; fluoxymesterone 2–10 mg/d orally. *Women*[a]: Ethinyl estradiol 20–25 µg/d orally, days 1–25; or conjugated estrogens, 0.3–1.25 mg/d orally, days 1–25, plus medroxyprogesterone acetate, 5–10 mg/d orally, days 16–25. (See Chaps. 100 and 236 for use of transdermal estrogen.) |
| Antidiuretic hormone | dDAVP, 5–40 µg/d intranasally[b]; oral dose may be 10-fold higher. |

[a]Full adult replacement doses; smaller doses gradually reaching these described can be used to induce puberty.
[b]Dosing by rhinal tube and spray are available—the latter requires a higher dose because the particles are less consistently absorbed.
(Adapted from Costin G. Endocrine disorders associated with tumors of the pituitary and hypothalamus. Pediatr Clin North Am 1979; 26:15.)

ever, they represent emergent but potentially treatable causes of hypopituitarism. Their diagnosis has been made much simpler with the confirmation provided by CT or MRI scanning and vascular contrast studies. Their treatment is mainly surgical.

Lymphocytic hypophysitis is rare, especially in children. It may be part of a multiple endocrine organ autoimmune syndrome or appear as an isolated condition (see Chap. 11). There are no specific clues to the diagnosis except when it is found in association with other endocrine gland dysfunction. However, this condition may be responsible for varying degrees of hypopituitarism postpartum, especially in women without an obvious hypotensive episode.

## DEPRIVATIONAL DWARFISM

The deprivational dwarfism syndrome (psychosocial dwarfism) is characterized by behavioral aberrations, emotional disturbances in association with growth failure, and abnormalities of pituitary function[30] (Fig. 18-7). These are transient and are reversed by changes in the child's home environment. As originally described, truly bizarre behavior (e.g., eating from garbage pails or dog dishes, drinking from toilet bowls, and exhibiting severe sleep disturbances) was common. Growth failure was invariant and, early after hospitalization, test results for GH and corticotropin (ACTH) reserve were usually abnormal. The transient nature of the hypopituitary state became obvious when these children grew and gained weight at phenomenal speed during hospitalization—a rate of 1 inch per month was not unusual. The results of pituitary function tests for GH and ACTH reserve often reverted to normal within days to weeks. Return to the same home environment can cause the syndrome to recur.

Dysfunction of central neurotransmitter function has been postulated to explain the hypopituitarism and the sleep disturbance. The role of malnutrition is controversial but probably is unimportant in those children older than 2 years of age who can fend for themselves, although in a disturbed manner. However, for younger infants, inadequate caloric intake may play some role.

The clinical presentations are inconstant but include variable age of onset, short stature, growth failure, bizarre eating and drinking (polydipsia) behavior, and sleep disturbance with nighttime roaming and foraging. The family social situation is best described as disorganized and disrupted. Often, only one member of a larger sibship is affected.

The diagnosis is clinical, based on the detailed history and observations of the growth failure in the child and the family's behavior. The results of endocrine tests for GH and ACTH (e.g., arginine and insulin tolerance tests) are likely to be abnormal during the first few days of hospitalization but may quickly revert to normal. There are no data concerning the use of direct tests of pituitary reserve by GHRH or corticotropin-releasing hormone.

Removal of such children from their environment is the only method of confirming the diagnosis and treating them. Truly remarkable acceleration of linear growth (catch-up growth) and

weight gain are not unusual during the first few months in a more nurturing environment. The prognosis for weight gain, growth, and pubertal development are excellent, provided these children remain outside the deleterious environment or that environment is sufficiently changed to become more nurturing. Long-term psychological therapy for both the parents and the child is often necessary.

## CUSHING DISEASE

Cushing disease is mentioned here not because the pituitary adenomas associated with this condition cause growth failure, but because the excessive circulating levels of cortisol in response to the elevated ACTH concentrations are potent inhibitors of growth. In fact, excess glucocorticoids from any source can adversely affect the growth rate by inhibiting both GH secretion and GH action. Diseases of glucocorticoid excess are considered in Chapters 75 and 83.

## DIAGNOSIS AND TREATMENT OF GROWTH FAILURE

The differential diagnosis of growth failure is broad; even when hypopituitarism is documented by proper testing in the appropriate clinical situation, the precise diagnosis may be elusive. The key features of the major disease entities and their criteria for diagnosis have been outlined in other chapters.

The treatment of hypopituitarism is dependent on the hormonal deficits and may include anterior and posterior pituitary hormones and some target-organ hormones or analogs. The replacement therapy strategy for diminished gonadotropin, thyroid-stimulating hormone, and ACTH concentrations is to use the target-gland hormones (Table 18-3). For diabetes insipidus, deamino-D-arginine vasopressin is preferred.

Until recently, the only therapeutic option for GH deficiency was to administer human cadaveric pituitary-derived material, usually at a dose of 1 to 2 U intramuscularly three times a week. With the more purified material produced within the last decade, the incidence of circulating antibody formation was low, and only rarely was the titer high enough to attenuate growth. However, because of the limited supply, not all children with hypopituitarism could be treated, and detailed pharmacologic studies to determine the optimal dose, route, and interdose interval could not be performed. With the recent concern over the transmission of Creutzfeldt-Jakob disease by materials derived from human brain, the recombinant DNA-produced GHs are the only agents presently available.

The last several years have been exciting in terms of the development of agents for the treatment of GH insufficiency. First, the human GH structural gene has been cloned and expressed in bacteria that can produce the hormone indefinitely. The purified product is available and as potent as the native hormone.

Second, GHRH has been extracted and purified, its structure determined, and large quantities of it and other stimulatory

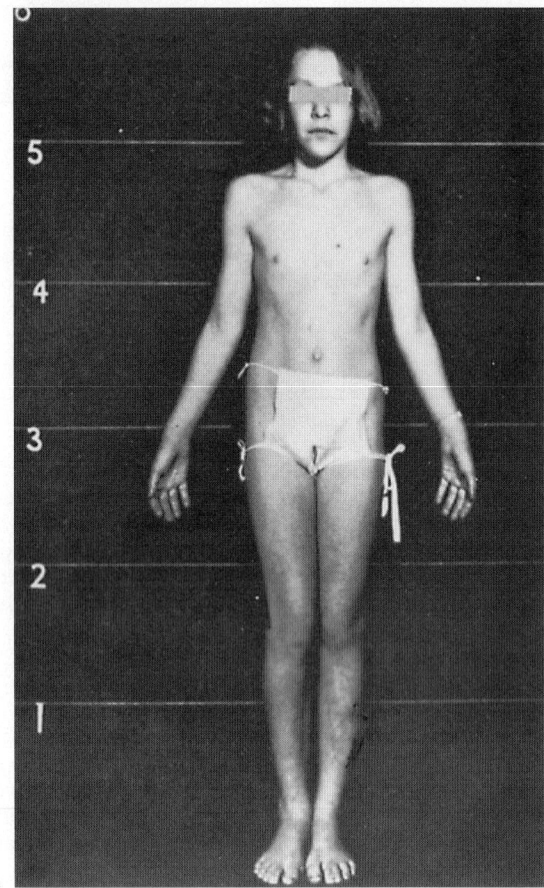

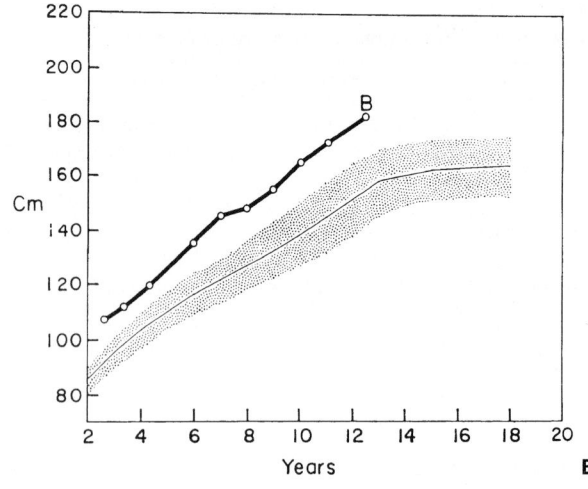

**FIGURE 18-8. A,** Patient with cerebral gigantism at age 11 years. **B,** Growth curve (mean and 2 SD) of the patient shown in (**A**). (From Hook EB, Reynolds JW. Cerebral gigantism: endocrinological and clinical observations of six patients including a congenital giant, concordant monozygotic twins, and a child who achieved adult gigantic size. J Pediatr 1967; 70:900.)

analogs produced. Early trials with subcutaneous administration in an intermittent, pulsatile fashion have proved efficacious.[31,32] Studies to determine the optimal form, dose, route, and frequency of administration are being vigorously pursued. More recent experience shows that GH-deficient children accelerate their growth when the GH dosage of 0.3 mg/kg per week is administered subcutaneously (typically subdivided into daily doses, e.g., 0.045 mg/kg per day) or when GHRH therapy is given subcutaneously (~8 μg/kg per dose twice daily) or using a portable minipump (2 μg/kg per dose every 3 hours).[33,34] Because most children with hypopituitarism, even those with structural lesions, have suprasellar defects, this form of therapy holds promise for large numbers of GH-deficient children.[35]

A hexapeptide, GH-releasing peptide (GHRP), has been developed synthetically but is not homologous to the GHRH-related peptides of 40 or 44 amino acids. Its activity in humans is not diminished by somatostatin, and its ability to cause release of GH when submaximal quantities of GHRH are present is at least additive and possibly synergistic. The role of this peptide or its analogs, or the native homolog if one exists, has not yet been defined, but preliminary data from a clinical trial with one analog are available.[36,37]

IGF-I is also available for therapeutic protocols in the treatment of GH-deficient patients. Its major use is in patients with GHIS and in patients with GH gene deletion treated with GH and producing anti–human GH antibodies. Preliminary data are consistent with growth rates in the range of 8 to 12 cm per year, similar to those among GH-deficient children treated with recombinant GH.

The other conditions (chromosomal defects, moderate to severe systemic illness, metabolic diseases, and chondrodystrophies)[38] are beyond the scope of this chapter. An extensive differential diagnosis of syndromes associated with short stature has been published.[39]

## TALL STATURE

### NONENDOCRINE DYSFUNCTION

Usually, children more than 2 to 3 SD above the mean height for age are considered tall. Most, of course, have a normal growth rate and are considered to be "constitutionally tall" without a pathologic cause. Many are the children of tall parents and are merely fulfilling their genetic potential.

In addition to constitutional tall stature, other *nonendocrine* conditions associated with tall stature or excessive growth rate are cerebral gigantism, Marfan syndrome, homocystinuria, and Beckwith-Wiedemann syndrome. *Endocrine dysfunctional* disorders include gigantism and aberrant sexual maturation (sexual precocity, hypogonadism). From a cultural viewpoint, excessively tall girls are more likely than boys to seek therapy to diminish their predicted adult height. Although, in girls, estrogen therapy in large doses has been used in the past, with some diminution from predicted adult height, the actual and potential side effects are severe enough that this form of therapy cannot be recommended except in particularly unusual circumstances.[40] Open discussion of the actions and potential deleterious effects of these potent sex steroids is often sufficient to dissuade their use.

### CEREBRAL GIGANTISM

Cerebral gigantism (Sotos syndrome) is a disorder in which a rapid growth rate and tall stature are noted in infancy and early childhood.[41] These children tend to be large at birth and grow excessively the first 3 or 4 years of life (Fig. 18-8). There are a number of dysmorphic features in addition to the tall stature: prominent forehead, high-arched palate, hypertelorism, and a long head are found in more than 80% of the children, who also are likely to be developmentally retarded. The excessive body and skeletal growth and the increased incidence of malignancies suggest that this condition is primarily a disorder of

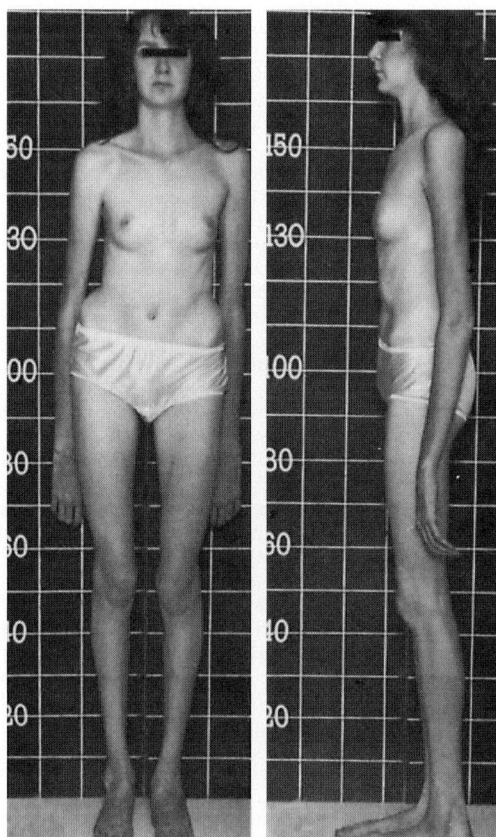

**FIGURE 18-9.** A 14-year-old girl with Marfan syndrome. There is excessive height (183 cm; 72 in.), a thin body habitus, and normal pubertal development. The face is long and thin, and the limbs, hands, and feet are elongated and spidery. Scoliosis necessitated the wearing of a body brace. There is muscle hypotonia and diminution of subcutaneous fat. There also was subluxation of the lenses. The patient was treated unsuccessfully with estrogen in an attempt to hasten skeletal maturation. Transmission of this condition is autosomal dominant. (From Rallison ML. Growth disorders in infants, children and adolescents. New York: Churchill Livingstone, 1986:330.)

growth factors, but there are no data relevant to the etiology and pathogenesis.

Diagnosis is based on the constellation of signs noted and cerebral ventricular widening on CT or MRI scans. The endocrine function is normal. No specific therapy exists, and although they become tall adults, few are excessively tall. The developmental delay and mental retardation do not progress.

### MARFAN SYNDROME

Marfan syndrome is a heritable disorder of connective tissue in which the patient tends to be tall and to have long slim limbs, arachnodactyly, lax joints, dislocation (subluxation) of the lens, and dilation with or without dissecting aneurysm of the ascending aorta[42] (see Chap. 189). During growth and development, there is a marked tendency to scoliosis (Fig. 18-9). The prognosis depends on the vascular complications. The diagnosis is clinical, with therapy directed toward the vascular lesions. The specific abnormality has now been identified.[43]

### HOMOCYSTINURIA

Homocystinuria, also a heritable disorder of connective tissue, is characterized by tall stature, fair complexion, mild mental retardation (inconstant), slim skeletal build, and arachnodactyly resembling Marfan syndrome but with severe osteoporosis and subluxation of the lens. The latter usually is not present at birth but has been described in patients 2 years old[42] (see Chap. 191).

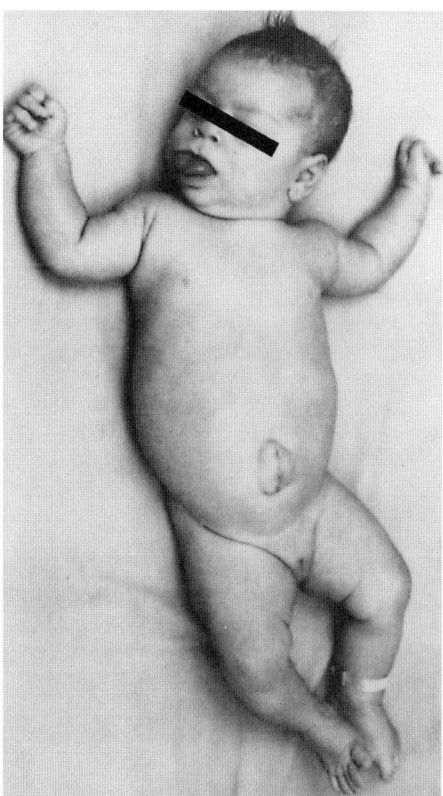

**FIGURE 18-10.** A 2.5-month old infant with Beckwith-Wiedemann syndrome. There was macroglossia at birth, and an omphalocele (congenital protrusion of omentum and intestine through an abdominal opening) necessitated surgical repair in the first 24 hours of life. It had been noted that the baby was big, had large facial features, and had mild weakness of the limbs. At the time this photograph was made, the infant was in the 97th percentile for weight and the 90th percentile for length. There were prominent inner canthal folds, marked enlargement of the tongue, and a high-arched palate. The nose was broad, and there was a long upper lip philtrum. There was a flat, red flame nevus in the center of the forehead and other nevi on the cheeks as well as on the eyelids. (The midline nevus as well as the bilateral double linear indentations of the ear lobes are typical.) Other findings in this infant included a short neck, large muscle mass, hepatosplenomegaly, and a residual ventral hernia. Occasionally girls with this syndrome may have clitoromegaly at birth, and some boys have cryptorchidism. The final adult height attained is relatively tall. Mild mental retardation is common, but not uniform. The relative tongue size may regress or may necessitate surgery. The condition usually appears sporadically, but autosomal-recessive transmission has been suspected. (From Filippi G, McKusick VA. The Beckwith-Wiedemann syndrome. Medicine [Baltimore] 1970; 49:279.)

The pathogenesis is cystathionine synthase deficiency, which is characterized by elevated plasma concentrations of methionine and homocystine and by the excretion of homocystine in the urine. The diagnosis is based on the clinical findings and the presence of homocystine in the urine. The prognosis depends on the marked tendency to form life-threatening arterial and venous thromboses. Many patients die of coronary or carotid occlusion in the second or third decade of life.[42]

The goals of dietary therapy are to eliminate potentially toxic substances accumulating proximal to the enzymatic deficiency and to supply those substances that are deficient distal to the defect.[44]

### BECKWITH-WIEDEMANN SYNDROME

Beckwith-Wiedemann syndrome is characterized by exomphalos (omphalocele), macroglossia, neonatal hypoglycemia, and postnatal gigantism[42] (Fig. 18-10). The birth weight usually is increased, but polyhydramnios and prematurity are common.

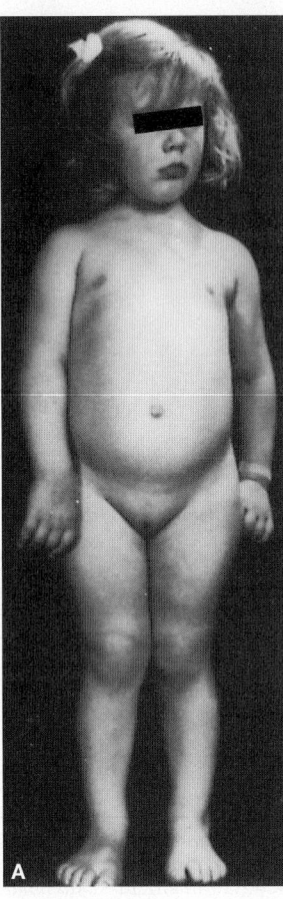
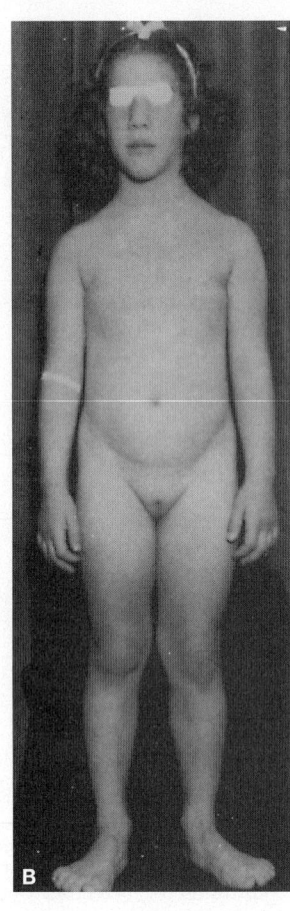
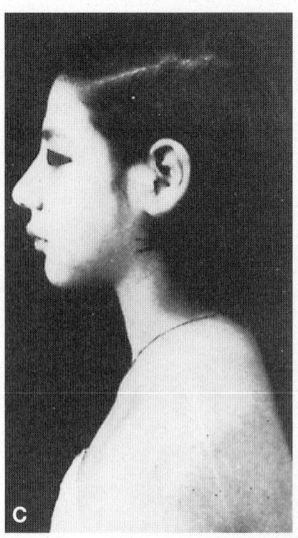

**FIGURE 18-11.** Pituitary gigantism in two children. Growth hormone excess before the fusion of the epiphyses is characterized predominantly by rapid growth rate and excessive size and weight for age. After epiphyseal closure, growth hormone excess induces acromegalic features, including overgrowth of soft tissue, thickening of skin, widening of bones, and prominence of acral parts of the body (face, hands, feet). Many pituitary giants exhibit both increased size and acral changes, particularly if the growth hormone excess persists into adulthood. Gigantism diagnosed during childhood also may show varying degrees of acromegaly. **A,** A 31-month-old girl with pituitary gigantism who began to grow rapidly in her second year of life. The rapid growth and large size had been noted by the parents, who also remarked on the excessive sweating and strong body odor. The height was 104 cm (41 in.), which was 5.5 cm (2.5 in.) greater than the estimated 97th percentile. The child resembled a 4-year-old. The facial features were normal, and the hands and feet were only slightly prominent. **B** and **C,** A girl who is 5 years, 8 months old with pituitary gigantism. Her height of 118 cm (50.5 in.) corresponds approximately to a height age of 8 years, 6 months. However, this child had considerably enlarged hands and feet and marked enlargement of the jaw, nose, and ears. (**A** from Espiner EA, Carter TA, Abbott GD, Wrightson P. Pituitary gigantism in a 31-month-old girl: endocrine studies and successful response to hypophysectomy. J Endocrinol Invest 1981; 4:445; **B** and **C** from Hurxthal LM. Pituitary gigantism in a child five years of age: effect of x-radiation, estrogen therapy and self-imposed starvation diet during an eleven year period. J Clin Endocrinol Metab 1961; 21:343.)

Although the early growth rate is often slow, these infants subsequently show accelerated growth with macrosomia, a large muscle mass, and thick subcutaneous tissue. Most children grow near the 90th percentile and have an advanced bone age. A characteristic face with macroglossia and a protruding tongue are prominent. Visceromegaly is invariant, and there is a susceptibility to abdominal malignancies because of the loss of heterozygosity of the chromosomal locus 11p15.5, an area that contains the genes for IGF-II and a tumor-suppressor gene. The most serious problem is neonatal hypoglycemia, usually with elevated circulating concentrations of insulin; however, as these infants mature, the episodes of hypoglycemia wane. The prognosis depends on the early control of the hypoglycemic episodes. This may require systemic glucocorticoid therapy for the first few months of life.

## ENDOCRINE DYSFUNCTION

### PITUITARY GIGANTISM

Pituitary gigantism (GH excess) is an extremely uncommon cause of accelerated growth and tall stature. The usual cause is a pituitary adenoma composed of somatotropes. However, excessive GHRH from the hypothalamus or from an ectopic source (e.g., a pancreatic islet cell tumor) may lead to a syndrome indistinguishable from that caused by a pituitary adenoma.[45,46] Theoretically, lack of somatostatin secretion or excessive secretory episodes of GHRH could cause an increased release of GH.

Clinically, the patients (often adolescents) have an augmented growth rate—crossing previously defined growth percentiles in an upward direction (Fig. 18-11). They may have evidence of the acral enlargement characteristic of an adult with acromegaly (see Chap. 12). Headache, visual field abnormalities (classically, bitemporal hemianopsia), decreased visual acuity, and other signs or symptoms of increased intracranial pressure may be prominent.

Laboratory confirmation of this basically clinical diagnosis includes high circulating levels of GH and especially IGF-I and failure of the elevated GH concentrations to be suppressed after an oral glucose load.

Standard CT imaging techniques with and without contrast medium, and especially MRI, are useful in defining the anatomic limits of the pituitary tumor (see Chap. 20). Transsphenoidal microsurgery often is curative, although some groups advocate radiation therapy, either as primary treatment or in addition to intracranial surgery. With large tumors, craniotomy with direct visualization and tumor removal is preferred (see Chap. 23).

### ABERRANT SEXUAL MATURATION

Aberrant sexual maturation, whether precocious in children or hypogonadal in adolescents, is associated with tall stature and an excessive growth rate[47,48] (see Chaps. 77 and 90 through 92). The more commonly encountered conditions are listed in Table 18-4.

**Precocious Sexual Development.** Sexual precocity occurs more commonly in girls than in boys and may be secondary to early maturation of the hypothalamic–pituitary–gonadal axis (precocious puberty) or a result of sex steroid production from the adrenal or gonad (sexual precocity, pseudoprecocious puberty). The signs of sexual maturation usually precede those of accelerated growth velocity, just as they do during normal pubertal development.

Precocious puberty may be caused by organic lesions (Fig. 18-12) or may be idiopathic (see Chap. 92).

The introduction of a long-acting gonadotropin-releasing hormone (GnRH) agonist, whose activity is based on the pharmacologic precept of down-regulation (desensitization) of the GnRH receptor on the gonadotropes, has made the goals for therapy of this condition realizable.[47–49] These goals are arrest or reversal of secondary sexual maturation; decrease of the linear growth rate to a normal prepubertal velocity; slowing of

## TABLE 18-4.
### Aberrant Sexual Maturation

**SEXUAL PRECOCITY**

*Isosexual*

    Precocious puberty

        Idiopathic

        Organic

    Precocious pseudopuberty

        Ovarian cysts and tumors

        McCune-Albright syndrome

        Testicular tumors

        Adrenal hyperplasia and tumors

        Testotoxicosis

*Heterosexual*

    Congenital virilizing adrenal hyperplasia

    Ovarian and adrenal tumors

**HYPOGONADISM**

*Hypogonadotropic*

    Kallmann syndrome

    Fertile eunuch syndrome

    Isolated gonadotropin deficiency

    Panhypopituitarism

*Hypergonadotropic*

    Klinefelter syndrome

    Turner syndrome and variants

    XX gonadal dysgenesis (pure)

    Androgen insensitivity

    Following radiation therapy and/or chemotherapy for malignant diseases

---

skeletal maturation to increase adult stature; preservation of fertility as an adult; and prevention or amelioration of any emotional disturbance. The therapy for organic lesions causing sexual precocity, including precocious puberty, is mainly surgery

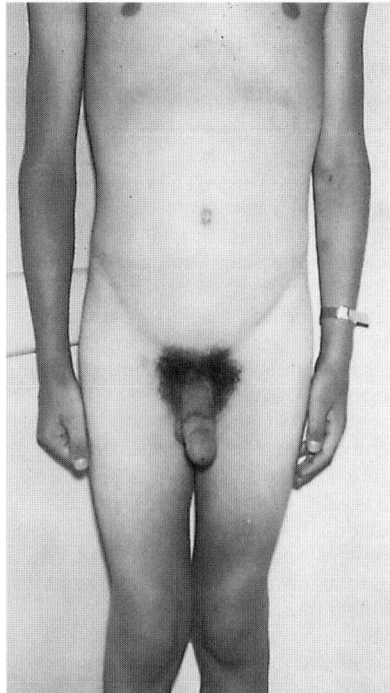

**FIGURE 18-12.** Nine-year-old boy with rapid growth and sexual precocity resulting from a hamartoma of the hypothalamus.

or radiation with, if needed, postoperative replacement of target-gland hormones.

The most common cause of heterosexual precocity in girls is congenital virilizing adrenal hyperplasia (adrenogenital syndrome; see Chap. 77). The excessive growth is caused by the failure of adequate ACTH suppression by cortisol and the subsequent overproduction of biologically active adrenal androgens. During the first few years, the goal of administering adequate but not excessive amounts of glucocorticoids is not always easily obtainable. Although children with inadequate adrenal suppression grow excessively, the bone age matures at an even greater rate, causing the patient to be tall as a child but to enter puberty early and become short as an adult.

**Hypogonadal Syndromes.** A number of hypogonadal syndromes—either hypogonadotropic or hypergonadotropic—exist. The pathophysiologic disturbance that leads to excessive stature and eunuchoid body proportions is failure of epiphyseal maturation (bone age) beyond ~13 years of age and, thus, continued, albeit often slow, growth into the third decade of life (see Chap. 115).[50] The therapy is mainly with gonadal steroids to produce secondary sexual characteristics and increased libido (see Table 18-3). Treatment of hypogonadotropic patients with GnRH or the gonadotropins themselves is appropriate when fertility is desired (see Chaps. 16, 97, and 115).

# REFERENCES

1. Wilkins L. The diagnosis and treatment of endocrine disorders in childhood and adolescence. Springfield, IL: Charles C Thomas Publisher, 1965.
2. Greulich WW, Pyle SI. Radiographic atlas of skeletal development of the hand-wrist, 2nd ed. Palo Alto, CA: Stanford University Press, 1959.
3. Laron Z. The hypothalamus and the pituitary gland. In: Hubble D, ed. Pediatric endocrinology. Oxford: Blackwell Scientific, 1969:35.
4. Rimoin DL, Schimke RN. Genetic disorders of the endocrine glands. St. Louis: Mosby, 1971:11.
5. Lieblich JM, Rogol AD, White BJ, Rosen SW. Syndrome of anosmia with hypogonadotropic hypogonadism (Kallmann syndrome). Am J Med 1982; 73:506.
6. Triulzi F, Scotti G, diNatale B, et al. Evidence of a congenital midline brain anomaly in pituitary dwarfs: a magnetic resonance imaging study in 101 patients. Pediatrics 1994; 93:409.
7. Lieblich JM, Rosen SW, Guyda H, et al. The syndrome of basal encephalocele and hypothalamic-pituitary dysfunction. Ann Intern Med 1978; 89:910.
8. Procter AM, Phillips JA III, Cooper DN. The molecular genetics of growth hormone deficiency. Hum Genet 1998; 103:255.
9. Rimoin DL. Hereditary forms of growth hormone deficiency and resistance. Birth Defects 1976; 12:15.
10. Phillips JA III. The growth hormone (hGH) gene and human disease. In: Banberry Report 14: Recombinant DNA applications to human disease. Cold Spring Harbor, NY: Cold Spring Harbor Laboratory, 1983; 305.
11. Rogol AD, Blizzard RM, Foley TP Jr, et al. Growth hormone releasing hormone and growth hormone: genetic studies in familial growth hormone deficiency. Pediatr Res 1985; 19:489.
12. Lovinger RD, Kaplan SL, Grumbach MM. Congenital hypopituitarism associated with neonatal hypoglycemia and microphallus: four cases secondary to hypothalamic hormone deficiencies. J Pediatr 1975; 87:1171.
13. Paja M, Lucas T, Garcia-Uria J, et al. Hypothalamic-pituitary dysfunction in patients with craniopharyngioma. Clin Endocrinol 1995; 42:467.
14. Burr IM, Slonim AE, Danish RK, et al. Diencephalic syndrome revisited. J Pediatr 1976; 88:439.
15. Tanabe M, Watanabe T, Hori T: Von Recklinghausen's disease with diencephalic syndrome in an adult: case report. J Neurosurg 1994; 80:556.
16. Rogol AD. Pituitary and parapituitary tumors of childhood and adolescence. In: Givens JR, ed. Hormone-secreting pituitary tumors. Chicago: Year Book Medical Publishers, 1982:349.
17. Kowarski AA, Schneider J, Ben-Galim E, et al. Growth failure with normal serum RIA-GH and low somatomedin activity: somatomedin restoration and growth acceleration after exogenous GH. J Clin Endocrinol Metab 1978; 47:461.
18. Valenta LJ, Sigel MB, Lesniak MA, et al. Pituitary dwarfism in a patient with circulating abnormal growth hormone polymers. N Engl J Med 1985; 312:214.
19. Takahashi Y, Kaji H, Okimura Y, et al. Short stature caused by a mutant growth hormone. N Engl J Med 1996; 334:432.
20. Duquesnoy P, Sobrier ML, Duriez B, et al. A single amino acid substitution in the extracytoplasmic domain of the human growth hormone (GH) receptor confirms familial GH resistance (Laron syndrome) with positive GH-binding activity by abolishing receptor homodimerization. EMBO J 1994; 13:1386.

21. Leung DW, Spencer SA, Cachianes G, et al. Growth hormone receptor and serum binding protein: purification, cloning and expression. Nature 1987; 330:537.

22. Eshet R, Laron Z, Pertzelan A, et al. Defect of human growth hormone receptors in the liver of two patients with Laron-type dwarfism. Isr J Med Sci 1984; 20:8.

23. Rosenfeld RG, Rosenbloom AL, Guevara-Aguirre J. Growth hormone (GH) insensitivity due to primary GH receptor deficiency. Endocr Rev 1994; 15:369.

24. Constine LS, Woolf PF, Cann D, et al. Hypothalamic-pituitary dysfunction after radiation for brain tumors. N Engl J Med 1993; 328:87.

25. Parker MW, Johanson AJ, Rogol AD, et al. Effect of testosterone on somatomedin C concentrations in pubertal boys. J Clin Endocrinol Metab 1984; 58:87.

26. Link K, Blizzard RM, Evans WS, et al. The effect of androgens on the pulsatile release and the twenty-four hour mean concentration of growth hormone in peripubertal males. J Clin Endocrinol Metab 1986; 62:159.

27. Mauras N, Blizzard RM, Link K, et al. Augmentation of growth hormone secretion during puberty: evidence for a pulse amplitude-modulated phenomenon. J Clin Endocrinol Metab 1987; 64:596.

28. Mauras N, Blizzard RM, Rogol AD. Androgen-dependent somatotroph function in a hypogonadal adolescent male: evidence for control of exogenous androgens on growth hormone release. Metabolism 1989; 38:286.

29. Blatt J, Bercu BB, Gillian C, et al. Reduced pulsatile growth hormone secretion in children after therapy for acute lymphoblastic leukemia. J Pediatr 1984; 104:182.

30. Powell GF, Brasel JA, Blizzard RM. Emotional deprivation and growth retardation simulating idiopathic hypopituitarism. I. Clinical evaluation of the syndrome. N Engl J Med 1967; 276:1271.

31. Thorner MO, Reschke J, Chitwood J, et al. Acceleration of growth in two children treated with human growth hormone-releasing factor. N Engl J Med 1985; 312:4.

32. Rogol AD, Blizzard RM, Vance ML, et al. Growth hormone releasing hormone: studies in vitro and in vivo. In: Hintz RL, Rosenfeld RG, eds. Growth abnormalities: contemporary issues in endocrinology and metabolism. New York: Churchill Livingstone, 1987; 4:13.

33. Frasier SD. Dose effect relationships and chronobiologic considerations in growth hormone administration. In: Laron Z, Butenandt O, Raiti S, eds. Clinical use of growth hormone: present and future aspects, Basel: Karger, 1987: 37. (Laron Z, ed. Pediatric and adolescent endocrinology, vol 16.)

34. Thorner MO, Rogol AD, Blizzard RM, et al. Acceleration of growth rate in growth hormone-deficient children treated with human growth hormone releasing hormone. Pediatr Res 1988; 24:145.

35. Thorner MO, Rochiccioli P, Colle M, et al. Once daily subcutaneous growth hormone-releasing hormone therapy accelerates growth in growth hormone-deficient children during the first year of therapy. J Clin Endocrinol Metab 1996; 81:1189.

36. Pihoker C, Badger TM, Reynolds GA, Bowers CY. Treatment effects of intranasal growth hormone releasing peptide-2 (GHRP-2) in children with growth hormone insufficiency. J Endocrinol 1997; 155:79.

37. Meriqa V, Merriam GR, Bowers CY, et al. Effects of eight months treatment with graded doses of a (GH)-releasing peptide in GH deficient children. J Clin Endocrinol Metab 1998; 83:2355.

38. Aceto T Jr, Bunger PF, Krell E, et al. Differential diagnosis of short stature and/or slow growth. Minn Med 1980; 63:469.

39. Bailey JA II. Disproportionate short stature, diagnosis and treatment. Philadelphia: WB Saunders, 1973.

40. Wettenhall HNB, Cahill C, Roche AF. Tall girls: a survey of 15 years of management and treatment. J Pediatr 1975; 86:602.

41. Sotos JF, Cutler EA, Dodge P. Cerebral gigantism. Am J Dis Child 1977; 131:625.

42. Maher ER, Reik W. Beckwith-Wiedemann syndrome: imprinting in clusters revisited. J Clin Invest 2000; 105:247.

43. Hayward C, Grook DJ. Fibrillin-1 mutations in Marfan's syndrome and other type-1 fibrillinopathies. Journal Hum Mutations 1997; 10:415.

44. Scriver CR, Rosenberg LE. Amino acid metabolism and its disorders. Philadelphia: WB Saunders, 1973.

45. Haigler ED, Hershman JM, Meador CK. Pituitary gigantism: a case report and review. Arch Intern Med 1973; 132:588.

46. Thorner MO, Perryman RL, Cronin MJ, et al. Somatotroph hyperplasia: successful treatment of acromegaly by removal of a pancreatic tumor secreting a growth hormone releasing factor. J Clin Invest 1982; 70:965.

47. Kaplan SL, Grumbach MM. Clinical review 14: pathophysiology and treatment of sexual precocity. J Clin Endocrinol Metab 1990; 71:785.

48. Kulin HE, Bourguignon JP. Central precocious puberty. In: Bardin CW, ed. Current therapy in endocrinology and metabolism. Toronto: Marcel Dekker, 1994.

49. Mansfield MJ, Beardsworth DE, Loughlen JS, et al. Long-term control of precocious puberty with a long-acting analogue of luteinizing hormone-releasing hormone. N Engl J Med 1983; 309:1286.

50. Van Dop C, Burstein S, Conte F, Grumbach MM. Isolated gonadotropin deficiency in boys: clinical characteristics and growth. J Pediatr 1987; 111:684.

# CHAPTER 19

# THE OPTIC CHIASM IN ENDOCRINOLOGIC DISORDERS

R. MICHAEL SIATKOWSKI AND JOEL S. GLASER

Situated in the floor of the third ventricle, in close proximity to the hypothalamus, hypophysial stalk, and pituitary gland, the optic chiasm is commonly involved by intracranial disease processes, many of which have endocrinologic manifestations. Such disorders include, but are not limited to, pituitary adenomas, optic gliomas, and congenital forebrain anomalies.

## ANATOMY AND EMBRYOLOGY OF THE OPTIC CHIASM

The optic chiasm may be considered the "Grand Central Station" of the vision sensory system, containing some 2.4 million afferent axons. Many of the disease processes that involve the intracranial optic nerves likewise involve the chiasm. Because of the relationship of the nerves and chiasm to the basal structures of the anterior and middle cranial fossae, pituitary adenomas and parasellar meningiomas frequently encroach on the anterior vision pathways. Failure of early diagnosis of chiasmal disorders may endanger the life of the patient and lessen the likelihood of reversal of visual deficits.

The chiasm is situated in the anteroinferior recess of the third ventricle. The inferior aspect of the chiasm usually is 8 to 13 mm above the nasotuberculum line (i.e., the plane of the diaphragma sellae or clinoid processes). The intracranial portion of the optic nerves is inclined as much as 45 degrees from the horizontal and measures $17 \pm 2.5$ mm in length (Fig. 19-1). The chiasm measures ~8 mm from anterior to posterior notch, 12 mm across, and 4 mm in height. The inferior surface of the chiasm projects more or less directly above the bony dorsum sellae (79%). When the chiasm lies more anteriorly over the diaphragm sellae, it is said to be prefixed (17%), and behind the dorsum, postfixed (4%).[1–3] The lateral aspect of the chiasm is embraced by the supraclinoid portion of the internal carotid artery. The anterior cerebral arteries of the circle of Willis (Fig. 19-2) pass over the dorsal surface of the optic nerves as they converge. The optic nerves are fixed at the intracranial entrance of the optic canals, the dorsal aspect of which is formed by an unyielding falciform fold of dura.

The pituitary gland lies within the sella turcica and is covered by the diaphragma sellae, through which the hypophysial stalk passes. The chiasmatic (suprasellar) cistern is the subarachnoid space between the chiasm and the pituitary gland into which pituitary macroadenomas grow, often becoming large before affecting the optic nerves or chiasm (see Chaps. 11 and 20).

Basal mass lesions, even of moderate size, do not necessarily encroach on the chiasm. For example, pituitary adenomas must extend well above the confines of the sella turcica to contact the chiasm. Conversely, in the presence of chiasmal visual field defects, advanced suprasellar extension of an adenoma may be predicted. Smaller tumors may be detected clinically only when signs of unilateral optic nerve compression evolve or when secretory manifestations accrue.

Although the anatomic variations in the position of the chiasm, as well as its arterial supply, have been studied,[3,4] it is difficult to draw conclusions regarding the preferential vulnerability of a particular portion of the chiasm based on blood supply. Moreover, it is unclear whether field defects are due to direct

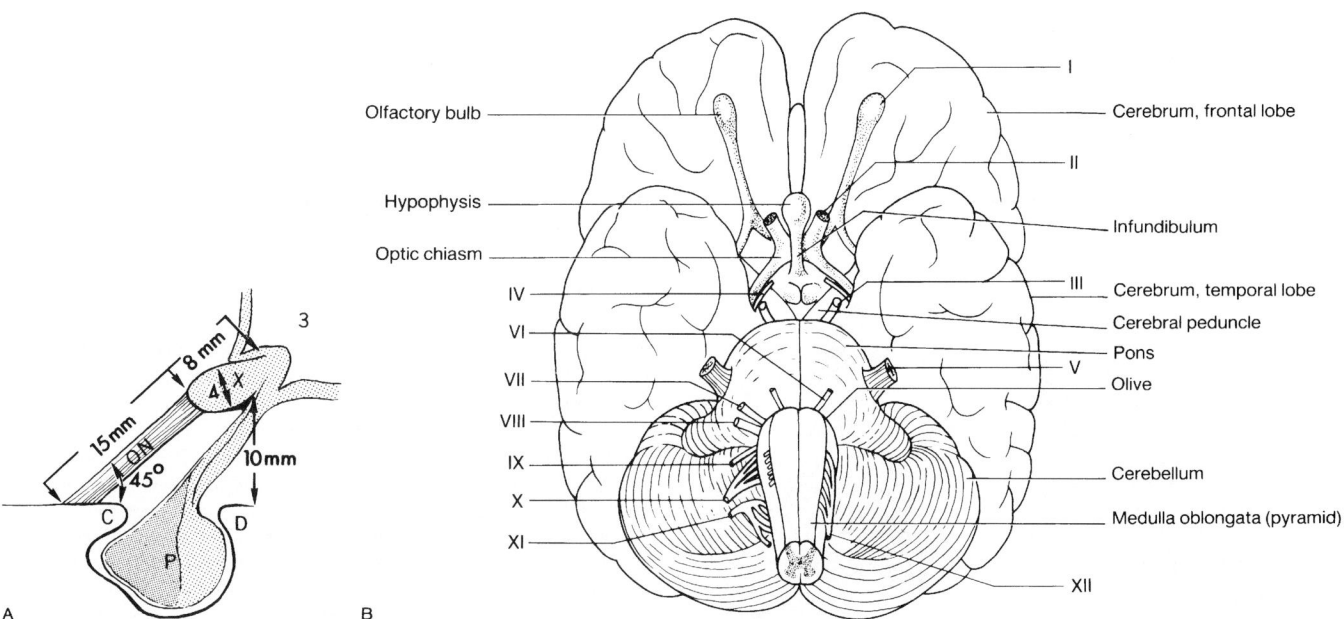

**FIGURE 19-1. A,** The relationships of the optic nerves (*ON*) and chiasm (*X*) to sellar structures and the third ventricle (*3*). (*C,* anterior clinoid; *D,* dorsum sellae; *P,* pituitary gland in sella.) **B,** Base of the brain, showing some of the pertinent anatomic structures. The cranial nerves are numbered. (**A,** From Glaser JS. Topical diagnosis: the optic chiasm. In: Glaser JS. Neuro-ophthalmology, 3rd ed. Philadelphia: Lippincott, 1999:81; **B,** From Akesson EJ, Loeb JA, Wilson-Pauwels L. Thompson's core textbook of anatomy, 2nd ed. Philadelphia: JB Lippincott, 1990:81.)

compression of vision axons or to interference with vasculature (or to both). At craniotomy, major stretching, distortion, and thinning of the nerves and chiasm are commonly encountered, shedding little light on the mechanisms of impairment of function.

The intrinsic nerve fiber anatomy of the optic nerves and chiasm provides the functional substrate for the clinical evolution of field defects. The retinal topographic pattern is preserved, even at the junction of the optic nerves with the chiasm (Fig. 19-3). Superior retinal quadrants are represented in the superior portion of the nerve, inferior retina below, with nasal and temporal retinal fibers maintaining their relative positions

in the optic nerve. Most axially located fibers within the optic nerves and chiasm are macular in origin. Some 2.4 million nerve fibers, ~1.2 million per nerve, enter the optic chiasm, with a crossed/uncrossed fibers ratio of 53:47.[5]

Macular axons constitute the largest portion of these fibers, which cross primarily in the central and posterior portions of the chiasm. The concept of *Wilbrand knee* (i.e., that contralateral, inferior nasal fibers cross in the anterior notch of the chiasm and loop forward into the terminal portion of the opposite optic nerve) is no longer universally accepted (see next paragraph). Superior nasal fibers cross more posteriorly in the chiasm. The lateral portions of

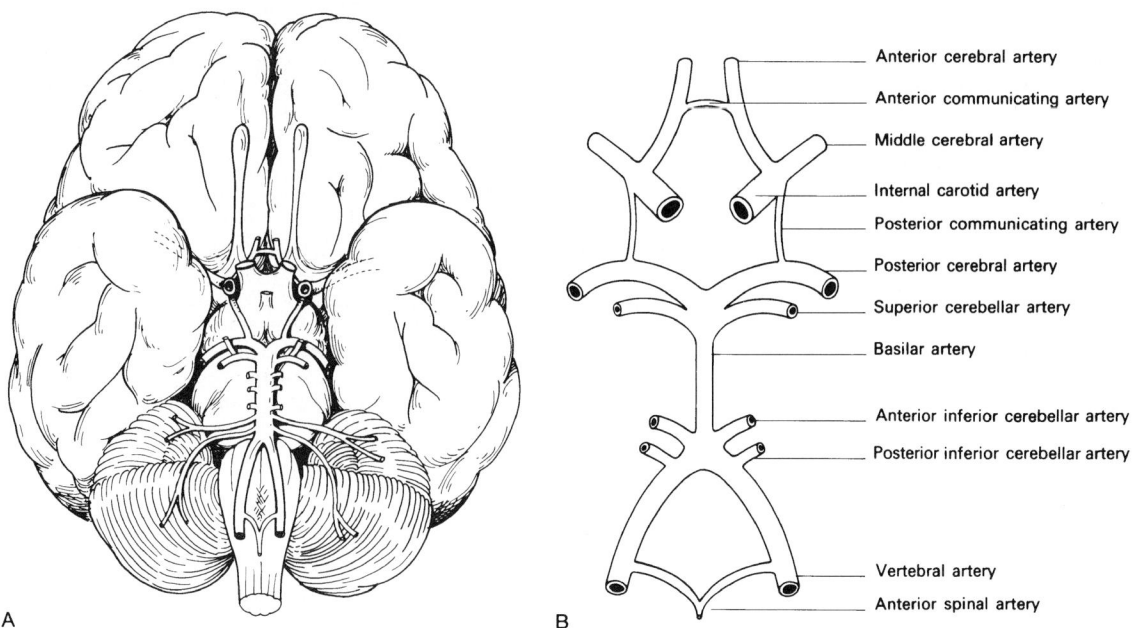

**FIGURE 19-2.** The circle of Willis and its environs. **A,** Relationship to intracranial contents, view from below. **B,** Anatomy of major intracranial arteries (caudal, top and dorsal, bottom). (From Akesson EJ, Loeb JA, Wilson-Pauwels L. Thompson's core textbook of anatomy, 2nd ed. Philadelphia: JB Lippincott, 1990:81.)

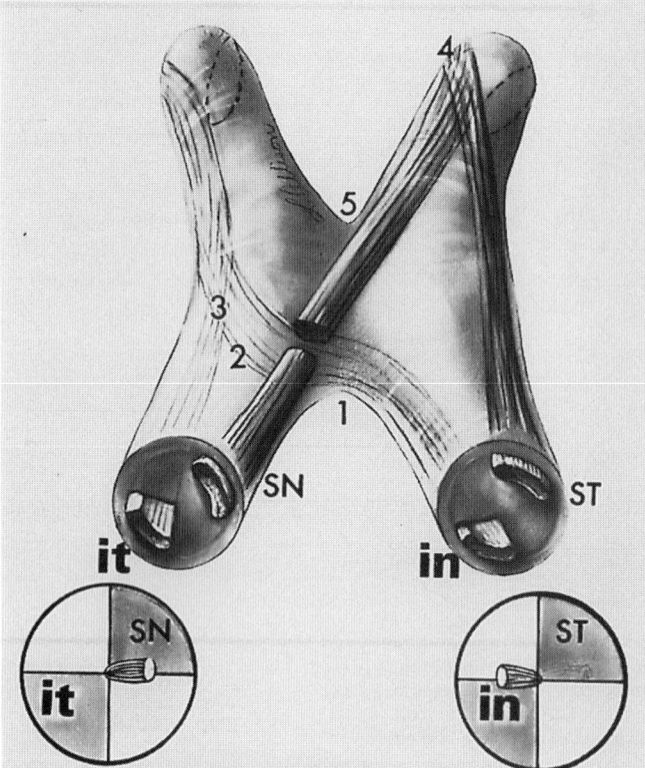

**FIGURE 19-3.** Retinotopic organization of visual fibers in the anterior visual pathways (after Hoyt). Diagram of homonymous retinal quadrants and their fiber projections, anterior aspect. (*SN*, superior nasal; *ST*, superior temporal; *it*, inferior temporal; *in*, inferior nasal.) Note: The superior fibers retain a superior course; the inferior fibers retain an inferior position; the anterior notch (*1*) is occupied by inferonasal (superior temporal field) fibers; inferior homonymous fibers, contralateral eye (*2*), and ipsilateral eye (*3*) converge in the chiasm, but superior homonymous fibers converge in the chiasm in the optic tract (*4*); the posterior notch (*5*) is occupied by the superior nasal (inferior temporal field) fibers as well as by macular fibers. (From Glaser JS. Topical diagnosis: the optic chiasm. In: Glaser JS. Neuro-ophthalmology, 3rd ed. Philadelphia: Lippincott, 1999:90.)

the chiasm are composed of uncrossed superior and inferior temporal retinal fibers.

Elegant anatomic autoradiography studies have been made of the chiasm in normal monkeys and in both monkey and human cadavers that had undergone monocular enucleation.[6] In normal monkeys, the optic nerve fibers cross the chiasm without entering the contralateral optic nerve, but after short-term monocular enucleation, fibers from the normal optic nerve begin to approach the entry zone of the degenerating optic nerve. Only after long-term enucleation (in both humans and monkeys) was "Wilbrand knee" identified. Thus, because Wilbrand knee does not occur in normal humans, the phenomenon of a superior temporal hemianopia in the so-called "junctional scotoma" must be due to "herniation" of optic nerve fibers subserving the superotemporal visual field into the chiasm after prolonged compression and subsequent neural atrophy.

The development of the embryonic optic chiasm begins between the fourth and sixth weeks of gestation (8- to 10-mm stage), when the optic nerves start to converge,[7] and a true chiasm is clearly evident by the end of the second month of gestation. The structures of the diencephalon, including the posterior lobe of the hypophysis, the tuber cinereum, and mammillary bodies, are well defined by the third month of gestation, but the infundibular pouch contacts the stomodeal hypophysial pouch even during the fourth week of development.

Congenital absence of the chiasm is a rare, but well-documented, phenomenon. It may occur in association with marked microphthalmia and aplasia of the optic nerves and tracts,[8] or, conversely, in children with normal eyeballs and only minimal optic nerve anomalies.[9] The latter cases are associated with strabismus and nystagmus and are likely to be secondary to developmental visuotopic misrouting.

## CLINICAL MANIFESTATIONS OF CHIASMAL SYNDROMES

### VISION CHANGES

Most chiasmal syndromes are caused by extrinsic tumors: classically, pituitary adenomas or suprasellar meningiomas and craniopharyngiomas. With few exceptions, these slow-growing tumors produce insidiously progressive visual deficits in the form of variations on a *bitemporal* theme (Fig. 19-4). Sophisticated neuroradiologic and psychophysical testing has attempted to correlate the degree of vision loss with the degree of anatomic displacement of the chiasm[10]; these studies have demonstrated that vision loss occurs well before it is detectable by conventional outpatient methods of assessing visual field and visual acuity.[11] *Asymmetry* of field loss is the rule, such that one eye may show advanced deficits, including reduced acuity, whereas only relative temporal field defects are present in the other eye. Unless acuity is diminished, patients report rather vague vision symptoms—for example, trouble seeing to the side, a history of fender accidents to their automobiles, or that, when passed by another automobile, the overtaking vehicle suddenly appears in their lane. The first clue to the presence of an hemianopic defect may be the manner in which acuity charts are read (i.e., with the right eye, only the left letters are seen, and with the left eye, only the right letters are seen). Progressive painless loss of peripheral field or central acuity (symmetric or asymmetric) may go unnoticed by many children as well as by some adults. Unilateral visual defects, especially in children, frequently are found during routine school vision tests. Rarely, vision may decrease precipitously when parachiasmal masses enlarge abruptly, as with infarction of an adenoma ("pituitary apoplexy"). Chiasmal visual field loss may differ depending on the anatomic area affected. Anterior lesions may cause an ipsilateral optic neuropathy with a contralateral superotemporal field deficit. Lesions in the body of the chiasm usually produce more symmetric bitemporal field loss, with normal visual acuity. Posterior lesions (with prefixed chiasm) may cause incongruous homonymous field loss secondary to involvement of the optic tract. Usually, many vision symptoms are vague and nonspecific until central acuity fails in one or both eyes. Unfortunately, it is all too common that visual field loss is already marked before initial perimetry is accomplished.

Vision loss of a chiasmal pattern during pregnancy should suggest the possibility of an enlargement of a preexisting pituitary adenoma or of an estrogen-dependent meningioma. There is little evidence to support the notion of a physiologic enlargement of a normal pituitary gland during pregnancy that is sufficient to encroach on the anterior visual pathways, nor is "lactation optic neuritis" a valid concept.

Even now, vision loss is the first palpable clinical manifestation of pituitary macroadenomas, but this symptom cannot be construed as an early sign. From the Mayo Clinic experience,[12] >40% of adenomas present as vision symptoms, and 70% show field defects.

### HEADACHE

Chronic headaches, mild or severe, are noted by most patients with pituitary adenomas.[13] Headache symptoms are variable but may be most marked where advancing pituitary adenomas are restrained by a taut diaphragma sellae. In acromegaly, chronic headaches may indicate paranasal sinus enlargement,

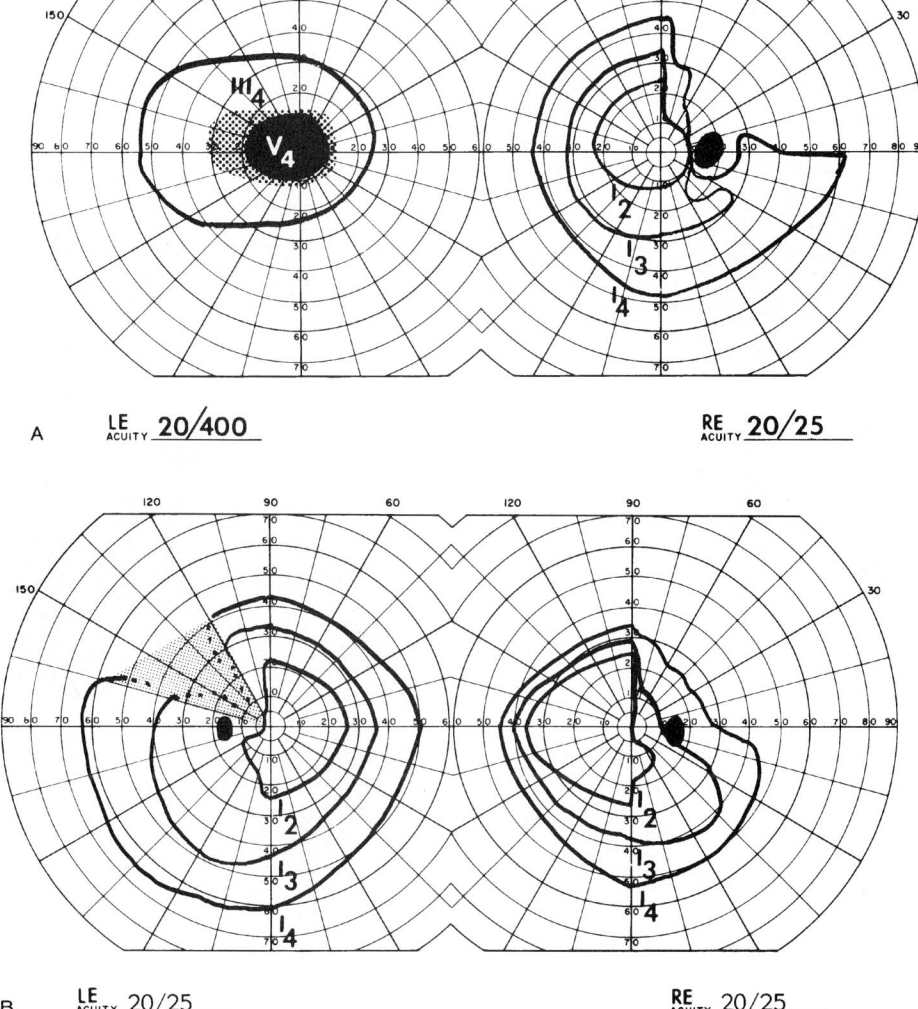

A  LE ACUITY 20/400          RE ACUITY 20/25

B  LE ACUITY 20/25          RE ACUITY 20/25

**FIGURE 19-4.** Chiasmal field defects. **A,** "Junctional scotoma" combines typical optic nerve defect (central scotoma) in left eye with temporal hemianopia in right (see also **C**). **B,** Classic bitemporal hemianopia. Riddoch phenomenon (movement perception) demonstrable in shaded area of the left field. *(continued)*

with or without active sinusitis. In children, headaches usually are not thoroughly evaluated until nausea, vomiting, and behavioral changes occur, at which point an intracranial lesion should be suspected. Additionally, obesity, precocious or delayed sexual development, somnolence, and diabetes insipidus should alert the clinician to hypothalamic dysfunction (see Chaps. 9, 18, and 26).

## SENSORY PHENOMENA

Peculiar sensory phenomena may be noted by patients with bitemporal field defects, resulting in a nonparetic form of strabismus or diplopia and in difficulty with visual tasks requiring depth perception (e.g., use of a screwdriver, threading a needle, and the like). Loss of portions of normally superimposed binocular fields results in the absence of corresponding points in visual space (and on the retina) and subsequently diminished fusional capacity. In essence, the patient has two free-floating nasal hemifields with no interhemispheral linkage to keep them aligned. Vertical and horizontal slippage produces doubling of images, gaps in otherwise continuous visual panorama, and steps in horizontal lines. A series of 260 patients with pituitary adenoma included some degree of double vision preoperatively in 98 patients, but a demonstrable ocular palsy was present in only 14.[13] Additionally, without temporal fields, objects beyond the point of binocular fix-

ation fall on nonseeing nasal hemiretina, so that a blind area exists with extinction of objects beyond the fixation point.

## EYE MOVEMENT DISORDERS

The association of extraocular muscle palsies with chiasmal field defects implies involvement of the structures in the cavernous sinus, usually a sign of rapid expansion of a pituitary adenoma. Only rarely is tumor diagnosis delayed sufficiently for obstruction of the ventricular system to occur, with elevation of intracranial pressure and unilateral or bilateral sixth nerve palsies (Figs. 19-5 and 19-6).

Patients with large parasellar masses may display "seesaw" nystagmus, with alternate depression and extorsion of one eye and elevation and intorsion of the other. This results from expansion of tumors within the third ventricle, with secondary midbrain compression, rather than from chiasmal involvement per se.[14]

## PALLOR OF THE OPTIC DISCS

Pallor of the optic discs, although an anticipated physical sign of chiasmal interference, is not a prerequisite for diagnosis. In a series of 156 cases of pituitary tumors, optic atrophy was found in only 155 of 312 eyes (50%)[15]; disc pallor was present in 34% of the adenomas studied at the Mayo Clinic.[12] Optic atrophy may not be

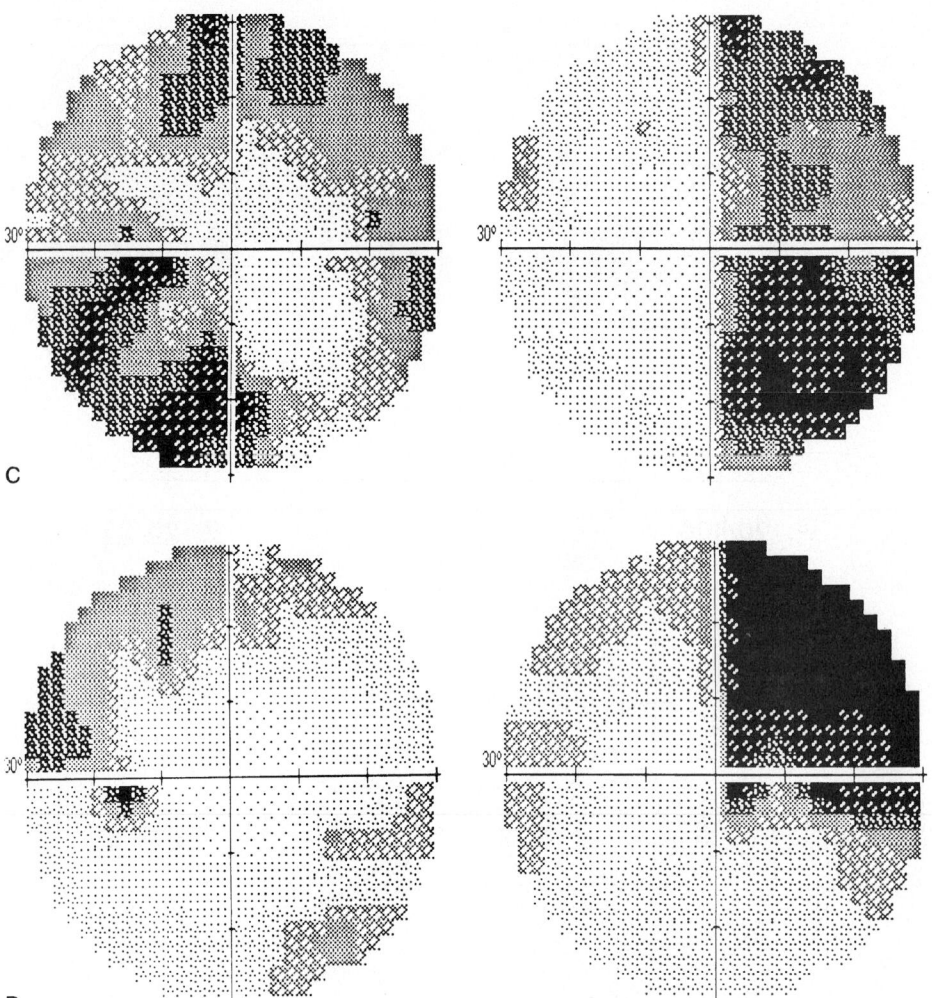

**FIGURE 19-4.** *(continued)* **C,** Automated perimetry (Humphrey) of a junction-type field defect demonstrates diffuse field loss in the left eye (*left*) and temporal hemianopia in the right (*right*). **D,** Automated perimetry from patient with pituitary tumor compressing chiasm from below demonstrates asymmetric bitemporal superior quadrantic defects. (*LE,* left eye; *RE,* right eye.)

present even when vision symptoms have lasted as long as 2 years.[16] Furthermore, extensive field loss in chiasmal syndromes may be associated with normal or minimally pale discs. Therefore, it is unwise to rely on the presence of optic atrophy as an indication of chiasmal interference; such findings are corroborative evidence at best, after the visual fields have been carefully evaluated.

It is somewhat risky to predict on the basis of disc appearance the ultimate level of vision anticipated after chiasmal decompression. As a rule, the more atrophic the disc, the less likely is the return of function in defective areas of field. However, vision recovery to surprisingly good levels may occur despite relatively advanced disc pallor.

Papilledema is a less common finding and results from large tumors compressing the third ventricle, with resultant hydrocephalus.

## EVALUATION OF FIELD DEFECTS

The importance of establishing that the vertical meridian forms the central border of the defect (see Fig. 19-4) is paramount in distinguishing chiasmal interference from deficits that mimic temporal hemianopia. Such mimicking conditions include tilted discs (congenital inferior scleral crescents); nasal sector retinitis pigmentosa; bilateral cecocentral scotomas; papilledema with greatly enlarged blind spots; nutritional optic neuropathy; retinal inflammatory disease; and redundant overhanging upper lid tissue.[17]

The endocrinologist should be aware of the general pattern of evolution of chiasmal field defects and of the useful screening procedures that are appropriate in the context of the general physical examination.

Visual field defects caused by chiasmal interference may be characterized by the following[17]: depressions initially occur in the *central* 20-degree field (therefore, exploration of the *periphery* is time-consuming and insensitive) (see Fig. 19-4); the central edge of the defect is aligned along the vertical meridian that passes through the point of visual fixation, in one or both eyes; the defect is more readily apparent with red targets than, for example, white against black (Fig. 19-7); and the loss of monocular acuity ("reading vision") that is not explained by uncorrected refractive error or ocular disease (cataract, macular degeneration, etc.) is evidence of prechiasmal optic nerve compression until proved otherwise. Three additional caveats are that normal visual fields do not preclude the presence of a parachiasmal lesion (e.g., a microadenoma does not cause field defects); the screening technique described does not replace other formal perimetric techniques, such as Goldmann or automated perimetry; and the assessment of visual fields in no way obviates the need for anatomic studies, that is, computed tomography (CT) or magnetic resonance imaging (MRI). Only limited information is available on plain films; subtle changes in the bony structures of the sella may be easily overlooked by the inexperienced. Radiologic measurements of the sella, whether linear or volumetric, are not intrinsically important. In marginal cases, such measurements are unreliable; in obvious cases, they are superfluous; and in neither case is the problem of suprasellar extension solved. Thus, plain films have little, if any, use today in the diagnostic evaluation of patients with parasellar disease.

The advent of thin-section CT and of gadolinium-enhanced MRI has greatly simplified the diagnosis of intracranial mass lesions. Pneumoencephalography no longer is indicated, and cerebral angiography is reserved for those patients in whom the

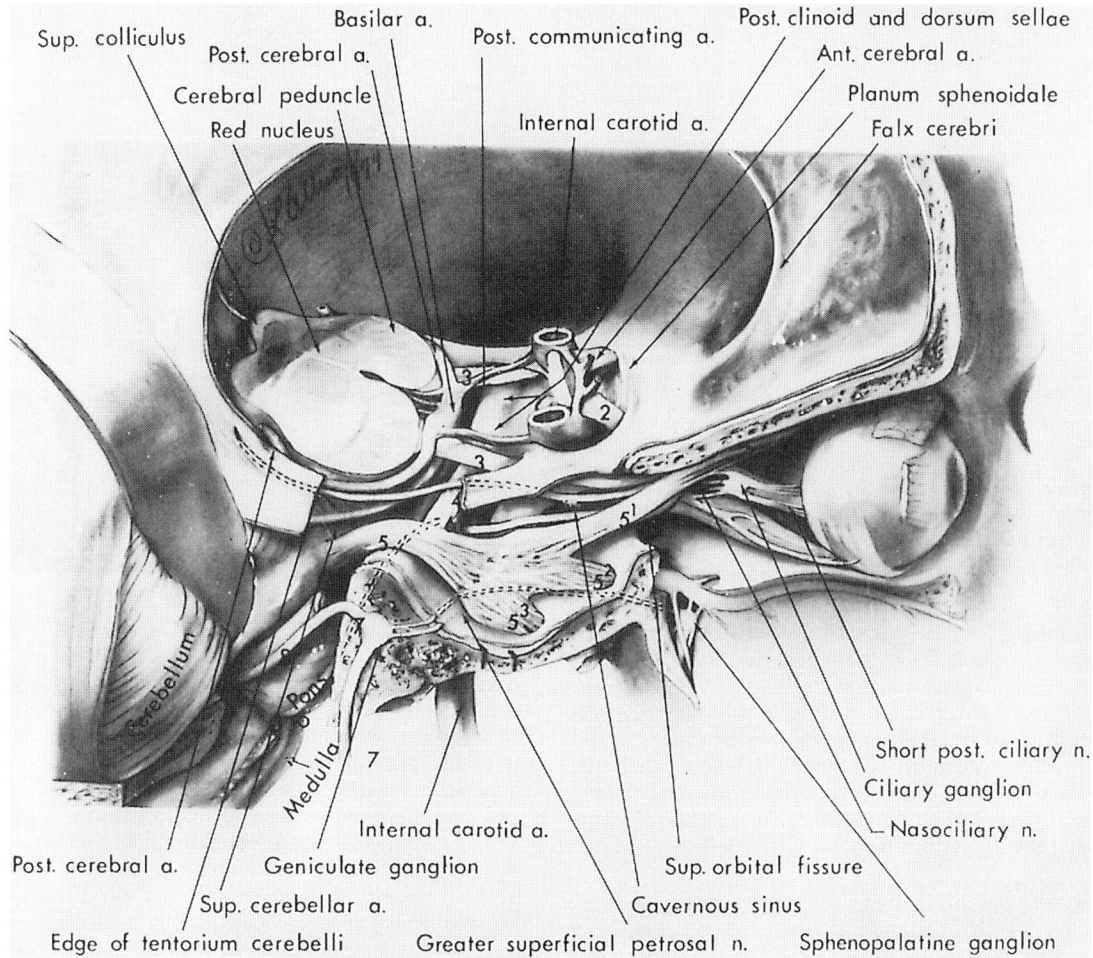

**FIGURE 19-5.** Diagram illustrating nerves and structures in and near the cavernous sinus. (*a*, artery; *ant.*, anterior; *n.*, nerve; *post.*, posterior; *sup.*, superior.) (From Glaser JS. Topical diagnosis: the optic chiasm. In: Glaser JS. Neuro-ophthalmology, 3rd ed. Philadelphia: Lippincott, 1999:408.)

precise configuration of neighboring vessels may be relevant to transsphenoidal or transcranial surgical approaches to intrasellar or suprasellar tumors. The question of "full" or "empty" sella is clearly settled by coronal-section MRI (Fig. 19-8).

## DEVELOPMENTAL CHIASMAL DYSPLASIAS

The chiasm is infrequently the site of developmental anomalies; at times, it is related to malformation of other diencephalic midline structures, including the third ventricle. Embryonic dysgenesis may result in the abnormal development of the primitive optic vesicles with resulting unilateral or bilateral anophthalmos (absent globe) or useless microphthalmic cysts. Such gross ocular abnormalities may occur in isolation or may be associated with a spectrum of neural defects, including major malformations that preclude survival.

Perhaps of greater clinical import are the more subtle ocular dysplasias that accompany those anterior forebrain malformations compatible with long life. Certain specific congenital anomalies of the optic disc may indicate the presence of otherwise occult forebrain malformations.

## DE MORSIER SYNDROME

The clinical constellation of pituitary dysfunction and optic nerve hypoplasia (Fig. 19-9) is recognized as the *de Morsier syndrome*.[18,19] Variable findings may include neonatal hypotonia; seizures; prolonged bilirubinemia; deficiencies of growth hormone, adrenocorticotropic hormone, or vasopressin; panhypo-

pituitarism; mental retardation; or a combination of these.[20] The association of this entity with midline cerebral anomalies (i.e., absence of septum pellucidum, agenesis of the corpus callosum) has been well documented.[21] Additional neuropathologic findings have included extensive atrophy of the optic nerves and chiasm, aplasia of olfactory bulbs and tracts, and hypoplasia of the hypophysial stalk and infundibulum.[22] Although the exact etiology of this condition has not been determined, it is well known to occur in association with maternal gestational diabetes and maternal use of phenytoin, quinine, alcohol, and lysergic acid.[19] Genetic defects—including partial deletion of chromosome 14[23] and mutations in the PAX3[24] and HESX1[25] genes—have been reported. Others have hypothesized that this group of defects represents a vascular disruption sequence.[26]

The wide clinical spectrum of patients with bilateral optic nerve hypoplasia is now well recognized. In one study, only 30 of 40 such children had coexistent central nervous system anomalies. Concomitant endocrinologic defects were associated with posterior pituitary ectopia rather than agenesis of the corpus callosum or other central nervous system abnormalities.[27] Some investigators feel that endocrine function may be predicted on the basis of pituitary appearance on MRI,[28] but others have documented normal-appearing glands in patients with central diabetes insipidus.[29] In 35 patients with bilateral optic nerve hypoplasia, endocrine dysfunction was seen in only 27% (growth hormone deficiency and hypothyroidism being most common), and abnormal neuroimaging in 46%.[30] Eighty percent of these patients were legally blind (34% had no light perception in either eye), but 10% of eyes had vision 20/60 or better. The "full-

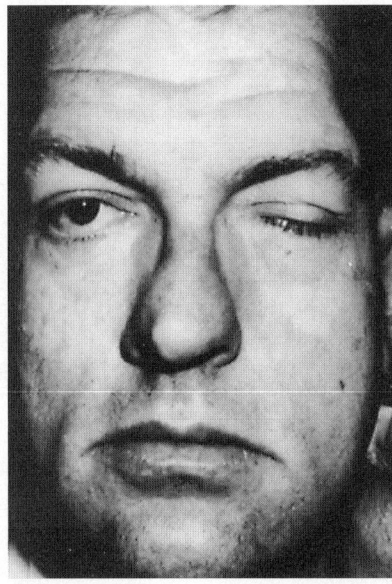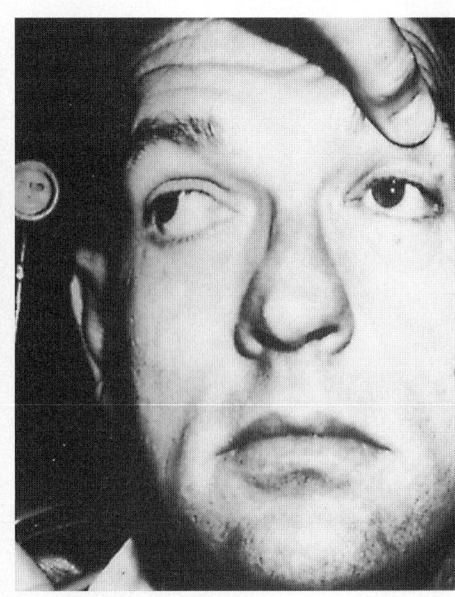

A,B

FIGURE 19-6. A, Acromegalic patient with involvement of left oculomotor nerve. B, Patient had reported a gradual onset of left-sided ptosis and diplopia with a mild headache.

blown" syndrome (i.e., septo-optic dysplasia with panhypopituitarism) occurred in only 11.5% of these patients.

An important clinical point is that children with such disorders are at risk for sudden death during febrile illnesses secondary to hypocortisolism, thermoregulatory disturbances, and dehydration.[31] The occurrence of segmental superior optic nerve hypoplasia has been observed in infants born to mothers with gestational diabetes[32]; this, perhaps, represents a forme fruste of the de Morsier syndrome.

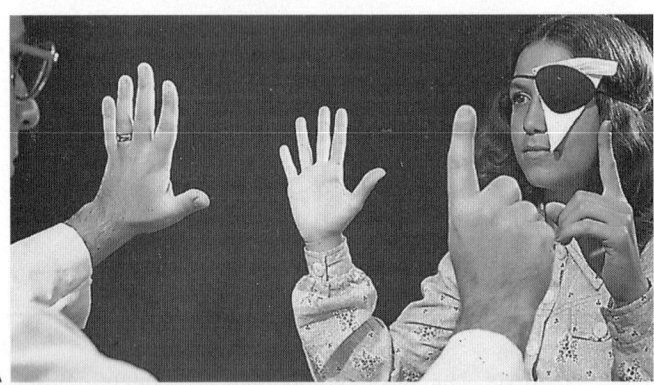

A

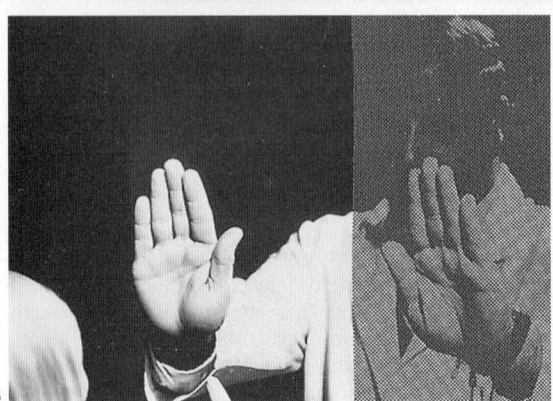

B

FIGURE 19-7. A, Finger-counting fields in adults. Four quadrants of each eye should be tested. Patient may name or hold up same number of fingers. Simultaneous finger counting may bring out subtle hemianopic defect. B, Hand comparison in hemianopic depression appears "darker," "in shadow," or "blurred." (From Glaser JS. Topical diagnosis: the optic chiasm. In: Glaser JS. Neuro-ophthalmology, 3rd ed. Philadelphia: Lippincott, 1999:31–33.)

## FOREBRAIN BASAL ENCEPHALOCELES

A variety of optic nerve abnormalities (hypoplasia, colobomata, peripapillary staphylomata, and the "morning glory" disc) may be associated with other developmental defects; principally, they take the form of midline craniofacial anomalies,[33,34] including hypertelorism; defects of the lip, palate, and maxilla; anencephaly[35] and prosencephaly[36]; skeletal malformations[37]; or combinations thereof. Of special neuro-ophthalmologic interest is the association of optic disc malformation with forebrain basal encephaloceles. Herniated brain tissue may present as pulsating exophthalmos (spheno-orbital encephalocele usually associated with neurofibromatosis), hypertelorism with a pulsatile nasopharyngeal mass (transsphenoidal encephalocele), or a frontonasal mass, with or without hypertelorism (frontoethmoidal encephalocele). Congenital disc anomalies, such as hypoplasia or the coloboma dysplasia variety[38] (Fig. 19-10), associated with hypertelorism or other midfacial malformation, are evidence of basal encephalocele until proved otherwise. There are also reports of isolated retinal colobomas, sparing the optic nerve, in association with sphenoethmoidal encephaloceles. The physical findings of transsphenoidal or transethmoidal basal encephalocele[39] are listed as follows:

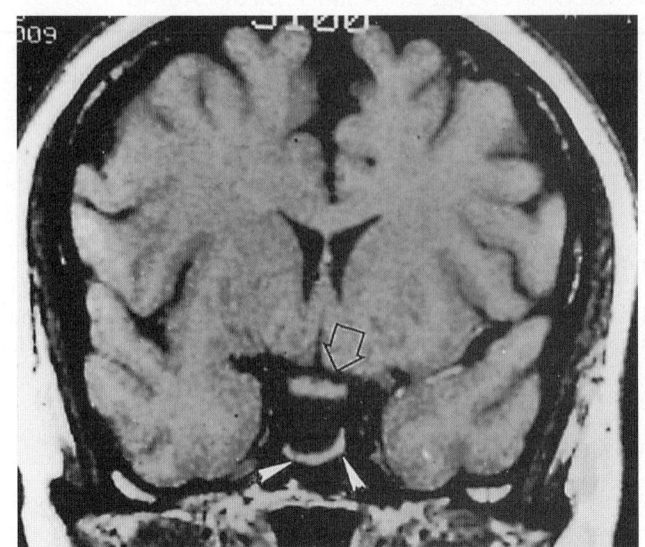

FIGURE 19-8. Empty sella syndrome. An MRI shows flattened remnant of pituitary (*arrowheads*) on sellar floor; chiasm above (*arrow*).

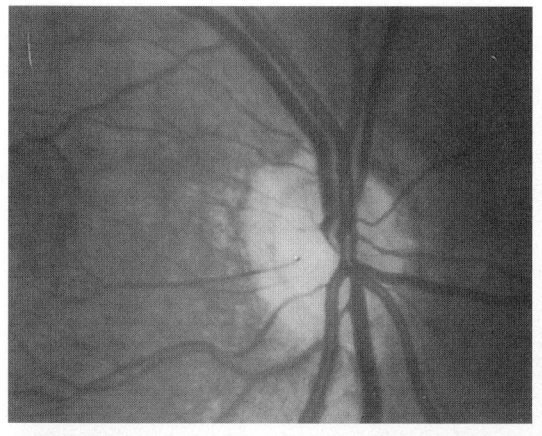
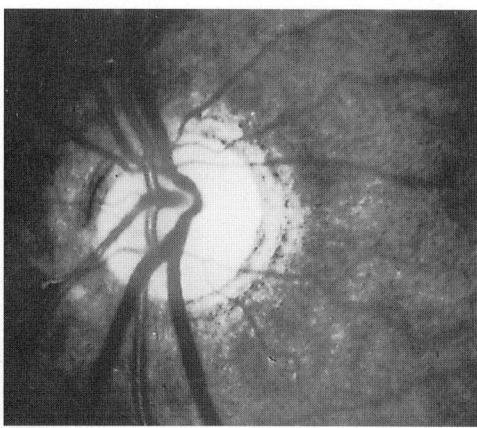

**A**

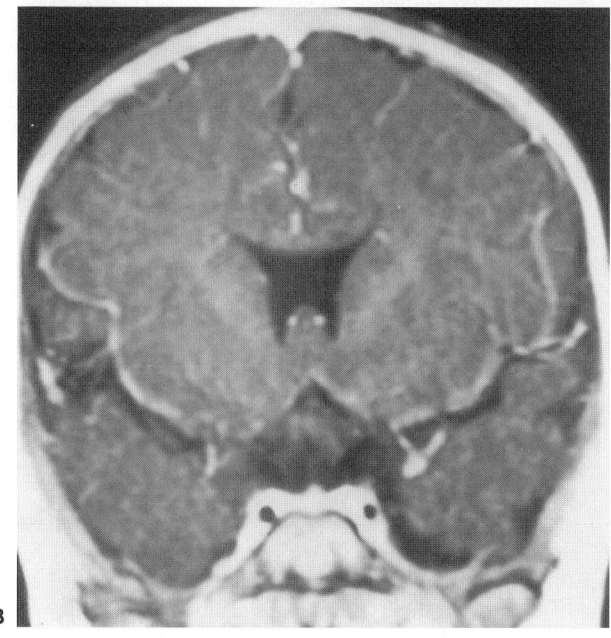

**B**

**FIGURE 19-9.** De Morsier syndrome. **A**, Hypoplastic optic discs. Note depigmented ring around discs. **B**, MRI, coronal view, demonstrates single ventricle with absence of septum pellucidum.

*Midline facial anomalies*: Broad nasal root, hypertelorism, midline lip defect, wide bitemporal skull diameter, cleft palate

*Nasopharyngeal mass*: Midline epipharyngeal space in location pulsatile; often symptoms of nasal obstruction may be confused with a nasal polyp; rare in infancy

*Hypopituitarism/dwarfism, ocular*: Congenital disc anomalies such as colobomatous dysplasias, chiasmal field defects, poor vision, exotropia

In the evaluation of basal encephalocele, neuroradiologic imaging of the cranial base is indicated. Biopsy or attempted resection

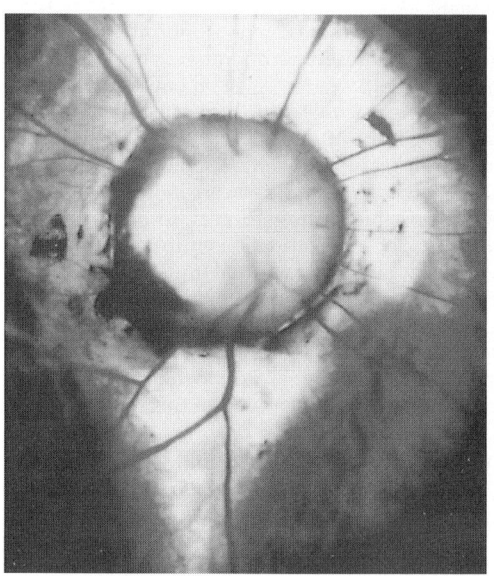
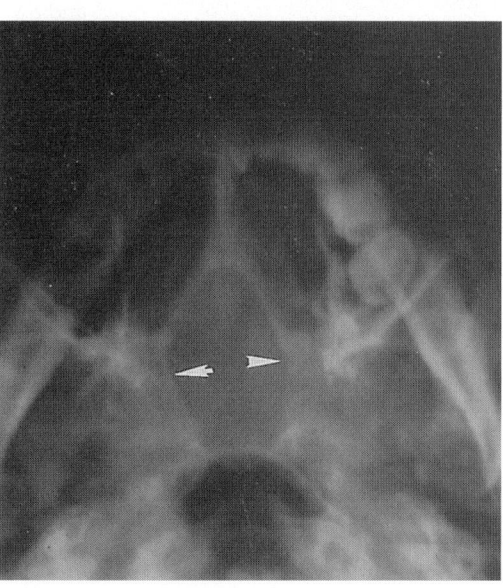

**A,B**

**FIGURE 19-10.** Transsphenoidal encephalocele. **A**, Large dysplastic optic disc (coloboma of nerve). **B**, Polytomogram demonstrates transsellar herniation of forebrain (*arrows*).

of posterior nasopharyngeal masses should be avoided because these masses invariably are encephalomeningoceles, and surgical manipulation may result in meningitis with tragic outcome.

Because both optic disc hypoplasia and colobomatous dysplasia may reflect developmental defects of the chiasm, it is essential to recognize that such ophthalmologic anomalies may be a clue to underlying brain and endocrine defects.

## HYPOGONADISM SYNDROMES

Hypogonadotropic hypogonadism (Kallmann syndrome) is an autosomal dominant disorder characterized by low levels of serum follicle-stimulating hormone and luteinizing hormone and by eunuchoid features[40] (see Chap. 115). Other pituitary hormone levels are usually normal, but midline facial anomalies and unilateral renal agenesis may be present. This disorder can be associated with anosmia, hypoplasia of the nose and eyes, hypogeusia (taste deficiency),[41] retinitis pigmentosa,[42] and Möbius syndrome (congenital facial diplegia and horizontal gaze palsies with esotropia) with peripheral neuropathy.[43,44] Hypoplastic development of the olfactory bulbs and the hypothalamus has been documented.

## PITUITARY DWARFISM

A large series[45] of 101 pituitary dwarfs revealed MRI evidence of posterior pituitary ectopia in 59. Pituitary volume did not change with hormonal therapy. There was a 3:1 male predominance, and a higher incidence of breech delivery (32% versus 7%) and congenital brain anomalies (12% versus 7%) in children with posterior pituitary ectopia. Defective induction of mediobasal brain structures in early embryonic life is the presumed cause, and mutation in the *PIT-1* gene may be implicated.

# PARACHIASMAL LESIONS

Most chiasmal syndromes are caused by extrinsic masses: classically, pituitary adenomas, suprasellar meningiomas, craniopharyngiomas, and internal carotid artery aneurysms. Although certain patterns of vision failure may suggest the location and type of lesion, such clinical impressions often prove fallible in the face of neuroradiologic procedures (and at craniotomy). At any rate, the diagnostic evaluation of all nontraumatic chiasmal syndromes is stereotyped: *to rule in or out the presence of a potentially treatable mass lesion.* Inflammatory or infectious causes are extremely rare, and chiasmal involvement by head trauma or radionecrosis is uncommon. The distinction is made by age-related incidence; accompanying signs and symptoms; and typical, if not diagnostic, radiologic appearance.

### OPTIC AND HYPOTHALAMIC GLIOMAS

Primary astrocytic tumors of the anterior visual pathways assume two major clinical forms: the relatively benign glioma (juvenile pilocytic astrocytoma) of childhood and the rare malignant glioblastoma of adulthood. With the exception of vision loss and anatomic location, these two groups have little in common, and the assumption that the progressive malignant form stems from the static childhood form is untenable.

For the indolent glioma of childhood, clinical presentation is predicated on the location and extent of the tumor. Gliomas may be separated into roughly three topographic groups: unilateral optic nerve (orbital, intracranial, or both, but not involving the chiasm); principally chiasmal mass; or simultaneous infiltration of the hypothalamus. Strictly intraorbital gliomas present as insidious proptosis of variable degree, and although vision is usually diminished, remarkably good vision function is not uncommon. Strabismus, disc pallor, or disc swelling may be observed. Progressive proptosis, even if abrupt, or increased

visual deficit does not imply an aggressive activity of the tumor, a hemorrhage, or necrosis. These tumors may rarely extend intracranially and have a low (~10%) mortality rate.[46]

Chiasmal gliomas are more common than the isolated orbital type. These tumors present with unilateral or bilateral vision loss, strabismus, optic atrophy, and/or infantile nystagmus. The nystagmus may mimic spasmus nutans (usually unilateral or asymmetric nystagmus), complete with head nodding and torticollis, or may show a coarse, conjugate mixed horizontal–rotary pattern, especially when vision is severely defective. "Seesaw" nystagmus may also rarely be seen in these patients.

Children with extensive basal tumors also show hydrocephalus and signs and symptoms of increased intracranial pressure. Hypothalamic signs include precocious puberty, obesity, dwarfism, hypersomnolence, and diabetes insipidus. Usually, the non-vision complications of extensive gliomas occur in infancy or early childhood, and onset of obstructive signs or hypothalamic involvement much beyond the age of 5 years is uncommon.

Gliomas of the optic nerves and chiasm may be associated with neurofibromatosis in 20% to 40% of cases; the patients either show other characteristic stigmata or have affected relatives.[47–49] Indeed, there is good evidence that children with neurofibromatosis type 1 and chiasmal gliomas have a better long-term prognosis than those with chiasmal gliomas alone.[46] Absence of neurofibromatosis, electrolyte abnormalities, and intracranial hypertension are all indicators of a poor prognosis.[50,51]

Treatment of benign optic gliomas in childhood is somewhat controversial, with most pediatric and neuro-ophthalmologists favoring a conservative approach. When there is documented progressive vision loss, significant tumor growth, or obstructive signs, intervention is obviously indicated. Debulking surgery, radiation therapy, and chemotherapy have all been advocated. Newer radiation techniques may allow a higher percentage of treated patients to grow normally,[52] and, when chemotherapy is indicated, reports suggest success with a combined carboplatin/vincristine regimen,[53] as well as oral etoposide (VP-16).[54]

## DIENCEPHALIC SYNDROME

When the hypothalamus is the site of childhood glioma, a *diencephalic syndrome* evolves.[55] Findings consist of emaciation, despite adequate food intake, that develops after a period of normal growth; hyperactivity and euphoria; skin pallor (without anemia); hypotension; and hypoglycemia. Other notable signs include nystagmus and disc pallor, to which may be added sexual precocity and laughing seizures.[56] Twelve cases of histologically proven opticochiasmatic glioma with diencephalic syndrome were culled from a 22-year review.[57] There were 6 men and 6 women, all with "failure to thrive" but with normal linear growth; none had stigmata of neurofibromatosis. Two patients died in the immediate postoperative period, and 10 patients received radiotherapy with "reversal of their diencephalic syndrome" (weight gain, deposition of subcutaneous fat, normal development). Six of 10 are alive, 3 being considered normal, and 3 are blind, retarded, or both. Clinical evidence of bilateral optic nerve involvement was seen in 10 of these 12 cases, but it was not possible during surgery to determine the origin of these tumors. The diencephalic syndrome appears to be related to the age at which the hypothalamus becomes compressed; none of the 12 patients (and only 4% of all published cases) had onset of symptoms after 2 years of age. Craniotomy with biopsy and radiotherapy is often indicated, as tumors involving the hypothalamus appear to be larger and more aggressive than other astrocytomas arising in this region.[58]

## RADIOLOGIC INVESTIGATION OF GLIOMAS

The radiologic investigation of suspected gliomas is now sophisticated to the extent that "neuroradiologic biopsy" may obviate tissue diagnosis. The typical, but variable, findings

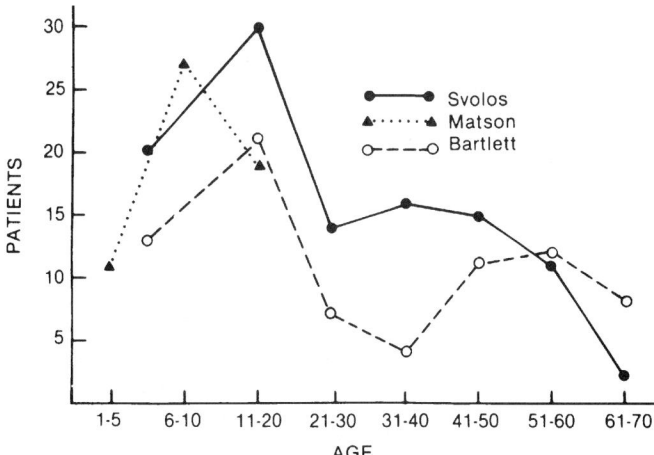

**FIGURE 19-11.** Age distribution of craniopharyngioma. (Data from Svolos D. Craniopharyngiomas: a study based on 108 verified cases. Acta Chir Scand Suppl 1969; 403:1; Matson DD, Crigler JF. Management of craniopharyngioma in childhood. J Neurosurg 1969; 30:377; Bartlett JR. Craniopharyngiomas: an analysis of some aspects of symptomatology, radiology and histology. Brain 1971; 94:725. Note: Matson and Crigler series limited to children younger than 16 years of age.)

include CT and MRI evidence of enlarged orbital or intracranial optic nerves; enlarged chiasm; a homogeneous hypothalamic mass; enlarged optic canals; and J-shaped or gourd-shaped sellae. The demonstration of such typical dysplastic changes of the sella turcica and optic canals, coupled with CT or MRI evidence of intrinsic chiasmal mass, so strongly suggests the diagnosis of glioma that histopathologic affirmation probably is superfluous and hazardous to vision.

Analysis of visual fields in patients with chiasmatic gliomas has shown no consistent relationship between the pattern of field defects and the location, size, or extent of tumor; in 12 of 20 patients, the putative bitemporal pattern of chiasmal involvement was absent.[59] Central scotomas or measurable depression of the central field occurred in 70% of the eyes; therefore, the absence of bitemporal hemianopia, or one of its variants, cannot be interpreted as a sign that the glioma does not involve the chiasm.

## CRANIOPHARYNGIOMAS

Craniopharyngiomas (see Chap. 11) are developmental tumors that arise from vestigial epidermoid remnants of Rathke pouch, scattered as cell nests in the infundibulohypophysial region. These tumors are usually admixtures of solid cellular components and variable-sized cysts containing oily mixtures of degenerated blood and desquamated epithelium or of necrotic tissue with cholesterol crystals. Calcification of such debris may be radiologically detectable, a helpful diagnostic sign. In rare instances, these tumors may present in the neonate, attesting to their congenital origin.[60] Craniopharyngiomas constitute 3% of all intracranial tumors (~15% in children), with two distinctive modes of presentation—in childhood and in adulthood—with a peak in the 40- to 70-year-old age range (Fig. 19-11).

The symptomatology of childhood craniopharyngioma is variable, depending on the position and mass of the tumor.[61,62] Frequently, progressive vision loss goes unnoticed until a level of severe impairment is reached, or unless headache, vomiting, or behavioral changes occur because of hydrocephalus. Obesity, delayed sexual development, somnolence, and diabetes insipidus attest to hypothalamic dysfunction, and other endocrinopathies may be present. Increased intracranial pressure is not uncommon, and papilledema may be observed. Some optic atrophy is usually present, but its absence does not conflict with the presence of chronic compression of the anterior visual

pathways, even with severe vision loss. Suprasellar or intrasellar calcification is a rather constant radiologic finding in childhood craniopharyngiomas, occurring in 80% to >90% of affected children. Cystic areas frequently occur in craniopharyngioma but rarely in opticochiasmatic gliomas. CT scanning retains special sensitivity in diagnosis, being superior to MRI in detecting calcifications and cyst formations. However, involvement of adjacent structures is more clearly defined by MRI.

In adults, defects in visual field or acuity are the initial symptoms, although increased intracranial pressure or endocrine dysfunction less frequently occur. Visual field defects often take the form of asymmetric bitemporal hemianopia or homonymous patterns, indicating optic tract involvement. Intracranial calcification is seen much less regularly in adults than in children.

The surgical therapy for craniopharyngiomas ranges from total (or at least radical) excision[63] or postoperative radiotherapy after partial removal of tumor, to radiation therapy administered after simple biopsy or cyst decompression.[64] Transsphenoidal decompression may be indicated for large tumors filling the sella. When possible, total removal of the tumor is ideal, but radical manipulations should not be attempted when adhesions to the optic nerves, chiasm, carotid arteries, or hypothalamus are present. The more conservative approach of simple decompression of the anterior visual pathways and relief of third-ventricle obstruction appears judicious, and postoperative radiation therapy has established efficacy. Endocrine replacement therapy is anticipated in the vast majority of cases, often for life.

As with pituitary adenoma and meningioma, craniopharyngiomas may enlarge abruptly during pregnancy.[65]

## RATHKE CLEFT CYSTS

Although previously regarded as a rare lesion in the sellar area, these cysts derive from Rathke cleft, an embryonic vestige of Rathke pouch. In a series of 18 patients with this lesion,[66] 7 presented with visual disturbance or bitemporal hemianopia, and 7 presented with a variety of endocrine dysfunctions. Unlike craniopharyngiomas, partial removal or decompression of these cysts with one procedure is usually sufficient, and regrowth is less common.

## ARACHNOID CYSTS

Enlarging loculations of cerebrospinal fluid (CSF) contained in arachnoidal cysts infrequently present as a chiasmal syndrome. These may arise, for example, in the floor of the third ventricle, causing chiasmal compression, a J-shaped sella, and occasional precocious puberty.[67] Women with benign intrasellar cysts have been reported,[68] showing bitemporal hemianopia, headache, optic atrophy, and panhypopituitarism. Another patient presented with obesity and amenorrhea but without visual defects.[69]

## SUPRASELLAR DYSGERMINOMA

Primary suprasellar dysgerminomas (atypical teratoma, "ectopic pinealoma") are rare causes of chiasmal interference, but they constitute a more or less distinguishable clinical syndrome. These tumors likely arise from cell rests in the anterior portion of the third ventricle and are not directly related to the pineal itself, although histologically, they resemble atypical pineal teratomas. A review of 64 cases[67] revealed that the classic triad consists of early diabetes insipidus; visual field loss, not necessarily of a clearly chiasmal pattern (owing to infiltration of the anterior visual pathways); and hypopituitarism. Symptoms commence at the end of the first or during the second decade of life. Girls are affected more frequently, with a peak incidence at 10 to 20 years of age. Usually, plain film radiology of the sella is normal, but MRI readily reveals the lesion. Frequently, there is growth retardation. The diagnosis is confirmed by CSF cytology, measurement of human chorionic gonadotropin, or both, but often biopsy is necessary.[70]

The radical excision of tumor invading the optic nerves and chiasm, infundibulum, and floor of third ventricle is not possible, but radiotherapy offers excellent palliation, if not a cure. Because subarachnoid seeding of the neuraxis is a distinct possibility, more extensive radiation may be indicated. Long-range endocrine replacement is critical.

## PITUITARY ADENOMAS

Asymptomatic pituitary adenomas occur in >20% of pituitary glands, and some degree of adenomatous hyperplasia can be found in almost every pituitary gland.[71] A postmortem study[72] of pituitaries removed from 120 patients without clinical evidence of pituitary tumors revealed a 27% incidence of microadenomas, of which 41% stained for prolactin, without gender difference. To generalize, >1 in 10 people in the general population dies harboring a prolactinoma. The incessant parade of this clinical syndrome is, therefore, not surprising. Tumor of the pituitary gland is the single most common intracranial neoplasm that produces neuro-ophthalmologic symptomatology, and chiasmal interference is overwhelmingly the most frequent presentation (see Chap. 11). Strictly speaking, a *microadenoma* refers to a tumor that is 10 mm or less in diameter and confined to the sella.

Symptomatic adenomas occur infrequently before 20 years of age but are common from the fourth through seventh decades of life. When these tumors do occur in childhood, most are asymptomatic. When symptoms are present, headache, visual field loss, and endocrinopathies are the most common. Dissimilar to adults, in children there is a definite male predominance, and many tumors are hemorrhagic.[73] Histologic staining characteristics alone do not correlate well with patterns of growth or clinical symptomatology. A functional classification of pituitary adenomas, as elaborated by electron microscopy and immunohistochemistry, has replaced the previous simplistic classification of "eosinophilic, basophilic, and nonfunctioning" (see Chap. 11).

## SYMPTOMATOLOGY

Nonocular symptoms include chronic headaches (severe or mild) in more than two-thirds of patients, fatigue, impotence or amenorrhea, sexual hair change, or other signs of gonadal, thyroid, or adrenal insufficiency (see Chap. 17). Prediagnostic signs and symptoms, affecting vision or otherwise, may exist for months to years before diagnosis is established.

## VISION CHANGES

With pituitary tumors, vision failure may take the form of a rather limited number of field patterns. As suprasellar extension evolves, a single optic nerve may be compromised, with resultant progressive monocular vision loss in the form of a central scotoma. More frequently, as the tumor splays apart the anterior chiasmal notch, superotemporal hemianopic defects occur (Wilbrand knee, as discussed previously). However, this well-touted superior bitemporal hemianopia is almost always accompanied by minor or major hemianopic scotomas approaching the fixational area along the vertical meridian (see Fig. 19-4). Asymmetry of field defects is common, the eye with the greater field deficit also being likely to show diminished central vision. Marked asymmetry is not uncommon, such that one eye may be blind and the other may show a temporal hemianopic defect, the so-called junctional scotoma; this combination is as exquisitely localizing to the chiasm as is the classic bitemporal hemianopia. Adenomas extending posteriorly produce incongruous homonymous hemianopias by optic tract involvement; central vision usually is diminished, at least in the ipsilateral eye. In late stages, the only suggestion of the chiasmal character of field defects may be minimal preservation of the nasal field of one eye.

The absence of field defects in patients undergoing evaluation for amenorrhea or a sella enlargement that is incidentally discovered does not imply the absence of an adenoma. For example, many patients with acromegaly do not show field defects, and microadenomas by definition do not escape the confines of the sella.

## EFFECT OF PREGNANCY

The effect of pregnancy on pituitary adenomas is of interest diagnostically and therapeutically. Enlargement of preexisting pituitary tumors during the third trimester of pregnancy may occur,[74] with reduction in size postpartum. That an otherwise normal pituitary gland may enlarge owing to the changes of pregnancy alone, causing symptoms affecting vision, is controversial.[75] Nevertheless, a 30-week pregnant woman with an enlarged pituitary and bitemporal hemianopia that regressed spontaneously postpartum was reported[76]; a retrospective diagnosis of lymphocytic hypophysitis was made.

## DIAGNOSIS

Many pituitary tumors deform the sella turcica sufficiently to be detected by plain film techniques, but, normal or otherwise, such procedures must be considered preliminary or superfluous. CT with contrast or gadolinium-enhanced MRI is mandatory when chiasmal lesions are suspected (see Chap. 20).

## THERAPY

The rational approach to treatment of pituitary adenomas has evolved radically over the past 2 decades with the advent of thin-section CT; MRI; transsphenoidal microsurgery; hormonal assays; and dopamine agonists (e.g., bromocriptine), potent inhibitors of pituitary synthesis and release of prolactin. The choice of treatment is open to discussion, with enthusiastic advocates in each camp, but the prime consideration is the ultimate well-being of the patient. Patients with high surgical risk, especially the elderly, should not be subjected to frontal craniotomy. After uncomplicated transsphenoidal surgery alone, vision recovery approaches 90%.[77] Radiation therapy, used either primarily or postoperatively, has great efficacy,[78] and stereotactic radiosurgery has been shown to be effective for select patient groups.[79]

The administration of bromocriptine may rapidly improve vision function when prolactinomas compress the chiasm. In a study[80] of 10 men with field defects caused by prolactinomas (initial prolactin level range 1535–14,200 ng/mL) who were treated with 7.5 to 30 mg per day bromocriptine, an increase in vision usually began within days of commencing therapy, and CT evidence of a decrease in tumor volume was documented somewhat later. Pregnancy apparently is not a contraindication for bromocriptine therapy.[81] An extraordinary, rare complication of chiasmal herniation from shrinkage of a pituitary tumor treated with bromocriptine has been reported; recovery of vision ensued after a decrease in the dosage.[82]

With the advent of pergolide, another ergot-derived dopamine agonist, comes another viable treatment alternative, with apparently fewer frequent side effects of hypotension, nausea, and headache. Also, cabergoline has a very long duration of action, as well as fewer adverse effects. Quinagolide, a non-ergot long-acting prolactin inhibitor, a pure $D_2$ agonist, is also useful.[83] Finally, the long-acting somatostatin analog octreotide may be effective in the treatment of somatotropic, thyrotropic, gonadotropic, and nonfunctioning adenomas.[84] In many cases, hormonal therapy of prolactinomas results in rapid improvement in vision function, often independently of decrease in tumor size.

## ACROMEGALY

Acromegaly is the relatively rare clinical condition related to adenomatous secretion of growth hormone, with resultant hypertrophy of bones, soft tissues, and viscera (see Chap. 12). Sellar changes, when present, are indistinguishable from those caused by other adenomas. Of 1000 pituitary adenomas, 144 of 228 acromegalic patients had visual field defects.[96] Possibly, this relatively high incidence of visual defects reflects delay in diagnosis in a series commenced 5 decades ago.

Diabetes mellitus in acromegaly may be associated with typical retinopathy.[85] Increase in corneal thickness and elevated ocular tension (glaucoma) has been reported,[86] and CT scan has revealed thickened extraocular muscles.[87]

An unusual developmental condition with a dominant inheritance pattern, the so-called ACL (*a*cromegaly, *c*utis verticis, *l*eukoma) syndrome, has been described.[88] This syndrome consists of acromegaloid features combined with severe ridging of the skin of the scalp (cutis verticis gyrata) and corneal whitening (leukoma). Pathologic examination of corneal leukoma has demonstrated a propensity for the nasal limbus, with whorl-like accumulations of disorganized collagen material and mucinous deposits.[89] Signs tend to increase with age, with variable family penetrance.

## PITUITARY APOPLEXY

Pituitary apoplexy—an acute change in adenoma volume resulting from hemorrhage, edematous swelling, or necrosis—is not rare, although the appropriate diagnosis may be elusive (see Chap. 17). Perhaps some 10% of pituitary adenomas undergo such acute or subacute changes,[90] with clinical signs and symptoms including change in headache pattern (often severe frontal cephalgia), rapid drop in visual function, unilateral or bilateral ophthalmoplegia, epistaxis or CSF rhinorrhea, and other complications of blood or necrotic debris in the CSF. In a review of 320 verified pituitary adenomas,[91] evidence of hemorrhage was found in 98 cases (18.1%). There was a high incidence of giant or large recurrent adenomas (41%). The mean age was 50 years (range, 17–71 years). The clinical course included acute apoplexy (7 cases); subacute apoplexy (11 cases); recent silent hemorrhages (13 cases); and old silent hemorrhages (27 cases). Sella enlargement was present in all patients.

These patients need not be stuporous, but rapid deterioration and obtundation are highly suggestive. There appears to be a tendency for such events to take place in intrasellar secretory adenomas confined by a competent diaphragma sellae. Ischemic necrosis causes sudden expansion of the tumor with acute compression of neighboring structures, including the optic nerves and chiasm and the ocular motor nerves in the cavernous sinus.

Although this syndrome should now be well known, delay in diagnosis is frequent. Common misdiagnoses usually include meningitis, ruptured intracerebral aneurysm, or sphenoidal mucocele. Almost all cases show abnormal sellae on plain skull series. The CT and MRI scans are typical, if not diagnostic.[92] MRI and CT scans distinguish between many tissue densities, and MRI can detect the presence of blood; the finding of acute or subacute bleeding within a tumor based in an enlarged sella is highly suggestive of pituitary apoplexy.

Although in a few cases (limited suprasellar extension and intact or improving vision) corticosteroid replacement and other expectant medical management may suffice, as a rule, rapid transsphenoidal decompression of the often hemorrhagic tumor should be accomplished without delay to minimize devastating visual consequences; final endocrine status is less likely to be affected.

## VISION ASPECTS OF THERAPY

The medical, surgical, and radiation therapies of pituitary adenomas are covered elsewhere (see Chaps. 21–24). The present role of irradiation of pituitary adenomas is problem-

atic, considering the palpable failure rate and question of untoward side effects. Radiation therapy does indeed appear to reduce the rate of recurrence of pituitary adenomas.[93] However, optic nerve and chiasm damage have occurred secondary to radiation necrosis anywhere from 2 months to 6 years after treatment.[94] Radiation retinopathy, empty sella syndrome, cranial neuropathies, and further pituitary–hypothalamic disturbances may result from radiation therapy of pituitary lesions. There are also anecdotal reports of sarcomas, gliomas, and meningiomas occurring after radiation treatment of pituitary adenomas.[95] The addition of bromocriptine before, during, or after radiotherapy may be helpful in controlling tumor secretion and size until the radiation treatment reaches its maximal effect.

After uncomplicated surgical decompression, visual acuity and fields may return rapidly within 24 to 48 hours or improve weekly (Fig. 19-12). Such restoration is dependent on the duration of visual morbidity and the degree of pallor of the optic discs. After surgery, if careful ophthalmoscopy reveals attrition of the retinal nerve fiber layer, corresponding field defects are permanent. For the most part, what vision returns does so by 3 to 4 months, although continued improvement to 1 year postoperatively is possible. Although fortunately the exception rather than the rule, vision loss is a well-known complication of both transsphenoidal surgery and craniotomy. Failure of vision recovery within the 24-48 hour postoperative interval is highly suggestive of occult hemorrhage in the tumor bed or from related vessels. MRI is essential and decompression may be necessary.

## FOLLOW-UP OF TREATED PITUITARY ADENOMAS

From the standpoint of detecting recurrence, the follow-up of treated adenomas has been problematic. Even as adenomas must be large initially to cause visual defects, so must recurrences be substantial before defects again evolve. Although progressive vision failure may be the incontestable impetus for reoperation, consecutive perimetry may not be counted on to reveal early tumor recurrence. One should obtain an anatomic assessment, as provided by CT scanning or MRI. Recurrence of vision failure may be caused by regrowth of tumor, arachnoidal adhesions associated with progressive empty sella syndrome, or delayed radionecrosis. Tumor recurrence is, by far, the most common mechanism of vision deterioration, but field examination alone may not make this distinction.

## EMPTY SELLA SYNDROME

Extension of the subarachnoid space into the sella turcica through a deficient sellar diaphragm may manifest itself clinically and radiologically as a syndrome mimicking pituitary adenoma. The empty sella may be defined as *nontumorous remodeling that results from a combination of incomplete diaphragma sellae and CSF fluid pressure.*[96]

Diaphragmal openings are common; in one study, defects >5 mm were found in 39% of normal autopsy cases.[97] The sella is characteristically enlarged, but an empty sella may be of normal size. *Primary empty sella* occurs spontaneously and may be associated with arachnoidal cysts or, possibly, infarction of the diaphragma and pituitary. *Secondary empty sella* follows pituitary surgery or radiotherapy (see Chaps. 11 and 17) and may also be seen in cases of elevated intracranial pressure (e.g., pseudotumor cerebri or hydrocephalus). Neuroradiographic evidence of a reversible empty sella syndrome after therapy for idiopathic intracranial hypertension has been reported.[98] Visual field defects, hypopituitarism, headaches, and spinal fluid rhinorrhea occasionally occur. A thorough review of the clinical and radiographic characteristics of primary empty sella[99] has revealed the following features: obese women predominate,

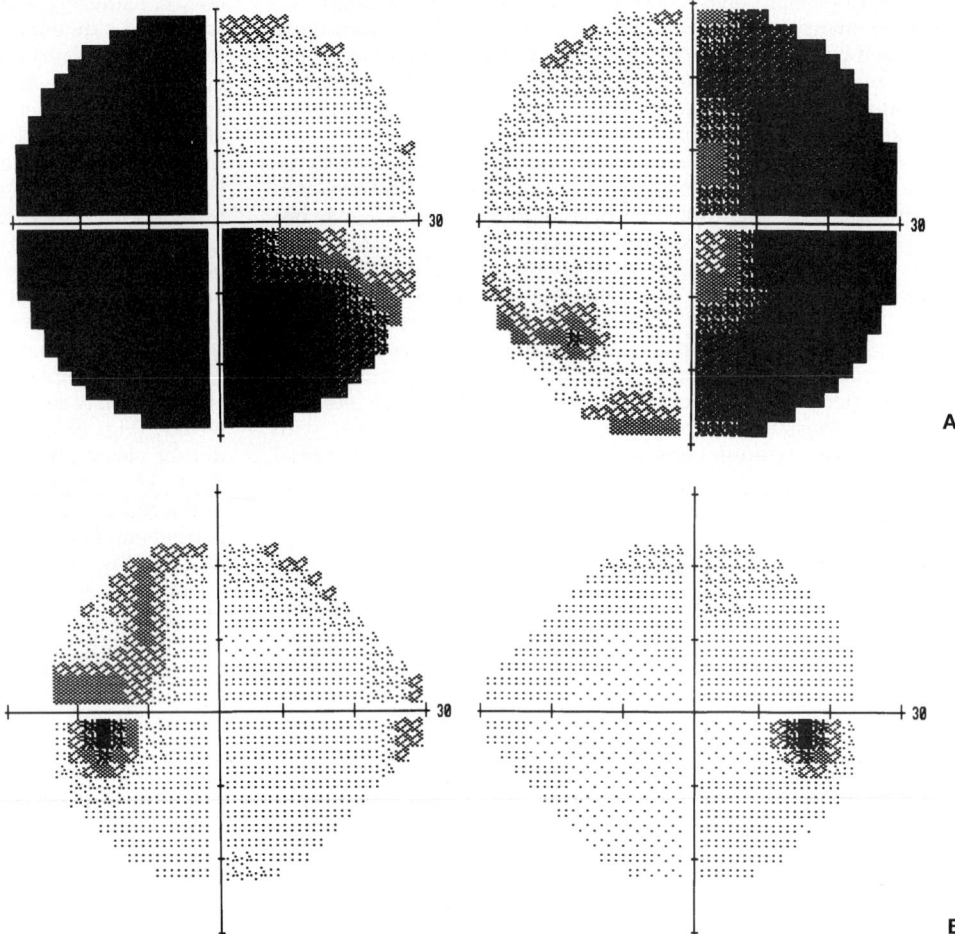

**FIGURE 19-12.** **A,** Preoperative automated visual fields from a 68-year-old man with a nonfunctioning pituitary adenoma. Note dense bitemporal defect. **B,** Same patient, 10 weeks after transsphenoidal decompression, enjoys dramatic recovery and near-normalization of visual fields. (*Left*, left eye; *right*, right eye.)

ranging in age from 27 to 72 years, with a mean age of 49 years; headache is a common symptom; there is no vision impairment because of chiasmal interference; usually, an enlarged sella turcica is found serendipitously on radiologic studies obtained for evaluation of headaches, syncope, or other symptoms; pseudotumor cerebri was present in 13% of patients; approximately two-thirds of the patients had normal pituitary function; and the remaining one-third demonstrated endocrine disturbances, including panhypopituitarism and growth hormone, gonadotropin, and thyrotropin deficiency. In another series of patients with primary empty sella,[100] the following features are noteworthy: all 19 were female; 12 patients initially reported headache; in 7, vision disturbances were prominent subjective symptoms (blurred vision, diplopia, micropsia); 3 patients had bilateral papilledema, and pseudotumor cerebri was diagnosed; and 2 patients demonstrated minimal, relative hemianopias without obvious cause. Additionally, visual field defects typical of those seen in glaucoma are well documented in patients with empty sella syndrome; the normal intraocular pressures implicate the empty sella syndrome as a potential cause of so-called *low-tension glaucoma*.[101]

Secondary empty sella occurs after pituitary surgery or radiotherapy, wherein adhesions form between the tumor "capsule" (or sellar diaphragm) and the nerves and chiasm. Retraction of these adhesions into the empty sella draws the chiasm and nerves downward, with resulting visual defects. Packing the sellar cavity to elevate the diaphragma (chiasmapexy) has been suggested for prophylactic purposes[102] or after the fact.

Primary empty sella may rarely occur in children in association with multiple congenital anomalies, including the *de Morsier syndrome*.[103]

## MISCELLANEOUS LESIONS OF THE OPTIC CHIASM

### TRAUMATIC CHIASMAL SYNDROME

Vision loss that follows closed-head trauma usually is attributed to contusion or laceration of the optic nerves occurring abruptly at the time of impact. Much less frequently, a chiasmal syndrome may be identified by the pattern of field loss and associated deficits, including diabetes insipidus, anosmia, CSF rhinorrhea, and fractures of the sphenoid bone. From a report of several such patients,[104] it was clear that neither the degree of vision loss nor the extent of diabetes insipidus was necessarily related to the severity of craniocerebral trauma. Transient diabetes insipidus was present in approximately one-half of these patients. Rarely, panhypopituitarism may occur.[105] The traumatic chiasmal syndrome may occur more commonly than recognized because of its frequent association with extensive basilar skull fractures and its concomitant altered level of consciousness and high mortality rate.[106]

Lesions of the hypophysial stalk and, more frequently, of the hypothalamus may follow blunt head trauma. Hypothalamic lesions have been noted in 42% of patients who died after head trauma.[107] Ischemic lesions and microhemorrhages were attributed to shearing of small perforating vessels.

### METASTATIC LESIONS

Pituitary metastases are uncommon manifestations of systemic cancer and, initially, may be difficult to distinguish from simple adenomas. To ascertain the incidence of pituitary tumors in cancer patients and to characterize the clinical presentations of metastases, the experience at Memorial Sloan-Kettering Cancer Center was reviewed.[108] Also, a series of 500 consecutive autopsies was analyzed, with inclusion of examination of the pituitary gland. In the clinical series, histologic diagnosis was made in 60% of patients. Radiologic evaluation, including polytomography and CT, did not reliably distinguish metastasis from adenoma, but the clinical syndromes were distinctive. In the metastasis group, the review[108] revealed an 82% incidence of diabetes insipidus but vision loss in only 11%. In the autopsy series, metastases were found in 36% of cases and adenomas in 1.8%. Two other reported cases[109] of sellar metastases showed diplopia resulting from palsies of the third, fourth, and sixth cranial nerves and eventually diabetes insipidus in one patient. In another report, a man with known colon carcinoma developed panhypopituitarism, hyperprolactinemia, chiasmal field loss, and a right third nerve palsy but no diabetes insipidus.[110]

Several generalizations emerge from these reports of metastatic involvement of the pituitary gland: either the anterior or posterior lobe may be involved; diabetes insipidus is more common than with simple adenoma; cranial nerve palsies are more common than simple adenomas; hyperprolactinemia may be seen, but the serum prolactin level usually is <200 ng/mL.

## INFLAMMATORY LESIONS

Chiasmal neuritis has been well documented and may occur in multiple sclerosis, systemic lupus erythematosus, and a variety of other vasculitic and autoimmune disorders. Such a case with positive serology for Lyme disease has been reported.[111] Sarcoidosis has a well-known predilection for leptomeninges at the base of the brain. The hypothalamus, pituitary, and optic chiasm all are involved in a variety of cases.[112]

Chiasmal arachnoiditis, secondary to tuberculosis or syphilis, is now a rare cause of the chiasmal syndrome in the United States but may be seen with increasing frequency in various immunodeficient states.

## VASCULAR ABNORMALITIES

Such lesions are indeed rare, but cavernous malformations appear to be the most common intrachiasmal vascular anomaly.[113] Suprasellar hemangioma with progressive vision loss has also been reported to occur in von Hippel-Lindau disease.[114]

## REFERENCES

1. Walker AE. The neurosurgical evaluation of the chiasmal syndromes. Am J Ophthalmol 1962; 54:563.
2. Schaeffer JP. Some points in the regional anatomy of the optic pathway, with special reference to tumors of the hypophysis cerebri and resulting in ocular changes. Anat Rec 1924; 28:243.
3. Bergland RM, Ray BS, Torack RM. Anatomical variations in the pituitary gland and adjacent structure in 225 human autopsy cases. J Neurosurg 1968; 28:93.
4. Bergland RM, Ray BS. The arterial supply of the human optic chiasm. J Neurosurg 1969; 31:327.
5. Kupfer C, Chumbley L, Downer J de C. Quantitative histology of optic nerve, optic tract and lateral geniculate nucleus of man. J Anat 1967; 101:393.
6. Horton JC. Wilbrand knee of the primate optic chiasm is an artefact of monocular enucleation. Trans Am Ophthalmol Soc 1997; 95:579.
7. Barber AN, Ronstrom GN, Muelling RJ Jr. Development of the visual pathway: optic chiasm. Arch Ophthalmol 1984; 52:447.
8. Scott IU, Warman R, Altman N. Bilateral aplasia of the optic nerves, chiasm, and tracts in an otherwise healthy infant. Am J Ophthalmol 1997; 124:409.
9. Apkarian P, Bour LJ, Barth PG, et al. Non-decussating retinal-fugal fibre syndrome. An inborn achiasmatic malformation associated with visuotopic misrouting, visual evoked potential ipsilateral asymmetry and nystagmus. Brain 1995; 118:1195.
10. Ikeda H, Yoshimoto T. Visual disturbances with pituitary adenoma. Acta Neurol Scand 1995; 92:157.

11. Gutowski NJ, Heron JR, Scase MO. Early impairment of foveal magno- and parvocellular pathways in juxta chiasmal tumours. Vision Research 1997; 37:1401.
12. Hollenhorst RW, Younge BR. Ocular manifestations produced by adenomas of the pituitary gland: analysis of 1000 cases. In: Kohler PO, Ross GT, eds. Diagnosis and treatment of pituitary tumors. Amsterdam: Excerpta Medica, 1973:53.
13. Elkington SG. Pituitary adenoma: preoperative symptomatology in a series of 260 patients. Br J Ophthalmol 1968; 52:322.
14. Schmidt D, Kommerell G. Schaukel-Nystagmus (see-saw nystagmus) mit bitemporaler Hemanopie als Folg von Schadelhirnstraumen. Graefes Arch Clin Exp Ophthalmol 1969; 178:349.
15. Chamlin M, Davidoff LM, Feiring EH. Ophthalmologic changes produced by pituitary tumors. Am J Ophthalmol 1955; 40:353.
16. Wilson P, Falconer MA. Patterns of visual failure with pituitary tumors: clinical and radiological correlations. Br J Ophthalmol 1968; 52:94.
17. Glaser JS. Neuro-ophthalmology. Hagerstown, MD: Harper & Row, 1978:135.
18. de Morsier G. Études sur les dysraphias cranio-encephaliques. III. Agenesie du septum lucidum avec malformation du tractus optique: la dysplasie septo-optique. Schweiz Arch Neurol Psychiatr 1956; 77:267.
19. Lambert SR, Hoyt CS, Narahara MH. Optic nerve hypoplasia. Surv Ophthalmol 1987; 32:1.
20. Glaser JS. The optic chiasm. In: Lessell S, van Dalen JTW, eds. Neuro-ophthalmology 1982. Amsterdam: Excerpta Medica, 1982:61.
21. de Morsier G. Median cranioencephalodysraphias and olfactogenital dysplasia. World Neurol 1962; 3:485.
22. Cagianut B, Sigg P, Isler W, Friede R. Dysplasia opticoseptalis. Klin Monatsbl Augenheilkd 1980; 176:699.
23. Lemyre E, Lemieux N, Decarie JC, Lambert M. Del (14)(q22.1q23.2) in a patient with anophthalmia and pituitary hypoplasia. Am J Med Genet 1998; 77:162.
24. Carey ML, Friedman TB, Asher JH Jr, Innis JW. Septo-optic dysplasia and WS1 in the proband of a WS1 family segregating for a novel mutation in PAX3 exon 7. J Med Genet 1998; 35:248.
25. Dattani MT, Martinez-Barbera JP, Thomsa PQ, et al. Mutations in the homeobox gene HESX1/Hesx1 associated with septo-optic dysplasia in human and mouse. Nat Genet 1998; 19:125.
26. Lubinsky MS. Hypothesis: septo-optic dysplasia is a vascular disruption sequence. Am J Med Genet 1997; 69:235.
27. Brodsky MC, Glasier CM. Optic nerve hypoplasia. Clinical significance of associated central nervous system abnormalities on magnetic resonance imaging. Arch Ophthalmol 1993; 111(1):66.
28. Sorkin JA, David PC, Meacham LR, et al. Optic nerve hypoplasia: absence of posterior pituitary bright signal on magnetic resonance imaging correlates with diabetes insipidus. Am J Ophthalmol 1996; 122:717.
29. Abernethy LJ, Qunibi MA, Smith CS. Normal MR appearances of the posterior pituitary in central diabetes insipidus associated with septo-optic dysplasia. Pediatr Radiol 1997; 27:45.
30. Siatkowski RM, Sanchez JC, Andrade R, Alvarez A. The clinical, neuroradiographic, and endocrinologic profile of patients with bilateral optic nerve hypoplasia. Ophthalmology 1997; 104:493.
31. Brodsky MC, Conte FA, Taylor D, et al. Sudden death in septo-optic dysplasia. Report of 5 cases. Arch Ophthalmol 1997; 115:66.
32. Landau K, Bajka JD, Kirchschlager BM. Topless optic disks in children of mothers with type I diabetes mellitus. Am J Ophthalmol 1998; 125:605.
33. Edward WC, Layden WE. Optic nerve hypoplasia. Am J Ophthalmol 1970, 70:950.
34. Walton DS, Robb RM. Optic nerve hypoplasia: a report of 20 cases. Arch Ophthalmol 1970; 84:572.
35. Boniuk V, Ho PK. Ocular findings in anencephaly. Am J Ophthalmol 1979; 88:613.
36. Greenfield PS, Wilcox LM Jr, Weiter JJ, Adelman L. Hypoplasia of the optic nerve in association with porencephaly. J Pediatr Ophthalmol Strabismus 1980; 17:75.
37. Lloyd L, Buncic JR. Hypoplasia of the optic nerve and disc. In: Smith JS, ed. Neuro-ophthalmology focus 1980. New York: Masson, 1979:85.
38. Apple DJ, Rabb MF, Walsh PM. Congenital anomalies of the optic disc. Surv Ophthalmol 1982; 27:3.
39. Pollack JA, Newton TH, Hoyt WF. Transsphenoidal and transethmoidal encephaloceles—a review of clinical and roentgen features of 8 cases. Radiology 1968; 90:442.
40. Males JS, Townsend JS, Schneider RA. Hypogonadotrophic hypogonadism with anosmia: Kallmann's syndrome. Arch Intern Med 1973; 131:501.
41. Bosma JF, Henkin RI, Christiansen RL, Herdt JR. Hypoplasia of the nose and eyes, hyposmia, hypogeusia, and hypogonadotrophic hypogonadism in two males. J Craniofac Genet Dev Biol 1981; 1:153.
42. Chang RJ, Davidson BJ, Carlson HE, et al. Hypogonadotrophic hypogonadism associated with retinitis pigmentosa in a female sibship: evidence for gonadotropin deficiency. J Clin Endocrinol Metab 1981; 53:1179.
43. Rubinstein AE, Lovelace RE, Behrens MM, Weisberg LA. Moebius syndrome in association with peripheral neuropathy and Kallmann syndrome. Arch Neurol 1975; 32:480.
44. Abid F, Hall R, Hudgson P, Weiser R. Moebius syndrome peripheral neuropathy and hypogonadotrophic hypogonadism. J Neurol Sci 1978; 35:309.

45. Triulzi F, Scott G, diNatale B, et al. Evidence of a congenital midline brain anomaly in pituitary dwarfs: a magnetic resonance imaging study in 101 patients. Pediatrics 1994; 93:409.

46. Alvord EC, Loftin S. Gliomas of optic nerve and chiasm: outcome by patients' age, tumor site, and treatment. J Neurosurg 1988; 68:85.

47. Blatt J, Jaffe R, Deutsch M, et al. Neurofibromatosis and childhood tumors. Cancer 1986; 57:1225.

48. Glaser JS, Topical diagnosis: the optic chiasm. In: Duane TD, Jaeger EA, eds. Clinical ophthalmology. Philadelphia: JB Lippincott, 1989:6.

49. Imes RK, Hoyt WF. Childhood chiasmal gliomas: update on the fate of patients in the 1969 San Francisco study. Br J Ophthalmol 1986; 70:179.

50. Shuper A, Horev G, Kornreich L, et al. Visual pathway glioma: an erratic tumour with therapeutic dilemmas. Arch Dis Child 1997; 76:259.

51. Optic chiasm astrocytomas of childhood. 1. Long-term follow-up. Pediatr Neurosurg 1997; 27:121.

52. Collet-Solberg PF, Sernyak H, Satin-Smith M, et al. Endocrine outcome in long-term survivors of low-grade hypothalamic/chiasmatic glioma. Clin Endocrinol (Oxf) 1997; 47:79.

53. Gropman AL, Packer RJ, Nicholson HS, et al. Treatment of diencephalic syndrome with chemotherapy: growth, tumor response, and long term control. Cancer 1998; 83:166.

54. Chamberlain MC, Grafe MR. Recurrent chiasmatic-hypothalamic glioma treated with oral etoposide. J Clin Oncol 1995; 13:2072.

55. Russell A. A diencephalic syndrome of emaciation in infancy and childhood. Arch Dis Child 1951; 26:274.

56. Pitlyk PJ, Miller RH, Johnson GM. Diencephalic syndrome of infancy presenting with anorexia and emaciation. Mayo Clin Proc 1965; 40:327.

57. De Sousa AC, Kalsbeck JE, Mealey J, Fitzgerald J. Diencephalic syndrome and its relation to optico-chiasmatic glioma: review of twelve cases. Neurosurgery 1979; 4:207.

58. Poussaint TY, Barnes PD, Nichols K, et al. Diencephalic syndrome: clinical features and imaging findings. AJNR Am J Neuroradiol 1997; 18:1499.

59. Glaser JS, Hoyt WF, Corbett J. Visual morbidity with chiasmal glioma: long-term studies of visual fields in untreated and irradiated cases. Arch Ophthalmol 1971; 85:3.

60. Tabaddor K, Shulman K, Del Canto MC. Neonatal craniopharyngioma. Am J Dis Child 1984; 128:381.

61. McLone DG, Raimondi AJ, Naidich TP. Craniopharyngiomas. Childs Brain 1982; 9:188.

62. Carmel PW, Antunes JS, Chang CH. Craniopharyngiomas in children. Neurosurgery 1982; 11:382.

63. Fischer EG, Welsh K, Belli JA, et al. Treatment of craniopharyngioma in children 1971–1980. J Neurosurg 1985; 62:496.

64. Hoffman HJ, Buncic JR. Craniopharyngioma in children. In: Smith JS, ed. Neuro-ophthalmology update. New York: Masson, 1977:241.

65. Sachs BP, Smith SK, Casser J, Van Iddekinge B. Rapid enlargement of craniopharyngioma in pregnancy. Br J Obstet Gynaecol 1978; 85:577

66. Sumid M, Uozimi T, Mukada K, et al. Rathke cleft cysts: correlation of enhanced MR and surgical findings. AJNR Am J Neuroradiol 1994; 15:525.

67. Bowman CB, Farris BK. Primary chiasmal germinoma: a case report and review of the literature. J Clin Neuro Ophthalmol 1990; 10:9.

68. Spanziante R, de Devitiis E, Stella L, et al. Benign intrasellar cysts. Surg Neurol 1981; 15:274.

69. Verier Mine O, Salomez-Granier F, Buvat J, et al. À propos d'un cas de kyste arachnoidien intrasellaire. Semaine Des Hôpitaux 1983; 59:408.

70. Izquierdo JM, Rougerie J, Lapras C, Sanz F. The so-called ectopic pinealomas: a cooperative study of 15 cases. Childs Brain 1979; 5:505.

71. Kernohan JW, Sayre GP. Tumors of the pituitary gland and infundibulum. In: Atlas of tumor pathology, ser 1, fascicle 36. Washington, DC: Armed Forces Institute of Pathology, 1956:15.

72. Burrow GN, Wortzman G, Rewcastle NB, et al. Microadenomas of the pituitary and abnormal sellar tomograms in unselected autopsy service. N Engl J Med 1981; 304:156.

73. Poussaint TY, Barnes PD, Anthony DC, et al. Hemorrhagic pituitary adenomas of adolescence. AJNR Am J Neuroradiol 1996; 17:1907.

74. Falconer MA, Stafford-Bell MA. Visual failure from pituitary and parasellar tumours occurring with favorable outcome in pregnant women. J Neurol Neurosurg Psychiatry 1975; 38:919.

75. Miller NR. Walsh and Hoyt's clinical neuro-ophthalmology, 4th ed. Baltimore: Williams & Wilkins, 1982:123.

76. Mikami T, Uozimi T, Yamamaka M. Lymphocytic adenohypophysitis: MRI findings of a suspected case. No Shinkei Geka 1989; 17:871.

77. Powell M. Recovery of vision following transsphenoidal surgery for pituitary adenomas. Br J Neurosurg 1995; 9:367.

78. McCord MW, Buatti JM, Fennell EM, et al. Radiotherapy for pituitary adenoma: long-term outcome and sequelae. Int J Radiat Oncol Biol Phys 1997; 39:437.

79. Yoon SC, Suh TS, Jang HS, et al. Clinical results of 24 pituitary macroadenomas with linac-based stereotactic radiosurgery. Int J Radiat Oncol Biol Phys 1998; 41:849.

80. Moster ML, Savino PJ, Schatz NJ, et al. Visual function in prolactinoma patients treated with bromocriptine. Ophthalmology 1985; 92:1332.

81. Crosignani P, Ferrari C, Mattei AM. Visual field defects and reduced visual acuity during pregnancy in two patients with prolactinoma: rapid regression of symptoms under bromocriptine. Case reports. Br J Obstet Gynaecol 1984; 91:821.

82. Taxel P, Waitzman DM, Harrington JF Jr, et al. Chiasmal herniation as a complication of bromocriptine therapy. J Neuro-ophthalmol 1996; 16:252.

83. Grochowicki M, Khalfallah Y, Vighetto A, et al. Ophthalmic results in patients with macroprolactinomas treated with a new prolactin inhibitor CV 205–502. Br J Ophthalmol 1993; 77:785.

84. Warnet A, Harris AG, Renard E, et al. A prospective multicenter trial of octreotide in 24 patients with visual defects caused by nonfunctioning and gonadotropin-secreting pituitary adenomas. Neurosurgery 1997; 41:786.

85. Amiya T, Toibana M, Hashimoto M, et al. Diabetic retinopathy in acromegaly. Ophthalmologica 1978; 176:74.

86. Bramsen T, Klauber A, Bjerre P. Central corneal thickness and intraocular tension in patients with acromegaly. Acta Ophthalmol 1980; 58:971.

87. Dal Pozzo G, Boschi MC. Extraocular muscle enlargement in acromegaly. J Comput Assist Tomogr 1982; 6:706.

88. Rosenthal JW, Kloepfer HW. An acromegaloid, cutis verticis gyrata, corneal leukoma syndrome: a new medical entity. Arch Ophthalmol 1962; 68:722.

89. Azar P, Rothschild H, Rosenthal JW, Ichinose H. Histopathology of corneal leukoma and fibroma in the ACL syndrome. Hum Pathol 1983; 14:188.

90. David NJ, Gargano FP, Glaser JS. Pituitary apoplexy in clinical perspective. In: Glaser JS, Smith JL, eds. Neuro-ophthalmology, vol 8. Symposium of the University of Miami and the Bascom Palmer Eye Institute. St. Louis: CV Mosby, 1975:140.

91. Symon L, Mohanty S. Haemorrhage in pituitary tumours. Acta Neurochir (Wien) 1982; 65:41.

92. Davis PC, Hoffman JC, Spencer T, et al. MR imaging of pituitary adenomas: CT, clinical, and surgical correlation. AJNR Am J Neuroradiol 1987; 8:107.

93. Grossman A, Cohen BL, Charlesworth M, et al. Treatment of prolactinomas with megavoltage radiotherapy. Br Med J 1984; 288:1105.

94. Warman R, Glaser JS. Radionecrosis of optico-hypothalamic glioma. Neuro-ophthalmology 1989; 9:299.

95. Capo H, Kupersmith M. Efficacy and complications of radiation therapy of anterior visual pathway tumors. Neurol Clin 1991; 9(1):179.

96. Kaufman B. The "empty" sella turcica, a manifestation of the intrasellar subarachnoid space. Radiology 1968; 90:931.

97. Bergland RM, Ray BS, Torack RM. Anatomical variations in the pituitary gland and adjacent structures in 225 human autopsy cases. J Neurosurg 1968; 28:93.

98. Zagardo MT, Cail WS, Kelman SE, Rothman MI. Reversible empty sella in idiopathic intracranial hypertension: an indicator of successful therapy? AJNR Am J Neuroradiol 1996; 17:1953.

99. Neelon FA, Goree JA, Lebovitz HE. The primary empty sella: clinical and radiographic characteristics and endocrine function. Medicine (Baltimore) 1973; 52:73.

100. Berke JP, Buxton LF, Kokmen E. The "empty" sella. Neurology 1975; 25:1137.

101. Beattie AM, Trope GE. Glaucomatous optic neuropathy and field loss in primary empty sella syndrome. Can J Ophthalmol 1991; 26(7):377.

102. Olson DR, Guiot G, Derome P. The symptomatic empty sella: prevention and correction via the transsphenoidal approach. J Neurosurg 1972; 37:533.

103. Wilkinson IA, Duck SC, Gager WE, Daniels DL. Empty sella syndrome: occurrences in childhood. Am J Dis Child 1982; 136:245.

104. Savino PJ, Glaser JS, Schatz NJ. Traumatic chiasmal syndrome. Neurology 1980; 30:963.

105. Gilad E, Dickerman Z, Laron Z, et al. Traumatic chiasmal syndrome with panhypopitituarism. Neuro Ophthalmol 1986; 6:79.

106. Heinz GW, Nunery WR, Grossman CB. Traumatic chiasmal syndrome associated with midline skull fractures. Am J Ophthalmol 1994; 117:90.

107. Crompton MR. Hypothalamic lesions followed closed head injury. Brain 1971; 94:165.

108. Max MB, Deck F, Rottenberg DA. Pituitary metastases: incidence in cancer patients and clinical differentiation from pituitary adenoma. Neurology 1981; 31:998.

109. Neeten SA, Mahler K, Bultinck J, Martin JJ. Sellar metastatic disease. Neuro Ophthalmol 1982; 2:255.

110. Leramo OB, Booth JD, Zinman B, et al. Hyperprolactinemia, hypopituitarism, and chiasmal compression due to carcinoma metastatic to the pituitary. Neurosurgery 1981; 8:477.

111. Scott IU, Silva-Lepe A, Siatkowski RM. Chiasmal optic neuritis in Lyme disease. Am J Ophthalmol 1997; 123:136.

112. Sherman JL, Stern B. Sarcoidosis of the CNS: comparison of unenhanced and enhanced MRI images. AJR Am J Roentgenol 1990; 155:1293.

113. Shibuya M, Baskaya MK, Saito K, et al. Cavernous malformations of the optic chiasm. Acta Neurochir (Wien) 1995; 136:29.

114. Balcer LJ, Galetta SL, Curtis M, et al. von Hippel-Lindau disease manifesting as a chiasmal syndrome. Surv Ophthalmol 1995; 39:302.

# CHAPTER 20

# DIAGNOSTIC IMAGING OF THE SELLAR REGION

ERIC BOUREKAS, MARY OEHLER, AND DONALD CHAKERES

Radiographic imaging of the sella and hypothalamic region is important in the overall evaluation of many patients with endocrine and metabolic disorders. Often, imaging is crucial, because different pathology in this region may present with similar clinical findings. Imaging can help identify a number of diagnostic entities based on anatomicopathologic characteristics. For example, in patients with hypopituitarism, one can often pinpoint the etiology more precisely, determining, for example, whether it is secondary to congenital absence of the gland, septo-optic dysplasia, transection of the pituitary stalk, a large pituitary mass, a suprasellar arachnoid cyst, a hypothalamic glioma, or an eosinophilic granuloma. In addition, in those patients who have known endocrine disorders such as acromegaly, imaging characterizes other important anatomic aspects of the pathology, such as the size of the mass and possible involvement of the optic chiasm or cavernous sinuses. Imaging of the venous drainage of the pituitary fossa is also used to allow for venous sinus sampling of blood for hormone analysis. Finally, imaging helps direct interventional procedures (i.e., surgery, radiotherapy) in the sellar region and plays a role in postoperative evaluation.

In this chapter, the various imaging modalities and their advantages and disadvantages are discussed in terms of their specific applications. A review is provided of the normal imaging anatomy and of the more commonly encountered pathologic entities, including normal variations, congenital anomalies, inflammations, neoplasms, trauma, and vascular disorders. The focus is primarily on disorders associated with endocrine malfunction.

## ADVANTAGES AND DISADVANTAGES OF IMAGING TECHNIQUES

Traditionally, the first imaging examination in the evaluation of the pituitary-sellar region was a *skull radiograph series*.[1] Plain radiographs offer the advantage of being noninvasive and inexpensive; they yield a certain amount of limited information about the adjacent bony structures (Fig. 20-1). However, potentially important secondary soft-tissue changes can only be inferred, although soft-tissue calcifications can be seen. Thus, in general, routine radiographs provide only minimal information related to the sella, and hence are generally not obtained.

*Computed tomography (CT)* was the first imaging modality to directly visualize the pituitary gland, hypothalamus, and optic chiasm.[2] The bony structures in this region can be well evaluated with CT (Fig. 20-2). It is more sensitive than either plain radiographs or *magnetic resonance imaging (MRI)* in the detection of calcifications within soft tissues. However, intravenous contrast agents frequently are necessary to improve the image contrast and to enhance the vasculature, and CT involves radiation exposure.

A major disadvantage of CT is that soft-tissue characterization is less than ideal. Artifacts from beam hardening, related to the dense bone in the skull base, obscure soft-tissue detail. Additionally, on direct coronal imaging, there often are artifacts that are due to metallic dental fillings. Intravenous contrast is used to improve soft-tissue contrast and highlight the vasculature, but the contrast agent may cause life-threatening reactions.

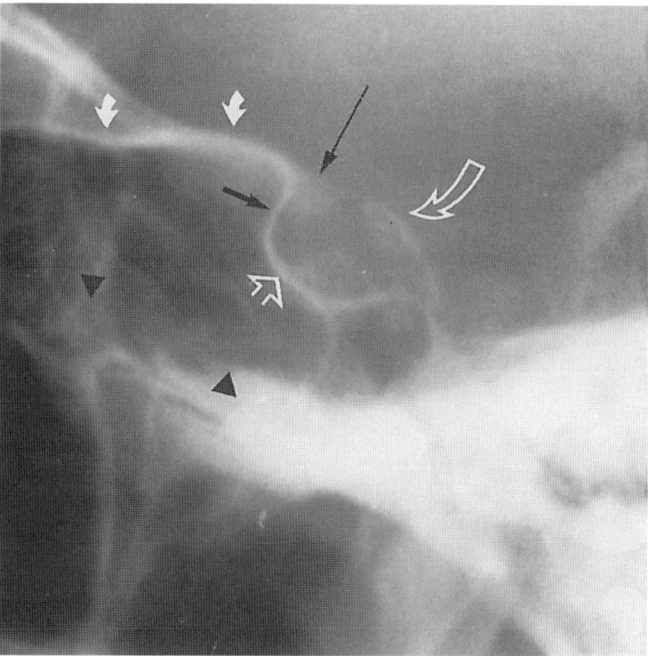

**FIGURE 20-1.** Lateral radiograph of sella. Labeled structures include planum sphenoidale (*curved solid white arrows*), tuberculum sella (*short black arrow*), lamina terminalis (*open white arrow*), sphenoid sinus (*black arrowheads*), anterior clinoid (*long thin black arrow*), and posterior clinoid (*open curved white arrow*). This patient has a relatively well-pneumatized sphenoid sinus. The chiasmatic sulcus is not well marginated.

MRI is the most important single overall imaging modality for the sellar region because it is effective in simultaneously characterizing the soft tissues, cerebrospinal fluid (CSF) spaces, and blood vessels (Fig. 20-3).[3] It is an extremely flexible imaging modality for which contrast can be extensively manipulated. The images may be acquired using a number of different techniques, each of which has specific advantages. For example, MRI (as *magnetic resonance angiography [MRA]*) can substitute for routine catheter angiography in most situations.

Although not hampered to the same extent as CT by artifacts, some magnetic susceptibility artifacts may be related to bone and air interfaces and to dental fillings; these are not as significant a problem with MRI as with CT. Moreover, MRI allows multiplanar acquisitions more readily than CT. There is no ionizing radiation with MRI, and the contrast agents are associated with far fewer serious reactions. Because of these advantages, MRI has become the method of choice for the evaluation of the pituitary gland and adjacent soft tissues, unless there is specific interest in the bone or in soft-tissue calcifications.

With precautions, the risks associated with MRI are low. Contraindications to MRI include cardiac pacemaker, a cerebral spring aneurysm clip, a metallic foreign body near a vital structure (e.g., within the eye, the spinal canal, or near a major blood vessel), neural stimulators, and some medical implants. For these patients, CT remains a possible alternative.

*Cerebral angiography* is still an important imaging technique and remains the gold standard for details of vasculature.[4] It is the examination of choice for the evaluation of aneurysms of the sellar/parasellar region and in the evaluation of profuse bleeding during or after transsphenoidal surgery, which may be secondary to injury of the sphenopalatine arteries or the internal carotids.[5] Inferior petrosal venous sinus angiography and blood sampling can also be helpful.[6] The main disadvantage of angiography is the risk of serious complications. In general, although the incidence of complications is low, the results can be catastrophic (infarcts and vascular occlusions). Even venous studies may have serious complications, such as brainstem infarction. The procedure is uncomfortable or painful for

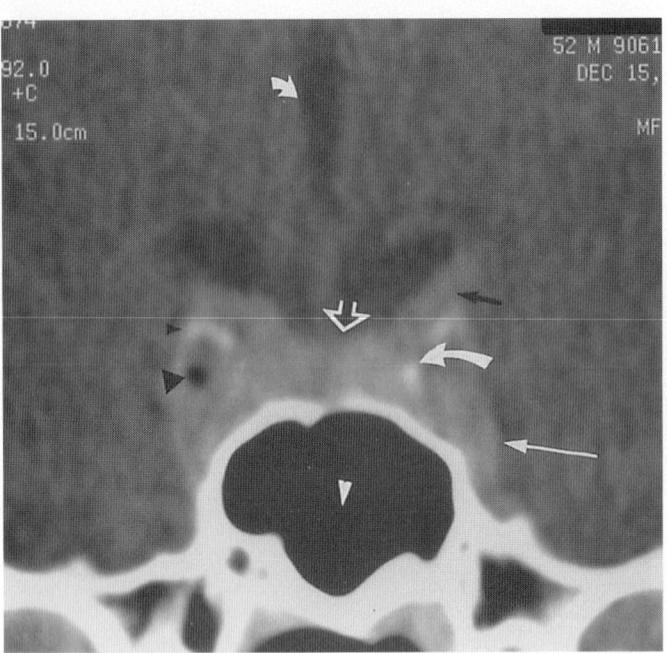 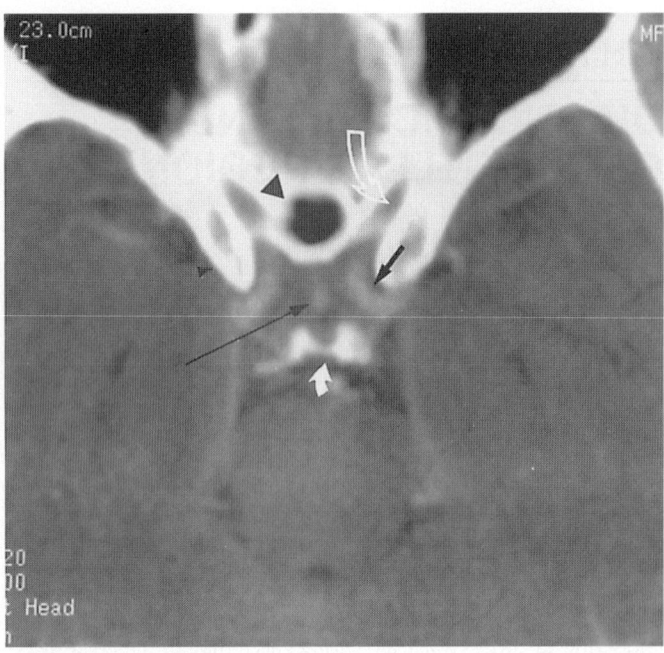

**FIGURE 20-2.** Normal sellar and suprasellar CT. **A,** Coronal CT scan obtained with contrast enhancement through the anterior third ventricle (*short curved solid white arrow*), supraclinoid carotid artery (*thick black arrow*), calcified cavernous carotid artery (*long curved solid white arrow*), pituitary gland (*open white arrow*), anterior clinoid (*small black arrowhead*), cavernous sinus (*long white arrow*), incidental fat in the cavernous sinus (*large black arrowhead*), and sphenoid sinus (*white arrowhead*). **B,** Axial CT scan made with contrast enhancement through the suprasellar cistern. The labeled structures include anterior clinoids (*small black arrowhead*), posterior clinoids (*curved solid white arrow*), optic canal (*curved open white arrow*), pneumatized planum sphenoidale (*large black arrowhead*), pituitary stalk (*long thin black arrow*), and supraclinoid carotid artery (*short black arrow*).

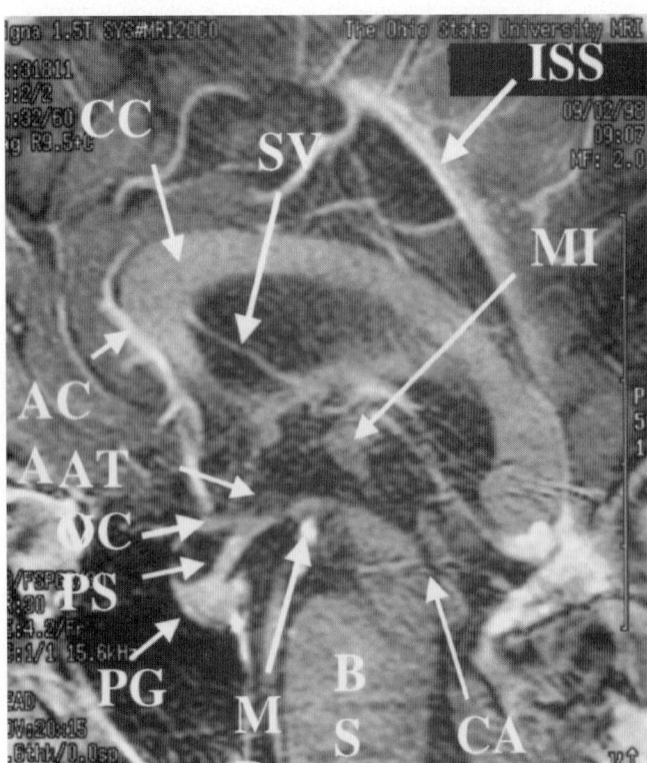 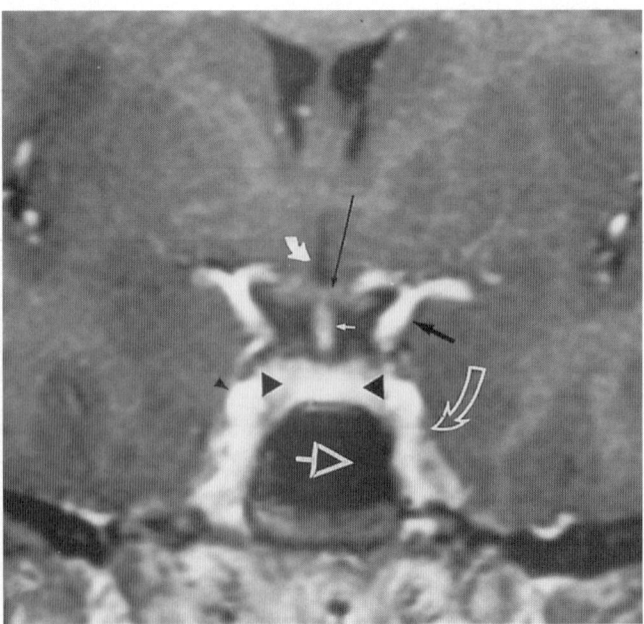

**FIGURE 20-3.** Normal sellar and suprasellar MRI. **A,** Sagittal contrast-enhanced T1-weighted 3D gradient echo image. Labeled structures include the pituitary gland (*PG*), pituitary stalk (*PS*), optic chiasm (*OC*), corpus callosum (*CC*), septal vein (*SV*), inferior sagittal sinus (*ISS*), massus intermedius (*MI*), anterior cerebral artery (*AC*), anterior third ventricle (*AAT*), brainstem (*BS*), cerebral aqueduct (*CA*), and mammillary body (*MB*). **B,** Coronal contrast-enhanced T1-weighted image with angiographic technique. Labeled structures include the cavernous carotid artery (*small black arrowhead*), supraclinoid carotid artery (*short black arrow*), pituitary stalk (*short white arrow*), optic chiasm (*long black arrow*), infundibular recess of the third ventricle (*curved solid white arrow*), sphenoid sinus (*open white arrow*), cavernous sinus (*curved open white arrow*), and pituitary gland (*large black arrowheads*). (*continued*)

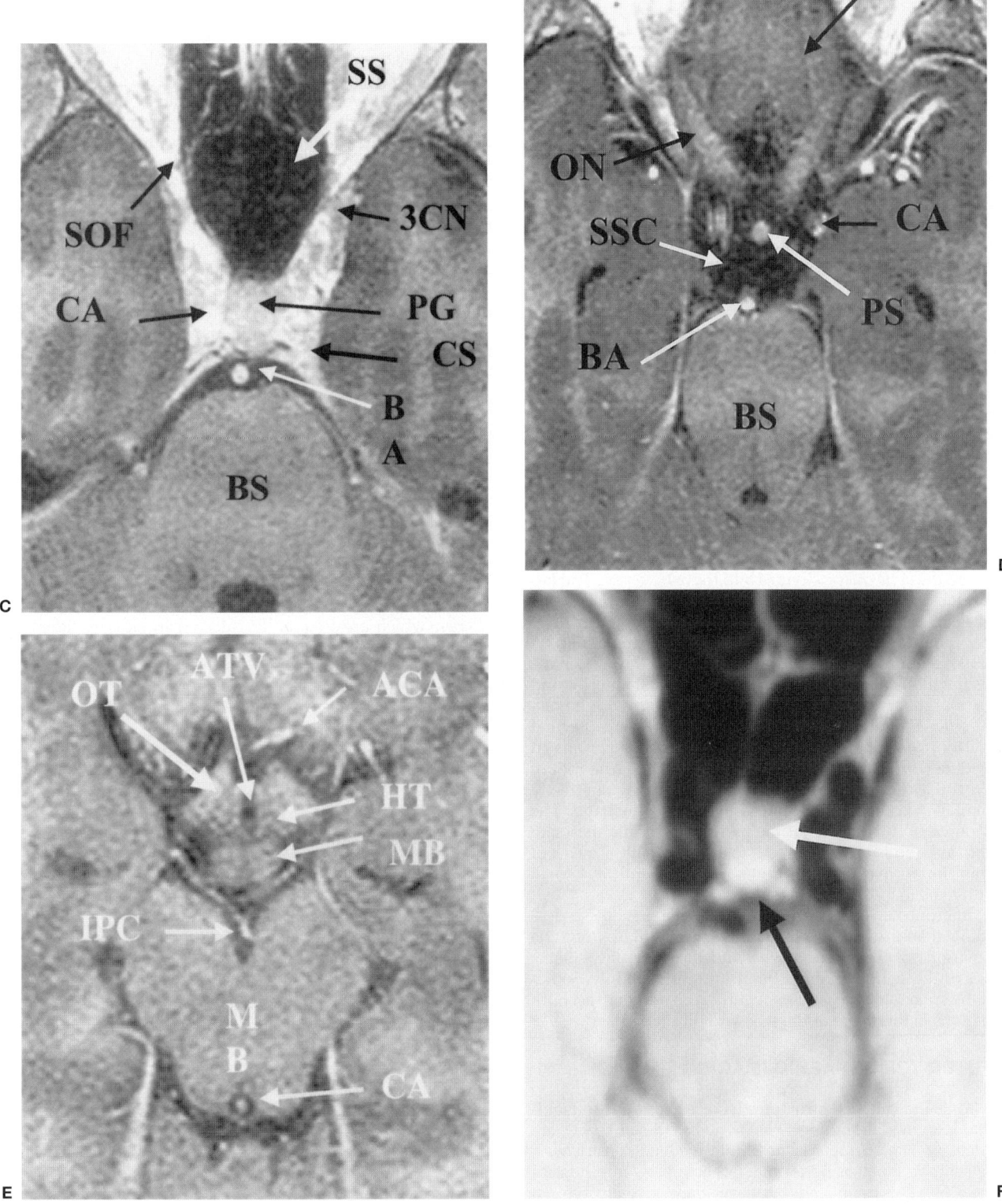

**FIGURE 20-3.** *Continued* **C,** Axial 3D gradient echo contrast-enhanced T1-weighted pituitary fossa. Labeled structures include the cavernous carotid artery (*CA*), sphenoid sinus (*SS*), cavernous sinus (*CS*), basilar artery (*BA*), third cranial nerve (*3CN*), superior orbital fissure (*SOF*), brainstem (*BS*), and pituitary gland (*PG*). **D,** Axial 3D gradient echo contrast-enhanced T1-weighted suprasellar cistern. Labeled structures include supraclinoid carotid artery (*CA*), suprasellar cistern (*SSC*), pituitary stalk (*PS*), basilar artery (*BA*), optic nerve (*ON*), rectus gyrus (*RG*), and brainstem (*BS*). **E,** Axial 3D gradient echo contrast-enhanced T1-weighted hypothalamus optic complex. Labeled structures include anterior cerebral artery (*ACA*), mammillary bodies (*MB*), anterior third ventricle (*ATV*), interpeduncular cistern (*IPC*), optic tract (*OT*), hypothalamus (*HT*), cerebral aqueduct (*CA*), and midbrain (*MB*). **F,** Axial spin-echo non–contrast-enhanced T1-weighted anterior posterior pituitary. Labeled structures include anterior pituitary (*white arrow*) and posterior pituitary (*black arrow*).

the patient and is associated with radiation exposure and potential contrast complications.

## NORMAL IMAGING ANATOMY

### SKULL RADIOGRAPHS

An evaluation of subtle changes of the bony architecture of the sella is not of great clinical use because there are many normal variations in the size, shape, and cortical margins of the sella. In part, this is due to differences in the configuration of the sphenoid bone and sphenoid sinus. It is important to realize that variations in the shape of the sella do not always reflect the pathology of the adjacent structures.

The sella is usually evaluated with lateral and posteroanterior plain radiographs (tomography has been largely replaced by CT). On the lateral projection, the *sella turcica* is a U-shaped structure that is seen as a crisp, dense cortical bone margin (see Fig. 20-1). Those segments of the sella that are outlined by the underlying air spaces of the sinuses exhibit a thin cortical margin, which is referred to as the *lamina dura*. If the sinus is opacified or not pneumatized and filled with bone marrow, the sellar margin is thicker.

The *planum sphenoidale* is a flat, thin bone that forms the roof of the anterosuperior sphenoid sinus and extends posteriorly to terminate in the *anterior clinoid processes*. Between the anterior clinoid processes, the planum sphenoidale ends at a small arc-shaped ridge of bone called the *limbus*; this forms the anterior margin of a small bony depression called the *chiasmatic sulcus* (which conforms to the optic chiasm and nerves). This concavity is where the *optic chiasm* divides into the *optic nerves*. The lateral margins of the chiasmatic depression extend into the *optic canals* that, in turn, extend anteriorly and laterally. Superior to the optic canals are the anterior clinoids, which are visible on lateral radiograph. The inferoposterior margin of the chiasmatic sulcus is the *tuberculum sella*, which forms the most anterior and superior margin of the *sella turcica (hypophyseal fossa)*. The *diaphragma sellae* is the superior dural covering of the sella that extends from the tuberculum sella to the *posterior clinoids*. It cannot be seen on plain radiographs, but marks the true roof of the sella turcica. Usually, the *floor of the sella* is not perfectly hemicircular in configuration, but is more oval in shape. The normal range of dimensions of the bony sella from anterior to posterior on lateral radiograph is 5 to 16 mm, with a mean of 10.6 mm. The normal range of dimensions in depth is 4 to 12 mm, with a mean of 8.1 mm.[7]

The anteroposterior projection of the sella usually is less informative than the lateral, but it may be useful in defining the lateral margins of the *sphenoid sinus* and the floor of the sella. The floor of the sella frequently bows inferiorly slightly. Septations of the sphenoid sinus are frequently seen and may account for variations in the shape of the sella and pituitary gland.

### COMPUTED TOMOGRAPHIC IMAGING

On CT, bone and calcified structures have a high density (similar to that seen in plain radiographs), whereas the air spaces are of low density. The CSF spaces are of intermediate density, with the fat structures (such as periorbital fat) being lower in density than the CSF. The brain and pituitary gland usually have a slightly higher density than the CSF. With the use of intravenous contrast agents, the blood vessels, cavernous sinus, pituitary gland, and pituitary stalk all enhance intensely, thus increasing their apparent density (see Fig. 20-2). This helps define the pituitary gland and the cranial nerves in the cavernous sinus. Rarely, intrathecal contrast is used for the evaluation of a CSF fistula.

In general, contrast-enhanced direct coronal CT images of the sella are the most informative, although axial sections are easier for patient positioning. If one is not able to perform direct coronal imaging, computer reconstructions of axial images into sag-

ittal and coronal sections can be obtained, although their detail is limited. On coronal CT, the bony sella is seen as a flat to minimally concave structure with the sphenoid sinus directly inferior (see Fig. 20-2A). The lateral walls of the sella are formed by the *cavernous sinuses,* which are visualized on enhanced CT as contrast-filled structures bounded laterally by dura. The individual *cranial nerves* (oculomotor, abducens, and trochlear) can be seen in the cavernous sinus. *Meckel cave,* which is a CSF space extending from the posterior fossa, contains the fifth cranial nerve. The dural margins of the cave enhance, while the CSF spaces are seen as low-density, vertical, oval cavities.

The lateral margins of the pituitary gland, which presents as an oval-shaped soft-tissue structure, may be difficult to differentiate from those of the cavernous sinus. The pituitary gland usually has a flat superior margin; however, it is common for adolescents and menstruation-aged women to have a slightly convex upward superior margin. This finding can also be seen in small tumors and is less common in men. The *infundibulum* or *pituitary stalk* is seen as a thin, usually midline tubular structure, extending inferiorly from the *median eminence* of the arc-shaped *hypothalamus* to insert on the superior margin of the *pituitary gland,* usually in the anterior third. Both the pituitary gland and the infundibulum enhance with intravenous contrast; this is partially due to the portal venous plexus and partially due to the lack of a blood–brain barrier. Directly superior to the infundibulum, in the anterior third of the sella turcica, is the *optic chiasm,* which is oriented horizontally across the top of the sella. The middle portion of the chiasm is rectangular in shape. Farther anteriorly, the chiasm is more figure-8 shaped as it divides into the individual optic nerves.

Axial CT images of the sella demonstrate the air-filled sphenoid inferiorly. Asymmetry of the floor is common. The *carotid arteries,* which are frequently calcified in elderly patients (see Fig. 20-2A), are seen lateral to the gland in the cavernous sinus. The cavernous sinuses form the lateral flat margins adjacent to the temporal lobes. Medially, the margins between the cavernous sinus and normal pituitary may not be clear. Incidental rests of fat are frequently seen in the cavernous sinus and should not be confused with air. The pituitary gland has a circular configuration, and the *suprasellar cistern* has a five-pointed-star configuration. Centrally, the pituitary stalk should be visible. The anterior and posterior clinoids are also well demonstrated on axial images (see Fig. 20-2B).

### MAGNETIC RESONANCE IMAGING

MRI is the examination of choice in the evaluation of the sella and parasellar regions. Unlike CT and plain radiographs, MRI does not use ionizing radiation to generate images; they are generated based on the intrinsic magnetic properties of hydrogen atoms. Respective parameters include proton density, relaxation times (T1 and T2), magnetic susceptibility, and motion. Importantly, only hydrogen atoms are detected with MRI. Regions of cortical bone or air have no signal (signal voids). The image contrast with MRI is plastic; thus, the tissues can have almost any type of signal. With routine, spin-echo, T1-weighted images, tissues with high triglyceride fat content (orbital fat, fatty bone marrow) have bright or high signal intensity. With T1-weighted images, the CSF has a low signal intensity, whereas the brain has an intermediate signal intensity. T2-weighted images demonstrate low signal intensity for fatty structures, intermediate signal intensity for the brain, and high signal intensity for tissues with high water content (e.g., CSF, cystic masses). Motion also has an imaging impact: The signal of moving atoms can have high, low, or misregistered signal intensities, depending on the type of motion and the pulse sequence.

On MRI (see Fig. 20-3), the bony portions of the sella lack signal, except for areas of fatty marrow that have a high signal intensity on T1-weighted images. The normal pituitary gland varies in size with age, growing linearly in the first years of life and developing physiologic hypertrophy at adolescence.[8] In fact, the gland tends to decrease in height and increase in width and anteroposterior dimension with age.[9] In adult patients younger than 50 years of age, the average height of the pituitary gland is 5.7 ± 1.4 mm, and the average length is 10.8 ± 1.2 mm.[10] In newborns younger than 6 weeks of age, the superior margin of the pituitary is usually concave, with an overall globular configuration.[9] In infants between the ages of 6 weeks and 2 years of age, the superior margin is convex in 46% and flat in 43%.[9] The superior margin is generally flat in adults, but in 56% of menstruating women, it may be convex.[8] In newborns younger than 6 weeks of age, both the anterior and posterior lobes of the pituitary are of high signal, whereas in infants 6 weeks to 2 years of age, the anterior lobe is of low signal in 52% and intermediate signal in 43%, and the posterior pituitary is of intermediate signal in 55% and of high signal in 37%.[9] In adults, the normal gland is isointense with white matter, while the *posterior pituitary* or *neurohypophysis* is usually of higher signal intensity on T1-weighted images[11] (see Fig. 20-3F). This is usually seen best on sagittal images as a bright spot posterior to the *adenohypophysis* of the gland, usually in the posterior one-third of the sella.

There has been much speculation about the cause of the high signal intensity within the posterior pituitary gland. It is probably related to neurosecretory granules. When the gland is ectopic, this bright spot is also seen proximally along the pituitary stalk, suggesting an accumulation of these substances in the hypothalamus.[11] The normal infundibulum is 3.5-mm thick near its origin from the hypothalamus and 2.8-mm thick at its midpoint.[12] On sagittal images, the stalk can be seen oriented slightly obliquely and inserting on the anterior one-third of the pituitary gland (see Fig. 20-3A). On coronal images, the stalk is usually midline and is seen extending from the hypothalamus to the upper margin of the pituitary (see Fig. 20-3B). With gadolinium enhancement, the pituitary gland and infundibulum enhance brightly because there is no normal blood–brain barrier in this region (see Fig. 20-3C and D). There is a characteristic enhancement pattern when one performs dynamic imaging with contrast flowing through the pituitary portal system. The enhancement starts in the infundibulum, proceeds to the central gland, and then spreads to involve the more lateral parts of the gland.[13] Dynamic gradient echo MRI has been shown to be superior to conventional contrast-enhanced spin-echo imaging in delineating the margins and extent of tumor.[14]

The optic chiasm and the hypothalamus are intimately associated and cannot be easily separated on axial images (see Fig. 20-3E). On coronal images (see Fig. 20-3B), the pituitary gland, infundibulum, and optic chiasm have a configuration similar to that seen on CT. On most spin-echo MRIs, the cavernous sinus contains tubular areas of low signal intensity related to flowing blood in the cavernous internal carotid arteries (see Fig. 20-3F). The signal can be high with some sequences. The most common pulse sequence is the time-of-flight MRA technique. With gadolinium enhancement, the remainder of the cavernous sinus enhances (except for the cranial nerves).

## NORMAL VARIANTS

### EMPTY SELLA

The sella may not be completely filled with tissue. When the sella is partially filled with CSF in the suprasellar cistern, it is referred to as an *empty sella* (Fig. 20-4). A partially empty sella is a common incidental finding and usually should be considered a normal variation in anatomy. The empty sella may be related to incomplete formation of the diaphragma sella, allowing CSF into the pituitary fossa (see Chap. 11). A partially empty sella can be seen in association with pseudotumor cerebri, hydrocephalus, previous pituitary surgery, or a previous pituitary mass that has shrunk. It can also be seen after irradiation, after trauma, or as

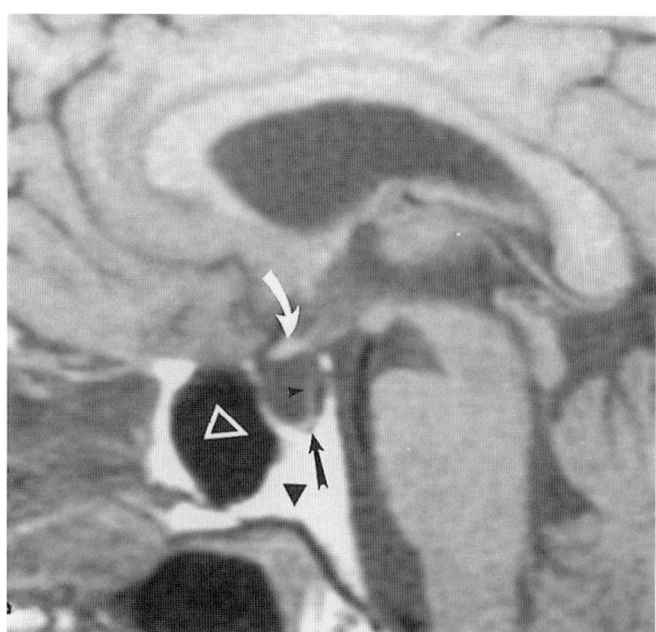

**A**

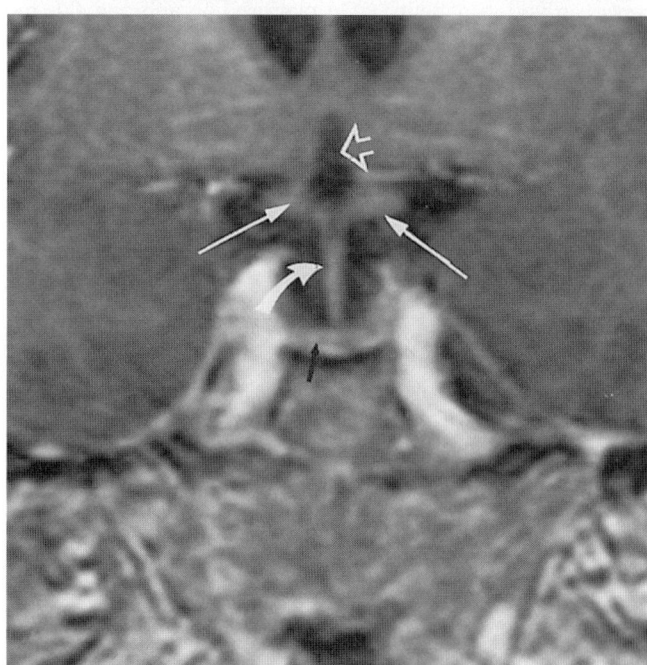

**B**

**FIGURE 20-4.** Empty sella. **A,** Sagittal T1-weighted non–contrast-enhanced image. Note that the pituitary stalk (*small black arrowhead*) extends all of the way to the floor of the sella (*thick black arrow*). The pituitary gland is very thin and not well marginated. In this case, the clivus (*large black arrowhead*) has a large amount of fat generating a high signal intensity region. The other normal structures include the optic chiasm (*curved white arrow*) and sphenoid sinus (*open white arrowhead*). **B,** Coronal contrast-enhanced T1-weighted image. The pituitary stalk (*curved white arrow*) is seen extending all of the way to the floor of the sella. The gland is seen as a thin, "crescent-shaped" structure (*thick black arrow*) at the base of the sella. Other labeled structures include the hypothalamus and optic chiasm (*white straight arrows*) and the anterior third ventricle (*open white arrow*).

sequela of apoplexy. Occasionally, an empty sella is associated with a CSF leak or fistula. The term *empty sella syndrome* has been used to describe a variable clinical constellation of findings, such as headache, endocrine dysfunction, and visual disturbances, which are seen in association with a partially empty sella.[15]

With an empty sella, the sellar bony margins may be expanded, forming an oval or J shape on plain radiograph or

CT. It is often of normal size. The CSF spaces extend into the sella; the pituitary gland may be normal, small, or large in size. The optic nerve, optic chiasm, and optic tracts may herniate into the empty sella. The main finding is visualization of the pituitary stalk extending into the fossa, which is the best way to distinguish an empty sella from a cystic mass.

## CONGENITAL ANOMALIES

### HYPOPLASTIC PITUITARY

The pituitary gland can be congenitally hypoplastic. Many of these patients present with a combination of endocrine deficiencies in childhood. Plain radiographs of the sella demonstrate a small sella turcica, which may measure only a few millimeters in dimension. The presence of a small bony cavity is a sign that the pituitary gland never developed to a normal size rather than an indication of some type of destructive process. Although CT and MRI confirm that the pituitary gland is small, the hypothalamus and other adjacent structures usually appear intact.

### ECTOPIC POSTERIOR PITUITARY GLAND

An ectopic posterior pituitary gland is a relatively common etiology for hypopituitarism and growth hormone (GH) disturbances in young patients.[16] On plain radiograph and CT, the pituitary fossa may be small or normal in size, with an ectopically placed pituitary gland. The pituitary gland itself may be hypoplastic or normal in appearance. Because CT and plain radiographs cannot differentiate the anterior and posterior lobes of the pituitary gland or demonstrate the nodule adjacent to the hypothalamus, there is really no role for these procedures in the evaluation of an ectopic posterior pituitary.

With T1-weighted MRI, the normal round or ovoid bright spot in the posterior sella, representing the posterior pituitary gland, is not seen. The ectopic posterior pituitary tissue is usually located in the region of the median eminence—the insertion of the infundibulum to the hypothalamus. Nevertheless, the posterior pituitary gland maintains its characteristic signal properties, appearing as a small, high signal nodule protruding from the undersurface of the hypothalamus on T1-weighted images (Fig. 20-5). This type of abnormality of the hypothalamus has been described in other entities, including pituitary dwarfism and traumatic transection of the infundibulum, and as a normal variant in asymptomatic patients.[16–18]

### RATHKE CLEFT CYST

Rathke cleft cysts are congenital variations derived from the embryologic precursors of the anterior lobe of the pituitary. The cysts have an epithelial lining and are rarely symptomatic. They may be seen incidentally and can mimic pituitary tumors. They usually occur in the midline of the anterior or superior sella. On plain radiographs of the skull, the sella is usually normal in appearance, although large Rathke cleft cysts can expand the sella. Rarely, calcifications may be seen.

On CT, the sella may be normal or slightly expanded. The cyst can usually be seen as an area of lower attenuation that is similar in signal intensity to CSF. Smaller cysts may be difficult to differentiate from small cystic tumors, and larger cysts may be confused with craniopharyngiomas. These lesions infrequently affect the cavernous sinus or optic chiasm. On MRI, Rathke cleft cysts are usually seen as small cysts displacing the normal enhancing gland. The cysts are usually isointense with CSF on all pulse sequences. Occasionally, they may have a more unusual signal that is due to hemorrhaging.

### ENCEPHALOCELE

Encephaloceles are defects in the skull and dura that may be associated with herniation of the brain or meninges. Encephaloceles can be congenital or acquired. When congenital, there is

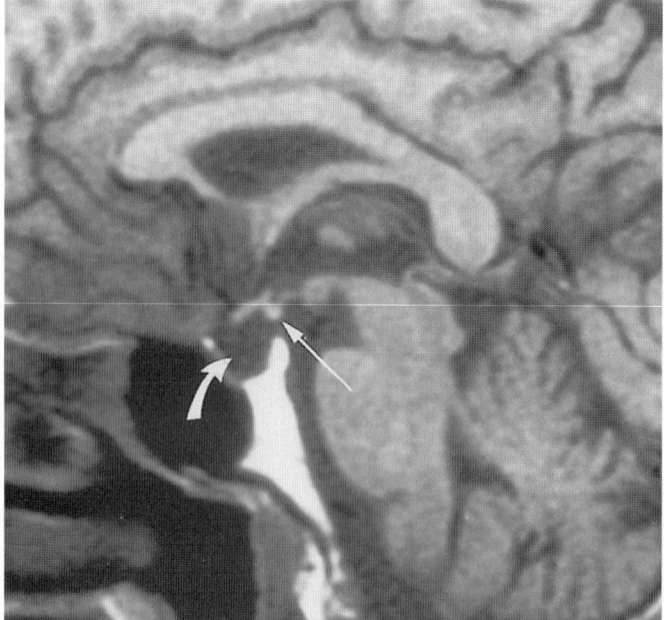

A

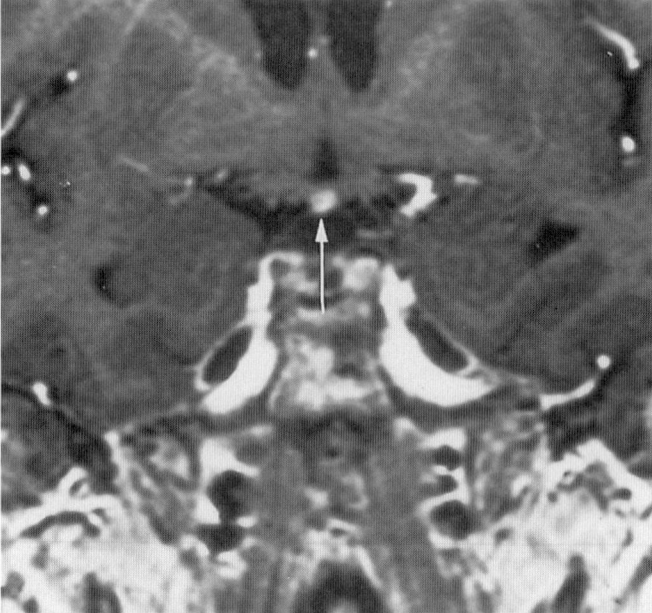

B

**FIGURE 20-5.** Ectopic posterior pituitary gland. **A,** Sagittal unenhanced T1-weighted image through the midline. Note the high signal "bright spot" of the ectopic posterior pituitary (*long straight white arrow*) at the junction of the posterior margin of the optic chiasm and hypothalamus. The sella (*curved white arrow*) is essentially empty, and the anterior pituitary and infundibulum are not well seen. **B,** Coronal contrast-enhanced T1-weighted image through the optic chiasm, hypothalamus, and the ectopic posterior pituitary (*long white arrow*). The infundibulum is not well seen, and the other adjacent structures appear normal.

an anomaly in the midline structures, resulting in a bony defect in the anterior cranial fossa, the superior nose, and the sella; this is a rare anomaly that is more common in the Asian population. An encephalocele may be associated with facial deformities as well.

On plain radiographs, the defect in the anterior cranial fossa and sella may be noted, but it often is small. On CT, the bony defect can usually be seen, and the brain can be observed to herniate into the sella. The findings on MRI are similar, but the detail of the brain is better seen, whereas the bony defect is less well seen.

Brain herniation and anomalous vessels must be distinguished from other abnormalities, such as nasal polyps or

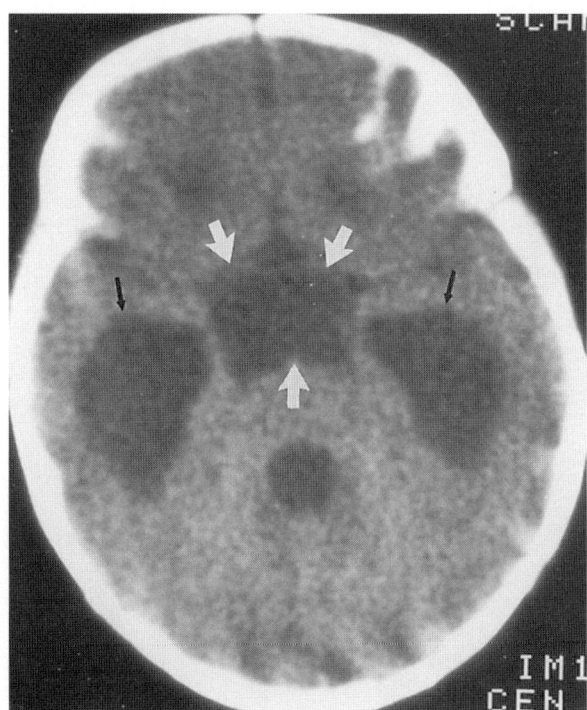

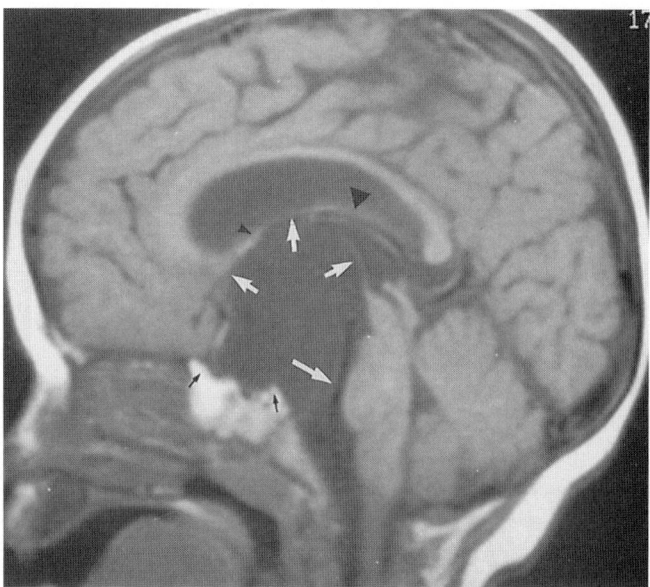

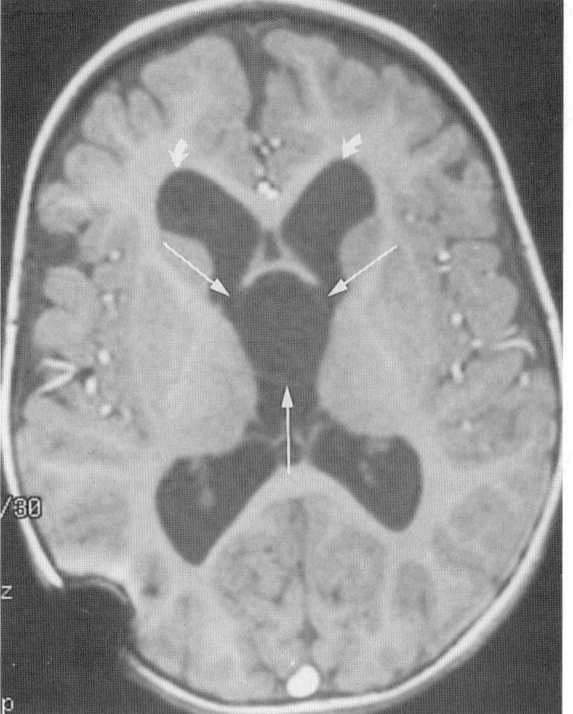

**FIGURE 20-6.** Suprasellar arachnoid cyst. **A,** Axial non–contrast-enhanced CT image of a young child with precocious puberty. The temporal horns are markedly dilated (*thin black arrows*). The suprasellar cistern is expanded (*thick white arrows*), but the cyst walls are not visible. **B,** Sagittal non–contrast-enhanced T1-weighted magnetic resonance image through the midline. The sella is small, and the clinoids are somewhat deformed (*short black arrows*). There is a large cerebrospinal fluid space filling the suprasellar region (*straight white arrows*). The third ventricle is inverted, and the brainstem is displaced posteriorly. The cyst extends all of the way to the foramen of Monro (*small black arrowhead*) and columns of the fornix (*large black arrowhead*). **C,** Axial contrast-enhanced T1-weighted image through the region of the foramen of Monro. The lateral ventricles are dilated (*curved white arrows*). The third ventricle is inverted and filled by the suprasellar cyst. The walls of the cyst are faintly seen as a thin septum (*long white arrows*).

masses, because inadvertent biopsy of an encephalocele that is mistaken for a nasal mass can be catastrophic.

### SUPRASELLAR ARACHNOID CYSTS

Suprasellar arachnoid cysts are parenchymal in origin and are caused by sequestered remnants of the arachnoid membrane. They can cause endocrine dysfunction, most commonly precocious puberty. On CT, these cysts may be seen to distort the chiasm, the floor of the sella, or the clinoids. They may cause hydrocephalus by compressing the third ventricle superiorly (Fig. 20-6). On plain radiographs, in skeletally immature patients, the sutures of the skull may be widened if hydrocephalus is present. The sella may also be expanded, and there may be dysplasia of the clinoid processes with remodeling but no destruction. These bony findings are also seen on CT, but additionally, the cyst is visualized as a low-density structure with an attenuation similar to CSF. When present, hydrocephalus is noted by the presence of

ventriculomegaly. It may be difficult to see the cyst as a separate structure when there is severe hydrocephalus (see Fig. 20-6A); thus, it is important to look for the membranous walls of the cyst, which may invert into the third ventricle.

On MRI, the findings are similar to CT, although the bony changes may be more difficult to see. MRI offers two advantages over CT in this setting. First, the margins of the cyst may be seen as separate from the ventricles; second, the additional planes of imaging may also help to delineate the cyst from the dilated ventricles (see Fig. 20-6B and C). Also, MRI is more sensitive than CT in the detection of transependymal migration of CSF as an indication of obstructive hydrocephalus.

### SEPTO-OPTIC DYSPLASIA

Septo-optic dysplasia is a congenital malformation of the midline structures with absence of the septum pellucidum and a hypoplasia of the optic nerves, optic chiasm, and pitu-

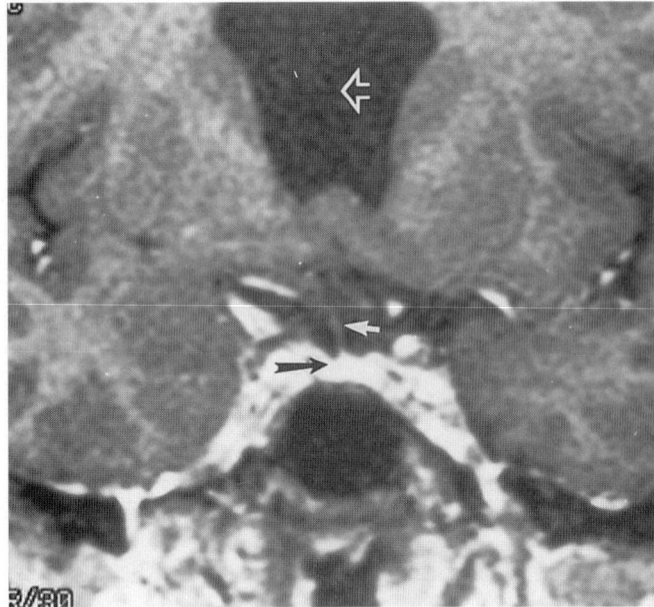

A

**FIGURE 20-7.** Septo-optic dysplasia. This adult presented with polydipsia, diabetes insipidus, and optic atrophy. **A,** Coronal contrast-enhanced T1-weighted image through the suprasellar region. The frontal horns are somewhat deformed, and the septum pellucidum is not visible in the midline (*open white arrow*). The pituitary gland (*black arrow*) is small. The infundibulum is also small (*solid white arrow*). The optic chiasm is not well seen. **B,** Axial proton-density image through the lateral ventricle. Again, the columns of the fornix and the septum pellucidum (*open white arrow*) are absent.

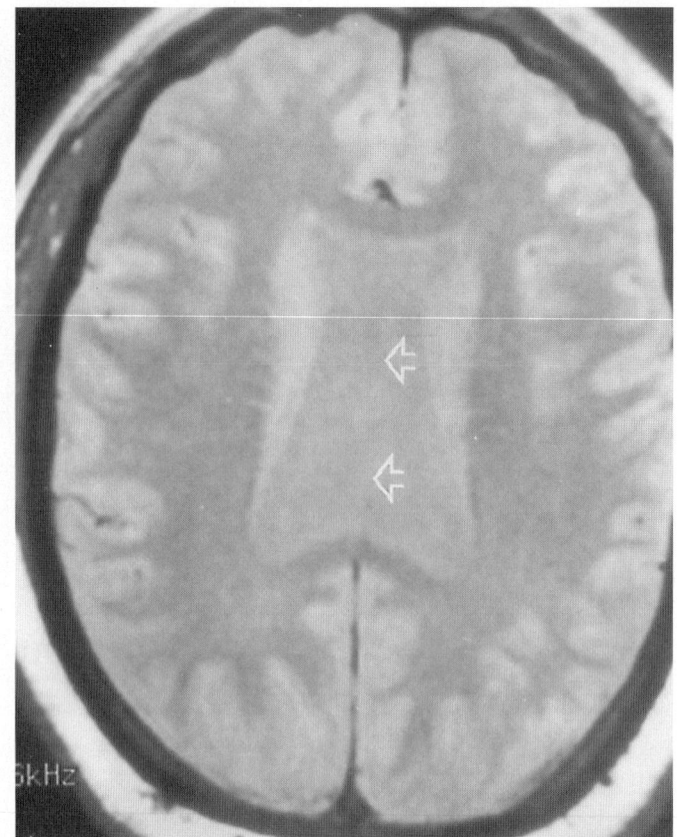

B

itary gland (Fig. 20-7). Septo-optic dysplasia can be considered the mildest form of holoprosencephaly. The patients have a variable degree of endocrine dysfunction, often including diabetes insipidus. Either vision or endocrine symptoms may predominate. Usually plain radiographs are normal, but the sella may be small. CT demonstrates the absence of the septum pellucidum. The optic chiasm is usually small, and the pituitary gland may be normal in size or hypoplastic. The findings on MRI are similar to those on CT, demonstrating an absence of the septum pellucidum and a small optic chiasm and optic nerves.

# NEOPLASMS

## CRANIOPHARYNGIOMA

Craniopharyngiomas (Figs. 20-8, 20-9, 20-10), which are formed from ectodermal elements of Rathke pouch, are composed of squamous epithelial structures. They can occur anywhere from the floor of the third ventricle (hypothalamus) to the pharyngeal tonsil, with the majority being found in the suprasellar region. These tumors have a bimodal incidence, with peaks in the first and fifth decades of life; they comprise 9% of pediatric brain tumors.[19] Clini-

**FIGURE 20-8.** Cystic craniopharyngioma. **A,** Contrast-enhanced sagittal T1-weighted image through the midline. A 2.5-cm inverted, pear-shaped cystic mass (*straight white arrows*) fills the sella and extends into the suprasellar cistern. The regions of the optic chiasm and pituitary stalk are not well demonstrated. There is no hydrocephalus. **B,** Axial T2-weighted image through the suprasellar cistern. The cystic craniopharyngioma demonstrates high signal intensity (*black straight arrows*) similar to that of cerebrospinal fluid. The suprasellar carotid arteries (*solid white arrow*) are seen as low signal intensity flow voids. They are displaced laterally by the mass.

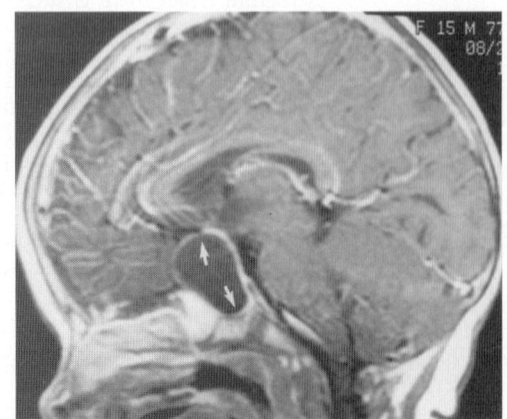

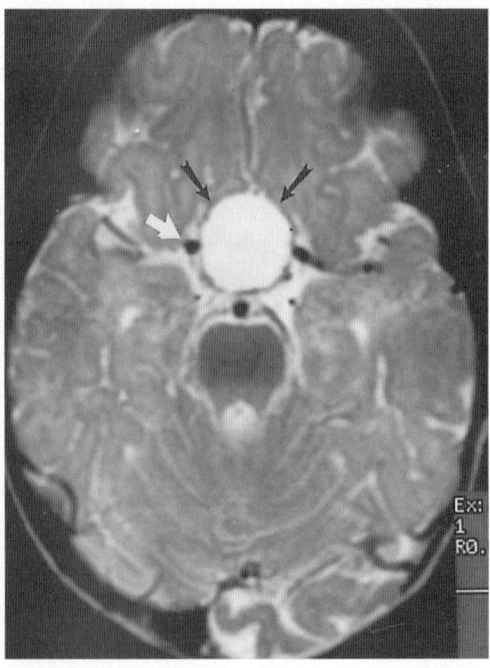

A,B

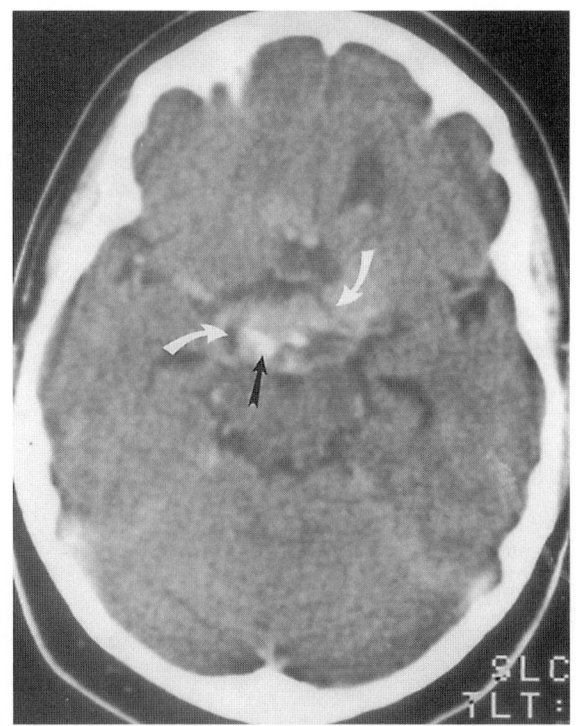

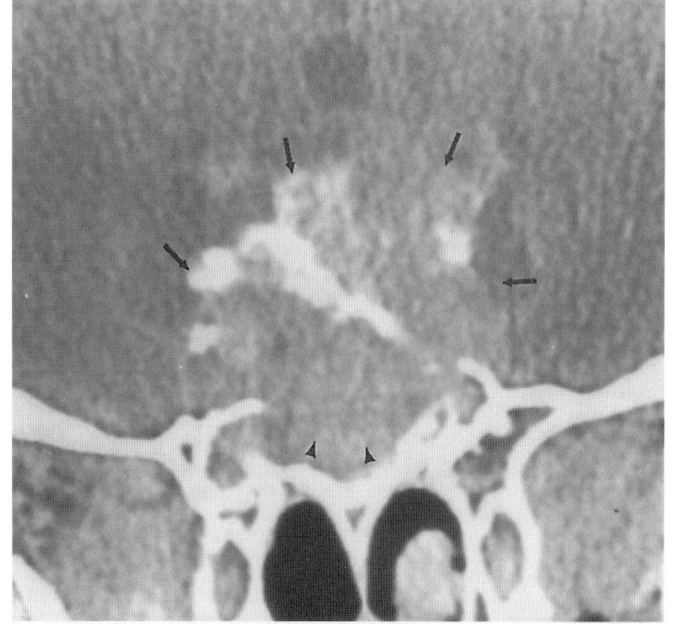

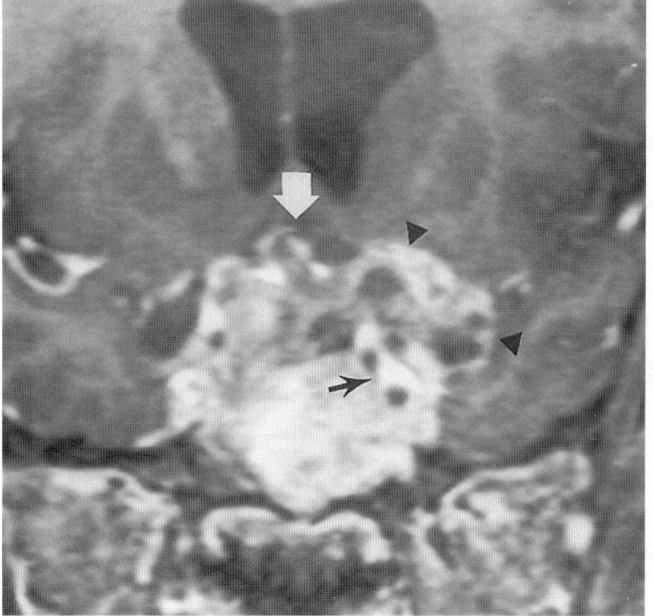

**FIGURE 20-9.** Mixed cystic and solid craniopharyngioma. This patient had a family history of multiple endocrine neoplasia syndrome type 1, with hypopituitarism. He did not have a primary pituitary tumor, but rather a craniopharyngioma. **A,** Axial contrast-enhanced CT scan through the suprasellar cistern. There is an irregular mixed-density mass filling most of the suprasellar cistern (*curved white arrows*). There are small calcifications (*thick black arrow*) within the central posterior portion of the mass. There is no hydrocephalus. **B,** Coronal CT scan through the region of the sella. The floor of the sella is completely destroyed (*small black arrowheads*), and the mass extends to fill much of the sphenoid sinus. The clinoids are not well defined, and there is a mixed-density, partially calcified mass in the suprasellar region (*small black arrows*). **C,** Coronal contrast-enhanced T1-weighted magnetic resonance image through the sella in a location similar to that of **B.** The mass demonstrates intense contrast enhancement. There is envelopment of the carotid artery on the left (*straight black arrow*). The lesion extends into the suprasellar cistern and obliterates the region of the optic chiasm and pituitary stalk (*solid white arrow*). The lesion also grows into the temporal and frontal lobes above the clinoids on the left (*black arrowheads*). The cystic spaces within the tumor are lower in signal intensity, similar to that of cerebrospinal fluid.

copathologically, two distinct subtypes are recognized: the *adamantinous*, which tend to occur in children, and the *squamous-papillary variants*, which tend to occur in adults.[20] Craniopharyngiomas may present because of a mass effect on the chiasm, headaches, hydrocephalus, or pituitary and hypothalamic dysfunction.

If the lesion is large enough, plain radiographs of the skull demonstrate remodeling of the sella turcica and clinoid processes. The amorphous or curvilinear calcifications, which are present in most pediatric tumors and half of adult tumors, are more readily detected by CT than on plain radiographs.

On CT, craniopharyngiomas can be mixed cystic and solid and often exhibit enhancement of the more solid portions (see Fig. 20-9). Hemorrhage is not an uncommon finding, particularly within cystic portions of the tumors. Most commonly, these tumors are suprasellar in location. Craniopharyngiomas may grow to displace the optic chiasm superiorly, to displace the normal pituitary gland and stalk, to extend into the cavernous sinuses, and even to encase or occlude the carotid arteries.

The imaging characteristics of craniopharyngiomas on MRI are variable, reflecting the wide range of components histologi-

cally composing these tumors. The tumors may be cystic (see Fig. 20-8), mixed cystic and solid (see Fig. 20-9), or primarily solid (see Fig. 20-10). High signal intensity on T1- and T2-weighted images is seen in cysts with high cholesterol content or with subacute hemorrhage. Craniopharyngiomas can also be of low signal intensity on T1-weighted images if the cyst contains a large amount of keratin.[21] Fluid levels can be seen in cystic regions. Adamantinous craniopharyngiomas tend to be primarily cystic or mixed cystic-solid lesions that occur in children and adults, whereas squamous-papillary subtypes tend to be predominantly solid or mixed solid-cystic and occur in adults. Distinguishing between the two has a prognostic significance, because *adamantinous tumors tend to recur.* MRI can be helpful in distinguishing between the two: Encasement of vessels, a lobulated shape, and the presence of hyperintense cysts is suggestive of adamantinous tumors; and a round shape, presence of hypointense cysts, and a predominantly solid appearance is seen with squamous-papillary tumors.[20] The overall sensitivity for detecting tumor is higher with MRI, and the potential for displaying anatomy in multiple planes pro-

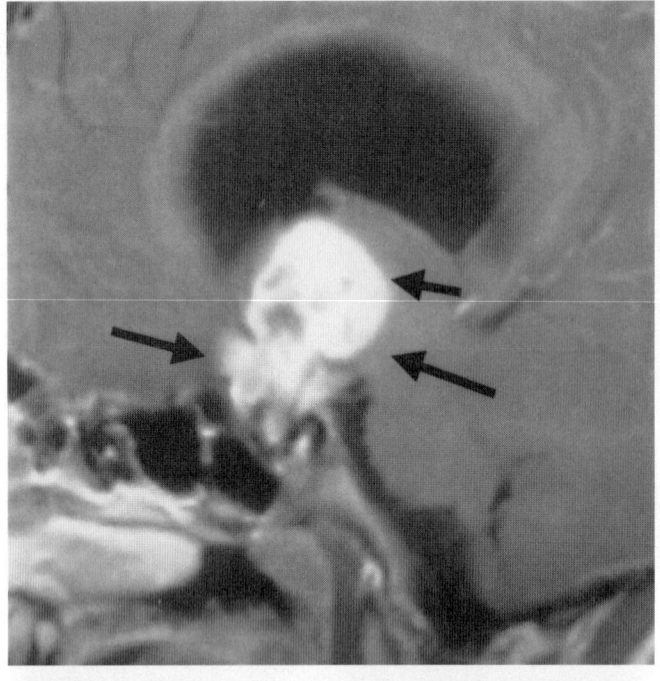

A

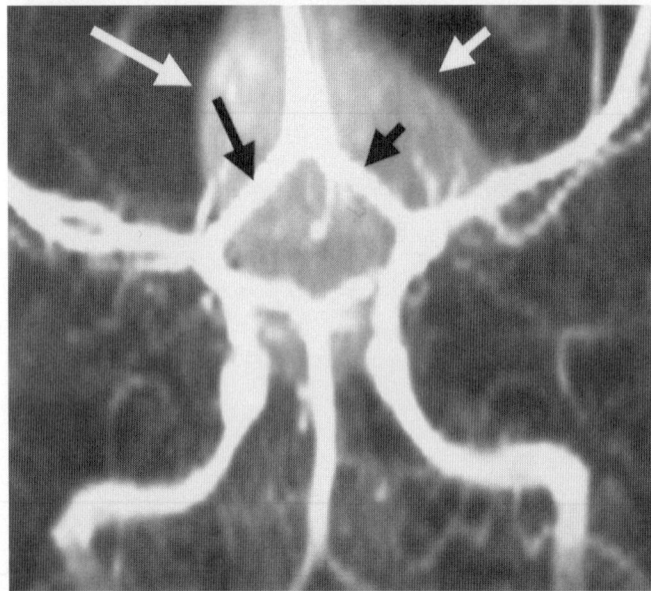

B

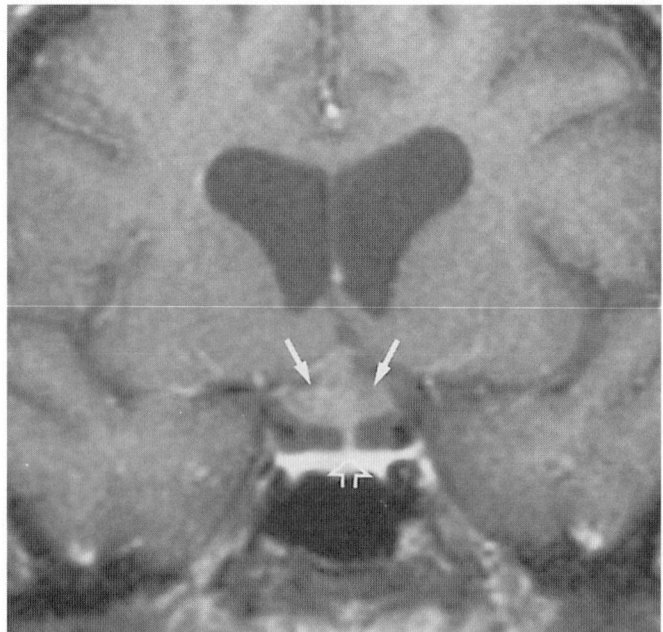

A

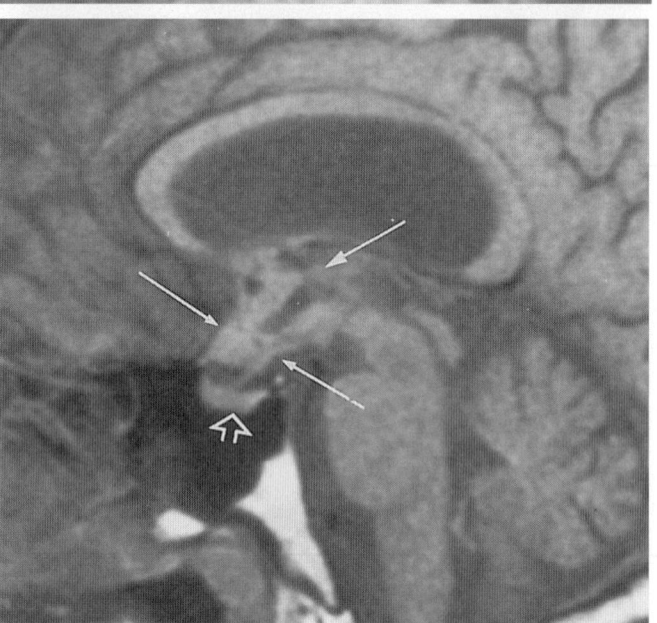

B

**FIGURE 20-10.** Solid sellar and suprasellar craniopharyngioma. **A,** Sagittal contrast-enhanced T1-weighted magnetic resonance imaging (*MRI*) scan through the midline demonstrates a large mushroom-shaped mass extending out of the deformed sella into the anterior third ventricle (*black arrows*). The mass obscures the optic chiasm and other anterior third ventricular structures. The mass is associated with hydrocephalus and expansion of the lateral ventricles and bowing of the corpus callosum. **B,** Anterior view reconstruction of a contrast-enhanced 3D gradient echo acquisition shows the large enhancing sellar and suprasellar mass (*white arrows*). The MR angiogram (*MRA*) demonstrates elevation of the anterior cerebral arteries bilaterally (*black arrows*).

**FIGURE 20-11.** Hypothalamic and optic pathway glioma. This young man presented with vision problems. He had a history of neurofibromatosis, type 1. **A,** Coronal contrast-enhanced T1-weighted magnetic resonance image. The optic chiasm and hypothalamus (*solid white arrows*) are thickened and globular in configuration. The anterior third ventricular recess is not well seen. The pituitary stalk and pituitary gland (*open white arrow*) are normal in configuration. **B,** Sagittal non–contrast-enhanced T1-weighted magnetic resonance image. An irregular mass fills the anterior third ventricle, optic chiasm, and hypothalamic area (*long thin white arrows*). A segment of the lesion may be cystic and appears as low signal regions. The pituitary gland and infundibulum are normal (*open white arrow*).

vides excellent data for surgical planning (see Fig. 20-10). Some lesions that can be confused with craniopharyngiomas include arachnoid cysts, dermoid tumors, meningiomas, and aneurysms (if calcified).

## OPTIC CHIASM AND HYPOTHALAMIC GLIOMAS

Gliomas involving the optic chiasm and hypothalamus present an imaging problem. It is often difficult or impossible to separate the origin of these tumors because of their intimate associa-

tion.[22] If there is extension of tumor along the optic tracts or optic nerves, it is much easier to determine the site of origin, because there is a characteristic growth pattern for optic pathway gliomas but not for hypothalamic gliomas. Histologically, these gliomas, which are more common in children, are slow-growing pilocytic astrocytomas. Optic gliomas are more common in patients with neurofibromatosis type 1 (Fig. 20-11). In adults, optic gliomas tend to be more aggressive and usually represent glioblastomas. Usually, plain radiographs are not helpful, except when the tumors extend along the optic nerves

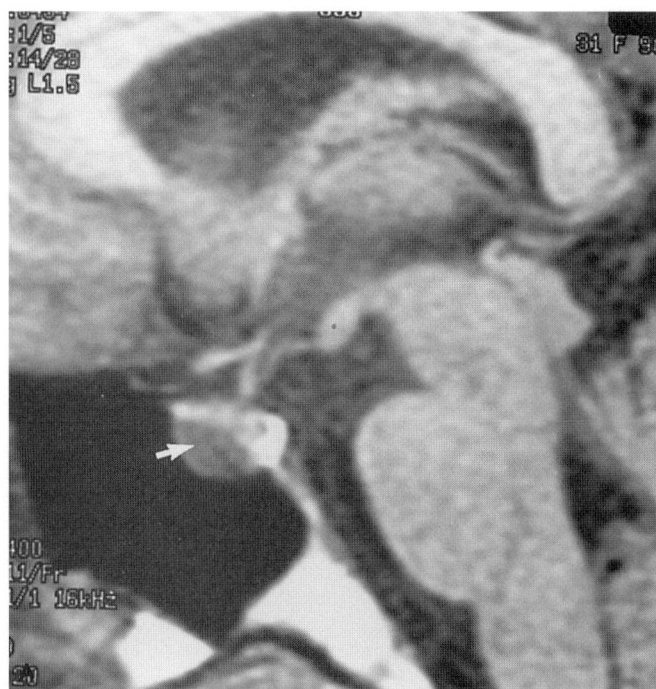

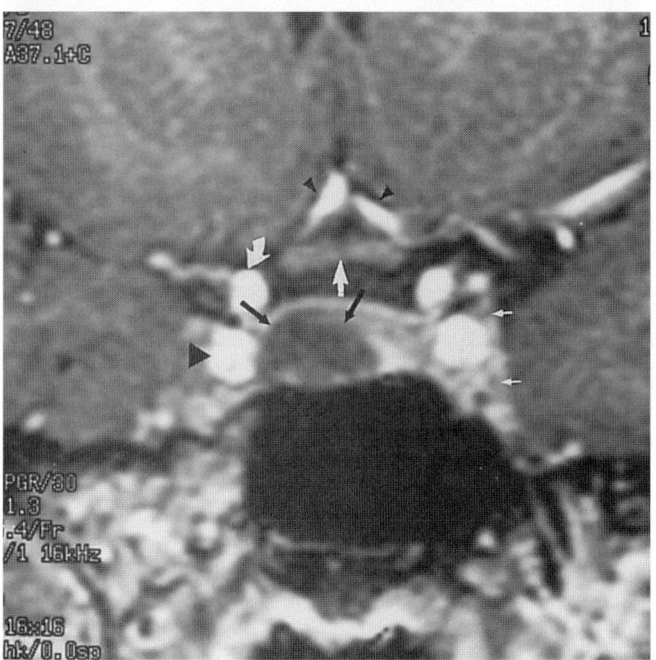

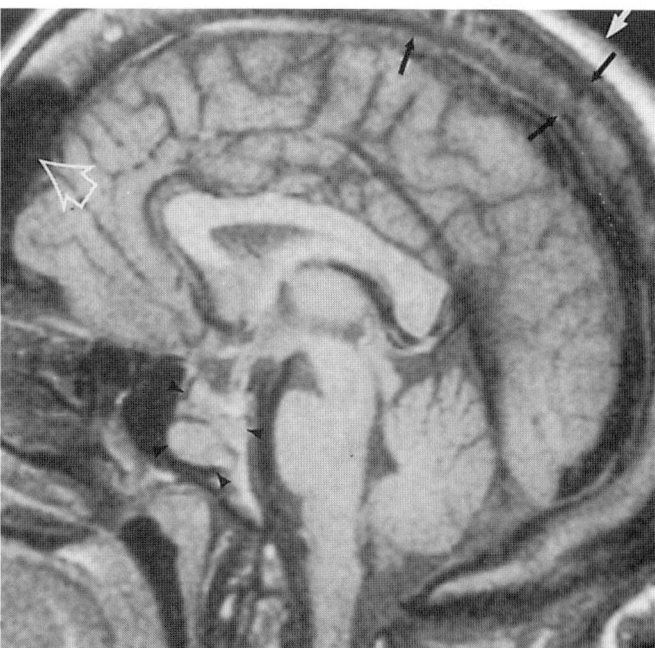

**FIGURE 20-13.** Acromegaly and macroadenoma of the pituitary. This is a sagittal non–contrast-enhanced T1-weighted image of the midline skull. The scalp is thickened (*solid white arrow*). The skull is also markedly thickened (*straight black arrows*). The frontal sinuses are expanded (*open white arrow*). The pituitary gland is enlarged (*small black arrowheads*) and fills much of the clivus and sphenoid sinus. It does not extend into the suprasellar cistern or involve the brainstem.

**FIGURE 20-12.** Pituitary microadenoma. This young woman presented with hyperprolactinemia. **A,** Sagittal T1-weighted non–contrast-enhanced magnetic resonance image. The anterior portion of the pituitary gland (*solid white arrow*) demonstrates slightly decreased signal. In general, the volume of the sella is not enlarged. The suprasellar structures are intact. **B,** Coronal contrast-enhanced T1-weighted image. The superior margin of the pituitary gland is slightly convex and asymmetrically enlarged on the right. The low signal microadenoma (measuring 8 × 5 mm) is seen on the right (*small black arrows*). The lesion crosses the midline. This section is anterior to the infundibulum and also shows the anterior cerebral arteries (*small black arrowheads*), the optic chiasm (*straight white arrow*), the supraclinoid carotid artery (*curved white arrow*), and the cavernous carotid arteries (*large black arrowhead*). A few of the cranial nerves in the cavernous sinus are also visible (*small white arrows*).

and cause expansion of the optic canals. CT and MRI demonstrate enlargement of the optic chiasm or hypothalamus, which is particularly well seen on coronal images (see Fig. 20-11*A*). These lesions usually enhance homogeneously with both CT and MRI contrast-enhanced images, and, in the case of optic nerve tumors, there may be extension of abnormal signal and enhancement along the optic tracts and radiations. The differential diagnosis includes craniopharyngiomas, sarcoid, metastases, or lymphomas.

## PITUITARY ADENOMAS

Pituitary adenomas can be classified according to function and size. Lesions smaller than 1 cm are classified as *microadenomas* (Fig. 20-12), and those larger than 1 cm are classified as *macroadenomas* (Figs. 20-13, 20-14, and 20-15). The most common functioning adenomas are prolactinomas (see Chap. 13). Other functioning adenomas include adrenocorticotropic hormone-secreting tumors, thyroid-stimulating hormone-secreting tumors, and GH-secreting tumors (see Chaps. 12, 14, and 15). Nonfunctioning adenomas account for ~40% of all pituitary adenomas. Adenocarcinomas of the pituitary gland are rare; in fact, metastasis to the gland is more common (see Chap. 11). Pituitary adenomas are usually seen in adults and are uncommon in children. When seen in childhood, they are usually seen in adolescent boys and are commonly macroadenomas, particularly prolactinomas that tend to be hemorrhagic.[23]

The imaging appearance of pituitary adenomas is nonspecific, and no inference to histology can be made from the sellar patterns. However, additional clues may be present, related to other secondary endocrine changes. For instance, with GH-secreting tumors, acromegaly occurs, and one may visualize thickening of the scalp or enlargement of the mandible on radiograph or physical examination (see Fig. 20-13); these tumors tend to be larger than 5 mm. Cushing adenomas usually are microadenomas, but compression vertebral fractures and a "buffalo hump" deformity may be clues. Prolactinomas are more variable in size; they usually are microadenomas, but may be macroadenomas. Nonfunctioning tumors tend to be large.

Enlargement of the pituitary gland may result from many etiologies, not just neoplasia. End-organ failure is a cause of gland enlargement, such as is seen with primary hypothyroid-

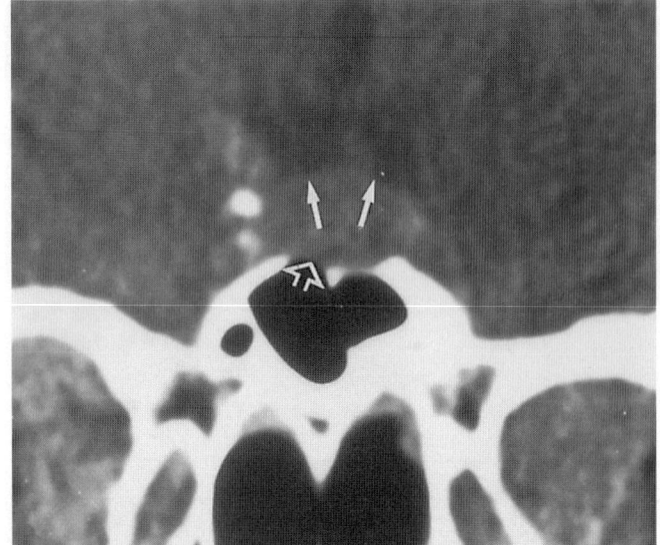

A

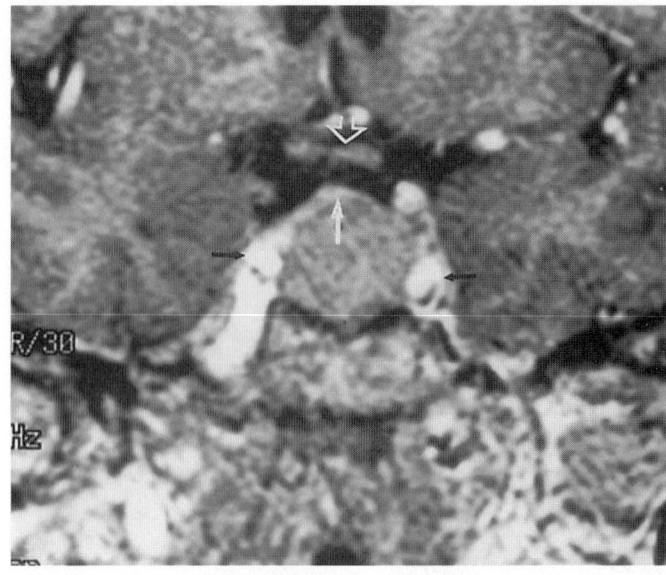

B

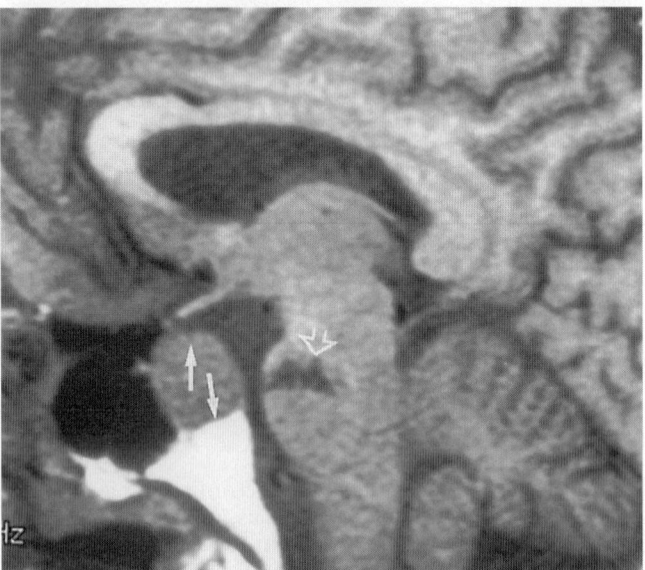

C

**FIGURE 20-14.** Pituitary macroadenoma. **A,** Coronal contrast-enhanced CT scan through the sella. The pituitary gland is slightly enlarged. The superior surface is bowed cephalad into the suprasellar cistern (*straight white arrows*). The optic chiasm and pituitary stalk are not significantly deformed. The floor of the sella may be partially eroded because there is no cortical margin (*open white arrow*). Involvement of the cavernous sinus and carotid arteries is not clearly demonstrated. **B,** Coronal magnetic resonance image at a level similar to that of Figure 20-14A. The soft-tissue contrast is much better. Again, the gland is slightly enlarged and measures >1 cm, with the superior margin (*solid white arrow*) protruding into the suprasellar cistern without coming in contact with the optic chiasm (*open white arrow*). The carotid arteries (*solid black arrows*) are displaced slightly laterally in the cavernous sinus regions. There does not appear to be clear-cut involvement of the cavernous sinus. **C,** Sagittal T1-weighted non–contrast-enhanced magnetic resonance image. Again, the small macroadenoma is seen filling the sella and remodeling the sella (*solid white arrows*). The clivus is slightly remodeled, and the posterior clinoids are not well defined. There is an incidental infarct in the pons (*open white arrow*).

ism or surgical removal of the adrenals (Nelson syndrome; see later in this chapter and Chap. 75). If the functional status of a suspected adenoma or pituitary mass is in question, venous sampling of the petrosal sinuses can be performed by means of a catheter placed from the femoral vein into the internal jugular vein and then advanced into the greater petrosal veins.[6] Analysis of blood samples can help determine the type of adenoma and the location of a lesion not detected by other imaging modalities. Sampling is also of value to demonstrate that the hormone originated from the gland rather than from an ectopic site. Although inferior petrosal sinus sampling is usually performed, it has been shown that bilateral, simultaneous *cavernous sinus* sampling, using corticotropin-releasing hormone, is as accurate as inferior petrosal sinus sampling in detecting Cushing disease and is perhaps more accurate in lateralizing the abnormality within the pituitary gland.[24]

The sella is usually normal in size with microadenomas and CT usually demonstrates no bony expansion, although there may be some asymmetry in the shape of the pituitary gland (see Fig. 20-12). CT, using thin-section coronal images and intravenous contrast, has been used successfully to detect microadenomas. The adenoma is identified as either a hypodense or hyperdense region in the gland after contrast enhancement. Cushing disease adenomas are more difficult to detect by CT,

possibly because of their relative enhancement with respect to the normal gland.[25]

The recommended modality for examining a pituitary adenoma is MRI, with coronal and sagittal imaging. Detection is best with high-resolution techniques, such as three-dimensional imaging. The coronal plane is the most sensitive imaging plane, and T1-weighted spin-echo and three-dimensional imaging sequences are the best pulse sequences. The use of gadolinium enhancement is somewhat controversial,[26,27] although the vast majority of radiologists believe that contrast is essential in the evaluation of the sella and parasellar regions. Usually, the tumors enhance less-than-normal tissue. Dynamic imaging can be of value in defining the abnormal segment of the gland.[13]

Of the pituitary macroadenomas, a higher percentage of these are nonfunctioning adenomas. Plain radiographs of the skull may demonstrate bony expansion or erosion of the sella; at times, the masses can be huge, with wide destruction of the skull base (to the extent that the site of origin is not clear). Calcifications are rare.

The sensitivity for detecting macroadenomas by CT is higher than for microadenomas; the CT examination should use thin-section coronal and axial imaging with intravenous contrast. Generally, the margins of the macroadenomas are more readily defined by MRI than by CT. Involvement of the optic chiasm, cavernous sinus, sphenoid sinus, orbit, temporal lobes, and

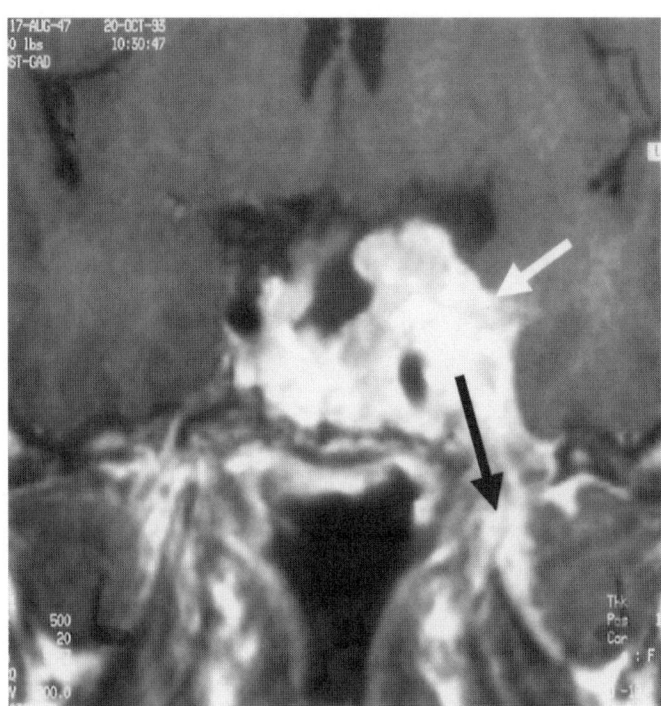

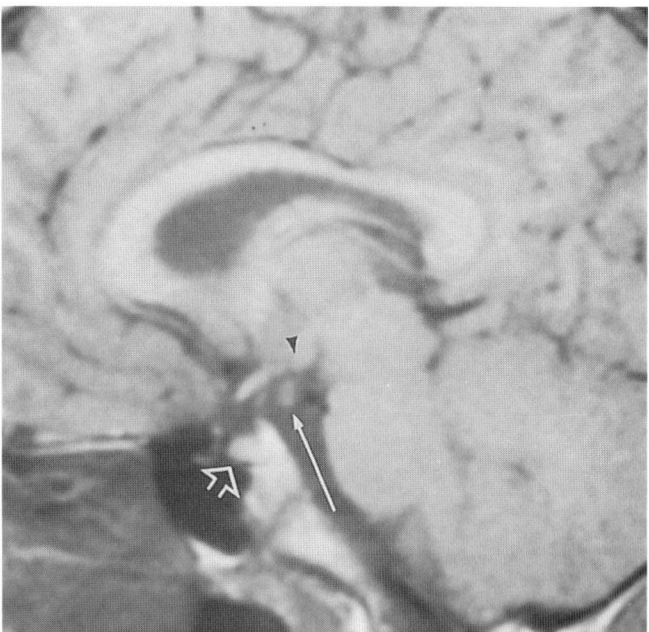

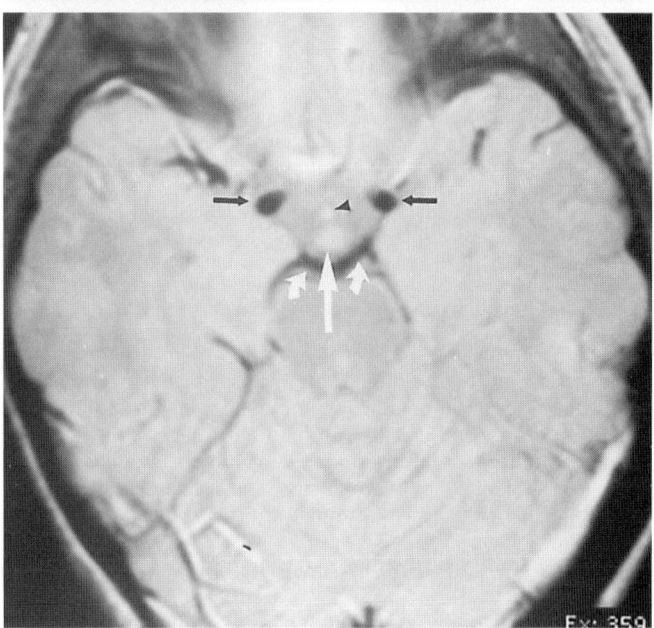

**FIGURE 20-15.** Invasive pituitary macroadenoma. This coronal contrast-enhanced 3D gradient echo magnetic resonance image through the sella demonstrates a large irregular aggressive skull-base mass (*white arrow*) with the pituitary gland enhancing diffusely. The pituitary stalk is displaced to the right. The low-signal-intensity left carotid artery (*black arrow*) is enveloped by the mass and is displaced inferiorly. The mass protrudes into the left suprasellar cistern. It is in contact with the left medial temporal lobe after breaking through the left cavernous sinus. The mass is extending through the left foramen ovale into the masticator space.

carotid arteries can all be seen using MRI. In prolactinomas, MRI is used to evaluate the patient's response to bromocriptine therapy. A decrease in tumor size can be seen as early as 1 week after the start of therapy. Additionally, MRI can detect posttherapy hemorrhage into macroadenomas and mass effect or inferior herniation of the chiasm as a result of a decrease in the tumor size.[28] In macroadenomas, subacute hemorrhage is readily detected by MRI because the breakdown products of hemoglobin have paramagnetic or diamagnetic effects, depending on their chemical composition. Moreover, MRI is good for evaluating invasion into the adjacent cavernous sinus and for documenting the patency of the carotid arteries (see Fig. 20-15).

## INFUNDIBULAR MASSES

The thickness of the normal pituitary stalk averages 3.5 mm at the median eminence and 2.8 mm near its midpoint. The normal stalk enhances markedly on CT with contrast and on MRI with gadolinium. The most common clinical problem associated with disease of the pituitary stalk is diabetes insipidus. When this is present, there usually is absence of the normal hyperintensity of the posterior pituitary. On T1-weighted MRI, diabetes insipidus may be found to occur as a result of transection of the pituitary stalk.

The differential diagnosis of a thickened stalk includes sarcoidosis, tuberculosis, histiocytosis X, and ectopic posterior pituitary as well as germinoma. A thickened stalk can also be due to an extension of a glioma within the hypothalamus.

In patients with neurosarcoidosis and tuberculous infiltration of the stalk, the chest radiograph is generally abnormal and may be helpful in the differentiation from histiocytosis X. Clinically, patients with histiocytosis X may have skin lesions, otitis media, or bone lesions in addition to interstitial lung disease.[12]

**FIGURE 20-16.** Hypothalamic hamartoma. This young girl presented with precocious puberty. **A,** Non–contrast-enhanced sagittal T1-weighted image through the midline. A small nodule measuring ~5 mm in dimension (*solid white arrow*) is seen protruding from the undersurface of the hypothalamus into the suprasellar cistern just anterior to the mammillary bodies (*small black arrowhead*). The pituitary gland and infundibulum are normal (*open white arrow*). There does not appear to be any deformity of the anterior third ventricle or invasion of the brain. **B,** Axial proton-density magnetic resonance image. The small hamartoma (*straight white arrow*) is just anterior to the bifurcation of the basilar artery in the suprasellar cistern. The infundibulum is seen directly anterior to this (*small black arrowhead*). Other labeled structures include the supraclinoid carotid arteries (*thin black arrows*) and the posterior cerebral arteries (*curved white arrows*).

## HYPOTHALAMIC HAMARTOMAS

A hamartoma of the tuber cinereum usually presents as precocious puberty in a young child.[29] It is important to differentiate this lesion from a hypothalamic glioma because the prognosis for hamartoma is much more favorable. Imaging is best with MRI thin-section coronal and sagittal planes (Fig. 20-16). The findings are usually characteristic: The mass arises from the

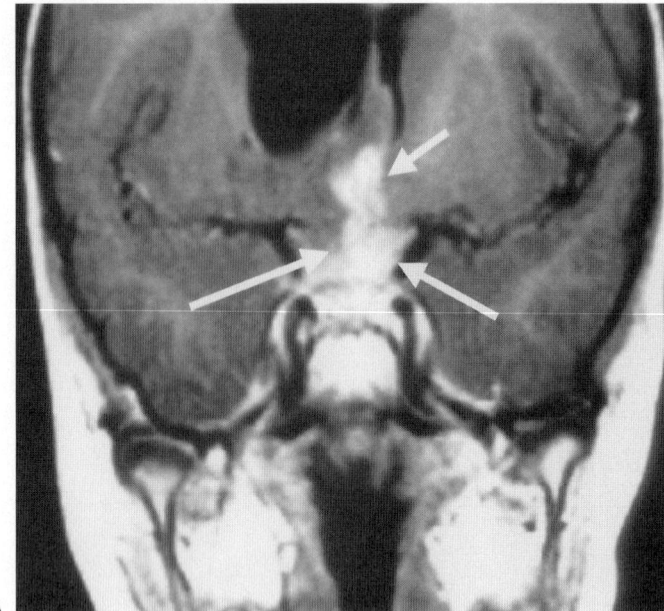

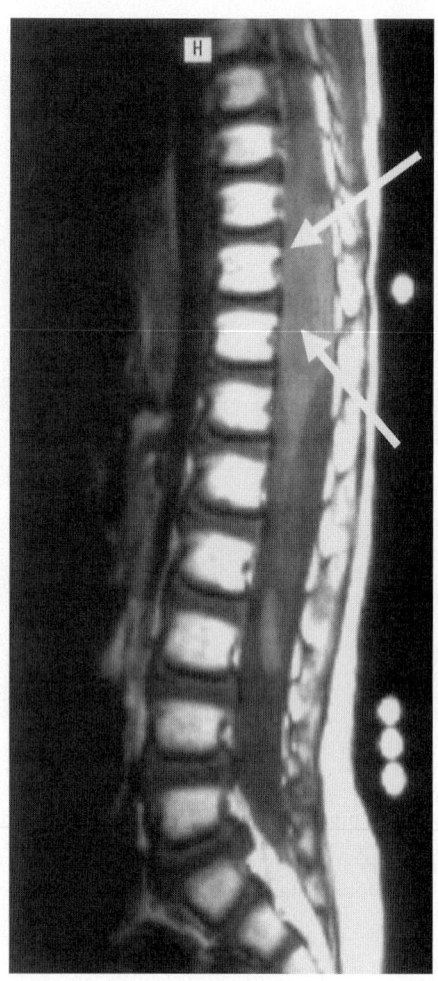

**FIGURE 20-17.** Metastatic suprasellar and pituitary ependymoma. **A,** Coronal contrast-enhanced magnetic resonance imaging scan through the sella. The pituitary gland, stalk, and hypothalamus are all infiltrated by an aggressive irregular mass (*white arrows*). This is a secondary CSF seeding metastasis from a primary ependymoma of the lower thoracic cord. This type of pattern can be seen in sarcoid, histiocytosis X, eosinophilic granuloma, lymphoma, leukemia, and carcinoma. It is not uncommon that the sellar metastasis presents before the spinal or other primary tumor site. **B,** Sagittal T1-weighted midline thoracolumbar spin-echo image. The primary conus ependymoma (*white arrows*) is seen as an isointense expansile mass of the conus. Note that there is also thickening of some of the lower lumbar roots consistent with other drop metastases.

undersurface of the hypothalamus and is exophytic. The nodular mass (<1 cm) hangs into the suprasellar cistern adjacent to the mammillary bodies. On T1-weighted images, the signal is isointense with normal brain; on T2-weighted images, there is mild hyperintensity or isointensity. These lesions usually do not enhance with contrast administration.

## SELLAR AND PARASELLAR MENINGIOMA

Meningiomas usually occur in the parasellar region rather than within the true sella. They are derived from meningeal cells and are intimately associated with the dura. They can arise from the planum sphenoidale, the diaphragma sella, the optic nerve sheaths, the clinoids, or within the cavernous sinuses. Meningiomas may demonstrate calcification on plain radiographs. On CT, they are usually hyperdense and may be mistaken for hemorrhagic lesions or aneurysms. Hyperostosis of the adjacent bones, including the clinoids, is characteristic, and there may be expansion of the sphenoid sinus by air. On MRI, meningiomas tend to be isointense with gray matter and may be difficult to see on T1-weighted images without gadolinium. With both iodinated CT contrast agents and gadolinium MRI agents, meningiomas usually demonstrate marked, homogeneous enhancement.

## SCHWANNOMAS AND NEUROFIBROMAS

Schwannomas, which are tumors derived from the myelin sheath of peripheral nerves, can be found involving the cranial nerves within the cavernous sinus and parasellar regions. In general, pituitary function is not affected; however, often the cranial nerves III, IV, V, and VI are affected within the cavernous sinuses or in the suprasellar and prepontine cisterns.

Schwannomas may remodel the foramina of the skull where the individual nerves exit. When multiple lesions are seen, neurofibromatosis should be considered.

On CT, schwannomas usually are hyperdense lesions with homogeneous enhancement, and they may be hard to differentiate from meningiomas. On MRI, they may be isointense or hyperintense to gray matter on T1-weighted images, and they enhance homogeneously.

## METASTASIS

Metastasis to the sellar, suprasellar, or parasellar regions may arise in the sphenoid bone or sinus, cavernous sinus, pituitary gland, hypothalamus, or surrounding soft tissues (Figs. 20-17 and 20-18). Endocrine symptoms are uncommon with pituitary metastasis but are often seen when the hypothalamus is involved. It may be difficult to distinguish a metastasis from a primary pituitary abnormality on the basis of imaging alone; however, the presence of bony destruction or the history of a known primary tumor may be helpful.

## GERM-CELL TUMORS

Suprasellar germ-cell tumors include seminomas (germinomas), teratomas, embryonal tumors, choriocarcinomas, and tumors of mixed histology. Some of these tumors are associated with simultaneous lesions in the pineal gland. These tumors are much more common in boys and tend to involve the pituitary stalk. When germ-cell tumors involve only the pituitary stalk, they can be difficult to differentiate from other primary processes involving the infundibulum (Fig. 20-19). If there is an associated pineal mass, it is virtually diagnostic of a germ-cell tumor.

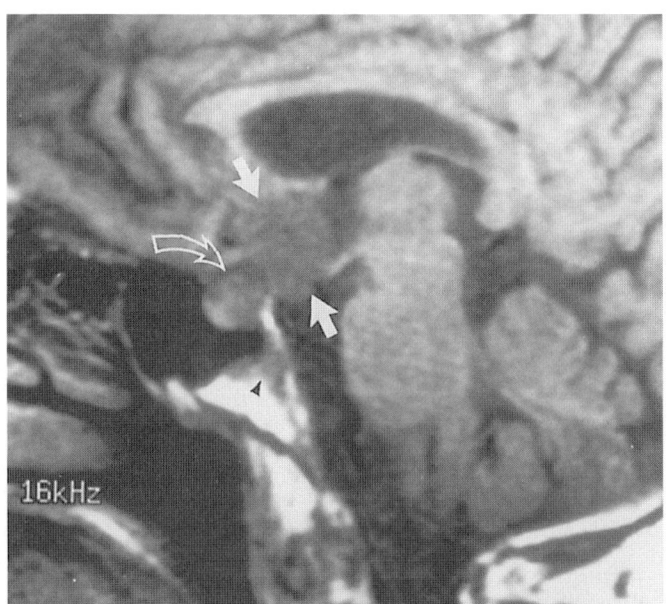

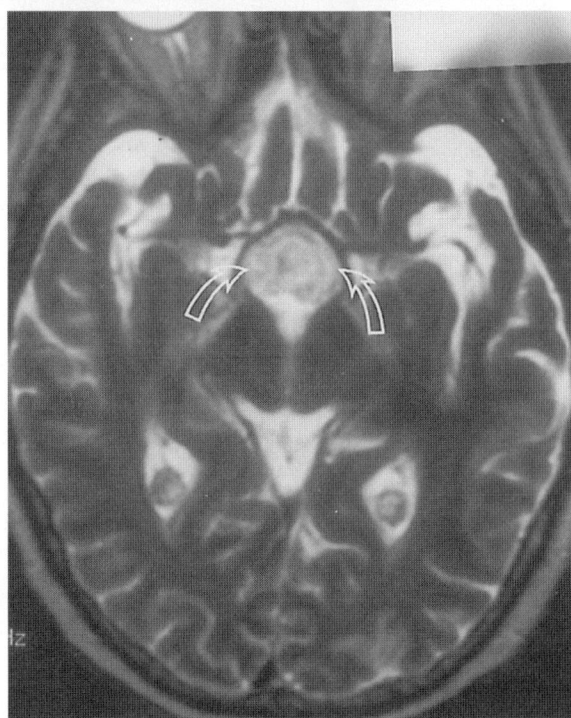

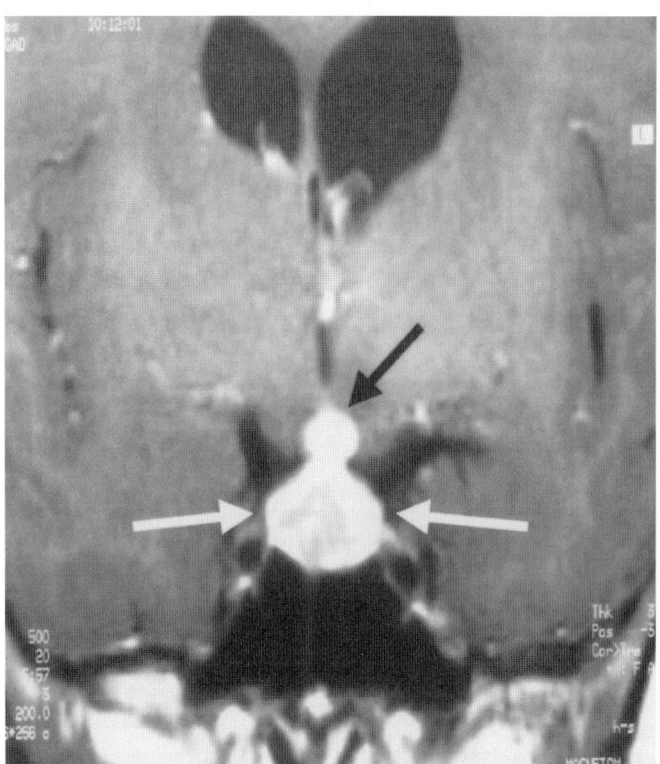

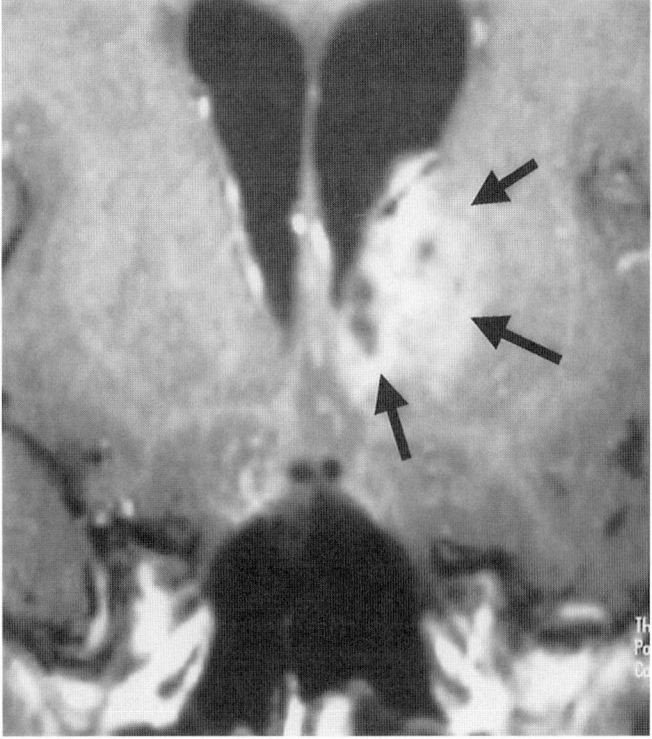

**FIGURE 20-18.** Hypothalamic and pituitary metastases. This patient presented with squamous cell carcinoma of the esophagus and diffuse metastatic bone disease. The patient became comatose. **A,** Sagittal non–contrast-enhanced T1-weighted magnetic resonance image. There is a 2-cm mass (*solid white arrows*) seen filling the anterior third ventricle and extending toward the pituitary. There is also deformity of the superior portion of the pituitary gland (*curved white arrow*). The low signal changes in the marrow of the clivus (*black arrowhead*) are secondary to metastatic disease in this area as well. **B,** T2-weighted axial image through the suprasellar region. There is an irregular mass (*open curved white arrows*) deforming the suprasellar cistern and displacing the adjacent vessels.

## MISCELLANEOUS ENTITIES

### PITUITARY APOPLEXY

Pituitary apoplexy is the result of necrosis of the anterior lobe of the pituitary. When seen in a postpartum woman, it is referred to as *Sheehan syndrome*. It is usually the result of hemorrhage into the gland, but may also be nonhemorrhagic in

**FIGURE 20-19.** Invasive pituitary germinoma. **A,** This coronal contrast-enhanced magnetic resonance imaging (*MRI*) spin-echo scan through the sella shows an expansile pituitary mass (*white arrows*) filling the sella. It protrudes into the suprasellar cistern (*black arrow*) and is displacing the adjacent brain structures cephalad. It does not appear to be invading the cavernous sinus. There is some odd contrast enhancement in the anterior third ventricle separate from the mass. **B,** Another coronal contrast-enhanced MRI spin-echo scan slightly farther anteriorly demonstrates that the germinoma is quite aggressive and is directly invading the left basal ganglion (*black arrows*).

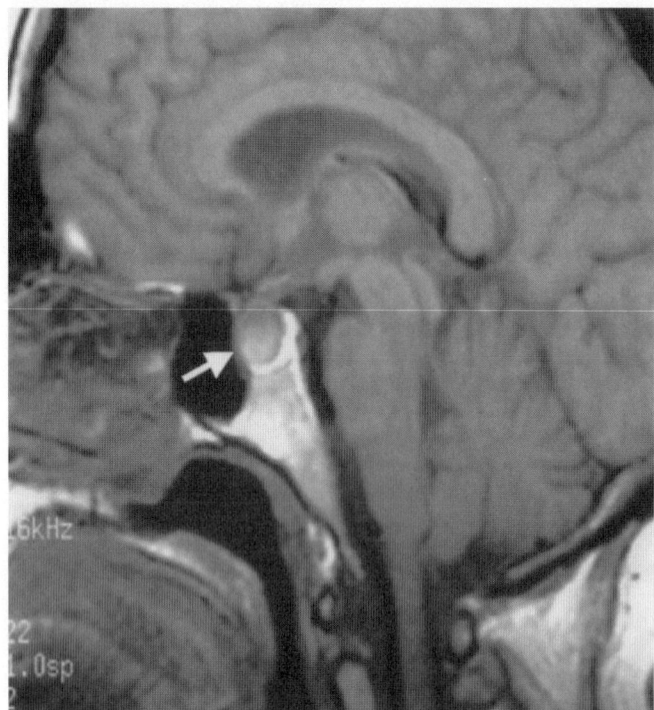

A

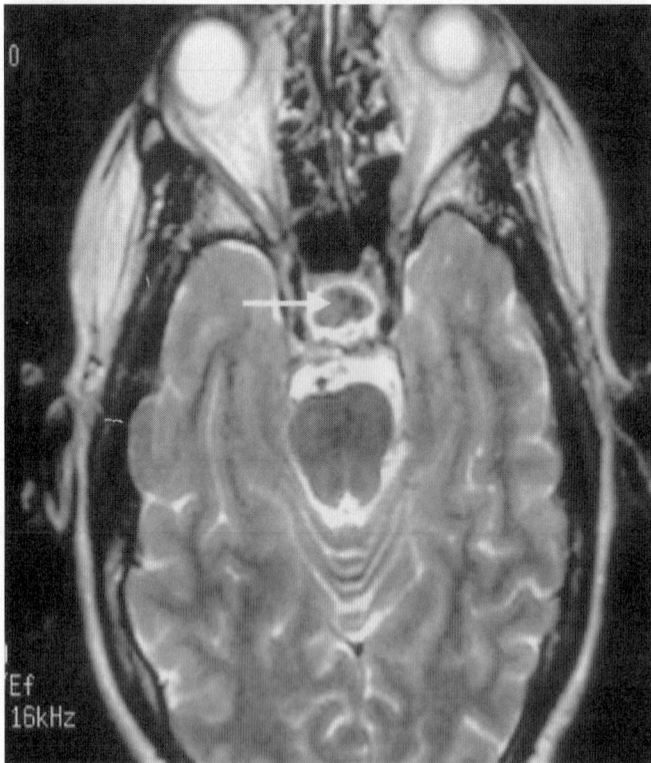

B

**FIGURE 20-20.** Hemorrhagic pituitary apoplexy. **A,** Sagittal T1-weighted spin-echo midline magnetic resonance imaging (*MRI*) demonstrates a high-signal-intensity abnormality of the sella (*white arrow*). It demonstrates bulging of the superior contour of the pituitary gland without major deformity of the optic chiasm. The high signal intensity without contrast suggests subacute hemorrhage. **B,** The pituitary apoplexy hemorrhage (*white arrow*) demonstrates low signal intensity on the T2-weighted axial image. This suggests that the hemorrhage is in the acute phase. Note the high-signal-intensity cerebro spinal fluid (*CSF*) spaces.

nature.[30] Pituitary apoplexy is usually associated with hemorrhage into a preexisting adenoma, although it can occur in a normal gland (Fig. 20-20).[30] Although CT in general is sensitive in making the diagnosis of acute hemorrhage, the changes in

the pituitary gland may be difficult to appreciate. The imaging modality of choice for evaluation of hemorrhage in the pituitary is MRI. Also, this allows for evaluation of the optic chiasm, which may be compressed.

## SPHENOID SINUS DISEASE

The sphenoid sinus can be involved with expansile (mucocele), inflammatory (Wegener granulomatosis), infectious (pyocele), or neoplastic (squamous cell carcinoma or lymphoma) processes. The inflammatory disease may cause irritation or may directly extend to involve the adjacent sella turcica. This is most severe with necrotizing infections (such as mucormycosis) in immunocompromised and diabetic patients. In this setting, it may be difficult to differentiate inflammatory from neoplastic disease, such as squamous cell or adenocarcinoma of the sphenoid sinus and chordoma of the clivus. Endocrine symptoms are rare.

## ANEURYSM

Aneurysms may involve any of the intracranial vessels and are usually found at branch points. Aneurysms of the cavernous supraclinoid carotid and anterior cerebral arteries may be located in the sella or suprasellar region (Fig. 20-21). Compressive symptoms of aneurysms depend on their location. Aneurysms that extend into the suprasellar region may compress the optic chiasm; thus, patients may present with bitemporal hemianopia. Aneurysms may also compress the pituitary or infundibulum and present with diabetes insipidus or other endocrine abnormalities. If there has been a subarachnoid hemorrhage, the patient may present with severe headache or with a neurologic deficit related to vasospasm.

On plain radiograph, curvilinear or ring-shaped calcifications may be seen in the wall of the aneurysm. Large aneurysms can remodel the skull base and erode the clinoids. On CT, these lesions tend to be of high density on unenhanced examinations, with marked enhancement after intravenous contrast. On spin-echo MRI images, aneurysms possess the characteristics of very low signal intensity or signal void and may demonstrate phase encoding or flow artifacts. MRA may be helpful in these cases, because it provides noninvasive screening for differentiating an aneurysm from some other causes of lesions of low signal intensity seen on the MRI (such as calcification). Arteriovenous malformations may also occur; they reveal characteristic large feeding arteries and several serpentine flow voids, representing the draining veins. Contrast angiography is still the gold standard for the evaluation of small aneurysms and arteriovenous malformations, but MRI can provide a good noninvasive screening examination in most cases. (See also refs. 30a and 30b.)

## SARCOIDOSIS

Neurosarcoidosis has a propensity to involve the basilar cisterns and the suprasellar region, specifically the infundibulum. This is best evaluated with MRI, which can show thickening and enhancement of the meninges in the basal cisterns and surrounding the suprasellar cisterns as well as thickening of the normal pituitary stalk. In 3% to 16% of patients with sarcoidosis, the nervous system is involved, and sarcoidosis can mimic almost any other lesion.[31,32]

## PRIMARY HYPOTHYROIDISM AND NELSON SYNDROME

Both primary hypothyroidism and Nelson syndrome[33] represent hypertrophic changes to the pituitary gland caused by end-organ failure. In the case of primary hypothyroidism, thyrotropin-releasing hormone is hypersecreted because of the lack of feed-

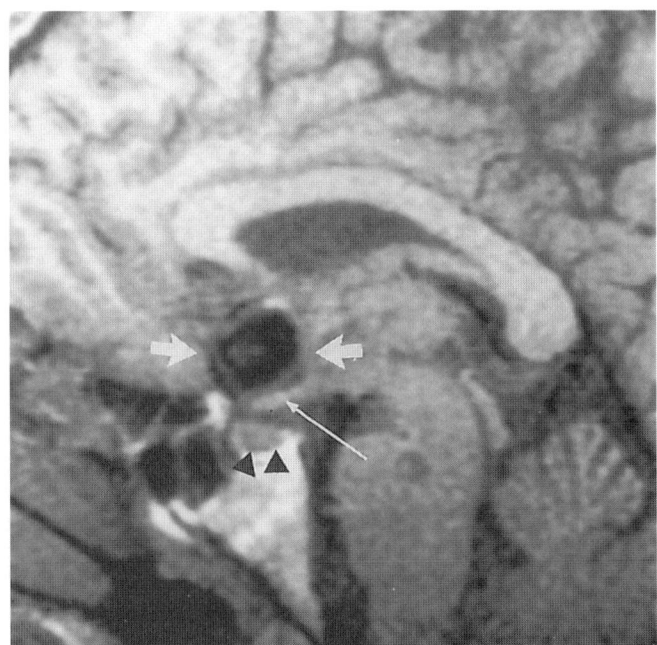

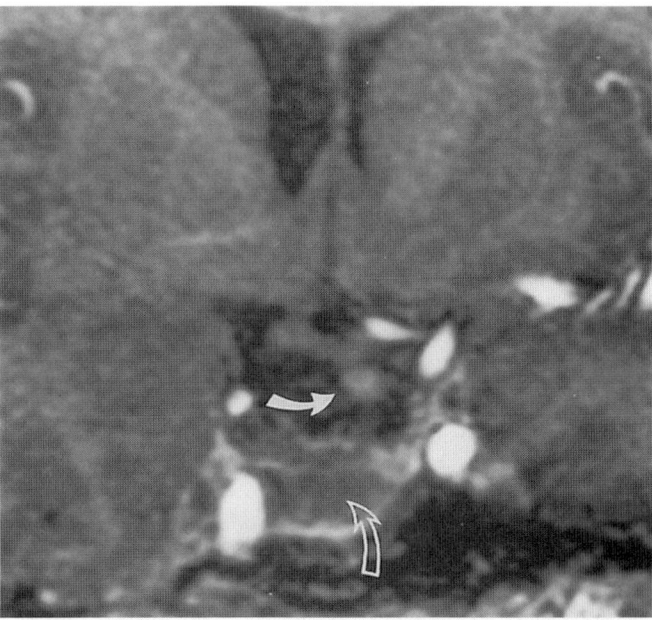

**FIGURE 20-22.** Postoperative changes. This patient had resection of a large pituitary adenoma. This coronal contrast-enhanced T1-weighted magnetic resonance image demonstrates displacement of the pituitary stalk to the left (*curved solid white arrow*). The floor of the sella is asymmetric and slopes inferiorly to the right. There is a cyst seen filling the residual sella (*open white curved arrow*). There is no mass displacing the stalk. This displacement is more likely related to postsurgical changes.

and tumorous enlargement of the pituitary gland that can appear to behave aggressively and even metastasize outside of the cranial cavity (see Chaps. 11, 14, and 75).

## POSTOPERATIVE CHANGES

Many pituitary resections are performed by means of a transsphenoidal approach. In the postoperative patient, the floor of the sella is generally found to be distorted. The sphenoid sinus may be filled with implanted gelatin foam or biologic materials, such as muscle or fat. The gland itself may have an unusual shape (including club-shaped), or it may be in a lateral position, and the infundibulum may be deviated with respect to the center of the fossa (Fig. 20-22). If a frontal approach has been used, skull defects may be noted, and there often are focal areas of increased water content in the frontal lobes, suggesting local injury to the brain.

The pituitary gland may be found to have regenerated to a normal shape and size. Large suprasellar masses can deform the optic chiasm, but the chiasm may return to its normal size and location after the mass is gone. The chiasm may have herniated into the sella after being stretched (Fig. 20-23). There may be residual or recurrent tumor, particularly if the preoperative evaluation reveals extension into or invasion of the cavernous sinus. The sella may be partially empty in the postoperative patient. Because of these dynamic postoperative changes, the recommended time for follow-up examination is ~4 to 6 months after surgery to allow for resolution of hematomas, fluid collections, and resorption of implant packing materials.[34,35]

## CONCLUSION

Imaging of the sella and pituitary fossa can be an important part of evaluating patients with endocrine or metabolic dysfunction. A review of the findings in both normal and diseased states has been presented. An emphasis has been placed on

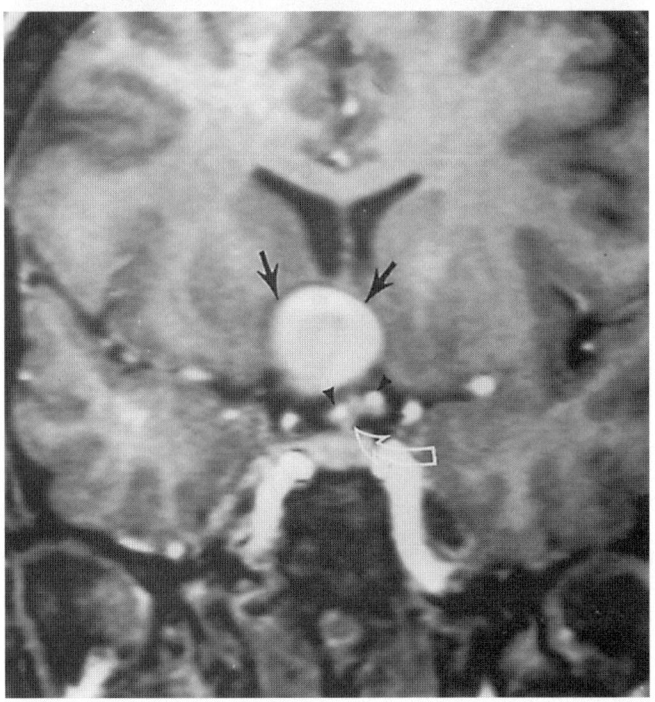

**FIGURE 20-21.** Supraclinoid internal carotid artery aneurysm. This patient presented with Cushing syndrome and no history of subarachnoid hemorrhage or headache. **A,** Sagittal non–contrast-enhanced T1-weighted image. There is a circular signal void measuring ~2 cm (*short white arrows*) in the suprasellar region. This is interposed between the optic chiasm (*long white arrows*) and the septal region of the frontal lobes. The pituitary gland (*large black arrowheads*) is essentially normal. **B,** Contrast-enhanced coronal T1-weighted magnetic resonance angiogram (*MRA*). The supraclinoid carotid aneurysm (*solid black arrows*) is seen to have a high signal rim at the periphery. This is related to the abnormal blood flow in aneurysms at the periphery rather than at the center of the lesion. The anterior cerebral arteries (*small black arrowheads*) and the pituitary stalk (*open curved white arrow*) are displaced to the left. The pituitary gland is normal.

back inhibition by thyroxine on the hypothalamus. The pituitary gland may be enlarged. In Nelson syndrome, adrenocorticotropic hormone is hypersecreted by a pituitary tumor, commonly after surgical removal of the adrenal glands for the treatment of Cushing syndrome. This causes hyperpigmentation of the skin

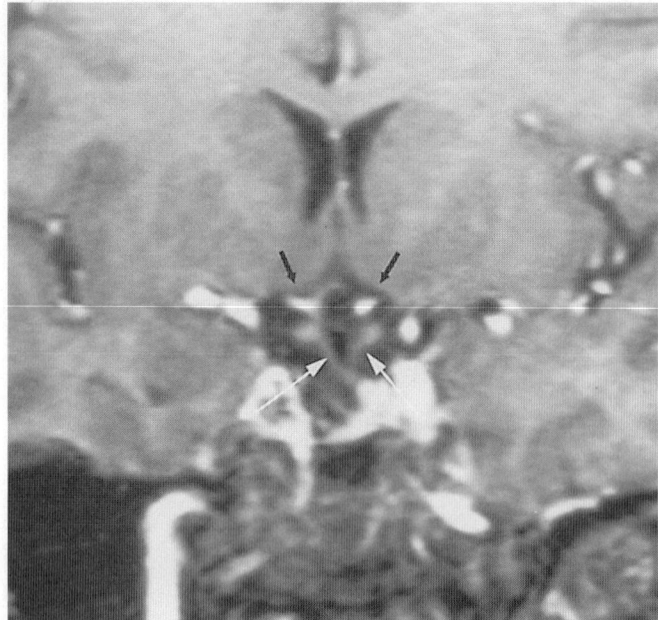

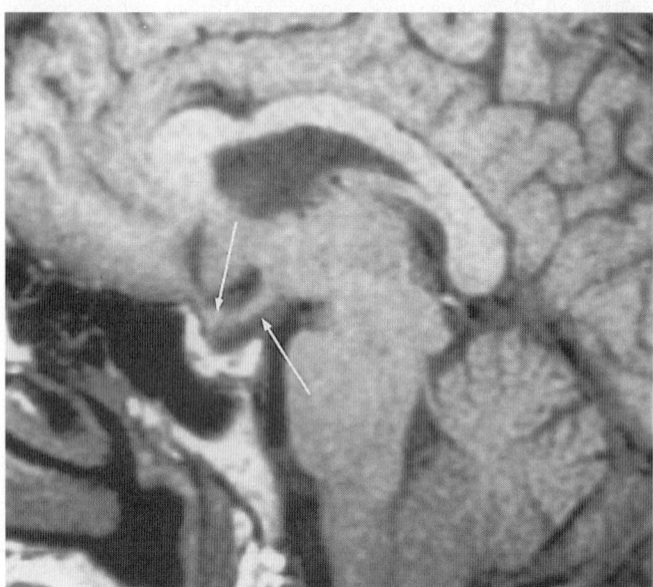

**FIGURE 20-23.** Postoperative sellar changes. **A,** Contrast-enhanced coronal T1-weighted magnetic resonance image. This patient had resection of a pituitary tumor. The anterior third ventricle and optic chiasm structures are herniated (*long white arrows*) into the region of the sellar surgical defect. The anterior cerebral arteries (*solid black arrows*) are displaced somewhat inferiorly as well. There is no residual mass. The floor of the sella is seen sloping far to the right. **B,** Sagittal non–contrast-enhanced T1-weighted magnetic resonance image. The hypothalamus and optic chiasm (*long white arrows*) are seen drooping in a J-like configuration into the surgical defect of the slightly expanded sella.

MRI, because in most cases, this has become the modality of choice for pituitary imaging.

## REFERENCES

1. Underwood LE, Radcliffe WB, Guinto FC Jr. New standards for the assessment of sella turcica volume in children. Radiology 1976; 126:651.
2. Reich NE, Zelch JV, Alfidi RJ, et al. Computed tomography in the detection of juxtasellar lesions. Radiology 1976; 118:333.
3. Elster AD. Modern imaging of the pituitary. Radiology 1993; 187:3.
4. Kishore PRS, Kaufman AB, Melichar FA. Intrasellar carotid anastomosis simulating pituitary microadenoma. Radiology 1979; 132:381.
5. Raymond J, Hardy J, Czepko R, Roy D. Arterial injuries in transsphenoidal surgery for pituitary adenoma: the role of angiography and endovascular treatment. AJNR Am J Neuroradiol 1997; 18:655.
6. Miller DL, Doppman JL, Nieman LK, et al. Petrosal sinus sampling: discordant lateralization of ACTH-secreting pituitary microadenomas before and after stimulation with corticotropin-releasing hormone. Radiology 1990; 176:429.
7. Lusted LB, Keats TE. Atlas of roentgenographic measurement, 4th ed. Chicago: Year Book Medical Publishers, 1978:59.
8. Elster AD, Chen M, Williams DW III, Key LL. Pituitary gland: MR imaging of physiologic hypertrophy in adolescence. Radiology 1990; 174:682.
9. Dietrich RB, Lis LE, Greensite FS, Pitt D. Normal appearance of the pituitary gland in the first 2 years of life. AJNR Am J Neuroradiol 1995; 16:1413.
10. Doraiswamy PM, Potts JM, Axelson DA, et al. MR assessment of pituitary gland morphology in healthy volunteers: age- and gender-related differences. AJNR Am J Neuroradiol 1992; 13:1297.
11. Mark LP, Haughton VM. The posterior sella bright spot: a perspective. AJNR Am J Neuroradiol 1990; 11:701.
12. Tien RD, Newton TH, McDermott MW, et al. Thickened pituitary stalk on MR images in patients with diabetes insipidus and Langerhans cell histiocytosis. AJNR Am J Neuroradiol 1990; 11:707.
13. Miki Y, Matsuo M, Nishizawa S, et al. Pituitary adenomas and normal pituitary tissue: enhancement patterns on Gadopentetate-enhanced MR imaging. Radiology 1990; 177:36.
14. Escott EJ, Rao VM, Ko WD, Guitierrez JE. Comparison of dynamic contrast-enhanced gradient-echo and spin-echo sequences in MR of head and neck neoplasms. AJNR Am J Neuroradiol 1997; 18:1411.
15. Chakeres DW, Curtin A, Ford G. Magnetic resonance imaging of pituitary and parasellar abnormalities. Radiol Clin North Am 1989; 27:267.
16. Kelly WM, Kucharczyk W, Kucharczyk J, et al. Posterior pituitary ectopia: an MR feature of pituitary dwarfism. AJNR Am J Neuroradiol 1988; 9:454.
17. Kurioiwa T, Okabe Y, Hasuo K, et al. MR imaging of pituitary dwarfism. AJNR Am J Neuroradiol 1991; 12:161.
18. Benshoff ER, Katz BH. Ectopia of the posterior pituitary gland as a normal variant: assessment with MR imaging. AJNR Am J Neuroradiol 1990; 11:711.
19. Young SC, Zimmerman REA, Nowell MA, et al. Giant cystic craniopharyngiomas. Neuroradiology 1987; 29:468.
20. Sartoretti-Schefer S, Wichman W, Aguzzi A, Valavanis A. MR differentiation of adamantinous and squamous-papillary craniopharyngiomas. AJNR Am J Neuroradiol 1997; 18:77.
21. Pusey E, Kortman KE, Flannigan BD, et al. MR of craniopharyngiomas: tumor delineation and characterization. AJNR Am J Neuroradiol 1987; 8:443.
22. Albert A, Lee BCP, Saint-Louis L, et al. Magnetic resonance imaging of optic chiasm and optic pathway. AJNR Am J Neuroradiol 1986; 7:255.
23. Poussaint TY, Barnes PD, Anthony DC, et al. Hemorrhagic pituitary adenomas in adolescence. AJNR Am J Neuroradiol 1996; 17:1907.
24. Oliverio PJ, Monsein LH, Wand GS, Debrun GM. Bilateral simultaneous cavernous sinus sampling using corticotropin-releasing hormone in the evaluation of Cushing disease. AJNR Am J Neuroradiol 1996; 17:1669.
25. Peck WW, Dillon WP, Norman D, et al. High-resolution MR imaging of pituitary microadenomas at 1.5 T: experience with Cushing disease. AJR Am J Roentgenol 1989; 9:149.
26. Stadnik T, Stevenaert A, Beckers A, et al. Pituitary microadenomas: diagnosis with two- and three-dimensional MR imaging at 1.5 T before and after injection of gadolinium. Radiology 1990; 176:422.
27. Chong BW, Kucharczk W, Singer W, et al. Pituitary gland MRI: a comparative study of healthy volunteers and patients with microadenomas. AJNR Am J Neuroradiol 1994; 15:675.
28. Lundin P, Bergstrom K, Nyman R, et al. Macroprolactinomas: serial MR imaging in long-term bromocriptine therapy. AJNR Am J Neuroradiol 1992; 13:1287.
29. Hahn FJ, Leinbrock LG, Huseman CA, Makos MM. The MR appearance of hypothalamic hamartoma. Neuroradiology 1988; 30:67.
30. Lavallee G, Marcos R, Palardy J. MR of nonhemorrhagic postpartum pituitary apoplexy. AJNR Am J Neuroradiol 1995; 16:1939.
30a. Jager HR, Grieve JP. Advances in non-invasive imaging of intracranial vascular disease. Ann R Coll Surg Engl 2000; 82:1.
30b. Wardlaw JM, White PM. The detection and management of unruptured intracranial aneurysms. Brain 2000; 123:265.
31. Hayes WS, Sherman JL, Stern BJ, et al. Magnetic resonance and CT evaluation of intracranial sarcoidosis. AJR Am J Roentgenol 1987; 8:1043.
32. Lexa FJ, Grossman RI. MR of sarcoidosis in the head and spine: spectrum of manifestations and radiographic response to steroid therapy. AJNR Am J Neuroradiol 1994; 15:973.
33. Nagesser SK, van Seters AP, Kievit J, et al. Long-term results of total adrenalectomy for Cushing's disease. World J Surg 2000; 24:108.
34. Steiner E, Knosp E, Herold CJ, et al. Pituitary adenomas: findings of postoperative MR imaging. Radiology 1992; 185:522.
35. Kaufman B, Tomsak RL, Kaufman BA, et al. Herniation of the suprasellar visual system and third ventricle into empty sellae: morphologic and clinical considerations. AJNR Am J Neuroradiol 1989; 10:65.

# CHAPTER 21

# MEDICAL TREATMENT OF PITUITARY TUMORS AND HYPERSECRETORY STATES

DAVID H. SARNE

## PROLACTIN HYPERSECRETION

### MICROPROLACTINOMAS

In women with microprolactinomas (tumor diameter of <10 mm) who require therapy for menstrual irregularities, infertility, or galactorrhea, bromocriptine is the treatment of choice.[1–3] A dose of 2.5 to 10 mg per day relieves the symptoms and normalizes serum prolactin in nearly 90% of patients. Approximately 10% of these patients fail to respond to bromocriptine regardless of the dosage, but many treatment failures are related to an inability to tolerate a sufficient dosage. With treatment, prolactin levels may normalize within a few days to several months. A reduction in microadenoma size has been reported in up to 75% of treated patients.

When bromocriptine is discontinued after 1 to 2 years, 20% of patients maintain normal prolactin levels.[4] In most patients, hyperprolactinemia recurs, although 25% have prolactin levels less than half the pretreatment value. No test predicts which patients will have sustained normalization. Prolactin levels usually reach a stable plateau within 2 months, but serum prolactin can reach the pretreatment level in <2 weeks. Some authors recommend that bromocriptine therapy be discontinued in patients with prolactin-secreting microadenomas after 1 to 2 years, with reinstitution of therapy only in those patients who again develop elevated levels.

The surgical treatment of microadenomas yields a high initial cure rate (85%), but the procedure is associated with complications. Moreover, with longer follow-up periods, half of these "cured" patients have a recurrence of hyperprolactinemia[5] (see Chaps. 13 and 23). Surgical treatment should be reserved for patients whose microadenomas fail to respond to bromocriptine or other dopaminergic agents or for those who are unable to tolerate the side effects of the drug regimen. Because studies of untreated patients have revealed that many microadenomas remain small for years, withholding treatment in patients with asymptomatic hyperprolactinemia may be reasonable.[6,7] Nevertheless, although patients may not be disturbed by amenorrhea or galactorrhea, prolonged hypogonadism increases the loss of skeletal mass, so bromocriptine therapy is recommended for these patients, although for women not interested in fertility, estrogen therapy is also an option.[3,8]

### MACROPROLACTINOMAS

The treatment of macroprolactinomas (tumor diameter of ≥10 mm) remains controversial. If the goal is to achieve lasting normalization of prolactin after discontinuing therapy, then surgery or radiation therapy is most effective; however, bromocriptine controls prolactin levels in more patients than does either surgery or radiation.[9]

A treatment regimen of 5 to 15 mg per day of bromocriptine causes serum prolactin levels to fall to <10% of the pretreatment value in 90% of patients and normalizes prolactin levels in ~66% of patients.[10] This decline in serum prolactin is usually accompanied by cessation of galactorrhea, return of normal menses in women, and improvement of libido in men. (The res-

olution of impotence in men occurs less frequently.) The maximal reduction of prolactin usually is seen after 2 to 3 months of therapy; however, some patients require up to 9 months of therapy for maximal suppression of prolactin. The gonadotropin abnormalities frequently found in these patients commonly improve with bromocriptine therapy.[11] Abnormal secretion of growth hormone, adrenocorticotropic hormone (ACTH), or thyroid-stimulating hormone (TSH) occurs less frequently than gonadotropin abnormalities but is less likely to resolve.

A reduction in tumor size is seen in 90% of treated patients; most exhibit a size reduction equal to or exceeding 50%.[10,12] The extent of the reduction cannot be predicted by either basal or treatment prolactin levels. Prolactin levels usually decline before a reduction in tumor size is noted. In some patients, despite an almost total disappearance of the lesion, serum prolactin levels remain mildly elevated. A significant reduction in tumor size may occur within 6 weeks, but such a reduction may not be evident for at least 6 months, and the process may continue for up to 1 year. In the absence of progressive tumor growth, bromocriptine should be administered for at least 6 months to 1 year before one concludes that it is ineffective. Usually, prolactin levels remain elevated if treatment with bromocriptine does not reduce the tumor's size. Rarely, the adenoma increases in size despite the suppression of serum prolactin levels.[13] When therapy is discontinued, hyperprolactinemia and an increase in tumor size usually follow.[14] Reexpansion of the adenoma can be rapid and dramatic. Therefore, treatment withdrawal should be undertaken cautiously and cannot be recommended routinely. If discontinuation of therapy is not accompanied by an increase in serum prolactin levels or by tumor regrowth, necrosis of the adenoma has probably occurred.

The role of bromocriptine in preparing patients for primary surgical treatment remains controversial.[15] Bromocriptine therapy should not be discontinued before surgery because rapid tumor reexpansion may result. In patients who are to undergo irradiation, treatment with bromocriptine for 1 to 2 years until the therapy is fully effective is associated with a more rapid improvement in hyperprolactinemia, amelioration of symptoms, and reduction in tumor growth. Bromocriptine is the treatment of choice in patients in whom both surgery and radiation therapy have failed.

### IDIOPATHIC HYPERPROLACTINEMIA

When treatment of idiopathic hyperprolactinemia is indicated, bromocriptine is the preferred mode of therapy.[16] A treatment regimen of 2.5 to 7.5 mg per day of bromocriptine restores normal prolactin levels, corrects gonadotropin dysfunction, and relieves symptoms in >90% of patients. Surgery and radiation therapy are not indicated for this condition.

### PROLACTIN HYPERSECRETION ASSOCIATED WITH OTHER LESIONS

Non–prolactin-secreting adenomas and other central nervous system lesions may increase prolactin levels by interfering with normal hypothalamic inhibition. Bromocriptine, 2.5 to 7.5 mg per day, usually normalizes serum prolactin levels in these patients. The normalization of prolactin is usually associated with the resolution of galactorrhea. Amenorrhea and infertility may also resolve with this mode of therapy; however, when the underlying lesion has disrupted the normal hypothalamic pituitary axis or has destroyed the gonadotropes, use of bromocriptine does not restore menses or fertility.

### DETAILS OF BROMOCRIPTINE THERAPY

Bromocriptine (2-Br-α-ergocryptine mesylate) is a semisynthetic ergot alkaloid. It specifically binds to and stimulates dopamine receptors.

One-third of an oral dose is absorbed, and peak serum levels are reached 1 to 3 hours after oral administration. It is extensively metabolized by the liver, with the metabolites being excreted almost entirely by biliary secretion.[17] Less than 5% of the drug is excreted in the urine. Maximal suppression of prolactin occurs 6 to 8 hours after a single dose, and suppression may be maintained for 12 to 14 hours.

Treatment with bromocriptine should be initiated with a dose of one-half of a 2.5-mg tablet taken with food just before bedtime, followed by a regimen of 1.25 mg given with food every 8 to 12 hours. Less than 1% of treated patients experience a first-dose phenomenon, characterized by marked faintness or dizziness. This is observed most commonly in elderly patients and in those with a previous history of fainting, peripheral vascular disease, or use of vasodilators. Increases in dosage should be gradual, no more than 2.5 to 5 mg within a period of a few days to 1 week. The total daily dose is usually divided and administered every 8 to 12 hours.

Side effects are usually dose related, with a rapid development of tolerance. Many side effects are potentiated by alcohol, the use of which should be avoided in sensitive patients. To tolerate bromocriptine therapy, some patients may need to begin with a dosage of 0.625 mg per day (one-fourth tablet), thereafter increasing the dosage at 1-week intervals.

Nausea is the most common side effect and occurs in up to 25% of treated patients. The nausea is usually mild, may be minimized by administration of the drug with food and by the initial use of low doses, and generally improves with time.[18] Constipation is also frequently reported, and some patients experience abdominal cramps. Seven patients receiving high doses of bromocriptine for the treatment of acromegaly were reported to have had major gastrointestinal hemorrhage associated with peptic ulcer disease (three of these episodes were fatal).[18] However, bromocriptine has not been associated with an increased incidence of peptic ulcer disease.

A slight decline in blood pressure is commonly observed in treated patients; however, patients usually remain asymptomatic. Mild orthostatic hypotension has also been noted.[18] The decrease in blood pressure is probably related to both a relaxation of vascular smooth muscle and central inhibition of sympathetic tone. As with the gastrointestinal side effects, symptomatic hypotension usually improves with time.

Vascular side effects, including digital vasospasm, livedo reticularis, and erythromelalgia, occur infrequently and are usually associated with bromocriptine doses that exceed those used in the treatment of hyperprolactinemia. Significant mental changes, including hallucinations, have been noted, most commonly in elderly patients receiving large doses of bromocriptine. In two patients, a dose of 5 to 7.5 mg of bromocriptine, administered for treatment of hyperprolactinemia, was reported to have caused psychotic delusions. However, one of these patients had a known history of schizophrenia in remission, and the other was under severe emotional stress. Other side effects of bromocriptine include nasal stuffiness, headache, and fatigue.

Women taking bromocriptine should be advised to use mechanical contraception and, if pregnancy is desired or suspected, to discontinue bromocriptine whenever expected menses are >2 days late. Visual fields should be evaluated regularly during pregnancy. If evidence of tumor enlargement is found, a choice is made between continued observation, treatment with bromocriptine, or transsphenoidal surgery, depending on the status of the individual patient. In the United States, women are usually advised to discontinue bromocriptine therapy during pregnancy; in Europe, however, treatment is commonly continued. A review of 1410 pregnancies in 1335 women who received bromocriptine while pregnant revealed that the incidence of spontaneous abortions (11.1%) and congenital anomalies (3.5%) was no higher than that seen in the general population.[19] In women not taking other fertility agents, a slightly increased incidence of twin pregnancies (1.8%) was seen. A retrospective study of 64 children born to 53 mothers who took bromocriptine while pregnant revealed no evidence of adverse effects on motor or psychological development.[20]

## THERAPY WITH OTHER DOPAMINERGIC AGONISTS

Several other dopamine agonists have been developed that may be useful in the treatment of hyperprolactinemia. A parenteral formulation of long-acting bromocriptine has been effective, with intramuscular injections given every 4 weeks. Pergolide is an ergoline derivative that can be given once daily in a dose of 50 to 100 µg.[21] Although it is similar to bromocriptine in its effectiveness and side effects, some patients who do not tolerate bromocriptine may tolerate pergolide.[22] The nonergot dopamine agonist quinagolide (CV 205-502) can be administered in dosages of 0.1 to 0.5 mg per day, with fewer side effects than bromocriptine or pergolide. Quinagolide was effective in patients who were unable to tolerate bromocriptine and in some patients who failed to respond adequately to bromocriptine.[23]

Cabergoline is a long-acting ergoline derivative that can be effective when given weekly or biweekly in doses of 0.5 to 2.0 mg. Its efficacy and side effects profile are similar to or better than those of bromocriptine.[24] In several studies, tumor shrinkage and normalization of prolactin levels have occurred in patients who could not tolerate bromocriptine or failed to respond adequately.[25–27]

# ADRENOCORTICOTROPIC HORMONE HYPERSECRETION

When Cushing syndrome is caused by a pituitary tumor (Cushing disease), transsphenoidal surgery is the treatment of choice.[3,28] Radiation therapy, by comparison, is less often successful and may take 1 to 2 years to be effective[3] (see Chap. 22). Drug treatment is generally not used as a primary mode of therapy except in patients who refuse surgery or irradiation. However, drug treatment may be appropriate in severely ill patients with marked hypokalemia, psychiatric disturbances, infection, or poor wound healing or in patients awaiting transsphenoidal surgery. Medical therapy is also useful in reducing cortisol levels and ameliorating symptoms until pituitary irradiation is fully effective. Finally, drug therapy may be useful in patients in whom surgery and radiation therapy have failed.

Patients with Cushing disease who are treated by adrenalectomy may develop large, ACTH-secreting, pituitary macroadenomas (Nelson syndrome). The response of such lesions to both surgery and irradiation has been disappointing.

Agents used in the treatment of ACTH hypersecretion can be divided into two classes—those that act centrally to reduce ACTH release and those that act peripherally to reduce cortisol production or block its effect (Table 21-1; see Chap. 75). Centrally acting agents are preferred if a drug is to be used for primary therapy; moreover, they are the only agents appropriate for the treatment of Nelson syndrome. Peripherally acting drugs are the preferred agents for rapid preoperative treatment of severely ill patients awaiting surgery. When the treatment regimen involves the chronic use of peripherally acting drugs, the resultant reduction in cortisol and in negative feedback may be followed by an increase in ACTH hypersecretion, thereby necessitating increased dosages of the drug.

## CENTRALLY ACTING DRUGS

### BROMOCRIPTINE

Unlike the excellent results achieved with bromocriptine therapy in patients with hyperprolactinemia, long-term administration of the drug, even at dosages of 20 to 30 mg per day, effectively reduces ACTH hypersecretion in only a few

**TABLE 21-1.**
**Treatment of Adrenocorticotropic Hormone Hypersecretion**

| | Metabolism | Excretion | Initial Dose | Maximum Dose | Major Side Effects |
|---|---|---|---|---|---|
| **CENTRALLY ACTING AGENTS** | | | | | |
| Bromocriptine (2.5-mg tablets, 5-mg capsules) | Liver | Liver | 1.25 mg bid | 60 mg/d | Nausea, hypotension |
| Cyproheptadine (4-mg tablets) | Liver | Kidney | 4 mg bid or tid | 32 mg/d | Drowsiness, hyperphagia, weight gain |
| Valproic acid (250-mg capsules) | Liver | Kidney | 250 mg tid | 1250 mg/d | Nausea and vomiting, hepatic failure, birth defects |
| **PERIPHERALLY ACTING AGENTS** | | | | | |
| Metyrapone (250-mg capsules) | Liver | Kidney | 250 mg tid | 4 g/d | Gastrointestinal irritation, hirsutism, acne |
| Mitotane (o,p'-DDD) (500-mg tablets) | Liver* | Liver and kidney | 500 mg tid | 6 g/d | Nausea and vomiting, diarrhea, ataxia, vertigo, somnolence, depression, pruritus, adrenal necrosis |
| Aminoglutethimide (250-mg tablets) | Liver† | Kidney | 250 mg qid | 2 g/d | Drowsiness, skin rash, nausea and vomiting, vertigo, depression, hypothyroidism, birth defects |
| Trilostane (30-mg and 60-mg capsules) | Liver | Kidney | 30 mg qid | 480 mg/d | Abdominal pain, nausea and vomiting, diarrhea, spontaneous abortion |
| Ketoconazole (200-mg tablets) | Liver | Liver (kidney) | 400 mg bid | 1200 mg/d | Nausea and vomiting, hepatotoxicity |

*bid*, twice a day; *tid*, three times a day; *qid*, four times a day.
*Large amounts of active drug are stored in fat.
†Most of the drug is not metabolized; primarily renal excretion.

patients.[29] Although a single 2.5-mg dose of bromocriptine reduces ACTH levels in ~40% of patients, many of these short-term responders fail to improve significantly with long-term treatment. Conversely, some patients who fail to respond to a single dose of bromocriptine demonstrate marked improvement in symptoms and in ACTH hypersecretion with prolonged therapy.[30] Neither the pretreatment ACTH and cortisol levels nor the tumor size can be used to predict accurately the response to therapy.

### CYPROHEPTADINE

The antiserotoninergic effect of cyproheptadine hydrochloride is thought to be the mechanism whereby ACTH secretion is reduced; however, this drug also has anticholinergic, antihistaminic, and antidopaminergic effects. Thirty percent to 50% of patients with Cushing disease achieve an initial clinical remission with this agent.[31] Usually, when the drug is discontinued, elevated cortisol levels and symptomatic disease promptly return. No clinical features can predict which patients will respond to cyproheptadine. Importantly, many authors report poor efficacy and significant side effects with this drug. Occasionally, patients with Nelson syndrome have been reported to improve with administration of cyproheptadine.

### VALPROIC ACID

The anticonvulsant agent valproic acid (and its derivatives) is a γ-aminobutyric acid transaminase inhibitor that decreases ACTH hypersecretion in some patients with Cushing disease or Nelson syndrome. Reduction of tumor size with valproate sodium has been reported in a single instance.[32]

The drug is highly protein bound and has a serum half-life of 6 to 16 hours. Capsules should be swallowed whole and not chewed to avoid local irritation to the mouth and pharynx. Nausea and vomiting are commonly experienced at the time therapy is initiated. Tolerance to these side effects develops rapidly, and symptoms may be reduced by administering the drug with meals. Fatal hepatic failure has occurred in several patients receiving this drug as an anticonvulsant agent. Liver function tests should be performed before the initiation of therapy and at regular intervals during the first year. The drug should not be used in patients with a history of liver disease and should be discontinued if evidence of hepatic dysfunction is found. However, hepatic dysfunction has been known to progress even after discontinuation of the drug. An increased incidence of neural tube defects has been reported in children whose mothers received this agent during the first trimester of pregnancy.

## PERIPHERALLY ACTING DRUGS

### METYRAPONE

Metyrapone reduces the production of cortisol by inhibiting 11-β-hydroxylation in the adrenal gland. The dosage is titrated to maintain normal serum cortisol levels (which should be evaluated at multiple intervals throughout the day) or titrated to keep the 24-hour urine free cortisol level within the physiologic range. The maintenance dosage varies from 250 mg three times a day to 1000 mg four times a day.[30,33] The metabolism of metyrapone is accelerated by administration of phenytoin (Dilantin).

The most common side effect is gastrointestinal irritation, which can be avoided by administering the drug with food. Despite improvement in serum cortisol levels, some women note worsening of hirsutism and acne during therapy.[33] Cost and side effects may be reduced and efficacy enhanced by combining metyrapone with aminoglutethimide, with 1 g per day of each administered in divided doses. Although the manufacture of metyrapone tablets has been discontinued, capsules remain available from the manufacturer.

### MITOTANE

Mitotane (1,1-dichloro-2-[o-chlorophenyl]-2-[p-chlorophenyl]-ethane or o,p'-DDD) suppresses the function of the zona fasciculata and zona reticularis of the adrenal cortex. The drug has been known to cause necrosis of the adrenal gland, producing acute adrenal insufficiency. Mitotane is inappropriate for rapid treatment because control of cortisol secretion requires 2 to 4 months of therapy.[34] It may be useful in the treatment of patients awaiting the full effect of radiation therapy or in those in whom surgery and irradiation have failed.[3,30]

### AMINOGLUTETHIMIDE

Aminoglutethimide reduces cortisol production by inhibiting the conversion of cholesterol to Δ5-pregnenolone. During short-term therapy, serum cortisol levels usually are suppressed to less than one-half of pretreatment values. In some patients, glucocorticoid insufficiency occurs, necessitating concurrent glucocorticoid replacement therapy. When aminoglutethimide is used to treat patients with Cushing disease, a secondary increase in ACTH levels frequently leads to escape from acceptable control.[30] Few patients have been treated for >3 months. Therapy is begun with administration of one 250-mg tablet every 6 hours. This dosage is then increased by 250 mg per day every 1 to 2 weeks until a total daily dose of 2 g is reached.

Significant side effects occur in two-thirds of patients treated with this agent. The most frequent effects of the drug include drowsiness, which occurs in 33% of patients; skin rashes, which affect 16%; and nausea and vomiting, which occur in 13%. Other significant side effects include vertigo and depression. In general, side effects decrease with smaller doses and often improve or disappear after 1 to 2 weeks of continued therapy. Skin rashes may represent allergic or hypersensitivity reactions; if these are severe or persistent, the drug should be discontinued. Interference with thyroid hormone synthesis may produce hypothyroidism. Decreased estrogen synthesis may produce menstrual irregularities and increased hirsutism and acne in some women. Two cases of pseudohermaphroditism were reported in female infants of mothers who took this drug while pregnant.

Because aminoglutethimide increases dexamethasone metabolism, hydrocortisone or cortisone acetate is preferred if glucocorticoid replacement therapy is needed. Inhibition of aldosterone synthesis may produce mineralocorticoid deficiency, presenting with orthostatic or persistent hypotension, which may require therapy with fludrocortisone acetate (Florinef).

### TRILOSTANE

Trilostane is an inhibitor of the 3-β-hydroxysteroid dehydrogenase: $\Delta^4,\Delta^5$-isomerase enzyme system. It is generally less effective than the agents described earlier, and results are highly variable.[35] Therapy is initiated with 30 mg of trilostane four times a day. This dosage is then increased as required to control serum cortisol and urinary cortisol levels, with an increase every 3 to 4 days until a total dose of 480 mg per day is reached. Significant side effects occur in half of treated patients. Gastrointestinal symptoms are the most common of these, with abdominal pain and discomfort being reported in 16% of patients, diarrhea in 17%, and nausea and vomiting in 5%. Trilostane has been reported to decrease progesterone levels, which has led to cervical dilation and termination of pregnancy in some women.

### KETOCONAZOLE

Ketoconazole is an antimycotic agent that decreases serum cortisol by inhibiting cholesterol synthesis through blockade of the 14-demethylation of lanosterol. Ketoconazole may also inhibit 11-hydroxylation and may decrease the binding of glucocorticoid to its receptor. This drug has been reported to be effective in the treatment of patients with Cushing disease in whom surgery and other drug therapy have proved unsuccessful.[3,30,36]

After oral administration, the drug is rapidly absorbed. An acid pH is required for absorption; therefore, in patients who are also taking antacids or antihistaminic $H_2$-inhibitors, the drug should be administered 2 hours after such therapy. Patients with achlorhydria may need to dissolve the tablets in aqueous hydrochloric acid. In serum, the drug is 99% protein bound.

In patients with Cushing disease, therapy is initiated with 400 mg of ketoconazole administered every 12 hours for 1 month; this dosage is then decreased to 400 to 600 mg per day. Urinary cortisol levels were reported to decline significantly within 1 day after onset of therapy. In patients receiving conventional antifungal doses (200–400 mg per day), the most common side effects are nausea and vomiting, occurring in 3%, and abdominal pain, occurring in 1.5%. Hepatotoxicity has been reported to occur in 1 in 10,000 treated patients; this condition usually resolves on discontinuation of the drug. However, one fatal case of hepatic necrosis that progressed despite discontinuation of the drug was reported.

### GLUCOCORTICOID RECEPTOR ANTAGONIST

Mifepristone (RU 486) is a synthetic steroid agonist antagonist that blocks the binding of glucocorticoids to their receptor. It is under investigation as a potential therapeutic agent in the treatment of Cushing disease.[37]

# GROWTH HORMONE HYPERSECRETION

Transsphenoidal surgery remains the treatment of choice for growth hormone–secreting adenomas (see Chap. 23). The overall rate of cure (defined as serum growth hormone levels of <5 ng/mL) is ~68% (88% of microadenomas and 59% of macroadenomas).[38] Approximately 75% of patients who undergo conventional radiation therapy eventually achieve normalization of serum growth hormone levels over several years (see Chap. 22). The cure rate with proton beam irradiation of tumors without extrasellar extension approaches 95%. Medical therapy has generally been reserved for those patients who refuse surgery or radiation therapy or in whom these treatment modalities have been unsuccessful as well as for those patients awaiting the full effects of irradiation. Pretreatment with somatostatin analogs may improve surgical outcomes.[39]

In patients with acromegaly secondary to paraneoplastic ("ectopic") growth hormone–releasing hormone secretion (see Chaps. 12 and 219), removal of the tumor secreting growth hormone–releasing hormone is the treatment of choice. If this is impossible, medical treatment may be indicated.

### BROMOCRIPTINE

Bromocriptine, at a dosage of 20 to 60 mg per day, is effective in many patients with acromegaly. At this dosage level, growth hormone levels are suppressed by more than half in ~70% of patients, but normalization is observed in <25%.[40,41] Symptomatic improvement (decreased sweating, decreased soft-tissue swelling, improvement of sexual functioning, and decreased joint swelling) and an improvement in glucose tolerance are noted in 80% to 90% of patients.[40,41] This discrepancy between growth hormone reduction and clinical improvement has been attributed to changes in the form of growth hormone secreted. Most authors recommend the use of insulin-like growth factor-I (IGF-I; also known as *somatomedin C*), rather than multiple determinations of growth hormone levels, to monitor therapy. In a few patients, a decrease in tumor size was observed. As with hyperprolactinemia, other dopamine agonists also appear to be effective in the treatment of acromegaly.[42,43]

Bromocriptine maintenance therapy in patients with acromegaly usually requires a minimum of 10 to 20 mg per day; and some patients require up to 80 mg per day. Bromocriptine dosage should be increased slowly to the maximum tolerated dose or until growth hormone levels normalize. Because the drug's half-life may vary, control may be assessed by measuring growth hormone levels three times the morning after a regular evening dose and then every 2 hours for 8 hours after the patient's usual morning dose. If serum growth hormone levels have not been suppressed significantly after several months of the maximum tolerated dosage, the drug should be discontinued.

Most patients who respond to long-term bromocriptine therapy exhibit a marked reduction in growth hormone levels within 4 to 8 hours after a single 2.5-mg dose. Patients have been treated for up to 5 years, with maintenance of growth hormone suppression and clinical improvement. Discontinuation of the drug is usually followed by a rapid increase in growth hormone to pretreatment levels and a return of symptoms. Because patients who have undergone previous radiation therapy may have a normal serum growth hormone level years after treatment, bromocriptine use in these patients should be discontinued for 4 to 8 weeks every 1 to 2 years to reevaluate growth hormone secretion.

## SOMATOSTATIN ANALOGS

Although somatostatin, a physiologic growth hormone inhibitor, lowers serum growth hormone levels in patients with acromegaly, it requires continuous infusion. In addition, the suppression of insulin secretion leads to hyperglycemia, and rebound growth hormone secretion is often observed after the infusion is discontinued. The longer-acting somatostatin analog octreotide acetate (SMS 201-995; see Chap. 169) is considerably more potent in the suppression of growth hormone. Growth hormone levels are suppressed for 8 to 12 hours after the subcutaneous administration of this analog. Octreotide has become the drug of choice for the medical therapy of acromegaly. It has been used successfully as primary therapy in patients with acromegaly[44] as well as in patients in whom surgery and radiation therapy have failed and in whom control has not been achieved with dopaminergic drugs.[3,45–47]

Therapy is initiated with 50 μg given subcutaneously every 12 hours, and the dose is increased based on the clinical and biochemical response. Many patients achieve a maximal response with a dosage of 100 μg three times per day, but some may require that octreotide be administered at higher doses or every 6 hours. Some have been treated with up to 500 μg three times per day or by continuous subcutaneous infusion. Symptomatic improvement is noted in 90% of patients within days to weeks. In patients who respond to the drug, growth hormone reductions are apparent after the first dose, and an IGF-I response is noted within 2 weeks. A reduction in growth hormone secretion occurs in 70% of patients, and mean growth hormone levels are usually normalized if the pretreatment value was <20.[45,46] IGF-I levels are reduced in 90% of patients and normalized in 60%.[45,46] Partial tumor shrinkage has been found in 20% to 50% of patients.[45,46] Some patients who do not respond adequately to either octreotide or a potent dopamine agonist have a greater response when the two agents are administered together.

Mild to moderate side effects are noted by one-third of patients, including pain at the injection site, abdominal pain, diarrhea and steatorrhea, vitamin $B_{12}$ malabsorption, gastritis, and worsening of glucose tolerance (although this also improved in many patients with effective therapy of the acromegaly).[45] Of greatest concern has been the development of gallstones, which may occur in up to 18% of patients. Some physicians administered a cholelitholytic agent with octreotide.[48] Gallstones resolved after octreotide was discontinued. No rebound increase in growth hormone levels after discontinuation of the drug has been reported.

Sandostatin LAR is a long-acting formulation of octreotide. Intramuscular injections of 20 to 30 mg every 4 weeks have been shown to be effective for up to 3 years in suppressing growth hormone and IGF-I levels and in inducing tumor shrinkage.[49,50] As with octreotide, side effects include pain at the injection site, gastrointestinal symptoms, and, infrequently, development of gallstones or $B_{12}$ malabsorption.[49,50]

Lanreotide is a depot preparation of somatostatin. Intramuscular injections of 30 mg every 10 to 14 days have also been shown to be effective in suppressing growth hormone and IGF-I levels and in inducing tumor shrinkage.[51,52] As with the other treatment modalities, symptomatic improvement may be greater than the changes in IGF-I or growth hormone. Side effects are similar to those of octreotide and Sandostatin LAR.[52a] Further studies are needed to determine which of the two long-acting preparations is more effective.[52b]

## ESTROGEN THERAPY

A decline in IGF-I levels in acromegalic patients treated with estrogen has suggested that this might be a useful therapy. However, estrogen appears to directly suppress IGF-I genera-

tion and does not decrease growth hormone or appreciably influence the symptomatology.

# GONADOTROPIN HYPERSECRETION

## GONADOTROPIN-SECRETING ADENOMAS

The standard therapy for gonadotropin-secreting adenomas is surgical resection, often followed by radiation therapy. However, this approach is rarely curative. Marked reductions (but not normalization) of follicle-stimulating hormone and α-subunit secretion have been seen in patients receiving bromocriptine after unsuccessful surgical therapy or as primary therapy.[53] Octreotide therapy has reduced α-subunit secretion and produced tumor shrinkage in a few patients.[54] Medical therapy should be considered only for those patients who refuse surgical and radiation therapy or in whom such treatment has failed.

Partial suppression of follicle-stimulating hormone was reported in male patients receiving testosterone or human chorionic gonadotropin (which increases endogenous testosterone).[53] Clomiphene citrate or estrogen failed to suppress gonadotropin secretion in these patients, and in one patient, estrogen therapy increased luteinizing hormone and α-subunit secretion.

## TRUE PRECOCIOUS PUBERTY

Previously, treatment of true precocious puberty was limited to the use of medroxyprogesterone acetate or cyproterone acetate. These agents failed to arrest bone age advancement adequately and were associated with significant side effects, including adrenal suppression, hypertension, and excessive weight gain. Moreover, they led to reduced fertility and an increased incidence of reproductive tumors in some patients.

Long-acting gonadotropin-releasing hormone agonists are effective in the management of central precocious puberty. These agents include leuprolide, nafarelin, and histrelin.[55,56] Although they initially stimulate further hormonal release, their continued use produces a marked suppression of spontaneous and stimulated gonadotropin release. This suppression is accompanied by a reduction in the circulating level of sex steroids (see Chaps. 16 and 225).

Although children treated with these agents continue to grow, a marked reduction in height velocity and a retardation in the advancement of bone age are seen. In some patients, an improvement in predicted attained height occurs. The gain in height is greatest with early initiation of therapy. In girls, a reduction in breast diameter, regression of pubic hair, and a cessation of menses (except for a menstrual period after the initial rapid rise and fall in estrogen level) may be seen.[55,56] By ultrasonography, uterine and ovarian size decrease, and ovarian cysts decrease or resolve. In boys, testicular volume is reduced and the frequency of erections and aggressive behavior is markedly decreased.[55,56] On discontinuation of therapy, serum gonadotropin and sex steroid levels rapidly return to pretreatment pubertal values, height velocity and bone age increase, and the development of secondary sexual characteristics progresses.[55,57]

Leuprolide, histrelin, and buserelin are administered as once-daily subcutaneous injections, but nafarelin is administered as a nasal spray; leuprolide is also available in a sustained-release preparation for depot intramuscular injections. Gonadotropin and sex steroid hormone levels are elevated during the first week of therapy but are then significantly reduced as long as therapy is maintained. If the plasma concentrations of sex steroids are not adequately suppressed in multiple samples obtained over several hours (estradiol level of <15 pg/mL in girls and testosterone level of <20 ng/dL in boys), the dosage is increased until adequate suppression is attained. The most common side effect is erythema at the injection site, seen in nearly one-third of treated patients. In two-thirds of these patients, the reaction does not progress. Two patients with erythema and wheal formation were desensitized and were treated with oral diphenhydramine hydrochloride (Benadryl). No patient developed immunoglobulin G antibodies against the analog. One-fourth of the girls treated with these agents developed hot flashes, which in one patient persisted for 2 years.

# HYPERSECRETION OF THYROID-STIMULATING HORMONE

## THYROID-STIMULATING HORMONE–SECRETING ADENOMA

The rare patients who have TSH-secreting adenoma present with increased serum levels of TSH and symptomatic thyrotoxicosis. They are usually treated surgically[58,59] (see Chaps. 15 and 42). Some suppression of TSH has been observed with bromocriptine therapy, but this has been inadequate to normalize thyroid hormone levels; a slight reduction in tumor size was reported in one patient. Conventional antithyroid therapy treats the thyrotoxicosis but not the primary lesion. Trials with octreotide acetate, however, appear promising.[47,60]

## ISOLATED PITUITARY RESISTANCE TO THYROID HORMONE

Patients with isolated pituitary resistance to thyroid hormone also present with TSH hypersecretion and symptomatic thyrotoxicosis, but have no demonstrable tumor. Unlike patients with TSH-secreting adenomas, TSH in these patients is suppressed by thyroid hormone administration.[58]

Because patients are thyrotoxic, treatment with conventional thyroid hormone is not suitable for long-term management. Treatment with propylthiouracil or methimazole reduces thyroid hormone levels but markedly increases TSH secretion. Bromocriptine therapy has been found to reduce TSH levels in some of these patients; usually, however, the serum TSH level remained elevated, and the patients continued to exhibit signs of mild thyrotoxicosis.[61] The combination of propylthiouracil and bromocriptine may produce euthyroidism with only a minimally elevated serum TSH. In one family, the use of 60 μg of triiodothyronine once daily led to TSH suppression, normalization of serum thyroxine, and amelioration of symptoms, but this mode of treatment was unsuccessful in other patients.[62] In one patient, the relatively inactive triiodothyronine metabolite triiodothyroacetic acid (TRIAC) was used to normalize TSH and thyroid hormone values.[63]

## NONSECRETORY ADENOMAS

The standard treatment modality for nonsecretory adenomas, if large, is transsphenoidal adenomectomy. However, in a series of 11 patients treated with bromocriptine (15 to 60 mg per day), 9 patients showed an average reduction in tumor size of 38%, whereas 2 patients exhibited a progressive increase in tumor size with treatment.[64] Bromocriptine and other dopamine agonists may be useful as adjunctive therapy in patients with nonsecretory lesions or in those who cannot tolerate surgery, but their use cannot be recommended routinely as primary therapy.

# REFERENCES

1. Vance ML, Thorner MO. Prolactinomas. Endocrinol Metab Clin North Am 1987; 16:731.
2. Colao A, Annunziato L. Treatment of prolactinomas. Ann Med 1998; 30:452.
3. Shimon I, Melmed S. Management of pituitary tumors. Ann Intern Med 1998; 129:472.
4. Moriondo P, Travaglini P, Nissim M, et al. Bromocriptine treatment of microprolactinomas: evidence of stable prolactin decrease after drug withdrawal. J Clin Endocrinol Metab 1985; 60:764.
5. Serri O, Rasio E, Beauregard H, et al. Recurrence of hyperprolactinemia after selective transsphenoidal adenomectomy in women with prolactinoma. N Engl J Med 1983; 309:280.
6. March CM, Kletzky OA, Davajan V, et al. Longitudinal evaluation of patients with untreated prolactin-secreting pituitary adenomas. Am J Obstet Gynecol 1981; 139:835.
7. Schlechte J, Dolan K, Sherman B, et al. The natural history of untreated hyperprolactinemia: a prospective analysis. J Clin Endocrinol Metab 1989; 68:412.
8. Greenspan SL, Neer RM, Ridgway EC, Klibanski A. Osteoporosis in men with hyperprolactinemic hypogonadism. Ann Intern Med 1986; 104:777.
9. Wollesen F, Bendsen BB. Effect rates of different modalities for treatment of prolactin adenomas. Am J Med 1985; 78:114.
10. Molitch ME, Elton RL, Blackwell RE, et al. Bromocriptine as primary therapy for prolactin-secreting macroadenomas: results of a prospective multicenter study. J Clin Endocrinol Metab 1985; 60:698.
11. Warfield A, Finkel DM, Schatz NJ, et al. Bromocriptine treatment of prolactin-secreting pituitary adenomas may restore pituitary function. Ann Intern Med 1984; 101:783.
12. Wass JAH, Williams J, Charlesworth M, et al. Bromocriptine in management of large pituitary tumours. BMJ 1982; 284:1908.
13. Dallabonzana D, Spelta B, Oppizzi G, et al. Reenlargement of macroprolactinomas during bromocriptine treatment: report of two cases. J Endocrinol Invest 1983; 6:47.
14. Thorner MO, Perryman RL, Rogol AD, et al. Rapid changes of prolactinoma volume after withdrawal and reinstitution of bromocriptine. J Clin Endocrinol Metab 1981; 53:480.
15. Landolt AM, Keller PJ, Froesch ER, Mueller J. Bromocriptine: does it jeopardize the result of later surgery for prolactinomas? Lancet 1982; 2:657.
16. Martin TL, Kim M, Malarkey WB. The natural history of idiopathic hyperprolactinemia. J Clin Endocrinol Metab 1985; 60:855.
17. Vance ML, Evans WS, Thorner MO. Bromocriptine. Ann Intern Med 1984; 100:78.
18. Spark RF, Dickstein G. Bromocriptine and endocrine disorders. Ann Intern Med 1979; 90:949.
19. Turkalj I, Braun P, Krupp P. Surveillance of bromocriptine in pregnancy. JAMA 1982; 247:1589.
20. Raymond JP, Goldstein E, Konopka P, et al. Follow-up of children born of bromocriptine-treated mothers. Horm Res 1985; 22:239.
21. Ciccarelli E, Grottoli S, Miola C, et al. Double blind randomized study using oral or injectable bromocriptine in patients with hyperprolactinemia. Clin Endocrinol 1994; 40:193.
22. Molitch ME. Pathologic hyperprolactinemia: neuroendocrine regulation of prolactin secretion. Endocrinol Metab Clin North Am 1992; 21:877.
23. Brue T, Pellegrini I, Gunz G, et al. Effects of the dopamine agonist CV 205-502 in human prolactinomas resistant to bromocriptine. J Clin Endocrinol Metab 1992; 74:577.
24. Webster J, Piscitelli G, Polli A. A comparison of cabergoline and bromocriptine in the treatment of hyperprolactinemic amenorrhea. N Engl J Med 1994; 331:904.
25. Colao A, Di Sarno A, Sarnacchiaro F, et al. Prolactinomas resistant to standard dopamine agonists respond to chronic cabergoline treatment. J Clin Endocrinol Metab 1997; 82:876.
26. Biller BM, Molitch ME, Vance ML, et al. Treatment of prolactin-secreting macroadenomas with the once-weekly dopamine agonist cabergoline. J Clin Endocrinol Metab 1996; 81:2338.
27. DeRosa M, Colao A, Di Sarno A, et al. Cabergoline treatment rapidly improves gonadal function in hyperprolactinemic males: a comparison with bromocriptine. Eur J Endocrinol 1998; 138(3):286.
28. Mampalam TJ, Tyrrell JB, Wilson CB. Transsphenoidal microsurgery for Cushing disease: a report of 216 cases. Ann Intern Med 1988; 109:487.
29. Boscaro M, Benato M, Mantero F. Effect of bromocriptine in pituitary-dependent Cushing's syndrome. Clin Endocrinol 1983; 19:485.
30. Miller JW, Crapo L. The medical treatment of Cushing's syndrome. Endocr Rev 1993; 14:443.
31. Krieger DT. Physiopathology of Cushing's disease. Endocr Rev 1983; 4:22.
32. Koppeschaar HPF, Croughs RJM, van't Verlatt JW, et al. Successful treatment with sodium valproate of a patient with Cushing's disease and gross enlargement of the pituitary. Acta Endocrinol 1984; 107:471.
33. Jeffcoate WJ, Rees LH, Tomlin S, et al. Metyrapone in long-term management of Cushing's disease. BMJ 1977; 2:215.
34. Luton JP, Mahoudeau JA, Bouchard P, et al. Treatment of Cushing's disease by o,p′ DDD. N Engl J Med 1979; 300:459.
35. Dewis P, Anderson DC, Builock DE, et al. Experience with trilostane in the treatment of Cushing's syndrome. Clin Endocrinol 1983; 18:533.
36. Sonino N. The use of ketoconazole as an inhibitor of steroid production. N Engl J Med 1987; 317:812.
37. Nieman LK, Chrousos GP, Kellner C, et al. Successful treatment of Cushing's syndrome with the glucocorticoid antagonist RU 486. J Clin Endocrinol Metab 1985; 61:536.
38. Serri O, Somma M, Comtois R, et al. Acromegaly: biochemical assessment of cure after long-term follow-up of transsphenoidal selective adenomectomy. J Clin Endocrinol Metab 1985; 61:1185.
39. Stevenaert A, Beckers A. Presurgical octreotide: treatment in acromegaly. Metabolism 1996;45:72.
40. Wass JAH, Thorner MO, Morris DV, et al. Long-term treatment of acromegaly with bromocriptine. BMJ 1977; 1:875.
41. Jaffe CA, Barkan AL. Treatment of acromegaly with dopamine agonists. Endocrinol Metab Clin North Am 1992; 21:713.

42. Cozzi R, Attanasio R, Barausse M, et al. Cabergoline in acromegaly: a renewed role for dopamine agonist treatment? Eur J Endocrinol 1998; 139(5):516.

43. Abs R, Verhelst J, Maiter D, et al. Cabergoline in the treatment of acromegaly: a study in 64 patients. J Clin Endocrinol Metab 1998; 83:374.

44. Newman CB, Melmed S, George A, et al. Octreotide as primary therapy for acromegaly. J Clin Endocrinol Metab 1998; 83:3034.

45. Lamberts SWJ, Uitterlinden P, Verschoor L. Long-term treatment of acromegaly with the somatostatin analogue SMS 201-995. N Engl J Med 1985; 313:1576.

46. Ezzat S, Snyder PJ, Young WF, et al. Octreotide treatment of acromegaly: a randomized, multicenter study. Ann Intern Med 1992; 117:711.

47. Comi RJ. Pharmacology and use in pituitary tumors. In: Gorden P, moderator. Somatostatin and somatostatin analog (SMS 201-995) in treatment of hormone-secreting tumors of the pituitary and gastrointestinal tract and non-neoplastic diseases of the gut. Ann Intern Med 1989; 110:35.

48. Montini M, Gianola D, Pagani MD. Cholelithiasis and acromegaly: therapeutic strategies. Clin Endocrinol 1994; 40:401.

49. Flogstad AK, Halse J, Bakke S, et al. Sandostatin LAR in acromegalic patients: long-term treatment. J Clin Endocrinol Metab 1997; 82:23.

50. Davies PH, Stewart SE, Lancranjan I, et al. Long-term therapy with long-acting octreotide (Sandostatin-LAR) for the management of acromegaly. Clin Endocrinol (Oxf) 1998; 48:311.

51. Caron P, Morange-Ramos I, Cogne M, Jaquet P. Three year follow-up of acromegalic patients treated with intramuscular slow-release lanreotide. J Clin Endocrinol Metab 1997; 82(1):18.

52. Giusti M, Gussoni G, Cuttica CM, Giordano G. Effectiveness and tolerability of slow release lanreotide treatment in active acromegaly: six-month report on an Italian multicenter study. J Clin Endocrinol Metab 1996; 81:2089.

52a. Turner HE, Lindsell DR, Vadivale A, et al. Differing effects on gall-bladder motility of lanreotide SR and octreotide LAR for the treatment of acromegaly. Eur J Endocrinol 1999; 141:590.

52b. Cozzi R, Dellabonzana D, Attonasio R, et al. A comparison between octreotide-LAR and lanreotide-SR in the chronic treatment of acromegaly. Eur J Endocrinol 1999; 141:267.

53. Snyder PJ. Clinically nonfunctioning pituitary adenomas. Endocrin Metab Clin North Am 1993; 22:163.

54. Katznelson L, Alexander JM, Klibanski A. Clinically nonfunctioning pituitary adenomas. J Clin Endocrinol Metab 1993; 76:1089.

55. Wheeler MD, Styne DM. The treatment of precocious puberty. Endocrinol Metab Clin North Am 1991; 20:183.

56. Lee PA. Advances in the management of precocious puberty. Clin Pediatr 1994; 33:54.

57. Manasco PK, Pescovitz OH, Feuillan PP, et al. Resumption of puberty after long-term luteinizing hormone–releasing hormone agonist treatment of central precocious puberty. J Clin Endocrinol Metab 1988; 67:638.

58. Beck-Peccoz P, Persani L, Mantivani S, et al. Thyrotropin-secreting pituitary adenomas. Metabolism 1996;45:75.

59. Brucker-Davis F, Oldfield EH, Skarulis MC, et al. Thyrotropin-secreting pituitary tumors: diagnostic criteria, thyroid hormone sensitivity, and treatment outcome in 25 patients followed at the National Institutes of Health. J Clin Endocrinol Metab 1999; 84:476.

60. Chanson P, Weintraub BD, Harris AG. Octreotide therapy for thyroid-stimulating hormone–secreting pituitary adenomas: a follow-up of 52 patients. Ann Intern Med 1993; 119:236.

61. Takamatsu J, Mozai T, Kuma K. Bromocriptine therapy for hyperthyroidism due to increased thyrotropin secretion. J Clin Endocrinol Metab 1984; 58:934.

62. Rosler A, Litvin Y, Hage C, et al. Familial hyperthyroidism due to inappropriate thyrotropin secretion successfully treated with triiodothyronine. J Clin Endocrinol Metab 1982; 54:76.

63. Beck-Peccoz P, Piscitelli G, Cattaneo MG, Faglia G. Successful treatment of hyperthyroidism due to nonneoplastic pituitary TSH hypersecretion with 3,5,3'-triiodothyroacetic acid (TRIAC). J Clin Endocrinol Invest 1983; 6:217.

64. Wollesen F, Andersen T, Karle A. Size reduction of extrasellar tumors during bromocriptine treatment. Ann Intern Med 1982; 96:281.

# CHAPTER 22

# RADIOTHERAPY OF PITUITARY-HYPOTHALAMIC TUMORS

MINESH P. MEHTA

Radiotherapeutic management of pituitary adenomas and tumors of the hypothalamus requires a thorough understanding of the various hypersecretory syndromes and their wide-spread clinical manifestations, a working knowledge of the diagnostic principles, and an appreciation for the roles of surgery and medical management. Treatment with external beam radiotherapy typically results in little radiographic change in the tumor itself, and endocrine changes may require years to become detectable or stabilized. Meaningful evaluation of pituitary or hypothalamic tumors requires long-term follow-up to assess response and to observe complications.

This chapter addresses the overall management of pituitary adenomas, craniopharyngiomas, hypothalamic tumors (including germ-cell neoplasms), parasellar meningiomas, and astrocytomas. This discussion emphasizes the role of and indications for radiotherapy. Standard external-beam techniques for radiotherapy are outlined, and less common techniques—such as intracavitary radioisotope instillation, brachytherapy, particle beam radiotherapy, and stereotactic radiosurgery—are discussed. The complications of conventional radiotherapy are also addressed.

## PITUITARY ADENOMAS

The role of radiotherapy in the management of pituitary adenomas remains poorly defined because of several factors, including the occasional need for emergent surgical decompression; the availability of competing therapeutic alternatives, such as transsphenoidal adenomectomy and medical treatment with dopamine agonists; the slow decline in hypersecretion after irradiation; the lack of large, well-controlled prospective randomized trials; concerns regarding possible long-term toxic effects of radiotherapy; and the *false belief that benign tumors are not effectively treated by radiation therapy.*

Available data typically represent experience with a small number of cases accrued over a period of several years or decades and contain the inherent bias of referral patterns at tertiary care centers. Most patients have not been observed for sufficiently long periods to allow adequate interpretation of response and toxicity. Despite these limitations, it has become clear that the role of radiotherapy in the management of pituitary neoplasms falls into two distinct categories: the control of hypersecretion when other modalities have failed or are contraindicated and the control of mass effects. For most pituitary adenomas, external beam irradiation, delivered in conventional fraction sizes of 1.8 to 2 Gy to a total of 45 Gy or more, appears to suffice. Newer techniques—such as radiosurgery, interstitial implantation, and particle beam therapy—are under investigation.

### PROLACTINOMAS

Prolactinomas, predominantly macroadenomas, were previously classified with the nonsecreting tumors as chromophobe adenomas; before the prolactin assay era, the major goal of radiotherapy was the control of the mass effect. With the availability of the prolactin assay, it became clear that some macroadenomas are functionally active. Prolactin-secreting microadenomas usually are effectively managed by bromocriptine or, rarely, by transsphenoidal adenomectomy. Long-term control of hyperprolactinemia after surgery alone is rare. Large tumors and tumors that persistently secrete prolactin despite resection can be treated medically with bromocriptine, a dopamine agonist that decreases prolactin levels and causes tumor shrinkage. The continued use of bromocriptine may be complicated by toxic effects, and its discontinuation often results in resumption of tumor growth and of prolactin hypersecretion. Despite prior therapy with bromocriptine, tumor growth may resume in women who become pregnant.

Radiotherapy is indicated if hyperprolactinemia persists despite transsphenoidal tumor resection or the use of bromocriptine. The results of several single-institution studies are summarized in Table 22-1.[1–9] Although irradiation causes a dramatic decrease in prolactin levels in some patients, the response

**TABLE 22-1.**
**Control of Prolactinomas with Radiotherapy**

| Investigation | Year | Number of Patients | Prolactin Level[#] PRE- | POST- | NL |
|---|---|---|---|---|---|
| Kleinberg[1*] | 1977 | 8 | 195 | 50 | — |
| Gomez[2*] | 1977 | 8 | 168 | 64 | — |
| Antunes[3†] | 1977 | 14 | 1683 | 153 | — |
| Sheline[4‡] | 1979 | 14 | 4700 | 820 | — |
| Sheline[4*] | 1979 | 4 | 387 | 192 | — |
| Frantz[5§] | 1981 | 26 | — | — | — |
| Mehta[6] | 1987 | 9 | — | — | 67% |
| Rush[7] | 1989 | 10 | — | — | 70% |
| Tran[8] | 1991 | 36 | — | — | 41% |
| Tsagarakis[9] | 1991 | 36 | 7000 | 1000 | 60% |

*Radiotherapy as the only treatment.
†Eight of 14 patients had surgery and radiotherapy, but there was no difference in the prolactin values for the two groups before or after treatment.
‡These were postop patients; the preprolactin values are postop values.
§Eleven of 26 patients had prior surgery. By 3 years, the mean prolactin had declined by 90%.
#Pre- and Post- indicate prolactin status before and after radiation therapy, and NL indicates the percentage of patients becoming normoprolactinemic.

is not always predictable. Serum assays obtained after radiotherapy have demonstrated a slow and variable decline in prolactin levels. Transient hyperprolactinemia, lasting as long as 2 years, has been described in patients irradiated for other pituitary-hypothalamic conditions.

After irradiation, prolactin levels decrease by an average of 60% by the end of the first year; after 3 or more years, the mean prolactin level decreases to one-tenth of the preirradiation value.[5] In another study, 16 (44%) of 36 prolactin-secreting adenomas were controlled after radiotherapy.[8] Another 36 female patients (12 with macroprolactinomas and 24 with microprolactinomas) were irradiated to a total dose of 45 Gy (1.8-Gy fractions) with a three-field technique.[9] All patients underwent baseline and periodic reassessment of anterior and posterior pituitary function at intervals of 1 year or less while off bromocriptine for at least 2 months; they also had dynamic screening with thyrotropin-releasing hormone and luteinizing hormone–releasing hormone and hypoglycemic stimulation every 2 to 3 years. The preirradiation prolactin levels ranged from 1150 to 34,000 mU/L. With a mean follow-up of 8.5 years (range, 3–14 years), the postirradiation serum prolactin levels fell to normal (i.e., <360 mU/L) in 18 patients (50%). Another 10 patients (28%) had prolactin levels just above the normal range (378–780 mU/L). Only 2 patients (6%) demonstrated an increase in prolactin levels; another patient had a radiographically confirmed recurrence. Neither the pretreatment prolactin level nor the size of the tumor influenced the outcome from radiotherapy.

In a smaller study, long-term control of hyperprolactinemia was achieved in 7 (70%) of 10 patients after a total dose of 45 Gy (1.8-Gy fractions) of radiation.[7] These studies elegantly demonstrated that radiotherapy and dopamine agonists are useful for long-term control of subtotally resected macroprolactinomas. Despite the paucity of long-term longitudinal studies of prolactin secretion after radiation therapy, studies indicate that over 2 to 13 years, prolactin levels return to normal or near-normal levels in >75% of irradiated patients.[7,9] However, physiologic symptoms, such as amenorrhea from markedly elevated prolactin production, persist even when these levels fall to baseline. For example, in a series of 24 patients with prolactin-secreting macroadenomas treated with transsphenoidal surgery, dopamine-agonist therapy, and 45 Gy radiotherapy, tumor control and prolactin reductions were achieved in all, but amenorrhea persisted in the majority.[10]

## GROWTH HORMONE–SECRETING TUMORS

Initial reports of the effectiveness of radiotherapy for the treatment of growth hormone (GH)–secreting tumors relied on clinical assessments of response, because direct measurements of GH levels were unavailable. Several investigators have reported clinical control rates of 80% to 90% after irradiation to doses of 40 Gy or more using conventional fraction sizes of 1.8 to 2 Gy per day.[11–14] Clinical experience also suggests a dose-response relationship; control improves with doses as great as 40 Gy, and toxic effects occur at doses higher than 50 to 54 Gy. In 105 patients with GH-secreting pituitary adenoma treated to a total dose of 42 to 55 Gy, no improvement in local control was found at doses higher than 45 Gy. Moreover, the advent of the serum GH assay revealed that the functional response by these tumors to radiotherapy occurred slowly. The current definition of cure requires a GH level of <5 mU/L (2 ng/mL), with the understanding that long-term survival is dependent on such a reduction. Although radiation-induced GH reduction requires a lag period, as opposed to the immediate decline seen after surgery, the hypothalamic effects of radiation abrogate the endogenous somatostatin tone, thereby abolishing several responses that may enhance GH secretion. In a 20-patient study, arginine increased GH hypersecretion in those with a prior history of acromegaly whose GH levels had normalized after surgery. This phenomenon could not be demonstrated in patients postradiation.[15]

Patients treated after incomplete pituitary adenomectomy with high-voltage or with proton beam irradiation achieved an 80% decrease in GH levels after 4.5 years.[14] In another report, control of GH secretion was achieved in 9 (60%) of 15 patients after irradiation.[8] For 56 acromegalic patients in whom surgery had been unsuccessful, treatment with 50 Gy of radiation brought a 50% reduction in preirradiation GH levels in 51 patients (91%) at 26 months; for 40 of these patients, there was a further 50% decrease in GH levels at 42 months.[16] At 2, 5, and 10 years after radiotherapy, endocrinologic control rates (defined by a drop in GH levels to <10 ng/mL) were 38%, 73%, and 81%, respectively.[13] These data suggest that in patients who respond to radiotherapy, the GH depression may follow a first-order reaction, with a half-life of just longer than 2 years.[16]

Because endocrinologic normalization can occur almost immediately after successful transsphenoidal resection, this approach has become the standard. Irradiation of GH-secreting pituitary microadenomas and most macroadenomas is limited to patients with persistent GH hypersecretion after resection and to those in whom surgery is otherwise contraindicated. Overall, ~75% of such patients achieve eventual control, defined as a GH level <10 ng/mL or a lack of progression of growth of the adenoma[4,8,11–14,17–23] (Table 22-2). Additionally, some data suggest that macroadenomas may have a higher failure rate after radiotherapy, as exemplified in a 21-patient series in which 5 of 6 failed patients had macroadenomas.[23]

## ADRENOCORTICOTROPIC HORMONE–SECRETING TUMORS

### CUSHING DISEASE

Cushing disease is typically associated with adrenocorticotropic hormone (ACTH)–secreting pituitary microadenomas. The standard management for this syndrome remains transsphenoidal adenomectomy, which yields a 75% success rate in the control of hypercortisolism (see Chaps. 23 and 75). Radiotherapy is restricted to inoperable patients or those in whom hypercortisolism persists after resection. Several reports of pituitary irradiation for Cushing disease are summarized in Table 22-3.[8,21–29] The control rates range from 50% to more than 80%. Although a dose-response relationship has not been established in a prospective, randomized trial, retrospective data suggest that the

**TABLE 22-2.**
**Control of Growth Hormone–Secreting Adenomas with Radiotherapy**

| Institution | Investigator | Year | Number of Patients | Control (%) |
|---|---|---|---|---|
| University of California, San Francisco | Sheline[11] | 1961 | 18 | 78* |
| Jefferson | Kramer[17] | 1973 | 25 | 86* |
| University of Kentucky | Williams[18] | 1975 | 6 | 67† |
| Stanford | Pistenma[19] | 1976 | 17 | 90* |
| National Institutes of Health | Eastman[13] | 1979 | 47 | 81 |
| University of California, San Francisco | Sheline[4] | 1979 | 27 | 85† |
| National Institutes of Health | Eastman[13] | 1979 | 5 | 80† |
| Several | Sheline[30] | 1983 | 24 | 92 |
| Karolinska | Werner[20] | 1985 | 19 | 84† |
| Mallinckrodt | Grigsby[21] | 1988 | 22 | 77* |
| Hamburg | Ludecke[14] | 1989 | 30 | 80† |
| University of California, Los Angeles | Tran[8] | 1991 | 15 | 60† |
| University of Florida | McCollough[12] | 1991 | 25 | 96* |
| Queensland | Hughes[22] | 1993 | 145 | 65* |
| Athens, Greece | Plataniotis[23] | 1998 | 21 | 72 |
| Overall | — | — | 446 | 76 |

*Control defined as lack of progression.
†Control defined as serum growth hormone <10 ng/mL.

**TABLE 22-3.**
**Control of Adrenocorticotropic Hormone–Secreting Adenomas with Radiotherapy**

| Investigation | Year | Number of Patients | Cure (%) | Remission (Months) |
|---|---|---|---|---|
| Dohan[24] | 1957 | 6 | 83 | 3–6 |
| Heuschele[25] | 1967 | 16 | 63 | 5–7 |
| Orth[26] | 1971 | 44 | 52 | — |
| Edmonds[27] | 1972 | 15 | 60 | 1–67 |
| Jennings[28] | 1977 | 15 | 80 | 9–18 |
| Grigsby[21] | 1988 | 6 | 100 | — |
| Howlett[29] | 1989 | 21 | 57 | 5–126 |
| Tran[8] | 1991 | 3 | 100 | — |
| Hughes[22] | 1993 | 40 | 59 | — |
| Overall | — | 166 | 63 | — |

control of hypercortisolism requires doses of 40 to 50 Gy. Cortisol levels normalized in 53% of patients treated with radiotherapy to the extent that no further treatment was required.[26]

In another study of 21 patients with Cushing disease for whom irradiation was the primary treatment, a total of 45 Gy in 25 fractions was delivered using a three-field technique, and patients were observed for 5.8 to 15.5 years (median of 9.5 years).[29] Initially, all patients were treated with metyrapone to normalize cortisol levels; at the latest follow-up evaluation, 57% had normal mean cortisol levels throughout the day and were off all therapy. Five patients required additional treatment with bilateral adrenalectomy or transsphenoidal hypophysectomy, yielding a failure rate for treatment of ACTH-secreting adenomas with radiotherapy of ~25%. The time to normalization of cortisol levels ranged from 0.7 to 10.5 years (median, 4 years).

In one study of 15 children with Cushing disease treated with radiotherapy, an 80% control rate was achieved.[28] The time to remission of hypercortisolism was only 9 to 18 months, in contrast to the substantially longer remission times for GH- and prolactin-secreting adenomas.

### NELSON SYNDROME

Nelson syndrome consists of hypersecretion of ACTH and melanocyte–stimulating hormone, with dermal hyperpigmentation and aggressive growth of a pituitary adenoma, after bilateral adrenalectomy. Limited data suggest that the syndrome can successfully be treated with megavoltage pituitary irradiation. In a series of 15 patients observed for a median of 9.6 years (range, 1.5–17.3 years), clinical, radiographic, and endocrinologic improvement was observed in 14 cases (93%) after 45 Gy of megavoltage irradiation.[29]

### NON-HORMONE–SECRETING TUMORS

The primary goal of therapy for endocrinologically inactive pituitary adenomas is control of the mass effect, which typically manifests with impaired vision, headaches, and pressure-

induced atrophic hypopituitarism. The mass effect primarily is a consequence of tumors that were previously referred to as chromophobe adenomas; occasionally, it is caused by GH-secreting macroadenomas. Modern pathologic assessment has demonstrated that some tumors that had been assumed to be nonfunctional chromophobe adenomas are instead prolactin-secreting tumors; these are discussed separately later. Other so-called nonfunctional tumors secrete gonadotropins or their subunits (see Chap. 16).

The consequences of a mass effect from pituitary adenomas can be quite severe. For example, in a report of 140 patients with macroadenomas, visual field deficits were identified in 92%; in 10%, the tumors invaded the brain or the nasopharynx.[30] In a subgroup of patients managed surgically without postoperative radiotherapy, the 5-, 10-, and 20-year recurrence-free survival rates were only 38%, 14%, and 0%, respectively. Postoperative radiotherapy increased the recurrence-free survival rates at 5, 10, and 20 years to 96%, 86%, and 73%, respectively. In that same study, 23 patients with relatively minor visual field deficits or with underlying medical conditions precluding surgery were selected for treatment with radiotherapy only; the 15-year recurrence-free survival rate was 93%.[30] Radiotherapy normalized visual field deficits in more than two-thirds of patients in whom one quadrant or less was affected, an outcome that compared favorably with the results obtained with surgery. However, in patients with more extensive visual loss, visual restoration was more rapid and effective after surgery than after radiotherapy. The potential for blindness from such large tumors mandates immediate surgical debulking if feasible; however, the probability of residual disease and late recurrence is significant.

Of 112 patients with nonfunctional pituitary adenomas, the actuarial progression-free survival rates after primary irradiation (25 patients) or postoperative irradiation (87 patients) was 97%, 89%, 87%, and 76% at 5, 10, 15, and 20 years, respectively.[31] No demonstrable difference in local control rates was identified between patients who underwent postoperative or primary irradiation. Because those data represent the experience of a single institution over more than 2 decades, radiotherapeutic techniques and doses varied. A further analysis of the dose-response relationship revealed no significant advantage in local control at dose levels that ranged between 35.7 and 62.3 Gy. Some data, however, do suggest the existence of a dose-response relationship; a 78% local control rate was obtained after 40 to 50 Gy, compared with a 56% local control rate after 30 to 40 Gy of radiation.[32] A summary of local control rates for nonfunctional adenomas after radiotherapy is presented in Table 22-4.[7,8,11,12,21,22,31,33,34]

Additional data supporting a role for radiotherapy in the preservation and improvement of vision in selected patients come from a report of 25 patients with pituitary macroadenomas causing vision impairment. These patients were treated

**TABLE 22-4.**
**Control of Nonfunctioning Pituitary Adenomas with Radiotherapy**

| Investigation | Year | Number of Patients | Local Control (%) 5 Year | 10 Year | >10 Year |
|---|---|---|---|---|---|
| Sheline[11] | 1961 | 97 | 95 | 87 | 73 |
| Grigsby[21] | 1988 | 19 | 90 | 80 | 80 |
| Chun[33] | 1988 | 43 | 93 | — | — |
| Flickinger[31] | 1989 | 112 | 97 | 89 | 87 |
| Rush[7] | 1989 | 19 | 93 | 93 | 93 |
| Tran[8] | 1991 | 36 | 87 | — | — |
| McCollough[12] | 1991 | 62 | 95 | 95 | 92 |
| Hughes[22] | 1993 | 121 | 90 | 82 | — |
| Fisher[34*] | 1993 | 25 | 84 | — | — |
| Total | — | 534 | 93 | 87 | 84 |

*All patients with giant pituitary adenomas.

**TABLE 22-5.**
**Survival Rates 5 and 10 Years after Three Therapeutic Approaches for Craniopharyngioma: Retrospective Data from 34 Reports**

| Treatment Outcomes | Total Resection | Subtotal Resection | Radiotherapy |
|---|---|---|---|
| 5-YEAR SURVIVAL | 81% | 53% | 89% |
| 10-YEAR SURVIVAL | 69% | 37% | 77% |
| RECURRENCE | 29% | 73% | 17% |

with radiation therapy alone. Twenty-three patients underwent neuro-ophthalmologic evaluation before and after radiation therapy. With a median follow-up of 3 years, 78% of patients whose pretreatment visual field deficits had less than dense hemianopia and who also did not have diffuse optic atrophy experienced visual field improvement. Only 1 patient experienced tumor progression.[35]

### GIANT PITUITARY ADENOMAS

The giant pituitary adenoma is a rare lesion, and its definition varies among case reports.[36] A study of 31 patients with this tumor reserved the term for lesions with 40 mm or more of suprasellar extension.[34] Eleven of the tumors were secretory, and 20 were nonfunctional. Four patients were treated with surgery, 2 with radiotherapy, and 25 with surgery plus radiotherapy. The patients who received combined-modality treatment were those with significant residual disease after surgery. With a mean follow-up of 8 years, the recurrence rate in either single-modality treatment group was 67% (4 of 6 patients). The use of combined-modality therapy yielded a local control rate of 84%. Based on limited experience, this rare subcategory of nonfunctional pituitary adenoma is best treated with surgery plus radiotherapy.

## CRANIOPHARYNGIOMAS

Craniopharyngiomas are relatively rare neoplasms that arise from epithelial remnants of the Rathke pouch and are typically found in the suprasellar region in children or adolescents; they account for ~5% of all intracranial neoplasms in childhood.[37] These tumors tend to grow slowly, and the patients often present with compression of adjacent neural structures, such as the optic chiasm. Hypopituitarism also may occur. Surgical decompression is the optimal treatment for symptom relief and immediate palliation. However, the location, proximity, and adhesiveness of the tumor to adjacent neural structures often preclude an effective total resection. Aggressive attempts at total resection carry high rates of morbidity and mortality.[38]

The management options for craniopharyngioma include total resection, which is applicable only to a very small proportion of patients; subtotal resection alone; or subtotal resection and postoperative radiotherapy. To understand the role of postoperative radiotherapy, it is necessary to compare the results for total or subtotal resection alone with subtotal resection plus postoperative radiotherapy. In the absence of a prospective randomized trial, the only data available for comparison are retrospective single-institution reports that span several decades. These suffer from the problems associated with such studies,

including an institutional bias regarding therapeutic preference and the impact of technologic advances on diagnosis, resection, and radiotherapy. Although flawed, this database represents the only opportunity to compare the various treatment options for the management of craniopharyngioma.

### OVERALL SURVIVAL

A review of the English language literature from the mid-1960s through 1998 yields 34 reports from which management and outcome data can be summarized[39] (Table 22-5). The data are broken down into three categories representing total resection, subtotal resection, and surgery plus postoperative radiotherapy. Actuarial 5- and 10-year survival rates after total resection were 81% and 69%. After subtotal resection alone, the survival rates were 53% and 37% at 5 and 10 years, and if radiotherapy was added, the survival rates were 89% and 77% at 5 and 10 years, respectively. There is a trend toward longer survival in later reports, which probably reflects improvements in neuroimaging, neurosurgery, radiotherapy, and overall medical management. Nonetheless, the outcome for patients undergoing subtotal resection is inferior to that of patients who also receive postoperative radiotherapy. Although the inferior outcome of patients who undergo subtotal resection could reflect a patient selection bias, the overall 5- and 10-year survival rates of 53% and 37% do not indicate a benign disease process.

### LOCAL RECURRENCE

Another important factor in the prognosis and management of craniopharyngioma is the local recurrence rate. A review of 31 published studies suggests that local recurrence rates are 29% (90 of 308 patients) after total resection, 73% (163 of 224) after subtotal resection, and 17% (104 of 596) after surgery plus radiotherapy. Even after aggressive resection, recurrences are reported for as many as one-third of patients.[40] The 20-year experience in childhood craniopharyngioma from the Joint Center for Radiation Therapy in Boston is a 10-year actuarial rate for freedom from progression of 31% after resection only, 100% after radiotherapy only, and 86% for patients treated with resection plus radiotherapy at the time of diagnosis. A point to consider is that surgical reports comment only on patients in whom resection was attempted. Patients in whom resection was not feasible were not reported as "failure of intent to resect." Reporting data for an "intent to resect" category could significantly lower the overall local control rates for this treatment approach.

### MORBIDITY AND MORTALITY

The morbidity and mortality rates that occur with total resection of craniopharyngiomas are significant. The operative mortality ranges from 2% to 43% (mean, 12%), and the morbidity ranges from 12% to 61% (mean, 30%). Surgical morbidity includes damage to the hypothalamus, which may result in diabetes insipidus or other endocrine anomalies (range, 30%–57%; mean, 40%), visual impairment (range, 10%–35%; mean, 19%), obesity, and memory impairment. In another report, 48% of patients developed obesity, and 57% developed memory impairment.[41] In the largest surgical series reported, the operative mortality for total resection was 17%, and the incidence of significant morbidity was 16%.[42] In contrast, subtotal resections carry a mortality of ~1%. The risk of late radiation damage to the hypothalamus, pituitary, and optic nerve is relatively low after conventionally fractionated irradiation (i.e., 1.8-Gy fractions to a total dose of 54 Gy). With these dose recommendations, visual impairment ranges between 1% and 1.5%.[43] The addition of radiotherapy to subtotal resection does not increase the mortality and adds little to morbidity.

The impairment of cognitive performance is difficult to assess, because few studies address the issue in detail and because the protocols for neuropsychologic evaluation are not standardized. In an analysis of 35 patients with craniopharyngioma who underwent neurologic and neuropsychologic assessment, a lower morbidity rate was observed after subtotal resection followed by radiotherapy than after attempted radical tumor resection alone.[44] From this experience, the researchers concluded that primary irradiation caused less frontal lobe dysfunction than radical subfrontal excision. Visual perceptual tests, visual acuity, and ocular motility improved in one-third of conservatively treated patients but deteriorated in patients who underwent radical tumor resection. A common deficit, independent of the treatment modality, was mild impairment of manual dexterity, which became evident in sequential tapping or in slow, smooth pursuit tasks. This deficit may represent the underlying basis for the awkwardness, the slowness, and the stiffness of gross motor function described in patients with craniopharyngioma.

An impairment of orbital-frontal lobe functions, which mainly manifests as persevering responses, was more pronounced in patients who had radical subfrontal excision than in those who had primary radiotherapy. This deficit persisted as long as 19 years after the resection. The intelligence quotients of the surgical and the radiotherapy groups remained within normal limits. Only 1 of the 18 patients in the primary irradiation group showed signs of frontal lobe disorder and had difficulty in school, but 2 patients required some tutoring for mild or moderate learning disability.[44] Most of the surgically treated patients were unable to maintain regular employment, achieve expected educational goals, or enjoy a normal family and social life. A review suggests that although total excisions may be appropriate for relatively small craniopharyngiomas, heroic attempts at total resection typically result only in partial resection with enhanced morbidity and mortality rates.[45] In light of the excellent results achieved after subtotal resection plus postoperative radiotherapy, this should be considered the standard management.

## DOSE CONSIDERATIONS

No prospective randomized trials analyzing dose-response relationships are available for the treatment of craniopharyngioma with radiotherapy. However, most institutions have routinely irradiated these patients to a total dose of 50 to 55 Gy in 1.8- to 2-Gy fractions. A long-term analysis (20 years) of dose-response data revealed a local failure rate of 50% with <54 Gy but only 15% with 54 Gy or higher doses.[46] In a retrospective analysis of patients treated with 51.3 to 70 Gy, a higher incidence of radiation-associated complications was identified in those who received >60 Gy (with an actuarial incidence of optic neuropathy of 30% and brain necrosis of 12.5%), without any concomitant improvement in tumor control.[47]

## RADIOTHERAPY FOR RECURRENT CRANIOPHARYNGIOMA

Limited data suggest that radiotherapy at recurrence, after prior resection, yields a 10-year progression-free survival rate of >70% for patients with craniopharyngiomas.[48] These results are similar to those obtained with subtotal resection and preliminary irradiation and suggest that radiotherapy may be delayed in very young children, in whom its toxic effects may be more pronounced. However, routinely delaying irradiation may entail additional morbidity from continued tumor growth, the possible requirement for repeat surgery, and irradiation of larger volumes at relapse. Delaying radiotherapy cannot be recommended for older children. Recurrences appear to occur from 3 to 192 months (median, 12 months) after subtotal resection.[43]

## HYPOTHALAMIC NEOPLASMS

### GERMINOMA

Germinomas typically arise in the floor of the third ventricle and have a propensity to invade and compress adjacent neural structures, such as the optic chiasm, or to spread in the periventricular space, which permits craniospinal seeding. Although germinomas are the most common embryonal cell tumors, choriocarcinoma, endodermal sinus tumors, and teratomas may also occur at this site. The initial intervention for tumors arising in the floor of the third ventricle is often surgical. Surgery is indicated for diagnosis and to decompress the ventricles or to relieve pressure on the chiasm or the pituitary stalk. The rare teratomas in this location are amenable to surgical cure.

Current staging recommendations include contrast-enhanced magnetic resonance imaging (MRI) of the entire craniospinal axis. The incidence of spinal seeding varies and is often a function of the thoroughness of the investigation. The author recommends the use of triple-strength contrast during spinal imaging to assist in the detection of seeding of the leptomeninges or the cauda equina. Cerebrospinal fluid and serum evaluation for $\alpha$-fetoprotein and the $\beta$-subunit of human chorionic gonadotropin ($\beta$-hCG) are recommended. Endodermal sinus tumors and, to a lesser extent, embryonal carcinomas cause elevations of $\alpha$-fetoprotein; choriocarcinomas cause elevations of $\beta$-hCG. If either marker is elevated, repeat levels should be obtained postoperatively, after allowing time for the markers to decline. These markers allow monitoring of the treatment and follow-up phases.

Historically, the standard management of germinomas has consisted of craniospinal irradiation. So dramatic is the response of these tumors to radiation therapy that some researchers recommended a low test dose of limited-field irradiation (to ~20 Gy) as a diagnostic test in place of a biopsy.[49] This practice is supported by a report that surgery is associated with a 41% incidence of spinal dissemination compared with a rate of only 2% in nonbiopsied patients.[50] Although the issues of total dose and whether the spinal axis should be prophylactically radiated remain controversial, the overall disease-free survival rate for patients with germinoma is usually in excess of 80%.[51] Of all patients with confirmed intracranial germ-cell tumors treated at the Hospital of Sick Children from 1952 to 1989, 25 patients with germinoma treated with radiotherapy had a 5-year survival rate of 85%, and 13 patients with nongerminoma germ-cell tumors treated with radiotherapy had a 5-year survival rate of 45.5%.[52]

The efficacy of chemotherapy for treatment of germ-cell neoplasms in other body sites has led to similar trials for intracranial germ-cell tumors. Preliminary results for treatment with platinum-based combination chemotherapy for 10 patients with intracranial germ-cell tumors are encouraging. Seven patients received primary chemotherapy consisting of vincristine, etoposide, and carboplatin before craniospinal axis irradiation; 3 patients had complete responses, 3 had partial responses, and 1 patient had stable disease. All 7 patients were alive and disease free at a median of 12 months after treatment. The author's treatment for germinomas, attaining complete response after two courses of chemotherapy, is a lowered radiation dose prescription, but nongerminomatous germ-cell tumors receive standard total dose irradiation.[53]

Because of its considerable morbidity, the value of craniospinal irradiation in very young children with nonseminomatous tumors (e.g., yolk sac tumors) is controversial.

## PARASELLAR AND SKULL BASE MENINGIOMA

Adjuvant postoperative external beam irradiation is effective treatment for parasellar meningiomas, because complete resections are usually impossible. Highly customized treatment fields, usually based on computed tomography (CT)- or MRI-guided treatment planning, are routinely used to minimize irradiation of normal tissues. Typically, the radiotherapy prescription is a dose of 54 Gy in 30 fractions of 1.8 Gy each.[54] In a series of 186 patients with meningiomas treated with megavoltage photon irradiation between 1963 and 1983, the 10-year actuarial cause-specific survival rate was 67%.[55] Radiotherapy alone resulted in improvement of neurologic performance in 12 (38%) of 32 patients with inoperable tumors. Multivariate analysis revealed that histology, extent of resection, and performance status at the time of presentation for radiotherapy were independent prognostic variables.

In a series of 115 patients with benign meningioma treated for primary or recurrent disease, 36 patients were treated by subtotal resection plus external beam irradiation, and 79 patients were treated by subtotal resection alone.[56] The progression-free survival rate for 17 patients irradiated after initial subtotal resection was 88% at 8 years, compared with 48% for a similar group of patients treated with surgery alone. Sixteen patients whose tumors were incompletely resected at the time of first recurrence were irradiated; 78% were progression free at 8 years. Only 11% of the patients treated with surgery alone were progression free at 8 years ($P = 0.001$). Twenty-five patients were irradiated with photons alone at doses of 45 to 60 Gy and at a median follow-up time of 57 months; 6 (24%) had recurrences. Eleven patients were treated with combined 10-MV photons and 160-MV protons using three-dimensional treatment planning. After 53 months, none of these patients had a recurrence.

These studies support a role for radiotherapy in the treatment of incompletely resected or inoperable meningioma of all histologic types.[55,56] Patients who undergo complete resection of the typical benign meningioma do not require adjuvant irradiation. The roles for stereotactically implanted high-activity iodine-125 seeds (i.e., brachytherapy), radiosurgery, or endocrinologic manipulation in the management of inoperable skull base meningioma are evolving, and these modalities should be considered when the indications are appropriate.[57–60]

## GLIOMA

The full histologic spectrum of gliomas, from the benign juvenile pilocytic variant to glioblastoma multiforme, is encountered in the hypothalamus; chiasmal gliomas may also invade the hypothalamus. Occasionally, oligodendroglioma, mixed tumors, and ganglioglioma may be encountered.

The management of juvenile pilocytic astrocytoma and ganglioglioma is surgical. When surgery fails, external beam radiotherapy provides highly effective adjuvant treatment. Other glial tumors usually are not amenable to total resection, and postoperative irradiation is frequently used as adjuvant treatment. In the management of 33 children with hypothalamic-chiasmatic gliomas, the median time to tumor progression was 70 months in patients who received irradiation and 30 months in those who did not ($P < 0.05$).[61] Nonirradiated patients who progressed were treated with irradiation. Clinical or radiographic improvement occurred in 11 (46%) of 24 irradiated patients. The 5- and 10-year survival rates for irradiated patients were 93% and 74%, respectively.[61]

To delay radiotherapy in very young children and to minimize the incidence of long-term complications, there is increasing interest in the initial treatment of histologically benign glial tumors with chemotherapy. In a study of 6 children with optic pathway gliomas who were treated with carboplatin at the time of progression, the median age at diagnosis was 2 years (range, 4 months to 7 years), and the interval between diagnosis and treatment with carboplatin ranged between 7 months and 6.5 years (median, 1.8 years).[62] Disease stabilization was observed in all patients, suggesting that carboplatin can arrest growth of progressive optic pathway gliomas in young children and may permit a delay in the use of radiotherapy.[62]

Among 19 children between the ages of 15 weeks and 15 years (median, 3.2 years) with chiasmal or hypothalamic gliomas who were treated with nitrosourea-based chemotherapy, 12 patients (7 juvenile pilocytic astrocytomas, 2 astrocytomas, 2 highly anaplastic astrocytomas, and 1 subependymal giant cell astrocytoma) received their chemotherapy immediately after diagnosis because of progressive symptoms.[63] Another 7 patients (all astrocytomas) received chemotherapy at the time of tumor progression. In 15 (83%) of 18 patients that could be evaluated, the tumor responded to or stabilized after chemotherapy. With a median follow-up of 79 weeks, median time to tumor progression had not been reached, and no tumor-related deaths had occurred. Improvement or stabilization of visual field function was observed in 16 patients. These results suggest that nitrosourea-based chemotherapy is useful for the initial treatment of children with chiasmal or hypothalamic gliomas and allows deferral of irradiation until such time as the tumor progresses.

## COMPLICATIONS OF BRAIN IRRADIATION

Modern megavoltage radiotherapy produces minimal acute toxicity, including temporary alopecia, mild dermatitis, and a serous otitis media if the middle ear is included in the treatment field. These acute toxic effects typically are grade 2 or less. The focus of the treatment planning process is to minimize late toxic effects, which are uncommon but can be devastating. Late toxic effects occur predominantly in tissue with a slow turnover time and reflect a combination of direct cellular and indirect vascular injury.

The factors that predict a higher rate of complications include very young age, large total dose, large fraction size, large irradiated volume of normal tissue, and underlying medical conditions. In an unselected series of 134 patients who had undergone pituitary-hypothalamic irradiation over an 18-year period, 97% of whom had been treated to 45 to 50 Gy, complications attributable to radiotherapy occurred in 7 patients (2 second malignancies, 2 auditory deteriorations, and 3 vision deteriorations), underscoring the 5% or less risk from a carefully prescribed course of radiotherapy.[64]

### ENDOCRINE COMPLICATIONS

Despite a low rate of cell proliferation in pituitary adenomas, the sequential assessment of hormone levels has demonstrated that the secretory functions of the pituitary gland are relatively susceptible to irradiation.[65] The incidence of hypopituitarism was analyzed in a group of 165 patients who underwent cranial irradiation to total doses of 37.5 to 42.5 Gy in 2.25- to 2.65-Gy fractions.[66] The analysis, which spanned a 10-year period, tested anterior pituitary function using insulin hypoglycemia or glucagon stimulation; thyrotropin-releasing hormone and luteinizing hormone–releasing hormone levels; and basal estimations of GH, prolactin, thyroid hormones, and testosterone or estradiol. Tests were repeated at 6- to 12-month intervals. Hyposecretion developed most rapidly for GH and least rapidly for thyroid-stimulating hormone; gonadotropins and

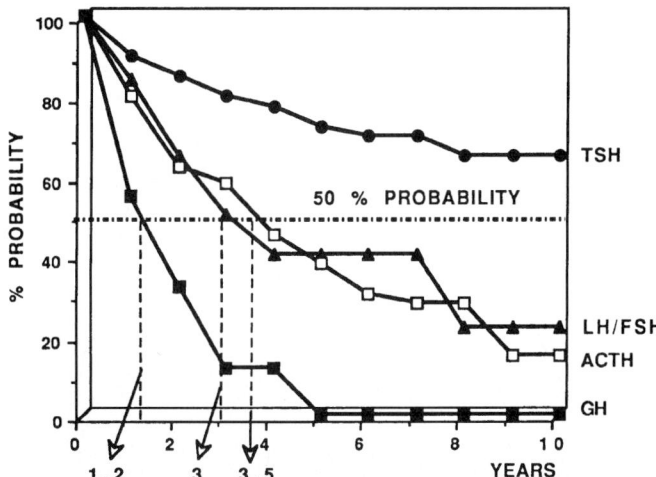

**FIGURE 22-1.** Actuarial probability of maintaining normal pituitary function. Growth hormone (*GH*) declines most rapidly, followed by luteinizing hormone (*LH*)/follicle-stimulating hormone (*FSH*) and adrenocorticotropic hormone (*ACTH*); thyroid-stimulating hormone (*TSH*) is most resistant to a decline. (Adapted from Littley MD, Shalet SM, Beardwell CG, et al. Hypopituitarism following external radiotherapy for pituitary tumors in adults. Q J Med 1989; 70:145.)

ACTH declined at an intermediate rate. The time required for 50% of patients with normal pituitary function to develop a hypofunctional pituitary was 1.2 years for GH, 3 years for luteinizing hormone and follicle-stimulating hormone (Fig. 22-1), and 3.2 years for ACTH. Almost two-thirds of patients exhibited the GH–luteinizing hormone/follicle-stimulating hormone–ACTH–thyroid-stimulating hormone sequence of hypopituitarism. In another report of 84 patients, radiotherapy resulted in local control of the majority of pituitary adenomas, but by 10 years of follow-up, the prevalence of hypopituitarism rose from 29% to 92%, suggesting that residual pituitary function is highly susceptible to long-term negation after radiotherapy. Patients should, therefore, be appropriately evaluated in follow-up and counseled regarding the almost universal need for hormone replacement after radiation.[66]

Before attributing hypopituitarism to irradiation, the clinician must consider that a large number of patients present with a compromised endocrine status before commencing radiotherapy and that the preexisting disease and the extent of tumor resection contribute significantly to this process. Additionally, radiation-induced hyperprolactinemia developed in 44% of patients; the mean prolactin rose from 227 to 369 mU/L by 2 years, but the level returned to normal in the following 2 years.[66]

## VISION SYSTEM COMPLICATIONS

Vision loss as a sequela of irradiation usually occurs within 2 years. When the literature was reviewed for reports of blindness as a complication of pituitary irradiation, only two cases of total vision loss were found when the fraction size was maintained below 2 Gy.[67] In a series of almost 500 patients with pituitary adenomas treated to a total dose of as much as 50 Gy in fraction sizes of 2 Gy or less, no optic nerve or chiasmal injury was reported.[30] A logistic regression dose-response analysis of injury to cranial nerves after proton beam radiation therapy delivered in 1.8-Gy equivalent fractions revealed that the risk of cranial nerve damage was 1% at a total dose equivalent to 60 Gy, and it increased to 5% at a 70-Gy equivalent dose.[68]

## POSTIRRADIATION BRAIN NECROSIS

Brain necrosis is an uncommon complication of cranial irradiation with modern radiotherapeutic technology, fraction size, and

total dose prescriptions. In a series of more than 650 patients, only 2 (0.3%) developed brain necrosis, and these cases were associated with the use of opposed lateral fields.[30] In the author's experience, opposed lateral fields are safe if used with very-high-energy photons (10 MV), small field sizes, fraction size no greater than 1.8 Gy, and total doses no higher than 50.4 Gy. Radiation necrosis most often occurs 9 months to 2 years after radiotherapy. The hallmarks of radiation necrosis include an elevated cerebrospinal fluid protein while glucose remains normal, a focal delta that slows on electroencephalography, and T1-weighted magnetic resonance images that show diffuse gadolinium-enhancing lesions in the optic chiasm and hypothalamus. After parasellar irradiation, patients with necrosis may present clinically with progressive vision impairment and dementia. Neurocognitive effects side effects may occur.[68a] Current treatment planning and dose prescription algorithms are aimed at maintaining the rate of clinically significant necrosis at <1%.

## VASCULAR COMPLICATIONS

Anecdotal reports have linked the occurrence of single or multiple intracranial aneurysms to irradiation for pituitary adenoma.[69] It has been suggested that postirradiation cerebral pathology—from localized to multifocal radiation necrosis and from localized to diffuse vasculopathy—is not rare in children, whose young nervous systems are particularly sensitive to ionizing radiation.[70] Of 156 patients irradiated for pituitary adenomas, 7 experienced cerebral strokes at intervals of 3.2 to 14.6 years after irradiation.[71] However, the observed incidence was not significantly greater than the expected value of 3.5 cerebral strokes ($P = 0.078$) for this population. No definitive data support the notion that irradiated patients are at a higher risk of developing strokes.

## RADIATION-INDUCED CARCINOGENESIS

To quantify the risk of second brain tumors after childhood cranial irradiation, a retrospective analysis of 305 patients treated for pituitary adenomas was performed. Four tumors, all gliomas, occurred within the radiation field after a latency period of 8 to 15 years. This group of patients had a 16 times greater relative risk of developing a malignant brain tumor than an age- and gender-adjusted population. The cumulative actuarial risk of a secondary glioma after radiation therapy was 1.7% at 10 years and 2.7% at 15 years. Meningiomas and sarcomas also have been reported to occur within the radiation field years after irradiation, including the low doses used for treatment of tinea capitis.[72]

# RADIATION TECHNIQUES

## GOALS OF RADIATION THERAPY AND CONVENTIONAL EXTERNAL BEAM TECHNIQUES

The primary goal of irradiation of tumors in the pituitary-hypothalamic region is delivery of the prescribed tumor dose with minimal exposure to critical normal surrounding structures, particularly the visual and auditory systems, brainstem, and temporal lobes, and to excessively large volumes of hypothalamus. The modern radiotherapeutic process is based on precise delineation of the target and critical structures, which is achieved using contrast-enhanced, thin-slice CT scanning. Further improvements in tumor localization are possible by correlation of CT and MRI data.[73]

The newer localization techniques can correct for the geometric distortion of MRI data sets and provide three-dimensional CT and magnetic resonance images and target volume correlation. Most patients with neuroendocrine tumors undergo the treatment planning process and the actual radiation treatments with a head immobilization device. The author's practice is to use a thermoplastic material that is molded to the patient's face and immobilized to a baseplate. The reproducibility of this device is within 2 to 3 mm on a daily basis during a conventional 5- to 6-week course of radiotherapy.

The treatment planning process itself is typically carried out at a workstation with three-dimensional capability. The objective of the treatment planning process is to evaluate the relative dose distribution to the tumor and surrounding normal tissues of a variety of field arrangements. The optimal plan is selected and is further refined by beam modulation with devices such as beam-attenuating wedges, compensators, or customized blocks. The use of two opposed lateral fields with low-energy photons is not recommended because of a slightly higher risk of temporal lobe radionecrosis. Satisfactory dose distribution generally is achieved with a three-field technique that uses two opposed lateral beams and a vertex or coronal field directed downward from the scalp to the pituitary fossa. This technique is less suitable for small tumors with minimal suprasellar extension, because the vertex field traverses a considerable amount of normal brain.

Other acceptable techniques include a four-field arrangement, which typically requires wedges in at least two fields, and the use of an arc technique. The bicoronal 110-degree arc technique with a reversing wedge filter moving in each beam is commonly used. With this setup, the linear accelerator rotates from the level of the ears superiorly to the midline, creating a 110-degree coronal arc. A similar arc is then created on the contralateral side. Although these arc fields can exhibit substantial nonuniformity of dose distribution because of the curvature of the skull, this can be corrected by using wedge filters in the field.

Similarly, an axial-oblique bilateral arc arrangement with wedges can be used if the patient's head can be flexed sufficiently to exclude the eyes from the treatment field. The author's standard practice is to generate multiple plans for each patient, evaluate the isodose distributions, and select the most appropriate treatment technique. With such refined treatment planning, the dose gradient within the tumor is typically <5%, and the dose falloff to surrounding critical structures is very sharp. An example of such an isodose distribution is presented in Figure 22-2, which illustrates an axial-oblique arc pair with 15-degree wedges.

The advent of three-dimensional treatment planning has introduced a new level of sophistication into the simulation process. Using 3-D techniques, three standard 2-D techniques (opposed-lateral two-field setup, 110-degree bilateral arcs, and a three-field technique) were compared with a single 330-degree rotational arc method (avoiding the eyes) and a four-field noncoplanar arc technique in an attempt to identify the optimal technique for minimizing exposure of normal tissues surrounding the pituitary.[74] These observations have significant practice implications. The two-field opposed-lateral technique using 6 MV photons resulted in the highest dose to the temporal lobes and, therefore, should not be used routinely. The dose to the temporal lobes could easily be reduced with this technique, simply by using a higher energy beam, such as 18 MV. The three-field technique was superior to the opposed-lateral technique in reducing temporal lobe dose. Both the bilateral arc and single 330-degree rotation technique further decreased temporal lobe dose, in comparison with the fixed two- and three-field techniques. The four-field noncoplanar arc technique yielded the lowest temporal lobe dose but also resulted in the highest lens dose.

After the treatment planning process, the exact field setup is determined during a simulation session. The patient is repositioned in the same configuration as used for the treatment-planning CT or MRI studies, and the central intersection point of the radiation fields, or isocenter, is determined using a coordinate transform system from the planning CT. The isocenter is verified with orthogonal radiographs. External reference land-

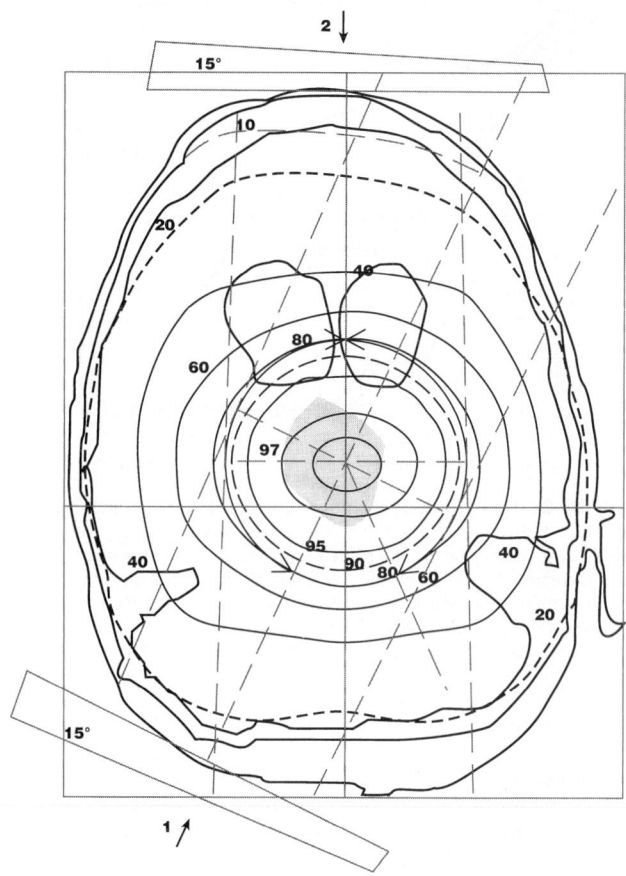

**FIGURE 22-2.** Isodose distribution using the arc technique (first setting) reveals a sharp dose falloff from the center of the target.

marks—specific points that had been selected at the time of the treatment-planning CT and that were visualized with barium strips or palates—are revisualized on the orthogonal films using radiopaque markers. These serve as external fiducial coordinate reference points that allow the transformation of CT location to orthogonal films. Because the thermoplastic mask provides rigid and reproducible immobilization, there is no need for skin marks; all necessary marks are placed directly on the mask. Daily alignment of the patient at the treatment machine is carried out using reference marks on the mask and a three-point laser system. At the first treatment session, verification portal images are obtained; in routine cases, weekly portal images are obtained. More complex setups using noncoplanar fields incorporate a portal verification imaging system.

The author uses a total dose of 45 Gy in 1.8-Gy fractions for patients with pituitary adenoma. This dose is delivered in five fractions per week over a 5-week period. Although a clear dose-response relationship has not been established, most reports suggest that 40 to 45 Gy in 1.8- to 2.25-Gy fraction sizes produces high local control rates for most pituitary microadenomas.[75] For craniopharyngioma and meningioma, the total dose is increased to 54 Gy. For low-grade glioma, the total dose is a function of the exact histologic type, the extent of residual disease, and the proximity of critical neural structures to the treatment field.

## INNOVATIVE RADIATION TECHNIQUES

### PARTICLE BEAM IRRADIATION OF THE PITUITARY GLAND

In the early 1950s, studies were performed with stereotactic-charged particles in patients with metastatic breast carcinoma to produce pituitary hormone suppression. Since then, more than 3500 patients have been treated worldwide to reduce primary pituitary tumors and to suppress pituitary function for the management of diabetic retinopathy, breast cancer, prostate cancer, and other conditions. Most of this experience was accrued at four institutions: the University of California at Berkeley, Massachusetts General Hospital, the Institute for Theoretical and Experimental Physics in Moscow, and the Institute of Nuclear Physics in St. Petersburg. The results in the management of more than 2000 patients with pituitary tumors have been excellent and are summarized in the following sections.

**Treatment of Acromegaly.** More than 200 patients with acromegaly have been treated with helium ion radiosurgery to a total dose of 30 to 50 Gy in four fractions delivered over 5 days. GH levels dropped more than two-thirds within the first year; by 4 years, the mean GH level had fallen below the normal value of 5 ng/mL. Although patients with microadenoma appeared to have an earlier and more dramatic decline, there was no difference by 4 years in GH levels between patients with microadenomas or macroadenomas.[76] Reported remission rates in acromegalic patients by 4 years have been 80% and 90%.[77,78]

**Treatment of Cushing Disease.** In a cohort of 44 patients with ACTH-secreting adenomas treated with stereotactic radiotherapy, the mean basal cortisol levels and dexamethasone suppression test results returned to normal within 1 year of treatment and remained normal during long-term follow-up. Although early failures were reported with a regimen of alternate-day irradiation, a total dose of 60 to 150 Gy in three to four fractions was successful in 40 of 42 patients. The mean ACTH level decreased from 90 pg/mL before treatment to 58 pg/mL 1 year after treatment. Plasma cortisol suppression by dexamethasone and plasma 11-deoxycortisol response to metyrapone normalized 1 year after treatment. Approximately two-thirds of 175 patients with Cushing disease treated with particle beam irradiation exhibited complete remission with restoration of clinical and laboratory parameters to normal.[77] Another 224 patients had similar responses.[78]

**Treatment of Prolactinomas.** In a cohort of 29 patients with prolactinoma treated with particle beam irradiation, 19 of 20 patients had marked decreases in their prolactin levels within 1 year. Partial or total remission of prolactin secretion was observed in 85% of patients after treatment with particle beam proton radiosurgery to doses ranging between 100 and 120 Gy.[79]

## RADIOSURGERY: PITUITARY ADENOMA AND CRANIOPHARYNGIOMA

Radiosurgery, a technique in which a single large fraction of radiation is deposited within a small intracranial target, has been used in several varieties of pituitary-hypothalamic tumors.[79a,79b] The appeal of this technique as compared with fractionated techniques includes a single fraction of radiation (as opposed to several weeks of fractionated radiotherapy), the ability to minimize exposure of surrounding normal brain tissue, and the possibility of a more rapid endocrine decline.

A major limitation to the use of stereotactic radiotherapy for the treatment of pituitary adenomas has been the low tolerance of the optic chiasm (probably <8 Gy) to radiation. Nevertheless, preliminary results using stereotactic radiosurgery have been reported. In an analysis of 77 patients, 42 (82%) of 51 patients with Cushing disease were described as cured.[80] Dose and tumor subtype may be critical factors in achieving an early response in secreting tumors. No endocrinologic response was observed with greater than 6 months follow-up in 14 patients having prolactinoma, Cushing syndrome, or Nelson syndrome after 8 to 20 Gy maximum dose, whereas significant hormonal declines occurred within 6 months in 14 acromegalic patients treated similarly.[81] In contrast, when higher doses—in the range of 25 to 60 Gy maximum—were used, endocrinologic normalization

occurred within 2 years in 36 of 37 patients, and major radiographic shrinkage occurred in all 13 patients observed for more than two years.[82] Similarly, in 27 patients treated with maximum doses of 25 to 75 Gy, 13 of 16 patients with secreting tumors experienced endocrinologic normalization or a >50% decrease within 10 months.[83] At lower maximum doses of 10 to 27 Gy, there was a significant endocrinologic response within 12 months in both prolactinomas and GH-secreting tumors, with 11 of 13 prolactinomas becoming normal within a year. Unlike the experience with fractionated radiation, a major radiographic response was observed in 15 of 21 patients with serial imaging studies.[84]

In perhaps the best comparison between single-fraction radiosurgery and fractionated radiotherapy,[85] the Mantel log-rank test was used to obtain the Kaplan-Meier estimate of time to GH normalization in 16 patients treated with radiosurgery (25 Gy minimum, 50 Gy maximum) and 40 patients treated with standard radiotherapy (40 Gy). The mean time to normalization was 1.4 years in the radiosurgery group as compared with 7.1 years in the fractionated radiotherapy group (P <0.0001).

Radiosurgical treatment has been reported for 61 patients with meningiomas (42 patients), craniopharyngiomas (4), pituitary adenomas (5), gliomas (3), and miscellaneous lesions in and around the cavernous sinus (7).[86] Long-term tumor control rates have not been analyzed, but an evaluation of toxicity revealed a 19% incidence of cranial neuropathies. Others have reported smaller series; the data are difficult to interpret because of short follow-up and patient heterogeneity. Clearly, these small experiences remain intriguing but need to be tested more rigorously through clinical trials.

## RADIOSURGERY: MENINGIOMA

Several reports indicate >90% local control rates for meningioma treated with subtotal resection and radiosurgery. These reports include parasellar meningioma as a subset of other intracranial meningiomas. One of the few reports specifically evaluating petroclival meningioma described the experience with 62 patients, of whom 39 (63%) had previously undergone surgical resection and 7 (11%) had received fractionated external beam radiation therapy.[87] The radiosurgery marginal dose ranged from 11 to 20 Gy. With a median follow-up of 37 months, the tumor volume decreased in 14 (23%), remained stable in 42 (68%), and increased in 5 patients (8%), for an overall control rate of 92%. Complications from radiosurgery were rare. Five patients (8%) developed new cranial nerve deficits within 24 months, which resolved completely in two patients within another 6 months.

In an Austrian report, 97 patients with skull base meningiomas were treated with radiosurgery; 53 had partial removal or recurrent growth and 44 underwent radiosurgery as primary treatment. The mean peripheral tumor dose was 13.8 Gy (range: 7–25 Gy). In 78 patients, follow-up scans were available. Follow-up imaging revealed decreased volume in 31 cases (40%), stabilization in 44 cases (56%), and progression in 3 cases (4%). In 8 cases, marked central tumor necrosis was seen.[88] When radiosurgery was performed on 50 patients with skull base meningiomas—5 sellar, 26 cavernous sinus, and 12 petroclival, with a mean peripheral dose of 18.0 Gy—the 1- and 2-year tumor control rates were 97% and 100%, respectively.[89]

In the largest linear-accelerator–based meningioma radiosurgery report to date, 127 patients with 155 meningiomas were observed for 31 months. The median marginal dose was 15 Gy, and 82 of the tumors were skull based. Freedom from progression was observed in 107 patients (84.3%) at a median time of 22.9 months. Actuarial tumor control for the patients with benign meningiomas was 100%, 92.9%, 89.3%, 89.3%, and 89.3% at 1, 2, 3, 4, and 5 years, respectively. Six patients (4.7%) had permanent complications attributable to the radiosurgery.[90]

Whereas the preliminary retrospective reports provide encouraging early data, many questions remain unanswered about the precise role of radiosurgery in these patients, especially in terms of patient selection, appropriate dose definition, and toxicity. As stated earlier, cranial neuropathies remain a concern. In a retrospective review, the endurance of the visual pathways and cranial nerves was evaluated after radiosurgery in 50 patients who had undergone radiosurgery for skull base tumors. With a mean follow-up of 40 months, the actuarial incidence of optic neuropathy was zero for patients who received <10 Gy, 26.7% for patients receiving <15 Gy, and 77.8% for those who received >15 Gy (P <0.0001). No neuropathy was seen in patients whose cavernous sinus cranial nerves received 5 to 30 Gy, suggesting that the visual pathways exhibit a much higher sensitivity to single-fraction radiation than do other cranial nerves.[91]

Yet another infrequent complication to consider is the development of radiation-induced edema. To evaluate the causative factors after radiosurgery, a retrospective study was performed in 34 patients. The minimum dose was 12 Gy, and the follow-up was 1 to 3 years. Edema developed preferentially in nonbasal tumors, especially those around the midline and sagittal sinus. In all but one case in which radiation-induced edema was observed, the marginal tumor dose was 18 Gy or more.[92]

## INTRACAVITARY INSTILLATION OF RADIOISOTOPES

Intracavitary instillation of isotopes such as yttrium-90, gold-198, and phosphorus-32 has been attempted for the treatment of cystic craniopharyngioma.[93] This therapeutic approach is attractive, because ~60% of craniopharyngiomas present as a single large cyst, and early refilling is frequent after drainage. Intermittent aspiration of the cyst by stereotactic puncture or drainage through an Ommaya reservoir is frequently necessary. Some reports have suggested that prognosis is worse for tumors with a large cystic component, reflecting the extensive attachment of the cyst wall to adjacent vital structures. The major advantage of intracystic radioisotope instillation is the reduced radiation dose to adjacent normal structures such as the optic chiasm, hypothalamus, and surrounding brain. Intracavitary radiotherapy can be used in patients who have previously been irradiated. The maximum range of particles from phosphorus-32 in soft tissue is ~8 mm, with more than one-half the dose absorbed within the first 1.5 mm, allowing ablation of secretory cells within the cyst wall without significant exposure of the surrounding brain to radiation. An acute inflammatory reaction has been reported after the procedure, leading some investigators to recommend the routine prophylactic use of corticosteroids. This treatment approach may be useful in the management of recurrent cystic craniopharyngioma.

Stereotactic instillation of radioisotopes into the cystic cavity of craniopharyngioma has been combined with radiosurgical treatment of the solid component.[94] With follow-up ranging from 10 to 23 years, 31 (74%) of 42 patients are alive. Moreover, the patients remained socially well adapted and maintained a high rate of full-time work and a low rate of intercurrent disease. The authors advocate a less aggressive surgical approach to craniopharyngioma.

Intracavitary yttrium-90 was used as primary treatment for 31 patients with craniopharyngioma, with an 84% overall survival rate for follow-up ranging from 2 to 80 months (median, 44 months). Visual acuity improved or stabilized in 42%, and visual fields improved in 48%.[95] Local control, defined as cyst stabilization (6 patients), reduction (12), or complete resolution (10), was observed in 28 (90%) of 31 patients. These results further support the use of intracavitary radioisotope instillation in the initial management of craniopharyngioma.

## INTERSTITIAL IMPLANTATION

The interstitial implantation of radioisotopes for the management of intracranial neoplasms has a long history, but technical difficulties have limited its widespread application in tumors of the pituitary-hypothalamic region. Permanent interstitial implantation of pituitary tumors was used in England in the 1960s. In the 1980s, the technique of transnasal transsphenoidal implantation of iodine-125 was introduced.[96] Iodine-125 implantation has the advantage of rapid dose attenuation outside the target volume, with the ability to minimize normal tissue complications. It also has several hypothetical radiobiologic advantages. Because implanting tumors in this location is complex, its role in the management of recurrent pituitary-hypothalamic tumors is based only on anecdotal reports.

## REFERENCES

1. Kleinberg DL, Noel GL, Frantz AG. Galactorrhea: a study of 235 cases, including 48 with pituitary tumors. N Engl J Med 1977; 296:589.
2. Gomez F, Reyes FI, Faiman C. Nonpuerperal galactorrhea and hyperprolactinemia: clinical findings, endocrine features and therapeutic responses in 56 cases. Am J Med 1977; 62:648.
3. Antunes JL, Housepian EM, Frantz AG, et al. Prolactin-secreting pituitary tumors. Ann Neurol 1977; 2:148.
4. Sheline GE. The role of conventional radiation therapy in the treatment of functional pituitary tumors. In: Linfoot JA, ed. Recent advances in the diagnosis and treatment of pituitary tumors. New York: Raven Press, 1979:289.
5. Frantz AG, Cogen EH, Chang H, et al. Long-term evaluation of the results of transsphenoidal surgery in radiotherapy in patients with prolactinoma. In: Chrosignani PG, Rueben BL, eds. Endocrinology of human infertility: new aspects. New York: Grune & Stratton, 1981:161.
6. Mehta AE, Reyes FL, Faiman C. Primary radiotherapy of prolactinomas. Am J Med 1987; 83:49.
7. Rush SC, Newal J. Pituitary adenoma: the efficacy of radiotherapy as the sole treatment. Int J Radiat Oncol Biol Phys 1989; 17:165.
8. Tran LM, Blount L, Horton D, et al. Radiation therapy of pituitary tumors results in 95 cases. Am J Clin Oncol 1991; 14:25.
9. Tsagarakis S, Grossman A, Plowman PN, et al. Megavoltage pituitary irradiation in the management of prolactinomas: long-term follow-up. Clin Endocrinol (Oxf) 1991; 34:399.
10. Rush S, Cooper PR. Symptom resolution, tumor control, and side effects following postoperative radiotherapy for pituitary macroadenomas. Int J Radiat Oncol Biol Phys 1997; 37:1031.
11. Sheline GE, Goldberg MB, Feldman R. Pituitary irradiation for acromegaly. Radiology 1961; 76:70.
12. McCollough WM, Markus RB, Rhoton AL, et al. Long-term follow-up of radiotherapy for pituitary adenoma: the absence of late recurrence after greater than or equal to 4500 cGy. Int J Radiat Oncol Biol Phys 1991; 21:607.
13. Eastman RC, Gorden P, Roth J. Conventional super-voltage in radiation is an effective treatment for acromegaly. J Clin Endocrinol Metab 1979; 48:931.
14. Ludecke DK, Lutz BS, Niedworok G. The choice of treatment after incomplete adenenomectomy in acromegaly: proton versus high voltage radiation. Acta Neurochir (Wien) 1989; 96:32.
15. Peacey SR, Toogood AA, Shalet SM. Hypothalamic dysfunction in "cured" acromegaly is treatment modality dependent. J Clin Endocrinol Metab 1998; 83:1682.
16. Trampe EA, Lundell G, Lax I, Werner S. External irradiational growth hormone in producing pituitary adenomas: prolactin as a marker of hypothalamic and pituitary effects. Int J Radiat Oncol Biol Phys 1991; 20:655.
17. Kramer S. Indications for, and results of, treatment of pituitary tumors by external radiation. In: Kohler PO, Ross GT, eds. Diagnosis and treatment of pituitary tumors. New York: Excerpta Medica, 1973:217.
18. Williams RA, Jacobs HS, Kurtz AB, et al. The treatment of acromegaly with special reference to transsphenoidal hypophysectomy. Q J Med 1975; 44:79.
19. Pistenma DA, Goffinet DR, Bagshaw MA, et al. Treatment of acromegaly with megavoltage radiation therapy. Int J Radiat Oncol Biol Phys 1976; 1:885.
20. Werner S, Trampe E, Palacios P, et al. Growth hormone producing pituitary adenomas with concomitant hypersecretion of prolactin are particularly sensitive to photon irradiation. Int J Radiat Oncol Biol Phys 1985; 11:1713.
21. Grigsby PW, Stokes S, Marks JE, Simpson JR. Prognostic factors and results of radiotherapy alone in the management of pituitary adenomas. Int J Radiat Oncol Biol Phys 1988; 15:1103.
22. Hughes MN, Llamas KJ, Yelland ME, et al. Pituitary adenomas: long-term results for radiotherapy alone and post-operative radiotherapy. Int J Radiat Oncol Biol Phys 1993; 27:1035.
23. Plataniotis GA, Kouvaris JR, Vlahos L, et al. Radiation therapy alone for growth hormone-producing pituitary adenomas. Acta Oncol 1998; 37:97.
24. Dohan FC, Raventos A, Boucot N, et al. Roentgen therapy in Cushing's syndrome without adrenocortical tumor. J Clin Endocrinol Metab 1957; 17:8.
25. Heuschele R, Lampe I. Pituitary irradiation for Cushing's syndrome. Radiol Clin Biol 1967; 36:27.

26. Orth DN, Liddle GW. Results of treatment in 108 patients with Cushing's syndrome. N Engl J Med 1971; 285:243.
27. Edmonds MW, Simpton WJK, Meakin JW. External irradiation of the hypophysis for Cushing's disease. C M A J 1972; 107:860.
28. Jennings AS, Liddle GW, Orth DN. Results of treating childhood Cushing's disease with pituitary irradiation. N Engl J Med 1977; 297:257.
29. Howlett TA, Plowman PN, Wass JAH, et al. Megavoltage pituitary irradiation in the management of Cushing's disease and Nelson's syndrome: long-term follow-up. Clin Endocrinol (Oxf) 1989; 31:309.
30. Sheline GE, Tyrrell B. Pituitary adenomas. In: Phillips TL, Pistenma DA, eds. Radiation oncology annual, 1983. New York: Raven Press, 1984:1.
31. Flickinger JC, Nelson PB, Martinez AJ, et al. Radiotherapy of non-functional adenomas with a pituitary gland: results with long-term follow-up. Cancer 1989; 63:2409.
32. Chang CH, Pool JL. The radiotherapy of pituitary chromophobe adenomas. Radiology 1967; 89:1005.
33. Chun M, Masko GB, Hetelekidis S. Radiotherapy in the treatment of pituitary adenomas. Int J Radiat Oncol Biol Phys 1988; 15:305.
34. Fisher BJ, Gaspar LE, Noon EB. Giant pituitary adenomas: a role of radiotherapy. Int J Radiat Oncol Biol Phys 1993; 25:677.
35. Rush SC, Kupersmith MJ, Lerch I, et al. Neuro-ophthalmological assessment of vision before and after radiation therapy alone for pituitary macroadenomas. J Neurosurg 1990; 72:594.
36. Jefferson G. Extrasellar extension of pituitary adenomas. Proc R Soc Med 1940; 33:433.
37. Laws ER. Craniopharyngiomas in children and young adults. Prog Exp Tumor Res 1987; 30:335.
38. Amacher AL. Craniopharyngioma: the controversy regarding radiotherapy. Childs Brain 1980; 6:57.
39. Brada M, Thomas DGT. Craniopharyngioma revisited. Int J Radiat Oncol Biol Phys 1993; 27:471.
40. Hoffman HJ, Silva DE, Humphries RP, et al. Aggressive surgical management of craniopharyngiomas in children. J Neurosurg 1992; 76:47.
41. Hetelekidis S, Barnes PD, Tao ML, et al. Twenty year experience in childhood craniopharyngioma. Int J Radiat Oncol Biol Phys 1993; 27:189.
42. Yasargil M, Curle M, Kis M, et al. Total removal of craniopharyngiomas: approaches and long-term results in 144 patients. J Neurosurg 1990; 73:3.
43. Weiss M, Sutton L, Marcialo V, et al. The role of radiation therapy in the management of childhood craniopharyngioma. Int J Radiat Oncol Biol Phys 1989; 17:1313.
44. Cavazzutti V, Fischer EG, Welch K, et al. Neurological and psychophysiological sequelae following different treatments of craniopharyngioma in children. J Neurosurg 1983; 59:409.
45. Rajan B, Ashley S, Gorman C, et al. Craniopharyngioma: long-term results following limited surgery and radiotherapy. Radiother Oncol 1993; 26:1.
46. Regine WF, Kramer S. Pediatric craniopharyngiomas: long-term results of combined treatment with surgery and radiation. Int J Radiat Oncol Biol Phys 1992; 24:611.
47. Flickinger JC, Lunsford LD, Singer J, et al. Megavoltage external beam irradiation of craniopharyngiomas: analysis of tumor control and morbidity. Int J Radiat Oncol Biol Phys 1990; 19:117.
48. Jose CC, Rajan B, Ashley S, et al. Radiotherapy for the treatment of recurrent craniopharyngioma. Clin Oncol (R Coll Radiol) 1992; 4:287.
49. Nakagawa K, Aoki Y, Akanuma A, et al. Radiation therapy of intracranial germ cell tumors with radiosensitivity assessment. Radiat Med 1992; 10:55.
50. Wara WW, Jenkin DT, Evans A. Tumors of the pineal and suprasellar region: Children's Cancer Study Group treatment results, 1960–1975. Cancer 1979; 43:698.
51. Linstadt D, Wara W, Edwards M, et al. Radiotherapy of primary intracranial germinomas: the case against routine craniospinal irradiation. Int J Radiat Oncol Biol Phys 1988; 15:291.
52. Hoffman HJ, Otsubo H, Hendrick EB, et al. Intracranial germ-cell tumors in children. J Neurosurg 1991; 74:545.
53. Sebag-Montefiore DJ, Douek E, Kingston JE, Plowman PN. Intracranial germ cell tumors: I. experience with platinum based chemotherapy and implications for curative chemoradiotherapy. Clin Oncol (R Coll Radiol) 1992; 4:345.
54. Schad LR, Gademann G, Knopp M, et al. Radiotherapy treatment planning of basal meningiomas: improved tumor localization by correlation of CT and MR imaging data. Radiother Oncol 1992; 25:56.
55. Glaholm J, Bloom HJ, Crow JH. The role of radiotherapy in the management of intracranial meningiomas: the Royal Marsden Hospital experience with 186 patients. Int J Radiat Oncol Biol Phys 1990; 18:755.
56. Miralbell R, Linggood RM, de la Monte S, et al. The role of radiotherapy in the treatment of subtotally resected benign meningiomas. J Neurooncol 1992; 13:157.
57. Capo H, Kupersmith MJ. Efficacy and complications of radiotherapy of anterior visual pathway tumors. Neurol Clin 1991; 9:179.
58. Kumar PP, Patil AA, Leibrock LG, et al. Brachytherapy: a viable alternative in the management of basal meningiomas. Neurosurgery 1991; 29:676.
59. Kondziolka D, Lunsford LD, Coffey RJ, Flickinger JC. Stereotactic radiosurgery of meningiomas. J Neurosurg 1991; 74:552.
60. Goodwin JW, Crowley J, Eyre HJ, et al. A phase II evaluation of tamoxifen in unresectable or refractory meningiomas: a Southwest Oncology Group study. J Neurooncol 1993; 15:75.
61. Rodriguez LA, Edwards MS, Levin VA. Management of hypothalamic gliomas in children: an analysis of 33 cases. Neurosurgery 1990; 26:242.
62. Moghrabi A, Friedman HS, Burger PC, et al. Carboplatin treatment of progressive optic pathway gliomas to delay radiotherapy. J Neurosurg 1993; 79:223.

63. Petronio J, Edwards MS, Prados M, et al. Management of chiasmal and hypothalamic gliomas of infancy and childhood with chemotherapy. J Neurosurg 1991; 74:701.
64. Fisher BJ, Gaspar LE, Noone B. Radiation therapy of pituitary adenoma: delayed sequelae. Radiology 1993; 187:843.
65. Colao A, Cerbone G, Cappabianca P, et al. Effect of surgery and radiotherapy on visual and endocrine function in nonfunctioning pituitary adenomas. J Endocrinol Invest 1998; 21:284.
66. Littley MD, Shalet SM, Beardwell CG, et al. Hypopituitarism following external radiotherapy for pituitary tumors in adults. Q J Med 1989; 70:145.
67. Millar JL, Spry NA, Lamb DS, Delahunt J. Blindness in patients after external beam irradiation for pituitary adenomas: two cases occurring after small daily fractional doses. Clin Oncol (R Coll Radiol) 1991; 13:291.
68. Urie MM, Fullerton B, Tatsuzaki H, et al. A dose-response analysis of injury to cranial nerves and/or nuclei following proton beam therapy. Int J Radiat Oncol Biol Phys 1992; 23:27.
68a. Meyers CA, Geara F, Wong PF, Morrison WH. Neurocognitive effects of therapeutic irradiation for base of skull tumors. Int J Radiat Oncol Biol Phys 2000; 46:51.
69. Matsukado Y, Hiraki T. Multiple intracranial aneurysms following radiation therapy for pituitary adenoma. Case report. Neurol Med Chir (Tokyo) 1987; 27:224.
70. Cantini R, Giorgetti W, Valleriani AM, et al. Radiation-induced cerebral lesions in childhood. Childs Nerv Syst 1989; 5:135.
71. Flickinger JC, Nelson PB, Taylor FH, Robinson A. Incidence of cerebral infarction after radiotherapy for pituitary adenoma. Cancer 1989; 63:2404.
72. Liwnicz BH, Berger TS, Liwnicz RG, Aron BS. Radiation-associated gliomas: a report of four cases and analysis of postirradiation tumors of the central nervous system. Neurosurgery 1985; 17:436.
73. Schad LR, Gademann G, Knopp M, et al. Radiotherapy treatment planning of basal meningiomas: improved tumor localization by correlation of CT and MR imaging data. Radiother Oncol 1992; 25:56.
74. Sohn JW, Dalzell JG, Suh JH, et al. Dose-volume histogram analysis of techniques for irradiating pituitary adenomas. Int J Radiat Oncol Biol Phys 1995; 32:831.
75. Zaugg M, Adaman O, Pescia R, Landolt AM. External irradiation of macroinvasive pituitary adenomas with telecobalt: a retrospective study with long-term follow-up in patients irradiated with doses mostly between 40–45 Gy. Int J Radiat Oncol Biol Phys 1995; 32:671.
76. Lawrence JH, Linfoot JA. Treatment of acromegaly, Cushing's disease and Nelson's syndrome. West J Med 1980; 133:197.
77. Kjellberg RN, Shintani A, Frantz AG. Proton beam therapy for acromegaly. N Engl J Med 1968; 278:689.
78. Minakova YEL, Kirpatovskaya LYE, Lyass FM. Proton beam therapy with pituitary tumors. Med Radiol (Mosk) 1983; 28:7.
79. Konnov B, Melnikov L, Zargarova O. Narrow proton beam therapy for intracranial lesions. In: Heikkinen E, Kiviniitty K, eds. International workshop on proton and narrow photon beam therapy. Oulu, Finland: University of Oulu, 1989:48.
79a. Friedman WA, Foote KD. Linear accelerator radiosurgery in the management of brain tumors. Ann Med 2000; 32:64.
79b. Inove HK, Kohga H, Hirato M, et al. Pituitary adenomas treated with or without gamma knife surgery: experience in 122 cases. Sterotact Funct Neurosurg 1999; 72 (suppl 1):125.
80. Rahn T, Thoren M, Werner S. Stereotactic radiosurgery in pituitary adenomas. In: Faglia G, Peck-Peccoz P, Abrosi B, eds. Pituitary adenomas: new trends in basic and clinical research. New York: Excerpta Medica, 1991:303.
81. Voges J, Sturm V, Deuss U, et al. LINAC-radiosurgery (LINAC-RS) in pituitary adenomas: preliminary results. Acta Neurochir (Wien) 1996; 65:41.
82. Ikeda H, Jokura H, Yoshimoto T. Gamma knife radiosurgery for pituitary adenomas: usefulness of combined transsphenoidal and gamma knife radiosurgery for adenomas invading the cavernous sinus. Radiat Oncol Investig 1998; 6:26.
83. Park YG, Chang JW, Kim EY, et al. Gamma knife surgery in pituitary microadenomas. Yonsei Med J 1996;37:165.
84. Yoon SC, Suh TS, Jang HS, et al. Clinical results of 24 pituitary macroadenomas with linac-based stereotactic radiosurgery. Int J Radiat Oncol Biol Phys 1998; 41:849.
85. Landolt AM, Haller D, Lomax N, et al. Stereotactic radiosurgery for recurrent surgically treated acromegaly: comparison with fractionated radiotherapy. J Neurosurg 1998; 88:1002.
86. Tishler RB, Loeffler JS, Lunsford LD, et al. Tolerance of cranial nerves of the cavernous sinus to radiosurgery. Int J Radiat Oncol Biol Phys 1993; 27:215.
87. Subach BR, Lunsford LD, Kondziolka D, et al. Management of petroclival meningiomas by stereotactic radiosurgery. Neurosurgery 1998; 42:437.
88. Pendl G, Schrottner O, Eustacchio S, et al. Stereotactic radiosurgery of skull base meningiomas. Minim Invasive Neurosurg 1997; 40:87.
89. Nicolato A, Ferraresi P, Foroni R, et al. Gamma knife radiosurgery in skull base meningiomas: preliminary experience with 50 cases. Stereotact Funct Neurosurg 1996; 66:112.
90. Hakim R, Alexander E III, Loeffler JS, et al. Results of linear accelerator-based radiosurgery for intracranial meningiomas. Neurosurgery 1998; 42:446.
91. Leber KA, Bergloff J, Pendl G. Dose-response tolerance of the visual pathways and cranial nerves of the cavernous sinus to stereotactic radiosurgery. J Neurosurg 1998; 88:43.
92. Ganz JC, Schrottner O, Pendl G. Radiation-induced edema after gamma knife treatment for meningiomas. Stereotact Funct Neurosurg 1996; 66:129.
93. Berg E, van den Berge JH, Blaauw G, et al. Intra-cavitary brachytherapy of cystic craniopharyngiomas. J Neurosurg 1992; 77:545.

94. Saaf M, Thoren M, Bergstrand CG, et al. Treatment of craniopharyngiomas—the stereotactic approach in a ten to twenty-three years' perspective. II. Psychosocial situation and pituitary function. Acta Neurochir (Wien) 1989; 99:97.

95. Van den Berge JH, Blaauw G, Breeman WA, et al. Intracavitary brachytherapy of cystic craniopharyngiomas. J Neurosurg 1992; 77:545.

96. Kumar PP, Good RR, Leibrock LG, et al. High activity iodine-125 endocurietherapy for recurrent skull base tumors. Cancer 1988; 61:1518.

# CHAPTER 23

# NEUROSURGICAL MANAGEMENT OF PITUITARY-HYPOTHALAMIC NEOPLASMS

DAVID S. BASKIN

Advances in endocrinology, neuroradiology, and microneurosurgery have revolutionized the care of patients with pituitary and hypothalamic tumors. With the development of accurate radioimmunoassays and an understanding of the interactions between the hypothalamus and the pituitary, sophisticated endocrine testing can be performed to define the nature of the dysfunction precisely. Neuroradiologic techniques, particularly high-resolution magnetic resonance imaging (MRI) and magnetic resonance angiography (MRA), enable the clinician to localize many structural abnormalities to within 1 to 2 mm. Improvements in neurosurgical technology, including the use of the operating microscope, special microinstrumentation, and minimally invasive techniques such as endoscopy and high-resolution ultrasonography enable the surgeon to secure total removal of the lesion, with preservation of endocrine function and significant lowering of morbidity and mortality.

The differential diagnosis of lesions in the sella and hypothalamic region is vast. Two common lesions are considered in this chapter: pituitary adenomas and craniopharyngiomas (see also Chaps. 11, 17, and 18).

## PITUITARY TUMORS

### CLASSIFICATION

The classic histologic designation of adenomas as chromophobic, eosinophilic, or basophilic on the basis of light microscopy is now obsolete and has been replaced by a system that classifies adenomas according to the hormones they secrete[1] (see Chap. 11). The term *chromophobe adenoma* has been replaced by terminology that designates two types of nonsecreting tumors: the *oncocytoma*, which is thought to be a neoplasm with transformed epithelial cells without endocrine potential, and the *null cell adenoma*, which may have an as yet unidentified secretory product.[2]

Patients with tumors of the pituitary present for treatment either because of *endocrinopathy* or because of *local mass effects*. Classification according to the *degree of sellar destruction* (*grade*) and *extrasellar extension* (*stage*) can assist the physician in determining the surgical prognosis[3] (Table 23-1).

### RADIOLOGIC EVALUATION

Before MRI scanning reached its present level of sophistication, the diagnosis of a pituitary tumor was based on thin-section

**TABLE 23-1.**
**Anatomic (Radiographic and Operative) Classification of Pituitary Adenomas**

**RELATIONSHIP OF ADENOMA TO SELLA AND SPHENOID SINUSES (GRADE)**

I: Sella normal or focally expanded; tumor <10 mm
II: Sella enlarged; tumor >10 mm
III: Localized perforation of sellar floor
IV: Diffuse destruction of sellar floor
V: Spread via cerebrospinal fluid or blood

**EXTRASELLAR EXTENSION (STAGE)**

*Suprasellar Extension*
O: None
A: Occupies suprasellar cistern
B: Recesses of third ventricle obliterated
C: Grossly displaced third ventricle

*Parasellar Extension*
D: Intracranial (intradural)*
E: Into or beneath cavernous sinus (extradural)

*Designate anterior ($D_1$), middle ($D_2$), or posterior ($D_3$) fossa.
(Adapted from Wilson CB. Neurosurgical management of large and invasive pituitary tumors. In: Tindall GT, Collins WF, eds. Clinical management of pituitary disorders. New York: Raven Press, 1979:335.)

polytomography of the sella, pneumoencephalography, computed tomography (CT) scanning, and bilateral carotid angiography. MRI scanning with and without gadolinium enhancement, with magnified images obtained in the axial, coronal, and sagittal planes, has made pneumoencephalography, CT scanning, and polytomography obsolete because it can more accurately diagnose pituitary adenomas in most cases (see Chap. 20). An MRI diagnosis of adenoma is based on the fact that both normal pituitary gland tissue and the adjacent cavernous sinuses enhance at a different time after the administration of intravenous paramagnetic contrast material than does an adenoma, which often enhances poorly, and usually late.[4] The timing of imaging is important. Most radiologists recommend imaging as soon as possible after the administration of the contrast. Other criteria suggestive of adenoma include a convex upper border of the pituitary gland (seen, however, in 2% of normal glands); increased height of the gland (>7 mm); lateral deviation of the pituitary stalk; and a focal area of altered attenuation relative to the normal gland, on either contrast or noncontrast studies. Usually, precise delineation between tumor and other important structures in the area can be accomplished (Fig. 23-1).

High-resolution MRI scanning with and without gadolinium enhancement is recommended for assessment of all suspected pituitary and hypothalamic lesions. Carotid angiography is reserved for those patients in whom an intrasellar aneurysm is suspected after high-quality MRI scans, including MRI angiography, have been performed. The author has not found it necessary to perform carotid angiography on the last 200 patients treated, now that high-resolution MRI angiography is available. CT scanning is no longer routinely performed in these patients. It can occasionally be helpful for patients in whom areas of hemorrhage, bony erosion, or calcification are being assessed or for patients with unusual bony sphenoid sinus anatomy, particularly those who have undergone previous transsphenoidal exploration.

### SURGICAL APPROACHES

Surgical approaches to pituitary adenomas have been described in detail.[5,6] The specific morphologic configuration of the neoplasm, rather than the endocrinologic syndrome, determines the choice between the *transcranial* and the *transsphenoidal approach*. The transsphenoidal approach is the technique of

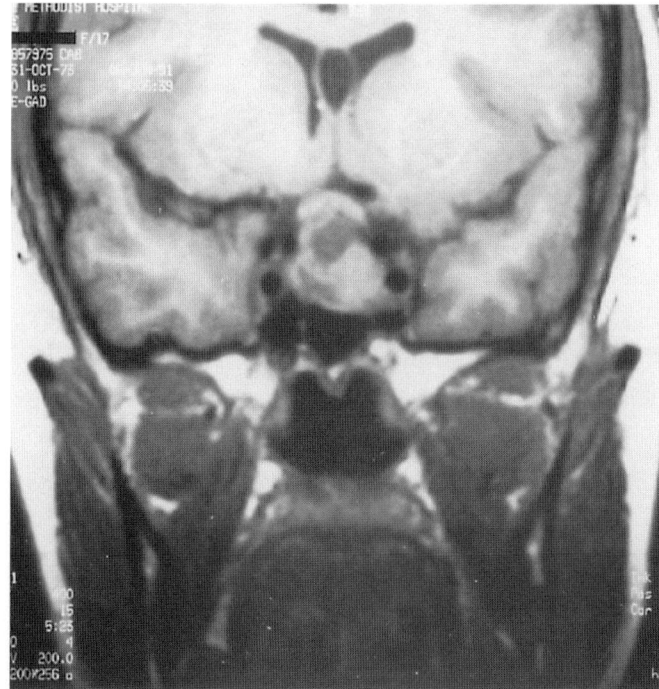

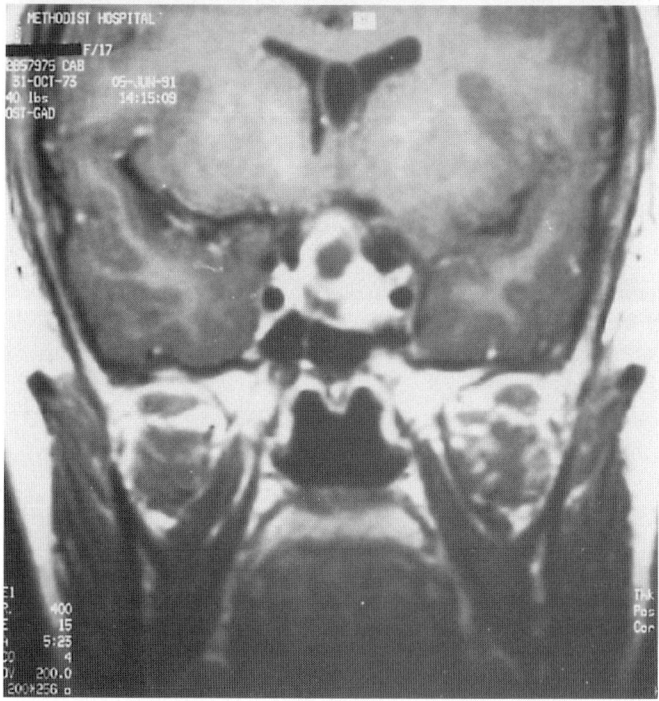

**FIGURE 23-1.** Magnetic resonance image without contrast (**A**) and with contrast (**B**) with direct coronal scans for a young woman with a pituitary macroprolactinoma. Note the low-density areas in the lesion on both scans. The surrounding tissue enhances after the administration of intravenous contrast, correlating well with the surgical finding of normal glandular tissue, rather than tumor, surrounding the low-density center. The tumor was precisely confined to the low-density area.

choice for tumors that occupy the sella, whether or not any extension has occurred into the sphenoid sinus (Figs. 23-2, 23-3, and 23-4). Tumors with vertical suprasellar extension without significant lateral extension are also well treated with this approach. The advantage of the transsphenoidal approach is that it usually allows selective excision of tumor with preservation of remaining normal pituitary gland, even when most of the sella is occupied by tumor. The approach involves no retraction of the cortex whatsoever, as opposed to the transcranial

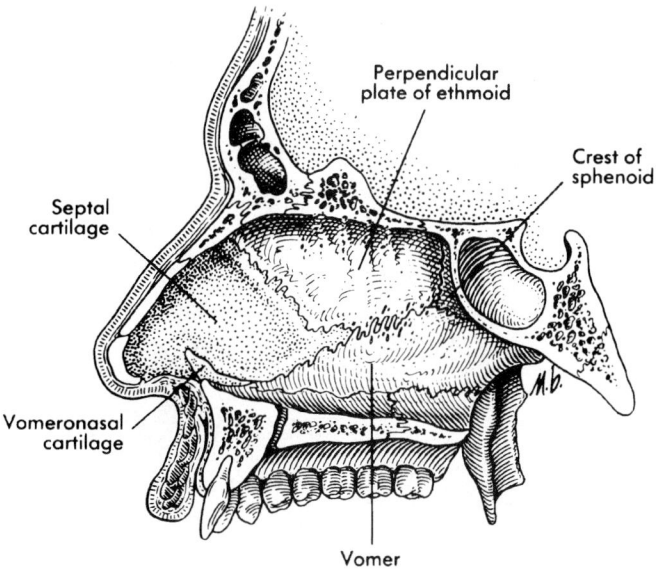

**FIGURE 23-2.** Bony and cartilaginous anatomy of the base of the skull, sphenoid sinus, and nasal areas. Note that the posterior wall of the sphenoid sinus is the floor of the sella turcica, making the transsphenoidal route uniquely suited for the removal of sellar lesions. (From Tindall GT, Barrow DL. Disorders of the pituitary. St. Louis: CV Mosby, 1986.)

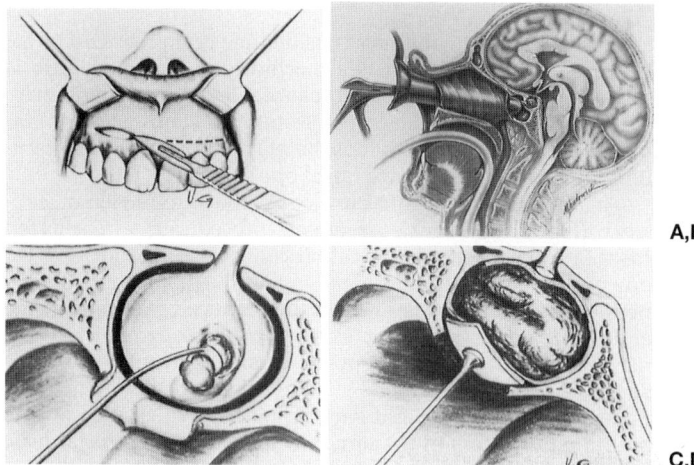

**FIGURE 23-3.** Diagrammatic summary of the transsphenoidal surgical approach. **A,** A linear incision is made from canine fossa to canine fossa. The entire surgical field lies within this incision. This provides a cosmetically favorable result because the scar is never visible externally. The nasal mucosa is dissected away from the cartilaginous and bony nasal septum. **B,** A speculum is then placed to expose the sphenoid sinus, and the posterior wall of the sphenoid sinus (the floor of the sella) is removed. Note the adenoma in the anterior aspect of the gland, where most of these lesions are located. This procedure is performed with the aid of an operating microscope, using a C-arm fluoroscope, which facilitates visualization of the area. **C,** Removal of the microadenoma. Using magnification and microdissection technique, the adenoma can be removed from the gland, sparing the normal gland tissue. **D,** Reconstitution of the sella after removal of the tumor or the gland. Fat is placed in the sella to prevent downward migration and herniation of the optic chiasm. A piece of nasal bone is then used to reconstitute the sellar floor, which later calcifies and forms new bone. (**A, C,** and **D** from Hardy J. Transsphenoidal operations on the pituitary. Codman and Shurtless, Inc. A division of Johnson and Johnson. 1983; **B** from Tindall GT, Barrow DL. Disorders of the pituitary. St. Louis, CV Mosby, 1986.)

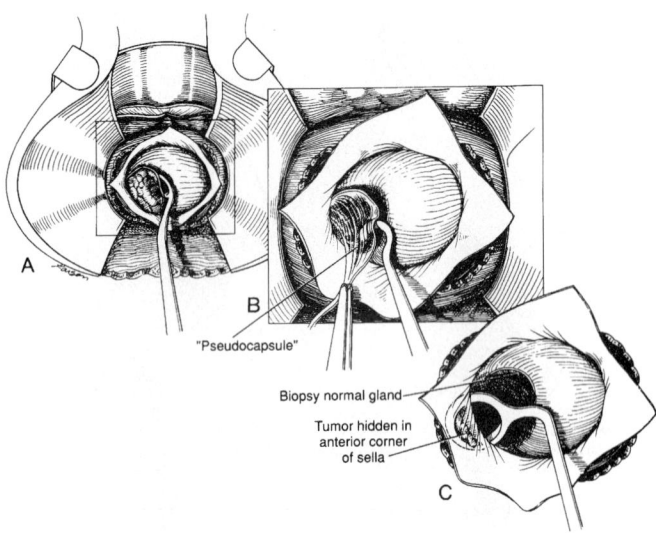

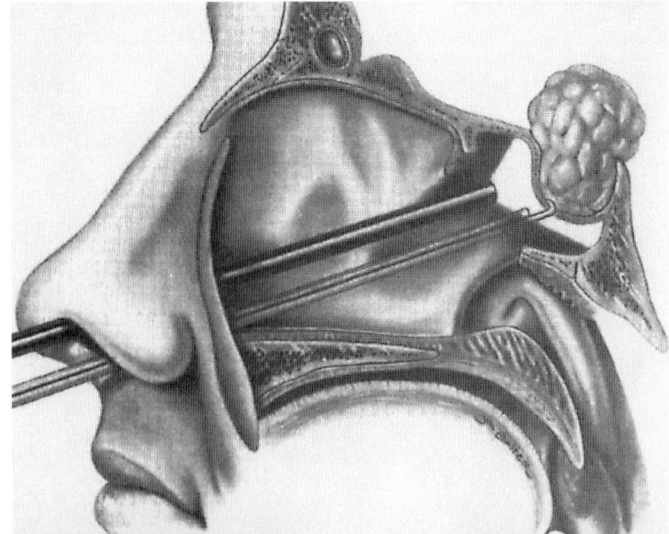

**FIGURE 23-4.** Technical details relating to removal of a microadenoma. **A,** Basic principles of tumor removal. Note the development of a plane between the tumor located laterally and the normal gland located medially. **B,** Dissection of the pseudocapsule, or the fibrous tissue surrounding the outer aspects of the tumor, which ensures a clean removal. **C,** Two important principles of microsurgical removal are illustrated. The first is to carefully inspect, or at least palpate, all hidden pockets. One can see tumor hidden in the anterior corner of the sella, which is extracted by the inserted curette. In addition, extracting the surrounding tissue for biopsy to confirm that it contains only normal gland and, therefore, that all tumor has been removed is usually advisable. (From Hardy J. Transsphenoidal approach to the sella. In: Wilson CB, ed. Neurosurgical procedures: personal approaches to classical operations. Philadelphia: Williams & Wilkins, 1992:30.)

approach, in which, at times, considerable brain retraction may be necessary. In addition, the morbidity of the procedure is exceedingly low, and it is well tolerated even by patients who would be considered unacceptable surgical candidates for craniotomy. In experienced hands, only 1% of patients with pituitary tumors require a transcranial operation.

An advance in surgical technology is the introduction of *endoscopy* (Fig. 23-5) into neurosurgical procedures.[6a] In selected cases, a transsphenoidal resection can now be performed via one nostril using the endoscope, so that the degree of invasiveness of the operation is even further reduced.[7] Moreover, the endoscope now permits the surgeon to "look around the corner" at angles that were not possible using conventional microsurgical techniques, thereby improving surgical outcome. Patients do not have nasal packing placed, which thus avoids both the numbness in the upper teeth that persists for at least several months and the nasal congestion and stuffiness that often occurs for several weeks after a standard transsphenoidal operation. In many cases, the patient can be discharged as early as the first postoperative day. A few patients have been given surgery on an outpatient basis with excellent outcomes.

Another advance is the refinement of intraoperative technology to permit the use of ultrasonography in the operating room to localize small tumors that might be otherwise difficult to visualize.[8] This is particularly useful for patients with Cushing disease for whom imaging studies have been normal or equivocal. The ultrasonic probe developed for this procedure is pencil thin and can therefore be used in the very small area that constitutes the surgical field.

## PROLACTIN-SECRETING ADENOMAS

Prolactin-secreting adenomas comprise the largest group of pituitary tumors. The behavior and relatively benign clinical

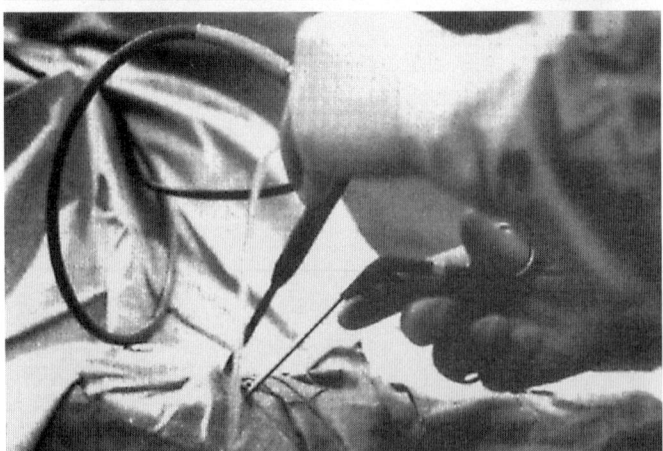

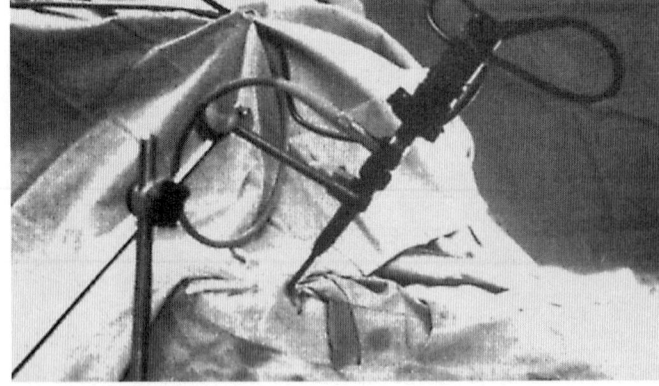

**FIGURE 23-5.** The use of the endoscope for transsphenoidal surgery. **A,** Diagram demonstrating an endoscopic endonasal approach to a sellar tumor. No septal, alar, or gingival incision is used, and no speculum or retractor is necessary. **B,** The endoscope is held in the surgeon's hand until an opening is made into the sphenoid sinus. **C,** The endoscope is mounted on a special holder, which provides the surgeon with a steady video image and frees both hands to use surgical instruments simultaneously. (From Jho HD, Carrau RL. Endoscopic endonasal transsphenoidal surgery: experience with 50 patients. J Neurosurg 1997; 87:44.)

manifestations of small prolactinomas distinguish them from the tumors that produce Cushing disease and acromegaly, two distinct endocrinopathies that are usually life-threatening. Whereas the clinical necessity of treating patients with either Cushing disease or acromegaly is clear, the indications for immediate treatment of patients harboring a small prolactin-secreting adenoma are less so (see Chaps. 13 and 21).

**TABLE 23-2.**
**Clinical Features of 121 Patients with Prolactinoma Treated by Transsphenoidal Surgery***

| Clinical Features | Female Series | | | Male Series |
| --- | --- | --- | --- | --- |
| | *Estrogen-Related Onset*[†] | *Spontaneous Onset* | *Primary Amenorrhea* | |
| Number of cases | 35 | 61 | 4 | 21 |
| Mean age at surgery (y) | 28.9 | 29 | 25.5 | 41.5 |
| Symptoms and signs | | | | |
| Amenorrhea | 32 | 48 | 4 | NA |
| Oligomenorrhea | 2 | 9 | — | NA |
| Galactorrhea | 33 | 46 | 2 | 2 |
| Headaches | 10 | 23 | — | 6 |
| Weight gain | 7 | 11 | — | 4 |
| Visual/ocular signs | — | 4 | — | 4 |
| Fatigue | 3 | 3 | — | 2 |
| Hirsutism | 1 | 3 | — | NA |
| Decreased libido/impotence | 2 | 2 | — | 9 |
| Acne | — | 1 | — | — |
| CSF leak | — | 1 | — | — |
| Multiple endocrine neoplasia, type 1 | 1 | 1 | 1 | — |
| Gynecomastia | NA | NA | NA | 5 |
| Delayed sexual development | — | — | — | 3 |
| Mean preoperative prolactin level (ng/mL) | 154 | 374 | 389 | 6130 |
| Mean tumor size (mm) | 9.4 | 10.6 | NA | NA |
| Number of macroadenomas (%) | 19 (54) | 37 (61) | 4 (100) | 20 (95) |
| Number of microadenomas (%) | 16 (46)[‡] | 24 (39)[‡] | 0 (0) | 1 (5) |

—, none; *NA*, not applicable; *CSF*, cerebrospinal fluid.
*Consecutive series including 100 females and 21 males with no prior operation or radiation therapy from 1980 to 1982.
[†]Onset following a prior pregnancy and administration of oral contraceptives.
[‡]Includes negative explorations.
(Adapted from Wilson CB. A decade of pituitary microsurgery: the Herbert Olivecrona lecture. J Neurosurg 1984; 61:814.)

## CLINICAL MANIFESTATIONS

In 1954, Forbes and colleagues[9] first reported that pituitary adenomas could produce amenorrhea and galactorrhea. However, only recently have these tumors been recognized as a frequent cause of secondary amenorrhea and galactorrhea. Among the women in one surgical series[5] (Table 23-2), 80% presented with secondary amenorrhea or galactorrhea, 10% with primary amenorrhea, and 10% with either oligomenorrhea and galactorrhea, secondary amenorrhea without galactorrhea, or secondary amenorrhea only. Among men, prolactinomas usually remain undetected until a large tumor produces either significant panhypopituitarism or compression and invasion of the parasellar structures. In the previously mentioned series,[5] only seven men had symptomatic hyperprolactinemia without abnormalities of additional pituitary hormones; either thyroid, adrenal, or gonadotropic function, or a combination of the three, was usually impaired as well. Many of these patients experience impotence early in the course of their disease, but this problem often does not lead to an investigation of the prolactin level. The author can recall seeing in his practice a 35-year-old man who received electroshock therapy for 10 years as "treatment" for his impotence; the patient presented with a prolactin level of >1000 ng/mL.

Hyperprolactinemia secondary to a pituitary adenoma has extragonadal manifestations. Recent rapid weight gain is a frequent complaint of hyperprolactinemic women and occurs with a frequency that suggests a correlation. Correction of hyperprolactinemia, either by surgery or by medical therapy, has been followed by impressive weight loss in many cases, despite no apparent change in dietary habits. Equally impressive is the incidence of emotional lability, which is often dramatically reversed after the correction of hyperprolactinemia. Studies demonstrate that the estrogen deficiency secondary to hyperprolactinemia causes bone demineralization, sometimes producing secondary complications.[10]

## LABORATORY EVALUATION

The first step in the evaluation of a patient with suspected hyperprolactinemia is to obtain a fasting serum prolactin level. The administration of thyrotropin-releasing hormone (TRH) does not consistently distinguish between functional hyperprolactinemia and actual prolactinoma[11] (see Chap. 13). In men whose basal prolactin values exceed 100 ng/mL, establishing a prolactinoma as the cause of the hyperprolactinemia is not difficult. In women, hyperprolactinemia (>200 ng/mL) almost invariably indicates a tumor. Caution must be exercised, because prolactin levels as high as 662 ng/mL have been observed to occur in nonsecreting tumors, presumably due to pronounced pressure on the pituitary stalk, which inhibits the transport of prolactin inhibitory factor to the pituitary gland.[12]

In the author's experience, the diagnosis of prolactinoma in a patient with basal prolactin levels <200 ng/mL requires radiographic identification of an intrasellar lesion. Even with unequivocal radiographic demonstration of such a lesion, transsphenoidal exploration occasionally reveals either a diffusely enlarged anterior lobe (*pituitary hyperplasia*) or a nonneoplastic intrasellar cyst, most often involving the pars intermedia. In such cases, the presence of the radiographic abnormality is usually not related to the elevated prolactin level. Patients must, therefore, be cautioned about this possibility, particularly now that the resolution of MRI imaging has become so good.

## SURGICAL DECISION MAKING

As experience with the use of the dopamine agonists (i.e., bromocriptine and cabergoline) accumulates, the indications for surgery in patients with prolactin-secreting tumors are changing. Currently, most patients who are referred for surgery have large and invasive tumors. Although a role exists for surgery in these patients, they are rarely cured by an operation alone, and usually require supplemental drug therapy, radiation therapy, or both.

The young and healthy patient with a microadenoma has an excellent chance to obtain a long-term remission with surgery; however, most are treated with medication and are never referred to a surgeon. In the author's opinion, surgery has a role in the treatment of these patients, as long as they are properly counseled regarding the options of medical and surgical therapy, and the pros and cons of either approach. Surgery provides the possibility of cure, obviating the need to take medication for years or for the patient's lifetime. Patients should be informed, however, that medical therapy is a perfectly acceptable treatment modality that in most cases provides adequate control of the tumor without the need for subsequent surgical intervention.

## VISION COMPROMISE IN PROLACTINOMA

Many would agree that medical therapy (bromocriptine or cabergoline) is indicated for the management of prolactinomas that are of sufficient size and invasiveness to produce serum prolactin levels of >600 ng/mL. (For such lesions, the cure rate with surgery, even in the most experienced hands, is only 10%.[10]) Medical therapy is usually effective for long-term control, with normalization of serum prolactin levels. On the other hand, the presence of vision loss complicates the management of such patients. This is because of the concern that such therapy either may fail or may take too long to produce sufficient reduction of tumor volume to relieve the compression of the vision system, which could result in further irreversible vision damage during the trial of medical treatment. Because vision compromise can reverse after surgical treatment, even when the compression is longstanding, some believe that vision compromise is not a contraindication to a trial of medical therapy. Substantial tumor shrinkage can occur within days, leading to improved vision.[13,14] Others,[5,6] including the author, believe that surgical intervention is indicated in these patients if they are otherwise healthy, because a risk exists of further permanent vision damage with the less rapid decompression provided by medical therapy. If medical therapy is selected for patients with vision compromise, careful monitoring of vision is essential.[13,14]

## PROLACTIN-PRODUCING MACROADENOMAS

For macroadenomas, operative removal is recommended if visual compromise is present and if the patient's overall medical condition justifies the small risks of surgical intervention. For macroadenomas without compression of the optic apparatus, surgery may be considered if the tumor is <2 cm and the prolactin level is <600 ng/mL, because surgical cure and a low complication rate are reasonable expectations under these conditions.[13] For tumors >2 cm and prolactin levels >600 ng/mL, medical therapy is recommended initially. A desire for pregnancy complicates matters, because pregnant patients with macroadenomas may develop complications related to accelerated tumor growth. Because of this concern, such patients may be candidates for surgery, even if no visual compromise is present.

## PROLACTIN-PRODUCING MICROADENOMAS

For microadenomas, opinions differ among surgeons concerning initial treatment. Some believe that all patients should be treated medically, except for those who develop unacceptable side effects to medical therapy or whose tumors are resistant to dopamine agonists.[15] Others believe that surgery should be the initial treatment for healthy patients with microadenomas and that bromocriptine, cabergoline, and irradiation should be reserved for cases of surgical failure or for those in whom the risk of surgery is high.[5,6]

Surgery does not always cure prolactin-producing microadenomas; in particular, tumors with higher prolactin levels have a greater likelihood of surgical treatment failure. Serious surgical complications can occur, although, in experienced hands, the complication rate is <1%. Still, medical management is not a perfect solution. Treatment with medication is a lifelong commitment. At effective doses, a significant number of patients have unpleasant side effects, although they may be able to tolerate these symptoms and continue to take the drug. Use of the dopamine agonist cabergoline has reduced some of the undesirable side effects associated with medical therapy. Some tumors are relatively resistant to bromocriptine, as indicated by either inadequate lowering of the prolactin levels or continued growth of the tumor. In such cases, the tumor may have a mixed population of cells, some of which are not responsive to bromocriptine (pseudoprolactinoma).[16] Well-documented cases have been seen of progressive enlargement of pituitary tumors, pituitary apoplexy, and even metastases of adenomas during bromocriptine therapy.[17–19] If nonsurgical management is chosen, a progressive elevation in prolactin levels approaching 200 ng/mL, or an enlargement of the tumor detected on MRI, represents a secondary indication for surgical intervention. Some believe that long-term treatment with medical therapy reduces the success of subsequent surgery; this effect has been reported to be due to the perivascular fibrosis that occurs when the tumor shrinks during drug treatment.[20]

## SURGICAL RESULTS

The surgical treatment of prolactin-secreting microadenomas results in a remission rate of 72% to 97%.[21–25] Remissions were experienced by 88% of patients who had preoperative prolactin levels of <100 ng/mL, whereas 50% of patients with prolactin levels of >100 ng/mL experienced remissions.[25] In long-term studies, remissions were observed in 93% of patients with microadenomas as well as in 88% of patients with tumors (regardless of size) confined to the sella or extending only moderately into the suprasellar region.[5] By contrast, remissions were seen in only 37% of female patients and in 15% of male patients who had significant extrasellar extension of tumor and were treated with surgery alone. In a series of patients receiving surgery for microprolactinoma who were followed for a mean of 70 months, only a 3% recurrence was observed.[22] Moreover, beyond 10 years after surgery, the cost of medical therapy exceeds that of surgery.

The value of surgery in treating macroadenomas without chiasmal compression in patients who have no special circumstances such as a desire for or presence of pregnancy, medication intolerance, or poor response to dopamine agonists is questionable. Surgery combined with dopamine agonists has been compared to use of dopamine agonists alone in the long-term treatment of macroprolactinomas.[23] Clearly, for this group of patients surgery did not improve the ultimate outcome for patients who responded to dopamine agonists. The situation is quite different for microadenomas. A study of surgery for microadenomas at an experienced center indicates a remission rate of 84%, even in patients followed for a median of 15.6 years. A 97% remission rate was seen in patients who received surgery using an improved microsurgical technique at a mean follow-up of 3.2 years.[24]

Even when the procedure is performed by experienced surgeons, prolactinomas have a higher recurrence rate than that of any other pituitary adenoma after primary successful surgery. Recurrence rates vary from 14% to 50% in published series[26,27] (Table 23-3). In part, the high recurrence rate may arise from the cause of the prolactin-secreting tumor, which is related to hypothalamic dysregulation. This dysregulation is unaltered after total resection of neoplasm, which leads to the growth of a new tumor rather than regrowth of residual tumor cells. In the author's experience, serum prolactin levels measured in the early postoperative period have prognostic value. A value of <5 ng/mL virtually assures a cure, whereas a prolactin level of >15

**TABLE 23-3.**
**Recurrences after Transsphenoidal Surgery for Prolactinomas: A Survey of the Recent Literature**

| Investigation | Reference | Number of Patients Followed | Follow-Up Period: Mean (Range), in Years | Recurrence Rate: Absolute (%) | Tumor Type |
|---|---|---|---|---|---|
| Faglia et al., 1983 | 67 | 39 | 3.5 (?–?) | 6/39 (15) | Microadenomas |
| Serri et al., 1983 | 27 | 24 | 6.2 (5–10) | 12/24 (50) | Microadenomas |
| Rodman et al., 1984 | 68 | 29 | 4.2 (0.9–6.7) | 5/29 (17) | Microadenomas |
| | | 5 | 3.4 (?–?) | 1/5 (20) | Microadenomas |
| Schlechte et al., 1986 | 69 | 31 | 5.0 (5–5) | 12/31 (39) | Micro- and macroadenomas |
| Maira et al., 1989 | 70 | 73 | ? (1–8) | 10/73 (14) | Micro- and macroadenomas |
| Ciccarelli et al., 1990 | 71 | 22 | 6.5 (4–9) | 8/22 (36) | Micro- and macroadenomas |
| Buchfelder et al., 1991 | 26 | 50 | 4.1 (3.3–13) | 8/50 (16) | Microadenomas |
| Turner et al., 1999 | 22 | 32 | 5.8 (0.2–16) | 1/31 (3) | Microadenomas |
| Tyrrell et al., 1999 | 24 | 121 | 15.6 (13–20) | 20/121 (16) | Micro- and macroadenomas |

(Modified from Buchfelder M, Fahlbusch R, Schott W, Honegger J. Long-term follow-up results in hormonally active pituitary adenomas after primary successful transsphenoidal surgery. Acta Neurochir 1991; Suppl 53:72.)

ng/mL is presumptive evidence of residual tumor and implies a probable regrowth.

## ACROMEGALY

By the time a patient with a growth hormone (GH)–secreting pituitary adenoma seeks the advice of a neurosurgeon, the diagnosis is usually obvious, and the need for therapy is urgent. Left untreated, this type of tumor produces metabolic disturbances with deleterious consequences and is associated with increased mortality.

The surgical options for the treatment of GH-secreting pituitary tumors include craniotomy or transsphenoidal surgery,[28,29] either for removal of the entire pituitary gland or for selective removal of adenomatous tissue. Irradiation, first used for the treatment of acromegaly in 1909, still provides an alternative to surgical intervention (see Chap. 22).

### ENDOCRINE EVALUATION

The evaluation of a patient with suspected acromegaly begins with a determination of the fasting GH level along with a complete assessment of anterior pituitary function (see Chap. 17). Additional testing should include the measurement of serum insulin-like growth factor-I (IGF-I, somatomedin C). Failure of suppression of GH levels to <3 ng/mL after oral administration of glucose can be helpful diagnostically, especially in patients with normal fasting GH or IGF-I levels who appear to be clinically symptomatic. A paradoxical rise in GH levels is seen after the intravenous administration of TRH in half of the patients. This test can be included in the preoperative evaluation.

### SURGICAL DECISION MAKING

First-line therapy for patients with acromegaly should be transsphenoidal surgery, especially if a microadenoma or small macroadenoma without invasion of the cavernous sinus is present.[30] Medical therapy as a primary treatment modality should be reserved for those in whom surgery cannot be safely undertaken.

### SURGICAL RESULTS

In the postoperative evaluation of the patient with acromegaly, the goals are a fasting GH level of <5 ng/mL and normalization of the IGF-I level. The restoration of normal GH dynamics, with a glucose-induced suppression of the serum GH level to <3 ng/mL after an oral glucose load, is desirable; however, in the author's experience, the absence of such normalization does not necessarily imply residual tumor or recurrence. Importantly, normalization of

GH and IGF-I levels may first occur as long as 3 to 6 months after surgery. Thus, if these values are elevated in the immediate postoperative period, a failure of surgery is not inevitable.

In experienced hands, transsphenoidal surgery is a highly effective treatment for the GH-secreting pituitary adenoma. Among 103 patients who underwent surgery during a 17-year period, the overall success rate of surgery alone was 82.4% in previously untreated patients, compared with 75% in patients with prior bromocriptine therapy and 63.6% in patients with prior radiation therapy.[31] Tumor stage was a strong predictor of outcome, with greater suprasellar extension associated with less favorable results. The tumor grade and the preoperative GH and IGF-I levels were also significant predictors of surgical success, with higher grade and higher preoperative serum hormonal levels associated with a less favorable outcome. In a study of 175 patients treated by transsphenoidal surgery during a period of 11 years, probability of remission after 5 years was 62.7%.[32] Moreover, the tumor size and the preoperative basal GH level correlated with outcome; a larger tumor size and a higher GH level were associated with less favorable results. Findings from the University of California in San Francisco[28,29] demonstrated long-term remission rates ranging from 80% to 90%, depending on the exact biochemical criteria used. Suprasellar extension, higher preoperative GH levels, and higher grade and stage also correlated with a less favorable outcome. Similar results were reported in another study,[33] which noted a 78% cure rate for enclosed adenomas in 100 acromegalic patients. This finding has been supported by a long-term study[34] in which patients were followed for at least 5 years. The cure rate for microadenomas was 88%. Similar results have been reported elsewhere with a long-term remission of 83%.[35]

Some authors have concluded that early postoperative GH dynamics do not clearly correlate with either long-term cure or recurrence. Thus, recurrence of acromegaly has been reported in three patients with normal postoperative GH dynamics.[36] Others have found that, although not all patients who have normal early postoperative GH levels but exhibit abnormal dynamics eventually experience relapse, such patients are nevertheless more likely to relapse than those who experience a complete biochemical remission.

Clearly the recurrence rate for acromegalic patients after selective adenomectomy is much lower than the rate that has been reported for prolactinomas. Although the reasons are not entirely clear, the suggestion has been made that most GH-secreting adenomas arise de novo in the pituitary gland and are not the result of underlying hypothalamic dysregulation. Table 23-4 summarizes reported recurrence rates seen after transsphenoidal surgery for acromegaly. Reoperation in these patients is successful in 88% if the MRI scan demonstrates a focal tumor recurrence within the sella.[37] Note that, for the endocrine-active tumors, the results of surgery are best in these circumstances.

**TABLE 23-4.**
**Recurrences after Transsphenoidal Surgery for Acromegaly: A Survey of the Recent Literature**

| Investigation | Reference | Number of Patients Followed | Follow-Up Period: Mean (Range), in Years | Recurrence Rate: Absolute (%) | Criteria of Remission |
|---|---|---|---|---|---|
| Serri et al., 1985 | 36 | 21 | 8.9 (5–11) | 3/21 (14) | Basal GH <5 ng/mL, GH (OGTT) <2.5 ng/mL |
| Roelfsema et al., 1985 | 72 | 43 | 3.3 (0.5–7) | 0/43 (0) | Basal GH <5 mU/L, GH (OGTT) ≤2.5 mU/L |
| Arafah et al., 1987 | 73 | 30 | 7.6 (?–?) | 5/30 (16) | Basal GH <5 ng/mL, GH (OGTT) <2 ng/mL |
|  |  | 21 | 8.1 (?–?) | 0/21 (0) |  |
| Artia et al., 1988 | 74 | 41 | ? (0.25–6.2) | 2/41 (5) | Basal GH <5 ng/mL, abnormal GH (TRH/LHRH) |
|  |  | 20 | ? (0.25–6.2) | 0/20 (0) | Basal GH <5 ng mL, normal GH (TRH/LHRH) |
| Grisoli et al., 1985 | 33 | 60 | ? (2–6) | 6/60 (10) | Basal GH <5 ng/mL, normal GH (TRH/LHRH) |
| Landolt et al., 1988 | 75 | 169 | 4.1 (0.1–14) | 4/169 (2) | Basal GH ≤5 ng/mL, or SmC ≤300 ng/mL |
| Losa et al., 1989 | 76 | 12 | 2.9 (0.5–3.8) | 0/12 (0) | GH (OGTT) <1 ng/mL |
| Buchfelder et al., 1991 | 77 | 61 | 6.1 (1.5–14) | 4/61 (7) | Basal GH <5 ng/mL, HG (OGTT) <2 ng/mL |
|  |  | 43 | 6.1 (1.5–14) | 0/43 (0) |  |
| Ross et al., 1988 | 29 | 174 | 6.3 (1–13.1) | 5/174 (3) | Basal GH <5 mg/mL |
| Freda et al., 1998 | 34 | 115 | 5 (1–15) | 6/115 (5) | Basal GH <5 ng/mL, GH (OGTT) <2 ng/mL, SmC <300 ng/mL |
| Abosch et al., 1998 | 78 | 129 | ? (6–24) | 9/129 (7) | Basal GH <5 ng/mL |
| Swearingen et al., 1998 | 35 | 149 | 7.8 (?–?) | 15/149 (10) | Basal GH <5 ng/mL or SmC <300 mg/mL |

*GH*, growth hormone; *OGTT*, oral glucose-tolerance test; *TRH*, thyrotropin-releasing hormone; *LHRH*, luteinizing hormone–releasing hormone; *SmC*, somatomedin C (insulin-like growth factor-I).
(Modified from Buchfelder M, Fahlbusch R, Schott W, Honegger J. Long term follow-up results in hormonally active pituitary adenomas after primary successful transsphenoidal surgery. Acta Neurochir 1991; Suppl 53:72.)

Although radiation therapy is highly effective as adjunctive treatment in patients with GH-secreting adenomas, its value as a primary therapeutic modality is less clear. A comparison of response rates indicates that the results obtained with transsphenoidal surgery are superior to those obtained with irradiation alone. Moreover, the response to transsphenoidal surgery is immediate, whereas a period of several years after the completion of radiation therapy is required before remission is obtained. During this time, the metabolic abnormalities associated with acromegaly continue unabated. Bromocriptine may be a useful adjunct in the treatment of some GH-secreting tumors, but except in rare cases, it is not effective as a primary mode of therapy[19] (see Chap. 21). The results of the International Multicenter Acromegaly Study Group using the somatostatin analog octreotide[38] do not compare favorably with the results of surgery. Although 88% of patients did show reduction in serum GH and IGF-I levels associated with clinical improvement, strict criteria used to define biochemical cure after surgery were met in less than half of the patients. Furthermore, unlike in the treatment of prolactinomas with bromocriptine, only 44% of patients treated with octreotide showed a decrease of tumor size, and only by 20%. Surgical results have been compared with octreotide treatment results in a series of patients who were first treated medically and then underwent surgery.[39] The effects on the levels of high-affinity GH–binding protein, GH, IGF-I, and insulin-like growth factor–binding protein-3 were determined. These markers did not normalize with octreotide therapy but did normalize after surgical removal of the tumor. Therefore, although somatostatin analogs hold promise for the future, they are presently indicated only as adjunctive treatment for patients for whom surgery, radiation therapy, or both have failed (see Chap. 169).

Of the therapeutic modalities available for the treatment of GH-secreting pituitary adenomas, only transsphenoidal surgery offers the unique combination of a low morbidity rate, a low incidence of postoperative hypopituitarism, and immediate remission.

## CUSHING DISEASE

Cushing disease has fascinated neurosurgeons ever since Harvey Cushing described the clinical syndrome and predicted that one cause of the disorder was a small pituitary adenoma.[40]

## ENDOCRINOLOGIC EVALUATION

No endocrinologic findings yield a 100% accuracy rate in the diagnosis of Cushing disease. The evaluation of patients suspected of having this condition should start with verification of sustained hypercortisolism. Morning and evening levels of serum cortisol as well as a 24-hour urine collection with measurement of urinary free cortisol levels should be determined. The diagnosis can generally be established by the demonstration of nonsuppressibility of corticosteroids in serum or urine after administration of low-dose dexamethasone but at least 50% suppressibility after administration of high-dose (8 mg) dexamethasone. A lack of suppression with high-dose dexamethasone can be seen in cases of macroadenoma and thus does not necessarily rule out an adrenocorticotropic hormone (ACTH)–secreting adenoma.[41] An elevated serum ACTH level in the presence of hypercortisolism provides additional supportive evidence.

Percutaneous transfemoral selective inferior petrosal venous sampling for ACTH before and after the administration of corticotropin-releasing factor has also been of help in equivocal cases.[42] If the diagnosis is uncertain and a paraneoplastic ("ectopic") source of ACTH secretion is suggested, selective venous sampling to determine a cephalic plasma ACTH gradient has proved to be diagnostically definitive.[5] When the samples have been obtained from the inferior petrosal sinus, no misleading results have been found. Sampling of another pituitary hormone along with ACTH is helpful to reduce confusion about results from various sites (see Chaps. 74, 75, and 219). Such sampling can be taken directly from the cavernous sinus, using a superselective microcatheterization technique.[43]

Experience indicates a high likelihood of cure after surgery if the serum cortisol values, measured at 8:00 a.m. and at least 24 hours after discontinuation of oral hydrocortisone therapy, either are unmeasurable or, if they are within the normal range, are shown to suppress fully during low-dose dexamethasone testing.[44–46] Some investigators have reported that Cushing disease has not recurred in any patient with undetectable serum cortisol in the early postoperative period,[44] although a normal cortisol level during this time does not necessarily imply failure. Measurement of ACTH levels during the operation does not accurately predict complete tumor resection.[47]

**TABLE 23-5.**
Surgical Outcome in Relation to Tumor Size, Extension, and Histologic Confirmation in 216 Patients with Cushing Disease

| Size and Confirmation | Grade* | Remission | Persistence | Recurrence | Total |
|---|---|---|---|---|---|
| Microadenomas | | | | | |
| Positive histologic findings | I–O | 113 | 5 | 0 | 118 |
| | I–A | 4 | 0 | 0 | 4 |
| | I–E | 1 | 6 | 4 | 11 |
| | III–O | 1 | 0 | 1 | 2 |
| Subtotal, no. (%; 95% CI) | — | 119 (88; 83–93) | 11 (8.2; 3.5–13) | 5 (3.7; 0.7–6.7) | 135 (100) |
| Negative histologic findings | I–O | 17 | 8 | 0 | 25 |
| | I–A | 2 | 0 | 0 | 2 |
| | EO | 1 | 7 | 0 | 8 |
| Subtotal, no. (%; 95% CI) | — | 20 (57; 41–73) | 15 (43; 27–59) | 0 (0; 0–10) | 35 (100) |
| Total microadenomas, no. (%; 95% CI) | | 139 (82; 76–88) | 26 (15; 10–20) | 5 (2.9; 0.4–5.4) | 170 (100) |
| Macroadenomas | | | | | |
| Positive histologic findings | II–O | 11 | 2 | 2 | 15 |
| | II–A to E | 4 | 8 | 2 | 14 |
| | III & IV | 4 | 3 | 0 | 7 |
| Subtotal, no. (%; 95% CI) | — | 19 (53; 37–69) | 13 (36; 20–52) | 4 (11; 1.2–21) | 36 (100) |
| Negative histologic findings | II–A | 2 | 0 | 0 | 2 |
| | II–E | 0 | 1 | 0 | 1 |
| Total macroadenomas, no. (%; 95% CI) | | 21 (54; 38–70) | 14 (36; 21–51) | 4 (10; 0.6–19) | 39 (100) |
| Ectopic source of ACTH | | 0 | 5 | 0 | 5 |
| Pituitary hyperplasia | | 2 | 0 | 0 | 2 |
| Series total, no. (%; 95% CI) | | 162 (75; 69–81) | 45 (21; 16–26) | 9 (4.2; 1.5–6.9) | 216 (100) |

*CI*, confidence intervals; *ACTH*, adrenocorticotropic hormone.
*Adenoma grading according to Wilson CB. Grade I: sella normal; tumor <10 mm. Grade II: sella enlarged; tumor, ≥10 mm or more. Grade III: localized perforation of sellar floor. Grade IV: diffuse destruction of sellar floor. Stage 0: no suprasellar extension. Stage A: occupies suprasellar cistern. Stage B: recesses of third ventricle obliterated. Stage C: third ventricle grossly displaced. Stage D: intracranial (intradural) extension. Stage E: into or beneath cavernous sinus (extradural).
(From Mampalam TJ, Tyrell JB, Wilson CB. Transsphenoidal microsurgical management of Cushing disease: a report of 216 cases. Ann Intern Med 1988, 109:487.)

## SURGICAL DECISION MAKING

Like patients with acromegaly, patients with Cushing disease require swift and efficacious therapeutic intervention (i.e., selective pituitary adenectomy). In adults, a total hypophysectomy is recommended if no abnormal tissue is identified during the transsphenoidal exploration. If no tumor is found in a child or in a young adult, postoperative radiation therapy or medical therapy is recommended instead of hypophysectomy. The rationale for this approach is that panhypopituitarism excludes procreation (except in rare cases after gonadotropin therapy) and that, even with synthetic GH, severe growth limitations occur in children.

## SURGICAL RESULTS

Once the pituitary has been established as the cause of a patient's hypercortisolism, the treatment of choice is transsphenoidal exploration. Patients who have negative imaging studies require careful systematic exploration of the intrasellar contents by an experienced pituitary surgeon.[48] Microadenomas secreting ACTH can often be small and located deep within the gland, so that the tumor is not immediately visualized when the dura is opened. Experience with systematic exploration, including microsurgical dissection and the ability to visualize areas that are technically difficult to reach, is essential to achieve optimal surgical results.[49] Although false localizing results that were based on sampling of the inferior petrosal sinus have been described, the author always first explores the side with the higher gradient in patients with negative imaging studies and no obvious tumor. In most cases, such exploration has been fruitful.

The results of surgical exploration in experienced hands are good, with remission rates ranging from 75% to 92%.[50–53] In a large surgical series, an 86% long-term remission rate was achieved for adenomas confined to the intrasellar compart-

ment, whereas only 46% of patients were successfully treated once the tumors had extrasellar extension.[50] Similarly, the recurrence rate was only 1.2% in those with intrasellar adenomas, whereas it was 15% in those with extrasellar adenomas. A high grade and stage of the tumor were associated with a low initial remission and a high recurrence rate. The results of this series are summarized in Table 23-5.

Unlike with other endocrine-active tumors, in 10% to 15% of patients with a preoperative diagnosis of Cushing disease, no tumor is found, even in the most experienced surgical hands. Some of these patients later are discovered to have paraneoplastic (ectopic) tumors, whereas others may be discovered to have a more obvious pituitary adenoma. Another small subgroup has an entity known as *pituitary hyperplasia* (hyperplasia of ACTH-secreting cells without obvious neoplasm). Such patients are candidates for either total hypophysectomy or, later, surgical (or medical) adrenalectomy. Pituitary irradiation also may be considered if the pituitary exploration does not reveal an adenoma. The final decision must be individualized. Young patients who desire pregnancy probably are better served by adrenalectomy, despite the risk of subsequent Nelson syndrome. Patients in whom the ability to conceive is not an issue and for whom total endocrine replacement does not produce an excessive burden are better served by total hypophysectomy.

In patients with ACTH-secreting pituitary adenomas, the recurrence rate ranges from 3% to 15% for the most experienced surgeons (Table 23-6). As with prolactin- and GH-secreting tumors, the most significant factor contributing to surgical failure is suprasellar or extrasellar extension of tumor. The absolute level of serum ACTH has not proved to be as reliable a prognostic indicator as are the prolactin or GH levels for the previously discussed adenomas. This may be attributed to variability in the values obtained with the radioimmunoassay for ACTH. Considering the morbidity and mortality associated with this disease, surgical treatment is a reasonable option.

**TABLE 23-6.**
**Recurrences after Transsphenoidal Surgery for Cushing Disease**

| Investigation | Reference | Number of Patients Followed | Follow-Up Period: Mean (Range), in Years | Recurrence Rate: Absolute (%) | Surgical Procedure |
|---|---|---|---|---|---|
| Hardy, 1982 | 79 | 63 | 1.75 (?–?) | 2/63 (3) | Selective adenomectomy or partial or total hypophysectomy |
| Nakane et al., 1987 | 53 | 86 | 3.2 (?–?) | 8/86 (9) | Selective adenomectomy |
| Derome et al., 1988 | 80 | 124 | 3.8 (0.5–17) | 19/124 (15) | Selective adenomectomy |
| Guilhaume et al., 1988 | 81 | 42 | 2.0 (0.5–7) | 6/42 (14) | Selective adenomectomy |
| Mampalam et al., 1988 | 50 | 141 | 3.9 (?–?) | 8/141 (6) | Selective adenomectomy |
| Pieters et al., 1989 | 82 | 16 | 4.0 (1.5–7.5) | 4/16 (25) | Selective adenomectomy |
| Buchfelder et al., 1991 | 77 | 66 | 8.2 (5–14) | 14/66 (21) | Selective adenomectomy |
| Mampalam et al., 1988 | 50 | 198 | 3.9 (1–7) | 9/198 (5) | Selective adenomectomy or total hypophysectomy (1 patient) |
| Knappe et al., 1996 | 83 | 55 | 1 (?–?) | (15.5) | Selective adenomectomy |
| Bochicchio et al., 1995 | 84 | 510 | 3.3 (0.5–8.6) | 65/510 (12) | Selective adenomectomy or partial or total hypophysectomy |

(Modified from Buchfelder M, Fahlbusch R, Schott W, Honegger J. Long term follow-up results in hormonally active pituitary adenomas after primary successful transsphenoidal surgery. Acta Neurochir 1991; [Suppl] 53:72.)

# CRANIOPHARYNGIOMA

Craniopharyngiomas have challenged neurologists and neurosurgeons since these tumors were first described in 1903.[54] With advances in microsurgical technique, the thought was that the total removal of these lesions would be achieved more readily. Although the results of such surgery have improved, most surgeons continue to find this procedure extremely difficult and fraught with morbidity and mortality. Subtotal removal often is the best that can be achieved, even with advanced microsurgical technology and superlative surgical skill.[55] Considerable debate exists about the surgical philosophy regarding craniopharyngioma: radical total removal in most cases versus a procedure that is more conservative and attempts to remove as much tumor as is possible, with the surgeon terminating the procedure when dense adherence to important neural or vascular structures is encountered. The problem is further complicated by the fact that adult and childhood craniopharyngiomas probably are different in this regard. That is, total removal is more easily achieved in children because the tumor has been present for a shorter period of time and, therefore, produces less inflammatory and gliotic reaction. In some cases total removal can be achieved with minimal morbidity, whereas in others such removal is not possible without damaging surrounding vital structures. Some of these neoplasms are densely adherent to the optic nerves, hypothalamus, and internal carotid artery; in these cases, an aggressive approach can produce a devastating outcome, even in the most experienced hands.

Radiation therapy plays an important adjunctive role in the treatment of this lesion. The MRI scan has been beneficial in resolving the controversy concerning which patients should undergo radiation therapy. Those patients with residual or recurrent tumor usually can be distinguished from those who have a clean surgical removal. Surgical intervention plus radiation therapy yield superior results compared with surgery alone in patients with obvious recurrent or residual tumor. This may be because the cells producing the secretions that form the cyst of this tumor have their secretory character altered by therapy. Therefore, radiation therapy is mandatory for optimal treatment of most incompletely removed tumors (see Chap. 22).

Unlike pituitary adenomas, many craniopharyngiomas require a transcranial approach because most of these lesions are located in the suprasellar region and often do not even extend into the sella. Furthermore, many of these tumors have a dense gliotic scar around them, which makes delivery of the suprasellar component of the tumor into the sella difficult without producing unacceptable damage to the suprasellar structures, including the hypothalamus and/or the optic apparatus. A transsphenoidal approach can be performed in a minority of patients, usually those in whom the tumor is confined largely to the sella. In these patients, the outcome is good, with less morbidity and frequent total tumor removal.[56,57]

## PREOPERATIVE EVALUATION

A complete assessment of the hypothalamic-pituitary axis is required for patients with a craniopharyngioma because often significant hypofunction of one or more of the pituitary hormones is present. Unlike with the pituitary adenomas, diabetes insipidus may be a presenting symptom for which patients should be evaluated.

Detailed assessment of visual function is critical. These tumors tend to be regionalized to the optic nerve, chiasm, and tract, and significant defects in visual function are common[58] (see Chap. 19).

## SURGICAL RESULTS

In 61 children with craniopharyngiomas who were treated with radiation therapy, surgery, or both, the addition of radiation therapy to surgical treatment or the use of radiation therapy alone provided a higher likelihood of regression of disease than did surgery alone.[59] In a study of 27 patients, total resection with no recurrence was achieved in 10 patients.[60] A 7% recurrence rate was reported among 144 patients, of whom 90% had complete resections.[61] Most of 173 patients treated at the Royal Marsden Hospital underwent incomplete or partial excision followed by treatment with radiation therapy.[62] The 10- and 20-year progression-free survival rates were 83% and 79%, respectively, supporting the concept that subtotal removal and radiation therapy can achieve excellent long-term tumor control and patient survival with low morbidity. In a series of 168 consecutive patients undergoing surgery between 1983 and 1997, total tumor removal was achieved in 45%.[57] Even with this modest attempt at total removal, mortality was 1.1% in primary cases and 10.5% in cases of tumor recurrence. No patient who underwent transsphenoidal surgery died. The rate of recurrence-free survival after total removal was 86% at 5 years and 81% at 10 years. The authors concluded that total tumor removal was preferable, but this was not always possible without hazardous intraoperative manipulation.

In a retrospective analysis[63] evaluating the neurologic and behavioral sequelae in 32 patients who underwent surgery, total excision was associated with greater immediate mortality and morbidity as well as a higher incidence of subsequent behavioral disability. In a series[55] of 74 patients with craniopharyngiomas treated during a 15-year period, an attempt was made to achieve a total removal. When this could not be achieved, the patients were treated with postoperative irradiation. Total removal was achieved in seven patients, six of whom have had no recurrence. However, of the entire series, 91% of treated patients were in long-term remission and fully functional.

Although total removal of a craniopharyngioma is possible in some patients in the adult population, this cannot always be achieved. A subtotal removal of tumor followed by radiation therapy has proved to be a satisfactory approach and has led to remission in most patients. With continued careful endocrine replacement therapy and monitoring, these patients can resume a normal functional life.

# ENDOCRINE-INACTIVE PITUITARY ADENOMAS

Endocrine-inactive pituitary adenomas produce clinical effects only as a direct consequence of their growth. Resulting clinical syndromes reflect either damage to the anterior pituitary gland and subsequent hypopituitarism, or compression of suprasellar and parasellar structures with development of associated neurologic deficits. Although these tumors have the necessary genetic information and cytoplasmic organelles to manufacture hormones and subunits, the products are secreted either in subclinical concentrations or in bioinactive forms; thus, these neoplasms are termed *endocrine-inactive*. When immunocytochemical and electron microscopic characteristics are taken into consideration, these tumors can be divided into null cell adenomas, oncocytomas, and glycoprotein-secreting adenomas.[64]

## CLINICAL PRESENTATION

Patients with endocrine-inactive pituitary adenomas generally present with visual impairment or hypopituitarism. Headaches are common and can be severe, relating to dural pressure. A variety of visual field defects can be seen, the most common being bitemporal hemianopia or bitemporal superior quadrantanopia. Extraocular dysfunction, related to lateral growth into the cavernous sinus, can occur, with consequent compression of the oculomotor, trochlear, or abducens nerves. Dementia and other symptoms associated with hydrocephalus also can occur when these tumors compress the third ventricular outflow, producing obstructive hydrocephalus.

These neoplasms can occasionally occur in children and adolescents. Presenting symptoms differ and usually include pubertal and growth delay and/or primary amenorrhea.[65] The tumor characteristics in this group of patients do not differ from those in the adult population.

## SURGICAL RESULTS

Surgical resection of these adenomas does not differ appreciably from the surgery for endocrine-active tumors, except that the tumors are more likely to be macroadenomas, with higher grades and stages. This results in a lower cure rate with surgery alone, which is related to size and extrasellar extension rather than to any innate biologic difference.

The goals of surgery include establishment of a diagnosis, decompression of adjacent structures, and an attempt at total surgical removal. Seventy-five percent to 80% of patients with visual compromise experience significant recovery of vision after transsphenoidal resection. Cure rates are low, ranging from 20% to 30%.[64] Although some recommend postoperative radiation therapy in all patients because of the low cure rate, others recommend careful serial MRI scanning, with radiation therapy reserved until obvious evidence is found of tumor regrowth. In support of the former approach is the reported 21% recurrence rate in a series of 126 patients with endocrine-inactive adenomas. All of these tumors except one were macroadenomas.[66]

Glycoprotein-secreting adenomas that may be associated with clinical symptoms (those producing thyroid-stimulating hormone, luteinizing hormone, and follicle-stimulating hormone) are discussed in Chapters 15, 16, and 42.

# CONCLUSION

In contrast to the results obtained in the past, the outcome of neurosurgical intervention for pituitary and hypothalamic neoplasms has improved greatly, due to both improvements in surgical technique and the use of the surgical microscope along with specialized micro-instrumentation. In most cases, the disabling and often life-threatening consequences of disease in this area can be improved significantly by surgical intervention. For pituitary adenomas, the development of the transsphenoidal technique and its subsequent refinement using endoscopy (see Fig. 23-5) and high-resolution ultrasonography has converted an operation with major morbidity and mortality into one with few complications and very good results.

# REFERENCES

1. Kovacs K, Horvath E, Ezrin E. Pituitary adenomas. Pathol Annu 1977; 2:341.
2. Kovacs K, Horvath E. Atlas of tumor pathology, series 2, fasc 21. Washington: Armed Forces Institute of Pathology, 1986.
3. Wilson CB. Neurosurgical management of large and invasive pituitary tumors. In: Tindall GT, Collins WF, eds. Clinical management of pituitary disorders. New York: Raven Press, 1979:335.
4. Davis PC, Gokhale KA, Joseph GJ, et al. Pituitary adenoma: correlation of half-dose gadolinium-enhanced MR imaging with surgical findings in 26 patients. Radiology 1991; 180:779.
5. Wilson CB. A decade of pituitary microsurgery: the Herbert Olivecrona Lecture. J Neurosurg 1984; 61:814.
6. Wilson CB. Role of surgery in the management of pituitary tumors. Neurosurg Clin North Am 1990; 1:139.
6a. Badie B, Nguyen P, Preston JK. Endoscopic-guided direct endonasal approach for pituitary surgery. Surg Neurol 2000; 53:168.
7. Jho HD, Carrau R. Endoscopic endonasal transsphenoidal surgery: experience with 50 patients. J Neurosurg 1997; 87:44.
8. Watson JC, Shawker TH, Nieman LK, et al. Localization of pituitary adenomas by using intraoperative ultrasound in patients with Cushing's disease and no demonstrable pituitary tumor on magnetic resonance imaging. J Neurosurg 1998; 89:927.
9. Forbes AP, Henneman PH, Griswold GC, Albright F. Syndrome characterized by galactorrhea, amenorrhea and low urinary FSH: comparison with acromegaly and normal lactation. J Clin Endocrinol Metab 1954; 14:265.
10. Klibanski A, Neer RM, Beitins IZ, et al. Decreased bone density in hyperprolactinemic women. N Engl J Med 1980; 303:1511.
11. Chang RJ, Keye WR Jr, Monroe SE, Jaffe RB. Prolactin-secreting pituitary adenomas in women. IV. Pituitary function in amenorrhea associated with normal or abnormal serum prolactin and sellar polytomography. J Clin Endocrinol Metab 1980; 51:830.
12. Albuquerque FC, Hinton DR, Weiss MH. Excessively high prolactin level in a patient with a nonprolactin-secreting adenoma. J Neurosurg 1998; 89:1043.
13. Weiss M. Pituitary tumors: an endocrinological and neurosurgical challenge. Clin Neurosurg 1992; 39:114.
14. Mbanya JCN, Mendelow AD, Crawford PJ, et al. Rapid resolution of visual abnormalities with medical therapy alone in patients with large prolactinomas. Br J Neurosurg 1993; 7:519.
15. Colao A, Annunziato L, Lombardi G. Treatment of prolactinomas. Ann Med 1998; 30:452.
16. Smith MV, Laws ER Jr. Magnetic resonance imaging measurements of pituitary stalk compression and deviation in patients with nonprolactin-secreting intrasellar and parasellar tumors: lack of correlation with serum prolactin levels. Neurosurgery 1994; 34:834.
17. Alhajje A, Lambert M, Crabbe J. Pituitary apoplexy in an acromegalic patient during bromocriptine therapy: case report. J Neurosurg 1985; 63:288.
18. Martin NA, Hales M, Wilson CB. Cerebellar metastasis from a prolactinoma during treatment with bromocriptine: case report. J Neurosurg 1981; 55:615.
19. Yamaji T, Ishibashi M, Kosaka K, et al. Pituitary apoplexy in acromegaly during bromocriptine therapy. Acta Endocrinol (Copenh) 1981; 98:171.
20. Landolt AM, Keller PJ, Froesch ER, Mueller J. Bromocriptine: does it jeopardize the result of later surgery for prolactinomas? Lancet 1982; 2 (8299):657.
21. Hardy J. Transsphenoidal microsurgery of prolactinomas. In: Black PM, Zervas NT, Ridgway EC, Martin JB, eds. Secretory tumors of the pituitary gland. New York: Raven Press, 1984:73.
22. Turner HE, Adams CB, Wass JA. Transsphenoidal surgery for microprolactinoma: an acceptable alternative to dopamine agonists? Eur J Endocrinol 1999; 140:43.
23. Hofle G, Gasser R, Mohsenipour I, et al. Surgery combined with dopamine agonists versus dopamine agonists alone in long-term treatment of macroprolactinoma: a retrospective study. Exp Clin Endocrinol Diabetes 1998; 106:211.
24. Tyrrell JB, Lamborn KR, Hannegan LT, et al. Transsphenoidal microsurgical therapy of prolactinomas: initial outcomes and long term results. Neurosurgery 1999; 44:254.
25. Randall RV, Laws ER, Abboud CF, et al. Transsphenoidal microsurgical treatment of prolactin-producing pituitary adenomas. Mayo Clin Proc 1983; 58:108.
26. Buchfelder M, Fahlbusch R, Schott W, Honegger J. Long-term follow-up results in hormonally active pituitary adenomas after primary successful transsphenoidal surgery. Acta Neurochirurgica 1991; (Suppl) 53:72.
27. Serri O, Rasio E, Beauregard H, et al. Recurrence of hyperprolactinemia after selective transsphenoidal adenomectomy in women with prolactinoma. N Engl J Med 1983; 309:280.
28. Baskin DS, Boggan JE, Wilson CB. Transsphenoidal microsurgical removal of growth hormone-secreting pituitary adenomas: a review of 137 cases. J Neurosurg 1982; 56:634.

29. Ross DA, Wilson CB. Results of transsphenoidal microsurgery for growth hormone–secreting pituitary adenoma in a series of 214 patients. J Neurosurg 1988; 68:854.

30. Melmed S, Jackson I, Kleinberg D. Current treatment guidelines for acromegaly. J Clin Endocrinol Metab 1998; 83:2646.

31. Tindall GT, Oyesiku NM, Watts NB, et al. Transsphenoidal adenomectomy for growth hormone-secreting pituitary adenomas in acromegaly: outcome analysis and determinants of failure. J Neurosurg 1993; 78:205.

32. Davis DH, Laws ER Jr, Ilstrup DM, et al. Results of surgical treatment for growth hormone–secreting pituitary adenomas. J Neurosurg 1993; 73:70.

33. Grisoli F, Leclercq T, Jaquet P, et al. Transsphenoidal surgery for acromegaly: long-term results in 100 patients. Surg Neurol 1985; 23:513.

34. Freda PU, Wardlaw SL, Post KD. Long term endocrinological follow-up evaluation in 115 patients who underwent transsphenoidal surgery for acromegaly. J Neurosurg 1998; 89:353.

35. Swearingen B, Barker FG II, Katznelson L, et al. Long-term mortality after transsphenoidal surgery and adjunctive therapy for acromegaly. J Clin Endocrinol Metab 1998; 83:3419.

36. Serri O, Somma M, Comtois R, et al. Acromegaly: biochemical assessment of cure after long term follow-up of transsphenoidal selective adenomectomy. J Clin Endocrinol Metab 1985; 61:1185.

37. Abe T, Ludecke DK. Recent results of secondary transnasal surgery for residual or recurring acromegaly. Neurosurgery 1998; 42:1013.

38. Vance ML, Harris AG. Long-term treatment of 189 acromegalic patients with the somatostatin analog octreotide. Arch Intern Med 1991; 151:1573.

39. Hernandez I, Soderlund D, Espinosa-de-los Monteros L, et al. Differential effects of octreotide treatment and transsphenoidal surgery on growth hormone-binding protein levels in patients with acromegaly. Neurosurg 1999; 90:647.

40. Cushing H. The basophil adenomas of the pituitary body and their clinical manifestations (pituitary basophilism). Bull Johns Hopkins Hosp 1932; 50:137.

41. Katznelson L, Bogan J, Thob J, et al. Biochemical assessment of Cushing's disease in patients with corticotroph macroadenomas. J Clin Endocrinol Metab 1998; 83:1619.

42. Oldfield EH, Chrousos GP, Schulte HM, et al. Preoperative lateralization of ACTH-secreting pituitary microadenomas by bilateral and simultaneous inferior petrosal venous sinus sampling. N Engl J Med 1985; 312:100.

43. Teramoto A, Yoshida Y, Sanno N, Nemoto S. Cavernous sinus sampling in patients with adrenocorticotrophic hormone dependent Cushing's syndrome with emphasis on inter and intracavernous adrenocorticotrophic hormone gradients. J Neurosurg 1998; 89:762.

44. Trainer PJ, Lawrie HS, Verheist J, et al. Transsphenoidal resection in Cushing's disease: undetectable serum cortisol as the definition of successful treatment. Clin Endocrinol 1993; 38:73.

45. McCance DR, Gordon DS, Fannin TF, et al. Assessment of endocrine function after transsphenoidal surgery for Cushing's disease. Clin Endocrinol 1993; 38:79.

46. Partington M, Davis D, Laws E, Scheithauer B. Pituitary adenomas in childhood and adolescence: results of transsphenoidal surgery. J Neurosurg 1994; 80:209.

47. Graham KE, Samuels MH, Raff H, Barnwell SL, Cook DM, et al. Intraoperative adrenocorticotropin levels during transsphenoidal surgery for Cushing's disease do not predict cure. J Clin Endocrinol Metab 1997; 82:1776.

48. Chandler WF, Schteingart DE, Lloyd RV, McKeever PE. Surgical treatment of Cushing's disease. J Neurosurg 1987; 66:204.

49. Chandler WF. Surgical treatment of pituitary adenomas. In: Lloyd RV, ed. Surgical pathology of the pituitary gland. Philadelphia: WB Saunders, 1993:235.

50. Mampalam TJ, Tyrrell JB, Wilson CB. Transsphenoidal microsurgery for Cushing's disease: a report of 216 cases. Ann Intern Med 1988; 109:487.

51. Tindall GT, Herring CJ, Clark RV, et al. Cushing's disease: results of transsphenoidal microsurgery with emphasis on surgical failures. J Neurosurg 1990; 72:363.

52. Fahlbusch R, Buchfelder M, Muller OA. Transsphenoidal surgery for Cushing's disease. J Royal Soc Med 1986; 79:262.

53. Nakane T, Kuwayama A, Watanabe M, et al. Long term results of transsphenoidal adenomectomy in patients with Cushing's disease. Neurosurgery 1987; 31:218.

54. Erdheim J. Zur normalen und pathologischen histologie der glandula thyreoidea parathyreoidea, und hypophysis. Beitr Path Anat Allge 1903; 33:158.

55. Baskin DS, Wilson CB. Surgical management of craniopharyngiomas: a review of 74 cases. J Neurosurg 1986; 65:22.

56. Abe T, Ludecke DK. Transnasal surgery for infradiaphragmatic craniopharyngiomas in pediatric patients. Neurosurgery 1999; 44:957.

57. Fahlbusch R, Honegger J, Paulus W, et al. Surgical treatment of craniopharyngiomas: experience with 168 patients. J Neurosurg 1999; 90:237.

58. Repka MX, Miller NR, Miller M. Visual outcome after surgical removal of craniopharyngiomas. Ophthalmology 1989; 96:195.

59. Hetelekidis S, Barnes PD, Tao ML, et al. 20-year experience in childhood craniopharyngioma. Int J Radiat Oncol Biophys 1993; 27:189.

60. Tomita T, McLone DG. Radical resections of childhood craniopharyngiomas. Pediatr Neurosurg 1993; 19:6.

61. Yasargil MG, Curcic M, Kis M, et al. Total removal of craniopharyngiomas: approaches and long-term results in 144 patients. J Neurosurg 1990; 73:3.

62. Rajan B, Ashley S, Gorman C, et al. Craniopharyngioma: long-term results following limited surgery and radiotherapy. Radiother Oncol 1993; 26:1.

63. Colangelo M, Ambrosio A, Ambrosio C. Neurological and behavioral sequelae following different approaches to craniopharyngioma: long term follow-up review and therapeutic guidelines. Childs Nerv Sys 1990; 6:379.

64. Wilson CB. Endocrine-inactive pituitary adenomas. Clin Neurosurg 1992; 38:10.

65. Abe T, Ludecke DK, Saeger W. Clinically nonsecreting pituitary adenomas in childhood and adolescence. Neurosurgery 1998; 42:744.

66. Comtois R, Beauregard H, Somma M, et al. The clinical and endocrine outcome to transsphenoidal microsurgery of nonsecreting pituitary adenoma. Cancer 1991; 68:860.

67. Faglia G, Monondo P, Travaglini P, Giovanelli MA. Influence of previous bromocriptine therapy on surgery for microprolactinoma. Lancet 1983; 1:133.

68. Rodrnan EF, Molitch ME, Post KD, et al. Long-term follow-up of transsphenoidal selective adenomectomy for prolactinoma. JAMA 1984; 252:921.

69. Schlechte JA, Sherman BM, Chapter FK, VanGilder J. Long term follow-up of women with surgically treated prolactin-secreting pituitary tumors. J Clin Endocrinol Metab 1986; 62:1296.

70. Maira G, Anile C, Do Mannis L, Barbanno A. Prolactin-secreting adenomas: surgical results and long-term follow-up. Neurosurgery 1989; 24:738.

71. Ciccarelli E, Ghigo E, Miola C, et al. Long-term follow-up of 'cured' prolactinoma patients after successful adenomectomy. Clin Endocrinol (Oxf) 1990; 32:583.

72. Roelfsema F, van Dutken H, Frolich M. Long-term results of transsphenoidal pituitary microsurgery in 60 acromegalic patients. Clin Endocrinol (Oxf) 1985; 23:555.

73. Arafah BM, Rosenzweig JL, Fenstermaker R, et al. Value of growth hormone dynamics and somatomedin C (insulin-like growth factor 1) levels in predicting the long-term benefit after transsphenoidal surgery for acromegaly. J Lab Clin Med 1987; 109:346W.

74. Artia N, Mon S, Saitoh Y, et al. Transsphenoidal surgery for acromegaly—follow-up results. In: Landolt AM, et al, eds. Progress in pituitary adenoma research. London: Pergammon Press, 1988:265.

75. Landolt AM, Illig R, Zapf J. Surgical treatment of acromegaly. In: Lamberts SWJ, ed. Sandostatin in the treatment of acromegaly. Berlin Heidelberg New York: Springer, 1988:22.

76. Lose M, Qeckter R, Schopohi J, et al. Evaluation of selective transsphenoidal adenomectomy by endocrinological testing and somatomedin-C measurement in acromegaly. J Neurosurg 1989; 70:561.

77. Buchfelder M, Brockmeier S, Fahlbusch R, et al. Recurrence following transsphenoidal surgery for acromegaly. Horm Res 1991; 35:113.

78. Abosch A, Tyrrell JB, Lamborn KR, et al. Transsphenoidal microsurgery for growth hormone-secreting pituitary adenomas: initial outcome and long-term results. J Clin Endocrinol Metab 1998; 83:3411.

79. Hardy J. Presidential address: XVII Canadian Congress of Neurological Sciences. Cushing's disease: 50 years later. Can J Neurol Sci 1982; 9:375.

80. Derome PJ, Delalande O, Bisot A, et al. Short and long term results after transsphenoidal surgery for Cushing's disease: incidence of recurrences. In: Landolt AM, et al, eds. Progress in pituitary adenoma research. London: Pergammon Press, 1988:375.

81. Gudhaume B, Bertagna X, Thomsen M, et al. Transsphenoidal pituitary surgery for the treatment of Cushing's disease: results in 64 patients and long term follow-up studies. J Clin Endocrinol Metab 1988; 66:1056.

82. Pieters GF, Hermus AR, Meijer E, et al. Predictive factors for initial cure and relapse rate after pituitary surgery for Cushing's disease. J Clin Endocrinol Metab 1989; 69:1122.

83. Knappe UJ, Ludecke DK. Transnasal microsurgery in children and adolescents with Cushing's disease. Neurosurgery 1996; 39:484.

84. Bochicchio D, Lose M, Buchfelder M. Factors influencing the immediate end late outcome of Cushing's disease treated by transsphenoidal surgery: a retrospective study by the European Cushing's Disease Survey Group. J Clin Endocrinol Metab 1995; 80:3114.

# CHAPTER 24

# PITUITARY TUMORS: OVERVIEW OF THERAPEUTIC OPTIONS

PHILIPPE CHANSON

Chapters 21, 22, and 23 discuss, respectively, medical, radiologic, and surgical therapies of pituitary tumors. This chapter reviews the current literature and draws on the author's own experience to systematically discuss and compare the different therapeutic options, their applicabilities, and their limitations. Whenever possible, an attempt has been made to categorize, in a statistical manner, response rates and recurrences.

Pituitary tumors are relatively common neoplasms of the adenohypophyseal cells; they represent ~15% of all intracranial tumors.[1,2] The prevalence of clinically recognizable pituitary adenomas is ~200 cases per million, and new cases number 15 per million per year.[3] However, asymptomatic adenomas (mostly microadenomas) are found in 6% to 20% (mean, 11%) of

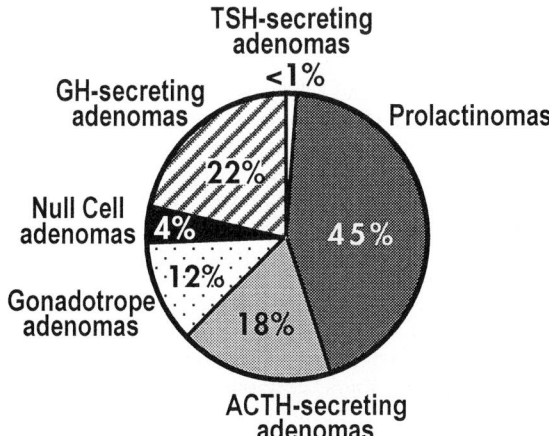

**FIGURE 24-1.** Distribution of the various types of pituitary adenomas in a surgical series. (*TSH*, thyroid-stimulating hormone; *GH*, growth hormone; *ACTH*, adrenocorticotropic hormone.) (From P. Derome, Hôpital Foch, Suresnes, France.)

presumably normal pituitary glands. This has been demonstrated by autopsy studies[4,5] and by systematic magnetic resonance imaging (MRI) studies.[6] Thus, pituitary adenomas—whether detected by clinical manifestations or by pituitary imaging that is performed for unrelated reasons (i.e., *incidentalomas*)—are becoming more frequently diagnosed. Therapeutic recommendations are based on previously reported studies that have evaluated results of various treatment strategies. However, few large comparative trials have been undertaken. Thus, therapeutic guidelines often are somewhat subjective.

An accurate classification of pituitary adenomas depends on *immunocytochemical studies* that are performed on tumoral tissue removed at surgery.[2] However, not all pituitary tumors require surgery. Thus, for practicality, and for simplification of therapeutic decisions, a *clinical classification* is used, which is based on the *presence or absence of a hypersecretion syndrome*. Generally, the clinical classification and the histopathologic classification concur (Fig. 24-1).

## CLINICAL CLASSIFICATION

1. *Growth hormone (GH)-secreting adenomas* are responsible for acromegaly. On immunocytochemical analysis, these adenomas may be purely GH-secreting or mixed (secreting GH and prolactin [PRL] or GH and α subunit).
2. *PRL-secreting adenomas* are responsible for hyperprolactinemia. Immunocytochemically, they can be composed of pure PRL-secreting adenomatous cells or can be mixed (secreting PRL and GH, or PRL and α subunit).
3. *Corticotropin-secreting adenomas* are associated with Cushing syndrome (when Cushing syndrome is due to a pituitary microadenoma, the condition is termed "Cushing disease"). On immunocytochemical analysis, these adenomatous cells stain for adrenocorticotropic hormone (ACTH), either alone or in association with other peptides.
4. *Thyrotropin* (thyroid-stimulating hormone, or TSH)–*secreting pituitary adenomas* are responsible for thyrotoxicosis, which occurs in conjunction with an inappropriate secretion of TSH. The TSH immunostaining may be isolated or may be associated with α subunit, GH, or PRL.
5. *Clinically nonfunctioning pituitary adenoma (NFPA)* is the preferred term for designating a pituitary adenoma that is not hormonally active (i.e., not associated with one of the above clinical syndromes); patients with NFPAs do not have acromegaly, a hyperprolactinemic syndrome, Cushing syndrome, or hyperthyroidism. Usually, the tumor has been found because of a tumor-mass effect or has been an inci-

dental discovery. The term "clinically NFPA" is preferred to "chromophobe" adenoma (the latter term was used before the routine use of immunocytochemical staining); it also is preferable to the term "nonsecreting adenoma," because immunocytochemical analysis has demonstrated that the majority of these lesions are, indeed, able to secrete one or more of the pituitary hormones. However, they may not be associated with increased plasma levels of the hormone (*silent adenoma*), or they may be associated with increased levels of a hormone that often does not produce a recognizable clinical hypersecretion syndrome (e.g., FSH, LH, or free α subunit). Whatever an immunocytochemical study of such surgically removed NFPA may reveal, the therapeutic management is the same.

The classification above is used in this chapter.

## GENERAL THERAPEUTIC PRINCIPLES OF SURGERY AND IRRADIATION

The management of pituitary tumors commences with a careful definition of the *location and extent* of the lesion and the *endocrinologic abnormalities*. The principles of therapy are based primarily on these factors and their clinical sequelae. Any direct effect of the mass (e.g., vision impairment) must be addressed, and any endocrinologic dysfunction must be corrected. Certain hormonal deficiencies, particularly those of cortisol or thyroid hormone, should be corrected immediately. Possible complications of therapy, most prominently hypopituitarism or tumor recurrence, can occur many years (up to 30 years) after therapy and must be carefully considered.

The choice of treatment modality is determined by several factors: (a) the need for immediate relief of a mass effect, (b) the need to relieve an endocrine abnormality, (c) the potential for obtaining long-term control, and (d) the character and frequency of possible associated morbidity.

*Surgery* and *radiotherapy* are the two main available tools for radical treatment of all types of pituitary adenomas. Their common technical characteristics and side effects are presented in this section. More specific *medical* modalities, applicable to certain types of pituitary tumors, are detailed in the later section, which deals with therapeutic options *according to the type of pituitary adenoma*.

### SURGERY

The purpose of surgery in the management of pituitary adenomas includes, according to the circumstances, the histologic confirmation of the diagnosis; the correction of tumor-mass effect; the complete excision of a microadenoma and, if possible, of a macroadenoma; and the reduction of the tumor bulk of an invasive adenoma. Whatever the immunocytochemical type, the greater the extent to which an adenoma is small, is enclosed, and is noninvasive, the better are the results of surgical removal. In most cases, either a *transsphenoidal* or a *subfrontal* transcranial approach is used[7–9] (see Chap. 23).

#### TRANSSPHENOIDAL TECHNIQUE

The transsphenoidal approach, via a sublabial incision, is now preferred by most pituitary neurosurgeons for the vast majority (>95%) of patients with pituitary tumors. This technique allows entry into the facial portion of the sphenoid sinus, through which access is gained to the pituitary fossa. Binocular surgical microscopy is coupled with fluoroscopic monitoring to obtain direct visualization of the surgical field. The transsphenoidal approach offers the capability of tumor destruction by resection, by coagulation, or by freezing. This technique is indicated for removal of a tumor that is confined to the sella turcica, removal of a tumor associated with cerebrospinal fluid (CSF) rhinorrhea or of a pituitary apoplexy, removal of a tumor with sphenoidal extension, removal of a tumor with only modest suprasellar extension, or removal of a tumor which has fluid

**TABLE 24-1.**
**Mortality and Morbidity of Transsphenoidal Surgery for Pituitary Adenomas**

| Complication | Percentage |
| --- | --- |
| **MORTALITY** | 0.6 |
| **MAJOR COMPLICATIONS** | 2.6 |
| CSF leaks | 1–8 |
| Early postoperative hemorrhage | 1 |
| Meningitis | <1 |
| Permanent diabetes insipidus | <1 |
| **TRANSIENT DIABETES INSIPIDUS** | 10 |
| **NEW DEFECT IN AT LEAST ONE PITUITARY HORMONE** | 20 |

(From Fahlbusch R, Honegger J, Buchfelder M. Surgical management of acromegaly. Endocrinol Metab Clin North Am 1992; 21:669; and from Tyrrell JB, Wilson CB. Cushing's disease. Therapy of pituitary adenomas. Endocrinol Metab Clin North Am 1994; 23:925.)

characteristics that allow the suprasellar part of the adenoma to flow down by gravity into the sellar cavity.

*Contraindications* to use of the transsphenoidal approach include the presence of dumbbell-shaped tumors with constriction at the diaphragma sellae, massive suprasellar tumors, lateral suprasellar extension of a tumor, and an incompletely pneumatized sphenoid bone. *Morbidities* include transient diabetes insipidus and, rarely, meningitis or persistent CSF rhinorrhea (Table 24-1). When a selective resection of an adenoma is possible, subsequent hypopituitarism is uncommon.

### SUBFRONTAL APPROACH

The subfrontal approach, via craniotomy, is limited to surgery for dumbbell-shaped lesions for which removal by a transsphenoidal approach is impossible; for tumors with suprasellar extension involving the chiasm; or for tumors involving the surrounding vascular structures. The disadvantages of the subfrontal approach include a high morbidity (increased duration of hospitalization, seizures, memory loss), and increased mortality resulting from damage to vital structures. Furthermore, a substantial incidence of postoperative hypopituitarism and diabetes insipidus is seen.

### COMBINED TRANSSPHENOIDAL AND SUBFRONTAL APPROACHES

When combined transsphenoidal and subfrontal approaches are used, due to the lower risk of side effects and complications with the transsphenoidal operation as compared with the subfrontal approach, transsphenoidal surgery may be used as the *primary surgery*, and the removal of a tumor remnant may be performed, when necessary, by a *subsequent* subfrontal route.

### IRRADIATION THERAPY[10–22]

Before the advent of transsphenoidal surgery, radiation therapy was extensively proposed as the primary treatment for pituitary adenomas. In general, such irradiation is external megavoltage photon therapy, although proton beams, cobalt-knife *radiosurgery*, and linear accelerator focal stereotactic technology are all potentially applicable to pituitary adenomas.[21,23,24] (The implantation of pellets containing radioactive isotopes [e.g., yttrium-90, gold-198] has been completely abandoned.)

The treatment techniques are variable. The dosage is tailored to the tumor volume, with a minimum dose being delivered to adjacent structures. Optimal techniques for conventional external radiotherapy include use of bilateral coaxial wedge fields plus a vertex field, moving arc fields, and 360° rotational fields[12,21,25] (see Chap. 22). Although the use of two bilateral opposed fields is occasionally necessary for large, asymmetric tumors, it is to be discouraged because of the large dose that is delivered to the temporal lobes. Modern radiotherapy simulator facilities together with current generation computed tomography (CT) or MRI scanning allow the

fields to be accurately molded around the tumor volume (*conformational irradiation*). The day-to-day reproducibility of the field setup should be within 2.0 mm. Optimum doses are based on evidence that doses <40 Gy provide a lower probability of tumor control; doses >50 Gy or fractions >2 Gy per day are associated with higher complication rates, including injury to the optic nerves or chiasm, and hypopituitarism. Thus, a dose of 50±5 Gy is advisable. If the bulk of the tumor is completely removed surgically, leaving only a minimum residue, and if the patient is young, 45 to 50 Gy is advisable. However, if a large residual lesion is present after surgical resection, if recurrent tumor is found, or if significant suprasellar extension is present, a higher dose (50 to 55 Gy depending on tumor bulk) is recommended.[12,21,25] As is the case with surgery, radiotherapy must be performed by skilled radiotherapists who have accumulated considerable experience in pituitary irradiation.

The major problem after pituitary irradiation (particularly when used as an adjunct to surgery) is the development of partial hypopituitarism or panhypopituitarism. Panhypopituitarism develops in approximately half of patients.[13] The variably quoted figures are 30% to 45% for ACTH deficiency, 40% to 50% for gonadotropin deficiency, and 5% to 20% for TSH deficiency.[12–14] The prevalence of deficiencies increases with the duration of follow-up: 100% of patients are GH deficient, 96% are gonadotropin deficient, 84% are ACTH deficient, and 49% are TSH deficient after a mean follow-up of 8 years.[16] Hypothalamic-pituitary dysfunction may take up to 20 years to develop.[20] The sensitivity of the hypothalamus and pituitary to the effects of radiation is well illustrated by the very frequent occurrence of endocrine dysfunction that is observed in patients irradiated for nasopharyngeal, extracranial, or primary brain tumors, even though these lesions were anatomically distinct from the hypothalamic-pituitary region.[19] Accordingly, prolonged and repeated assessment of pituitary function is mandatory after irradiation therapy. This should permit a precise detection of pituitary deficiencies and the selection of appropriate replacement therapy. Nevertheless, one should emphasize that hormonal side effects of irradiation therapy, if diagnosed early, are easily managed.

Other disadvantages of radiotherapy include a delayed therapeutic benefit for patients who have hormonally active tumors, irradiation-induced optic neuropathy, cortical injury, and, rarely, irradiation-induced malignancies (e.g., meningioma, astrocytoma).[15,26]

The term "radiosurgery" is applied to high-precision localized irradiation, given in one session. The "gamma knife" is one of these techniques and uses cobalt sources arranged in a hemisphere and focused onto a central target. High-precision stereotactic radiosurgery may also be delivered by adjusted linear accelerators. The aim of radiosurgery is to deliver a high dose of irradiation that is more localized than would be achieved with conventional radiotherapy. However, this is possible only for relatively small adenomas (<3–4 cm in diameter) and when the margins of the tumor are distant by >5 mm from the optic chiasm or optic nerves (due to the risk of irradiation-induced optic neuropathy that causes visual impairment). The long-term results of radiosurgery on hypersecretion, as on subsequent tumor growth, are presently unknown[27] (also see Chap. 22).

## THERAPEUTIC OPTIONS AND RESULTS BY TYPE OF PITUITARY ADENOMA

The recommendations for treatment of the different types of adenomas are summarized in Table 24-2.

### GROWTH HORMONE–SECRETING PITUITARY ADENOMAS

#### THERAPEUTIC OPTIONS

**Surgery and Radiotherapy.**   Surgery and radiotherapy, as previously summarized, are commonly used in the treatment of acromegaly.

**TABLE 24-2.**
**Multidisciplinary Treatment Decisions Based on Tumor Type in Pituitary Adenomas**

| | Surgery | | Chemotherapy | | Radiation Therapy |
|---|---|---|---|---|---|
| **PRL-SECRETING ADENOMAS** | | | | | |
| Microadenoma | TSS | or | DA agonists* | | NR |
| Macroadenoma | ** | | DA agonists | | ** |
| **GH-SECRETING ADENOMAS** | | | | | |
| Microadenoma | TSS | | | | |
| Macroadenoma | TSS | and/or | Somatostatin analogs‡ | and/or | ART‡ |
| **ACTH-SECRETING ADENOMAS** | | | | | |
| Microadenoma | TSS | | Mitotane§ | and/or | ART§ |
| Macroadenoma | TSS | and | Mitotane | and | ART |
| **CLINICALLY NFPA** | | | | | |
| Microadenoma | TSS | | | | |
| Macroadenoma | TSS | | | and | ART¶ |

*PRL*, prolactin; *TSS*, transsphenoidal surgery; *DA*, dopamine; *NR*, not recommended; *GH*, growth hormone; *ACTH*, adrenocorticotropic hormone; *ART*, adjuvant radiotherapy; *NFPA*, nonfunctioning pituitary adenoma.
*DA agonists, either as first-line therapy or, in case of persistent hyperprolactinemia, after surgery.
**TSS not recommended as first-line treatment. May be proposed in case of resistance to DA agonists, often followed by radiation therapy.
‡Somatostatin analogs and/or radiation therapy are proposed when surgery has failed to cure GH hypersecretion.
§Mitotane, either alone or in combination with radiation therapy, is proposed when surgery has failed to cure Cushing disease.
¶ART is proposed in cases of invasive tumor postoperative remnant.

**Medical Treatment.** *Bromocriptine and other dopamine agonists* are able to improve symptoms of acromegaly in a few patients and to decrease GH secretion.[28,29]

*Somatostatin*, the hypothalamic GH-release inhibitory factor and its analogs, SMS 201-995 (octreotide) and BIM 23014 (lanreotide), are able to reduce GH secretion. The native somatostatin peptide has a half-life that is too short for it to be administered easily. However, octreotide, given subcutaneously three times daily, has been shown to control GH hypersecretion and to decrease tumor volume in a significant proportion of patients with acromegaly with relatively few side effects.[30–36] The availability of a long-acting form of octreotide allows once-monthly intramuscular injections with the same efficacy.[37] Another somatostatin analog, lanreotide, when encapsulated in microspheres, has a prolonged release; it has proved to be effective in lowering levels of GH and insulin-like growth factor-I (IGF-I), and often in decreasing the tumor mass of acromegalic patients, in a manner comparable to that of octreotide.[38–41] The side effects of somatostatin analogs are benign. Digestive problems (i.e., abdominal cramps, diarrhea, flatulence) are minor and most often transitory. Cholelithiasis occurs in 10% to 55% of patients, with the incidence related to the duration of the study.[30,33,34,36] Generally, it is asymptomatic and is treated conservatively. Despite the reduction in insulin secretion due to the use of somatostatin analogs, glucose-tolerance alterations are of minor significance. Somatostatin analogs are very expensive drugs and need to be given for the remainder of life.

Importantly, *scintigraphy* after administration of labeled octreotide (*somatostatin-receptor scintigraphy*) allows for the visualization of pituitary tumors.[42] The resulting images are thought to reflect the concentration of the somatostatin receptors that are present at the surface of the tumor cells. However, scintigraphic findings are poor predictors of long-term results of treatment with somatostatin analog, regardless of the type of pituitary adenoma[43] (also see Chap. 169).

### CRITERIA OF CURE OF ACROMEGALY

The results of the various modes of therapy for acromegaly should be analyzed according to stringent criteria. Currently, "cure" (or good control) of acromegaly is defined by plasma GH levels: the mean of sequential sampling or the nadir after oral glucose administration should be <2.5 µg/L and the IGF-I level should be normal.[44,45] Indeed, when these goals are achieved, the life expectancy of patients with acromegaly seems comparable to that of the general population.[46–51] In the future, even more stringent criteria (nadir GH after oral glucose administration of <1 µg/L, and age- and sex-normalized IGF-I levels without clinical indications of activity) will probably be proposed for defining good therapeutic control of acromegaly.[52] In the interim, the following section, using the currently accepted criteria for good control (plasma GH of <2.5 µg/L and normal IGF-I level), compares the effects of the different treatments as indicated by several studies.

### RESULTS OF TREATMENT

**Transsphenoidal Surgery.** According to the stringent criteria indicated above, 42% to 62% of patients can be considered to have their disease "well controlled" by surgery alone.[8,45,48,50,53–58] (Table 24-3). The results depend on the size of the tumor: surgery is able to cure 61% to 91% of patients with microadenomas and 26% to 60% of those with macroadenomas. When the macroadenoma is very large, or when parasellar or sphenoid sinus invasion has occurred, the cure rate decreases to 17% and 40%, respectively.[8] Also, the success rate of surgery in patients with acromegaly varies according to preoperative GH levels: surgical treatment is successful in ~70% of patients with preoperative GH levels of <10 µg/L, 43% to 55% of those with GH levels of 10 to 50 µg/L, and 18% to 40% of those with GH levels of >50 µg/L.[8,54] The relapse rate after surgical cure is <3%.[53,54,59,60] (also see Chaps. 12 and 23).

**Irradiation Therapy.** Irradiation therapy is able to decrease GH levels in a large proportion of patients. Mean plasma GH levels of <5 µg/L are obtained in ~50% of patients (40% to 80%, depending on the length of follow-up).[18,22,61–66] However, when more stringent criteria for cure (as stated earlier) are applied, radiation therapy leads to cure of the disease in only 5% to 38% of the cases after a median follow-up of ~7 years [22,65,66] (Table 24-4). Irradiation is almost always followed by hypopituitarism, however, and the full impact on GH hypersecretion is delayed for many years. Preliminary results with *radiosurgery* are now available, but the follow-up is short. In one study,[67] at 20 months, 20% of patients had "normalized" GH and IGF-I levels after radiosurgery, and the mean delay for "normalization" of hormonal parameters was reduced (1.4 years as

**TABLE 24-3.**
**Results of Transsphenoidal Surgery for Treatment of Acromegaly with Stringent Criteria of Cure**

| Author (Year) | Reference | Type of Adenoma | N | Patients with GH <2.5 µg/L | Patients with GH <2.5 µg/L and Normal IGF-I |
|---|---|---|---|---|---|
| Roelfsema et al. (1985) | 53 | Microadenoma | 9 | 6 (66%) | |
| | | Macroadenoma | 51 | 31 (60%) | |
| | | TOTAL | 60 | 37 (62%) | |
| Fahlbusch et al. (1992) | 8 | Microadenoma | 74 | 53 (72%) | |
| | | Macroadenoma | 170 | 73 (43%) | |
| | | TOTAL | 244 | 126 (51%) | |
| Yamada et al. (1996) | 55 | TOTAL | 61 | | 34 (56%) |
| Sheaves et al. (1996) | 54 | Microadenoma | 44 | 27 (61%) | |
| | | Macroadenoma | 56 | 15 (26%) | |
| | | TOTAL | 100 | 42 (42%) | |
| Colao et al. (1997) | 57 | TOTAL | 86 | | 37 (62%) |
| Derome et al. (1998) | Personal communication | Microadenoma | 44 | | 38 (86%) |
| | | Macroadenoma | 96 | | 44 (46%) |
| | | TOTAL | 140 | | 82 (59%) |
| Freda et al. (1998) | 58 | Microadenoma | 25 | | 22 (88%) |
| | | Macroadenoma | 90 | | 48 (53%) |
| | | TOTAL | 115 | | 70 (61%) |
| Abosch et al. (1998) | 48 | TOTAL | 120 | 101 (84%) | |
| Swearingen et al. (1998) | 50 | Microadenoma | 33 | | 30 (91%) |
| | | Macroadenoma | 129 | | 62 (48%) |
| | | TOTAL | 162 | | 92 (57%) |

*N*, number of patients; *GH*, growth hormone; *IGF-I*, insulin-like growth factor-I.

opposed to 7.1 years after conventional radiotherapy).[68] Studies involving a higher number of patients followed for a longer period of time and assessed with more stringent criteria of cure are needed before one can conclude that radiosurgery is superior to conventional radiotherapy.

**Therapy with Bromocriptine and Other Dopaminergic Agonists.** Treatment with bromocriptine or other dopaminergic agonists produces improvement in clinical symptoms of acromegaly in half of the patients. These drugs substantially decrease GH levels in some patients but only rarely normalize GH and IGF-I levels (i.e., in <10% of cases).[28] Better results seem to be obtained with cabergoline than with bromocriptine, however; in a multicenter study, nearly 40% of patients acromegaly treated with cabergoline were reported to have normalized IGF-I levels.[29]

**Therapy with Somatostatin Analogs.** Somatostatin-analog therapy has now gained wide acceptance in the medical treatment of acromegaly. GH levels are decreased in 50% to 80% of patients treated with octreotide subcutaneously three times daily.[30,33–36,45,69,70] With this treatment, up to 50% of acromegalic patients may be considered as "cured" (GH plasma levels of <2 µg/L [20–30% of cases] and/or normal IGF-I [20–60% of cases]) (Table 24-5). Similar results are obtained with lanreotide LAR (long-acting release), 30 mg administered intramuscularly every 10 or 14 days (GH plasma levels of <2 µg/L [30–70% of cases] and/or normal IGF-I [40–70% of patients]),[38–41] or with octreotide LAR. This latter drug has been administered intramuscularly every month at a dose of 20 to 30 mg (yielding GH plasma levels of <2 µg/L [50–60% of patients] and/or normal IGF-I [60–90% of cases])[37,71–73] (see Table 24-5). Such variations in the data obtained from one study to another is probably explained by differences in the methods used for IGF-I assay and by differences in the inclusion criteria used. Thus, in some of the studies assessing the efficiency of long-acting forms of somatostatin analogs, patients were included if they had previously been shown to be responsive to subcutaneous octreotide, whereas in others, patients were entered blindly, without any knowledge of whether or not they were responsive. As demonstrated by a multicenter prospective study, the efficacy of octreotide as primary treatment (in 26 previously untreated patients) proved to be equivalent to that of secondary treatment (in 81 patients previously treated with surgery and/or radiotherapy).[70]

A small reduction in tumor volume may be observed (in general at the level of the suprasellar expansion) in 15% to 70% of patients with acromegaly[30,33–37,39–41,45,69–73] (see Table 24-5).

Administration of a *combination* of a dopamine agonist and a somatostatin analog may be beneficial for some patients, but long-term studies assessing this therapeutic association are not currently available.

**TABLE 24-4.**
**Success Rate of Radiation Therapy for Acromegaly with Different Criteria of Cure**

| Author (Year) | Reference | N | Patients with GH <10 µg/L | Patients with GH <5 µg/L | Patients with GH <2.5 µg/L and Normal IGF-I |
|---|---|---|---|---|---|
| Lamberg et al. (1976) | 61 | 31 | | 50% | |
| Feek et al. (1984) | 62 | 48 | 62% | 42% | |
| Kliman et al. (1986) | 63 | 435 | 78% | 44% | |
| Speirs et al. (1990) | 64 | 17 | | 46% | |
| Eastman et al. (1992) | 18 | 87 | 92% | 80% | |
| Barkan et al. (1997) | 22 | 38 | | 65% | 5% |
| Chanson et al. (1997) | 65 | 34 | | 71% | 35% |
| Thalassinos et al. (1998) | 66 | 46 | | 31% | 20% |

*N*, number of patients; *GH*, growth hormone; *IGF-I*, insulin-like growth factor-I.

**TABLE 24-5.**
**Effects of Long-Term Treatment of Acromegaly with the Somatostatin Analogs Octreotide and Lanreotide with Various Modes of Preparation and Administration and Different Criteria of Cure**

| Author (Year) | Reference | N | Type of Treatment (Dose) | Percentage of Patients with GH <5 µg/L | Percentage of Patients with GH <2.5 µg/L (GH) and/or Normal IGF-I (IGF-I) | Percentage of Patients with >20% Reduction in Tumor Volume |
|---|---|---|---|---|---|---|
| Sassolas et al. (1990) | 33 | 58 | Octreotide sc (300–1500 µg/d) | 43 | 29 (GH) | 47 |
| Vance & Harris (1991) | 34 | 189 | Octreotide sc (50–500 µg/d) | 45 | 46 (IGF-I) | 44 |
| Ezzat et al. (1992) | 35 | 115 | Octreotide sc (300–750 µg/d) | 51 | 18 (GH); 61 (IGF-I) | 28 |
| Arosio et al. (1995) | 69 | 68 | Octreotide sc (300–600 µg/d) | | 20 (IGF-I) | 27 |
| Newman et al. (1998) | 70 | 26* 81† | Octreotide sc (100–1750 µg/d) | | 43 (GH); 68 (IGF-I)* 22 (GH); 62 (IGF-I)† | 23* |
| Morange et al. (1994) | 39 | 19 | Lanreotide PR im (30 mg q 10–14 d) | 89 | 68 (IGF-I) | |
| Giusti et al. (1996) | 40 | 57 | Lanreotide PR im (30 mg q 10–14 d) | 85 | 76 (GH); 38 (IGF-I) | 17 |
| Caron et al. (1997) | 41 | 22 | Lanreotide PR im (30 mg q 10–14 d) | 68 | 27 (GH); 63 (IGF-I) | 13 |
| Stewart et al. (1995) | 73 | 8 | Octreotide LAR im (20–40 mg q 28–42 d) | 100 | 63 (GH); 88 (IGF-I) | 43 |
| Lancranjan et al. (1996) | 72 | 101 | Octreotide LAR im (20–40 mg q 28 d) | 94 | 54 (GH); 65 (IGF-I) | 72 |
| Fløgstad et al. (1997) | 71 | 14 | Octreotide LAR im (20–40 mg q 28 d) | 86 | 64 (GH); 64 (IGF-I) | 29 |

N, number of patients; GH, growth hormone; IGF-I, insulin-like growth factor-I; LAR, long-acting release; PR, prolonged release.
*Octreotide as primary treatment.
†Octreotide as secondary treatment, administered after surgery and/or radiotherapy.

*GH-receptor antagonist therapy* may be effective in the control of the clinical symptoms of acromegaly and normalizes IGF-I levels in a substantial number of patients.

## SUMMARY OF RECOMMENDATIONS FOR TREATMENT OF GROWTH HORMONE–SECRETING ADENOMAS

Table 24-2 summarizes the treatment decisions for GH-secreting adenomas.

1. Transsphenoidal surgery is the first-line therapy, except when a macroadenoma is extremely large or when surgery is contraindicated.
2. Postoperative radiation therapy (50 to 55 Gy) is performed for partially resected tumors or when GH levels remain elevated after a trial of a somatostatin analog.
3. Somatostatin analogs are best used when surgery is contraindicated or when the surgery has failed to normalize GH levels. These drugs are also used when waiting for the delayed effects of radiation therapy. Somatostatin analogs may be a reasonable primary therapeutic modality if the possibility of surgical cure is low (as in patients with large and/or invasive tumors), provided that the tumor does not threaten vision or neurologic function.

## PROLACTIN-SECRETING TUMORS

### THERAPEUTIC OPTIONS

Occasionally, *surgery* and, more rarely, *radiotherapy* may be used. Their techniques and side effects have been detailed in the first section (see earlier).

In the vast majority of cases, however, medical therapy with *dopamine agonists* is chosen. Bromocriptine or other ergot derivatives with dopaminergic properties (e.g., pergolide, quinagolide, cabergoline) are used. Bromocriptine effectively reduces elevated serum PRL levels in most patients with PRL-secreting

pituitary adenomas.[74–76] Thus, it is the primary treatment for microadenomas. Furthermore, macroprolactinomas have also been successfully managed medically.[74,77–79] Bromocriptine not only decreases PRL levels but also is able to produce a dramatic reduction in tumor volume. This antitumor effect of bromocriptine may be very rapid. In the presence of chiasmal compression by a macroadenoma, visual improvement often occurs within the first hours after the initiation of bromocriptine therapy. Ovulatory and menstrual cycles may resume in 75% to 80% of female patients.[74,78] Patients with macroadenomas who become pregnant are at risk for complications related to tumor growth. For these patients, pregnancy should be delayed by contraceptive methods, while shrinkage is attempted with bromocriptine. Definitive ablative therapy of macroadenomas may be performed before pregnancy.[74,78] However, patients with intrasellar microadenomas or macroadenomas of <12 mm are at <6% risk for any substantial tumor growth or associated complications.[80–82] Bromocriptine should be discontinued when pregnancy is confirmed, although early concerns regarding the teratogenicity of this drug have not, to date, been substantiated.[74] Quinagolide and cabergoline are two other dopamine agonists now available in the United States and/or in Europe. Quinagolide is not an ergot derivative; it binds specifically to dopamine type 2 receptors. It is at least as effective as bromocriptine[83] and may be useful in rare cases of resistance[84–86] or intolerance[86] to bromocriptine. It offers the advantage of once-daily administration. Cabergoline is notable for its very long duration of action (half-life is ~70 hours). This allows a once- or twice-weekly oral administration.[87] The efficacy of cabergoline is at least equal to that of bromocriptine and tolerance to it is better.[87,88] In patients with macroprolactinoma, cabergoline is quite effective in reducing PRL levels and in producing tumor shrinkage.[89–91] Furthermore, cabergoline normalizes serum PRL levels in a significant number of patients who are resistant to bromocriptine and/or quinagolide[90] (see Chap. 13).

## RESULTS OF TREATMENT

### Transsphenoidal Surgery

MICROADENOMA.    In a compilation of various studies involving a total of 1224 patients, transsphenoidal resection was found to normalize PRL levels in 71.2% of patients.[74] Cure rates vary according to preoperative serum PRL level; when the PRL level is >200 μg/L, the cure rate decreases to 13%. After surgery, up to 88% of women desiring conception conceived within 1 year.[74,92] Initially, the recurrence rate after surgical success was thought to be as high as 50%; however, more recent studies report a recurrence rate from 5% to 18% after a 10-year follow-up.[74,92,93] Nonetheless, even if hyperprolactinemia should relapse, it tends to remain mild and usually without any clinical consequences. Ten years after surgery, 55% to 73% of patients have normal serum PRL levels, and 75% have normal menstrual cycles.[92-94]

MACROADENOMA.    The success rate for transsphenoidal surgery is much lower for macroadenomas. According to a compilation of 1256 such patients from reported series, the mean cure rate was 31.8%.[74] Moreover, after apparent initial cure, 18% of patients relapsed. Surgical results were proportional to the preoperative size of the tumor and to the initial level of serum PRL. When the adenoma size was >20 mm and the serum PRL levels were >200 μg/L, the cure rate was <15%.[74]

**Medical Therapy.**    Dopamine agonists are able to decrease PRL levels in 73% to 95% of patients, whatever the size of their adenomas; moreover, the drugs produce a decrease in tumor volume in 77% of patients with a macroprolactinoma.[74,77,79,83,89,91] This tumor shrinkage may be dramatic (>50% of initial volume in half of the patients). Treatment with dopamine agonists is prolonged and often lifelong. Indeed, after withdrawal of treatment, the tumor usually returns to its original size, often within days to weeks, and the serum PRL levels again rise.

In patients who are resistant to bromocriptine, other dopamine agonists such as quinagolide or cabergoline may be a useful alternative; quinagolide allows normalization of PRL levels in 16% to 20% of cases, and cabergoline in 80% of patients.[84-86,90] In cases of intolerance of bromocriptine, PRL may be normalized by quinagolide in more than half of patients.[86] Tolerance of cabergoline has proven to be better than tolerance of bromocriptine, so that larger doses can be used in cases of incomplete response.[87-91]

**Irradiation Therapy.**    Irradiation therapy is indicated only in rare cases of surgical failure in which the patient has subsequently been found to be intolerant of or resistant to dopamine agonists 20% to 30%,[12,74,95,96] and only half of such patients have normal serum PRL levels 3 to 4 years and 8 years after irradiation therapy, respectively.[97]

## SUMMARY OF RECOMMENDATIONS FOR TREATMENT OF PROLACTIN-SECRETING PITUITARY ADENOMAS

Table 24-2 summarizes the treatment decisions for prolactin-secreting pituitary adenomas.

1. Selected hyperprolactinemic patients with microadenomas may be carefully followed without treatment if regular ovulatory cycles occur, or if the patient is postmenopausal.
2. Patients with microadenomas are usually treated with dopamine agonists. In the uncommon circumstance that transsphenoidal surgery was the initial choice, dopamine agonists may be useful if the serum PRL levels remain elevated postoperatively. When medical therapy with dopamine agonists is the primary treatment, secondary surgery may occasionally be proposed in cases of resistance to or intolerance of these drugs. In dopamine-treated microprolactinoma patients, pregnancy can be permitted, and the dopamine agonists are generally interrupted as soon as the pregnancy is confirmed.
3. In patients with macroadenomas, even in the presence of a chiasmatic syndrome, dopamine agonists are the best primary treatment. Improvement in the visual disturbance is often very rapid, and tumor shrinkage is usually very significant. Thus, the results provided by dopamine agonists are generally much better than those obtained with surgery, even when it is performed by a highly skilled surgeon. If dopamine agonists are not rapidly effective, however, surgery is recommended. In such cases, if serum PRL levels remain high postoperatively (which is likely the case for macroadenomas, particularly when they are large), dopamine agonists are given. When pregnancy is planned in patients with macroprolactinomas, one might propose to pursue treatment with dopamine agonists during the entire pregnancy. Alternatively, before pregnancy, surgery may be selected with the goal of removing much of or the entire lesion. Thereafter, dopamine agonists are given to those patients with remaining hyperprolactinemia until the onset of pregnancy; at that time, the drugs are halted.
4. Currently, radiotherapy is an option that is very seldom used. This treatment must be limited to the rare patients with large, incompletely resected tumors who continue to have high serum PRL levels, are resistant to dopamine agonists, and experience amenorrhea or mass effects of the lesion.

## ADRENOCORTICOTROPIC HORMONE–SECRETING ADENOMAS

Most ACTH-secreting adenomas (90%) are microadenomas. The principal therapeutic difficulty caused by these lesions are their small size, which may hamper their preoperative visualization by imaging studies and their subsequent surgical resection. When a rare macroadenoma occurs, it usually is large and invasive; in such a case, total surgical resection may be difficult. Due to the poor prognosis of persistent hypercortisolism, adjuvant therapy with drug therapy is frequently required.

### THERAPEUTIC OPTIONS

*Transsphenoidal surgery* and/or *radiotherapy* are the main therapeutic options; their techniques and side effects have been described.

*Medical treatment* has an important place as an adjuvant therapy.

Although a few case reports of cyproheptadine-induced remission of Cushing disease have been described, in the vast majority of patients no beneficial effect or only a moderate improvement has been observed with cyproheptadine administration,[98] and its use has been abandoned.

Octreotide and lanreotide have no established place in the treatment of Cushing disease, although a few patients may respond with a decrease in ACTH secretion.[98]

Medical therapy in Cushing disease is currently limited to the use of compounds directed to the adrenal that are able to inhibit steroidogenesis (i.e., mitotane, ketoconazole, metyrapone, etomidate, trilostane, or aminoglutethimide).[98,99] The adrenolytic agent mitotane (1,1-dichloro-2-[o-chlorophenyl]-2-[p-chlorophenyl]-ethane or o,p'-DDD) inhibits 11β-hydroxylase and cholesterol side-chain cleavage enzymes and destroys adrenocortical cells. The drug is given orally at a dosage of 6 to 12 g per day. Principal side effects of mitotane are gastrointestinal symptoms (nausea, loss of appetite), hypercholesterolemia, and gynecomastia. Neurologic side effects and skin rashes rarely occur. True drug-induced hepatitis (with increased levels of serum transaminases), which requires discontinuation of the drug, is rare; this must be distinguished from increased levels of γ-glutaryl transferase, which is frequent and benign and occurs in the setting of a fatty liver associated with the obesity of Cushing syndrome. Due to its marked liver enzyme–inducing effect, increased pro-

TABLE 24-6.
Results of Transsphenoidal Surgery for Treatment of Cushing Disease

| Author (Year) | Reference | Success Rate (%) | Recurrences (%) | Mean Follow-Up (Months) |
|---|---|---|---|---|
| Guilhaume et al. (1988) | 103 | 42/61 (69%) | 6/42 (14.3%) | 24 |
| Mampalam et al. (1988) | 104 | 171/216 (79%) | 9/171 (5.3%) | 46 |
| Arnott et al. (1990) | 100 | 24/28 (85%) | 3/24 (12.5%) | 22 |
| Burke et al. (1990) | 105 | 44/54 (81%) | 2/44 (4.5%) | 56 |
| Post & Habas (1990) | 106 | 29/37 (78%) | 1/29 (3.4%) | ? |
| Tindall et al. (1990) | 107 | 46/53 (86%) | 1/46 (2.1%) | 57 |
| Robert & Hardy (1991) | 108 | 60/78 (77%) | 5/60 (8.3%) | 77 |
| Tahir & Sheeler (1992) | 109 | 34/45 (75%) | 7/34 (20.6%) | 69 |
| Trainer et al. (1993) | 110 | 39/48 (81%) | 3/39 (7.7%) | ? |
| Ram et al. (1994) | 111 | 205/222 (92%) | ? | ? |
| Bochicchio et al. (1995) | 102 | 510/668 (76%) | 65/510 (12.7%) | 46 |

duction of several binding proteins (in particular transcortin, the cortisol-binding globulin) occurs during mitotane therapy. Thus, the efficacy of the drug needs to be monitored; assessment should not be based on total plasma cortisol levels (which remain artifactually increased) but on free urinary cortisol or on salivary cortisol. These latter tests reflect the serum levels of the free, unbound cortisol. Doses of hydrocortisone given for replacement therapy, if required, may for the same reason show superior effects to those generally used for the replacement therapy of adrenal insufficiency. With prolonged administration at high doses, mitotane is able to produce permanent destruction of adrenocortical cells and result in glucocorticoid insufficiency; this may be associated with hypoaldosteronism (see Chap. 75).

Ketoconazole, an imidazole-derivative antimycotic agent, inhibits various cytochrome P450 enzymes, including the side-chain cleavage enzymes 17,20 lyase, 11β-hydroxylase, and 17-hydroxylase. Ketoconazole is administered at a dosage of 600 to 800 mg twice daily. Reported side effects are hepatitis, gynecomastia, and gastrointestinal symptoms. Another imidazole derivative, the anesthetic drug etomidate, when given intravenously at a nonhypnotic dose (3 mg/kg body weight per hour) has an immediate cortisol-lowering effect. Metyrapone, administered at a dosage of 2 to 4 g per day, inhibits 11β-hydroxylase and also may be used in the treatment of hypercortisolism. Nausea, vomiting, and neurologic symptoms are the most commonly reported side effects of metyrapone therapy. Aminoglutethimide (750 mg per day) inhibits several cytochrome p450 steroidogenic enzymes and efficiently controls hypercortisolism, but it may cause sedation, nausea, and rash; the same is true for trilostane (200–1000 mg per day), a carbonitrile derivative that inhibits conversion of pregnenolone to progesterone.

Except in the rare cases in which medical treatment is poorly tolerated or produces severe side effects (hepatitis), bilateral adrenalectomy is no longer used as therapy for Cushing disease because of substantial morbidity and mortality, the need for permanent replacement therapy with corticosteroids, and the subsequent (albeit low) risk for development of Nelson syndrome.

### RESULTS OF TREATMENT

In the hands of skilled neurosurgeons, the apparent cure rate achieved by *transsphenoidal surgery* for Cushing disease due to microadenoma is 70% to 80%.[98,100–111] The criteria for cure are an undetectable morning serum cortisol concentration and a plasma ACTH concentration of <5 pg/mL 4 to 7 days after surgery.[101] Less strict criteria result in higher rates of apparent cure but a higher rate of recurrence (Table 24-6).

The recurrence rate of Cushing disease after surgery for a microadenoma is more frequent than was previously thought; a progressive upward trend is seen with time.[103] In most series, the recurrence rate is 10% to 20% (see Table 24-6).

Only 50% of patients with macroadenomas achieve remissions after initial pituitary microsurgery.

In children, the rate of cure after transsphenoidal surgery is 70% to 86%[104,112–114] and even reached 97% for one team.[115] As is the case with adults, however, after extended follow-up and using the more stringent criteria now applied, these results will probably prove to be less favorable, probably in the range of 50% to 75%.[113,114]

In case of surgical failure, *secondary irradiation therapy* is able to produce remission in 56%[116] to 83%[117] of patients with Cushing disease after a median follow-up of ~3 years. *Primary radiotherapy* for Cushing disease is effective in 50% to 60% of adults and 85% of children.[21,98,99,118]

During the months or years required to achieve maximal benefits from irradiation, hypercortisolism usually can be controlled with *adrenal enzyme inhibitors*.[98,99] After 8 months of therapy, remission of hypercortisolism is achieved in 83% of patients treated with mitotane. Combined with pituitary irradiation, mitotane produces remission of hypercortisolism in 80% to 100% of patients, but discontinuation of the drug leads to recurrence of the hypercortisolism in 30% to 50% of cases. Use of ketoconazole rapidly normalizes serum cortisol levels, but an escape from the effect of the steroidogenic agent is generally observed after a few months of treatment; this prevents long-term administration. Metyrapone is able to rapidly normalize plasma cortisol in 50% to 75% of patients with Cushing disease. Its interruption leads to recurrence of hypercortisolism. Aminoglutethimide only appears to be effective in controlling hypercortisolism in <50% of cases.

### SUMMARY OF RECOMMENDATIONS FOR TREATMENT OF ADRENOCORTICOTROPIC HORMONE–SECRETING ADENOMAS

Table 24-2 summarizes the treatment decisions for Adrenocorticotropic Hormone–Secreting Adenomas.

1. The primary therapy for children and adults is generally transsphenoidal surgery.
2. Radiotherapy (50 Gy) is reserved for patients who have undergone only subtotal resection or who remain hypersecretory after surgery.
3. While one waits for the effects of radiotherapy, or if it is contraindicated, adrenal steroidogenesis inhibitors (in particular, mitotane) may be indicated.

### THYROID-STIMULATING HORMONE–SECRETING ADENOMAS

#### THERAPEUTIC OPTIONS

*Surgery* and *radiotherapy* are the usual therapeutic tools for treating TSH-secreting adenomas. They have been described in detail earlier in this chapter.

TABLE 24-7.
Recurrence Rate According to Therapy for Nonfunctioning Pituitary Adenomas

| Author | Reference | Surgical Therapy Alone | | Surgery + Radiation Therapy | |
|--------|-----------|------------------------|--|-----------------------------|--|
| | | *Total Number* | *Recurrences (%)* | *Total Number* | *Recurrences (%)* |
| Ebersold et al. (1986) | 125 | 42 | 5 (12%) | 50 | 9 (18%) |
| Jaffrain-Rea et al. (1993) | 133 | 33 | 9 (27%) | 24 | 2 (8.8%) |
| Hayes et al. (1971) | 130 | 29 | 13 (45%) | 42 | 9 (21%) |
| Sheline et al. (1974) | 25 | 29 | 20 (69%) | 80 | 9 (11%) |
| Ciric et al. (1983) | 131 | 32 | 9 (28%) | 67 | 4 (6%) |
| Chun et al. (1988) | 10 | 60 | 9 (15%) | 54 | 4 (7%) |
| Vlahovitch et al. (1988) | 132 | 89 | 14 (16%) | 46 | 4 (8%) |
| Gittoes et al. (1998) | 135 | 63 | 20 (66%) | 63 | 4 (7%) |
| TOTAL | | 377 | 99 (26%) | 426 | 45 (11%) |

*Medical adjuvant therapy with somatostatin analogs* has proven to be very useful. Octreotide and lanreotide are quite effective in reducing TSH levels in patients with TSH-secreting adenomas, thus allowing normalization of plasma thyroid hormone levels in a high proportion of patients.[119,120] The associated side effects are similar to those of somatostatin analogs used in the treatment of acromegaly.

### RESULTS OF TREATMENT

Forty percent of patients with TSH-secreting adenomas are not cured by surgery, even when it is combined with radiation therapy. In these patients, thyrotoxicosis persists.[121]

Octreotide, the somatostatin analog, is able to reduce serum TSH and α subunit levels in 91% of patients and normalizes thyroid hormone levels in 73% of patients.[119] The reduction in tumor volume is similar to that obtained in acromegalic patients treated with octreotide. Lanreotide has very similar effects.[120]

### SUMMARY OF RECOMMENDATIONS FOR TREATMENT OF THYROID-STIMULATING HORMONE–SECRETING ADENOMAS

Treatment decisions for TSH-secreting adenomas are summarized as follows:

1. The primary therapy is transsphenoidal surgery, regardless of the size of the tumor.
2. Irradiation therapy (40–50 Gy) is generally proposed only in the case of incomplete resection, particularly when the remnant is invasive.
3. Somatostatin analogs are indicated in cases of persistent postoperative hyperthyroidism, while the effects of radiotherapy are being awaited.

### CLINICALLY NONFUNCTIONING PITUITARY ADENOMAS

The majority of NFPAs are gonadotrope cell adenomas. Indeed, among all the types of macroadenomas, NFPAs are the most frequent. Despite their gonadotrope nature, as demonstrated by immunocytochemical staining, NFPAs are only rarely associated with increased levels of dimeric LH or FSH. However, increased levels of uncombined subunits (free α subunit primarily, LH-β subunit more rarely) are more frequently encountered but are generally modest in titer. The posttreatment assessment of cure usually is based on morphologic changes; hormonal monitoring is not usually helpful for this assessment. The main problems raised by NFPAs are the mass effects, mainly optic chiasm compression and/or deficient hormone secretion resulting from compression of normal anterior pituitary cells.

### THERAPEUTIC OPTIONS

*Surgery* and *radiotherapy* are the only really effective therapeutic options available for NFPA; technical aspects and side effects have been discussed earlier.

Various *medical treatments* have been tried (i.e., administration of dopamine agonists, gonadotropin-releasing hormone [GnRH] analogs), but none has proven to be sufficiently effective as a reasonable therapeutic option. In occasional patients, the somatostatin analog octreotide may minimally improve visual defects due to chiasmal compression.[122,123]

### RESULTS OF TREATMENT

The strategy of *observation only* for patients with incidentally discovered pituitary adenomas (*incidentalomas*) may be appropriate provided the tumor is well delimited, small, and has no suprasellar or lateral extension that risks neurologic or visual chiasm compression, and a meticulous hormonal work-up has ruled out the possibility that the hormonal hypersecretion is sufficient to produce a clinical syndrome.[124] In all other cases, clinically evident, but apparently inactive, pituitary adenomas require surgery.

*Transsphenoidal surgery* allows improvement in visual disturbances due to chiasmal syndrome in 44% to 70% of patients.[125–129] When the NFPA is a gonadotropin-secreting adenoma associated with supranormal levels of gonadotropins or free subunits, surgery almost always reduces supranormal plasma FSH and/or α subunit levels and normalizes them,[129] despite the persistence of a tumor remnant. When an NFPA is responsible for pituitary failure, surgery is able to improve pituitary function in 15% to 50% of cases. On the other hand, surgery may aggravate the preoperative pituitary deficiency.

After surgery alone, nearly 30% (from 10% to 69%) of patients relapse within 5 to 10 years.[10,25,125,127,129–135] The variability in these data reflect differences in neurosurgical expertise, as well as the differing quality of the imaging techniques used postoperatively to assess the extent of tumor excision (Table 24-7).

*Radiotherapy* is proposed either as a systematic adjunct or if a significant remnant persists. Use of systematic radiation therapy is supported by the low relapse rate (mean, 11%; range, 6%–21%) that is observed when irradiation is routinely combined with surgery[10,20,25,125,129–135] (see Table 24-7). However, irradiation is almost always followed by hypopituitarism, and several epidemiologic studies have demonstrated that postirradiation hypopituitarism might be associated with a reduction in life expectancy, despite appropriate replacement therapy[136–138] (see Prognosis section).

Results of *medical treatment* are disappointing. Bromocriptine is not very effective in reducing levels of supranormal gonadotropins and free subunits, and only rarely produces a minimal tumor shrinkage.[79,139] Somatostatin analogs are able to improve visual problems minimally in 20% to 40% of cases, but reports of reduction in tumor volume is anecdotal.[122,123] Use of GnRH agonists is generally ineffective[139] and may be hazardous.[140] Prolonged administration of a GnRH antagonist to a small number of patients with a secreting gonadotrope cell adenoma

**TABLE 24-8.**
**Epidemiologic Studies Demonstrating an Increased Mortality in Patients with Hypopituitarism**

| Author (Year) | Reference | N | SMR (95% Confidence Interval) | | | SMR from Total Cardiac and Vascular Causes | | | SMR from Cerebrovascular Causes | | | SMR from Malignancy |
|---|---|---|---|---|---|---|---|---|---|---|---|---|
| | | | Total | Male | Female | Total | Male | Female | Total | Male | Female | Total |
| Rosen et al. (1990) | 136 | 333 | 1.81* | 1.46 | 2.82 | 1.94* | 1.70 | 2.70 | | | | 0.49* |
| Bates et al. (1996) | 137 | 172 | 1.73 (1.28– 2.28)* | 1.50 (1.02– 2.13)* | 2.29 (1.37– 3.58)* | 1.35 (0.84– 2.07) | 1.32 (0.94– 2.17) | 1.46 (0.50– 3.20) | | | | 1.41 (0.73–2.47) |
| Bülow et al. (1997) | 138 | 344 | 2.17 (1.88– 2.51)* | 1.91 (1.59– 2.28)* | 2.93 (2.28– 3.75)* | 1.75 (1.40– 2.19)* | 1.54 (1.16– 2.03)* | 2.39 (1.60– 3.52)* | 3.39 (2.27– 4.99)* | 2.64 (1.44– 4.42)* | 4.91 (2.62– 8.40)* | 1.71 (1.21– 2.37)* |

*SMR*, standardized mortality ratio, calculated by dividing observed mortality by expected mortality in an age- and sex-matched control population; when available, 95% confidence interval is given; *N*, number of patients.
*Statistically significant.

has been reported to reduce supranormal gonadotropin levels but did not produce any change in tumor size.[141]

### THERAPEUTIC RECOMMENDATIONS FOR TREATMENT OF CLINICALLY NONFUNCTIONING ADENOMAS

Table 24-2 summarizes recommendations for the treatment of NFPAs.

Transsphenoidal surgery with or without postoperative radiation therapy (50 Gy) is performed for almost all patients, irrespective of whether they have visual consequences of their tumor. Selected patients with small, incidentally discovered microadenomas may be carefully followed without immediate therapy.

## PROGNOSIS OF PITUITARY ADENOMAS AND THERAPEUTIC PERSPECTIVES

### PROGNOSIS

Prognosis depends on the type of tumor and a combination of other factors, including (a) the severity of the endocrinologic disturbance or mass-related symptoms and signs, (b) the size and extent of the tumor as indicated earlier, (c) the success of therapy in reversing these abnormalities, (d) morbidities due to therapy, and (e) permanence of the therapeutic response. Although pituitary tumors are generally benign, the failure to provide adequate therapy can lead to severe functional deficits and death. Optimal therapy can greatly improve quality and duration of life.

### ACROMEGALY

If patients with acromegaly remain untreated, they have a 10-year reduction in life expectancy, in particular due to cardiovascular and respiratory problems and to the increased risk of neoplasms. The *standardized mortality ratio* (SMR, the observed mortality divided by the expected mortality in a sex- and age-matched control population) is from 1.8 to 3.[46,48–50] The most important predictive factor of mortality is the "final" posttherapeutic serum GH level.[46–50] When the "final" serum GH level is <2.5 μg/L, the mortality is not significantly different from that of the general population. When the final serum GH level is >2.5 μg/L, the SMR is between 1.4 and 2, which signifies a statistically different mortality from that of the general population. This indicates that application of the more stringent definition of cure or successful outcome in acromegaly which is currently used (i.e., serum GH levels of <2.5 μg/L) is probably associated with better survival than were the criteria previously used (i.e., serum GH <5 μg/L or <10 μg/L).

### CUSHING DISEASE

The mortality in patients with Cushing disease is higher than that expected for the control population (SMR, 3.8; 95% confidence limits, 2.5–17.9). The most common cause of death is vascular disease. Advanced age, persistence of hypertension, and abnormalities in glucose metabolism after treatment are independent predictors of mortality.[142]

### HYPOPITUITARISM

Hypopituitarism, particularly after surgery and/or radiation therapy for NFPA, is also associated with an increase in mortality (SMR, 1.70–2.10), according to the very concordant results of three studies.[136–138] Death was reported to be due mainly to an increase in cardiovascular deaths in some studies[136–138] but not in others[137] (Table 24-8). GH deficiency was cited as a potential cause of the increased mortality in these patients; presumably, they were given adequate replacement therapy for other pituitary hormones but had not received GH-replacement therapy. This assertion remains highly questionable, however, because GH deficiency was not proven in all the patients in these studies and because often evidence was found of a long-term lack of pituitary hormones or of an inadequacy of hormonal substitution in many of them. GH treatment in patients with GH deficiency has been reported to be associated with numerous, albeit modest, increases in lean body mass, improved quality of life, amelioration of lipid abnormalities, and increased bone mineral content.[143] However, whether or not a substitutive therapy with GH would improve the prognosis for hypopituitarism in adults is presently unknown.

### PROLONGED (LIFELONG) SURVEILLANCE

Regular assessment for many years of the pituitary function of patients treated for pituitary adenomas is essential to allow rapid adequate replacement therapy in patients who develop hypopituitarism. Hypopituitarism may occur up to 30 years after radiation therapy.

### CONCLUSIONS AND PERSPECTIVES CONCERNING TREATMENT OF PITUITARY ADENOMAS

Although progress in imaging techniques has greatly improved the ease of diagnosing and localizing pituitary lesions, it has also been responsible for more frequent detection of incidental and clinically innocent lesions. The appropriate management of such pituitary incidentalomas, taking into account the cost, possible benefits, and complications of potential therapy, needs to be determined more precisely.

The early recognition of acromegaly, a condition that is responsible for important morbidity and cosmetic consequences, needs to be improved.

The management of pituitary adenomas is currently well defined. According to the type of tumor and the clinical situation, options include surgery, irradiation, and/or drugs.[144]

Surgical resection by the transsphenoidal route carries a very low morbidity and mortality. In skilled hands, it often allows a complete cure of the disease. Improvement is needed in surgical techniques to obtain a better removal of invasive tumors. Whether endoscopic techniques or the use of intraoperative MRI or intraoperative computer-assisted neuronavigation with robots would improve the outcome is presently unknown.

Diagnostic challenges are rare, except in the case of Cushing disease. Here, Cushing syndrome due to occult ectopic ACTH-secreting tumors (often bronchial carcinoids) may be misconstrued as being due to a nonvisible corticotropic microadenoma. This may delay appropriate treatment. Further improvements in imaging techniques are unlikely to allow better definition of these pituitary microadenomas. When Cushing disease is suspected, bilateral inferior petrosal sinus catheterization generally confirms or rules out a pituitary causation.

Histopathologic techniques (particularly immunocytochemistry) have greatly assisted the classification of pituitary adenomas. However, no markers of invasiveness or aggressiveness have been identified that can be routinely applied to tumor specimens removed at surgery. In this respect, prospective studies of molecular genetic alterations that have been demonstrated in pituitary adenomas[144] will determine whether they are truly predictive of subsequent behavior and can be used to aid clinical management in a manner not possible with current histologic criteria. Conceivably, this may assist in decisions regarding which patients might need postoperative irradiation therapy.

# REFERENCES

1. Kovacs K, Horvath E. Tumors of the pituitary gland. In: Hartman WH, ed. Atlas tumor of pathology, 2nd series, Fascicle XXI. Washington: Armed Forces Institute of Pathology, 1986:1.
2. Horvath E, Kovacs K. The adenohypophysis. In: Kovacs K, Asa L, eds. Functional endocrine pathology. Boston: Blackwell Science, 1998:247.
3. Ambrosi B, Faglia G. Epidemiology of pituitary tumors. In: Faglia G, Beck-Peccoz P, Ambrosi B, Travaglini P, Spada A, eds. Pituitary adenomas : new trends in basic and clinical research. Amsterdam: Excerpta Medica, 1991:159.
4. Molitch ME, Russell EJ. The pituitary "incidentaloma." Ann Intern Med 1990; 112:925.
5. Teramoto A, Hirakawa K, Sanno N, Osamura Y. Incidental pituitary lesions in 1,000 unselected autopsy specimens. Radiology 1994; 193:161.
6. Hall WA, Luciano MG, Doppman JL, et al. Pituitary magnetic resonance imaging in normal human volunteers: occult adenomas in the general population. Ann Intern Med 1994; 120:817.
7. Laws ER Jr, Thapar K. Surgical management of pituitary adenomas. Baillières Clin Endocrinol Metab 1995; 9:391.
8. Fahlbusch R, Honegger J, Buchfelder M. Surgical management of acromegaly. Endocrinol Metab Clin North Am 1992; 21:669.
9. Wilson CB. Extensive clinical experience: surgical management of pituitary tumors. J Clin Endocrinol Metab 1997; 82:2381.
10. Chun M, Masko GB, Hetelekidis S. Radiotherapy in the treatment of pituitary adenomas. Int J Radiat Oncol Biol Phys 1988; 15:305.
11. Grigsby PW, Stokes S, Marks JE, Simpson JR. Prognostic factors and results of radiotherapy alone in the management of pituitary adenomas. Int J Radiat Oncol Biol Phys 1988; 15:1103.
12. Sheline G, Tyrrell J. Pituitary tumors. In: Perez C, Brady L, eds. Principles and practice of radiation oncology. Philadelphia: JB Lippincott, 1987:1108.
13. Nelson PB, Goodman ML, Flickenger JC, et al. Endocrine function in patients with large pituitary tumors treated with operative decompression and radiation therapy. Neurosurgery 1989; 24:398.
14. Snyder PJ, Fowble BF, Schatz NJ, et al. Hypopituitarism following radiation therapy of pituitary adenomas. Am J Med 1986; 81:457.
15. Brada M, Ford D, Ashley S, et al. Risk of second brain tumour after conservative surgery and radiotherapy for pituitary adenoma. BMJ 1992; 304:1343.
16. Littley MD, Shalet SM, Beardwell CG, et al. Hypopituitarism following external radiotherapy for pituitary tumours in adults. Q J Med 1989; 262:145.
17. Linfoot JA. Heavy ion therapy. In: Linfoot JA, ed. Recent advances in the diagnosis and treatment of pituitary tumors. New York: Raven Press, 1979:245.
18. Eastman RC, Gorden P, Glatstein E, Roth J. Radiation therapy of acromegaly. Endocrinol Metab Clin North Am 1992; 21:693.
19. Constine LS, Woolf PD, Cann D, et al. Hypothalamic-pituitary dysfunction after radiation for brain tumors. N Engl J Med 1993; 328:87.
20. Brada M, Rajan B, Traish D, et al. The long-term efficacy of conservative surgery and radiotherapy in the control of pituitary adenomas. Clin Endocrinol (Oxf) 1993; 38:571.
21. Plowman PN. Radiotherapy for pituitary tumours. Baillières Clin Endocrinol Metab 1995; 9:407.
22. Barkan AL, Halasz I, Dornfeld KJ, et al. Pituitary irradiation is ineffective in normalizing plasma insulin-like growth factor I in patients with acromegaly. J Clin Endocrinol Metab 1997; 82:3187.
23. Thorén M, Rähn T, Guo WY, Werner S. Stereotactic radiosurgery with the cobalt-60 gamma unit in the treatment of growth hormone-producing pituitary tumors. Neurosurgery 1991; 29:663.
24. Pollock BE, Kondziolka D, Lunsford LD, Flickinger JC. Stereotactic radiosurgery for pituitary adenomas: imaging, visual and endocrine results. Acta Neurochir Suppl (Wien) 1994; 62:33.
25. Sheline GE. Proceedings: treatment of nonfunctioning chromophobe adenomas of the pituitary. Am J Roentgenol Radium Ther Nucl Med 1974; 120:553.
26. Tsang RW, Laperriere NJ, Simpson WJ, et al. Glioma arising after radiation therapy for pituitary adenoma. A report of four patients and estimation of risk. Cancer 1993; 72:2227.
27. Brada M, Cruickshank G. Radiosurgery for brain tumours. BMJ 1999; 318:411.
28. Jaffe CA, Barkan AL. Treatment of acromegaly with dopamine agonists. Endocrinol Metab Clin North Am 1992; 21:713.
29. Abs R, Verhelst J, Maiter D, et al. Cabergoline in the treatment of acromegaly: a study in 64 patients. J Clin Endocrinol Metab 1998; 83:374.
30. Chanson P, Timsit J, Harris AG. Clinical pharmacokinetics of octreotide. Therapeutic applications in patients with pituitary tumours. Clin Pharmacokinet 1993; 25:375.
31. Lamberts SW, Hofland LJ, de Herder WW, et al. Octreotide and related somatostatin analogs in the diagnosis and treatment of pituitary disease and somatostatin receptor scintigraphy. Front Neuroendocrinol 1993; 14:27.
32. Lamberts SW, van der Lely AJ, de Herder WW, Hofland LJ. Octreotide. N Engl J Med 1996; 334:246.
33. Sassolas G, Harris AG, James-Deidier A. Long term effect of incremental doses of the somatostatin analog SMS 201-995 in 58 acromegalic patients. French SMS 201-995 Acromegaly Study Group. J Clin Endocrinol Metab 1990; 71:391.
34. Vance ML, Harris AG. Long-term treatment of 189 acromegalic patients with the somatostatin analog octreotide. Results of the International Multicenter Acromegaly Study Group. Arch Intern Med 1991; 151:1573.
35. Ezzat S, Snyder PJ, Young WF, et al. Octreotide treatment of acromegaly. A randomized, multicenter study. Ann Intern Med 1992; 117:711.
36. Newman CB, Melmed S, Snyder PJ, et al. Safety and efficacy of long-term octreotide therapy of acromegaly: results of a multicenter trial in 103 patients—a clinical research center study. J Clin Endocrinol Metab 1995; 80:2768.
37. Gillis JC, Noble S, Goa KL. Octreotide long-acting release (LAR). A review of its pharmacological properties and therapeutic use in the management of acromegaly. Drugs 1997; 53:681.
38. Heron I, Thomas F, Dero M, et al. Pharmacokinetics and efficacy of a long-acting formulation of the new somatostatin analog BIM 23014 in patients with acromegaly. J Clin Endocrinol Metab 1993; 76:721.
39. Morange I, De Boisvilliers F, Chanson P, et al. Slow release lanreotide treatment in acromegalic patients previously normalized by octreotide. J Clin Endocrinol Metab 1994; 79:145.
40. Giusti M, Gussoni G, Cuttica CM, Giordano G. Effectiveness and tolerability of slow release lanreotide treatment in active acromegaly: six-month report on an Italian multicenter study. Italian Multicenter Slow Release Lanreotide Study Group. J Clin Endocrinol Metab 1996; 81:2089.
41. Caron P, Morange-Ramos I, Cogne M, Jaquet P. Three year follow-up of acromegalic patients treated with intramuscular slow-release lanreotide. J Clin Endocrinol Metab 1997; 82:18.
42. Krenning EP, Kwekkeboom DJ, Bakker WH, et al. Somatostatin receptor scintigraphy with [111In-DTPA-D-Phe1]- and [123I-Tyr3]-octreotide: the Rotterdam experience with more than 1000 patients. Eur J Nucl Med 1993; 20:716.
43. Chanson P. Predicting the effects of long-term medical treatment in acromegaly. At what cost? For what benefits? Eur J Endocrinol 1997; 136:359.
44. Frohman LA. Acromegaly: what constitutes optimal therapy? J Clin Endocrinol Metab 1996; 81:443.
45. Melmed S, Ho K, Klibanski A, et al. Clinical review 75: recent advances in pathogenesis, diagnosis, and management of acromegaly. J Clin Endocrinol Metab 1995; 80:3395.
46. Bates AS, Van't Hoff W, Jones JM, Clayton RN. An audit of outcome of treatment in acromegaly. Q J Med 1993; 86:293.
47. Rajasoorya C, Holdaway IM, Wrightson P, et al. Determinants of clinical outcome and survival in acromegaly. Clin Endocrinol (Oxf) 1994; 41:95.
48. Abosch A, Tyrrell JB, Lamborn KR, et al. Transsphenoidal microsurgery for growth hormone-secreting pituitary adenomas: initial outcome and long-term results. J Clin Endocrinol Metab 1998; 83:3411.

49. Orme SM, McNally RJ, Cartwright RA, Belchetz PE. Mortality and cancer incidence in acromegaly: a retrospective cohort study. United Kingdom Acromegaly Study Group. J Clin Endocrinol Metab 1998; 83:2730.

50. Swearingen B, Barker FGN, Katznelson L, et al. Long-term mortality after transsphenoidal surgery and adjunctive therapy for acromegaly. J Clin Endocrinol Metab 1998; 83:3419.

51. Melmed S. Tight control of growth hormone: an attainable outcome for acromegaly treatment. J Clin Endocrinol Metab 1998; 83:3409.

52. Giustina A, Barkan A, Casanueva FF, et al. Criteria for cure in acromegaly: a consensus statement. J Clin Endocrinol Metab 2000; 85:526.

53. Roelfsema F, van Dulken H, Frolich M. Long-term results of transsphenoidal pituitary microsurgery in 60 acromegalic patients. Clin Endocrinol (Oxf) 1985; 23:555.

54. Sheaves R, Jenkins P, Blackburn P, et al. Outcome of transsphenoidal surgery for acromegaly using strict criteria for surgical cure. Clin Endocrinol (Oxf) 1996; 45:407.

55. Yamada S, Aiba T, Takada K, et al. Retrospective analysis of long-term surgical results in acromegaly: preoperative and postoperative factors predicting outcome. Clin Endocrinol (Oxf) 1996; 45:291.

56. Colao A, Ferone D, Cappabianca P, et al. Effect of octreotide pretreatment on surgical outcome in acromegaly. J Clin Endocrinol Metab 1997; 82:3308.

57. Colao A, Merola B, Ferone D, Lombardi G. Acromegaly. J Clin Endocrinol Metab 1997; 82:2777.

58. Freda PU, Wardlaw SL, Post KD. Long-term endocrinological follow-up evaluation in 115 patients who underwent transsphenoidal surgery for acromegaly. J Neurosurg 1998; 89:353.

59. Buchfelder M, Brockmeier S, Fahlbusch R, et al. Recurrence following transsphenoidal surgery for acromegaly. Horm Res 1991; 35:113.

60. Losa M, Oeckler R, Schopohl J, et al. Evaluation of selective transsphenoidal adenomectomy by endocrinological testing and somatomedin-C measurement in acromegaly. J Neurosurg 1989; 70:561.

61. Lamberg BA, Kivikangas V, Vartianen J, et al. Conventional pituitary irradiation in acromegaly. Effect on growth hormone and TSH secretion. Acta Endocrinol 1976; 82:267.

62. Feek CM, McLelland J, Seth J, et al. How effective is external pituitary irradiation for growth hormone-secreting pituitary tumors? Clin Endocrinol (Oxf) 1984; 20:401.

63. Kliman B, Kjellberg RN, Swisher B, Butler W. Long-term effects of proton-beam therapy for acromegaly. In: Robbins RJ, Melmed S, eds. Acromegaly. New York: Plenum Press, 1986:221.

64. Speirs CJ, Reed PI, Morrison R, et al. The effectiveness of external beam radiotherapy for acromegaly is not affected by previous pituitary ablative treatments. Acta Endocrinol (Copenh) 1990; 122:559.

65. Chanson P, Grellier-Fouqueray P, Young J, et al. Comment et avec quelle efficacité traite-t-on l'acromégalie en 1997? Enquête transversale sur une population de 74 acromégales. (Abstract). Ann Endocrinol (Paris) 1997; 58(Suppl 2):2S69.

66. Thalassinos NC, Tsagarakis S, Ioannides G, et al. Megavoltage pituitary irradiation lowers but seldom leads to safe GH levels in acromegaly: a long-term follow-up study. Eur J Endocrinol 1998; 138:160.

67. Morange-Ramos I, Regis J, Dufour H, et al. Gamma-knife surgery for secreting pituitary adenomas. Acta Neurochir (Wien) 1998; 140:437.

68. Landolt AM, Haller D, Lomax N, et al. Stereotactic radiosurgery for recurrent surgically treated acromegaly: comparison with fractionated radiotherapy. J Neurosurg 1998; 88:1002.

69. Arosio M, Macchelli S, Rossi CM, et al. Effects of treatment with octreotide in acromegalic patients—a multicenter Italian study. Italian Multicenter Octreotide Study Group. Eur J Endocrinol 1995; 133:430.

70. Newman CB, Melmed S, George A, et al. Octreotide as primary therapy for acromegaly. J Clin Endocrinol Metab 1998; 83:3034.

71. Fløgstad AK, Halse J, Bakke S, et al. Sandostatin LAR in acromegalic patients: long-term treatment. J Clin Endocrinol Metab 1997; 82:23.

72. Lancranjan I, Bruns C, Grass P, et al. Sandostatin LAR: a promising therapeutic tool in the management of acromegalic patients. Metabolism 1996; 45:67.

73. Stewart PM, Kane KF, Stewart SE, et al. Depot long-acting somatostatin analog (Sandostatin-LAR) is an effective treatment for acromegaly. J Clin Endocrinol Metab 1995; 80:3267.

74. Molitch M. Prolactinoma. In: Melmed S, ed. The pituitary. Boston: Blackwell Science, 1995:443.

75. Thorner M, Vance ML, Laws ER Jr, et al. The anterior pituitary. In: Wilson JD, Foster DW, Kronenberg HM, Larsen PR, eds. Williams textbook of endocrinology. Philadelphia: WB Saunders, 1998:249.

76. Vance ML, Evans WS, Thorner MO. Drugs five years later. Bromocriptine. Ann Intern Med 1984; 100:78.

77. Liuzzi A, Dallabonzana D, Oppizzi G, et al. Low doses of dopamine agonists in the long-term treatment of macroprolactinomas. N Engl J Med 1985; 313:656.

78. Molitch ME, Thorner MO, Wilson C. Management of prolactinomas. J Clin Endocrinol Metab 1997; 82:996.

79. Bevan JS, Webster J, Burke CW, Scanlon MF. Dopamine agonists and pituitary tumor shrinkage. Endocr Rev 1992; 13:220.

80. Molitch ME. Pregnancy and the hyperprolactinemic woman. N Engl J Med 1985; 312:1364.

81. Kupersmith MJ, Rosenberg C, Kleinberg D. Visual loss in pregnant women with pituitary adenomas. Ann Intern Med 1994; 121:473.

82. Gemzell C, Wang CF. Outcome of pregnancy in women with pituitary adenoma. Fertil Steril 1979; 31:363.

83. van't Verlaat JW, Croughs RJ, Brownell J. Treatment of macroprolactinomas with a new non-ergot, long-acting dopaminergic drug, CV 205-502. Clin Endocrinol (Oxf) 1990; 33:619.

84. Duranteau L, Chanson P, Lavoinne A, et al. Effect of the new dopaminergic agonist CV 205-502 on plasma prolactin levels and tumour size in bromocriptine-resistant prolactinomas. Clin Endocrinol (Oxf) 1991; 34:25.

85. Brue T, Pellegrini I, Gunz G, et al. Effects of the dopamine agonist CV 205-502 in human prolactinomas resistant to bromocriptine. J Clin Endocrinol Metab 1992; 74:577.

86. Vilar L, Burke CW. Quinagolide efficacy and tolerability in hyperprolactinaemic patients who are resistant to or intolerant of bromocriptine. Clin Endocrinol (Oxf) 1994; 41:821.

87. Rains CP, Bryson HM, Fitton A. Cabergoline: a review of its pharmacological properties and therapeutic potential in the treatment of hyperprolactinaemia and inhibition of lactation. Drugs 1995; 49:255.

88. Webster J, Piscitelli G, Polli A, et al. A comparison of cabergoline and bromocriptine in the treatment of hyperprolactinemic amenorrhea. Cabergoline Comparative Study Group. N Engl J Med 1994; 331:904.

89. Biller BM, Molitch ME, Vance ML, et al. Treatment of prolactin-secreting macroadenomas with the once-weekly dopamine agonist cabergoline. J Clin Endocrinol Metab 1996; 81:2338.

90. Colao A, Di Sarno A, Sarnacchiaro F, et al. Prolactinomas resistant to standard dopamine agonists respond to chronic cabergoline treatment. J Clin Endocrinol Metab 1997; 82:876.

91. Colao A, Di Sarno A, Landi ML, et al. Long-term and low-dose treatment with cabergoline induces macroprolactinoma shrinkage. J Clin Endocrinol Metab 1997; 82:3574.

92. Feigenbaum SL, Downey DE, Wilson CB, Jaffe RB. Transsphenoidal pituitary resection for preoperative diagnosis of prolactin-secreting pituitary adenoma in women: long term follow-up. J Clin Endocrinol Metab 1996; 81:1711.

93. Thomson JA, Davies DL, McLaren EH, Teasdale GM. Ten year follow up of microprolactinoma treated by transsphenoidal surgery. BMJ 1994; 309:1409.

94. Serri O, Hardy J, Massoud F. Relapse of hyperprolactinemia revisited. N Engl J Med 1993; 329:1357.

95. Grossman A, Cohen BL, Charlesworth M, et al. Treatment of prolactinomas with megavoltage radiotherapy. BMJ 1984; 288:1105.

96. Nabarro JD. Pituitary prolactinomas. Clin Endocrinol (Oxf) 1982; 17:129.

97. Tsagarakis S, Grossman A, Plowman PN, et al. Megavoltage pituitary irradiation in the management of prolactinomas: long-term follow-up. Clin Endocrinol (Oxf) 1991; 34:399.

98. Miller JW, Crapo L. The medical treatment of Cushing's syndrome. Endocr Rev 1993; 14:443.

99. Bertagna X, Raux-Demay MC, Guilhaume B, et al. Cushing's disease. In: Melmed S, ed. The pituitary. Boston: Blackwell Science, 1995:478.

100. Arnott RD, Pestell RG, McKelvie PA, et al. A critical evaluation of transsphenoidal surgery in the treatment of Cushing's disease: prediction of outcome. Acta Endocrinol (Copenh) 1990; 123:423.

101. Orth DN. Cushing's syndrome. N Engl J Med 1995; 332:791.

102. Bochicchio D, Losa M, Buchfelder M. Factors influencing the immediate and late outcome of Cushing's disease treated by transsphenoidal surgery: a retrospective study by the European Cushing's Disease Survey Group. J Clin Endocrinol Metab 1995; 80:3114.

103. Guilhaume B, Bertagna X, Thomsen M, et al. Transsphenoidal pituitary surgery for the treatment of Cushing's disease: results in 64 patients and long term follow-up studies. J Clin Endocrinol Metab 1988; 66:1056.

104. Mampalam TJ, Tyrrell JB, Wilson CB. Transsphenoidal microsurgery for Cushing disease. A report of 216 cases. Ann Intern Med 1988; 109:487.

105. Burke CW, Adams CB, Esiri MM, et al. Transsphenoidal surgery for Cushing's disease: does what is removed determine the endocrine outcome? Clin Endocrinol (Oxf) 1990; 33:525.

106. Post KD, Habas JE. Comparison of long term results between prolactin secreting adenomas and ACTH secreting adenomas. Can J Neurol Sci 1990; 17:74.

107. Tindall GT, Herring CJ, Clark RV, et al. Cushing's disease: results of transsphenoidal microsurgery with emphasis on surgical failures. J Neurosurg 1990; 72:363.

108. Robert F, Hardy J. Cushing's disease: a correlation of radiological, surgical and pathological findings with therapeutic results. Pathol Res Pract 1991; 187:617.

109. Tahir AH, Sheeler LR. Recurrent Cushing's disease after transsphenoidal surgery. Arch Intern Med 1992; 152:977.

110. Trainer PJ, Lawrie HS, Verhelst J, et al. Transsphenoidal resection in Cushing's disease: undetectable serum cortisol as the definition of successful treatment. Clin Endocrinol (Oxf) 1993; 38:73.

111. Ram Z, Nieman LK, Cutler GB Jr, et al. Early repeat surgery for persistent Cushing's disease. J Neurosurg 1994; 80:37.

112. Styne DM, Grumbach MM, Kaplan SL, et al. Treatment of Cushing's disease in childhood and adolescence by transsphenoidal microadenomectomy. N Engl J Med 1984; 310:889.

113. Dyer EH, Civit T, Visot A, et al. Transsphenoidal surgery for pituitary adenomas in children. Neurosurgery 1994; 34:207.

114. Leinung MC, Kane LA, Scheithauer BW, et al. Long term follow-up of transsphenoidal surgery for the treatment of Cushing's disease in childhood. J Clin Endocrinol Metab 1995; 80:2475.

115. Magiakou MA, Mastorakos G, Oldfield EH, et al. Cushing's syndrome in children and adolescents. Presentation, diagnosis, and therapy. N Engl J Med 1994; 331:629.

116. Howlett TA, Plowman PN, Wass JA, et al. Megavoltage pituitary irradiation in the management of Cushing's disease and Nelson's syndrome: long-term follow-up. Clin Endocrinol (Oxf) 1989; 31:309.

117. Estrada J, Boronat M, Mielgo M, et al. The long-term outcome of pituitary irradiation after unsuccessful transsphenoidal surgery in Cushing's disease. N Engl J Med 1997; 336:172.

118. Tyrrell JB, Wilson CB. Cushing's disease. Therapy of pituitary adenomas. Endocrinol Metab Clin North Am 1994; 23:925.

119. Chanson P, Weintraub BD, Harris AG. Octreotide therapy for thyroid-stimulating hormone-secreting pituitary adenomas. A follow-up of 52 patients. Ann Intern Med 1993; 119:236.

120. Gancel A, Vuillermet P, Legrand A, et al. Effects of a slow-release formulation of the new somatostatin analogue lanreotide in TSH-secreting pituitary adenomas. Clin Endocrinol (Oxf) 1994; 40:421.

121. Beck-Peccoz P, Brucker-Davis F, Persani L, et al. Thyrotropin-secreting pituitary adenomas. Endocr Rev 1996; 17:610.

122. Warnet A, Timsit J, Chanson P, et al. The effect of somatostatin analogue on chiasmal dysfunction from pituitary macroadenomas. J Neurosurg 1989; 71:687.

123. Warnet A, Harris AG, Renard E, et al. A prospective multicenter trial of octreotide in 24 patients with visual defects caused by nonfunctioning and gonadotropin-secreting pituitary adenomas. Neurosurgery 1997; 41:786.

124. Molitch ME. Evaluation and treatment of the patient with a pituitary incidentaloma. J Clin Endocrinol Metab 1995; 80:3.

125. Ebersold MJ, Quast LM, Laws ER Jr, et al. Long-term results in transsphenoidal removal of nonfunctioning pituitary adenomas. J Neurosurg 1986; 64:713.

126. Harris PE, Afshar F, Coates P, et al. The effects of transsphenoidal surgery on endocrine function and visual fields in patients with functionless pituitary tumours. Q J Med 1989; 71:417.

127. Comtois R, Beauregard H, Somma M, et al. The clinical and endocrine outcome to transphenoidal microsurgery of non secreting pituitary adenomas. Cancer 1991; 68:860.

128. Sassolas G, Trouillas J, Treluyer C, Perrin G. Management of non-functioning pituitary adenomas. Acta Endocrinol 1993; 129(Suppl 1):21.

129. Chanson P. Les adénomes hypophysaires non-fonctionnels. Paris: John Libbey Eurotext, 1998.

130. Hayes TP, Davis RA, Raventos A. The treatment of pituitary chromophobe adenomas. Radiology 1971; 98:149.

131. Ciric I, Mikhael M, Stafford T, et al. Transsphenoidal microsurgery of pituitary macroadenomas with long-term follow-up results. J Neurosurg 1983; 59:395.

132. Vlahovitch B, Reynaud C, Rhiati J, et al. Treatment and recurrences in 135 pituitary adenomas. Acta Neurochir 1988; 42(Suppl):120.

133. Jaffrain-Rea ML, Derome P, Bataini JP, et al. Influence of radiotherapy on long-term relapse in clinically non-secreting pituitary adenomas. A retrospective study (1970–1988). Eur J Med 1993; 2:398.

134. Bradley KM, Adams CBT, Potter CPS, et al. An audit of selected patients with non-functioning pituitary adenoma treated by transsphenoidal surgery without irradiation. Clin Endocrinol (Oxf) 1994; 41:655.

135. Gittoes NJL, Bates AS, Tse W, et al. Radiotherapy for non-functioning pituitary tumours. Clin Endocrinol (Oxf) 1998; 48:331.

136. Rosen T, Bengtsson A-G. Premature mortality due to cardiovascular disease in hypopituitarism. Lancet 1990; 336:285.

137. Bates AS, Van't Hoff W, Jones PJ, Clayton RN. The effects of hypopituitarism on life expectancy. J Clin Endocrinol Metab 1996; 81:1169.

138. Bülow B, Hagmar L, Mikoczy Z, et al. Increased cerebrovascular mortality in patients with hypopituitarism. Clin Endocrinol (Oxf) 1997; 46:75.

139. Liuzzi A, Dallabonzana D, Oppizzi G, et al. Is there a real medical treatment for "non-secreting" pituitary adenoma? In: Faglia G, Beck-Peccoz P, Ambrosi P, Travaglini P, Spada A, eds. Pituitary adenomas: new trends in basic and clinical research. Amsterdam: Excerpta Medica, 1991:383.

140. Chanson P, Schaison G. Pituitary apoplexy caused by GnRH-agonist treatment revealing gonadotroph adenoma. J Clin Endocrinol Metab 1995; 80:2267.

141. McGrath GA, Goncalves RJ, Voupa JK, et al. New technique for quantitation of pituitary adenoma size: use in evaluating treatment of gonadotroph adenomas with a gonadotropin-releasing hormone antagonist. J Clin Endocrinol Metab 1993; 76:1363.

142. Etxabe J, Vazquez JA. Morbidity and mortality in Cushing's disease: an epidemiological approach. Clin Endocrinol (Oxf) 1994; 40:479.

143. Carroll PV, Christ ER, Bengtsson BA, et al. Growth hormone deficiency in adulthood and the effects of growth hormone replacement: a review. Growth Hormone Research Society Scientific Committee. J Clin Endocrinol Metab 1998; 83:382.

144. Orrego JJ, Barkan AL. Pituitary disorders. Drug treatment options. Drugs 2000; 59:93.

145. Bates AS, Farrell WE, Bicknell EJ, et al. Allelic deletion in pituitary adenomas reflects aggressive biological activity and has potential value as a prognostic marker. J Clin Endocrinol Metab 1997; 82:818.

# SECTION B

# NEUROHYPOPHYSIAL SYSTEM

## CHAPTER 25

# PHYSIOLOGY OF VASOPRESSIN, OXYTOCIN, AND THIRST

GARY L. ROBERTSON

## ANATOMY OF THE NEUROHYPOPHYSIS

### GROSS FEATURES

The neurohypophysis, an extension of the ventral hypothalamus, attaches to the dorsal and caudal surface of the adenohypophysis[1] (Fig. 25-1). In adult men and women, it weighs ~100 mg. It is divided by the diaphragma sellae into an upper part, called the *infundibulum* or *median eminence,* and a lower part, known as the *infundibular process* or *pars nervosa.* The two parts are supplied

with blood by branches from the superior and inferior hypophyseal arteries. In the pars nervosa, the arterioles break up into localized capillary networks that drain directly into the jugular vein through the sellar, cavernous, and lateral venous sinuses. In the infundibulum, the primary capillary networks coalesce into another system, the portal veins, which perfuse the adenohypophysis before discharging into the systemic circulation.

### MICROSCOPIC FEATURES

On microscopic examination, the neurohypophysis appears as a densely interwoven network of capillaries, pituicytes, and nonmyelinated nerve fibers containing many electron-dense neurosecretory granules. These neurosecretory neurons terminate as bulbous enlargements on capillary networks located at all levels of the neurohypophysis, including the stalk and infundibulum. The vasopressin-containing neurosecretory neurons that form the pars nervosa originate primarily in the supraoptic nuclei[2] and probably provide most, if not all, of the vasopressin and oxytocin in the peripheral plasma. Those that terminate in the median eminence originate primarily in the paraventricular or other hypothalamic nuclei,[2] probably releasing their hormones into the portal blood supply of the anterior pituitary. Other,

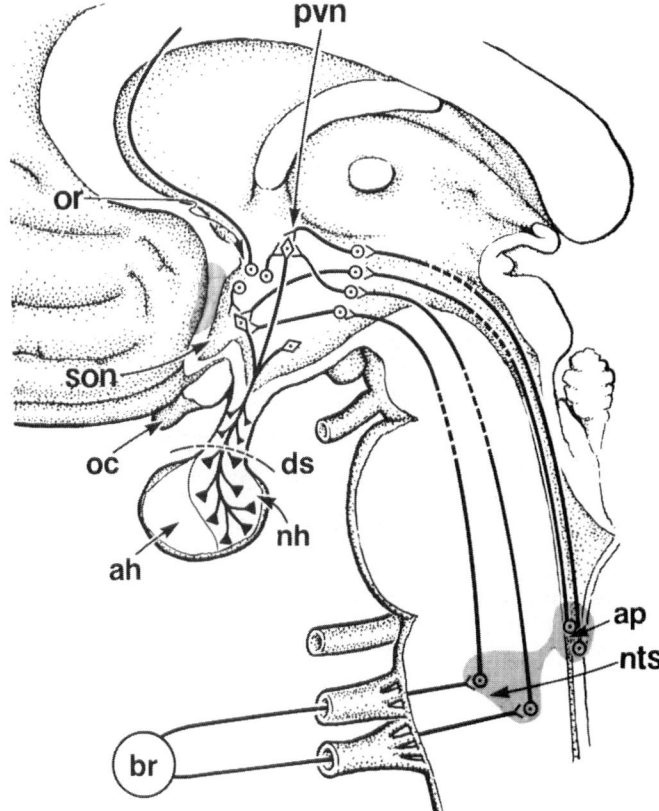

**FIGURE 25-1.** The neurohypophysis and its principal regulatory afferents are illustrated. (*pvn*, paraventricular nucleus; *or*, osmoreceptor; *son*, supraoptic nucleus; *oc*, optic chiasm; *ds*, diaphragma sellae; *ah*, adenohypophysis; *nh*, neurohypophysis; *br*, volume and baroreceptors; *ap*, area postrema [emetic center]; *nts*, nucleus tractus solitarii.) (From Robertson GL. Disorders of the posterior pituitary. In: Stein JH, ed. Internal medicine. Boston: Little, Brown and Company, 1983:1728.)

smaller groups of vasopressinergic neurons project from the paraventricular nucleus to the medulla, amygdala, spinal cord, and the walls of the lateral and third ventricles.[2] The latter may secrete directly into the cerebrospinal fluid (CSF).[3]

Oxytocinergic cell bodies appear to be less numerous than those containing vasopressin.[2] They are found primarily in discrete areas in or around the paraventricular nuclei and, to a lesser extent, the supraoptic nuclei. Most oxytocinergic neurons project to the pars nervosa, but many also terminate in the organum vasculosum or the median eminence. In addition, a relatively large paraventricular division runs parallel to the vasopressinergic fibers that connect to the medulla and spinal cord (see Chaps. 8 and 9).

## CHEMISTRY

Vasopressin and oxytocin are the only hormones known to be secreted in significant amounts by the neurohypophysis. As first shown by du Vigneaud and coworkers,[4] the two hormones have similar structures (Fig. 25-2), being nonapeptides that contain six-membered disulfide rings and the same amino acid residues in seven of the nine positions. They are stored in neurosecretory granules as insoluble complexes with specific carrier proteins known as *neurophysins*.[5] The neurophysins associated with vasopressin and oxytocin also have similar structures, each having ~100 amino-acid residues with extensive areas of homology. Binding of the hormones to their neurophysins has a pH optima (5.2–5.8) and dissociation constant (Kd) (~5 × 10$^5$) that favor asso-

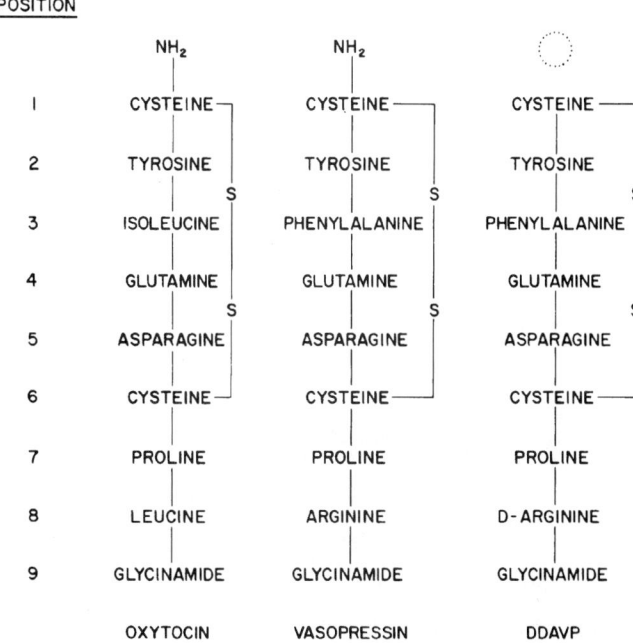

**FIGURE 25-2.** Structure of oxytocin, vasopressin, and 1-deamino-(8-D-arginine)-vasopressin (*DDAVP*). (*S*, sulfur.)

ciation in neurosecretory granules but ensures almost complete dissociation in plasma and other body fluids.

## BIOSYNTHESIS AND RELEASE OF VASOPRESSIN AND OXYTOCIN

Vasopressin and oxytocin are synthesized through protein precursors encoded by single-copy genes that are located near each other on chromosome 20 in humans[6–9] (Fig. 25-3). The gene for the vasopressin precursor, known as *propressophysin* or *vasopressin neurophysin II*, is ~2-kb long. It contains three exons that encode, respectively, (a) a signal peptide, vasopressin, and the variable amino-terminal end of neurophysin; (b) the highly conserved middle portion of neurophysin; and (c) the variable, carboxy-terminal end of neurophysin and copeptin, a glycosylated peptide of unknown function. The gene for the oxytocin precursor is similar except that exon C is shorter and codes only

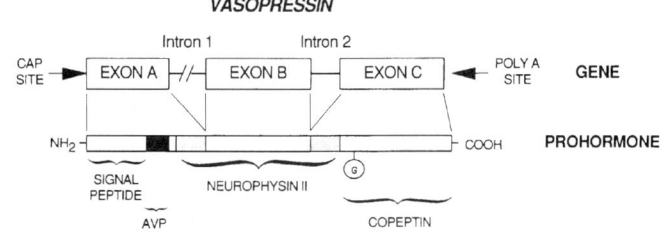

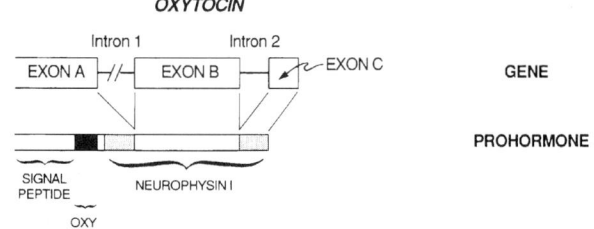

**FIGURE 25-3.** Structure of the vasopressin and oxytocin prohormones and the genes that encode them. (*AVP*, arginine vasopressin; *G*, glycosylation.)

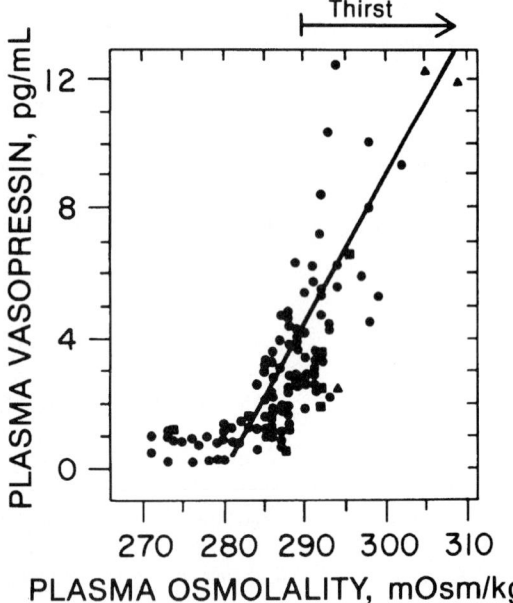

**FIGURE 25-4.** The relationship of thirst and plasma vasopressin to plasma osmolality in healthy adults under varying conditions of water balance. (From Robertson GL. Thirst and vasopressin function in normal and disordered states of water balance. J Lab Clin Med 1983; 101:351.)

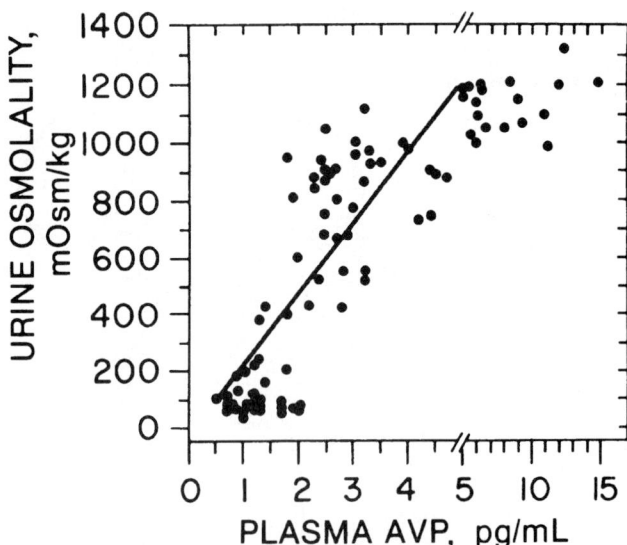

**FIGURE 25-5.** The relation of urine osmolality to plasma vasopressin in healthy adults under varying conditions of water balance. (*AVP,* arginine vasopressin.) (From Robertson GL. Thirst and vasopressin function in normal and disordered states of water balance. J Lab Clin Med 1983; 101:351.)

for the variable carboxy terminus of neurophysin and a single histidine residue. The copeptin moiety is absent.

In humans and other mammals, the vasopressin and oxytocin genes are expressed in different magnocellular neurons. After transcription and translation in cell bodies within the supraoptic and paraventricular nuclei, the preprohormones are translocated into the endoplasmic reticulum, where the signal peptide is removed and the prohormones fold and self-associate before moving through the Golgi apparatus and on into the neurosecretory granules. There they are transported down the axons and cleaved into the intact hormone, neurophysin, and, in the case of vasopressin, *copeptin.* This process is critically dependent on correct folding and self-association of the prohormone in the endoplasmic reticulum, because genetic mutations predicted to alter amino acids important for correct folding severely disrupt transport and destroy the neurons, producing the autosomal dominant form of familial neurohypophyseal diabetes insipidus.

Release of the hormones and their associated neurophysins occurs via a calcium-dependent exocytotic process similar to that described for other neurosecretory systems.[10] An electrical impulse propagated along the neuron depolarizes the cell membrane, causing an influx of calcium, fusion of secretory granules with the outer cell membranes, and extrusion of their contents.

## REGULATION OF VASOPRESSIN SECRETION

### OSMOTIC REGULATION

The secretion of vasopressin is influenced by a number of variables.[11–15] The most important under physiologic conditions is the effective osmotic pressure of plasma. This influence is mediated by specialized cells called *osmoreceptors.* These osmoreceptors appear to be concentrated in the anterolateral hypothalamus,[16–18] in an area that is near, but separate from, the supraoptic nuclei (see Fig. 25-1). This area is supplied with blood by small perforating branches of the anterior cerebral or communicating arteries.[1]

The basic structure, modus operandi, and organization of the individual osmoreceptors have not yet been determined. However, the system as a whole functions like a discontinuous or setpoint receptor (Fig. 25-4). Thus, at plasma osmolalities below a certain minimum or threshold level, plasma vasopressin is sup-

pressed to low or undetectable concentrations. Above this setpoint, plasma vasopressin rises steeply in direct proportion to plasma osmolality. The slope of the relationship indicates that a change in plasma osmolality of only 1% alters plasma vasopressin by an average of 1 pg/mL, an amount sufficient to significantly affect the urinary concentration and flow (Fig. 25-5).

The sensitivity and "set" of the osmoregulatory system varies considerably among healthy adults. The interindividual differences in sensitivity are large (up to 10-fold), are constant over long periods of time, and appear to be genetically determined.[19] However, they can be altered slightly by a variety of pharmacologic or pathologic influences.[20] The interindividual differences in setpoint are not as large (275–290 mOsm/kg) or as constant over time but also appear to have a significant genetic component.[19] They are more subject to alteration by a variety of physiologic factors, including posture, pregnancy, and the phase of the menstrual cycle,[20,21] all of which lower the osmotic threshold or setpoint.

The sensitivity of the osmoregulatory system also varies for different plasma solutes (Fig. 25-6). Sodium and its anions, which normally contribute >95% of the osmotic pressure of plasma, are the most potent solutes known in terms of their capacity to stimulate vasopressin release.[20] Certain sugars, such as sucrose and mannitol, appear to be nearly as potent. However, a rise in plasma osmolality secondary to urea or glucose causes little or no increase in plasma vasopressin in healthy adults or animals. These differences in response to various plasma solutes are independent of any recognized nonosmotic influence and probably reflect some property of the osmoregulatory mechanism. Precisely how the osmoreceptor discriminates so effectively between different kinds of plasma solutes still is unresolved. According to current concepts, the signal that stimulates the osmoreceptor is an osmotically induced decrease in the water content of the cell. If this hypothesis is correct, the capacity of a given solute to stimulate vasopressin secretion should be inversely related to the rate at which it passes from plasma into the osmoreceptor. This concept agrees well with the observed inverse relationship between the stimulatory effect of certain solutes, such as sodium, mannitol, and glucose, and the rate at which they penetrate the blood–brain barrier. However, urea is an exception because it penetrates the blood–brain barrier slowly yet is a relatively weak stimulus for thirst and vasopressin. This singular disparity suggests that most, if not all, of the osmorecep-

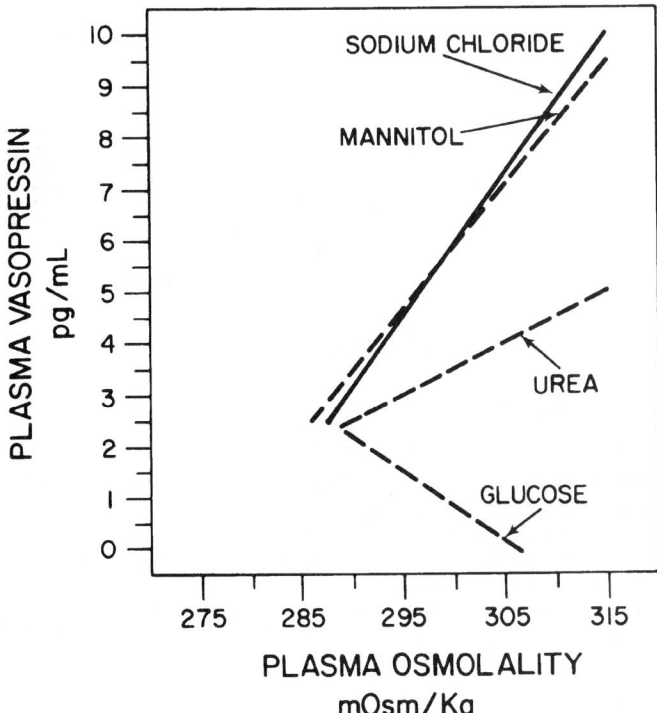

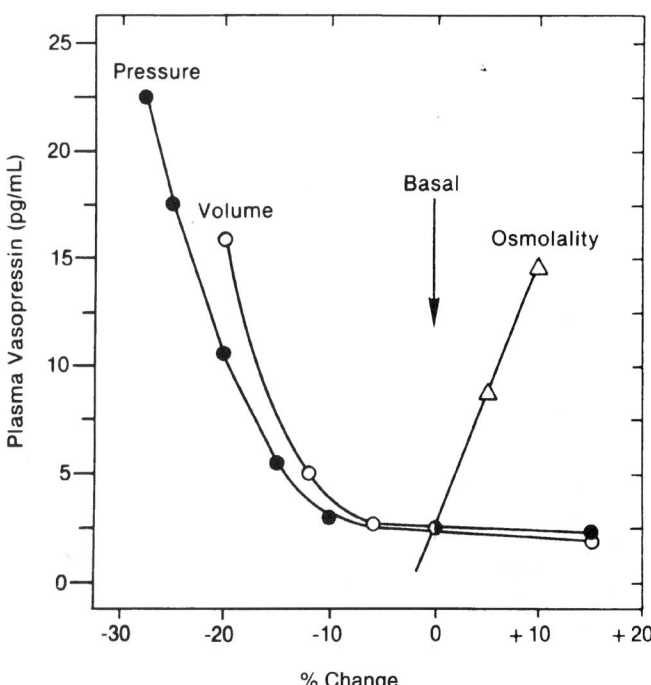

**FIGURE 25-6.** The relationship of plasma vasopressin to plasma osmolality in healthy adults during the infusion of hypertonic solutions of different solutes. (From Robertson GL. Disorders of the posterior pituitary. In: Stein JH, ed. Internal medicine. Boston: Little, Brown and Company, 1983:1728.)

**FIGURE 25-7.** Schematic representation of the relationship between plasma vasopressin and percentage of change in plasma osmolality, blood volume, or blood pressure in healthy adults. (From Robertson GL. Diseases of the posterior pituitary. In: Felig P, Baxter J, Brodus A, Frohman L, eds. Endocrinology and metabolism. New York: McGraw-Hill, 1981:251.)

tors are located outside of the blood–brain barrier and that another factor (most likely, the permeability of the osmoreceptor cell itself) determines the solute specificity of the system.

The solute specificity of the osmoregulatory system is also subject to change. Thus, its sensitivity to stimulation by glucose increases when insulin is deficient.[20] This change probably results from decreased permeability of the osmoreceptors to glucose and indicates that these cells are insulin dependent. It may also explain the hyperdipsia and at least part of the hypervasopressinemia that occurs in many patients with uncontrolled type 1 diabetes mellitus.

### HEMODYNAMIC REGULATION

The secretion of vasopressin is also affected by changes in blood volume, pressure, or both.[11,12,14,15,22] These hemodynamic influences are mediated largely, if not exclusively, by neurogenic afferents that arise in pressure-sensitive receptors in the heart and large arteries and that travel by way of the vagal and glossopharyngeal nerves to primary synapses in the nucleus tractus solitarius in the brainstem (see Fig. 25-1). From there, postsynaptic pathways project to the region of the paraventricular and supraoptic nuclei. At least one of the links in the afferent chain for volume control involves opioid receptors in the lateral parabrachial nucleus, because administration of selective as well as nonselective antagonists in this area almost totally inhibits the vasopressin response to an acute hypovolemic stimulus.[23–25]

The functional properties of the baroregulatory system also differ from those of the osmoregulatory mechanism (Fig. 25-7). In healthy adults and animals, acutely lowering blood pressure increases plasma vasopressin in proportion to the degree of hypotension achieved. However, this stimulus-response relationship follows a distinctly exponential pattern. Thus, small decreases in blood pressure of 5% to 10% usually have little effect on plasma vasopressin, whereas decreases in blood pressure of 20% to 30% result in hormone levels many times those required to produce maximal antidiuresis. The vasopressin

response to changes in blood volume has not been well defined but appears to be quantitatively and qualitatively similar to the vasopressin response to changes in blood pressure. An acute rise in blood volume or pressure appears to suppress vasopressin secretion.

The failure of small changes in blood volume and pressure to alter vasopressin secretion contrasts markedly with the extraordinary sensitivity of the osmoregulatory system (see Fig. 25-7). The recognition of this difference is essential for understanding the relative contribution of each system to the control of the hormone under both physiologic and pathologic conditions. Because day-to-day variations of total body water rarely exceed 2% to 3%, their effect on vasopressin secretion must be mediated largely, if not exclusively, by the osmoregulatory system. For this reason, patients with destruction of the osmoreceptor exhibit a markedly subnormal vasopressin response to changes in water balance, even though baroregulatory mechanisms are completely intact. On the other hand, baroregulatory input appears to mediate the effects of a large number of pharmacologic agents and pathologic conditions (Table 25-1). Among these are diuretics, isoproterenol, nicotine, prostaglandins, nitroprusside, trimethaphan camsylate, histamine, morphine, and bradykinin, all of which stimulate vasopressin secretion, at least in part, by lowering blood volume or pressure. In addition, norepinephrine and aldosterone suppress vasopressin secretion by raising blood volume, pressure, or both. In addition, upright posture, sodium depletion, congestive failure, cirrhosis, and nephrosis stimulate vasopressin secretion, probably by reducing total or effective blood volume, whereas orthostatic hypotension, vasovagal reactions, and other forms of syncope markedly stimulate secretion of the hormone by reducing blood pressure. This list probably could be extended to include almost every other hormone, drug, and condition known to affect blood volume or pressure. The only recognized exception is a form of orthostatic hypotension associated with the loss of afferent baroregulatory function.[26]

**TABLE 25-1.**
**Variables That Influence Vasopressin Secretion**

---

**OSMOTIC**
  Plasma osmolality
    Changes in water balance
    Infusion of hypertonic, hypotonic solutions
    Hyperglycemia (diabetics)
**HEMODYNAMIC**
  Blood volume (total or effective)
    Posture
    Hemorrhage
    Aldosterone deficiency or excess
    Gastroenteritis
    Congestive failure
    Cirrhosis
    Nephrosis
    Positive pressure breathing
    Diuretics
  Blood pressure
    Orthostatic hypotension
    Vasovagal reaction
    Drugs (isoproterenol, norepinephrine, nicotine, nitroprusside, trimethaphan, histamine, bradykinin, morphine)
**EMETIC**
  Nausea
    Drugs (apomorphine, morphine, nicotine)
    Motion sickness
**GLUCOPENIC**
  Intracellular hypoglycemia
    Drugs (insulin, 2-deoxyglucose)
**OTHER**
  Angiotensin
  $P_{CO_2}$, $P_{O_2}$, pH
  Drugs
  Stress (?)
  Temperature (?)

---

Changes in blood volume or pressure that are large enough to affect vasopressin secretion do not necessarily interfere with osmoregulation of the hormone.[12–15] Instead, they appear to act by shifting the setpoint of the system in such a way as to increase or decrease the effect on vasopressin of a given osmotic stimulus (Fig. 25-8). This kind of interaction ensures that, even in the presence of hemodynamic stimuli, the capacity to osmoregulate is not lost. How this integration occurs is unknown, but it probably involves one or more interneurons that link the osmoreceptor to neurosecretory neurons.

**EMESIS**

Nausea is an extremely potent stimulus for vasopressin secretion in humans.[15] The pathway that mediates this effect probably involves the chemoreceptor trigger zone in the area postrema of the medulla (see Fig. 25-1). It can be activated by a variety of drugs and conditions, including apomorphine, morphine, nicotine, alcohol, and motion sickness.[15] Its effect on vasopressin secretion is instantaneous and extremely potent (Fig. 25-9). Increases in vasopressin of 100 to 1000 times basal levels are not unusual, even when the nausea is transient and unaccompanied by vomiting or changes in blood pressure. Pretreatment with fluphenazine, haloperidol, or promethazine in doses sufficient to prevent nausea completely abolishes the vasopressin response.[27] The inhibitory effect of these dopamine antagonists is specific for emetic stimuli because they do not alter the vasopressin response to hyperosmolality, hypovolemia, or hypotension.

Water loading blunts, but does not abolish, the effect of nausea on vasopressin release, a finding which suggests that

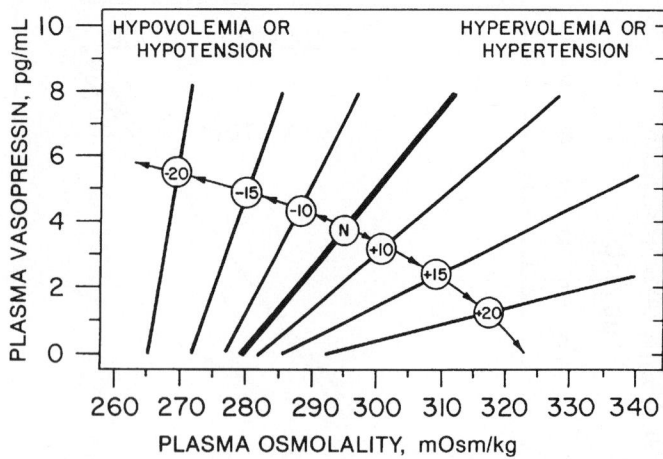

**FIGURE 25-8.** The relationship between plasma vasopressin and plasma osmolality in the presence of different states of blood volume or pressure. The oblique heavy line, labeled *N*, represents normovolemic, normotensive conditions. Lines labeled with negative numbers (*to the left*) or positive numbers (*to the right*) indicate, respectively, the percentage of decrease or increase in blood volume or pressure. (From Robertson GL. Disorders of the posterior pituitary. In: Stein JH, ed. Internal medicine. Boston: Little, Brown and Company, 1983:1728.)

osmotic and emetic influences interact in a manner similar to osmotic and hemodynamic pathways.[27] Emetic stimuli probably mediate many pharmacologic and pathologic effects on vasopressin secretion. For example, emetic stimulation may be at least partially responsible for the increase in vasopressin secretion that has been observed with intravenous administration of cyclophosphamide, vasovagal reactions, ketoacidosis, acute hypoxia, and motion sickness. Because nausea and vomiting are frequent side effects of many other drugs and diseases, additional examples of emetically mediated vasopressin secretion doubtlessly could be demonstrated.

**OTHER STIMULI**

**Hypoglycemia.** Acute hypoglycemia is a relatively weak stimulus for vasopressin release.[28] The receptor and pathway that mediate this effect are unknown but must be separate from those of other recognized stimuli because hypoglycemia stimulates vasopressin secretion in patients who have lost the capacity to respond selectively to osmotic, hemodynamic, or emetic stimuli. However, the vasopressin response to hypoglycemia is

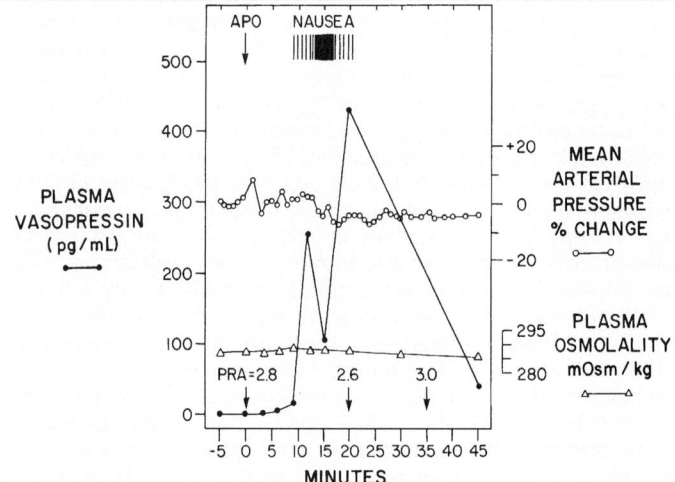

**FIGURE 25-9.** Effect of nausea on plasma vasopressin in a healthy adult. (*APO,* apomorphine; *PRA,* plasma renin activity.) (From Robertson GL. The regulation of vasopressin function in health and disease. Recent Prog Horm Res 1977; 33:333.)

accentuated by dehydration and is abolished by water loading. Thus, glucopenic stimuli probably act in concert with osmotic influences, even though the osmoreceptors are unnecessary for the response. Vasopressin release may be triggered by an intracellular deficiency of glucose or one of its metabolites because 2-deoxyglucose is also an effective stimulus.[29]

**Angiotensin.** The renin angiotensin system has also been implicated in the control of vasopressin secretion.[30] The precise site and mechanism of action have not been defined, but central receptors are likely to be involved because angiotensin is most effective when injected directly into brain ventricles or cranial arteries. The levels of plasma renin or angiotensin required to stimulate vasopressin release have not been determined but probably are high. When administered intravenously, pressor doses of angiotensin increase plasma vasopressin twofold to fourfold. The magnitude of the vasopressin response may depend on the concurrent osmotic stimulus, because angiotensin increases the sensitivity of the osmoregulatory system.[31] This dependency on osmotic influences resembles that seen with glucopenic stimuli and may account for the inconsistency of the vasopressin response to exogenous angiotensin.

### STRESS, TEMPERATURE, AND HYPOXIA

Nonspecific stress caused by pain, emotion, or physical exercise has long been thought to cause the release of vasopressin.[32] However, this effect now appears likely to be secondary to other stimuli, such as hypotension or nausea, which usually accompanies stress-induced vasovagal reactions. In the absence of hypotension or nausea, pain sufficient to stimulate the pituitary-adrenal axis has no effect on vasopressin secretion in humans.[33]

Acute hypoxia or hypercapnia also stimulates vasopressin release.[34] In conscious humans, however, the stimulatory effect of moderate hypoxia is inconsistent and appears to occur only in subjects who develop nausea or hypotension.[35] Severe hypoxia probably has a greater effect on vasopressin secretion and may be responsible for the osmotically inappropriate hormonal elevations noted in some patients with acute respiratory failure. Whether or not hypercapnia has similar effects on vasopressin secretion in conscious persons is not known.

### OROPHARYNGEAL INFLUENCES

Vasopressin secretion is inhibited by drinking before any detectable decrease in plasma osmolality is seen.[36] This inhibition can override a moderately strong osmotic stimulus but is not sustained unless it is followed by a prompt decline in plasma osmolality. The mechanism has not been determined, but it probably involves some kind of oropharyngeal receptor.

### OTHER HORMONES AND DRUGS

Many hormones and drugs influence vasopressin secretion.[37] Those that have a *stimulatory effect* include acetylcholine, nicotine, apomorphine, morphine (high doses), epinephrine, isoproterenol, histamine, bradykinin, prostaglandins, β-endorphin, intravenous cyclophosphamide, vincristine, insulin, 2-deoxyglucose, angiotensin, lithium, and possibly chlorpropamide and clofibrate. Those that have an *inhibitory effect* include norepinephrine, fluphenazine, haloperidol, promethazine, oxilorphan, butorphanol, morphine (low doses), alcohol, carbamazepine, glucocorticoids, clonidine hydrochloride, muscimol, and possibly phenytoin. Many stimulants, such as isoproterenol, nicotine, and high doses of morphine, undoubtedly act by lowering blood pressure or producing nausea. Others, such as substance P, prostaglandin, endorphin, and other opioids, also probably exert their influence by one or both of the same mechanisms. Insulin and 2-deoxyglucose appear to act by producing intracellular glucopenia, whereas angiotensin has an undefined but probably independent central effect. Vincristine may act by exerting a direct effect on the neurohypophysis or on peripheral neurons involved in the regulation of vasopressin secretion.

Lithium, which antagonizes the antidiuretic effect of vasopressin, also increases secretion of the hormone. This effect is independent of changes in water balance and appears to result from an increase in sensitivity of the osmoregulatory system. The stimulatory effects of chlorpropamide and clofibrate are still controversial. Carbamazepine inhibits vasopressin secretion by diminishing the sensitivity of the osmoregulatory system. This effect occurs independently of changes in blood volume, blood pressure, or blood glucose levels and suggests that the ability of carbamazepine to produce antidiuresis in patients with neurogenic diabetes insipidus is the result of action on the kidney.

Vasopressor drugs, such as norepinephrine, inhibit vasopressin secretion indirectly by raising arterial pressure. Dopaminergic antagonists, such as fluphenazine, haloperidol, and promethazine, probably act by suppressing the emetic center because they inhibit the vasopressin response to emetic stimuli only, not to osmotic or hemodynamic stimuli. In low doses, a variety of opioids, including morphine, butorphanol, and oxilorphan, inhibit vasopressin secretion, apparently by increasing the osmotic threshold for vasopressin release. The inhibitory effect of alcohol may be mediated by endogenous opiates; this effect also may be attributable to an elevation in the osmotic threshold for vasopressin release and can be blocked in part by treatment with naloxone hydrochloride. Other drugs that can inhibit vasopressin secretion include clonidine, which appears to act through both central and peripheral adrenoreceptors, and muscimol, which is postulated to act as a γ-aminobutyric acid antagonist. Vasopressin and oxytocin may also exert a feedback effect, inhibiting or facilitating their own secretion. In the case of vasopressin, feedback inhibition occurs after systemic or central administration of relatively large doses of the hormone.

## REGULATION OF OXYTOCIN SECRETION

In humans, the only stimulus known to reproducibly increase plasma oxytocin is suckling or other stimulation of the nipple in lactating women.[38] This stimulus may also cause the release of oxytocin in nonlactating women, but the effect is less consistent. No recognized stimulus has been found for oxytocin secretion in men. In rats, but not in humans, oxytocin secretion is induced by osmotic, hemodynamic, and emetic stimuli, which indicates that this hormone is regulated quite differently in the two species.

## DISTRIBUTION AND CLEARANCE OF VASOPRESSIN AND OXYTOCIN

In healthy adults, vasopressin and oxytocin distribute rapidly into a space roughly equivalent in volume to the extracellular compartment.[12,39] This initial mixing phase has a half-time of 4 to 8 minutes and is virtually complete in 10 to 15 minutes. This rapid mixing phase is followed by a second, slower decline that probably corresponds to the metabolic or irreversible phase of clearance. The half-time of the metabolic phase varies considerably from person to person but is in the range of 10 to 20 minutes. The metabolic clearance rate determined by steady-state as well as non–steady-state methods is largely independent of the plasma concentration within the physiologic range (ranging from 5 to 20 mL/kg per minute for vasopressin[12,39] and from 10 to 23 mL/kg per minute for oxytocin).[40] In pregnant women, the metabolic clearance rate of vasopressin is increased threefold to fourfold.[21]

Many tissues have the capacity to inactivate vasopressin in vitro, but most metabolism in vivo probably occurs in the liver and kidney. The plasma of pregnant women contains an enzyme that is capable of rapidly degrading the hormones in vitro, and it may also be active in vivo.[21]

Vasopressin and oxytocin are also excreted in urine, but the amounts are generally <10% of the total clearance.[12,40,41] The mechanisms involved in the excretion of vasopressin probably involve filtration at the glomerulus and variable reabsorption at one or more sites along the tubule. The latter process may be linked in some way to the handling of sodium in the proximal nephron because the urinary clearance of vasopressin varies by as much as 20-fold in a direct relationship with solute clearance. Consequently, measurements of urinary vasopressin do not provide a reliable index of changes in plasma vasopressin unless glomerular filtration and solute clearance are normal. The dependence of urinary oxytocin excretion on solute clearance has not been determined but is probably similar.

Vasopressin is also secreted into CSF[3] and the portal venous system of the anterior pituitary.[2] The concentration of vasopressin in the lumbar cistern is usually lower than that in plasma, but the two values tend to change in a parallel manner, a finding that suggests that they are subject to most, if not all, of the same regulatory influences. The two compartments must receive the hormone from different groups of neurons, however, because patients with neurogenic diabetes insipidus often have normal or increased CSF concentrations of vasopressin. The concentration of vasopressin in adenohypophyseal portal blood is much higher than that in peripheral veins but appears to be subject to some of the same regulatory influences (e.g., hypotension and hypovolemia).

## BIOLOGIC ACTIONS

### VASOPRESSIN

#### RENAL ACTION

The most important action of vasopressin is to *conserve body water* by reducing the rate of urinary, solute-free water excretion.[39] This antidiuretic effect is achieved by promoting the reabsorption of solute-free water from urine as it passes through the distal or collecting tubules of the kidney (Fig. 25-10) (see Chap. 206). In the absence of vasopressin, the membranes lining this portion of the nephron are impermeable to water as well as to solutes. Hence, hypotonic filtrate formed in the more proximal part of the nephron passes unmodified through the distal tubule and collecting duct. In this condition, which is known as *water diuresis*, urine osmolality and flow in a healthy adult usually approximate 40 to 60 mOsm/kg and 15 to 20 mL per minute, respectively. In the presence of vasopressin, the hydroosmotic permeability of the distal and collecting tubules increases, which allows water to back-diffuse down the osmotic gradient that normally exists between tubular fluid and the isotonic or hypertonic milieu of the renal cortex and medulla. Because water is reabsorbed without solute, the urine that remains has an increased osmotic pressure as well as a decreased volume or flow rate. The degree of urinary concentration is proportional to the plasma vasopressin concentration, and in healthy adults, it is usually maximal at hormone concentrations of 5 pg/mL or less (see Fig. 25-5).

The effect of vasopressin on urinary concentration and flow can be influenced markedly by changes in the volume of filtrate presented to the distal tubule. If the intake of salt is high, or if a poorly reabsorbed solute, such as mannitol, urea, or glucose, is filtered in increased amounts, the resultant decreased reabsorption in the proximal tubule may overwhelm the limited capacity of the distal nephron to reabsorb water and electrolytes. As a consequence, urine osmolality decreases, and the rate of flow rises, even in the presence of supranormal levels of vasopressin. This type of polyuria is referred to as *solute diuresis* to distinguish it from that resulting from a deficiency of vasopressin action. Conversely, in clinical conditions, such as congestive failure, in which the proximal nephron reabsorbs increased amounts of filtrate, the capacity to excrete solute-free water is greatly reduced, even in the absence of vasopressin.

The antidiuretic effect of vasopressin also may be inhibited by the dissipation of the medullary concentration gradient. The latter

may result from such diverse causes as chronic water diuresis, reduced medullary blood flow, or protein deficiency. However, probably because the bulk of the fluid issuing from the Henle loop can still be reabsorbed isotonically in the distal convoluted tubule or proximal collecting duct, the loss of the medullary concentration gradient alone rarely results in marked polyuria.

The cellular receptors that mediate the antidiuretic effect of vasopressin are located on the serosal surface of renal tubular epithelia in the collecting ducts. They are known as $V_2$ receptors and have a structure similar to that of other G protein–coupled receptors.[42] Binding of these receptors activates adenylate cyclase, which in turn increases the hydroosmotic permeability of the mucosal surface by inserting preformed water channels composed of a protein known as *aquaporin-2*,[43] a nonpeptide antagonist that binds selectively to $V_2$ receptors and blocks the antidiuretic action of vasopressin in humans that has been developed[44a,44b] and may prove useful in treating clinical disorders of water balance resulting from osmotically inappropriate secretion of vasopressin (see Chap. 27). A number of different mutations in the genes that encode the $V_2$ receptor protein or the aquaporin-2 proteins impair the urinary concentration and results in the clinical syndrome of congenital nephrogenic diabetes insipidus.[45]

### EXTRARENAL ACTION

Vasopressin has been implicated in the control of other physiologic functions such as blood pressure, temperature, insensible water loss, adrenocorticotropic hormone (ACTH) secretion, glycogenolysis, platelet function, CSF formation, and memory.

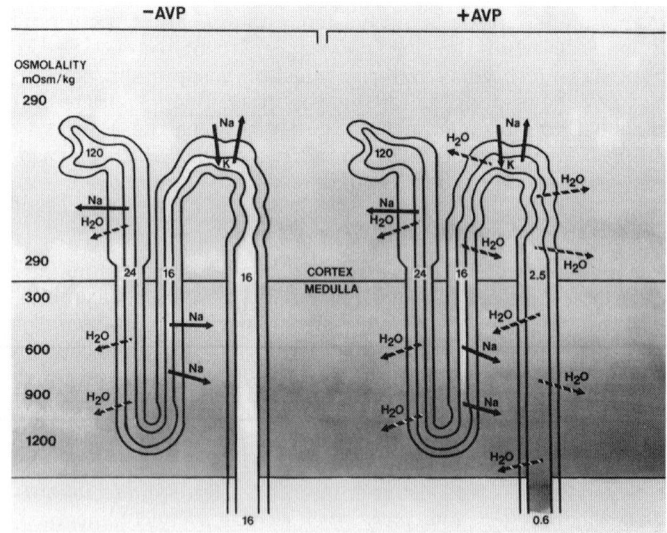

**FIGURE 25-10.** Schematic representation of the effect of vasopressin (*AVP*) on the formation of urine by the nephron. The osmotic pressure of tissue and tubular fluid is indicated by the density of the shading. The numbers within the lumen of the nephron indicate typical rates of flow in milliliters per minute. Arrows indicate reabsorption of sodium (*Na*) or water ($H_2O$) by active (*solid*) or passive (*broken*) processes. Note that vasopressin acts only on the distal nephron, where it increases the hydroosmotic permeability of tubular membranes. The fluid that reaches this part of the nephron normally amounts to 10% to 15% of the total filtrate and is hypotonic, owing to selective reabsorption of sodium in the ascending limb of the Henle loop. In the absence of vasopressin, the membranes of the distal nephron remain relatively impermeable to water as well as to solute, and the fluid issuing from the Henle loop is excreted essentially unmodified as urine. With maximum vasopressin action, all but 5% to 10% of the water in this fluid is reabsorbed passively down the osmotic gradient that normally exists with the surrounding tissue. (From Robertson GL. Diseases of the posterior pituitary. In: Felig P, Baxter J, Brodus A, Frohman L, eds. Endocrinology and metabolism. New York: McGraw-Hill, 1986:351.)

Most of these effects are thought to be mediated by different receptors, known as $V_{1a}$ and $V_{1b}$,[46,47] which are present in several parts of the body, including the brain.[48,49] For the most part, however, these extrarenal effects of vasopressin have been demonstrated only at relatively high concentrations of the hormone in experimental animals, and their putative role in human physiology or pathophysiology is still uncertain.

## OXYTOCIN

The major physiologic action of oxytocin is to facilitate nursing by stimulating the contraction of myoepithelial cells in the lactating mammary gland (see Chap. 106). Oxytocin may also aid in parturition by stimulating contraction of the uterus (see Chap. 109).[49a] These effects are mediated via a specific oxytocin receptor,[50] which may be up-regulated during pregnancy. Whether the hormone has any significant physiologic role in men is unknown. At supraphysiologic concentrations approaching those achieved during the infusion of Pitocin (oxytocin) to induce labor, oxytocin exerts a significant antidiuretic effect[51] in humans, probably by stimulating vasopressin $V_2$ receptors.[52]

## THIRST MECHANISM

The thirst mechanism provides an indispensable adjunct to the antidiuretic control of water balance in humans (see Chaps. 26 and 27). Thirst is stimulated by many of the same variables that cause vasopressin release,[53] the most potent of which appears to be hypertonicity. In healthy adults, a rise in effective plasma osmolality to 2% to 3% above basal levels produces a strong desire to drink. The absolute level of plasma osmolality at which a desire for water is first perceived may be termed the *osmotic threshold for thirst*. This threshold varies appreciably, but among healthy adults, it averages ~295 mOsm/kg (see Fig. 25-4). This level is higher than the osmotic threshold for vasopressin release and closely approximates the level at which the amount of hormone secreted is sufficient to produce maximal concentration of the urine (see Fig. 25-5). The osmoreceptors that regulate thirst appear to be located in the anterolateral hypothalamus near, but not totally coincident with, those responsible for vasopressin release.[54] The sensitivity and solute specificity of the thirst and vasopressin osmoreceptors also appear to be similar. Thus, the intensity of thirst and the amount of water ingested increase rapidly in direct proportion to plasma sodium or osmolality. As with vasopressin secretion, thirst is not stimulated in healthy adults when the rise in plasma osmolality is secondary to urea or glucose. However, thirst, as well as vasopressin release, is stimulated by hyperglycemia in insulin-deficient diabetics, probably because insulin is necessary for uptake of glucose by both types of osmoreceptor.

Hypovolemia and hypotension are also dipsogenic.[55] The degree of hypovolemia or hypotension required to produce thirst appears to be greater than the degree at which vasopressin release is affected. The pathways by which hypovolemia and hypotension produce thirst are uncertain, but they probably are similar, if not identical, to those that mediate the baroregulation of vasopressin. Hemodynamic stimuli also reset the osmotic threshold for thirst, just as they do for vasopressin.[56]

## WATER HOMEOSTASIS

### VOLUME, COMPOSITION, DISTRIBUTION, AND BALANCE

Water is by far the largest constituent of the human body. In lean, healthy adults, it constitutes 55% to 65% of body weight, and in infants and young children, it represents an even larger proportion.[57] Approximately two-thirds of body water is intracellular. The rest is extracellular and is divided further into the intravascular (plasma) and extravascular (interstitial) compartments. Plasma is much the smaller of the two, constituting only approximately one-fourth of the total extracellular volume.

The solute composition of intracellular and extracellular fluid differs markedly because most cell membranes possess an array of transport systems that actively accumulate or expel specific solutes.[58] However, the *total solute concentration* of the extracellular and the intracellular fluid is always the same because most cell membranes are freely permeable to water. Thus, distribution of water between the intracellular and extracellular compartments is determined by osmotic pressure resulting from differences in the solute content of the two compartments. If the total solute concentration of one compartment changes, the difference in osmotic pressure induces a rapid efflux or influx of water from the neighboring compartments until osmotic equilibrium is restored.[59,60] Similarly, the distribution of extracellular water between the intravascular and interstitial compartments is determined largely by the balance of hemodynamic and oncotic pressure.

The total amount of water in the body is determined by the balance between intake and loss to the environment. The latter occurs via two routes; urination and evaporation, mostly from skin and lungs. The amounts lost via either route can vary markedly depending on antidiuretic function, solute load, physical activity, and temperature. However, even when conservation is maximum, the total amount of water lost by a healthy 70-kg adult cannot be reduced below ~1000 mL a day. Part of this obligatory loss can be replaced by the metabolism of fat (~300 mL per day in the average adult). The rest must come from the ingestion of water either as food or beverage. Thus, the mechanisms for ensuring an adequate intake of water are the most important for maintaining normal hydration.

### OSMOREGULATION

Despite large daily variations in sodium intake and water output, plasma osmolality and its principal determinant—plasma sodium concentration—normally are maintained within a remarkably narrow range (Fig. 25-11). The only perceptible changes occur after meals when plasma osmolality rises transiently as a result of the absorption of sodium, glucose, and other solutes. This stability is achieved largely by keeping total body water in balance with sodium through the osmoregulation of thirst and vasopressin secretion. Thus, a reduction in osmotic pressure of only 1% or 2% inhibits vasopressin secretion, thereby decreasing the urine concentration and increasing the urine flow. Concomitantly, fluid intake is reduced,[53] apparently because a sense of satiety develops. Conversely, a rise in the osmotic pressure of body fluids of 1% to 2% stimulates vasopressin secretion and thirst, thereby decreasing urinary water excretion and increasing oral water intake.

The ability of the thirst or vasopressin mechanisms to effect very large changes in the rate of water intake or excretion provides almost insurmountable barriers to excessive overhydration or underhydration even in certain conditions in which one or the other control mechanism malfunctions. Thus, if plasma osmolality falls enough to maximally inhibit vasopressin secretion (and renal function and solute excretion are normal), the rate of water excretion rises to levels that can equal or surpass all but the most pathologically excessive rates of water intake (as in many patients with severe primary polydipsia). In this situation, the osmotic threshold for vasopressin secretion effectively determines the lower limit to which the osmotic pressure of body fluids can be depressed. If the diuretic control system is inoperable (as in patients treated with antidiuretic hormone), the thirst mechanism can compensate by down-regulating water intake to keep it in balance with even minimal rates of urine output. On the other hand, if plasma osmolality rises sufficiently to stimulate

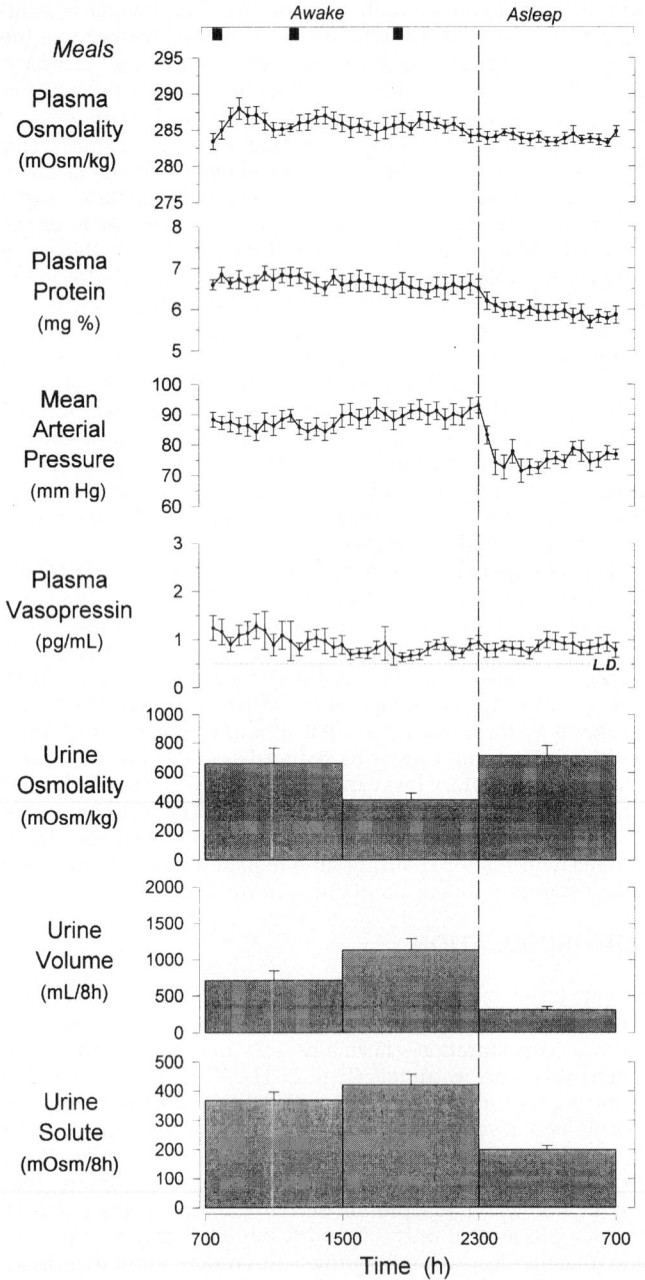

**FIGURE 25-11.** Circadian pattern of urine output, plasma vasopressin, and its recognized influences in healthy young adults. Each value represents the mean ± standard error of the mean of nine subjects. Note that urine volume decreases by ~50% during sleep, owing largely to a decrease in the rate of solute excretion and a resultant rise in urine osmolality. Plasma vasopressin changes relatively little throughout the day except for transient small increases that occur after meals, coincident with small increases in plasma osmolality and sodium. The 15% to 20% fall in mean arterial pressure that occurs during sleep has no appreciable effect on vasopressin secretion, possibly because this stimulus is counteracted by an increase in plasma volume that results from a net influx of fluid from the interstitial space. (From Robertson GL. The regulation of vasopressin secretion. In: Seldin DW, Giebisch G, ed. The kidney: physiology and pathophysiology. Philadelphia: Lippincott–Raven, 2000; in press.)

thirst (and access to fresh water is unrestricted), the rate of water intake can rise to levels sufficient to replace all but the most extraordinary rates of loss (as in many patients with severe pituitary or nephrogenic diabetes insipidus). In this situation, the osmotic threshold for thirst effectively determines the highest levels to which plasma osmolality is allowed to rise. However, if the thirst mechanism fails, the antidiuretic mechanism cannot

compensate because it cannot generate water to offset even minimal obligatory losses caused by urination and evaporation.

## HEMODYNAMIC INFLUENCES

In humans, blood pressure and volume vary appreciably throughout the day (see Fig. 25-11). However, because the stimulus response curve is curvilinear (see Fig. 25-7), these hemodynamic changes are usually too small to affect thirst or vasopressin secretion. Even if the hemodynamic changes reach levels sufficient to affect thirst or vasopressin secretion, the fundamental nature of the osmoregulatory system is not compromised because they merely raise or lower the setpoint a few percent, depending on whether blood pressure, effective blood volume, or both are rising or falling. This constant resetting has the effect of slightly widening the range over which plasma osmolality is allowed to fluctuate, but it does not jeopardize the essential osmoregulatory system. Consequently, plasma vasopressin as well as plasma osmolality remain relatively constant throughout the day except for the small, transient increases that occur after meals (see Fig. 25-11). Urine osmolality and flow, on the other hand, show considerable circadian variation owing largely to changes in the rate of solute excretion throughout the day.

The contributions of vasopressin and thirst to the regulation of blood volume and pressure are trivial and occur largely as an indirect consequence of efforts to preserve osmolality. Indeed, in situations in which total body sodium is increased abnormally, thirst and vasopressin act in such a way as to aggravate, instead of ameliorate, the underlying hypervolemia. The responsibility for coping with disturbances in volume rests primarily with those elements of the renal and endocrine systems that regulate sodium excretion. This distinction is useful to bear in mind when considering the pathogenesis of clinical disorders of salt and water balance.

## REFERENCES

1. Haymaker W. Hypothalamo-pituitary neural pathways and the circulatory system of the pituitary. In: Haymaker W, et al., eds. The hypothalamus. Springfield: Charles C Thomas, 1969:219.
2. Zimmerman EA. The organization of oxytocin and vasopressin pathways. In: Martin JB, Reichlin S, Bick KL, eds. Neurosecretion and brain peptides. New York: Raven Press, 1981:63.
3. Luerssen TG, Robertson GL. Cerebrospinal fluid vasopressin and vasotocin in health and disease. In: Wood JH, ed. Neurobiology and cerebrospinal fluid, vol 1. New York: Plenum Publishing, 1980:613.
4. du Vigneaud V, Shorr E, Bing RJ, et al. Hormones of the posterior pituitary gland: oxytocin and vasopressin. In: Harvey Lectures, 1954–1955. New York: Academic Press, 1956.
5. Breslow E. The neurophysins. Adv Enzymol 1974; 40:271.
6. Richter D. Molecular events in expression of vasopressin and oxytocin and their cognate receptors. Am J Physiol 1988; 255:F207.
7. Sausville E, Carney D, Battey J. The human vasopressin gene is linked to the oxytocin gene and is selectively expressed in a cultured lung cancer cell line. J Biol Chem 1985; 260:10236.
8. Riddell DC, Mallonee R, Phillips JA, et al. Chromosomal assignment of human sequences encoding arginine vasopressin-neurophysin ii and growth hormone. Somat Cell Mol Genet 1985; 11:189.
9. Hansen L, Rittig S, Robertson GL. The genetic basis of familial neurohypophyseal diabetes insipidus. Trends Endocrinol Metab 1997; 8:363.
10. Douglass WW. How do neurons secrete peptides? Exocytosis and its consequences including synaptic vesicle formation in the hypothalamo-neurohypophyseal system. Prog Brain Res 1973; 39:21.
11. Verney EB. Antidiuretic hormone and the factors which determine its release. Proc R Soc Lond [Biol] 1947; 135:25.
12. Robertson GL. The regulation of vasopressin function in health and disease. Recent Prog Horm Res 1977; 33:333.
13. Robertson GL, Athar S, Shelton RL. Osmotic control of vasopressin function. In: Andreoli TE, Grantham JJ, Rector FC, eds. Disturbances in body fluid osmolality. Bethesda, MD: American Physiological Society, 1977:125.
14. Schrier RW, Berl T, Anderson RJ. Osmotic and nonosmotic control of vasopressin release. Am J Physiol 1979; 236:F321.
15. Robertson GL. Thirst and vasopressin function in normal and disordered states of water balance. J Lab Clin Med 1983; 101:351.
16. Jewell PA, Verney EB. An experimental attempt to determine the site of the neurohypophyseal osmoreceptors in the dog. Philos Trans R Soc Lond [Biol] 1957; 240:197.

17. Andersson B. Thirst and brain control of water balance. Am Sci 1971; 59:408.
18. Oldfield BJ, Miselis RR, McKinley MJ. Median preoptic nucleus projections to vasopressin-containing neurones of the supraoptic nucleus in sheep: a light and electron microscopic study. Brain Res 1991; 542:193.
19. Zerbe RL, Miller JZ, Robertson GL. The reproducibility and heritability of individual differences in osmoregulatory function in normal human subjects. J Lab Clin Med 1991; 117:51.
20. Robertson GL. Physiology of ADH secretion. Kidney Int 1987; 32:3.
21. Lindheimer MD, Davison JM. Osmoregulation, the secretion of arginine vasopressin and its metabolism during pregnancy. Eur J Endocrinol 1995; 132:133.
22. Schrier RW, Bert T, Anderson RJ, McDonald KM. Nonosmolar control of renal water excretion. In: Andreoli TE, Giantham JJ, Rector FC, eds. Disturbances in body fluid osmolality. Bethesda, MD: American Physiological Society, 1977:149.
23. Iwasaki Y, Gaskill MB, Boss CA, Robertson GL. The effect of the nonselective opioid antagonist diprenorphine on vasopressin secretion in the rat. Endocrinology 1994; 134:48.
24. Iwasaki Y, Gaskill MB, Robertson GL. The effect of selective opioid antagonists on vasopressin secretion in the rat. Endocrinology 1994; 134:55.
25. Iwasaki Y, Gaskill MB, Fu R, et al. Opioid antagonist diprenorphine microinjected into parabrachial nucleus selectively inhibits vasopressin response to hypovolemic stimuli in the rat. J Clin Invest 1993; 92:2230.
26. Zerbe RL, Henry DP, Robertson GL. Vasopressin response to orthostatic hypotension: etiological and clinical implications. Am J Med 1983; 74:265.
27. Rowe JW, Shelton RL, Helderman JH, et al. Influence of the emetic reflex on vasopressin release in man. Kidney Int 1979; 16:729.
28. Baylis PH, Zerbe RL, Robertson GL. Arginine vasopressin response to insulin-induced hypoglycemia in man. J Clin Endocrinol Metab 1981; 53:935.
29. Thompson DA, Cambell RG, Lilavivat U, et al. Increased thirst and plasma arginine vasopressin levels during 2-deoxy-D-glucose-induced glucoprivation in humans. J Clin Invest 1981; 67:1083.
30. Mouw D, Bonjour JP, Malvin RL, Vander A. Central action of angiotensin in stimulating ADH release. Am J Physiol 1971; 220:239.
31. Shimizu K, Share L, Claybaugh JR. Potentiation of angiotensin II of the vasopressin response to an increasing plasma osmolality. Endocrinology 1973; 93:42.
32. Rydin H, Verney EB. The inhibition of water-diuresis by emotional stress and by muscular exercise. Q J Exp Physiol 1938; 27:343.
33. Edelson JT, Robertson GL. The effect of the cold pressor test on vasopressin secretion in man. Psychoneuroendocrinology 1985; 11:307.
34. Rose CE Jr, Anderson RJ, Carey RM. Antidiuresis and vasopressin release with hypoxemia and hypercapnia in conscious dogs. Am J Physiol 1984; 247:R127.
35. Heyes MP, Farber MO, Manfredi F, et al. Effect of hypoxia on renal and endocrine function in normal humans. Am J Physiol 1982; 243:R265.
36. Thompson CJ, Burd JM, Baylis PH. Acute suppression of plasma vasopressin and thirst after drinking in hypernatremic humans. Am J Physiol 1987; 252:R1138.
37. Robertson GL, Berl T. Water metabolism. In: Brenner BM, Rector FC, eds. The kidney, 3rd ed. Philadelphia: WB Saunders, 1985:385.
38. Amico JA, Finley BE. Breast stimulation in cycling women, pregnant women and a woman with induced lactation: pattern of release of oxytocin, prolactin and luteinizing hormone. Clin Endocrinol 1986; 25:97.
39. Lauson HD. Metabolism of neurohypophysial hormones. In: Handbook of physiology, vol 6, section 7. Endocrinology. Bethesda, MD: American Physiologic Society, 1971:287.
40. Amico JA, Ulbrecht JS, Robinson AG. Clearance studies of oxytocin in humans using radioimmunoassay measurements of the hormone in plasma and urine. J Clin Endocrinol Metab 1987; 64:340.
41. Berliner BW, Levinsky NG, Davidson DG, Eden M. Dilution and concentration of the urine and the action of antidiuretic hormone. Am J Med 1958; 24:730.
42. Bimbaumer M, Seibold A, Gilbert S, et al. Molecular cloning of the receptor for human antidiuretic hormone. Nature 1992: 357:333.
43. Knepper MA. Molecular physiology of urinary concentrating mechanism: regulation of aquaporin water channels by vasopressin. Am J Physiol 1997; 272:F3.
44a. Ohnishi A, Orita Y, Okahara R, et al. Potent aquaretic agent: a novel nonpeptide selective vasopressin 2 antagonist (OPC-3 1260) in men. J Clin Invest 1993; 92:2653.
44b. Tahara A, Saito M, Sugimoto T, et al. Pharmacological characterization of YM087, a potent, nonpeptide human vasopressin $V_{1a}$ and $V_2$ receptor antagonist. Naunyn-Schmiedeberg's Arch Pharmacol 1998; 357:63.
45. Bichet DG, Fujiwara MT. Diversity of nephrogenic diabetes insipidus mutations and importance of early recognition and treatment. Clin Exp Nephrol 1998; 2:253.
46. Morel A, O'Carrol AM, Brownstein MJ, Lolait S. Molecular cloning and expression of a rat $V_{1a}$ arginine vasopressin receptor. Nature 1992; 356:523.
47. Sugimoto T, Saito M, Mockzuki S, et al. Molecular cloning and functional expression of a cDNA encoding the human $V_{1b}$ receptor. J Biol Chem 1994; 269:27088.
48. Vaccari C, Lolait S, Ostrowski NL. Comparative distribution of vasopressin $V_{1b}$ and oxytocin receptor messenger ribonucleic acids in brain. Endocrinology 1998; 139:5015.
49. Hurbin A, Boissin-Agasse L, Orcel H, et al. The $V_{1a}$ and $V_{1b}$ but not the $V_2$ vasopressin receptor genes are expressed in the supraoptic nucleus of the rat hypothalamus and the transcripts are essentially colocalized in the vasopressingeric magnocellular neurons. Endocrinology 1998; 139:4701.
49a. Voutsos L, Cantor D. Randomized, double-masked comparison of oxytocin dosage in induction and augmentyation of labor. Obstet Gynecol 2000; 95:472.
50. Kimura T, Tanizawa O, Mon K, et al. Structure and expression of a Human Oxytocin Receptor. Nature 1992; 356:526.
51. Kelly S, Robertson GL, Amico J. Antidiuretic action of oxytocin in humans. Clin Res 1992; 40:711A.
52. Chou CL, DiGiovanni SR, Luther A, et al. Oxytocin as an antidiuretic hormone ii: role of $V_2$ vasopressin receptor. Am J Physiol 1995; 269:F78.
53. Robertson GL. Disorders of thirst in man. In: Ramsay DJ, Booth DA, eds. Thirst: physiological and psychological aspects. London: Springer-Verlag, 1991:453.
54. McKinley MJ. Osmoreceptors for thirst. In: Ramsay DJ, Booth DA, eds. Thirst: physiological and psychological aspects. London: Springer-Verlag, 1991:77.
55. Thrasher TN. Volume receptors and the stimulation of water intake. In: Ramsay DJ, Booth DA, eds. Thirst: physiological and psychological aspects. London: Springer-Verlag, 1991:91.
56. Kozlowski S, Szczepanska-Sadowska E. Antagonistic effects of vasopressin and hypervolemia on osmotic reactivity of the thirst mechanism in dogs. Pflugers Arch 1975; 353:59.
57. Altman PL, Dittmer DS, eds. Blood and other body fluids. Washington, DC: American Society for Experimental Biology, 1961.
58. Wolf AV, McDowell ME. Apparent and osmotic volumes of distribution of sodium, chloride, sulfate and urea. Am J Physiol 1954; 176:207.
59. Darrow DC, Yanett H. Changes in distribution of body water accompanying increase and decrease in extracellular electrolytes. J Clin Invest 1935; 14:266.
60. Leaf A, Chatillon JY, Wrong O, Tuttle EP Jr. The mechanism of the osmotic adjustment of body cells as determined in vivo by the volume of distribution of a large water load. J Clin Invest 1954; 33:1261.

# CHAPTER 26

# DIABETES INSIPIDUS AND HYPEROSMOLAR SYNDROMES

PETER H. BAYLIS AND CHRISTOPHER J. THOMPSON

Blood osmolality in healthy persons is maintained within narrow limits by a series of mechanisms that are described in detail in Chapter 25. Adjustments in water balance determine the constancy of blood osmolality, which is mediated by delicate alterations in thirst appreciation (with consequent promotion of drinking) plus the enormous capacity of the kidney to alter urine flow rates and urine osmolality in response to relatively small changes in the plasma vasopressin concentration (see Chap. 206). Thus, healthy humans are able to conserve their osmotic internal milieu despite extremes in climatic conditions, sustained severe exertion, or, to a certain degree, an inadequate supply of water.

Aberrations of the intricate mechanisms involved in maintaining osmoregulation can lead to the inappropriate accumulation of water, which is recognized as one of the hypoosmolar states, or to the loss of renal water, which usually is clinically apparent as polyuria but also may be manifested as one of the hyperosmolar syndromes. This chapter is concerned with clinical situations associated with polyuria and, on occasion, abnormalities of thirst appreciation.

## DEFINITIONS

*Diabetes insipidus* refers to the passage of copious volumes of dilute urine and is synonymous with polyuria. In adults, the urine volume exceeds 2.5 L per 24 hours (>40 mL/kg per 24 hours), while in children the output is greater (>100 mL/kg per 24 hours).

Three pathophysiologic conditions result in diabetes insipidus. An absolute or partial deficiency of vasopressin secretion from the neurohypophysis in response to normal osmotic stimulation is termed *hypothalamic diabetes insipidus*. This disorder is also known as cranial, central, or neurogenic diabetes insipidus. Patients with hypothalamic diabetes insipidus generally have normal thirst sensation. Their basic abnormality is insufficient circulating antidiuretic activity, which is the principal, but not the sole, cause of their polyuria. Diabetes insipidus secondary to decreased renal sensitivity to the antidiuretic effect of vasopressin circulating in normal or high concentrations is usually called *nephrogenic diabetes insipidus*. Again, these patients rely on normal thirst sensation to regulate water balance. The third mechanism leading to diabetes insipidus is the ingestion of excessive volumes of fluid, which results in suppression of vasopressin release and consequent polyuria. This condition is referred to as *dipsogenic diabetes insipidus*, sometimes termed *primary polydipsia*.

A decrease in maximal urine-concentrating ability occurs after prolonged periods of polyuria, regardless of the primary cause. The passage of large amounts of dilute urine through the distal nephron removes solute from the renal medullary interstitium, a process known as the washout phenomenon.[1,2] The osmotic gradient across the collecting tubular cell, which is essential for the antidiuretic action of vasopressin, is decreased. Thus, any of the three pathophysiologic mechanisms responsible for diabetes insipidus may lead to an additional defect that complicates the interpretation of diagnostic tests based on indirect assessment of the antidiuretic action of vasopressin.

In contrast to hypothalamic diabetes insipidus, which is usually the result of a loss of neurosecretory neurons, the chronic hyperosmolar syndromes are frequently the consequence of a defective thirst mechanism. Thirst osmoreceptors may fail to respond to hypertonicity, which results in hypodipsia. Because the putative thirst osmoreceptors are believed to be in proximity to the osmoreceptors that regulate vasopressin secretion, a defect in osmotically mediated vasopressin release is often associated with hypodipsia. Polyuria is rarely a feature of hyperosmolar syndromes, because many patients secrete small amounts of vasopressin that are sufficient to concentrate urine to some extent, and nonosmotic factors regulating vasopressin secretion often remain intact. In view of this characteristic difference between diabetes insipidus and hyperosmolar syndromes, these conditions are discussed separately.

# DIABETES INSIPIDUS

## ETIOLOGY

In theory, any of a series of defects in the vasopressin neurosecretory process can be implicated as the cause of hypothalamic diabetes insipidus.[3] Abnormalities may arise in the osmoreceptor that controls vasopressin secretion, even when the thirst osmoreceptor is spared. Alternatively, abnormalities may involve the synthesis and packaging of vasopressin (including genetic defects), damage to the vasopressinergic neurons, or disorders of neurohypophyseal hormone release. Enhanced inactivation of vasopressin by circulating degrading enzymes or antibodies is another potential cause of decreased antidiuretic activity.

In practice, however, most cases of permanent hypothalamic diabetes insipidus are caused by damage to the hypothalamo-neurohypophyseal area. The most common causes of this condition are listed in Table 26-1.[4]

## FAMILIAL ABNORMALITIES

Studies have revealed exciting data regarding a variety of genetic abnormalities found on chromosome 20 in several kindreds with autosomal dominant hypothalamic diabetes insipidus. The first report on different families showed single nucleotide substitutions in the region coding for neurophysin (glycine to serine at position 57).[5] This mutation is presumed to interfere with the normal vasopressin-neurophysin tetramer complex formation that occurs in the packaging and transport of vasopressin to the neurohypophysis. Two groups investigating another extended family discovered a nucleotide substitu-

**TABLE 26-1.**
**Causes of Diabetes Insipidus**

**HYPOTHALAMIC DIABETES INSIPIDUS**
*Familial*
  Hereditary (usually autosomal dominant)
  Association of diabetes insipidus with diabetes mellitus, optic atrophy, nerve deafness, atonia of bladder and ureters (DIDMOAD)
*Acquired*
  Head trauma
  Neurosurgery
  Tumors (craniopharyngioma, germinoma, metastatic deposits in hypothalamus)
  Granulomatous disease (tuberculosis, histiocytosis, sarcoidosis, Wegener granulomatosis)
  Infections (encephalitis, meningitis)
  Infundibuloneurohypophysitis
  Vascular disorders (Sheehan syndrome, aneurysms, thrombotic thrombocytopenic purpura)
  Circulating antibodies to vasopressin (secondary to Pitressin injection)
  Pregnancy
  Autoimmunity
  Idiopathic
**NEPHROGENIC DIABETES INSIPIDUS**
*Familial*
  X-linked recessive: $V_2$ receptor gene
  Autosomal recessive: aquaporin-2 gene
*Acquired*
  Chronic renal disease
  Metabolic disease (hypokalemia, hypercalcemia)
  Drugs (lithium, demeclocycline)
  Osmotic diuresis
  Pregnancy
**DIPSOGENIC DIABETES INSIPIDUS**
  Idiopathic
  Associated with psychosis
  Sarcoidosis
  Autoimmune (multiple sclerosis)
  Drug induced (lithium, tricyclic antidepressants)

tion in the signal peptide (alanine to threonine at position −1).[6,7] The signal peptide directs the prohormone to the endoplasmic reticulum, where it is cleaved. Both groups speculate that the mutation alters the cleavage mechanism, resulting in abnormal processing of the prohormone. After the description of the first genetic abnormalities causing familial hypothalamic diabetes insipidus, more than 22 different kindreds with unique genetic mistakes have been documented[8] (Fig. 26-1).

The genetic basis of the DIDMOAD (diabetes insipidus, diabetes mellitus, optic atrophy, deafness), or Wolfram, syndrome is less well understood, although some evidence exists that it is a disorder of mitochondrial DNA.[9,10]

## TRAUMA

Closed head trauma or frank damage to the pituitary stalk or hypothalamus as a result of surgical intervention is often the cause of a form of diabetes insipidus that usually presents within 24 hours of injury. In ~50% of cases of post-traumatic diabetes insipidus, the condition resolves spontaneously within a few days. Permanent diabetes insipidus develops in another 30% to 40% of these patients, and the remainder exhibit a *triphasic response to injury*. In the last group, the onset of polyuria is abrupt and the condition lasts a few days. It is followed by a period of antidiuresis that may last 2 to 14 days before permanent diabetes insipidus develops. This triple response to injury is believed to be attributable to release of the vasopressin that is stored in granules.[11] Recognition of this entity by clinicians

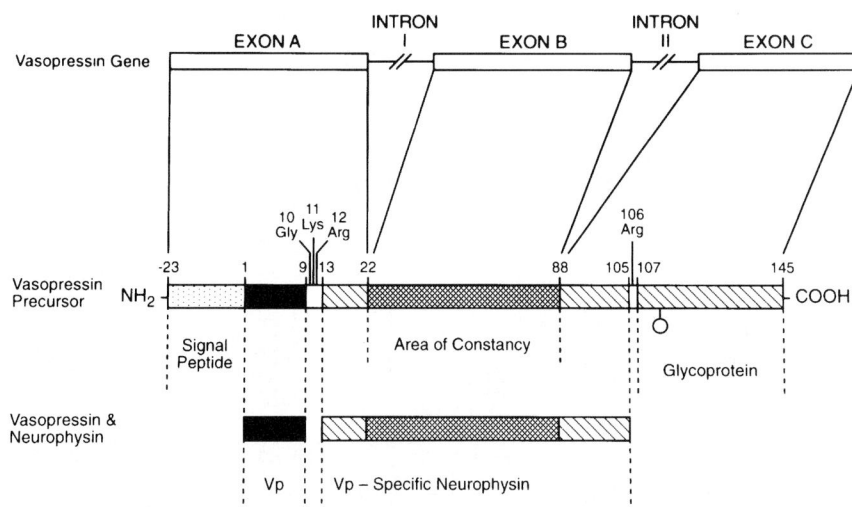

**FIGURE 26-1.** Vasopressin gene, vasopressin precursor molecule, and vasopressin with its specific neurophysin. Three exons encode for the precursor molecule, which comprises a signal protein, vasopressin hormone, neurophysin, and a glycoprotein moiety coupled by amino acids. Mutations in the vasopressin gene have been located in all parts of the precursor molecule except vasopressin itself. (*Vp*, vasopressin.)

should help to prevent inappropriate treatment that would result in hyponatremia during the second of the three phases.

## TUMORS

Tumors of the anterior pituitary rarely cause diabetes insipidus. In a series of >100 cases of hypothalamic diabetes insipidus, 13% were attributable to tumors, which included glioma, germinoma, and craniopharyngioma.[12] In children, a central tumor is a frequent cause of hypothalamic diabetes insipidus, accounting for ~25% of cases; in this population, the most common intracranial tumor is germinoma.[13] Metastatic deposits in the hypothalamus causing diabetes insipidus usually arise from carcinoma of the breast or bronchus.

## GRANULOMATOUS DISEASE

Granulomatous disease accounts for only a few cases of diabetes insipidus in adults (i.e., sarcoidosis, tuberculosis). However, in children with granulomatous disease, histiocytosis X may cause as many as 40% of pediatric cases.

## IDIOPATHIC

Idiopathic hypothalamic diabetes accounts for ~25% of all cases.[12] One-third of patients with apparent idiopathic disease have circulating antibodies to the vasopressin-producing cells in the hypothalamus, a finding which suggests an autoimmune origin for the disorder.[14] Some patients have an acute lymphocytic infiltration of the infundibulum and neurohypophysis that can be demonstrated on open biopsy and subsequently resolves.[15]

## NEPHROGENIC DIABETES INSIPIDUS

Mild forms of nephrogenic diabetes insipidus are relatively common (see Table 26-1). Mechanisms responsible for renal resistance to the antidiuretic effect of vasopressin may occur at one or more of the many different sites in the chain of biochemical responses to vasopressin.[11,15a] Chronic renal disease secondary to numerous conditions, many drugs (e.g., lithium[15b]), prolonged electrolyte disturbances from hypokalemia, and hypercalcemia account for most cases of nephrogenic diabetes insipidus. The inherited forms of nephrogenic diabetes insipidus are rare, and cause severe polyuria, dehydration, and failure to thrive in the young. With the identification of the $V_2$ (antidiuretic) receptor gene on the X chromosome, a variety of substitutions, mutations, or premature stops have been isolated in kindreds with this disorder that cause defects in the transmembrane $V_2$ receptor.[16] Studies involving three other families with congenital nephrogenic diabetes insipidus have shown

autosomal inheritance of the disorder, in contrast to the more common X-linked form due to genetic mutations of the $V_2$ receptor gene localized to the Xq28 region of the long arm of the X chromosome. The autosomal form is due to novel genetic mutations of the gene encoded for the vasopressin-sensitive water channel protein, *aquaporin-2*, which is located in the collecting tubules.[17]

## DIPSOGENIC DIABETES INSIPIDUS

Dipsogenic diabetes insipidus, also called *primary polydipsia* or *habitual water drinking*, is often psychogenic in origin. The course of polyuria in psychotic patients is variable, with fluctuations in polydipsia and urine volumes occurring over the years. Occasional patients with hypothalamic diabetes insipidus who are treated with antidiuretic preparations continue to have polydipsia and, consequently, run the risk of developing hyponatremia. Whether these patients continue to drink because of habit or because of a hypothalamic lesion affecting the thirst osmoreceptor is unknown. A few structural abnormalities resulting in increased thirst have been reported. Drugs that cause dryness of the mouth (e.g., thioridazine hydrochloride) may increase drinking but do not result in true polydipsia, in contrast to lithium, which can stimulate thirst directly.

## CLINICAL FEATURES

In adults, the major clinical manifestations of diabetes insipidus include the frequent passage of large volumes of dilute urine (often both day and night), excessive thirst, and increased fluid ingestion. Patients with mild degrees of diabetes insipidus may consider their symptoms to be so minimal that they fail to seek medical attention. However, the severity of diabetes insipidus varies widely, with 24-hour urine volumes ranging from 2.5 to 20 L. Even with the most extreme forms of the disorder, patients maintain their water balance as long as thirst appreciation remains intact and adequate volumes of fluid are ingested.

The onset of the disease occurs at any time from the neonatal period to old age, and the sex distribution is approximately equal, although one large review of adults with hypothalamic diabetes insipidus reported a slight male preponderance (60%:40%).[12] In infants, diabetes insipidus usually presents with evidence of chronic dehydration, unexplained fever, vomiting, neurologic disturbance, and failure to thrive.[13] Enuresis, sleep disturbances, and difficulties at school are the most common presenting complaints in older children. Usually, no growth retardation or failure to enter puberty occurs. Affected children from families with histories of diabetes insipidus often do not complain; they regard their polydipsia and polyuria as the norm. Once hypothalamic diabetes insipidus develops, it rarely goes into remission spontaneously.

Patients with hypothalamic diabetes insipidus also may have anterior pituitary dysfunction (see Chap. 17), particularly if their disorder resulted from trauma to or a tumor in the hypothalamo-neurohypophyseal area. Even patients with the idiopathic form of the disease frequently have endocrinologic evidence of anterior pituitary dysfunction, which suggests a more generalized hypothalamic disorder.[12] Glucocorticoid deficiency secondary to impaired corticotropin secretion or to primary adrenal disease leads to impairment of the ability of the kidneys to excrete a water load and to dilute urine maximally. At least two mechanisms are responsible for this defect. One involves the distal nephron, which remains partially impermeable to water in the absence of glucocorticoid; the other involves persistent vasopressin secretion, possibly secondary to a resetting of the osmostat. A similar abnormality of water excretion has been reported with severe thyroid hormone deficiency (see Chap. 45). Thus, impairment of anterior pituitary function can mask hypothalamic diabetes insipidus, which becomes apparent only when the hypopituitarism is adequately treated.

Routine skull radiographs are rarely helpful in patients with hypothalamic diabetes insipidus but nuclear magnetic resonance imaging (MRI) can be extremely useful. T1-weighted magnetic resonance imaging of the neurohypophysis produces a characteristic hyperintense signal in healthy persons that disappears in most patients with hypothalamic diabetes insipidus.[18] The infundibular stalk frequently is thickened in the early phase of the idiopathic form of the disorder, as demonstrated by both MRI and computed tomographic scanning.[15]

## DIFFERENTIAL DIAGNOSIS

Polyuria may be defined as the excretion of >2.5 L of urine per 24 hours on two consecutive days, provided that patients are allowed free access to and drink water ad libitum. Once polyuria has been demonstrated, the clinician's first responsibility is to establish the pathophysiologic mechanism—dipsogenic diabetes insipidus, hypothalamic diabetes insipidus, or nephrogenic diabetes insipidus. Defining the underlying disease process is then important.

### INDIRECT TESTS

Before the development of plasma assays that were capable of detecting low physiologic concentrations of vasopressin, indirect methods were used to assess the antidiuretic activity of the hormone.

The classic diagnostic approach is to measure the responses of urinary osmolality and flow rate to a period of dehydration and, subsequently, to the administration of an exogenous vasopressin preparation. Various dehydration tests have been described in which changes in plasma and urine osmolalities in patients with polyuria were compared to the responses of healthy persons.[19–21] In theory, differentiation between hypothalamic diabetes insipidus, nephrogenic diabetes insipidus, and dipsogenic diabetes insipidus should be readily possible, but the disorders actually can be diagnosed correctly only in certain circumstances. Frequently, tests yield equivocal results. For example, although patients with primary polydipsia might be anticipated to have significantly lower plasma osmolalities and sodium concentrations than patients with hypothalamic or nephrogenic diabetes insipidus, such a distinction is useful diagnostically in only a few cases.[22] The reason for the lack of differentiation is the wide variation in the setpoint of the osmoregulatory mechanisms for thirst and vasopressin secretion. Even after fluid deprivation and the administration of exogenous vasopressin, urine osmolality frequently fails to attain normal values (Fig. 26-2) because of the secondary nephrogenic diabetes insipidus induced by prolonged polyuria, as explained earlier. A similar ambiguity arises in the interpretation of

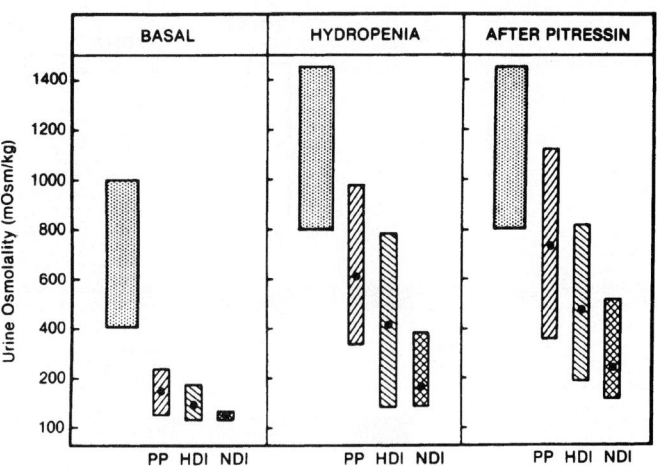

**FIGURE 26-2.** Urine osmolality is depicted under basal conditions after a period of fluid deprivation (hydropenia) designed to attain maximum urinary concentration, and after intramuscular injection of 5 U of vasopressin (Pitressin). The test group included healthy subjects (*stippled area*) and patients with dipsogenic diabetes insipidus (primary polydipsia, *PP*), hypothalamic diabetes insipidus (*HDI*), or nephrogenic diabetes insipidus (*NDI*). The bars represent the range of results and the closed circle indicates the mean value for the group. (Adapted from Robertson, GL. Diagnosis of diabetes insipidus. In: Czernichow P, Robinson AG, eds. Diabetes insipidus in man. Frontiers of hormone research, vol 13. Basel: S Karger, 1985:176.)

results from patients with hypothalamic diabetes insipidus. In theory, these patients, who have low circulating concentrations of vasopressin, should demonstrate a substantial increase in urine osmolality to the normal range in response to exogenous vasopressin. In practice, however, they fail to do so (see Fig. 26-2). Again, the reason for the inadequate urinary response lies in the washout of solute from the renal medullary interstitium. The greater the 24-hour urine volume, the greater is the degree of renal resistance to antidiuretic activity.[2] The large overlap in urine osmolality values with these tests is illustrated explicitly in Figure 26-2. The refinement of dehydration tests by calculation of free water clearance adds little to their ability to distinguish among the causes of diabetes insipidus. Other means of evaluating the osmoregulatory system using indirect methods to assess antidiuretic activity in an attempt to identify the cause of polyuria (i.e., infusion of hypertonic saline[23]) also fail to establish an unequivocal diagnosis for the reasons described earlier, as well as because the saline load induces a solute diuresis. Thus, indirect tests of vasopressin function are considerably limited in their ability to establish the cause of polyuria.

### DIRECT TESTS

The introduction of sensitive and specific radioimmunoassays capable of detecting low physiologic concentrations of vasopressin in plasma not only has clarified and simplified the diagnosis of diabetes insipidus, but also has extended the understanding of its underlying pathophysiologic mechanisms. The measurement of plasma vasopressin, plasma osmolality, and urine osmolality under basal conditions affords little diagnostic discrimination. However, after osmotic stimulation by a period of fluid deprivation, an infusion of hypertonic saline, or both, the estimation of these indices provides a precise diagnosis.

### PLASMA VASOPRESSIN IN THE DIAGNOSIS OF DIABETES INSIPIDUS

**Hypothalamic Diabetes Insipidus.** Hypothalamic diabetes insipidus is recognized by the subnormal plasma concentrations of vasopressin in relation to plasma osmolality that occur in affected persons (Fig. 26-3A). A clear distinction may be made between patients with hypothalamic diabetes insipidus, patients with nephrogenic diabetes insipidus or dipsogenic dia-

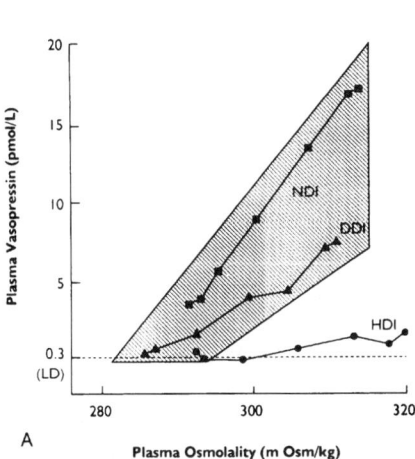

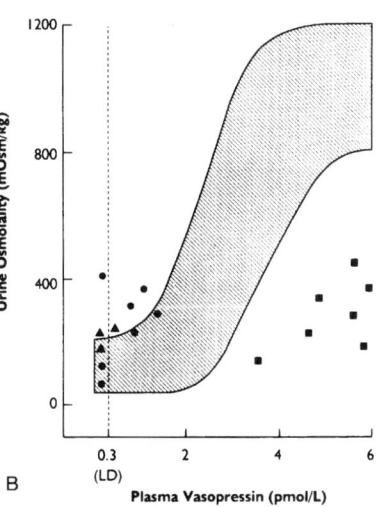

FIGURE 26-3. **A,** Plasma osmolality and vaso-pressin responses to infusion of 5% hypertonic saline solution in representative patients with hypothalamic diabetes insipidus (*HDI*, ●—●), nephrogenic diabetes insipidus (*NDI*, ■—■ ), and dipsogenic diabetes insipidus (*DDI*, ▲—▲). **B,** Plasma vasopressin and urine osmolality responses to a period of dehydration in patients with hypothalamic diabetes insipidus (●), nephro-genic diabetes insipidus (■), and dipsogenic diabetes insipidus (▲). The responses of healthy subjects are indicated by the stippled areas. The limit of detection of the vasopressin assay (*LD*) was 0.3 pmol/L (1 pmol/L ≡ 1.1 pg/mL).

betes insipidus, and healthy persons by assessing plasma osmolality as it is increased by the infusion of hypertonic saline.[24] Many patients with diabetes insipidus have detectable plasma vasopressin, which represents the partial form of the disorder. The ability to secrete vasopressin at high plasma osmolality levels partially explains the ability of some patients to generate a concentrated, if submaximal, urine after fluid dep-rivation. A few patients fail to exhibit detectable immunoreac-tive plasma vasopressin, despite marked increases in plasma osmolality. However, some of these patients still manage to concentrate their urine to some extent, suggesting that their kidneys are particularly sensitive to very low concentrations of vasopressin. Occasionally, patients with hypothalamic diabetes insipidus clearly demonstrate osmotically regulated vaso-pressin release (see Fig. 26-3*A*). In such patients, the theoretic threshold for vasopressin release, obtained from the abscissal intercept of the osmoregulatory line (the function relating plasma, vasopressin to plasma osmolality), is normal, but the slope that defines the sensitivity of osmotically regulated vaso-pressin release is significantly reduced. Thus, the osmoreceptor controlling vasopressin secretion is probably intact in this group of patients.

Some patients who have been treated with parenteral neuro-hypophyseal extract (Pitressin) have developed antibodies to vasopressin. These patients exhibit "vasopressin" in their plasma as a direct result of assay interference, but this can be recognized by laboratory testing simply through detection of plasma-binding activity to synthetic vasopressin. Therefore, screening for vasopressin antibodies in all patients treated with Pitressin is wise to prevent spurious plasma results.

After hypertonic saline infusion, patients with primary poly-dipsia or nephrogenic diabetes insipidus have plasma vaso-pressin and plasma osmolality values that fall within the normal reference range (see Fig. 26-3*A*). A supranormal plasma vasopressin response to rising plasma osmolality has been demonstrated in a few patients. Whether this response is attrib-utable to a state of chronic underhydration is not known. Thus, hypothalamic diabetes insipidus is clearly distinguishable from other forms of diabetes insipidus by relating plasma vaso-pressin to plasma osmolality after osmotic stimulation.

**Nephrogenic Diabetes Insipidus Versus Primary Polydip-sia.** Analysis of the relationship between plasma vasopressin and urine osmolality after a period of fluid deprivation offers a potential means of differentiating nephrogenic diabetes insipidus from dipsogenic diabetes insipidus (see Fig. 26-3*B*). Patients with nephrogenic diabetes insipidus have plasma vasopressin concen-trations that are inappropriately high in relation to urine osmolal-ity. However, prolonged polyuria from any cause can induce renal resistance to vasopressin, with blunting of the maximal uri-

nary concentration in response to vasopressin. This difficulty can be partially overcome by examining the basal values of plasma vasopressin and urine osmolality. Plasma vasopressin tends to be detectable or even elevated in nephrogenic diabetes insipidus, whereas immunoreactive vasopressin is generally undetectable in primary polydipsia[2] (see Fig. 26-3*B*). The administration of exogenous vasopressin after a period of fluid deprivation does not help to discriminate further between the causes of polyuria.

Close examination of the data regarding plasma vasopressin and urine osmolality in patients with partial hypothalamic dia-betes insipidus reveals an inappropriately high urine osmolal-ity in relation to the low plasma vasopressin concentrations (see Fig. 26-3*B*). This observation confirms the earlier impression that the renal tubule may become extraordinarily sensitive to vasopressin. Because sustained polyuria from any cause induces a state of secondary partial nephrogenic diabetes insip-idus, the administration of exogenous vasopressin to patients with partial hypothalamic diabetes insipidus fails to induce maximal urinary osmolality.

A systematic study to compare the diagnostic efficacy of indirect tests with direct measurement of osmotically stimu-lated vasopressin release has clearly demonstrated that direct plasma vasopressin measurement methods are superior.[25]

If the clinician does not have ready access to suitable assays for plasma vasopressin measurement, a satisfactory diagnosis may be established using a closely monitored, prolonged thera-peutic trial with desmopressin, administered intramuscularly in daily dosages of 1 μg for as long as 7 days, preferably while patients are hospitalized. Patients with hypothalamic diabetes insipidus who undergo this regimen show an improvement in the degree of polyuria and a reduction in polydipsia. At the end of the trial, a standard water deprivation test, followed by the administration of exogenous vasopressin using indirect assess-ment methods, may demonstrate maximal urinary concentra-tions that are within the normal reference range. This is because, during the period of the trial, the renal medullary interstitial solute concentration was restored. Patients with pri-mary polydipsia experience progressive hyponatremia and gain weight because they continue to drink fluid despite persis-tent antidiuresis. Some of these patients run the risk of neuro-logic disturbances, particularly seizures, secondary to the development of sudden, profound hyponatremia. Finally, patients with nephrogenic diabetes exhibit little, if any, improvement in thirst or polyuria.

Even the most carefully conducted therapeutic trial, how-ever, can yield misleading results. For example, a few patients who have had severe hypothalamic diabetes insipidus for many years develop water intoxication when first treated with vasopressin because they initially fail to reduce their water intake appropriately, and therefore they appear to have primary polydipsia. Thus, with the currently available diagnostic investigations, the measurement of plasma vasopressin levels with plasma and urine osmolalities during osmotic stimulation provides the most reliable method for determining the cause of polyuria.

## THIRST IN HYPOTHALAMIC DIABETES INSIPIDUS

The thirst mechanism in patients with hypothalamic and nephrogenic diabetes insipidus generally operates normally.[26] Such patients rely on an intact thirst appreciation to maintain water balance. In one study that documented the osmolar threshold for the onset of thirst, no significant difference was found between the mean value for a group of 11 patients with hypothalamic diabetes insipidus and that for 11 healthy persons; however, the range of values was wider in the affected patients. Only a few patients who are treated with vasopressin and who have inappropriate persistent thirst develop episodes of hyponatremia. When thirst appreciation is blunted, hypernatremia develops.

## DIABETES INSIPIDUS AND PREGNANCY

Normal human pregnancy is associated with subtle changes in osmoregulation. Plasma osmolality falls by 8 to 10 mOsm/kg due to a lowering of the osmolar thresholds for both thirst and vasopressin release,[27] and a small reduction occurs in maximal urinary concentrating ability.

Established hypothalamic diabetes insipidus appears to have little effect on fertility, gestation, delivery, and lactation in humans.[28] A few studies have demonstrated that the secretion of oxytocin is normal in patients with diabetes insipidus. By contrast, many pregnant patients with hypothalamic diabetes insipidus notice a worsening of their polyuria and polydipsia.[29] The mechanisms responsible for this may include depression of the osmolar thirst threshold to levels at which vasopressin secretion is suppressed further; circulating vasopressin that is degraded by the placental enzyme cystine aminopeptidase; and renal resistance to vasopressin, which is increased. Some patients show no change in their polyuria, whereas a few improve.

Transient central and nephrogenic diabetes insipidus associated with pregnancy has been documented in some patients[30,31] and has been found to recur in subsequent pregnancies. Whether this is attributable to an exaggeration of normal physiologic adaptation to pregnancy or represents a distinct disease entity remains unresolved.

## TREATMENT

Hypothalamic diabetes insipidus can be treated by the ingestion of adequate volumes of water, with patients relying on the quenching of thirst as the sole indicator of sufficient intake. Some patients who have had severe polyuria since childhood may prefer to manage their symptoms in this manner, thereby avoiding the need for medication. They organize their lives around the inconveniences of frequent micturition and copious drinking. However, good reasons exist why all patients with moderate to severe polyuria should be treated more actively. Prolonged, severe polyuria can result in distention and atonia of the bladder and hydroureter, and, eventually, in hydronephrosis with consequent renal damage. Susceptibility to potassium deficiency is another potential risk. Furthermore, untreated patients, if deprived of fluid for any reason, are at risk for the development of life-threatening hypernatremia and dehydration. In young children, withholding therapy may lead to failure to thrive. For these reasons, as well as for the relief of symptoms, antidiuretic treatment is advised for patients with 24-hour urine volumes exceeding 4 L.

Hormone replacement therapy using arginine vasopressin, a natural endogenous peptide, is inappropriate for most patients with hypothalamic diabetes, regardless of whether it is administered parenterally or intranasally. The peptide has a short half-life and may be associated with significant pressor side effects that render the use of aqueous vasopressin preparations impractical. However, during the last three decades, considerable advances have been made in the development of synthetic vasopressin analogs with various agonist and antagonist activities to the pressor ($V_1$) and antidiuretic ($V_2$) receptors. One class of analogs with minimal pressor activity but increased antidiuretic potency and some resistance to degradation in vivo has been developed to treat hypothalamic diabetes insipidus. The current drug of choice is desmopressin.[32,33] For adults, it can be administered orally, 50 to 400 µg one to three times daily; intranasally, 5 to 40 µg once or twice daily; or parenterally, 0.5 to 2.0 µg daily. A wide variation is seen in individual desmopressin requirements for the control of polyuria. For children, the dosage is halved. Desmopressin is not associated with pressor agonist side effects but carries the potential hazard of dilutional hyponatremia if patients continue to drink inappropriately despite persistent antidiuresis.

If desmopressin proves to be too potent, it can be diluted. Alternatively, a shorter-acting preparation—lysine vasopressin—can be administered intranasally. However, because it possesses pressor activity, it may induce vasoconstriction, angina, or renal and intestinal colic when taken in excess. If desmopressin is unavailable, it still may be possible to obtain vasopressin tannate in oil, a crude extract of bovine neurohypophysis containing arginine vasopressin suspended in peanut oil. Before intramuscular injection, this preparation should be warmed and shaken vigorously until the extract is evenly distributed in the oil. A single dose of 5 to 10 IU provides as much as 72 hours of antidiuresis. However, this agent is associated with pressor side effects similar to those of lysine vasopressin, an erratic absorption rate, and the formation of sterile abscesses. Pitressin also has been administered as a nasal insufflation.

Now that desmopressin is established as the drug of choice, little need exists to prescribe the partially effective oral agents—chlorpropamide, carbamazepine, clofibrate, or thiazide diuretics—because all are associated with significant and sometimes dangerous side effects.

Rarely, direct treatment of the underlying cause of hypothalamic diabetes insipidus relieves the symptoms. Documented examples include corticosteroid therapy for hypothalamic sarcoidosis, cyclophosphamide therapy for Wegener granulomatosis, and radiotherapy for metastatic disease of the hypothalamus.

Effective treatment of nephrogenic diabetes insipidus still poses problems, except for the forms that are drug induced or related to metabolic disorders (see Table 26-1). The latter are frequently reversible after withdrawal of the drug or correction of the metabolic disturbance. Profound polyuria secondary to the familial forms of this disease is particularly difficult to treat. Restriction of sodium intake, combined with the administration of a thiazide diuretic, reduces urine output by almost 40% in infants. A similar reduction in urine flow may be achieved with the prostaglandin synthetase inhibitor indomethacin when it is administered in dosages of 1.5 to 3.0 mg/kg. The most promising results are achieved with the administration of a combined regimen of thiazide, indomethacin, and desmopressin, which reduces diuresis by as much as 80%.

## HYPEROSMOLAR SYNDROMES

Hyperosmolar or hypernatremic syndromes may be defined as plasma osmolality levels and sodium concentrations of >300 mOsm/kg and >145 mEq/L (145 mmol/L), respectively. Although rare, they constitute a major management challenge.

**TABLE 26-2.**
**Specific Causes of Hypodipsic Hypernatremia**

**VASCULAR**
Anterior communicating artery aneurysm (ligation)
Intrahypothalamic hemorrhage
Internal carotid artery ligation
**NEOPLASTIC**
Primary (craniopharyngioma, pinealoma, meningioma, chromophobe adenoma)
Metastatic (lung, breast)
**GRANULOMATOUS**
Histiocytosis
Sarcoidosis
Tuberculosis
**MISCELLANEOUS**
Hydrocephalus
Head injury
Toluene exposure
Idiopathic
Old age

(Adapted from Robertson GL, Aycinena P, Zerbe RL. Neurogenic disorders of osmoregulation. Am J Med 1982; 72:339.)

## ETIOLOGY

Transient hyperosmolality may occur after the ingestion of large amounts of salt,[34] but most hypernatremic states occur after inadequate water intake. This can occur in any healthy individual in whom the combination of excess fluid loss—from skin, gastrointestinal tract, lungs, or kidneys—and inadequate access to water is found. This occurs most commonly in acute illness in which water intake is compromised by vomiting or impaired consciousness and most vividly in patients with diabetes insipidus, before treatment, or when access to water is denied. In other cases, however, hypernatremia reflects a primary disorder of thirst deficiency (hypodipsia).

A number of conditions are associated with hypodipsia (Table 26-2). One of the more common causes of hypodipsic hypernatremia that the authors have seen is ligation of the anterior communicating artery, after subarachnoid hemorrhage from a berry aneurysm. Other centers have reported that neoplasms account for 50% of such cases.[35] Craniopharyngiomas are particularly associated with hypodipsic diabetes insipidus, sometimes in conjunction with other hypothalamus-related disorders, such as polyphagia, weight gain, and abnormal thermoregulation. Survivors of diabetic hyperosmolar coma have been shown to have impaired osmoregulated thirst,[35] which suggests that hypodipsia contributes to the development of the hypernatremia, which is characteristic of the condition. In almost every case of hypodipsia, associated abnormalities of vasopressin secretion are seen, a finding that reflects the close anatomic proximity of the osmoreceptors for vasopressin secretion and thirst.

## CLINICAL FEATURES

In young children and the elderly, hypernatremia may be associated with significant degrees of dehydration.[36] Infants are at particular risk, and the mortality is high. In this clinical situation, signs are seen of extracellular fluid loss, decreased skin turgor and elasticity, dry and shrunken tongue, tachycardia, and orthostatic hypotension. Affected infants have depressed fontanelles and tachypnea, and their respirations are deep and rapid. Fever is often present, and the temperature may be as high as 40.5°C (105°F). Adults with mild hypernatremia may have no symptoms, but as plasma sodium levels rise above 160 mEq/L, neurologic signs become apparent.[36,37] Early symptoms

include lethargy, nausea, and tremor, which progress to irritability, drowsiness, and confusion. Later features of muscular rigidity, opisthotonus, seizures, and coma reflect generalized cerebral and neuromuscular dysfunction. The most severe neurologic disturbances are seen at both ends of the age spectrum. The severity of such disturbances is also related to the rate at which hypernatremia develops, as well as to the absolute degree of hyperosmolality. Intracerebral vascular lesions are often the cause of death.

In contrast to patients with the life-threatening clinical features of hypernatremic dehydration, patients with long-standing, moderate hypernatremia (plasma sodium concentrations of 145 to 160 mEq/L) may have few manifestations of the disorder other than lack of thirst. Hypodipsia is the crucial symptom, but it is often overlooked in the clinical setting because patients fail to complain of lack of thirst. However, careful evaluation of these patients reveals that some have no desire to drink any fluid under any circumstances, which suggests a total loss of the thirst osmoreceptor function. Others have only minimal thirst with marked hypertonicity, whereas a third group eventually experiences a normal thirst sensation, but only at high plasma osmolality levels.

The key to recognizing subtle differences in thirst appreciation rests with a satisfactory measure of thirst. Visual analog scales for measuring thirst during dynamic tests of osmoregulation[38,39] have been shown to produce highly reproducible results.[40] When these scales are used in evaluating healthy persons, a linear increase is noted in the degree of thirst and fluid intake with increase in plasma osmolality, and an osmolar threshold for thirst is seen that is a few milliosmoles per kilogram higher than the osmolar threshold for vasopressin secretion.[39] The application of these techniques to patients with chronic hypernatremia has disclosed numerous disorders of osmoregulation.

## OSMOREGULATORY DEFECTS IN CHRONIC HYPERNATREMIA

Chronic hypernatremia is characterized by inappropriate lack of thirst despite increased plasma osmolality and mild hypovolemia. Plasma sodium concentrations are typically elevated (150–160 mmol/L) and may reach extremely high concentrations during intercurrent illnesses (e.g., gastroenteritis) in which body water deficits increase. Although adipsic hypernatremia is uncommon, four distinct patterns of abnormal osmoregulatory function have been described.

**Type 1 Adipsia.** The characteristic abnormalities in type 1 adipsia are subnormal vasopressin levels and thirst responses to osmotic stimulation (Fig. 26-4). The sensitivity of the osmoreceptors is decreased, producing partial diabetes insipidus and relative hypodipsia. Because some capacity remains to secrete vasopressin and experience thirst, such patients are protected from extremes of hypernatremia, as they can produce near-maximal antidiuresis as plasma osmolality increases. Patients with this type of adipsia usually have normal vasopressin responses to hypotension and hypoglycemia, and show suppression of vasopressin secretion, with the development of hypotonic diuresis in response to water loading.

**Type 2 Adipsia.** Total ablation of the osmoreceptors produces complete diabetes insipidus and absence of thirst in response to hyperosmolality. This is the pattern of osmoregulatory abnormality seen after surgical clipping of aneurysms of the anterior communicating artery,[41,42] and despite the complete absence of osmoregulated thirst and vasopressin release, thirst and vasopressin responses to hypotension and apomorphine are preserved.[41,43] Some patients also develop this type of osmoregulatory dysfunction after surgery for large, suprasellar craniopharyngiomas. Interestingly, these patients also have absent baroregulated thirst and vasopressin secretion—presumably because the extent of surgical injury is such that both

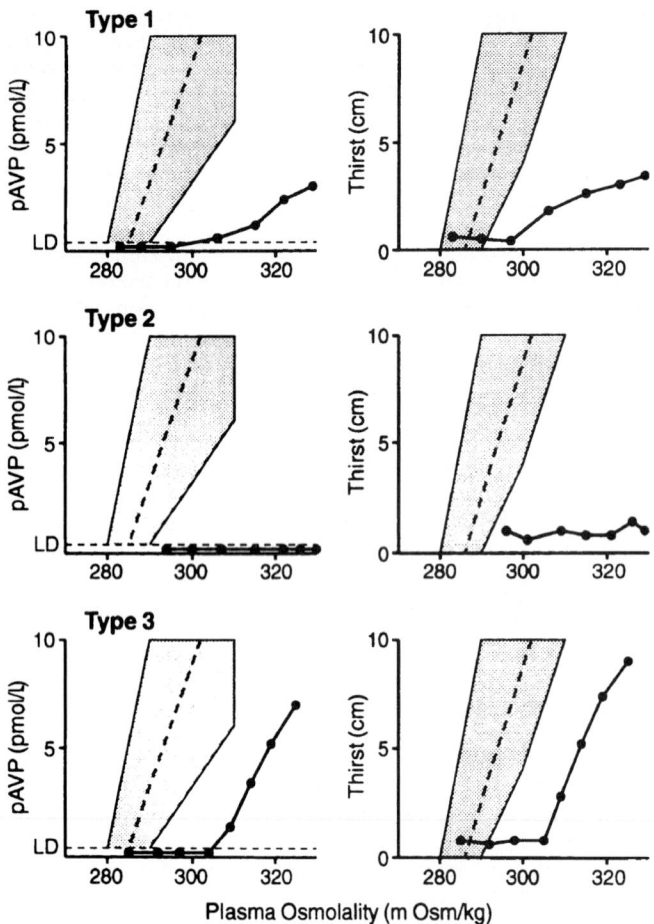

**FIGURE 26-4.** Thirst and vasopressin responses to osmotic stimulation in adipsic hypernatremia. Type 1: subnormal response of both thirst and vasopressin secretion. Type 2: total lack of response of thirst and vasopressin secretion. Type 3: reset of osmostat for vasopressin release and thirst to the right of normal. Shaded areas indicate the response ranges in healthy control subjects; the dotted lines are the mean regression lines. (*pAVP*, plasma arginine vasopressin; *LD*, limit of detection of the pAVP assay [0.3 pmol/L]).

the osmoreceptors and the paraventricular and supraoptic nuclei are damaged. Patients with complete adipsic diabetes insipidus have no defense against dehydration, and unless they are closely supervised and trained to drink even in the absence of thirst, they can develop profound hypernatremic dehydration, even in the absence of intercurrent illness.

Interest has been shown in the concept that osmoreceptor activity is under bimodal control; that is, a specific stimulus is required to *switch off* vasopressin secretion in the same way that elevation of plasma osmolality stimulates vasopressin secretion. Patients with complete osmoreceptor ablation clearly are unable to respond to inhibitory inputs; this has been demonstrated in clinical studies in which complete suppression of the secretion of the small quantities of radioimmunoassayable vasopressin or the achievement of maximal free water clearance during water loading was impossible in a patient with this type of osmoregulatory dysfunction.[44] Therefore, in some patients vasopressin secretion may not be entirely suppressed during fluid loads, resulting in significant hyponatremia.

**Type 3 Adipsia.**   The osmostats for thirst and vasopressin release may be reset to the right of normal (type 3 in Fig. 26-4), such that vasopressin secretion and thirst do not occur until higher plasma osmolalities are reached. Thereafter, the slope of the osmoregulatory lines are normal. This pattern is found in conjunction with a number of cases of "essential" hypernatremia, although type 1 defects have also been reported.[45–47]

Patients also have intact nonosmotic release of vasopressin and increased renal sensitivity to vasopressin, so that renal concentrating ability may be reasonably well maintained.

**Miscellaneous Causes of Adipsia.**   Osmoregulatory dysfunction has also been reported in elderly patients, who have diminished thirst in response to hypernatremia.[38] Although the defect in thirst appreciation is similar to that in type 1 dysfunction, vasopressin responses have variously been reported as being subnormal, normal, or enhanced. Survivors of diabetic hyperosmolar, nonketotic coma have also been reported to have hypodipsia with exaggerated vasopressin secretion.[35] In addition, a single case has been reported of a young patient who had hypodipsia but a normal osmotically regulated vasopressin release.[48] All of these reports lend support to the hypothesis that the osmoreceptors subserving vasopressin release are anatomically and functionally distinct from those controlling thirst.

## TREATMENT

Water replacement is the basic therapy for patients with hyperosmolar states associated with dehydration. The oral route is preferred, but if the clinical situation warrants urgent treatment, the infusion of hypotonic solutions may be necessary. However, overzealous rehydration with hypotonic fluids may result in seizures, neurologic deterioration, coma, and even death secondary to cerebral edema.[34,37] Therefore, the decision to treat with hypotonic intravenous fluids should not be made lightly, and rehydration to a euosmolar state should proceed cautiously over at least 72 hours. As plasma osmolality falls, polyuria indicative of hypothalamic diabetes insipidus may develop; this responds to administration of desmopressin.

For patients with chronic hyperosmolar syndromes (see Fig. 26-4), longer-term therapy must be considered. Patients with type 3 defects rarely need specific therapy because their osmoregulatory system is essentially intact but operates around a higher than normal plasma osmolality. Patients with type 1 defects (involving partial destruction of the osmoreceptor) should be treated with a regimen of increased water intake (2–4 L every 24 hours). If this leads to persistent polyuria, a small dose of desmopressin can be administered, but plasma osmolality or sodium levels must then be monitored regularly.

Considerable difficulties arise in treating patients who have complete destruction of their osmoreceptors (type 2 defect), because these patients cannot protect themselves from extremes of dehydration and overhydration. Most patients need between 2 and 4 L of fluid per day, but the precise amount varies according to seasonal climatic changes, and the body weight must be monitored daily to provide an index of fluid balance.[44] Regular (usually weekly) measurements of plasma osmolality or sodium are needed to ensure that no significant fluctuations occur in body water, and constant supervision is required to make certain the requisite volume of water is consumed. Despite the most vigorous supervision, such patients are extremely vulnerable to swings in plasma osmolality and are particularly prone to severe hypernatremic dehydration.

## REFERENCES

1. De Wardener HE, Herxheimer A. The effect of high water intake on the kidneys' ability to concentrate urine in man. J Physiol (Lond) 1957; 139:42.
2. Robertson GL. Diagnosis of diabetes insipidus. In: Czernichow P, Robinson AG, eds. Diabetes insipidus in man. Frontiers of hormone research, vol 13. Basel: S Karger, 1985:176.
3. Maffly RH. Diabetes insipidus. In: Andreoli TE, Grantham JJ, Rector FCJ, eds. Disturbances in body fluid osmolality. Bethesda, MD: American Physiology Society, 1977:285.
4. Robertson GL. Diabetes insipidus. Endocrinol Metab Clin North Am 1995; 24:549.
5. Ito M, Mori Y, Oiso Y, Saito H. A single base substitution in the coding region for neurophysin II associated with familial central diabetes insipidus. J Clin Invest 1991; 87:725.

6. Krishnamani MRS, Philips PA III, Copeland KC. Detection of a novel arginine vasopressin defect by dideoxy fingerprinting. J Clin Endocrinol Metab 1993; 77:596.

7. McLeod JF, Kovacs L, Gaskill MB, et al. Familial neurohypophyseal diabetes insipidus associated with a signal peptide mutation. J Clin Endocrinol Metab 1993; 77:599A.

8. Heppner C, Kotzka J, Bullmann C, et al. Identification of mutations of the arginine vasopressin-neurophysin II gene in two kindreds with familial central diabetes insipidus. J Clin Endocrinol Metab 1998; 83:693.

9. Rotig A, Cormier V, Chatelain P. Deletion of the mitochondrial DNA in a case of early-onset diabetes mellitus, optic atrophy and deafness, Wolfram syndrome (MIM 222300). J Clin Invest 1993; 91:1095.

10. Barrett TG, Bundey SE. Wolfram (DIDMOAD) syndrome. J Med Genet 1997; 34:838.

11. Verbalis JG, Robinson AG, Moses AM. Postoperative and post-traumatic diabetes insipidus. In: Czernichow P, Robinson AG, eds. Diabetes insipidus in man. Frontiers of hormone research, vol 13. Basel: S Karger, 1985:247.

12. Moses AM. Clinical and laboratory observations in the adult with diabetes insipidus and related syndromes. In: Czernichow P, Robinson AG, eds. Diabetes insipidus in man. Frontiers of hormone research, vol 13. Basel: S Karger, 1985:156.

13. Baylis PH, Cheetham T. Diabetes insipidus. Arch Dis Child 1998; 79:84.

14. Scherbaum WA, Bottazzo GF. Autoantibodies to vasopressin cells in idiopathic diabetes insipidus: evidence for an autoimmune variant. Lancet 1983; 1:897.

15. Imura H, Nakao K, Shimatsu A, et al. Lymphocytic infundibuloneurohypophysitis as a cause of central diabetes insipidus. N Engl J Med 1993; 329:683.

15a. Knoers NV, Monnens LL. Nephrogenic diabetes insipidus. Semin Nephrol 1999; 19:344.

15b. Bendz H, Aurell M. Drug-induced diabetes insipidus. Drug Saf 1999; 21:449.

16. Bichet DG, Birnbaumer M, Louergan M, et al. Nature and recurrence of AVPR2 mutations in X-linked nephrogenic diabetes insipidus. Am J Hum Genet 1994; 55:278.

17. Hochberg Z, van Lieburg A, Even L, et al. Autosomal recessive nephrogenic diabetes insipidus caused by an aquaporin-2 mutation. J Clin Endocrinol Metab 1997; 82:686.

18. Sato N, Ishizaka H, Yagi H, et al. Posterior lobe of the pituitary in diabetes insipidus: dynamic MR imaging. Radiology 1993; 186:357.

19. Dashe AM, Cramm RE, Crist CA, et al. A water deprivation test for the differential diagnosis of polyuria. JAMA 1963; 185:699.

20. Miller MT, Dalakos T, Moses AM, et al. Recognition of partial defects in antidiuretic hormone secretion. Ann Intern Med 1970; 73:721.

21. Baylis PH. Diabetes insipidus. Medicine 1997; 25:9.

22. Robertson GL. The regulation of vasopressin function in health and disease. Recent Prog Horm Res 1977; 33:333.

23. Moses A, Streeten D. Differentiation of polyuric states by measurement of responses to changes in plasma osmolality induced by hypertonic saline infusions. Am J Med 1967; 42:368.

24. Baylis PH, Robertson GL. Vasopressin response to hypertonic saline infusion to assess posterior pituitary function. J R Soc Med 1980; 73:255.

25. Zerbe RL, Robertson GL. A comparison of plasma vasopressin measurement with a standard indirect test in the differential diagnosis of polyuria. N Engl J Med 1981; 305:1539.

26. Thompson CJ, Baylis PH. Thirst in diabetes insipidus: clinical relevance of quantitative assessment. Q J Med 1987; 65:853.

27. Davison JM, Gilmore EA, Dürr J, et al. Altered osmotic thresholds for vasopressin secretion and thirst in human pregnancy. Am J Physiol 1984; 246:F105.

28. Amico J. Diabetes insipidus in pregnancy. In: Czernichow P, Robinson AG, eds. Diabetes insipidus in man. Frontiers in hormone research, vol 13. Basel: S Karger, 1985:266.

29. Hime MC, Richardson JA. Diabetes insipidus and pregnancy: case report, incidence and review of the literature. Obstet Gynecol Surv 1978; 33:375.

30. Barron WM, Cohen LH, Ulland LA, et al. Transient vasopressin-resistant diabetes insipidus of pregnancy. N Engl J Med 1984; 310:442.

31. Hughes JM, Barron WM, Vance ML. Recurrent diabetes insipidus associated with pregnancy: pathophysiology and therapy. Obstet Gynecol 1989; 73:462.

32. Cobb WE, Spare S, Reichlin S. Diabetes insipidus: management with DDAVP (1-desamino-8-D-arginine vasopressin). Ann Intern Med 1978; 88:183.

33. Williams TDM, Dungar DB, Lyon CC, et al. Antidiuretic effect and pharmacokinetics of oral 1-desamino-8-D-arginine vasopressin. 1. Studies in adults and children. J Clin Endocrinol Metab 1986; 63:129.

34. Ross EJ, Christie SBM. Hypernatremia. Medicine (Baltimore) 1969; 48:441.

35. McKenna K, Morris AM, Azam H, et al. Subnormal osmotically stimulated thirst and exaggerated vasopressin release in human survivors of hyperosmolar coma. Diabetologia May 1999; 42:538.

36. Robertson GL, Aycinena P, Zerbe RL. Neurogenic disorders of osmoregulation. Am J Med 1982; 72:339.

37. Arieff AL, Guisado R. Effects on the central nervous system of hypernatremic and hyponatremic states. Kidney Int 1976; 10:104.

38. Phillips PA, Rolls BJ, Ledingham JGG, et al. Reduced thirst after water deprivation in healthy elderly men. N Engl J Med 1984; 311:753.

39. Thompson CJ, Thompson J, Burd J, Baylis PH. The osmotic threshold for thirst and vasopressin release are similar in healthy men. Clin Sci 1986; 71:651.

40. Thompson CJ, Selby P, Baylis PH. Reproducibility of osmotic and nonosmotic tests of vasopressin secretion in men. Am J Physiol 1991; 260:R533.

41. Pearce SHS, Argent NB, Baylis PH. Chronic hypernatremia due to impaired osmoregulated thirst and vasopressin secretion. Acta Endocrinol (Copenh) 1991; 125:234.

42. McIver B, Connacher A, Whittle A, et al. Adipsic diabetes insipidus after clipping of anterior communicating artery aneurysm. BMJ 1991; 303:1465.

43. Teelucksingh S, Steer CR, Thompson CJ, et al. Hypothalamic syndrome and central sleep apnea associated with toluene exposure. Q J Med 1991; 286:185.

44. Ball SG, Vaidja B, Baylis PH. Hypothalamic adipsic syndrome: diagnosis and management. Clin Endocrinol 1997; 47:405.

45. De Rubertis FR, Michelis MF, Beck N, et al. "Essential" hypernatremia due to ineffective osmotic and intact volume regulation of vasopressin secretion. J Clin Invest 1971; 50:97.

46. Dunger DB, Seckl JR, Lightman SL. Increased renal sensitivity to vasopressin in two patients with essential hypernatremia. J Clin Endocrinol Metab 1987; 64:185.

47. Gill G, Baylis PH, Burn J. A case of "essential" hypernatremia due to resetting of the osmostat. Clin Endocrinol (Oxf) 1985; 22:545.

48. Hammond DN, Moll GW, Robertson GL, Chelmicks-Schorr E. Hypodipsic hypernatremia with normal osmoregulation of vasopressin. N Engl J Med 1986; 315:433.

# CHAPTER 27

# INAPPROPRIATE ANTIDIURESIS AND OTHER HYPOOSMOLAR STATES

JOSEPH G. VERBALIS

## FREQUENCY AND SIGNIFICANCE OF HYPOOSMOLALITY

Hypoosmolality of plasma is relatively common in hospitalized patients. The incidence and prevalence of hypoosmolar disorders depend on the nature of the patient population being studied and on the laboratory methods and diagnostic criteria used. Most investigators have used the serum sodium concentration ([Na+]) to determine the clinical incidence of hypoosmolality. When hyponatremia is defined as a serum [Na+] of <135 mEq/L, an incidence as high as 15% to 30% has been observed in patients hospitalized for both short[1] and longer[2] periods. However, the incidence decreases to a range of 1% to 4% when only patients with a serum [Na+] of <130 to 131 mEq/L are included,[1,3] although even when these more stringent criteria are used, incidences of 7% to 30% have been reported in hospitalized geriatric patients.[2] Interestingly, many studies have noted a high incidence of *iatrogenic* or *hospital-acquired hyponatremia,* which accounts for 40% to 75% of all cases examined.[3,4] Furthermore, a frequency analysis of a large group of hospitalized patients demonstrated serum sodium and chloride concentrations that were ~5 mEq/L lower than those in a control group of healthy, nonhospitalized subjects.[5] Consequently, the conclusion can be drawn that most cases of hypoosmolality are relatively mild and that it is often acquired during hospitalization. Although this might appear to signify that hypoosmolality generally is of little clinical significance, this conclusion is unwarranted for several reasons. First, severe hypoosmolality (serum [Na+] level of <125 mEq/L), although relatively uncommon, is associated with substantial morbidity and mortality. Second, even relatively mild hypoosmolality can progress to more dangerous levels during the therapeutic management of other disorders. Finally, the observation has been made that mortality is as much as 60-fold higher in patients with even asymptomatic degrees of hypoosmolality than in normonatremic patients.[3] Although this probably indicates that hypoosmolality is more an indicator of the severity of many underlying illnesses than an independent factor contributing to mortality, this presumption may not be true in all cases. These considerations, therefore, emphasize the importance of a careful evaluation of all hyponatremic patients, regardless of the clinical setting.

## DEFINITION OF HYPOOSMOLALITY

The only clinical abnormality known to result from increased secretion of arginine vasopressin (AVP) is a decrease in the osmotic pressure of body fluids. Hence it is appropriate to begin this chapter by considering how osmotic pressure, or osmolality, is determined and the factors that can influence these measurements.

The osmolality of body fluid normally is maintained within narrow limits by osmotically regulated AVP secretion and thirst (see Chap. 25). Although basal plasma osmolality can vary appreciably among individuals, under conditions of normal hydration, the range in the general population lies between 275 and 295 mOsm/kg $H_2O$. Plasma osmolality can be determined by direct measurement using either freezing-point depression or vapor pressure. Alternatively, it can be calculated from the concentrations of the major solutes in serum:

$$pOsm\ (mOsm/kg\ H_2O) = 2 \times [Na^+]\ (mEq/L) + glucose\ (mg/dL)/18 + blood\ urea\ nitrogen\ (mg/dL)/2.8$$

The two methods produce comparable results under most conditions. Although these methods yield valid measures of *total* osmolality, however, this is not always equivalent to *effective* osmolality, sometimes referred to as the *tonicity* of the fluid.[6] Only those solutes that remain relatively compartmentalized within the extracellular fluid (ECF) space (e.g., sodium and chloride) are considered to be effective solutes, because they create osmotic gradients across cell membranes and thus are capable of causing osmotic movement of water from the intracellular fluid (ICF) compartment to the ECF compartment. In contrast, solutes that readily permeate cell membranes (e.g., urea, ethanol, methanol) are not effective solutes, because they do not create osmotic gradients across cell membranes and thus are not capable of causing water movement between fluid compartments. Consequently, only the concentration of effective solutes in serum should be used to define clinically significant hypoosmolality or hyperosmolality of serum, because these are the only solutes that affect cellular hydration.

### SITUATIONS IN WHICH HYPONATREMIA DOES NOT REFLECT TRUE HYPOOSMOLALITY

Because sodium and its accompanying anions represent the major effective serum solutes, hyponatremia and hypoosmolality are usually synonymous. However, two situations exist in which hyponatremia does not reflect true hypoosmolality. The first is *pseudohyponatremia*, produced by marked elevations of bulky solutes such as lipids or proteins in serum. In such cases, the concentration of sodium per liter of serum *water* is unchanged, but the concentration of sodium per liter of *serum* is artifactually decreased because of the increased relative proportion of serum volume that is occupied by the lipids or proteins. Because the increase in lipids or proteins does not appreciably increase the total number of solute particles in solution, however, the measured plasma osmolality is *not* affected significantly. In addition, measurement of serum $[Na^+]$ by ion-specific electrode, a method currently used by most clinical laboratories,

is less influenced by high concentrations of lipids or proteins than was measurement of serum $[Na^+]$ by flame photometry.[7]

The second situation in which hyponatremia does not reflect true plasma hypoosmolality occurs when high concentrations of effective solutes other than sodium are present in the ECF, causing relative decreases in serum $[Na^+]$ despite an unchanged total effective osmolality. This effect usually is seen with hyperglycemia and represents a very common cause of hyponatremia, accounting for 10% to 20% of cases in hospitalized patients.[3] Misdiagnosis of hypoosmolality in such cases can again be avoided by measuring plasma osmolality directly or, alternatively, by correcting the measured serum $[Na^+]$ by 1.6 mEq/L for each 100 mg/dL-increase in serum glucose concentration above normal levels.[6]

### INFLUENCE OF UNMEASURED SOLUTES

Plasma osmolality cannot be calculated when the ECF contains significant amounts of unmeasured solutes, such as osmotic diuretics, radiographic contrast agents, and some toxins (ethanol, methanol, and ethylene glycol). In these situations, plasma osmolality is better ascertained by direct measurement, although even this method does not yield an accurate measure of the true effective plasma osmolality if the unmeasured solutes are noneffective solutes, such as ethanol, that freely permeate cells.

As a result of these considerations, the ascertainment of true hypoosmolality can sometimes be difficult. Nevertheless, a straightforward and relatively simple approach suffices in most cases. This entails initially calculating the *effective* plasma osmolality from the measured serum $[Na^+]$ and glucose concentrations ($2 \times [Na^+]$ + glucose ÷ 18) or, alternatively, simply correcting the serum $[Na^+]$ for elevations of serum glucose, as described previously. If the calculated effective osmolality is <275 mOsm/kg $H_2O$, or the corrected serum $[Na^+]$ is <135 mEq/L, significant hypoosmolality is present, *assuming* that significant concentrations of unmeasured solutes or pseudohyponatremia from hyperlipidemia or hyperproteinemia are not present. *If uncertainty exists about either of these latter points, the plasma osmolality should also be measured directly.*

The absence of a significant discrepancy (<10 mOsm/kg $H_2O$) between the measured and calculated total plasma osmolality (called the *osmolar gap*) confirms the absence of significant amounts of unmeasured solutes, such as osmotic diuretics, radiocontrast agents, or alcohol. However, if a significant discrepancy between these measures is found, appropriate tests must then be conducted to rule out pseudohyponatremia or to identify possible unmeasured serum solutes. Whether significant hypoosmolality exists in the latter case depends on the nature of the unmeasured solutes. Although this determination may not always be possible, in such cases the clinician at least is alerted to the uncertainty of true hypoosmolality.

## PATHOGENESIS OF HYPOOSMOLALITY

The presence of true hypoosmolality *always* signifies an excess of water relative to solute in the ECF. Because water moves freely across most cell membranes between the ICF and ECF, this usually also implies an excess of total body water relative to total body solute. As shown in Table 27-1, an imbalance between water and solute can be generated either by a *depletion* of total body solute in excess of concurrent body water losses, or by a *dilution* of total body solute secondary to increases in total body water. This classification represents an obvious oversimplification, because most hypoosmolar states have components of both solute depletion and water retention. Nonetheless, it represents a valid starting point for understanding the mechanisms underlying the pathogenesis of hypoosmolality and also provides a useful framework for discussing the treatment of hypoosmolar disorders.

**TABLE 27-1.**
Pathogenesis of Hypoosmolar Disorders

**DEPLETION (PRIMARY DECREASES IN TOTAL BODY SOLUTE + SECONDARY WATER RETENTION)**

*Renal Solute Loss*
  Diuretic use
  Solute diuresis (glucose, mannitol)
  Salt-wasting nephropathy
  Mineralocorticoid deficiency

*Nonrenal Solute Loss*
  Gastrointestinal (diarrhea, vomiting, pancreatitis, bowel obstruction)
  Cutaneous (sweating, burns)
  Blood loss

**DILUTION (PRIMARY INCREASES IN TOTAL BODY WATER + SECONDARY SOLUTE DEPLETION)**

*Impaired Renal Free Water Excretion*
  **Increased Proximal Reabsorption**
    Hypothyroidism
  **Impaired Distal Dilution**
    Syndrome of inappropriate antidiuresis hormone secretion
    Glucocorticoid deficiency
  **Combined Increased Proximal Reabsorption and Impaired Distal Dilution**
    Congestive heart failure
    Cirrhosis
    Nephrotic syndrome
  **Decreased Urinary Solute Excretion**
    Beer potomania

*Excess Water Intake*
  Primary polydipsia
  Dilute infant formula

## SOLUTE DEPLETION

Depletion of body solute can result from any significant ECF losses. Whether by renal or nonrenal routes, the fluid loss itself rarely causes hypoosmolality because excreted or secreted fluid usually is isotonic or hypotonic relative to serum. Therefore, when hypoosmolality accompanies ECF losses, it is generally the result of replacement of the fluid losses by hypotonic solutions, causing dilution of the remaining body solutes. This usually occurs when patients drink only water in response to ongoing solute and water losses, but it can also occur when hypotonic fluids are administered intravenously to hospitalized patients. When solute losses are marked, these patients show obvious signs of volume depletion (e.g., addisonian crisis; see Chap. 76). However, such patients often have a more deceptive clinical picture because their volume deficits may be partially replaced. Moreover, they may not manifest signs or symptoms of cellular dehydration because osmotic gradients act to draw water into the relatively hypertonic ICF compartment, causing cellular volume expansion. Consequently, although clinical evidence of hypovolemia strongly supports solute depletion as the cause of plasma hypoosmolality, the absence of clinically evident hypovolemia never completely eliminates this possibility. Although ECF solute loss is responsible for most cases of depletion-induced hypoosmolality, ICF solute loss can also lead to hypoosmolality as a result of osmotic water shifts into the ECF. This mechanism likely contributes to the hypoosmolality that is observed in some cases of diuretic-induced hypoosmolality in which marked depletion of total body potassium occurs.[8]

## WATER RETENTION

Despite the importance of solute depletion in some patients, most cases of clinically significant hypoosmolality are caused by increases in total body water rather than by losses of extracellular solute. Theoretically, this can occur because of either *impaired renal free water excretion* or *excessive free water intake*. However, the former accounts for most hypoosmolar disorders because normal kidneys have sufficient diluting capacity to allow excretion of 20 to 30 L per day of free water.[9] Intakes of this magnitude are occasionally seen in psychiatric patients, but not in most patients with primary polydipsia. Furthermore, studies have demonstrated that psychotic patients with polydipsia and hyponatremia also have abnormalities of free water excretion.[10] Consequently, dilutional hypoosmolality usually implies an abnormality of renal free water excretion. The renal mechanisms responsible for impairments in free water excretion are commonly classified according to whether the major effect occurs in the proximal or distal nephron (see Table 27-1).

Any disorder that leads to a decrease in glomerular filtration rate (GFR) causes increased reabsorption of both sodium and water in the proximal tubule. Consequently, the ability to excrete free water is limited because of decreased delivery of tubular fluid to the distal nephron. Disorders causing solute depletion through nonrenal mechanisms also produce the same effect.

Disorders that cause a decreased glomerular filtration rate in the absence of significant ECF fluid losses are, for the most part, edema-forming states associated with decreased effective intravascular volume and secondary hyperaldosteronism. Severe hypothyroidism causes a similar effect, but does so through mechanisms that have not been delineated fully. However, even though these conditions traditionally have been considered to be primarily disorders of excess proximal fluid reabsorption, convincing evidence now exists that water retention also results from increased distal reabsorption caused by hemodynamically stimulated increases in serum AVP levels.[11]

Distal nephron impairments in free water excretion are characterized by an inability to dilute tubular fluid maximally. Such disorders are usually associated with abnormalities in AVP secretion, as depicted in Table 27-1.

Just as depletion-induced hypoosmolar disorders usually include an important component of *secondary* impairment of free water excretion, so do most dilution-induced hypoosmolar disorders involve a component of *secondary* solute depletion. This effect has been recognized ever since early studies of the effects of AVP on water retention demonstrated that renal sodium excretion in such subjects was predominantly a result of ECF volume expansion from retained water.[12] *Thus, after sustained increases in total body water caused by inappropriately elevated AVP levels, sufficient secondary solute losses can occur to lower plasma osmolality further or, more often, to allow the maintenance of a lowered plasma osmolality with lesser degrees of ECF volume expansion from retained water.*[13] The actual contribution of solute losses to the hypoosmolality of inappropriate antidiuresis is variable and in experimental[14,15] and clinical[16] studies has been shown to depend on both the rate and the volume of AVP-induced ECF water expansion.

Some dilutional disorders do not fit well into either category. Among these is the hyponatremia that sometimes occurs in patients who ingest large volumes of beer with little food intake for prolonged periods, frequently called "beer potomania." Even though the volume of fluid ingested may not seem sufficiently excessive to overwhelm renal-diluting mechanisms, in these cases free water excretion is limited by very low urinary solute excretion, thereby causing water retention and dilutional hyponatremia. However, because such patients also have very little food intake, relative depletion of body sodium stores probably also is a contributing factor to the hypoosmolality in some cases.

## CELLULAR INACTIVATION OF SOLUTE

Even the combined effects of water retention plus urinary solute excretion cannot adequately explain the degree of plasma

**TABLE 27-2.**
**Differential Diagnosis of Hypoosmolar Disorders**

| Extracellular Fluid Volume | Urinary [Na+]* | Presumptive Diagnosis |
|---|---|---|
| *Decreased* | LOW | **Depletion (Nonrenal):** Gastrointestinal, cutaneous, or blood ECF loss |
| | HIGH | **Depletion (Renal):** Diuretics, mineralocorticoid insufficiency (Addison disease), salt-losing nephropathy |
| *Normal* | LOW | **Depletion (Nonrenal):** Any cause + hypotonic fluid replacement |
| | | **Dilution (Proximal):** Hypothyroidism, early decreased effective arterial blood volume |
| | | **Dilution (Distal):** SIAD + fluid restriction |
| | HIGH | **Dilution (Distal):** SIAD, glucocorticoid insufficiency |
| | | **Depletion (Renal):** Any cause + hypotonic fluid replacement (especially diuretic treatment) |
| *Increased* | LOW | **Dilution (Proximal):** Decreased effective arterial blood volume (CHF, cirrhosis, nephrosis) |
| | HIGH | **Dilution (Proximal):** Any cause + diuretics, improvement in underlying disease, renal failure |

[Na+], sodium concentration; *ECF*, extracellular fluid; *SIAD*, syndrome of inappropriate antidiuresis; *CHF*, congestive heart failure.
*Urine [Na+] values <30 mEq/L are generally considered to be low, and values ≥30 mEq/d to be high, based on studies of responses of hyponatremic patients to infusions of isotonic saline.[24]

hypoosmolality observed in some patients.[17] This observation led to the theory of *cellular inactivation of solute*. Simply stated, this theory maintains that, as ECF osmolality falls, water moves into cells along osmotic gradients, causing the cells to swell. At some point during volume expansion, these cells osmotically inactivate some of the intracellular solutes as a defense mechanism to prevent continued cellular swelling and subsequent detrimental effects on cell function. With this decrease in intracellular osmolality, some water then shifts back out of the ICF into the ECF, but at the cost of worsening the dilution-induced ECF hypoosmolality. Despite the appeal of this theory, its validity has never been demonstrated conclusively in either human or animal studies. In part, this is because the production of unexplained hypoosmolality has generally been observed only with severe degrees of hypoosmolality (i.e., serum osmolalities of <240 mOsm/kg H₂O), which is difficult to study clinically. However, animal studies have failed to demonstrate this effect even with severe, sustained hypoosmolality.[18] An alternative theory has been suggested by in vitro studies of cultured cells, which regulate cell volume in response to hypoosmolar conditions by *extrusion* of potassium rather than osmotic inactivation of cellular solute.[19] Subsequent animal studies confirmed that after long periods of sustained hypoosmolality, the brain regulates its volume back to normal levels[20]; moreover, this process is accompanied by marked losses of organic solutes, called *organic osmolytes*,[21] as well as electrolytes[22] from the brain. Consequently, cellular volume regulation in vivo is more likely to occur predominantly through a process of *depletion*, rather than inactivation, of a variety of intracellular solutes.[13,23]

## DIFFERENTIAL DIAGNOSIS OF HYPOOSMOLALITY

The diagnostic approach to patients with hypoosmolality includes a careful history-taking (especially with regard to medications); clinical assessment of ECF volume status; a complete neurologic evaluation; measurement of serum electrolytes, glucose, blood urea nitrogen and creatinine; calculated or direct measurements of plasma osmolality, or both; and simultaneous measurement of urinary electrolytes and osmolality. Because of the multiplicity of disorders that can cause hypoosmolality and the fact that many involve more than one pathologic mechanism, a definitive diagnosis is not always possible at the time of presentation. Nonetheless, a relatively simple evaluation with a careful interpretation of laboratory results provides a sufficient categorization of the underlying cause in most cases to allow appropriate decisions regarding initial therapy. Table 27-2 summarizes a method for the differential diagnosis of hypoosmolality based on the commonly used parameters of ECF volume

status and spot urine sodium concentration (urine osmolality generally is elevated to varying degrees in most of these disorders and, therefore, is of limited value in differential diagnosis).

### DECREASED EXTRACELLULAR FLUID VOLUME (HYPOVOLEMIA)

The presence of clinically detectable hypovolemia always implies total body solute depletion. If the urine [Na+] is low, a nonrenal cause of solute depletion should be sought. If the urine [Na+] is high despite hypoosmolality, renal causes of solute depletion are likely responsible, most commonly attributable to diuretic therapy. In such cases the possibility of adrenal insufficiency must always be considered as well, especially in the presence of hyperkalemia, hypoglycemia, or clinical signs of Addison disease or hypopituitarism (see Chaps. 17 and 76). Finally, in hypovolemic patients not receiving diuretics and without evidence of adrenal insufficiency, salt-wasting nephropathy is possible (e.g., polycystic kidney disease, chronic interstitial nephritis), and usually requires further, more extensive evaluation of renal function for definitive diagnosis.

### INCREASED EXTRACELLULAR FLUID VOLUME (EDEMA, ASCITES)

The presence of clinically detectable hypervolemia implies a total body sodium excess. In these patients, hypoosmolality results from an even greater expansion of total body water caused by a marked reduction in the rate of water excretion (and sometimes an increased rate of ingestion). The impairment in water excretion is caused by a decreased effective arterial blood volume, which increases the reabsorption of glomerular filtrate not only in the proximal nephron but also in the distal and collecting tubule by stimulating AVP secretion.[11] By the time most of these disorders cause significant hypoosmolality, they are usually readily apparent; however, occasionally, hypoosmolality occurs during early stages, with relatively mild clinical manifestations of the underlying disease. These patients have a low urine [Na+] because of secondary hyperaldosteronism, which is also a product of decreased effective intravascular volume. However, under certain conditions, urine [Na+] may be elevated, usually secondary to concurrent diuretic therapy, but also sometimes because of a solute diuresis (e.g., glucosuria in diabetics) or after successful treatment of the underlying disease (e.g., ionotropic therapy in patients with congestive heart failure). One must recognize that *primary polydipsia does not cause signs of hypervolemia*, because water ingestion alone, without sodium retention, does not produce clinically apparent degrees of ECF volume expansion.

One other important disorder that can produce hypoosmolality and hypervolemia is acute or chronic renal failure with fluid overload. Urine [Na$^+$] in these cases is usually elevated, but it can be variable, depending on the stage of renal failure. This should not represent a diagnostic problem, except perhaps in the early stages of acute tubular necrosis before significant elevations of blood urea nitrogen and creatinine have occurred.

## NORMAL EXTRACELLULAR FLUID VOLUME (EUVOLEMIA)

Hypoosmolality in the clinically euvolemic patient represents the greatest diagnostic challenge, because detecting modest changes in volume status is difficult using standard methods of clinical assessment. In such cases, the determination of urine [Na$^+$] is an especially important first step.[24] A high urine [Na$^+$] in euvolemic patients usually implies a distally mediated, dilution-induced hypoosmolality, such as the syndrome of inappropriate antidiuresis (SIAD). Glucocorticoid deficiency can mimic SIAD so closely that these two disorders may be indistinguishable in terms of evaluation of water balance. This is because glucocorticoid deficiency can produce elevated serum AVP levels and, in addition, exerts a direct effect on the distal nephron to prevent maximal urinary dilution even in the absence of AVP.[25] Clinically, this phenomenon is well known by virtue of the observation that cortisol insufficiency can mask diabetes insipidus in patients who have both disorders. Therefore, both primary and secondary adrenal insufficiency must be ruled out before a diagnosis of inappropriate antidiuresis is established. This is most easily accomplished with a rapid adrenocorticotropic hormone stimulation test (see Chap. 74). A low urine [Na$^+$] suggests depletion-induced hypoosmolality secondary to ECF losses with subsequent volume replacement by water or other hypotonic fluids. The solute loss often is nonrenal in origin. An important exception is recent cessation of diuretic therapy, because urine [Na$^+$] can quickly decrease again to low levels within 12 to 24 hours after discontinuation of the diuretic drug. Low urine [Na$^+$] also can be seen in some cases of hypothyroidism, in the early stages of decreased effective intravascular volume (before the development of clinically apparent salt retention and fluid overload), or during the recovery phase of SIAD. Hence, a low urine sodium is less meaningful diagnostically than a high value.

Hyponatremia caused by diuretic use can present without clinically evident hypovolemia, and urine [Na$^+$] can be elevated in such cases because of the renal effects of the diuretics. The presence of a low serum [K$^+$] is an important clue to diuretic use, because none of the other disorders that cause hypoosmolality are associated with significant hypokalemia. However, even in the absence of hypokalemia, any hypoosmolar, clinically euvolemic patient taking diuretics should be *assumed* to have solute depletion and should be treated accordingly. Subsequent failure to correct the hypoosmolality with isotonic saline administration and a persistence of an elevated urine [Na$^+$] after discontinuation of diuretics then changes the diagnosis to a dilution-induced hypoosmolality by exclusion.

## SYNDROME OF INAPPROPRIATE ANTIDIURESIS

### DIAGNOSTIC CRITERIA

The syndrome of inappropriate antidiuresis is the most common cause of euvolemic hypoosmolality. It is also the most prevalent cause of hypoosmolality of all etiologies encountered in clinical practice today, with an incidence of 30% to 40% among all hypoosmolar patients.[2,3] The clinical criteria necessary for a diagnosis of SIAD remain basically as set forth by Bartter and Schwartz in 1967.[26] A modified summary of these criteria is presented in Table 27-3 along with other findings that support this diagnosis.

**TABLE 27-3.**
**Syndrome of Inappropriate Antidiuresis: Diagnostic Criteria**

**ESSENTIAL REQUIREMENTS**

Decreased effective osmolality of the extracellular fluid (P$_{osm}$ <275 mOsm/kg H$_2$O).

Inappropriate urinary concentration (U$_{osm}$ > 100 mOsm/kg H$_2$O with normal renal function) at some level of hypoosmolality.

Clinical euvolemia, as defined by the absence of signs either of hypovolemia (orthostasis, tachycardia, decreased skin turgor, dry mucous membranes) or of hypervolemia (subcutaneous edema, ascites).

Elevated urinary sodium excretion while on a normal salt and water intake.

Absence of other potential causes of euvolemic hypoosmolality: hypothyroidism, hypocortisolism (Addison disease or pituitary ACTH insufficiency), or recent diuretic use.

**SUPPLEMENTAL CRITERIA**

Abnormal water-load test (inability to excrete at least 90% of a 20-mL/kg water load in 4 hours and/or failure to dilute U$_{osm}$ to <100 mOsm/kg H$_2$O).

Plasma AVP level inappropriately elevated relative to plasma osmolality.

No significant correction of serum [Na$^+$] with volume expansion but improvement after fluid restriction.

*P$_{osm}$,* plasma osmolality; *U$_{osm}$,* urine osmolality; *ACTH,* adrenocorticotropic hormone; *AVP,* arginine vasopressin; *[Na$^+$],* sodium concentration.

Several of these criteria deserve emphasis or qualification. First, true hypoosmolality must be present. Hyponatremia secondary to pseudohyponatremia or hyperglycemia alone must be excluded. Second, urinary concentration (osmolality) must be inappropriate for plasma hypoosmolality. This does *not* mean that urine osmolality must be greater than plasma osmolality (a common misinterpretation of this criterion), but simply that the urine osmolality must be greater than *maximally* dilute (maximal dilution in normal adults is <100 mOsm/kg H$_2$O). One must also remember that urine osmolality need not be elevated inappropriately at *all* levels of plasma osmolality because in one form of SIAD, the *reset osmostat variant,* AVP secretion can be suppressed and maximal urinary dilution and free water excretion can occur if plasma osmolality is decreased to sufficiently low levels. Hence, satisfaction of criteria for the diagnosis of SIAD requires only that urine osmolality (or serum AVP) be inadequately suppressed at some level of plasma osmolality below 275 mOsm/kg H$_2$O. Third, clinical euvolemia *must* be present to establish a diagnosis of SIAD, because both hypovolemia and hypervolemia strongly suggest different causes of hypoosmolality. *This does not mean that patients with SIAD cannot become hypovolemic or hypervolemic for other reasons, but in such cases, the underlying inappropriate antidiuresis cannot be diagnosed until the patient is rendered euvolemic and is found to have persistent hypoosmolality.* The fourth criterion, renal salt wasting, has probably caused the most confusion over the years regarding the diagnosis of SIAD. This criterion is included primarily because of its usefulness in differentiating between hypoosmolality caused by a decreased effective extracellular volume (in which case renal sodium conservation occurs) and distally mediated dilution-induced disorders, in which urinary sodium excretion is normal or increased secondary to ECF volume expansion. However, two important qualifications limit the utility of urine [Na$^+$] measurement in hypoosmolar patients: (a) urine [Na$^+$] also is high when solute depletion is of renal origin, as with diuretic use or Addison disease, and (b) patients with SIAD can have low urinary sodium excretion if they subsequently become hypovolemic or solute depleted, conditions that sometime follow severe salt and water restriction. Consequently, although high urinary sodium excretion is the rule in most patients with SIAD, its presence certainly does not guarantee this diagnosis, and, conversely, its absence does not necessarily rule out the diagnosis. The fifth criterion emphasizes that, in many ways, SIAD remains a diagnosis of exclusion. Thus, the presence of other potential causes of euvolemic hypoosmolality must always be excluded. This includes not only thyroid and adrenal dysfunction, but also diuretic use, because this also often presents as euvolemic hypoosmolality.

Table 27-3 lists three other criteria that support, but are not essential for, the diagnosis of SIAD. The first of these criteria, water loading, is of value when uncertainty exists regarding the cause of modest degrees of hypoosmolality in euvolemic patients (it does not add useful information if the plasma osmolality is already significantly lower than 275 mOsm/kg $H_2O$). An inability to excrete a standard water load normally (with normal excretion defined as a cumulative urine output of at least 90% of the administered water load within 4 hours and suppression of urine osmolality to <100 mOsm/kg $H_2O$[27]) confirms the presence of an underlying defect in free water excretion. Unfortunately, water loading is abnormal in almost *all* disorders that cause hypoosmolality, whether dilutional or depletion induced with secondary impairments in free water excretion. Two exceptions to this are primary polydipsia, in which hypoosmolality can rarely be secondary to excessive water intake alone, and the reset osmostat variant of SIAD, in which normal excretion of a water load can occur once plasma osmolality falls below the new setpoint for AVP secretion. The water-load test is also useful to assess water excretion after treatment of an underlying disorder thought to be causing SIAD. For example, after discontinuation of a drug associated with SIAD in a patient who has already achieved a normal plasma osmolality by fluid restriction, a normal water-load test can confirm the absence of persistent inappropriate antidiuresis much more quickly than can simple monitoring of the serum [Na⁺] during ad libitum fluid intake. Despite its limitations as a diagnostic clinical test, water loading remains an extremely useful tool in clinical research for quantitating changes in free water excretion in response to physiologic or pharmacologic manipulations.

The second supportive criterion for a diagnosis of SIAD is an inappropriately elevated AVP level in relation to plasma osmolality. At the time that SIAD was originally described, inappropriately elevated levels of AVP were merely postulated, because the measurement of serum levels of AVP was limited to relatively insensitive bioassays. With the development of sensitive AVP radioimmunoassays capable of detecting the small physiologic concentrations of this peptide that circulate in serum, the hope was that the accurate measurement of serum AVP levels might supplant the classic criteria and become the definitive test for diagnosing SIAD. This has not occurred for several reasons. First, although serum AVP levels are elevated in most patients with this syndrome, the elevations generally remain within the normal physiologic range and are abnormal only in relation to plasma hypoosmolality. This is demonstrated in Figure 27-1.[28] Thus, *AVP levels can be interpreted only in conjunction with a simultaneous plasma osmolality and a knowledge of the relation between AVP levels and plasma osmolality in normal subjects.* Second, 10% to 20% of patients with SIAD do not have measurably elevated AVP levels. As shown in Figure 27-1, many patients have AVP levels that are precisely at, or even below, the limits of detection by radioimmunoassay. Whether these cases are true examples of inappropriate antidiuresis in the absence of AVP, possibly secondary to abnormal regulation of the aquaporin-2 water channels that mediate AVP-stimulated water reabsorption in the collecting ducts,[29] or whether they simply represent inappropriate AVP levels that fall below the limits of detection by radioimmunoassay is not clear at this time. For this reason, it is more accurate to use the term SIAD than the originally proposed designation of *syndrome of inappropriate antidiuretic hormone secretion (SIADH)* to describe this entire group of disorders.[30] Third, just as water loading fails to distinguish between various causes of hypoosmolality, so do AVP levels. Many disorders causing solute and volume depletion are associated with elevations of serum AVP levels secondary to nonosmotic hemodynamic stimuli. For similar reasons, patients with disorders that cause decreased effective volume, such as congestive heart failure and

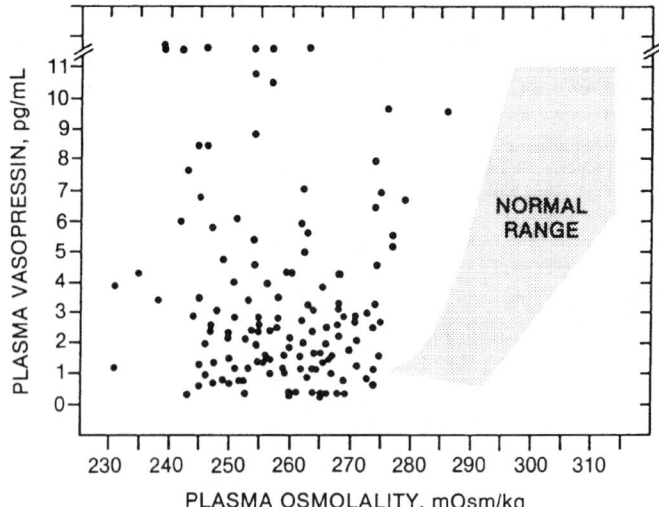

**FIGURE 27-1.** Plasma vasopressin (*AVP*) levels are shown as a function of plasma osmolality in patients with the syndrome of inappropriate antidiuresis. Each point depicts one patient. The shaded area represents AVP levels in normal subjects over physiologic ranges of plasma osmolality. (From Robertson GL, Aycinena P, Zerbe RL. Neurogenic disorders of osmoregulation. Am J Med 1982; 72:339.)

cirrhosis, also have elevated AVP levels.[11] Even glucocorticoid insufficiency has been associated with inappropriately elevated AVP levels in animal studies, although experience in humans is limited. Thus, many different disorders can cause stimulation of AVP secretion through nonosmotic mechanisms.

The final supportive criterion, an improvement in plasma osmolality with fluid restriction but not with volume expansion, can be helpful in differentiating between disorders causing solute depletion and those associated with dilution-induced hypoosmolality. The infusion of isotonic sodium chloride in patients with SIAD is well known to provoke a natriuresis with little correction of osmolality,[17,26] whereas fluid restriction allows such patients to achieve solute and water balance gradually through insensible free water losses. In contrast, isotonic saline is the treatment of choice in disorders of solute depletion, because once volume deficits are corrected, the stimulus to AVP secretion and free water retention is eliminated. The diagnostic value of this therapeutic response is limited somewhat by the fact that patients with proximal types of dilution-induced disorders may show a response similar to that found in patients with SIAD. The major drawback of this criterion, however, is that it represents a retrospective test in a situation in which establishing a diagnosis before making a decision regarding treatment options would be preferable. Nonetheless, in difficult cases of *euvolemic* hypoosmolality, an appropriate therapeutic response can sometimes be helpful in diagnosing SIAD.

## ETIOLOGY

Disorders associated with SIAD can be divided into several major etiologic groups. These groups are summarized in Table 27-4.

### TUMORS

The most common cause of SIAD is a tumor. Although several different types of tumors are listed in Table 27-4, bronchogenic carcinoma of the lung has been uniquely associated with SIAD since the first description of this disorder in 1957.[17] In virtually all cases, the bronchogenic carcinomas causing this syndrome have been of the small cell (or oat cell) variety (a few squamous cell types have been described, but these are rare). The unusually high incidence of small cell carcinoma of the lung in

**TABLE 27-4.**
**Syndrome of Inappropriate Antidiuresis: Etiologies**

**TUMORS**

 **Pulmonary/mediastinal** (bronchogenic carcinoma; mesothelioma; thymoma)
 **Nonchest** (duodenal carcinoma; pancreatic carcinoma; ureteral/prostate carcinoma; uterine carcinoma; nasopharyngeal carcinoma; leukemia)

**CENTRAL NERVOUS SYSTEM DISORDERS**

 **Mass lesions** (tumors; brain abscesses; subdural hematoma)
 **Inflammatory diseases** (encephalitis; meningitis; systemic lupus erythematosus; acute intermittent porphyria)
 **Degenerative/demyelinative diseases** (Guillain-Barré syndrome; spinal cord lesions)
 **Miscellaneous** (subarachnoid hemorrhage; head trauma; acute psychosis; delirium tremens; transsphenoidal hypophysectomy)

**DRUG EFFECTS**

 **Stimulated AVP release** (nicotine; phenothiazines; tricyclic antidepressants)
 **Direct renal effects and/or potentiation of AVP antidiuretic effects** (DDAVP; oxytocin; prostaglandin synthesis inhibitors)
 **Mixed or uncertain actions** (chlorpropamide; clofibrate; carbamazepine and oxcarbazepine; cyclophosphamide; vincristine; lisinopril; clozapine; serotonin reuptake inhibitors)

**PULMONARY DISEASES**

 **Infections** (tuberculosis; acute bacterial and viral pneumonia; aspergillosis; empyema)
 **Mechanical/ventilatory** (acute respiratory failure; COPD; positive-pressure ventilation)

**OTHER CAUSES**

 **Acquired immunodeficiency syndrome (AIDS) and AIDS-related complex**
 **Senile atrophy**
 **Idiopathic**

*AVP*, arginine vasopressin; *DDAVP*, desmopressin; *COPD*, chronic obstructive pulmonary disease.

---

patients with SIAD, together with the relatively favorable therapeutic response of this type of tumor, makes it *imperative* that all adult patients presenting with an otherwise unexplained SIAD be investigated thoroughly and aggressively for a possible tumor. The evaluation should include a chest computed tomographic scan or magnetic resonance imaging study, with bronchoscopy and cytologic analysis of bronchial washings in any suspicious cases. The reason for this approach is that several studies have reported hypoosmolality that predated any radiographically evident abnormality in patients who developed bronchogenic carcinoma 3 to 12 months later (see Chap. 219).

### CENTRAL NERVOUS SYSTEM DISORDERS

The second major etiologic group of disorders causing SIAD has its origins in the central nervous system (CNS). Despite the diversity of CNS disorders associated with SIAD, no apparent common denominator links them. This is not surprising when one considers the neuroanatomy of neurohypophyseal innervation. As discussed in Chapter 25, the magnocellular AVP neurons receive excitatory input from osmoreceptor cells of the anterior hypothalamus as well as major innervation from brainstem cardiovascular regulatory centers. Although these pathways have yet to be elucidated fully, at least some of them appear to be inhibitory. Any diffuse CNS disorder can potentially disrupt this long and probably multisynaptic pathway from the brain stem to the hypothalamus and, in so doing, can cause AVP hypersecretion and SIAD as a result of a decrease in inhibitory tone originating from these pathways.[30a] Consequently, a variety of CNS disorders can cause this syndrome, but only destructive lesions involving the hypothalamus or pituitary cause diabetes insipidus. An interesting cause of transient CNS SIAD has been described after pituitary surgery. As many as 33% of patients have been found to develop moderate hyponatremia 5 to 7 days after transsphenoidal resection of pituitary adenomas due to inappropriate AVP secretion as a result of neural lobe/pituitary

stalk damage.[31] This had largely gone unnoticed in the past, not only because most patients are discharged before this time, but also because, although most patients develop some degree of inappropriate AVP secretion (as documented by impaired water-loading tests),[32] only those few who continue to ingest large volumes of fluid actually develop symptomatic hyponatremia and come to medical attention.

### DRUGS

The third major category, drug-induced SIAD, is rapidly becoming the most common cause of hypoosmolality.[32a] In general, pharmacologic agents cause this syndrome by directly stimulating AVP secretion, by directly activating AVP renal receptors to cause antidiuresis, or by potentiating the effect of AVP on the kidney. Not all of the drug effects associated with inappropriate antidiuresis are fully understood, however; indeed, many agents may work by means of a combination of mechanisms.[33] For example, chlorpropamide appears to have both a direct pituitary and a renal stimulatory effect. Newly developed drugs are regularly being added to the list of agents that induce SIAD, particularly psychotropic drugs such as selective serotonin reuptake inhibitors used to treat depression; these have been reported to cause hyponatremia in up to 22% to 28% of elderly patients.[34] Agents that cause AVP secretion primarily through solute depletion are best considered to cause depletion-induced hypoosmolality rather than true SIAD.

### PULMONARY DISORDERS

Pulmonary disorders, as a group, represent an often-mentioned but largely misunderstood cause of SIAD. A variety of pulmonary disorders have been associated with this syndrome, but except in tuberculosis, advanced chronic obstructive lung disease, and acute pneumonias, the occurrence of hypoosmolality has been noted only in sporadic case reports. A review of these reports reveals that virtually all cases of nontuberculous pulmonary SIAD have occurred in the setting of acute respiratory failure with marked hypoxia, hypercapnia, or both. When such patients were evaluated serially, the inappropriate AVP secretion was found to be limited to the initial days of hospitalization, when respiratory failure was most marked or when patients were ventilated by mechanical means. Even the cases of tubercular SIAD uniformly occurred in patients with far-advanced, active pulmonary tuberculosis. Therefore, although SIAD may occur fairly commonly with non–tumor-related pulmonary disease, two factors should be remembered: (a) in all cases, the pulmonary disease is obvious as a result of severe dyspnea or extensive, radiographically evident infiltrates; and (b) the inappropriate antidiuresis is usually limited to the period of respiratory failure. Once clinical improvement has begun, free water excretion generally improves rapidly. Mechanical ventilation can cause inappropriate AVP secretion, or it can worsen any SIAD caused by other factors. This phenomenon has been associated most often with continuous positive-pressure ventilation, but it can also occur with the use of positive end-expiratory pressure.

### UNEXPLAINED (IDIOPATHIC) OR MULTIFACTORIAL CAUSES

Unexplained or idiopathic SIAD accounts for a small number of cases. Although the cause of the syndrome may not be readily diagnosed initially, the number of patients in whom an apparent cause cannot be established after consistent follow-up over time is relatively low.

Hospitalized patients with acquired immunodeficiency syndrome (AIDS) have been recognized to have a high incidence of hyponatremia, as high as 30% to 50% in some series.[35] This represents perhaps the most classic example of a truly multifactorial hyponatremia. Approximately half of such patients have a depletional hyponatremia from primary solute losses, both from diarrheal fluid losses and (in some patients) from adrenal insufficiency due to cytomegalovirus adrenalitis (see Chaps. 76 and 214); others have true SIAD from an acute pneumonia, typically due to *Pneumocystis carinii*; a smaller subset have drug-induced SIAD; and still others with CNS human immunodeficiency virus (HIV) or opportunistic infections have SIAD from disordered AVP regulation. Clearly, many potential etiologies must be considered in the differential diagnosis of hyponatremic patients with HIV infections.

Some known stimuli to AVP secretion are notable because of their exclusion from Table 27-4. Despite stimulation of AVP secretion by nicotine (see Chap. 234), cigarette smoking has not been associated with SIAD, presumably because of chronic adaptation. Similarly, although nausea is the most potent known stimulus to AVP secretion, and although the AVP secreted in response to nausea clearly is bioactive,[36] in the absence of vomiting, with subsequent ECF and solute depletion, chronic nausea is generally not associated with hypoosmolality. This is probably attributable to the fact that such patients are not inclined to drink fluids under such circumstances (however, hyponatremia can occur when such patients are infused with high volumes of hypotonic fluids). Finally, a causal relation between chronic stress (either physical or mental) and SIAD has not been established. This underscores the fact that stress, independent of nausea or hypotension, has *never* been clearly shown to cause significantly elevated AVP levels and, in fact, has been found to suppress AVP secretion in animals.

## PATHOPHYSIOLOGY

Disorders that cause inappropriate antidiuresis secondary to elevated serum AVP levels can be subdivided into those associated with either paraneoplastic ("ectopic") or pituitary AVP hypersecretion. Most ectopic production is from tumors, and conclusive, cumulative evidence exists that tumor tissue can, in fact, synthesize AVP. Evidence of such synthesis has been derived from several findings: (a) tumor extracts have been found to possess antidiuretic hormone bioactivity and immunologically recognizable AVP and neurophysin, (b) electron microscopy has revealed that many tumors possess secretory granules, and (c) cultured tumor tissue has been shown to synthesize not only AVP but also the entire AVP prohormone (provasopressin). Although clearly some tumors can produce AVP, whether or not *all* tumors associated with SIAD do so is not certain, because only approximately half of small cell carcinomas have been found to contain AVP immunoreactivity,[37] and many of the tumors listed in Table 27-4 have not been studied as extensively as have bronchogenic carcinomas. Studies of tissue cultures from hyponatremic patients with small cell lung cancers have shown that many tumor cell lines produce mRNA for atrial natriuretic peptide (ANP) in addition to, or instead of, AVP mRNA,[38] raising the possibility of ectopic ANP secretion. Clinical studies have verified the importance of elevated serum AVP levels in most hyponatremic patients with small cell lung cancers, but have also demonstrated elevated serum ANP levels, a finding which suggests that ANP might contribute to the hyponatremia in such patients by virtue of aggravating solute depletion as a result of increased natriuresis.[39]

The only nonneoplastic disorder that has been proven to cause SIAD by means of ectopic AVP production is tuberculosis. However, this conclusion is based on studies of a single patient in whom extracts of tuberculous lung were shown by bioassay to possess antidiuretic activity.[40]

Studies of serum AVP levels in patients with SIAD during graded increases in plasma osmolality produced by hypertonic saline administration have suggested four patterns of secretion (Fig. 27-2): (a) random hypersecretion of AVP; (b) a "reset osmostat," whereby AVP is secreted at an abnormally low threshold of plasma osmolality but otherwise displays a normal response to relative changes in osmolality; (c) inappropriate hypersecretion below the normal threshold for AVP release, but

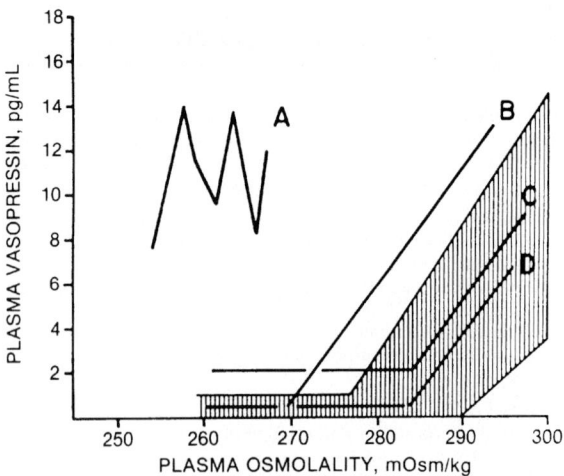

**FIGURE 27-2.** Schematic summary is shown of different patterns of vasopressin (*AVP*) secretion observed in patients with the syndrome of inappropriate antidiuresis. Each line (*A–D*) represents the relation between serum AVP and plasma osmolality of individual subjects in whom osmolality was increased via hypertonic saline infusions. The shaded area represents serum AVP levels in normal subjects over physiologic ranges of plasma osmolality. (From Robertson GL, Aycinena P, Zerbe RL. Neurogenic disorders of osmoregulation. Am J Med 1982; 72:339.)

normal secretion in response to osmolar changes within normal ranges of plasma osmolality; and (d) low or undetectable serum AVP levels despite clinical characteristics of SIAD.[30]

The first pattern simply represents unregulated AVP secretion, which is often observed in patients exhibiting paraneoplastic AVP production. Nonosmotic resetting of the osmotic threshold for AVP secretion has been well described with volume depletion[27] and also has been shown to occur in congestive heart failure, presumably as a result of decreases in effective arterial blood volume. However, many patients with a reset osmostat are clinically euvolemic; therefore, it has been suggested that chronic hypoosmolality itself may reset the intracellular threshold for osmoreceptor firing, although studies in hyponatremic animals have not supported a major role for this mechanism.[41] Perhaps the most perplexing aspect of the reset osmostat pattern is its occurrence in some patients with tumors,[28,30] which suggests that some of these cases represent tumor-stimulated pituitary AVP secretion rather than ectopic AVP production. The pattern of SIAD that occurs without measurable AVP secretion is not yet understood. This form of the syndrome may be attributable to the secretion of AVP with some bioactivity but altered immunoreactivity, to the presence of other circulating antidiuretic factors, to increased renal sensitivity to very low circulating levels of AVP, to abnormalities of kidney aquaporin-2 regulation,[29] or in some cases to ANP-induced natriuresis.[38,39] To date, a sufficient number of patients with this form of the disorder have not been studied adequately to form any basis for discrimination among these possibilities (although on theoretic grounds, increased renal sensitivity to low levels of AVP appears most plausible). Despite these well-described patterns of inappropriate AVP secretion in SIAD, however, the fact that no correlation has been found between any of these four patterns and the various causes of the syndrome is surprising.[30]

## CLINICAL MANIFESTATIONS OF HYPOOSMOLALITY

Hypoosmolality is associated with a broad spectrum of neurologic manifestations, ranging from mild nonspecific symptoms (e.g., headache, nausea) to more significant disorders (e.g., disorienta-

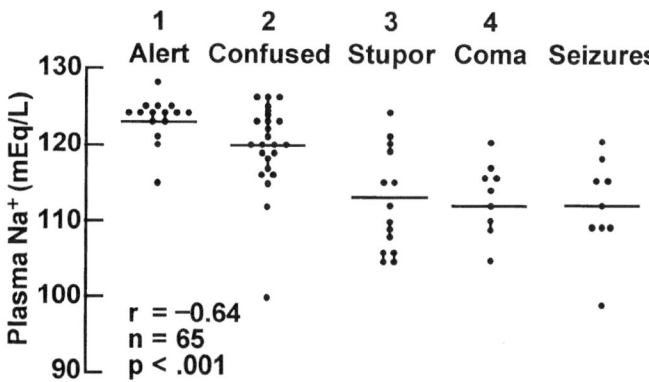

**FIGURE 27-3.** The relationship between serum sodium concentration [Na$^+$] and central nervous system (*CNS*) symptoms in *hypoosmolar* patients is depicted. Each point represents a different patient. Correlation is expressed between serum [Na$^+$] levels and the level of CNS depression, as indicated by the scale at the top. (From Arieff AJ, Llach F, Massy SG. Neurological manifestations and morbidity of hyponatremia: correlation with brain water and electrolytes. Medicine [Baltimore] 1976; 55:121.)

tion, confusion, obtundation, and seizures). In the most severe cases, death can result from respiratory arrest after tentorial cerebral herniation and brainstem compression. This neurologic symptom complex has been termed *hyponatremic encephalopathy* and primarily reflects brain edema resulting from osmotic water shifts into the brain because of decreased effective plasma osmolality. Significant symptoms generally do not occur until the serum [Na$^+$] falls below 125 mEq/L, and the severity of symptoms can be roughly correlated with the degree of hypoosmolality[4] (Fig. 27-3). Individual variability is marked, however, and for any single patient, the level of serum [Na$^+$] at which symptoms appear cannot be predicted with great accuracy. Furthermore, several factors other than the severity of the hypoosmolality also affect the degree of neurologic dysfunction. Most important is the period over which hypoosmolality develops. Rapid development of severe hypoosmolality is frequently associated with marked neurologic symptoms, whereas gradual development over several days or weeks is often associated with relatively mild symptomatology despite profound degrees of hypoosmolality. This is because the brain can counteract osmotic swelling by excreting intracellular solutes (including potassium[4] and organic osmolytes[22]), an adaptive process known as *volume regulation*.[21] Because this is a time-dependent process, rapid development of hypoosmolality can result in brain edema before this adaptation occurs, but with slower development of the same degree of hypoosmolality, brain cells can lose solute sufficiently rapidly to prevent brain edema and neurologic dysfunction.[42] This accounts for the much higher incidence of neurologic symptoms as well as higher mortality rates in patients with acute hyponatremia than in those with chronic hyponatremia.[4] A striking example of this is the fact that the most dramatic cases of death due to hyponatremic encephalopathy have generally been reported in postoperative patients,[43] in whom hyponatremia can develop rapidly as a result of postoperative retention of hypotonic fluid infusions.

Underlying neurologic disease also affects the level of hypoosmolality at which CNS symptoms appear; for example, moderate hypoosmolality is generally of little concern in an otherwise healthy patient but can cause morbidity in a patient with an underlying seizure disorder. Nonneurologic metabolic disorders (e.g., hypoxia, hypercapnia, acidosis, hypercalcemia) similarly can affect the level of plasma osmolality at which CNS symptoms occur. Clinical studies have suggested that menstruating women[43] and young children[44] may be particularly susceptible to the development of neurologic morbidity and mortality during hyponatremia, especially in the acute postoperative setting. The true clinical incidence,[45] as well as the

underlying mechanisms responsible for these sometimes catastrophic cases, remains to be determined.[42] One final consideration is that nausea and vomiting are frequently overlooked as potential signs of increased intracranial pressure in hypoosmolar patients. *Because hypoosmolality does not cause any known direct effects on the gastrointestinal tract, the presence of unexplained nausea or vomiting in a hypoosmolar patient must be assumed to be of CNS origin, and the patient should be treated appropriately for symptomatic hypoosmolality.*

## THERAPEUTIC APPROACH TO HYPOOSMOLALITY

Despite continuing controversy concerning the rapid correction of osmolality in hypoosmolar patients, relative consensus exists regarding appropriate treatment of this disorder (Fig. 27-4). Once true hypoosmolality is verified, the ECF volume status of the patient should be assessed by careful clinical examination. If fluid retention is present, the treatment of the underlying disease should take precedence over the correction of plasma osmolality. Often, this involves treatment with diuretics, which, by virtue of the excretion of hypotonic urine, should simultaneously improve serum tonicity. If any degree of hypovolemia is present, the patient *must* be considered to have depletion-induced hypoosmolality, in which case volume repletion with isotonic saline (0.9% sodium chloride) at a rate appropriate for the estimated volume depletion should be initiated immediately. If diuretic use is known or suspected, the isotonic saline should be supplemented with potassium (30 to 40 mEq/L), even if the serum [K$^+$] is not low, because of the propensity of such patients to develop total body potassium depletion. Most often, the hypoosmolar patient is clinically euvolemic, in which case the evaluation should include the measurement of urine osmolality and [Na$^+$]. Several situations dictate the reconsideration of solute depletion as a potential diagnosis, even in the patient without clinically apparent hypovolemia. These include a decreased urine [Na$^+$], *any* history of recent diuretic use, and *any* suggestion of primary adrenal insufficiency. In fact, *whenever a reasonable possibility of depletion-induced, rather than dilution-induced, hypoosmolality exists, the patient is most appropriately treated initially with isotonic saline, regardless of whether signs of hypovolemia are present.* An improvement in and eventual correction of osmolality support a diagnosis of solute and volume depletion,[24] although SIAD may also resolve spontaneously. If the patient has SIAD rather than solute depletion, no harm comes from administration of a limited amount (i.e., 1–2 L) of isotonic saline, because such patients simply excrete excess sodium chloride without a significant change in plasma osmolality.[17]

The approach to patients with SIAD varies according to the clinical situation. A patient who meets all essential criteria for the syndrome but has a low urine osmolality should be observed on a trial of modest fluid restriction. If the hypoosmolality is attributable to transient SIAD or severe polydipsia, the urine will remain dilute, and the plasma osmolality will be corrected as free water is excreted. If, however, the patient has the reset osmostat form of the disorder, then the urine will become concentrated at some point before the plasma osmolality and serum [Na$^+$] return to normal ranges. If either primary or secondary adrenal insufficiency is suspected, glucocorticoid replacement should be initiated immediately after the completion of a rapid adrenocorticotropic hormone stimulation test. A prompt water diuresis after initiation of glucocorticoid treatment supports a diagnosis of glucocorticoid deficiency. However, the absence of a quick response does not necessarily negate this diagnosis because several days of glucocorticoid replacement are sometimes required for normalization of plasma osmolality. If hypothyroidism is suspected, thyroid function tests should be conducted and a serum thyroid-stimu-

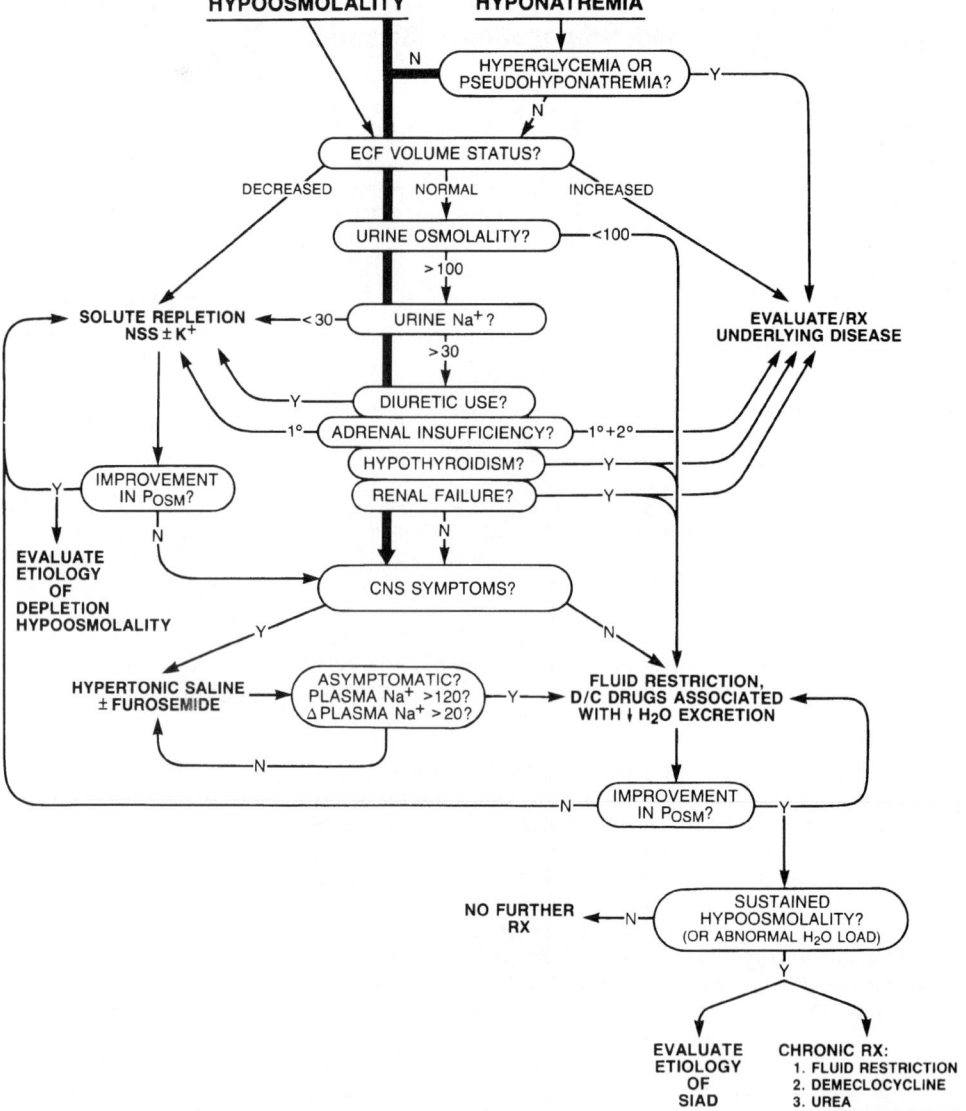

**FIGURE 27-4.** Schematic summary of the evaluation and treatment of hypoosmolar patients is presented. The dark black arrow indicates that central nervous system (*CNS*) symptomatology should always be evaluated immediately in *all* hypoosmolar patients, even while the outlined diagnostic evaluation is still proceeding. (*N*, no; *Y*, yes; *ECF*, extracellular fluid; *NSS*, normal saline solution [0.9% NaCl]; *RX*, treat/treatment; $P_{osm}$, plasma osmolality; *D/C*, discontinue; *AVP*, arginine vasopressin; *SIAD*, syndrome of inappropriate antidiuresis.)

lating hormone level should be obtained; usually, however, thyroid replacement therapy is withheld pending these results unless the patient is obviously myxedematous (see Chap. 45). The presence of renal failure in a patient with hypoosmolality generally requires a more extensive evaluation of renal function before treatment is initiated.

## ACUTE TREATMENT OF HYPOOSMOLALITY

In any significantly hypoosmolar patient, one is immediately faced with the question of how quickly the plasma osmolality should be corrected. Although hyponatremia is associated with a broad spectrum of neurologic symptoms,[4] sometimes leading to death in severe cases,[43,44] too rapid correction of severe hyponatremia can produce pontine and extrapontine myelinolysis, a brain demyelinating disease that also can cause substantial neurologic morbidity and mortality.[46,47] Furthermore, some studies have suggested that the morbidity and mortality associated with even symptomatic hyponatremia may not be as high as previously thought.[48] Reviews of clinical and experimental results have suggested that optimal treatment of hyponatremic patients must, therefore, entail balancing the risks of hyponatremia against the risks of correction for each patient.[42,49–52] Although individual variability in response remains great, and consequently which patients will develop neurologic complications

from either hyponatremia or its correction cannot always be accurately predicted, consensus guidelines for treating hypoosmolar patients allow a rational approach that minimizes the risks of both these complications. Implicit in these guidelines is the concept that treatment must be tailored to the patient's clinical presentation: *appropriate therapy for one patient may be inappropriate for another patient despite equivalent degrees of hypoosmolality.*

Three major factors should be taken into consideration when making a treatment decision with regard to a hypoosmolar patient: the severity of the hyponatremia, the duration of the hyponatremia, and the patient's neurologic symptomatology. The severity of the hypoosmolality is an important consideration because neither sequelae from hyponatremia itself nor myelinolysis after therapy are likely in patients whose serum [Na+] remains ≥120 mEq/L (although significant symptoms can develop even at higher serum [Na+] levels if the rate of fall of plasma osmolality is particularly rapid). The importance of duration and symptomatology relate to how well the brain has volume-adapted to the hyponatremia and consequently its degree of risk for subsequent demyelination with rapid correction.[42] Cases of acute hyponatremia (defined as ≤48 hours in duration) are usually symptomatic if the hyponatremia is severe (i.e., ≤120 mEq/L). These patients are at greatest risk for neurologic complications from the hyponatremia, and their serum [Na+] should be corrected to higher levels promptly.

Postoperative patients, particularly young women and children,[43,44] appear to be at greatest risk for rapidly progressing hyponatremic encephalopathy and should be evaluated carefully for any neurologic symptomatology. The dark black arrow in Figure 27-4 emphasizes that *hyposmolar patients should always be evaluated quickly for the presence of neurologic symptoms so that appropriate therapy can be initiated, if indicated, even while other results are still pending.* Several studies have documented that rapid correction of serum [Na$^+$] in patients with *acute* hyponatremia carries little, if any, risk of demyelination,[53] presumably because sufficient brain volume regulation has not yet occurred to increase brain susceptibility to osmotic dehydration with the correction.[42] Conversely, patients with more chronic hyponatremia (defined as >48 hours in duration) who have minimal neurologic symptomatology are at little risk from complications of hyponatremia itself but can develop demyelination after rapid correction because of greater degrees of brain volume regulation through electrolyte and osmolyte losses.[54] *No indication exists to correct these patients rapidly, regardless of the initial serum [Na$^+$], and they should be treated using slower-acting therapies, such as fluid restriction.*

Although these extremes have clear treatment indications, the hyponatremia of most patients is of indeterminate duration and produces varying degrees of milder neurologic symptomatology. This group of patients is the most challenging to treat because the hyponatremia will have been present sufficiently long to allow some degree of brain volume regulation, but not long enough to prevent some brain edema and neurologic symptomatology. Most clinicians recommend prompt treatment of such patients because of their symptoms, using methods that allow a *controlled and limited correction* of their hypoosmolality. Some clinicians have suggested that correction parameters should consist of a maximal rate of correction of serum [Na$^+$] in the range of 1 to 2 mEq/L per hour as long as the total magnitude of correction does not exceed 25 mEq/L over the first 48 hours.[55] Other clinicians argue that these parameters should be more conservative, with maximal correction rates of 0.5 mEq/L per hour or less and magnitudes of correction that do not exceed 12 mEq/L in the first 24-hour period and 18 mEq/L in the first 48-hour period.[49] A reasonable approach for treatment of individual patients would therefore entail choosing correction parameters within these limits depending on the patient's symptomatology[13,42]: when patients are only moderately symptomatic, one should proceed at the lower recommended limits of 0.5 mEq/L per hour or less, whereas when patients manifest more severe neurologic symptoms, an initial correction at a rate of 1 to 2 mEq/L per hour would be more appropriate. *Regardless of the initial rate of correction chosen, acute treatment should be interrupted as soon as any of the following three end points is reached:* (a) the patient's symptoms are abolished, (b) a safe serum [Na$^+$] (generally ≥120 mEq/L) is achieved, or (c) a total magnitude of correction of 15 to 20 mEq/L is achieved. Once any of these end points is achieved, the active correction should be stopped and the patient treated with slower-acting therapies, such as oral rehydration or fluid restriction, depending on the cause of the hypoosmolality. It follows from these recommendations that serum [Na$^+$] levels must be carefully monitored at frequent intervals (at least every 4 hours) during the active phases of treatment to adjust therapy to keep the correction parameters within these guidelines.

Controlled limited corrections can be accomplished with either isotonic or hypertonic saline infusions, depending on the cause of the hypoosmolality. Patients with volume depletion hypoosmolality (e.g., clinical hypovolemia, history of diuretic use, or urine [Na$^+$] ≤30 mEq/L[24]) usually respond well to isotonic (0.9%) sodium chloride. Patients with euvolemic hypoosmolality (including patients with SIAD) do not respond to isotonic sodium chloride and are best treated with hypertonic (3%) sodium chloride solution given by continuous infusion.

An initial infusion rate can be estimated by multiplying the patient's body weight in kilograms by the desired rate of increase in serum [Na$^+$] in milliequivalents per liter per hour (e.g., in a 70-kg patient an infusion of 3% sodium chloride at 70 mL per hour will increase serum [Na$^+$] by ~1 mEq/L per hour, whereas an infusion of 35 mL per hour will increase serum [Na$^+$] by ~0.5 mEq/L per hour). Furosemide should be used to treat volume overload, in some cases anticipatorily in patients with known cardiovascular disease. *Regardless of the therapy or rate initially chosen, one cannot emphasize too strongly that the plasma osmolality need be corrected acutely only to a safe range rather than completely to normonatremia.*

Rarely, hyponatremia may be spontaneously corrected by means of a water diuresis. If the hyponatremia is acute (e.g., psychogenic polydipsia with water intoxication), these patients do not appear to be at risk for subsequent demyelination.[53] However, in cases in which the hyponatremia has been chronic (e.g., hypocortisolism), such patients are at some risk of demyelination, and intervention (e.g., administration of desmopressin) should be considered to limit the rate and magnitude of correction of serum [Na$^+$], with use of the same end points as described previously for active corrections.[13,42] Finally, any potassium deficits in hyponatremic patients should be corrected promptly, because hypokalemic patients appear to be at significantly greater risk for demyelination after correction of hyponatremia.[56]

## LONG-TERM TREATMENT OF HYPOOSMOLALITY

If SIAD persists, then investigation of other potential causes should be pursued (see Table 27-4), and long-term therapy should be instituted. The treatment of chronic SIAD entails choosing among several suboptimal therapeutic regimens. Continued fluid restriction represents the least toxic treatment choice and is the preferred treatment for most cases of mild to moderate SIAD. Several points should be remembered when using this approach: (a) all fluids, not only water, must be included in the restriction; (b) the degree of restriction required depends on urine output plus insensible fluid loss (generally, discretionary, i.e., nonfood, fluids should be limited to 500 mL a day below the average daily urine volume); (c) several days of restriction are usually necessary before a significant increase in plasma osmolality occurs; and (d) only fluid, not salt, should be restricted. Because of the ongoing natriuresis, these patients often have a negative total body sodium balance and therefore should be maintained on a relatively high sodium chloride intake unless otherwise contraindicated. However, just as failure to correct a presumed depletion-induced hyponatremia with isotonic saline should lead one to consider the possibility of a dilution-induced hypoosmolality, so should the failure of significant fluid restriction after several days of a *confirmed* negative fluid balance prompt reconsideration of other possible causes, including solute depletion and clinically inapparent hypovolemia. At the time that fluid restriction is first initiated, any drugs known to be associated with SIAD should be discontinued or changed (e.g., second-generation hypoglycemic agents such as glyburide should be substituted for first-generation agents such as chlorpropamide). Fluid restriction should *always* be tried as the initial therapy for patients with chronic SIAD, with pharmacologic intervention reserved for refractory cases in which the degree of fluid restriction required to avoid hypoosmolality is so severe that the patient is unable, or unwilling, to maintain it. In such cases, reasonable efforts should be made to ameliorate thirst, such as substituting hard candy or ice chips for fluid drinking. However, alternative pharmacologic management is often necessary. Pharmacologic intervention should also be avoided initially in patients with SIAD that is secondary to tumors, because successful treatment of the underlying malignant lesion often eliminates or reduces the inappropriate AVP secretion. If pharmacologic treatment is necessary, the preferred drug currently is the tetracycline derivative demeclocycline. This agent causes a nephrogenic form of diabetes insipidus, with decreased urine concentration even in the presence of high serum AVP levels. An appropriate dosage of demeclocycline ranges from 600 to 1200 mg per day, administered in divided doses. Treatment must be continued for several days to achieve maximal diuretic effects; consequently, one should wait 3 to 4 days before increasing the dosage. Demeclocycline can cause nephrotoxicity, especially in patients with cirrhosis, although this is generally reversible. Renal function should therefore be monitored on a regular basis and the medication discontinued if increasing azotemia is noted.

Other agents, such as lithium, have similar effects, but their use is less desirable because of inconsistent results and significant side effects. Urea has been described as an alternative mode of treatment for SIAD.[57] Although it has long been recognized that any osmotic diuretic can be used to treat hypoosmolality by virtue of increasing free water excretion, such therapeutic modalities have generally proved impractical for long-term ambulatory use. Urea is an exception because it can be administered orally; furthermore, it corrects hypoosmolality not only by increasing free water excretion but also by decreasing urinary sodium excretion. Dosages of 30 g per day are generally effective. (Dissolving the urea in orange juice or some other strongly flavored liquid to camouflage the taste is advisable.) Even if completely normal water balance is not achieved, the patient can often be allowed to maintain a less strict regimen of fluid restriction while receiving urea. The disadvantages associated with the use of urea include poor palatability, the development of azotemia at higher doses, and unavailability of a convenient form of the agent.

Several other drugs that have been described appear to decrease AVP hypersecretion in some cases (e.g., diphenylhydantoin, opiates, ethanol), but responses are erratic and unpredictable. Much better therapeutic agents for chronic SIAD will probably soon be available, because the synthesis of a variety of analogs to AVP has yielded potent AVP-receptor antagonists. Particularly promising is the synthesis of several potent nonpeptide antagonists that are selective for AVP $V_2$ (antidiuretic) rather than $V_1$ (pressor) receptors,[58] or combine both activities.[59] Clinical studies using one such agent have confirmed its efficacy in patients with SIAD.[60] If such compounds prove to be effective and safe for human use in larger clinical trials, they undoubtedly will become the drugs of choice for euvolemic, and possibly hypervolemic, hypoosmolar patients, rendering all other modes of pharmacologic therapy obsolete.

# REFERENCES

1. Flear CTG, Gill GV, Burn J. Hyponatremia: mechanisms and management. Lancet 1981; 2:26.
2. Kleinfeld M, Casimir M, Borra S. Hyponatremia as observed in a chronic disease facility. J Am Geriatr Soc 1979; 27:156.
3. Anderson RJ, Chung H, Kluge R, Schrier RW. Hyponatremia: a prospective analysis of its epidemiology and the pathogenetic role of vasopressin. Ann Intern Med 1985; 102:164.
4. Arieff AI, Llach F, Massry SG. Neurological manifestations and morbidity of hyponatremia: correlation with brain water and electrolytes. Medicine (Baltimore) 1976; 55:121.
5. Owen JA, Campbell DG. A comparison of plasma electrolyte and urea values in healthy persons and in hospital patients. Clin Chim Acta 1968; 22:611.
6. Alvis R, Geheb M, Cox M. Hypo- and hyperosmolar states: diagnostic approaches. In: Arieff AI, DeFronzo RA, eds. Fluid, electrolyte, and acid-base disorders, vol 2. New York: Churchill Livingstone, 1985:185.
7. Ladenson JH, Apple FS, Koch DD. Misleading hyponatremia due to hyperlipemia: a method-dependent error. Ann Intern Med 1981; 95:707.
8. Fichman MP, Vorherr H, Kleeman CR, Telfer N. Diuretic-induced hyponatremia. Ann Intern Med 1971; 75:853.
9. Robertson GL. Psychogenic polydipsia and inappropriate antidiuresis. Arch Intern Med 1980; 140:1574.
10. Goldman MB, Luchins DJ, Robertson GL. Mechanisms of altered water metabolism in psychotic patients with polydipsia and hyponatremia. N Engl J Med 1988; 318:397.

11. Schrier RW. Pathogenesis of sodium and water retention in high-output and low-output cardiac failure, nephrotic syndrome, cirrhosis and pregnancy. N Engl J Med 1988; 319:1065.
12. Leaf A, Bartter FC, Santos RF, Wrong O. Evidence in man that urinary electrolyte loss induced by Pitressin is a function of water retention. J Clin Invest 1953; 32:868.
13. Verbalis JG. The syndrome of inappropriate hormone secretion and other hypoosmolar disorders. In: Schrier RW, Gottschalk CW, eds. Diseases of the kidney. Boston: Little, Brown and Company 1998:2393.
14. Verbalis JG. Pathogenesis of hyponatremia in an experimental model of the syndrome of inappropriate antidiuresis. Am J Physiol 1994; 267:R1617.
15. Smith MJ Jr, Cowley AW Jr, Guyton AC, Manning RD Jr. Acute and chronic effects of vasopressin on blood pressure, electrolytes, and fluid volumes. Am J Physiol 1979; 237:F232.
16. Nolph KD, Schrier RW. Sodium, potassium and water metabolism in the syndrome of inappropriate antidiuretic hormone secretion. Am J Med 1970; 49:534.
17. Schwartz WB, Bennett W, Curelop S, Bartter FC. A syndrome of renal sodium loss and hyponatremia probably resulting from inappropriate secretion of antidiuretic hormone. Am J Med 1957; 23:529.
18. Gross PA, Anderson RJ. Effects of DDAVP and AVP on sodium and water balance in conscious rat. Am J Physiol 1982; 243:R512.
19. Grantham JJ. Pathophysiology of hypo-osmolar conditions: a cellular perspective. In: Andreoli TE, Grantham JJ, Rector FC Jr, eds. Disturbances in body fluid osmolality. Bethesda, MD: American Physiological Society, 1977:217.
20. Verbalis JG, Drutarosky MD. Adaptation to chronic hypoosmolality in rats. Kidney Int 1988; 34:351.
21. Gullans SR, Verbalis JG. Control of brain volume during hyperosmolar and hypoosmolar conditions. Annu Rev Med 1993; 44:289.
22. Verbalis JG, Gullans SR. Hyponatremia causes large sustained reductions in brain content of multiple organic osmolytes in rats. Brain Res 1991; 567:274.
23. Strange K. Regulation of solute and water balance and cell volume in the central nervous system. J Am Soc Nephrol 1992; 3:12.
24. Chung H-M, Kluge R, Schrier RW, Anderson RJ. Clinical assessment of extracellular fluid volume in hyponatremia. Am J Med 1987; 83:905.
25. Linas SL, Berl T, Robertson GL, et al. Role of vasopressin in the impaired water excretion of glucocorticoid deficiency. Kidney Int 1980; 18:58.
26. Bartter FC, Schwartz WB. The syndrome of inappropriate secretion of antidiuretic hormone. Am J Med 1967; 42:790.
27. Robertson GL. Diseases of the posterior pituitary. In: Felig P, Baxter JD, Frohman LA, eds. Endocrinology and metabolism. New York: McGraw-Hill, 1995:385.
28. Robertson GL, Aycinena P, Zerbe RL. Neurogenic disorders of osmoregulation. Am J Med 1982; 72:339.
29. Knepper MA. Molecular physiology of urinary concentrating mechanism: regulation of aquaporin water channels by vasopressin. Am J Physiol 1997; 272:F3.
30. Zerbe R, Stropes L, Robertson G. Vasopressin function in the syndrome of inappropriate antidiuresis. Annu Rev Med 1980; 31:315.
30a. Liamis G, Elisaf M. Syndrome of inappropriate antidiuresis associated with multiple sclerosis. Neurol Sci 2000; 172:38.
31. Miller M, Moses AM. Drug-induced states of impaired water excretion. Kidney Int 1976; 10:96.
32. Strachan J, Shepherd J. Hyponatremia associated with the use of selective serotonin re-uptake inhibitors. Aust NZJ Psychiatry 1998; 32:295.
32a. Belton K, Thomas SH. Drug-induced syndrome of innapropriate antidiuretic hormone secretion. Postgrad Med J 1999; 75:509.
33. Olson BR, Rubino D, Gumowski J, Oldfield EH. Isolated hyponatremia after transsphenoidal pituitary surgery. J Clin Endocrinol Metab 1995; 80:85.
34. Olson BR, Gumowski J, Rubino D, Oldfield EH. Pathophysiology of hyponatremia after transsphenoidal pituitary surgery. J Neurosurg 1997; 87:499.
35. Bevilacqua M. Hyponatraemia in AIDS. Baillieres Clin Endocrinol Metab 1994; 8:837.
36. Rowe JW, Shelton RL, Helderman JH, et al. Influence of the emetic reflex on vasopressin release in man. Kidney Int 1979; 16:729.
37. Vorherr H, Massry SG, Utiger RD, Kleeman CR. Antidiuretic principle in malignant tumor extracts from patients with inappropriate ADH syndrome. J Clin Endocrinol Metab 1968; 28:162.
38. Gross AJ, Steinberg SM, Reilly JG, et al. Atrial natriuretic factor and arginine vasopressin production in tumor cell lines from patients with lung cancer and their relationship to serum sodium. Cancer Res 1993; 53:67.
39. Johnson BE, Chute BP, Rushin J, et al. A prospective study of patients with lung cancer and hyponatremia of malignancy. Am J Respir Crit Care Med 1997; 156:1669.
40. Vorherr H, Massry SG, Fallet R, et al. Antidiuretic principle in tuberculous lung tissue of a patient with pulmonary tuberculosis and hyponatremia. Ann Intern Med 1970; 72:383.
41. Verbalis JG, Dohanics J. Vasopressin and oxytocin secretion in chronically hypoosmolar rats. Am J Physiol 1991; 261:R1028.
42. Verbalis JG. Adaptation to acute and chronic hyponatremia: implications for symptomatology, diagnosis, and therapy. Semin Nephrol 1998; 18:3.
43. Ayus JC, Wheeler JM, Arieff AI. Postoperative hyponatremic encephalopathy in menstruant women. Ann Intern Med 1992; 117:891.
44. Arieff AI, Ayus JC, Fraser CL. Hyponatraemia and death or permanent brain damage in healthy children. BMJ 1992; 304:1218.
45. Wijdicks EF, Larson TS. Absence of postoperative hyponatremia syndrome in young, healthy females. Ann Neurol 1994; 35:626.

46. Sterns RH, Riggs JE, Schochet SS Jr. Osmotic demyelination syndrome following correction of hyponatremia. N Engl J Med 1986; 314:1535.
47. Karp BI, Laureno R. Pontine and extra pontine myelinolysis: a neurologic disorder following rapid correction of hyponatremia. Medicine (Baltimore) 1993; 72:359.
48. Sterns RH. Severe symptomatic hyponatremia: treatment and outcome. Ann Intern Med 1987; 107:656.
49. Sterns RH, Cappuccio JD, Silver SM, Cohen EP. Neurologic sequelae after treatment of severe hyponatremia: a multicenter perspective. J Am Soc Nephrol 1994; 4:1522.
50. Lauriat SM, Berl T. The hyponatremic patient: practical focus on therapy. J Am Soc Nephrol 1997; 8:1599.
51. Fraser CL, Arieff AI. Epidemiology, pathophysiology, and management of hyponatremic encephalopathy. Am J Med 1997; 102:67.
52. Gross P, Reimann D, Neidel J, et al. The treatment of severe hyponatremia. Kidney Int 1998; 64:S6.
53. Cheng JC, Zikos D, Skopicki HA, et al. Long term neurologic outcome in psychogenic water drinkers with severe symptomatic hyponatremia: the effect of rapid correction. Am J Med 1990; 88:561.
54. Verbalis JG, Gullans SR. Rapid correction of hyponatremia produces differential effects on brain osmolyte and electrolyte reaccumulation in rats. Brain Res 1993; 606:19.
55. Ayus JC, Krothapalli RK, Arieff AI. Treatment of symptomatic hyponatremia and its relation to brain damage: a prospective study. N Engl J Med 1987; 317:1190.
56. Lohr JW. Osmotic demyelination syndrome following correction of hyponatremia: association with hypokalemia. Am J Med 1994; 96:408.
57. Decaux G, Brimioulle S, Fenette F, Mockel J. Treatment of the syndrome of inappropriate secretion of antidiuretic hormone by urea. Am J Med 1980; 69:99.
58. Ohnishi A, Orita Y, Okahara R, et al. Potent aquaretic agent: a novel nonpeptide selective vasopressin antagonist (OPC-31260) in men. J Clin Invest 1993; 92:2653.
59. Yatsu T, Tomura Y, Tahara A, et al. Pharmacological profile of ym087, a novel nonpeptide dual vasopressin V1a and V2 receptor antagonist, in dogs. Eur J Pharmacol 1997; 321:225.
60. Saito T, Ishikawa S, Abe K, et al. Acute aquaresis by the nonpeptide arginine vasopressin (AVP) antagonist OPC-31260 improves hyponatremia in patients with syndrome of inappropriate secretion of antidiuretic hormone (SIADH). J Clin Endocrinol Metab 1997; 82:1054.

# THE THYROID GLAND

LEONARD WARTOFSKY, EDITOR

# CHAPTER 28

# APPROACH TO THE PATIENT WITH THYROID DISEASE

LEONARD WARTOFSKY

The following chapters on the thyroid were written with the clinician in mind. Adequate basic information is provided to serve as a background or rationale for positions taken on controversial issues, as well as to keep the reader abreast of the latest developments. The primary intention of this section, however, is to present expert critical appraisals of all important aspects of each clinical problem in a most current, factual, readable, and comprehensible format.

## MEDICAL HISTORY OF THE THYROID GLAND

The naming of the thyroid gland has been attributed to Wharton[1] in 1656, but an endocrine function was not proposed until almost 200 years later.[2] Appreciation of the clinical disorders affecting the thyroid followed, the earliest descriptions of which appeared in the following order: thyroid cancer in 1811[3]; diffuse toxic goiter by Parry in 1825,[4] Graves in 1835,[5] and von Basedow in 1840[6]; cretinism in 1871[7]; myxedema in 1874[8]; thyroidectomy for the treatment of toxic goiter in 1884[9]; thyroid extract therapy for myxedema in 1891[10]; Hashimoto disease in 1912[11]; subacute (de Quervain) thyroiditis in 1936[12]; the structure of thyroxine ($T_4$) in 1926[13]; identification of triiodothyronine ($T_3$) in 1952[14]; the presence of thyroid autoantibodies in Hashimoto disease in 1957[15]; the earliest evidence of the thyroid-stimulating antibodies of Graves disease in 1956[16]; recognition of medullary thyroid carcinoma as a distinct entity in 1959[17]; and reports of cases of postpartum thyroiditis with hypothyroidism[18] or thyrotoxicosis[19] only since 1976 to 1977.

Other subsequent milestones included the first description of resistance to thyroid hormone in 1967[20]; substantiation that circulating $T_3$ was derived largely from peripheral monodeiodination of $T_4$ in 1970[21]; identification of $T_3$-binding receptors in tissues in 1972[22] and their homology to the viral oncogene *erb*A in 1986[23,24]; and demonstrations that point mutations in the thyroid-hormone receptor accounted for hormone resistance in 1989 and 1990.[25,26]

The thyrotropin (TSH) receptor was cloned in 1989[27,28]; studies since have identified both loss of function and gain of function mutations in the TSH receptor that account for specific

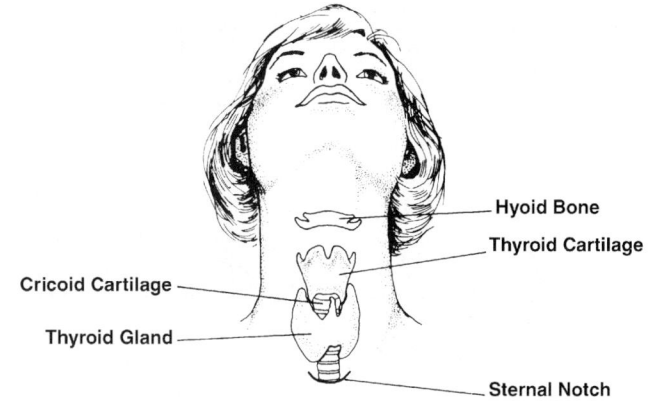

**FIGURE 28-1.** Landmarks for the anatomic location of the thyroid gland.

types of hypothyroidism and hyperthyroidism, respectively.[29] The gene for the β subunit of TSH was then cloned,[30] facilitating the development of human recombinant TSH (rhTSH); this agent has great clinical utility for the diagnosis and treatment of thyroid cancer.[31,32]

## EVALUATION OF THE PATIENT WITH THYROID DISEASE

The location of the thyroid makes it readily accessible to both inspection and palpation (Fig. 28-1). Often, the casual detection of a lump or mass in the thyroid by either the patient, a spouse, or an acquaintance first brings the patient in for evaluation. The thyroid examination is a mandatory and routine component of any complete history and physical examination. Aspects of the patient's clinical history may suggest thyroid dysfunction, in which case a careful thyroid examination is warranted. Symptoms of thyroid dysfunction may be caused by either hypofunction or hyperfunction of the thyroid, or they may be related to neck symptoms resulting from an enlarging nodule or goiter. The clinician then must assess the significance of the patient's complaints by simultaneously ascertaining both a functional and an anatomic diagnosis. The functional evaluation is based on various components of the history and physical examination, as well as the results of thyroid function tests (which, in general, are outlined in several chapters within this section; specific tests are described in relation to individual disorders that are discussed in separate chapters). The symptoms associated with deficient or excessive thyroid hormone production (Table 28-1) represent the most important and relevant information to be obtained

**TABLE 28-1.**
**Symptoms and Signs Relevant to Disordered Thyroid Function**

| Body System | Hyperthyroidism | Hypothyroidism |
|---|---|---|
| CENTRAL NERVOUS SYSTEM | Irritability, anxiety, depression, insomnia, agitation, heat intolerance | Memory loss, somnolence, depression, cold intolerance |
| EYES, EARS, NOSE, AND THROAT | Eye grittiness, tearing, proptosis | Periorbital edema, hoarseness |
| CARDIORESPIRATORY | Dyspnea, palpitations | Chest pain, peripheral edema |
| GASTROINTESTINAL | Increased appetite, weight loss, dysphagia, hyperdefecation, diarrhea | Decreased appetite, weight gain, constipation |
| SKIN | Increased sweating, hair loss, pruritus | Decreased sweating, dry coarse skin, coarse hair, hair loss |
| GENITOURINARY | Polyuria, polydipsia, amenorrhea, decreased libido, impotence | Menorrhagia, decreased libido |
| MUSCULOSKELETAL | Fatigue, muscle weakness, tremor | Fatigue, arthralgias, myalgias |

on history-taking. When taking a history, the clinician should be attentive to the quality of the patient's voice: the presence of hoarseness suggests involvement of the recurrent laryngeal nerve, slow husky speech is characteristic of hypothyroidism, and rapid, more staccato cadences often are present in thyrotoxic individuals. Occasionally, patients may have a serum TSH value that is below or above the normal range, suggestive of hyperthyroidism or hypothyroidism, respectively, but have no complaints or discernible symptoms. Often, this represents early or mild disease, which has not yet progressed to either overt symptoms or abnormalities in the levels of thyroid hormones and has been called "chemical," "subclinical," or "minimally symptomatic" thyroid disease.[33,34] This entity is discussed further in Chapters 42 and 45. Important aspects of the clinical history in a patient with a goiter or a thyroid mass are discussed in Chapters 38 through 41.

## EXAMINATION OF THE THYROID GLAND

Some features of the general physical examination are of particular interest in a patient with a suspected thyroid disorder. These include the texture and temperature of the skin, the degree of perspiration, the pulse rate, the deep tendon reflex relaxation time, hoarseness of the voice, facial or periorbital puffiness, ophthalmopathy, edema, apparent weight loss, tremor, and reduced muscle mass or muscle weakness.

Examination of the thyroid is facilitated by the ready availability of water to expedite swallowing. Many patients tend to hyperextend their necks at the beginning of the examination, thinking that this simplifies the palpation when it actually makes it more difficult. The patient's neck should be flexed only slightly, so as to relax the sternocleidomastoid muscles. The neck is inspected for visible goiter or masses, both at rest and during swallowing. Nonthyroidal masses do not move up and down with swallowing because they do not lie within the fascial sheathing of the trachea. That a midline mass may represent a thyroglossal duct cyst (with embryologic derivation from the hypoglossal region) may be inferred from its cephalad excursion on protrusion of the tongue. Plethoric suffusion of the face on raising both arms to the sides of the head (Pemberton sign) suggests a retrosternal goiter brought up into a thoracic inlet narrowed by the goiter and causing obstruction to venous return.

Palpation of the thyroid is performed best from behind, with the patient in a seated position (Fig. 28-2). The author does not concur with earlier dogma that maintained that a palpable thyroid indicated goiter or disease because the normal gland usually could not be palpated; with patience and experience, a normal gland can be palpated. The size of the normal thyroid varies directly with body size. The average thyroid gland weighs 14 to 18 g. Those physicians who estimate the weight of enlarged glands usually do so on the basis of a comparison to the weight of the normal gland. That is, a gland that is thought to be approximately three times larger than normal would be described as weighing 45 to 55 g.

Using the fingertips of both hands, the examiner first evaluates the surface of the lateral lobes (see Fig. 28-2A). The fingertips then are moved progressively (see Fig. 28-2B through D) to outline the lateral and medial extent of each lobe, and thence to the connecting thyroid isthmus, which lies just below the cricoid cartilage. A pyramidal lobe most often is identified extending up from the isthmus and, when enlarged, may suggest either Hashimoto thyroiditis or Graves disease. Sometimes, a thyroid gland that appears to be enlarged on inspection proves to be of normal size on palpation. Such cases often represent *pseudogoiter,*[35] which occurs when the gland is located higher than usual over the thyroid cartilage.

In addition to size, the examiner should attempt to ascertain the consistency of the gland. The thyroid in a patient with Graves disease typically is soft, spongy, and as malleable as an uncooked sirloin steak but becomes progressively more firm after iodine exposure. This increase in firmness is attributable to involutional changes and an increased ratio of colloid to cellular mass. In general, a continued progression to increasing hardness is seen from Graves disease, to colloid goiter, to early Hashimoto disease with lymphocytic infiltration, to adenomatous and multinodular goiter, to late Hashimoto disease with fibrosis, to infiltrating thyroid malignant disease, and, finally, to Riedel (fibrosing) thyroiditis. An extremely hard consistency in a single thyroid nodule often, but not invariably, signals a malignant lesion; the hard texture may be attributable in part to psammoma bodies in papillary carcinoma or to the dense calcification seen with medullary thyroid cancer. In a patient with an obese or muscular neck, full delineation of the lateral lobes may be difficult. A useful maneuver in such a case is to displace the thyroid cartilage first to one side and then to the other with lateral pressure from the fingertips. This serves to displace the lobe outwardly on the contralateral side, making it more accessible to examination (see Fig. 28-2C).

On palpation, the size and position, as well as the consistency, of any thyroid nodules should be noted. Transillumination may be helpful in establishing whether a nodule is cystic; the amount of light transmitted by a penlight pressed against a nodule (in a darkened room) is compared to that transmitted on the contralateral (normal) side. The size of a nodule can be estimated by direct measurement after marking the overlying skin, or by outlining the nodule on a 3- to 4-inch wide strip of adhesive tape placed over the nodule. This tape then can be removed and inserted into the patient's record to be used for future comparisons as a substitute for or adjunct to the precise sizing that may be achieved with ultrasonography. Alternatively, the size of a nodule may be estimated easily on the basis of the width of the examiner's index finger (i.e., usually 1.0–1.5 cm) by determining how much of the nodule is covered by the examining finger. Uniformly enlarged goiters may be monitored by comparing periodic measurements of neck circumference. This method involves the use of a tape measure and notations regarding fixed landmarks, such as the spine of the seventh cervical vertebra posteriorly and the midpoint of the isthmus anteriorly.

Examination of the thyroid also should include a determination of the presence or absence of lymphadenopathy, particularly in the central cricoid area, where an enlarged Delphian node may be the earliest indication of metastatic papillary cancer. Occasionally, lymphadenopathy, which returns to normal after therapy, may be observed in a patient with Graves disease, and enlarged benign nodes may be seen more rarely in a patient with Hashimoto disease. The presence of a palpable thrill over the gland suggests increased vascularity, as seen in Graves disease, and should correlate with an audible bruit on auscultation. Gland tenderness indicates possible subacute thyroiditis, hemorrhage within a nodule, or malignant disease. Extremely rarely, this sign is observed in a patient with Hashimoto thyroiditis; however, it occurs commonly in the rare acute suppurative form of thyroiditis. Imaging studies, such as sonography, radioisotope scanning, or magnetic resonance imaging/computed tomography, may be useful to complement the physical examination (see Chaps. 34 and 35).

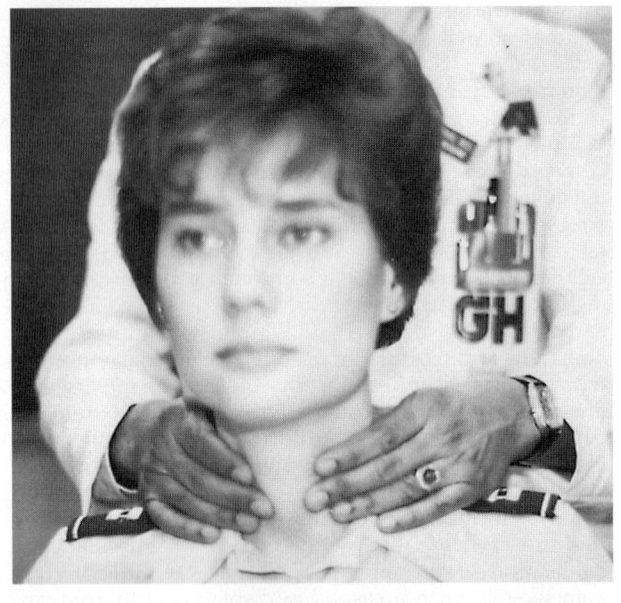
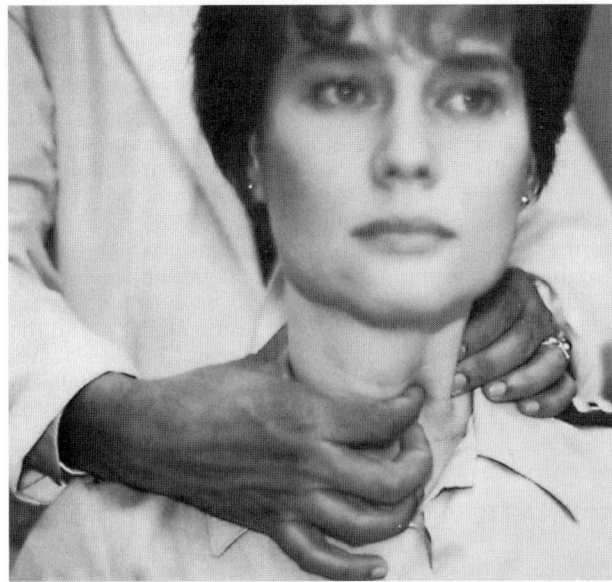
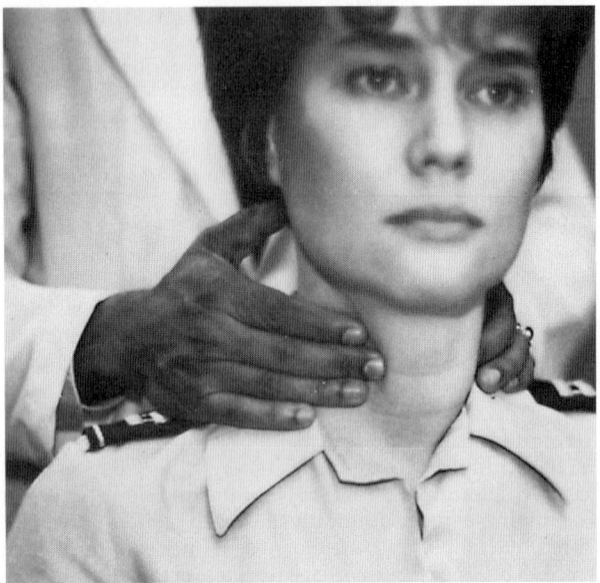
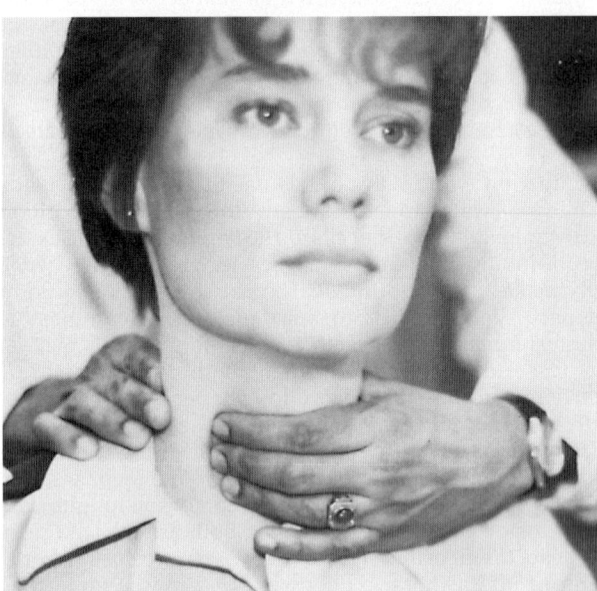

**FIGURE 28-2.** Technique for physical examination of the thyroid gland. **A,** The thyroid is examined from behind, with the patient in a sitting position, avoiding hyperextension of the neck. **B,** The exploring fingers determine the extent of the gland, after which attention is directed to the size, consistency, and presence of any nodules. **C,** By using the fingertips alternately to displace the gland to the contralateral side, an appreciation of deeper abnormalities may be gained. This is particularly effective when the sternocleidomastoid muscle is thickened, in which case direct palpation would be difficult. **D,** Examination for lymphadenopathy is conducted in a routine manner but should be especially thorough in the presence of a thyroid nodule.

# REFERENCES

1. Rolleston HD. The endocrine organs in health and disease. London: Oxford University Press, 1936.
2. King TW. Observations on the thyroid gland. Guy's Hosp Rep 1836; 1:429.
3. Burns P. Observations on the surgical anatomy of the head and neck. Edinburgh: Bryce, 1811:207.
4. Parry CH. Collections from the unpublished papers of the late Caleb Hillier Parry, vol 2. London: 1825:111.
5. Graves RJ. Clinical lectures. Lond Med Surg J (Part II) 1835; 7:516.
6. von Basedow CA. Exophthalmos durch hypertrophie des Zellgewebes in der Augen hohle. Wochenschr Heilk 1840; 6:197.
7. Fagge CH. On sporadic cretinism occurring in England. BMJ 1871; 1:279.
8. Gull WW. On a cretinoid state supervening in adult life in women. Trans Clin Soc (Lond) 1874; 7:180.
9. Rehn L. Uber die extirpation des Kropfs bei morbus Basedowii. Berlin Klin Wochenschr 1884; 21:163.
10. Murray GR. Note on the treatment of myxoedema by hypodermic injections of an extract of the thyroid gland of a sheep. BMJ 1891; 2:796.
11. Hashimoto H. Zur kenntnis der lymphomatoser veranderung der schildruse (struma lymphomatosa). Arch Klin Chir 1912; 97:219.
12. De Quervain F, Giordanengo G. Die akute und subakute nichteitrige thyreoditis. Mitt Grenzgeb Med Chir 1936; 44:538.
13. Harington CR. Chemistry of thyroxine I. Isolation of thyroxine from the thyroid gland. Biochem J 1926; 20:293.
14. Gross J, Pitt-Rivers R. The identification of 3:5:3'-1-triido-thyronine in human plasma. Lancet 1952; 1:439.
15. Doniach D, Roitt IM. Autoimmunity in Hashimoto's disease and its implications. J Clin Endocrinol Metab 1957; 17:1293.
16. Adams DD, Purves HD. Abnormal responses in the assay of thyrotrophin. Proc Univ Otago Med Sch 1956; 34:11.
17. Hazard JB, Hawk WA, Crile G Jr. Medullary (solid) carcinoma of the thyroid: a clinicopathologic entity. J Clin Endocrinol Metab 1959; 19:152.
18. Amino N, Miyai K, Onishi T, et al. Transient hypothyroidism after delivery in autoimmune thyroiditis. J Clin Endocrinol Metab 1976; 42:296.

19. Ginsberg J, Walfish PG. Post-partum transient thyrotoxicosis with painless thyroiditis. Lancet 1977; 1:1125.
20. Refetoff S, DeWind LT, DeGroot LJ. Familial syndrome combining deaf-mutism, stippled epiphyses, goiter, and abnormally high PBI: possible target organ refractoriness to thyroid hormone. J Clin Endocrinol Metab 1967; 27:279.
21. Braverman LE, Ingbar SH, Sterling K. Conversion of thyroxine ($T_4$) to tri-iodothyronine ($T_3$) in athyreotic human subjects. J Clin Invest 1970; 49:855.
22. Oppenheimer JH, Koerner D, Schwartz HL, Surks MI. Specific nuclear tri-iodothyronine binding sites in rat liver and kidney. J Clin Endocrinol Metab 1972; 35:330.
23. Sap J, Munoz A, Damm K, et al. The c-erbA protein is a high-affinity recep-tor for thyroid hormone. Nature 1986; 324:635.
24. Weinberger C, Thompson CC, Ong ES, et al. The c-erbA gene encodes a thyroid hormone receptor. Nature 1986; 324:641.
25. Sakurai A, Takeda K, Ain K, et al. Generalized resistance to thyroid hor-mone associated with a mutation in the ligand-binding domain of the human thyroid hormone receptor β. Proc Natl Acad Sci U S A 1989; 86:8977.
26. Usala SJ, Tennyson GE, Bale AE, et al. A base mutation of the c-erbA β thy-roid hormone receptor in a kindred with generalized thyroid hormone resistance. Molecular heterogeneity in two other kindreds. J Clin Invest 1990; 85:93.
27. Parmentier M, Libert F, Maenhaut C, et al. Molecular cloning of the thy-rotropin receptor. Science 1989; 246:1620.
28. Nagayama Y, Kaufman KD, Seto P, Rapoport B. Molecular cloning, sequence and functional expression of the cDNA for the human thyrotro-pin receptor. Biochem Biophys Res Commun 1989; 165:1184.
29. Morris JC. The clinical expression of thyrotropin receptor mutations. The Endocrinologist 1998; 8:195.
30. Wondisford FE, Radovick S, Moates JM, et al. Isolation and characterization of the human thyrotropin beta-subunit gene. J Biol Chem 1988; 263:12538.
31. Meier CA, Braverman LE, Ebner SA, et al. Diagnostic use of recombinant human thyrotropin in patients with thyroid carcinoma (Phase I/II study). J Clin Endocrinol Metab 1994; 78:188.
32. Ladenson PW, Braverman LE, Mazzaferri EL, et al. Comparison of admin-istration of recombinant human thyrotropin with withdrawal of thyroid hormone for radioactive iodine scanning in patients with thyroid carci-noma. N Engl J Med 1997; 337:888.
33. Haden ST, Marqusee E, Utiger RD. Subclinical hyperthyroidism. The Endocrinologist 1996; 6:322.
34. Ayala A, Wartofsky L. Minimally symptomatic (subclinical) hypothyroid-ism. The Endocrinologist 1997; 7:44.
35. Gwinup G, Morton E. The high lying thyroid: a cause of pseudogoiter. J Clin Endocrinol Metab 1975; 40:37.

# CHAPTER 29

# MORPHOLOGY OF THE THYROID GLAND

VIRGINIA A. LIVOLSI

## EMBRYOLOGY OF THE THYROID

To understand and evaluate the morphologic and clinical aspects of thyroid disease, knowing the embryology, anatomy, cytology, and immunohistochemistry of the thyroid gland is essential. The embryologic development of the human thyroid gland can be understood by distinguishing between the origin of the medial portions of the gland and the lateral lobes (see Chap. 47). The medial portion of the thyroid arises as a bilobed vesicular struc-ture at the *foramen cecum* of the tongue; it is attached to the tongue by the *thyroglossal duct.* Beginning in approximately the *fifth* week of fetal life, as the heart and great vessels move caudally, the thy-roid gland descends until it reaches its adult location in the lower anterior neck. This descent of thyroid tissue is accompanied by the elongation of the thyroglossal duct, which normally atro-phies. Remnants of thyroid tissue may persist anywhere along this pathway of descent. If the thyroglossal duct does not atro-phy, it may become cystic, dilated, or even cancerous.[1]

The lateral portions of the thyroid are derived embryologi-cally from a portion of the ultimobranchial body, a component of the *fifth* branchial pouch. From this embryologic structure the

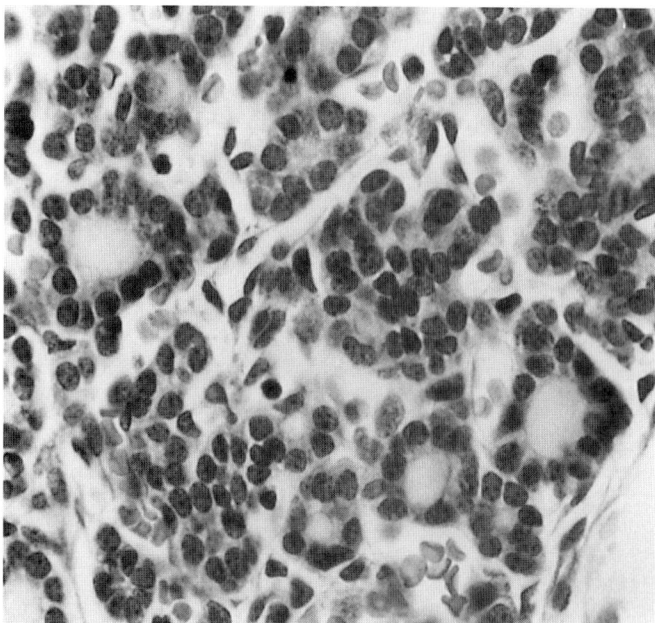

**FIGURE 29-1.** Thyroid tissue from an 18-week-old fetus. Note the uni-form pattern of microfollicles, some of which contain colloid. (Hema-toxylin and eosin; ×250)

parafollicular or C cells are derived. The ultimobranchial bod-ies fuse with the medial anlage of the thyroid in its upper lat-eral aspects; hence, in humans, this is the area where the C cells are found (see Chap. 53).

In early fetal life the histology of the thyroid is characterized by solid cords or clusters of cells with scant, rough, endoplas-mic reticulum. At the 50-mm stage, intercellular clefts form and, eventually, follicles are produced (Fig. 29-1). Rough endoplas-mic reticulum and Golgi apparatuses are extensive, lysosomes become abundant, and thyroglobulin synthesis begins.[1a,2]

## CLINICAL IMPLICATIONS OF THYROID EMBRYOLOGY

### NONDESCENT AND MALDESCENT

Abnormal migration of the median thyroid anlage may take the form of either *nondescent* or *maldescent.* Nondescent of the thyroid produces the clinical syndrome of *lingual thyroid,* in which the entire tissue is located at the base of the tongue[3–6] (see Chap. 47). Maldescent may cause thyroid tissue to remain along the path-way of the thyroglossal duct or in the trachea, larynx, or poste-rior pharynx.[4,5] Elongated descent into the superior mediastinum may lead to substernal, preaortic, or pericardial thyroid.[3,7]

When the thyroid is diffusely involved by a disease process such as nodular goiter or thyroiditis, the remnants of thyroid along the medial aspects of the gland's descent also may be involved, may enlarge, or may produce nodules or mass lesions that are separate from the thyroid (i.e., in skeletal muscle). Such lesions may be confused clinically and surgically with neoplas-tic disease.

### LATERAL ABERRANT THYROID

The lateral aberrant thyroid, which has been the subject of contro-versy for many years, has been defined in several ways. The most acceptable definition is that it is thyroid tissue that is located lat-eral to the jugular vein. Thyroid tissue that is unassociated with a lymph node and located lateral to the jugular vein may be seen as a component of anomalous development (especially when the thyroid is involved by thyroiditis or nodular goiter), after neck surgery, or after trauma to the neck, in which case dislodged portions of the thyroid may implant in the lateral aspects of the neck. Unfortunately, the term "lateral aberrant thyroid" has also been used to describe thyroid tissue in lymph nodes lateral to the jugular vein. It is widely recognized that normal-appearing thyroid follicles within lymph nodes lateral to the jugular vein represent *metastatic thyroid carcinoma,* not a developmental anomaly. The possibility that normal thyroid follicles may be present as an embryologic rest within capsules of *medially* located lymph nodes remains disputed, although many pathologists agree with this concept. Others, however, insist that any thyroid follicles present within a lymph node, regardless of their location, represent metastatic thyroid cancer to that node.[7,8]

## DIGEORGE SYNDROME

Abnormalities in the development of the fifth branchial pouch are associated with partial or total absence of C cells. Frequently accompanying this are abnormal or absent parathyroid glands and thymus, known as DiGeorge syndrome[9] (see Chap. 60).

## THYROID INCLUSIONS

The thyroid itself may contain inclusions, especially in its lateral aspects, from numerous branchial or pharyngeal pouches. Thus, intrathyroidal parathyroids, salivary gland remnants, or thymic tissue remnants may be identified. Solid cell nests, probably representing rests of ultimobranchial body, may also be seen.[10,11] Solid cell nests are found in the posterolateral or posteromedial portion of the lateral lobes of the thyroid. They can be found in up to 21% of adult glands and in between 33% and 89% of fetal and neonatal glands.[10,13] These nests are composed of epidermoid cells with palisading at the edges of the nests.[10] Mucin may be found in some of these cells. Some of these nests contain groups of C cells. In chronic lymphocytic thyroiditis, especially the fibrous variant, these solid cell nests become prominent.[14] In two reported cases, C-cell hyperplasia and elevated serum calcitonin levels were found in lymphocytic thyroiditis.[15,16] In addition, the intimate association of the thyroid with the developing mesodermal structures of the neck may lead to the finding of normal thyroid tissue within skeletal muscle or within fat. This is not neoplastic growth but merely a normal variant of thyroid anatomy.

## GROSS ANATOMY OF THE THYROID

The normal adult thyroid gland consists of two lobes connected by an isthmus. Thyroid tissue is light brown, and the cut surface often glistens. The normal gland is surrounded by a delicate fibrous capsule and weighs 15 to 25 g. The normal thyroid is attached loosely to neighboring structures, and the fascial planes are distinct. Nodules, which are common in the adult gland, can be seen grossly in ~10% of the population in the United States.[17]

The vascular supply to the thyroid is derived from the superior and inferior thyroidal arteries; venous blood drains through thyroidal veins into the external jugular vein. The thyroid contains a rich lymphatic network; intraglandular and subcapsular lymphatics drain into the internal jugular lymph nodes.[18]

On microscopic examination, the thyroid is divided into lobules composed of 20 to 40 *follicles* (Fig. 29-2). Each lobule is supplied by an intralobular artery and vein. The follicles are lined by epithelial cells that surround central deposits of *colloid* (Fig. 29-3). In general, the follicles are uniform in size (ranging from 50 to 500 μm); however, the plane of section may give the appearance of small follicles interspersed with large ones. Studies using serial sections disclose that small follicles, or clusters of epithelial cells that apparently lie between follicles, represent the edges of follicles whose maximum diameter is situated at another level.[19] Estimates are that, in human adults, ~3 million

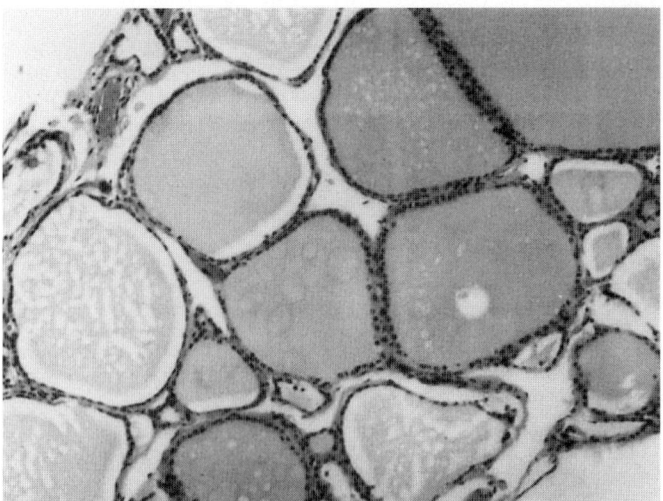

**FIGURE 29-2.** A portion of a thyroid lobule. Note the relatively uniform size of the individual follicles. Smaller units represent edges of follicles whose maximum diameter lies at another level of sectioning. (Hematoxylin and eosin; ×100)

follicles are present in the thyroid. Follicular cells have a definite polarity; their apices are directed toward the lumen of the follicle, whereas their bases are positioned toward the basement membrane. The colloid found within the follicular lumen also can be seen on the cell surfaces. The periodic acid–Schiff stain (which stains glycogen) reveals that the cytoplasm of follicular cells may contain numerous small to large (0.5 to 2.0 μm) inclusions, representing colloid (glycoprotein) droplets.

## ELECTRON MICROSCOPY OF THE THYROID

Ultrastructural studies of normal thyroid disclose that the follicular cells are arranged in a single layer. The apical surface contains microvilli that extend into a central lumen (Fig. 29-4); one to four cilia project from the central portion of each follicular cell. The cilia may alter the physical properties of the colloid, allowing for its ingestion by the apical portion of the follicular cell.[20–22] Within the cytoplasm, lysosomes are promi-

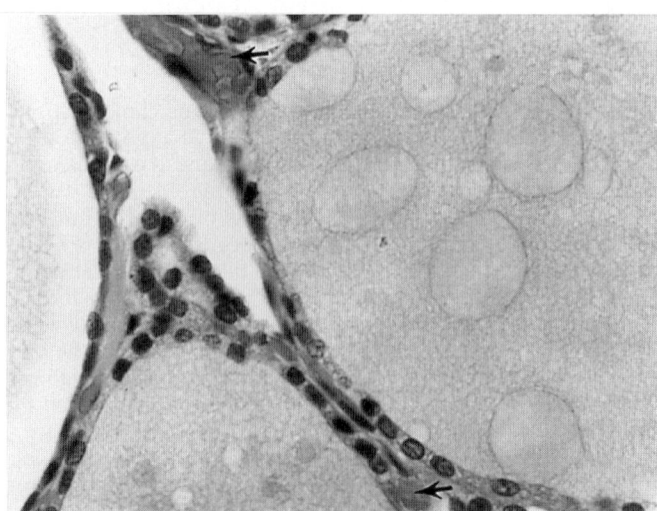

**FIGURE 29-3.** Follicular epithelium is cuboidal in the normal state. Note the interfollicular capillaries (*arrows*). (The circles in the colloid are artifacts of fixation.) (Hematoxylin and eosin; ×250)

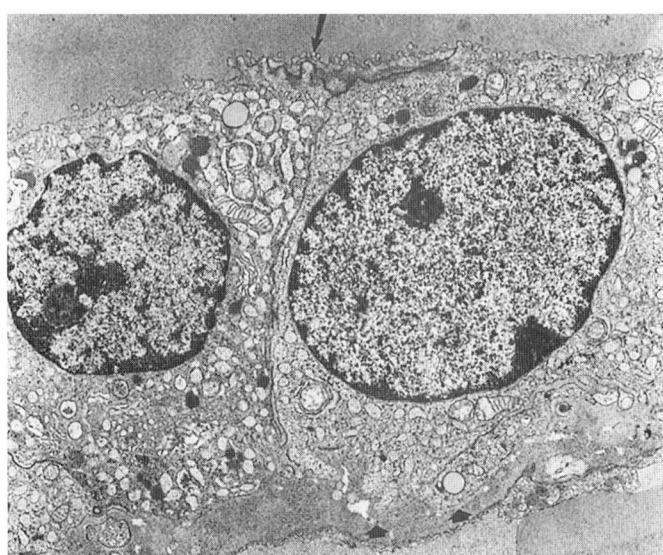

**FIGURE 29-4.** A normal thyroid follicle at the ultrastructural level. Note the cytoplasm, which is rich in organelles. Microvilli are visible at the cell–colloid interface (*arrow*) and in the basement membrane (*arrowheads*). ×10,600

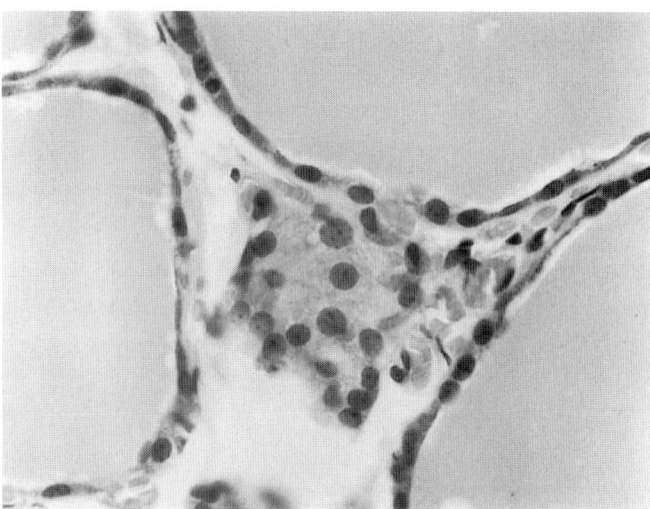

**FIGURE 29-5.** A cluster of C cells in the interfollicular stroma. Note the large size and abundant cytoplasm of these cells as compared with normal follicular elements. (Hematoxylin and eosin; ×250)

nent and endoplasmic reticulum and small mitochondria are seen. Well-developed desmosomes and terminal bars are found between cells. The basal surface is separated from the interfollicular space by a basement membrane that is 35 to 40 nm thick. In the interstitium, fenestrated capillaries and collagen fibers are noted.

Scanning electron microscopic studies indicate that, within each follicle, some individual cells or groups of cells appear to be different from neighboring ones. Thus, the apical morphology and density of microvilli differ; these differences may reflect different functional states. Experiments with cultured dog thyroid indicate that morphologic changes result from thyroid-stimulating hormone stimulation. Scanning electron microscopy has demonstrated that 15 minutes to 4 hours after administration of thyroid-stimulating hormone, thickening of the cell border occurs with subsequent development of cytoplasmic projections and an increase in the number of microvilli.[23]

In the interfollicular stroma, and occasionally abutting between the follicular epithelial cells, individual or scattered small groups of C cells are present (Fig. 29-5). Usually, on sections stained with hematoxylin and eosin, identification of C cells is difficult; calcitonin immunostaining may be necessary to disclose their location (Fig. 29-6). C cells are large, polygonal elements with centrally placed nuclei and pale-staining granular cytoplasm. In children younger than 6 years of age, the C cells are abundant, whereas in adults, they are scattered individually or appear in groups of three to five cells.[24] The normal adult complement of C cells remains debated.[24,25] The currently proposed estimate of C-cell number in adult human thyroid is no greater than 40 C cells/mm[2].[24,25]

On electron microscopy, the cytoplasm of C cells is occupied by numerous membrane-bound (neurosecretory) granules. On immunoelectron microscopic examination, these granules have been shown to contain calcitonin.[26]

## IMMUNOHISTOCHEMISTRY OF THE THYROID

Immunoperoxidase techniques have improved our understanding of the substances, especially hormones, that are contained in normal and abnormal thyroid cells.[26a] Antisera to thyroglobulin demonstrate this protein both within colloid and in follicular epithelium. Immunoelectron microscopic studies

indicate that thyroglobulin is present in the rough endoplasmic reticulum, the Golgi apparatus, and the apical cell border.[27]

The expression and distribution of intermediate filament proteins vary in normal and diseased thyroids.[28] Thus, normal follicular epithelium contains cytokeratin and, rarely, epidermal prekeratin. By contrast, cells in papillary carcinoma contain large amounts of prekeratin, as demonstrated by staining with antiprekeratin antibodies.[21]

C cells that contain neurosecretory granules may be stained by nonspecific silver techniques (Grimelius, Sevier-Munger).[29] Specific immune staining is appropriate for calcitonin (see Fig. 29-6).

## FINE-NEEDLE ASPIRATION

Fine-needle aspiration cytology of the thyroid has proven to be a safe and effective screening and diagnostic method for the evaluation of thyroid nodules (see Chap. 39). To understand changes seen in pathologic conditions, one must be aware of the range of normal results with such needle aspirations. In aspirates from nor-

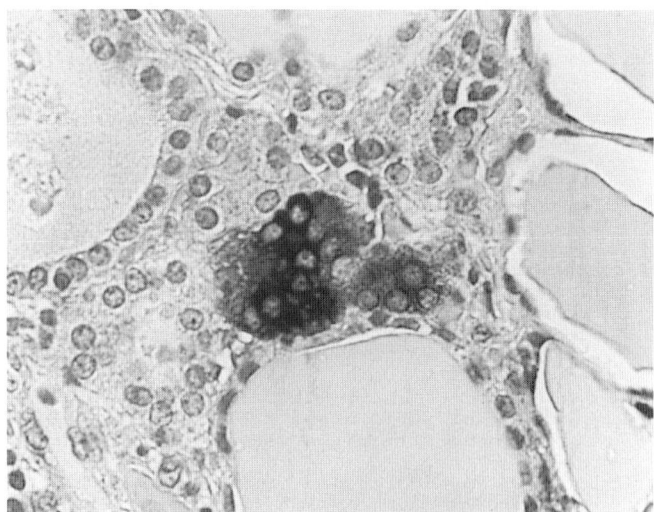

**FIGURE 29-6.** Immunoperoxidase stain with anticalcitonin antisera has been used to stain this C-cell cluster (*center*). (Immunoperoxidase-diaminobenzidine [*DAB*] with hematoxylin nuclear counterstain; ×200)

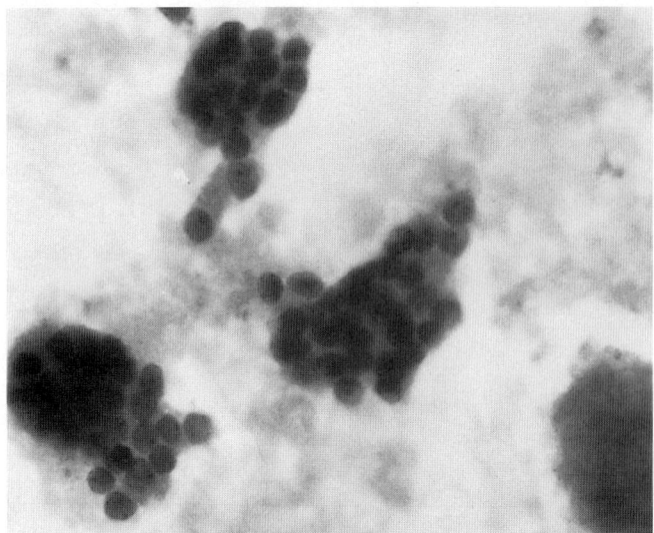

**FIGURE 29-7.** This specimen was obtained by needle aspiration from a normal thyroid lobe after surgery for laryngeal cancer. Note the rounded clusters of uniform follicular cells. The wispy material visible in the smear background and lower right is colloid. (Hematoxylin and eosin; ×400)

mal glands, uniform epithelial cells, often forming follicles surrounding drops of colloid, may be seen (Fig. 29-7). When seen en face, a honeycomb pattern is observed. The follicular cells are round to oval, measuring 8 to 10 μm in diameter; a central nucleus and pale cytoplasm are present. The nuclear chromatin is uniform and finely granular.[30] Variations occur in normal glands as a part of the aging process. Nuclear size is increased significantly in thyrocytes from normal glands of subjects 60 years of age or older in comparison with the size of those in individuals younger than 30 years of age.[31] These variations are important to recognize to avoid the diagnosis of atypical follicular epithelium from fine-needle aspiration samples solely on the basis of size.

## REFERENCES

1. Yang YJ, Haghir S, Wanamaker JR, Powers CN. Diagnosis of papillary carcinoma in a thyroglossal duct cyst by fine needle aspiration biopsy. Arch Pathol Lab Med 2000; 124:139.
1a. Chan AS. Ultrastructural observations on the formation of follicles in the human fetal thyroid. Cell Tissue Res 1983; 233:693.
2. Garcia-Bunuel R, Anton B, Brandes D. The development of lysosomes in the fetal thyroid in correlation with the onset of functional maturation. Endocrinology 1971; 91:438.
3. Larochelle D, Arcand P, Belzile M, Gagnon NB. Ectopic thyroid tissue—a review of the literature. J Otolaryngol 1979; 8:523.
4. Nienas FW, Gorman CA, Devine KD, Woolner LB. Lingual thyroid. Clinical characteristics of 15 cases. Ann Intern Med 1973; 79:205.
5. Wong RJ, Cunningham MJ, Curtin HD. Cervical ectopic thyroid. Am J Otolaryngol 1998; 19:397.
6. Prasad KC, Bhat V. Surgical management of lingual thyroid: a report of four cases. J Oral Maxillofac Surg 2000; 58:223.
7. LiVolsi VA, Perzin K, Savetsky L. Carcinoma arising in median ectopic thyroid (including thyroglossal duct tissue). Cancer 1974; 34:1303.
8. Rabinov CR, Ward PH, Pusheck T. Evolution and evaluation of lateral cystic neck masses containing thyroid tissue: "lateral aberrant thyroid" revisited. Am J Otolaryngol 1996; 17:12.
9. Robinson HB. DiGeorge's or the III–IV pharyngeal pouch syndrome: pathology and a theory of pathogenesis. In: Rosenberg HS, Bolande RP, eds. Perspectives in pediatric pathology, vol 2. Chicago: Year Book Medical Publishers, 1975:173.
10. Harach HR. Solid cell nests of the thyroid. Acta Anat (Basel) 1985; 122:249.
11. Autelitano F, Santeusanio G, Tondo UD, et al. Immunohistochemical study of solid cell nests of the thyroid gland found from an autopsy study. Cancer 1987; 59:477.
12. Bechner ME, Shulz MS, Richardson T. Solid and cystic ultimobranchial body remnants in the thyroid. Arch Pathol Lab Med 1990; 114:1049.
13. Harach HR, Day ES, Franssila KO. Thyroid spindle cell tumor with mucous cysts: an intrathyroid thymoma? Am J Surg Pathol 1985; 8:525.
14. Janzer RC, Weber E, Hedinger C. The relation between solid cell nests and C-cells of the thyroid gland. Cell Tissue Res 1979; 197:295.
15. Biddinger PW, Brennan MR, Rosen PP. Symptomatic C cell hyperplasia associated with chronic lymphocytic thyroiditis. Am J Surg Pathol 1991; 15:599.
16. Libbey NP, Nowakowski KJ, Tucci JR. C-cell hyperplasia of the thyroid in a patient with goitrous hypothyroidism and Hashimoto's thyroiditis. Am J Surg Pathol 1989; 13:71.
17. DeHaven JW, Sherwin RS. The thyroid nodule: approach to diagnosis and therapy. Conn Med 1979; 43:761.
18. Romanes GJ. Cunningham's textbook of anatomy. London: Oxford University Press, 1964:537.
19. Rienhoff WF. Gross and microscopic structure of thyroid gland in man. Contrib Embryol 1930; 21:99.
20. Sobrinho-Simoes M, Johannesson JV. Scanning electron microscopy of the normal human thyroid. J Submicrosc Cytol 1981; 13:209.
21. Echeverria OM, Hernandez-Pando R, Vasquez-Nin GH. Ultrastructural, cytochemical and immunohistochemical study of nuclei and cytoskeleton of thyroid papillary carcinoma cells. Ultrastruct Pathol 1998; 22:185.
22. Gould VE, Johannessen JV, Sobrinho-Simoes M. The thyroid gland. In: Johannessen JV, ed. Electron microscopy in human medicine, vol 10. New York: McGraw-Hill, 1981.
23. Rapoport B, Jones AL. Acute effects of thyroid stimulating hormone on cultured thyroid cell morphology. Endocrinology 1978; 102:175.
24. Guyetant S, Wion-Barbot N, Rousselot MC, et al. C-cell hyperplasia associated with chronic lymphocytic thyroiditis. Hum Pathol 1994; 25:514.
25. Guyetant S, Rousselot M, Durison M, et al. Sex-related C-cell hyperplasia in the normal human thyroid: a quantitative autopsy study. J Clin Endocrinol Metab 1997; 82:42.
26. Wolfe HF, Voelkel EF, Tashjian AJ. Distribution of calcitonin-containing cells in the normal adult human thyroid gland: a correlation of morphology and peptide content. J Clin Endocrinol Metab 1974; 38:688.
26a. DeMicco C, Kopp F, Vassko V, Grino M. In situ hybridization and immunohistochemistry study of thyroid peroxidase expression in thyroid tumors. Thyroid 2000: 10:109.
27. Ide M. Immunoelectron microscopic localization of thyroglobulin in the human thyroid gland. Acta Pathol Jpn 1984; 34:575.
28. Miettinen M, Franssila K, Lehto V-P, et al. Expression of intermediate filament proteins in thyroid gland and thyroid tumors. Lab Invest 1984; 50:262.
29. Wilander E, Justti-Berggren L, Lundqvist M, Grimelius L. Staining of rat thyroid parafollicular (C) cells with the Sevier-Munger silver technique. Acta Pathol Microbiol Immunol Scand [A] 1980; 88:339.
30. Kini SR. Guidelines to clinical aspiration cytology: thyroid. New York: Igaku-Shoin, 1987.
31. Ferchter GE, Goerthler K. Age related nuclear size variability of thyrocytes in thyroid aspirates. Anal Quant Cytol 1983; 5:75.

## CHAPTER 30

# THYROID PHYSIOLOGY: SYNTHESIS AND RELEASE, IODINE METABOLISM, BINDING AND TRANSPORT

H. LESTER REED

The thyroid hormones, L-3,5,3',5'-tetraiodothyronine (L-thyroxine [$T_4$]) and, to a much less extent, L-3,5,3'-triiodothyronine (L-triiodothyronine [$T_3$]) are synthesized by the follicular epithelial cells of the thyroid gland. This synthesis requires the availability of iodine and is increased by thyroid-stimulating hormone (thyrotropin; TSH) from the anterior pituitary gland through a specific thyroidal receptor.

Small amounts of thyroid hormone are secreted continuously into the blood and are almost entirely bound (in a large circulating reservoir) to plasma proteins (Table 30-1), with a very small percentage remaining unbound or free. The speculation is that the free hormones (free $T_4$ and $T_3$), principally derived from circulating $T_4$, enter the cell and mediate their effects through specific nuclear receptors (see Chap. 31), which are heterogeneously distributed among tissues. The hypothalamic–pituitary–thyroid axis is regulated by autocrine, paracrine, hemocrine, and environmental factors to maintain steady-state hormone economy.

**TABLE 30-1.**
**Thyroid Hormone–Binding Proteins**

| | Thyroxine-Binding Globulin | Transthyretin | Albumin |
|---|---|---|---|
| **A. PHYSIOLOGIC CHARACTERISTICS** | | | |
| Serum (µmol/L) | 0.3 | 4.6 | 650 |
| Binding sites (no.) | 1 | 2 | 5–6 |
| $K_a$ (mol/L) | | | |
| $T_4$ | $1.0 \times 10^{10}$ | $\sim1.0 \times 10^8$ | $\sim1.0 \times 10^6$ |
| $T_3$ | $0.5 \times 10^9$ | $1.0 \times 10^7$ | $1.0 \times 10^5$ |
| *Distribution of Iodothyronines between Proteins (% of Total)* | | | |
| $T_4$ | 70–75 | 10–25 | 10–20 |
| $T_3$ | 70–80 | ≤10 | 10–20 |
| **B. INFLUENTIAL CLINICAL CONDITIONS** | | | |
| Hypothyroidism | ↑ | ↑ | ↑ |
| Hyperthyroidism | ↓ | ↓ | NC |
| Estrogen | ↑ | ↑ | NC |
| Androgens | ↓ | ↓ | NC |
| Hepatitis | ↑ | ↓ | ↓ |
| Porphyria | ↑ | ? | NC |
| Cirrhosis | ↓ | ↓ | ↓ |
| Familial | ↓/↑ | ↓/↑ | ↑ |
| Malnutrition | ↓ | ↓ | ↓ |

NC, no change; $K_a$, association constant for binding; for multiple sites, the $K_a$ is provided for the highest affinity site and represents the mean from several sources; $T_4$, thyroxine; $T_3$, triiodothyronine.

## IODINE METABOLISM

Iodine is essential for the synthesis of thyroid hormones. With four iodines per molecule of $T_4$, iodine comprises 66% of $T_4$ by weight; with three iodines, $T_3$ is 58% iodine (Fig. 30-1). Normally, ~90 µg (~120 nmol) of $T_4$ and 6.5 µg (~10 nmol) of $T_3$ are

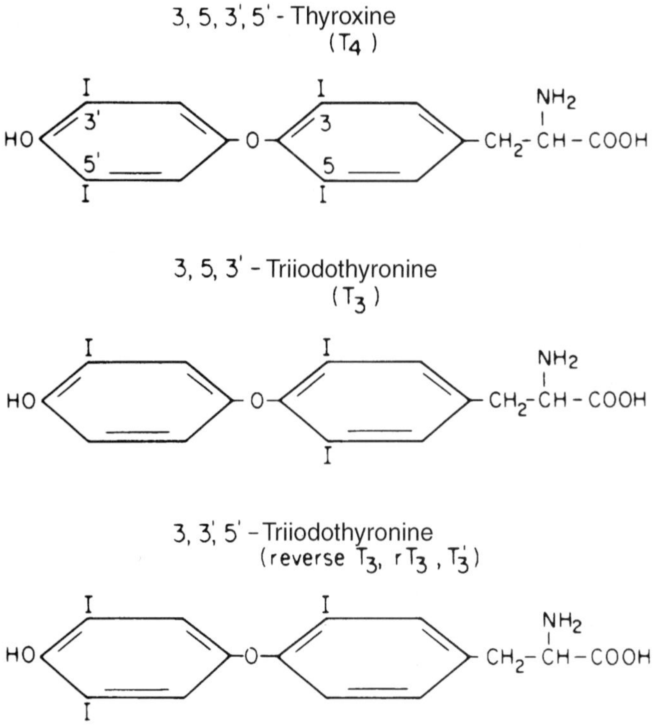

**FIGURE 30-1.** Chemical structures of L-thyroxine ($T_4$), L-triiodothyronine ($T_3$), and reverse $T_3$ ($rT_3$). (From Hershman JM. Endocrine pathophysiology. Philadelphia: Lea & Febiger, 1980.)

secreted daily by the thyroid gland. Thus, 60 to 80 µg (~550 nmol) of iodine must be transported into the gland daily to maintain normal daily hormone production.[1]

Iodine is not always present in sufficient quantities from dietary sources in the environment. Surprisingly, even in the United States, the daily iodine intake has been declining.[2] Accumulation of the absolute iodine requirement for thyroid hormone synthesis is facilitated by an efficient system for concentrating and conserving iodine in the thyroid gland. Between 5000 and 10,000 µg of hormonal iodine is stored within the gland.[1] This pool constitutes a protective reserve against periods of dietary iodine deficiency.

### IODIDE CLEARANCE

Within a certain range, the thyroid gland can adjust to variation in dietary iodine with changes in its clearance of iodide from plasma. However, either chronic dietary deficiency of iodine or conditions of severe iodine excess often exceed the capacity for regulation, resulting in disease states (see Chaps. 37 and 38).

Virtually all of dietary iodine is reduced to iodide and absorbed in the small intestine. Circulating iodide is cleared from the blood principally by the kidney (80%) and by the thyroid (20%).[1] Renal excretion, measured with a 24-hour collection, varies with filtered load and reflects 97% of dietary intake; only ~3% is lost in the stool.[1] Renal iodide is passively reabsorbed; thus, the renal clearance depends on glomerular filtration rate and is apparently unaffected by serum iodide concentration. Patients with end-stage renal disease (ESRD) have decreased renal iodide clearance and elevated serum iodide concentrations.[3] Iodide excess is a proposed mechanism for the increased incidence of hypothyroidism, thyroid nodules, and goiter, whereas the mechanisms for increased thyroid cancer with ESRD are unknown.[3] In contrast, thyroidal iodide clearance changes inversely with dietary intake and intrathyroidal iodine stores, increasing as much as five-fold under conditions of iodine deficiency.[1]

In addition to the thyroid gland, the salivary glands, gastric mucosa, choroid plexus, and mammary glands may concentrate iodine, which can be detected with radioiodine scintigraphy[1]; however, only in the thyroid is this function influenced by TSH. Therefore, although radiation-induced salivary gland inflammation and breast milk contamination are possible complications of treatment with radioactive iodine, they should not be worsened by recombinant human TSH administration.[4]

### IODIDE EXCESS

The amount of iodine in the American diet, with its iodine-enriched foods, usually greatly exceeds the recommended 150 µg/day of iodine in most areas. Nonetheless, a decline in dietary iodine has been noted over the last 20 years, with ~10% of the U.S. population being at risk for iodine deficiency.[2] The American diet contrasts with diets in many other areas of the world, such as central Africa,[2,3] where the percentage of people at risk for deficiency is much higher.[5,6] Additional dietary iodine from many common agents such as cough medicines, vitamins, kelp, iodinated contrast agents (iopanoic acid, sodium ipodate), antiarrhythmics (amiodarone), antiseptics (iodoform gauze), and water purification tablets (tetraglycine hydroperiodide) is often unexpected (see Chap. 37). In normal individuals, as well as patients with ESRD, an increased iodine load can decrease radioiodine uptake and increase serum TSH and thyroidal size (see Chap. 37).[3] High doses of iodine dilute diagnostic radioiodine tracers and thereby reduce fractional thyroidal uptake of the tracer; this causes low radioiodine uptake and diminished ability to image the thyroid by scintiscan. Further, depending on the amount, excess iodine inhibits uptake, organification, and release of the hormones (Fig. 30-2) and decreases thyroidal blood flow.[7] An intrinsically abnormal

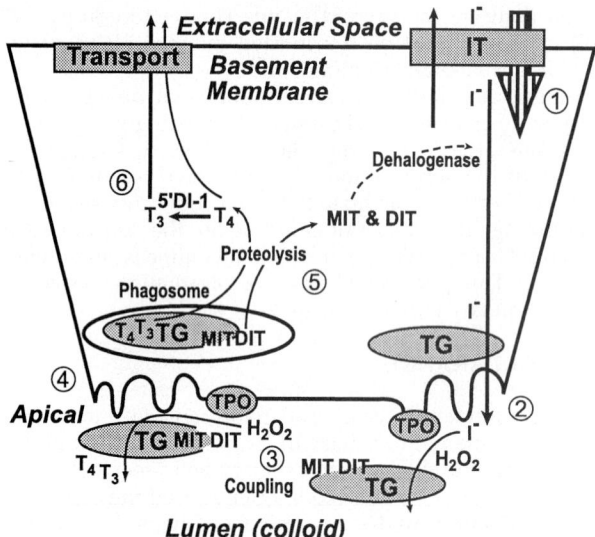

**FIGURE 30-2.** Thyroid hormone synthesis. Iodide (*I⁻*) is transported by the iodide transporter (*IT*) from the plasma into the thyroid cell and then I⁻ moves to the apical membrane, where it is organified and coupled under the influence of thyroid peroxidase (*TPO*) to thyroglobulin (*Tg*), which is synthesized within the cell. Hormone stored as colloid reenters the cell through endocytosis and moves back toward the basal membrane, where $T_4$ and $T_3$ are secreted. Nonhormonal iodide is recycled. Hormone synthesis may be inhibited at: (1) *iodine transport* by thiocyanate, perchlorate, interleukin-1, and tumor necrosis factor-α; (2) *organification* and (3) *coupling* by propylthiouracil (*PTU*) and methimazole and through decreasing TPO by interferon-γ and interleukin-1; (4) *endocytosis* by lithium and iodide; (5) *thyroglobulin proteolysis* by iodide; and (6) *intrathyroidal deiodination* by PTU and tumor necrosis factor-α.

gland is less likely to adjust successfully to these changes in dietary or pharmaceutical iodine and, thus, may present with clinical disease[1] (see Chaps. 37 and 38).

## TRANSPORT OF IODIDE

Thyroid cells actively transport iodide and other monovalent anions such as *perchlorate* and *pertechnetate* (see Chap. 33) from the plasma into their cytoplasm. This adenosine triphosphatase (ATPase)–dependent sodium-iodide cotransporter or symporter has been isolated and cloned (see Chap. 34).[8] Although the transport system, often called *trapping*, can be saturated, its capacity is above that of typical plasma iodide levels. Thus, small increases in available iodide are followed by increased transport. This *trapping* by the symporter is rate-limiting to thyroid hormone synthesis and is regulated by the TSH receptor. It can move iodide against a gradient and increase thyroidal iodide 30-fold over blood concentrations.

Iodine is stored in the thyroid gland in thyroglobulin (Tg), a large glycoprotein essential to the synthesis and storage of the thyroid hormones (see Thyroglobulin section later in this chapter).

## THYROID HORMONE SYNTHESIS

The major synthetic steps regulated by TSH are transport of iodide, organification, coupling, Tg synthesis, and endocytotic secretion. Under the stimulation of TSH, the thyroid cells remove iodide from the capillary network at the base of the cell (see Fig. 30-2) and move the iodide to the apex of the cell, where it is joined with molecules of tyrosine to make mostly $T_4$ and some $T_3$. $T_4$ and $T_3$ are stored in colloid within the follicles of the gland. They are then released together, or some $T_4$ is further deiodinated to $T_3$ before release (see Fig. 30-2). These two steps

are also under the influence of TSH or other proteins that bind to the TSH receptor. Mutations of this TSH receptor are continuously activated in some toxic adenomas and multinodular goiters.[9] A small but measurable amount of non–TSH-dependent $T_4$ secretion also occurs normally.

## ORGANIFICATION

Iodide ions transported into the thyroid cell are oxidized before being used for iodinating tyrosyl residues present in the Tg molecules. This process, called *organification*, takes place at the apex of the cell (see Fig. 30-2) and requires the enzyme thyroid peroxidase (TPO). The decrease in peroxidase activity and organification that follows iodine excess, known as the *Wolff-Chaikoff effect*, may protect against hyperthyroidism. The effect is transient, and "escape" occurs within several days. Failure to escape from the Wolff-Chaikoff effect is common in certain diseased glands; therefore, the reduction in organification due to iodine excess is perpetuated, leading to hypothyroidism[1] (see Chap. 37). The activity of TPO may be deficient on a congenital basis and is reduced by antimicrosomal antibodies directed against it (see Chaps. 46 and 197) or with administration of thiourea drugs, such as propylthiouracil (PTU), which is commonly used to treat hyperthyroidism (see Chap. 42).

## THYROGLOBULIN

The tyrosine residues to which the iodine is joined in the organification process are part of the Tg molecule, a 660-kDa glycoprotein. Defects in Tg synthesis have been proposed to cause some cases of goiter, although such cases are rare. Thus far, therapeutic interference with the synthesis of Tg has not been possible. Serum values of Tg are extremely useful in the management of well-differentiated thyroid cancer as an indicator of biologic activity or recurrence.[10]

Iodination of the tyrosyl residues within Tg (i.e., organification of the iodine) involves substitution on the tyrosyl ring. If one iodine replaces a hydrogen, then monoiodotyrosine (MIT) is formed; if two iodines are joined to tyrosine, diiodotyrosine (DIT) is formed. The MIT/DIT ratio depends on iodine availability; during iodine deficiency, for example, relatively more MIT is formed.

## COUPLING

The iodothyronines are formed by coupling of two DITs to form $T_4$ and one MIT and one DIT to form $T_3$. The coupling process is catalyzed by TPO, blocked by thiourea drugs and excess iodine, and stimulated by TSH (see Fig. 30-2). Congenital defects in MIT and DIT coupling result in decreased hormone synthesis and goiter. Because the MIT/DIT ratio varies inversely with iodine availability, relatively more $T_3$ is formed with iodine deficiency and relatively more $T_4$ with iodine surfeit.

## HORMONE STORAGE AND SECRETION

Thyroglobulin is contained within cytoplasmic bodies called *vesicles* that fuse with the apical membrane of the cell and extrude their Tg content into the colloid space at the center of the thyroid follicle (see Fig. 30-2). This space is bounded by the apical membranes of adjacent follicle cells and is inaccessible to the circulation. Here, hormone is stored in colloid. Ordinarily, only a very small fraction of stored hormone, ~1%, turns over each day. Under TSH stimulation, hormones are secreted, and less colloid is stored. The process of hormone secretion moves in the opposite direction back to the basal membrane of the cell. Each step is controlled by TSH. First, pseudopods of the apical cell membrane enclose colloid and form a droplet that merges with the apical membrane and moves into the cell. This process of endocytosis occurs within minutes of TSH stimulation.

**TABLE 30-2.**
**Kinetic Characteristics of Thyroid Hormones**

|  | $T_4$ | $T_3$ | $rT_3$ |
|---|---|---|---|
| Serum (nmol/L) | 90 | 2.0 | 0.3 |
| Free fraction (%) | 0.03 | 0.3 | 0.13 |
| PAR (nmol/d/70 kg) | 120 | 47 | 50 |
| $V_D$ (L/70 kg) | 10 | 38 | 34 |
| PCR (L/d/70 kg) | 1.2 | 24 | 120 |
| $Q_{tot}$ (nmol/70 kg) | 850 | 76 | 18 |
| **COMPARTMENTAL DISTRIBUTION (%)** | | | |
| Serum | 28.8 | 14.7 | 13.8 |
| Rapid exchange* | 25.6 | 8.3 | 36.9 |
| Slow exchange* | 45.6 | 76.9 | 49.3 |
| **INFLUENTIAL CLINICAL CONDITIONS[23]** | | | |
| Undernutrition[5,12] | NS PAR | ↓ PAR | ↓ PCR |
| Overnutrition[5] | NS PAR | ↑ PAR | ↑ PCR |
| Exercise[33] | Slight ↓ PCR | ↑ PAR; ↑ PCR | ? |
| Pregnancy[32] | ↑ PAR | ? | ? |

$T_4$, thyroxine; $T_3$, triiodothyronine; $rT_3$, reverse $T_3$; *PAR*, plasma appearance rate; $V_D$, volume of distribution; *PCR*, plasma clearance rate; $Q_{tot}$, total hormone mass; *NS*, not significant; $T_4$, 1 nmol = 0.78 μg; $T_3$, 1 nmol = 0.65 μg.

*Rapid exchange compartments may include liver and kidney, whereas slow exchange compartments may include muscle and adipose.[13]

(Data are pooled from several references[11–13] utilizing compartmental analysis in human subjects and may be considered to have ±10–20% variation.)

In the interior of the cell, the colloid droplet is joined by a lysosome, forming a phagolysosome. As the phagolysosome moves toward the base of the cell, the Tg molecule is digested. Amino acids and nonhormone iodine are recovered in the cell for recycling. $T_4$ and $T_3$ are secreted into the capillaries at the base of the cell in proportion to their presence in Tg. Most $T_3$ is derived from extrathyroidal conversion of $T_4$ by 5'monodeiodinase type I (5'D-I) in peripheral tissues. However, a 27-kDa protein with 5'D-I activity has been found within human thyroid glands.[1,6] It is regulated by TSH, has higher activity in Graves disease and follicular adenomas, and has lower activity in papillary carcinoma.

## THYROID HORMONE CIRCULATION AND TRANSPORT

Approximately 120 nmol of $T_4$, 47 nmol of $T_3$, and 50 nmol of reverse $T_3$ ($rT_3$) appear in the serum each day in a typical 70-kg person[11–13] (Table 30-2). The balance between production and degradation is mediated by, among other things, nutrition, nonthyroidal illness, exercise, pregnancy, and medications. At steady-state conditions, this balance is reflected by serum values that represent only ~29% of $T_4$, 14% of $T_3$, and 14% of $rT_3$ total body hormone stores or pool ($Q_{tot}$). Less than 1% of the total circulating amount of each hormone is free in the plasma (see Table 30-2). This extraordinary degree of binding to transport proteins has several important consequences: (a) The plasma contains a large capacity to store hormone, serving as a reservoir or a buffer against fluctuations in blood levels; (b) Little hormone is lost through the kidneys by glomerular filtration of free hormone; and (c) Changes in binding proteins affect the serum reservoir but do not affect the amount of free hormone, presumably not altering the physiologic actions of the hormone (see Table 30-1). Either the binding protein capacity, the free hormone concentration, or the binding protein concentration may be measured to clarify the changes in circulating $T_4$ or $T_3$ concentrations that accompany genetic or acquired aberrations in the binding proteins (also see Chap. 33 and ref. 13a).

Table 30-2 shows some of the similarities and differences between the major iodothyronines. $T_3$ has 10% and $rT_3$ has only 2% of $Q_{tot}$ compared with $T_4$. Although ~50% of $T_4$ and $rT_3$ cir-

culates in the blood and other rapidly equilibrating tissues, such as liver and kidney, only ~25% of $T_3$ is found in these same kinetic compartments. Hormone stores are turned over at a rate of ~10% per day for $T_4$, 70% per day for $T_3$, and 350% per day for $rT_3$. Thus, with inhibited production of *endogenous* hormone (see Table 30-2) or increased appearance of *exogenous* hormone (e.g., increased dosage), the new steady-state conditions are reached within weeks for $T_4$, within days for $T_3$, and within hours for $rT_3$.[11,12] Compared with $T_3$, $T_4$ has a higher binding affinity (see Table 30-1) and slower plasma clearance rate (relative to the distribution volume [$V_D$]), making $T_4$ a stable circulating hormone reservoir and substrate for $T_3$ formation. The rapid plasma clearance rate of $T_3$, relative to its $V_D$, is associated with more labile equilibration or disequilibration, reflecting shorter response times of circulating $T_3$ to environmental and nutritional influences.

## BINDING PROTEINS

$T_4$ and $T_3$ are reversibly bound to several proteins synthesized by the liver (see Table 30-1). The variety of relative serum concentrations, hormone affinity constants ($K_a$), and dissociation constants ($K_d$) help provide a buffered, stable plasma pool and a homogeneous distribution of free hormone during capillary transport.[14] *Transthyretin* (TTR), previously known as *thyroid-binding prealbumin* (TBPA), has a low affinity and rapid $K_d$; therefore, it plays a greater role in delivering iodothyronines to tissues than do circulating proteins with higher binding affinity.[14,15] Specifically, TTR is the major $T_4$-binding protein in the cerebrospinal fluid and is thought to be a major mechanism for homogenous central nervous system hormone distribution.[1] Some evidence dates this mechanism to more than 300 million years.[15] Thyroxine-binding globulin (TBG), however, with its relatively high binding affinity and slower dissociation, provides a stable hormone reservoir in the plasma. Changes in the glycoprotein nature of TBG slow its removal in certain physiologic conditions such as pregnancy. Albumin, with its relatively high serum concentration, has multiple binding sites with a low binding affinity and, thus, like TTR, may contribute to tissue delivery of the free hormone. Lipoproteins bind small amounts of thyroid hormones, but their physiologic significance is unknown.[14] Increased binding to albumin from a hereditary cause is associated with increased production of both $T_4$ and $T_3$, which suggests increased tissue delivery by this protein deiodination.[16]

Under normal conditions, only ~25% of TBG and 0.3% of TTR molecules carry $T_4$. The hormone distribution among the carrying proteins is listed in Table 30-1. Over a wide range of binding protein concentrations, steady-state free hormone concentration, and production rates remain nearly constant.[14,16] Thus, the measurement of free $T_4$ or free $T_3$ concentrations by equilibrium dialysis or a comparable method is critical in clinical circumstances when changes in the transport proteins are present (see Table 30-1).[14] Genetic or induced alterations of TBG are important because this protein carries 75% of $T_4$ and 80% of $T_3$, and because these bound iodothyronines have the greatest impact on measured values of circulating total thyroid hormone by routine analysis.

Clearance of TBG is decreased by an increased sialic acid content of the terminal sugar of its polysaccharide chain. Sialic acid content is increased in pregnancy; the resultant decreased clearance of TBG, along with increased production of the protein, contributes to elevated serum TBG.

Inherited conditions may affect TBG, TTR, and albumin. Familial increases and decreases of TBG, increased TTR binding of $T_4$, decreased TBG affinity for $T_4$, and abnormal $T_4$ binding to albumin have all been described. Generally, these variations are associated with an asymptomatic euthyroid condition.[14,16] Nonthyroidal illness may be associated with circulating inhibitors to hormone binding to these carrier proteins (see Chap. 36).

TABLE 30-3.
Thyroid Hormone Deiodinase Characteristics

| | Type I | Type II | Type III |
|---|---|---|---|
| Deiodination site* | Outer and inner rings | Outer ring | Inner ring |
| Substrate preference† | $rT_3 > T_4 > T_3$ | $T_4 > rT_3$ | $T_3, T_4$ |
| Location | Liver, kidney, thyroid | Brain, brown adipose tissue, pituitary, pineal; cardiac and skeletal muscle; placenta | Brain, skin, placenta |
| Seleno-protein | Yes | Yes | Yes |
| Sensitive to dietary selenium deficiency | Yes | No | Yes |
| Optimal pH | Outer ring, 6.5–7.5; inner ring, 8.0–8.5 | 6.5–7.5 | 8.0–8.5 |
| Response to ↑ $T_4$ | ↑ Activity | ↓ Activity | ↑ Activity |
| Response to ↓ $T_4$ | ↓ Activity | ↑ Activity | ↓ Activity |
| Response to fasting | ↓ Activity | Little effect | Little effect |
| Response to propylthiouracil | ↓ Activity | Little to no effect | Little effect |
| Response to iopanoic acid | ↓ Activity | ↓ Activity | ? |
| Characterized | 27-kDa subunit; cloned | 29-kDa subunit; cloned | 32-kDa subunit; cloned |

$rT_3$, reverse triiodothyronine; $T_4$, thyroxine; $T_3$, triiodothyronine.
*Inner ring deiodination may increase maximal velocity($V_{max}$)/apparent michaZelis-manten constant($K_m$) by 50- to 200-fold under the influence of the sulfate substrate.[6,20,21]
†Substrate preference may be changed for type I deiodination with sulfation of the substrate.

# PERIPHERAL METABOLISM OF THYROID HORMONES

$T_4$ is metabolized by the sequential removal of iodine atoms. Although most human tissues have the ability to perform this enzymatic step, liver and kidney are the most important sites of deiodination.

The stepwise removal of iodine atoms from thyroxine has been well described.[11] The process is enzymatic and depends on available sulfhydryl compounds. First, a hydrogen atom replaces iodine at one of four positions on $T_4$. Subsequently, further iodine atoms are removed, yielding thyronines with two, one, and, finally, no iodine atoms. Iodine may be removed from the inner (tyrosyl) or outer (phenolic) ring. The entire process is referred to as *sequential deiodination* and is mediated by a family of enzymes listed in Table 30-3.

Removing either iodine atom from the *outer ring* (designated as the 3' or 5' position) of $T_4$ yields $T_3$. By convention, this pathway is referred to as *5'-deiodination*. Two distinct enzymes are known to catalyze this process, monodeiodinase type I (5'D-I) and type II (5'D-II), both of which are described in Table 30-3. Because $T_3$ has more metabolic activity than $T_4$, this pathway represents activation. Intrapituitary conversion of $T_4$ to $T_3$ is important in the regulation of TSH secretion.

Removing either iodine atom from the *inner ring* (the 3 or 5 position) of $T_4$ yields $rT_3$. Reverse $T_3$ has no known metabolic activity. It does not prevent goiter but is a competitive inhibitor of 5'D-I. Therefore, the 5-deiodination pathway catalyzed both by 5'D-I, at a different pH optima from that for phenolic ring deiodination, and by a type III seleno-enzyme (see Table 30-3) that is found in placenta, brain, and skin, constitutes an inactivation. Substrate conjugation with sulfate can increase the tyrosyl ring deiodination of $T_4$ and $T_3$ by 5'D-I several hundred-fold, thereby inactivating these hormones.[17] $T_3$ sulfate is produced in peripheral tissues and does not suppress TSH in normal humans. It may account for facilitated 5'D-I or augmented biliary losses in disease states.[18] The sequential deiodination continues to yield thyronine and a family of diiodothyronines and monoiodothyronines that have uncertain bioactivity (see Fig. 30-1).

Peripheral $T_4$ deiodination contributes 80% to 85% of the $T_3$ plasma appearance rate (PAR). This conversion occurs mostly in the liver and kidney. The thyroid gland may secrete ~15% of the $T_3$ total PAR directly in the form of $T_3$. The role of thyroidal 5'D-I as a contributing mechanism of peripheral $T_4$ deiodination is presently under investigation. Nearly 100% of $rT_3$ comes from peripheral $T_4$ deiodination, although not necessarily from hepatic or renal sources.

5'D-I is a selenium-dependent enzyme found in human thyroid, liver, and kidney; it has decreased activity in hypothyroidism, undernutrition, nonthyroidal illness, and selenium deficiency, and after PTU administration.[6,12,19] When phenolic ring deiodination (5'D-I) activity is decreased, both the production of $T_3$ and the degradation of $rT_3$ decline.[12] These changes result in an increase in plasma $rT_3$ and a decrease in $T_3$ concentration as found with fasting and some nonthyroidal illnesses.[13,19] Many other situations may also have a similar profile consisting of a low serum level of $T_3$ and high $rT_3$, including drug administration (e.g., glucocorticoids, β-blockers, thionamides, oral cholecystographic dyes), chronic illness (cirrhosis, renal failure, malignancy), and acute illness (e.g., myocardial infarction, sepsis, uncontrolled diabetes mellitus, severe burns) (see Chap. 36). However, in human immunodeficiency virus (HIV) infection, the $rT_3$ is paradoxically decreased and $T_3$ is normal or increased, suggesting another mechanism during nonthyroidal illness (NTI) to that previously described (see Chap. 36).

In central Africa, myxedematous cretinism associated with iodine deficiency predominates, with little incidence of neurologic cretinism.[6] Some of these regions have coexistent iodine and selenium deficiency. The resultant hypothyroidism that occurs in these locations is associated with a decreased selenium-dependent activity of 5'D-I that may attenuate the frequency of neurologic cretinism.[6] Fetal brain $T_4$ acts as the major source of brain $T_3$ converted by 5'D-II that is a seleno-protein but is resistant to dietary selenium deficiency[20] (see Table 30-3). Placental type III deiodinase (see Table 30-3) shares a similar resistance to dietary selenium deficiency that may reflect tissue specific preservation of selenium stores.[21] The presence of more circulating fetal $T_4$ that has not been converted to $T_3$ by 5'D-I, an extremely selenium sensitive enzyme, results in increased serum $T_4$ available for uptake by the fetal brain during early pregnancy. Thus, the selenium-mediated decrease in $T_4$ peripheral deiodination may help reduce the incidence of neurologic cretinism. Iodine should be replaced first in this particular circumstance to avoid premature activation of 5'D-I by selenium replacement, thus predisposing to a further lowering of serum $T_4$.[6,20]

Other pathways for the disposal of thyroid hormones exist. The ether bond may be broken or the alanine side chain of $T_4$ and $T_3$ may be oxidized. *Tetraiodoacetic acid* (tetrac) and *triiodoacetic acid*

(TRIAC) are formed by this oxidation. These compounds have some metabolic activity, and their clinical role is being investigated. Sulfoconjugation of iodothyronines facilitates tyrosyl (inner ring) deiodination except possibly of $rT_3$, which is already a very favored substrate for phenolic (outer ring) deiodination. Glucuronide conjugates of iodothyronines are more hydrophilic and are consequently excreted more readily in the bile. In humans, changing this enterohepatic circulation with an anion exchange resin (cholestyramine) lowers serum $T_4$ in postabsorptive states, after excessive thyroxine ingestion, and in Graves disease.[22]

The intrapituitary generation of $T_3$ from $T_4$ by 5'D-II helps maintain regulation of TSH release. In contradistinction to 5'D-I, as the substrate level of $T_4$ declines, the activity of this form of phenolic ring deiodination increases, and fasting and PTU do not inhibit its activity (see Table 30-3).

Pharmacologic inhibition of 5'D-I conversion of $T_4$ to $T_3$ with the use of iodinated radiographic contrast agents (e.g., iopanoic acid) and thiourea compounds (e.g., PTU) is an effective means of rapidly decreasing $T_3$ production in hyperthyroid patients (see Table 30-3 and Fig. 30-2) (see Chap. 42).

# REGULATION OF THYROID HORMONE ECONOMY

Thyroid hormone regulation is directed through the neuroendocrine–hypothalamic–pituitary–thyroid–peripheral tissue axis (Fig. 30-3). This system has autocrine (e.g., enzyme autoregulation), paracrine (e.g., somatostatin, thyrotropin-releasing hormone [TRH]), and endocrine (e.g., $T_4$, $T_3$) autoregulation that is also influenced by environmental factors (e.g., energy balance, circadian variation, illness).

## NEUROENDOCRINE MODULATION

Serum TSH secretion has a diurnal rhythm: values peak after midnight (nearly 50% over the 24-hr mean or mesor) and are lowest in midafternoon. The core body temperature rhythm is highly associated with this serum TSH rhythm.[23] Advancing age may blunt this nocturnal surge in TSH.[24] In rodents and human infants, cold stimulates TSH secretion.[23] Hypothyroid patients administered a constant $T_4$ dose have a slight decline in serum $T_4$, unchanged $T_3$, and increased TSH response to TRH in winter months.[23] Several factors are well recognized to increase the release of TSH (e.g., estrogens, α-adrenergic agonists, dopamine antagonists, sleep deprivation) or decrease it (e.g., thyroid hormones, glucocorticoids, dopamine, growth hormone, somatostatin, tumor necrosis factor, sleep initiation)[23,25,26] (see Fig. 30-3).

## HYPOTHALAMUS

To maintain thyroid hormone production, the tonic stimulation by TRH is required. Severe hypothalamic injury or separation of the pituitary from the hypothalamus by stalk section results in hypothyroidism. TRH is a tripeptide (Glu-His-Pro) synthesized in the paraventricular nucleus of the hypothalamus, and its mRNA concentration is inversely related to concentrations of circulating thyroid hormones. TRH is transported down nerve endings to the median eminence and reaches the anterior pituitary through the portal capillary plexus. Somatostatin, found in the anterior periventricular region, inhibits TSH release. Administration of somatostatin decreases the TSH response to TRH, nocturnal TSH rise, and the TSH elevations seen in primary hypothyroidism (see Chap. 15). Tumor necrosis factor-α (TNF-α) and interleukin-1 (IL-1) decrease TSH, and some of that effect is possibly mediated through TRH.

TRH binds to high-affinity receptors on the surface of TSH-producing cells (thyrotropes) and leads to a prompt release of stored TSH. With more prolonged stimulation, new synthesis and release of TSH occur. As a diagnostic procedure, the provocation of

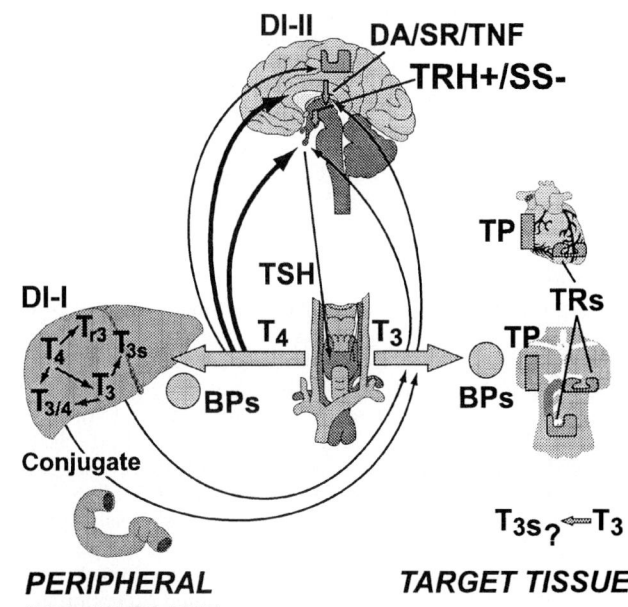

**FIGURE 30-3.** Major steps in thyroid hormone regulation. Thyrotropin-releasing hormone (*TRH*) from the hypothalamus stimulates and somatostatin (*SS*) inhibits thyroid-stimulating hormone (*TSH*) release under the influence of such neurotransmitters as dopamine (*DA*), serotonin (*SR*), and tumor necrosis factor (*TNF*). The pituitary secretes TSH that leads to regulation of the thyroid gland. Peripheral monodeiodination by monodeiodinase type I (*DI-I*) or type II (*DI-II*)[6,20] yields triiodothyronine (*$T_3$*) and other iodothyronines that may enter the bowel[22] or may be further deiodinated after sulfur (*$T_{3S}$*) or other conjugates (*$T_{3/4\ conjugates}$*) are formed. Thyroid hormones may be actively transported into cells by a transport protein (*TP*).[19] $T_3$ initiates action in target tissues through a variety of thyroid-hormone receptors (*TRs*), which differ between tissues. Circulating thyroxine (*$T_4$*) principally (*heavy arrows*) and $T_3$ are transported by binding proteins (*BPs*)[14,15] and have inhibitory action, primarily on the pituitary but also on the hypothalamus. (The images used here were obtained from ISMI's master clip collection, 1895 Francisco Blvd East, San Rafael, CA 94901-5506, USA.)

TSH secretion by injecting TRH has limited utility because free $T_4$ assays and sensitive TSH assays are readily available[27] (see Chap. 33). Direct measurement of serum TRH is not yet clinically feasible.

## PITUITARY GLAND

TSH is a glycoprotein synthesized in the anterior pituitary gland. It has a molecular mass of 28 kDa and is composed of two subunits, designated as the α and β chains, whose bioactivity may depend on the attached carbohydrate moiety. This two-subunit structure is similar to that of follicle-stimulating hormone, luteinizing hormone, and human chorionic gonadotropin (see Chaps. 11, 15, and 16); in fact, these regulatory hormones all share a common structure for the α subunit. Excess α subunit is synthesized by the pituitary cells. The rate-limiting step in TSH synthesis is production of the β subunit, which also confers specificity in stimulation of target organs.

Only intact TSH is routinely measured in the serum, but measurement of subunits may be useful in syndromes of inappropriate TSH secretion. TSH-producing pituitary tumors may be associated with disproportionately elevated serum α-subunit levels (see Chaps. 15 and 42).

Two major factors regulate TSH synthesis and secretion: inhibitory, negative feedback at the anterior pituitary, from circulating thyroid hormones and hypothalamic mediators, such as somatostatin and dopamine; and stimulation by TRH from the hypothalamus (see Fig. 30-3).

High circulating levels of $T_4$ or $T_3$ suppress TSH synthesis and release by negative feedback. Either excess endogenous hormone from primary hyperthyroidism or exogenous $T_4$ or $T_3$ from hormone administration should lead to low serum TSH levels; otherwise, a measurable TSH concentration in the face of elevated levels of free $T_4$ and $T_3$ is considered inappropriately elevated and may suggest a TSH-secreting pituitary tumor. Physiologically, small changes in the levels of free $T_4$ or $T_3$ lead to a small inverse-logarithmic change in serum TSH concentration, sufficient to return the free hormone level to its prior level.[26] These changes in TSH between 0.1 and 10.0 mU/L have been inversely correlated with free $T_4$ and a 15% change in resting energy expenditure.[28]

Intrapituitary $T_3$ and, thus, TSH regulation are derived principally by 5'D-II (see Table 30-3) from circulating $T_4$. TSH, therefore, may be seen to rise if serum $T_4$ is decreased, even though serum $T_3$ is in the normal or slightly elevated range. This situation is found during primary hypothyroidism or iodine deficiency, in which the TSH-secretion rate may increase 20-fold (see Chap. 45). However, with excess $T_3$ administration, TSH secretion and thyroidal iodine uptake can be greatly inhibited; this inhibition is the basis for the $T_3$ suppression test (see Chap. 33). Consequently, most $T_3$ used by the pituitary is generated locally. This is in contrast to most other human tissues, which obtain their supplies of $T_3$ from the circulation. A noted exception is the brown adipose tissue that is found in human infants and in both adult and infant rodents, which has a high activity of 5'D-II.

## THYROID GLAND

Production of $T_3$ and $T_4$ by the thyroid gland is regulated primarily by circulating TSH. A small fraction of thyroidal activity and $T_4$ release, however, has been described as non–TSH dependent. TSH binds to specific membrane receptors on the surface of thyroid cells, activates intracellular adenylate cyclase, and mediates most of its action through increased cyclic adenosine monophosphate. This receptor may also be engaged by proteins found in autoimmune thyroid disease that activate or block postreceptor effects (see Chaps. 196 and 197). TSH stimulation induces thyroid growth and differentiation and all phases of iodine metabolism from uptake to secretion of $T_3$ and $T_4$. In addition, there is some autoregulation of thyroid cells by iodide; however, the principal regulation of the thyroid gland is from the pituitary. Recombinant human TSH, which has now been commercially manufactured and has a longer half-life than endogenous TSH, increases serum Tg, $T_4$, and $T_3$ after its administration to normal volunteers.[4] This difference is probably due to increased sialylation of the recombinant form. When available for clinical use, recombinant human TSH will expand our understanding of thyroid gland responses to TSH and be of major benefit in the management of thyroid cancer patients.

## PERIPHERAL THYROID METABOLISM

Many disease states result in decreased $T_4$ to $T_3$ conversion.[11,13] Although $T_3$ levels may be markedly depressed, serum TSH does not rise in this setting. A dissociation of peripheral (hepatic, 5'D-I) and central (pituitary, 5'D-II) generation of $T_3$, as outlined in Table 30-3, or tissue specific hormone uptake,[19] may help explain this observation. Very severe NTI may depress total $T_4$ to nearly undetectable levels and elevate free $T_4$, which suggests a decreased binding to carrier proteins (see Chap. 36). Intracellular free $T_3$ binds to several types of specific nuclear receptors. These receptors may activate or inactivate postreceptor responses depending on the isoform of the receptor (see Chap. 31). The intracellular free $T_3$ concentration is mediated by both passive and active tissue uptake, possible conjugation and deiodination locally, and efflux of $T_3$ from the tissue.[1,29] These combined mechanisms allow for a diverse tissue specific delivery and effect of thyroid hormones. One contribution to tissue heterogeneity is the uncoupling protein-3 (UCP-3), which may be linked to some metabolic actions of $T_3$.[30] Therefore, it is not surprising to find

thyroid hormone analogs that have augmented hepatic and skeletal effects when compared with equivalent changes in serum TSH caused by thyroxine.[31] This type of physiology may be analogous to the tissue specific effects of estrogen receptor agonists and antagonists. Increased tissue requirements of thyroid hormones may occur during pregnancy in hypothyroid women[32] and also may occur with extensive exercise.[33] These variations in normal physiology depend on energy balance, tissue hormone use, and systemic and local responses, so that thyroid hormone delivery can fluctuate over a wide range (see Chap. 36).

## REFERENCES

1. Cavalieri RR. Iodine metabolism and thyroid physiology: current concepts. Thyroid 1997; 7:177.
2. Hollowell JG, Staehling NW, Hannon H, et al. Iodine nutrition in the United States. Trends and public health implications: iodine excretion data from National Health and Nutrition Examination Surveys I and III (1971–1974 and 1988–1994). J Clin Endocrinol Metab 1998; 83:3401.
3. Kaptein EM. Thyroid hormone metabolism and thyroid disease in chronic renal failure. Endocr Rev 1996; 17:45.
4. Ramirez L, Braverman LE, White B, Emerson CH. Recombinant human thyrotropin is a potent stimulator of thyroid function in normal subjects. J Clin Endocrinol Metab 1997; 82:2836.
5. Danforth E, Burger AG. The impact of nutrition on thyroid hormone physiology and action. Annu Rev Nutr 1989; 9:201.
6. Berry MJ, Larsen PR. The role of selenium in thyroid hormone action. Endocr Rev 1992; 13:207.
7. Arntzenius AB, Smit LJ, Schipper J, et al. Inverse relation between iodine intake and thyroid blood flow: color doppler flow imaging in euthyroid humans. J Clin Endocrinol Metab 1991; 73:1051.
8. Dai G, Levy O, Carrasco N. Cloning and characterization of the thyroid iodide transporter. Nature 1996; 379:458.
9. Tonacchera M, Chiovato L, Pinchera A, et al. Hyperfunctioning thyroid nodules in toxic multinodular goiter share activating thyrotropin receptor mutations with solitary toxic adenoma. J Clin Endocrinol Metab 1998; 83:492.
10. Burmeister LA, Goumaz MO, Mariash CN, Oppenheimer JH. Levothyroxine dose requirements for thyrotropin suppression in the treatment of differentiated thyroid cancer. J Clin Endocrinol Metab 1992; 75:344.
11. Engler D, Burger AG. The deiodination of the iodothyronines and of their derivatives in man. Endocrine Rev 1984; 5:151.
12. LoPresti JS, Gray D, Nicoloff JT. Influence of fasting and refeeding on 3,3',5'-triiodothyronine metabolism in man. J Clin Endocrinol Metab 1991; 72:130.
13. Kaptein EM, Kaptein JS, Chang EI, et al. Thyroxine transfer and distribution in critical nonthyroidal illnesses, chronic renal failure, and chronic ethanol abuse. J Clin Endocrinol Metab 1987; 65:606.
13a. Schussler GC. The thyroxine binding proteins. Thyroid 2000; 10:141.
14. Robbins J. Thyroid hormone transport proteins and the physiology of hormone binding. In: Braverman LE, Utiger RD, eds. Werner and Ingbar's the thyroid: a fundamental and clinical text, 7th ed. Philadelphia: Lippincott–Raven, 1996:96.
15. Schreiber G, Southwell BR, Richardson SJ. Hormone delivery systems to the brain-transthyretin. Exp Clin Endocrinol Diabetes 1995; 103:75.
16. Bianchi R, Iervasi G, Pilo A, et al. Role of serum carrier proteins in the peripheral metabolism and tissue distribution of thyroid hormones in familial dysalbuminemic hyperthyroxinemia and congenital elevation of thyroxine-binding globulin. J Clin Invest 1987; 80:522.
17. Mol JA, Visser TJ. Rapid and selective inner ring deiodination of thyroxine sulfate by rat liver deiodinase. Endocrinology 1985; 117:8.
18. LoPresti JS, Nicoloff JT. 3,5,3'-Triiodothyronine ($T_3$) sulfate: a major metabolite in $T_3$ metabolism in man. J Clin Endocrinol Metab 1994; 78:688.
19. Everts ME, deJong M, Lim C, et al. Different regulation of thyroid hormone transport in liver and pituitary: its possible role in the maintenance of low $T_3$ production during nonthyroidal illness and fasting in man. Thyroid 1996; 6:359.
20. Croteau W, Davey JC, Galton VA, St Germain DL. Cloning of the mammalian type II iodothyronine deiodinase. A selenoprotein differentially expressed and regulated in human and rat brain and other tissues. J Clin Invest 1996; 98:405.
21. Croteau W, Whittemore SL, Schneider MJ, St Germain DL. Cloning and expression of a cDNA for mammalian type III iodothyronine deiodinase. J Biol Chem 1995; 270:16569.
22. Solomon BL, Wartofsky L, Burman KD. Adjunctive cholestyramine therapy for thyrotoxicosis. Clin Endocrinol 1993; 38:39.
23. Reed HL. Environmental influences on thyroid hormone regulation. In: Braverman LE, Utiger RD, eds. Werner and Ingbar's the thyroid: a fundamental and clinical text, 7th ed. Philadelphia: Lippincott–Raven, 1996:259.
24. Greenspan SL, Klibanski A, Rowe JW, Elahi D. Age-related alterations in pulsatile secretion of TSH: role of dopaminergic regulation. Am J Physiol 1991; 260:E486.

25. Maes M, Mommen K, Hendrickx D, et al. Components of biological variation, including seasonality, in blood concentrations of TSH, $TT_3$, $FT_4$, PRL, cortisol and testosterone in healthy volunteers. Clin Endocrinol (Oxf) 1997; 46:587.

26. Morley JE. Neuroendocrine control of thyrotropin secretion. Endocr Rev 1981; 2:396.

27. Spencer CA, LoPresti JS, Patel A, et al. Applications of a new chemiluminometric thyrotropin assay to subnormal measurement. J Clin Endocrinol Metab 1990; 70:453.

28. al-Adsani H, Hoffer LJ, Silva JE. Resting energy expenditure is sensitive to small dose changes in patients on chronic thyroid hormone replacement. J Clin Endocrinol Metab 1997; 82:1118.

29. Ribeiro RC, Cavalieri RR, Lomri N, et al. Thyroid hormone export regulates cellular hormone content and response. J Biol Chem 1996; 271:17147.

30. Freake HC. Uncoupling proteins: beyond brown adipose tissue. Nutr Rev 1998; 56:185.

31. Sherman SI, Ringel MD, Smith MJ, et al. Augmented hepatic and skeletal thyromimetic effects of tiratricol in comparison with levothyroxine. J Clin Endocrinol Metab 1997; 82:2153.

32. Mandel SJ, Larsen PR, Seely EW, Brent GA. Increased need for thyroxine during pregnancy in women with primary hypothyroidism. N Engl J Med 1990; 323:91.

33. Rone JK, Dons RF, Reed HL. The effect of endurance training on serum triiodothyronine kinetics in man: physical conditioning marked by enhanced thyroid hormone metabolism. Clin Endocrinol 1992; 37:325.

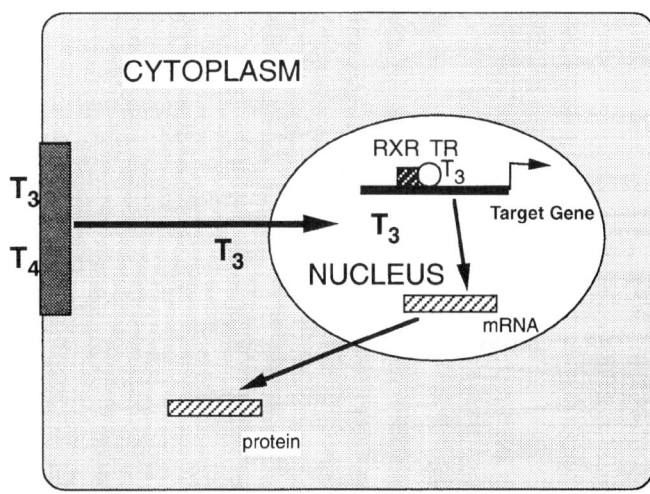

**FIGURE 31-1.** General model for thyroid hormone action in the nucleus. (*mRNA*, messenger RNA; *RXR*, retinoid X receptor; *TR*, thyroid-hormone receptor; $T_3$, triiodothyronine; $T_4$, thyroxine.)

# CHAPTER 31

# THYROID PHYSIOLOGY: HORMONE ACTION, RECEPTORS, AND POSTRECEPTOR EVENTS

PAUL M. YEN

## TARGET GENE REGULATION BY THYROID HORMONE

The effects of thyroid hormone (TH; L-thyroxine, $T_4$; L-triiodothyronine, $T_3$) on cellular growth, development, and metabolism are legion and diverse. TH exerts its major effects at the genomic level; however, examples have been found of nongenomic action in the cytoplasm, plasma membrane, and mitochondrion.[1] Early studies clearly demonstrated that TH could bind to nuclear sites and stimulate transcription and translation of new proteins.[2] These early studies led to a model for genomic TH action for which the general features have been confirmed, but for which much refinement has occurred as the molecular details of TH action have been elucidated. As seen in Figure 31-1, circulating free TH enters the cell by passive diffusion, and in some tissues is converted from $T_4$ to the more biologically potent $T_3$ by deiodinase activity. TH then enters the nucleus and specifically binds to nuclear thyroid-hormone receptors (TRs). TRs have been shown to be intimately associated with chromatin, and ligand binding to TRs stimulates transcription of target genes and protein synthesis in a concentration- and time-dependent manner.

This model of TH action is based on the notion that the amount of $T_3$ binding to nuclear receptors correlates with gene activation. In the euthyroid rat, research has shown that ~50% of $T_3$ nuclear receptors are bound to TH.[2] In the hyperthyroid state, a corresponding increase in $T_3$ occupancy is seen. In general, receptor occupancy correlates well with gene activation for those genes that have been characterized.

Approximately 30 genes have been described that are regulated by TH.[3] Most of these genes are positively regulated, but interestingly, some genes are negatively regulated by TH. A partial list of some of the better-characterized genes, which have contributed to our understanding of TH action, is included in Table 31-1. Transcriptional regulation by TH can occur via effects on the rate of transcription (rate of nuclear RNA synthesis) and/or stabilization of mRNA. In most cases, TH appears to regulate the transcriptional rate directly, although TH can modulate mRNA stability in certain instances (e.g., malic enzyme and thyroid-stimulating hormone β subunit [TSH-β] genes).[4,5]

## THYROID-HORMONE RECEPTORS AND THEIR STRUCTURE

Two related TRs, which have been identified, bind TH with high affinity and specificity[6,7]; these TRs, initially called c-*erb*As, are protooncogenes of a previously described viral oncogene product, v-*erb*A, that causes erythroblastosis in chicks. On the basis of amino-acid sequence homology and similarity in the organization of functional domains of receptors, TRs belong to a large superfamily of nuclear-hormone receptors that include the steroid hormone, vitamin D, and retinoic acid receptors.

Like the other family members, TRs contain a central DNA-binding domain with two "zinc finger" motifs and a carboxy-terminal ligand-binding domain[8,9] (Fig. 31-2). The ligand-binding domain is important for ligand binding and also for transactivation and dimerization. X-ray crystallographic studies of liganded

**TABLE 31-1.**
**Genes Regulated by Thyroid Hormone**

**POSITIVELY REGULATED BY $T_3$**

Sarcoplasmic reticulum calcium ATPase

α-Myosin heavy chain

Spot 14

Malic enzyme

Myelin basic protein

Rat growth hormone

Chicken lysozyme silencer

**NEGATIVELY REGULATED BY $T_3$**

μ-Glycoprotein hormone α subunit

TSH-β subunit

β-Myosin heavy chain

$T_3$, triiodothyronine; *ATPase*, adenosine triphosphatase; *TSH*, thyroid-stimulating hormone.

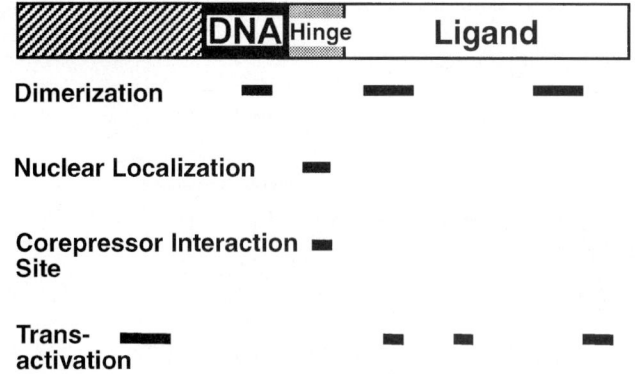

**FIGURE 31-2.** General organization of major thyroid-hormone receptor domains and functional subregions.

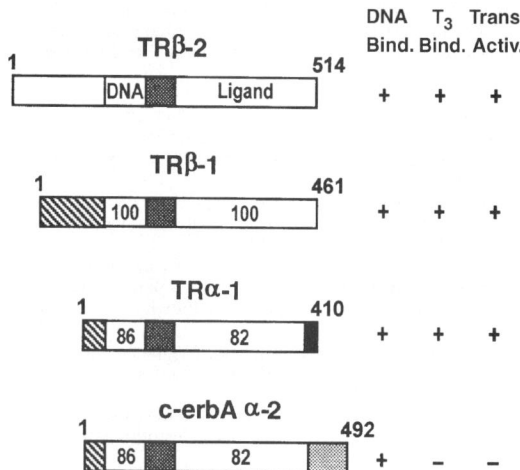

**FIGURE 31-3.** Comparison of amino-acid homologies and their functional properties among thyroid-hormone receptor (*TR*) isoforms; length of receptors is indicated just above receptor diagrams and percentage amino-acid homology with TRβ-2 is included within the receptor diagrams. ($T_3$, triiodothyronine.)

TR have shown that TH is embedded in a hydrophobic pocket flanked by discontinuous stretches of the ligand-binding domain.[10] A subregion important for transcriptional activation (AF-2)[11,12] also exists at the extreme carboxy terminus. This subregion is highly conserved within the nuclear-hormone receptor superfamily and appears to undergo a major conformational change on ligand binding.[11,12] The ligand-binding domain contains at least nine hydrophobic, heptad repeats, which potentially may be involved in TR homo- and heterodimerization.[13] Mutations in the ninth heptad region abrogates TR heterodimerization, thus suggesting that this may be a particularly important region for dimerization. The hinge region between the DNA- and TH-binding domains contains a nuclear-localization motif common among nuclear-hormone receptors.[8,9] However, unlike steroid-hormone receptors, which associate with cytoplasmic heat shock proteins in the absence of ligand, TRs are localized predominantly in the nucleus and bind DNA even in the absence of ligand.

## THYROID-HORMONE RECEPTOR ISOFORMS

There are two genes encoding TRs, α and β, which are located on human chromosomes 17 and 3.[8,9] These genes encode TR isoforms (TRs α-1, β-1, β-2) that bind $T_3$ with similar affinity (reported dissociation constant [$K_d$] between $10^{-10}$ to $10^{-11}$ mol/L) and mediate TH-regulated gene expression. These TR isoforms range from 400 to slightly more than 500 amino acids in size.[8,9] The DNA-binding and ligand-binding domains are highly conserved among the isoforms and also among different mammalian species (Fig. 31-3). By alternative splicing, the TRβ gene generates two mRNAs that encode two proteins: TRα-1 and c-*erb*A α-2, which differ only in the coding region of the last exon (see Fig. 31-3). Because this region is critical for ligand binding, c-*erb*A α-2 cannot bind TH. In cotransfection experiments, c-*erb*A α-2 blocks the transcriptional activity of TRs, so this alternative splice product may antagonize TR action.

The TRβ gene encodes two TRs, TRβ-1 and TRβ-2, that are generated by alternative promoter choice and/or mRNA splicing.[8,9] These receptors have different amino-terminal regions but are otherwise identical. They appear to have similar TH binding affinity and transcriptional activity. TRα-1 and TRβ-1 are expressed in almost all tissues; in contrast, TRβ-2 is selectively expressed in the anterior pituitary gland and specific areas of the hypothalamus, as well as in the developing brain and inner ear.[14]

The specific roles of these isoforms are poorly understood. Cotransfection and knockout-mouse studies suggest that many TH-regulated effects are redundant and may be regulated by either TRα or TRβ. However, some studies suggest that TRβ-2 may be involved in the negative regulation of anterior-pituitary genes such as TSH-β,[15] and that TRβ may play important roles in brain and inner ear development.[14] During development, important differences are seen in the timing of expression of these iso-

forms, as TRα-1 mRNA is expressed in the rat fetal brain whereas TRβ-1 mRNA is induced in the brain just before birth.[2]

The regulation of the TR mRNAs is isoform- and cell-type dependent. In the intact rat pituitary, $T_3$ decreases TRβ-2 mRNA, modestly decreases TRα-1 mRNA, and slightly increases rat TRβ-1 mRNA.[16] This results in a 30% decrease in total $T_3$ binding in the $T_3$-treated rat pituitary. In other rat tissues, $T_3$ slightly decreases TRα-1 and c-erb α-2 mRNA except in the brain, where c-erbA α-2 levels are not affected. TRβ-1 mRNA is affected minimally in nonpituitary tissues. In patients with nonthyroidal illness who have decreased free $T_3$ and $T_4$ serum levels, increased TRα and TRβ mRNA levels have been observed in peripheral mononuclear cells and liver biopsy specimens.[17] Thus, induction of TR expression may compensate for decreased circulating TH levels in some of these patients.

## THYROID HORMONE RESPONSE ELEMENTS

TRs are ligand-dependent transcription factors that bind to distinct DNA sequences, generally in the promoter region of target genes. TRs frequently positively regulate target genes by stimulating gene transcription in the presence of TH; however, they also can negatively regulate transcription of certain genes (e.g., TSH-β, a glycoprotein subunit, and thyrotropin-releasing hormone). In vitro binding and functional analyses of thyroid hormone response elements (TREs) from positively regulated target genes have demonstrated that TREs generally contain a hexamer half-site sequence of AGGT(C/A)A arranged as two or more tandem repeats.[3] Similar to steroid-hormone receptors, TRs bind to TREs as dimers. However, unlike steroid-hormone receptors, which bind to two well-conserved palindromic half-sites, TRs bind to TREs that vary in their primary nucleotide sequence as well as the number, spacing, and orientation of their half-sites.[3,9,18] In particular, TRs bind to TREs in which half-sites are arranged as direct repeats, inverted palindromes, and palindromes (Fig. 31-4). Of the ~30 natural TREs that have been characterized, most are arranged as direct repeats, followed by inverted palindromes, and then palindromes. In simple TREs containing two half-sites, the optimal spacings of half-sites in these arrangements are four, six, and zero nucleotides, respectively.[3,8,9,18] Several studies have shown that flanking sequences around the half-sites also can contribute to transcriptional activity.[18]

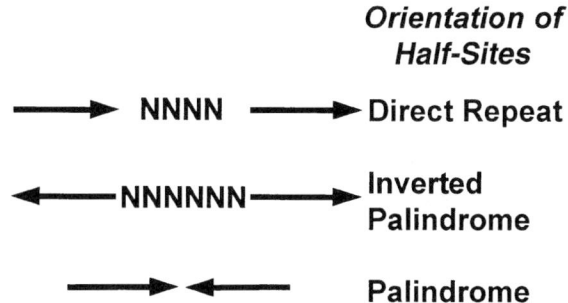

***Orientation of
Half-Sites***

NNNN → Direct Repeat

←NNNNNN→ Inverted Palindrome

Palindrome

**FIGURE 31-4.** Half-site orientations and optimal nucleotide spacing between half-sites. *N* refers to nucleotides and arrows indicate directions to half-sites on the sense strand.

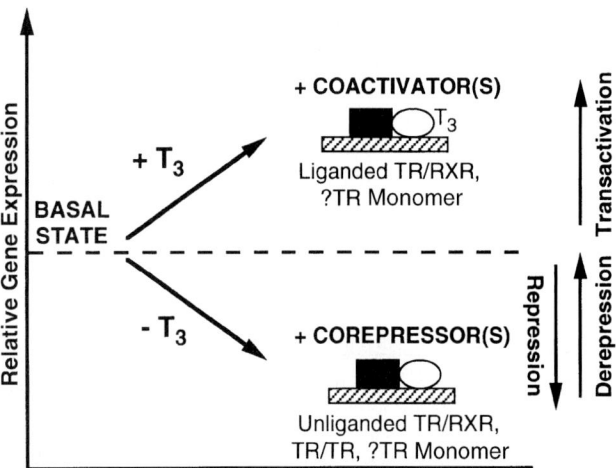

**FIGURE 31-5.** Model for repression, derepression, and transcriptional activation by thyroid-hormone receptor (*TR*). (*RXR*, retinoid X receptor; $T_3$, triiodothyronine.)

## THYROID-HORMONE RECEPTOR BINDING TO THYROID HORMONE RESPONSE ELEMENTS

TRs bind to TREs as monomers, dimers, and heterodimers in vitro.[8,9,18] However, the functional roles of these putative complexes in transcriptional regulation are not well understood. Although TRs can form heterodimers with several other family members on TREs, their major heterodimer partner appears to be the retinoid X receptor (RXR), which bears some amino-acid homology with the retinoic acid receptor and binds 9-*cis* retinoic acid.[8,9,18] At least three major isoforms of RXR exist, so possibly different TR/RXR-isoform complexes may have differential affinities for TREs and/or abilities to transactivate target genes.

TR/RXR heterodimers are likely to be involved in TH-mediated transcriptional regulation. In in vitro experiments, $T_3$ caused rapid dissociation of TR homodimers from TREs (direct repeats and inverted palindrome) but had little effect on the binding of TR/RXR heterodimer to TREs,[9] results which suggest that the latter complexes may be involved in transcriptional activation. On the other hand, both TR homo- and heterodimers bind to TREs in the absence of ligand and, thus, could be involved in repression of basal transcription by TRs (see the following).

## REPRESSION OF BASAL TRANSCRIPTION/COREPRESSORS

Unliganded TRs bind to TREs and can repress transcription of positively regulated target genes (Fig. 31-5). Although the physiologic significance of this basal repression is not known, it may influence target-gene expression during early fetal development when the fetal thyroid gland is incapable of producing TH. The basal repression may be due, in part, to interactions with the basal transcription machinery as unliganded TRs can interact with transcription factor IIB (TFIIB), a key component of the basal transcription complex.[19] However, several laboratories have cloned proteins that interact with TR and retinoic acid receptor (RAR) in the absence of their cognate ligands.[11,12] These proteins repressed basal transcription by TR and RAR and have been termed *corepressors*. One of these corepressors is a 270-kDa protein termed *nuclear-receptor corepressor* (N-CoR). It has two transferable repression domains and a carboxy-terminal α-helical interaction domain. A truncated version of N-CoR, N-CoRi, which is missing the repressor region, also has been identified and may represent an alternative-splice variant of N-CoR.[20] This protein blocks basal repression by N-CoR and thus may serve as a natural antagonist for N-CoR. Another corepressor, silencing mediator for RAR and TR (SMRT), is a 168-kDa protein that has some homology with N-CoR.[11,12]

The hinge region of TR (located between the DNA- and ligand-binding domains) is important for interactions with corepressors. Mutations in this region decrease interactions with corepressors and abrogate basal repression, without affecting transcriptional activation.[11,12] Several groups showed that corepressors can complex with another putative corepressor, mSin3, and histone deacetylase.[21,22] These findings suggest that local histone deacetylation may play an important role in basal repression by altering the local chromatin structure near the minimal promoter region (where transcription is initiated).

In negatively regulated target genes, ligand-independent activation of transcription occurs in the absence of TH.[23,24] This activation may determine a "set point" from which ligand-dependent negative regulation begins. The mechanism of the ligand-independent activation is not known but may also involve TR interaction with corepressors.[20,23]

## TRANSCRIPTIONAL ACTIVATION BY THYROID HORMONE COACTIVATORS

Many factors potentially can modulate TH-mediated transcription. These include variability among TR isoforms, TR complexes, heterodimerization partners, nature of TREs, and TR phosphorylation state.[8,23a,23b] These factors likely influence interactions of liganded TR with TR-associated nuclear proteins called *coactivators*. Several such proteins have been identified that interact with liganded TR and enhance TH-mediated transcriptional activation.[11,12] A 160-kDa protein called *steroid receptor coactivator-1* (SRC-1)[25] has been identified that interacts with steroid-hormone receptors and TR. SRC-1 mRNA undergoes alternative splicing to generate multiple SRC-1 isoforms, although the functional significance of these SRC-1 isoforms currently is not known.[26] Several other 160-kDa proteins also interact with liganded nuclear-hormone receptors and TRs, as well as share partial sequence homology with SRC-1. These findings suggest that a family of coactivators related to SRC-1 may exist.[11,12] Some studies have suggested that interaction of coactivators with nuclear-hormone receptors involves the carboxy-terminal AF-2 subregion, although other subregions of the TR ligand-binding domain also may be involved.

As seen in Figure 31-6, these putative coactivators have several common features. First, multiple putative nuclear-hormone receptor interaction sites are present, which have a signature LXXLL sequence motif.[11,12] Several coactivators also have a polyglutamine region, similar to that found in androgen receptors. In addition, a bHLH motif is seen in the amino-terminal region, suggesting that these coactivators may bind to DNA. Also

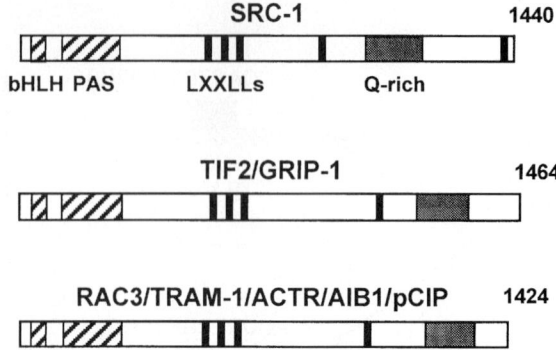

**FIGURE 31-6.** Comparison of the organization and structure of putative nuclear-hormone receptor coactivators. (*SRC-1*, steroid receptor coactivator-1; *TIF-2*, transcription intermediary factor 2; *GRIP-1*, glucocorticoid receptor interacting protein; *RAC-3*, receptor-associated coactivator 3; *TRAM-1*, thyroid receptor activator molecule 1; *ACTR*, activator of thyroid receptor; *AIB-1*, amplified in breast-1; *PCIP*, p300/CBP cointegrator-associated protein.)

located in this region is the PAS (Per/Arnt/Sim) domain, which is shared by a number of hypothalamic genes that regulate circadian rhythm and may serve as a dimer interface with other cofactors. Finally, in addition to the SRC-1 family, other cofactors may be associated with liganded TR.[11,12,27] The functional roles of these proteins are not well understood.

SRC-1 can interact with the cyclic AMP response element binding protein (CREB)–binding protein (CBP), the putative coactivator for cyclic adenosine monophosphate–stimulated transcription as well as the related protein, p300, which interacts with the viral coactivator E1A.[11,12] These proteins might serve as integrator molecules for different signaling inputs such as protein kinase A- and C-pathway–mediated transcription as well as bridge-liganded TRs with other adapter molecules and/or the basal transcriptional machinery[11,12,28] (see Fig. 31-6). In addition, TRs, coactivators, CBP, and the histone acetylase, p300, and CBP-associated factor (PCAF) can form a complex that can remodel local chromatin structure. Indeed, CBP and PCAF as well as SRC-1[11,12] have intrinsic histone acetylase activity, although the histone substrates are different for these proteins.

## MODEL OF THYROID-HORMONE RECEPTOR ACTION

On the basis of these findings, a model for the mechanism of basal repression and transcriptional activation has emerged (Fig. 31-7). When ligand is absent, TR homodimers or TR/RXR heterodimers bind to the TRE and complex with corepressor, which, in turn, interacts with mSin3 or a related protein, and histone deacetylase. This complex may keep surrounding histones deacetylated and maintain chromatin near the TRE in a transcriptionally repressed state. When ligand is present, the TR/corepressor complex dissociates and is replaced by a coactivator complex that likely contains CBP and the histone acetylase p300/CBP associated factor (PCAF). These changes result in remodeling of chromatin structure and nucleosome positioning. The subsequent recruitment of RNA polymerase II to the transcription initiation site within the minimal promoter results in transcriptional activation. This model is probably an oversimplification as other proteins likely exist that form the TR/coactivator complex,[29,30] which may interact directly with the basal-transcriptional machinery or other transcription factors. The identities of these proteins and their protein/protein interactions remain to be elucidated.

Our understanding of TR action has grown at an accelerating pace and has shed light on both nuclear-hormone receptor action

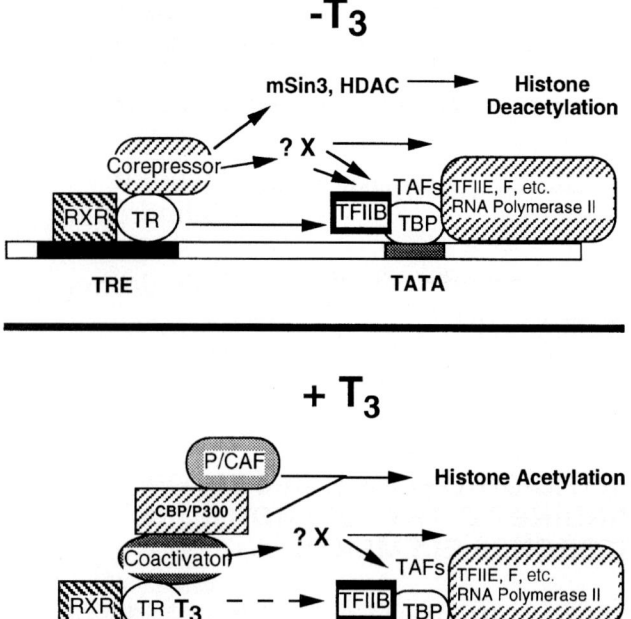

**FIGURE 31-7.** Molecular model for basal repression in the absence of triiodothyronine ($T_3$) and transcriptional activation in the presence of $T_3$. X refers to possible additional cofactors that remain to be identified. (See text for details.) (*HDAC*, histone deacetylase; *TAF*, TBP-associated factors; *TFIIE*, transcription factor IIE; *RXR*, retinoid X receptor; *TR*, thyroid-hormone receptor; *TFIIB*, transcription factor IIB; *TBP*, TATA-binding protein; *TRE*, thyroid hormone response element; *TATA*, tumor-associated transplantation antigen; *P/CAF*, p300/CBP associated factor; *CBP*, CREB-binding protein.)

and general mechanisms of transcriptional regulation.[31a] As more of the molecular details of TR action have become known, so has the molecular basis of human diseases that involve TRs and coactivators. As is discussed in the next chapter (Chap. 32), mutations of TRβ-1 have been associated with resistance to TH, an autosomal disorder in which patients have elevated serum concentrations of TH and inappropriately normal thyrotropin levels. Almost all of these patients have mutations in the TRβ-1 ligand-binding domain that decrease TH-binding affinity but still allow the TR to bind to DNA.[31] These receptors block the transcriptional activity of wild-type receptors (dominant negative activity). These mutant receptors may have defects in corepressor release and interactions with coactivators.[32,33] In addition, mutations in CBP have been associated with Rubinstein-Taybi syndrome, a congenital neurologic disorder.[34] Last, amplification and overexpression of the coactivator AIB-1 may be associated with primary human breast cancer.[35] New knowledge of TR action should provide further insight into the molecular basis of these and other diseases involving nuclear-hormone receptors.

## REFERENCES

1. Davis PJ, Davis FB. Nongenomic actions of thyroid hormone. Thyroid 1996; 6:497.
2. Oppenheimer J, Schwartz H, Strait K. An integrated view of thyroid hormone actions in vivo. In: Weintraub B, ed. Molecular endocrinology: basic concepts and clinical correlations. New York: Raven Press, 1995:249.
3. Williams G, Brent G. Thyroid hormone response elements. In: Weintraub B, ed. Molecular endocrinology: basic concepts and clinical correlations. New York: Raven Press, 1995:217.
4. Leedman PJ, Stein AR, Chin WW. Regulated specific protein binding to a conserved region of the 3'- untranslated region of thyrotropin beta-subunit mRNA. Mol Endocrinol 1995; 9:375.

5. Oppenheimer J, Schwartz H, Mariash C, et al. Advances in our understanding of thyroid hormone action at the cellular level. Endocr Rev 1987; 8:288.

6. Weinberger C, Thompson C, Ong E, et al. The c-erbA gene encodes a thyroid hormone receptor. Nature 1986; 324:641.

7. Sap J, Munoz A, Damm K, Vennstrom B. The c-erbA protein is a high affinity receptor for thyroid hormone. Nature 1986; 324:635.

8. Lazar M. Recent progress in understanding thyroid hormone action. Thyroid Today 1997; 20:1.

9. Yen P, Chin W. New advances in understanding the molecular mechanisms of thyroid hormone action. Trends Endocrinol Metab 1994; 5:65.

10. Wagner R, Apriletti J, McGrath M, et al. A structural role for hormone in the thyroid hormone receptor. Nature 1995; 378:690.

11. Torchia J, Glass C, Rosenfeld M. Co-activators and co-repressors in the integration of transcriptional responses. Curr Opin Cell Biol 1998; 10:373.

12. McKenna N, Lanz R, O'Malley B. Nuclear receptor co-regulators. Cell Mol Biol 1999; 20:321.

13. Forman B, Yang C, Au M, et al. A domain continuing leucine-zipper-like motifs mediate novel in vivo interactions between the thyroid hormone and retinoic acid receptors. Mol Endocrinol 1989; 3:1610.

14. Forrest D, Golarai G, Connor J, Curran T. Genetic analysis of thyroid hormone receptors in development and disease. Recent Prog Horm Res 1996; 51:1.

15. Langlois MF, Zanger K, Monden T, et al. A unique role of the beta thyroid hormone receptor isoform in negative regulation by thyroid hormone. Mapping of a novel amino-terminal domain important for ligand-independent activation. J Biol Chem 1997; 272:24927.

16. Hodin R, Lazar M, Chin W. Differential and tissue-specific regulation of the multiple rat c-erbA mRNA species by thyroid hormone. J Clin Invest 1990; 85:101.

17. Williams G, Franklyn J, Neuberger J, Sheppard M. Thyroid hormone receptor expression in the "sick euthyroid" syndrome. Lancet 1989; 2:1477.

18. Glass C. Differential recognition of target genes by nuclear receptor monomers, dimers and heterodimers. Endocr Rev 1994; 15:391.

19. Baniahmad A, Ha I, Reinberg D, et al. Interaction of human thyroid hormone receptor β with transcription factor TFIIB may mediate target gene derepression and activation by thyroid hormone. Proc Natl Acad Sci U S A 1993; 90:8832.

20. Hollenberg A, Monden T, Madura J, et al. Function of nuclear co-repressor protein on thyroid hormone response elements is regulated by the receptor A/B domain. J Biol Chem 1996; 271:28516.

21. Alland L, Muhle R, Hou H Jr, et al. Role for N-CoR and histone deacetylase in Sin3-mediated transcriptional repression. Nature 1997; 387:49.

22. Heinzel T, Lavinsky RM, Mullen TM, et al. A complex containing N-CoR, mSin3 and histone deacetylase mediates transcriptional repression. Nature 1997; 387:43.

23. Tagami T, Madison LD, Nagaya T, Jameson JL. Nuclear receptor corepressors activate rather than suppress basal transcription of genes that are negatively regulated by thyroid hormone. Mol Cell Biol 1997; 17:2642.

23a. Takeda T, Nagasawa T, Miyamoto T, et al. Quantitative analysis of DNA binding affinity and dimerization properties of wild-type and mutant thyroid hormone receptor β1. Thyroid 2000; 10:11.

23b. Forrest D, Vennström B. Functions of thyroid hormone receptors in mice. Thyroid 2000; 10:11.

24. Hollenberg A, Monden T, Flynn T, et al. The human thyrotropin-releasing hormone gene is regulated by thyroid hormone through two distinct classes of negative thyroid hormone response elements. Mol Endocrinol 1995; 9:540.

25. Onate S, Tsai S, Tsai M, O'Malley B. Sequence and characterization of a coactivator for the steroid hormone receptor superfamily. Science 1995; 270:1354.

26. Kamei Y, Xu L, Heinzel T, et al. A CBP integrator complex mediates transcriptional activation and AP-1 inhibition by nuclear receptors. Cell 1996; 85:403.

27. Lee J, Choi H, Gyuris J, et al. Two classes of proteins dependent on either the presence or absence of thyroid hormone for interaction with the thyroid hormone receptor. Mol Endocrinol 1995; 9:243.

28. Korzus E, Torchia J, Rose DW, et al. Transcription factor–specific requirements for coactivators and their acetyltransferase functions. Science 1998; 279:703.

29. Fondell J, Ge J, Roeder R. Ligand induction of a transcriptionally active thyroid hormone receptor coactivator complex. Proc Natl Acad Sci U S A 1996; 93:8329.

30. Freedman L. Increasing the complexity of coactivation in nuclear receptor signaling. Cell 1999; 97:5.

31. Refetoff S, Weiss R, Usala S. The syndromes of resistance to thyroid hormone. Endocr Rev 1993; 14:348.

31a. Pohlenz J, Manders L, Sadow PM, et al. A novel point mutation in cluster 3 of the thyroid hormone receptor beta gene (P247L) causing mild resistance to thyroid hormone. Thyroid 1999; 9:1195.

32. Yoh SM, Chatterjee VK, Privalsky ML. Thyroid hormone resistance syndrome manifests as an aberrant interaction between mutant T$_3$ receptors and transcriptional corepressors. Mol Endocrinol 1997; 11:470.

33. Liu Y, Takeshita A, Misiti S, et al. Lack of coactivator interaction can be a mechanism for dominant negative activity by mutant thyroid hormone receptors. Endocrinology 1998; 139:4197.

34. Petrij F, Giles R, Dauwerse H, et al. Rubinstein-Taybi syndrome caused by mutations in the transcriptional co-activator CBP. Nature 1995; 376:348.

35. Anzick SL, Kononen J, Walker RL, et al. AIB1, a steroid receptor coactivator amplified in breast and ovarian cancer. Science 1997; 277:965.

# CHAPTER 32

# THYROID HORMONE RESISTANCE SYNDROMES

STEPHEN JON USALA

## CLINICAL FORMS OF RESISTANCE TO THYROID HORMONE

In 1967, a bizarre finding in two young deaf-mute patients was reported by Refetoff and coworkers.[1] These patients had delayed bone ages and stippled epiphyses consistent with juvenile hypothyroidism but, paradoxically, significantly elevated levels of circulating thyroid hormones. It was concluded that these patients had a tissue-specific combination of hypothyroidism, hyperthyroidism, and euthyroidism. Because tissues such as bone and brain were judged to lack the appropriate sensitivity to the high levels of thyroid hormone and the patients failed to manifest other common symptoms and signs of hyperthyroidism, the proposal was made that the Refetoff patients were the first examples of *thyroid hormone resistance*.

Time has validated this conclusion. Many kindreds and sporadic patients with thyroid hormone resistance syndromes have been studied. The most common form of thyroid hormone resistance is called *generalized resistance to thyroid hormone*[2] (Fig. 32-1). Patients with this form must satisfy three criteria: elevated serum levels of free thyroid hormones (i.e., free triiodothyronine [T$_3$] and free thyroxine [T$_4$]), inappropriately normal levels of serum thyroid-stimulating hormone (TSH), and clinical euthyroidism.

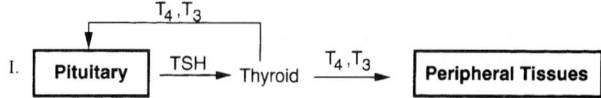

*Generalized Resistance to Thyroid Hormone*

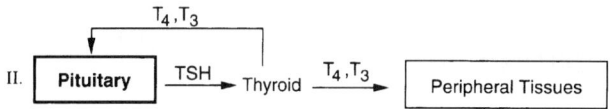

*Selective Pituitary Resistance to Thyroid Hormone*

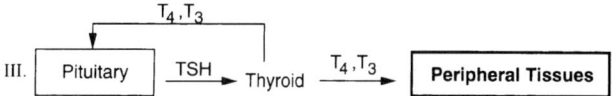

**FIGURE 32-1.** Three clinical forms of thyroid hormone resistance in humans. The first shows blockage of the biologic responses to thyroxine (*T$_4$*) and triiodothyronine (*T$_3$*) in the pituitary and peripheral tissues, which is characteristic of generalized resistance to thyroid hormone. The second shows selective blockage at the pituitary, which is characteristic of selective pituitary resistance to thyroid hormone. The third shows selective blockage at the peripheral tissues, as described in one patient with selective peripheral resistance to thyroid hormone. Patients with identical mutations in the c-*erb*Aβ thyroid-hormone receptor can present clinically with generalized or selective pituitary resistance. TSH, thyroid-stimulating hormone. (Modified from Usala SJ, Weintraub BD. Familial thyroid hormone resistance: clinical and molecular studies. In: Mazzaferri E, Kreisberg RA, Bar RS, eds. Advances in endocrinology and metabolism, vol 2. Chicago: Mosby–Year Book, 1991:59.)

Patients with the syndrome of generalized resistance to thyroid hormone manifest a proportional decrease in sensitivity to thyroid hormone in the pituitary and many of the peripheral tissues. As manifested by the Refetoff patients, the degree of tissue sensitivity to thyroid hormone may vary. In other examples, patients with generalized resistance to thyroid hormone are affected in the brain (i.e., reduced intelligence quotient resulting in part from resistance) but have no evidence of resistance in the bone compartment (i.e., normal final adult height).[2] The variable tissue resistances are reflected in the different phenotypes of generalized resistance to thyroid hormone. By definition, however, the patients lack the clinical signs and symptoms of hyperthyroidism, such as weight loss, heat intolerance, nervousness, and hyperkinesis, and the compensatory elevation of thyroid hormone is such that the patients do not have complaints of hypothyroidism. In 108 different kindreds with generalized resistance to thyroid hormone, most patients were identified after screening for goiter.[2]

A less common form of resistance is *selective pituitary resistance to thyroid hormone*, in which the sensitivity to thyroid hormone is decreased in the pituitary relative to peripheral tissues (see Fig. 32-1). Most of the patients with this syndrome have inappropriately normal TSH at elevated levels of free thyroid hormone, as in generalized resistance to thyroid hormone, but with signs and symptoms of hyperthyroidism.[2,3] The last criterion is often a subjective one; the assignment of selective pituitary resistance or generalized resistance to thyroid hormone may be less than rigorous. Because the phenotypic borders are often not sharp, differentiating selective pituitary resistance from generalized resistance to thyroid hormone can be a problem.[2,3]

Another form of resistance is *selective peripheral resistance to thyroid hormone*, which is of more theoretical than therapeutic significance.[2,4] In this form, the sensitivity of peripheral tissues to thyroid hormones is decreased relative to that of the pituitary, to the point of clinical hypothyroidism; thyrotropic resistance to thyroid hormone is nonexistent or inadequate, and the TSH secretion is not increased to compensate for the increased peripheral resistance (see Fig. 32-1). One well-studied patient taking large doses of exogenous $T_3$ had clinical hypothyroidism and suppressed TSH.[4] The possibility exists that selective peripheral resistance to thyroid hormones is more common than indicated by this one patient and escapes diagnosis. Making this diagnosis is difficult, because the markers of thyroid hormone action in humans, with the exception of TSH levels, lack quantitativeness.

## GENETIC MUTATIONS IN THYROID HORMONE RESISTANCE SYNDROMES

Generalized resistance to thyroid hormone is a genetic disease. Most reported cases belong to families with multiple affected members, and inspection of these pedigrees reveals that, in all but the original Refetoff kindred, the abnormal trait is transmitted dominantly.[2] Compelling evidence that generalized resistance to thyroid hormone is a disease of the c-erbAβ thyroid-hormone receptor gene has come from linkage studies.[2,5,6] Restriction fragment length polymorphisms (RFLPs) have been used to establish tight linkage between the β receptor gene and the syndrome of generalized resistance to thyroid hormone. Given the dominant inheritance pattern of pedigrees of generalized resistance to thyroid hormone, it was originally postulated that resistance occurred because mutant β receptors inhibited the activity of the normal β and α1 receptors (from one and two alleles, respectively).[6] This hypothesis was convincingly proved in humans from the recessive kindred that has been extensively studied by Refetoff and coworkers.[7,8] Sixty-five different mutations in the c-erbAβ gene have been identified in 115 families with either generalized or selective pituitary resistance to thyroid hormone[9] (Fig. 32-2). These mutations exist as single (i.e., heterozygous) alleles, except in the Refetoff and Bercu patients.[7,8,10,11] The majority of the c-erbAβ mutations is located in the penultimate and final exons of the gene and reduce $T_3$-binding affinity; these mutations cluster

within two hot spots in the $T_3$-binding domain between amino acids 310-353 and 429-461.[2,9]

Presently, only one exception exists to the c-erbAβ rule. A kindred has been reported in whom the resistance phenotype is not linked to the c-erbAα gene and who has no c-erbAβ1 or c-erbAβ2 defect.[12] These data suggest that other factors that mediate thyroid hormone action may be defective, resulting in thyroid hormone resistance.

### HOMOZYGOUS C-*ERBA*β MUTATIONS IN REFETOFF AND BERCU PATIENTS

Two humans with mutations, the Refetoff and Bercu patients, provide important information on the interrelationships of the α and β receptors in mediating thyroid hormone action in humans (Fig. 32-3). These patients with mutations are homozygous for very different abnormalities in c-erbAβ and have very different phenotypes.

The resistance syndrome of the Refetoff patient is considerably milder than that of the Bercu patient (see Fig. 32-3). Although the original bone radiographs of the first Refetoff patient suggested juvenile hypothyroidism, the final adult height in affected members was above the parental mean. The intelligence quotients of the Refetoff patients were normal compared with the ranges seen in hearing-impaired individuals.[13] The Refetoff patients had a major deletion in both β receptor alleles and had only functional α receptors.[7,8] Significantly, the obligate heterozygotes in the Refetoff kindred were phenotypically normal; these heterozygotes had normal TSH and thyroid hormone levels. Several conclusions can be drawn from the Refetoff patients: that only one β-receptor allele is necessary (with two α receptor alleles) for normal thyroid hormone action in humans; most, or at least life-sustaining, thyroid hormone action can be mediated solely through the α receptor; and the heterozygous, mutant c-erbAβ alleles in resistance patients act as dominant negative genes. The obligate heterozygotes demonstrate that it is not the loss of function of a β-receptor allele that results in thyroid hormone resistance.

The Bercu patient (see Fig. 32-3) had a complex pattern of hyperthyroidism and hypothyroidism resulting from homozygosity of a dominant negative allele.[10,11] This patient manifested severe pituitary resistance with strikingly elevated TSH levels in the setting of high free thyroid hormone levels. Significant growth retardation and profound bone retardation suggested hypothyroidism. However, this patient was tachycardic and appeared to be hypermetabolic, consistent with hyperthyroidism. The patient was severely mentally retarded, although it is not clear whether this was secondary to hyperthyroidism or hypothyroidism or both conditions in distinct regions of the brain.[14] Because the Bercu patient was clinically much more severely affected than the Refetoff patients, it follows that dominant negative forms of c-erbAβ inhibit at least some thyroid hormone action mediated through the α receptor. The severity of the Bercu patient phenotype may also be due to the silencing activity (active repression) by the "double dose" of mutant c-erbAβ receptor. The variable thyroidal states in the Bercu patient highlights the fact that different tissues are regulated by different relative concentrations of α and β receptors.

### MOLECULAR MECHANISMS WITH DOMINANT NEGATIVE β RECEPTORS

The molecular genetics of the syndrome of generalized resistance to thyroid hormone indicated that the mutant c-erbAβ receptors antagonized the normal regulation of gene expression by wild-type α and β receptors. Most of the mutant β1 receptors that have been cloned and synthesized in vitro have compromised $T_3$ binding and transactivating ability, although a broad spectrum of defects exists.[15] For example, the mutant S receptor of the Bercu patient has no detectable $T_3$-binding activity and cannot induce expression from heterologous promoters containing thyroid hormone response element (TREs) with exposure to $T_3$ in transient expression experiments.[16] However, other

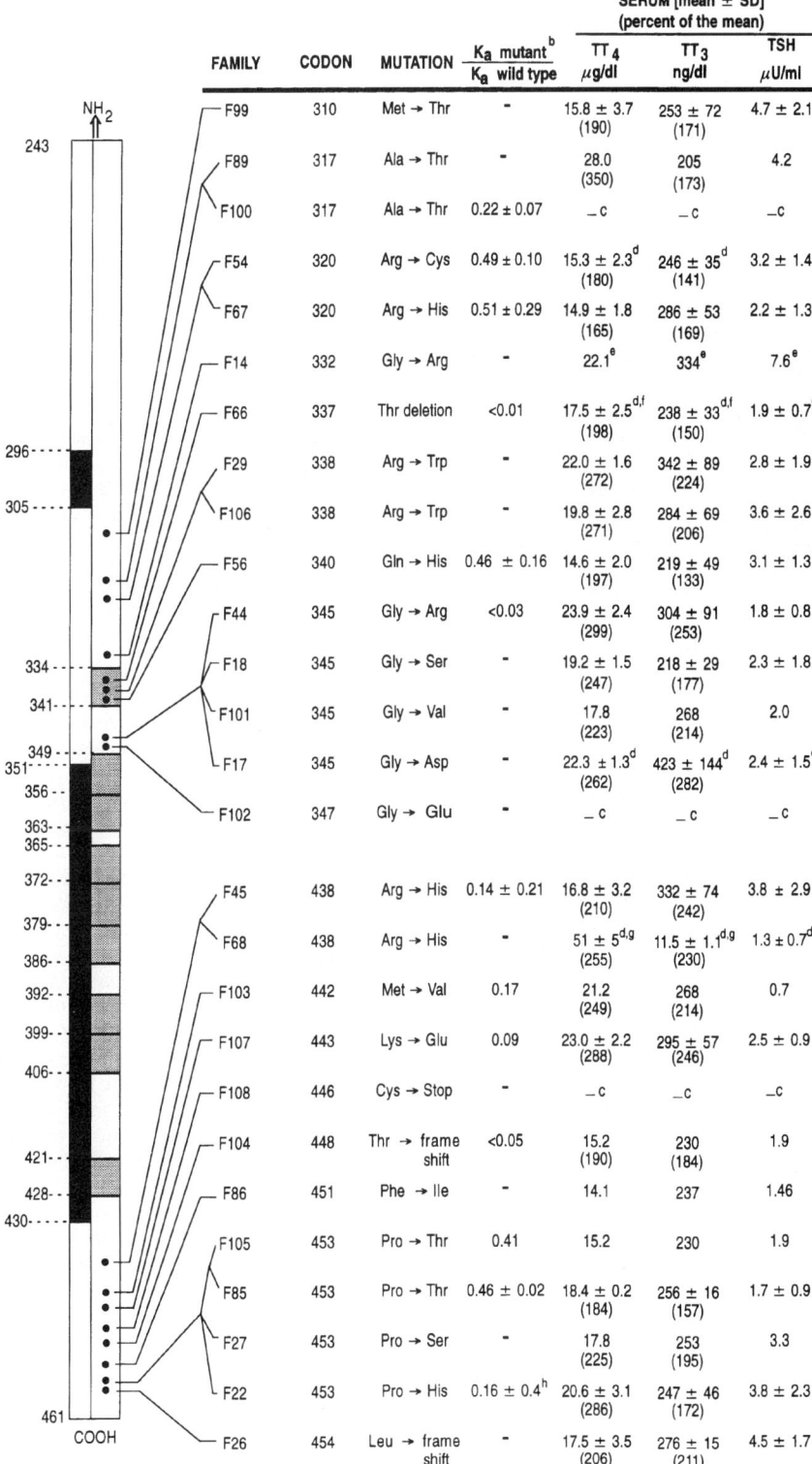

| FAMILY | CODON | MUTATION | $\dfrac{K_a \text{ mutant}^b}{K_a \text{ wild type}}$ | SERUM [mean ± SD] (percent of the mean) | | |
|---|---|---|---|---|---|---|
| | | | | $TT_4$ μg/dl | $TT_3$ ng/dl | TSH μU/ml |
| F99 | 310 | Met → Thr | - | 15.8 ± 3.7 (190) | 253 ± 72 (171) | 4.7 ± 2.1 |
| F89 | 317 | Ala → Thr | - | 28.0 (350) | 205 (173) | 4.2 |
| F100 | 317 | Ala → Thr | 0.22 ± 0.07 | _c | _c | _c |
| F54 | 320 | Arg → Cys | 0.49 ± 0.10 | 15.3 ± 2.3$^d$ (180) | 246 ± 35$^d$ (141) | 3.2 ± 1.4$^d$ |
| F67 | 320 | Arg → His | 0.51 ± 0.29 | 14.9 ± 1.8 (165) | 286 ± 53 (169) | 2.2 ± 1.3 |
| F14 | 332 | Gly → Arg | - | 22.1$^e$ | 334$^e$ | 7.6$^e$ |
| F66 | 337 | Thr deletion | <0.01 | 17.5 ± 2.5$^{d,f}$ (198) | 238 ± 33$^{d,f}$ (150) | 1.9 ± 0.7$^{d,f}$ |
| F29 | 338 | Arg → Trp | - | 22.0 ± 1.6 (272) | 342 ± 89 (224) | 2.8 ± 1.9 |
| F106 | 338 | Arg → Trp | - | 19.8 ± 2.8 (271) | 284 ± 69 (206) | 3.6 ± 2.6 |
| F56 | 340 | Gln → His | 0.46 ± 0.16 | 14.6 ± 2.0 (197) | 219 ± 49 (133) | 3.1 ± 1.3 |
| F44 | 345 | Gly → Arg | <0.03 | 23.9 ± 2.4 (299) | 304 ± 91 (253) | 1.8 ± 0.8 |
| F18 | 345 | Gly → Ser | - | 19.2 ± 1.5 (247) | 218 ± 29 (177) | 2.3 ± 1.8 |
| F101 | 345 | Gly → Val | - | 17.8 (223) | 268 (214) | 2.0 |
| F17 | 345 | Gly → Asp | - | 22.3 ± 1.3$^d$ (262) | 423 ± 144$^d$ (282) | 2.4 ± 1.5$^d$ |
| F102 | 347 | Gly → Glu | - | _c | _c | _c |
| F45 | 438 | Arg → His | 0.14 ± 0.21 | 16.8 ± 3.2 (210) | 332 ± 74 (242) | 3.8 ± 2.9 |
| F68 | 438 | Arg → His | - | 51 ± 5$^{d,g}$ (255) | 11.5 ± 1.1$^{d,g}$ (230) | 1.3 ± 0.7$^d$ |
| F103 | 442 | Met → Val | 0.17 | 21.2 (249) | 268 (214) | 0.7 |
| F107 | 443 | Lys → Glu | 0.09 | 23.0 ± 2.2 (288) | 295 ± 57 (246) | 2.5 ± 0.9 |
| F108 | 446 | Cys → Stop | - | _c | _c | _c |
| F104 | 448 | Thr → frame shift | <0.05 | 15.2 (190) | 230 (184) | 1.9 |
| F86 | 451 | Phe → Ile | - | 14.1 | 237 | 1.46 |
| F105 | 453 | Pro → Thr | 0.41 | 15.2 | 230 | 1.9 |
| F85 | 453 | Pro → Thr | 0.46 ± 0.02 | 18.4 ± 0.2 (184) | 256 ± 16 (157) | 1.7 ± 0.9 |
| F27 | 453 | Pro → Ser | - | 17.8 (225) | 253 (195) | 3.3 |
| F22 | 453 | Pro → His | 0.16 ± 0.4$^h$ | 20.6 ± 3.1 (286) | 247 ± 46 (172) | 3.8 ± 2.3 |
| F26 | 454 | Leu → frame shift | - | 17.5 ± 3.5 (206) | 276 ± 15 (211) | 4.5 ± 1.7 |

**FIGURE 32-2.** Mutations in the c-*erb*Aβ thyroid-hormone receptor gene responsible for generalized thyroid hormone resistance. The relative sites of the mutations in the triiodothyronine ($T_3$)-binding domain of the receptor with the alterations in amino acids are indicated. The last three exons of the β gene comprise amino acids 247–295, 296–381, and 382–461. The relative deficiencies in the $T_3$-binding affinities of the mutant receptors measured in vitro (1.0 = no defect, 0.01 = 100-fold reduction in $K_a$) are shown ($K_a$ mutant/$K_a$ wild-type). The mean total thyroxine ($TT_4$), total $T_3$ ($TT_3$), and thyroid-stimulating hormone (*TSH*) levels for the patients are listed; the results in brackets are mean values expressed as a percent of the corresponding mean levels of unaffected family members or the mean value for the laboratory. F100, F102, and F108 had prior (inappropriate) ablative therapy and were on $T_3$ therapy. Values for F68 are free $T_4$ and free $T_3$ given in picomoles per liter. The $T_3$-binding domain of c-*erb*Aβ spans amino acids 243–461, at the COOH terminus. The *black bars* represent areas that interact with thyroid hormone auxiliary proteins (*RXR*) and stabilize RXR-receptor heterodimers. Some of these regions may stabilize homodimers of c-*erb*Aβ as well. The 349–428 region contains heptad repeats (*gray boxes*) with hydrophobic amino acids that form a leucine zipper structure, which is involved in receptor dimerization. Some of these heptads appear to be critical for the dominant negative function of mutant c-*erb*Aβ1 receptors, although other domains may be involved. (*SD*, standard deviation.) (From Refetoff S, Weiss RE, Usala SJ. The syndrome of resistance to thyroid hormones. Endocr Rev 1993; 14:348.)

human mutant receptors do have demonstrable $T_3$-binding activity and can up-regulate gene expression at high levels of thyroid hormone.[15,16] The DNA-binding function of the mutant receptors appears to be required for dominant negative activity.[17]

No human DNA-binding mutations are found in the β thyroid-hormone receptor gene, except for the total deletion of the β alleles in the Refetoff patients, which is not dominant negative. The hypothesis has been made that the dominant negative activity of the human mutant receptors may result from competitive inhibition by mutant homodimers or heterodimers with wild-type receptors.[2] This would be a form of passive repression. Mutant receptors as homodimers or heterodimers may also block formation of the transcriptional preinitiation complex and silence gene transcription.[18–20] This could result in repression of basal gene expression.

Novel mutant c-*erb*Aβ receptors with relatively normal $T_3$-binding affinities have been isolated from kindreds with pro-

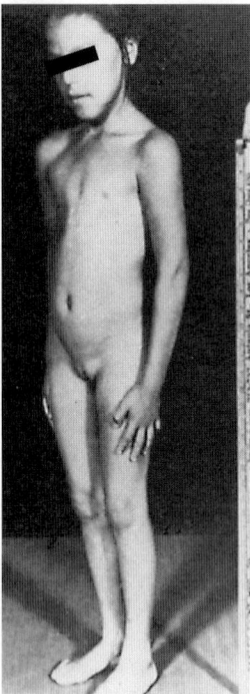 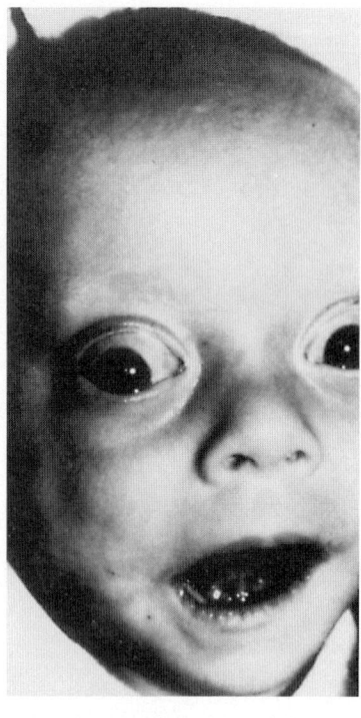

**A,B**

FIGURE 32-3. The Refetoff patient at 8.5 years of age (A) and the Bercu patient at 3.5 weeks of age (B). The Refetoff patient has a complete absence of functional β receptors. A bird-like facies and a pigeon chest are present. The Bercu patient is homozygous for a dominant negative β receptor (i.e., S receptor). Note the exophthalmos. (From Refetoff S, DeWind LD, DeGroot LJ. Familial syndrome combining deaf-mutism, stippled epiphyses, goiter, and abnormally high PBI: possible target organ refractoriness to thyroid hormone. J Clin Endocrinol Metab 1967; 27:279; and from Ono S, Schwartz ID, Mueller OT, et al. Homozygosity for a dominant negative thyroid hormone receptor gene responsible for generalized thyroid hormone resistance. J Clin Endocrinol Metab 1991; 73:990.)

nounced clinical manifestations of thyroid hormone resistance.[21,22] The R243Q and R243W c-*erb*Aβ mutations may create thyroid hormone resistance in part by increasing mutant homodimer formation or by reducing the receptor affinity for $T_3$ only after it binds to DNA.[21] An R383H mutant receptor has been shown to impair release of a corepressor factor in the context of TSHα and TRH promoters.[22]

### CLINICAL HETEROGENEITY IN THYROID HORMONE RESISTANCE SYNDROMES

The reasons for clinical heterogeneity in thyroid hormone resistance syndromes are complex. The correlation between the degree of functional impairment of the mutant c-*erb*Aβ receptor and the phenotype of resistance to thyroid hormone is not precise. Several explanations have been advocated.

In fibroblasts from one kindred, an increased proportion of mutant receptor messenger RNA (mRNA) was found that was associated with short stature.[23] In other kindreds in whom the mutant versus wild-type β1 receptor mRNA was quantitated, levels were approximately equivalent.[24,25]

Another gene or genes could affect the phenotypic expression of a mutant c-*erb*Aβ allele.[26] Although the mutant c-*erb*Aβ allele might be the most "dominant gene," its bioeffects could be modulated by other genes such as those for corepressors and coactivators.[27] That genetic factors modulate the expression of the resistance phenotype is suggested by comparison of thyroid function tests in unaffected first-degree relatives and relatives by marriage between kindreds with identical c-*erb*Aβ mutations.[28] For example, among members of a kindred with an R32OC mutation, higher concentrations of free $T_4$ were necessary to maintain a normal TSH level in affected subjects and

unaffected first-degree relatives (siblings and children of affected patients) but not relatives by marriage.[28]

The molecular analysis of thyroid hormone resistance syndromes has revealed that selective pituitary resistance to thyroid hormone can also result from mutations in c-*erb*Aβ.[29,30] Identical mutations have been found in different patients classified with generalized resistance and selective pituitary resistance to thyroid hormone.[2,3,29,30] This clinical discrepancy may result in part from the difficulty in discriminating selective pituitary resistance from generalized resistance. Patients with nervousness and tachycardia as their only thyrotoxic symptom and sign have been variously diagnosed as having selective pituitary resistance or generalized resistance to thyroid hormone. However, other genetic or acquired factors may play a role in determining the relative levels of resistance between pituitary and peripheral tissues. For example, a bona fide case of selective pituitary resistance to thyroid hormone was seen in the proband of a "Kindred G-H" with the ARG-316-HIS mutation in c-*erb*Aβ; this patient had unusually high thyroid hormone levels compared with other kindred members with the identical mutant allele.[29,31] Interestingly, thyroid hormone resistance has been diagnosed prenatally.[31a]

## TREATMENT CONSIDERATIONS FOR THYROID HORMONE RESISTANCE

The diagnosis of generalized resistance or selective pituitary resistance to thyroid hormone does have a bearing on treatment. For the patient with generalized resistance who is clinically euthyroid, antithyroid medications, thyroidectomy, and radioiodine treatment are to be strictly avoided.[2] In generalized resistance to thyroid hormone, the patient's own hypothalamic–pituitary–thyroid axis is allowed to render the appropriate level of thyroid hormone. However, in cases of concomitant primary hypothyroidism with elevation in serum TSH, the patient should be treated with thyroid hormone. Patients with generalized resistance who have been inappropriately treated with radioiodine or thyroidectomy may have striking elevations in TSH; for poorly understood reasons, in these patients completely normalizing the serum TSH level and avoiding signs and symptoms of thyrotoxicosis with $T_4$ may be difficult.

A minority of adolescents with generalized resistance demonstrate significant bone resistance and subnormal growth.[32] The suggestion has been made that exogenous $T_4$ or $T_3$ may augment growth.[2,32] For patients receiving thyroid hormone, it should be administered cautiously, with special attention given to cardiac and neurologic status.

The treatment of selective pituitary resistance to thyroid hormone is somewhat controversial. This condition must be differentiated from a TSH-secreting adenoma, because the treatment of the latter is surgical.[33,34] Radiologic visualization by magnetic resonance imaging or computed tomographic scan is primarily used in the diagnosis. The molar ratio of α-subunit to TSH is often elevated in patients with TSH-secreting adenoma.[33,34] Therapy for pituitary resistance has included β-blockers such as propranolol, bromocriptine, methimazole, or propylthiouracil, 3,5,5'-triiodothyroacetic acid (i.e., TRIAC), somatostatin, and thyroidectomy.[2,3,34–36a] Many cases are mild, and no intervention other than observation is required, because the level of symptomatic thyrotoxicosis can abate with time.[3] One severely thyrotoxic patient has been successfully treated for several years with methimazole.[36]

*Attention deficit hyperactivity disorder* (ADHD) is commonly found in patients with thyroid hormone resistance syndromes.[37–39] Indicative of learning disabilities, discrepancies often exist between achievement and visual-motor development scores, and intelligence quotients. In one study of 49 affected (generalized resistance syndrome) and 55 unaffected members of kindreds, 50% of affected adults met the criteria for ADHD, and 70% of affected children were diagnosed with ADHD.[38] However, the converse study, which examined 277 children with ADHD, found no thyroid hormone resistance, although the prevalence of other thyroid abnormalities was 5.4%.[39] Thyroid hormone resistance syndromes are a very rare cause of ADHD, although perhaps TSH and free $T_4$ measurements are advisable in children with ADHD given the high prevalence of other thyroid diseases.[39] Children with resistance to thyroid hormone have weaker abilities of perceptual organization and lower school achievement compared to those with ADHD, indicating a more severe neurobehavioral impairment than with ADHD.[40] In children with resistance to thyroid hormone and ADHD (but not in unaffected children with ADHD), administration of $T_3$ in supraphysiologic doses (25–75 µg per day) may be beneficial in reducing hyperactivity and impulsivity.[41]

# REFERENCES

1. Refetoff S, DeWind LT, DeGroot LJ. Familial syndrome combining deaf-mutism, stippled epiphyses, goiter, and abnormally high PBI: possible target organ refractoriness to thyroid hormone. J Clin Endocrinol Metab 1967; 27:279.
2. Refetoff S, Weiss RE, Usala SJ. The syndrome of resistance to thyroid hormones. Endocr Rev 1993; 14:348.
3. Beck-Peccoz P, Chatterjee VKK. The variable clinical phenotype in thyroid hormone resistance syndrome. Thyroid 1994; 4:225.
4. Kaplan MM, Swartz SL, Larsen PR. Partial peripheral resistance thyroid hormone. Am J Med 1981; 70:1115.
5. Usala SJ, Weintraub BD. Familial thyroid hormone resistance: clinical and molecular studies. In: Mazzaferri E, Kreisberg RA, Bar RS, eds. Advances in endocrinology and metabolism, vol 2. Chicago: Mosby–Year Book, 1991:59.
6. Usala SJ, Bale AE, Gesundheit N, et al. Tight linkage between the syndrome of generalized thyroid hormone resistance and the human c-erbAβ gene. Mol Endocrinol 1988; 1:1217.
7. Takeda A, Balzano S, Sakurai A, et al. Screening of nineteen unrelated families with generalized resistance to thyroid hormone for known point mutations in the thyroid-hormone receptor β gene and the detection of a new mutation. J Clin Invest 1991; 87:496.
8. Takeda K, Sakurai A, DeGroot LJ, Refetoff S. Recessive inheritance of thyroid hormone resistance caused by complete deletion of the protein-coding region of the thyroid hormone receptor-β gene. J Clin Endocrinol Metab 1992; 74:49.
9. Announcement 1994. A registry for resistance to thyroid hormone. Mol Endocrinol 1994; 8:1558.
10. Ono S, Schwartz ID, Mueller OT, et al. Homozygosity for a dominant negative thyroid hormone receptor gene responsible for generalized thyroid hormone resistance. J Clin Endocrinol Metab 1991; 73:990.
11. Usala SJ, Menke JB, Watson TL, et al. A homozygous deletion in the c-erbAβ thyroid hormone receptor gene in a patient with generalized thyroid hormone resistance: isolation and characterization of the mutant receptor. Mol Endocrinol 1991; 5:327.
12. Weiss RE, Hayashi Y, Nagaya T, et al. Dominant inheritance of resistance to thyroid hormone not linked to defects in the thyroid hormone receptor α or β genes may be due to a defective cofactor. J Clin Endocrinol Metab 1996; 81:4196.
13. Refetoff S, DeGroot LJ, Bernard B, DeWind LT. Studies of a sibship with apparent hereditary resistance to the intracellular action of thyroid hormone. Metabolism 1972; 21:723.
14. Stein SA, Nici JA, Gamache MP, et al. Preliminary characterization of the neurological and neuropsychological abnormalities in a homozygote and heterozygotes of kindred S with generalized thyroid hormone resistance syndrome. Thyroid 1991; 1(Suppl):5.
15. Hayashi Y, Weiss RE, Sarne DH, et al. Do clinical manifestations of resistance to thyroid hormone correlate with the functional alterations of the corresponding mutant thyroid hormone-β receptors? J Clin Endocrinol Metab 1995; 80:3246.
16. Meier CA, Dickstein BM, Ashizawa K, et al. Variable transcriptional activity and ligand binding of mutant $β_1,T_3$ receptors from four families with generalized resistance to thyroid hormone. Mol Endocrinol 1992; 6:248.
17. Nagaya T, Madison LD, Jameson JL. Thyroid hormone receptor mutant that causes resistance to thyroid hormone. J Biol Chem 1992; 267:13014.
18. Baniahmad A, Tsai SY, O'Malley BW, Tsai MJ. Kindred S thyroid hormone receptor is an active and constitutive silencer and repressor for thyroid hormone and retinoic acid responses. Proc Natl Acad Sci U S A 1992; 89:10633.
19. Fondell JD, Roy AL, Roeder RG. Unliganded thyroid hormone receptor inhibits formation of a functional preinitiation complex: implications for active repression. Genes Dev 1992; 7:1400.
20. Baniahmad A, Ha I, Reinberg D, et al. Interaction of human thyroid hormone receptor β with transcription factor TFIIB may mediate target gene derepression and activation by thyroid hormone. Proc Natl Acad Sci U S A 1993; 90:8832.
21. Yagi H, Pohlenz J, Hayashi Y, et al. Resistance to thyroid hormone caused by two mutant thyroid hormone receptors β, R243Q and R243W, with impairment of function that cannot be explained by altered in vitro 3,5,3'-triiodothyronine-binding affinity. J Clin Endocrinol Metab 1997; 82:1608.
22. Clifton-Bligh RJ, de Zegher F, Wagner RL, et al. A novel TRβ mutation (R383H) in resistance to thyroid hormone syndrome predominantly impairs corepressor release and negative transcriptional regulation. Mol Endocrinol 1998; 12:609.
23. Mixson AJ, Hauser P, Tennyson G, et al. Differential expression of mutant and normal beta $T_3$ receptor alleles in kindreds with generalized resistance to thyroid hormone. J Clin Invest 1993; 91:2296.
24. Hayashi Y, Janssen OE, Weiss RE, et al. The relative expression of mutant and normal thyroid hormone receptor genes in patients with generalized resistance to thyroid hormones determined by estimation of their specific messenger RNA products. J Clin Endocrinol Metab 1993; 76:64.
25. Klann RC, Torres B, Menke JB, et al. Competitive PCR quantitation of c-erbAβ1, c-erbAα1, and c-erbα2 messenger RNA levels in normal heterozygous and homozygous fibroblasts of kindred S with thyroid hormone resistance. J Clin Endocrinol Metab 1993; 77:969.
26. Weiss RE, Marcocci C, Bruno-Bossio G, Refetoff S. Multiple genetic factors in the heterogeneity of thyroid hormone resistance. J Clin Endocrinol Metab 1993; 76:257.
27. Koenig RJ. Thyroid hormone receptor coactivators and corepressors. Thyroid 1998; 8:703.
28. Weiss RE, Tunca H, Knapple WL, et al. Phenotype differences of resistance to thyroid hormone in two unrelated families with an identical mutation in the thyroid hormone receptor β gene (R320C). Thyroid 1997; 7:35.
29. Geffner ME, Su F, Ross NS, et al. An arginine to histidine mutation in codon 311 of the c-erbAβ gene results in a mutant receptor which does not mediate a dominant negative phenotype. J Clin Invest 1993; 91:538.
30. Mixson AJ, Renault JC, Ransom S, et al. Identification of a novel mutation in the gene encoding the β-triiodothyronine receptor in a patient with apparent selective pituitary resistance to thyroid hormone. Clin Endocrinol 1993; 38:227.
31. Hao E, Menke JB, Smith AM, et al. Divergent dimerization properties of mutant β1 thyroid hormone receptors are associated with different dominant negative activities. Mol Endocrinol 1994; 8:841.
31a. Asteria C, Rajanayagam O, Collingwood T, et al. Prenatal diagnosis of thyroid hormone resistance. J Clin Endocrinol Metab 1999; 84:405.
32. Gesundheit N, Gyves PW, Okihiro MM, et al. Short stature in children with generalized thyroid hormone resistance: clinical and biochemical features in eight patients from three kindreds. (Abstract). Endocrinol 1988; 121(Suppl):T-36.
33. Magner JA. TSH-mediated hyperthyroidism. Endocrinologist 1993; 3:289.
34. Beck-Peccoz P, Mariotti S, Guillausseau PJ. Treatment of hyperthyroidism due to inappropriate secretion of thyrotropin with the somatostatin analog SMS 201–995. J Clin Endocrinol Metab 1989; 68:208.
35. Kunitake JM, Hartman N, Henson LC, et al. 3,5,3'-triiodothyroacetic acid therapy for thyroid hormone resistance. J Clin Endocrinol Metab 1989; 69:461.
36. Dulgeroff AJ, Geffner ME, Koyal SN, et al. Bromocriptine and Triac therapy for hyperthyroidism due to pituitary resistance to thyroid hormone. J Clin Endocrinol Metab 1992; 75:1071.
36a. Weiss RE, Refetoff S. Treatment of resistance to thyroid hormone-primum non nocere. J Clin Endocrinol Metab 1999; 84:401.
37. Cugini CD Jr, Leidy JW Jr, Chertow BS, et al. An arginine to histidine mutation in codon 315 of the c-erbAβ thyroid hormone receptor in a kindred with generalized resistance to thyroid hormones results in a receptor with significant 3,5,3'-triiodothyronine binding activity. J Clin Endocrinol Metabol 1992; 74:1164.
38. Hauser P, Zametkin AJ, Martinez P. Attention deficit-hyperactivity disorder in people with generalized resistance to thyroid hormone. N Engl J Med 1993; 328:997.
39. Weiss RE, Skin M, Trommer B, Refetoff S. Attention deficit hyperactivity disorder and thyroid function. J Pediatr 1993; 123:539.
40. Stein MA, Weiss RE, Refetoff S. Neurocognitive characteristics of individuals with resistance to thyroid hormone: comparisons with individuals with attention-deficit hyperactivity disorder. Dev Behav Pediatr 1995; 16:406.
41. Weiss RE, Stein MA, Refetoff S. Behavioral effects of Liothyronine (L-T3) in children with attention deficit hyperactivity disorder in the presence and absence of resistance to thyroid hormone. Thyroid 1997; 7:389.

---

# CHAPTER 33

---

# THYROID FUNCTION TESTS

ROBERT C. SMALLRIDGE

The determination of circulating levels of thyroid hormones is essential for an accurate assessment of the functional status of patients. By means of specific competitive immunoassays (radioimmunoassays [RIAs], enzyme or chemiluminescent immunoassays [EIAs; CLIAs], or immunoradiometric assays

**TABLE 33-1.**
**Effects of Some Drugs on Thyroid Hormone Tests**

**INCREASE IN BINDING PROTEIN CONCENTRATIONS**
($\uparrow$ $T_4$ and $T_3$; N, $\uparrow$ $FT_4$; normal TSH)
  Estrogens
  Clofibrate
  Opiates (heroin, methadone)
  5-Fluorouracil
**DECREASE IN BINDING PROTEIN CONCENTRATIONS**
($\downarrow$ $T_4$ and $T_3$; normal $FT_4$, $FT_3$, TSH)
  Androgens
  Glucocorticoids
  Danazol
  L-Asparaginase
  Colestipol–niacin combination
**INHIBITION OF BINDING TO TRANSPORT PROTEINS**
($\downarrow$ $T_4$ and $T_3$; $\uparrow$, $\downarrow$ $FT_4$ and $FT_3$; N, $\downarrow$ TSH)
  Salicylates, salsalate
  Phenylbutazone
  Diphenylhydantoin
  Furosemide
  Sulfonylureas
  Diazepam
  Heparin
  Chloral hydrate
  Fenclofenac
**INHIBITION OF THYROID FUNCTION**
($\downarrow$ $T_4$ and $T_3$; $\downarrow$ $FT_4$; $\uparrow$ TSH)
  Iodine
  Lithium
  Sulfonylureas
  Interleukin-2
**INHIBITION OF $T_4$ TO $T_3$ CONVERSION**
($\downarrow$ $T_3$; $\downarrow$, N, $\uparrow$ $T_4$ and $FT_4$; $\uparrow$ $rT_3$; N, $\uparrow$ TSH)
  Glucocorticoids
  Ipodate, iopanoic acid
  Propranolol
  Amiodarone
  Propylthiouracil
**INCREASE IN TSH CONCENTRATION**
($\downarrow$, N $T_4$; $\downarrow$, N $T_3$)
  Iodine
  Lithium
  Dopamine antagonists
  Cimetidine
**DECREASE IN TSH CONCENTRATION**
(N, $\downarrow$ $T_4$; $\downarrow$ $T_3$; $\downarrow$ TSH)
  Glucocorticoids
  Dopamine agonists
  Somatostatin
**INHIBITION OF GI ABSORPTION OF EXOGENOUS HORMONE**
($\downarrow$ $T_4$ and $FT_4$; $\uparrow$ TSH)
  Cholestyramine
  Colestipol
  Soybean flour
  Iron
  Sucralfate

$\downarrow$, reduced serum hormone level; *N*, no change; $\uparrow$, increased serum hormone level; $T_4$, thyroxine; $T_3$, triiodothyronine; $FT_4$, free $T_4$; $FT_3$, free $T_3$; *TSH*, thyrotropin (thyroid-stimulating hormone); $rT_3$, reverse $T_3$; *GI*, gastrointestinal.
Note: Thyroid test results in parentheses indicate the types of changes reported. Not every test result is produced by every drug in a specific category.

[IRMAs]), small quantities of these and other hormones can be detected, enabling physicians to diagnose even mild degrees of thyroid dysfunction. RIA methodology involves a reaction between a specific antibody and two antigens, one of which is radiolabeled (see Chap. 237). In addition, various other laboratory procedures are available for examining thyroid disorders.

Numerous factors may affect the function of the hypothalamic–pituitary–thyroid axis. These include *physiologic* factors (age, pregnancy, stress, temperature, genetics), *pathologic* factors (hyper- or hypothyroidism, systemic illness, surgery, starva-

tion), and *pharmacologic* factors (Table 33-1). Some of these conditions produce a bewildering array of alterations in serum concentrations of these hormones, and a carefully selected set of tests may be required to establish the correct diagnosis. These tests are discussed in this chapter.

Preanalytical factors affecting thyroid function tests include not only the ones just mentioned, but also variables directly affecting the specimen (e.g., hemolysis, bilirubin, free fatty acids).[1] Assay performance is also affected by many analytical characteristics (e.g., bias, specificity, sensitivity and working range, presence of interfering substances, imprecision, recovery, calibration, and parallelism).[2]

# IODOTHYRONINES

## PROTEIN BOUND CONCENTRATIONS

Serum thyroxine ($T_4$) concentration was, for many years, the most useful first-line test of thyroid function. Historically, $T_4$ was estimated by measuring the serum protein bound iodine or the butanol extractable iodine; these measures are no longer used. (In suspected iodide ingestion, the protein bound iodine is much greater than the $T_4$.) Serum $T_4$ is determined almost exclusively by RIA; values in euthyroid patients range between 5 and 12 $\mu$g/dL. In hyperthyroidism, higher levels are present, and in hypothyroidism, lower levels are seen.

In general, the level of serum triiodothyronine ($T_3$), the most active thyroid hormone, varies in parallel with the $T_4$ level. Healthy subjects have values of 80 to 200 ng/dL, with higher levels occurring in hyperthyroidism. Indeed, the $T_3$ levels may increase despite a normal serum $T_4$ level, a condition known as $T_3$ *toxicosis*. Whereas $T_4$ is usually low in hypothyroidism, serum $T_3$ is often in the normal range, possibly owing to increased conversion of $T_4$ to $T_3$. Also, the peripheral conversion of $T_4$ to $T_3$ is exquisitely sensitive to acute stresses of many causes. Thus, a low serum $T_3$ level is to be expected in many nonthyroidal illnesses,[3] whereas serum $T_4$ levels may be low, normal, or elevated.

Serum reverse $T_3$ ($rT_3$) ranges from 10 to 60 ng/dL in euthyroid patients. Like $T_4$, serum $rT_3$ level is high in hyperthyroidism and low in hypothyroidism. In nonthyroidal illness, serum $rT_3$ concentrations are often elevated,[4] whereas $T_4$ levels are normal or low, and $T_3$ levels are reduced. The discrepant results for $T_3$ and $rT_3$ in such disorders have made $rT_3$ measurements clinically useful in differentiating primary hypothyroidism from acute illness.

Although RIAs have been developed for the diiodothyronines,[4] monoiodothyronines,[5,6] and $T_4$ and $T_3$ sulfates,[7,8] measurement of these iodothyronine metabolites has no current clinical utility.

Several of the iodothyronines have been measured in the urine,[9] but their clinical applicability is limited.

## FREE THYROXINE AND TRIIODOTHYRONINE BY EQUILIBRIUM DIALYSIS

*To assess the patient's true metabolic status, estimation of the concentration of free $T_4$ or free $T_3$—the "active" hormones—is advisable.* The most precise determination is obtained by *equilibrium dialysis*.[10] In this procedure, a diluted serum sample is incubated with $T_4$ labeled with iodine-125 ($^{125}$I) in a dialysis system. The free fraction of hormone (both the patient's $T_4$ and the $^{125}$I-$T_4$ tracer) achieves equilibrium by diffusing across a semipermeable membrane, whereas the protein bound hormone remains inside the dialysis tubing. The small percentage of dialyzable $T_4$ (percentage of free $T_4$) is determined directly, and the total $T_4$ is measured by RIA. Multiplying the total $T_4$ by the percentage of free $T_4$ yields the free $T_4$ value. Free $T_3$ is measured in an analogous manner. A reliable commercial assay for free $T_4$ by equilibrium dialysis is available[2,11] with a normal range of 0.8 to 2.7 ng/dL. Commercial assays for free $T_3$ may be unreliable in patients with nonthyroidal illnesses or those taking amiodarone.[12,13]

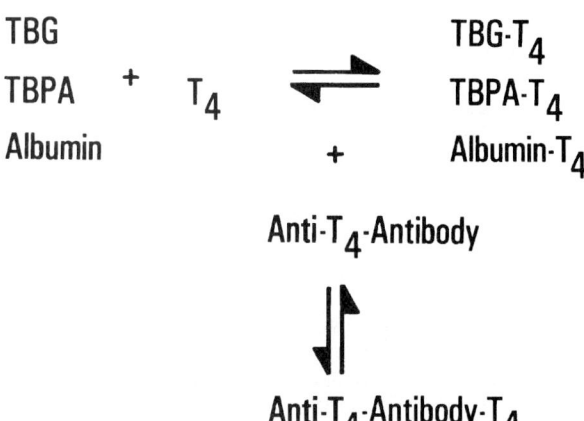

**FIGURE 33-1.** Free thyroxine ($T_4$) measurement by immunoassay. Antibody extraction assays involve the incubation of patient serum samples with anti-$T_4$ antibody, during which time $T_4$ approaches a new equilibrium with all the binders present. (*TBG*, thyroxine-binding globulin; *TBPA*, thyroxine-binding prealbumin.) (From Witherspoon LR, Shuler SE. Estimation of free thyroxine concentration: clinical methods and pitfalls. J Clin Immunoassay 1984; 7:192.)

## FREE THYROXINE: TWO-STEP AND ANALOG METHODS

A variety of commercial RIA kits have become available for measuring free $T_4$.[11,14–16] A patient's serum is incubated with an anti-$T_4$ antibody, and the $T_4$ is allowed to reach a new equilibrium among endogenous serum binding proteins and the added antibody (Fig. 33-1). The amount of $T_4$ extracted from the serum and bound to the anti-$T_4$ antibody is quantified and related to known serum calibrators, which are similarly extracted. The antibody bound $T_4$ can be quantified in several ways. Some assays require two steps and entail removal of serum and $T_4$ binders. Another method necessitates only a single incubation and includes the addition of a $T_4$ analogue to the incubation system. The *two-step procedure* for free $T_4$ has proved comparable to equilibrium dialysis in evaluating many clinical disorders. In contrast, the *analog method* has yielded inaccurate results in situations in which there may be an aberrant increase in $T_4$ binding to albumin or thyroxine-binding prealbumin (TBPA; transthyretin [TTR]). A comparison of the methods for estimating serum free $T_4$ is given in Table 33-2.

The free hormone hypothesis has been extensively reviewed, as have the various methods available for measurement.[17,17a] Several assays have been useful in measuring free $T_4$ in patients with abnormal thyroid hormone–binding proteins or with nonthyroidal illness,[11,14,15] although low values are reported in some assays. Measurement of free $T_4$ by ultrafiltration, which avoids serum dilution, may be more accurate in certain situations.[18,19]

## SERUM BINDING PROTEINS

Thyroid hormones are bound to three circulating proteins: thyroxine-binding globulin (TBG); TBPA, or TTR; and albumin. Routine serum $T_4$ and $T_3$ determinations measure the total amount of the hormones, of which more than 99% is protein bound. Many factors influence the levels of TBG and TBPA; thus, a total $T_4$ or $T_3$ level may deviate from euthyroid levels. Therefore, examining the status of these binding proteins is important.

### TRIIODOTHYRONINE UPTAKE AND FREE THYROXINE INDEX

Several methods are used to evaluate binding proteins and to estimate the free $T_4$ concentration. A commonly used test is the $T_3$ uptake ($T_3U$) test.[10] In this procedure, a patient's serum sample is placed in a test tube to which is added a tracer amount of $^{125}I$-$T_3$ and a resin or other solid phase matrix. During incubation, binding sites on the resin and on the patient's serum binding proteins compete for the $^{125}I$-$T_3$ until equilibrium is achieved. When the serum has an increased number of unoccupied binding sites, a greater percentage of the $^{125}I$-$T_3$ binds to these serum proteins. When the resin is separated and counted for radioactivity, the decreased percentage of $^{125}I$-$T_3$ resin uptake indicates an increased number of unoccupied TBG-binding sites. In contrast, when the patient's TBG-binding sites are nearly saturated, the $T_3U$ is elevated. The free thyroxine index ($FT_4I$) is calculated by multiplying the serum total $T_4$ by the percentage of resin uptake.

Several modifications have evolved in $FT_4I$ determinations. To permit comparisons of varying methods, a thyroid hormone–binding ratio (THBR) can be derived by dividing the patient's $T_3U$ by the mean of a reference population. Multiplying the THBR by the total $T_4$ gives the $FT_4I$. A second change has been the development of nonisotopic automated methods. Rather than using $T_3$, $T_4$ is labeled (enzyme or fluorescein). This assay method is called a "T-uptake".[20]

Table 33-3 illustrates the directional changes observed in the more common derangements of thyroid function. Whenever total $T_4$ and $T_3U$ values diverge and the $FT_4I$ is normal, binding protein concentrations of TBG are probably abnormal. In these settings, an excellent correlation is found between the $FT_4I$ and the free $T_4$ determined by equilibrium dialysis. Unfortunately, numerous conditions may alter the binding proteins to produce a spurious $FT_4I$ estimate of the free $T_4$.

A free $T_3$ index, calculated as a product of the total $T_3$ and the $T_3U$ ratio, provides a reasonable estimate of serum free $T_3$. It may aid in the diagnosis of $T_3$ toxicosis when the serum $T_4$ is normal[21] (see Chap. 42).

**TABLE 33-2.**
**Methods for Estimating Serum Free Thyroxine in Thyroid Diseases**

| Condition | Equilibrium Dialysis | $FT_4$ Index | $T_4$-Antibody Extraction | |
| --- | --- | --- | --- | --- |
| | | | Two-Step | Analog |
| Euthyroidism | N | N | N | N |
| Hyperthyroidism | ↑ | ↑ | ↑ | ↑ |
| Hypothyroidism | ↓ | ↓ | ↓ | ↓ |
| Increased TBG | N | N, ↑ | N | N |
| Decreased TBG | N | N, ↓ | N | N |
| Nonthyroidal illness | N | ↓ | N, ↓ | ↓ |
| Familial dysalbuminemic hyperthyroxinemia | N | ↑ | N | ↑ |
| Thyroid hormone autoantibodies | N | ↑, ↓* | N | ↑ |

*N*, normal; ↑, increase; ↓, decrease; $T_4$, thyroxine; $FT_4$, free $T_4$; *TBG*, thyroxine-binding globulin.
*Depends on method of separating bound from free hormone in $T_4$ radioimmunoassay (see text).

**TABLE 33-3.**
**Diagnostic Utility of the Free Thyroxine Index Values**

| | Total $T_4$ | $T_3$ Uptake | $FT_4$ Index |
| --- | --- | --- | --- |
| Euthyroidism | N | N | N |
| Hyperthyroidism | ↑ | ↑ | ↑ |
| Hypothyroidism | ↓ | ↓ | ↓ |
| Increased TBG | ↑ | ↓ | N |
| Decreased TBG | ↓ | ↑ | N |

*N*, normal; ↑, increase; ↓, decrease; $T_4$, thyroxine; $T_3$, triiodothyronine; $FT_4$, free $T_4$; *TBG*, thyroxine-binding globulin.

## THYROXINE/THYROXINE-BINDING GLOBULIN RATIO

A second method of examining thyroid hormone–binding proteins is to measure TBG by RIA and calculate a $T_4$/TBG ratio. TBG can be measured by sensitive immunoelectrophoresis techniques.[22] This method correlates well with the usual clinical state.

The $FT_4I$ has been calculated using five nonisotopic T-uptake assays, the $T_3U$ method, and TBG.[20] All methods performed comparably in patients with hyper- or hypothyroidism or nonthyroidal illnesses. However, all were affected by sera containing increased concentrations of TBG (see also ref. 22a).

## EFFECTS OF DRUGS

Numerous drugs affect the measurement of total and free thyroid hormones.[23] Many of these changes result from altered binding of $T_4$ and $T_3$ to their carrier proteins. Other drugs may act on the hypothalamus, the pituitary, or the thyroid gland. The patient's thyroid status depends on the number and severity of effects evoked. The myriad changes induced by commonly used drugs are summarized in Table 33-1.

## THYROTROPIN

Serum thyrotropin (thyroid-stimulating hormone, TSH) has been a reliable indicator of primary hypothyroidism, with levels rising even when thyroid deficiency is mild and the $T_4$ level is still normal (see Chaps. 15 and 45). Distinguishing euthyroid patients from those with mild hyperthyroidism based on a suppressed TSH level has been encumbered by inadequate assay sensitivity. Although RIAs were developed that could detect TSH concentrations of 0.1 to 0.3 μU/mL, this sensitivity was achieved by extensive purification of the radioligand and concentration of specimens. Commercially available RIAs have not provided quantitative values below 1 μU/mL.

Many second-generation assays detect TSH in the range of 0.1 to 0.5 μU/mL, and third-generation assays have an even 10-fold greater functional sensitivity[24–26] (Fig. 33-2). The first-generation RIA relies on a radiolabeled antigen and a single polyclonal antibody. The newer IRMAs use two or three antibodies (one or two are radiolabeled). These monoclonal antibodies are directed at the TSH subunits or at some specific epitopes on the TSH mole-

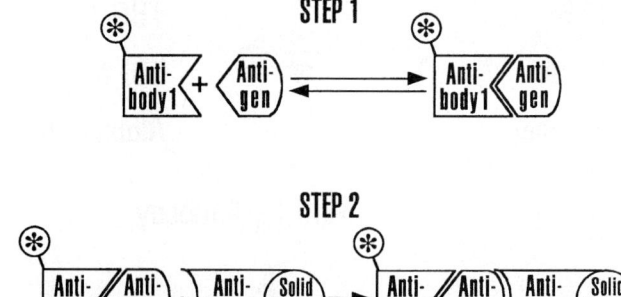

**FIGURE 33-3.** Principles of immunoradiometric assay. In step 1, a radiolabeled monoclonal antibody reacts with a specific antigen. In step 2, a second monoclonal antibody reacts with a different unique antigenic binding site. The second antibody is bound to a solid phase carrier, which is then washed to remove unbound radiolabeled antibody from the reaction. The complex bound to the solid matrix is then counted in a gamma spectrometer, and the concentration of antigen is determined by comparing the results to a simultaneously constructed standard curve.

cule (Fig. 33-3). This provides a more stable radioligand and a higher assay sensitivity. EIAs for TSH also use several monoclonal antibodies and have similar performance characteristics. They rely on colorimetry, however, and are affected by lipemic and hemolyzed samples.

These assays usually show undetectable TSH levels in hyperthyroid patients (Fig. 33-4) and in patients taking sufficient doses of $T_4$ to suppress the TSH response to thyrotropin-releasing hormone. Thus, a suppressed basal TSH determination may be sufficient to diagnose hyperthyroidism in more than 95% of cases. This obviates the need for thyrotropin-releasing hormone stimulation tests in the diagnosis of mild hyperthyroidism or determination of the adequacy of suppressive thyroid hormone therapy.

Assays may vary in their characteristics, and standard criteria for performance have been proposed.[26] For clinical use, the recommendation is that the lower limit of the assay be determined by its functional sensitivity; that is, the concentration at which the interassay precision CV = 20%.[26] This level is higher than the analytical sensitivity, but provides greater assurance that the TSH value reported is a real number. Although sensitivity is the most critical factor involved in selection of a TSH assay, specificity may be influenced by epitope differences in the TSH antibodies, and interference in the assay by heterophile antibodies.[26,27]

## THYROGLOBULIN AND THYROGLOBULIN ANTIBODIES

Serum thyroglobulin (Tg) measurements are useful in the follow-up of patients with thyroid cancer[28,29] (see Chap. 40). Numerous studies have shown that very low or undetectable Tg levels are found in patients who have been successfully treated and have no evidence of residual thyroid tissue. The performance characteristics of the assay used are important. Five problems complicating current Tg assay methods have been evaluated for six different Tg assays.[29] First, standardization has been lacking, although a Tg reference standard has now been adopted. Second, functional sensitivity in some assays is suboptimal: Small amounts of residual thyroid tissue may go undetected. Third, poor precision of repeated interassay measurements, over a relevant clinical time frame of 6 to 12 months, may limit the ability to detect cancer recurrences or progression. Fourth, the "hook" effect may lead to a report of falsely normal or low Tg values in sera with very high Tg concentrations, especially in an

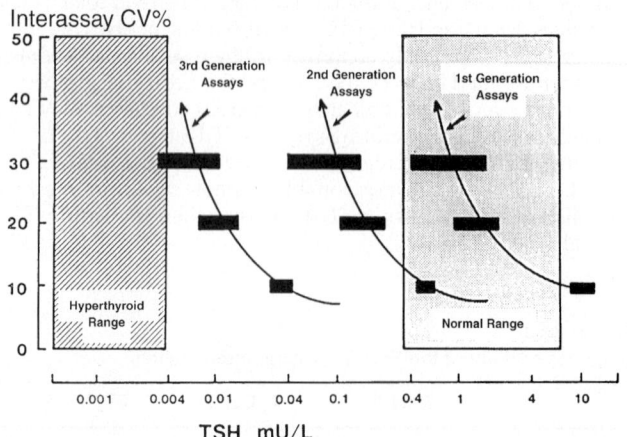

**FIGURE 33-2.** Schematic representation of the generation system of nomenclature designation for thyroid-stimulating hormone (*TSH*) assays based on interassay precision [percent coefficient of variation (*CV*)]. Each generation represents a ten-fold improvement in functional sensitivity (20% interassay CV value). The black bars denote the 95% confidence limits of measurement at different TSH levels. (From Nicoloff JT, Spencer CA. The use and misuse of the sensitive thyrotropin assays. J Clin Endocrinol Metab 1990; 71:553.)

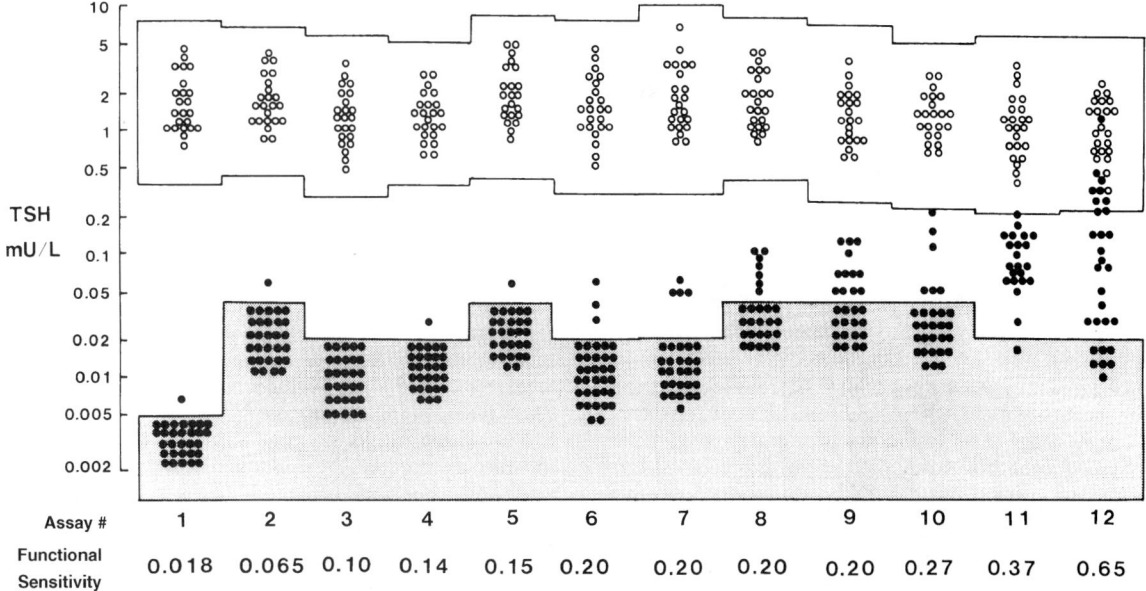

**FIGURE 33-4.** Comparative evaluation of sera from the same group of normal (*open symbols*) and hyperthyroid (*solid symbols*) patients measured by different commercially available thyroid-stimulating hormone (*TSH*) immunometric assays, ordered (*left to right*) relative to their functional sensitivities (20% interassay). The normal reference ranges (mean ± 3 standard deviations of log values) are shown by the open box, and the analytic (intraassay) sensitivity limits are depicted by the shaded area. Assay 1 exhibits third-generation functional performance, whereas assays 2 through 9 exhibit second-generation performance. Assays 10 through 12, although cited by their manufacturers as being sensitive TSH assays, only meet first-generation performance criteria and do not qualify as sensitive TSH assays. (From Nicoloff JT, Spencer CA. The use and misuse of the sensitive thyrotropin assays. J Clin Endocrinol Metab 1990; 71:553.)

immunoradiometric assay (IRMA). Samples should be run undiluted and at a 1:10 dilution to avoid this potentially serious mistake. Fifth, Tg antibodies can overestimate the Tg level in double-antibody RIAs, whereas IRMAs underestimate the true value. Sera should be screened for the presence of Tg antibodies, which should be reported to the clinician.[29]

## THYROID PEROXIDASE ANTIBODIES

Patients with autoimmune thyroid disease commonly develop antibodies to thyroid antigens. Thyroid microsomal antibodies frequently are present in patients with chronic lymphocytic thyroiditis, and Tg antibodies develop in a few patients. Passive hemagglutination tests have often been used clinically. In such tests, sheep erythrocytes are coated with either thyroid microsomal proteins or Tg. These cells are exposed to serial dilutions of serum, and the presence of antibodies is indicated by observing hemagglutination in the test tube. These antibodies may also be detected by several other techniques, including immunofluorescence, complement fixation, EIA, IRMA, and RIA (see Chap. 46). Antithyroid peroxidase antibody measurements are more sensitive and specific for autoimmune thyroid disease[30] and are replacing microsomal antibody determinations.

## THYROID HORMONE ANTIBODIES

Occasional patients have autoantibodies to $T_4$, $T_3$, or both.[27,31,32] Depending on the method used to separate bound from free hormone in the RIA, these patients may have spuriously high or low $T_4$ or $T_3$ values (Fig. 33-5). These antibodies are usually immunoglobulin G and can be identified by a variety of techniques, including affinity chromatography, immunoprecipitation, immunoelectrophoresis, and RIA. The presence of such

antibodies should be considered when serum $T_4$ or $T_3$ measurements conflict with the clinical presentation.

## THYROTROPIN RECEPTOR ANTIBODIES

Certain thyroid disorders have been associated with an immunologic abnormality. Early bioassays, such as the long-acting thyroid stimulator and its protector assay, demonstrated that the immunoglobulin of patients with Graves disease stimulates thyroid hormone secretion. Several functional types of antibodies are now recognized to exist (see Chap. 42). Although these antibodies appear to interact with thyroid follicular cell receptors, their effects are varied. Some antibodies promote thyroid gland function (thyroid-stimulating antibodies), some inhibit the binding of TSH to its receptor (thyroid-binding inhibitory immunoglobulins), and some enhance or inhibit thyroid growth. These antibodies are measured by a variety of bioassays and receptor assays.[33–35] Patients may present with hyperthyroidism, hypothyroidism, goiter, or thyroid atrophy. Pregnant women with high titers of these antibodies may give birth to infants with transient hyperthyroidism or hypothyroidism.[36]

### PERIPHERAL INDICES OF THYROID FUNCTION

Serum thyroid hormone measurements are essential for making the diagnosis of thyroid dysfunction. Usually, altered levels of $T_4$ and $T_3$ correlate well with the patient's clinical presentation, and the diagnosis of hyperthyroidism or hypothyroidism is readily made. In some situations, however, the patient's metabolic status is not apparent from the thyroid blood tests. Such occurrences are expected in euthyroid hyperthyroxinemia[37] and nonthyroidal illnesses[3] (see Chap. 36). For instance, patients with thyroid hormone resistance have high serum $T_4$ and $T_3$ levels yet may appear euthyroid. The recommendation is that

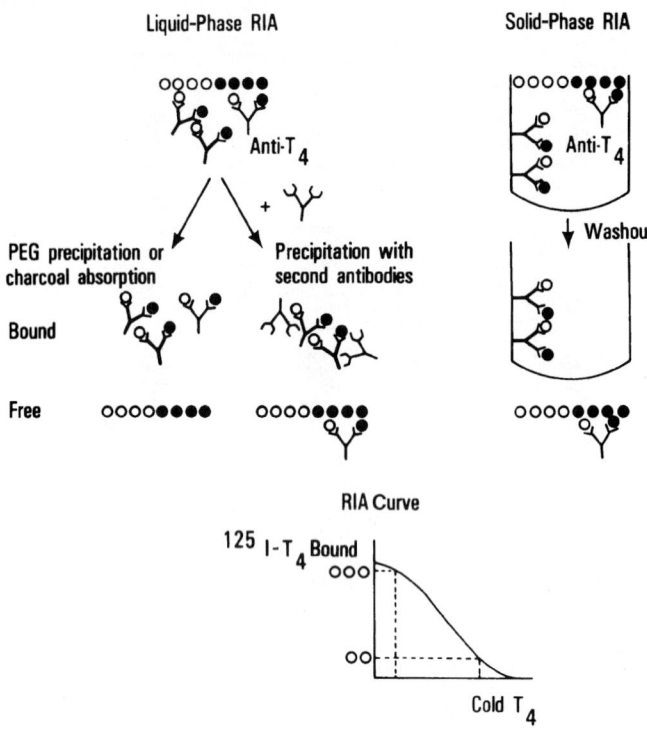

**FIGURE 33-5.** Schematic representations of how antithyroxine (*anti-T$_4$*) autoantibodies in patient's serum interfere with liquid-phase (single- or double-antibody methods) and solid-phase radioimmunoassays (*RIAs*). Thus, the bound $^{125}$I-T$_4$ would be increased in single-antibody methods, leading to a falsely low value, whereas the liquid-phase RIA using second antibodies or the solid-phase RIA would yield a falsely high value. Identical situations occur in RIAs for triiodothyronine. *Open circles* represent $^{125}$I-labeled T$_4$; *solid circles* represent "cold" T$_4$. (*PEG*, polyethylene glycol.) (From Sakata S, Nakamura S, Miura K. Autoantibodies against thyroid hormones or iodothyronine. Ann Intern Med 1985; 103:579.)

many target organs be evaluated clinically because tissue responses may be in the hyperthyroid, euthyroid, or hypothyroid range owing to heterogeneity of tissue resistance.[38,39] Patients with nonthyroidal illness have low serum T$_3$ levels and sometimes low T$_4$ levels as well. No consensus yet exists about whether these patients are completely euthyroid or whether their tissues are hypothyroid, perhaps as a protective response to conserve precious energy stores.

A variety of tests demonstrate the effects of thyroid hormone on peripheral tissues (Table 33-4). Occasionally, these tests reflect a relatively specific direct effect of thyroid hormone on an organ system. Examples are increased production of specific proteins, enhanced enzyme activity, and augmented cardiac contractility. Other tests are affected because of a change in the metabolism of the particular substance being analyzed, such as an elevated serum creatine phosphokinase (CPK) level in hypothyroidism.

Although tests reflecting peripheral action of thyroid hormone are not indicated in the evaluation of most patients, occasionally one or more of these tests may be informative.

## BLOOD TESTS

The influence of thyroid hormone status on several enzymes in the erythrocyte has been extensively studied. Red blood cell Na$^+$/K$^+$ adenosine triphosphatase is decreased in hyperthyroidism, and consequently intracellular sodium is increased; opposite changes occur in hypothyroidism.[40] Glucose-6-phosphate dehydrogenase activity is increased in half of hyperthyroid patients and is modestly reduced in hypothyroidism.[41] Transke-

**TABLE 33-4.**
**Peripheral Indices of Thyroid Function**

| Tests | Hyperthyroid | Hypothyroid |
|---|---|---|
| **BLOOD TESTS** | | |
| Erythrocyte | | |
| Na$^+$/K$^+$ adenosine triphosphatase | ↓ | ↑ |
| Sodium content | ↑ | ↓ |
| Glucose-6-phosphate dehydrogenase | ↑ | ↓ |
| Carbonic anhydrase | ↓ | ↑, N |
| Transketolase | ↓ | N |
| Serum | | |
| Creatine phosphokinase | ↓ | ↑ |
| Tyrosine | ↑ | ↓ |
| Cholesterol; lipoprotein (a) | ↓ | ↑ |
| Sex hormone–binding globulin | ↑ | ↓ |
| Ferritin | ↑ | N |
| Factor VIII activity | ↑ | ↓ |
| Angiotensin-converting enzyme | ↑ | ↓ |
| Cyclic adenosine monophosphate | ↑ | N |
| Fibronectin | ↑ | ↓ |
| Osteocalcin | ↑ | ND |
| Soluble interleukin-2 receptor | ↑ | ND |
| **OTHER TESTS** | | |
| Basal metabolic rate | ↑ | ↓ |
| Cardiac contractility | | |
| QK$_d$ | ↓ | ↑ |
| Preejection period/left ventricular ejection time ratio | ↓ | ↑ |
| Deep tendon reflex (relaxation time) | ↓ | ↑ |

*N*, normal; ↑, increase; ↓, decrease; *ND*, not done.

tolase and carbonic anhydrase activities are low in hyperthyroidism, and the latter is elevated in hypothyroid patients.[42]

CPK levels may be increased, sometimes to extremely high values, in myxedema. Isoenzyme studies have shown this CPK to be of skeletal muscle origin,[43] and the elevation probably results from impaired clearance. The low levels in hyperthyroidism are the result of an increased disappearance rate. Plasma tyrosine levels, basally and in response to oral tyrosine ingestion, are elevated in hyperthyroidism and decreased in hypothyroidism.[44]

Cholesterol levels are high in hypothyroid patients and low in hyperthyroid patients. Thyroid dysfunction influences numerous components of the lipoproteins, whether high-density, low-density, or very-low-density lipoproteins. Additionally, changes occur in the phospholipids, apoproteins, and hepatic lipase activities.[45,46] Sex hormone–binding globulin, a hepatic protein, is increased in hyperthyroidism and decreased in hypothyroidism. In patients with thyroid hormone resistance, sex hormone–binding globulin may be inappropriately normal,[38] suggesting that the liver shares the tissue resistance. Ferritin, an iron-storage protein synthesized by erythrocyte precursors and reticuloendothelial cells, is increased in hyperthyroidism.[47] Similar results have been reported for plasma cyclic adenosine monophosphate.[48] Angiotensin-converting enzyme activity[49] varies directly with the thyroid status, whereas plasma levels of several other endothelium-derived proteins (fibronectin and factor VIII–related antigen) are increased in hyperthyroidism.[50] Increased serum osteocalcin (bone Gla protein), and urinary pyridinoline cross-link excretion, markers of bone metabolism, are observed with elevated thyroid hormone levels.[51] Soluble interleukin-2 receptor is increased in hyperthyroidism and decreases with antithyroid drug therapy.[52]

## OTHER TESTS

Measurement of the basal metabolic rate (BMR) takes advantage of the correlation between energy expenditure at rest and the metabolic response to thyroid hormone. When BMR is measured under carefully controlled conditions, low values are compatible with the diagnosis of hypothyroidism and high values with hyperthyroidism. The normal range is –20% to +5%. Test conditions must be rigorously controlled because numerous pathophysiologic conditions and drugs can influence the BMR test. A more contemporary test, the basal oxygen uptake, correlates directly with thyroid status.[53]

Cardiac contractility is influenced by thyroid hormone. The clinician has two noninvasive measures for examining a patient's cardiac status. One test, the $QK_d$ interval, measures the time from the onset of the Q wave of the electrocardiogram to the Korotkoff sound recorded over the brachial artery. Euthyroid patients have a value of 205 ± 12 milliseconds. This interval is shortened in hyperthyroidism and lengthened in hypothyroidism.[54] Unfortunately, this test is not available in many hospitals. An alternative estimate of contractility can be obtained using *systolic time intervals* determined by echocardiography. This procedure measures the preejection period and the left ventricular ejection time; an inverse relation is seen between thyroid function and the preejection period/left ventricular ejection time ratio.[55]

The Achilles tendon reflex is a measure of the muscular activity of the deep tendon reflexes and may be quantified with the aid of a photoelectric cell and electrocardiogram. A prolonged relaxation time, although not pathognomonic, is a characteristic physical finding in ~60% of patients with myxedema. The instruments are less reliable in documenting the rapid reflexes that occur in hyperthyroidism.[56]

## EVALUATION OF THE PATIENT

The clinician has available a large number of tests for evaluating a patient's thyroid status.[57] In many instances, a serum free $T_4$ estimate and a serum TSH level provide sufficient information for adequate diagnosis and management. However, a number of conditions (e.g., drug use, acute illness, dysproteinemias, autoimmunity, resistance disorders) require additional laboratory procedures for confirmation. Fortunately, a broad spectrum of ancillary tests are available to assist the physician.

Some authors have proposed TSH as the first-line test. One group has recommended a TSH test only, with free $T_4$ measured when TSH is <0.1 or >5.0 mIU/L,[58] whereas another group[59] has shown an economic savings using a TSH algorithm, with a diagnostic failure rate of 2.7%.

## REFERENCES

1. Keffer JH. Preanalytical considerations in testing thyroid function. Clin Chem 1996; 42:125.
2. Nelson JC, Wilcox RB. Analytical performance of free and total thyroxine assays. Clin Chem 1996; 42:146.
3. De Groot LJ. Dangerous dogmas in medicine: the nonthyroidal illness syndrome. J Clin Endocrinol Metab 1999; 84:151.
4. Engler D, Burger AG. The deiodination of the iodothyronines and of their derivatives in man. Endocr Rev 1984; 5:151.
5. Smallridge RC, Wartofsky L, Green BJ, et al. 3'-L-Monoiodothyronine: development of a radioimmunoassay and demonstration of in vivo conversion from 3',5'-diiodothyronine. J Clin Endocrinol Metab 1979; 48:32.
6. Corcoran JM, Eastman CJ. Radioimmunoassay of 3-l-monoiodothyronine: application in normal human physiology and thyroid disease. J Clin Endocrinol Metab 1983; 57:66.
7. Chopra IJ, Santini F, Hurd RE, Chua Teco GN. A radioimmunoassay for measurement of thyroxine sulfate. J Clin Endocrinol Metab 1993; 76:145.
8. Chopra IJ, Wu S-Y, Chua Teco GN, Santini F. A radioimmunoassay for measurement of 3,5,3'-triiodothyronine sulfate: studies in thyroidal and nonthyroidal diseases, pregnancy, and neonatal life. J Clin Endocrinol Metab 1992; 75:189.
9. Faber J, Busch-Sorensen M, Rogowski P, et al. Urinary excretion of free and conjugated 3',5'-diiodothyronine and 3,3'-diiodothyronine. J Clin Endocrinol Metab 1981; 53:587.
10. Witherspoon LR, Shuler SE. Estimation of free thyroxine concentration: clinical methods and pitfalls. J Clin Immunoassay 1984; 7:192.
11. Nelson JC, Weiss RM, Wilcox RB. Underestimates of serum free thyroxine ($T_4$) concentrations by free $T_4$ immunoassays. J Clin Endocrinol Metab 1994; 79:76.
12. Sapin R, Schlienger J-L, Kaltenbach G, et al. Determination of free triiodothyronine by six different methods in patients with non-thyroidal illness and in patients treated with amiodarone. Ann Clin Biochem 1995; 32:314.
13. Piketty M-L, d'Herbomez M, Le Guillouzic D, et al. Clinical comparison of three labeled-antibody immunoassays of free triiodothyronine. Clin Chem 1996; 42:933.
14. Wong TK, Pekary AE, Hoo GS, et al. Comparison of methods for measuring free thyroxine in nonthyroidal illness. Clin Chem 1992; 38:720.
15. Docter R, van Toor H, Krenning EP, et al. Free thyroxine assessed with three assays in sera of patients with nonthyroidal illness and of subjects with abnormal concentrations of thyroxine-binding proteins. Clin Chem 1993; 39:1668.
16. Van Blerk M, Smitz J, Rozenski E, et al. Four radioisotopic immunoassays of free thyroxine compared. Ann Clin Biochem 1996; 33:335.
17. Ekins R. Measurement of free hormones in blood. Endocr Rev 1990; 11:5.
17a. Wang R, Nelson JC, Weiss RM, Wilcox RB. Accuracy of free thyroxine measurements across natural ranges of thyroxine binding to serum proteins. Thyroid 2000; 10:31.
18. Faber J, Waetjen I, Siersbaek-Nielsen K. Free thyroxine measured in undiluted serum by dialysis and ultrafiltration: effects of non-thyroidal illness, and an acute load of salicylate or heparin. Clin Chim Acta 1993; 223:159.
19. Surks MI, DeFesi CR. Normal serum free thyroid hormone concentrations in patients treated with phenytoin or carbamazepine: a paradox resolved. JAMA 1996; 275:1495.
20. Faix JD, Rosen HN, Velazquez FR. Indirect estimation of thyroid hormone-binding proteins to calculate free thyroxine index: comparison of nonisotopic methods that use labeled thyroxine ("T-Uptake"). Clin Chem 1995; 41:41.
21. Sawin T, Chopra D, Albano J, Azizi F. The free triiodothyronine ($T_3$) index. Ann Intern Med 1978; 88:474.
22. Copping S, Byfield PGH. Thyroxine-binding globulin deficiency reexamined. Clin Endocrinol 1988; 28:45.
22a. Schussler GC. The thyroxine-binding proteins. Thyroid 2000; 10:141.
23. Surks MI, Sievert R. Drugs and thyroid function. N Engl J Med 1995; 333:1688.
24. Nicoloff JT, Spencer CA. The use and misuse of the sensitive thyrotropin assays. J Clin Endocrinol Metab 1990; 71:553.
25. Franklyn JA, Black EG, Betteridge J, Sheppard MC. Comparison of second and third generation methods for measurement of serum thyrotropin in patients with overt hyperthyroidism, patients receiving thyroxine therapy, and those with nonthyroidal illness. J Clin Endocrinol Metab 1994; 78:1368.
26. Spencer CA, Takeuchi M, Kazarosyan M. Current status and performance goals for serum thyrotropin (TSH) assays. Clin Chem 1996; 42:140.
27. Despres N, Grant AM. Antibody interference in thyroid assays: a potential for clinical misinformation. Clin Chem 1998; 44:440.
28. Ozata M, Suzuki S, Miamoto T, et al. Serum thyroglobulin in the follow-up of patients with treated differentiated thyroid cancer. J Clin Endocrinol Metab 1994; 79:98.
29. Spencer CA, Takeuchi M, Kazarosyan M. Current status and performance goals for serum thyroglobulin assays. Clin Chem 1996; 42:164.
30. McLachlan SM, Rapoport B. The molecular biology of thyroid peroxidase: cloning, expression and role as autoantigen in autoimmune thyroid disease. Endocr Rev 1992; 13:192.
31. Sakata S, Nakamura S, Miura K. Autoantibodies against thyroid hormones and iodothyronine. Ann Intern Med 1985; 103:579.
32. Sakata S. Autoimmunity against thyroid hormones. Crit Rev Immunol 1994; 14:157.
33. Vitti P, Elisei R, Tonacchera M, et al. Detection of thyroid-stimulating antibody using Chinese hamster ovary cells transfected with cloned human thyrotropin receptor. J Clin Endocrinol Metab 1993; 76:499.
34. Weetman AP, McGregor AM. Autoimmune thyroid disease: further developments in our understanding. Endocr Rev 1994; 15:788.
35. Costagliola S, Morgenthaler NG, Hoermann R, et al. Second generation assay for thyrotropin receptor antibodies has superior diagnostic sensitivity for Graves' disease. J Clin Endocrinol Metab 1999; 84:90.
36. McKenzie JM, Zakarija M. Fetal and neonatal hyperthyroidism and hypothyroidism due to maternal TSH receptor antibodies. Thyroid 1992; 2:155.
37. Borst GC, Eil C, Burman KD. Euthyroid hyperthyroxinemia. Ann Intern Med 1983; 98:366.
38. Smallridge RC, Parker RA, Wiggs EA, et al. Thyroid hormone resistance in a large kindred: physiologic, biochemical, pharmacologic, and neuropsychologic studies. Am J Med 1989; 86:289.
39. Refetoff S, Weiss RE, Usala SJ. The syndromes of resistance to thyroid hormone. Endocr Rev 1993; 14:348.
40. Dasmahapatra A, Cohen MP, Grossman SD, Lasker N. Erythrocyte sodium/potassium adenosine triphosphatase in thyroid disease and nonthyroidal illness. J Clin Endocrinol Metab 1985; 61:110.
41. Viherkoski M, Lamberg BA. The glucose-6-phosphate dehydrogenase activity (G-6-PD) of the red blood cells in hyperthyroidism and hypothyroidism. Scand J Clin Lab Invest 1970; 25:137.
42. Kiso Y, Yoshida K, Kaise K, et al. Erythrocyte carbonic anhydrase-I concentrations in patients with Graves' disease and subacute thyroiditis reflect inte-

grated thyroid hormone levels over the previous few months. J Clin Endocrinol Metab 1991; 72:515.

43. Docherty I, Harrop JS, Hine KR, et al. Myoglobin concentration, creatine kinase activity, and creatine kinase B subunit concentrations in serum during thyroid disease. Clin Chem 1984; 30:42.

44. Belanger R, Chandramohan N, Misbin R, Rivlin RS. Tyrosine and glutamic acid in plasma and urine of patients with altered thyroid function. Metabolism 1972; 21:855.

45. de Bruin TWA, van Barlingen H, van Linde-Sibenius Trip M, et al. Lipoprotein (a) and apolipoprotein B plasma concentrations in hypothyroid, euthyroid, and hyperthyroid subjects. J Clin Endocrinol Metab 1993; 76:121.

46. Tan KCB, Shiu SWM, Kung AWC. Effect of thyroid dysfunction on high-density lipoprotein subfraction metabolism: roles of hepatic lipase and cholesteryl ester transfer protein. J Clin Endocrinol Metab 1998; 83:2921.

47. Takamatsu J, Majima M, Miki K, et al. Serum ferritin as a marker of thyroid hormone action on peripheral tissues. J Clin Endocrinol Metab 1985; 61:672.

48. Peracchi M, Bamonti-Catena F, Lombardi L, et al. Plasma and urine cyclic nucleotide levels in patients with hyperthyroidism and hypothyroidism. J Endocrinol Invest 1983; 6:173.

49. Smallridge RC, Rogers J, Verma PS. Serum angiotensin-converting enzyme: alterations in hyperthyroidism, hypothyroidism, and subacute thyroiditis. JAMA 1983; 250:2489.

50. Graninger W, Pirich KR, Speiser W, et al. Effect of thyroid hormones on plasma protein concentrations in man. J Clin Endocrinol Metab 1986; 63:407.

51. Garnero P, Vassy V, Bertholin A, et al. Markers of bone turnover in hyperthyroidism and the effects of treatment. J Clin Endocrinol Metab 1994; 78:955.

52. Smallridge RC, Tsokos GC, Burman KD, et al. Soluble interleukin-2 receptor is a thyroid hormone–dependent early-response marker in the treatment of thyrotoxicosis. Clin Diagn Lab Immunol 1997; 4:583.

53. Lim VS, Zavala DC, Flanigan MJ, Freeman RM. Basal oxygen uptake: a new technique for an old test. J Clin Endocrinol Metab 1986; 62:863.

54. Young RT, Van Herle AJ, Rodbard D. Improved diagnosis and management of hyper- and hypothyroidism by timing the arterial sounds. J Clin Endocrinol Metab 1976; 42:330.

55. Tseng KH, Walfish PG, Persaud JA, Gilbert BW. Concurrent aortic and mitral valve echocardiography permits measurement of systolic time intervals as an index of peripheral tissue thyroid functional status. J Clin Endocrinol Metab 1989; 69:633.

56. Ballantyne GH, Croxson MS. The effect of exercise, thyroid status and insulin-induced hypoglycemia on the Achilles tendon reflex time in man. Eur J Appl Physiol 1981; 46:77.

57. Larsen PR, Alexander NM, Chopra IJ, et al. Revised nomenclature for tests of thyroid hormones and thyroid-related proteins in serum. J Clin Endocrinol Metab 1987; 64:1089.

58. Klee GG, Hay ID. Biochemical testing of thyroid function. Endocrinol Metab Clin North Am 1997; 26:763.

59. Davey RX, Clarke MI, Webster AR. Thyroid function testing based on assay of thyroid-stimulating hormone: assessing an algorithm's reliability. Med J Aust 1996; 164:329.

**TABLE 34-1.**
**Thyroid Radiopharmaceuticals**

| Radiopharmaceutical | Physical Half-Life | Imaging Interval | Millicuries Administered | | Average Dose (rad) to Thyroid per Scan |
| --- | --- | --- | --- | --- | --- |
| | | | *For Imaging* | *For Uptake* | |
| **Iodine-131** (sodium iodide) | 8 d | 24 h | 0.030* | 0.005 | 50 |
| **Iodine-123** (sodium iodide) | 13 h | 4–24 h | 0.4 | 0.100 | 5 |
| **Technetium-99m** (pertechnetate) | 6 h | 20–30 min | 5.0 | — | 1 |

*Amounts administered are about 2 mCi for thyroid cancer investigation (see text).

However, $^{99m}$Tc pertechnetate is not optimally suited for imaging of metastatic differentiated thyroid cancer. Cancer tissue functions relatively poorly compared with normal thyroid tissue, and $^{99m}$Tc pertechnetate is usually not accumulated by such tissue in sufficient amounts relative to background for external imaging. Iodine-123, with higher target/background activity ratios, allows imaging of metastases and is being used increasingly as an alternative to $^{131}$I, the traditional radiopharmaceutical for the evaluation of metastatic disease. Fluorine-18 fluorodeoxyglucose ($^{18}$F-FDG) is the newest radiotracer to be used in evaluating thyroid cancer. It may help image metastases not detected with $^{131}$I and, therefore, appears to be complementary to the use of radioiodine. For thyroid uptake measurements, $^{131}$I continues to be used widely because it is inexpensive, the methodology is simple, and the radiation exposure from the small amount of radioactivity required for this test is low (Table 34-1).

Imaging instrumentation in nuclear medicine also has greatly improved. Rectilinear scanners equipped with detector heads that move back and forth across the organ to be imaged have been replaced by stationary scintillation cameras that afford higher count rates and superior image resolution.

# CHAPTER 34

# THYROID UPTAKE AND IMAGING

SALIL D. SARKAR AND DAVID V. BECKER

Thyroid radionuclide uptake and imaging play an important part in the clinical management of thyroid disease when used in conjunction with a physical examination and laboratory tests. The proper use of radionuclide techniques requires a basic knowledge of their underlying principles and of their clinical advantages and limitations.

Major changes have occurred in the last two decades in the choice of radiopharmaceuticals for thyroid imaging. Iodine-131 ($^{131}$I), used routinely in the past, is associated with a relatively high radiation absorbed dose to the thyroid. Although no evidence exists of any deleterious radiation effect,[1] the use of $^{131}$I has been replaced by the use of technetium-99m ($^{99m}$Tc) pertechnetate and iodine-123 ($^{123}$I) for routine thyroid imaging. Both $^{99m}$Tc pertechnetate and $^{123}$I deliver a much lower radiation dose per μCi deposited, permitting the administration of larger radiotracer amounts that provide higher count rates and improved image resolution.

# RADIOPHARMACEUTICALS

## IODINE-131

Iodine-131, produced in a nuclear reactor, is selectively localized by thyroid tissue and is metabolized in the same manner as stable iodine ($^{127}$I). The biologic half-life of iodine is ~80 days in the normally functioning thyroid gland, and its physical half-life is 8 days. Because of the relatively long half-life and energetic β-emission, the thyroidal radiation absorbed dose is proportionately high.[2,3] Therefore, in benign thyroid disease in which every attempt is made to keep the radiation dose as low as possible, the diagnostic use of $^{131}$I generally is limited to the measurement of thyroid uptake, a nonimaging test that requires only a small amount of radiotracer, ~0.005 mCi. In thyroid cancer, however, larger amounts (~2 mCi) of $^{131}$I are used to improve the ability to detect metastatic foci. Such amounts, however, are associated with a higher radiation dose and may cause "stunning" of residual thyroid tissue, so that the efficacy of a subsequent ablative $^{131}$I dose is diminished. If stunning is a concern, $^{123}$I may be used instead for the diagnostic workup (see later).[4–6] Finally, and perhaps most important, $^{131}$I still has a key role in the treatment of hyperthyroidism and differentiated thyroid cancer by virtue of its selective accumulation by follicular cells and its high radiation dose to thyroid tissue (see Chaps. 40 and 42).

## TECHNETIUM-99M PERTECHNETATE

$^{99m}$Tc pertechnetate is conveniently available from reactor-produced molybdenum-99 generators. $^{99m}$Tc pertechnetate is trapped by the thyroid, but unlike $^{131}$I, it does not participate in hormonogenesis; therefore, its biologic half-life in the thyroid is short. The physical half-life also is short (6 hours), and no β-rays are emitted. Consequently, the radiation absorbed dose to the thyroid is low,[7,7a] permitting the use of this radiopharmaceutical for routine imaging of the thyroid gland. Furthermore, because of its short half-life, $^{99m}$Tc pertechnetate may be used in a lactating patient with only temporary interruption of breast-feeding.[8] Maximum uptake of $^{99m}$Tc occurs early; therefore, imaging is performed 20 to 30 minutes after tracer administration. The thyroid uptake of $^{99m}$Tc pertechnetate is much lower than that of $^{123}$I, the alternative radiopharmaceutical for routine thyroid imaging (see later). However, the lower uptake of $^{99m}$Tc pertechnetate is offset by higher count rates from larger administered radiotracer amounts. As alluded to earlier, $^{99m}$Tc pertechnetate is suitable primarily for imaging of the in situ thyroid gland because the target/background uptake ratios do not permit imaging of metastases, which accumulate radiotracer poorly relative to normal thyroid tissue.

## IODINE-123

$^{123}$I, a cyclotron product, has biodistribution properties identical to those of $^{131}$I but a much shorter physical half-life (13 hours). Thus, high thyroid/background ratios are achieved at low radiation doses.[2] Overall image quality and detection of hypoactive thyroid lesions with $^{123}$I are comparable to those with $^{99m}$Tc pertechnetate,[9,10] although imaging time per view is longer with $^{123}$I because the administered activity is lower. $^{123}$I may be considered the ideal "physiologic" imaging agent for the thyroid, but it is not used universally because of its high cost (roughly 10-fold greater than $^{99m}$Tc pertechnetate per patient) and more complex logistics. $^{123}$I also may be used for thyroid uptake measurements, particularly when uptake is combined with imaging, although, as noted earlier, $^{131}$I is more widely used for this purpose.

In thyroid cancer, the diagnostic use of $^{123}$I as an alternative to $^{131}$I is being investigated.

## FLUORINE-18 FLUORODEOXYGLUCOSE

Physiologic substrates, including glucose, can be labeled with a positron-emitting radionuclide such as fluorine-18. Malignant tumors have increased rates of glycolysis and glucose utilization and, consequently, are associated with increased uptake of $^{18}$F-FDG. $^{18}$F-FDG undergoes phosphorylation by hexokinase but does not undergo further metabolism. Its biodistribution can be imaged with specialized detectors, and the procedure is referred to as *positron emission tomography* (PET). Preliminary reports suggest that PET with $^{18}$F-FDG may be a valuable adjunct in the management of differentiated thyroid cancer.[11–14] PET frequently detects metastases not visualized by routine radioiodine scanning and may be particularly helpful in evaluating patients with negative scans and positive serum thyroglobulin levels. To date, however, the use of this diagnostic modality has been limited because of the high cost of PET detectors. The introduction of lower-cost "hybrid" cameras capable of both standard gamma imaging and PET is expected to increase the use of $^{18}$F-FDG in thyroid cancer cases.

## THALLIUM-201 CHLORIDE, TECHNETIUM-99M SESTAMIBI, TECHNETIUM-99M TETROFOSMIN

Thallium-201 chloride, $^{99m}$Tc sestamibi, and $^{99m}$Tc tetrofosmin, widely used for myocardial perfusion studies, have been used for the evaluation of thyroid cancer. As nonspecific tumor markers, these radiotracers may help detect recurrent or metastatic thyroid cancer not visualized by radioiodine imaging.[15,16] However, their routine use as

adjuncts to whole body radioiodine imaging is still not widely accepted.

# INSTRUMENTATION

## SCINTILLATION SCANNER AND CAMERA

The rectilinear scanner was the first nuclear imaging instrument devised.[17] This highly focused detector views a small area of the organ at a time; it images successive areas by a transverse back-and-forth motion until the entire organ is imaged. Because the detector head points in only one direction, oblique and lateral views of the thyroid are difficult to obtain. Image resolution is relatively poor compared with that of contemporary scintillation cameras. The principal advantage of the rectilinear scanner is the ability to obtain a full-sized 1:1 image, which facilitates precise in vivo location of neck masses. However, this instrument is not readily available presently.

The scintillation camera is the standard imaging instrument in nuclear medicine.[18] The detector is capable of viewing either a small region of interest such as the thyroid, or a large area such as the abdomen or chest, with the use of appropriate collimators (see later). In addition, the detector can be easily rotated for lateral and oblique views.

Incoming gamma rays interact with a crystal in the scintillation detector to produce flashes of light. The crystal is in contact with photomultiplier tubes that detect, amplify, and locate the light signals electronically. Scintillation crystals generally are $^1/_4$ inch or $^3/_8$ inch thick. The $^1/_4$-inch crystal is suitable for only low energy radionuclides such as $^{99m}$Tc and $^{123}$I, whereas the thicker $^3/_8$-inch crystal provides adequate interactions with higher energy gamma rays such as $^{131}$I. In addition, detectors are fitted with a collimator, generally a removable lead plate with many holes or a lead cone with a single small hole at the tip (pinhole collimator). Detector heads and fields of view are smaller for the portable cameras as compared to the standard wide-field-of-view cameras.

Collimators with multiple holes that are parallel to each other are routinely used with cameras to view a large area of the body. The lead septa between the holes in a parallel hole collimator allow primarily those rays originating directly below each hole to enter through that hole, thereby narrowing the view of each photomultiplier tube and assisting it in locating the origin of the gamma radiation in the field of view. To prevent septal penetration of gamma rays, a "high energy collimator," that is, one with thick septa, is used to image a radionuclide with high energy gamma emissions such as $^{131}$I. Conversely, a "low energy collimator" with thin septa is used for low energy gamma emissions as with $^{123}$I. Parallel hole collimators, with the wide-field-of-view camera, are the mainstay of clinical nuclear imaging and are particularly suitable for whole body imaging for thyroid cancer metastases.

Pinhole collimators are used with scintillation cameras to provide a detailed picture of small areas and, therefore, are suitable for imaging such organs as the thyroid.[19,20] This method may detect areas of localized variations in function within thyroid tissue that often are not palpable as discrete abnormalities. A disadvantage of the pinhole collimator is that it introduces spatial distortion, making it more difficult to correlate the image with physical landmarks. For the same reason, measurement of gland size using a calibrated marker next to the thyroid is unreliable. Pinhole collimator imaging of the thyroid is feasible using cameras with both small and large fields of view.

## THYROID PROBE

The thyroid probe is a small, portable scintillation detector used to measure thyroid uptake. It consists of a scintillation crystal

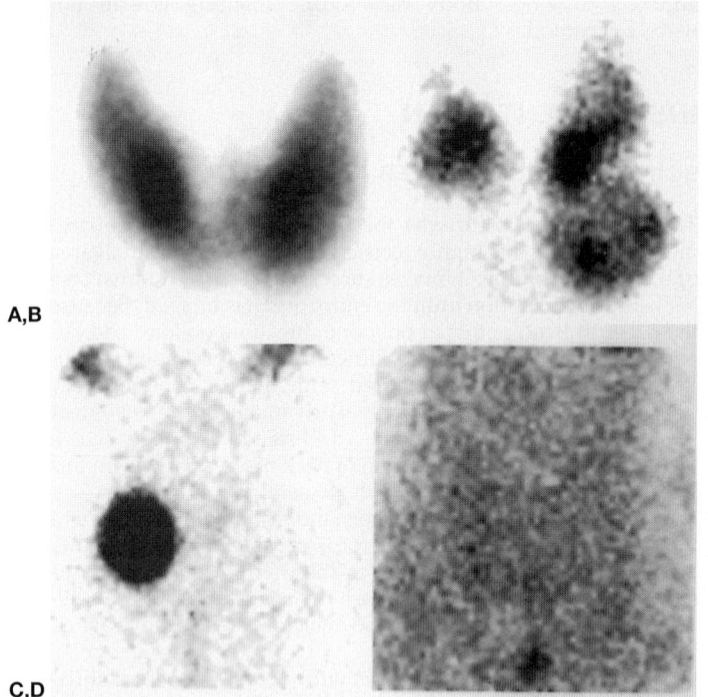

A,B

C,D

**FIGURE 34-1.** Typical images in (**A**) Graves disease; (**B**) toxic multinodular goiter; (**C**) solitary hyperfunctioning nodule; (**D**) destructive thyroiditis.

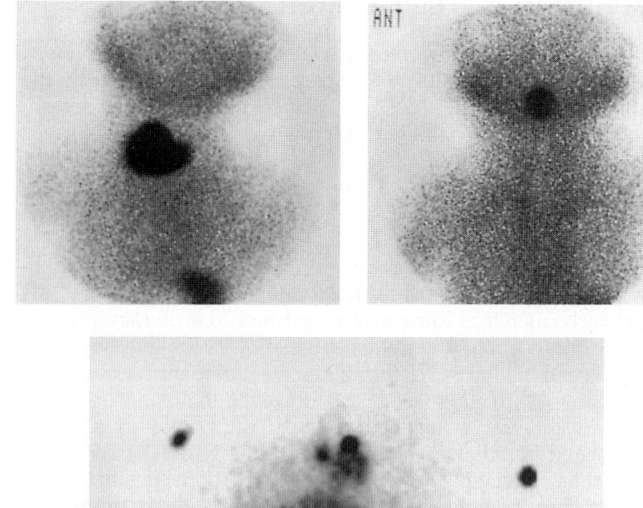

**FIGURE 34-2.** *Upper left,* normally located thyroid gland in infant. *Upper right,* lingual thyroid in infant. *Below,* large mediastinal thyroid in elderly woman (markers at shoulders and suprasternal notch).

and a single photomultiplier tube housed in a cylindrical lead casing. This probe, placed at a distance from the neck, is capable of measuring or counting radioactivity.[21] It does not produce an image of the organ.

## APPLICATIONS, TECHNIQUES, AND INTERPRETATION OF RADIONUCLIDE IMAGING

### APPLICATIONS OF IMAGING

Imaging is of value in distinguishing Graves disease from toxic nodular goiter, assessing the function of nodules, differentiating subacute thyroiditis and related conditions from Graves disease and toxic nodular goiter, defining occult thyroid lesions, determining the location and size of functional thyroid tissue, and detecting metastases from differentiated thyroid cancer. Perhaps the most frequent application of thyroid imaging is in evaluating the function of palpable nodules. A *nodule* is a palpatory or pathologic finding and cannot be defined by thyroid imaging alone. The imaging of palpable nodules allows normally functioning tissue to be distinguished from hypofunctioning ("cold") or hyperfunctioning ("hot") lesions. Hyperfunctional nodules (Fig. 34-1) may be associated with clinical or subclinical hyperthyroidism and are unlikely to be cancer. Hypofunctional nodules may be associated with a higher incidence of malignancy (see Chaps. 39 and 40).

Imaging with or without an uptake measurement may help differentiate hyperthyroidism due to thyroiditis (viral, postpartum, or amiodarone related), from hyperthyroidism due to Graves disease or nodular goiter (see Fig. 34-1).

Occult or nonpalpable thyroid lesions may be a clinical consideration in some patients without known primary tumors and in patients exposed to therapeutic x-rays or other radiation in infancy and childhood, who are at risk of developing a thyroid neoplasm later in life.[22,23]

Thyroid size generally is estimated by palpation or by ultrasonography. Size also may be assessed scintigraphically, using a rectilinear scanner that provides a full-sized 1:1 image.[24] Estimates of the size of the thyroid gland or thyroid nodule are usually used to calculate the amount of therapeutic radioiodine to be administered in hyperthyroidism and to assess the response to radioiodine or suppressive therapy. The use of ultrasonography to measure thyroid volume is discussed in Chapter 35.

Imaging may help establish the presence of a nonpalpable thyroid gland, for instance in hypothyroid infants, and may help localize mediastinal, lingual, or other ectopic thyroid tissue[25,26] (Fig. 34-2). Mediastinal imaging is useful to locate aberrant thyroid tissue that might manifest as a substernal mass on a chest radiograph, often with tracheal deviation.

Whole body radioiodine imaging, together with serum thyroglobulin determinations, is used to identify, locate, and monitor differentiated thyroid cancer (see Chap. 40).

### TECHNIQUES OF IMAGING

#### IMAGING OF THE THYROID GLAND

The radiopharmaceuticals of choice are $^{123}$I and $^{99m}$Tc pertechnetate. For mediastinal thyroid tissue, $^{123}$I imaging at 24 hours may have advantages over $^{99m}$Tc imaging because activity in the heart blood pool on the $^{99m}$Tc image may preclude optimal visualization of overlying thyroid tissue. Imaging with $^{99m}$Tc, however, may suffice for most goiters with substernal extensions and, hence, can be used for the initial evaluation. $^{131}$I may be used in lieu of $^{123}$I, if the latter is not available. $^{131}$I offers the same advantage as $^{123}$I, and its more energetic gamma rays are less likely to be absorbed by the overlying sternum.

$^{123}$I has theoretical advantages over $^{99m}$Tc for the evaluation of lingual thyroid tissue because of the absence of significant $^{123}$I accumulation in the salivary glands, which may interfere with interpretation (the salivary glands trap but do not bind

[99m]Tc or iodine, so only early imaging, as with [99m]Tc, shows accumulation of radioactivity). Nonetheless, [99m]Tc has been used successfully in assessing ectopic thyroid tissue.[26]

Imaging is performed 4 or 24 hours after the administration of 0.3 to 0.4 mCi of [123]I orally, or 24 hours after the oral ingestion of 0.03 to 0.05 mCi of [131]I, or 20 to 30 minutes after the intravenous injection of ~5 mCi of [99m]Tc pertechnetate. Standard imaging projections are anterior, left anterior oblique, and right anterior oblique.

Prior exposure to stable iodine in iodinated contrast radiographic dyes and iodine-rich foods, or to thyroid hormone, may depress the thyroidal uptake of radioiodine or [99m]Tc for 2 to 10 weeks, depending on the nature of the interfering substance and thyroid function.[27–29] After prior exposure to stable iodine, it may be possible to obtain an adequate image in 7 to 10 days if the radiopharmaceutical amount is increased (e.g., 10 mCi of [99m]Tc).

The standard imaging instrument is the scintillation camera with a pinhole collimator. Single photon emission computed tomography with the camera and a parallel hole collimator may allow three-dimensional evaluation of the thyroid, but the clinical application of this technique is limited because of its complexity and cost.[30]

When hypothyroid infants are imaged, the stomach also should be imaged because there may be a trapping defect in the thyroid associated with a similar defect in the salivary glands and gastric mucosa.[31] The imaging time per camera view is ~5 minutes for [99m]Tc pertechnetate and ~10 minutes for [123]I, and varies with the thyroid uptake of radiotracer and administered amount of radiotracer. The location on the scintillation camera image of a palpable mass may be determined by placing a small radioactive source over the center of the mass or at several points around it.

### EXTENDED BODY IMAGING FOR DIFFERENTIATED THYROID CANCER

For optimal imaging of metastatic differentiated thyroid carcinoma, patient preparation is crucial. All patients will have undergone surgical or radioiodine ablation of normal thyroid tissue to remove competing functioning normal tissue. High levels of thyroid-stimulating hormone (TSH) maximize radioiodine uptake in thyroid tissues and facilitate their visualization.[32,33] Sustained elevation of endogenous serum TSH can be achieved by one of two regimens. In the first regimen, all thyroid hormone preparations are withheld for 6 weeks before imaging; alternatively, triiodothyronine ($T_3$) is substituted for thyroxine ($T_4$) in patients receiving long-term $T_4$ therapy 6 weeks in advance and is discontinued 2 to 3 weeks before imaging, thereby shortening the period of symptomatic hypothyroidism.[32,34] Recombinant human TSH may be used in selected patients in lieu of prolonged thyroid hormone withdrawal.[35,36] The prior use of iodinated contrast radiographic dyes, therapeutic iodide-containing preparations including amiodarone, vitamins, and kelp should be avoided. In addition, an iodine-poor diet instituted a week before the test may enhance radiotracer uptake by thyroid tissue.[37,38] Foods rich in iodine include certain seafood (ocean fish, shrimp, lobster, clams, oysters, seaweed); milk, cured and spicy meats (ham, bacon, salami, pastrami); certain commercial food preparations (pizza, chili, potato chips, pretzels, nuts), and canned fruits and vegetables. Diuretics such as hydrochlorothiazide and furosemide have been used to help deplete body iodine stores before imaging. Although radioiodine uptake by tumor tissue may be increased by diuretics, the renal clearance of radioiodine is decreased, resulting in [131]I retention and increased total body radiation dose.[39]

[131]I is the traditional radiopharmaceutical for the imaging of differentiated thyroid cancer, although [123]I has been proposed as an alternative. The administered amount of [131]I usually is ~2 mCi. Larger amounts—up to 10 mCi—have been used in an attempt to visualize more metastatic sites.[40] Their use, however, is controversial because subsequent uptake of therapeutic [131]I may be impaired due to "stunning" of thyroid tissue.[4–6] If [123]I is used, ~2 mCi of the radiotracer may be administered. Imaging after [131]I therapy, optimally at 7 to 10 days, often helps discover tumor foci not visualized on the pretherapy scan.[41,42]

Body imaging is best performed with a wide-field-of-view scintillation camera and a parallel hole collimator that is appropriate for the energy of the radionuclide used, that is, a "high energy" collimator for [131]I and "low energy" collimator for [123]I. If a significant amount of radioactivity is present in residual tissue in the thyroid bed, the thyroid bed should be covered with a lead shield during imaging, or the halo or "flare" from this radioactivity may obscure smaller amounts of abnormal uptake in adjacent areas. Despite this precaution, however, the presence of large thyroid remnants may well preclude optimal visualization of the lungs, necessitating additional evaluation with CT. Anterior and posterior views of the head/neck, thorax, abdomen/pelvis, and proximal femurs are obtained routinely. In addition, images of the anterior neck taken with a pinhole collimator facilitate the evaluation of thyroid remnants and cervical lymph node metastases. Quantitation of uptake in residual thyroid tissue may be used to determine the ablative [131]I dose. Such uptakes have been traditionally measured with the thyroid probe but can be derived more accurately from the camera images with the use of suitable regions of interest.[43] Quantitative techniques are being developed to allow the prediction of absorbed radiation dose actually delivered to the tumor.[44]

## INTERPRETATION OF IMAGES

The assessment of function in a thyroid nodule is generally straightforward. Occasionally, one encounters the entity known as *discrepant nodule,* a nodule that appears to be functioning, or hot, on the early [99m]Tc image but is hypoactive on the relatively delayed radioiodine image[45,46] (Fig. 34-3). This discrepancy may be explained by the preservation within the nodule of the trapping mechanism, but the loss of organification. Discrepant nodules do not represent a specific histopathologic entity and comprise a variety of benign and malignant lesions.[46]

Subacute thyroiditis is characterized by sharply decreased radiotracer accumulation in the thyroid gland and, therefore, can be easily distinguished from hyperthyroidism due to overproduction of hormone (Graves/toxic nodular disease), which is associated with increased radiotracer uptake (see Fig. 34-1). Mediastinal thyroid tissue occasionally does not collect enough radioactivity to be adequately visible, although prior stimulation with exogenous TSH may improve the likelihood of imaging this tissue. If the pinhole collimator is not positioned directly over the mediastinal tissue, this tissue may appear to be above the suprasternal notch because of parallax error.[47] Extension of the neck, as required for imaging, may move the thyroid cephalad so that

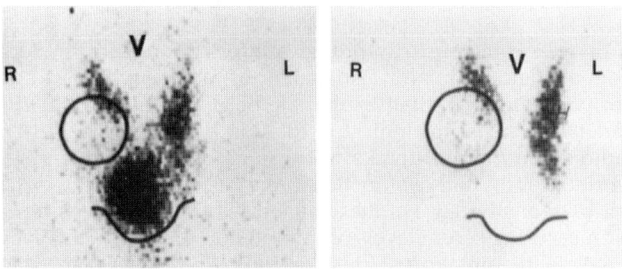

**FIGURE 34-3.** *Left,* [99m]Tc image shows decreased uptake in a nodule in the right lobe and increased uptake in a nodule in the isthmus. *Right,* [131]I image shows decreased uptake in the right lobe nodule, as with [99m]Tc, and discrepant (decreased) uptake in the isthmic nodule. Both nodules were benign on histopathologic examination.

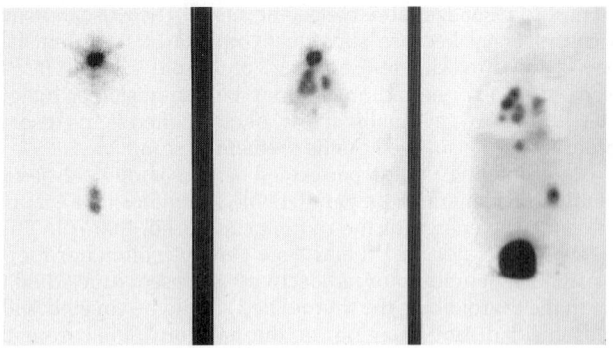

**FIGURE 34-4.** Whole-body images in metastatic differentiated thyroid cancer. *Left*, [131]I image before therapy shows uptake in large thyroid remnant in the neck and no metastases. *Middle*, image after therapy dose of [131]I shows uptake in thyroid remnant, and mediastinal/lung and abdominal metastases. *Right*, image with [18]F-fluorodeoxyglucose shows mediastinal/lung and abdominal metastases.

partly substernal thyroids may appear to lie entirely above the suprasternal notch. Activity adjacent to the thyroid occasionally is seen in a pyramidal lobe or in the esophagus. The former often is observed in Graves disease, whereas the latter is due to radioactivity in swallowed saliva and should not be mistaken for substernal extension of the thyroid. Esophageal activity usually diminishes after the patient drinks water. Visualization of thyroglossal duct cysts is unusual in euthyroid patients, although far more common in thyroidectomized patients with high TSH levels (see later). Rarely, metastatic cervical nodes are detected in a patient with an intact thyroid gland.[48]

Whole body imaging with radioiodine for metastases (Fig. 34-4) usually shows concomitant uptake in the salivary glands and stomach, reflecting trapping of the radioiodine. In the presence of thyroid tissue—benign or malignant—uptake may also be seen in the liver, reflecting accumulation and metabolism of labeled thyroid hormone. A hypertrophied thyroglossal duct remnant is often visualized, because of the hypothyroid state and elevated serum TSH levels. Contamination of clothing or skin by saliva and accumulation of radiotracer in bronchopulmonary secretions may mimic metastases.[49–51] Uncommon sites of uptake worth noting include the thymus, gallbladder, sebaceous cyst, Meckel's diverticulum, breast cyst, and such neoplasms as gastric cancer, lung cancer, and Warthin tumor.[49,51]

With careful attention to patient preparation and methodology, metastases from differentiated thyroid carcinoma are detected with ~80% accuracy. Anaplastic and medullary thyroid cancers concentrate radioiodine poorly.

# APPLICATIONS, TECHNIQUES, AND INTERPRETATION OF THYROID UPTAKE

## APPLICATIONS OF UPTAKE MEASUREMENTS

A thyroid scan primarily provides information as to the location, configuration, and distribution of radioactivity, but does not provide a quantitative estimate of global thyroid function and therefore is not indicated for this purpose. The 24-hour radioiodine thyroid uptake test was an important part of the workup for thyroid dysfunction in the past; however, it is not as critical today because of the availability of sensitive techniques for measuring serum levels of thyroid hormone and TSH. Nevertheless, the uptake test, together with the thyroid scan, plays an important role in the diagnosis of hyperthyroidism due to destructive thyroiditis, which is characterized by very low uptake of radioiodine and [99m]Tc pertechnetate. More importantly, the radioiodine uptake is also used in calculating the

therapeutic amount of radioiodine to be administered in Graves disease and toxic nodular disease (see Chap. 42). Its occasional use in the $T_3$ suppression and perchlorate discharge tests is described later.

## TECHNIQUES OF UPTAKE MEASUREMENTS

The uptake test consists of the administration of ~0.005 mCi of [131]I or 0.100 mCi of [123]I orally and measurement of the percentage of the administered amount in the neck (thyroid) 24 hours later, using the thyroid probe.[52] Methods using [99m]Tc are available but require a scintillation camera and are somewhat cumbersome.[53]

## INTERPRETATION OF UPTAKES

The normal 24-hour radioiodine uptake ranges from 10% to 35%; regional variations due to differences in iodine intake may occur.[54,55] The uptake in hypothyroid patients tends to overlap with the low range of normal, but values in overtly hyperthyroid patients usually are distinctively high. Among hyperthyroid patients, those with Graves disease usually have higher 24-hour uptakes than those with autonomously functioning toxic nodules. Patients with hyperthyroidism due to thyroiditis (viral, postpartum, amiodarone/cytokine related) and those with struma ovarii typically have low thyroid uptakes. In contrast, some disorders, including Hashimoto (autoimmune) disease and iodine deficiency, may be associated with high uptake despite euthyroid or even hypothyroid status.[27]

As with thyroid imaging, the prior intake of exogenous iodide or thyroid hormone interferes with the thyroid uptake test. However, the results of the uptake test still may be of value. For instance, a low uptake in cases of suspected subacute thyroiditis may not be diagnostic, but a normal or high uptake despite the prior intake of iodine or thyroid hormone makes the diagnosis unlikely.

# PHARMACOLOGIC MANIPULATIONS

Tests that use the thyroid scan or uptake, in conjunction with pharmacologic manipulation of the hypothalamic–pituitary–thyroid axis, may provide additional diagnostic information in certain disorders. Three such tests involving the use of $T_3$, potassium perchlorate, and TSH are discussed next.

## TRIIODOTHYRONINE SUPPRESSION TEST

The $T_3$ suppression test is based on the finding that the administration of $T_3$ (75–100 µg per day for 8–10 days) suppresses the uptake of radioiodine in the normal thyroid gland by at least 50% but does not suppress uptake in Graves disease or toxic nodular goiter because the thyroid glands in the latter are autonomous and not dependent on pituitary TSH.[56,57] The $T_3$ suppression test, once popular for the diagnosis of borderline hyperthyroidism, is only occasionally used today in conjunction with imaging to determine thyroid nodular autonomy. Modifications of the standard $T_3$ suppression test are necessary in some conditions. Occasional patients, particularly those with nodular thyroids, may exhibit autonomous increase in thyroid function while receiving long-term replacement therapy with $T_4$.[58] This may be confirmed by measuring the thyroid uptake without discontinuing $T_4$ and without the addition of $T_3$. Such uptake measurements normally should be no more than 1% to 2%. The adequacy of suppressive thyroid hormone therapy can be evaluated in the same manner, although the ultrasensitive TSH assays and the thyrotropin-releasing hormone stimulation test offer alternative methods (see Chap. 15).

## PERCHLORATE DISCHARGE TEST

Impaired organic iodination within the thyroid in certain disorders results in increased unbound iodide. The administration of potassium perchlorate, a competitive inhibitor of iodide trapping, to patients with these disorders causes discharge of the unbound iodide. In healthy subjects, the thyroidal iodide content does not change significantly after perchlorate administration because most of the iodide is bound and cannot be discharged.

A change in thyroidal iodide content after perchlorate administration can be inferred from a change in the thyroidal content of previously administered [131]I. The test involves baseline measurement of thyroid uptake 2 hours after [131]I administration. Then, 600 to 1000 mg of potassium perchlorate is given orally, followed 1 hour later by a second measurement of thyroid uptake. A 5% or greater decrease in the thyroid counts suggests impaired organic iodination.[59] The test may be enhanced by use of carrier iodide.[60]

## THYROID-STIMULATING HORMONE STIMULATION

The intramuscular or subcutaneous injection of TSH increases the uptake of $^{99m}$Tc or radioiodine by the thyroid gland. Recombinant human TSH could potentially be used to visualize hypoactive retrosternal thyroid tissue, enhance radiotracer uptake in nodular goiters before [131]I therapy, and distinguish primary from secondary hypothyroidism.[61] It is also very useful in the management of differentiated thyroid cancer.[35,35a,36]

## REFERENCES

1. Becker DV. Choice of therapy for Graves' hyperthyroidism. N Engl J Med 1984; 311:464.
2. MIRD/Dose Estimate Report no. 5: summary of current radiation dose estimates to human from I-123, I-124, I-125, I-126, I-130, I-131 and I-132 as sodium iodide. J Nucl Med 1975; 16:857.
3. Dunning DE, Schwartz G. Variability of human thyroid characteristics and estimates of dose from ingested I-131. Health Phys 1981; 40:661.
4. Jeevanram RK, Shah DH, Sharma SM, et al. Influence of initial large dose on subsequent uptake of therapeutic radioiodine in thyroid cancer patients. Nucl Med Biol 1986; 13:277.
5. Park HM, Park YH, Zhou XH. Detection of thyroid remnant/metastases without stunning: an ongoing dilemma. Thyroid 1997; 7:277.
6. Kao CH, Yen TC. Stunning effects after a diagnostic dose of iodine-131. Nuklearmedizin 1998; 37:30.
7. MIRD/Dose Estimate Report no. 8: summary of current radiation dose estimates to normal humans from Tc-99m as sodium pertechnetate. J Nucl Med 1976; 17:74.
7a. Sfakianakis GN, Ezuddin SH, Sanchez JE, et al. Pertechnetate scintigraphy in primary congenital hypothyroidism. J Nucl Med 1999; 40:799.
8. Romney B, Nickoloff EL, Esser PD. Excretion of radioiodine in breast milk. J Nucl Med 1989; 30:124.
9. Ryo UY, Vaidya P, Schneider AB, et al. Thyroid imaging agents: a comparison of I-123 and Tc-99m pertechnetate. Radiology 1983; 148:819.
10. Arnold JE, Pinsky S. Comparison of Tc-99m and I-123 for thyroid imaging. J Nucl Med 1976; 17:361.
11. Sisson JC, Ackerman RJ, Meyer MA, et al. Uptake of 18-fluoro-2-deoxy-D-glucose by thyroid cancer: implication for diagnosis and therapy. J Clin Endocrinol Metab 1993; 77:1090.
12. Feine U, Lietzenmayer R, Hanke JP, et al. Fluorine-18-FDG and Iodine-131 iodide uptake in thyroid cancer. J Nucl Med 1996; 37:1468.
13. Dietlein M, Scheidhauer K, Voth E, et al. Fluorine-18-fluorodeoxyglucose positron emission tomography and iodine-131 whole-body scintigraphy in the followup of differentiated thyroid cancer. Eur J Nucl Med 1997; 24:1342.
14. Altenvoerde G, Lerch H, Kuwert T, et al. Positron emission tomography with F-18-deoxyglucose in patients with differentiated thyroid carcinoma, elevated thyroglobulin levels, and negative iodine scans. Langenbacks Archives of Surgery 1998; 383:160.
15. Ugur O, Kostakoglu L, Caner B, et al. Comparison of $^{201}$Tl, 99mTc-MIBI and $^{131}$I imaging in the followup of patients with well-differentiated thyroid carcinoma. Nucl Med Commun 1996; 17:373.
16. Gallowitsch HJ, Mikosch P, Kresnik E, et al. Thyroglobulin and low-dose Iodine-131 and Technetium-99m-Tetrofosmin whole-body scintigraphy in differentiated thyroid carcinoma. J Nucl Med 1998; 39:870.
17. Brownell GL, Aronow S, Hine GJ. Radioisotope scanning. In: Hine GJ, ed. Instrumentation in nuclear medicine, vol 1. New York: Academic Press, 1967:381.
18. McIntyre WJ, Saha GB, Go RT. Planar imaging with single-head large-field-of-view cameras: are they still the workhorse? Semin Nucl Med 1994; 24(1):11.
19. Sarkar SD. In vivo thyroid studies. In: Gottschalk AA, Hoffer PB, Potchen EJ, eds. Diagnostic nuclear medicine, 2nd ed. Baltimore: Williams & Wilkins, 1988:756.
20. Pinsky SM, Ryo UY. Technique and utility of thyroid scans. In: DeGroot L, Frohman LA, Kaplan EL, Refetoff S, eds. Radiation associated thyroid carcinoma. New York: Grune & Stratton, 1977:297.
21. Hine GJ, Williams JB. Thyroid radioiodine uptake measurements. In: Hine GJ, ed. Instrumentation in nuclear medicine, vol 1. New York: Academic Press, 1967:327.
22. Schneider AB, Ron E, Lubin J, et al. Dose-response relationships for radiation-induced thyroid cancer and thyroid nodules: evidence for the prolonged effects of radiation on the thyroid. J Clin Endocrinol Metab 1993; 77:362.
23. Cicerio G, Frohman LA, Bekerman C, et al. Scintigraphic thyroid abnormalities after radiation: a controlled study with Tc-99m pertechnetate scanning. Ann Intern Med 1982; 97:55.
24. Mandart G, Erbsmann F. Estimation of thyroid weight by scintigraphy. Int J Nucl Med Biol 1975; 2:185.
25. Schoen EJ, Dos Remedios LV, Backstrom M. Heterogeneity of congenital primary hypothyroidism: the importance of thyroid scintigraphy. J Perinat Med 1987; 15:137.
26. Verelst J, Chanoine JP, Delange F. Radionuclide imaging in primary permanent congenital hypothyroidism. Clin Nucl Med 1991; 16:652.
27. Grayson RR. Factors which influence the radioactive iodine thyroidal uptake test. Am J Med 1960; 28:397.
28. Krugman LC, Hershman JM, Chopra IJ, et al. Patterns of recovery of the hypothalamic-pituitary-thyroid axis in patients taken off chronic thyroid therapy. J Clin Endocrinol Metab 1975; 41:70.
29. Laurie AJ, Lyon SG, Lasser EC. Contrast material iodides: potential effects on radioactive iodine thyroid uptake. J Nucl Med 1992; 33:237.
30. Chen JJS, LaFrance ND, Allo MD, et al. Single photon emission computed tomography of the thyroid. J Clin Endocrinol Metab 1988; 66:1240.
31. Lever EG, Medeiros-Neto GA, DeGroot LJ. Inherited disorders of thyroid metabolism. Endocr Rev 1983; 4:213.
32. Beierwaltes WH. The treatment of thyroid carcinoma with radioactive iodine. Semin Nucl Med 1978; 3:79.
33. Sarkar SD, Torres MA, Manalili E, et al. Iodine-131 effects on thyroid remnant function: influence of serum TSH levels. Radiology 1998; 209P:404.
34. Schneider AB, Line BR, Goldman JM, Robbins J. Sequential serum thyroglobulin determinations, I-131 scans, and I-131 uptakes after triiodothyronine withdrawal in patients with thyroid cancer. J Clin Endocrinol Metab 1981; 53:1199.
35. Ladenson PW, Braverman LE, Mazzaferri EL, et al. Comparison of administration of recombinant human thyrotropin with withdrawal of thyroid hormone for radioactive iodine scanning in patients with thyroid carcinoma. N Engl J Med 1997; 337:888.
35a. Haugen BR, Pacini F, Reiners C, et al. A comparison of recombinant human thyrotropin and thyroid hormone withdrawal for the detection of thyroid remnant or cancer. J Clin Endocrinol Metab 1999; 84:3877.
36. Adler ML, Macapinlac HA, Robbins RJ. Radioiodine treatment of thyroid cancer with the aid of recombinant human thyrotropin. Endocr Pract 1998; 4:282.
37. Lakshmanan M, Schaffer A, Robbins J, et al. A simplified low iodine diet in I-131 scanning and therapy of thyroid cancer. Clin Nucl Med 1988; 13:866.
38. Maxon HR, Thomas SR, Boehringer A, et al. Low iodine diet in I-131 ablation of thyroid remnants. Clin Nucl Med 1983; 8:123.
39. Maruca J, Santner S, Miller K, Santen J. Prolonged iodine clearance with a depletion regimen for thyroid carcinoma. J Nucl Med 1984; 25:1089.
40. Halpern SE, Preisman R, Hagan PL. Scanning dose and the detection of thyroid metastases. J Nucl Med 1979; 20:1099.
41. Sherman SI, Tielens ET, Sostre S, et al. Clinical utility of posttreatment radioiodine scans in the management of patients with thyroid carcinoma. J Clin Endocrinol Metab 1994; 78:629.
42. Pacini F, Hippi F, Formica N, et al. Therapeutic doses of iodine-131 reveal undiagnosed metastases in thyroid cancer patients with detectable serum thyroglobulin levels. J Nucl Med 1987; 28:1888.
43. Sarkar SD, Leveque FC, Palestro CJ, Afriyie MO. Comparison of the thyroid probe and scintillation camera for uptake measurements in thyroid remnants. J Nucl Med 1999; in press. J Nucl Med 1999; 40:208P.
44. Maxon HR, Thomas SR, Samaratunga RC, et al. Dosimetric considerations in the radioiodine treatment of macrometastases and micrometastases from differentiated thyroid cancer. Thyroid 1997; 7:183.
45. Demeester-Mirkine N, Van Sande J, Corvilain J, Dumont J. Benign thyroid nodule with normal iodide trap and defective organification. J Clin Endocrinol Metab 1975; 41:1169.
46. Kusic Z, Becker DV, Sanger EL, et al. Comparison of technetium-99m and iodine-123 imaging of thyroid nodules: correlation with pathologic findings. J Nucl Med 1990; 31:393.
47. McKitrick WL, Park HM, Kosegi JE. Parallax error in pinhole thyroid scintigraphy: a critical consideration in the evaluation of substernal goiters. J Nucl Med 1985; 26:418.
48. Ryo UY, Stachura ME, Schneider AB, et al. Significance of extrathyroidal uptake of Tc-99m and I-123 in the thyroid scan. J Nucl Med 1981; 22:1039.
49. Brucker-Davis F, Reynolds JC, Skarulis MC, et al. False-positive iodine-131 whole-body scans due to cholecystitis and sebaceous cyst. J Nucl Med 1996; 37:1690.
50. Kappes RS, Sarkar SD, Har-El G, et al. Iodine-131 therapy of thyroid cancer: extensive contamination of the hospital room in a patient with tracheostomy. J Nucl Med 1994; 35:2053.
51. Serafini A, Sfakianakis G, Michalakis G, et al. Breast cyst simulating metastases on Iodine-131 imaging in thyroid carcinoma. J Nucl Med 198; 39:1910.

52. Becker DV, Charkes ND, Dworkin H, et al. Procedure guideline for thyroid uptake measurement. J Nucl Med 1996; 37:1266.
53. Smith JJ, Croft BY, Brookeman VA, Teates CD. Estimation of 24-hour thyroid uptake of I-131 sodium iodide using a 5-minute uptake of technetium-99m pertechnetate. Clin Nucl Med 1990; 15:80.
54. Robertson JS, Nolan NG, Wahner HW, McConahey WM. Thyroid radioiodine uptakes and scans in euthyroid patients. Mayo Clin Proc 1975; 50:79.
55. Hooper PL, Turner JR, Conway MJ, Plymate SR. Thyroid uptake of I-123 in a normal population. Arch Intern Med 1980; 140:757.
56. Burke G. The triiodothyronine suppression test. Am J Med 1967; 42:600.
57. Blum M, Seltzer TF, Campbell CC, Burroughs VJ. Evaluation of euthyroid solitary autonomous nodule of the thyroid gland: importance of scintillation scanning and thyrotropin releasing hormone testing. JAMA 1982; 247:1991.
58. Dymling JF, Becker DV. Occurrence of hyperthyroidism in patients receiving thyroid hormone. J Clin Endocrinol Metab 1967; 27:1487.
59. Baschieri L, Benedetti G, DeLuca F, Negri M. Evaluation and limitations of the perchlorate test in the study of thyroid function. J Clin Endocrinol Metab 1963; 23:786.
60. Stewart RDH, Murray IPC. Effect of small doses of carrier iodide upon the organic binding of radioactive iodine by the human thyroid gland. J Clin Endocrinol Metab 1967; 27:500.
61. Ramirez L, Braverman LE, White B, et al. Recombinant human thyrotropin is a potent stimulator of thyroid function in normal subjects. J Clin Endocrinol Metab 1997; 82:2836.

# CHAPTER 35

# THYROID SONOGRAPHY, COMPUTED TOMOGRAPHY, AND MAGNETIC RESONANCE IMAGING

MANFRED BLUM

Thyroid goiters and nodules are common disorders, whereas thyroid malignancies are relatively rare. The main purpose of sonography (ultrasonography), computed tomography (CT), and magnetic resonance imaging (MRI) of the thyroid gland is to help to confirm the diagnosis and to assist in planning therapy. Imaging should not be used routinely in screening procedures because it is not efficient in establishing the likelihood of cancer in a thyroid nodule. Although percutaneous needle biopsy is the most specific diagnostic tool for this purpose, its limitations are evident. Decision analysis has indicated that no single test is best; therefore, several tests continue to be needed.[1] Appropriate clinical diagnosis and management depend on a familiarity with these tests and their applicability.

Technologic advances have provided several methods that image the thyroid gland and surrounding tissues. In an era of cost containment, the physician must choose diagnostic tests carefully, selecting only those that contribute meaningfully to management.[2] The imaging findings complement information gained from the history and physical examination; these techniques do not supplant good clinical skills. Indeed, the results of these tests may be confusing and may lead to an erroneous diagnosis when taken out of clinical context; however, when appropriately used and interpreted, they are extremely useful.

All imaging techniques represent anatomic mapping. The scintiscan examines the accumulation by thyroid tissues of iodine or its partial analog, pertechnetate, to provide a "functional" map of where iodine is taken up and metabolized (see Chap. 34). Ultrasonography, CT, and MRI, whose suggested use is shown in Table 35-1, provide topographic maps; none of these techniques differentiates benign from malignant lesions. Diagnosing histopathology is not possible with these methods, except by inference and by correlation with other data. Evidence of gross fixation of structures and loss of tissue planes may be demonstrated on an image, but invasion that is obvious at surgery may have escaped detection by the best of imaging studies.

## SONOGRAPHY (ECHOGRAPHY) OF THE THYROID

In ultrasonography, high-frequency sound waves enter the body and are transmitted or reflected by tissue interfaces to produce a photographic image of the internal structure. With current high-resolution equipment, nodules as small as 2 to 3 mm can be identified by using a signal with a frequency of 7.5 to 10 MHz that penetrates <5 cm. The deeper penetration that is achieved by lower-frequency sound waves seldom is necessary for the evaluation of thyroid structures.[3,4,4a]

Patients are examined in the supine position with the neck hyperextended. For full imaging of the thyroid gland and appropriate landmarks, the neck must be surveyed in the sagittal, transverse, and oblique planes. The images are produced quickly and assembled in rapid sequence in "real time", much as in a motion picture. Swallowing may facilitate identification of the esophagus; swallowing also elevates the thyroid so that its lower poles can be examined. A useful advance in thyroid ultrasonography is color flow Doppler imaging, which adds dynamic flow information to a static gray-scale image.[4b] Color-encoded signals differentiate a fluid-filled cystic space and vasculature, indicating the direction and the velocity of blood flow and the degree of vascularity.[5] The assignment of color is arbitrary; arterial signals can be assigned the color red and the companion venous signals, blue, assuming that venous flow is parallel to, but in the opposite direction of, arterial flow. However, because vessels may be tortuous, portions of the same vessel may display in different colors depending on the direction of flow in relation to the transducer, even if the true direction of flow has not changed. The shade of a color is related roughly to flow velocity. The ultrasonography operator must be experienced and must be aware of the clinical question that has been posed by the clinician to provide an appropriate answer. Routine protocols for scanning are unsatisfactory.

Ultrasonography is safe and relatively inexpensive. No ionizing radiation is present, and damage to tissues has not been reported. The procedure permits continuation of suppressive therapy with thyroid hormone. Use of contrast material and patient preparation are unnecessary. Ultrasonography is of limited value adjacent to the trachea, is hard to interpret in the upper jugular region, and is not useful just behind the air-filled trachea or substernally.

### NORMAL THYROID GLAND

The thyroid gland (Fig. 35-1) is characterized by homogeneous echoes, which give the gland a uniform ground-glass appearance. The surrounding muscles are of lower echogenicity. Medial to the thyroid lobes is the air-filled trachea, which does not transmit ultrasonic waves and is, therefore, poorly imaged. A calcified tracheal ring is represented anteriorly by dense echoes. The tubular carotid artery is echo free. Lateral and anterior to the carotid is the jugular vein, which can be identified when it is distended during a Valsalva maneuver. Behind the thyroid and anteromedial to the longus colli muscle is the esophagus, which can be identified as the patient swallows. The neurovascular bundle containing the inferior thyroid artery and recurrent laryngeal nerve may sometimes be identified, and blood vessels as small as 1 to 2 mm can occasionally be seen on the surface of the thyroid.

### THYROID NODULE

Thyroid nodules distort the uniform echo pattern of the normal gland. Seventy-five percent of nodules are of lower echogenicity and 15% are of higher echogenicity than normal thyroid tissue, but this

**TABLE 35-1.**
**Suggested Clinical Use of Nonisotopic Thyroid Imaging**

| Clinical Circumstance | US | MRI | CT |
|---|---|---|---|
| **I. NO THYROID NODULE** | | | |
| A. Identifies a nonpalpable nodule when risk of thyroid neoplasm is high | Yes | NA | NA |
| **II. COLD THYROID NODULE** | | | |
| A. Initial diagnosis | | | |
| 1. Palpable nodule 2–5 cm | NA | NA | NA |
| 2. Large nodule: differentiates solid, degenerated, and simple cyst | Opt | NA | NA |
| 3. Examines for a nonpalpable multinodular process in a patient with a clinically solitary nodule | Opt | NA | NA |
| 4. Evaluates distortion of regional architecture | Opt | PRN | PRN2 |
| 5. Identifies adenopathy | Yes | PRN | PRN2 |
| B. In conjunction with needle biopsy | | | |
| 1. Palpable nodule | | | |
| a. Localizes the solid component for aspiration cytology | Yes | NA | NA |
| b. Localizes fluid-filled areas so that they may be aspirated | Yes | NA | NA |
| 2. Nonpalpable nodule identification | Yes | NA | NA |
| C. In conjunction with suppressive therapy and long-term follow-up | | | |
| 1. Provides an objective assessment of size | Yes | NA | NA |
| 2. Identifies the cause of shrinkage of a nodule: resolution of tumor or absorption of fluid | Yes | PRN | NA |
| 3. Identifies the cause of enlargement: growth of tumor or accumulation of fluid | Yes | PRN | NA |
| **III. HOT NODULE** | | | |
| A. Identifies the presence of the dormant contralateral lobe to rule out hemiagenesis | Yes | NA | NA |
| B. Documents the size of a nodule | Opt | NA | NA |
| C. Attributes a cold area in the hot nodule to hemorrhagic degeneration or a solid change in the nodule that might be malignant | Yes | NA | NA |
| **IV. GOITER** | | | |
| A. Assesses the size of a hyperthyroid gland for dosimetry with iodine-131 | PRN | NA | NA |
| B. Attributes changes in the size of a goiter to a new nodule that could be a tumor, hemorrhage, or goiter growth | Yes | PRN | NA |
| C. Identifies a discrete suspicious nodule in an otherwise multinodular goiter | Yes | NA | NA |
| D. Identifies changes that suggest lymphoma or tumor in thyroiditis | Yes | PRN | NA |
| E. Identifies mediastinal extension of nodule or goiter | NA | Yes | PRN |
| F. Locates thyroid gland versus athyreosis in a neonate | Yes | NA | NA |
| **V. CANCER** | | | |
| A. Assesses the extent of tumor | Yes | PRN | PRN2 |
| B. Detects multifocal disease | Yes | PRN | PRN2 |
| C. Identifies lymphadenopathy | Yes | PRN | PRN2 |
| D. May detect a nonpalpable primary lesion within the thyroid when the clinical presenting finding is adenopathy elsewhere in the neck | Yes | PRN | PRN2 |
| E. Is used to monitor the postoperative situation | Yes | PRN | PRN2 |
| F. Shows postoperative recurrence early, before it becomes palpable | Yes | PRN | PRN2 |
| G. Characteristics of adenopathy may hint at pathology (infection versus tumor) | Yes | PRN | PRN2 |
| H. May locate lesion in neck when thyroglobulin increases after thyroidectomy | Yes | PRN | PRN2 |
| **VI. VASCULATURE** | | | |
| A. Differentiates blood vessel and cystic space | DOP | Future | PRN |
| B. Demonstrates blood flow/perfusion: may correlate physiology/pathology | DOP | Future | NA |

US, ultrasonography; MRI, magnetic resonance imaging; CT, computed tomography; Yes, useful, advised; NA, not advised; Opt, optional; PRN, only if needed; PRN2, only if needed, secondary; DOP, Doppler ultrasonography; Future, development in the future is anticipated.

characteristic has limited diagnostic value because most thyroid cancers are less echo-dense than normal tissue, and benign nodules may be more or less dense.[4] The nodules may contain echo-dense deposits of calcium. Some nodules have a sonolucent rim called a *halo* (Fig. 35-2). Within small nodules, the echo texture tends to be uniform, but nodules larger than 2.5 cm usually have irregular, echo-free zones that represent cystic or hemorrhagic degeneration. These degenerative changes in a nodule may almost completely replace the solid structure, and careful examination in various planes is necessary to discern internal echoes that represent septa or small solid regions (Fig. 35-3). These complex "cystic" nodules are extremely common and must be differentiated from the rare true thyroid cyst, which is encountered in ~1 in 500 to 1000 nodules[4] (Fig. 35-4). A thyroid cyst is globular, smooth walled, and without internal echoes.

Ultrasonography cannot differentiate benign from malignant solitary nodules. However, a true simple cyst is almost invariably benign. Because almost 90% of all solitary nodules

are benign, the discovery of a solitary nodule should not cause undue alarm. Nevertheless, ~10% of solitary nodules in an otherwise normal gland are malignant, and they can be solid or can have degenerative changes. Large deposits of calcium signify healing of an old degenerative change or hemorrhage and may be seen in benign or malignant nodules. Punctate calcifications frequently represent psammoma bodies in papillary cancer, whereas more dense calcification may represent medullary carcinoma. A low echo halo that is seen around certain nodules signifies a boundary, perhaps a capsule. Doppler technique may demonstrate blood vessels within this rim. A halo may be seen in either benign or malignant conditions.[4]

Improved technology has permitted the detection of nodules in the millimeter range (Fig. 35-5); although this is an enormous advance, it is also the source of a problem.[3] As many as 20% of all people have nonpalpable micronodules of indeterminate significance.[3,6] Indeed, some of these lesions may represent occult thy-

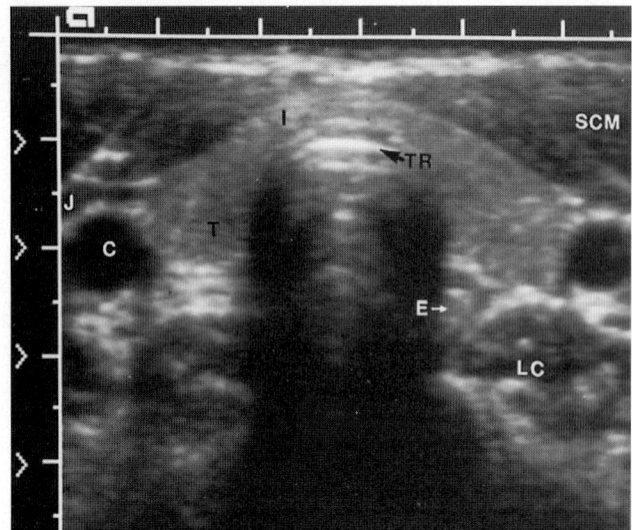

**FIGURE 35-1.** Sonogram of normal thyroid gland showing a transverse section of the lower anterior neck. Both lobes of the thyroid gland (*T*) are seen; they have a uniform, ground-glass appearance. The isthmus (*I*) is located anterior to the echo-dense tracheal ring (*TR*); behind that are artifactual reverberations of the sound waves. The carotid artery (*C*) and jugular veins (*J*) are found laterally. The sternocleidomastoid muscles (*SCM*) are anterior, and the longus colli muscles (*LC*) are posterior. The esophagus (*E*) is anteromedial to the left longus colli muscle.

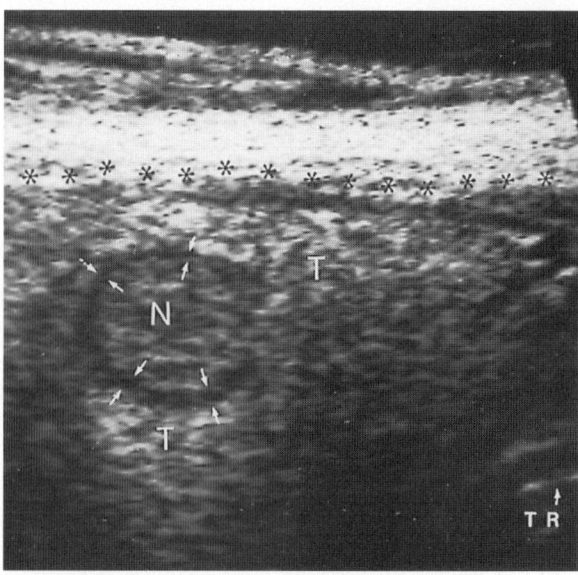

**FIGURE 35-2.** Sonogram of solid thyroid nodule showing the right thyroid lobe (*T*) of a patient who had a cold nodule (*N*). The nodule is of slightly lower echogenicity than the rest of the lobe and is surrounded by a halo (*arrows*) that is almost sonolucent. The lesion was a follicular adenoma. Asterisks indicate the anterior border of the thyroid lobe. (*TR*, a portion of a tracheal ring.)

roid cancer, the incidence of which varies from a few percent in this country to as much as 20% in other parts of the world. Clinical experience has indicated that these lesions are of little biologic consequence in most patients, and their discovery during echography may cause needless concern and therapy. Yet some small carcinomas do metastasize and may ultimately cause death.[7] Therefore, the finding of a minute tumor cannot be dismissed. Future investigation must determine the proper treatment for these patients, including the role of periodic ultrasonography to monitor changes in the size of the nodule and the appropriateness of suppressive therapy with thyroid hormone. Identification of a nonpalpable nodule may have greatest clinical value in a

patient who underwent therapeutic irradiation in youth (see Fig. 35-5). Another clinical challenge raised by ultrasonography pertains to the discovery of nonpalpable nodularity of the thyroid gland when only a solitary nodule is palpable (Fig. 35-6B). This is a common occurrence in patients with a palpable solitary nodule and should be approached in the same way as a dominant nodule in a patient with clinical multinodularity. By current consensus, fine-needle aspiration biopsy of the dominant nodule appears to be the most cost-effective approach when the nodule is "cold" on isotope scanning.

Ultrasonography can be used with great accuracy and objectivity to assess the size of the thyroid gland[8] or of a nodule periodically

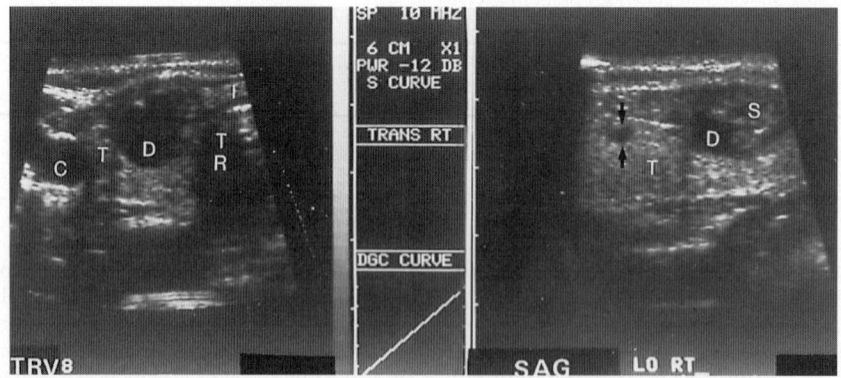

**FIGURE 35-3.** Sonogram of complex thyroid nodule. Sonograms in the transverse (*TRV*) and sagittal (*SAG*) planes of the right thyroid lobe (*T*) in a patient with a cold right thyroid nodule on radionuclide imaging. Previous aspiration yielded nondiagnostic debris. The sonograms show extensive degeneration (*D*) of the nodule. The lesion could easily be mistaken for a cyst in the transverse view. However, in the sagittal view, the solid component (*S*) is seen at the lower pole. This view was used as a guide to insert a needle into the solid component. The aspirate was consistent with a benign nodular thyroid. A second, low-echogenicity, 2 × 3 mm nonpalpable nodule higher in the right lobe in the sagittal view (*arrows*) suggests that this is a multinodular goiter. The increased acoustic shadowing behind the fluid-filled space in both views is caused by enhanced transmission of sound waves through fluid. The carotid artery (*C*), thyroid isthmus (*I*), and trachea (*TR*) are seen. The patient was given suppressive therapy after the fluid was aspirated. The solid component shrank, and the fluid did not reaccumulate. (From Blum M. Practical application of modern technology in thyroid evaluation. In: Van Middlesworth L, ed. The thyroid gland: practical clinical treatise. Chicago: Year Book Medical Publishers, 1986:58.)

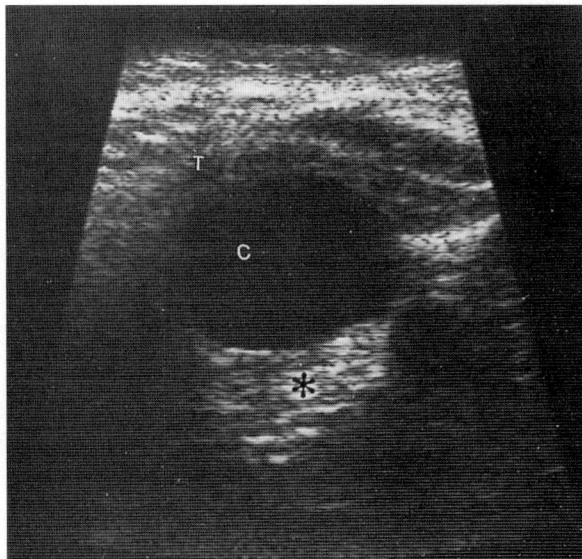

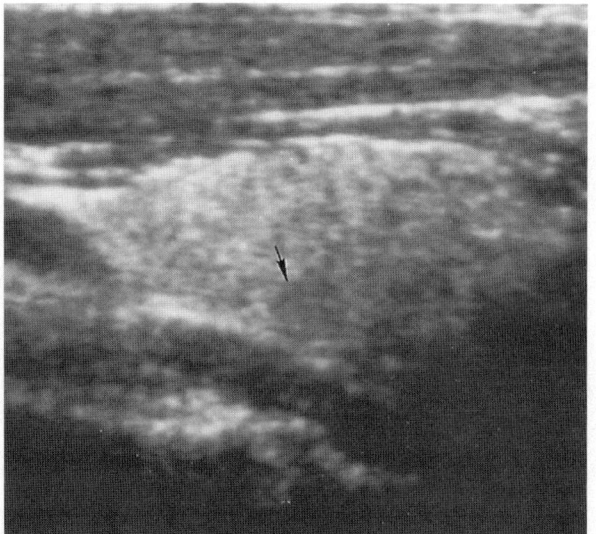

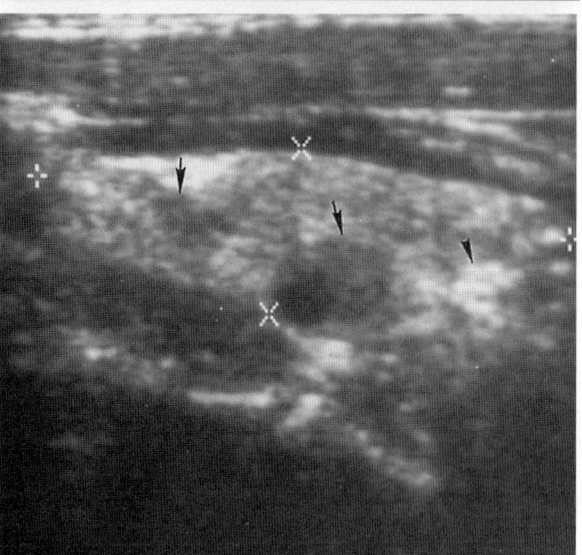

**FIGURE 35-4.** Sonogram showing a cyst (*C*) in the thyroid lobe (*T*). Dense echoes behind the cyst (*) signify enhanced transmission of the sound waves through the fluid-filled structure. No internal echoes are seen within the cyst space; it is globular in shape and has smooth walls.

during the course of therapy. Because patients are likely to change physicians over the years, an objective assessment of thyroid size may be invaluable to facilitate continuity of care. Comparison of serial ultrasonographic scans may lead to surgery if a nodule grows despite suppressive therapy. Figure 35-6 shows evolution of a nodular goiter. Resolution of a nodules is shown in Figure 35-7.

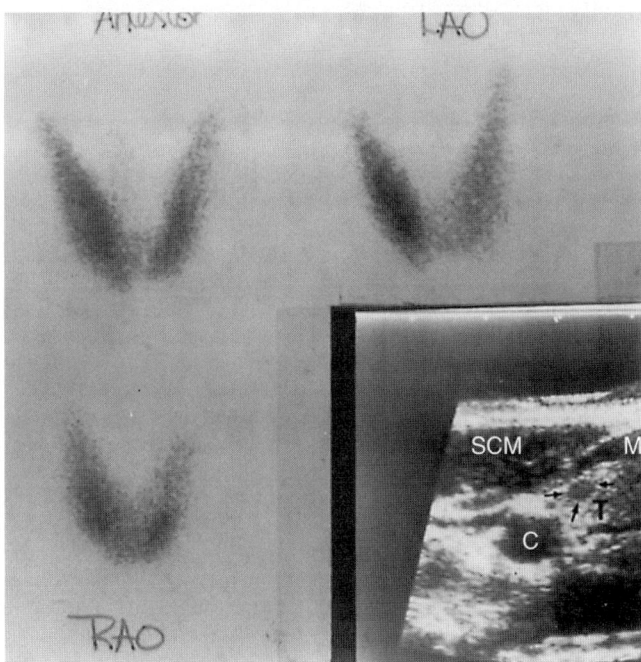

**FIGURE 35-5.** Sonogram of nonpalpable thyroid nodule. Imaging findings in an asymptomatic 46-year-old man who underwent radiation therapy for acne during his midteens. The thyroid gland was normal to palpation. An iodine-123 scintillation scan was normal in the anterior, left anterior oblique (*LAO*), and right anterior oblique (*RAO*) projections. *Inset*, 10-MHz thyroid sonogram showing a 2 × 4 mm hypoechoic nodule (*arrow*) in the right lobe of the thyroid gland (*T*). (*SCM*, sternocleidomastoid muscle; *M*, strap muscles; *C*, carotid artery.) (From Blum M. Practical application of modern technology in thyroid evaluation. In: Van Middlesworth L, ed. The thyroid gland: practical clinical treatise. Chicago: Year Book Medical Publishers, 1986:59.)

**FIGURE 35-6.** The use of periodic ultrasonography in a patient with a thyroid nodule, showing the evolution of a nodular goiter. A 50-year-old man had annual sonograms because of a small nodule in the left thyroid lobe. He was euthyroid. Antithyroglobulin and antithyroid peroxidase antibodies were not detected. The concentrations of thyroglobulin and calcitonin were not elevated. The patient had no history of exposure to therapeutic radiation, but he had a strong family history of goiter. Fine-needle aspiration biopsy showed colloid and unremarkable thyroid cells, consistent with an adenomatous goiter. The patient elected observation without intervention. **A,** An image in the sagittal plane from the sonogram shows a 1.7 × 1.5 × 1.2 cm solitary nodule in the posterior portion of the left thyroid lobe (*arrow*). Activity throughout the rest of the thyroid was uniform. The sonogram was repeated after a 7-month interval and was unchanged. However, another sonogram (**B**) obtained 1 year later showed several new nodules in the left lobe (*arrows*). The lower part of the original nodule now has an area of cystic degeneration (lower *X*). Only this nodule was clinically palpable. The rest of the lobe is sonographically heterogeneous. Suppressive therapy with L-thyroxine was advised, and continued observation is planned.

## GOITER

Sonography can identify a goiter by showing an enlarged thyroid gland and heterogeneity of the echo pattern. These findings are not specific for any particular type of pathology. However, generalized low echogenicity may suggest Hashimoto thyroiditis[9]; subacute thyroiditis usually exhibits very low echogenicity.[10] Examination of a goiter with Doppler tech-

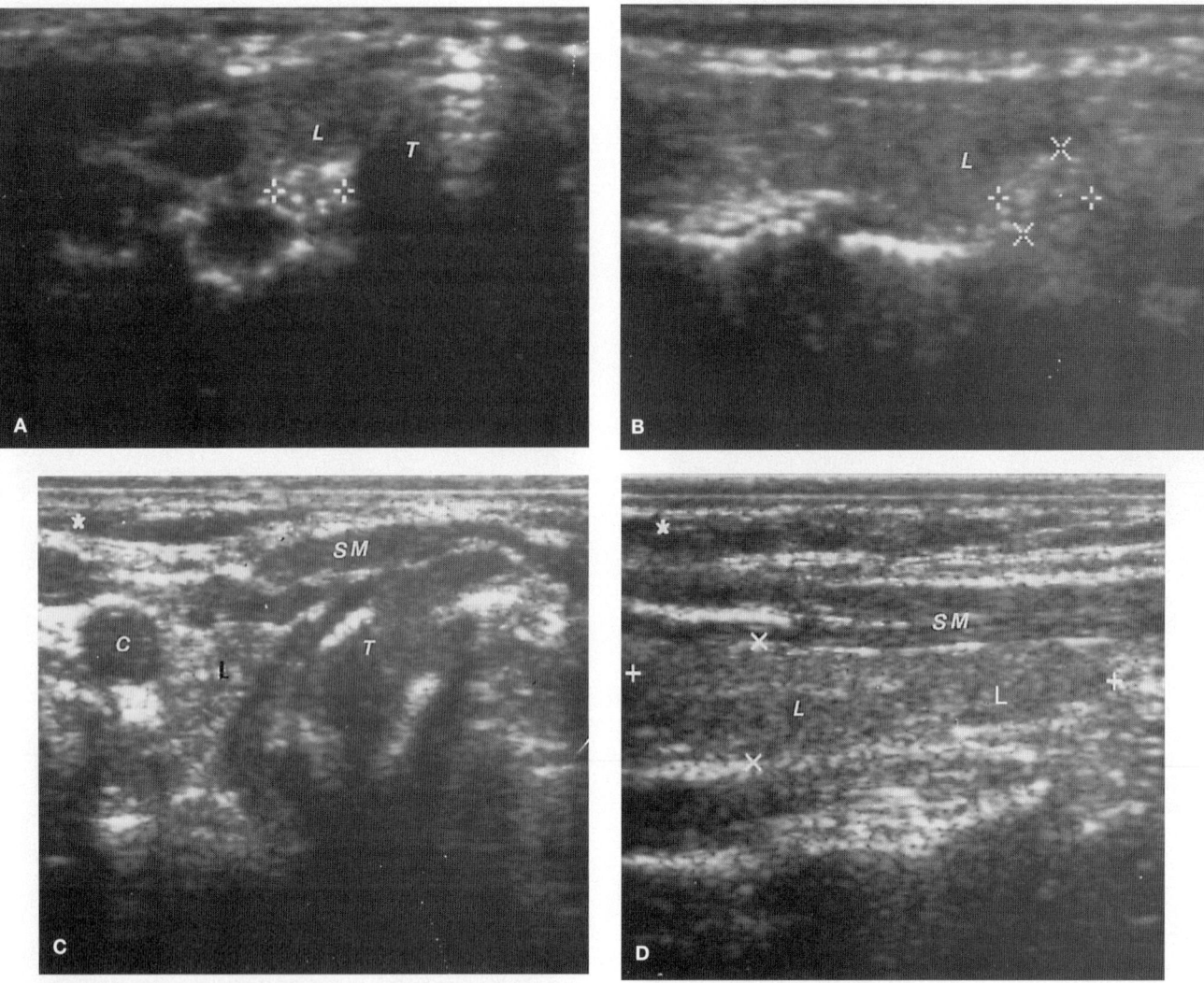

**FIGURE 35-7.** The use of periodic ultrasonography in a patient with a thyroid nodule showing resolution of the nodule. A 38-year-old euthyroid woman was found to have a small palpable nodule in the inferior portion of the right thyroid lobe. Iodine-123 scan showed that the nodule was cold and a needle biopsy showed evidence of adenomatous hyperplasia. Ultrasonography that was performed in the transverse plane (**A**) and in the sagittal plane (**B**) showed a 0.9 × 0.9 cm nodule in the lower portion of the right thyroid lobe (+, X, +). Suppressive therapy with L-thyroxine was given. Ultrasonography was repeated 5.5 months later and used multiple cuts through the thyroid region in the transverse and sagittal planes (**C** and **D**); a nodule was not evident, and none was palpated clinically. (*L*, thyroid lobe; *T*, trachea and associated artifacts; *C*, carotid artery; *SM*, strap muscles.)

nique may demonstrate enhanced blood flow, especially in Graves disease. In a uniform goiter, the sonogram can show a region whose echo pattern is different from that of the rest of the gland, suggesting a second lesion, especially if it is surrounded by a halo. The author has observed several patients with Hashimoto disease in whom such a focal lesion led to the demonstration by needle biopsy of a neoplasm (Fig. 35-8). Because ultrasonography can be used to measure the size of a goiter, it also may be useful in calculating the dose of iodine-131 for the treatment of hyperthyroidism.

## LYMPHADENOPATHY

Normal lymph nodes are rarely seen on sonograms. When nodes are slightly enlarged due to inflammation, they are thin and oval in shape and have a central echogenic hilus.[11] In distinction, nodes involved with malignancy more commonly are rounded, having a widened cortex and a narrowed or absent hilus. Thus, the ratio of the longitudinal to transverse diameter (L/T ratio) has been reported as <1.5 in 62% of nodes con-

taining metastases and as >2 in 79% of benign reactive nodes.[12] However, no significant differences in size are seen between benign and malignant nodes. When color and spectral Doppler techniques are used, malignant nodes frequently demonstrate a high ratio of systolic to diastolic blood flow (*resistive index*), with a mean of 0.92, whereas benign reactive nodes tend to be characterized by an index of <0.6.[13] Therefore, ultrasonography is useful in the diagnosis of patients who have lymphadenopathy (especially if they are suspected of having thyroid cancer, if they have a history of therapeutic irradiation in youth, or if they have had a thyroidectomy for cancer or an adenoma.) However, even in patients with thyroid cancer, enlarged benign nodes are more common than malignant ones.

## SONOGRAPHY IN THE PATIENT WITH KNOWN THYROID CANCER

Sonography is helpful in the management of a patient with thyroid carcinoma.[4] Periodic ultrasonographic studies may dis-

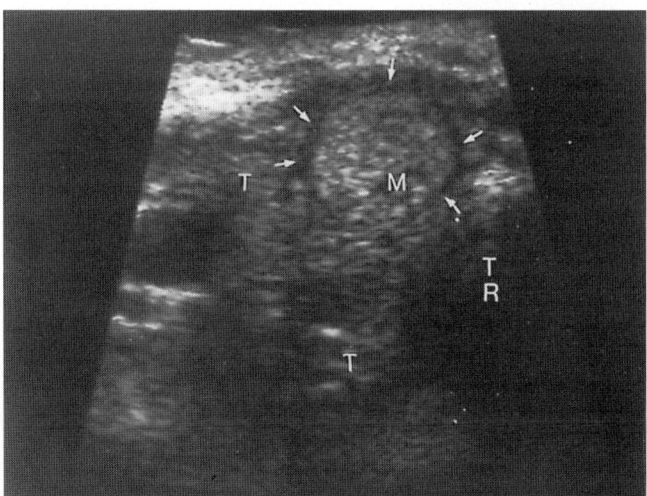

**FIGURE 35-8.** Sonogram of a nodule in Hashimoto thyroiditis. Sonogram of a patient with an enlarged multinodular thyroid. The antithyroid microsomal antibody titer was 1:25,600, indicative of Hashimoto (chronic lymphocytic) thyroiditis. An isotope scintiscan showed generalized heterogeneity of activity. The sonogram shows an echo-dense focal area (*M*) surrounded by a halo (*arrows*) in the right thyroid lobe (*T*). A needle biopsy of this mass revealed follicular carcinoma, which was confirmed at surgery. The rest of the thyroid has a low-echogenicity irregular echo pattern that is typical of Hashimoto thyroiditis and is enlarged. (*TR,* trachea.)

close recurrent, nonpalpable carcinoma in the thyroid bed or in lymph nodes (Fig. 35-9). Ultrasonography can be performed during suppressive therapy, so that the inconvenience and risks of hypothyroidism associated with radionuclide scintigraphy are avoided. In patients with cervical adenopathy due to thyroid cancer but with a nonpalpable primary lesion, ultrasonography may disclose a mass in the thyroid gland, even if the scintiscan is normal.

### SONOGRAPHY IN CONJUNCTION WITH NEEDLE BIOPSY

Fine-needle aspiration biopsy of thyroid nodules has become a major diagnostic tool. For most needle biopsies, prior ultrasonography is not needed. The procedure is safe and inexpensive, and its accuracy may be as high as 97% when an expert performs the puncture and an experienced cytologist interprets the specimen. However, the accuracy declines to 50% with inexperience.[2] Other factors that detract from accuracy include a low yield in complex, degenerated nodules, when fluid and necrotic debris are aspirated rather than the cellular component. Particularly when the nodule is deep or in a goiter, sampling errors are common in nodules <1 cm or in nodules >2.5 cm, which usually have degenerated zones.

In an attempt to reduce these sources of error, and for nonpalpable nodules, ultrasonography-guided biopsy has been used.[14–16] A special echographic transducer to guide the needle is available but is not essential. Rather, it is easier to locate the nodule or node freehand, applying the transducer from one angle and inserting the needle from another direction. Ultrasonography-guided biopsy does not negate the importance of multiple punctures of a nodule or goiter to improve the diagnostic yield.

For complex nodules, the solid component is identified and the needle inserted into that area (Fig. 35-10; see Fig. 35-3). Thereafter, the fluid component can be aspirated to collapse the cystic space if desired. Aspirating the fluid first and then sam-

pling the solid component is less satisfactory because the remnant may be small and difficult to find.

## SECTIONAL THYROID IMAGING

Sectional imaging, which includes CT and MRI, is used to depict the regional anatomy of the neck and the superior mediastinum, but it plays no role in the diagnosis of the patient with a solitary thyroid nodule or goiter.[17–19] Nevertheless, when these tests are done for other indications, the asymptomatic and unsuspected thyroid lesions that are often revealed need to be managed.

As is shown in Table 35-1, however, some circumstances exist for which these imaging techniques are the only means available for the proper clinical evaluation of patients. In selected instances, sectional imaging may be used to assess the extent of an unusually large or obstructive thyroid gland or nodule, a cancer (Fig. 35-11), or a substernal goiter (Fig. 35-12), especially before surgery. Furthermore, when the postsurgical clinical findings are confusing, sectional imaging can provide accurate and essential management information. A detailed knowledge of the regional anatomy and experience with the techniques are required for the optimal interpretation of the images. Consultation between the clinician and the radiologist is important in this situation, as with all other imaging methods. Although the early identification of a recurrence of a tumor using this technique is possible, sonography is more sensitive for small lesions, less costly, more convenient, and safer. The periodic repetition of sectional imaging as a screening tool is rarely warranted.[17,19,20]

## MAGNETIC RESONANCE IMAGING OF THE THYROID

MRI depicts the interactions that occur between the hydrogen atoms (protons) in different tissues in the patient's body and an externally applied magnetic field (radiowaves of a specific frequency). Different properties (relaxation times) of the hydrogen atoms, termed *T1* and *T2,* can be selectively emphasized. Because the hydrogen atoms of different tissues have different T1 and T2 properties, a computer-assisted analysis of T1-weighted and T2-weighted signals is used to differentiate the thyroid gland from skeletal muscle, blood vessels, or regional lymph nodes. Normal thyroid tissue tends to be slightly more intense than muscle on a T1-weighted image, and tumors frequently appear even more intense. The intravenous administration of noniodinated contrast agents, such as gadolinium-DTPA (pentetic acid), may further enhance the characterization of tissue and organs, as may suppressing the signal that is derived from fat (short tau inversion, or STIR).

The test is uncomfortable; claustrophobic reactions occur, and considerable noise is inherent to the technique. Generally, the patient's entire body must be inserted into a large cylinder. Advances such as the use of special surface electromagnets over the neck provide impressive images and, thus, may increase the usefulness of MRI for thyroid evaluation. The equipment is costly and in great competitive demand for other types of examinations. The guidelines for use were discussed earlier in Sectional Thyroid Imaging. Figure 35-9 shows the evaluation of a suspicious ultrasonographic finding, and Figure 35-12 demonstrates the use of MRI to show the extent of a large obstructive goiter and to help plan a surgical approach. Occasionally, in this setting, sectional imaging may help the physician to choose between medical management and surgery. In Figure 35-13, an MRI shows the size and extent of postsurgery cancer. Figure 35-14 demonstrates the use of MRI to examine enlarged upper cervical lymph nodes in a patient with thyroid cancer. Figure

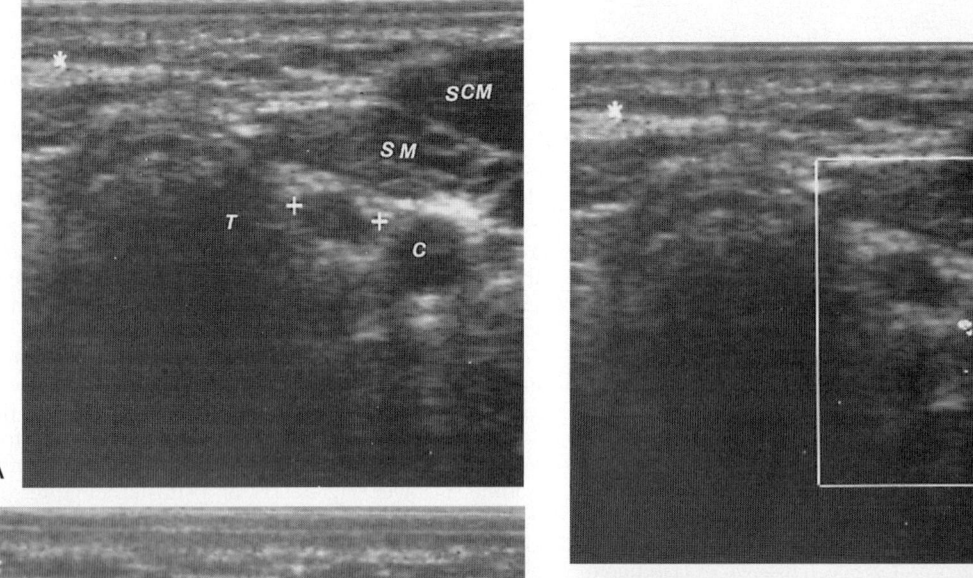

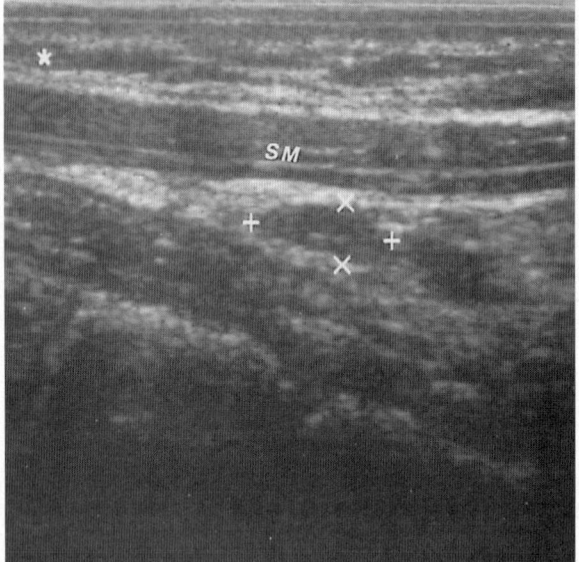

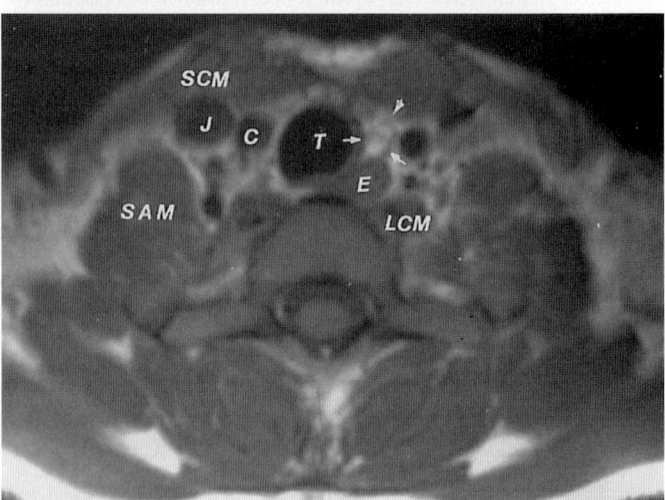

**FIGURE 35-9.** Routine follow-up of a patient with a history of thyroid cancer and a normal examination with ultrasonography. Magnetic resonance imaging (MRI), a more costly and cumbersome procedure, was used to confirm a suspicious finding, leading to surgery. This 28-year-old woman had a left hemithyroidectomy and isthmusectomy for a 1.2-cm encapsulated papillary carcinoma without adenopathy and was taking suppressive therapy with L-thyroxine. Thyroid-stimulating hormone was undetectable by third-generation assay, and the concentration of thyroglobulin was <1.5 ng/mL. The examination did not reveal a nodule. Annual sonography (**A,** in the transverse plane; **B,** the same with Doppler added; and **C,** longitudinal plane) showed a new nodule in the bed of the left lobe. **B,** with Doppler added, highlights the carotid artery (*bright circle*), whereas the image of the nodule remains unchanged. The patient was reluctant to undergo another operation because a nodule was not palpable by several physicians and the concentration of thyroglobulin remained low. Therefore, MRI of the neck was performed 1.5 months after the initial ultrasonography to see if the sonographic findings could be verified with another imaging modality. The MRI confirmed the masses. **D,** A T1-weighted MRI scan that shows a 1-cm nodule whose appearance is more intense than muscle. It remained markedly hyperintense on the prolonged repetition time (RT) sequences and short tau inversion images (a technique that is used to enhance contrast by suppressing the signal that is derived from fat), which is not usual for normal thyroid tissue. A total thyroidectomy was performed, revealing that the nodule was papillary carcinoma. (*Arrowhead* on MRI scan, cancerous nodule; *SCM,* sternocleidomastoid muscle; *SM,* strap muscles; *T,* trachea and associated artifacts; *C,* carotid artery; *J,* jugular vein; *L,* thyroid lobe; *E,* esophagus; *SAM,* scalenus anticus muscle; *LCM,* longus colli muscle.)

35-15 shows an MRI that helped the physician to diagnose a complex clinical problem. Several studies have suggested new directions for future research, including correlation of images with the biochemistry and histopathology of tissue.[21,22] Qualitative and quantitative similarities of the proton response of thyroid tissue in the neck and chest have been demonstrated,[23] and differences in these characteristics in malignant and benign thyroid tissues have been studied in vitro.[24]

## COMPUTED TOMOGRAPHY OF THE THYROID

The characterization of tissue and organs by CT is accomplished by computer-assisted analysis of the attenuation of x-rays that are transmitted through the patient. For some purposes, the images may be examined directly because the thyroid gland is somewhat more radiopaque than the rest of

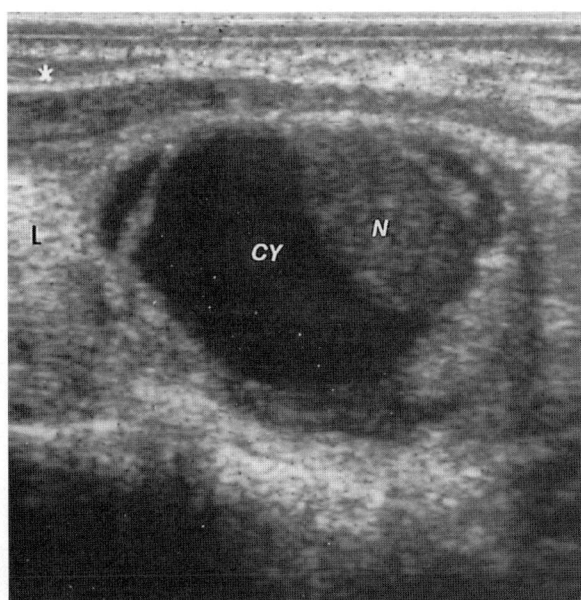

**A**

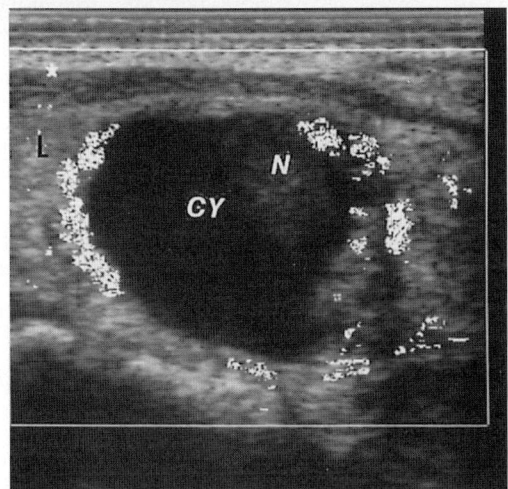

**B**

**FIGURE 35-10.** The use of ultrasonography to help with a differential diagnosis in a patient who had a hemithyroidectomy for adenoma and a new clinical finding. This 24-year-old woman had a left thyroid lobectomy 2 years earlier because of a toxic autonomous thyroid nodule, which was reported to be a follicular adenoma. She was not given suppressive therapy and remained euthyroid. Enlargement of the right lobe was detected. Ultrasonography was performed to try to differentiate compensatory hypertrophy from a focal lesion. **A,** The sonogram showed a uniform-appearing right thyroid lobe (L) with a 3.1 × 2.2 × 1.4 cm nodule (N) that was mainly cystic (CY) and had a small solid component. **B,** A flow Doppler study showed a vascular halo at the periphery of the nodule. All of these findings suggested tumor and not hypertrophy. Iodine-123 scan did not show a hyperfunctioning area in the zone that was solid tissue. Fine-needle aspiration biopsy of a solid portion of the new nodule, using the sonogram as a guide, showed sheets of uniform follicular cells without colloid. Surgery disclosed a follicular adenoma.

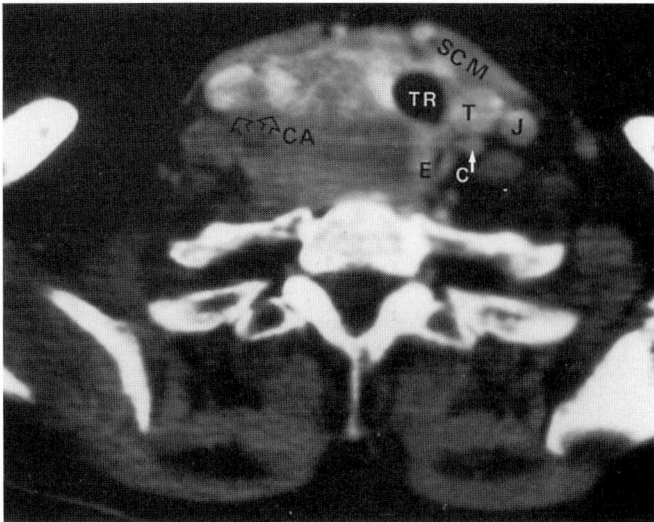

**FIGURE 35-11.** Computed tomographic (CT) scan of neck containing extensive thyroid cancer. CT scan with contrast agent enhancement. Anaplastic thyroid cancer (CA) encased the right carotid artery and jugular vein (open arrows). The trachea (TR) is displaced and indented, the right wall of the esophagus (E) is involved, and muscle tissue planes are lost. (SCM, left sternocleidomastoid muscle; T, left thyroid lobe; J, left jugular vein; C, left carotid artery.) (From Blum M. Practical application of modern technology in thyroid evaluation. In: Van Middlesworth L, ed. The thyroid gland: practical clinical treatise. Chicago: Year Book Medical Publishers, 1986:61.)

nal lymph nodes (stage I, 1.5 cm in diameter),[25] is more reliable than MRI in the detection of small pulmonary nodules,[26] is more appropriate for the unstable or claustrophobic patient, and is the only study possible in those patients with cardiac pacemakers or other biomechanical devices, who require sec-

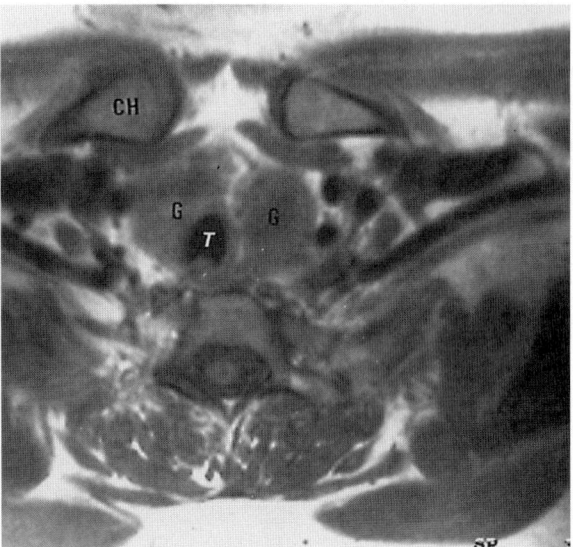

**FIGURE 35-12.** The selective use of magnetic resonance imaging (MRI) to show the extent of a large goiter. This 40-year-old woman had a large goiter and clinical evidence of mild obstruction of the thoracic inlet only when she raised her arms and flexed her head forward. MRI of the neck and superior mediastinum was performed to evaluate for evidence of tracheal involvement and substernal extension. This image shows a large goiter (G) at the level of the thoracic inlet. The thyroid capsule was intact. Slight compression of the trachea (T) was present at the level of the clavicular heads (CH), but no tracheal invasion was seen. Other images (not shown here) demonstrated extension of the goiter to the level of the aortic arch. The thyroid surgeon alerted a thoracic surgeon to be available if the goiter could not be delivered through a low collar incision.

the soft-tissue structures of the neck due to its high iodine content. More often, the contrast must be enhanced by the intravenous administration of iodinated material. Unfortunately, however, the iodine in the dye may be counterproductive to further diagnostic testing and to the treatment of thyroid disorders. Therefore, in most centers, CT has assumed a role in the diagnosis and management of thyroid problems that is complementary to that of MRI.[14,17] CT should be used selectively and only in response to a specific clinical question that cannot be answered in a more cost-effective way. CT is more sensitive than MRI in detecting small metastases to cervical or mediasti-

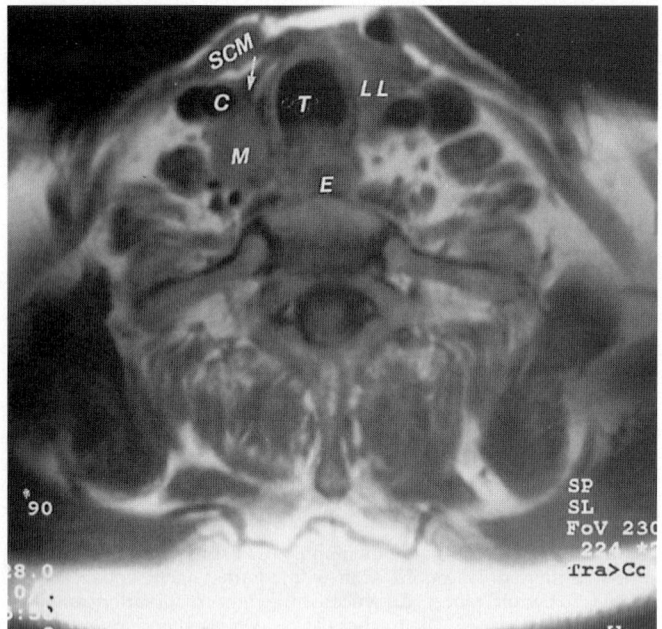

**FIGURE 35-13.** The use of magnetic resonance imaging (*MRI*) to show the extent of a residual thyroid cancer after surgery, as a guide to possible additional therapy. MRI of a 72-year-old man with a history of several myocardial infarctions, coronary artery surgery, and a right thyroid lobectomy because of an invasive multifocal Hürthle cell carcinoma of the thyroid. An attempt to remove the lesion resulted in the sacrifice of the right laryngeal nerve, but the tumor could not be completely excised. The left lobe (*LL*) was not removed for technical reasons. Iodine-131 ($^{131}$I) whole body scan showed that the mass did not take up radioiodine in the presence of the left lobe. $^{131}$I therapy was rejected by the patient. The concentration of thyroglobulin has remained stable in the 10- to 17-ng/mL range for 2 years. Thyroid-stimulating hormone level has remained low, consistent with cardiovascular tolerance. Clinical examination revealed an ill-defined and deep right paratracheal mass that had not grossly changed. Sonography in the past had not clearly revealed the extent of the mass. MRI was performed to evaluate the size of the mass and possible progression, which would lead to radiation therapy. The MRI scan shows a right paratracheal mass (*M*) that is unchanged in size and extent from the previous MRI study. The *arrow* points to the region where the cancer partly encases the carotid artery (*C*), as before. The management was not changed. Note that on this T1-weighted image, the cancer is characteristically brighter than the left thyroid lobe (*LL*) or muscle tissue (*SCM*). (*T*, trachea; *E*, esophagus.)

tional imaging.[27] Pragmatically, access to CT is greater than access to MRI because of the larger number of CT scanners available and because the cost of a CT examination is lower than that of an MRI examination. Therefore, in some centers, CT is used in a manner similar to that described for MRI. An example of CT imaging for a patient with extensive thyroid cancer is shown in Figure 35-11.

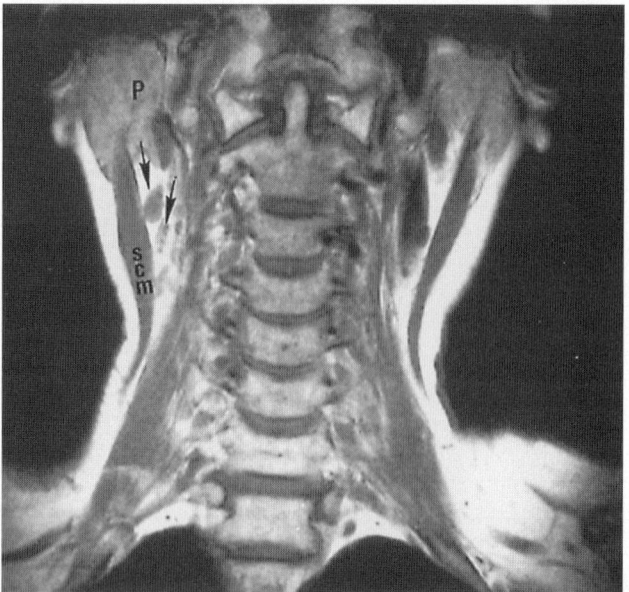

**FIGURE 35-14.** Magnetic resonance imaging (*MRI*) scan of the neck that was made to obtain information about possible tumor involvement of lymph nodes that had been detected with a sonogram. Ten years previously, this 57-year-old woman had a right hemithyroidectomy and removal of the isthmus because of a 1.5-cm encapsulated noninvasive papillary carcinoma of the thyroid. Her serum thyroglobulin was not elevated, and a postoperative sonogram showed a normal-appearing left thyroid lobe without adenopathy. Suppressive therapy has been maintained, and the thyroid-stimulating hormone has been undetectable. The serum thyroglobulin has not risen (1.7 ng/mL). The current examination suggested left upper jugular adenopathy but no nodule in the thyroid region. No clinical evidence of an infection was present, but the patient had considerable disease of the gingiva and a flare of her psoriasis. Ultrasonography showed two new anterior cervical lymph nodes, each 1.5 cm in size. The left thyroid lobe was <1.5 cm in length and was uniform. The right thyroid bed showed no nodules or nodes. MRI of the neck was performed to better define the uniformity of the lymph nodes. This T1-weighted coronal image shows upper internal jugular chain lymph nodes (*arrows*) with a homogeneous display of signal pattern on all pulse sequences. The nodes are not brighter than muscle (*SCM*), which is more compatible with hyperplastic nodes than with cancer. Six months later, clinical examination and sonography failed to disclose the nodes. Clinical follow-up is in progress. (*P*, parotid gland.)

## CONCLUSION

No best method exists for evaluating thyroid masses. The history, physical examination, imaging techniques, and percutaneous biopsy all contribute to management.[28] The diagnostic tests must be used selectively, with good judgment, and in a cost-effective fashion to answer specific questions that are posed by the clinical

**FIGURE 35-15.** Magnetic resonance image (MRI) of neck at thoracic inlet showing a thyroid tumor in the neck and primary cancer of the lung rather than a single primary lesion and metastases. The patient had a large left thyroid tumor that extended substernally. Clinically, the lesion was continuous across the superior mediastinum with a mass that extended into the right superior hemithorax. Computed tomography could not exclude a connection between the two sides of the mass. This MRI shows two separate and distinct masses. (*T*, thyroid mass; *L*, mass of higher signal intensity in the anterior segment of the right upper lobe of the lung that extends through the chest wall—an adenocarcinoma of the lung.) The difference in the signal characteristics of the two masses connotes tissue differences and suggests two tumors. (Courtesy of Dr. Deborah L. Reede.)

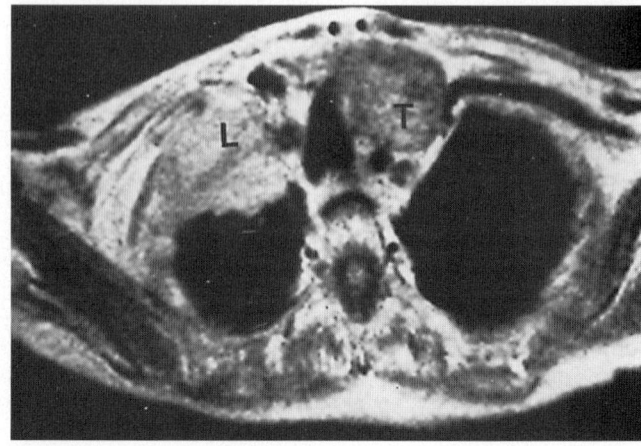

circumstance. The imaging methods provide information about gross anatomy—in the case of ultrasonography, down to the millimeter range. Ultrasonography is the primary imaging method used to identify the solid component of a complex nodule for performing guided fine-needle aspiration, to determine the comparative size of nodules in patients who are under observation (especially when they are taking thyroid-stimulating hormone–suppressive therapy), to detect a small nodule in patients who were exposed to therapeutic irradiation of the head or neck, and to search for a recurrence of thyroid cancer after surgery.

## REFERENCES

1. Molitch ME, Beck JR, Dreisman M, et al. The cold thyroid nodule: an analysis of the diagnostic and therapeutic options. Endocr Rev 1984; 5:185.
2. Van Herle AJ, Rich P, Ljung BME, et al. The thyroid nodule. Ann Intern Med 1982; 96:221.
3. Leopold GR. Ultrasonography of superficially located structures. Radiol Clin North Am 1980; 18:161.
4. Butch RJ, Simeone JF, Mueller PR. Thyroid and parathyroid ultrasonography. Radiol Clin North Am 1985; 23:57.
4a. Barraclough BM, Barraclough BH. Ultrasound of the thyroid and parathyroid glands. World J Surg 2000; 24:158.
4b. Hiromatsu Y, Ishibashi M, Miyaki I, et al. Color doppler ultrasonography in patients with subacute thyroiditis. Thyroid 1999; 9:1189.
5. Foley WD. Color Doppler flow imaging. Boston: Andover Medical Publishers, 1991.
6. Tan GH, Gharib H. Thyroid incidentalomas: management approaches to nonpalpable nodules discovered incidentally on thyroid imaging. Ann Intern Med 1997; 126:226.
7. Boehm TM, Rothouse L, Wartofsky L. Occult follicular carcinoma of the thyroid with a solitary slowly growing metastasis. JAMA 1976; 235:2420.
8. Hegedus L. Decreased thyroid gland volume in alcoholic cirrhosis of the liver. J Clin Endocrinol Metab 1984; 58:930.
9. Marcocci C, Vitti P, Cetani F, et al. Thyroid ultrasonography helps to identify patients with diffuse lymphocytic thyroiditis who are prone to develop hypothyroidism. J Clin Endocrinol Metab 1991; 72:209.
10. Blum M, Passalaqua AM, Sackler J, Pudiowski R. Thyroid echography of subacute thyroiditis. Radiology 1977; 124:795.
11. Solbiati L, Rizzatto G, Bellotti E, et al. High resolution sonography of cervical lymph nodes in head and neck cancer: criteria for differentiation of reactive versus malignant nodes (abstract). Radiology 1988; 169(P):113.
12. Vassallo P, Wernecke K, Roos N, Peters PE. Differentiation of benign from malignant superficial lymphadenopathy: the role of high-resolution US. Radiology 1992; 183:215.
13. Choi M, Lee JW, Jang KJ. Distinction between benign and malignant causes of cervical, axillary, and inguinal adenopathy: value of Doppler spectral waveform analysis. AJR Am J Roentgenol 1995; 165:981.
14. Blum M. Practical application of modern technology in thyroid evaluation. In: Van Middlesworth L, ed. The thyroid gland: practical clinical treatise. Chicago: Year Book Medical Publishers, 1986:47.
15. Boland GW, Lee MJ, Mueller PR, et al. Efficacy of sonographically guided biopsy of thyroid masses and cervical lymph nodes. AJR Am J Roentgenol 1993; 161:1053.
16. Gharib H, Goellner JR, Johnson DA. FNA cytology of the thyroid: a 12 year experience with 11,000 biopsies. Clin Lab Med 1995; 13:699.
17. Blum M, Reede DL, Seltzer TF, et al. Computerized axial tomography in the diagnosis and management of thyroid and parathyroid disorders. Am J Med Sci 1984; 287:34.
18. Blum M, Holliday RA, Yee JM. Non-isotopic imaging of the thyroid. In: Wagner HN Jr, ed. Nuclear medicine. Philadelphia: WB Saunders, 1995:595.
19. Bahist B, Ellis K, Gold RP. Computed tomography of intrathoracic goiters. AJR Am J Roentgenol 1983; 140:455.
20. Higgins CB, Auffermann W. MR imaging of thyroid and parathyroid glands: a review of current status. AJR Am J Roentgenol 1988; 151:1095.
21. Charkes ND, Maurer AH, Siegel JA, et al. MR imaging in thyroid disorders: correlation of signal intensity with Graves disease activity. Radiology 1987; 164(2):491.
22. Mountz JM, Glazer GM, Dmuchowski C, Sisson JC. MR imaging of the thyroid: comparison with scintigraphy in the normal and diseased gland. J Comput Assist Tomogr 1987; 11(4):612.
23. Sandler MP, Putton JA, Sacks GA, et al. Evaluation of intrathoracic goiter with I-123 scintigraphy and nuclear magnetic resonance imaging. J Nucl Med 1984; 25:874.
24. Tennvall J, Biorklund A, Moller T, et al. Studies of MRI relaxation times in malignant and normal tissues of the human thyroid gland. Prog Nucl Med 1984; 8:142.
25. Yousem DM, Som PM, Hackney DB, et al. Central nodal necrosis and extracapsular neoplastic spread in cervical lymph nodes: MR imaging versus CT. Radiology 1992; 182:753.
26. Webb WR, Sostman HD. MR imaging of thoracic disease: clinical uses. Radiology 1992; 182:621.
27. Shellock FG. MR imaging of metallic implants and materials: a compilation of the literature. AJR Am J Roentgenol 1988; 151:811.
28. Ghaarib H. Fine-needle aspiration biopsy of thyroid nodules: advantages, limitations, and effects. Mayo Clin Proc 1994; 69:44.

# CHAPTER 36

# ABNORMAL THYROID FUNCTION TEST RESULTS IN EUTHYROID PERSONS

HENRY B. BURCH

## EFFECTS OF ILLNESS ON INDICES OF THYROID FUNCTION

The frequency with which thyroid disease is encountered in the general population, the ease with which it is excluded in otherwise healthy persons, and the poor specificity of the individual signs and symptoms of thyroid dysfunction all have contributed to the practice of screening for thyroid disease in patients with nonthyroidal illness (NTI), in the search for a readily reversible component to the presenting illness. The resultant recognition of multiple abnormalities in *parameters* of thyroid function in patients who ultimately are deemed to be euthyroid has engendered the term *euthyroid sick syndrome* to describe these persons.[1,2] Although early cross-sectional studies in such patients had revealed a baffling collection of low, normal, or high values for total and free thyroid hormones, subsequent work has suggested a continuum of change, within which a given patient's status is determined by the severity and duration of illness as well as the presence of mitigating influences that are associated with the specific underlying disorder. Hence, an early and dramatic reduction in serum total and free triiodothyronine ($T_3$) levels occurs, followed, in cases of sufficient severity, by a depression in serum total thyroxine ($T_4$) and variable changes in serum free thyroxine ($FT_4$) levels. Concurrent with decrements in levels of circulating thyroid hormones, a seemingly inept response is seen at the hypothalamic-pituitary level; this persists until the recovery phase of the underlying illness, at which time a rise in thyroid-stimulating hormone (TSH) to even supranormal levels may be seen that coincides with a rapid recovery in $T_4$ and $T_3$ levels[3] (Fig. 36-1).

## CHANGES IN INDIVIDUAL PARAMETERS OF THYROID FUNCTION

### TRIIODOTHYRONINE AND REVERSE TRIIODOTHYRONINE

The most prevalent and pronounced anomaly in the parameters of thyroid function during NTI is a depression in the serum total and free $T_3$ levels. This manifestation, which is present in 70% or more of hospitalized patients, may be considered, with a few notable exceptions (discussed later), the sine qua non of the euthyroid sick syndrome.[4,5] The likelihood of finding a depression of serum $T_3$ varies with the severity of the NTI; in one study, it occurred in 23% of patients on regular hospital wards, 56% of those in intensive care units, 76% of those undergoing coronary artery bypass, and 86% of those receiving heart transplants.[5] The depression in serum $T_3$ may be pronounced, achieving levels below those seen in hypothyroid persons.[6,7] Concomitant reductions in thyroid hormone–binding proteins account for less than one-third of the observed decrease in serum $T_3$ level[4]; much of the remainder is attributable to a decreased peripheral monodeiodination of serum $T_4$ (discussed later). Serum free $T_3$, as measured by equilibrium dialysis, also is decreased in as many as 50% of patients with NTI. Given the frequency and magnitude of the $T_3$ depression during severe

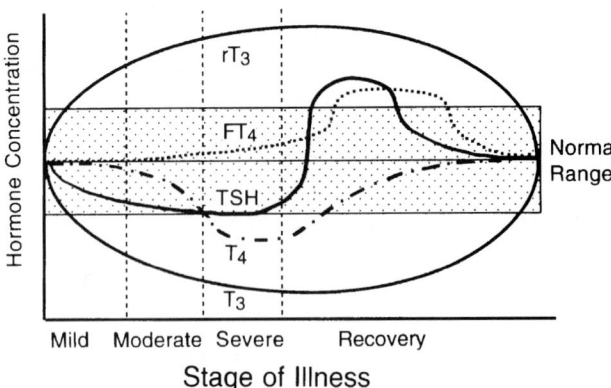

**FIGURE 36-1.** Influence of the stage and the severity of nonthyroidal illness (*NTI*) on the parameters of thyroid function. Early in the course of illness, marked decreases in triiodothyronine ($T_3$) are accompanied by reciprocal changes in reverse $T_3$ ($rT_3$). The free thyroxine ($FT_4$) and thyroid-stimulating hormone (*TSH*) generally remain within normal limits but may transiently exceed this range, particularly during the recovery phase. The total thyroxine ($T_4$), which generally is normal during mild to moderate NTI, falls progressively with increasing disease severity. Recovery is accompanied by gradual normalization of $T_4$, followed by normalization of $T_3$ and reverse $T_3$, as well as of TSH. (Adapted from Nicoloff JT, LoPresti JS. Extrinsic and intrinsic variables: nonthyroidal illness. In: Braverman LE, Utiger RD, eds. Werner and Ingbar's the thyroid. A fundamental and clinical text, 7th ed. Philadelphia: JB Lippincott, 1996:289.)

NTI, the finding of a normal or elevated $T_3$ concentration in this setting occasionally is the first indication of a coexistent thyrotoxicosis.[8] Serum *reverse* $T_3$ ($rT_3$), a metabolically inert metabolite of $T_4$ obtained through 5-deiodination, has long been valued as a diagnostic tool in the distinction of sick euthyroid patients (elevated $rT_3$) from patients with hypothyroidism (depressed $rT_3$), although this is not always reliable.[9,10] As with $T_4$ and $T_3$, serum $rT_3$ is predominantly protein bound in the circulation. Beyond its role as the "alternate" metabolite of $T_4$, $rT_3$ has the ability to act as both substrate and inhibitor of type I and type II 5'-monodeiodinases, thereby potentially contributing to the decreased production of $T_3$ seen in NTI.[11]

## TOTAL THYROXINE

Thyroxine levels enjoy a greater degree of stability than do $T_3$ levels during NTI of mild or moderate severity. However, with increasing gravity of the underlying illness, the serum total $T_4$ levels may be subnormal in as many as 20% to 50% of hospitalized patients.[5–7,12,13] Extremely low serum $T_4$ levels portend a fatal outcome to an extent that rivals traditional prognostic indices (see later). Conversely, a rise in $T_4$ levels accompanies the recovery phase of illness in patients who survive critical illness (see Fig. 36-1). Hyperthyroxinemia may be seen occasionally in NTI, although this generally occurs in a predictable fashion in association with certain hepatic disorders or acute psychiatric illnesses, or in conjunction with specific medications (see later).

## FREE THYROXINE

In view of the described abnormalities in serum $T_4$ and $T_3$, an accurate assessment of circulating $FT_4$ levels assumes a critical role in the metabolic evaluation of patients with NTI. Likewise, the measurement of serum $FT_4$ is essential to the understanding of the apparently euthyroid status that is observed in these patients despite the profound changes in other parameters of thyroid function. Unfortunately, several features inherent to NTI serve to undermine attempts to measure and interpret serum $FT_4$ levels accurately. These include postulated circulating inhibitors to $T_4$ binding, the effects of commonly used drugs

on hormone binding and on the hypothalamic–pituitary–thyroid axis, and the frequent finding of spuriously low serum $FT_4$ values during NTI when these are assessed using $FT_4$ *indices* or are measured by several of the indirect $FT_4$ techniques in common use.[14] Serum $FT_4$ index calculations, which depend on the resin uptake of labeled $T_3$ or $T_4$, generally underestimate serum $FT_4$ levels during NTI, perhaps as a result of the presence of circulating inhibitors to thyroid hormone binding. This artifact may be particularly pronounced in patients who have low total $T_4$ levels.[12] Serum $FT_4$ assays that use synthetic $T_4$ analogs also may yield falsely low $FT_4$ levels because of undesired protein binding of the analog; this occurs despite attempts to design agents that minimize such effects.[14] As a result, these methodologies are (paradoxically) dependent on concentrations of thyroid hormone–binding proteins as well as on serum dilution.[15] When assessed by equilibrium dialysis, serum $FT_4$ has been found to be normal or minimally elevated in most patients with NTI.[7,14,16] However, the high cost and technical demands that are associated with equilibrium dialysis generally have limited the utility of this measurement in clinical practice. Measurement of serum $FT_4$ by direct equilibrium dialysis using undiluted serum[3,17] has revealed normal $FT_4$ values in most patients with NTI.[18] This method and similar techniques ultimately may serve to increase the feasibility and accuracy of serum $FT_4$ measurement in patients with NTI.

## THYROID-STIMULATING HORMONE

The response of serum TSH to the marked reduction in levels of free and total $T_3$ has been viewed alternatively as either inappropriately blunted or indicative of normal intracellular thyroid hormone effects. A normal serum TSH level in the setting of NTI frequently is offered as evidence for euthyroidism. However, current experimental evidence suggests the presence of a complicity at the hypothalamic-pituitary level in the thyroidal alterations that occur in NTI. For example, an abrupt decline in serum TSH occurs in acutely ill or stressed patients, such as during fasting,[19] after major surgery,[5] or after bone marrow transplantation.[13] Furthermore, the subsequent rise in serum TSH that coincides with the normalization of serum $T_4$ suggests an amelioration of a relative central hypothyroidism in these patients.[3] Moreover, although the responsiveness of the pituitary thyrotrope to exogenous thyrotropin-releasing hormone (TRH) generally is maintained during NTI,[16,20,21] an inability to augment this response appropriately has been demonstrated,[22] and a *relative* blunting of the serum TSH peak occurs in critical illness[23] and with acute caloric deprivation.[24] The nocturnal surge that occurs in serum TSH levels in healthy persons also is diminished during NTI.[20,25] Alterations in serum TSH levels in hospitalized patients with NTI have been examined using a second-generation sensitive TSH assay.[26] Of 1580 hospitalized patients, 33% were found to have abnormal serum TSH values, and 15% had levels more than 3 standard deviations above or below the mean for control subjects. When a subgroup of these patients was followed longitudinally, 84% had NTI or recent glucocorticoid use as the sole explanation for their abnormal serum TSH value; this included 76% of patients who had an undetectable serum TSH and 50% of patients who had a serum TSH of more than 20 mIU/mL (Fig. 36-2). Interestingly, 86% of patients with NTI who had undetectable serum TSH levels by a second-generation assay (<0.1 mIU/mL) had detectable levels (>0.01 mIU/mL) using a third-generation TSH assay.[27] These results have been duplicated elsewhere.[28]

Although cross-sectional analysis reveals a high frequency of abnormalities in thyroid function test results during NTI, changes beyond the reference range for serum TSH and $FT_4$, when present, generally are small and may be best accounted for by a broadening of the range accepted as "normal" during NTI[5,26] (as discussed later).

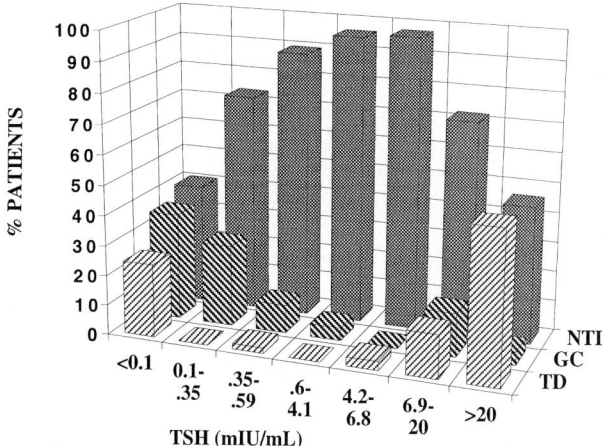

**FIGURE 36-2.** Etiology of abnormal values in sensitive assays for thyroid-stimulating hormone (*TSH*) values in hospitalized patients. A cohort of 329 individuals selected from 1580 hospitalized patients and categorized on the basis of TSH level were reevaluated after recovery from nonthyroidal illness to determine the true thyroid status. The percentage of patients in each TSH category who were ultimately found to have thyroid disease (*TD*), nonthyroidal illness (*NTI*), or glucocorticoid use (*GC*) as the explanation for the baseline TSH is shown. Patients in each category included: TSH <0.1 mIU/mL (*n* = 45); 0.1–0.34 (*n* = 70); 0.35–0.59 (*n* = 54); 0.60–4.1 (*n* = 70); 4.2–6.8 (*n* = 33); 6.9–20.0 (*n* = 35); and >20 mIU/mL (*n* = 22). Most notable is the high percentage of patients with TSH <0.1 mIU/mL or >20 mIU/mL who were ultimately found to be free of thyroid dysfunction (76% and 50%, respectively). (Data derived from Spencer CA, Eigen A, Shen D, et al. Specificity of sensitive assays of thyrotropin used to screen for thyroid disease in hospitalized patients. Clin Chem 1987; 33:1391.)

## DISEASE-SPECIFIC VARIATION

A wide variety of severe illnesses, including poorly controlled diabetes mellitus, infection, malignancy, acute myocardial infarction, stroke, major surgery or injury, and malnutrition, may lead to characteristic patterns of altered thyroid hormone indices. This section reviews selected nonthyroidal disorders, with an emphasis on caloric deprivation as both a model and a common component of diverse forms of NTI. In addition, disorders in which the usual pattern of NTI has been modified because of the superimposition of effects unique to the underlying disease state are discussed.

### CALORIC DEPRIVATION

The effect of prolonged fasting on the parameters of thyroid function is a well-studied model for NTI. With this model, the myriad of interfering influences that are present in many hospitalized ill patients are avoided. During acute caloric deprivation, serum total and free $T_3$ levels begin to descend within the first 24 hours and reach a plateau within 1 to 2 weeks. The concentration of serum $rT_3$ rises, and it plateaus at nearly double basal levels during this period.[29] Serum $T_4$ levels generally remain stable during fasting, and $FT_4$ levels are either normal or slightly increased. Serum TSH levels decrease slightly during the initial fasting period and return to baseline within 96 hours.[19] The pituitary response to TRH is blunted during a fast relative to the fed state, but generally remains in a range that is appropriate to the true thyroid state.[24,30] Interestingly, the effect of fasting on thyroid indices is ameliorated when as little as 50 g of glucose or protein is given, but not when fat is the sole source of the caloric supplement.[1,30] The concept that these changes are homeostatic in nature has been strengthened by the observation that the administration of $T_3$ in this setting increases gluconeogenesis

at the expense of muscle protein catabolism and thereby promotes depletion of lean body mass.[31]

## RENAL FAILURE

Patients with end-stage renal disease have a higher incidence of both goiter and primary hypothyroidism than do hospitalized control patients.[32] Like patients with other serious NTIs, patients with chronic renal failure have depressions in serum $T_3$ and $T_4$ levels, normal $FT_4$ levels, normal TSH levels, and *elevated free* $rT_3$ levels.[32,32a] However, in contrast to other disorders, serum *total* $rT_3$ levels generally are *normal* rather than elevated in renal failure. Multiple differences in $rT_3$ handling account for this observation, including a normal rather than a decreased $rT_3$ metabolic clearance rate, a decreased protein binding of $rT_3$, an enhanced exit rate of $rT_3$ from the serum into tissue, and enhanced tissue $rT_3$ binding.[32] Patients with the nephrotic syndrome have enhanced urinary $T_4$ and $T_3$ losses; much of this is accounted for by the concurrent loss of thyroid-binding globulin (TBG) in the urine. Despite this finding, these patients usually have changes in their thyroid indices similar to those of patients with chronic renal failure. Shortly after the initiation of dialysis, patients with renal failure may experience improvement in serum $T_4$ and $T_3$ levels; this may be only temporary, because patients undergoing long-term dialysis generally have persistent decrements in these levels.[1,32]

## HEPATIC DISORDERS

The liver supports several key aspects of thyroid function, including the biosynthesis of each of the three principal binding proteins, the peripheral conversion of $T_4$ to $T_3$, and the provision of a reservoir for $T_4$ and $T_3$. Therefore, the fact that disorders of hepatic function compound the defects in thyroid economy that typically are observed in NTI is not unexpected. Patients with *hepatic cirrhosis* generally have normal or decreased serum $T_4$ values and depressed $T_3$ levels. The decrease in serum $T_4$, when present, does not appear to be a result of reductions in serum TBG levels (which generally are normal) but may be due in part to decreases in thyroxine-binding prealbumin and albumin concentrations, both of which are lower than normal in this population. Serum $FT_4$ and free $T_3$ levels usually are within the normal range in cirrhosis. TSH levels frequently are normal but occasionally may be increased in patients with cirrhosis.[6,33] An elevation, rather than a depression, in $T_3$ and $T_4$ levels distinguishes patients with *acute infectious hepatitis, chronic active hepatitis,* and *primary biliary cirrhosis* from those with the pattern that is more typical of NTI.[33,34] An increased synthesis and release of TBG occurs in these disorders, resulting in elevations of both $T_4$ and $T_3$. The serum $FT_4$ generally remains in the normal range. Occasionally, the serum TSH may be elevated in patients with chronic active hepatitis or primary biliary cirrhosis, but this probably is related to the higher prevalence of Hashimoto thyroiditis and associated primary thyroid failure in patients with these conditions.[34]

## ACQUIRED IMMUNODEFICIENCY SYNDROME AND ACQUIRED IMMUNODEFICIENCY SYNDROME–RELATED COMPLEX

Persons infected with the human immunodeficiency virus (HIV) have an atypical pattern of change in the indices of thyroid function that varies with the severity of illness.[35,36] An unexplained rise in serum TBG levels occurs with HIV infection; this is associated with a rise in serum total $T_4$ values, but normal $FT_4$ values and normal rather than decreased $T_3$ levels in ambulatory patients. With hospitalization or progressive illness, however, serum $T_3$ levels fall.[36] In addition, patients with acquired immunodeficiency syndrome (AIDS) may have unexpectedly normal or even low $rT_3$ values relative to healthy con-

**TABLE 36-1.**
**The Effect of Various Clinical Conditions or Illnesses on Indices of Thyroid Function**

| Disorder | $T_4$ | $FT_4$ | $T_3$ | $rT_3$ | TSH | TRH Stim | Comment |
|---|---|---|---|---|---|---|---|
| Malnutrition | N | N | ↓ | ↑ | N | N or ↓ | CHO-responsive |
| Chronic renal failure | N or ↓ | N | ↓ | N | N | N | Transient improvement after dialysis |
| Hepatitis (acute infectious) | N or ↑ | N | ↑ | ↑ | N | N | Increased TBG synthesis and release |
| Hepatitis (chronic active) | N or ↑ | N | ↑ | N | N or ↑ | N or ↑ | Increased incidence of AITD |
| Cirrhosis | N or ↓ | N | ↓ | ↑ | N or ↑ | N | — |
| Surgery | ↓ | N | ↓ | ↑ | N or ↓ | N or ↑ | Immediate postop |
| Myocardial infarction | N | N | ↓ | ↑ | N or ↑ | NS | 1–3 Days after infarction |
| AIDS | ↑ | N | N | N or ↓ | N | N or ↓ | Changes proportional to stage until critically ill |
| Acute psychiatric disorder | N or ↑ | N or ↑ | N or ↑ | ↑ | N or ↑ | N or ↓ | — |
| Critical illness | N or ↓ | N or ↓* | ↓ | ↑ | N or ↓* | N or ↓ | Consider drug effects |

N, normal; NS, not studied; ↑, increased; ↓, decreased; $T_4$, thyroxine; $FT_4$, free thyroxine; $T_3$, triiodothyronine; $rT_3$, reverse triiodothyronine; TSH, thyroid-stimulating hormone; *TRH stim*, thyrotropin-releasing hormone stimulation; CHO, carbohydrate; TBG, thyroxine-binding globulin; AITD, autoimmune thyroid disease; *postop*, postoperative; AIDS, acquired immunodeficiency syndrome.
*Commonly decreased with dopamine therapy.
(Adapted from Wartofsky L, Burman KD. Alterations in thyroid function in patients with systemic illness: the "euthyroid sick" syndrome. Endocr Rev 1982; 3[1]:164.)

trol subjects.[35,37,38] The serum TBG rises progressively in HIV infection as the disease advances from the asymptomatic carrier stage to AIDS-related complex and, finally, to AIDS. The TBG levels have been found to correlate inversely with the CD4 count in these persons.[38] The serum TSH may be higher than in healthy control subjects, but remains within the normal range and responds with a normal or slightly exaggerated response to the injection of TRH.[37] The paradoxically normal or even high serum $T_3$ level in HIV-infected patients has been postulated to contribute to the extreme cachexia that is seen with this disorder, but no correlation has been found between weight loss and relative serum $T_3$ elevation in these patients.[36] Patients with advanced AIDS ultimately may manifest decreases in serum $T_3$ and $T_4$, which signify a preterminal state.[35]

## PSYCHIATRIC DISTURBANCE

Thyroid hormone levels have been examined extensively in patients hospitalized with acute psychiatric illness. In various studies, between 10% and 33% of such patients have elevated serum $T_4$ levels at the time of admission.[39–41] The serum $FT_4$ index is elevated in 3% to 18% of such patients, and the $FT_4$ value is either normal or supranormal.[39] Serum $T_3$ concentrations generally are normal[39] or minimally elevated,[41] and $rT_3$ levels are increased. The serum TSH, as assessed using a sensitive assay, is elevated in as many as 17% of such cases, prompting the speculation that hyperthyroxinemia in these patients is driven centrally.[41] However, little correlation exists between the serum total $T_4$ or $FT_4$ index and the TSH level in patients who experience hyperthyroxinemia during their psychiatric illness.[40,41] TRH responsiveness was found to be blunted in more than one-half of the patients in one study,[39] but in none of four patients in another report.[41] The response to TRH in depressed patients has been found to be directly proportional to the basal serum TSH level and provides little additional diagnostic value.[42] Rapid improvement in each of these parameters has been demonstrated repeatedly in most hospitalized psychiatric patients. Therefore, the utility of thyroid function testing in these patients at the time of hospital admission has been legitimately questioned. However, in most cases, with the combined use of a sensitive TSH assay and a measured or estimated serum $FT_4$, true thyroid dysfunction should be readily distinguished from the transient effects of the psychiatric disturbance.

The exceptions notwithstanding, diverse NTIs have a surprisingly predictable influence on parameters of thyroid economy. The *severity* of the illness rather than the *type* of illness appears to determine the presence and magnitude of the observed change. The perturbations in indices of thyroid func-

tion observed in these and other common medical conditions are outlined in Table 36-1.

## PATHOPHYSIOLOGY

### SITES OF NONTHYROIDAL ILLNESS INTERACTION WITH THYROID ECONOMY

Every accessible point in thyroid hormone homeostasis has been examined or considered as a potential contributor to the thyroidal effects of NTI (Fig. 36-3). A number of studies have examined the role of cytokines in the mediation of these effects (discussed later). At the *hypothalamic-pituitary level*, decreases in mRNA for TRH have been noted in the hypothalamus obtained at autopsy from patients succumbing to an NTI.[43] In these patients, TRH gene expression was inversely correlated with antemortem serum $T_3$ levels. Other endogenous modulators of the hypothalamic–pituitary–thyroid axis that potentially are activated during NTI include cortisol, somatostatin, dopamine, and the β-endorphins. *Within the pituitary*, several potential

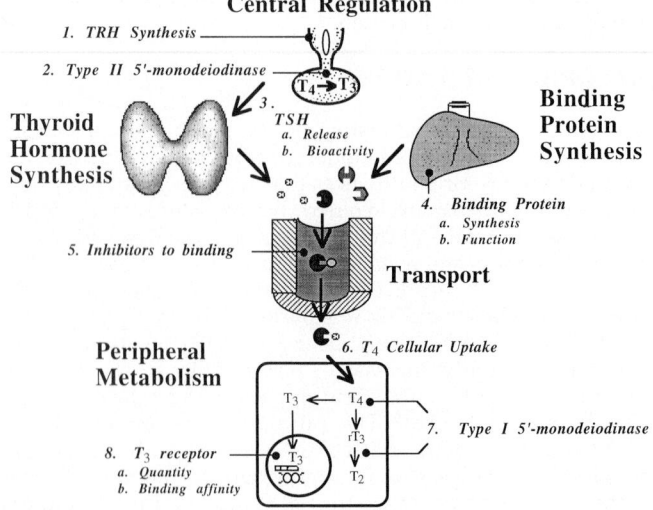

**FIGURE 36-3.** Potential sites of interaction between thyroid economy and nonthyroidal illness. Interaction at multiple levels of regulation has been demonstrated or hypothesized (see text). (TRH, thyrotropin-releasing hormone; $T_4$, thyroxine; $T_3$, triiodothyronine; TSH, thyroid-stimulating hormone; $rT_3$, reverse $T_3$; $T_2$, diiodothyronine.)

defects, including altered tissue levels of $T_3$[44] or of the $T_3$ receptor[45]; enhanced activity of the type II 5'-monodeiodinase enzyme[13]; and diminished synthesis,[46] release,[19] or bioactivity[47,48] of TSH, have been considered as possible explanations for the apparently blunted pituitary responsiveness that occurs in NTI. Multiple disturbances, rather than any single defect, probably account for the diverse changes in the hypothalamic-pituitary control of thyroid function observed in NTI.

Much has been learned about *thyroid hormone production, binding defects,* and *peripheral metabolism* in NTI. Decrements in circulating thyroid hormone levels are well-established features of NTI, yet the production and release of serum $T_4$ is normal in these disorders. Furthermore, a decreased production or an accelerated loss (nephrotic syndrome) of binding proteins accounts for only a small portion of the observed decreases in serum $T_4$ and $T_3$ levels. *Circulating inhibitors of thyroid hormone binding* have been postulated to contribute to the lowering of serum total $T_4$ levels[12] and the decreased $T_4$/TBG ratio[49] that occurs in NTI in the face of normal or high serum $FT_4$ concentrations. Free fatty acids have been investigated in this regard.[10] However, the nature and even the existence of these inhibitors remains controversial, and alternative explanations have been proposed for the binding abnormality in NTI.[50] *Defects in TBG* itself, as evidenced by relative increases in an isoform that has an altered electrophoretic motility, have been reported to affect thyroid hormone levels in NTI.[51] *Altered metabolism of $T_4$* resulting from decreased activity of type I 5'-monodeiodinase activity is the best known, yet still incompletely understood, phenomenon noted in NTI. The result of this enzymatic inhibition is the striking decrease in serum $T_3$ and elevation in $rT_3$ that is characteristic of the euthyroid sick syndrome. Diminished hepatic uptake of $T_4$ may also contribute to decreased peripheral production of $T_3$ in patients with NTI.[52] Interestingly, $rT_3$ may compete with $T_4$ as a substrate for both type I and type II 5'-monodeiodinases, compounding the defect in $T_4$-to-$T_3$ conversion.[11] Other nonpharmacologic mechanisms contributing to the inhibition of 5'-monodeiodination that occurs during NTI remain to be elucidated. The cloning of the complementary DNA for human type I 5'-monodeiodinase[53] has allowed the demonstration of decreased expression of this gene in an animal model of NTI.[54]

*Tissue levels of thyroid hormones* are likely to be important determinants of the true metabolic state in NTI but are not readily measured. The existing studies suggest that decreased tissue levels of thyroid hormones are present in patients who succumb to a wasting illness as compared to patients who experience sudden death.[45] The uptake of $T_4$ into cultured rat hepatocytes[52] or human hepatoma cells[55] is lower in the presence of sera from patients with NTI than in control sera. $T_3$ receptor mRNA is increased in peripheral leukocytes and liver cells from patients with NTI, and the increments in hepatic $T_3$ receptor are partially reversed after liver transplantation.[56] These findings suggest a mechanism for an intact cellular response to $T_3$ in the face of decreases in cellular uptake and tissue levels of thyroid hormones. Finally, the ultimate assessment of the integrity of thyroid hormone economy during NTI is measurement of the transcription and translation products from thyroid hormone–responsive genes. Circulating markers of thyroid hormone action, such as levels of TSH, ferritin, osteocalcin, sex hormone–binding protein, and angiotensin-converting enzyme, are generally normal in NTI,[57] as is the production rate of $rT_3$, a finding consistent with euthyroidism at the target organ level.[15] Similarly, clinical indicators of thyroid status, such as basal metabolic rate, $QK_d$ interval (a measure of cardiac contractility), and deep tendon reflex relaxation times, are most consistent with a euthyroid state in these patients.[15]

The role of cytokines in the modulation of the thyroid hormone changes seen in NTI has received considerable attention.[58] Interpretation of these studies is hampered by the complexity and redundancy of the cytokine network, the flulike

illness (and accompanying NTI-related thyroid changes) associated with experimental infusion of these agents, and the difficulty in discerning causation from mere association when concurrent changes are observed in both thyroid hormone and cytokine levels. Further compounding this difficulty is the lack of measurable changes in circulating levels of those cytokines that act through paracrine mechanisms, such as TNF-α. Despite these obstacles, several interesting findings have emerged. At the hypothalamic-pituitary level, interleukin-1β (IL-1β) decreases the levels of TRH mRNA in the rat,[59] and TNF-α, IL-1β, and interleukin-6 (IL-6) decrease serum levels of TSH in human subjects. At the thyrocyte level, TNF-α, interleukin-1α (IL-1α), IL-1β, IL-6, and interferon-γ display inhibitory effects in vitro, and TNF-α, IL-1β, and IL-6 decrease thyroid hormone levels in experimental animals.[58,60–62] A strong correlation has been noted between serum IL-6 levels and $T_3$ (inversely correlated) and $rT_3$ levels,[63,64] but as noted earlier, this does not prove causation. For example, although IL-6 knock-out mice have diminished NTI-related thyroid hormone changes,[65] the reduction of IL-6 after mouse liver macrophage depletion does not prevent the development of NTI changes in thyroid hormones.[66] Likewise, although IL-6 infusion in humans acutely decreases both $T_3$ and TSH, these latter changes remit with chronic IL-6 administration.[67] Lastly, incubation of rat hepatocytes with the cytokines and IL-6, TNF-α, or IL-1β inexplicably increases 5'-monodeiodinase activity in rat hepatocytes.[61] Hence, although cytokines are likely to contribute to the thyroid hormone changes associated with NTI, the extent of this participation remains to be determined.

## DIFFERENTIATION FROM PRIMARY THYROID DYSFUNCTION

### NONTHYROIDAL ILLNESS SIMULATING THYROID DYSFUNCTION

A timely distinction between the alterations in thyroid indices that are due to NTI alone and those that are related to true thyroid dysfunction is critical both to the prevention of inappropriate intervention and to the identification of patients with myxedema or thyrotoxicosis, in whom metabolic correction may have a profound influence on disease outcome. A knowledge of the previously outlined patterns of change typically seen in NTI, as well as an awareness of the pitfalls associated with strict reliance on "normal" ranges for thyroid function tests in NTI, better equips the clinician to make this distinction. Advances in serum TSH assays have greatly increased the sensitivity and specificity of these assays for detecting thyroid hormone excess and deficiency states. However, applying the normal range designed to distinguish euthyroidism from thyroid hormone excess or thyroid hormone deficiency to patients with NTI results in a loss of specificity.[26] This is particularly true for patients with serum TSH values only slightly above or below the normal range. When the "euthyroid" range for serum TSH is broadened to encompass values between 0.1 and 20.0 mIU/mL in patients with NTI, the specificity of this test is enhanced to 97%.[26] However, the fact that even patients with NTI who have serum TSH values that are undetectable or greater than 20 mIU/mL are still likely to be found ultimately to be euthyroid underscores the peril of relying on any single thyroid function test in these cases.[26]

The combined measurement of serum $FT_4$ and TSH is prudent in patients with NTI in whom thyroid dysfunction is suspected. Although deviation from the reference range commonly occurs when either of these assays is used in patients with NTI, the concurrence of a low serum $FT_4$ and a high TSH ("hypothyroid" pattern) or of a high serum $FT_4$ and a low TSH ("hyperthyroid" pattern) is distinctly uncommon as a manifestation of NTI alone[5,68] (Fig. 36-4). Clinicians must be familiar with the

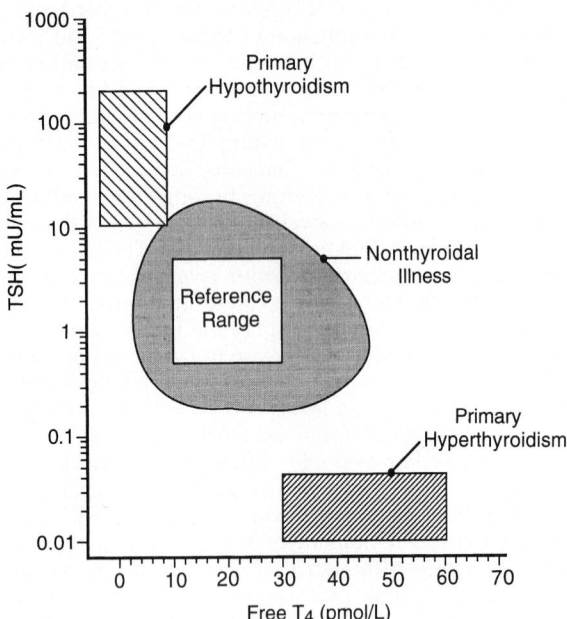

**FIGURE 36-4.** Distinguishing true thyroid dysfunction from the effects of nonthyroidal illness (*NTI*). Although both the free thyroxine ($T_4$) and thyroid-stimulating hormone (*TSH*) values may deviate from the reference range during NTI, the combined use of these parameters generally allows for the accurate distinction from primary thyroid dysfunction. Patients with NTI who have abnormal values for either $FT_4$ or TSH (or both) are likely to occupy positions above and to the right of the reference range as shown in this nomogram. This is distinct from the pattern seen in patients experiencing either primary hypothyroidism (*above and to the left*) or hyperthyroidism (*below and to the right*). (Adapted from Kaptein EM. Clinical application of free thyroxine determinations. Clin Lab Med 1993; 13:653.)

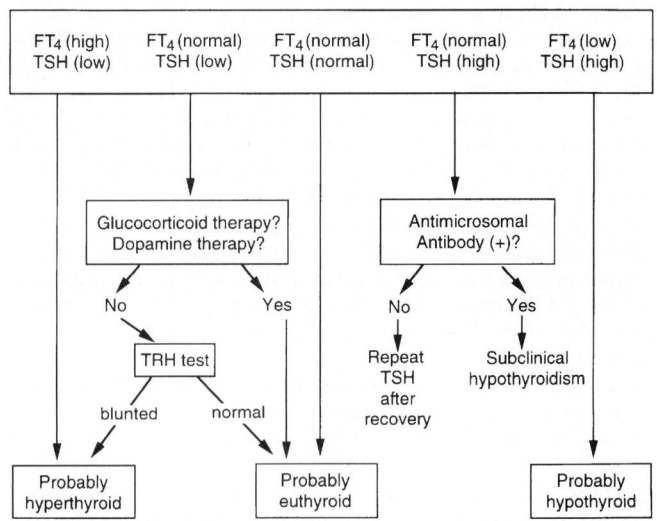

**FIGURE 36-5.** An approach to thyroid function testing in hospitalized patients. The combined use of free thyroxine ($FT_4$) and a sensitive thyroid-stimulating hormone (*TSH*) assay suggests primary thyroid dysfunction when these two parameters deviate in opposite directions from the reference range. Conversely, thyroid dysfunction is unlikely when both $FT_4$ and TSH are normal. When only one of these parameters is normal, further information or testing is needed to distinguish non-thyroidal illness (*NTI*) from true thyroid dysfunction. A normal $FT_4$ but subnormal TSH in patients receiving glucocorticoids or dopamine is likely to be explicable as a drug effect alone. In the absence of these medications, this pattern may represent a subclinical hyperthyroidism that will yield a blunted TSH response to thyrotropin-releasing hormone (*TRH*) testing. A normal $FT_4$ but high TSH may be seen in both subclinical hypothyroidism and NTI. The presence of significant (>1:400) microsomal antibody (*MA*) titers increases the likelihood of the former; negative MA titers increase the likelihood that the TSH elevation is the result of NTI alone. Testing should be performed again to verify this interpretation after recovery from illness. (From Spencer CA. Serum TSH measurement: a 1990 status report. Thyroid Today 1990; 13:1.)

techniques used at their institutions to measure or to estimate $FT_4$. Indices, as well as analog methodologies, are likely to underestimate serum $FT_4$ values during NTI. Newer, simplified methods for measuring $FT_4$ by direct equilibrium dialysis should provide the needed supplement to a sensitive TSH assay in this setting. For patients for whom diagnostic uncertainty remains, the measurement of significant antibody titers against thyroid peroxidase (microsomal antigen) appears to enhance the likelihood of finding underlying thyroid disease.[26] This possibility also is greater in patients who are older than 60 years of age and in those who have other autoimmune disorders.[15] Similarly, an abnormal TSH response to TRH further increases the likelihood that true thyroid dysfunction is present. A diagnostic approach encompassing these concepts in hospitalized patients with NTI is illustrated in Figure 36-5. A comparison of thyroid function indices found in NTI to those observed in primary hypothyroidism is provided in Table 36-2.

This discussion has dealt primarily with distinguishing NTI from primary thyroid dysfunction. Other, rarer causes of diagnostic uncertainty in critically ill patients include central hypothyroidism (in which other clinical evidence that is suggestive of hypothalamic-pituitary dysfunction may be evident) and disorders of inappropriate TSH secretion, including TSH-secreting pituitary adenomas and syndromes of thyroid hormone resistance.

## NONTHYROIDAL ILLNESS MASKING THYROID DYSFUNCTION

Occasionally, the superimposition of NTI on an established thyroid disorder results in the transient normalization of thyroid indices, thereby masking true thyroid dysfunction. The most common example of this occurrence is the depression of serum

TSH from a clearly hypothyroid value toward one that might easily be attributed to NTI alone.[5,69] Another example is a decrease of serum $T_3$ and $T_4$ in a thyrotoxic patient to the euthyroid range during an NTI, with subsequent unmasking of the toxic state after recovery from the disease.[8,70] These examples point to the need for careful follow-up of patients who are found

**TABLE 36-2.**

**Comparison of Laboratory Findings in Nonthyroidal Illness and Primary Hypothyroidism**

| Laboratory Test | Nonthyroidal Illness | Overt Hypothyroidism |
|---|---|---|
| Total $T_4$ | ↓ | ↓ |
| Free $T_4$ index | ↓ | ↓ |
| Free $T_4$ (equilibrium dialysis)* | N or ↑ | ↓ |
| Total $T_3$ | ↓ | N or ↓ |
| Free $T_3$ | N or ↓ | N or ↓ |
| $rT_3$* | ↑ | ↓ |
| TBG | N or ↓ | N or ↑ |
| TSH, basal | N or ↓ or ↑† | ↑ |
| TSH, response to TRH* | N or ↓ | ↑ |
| Microsomal (anti-thyroid peroxidase) antibody* | Negative (titer <1:400) | Positive (titer >1:400) |

N, normal; ↑, increased; ↓, decreased; $T_4$, thyroxine; $T_3$, triiodothyronine; $rT_3$, reverse triiodothyronine; TBG, thyroxine-binding globulin; TSH, thyroid-stimulating hormone; TRH, thyrotropin-releasing hormone.

*These tests provide the best differentiation between nonthyroidal illness and hypothyroidism.

†"Expanded" normal range increases specificity in nonthyroidal illness (see text).

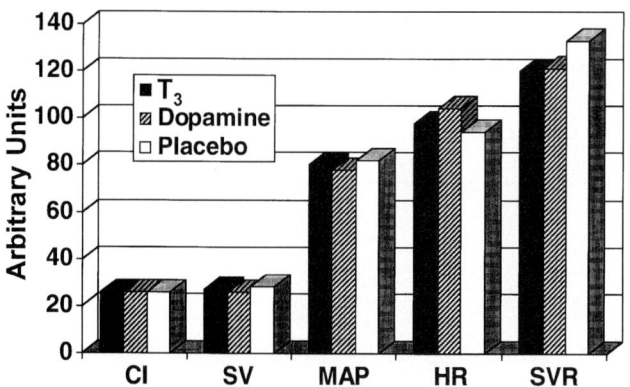

**FIGURE 36-6.** Lack of effect of triiodothyronine ($T_3$) treatment on cardiovascular parameters in patients undergoing coronary artery bypass graft surgery. Values shown represent readings taken at 4 hours after the start of administration of $T_3$ (0.8 µg/kg intravenous bolus followed by 0.12 µg/kg/hour continuous infusion) or dopamine (5 µg/kg/minute continuous infusion) or normal saline alone (placebo). Cardiac index (*CI*) shown as $10 \times (L/min)/m^2$; stroke volume (*SV*) shown in mL; mean arterial blood pressure (*MAP*) shown as mm Hg; heart rate (*HR*) shown as beats per minute; and systemic vascular resistance (*SVR*) shown as $0.1 \times dyne \times s \times cm^{-5}$. (Adapted from Bennett-Guerrero E, Jimenez JL, White WD, D'Amico EB, Baldwin BI, Schwinn DA. Cardiovascular effects of intravenous triiodothyronine in patients undergoing coronary artery bypass graft surgery. A randomized, double-blind, placebo-controlled trial. Duke $T_3$ study group. JAMA 1996; 275:687.)

to have incongruous thyroid indices or who manifest equivocal clinical findings during the course of an NTI. Thus, values should be measured again 2 to 4 weeks after recovery from the disease, or at any time during the course of an illness that the clinical findings become suggestive of true thyroid dysfunction.

## PROGNOSTIC IMPLICATIONS AND ROLE OF THYROID HORMONE THERAPY

In critically ill patients, a strong correlation has been found between the serum $T_4$ level at the time of hospital admission and the mortality rate. Given that the magnitude of depression in thyroid hormones corresponds to the severity of the underlying NTI, the fact that patients who have the greatest thyroid hormone depression have the worst prognosis is not unexpected. A particularly high mortality rate has been noted in critically ill patients with levels of serum $T_4$ and TSH that remain depressed for >1 week after admission to hospital.[5] The serum $T_4$ depression correlates negatively with survival in a manner that parallels the traditional Acute Physiology and Chronic Health Evaluation II (APACHE-II) prognostic score. Critically ill elderly patients with high serum IL-6 values and low serum albumin levels are more likely to have NTI-related thyroid alterations and have a higher likelihood of dying from their acute illness.[71]

Although the thyroid changes associated with NTI are generally believed to be adaptive in nature and to conserve energy for the organism as a whole, the possibility exists that organ or tissue-specific hypothyroidism is present,[72] the correction of which might lead to clinical improvement. Several studies have assessed the utility of replacement therapy in critically ill patients or laboratory animals who had depressed levels of thyroid hormones. Early controlled studies in humans, using either $T_3$ or $T_4$, failed to demonstrate beneficial effects on survival. Two prospective randomized trials have examined the use of $T_3$ to treat patients undergoing coronary artery bypass surgery.[73,74] Despite improvement in cardiac index and decreased vascular resistance in one of these trials,[74] no differences were observed in either study with respect to multiple

outcome variables, including the requirement for inotropic agents, the incidence of postoperative arrhythmia, time in the intensive care unit, or mortality rate (Fig. 36-6). On the basis of these studies, little role appears to exist for the administration of $T_3$ or $T_4$ to patients with a NTI.

In patients being evaluated for possible myxedema, in whom the mitigating influences of an NTI, the use of medication, and an equivocal clinical assessment prevent the exclusion of hypothyroidism, the judicious administration of thyroid hormone while awaiting the results of serum $FT_4$ and TSH measurements is unlikely to cause acute harm in patients with NTI and significantly improves the outcome in patients with myxedema.

## EUTHYROID HYPERTHYROXINEMIA

Numerous disorders result in elevations of circulating $T_4$ levels without true thyrotoxicosis. These can be grouped into four large categories, including *abnormalities in the concentration or function of thyroid hormone–binding proteins, the effects of pharmacologic agents, syndromes of generalized or peripheral thyroid hormone resistance,* and *variants of NTI.* These conditions are summarized in Table 36-3. Among patients with disorders involving thyroid hormone–binding proteins, those with familial dysalbuminemic hyperthyroxinemia and serum thyroxine-binding prealbumin elevations have a falsely elevated serum $FT_4$ index resulting from normal binding of the radiolabeled $T_3$ that is used in most thyroid hormone–binding resin or $T_3$-resin uptake assays. In addition, patients with familial dysalbuminemic hyperthyroxinemia,[74a] as well as persons with $T_4$ autoantibodies, may have falsely elevated serum $FT_4$ values, when determined using some $FT_4$ methodologies. The elevation in serum $T_4$ levels that is seen after the use of oral contrast agents and amiodarone in healthy persons

**TABLE 36-3.**
**Causes of Euthyroid Hyperthyroxinemia**

**ALTERED SERUM OR PROTEIN BINDING**
 Congenital binding defects
 Familial dysalbuminemic hyperthyroxinemia
 Increased thyroxine-binding globulin
 Increased transthyretin (thyroxine-binding prealbumin, TBPA)
 Acquired binding defects (physiologic)
 Pregnancy
 Neonatal state
 Presence of $T_4$ autoantibodies
 Miscellaneous
**PHARMACOLOGIC AGENTS**
 Estrogen replacement therapy
 Oral contraceptives
 Heroin and methadone
 Clofibrate
 Amiodarone
 Ipodate and iopanoic acid
 Propranolol (high dose)
 5-Fluorouracil
**THYROID HORMONE RESISTANCE SYNDROMES**
 Generalized resistance
 Peripheral resistance
**VARIANTS OF NONTHYROIDAL ILLNESS**
 Infectious hepatitis
 Chronic active hepatitis
 Primary biliary cirrhosis
 Acute psychiatric disorders
 Acute intermittent porphyria
 Hyperemesis gravidarum

**TABLE 36-4.**
**Potential Effects of Various Drugs on Parameters of Thyroid Function**

| Drug | ↓TSH or Response to TRH | ↓Synthesis or Release of Thyroid Hormone | ↑TBG | ↓TBG | $T_4 \rightarrow T_3$ | Inhibit Protein Binding | ↓GI Absorption or ↑MCR Thyroid Hormone |
|---|---|---|---|---|---|---|---|
| Amiodarone*† | | √ | | | √ | | |
| Calcium carbonate | | | | | | | √ |
| Carbamazepine | √ | | | | | √ | √ |
| Cholestyramine | | | | | | | √ |
| Diazepam‡ | | | | | | √ | |
| Dopamine | √ | | | | | | |
| Ferrous sulfate | | | | | | | √ |
| Furosemide | | | | | | √ | |
| Glucocorticoids | √ | | | √ | √ | | |
| Heparin‡ | | | | | | √ | |
| Interferon-α§ | | √ | | | | | |
| Interleukin-2§ | | √ | | | | | |
| Iodine | | √ | | | | | |
| Ipodate/iopanoic acid | | √ | | | √ | | |
| L-Asparaginase | | | | √ | | | |
| Lithium | | √ | | | | | |
| Opiates | √ | | √ | | | | |
| Phenobarbital | | | | | | | √ |
| Phenytoin†¶ | √ | | | | | √ | √ |
| Propranolol | | | | | √ | | |
| Propylthiouracil | | √ | | | √ | | |
| Rifampin | | | | | | | √ |
| Salicylates/salsalate | √ | | | | | √ | |
| Sertraline | | | | | | | ?√ |
| Sulfonamides‡ | | √ | | | | √ | |
| Testosterone | | | | √ | | | |

*TSH*, thyroid-stimulating hormone; *TRH*, thyrotropin-releasing hormone; *TBG*, thyroxine-binding globulin; $T_4$, thyroxine; $T_3$, triiodothyronine; *GI*, gastrointestinal; *MCR*, metabolic clearance rate.
*May cause thyroiditis and hyperthyroxinemia.
†May exhibit antagonist or partial agonist binding properties with the $T_3$-receptor.
‡In vitro effects only.
§Effects primarily seen in patients predisposed to thyroid autoimmunity.
¶Also augments $T_4$ to $T_3$ conversion.

must be distinguished from the true hyperthyroidism that may occur through jodbasedow mechanisms in the subset of patients who are susceptible to this phenomenon (see Chap. 37).

Generalized resistance to thyroid hormone, a disorder caused by mutations in the c-*erb*A β gene for the $T_3$ receptor, is characterized by a heterogeneity in tissue responsiveness to the elevated levels of thyroid hormone; this may impede attempts to exclude thyroid dysfunction (see Chap. 32). Despite the variable tissue response to thyroid hormone in this disorder, most patients with generalized resistance to thyroid hormone are asymptomatic and have similarly affected family members, which facilitates the establishment of the correct diagnosis. Patients with pituitary-selective thyroid hormone resistance are truly hyperthyroid and, therefore, are not included in this section. (Common NTIs in which patients may present with elevated—rather than normal or depressed—thyroid hormone levels have been discussed previously.) The true metabolic state in hyperemesis gravidarum is somewhat controversial[75]; some argue for a human chorionic gonadotropin–mediated thyrotoxicosis in this common disorder.

## DRUGS AFFECTING PARAMETERS OF THYROID FUNCTION

Many medications may exert unwanted effects at one or more levels of thyroid hormone economy.[76] Of particular importance

are those agents that are commonly used in the diagnosis or treatment of critically ill patients, such as iodinated contrast agents, dopamine, corticosteroids, heparin, and furosemide. In addition, a number of common medications such as calcium carbonate,[77] ferrous sulfate,[78] aluminum hydroxide,[79] sucralfate,[80] and cholestyramine[81] may adversely affect gastrointestinal absorption of L-thyroxine. The effects of NTI on thyroid economy are compounded by the addition of these drugs and make the distinction from true thyroid dysfunction even more challenging to discern. Although certain of these changes are purely in vitro phenomena, such as the heparin-induced interference with thyroid hormone binding, other manifestations, such as the impairment of pituitary responsiveness that is caused by dopamine therapy, can lead to decreases in $FT_4$ to hypothyroid levels in the setting of critical illness. Table 36-4 provides a list of common medications known to affect thyroid economy, as well as the known or hypothesized mechanisms underlying these interactions.

## REFERENCES

1. Wartofsky L, Burman KD. Alterations in thyroid function in patients with systemic illness: the "euthyroid sick" syndrome. Endocr Rev 1982; 3:164.
2. Wartofsky L. The low $T_3$ of "euthyroid sick syndrome": update 1994. In: Braverman LE, Refetoff S, eds. Endocrine review monographs. 3. Clinical and molecular aspects of diseases of the thyroid. Bethesda, MD: Endocrine Society Monographs, 1994:248.

3. Hamblin PS, Dyer SA, Mohr VS, et al. Relationship between thyrotropin and thyroxine changes during recovery from severe hypothyroxinemia of critical illness. J Clin Endocrinol Metab 1986; 62:717.

4. Bermudez F, Surks MI, Oppenheimer JH. High incidence of decreased serum triiodothyronine concentration in patients with nonthyroidal disease. J Clin Endocrinol Metab 1975; 41:27.

5. Bayer MF, Macoviak JA, McDougall IR. Diagnostic performance of sensitive measurements of serum thyrotropin during severe nonthyroidal illness: their role in the diagnosis of hyperthyroidism. Clin Chem 1987; 33:2178.

6. Melmed S, Geola FL, Reed AW, et al. A comparison of methods for assessing thyroid function in nonthyroidal illness. J Clin Endocrinol Metab 1982; 54:300.

7. Surks MI, Hupart KH, Pan C, Shapiro LE. Normal free thyroxine in critical nonthyroidal illnesses measured by ultrafiltration of undiluted serum and equilibrium dialysis. J Clin Endocrinol Metab 1988; 67:1031.

8. Lum SMC, Kaptein EM, Nicoloff JT. Influence of nonthyroidal illness on serum thyroid hormone indices in hyperthyroidism. West J Med 1983; 138:670.

9. Burmeister LA. Reverse $T_3$ does not reliably differentiate hypothyroid sick syndrome from euthyroid sick syndrome. Thyroid 1995; 5:435.

10. Chopra IJ. Clinical review 86. Euthyroid sick syndrome: is it a misnomer? J Clin Endocrinol Metab 1997; 82:329.

11. Hurd RE, Chopra IJ. Reverse $T_3$. Endocrinologist 1993; 3:365.

12. Chopra IJ, Solomon DH, Hepner GW, Morgenstein AA. Misleadingly low free thyroxine index and usefulness of reverse triiodothyronine measurement in nonthyroidal illness. Ann Intern Med 1979; 90:905.

13. Wehmann RE, Gregerman RI, Burns WH, et al. Suppression of thyrotropin in the low-thyroxine state of severe nonthyroidal illness. N Engl J Med 1985; 312:546.

14. Hay ID, Bayer MF, Kaplan MM, et al. American Thyroid Association assessment of current free thyroid hormone measurements and guidelines for future clinical assays. Clin Chem 1991; 37:2002.

15. Kaptein EM. Clinical application of free thyroxine determinations. Clin Lab Med 1993; 13:653.

16. Faber J, Kirkegaard C, Rasmussen B, et al. Pituitary-thyroid axis in critical illness. J Clin Endocrinol Metab 1987; 65:315.

17. Nelson JC, Tomei RT. Direct determination of free thyroxine in undiluted serum by equilibrium dialysis/radioimmunoassay. Clin Chem 1988; 34:1737.

18. Chopra IJ. Simultaneous measurement of free thyroxine and free 3,5,3′-triiodothyronine in undiluted serum by direct equilibrium dialysis/radioimmunoassay: evidence that free triiodothyronine and free thyroxine are normal in many patients with the low triiodothyronine syndrome. Thyroid 1998; 8:249.

19. Spencer CA, Lum SMC, Wilber JF, et al. Dynamics of serum thyrotropin and thyroid hormone changes in fasting. J Clin Endocrinol Metab 1983; 56:883.

20. Romijn JA, Wiersinga WM. Decreased nocturnal surge of thyrotropin in nonthyroidal illness. J Clin Endocrinol Metab 1990; 70:35.

21. Spencer CA, Schwarzbein D, Guttler RB, et al. Thyrotropin-releasing hormone stimulation test responses employing third and fourth generation TSH assays. J Clin Endocrinol Metab 1993; 76:494.

22. Maturlo SJ, Rosenbaum RL, Surks MI. Variable thyrotropin response to thyrotropin-releasing hormone after small decreases in plasma free thyroid hormone concentrations in patients with nonthyroidal illness. J Clin Invest 1980; 66:451.

23. Sumita S, Ujike Y, Namiki A, et al. Suppression of the thyrotropin response to thyrotropin-releasing hormone and its association with severity of critical illness. Crit Care Med 1994; 22:1603.

24. Borst GC, Osborne RC, O'Brian JT, et al. Fasting decreases thyrotropin responsiveness to thyrotropin-releasing hormone: a potential cause of misinterpretation of thyroid function tests in the critically ill. J Clin Endocrinol Metab 1983; 57:380.

25. Adriaanse R, Romijn JA, Brabant G, et al. Pulsatile thyrotropin secretion in nonthyroidal illness. J Clin Endocrinol Metab 1993; 77:1313.

26. Spencer C, Eigen A, Shen D, et al. Specificity of sensitive assays of thyrotropin used to screen for thyroid disease in hospitalized patients. Clin Chem 1987; 33:1391.

27. Spencer CA, LoPresti JS, Patel A, et al. Applications of a new chemiluminometric thyrotropin assay to subnormal measurement. J Clin Endocrinol Metab 1990; 70:453.

28. Franklyn JA, Black EG, Betteridge J, Sheppard MC. Comparison of second and third generation methods for measurement of serum thyrotropin in patients with overt hyperthyroidism, patients receiving thyroxine therapy, and those with nonthyroidal illness. J Clin Endocrinol Metab 1994; 78:1368.

29. LoPresti JS, Gray D, Nicoloff JT. Influence of fasting and refeeding on 3,3′,5′-triiodothyronine metabolism in man. J Clin Endocrinol Metab 1991; 72:130.

30. Burman KD, Dimond RC, Harvey GS, et al. Glucose modulation of alterations in serum iodothyronines induced by fasting. Metabolism 1979; 28:291.

31. Burman KD, Wartofsky L, Dinterman RE, et al. The effect of $T_3$ and reverse $T_3$ on muscle protein catabolism during fasting as measured by 3-methylhistidine excretion. Metabolism 1979; 28:805.

32. Kaptein EM. Thyroid hormone metabolism and thyroid diseases in chronic renal failure. Endocr Rev 1996; 17:45.

32a. Acker CG, Singh AR, Flick RP, et al. A trial of thyroxine in acute renal failure. Kidney Int 2000; 57:293.

33. John R, Evans PE, Scanlon MF, Hall R. Clinical value of immunoradiometric assay of thyrotropin for patients with nonthyroidal illness and taking various drugs. Clin Chem 1987; 33:566.

34. Schussler GC, Schaffner F, Korn F. Increased serum thyroid hormone binding and decreased free hormone in chronic active liver disease. N Engl J Med 1978; 299:510.

35. LoPresti JS, Fried JC, Spencer CA, Nicoloff JT. Unique alterations of thyroid hormone indices in the acquired immunodeficiency syndrome. Ann Intern Med 1989; 110:970.

36. Sellmeyer DE, Grunfeld C. Endocrine and metabolic disturbances in human immunodeficiency virus infection and the acquired immune deficiency syndrome. Endocr Rev 1996; 17:518.

37. Hommes MJT, Romijn JA, Endert E, et al. Hypothyroid-like regulation of the pituitary-thyroid axis in stable human immunodeficiency virus infection. Metabolism 1993; 42:556.

38. Lambert M, Zech F, De Nayer P, et al. Elevation of serum thyroxine-binding globulin (but not of cortisol-binding globulin and sex hormone–binding globulin) associated with the progression of human immunodeficiency virus infection. Am J Med 1990; 89:748.

39. Spratt DI, Pont A, Miller MB, et al. Hyperthyroxinemia in patients with acute psychiatric disorders. Am J Med 1982; 73:41.

40. Nader S, Warner MD, Doyle S, Peabody CA. Euthyroid sick syndrome in psychiatric inpatients. Biol Psychiatry 1996; 40:1288.

41. Chopra IJ, Solomon DH, Huang T-S. Serum thyrotropin in hospitalized patients: evidence for hyperthyroxinemia as measured by an ultrasensitive thyrotropin assay. Metabolism 1990; 39:538.

42. Maes M, Schotte C, Vandewoude M, et al. TSH responses to TRH as a function of basal serum TSH: relevance for unipolar depression in females—a multivariate study. Pharmacopsychiatry 1992; 25:136.

43. Fliers E, Guldenaar SE, Wiersinga WM, Swaab DF. Decreased hypothalamic thyrotropin-releasing hormone gene expression in patients with nonthyroidal illness. J Clin Endocrinol Metab 1997; 82:4032.

44. Arem R, Wiener GJ, Kaplan SG, et al. Reduced tissue thyroid hormone levels in fatal illness. Metabolism 1993; 42:1102.

45. Hupart KH, De Fesi CR, Katz C?, et al. Decreased anterior pituitary $T_3$ nuclear receptors in a Walker 256 carcinoma–bearing rat model of nonthyroidal disease. Acta Endocrinol (Copenh) 1989; 121:811.

46. Boado R, Chopra IJ, Huang T-S, et al. A study of pituitary thyrotropin, its subunits, and messenger ribonucleic acids in nonthyroidal illness. Metabolism 1988; 37:395.

47. Lee H-Y, Suhl J, Pekary AE, Hershman JM. Secretion of thyrotropin with reduced concanavalin-A–binding activity in patients with nonthyroidal illness. J Clin Endocrinol Metab 1987; 65:942.

48. Magner J, Roy P, Fainter L, et al. Transiently decreased sialylation of thyrotropin (TSH) in a patient with the euthyroid sick syndrome. Thyroid 1997; 7:55.

49. Pandian MR, Morgan C, Nelson JC, Fisher DA. Differentiating various abnormalities of thyroxine binding to serum proteins by radioelectrophoresis of thyroxine and immunoassay of binding proteins. Clin Chem 1990; 36:457.

50. Mendel CM, Laughton CW, McMahon FA, Cavalerri RR. Inability to detect an inhibitor of thyroxine-serum protein binding in sera from patients with nonthyroid illness. Metabolism 1991; 40:491.

51. Reilly CP, Wellby ML. Slow thyroxine binding globulin in the pathogenesis of increased dialysable fraction of thyroxine in nonthyroidal illness. J Clin Endocrinol Metab 1983; 57:15.

52. Lim CF, Docter R, Visser TJ, et al. Inhibition of thyroxine transport into cultured rat hepatocytes by serum of nonuremic critically ill patients: effects of bilirubin and nonesterified fatty acids. J Clin Endocrinol Metab 1993; 76:1165.

53. Mandel SJ, Berry MJ, Kieffer JD, et al. Cloning and in vitro expression of the human selenoprotein type I iodothyronine deiodinase. J Clin Endocrinol Metab 1992; 75:1133.

54. Boelen A, Platvoetter Schiphorst MC, Wiersinga WM. Immunoneutralization of interleukin-1, tumor necrosis factor, interleukin-6 or interferon does not prevent the LPS-induced sick euthyroid syndrome in mice. J Endocrinol 1997; 153:115.

55. Sarne DH, Refetoff S. Measurement of thyroxine uptake from serum by cultured human hepatocytes as an index of thyroid status: reduced thyroxine uptake from serum of patients with nonthyroidal illness. J Clin Endocrinol Metab 1985; 61:1046.

56. Williams GR, Neubauer JM, Franklin JA, Sheppard MC. Thyroid hormone receptor expression in the "sick euthyroid" syndrome. Lancet 1989; 2:1477.

57. Seppel T, Becker A, Lippert F, Schlaghecke R. Serum sex hormone–binding globulin and osteocalcin in systemic nonthyroidal illness associated with low thyroid hormone concentrations. J Clin Endocrinol Metab 1996; 81:1663.

58. Bartalena L, Bogazzi F, Brogioni S, et al. Role of cytokines in the pathogenesis of the euthyroid sick syndrome. Eur J Endocrinol 1998; 138:603.

59. Kakucska I, Romero LI, Clark BD, et al. Suppression of thyrotropin-releasing hormone gene expression by interleukin-1-beta in the rat: implications for nonthyroidal illness. Neuroendocrinology 1994; 59:129.

60. Poth M, Tseng YC, Wartofsky L. Inhibition of TSH activation of human thyroid cells by tumor necrosis factor: an explanation for decreased thyroid function in systemic illness? Thyroid 1991; 1:235.

61. Davies PH, Sheppard MC, Franklyn JA. Inflammatory cytokines and type I 5′-deiodinase expression in phi1 rat liver cells. Mol Cell Endocrinol 1997; 129:191.

62. Jones TH, Wadler S, Hupart KH. Endocrine-mediated mechanisms of fatigue during treatment with interferon-alpha. Semin Oncol 1998; 25(Suppl 1):54.
63. Boelen A, Platvoet-Ter Schiphorst MC, Wiersinga WM. Soluble cytokine receptors and the low 3,5,3'-triiodothyronine syndrome in patients with nonthyroidal disease. J Clin Endocrinol Metab 1995; 80:971.
64. Bartalena L, Brogioni S, Grasso L, et al. Relationship between the increased serum interleukin-6 concentration to changes in thyroid function in nonthyroidal illness. J Endocrinol Invest 1994; 17:269.
65. Boelen A, Maas MA, Lowik CW, et al. Induced illness in interleukin-6 (IL-6) knock-out mice: a causal role of IL-6 in the development of the low 3,5,3'-triiodothyronine syndrome. Endocrinology 1996; 137:5250.
66. Boelen A, Platvoet-Ter Schiphorst MC, van Rooijen N, Wiersinga WM. Selective macrophage depletion in the liver does not prevent the development of the sick euthyroid syndrome in the mouse. Eur J Endocrinol 1996; 134:513.
67. Stouthard JM, van der Poll T, Endert E, et al. Effects of acute and chronic interleukin-6 administration on thyroid hormone metabolism in humans. J Clin Endocrinol Metab 1994; 79:1342.
68. Midgley JEM, Sheehan CP, Christofides ND, et al. Concentrations of free thyroxine and albumin in serum in severe nonthyroidal illness: assay artifacts and physiologic influences. Clin Chem 1990; 36:765.
69. Van den Berghe G, de Zegher F, Lauwers P. Dopamine and the sick euthyroid syndrome in critical illness. Clin Endocrinol (Oxf) 1994; 41:731.
70. Archambeaud-Mouveroux F, Dejax C, DeBuhan B, Bonnaud F. Hyperthyroidism without elevated levels of thyroxine and triiodothyronine in a patient with pulmonary TB. South Med J 1989; 82:907.
71. Girvent M, Maestro S, Hernandez R, et al. Euthyroid sick syndrome, associated endocrine abnormalities, and outcome in elderly patients undergoing emergency operation. Surgery 1998; 123:560.
72. Brennan MD, Bahn RS. Thyroid hormone and illness. Endocr Pract 1998; 4:396.
73. Bennett-Guerrero E, Jimenez JL, White WD, et al. Cardiovascular effects of intravenous triiodothyronine in patients undergoing coronary artery bypass graft surgery. A randomized, double-blind, placebo-controlled trial. Duke T$_3$ study group. JAMA 1996; 275:687.
74. Klemperer JD, Klein I, Gomez M, et al. Thyroid hormone treatment after coronary-artery bypass surgery. N Engl J Med 1995; 333:1522.
74a. Tang KT, Yang HJ, Choo KB, et al. A point mutation in the albumin gene in a Chinese patient with familial dysalbuminemic hyperthyroxinemia. Eur J Endocrinol 1999; 141:374.
75. Burrow GN. Thyroid function and hyperfunction during gestation. Endocr Rev 1993; 14:194.
76. Surks MI, Sievert R. Drugs and thyroid function. N Engl J Med 1995; 333:1688.
77. Schneyer CR. Calcium carbonate and reduction of levothyroxine efficacy. (Letter). JAMA 1998; 279:750.
78. Campbell NRC, Hasinoff BB, Stalts H, et al. Ferrous sulfate reduces thyroxine efficacy in patients with hypothyroidism. Ann Intern Med 1992; 117:1010.
79. Liel Y, Sperber AD, Shany S. Nonspecific intestinal adsorption of levothyroxine by aluminum hydroxide. Am J Med 1994; 97:363.
80. Sherman SI, Tielens ET, Ladenson PW. Sucralfate causes malabsorption of L-thyroxine. Am J Med 1994; 96:531.
81. Solomon BL, Wartofsky L, Burman KD. Adjunctive cholestyramine therapy for thyrotoxicosis. Clin Endocrinol (Oxf) 1993; 38:39.

# CHAPTER 37

# ADVERSE EFFECTS OF IODIDE

JENNIFER A. NUOVO AND LEONARD WARTOFSKY

## POPULATION EXPOSURE TO IODIDE

Iodine is a requisite part of the thyroid hormone molecule, and a deficiency or excess of iodine can dramatically affect thyroid gland function. In 1820, iodide therapy was being used in Europe for the treatment of goiter; shortly thereafter, cases of probable thyrotoxicosis were reported in a few patients receiving this treatment. Although iodide supplementation has been adopted worldwide in the past 50 years, concern remains over the danger this poses to certain susceptible individuals.[1,2]

*Iodine deficiency* and goiter remain major health problems in many parts of the world. During the two decades from 1965 to 1985 in the United States, however, iodine supplementation resulted in an increased prevalence of disordered thyroid regulation resulting from *iodine excess.*[1-3] Although the normal thyroid gland usually adapts readily to extremes of iodine intake, some persons are vulnerable to the induction of goiter, hypothyroidism, or hyperthyroidism with exposure to excess iodine. This risk may be diminishing, for it appears that iodine intake in North America is on the decline, conceivably secondary to a reduction in its use as a preservative and disinfectant in the food and dairy industry.[4]

The physiology of iodine metabolism is discussed in Chapter 30 and has been reviewed.[5] Normal thyroid economy can be maintained with an iodine intake of only 50 to 70 µg per day because some iodine is available internally from the leak of nonhormonal iodine from the thyroid and from the peripheral deiodination of thyroxine (T$_4$) and triiodothyronine (T$_3$). Urinary iodide excretion fairly accurately reflects dietary (and nondietary) intake. Urinary iodide excretion may vary from 45 to 700 µg per 24 hours in areas of iodide sufficiency but be as low as 3 µg per 24 hours in regions of endemic goiter.[6] In addition to dietary sources, large amounts of iodine are available in drugs, intravenous and oral radiologic contrast agents, and supplements from "health"-food stores. With increasing frequency, such exposures to iodine excess are being recognized as having adverse effects on thyroid function. Speculation also exists that the chronically high levels of iodine intake observed in Western countries may contribute to the increasing prevalence of autoimmune thyroid disease.

## ADVERSE EFFECTS OF IODIDE

### EXTRATHYROIDAL EFFECTS

The adverse effects of iodides may be classified as *extrathyroidal* or *intrathyroidal.* Extrathyroidal effects are uncommon; the most frequently encountered is sialoadenitis, which occurs after the administration of large doses of iodide. (Therapeutic doses of radioactive iodine also may cause sialoadenitis; however, this depends on the radiation dose rather than on the extremely small amount of stable iodine administered.) The acute, painful swelling of the parotid and other salivary glands resolves shortly after iodide therapy is discontinued. Severe skin eruptions have been reported after topical and enteral iodine exposure. In addition, "iodism" may occur, which is marked by symptoms of metallic taste, acneiform skin lesions, mucous membrane irritation, nausea, and salivary gland swelling. These symptoms subside on withdrawal of iodide. Various allergic reactions, including a syndrome similar to polyarteritis nodosa, eosinophilia, and fever, also have been reported. Drug sensitivity rashes, including dermatitis herpetiformis and hypocomplementemic vasculitis, can occur after iodide exposure but are rare.[7]

### INTRATHYROIDAL EFFECTS

Iodide exposure causes three primary types of intrathyroidal effects. The first is *iodide-induced thyroiditis,* which sometimes causes painful inflammation of the thyroid that occurs after the receipt of large doses of iodide and usually resolves rapidly and spontaneously within a few days after the exposure[8]; however, experimental evidence exists for an iodide-induced autoimmune thyroiditis as well.[9,10] The second intrathyroidal iodide effect is *iodide goiter with hypothyroidism* or, more commonly, *goiter alone* without hypothyroidism. This usually occurs after prolonged exposure to dietary or drug-containing iodides.[11,12] Ultrasonographic techniques, however, have detected significant increases in thyroid size after only 4 weeks of excess iodine supplementation.[13] The third effect of iodide on the thyroid is *iodide-induced thyrotoxicosis,* which is seen after excess iodine exposure in four patient groups: patients from areas of endemic (iodide-deficiency)

**TABLE 37-1.**
Iodine Content of Iodinated Radiologic Dyes and Some Iodine-Containing Drugs

| Substance | Iodine Content | Usual Dose | Total Dose of Iodine (mg) |
|---|---|---|---|
| **RADIOLOGIC CONTRAST DYES** | | | |
| *Cholecystographic dyes* | | | |
| Iopanoate, ipodate, tyropanoate, iodoxamate | 55–70% | 3–9 g | 1650–6300 |
| Diatrizoate, iodamide, iothalamate | 45–60% | 1–70 g | 450–4200 |
| *Lymphangiographic dye* | | | |
| Lipiodol (iodized poppyseed oil) | 45–60% | 1–70 g | 450–4200 |
| *Myelographic dye* | | | |
| Metrizamide | 48% | 5–15 mL | 1100–3000 |
| **IODINE-CONTAINING DRUGS** | | | |
| *Oral agents* | | | |
| Amiodarone | 75 mg/200 mg tablet | 300–1200 mg/d (initial) | 75–300/d |
| Benziodarone | 49 mg/100 mg tablet | 100–200 mg/d | 49–98/d |
| Iodine-containing cough medications | 15–325 mg/teaspoon | 1–2 teaspoon/q4h | 90–3900/d |
| Potassium iodide | | | |
| Calcium iodide | | | |
| Iodinate glycerol | | | |
| Iodochlorhydroxyquin (antiamebic) | 104 mg/tablet | 600–650 mg tid × 20 d | 312/d |
| Iodine-containing vitamins (prenatal vitamins) | 0.15 mg/tablet | 1/d | 0.15/d |
| Quadrinal (KI) | 320 mg/tablet 160 mg/5 mL | 1 tablet qid or 10 mL q4h | 1280–1920/d |
| Kelp tablets | 0.15 mg/tablet | 1 or more/d | ≥0.15/d |
| Antithyroidal preparations | | | |
| Lugol solution | 8.4 mg/drop* | 15 drops qid | 378/d* |
| SSKI | 38 mg/drop* | 5 drops qid | 760/d* |
| *Topical iodine preparations* | | | |
| Iodohydroxyquinolone | 12 mg/g | 4 g/d | 4800/d |
| Povidone-iodine (Betadine) | 10 mg/mL | Variable | |
| Ophthalmic solution | | | |
| Echothiophate iodide | 5–40 µg/drop* | 2 drops qid | 0.40–0.320/d* |
| Idoxuridine solution | 18 µg/drop* | 2 drops qid | 0.144/d* |

*Varies according to drop size.

goiter; patients not from endemic areas with known goiters; euthyroid patients with autonomous hyperfunctioning nodules or histories of prior hyperthyroidism or Graves disease; and, rarely, patients with no underlying thyroid disorders.[14,15]

## IODIDE SOURCES

### AVERAGE IODIDE INTAKE

The normal thyroid adapts easily to iodide excess or deficiency. Hyperthyroidism or hypothyroidism resulting from abnormal amounts of dietary iodine is unusual. In the United States, dietary iodide intake is estimated to average 350 to 650 µg per day, although it may exceed 1 mg per day in some areas. Some of the major sources are iodinated feed used in the dairy industry (secreted as iodine in cow's milk), iodates used as dough conditioners in bread baking, iodide in drinking water, and iodide supplements in salt.[15a] An average of 10 g of iodine-supplemented table salt per day in the American diet provides 76 µg of iodine.[16] In some parts of Africa, South America, Europe, the Middle East, and Asia, where iodide-deficiency goiter is prevalent, iodine intake may still average <50 µg per day. By contrast, in Japan and other Asian nations, a diet rich in fish and often supplemented with iodide-rich seaweed (kelp) results in an intake of several milligrams per day.[11] Elemental iodine or inorganic iodide salts, once ingested, are reduced to iodide, thereafter becoming available for uptake by the thyroid.

Iodine is a substantial component of many commonly available oral and topical medications, as well as oral and intravenous contrast agents. Table 37-1 lists commonly used iodide-containing compounds, and the iodine dose expected with routine use.

### RADIOGRAPHIC CONTRAST AGENTS

Between 180,000 and 320,000 µg of iodine is derived from the radiographic contrast agent given for routine oral cholecystography, and intravenous pyelography presents a dose of >10^6 µg of iodine. Although most of the iodine in radiologic contrast media is in the form of organic iodine, large amounts of free iodide also are present. These organic iodine compounds may be taken up by peripheral tissues, particularly the liver, where deiodination generates free iodide that can be trapped by the thyroid. Much of the iodine becomes protein bound and circulates in serum, remaining available to the thyroid for prolonged periods after a single exposure. Blood iodide content may increase to 200 times baseline levels after oral cholecystography or intravenous pyelography and remains elevated for days to weeks.[14,17]

Although the thyroidal uptake of even a small amount of the circulating iodide load after a dye study may be significant, normal thyroidal autoregulation results in a reduced fractional uptake and iodide clearance; this serves to regulate thyroid function and maintain homeostasis. In this context, therefore, it is not surprising that, despite the 4 million intravenous pyelography procedures and 4 million oral cholecystography procedures that are done yearly in the United States, clinically significant iodine-induced alteration in thyroid function is uncommon. Some radiologic contrast agents (those containing ipodate) have additional specific actions, such as inhibiting peripheral conversion of $T_4$ to $T_3$.

## IODIDE-CONTAINING DRUGS

Common iodide-containing drugs are listed in Table 37-1. Until recently, reports of iodine-induced goiter and hyperthyroidism were related exclusively to iodide-containing cough syrups and expectorants. Potassium iodide, calcium iodide, and iodinated glycerol usually are combined with antihistamines, decongestants, or bronchodilators as mucolytic agents in cough preparations and asthma medications. These antitussives contain 15 to 325 mg of iodine per teaspoon and are taken in doses of 1 to 2 teaspoons every 4 hours, imposing a typical exogenous iodine dose of 90 to 3900 mg per day.

Iodochlorhydroxyquin is compounded in creams as a topical antifungal and bacteriostatic agent. Povidone-iodine solution (Betadine) is widely used as a topical antiseptic. When this agent has been applied directly to open wounds or burns, or has been used as a vaginal douche, high blood iodide levels have been reported that occasionally cause iodide toxicity.[14,18–20] The antiamebic drugs with the active compound iodoquinol contain 64% organic iodine and, in typical dosages, provide 19.5 g of iodine daily, usually for a 20-day course.

Amiodarone is an antiarrhythmic agent, which is widely used in both Europe and the United States. The drug contains 37.2% iodine and is prescribed initially in dosages of 300 to 1200 mg per day, providing 100 to 400 mg of iodine and an estimated 900 μg of free iodine.[14] Amiodarone can have both acute and chronic effects on thyroid function, as well as the unique effect of inhibiting peripheral conversion of $T_4$ to $T_3$; the drug has been implicated in both hypothyroidism and hyperthyroidism.[21,22] Increased serum reverse $T_3$ levels and decreased $T_3$ levels may be seen, as well as increased or decreased thyroid gland $T_4$ production and release.[23] Amiodarone causes problems of clinical significance more commonly than do the other drugs mentioned. Reports from France describe a particularly high incidence of abnormalities, perhaps because of widespread use, and also perhaps because the dietary iodine intake is borderline low, resulting in a high incidence of endemic goiter and a susceptibility to thyroid abnormalities after iodine exposure.[14,24] The use of benziodarone, a uricosuric available in Europe, has prompted similar reports of iodine-related thyroid abnormalities.

## MECHANISM OF ACTION OF EXCESS IODIDE

When a small amount of iodide (100–250 μg per day) is administered along with the usual dietary intake, there is *no* appreciable change in iodine-131 ($^{131}I$) uptake, and no change in thyroidal organic iodine or in the amount of iodotyrosines and iodothyronines produced.[25] After larger, single iodide doses (several milligrams), the formation of organic iodine within the thyroid decreases and the monoiodotyrosine/diiodotyrosine ratio increases, resulting in decreased $T_4$ and $T_3$ formation.[16,26] This inhibitory effect of iodide on *organification and thyroid hormone formation* is known as the *Wolff-Chaikoff effect.* A high concentration of inorganic iodide within the thyroid is necessary for this effect to occur. This inhibition serves as temporary protection against the production of excess amounts of thyroid hormone in the period after the excess ingestion. The inhibitory effect is temporary because the intrathyroidal iodine concentration ultimately decreases as a result of reduced iodide transport; the result is resumption of organic iodine formation and "escape" from the Wolff-Chaikoff effect. Larger doses, including those in normal daily intake of iodide,[27] have an additional independent effect on the thyroid gland to block the *release* of thyroid hormone. Intrathy-

roidal excess iodide appears to inhibit proteolysis of thyroglobulin, thereby inhibiting the release of stored $T_4$ and $T_3$ into the circulation. Although this effect may be seen in healthy persons, the diminished hormonal release does not result in hypothyroidism because a decreasing peripheral $T_4$ level stimulates a rise in serum thyroid-stimulating hormone (TSH) and augmented $T_4$ production from the thyroid. Large doses of stable iodine induce an acute reduction in $T_4$ release from the thyroid gland and are used as effective short-term therapy for Graves hyperthyroidism (see Chap. 42). This acute inhibitory effect of iodide is of therapeutic value when a rapid reduction in thyroid hormone secretion is desirable, as in severe hyperthyroid states, in preparation for surgery, or in the treatment of thyroid storm. Five drops of SSKI (190 mg of iodine) or 15 drops of Lugol solution (135 mg of iodine), given two to three times a day, quickly and dramatically decreases thyroid hormone release.[28] Although these dosages also block organification, the major effect is on hormone secretion. The use of iodides as the only antithyroidal drug in hyperthyroidism is not recommended, because they are only partially and transiently effective in reducing serum hormone levels. A period of 10 to 14 days is required before the thyroid gland adapts, and the production and release of $T_4$ resume.

## RESULTS OF CHRONIC IODIDE EXCESS IN HEALTHY PERSONS

The long-term administration of iodides results in *escape from* or *adaptation to* the iodide concentration. Organic binding is no longer inhibited, and iodothyronine formation proceeds at the expected accelerated rate because of the excess iodine present. Despite excess organic iodine, the serum $T_4$ level usually does not increase measurably in healthy persons, although such an effect has been described.[15] In the normal gland, an inhibition of $T_4$ and $T_3$ release by acute, large doses of iodide is more likely to be seen, although it will be overcome by an increase in TSH. Thus, as peripheral iodothyronine levels decrease, hormone release normalizes. Probably because the gland remains responsive to TSH, hypothyroidism is prevented in most populations with high iodine ingestion.[14,15]

## PREEXISTING FACTORS

Patients may be exposed to excess iodine in health foods, seaweed, expectorants, amiodarone, and iodine-containing intravenous and oral contrast dyes. Although the incidence of goiter, hyperthyroidism, and hypothyroidism caused by this exposure is small, it should be considered carefully whenever goiter or altered thyroid function is seen in patients given iodide diagnostically or therapeutically. Although iodine-induced thyroid disease probably occurs in the setting of a preexisting thyroid abnormality that prevents the normal adaptation to excess iodine, iodide-induced thyroid abnormalities have been noted in seemingly healthy persons.

## IODINE-INDUCED GOITER AND HYPOTHYROIDISM

Iodine-induced goiter was first reported in 1938; since then, >200 cases have been described. Of 154 cases reviewed, euthyroid goiter accounted for 39%, hypothyroidism without goiter for 17%, and hypothyroidism with goiter for the remaining cases.[11] Such goiters, often associated with hypothyroidism, have been reported sporadically in the United States for many years and more commonly in Europe. In the past, the problem was seen most often after the use of iodide-containing expectorants. Amiodarone use has been associated with hypothyroidism and, in several cases, goiter has developed with benziodarone use. The high incidence of antithyroidal antibodies in patients with goiter development suggests that these

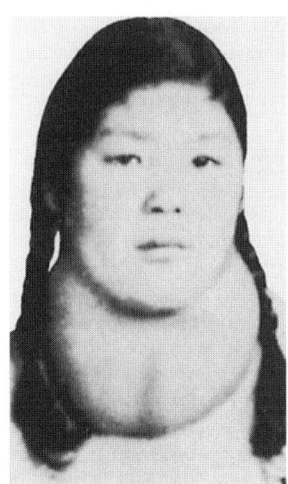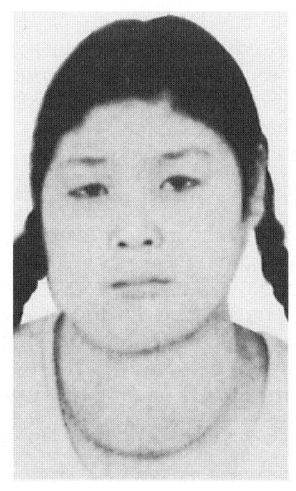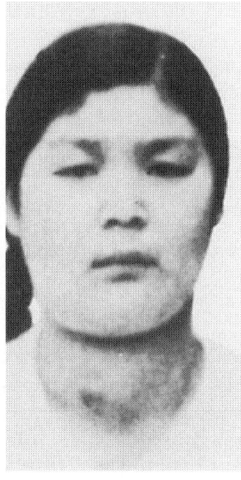

**A–C**

**FIGURE 37-1.** A 14-year-old patient from Hokkaido, Japan, with usual daily diet of 50 to 80 mg of iodine derived from seaweed (kelp). **A,** Appearance at time of first presentation with "coast goiter." **B,** Appearance 3 weeks after removal of seaweed from the diet. **C,** Appearance after 2 months of treatment with thyroid hormone. The goiter has regressed further. (From Suzuki H, Higuchi T, Sawa K, et al. Endemic coast goiter in Hokkaido, Japan. Acta Endocrinol [Copenh] 1965; 50:161.)

patients have underlying Hashimoto thyroiditis with abnormal hormone synthesis and a unique sensitivity to the effects of iodine.[29] It may be that iodide-induced goiter or hypothyroidism occurs only in the presence of thyroid dysfunction. The true incidence of goiter in patients exposed to iodides is unknown. The incidence is higher in women than in men, and most patients have received large amounts of iodide (several milligrams to >1 g) daily for long periods.[3] Goiter also has been seen after therapy with small amounts of iodide, however.[12] The interval from the institution of therapy with iodine-containing compounds to the appearance of goiter or hypothyroidism varies widely, from a few months to several years.

## EFFECTS DURING PREGNANCY

Iodides cross the placenta easily; therefore, one should expect that goiter may be seen in neonates whose mothers received iodide-containing drugs during pregnancy. *Congenital goiter* and *neonatal hypothyroidism* resulting from long-term maternal iodide use are rare and have similar manifestations as in adults, but the consequences for infants are severe and include asphyxiation from tracheal compression and potential mental retardation if the condition is not treated. Death from asphyxiation was reported in 8 of 22 infants born with goiter.[11] Surgical intervention may be warranted in selected cases, although the goiters resolve over a few months in asymptomatic infants. Generally, the mothers have had no manifestations of goiter or hypothyroidism.

## NEONATAL PERIOD

The frequency or magnitude of the problem of neonatal iodide-induced goiter or hypothyroidism is unknown. Iodides are secreted into breast milk, and hypothyroidism or goiter may be seen in breast-fed infants of mothers chronically exposed to high doses of iodides.[11,30] Prenatal vitamins usually contain 150 µg of iodine, which should not constitute a hazard but does pose an additional risk in pregnant women who already are ingesting iodides from other sources. In an intensive care unit setting, within 1 month after the extensive topical use of 1% iodine and 3.9% iodine solutions (Polyvidone) for 4 to 8 days, goiter and hypothyroidism developed in 5 of 30 neonates.[31] The affected infants had significantly increased ioduria, whereas the other infants did not, which suggests a difference in skin permeability. In all cases, the goiter resolved after brief therapy with thyroid hormone, and neither hypothyroidism nor goiter recurred subsequently. These observations suggest inadequate or undeveloped ability of the neonatal thyroid gland to "autoregulate" or control iodide

uptake and binding, resulting in saturation and suppression of hormone synthesis and secretion.

## "COAST GOITER"

"Coast goiter," the endemic iodide goiter seen in the northern Japanese island of Hokkaido, is the most common form of iodide goiter.[12,32] It occurs in 6% to 12% of that population, most commonly among the seaweed harvesters and their families, who may consume 50 to 200 mg of iodide daily. In a survey of schoolchildren, 508 goiters were found, 330 in girls and 178 in boys. Nearly all the glands (97.4%) were diffusely enlarged, and a histologic diagnosis of colloid goiter was rendered in the seven glands that underwent biopsy. Despite having extremely large goiters, these patients all were euthyroid. When seaweed was withdrawn from the diet, the elevated plasma and urinary iodide levels returned toward normal, resulting in a rebound increase of [131]I uptake 1 to 2 weeks later.[32] In the few patients studied, the goiters disappeared or significantly decreased in size after seaweed withdrawal (Fig. 37-1). In 75% of 50 patients treated with thyroid hormone who maintained their usual dietary habits, the goiters decreased in size or resolved.[33] The mechanism underlying the absence of hypothyroidism in these patients is not well understood, but they appear to reach a new steady state, manifested by a normal serum $T_4$ level and goiter, presumably maintained by TSH. The erratic availability of seaweed also may be important because seaweed is a significant part of the diet only during good harvesting weather.[12] A similar incidence of hyperthyroidism in five coastal regions of Japan has been reported, along with a widely varying incidence of hypothyroidism (0–9.7%). High urinary iodine concentration correlated with antibody-negative hypothyroidism.[34]

## PREDISPOSITION TO INDUCED HYPOTHYROIDISM

Congenital and acquired defects in intrathyroidal organification increase the risk of induced hypothyroidism with iodine exposure. Patients with simple goiter resulting from organification defects appear to be highly susceptible to iodide-induced hypothyroidism. A prospective study of biochemically euthyroid patients with Hashimoto thyroiditis who were treated with iodides revealed a high incidence of iodide-related hypothyroidism that was reversible on cessation of iodides.[29] These thyroid glands probably fail to escape from the acute inhibitory effect of iodide on the organification process and manifest a persistence of the Wolff-Chaikoff effect. The increasing incidence of Hashimoto thyroiditis with hypothyroidism or goiter in the United States may be the result of an unmasking of the organification defect with a chronically high dietary iodine intake.

Hypothyroidism also has been seen in euthyroid patients given iodides who previously underwent [131]I or surgical therapy for Graves disease.[11,35] With withdrawal of iodides, the euthyroid state was restored, and TSH levels normalized. The speculation is that this phenomenon is the result of an organification defect caused by the radiation therapy. Although hypothyroidism after iodide exposure was seen in all patients treated with [131]I, it also was seen in 40% of surgically treated patients.[35] Thus, an underlying defect related to Graves disease that can be compounded by a radiation-induced sensitivity of the thyroid gland to an iodide load appears to exist.

## CLINICAL FEATURES OF IODIDE-INDUCED HYPOTHYROIDISM

The clinical presentation of iodide-induced hypothyroidism is variable. Goiter alone is much more common than is hypothyroidism, and the thyroid gland may be modestly or significantly enlarged. Generally, the goiter is diffuse, but in the context of antithyroidal antibodies, a nodular gland may be present. A history of previous Hashimoto disease, Graves disease, or goiter should raise the suspicion of an iodide-induced abnormality of thyroid function. The symptoms and signs of hypothyroidism may be subtle or absent.[10,34,36] In the presence of normal to marginal values for serum $T_4$ and basal TSH, the serum TSH response to thyrotropin-releasing hormone affords the most sensitive indicator of hypothyroidism. Iodine-131 uptake may not be a helpful measure, depending on the amount of exogenous iodide ingested and the functional capabilities of the thyroid gland. In a setting of high iodide intake, a low uptake of radioiodine is expected. Low, normal, and elevated uptakes have all been seen, however, with iodide-induced goiter. An early peak in [131]I uptake has been described, with the 4-hour or 6-hour uptake higher than the 24-hour uptake, a typical finding in patients with organification defects.

The best evidence that goiter or hypothyroidism is related to excess iodides is return to normal function and size of the gland on withdrawal of exogenous iodide. Patients at highest risk are those with underlying thyroid abnormalities, Hashimoto disease, or previously treated Graves disease. A Japanese study of iodine-induced hypothyroidism indicated that patients with hypothyroidism that was reversible after iodine withdrawal had underlying focal lymphocytic thyroiditis, whereas those with irreversible hypothyroidism had more severe destruction of the thyroid gland.[37]

## IODIDE-INDUCED THYROTOXICOSIS

The occurrence of hyperthyroidism after iodide administration has been reported throughout the world since this element was first used to treat endemic iodine-deficient goiter. The first case report of thyrotoxicosis after iodine supplementation was published in 1821. Iodide-induced hyperthyroidism subsequently has been referred to as the *jodbasedow phenomenon*. Thyrotoxicosis occurring after iodide supplementation for endemic goiter in iodine-deficient areas is frequently reported. The mechanism underlying this phenomenon may relate to the rapid iodination and proteolysis of previously iodine-poor thyroglobulin, or to the presence of a subpopulation of patients with goiters who have gross or microscopic autonomous areas of functioning tissue. The latter hypothesis is supported by the observation that hyperthyroidism may develop after an iodine load in euthyroid patients with solitary autonomous nodules.[38] Four populations—in Holland, Tasmania, Yugoslavia, and Australia—were observed closely for the prevalence of thyrotoxicosis before and after iodide supplementation. The incidence of thyrotoxicosis after iodide supplementation ranged from .01% to .04%.[14] The incidence of thyrotoxicosis in a population rises 6 months after long-term iodine exposure begins, peaks at 1 to 3 years, and

returns to baseline by 6 to 10 years. Although several reports have indicated no increased incidence of thyrotoxicosis in some populations given iodine prophylactically, these follow-up studies may have been conducted too late to detect transient hyperthyroidism.

Reviews have addressed the prevention of iodine-induced thyrotoxicosis[39] and its epidemiology in Europe and worldwide.[40] Iodine-induced thyrotoxicosis has been reported from areas of endemic iodine deficiency in Germany after the use of iodine-containing drugs or contrast media, in much the same manner as was seen when iodine was added as a dietary supplement.[41] The reported 5% to 30% incidence in this area of endemic goiter in Germany is much higher than that seen in iodine-sufficient areas. Follow-up studies on patients exposed to iodine-containing drugs or dyes indicate that serum iodothyronine concentrations increase rapidly in relation to iodine dose, with a doubling of free $T_4$ index and a 53% increase in serum $T_3$ at a time when urinary iodine excretion is increased 5-fold to 10-fold over baseline.[42] Additional exposure to excess iodine intake further increased serum iodothyronine concentrations, albeit less dramatically.[42] In addition, the incidence of $T_3$ toxicosis relative to that of $T_4$ toxicosis declined with increasing iodine intake.

In the United States, concern exists that iodine-induced thyrotoxicosis may occur in persons without any underlying goiter or thyroid function abnormality. The incidence of goiter is ~3% in this country, and no areas of iodine deficiency are found. Dozens of cases of drug-induced thyrotoxicosis have been reported in the United States. Far more cases have come from Europe, although these may be from areas of relative dietary iodine deficiency. Several of the patients described in the United States have had preexisting thyroid disorders, most have had multinodular goiters, and most have been women. Drug-induced thyrotoxicosis has been seen after the use of potassium iodide, oral and intravenous contrast agents, the iodine-containing antiarrhythmic amiodarone (see preceding), and the topical antiinfective iodochlorhydroxyquin. Hyperthyroidism has been observed to develop 4 days to 4 months after iodine exposure. The thyrotoxicosis may persist for 1 to 6 months and usually is self-limited.

In one study, thyrotoxicosis developed in four of eight patients with goiter after a 180-mg daily dose of potassium iodide, and the suggestion was made that thyrotoxicosis may be a common outcome in patients from nonendemic areas with goiter who are exposed to iodides.[43] The authors recommended that caution be exercised in administering iodine-containing drugs or performing radiographic contrast procedures in persons with goiter. Patients with multinodular goiter are at some increased risk for iodine-induced thyrotoxicosis. The risk may be overstated, however; despite the high prevalence of goiter and the several million dye studies that are done yearly in this country, an epidemic of thyrotoxicosis has not occurred. Thus, most patients with goiter are not clinically affected by iodine exposure, and goiter should not be considered a contraindication to the use of necessary iodine-containing drugs or contrast media. In a study of 10 women who were in remission after a prior history of Graves thyrotoxicosis, the administration of SSKI caused recurrence of thyrotoxicosis in two patients and blunting of the thyrotropin-releasing hormone stimulation test in two others.[44] Iodine-induced thyrotoxicosis also has occurred with metastatic thyroid carcinoma after earlier thyroidectomy.[45]

## CLINICAL FEATURES OF IODIDE-INDUCED THYROTOXICOSIS

The clinical features of iodide-induced thyrotoxicosis in endemic goiter are similar to those seen in Graves disease with thyrotoxicosis. In the former case patients tend to be older, however, and to have long histories of iodide deprivation preceding the addition of iodine. Some predisposition may be present with advancing age, because thyrotoxicosis occurred in none of 50,000 children in this country who were treated with iodides in the 1920s. The ratio of men to women affected may also be different from the ratio in Graves disease. In Yugoslavia, the ratio of men to women with thyrotoxicosis increased from 1:10 to 1:6 after iodine supplementation. In Holland, 15% of the cases of hyperthyroidism occurred in men before iodine supplementation, compared to 31% after iodine supplementation. Exophthalmos is not encountered, and thyroid antibodies are not detected. Among patients with iodide-induced thyrotoxicosis from iodide-deficient areas, most patients had long-standing nodular goiter; however, 15% to 30% of patients had minimal to no goiter, and many persons with goiter did not have nodules.

The clinical manifestations of drug-induced thyrotoxicosis are similar to those of Graves hyperthyroidism and include tremor, tachycardia, palpitations, weight loss, heat intolerance, concentration difficulties, and mental status changes.[19] There is no tenderness of the thyroid gland such as is seen in granulomatous thyroiditis; there is no exophthalmos such as is seen in Graves disease. The serum $T_4$ and free $T_4$ values and the free $T_4$ index are elevated. Typically, the 24-hour $^{131}$I uptake is reduced, and the technetium thyroid scan may show reduced or patchy uptake. Generally, the $T_3$ level also is elevated; however, with amiodarone and the oral cholecystographic dye ipodate, the peripheral conversion of $T_4$ to $T_3$ is blocked, and the serum $T_3$ level may be disproportionately low compared to the elevated serum $T_4$ level.

## TREATMENT OF IODIDE-INDUCED THYROTOXICOSIS

The treatment of thyrotoxicosis is discussed in Chapter 42. The major difference in the approach to treating iodide-induced hyperthyroidism as opposed to Graves disease relates to the self-limited nature of the former, with resolution occurring after removal of the source of excess iodine and clearance of iodine from the circulation. The thyrotoxicosis, although usually self-limited, may persist for weeks to months because of the increased thyroidal iodine stores and increased plasma iodide. Mildly symptomatic patients may be treated with β-blockade therapy alone; more specific antithyroid drugs may be necessary in severely affected patients, but ablative therapy should not be required.

Amiodarone iodine-induced thyrotoxicosis may be resistant to the usual antithyroidal therapy.[46] A study of 58 patients with amiodarone-induced thyrotoxicosis showed persistent thyrotoxicosis at 6 to 9 months in more than one-half of those who were not treated. The use of methimazole in high doses proved ineffective in most patients. Euthyroidism was restored, however, in all patients who were treated with a combination of methimazole and potassium perchlorate (1 g per day). Other authors have found prolonged persistent thyrotoxicosis even with the addition of potassium perchlorate to propylthiouracil.[47] Successful resolution of the hyperthyroidism may require prolonged therapy. Of note for those cases in which the underlying cardiac dysrhythmia precludes safe discontinuation of the drug, the thyrotoxicosis was treated successfully in five patients by adding only thiourea.[48] Although most cases of amiodarone-induced thyrotoxicosis are related to the provision of its rich iodine content to patients who have thyroid glands with underlying autonomous function (e.g., hyperfunctioning nodules), a variant of the syndrome that is akin to destructive thyroiditis exists.[49] Patients with this condition, who may have low radioiodine uptake and elevated serum interleukin-6 levels,[50] should be treated with glucocorticoids rather than methimazole.[51]

## IODINE-INDUCED AUTOIMMUNITY

Investigators have speculated that increased iodine intake may contribute to the prevalence of autoimmune thyroid disease. Individuals with Hashimoto disease are well known to be sensitive to the effects of iodine and vulnerable to iodine-induced hypothyroidism. Less well known is that iodine exposure may induce a lymphocytic thyroiditis in a variety of experimental animals (rat, hamster, dog) as well as in humans.[9,52] A few studies have examined the greater prevalence of thyroid antibodies after increases in iodine exposure.[53] Specific histologic features of iodine-induced goiter have been described in one study of 28 patients, with half the biopsies also showing typical lymphocytic infiltration.[54]

Persons with preexisting thyroid disease who live in areas of iodide deficiency may be predisposed to the development of iodine-induced thyrotoxicosis.[52] Iodine-rich thyroglobulin has been shown to be more immunogenic,[55] and a greater proliferation of T cells is seen in patients with chronic thyroiditis after exposure to normally iodinated thyroglobulin, whereas noniodinated thyroglobulin elicits no response.[56] In some unknown manner, iodine may relate to the development of thyroid growth-stimulating immunoglobulins.[57] In this regard, iodide has been shown to enhance immunoglobulin G release into the media of cultured human lymphocytes,[58] but other mechanisms of immune stimulation may exist.[56] Controversy exists as to whether amiodarone may induce autoimmunity and, if so, whether the drug itself or its iodine content is responsible. Thirty percent to 50% of patients who become hypothyroid during amiodarone treatment have antithyroid antibodies in their serum. In one prospective study, antibodies developed in 6 of 13 patients given amiodarone, compared to none of 22 control subjects.[59] The proposal has been made that amiodarone alters T-cell subsets with enhanced T-cell expression of Ia antigen, consistent with precipitation of organ-specific autoimmunity in susceptible persons.[60]

## REFERENCES

1. Braverman LE. Iodine and the thyroid: 33 years of study. Thyroid 1994; 4:351.
2. Koutras DA. Control of efficiency and results and adverse effects of excess iodine administration on thyroid function. Ann Endocrinol (Paris) 1996; 57:463.
3. Khan LK, Li R, Gootnick D, et al. Thyroid abnormalities related to iodine excess from water purification units. Lancet 1998; 352:1519.
4. Hollowell JG, Staehling NW, Hannon WH, et al. Iodine nutrition in the United States. Trends and public health implications: iodine excretion data from national health and nutrition examination surveys I and III (1971–1974 and 1988–1994). J Clin Endocrinol Metab 1998; 83:3401.
5. Cavalieri RR. Iodine metabolism and thyroid physiology: current concepts. Thyroid 1997; 7:177.
6. Ermans AM. Disorders of iodine deficiency. In: Ingbar SH, Braverman LE, eds. The thyroid: a fundamental and clinical text. Philadelphia: JB Lippincott, 1986:707.
7. Peacock I, Davison H. Observations of iodide sensitivity. Ann Allergy 1958; 16:158.
8. Edmunds HT. Acute thyroiditis from potassium iodide. BMJ 1955; 1:354.
9. Bagchi N, Brown TR, Urdanivia E, Sundick RS. Induction of autoimmune thyroiditis in chickens by dietary iodine. Science 1985; 230:325.
10. Sato K, Okamura K, Hirata T, et al. Immunological and chemical types of reversible hypothyroidism; clinical characteristics and long-term prognosis. Clin Endocrinol 1996; 45:519.
11. Vagenakis AG, Braverman LE. Adverse effects of iodides on thyroid function. Med Clin North Am 1975; 59:1075.
12. Wolff J. Iodide goiter and the pharmacologic effects of excess iodide. Am J Med 1969; 47:101.
13. Namba H, Yamashita S, Kimura H, et al. Evidence of thyroid volume increase in normal subjects receiving excess iodide. J Clin Endocrinol Metab 1993; 76:605.
14. Fradkin JE, Wolff J. Iodide induced thyrotoxicosis. Medicine (Baltimore) 1983; 62:1.
15. Savoie J-C, Massin JP, Thomopoulos P, Leger F. Iodine induced thyrotoxicosis in apparently normal glands. J Clin Endocrinol Metab 1975; 4:685.
15a. Jooste PL, Weight MJ, Lombard CJ. Short-term effectiveness of mandatory iodization of table salt, at an elevated iodine concentration, on the iodine and goiter status of school children with endemic goiter. Am J Clin Nutr 2000; 71:75.
16. Park YK, Harland BF, Vandervein JE, et al. Estimation of dietary iodine intake of Americans in recent years. J Am Diet Assoc 1981; 79:17.
17. Burgi H, Wimpfheimer C, Burger A, et al. Changes of circulating thyroxine, triiodothyronine, and reverse triiodothyronine after radiographic contrast agents. J Clin Endocrinol Metab 1976; 43:1203.
18. Nagataki S. Effect of excess quantities of iodide. In: Greer MA, Solomon DH, eds. Handbook of physiology, section 7, Endocrinology, VIII. Baltimore: Williams & Wilkins, 1974:329.
19. Safran M, Braverman LE. Effect of chronic douching with polyvinyl-pyrrolidone-iodine on iodine absorption and thyroid function. Obstet Gynecol 1982; 60:35.

20. Rajatanavin R, Safran M, Stoller WA, et al. Five patients with iodine-induced hyperthyroidism. Am J Med 1984; 77:378.
21. Loh KC. Amiodarone-induced thyroid disorders: a clinical review. Postgrad Med J 2000; 76:133.
22. Harjai KJ, Licata AA. Effects of amiodarone on thyroid function. Ann Intern Med 1997; 126:63.
23. Iudica-Souza C, Burch HB. Amiodarone-induced thyroid dysfunction. The Endocrinologist 1999; in press.
24. Leger AF, Massin JP, Laurent ME, et al. Iodine-induced thyrotoxicosis: analysis of eighty-five consecutive cases. Eur J Clin Invest 1984; 14:449.
25. Paul T, Myers B, Witorsch RJ, et al. The effect of small increases in dietary iodine on thyroid function in euthyroid subjects. Metabolism 1988; 37:121.
26. Wolff J, Chaikoff IL. Plasma inorganic iodide as a homeostatic regulator of thyroid function. J Biol Chem 1948; 174:555.
27. Gardner DF, Centor RM, Utiger RD. Effects of low dose oral iodide supplementation on thyroid function in normal men. Clin Endocrinol (Oxf) 1988; 28:283.
28. Wartofsky L, Ransil BJ, Ingbar SH. Inhibition by iodine of the release of thyroxine from the thyroid glands of normal subjects and patients with thyrotoxicosis. J Clin Invest 1970; 49:78.
29. Braverman LE, Ingbar SH, Vagenakis AG. Enhanced susceptibility to iodide myxedema in patients with Hashimoto's disease. J Clin Endocrinol Metab 1971; 32:515.
30. DeLange F, Chanoine JP, Abrassart C, Bourdoux P. Topical iodine, breast-feeding, and neonatal hypothyroidism. Arch Dis Child 1988; 63:106.
31. Chabrolle JP, Rossier A. Goiter and hypothyroidism in the newborn after cutaneous absorption of iodine. Arch Dis Child 1978; 53:495.
32. Suzuki H, Higuchi T, Sawa K, et al. Endemic coast goiter in Hokkaido, Japan. Acta Endocrinol (Copenh) 1965; 50:161.
33. Higuchi T. The study of endemic seashore goiter in Hokkaido. Folia Endocrinol Jpn 1964; 40:982.
34. Konno N, Makita H, Yuri K, et al. Association between dietary iodine intake and prevalence of subclinical hypothyroidism in the coastal regions of Japan. J Clin Endocrinol Metab 1994; 78:393.
35. Braverman LE, Walker KA, Ingbar SH. Induction of myxedema by iodide in patients euthyroid after radioiodine or surgical treatment of diffuse toxic goiter. N Engl J Med 1969; 281:816.
36. Lesher JL Jr, Fitch MH, Dunlap DB. Subclinical hypothyroidism during potassium iodide therapy for lymphocutaneous sporotrichosis. Cutis 1994; 53:128.
37. Tajiri J, Higashi K, Morita M, et al. Studies of hypothyroidism in patients with high iodine intake. J Clin Endocrinol Metab 1986; 63:412.
38. Ermans AM, Camus M. Modification of thyroid function induced by chronic administration of iodide in the presence of "autonomous" thyroid tissue. Acta Endocrinol (Copenh) 1972; 70:463.
39. Dunn JT, Semigran MJ, Delange F. The prevention and management of iodine-induced hyperthyroidism and its cardiac features. Thyroid 1998; 8:101.
40. Stanbury JB, Ermans AE, Bourdoux P, et al. Iodine-induced hyperthyroidism: occurrence and epidemiology. Thyroid 1998; 8:83.
41. Kallee E, Wahl R, Bohner J, et al. Thyrotoxicosis induced by iodine-containing drugs. J Mol Med 1980; 4:221.
42. Emrich D, Karkavitsas N, Facorro U, et al. Influence of increasing iodine intake on thyroid function in euthyroid and hyperthyroid states. J Clin Endocrinol Metab 1982; 54:1236.
43. Vagenakis AG, Wang C, Burger A, et al. Iodide-induced thyrotoxicosis in Boston. N Engl J Med 1972; 287:524.
44. Roti E, Gardini E, Minelli R, et al. Effects of chronic iodine administration on thyroid status in euthyroid subjects previously treated with antithyroid drugs for Graves' hyperthyroidism. J Clin Endocrinol Metab 1993; 76:928.
45. Yoshinari M, Tokuyama T, Okamura K, et al. Iodide-induced thyrotoxicosis in a thyroidectomized patient with metastatic thyroid carcinoma. Cancer 1988; 61:1674.
46. Martino E, Aghini-Lombardi F, Mariotti S, et al. Amiodarone: a common source of iodine-induced thyrotoxicosis. Horm Res 1987; 26:158.
47. Newnham HH, Topliss BJ, LeGrand BA, et al. Amiodarone-induced hyperthyroidism: assessment of the predictive value of biochemical testing and response to combined therapy using propylthiouracil and potassium perchlorate. Aust N Z J Med 1988; 18:37.
48. Davies PH, Franklyn JA, Sheppard MC. Treatment of amiodarone induced thyrotoxicosis with carbimazole alone and continuation of amiodarone. BMJ 1992; 305:224.
49. Smyrk TC, Goellner JR, Brennan MD, Carnei JA. Pathology of the thyroid in amiodarone-associated thyrotoxicosis. Am J Surg Pathol 1987; 11:197.
50. Bartalena L, Grasso L, Brogioni S, et al. Serum interleukin-6 in amiodarone-induced thyrotoxicosis. J Clin Endocrinol Metab 1994; 78:423.
51. Bartalena L, Brogioni S, Grasso L, et al. Treatment of amiodarone-induced thyrotoxicosis, a difficult challenge: results of a prospective study. J Clin Endocrinol Metab 1996; 81:2930.
52. Harach HR, Escalante DA, Onativia A, et al. Thyroid carcinoma and thyroiditis in an endemic goitre region before and after iodine prophylaxis. Acta Endocrinol (Copenh) 1985; 108:55.
53. Koutras DA, Karaiskos KS, Evangelopoulou K, et al. Thyroid antibodies after iodine supplementation. In: Drexhage HA, Wiersinga WM, eds. The thyroid and autoimmunity. Amsterdam: Excerpta Medica, 1986:211.
54. Mizukami Y, Michigishi T, Nonomura A, et al. Iodine-induced hypothyroidism: a clinical and histological study of 28 patients. J Clin Endocrinol Metab 1993; 76:466.
55. Sundick RS, Herdegen DM, Brown TR, Bagchi N. The incorporation of dietary iodine into thyroglobulin increases its immunogenicity. Endocrinology 1987; 120:2078.
56. Rose NR, Saboori AM, Rasooly L, Burek CL. The role of iodine in autoimmune thyroiditis. Crit Rev Immunol 1997; 17:511.
57. Medeiros-Neto GA, Halpern A, Cozzi ZS, et al. Thyroid growth immunoglobulins in large multinodular endemic goiters: effect of iodized oil. J Clin Endocrinol Metab 1986; 63:644.
58. Weetman AP, McGregor AM, Campbell H, et al. Iodide enhances IgG synthesis by human peripheral blood lymphocytes in vitro. Acta Endocrinol (Copenh) 1983; 103:210.
59. Monteiro E, Galvao Teles A, Santos ML, et al. Antithyroid antibodies as an early marker for thyroid disease induced by amiodarone. BMJ 1986; 292:227.
60. Rabinowe SL, Larsen PR, Antman EM, et al. Amiodarone therapy and autoimmune thyroid disease. Am J Med 1986; 81:53.

# CHAPTER 38

# NONTOXIC GOITER

PAUL J. DAVIS AND FAITH B. DAVIS

*Goiter* (L. *guttur*, throat) is a clinical term denoting thyroid gland enlargement to twice normal size or larger (see also ref. 1). The term implies no specific etiology, although the mechanisms of certain toxic and nontoxic (eumetabolic) goitrous states are understood. The prevalence of nontoxic goiter in the United States is ~5%,[1a] with a predominance among females. In the Framingham, Massachusetts, study, the prevalence of nontoxic goiter was 4.2%, with a 4:1 female to male ratio.[2]

## PATHOGENESIS OF NONTOXIC GOITER

Nontoxic goiter is the result of an interplay of factors intrinsic and extrinsic to the thyroid. In most patients, subtle limitations on hormonogenesis—imposed, for example, by iodine insufficiency or constitutional biochemical abnormalities in the gland—lead to nontoxic goiter when permissive normal or increased circulating levels of thyroid-stimulating hormone (TSH, thyrotropin) foster gland enlargement. Impaired hormonogenesis, TSH-dependent goiter, and eumetabolism may also reflect the presence of Hashimoto thyroiditis or the ingestion of goitrogens. In the absence of TSH, as in hypopituitarism, nontoxic goiter is rare.

Some have argued that the mechanisms of *diffuse* and *nodular* nontoxic goiter are different, with the latter reflecting an autonomous state independent of the permissive effect of TSH.[3] Although gland autonomy is present in certain patients with nontoxic nodular goiters, it occurs in few such patients, and whether autonomy develops early or late in the course of goitrogenesis is unknown.[4] The suggestion has also been made that the cyclic hypersecretion of TSH in response to periodic underproduction of hormone by the thyroid gland is essential to the development of nodular goiter. Formation of fibrous strands or scar tissue (consequent to cyclic follicular hyperplasia, microscopic hemorrhage, and necrosis) has been postulated to impose the anatomical limits within which nodules form.[5] Nevertheless, the possibility seems likely that subtle constitutional derangements of hormonogenesis and the permissive action of circulating TSH act together to produce both diffuse and nodular nontoxic goiter.

Various abnormalities of hormone production have been described in cases of nontoxic goiter (Table 38-1).[6–12,12a] These biochemical abnormalities, or altered sensitivity to TSH, might be expressed only in certain follicles (biochemical follicular heterogeneity), which would explain the occurrence of nodular

**TABLE 38-1.**
**Biochemical Findings Described in Nontoxic Goitrous Tissue**

| Clinical Pattern | Basal State | Stimulation/Suppression | Reference |
|---|---|---|---|
| Multinodular goiter | Heterogeneity among follicles of: Iodination of proteins Peroxidase activity [$^3$H]thyroxine labeling TSH endocytosis | Variable response of growth and function of cells within follicles after $T_4$ suppression, TSH stimulation in vivo | 6 |
| Multinodular goiter | Iodide-peroxidase activity correlated directly with radioiodine uptake in cold and warm nodules | | 7 |
| Benign nonfunctioning nodule | Decreased iodide accumulation in vitro* | TSH in vitro: increased iodide organification | 8 |
| | Decreased iodide organification | | |
| | Normal MIT/DIT ratio | | |
| | Decreased $T_4$ content | | |
| | Increased adenylate cyclase | TSH in vitro: increase in adenylate cyclase | |
| | Na–K ATPase activity normal | | |
| | ATP concentrations normal | | |
| Autonomous nodule | Increased $T_4$ and $T_3$ release; $T_4/T_3$ ratios unchanged | TSH in vitro: no effect on hormone release | 9 |
| Autonomous nodule | Increased $T_3$ concentration in autonomous nodule; $T_4$ not increased | | 10 |
| Autonomous nodule | Decreased $T_4/T_3$ ratio | TSH-dependent iodothyronine release absent | 11 |
| | Decreased iodine content of thyroglobulin | | |
| | Normal basal cAMP, cGMP, phosphodiesterase, and protein kinase | Decreased TSH-dependent cAMP accumulation | |
| Multinodular goiter | Normal high- and low-affinity TSH receptors | | 12 |
| | Normal basal adenylate cyclase activity | Normal stimulation of cyclase by NaF, GTP, PGE$_1$, and TSH | |
| Adenoma | Decreased low-affinity TSH receptors | | 12 |
| | Normal basal adenylate cyclase activity | Enhanced stimulation of cyclase by NaF, GTP, PGE$_1$, and TSH | |

$T_4$, thyroxine; *TSH*, thyroid-stimulating hormone; *MIT*, monoiodotyrosine; *DIT*, diiodotyrosine; *ATPase*, adenosine triphosphatase; *ATP*, adenosine triphosphate; $T_3$, triiodothyronine; *cAMP*, cyclic adenosine monophosphate; *cGMP*, cyclic guanosine monophosphate; *NaF*, sodium fluoride; *GTP*, guanosine 5'-triphosphate; *PGE$_1$*, prostaglandin E$_1$.
*In these studies, nodular or adenomatous tissue was compared with normal and/or paranodular thyroid tissue.

goiter. Excluded from Table 38-1 are genetically determined biochemical lesions that exist in familial goiter with hypothyroidism (see Chap. 47).

Other mechanisms leading to the development of goiter are infiltrative diseases of the thyroid, such as amyloidosis or granulomatous diseases, and the action of nonpituitary thyrotropic substances. Among the latter are polypeptides that circulate in pregnancy (human chorionic gonadotropin [hCG] and, less importantly, a placental TSH-like substance[13]) and thyroid-stimulating antibodies (see Chap. 197). Some of these thyroid-stimulating immunoglobulins (hTSI) have been identified in human serum[14-22] and act either through the thyroid cell membrane TSH receptor or by enhancing thyroid cell activity independently of the TSH receptor. The hTSIs that interact with the TSH receptor are recognized in vitro in a competitive binding assay involving radiolabeled TSH and thyroid cell membranes (TSH-binding inhibitory immunoglobulin [TBII] assay). Thyroid-stimulating antibodies that are inactive in the TBII assay are recognized by their "growth" effects, measured in vitro by sensitive histocytochemical methods or other methods. The hTSIs that cross-react with an antigenic site at the TSH receptor are probably unimportant in the pathogenesis of nontoxic goiter,[15] although they play a role in diffuse toxic goiter. On the other hand, thyroid-stimulating antibodies that act independently of the TSH site are found in the sera of more than 50% of patients with nontoxic goiter. Although these observations support an autoimmune contribution to the pathogenesis of nontoxic goiter, a search for helper T lymphocytes sensitized to thyroid membrane antigens in the peripheral blood of patients with nontoxic nodular goiter yielded negative results.[15] Hence, the importance of hTSIs in the formation of nontoxic goiter is not yet clear.

Certain cytokines have been implicated in the pathogenesis of nontoxic goiter. For example, the content of insulin-like growth factor-I (IGF-I) is increased more than two-fold in thyroid nodules compared with normal tissue obtained from the same gland.[17] Thyroid glands from patients with Graves disease and Hashimoto thyroiditis show no increase in IGF-I. Transforming growth factor-β (TGF-β) has been proposed to be an autocrine growth inhibitor in thyroid follicular cells, at least in the setting of iodide deficiency.[18] TGF-β blocks the growth stimulation, measured as thymidine incorporation, imposed on thyroid follicular cells in vitro by IGF-I, epidermal growth factor, and TGF-α, and endogenous TGF-β levels are decreased in iodide-deficient nontoxic goiter.[18] Although these studies suggest that cytokines can promote or mediate goiter formation, evidence exists that at least in goiter due to iodine-insufficiency, thyroid growth–promoting factors are not detectable in serum.[23]

The goiter of pregnancy may be a response both to placental TSHs and to maternal iodide insufficiency. The latter is a complex function of increased maternal renal iodide clearance, iodide parasitism by the fetus, and maternal losses during lactation.

## SPECIFIC ETIOLOGIES OF GOITER

### CONGENITAL GOITER

Congenital goiter is either *familial*—that is, an expression of genetic disorders of intrathyroidal hormonogenesis (see Chap. 47)—or *sporadic*. In the neonate, sporadic congenital goiter reflects intrauterine iodide insufficiency or fetal exposure to goitrogens. Maternal consumption of naturally occurring goitrogens is rarely the cause of thyroid enlargement in the neonate; this contrasts with endemic goiter, in which community-wide ingestion of a goitrogen occurs. Use of antithyroid medications is a significant cause of sporadic congenital goiter (i.e., thionamide administration to pregnant thyrotoxic women). Thionamides cross the placental barrier and limit fetal hormonogenesis after the 12th week of gestation. The requisites for such a congenital goiter include fetal TSH production, maturation of the fetal thyroid to the point of TSH responsiveness, and sensitivity of the pituitary to low levels of thyroid hormone. Because insubstantial quantities of maternal thyroxine ($T_4$) or triiodothyronine ($T_3$) cross the placenta, the maternal ingestion of $T_4$ or $T_3$ concomitantly with thionamides does not prevent fetal goiter. A specialized metabolically active analog, 3,5-dimethyl-3'-isopropyl-L-thyronine (DIMIT),[24] does cross the placenta, but it is not available for clinical use. Other iatrogenic goitrogens, such as aminoglutethimide and carbutamide, do not appear to cause fetal goiter, and neither agent is likely to be prescribed to pregnant women. Lithium and amiodarone, both potential causes of fetal goiter, are contraindicated during pregnancy.

## ENDEMIC GOITER

Iodine deficiency has been extensively studied as a cause of endemic goiter.[25] Before the introduction of iodized salt in 1925, "goiter belts" of low iodine content in water supplies existed in the United States near the Great Lakes, in the Appalachian region, and elsewhere.[26] During World War I, a 5% incidence of goiter was seen among U.S. Army inductees,[27] presumably reflecting widespread iodine deficiency. By World War II, the nationwide effort to increase dietary iodine had reduced the incidence of goiter in military recruits to 0.06%. Dietary iodine insufficiency no longer is a significant cause of euthyroid goiter in the United States but persists in enclaves in South America, Africa, and Asia,[1,28] and as many as 200 million people worldwide are estimated to experience iodine-deficiency goiter.

The excessive dietary intake of iodine is an occasional but nonendemic cause of goiter in the United States. In a localized region in Japan, however, high iodine intake has caused endemic goiter. The inhibition of thyroid hormonogenesis by excess iodine is termed the Wolff-Chaikoff effect.

Severe fetal iodine deprivation culminates in *endemic and sporadic cretinism* (see Chap. 47), with distinctive clinical findings. Moderate fetal iodine insufficiency results in euthyroid fetal goiter. Iodide crosses the placenta, and parasitism of maternal iodide by the fetus contributes to the "goiter of pregnancy" in women whose dietary iodine intake is marginal.

Both well-characterized and poorly characterized dietary goitrogens have been reported in a variety of epidemiologic studies. Water supplies have been a frequent source.[29] Certain vegetables (e.g., cabbage and other members of the *Brassica* family—turnip, kale, rape) contain thionamide-like substances.[1] Cassava is an important goitrogen in Africa, but no evidence exists for dietary goitrogens as a cause of endemic goiter in the United States.

Most patients with endemic goiter have no constitutional abnormalities of thyroid hormonogenesis. The goiter formation reflects either extrinsic iodine deficiency or goitrogen ingestion.

## SPORADIC GOITER

As with endemic goiter, sporadic goiter may reflect variations in iodide intake[30] and dietary goitrogen content. Although iodine insufficiency rarely causes thyroid enlargement in the United States, iodine excess can lead to goiter in two settings. First, although the thyroid gland escapes from the Wolff-Chaikoff effect in normal subjects after several weeks of excessive iodine intake, the thyroid in some patients does not. Resulting defective hormonogenesis and release cause increased pituitary TSH secretion and goiter formation. A new steady state is achieved in which the enlarged, inefficient gland produces sufficient hormone to maintain euthyroidism. This proposed pathogenetic sequence, based on increased TSH production, seems likely, but this hypothesis has not been validated by prospective application of sensitive serum TSH assays to populations at risk. Patients at risk for goiter, due to failure to escape from iodine inhibition of thyroid hormonogenesis, are those with Hashimoto thyroiditis or with other gland damage syndromes, such as those due to thyroid surgery or radiation of the neck.[31]

**TABLE 38-2.**
**Drugs Reported to Cause Goiter in Humans**

| Agent | Mechanism | Reference |
|---|---|---|
| Iodide | Inhibition of thyroid hormone release and synthesis | 33 |
| Thionamides | Inhibition of tyrosyl iodination and coupling | 34 |
| Aminoglutethimide | Inhibition of iodide organification | 35 |
| Lithium | Inhibition of thyroid hormone release | 36 |
| Amiodarone | Inhibition of thyroid hormone synthesis (effect mediated by iodide) | 37 |
| Fluoride | Exacerbation of effects of iodide deficiency* | 38 |
| Carbutamide | Decreased iodide uptake and inhibition of thyroid hormone synthesis | 39 |

*Excess calcium intake (increased hardness of potable water) also correlates with goiter formation in areas of marginal iodine intake.

A second setting in which goiter occurs with excess iodine administration is *jodbasedow*,[32] a syndrome of latent hyperthyroidism that is rare in the United States (see Chap. 37). Increasing iodine intake promotes goiter and, nearly concomitantly, thyrotoxicosis.

The source of increased iodine intake in goitrous patients is either medicinal—for example, saturated solution of potassium iodide (SSKI) continues to be used by some physicians as a mucolytic agent in patients with chronic lung disease, despite its clinical ineffectiveness—or paramedicinal—for example, from kelp ingestion. Radiologic contrast media and skin antiseptics contain iodine, but, because of their short-term use, are not causes of goiter. Long-term iodine excess followed by the acute interruption of iodine intake can have a distinct effect on thyroid function tests.

A variety of medications have antithyroid and goitrogenic effects (Table 38-2).[33–39] The mechanisms of the antithyroid actions of these agents can be interference with hormonogenesis at the level of organification of iodide or inhibition of hormone release or both. Lithium, a monovalent cation, has an effect on the thyroid similar to that of the anion iodide: hormone release is inhibited after the drug is concentrated in the gland.[36,40] Amiodarone, an antiarrhythmic drug, has been associated with the induction of hyperthyroidism and hypothyroidism.[37] Most patients who receive the drug remain euthyroid. The effects of amiodarone appear to be largely due to its iodine content, and this agent appears to promote hyperthyroidism in patients with limited, possibly insufficient, iodine intake. Aminoglutethimide[35] and oral sulfonylureas[39] interfere with hormonogenesis. Among the sulfonylureas, only carbutamide, which is used in Europe, causes goiter. Aminoglutethimide, an antiadrenal agent used as medical treatment of states of excess adrenocortical hormone production, can cause hypothyroidism and goiter.

Thyroiditis syndromes may be associated with goiter (see Chap. 46). The thyroid gland in these conditions is frequently symptomatic locally, and the glandular enlargement may be due to inflammatory infiltration rather than to TSH. The differential diagnosis of nontoxic goiter must always include early hyperthyroidism or, particularly in elderly subjects, *monosystemic* or *apathetic hyperthyroidism*. In these states, clinical hypermetabolism may be absent and isolated features such as myopathy, cardiomyopathy, or weight loss may be encountered[41] (see Chap. 199). Pregnancy is also a cause of nontoxic goiter, which usually remits postpartum. After multiple pregnancies, substantive thyromegaly may occur.

The possible contributions of other environmental factors to the development of nontoxic goiter are more difficult to evaluate. For example, cigarette smoking—the inhalation of thiocyanate—

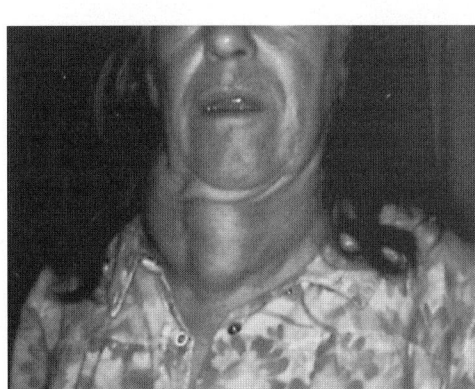
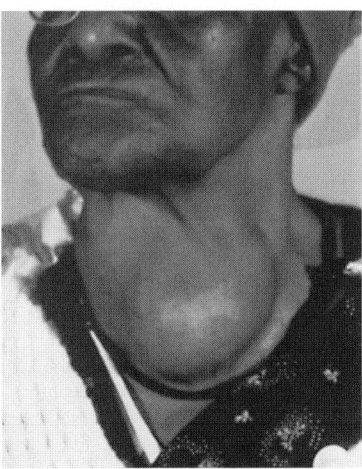
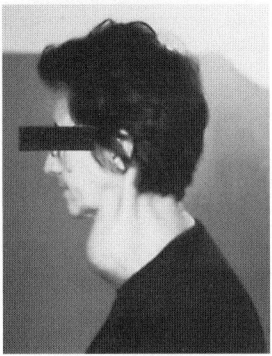
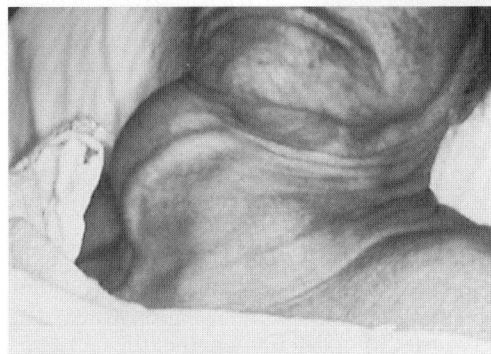

**FIGURE 38-1.** Examples of nontoxic goiter. *Top left,* Sporadic multinodular goiter in an 85-year-old woman. No local symptoms were present. *Top right,* 65-year-old woman with a 40-year history of nontoxic goiter and thyrotoxicosis of recent onset. Multiple ablative doses of [131]I controlled the hyperthyroidism but had no appreciable effect on thyroid gland size. *Bottom right,* Multinodular goiter with clinical findings of thoracic inlet obstruction and tracheal compression syndrome in a 70-year-old woman. The goiter was treated surgically to relieve obstructive symptoms. *Bottom left,* Endemic goiter in a 45-year-old Peruvian woman.

has been implicated in goitrogenesis,[42] and serum thyroglobulin levels appear to be higher in smokers than in nonsmokers.

The incidence of goiter in patients with end-stage renal disease is variable[43] and unlikely to be explained by a single factor. The variability in incidence appears to be regional and may relate to diet or to the use in dialysis baths of tap water that contains ions or other factors that are goitrogenic.

## CLINICAL FEATURES OF NONTOXIC GOITER

### HISTORY AND PHYSICAL FINDINGS

Patients with nontoxic goiter have no systemic symptoms, and the goiter is usually found on routine physical examination or is detected by the patient as a neck mass. Local symptoms occasionally include those due to tracheal compression (stridor or respiratory distress) and/or displacement of the esophagus (dysphagia). Rarely, substernal extension of nontoxic goiter may lead to recurrent laryngeal nerve entrapment and hoarseness. Spontaneous hemorrhage into a goiter manifests as local pain and tenderness in one thyroidal lobe. When Hashimoto thyroiditis causes nontoxic thyroidal enlargement, the gland is usually without local symptoms but diffuse tenderness or adenopathy occasionally occurs (see Chap. 46).

History-taking from patients with nontoxic goiter includes a focused review of possible environmental or genetic factors that may be causative. The emphasis is on dietary or medicinal sources of excessive iodine intake, antithyroid drugs, or, in regions of the world where iodine deficiency or naturally occurring dietary goitrogens are common, on establishment of a possible role for these factors. Goiter during pregnancy or the enhancement of established thyromegaly in successive pregnancies should raise the possibility of marginal iodine deficiency. Low-dose head-and-neck irradiation in childhood increases the risk of nodular goiter and thyroid carcinoma.[44] Systemic illnesses

such as sarcoidosis or amyloidosis raise the rare possibility of infiltrative disease of the thyroid. Isolated thyroid nodules in the euthyroid patient often indicate adenomas or cysts (see Chap. 39). Cancer originating in other organs may (rarely) metastasize to the thyroid.[45] At autopsy, infection of the thyroid is relatively common in patients who have succumbed to septicemia, but such involvement is seldom clinically apparent before death.[46]

Physical examination of the nontoxic goiter should include the following: size, consistency, the absence or presence of nodularity, bruit, tenderness, and concomitant anterior cervical lymphadenopathy. The clinical and etiologic implications of each of these factors are controversial, but their accurate description is useful in the subsequent evaluation of the patient.

Extreme firmness of a diffuse goiter is suggestive of infiltrative disease (amyloidosis, Riedel struma) or intense TSH stimulation (Hashimoto thyroiditis); firmness of a nodule has been suggested to be a sign of thyroid cancer. However, in the individual patient these generalizations are frequently incorrect.

Tenderness of the thyroid gland can be a useful clinical finding, indicating inflammatory disease or intrathyroidal hemorrhage, usually into a preexisting cyst. Tenderness may also reflect acute thyroiditis contiguous with intercurrent tracheitis and occasionally is encountered in Hashimoto thyroiditis. Granulomatous or subacute thyroiditis is usually associated with exquisite thyroidal tenderness and pain radiating to the mandible.

In all age groups, anterior cervical and supraclavicular adenopathy is a hallmark of locally metastatic papillary thyroid carcinoma (see Chap. 40). Because a centrally located node immediately above the isthmus of the thyroid gland drains both lobes, it has been ascribed "oracular" qualities (*delphian node*), usually reflecting the presence of thyroid cancer. However, this node is sometimes enlarged in patients with Hashimoto thyroiditis. Dullness to percussion over the upper sternum may be noted when a large substernal goiter is present.

Instructive examples of nontoxic goiters are shown in Figure 38-1, and radiologic findings associated with substernal goiter are depicted in Figure 38-2.

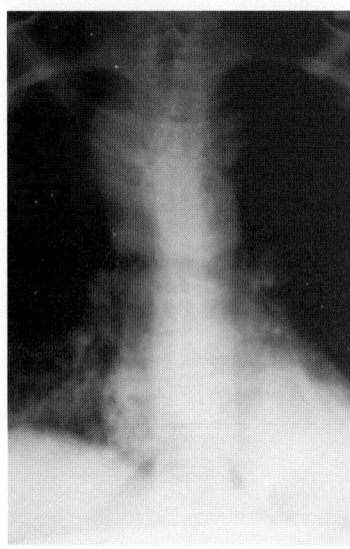 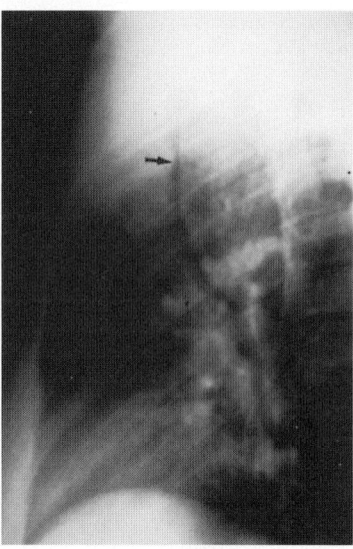 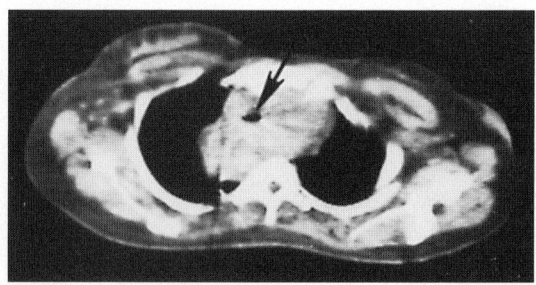

**FIGURE 38-2.** Radiographic and imaging studies in substernal goiter. Patient was a 28-year-old woman who presented with acute bronchitis. *Left,* Posteroanterior chest roentgenogram revealed right paratracheal mass contiguous with the aortic arch. *Middle,* Lateral roentgenogram of the chest showed tracheal compression *(arrow)* by anterior mediastinal mass. *Right,* Transverse superior mediastinal computed tomographic scan. The trachea *(arrow)* is enveloped and compressed by goiter, which extended posteriorly to the vertebral body.

## NONTHYROIDAL ANTERIOR CERVICAL NECK MASSES

The thyroidal origin of neck masses is usually apparent from their location and their movement with the thyroid gland on deglutition. Previous neck surgery, obesity, and hypertrophied bellies of sternocleidomastoid muscles can obscure the thyroidal nature of neck masses. Included in the differential diagnosis of neck lesions are *branchial cleft cyst* and *thyroglossal duct cyst* (Fig. 38-3). Branchial cleft cysts are anterolateral, whereas thyroglossal duct cysts are midline and are found at any point between the isthmus and the area above the laryngeal prominence (cartilage). When thyroglossal duct cysts remain contiguous with the base of the tongue (foramen caecum linguae), they move upward with voluntary protrusion of the tongue. Cystic hygroma (diffuse, fluid-filled, multiloculated lymphangioma that is present at birth) arises from the supraclavicular fossa and should not be confused with goiter.

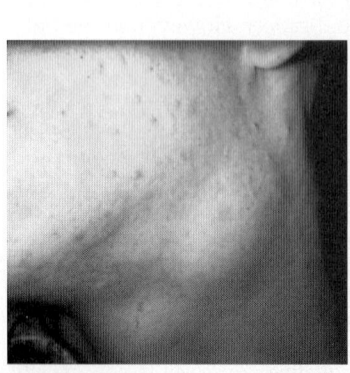 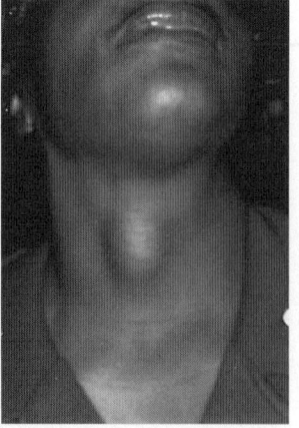

**FIGURE 38-3.** Abnormal nonthyroidal cervical structures included in the differential diagnosis of goiter. *Left,* Infected branchial cleft cyst in a 28-year-old woman with a neck mass and fever. The lateral, superior location in the neck is typical for this lesion. *Right,* Thyroglossal duct cyst in an asymptomatic 42-year-old woman. Lesion was smooth and moved with deglutition and with protrusion of the tongue. The midline or near-midline location and cystic consistency are typical for this lesion. The thyroid gland was not enlarged.

## LABORATORY EVALUATION OF THE PATIENT WITH GOITER

The principles of diagnostic evaluation of the patient with nontoxic goiter are: (a) confirmation of eumetabolism; (b) establishment of the cause, insofar as doing so is cost effective; and (c) determination of the impact of the lesion on important nonthyroidal structures in the neck or upper mediastinum.

Confirmation of the euthyroid state is essential, regardless of the chronicity of the goiter and its historically eumetabolic nature. The development of hyperthyroidism in the setting of long-standing nontoxic goiter is frequent—thyrotoxicosis may develop in as many as one-third of patients with a large nontoxic goiter of 30 years' duration. Nevertheless, in a large series of elderly subjects with hyperthyroidism,[41] patients with long-standing goiter comprised <10% of the subject population. Because diffuse nontoxic goiter, and occasionally nodular goiter, can reflect the presence of Hashimoto thyroiditis, the hypothyroid state may emerge insidiously during the course of a "euthyroid goiter." Tests of serum thyroid function in the patient with nontoxic goiter should include TSH measurement. In patients with normal serum $T_4$ concentrations, mild $T_3$ toxicosis should be ruled out. Thyrotropin-releasing hormone testing is only rarely required to demonstrate euthyroidism in goitrous patients with nondiagnostic serum free $T_4$ and total $T_3$ values and low, but not fully suppressed, serum TSH levels.

A substantial minority (39%) of patients with nontoxic goiter have abnormal esophageal transit times.[47] This observation is not an indication for routine evaluation of esophageal function in goiter patients, because symptoms or medical consequences of the transit abnormality appear to be minimal,[47] unless the goiter is very large.

## ESTABLISHMENT OF THE CAUSE OF NONTOXIC GOITER

Serum antithyroid antibody titers should be measured in all patients with nontoxic goiter. Elevated antibody titers (e.g., antithyroglobulin and anti–thyroid peroxidase [anti-TPO, "microsomal"] antibodies) are prima facie evidence of an autoimmune basis for goiter formation in the euthyroid patient (e.g., those with Hashimoto thyroiditis). Elevated titers occur in up to 90% of such patients.[48]

In antibody-negative patients with nontoxic goiter, thyroidal radioiodide uptake and scan (iodine-123) may be helpful diagnostically. An elevated uptake is consistent with increased TSH action (e.g., antibody-negative Hashimoto thyroiditis or iodide deficiency) or with the action of non-TSH thyroid stimulators. Extremely low or undetectable radioiodide uptake by the thyroid is an important finding in the goitrous patient; the differential diagnosis includes excessive iodide intake, lymphocytic thyroiditis ("painless thyroiditis," usually with transient hyperthyroidism), and granulomatous thyroiditis. Struma ovarii and factitious hyperthyroidism are also associated with extremely low or undetectable radioiodide uptake, but no goiter is present. The normalization of a previously high iodine intake in patients with iodine-induced hypothyroidism may result in an acute elevation of thyroidal radioiodide uptake, although serum $T_4$ values remain low. A "patchy" uptake pattern on scan is frequently encountered in Hashimoto thyroiditis. Localized areas of reduced or absent uptake are difficult to interpret. They are associated with a 0% to 30% risk of carcinoma in various reports but most commonly represent adenoma or cyst. Areas of increased uptake are associated with an extraordinarily low risk of cancer (see Chap. 34). The estimation of iodide intake by measurement of 24-hour urinary iodide excretion is seldom necessary in the United States.

Serum thyroglobulin levels are elevated in one-third of patients with nontoxic goiter and are not helpful in establishing a cause. Plasma calcitonin levels are normal in patients with benign nontoxic goiter.[49]

Ultrasonography of the thyroid is useful in distinguishing cystic from solid nodules in nontoxic goiter (see Chap. 35).

Needle biopsy and aspiration cytology of the thyroid gland are valuable techniques for establishing certain pathologic states of the thyroid gland (see Chap. 39).[50] In antibody-negative patients with Hashimoto thyroiditis, needle biopsy is useful in establishing the diagnosis. Both needle biopsy and aspiration cytology are important tools in assessing a nontoxic goiter for the possible presence of cancer.

In patients with large goiters or local symptoms attributable to goiter, the extent of the goiter can be determined in several ways. Routine chest radiographs reveal a paratracheal mass and tracheal deviation (posteroanterior view) and obliteration of the superior retrosternal space (lateral view). Radionuclide scintigraphy of the thyroid usually shows the retrosternal extent of the gland. Iodine-123 is inadequate for substernal scanning; therefore, iodine-131 ($^{131}$I) should be requested when a substernal goiter is a possibility. Technetium-99m pertechnetate has also been used, although less successfully, to evaluate the extent of substernal glands. Flow-loop studies of the upper airway[51] and barium pharyngoesophagography are valuable in detecting tracheal and esophageal obstruction due to goitrous encroachment. Flow-loop studies do not necessarily correlate with clinical symptoms, because the latter may reflect the patient's anxiety. The marked distensibility of the esophagus minimizes, as noted earlier, the clinical impact of goiter on swallowing.

## PROGNOSIS OF NONTOXIC GOITER

In young or middle-aged patients, particularly those with nontoxic gland enlargement due to Hashimoto thyroiditis, goiter may remit spontaneously. Goiter due to severe Hashimoto thyroiditis is thought to lead to progressive thyroid atrophy ("remission of goiter") and eventual hypothyroidism. Mild thyroiditis usually has no metabolic sequelae. As many as one-third of autonomous ("warm" or "hot") solitary nodules may remit spontaneously ("burn out").[52]

The natural course of nontoxic goiter, however, ordinarily is further enlargement of the gland and the appearance of benign nodularity, estimated at 4.5% increase in size annually.[53] Indeed, even normal thyroids, over the life span, often develop micronodularity or macronodularity. Except in the case of patients who have

received low-energy head-and-neck irradiation, the risk of development of thyroid carcinoma in a nontoxic goiter is low (<1%). The overall risk of thyroid cancer in patients who have had head-and-neck irradiation may be as high as 8%.[54] As indicated earlier, long-term follow-up of patients with large nontoxic goiter reveals a strong incidence (33%) of development of thyrotoxicosis. The rate of hyperthyroidism in patients with previously nontoxic goiter depends on duration of follow-up, for example, 15% at 12 years[55] compared with the higher incidence cited earlier at 30 years. Thus, the prognostic spectrum of nontoxic goiter is broad, and the histopathology is usually benign.

The interesting possibility has been raised that a substantial number of patients with nontoxic goiter have (extrapituitary) "tissue overexposure" to thyroid hormone.[56] That is, the lower the level of circulating TSH in such patients, the more likely that indices of thyroid hormone action on bone or liver are elevated. The indices measured were, respectively, plasma concentration of bone γ-carboxyglutamic acid–containing protein (Gla protein) and plasma sex hormone–binding globulin.[56] The long-term implications of the presence of low-grade, minimally excessive levels of thyroid hormone, as inferred from Gla protein and sex hormone–binding globulin levels, are unknown, although patients may be at increased risk for atrial fibrillation.[57]

## TREATMENT OF NONTOXIC GOITER

The approach to managing nontoxic goiter involves (a) prevention of progressive enlargement of the thyroid gland; (b) anticipation, where appropriate, of hyperthyroidism or hypothyroidism; (c) reduction of the risk of carcinoma in the gland; and (d) relief of local symptoms attributable to goiter. Annual clinical evaluation of the patient with nontoxic goiter is a cornerstone of management, as is routine instruction of the patient to contact the treating physician if local symptoms emerge or change, or if systemic symptoms develop that are consistent with hypothyroidism or hyperthyroidism.

Because nontoxic goiter is a state in which the permissive or directorial role of TSH is expressed, suppression of endogenous TSH secretion with exogenous thyroid hormone (L-thyroxine, $T_4$) prevents further enlargement of the gland.[58] Two-thirds of sporadic nontoxic goiters shrink when endogenous TSH is suppressed by exogenous thyroid hormone.[59] This rate of success is less likely for nodular goiters than for diffuse goiters.[59] Modest goiter, particularly that associated with Hashimoto thyroiditis, predictably responds to TSH suppression with a return of the gland to normal or near-normal size. Nodular goiter responds to suppression therapy in a nonpredictable manner. Sometimes normal thyroid tissue located between multiple nodules atrophies when endogenous TSH is suppressed, bringing the nodules into greater relief. This change can be misinterpreted as an increase in nodule size in the face of suppression. The effectiveness of the strategy of TSH suppression in management of nodular goiter is under review by several groups. Nodular or nonnodular, very large nontoxic goiters are unlikely to respond to suppressive treatment, and aggressive suppression of TSH places such patients at risk for iatrogenic hyperthyroidism.

Although the suggestion has been made that $T_3$ may be more effective than $T_4$ in reducing goiter size,[60] use of $T_4$ is preferable because $T_4$ has a long half-life and it does not lead to the transient episodes of elevated circulating $T_3$ levels that occur with daily $T_3$ therapy. TSH is suppressed in hypothyroid patients by 1.8 μg/kg body weight per day, and by 2.2 to 2.5 μg/kg per day in thyroid cancer patients.[61] Although a definitive study of the suppressibility by $T_4$ of TSH in nontoxic goiter patients using a sensitive TSH assay has not been conducted, a dose of 2 to 2.5 μg/kg per day suffices in these patients.

Avoidance of overtreatment with exogenous thyroid hormone is desirable, particularly in the elderly. The increasing availability of sensitive TSH assays that readily distinguish between suppressed and normal levels of TSH should help in determining the lowest suppressive dose of $T_4$.[62] The risk of bone demineralization in the course of $T_4$ administration to suppress endogenous TSH secretion has been widely discussed, although its clinical impact, particularly in the setting of treatment of nontoxic goiter, is not clear.[63] Another apparent complication of long-term $T_4$ treatment of nontoxic goiter patients may be increased left ventricular cardiac mass and diastolic dysfunction.[64] The frequency and significance of these echocardiographic findings have not yet been determined. Autonomous nodular goiter should not be treated with $T_4$; the additional hormonal load may result in clinical hyperthyroidism.

In clinically euthyroid patients with goiter whose serum $T_4$ levels are in the lower 25% of the normal range and whose serum TSH concentrations are moderately elevated, hypothyroidism is incipient (subclinical hypothyroidism) and should be managed expectantly with replacement doses of $T_4$ (<0.10 to 0.15 mg per day).[65] A distinction is made here between *replacement* therapy and *suppressive* therapy. The latter is intended to remove the thyroid gland from the influence of endogenous TSH and to raise serum $T_4$ levels to the normal range but above the pretreatment level. However, in incipient hypothyroidism with goiter, the intent is to raise the low serum thyroid hormone levels to the patient's normal range and to normalize serum TSH levels. The first .025-mg (25-µg) increment (at 2- to 4-week intervals) of daily $T_4$ replacement that normalizes serum TSH defines full replacement.[65–67]

The risk of occurrence of carcinoma in nontoxic goiter appears to be low. Suppression of endogenous TSH reduces the possibility even further. TSH is a permissive factor in the emergence of thyroid cancer, particularly, papillary carcinoma.[68] The suppression of endogenous TSH in patients who have had prior head-and-neck irradiation has been presumed to reduce the risk of the emergence of thyroid cancer. However, patients who develop palpable abnormalities of the thyroid after irradiation should undergo thyroidectomy.[69]

Interest is increasing in the management of sporadic nontoxic goiter in older patients with [131]I. In one study, 27 patients who received 507–3700 MBq of [131]I experienced a mean reduction in thyroid gland volume of 34% 1 year posttreatment.[70] A review of multiple studies of this strategy confirmed the 1-year success rate and concluded that a 50% to 60% reduction in gland volume was achieved by 3 to 5 years after isotope administration.[71] Estimates of the volume changes of the thyroid gland in such studies have been made ultrasonographically and with magnetic resonance imaging. The complications of this approach include hypothyroidism (20% to 30% incidence at 5 years after treatment) and radiation thyroiditis shortly after treatment. Radiation thyroiditis may be associated with transient hyperthyroidism. The risk of fatal and nonfatal thyroid cancer is also present but has not been precisely established. Thus, the approach is not endorsed in younger patients. A particularly interesting, but infrequent, complication of [131]I treatment of nontoxic goiter is transient Graves-like hyperthyroidism associated with circulating levels of TSH receptor antibody.[72] This syndrome appears to be distinct from radiation thyroiditis–related release of stored thyroid hormone from the gland, but measurement of anti-TPO titers before [131]I administration appeared to predict both radiation thyroiditis and hyperthyroidism associated with TSH receptor antibody.

Large nontoxic goiters may induce substantial local symptoms and may be cosmetically unacceptable. In long-standing goiters of large size, fibrosis and hemorrhage may significantly reduce the amount of TSH-responsive glandular epithelium. Hence, in these patients, the suppression of endogenous TSH with exogenous thyroid hormone has little effect on gland size. Similarly, attempts to reduce the size of large nontoxic goiters by [131]I ablation usually are disappointing, at least in cosmetic terms. For radioablation to succeed, residual glandular epithelium must comprise a significant proportion of the goiter. Treatment of large nontoxic goiters with [131]I can relieve tracheal

**TABLE 38-3.**
**Clinical Features of Patients with Substernal Goiter**

| Feature | Incidence |
|---|---|
| Age at diagnosis | Sixth decade |
| Female/male ratio | 1.6:1 to 3.2:1 |
| Symptoms | |
| Dysphagia | 30% |
| Dyspnea | 35% |
| Hoarseness | 8% |
| None | 15–50% |
| Enlarged cervical thyroid | 90% |
| Euthyroid metabolic state | 95% |
| Radiologic findings | |
| Tracheal deviation | 80% |
| Soft-tissue mass | 56% |
| Pathology | |
| Multinodular goiter | 50% |
| Follicular adenoma | 40% |
| Hashimoto thyroiditis | 5% |
| Papillary carcinoma | 2–16% |

(Data summarized from Katlic MR, Wang CA, Grillo HC. Substernal goiter. Ann Thorac Surg 1985; 39:391; Katlic MR, Grillo HC, Wang CA. Substernal goiter: analysis of 80 patients from Massachusetts General Hospital. Am J Surg 1985; 149:283; Allo MD, Thompson NW. Rationale for the operative management of substernal goiters. Surgery 1983; 94:969; and Davis PJ, Davis FB. Hyperthyroidism in patients over the age of 60 years: clinical features in 85 patients. Medicine [Baltimore] 1974; 53:161.)

compression,[71] as confirmed by magnetic resonance imaging; this may be the case even when the extent of gland shrinkage in a large goiter is only 5% to 10%.[73]

Large goiters accompanied by substantial local symptoms or unacceptable cosmesis should usually be treated surgically. Surgery may be difficult if a large and vascular goiter has involved vital structures in the neck. The incidence of tracheomalacia in large goiters has been overemphasized. When it does occur, however, it is a life-threatening complication and must be promptly managed with tracheal intubation or tracheotomy. Long-term serial measurement of serum thyroglobulin in one surgical series predicted growth activity of thyroid remnants in patients who had undergone resection of nontoxic goiter.[74]

## SUBSTERNAL GOITER

Substernal goiter refers to thyroidal enlargement, the major portion of which is inferior to the thoracic inlet.[75] Most substernal goiters are contiguous with an enlarged cervical thyroid; only very rarely is ectopic goitrous thyroid found in the mediastinum in the absence of cervical thyroid tissue. The clinical features of substernal goiter are summarized in Table 38-3 and illustrated in Figure 38-2. It most often occurs in older women and is frequently asymptomatic, in which case it appears on routine chest radiographs as a tracheal deviation or as a right paratracheal soft-tissue mass. Symptomatic substernal goiter may be associated with dyspnea or dysphagia. The severity of dyspnea may not correlate well with objective measurements of airway patency by flow-loop studies. Occasionally, superior vena caval obstruction may result from a substernal goiter.[76] Patients with substernal goiter are usually euthyroid[77] but occasionally are thyrotoxic.[41] The mediastinal extent of goiter may be demonstrated by radionuclide study or by computed tomography (see Fig. 38-2).

The management of large substernal goiter is surgical. Virtually all such goiters may be removed through a standard cervical collar incision without a sternotomy.[78] Ablative radioactive iodine administration offers little to the euthyroid patient with substernal goiter. Therapy with L-thyroxine to suppress endogenous TSH may prevent further gland enlargement but does not reduce gland size, except in the very rare patient with hypothyroidism.

An important issue in the therapy of substernal goiter is the role and timing of surgery. Symptomatic patients and those with known tracheal, esophageal, or vena caval encroachment by the goiter are candidates for early surgery. The surgical literature indicates some bias for routine surgical excision of all substernal goiters because of the small risk of progression of the lesion to significant airway obstruction and because of a variable risk of there being cancer in the gland,[77,78] compounded by the inaccessibility of the gland to diagnostic needle aspiration. Surgical removal of substernal goiter through a cervical collar incision has an extraordinarily low complication rate when performed by experienced surgeons.[78,79] However, in otherwise healthy patients in the sixth and seventh decades of life, such surgery is recommended only when computed tomography or flow-loop studies indicate the presence of significant tracheal narrowing.

# REFERENCES

1. Peterson S, Sanga A, Eklöf H, et al. Classification of thyroid size by palpation and ultrasonography in field surveys. Lancet 2000; 355:106.
1a. Matovinovic J. Endemic goiter and cretinism at the dawn of the third millennium. Annu Rev Nutr 1983; 3:341.
2. Vander JB, Gaston EA, Dawber TR. The significance of nontoxic thyroid nodules. Ann Intern Med 1968; 69:537.
3. Toft AD, Irvine WJ, Hunter WM. A comparison of plasma TSH levels in patients with diffuse and nodular non-toxic goiter. J Clin Endocrinol Metab 1976; 42:973.
4. Bregengard C, Kirkegaard C, Faber J, et al. Relationships between serum thyrotropin, serum free thyroxine (T₄), and 3,5,3′-triiodothyronine (T₃) and the daily T₄ and T₃ production rates in euthyroid patients with multinodular goiter. J Clin Endocrinol Metab 1987; 65:258.
5. Romelli F, Stoder H, Bruggisser D. Pathogenesis of thyroid nodules in multinodular goiter. Am J Pathol 1982; 109:215.
6. Peter HJ, Studer H, Forster R, Gerber H. The pathogenesis of "hot" and "cold" follicles in multinodular goiters. J Clin Endocrinol Metab 1982; 55:941.
7. Niepomniszcze H, Altschuler N, Korob MH, Degrossi OJ. Iodide-peroxidase activity in human thyroid: I. Studies on non-toxic nodular goiter. Acta Endocrinol (Copenh) 1969; 62:193.
8. Field JB, Larsen PR, Yamashita K, et al. Demonstration of iodide transport defect but normal iodide organification in nonfunctioning nodules of human thyroid glands. J Clin Invest 1973; 52:2404.
9. Sugenoya A, Yamada Y, Kaneko G, et al. In vitro study on release of thyroid hormone in solitary autonomously functioning thyroid nodules using cell culture method. Endocrinol Jpn 1984; 31:749.
10. Gheri RG, Berrelli D, Cicchi P, et al. Thyroxine and triiodothyronine levels in thyroid vein blood and in thyroid tissue of patients with autonomous adenomas. Clin Endocrinol (Oxf) 1981; 15:485.
11. Toccafondi R, Rotella CM, Tanini A, et al. Effects of TSH on cAMP levels and thyroid hormone release in human thyroid "autonomous" nodules: relationship with iodothyronine and iodine content in thyroglobulin. Clin Endocrinol (Oxf) 1982; 17:537.
12. Thomas CG Jr, Combest W, McQuade R, et al. Biological characteristics of adenomatous nodules, adenomas, and hyperfunctioning nodules as defined by adenylate cyclase activity and TSH receptors. World J Surg 1984; 8:445.
12a. Schuppert F, Ehrenthal D, Frilling A, et al. Increased major histocompatibility complex (MHC) expression in nontoxic goiters. J Clin Endocrinol Metab 2000; 85:858.
13. Cooper DS, Ridgway EC, Maloof F. Unusual types of hyperthyroidism. Clin Endocrinol Metab 1978; 7:199.
14. Drexhage HA, Bolcazzo GF, Doniach D, et al. Evidence for thyroid growth stimulating immunoglobulins in some goitrous thyroid diseases. Lancet 1980; 2:287.
15. van der Gaag RD, Drexhage HA, Wiersinga WM, et al. Further studies on thyroid growth-stimulating immunoglobulins in euthyroid nonendemic goiter. J Clin Endocrinol Metab 1985; 60:972.
16. Aguayo J, Sakatsume Y, Jamieson C, et al. Nontoxic nodular goiter and papillary thyroid carcinoma are not associated with peripheral blood lymphocyte sensitization to thyroid cells. J Clin Endocrinol Metab 1989; 68:145.
17. Minuto F, Barreca A, Del Monte P, et al. Immunoreactive insulin-like growth factor I (IGF-I) and IGF-I binding protein content in human thyroid tissue. J Clin Endocrinol Metab 1989; 68:621.
18. Grubeck-Loebenstein B, Buchan G, Sadeghi R, et al. Transforming growth factor β regulates thyroid growth. Role in the pathogenesis of nontoxic goiter. J Clin Invest 1989; 83:764.
19. Smyth PPA, Neylan D, O'Donovan DK. The prevalence of thyroid-stimulating antibodies in goitrous disease assessed by cytochemical section bioassay. J Clin Endocrinol Metab 1982; 54:357.
20. Valente WA, Vitti P, Rotella CM, et al. Antibodies that promote thyroid growth: a distinct population of thyroid-stimulating autoantibodies. N Engl J Med 1983; 309:1028.
21. Rapoport B, Greenspan FS, Filetti S, Pepitone M. Clinical experience with a human thyroid cell bioassay for thyroid-stimulating immunoglobulin. J Clin Endocrinol Metab 1984; 58:332.
22. Etienne Decerf J, Winand RJ. A sensitive technique for determination of thyroid-stimulating immunoglobulin (TSI) in unfractionated serum. Clin Endocrinol (Oxf) 1981; 14:83.
23. Vitti P, Chiovato L, Tonacchera M, et al. Failure to detect thyroid growth-promoting activity in immunoglobulin G of patients with endemic goiter. J Clin Endocrinol Metab 1994; 78:1020.
24. Comite F, Burrow GN, Jorgensen EC. Thyroid hormone analogs and fetal goiter. Endocrinology 1978; 102:1670.
25. Henneman G. Non-toxic goiter. Clin Endocrinol Metab 1979; 8:167.
26. Oddie TH, Fisher DH, McConahey WM, Thompson CS. Iodine intake in the United States: a reassessment. J Clin Endocrinol Metab 1970; 30:659.
27. Kelly FC, Snedden WW. Prevalence and geographic distribution of endemic goitre. In: Endemic goitre. Monograph series no. 44. Geneva: World Health Organization, 1960:27.
28. Stanbury JB, Kroc RL, eds. Human development and the thyroid gland. Adv Exp Med Biol 1972; 30:3.
29. Langer P, Greer MA. Antithyroid substances and naturally occurring goitrogens. Basel: S Karger, 1977:79.
30. Agerboek H. Non-toxic goitre: the role of iodine deficiency in goitre formation in a non-endemic area. Acta Endocrinol (Copenh) 1974; 76:74.
31. Braverman LE, Woeber KA, Ingbar SH. Induction of myxedema by iodide in patients euthyroid after radioiodine or surgical treatment of diffuse toxic goiter. N Engl J Med 1969; 281:816.
32. Vagenakis AG, Wang C, Burger A, et al. Iodide-induced thyrotoxicosis in Boston. N Engl J Med 1972; 287:523.
33. Wartofsky L, Ransil BJ, Ingbar SH. Inhibition by iodine of release of thyroxine from the thyroid glands of patients with thyrotoxicosis. J Clin Invest 1970; 49:78.
34. Braverman LE. Therapeutic considerations. Clin Endocrinol Metab 1978; 7:221.
35. Rallison MI, Kumagai LF, Tyler FH. Goitrous hypothyroidism induced by aminoglutethimide, anticonvulsant drug. J Clin Endocrinol Metab 1967; 27:265.
36. Spaulding SW, Burrow GN, Bermudez F, Himmelhoch JM. The inhibitory effect of lithium on thyroid hormone release in both euthyroid and thyrotoxic patients. J Clin Endocrinol Metab 1972; 35:905.
37. Singh BN, Nademanee K. Amiodarone and thyroid function: clinical implications during antiarrhythmic therapy. Am Heart J 1983; 106:857.
38. Day TK, Powell-Jackson PR. Fluoride, water hardness, and endemic goitre. Lancet 1972; 1:1135.
39. Brown J, Solomon DH. Effects of tolbutamide and carbutamide on thyroid function. Metabolism 1956; 5:813.
40. Martino E, Placidi GF, Sardano G, et al. High incidence of goiter in patients treated with lithium carbonate. Ann Endocrinol (Paris) 1982; 43:269.
41. Davis PJ, Davis FB. Hyperthyroidism in patients over the age of 60 years: clinical features in 85 patients. Medicine (Baltimore) 1974; 53:161.
42. Borup Christensen S, Ericsson U-B, Janzon L, et al. Influence of cigarette smoking on goiter formation, thyroglobulin, and thyroid hormone levels in women. J Clin Endocrinol Metab 1984; 58:615.
43. Spector DA, Davis PJ, Helderman JH, et al. Thyroid function and metabolic state in chronic renal failure. Ann Intern Med 1976; 85:724.
44. Favus MJ, Schneider AB, Stachura ME, et al. Thyroid cancer occurring as a late consequence of head-and-neck irradiation. N Engl J Med 1976; 294:1019.
45. Ivy HK. Cancer metastatic to the thyroid: a diagnostic problem. Mayo Clin Proc 1984; 59:856.
46. Hazard JB. Thyroiditis: a review. Am J Clin Pathol 1955; 25:289.
47. Glinoer D, Verelst J, Ham HR. Abnormalities of esophageal transit in patients with sporadic nontoxic goiter. Eur J Nucl Med 1987; 13:239.
48. Strakosch CR, Wenzel BE, Row VV, Volpe R. Immunology of autoimmune thyroid diseases. N Engl J Med 1982; 307:1499.
49. Levine GA, Hershman JM, Van Herle AJ, et al. Thyroglobulin and calcitonin in patients with nontoxic goiter. JAMA 1978; 240:2282.
50. Tani EM, Skoog L, Lowhagen T. Clinical utility of fine needle aspiration cytology of the thyroid. Annu Rev Med 1988; 39:255.
51. Jauregui R, Lilker ES, Bayley A. Upper airway obstruction in euthyroid goiter. JAMA 1977; 238:2163.
52. Silverstein GE, Burke G, Cogan R. The natural history of the autonomous hyperfunctioning thyroid nodule. Ann Intern Med 1967; 67:539.
53. Berghout A, Wiersinga WM, Smits NJ, Touber JL. Interrelationships between age, thyroid volume, thyroid nodularity and thyroid function in patients with sporadic nontoxic goiter. Am J Med 1990; 89:602.
54. Refetoff S, Harrison J, Karanfilski BT, et al. Continuing occurrence of thyroid carcinoma after irradiation to the neck in infancy and childhood. N Engl J Med 1975; 292:171.
55. Wiersinga WM. Determinants of outcome in sporadic nontoxic goiter. Thyroidol Clin Exp 1992; 4:41.
56. Faber J, Perrild H, Johansen JS. Bone Gla protein and sex hormone–binding globulin in nontoxic goiter: parameters for metabolic status at the tissue level. J Clin Endocrinol Metab 1990; 70:49.
57. Sawin CT, Geller A, Wolf PA, et al. Low serum thyrotropin concentrations as a risk factor for atrial fibrillation in older persons. N Engl J Med 1994; 331:1249.
58. Astwood EB, Cassidy CE, Aurbach GD. Treatment of goiter and thyroid nodules with thyroid. JAMA 1960; 174:459.

59. Ross DS. Thyroid hormone suppressive therapy of sporadic nontoxic goiter. Thyroid 1992; 2:263.
60. Shimaoka K, Sokal JE. Suppressive therapy of nontoxic goiter. Am J Med 1974; 57:576.
61. Burmeister LA, Goumaz MO, Mariash CN, Oppenheimer JH. Levothyroxine dose requirements for thyrotropin suppression in the treatment of differentiated thyroid cancer. J Clin Endocrinol Metab 1992; 75:344.
62. Spencer CA, LoPresti JS, Patel A, et al. Applications of a new chemiluminometric thyrotropin assay to subnormal measurement. J Clin Endocrinol Metab 1990; 70:453.
63. Müller CG, Bayley TA, Harrison JE, Tsang R. Possible limited bone loss with suppressive thyroxine therapy is unlikely to have clinical relevance. Thyroid 1995; 5:81.
64. Fazio S, Biondi B, Carella C, et al. Diastolic dysfunction in patients on thyroid-stimulating hormone suppressive therapy with levothyroxine: beneficial effect of beta-blockade. J Clin Endocrinol Metab 1995; 80:2222.
65. Davis FB, LaMantia RS, Spaulding SW, et al. Estimation of a physiologic replacement dose of levothyroxine in elderly patients with hypothyroidism. Arch Intern Med 1984; 144:1752.
66. Hennessey JV, Evaul JE, Tseng Y-C, et al. L-thyroxine dosage: a reevaluation of therapy with contemporary preparations. Ann Intern Med 1986; 105:11.
67. Wartofsky L. Diffuse nontoxic and multinodular goiter. In: Current therapy in endocrinology and metabolism 1985–1986. Toronto: BC Decker, 1986:75.
68. Rojeski MT, Gharib H. Nodular thyroid disease: evaluation and management. N Engl J Med 1985; 313:428.
69. McConahey WM, Hayles AB. Radiation and thyroid neoplasia. Ann Intern Med 1976; 84:749.
70. deKlerk JM, van Isselt JW, van Kijk A, et al. Iodine-131 therapy in sporadic nontoxic goiter. J Nucl Med 1997; 38:372.
71. Huysmans D, Hermus A, Edelbroek M, et al. Radioiodine for nontoxic multinodular goiter. Thyroid 1997; 7:235.
72. Nygaard B, Knudsen JH, Hegedus L, et al. Thyrotropin receptor antibodies and Graves' disease, a side effect of $^{131}$I treatment in patients with nontoxic goiter. J Clin Endocrinol Metab 1997; 82:2926.
73. Kay TWH, d'Eurden MC, Andrews JT, Martin FR. Treatment of nontoxic multinodular goiter with radioactive iodine. Am J Med 1988; 84:19.
74. Date J, Feldt-Rasmussen U, Blichert-Toft M, et al. Long-term observation of serum thyroglobulin after resection of nontoxic goiter and relation to ultrasonographically demonstrated relapse. World J Surg 1996; 20:351.
75. Katlic MR, Wang CA, Grillo HC. Substernal goiter. Ann Thorac Surg 1985; 39:391.
76. McKellar DP, Verazin GT, Lim KM, et al. Superior vena cava syndrome and tracheal obstruction due to multinodular goiter. Head Neck 1994; 16:72.
77. Allo MD, Thompson NW. Rationale for the operative management of substernal goiters. Surgery 1983; 94:969.
78. Katlic MR, Grillo HC, Wang CA. Substernal goiter: analysis of 80 patients from Massachusetts General Hospital. Am J Surg 1985; 149:283.
79. Melliere D, Saada F, Etienne G, et al. Goiter with severe respiratory compromise: evaluation and treatment. Surgery 1988; 103:367.

# CHAPTER 39

# THE THYROID NODULE

LEONARD WARTOFSKY AND ANDREW J. AHMANN

The clinical management of nodular thyroid disease is controversial.[1–12] The finding of a thyroid nodule poses considerable anxiety for patient and physician alike, despite the modest probability of malignancy and the likelihood that a tumor, if present, will follow a relatively benign course. In the evaluation of thyroid nodules, the physician has the opportunity to use a growing number of diagnostic tools, no single one of which provides the desired accuracy in identifying all cases of carcinoma requiring surgical intervention. Some consensus has been reached, however, on guidelines for the diagnosis and management of thyroid nodules.[13]

## PREVALENCE OF THYROID NODULES

The prevalence of thyroid nodules must be considered from several perspectives. As many as 1.5% of adolescents may have

**TABLE 39-1.**
**Differential Diagnosis of Apparent Thyroid Nodules**

**BENIGN THYROID NEOPLASMS**
Follicular adenoma
Colloid (macrofollicular)
Simple
Fetal (microfollicular)
Embryonal (trabecular)
Hürthle cell
Papillary adenoma (?)
Teratoma
Lipoma
Dermoid cyst
**MALIGNANT THYROID NEOPLASMS**
Papillary carcinoma
Follicular carcinoma
Medullary thyroid carcinoma
Anaplastic carcinoma
Metastatic carcinoma
Sarcoma
Lymphoma
**OTHER THYROID ABNORMALITIES**
Thyroiditis
Thyroid cyst
Hemiagenesis of thyroid
Infection
Granulomatous disease (e.g., sarcoidosis)
**NONTHYROID LESIONS**
Lymphadenopathy
Aneurysm
Thyroglossal duct cyst
Parathyroid cyst
Parathyroid adenoma
Laryngocele
Cystic hygroma

palpable thyroid nodules, and the frequency increases linearly with age.[11] In large population studies, nodules have been reported in 3% to 7% of adults, with a 5:1 female/male ratio. Many of these reports have failed to distinguish *solitary* nodules from *multiple* thyroid nodules; on histologic examination, many single, palpable nodules are found to be within a multinodular thyroid gland. Some autopsy series report thyroid nodules in more than one-half of consecutive cases, although many may be small, nonpalpable lesions, and multinodularity occurs in up to 75% of these.[1,3,4] High-resolution ultrasonography has identified nodules in 13% to 40% of patients undergoing evaluation for nonthyroidal problems.[14–17] Thus, a discrepancy exists between the true prevalence of thyroid nodules and the number that are apparent by physical examination. Normally, nodules must approach 1 cm in diameter to be consistently recognized on palpation, although this size varies according to the location of the nodule within the gland and the anatomy of the neck. Nonpalpable nodules, such as those incidentally seen on ultrasonographic studies for nonthyroidal neck evaluation, are of unknown clinical significance.

## DIFFERENTIAL DIAGNOSIS OF THYROID NODULES

The differential diagnosis of apparent thyroid nodules covers a wide range of pathology[1–5] (Table 39-1). The usual diagnostic challenge is to distinguish malignant from benign lesions. Most true intrathyroidal nodules are colloid adenomas (27–60%) or simple follicular adenomas (26–40%), although fully reliable figures are not available.[18] Follicular adenomas introduce significant uncertainty in the diagnosis and treatment because no available measures short of surgical resection with detailed histologic examination allow the separation of well-differentiated follicular carcinomas from adenomas. Instead, the distinction depends on the presence or absence of capsular or vascular invasion by the tumor; cellular detail is of little value.[19] Hürthle cell tumors are a subset of follicular lesions composed of oval to polygonal cells with dense, granular, acidophilic cytoplasm and a prominent macronucleolus. The malignant potential of histologically benign Hürthle cell tumors and the natural history of Hürthle cell malignancies continue to be subjects of controversy.[20,21]

Although the functional activity of thyroid adenomas varies, most appear to have defects in the iodine symporter resulting in reduced iodide accumulation and/or organification; this may be demonstrated by reduced trapping of radionuclide, leading to the designation of "cold" nodules. Five percent to 15% of thyroid nodules are classified as "hot" on the basis of a relatively increased ability to trap iodide. Most of these hot nodules are autonomously functioning (see Chaps. 34 and 42). The patients are usually clinically euthyroid, although more than one-half of those older than 60 years of age may be hyperthyroid. Whether or not hyperthyroidism is present is related to the size of the hyperfunctioning nodules. Nodules >3 cm in diameter are associated with hyperthyroidism in 20% of cases, whereas <2% of smaller lesions produce a toxic state.[22,23] The thyrotoxicosis associated with a hot nodule may be transient, arising from acute hemorrhage, or, more commonly, after exposure to a high iodine load (see Chap. 37). Although most toxic, autonomous nodules secrete both thyroxine ($T_4$) and triiodothyronine ($T_3$), occasionally they may elevate serum $T_3$ alone or, rarely, serum $T_4$ alone. Moreover, even when levels of circulating thyroid hormones are normal, a blunted response of thyroid-stimulating hormone (TSH) to thyrotropin-releasing hormone (TRH) stimulation is common, suggesting supraphysiologic iodothyronine production. Progression to a relatively mild toxic state is usually insidious. Autonomous adenomas have no unique histologic characteristics. Clinically, the functional distinction is important because of the natural history of these nodules: hot nodules have a much lower malignancy potential than hypofunctioning lesions. Constitutive activating mutations of the TSH receptor gene have been identified as the probable basis for many hot nodules.[24–27]

The absence of function in a thyroid nodule should arouse a greater suspicion of cancer. More than 60% of malignant lesions of the thyroid are papillary carcinomas, with follicular and anaplastic lesions being the next most common histologic types (see Chap. 40). Medullary thyroid carcinomas[28,29] account for 5% of malignant thyroid nodules, and other categories represent <5% of such nodules.[3,7] A cold thyroid nodule occasionally represents metastasis. The malignancies most likely to metastasize to the thyroid are malignant melanoma, bronchogenic carcinoma, renal cell carcinoma, breast carcinoma, and lymphoma. Presently, ~17,200 new thyroid cancer cases are diagnosed annually in the United States, and 1200 thyroid cancer–related deaths occur.[30] Although the probability at birth of eventually dying from thyroid cancer is <0.1%, the management of potentially malignant thyroid nodules may lead to 50,000 thyroid operations yearly. Studies have revealed occult thyroid cancer in 6% of autopsy cases in North American series; clinically significant cancers are found in 10% to 14% of patients with palpable thyroid nodules, and the incidence has increased in the past 50 years.[1,3,7] As with benign nodules and many other thyroid diseases, thyroid cancer is more common in women than in men; however, among men with nodules, the probability of cancer is higher. The incidence of thyroid cancer increases with age, but a greater percentage of nodules in patients younger than 20 years of age represents malignancy.[31–33] Although data are conflicting on the increased risk of malignancy in new nodules in patients older than 60 years of age, the incidence of anaplastic carcinoma is higher in this group.

# IRRADIATION-RELATED THYROID NEOPLASIA

Many causative factors in the development of thyroid nodules, especially thyroid carcinomas, are uncertain. One undisputed factor, however, is radiation exposure. Animal studies have consistently confirmed radiation induction of thyroid neoplasia, which can be further promoted by TSH. By 1950, many children with thyroid carcinoma were known previously to have received radiation to the neck as treatment for benign conditions, including enlarged thymus, chronic tonsillitis, acne, and cervical adenitis. Numerous studies have now confirmed a linear relationship between radiation dose (for doses up to 1500 rad) and the incidence of thyroid nodules and thyroid cancer.

Some 40 million Ci of iodine-131 ($^{131}$I) and another 100 million Ci of shorter-lived isotopes of iodine were released into the atmosphere by the nuclear reactor accident at Chernobyl in the Belarus in April 1986. The number of new cases of thyroid cancer appearing in patients who were exposed to the fallout as young children in 1986 has shown a dramatic increase between 1989 and the present.[34,35] Similar associations were demonstrated for radioactive fallout after the World War II experience in Japan and the atomic test explosions in the Marshall Islands. Nasopharyngeal radium implants appear to add little risk of cancer.

Childhood radiation exposure is more likely to produce thyroid neoplasms than similar exposure at a later age, possibly because of greater cellular mitotic activity at the earlier age. In the United States, palpable nodules are found in 16% to 29% of persons who received low-dose head and neck irradiation in childhood, and carcinoma is found in one-third of these patients with nodules.[36] Lesions can occur within several years of exposure, but the peak incidence after external radiation exposure for both benign and malignant nodules occurs after a latency period of 20 to 30 years, and the risk may exist for more than 35 years. Approximately 85% of radiation-induced cancers are pure papillary or papillary-follicular lesions and have a favorable prognosis; anaplastic lesions are rare. At least one-third of the carcinomas associated with earlier irradiation to the head and neck are <1 cm in diameter. The lymph nodes are involved in 25% to 30% of patients, including many with nonpalpable primary lesions. The irradiated thyroid gland often presents with multiple nodules, and at surgery, the lesion of initial concern may prove to be benign, whereas one or more carcinomas may be found elsewhere in the gland. Thus, multicentricity is common, and most cancers coexist with benign adenomas. Contrary to usual circumstances, those nodules associated with previous radiation therapy do not demonstrate a marked reduction in cancer risk when the thyroid contains multiple nodules. The thyroid cancers seen after the Chernobyl accident have appeared after a much shorter latency period, but they, too, were largely papillary in nature.

The consequences of high-dose external head and neck irradiation (>2000 rad) are not well defined because of relatively short follow-up in reported series. Although low-dose irradiation does not produce hypothyroidism, larger doses, such as those used for Hodgkin disease, are associated with a high rate of thyroid dysfunction, as manifested by elevated serum TSH levels, with or without hypothyroxinemia.[37] Despite a postulated inducer effect of elevated TSH levels, and despite some reports of nodular thyroid disease, including carcinoma, in patients who have received high-dose irradiation, no definitive evidence exists of an increased incidence of carcinoma in this group. Consideration of isodose curves, penumbra effect, backscatter, and specifics of the employed field suggests that in many of the reported cases thyroid lesions occurring after higher dose radiation therapy actually have been associated with low-dose exposure of the thyroid.[38]

As with high-dose external irradiation, $^{131}$I therapy does not appear to be causally related to subsequent thyroid carcinoma.

In both cases, the high-dose thyroid exposure with attendant cell destruction, fibrosis, and hypothyroidism may serve to attenuate any carcinogenic effect.

# DIAGNOSTIC EVALUATION OF THE THYROID NODULE

Because most thyroid nodule morbidity is related to cancerous lesions, clinical evaluation focuses on the identification of malignant nodules. Numerous methods have evolved to better define the probability of cancer in a given lesion.

## HISTORY AND PHYSICAL EXAMINATION

The single most important historical risk factor for cancer is irradiation. The age at exposure, the type and site of therapy, and, if possible, the radiation dose to the thyroid should be determined. A family history of pheochromocytoma, hypercalcemia, mucosal abnormalities, or medullary thyroid carcinoma should raise suspicion of the latter diagnosis as part of the multiple endocrine neoplasia syndrome (see Chap. 188). A family history of benign goiter may be reassuring, although the rare Pendred syndrome (familial goiter and deaf-mutism) is associated with a higher cancer risk.[1,3] Nodules in men are more likely to be malignant than those in women; nodules in children are more likely to be malignant than those in adults. The diagnosis of thyroid lymphoma should be considered in patients with a previous diagnosis of Hashimoto thyroiditis, especially in women older than 50 years of age.

The following clinical findings are thought to be more common in malignant than benign nodules: a history of radiation therapy, a family history of multiple endocrine neoplasia type 2A or 2B, rapid growth, hoarseness, pain, dysphagia, respiratory obstructive symptoms, and growth of the nodule despite $T_4$ medication; and physical examination findings of cervical lymphadenopathy, firmness, documented nodule growth, vocal cord paralysis, fixation, and Horner syndrome. In general, signs and symptoms alone are not sufficiently sensitive or specific to allow selection of candidates for surgery. However, patients with advanced disease may present with lymphadenopathy, recent growth of hard nodules, and vocal cord paralysis, all of which suggest malignancy; the presence of obstructive symptoms is less reliable.[1,39] As indicated, identification of a single nodule renders the patient at higher risk than does multinodularity.[40]

## LABORATORY TESTS

The commonly used blood thyroid function tests often are of limited value in the evaluation of thyroid nodules. Functional thyroid parameters, including serum $T_3$ and $T_4$ or TRH stimulation (see Chaps. 15 and 33) are useful in evaluating possible toxic adenomas. Thyroglobulin levels may be elevated in patients with thyroid malignancy but do not differentiate malignant adenomas from benign adenomas or from thyroiditis.[41,42] Serum levels of antithyroglobulin and antimicrosomal antibodies also are of limited value.[1,3] An increased basal plasma calcitonin level is reasonably sensitive and specific for medullary thyroid carcinoma in the setting of a thyroid nodule, although abnormal calcium and pentagastrin stimulation tests or detection of mutations in the *ret* protooncogene provide the greatest sensitivity[43] (see Chaps. 40, 53, and 188). In one large series, an elevated plasma calcitonin level was found in 0.5% of all patients with thyroid nodules and in 15.7% of those with thyroid carcinomas, a finding that led the authors to recommend routine measurement in the evaluation of thyroid nodules.[44] Serum carcinoembryonic antigen levels are also elevated in most patients with medullary thyroid carcinoma, but they may be increased in patients with other thyroid carcinomas as well.[1,4,7,45] None of these tests intended to detect medullary thyroid carcinoma is cost-effective for the initial evaluation of the nodular thyroid.

## THYROID SCANNING

### RADIONUCLIDE UPTAKE

Based on the pattern of radionuclide uptake (see Chap. 34), nodules may be classified as hot (hyperfunctioning) or cold. Hyperfunctioning nodules rarely represent malignancy, nondelineated or hypofunctioning lesions carry an intermediate risk, and nonfunctioning (cold) nodules have the highest risk.[2,4,7] More than 80% of nonfunctioning nodules, however, still represent benign pathology. Therefore, radioisotope scans are of low diagnostic specificity despite their high sensitivity for nodules >1 cm in diameter. Scanning usually is done with iodine-123 ($^{123}$I) or technetium-99m ($^{99m}$Tc) pertechnetate. Despite some limitations, the advantages of low radiation dose, low cost, short scanning time, and reliability have led to the wide use of $^{99m}$Tc. $^{123}$I also delivers low radiation and is the preferred iodine-scanning agent. In addition to functional information, scans may reveal multinodularity in up to one-third of clinically palpable solitary lesions, a finding that decreases the likelihood of malignancy. Nuclear imaging with radioiodine and other isotopes plays an important role in the follow-up evaluation and treatment of patients proven to have thyroid cancer.[46]

### FLUORESCENT THYROID SCANNING

Fluorescent thyroid scanning uses americium-241, which can excite thyroidal iodine, causing the release of x-rays; this release correlates quantitatively with iodine content of the imaged tissue. Fluorescent scanning is rapid and provides minimal radiation exposure, thereby offering special advantages for children and pregnant women. The procedure is nearly 100% sensitive but only 64% specific when areas of low iodine content are taken as positive results. However, a large series has indicated that the converse analysis may be more reliable because areas with an iodine content ratio above 0.60 yielded 63% sensitivity and 99% specificity for benign lesions.[47] Unfortunately, the required equipment is not widely available, and accumulated data remain too limited for this technique to be used routinely.

The use of other radionuclides, including thallium-201, selenomethionine-75, gallium-67, and cesium-131, for differentiating benign from malignant lesions of the thyroid has been investigated. None of these has proved to be a reliable indicator of malignancy.

### OTHER THYROID IMAGING TECHNIQUES

**Radiography.** *Routine radiographic techniques* have long been used in an attempt to identify calcifications characteristic of malignancy, but they are of limited value. Shell-like calcifications are most typical of benign cysts, stippled (psammomatous) calcifications have high specificity for papillary carcinoma, and flocculent deposits are more characteristic of medullary carcinoma, but other descriptive terms of calcification have minimal predictive value.[1,2]

**Ultrasonography.** *Ultrasonography* is frequently used to evaluate the thyroid. Conventional ultrasonographic techniques are most valuable in differentiating solid from cystic lesions.[48] This differentiation is important because solid lesions have a higher malignant potential and require different therapy. However, cystic lesions larger than 4 cm in diameter may pose a significant cancer risk.[1] Modern high-resolution ultrasonography provides detailed information and can demonstrate lesions as small as 2 mm; this increased sensitivity has revealed that pure simple cysts are exceedingly rare because most cystic lesions contain some solid components.[49] Although high-resolution ultrasonography discloses multinodularity in up to 40%

of glands presumed to have a single palpable nodule, whether this "subclinical" multinodularity has the same favorable connotation as multinodularity detected with the less sensitive techniques of physical examination or radionuclide scanning is unclear (see Chap. 35). However, it does appear that the majority of small "incidentalomas" of the thyroid detected by high resolution ultrasonography are benign.[50]

Ultrasonography may be used for the following purposes: to differentiate solid from cystic nodules, to detect multinodularity, to detect occult thyroid malignancy in cases of metastatic cervical lymphadenopathy from an unknown primary, to monitor the size of a nodule (including any response to suppressive therapy), to differentiate solid from hemorrhagic expansion in fast-growing thyroid lesions, to guide needle biopsy in selected cases, to monitor irradiated thyroids, and to monitor the local recurrence of thyroid carcinoma. Unfortunately, the value of ultrasonography in specifically identifying malignancy is limited. Carcinomas are usually hypoechoic, but many adenomas have a similar echogenicity. The appearance of a 1- to 2-mm, decreased echogenic halo surrounding nodules strongly favors follicular adenoma as the diagnosis, but this also has been found in a few carcinomas.[49,51]

**Other Imaging Techniques.** Two other imaging techniques deserve mention. *Computed tomography* (CT) can provide descriptive information similar to that achieved with ultrasonography but offers no advantages except in cases of mediastinal extension.[51] CT is associated with high doses of ionizing radiation, is more expensive, and requires iodine contrast media for maximal visualization. Ultrasonography is preferable to CT as a thyroid imaging method in most cases. *Magnetic resonance imaging* of the thyroid does not require iodine contrast or involve radiation exposure and provides superior vascular imaging and substernal views as compared with CT, but both CT and magnetic resonance imaging are useful for substernal goiter and for both initial presentation and recurrence of thyroid malignancies (see Chap. 35). Use of a number of other isotopes and the technique of *positron emission tomography* scanning have been applied to the assessment of thyroid nodules and thyroid malignancies.[52,53]

## THYROID HORMONE SUPPRESSION

Thyroid hormone has been used for many years to reduce the size of thyroid lesions thought to be dependent on TSH stimulation. In using hormone administration as a diagnostic test for thyroid nodules, the assumption is that benign lesions will show preferential reduction in size. Typically, patients are given a 3- to 6-month trial of $T_4$ at a dose titrated to result in undetectable serum TSH in an ultrasensitive assay or unresponsiveness of TSH to TRH stimulation, but without induction of clinical hyperthyroidism. Continued growth of a nodule or lack of reduction in size during therapy increases the suspicion of malignancy. However, an absolute reduction in size sufficient to denote benignancy has not been determined, and various investigators have adopted different criteria for response, which renders the interpretation of results more difficult. A partial response to treatment is not particularly reassuring because of the possibility of inconsistency in palpated size and/or a misleading apparent reduction in size of a nodule due to regression of surrounding normal tissue. Seven percent to 16% of nonresponding lesions harbor carcinoma, and an occasional carcinoma has exhibited partial regression.[2] Largely uncontrolled studies have suggested that a complete response to suppressive therapy occurs in <10% of cases, whereas a 50% reduction in size is seen in ~30% of cases.[7] However, one double-blind controlled study found no significant difference in sonographically measured colloid nodule size reduction between a group of patients treated with suppressive doses of $T_4$ and those treated with placebo.[54] Although 21% of thyroid hormone–treated nodules decreased >30% in volume over 6 months, equivalent size reductions were noted in nodules in the placebo-treated group. Some confirmation of these findings was provided by the failure to observe significant shrinkage of nodules on $T_4$ therapy in two other studies.[55,56] On the other hand, other workers continue to suggest that suppressive therapy may shrink both nontoxic goiter[57] and thyroid nodules.[58–61]

One review of relevant studies on the efficacy of L-thyroxine in suppressing thyroid nodules concluded that therapy provided benefit for only 10% to 20% of lesions proven benign by fine-needle aspiration cytology.[9] Results of other studies suggest that the smaller lesions in younger patients are the ones that are more likely to shrink with suppression.[62,63] But in spite of decades of such therapy and numerous published reports, one can conclude that additional carefully controlled studies of large numbers of patients are required to clarify the management of thyroid nodules with suppression therapy.[10] The increasing concern about possible risk of osteopenia after long-term suppressive doses of thyroid hormone has been allayed somewhat by careful analyses of the data.[64] Use of prudent suppression doses of $T_4$ has not been shown to contribute to osteopenia.[65] Moreover, supplementation of $T_4$ with estrogen replacement in postmenopausal women may obviate any potential risk of osteopenia.[66,67]

Failure of suppression appears to minimally increase the probability of cancer, whereas successful suppression reduces the probability by ~25%.[7] An unusual category of lesions that may carry an exceptionally high risk of carcinoma comprises those that respond initially to thyroid hormone but later grow.[7] A trial of thyroid hormone suppression therapy alone is neither sensitive nor specific but may have utility as an adjunct to other modalities of evaluation. This therapy requires periodic and regular follow-up.

## THYROID NEEDLE ASPIRATION AND BIOPSY

Obtaining tissue or cells from a thyroid nodule by some form of biopsy technique is the best single method to identify malignancy.[68–70] Biopsies can be performed by fine-needle (22- to 27-gauge) aspiration (FNA), large-needle (16- to 18-gauge) aspiration, or cutting-needle biopsy (14-gauge Tru-Cut or Silverman needle). Most clinicians have found FNA to provide the highest incidence of successful samples and the lowest incidence of complications while yielding a diagnostic precision equal to or better than that of other methods.[2] This technique is shown in Figure 39-1. In selected large lesions for which FNA has failed to provide a satisfactory diagnosis, some other aspiration method may be used.

FNA has been popular in Europe for decades and now has attained similar acceptance in the United States. The ability to obtain adequate samples improves with experience, and the success rate approaches 95%. However, the collecting technique appears less critical than the ability of the pathologist to interpret the cytologic specimens correctly. Because of these two primary factors, this procedure is best limited to situations in which the operator and pathologist each have considerable experience.[71–73] Ultrasonography-guided FNA has proven a useful technique for biopsy of low-lying nodules or those that are detected by ultrasonography but are difficult to palpate.[74,75]

FNA results may yield a variety of descriptive diagnoses.[76,77] The most common and important categories are typically *benign, suspicious for malignancy, malignancy,* and *inadequate for diagnosis.* Examples of cytologic and histologic features are shown in Figure 39-2. At least 60% of aspirates are categorized as benign. The determination of sensitivity and specificity depends on whether suspicious lesions are considered positive. This latter group is primarily composed of highly cellular lesions, which represent

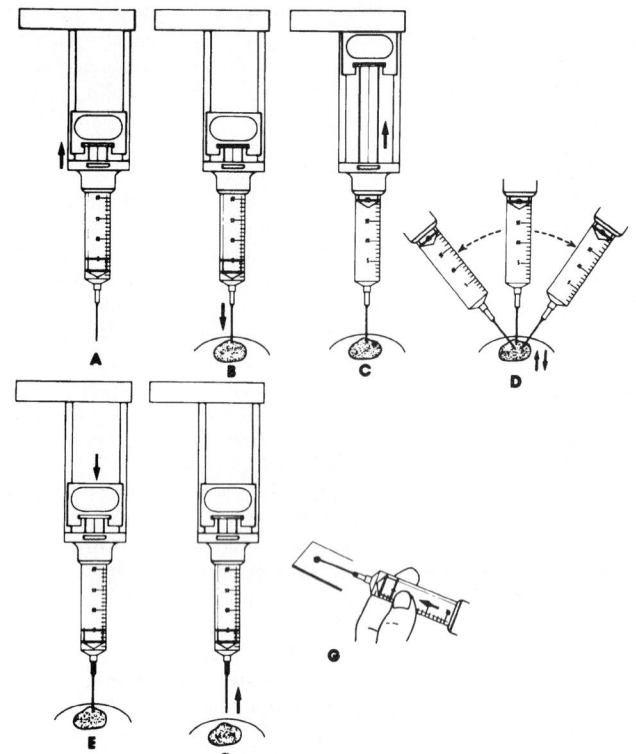

**FIGURE 39-1.** Technique for fine-needle aspiration biopsy. **A,** Aspirate 1 to 2 mL of air into syringe to loosen plunger and facilitate expiration of contents after aspiration. **B,** Insert needle into lesion without aspiration. **C,** Retract syringe piston to provide maximum suction. **D,** Make several passes at different angles, withdrawing needle to near the surface before redirecting. **E,** Release suction passively. **F,** Withdraw needle. **G,** Express needle contents onto a glass slide.

~20% of aspirations, of which 20% are cases of malignancy.[77] When all suspicious lesions are taken to surgery, the sensitivity of FNA exceeds 90%, with specificity approximating 70%.[68–70] The specificity of FNA for the malignant aspirates probably exceeds 95%. The use of FNA has decreased the frequency of surgery by 50% while doubling the rate of finding carcinoma in patients undergoing surgery. The relative economic advantage of this technique has been documented.[3,4,6]

Difficulties in interpretation of FNA biopsy specimens involve the differentiation of cellular specimens from possible Hürthle cell tumors, low-grade carcinomas, cellular adenomas, and Hashimoto thyroiditis. A few clinicians have performed quantitative DNA analyses on aspirated thyroid cells in an attempt to distinguish benign from malignant lesions.[78] DNA measurements have been unsuccessful, although the technique may provide prognostic indications of malignant tumor aggressiveness, with correlation to outcome and survival.[79] Another approach being evaluated is to perform immunohistochemical analysis on the FNA sample.[80]

Hashimoto disease also may be difficult to differentiate from lymphoma or from carcinoma with background Hashimoto changes. Anaplastic carcinomas may resemble poorly differentiated lymphoma or granulomatous thyroiditis.

Cysts pose several diagnostic difficulties.[48,51] Attempts to correlate characteristics of aspirated fluid with pathologic diagnosis have proved unreliable, although the occasional finding of clear, colorless fluid is typical of parathyroid cysts.[2] Cystic fluid may be difficult to aspirate unless a large needle is used. Cells obtained by centrifugation of cyst fluid may provide insufficient or confusing information.[76] Any solid remnant that follows initial cyst aspiration should be subjected to cautious follow-up and consideration for repeat aspiration. Finally, solid nodules <1 cm or >4 cm in diameter may be associated with an increased sampling error.

FNA carries minimal risk when properly performed. Concerns have been raised as to the possibility of severe local hemorrhage with airway obstruction and recurrent laryngeal nerve damage, but such complications are not documented in large reported series of FNA.[2,70] Bleeding complications are unusual and almost always self-limited. However, core biopsy has been associated with occasional severe bleeding and rare reports of tumor seeding.

## INTEGRATED APPROACH TO MANAGEMENT OF THYROID NODULES

The clinical challenge in thyroid nodule management is to define a diagnostic protocol that will produce the most accurate and cost-effective use of the various diagnostic methods. The implementation of decision analysis appears to highlight the difficulty in attaining this goal because consideration of all possible combinations of tests would require unmanageable decision trees, and the calculation of individual occurrence probabilities depends on an inconsistent literature. Limited decision analysis has suggested that FNA biopsy, the most accurate single evaluation technique, provides a minimal advantage in quality-adjusted life expectancy over the use of the usually inexact trial of thyroid suppression in patients already known to have solid, cold thyroid nodules. Either of these latter approaches appears slightly superior to a decision tree selecting immediate surgery when life expectancy is used as the gauge, but the differences may not be significant.[7] On the other hand, analysis of the selection of radionuclide scanning indicates questionable benefit because initial aspiration can provide equal sensitivity and specificity at a lower cost.[3,4,6,69]

Figure 39-3 suggests an algorithm that may be useful in a practice in which FNA biopsy is frequently used and experienced cytopathologic support is available. Many factors may alter the protocol for individual patients or clinical practice situations. At present, no right or wrong approach exists, and many physicians prefer radionuclide imaging as the initial step. However, this may increase costs because only 5% to 10% of scans obviate the need for aspiration, whereas 60% of 80% of FNA biopsies eliminate scan requirements. The use of scans in identifying multinodularity is largely negated by the high incidence of benign cytology results in these cases. Aspiration and biopsy identify predominantly cystic lesions, which rarely are simple cysts; therefore, ultrasonography has limited use initially but may be of significant value in monitoring the results of suppressive therapy, especially in patients with suspicious lesions and in practices in which the patient may see different clinicians on follow-up. The argument can be made that the 20% to 25% cancer risk in suspicious lesions should lead to immediate surgery in all cases, but a trial of suppressive therapy may still be warranted in selected patients. In many borderline clinical situations, the patient's strong preference or surgical risk factors may be important considerations. When a trial of suppressive therapy is undertaken, the approximate dosage required is >1.7 µg/kg per day of $T_4$.[81] The dose is increased incrementally by 0.025 mg per day every 5 to 6 weeks with TSH monitoring until TSH levels are reduced to the desired range. Usually the degree of TSH suppression need not be to an undetectable level but rather to a level of 0.1 to 0.3 mU/L. This should be the case particularly in postmenopausal women, in whom possible adverse effects of a fully suppressive dosage on bone mineral density are to be avoided. Nodules are assessed for change in size by physical examination (or ultrasonography if required) every 6 weeks for the first 6 months. The follow-up intervals may be more prolonged when significant decreases in size are observed, extending eventually to annual follow-up.

FNA biopsy should be repeated immediately when a nodule is found to be enlarging on suppressive therapy, with surgical exploration likely to be inevitable unless cystic fluid or hemor-

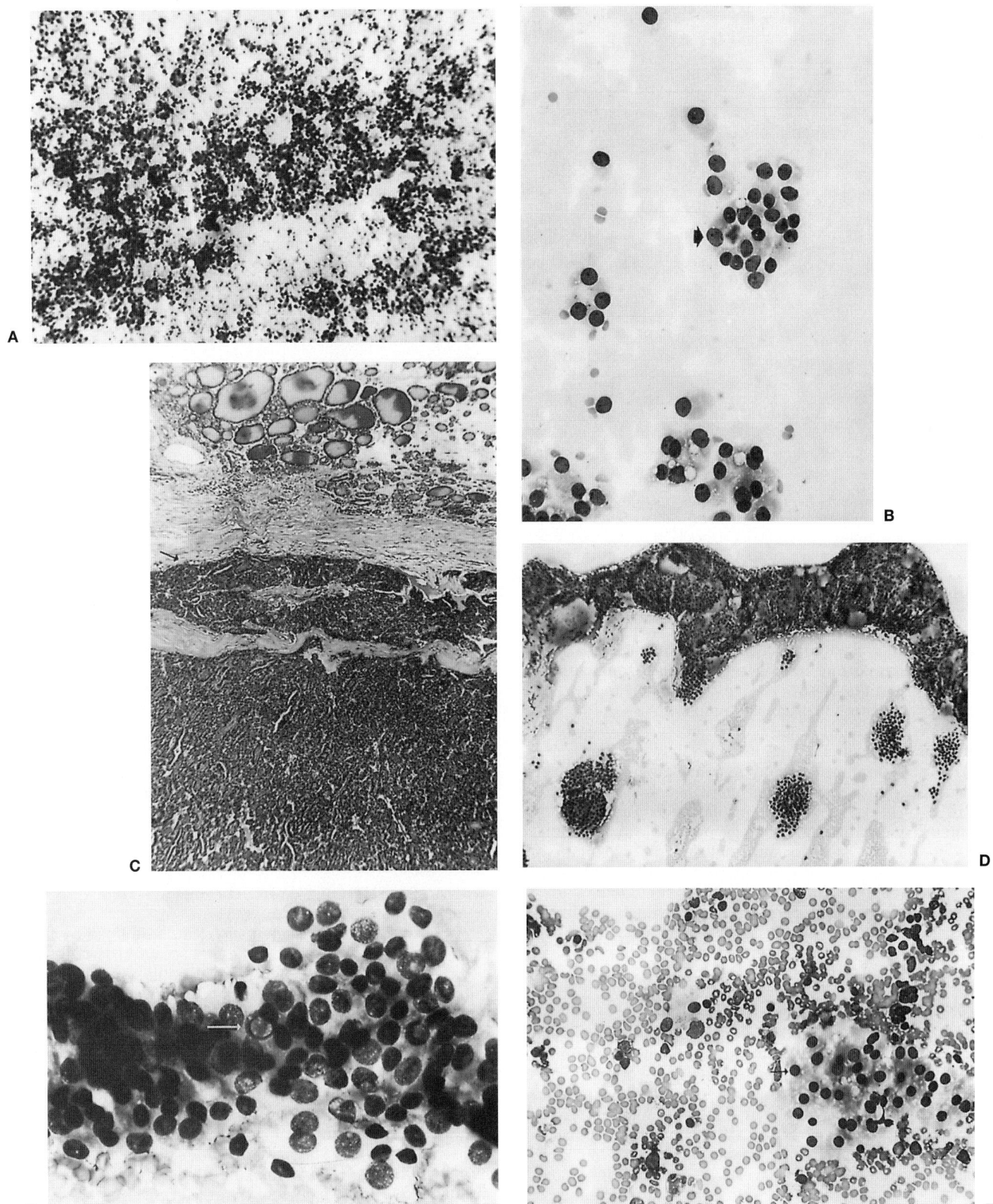

**FIGURE 39-2. A,** Fine-needle aspirate (*FNA*) of follicular neoplasm showing hypercellular specimen consisting of follicular epithelium. ×150 **B,** Microfollicular structures with centrally located colloid (*arrow*). Follicular cell nuclei are enlarged and pleomorphic (FNA of follicular neoplasm, ×540). **C,** Follicular carcinoma (histology). Note well-defined capsule with invasion (*arrow*). Residual normal thyroid gland is present at top of the field. ×95 **D,** Papillary carcinoma (FNA). Specimen is hypercellular, with numerous papillary clusters. ×150 **E,** Papillary cluster with diagnostic intranuclear inclusions at *arrow.* ×960 **F,** Hashimoto thyroiditis (FNA). Note chronic inflammatory background with reactive lymphocytes. A follicular epithelial group showing oxyphilic metaplasia is seen in the background. Note enlarged nuclei and granular cytoplasm of these cells (*arrow*). ×480 (Slides and legend text courtesy of Dr. Sanford Robbins. Photography courtesy of Charles Brown, M.S. From the Department of Pathology, Walter Reed Army Medical Center, Washington, DC.)

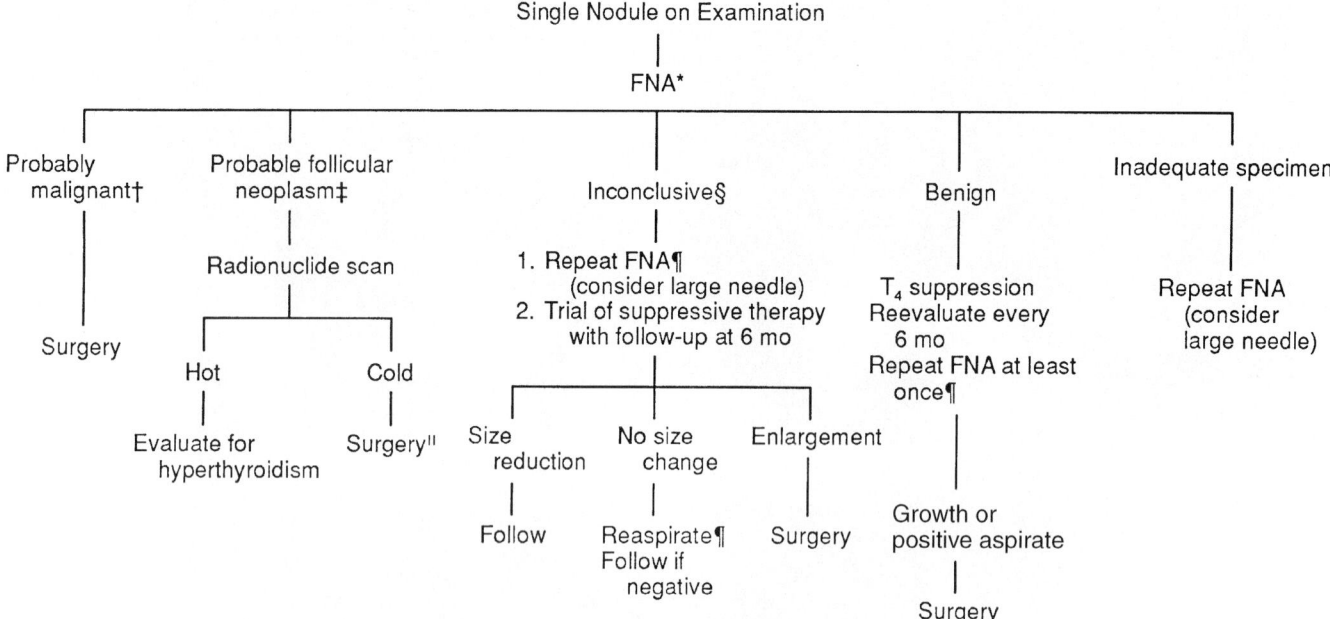

**FIGURE 39-3.** Approach to the solitary nodule. *22- to 25-gauge needle, repeated with 18-gauge needle if fluid is obtained. †Evidence of carcinoma (papillary, medullary, poorly differentiated, follicular) or lymphoma. ‡For example, sheets of follicular cells. §For example, small groups of uniform follicular cells with little colloid. ‖Selected patients with above-normal surgical risk or other extenuating circumstances may be followed closely with suppressive therapy. ¶Changes in cytologic findings redirect clinician to the appropriate arm of the algorithm. (*FNA*, fine-needle aspiration; *T₄*, thyroxine.)

rhage with benign cytology is found. FNA should also be repeated if no significant reduction in nodule size is obtained after 6 to 12 months of suppressive therapy. Of repeat FNA biopsies, 98% confirm the original diagnosis.[82]

Lesions with benign cytology on initial FNA biopsy may be identified as malignancies in only a very few cases on subsequent repeat aspiration.[72,82] However, the prognosis for neoplasms discovered during a later evaluation is unlikely to be different from the prognosis for neoplasms discovered earlier. The authors believe that reaspiration is preferable to the requirement of nodule size reduction as a confirmation of benignity in such cases and that use of this management approach significantly reduces the frequency of unnecessary surgery.

Patients with a history of irradiation present a special situation.[83] Historically, these patients have been immediately referred for surgery because of their high cancer rate. Some clinicians now advocate FNA biopsy in the management of these patients, although sufficient evidence for the reliability of benign results is still lacking.

The surgical approach to thyroid nodules varies. An ipsilateral lobectomy and isthmusectomy are commonly used for single nodules when the preoperative diagnosis is uncertain. Frequently, histologic evaluation of frozen sections is inconclusive or unreliable, and the final diagnosis requires careful examination of permanent sections. When the ultimate diagnosis is carcinoma, the customary practice is to complete a near-total thyroidectomy within 1 week of the first operation.[84] Near-total thyroidectomy is the initial procedure of choice in patients with thyroid nodules and a history of thyroid irradiation (see Chap. 44). When only a lobectomy, or lobectomy and isthmusectomy, is adequate (i.e., with benign histopathology), a question of indication for postoperative T₄ therapy often arises. In one group of patients with a history of neck irradiation who underwent partial thyroidectomy for nodules, the T₄-treated patients had a nodule recurrence rate of 8.4%, compared with a rate of 35.8% in untreated patients.[85] However, T₄ therapy may not prevent postoperative recurrence of nontoxic goiter.[86,87] The importance of referral to a surgeon highly skilled and experi-

enced in thyroid surgery cannot be overemphasized.[88] An alternative nonsurgical approach popularized in Europe is the percutaneous injection of 95% ethanol into thyroid nodules previously proved benign by FNA. This approach has been applied to benign thyroid cysts and hyperfunctioning nodules[89,90]; it also has been applied to cold nodules.[91–95] The procedure can be very painful for the patient and has been associated with transient increases in serum thyroglobulin and the thyroid hormones, with self-limited thyrotoxicosis. Fever, local pain, hematomata, and vocal cord paralysis are also possible in inexperienced hands.

## MANAGEMENT OF THYROID CYSTS

Simple thyroid cysts are often successfully drained by thyroid aspiration. In many cases, a single aspiration is curative; in other cases, cysts recur even after multiple aspirations. If the initial aspiration leaves no solid residual, the risk of cancer is very low; an additional therapeutic effect can be obtained in recurrent lesions by instilling sclerosing agents such as tetracycline[96] or ethanol.[89] No convincing evidence exists that thyroid hormone therapy reduces the likelihood of recurrence. Surgery is usually reserved for cysts >4 cm in diameter or for recurrent cysts that produce local symptoms. In cysts defined only by needle aspiration of at least 1 mL of fluid, it may be prudent to consider surgery for lesions that recur after two or more aspirations, especially if the fluid is hemorrhagic, if the nodules are >3 cm in diameter, or if a residual abnormality remains after maximum drainage.[97]

## MANAGEMENT OF AUTONOMOUS NODULES

Hot nodules are commonly identified by thyroid scanning.[98] The need for definitive treatment is determined by the degree of functional activity of the nodules rather than by their malignant potential. Nontoxic hot nodules are most often followed clinically. Toxic nodules may be treated with antithyroid drugs temporarily but require definitive therapy with [131]I or surgery. The choice between these two modalities remains controversial. Surgery is recommended for those with a history of radiation, for children, and for women of childbearing age. The use of $^{131}$I usually reduces the nodule's functional activity, but palpable nodules often persist.[99] For patients with toxic nodules, doses of $^{131}$I (5–20 mCi) appear to be successful in rendering patients euthyroid, but this may depend on the ratio of dose to nodular area[100]; higher doses—especially when given to euthyroid patients with autonomous nodules—produce hypothyroidism[101] (see Chap. 45). Percutaneous injection of ethanol (see earlier) has also been used with some success.[90,102]

# REFERENCES

1. Ashcraft MW, VanHerle AJ. Management of thyroid nodules. I. History and physical examination, blood tests, x-ray tests, and ultrasonography. Head Neck Surg 1981; 3:216.
2. Ashcraft MW, VanHerle AJ. Management of thyroid nodules. II. Scanning techniques, thyroid suppressive therapy, and fine needle aspiration. Head Neck Surg 1981; 3:297.
3. Mazzaferri EL. Management of a solitary thyroid nodule. N Engl J Med 1993; 328:553.
4. Burch HB. Evaluation and management of the solid thyroid nodule. Endocrinol Metab Clin North Am 1995; 24:663.
5. Sheppard MC, Franklyn JA. Management of the single thyroid nodule. Clin Endocrinol 1992; 37:398.
6. Ridgway EC. Clinical review 30: clinician's evaluation of a solitary thyroid nodule. J Clin Endocrinol Metab 1992; 74:231.
7. Molitch ME, Beck JR, Dreisman M, et al. The cold thyroid nodule: an analysis of diagnostic and therapeutic options. Endocr Rev 1984; 5:185.
8. Hermus AR, Huysmans DA. Treatment of benign nodular thyroid disease. N Engl J Med 1998; 338:1438.
9. Gharib H, Mazzaferri EL. Thyroxine suppressive therapy in patients with nodular thyroid disease. Ann Intern Med 1998; 128:386.
10. Ridgway EC. Medical treatment of benign thyroid nodules: have we defined a benefit? Ann Intern Med 1998; 128:403.
11. Rallison ML, Dobyns BM, Meikle AW, et al. Natural history of thyroid abnormalities: prevalence, incidence, and regression of thyroid diseases in adolescents and young adults. Am J Med 1991; 91:363.
12. Jackson SG, Wartofsky L. The thyroid nodule. In: Monaco F, ed. Thyroid diseases: clinical fundamentals and therapy. Boca Raton, FL: CRC Press, 1993:chap VIIA,253.
13. Singer PA, Cooper DA, Daniels GH, et al. Treatment guidelines for patients with thyroid nodules and well differentiated thyroid cancer. Arch Intern Med 1996; 156:2165.
14. Brander A, Viikinkoski P, Nickels J, Kivisaari L. Thyroid gland: US screening in a random adult population. Radiology 1991; 181:683.
15. Carroll BA. Asymptomatic thyroid nodules: incidental sonographic detection. AJR Am J Roentgenol 1982; 138:499.
16. Horlocker TT, Hay JE, James EM. Prevalence of incidental nodular thyroid disease detected during high resolution parathyroid ultrasonography. In: Medeiros-Neto G, Gaitan E, eds. Frontiers in thyroidology, vol 1. New York: Plenum Press, 1986:1309.
17. Brander A, Viikinkoski P, Nickels J, Kivisaari L. Thyroid gland: ultrasound screening in middle aged women with no previous thyroid disease. Radiology 1989; 173:507.
18. Walfish AG, Hazani E, Strawbridge HTG, et al. Combined ultrasound and needle aspiration cytology in the assessment and management of hypofunctioning thyroid nodules. Ann Intern Med 1977; 87:270.
19. Brown CL. Pathology of the cold nodule. Clin Endocrinol Metab 1981; 10:235.
20. Cooper DS, Schneyer CR. Follicular and Hürthle cell carcinoma of the thyroid. Endocrinol Metab Clin North Am 1990; 19:577.
21. Goldman ND, Coniglio JU, Falk SA. Thyroid cancers I: papillary, follicular, and Hürthle cell. Otolaryngol Clin North Am 1996; 29:593.
22. Hamburger JI. Evolution of toxicity in solitary nontoxic autonomously functioning thyroid nodules. J Clin Endocrinol Metab 1980; 50:1089.
23. Hamburger JI. The autonomously functioning thyroid nodule: Goetsch's disease. Endocr Rev 1987; 8:439.
24. Porcellini A, Ciollo I, Laviola L, et al. Novel mutations of thyrotropin receptor gene in thyroid hyperfunctioning adenomas. J Clin Endocrinol Metab 1994; 76:657.
25. Paschke R, Ludgate M. The thyrotropin receptor in thyroid diseases. N Engl J Med 1997; 337:1675.
26. Duprez L, Hermans J, Van Sande J, et al. Two autonomous nodules of a patient with multinodular goiter harbor different activating mutations of the thyrotropin receptor gene. J Clin Endocrinol Metab 1997; 82:306.
27. Russo D, Arturi F, Suarez HG, et al. Thyrotropin receptor gene alterations in thyroid hyperfunctioning adenomas. J Clin Endocrinol Metab 1996; 1548.
28. Marsh DJ, Learoyd DL, Robinson BG, et al. Medullary thyroid carcinoma: recent advances and management update. Thyroid 1995; 5:407.
29. Heshmati HM, Gharib H, van Heerden JA, Sizemore GW. Advances and controversies in the diagnosis and management of medullary thyroid carcinoma. Am J Med 1997; 103:60.
30. Landis SH, Murray T, Bolden S, Wingo PA. Cancer statistics, 1998. CA Cancer J Clin 1998; 48:6.
31. McHenry C, Smith M, Lawrence AM, et al. Nodular thyroid disease in children and adolescents: a high incidence of carcinoma. Am Surg 1988; 54:444.
32. Gorlin JB, Sallan SE. Thyroid cancer in childhood. Endocrinol Metab Clin North Am 1990; 19:649.
33. Hung W. Nodular thyroid disease and thyroid carcinoma. Pediatr Ann 1992; 21:50.
34. Robbins J. Lessons from Chernobyl: the event, the aftermath fallout: radioactive, political, social. Thyroid 1997; 7:189.
35. Becker DV, Robbins J, Beebe GW, et al. Childhood thyroid cancer following the Chernobyl accident. A status report. Endocrinol Metab Clin North Am 1996; 25:197.
36. Sarne D, Schneider AB. External radiation and thyroid neoplasia. Endocrinol Metab Clin North Am 1996; 25:181.
37. Smith RE, Adler RA, Clark P, et al. Thyroid function after mantle irradiation in Hodgkin's disease. JAMA 1981; 245:46.
38. Rosen IB, Simpson JA, Sutcliff S, et al. High-dose radiation and the emergence of thyroid nodular disease. Surgery 1984; 96:988.
39. Blum M, Rothschild M. Improved nonoperative diagnosis of the solitary cold thyroid nodule. JAMA 1980; 243:242.
40. Belfiore A, LaRosa GL, LaPorta GA, et al. Cancer risk in patients with cold thyroid nodules: relevance of iodine intake, sex, age, and multinodularity. Am J Med 1992; 93:363.
41. Spencer CA, Wang C-C. Thyroglobulin measurement: techniques, clinical benefits, and pitfalls. Endocrinol Metab Clin North Am 1995; 24:841.
42. Torrens JI, Burch HB. Serum thyroglobulin measurement: utility in clinical practice. Endocrinologist 1996; 6:125.
43. Vierhapper H, Raber W, Bieglmayer C, et al. Routine measurement of plasma calcitonin in nodular thyroid disease. J Clin Endocrinol Metab 1997; 82:1589.
44. Pacini F, Fontanelli M, Fugazzola L, et al. Routine measurement of serum calcitonin in nodular thyroid diseases allows the preoperative diagnosis of unsuspected sporadic medullary thyroid carcinoma. J Clin Endocrinol Metab 1994; 78:826.
45. Saad MF, Fritsche HA Jr, Samaan NA. Diagnostic and prognostic values of carcinoembryonic antigen in medullary carcinoma of the thyroid. J Clin Endocrinol Metab 1984; 58:889.
46. Cavalieri RR. Nuclear imaging in the management of thyroid carcinoma. Thyroid 1996; 6:485.
47. Patton JA, Sandler MP, Partain CL. Prediction of benignancy of the solitary "cold" thyroid nodule by fluorescent scanning. J Nucl Med 1985; 26:461.
48. de los Santos ET, Keyhani-Rofagha S, Cunningham JJ, Mazzaferri EL. Cystic thyroid nodules: the dilemma of malignant lesions. Arch Intern Med 1990; 150:1422.
49. Simeone JF, Daniels GH, Mueller PR, et al. High-resolution real-time sonography of the thyroid. Radiology 1982; 145:431.
50. Tan GH, Gharib H. Thyroid incidentalomas: management approaches to nonpalpable nodules discovered incidentally on thyroid imaging. Ann Intern Med 1997; 126:226.
51. Blum M. Non-isotopic imaging of the neck in patients with thyroid nodules or cancer. In: Thyroid cancer: clinical management. Totowa, NJ: Humana Press, 2000, 9.
52. Bloom AD, Adler LP, Shuck JM. Determination of malignancy of thyroid nodules with positron emission tomography. Surgery 1993; 114:728.
53. Wartofsky L. Management of patients with scan negative, thyroglobulin positive differentiated thyroid carcinoma. In: Wartofsky L, Sherman SI, Gopal J, Schlumberger M, Hay ID, eds. The use of radioactive iodine in patients with papillary and follicular thyroid cancer. J Clin Endocrinol Metab 1998; 83:4195.
54. Gharib H, James EM, Charboneau JW, et al. Suppressive therapy with levothyroxine for solitary nodules. N Engl J Med 1987; 317:70.
55. Cheung PSY, Lee JMH, Boey JH. Thyroxine suppressive therapy of benign solitary thyroid nodules: a prospective randomized study. World J Surg 1989; 13:818.
56. Reverter JL, Lucas A, Salinas I, et al. Suppressive therapy with levothyroxine for solitary thyroid nodules. Clin Endocrinol 1992; 36:25.
57. Berghout A, Wiersinga WM, Drexhage HA, et al. Comparison of placebo with L-thyroxine alone or with carbimazole for treatment of sporadic nontoxic goitre. Lancet 1990; 336:193.
58. Celani MF, Mariani M, Mariani G. On the usefulness of levothyroxine suppressive therapy in the medical treatment of benign solitary, solid, or predominantly solid thyroid nodules. Acta Endocrinol 1990; 123:603.
59. Papini E, Bacci B, Panunzi C, et al. A prospective randomized trial of levothyroxine suppressive therapy for solitary thyroid nodules. Clin Endocrinol 1993; 38:507.
60. LaRosa GL, Lupo L, Giuffrida D, et al. Levothyroxine and potassium iodide are both effective in treating benign solitary solid cold nodules of the thyroid. Ann Intern Med 1995; 122:1.
61. Zelmanovitz F, Genro S, Gross JL. Suppressive therapy with levothyroxine for solitary thyroid nodules: a double-blind controlled clinical study and cumulative meta-analyses. J Clin Endocrinol Metab 1998; 83:3881.
62. Papini E, Petrucci L, Guglielmi R, et al. Long-term changes in nodular goiter: a 5-year prospective randomized trial of levothyroxine suppressive

therapy for benign cold thyroid nodules. J Clin Endocrinol Metab 1998; 83:780.

63. Lima N, Knobel M, Cavaliere H, et al. Levothyroxine suppressive therapy is partially effective in treating patients with benign, solid thyroid nodules and multinodular goiters. Thyroid 1997; 7:691.

64. Wartofsky L. Does replacement L-thyroxine therapy cause osteoporosis? Adv Endocrinol Metab 1993; 4:157.

65. Marcocci C, Golia F, Bruno-Bossio G, et al. Carefully monitored levothyroxine suppressive therapy is not associated with bone loss in premenopausal women. J Clin Endocrinol Metab 1994; 78:818.

66. Schneider DL, Barrett-Connor EL, Morton DJ. Thyroid hormone use and bone mineral density in elderly women. JAMA 1994; 271:1245.

67. Franklyn J, Betteridge J, Holder R, Sheppard MC. Effect of estrogen replacement therapy upon bone mineral density in thyroxine treated postmenopausal women with a past history of thyrotoxicosis. Thyroid 1995; 5:359.

68. Oertel YC. Fine needle aspiration and the diagnosis of thyroid cancer. Endocrinol Metab Clin North Am 1996; 25:69.

69. Gharib H, Goellner JR. Fine needle aspiration biopsy of the thyroid: an appraisal. Ann Intern Med 1993; 118:282.

70. Gharib H, Goellner JR, Johnson DA. Fine-needle aspiration cytology of the thyroid. A 12-year experience with 11,000 biopsies. Clin Lab Med 1993; 13:699.

71. Hall TL, Layfield LJ, Philippe A, Rosenthal DL. Sources of diagnostic error in fine needle aspiration of the thyroid. Cancer 1989; 63:718.

72. Hamburger JI, Husain M, Nishiyama R, et al. Increasing the accuracy of fine-needle biopsy for thyroid nodules. Arch Pathol Lab Med 1989; 113:1035.

73. Caraway NP, Sneige N, Samaan NA. Diagnostic pitfalls in thyroid fine-needle aspiration: a review of 394 cases. Diagn Cytopathol 1993; 9:345.

74. Leenhardt L, Hejblum G, Franc B, et al. Indications and limits of ultrasound-guided cytology in the management of nonpalpable thyroid nodules. J Clin Endocrinol Metab 1999; 84:24.

75. Hatada T, Okada K, Ishii H, et al. Evaluation of ultrasound-guided fine-needle aspiration biopsy for thyroid nodules. Am J Surg 1998; 175:133.

76. Wartofsky L, Oertel Y. Fine needle aspiration biopsy of thyroid nodules. In: Van Nostrand D, ed. Nuclear medicine atlas. Philadelphia: JB Lippincott, 1988:193.

77. Tani EM, Skoog L, Löwhagen T. Clinical utility of fine-needle aspiration cytology of the thyroid. Annu Rev Med 1988; 39:255.

78. Bäckdahl M, Wallin G, Löwhagen T, et al. Fine-needle biopsy cytology and DNA analysis. Surg Clin North Am 1987; 67:197.

79. Pasielka JL, Zedenius J, Auer G, et al. Addition of nuclear DNA content to the AMES-risk group classification for papillary thyroid cancer. Surgery 1992; 112:1154.

80. Davila RM, Bedrossian CWM, Silverberg AB. Immunocytochemistry of the thyroid in surgical and cytologic specimens. Arch Pathol Lab Med 1988; 42:51.

81. Hennessey JV, Evaul JE, Tseng YL, et al. L-Thyroxine dosage: a reevaluation of therapy with contemporary preparations. Ann Intern Med 1986; 105:11.

82. Erdogan MF, Kamel N, Aras D, et al. Value of re-aspirations in benign nodular thyroid disease. Thyroid 1998; 8:1087.

83. DeGroot LJ. Clinical review 2: diagnostic approach and management of patients exposed to irradiation to the thyroid. J Clin Endocrinol Metab 1989; 69:925.

84. Brooks JR, Starnes HF, Brooks DC, Pelkey JN. Surgical therapy for thyroid carcinoma: a review of 1249 solitary thyroid nodules. Surgery 1988; 104:940.

85. Fogelfeld L, Wiviott MBT, Shore-Freedman E, et al. Recurrence of thyroid nodules after surgical removal in patients irradiated in childhood for benign conditions. N Engl J Med 1989; 320:835.

86. Anderson PE, Hurley PR, Rosswick P. Conservative treatment and long term prophylactic thyroxine in the prevention of recurrence of multinodular goiter. Surg Gynecol Obstet 1990; 171:309.

87. Hegedus L, Hansen JM, Veiergang D, Karstrup S. Does prophylactic thyroxine treatment after operation for non-toxic goitre influence thyroid size? BMJ 1987; 294:801.

88. Sosa JA, Bowman HM, Tielsch JM, et al. The importance of surgeon experience for clinical and economic outcomes from thyroidectomy. Ann Surg 1998; 228:320.

89. Lippi F, Ferrari C, Manetti L, et al. Treatment of solitary autonomous thyroid nodules by percutaneous ethanol injection: results of an Italian multicenter study. J Clin Endocrinol Metab 1996; 81:3261.

90. Cho YS, Lee HK, Ahn IM, et al. Sonographically guided ethanol sclerotherapy for benign thyroid cysts: results in 22 patients. AJR Am J Roentgenol 2000; 174:213.

91. Papini E, Pacella CM, Verde G. Percutaneous ethanol injection (PEI): what is its role in the treatment of benign thyroid nodules? Thyroid 1995; 5:147.

92. Caraccio N, Goletti O, Lippolis PV, et al. Is percutaneous ethanol injection a useful alternative for the treatment of the cold benign thyroid nodule? Five years experience. Thyroid 1997; 7:699.

93. Bennedbæk FN, Nielsen LK, Hegedus L. Effect of percutaneous ethanol injection therapy versus suppressive doses of L-thyroxine on benign solitary solid cold thyroid nodules: a randomized trial. J Clin Endocrinol Metab 1998; 83:830.

94. Goletti O, Monzani F, Lenziardi M, et al. Cold thyroid nodules: a new application of percutaneous ethanol injection treatment. J Clin Ultrasound 1994; 22:175.

95. Zingrillo M, Collura D, Ghiggi MR, et al. Treatment of large cold benign thyroid nodules not eligible for surgery with percutaneous ethanol injection. J Clin Endocrinol Metab 1998; 83:3905.

96. Treece GL, Georgitis WJ, Hofeldt FD. Resolution of recurrent thyroid cysts with tetracycline instillation. Arch Intern Med 1983; 140:2285.

97. Rosen IB, Provias JP, Walfish PG. Pathologic nature of cystic thyroid nodules selected for surgery by needle aspiration biopsy. Surgery 1986; 100:606.

98. Hamburger JI. The autonomously functioning thyroid nodule: Goetsch's disease. Endocr Rev 1987; 8:439.

99. Goldstein R, Hart IR. Follow-up of solitary autonomous thyroid nodules treated with $^{131}$I. N Engl J Med 1983; 309:1473.

100. Estour B, Millot L, Vergely N, et al. Efficacy of low doses of radioiodine in the treatment of autonomous thyroid nodules: importance of dose/area ratio. Thyroid 1997; 7:357.

101. Ross DS, Ridgway EC, Daniels GH. Successful treatment of solitary toxic thyroid nodules with relatively low-dose iodine 131, with low prevalence of hypothyroidism. Ann Intern Med 1984; 101:488.

102. Tarantino L, Giorgio A, Mariniello N, et al. Percutaneous ethanol injection of large autonomous hyperfunctioning thyroid nodules. Radiology 2000; 214:143.

# CHAPTER 40

# THYROID CANCER

ERNEST L. MAZZAFERRI

Approximately 18,100 new cases of thyroid carcinoma were diagnosed in the United States in 1999, ranking it 22nd in incidence among the major malignancies.[1] Its frequency varies with gender and age and is highest among women between the ages of 30 and 70 years. The lifetime risk of being diagnosed with thyroid cancer is ~0.64% for women and 0.25% for men.[2] In 1998, ~1200 of the 135,000 persons with thyroid carcinoma in the United States died of their disease.[1] Between 1973 and 1992, its incidence among all ages rose steadily (almost 28%), whereas its mortality rates dropped more than 23%.[2] The declining mortality rates are largely due to early diagnosis and effective therapy applied at an early tumor stage when it is most amenable to surgery and $^{131}$I therapy.[3]

## RADIATION AND THYROID CARCINOMA

Thyroid carcinoma may be caused by exposure to ionizing radiation. It was the first solid tumor found to have a significantly increased incidence in A-bomb survivors, but only among those younger than 20 years of age at the time of exposure.[4]

**External Radiation.** The risk of developing papillary thyroid cancer after therapeutic external radiation, used in the past to treat children with benign head and neck conditions, is well known.[5] Exposure before the age of 15 years poses a major risk that becomes progressively greater with increasing amounts of radiation between 0.10 Gy (10 rad) and 10 Gy (1000 rad). This increases the incidence of thyroid carcinoma within 5 years of exposure, and this increased incidence continues for 30 years, at which time it begins to decline.[5] Girls are only slightly more likely than boys to develop thyroid carcinoma after irradiation.[5]

**Radioiodine-Induced Thyroid Carcinoma.** Until recently, most studies have suggested that $^{131}$I is less effective than external gamma radiation in inducing thyroid cancer.[4] A slightly elevated risk of thyroid cancer found in a large Swedish population exposed to diagnostic doses of $^{131}$I was attributed to cancers found among those examined for a suspected thyroid tumor.[4] Another study from the United States reported a slight elevation

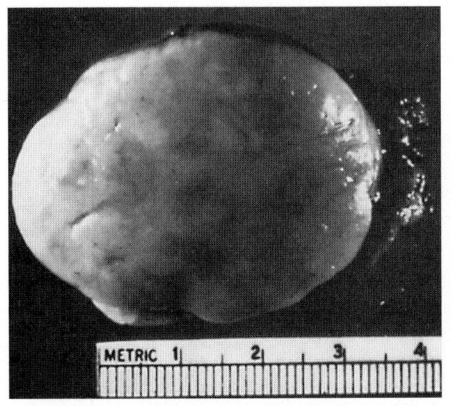
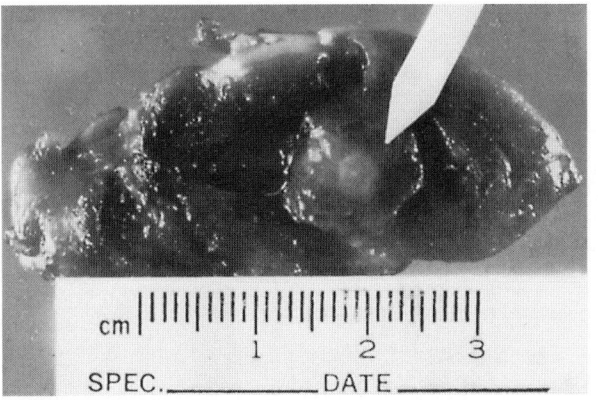

**FIGURE 40-1.** Papillary thyroid carcinoma: gross pathology. **A,** Large papillary thyroid carcinoma completely replacing right thyroid lobe and extending beyond the thyroid capsule. Such lesions are associated with high recurrence and mortality rates. **B,** Occult papillary thyroid carcinoma found incidentally at surgery. This lesion almost invariably has a benign clinical course.

of thyroid cancer mortality after treatment of hyperthyroidism with [131]I, but the absolute risk was small, and the underlying thyroid disease appeared to play a role.[6,6a] However, most of these studies involved adults. When a large number of children developed thyroid carcinoma after being exposed to radioiodine fallout from the Chernobyl nuclear reactor accident in 1986, it became clear that [131]I and other short-lived radioiodines were potent thyroid carcinogens in children, particularly those exposed when younger than age 10 years.[7]

**Nuclear Weapon Fallout.** Nuclear weapons that were tested above ground in Nevada between 1951 and 1963 resulted in radiation exposure to individuals across the continental United States. The chance of a significant exposure was highest in the 1950s for children who routinely drank milk from a backyard cow or goat that had ingested grass contaminated with radioactive fallout. The average cumulative thyroid dose from radioiodine fallout was 0.02 Gy (2 rad) for the American population collectively and 0.1 Gy (10 rad) for those younger than age 20 years at the time of exposure in the range known to cause thyroid carcinoma in children.[5,8] Approximately 50,000 cases of thyroid cancer are likely to result from these exposures—nearly half of which have probably already appeared—but these are highly uncertain estimates.[9] Nevertheless, a large study found an association between thyroid carcinoma and exposure to radioiodine fallout from nuclear tests in Nevada for children exposed at younger than 1 year of age and for those in the 1950 to 1959 birth cohort.[10] Screening for thyroid disease that is due to fallout exposure is not recommended, but physicians should discuss the risk and palpate the neck of concerned patients.[9]

# PAPILLARY THYROID CARCINOMA

## PREVALENCE

Thyroid carcinoma is classified into four major types, which in decreasing order of frequency are *papillary, follicular, medullary,* and *anaplastic* carcinomas. Papillary and follicular carcinomas—often termed *differentiated thyroid carcinomas*—arise from follicular cells, synthesize thyroglobulin (Tg), and tend to be slow growing. Medullary carcinoma, which originates from thyroidal C cells that secrete calcitonin, may be sporadic or familial. Anaplastic carcinoma usually arises from well-differentiated thyroid tumors and is almost invariably fatal within a brief period (see Chap. 41).

Papillary thyroid carcinoma accounts for ~80% of all thyroid cancers in the United States,[11] including those induced by radiation.[12] It is diagnosed in ~1 in 17,000 people in the United States annually, although occult microscopic papillary thyroid carcinoma is found in 10% or more of autopsy and surgical thyroid specimens from men and women throughout adult life.[13] In contrast, clinically manifest papillary thyroid carci-

noma has a peak incidence in the fourth decade and is three times more frequent in women than in men. In children, the sex ratio is nearly equal, which may reflect radiation-induced disease.

## FAMILIAL PAPILLARY CARCINOMA

Approximately 5% of papillary carcinomas are familial tumors, which are sometimes inherited as an autosomal dominant trait.[14,15,15a] Others are inherited as a component of familial adenomatous polyposis (*Gardner syndrome*), occurring at a young age as bilateral, multicentric tumors with an excellent prognosis, particularly those with ret-PTC activation.[16,17] *Cowden disease* is an autosomal dominant syndrome characterized by multiple mucocutaneous hamartomas, keratoses, fibrocystic breast disease or breast cancer, and well-differentiated thyroid cancer.[18,19] *Carney complex*—a syndrome with spotty skin pigmentation, myxomas, schwannomas, and multiple neoplasia that affects multiple glands—also includes thyroid carcinoma.[20]

## PATHOLOGY

**Gross Tumor.** Papillary carcinoma usually is an unencapsulated and invasive tumor with ill-defined margins that is 2 to 3 cm when diagnosed, but this varies widely (Fig. 40-1*A*).[3] Approximately 10% extend through the thyroid capsule into surrounding neck tissues, and another 10% are fully encapsulated.[21] They typically are firm and solid, but some develop chronic hemorrhagic necrosis, yielding a thick brownish fluid on needle biopsy that may be mistaken for a benign cyst.[22] Small tumors as large as 1.0 cm that often have a stellate appearance, termed *microcarcinomas,* usually are found by serendipity but rarely are invasive or metastasize (see Fig. 40-1*B*).[23]

**Architectural Features.** Most papillary carcinomas contain complex branching papillae with a fibrovascular core covered by a single layer of tumor cells, intermingled with follicular structures (Fig. 40-2*A*), although some have a pure follicular or trabecular appearance.[24] The term *mixed papillary–follicular carcinoma* has no clinical value because the follicular component does not alter [131]I uptake or prognosis.[25] Moreover, a tumor's nuclear features are more important than its architectural appearance in establishing a diagnosis of papillary carcinoma. Those with cellular features of papillary carcinoma but a pure follicular pattern are termed *follicular variant papillary carcinoma* (see Fig. 40-2*D*), which some argue comprise most tumors diagnosed as follicular carcinoma.[26]

**Cytology Features.** Papillary carcinoma has cellular features that distinguish it from other thyroid neoplasms regardless of its architecture, permitting an accurate diagnosis by fine-needle aspiration (FNA) (see Fig. 40-2*C*). The cells are large and contain pink to amphophilic finely granular cytoplasm and

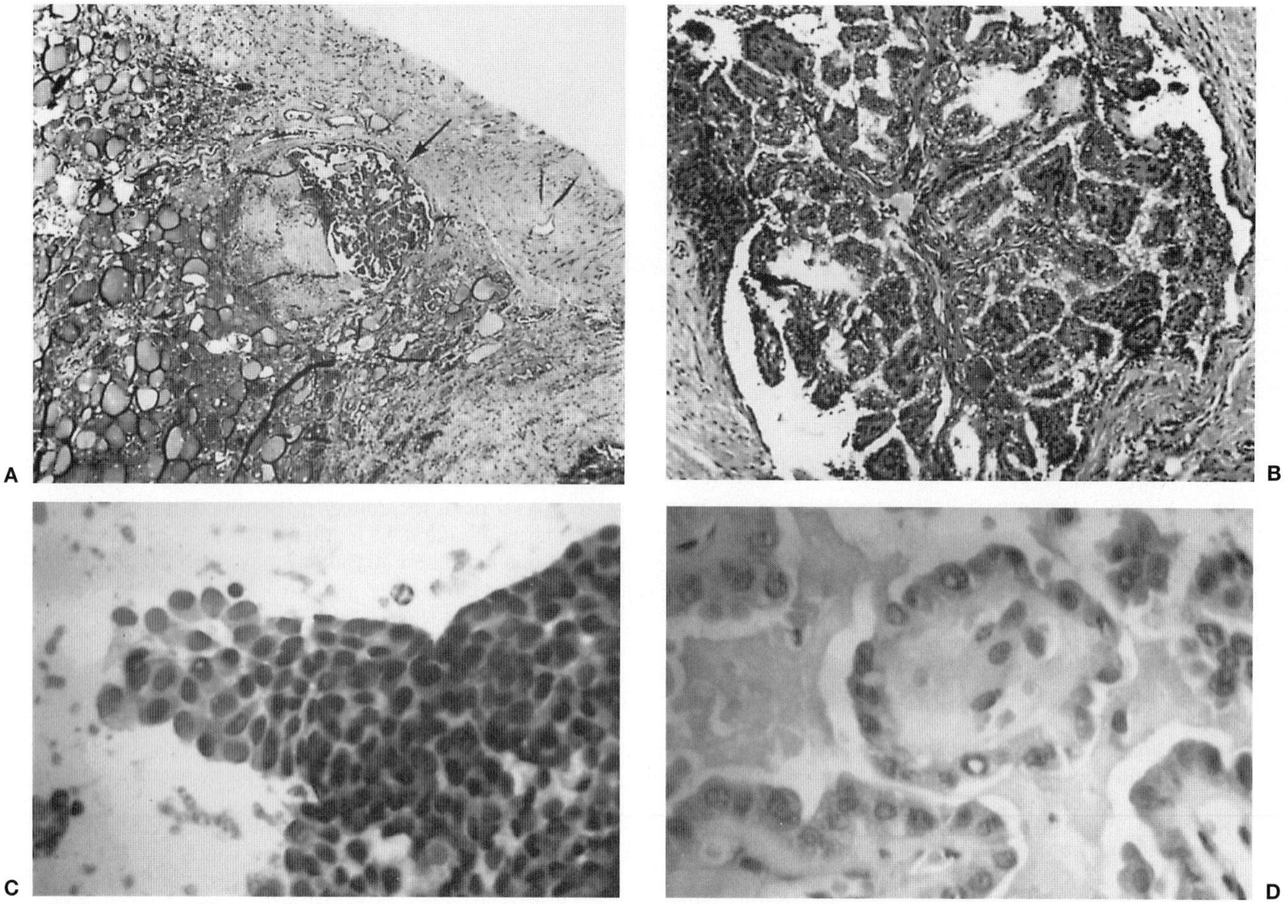

A

B

C

D

**FIGURE 40-2.** Papillary thyroid carcinoma: histology. **A,** Microscopic papillary thyroid carcinoma (*arrow*) showing a mixed papillary and follicular architecture, and encapsulation. Isolated microscopic papillary carcinomas, found in ~10% of the general population, are incidental findings at surgery or autopsy and almost never are of clinical significance. ×20 **B,** Papillary thyroid carcinoma with typical papillae containing a fibrovascular core, and cells with large, pale-staining nuclei that appear crowded and overlapping. ×100 **C,** Fine-needle aspiration biopsy specimen of papillary thyroid carcinoma showing typical cytologic features of the tumor. ×400 **D,** High-power magnification of follicular variant papillary thyroid carcinoma showing characteristic cellular features, including nuclear inclusions, irregularly placed, pale-staining nuclei, and abundant cytoplasm. ×400

large pale nuclei ("Orphan Annie eye" nuclei) with inclusion bodies and nuclear grooves that identify the tumor as papillary carcinoma (see Fig. 40-2D). Psammoma bodies (Fig. 40-3)—the "ghosts" of infarcted papillae that are virtually pathognomonic of papillary carcinoma—are calcified, concentric lamellated spheres found in approximately half the cases within or near the tumor and lymph nodes or in cytology specimens.[27] Lymphocytic infiltration—ranging from focal areas of lymphocytes and plasma cells to classic Hashimoto disease (see Chap. 46)—is often seen in papillary carcinoma. Papillary carcinomas are commonly found in multiple sites within the thyroid gland, which are generally thought to be intraglandular metastases. Multiple microscopic tumor foci are found in as many as 80% of cases when the gland is examined in considerable detail, but in routine clinical practice their frequency is as high as 45%, and they usually are bilateral (Fig. 40-4).[11]

**Lymph Node Metastases.**   Papillary carcinoma commonly metastasizes to lymph nodes in the lateral neck, central neck compartment, and mediastinum. Gross lymph node metastases are present in approximately half the cases at the time of diagnosis, while even more—as many as 85% in studies from Japan[28,29]—have microscopic nodal metastases.[25] Their number rises as primary tumor size increases. Nodal metastases tend to be bilateral when the isthmus or both thyroid lobes are involved with tumor, or they may extend into the mediastinum

or extend beyond the lymph node capsule into soft tissues, which are all poor prognostic signs.[25,30]

**Distant Metastases.**   Fewer than 5% of patients have distant metastases at the time of diagnosis, and another 5% develop them later.[11] In a review of 1231 patients with distant metastases,

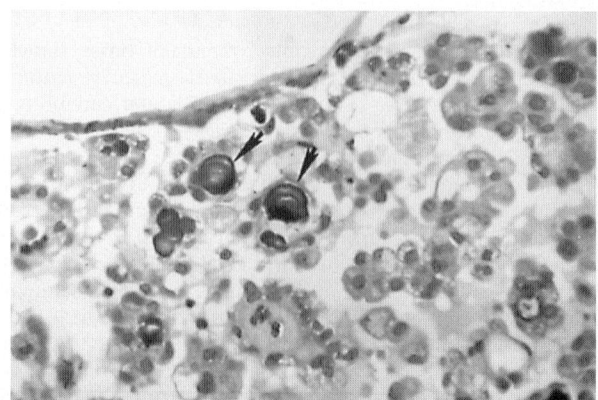

**FIGURE 40-3.** Psammoma bodies of papillary carcinoma (*arrows*) are calcified, dark-staining, lamellated spheres that are virtually pathognomonic of papillary thyroid carcinoma. ×400

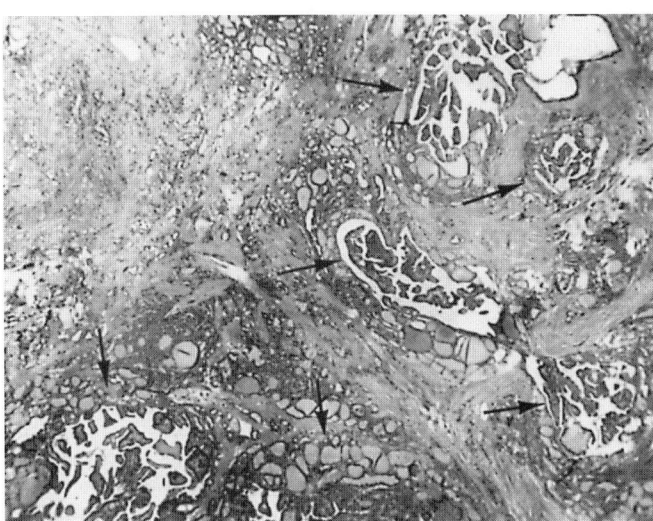

**FIGURE 40-4.** Microscopically multifocal papillary thyroid carcinoma (*arrows*) usually represents intraglandular metastases. ×20

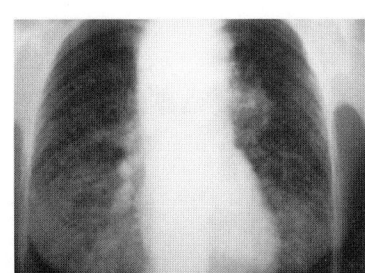
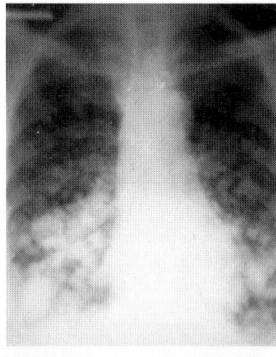

A,B

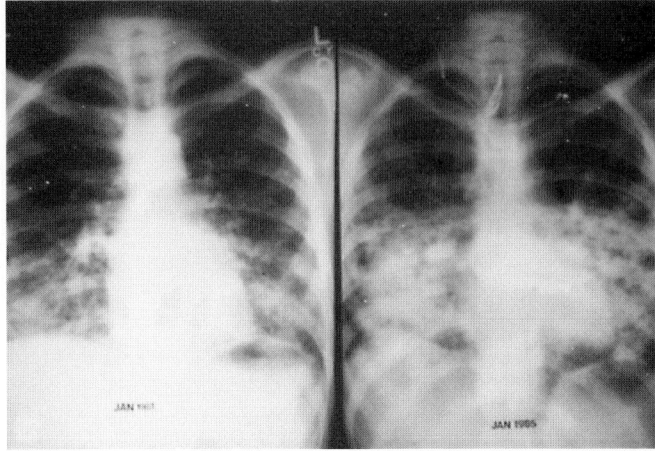

C

**FIGURE 40-5.** Distant metastases of papillary thyroid carcinoma. **A,** Papillary thyroid carcinoma with diffuse lymphangitic spread of tumor giving a typical "snowflake" appearance on the chest radiograph. Such tumors typically concentrate [131]I in younger patients and tend to have a good prognosis. **B,** Papillary thyroid carcinoma with diffuse nodular infiltrates that concentrated [131]I poorly. This patient had pulmonary metastases at the time of initial diagnosis. **C,** Papillary thyroid carcinoma (*left*) in a young woman that did not concentrate [131]I and grew steadily over a 4-year period (*right*).

49% were in the lung, 25% were in bone, 15% were in lung and bone, and 12% were in the central nervous system or in multiple organs.[11] Pulmonary metastases may be large discrete nodules or may have a "snowflake" appearance caused by diffuse lymphangitic tumor spread (Fig. 40-5A, B, and C). Pulmonary metastases not seen on radiographs may be detected only with whole body scanning done after therapeutic doses of [131]I have been administered.[31–34]

**Thyroglossal Duct.** Papillary thyroid carcinoma arising within a thyroglossal duct is almost always small and usually has a benign course.[35]

**Papillary Microcarcinoma.** Different histologic variants or subtypes of papillary carcinoma have distinct biologic behaviors (Table 40-1). Five histologic subtypes or variants were recognized in the 1988 World Health Organization classification,[24] and at least five others have been described since then.[36,37] Papillary microcarcinoma is a tumor 1.0 cm or smaller. Approximately 20% are multifocal, and as many as 60% have cervical lymph node metastases,[29] which may be their presenting feature.[23] Lung metastases occur rarely with multifocal tumors that have bulky cervical metastases; these are the only microcarcinomas with significant morbidity and mortality.[23,37] Otherwise, the recurrence and cancer-specific mortality rates are near zero.[13,23]

**Encapsulated Papillary Carcinoma.** Encapsulated papillary carcinoma is an otherwise typical tumor completely surrounded by a fibrous capsule. It accounts for ~10% of papillary carcinomas and is approximately half as likely to metastasize as is typical papillary carcinoma.[37] Tumor recurrence is lower than usual, and death that is due to cancer almost never occurs with these tumors.[27,37]

**Follicular Variant Papillary Carcinoma.** Follicular variant papillary carcinoma accounts for ~10% of papillary carcinomas.[37] Usually not encapsulated, its microfollicular architectural pattern is otherwise indistinguishable from follicular carcinoma, but the typical nuclear features of papillary carcinoma identify its true nature, which can be diagnosed by FNA cytology.[27] Its metastases often have psammoma bodies and may show the typical features of papillary carcinoma. Some claim that its prognosis is similar to the usual papillary carcinoma, and others suggest that distant metastases are more likely and that long-term outcome may be unfavorable with this tumor.[36–38]

**Diffuse Macrofollicular Variant Papillary Carcinoma.** Diffuse macrofollicular variant papillary carcinoma is an uncommon tumor that can be confused with goiter or macrofollicular adenoma on frozen section.[36] It occurs predominantly in women with goiter, approximately one-third of whom have hyperthyroidism. Most have distant metastases with very high mortality rates.[36]

**Tall Cell Variant.** Approximately 10% of papillary thyroid carcinomas show extensive papillae formation with cells twice as tall as they are wide that comprise at least 30% of the tumor.[36] Compared with typical papillary carcinoma, tall cell tumors tend to be diagnosed approximately two decades later (in the mid-50s), are larger tumors associated with significantly more invasion into extrathyroidal soft tissues, and have more distant metastases.[18,36,37] The tumor, which can be identified on a cytology specimen from fine-needle biopsy, often expresses the p53 suppressor oncogene, perhaps accounting for its frequent loss of [131]I uptake and long-term mortality rates that are two- to threefold those of typical papillary carcinomas.[18,37]

**Columnar Cell Variant.** Columnar cell variant is a rare variant possibly related to tall cell carcinoma. It occurs mainly in men and is composed of rectangular cells with clear cytoplasm.[36] More than 90% develop distant metastases, which usually are unresponsive to [131]I therapy or chemotherapy and result in death.[36,37] When encapsulated, it has a much better prognosis.[21]

**Diffuse Sclerosis Variant.** Approximately 5% of papillary carcinomas are of the diffuse sclerosis variant type, which is even more common in children and adolescents.[36,37] Approxi-

**TABLE 40-1.**
**Tumor Histologic Variants That Influence Prognosis in Papillary and Follicular Thyroid Carcinoma**

| | PROGNOSIS | | |
|---|---|---|---|
| *Better* | *Worse* | *Possibly Worse* | *Too Few Cases Reported to Assess* |
| **PAPILLARY THYROID CARCINOMA** | | | |
| Encapsulated variant | Tall cell variant | Follicular variant | PTC with lipomatous stroma |
| Cystic variant | Columnar variant | Solid variant | PTC with fasciitislike stroma |
| Microcarcinoma variant | Diffuse sclerosis variant | Oncocytic (Hürthle cell) variant | Myxoid variant |
| Macrocarcinoma variant | Diffuse macrofollicular variant | Associated with Graves disease | Cribriform variant |
| | Insular cell variant | | |
| | PTC with de-differentiation | | |
| **FOLLICULAR THYROID CARCINOMA** | | | |
| | Oncocytic (Hürthle cell) variant | | |
| | Insular cell variant | | |

PTC, papillary thyroid carcinoma.
(Modified from LiVolsi VA. Unusual variants of papillary thyroid carcinoma. In: Mazzaferri EL, ed. Advances in endocrinology and metabolism, vol. 6. St. Louis: Mosby–Year Book, Inc., 1995:39.)

mately 10% of the tumors in the children of Chernobyl are of this type.[39] Usually involving both lobes, diffuse sclerosis variant presents as a goiter with extensive squamous metaplasia, sclerosis, abundant psammoma bodies, and lymphatic invasion involving the whole thyroid gland. Lymph node metastases are almost always present, and ~25% have lung metastases.[36,37] Cytology specimens reveal squamous metaplasia, inflammatory cells, and psammoma bodies, but may be difficult to differentiate from thyroiditis. Although it has a higher incidence of local and pulmonary metastases than typical papillary carcinomas, there is some disagreement about whether its long-term prognosis is worse than usual.[36,37]

**Oxyphilic (Hürthle Cell) Variant.** Approximately 2% of papillary carcinomas have nuclei resembling those of Hürthle cell follicular carcinomas.[40] Multiple oxyphilic thyroid tumors and a familial occurrence have been noted in some cases.[41] This tumor cannot be identified by FNA cytology but is recognized by its papillary architecture on the final histologic sections. Compared with typical papillary carcinomas, oxyphilic carcinomas have fewer neck nodal metastases at diagnosis but have higher rates of recurrence and cause-specific mortality; in this respect, they resemble oxyphilic follicular carcinoma.[37,40]

**Solid or Trabecular Variant.** A tumor with a predominantly (>75%) solid architectural pattern that maintains the typical nuclear features of papillary carcinoma, the solid or trabecular variant has a propensity for extrathyroidal spread and lung metastases.[36,37] Some, however, find it to be more common in children and report that its prognosis is the same as with typical papillary carcinoma.[42]

**Insular Carcinoma.** Approximately 5% of all thyroid carcinomas show solid clusters of cells with small follicles that contain Tg but resemble pancreatic islet cells. This is often categorized as a variant of follicular carcinoma, but it may show papillary differentiation, and it has been suggested that it should be considered a separate entity derived from follicular

epithelium.[43] Insular carcinomas usually are large and highly invasive tumors that grow through the tumor capsule and into tumor blood vessels. Compared with differentiated thyroid carcinoma, insular carcinoma presents at an older age (54 vs. 36 years); with larger tumors (4.7 vs. 2.5 cm); with fewer neck metastases (36% vs. 50%) but more distant metastases (26% vs. 2%); and has a worse 30-year cancer-specific mortality rate (25% vs. 8%).[18] Insular carcinoma also displays aggressive behavior in children.[44]

## DIAGNOSIS

**History.** In the past, many papillary carcinomas were large and invasive when first diagnosed; however, with the use of FNA, most are small tumors found at an early stage as an asymptomatic thyroid nodule on routine examination or in screening programs of patients with head and neck irradiation.[3] The timeliness of diagnosis affects the prognosis (see Prognosis).[3] Occasionally, it causes pain, hoarseness, dysphagia, or hemoptysis, or it infiltrates surrounding structures or grows rapidly—findings that are associated with high mortality rates. However, only a few patients have such symptoms. A history of irradiation is important, but only 30% of patients develop palpable thyroid nodules after irradiation, and of these, only one-third are malignant.[45] Thyroid nodules that appear after radiation should undergo an evaluation similar to that used for nodules that occur spontaneously.

**Physical Examination.** Papillary carcinoma usually is manifest as a palpably discrete thyroid nodule that moves upward when the patient swallows, but a cervical lymph node metastasis may be its only sign. A midline mass above the thyroid isthmus may be a metastatic lymph (Delphian) node or may be carcinoma within a thyroglossal duct that can be identified from its upward movement when the tongue is protruded. Papillary carcinoma may be a firm, nontender, discrete mass, but many are soft and cystic or diffusely infiltrate one lobe or the entire thyroid. Distant metastases are found less often at the time of diagnosis of papillary carcinoma than follicular carcinoma, but when they are found, the primary tumor is almost invariably large (see Figs. 40-1A and 40-5B).

**Fine-Needle Aspiration.** Approximately 10% of thyroid nodules show clear evidence of malignancy, such as vocal cord paralysis, signs of invasion, or bulky lymph node metastases, whereas the others appear benign on examination. Neither the history nor the physical examination offers sufficient evidence of a nodule's benign nature that further testing can be deferred (see Chaps. 34, 35, and 39). The first test in a clinically euthyroid patient is FNA.[46] Other tests are too nonspecific to be used first. Except for hyperfunctional ("hot") nodules that are rarely malignant, most thyroid nodules—whether single in an otherwise normal gland or a dominant nodule in a multinodular goiter—require FNA for diagnosis. Although large-needle cutting biopsies can be done, FNA is considerably safer and is highly effective in obtaining sufficient cytology to identify the distinctive features of papillary carcinoma, including most of its variants[46] (see Chap. 39). Nodules that yield diagnostic or suspicious cytology are excised; the others are scanned to exclude hot nodules, whereas benign nodules are simply observed or sometimes treated with thyroxine-suppressive therapy. Thyroxine suppression should not be done without prior FNA and should not be used as a diagnostic test, because thyroid carcinomas may appear to shrink.[46]

**Prior Neck Irradiation.** FNA should be the first test performed on a palpable thyroid nodule in a euthyroid patient with a history of head-and-neck irradiation. An asymptomatic patient with a palpably normal thyroid gland who has history of head and neck irradiation should not undergo ultrasonography because nearly 90% of such patients have thyroid nodules found by this test, most of which are benign.[9,47]

Ultrasonography reveals thyroid lesions <1 cm in ~50% of the healthy middle-aged population.[48,49] Thyroid hormone does not prevent the appearance of thyroid nodules or cancer in previously irradiated patients with a palpably normal thyroid gland,[45] but it does reduce the recurrence of nodules in irradiated patients who have undergone thyroid surgery for benign thyroid nodules.[50]

## FACTORS INFLUENCING PROGNOSIS

Once the diagnosis is established, the prognosis is determined by an interaction of three variables: tumor stage, the patient's age, and therapy. The cancer-specific mortality rate is <10% over three decades, but distant metastases or serious local recurrences can occur many years after initial therapy.[3,11]

**Delay in Diagnosis.** The author of this chapter has found that the median time from the first manifestation of thyroid cancer—nearly always a neck mass—to initial therapy was 4 months in patients who survived and 18 months in those who died of cancer ($P$ <.001).[3] The 30-year cancer mortality was nearly twice as high when therapy was delayed for longer than a year than when it was done within 12 months of a nodule's discovery (13% vs. 6%, $P$ <.001).[3]

**Age at Time of Diagnosis.** Age is the most important prognostic factor. The adverse effect of age appears at ~40 years and becomes progressively worse thereafter, increasing at a steep rate after age 60 years, when men have the worst prognosis.[3,11] The response to therapy is most favorable in younger patients whose tumors concentrate [131]I.[51-53]

**Prognosis in Children.** Outcome is usually favorable in children, although their tumors are typically at a more advanced stage, with more local and distant metastases than are those of adults at the time of diagnosis.[51,53-55] Recurrence rates in children are ~40% over several decades compared with 20% in adults.[3,53] The rate of pulmonary metastases in children is almost twice that in adults, reaching more than 20% in some series.[3,11,54] Their prognosis for survival is, however, excellent, with or without a history of irradiation, except for those younger than age 10 years, who have high mortality rates.[51-53] Nonetheless, despite the relatively good prognosis in children, one study found that children with thyroid cancer had, as a group, poorer long-term survival rates than did normal children.[56]

**Gender.** Men tend to have higher recurrence and cancer-specific mortality rates than do women.[37] I found that the 30-year cancer-specific mortality rate for men with papillary carcinoma was nearly twice that of women (7.8% vs. 4%, $P$ <.01) and that gender was an independent prognostic factor.[3] Although estrogen and progesterone receptors are expressed in as many as 50% of papillary carcinomas, this does not explain the divergent risks imposed by gender.

**Tumor Size.** The tumor features affecting prognosis are summarized in Tables 40-1 and 40-2. Primary tumors <1.5 cm in diameter rarely recur or cause death, whereas those >4.5 cm are associated with high mortality rates.[3,11] In the author's study, tumors stratified as <1.5 cm, 1.5 to 4.4 cm, and ≥4.5 cm, respectively, were associated with distant metastases in 4%, 10%, and 17% of patients and had 30-year cancer-specific mortality rates of 0.5%, 8%, and 22%.[3] The 20-year cause-specific mortality rates in the large Mayo Clinic series for tumors 2 to 3.9 cm, 4 to 6.9 cm, and ≥7 cm were 6%, 16%, and 50%; respectively.[57]

**Multicentricity.** Among those undergoing completion thyroidectomy for recurrent cancer, multifocal disease in the thyroid lobe excised first is almost always associated with bilateral thyroid cancer.[58] Nonetheless, some report almost no tumor recurrences in the thyroid remnant,[59,60] while others find that the rate of recurrence of locally persistent disease is significantly higher after less than near-total thyroidectomy.[61-65] One study reported a 1.7-fold higher risk of recurrence in multifocal compared with unifocal tumors.[66] Another

## TABLE 40-2.
### Factors Influencing the Prognosis of Papillary and Follicular Thyroid Cancer

**PAPILLARY THYROID CANCER**

*Most Aggressive Tumor Behavior*
Large primary tumors (>4.5 cm in diameter)
Tumor invasion into neck
Symptomatic primary tumors with aggressive growth characteristics
Anaplastic transformation
Age ≥40 years at the time of diagnosis
Mediastinal lymph node metastases
Bone metastases
Large solitary pulmonary metastases
Distant metastases that do not effectively concentrate [131]I

*Less Aggressive but More Unpredictable Tumor Behavior*
Primary tumors of intermediate size (1.5–4.5 cm)
Microscopic multicentric primary tumors*
Bilateral cervical lymph node metastases*
Male gender*
Tumors occurring after head and neck irradiation*
Pulmonary metastases that are diffuse *and* concentrate [131]I seen only on [131]I diagnostic or posttherapy scan

*Least Aggressive Tumor Behavior*
Small primary tumors (<1.5 cm in diameter)
Young patients (10–40 years)
Lymphocytic infiltration of tumor
Encapsulated primary tumors
Thyroglossal duct tumors

**FOLLICULAR THYROID CANCER**

*Most Aggressive Tumor Behavior*
Large primary tumors (>4 cm in diameter)†
Tumor invasion of cervical structures
Moderate to extensive vascular and capsular invasion†
Oxyphilic tumors (Hürthle cell carcinoma)†
Anaplastic transformation or marked cellular atypia
Age ≥40 years at the time of diagnosis
Male patients (slight preponderance)†
Distant metastases

*Least Aggressive Tumor Behavior*
Medium-sized or large tumor follicles
Minimal vascular or capsular tumor invasion†

*Features about which the most controversy or uncertainty exists concerning the influence on prognosis.
†See text for explanation.

study found that the only two parameters significantly influencing tumor recurrence of papillary microcarcinomas were the number of histologic foci ($P$ <.002) and the extent of initial thyroid surgery.[23]

**Lymph Node Metastases.** When lymph nodes are meticulously examined, as many as 85% of cases contain metastatic deposits that correlate with primary tumor size and the presence of multicentric tumor, and reflect aggressive tumor behavior.[37] Some find that metastatic lymph nodes have no impact on recurrence or survival.[59,67] Others report an increased risk for local tumor recurrence when cervical lymph node metastases are present.[3,62,68,69] The prognosis is less favorable with bilateral metastases, mediastinal lymph node metastases, or when tumor is invading through the lymph node capsule into surrounding tissues; these findings correlate with high cancer-specific mortality rates.[3,30,70-73]

**Thyroid Capsular Invasion and Extrathyroidal Extension.** As many as one-third of the papillary carcinomas may invade the thyroid capsule, which in its most severe form results in tracheal or spinal cord invasion and compromise of the major vessels. When this occurs, the mortality rate is ~20% at 5 years, which is a 10-fold increase over that of noninvasive tumors.[3,11]

**Distant Metastases.** Distant metastases are the main cause of death from papillary carcinoma. The 5-year survival rate of 1231 patients with distant metastases was 53%.[11] Long-term survival is common in children and young adults with pulmonary metastases and is most favorable when they are discovered early, are small, and concentrate [131]I (see Fig. 40-5).[54,74] For example, 10-year survival rates are ~80% in young patients with micronodular pulmonary metastases that concentrate [131]I, but are only ~20% with macronodular lung or bone metastases.[75] Early scintigraphic diagnoses before the metastases are apparent on chest roentgenograms and their treatment with [131]I appear to be the most important elements in prolonging disease-free survival and improving the survival rate.[76] Widespread distant metastases may cause thyrotoxicosis, which usually has a poor prognosis.

**Other Tumor Factors.** The histologic variants of this tumor affect prognosis (see Tables 40-1 and 40-2).[18,36] Coexistent Hashimoto thyroiditis is associated with a low tumor stage and may be an independent predictor of a favorable prognosis.[77,78] Anaplastic transformation occurs in well-differentiated thyroid carcinoma, dramatically altering its course and resulting in aggressive local invasion of tumor and widespread, rapidly fatal metastases that do not concentrate [131]I.[37]

**Irradiation-Induced Papillary Carcinomas.** Often, although large multicentric tumors are associated with more frequent recurrences than are spontaneously occurring papillary carcinomas, their cancer-specific mortality rates are similar.[45,79]

**Graves Disease.** The serum of patients with Graves disease stimulates thyroid follicular cells in vitro and can produce progression of thyroid carcinoma.[80] One study of papillary carcinoma associated with Graves disease found the tumors were more often multifocal and that the rate of distant metastases was four times higher than usual.[81] Other studies have failed to show this effect.[57] However, on balance the literature suggests that thyroid cancer occuring with Graves disease is more aggressive than usual.[18a]

**Oncogenes.** Several oncogenes, including the novel PTC oncogenes that are specific for papillary thyroid carcinoma, have been identified.[82–84] The PTC oncogene, which has been found in many papillary carcinomas in the children of Chernobyl,[85] induces the formation of papillary thyroid carcinoma in transgenic mice, showing that it is specific to the development of this tumor.[86,87] To date, no convincing evidence exists that prognosis can be predicted on the basis of a tumor's genetic makeup.

## STAGING SYSTEMS

Several staging systems and prognostic scoring systems have been devised to discriminate between low-risk patients who are anticipated to have a good outcome, thus requiring less aggressive therapy, and higher-risk patients who require the most aggressive therapy to avoid morbidity and/or mortality from thyroid carcinoma.[88] Most do not identify the variants of papillary and follicular carcinoma, which have remarkably different behaviors. Their greatest utility is in epidemiology studies and as tools to stratify patients for prospective therapy trials.[37] They are least useful in determining treatment for individual patients.

## CONSENSUS VIEWS CONCERNING THERAPY

Three studies have shed light on the current practice. At an international symposium held in 1987 in the Netherlands, 160 specialists from 13 countries recommended total thyroidectomy followed by postoperative [131]I thyroid remnant ablation for most patients with differentiated thyroid carcinoma, regardless of their age.[89] A second study was based on the responses of

157 thyroid experts to a questionnaire regarding the management of a hypothetical patient with a solitary thyroid nodule.[90] The majority recommended total or near-total thyroidectomy followed by [131]I ablation of the thyroid remnant; most did not recommend altering this for different tumor histologic types. The third study was based on a survey of the clinical members of the American Thyroid Association who were queried about their long-term management of a hypothetical patient with papillary thyroid carcinoma.[91] Most recommended near-total thyroidectomy and [131]I ablation, and almost everyone preferred long-term levothyroxine ($T_4$) therapy in doses sufficient to lower the thyroid-stimulating hormone (TSH) levels to 0.01 to 0.5 μU/mL. The majority did not alter therapy for patients with a history of radiation, extremes of age, the presence of a nodule <1 cm, multiple foci in the contralateral lobe, or capsular invasion of the nodule.

## SURGERY

When papillary thyroid carcinoma is diagnosed on FNA, total thyroidectomy can be done without frozen section because of the high specificity of FNA for papillary carcinoma. If the FNA is suspicious for papillary carcinoma, frozen section of the tumor should be done at surgery. When either gross findings or frozen sections suggest malignancy, total thyroidectomy can be performed, because almost all such cases have cancer. If frozen section is not diagnostic of malignancy, a thyroid lobectomy with or without isthmusectomy is recommended, because ~75% are benign lesions.[92]

**Extent of Thyroid Resection.** Some prefer lobectomy and regional lymph node dissection as the initial surgery for nearly all patients.[93] Others advise total or near-total thyroidectomy for most patients.[94,95] Guidelines from the National Cancer Center Consortium advise total thyroidectomy for most patients with papillary and follicular thyroid cancer.[95a] In most cases, more extensive thyroid surgery should be done, because disease-free survival is improved, even in children and adults with low-risk tumors.[95–98] In addition to removing multifocal and bilateral carcinoma, total thyroidectomy affords the opportunity to ablate residual uptake in the thyroid bed with small doses of [131]I, facilitating subsequent follow-up.

**Subtotal Thyroidectomy.** Resection of less than a thyroid lobe often done as a nodulectomy is inadequate therapy and is not the current standard of practice.[37,99] Even microscopic thyroid carcinoma requires more surgery than subtotal lobectomy.[13,23,100] Ipsilateral lobectomy and isthmusectomy may be adequate for microcarcinomas discovered postoperatively on study of the final histologic sections, providing they are unifocal tumors confined to the thyroid in a patient who has not been exposed to significant radiation.[3,13,23,100] Complications with this procedure are few, and survival in this group is virtually assured.[3,13,23,100]

**Tumor Recurrence after Subtotal Thyroidectomy.** Tumors treated by lobectomy alone have a recurrence rate in the opposite lobe of as much as 10% and have the highest frequency (11%) of subsequent pulmonary metastases, compared with 1% recurrence rates after total thyroidectomy and [131]I therapy.[11,65] Higher recurrence rates are observed with cervical node metastases and multicentric tumors, justifying a more aggressive surgical approach, particularly in those older than 40 years (see Chap. 43).[3]

**Near-Total or Total Thyroidectomy.** At least near-total thyroidectomy (ipsilateral total lobectomy, isthmusectomy, and nearly total contralateral lobectomy) should be performed for tumors that are either ≥1.5 cm in diameter or multicentric (any size), or are either metastatic or invade the thyroid capsule. Modified neck dissection that preserves the sternocleidomastoid muscle is done for involved lateral cervical lymph nodes. Radical neck dissection is only done for tumors extensively invading the strap muscles.[25]

**Completion Thyroidectomy.** If only partial lobectomy has been performed, it is best to consider completion thyroidectomy for lesions that are anticipated to have the potential for recurrence, because large thyroid remnants are difficult to ablate with [131]I.[101] Completion thyroidectomy has a low complication rate and is appropriate to perform routinely for tumors ≥1 cm, because as many as 40% of patients have residual carcinoma in the contralateral thyroid lobe.[102,103] When there has been a local or distant tumor recurrence, carcinoma is found in >60% of the excised contralateral lobes.[58] A study of children from Chernobyl found that completion thyroidectomy allowed for the diagnosis and treatment of recurrent cancer and lung or lymph node metastases in 61% of patients in whom residual carcinoma was not preoperatively recognized.[97] In another study, patients who underwent completion thyroidectomy within 6 months of their primary operation developed significantly fewer lymph node and hematogenous recurrences and survived significantly longer than those in whom the second operation was delayed for longer than 6 months.[104]

**Radioiodine-Assisted Surgery.** The completeness of surgical excision of recurrent or persistent disease can be improved by giving 100 mCi [131]I to patients with functioning lymph node metastases and locating the tumor with the aid of an intraoperative probe.[105] In one study, it detected both suspected and unsuspected lesions in 56% of the patients, although ~25% had nodal metastases that were undetected by this and other techniques.[105]

**Surgical Complications.** Hypoparathyroidism and damage to the recurrent laryngeal nerve are the main surgical complications, which are highest after total thyroidectomy. Rates of hypoparathyroidism as high as 5% are reported in adults,[106] and even higher rates are reported in children[97,107] undergoing total thyroidectomy. However, one study reported a 5.4% rate of hypocalcemia after total thyroidectomy that persisted in only 0.5% of the patients 1 year after surgery.[108] In a review of seven published surgical series, the mean rates of permanent recurrent laryngeal nerve injury and hypoparathyroidism, respectively, were 3% and 2.6% after total thyroidectomy and 1.9% and 0.2% after subtotal thyroidectomy.[109] Hypoparathyroidism occurs at a lower rate when experienced surgeons perform the surgery and the posterior thyroid capsule is left intact on the contralateral side. A study of 5860 patients found that surgeons who performed more than 100 thyroidectomies a year had the lowest complication rates (4.3%), which were four-fold lower than those who performed <10 cases annually.[110]

**Thyroidectomy During Pregnancy.** Thyroid carcinoma during pregnancy may occasionally progress rapidly, perhaps because of high maternal β-human chorionic gonadotropin levels that have a TSH-like effect.[111] Nonetheless, most tumors are slow growing and have an excellent prognosis during pregnancy, and surgery can be delayed until delivery in most women.[112]

## RADIOIODINE THERAPY

**Sodium-Iodide Symporters.** Iodide is concentrated much less avidly by differentiated thyroid carcinoma than by normal thyroid tissue, perhaps because of abnormalities in the sodium-iodide symporters (NIS) that have been identified in differentiated thyroid carcinomas. One study found increased NIS activity in papillary carcinoma,[113] and others have found reduced NIS activity and heterogeneous immunohistochemical NIS staining in differentiated thyroid carcinoma.[114,115]

**Preparation for [131]I Therapy.** In preparation for [131]I therapy, all women of childbearing age must have a pregnancy test unless they have undergone a tubal ligation or hysterectomy. Recombinant human TSH (rhTSH) can be given to raise the serum TSH sufficiently to perform a postoperative total-body [131]I scan (see Follow-Up) but is not yet approved for use in [131]I therapy. However, in special cases in which thyroid hormone withdrawal is not possible or is ineffective, rhTSH may be used successfully in the preparation of patients for [131]I therapy.[115a,115b] Radioiodine is given ~6 weeks after surgery when serum TSH levels have risen enough (>30 μU/mL) to stimulate neoplastic and normal thyroid tissues to concentrate [131]I maximally. Triiodothyronine (Cytomel), 1 μg/kg per day (~25 μg orally, two or three times daily) is given for the first 4 weeks after surgery, then is discontinued for 2 weeks, and serum TSH usually rises above 30 μU/mL.[116] The patient must avoid iodine during this period, especially in the form of drugs and iodine-rich foods. During the last 2 weeks, a low-iodine diet should be ingested[117] and the serum TSH and Tg levels should be measured just before performing the diagnostic [131]I scan.

**Lithium.** Tumor [131]I retention is enhanced by lithium, which decreases the release of iodine from normal thyroid and tumor cells.[118] Given at a dosage of 400 to 800 mg daily in divided doses (10 mg/kg) for 7 days, it increases [131]I uptake in metastatic lesions while only slightly increasing uptake in normal tissue.[118] Blood lithium levels should be measured daily and maintained between 0.8 and 1.2 nmol/L, which prolongs the biologic half-life of [131]I without altering the amount of whole-body radiation. Lithium was found to increase [131]I retention in 24 of 31 metastatic lesions and in 6 of 7 thyroid remnants. Comparing [131]I retention during lithium treatment with that during the control period showed that the mean increase in the retention half-life was 50% in tumors and 90% in remnants. An increase in the accumulated [131]I and the lengthening of the effective half-life (biologic turnover and isotope decay) combined to increase the estimated [131]I radiation dose in metastatic tumor by an average of more than two-fold, which was greatest in tumors with initially low [131]I uptake.[118a] Radiation to tumors with a short biologic half-life (<6 days) is maximized without increasing radiation to other organs.

**Whole-Body [131]I Scan and the Stunning Effect.** A whole-body scan is obtained 24 to 72 hours after giving 2 to 4 mCi of [131]I. Larger scanning doses should not be given, because focal abnormalities not seen with 2 to 4 mCi doses are unlikely to be ablated successfully.[119] Moreover, [131]I doses as small as 3 mCi diminish the subsequent uptake of therapeutic doses of [131]I.[120] Termed the *stunning effect*, this is presumably due to follicular cell damage induced by large scanning doses of [131]I that decrease uptake in the thyroid remnant or metastases for several weeks, thus impairing the therapeutic efficacy of [131]I.[121] After a large scanning dose of [131]I is given, there is an increase in serum Tg that is associated with a higher rate of incomplete ablation, perhaps reflecting a stunning effect on the thyroid remnant.[122] However, 2- or 3-mCi doses of [131]I or the use of [131]I that avoids the stunning effect are slightly less sensitive than larger scanning [131]I doses in identifying thyroid remnants.[121,122]

**Thyroid Remnant Ablation.** Because it is nearly impossible to remove all thyroid tissue with routine surgery, uptake of [131]I is almost always seen in the thyroid bed postoperatively, which must be ablated before [131]I will optimally concentrate in metastatic deposits.[97,123] There are three compelling reasons to ablate a thyroid remnant. First, a large thyroid remnant can obscure [131]I uptake in cervical or lung metastases because they accumulate [131]I optimally only in the absence of normal thyroid tissue.[123] Second, high levels of circulating TSH are necessary to enhance tumor [131]I uptake, which cannot be achieved with a large thyroid remnant.[116] Third, serum Tg measurements are the most sensitive test for carcinoma when they are measured during hypothyroidism after the thyroid bed uptake has been ablated.[124] Nonetheless, there continues to be debate concerning the use of [131]I to ablate uptake in the thyroid bed after near-total thyroidectomy.[57,64]

**Recurrence after $^{131}$I Ablation.**    Patients with tumors who have the potential for recurrence are given $^{131}$I postoperatively to ablate the thyroid remnant.[64] A large and growing number of studies demonstrate decreased recurrence of papillary carcinoma and decreased disease-specific mortality attributable to $^{131}$I therapy (Fig. 40-6).[3,63,64,68,125–128] The lowest incidence of pulmonary metastases occurs after total thyroidectomy and $^{131}$I. In one study, recurrences in the form of pulmonary metastases, analyzed as a function of initial therapy of papillary or follicular carcinoma, was reported to be as follows: thyroidectomy plus $^{131}$I (ablation dose of 100 mCi), 1.3%; thyroidectomy alone, 3%; partial thyroidectomy plus $^{131}$I, 5%; and partial thyroidectomy alone, 11%.[65]

**$^{131}$I Dose for Thyroid Remnant Ablation.**    Thyroid remnant ablation usually can be achieved with a dose of 30 to 50 mCi of $^{131}$I, which appears to be as effective as larger doses in preventing tumor recurrence.[3,125,129] This has been a popular way to avoid hospitalization, but is no longer necessary in most states because of a change in federal regulations that permits the use of much larger $^{131}$I doses in ambulatory patients.[130] Nonetheless, considering the large differences in cost and radiation exposure and the fact that doses >50 mCi do not substantially improve the rate of successful ablation, it is reasonable to use a 30- to 50-mCi dose for remnant ablation.[129] Some use a dosimetry calculation (see Quantitative Tumor Dosimetry) that delivers 30,000 rad to the thyroid remnants; in one study, this was achieved with a mean $^{131}$I dose of almost 87 mCi that completely ablated 86% of the remnants.[101] Increasing the $^{131}$I dose to deliver >30,000 rad does not increase the success rate.[101,129] Response rates are significantly lower when patients have less than a total or near-total thyroidectomy or have a thyroid remnant calculated to be >2 g.[101]

**Therapeutic $^{131}$I for Residual or Recurrent Carcinoma.**    Residual or recurrent carcinoma should be treated surgically whenever possible; however, only ~50% to 75% of differentiated thyroid carcinomas and their metastases and approximately one-third of Hürthle cell carcinomas concentrate $^{131}$I.[131–133] One study found that two-thirds of 283 patients with lung or bone metastases had tumors that concentrated $^{131}$I.[134] This is crucial to survival. For example, 10-year survival rates in one study were 83% or 0%, respectively, depending on whether pulmonary metastases did or did not concentrate $^{131}$I.[75] The lung metastases that concentrate $^{131}$I best are the smallest lesions found in young patients.[75]

**Empiric Fixed Doses.**    There are basically three approaches to therapy: empiric fixed doses, upper bound limits set by blood dosimetry, and quantitative dosimetry.[130] With the first, a fixed amount of $^{131}$I is given based on what is being treated. For example, 30 to 50 mCi are given to ablate thyroid remnants, 150 to 175 mCi for residual carcinoma in cervical nodes or neck tissues, and 200 mCi or more for distant metastases. Tumor $^{131}$I uptake in amounts adequate for imaging with 4-mCi scanning doses is usually sufficient for $^{131}$I therapy, using empiric doses from 30 to 200 mCi.[135]

**Upper Bound Limits Set by Blood Dosimetry.**    Blood dosimetry is done to establish an upper limit on the amount of $^{131}$I that can be given safely, which is generally considered to be 200 rad to the whole blood from a single dose.[136]

**Quantitative Tumor Dosimetry.**    The third approach is to calculate the dose of $^{131}$I that is required to deliver 30,000 rad to ablate the thyroid remnant or 8000 to 12,000 rad to treat nodal or discrete soft tissue metastases. For pulmonary metastases, the amount of $^{131}$I is administered that delivers 200 rad to whole blood with no more than 80 mCi of whole blood retention at 48 hours.[130] The two most important factors in determining success are the mass of residual tissue and the effective half-time of $^{131}$I in that tissue.[130] An 80% response was found in tumor deposits that received at least 8000 rad.[101] Lesions that receive <3000 to 4000 rad from 150 to 200 mCi $^{131}$I should be considered for alternative therapy.

**Repeat $^{131}$I Treatments.**    As long as metastatic deposits concentrate $^{131}$I, treatment should be continued every 6 to 12 months until the tumor has been ablated or adverse effects are seen. Repeat doses of $^{131}$I should not be given until the bone marrow has fully recovered from the previous dose. Few adverse effects occur with this approach to $^{131}$I therapy.[137]

**Immediate Risks of $^{131}$I Therapy.**    There are few immediate serious risks of $^{131}$I therapy, except when brain or spinal cord metastases are present that can undergo edema and hemorrhage 12 hours to 2 weeks after treatment.[138] Severe radiation thyroiditis can occur within a week of administering a large dose of $^{131}$I to a patient who has undergone only lobectomy, causing pain, swelling, and (rarely) airway compromise that may require prednisone therapy.[139] Thyroid storm, a rare occurrence, may appear ~2 to 10 days after administering a therapeutic dose of $^{131}$I to a patient with a large functioning tumor burden.[130] Some experience acute bone pain after being treated with $^{131}$I. Approximately 4 to 12 hours after the oral administration of 200 mCi or more of $^{131}$I, two-thirds of patients develop mild radiation sickness characterized by headache, nausea, and occasional vomiting that resolves in ~24 hours.[130] This is rarely seen with $^{131}$I doses <200 mCi. Patients with extensive tumor may rarely develop transient vocal cord paralysis.[130] Facial nerve paralysis has been reported in one patient given a very high dose of $^{131}$I.[130] Radiation cystitis does not occur if the patient is well hydrated. Mild radiation sialadenitis, leukopenia, and a slight drop in the number of platelets often occur ~6 weeks after therapy, but ordinarily these effects are mild and usually transient.[140]

**Parotid Dysfunction.**    Having the patient suck on hard lemon candy increases salivary flow, which decreases but does not prevent the effects of salivary gland $^{131}$I radiation. Transient parotid swelling reminiscent of Stensen duct obstruction may occur for nearly a year after $^{131}$I therapy. In one study, ~60% of patients reported side effects lasting >3 months, including sialoadenitis (33%) and transient loss of taste or smell (27%).[141] More than a year after the last $^{131}$I treatment, 43% experienced reduced salivary gland function, and more than 4% had complete xerostomia, both of which were related to the cumulative dose of $^{131}$I.[141] Nearly 23% of the patients reported chronic or recurrent conjunctivitis.[141]

**Radiation Pneumonitis.**    Pulmonary fibrosis may occur after $^{131}$I therapy for widespread pulmonary metastases, but this is rare when the whole body retention is <80 mCi 48 hours

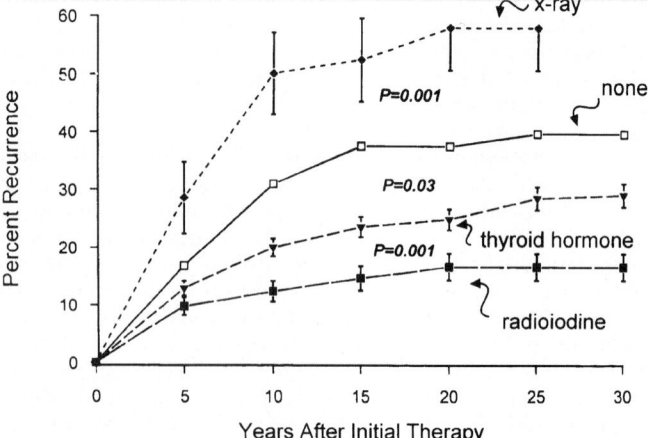

**FIGURE 40-6.** Differentiated thyroid carcinoma recurrence rates after different types of medical therapy. (Adapted from data published in Mazzaferri EL, Jhiang SM. Long term impact of initial surgical and medical therapy on papillary and follicular thyroid cancer. Am J Med 1994; 97:418.)

after treatment. Most diffuse pulmonary metastases can be treated with 150 mCi [131]I without risking pulmonary fibrosis.[142] Smaller [131]I doses ~100 mCi can be given when there is diffuse and intense uptake of the scanning dose in the lungs.[33]

**Leukemia and Other Bone Marrow Effects.** There is a small risk of developing acute myelogenous leukemia after [131]I therapy, estimated at 3 to 22 excess cases per 1000 patients treated with [131]I, depending on the cumulative dose.[130,137] However, the lower estimate seems more likely based on a Swedish study that found two leukemia cases among 834 thyroid carcinoma patients treated with [131]I, which was not statistically significant.[143] When [131]I doses are given at 12-month intervals and total cumulative doses are limited to 500 mCi in children and 800 mCi in adults, long-term effects on the bone marrow are minimal, and few cases of leukemia occur.[137,144,145] In practice, this is usually not a problem, because tumor tissue that concentrates [131]I is likely to be ablated by several treatments, leaving either no residual tumor or metastases that do not concentrate [131]I. Cumulative doses >800 mCi are given to patients with extensive metastatic disease, because the risk posed by the thyroid cancer outweighs that due to radiation. Trivial uptake of [131]I in the neck or elsewhere that cannot be ablated is not a reason for administering large cumulative [131]I doses.

**Cancer Caused by [131]I Therapy.** Small increases in the incidence of colon, breast, bladder, and salivary cancer have been found in some studies of [131]I therapy for thyroid carcinoma, but not in others.[130,143] This underscores the need for laxatives and hydration after [131]I treatment, especially for hypothyroid patients.

**Infertility and Gonadal Failure.** Large doses of [131]I are a risk to gonadal damage, but it is infrequently observed.[130,146] A European study of 2113 pregnancies in women with thyroid carcinoma who had been treated with surgery and [131]I found that the miscarriage rate increased from 11% before surgery to 20% after surgery and remained at this level after [131]I therapy.[147] Miscarriages were more frequent in women who were treated during the year preceding conception, but whether this was related to gonadal irradiation or to insufficient control of hormonal thyroid status was uncertain.[147] Testicular germinal cell function may be transiently impaired when men are given [131]I therapy for thyroid carcinoma.[148] Because this occasionally is permanent, it seems prudent to advise young men to bank their sperm before therapy.

## THYROID HORMONE THERAPY

**Levothyroxine Thyroid-Stimulating Hormone Suppression.** Differentiated thyroid carcinomas contain TSH receptors, and TSH stimulates their growth.[80] Therapy with $T_4$ significantly reduces recurrence rates and cancer-specific mortality rates (see Fig. 40-6).[3] The $T_4$ dose needed to attain serum TSH levels in the euthyroid range is greater in those with thyroid cancer (2.11 μg/kg per day) than in patients with primary hypothyroidism associated with nonmalignant disease (1.62 μg/kg per day).[149] For patients who have undergone total thyroid ablation for thyroid carcinoma, the $T_4$ dosage necessary to achieve an undetectable basal serum TSH level that does not increase after thyrotropin-releasing hormone administration is 2.7 ± 0.4 (SD) μg/kg per day.[150] One study found that a constantly suppressed TSH (≤.05 μU/mL) was associated with a longer relapse-free survival than serum TSH levels that were always ≥1 μU/mL, and that the degree of TSH suppression was an independent predictor of recurrence.[151] However, a prospective study of 617 patients in the National Thyroid Cancer Treatment Cooperative Study found that disease stage, patient age, and [131]I therapy independently predicted disease progression, but the degree of TSH suppression did not.[152] Hence, these data do not support the concept that great degrees of TSH suppression are required to prevent disease progression. As a

practical matter, the most appropriate dose of $T_4$ for most patients with thyroid carcinoma is that which reduces the serum concentration to just below the lower limit of the normal range for the assay being used.

**Complications.** Cardiovascular abnormalities, which are well recognized in overt thyrotoxicosis, also occur in those taking suppressive doses of $T_4$.[153] Among the cardiovascular problems associated with subclinical thyrotoxicosis are an increased risk of atrial fibrillation,[154] a higher 24-hour heart rate, more atrial premature contractions per day, and not only increased cardiac contractility but also ventricular hypertrophy.[153,155,156]

Patients with thyroid carcinoma treated with suppressive doses of $T_4$ have a high rate of bone turnover that decreases acutely after withdrawing treatment.[157] This is of most concern in postmenopausal women, but using the smallest $T_4$ dose necessary to suppress TSH has been shown to have no significant effects on bone metabolism and bone mass in men or women with thyroid carcinoma.[158]

## OTHER THERAPY

**Retinoic Acid.** A few patients may benefit from retinoic acid, a drug that in vitro partly redifferentiates follicular thyroid carcinoma. In one study, retinoic acid given orally (1.18 ± 0.37 mg/kg) for at least 2 months to 12 patients with differentiated carcinoma that could not be treated with other modalities induced significant [131]I uptake in two patients.[159] This response was associated with a rise in serum Tg concentration, suggesting tumor redifferentiation.

**Surgical Excision of Metastases.** Focal lesions that do not concentrate [131]I adequately and isolated skeletal metastases should be considered for surgical excision or external irradiation.[68] Life-threatening tumor refractory to all other forms of therapy may be palliatively treated with doxorubicin (Adriamycin), although the response rate is poor.[11]

## FOLLOW-UP

Follow-up consists of examination; neck ultrasonography; chest radiography; and, if postoperative thyroid [131]I ablation has been performed, whole-body [131]I scans and serum Tg determinations (Fig. 40-7). Patients with clinically significant tumors (>1.5 cm) should be evaluated every 6 to 12 months for 10 years. Whole-body [131]I scan performed 12 months after surgery and [131]I ablation often can document complete absence of tumor. Thereafter, scanning can be done at infrequent intervals unless there is a change in the examination or a rise in Tg.

### RECOMBINANT HUMAN THYROID-STIMULATING HORMONE

Periodic withdrawal of thyroid hormone therapy is required during follow-up. This causes symptomatic hypothyroidism to raise the serum TSH concentrations sufficiently to stimulate thyroid tissue so that [131]I scanning and serum Tg measurements can be obtained. Intramuscular administration of rhTSH stimulates thyroidal [131]I uptake and Tg release while the patient continues thyroid hormone suppression therapy, thus avoiding symptomatic hypothyroidism.[160,161] Now approved for diagnostic use, rhTSH has been tested in two large international multicenter studies. The first study found that whole-body [131]I scan results done after two 0.9-mg doses of rhTSH (while thyroid hormone therapy was continued) were of good quality; they were equivalent to the scans obtained after thyroid hormone withdrawal in 66% of the patients, superior in 5%, and inferior in 29%.[161] This study found that rhTSH stimulates [131]I uptake for whole-body scanning, but the sensitivity of scanning after rhTSH administration was less than after the withdrawal of thyroid hormone.[161] Scanning with rhTSH was associated with significantly fewer symptoms and dysphoric mood states.

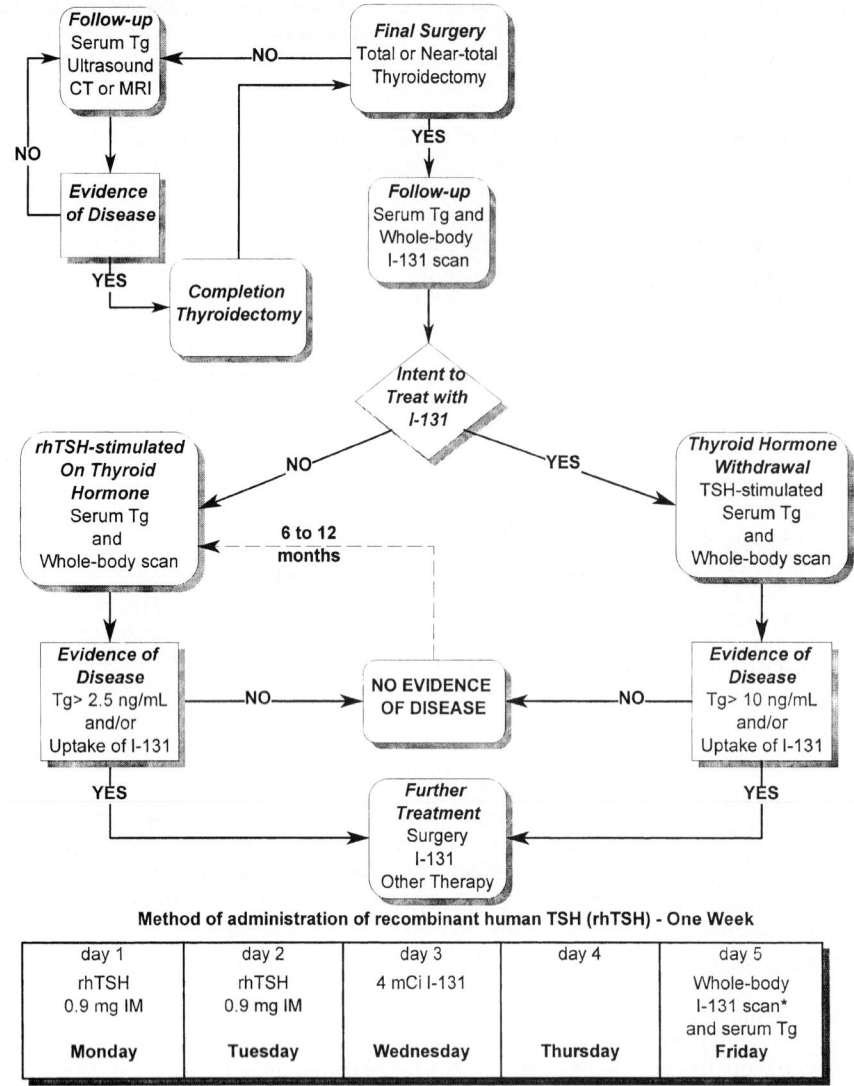

**Method of administration of recombinant human TSH (rhTSH) - One Week**

| day 1 | day 2 | day 3 | day 4 | day 5 |
|---|---|---|---|---|
| rhTSH 0.9 mg IM | rhTSH 0.9 mg IM | 4 mCi I-131 | | Whole-body I-131 scan* and serum Tg |
| **Monday** | **Tuesday** | **Wednesday** | **Thursday** | **Friday** |

* scan for 30 minutes or until 140,000 counts are obtained

**Method of Thyroid Hormone Withdrawal - Six Weeks**

| Week 1 | Week 2 | Week 3 | Week 4 | Week 5 | Week 6 **Scan and Tg** |
|---|---|---|---|---|---|
| Cytomel 25 µg BID or TID | Cytomel 25 µg BID or TID | Cytomel 25 µg BID or TID | Cytomel 25 µg BID or TID | No Thyroid Hormone Low Iodine Diet | No Thyroid Hormone Low Iodine Diet |

**FIGURE 40-7.** Use of recombinant human thyroid-stimulating hormone (*TSH*) in the management of differentiated thyroid carcinoma. Top shows method of recombinant human TSH (*rhTSH*) administration, and bottom shows algorithm for its use. (*CT*, computed tomography; *IM*, intramuscularly; *MRI*, magnetic resonance imaging; *Tg*, thyroglobulin.)

A second multicenter international study was done to test two dosing schedules of rhTSH on the results of whole-body scans and serum Tg levels compared with those obtained after thyroid hormone withdrawal. The whole-body $^{131}$I scanning method was more carefully standardized in the second study than in the first.[162] The scans in this study were concordant in 89% of the patients, with superior whole-body scans seen in 4% of the subjects after rhTSH and in 8% after thyroid hormone withdrawal, differences that were not statistically significant. The combination of whole-body scanning and serum Tg measurements detected 93% of the patients with disease or tissue limited to the thyroid bed and detected 100% of the patients with metastatic carcinoma.[162] Although not yet approved for preparation of patients for $^{131}$I therapy, rhTSH has been used successfully for this purpose.[163]

Recombinant human TSH, 0.9 mg, is given intramuscularly every day for 2 days, followed by a minimum of 4 mCi of $^{131}$I on the third day and a whole-body scan and Tg measurements on the fifth day (see Fig. 40-7). Whole-body $^{131}$I images are acquired after 30 minutes of scanning or after obtaining 140,000 counts. A serum Tg of ≥2.0 ng/mL obtained 72 hours after the last rhTSH injection indicates that thyroid tissue or thyroid carcinoma is present, which almost always can be identified on the rhTSH-stimulated whole-body scan using the indicated scanning method.[162] The drug is well tolerated, with mild headache and nausea being its main adverse effects.

**Serum Thyroglobulin Measurement.**   Serum Tg determinations and whole-body $^{131}$I imaging together detect recurrent or residual disease in most patients who have undergone total thyroid ablation. The serum Tg concentration reflects the mass of normal thyroid tissue or differentiated thyroid carcinoma, the degree of thyroid physical damage or inflammation, and the level of TSH receptor stimulation.[164] Serum anti-Tg antibodies should be measured in the sample obtained for serum Tg assay because these antibodies, which are found in as many as 25% of patients with thyroid carcinoma, invalidate serum Tg measurements in most assays.[124,165] Tg measurement is more sensitive when $T_4$ has been stopped or rhTSH is given to elevate the serum TSH.[31,162] Under these circumstances, serum Tg has a lower false-negative rate than whole-body [131]I scanning.[31,162] Detecting serum Tg by a newly introduced Tg mRNA method is a more sensitive marker of residual thyroid tissue or cancer than measuring Tg by immunometric assay, particularly when Tg mRNA is detected during $T_4$ treatment or with circulating anti-Tg antibodies.[166]

The author uses a sensitive Tg immunometric assay with a detection limit of 0.5 ng/mL. A serum Tg above this level during $T_4$ therapy after total or near-total thyroidectomy and [131]I ablation has been achieved is a sign of persistent normal tissue or differentiated thyroid carcinoma, which is an indication for repeat scanning when there is no other evidence of disease (see Fig. 40-7). If serum Tg rises above 10 ng/mL after $T_4$ is discontinued or rises above 2.5 ng/mL after rhTSH is administered, normal or malignant thyroid tissue is usually present, even if the 2- to 4-mCi [131]I diagnostic scan is negative (i.e., <1% [131]I uptake).[94,162,164] In this case, neck ultrasonography, magnetic resonance imaging, or other scans are performed to detect occult tumor that can be excised. However, if tumor is not found and the serum Tg is >10 ng/mL, the author gives a therapeutic dose of [131]I, usually 100 to 150 mCi, and perform a posttreatment scan. In the author's experience, ~20% of such patients have lung metastases. Others use different cutoff values and different doses of [131]I, but the Tg level to trigger treatment has gradually come down.[34]

**Scanning Patients with High Serum Thyroglobulin Concentrations and Negative [131]I Scans.** Several radionuclide scanning techniques may be used to identify the location of tumor in patients with high serum Tg levels, negative diagnostic [131]I scans, and negative neck ultrasonography.

**Thallium-201.** Thallium-201 ([201]Tl) scintigraphy may identify metastases or uptake in the neck when the serum Tg is elevated but the diagnostic whole-body [131]I scan is negative.[167] In a study comparing [201]Tl and [131]I scans, the sensitivities and specificities, respectively, were 94% and 96% for [201]Tl, and 29% and 100% for [131]I.[168] However, another study found that [131]I is much more sensitive than [201]Tl in demonstrating residual thyroid tissue after surgery (100% and 33%, respectively).[169] Others also find that [131]I scintigraphy is more sensitive and more specific than [201]Tl scintigraphy in identifying both residual neck uptake and metastases.[170] In a study of 36 paired whole-body [131]I and [201]Tl scan results, residual uptake in the neck was seen on all the [131]I scans but on only 17% of the [201]Tl scans.[170] In this study, multiple metastatic lesions identified on 14 [131]I scans were interpreted as negative or nonspecific, or as showing fewer lesions on the corresponding [201]Tl scans. Sixteen [201]Tl scans gave false-positive results. The authors concluded that [131]I scintigraphy is more sensitive and more specific than [201]Tl scintigraphy for detecting distant metastases and for identifying residual activity in the neck after thyroidectomy.[170] Other studies have found the two scanning techniques approximately equally useful in detecting local recurrences or distant metastases.[171]

**Technetium-99m.** Technetium-99m ([99m]Tc) may localize differentiated thyroid carcinoma. One study found that the sensitivities of [201]Tl, [99m]Tc-tetrofosmin, and [131]I in identifying distant metastases were comparable (85%, 85%, and 78%, respectively).[169] However, [131]I was much more sensitive than [99m]Tc-tetrofosmin for demonstrating remnant thyroid tissue after surgery (100% and 33%, respectively).[169] Scanning with [99m]Tc-methoxyisobutyl isonitrile ([99m]Tc-MIBI) also detects metastases of thyroid carcinoma and may be useful in the postoperative follow-up. One large study found increased accumulation of [99m]Tc-MIBI in 75% of the patients with lung metastases, in 100% of those with lymph node metastases, and in 94% of the patients with bone metastases.[172] The [99m]Tc-MIBI

scans identified more lesions in the lung than did [201]Tl or [131]I scans, which, respectively, were positive in 80% and 85% of patients with lung metastases, in 100% and 42% of patients with lymph node metastases, and in 90% and 87% of patients with bone metastases.[172]

**Whole-Body Positron Emission Tomography.** Whole-body positron emission tomography (PET) with [18]F-fluorodeoxyglucose (FDG) may identify differentiated thyroid carcinoma metastasis that cannot be identified by scintigraphy with [131]I or [99m]Tc. Although PET has better sensitivity, resolution imaging, and spatial localization, this has to be balanced with its higher cost when compared with thallium scintigraphy.[173] False-positive [18]F-fluorodeoxyglucose uptake may occur with benign lung disease.[174] FDG-PET scans are useful in predicting survival in differentiated thyroid cancer. In one study, multivariate analysis demonstrated that the single strongest predictor of survival was the volume of disease that displayed avidity for FDG-PET. The probability of surviving 3 years with FDG volumes of 125 mL or less was 96% compared with 18% in those with a FDG volume >125 mL. All of the 10 patients with distant metastases and negative PET scans were alive and well at the end of the study, whereas those with positive PET scans were more likely to die of disease.[174a]

**False-Positive [131]I Scans.** Body secretions, transudates, inflammation, nonspecific mediastinal uptake, and neoplasms of nonthyroidal origin may concentrate [131]I.[175] This also can be seen with physiologic secretion of [131]I from the nasopharynx, salivary and sweat glands, stomach, genitourinary tract, and from skin contamination with sputum or tears.[176] Pathologic pulmonary transudates and inflammation that is due to cysts, as well as lung lesions caused by fungal and other inflammatory disease, may produce false-positive scans. Diffuse hepatic uptake of [131]I is rarely due to occult liver metastases but usually is from hepatic clearance of Tg labeled with [131]I by functioning thyroid remnants or extrahepatic thyroid cancer metastases. The more [131]I uptake that appears in the residual thyroid tissue, the more it appears in the liver. In one large study,[177] diffuse hepatic [131]I uptake was seen in 60% of 399 patients undergoing [131]I scans and in nearly 36% of 1115 [131]I scintigraphy studies. Twelve percent of the diagnostic scans in this study showed uptake in the liver. The frequency of hepatic uptake in the posttherapy scans was related to the dose of [131]I as follows: 39% with 30 mCi; 61.5% with 75 to 100 mCi; and 71.3% with 150 to 200 mCi.[177] Patients whose [131]I scans show hepatic uptake without uptake in the thyroid bed or in extrahepatic metastases, however, often have occult liver metastases.[177]

**[131]I Treatment of Patients with Negative [131]I Scans and High Serum Thyroglobulin.** When the serum Tg level is elevated and a tumor cannot be found by localizing techniques, pulmonary metastases are sometimes found only after administrating therapeutic doses of [131]I.[34,178] The Tg cutoff level has been gradually coming down for treating patients with large doses of [131]I whose only evidence of disease is an elevated serum Tg. It was ~30 or 40 ng/mL 10 years ago, but now is closer to 10 ng/mL when the patient is off thyroid hormone.[34] There is increasing evidence that this treatment is beneficial. Multivariate analyses have shown the prognostic importance of the size of pulmonary metastases at the time of discovery.[179] Another multivariate analysis of prognostic factors in 134 patients with pulmonary metastases showed that early (normal chest roentgenogram) scintigraphic diagnosis and [131]I therapy for lung metastases were the most important elements in obtaining both a significant improvement in survival rate and a prolonged disease-free time interval.[76]

Two studies[32,33] found beneficial effects of [131]I therapy for patients with high serum Tg levels, a normal chest roentgenogram, and a negative diagnostic [131]I scan. Of the patients reported in these two series, 80% achieved a negative [131]I on posttherapy scan, 60% had a serum Tg <5 ng/mL off thyroid hormone, six of eight patients had a normalization of the com-

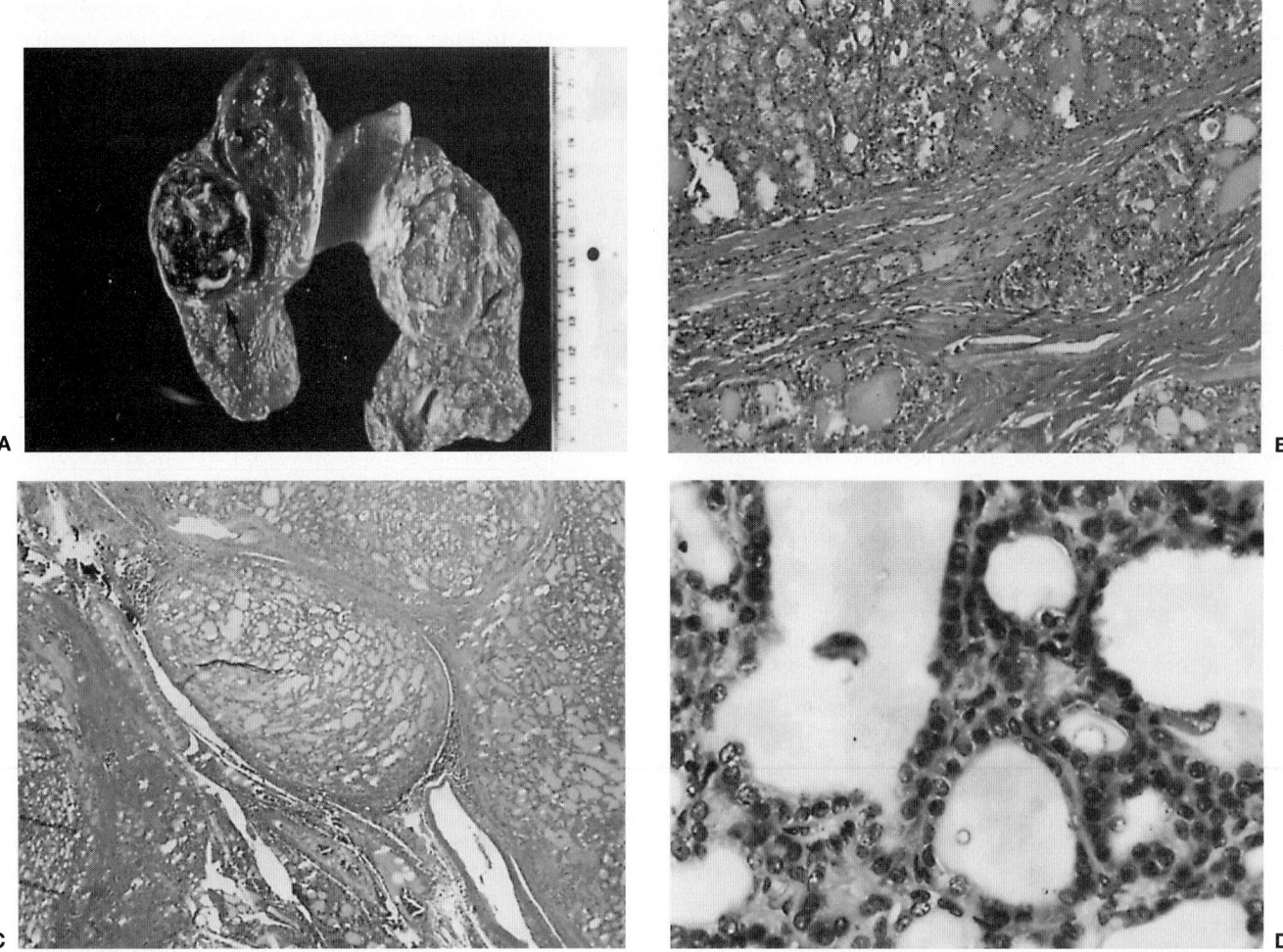

**FIGURE 40-8.** Follicular thyroid carcinoma. **A,** Large follicular thyroid carcinoma (*arrow*) with satellite lesions above the primary. The primary tumor contains areas of hemorrhagic necrosis. **B,** Follicular thyroid carcinoma showing capsular invasion. The tumor, at the top of the photomicrograph, shows a finger-like extension into the capsule and small areas of tumor just below the capsule near its center. ×100 **C,** Follicular thyroid carcinoma showing capsular and vascular invasion. There is a large vessel engorged with tumor in the center of the photo. ×100 **D,** High-power view of follicular thyroid carcinoma containing microfollicles and cells with small, fairly uniform nuclei, which on high power show multiple mitotic figures. ×400

puted tomography scan, and two patients had negative lung biopsies.[32,33] This may occur with one or two [131]I treatments, although complete resolution of pulmonary metastases after [131]I therapy is difficult to achieve.[54] When a partial response with reduction of metastatic disease is achieved, patients usually have a good quality of life with no further disease progression and a low mortality rate.[54]

## FOLLICULAR THYROID CARCINOMA

### PREVALENCE

Follicular thyroid carcinoma accounts for ~5% to 10% of all thyroid cancers in the United States.[11] It occurs at a slightly older age than papillary carcinoma but in recent years has been diagnosed earlier; in some studies, almost half of patients are younger than 40 years of age at the time of diagnosis.[180] This tumor is rare in children, occurs infrequently after head and neck irradiation, and is not commonly found at autopsy as an occult tumor.

## PATHOLOGY

Follicular carcinoma, which is usually encapsulated even when it is aggressive, may initially appear benign on FNA, gross tumor inspection, and frozen-section study; this must be differentiated from follicular variant papillary carcinoma and follicular adenoma.[11] Aggressive tumors show extensive vascular invasion or gross capsular penetration and satellite tumor foci around the periphery of the neoplasm (Fig. 40-8A). Most are single lesions that usually do not show necrotic degeneration. Large aggressive tumors extend into the opposite lobe or may lie in adjacent cervical tissue; they should not be mistaken for lymph node metastases, which ordinarily occur only in the more advanced cases with distant metastases.

Microscopically, these are usually compact, highly cellular tumors composed of microfollicles, trabeculae, and solid masses of cells (see Fig. 40-8B, C, and D). Less often, follicular carcinoma has medium-sized or large follicles and such low invasive characteristics that it is difficult to differentiate from a benign adenoma. Such carcinomas have an excellent prognosis.[11] Follicular carcinoma has compact, dark-staining, round nuclei that are more uniform in shape, size, and location than the nuclei of papillary carcinoma and are difficult or impossible to identify as carcinoma by FNA.[11,46]

**Hürthle Cell Carcinoma.** Oxyphilic cells, termed *Hürthle* or *Askanazy cells,* which contain increased amounts of acidophilic cytoplasm with numerous mitochondria on electron microscopy, may constitute most or all of a follicular carcinoma. Some consider Hürthle cell neoplasms to be a distinct clinicopathologic entity; others consider them to be variants of follicular thyroid cancer.[26] Regardless of their classification, Hürthle cell carcinomas have a less favorable prognosis than nonoxyphilic follicular carcinomas, although they initially may not appear less differentiated or more invasive.[11]

**Classification.** Follicular carcinoma can be classified as minimally or highly invasive. Minimally invasive tumors show just enough evidence—slight penetration of the tumor capsule—to make a diagnosis of carcinoma. Others contain multiple foci of vascular and capsular penetration but are fairly discrete masses. Highly invasive tumors have satellite nodules.

**Distant Metastases.** Follicular carcinoma tends to metastasize to lung, bone, the central nervous system, and other soft tissues with greater frequency than does papillary carcinoma, and the metastases often avidly concentrate $^{131}$I (Figs. 40-9 and 40-10). Also, unlike papillary carcinoma, small lesions can metastasize widely, although tumors >4 cm are associated with a much higher mortality rate.[181]

## DIAGNOSIS

Follicular carcinoma may present as an asymptomatic neck mass, usually without palpable cervical lymph nodes, or a distant metastasis may be the first sign of tumor. Metastases may appear as large discrete pulmonary nodules, osteolytic bone lesions causing pathologic fractures, or as central nervous system tumors with serious neurologic sequelae, which are rarely seen in the absence of a palpable thyroid lesion.[11] Bulky metastatic lesions may be functional and can cause thyrotoxicosis, which can be triiodothyronine toxicosis (see Chap. 42).

The diagnostic evaluation is similar to that for papillary thyroid carcinoma, except a problem is usually encountered in differentiating benign Hürthle cell tumors and follicular adenomas from their malignant counterparts by FNA or by study of the frozen sections at surgery.[95a] Typically, such tumors are simply designated as follicular neoplasms, because their benign or malignant character cannot be determined. Large-needle aspiration biopsies and cutting-needle biopsies usually

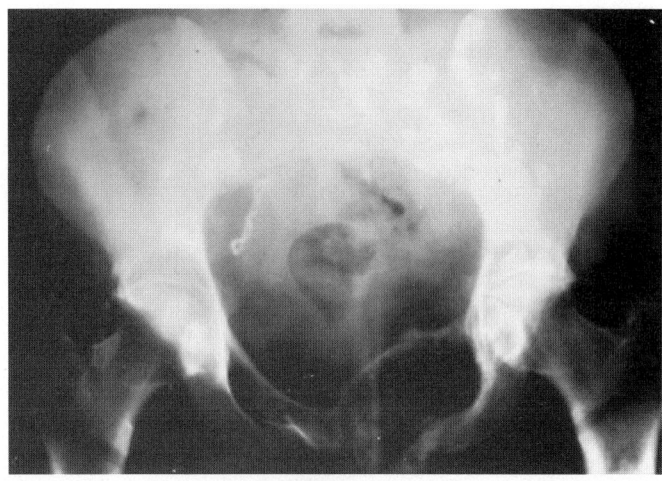

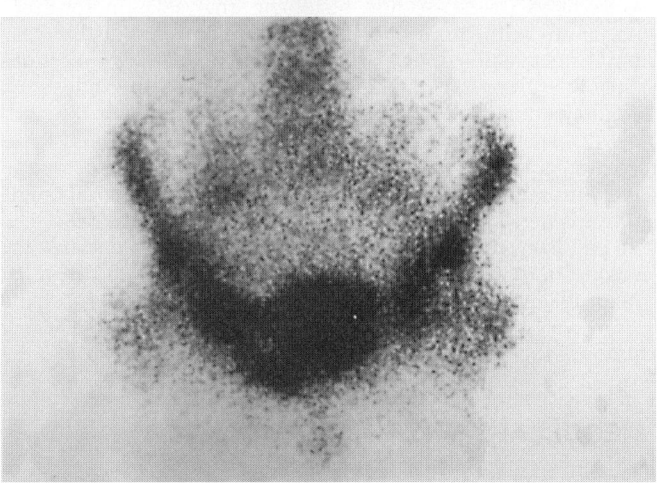

**FIGURE 40-10.** Follicular carcinoma metastatic to pelvis. **A,** Radiograph showing large osteolytic lesions of pubic bones. **B,** Follicular carcinoma, $^{131}$I uptake in lesions shown in **A.** Note that $^{131}$I uptake is more extensive than might be predicted from the radiograph.

yield results similar to those of FNA but have more serious complications.[46] Some physicians suggest that large-needle biopsy, if it can be done efficiently and safely, may be diagnostically useful for follicular nodules ≥3 cm that demonstrate suspicious cytology on FNA. However, most recommend surgical excision of thyroid nodules that are suspicious on FNA[46,95a] (see Chap. 39).

## FACTORS INFLUENCING PROGNOSIS

The 10-year mortality from follicular carcinoma is ~10%[182] but ranges to 50%, depending on the degree of vascular invasion and capsular penetration by the tumor.[11,182–184] Hürthle cell carcinomas have the worst prognosis.[183] Tumor recurrence in distant sites is seen more often with follicular than with papillary carcinomas and occurs most frequently with highly invasive tumors, when the primary lesions are >4 cm, and in Hürthle cell carcinomas.[11,180,181,183] Marked cellular atypia or frank anaplastic transformation is also associated with a poor prognosis. Women with this tumor may fare better than men do, but age has the most important influence on prognosis. Patients younger than 40 years of age at the time of diagnosis have the best prognosis, whereas older patients tend to have higher recurrence and mortality rates from tumors that often do not concentrate $^{131}$I.[11] Ten- and 15-year survival rates with distant metastases (~30% and 10%, respectively) are lowest among patients older than 40 years of age.[11,181]

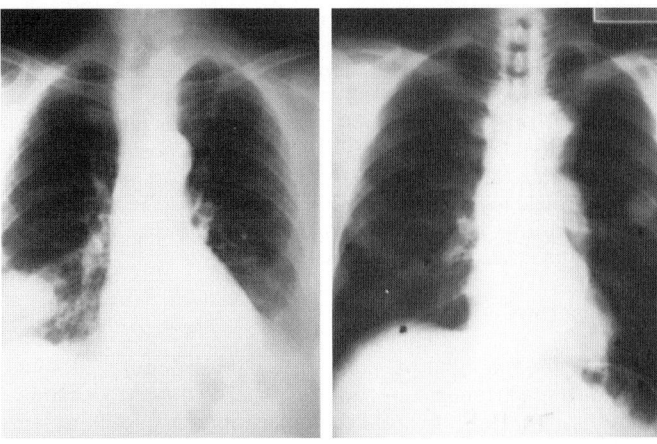

**FIGURE 40-9. A,** Follicular thyroid carcinoma with a large isolated nodular pulmonary metastasis. **B,** Hürthle cell carcinoma with multiple nodular pulmonary and bone metastases that did not concentrate $^{131}$I.

## THERAPY

Appropriate treatment can improve survival with this tumor. Relapse, which occurs less often with surgery followed by $^{131}$I therapy,[11,180] is seen least often in distant sites after total thyroidectomy and $^{131}$I therapy.[65] Survival rates are best if the tumor initially concentrates $^{131}$I and can be completely ablated with the initial surgery and $^{131}$I therapy.[11]

The argument for total or near-total thyroidectomy for follicular carcinoma is stronger for tumors that are more highly invasive, for Hürthle cell carcinomas, and for primary tumors >4 cm in diameter.[11,181,184] Less extensive thyroid surgery may be adequate for tumors that are minimally invasive, because such tumors ordinarily have an excellent prognosis[95a,185]; however, because this distinction cannot be made preoperatively, most clinicians prefer total thyroidectomy for follicular carcinoma.

When the diagnosis of follicular carcinoma is not initially appreciated (frozen-section histologic analysis is notoriously inaccurate with this tumor), only lobectomy and isthmusectomy are usually done. If the permanent histologic sections show the tumor to be malignant, then complete thyroidectomy should be done within 2 to 3 days.[11]

In most clinics, patients with moderately to extensively invasive follicular carcinomas are routinely given $^{131}$I postoperatively to ablate residual $^{131}$I uptake in the thyroid bed. When the tumor is metastatic, the principal treatment is $^{131}$I, as described for papillary carcinoma, provided the tumor concentrates the isotope. If it does not, treatment with external radiation or doxorubicin may be effective.[95a] Thyroid hormone suppression is always given unless the patient is thyrotoxic from metastatic tumor tissue, which produces thyroid hormone.

## MEDULLARY THYROID CARCINOMA

Medullary thyroid carcinoma (MTC), first recognized in 1959, is a pleomorphic neoplasm with amyloid stroma that arises from the calcitonin-secreting C cells of the thyroid. Approximately 20% are familial tumors that are transmitted as an autosomal dominant trait and are often associated with other endocrine neoplasms. The genes responsible for the familial forms of MTC map to the pericentromeric region of chromosome 10.[186]

### MULTIPLE ENDOCRINE NEOPLASIA TYPE 2 SYNDROMES

MTC may occur in four settings. *Sporadic MTC* is a unilateral thyroid tumor with no somatic lesions other than the neoplasm. *Multiple endocrine neoplasia type 2A (MEN2A)* is familial, bilateral MTC with hyperparathyroidism and bilateral pheochromocytoma. *Multiple endocrine neoplasia type 2B (MEN2B)* may be sporadic or familial and features bilateral MTC, bilateral pheochromocytoma, an abnormal phenotype with multiple mucosal ganglioneuromas, and musculoskeletal abnormalities suggestive of the marfanoid habitus. *Familial non-MEN MTC (FMTC)* comprises bilateral MTC with no other endocrine tumors or somatic abnormalities.[187] MEN2A is always inherited as an autosomal dominant trait, whereas MEN2B may be similarly transmitted or can occur sporadically. FMTC is an autosomal dominant trait that is the least common form, and manifests at a later age.[187]

**Medullary Thyroid Carcinoma.**   The MTC in both MEN2 syndromes is generally bilateral and multicentric, as opposed to sporadic MTC, which is usually unilateral. The C cells are normally located in the upper and middle thirds of the lateral thyroid lobes. In MEN2, the C cells initially undergo hyperplasia, which precedes the development of MTC.

**Parathyroid Disease.**   One-third to one-half of the patients with the MEN2A syndrome have hyperparathyroidism, most of whom (85%) have parathyroid hyperplasia.[188] In contrast, almost no patients with MEN2B have parathyroid disease.[189] Patients with MEN2A seldom present with symptoms of hypercalcemia but often form kidney stones. Parathyroid hyperplasia is discovered during MTC surgery in most MEN2A patients, even those without clinical or biochemical evidence of hyperparathyroidism.[189]

**Pheochromocytoma.**   Adrenal medullary disease, ranging from diffuse or nodular hyperplasia to large bilateral multilobular pheochromocytomas, occurs in both MEN2 syndromes. Pheochromocytomas or medullary hyperplasia is typically bilateral and occurs in ~40% of patients, with a range of 6% to 100% in different kindreds.[188] The symptoms are typically subtler than those encountered with sporadic pheochromocytoma.[190] The diagnosis is usually established by demonstrating high urinary or plasma catecholamine levels, but the total urinary catecholamines may be normal, with only an increased epinephrine:norepinephrine ratio, particularly in those with adrenal medullary hyperplasia[190] (see Chap. 86).

**Multiple Endocrine Neoplasia Type 2B.**   MEN2B is characterized by a constellation of somatic abnormalities consisting of ganglioneuromas of the tarsal plates and the anterior third of the tongue, and a marfanoid habitus. Nodules may occur in the lips, causing them to appear lumpy and patulous. Ganglioneuromas in the alimentary tract may be associated with constipation, diarrhea, and megacolon. The marfanoid characteristics include long limbs, hyperextensible joints, scoliosis, and anterior chest deformities, but not ectopic lens or cardiovascular abnormalities[189] (see Chap. 188).

Point mutations of the RET protooncogene have been identified in germline and tumor DNA of unrelated patients from kindreds with MEN2A, MEN2B, and FMTC.[186,191,192] A relationship exists between specific RET protooncogene mutations and the disease phenotype in MEN2.[192] Although several different and independent point mutations in the genomic sequence of the RET protooncogene have been identified, all involving codons for cysteine residues, the normal function of RET is not yet known, and its role in the development of these inherited neoplasms remains unclear. Nevertheless, the identification of point mutations provides an important direct means of identifying affected MEN and FMTC kindreds.

### PREVALENCE

MTC accounts for ~10% of all thyroid malignancies. Approximately 80% to 90% of MTC cases occur sporadically, and 10% to 20% are inherited. MTC may occur at any age, but sporadic disease is diagnosed later in life than is familial MTC. The median age of patients seen at the Mayo Clinic with sporadic MTC was 51 years, compared with 21 years for those with familial tumors.[190] MEN2A and FMTC are both characterized by the development of bilateral MTC, but the age at onset of FMTC is usually later, ranging from 40 to 50 years, as compared with an average of 20 to 30 years for MEN2A. Familial MTC occurs with equal frequency in both sexes, while sporadic MTC has a female-male ratio of 1.5:1.

### PATHOLOGY

Sporadic and familial MTC are histologically similar, although a wider spectrum of appearances is encountered in familial tumors, ranging from isolated hypertrophied C cells to large bilateral multicentric tumors that are usually in the superior portions of the thyroid lobes. Typically, the tumor is composed of fusiform or polygonal cells surrounded by irregular masses of amyloid and abundant collagen (Fig. 40-11). Calcifications

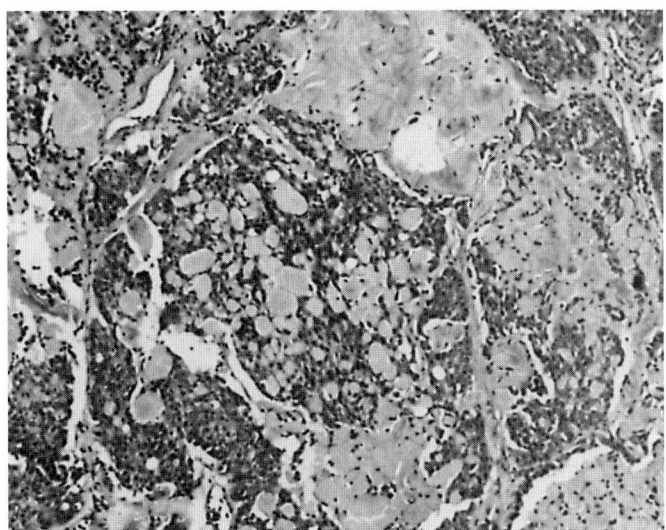

**FIGURE 40-11.** Medullary thyroid carcinoma showing trabecular architecture with spindle and round cells and abundant stroma that stained positively with Congo red, for amyloid. ×100

are present in approximately one-half of the tumors, and occasionally trabecular bone formation is seen. Calcitonin can usually be demonstrated in the tumor by immunohistochemical studies.

Cervical node metastases occur early in the disease and can be seen with primary lesions as small as several millimeters. Tumors >1.5 cm in diameter are more likely to metastasize to distant sites.

The pattern of tissue calcitonin staining may differentiate virulent from less aggressive tumors. In one study, patients with primary tumors that showed intense homogeneous calcitonin staining were all clinically well on follow-up examination, whereas patients whose tumors showed patchy localization of calcitonin either developed metastatic disease or died of cancer within 6 months to 5 years of initial surgery.[193]

## DIAGNOSIS

**Clinical Features.** Patients with sporadic disease or previously unrecognized familial MTC usually present with one or more painless thyroid nodules in an otherwise normal gland, but the tumor may cause pain, dysphagia, and hoarseness. The dominant sign may be enlarged cervical lymph nodes or, occasionally, distant metastases, most commonly to the lung, followed in frequency by metastases to the liver, bone (osteolytic or osteoblastic lesions), and brain. In approximately one-half of patients with sporadic MTC, cervical lymph node metastases are present at the time of diagnosis. The thyroid nodule may be cold or normal on radionuclide imaging and is usually solid on echography and malignant on FNA. Radiographs may show dense, irregular calcifications of the primary tumor and cervical nodes, and mediastinal widening that is due to metastases. Rarely, an abnormal phenotype may correctly identify the tumor, or a paraneoplastic syndrome may be the presenting manifestation.

**Hormonal Features.** In addition to calcitonin, MTC may synthesize calcitonin gene-related peptide, L-dopa decarboxylase, serotonin, prostaglandins, adrenocorticotropin, histaminase, carcinoembryonic antigen, nerve growth factor, and substance P.[190] Elevated calcitonin, histaminase, L-dopa decarboxylase, and carcinoembryonic antigen serum levels occur frequently in MTC patients, but not in other thyroid cancers. Approximately 10% of MTC patients have episodes of flushing

often induced by alcohol ingestion, calcium infusion, and pentagastrin injection; these episodes may be due to tumor release of prostaglandins and serotonin.[190] The only recognized clinical manifestation of high circulating calcitonin levels is a secretory diarrhea that occurs in ~30% of patients and is usually seen only with advanced tumors. Because of the indolent course of MTC, the secretion of adrenocorticotropin by the tumor may cause typical Cushing syndrome (see Chaps. 75 and 219).

**Calcitonin Determination.** Assay of plasma calcitonin is helpful in the early diagnosis of C-cell hyperplasia and MTC and has influenced the management of these disorders, particularly the MEN2 syndromes. Elevated basal plasma calcitonin levels are found in almost all patients with a palpable MTC and correlate directly with tumor mass.[190] Basal calcitonin may not be elevated in patients with small tumors and is almost invariably normal in those with C-cell hyperplasia; however, the plasma calcitonin levels increase to abnormally high levels after stimulation with calcium or pentagastrin. Pentagastrin, 0.5 μg/kg, is given intravenously over 5 seconds, and blood samples are taken at 0, 2, and 5 minutes. Depending on the calcitonin antibody used, this stimulus causes calcitonin levels to rise approximately three- to fivefold with MTC or C-cell hyperplasia.[190] Calcium and pentagastrin infused together is more reliable than either used alone because some patients respond to one but not the other. In the combined test, 2 mg/kg of elemental calcium is infused over 60 seconds, followed by 0.5 μg/kg of pentagastrin infused over 5 to 10 seconds, and plasma calcitonin is measured before and 1, 2, 3, 5, and 10 minutes after infusion. Depending on the calcitonin antibody used, the plasma calcitonin level rises approximately five-fold with MTC or C-cell hyperplasia if the basal calcitonin level is minimally elevated. Diagnosis of familial cases is now possible with genetic screening long before the thyroid tumor is clinically manifest or calcitonin levels are elevated (see Factors Influencing Prognosis).

Hypercalcitoninemia is not absolutely diagnostic of MTC because it occurs in other conditions.[190] When the differential diagnosis of a high plasma calcitonin value is between MTC and another malignancy, a higher calcitonin value and a palpable thyroid tumor usually can identify patients with MTC. In addition, calcitonin secretion by other cancers is poorly stimulated by pentagastrin[190] (see Chap. 53).

## FACTORS INFLUENCING PROGNOSIS

MTC is much more aggressive than papillary and follicular carcinoma and has a cancer-specific mortality of ~20% at 10 years.[182] Also, a significant number of deaths occur from pheochromocytoma.[194] The survival rate is substantially worse with sporadic tumors or when metastases are found at the time of diagnosis, with the MEN2B phenotype, and among patients older than 50 years of age at the time of diagnosis. However, the most important prognostic factors are age and tumor stage at the time of diagnosis and the presence of residual disease postoperatively.[195,196,196a]

Prognosis is best with FMTC and MEN2A. Early detection and treatment has a profound impact on the clinical course of MTC. The 10-year survival rates are nearly similar to those in unaffected subjects when nodal metastases are not present, but fall to ~45% with nodal metastases.[190]

Patients operated on during the first decade of life generally have no evidence of residual disease postoperatively.[190] However, persistent or recurrent disease is seen in approximately one-third of patients operated on in the second decade and gradually increases in frequency with age until the seventh decade, when approximately two-thirds of patients have persistent disease after surgery.[190] This is largely due to the clinical stage of the disease at the time of surgery.[195,196,196a]

Before 1970, MTC was usually diagnosed in the fifth or sixth decade. With periodic calcitonin screening, affected patients with MEN kindred have been diagnosed at a much earlier age, usually in the second decade or earlier, when they have C-cell hyperplasia or microscopic carcinoma confined to the thyroid.[197] Now, with the availability of genetic testing, affected patients can be identified at birth.[198] However, the sensitivity of genetic screening for MEN2A offered by diagnostic laboratories that limit RET analysis to exons 10 and 11 is ~83%.[199] Genetic testing that includes RET exon 14 results in a more complete and accurate analysis with a sensitivity approaching 95%.[199] It is recommended that clinicians confirm the comprehensiveness of a laboratory's genetic screening approach for MEN2A to ensure thoroughness of sample analysis.

## THERAPY

**Initial Surgery.** Surgery offers the only chance for cure and should be performed as soon as the disease is detected.[195,196] Before thyroidectomy, however, pheochromocytoma must be rigorously searched for and excised. The treatment of MTC confined to the neck is total thyroidectomy because the disease is often multicentric, even in patients with a negative family history who are often unsuspected relatives of affected MEN2 kindred.[195,196] Because cervical node metastases occur early and adversely influence survival, all patients with palpable MTC or clinically occult disease that is visible on cut section of the thyroid should undergo routine dissection of lymph nodes in the central neck compartment. The lateral lymph nodes should be dissected when they contain tumor, but radical neck dissection is not recommended unless the jugular vein, accessory nerve, or sternocleidomastoid muscle is invaded by tumor.[107]

**Residual or Recurrent Medullary Thyroid Carcinoma.** Residual or recurrent MTC, manifested by elevated calcitonin levels, occurs commonly after primary treatment of the tumor. Reoperation in appropriately selected patients is the only treatment that consistently and reliably reduces calcitonin levels and may result in excellent local disease control. Although reoperative neck microdissections can normalize calcitonin levels when metastatic MTC is confined to regional lymph nodes, there is no curative therapy for widely metastatic disease. Improved results are reported with surgical management of recurrent MTC, mainly through better preoperative selection of patients and the institution of routine laparoscopic liver examination preoperatively, which identifies distant metastases in patients with normal computed tomography and magnetic resonance imaging.[200] Patients with widely metastatic MTC often live for years, but many develop symptoms secondary to tumor persistence or progression. Judicious palliative, reoperative resection of discrete, symptomatic lesions provides significant long-term relief of symptoms with minimal operative mortality and morbidity.[201] Patients with metastatic MTC causing significant symptoms or physical compromise may respond to palliative reoperative resection despite the presence of widespread incurable metastatic disease.[201]

**Inoperable Disease.** Patients with inoperable disease are often given palliative treatment, with external radiation for localized disease, or with doxorubicin or other chemotherapy combinations for widespread, life-threatening disease, which is of limited benefit. Radiolabeled metaiodobenzylguanidine and [111]In-octreotide are potentially useful in palliative care. Octreotide does not improve the natural course of advanced stages of MTC.[202] Initial reports of the aggressive use of radioimmunotherapy with radiolabeled monoclonal antibodies against carcinoembryonic antigen in patients with far advanced disease appear hopeful. The phase I studies, which show the safety of administering high myeloablative doses of $^{131}$I-MN-14 F(ab)$_2$ labeled carcinoembryonic antigen, are encouraging but require confirmation.[202a]

## FOLLOW-UP

The efficacy of surgery for MTC is assessed postoperatively by measurement of plasma calcitonin levels, which may require as long as 6 months to normalize. A normal basal and provoked calcitonin level after surgery indicates cure in most cases. Persistent modest basal calcitonin elevation is often seen after surgery in patients who may remain well for many years, particularly those from a MEN2A kindred who should be observed without further aggressive therapy. When plasma calcitonin levels are extremely high or when diarrhea occurs postoperatively, metastases can be localized by neck palpation, chest radiography, computed tomography, isotope bone (but not liver) scans, liver biopsy, angiography, and venous catheterization with calcitonin measurement. Both $^{99m}$Tc-dimercaptosuccinic acid and $^{111}$In-octreotide studies have similar sensitivity to localized primary MTC; however, these scans do not detect small lymph node involvement (micrometastases) before initial surgery.[203] Unfortunately, both scans have no clinical implication for preoperative MTC staging.

## FAMILY SCREENING

**Genetic Screening.** Genetic screening should be done in all first-degree relatives of any patient who tests positive for a MEN2 or FMTC mutation. One study found that without genetic testing, even when the mean age at the time of thyroidectomy was ~10 years, a significant number of patients (21%) with MEN2A or MEN2B have persistent or recurrent MTC over a follow-up time of approximately a decade.[204]

**Prophylactic Total Thyroidectomy.** In 1993, when mutations of the RET protooncogene were found to account for hereditary MTC, surgeons gained the opportunity to prophylactically operate on patients at an asymptomatic stage or before the disease became clinically manifest. With this approach, microscopic or grossly evident MTC is often present in the excised thyroid glands, but almost none of the patients have metastasis of their MTC to regional lymph nodes at the time of surgery.[198] Almost all patients are biochemically cured with prophylactic total thyroidectomy, which can be performed safely in experienced centers.[107]

Prophylactic total thyroidectomy done by an experienced surgeon is recommended at age 6 years for patients who test genetically positive for MEN2A.[107,205] Thyroidectomy should be done at an even earlier age for children who test positive for MEN2B, because of its aggressive behavior.[204,206] Central neck lymph node dissection should be included when calcitonin levels are elevated or if patients are older than 10 years.[107]

**Surgical Management of Hyperparathyroidism.** Surgical management of hyperparathyroidism in those with MEN2A is controversial. Some advocate total parathyroidectomy and heterotopic autotransplantation for all MEN2A patients with hyperparathyroidism.[207] Others advocate preservation of the parathyroids, which obviates the potential morbidity associated with total parathyroidectomy and autotransplantation.[208,209]

**Screening for Pheochromocytoma.** Before thyroidectomy is performed, those with MEN2 also should have catecholamine and metanephrine measurements. All patients with MTC require postoperative follow-up of serum calcitonin levels.

## REFERENCES

1. Landis SH, Murray T, Bolden S, Wingo PA. Cancer statistics, 1999. CA Cancer J 1999; 49:8.
2. Kosary CL, Ries LAG, Miller BA, et al. SEER cancer statistic review, 1973–1992: tables and graphs. Bethesda, MD: National Cancer Institute. NIH Pub. No. 96-2789, 1995.

3. Mazzaferri EL, Jhiang SM. Long-term impact of initial surgical and medical therapy on papillary and follicular thyroid cancer. Am J Med 1994; 97:418.
4. Hall P, Holm LE. Radiation-associated thyroid cancer: facts and fiction. Acta Oncol 1998; 37:325.
5. Ron E, Lubin JH, Shore RE, et al. Thyroid cancer after exposure to external radiation: a pooled analysis of seven studies. Radiat Res 1995; 141:259.
6. Ron E, Doddy MM, Becker DV, et al. Cancer mortality following treatment for adult hyperthyroidism. JAMA 1998; 280:347.
6a. Franklyn JA, Maisonneuve P, Sheppard M, et al. Cancer incidence and mortality after radioiodine treatment for hyperthyroidism: a population-based cohort study. Lancet 1999; 353:2111.
7. Jacob P, Goulko G, Heidenreich WF, et al. Thyroid cancer risk to children calculated. Nature 1998; 392:31.
8. National Cancer Institute. Estimated exposures and thyroid doses received by the American people from iodine-131 in fallout following nuclear atmospheric nuclear bomb tests: a report from the National Cancer Institute. Washington, DC: US Department of Health and Human Services, National Institutes of Health, National Cancer Institute, 1997.
9. Institute of Medicine. Committee on exposure of the American people to I-131 from the Nevada atomic-bomb test: implications for public health. Washington, DC: National Academy Press, 1999.
10. Gilbert ES, Tarone R, Bouville A, Ron E. Thyroid cancer rates and [131]I doses from Nevada atmospheric nuclear bomb tests. Am J Med 1998; 90:1654.
11. Mazzaferri EL. Thyroid carcinoma: papillary and follicular. In: Mazzaferri EL, Samaan N, eds. Endocrine tumors. Cambridge, England: Blackwell Scientific Publications Inc., 1993:278.
12. Robbins J, Schneider AB. Radioiodine-induced thyroid cancer: studies in the aftermath of the accident at Chernobyl. Trends 1998; 9:87.
13. Moosa M, Mazzaferri EL. Occult thyroid carcinoma. Cancer J 1997; 10:180.
14. Burgess JR, Duffield A, Wilkinson SJ, et al. Two families with an autosomal dominant inheritance pattern for papillary carcinoma of the thyroid. J Clin Endocrinol Metab 1997; 82:345.
15. Malchoff CD, Sarfarazi M, Tendler B, et al. Familial papillary thyroid carcinoma is genetically distinct from familial adenomatous polyposis coli. Thyroid 1999; 9:247.
15a. Lupoli G, Vitale G, Caraglia M, et al. Familial papillary thyroid microcarcinoma: a new clinical entity. Lancet 1999; 353:37.
16. Bell B, Mazzaferri EL. Familial adenomatous polyposis (Gardner's syndrome) and thyroid carcinoma: a case report and review of the literature. Dig Dis Sci 1993; 38:185.
17. Cetta F, Olschwang S, Petracci M, et al. Genetic alterations in thyroid carcinoma associated with familial adenomatous polyposis: clinical implications and suggestions for early detection. World J Surg 1998; 22:1231.
18. Burman KD, Ringel MD, Wartofsky L. Unusual types of thyroid neoplasms. Endocrinol Metab Clin North Am 1996; 25:49.
19. Dahia PLM, Marsh DJ, Zheng ZM, et al. Somatic deletions and mutations in the Cowden disease gene, PTEN, in sporadic thyroid tumors. Cancer Res 1997; 57:4710.
20. Stratakis CA, Courcoutsakis NA, Abati A, et al. Thyroid gland abnormalities in patients with the syndrome of spotty skin pigmentation, myxomas, endocrine overactivity, and schwannomas (Carney complex). J Clin Endocrinol Metab 1997; 82:2037.
21. Evans HL. Encapsulated columnar-cell neoplasms of the thyroid: a report of four cases suggesting a favorable prognosis. Am J Surg Pathol 1996; 20:1205.
22. de los Santos ET, Keyhani-Rofagha S, Cunningham JJ, Mazzaferri EL. Cystic thyroid nodules: the dilemma of malignant lesions. Arch Intern Med 1990; 150:1422.
23. Baudin E, Travagli JP, Ropers J, et al. Microcarcinoma of the thyroid gland: the Gustave-Roussy Institute experience. Cancer 1998; 83:553.
24. Hedinger C, Williams ED, Sobin LH. The WHO histological classification of thyroid tumors: a commentary on the second edition. Cancer 1989; 63:908.
25. Mazzaferri EL, Young RL, Oertel JE, et al. Papillary thyroid carcinoma: the impact of therapy in 576 patients. Medicine (Baltimore) 1977; 56:171.
26. LiVolsi V, Asa SL. The demise of follicular carcinoma of the thyroid gland. Thyroid 1994; 4:233.
27. LiVolsi VA. Papillary lesions of the thyroid. In: LiVolsi VA, ed. Surgical pathology of the thyroid. Philadelphia: WB Saunders, 1990.
28. Noguchi M, Yamada H, Ohta N, et al. Regional lymph node metastases in well-differentiated thyroid carcinoma. Int Surg 1987; 72:100.
29. Sugino K, Ito K Jr, Ozaki O, et al. Papillary microcarcinoma of the thyroid. J Endocrinol Invest 1998; 21:445.
30. Yamashita H, Noguchi S, Murakami N, et al. Extracapsular invasion of lymph node metastasis is an indicator of distant metastasis and poor prognosis in patients with thyroid papillary carcinoma. Cancer 1997; 80:2268.
31. Pacini F, Lari R, Mazzeo S, et al. Diagnostic value of a single serum thyroglobulin determination on and off thyroid suppressive therapy in the follow-up of patients with differentiated thyroid cancer. Clin Endocrinol 1985; 23:405.
32. Pineda JD, Lee T, Ain K, et al. Iodine-131 therapy for thyroid cancer patients with elevated thyroglobulin and negative diagnostic scan. J Clin Endocrinol Metab 1995; 80:1488.
33. Schlumberger M, Arcangioli O, Piekarski JD, et al. Detection and treatment of lung metastases of differentiated thyroid carcinoma in patients with normal chest X-rays. J Nucl Med 1988; 29:1790.
34. Schlumberger M, Mancusi F, Baudin E, Pacini F. 131-I therapy for elevated thyroglobulin levels. Thyroid 1997; 7:273.
35. Yoo KS, Chengazi VU, O'Mara RE. Thyroglossal duct cyst with papillary carcinoma in an 11-year-old girl. J Pediatr Surg 1998; 33:745.
36. LiVolsi VA. Unusual variants of papillary thyroid carcinoma. In: Mazzaferri EL, Kreisberg RA, Bar RS, eds. Advances in endocrinology and metabolism, 6th ed. St. Louis: Mosby-Year Book, Inc., 1995:39.
37. Ain KB. Papillary thyroid carcinoma etiology, assessment, and therapy. Endocrinol Metab Clin North Am 1995; 24:711.
38. Sobrinho-Simoes M, Soares J, Carneiro F. Diffuse follicular variant of papillary carcinoma of the thyroid: report of eight cases of a distinct aggressive type of tumor. Surg Path 1990; 3:189.
39. Nikiforov Y, Gnepp DR. Pediatric thyroid cancer after the Chernobyl disaster: pathomorphologic study of 84 cases (1991–1992) from the Republic of Belarus. Cancer 1994; 74:748.
40. Herrera MF, Hay ID, Wu PS, et al. Hürthle cell (oxyphilic) papillary thyroid carcinoma: a variant with more aggressive biologic behavior. World J Surg 1994; 16:669.
41. Katoh R, Harach HR, Williams ED. Solitary, multiple, and familial oxyphil tumours of the thyroid gland. J Pathol 1998; 186:292.
42. Rosai J. Papillary carcinoma. Monogr Pathol 1993; 138.
43. LiVolsi VA. Follicular lesions of the thyroid. In: LiVolsi VA, ed. Surgical pathology of the thyroid. Philadelphia: WB Saunders, 1990:173.
44. Hassoun AAK, Hay ID, Goellner JR, Zimmerman D. Insular thyroid carcinoma in adolescents: a potentially lethal endocrine malignancy. Cancer 1997; 79:1044.
45. Schneider AB, Shore-Freedman E, Ryo UY, et al. Radiation-induced tumors of the head and neck following childhood irradiation: prospective studies. Medicine (Baltimore) 1985; 64:1.
46. Mazzaferri EL. Management of a solitary thyroid nodule. N Engl J Med 1993; 328:553.
47. Schneider AB, Bekerman C, Leland J, et al. Thyroid nodules in the follow-up of irradiated individuals: comparison of thyroid ultrasound with scanning and palpation. J Clin Endocrinol Metab 1997; 82:4020.
48. Ezzat S, Sarti DA, Cain DR, Braunstein GD. Thyroid incidentalomas: prevalence by palpation and ultrasonography. Arch Intern Med 1994; 154:1838.
49. Tan GH, Gharib H. Thyroid incidentalomas: management approaches to nonpalpable nodules discovered incidentally on thyroid imaging. Ann Intern Med 1997; 126:226.
50. Fogelfeld L, Wiviott MBT, Shore-Freedman E, et al. Recurrence of thyroid nodules after surgical removal in patients irradiated in childhood for benign conditions. N Engl J Med 1989; 320:835.
51. Dottorini ME, Vignati A, Mazzucchelli L, et al. Differentiated thyroid carcinoma in children and adolescents: a 37-year experience in 85 patients. J Nucl Med 1997; 38:669.
52. Harach HR, Williams ED. Childhood thyroid cancer in England and Wales. Br J Cancer 1995; 72:777.
53. Hung W. Well-differentiated thyroid carcinomas in children and adolescents: a review. Endocrinologist 1994; 4:117.
54. Samuel AM, Rajashekharrao B, Shah DH. Pulmonary metastases in children and adolescents with well-differentiated thyroid cancer. J Nucl Med 1998; 39:1531.
55. Zimmerman D, Hay ID, Gough IR, et al. Papillary thyroid carcinoma in children and adults: long-term follow-up of 1039 patients conservatively treated at one institution during three decades. Surgery 1988; 104:1157.
56. Schlumberger M, De Vathaire F, Travagli JP, et al. Differentiated thyroid carcinoma in childhood: long term follow-up of 72 patients. J Clin Endocrinol Metab 1987; 65:1088.
57. Hay ID. Papillary thyroid carcinoma. Endocrinol Metab Clin North Am 1990; 19:545.
58. Pasieka JL, Thompson NW, McLeod MK, et al. The incidence of bilateral well-differentiated thyroid cancer found at completion thyroidectomy. World J Surg 1992; 16:711.
59. Shaha AR, Loree TR, Shah JP. Prognostic factors and risk group analysis in follicular carcinoma of the thyroid. Surgery 1995; 118:1131.
60. Sanders LE, Cady B. Differentiated thyroid cancer: reexamination of risk groups and outcome of treatment. Arch Surg 1998; 133:419.
61. Sarda AK, Bal S, Kapur MM. Near-total thyroidectomy for carcinoma of the thyroid. Br J Surg 1989; 76:90.
62. DeGroot LJ, Kaplan EL, McCormick M, Straus FH. Natural history, treatment, and course of papillary thyroid carcinoma. J Clin Endocrinol Metab 1990; 71:414.
63. Taylor T, Specker B, Robbins J, et al. Outcome after treatment of high-risk papillary and non-Hürthle-cell follicular thyroid carcinoma. Ann Intern Med 1998; 129:622.
64. Mazzaferri EL. Thyroid remnant [131]I ablation for papillary and follicular thyroid carcioma. Thyroid 1997; 7:265.
65. Massin JP, Savoie JC, Garnier H, et al. Pulmonary metastases in differentiated thyroid carcinoma: study of 58 cases with implications for the primary tumor treatment. Cancer 1984; 53:982.
66. Loh KC, Greenspan FS, Gee L, et al. Pathological tumor-node-metastasis (pTNM) staging for papillary and follicular thyroid carcinomas: a retrospective analysis of 700 patients. J Clin Endocrinol Metab 1997; 82:3553.
67. Cady B. Staging in thyroid carcinoma. Cancer 1998; 83:844.
68. Tsang TW, Brierley JD, Simpson WJ, et al. The effects of surgery, radioiodine, and external radiation therapy on the clinical outcome of patients with differentiated thyroid carcinoma. Cancer 1998; 82:375.

69. Simpson WJ, McKinney SE, Carruthers JS, et al. Papillary and follicular thyroid cancer: prognostic factors in 1578 patients. Am J Med 1987; 83:479.

70. Kurozumi K, Nakao I, Nishida T, et al. Significance of biologic aggressiveness and proliferating activity in papillary thyroid carcinoma. World J Surg 1998; 22:1237.

71. Sugitani I, Yanagisawa A, Shimizu A, et al. Clinicopathologic and immunohistochemical studies of papillary thyroid microcarcinoma presenting with cervical lymphadenopathy. World J Surg 1998; 22:731.

72. Akslen LA, Varhaug JE. Oncoproteins and tumor progression in papillary thyroid carcinoma: presence of epidermal growth factor receptor, c-erbB-2 protein, estrogen receptor related protein, p21-ras protein, and proliferation indicators in relation to tumor recurrences and patient survival. Cancer 1995; 76:1643.

73. Sellers M, Beenken S, Blankenship A, et al. Prognostic significance of cervical lymph node metastases in differentiated thyroid cancer. Am J Surg 1992; 164:578.

74. Sisson JC, Giordano TJ, Jamadar DA, et al. [131]I treatment of micronodular pulmonary metastases from papillary thyroid carcinoma. Cancer 1996; 78:2184.

75. Nêmec J, Zamrazil V, Pohunková D, Röhling S. Radioiodide treatment of pulmonary metastases of differentiated thyroid cancer: results and prognostic factors. Nuklearmedizin 1979; 18:86.

76. Casara D, Rubello D, Saladini G, et al. Different features of pulmonary metastases in differentiated thyroid cancer: natural history and multivariate statistical analysis of prognostic variables. J Nucl Med 1993; 34:1626.

77. Kashima K, Yokoyama S, Noguchi S, et al. Chronic thyroiditis as a favorable prognostic factor in papillary thyroid carcinoma. Thyroid 1998; 8:197.

78. Schäffler A, Palitzsch KD, Seiffarth C, et al. Coexistent thyroiditis is associated with lower tumour stage in thyroid carcinoma. Eur J Clin Invest 1998; 28:838.

79. Viswanathan K, Gierlowski TC, Schneider AB. Childhood thyroid cancer: characteristics and long-term outcome in children irradiated for benign conditions of the head and neck. Am J Dis Child 1994; 148:260.

80. Filetti S, Belfiore A, Amir SM, et al. The role of thyroid-stimulating antibodies of Graves' disease in differentiated thyroid cancer. N Engl J Med 1988; 318:753.

81. Belfiore A, Garofalo MR, Giuffrida D, et al. Increased aggressiveness of thyroid cancer in patients with Graves' disease. J Clin Endocrinol Metab 1990; 70:830.

81a. Mazzaferri EL. Thyroid cancer and Graves' disease: the controversy ten years later. Endocrine Practice 2000; 6:221.

82. Fusco A, Grieco M, Santoro M, et al. A new oncogene in human thyroid papillary carcinomas and their lymph-nodal metastases. Nature 1987; 328:170.

83. Donghi R, Sozzi G, Pierotti MA, et al. The oncogene associated with human papillary thyroid carcinoma (PTC) is assigned to chromosome 10 q11-q12 in the same region as multiple endocrine neoplasia type 2A (MEN2A). Oncogene 1989; 4:521.

84. Smanik PA, Furminger TL, Mazzaferri EL, Jhiang SM. Breakpoint characterization of the ret/PTC oncogene in human papillary thyroid carcinoma. Hum Mol Genet 1995; 4:2313.

85. Nikiforov YE, Nikiforova M, Fagin JA. Radiation-induced post-Chernobyl pediatric thyroid carcinomas. Oncogene 1998; 17:1983.

86. Jhiang SM, Sagartz JE, Tong Q, et al. Targeted expression of the *ret*/PTC1 oncogene induces papillary thyroid carcinomas. Endocrinology 1996; 137:375.

87. Santoro M, Chiappetta G, Cerrato A, et al. Development of thyroid papillary carcinomas secondary to tissue-specific expression of the RET/PTC1 oncogene in transgenic mice. Oncogene 1996; 12:1821.

88. American Joint Committee on Cancer. Head and neck tumors: thyroid gland. In: Beahrs OH, Henson DE, Hutter RVP, Myers MH, eds. Manual for staging of cancer, 4th ed. Philadelphia: JB Lippincott, 1992:53.

89. Van De Velde CJH, Hamming JF, Goslings BM, et al. Report of the consensus development conference on the management of differentiated thyroid cancer in the Netherlands. Eur J Cancer Clin Oncol 1988; 24:287.

90. Baldet L, Manderscheid JC, Glinoer D, et al. The management of differentiated thyroid cancer in Europe in 1988: results of an international survey. Acta Endocrinol (Copenh) 1989; 120:547.

91. Solomon BL, Wartofsky L, Burman KD. Current trends in the management of well differentiated papillary thyroid carcinoma. J Clin 1996; 81:333.

92. Chen H, Zeiger MA, Clark DP, et al. Papillary carcinoma of the thyroid: can operative management be based solely on fine-needle aspiration? J Am Coll Surg 1997; 184:605.

93. Cady B. Our AMES is true: how an old concept still hits the mark: or, risk group assignment points the arrow to rational therapy selection in differentiated thyroid cancer. Am J Surg 1997; 174:462.

94. Schlumberger MJ. Medical progress: papillary and follicular thyroid carcinoma. N Engl J Med 1998; 338:297.

95. Mazzaferri EL. Treating differentiated thyroid carcinoma: where do we draw the line? Mayo Clin Proc 1991; 66:105.

95a. Mazzaferri EL. NCCN thyroid carcinoma practice guidelines. Oncology 1999; 13:391.

96. Newman KD, Black T, Heller G, et al. Differentiated thyroid cancer: determinants of disease progression in patients <21 years of age at diagnosis: a report from the Surgical Discipline Committee of the Children's Cancer Group. Ann Surg 1998; 227:533.

97. Miccoli P, Antonelli A, Spinelli C, et al. Completion total thyroidectomy in children with thyroid cancer secondary to the Chernobyl accident. Arch Surg 1998; 133:89.

98. Hay ID, Grant CS, Bergstralh EJ, et al. Unilateral total lobectomy: is it sufficient surgical treatment for patients with AMES low-risk papillary thyroid carcinoma? Surgery 1998; 124:958.

99. Pasieka JL, Rotstein LE. Consensus conference on well-differentiated thyroid cancer: a summary. Can J Surg 1999; 36:298.

100. Tourniaire J, Bernard MH, Bizollon-Roblin MH, et al. Thyroid papillary microcarcinoma: 179 cases since 1973. Presse Med 1998; 27:1467.

101. Maxon HR, Englaro EE, Thomas SR, et al. Radioiodine-131 therapy for well-differentiated thyroid cancer: a quantitative radiation dosimetric approach: outcome and validation in 85 patients. J Nucl Med 1992; 33:1132.

102. Chao TC, Jeng LB, Lin JD, Chen MF. Completion thyroidectomy for differentiated thyroid carcinoma. Otolaryngol Head Neck Surg 1998; 118:896.

103. DeGroot LJ, Kaplan EL. Second operations for "completion" of thyroidectomy in treatment of differentiated thyroid cancer. Surgery 1991; 110:936.

104. Scheumann GFW, Seeliger H, Musholt TJ, et al. Completion thyroidectomy in 131 patients with differentiated thyroid carcinoma. Eur J Surg 1996; 162:677.

105. Travagli JP, Cailleux AF, Ricard M, et al. Combination of radioiodine ([131]I) and probe-guided surgery for persistent or recurrent thyroid carcinoma. J Clin Endocrinol Metab 1998; 83:2675.

106. Burge MR, Zeise TM, Johnsen MW, et al. Risks of complication following thyroidectomy. J Gen Intern Med 1998; 13:24.

107. Dralle H, Gimm O, Simon D, et al. Prophylactic thyroidectomy in 75 children and adolescents with hereditary medullary thyroid carcinoma: German and Austrian experience. World J Surg 1998; 22:744.

108. Pattou F, Combemale F, Fabre S, et al. Hypocalcemia following thyroid surgery: incidence and prediction of outcome. World J Surg 1998; 22:718.

109. Udelsman R, Lakatos E, Ladenson P. Optimal surgery for papillary thyroid carcinoma. World J Surg 1996; 20:88.

110. Sosa JA, Bowman HM, Tielsch JM, et al. The importance of surgeon experience for clinical and economic outcomes from thyroidectomy. Ann Surg 1998; 228:320.

111. Driggers RW, Kopelman JN, Satin AJ. Delaying surgery for thyroid cancer in pregnancy: a case report. J Reprod Med 1998; 43:909.

112. Moosa M, Mazzaferri EL. Outcome of differentiated thyroid cancer diagnosed in pregnant women. J Clin Endocrinol Metab 1997; 82:2862.

113. Saito T, Endo T, Kawaguchi A, et al. Increased expression of the sodium/iodide symporter in papillary thyroid carcinomas. J Clin Invest 1998; 101:1296.

114. Arturi F, Russo D, Schlumberger M, et al. Iodide symporter gene expression in human thyroid tumors. J Clin Endocrinol Metab 1998; 83:2493.

115. Jhiang SM, Cho JY, Ryu K-Y, et al. An immunohistochemical study of Na[+]/I[−] symporter in human thyroid tissues and salivary gland tissues. Endocrinology 1998; 139:4416.

115a. Rotman-Pikielny P, Reynolds JC, Barker WC, et al. Recombinant human thyrotropin for the diagnosis and treatment of a highly functional metastatic struma ovarii. J Clin Endocrinol Metab 2000; 85:237.

115b. Rudavsky AZ, Freeman LM. Treatment of scan-negative, thyroglobulin-positive metastatic thyroid cancer using radioiodine [131]I and recombinant human thyroid stimulating hormone. J Clin Endocrinol Metab 1997; 82:11.

116. Goldman JM, Line BR, Aamodt RL, Robbins J. Influence of triiodothyronine withdrawal time on 131-I uptake postthyroidectomy for thyroid cancer. J Clin Endocrinol Metab 1980; 50:734.

117. Lakshmanan M, Schaffer A, Robbins J, et al. A simplified low iodine diet in I-131 scanning and therapy of thyroid cancer. Clin Nucl Med 1988; 2:866.

118. Pons F, Carrio I, Estorch M, et al. Lithium as an adjuvant of iodine-131 uptake when treating patients with well-differentiated thyroid carcinoma. Clin Nucl Med 1987; 8:644.

118a. Koong SS, Reynolds JC, Movius EG, Keenan AM, et al. Lithium as a potential adjuvant to [131]I therapy of metastatic, well-differentiated thyroid carcinoma. J Clin Endocrinol Metab 1999; 84:912.

119. Maxon HR, Thomas SR, Hertzberg VS, et al. Relation between effective radiation dose and outcome of radioiodine therapy for thyroid cancer. N Engl J Med 1983; 309:937.

120. Park HM, Perkins OW, Edmondson JW, et al. Influence of diagnostic radioiodines on the uptake of ablative dose of iodine. Thyroid 1994; 4:49.

121. Leger FA, Izembart M, Dagousset F, et al. Decreased uptake of therapeutic doses of iodine-131 after 185-MBq iodine-131 diagnostic imaging for thyroid remnants in differentiated thyroid carcinoma. Eur J Nucl Med 1998; 25:242.

122. Muratet JP, Giraud P, Daver A, et al. Predicting the efficacy of first iodine-131 treatment in differentiated thyroid carcinoma. J Nucl Med 1997; 38:1362.

123. Vassilopoulou-Sellin R, Klein MJ, Smith TH, et al. Pulmonary metastases in children and young adults with differentiated thyroid cancer. Cancer 1993; 71:1348.

124. Spencer CA, Takeuchi M, Kazarosyan M, et al. Serum thyroglobulin autoantibodies: prevalence, influence on serum thyroglobulin measure-

ment, and prognostic significance in patients with differentiated thyroid carcinoma. J Clin Endocrinol Metab 1998; 83:1121.

125. Hodgson DC, Brierley JD, Tsang RW, Panzarella T. Prescribing [131]iodine based on neck uptake produces effective thyroid ablation and reduced hospital stay. Radiother Oncol 1998; 47:325.

126. Cunningham MP, Duda RB, Recant W, et al. Survival discriminants for differentiated thyroid cancer. Am J Surg 1990; 160:344.

127. DeGroot LJ, Kaplan EL, Straus FH, Shukla MS. Does the method of management of papillary thyroid carcinoma make a difference in outcome? World J Surg 1994; 18:123.

128. Samaan NA, Maheshwari YK, Nader S, et al. Impact of therapy for differentiated carcinoma of the thyroid: an analysis of 706 cases. J Clin Endocrinol Metab 1983; 56:1131.

129. Bal C, Padhy AK, Jana S, et al. Prospective randomized clinical trial to evaluate the optimal dose of [131]I for remnant ablation in patients with differentiated thyroid carcinoma. Cancer 1996; 77:2574.

130. Brierley J, Maxon HR. Radioiodine and external radiation therapy. In: Fagin JA, ed. Thyroid cancer, 1st ed. Boston/Dordrecht/London: Kluwer Academic Publishers, 1998:285.

131. Simpson WJ, Panzarella T, Carruthers JS, et al. Papillary and follicular thyroid cancer: impact of treatment in 1578 patients. Int J Radiat Oncol Biol Phys 1988; 14:1063.

132. Samaan NA, Schultz PN, Haynie TP, Ordonez NG. Pulmonary metastasis of differentiated thyroid carcinoma: treatment results in 101 patients. J Clin Endocrinol Metab 1985; 60:376.

133. Ruegemer JJ, Hay ID, Bergstralh EJ, et al. Distant metastases in differentiated thyroid carcinoma: a multivariate analysis of prognostic variables. J Clin Endocrinol Metab 1988; 67:501.

134. Schlumberger M, Tubiana M, De Vathaire F, et al. Long-term results of treatment of 283 patients with lung and bone metastases from differentiated thyroid carcinoma. J Clin Endocrinol Metab 1986; 63:960.

135. Mazzaferri EL. Carcinoma of follicular epithelium: radioiodine and other treatment outcomes. In: Braverman LE, Utiger RD, eds. The thyroid: a fundamental and clinical text, 7th ed. Philadelphia: Lippincott-Raven, 1996:922.

136. Benua RS, Cicale NR, Sonenberg M, et al. The relation of radioiodine dosimetry to results and complications in the treatment of metastatic thyroid cancer. AJR Am J Roentgenol 1962; 87:171.

137. Maxon H III, Smith HS. Radioiodine-131 in the diagnosis and treatment of metastatic well differentiated thyroid cancer. Endocrinol Metab Clin North Am 1990; 19:685.

138. Datz FL. Cerebral edema following iodine-131 therapy for thyroid carcinoma metastatic to the brain. J Nucl Med 1986; 27:637.

139. DiRusso G, Kern KA. Comparative analysis of complications from I-131 radioablation for well-differentiated thyroid cancer. Surgery 1994; 116:1024.

140. Allweiss P, Braunstein GD, Katz A, Waxman A. Sialadenitis following I-131 therapy for thyroid carcinoma: concise communication. J Nucl Med 1984; 25:755.

141. Alexander C, Bader JB, Schaefer A, et al. Intermediate and long-term side effects of high-dose radioiodine therapy for thyroid carcinoma. J Nucl Med 1998; 39:1551.

142. Brown AP, Greening WP, McCready VR, et al. Radioiodine treatment of metastatic thyroid carcinoma: the Royal Marsden Hospital experience. Br J Radiol 1984; 57:323.

143. Hall P, Holm L-E. Cancer in iodine-131 exposed patients. J Endocrinol Invest 1995; 18:147.

144. Van Nostrand D, Neutze J, Atkins F. Side effects of "rational dose" iodine-131 therapy for metastatic well-differentiated thyroid cancer. J Nucl Med 1986; 27:1519.

145. De Vathaire F, Schlumberger M, Delisle MJ, et al. Leukaemias and cancers following iodine-131 administration for thyroid cancer. Br J Cancer 1997; 75:734.

146. Schlumberger M, De Vathaire F, Ceccarelli C, et al. Outcome of pregnancy in women with thyroid carcinoma. J Endocrinol Invest 1995; 18:150.

147. Schlumberger M, De Vathaire F, Ceccarelli C, et al. Exposure to radioactive iodine-131 for scintigraphy or therapy does not preclude pregnancy in thyroid cancer patients. J Nucl Med 1996; 37:606.

148. Pacini F, Gasperi M, Fugazzola L, et al. Testicular function in patients with differentiated thyroid carcinoma treated with radioiodine. J Nucl Med 1994; 35:1418.

149. Burmeister LA, Goumaz MO, Mariash CN, Oppenheimer JH. Levothyroxine dose requirements for thyrotropin suppression in the treatment of differentiated thyroid cancer. J Clin Endocrinol Metab 1992; 75:344.

150. Bartalena L, Martino E, Pacchiarotti A, et al. Factors affecting suppression of endogenous thyrotropin secretion by thyroxine treatment: retrospective analysis in athyreotic and goitrous patients. J Clin Endocrinol Metab 1987; 64:849.

151. Pujol P, Daures JP, Nsakala N, et al. Degree of thyrotropin suppression as a prognostic determinant in differentiated thyroid cancer. J Clin Endocrinol Metab 1996; 81:4318.

152. Cooper DS, Specker B, Ho M, et al. Thyrotropin suppression and disease progression in patients with differentiated thyroid cancer: results from the National Thyroid Cancer Treatment Cooperative Registry. Thyroid 1999; 8:737.

153. Biondi B, Fazio S, Carella C, et al. Cardiac effects of long term thyrotropin-suppressive therapy with levothyroxine. J Clin Endocrinol Metab 1993; 77:334.

154. Sawin CT, Geller A, Wolf PA, et al. Low serum thyrotropin concentrations as a risk factor for atrial fibrillation in older persons. N Engl J Med 1994; 331:1249.

155. Fazio S, Biondi B, Carella C, et al. Diastolic dysfunction in patients on thyroid-stimulating hormone suppressive therapy with levothyroxine: beneficial effect of β-blockade. J Clin Endocrinol Metab 1995; 80:2222.

156. Shapiro LE, Sievert R, Ong L, et al. Minimal cardiac effects in asymptomatic athyreotic patients chronically treated with thyrotropin-suppressive doses of L-thyroxine. J Clin Endocrinol Metab 1997; 82:2592.

157. Toivonen J, Tahtela R, Laitinen K, et al. Markers of bone turnover in patients with differentiated thyroid cancer with and following withdrawal of thyroxine suppressive therapy. Eur J Endocrinol 1998; 138:667.

158. Marcocci C, Golia F, Vignali E, Pinchera A. Skeletal integrity in men chronically treated with suppressive doses of L-thyroxine. J Bone Miner Res 1997; 12:72.

159. Grünwald F, Menzel C, Bender H, et al. Redifferentiation therapy-induced radioiodine uptake in thyroid cancer. J Nucl Med 1998; 39:1903.

160. Meier CA, Braverman LE, Ebner SA, et al. Diagnostic use of recombinant human thyrotropin in patients with thyroid carcinoma (phase I/II study). J Clin Endocrinol Metab 1994; 78:188.

161. Ladenson PW, Braverman LE, Mazzaferri EL, et al. Comparison of administration of recombinant human thyrotropin with withdrawal of thyroid hormone for radioactive iodine scanning in patients with thyroid carcinoma. N Engl J Med 1997; 337:888.

162. Haugen B, Pacini F, Reiners C, et al. A comparison of recombinant human thyrotropin and thyroid hormone withdrawal for the detection of thyroid remnant or cancer. J Clin Endocrinol Metab 1999; 84:3877.

163. Rudavsky AZ, Freeman LM. Treatment of scan-negative, thyroglobulin-positive metastatic thyroid cancer using radioiodine [131]I and recombinant human thyroid stimulating hormone. J Clin Endocrinol Metab 1997; 82:11.

164. Spencer CA, Wang CC. Thyroglobulin measurement: techniques, clinical benefits, and pitfalls. Endocrinol Metab Clin North Am 1995; 24:841.

165. Spencer CA. Recoveries cannot be used to authenticate thyroglobulin (Tg) measurements when sera contain Tg autoantibodies. Clin Chem 1996; 42:661.

166. Ringel M, Ladenson P, Levine MA. Molecular diagnosis of residual and recurrent thyroid cancer by amplification of thyroglobulin messenger ribonucleic acid in peripheral blood. J Clin Endocrinol Metab 1998; 83:4435.

167. Nakada K, Katoh C, Kanegae K, et al. Thallium-201 scintigraphy to predict therapeutic outcome of iodine-131 therapy of metastatic thyroid carcinoma. J Nucl Med 1998; 39:807.

168. Carril JM, Quirce R, Serrano J, et al. Total-body scintigraphy with thallium-201 and iodine-131 in the follow-up of differentiated thyroid cancer. J Nucl Med 1997; 38:686.

169. Ünal S, Menda Y, Adalet I, et al. Thallium-201, technetium-99m-tetrofosmin and iodine-131 in detecting differentiated thyroid carcinoma metastases. J Nucl Med 1998; 39:1897.

170. Lorberboym M, Murthy S, Mechanick JI, et al. Thallium-201 and iodine-131 scintigraphy in differentiated thyroid carcinoma. J Nucl Med 1996; 37:1487.

171. Lin JD, Kao PF, Weng HF, et al. Relative value of thallium-201 and iodine-131 scans in the detection of recurrence or distant metastasis of well differentiated thyroid carcinoma. Eur J Nucl Med 1998; 25:695.

172. Miyamoto S, Kasagi K, Misaki T, et al. Evaluation of technetium-99m-MIBI scintigraphy in metastatic differentiated thyroid carcinoma. J Nucl Med 1997; 38:352.

173. Huang TS, Chieng PU, Chang CC, Yen RF. Positron emission tomography for detecting iodine-131 nonvisualized metastasis of well-differentiated thyroid carcinoma: two case reports. J Endocrinol Invest 1998; 21:392.

174. Bakheet SMB, Powe J. Fluorine-18-fluorodeoxyglucose uptake in rheumatoid arthritis-associated lung disease in a patient with thyroid cancer. J Nucl Med 1998; 39:234.

174a. Wang W, Larson SM, Fazzari M, et al. Prognostic value of [18F]fluorodeoxyglucose positron emission tomographic scanning in patients with thyroid cancer. J Clin Endocrinol Metab 2000; 85:1107.

175. Greenler DP, Klein HA. The scope of false-positive iodine-131 images for thyroid carcinoma. Clin Nucl Med 1989; 14:111.

176. Bakheet SMB, Hammami MM, Hemidan A, et al. Radioiodine secretion in tears. J Nucl Med 1998; 39:1452.

177. Chung JK, Lee YJ, Jeong JM, et al. Clinical significance of hepatic visualization on iodine-131 whole-body scan in patients with thyroid carcinoma. J Nucl Med 1997; 38:1191.

178. Mazzaferri EL. Treating high thyroglobulins with radioiodine: a magic bullet or a shot in the dark? J Clin Endocrinol Metab 1995; 80:1485.

179. Schlumberger M, Challeton C, De Vathaire F, et al. Radioactive iodine treatment and external radiotherapy for lung and bone metastases from thyroid carcinoma. J Nucl Med 1996; 37:598.

180. Young RL, Mazzaferri EL, Rahe AJ, Dorfman SG. Pure follicular thyroid carcinoma: impact of therapy in 214 patients. J Nucl Med 1980; 21:733.

181. Lin JD, Chao TC, Ho J, et al. Poor prognosis of 56 follicular thyroid carcinomas with distant metastases at the time of diagnosis. Cancer J 1998; 11:190.

182. Gilliland FD, Hunt WC, Morris DM, Key CR. Prognostic factors for thyroid carcinoma: a population-based study of 15,698 cases from the surveillance, epidemiology and end results (SEER) program 1973. Cancer 1997; 79:564.

183. Samaan NA, Schultz PN, Hickey RC, et al. Well-differentiated thyroid carcinoma and the results of various modalities of treatment. A retrospective review of 1599 patients. J Clin Endocrinol Metab 1992; 75:714.

184. Brennan MD, Bergstralh EJ, van Heerden JA, McConahey WM. Follicular thyroid cancer treated at the Mayo Clinic, 1946 through 1970: initial manifestations, pathologic findings, therapy, and outcome. Mayo Clin Proc 1991; 66:11.

185. Tennvall J, Biorklund A, Moller T, et al. Prognostic factors of papillary, follicular and medullary carcinomas of the thyroid gland: retrospective multivariate analysis of 216 patients with a median follow-up of 11 years. Acta Radiologica Oncol 1985; 24:17.

186. Mulligan LM, Kwok JBJ, Healey CS, et al. Germ-line mutations of the RET proto-oncogene in multiple endocrine neoplasia type 2A. Nature 1993; 363:458.

187. Gagel RF, Robinson MF, Donovan DT, Alford BR. Medullary thyroid carcinoma: recent progress. J Clin Endocrinol Metab 1993; 76:809.

188. Howe JR, Norton JA, Wells SA Jr. Prevalence of pheochromocytoma and hyperparathyroidism in multiple endocrine neoplasia type 2A: results of long-term follow-up. Surgery 1993; 114:1070.

189. Raue F, Zink A. Clinical features of multiple endocrine neoplasia type 1 and type 2. Horm Res 1992; 38 (Suppl2):31.

190. Sizemore GW. Medullary carcinoma of the thyroid gland. Semin Oncol 1987; 14:306.

191. Donis Keller H, Dou S, Chi D, et al. Mutations in the RET protooncogene are associated with MEN 2A and FMTC. Hum Mol Genet 1993; 2:851.

192. Eng C, Clayton D, Schufenecker I, et al. The relationship between specific RET proto-oncogene mutations and disease phenotype in multiple endocrine neoplasia type 2: international RET mutation consortium analysis. JAMA 1996; 276:1575.

193. Mendelsohn G. Markers as prognostic indicators in medullary thyroid carcinoma. Am J Clin Pathol 1991; 95:297.

194. Cohen R, Buchsenschutz B, Estrade P, et al. Causes of death in patients suffering from medullary thyroid carcinoma: report of 119 cases. Presse Med 1996; 25:1819.

195. Modigliani E, Cohen R, Campos JM, et al. Prognostic factors for survival and for biochemical cure in medullary thyroid carcinoma: results in 899 patients. Clin Endocrinol (Oxf ) 1998; 48:265.

196. Dottorini ME, Assi A, Sironi M, et al. Multivariate analysis of patients with medullary thyroid carcinoma: prognostic significance and impact on treatment of clinical and pathologic variables. Cancer 1996; 77:1556.

196a. Kebebew E, Ituarte PH, Siperstein AE, et al. Medullary thyroid carcinoma: clinical characteristics, treatment, prognostic factors, and a comparison of staging systems. Cancer 2000; 88:1139.

197. Wells SA, Baylin SB, Leight G, et al. The importance of early diagnosis in patients with hereditary medullary thyroid carcinoma. Ann Surg 1982; 195:204.

198. Wells SA Jr, Skinner MA. Prophylactic thyroidectomy, based on direct genetic testing, in patients at risk for the multiple endocrine neoplasia type 2 syndromes. Exp Clin Endocrinol Diabetes 1998; 106:29.

199. Decker RA, Peacock ML. Update on the profile of multiple endocrine neoplasia type 2a RET mutations: practical issues and implications for genetic testing. Cancer 1997; 80:557.

200. Moley JF, DeBenedetti MK, Dilley WG, et al. Surgical management of patients with persistent or recurrent medullary thyroid cancer. J Intern Med 1998; 243:521.

201. Chen HB, Roberts JR, Ball DW, et al. Effective long-term palliation of symptomatic, incurable metastatic medullary thyroid cancer by operative resection. Ann Surg 1998; 227:887.

202. Frank-Raue K, Ziegler R, Raue F. The use of octreotide in the treatment of medullary thyroid carcinoma. Horm Metab Res 1993; 27(Suppl):44.

202a. Juweid ME, Hajjar G, Stein R, et al. Initial experience with high-dose radioimmunotherapy of metastatic medullary thyroid cancer using [131]I-MN-14 F(ab)2 anti-carcinoembryonic antigen MAb and AHSCR [see comments]. J Nucl Med 2000; 41:93.

203. Kurtaran A, Scheuba C, Kaserer K, et al. Indium-111-DTPA-D-Phe-1-octreotide and technetium-99m-(V)-dimercaptosuccinic acid scanning in the preoperative staging of medullary thyroid carcinoma. J Nucl Med 1998; 39:1907.

204. Skinner MA, DeBenedetti MK, Moley JF, et al. Medullary thyroid carcinoma in children with multiple endocrine neoplasia types 2A and 2B. J Pediatr Surg 1996; 31:177.

205. Ledger GA, Khosla S, Lindor NM, et al. Genetic testing in the diagnosis and management of multiple endocrine neoplasia type II. Ann Intern Med 1995; 122:118.

206. O'Riordain DS, O'Brien T, Weaver AL, et al. Medullary thyroid carcinoma in multiple endocrine neoplasia types 2A and 2B. Surgery 1994; 116:1017.

207. Coustan DR, Carpenter MW. The diagnosis of gestational diabetes. Diabetes Care 1998; 21:B5.

208. Decker RA, Geiger JD, Cox CE, et al. Prophylactic surgery for multiple endocrine neoplasia type IIa after genetic diagnosis: is parathyroid transplantation indicated? World J Surg 1996; 20:814.

209. Kraimps JL, Denizot A, Carnaille B, et al. Primary hyperparathyroidism in multiple endocrine neoplasia type IIa: retrospective French multicentric study. World J Surg 1996; 20:808.

# CHAPTER 41

# UNUSUAL THYROID CANCERS

MATTHEW D. RINGEL

Approximately 10% of thyroid cancers are either poorly differentiated epithelial tumors or nonepithelial malignancies that are included in the World Health Organization (WHO) classification of thyroid tumors.[1] The variants of epithelial tumors, including anaplastic, squamous cell, tall cell, insular, and other poorly differentiated types of thyroid cancer, are characterized by more aggressive courses than are well-differentiated histologic subtypes. In addition, nonepithelial malignancies (e.g., lymphomas, sarcomas, and others) and tumors that metastasize to the thyroid occur and can now be recognized by fine-needle aspiration (FNA). The clinician must recognize these uncommon tumors because they are treated differently from the typical epithelial thyroid cancers. The clinical presentation, treatment, and prognosis of these unusual thyroid malignancies are discussed in this chapter. More common thyroid malignancies are discussed in Chapter 40.

## ANAPLASTIC THYROID CARCINOMA

Anaplastic cancer is a rare, aggressive malignancy with mean survival rates of <1 year. These tumors are comprised of large, pleomorphic cells with mitoses and bizarre nuclei. The cytologic pattern can range from large cells to spindle cells that conform to a variety of different histologic patterns.[2,3] All of these tumors share similar clinical characteristics; therefore, clinical presentation, management, and prognosis are considered together. In the past, small cell carcinomas of the thyroid were also considered a variant of anaplastic carcinoma; however, these have been reclassified as thyroid lymphomas, typically respond to lymphoma therapy, and are considered in a separate section.

### DEMOGRAPHICS AND PATHOGENESIS

The annual incidence of anaplastic carcinoma is estimated to be two per million in the United States.[4,5] Anaplastic carcinomas are more frequently identified in regions of iodine deficiency,[6] and the incidence decreases with introduction of iodine prophylaxis. In all populations studied, the incidence rises with increasing age. Demographically, anaplastic thyroid cancer shows a predominance among females, with a median age of onset in the sixth and seventh decades.[2–4,7]

The pathogenesis of anaplastic thyroid cancer is not entirely clear. A stepwise "multi-hit" hypothesis for thyroid tumor dedifferentiation has been proposed,[8] based on the high frequency of concurrent well-differentiated and anaplastic carcinoma, and epidemiologic data showing that as many as 30% of patients with anaplastic cancer have a history of well-differentiated carcinoma.[2–4,7] In support of this model, poorly differentiated thyroid tumors have a higher incidence of mutations of the genes encoding p53, other tumor suppressors, and oncogenes associated with aggressive cancers. Thus, the general belief is that anaplastic thyroid cancers rarely occur de novo.

Other factors proposed to be involved in the development of anaplastic thyroid cancer include a history of neck/mantle external radiation and prior iodine-131 ([131]I) therapy. Although it is associated with development of nodules and hypothyroidism, no convincing data other than several case reports exist linking external irradiation to anaplastic thyroid cancer. Similarly, [131]I therapy does not appear to cause anaplastic thyroid cancer.[9]

## CLINICAL PRESENTATION AND DIAGNOSIS

Patients with anaplastic cancer classically tend to be older, with a prior history of multinodular goiter that manifests as a rapid enlargement of a nodule or appearance of a lymph node and is characterized by severe pain, dysphagia or odynophagia, and airway compression. The rapid enlargement is often due to hemorrhage into a preexistent tumor.[2–4,7] Superior vena cava syndrome from extensive cervical disease and/or symptoms from distant metastases are sometimes present at initial evaluation. Dense fibrosis and calcifications are also well described.[10] Anaplastic carcinoma can also be found in more typical nodules that are not rapidly enlarging and within large compressive multinodular goiters that do not have the rapid enlargement noted above.

In addition, paraneoplastic syndromes also occur with anaplastic thyroid cancer and primary squamous cell thyroid cancer (discussed later). Patients with humoral hypercalcemia of malignancy due to production of parathyroid hormone–related protein (PTHrP) and leukocytosis caused by production of granulocyte colony stimulating factor (G-CSF) have been described. Moreover, cell lines derived from these tumors have been shown to produce these two factors.[11,12]

Evaluation of thyroid masses typically includes initial FNA. The accuracy of FNA in diagnosing anaplastic thyroid cancer is reported to range from 89% to 100%.[2,3] Despite these studies, and the use of flow cytometry to help exclude lymphoma, many centers perform open biopsy to confirm the diagnosis of anaplastic carcinoma, because the distinction from lymphoma is critical to management and prognosis.

Frequently, the clinician is confronted with a patient with a large tumor mostly comprised of well-differentiated cancer that contains a small focus of anaplastic cancer. The prognosis of the patient seems to be related to the presence of any focus of anaplastic carcinoma; thus, in the thyroid node metastasis (TNM) and other staging systems, the presence of anaplastic carcinoma defines a stage 4 lesion, regardless of patient age, tumor size, or lymph node spread.

## TREATMENT

Therapy for anaplastic carcinoma differs from that for other epithelial thyroid malignancies due to the absence of thyroid-stimulating hormone (TSH) receptor expression and iodine uptake. Therefore, radioiodine and TSH suppression are usually ineffective. TSH should be maintained in the lower part of the normal range but should not be suppressed, because nutritional status and weight are critical in chemotherapy. In addition, one of the frequently used chemotherapy medications, doxorubicin hydrochloride (Adriamycin), has cardiotoxic side effects, further limiting a role for TSH-suppression therapy. Thus, treatment paradigms are more similar to those for nonthyroidal poorly differentiated cancers.

## CONTROL OF LOCAL CERVICAL TUMOR

Preservation of vital neck structures to prevent airway and esophageal disasters is the initial focus of anaplastic thyroid cancer management. Preoperative panendoscopy is often performed, as in other head/neck cancers. Initial surgery should be performed with as complete a resection as possible. This may include neck dissection. In cases of smaller, intrathyroidal tumors, or ones with lymph node metastases without invasion into local structures, the surgeon may be able to avoid tracheostomy at this time. In cases in which tumor is invading local structures and gross disease remains, placing a tracheostomy at the time of primary surgery is reasonable. In addition, if periesophageal disease or loss of swallowing reflexes is identified, a percutaneous gastric feeding tube may be placed for either immediate or later use.

After surgery, external beam radiation is frequently performed. As with other head and neck cancers, treatment with 5000 to 6000 rads is typical and is associated with significant side effects including esophagitis, malnutrition, and stomatitis. Most patients with anaplastic carcinoma receive postoperative radiation therapy to control gross or microscopic residual disease. Several studies have evaluated the usefulness of radiation-sensitizing chemotherapy agents to reduce the dose of radiation needed. In some of these trials, patients with inoperable disease were treated with combined radiation and chemotherapy before surgery and treatment then continued with the combination therapy after thyroidectomy.[2–4,7,13–16] Although local control was frequently obtained, overall survival was not improved. Long-term survival was seen only in patents with no measurable disease after surgery. In general, aggressive surgical resection of the primary tumor is performed, usually without preoperative radiation therapy, although other approaches may be appropriate in selected cases.

## TREATMENT OF METASTATIC DISEASE

Treatment of metastatic anaplastic thyroid cancer has been largely ineffective despite the use of a wide variety of chemotherapy regimens.[8,13,15–17] Partial response rates as high as 20% to 30% have been described, but median and mean survival times still range between 4 and 18 months, consistent with the natural history of the disease.[18] The most active agents appear to be doxorubicin (alone or in combination with cisplatin) and perhaps paclitaxel (Taxol) and other taxanes, although the results of phase 1 and 2 clinical trials are not yet complete. Combination chemotherapy with bleomycin, cyclophosphamide, and 5-fluorouracil has also been used, but with similar results and greater toxicity. Several newer agents are under evaluation in phase 1 trials, including antiangiogenic factors and immunomodulators, but results have not yet been reported.[2,19] Autologous or allogeneic transplantation has not been used, probably because of the older age of most of the patients and the poor response to chemotherapy.

Because of the absence of data supporting an improvement in length of survival, a decision to use chemotherapy must be made jointly with the patient, with a clear understanding of the quality-of-life issues. After initial surgery and radiation (with or without chemotherapy), patients with measurable metastatic disease who also have a reasonable performance status are appropriate candidates for chemotherapy.

## PROGNOSIS

The overall prognosis for patients with anaplastic thyroid cancer remains dismal and has been largely unaffected by chemotherapy or radiation therapy. Mean and median survival is still measured in months despite aggressive therapy. Most patients can be protected from death due to local airway compression and hemorrhage with aggressive surgery, radiation therapy, and chemotherapy. In two cohorts, more complete surgical resections provided a significant survival advantage for younger individuals presenting with smaller tumors confined to the thyroid.[4,7] The 14% of patients in the second cohort[7] who were alive 24 months after diagnosis were younger, had smaller tumors, and were treated aggressively with both surgery and radiation therapy.

## SUMMARY

Anaplastic thyroid cancer is one of the most virulent tumors known to humans. Aggressive therapy to control local disease, particularly in individuals with no measurable metastases at the time of diagnosis, is appropriate to attain control of local disease and to create an opportunity for long-term survival. The side effects and potential effects on quality of life need to be openly discussed with the patient and the family preoperatively when possible. Systemic chemotherapy for metastatic disease is more controversial but is often attempted in younger patients with doxorubicin- or taxane-based regimens. Further clinical and basic research is needed to better understand the pathogenesis of anaplastic thyroid cancer and to develop more effective therapies.

# POORLY DIFFERENTIATED ("INSULAR") CARCINOMA

Insular thyroid carcinoma was originally described as *Wuchernde Struma*[20] and later became known as *insular carcinoma* because of the tendency of the polygonal cancer cells to grow in nests or insulae.[21] The growth pattern of insular carcinoma is distinct from that of the usual forms of thyroid carcinoma. The cells lack the nuclear features of papillary cancer; thus, these tumors are generally considered variants of follicular carcinoma. However, small foci of more typical well-differentiated cancers, including papillary cancer, are occasionally identified within or adjacent to the poorly differentiated component. The histologic patterns of poorly differentiated follicular cancers can vary from solid, to insular, to trabecular. Frequently, all three histologic patterns are seen within the same tumor. The exact percentage of tumor in the poorly differentiated pattern required for diagnosis is not clear because similar prognoses have been identified for patients with a predominantly poorly differentiated pattern and for those with a predominantly well-differentiated pattern.[22]

## DEMOGRAPHICS AND PATHOGENESIS

Patients with poorly differentiated carcinomas tend to be older (mean of 54 years) than those with well-differentiated tumors, and their tumors tend to be larger.[23] Insular carcinomas are uncommon, representing 1% to 2% of all thyroid cancers. The absence of a clear pathologic definition for this tumor (e.g., the amount of tumor required to be categorized as this pattern) make incidence studies difficult to interpret.

Poorly differentiated carcinomas are thought to represent an intermediate step in the progression of well-differentiated cancer to anaplastic cancer. Indeed, mutations in genes associated with aggressive cancer are reported to be more common in these tumors than in well-differentiated tumors.[10] Insular cancer is frequently diagnosed along with well-differentiated cancer in the same nodule; in addition, regions of poorly differentiated histology are often identified in the transition areas from well-differentiated to anaplastic cancer. Most insular carcinomas concentrate iodine and express thyroglobulin but have a prognosis that is intermediate between those of well-differentiated and anaplastic carcinoma.[24,25] These factors further support the notion that they represent tumors of moderate dedifferentiation.

## CLINICAL PRESENTATION AND DIAGNOSIS

As previously noted, patients with insular carcinomas tend to be older, have larger tumors, and are more likely to present with metastases as compared to patients with well-differentiated cancers. The male to female ratio is also preserved.[23] Most commonly, these tumors present as enlarging masses that may be slow growing, often in the setting of a multinodular goiter. Occasionally they may rapidly enlarge from hemorrhage or anaplastic transformation. FNA results often are suspicious for poorly differentiated carcinoma on the basis of the enlarged, polygonal cells.[26] Children with insular carcinoma tend to present with early nodal or distant metastases.

## TREATMENT AND PROGNOSIS

Treatment of poorly differentiated thyroid cancers is similar to that for well-differentiated tumors because they usually concentrate radioiodine. Near-total thyroidectomy should be performed in all patients with these tumors to maximize the effectiveness of postoperative therapy and monitoring. Treatment with radioiodine and thyroxine suppression should be performed, with a goal of undetectable circulating levels of TSH and the complete ablation of iodine-avid tissue on diagnostic scan. This approach may require multiple treatments with radioiodine at 10- to 12-month intervals. Magnetic resonance imaging (MRI), computed tomography (CT), and ultrasonography may also be helpful in defining metastases, particularly in the neck, that may be amenable to surgical excision. In occasional cases with extensive direct local invasion, external beam radiation may also be useful to control neck disease locally.

No proven chemotherapy regimens exist for these tumors if they progress despite radioiodine therapy. Successful redifferentiation therapy with retinoids has been reported, but only in a few cases.[27] Thus, the use of retinoids is considered experimental.

The prognosis for patients with poorly differentiated thyroid cancer appears to relate mostly to the stage of disease at the time of diagnosis. In one review, 26% of patients with insular cancer presented with distant metastases, and 36% had cervical metastases.[23] During the course of follow-up (means of 3.5 to 7 years), 25% of patients died of poorly differentiated cancer and an additional 25% had residual or recurrent disease—figures much higher than those typically reported for well-differentiated cancer. Most of these patients had metastases at the time of diagnosis and were treated with the aggressive paradigm previously suggested.

## SUMMARY

Insular and other poorly differentiated thyroid cancers appear to be more aggressive tumors than well-differentiated thyroid malignancies; they present with later-stage disease and larger tumors, and have a worse prognosis. The majority are iodine avid; therefore, aggressive surgical therapy followed by radioiodine therapy and TSH suppression is recommended. Careful monitoring with measurement of serum levels of thyroglobulin, yearly radioiodine scanning, and neck and chest imaging are appropriate.

# TALL CELL VARIANT OF PAPILLARY CARCINOMA

The tall cell variant of papillary cancer (TCV) was first identified in a subgroup of papillary cancers of which at least 30% were comprised of large papillary structures—with cells characterized by a height at least twice the width, an oxyphilic cytoplasm, and hyperchromic basal nuclei.[28] These characteristic patterns were present in nearly 10% of all papillary cancers. As with poorly differentiated carcinomas, these tumors are believed to represent dedifferentiated cancer cells; however, the prognostic implications of TCV have been controversial.

## DEMOGRAPHICS AND PATHOGENESIS

Most studies report that TCV accounts for 5% to 10% of papillary carcinomas, although the percentage of TCV in the tumor required for a diagnosis has not been entirely consistent. In addition, the TCV must be differentiated from the similar columnar cell variant characterized by similar "tall cells" that have stratified rather than basal nuclei. The reported cooccurrence of TCV and columnar cell variants suggests a similar pathogenesis for both tumors. TCV has also been associated with anaplastic carcinomas in a manner similar to that of insular carcinoma. In addition, a high incidence of mutations in the p53 tumor-suppressor gene has been reported in TCV, further supporting its "transitional" nature.

Patients with TCV, like those with other dedifferentiated tumors, tend to be older and present with larger tumors. They are also more likely to present with local invasion or metastases.[23] The typical female predominance of thyroid cancer is seen for TCV.

## CLINICAL PRESENTATION AND DIAGNOSIS

Patients with TCV tend to present in a similar manner to those with well-differentiated papillary cancer, albeit at a later age. The frequency of local metastases is relatively high, and distant metastases are more common than for papillary carcinoma (19%).[23,29–31,31a] Occasionally, young individuals with small intrathyroidal TCV cancers are identified. Much controversy exists regarding the natural history of these tumors.

Typically, patients with TCV present with a solitary thyroid nodule or a dominant nodule in a multinodular goiter and then are evaluated by FNA. The cytopathology of TCV generally reflects the papillary origin of the tumor with nuclear grooves, cytoplasmic inclusions, papillary fronds, and occasional psammoma bodies.[32] Cells with basilar nuclei and abundant oxyphilic cytoplasm may suggest TCV, but usually the FNA is diagnostic for papillary cancer and the diagnosis is made on final surgical histology.

## TREATMENT AND PROGNOSIS

The management of patients with TCV is similar to that for patients with other poorly differentiated tumors. These tumors are iodine avid and express thyroglobulin. Therefore, near-total thyroidectomy, aggressive radioiodine therapy, and TSH suppression are appropriate. Occasionally, external beam radiation is used for control of local disease.

Patients are monitored with serum thyroglobulin measurement and radioiodine scanning. The use of neck CT, MRI, or ultrasonography is reasonable for patients with locally recurrent or invasive disease or those individuals with elevated levels of thyroglobulin to determine if their disease can be managed with surgical removal of the recurrence.

Drawing conclusions regarding the prognosis of TCV is difficult due to the absence of large, long-term prospective or retrospective studies. Most published studies are small and retrospective with discordant outcomes. The author and colleagues have attempted to define an overall sense of the prognosis of TCV based on the published data.[23] The prognosis of patients with TCV appears to be related to the stage of disease and the age at diagnosis. Patients older than 50 years of age tend to have larger tumors and present with more aggressive disease, and are more likely to have recurrence and to die of their disease than are similarly aged patients with well-differentiated cancer.[23,29–31] Conversely, patients younger than 50 years of age tend to present with early-stage disease and have a prognosis similar to that for patients with well-differentiated cancer, although the follow-up time has been much shorter and the treatments have not been consistent. However, a review has described young patients with small primary tumors and agressive disease.[31a] Thus, although it seems relatively clear that older patients with TCV have a worse prognosis, in younger patients, the biologic behavior of TCV may be more similar to that of

well-differentiated thyroid cancer. However, short lengths of follow-up as well as inconsistencies in treatment regimens may cause underestimation of the true aggressiveness of TCV in young patients. Therefore, the author recommends treating young patients who have TCV with the aggressive protocol previously mentioned unless they have small intrathyroidal primary tumors, in which case they can be treated like other young patients with well-differentiated papillary carcinoma.

## SUMMARY

TCV probably represents a poorly differentiated subtype of papillary cancer that tends to present with later-stage disease in older patients. The biologic behavior in younger patients with smaller tumors appears to be less aggressive. TCV tumors contain molecular characteristics suggesting its role as a "transitional" tumor in the dedifferentiation of well-differentiated to anaplastic thyroid cancer. Treatment usually includes radioiodine therapy and TSH suppression because most of the tumors concentrate iodine. Additional studies will help clarify the biologic behavior of TCV, particularly in younger patients.

# COLUMNAR CELL VARIANT OF PAPILLARY CARCINOMA

Columnar cell variant is similar to TCV in that it appears to be a dedifferentiated subtype characterized by "tall cells." The distinction between the two is generally based on the *nuclear stratification of the columnar cell versus the basal nuclei typical of TCV and the presence of clear rather than pink cytoplasm.* Columnar cell carcinoma is much less common than TCV, with only 24 reported cases. It has been associated with anaplastic carcinoma, well-differentiated thyroid cancer, and TCV.[33,34]

## CLINICAL PRESENTATION AND DIAGNOSIS

The mean age of the reported cases of columnar cell carcinoma is 45 years; the female-male ratio is 1.4:1.0. The majority of the reported cases occurred in older individuals with locally invasive tumors that rapidly enlarged. Several young patients with smaller, less aggressive tumors have been described. Distant metastases, including pulmonary, bone, and brain metastases, were present in 29% of the reported patients at the time of diagnosis.

As with TCV, several clues may suggest a columnar cell carcinoma on FNA, but usually the aspirate is diagnostic for papillary cancer. Histologic analysis is usually required to make the diagnosis.

## TREATMENT AND PROGNOSIS

In the reported patients, most of the tumors were iodine avid, and patients were treated with thyroidectomy, radioiodine, and TSH suppression. Several patients also received external beam radiation to the neck to control local spread.[34] In the short periods of follow-up included in the reports, 38% of patients died of the cancer and 58% were free of disease at last follow-up, although the monitoring methods used are not clear.

## SUMMARY

Columnar cell carcinoma is a rare variant of papillary cancer that likely represents a dedifferentiated subtype with an aggressive clinical course distinct from TCV. Cure seems possible for patients with small, intrathyroidal tumors, although the reported follow-up times have been short. Treatment with surgery, radioiodine, and TSH-suppression with external radiation for local disease is appropriate.

# DIFFUSE SCLEROSING PAPILLARY THYROID CANCER

Although initially described in 1953,[35] the diffuse sclerosing variant of papillary cancer was first formally defined in 1985 when it was identified as a subset of papillary cancers characterized by typical papillary cells, dense sclerosis, abundant psammoma bodies, squamous metaplasia, and significant lymphocytic infiltration.[36] Subsequent reviews of papillary carcinomas have identified these tumors in 1% to 3% of cases.[35-37]

Based on the small number of reported cases, these tumors are typically large and often diffusely involve both lobes. They tend to occur in younger patients (mean age in the 30s) and show predominance among females. Cervical adenopathy is nearly uniformly present at diagnosis, and distant metastases and tumor recurrence are more common than in typical papillary cancer. Despite the apparent aggressive nature of the tumor at presentation, tumor-related mortality has not been reported, and patients surviving decades after diagnosis are well described. This may be related to the lymphocytic response to the tumor. Treatment with near-total thyroidectomy, lymph node removal, and radioiodine all are appropriate. Longer follow-up will be required to better define the clinical course of this disease.

# SQUAMOUS CELL CARCINOMA OF THE THYROID

Primary squamous cell carcinoma of the thyroid is defined by the WHO classification as a tumor comprised "entirely of cells showing so-called intracellular bridges and/or forming keratin."[1] The squamous cells are of uncertain origin.[38] When this definition of "pure" squamous cell carcinoma is used, rather than that of tumors with an adenosquamous appearance or tumors with squamous metaplasia, the incidence is <1% of all thyroid malignancies.[39] Before therapy, the clinician must be certain that the tumor does not represent metastases from head and neck or lung cancers.

## DEMOGRAPHICS AND PATHOGENESIS

Forty-five individuals have been identified by MEDLINE review who clearly had tumors meeting the WHO definition of "pure" squamous cell carcinoma. The median age of 45 years at presentation is younger than that for anaplastic carcinoma but older than that for well-differentiated cancer. Female-male predominance is 1.8:1.

As noted previously, the origin of the squamous cells remains quite controversial. The relatively high frequency of squamous cell carcinoma of thyroglossal duct remnants raises the possibility that small nests of squamous cells exist in the thyroid glands. Indeed, a small subset of thyroid squamous cells with high basal cell proliferation has been identified.[40] The relatively common finding of squamous metaplasia does not typically occur in association with squamous cell carcinoma, and the pattern of evolution of squamous metaplasia to carcinoma is not characteristic of other squamous cell cancers. Thus, squamous metaplasia is unlikely to represent a premalignant lesion.

## CLINICAL PRESENTATION AND DIAGNOSIS

Most patients with squamous cell thyroid carcinoma present with a rapidly enlarging mass arising within a multinodular goiter, as in anaplastic cancer. Tumor production of PTHrP and G-CSF has been described.[12] Rarely, this cancer has been described to occur in conjunction with other thyroid malignancies. Squamous cell carcinomas are difficult to diagnose on FNA because of the difficulty in differentiating metaplasia from carcinoma. Some patients present with distant metastases, but more typically, these tumors are locally invasive in the neck. Squamous carcinomas may be more common in thyroglossal duct remnants and account for 7% of all primary thyroglossal duct carcinomas.[23]

## TREATMENT AND PROGNOSIS

The management of squamous cell carcinoma of the thyroid is similar to that of other squamous cell tumors of the head and neck and anaplastic thyroid carcinoma. No role exists for radioiodine therapy because these tumors do not concentrate iodine, and TSH suppression is not known to be beneficial. A complete surgical resection, often including bilateral neck dissections, is performed. After surgery, local control is paramount, and patients are typically treated with external beam radiation to control local recurrence. Distant metastases have been treated with a variety of chemotherapy regimens including bleomycin, cisplatin, and doxorubicin, with disappointing results. Overall, survival of patients with squamous cell cancer is low, with nearly all patients dying within 16 months of diagnosis. Long-term survival appears to be possible for patients with smaller tumors that are amenable to complete surgical resection.

# MUCOEPIDERMOID CARCINOMA

Mucoepidermoid cancer is a rare tumor (~40 cases) that is associated with epithelial thyroid cancers and lymphocytic thyroiditis.[41] These tumors may be cystic or mucin filled and present as a typical thyroid nodule. FNA is often nondiagnostic or suggestive of carcinoma, but not of mucoepidermoid cancer; therefore, the diagnosis is made on the basis of surgical histology. Many of the reported cases had metastases (55%), but these were generally confined to the neck. Thyroidectomy, lymph node dissection, and external beam radiation therapy appear to be effective, but the duration of follow-up has been short. The role of radioiodine therapy and TSH suppression has not been explored.

# MIXED MEDULLARY-FOLLICULAR AND MEDULLARY-PAPILLARY CARCINOMA

Rarely, thyroid cancers may display features of both medullary and follicular carcinoma.[42] These tumors are distinct from medullary cancer with normal "trapped" follicles and are characterized by distinct regions of medullary carcinomas adjacent to follicular or papillary cancer. The pathogenesis of these tumors is not clear. Their occurrence suggests a similar response of follicular and parafollicular cells to an oncogenic stimulus rather than the presence of a common progenitor cell. However, cells expressing both thyroglobulin and calcitonin have been identified.[42] The presence of mutations in the *ret* oncogene, typical of medullary cancer, have not been studied, but familial occurrence of these tumors has been described.[43,44]

# THYROID SARCOMAS

True sarcomas of the thyroid are quite rare and must be differentiated from anaplastic cancers with sarcomatoid features. Careful analysis has disclosed several cases of thyroid sarcoma, including leiomyosarcomas, osteosarcomas, chondrosarcomas, fibrosarcomas, and angiosarcomas.[45,46] Of these subtypes, angiosarcomas are most common and are found most frequently in regions of iodine deficiency (another term is *hemangioepitheliomas*).

These tumors, particularly the angiosarcomas, tend to occur in older patients with long-standing goiters. Careful immuno-histochemical analysis must be performed to separate these tumors from carcinomas. The markers should confirm endothelial lineage (e.g., CD34, CD31, and factor VII–related antigen) rather than epithelial lineage.

The prognosis for thyroid sarcomas, regardless of subtype, is poor. Most patients have large tumors with local invasion and metastases on diagnosis. Rare cures in cases of small intrathyroidal tumors have been described. Patients are treated with surgery, external irradiation, and chemotherapy regimens used for sarcomas arising from other organs. In addition to primary thyroid sarcomas, Kaposi sarcoma infiltrating the thyroid has been described in the setting of acquired immunodeficiency syndrome (AIDS)[47] and should be considered in the AIDS patient group.

# THYROID TERATOMA

Thyroid teratomas are rare, usually benign, and most frequently diagnosed in childhood. Teratomas of the thyroid, like teratomas at any location, are characterized by the presence of cells arising from all three germ cell layers. Thyroidal origin is determined by identification of the blood supply leading to the tumor.

Malignant teratomas are extremely rare and, when considered as a percentage of all teratomas, are more common in adults. A review has determined that mean age at diagnosis is 31.2 years, size is large (up to 17 cm), and prognosis is poor.[48] All patients had metastases, all were treated surgically and with external beam radiation, and all died within 22 months of diagnosis with the exception of one patient for whom only a 7-month follow-up was reported.

# THYROID LYMPHOMA

Classically, primary thyroid lymphomas occur in patients with Hashimoto thyroiditis and are usually non-Hodgkin B-cell lymphomas. Lymphomas include the "small cell" anaplastic carcinoma that has been determined to represent a small B-cell lymphoma.

## DEMOGRAPHICS AND PATHOGENESIS

As previously noted, thyroid lymphoma generally occurs in patients with Hashimoto thyroiditis. Therefore, this malignancy is more common in women. It typically occurs in the fifth and sixth decades of life, but patients younger than 40 years have been reported.[23,49,50] Nearly all patients have histologic evidence of Hashimoto thyroiditis and approximately two-thirds have detectable serum levels of antithyroid peroxidase or antithyroglobulin antibodies. Most patients are euthyroid at the time of diagnosis, although hypothyroidism is common. Primary thyroid lymphomas account for only a small percentage of lymphomas or thyroid cancers, but the tumors tend to respond well to appropriate therapy; thus, early and accurate diagnosis is critical.

The pathogenesis of thyroid lymphoma is unclear. The association with thyroiditis has given rise to the hypothesis that thyroid lymphoma may be a variety of MALT (mucosa-associated lymphoid tissue) lymphomas. The cells of MALT lymphomas typically resemble cells that surround lymphoid follicles (centrocyte-like); they can undergo plasmacytic change—as has been described in thyroid lymphomas[51]—and can progress to high-grade lymphoma. Thyroid lymphomas are comprised of a population of monotonous lymphoid cells that replace the thyroid parenchyma, with additional evidence of prior Hashimoto thyroiditis.

## CLINICAL PRESENTATION AND DIAGNOSIS

Most patients with thyroid lymphoma have hypothyroidism or a preexisting goiter that begins to grow, sometimes rapidly and with pain.[49] Local symptoms such as dysphonia and dysphagia occur but are uncommon. The classic "B symptoms" of lymphoma are also usually absent.

Presurgical diagnosis is often possible by FNA, provided the clinician's index of suspicion is high before performing the procedure. Flow cytometric analysis of the aspirated cells has been shown to be quite accurate, with a high specificity and sensitivity.[49,50] In addition, typical ultrasonographic findings of a "pseudocystic" pattern[50] have been identified in thyroid lymphoma; this pattern is present in only 10% of patients with Hashimoto thyroiditis without lymphoma. These methods are dependent on the expertise of the pathologists and radiologists at a given institution. Therefore, even with these advances, open surgical biopsy, tumor debulking, or thyroidectomy is frequently required to confirm the diagnosis before therapy. Gallium scanning may also be helpful in diagnosing lymphoma.

## TREATMENT AND PROGNOSIS

The treatment of patients with thyroid lymphoma has been controversial, specifically with regard to the need for near total thyroidectomy in all patients. One large study reported 8-year disease-free survivals of 100% in 16 individuals treated with cyclophosphamide, doxorubicin, vincristine, and prednisone (CHOP) for one cycle, followed by 40 to 60 Gy of external radiation and then an additional five cycles of CHOP without a surgical thyroidectomy.[50] These results are better than the previously reported cure rates, which approach 80% in the studies that used combined-modality therapy.[49] The role for thyroidectomy is not clear, and its routine use in patients with thyroid lymphoma is debated. The physician must have complete confidence in the diagnosis of lymphoma before initiating therapy because the treatment differs dramatically from that for any other thyroid malignancy. If a core sample is required in addition to the FNA, performing a lobectomy or near-total thyroidectomy may be reasonable if the surgical risk is acceptably low. Alternatively, a core biopsy could be performed, and if the results are consistent with lymphoma, treatment could be initiated without waiting several weeks for the patient to recover fully from a thyroidectomy.

## SUMMARY

Thyroid lymphoma is an uncommon malignancy that generally occurs in individuals with preexisting Hashimoto thyroiditis; it presents as an enlarging, tender gland, often with local symptoms. Diagnosis is based on a high level of clinical suspicion and often requires histologic confirmation with a core biopsy of partial or total thyroidectomy. Treatment is based on combined chemotherapy and radiation therapy. Reports for aggressive high-dose therapy suggest a good long-term prognosis.

# METASTATIC CANCERS IN THE THYROID

Clinically evident metastases to the thyroid are rare occurrences. They generally present as typical solitary thyroid nodules and are most commonly due to renal cell carcinoma, breast cancer, lung cancer, and malignant melanoma. Usually, widespread disease is evident, but occasionally, thyroid metastases may be the sentinels for metastatic disease.

## CLINICAL PRESENTATION AND DIAGNOSIS

In one study, 40 of 43 patients with cancer metastatic to the thyroid gland presented with nodular disease (solitary or multinodular), and 3 presented with compression of local structures.[52] FNA is often adequate to confirm the diagnosis if the patient has widespread metastatic disease at the time of the procedure and the cells resemble those of the original tumor. Rarely, a patient may develop a nodule many years after therapy for the primary tumor. This occurs most commonly with renal cell carcinoma. In this situation, surgical lobectomy may be required to confirm the diagnosis.

The tissue of origin for the tumors that metastasize is most commonly renal cell carcinoma, followed by lung cancer, and breast cancer. Spread from adjacent head and neck cancers as well as parathyroid carcinomas is also well described. Hematologic malignancies (i.e., lymphoma, leukemia, and myeloma) can metastasize or infiltrate the thyroid. Kaposi sarcoma metastatic to the thyroid has also been reported.[47]

## TREATMENT AND PROGNOSIS

The treatment and prognosis of metastatic cancer to the thyroid gland relates to the primary tumor and not to the thyroid metastases. In selected cases, thyroidectomy may be beneficial, but generally, metastases to the thyroid occur in the setting of other metastatic disease. A discussion of the prognosis of the metastatic cancer should be held with patients, their families, and the physicians (including a medical oncologist), because the outcome is generally poor.

## CONCLUSION

This chapter has reviewed a variety of unusual thyroid malignancies. For many of these tumors, too few cases exist for definitive recommendations to be made; however, many, if not all, of these tumors are seen in clinical practice. Therefore, these patients should be diagnosed and treated in a rational manner based on the biology and prognosis of the individual cancer. Clinical trials, which are ongoing in evaluating the use of new treatments for many of these tumors, hopefully will improve clinical outcomes in the next several years.

## REFERENCES

1. Hedinger C, Williams ED, Sobin LH. Histological typing of thyroid tumors. Berlin: Springer-Verlag, 1988.
2. Ain KB. Anaplastic thyroid carcinoma: behavior, biology, and therapeutic approaches. Thyroid 1997; 8:715.
3. Samaan NA, Ordoñez NG. Uncommon types of thyroid cancer. Endocrinol Metab Clin North Am 1990; 19:637.
4. Tan RK, Finley RK, Driscoll D, et al. Anaplastic carcinoma of the thyroid: a 24 year experience. Head Neck 1995; 17:41.
5. dos Santos Silva I, Swerdlow AJ. Thyroid cancer epidemiology in England and Wales: time trends and geographical distribution. Br J Cancer 1993; 67:330.
6. Harach HR, Escalante DA, Onativa A, et al. Thyroid carcinoma and thyroiditis in an endemic goitre region before and after iodine prophylaxis. Acta Endocrinol 1985; 108:55.
7. Vanketesh YSS, Ordoñez NG, Schultz PN, et al. Anaplastic carcinoma of the thyroid: a clinicopathologic study of 121 cases. Cancer 1990; 66:321.
8. Fagin JA. Genetic basis of endocrine disease 3: molecular defects in thyroid gland neoplasia. J Clin Endocrinol Metab 1992; 75:1398.
9. Ron E, Doody MM, Becker DV, et al. Cancer mortality following treatment for adult hyperthyroidism. JAMA 1998; 280:347.
10. LiVolsi VA, Brooks JJ, Arendash Durand B. Anaplastic thyroid tumors. Immunohistology. Am J Clin Pathol 1987; 87:434.
11. Yazawa S, Toshimori H, Nakatsuru K, et al. Thyroid anaplastic carcinoma producing granulocyte-colony-stimulating factor and parathyroid hormone-related protein. Int Med 1995; 34:584.
12. Saito K, Kuratomi Y, Yamamoto K, et al. Primary squamous cell carcinoma of the thyroid associated with marked leukocytosis and hypercalcemia. Cancer 1981; 48:2080.
13. Kim JH, Leeper RD. Treatment of locally advanced thyroid carcinoma with combination doxorubicin and radiation therapy. Cancer 1987; 60:2372.
14. Junor EJ, Paul J, Reed NS. Anaplastic thyroid carcinoma: 91 patients treated by surgery and radiotherapy. Eur J Surg Oncol 1992; 18:83.
15. Tennvall J, Lundell G, Hallquist A, et al. Combined doxorubicin, hyperfractionated radiotherapy, and surgery in anaplastic thyroid carcinoma: report on two protocols. Cancer 1994; 74:1348.
16. Schlumberger M, Parmentier C, Delisle M-J, et al. Combination therapy for anaplastic giant cell thyroid carcinoma. Cancer 1991; 67:564.
17. Shimaoka K, Schoenfeld DA, DeWys WD, et al. A randomized trial of doxorubicin versus doxorubicin plus cisplatin in patients with advanced thyroid carcinoma. Cancer 1985; 56:2155.
18. Woolner LB, Beahrs OH, Black BM, et al. Classification and prognosis of thyroid carcinoma: a study of 885 cases observed in a thirty year period. Am J Surg 1961; 102:354.
19. Ain KB, Tofiq S, Taylor KD. Antineoplastic activity of Taxol against human anaplastic thyroid carcinoma cell lines in vitro and in vivo. J Clin Endocrinol Metab 1996; 81:3650.
20. Langhans T. Über die epithelialen formen der malignen struma. Virchows Arch (Pathol Anat) 1907; 385:125.
21. Carcangiu ML, Zampi G, Rosai J. Poorly differentiated ("insular") thyroid carcinoma. Am J Surg Pathol 1984; 8:655.
22. Papotti M, Botto Mica F, Favero A, et al. Poorly differentiated thyroid carcinomas with primordial cell component: a group of aggressive lesions sharing insular, trabecular, and solid patterns. Am J Surg Pathol 1993; 17:291.
23. Burman KD, Ringel MD, Wartofsky L. Unusual types of thyroid neoplasms. Endocrinol Metab Clin North Am 1996; 25:49.
24. Justin EP, Seabold JE, Robinson RA, et al. Insular carcinoma: a distinct thyroid carcinoma associated with iodine-131 localization. J Nucl Med 1991; 32:1358.
25. Ashfaq R, Vuitch F, Delgado R, Albores-Saavedra J. Papillary and follicular carcinomas with an insular component. Cancer 1994; 73:416.
26. Pietribiasi F, Sapino A, Papotti M, Bussolati G. Cytologic features of poorly differentiated "insular" carcinoma of the thyroid, as revealed by fine-needle aspiration biopsy. Am J Clin Pathol 1990; 94:687.
27. Grunwald F, Menzel C, Bender H, et al. Redifferentiation therapy-induced radioiodine uptake in thyroid cancer. J Nucl Med 1998; 39:1903.
28. Hawk WA, Hazard JB. The many appearances of papillary carcinoma of the thyroid. Cleve Clin Q 1976; 45:207.
29. Terry JH, St John SA, Karkowski FJ, et al. Tall cell papillary thyroid carcinoma: incidence and prognosis. Am J Surg 1994; 168:459.
30. Johnson TL, Lloyd RV, Thompson NW, et al. Prognostic implications of the tall cell variant of papillary thyroid cancer. Am J Surg Pathol 1988; 12:22.
31. Ain KB. Papillary thyroid carcinoma: etiology, assessment, and therapy. Endocrinol Metab Clin North Am 1995; 24:711.
31a. Prendiville S, Burman KD, Ringel MD, et al. Tall cell variant: an agressive form of papillary thyroid cancer. Otolaryngol Head Neck Surg 2000; 122:352.
32. Harach HR, Zusman SB. Cytopathology of the tall cell variant of thyroid papillary carcinoma. Acta Cytol 1992; 36:895.
33. Asklen LA, Verhaug JE. Thyroid carcinoma with mixed tall-cell and columnar-cell features. Am J Clin Pathol 1990; 94:442.
34. Mizukami Y, Nonomura A, Michigishi T, et al. Columnar cell carcinoma of the thyroid gland: a case report and review of the literature. Hum Pathol 1994; 25:1098.
35. Crile G Jr, Fisher ER. Simultaneous occurrence of thyroiditis and papillary carcinoma. Report of two cases. Cancer 1953; 6:57.
36. Vickery AL, Carcangiu ML, Johannessen JV, Sobrinho-Simoes M. Papillary carcinoma. Session I of thyroid tumor pathology. Semin Diagn Pathol 1985; 2:909.
37. Caplan RH, Wester S, Kisken WA. Diffuse sclerosing variant of papillary thyroid carcinoma: case report and review of the literature. Endocr Pract 1997; 3: 287.
38. LiVolsi VA, Merino MJ. Squamous cells in the thyroid gland. Am J Surg Pathol 1978; 2:133.
39. Misonou J, Aizawa M, Kanda M, et al. Pure squamous cell carcinoma of the thyroid gland—report of an autopsy case and review of the literature. Jpn J Surg 1988; 18:469.
40. Bond JA, Wyllie FS, Ivan M, et al. A variant epithelial sub-population in normal thyroid with high proliferative capacity in vitro. Mol Cell Endocrinol 1993; 93:175.
41. Wenig BM, Adair CF, Heffess CS. Primary mucoepidermoid carcinoma of the thyroid gland: a report of six cases and a review of the literature of a follicular epithelial-derived tumor. Hum Pathol 1995; 26:1099.
42. Papotti M, Negro F, Carney JA, et al. Mixed medullary-follicular carcinoma of the thyroid. A morphological, immunohistochemical and in situ hybridization analysis of 11 cases. Virchows Arch (Pathol Anat) 1997; 430:397.
43. Mizukami Y, Michigishi T, Nonomura A, et al. Mixed medullary-follicular carcinoma of the thyroid occurring in the familial form. Histopathology 1993; 22:284.
44. Lamberg BA, Reissel P, Stenman S, et al. Concurrent medullary and papillary thyroid carcinoma in the same thyroid lobe and in siblings. Acta Med Scand 1981; 209:421.

45. Thompson LDR, Wenig BM, Adair CF, et al. Primary smooth muscle tumors of the thyroid gland. Cancer 1997; 79:579.
46. Syrjänen KJ. An osteogenic sarcoma of the thyroid gland (report of a case and survey of the literature). Neoplasma 1979; 26:623.
47. Mollison LC, Mijch A, McBride G, Dwyer B. Hypothyroidism due to destruction of the thyroid by Kaposi's sarcoma. Rev Infect Dis 1991; 13:826.
48. Bowker CM, Whittaker RS. Malignant teratoma of the thyroid: case report and literature review of thyroid teratoma in adults. Histopathology 1992; 21:81.
49. Weinstein LJ, Ain KB. Primary thyroid lymphoma: a comprehensive assessment and clinical approach. Endocrinologist 1999; 9:45.
50. Matsuzuka F, Miyauchi A, Katayama S, et al. Clinical aspects of primary thyroid lymphoma: diagnosis and treatment based on our experience of 119 cases. Thyroid 1993; 3:93.
51. Isaacson PG. Lymphomas of mucosa-associated lymphoid tissue (MALT). Histopathology 1990; 16: 617.
52. Nakhjavani MK, Gharib H, Goellner JR, van Heerden JA. Metastasis to the thyroid gland. A report of 43 cases. Cancer 1997; 79: 574.

# CHAPTER 42

# HYPERTHYROIDISM

KENNETH D. BURMAN

Of the several varieties of hyperthyroidism, one of the most common is Graves disease. Graves disease is an autoimmune disease in which thyroid-stimulating hormone (TSH) receptor antibodies bind to and stimulate the thyroid gland, causing the excessive secretion of thyroxine ($T_4$) or triiodothyronine ($T_3$) or both, resulting in the clinical manifestations of thyrotoxicosis.[1-6] Graves disease has fascinated clinicians because of its possible relationship to stress, its unusual and varied manifestations (e.g., eye involvement, pretibial myxedema), and its unpredictable course, characterized by relapses and exacerbations.

## PATHOGENESIS OF GRAVES DISEASE

Graves disease is associated with TSH receptor antibodies that stimulate the thyroid gland.[1-6] In most patients, the population of TSH receptor antibodies is heterogeneous, with some antibodies that stimulate and others that inhibit TSH receptor-mediated action. Patients have been described with even more complex antibodies in their serum, as determined by binding or stimulating actions on the TSH receptors in thyroid membrane or guinea pig fat membrane preparations.[7]

There are four major hypotheses as to the etiology of Graves disease (Fig. 42-1):

1. A basic *defect in antigen-specific suppressor T cells* allows an imbalance in helper cell action versus suppressor cell function, resulting in the excessive generation or unregulated synthesis of TSH receptor antibodies.[8-10] Abnormal macrophage migration inhibition and monocyte procoagulant activities in patients with Graves disease represent relatively specific defects observed only with peripheral mononuclear cells of these patients in the presence of thyroidal antigens.[11] These same peripheral mononuclear cells are capable of correcting the pancreatic islet cell specific antigen defect found in diabetic mononuclear cells. Although this theory is appealing, it does not explain the etiologic mechanism of the antigen-specific suppressor cell defect,[12,13] nor does it explain the polyclonal B- and T-cell patterns observed with molecular probes.[14]

2. A defect may exist in the *mechanism by which thyrocytes and T cells initiate helper T-cell activation.* Thyrocytes themselves can express human leukocyte antigen (HLA) class II antigens, and it is speculated that HLA antigens, as well as thyroid-specific antigen, interact with helper cells, presumably through the T-cell $T_3$ receptor complex.[15] Although the thyroid gland's ability to present HLA antigens is thought by some to be a primary event, others believe that the expression of D-related (DR) antigens is secondary to the presence of a small number of intrathyroidal lymphocytes that are activated and thus secrete interleukin-2, which is known to cause HLA-DR expres-

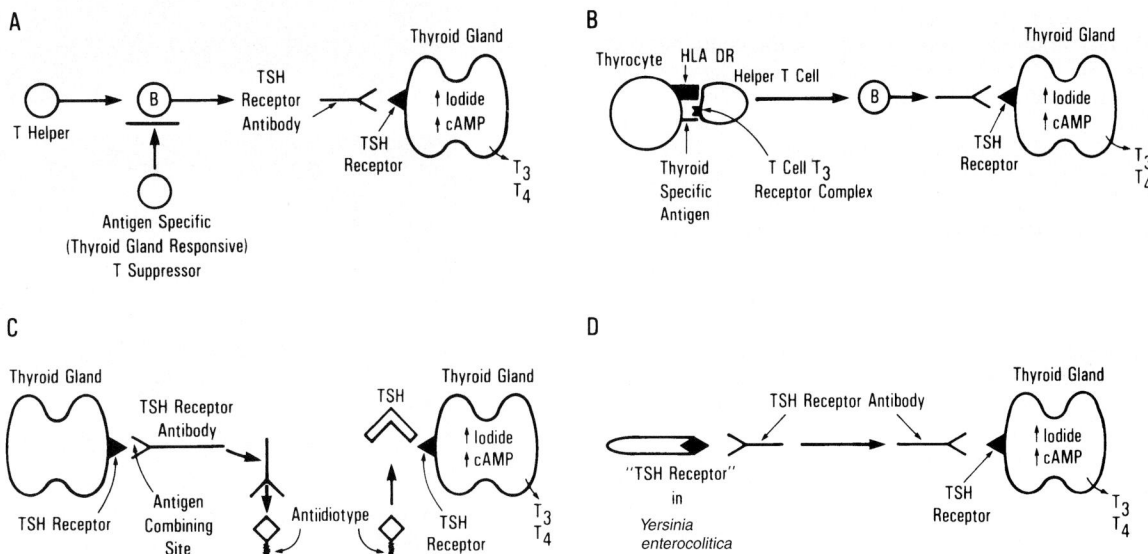

**FIGURE 42-1.** **A** through **D,** Theoretical explanations for the initiation or propagation of Graves disease (see text). $T_3$ receptor complex refers to the T-cell antigen receptor, of which the CD3 molecule is a component. $T_3$ and $T_4$ refer to triiodothyronine and thyroxine derived from thyroidal secretion. (*cAMP,* cyclic adenosine monophosphate; *TSH,* thyroid-stimulating hormone.) (From Burman KD, Baker JR Jr. Immune mechanisms in Graves disease. Endocr Rev 1985; 6:183. Reproduced by permission of The Endocrine Society.)

**TABLE 42-1.**
**Effects of Thyrotoxicosis**

| System | Effects |
|---|---|
| General | Nervousness, insomnia, fatigue, tremulousness, heat intolerance, weight loss |
| Skin | Warm and moist, hyperhidrosis, alopecia, hyperpigmentation, onycholysis, acropachy, pretibial myxedema, preradial myxedema, urticaria, pruritus, vitiligo |
| Eyes | Exophthalmos, conjunctivitis, chemosis, ophthalmoplegia, optic nerve involvement |
| Cardiovascular | Tachycardia, shortness of breath, palpitations, atrial fibrillation, heart block, high-output congestive heart failure, angina pectoris, increased pulse pressure, Means-Lerman "scratch" murmur |
| Gastrointestinal | Tremor of tongue, hyperphagia, increased thirst, diarrhea or hyperdefecation, elevated liver function tests, hepatomegaly |
| Metabolic | Elevated serum calcium, decreased serum magnesium, increased osseous alkaline phosphatase, hypercalciuria |
| Neuromuscular | Fine tremor of hands, weakness of proximal muscles, myopathy, muscle atrophy, creatinuria, periodic paralysis |
| Osseous | Osteoporosis |
| Neurologic | Fever, delirium, stupor, coma, syncope, choreoathetosis |
| Reproductive/ sexual | Irregular menses, gynecomastia, decreased fertility |
| Hematopoietic | Anemia (usually normochromic, normocytic), lymphocytosis, lymphadenopathy, enlarged thymus, splenomegaly |
| Mental | Restlessness, irritability, anxiety, inability to concentrate, lability, depression, psychiatric reactions |
| Influence on vitamins | Decreased serum vitamin A, prealbumin, and retinol-binding protein; increased requirement for pyridoxine and thiamine; decreased serum 1,25-vitamin $D_2$ |

sion.[16] This hypothesis does not explain the mechanism involved in T-cell activation.

3. According to the *idiotypic-antiidiotypic network theory,* antibodies themselves initiate the development of secondary antibodies against the idiotypic combining sites of the primary antibody.[17] This sequence of secondarily developing antibodies results in a cascade by which the body can modulate or regulate antibody formation. As applied to Graves disease, TSH receptor antibodies would provoke secondary antibodies directed against the combining site of the TSH receptor antibodies. These secondary antiidiotypic antibodies would look like a mirror image of the TSH receptor antibody-combining site and thus would bind both TSH and TSH receptor antibodies. The observation that antiidiotypic antibodies are present in the serum of patients with Graves disease is consistent with an alteration in the "network cascade," at least in some patients.[18]

The fourth hypothesis relates to the presence of TSH receptor-"like" antigens in various bacteria or parasites. *Yersinia enterocolitica* possesses a specific TSH-binding site that has binding characteristics similar to those of the thyroidal TSH receptor.[19] Iodine-125–labeled TSH bound to the "receptor" could be displaced by unlabeled TSH but not by other glycoprotein hormones. The identification of this TSH "receptor" in other bacteria (e.g., *Mycoplasma*) or parasites has led to the hypothesis that *infection with agents possessing these TSH "receptors"* could result in the formation of antibodies directed against the thyroidal TSH receptor, causing stimulation (or blockade).[19,20] Alternatively, these bacteria or parasites could be engulfed by macrophages and could then be processed and presented on the macrophage surface to initiate T-cell activation in genetically susceptible patients. A potentially very important finding is that the peripheral lymphocytes from patients with Graves disease may contain human spumaretro-

virus-related sequences.[21] In other work, the TSH receptor has been found to have mutations, especially if ophthalmopathy is present.[22] Further work is required to determine the importance of these and other findings and their relevance to the initiation or propagation of autoimmune thyroid disease.

## CLINICAL MANIFESTATIONS OF GRAVES DISEASE

The clinical manifestations of Graves disease are myriad and can involve almost any organ system (Table 42-1; Figs. 42-2, 42-3, and 42-44).[23–33] Usually, there is a palpable, diffusely enlarged, smooth goiter that initially may be soft but becomes progressively firmer. Because of the increased vascularity of the gland, there may be a systolic bruit heard with the stethoscope. Patients commonly report nervousness, malaise, irritability, inability to concentrate, hand tremor, weight loss, and burning or itching eyes. Unilateral or bilateral proptosis is frequent, and

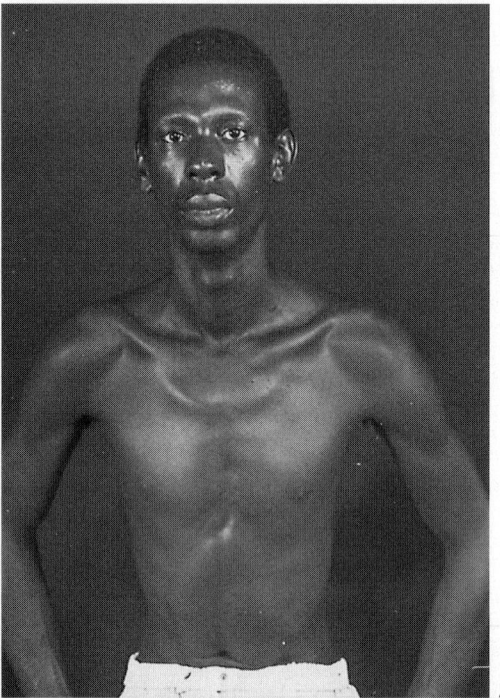

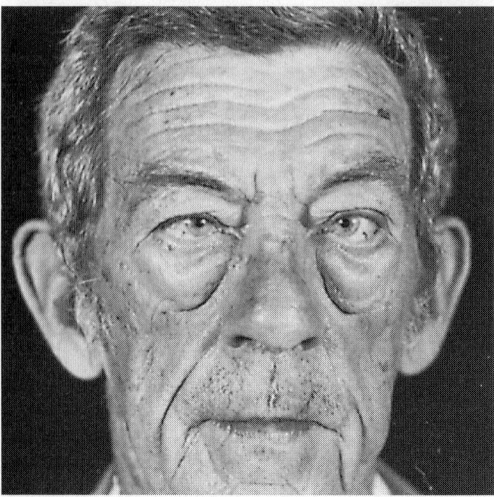

**FIGURE 42-2. A,** Severe weight loss, nervousness, and sweating in a thyrotoxic man. **B,** This 57-year-old man with Graves disease reported diplopia and tachycardia.

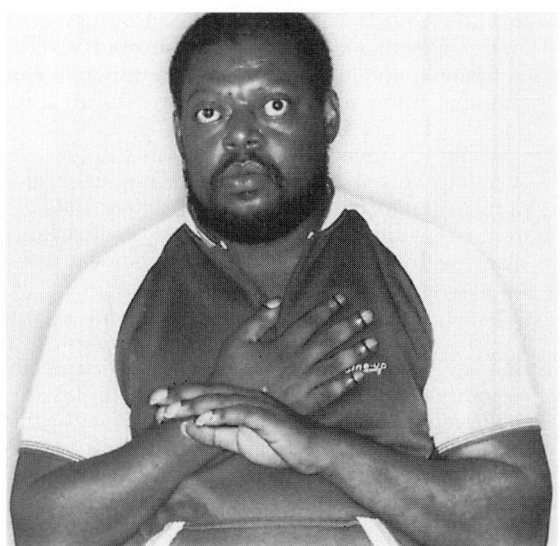
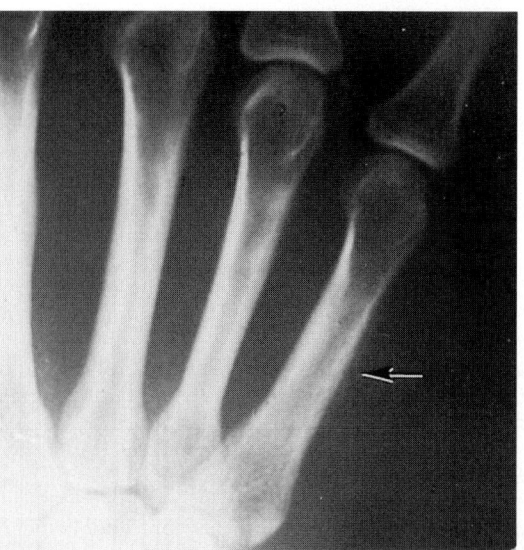

**FIGURE 42-3. A,** Graves disease in a 33-year-old man manifested by bilateral exophthalmos, acropachy (clubbing), extensive pretibial myxedema, and insulin-dependent diabetes mellitus. When this photograph was taken, he already had been treated with [131]I, had become hypothyroid, and was receiving replacement therapy with exogenous L-thyroxine. **B,** Radiograph in same patient showing phalangeal periosteal reaction (*arrow*).

vitiligo, pruritus, osteoporosis, and gynecomastia can occur. Choreoathetosis and ataxia are rare presenting signs or symptoms.[27] A severe, incapacitating, elephantiasis-like syndrome with pretibial myxedema and acropachy is also seen rarely and may be exacerbated by local trauma (see Figs. 42-3 and 42-4).[28]

Patients with Graves disease are more likely to have or to acquire several other disorders, such as Addison disease, diabetes mellitus, idiopathic thrombocytopenic purpura, myasthenia gravis, pernicious anemia, rheumatoid arthritis, scleroderma, systemic lupus erythematosus, vitiligo, dermatitis herpetiformis, thymic hyperplasia, and Albright syndrome (cutaneous pigmentation, precocious puberty, and polyostotic fibrous dysplasia of bones).[23–31]

Myopathies that are mild or moderate occur frequently in Graves disease, affecting skeletal or ocular muscles. Muscle weakness involving the shoulders, limbs, and particularly the quadriceps muscles is quite common and occasionally profound. Thyrotoxicosis with periodic paralysis occurs rarely; it is characterized by sporadic attacks, most commonly involving flaccidity and paralysis of the legs, arms, and trunk, although any muscle (e.g., facial) can be involved (see Chap. 210). Respiratory muscles can be affected, but the heart is usually not involved. These attacks may last from minutes to many hours and can occur spontaneously or after the ingestion of carbohydrates or after exercise. Occasionally the serum potassium concentration is decreased. Treatment of

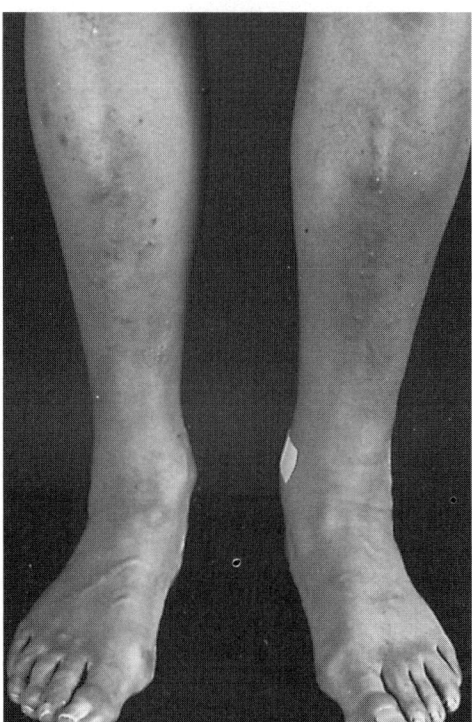
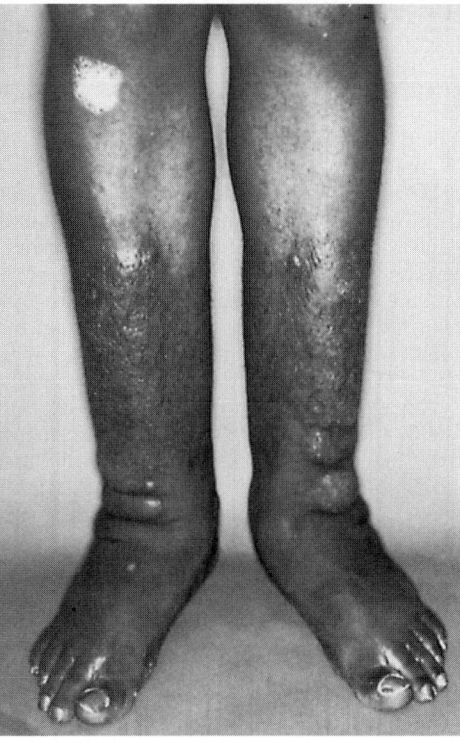

**FIGURE 42-4. A** and **B,** Different degrees of involvement of the tissues in pretibial myxedema. Patient in **B** also shows a patch of vitiligo.

thyrotoxicosis with periodic paralysis entails restoration of euthyroidism with antithyroid drugs. Administration of β-adrenergic blockers sometimes rapidly stops the attack, and potassium should be administered when serum levels are low. Thyrotoxicosis with periodic paralysis occurs most frequently in Asians. Changes in bone parameters can also occur.[31a]

Patients with Graves disease may also have myxedema in the pretibial or preradial area. This accumulation of fluid and mucopolysaccharides can be mild and clinically inconsequential or severe and incapacitating. The causes of these connective tissue effects are unknown but may be related to abnormal T- or B-cell stimulation or to cross-reacting epitopes in these tissues and serum antithyroid antibodies. The onset and progression of these problems may not correlate with the severity or progression of the thyrotoxicosis.

## OCULAR MANIFESTATIONS

The onset of Graves ophthalmopathy may precede, coincide with, or follow the thyrotoxicosis,[29,30] and sometimes its clinical course appears unrelated to the thyrotoxicosis. Nevertheless, it is a clinical dictum that rapid restoration of the euthyroid state is an important component of the management of ophthalmopathy (see Chap. 43). The pathogenesis of Graves ophthalmopathy and its relationship to the thyroidal manifestations are unclear, but it appears that retroocular fibroblasts contain TSH-receptor transcripts and, perhaps, receptor protein. It is speculated that TSH-receptor antibodies may bind to the TSH receptor within the fibroblasts, mediating or propagating the immune response. Extraocular muscle antigens may also be involved in the pathogenetic process.

# LABORATORY ASSESSMENT OF GRAVES DISEASE

The initial laboratory assessment of a patient with thyrotoxic Graves disease should include measurement of hemoglobin, hematocrit, white blood cell count, liver profile (serum alkaline phosphatase, transaminases, and bilirubin), calcium, blood urea nitrogen, creatinine, and electrolytes, as well as thyroid function tests.[32,33]

## THYROID FUNCTION TESTS

Serum TSH should be undetectable in patients with active hyperthyroidism; serum total and free $T_4$ and $T_3$ may be measured and are usually elevated. Although there may be different approaches based on background and clinical practice, most patients with suspected Graves disease should have free $T_4$, total triiodothyronine ($TT_3$), and TSH determined initially to help confirm the diagnosis. When patients with known Graves disease are observed, usually free $T_4$ and $TT_3$ are determined, and occasionally TSH may be useful. Evaluation of $TT_3$ levels should be routine, but may be especially useful when the clinical signs or symptoms are marked and seemingly disproportionate to the free $T_4$ elevation.[34,35] $T_3$ toxicosis, a condition of clinical thyrotoxicosis with a normal serum $T_4$ level but an elevated $TT_3$ level, is relatively unusual; it is more likely to occur in patients with an autonomous nodule, early Graves disease, or recurrent disease. To develop tests that would not be influenced by binding proteins, investigators have developed free $T_4$ and free $T_3$ measurements that are sensitive and applicable to clinical use.[35-38] Free $T_4$ should replace the more traditional total $T_4$ and resin $T_3$ uptake tests given that it is not influenced by alterations in binding proteins and because it is now widely available. However, free $T_3$ is not yet readily available commercially with a rapid turnaround time; therefore, it is still appropriate to obtain a $TT_3$ level, although it must be remembered

that $TT_3$ levels are increased when there are elevations of $T_4$-binding globulin (e.g., pregnancy, estrogen).

Serum thyroglobulin levels and antithyroglobulin or antimicrosomal antibodies need not be measured routinely in a patient with Graves disease.

In most patients with Graves disease (except pregnant or lactating women), the 24-hour (or 6-hour) radioactive iodine uptake should be determined to differentiate Graves disease from thyroiditis (subacute, painless, postpartum). In painless subacute thyroiditis, the radioactive iodine uptake is <5% when the patient is hyperthyroid with elevated free $T_4$ and $TT_3$ in conjunction with a decreased TSH level. However, the physician also should consider postpartum thyroiditis, subacute thyroiditis, recent exposure to excessive iodide in drugs, and amiodarone use or radiopaque dyes (as used in computed tomography scans or angiograms) that may artifactually lower the uptake. A radioisotopic thyroid scan in a thyrotoxic patient helps confirm that a patient has Graves disease when the scan shows diffuse homogeneous uptake of tracer, although such a scan is not always necessary. However, a palpable thyroid nodule or other unusual finding (e.g., lymphadenopathy) or worrisome signs or symptoms (e.g., pain, rapid growth of thyroid gland) are indications for a radioisotopic thyroid scan to help rule out concomitant neoplasm. Of course, fine-needle aspiration of suspicious or abnormal nodules (intrathyroidally or extrathyroidally) or nodes should be performed as appropriate to help determine the nature of these abnormalities.

Occasionally it is difficult to determine clinically that a patient is thyrotoxic, especially when the thyroid gland is only minimally enlarged and the serum $T_4$ or free $T_4$ value is normal or marginally elevated. A thyrotropin-releasing hormone (TRH) stimulation test—in which serum TSH is measured 0, 15, and 30 minutes after the administration of 200 to 500 μg of TRH by intravenous bolus—may then be indicated. An increase in the TSH level of 2 to 3 μU/mL or more after TRH administration excludes hyperthyroidism. With the exception of hypopituitarism, a blunted response almost always indicates hyperthyroidism, although psychiatric patients, patients with hyperemesis gravidarum, or elderly patients may have a blunted or minimal rise in TSH after TRH stimulation, even when they are euthyroid (see Chap. 15). Use of a highly sensitive TSH assay has obviated the utility of most TRH tests. Third-generation TSH assays have a sensitivity of ~0.01 μU/mL, and these assays can discriminate subnormal from undetectable TSH concentrations. Thus, thyrotoxic patients have an undetectable TSH level, except in rare instances of a TSH-secreting pituitary tumor.[37,38] Serum $T_4$ levels may be elevated in other conditions that can be classified as "euthyroid hyperthyroxinemia" (see Chap. 36).[39]

Several other laboratory tests not commonly required in the evaluation of a thyrotoxic patient are occasionally helpful. A 24-hour urinary iodide excretion test may help identify hyperthyroid patients who have a low radioactive iodine uptake secondary to exogenous iodide ingestion. A patient ingesting a normal diet may excrete 500 to 1000 μg of iodide in the urine daily. The minimal daily requirement of iodine is ~150 μg per day. A patient with a low (<5%) radioactive iodine uptake secondary to exogenous iodine intake usually excretes >1000 μg of iodine a day. Serum $T_4$-binding globulin levels may be helpful in selected patients but are unnecessary if there is an obvious cause of the elevated $T_4$-binding globulin (e.g., use of birth control pills) associated with elevated $T_4$ levels and a decreased resin $T_3$ uptake.

## TSH RECEPTOR ANTIBODY MEASUREMENTS

Occasionally it may be important to measure TSH receptor antibodies. TSH receptor antibodies in the sera may be measured by bioassays that detect cyclic adenosine monophosphate production by immunoglobulin G (IgG) isolated from patients with Graves disease (thyroid-stimulating immunoglobulin

**TABLE 42-2.**
**Thyroid-Stimulating Hormone Receptor Antibody Measurements**

| Method | Nomenclature | Frequency in Graves Disease (%) | Frequency in Normal Sera (%) | Frequency in Autoimmune Thyroiditis (%) | Advantages | Disadvantages |
|---|---|---|---|---|---|---|
| Cyclic adenosine mono-phosphate production in thyroid membrane or thyrocytes | Thyroid-stimulating immunoglobulins | 80–100 | 0–10 | 0–20 | Relatively specific for Graves disease; detects stimulatory antibodies | Difficult to perform |
| Displacement of $^{125}$I-TSH binding to thyroid membranes | TSH receptor bind-ing inhibitory immunoglobulins | 70–90 | 0–10 | 0–20 | Easy to perform | Antibodies that bind to TSH receptor may not be stimu-latory in vivo |
| Enzyme-linked immuno-sorbent assay | — | 80–90 | 0–10 | 10–30 | Easy to perform; does not require immuno-globulin G extrac-tion from sera | Antibodies that bind to TSH receptors may not be stimu-latory in vivo |

*TSH*, thyroid-stimulating hormone.
(Adapted from Burman KD, et al. Immune mechanisms in Graves' disease. Endocr Rev 1985; 6:183. Reproduced by permission of The Endocrine Society.)

[TSI] assay), by the ability of Graves IgG to inhibit $^{125}$I-TSH binding to thyroid-binding inhibitory immunoglobulins (TBII) of thyroid membranes (TBII assay), or by the ability of sera to bind to TSH receptors in enzyme-linked immunosorbent assay (ELISA) (Table 42-2).[1,40–42] TSH receptor antibodies are usually of the IgG class. In general, assays that detect stimulatory antibodies are preferable. Assays that measure binding to TSH receptors (TBII or ELISA) are easier to perform but may detect antibodies that are not stimulatory and, thus, may have less clinical relevance to Graves thyrotoxicosis. TSI assays have been improved by the use of recombinant TSH receptor. Inhibitory (blocking) TSH receptor antibodies may be found in ~20% of patients with primary hypothyroidism. Some infants may become hypothyroid in the first 3 months of life because of the transplacental passage of these inhibitory antibodies. TSH receptor antibody assays can be modified to detect inhibitory immunoglobulins by assessing the ability of the patient's IgG to inhibit TSH-mediated rises in cyclic adenosine monophosphate. Clinical circumstances in which measurement of TSH receptor antibody may be helpful include differentiation of autoimmune thyroid disease from thyrotoxicosis that is due to other causes; diagnosis of euthyroid Graves disease; prediction of the likelihood that a pregnant woman who has autoimmune thyroid disease will deliver a neonate with thyrotoxicosis; helping to predict the likelihood of relapse or remission; and helping to predict if the thyrotoxicosis in the postpartum period will be transient or persistent.

Other than the TSH measurement, which reflects thyroid action at the level of the hypothalamic-pituitary axis, there are presently no clinically available laboratory tests that directly and reliably reflect the effect of $T_4$ or $T_3$ on tissues (see Chap. 33).

## OTHER LABORATORY TESTS IN GRAVES DISEASE

In long-standing Graves disease, anemia, which can be normochromic or mildly hypochromic, may be noted. Occasionally there is a mild neutropenia and lymphocytosis. Rarely, thrombocytopenia may occur. Commonly, the serum cholesterol level is decreased and there may be a minimal increase of the serum aspartate aminotransferase value.

Perhaps 5% to 10% of patients with thyrotoxicosis manifest elevations in total serum calcium value.[32] These elevations, which are due to increased bone resorption, are usually mild. The serum phosphate value is normal; the urinary hydroxyproline level is elevated. The hypercalcemia usually resolves as the serum $T_4$ level decreases. Initially, β-adrenergic blockers may hasten the return to normocalcemia. Rarely, the serum calcium level remains elevated and is found to be associated with coex-

isting hyperparathyroidism. Similarly, the decreased serum magnesium, elevated serum alkaline phosphatase, and abnormal liver function tests should resolve as the thyrotoxicosis is controlled.

# DIFFERENTIAL DIAGNOSIS OF HYPERTHYROIDISM

## GRAVES DISEASE

Graves disease occurs most frequently in young women (~5:1 female to male ratio) but is not uncommon in any age group or in any geographic population.[1–3,5] No single clinical sign or symptom differentiates Graves disease from other causes of thyrotoxicosis, although the presence of ophthalmopathy, a diffusely enlarged and firm thyroid gland, and pretibial myxedema or acropachy strongly suggests this illness. The cooccurrence of another autoimmune disease in the patient (e.g., myasthenia gravis) or a family history of Hashimoto or Graves disease or of any other autoimmune disease is a frequent accompaniment of this condition. Graves disease is found more frequently in patients with HLA-DR3 antigens. The laboratory diagnosis is supported by the presence of stimulatory TSH receptor antibodies in a thyrotoxic patient.[1–3,43] However, the measurement of TSH receptor antibodies is not indicated in most patients, as usually the diagnosis can be made on the basis of the previously listed clinical characteristics.

Although rarely indicated, the thyroid gland may be imaged in such patients by a radioisotopic thyroid scan, CT, magnetic resonance imaging (MRI), or fluorescent iodide scan (Figs. 42-5, 42-6, and 42-7) (see Chaps. 34, 35, and 39). The differential diagnosis of hyperthyroidism includes more than a dozen other conditions (Table 42-3).

## SURREPTITIOUS INGESTION OF THYROXINE OR TRIIODOTHYRONINE

Hyperthyroidism that is due to the administration of thyroid hormones is not uncommon, as exogenous thyroid hormone is easily obtained. This medication is often taken by persons who wish to lose weight. The surreptitious ingestion of $T_4$ or $T_3$ (thyrotoxicosis factitia) can be inferred from the measurement of inappropriately low levels of serum thyroglobulin. Because thyroglobulin is normally secreted by the thyroid gland in concert with $T_4$ and $T_3$, its levels should be elevated in cases of thyroidal hyperfunction, whereas its levels are suppressed with ingestion of exogenous thyroid hormones.[44] In addition, the

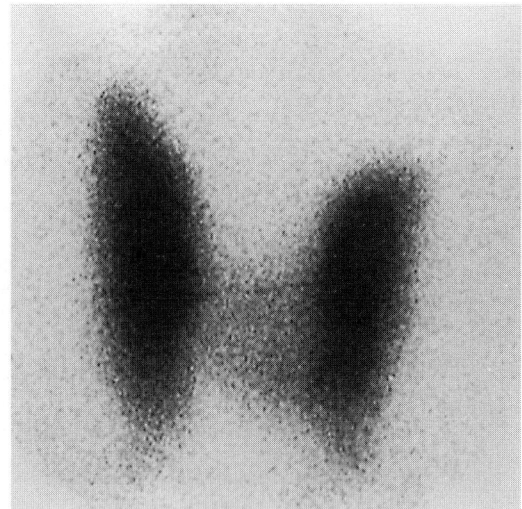

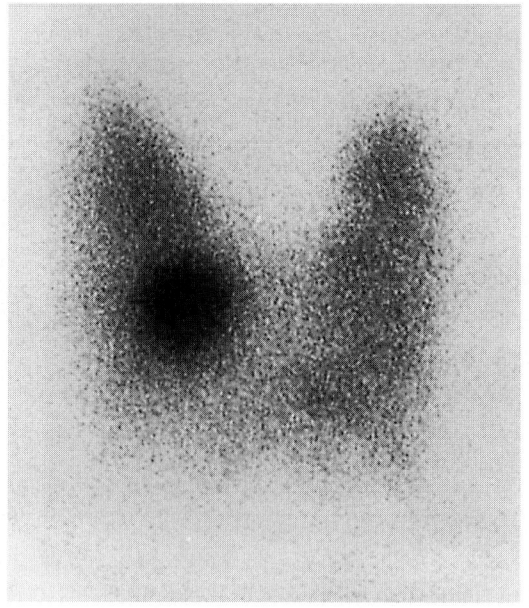

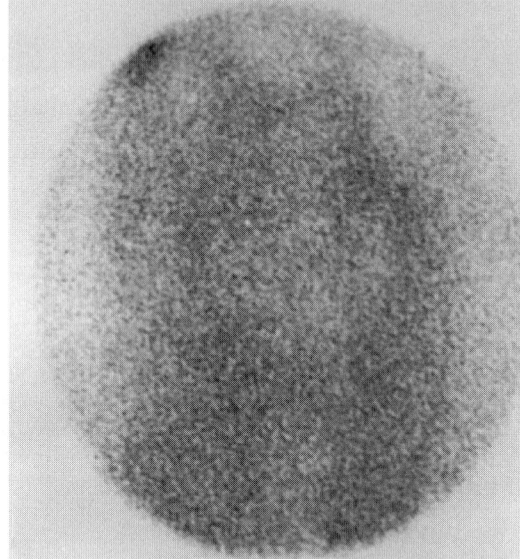

**FIGURE 42-5.** Technetium thyroid scans (anterior views). **A,** Scan of a normal subject. Note the bilateral, relatively homogeneous tracer distribution (imaging time, 134 seconds). **B,** Scan illustrating a dominant hyperfunctioning right lower pole thyroid nodule (imaging time, 235 seconds). The nodule was not hyperfunctioning sufficiently to completely suppress the remainder of the thyroid gland, but there was no serum thyroid-stimulating hormone rise after thyrotropin-releasing hormone stimulation, and clinically the patient was mildly thyrotoxic. **C,** Scan of a 50-year-old thyrotoxic patient with subacute thyroiditis. The 24-hour radioactive iodine uptake was <1%. The thyroid scan barely shows a faint outline of thyroid tissue (imaging time, 563 seconds). This patient had painful thyroiditis, a serum thyroxine level of 15.9 μg/dL, a resin triiodothyronine uptake of 46%, an erythrocyte sedimentation rate of 32 mm/h, and no serum thyroid-stimulating hormone response to thyrotropin-releasing hormone stimulation.

thyroid radioiodine uptake is depressed. If the patient is taking $T_4$, serum values of this hormone are typically increased more than those of $T_3$. If the patient is taking $T_3$, the serum $T_3$ level may be preferentially increased, with the $T_4$ level being decreased. The extent of serum $T_3$ changes in these patients depends on the dose ingested and how long after ingestion the blood is obtained. Thyroid extract ingestion may be associated with elevations of both $T_4$ and/or $T_3$, depending on the preparation used and the time interval since ingestion.

## TOXIC MULTINODULAR GOITER

Toxic multinodular goiters that cause thyrotoxicosis are usually very large. Patients with thyrotoxicosis that is due to a multinodular gland do not undergo spontaneous exacerbations and remissions, and definitive therapy ($^{131}$I or surgery) is usually required. Thyroid scans show diffuse inhomogeneous tracer uptake, reflecting areas of hyperfunction and hypofunction within the gland. Occasionally, CT or MRI of the neck may be helpful in delineating the size of a thyroid gland and in assessing impingement on surrounding structures (see Fig. 42-6). As stated in Chapter 37, the iodine contained in radiocontrast agents used with CT scans may cause thyroid dysfunction. On physical examination, the thyroid glands are multinodular and enlarged. The nodules usually are benign follicular adenomas. Toxic nodular goiters occur equally in men and women and can appear at any age,

although they most frequently occur in patients older than 40 years. Usually, there is no exophthalmos, acropachy, onycholysis, or pretibial myxedema. Toxic nodular goiters are not believed to have an autoimmune etiology, because serum TSH receptor antibodies are absent. Antibodies that stimulate thyroid growth may be important in these disorders,[45] but this finding is controversial. Low-titer antithyroglobulin or antimicrosomal antibodies may be present. Occasionally, eye findings may also be present. This presentation of stigmata of Graves disease with a nodular rather than diffuse goiter has been termed the *Marine-Lenhart syndrome.*

## SOLITARY AUTONOMOUS NODULE

Patients who have a solitary autonomous nodule (toxic adenoma, Plummer disease) (see Fig. 42-5 and Chap. 39) as the cause of their thyrotoxicosis generally have a palpable thyroid nodule that, on thyroid scan, is seen to be suppressing the function of the extranodular tissue. However, solitary autonomous nodules usually do not secrete sufficient hormone to cause clinical thyrotoxicosis, although an undetectable $T_3$ may be seen. Most autonomous nodules continue to function at the same rate over time, but 10% to 20% gradually enlarge, and their secretion is increased sufficiently to cause clinical thyrotoxicosis. Nodules more than 3 cm in diameter evolve to cause clinical thyrotoxicosis more frequently than do smaller nodules. Thyroid function tests often are only mildly abnormal. When

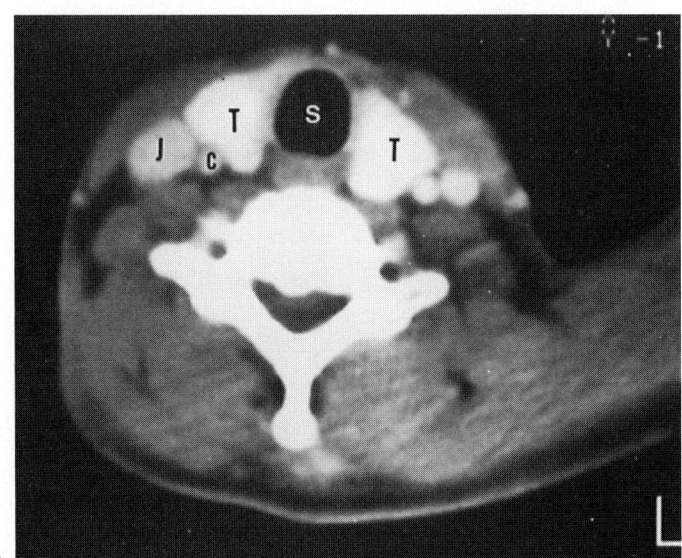

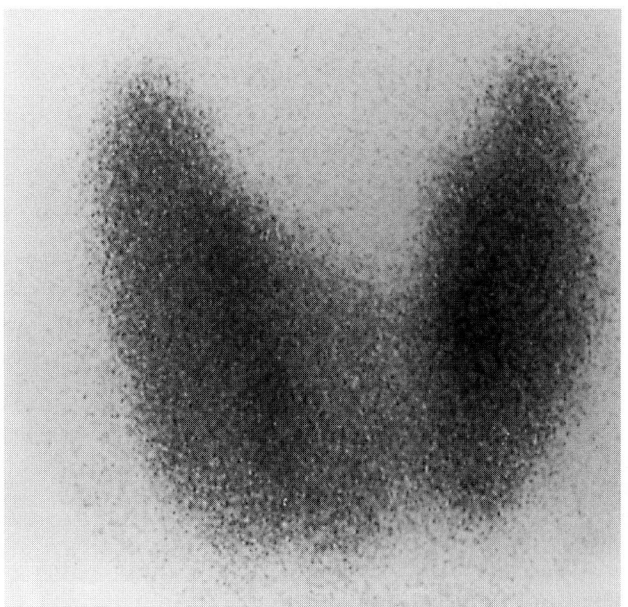

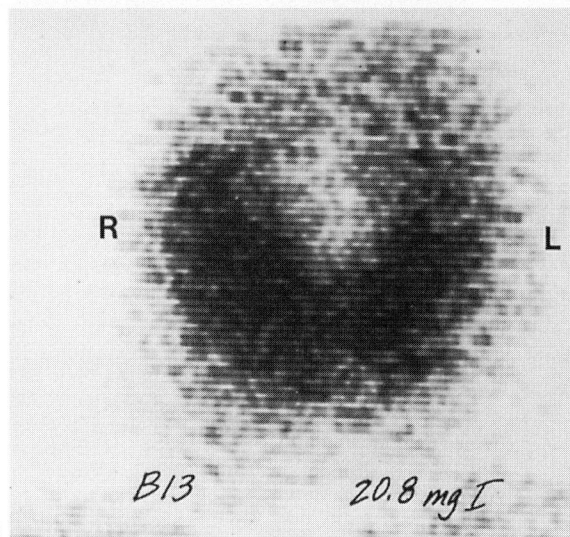

**FIGURE 42-6.** **A,** Computed tomography scan of the neck in a patient with Graves disease. Note mildly enlarged thyroid gland that does not impinge on the subglottic trachea. Asymmetric jugular veins often are observed in normal subjects and are considered a nonpathologic variant. (*C,* carotid artery; *J,* external jugular vein; *S,* subglottic trachea; *T,* thyroid gland.) **B,** Technetium thyroid scan of the same patient showing bilateral, relatively homogeneous uptake. The 24-hour radioactive iodine uptake was 31% (imaging time, 152 seconds). **C,** Fluorescent thyroid scan in the same patient. The thyroid gland had a content of 20.8 mg iodine (normal, 5–15 mg).

hyperthyroidism occurs, therapy with [131]I or surgery is indicated. As in toxic multinodular goiter, surgery seems preferable in young adults and children, whereas radioactive iodine therapy is preferable in older patients. In general, 10 to 15 mCi of [131]I is given to patients with autonomous nodules and 15 to 25 mCi of [131]I to those with multinodular goiters. Because it is mainly the hyperactive tissue that traps the radioiodine and not the suppressed tissue, radioiodine therapy may not result in hypothyroidism, although these patients have to be observed indefinitely for the development of thyroid dysfunction.

The differential diagnosis between toxic nodular goiter and Graves disease usually poses no difficulty, with the distinction resting on the anatomy of the thyroid by physical and scan examination and the presence or absence of other signs of Graves disease. In general, definitive therapy usually should not be administered while the patient is clinically thyrotoxic, particularly in older patients. Rather, antithyroid drugs should be given initially to render the patient euthyroid; these latter drugs do not cure the condition.

## EXOGENOUS IODINE EXCESS

Exogenous iodine excess (e.g., iodide supplementation with radiocontrast agents or amiodarone) may induce hyperthyroid-

ism in some individuals with autonomously functioning tissue; hence, this may occur in both Graves disease and nodular goiter (see Chap. 37). A history of iodide excess strongly suggests iodide-induced disease; and the radioactive iodine uptake may be suppressed because of dilution. A low radioactive iodine uptake may also be seen with subacute, silent, or postpartum thyroiditis, although in these circumstances it is thought to be due to impaired ability to trap iodine.[5,46–48] A fluorescent iodine scan (see Chap. 39) may be useful in assessing intrathyroidal iodine content, which is usually increased in Graves disease and iodide-induced hyperthyroidism, and decreased in the hyperthyroidism of subacute thyroiditis (see Fig. 42-6C).

## SUBACUTE (GRANULOMATOUS) THYROIDITIS

Subacute (granulomatous) thyroiditis is a spontaneously resolving inflammation of the thyroid gland that can have a varied course and clinical presentation (see Fig. 42-5C and Chap. 46). Viral infections of the thyroid gland are thought to cause or predispose to this disease (see Chap. 213).[46] Although it may present at any age, women and men between the ages of 20 and 50 are most frequently affected. Often, the disorder evolves through a characteristic pattern, from thyrotoxicosis to hypothy-

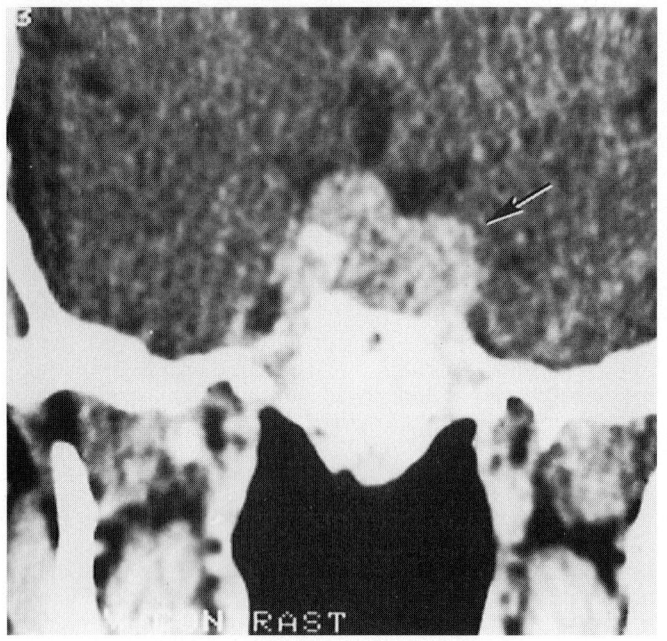

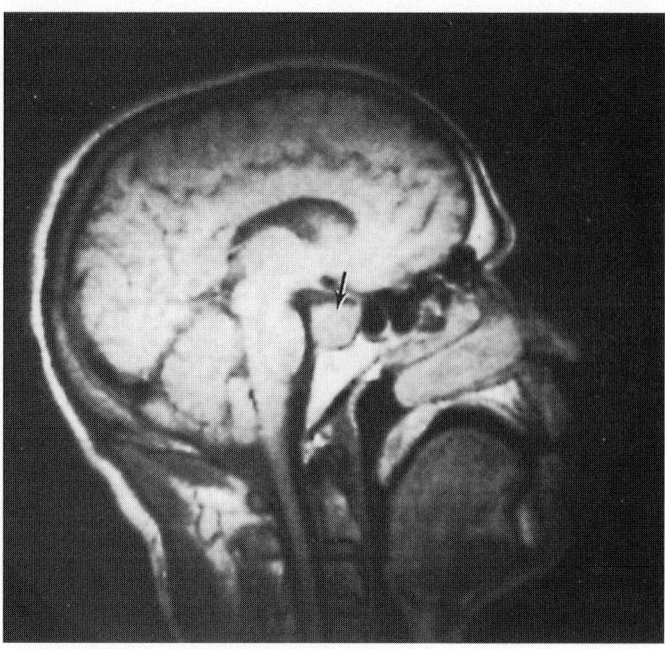

**FIGURE 42-7. A,** Computed tomography scan showing a suprasellar pituitary tumor (*arrow*) in a thyrotoxic patient with a thyroid-stimulating hormone–secreting pituitary tumor. These tumors frequently secrete α subunit disproportionately to thyroid stimulating hormone. **B,** Magnetic resonance image (T1-weighted) in the same patient showing a 2 × 2-cm pituitary tumor (*arrow*). T1-weighted images are favorable for demonstrating anatomical detail. (Adapted from Smallridge RC. Thyrotropin-secreting pituitary tumors. Endocrinol Metab Clin North Am 1987; 16:3.)

**TABLE 42-3.**
**Disorders That Can Cause Thyrotoxicosis\***

| Disorder | Comments | Disorder | Comments |
|---|---|---|---|
| Graves disease | Elevated RAI uptake, eye findings, pretibial myxedema, TSH receptor antibodies | "Hashitoxicosis" | High-titer antithyroglobulin and antimicrosomal antibodies, usually transient thyrotoxicosis, increased RAI uptake |
| Surreptitious (or iatrogenic) | No goiter, no exophthalmos; patient may be emotionally disturbed; decreased serum thyroglobulin by RIA | Trophoblastic tumors | Elevated hCG level; nodule may be palpable in testes; may occur with pregnancy |
| Toxic multinodular goiter | Nodular enlarged thyroid gland for several years, nonhomogeneous scan, lack of eye findings† | Struma ovarii | 24-h thyroid RAI uptake <5%, usually mild hyperthyroidism, no exophthalmos, may have palpable abnormality in ovary |
| Solitary autonomous nodule | Single large hyperfunctioning nodule on thyroid scan, often of long duration; may preferentially secrete $T_3$ rather than $T_4$ | TSH-secreting pituitary tumor | Mild hyperthyroidism; no exophthalmos; neurologic symptoms may be present; may have headache or bitemporal hemianopsia; tumor usually large and seen on CT or MRI, sometimes on skull radiographs; should be considered if thyroid gland regrows after prior subtotal thyroidectomy or radioactive iodine; abnormal α subunit to entire TSH ratio (molar) |
| Exogenous iodine excess | History of exposure to excessive iodide (including amiodarone); usually underlying goitrous thyroid disease; 24-h RAI uptake <5%; 24-h urine iodide excretion >1000 μg/d | Metastatic thyroid cancer | Usually obvious extensive metastases |
| Subacute (granulomatous) thyroiditis | May have tenderness in neck area; may have fever and malaise; 24-h RAI uptake <5% while thyrotoxic; may evolve into hypothyroidism or euthyroidism | "Hamburger" thyrotoxicosis | History of ingestion of hamburger or meat containing thyroid tissue; several persons involved, no goiter. Increased serum iodothyronines, but low RAI uptake; spontaneous resolution in 1–2 wk |
| Spontaneously resolving thyroiditis | Thyroid usually not tender; patients may have elevated $T_4$ and clinical thyrotoxicosis with 24-h RAIU <5%; spontaneous remissions; may proceed to hypothyroidism | Interleukin-2, α-interferon administration | Causes thyroiditis; patient usually hypothyroid although also may become hyperthyroid |
| Postpartum thyroiditis | May present as hypothyroidism or thyrotoxicosis; evolves into euthyroidism in most cases; usually painless; most patients have positive antithyroglobulin or antimicrosomal antibodies | Hyperemesis gravidarum | Correlated with hCG levels; symptoms tend to resolve at 12–15 weeks of gestation; TSH undetectable or suppressed; difficult to distinguish from Graves disease during pregnancy |

*CT*, computed tomography; *hCG*, human chorionic gonadotropin; *MRI*, magnetic resonance imaging; *RAI*, radioactive iodine; *RAIU*, radioactive iodine uptake; *RIA*, radioimmunoassay; $T_3$, triiodothyronine; $T_4$, thyroxine; *TSH*, thyroid-stimulating hormone.
\*Each of these conditions can cause clinical thyrotoxicosis and elevated serum $T_4$, resin $T_3$ uptake test (r$T_3$U), $T_3$(RIA), and free $T_4$ levels.
†Rarely, thyrotoxicosis that is due to a hyperfunctioning multinodular gland can be accompanied by eye findings (e.g., chemosis, conjunctivitis) and is referred to as Marine-Lenhart syndrome.

roidism to the euthyroid state. Each phase may last ~2 to 10 weeks, and any or all of the clinical phases may be seen in individual patients. The distinction between this disorder and other causes of hyperthyroidism is usually not difficult (Table 42-4). The hyperthyroid phase may be accompanied by fever, pain in the thyroid area that radiates to the neck or jaw, myalgias, tachycardia, nervousness, and palpitations. The thyroid gland is usually enlarged, firm, and tender, and the erythrocyte sedimentation rate is usually elevated. Despite elevated serum $T_4$ and $T_3$ concentrations, the radioactive iodine uptake is very low (<5%). Because the thyrotoxic phase gradually resolves spontaneously, only temporary or palliative treatment is usually required. Some patients may require aspirin or corticosteroids to control the thyroidal pain, and the clinical hyperthyroidism can be treated with β-adrenergic blockers. Subacute thyroiditis may occur in otherwise normal thyroid glands or in patients with preexisting multinodular goiter or Hashimoto thyroiditis.

## SPONTANEOUSLY RESOLVING THYROIDITIS

In spontaneously resolving thyroiditis,[46] the thyroid gland is usually painless and there is little evidence of acute inflammation. The thyrotoxicosis is mild; the 24-hour radioactive iodine uptake is low, and serum iodothyronine concentrations are increased. Thyroid glands demonstrate focal or diffuse lymphocytic infiltrations with varying fibrosis. There are no giant cells (which would be indicative of subacute granulomatous thyroiditis). The clinical course usually evolves from thyrotoxicosis to euthyroidism, with or without transient hypothyroidism. As with granulomatous thyroiditis, treatment is usually supportive, although control of the thyrotoxic signs or symptoms with β-adrenergic blockers is occasionally required.

## POSTPARTUM THYROIDITIS

Postpartum thyroiditis occurs in 5% to 10% of women within the first year after parturition.[47,49,50] This disease may evolve through a thyrotoxic, hypothyroid, and euthyroid recovery phase or may simply manifest with either hypothyroidism or thyrotoxicosis that spontaneously and gradually returns to euthyroidism. Approximately 67% of women with positive antimicrosomal thyroid antibodies develop thyroid dysfunction.[49] Patients without detectable thyroid antibodies at delivery can also develop postpartum thyroiditis.[50] Present knowledge suggests that pregnancy decreases immunologic responsiveness and that there is a "rebound effect" during the postpartum period; the thyroidal injury observed may be related to increased natural killer cell activity. Treatment of the thyrotoxic symptoms may not be necessary because of their mild elevation and evanescent pattern. Although the thyroid disease resolves spontaneously in many patients, the hypothyroidism or thyrotoxicosis may persist for more than a year after parturition, thus suggesting an unmasking of preexisting thyroid disease. When spontaneous remission does occur, the patient tends to have similar disease progression during each subsequent pregnancy. Moreover, evidence indicates that women with thyroid antibodies during pregnancy may develop gestational hypothyroidism; therefore, periodic monitoring of these women may be indicated.[51]

## "HASHITOXICOSIS"

"Hashitoxicosis" is a rare cause of hyperthyroidism in which the radioactive iodine uptake is typically increased or within the normal range, serum iodothyronine levels are elevated with an undetectable TSH, and the patient is clinically thyrotoxic. The pathologic findings in the thyroid resemble those of Hashimoto disease, with lymphocytic infiltration, fibrosis, and few or no enlarged follicles. Antimicrosomal and antithyroglobulin antibodies are present in high titer. It is believed that in some patients the condition evolves into hypothyroidism as the thyroid gland undergoes fibrosis and as destruction proceeds.

## TROPHOBLASTIC TUMORS

Thyrotoxicosis that is usually mild, but can be severe, is seen in 10% to 20% of patients with trophoblastic tumors such as benign hydatidiform mole, malignant choriocarcinoma, or embryonal carcinoma of the testis. These tumors cause thyroidal hyperfunction by secretion of human chorionic gonadotropin (hCG), which may be capable of direct thyroid gland stimulation.[48,52] There may be no goiter, or only mild thyroidal enlargement may be present. In some cases of choriocarcinoma, the original tumor may be small and difficult to find, but hCG levels in blood or urine are elevated. More patients have abnormal thyroid function tests than have clinical thyrotoxicosis. Treatment of the hyperthyroidism includes β-blockers, iodides, and, on occasion, antithyroidal agents. Therapy for the trophoblastic lesion is discussed in Chapters 111 and 112.

## STRUMA OVARII

Struma ovarii denotes thyroid hormone secretion by embryonic rests of thyroidal tissue in the ovary (see Chap. 102). This extrathyroidal source of thyroid hormone is associated with rel-

**TABLE 42-4.**
**Clinical and Laboratory Findings in Various Types of Thyroiditis**

| Parameter | Subacute Granulomatous Thyroiditis | Spontaneously Resolving Thyroiditis | Postpartum Thyroiditis |
|---|---|---|---|
| Sex predilection | Female > Male | About equal | Female only |
| Temperature | May be elevated | Afebrile | Afebrile |
| ESR and WBC | Very high ESR; WBC usually normal, may be increased | Normal or slightly elevated | Normal |
| Thyroid gland | Painful, large, indurated | Painless, usually large | Painless, usually enlarged |
| Radioactive iodine uptake in thyrotoxic phase | <5% | <5% | Usually decreased |
| Thyroid autoantibodies | Low titer or absent | Low titer or absent | Low to high titer; titer rises progressively in postpartum period |
| Spontaneous resolution | Yes | Yes | Sometimes; disease may still be present 1–2 yr later |
| Recurrences after spontaneous resolution | Rare | Rare | After each pregnancy |
| Thyroid pathology | Granuloma, giant cell infiltration | Lymphocytic infiltration | Lymphocytic infiltration |

*ESR*, erythrocyte sedimentation rate; *WBC*, white blood cell count.

atively suppressed thyroid gland activity, manifested by a low 24-hour radioactive iodine uptake over the cervical area.[53] Struma ovarii is extremely rare but should be considered in a thyrotoxic woman without a goiter and with a low radioactive iodine uptake in the neck. The diagnosis can be confirmed by pelvic scan with radioiodine. The primary treatment is surgical with restoration of euthyroidism, if possible, before surgery.

## THYROID-STIMULATING-HORMONE–SECRETING PITUITARY TUMOR

TSH-secreting pituitary tumors are a very unusual cause of thyrotoxicosis (see Fig. 42-7).[54–56] These tumors occur equally in men and women. The diagnosis should be considered if the thyroid gland regrows after an ablative procedure or in patients with thyrotoxicosis and headaches or visual disturbances. Unilateral proptosis, galactorrhea, amenorrhea, or associated acromegaly may also occur. In contrast to primary thyroidal hyperthyroidism, serum TSH levels are detectable or even elevated (see Chap. 15). A CT scan or MRI of the pituitary is often abnormal. Serum studies show a disproportionately elevated $\alpha$ subunit of TSH. TSH is poorly responsive to TRH stimulation or to $T_4$ suppression. Although rare, the diagnosis should be considered in the previously mentioned circumstances, because the mass effect of the pituitary tumor can be damaging. The treatment is pituitary surgery, irradiation, or both. External radiation alone may be helpful but is not considered curative. Studies suggest that somatostatin analogs have a role in therapy.[56] Pituitary tumors that secrete TSH may also secrete other pituitary hormones (growth hormone in particular); therefore, such patients should be screened appropriately. In a report summarizing the experience of the National Institutes of Health,[55] in 25 patients with a TSH-secreting pituitary tumor, thyrotoxic symptoms were present in 22 subjects and absent in 3. In 14 patients previously untreated for their pituitary tumor, an elevated $\alpha$ subunit to TSH molar ratio was present in 12 cases, giving 83% sensitivity. Considering all cases, apparent cure was noted in 35% of patients with surgery alone and in an additional 22% with a combined approach. Three deaths were noted, including one with metastatic pituitary cancer. Five of six patients with residual tumor had their hyperthyroidism controlled with octreotide therapy.

## METASTATIC THYROID CANCER

Metastatic thyroid cancer must be widespread before there is sufficient mass to secrete enough iodothyronine to cause hyperthyroidism.[57] Follicular carcinoma is the tumor type most likely to produce this syndrome. The diagnosis of this entity derives from finding extensive radioactive iodine uptake outside the thyroid bed on thyroid scan and elevated serum thyroglobulin levels. Usually, there is a history of known thyroid cancer. Treatment consists of $^{131}$I administration and the temporary administration of antithyroid drugs and β-blockers. Of interest, tumors (e.g., lymphoma, pancreas, breast, malignant thymoma) that are metastatic to the thyroid gland can also cause hyperthyroidism, probably by local injury and release of cytokines.

## "HAMBURGER" THYROTOXICOSIS

"Hamburger" thyrotoxicosis is a fascinating syndrome that was described by astute investigators who noted a regional outbreak of hyperthyroidism. Further study revealed that local abattoirs were including thyroid glands with the other meats obtained from cattle. The iodothyronines in the meat were ingested by individuals, who then exhibited elevated serum $T_4$ and $T_3$ levels and clinical thyrotoxicosis. The limitation of this entity to one geographic area was related to the meat distribution pattern from one local abattoir.[58] The clinical manifestations included thyrotoxicosis and elevated serum $T_4$ and $T_3$

levels but low radioactive iodine uptake, similar to what is seen with surreptitious ingestion of thyroid hormone. Although inclusion of the thyroid gland in meat products is now banned in several states, this entity should be considered when patients present with elevated serum iodothyronine levels and a low radioactive iodine uptake. Furthermore, it is possible that similar geographic outbreaks have occurred before and may have accounted for some previously reported cases of spontaneously resolving thyroiditis.

## NATURAL HISTORY OF GRAVES DISEASE

Although our understanding of the pathogenesis of Graves disease is progressing rapidly, we still cannot accurately predict the natural history in a given patient. Virtually all patients with Graves disease can be treated effectively with antithyroid drugs, $^{131}$I, or surgery. Most patients treated with $^{131}$I or surgery eventually become hypothyroid and require L-$T_4$ therapy. Therefore, if a patient does not become endogenously hypothyroid within the first several months after radioactive iodine therapy, he or she will need clinical and laboratory examination once or twice yearly thereafter. Although most patients who do manifest radioiodine-induced hypothyroidism have no recurrences of thyrotoxicosis, an occasional patient with documented hypothyroidism may again develop thyrotoxic Graves disease and require definitive antithyroid therapy. These patients probably have heterogeneous anti-TSH receptor antibodies in their serum, with earlier predominance of the blocking antibodies,[40] after which the character or affinity of the antibodies changes to predominantly stimulating antibodies. Patients with stimulating TSH receptor antibodies in high titer or affinity may have particularly aggressive disease, which may include resistance of thyrotoxicosis to two or three standard doses of $^{131}$I therapy or recurrence after a near-total thyroidectomy.

Some insight into the natural history of Graves disease came from a study of 15 patients who had undergone a course of antithyroid medication with restoration of the euthyroid status 20 to 27 years earlier and who had no subsequent therapy with antithyroid or thyroid medications.[59] Four patients had become hypothyroid, and one developed recurrent thyrotoxicosis 25 years after the initial diagnosis; 5 of 10 patients had an abnormal iodide perchlorate discharge test, and 12 of 15 had elevated antimicrosomal antibody titers. These results suggest that patients with Graves disease require medical follow-up throughout their lives.

## TREATMENT OF GRAVES DISEASE

The three major modalities of treatment for a thyrotoxic patient with Graves disease are antithyroid medications, $^{131}$I, and thyroidectomy.

### ANTITHYROID DRUGS

Either propylthiouracil (PTU) or methimazole (methylmercaptoimidazole, MMI) is considered a first-line agent in the treatment of thyrotoxic Graves disease (Table 42-5).[60–64] PTU and MMI inhibit iodination of thyroglobulin, iodotyrosine coupling, thyroglobulin synthesis, and lymphocyte in vitro responsiveness. PTU, but not MMI, inhibits conversion of $T_4$ to $T_3$.[62] Other possible actions of MMI, which have been suggested for PTU, include inhibition of synthesis of anti-TSH receptor antibodies and inhibition of thyroglobulin-primed antigen-presenting cells.[62]

Before PTU or MMI therapy is begun, the radioactive iodine uptake should be measured; this can also be accomplished during the first week of therapy if the patient's clinical status requires immediate treatment.

**TABLE 42-5.**
**Pharmacology of Agents Used to Treat Hyperthyroidism***

| Agent | Maintenance Dose | Mechanism of Action | Common or Serious Adverse Affects |
|---|---|---|---|
| **COMMONLY USED** | | | |
| Propylthiouracil (6-pro-pyl-2-thiouracil) | 50–300 mg tid, PO | Inhibition of thyroid hormone synthesis; inhibits $T_4$ extrathyroidal conversion to $T_3$ | Rash, nausea, epigastric distress, agranulocytosis, granulocytopenia, hepatitis, lupus-like syndrome |
| Methimazole (1-methyl-2-mercapto-imidazole) | 5–30 mg tid, PO | Inhibition of thyroid hormone synthesis | As above |
| Propranolol[†] | 10–80 qid, PO | Decreases β-adrenergic–mediated activity and helps ameliorate signs and symptoms of thyrotoxicosis | Cardiovascular, bradycardia, decreased cardiac output, bronchospasm, short-term memory loss, mental depression; must be used with care in patients with congestive heart failure or asthma; short-acting agents should not be discontinued abruptly |
| Atenolol | 50–100 mg/d, PO | | |
| Nadolol | 80–160 mg/d, PO | | |
| Metoprolol | 100–200 mg/d, PO | | |
| **NONROUTINE AGENTS[‡]** | | | |
| Iodides[§] | 5 drops SSKI tid, PO or 5 drops Lugol's solution tid, PO | Decreases thyroid secretion | Parotitis or rash or serum sickness–like reaction; prolonged use may lead to unabated hypersecretion of thyroid hormone; should not be used in patient with known history of iodide allergy |
| Ipodate sodium[§] | 3 g PO every 2–3 d or 0.5 g/d | Decreases thyroidal secretion and diminishes extrathyroidal $T_4$ to $T_3$ conversion | Rash, agranulocytosis, liver disease; should not be used in patient with history of iodide allergy |
| Lithium carbonate | 300 mg tid or qid, PO, to produce blood levels of 0.6–1.2 mEq/L | Probably decreases thyroidal secretion and possibly inhibits extrathyroidal $T_4$ to $T_3$ conversion | Hand tremor, polyuria, drowsiness, lack of coordination, ataxia, blurred vision; may increase thyroid size; may cause hypothyroidism or thyrotoxicosis |

*PO*, by mouth; *qid*, four times a day; *SSKI*, saturated solution of potassium iodide; $T_3$, triiodothyronine; $T_4$, thyroxine; *tid*, three times a day.
*The prescribing physician should know the mechanisms of action and potential warnings and potential side effects of these agents. Appropriate textbooks or articles should be consulted before their use.
†A long-acting cardioselective agent is preferable. Pindolol should not be used because it has intrinsic sympathomimetic activity. Atenolol and metoprolol are relatively cardioselective; atenolol and nadolol are longer acting. Precise doses should be titrated with desired pulse rate.
‡None of these agents has been studied adequately in the prolonged treatment of hyperthyroidism. As a general rule, these agents should not be used for longer than 1 month, because the potential complications have not been investigated and the likelihood of causing unabated thyrotoxicosis exists, especially with iodide-containing substances. Lithium and ipodate are not presently approved by the Food and Drug Administration for treatment of Graves disease.
§SSKI (1 g/mL) contains 76.4% iodine. Five drops 3 times a day (assuming 20 drops/mL) contain about 573 mg iodine. Lugol's solution (125 mg/mL of total iodine) contains, in each 100 mL, 5 g of iodine and 10 g of potassium iodide. Five drops 3 times a day contain about 126 mg of iodine. The antithyroid action of ipodate is related partly to the release of iodides and partly to the ipodate molecule itself. Ipodate contains 61.4% iodine, so one 3-g dose of ipodate contains 1842 mg iodine. (For the purposes of this chapter, "iodide" and "iodine" are used interchangeably.)
(Adapted from Burman KD. Thyroid hormones. In: Chernow B, Lake CR, eds. The pharmacological approach to the critically ill patient. Baltimore: Williams & Wilkins, 1983:592.)

PTU and MMI are well absorbed by the gastrointestinal tract. Both drugs are immediately concentrated by the thyroid gland and have a more prolonged biologic effect than indicated by their serum half-lives (PTU, 1 hour; MMI, 5 hours). PTU should be administered 2 or 3 times daily, whereas MMI can be given once daily. The customary starting dose of PTU in a slightly thyrotoxic subject may be 100 to 300 mg per day in divided doses; in a moderately thyrotoxic patient, 300 to 800 mg per day; and in a very thyrotoxic patient, 800 to as high as 1200 mg per day. Patients should be examined periodically to determine the effect of the medications. Serum $T_4$ or free $T_4$ should also be measured, and the dose of PTU or MMI is tapered gradually as the serum hormone levels fall. The aim is to restore the euthyroid state within 1 to 2 months. Because a thyrotoxic patient may have rich hormonal stores in the thyroid gland that continue to be secreted during antithyroid therapy, and because the $T_4$ half-life in these patients is ~5 days, even maximal doses of MMI or PTU may not restore euthyroidism quickly, so 4 to 8 weeks may be required for the serum $T_4$ and $T_3$ levels to normalize. The pathophysiology of Graves disease and treatment options are discussed with each patient. It is stressed that antithyroid agents help treat the thyrotoxic state but usually are not curative and that surgery or $^{131}I$ may be required.[64]

A complete blood cell count and chemistry profile (particularly calcium and liver function tests) may be obtained initially and perhaps every 1 to 2 months during treatment, although agranulocytosis or drug-related hepatitis cannot be accurately predicted by these tests. All patients are informed of the potentially adverse effects of PTU or MMI (Table 42-6)[62] and are cautioned that a fever, rash, urticaria, arthralgia, or sore throat should be reported. Agranulocytosis occurs in ~1 of every 200 patients treated with PTU or MMI; most frequently it develops in the first several months of drug administration in patients older than age 40 and in patients taking larger doses of PTU or MMI (e.g., >400 mg per day or 40 mg per day, respectively). If there is any question that PTU or MMI may be causing an adverse effect, the individual drug should be discontinued and the patient either observed without medication for a short time or the alternative agent substituted if needed. If there was a serious adverse reaction to one agent, the alternative agent should probably not be used. There is an estimated 20% to 50% likelihood that a patient with a reaction to one agent (e.g., PTU) will have an adverse reaction to the other (i.e., MMI). There has been interest in the use of recombinant human granulocyte colony-stimulating factor in the treatment of antithyroid agent-induced agranulocytosis.[64,64a] In a review of generalized reactions to PTU or MMI, fewer than 100 cases had been reported since 1945.[65] The most common, generalized reactions included vasculitis, lupus erythematosus, and polyarthritis. Reactions were more common with PTU than with MMI, but occasionally, even with discontinuation of the medication, fatality can occur. Cross-reactions to PTU and MMI may occur.

Most patients tolerate PTU or MMI, and therapy is continued as biochemical and clinical euthyroidism returns. At this time a decision is made whether to continue the antithyroid medications (Fig. 42-8). Some physicians maintain patients on PTU or MMI for ~1 year in an effort to "induce" a remission (Tables 42-7 and 42-8). In the United States, it is likely that only

**TABLE 42-6.**
**Potential Side Effects of Antithyroid Medications**

**PROPYLTHIOURACIL OR METHIMAZOLE**
  Rash
  Adverse taste in mouth (especially propylthiouracil)
  Nausea
  Epigastric distress
  Vomiting
  Drug-induced fever
  Lupus-like syndrome
  Arthralgias
  Hepatitis
  Glucagon- or insulin-binding antibodies
  Agranulocytosis
  Granulocytopenia
  Leukopenia
  Aplastic anemia
  Thrombocytopenia
  Nephrotic syndrome
  Hypoprothrombinemia
**IODIDES**
  Parotitis
  Urticaria
  Rash
  Drug-induced fever
  Iodide-induced or iodide-associated thyrotoxicosis
  Serum sickness–like reaction
**IPODATE**
  Same as iodide
  Agranulocytosis
  Liver disease
**LITHIUM**
  Neurologic findings (e.g., ataxia, slurred speech)
  Hand tremor, muscle weakness
  Polyuria
  Drowsiness
  Blurred vision, hypercalcemia
  Goiter, hypothyroidism (rarely, can induce hyperthyroidism in suscepti-
    ble subjects)
**β-BLOCKERS**
  Induce or aggravate asthma and congestive heart failure

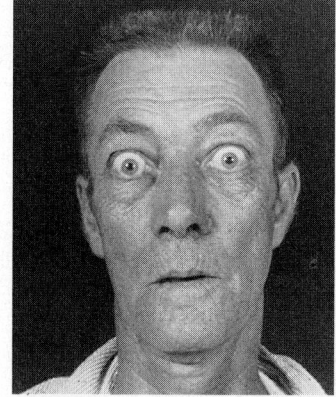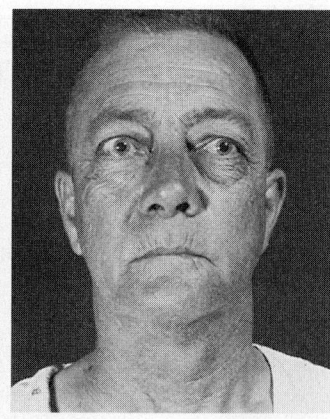
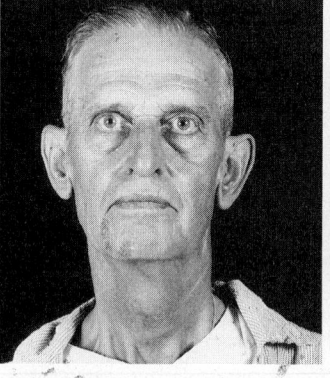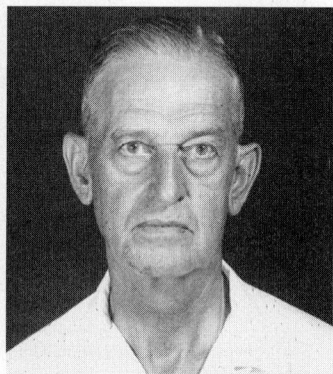

**FIGURE 42-8.** *Upper panel*: Patient with Graves disease treated with antithyroid drug. *Left*: Appearance before therapy. *Right*: Four months after commencement of therapy. Note the markedly decreased stare and the weight gain. *Lower panel*: Patient with Graves disease treated with radioiodine. *Left*: Before therapy. *Right*: Six months later.

20% to 40% of patients will have a remission; a small goiter size, response to low doses of PTU or MMI, mild thyrotoxicosis at presentation, and perhaps low-titer TSH receptor antibodies and lack of HLA-Dw3 and B8 antigens all increase the likelihood of remission (Table 42-9). Different geographic areas with variable iodine intake may be associated with different remission rates. In one multicenter study, the efficiency of 40 mg versus 10 mg of MMI was compared in the treatment of Graves disease.[60] In this study, 196 of 309 (63%) patients achieved a remission, with the differences in the two groups not being significantly different. Adverse reactions occurred in 16% of the group taking 10 mg and in 26% of the group taking 40 mg, with ~0.8% having a serious hematologic abnormality.

### β-BLOCKERS AND OTHER AGENTS

When a thyrotoxic patient is symptomatic, a β-adrenergic blocker is often prescribed at the same time PTU or MMI therapy is initiated (see Table 42-5).[66] β-Blockers improve many of the symptoms of thyrotoxicosis, improve myocardial efficiency, reduce myocardial oxygen demand, and may decrease nitrogen loss. It may be advisable to recommend that a hyperthyroid patient receiving a β-blocker record his or her pulse several times daily. The time-honored β-blocker is propranolol, and the

oral dose range is 20 to 40 mg every 8 hours for mild to moderate thyrotoxicosis and as high as 60 to 80 mg four times a day for more severe cases. The therapeutic objective is subjective improvement and the restoration of the pulse rate to ~80 beats

**TABLE 42-7.**
**Indications for the Different Therapies of Graves Disease**

**ANTITHYROID MEDICATIONS**
  Patient preference
  Induce euthyroidism before surgery or [131]I therapy
  Induce a remission by maintenance therapy for approximately 12 months
  Occasionally used to treat thyrotoxicosis for prolonged periods (i.e., years);
    dose of propylthiouracil in this instance generally ≤150 mg/d, and of
    methimazole, ≤15 mg/d
  Thyroid storm
  Childhood Graves disease*
  Pregnant Graves disease patients
**[131]I THERAPY**
  Patient preference
  Relapse after discontinuance of antithyroid medication
  Relapse after thyroidectomy
  Consider for patients older than 20 years; obtain negative pregnancy test
    in women
**THYROIDECTOMY**
  Patient preference
  Relapse after discontinuation of antithyroid drugs
  Relapse after previous thyroidectomy
  Pregnancy
  Childhood

  *Age range guidelines are arbitrary and vary in different clinics.

**TABLE 42-8.**
**Complications of Therapies for Graves Disease**

**ANTITHYROID MEDICATION**

See Table 42-6.

**$^{131}$I THERAPY***

Thyroid storm

Transient neck pain

Sialadenitis

Fetal hypothyroidism or malformation if administered during pregnancy

Hypothyroidism

Genetic effects still under evaluation

Carcinogenic effects still under evaluation

**THYROIDECTOMY**

Hypothyroidism

Anesthetic complication

Hypoparathyroidism

Postoperative hypocalcemia ("hungry bones")

Recurrent or superior laryngeal nerve injury

Hemorrhage

Thyroid storm (especially in the medically unprepared patient)

Recurrent thyrotoxicosis

Jugular vein or carotid artery damage

Infection

*$^{131}$I therapy may aggravate thyrotoxicosis, especially in the absence of β blockade or in elderly patients.

**TABLE 42-9.**
**Long-Term Antithyroid Medication as a Treatment for Graves Disease**

**FACTORS INCREASING LIKELIHOOD OF LONG-TERM REMISSION**

Mild thyrotoxicosis at presentation

Minimally enlarged thyroid gland

Low levels of serum TSH receptor antibodies

Low dose propylthiouracil or methimazole sufficient to maintain euthyroidism

Return of normal hypothalamic–pituitary–thyroid axis (e.g., $T_3$ suppressibility or thyrotropin-releasing hormone responsiveness)

**FACTORS INCREASING LIKELIHOOD OF RELAPSE**

Severe thyrotoxicosis at presentation

Markedly enlarged thyroid gland

High titer of serum TSH receptor antibodies

High dosages of propylthiouracil or methimazole required to maintain euthyroidism

HLA-DR3 or HLA-DR4 (controversial)

Maintenance of abnormal hypothalamic–pituitary–thyroid axis (e.g., no TRH response, $T_3$ nonsuppressible)

$T_3$, triiodothyronine; *TRH*, thyrotropin-releasing hormone; *TSH*, thyroid-stimulating hormone.

per minute. Newer β-blocking agents have the advantages of cardioselectivity and longer duration of action. A thyrotoxic patient responds very rapidly to the administration of β-blockers. If no clinical or subjective response is noted in 2 to 3 days, the dose should be increased. β-Blockers have no direct effect on radioactive iodine uptake or the synthesis or secretion of $T_4$ or $T_3$. These agents should be given with caution, if at all, to patients with a history of asthma. High-output cardiac failure may be improved by β-blockers, but their use in such patients should be judicious. It is usually not prudent to use long-term β-blockers as the sole therapy in the treatment of Graves disease.

Because β-blockers do not alter $T_4$ or $T_3$ synthesis or secretion, the underlying thyrotoxicosis may worsen while a patient is taking β-blockers alone. If a patient is allergic to both PTU and MMI, if the thyrotoxicosis has not responded appropriately, or if the thyrotoxicosis requires more rapid restoration of the euthyroid state, alternative agents such as ipodate, other iodides, or lithium carbonate should be considered (see Table 42-5).[64,67–69] Patients taking one of these latter antithyroid agents usually need closer medical supervision and possibly hospitalization.

## IODIDES

Iodides may be very effective antithyroid agents but should be used in thyrotoxicosis only when specific indications exist.[70] Iodides should usually not be used as customary or sole therapy because there can be an "escape" from their inhibitory effects, and the resultant exacerbation in thyrotoxicosis may be extremely difficult to control. For this reason, iodides are typically used in combination with thioureas, and therapy is not instituted until a patient has been started on PTU or MMI. Iodides can decrease serum $T_4$ and $T_3$ levels by 30% to 50% in 10 days; iodide and lithium may have an additive effect on decreasing serum $T_4$.[68,69] A thorough medical history, with specific inquiry as to allergies to iodides, should be taken before initiating therapy with ipodate or other iodides. The doses of iodides given with these agents are enormous when compared with the minimal daily requirement, and the consequent suppression of radioactive iodine uptake compromises the ability to use radioiodine for either diagnostic studies or therapy. Data

suggest that $^{131}$I can probably be used effectively again as early as 4 to 6 weeks after ipodate is discontinued,[67] but this area requires further investigation. Iodide (or ipodate) does not interfere technically with the measurement of serum iodothyronines or TSH.

Iodides, ipodate, and lithium are especially useful in lowering the serum $T_4$ and $T_3$ levels, and thus decrease the chance of thyroid storm when a thyrotoxic patient is being prepared for surgery and there is insufficient time to administer PTU or MMI alone for several weeks. Of the three agents noted, ipodate is a good choice in nonpregnant individuals; lithium therapy requires extremely close observation with frequent serum monitoring of electrolytes, liver function tests, and lithium levels.

Ipodate is an iodide-containing radiocontrast agent that is very effective in the treatment of thyrotoxicosis.[67] The ipodate molecule inhibits extrathyroidal $T_4$ to $T_3$ conversion, and a dose of 0.5 to 3 g decreases the serum $T_3$ level by 50% within several days. The iodide released from ipodate may help decrease thyroidal secretion when used for short periods (i.e., <1 month). Ipodate has been shown to be safe, with few adverse effects; it may be effective for as long as 6 months; however, its prolonged use in this manner requires a careful assessment. Escape from the antithyroid effects of both ipodate and other iodides may occur, especially after chronic administration. Although the use of ipodate in conjunction with PTU or MMI and β-blockers is gaining acceptance, the drug has not yet been approved by the U.S. Food and Drug Administration for this indication. In a typical nonpregnant patient before thyroid surgery, 0.5 to 1.0 g of ipodate on preoperative days 10, 7, 4, and 1 can be recommended. Serum complete blood count, liver function tests, and thyroid function tests should be measured frequently in a patient receiving ipodate.

## LITHIUM CARBONATE

Lithium carbonate is another second-line agent that can be effective in the treatment of thyrotoxicosis.[68,69] Commonly, the drug is first used in hospitalized patients to closely monitor serum lithium levels (therapeutic range, 0.5 to 1.2 mEq/L). Lithium acts on the thyroid gland to decrease the secretion of iodothyronines, without a major effect on iodide uptake. The frequency of adverse effects, such as ataxia and drowsiness, is much reduced when serum levels are maintained within the therapeutic range. The customary antithyroid effect of lithium is seen with doses of 600 to 900 mg per day. Lithium carbonate lowers serum $T_4$ levels by 30% to 50% in ~10 days. Paradoxically, there have been cases of lithium-associated thyrotoxicosis.[71] This potential untoward effect of lithium may be related to increases in thyroidal iodine and appears to be less likely when lithium is administered for <1 month.

## RADIOACTIVE IODINE THERAPY

Iodine-131 has been used to treat Graves disease since the 1940s, and its use has enjoyed increasing popularity because of its efficacy and few side effects (see Table 42-7 and Fig. 42-8).[72] Follow-up studies have not implicated [131]I therapy in a higher risk of carcinoma in general, leukemia, or lymphoma.[73] Therapy with [131]I does increase the gonadal radiation exposure, but a higher risk of fetal malformation in subsequent pregnancies has not been demonstrated. Nevertheless, [131]I therapy should be administered with caution to any female patient of childbearing age. A retrospective collaborative study analyzed ~35,000 hyperthyroid patients treated with radioiodine between 1946 and 1964.[74] Radioiodine therapy and hyperthyroidism itself were not associated with increased cancer mortality. However, thyroid cancer mortality was slightly increased in patients receiving radioiodine. The absolute number of excess deaths was slight, but was statistically significant, throughout the duration of the study. This study can be criticized, however, for several reasons: It is retrospective; patients were not randomly allocated to a given treatment group; initial and follow-up evaluation did not include sonograms, aspirations, or reports of $T_4$ and TSH; many patients required two doses of radioiodine; it cannot be discerned which patients became hypothyroid and required L-$T_4$ therapy; and the histologic diagnosis of thyroid cancer was determined from death certificates rather than from examination of the original slides. It also is conceivable that the risk of thyroid cancer occurring would be decreased if the patients had become hypothyroid within several months after radioiodine therapy. Lastly, the age at which patients received radioiodine and subsequently had thyroid cancer cannot be determined. Another study[5] retrospectively analyzed 7209 thyrotoxic patients and noted that the standardized mortality rate was increased slightly, but significantly, for deaths from thyroid disease, cerebrovascular disease, and fracture of the femur. The increased mortality was observed mainly within the initial year after radioiodine therapy. It is possible that these early deaths were related to lack of adequate control of the hyperthyroidism and follow-up issues rather than the radioiodine itself; furthermore, the control group to which the thyrotoxic patients were compared can be questioned. When these two studies are considered in context with earlier studies,[5,73,74] it still seems that radioiodine therapy is a relatively safe and effective therapy for Graves disease, and these two studies[5,74] do not directly influence the choices of therapy. It is important, however, to discuss these issues and review these reports with patients and to emphasize that further studies in these areas would be useful.

A thorough menstrual history and a serum β-hCG level should be obtained to rule out pregnancy just before a [131]I dose. [131]I crosses the placenta and may damage fetal thyroid gland development. Potential harmful effects of [131]I depend on the dose and the time during pregnancy when it is given. Because the fetal thyroid develops during weeks 10 to 15, there is little [131]I trapping before that time. Rarely, the issue of how to treat a pregnant woman who inadvertently received radioactive iodine therapy during pregnancy arises. The intraamniotic administration of L-$T_4$ to treat the potentially hypothyroid fetus has been suggested;[75] however, this is not approved by the Food and Drug Administration. In my clinic, it is recommended that a woman avoid becoming pregnant for 6 to 12 months after a therapeutic dose of radioactive iodine. In the treatment of Graves disease, the dose of [131]I can be calculated by a variety of techniques. In one method, the product of the thyroid weight and the customary dose rate (80 to 120 μCi/g) is divided by the radioactive iodine uptake. For example, a patient with a 60-g

goiter and a 60% radioactive iodine uptake would receive 8 to 12 mCi. For calculation of the dose, the author prefers to measure the radioactive iodine uptake 1 to 2 weeks before therapy; on an empirical basis, a higher dose is used if it is thought necessary to ensure a cure of the hyperthyroidism. In the author's hands, a typical patient with Graves disease would perhaps receive 10 to 15 mCi radioactive iodine. PTU or MMI should be discontinued for several days before and after [131]I therapy.[76] Probably, prior antithyroid agent administration confers relative resistance to a given dose of radioactive iodine; therefore, a relatively higher dose of radioactive iodine is used in these circumstances. Given that Graves hyperthyroidism is mediated by TSH receptor antibodies that are largely unaltered by radioactive iodine administration, the author believes that the optimal and desired goal of [131]I therapy is the development of hypothyroidism as rapidly as possible. Thereafter, the patient is given L-$T_4$ therapy and observed on a lifelong basis.

The decision to treat a hyperthyroid patient with radioactive iodine early in the disease course (i.e., within several weeks of diagnosis) or to treat the patient initially with several weeks or months of antithyroid agents before radioactive iodine therapy to render the patient euthyroid is a difficult decision. The clinical context, severity of hyperthyroidism, extent of iodothyronine elevation, and presence of associated medical and endocrine conditions (e.g., cardiac arrhythmias, ophthalmopathy) are relevant to this decision. In the author's practice, ~70% of patients are treated with radioactive iodine early in their course before the administration of antithyroid agents. The patient—and frequently, the family—should participate in this decision. It should be remembered that hyperthyroid patients may not make decisions in as reasonable a manner as they would if they were euthyroid.

[131]I therapy may aggravate uncontrolled thyrotoxicosis, can precipitate thyroid storm, and can exacerbate ophthalmopathy (especially if moderate or severe).[77,78] The serum $T_4$ level is rarely increased significantly by [131]I therapy, but one cannot predict which patients will have a marked $T_4$ rise.[76] Radioiodine may make ophthalmopathy worse, particularly if the serum $T_3$ level is increased.[78] A study of 443 patients with Graves hyperthyroidism (slight or no ophthalmopathy) randomized them to receive radioiodine, to receive radioiodine followed by a 90-day course of prednisone, or to receive MMI for 18 months.[78] After 6 months of radioiodine treatment, 15% of 150 patients developed or had exacerbated ophthalmopathy (transient in 15/23), and none of 55 improved. Of 145 patients treated with radioiodine and prednisone, 75% of those with baseline ophthalmopathy (67%) had improvement; none had progression. Of 148 patients treated with MMI, 141 had no change in their ophthalmopathy, whereas 3 patients (2%) had improvement in baseline ophthalmopathy and 4 patients (3%) had exacerbation. In summary, this prospective study suggests that radioiodine is associated with the presence or exacerbation of ophthalmopathy more frequently than is MMI therapy. Nevertheless, the frequency of the worsening of ophthalmopathy with radioiodine therapy is ~15%, only being persistent ~33% of the time. Prednisone essentially prevented the radioiodine-induced worsening of ophthalmopathy. A patient with moderate or severe thyrotoxic Graves disease is typically treated with PTU or MMI and β-blockers for 1 to 2 months before treatment with [131]I is initiated. During this period, the patient is seen frequently, and the other potential therapeutic modalities are discussed, with special emphasis on the potential risks and benefits of [131]I treatment. Once treatment with [131]I has been agreed to, the PTU or MMI (but not the β-blocker) is discontinued 2 to 3 days before therapy. A negative β-hCG value is required in women of childbearing potential. After informed consent has been obtained and a [131]I uptake study has been performed, the patient receives [131]I therapy and is cautioned to return if an exacerbation of symptoms is perceived. Patients with persistent mild symptoms are continued on a β-blocker

until they become euthyroid. In more symptomatic patients, in patients with potentially serious concomitant medical disorders, and in those with a labile condition in whom hyperthyroxinemia is likely to return before maximal radioiodine effect is achieved, PTU or MMI is restarted 2 to 3 days after $^{131}$I therapy. After $^{131}$I therapy, patients are examined, and serum $T_4$ and $T_3$ levels are determined periodically. Based on the progressive improvement, indicated by the results of the physical examination and thyroid function tests, the PTU or MMI dosage is gradually tapered and discontinued, usually within 2 months after the $^{131}$I dose. It is controversial whether patients with Graves disease with moderate or severe ophthalmopathy should receive corticosteroids to minimize the possible adverse effect of $^{131}$I on ophthalmopathy.[29,30,78] The author discusses the issue with the patient, considers the potential risks of corticosteroid therapy, and analyzes the severity of the ophthalmopathy. Patients are frequently referred to an ophthalmologist who is familiar with thyroid-related eye disease, and medical and/or surgical considerations and decisions are discussed. When appropriate (generally including patients with moderate or severe ophthalmopathy), the author considers treating individual patients with 40 mg prednisone for 7 days before $^{131}$I therapy, continuing this dose of prednisone for 14 to 28 days after therapy, and then tapering the dose with the purpose of discontinuing the medication within 4 to 8 weeks after radioiodine administration.

The patients are followed up closely after the discontinuation of PTU or MMI at least 3 to 4 months after the radioiodine administration, depending on the laboratory and clinical evaluation. An increase in serum $T_4$ and $T_3$ levels to above normal (after PTU or MMI discontinuation) indicates that another dose of radioiodine may be required, although, generally, the second dose is not administered until at least 6 months have elapsed since the initial dose. In this circumstance, the TSH value must be interpreted in conjunction with the serum iodothyronine levels and the clinical context. Occasionally, the hypothalamic pituitary axis, as manifest by serum TSH, may not respond appropriately to the serum iodothyronine levels in patients who have had Graves hyperthyroidism within the recent past. If the serum $T_4$ level decreases to below normal and the serum TSH is elevated, L-$T_4$ therapy is initiated. Approximately 80% of patients with Graves disease become euthyroid or hypothyroid after one dose of $^{131}$I; 15% require two doses of $^{131}$I, and 5% require three or more doses. Patients who remain biochemically and clinically euthyroid after $^{131}$I therapy are observed for life with thyroid function studies and are advised that hypothyroidism or recurrent hyperthyroidism could occur at any time. $^{131}$I therapy is generally considered for persons older than 20 years of age. However, many factors enter into the decision for a choice of therapy, and it is most important that each patient be counseled about the options and risks so that he or she can participate in the treatment decisions. Patients should be encouraged to obtain information regarding Graves disease from a variety of sources, especially Internet sites sponsored by medical organizations.

Although hypothyroidism is an expected and even desirable result of $^{131}$I treatment, some physicians prefer to administer several small doses of $^{131}$I to achieve euthyroidism and avoid hypothyroidism. The author does not subscribe to this approach. $^{131}$I is the isotope most commonly used to treat Graves disease.

After radiotherapy, patients are counseled not to have close contact with family members for ~7 days and, because of salivary radioiodine, should not share eating or drinking utensils. Particular care should be exercised if there is a pregnant woman or a child in the household. For purposes of comparison, a typical dose of $^{131}$I for therapy for Graves disease is 5 to 15 mCi, but the dosage for therapy for thyroid cancer is often ~100 to 150 mCi. The Nuclear Regulatory Commission guidelines have indicated that a patient given a dose of $^{131}$I >30 mCi usually should be hospitalized, whereas lesser doses may be administered to outpatients.

## SURGERY

Although surgery is considered primary definitive therapy by fewer physicians now than in the past, it still is important in the treatment of some patients with Graves disease (see Chap. 44).[79] Surgery, rather than $^{131}$I therapy, should be considered in a patient of any age if any aspect of the case suggests possible malignancy, such as a palpable thyroid nodule, cervical lymphadenopathy, hoarseness (recurrent laryngeal nerve involvement), pain or tenderness, or rapid growth of the goiter. There is a question as to whether thyroid cancer that does occur in conjunction with Graves disease has a more aggressive course (e.g., increased frequency of local invasion and metastases to lymph nodes and distant sites) as compared with thyroid cancer in a patient without Graves disease.[80] Severe or advancing ophthalmopathy may also favor surgery, because some studies suggest that $^{131}$I (especially in high doses) may aggravate eye findings. Also, surgery lowers serum $T_4$ and $T_3$ values to normal more quickly than does $^{131}$I therapy. Surgery may also be the best choice in a pregnant patient with hyperthyroidism that is difficult to control and in whom $^{131}$I therapy is contraindicated. Specific thyroid nodules, detected by physical examination or sonography, or when suggested by radioisotope scan, should usually be aspirated before a decision regarding therapy for the hyperthyroidism, and the results must, obviously, be considered an integral part of the therapeutic decision.

Patients with Graves disease who are being considered for surgery should usually be rendered euthyroid with PTU or MMI before surgery is undertaken. Iodides (e.g., saturated solution of potassium iodide or Lugol's solution or ipodate) are generally not required except in moderate to severe cases, although some authorities administer them in a routine manner before surgery (assuming no contraindications) to decrease thyroidal iodothyronine stores and secretion and to decrease gland vascularity (see Chap. 44). Only an experienced surgeon and anesthesiologist should perform or participate in the surgery. A near-total thyroidectomy, leaving 5 to 10 g of thyroid tissue, is usually performed, with care taken to preserve parathyroid and recurrent laryngeal nerve integrity. There is high likelihood that a patient will become hypothyroid after this procedure. Other complications are listed in Table 42-8. Transient laryngeal nerve palsy may occur in ~5% of patients, but <1% of patients should sustain permanent damage. The usually transient hypocalcemia after surgery may not necessarily be due to parathyroid compromise. The syndrome of "bone hunger," or increased calcium removal from serum with increased deposition in bone,[81] is often short-lived but may persist for 6 to 12 months after surgery; calcium supplements may be needed during this time. A prospective analysis comparing the treatment modalities for 174 Graves disease patients[82] showed that patients were generally pleased with whichever therapy they received, and, of interest, the cost estimate for medical therapy (including costs of relapse) was $2284. Surgery and radioactive iodine therapy were each ~1.5 times as expensive as medical therapy.

## GRAVES DISEASE IN SPECIAL SITUATIONS

### PREGNANCY AND GRAVES DISEASE

The diagnosis of thyrotoxic Graves disease in a pregnant patient is especially difficult, because euthyroid pregnant women may share many signs and symptoms considered indicative of hyperthyroidism, including nervousness, irritability, warm skin, hand tremor, palmar erythema, diaphoresis, goiter, widened pulse pressure, and fatigue.[83] No signs or symptoms are absolutely discriminatory of the thyrotoxic state, but clinical emphasis should be placed on (a) an inability to gain weight normally while pregnant; (b) a firm thyroid gland weighing more than 40 g and which may demonstrate a bruit; (c) a prior history of Graves disease; and (d) ophthalmopathy with conjunctivitis, chemosis, or proptosis. The total serum $T_4$ level rarely increases to higher than 20 µg/dL in euthyroid pregnant women, and the serum free $T_4$ level should not be elevated. TSH receptor antibodies should not be detectable in a euthyroid pregnant woman. The proper interpretation depends on whether binding inhibition or stimulatory assays are performed. Stimulatory TSH receptor antibodies are more supportive of the diagnosis of thyrotoxic Graves disease, whereas positive binding inhibition assays may indicate Graves disease or autoimmune thyroid disease but not necessarily hyperthyroidism. The laboratory evaluation of a pregnant woman should not entail exposure to isotopes or radiation. The use of third-generation TSH assays preclude the necessity of performing a TRH assay in most patients.

Moderate to severe thyrotoxic Graves disease in a pregnant woman requires treatment. If it is difficult to distinguish between euthyroidism or mild thyrotoxicosis, the decision to treat with antithyroid medications is more difficult, because mild thyrotoxicosis in some instances may pose less of a risk to the mother and fetus than the administration of antithyroid medications.[84,85]

Thyrotoxicosis often improves during pregnancy, and antithyroid medication dosages may be less than those required during the nonpregnant state. Occasionally, however, thyrotoxicosis may be severe and difficult to control. It is important to render these women euthyroid, but it is also important not to administer very large PTU or MMI doses, because the antithyroid medications cross the placenta and can cause fetal goiter or hypothyroidism. The author believes there is greater confidence and experience with the use of PTU than with MMI during pregnancy and so consider it the agent of choice. Furthermore, MMI has been reported to cause aplasia cutis, a scalp condition in neonates. The infant's thyroid function should be checked immediately after birth and probably again in 1 to 2 months. Although some complications occur, in general, antithyroid agents do not appear to be highly teratogenic.[85–87] PTU doses of <300 mg per day and MMI doses of <30 mg per day rarely seem to have adverse effects on the fetus. In one study, the neonatal malformation rate was higher in thyrotoxic mothers than in euthyroid mothers, and the restoration of maternal euthyroidism with the use of antithyroid medication had a beneficial effect in decreasing the frequency of the malformations.[85] There was no correlation between MMI dose and the frequency or type of malformation. Thus, uncontrolled hyperthyroidism in the mother may be a more important factor in causing malformations than the antithyroid drugs themselves.

It is believed the pregnancy itself may decrease the immunologic responses involved in causing Graves disease, and, commonly, improvement or even remission occurs during pregnancy. Unfortunately, however, after delivery the Graves disease often relapses.

The therapeutic goal is clinical euthyroidism, a serum $T_4$ level within the normal range for pregnancy (i.e., 10 to 16 µg/dL),[84] and a normal free $T_4$. It is preferable to monitor free $T_4$ and $T_3$ when observing a hyperthyroid pregnant patient. On the other hand, if larger doses of PTU or MMI are necessary to restore the euthyroid state, or if the condition cannot be well controlled with antithyroid medications, surgical thyroidectomy then becomes a treatment option and is optimally performed in the second trimester.[79,83,88] A patient with uncontrolled or poorly controlled thyrotoxicosis should usually be monitored closely for 1 to 2 weeks before thyroidectomy to ensure compliance with medications. Because of the brief period involved, daily doses of PTU of as much as 600 mg (or 60 mg of MMI) may need to be given for a very short time preoperatively. The addition of stable iodine for 7 days or less may be necessary if the thyrotoxicosis is extremely poorly controlled. Extreme caution must be exercised,

because iodides, especially when given for longer periods, may cause massive enlargement of the fetal thyroid gland, resulting rarely in asphyxiation. Management of a pregnant Graves disease patient who is severely hyperthyroid should be performed by physicians familiar with this condition. Similarly, thyroidectomy should not generally be undertaken unless an experienced surgeon and anesthesiologist are available and the patient is in nearly a euthyroid condition (see also Chap. 110).

When the use of a β-adrenergic blocker is deemed necessary in a pregnant patient with Graves disease, propranolol is preferred because of the extensive experience with this agent.[83,84,86–89] Although propranolol is generally safe, intrauterine growth retardation and fetal bradycardia have been associated with its use. Hence, propranolol should be reserved for severely thyrotoxic pregnant subjects and used judiciously, with careful monitoring of the patient and fetus.

The measurement of serum TSH receptor antibody is indicated in most pregnant patients with Graves disease, with or without active thyrotoxicosis. A maternal level of stimulatory TSH receptor antibody more than five times higher than control in the third trimester accurately predicts neonatal thyrotoxicosis.[88] If the titer is very high, the fetus is monitored closely, and the neonate is carefully examined at birth, with determination of serum iodothyronines and TSH levels. An apparently euthyroid infant should nevertheless be monitored closely for the development of thyrotoxicosis during the first 3 months of life (see Chap. 47). There is no safe and effective method of treating a thyrotoxic fetus in utero, although this has been done successfully in one reported case.[89]

It is controversial whether postpartum women with Graves disease who are receiving antithyroid drugs should breast-feed their infants, because the potential harm to the neonates' thyroid gland of such therapy is uncertain. PTU may be preferred over MMI in breast-feeding women.[62] Because of its known effect on the neonatal thyroid gland, administration of $^{131}I$, whether therapeutic or diagnostic, should be avoided in the nursing woman. If radioiodine therapy must be administered, breast-feeding should be avoided for 3 or 4 months. If a diagnostic radioisotope study must be performed, interruption of the nursing may be done for the following periods: 7 to 10 µCi $^{131}I$, 3 to 4 weeks; 50 µCi $^{131}I$, 7 to 8 weeks; 10 mCi technetium-99m, 24 hours; 100 µCi $^{123}I$, 3 to 4 weeks.[90]

Elevated hCG levels may increase thyroid hormone secretion during pregnancy and, as a result, hyperemesis gravidarum may be associated with elevated serum free $T_4$ and free $T_3$ with a suppressed TSH.[91] This entity is difficult to diagnose, and some authorities recommend short-term antithyroid therapy if the signs, symptoms, and thyroid test results are markedly abnormal. Antithyroid agents for this condition of transient hyperthyroxinemia are seldom indicated. As the hCG levels decline, this condition also tends to resolve.

## THYROID STORM

Thyroid storm is a life-threatening condition in which the customary signs and symptoms of thyrotoxic Graves disease are exaggerated; many patients also have vomiting, diarrhea, dehydration, fever, disorientation or impaired mentation, and, rarely, jaundice.[92] Frequently, they have severe tachycardia and may manifest heart failure. The extreme restlessness and adrenergic hyperactivity may proceed to mania. Coma may occur. Thyroid storm is not associated with disproportionately elevated serum total iodothyronine levels compared with other thyrotoxic patients. Thus, it is believed that other factors—such as increased receptor occupancy or increased free and tissue iodothyronine levels—must contribute to this condition.

Thyroid storm should not be viewed as an entity distinct from thyrotoxicosis but as one end of a continuum of severity of hyperthyroidism. Indeed, authorities may disagree as to what the specific definition or clinical requirements for thyroid storm may be. Although thyroid storm may occur without a known precipitating event, it most frequently occurs during or after thyroidal or nonthyroidal surgery; in the peripartum or postpartum period; after [131]I therapy; after administration of iodine-containing materials; or after infections, such as pharyngitis or pneumonitis. The best treatment is prophylactic. Thyroid storm is rare if a patient has received adequate therapy with PTU or MMI before known precipitating events, such as surgery or delivery of a neonate.

Because the outcome may be so serious, patients thought to have thyroid storm should usually be treated as if they do have the condition. The diagnosis is particularly difficult to establish in a thyrotoxic patient with a superimposed infectious illness. The customary therapy consists of administration of β-blockers, corticosteroids, iodide or ipodate, and PTU or MMI (Table 42-10). No parenteral preparation of PTU or MMI is available, but MMI or PTU may be administered intrarectally by enema.[93] Alternatively, and probably more reliably, the PTU or MMI tablets may be crushed and administered through a nasogastric tube. Antithyroid drugs should be given several hours before the administration of iodides. Hyperactive patients require sedation, and severely pyrexic patients should be treated with acetaminophen and a cooling blanket. If this customary therapy is not effective, peritoneal dialysis, resin or charcoal hemoperfusion, or plasmapheresis can be attempted if the patient is seriously ill.[94]

## EUTHYROID GRAVES DISEASE

Euthyroid Graves disease refers to clinically euthyroid patients who may have detectable serum TSH receptor antibodies and also may have other signs of autoimmune thyroid disease, such as ophthalmopathy.[95,96] These euthyroid patients may present with unilateral proptosis, and the clinician must determine whether autoimmune Graves disease is present (see Chap. 43). A thorough medical history and physical examination may uncover data suggesting an earlier occurrence of Graves disease. Serum total, free $T_4$ and $T_3$, and a third-generation TSH may be normal (see Chap. 15). Measurement of TSH receptor antibodies may also be helpful. Because a rare patient may have euthyroid Graves disease and a coexisting retroorbital or brain tumor causing proptosis, orbital and head CT (noncontrast) or MRI may be indicated and could disclose thickening of the orbital muscles or other findings consistent with Graves disease, thereby confirming the presence of autoimmune thyroid eye disease. It should be kept in mind that a CT study with radiopaque dye influences the thyroidal iodine transport system and the ability to perform a radioactive iodine uptake study or treatment with [131]I.

The diagnosis of euthyroid Graves disease is based on inference and exclusion. The natural history of euthyroid Graves disease is unpredictable, with some patients remaining euthyroid and others becoming thyrotoxic or even hypothyroid. Some may have euthyroid Graves disease without marked clinical eye findings. The distinction between euthyroid Graves disease and Graves disease in remission is difficult. "Latent" euthyroid Graves disease may be associated with an abnormal TRH test and/or abnormal $T_3$-suppression test. The author rarely performs these tests, especially because a third-generation TSH assay abrogates the necessity for TRH stimulation tests, and a $T_3$-suppression test may be dangerous, without being particularly helpful if TSH receptor antibodies have been measured.

## HASHIMOTO THYROIDITIS VERSUS GRAVES DISEASE

Although earlier studies suggested that Hashimoto and Graves disease were separate entities, there is evidence of some overlap. Thus, antithyroglobulin and peroxidase antibodies may be seen in Graves disease, and some patients with Hashimoto disease may have TSH receptor antibodies.[97,98] It has been sug-

## TABLE 42-10.
### Treatment of Thyroid Storm*

| Drug | Dosage |
|---|---|
| Propranolol | 60–80 mg q6h PO; or 1–3 mg IV, slowly, q4h prn |
| Hydrocortisone | 100–500 mg IV q12h |
| Sodium iodide | 1 g in 1 L saline q12h |
| or | |
| SSKI | 5 drops tid PO |
| or | |
| Lugol's solution | 5 drops tid PO |
| or | |
| Ipodate | 0.5 g PO daily or 3.0 g PO every 2 to 3 days |
| Propylthiouracil | 100–200 mg q4h PO |
| or | |
| Methimazole | 10–20 mg q4h PO |

*IV*, intravenously; *PO*, by mouth; *prn*, as circumstances require; *q4h*, every 4 hours; *q6h*, every 6 hours; *q12h*, every 12 hours; *SSKI*, saturated solution of potassium iodide; *tid*, three times a day.
*Use supportive measures such as mild sedation, fluid replacement, oxygen, vitamins, cooling, and antibiotics, as needed.

gested that autoantibodies against thyroid peroxidase may react to different epitopes, depending on whether Graves disease or Hashimoto thyroiditis is present. Furthermore, patients with Hashimoto thyroiditis may present with thyrotoxicosis, and patients with Graves disease may present with hypothyroidism. Patients with either disease may have blocking antibodies directed against the TSH receptor, and there is preliminary evidence that serum in either disease may contain antibodies that recognize identical or similar antigens in thyroid membranes. It is not known whether the causes of Graves disease and Hashimoto disease are similar and whether these two diseases reflect a varied spectrum of the same pathologic process. Nevertheless, one of the relevant clinical findings is that a condition diagnosed as hypothyroid Hashimoto disease rarely may evolve into thyrotoxicosis, necessitating an evaluation on an annual basis of hypothyroid patients receiving L-$T_4$ replacement therapy. One should not presume that a thyrotoxic patient with high-titer microsomal antibodies has a self-limited variant of hyperthyroidism such as "hashitoxicosis," because it is possible that serum $T_4$ levels will remain elevated and that the patient will ultimately need definitive therapy. Patients with Graves disease and high-titer antithyroid (peroxidase or thyroglobulin) antibodies are probably more likely to have thyroid hypofunction after either medical or ablative therapy. The presence of very-high-titer anti-TSH receptor antibodies in a pregnant woman presumed to have Hashimoto disease is particularly worrisome, because these antibodies can cross the placenta to cause either thyrotoxicosis or hypothyroidism in the neonate.[97] Finally, postpartum thyroiditis (with thyrotoxicosis) occurs mainly in patients with significant antimicrosomal (antiperoxidase) or antithyroglobulin antibody titers.[97]

## GRAVES DISEASE IN CHILDREN

Graves disease rarely occurs before age 18. Many of the clinical signs and symptoms, laboratory assessments, and treatment protocols in adults and children are similar (see Chap. 47).[98] Because it is likely to be more successful, and because of the reluctance to recommend ablative therapy in a child, most patients with Graves disease younger than age 18 are given PTU or MMI for a year in an effort to induce remission. In some subjects with persistent disease who respond to small doses of PTU or MMI, these medications may be continued until the patients are judged to be old enough (or sufficiently mature) to understand the therapeutic options of receiving [131]I or undergoing thyroidectomy.

The major controversy in the treatment of childhood Graves disease that does not remit with antithyroid drugs concerns the choice between surgery and [131]I treatment. Thyroidectomy can be performed in children with the same comparably low complication rates as in adults. Authorities disagree, however, as to whether children and adolescents should be treated with radioactive [131]I. In addition to the arguments already noted, young persons are at risk for the development of [131]I-related effects for a longer interval than adults so treated, and there is some evidence that children treated with [131]I are more likely to develop benign thyroid nodules.

In general, the same guidelines for treatment apply as in adults. Given the advantages and disadvantages of each form of therapy, these guidelines should be individualized to the wishes of the child and his or her parents.

## GRAVES DISEASE IN THE AGED

The elderly patient with Graves disease often does not have hyperkinetic symptomatology despite the occasional presence of severe disease (see Chap. 199). Exophthalmos is often absent, and the goiter may be minimal or absent. Instead of an increased appetite and diarrhea, anorexia and constipation may be present. It is not uncommon for these patients to present with manifestations that may be unusual in younger subjects, such as myopathy, arrhythmia, or heart failure.[24–26] The issue of the risk of thromboembolism occurring in hyperthyroid patients with atrial fibrillation is important. In one retrospective study, 30 of 142 thyrotoxic patients (21%) had atrial fibrillation, and 12 of these patients had thromboemboli.[99] None of 112 thyrotoxic patients without atrial fibrillation had emboli.

Although these data need to be confirmed, many clinicians prescribe anticoagulants for thyrotoxic patients with atrial fibrillation, assuming there are no contraindications; in an individual patient, the benefits are thought to outweigh the potential disadvantages. This decision also depends on factors such as the presence or absence of other underlying cardiac disease, the results of the echocardiogram, and the entire clinical situation. Close monitoring is essential.[100] Patients with a placid facies and withdrawn behavior, limited attention span, or depression have been described as having *"apathetic" hyperthyroidism.* The term *masked* or *monosymptomatic hyperthyroidism* has been used for those patients who have only one predominant symptom, such as severe weight loss mimicking a malignancy or severe hypomagnesemia (Fig. 42-9). The elderly hyperthyroid patient requires close follow-up and usually nonsurgical therapy.

## L-THYROXINE ADMINISTRATION IN TREATED GRAVES DISEASE

Reports have suggested that it might be useful to administer L-$T_4$ supplementation to Graves disease patients after they have been rendered euthyroid by MMI.[101,102] In a controlled study from Japan, patients administered MMI plus L-$T_4$ had lower levels of TSH receptor antibodies and a lower incidence of disease recurrence when observed for as long as 3 years after discontinuation of MMI, as compared with the group treated with MMI alone. The mechanism for this potential effect is unknown. The same investigators also reported that $T_4$ administration during pregnancy and in the postpartum period prevented a recurrence of postpartum hyperthyroidism.[101] These studies are of interest, but most authorities believe this therapy should not yet be used in the routine treatment of Graves disease. Indeed, studies have not been able to confirm the potential benefit of L-$T_4$ supplementation in this circumstance.[102]

## SUPPRESSED SERUM THYROID-STIMULATING HORMONE

Because of the development of highly sensitive TSH assays, many individuals have been found with *normal total $T_4$ and a*

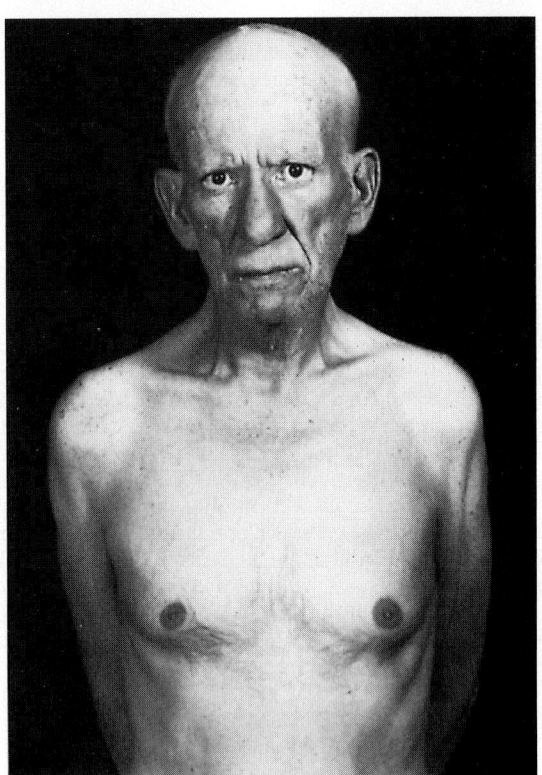

**FIGURE 42-9.** "Masked" hyperthyroidism in a 65-year-old man whose principal symptom was weight loss. No goiter was palpable. Note the gynecomastia.

*TSH of <0.1 µU/mL in the context of clinical euthyroidism.* The precise pathophysiology of this occurrence is unknown, and the natural history is undefined. On occasion, these individuals develop overt hyperthyroidism, whereas in others, transient decrements in TSH return to normal. Many subjects have persistent suppression of TSH with normal total and free $T_4$ and $T_3$. Further studies are needed to determine the proper approach to these patients. However, it appears reasonable to perform a thorough history and physical examination, to obtain a total $T_3$ and free $T_4$ measurement, and, in some instances, to obtain radioactive iodine uptake and a free $T_3$. These patients should be evaluated periodically—especially elderly individuals—for the development of atrial fibrillation.[103–105] One approach is to measure free $T_4$ and $T_3$ and TSH (third generation) monthly for 3 months to ensure that the perturbations are not transient. If the repeat laboratory studies show persistent TSH levels that are undetectable in conjunction with a normal free $T_4$ and free $T_3$, a radioactive iodine uptake and scan are performed and serum TSI levels are obtained to assess the likelihood of overt hyperthyroidism developing. Occasionally, a thyroid sonogram is also performed to determine whether the thyroid gland contains nonpalpable nodules. Assuming these tests are normal or only mildly abnormal, one may consider therapy for these patients to decrease the risk of cardiac arrhythmias and possible bone loss over an extended time. The consideration of therapy depends on the clinical context and the patient's desires, but, in general, antithyroid treatment is the primary choice, rather than more definitive therapy such as radioactive iodine or surgery. For example, 5 mg MMI may be given as a therapeutic trial for 6 to 12 months, with monitoring of complete blood count, liver function test, and thyroid function tests perhaps every 4 to 6 weeks. It is unknown if this condition represents a singular entity or is a manifestation of a different disorder. It is also unknown if such patients are at higher risk for complications if they require nonthyroidal surgery. Future studies addressing these issues are required.

# REFERENCES

1. Burman KD, Baker JR Jr. Immune mechanisms in Graves disease. Endocr Rev 1985; 6:183.
2. Weetman AP, McGregor AM. Autoimmune thyroid disease: developments in our understanding. Endocr Rev 1984; 5:309.
3. Baker JR Jr. Dissecting the immune response to the thyrotropin receptor in autoimmune thyroid disease. J Clin Endocrinol Metab 1993; 77:16.
4. Ajjan RA, Findlay C, Metcalfe RA, et al. The modulation of the human sodium iodide symporter activity by Graves' disease sera. J Clin Endocrinol Metab 1998; 83:1217.
5. Franklyn JA, Maisonneuve P, Sheppard MC, et al. Mortality after the treatment of hyperthyroidism with radioactive iodine. N Engl J Med 1998; 338:712.
6. Jaspan JB, Luo H, Ahmed B, et al. Evidence for a retroviral trigger in Graves' disease. Autoimmunity 1995; 20:135.
7. Zakarija M, McKenzie JM, Munro DS. Immunoglobulin G inhibitor of thyroid-stimulating antibody is a cause of delay in the onset of neonatal Graves disease. J Clin Invest 1983; 72:1352.
8. Ahmann AJ, Burman KD. The role of T lymphocytes in autoimmune thyroid disease. Endocrinol Metab Clin North Am 1987; 16:287.
9. Iitaka M, Aguayo JF, Iwatani Y, et al. Studies of the effect of suppressor T lymphocytes on the induction of antithyroid microsomal antibody-secreting cells in autoimmune thyroid disease. J Clin Endocrinol Metab 1988; 66:708.
10. Dayan CM, Londei M, Corcoran AE, et al. Autoantigen recognition by thyroid-infiltrating T cells in Graves disease. Proc Natl Acad Sci U S A 1991; 88:7415.
11. Topliss D, How J, Lewis M, et al. Evidence for cell-mediated immunity and specific suppressor T lymphocyte dysfunction in Graves disease and diabetes mellitus. J Clin Endocrinol Metab 1983; 57:700.
12. Vento S, Hegarty JE, Bottazzo GF, et al. Antigen-specific suppressor cell function in autoimmune chronic active hepatitis. Lancet 1984; 1:1200.
13. Ludgate ME, Ratanachaiyavong S, Weetman AP, et al. Failure to demonstrate cell-mediated immune responses to thyroid antigens in Graves disease using in vitro assays of lymphokine-mediated migration inhibition. J Clin Endocrinol Metab 1985; 60:98.
14. Kaulfersch W, Baker JR, Burman KD, et al. Immunoglobulin and T cell gene rearrangements demonstrate that the immune response in autoimmune thyroid disease is polyclonal in nature. J Clin Endocrinol Metab 1988; 66:958.
15. Melver B, Morris JC. The pathogenesis of Graves' disease. Endocrinol Metab Clin North Am 1998; 27:73.
16. Weetman AP, Volkman DJ, Burman KD, et al. The in vitro regulation of human thyrocyte HLA-DR antigen expression. J Clin Endocrinol Metab 1985; 61:817.
17. Jerne NK. Towards a network theory of the immune system. Ann Immunol (Paris) 1974; 125:373.
18. Raines KB, Baker JR Jr, Lukes YG, et al. Antithyrotropin antibodies in the sera of Graves disease patients. J Clin Endocrinol Metab 1985; 61:217.
19. Weiss M, Ingbar SH, Winblad S, Kasper DL. Demonstration of a saturable binding site for thyrotropin in Yersinia enterocolitica. Science 1983; 219:1331.
20. Sack J, Zilberstein D, Barile MF, et al. Binding of thyrotropin to selected Mycoplasma species: detection of serum antibodies against a specific Mycoplasma membrane antigen in patients with autoimmune thyroid disease. J Endocrinol Invest 1989; 12:77.
21. Lagaye S, Vexiau P, Morozov V, et al. Human spumaretrovirus–related sequences in the DNA of leukocytes from patients with Graves' disease. Proc Natl Acad Sci U S A 1992; 89:10070.
22. Bahn RS, Dutton CM, Heufelder AE, Sarkar G. A genomic point mutation in the extracellular domain of the thyrotropin receptor in patients with Graves ophthalmopathy. J Clin Endocrinol Metab 1994; 78:256.
23. Gorman CA. Unusual manifestation of Graves disease. Mayo Clin Proc 1972; 47:926.
24. Davis PJ, Davis FB. Hyperthyroidism in patients over the age of 60 years: clinical features in 85 patients. Medicine (Baltimore) 1974; 53:161.
25. Parker JLW, Lawson DH. Death from thyrotoxicosis. Lancet 1973; 2:894.
26. Thomas FB, Mazzaferri EL, Skillman TG. Apathetic thyrotoxicosis: a distinctive clinical and laboratory entity. Ann Intern Med 1970; 72:679.
27. Heffron W, Eaton RP. Thyrotoxicosis presenting as choreoathetosis. Ann Intern Med 1970; 73:425.
28. Singh SP, Ellyin F, Singh SK, Yoon B. Elephantiasis-like appearance of upper and lower extremities in Graves dermopathy. Am J Med Sci 1985; 290:73.
29. Burch HB, Wartofsky L. Graves ophthalmopathy: current concepts regarding pathogenesis and management. Endocr Rev 1993; 14:747.
30. Bahn RS, Heufelder AE. Pathogenesis of Graves ophthalmopathy. N Engl J Med 1993; 329:1468.
31. Cunningham M, Zone JJ. Thyroid abnormalities in dermatitis herpetiformis. Ann Intern Med 1985; 102:194.
31a. Pantazi H, Papapetrou PD. Changes in parameters of bone and mineral metabolism during therapy for hyperthyroidism. J Clin Endocrinol Metab 2000; 85:1099.
32. Burman KD, Monchik J, Earll JM, Wartofsky L. Total and ionized calcium and parathyroid hormone in hyperthyroidism. Ann Intern Med 1976; 84:668.
33. Thompson P Jr, Strum D, Boehm T, Wartofsky L. Abnormalities of liver function tests in thyrotoxicosis. Mil Med 1978; 143:548.
34. Sterling K, Refetoff S, Selenkow HA. T$_3$ thyrotoxicosis: thyrotoxicosis due to elevated serum triiodothyronine levels. JAMA 1970; 213:571.
35. Hay ID, Bayer MF, Kaplan MM, et al, for the Committee on Nomenclature of the American Thyroid Association. American Thyroid Association assessment of current free thyroid hormone and thyrotropin measurements and guidelines for future clinical assays. Clin Chem 1991; 37:2002.
36. Sturgess ML, Weeks I, Evans PJ, et al. An immunochemiluminometric assay for serum free thyroxine. Clinical Endocrinol (Oxf) 1987; 27:383.
37. Symposium on Sensitive TSH Assays. Mayo Clin Proc 1988; 63:1026, 1123, 1214.
38. Cooper DS. Subclinical thyroid disease. Ann Intern Med 1998; 129:135.
39. Wartofsky L, Burman KD. Alterations in thyroid function in patients with systemic illness: the "euthyroid sick syndrome." Endocr Rev 1982; 3:164.
40. Patibandla SA, Dallas JS, Seetharamaiah GS, et al. Flow cytometric analysis of antibody binding to Chinese hamster ovary cells expressing human thyrotropin receptor. J Clin Endocrinol Metab 1997; 82:1885.
41. Morris JC, Hay ID, Nelson RE, Jiang N-S. Clinical utility of thyrotropin-receptor assays: comparison of radioreceptor and bioassay methods. Mayo Clin Proc 1988; 63:707.
42. Burman KD, Pandian R. Clinical utility of assays for TSH receptor antibodies. The Endocrinologist 1998; 8:284.
43. Kim WB, Chung HK, Lee HK, et al. Changes in epitopes for thyroid-stimulating antibodies in Graves' disease sera during treatment of hyperthyroidism: therapeutic implications. J Clin Endocrinol Metab 1997; 82:1953.
44. Mariotti S, Martino E, Cupini C, et al. Low serum thyroglobulin as a clue to the diagnosis of thyrotoxicosis factitia. N Engl J Med 1982; 307:410.
45. Kraiem Z, Glaser B, Yigla M, et al. Toxic multinodular goiter: a variant of autoimmune hyperthyroidism. J Clin Endocrinol Metab 1987; 65:659.
46. Hay ID, Thyroiditis: a clinical update. Mayo Clin Proc 1985; 60:836.
47. Amino N, Mori H, Iwatani Y, et al. High prevalence of transient postpartum thyrotoxicosis and hypothyroidism. N Engl J Med 1982; 306:849.
48. Stanbury JB, Eermans AE, Bourdoux P, et al. Iodine-induced hyperthyroidism: occurrence and epidemiology. Thyroid 1998; 8:83.
49. Hayslip CC, Fein HG, O'Donnell VM, et al. The value of serum antimicrosomal antibody testing in screening for symptomatic postpartum thyroid dysfunction. Am J Obstet Gynecol 1988; 159:203.
50. Waterman EA, Watson PF, Lazarus JH, et al. A study of the association between a polymorphism in the CTLA-4 gene and postpartum thyroiditis. Clin Endocrinol 1998; 49:251.
51. Glinoer D, Riahi M, Grün J-P, Kinthaert J. Risk of subclinical hypothyroidism in pregnant women with asymptomatic autoimmune thyroid disorders. J Clin Endocrinol Metab 1994; 79:197.
52. Rajanatavin R, Chailurkit L, Srisupandit S, et al. Trophoblastic hyperthyroidism: clinical and biochemical features of five cases. Am J Med 1988; 85:237.
53. Kempers RD, Dockerty MB, Hoffman DL, Bartholomew LG. Struma ovarii, ascitic hyperthyroid, and asymptomatic syndromes. Ann Intern Med 1970; 72:883.
54. Smallridge RC. Thyrotropin-secreting pituitary tumors. Endocrinol Metab Clin North Am 1987; 16:765.
55. Brucker-Davis F, Oldfield EH, Skarulis MC, et al. Thyrotropin-secreting pituitary tumors: diagnostic criteria, thyroid hormone sensitivity, and treatment outcome in 25 patients followed at the National Institutes of Health. J Clin Endocrinol Metab 1999; 84:476.
56. Chanson P, Weintraub BD, Harris AG. Octreotide therapy for thyroid-stimulating hormone-secreting pituitary adenoma: a follow-up of 52 patients. Ann Intern Med 1993; 119:236.
57. Kasagi K, Takeuchi R, Miyamoto S, et al. Metastatic thyroid cancer presenting as thyrotoxicosis. Clin Endocrinol (Oxf) 1994; 40:429.
58. Hedberg CW, Fishbein DB, Janssen RS, et al. An outbreak of thyrotoxicosis caused by the consumption of bovine thyroid gland in ground beef. N Engl J Med 1987; 316:993.
59. Wood LC, Ingbar SH. Hypothyroidism as a late sequela in patients with Graves disease treated with antithyroid agents. J Clin Invest 1979; 64:1429.
60. Reinwein D, Benker G, Lazarus JH, Alexander WD, and the European Multicenter Study Group on Antithyroid Drug Treatment. A prospective randomized trial of antithyroid drug dose in Graves disease therapy. J Clin Endocrinol Metab 1993; 76:1516.
61. Singer PA, Cooper DS, Levy EG, et al. Treatment guidelines for patients with hyperthyroidism and hypothyroidism: Standards of care committee, American Thyroid Association. JAMA 1995; 273:808. .
62. Cooper DS. Antithyroid drugs. N Engl J Med 1984; 311:1353.
63. Solomon BL, Evaul JE, Burman KD, Wartofsky L. Remission rates with antithyroid drug therapy: continuing influence of iodine intake? Ann Intern Med 1987; 107:510.
64. Mezquita P, Luna V, Munoz-Torres M, et al. Methimazole-induced aplastic anemia in third exposure: successful treatment with recombinant human granulocyte colony-stimulating factor. Thyroid 1998; 8:791.
64a. Mylonakis E, Akhtar MS, Lopez F, et al. Resolution of drug-induced agranulocytosis. Geriatrics 2000; 55:89.
65. Mathieu E, Fain O, Sitbon M, Thomas M. Systemic adverse effect of antithyroid drugs. Clin Rheumatol 1999; 18:66.
66. Burman KD. Thyroid hormones. In: Chernow B, ed. The pharmacologic approach to the critically ill patient. Baltimore: Williams & Wilkins, 1988:586.
67. Shen D-C, Wu S-Y, Chopra IJ, et al. Long-term treatment of Graves hyperthyroidism with sodium ipodate. J Clin Endocrinol Metab 1985; 61:723.
68. Boehm TM, Burman KD, Barnes S, Wartofsky L. Synergism of lithium and iodine in the treatment of thyrotoxicosis. Acta Endocrinol (Copenh) 1980; 94:174.
69. Kushner JP, Wartofsky L. Lithium thyroid interactions. In: Johnson FN, ed. Lithium therapy monographs, vol 2. Basel: Karger, 1988:74.

70. Wartofsky L, Ransil BJ, Ingbar SH. Inhibition by iodine of the release of thyroxine from the thyroid glands of patients with thyrotoxicosis. J Clin Invest 1970; 49:78.
71. McDermott MT, Burman KD, Hofeldt FD, Kidd GS. Lithium-associated thyrotoxicosis. Am J Med 1986; 80:1245.
72. Graham DG, Burman KD. Radioiodine treatment of Graves disease. Ann Intern Med 1986; 105:900.
73. Saenger EL, Thoma GE, Tompkins EA. Incidence of leukemia following treatment of hyperthyroidism. JAMA 1968; 205:147.
74. Ron E, Doody MM, Becker DV, et al. Cancer-mortality following treatment for adult hyperthyroidism: cooperative thyrotoxicosis therapy follow-up study group. JAMA 1998; 280:375.
75. Klein AH, Hobel CJ, Sack J, Fisher DA. Effect of intra-amniotic fluid thyroxine injection on fetal serum and amniotic fluid iodothyronine concentrations. J Clin Endocrinol Metab 1978; 47:1034.
76. Burch HB, Solomon BL, Wartofsky L, Burman KD. Discontinuing antithyroid drug therapy before ablation with radioiodine in Graves disease. Ann Intern Med 1994; 121:553.
77. McDermott MT, Kidd GS, Dodson LE, Hofeldt FD. Radioiodine-induced thyroid storm. Arch Intern Med 1983; 75:353.
78. Bartalena L, Marcocci C, Bogazzi F, et al. Relation between therapy for hyperthyroidism and the course of Graves' ophthalmopathy. N Engl J Med 1998; 338:73.
79. Hershman JM. The treatment of hyperthyroidism. Ann Intern Med 1966; 64:1306.
80. Pellegriti G, Belfiiore A, Giuffrida D, et al. Outcome of differentiated thyroid cancer in Graves' disease. J Clin Endocrinol Metab 1998; 83:2805.
81. Dent CE, Harper CM. Hypoparathyroid tetany (following thyroidectomy) apparently resistant to vitamin D. Proc R Soc Med 1958; 51:489.
82. Ljunggren JG, Torring O, Wallin G, et al. Quality of life aspects and costs in treatment of Graves' hyperthyroidism with antithyroid drugs, surgery, or radioiodine: results from a prospective, randomized study. Thyroid 1998; 8:653.
83. Glinoer D. Thyroid hyperfunction during pregnancy. Thyroid 1998; 8:859.
84. Momotani N, Noh J, Oyanagi H, et al. Antithyroid drug therapy for Graves disease during pregnancy: optional regimen for fetal thyroid status. N Engl J Med 1986; 315:24.
85. Momotani N, Ito K, Hamada N, et al. Maternal hyperthyroidism and congenital malformation in the offspring. Clin Endocrinol (Oxf) 1984; 20:695.
86. Rubin PC. Beta-blockers in pregnancy. N Engl J Med 1981; 305:1323.
87. Van Dijke CP, Heydendael RJ, DeKleine MJ. Methimazole, carbimazole, and congenital skin defects. Ann Intern Med 1987; 106:60.
88. Zakarija M, McKenzie JM. Pregnancy associated changes in the thyroid-stimulating antibody and the relationship to neonatal hyperthyroidism. J Clin Endocrinol Metab 1982; 57:1036.
89. Volpé R, Ehrlich R, Steiner G, Row VV. Graves disease in pregnancy years after hypothyroidism with recurrent passive-transfer neonatal Graves disease in offspring: therapeutic considerations. Am J Med 1984; 77:572.
90. Dydek GJ, Blue PW. Human breast milk excretion of iodine-131 following diagnostic and therapeutic administration to a lactating patient with Graves disease. J Nucl Med 1988; 29:407.
91. Davis LE, Lucas MJ, Hankins DV, et al. Thyrotoxicosis complicating pregnancy. Am J Obstet Gynecol 1989; 160:63.
92. Burch HB, Wartofsky L. Life-threatening thyrotoxicosis. Endocrinol Metab Clin North Am 1993; 22:263.
93. Nabil N, Miner DJ, Amatruda JM. Methimazole: an alternative route of administration. J Clin Endocrinol Metab 1982; 54:180.
94. Tajiri J, Katsuya H, Kiyokawa T, et al. Successful treatment of thyrotoxic crisis with plasma exchange. Crit Care Med 1984; 12:536.
95. Franco PS, Hershman JM, Haigler ED Jr, Pittman JA Jr. Response to thyrotropin-releasing hormone compared with thyroid suppression tests in euthyroid Graves disease. Metabolism 1973; 22:1357.
96. Solomon DH, Chopra IJ, Chopra U, Smith FJ. Identification of subgroups of euthyroid Graves ophthalmopathy. N Engl J Med 1977; 296:181.
97. Ueta Y, Fukui H, Murakami H, et al. Development of primary hypothyroidism with the appearance of blocking-type antibody to thyrotropin receptor in Graves' disease in late pregnancy. Thyroid 1999; 9:179.
98. Rivkees SA, Sklar C, Freemark M. Clinical review: the management of Graves' disease in children, with special emphasis on radioiodine treatment. J Clin Endocrinol Metab 1998; 83:3767.
99. Bar-Sela S, Ehrenfeld M, Eliakim M. Arterial embolism in thyrotoxicosis with atrial fibrillation. Arch Intern Med 1981; 141:1191.
100. Woeber KA. Thyrotoxicosis and the heart. N Engl J Med 1992; 327:94.
101. Hashizume K, Ichikawa K, Nishii Y, et al. Effect of administration of thyroxine on the risk of postpartum recurrence of hyperthyroid Graves disease. J Clin Endocrinol Metab 1992; 75:6.
102. Rittmaster RS, Zwicker H, Abbott EC, et al. Effect of methimazole with or without L-thyroxine on serum concentrations of thyrotropin (TSH) receptor antibodies on patients with Graves' disease. J Clin Endocrinol Metab 1996; 81:3283.
103. Cooper, DS. Subclinical thyroid disease: a clinician's perspective. Ann Intern Med 1998; 129(2):135.
104. Marqusee E, Haden ST, Utiger RD. Subclinical thyrotoxicosis. Endocrinol Metab Clin North Am 1998; 27:37.
105. Samuels MH. Subclinical thyroid disease in the elderly. Thyroid 1998; 8(9):803.

# CHAPTER 43

# ENDOCRINE OPHTHALMOPATHY

MELVIN G. ALPER AND LEONARD WARTOFSKY

## DEFINITION

Endocrine ophthalmopathy is a complex orbital disease of unknown cause characterized by round-cell infiltration, edema, and proliferation of connective tissue. These changes affect predominantly the extraocular muscles and to a lesser degree the lacrimal glands and retrobulbar fat. Usually, exophthalmos, or protrusion of the eyeballs, is present. Endocrine ophthalmopathy may occur alone, in association with diffuse thyrotoxic goiter or pretibial myxedema, or with both conditions. These findings form part of the symptom complex that is termed *Graves disease* (see Chap. 42).

Endocrine ophthalmopathy, or *endocrine exophthalmos*, the latter term coined by Brain[1] in 1959, is a useful but somewhat misleading appellation because the orbital changes may occur without endocrine abnormalities. McKenzie[2] defined the association of ophthalmopathy with endocrinopathy as a "multisystem disorder of unknown etiology, characterized by one or more of three clinical entities: (a) hyperthyroidism associated with diffuse hyperplasia of the thyroid gland, (b) infiltrative ophthalmopathy, and (c) infiltrative dermopathy (localized pretibial myxedema)." The condition is more common in women, but often the most severe cases are encountered in men. The genetics of ophthalmopathy appear to be linked to those of Graves disease, with severity of disease distinguished by certain human leukocyte antigen (HLA) types.[3] Reported estimates of the prevalence of ophthalmopathy in Graves disease vary widely from 4% to 60%, probably owing to variation in both definition and the sensitivity of detection techniques. Excluding eyelid signs, only 5% to 20% of Graves patients have ophthalmopathy, but the rate rises to 60% or more when computed tomography (CT) or magnetic resonance imaging (MRI) techniques are used to uncover otherwise unapparent muscle involvement.

Werner[4] devised a classification of the eye changes of Graves disease:

*Class 0*: No signs or symptoms
*Class 1*: Only signs, no symptoms (signs limited to upper eyelid; retraction and stare, with or without eyelid lag and proptosis)
*Class 2*: Soft-tissue involvement (symptoms and signs)
*Class 3*: Proptosis
*Class 4*: Extraocular muscle involvement
*Class 5*: Corneal involvement
*Class 6*: Sight loss (optic nerve involvement)

The progression of eye changes need not be sequential through each of the classes. The principal usefulness of the system relates to its ability to describe and transmit information to other observers about the clinical details of the ocular changes of Graves disease, but it has limitations as a guide for quantitating such changes. As a result, a number of other workers have devised, modified, and revised classifications that provide increased utility.[5] Aspects of a typical clinical presentation, characteristics of the natural history with time, and long-term follow-up have been described.[6-12] Diagnostic criteria have been described for Graves patients with either new, evolving, or worsening ophthalmopathy.[8,11,12]

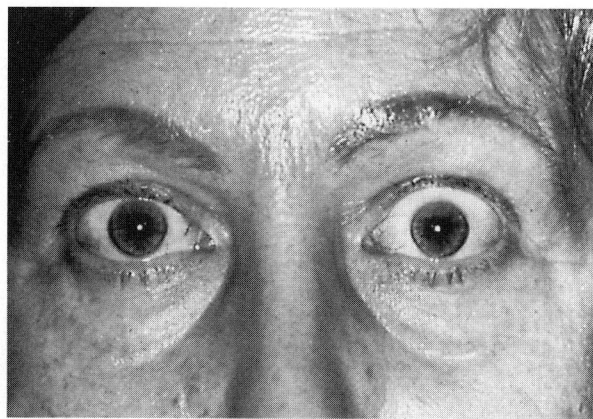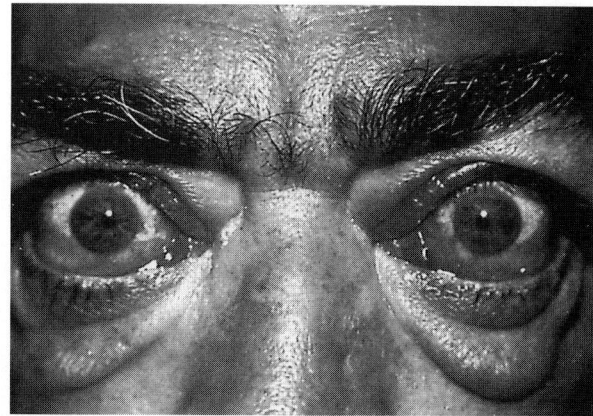

**FIGURE 43-1. A,** A 38-year-old woman with Graves hyperthyroidism. Note widened palpebral fissures, left greater than right, giving appearance of left unilateral exophthalmos. Measurements showed no proptosis. Both upper eyelids are retracted, baring sclera above the limbus in each eye, in left greater than in right (class 1 of Werner's abridged classification of ocular changes of Graves disease). **B,** A 56-year-old man with recent onset of class 3 ocular changes 2 years after treatment with radioactive iodine for Graves hyperthyroidism. The patient developed hypothyroidism after therapy and was receiving replacement thyroxine. Proptosis was present; Hertel exophthalmometry measured 33 mm in each eye. Note the soft-tissue involvement with fullness and edema of eyelids, chemosis, edema of caruncles, and conjunctival injection. Both upper lids are retracted. Herniation of retrobulbar fat through the orbital septal spaces of Charpey is present.

## ETIOLOGY

Proptosis, soft-tissue involvement, and ophthalmoplegia occurring in a patient with concurrent thyrotoxicosis or a past history of hyperthyroidism suggests dysfunction of the thyroid. Occasionally, Hashimoto thyroiditis, with or without clinical hypothyroidism, may be coexistent. When the eye changes occur in apparently euthyroid patients, not only Graves ophthalmopathy but also other primary orbital diseases must be considered.

Although the fundamental cause of Graves disease is unknown, the hyperthyroidism is generally accepted to be caused by a group of thyroid-stimulating immunoglobulins directed toward thyroid-stimulating hormone (TSH) receptors.[13-17] Whether or not these same antibodies also are responsible for the ophthalmopathy and associated immune syndromes remains to be determined,[18-20] although B lymphocytes represent a minor fraction of the cells infiltrating orbital connective tissue and muscle. Although no studies have demonstrated in vivo binding of TSH-receptor antibodies to TSH receptor in retroocular tissues, findings of TSH-receptor transcripts and TSH receptor–like proteins in orbital fibroblasts suggest an important link to the pathogenesis,[21,22] albeit possibly to only a portion of the TSH receptor.[23] Some in vitro evidence of cytotoxic responses against eye muscle antigens exists, but no histologic evidence of cytotoxicity against eye muscle has been demonstrated. A 64-kDa protein has been identified that may be a shared eye muscle and thyroid antigen, but its specificity to Graves ophthalmopathy patients has not been established.

One hypothesis is that autoreactive CD4+ T lymphocytes are activated by thyroid antigen in Graves disease, leading to the immune response against the TSH receptor and T-cell infiltration in the orbit. T lymphocytes are the predominant cells infiltrating eye muscle and are drawn to the eye by a complex interaction involving expression by retroocular fibroblasts of intercellular adhesion molecule-1 along with vascular and endothelial adhesion molecules.[24] A variety of other cytokines (interferon-γ, transforming growth factor-β, interleukin-1, tumor necrosis factor, and other fibroblast growth and activating factors) are also involved.[25] The cytokines stimulate the fibroblasts to release glycosaminoglycans, which, because of their hydrophilic nature, lead to interstitial edema.[26] Progression of the autoimmune response with more intense lymphocyte infiltration, fibroblast proliferation, and edema leads to increased orbital tissue volume, protrusion of the globe, exposure keratopathy, and venous compression, which in turn results in more edema. What initiates the entire process in genetically susceptible people is under intense study. The possible role played by the release of thyroid antigen, such as occurs after radioiodine therapy,[27-32] and by eye muscle as antigen,[33] as well as by other exogenous factors, has been reviewed. Superoxide (oxygen free) radicals have been implicated as well, with the proliferative response from orbital fibroblasts being caused by conditions of oxidative stress.[34] One such stress may be tobacco smoking, which has been associated with worsening ophthalmopathy.[13,14,35-37]

The possibility that patients receiving radioiodine may experience exacerbated ophthalmopathy has been evaluated by frequency comparisons with the outcomes for patients treated with thyroidectomy or antithyroid drugs;[27-32,38-40] some of the evidence is compelling. The mechanism appears to be antigenic release of TSH receptor from the thyroid, with activation of T and B lymphocytes leading to increases in serum TSH-receptor antibodies. Until the issue is resolved with a large, well-controlled prospective study, physicians should counsel patients who appear to be at highest risk of worsening ophthalmopathy after radioiodine (e.g., those with more severe thyrotoxicosis, smokers, and those with preexistent ophthalmopathy). If antithyroid drugs or thyroidectomy are not viable alternatives, concomitant therapy with corticosteroids should be considered.[39,41]

In addition to varying in presentation, the ophthalmopathy of Graves disease may vary in severity. The degree of exophthalmos often is unrelated to the severity of the thyrotoxicosis and, paradoxically, may occasionally appear after the hyperthyroidism is controlled.[9,12,29,42,43] The severity of eye changes may vary (Fig. 43-1), but the basic pathogenetic process is the same.

## PATHOLOGY

The major pathologic changes that occur in Graves disease are inflammatory infiltration by lymphocytes and chronic inflammatory cells in all orbital tissues with proliferation of the connective tissue (Table 43-1). Because autopsy findings are rare in this condition, precise clinicopathologic correlation has not been made for each of the physical signs that are described. Most of the material examined by pathologists is obtained at

**TABLE 43-1.**
**Pathogenesis of Graves Ophthalmopathy**

| Stage | Description |
| --- | --- |
| Autoreactive T cell | Autoreactive T cells may arise through an escape from clonal deletion, failure of suppressor T-cell activity, or molecular mimicry. |
| Thyroid damage | Thyroid damage may occur through chronic thyroiditis, external beam radiation, smoking, or radioiodine therapy, resulting in the release of thyroid antigen. |
| Amplification | The autoimmune process, activated through thyroid antigen release, undergoes amplification, resulting in a proliferation of activated T lymphocytes and stimulation of humoral immunity. |
| Thyrotoxicosis | Stimulating antibodies directed against the TSH receptor cause hyperthyroidism with release of thyroid hormone as well as additional thyroid antigen. Concurrent reduced reserve or blocking antibodies may limit thyrotoxic response in some patients. |
| Ocular infiltration | Activated T lymphocytes enter the orbital connective tissue through interaction with circulating and cell-surface adhesion molecules. Local humoral immunity may precede or follow infiltration of T lymphocytes. |
| Fibroblast activity | Retroorbital fibroblast proliferation is mediated through humoral and cellular immune processes. Synthesis and release of glycosaminoglycans into connective tissue matrix occur. |
| Perpetuation | Perpetuation of the retroorbital autoimmune response occurs through lymphokine release and activation of fibroblasts. Shared eye–thyroid antigens such as the thyrotropin receptor are presented and/or released. |
| Mass-volume effect | Retroocular and perimysial connective tissue becomes increasingly hypercellular and edematous. Retroocular mass increases disproportionate to volume expansion. |

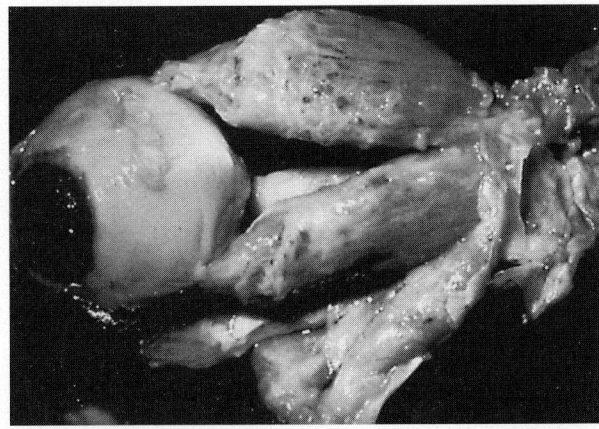

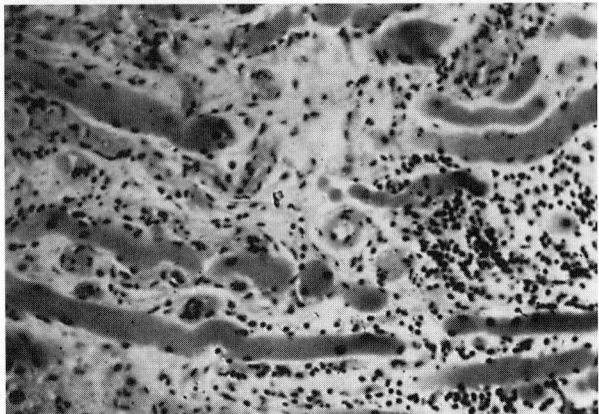

**FIGURE 43-2.** **A,** Orbital contents obtained at autopsy from a 47-year-old man with an 8-month history of Graves hyperthyroidism. Bilateral vision loss had been present for 2 months. While hospitalized for high-dose prednisone and orbital radiotherapy, he experienced acute myocardial infarction. Note massive enlargement of extraocular muscles surrounding the optic nerve. Orbital fat has been removed. **B,** Photomicrograph of a muscle biopsy from inferior rectus muscle of a 58-year-old woman with endocrine ophthalmopathy. Note focal collection of lymphocytes. Muscle fibers appear normal. ×60 (**A** from Hufnagel TH, Hickey WF, Cobbs WH, et al. Immunohistochemical and ultrastructure studies on the exenterated orbital tissue of a patient with Graves' disease. Ophthalmology 1984; 91:1411. Published courtesy of Ophthalmology.)

the time of surgery for orbital decompression or correction of extraocular muscle difficulties. Thus, the earliest changes in the orbital tissues are rarely studied, whereas abundant reports exist of some of the pathologic findings in the more severe forms of ophthalmopathy.

All orbital structures, including lacrimal glands, are affected. Massive swelling of the extraocular muscles is commonly seen; occasionally, they may become 8 to 10 times their normal volume (Fig. 43-2). Histologically, marked interstitial inflammatory edema and focal lymphocytic infiltration of the muscles is noted. The myofibrillar structure remains normal, but loss of striations and disorganization may occur later. With thyrotoxicosis, a diffuse increase in orbital fat content may be present, and a deposition of adipose tissue cells lying in strands between the muscle fibers may be noted. In the absence of thyrotoxicosis, the fat content is decreased and is replaced by connective tissue. The mucopolysaccharide and water content of the tissues increases, and large numbers of mast cells are seen in the perivascular areas.

As the volume of the orbital tissues increases, proptosis occurs. The swollen muscles become increasingly immobile, and

the globe may deviate, often in a downward direction. Fibrosis of the muscles may ensue, causing permanent limitation of motion. As proptosis progresses, corneal exposure with subsequent ulceration may appear (Fig. 43-3). The pressure in the posterior orbit may be so great that venous drainage is impaired, leading to conjunctival injection initially, edema (chemosis), and eventually optic disc swelling (Fig. 43-4). Occlusion of the central retinal vein or artery may occur if the pressure is sufficient. Optic neuropathy with loss of central vision may appear at any time during the course of the ophthalmopathy. Some patients without marked proptosis have normal-appearing optic nerve discs but have vision loss. The cause of the loss of vision in these patients is probably mechanical compression from the massively swollen extraocular muscles pressing on the optic nerve at the apex of the orbit.[44] CT scanning confirms this occurrence.[45] Prompt recovery of vision after surgical decompression of the orbit and altitudinal visual field defects suggest that vascular compression also may be a factor.[46]

## CLINICAL COURSE

Retraction of the upper eyelids is the most important clinical clue and produces a triad that is nearly pathognomonic of

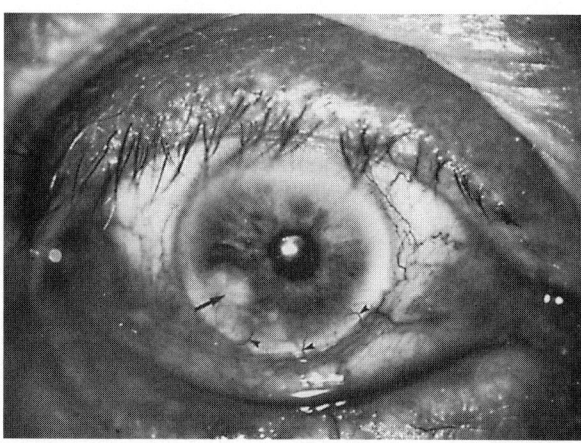

**FIGURE 43-3.** Eye of a 60-year-old man with severe endocrine ophthalmopathy causing marked proptosis, extraocular muscle tethering, and corneal exposure. Marked visual loss was present secondary to corneal ulceration in the right eye (class 5 Werner's abridged classification of ocular changes of Graves disease). Note the opacification (*arrow*) and vascularization of cornea (*arrowheads*).

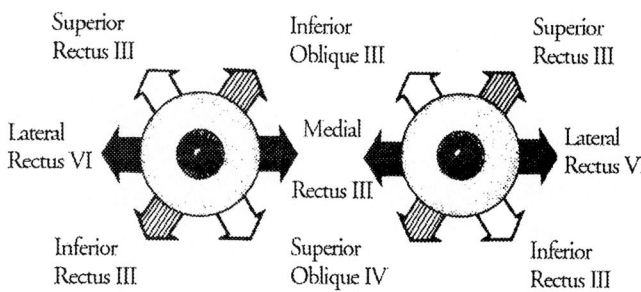

**FIGURE 43-5.** Extraocular movements, the muscles involved, and their controlling nerves. (From Judge RD, et al. Clinical diagnosis, a physiologic approach. Boston: Little, Brown, 1982:107.)

endocrine ophthalmopathy: widened palpebral fissures, lid lag on downward gaze, and infrequent blinking (see Fig. 43-1A).

Normally, the upper lid covers the upper limbus so that the free border rests at the upper edge of the pupil. Many factors change this relation, and care must be taken in assuming that the upper lid retraction is abnormal. Lid retraction exists if, when the eyes are directed horizontally forward without staring, a band of white sclera is seen above the iris. Because of the cosmetic changes created by this phenomenon, concern over appearance usually is the presenting complaint. In some instances, only one eyelid is retracted, and the patient may complain that the other upper lid is drooped. Lid lag accompanies the retraction of the upper eyelid and is manifested as a failure of the lid to accompany the descent of the globe on downward gaze, with the appearance of a white band of sclera above the upper limbus.

These phenomena (lid retraction and lid lag) give the impression of exophthalmos, but in the early stages, usually little or no measurable proptosis is present. In the mild form of orbital involvement, as the process continues, actual exophthalmos may occur. The forward position of the globe is appreciated best by direct measurements but can be suggested by retraction of the lower lid.

If the soft tissues of the orbit become involved, symptoms of lacrimation, foreign-body sensation, and tenseness around the eyes appear. The eyelids become edematous and full, and the conjunctiva develop chemosis in the lower cul-de-sac. Conjunctival injection and dilated epibulbar blood vessels overlying the lateral rectus muscles appear, indicating an increase in orbital pressure and venostasis (see Fig. 43-1B). In some patients, the lacrimal gland may become enlarged, reaching enormous size. It may be prominent on physical examination and also appears as a large mass on CT scanning.

Involvement of the extraocular muscles with limitation of ocular motility may occur in one or both eyes and, because of the resultant diplopia, may represent the most common major disability of this condition. (Fig. 43-5 is a diagrammatic representation of extraocular movements, the muscles involved, and their controlling nerves.) Typically, limitation of upward gaze is the most common finding and gives the false impression of paralysis of elevation. It is caused, however, by tethering of the inferior rectus muscle by inflammatory infiltration and subsequent fibrosis. The patient often tilts the chin upward to gain fusion in the lower fields of vision. Eventually, as fibrosis progresses, a unilaterally proptosed eye may become fixed in a downward and inward position owing to contracture of the damaged inferior rectus muscle. Then, enophthalmos may replace the former exophthalmos.

Less commonly, involvement of the medial rectus muscle causes limitation of lateral gaze, simulating a lateral rectus muscle paralysis (Fig. 43-6). Uncommonly, involvement of the superior rectus muscle causes restriction of motility on downward gaze.

Myasthenia gravis must be considered as a possible cause of extraocular muscle limitation, because 0.2% of patients with Graves disease develop myasthenia and 5% of myasthenic patients have associated Graves disease. In addition to the edrophonium chloride (Tensilon) test, the forced-duction test is helpful in ruling out this condition. It can be conducted with topical anesthesia; one applies either forceps or a suction cup to the globe and attempts to move the eye in a direction against the field of action of the involved muscle. A positive test result (indicative of a restrictive mechanical process, not a neurologic disease) is one in which marked resistance is encountered during this maneuver, such that the globe cannot be moved.

An elevation of intraocular pressure to glaucomatous levels on attempted upward gaze, when compared with readings taken with the globe in the straight-ahead position, frequently accompanies a slight tethering of the inferior rectus muscle. This may be the first sign of ophthalmopathy and a means for early clinical detection of Graves disease.[47] Upward gaze–

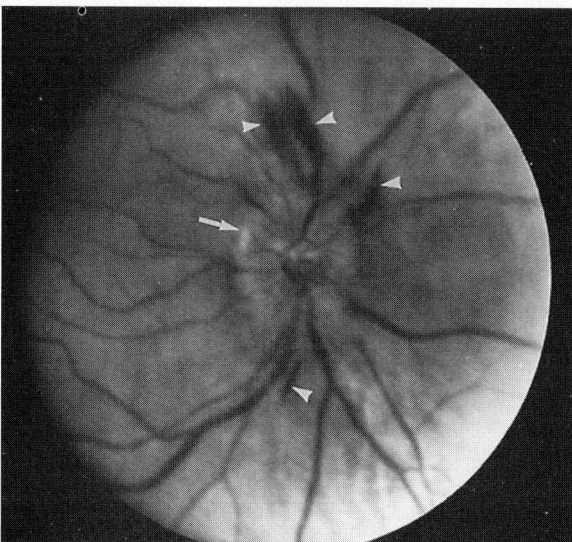

**FIGURE 43-4.** Funduscopic view of the right eye of a 58-year-old woman with severe Graves ophthalmopathy. Marked loss of vision occurred because of optic nerve neuropathy. The funduscopic examination shows a swollen optic disc (*arrow*) with hemorrhages (*arrowheads*). The patient was treated with megadose corticosteroids; the process resolved, and vision was restored.

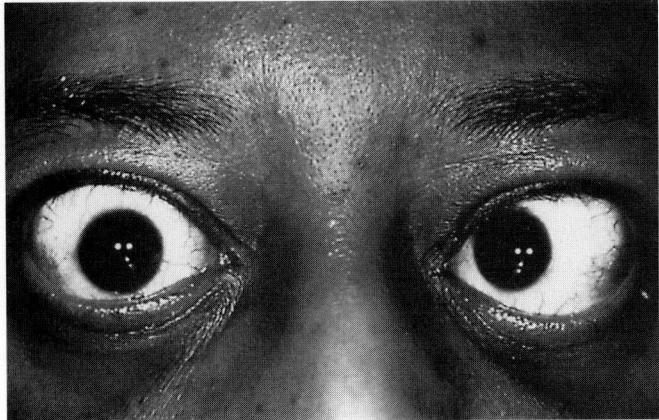

**FIGURE 43-6.** Patient is looking to the right. Note the limitation of abduction of the right eye.

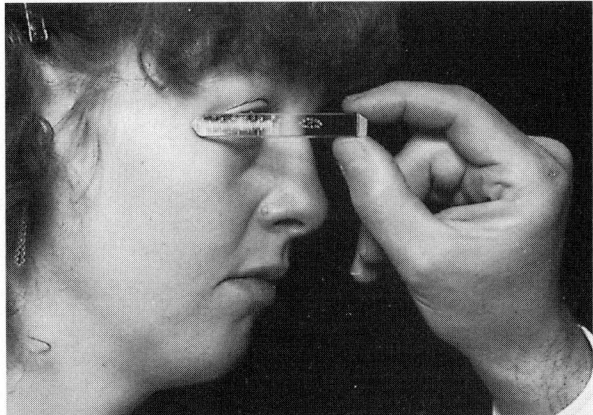

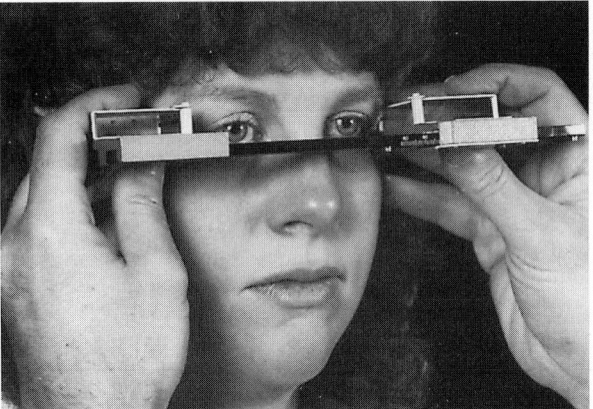

**FIGURE 43-7.** Measuring devices to quantitate exophthalmos. **A,** Luedde exophthalmometer. **B,** Hertel exophthalmometer.

evoked elevation of intraocular pressure does not require treatment if the pressure is normal in downward gaze.

## COMPLICATIONS

With increasing exophthalmos, the globe may be proptosed through the eyelids so that exposure of the cornea occurs. Ulceration, with scarring or spontaneous perforation, may lead to vision loss or even loss of the eye.

Occasionally, the optic nerve becomes involved; an unusual neuropathy may develop that threatens vision, causing central scotomas and other visual field losses. This neuropathy may present either as a normal or a swollen optic disc and eventually may progress to optic atrophy. Disc swelling may occur without vision loss as a result of increased posterior orbital pressure. The optic neuropathy with vision loss can occur in the absence of clinical signs of markedly increased intraorbital pressure, but in these patients, CT scanning usually reveals enlarged extraocular muscles at the orbital apex. Asymptomatic optic nerve involvement may be detected by measurement of visual evoked cortical potentials.[48]

## PHYSICAL EXAMINATION AND MENSURATION

The purpose of physical examination and mensuration in orbital disease initially is to establish the position of the eyes relative to each other and to the bony landmarks of the orbit. Orbital disease processes usually affect only the soft tissue of the orbit so that, with very few exceptions, the bony margins remain constant. Thus, measuring devices relate the globe to the fixed bony points of reference.

Physical examination of the exophthalmic patient begins with inspection, but direct viewing of the subject can be misleading. The best method of determining if proptosis exists is to stand behind the seated patient and evaluate the position of the eyes by looking down over the brows. The patient is then placed in a supine position, and the position of the eyes is reassessed while the physician is standing above and behind the patient. In normal people, the globe sinks back when the patient is recumbent. In such circumstances, exophthalmometric measurements are reduced from the erect position by 1 to 3 mm.[49] This retraction does not occur in the seemingly unaffected eye of patients with Graves disease even though the exophthalmos may appear to be unilateral. However, in cases of exophthalmos resulting from a unilateral orbital tumor, the normal postural difference of the unaffected eye is noted; there-

fore, this may be used as a method of differential diagnosis between seemingly unilateral endocrine exophthalmos and a unilateral orbital tumor.

These techniques merely provide the observer with an impression of exophthalmos, but more accurate measurements are needed to establish a baseline and to follow the progress of a patient with the ophthalmopathy of Graves disease. A measuring device, therefore, is necessary.

When a measuring device is used, the most commonly accepted reference points are the cornea and the lateral rim of the orbit. With the eye viewed from the side, a transparent ruler may be held against the lateral bony rim of the orbit; the distance to the cornea may be seen and directly measured. The Luedde exophthalmometer is one such device, which can give approximate results; the measurements with this device are less accurate than those obtained with the instrument devised by Hertel (Fig. 43-7). The latter consists of a system of mirrors or prisms that projects a lateral view of the eye forward and superimposes a millimeter rule measuring from the anterior rim of the lateral orbital wall onto the viewing mirror. Certain errors are inherent in the use of this instrument because of factors such as thickness of tissue over the lateral orbital margins, parallax, and facial asymmetry. In practice, the instrument is placed beneath the lateral canthal tendon, pressed firmly against the lateral bony rim, and stabilized in a vertical plane held parallel to the ground. Readings of the position of the anterior aspect of each eye are recorded with the interorbital distance, which is noted on the base scale and varies from patient to patient. Normal readings range from 15 to 20 mm, and the difference between the eyes usually does not exceed 1 mm. A difference of up to 2 mm may occur with extraocular muscle paralysis, but differences of more than 2.5 mm usually indicate a pathologic process in the orbit. Frequently, an iso-

**TABLE 43-2.**
**Investigative Studies for Unilateral Exophthalmos**

**A. NONINVASIVE STUDIES**
  1. Establish presence of unilateral exophthalmos
  2. Rule out Graves disease (e.g., serum thyroxine, triiodothyronine [$T_3$], $T_3$ resin uptake, sensitive TSH, TRH stimulation test)
  3. Conventional radiographic films of orbits, optic foramina, sphenoid ridges, and paranasal sinuses
  4. Medical imaging (ultrasonography, CT, MRI)

**B. INVASIVE STUDIES**
  1. Orbital venography
  2. Cerebral angiography
  3. Trial of corticosteroids
  4. Orbital biopsy
     a. Fine-needle aspiration
     b. Orbitotomy

*TSH,* thyroid-stimulating hormone; *TRH,* thyrotropin-releasing hormone; *CT,* computed tomography; *MRI,* magnetic resonance imaging.

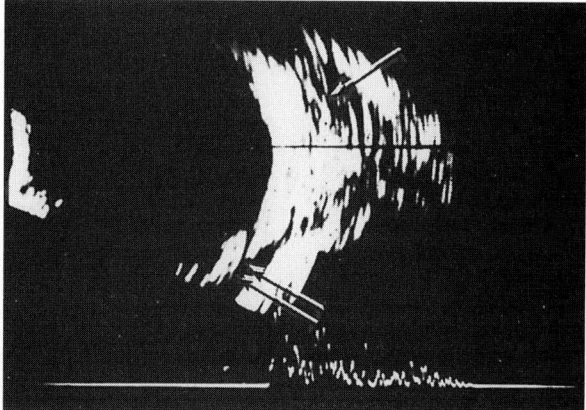

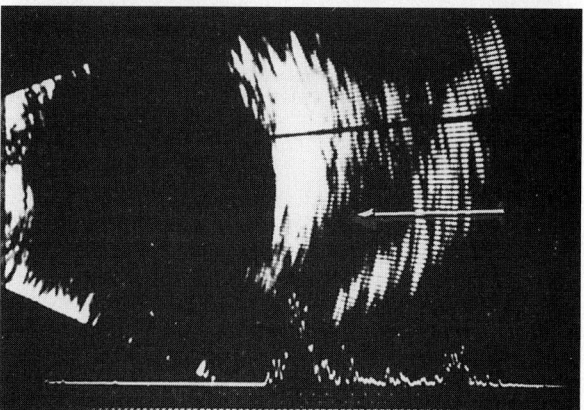

**FIGURE 43-8. A,** Normal B-scan ultrasonogram demonstrates superior (*single arrow*) and inferior (*double arrows*) rectus muscles. Optic nerve is denoted by vector. A-scan ultrasonogram is superimposed at bottom of picture. **B,** Abnormal B-scan ultrasonogram of patient with Graves ophthalmopathy. Because of technicalities in positioning the ultrasonic probe, the superior rectus muscle (*arrow*) in this scan appears below the vector through the optic nerve. Compare size of this enlarged muscle to the normal size muscle in **A.**

lated reading is inconclusive, but repeated examinations may reveal a progressive exophthalmic process.

Other methods of demonstrating exophthalmos are more complex and expensive. One radiographic method places a radiopaque contact lens on the eye and measures its distance from the anterior clinoid process on a lateral view. CT scanning is a useful adaptation of radiographic techniques. Care must be taken with radiographic techniques to maintain the head in the same position each time a measurement is taken. The Hertel exophthalmometer remains the most practical and accurate method of measuring exophthalmos. Palpation of the orbit may indicate a moderate to severe degree of retrobulbar resistance. Orbitonometers, however, invented to calibrate the force of orbital resistance, have proved to be of little clinical value.

## DIFFERENTIAL DIAGNOSIS

When exophthalmos occurs bilaterally and is accompanied by retraction of the upper lid, with lid lag and limitation of upward gaze, little difficulty is encountered in establishing the diagnosis of Graves ophthalmopathy, even if thyrotoxicosis is absent.[6,11,12,50] If proptosis is unilateral, this entity is still the most common cause, but other conditions must be ruled out. A logical, sequential evaluation of the orbit should include studies to separate orbital from periorbital and intracranial lesions and should proceed in a rational fashion without risk to the patient.[51] A team effort is necessary that may include the ophthalmologist, endocrinologist, otolaryngologist, nuclear medicine specialist, and neuroradiologist. Table 43-2 shows a useful scheme for the diagnostic evaluation of unilateral exophthalmos. The evaluation of thyroid function is discussed in Chapters 33 through 36.

Conventional radiographic films disclose a great variety of diseases in the orbit, paranasal sinuses, and intracranial cavity, but they reveal little information about the soft-tissue changes of Graves disease; such changes can be visualized with techniques for imaging the orbit, such as ultrasonography, CT, and MRI.[52]

Ultrasonography measures the reflectivity of sound waves as they pass through a given slice of tissue. B-scan ultrasonography demonstrates the inflammatory changes that occur in the ophthalmopathy of Graves disease and may differentiate it from normal (Fig. 43-8*A*), from inflammatory pseudotumor, or from expanding orbital masses (see Fig. 43-8*B*).

A CT scan measures the absorption of x-rays as they pass through a given section of tissue. By use of high-resolution instruments, the CT characteristics of pathologic features of Graves ophthalmopathy have been defined (Fig. 43-9). A clas-

sic CT scan of Graves ophthalmopathy demonstrates exophthalmos, herniation of retrobulbar fat through the orbital septum, enlargement of extraocular muscles with normal tendons, bilateral involvement, and, frequently, enlargement of the lacrimal glands.

MRI is a nonionizing technique that measures the resonance of hydrogen ions in a given section of tissue when subjected to a magnetic field.[51,52] Excellent contrast between pathologic and normal anatomic structures has been demonstrated in Graves ophthalmopathy (Fig. 43-10). MRI scans are as useful as those obtained from high-resolution thin-section CT of the orbit. However, because of the greater availability and cheaper cost, CT is the medical imaging technique of choice.

Other conditions that may be confused with Graves ophthalmopathy and that may be diagnosed by these visualizing techniques include orbital tumors, axial myopia, inflammatory granulomas, cysts, arteriovenous aneurysms, lymphomas, and aberrant third-nerve regeneration (in patients who demonstrate lid retraction on downward gaze).

A common error in clinical diagnosis is failure to recognize meningioma en plaque because of the exophthalmos and brawny edema of the eyelids that may occur in this condition. In meningioma, however, the edema of the lower lid has a characteristic unilateral "baggy" appearance, and no lid retraction is seen. A frequent source of confusion in the differential diagnosis is axial myopia, a common cause of unilateral exophthalmos. Retinoscopy and A-scan ultrasonography reveal this condition. Inflammatory pseudotumor is a condition simulating orbital neoplasm that usually affects the orbital floor struc-

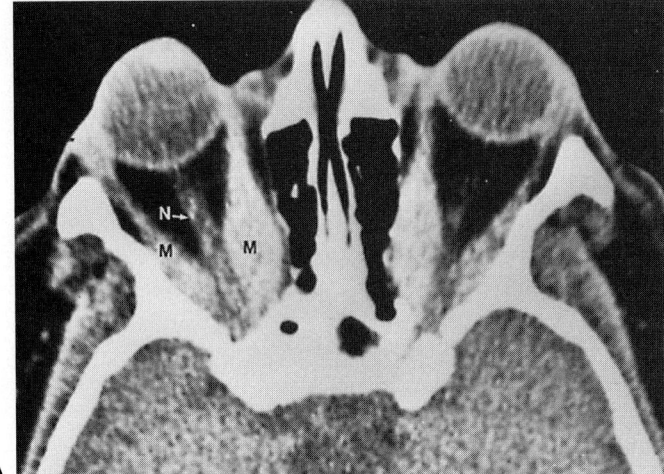

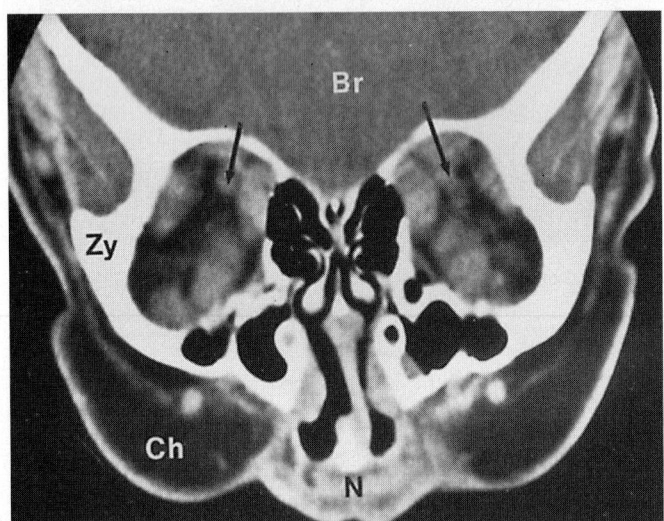

**FIGURE 43-9. A,** Transaxial computed tomographic (*CT*) scan of a 50-year-old woman with severe endocrine ophthalmopathy. Optic nerve neuropathy was present in each eye. Note bilateral involvement with exophthalmos, enlarged medial and lateral rectus muscles (*M*), normal tendinous insertions, moulding of the medial rectus muscle into the ethmoid bones and sinuses bilaterally, and compression of the optic nerves (*N*) at the orbital apex bilaterally. **B,** Coronal CT scan through midorbit demonstrates enlarged extraocular muscles. Note that optic nerves (*arrows*) can be distinguished as separate structures and are not compressed in this plane. (*Zy,* zygomatic arches; *Ch,* cheeks; *Br,* brain.)

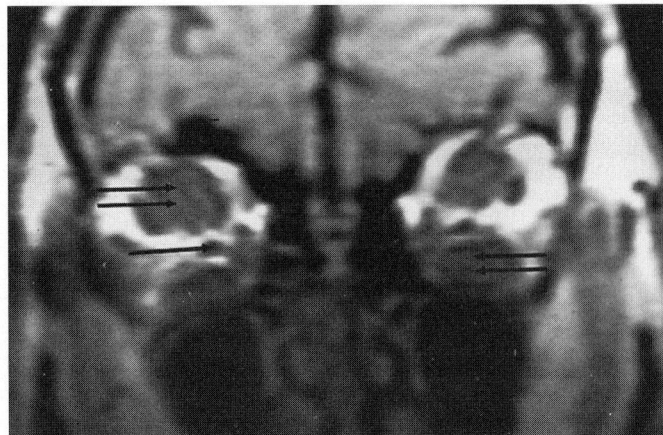

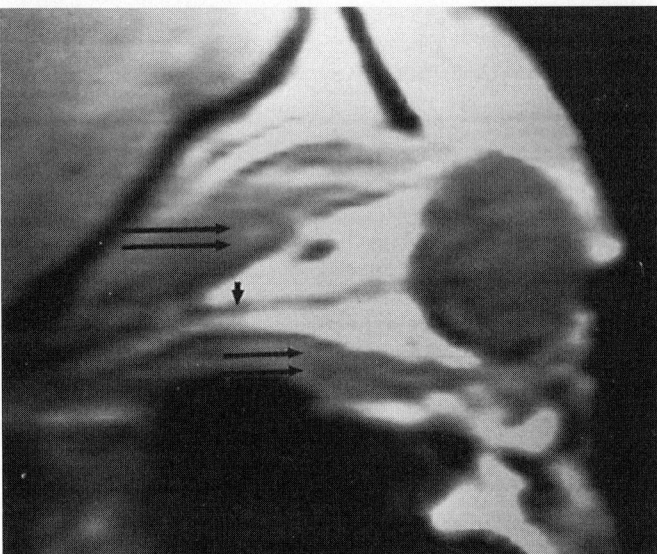

**FIGURE 43-10. A,** Coronal magnetic resonance imaging (*MRI*) scan of a 59-year-old man with severe Graves ophthalmopathy. Bilateral optic nerve neuropathy was present. Note the markedly enlarged superior and inferior rectus muscles (*double arrows*) encroaching on the optic nerve (*single arrow*). Orbital fat gives a white signal in this T1 sequence. **B,** Sagittal MRI scan shows markedly enlarged superior and inferior rectus muscles (*double arrows*) converging on and compressing the optic nerve (*single arrow*) at the orbital apex. In this T1 sequence, retrobulbar fat is seen as a white signal.

tures; it presents with sudden proptosis, lid edema, pain, ophthalmoplegia, and vision loss at the onset of the disease. The exquisite sensitivity to corticosteroids that generally accompanies this condition has been used as an aid in the differential diagnosis. Differentiation of Graves ophthalmopathy from inflammatory orbital pseudotumor often presents a diagnostic challenge clinically, but it is readily accomplished by CT scanning. In pseudotumor, a classic CT scan shows (a) exophthalmos; (b) enhancement of the sclerouveal rim by contrast media ("rim sign"); (c) enlarged extraocular muscles with abnormal tendons; (d) "feathery" infiltration of the retrobulbar fat, especially in the anterior third of the orbit; and (e) unilateral involvement (Fig. 43-11).

A carotid cavernous aneurysm may produce exophthalmos similar to that seen in patients with unilateral proptosis of Graves ophthalmopathy. In an aneurysm, however, the episcleral veins are distended, a bruit is heard overlying the globe, and the patient hears noises that are synchronous with the pulse. Furthermore, medical imaging demonstrates an enlarged or distended superior ophthalmic vein due to arterial blood

shunted by the aneurysm. Lymphomas may cause either bilateral or unilateral exophthalmos. A CT scan demonstrates retrobulbar masses that mold to the posterior aspect of the globe and to the muscle cone. Fine-needle aspiration biopsy under ultrasonographic guidance may yield the diagnosis.

## TREATMENT

Treatment of the eye changes of Graves disease is primarily palliative. The patient should be reassured that the ophthalmopathy is usually self-limited. Above all, if thyroid dysfunction is present, the patient must be rapidly treated and maintained in a euthyroid state. Subsequent hypothyroidism should be avoided (see Chap. 45). Initially, during the acute phase of the disease, elevation of the head of the bed and diuretic use may reduce the periorbital edema. A controversy has existed for some time regarding whether any of the three treatments for Graves disease (antithyroid drugs, radioiodine therapy, or thyroidectomy) was associated with greater benefit in preventing

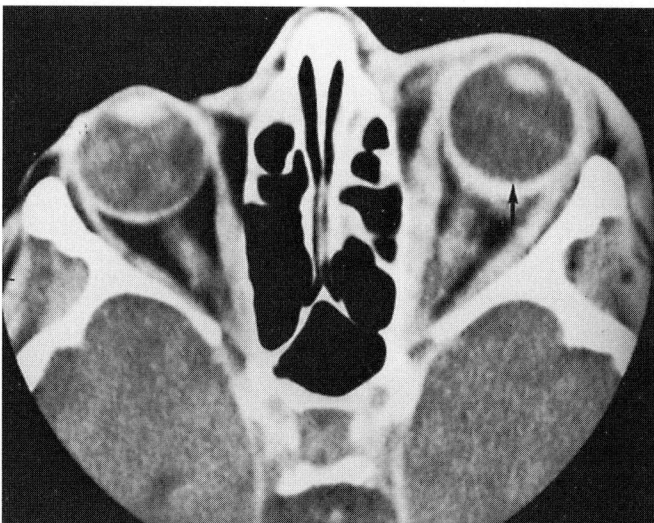

**FIGURE 43-11.** Transaxial computed tomographic (CT) scan of a 52-year-old woman with classic inflammatory orbital pseudotumor of left orbit. Note unilateral involvement with left exophthalmos, enlargement of left medial and lateral rectus muscles, thickened abnormal tendons, enhancement of sclerouveal rim (*arrow*) by contrast media ("rim sign"), and "feathery" infiltration of fat in the retrobulbar and perineural areas. Prompt resolution was obtained with corticosteroid therapy.

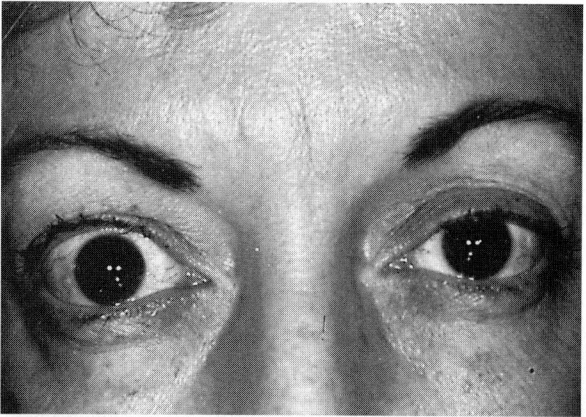

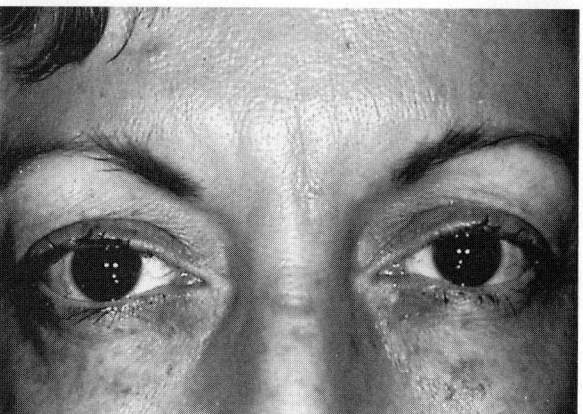

**FIGURE 43-12. A,** Right upper lid retraction in a 42-year-old woman with Graves hyperthyroidism. **B,** Postoperative appearance after myectomy of Müller muscle of right upper lid.

onset or exacerbation of ophthalmopathy.[13,27–32,53] Most of these earlier studies were poorly controlled. Three randomized clinical trials have suggested that ophthalmopathy may be more common after treatment with radioactive iodine than after medical or surgical treatment.[29,39,41]

A clear understanding by the patient that a protracted period of therapy is necessary helps to foster a good patient-doctor relationship. Encouragement that the therapy usually prevents loss of vision and maintains function is helpful for the patient's peace of mind. Many patients are concerned about cosmetic disfigurement caused by the disease. Reassurance that this also can be managed to a considerable degree builds confidence.

Treatment of the ophthalmopathy is indicated for functional and cosmetic reasons, which frequently overlap.[54] These disabilities relate to lid retraction, extraocular muscle myopathy, exophthalmos, protrusion of retrobulbar fat through the orbital septum, and optic nerve neuropathy.[55]

Functional disability may result from extraocular muscle malalignment causing diplopia, from vision loss because of corneal exposure owing to exophthalmos or lid retraction, or from optic nerve neuropathy. Also, soft-tissue involvement can cause severe discomfort. Cosmetic deficit may arise from upper eyelid retraction, eyeball malposition, exophthalmos, herniation of retrobulbar fat through the spaces of Charpey in the orbital septum, or soft-tissue involvement.

Lid retraction may cause both a cosmetic and functional problem. Drying of the eye from exposure, especially during sleep, leads to keratitis with constant redness, foreign-body sensation, and photophobia. In the early stages, eyedrops of 5% guanethidine (Ismelin), a sympatholytic agent, may relieve lid retraction. This drug has not been approved by the U.S. Food and Drug Administration but is available for use in Europe. Some symptomatic relief may be obtained by increasing the humidity in the home environment, wearing sunglasses when outdoors, using artificial tears (1% methylcellulose) during the day, and applying emollients to lubricate the eyes at bedtime. If these measures fail to relieve the symptoms, or if the disfigurement is too great, one may turn to surgery. However, surgery should not be performed until the patient is stabilized in the euthyroid state.

Myectomy of the Müller muscle is effective in relieving lid retraction in many cases (Fig. 43-12). The operation is not indicated, however, in cases of lid retraction secondary to tethering

of the inferior rectus muscle (Collier sign) or when organic changes have occurred in the superior levator muscle. When this latter muscle becomes involved by morphologic changes, it becomes tethered so that the upper lid does not close, even under general anesthesia. A technique for testing for this is to grasp the upper eyelashes and pull inferiorly in a direction opposite the field of action of the levator muscle. When the result of this forced duction test is positive, myectomy of the Müller muscle will not alleviate the lid retraction. In this event, one must perform recession of the superior levator muscle with or without the use of some kind of donor material (preserved sclera, Tenon fascia, or preserved dura) as a spacer between the tarsus and muscle. In rare cases, the injection of a soluble corticosteroid (triamcinolone) adjacent to the levator, under ultrasonographic control, has been successful.

Tethering of the inferior rectus muscle causes not only vertical diplopia, which probably is the most common functional disability, but also malposition of the eyeball, which can be cosmetically disfiguring. Recession of the muscle and lysis of adhesions between it and the lower lid retractors often restores single binocular vision. Just as often, the lower lid sags postoperatively, which necessitates another operation to elevate the lower lid to prevent exposure of the lower one-third of the globe.

Tethering of the medial rectus is not as common as inferior rectus tethering but is equally disabling. It simulates lateral rectus muscle palsy and causes horizontal diplopia and cosmetic disfigurement by eyeball malalignment (see Fig. 43-6). Surgical recession of the medial rectus muscles restores single binocular vision and corrects the disfigurement.

Progressive soft-tissue involvement may cause marked functional and cosmetic deficits. These patients may be discomforted by pain, epiphora, and photophobia, becoming functionally disabled, although no vision loss may occur. They may be markedly disfigured, with exophthalmos, lid edema, chemosis edema of the caruncle, and conjunctival injection (see Fig. 43-1*B*). Ultimately, compressive neuropathy of the optic nerve at the orbital apex resulting from the enlarged extraocular muscles may ensue, and blindness becomes a distinct danger.

Therapeutic options for progressive ophthalmopathy include (a) corticosteroid therapy, (b) supervoltage orbital radiotherapy, (c) surgical decompression of the orbit, and (d) combinations of these methods.

## IMMUNOMODULATORY THERAPY

### CORTICOSTEROIDS

A large number of immunomodulatory agents have been used in the treatment of Graves ophthalmopathy, but no single agent seems to have a clear advantage over corticosteroids.[56] Corticosteroid use may produce dramatic relief of the signs and symptoms of progressive inflammatory changes. The dosage is tailored to the severity of involvement and may range from 40 to 120 mg per day of prednisone, which then is gradually tapered as improvement occurs.

When the optic nerve becomes involved, larger doses of corticosteroids are needed to restore function and save vision. The patient may need to be hospitalized if large doses of prednisone are administered (e.g., 120–140 mg per day). If adverse reactions occur, the dosage sometimes must be reduced and the treatment augmented with subtenon or retrobulbar injections of triamcinolone or methylprednisolone. As soon as the vision is restored (usually after 7 to 10 days of this therapy), the prednisone dosage is reduced. Sometimes, exacerbations occur when the dose level reaches 40 mg per day. In this event, larger doses once again must be administered. Pulse methylprednisolone treatment has been reported to be effective, with documented clinical improvement and reduced muscle size on CT scan.[13] A prospective study indicates that corticosteroids may prevent worsening of ophthalmopathy in patients treated with radioiodine, but this remains controversial.[39,41]

### CYCLOSPORINE

Cyclosporine therapy was applied to Graves ophthalmopathy in view of the drug's immunomodulatory effects directed at several points in the presumed pathogenesis of the disease (see Table 43-1). The drug inhibits early induction of T helper cell proliferation, permits activation of T-suppressor cells, blocks activation of cytotoxic T cells and production of cytokines, and may also inhibit synthesis of TSH-receptor antibodies by B lymphocytes.[57] Several early reports showed mixed but encouraging results, which led to two prospective randomized studies of note. A comparison of cyclosporine plus prednisone to prednisone alone in 40 patients showed that patients on combined treatment had a faster and more long-lasting response with fewer recurrences. Objective improvement attributed to cyclosporine included reduced eye muscle thickness.[58] In a study of 36 patients randomized to receive either prednisone or cyclosporine, 61% of patients responded to prednisone alone, compared with only 22% who showed good responses to cyclosporine. However, 59% of the treatment failures responded to a second course of both drugs in combination.[59] Thus, it appears that cyclosporine may provide an added benefit to corticosteroid therapy and shorten the course of the disease. The obvious drawbacks to both corticosteroids and cyclosporine are their potential adverse side effects. Renal function and liver function must be monitored during cyclosporine treatment, with the daily dose kept between 2.5 and 5 mg/kg of body weight.

### SOMATOSTATIN

Trials of somatostatin therapy for ophthalmopathy were undertaken because of the detection of somatostatin receptors in orbital fibroblasts and lymphocytes. The mechanism of action is presumed to be based on reduction of edema mediated by insulin-like growth factor-I and reduction of autoreactivity of T cells via inhibition by somatostatin of proliferation of activated T cells. Octreotide has also been shown to reduce serum levels of *intercellular adhesion molecule-1* (sICAM-1),[60] thought to be a marker for orbital fibroblast activation that correlates with inflammatory changes.[61] Various analogs of somatostatin, including indium-labeled octreotide and pentetreotide, have been used effectively with single photon emission computed tomography (SPECT) to scintigraphically image active ophthalmopathy.[62–66] A drawback of somatostatin therapy had been the need to give multiple daily subcutaneous injections due to its brief half-life, but longer lasting analogs are now available. One such analog, lanreotide, is given only once every 2 weeks and has been associated with comparable clinical benefit in preliminary trials.[67] In one comparison between somatostatin therapy and corticosteroid therapy, the former was as effective in relieving symptoms and soft-tissue inflammation, but not in reducing muscle size.[68] On the other hand, a correlation may exist between intensity of octreotide uptake on scintiscan and clinical responsiveness to corticosteroids.[69]

### OTHER IMMUNOMODULATORY AGENTS

Plasma exchange or plasmapheresis with or without administration of immunosuppressive agents has been used without striking success. Other antiimmune therapies that have been used with mixed success include cyclophosphamide, ciamexone, and azathioprine as well as infusions of high-dose intravenous immunoglobulin. The results have not been promising.[13] One advantage of intravenous immunoglobulin over corticosteroids is the much lower incidence of adverse side effects.[70,71] Strategies are currently under way for the development of cytokine antagonists to be applied to the pathophysiology underlying Graves ophthalmopathy.[72] One limited clinical study describes a salutary effect achieved by pentoxifylline, a drug that in vitro has been shown to inhibit glycosaminoglycan synthesis and HLA-DR expression in orbital fibroblasts.[73]

## SUPERVOLTAGE THERAPY

Because of adverse side effects of corticosteroids and the inadvisability of long-term therapy, the physician may need to turn to supervoltage orbital radiotherapy or to surgical decompression. Indications for supervoltage therapy are (a) progression of exophthalmos under medical observation, (b) functional incapacitation because of progressive soft-tissue signs, (c) failure of corticosteroid therapy, (d) optic nerve neuropathy, and (e) as an adjunct to surgical decompression. The radiotherapy technique uses a 4-MeV linear accelerator to deliver 1800 to 2000 rad over 2 weeks.[74] In an extensive series of 311 patients (one-third of whom also received corticosteroids), 80% had soft-tissue improvement, 51% experienced a reduction in proptosis, 67% had improved vision, and 56% showed some improvement in eye muscle function.[75] A combination of prednisone, 40 to 80 mg, and supervoltage radiotherapy may be used as the initial treatment. Soft-tissue signs subside in an average of 6 weeks, and maximal improvement occurs by 3 months (Fig. 43-13). Patients who have short-term disease have the best response, whereas patients who have more chronic disease with significant proptosis and muscle dysfunction due to fibrosis are unlikely to receive any benefit. A diminution in exophthalmos and improvement in muscle balance may be seen, but approximately one-third of patients still require muscle surgery. Lid signs and herniation of retrobulbar fat through the orbital septum do not improve. Also, orbital radiotherapy is ineffective for proptosis without muscle enlargement or for long-standing ophthalmoplegia. Nevertheless, radiation is a safe, effective therapy that may reduce the time required to attain sufficient

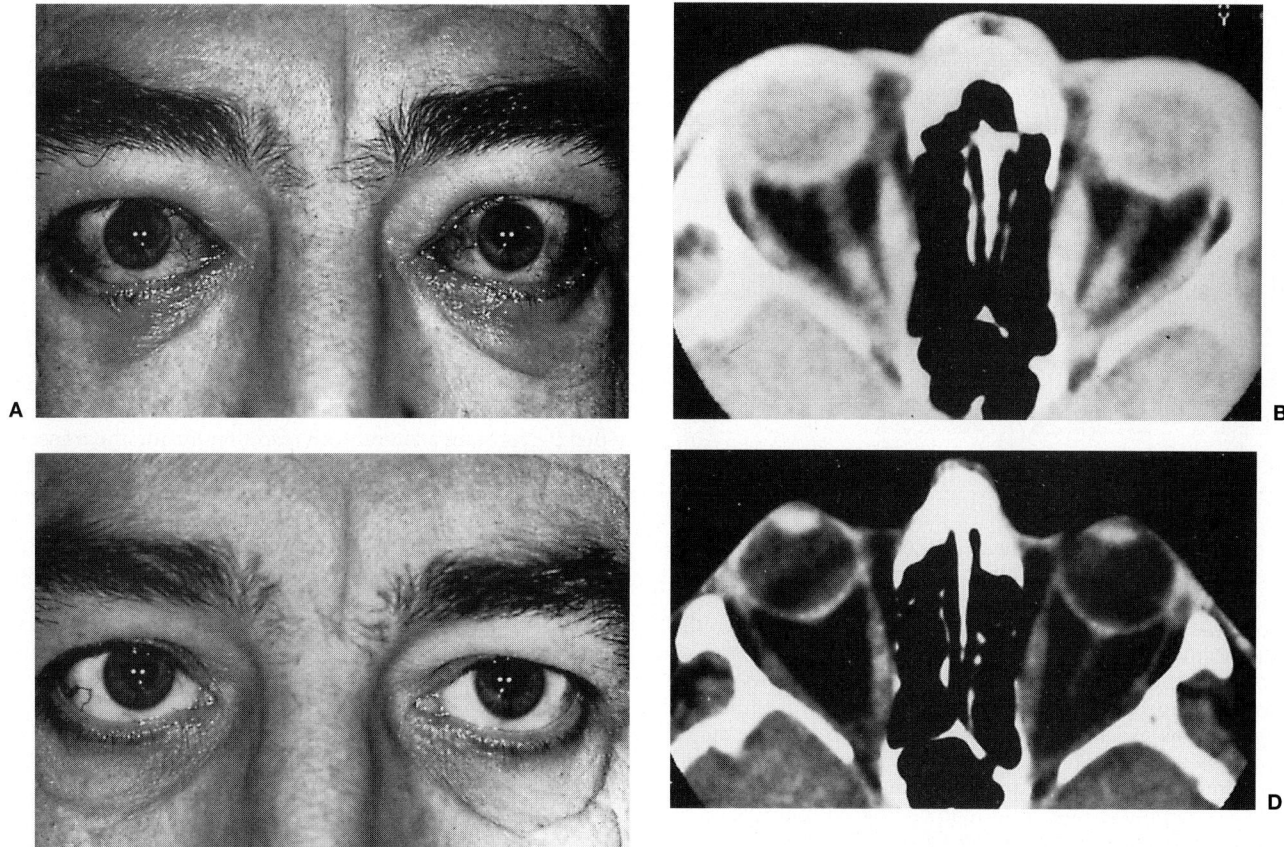

**FIGURE 43-13. A,** This 48-year-old man with Graves ophthalmopathy was vocationally incapacitated because of involvement of soft tissue and extraocular muscle. Note marked hyperemia and widened palpebral fissures in this view with eyes fixed in primary gaze. On attempted upward gaze, a marked restriction of elevation occurred because of tethered inferior rectus muscles in each eye. **B,** Transaxial computed tomographic (*CT*) scan of the patient. Note characteristic enlargement of extraocular muscles noted in endocrine ophthalmopathy. **C,** Appearance in primary gaze 3 months after orbital radiotherapy. The patient received 2000 rad in 10 fractional doses delivered over a period of 2 weeks by a 6-MeV linear accelerator using the technique of Kriss et al.[74] Note diminution of hyperemia and soft-tissue signs. Almost full extraocular motility was restored, and the patient was vocationally rehabilitated. **D,** The transaxial CT scan after orbital radiotherapy demonstrates marked diminution in size of extraocular muscles.

stability to allow surgical intervention. In one study[76] of the effects of orbital radiation plus corticosteroid therapy compared to corticosteroid use alone, the combination therapy was far more effective, particularly in those patients with disease of relatively short duration. An experienced radiotherapist should supervise this treatment to minimize the hazards of radiation retinitis and optic nerve necrosis.

The efficacy of orbital radiation therapy is putatively due to the radiosensitivity of lymphocytes infiltrating the orbit as well as to reduced proliferation and glycosaminoglycans production by orbital fibroblasts. The most remarkable improvement occurs within 1 year of onset or aggravation of the ophthalmopathy; it is primarily manifest in soft-tissue changes and minimally reduced proptosis, with little beneficial effect on the function of extraocular muscles. Such improvement is associated with the ability to discontinue use of corticosteroids within a few months in as many as 75% of patients. However, approximately one-third of patients still require posttreatment corrective eye surgery.

The excellent results observed when systemic corticosteroids are administered with retrobulbar irradiation[76] have led to some popularization of this combined modality of therapy in the past decade. In a randomized double-blind study of orbital irradiation versus corticosteroid use,[77] after 6 months, significant improvement was noted in approximately one-half of both treatment groups, results that lead to the conclusion that the therapies were equally effective. Follow-up for longer than 6 months would be of interest because one group has reported that the acute improvement in soft-tissue signs after irradiation may not translate into any apparent long-term benefit.[78] Proposed indications for retrobulbar irradiation and guidelines for management[13] will have to remain acceptable until availability of more definitive results dictates otherwise.

## SURGICAL DECOMPRESSION OF ORBIT

Relatively conservative orbital decompression can be accomplished with minimal invasiveness by removal of orbital fat.[79,80] More aggressive surgical decompression of the orbit may need to be the next step in therapy when fat removal and medical therapy with corticosteroids fail. This operation should be reserved for (a) severe proptosis with corneal exposure or ulceration, (b) optic neuropathy unresponsive to corticosteroid or orbital radiotherapy, (c) marked optic neuropathy in patients who cannot tolerate corticosteroids, and (d) cosmesis.

Historically, several decompressive operations of the orbit have been used, in which different regions of the bony orbit have been removed (Fig. 43-14). Currently, many ophthalmologists perform surgical decompression by a *transorbital approach* (Fig. 43-15) in which three walls of the orbit are removed; the lateral

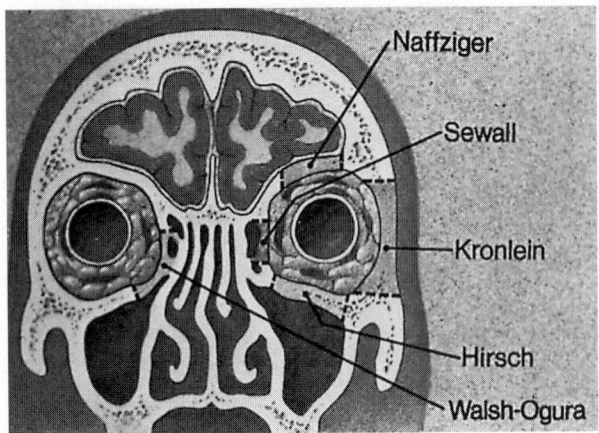

**FIGURE 43-14.** Schematic representation of region of bony orbit removed in several historical decompressive procedures.

wall, the floor, and the medial wall of the orbit may be removed in one stage. The otolaryngologist performs decompression by the *transantral approach*, removing the floor and medial wall.[81] Both of these approaches decompress the orbital contents into the paranasal sinuses. The transantral route allows better decompression of the orbital apex than does the transorbital procedure. Some neurosurgeons decompress the orbit by removal of the roof through a *transcranial or coronal approach*.[82] Both orbits may be decompressed in one stage by either the transcranial or transantral technique, if indicated. In the transorbital route, the surgeon usually decompresses one orbit, followed by decompression of the other, if needed, after 1 week (see Chap. 215).

A comparable degree of decompression has been reported with a *transnasal* endoscopic technique.[83] Chronic sinusitis is a contraindication to decompression into the paranasal sinuses. Restoration of visual acuity is comparable after either transantral or transcranial decompression, whereas the transorbital technique may require adjunctive orbital radiotherapy. All are equally effective in diminishing proptosis.

The transcranial approach has the highest morbidity. Transantral decompression is followed by increased diplopia caused by entrapment of the medial rectus muscles into the ethmoid sinuses in approximately two-thirds of cases, which requires further muscle surgery. Cerebrospinal fluid leaks are reported in a small percentage of patients undergoing transantral decompression resulting from penetration of the cribriform plate. Damage to the infraorbital sensory nerve may occur with either the transantral or orbital approach, resulting in permanent anesthesia of the upper lip and gum. Pain in the jaw when eating or chewing frequently occurs if the temporalis muscle is severed when performing a lateral wall resection during the transorbital approach. Pulsation of the orbital structures may be noted after transcranial decompression. Pneumoproptosis may occur with either transorbital or transantral decompression if an ethmoid air cell ruptures into the orbital tissues after removal of the medial wall. To avoid this frightening experience, patients undergoing this procedure should be warned not to blow their noses forcefully. However, the air rapidly absorbs, and the proptosis subsides. A history of sudden proptosis and crepitation with confirmation by CT scan confirms this diagnosis.

## REFERENCES

1. Brain R. Pathogenesis and treatment of endocrine exophthalmos. Lancet 1959; 1:109.
2. McKenzie JM. Humoral factors in the pathogenesis of Graves' disease. Physiol Rev 1968; 48:252.

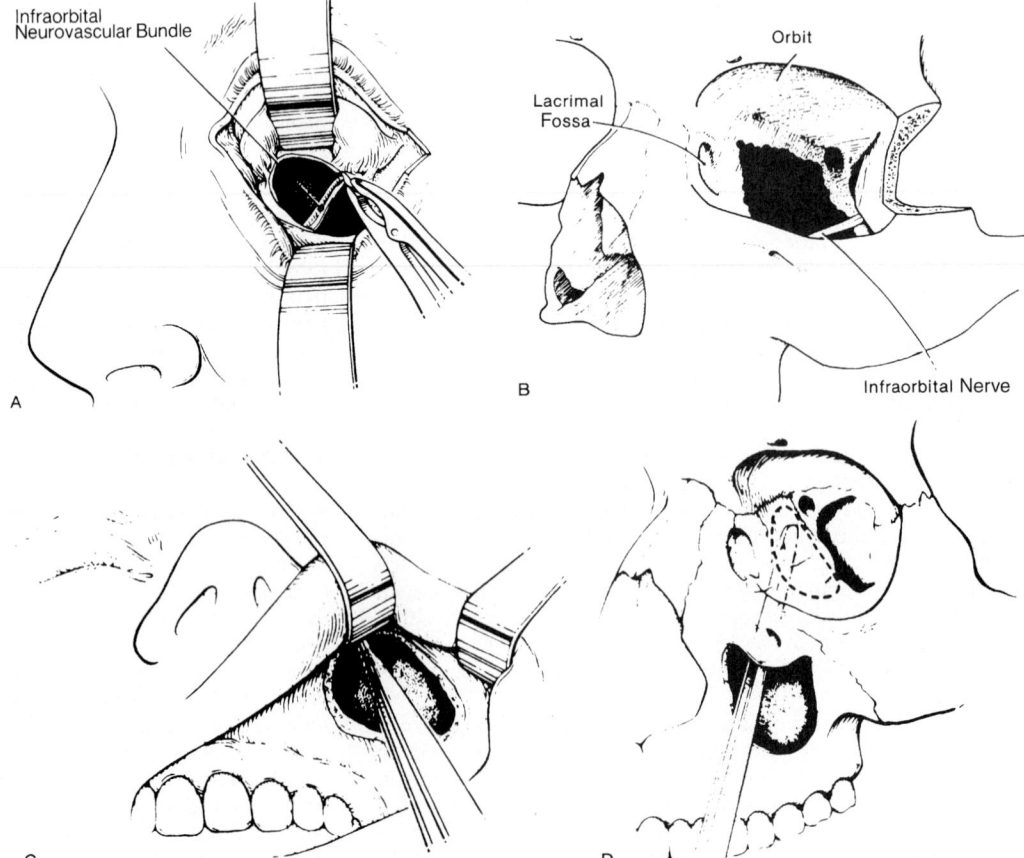

**FIGURE 43-15.** Commonly used orbital decompression procedures. **A,** *Transorbital approach,* followed by **B,** removal of the lateral wall, medial wall, and floor. **C,** *Transantral approach,* involving a buccogingival incision, followed by **D,** removal of the floor and medial wall of the orbit through the antrum and ethmoids. **A,** copyrighted by Emory, 1983.

3. Farid NR, Balazs C. The genetics of thyroid associated ophthalmopathy. Thyroid 1998; 8:407.

4. Werner SC. Modification of the classification of the eye changes of Graves' disease: recommendations of the Ad Hoc Committee of the American Thyroid Association. J Clin Endocrinol Metab 1977; 44:203.

5. Bartley GB. Evolution of classification systems for Graves' ophthalmopathy. Ophthal Plas Reconstr Surg 1995; 11:229.

6. Kendall-Taylor P, Perros P. Clinical presentation of thyroid associated orbitopathy. Thyroid 1998; 8:427.

7. Perros P, Kendall-Taylor P. Natural history of thyroid eye disease. Thyroid 1998; 8:423.

8. Bartley GB, Fatourechi V, Kkadrmas EF, et al. Clinical features of Graves' ophthalmopathy in an incidence cohort. Am J Ophthal 1996; 121:284.

9. Bartley GB, Fatourechi V, Kkadrmas EF, et al. The chronology of Graves' ophthalmopathy in an incidence cohort. Am J Ophthal 1996; 121:426.

10. Bartley GB, Fatourechi V, Kkadrmas EF, et al. Long-term follow-up of Graves' ophthalmopathy in an incidence cohort. Ophthal 1996; 103:958.

11. Bartley GB, Gorman CA. Diagnostic criteria for Graves' ophthalmopathy. Am J Ophthal 1995; 119:792.

12. Gorman CA. The measurement of change in Graves' ophthalmopathy. Thyroid 1998; 8:539.

13. Burch HB, Wartofsky L. Graves' ophthalmopathy: current concepts regarding pathogenesis and management. Endocr Rev 1993; 14:747.

14. Bahn RS, Heufelder AE. Pathogenesis of Graves' ophthalmopathy. N Engl J Med 1993; 329:1468.

15. Gorman CA. Pathogenesis of Graves' ophthalmopathy. Thyroid 1994; 4:379.

16. Ludgate M, Crisp M, Lane C, et al. The thyrotropin receptor in thyroid eye disease. Thyroid 1998; 8:411.

17. Bahn RS, Dutton CM, Heufelder AE, Sarkar G. A genomic point mutation in the extracellular domain of the thyrotropin receptor in patients with Graves' ophthalmopathy. J Clin Endocrinol Metab 1994; 78:256.

18. Burch HB, Sellitti D, Barnes SG, et al. Thyrotropin receptor antisera for the detection of immunoreactive protein species in retroocular fibroblasts obtained from patients with Graves' ophthalmopathy. J Clin Endocrinol Metab 1994; 78:1384.

19. Baker JR Jr. Dissecting the immune response to the thyrotropin receptor in autoimmune thyroid disease. (Editorial). J Clin Endocrinol Metab 1993; 77:16.

20. Davies TF. The thyrotropin receptors spread themselves around. (Editorial). J Clin Endocrinol Metab 1994; 79:1232.

21. Spitzweg C, Joba W, Hunt N, Heufelder AE. Analysis of human thyrotropin receptor gene expression and immunoreactivity in human orbital tissue. Eur J Endocrinol 1997; 136:599.

22. Burman KD. Graves' ophthalmopathy: what is the initial abnormality? Eur J Endocrinol 1997; 136:583.

23. Paschke R, Metcalfe A, Alcalde L, et al. Presence of nonfunctional thyrotropin receptor variant transcripts in retroocular and other tissues. J Clin Endocrinol Metab 1994; 79:1234.

24. Heufelder AE, Bahn RS. Soluble intercellular adhesion molecule-1 (sICAM-1) in sera of patients with Graves' ophthalmopathy and thyroid diseases. Clin Exp Immunol 1993; 92:296.

25. Bahn RS. Cytokines in thyroid eye disease: potential for anticytokine therapy. Thyroid 1998; 8:415.

26. Kahaly G, Forster G, Hansen C. Glycosaminoglycans in thyroid eye disease. Thyroid 1998; 8:429.

27. Marcocci C, Bartalena L, Bogazzi F, et al. Relationship between Graves' ophthalmopathy and type of treatment of Graves' hyperthyroidism. Thyroid 1992; 2:171.

28. Manso PG, Furlanetto RP, Wolosker AMB, et al. Prospective and controlled study of ophthalmopathy after radioiodine therapy for Graves' hyperthyroidism. Thyroid 1998; 8:49.

29. Tallstedt L, Lundell G, Torring O, et al. Occurrence of ophthalmopathy after treatment for Graves' hyperthyroidism. N Engl J Med 1992; 326:1733.

30. Kung AWC, Yau CC, Cheng A. The incidence of ophthalmopathy after radioiodine therapy for Graves' disease: prognostic factors and the role of methimazole. J Clin Endocrinol Metab 1994; 79:542.

31. Burmeister LA, Beatty RL, Wall JR. Malignant ophthalmopathy presenting one week after radioiodine treatment of hyperthyroidism. Thyroid 1999; 9:189.

32. Soliman M, Kaplan E, Abdel-Latif A, et al. Does thyroidectomy, radioactive iodine therapy, or antithyroid drug treatment alter reactivity of patients' T cells to epitopes of thyrotropin receptor in autoimmune thyroid diseases? J Clin Endocrinol Metab 1995; 80:2312.

33. Gunji K, Kubota S, Swanson JIL, et al. Role of the eye muscles in thyroid eye disease: identification of the principal autoantigens. Thyroid 1998; 8:553.

34. Burch HB, Lahiri S, Bahn RS, Barnes S. Superoxide radical production stimulates retroocular fibroblast proliferation in Graves' ophthalmopathy. Exp Eye Res 1997; 65:311.

35. Bertelsen JB, Hegedus L. Cigarette smoking and the thyroid. Thyroid 1994; 4:327.

36. Bartalena L, Marcocci C, Tanda ML, et al. Cigarette smoking and treatment outcomes in Graves' ophthalmopathy. Ann Intern Med 1998; 129:632.

37. Hofbauer LC, Muhlberg T, Konig A, et al. Soluble IL-1 receptor antagonist serum levels in smokers and nonsmokers with Graves' ophthalmopathy undergoing orbital radiotherapy. J Clin Endocrinol Metab 1997; 82:2244.

38. Fernandez-Sanchez JR, Pradas JR, Martinez OC, et al. Graves' ophthalmopathy after subtotal thyroidectomy and radioiodine therapy. Br J Surg 1993; 80:1134.

39. Bartalena L, Marcocci C, Bogazzi F, et al. Relation between therapy for hyperthyroidism and the course of Graves' ophthalmopathy. N Engl J Med 1998; 338:73.

40. Sridama V, DeGroot LJ. Treatment of Graves' disease and the course of ophthalmopathy. Am J Med 1989; 87:70.

41. Bartalena L, Marcocci C, Bogazzi F, et al. Use of corticosteroids to prevent progression of Graves' ophthalmopathy after radioiodine therapy for hyperthyroidism. N Engl J Med 1989; 321:349.

42. Gorman CA. Temporal relationship between onset of Graves' ophthalmopathy and diagnosis of thyrotoxicosis. Mayo Clin Proc 1983; 58:515.

43. Wiersinga WM, Smit T, VanderGaag R, Koorneef L. Temporal relationship between onset of Graves' ophthalmopathy and onset of thyroidal Graves' disease. J Endocrinol Invest 1988; 11:615.

44. Hufnagel TH, Hickey WF, Cobbs WH, et al. Immunohistochemical and ultrastructural studies on the exenterated orbital tissues of a patient with Graves' disease. Ophthalmology 1984; 91:1411.

45. Trokel SL, Jakobiec FA. Correlation of CT scanning and pathologic features of ophthalmic Graves' disease. Ophthalmology 1981; 88:553.

46. Trobe JD. Optic nerve involvement in dysthyroidism. Ophthalmology 1981; 88:488.

47. Gamblin GT, Harper DG, Galentine P, et al. Screening for elevated intraocular pressure in Graves' disease: evidence of frequent subclinical ophthalmology. N Engl J Med 1983; 208:420.

48. Salvi M, Spaggiari E, Neri F, et al. The study of visual evoked potentials in patients with thyroid-associated ophthalmopathy identifies asymptomatic optic nerve involvement. J Clin Endocrinol Metab 1997; 82:1027.

49. Hauer J. Additional clinical signs of "unilateral" endocrine exophthalmos. Br J Ophthalmol 1969; 53:210.

50. Bartley GB. The differential diagnosis and classification of eyelid retraction. Ophthalmol 1996; 103:168.

51. Bailey CC, Kabala J, Laitt R, et al. Magnetic resonance imaging in thyroid eye disease. Eye 1996; 10:617.

52. Nianiaris N, Hurwitz JJ, Chen JC, Wortzman G. Correlation between computed tomography and magnetic resonance imaging in Graves' orbitopathy. Can J Ophthalmol 1994; 29:9.

53. DeGroot JJ, Gorman CA, Pinchera A, et al. Therapeutic controversies: radiation and Graves' ophthalmopathy. J Clin Endocrinol Metab 1995; 80:339.

54. Bahn RS, Gorman CA. Choice of therapy and criteria for assessing treatment outcome in thyroid-associated ophthalmopathy. Endocrinol Metab Clin North Am 1987; 16:391.

55. Tallstedt L. Surgical treatment of thyroid eye disease. Thyroid 1998; 8:447.

56. Prummel MF, Wiersinga WM. Immunomodulatory treatment of Graves' ophthalmopathy. Thyroid 1998; 8:545.

57. Wiersinga WM. Novel drugs for the therapy of Graves' ophthalmopathy. In: Wall JR, How J, eds. Graves' ophthalmopathy. Cambridge, MA: Blackwell Scientific, 1990:111.

58. Kahaly G, Schrezenmeir J, Krause U, et al. Cyclosporine and prednisone in treatment of Graves' ophthalmopathy: a controlled, randomized and prospective study. Eur J Clin Invest 1986; 16:415.

59. Prummel MF, Mourits MP, Berghout A, et al. Prednisone and cyclosporine in the treatment of severe Graves' ophthalmopathy. N Engl J Med 1989; 321:1353.

60. Ozata M, Bolu E, Sengul A, et al. Effects of octreotide treatment on Graves' ophthalmopathy and circulating sICAM-1 levels. Thyroid 1996; 6:283.

61. DeBellis A, SiMartino S, Fiordelisi F, et al. Soluble intercellular adhesion molecule-1 (sICAM-1) concentrations in Graves' disease patients followed up for development of ophthalmopathy. J Clin Endocrinol Metab 1998; 83:1222.

62. Kahaly GJ, Gorges R, Diaz M, et al. Indium-111-pentreotide in Graves' disease. J Nucl Med 1998; 39:533.

63. Wiersinga WM, Gerding MN, Prummel MF, Krenning EP. Octreotide scintigraphy in thyroidal and orbital Graves' disease. Thyroid 1998; 8:433.

64. Postema PTE, Krenning EP, Wijngaarde R, et al. [111In-DTPA-D-phe1]-Octreotide scintigraphy in thyroidal and orbital Graves' disease: a parameter for disease activity. J Clin Endocrinol Metab 1994; 79:1845.

65. Kahaly GJ, Forster GJ. Somatostatin receptor scintigraphy in thyroid eye disease. Thyroid 1998; 8:549.

66. Krassas GE. Somatostatin analogues in the treatment of thyroid eye disease. Thyroid 1998; 8:443.

67. Krassas GE, Kaltsas T, Dumas A, et al. Lanreotide in the treatment of patients with thyroid eye disease. Eur J Endocrinol 1997; 136:416.

68. Kung AWC, Michon J, Tai KS, Chan FL. The effect of somatostatin versus corticosteroid in the treatment of Graves' ophthalmopathy. Thyroid 1996; 6:381, 489.

69. Colao A, Lastoria S, Ferone D, et al. Orbital scintigraphy with [111In-diethylenetriamine pentaacetic acid-D-phe1]-Octreotide predicts the clinical response to corticosteroid therapy in patients with Graves' ophthalmopathy. J Clin Endocrinol Metab 1998; 83:3790.

70. Kahaly GJ, Pitz S, Muller-Forell W, Hommel G. Randomized trial of intravenous immunoglobulins versus prednisolone in Graves' ophthalmopathy. Clin Exp Immunol 1996; 106:197.

71. Baschieri L, Antonelli A, Nardi S, et al. Intravenous immunoglobulin versus corticosteroid in treatment of Graves' ophthalmopathy. Thyroid 1997; 7:579.

72. Bartalena L, Marcocci C, Pinchera A. Cytokine antagonists: new ideas for the management of Graves' ophthalmopathy. (Editorial). J Clin Endocrinol Metab 1996; 81:446.

73. Balazs C, Kiss E, Vamos A, et al. Beneficial effect of pentoxifylline on thyroid associated ophthalmopathy: a pilot study. J Clin Endocrinol Metab 1997; 82:1999.

74. Kriss JP, McDougall IR, Donaldson SS. Graves ophthalmopathy. In: Krieger DT, Bardin W, eds. Current therapy in endocrinology 1983-84. New York: Decker, 1984:104.

75. Peterson IA, Kriss JP, McDougall IR, Donaldson SS. Prognostic factors in the radiotherapy of Graves' ophthalmopathy. Int J Radiat Oncol Biol Phys 1990; 19:259.

76. Bartalena L, Marcocci C, Chiovato L, et al. Orbital cobalt irradiation combined with systemic corticosteroids for Graves' ophthalmopathy: comparison with systemic corticosteroids alone. J Clin Endocrinol Metab 1983; 56:1139.

77. Prummel MF, Mourits MP, Blank L, et al. Randomized double-blind trial of prednisone versus radiotherapy in Graves' ophthalmopathy. Lancet 1993; 342:949.

78. Kao SCS, Kendler DL, Nugent RA, et al. Radiotherapy in the management of thyroid orbitopathy. Arch Ophthalmol 1993; 111:819.

79. Trokel S, Kazim M, Moore S. Orbital fat removal: decompression for Graves' ophthalmopathy. Ophthalmology 1993; 100:674.

80. Adenis JP, Robert PY, Lasudry JG, Dalloul Z. Treatment of proptosis with fat removal orbital decompression in Graves' ophthalmopathy. Eur J Ophthal 1998; 8:246.

81. Garrity JA, Fatourechi V, Bergstralh EJ, et al. Results of transantral orbital decompression in 428 patients with severe Graves' ophthalmopathy. Am J Ophthal 1993; 116:533.

82. Kalmann R, Mourits MP, van der Pol JP, Koornneef L. Coronal approach for rehabilitative orbital decompression in Graves' ophthalmopathy. Br J Ophthalmol 1997; 81:41.

83. Lund VJ, Larkin G, Fells P, Adams G. Orbital decompression for thyroid eye disease: a comparison of external and endoscopic techniques. J Laryngol Otol 1997; 111:1051.

# CHAPTER 44

# SURGERY OF THE THYROID GLAND

EDWIN L. KAPLAN

The modern era of thyroid surgery began in the 1860s with the work of Billroth and colleagues.[1] Operative techniques and results were so greatly advanced by Kocher[2] and others that, by 1920, Halsted[3] referred to thyroidectomy as a "feat which today can be accomplished by any competent operator without danger of mishap." Decades later, some complications still occur. Nevertheless, with advances in diagnosis and surgical technique, thyroidectomy is one of the safest and most effective major operations performed today.

## PREPARATION FOR SURGERY

Most patients undergoing thyroid surgery are euthyroid and require no specific preoperative preparation other than standard preoperative examination and a few tests. A serum calcium value should be determined, and fiberoptic laryngoscopy should be performed, especially in those patients who have had previous thyroid or parathyroid operations, to detect an unrecognized recurrent laryngeal nerve injury.

## HYPOTHYROIDISM

Myxedema creates great potential for morbidity and even mortality from the effects of both the anesthesia and the operation.[4] Severely hypothyroid patients have a higher incidence of perioperative hypotension, gastrointestinal hypomotility, prolonged anesthetic recovery, and neuropsychiatric disturbances. In addition, they are very sensitive to preoperative medication. Thus, when severe myxedema is present, deferring elective surgery until a euthyroid state is achieved is preferable. Urgent surgery need not be postponed simply for repletion of thyroid hormone, however. Guidelines for thyroxine therapy appear in Chapter 45.

## HYPERTHYROIDISM

A number of different regimens are available for the preoperative preparation of patients with thyrotoxicosis; for example, iodine alone; propylthiouracil (PTU) plus iodine; PTU or methimazole (Tapazole) plus thyroxine plus iodine; PTU plus propranolol plus iodine; propranolol plus iodine; and propranolol alone. The author's patients are typically prepared for operation by the use of PTU or methimazole, plus iodine, with or without the addition of propranolol. Each treatment has advantages and disadvantages; however, the preoperative restoration of euthyroidism is recommended.[5] Most patients are treated initially with an antithyroid drug, PTU or methimazole, until they approach a normal thyroid state. Many surgeons then prefer to administer several drops of iodine (saturated solution of potassium iodide, or SSKI), two to three times a day, for 8 to 10 days or longer before surgery. The iodine decreases the vascularity and increases the firmness of the gland.

The β-adrenergic receptor blockers, such as propranolol, are useful in the control of tremor, tachycardia, and cardiac arrhythmias. Many surgeons have had excellent results with the use of propranolol, alone[6] or with iodine, as preoperative treatment of Graves disease, citing ease and speed of preparation as the major advantages.[7] However, reliance on this drug alone may be hazardous,[8] and reserving the use of propranolol alone (or with iodine) for selected patients who are allergic to antithyroid medications may be wise. When patients are treated with propranolol alone preoperatively, this drug must be continued into the postoperative period as well, because such patients are still thyrotoxic at that time.

The medical management of Graves disease has been discussed in detail in Chapter 42. However, the advantages and disadvantages of the two ablative approaches to treatment (i.e., surgery or radioiodine therapy) are listed in Table 44-1. The author uses subtotal thyroidectomy in young patients with Graves disease, primarily because it rapidly corrects the thyrotoxic state with decreased risk of hypothyroidism, while avoiding the potential risks of radioiodine therapy.[5] Operations include bilateral subtotal lobectomies or unilateral lobectomy with contralateral subtotal lobectomy. To minimize the recurrence of disease, only several grams of thyroid tissue are left. When the surgery is to treat ophthalmopathy, however, a near-total or total thyroidectomy should be performed.

## SURGICAL APPROACH TO THYROID NODULES

### NON-IRRADIATED PATIENTS

Fine-needle aspiration with cytologic examination is heavily relied on when choosing patients for surgery. Generally, any nodule suspected of being a carcinoma should be completely removed, along with surrounding tissue; thus, a total lobectomy (or lobectomy with isthmusectomy) is the initial operation of choice in most patients. A frozen section should be obtained intraoperatively. If the diagnosis of a colloid nodule is made, the surgery is terminated. If a diagnosis of an adenoma is made, then difficulty arises of differentiating, on frozen section,

**TABLE 44-1.**
**Ablative Treatment of Graves Disease with Thyrotoxicosis**

| Method | Dose or Extent of Surgery | Onset of Response | Complications | Remarks |
|---|---|---|---|---|
| **Surgery** | Subtotal (90–95%) excision of gland | Immediate | Mortality: <1% <br> Permanent hypothyroidism: 20–30% <br> Recurrent hyperthyroidism: <10% <br> Vocal cord paralysis: ~1% <br> Hypoparathyroidism: ~1% | Applicable in younger patients and pregnant women |
| **Radioiodine ($^{131}$I)** | 5–10 mCi | Several weeks to months | Permanent hypothyroidism: 50%–70%, often with delayed onset <br> Multiple treatments sometimes necessary <br> Recurrence possible | Potential risks require ongoing study <br> Close long-term follow-up needed <br> Avoid in pregnant women and use carefully in children |

a follicular adenoma from a follicular carcinoma, or a benign Hürthle cell tumor from a Hürthle cell carcinoma.[9] These diagnoses require the careful assessment of cellular morphology as well as capsular and vascular invasion, which are often difficult to evaluate on frozen section analyses. To aid in the diagnosis, enlarged lymph nodes of the central compartment are sampled and a biopsy of the jugular nodes is also performed. If the results are negative, two options exist: (a) stopping the surgery after lobectomy, with the understanding that a second operation may be necessary to complete the thyroidectomy if a carcinoma is ultimately found, or (b) performing a subtotal resection of the contralateral lobe. This latter approach is often used if the patient consents, particularly when a preoperative needle aspiration suggests that a follicular lesion will be encountered intraoperatively (see Chap. 39).[10]

## IRRADIATED PATIENTS

In patients who have been exposed to low-dose, external radiation to the head and neck during infancy, childhood, or adolescence, because of the frequency of bilateral disease, the known coincidence of benign and malignant nodules in the same gland, and the prevalence of papillary carcinoma in 35% to 40% of patients, a near-total resection of the thyroid gland with a biopsy of the jugular nodes is usually performed, even if a frozen section of the dominant nodule is benign.[11] This therapy is thought to be advantageous because the remaining thyroid remnant of these patients can usually be ablated with one 30-mCi dose of radioiodine given on an outpatient basis if a carcinoma is found later.[12] Of course, if a carcinoma is diagnosed on frozen section, a total thyroidectomy is attempted. In any event, these patients require therapy with thyroid hormone. Patients who have received high-dose radiation to the thyroid bed, such as those treated with mantle radiation for Hodgkin disease, are also at greater risk for developing thyroid carcinomas years later; they should be followed carefully and their disease should be treated aggressively.

# SURGICAL APPROACH TO THYROID CANCER

## PAPILLARY CARCINOMA

The surgical treatment of papillary carcinoma (see Chap. 40) is best divided into two categories, based on the clinical characteristics and virulence of these lesions.

### MINIMAL PAPILLARY CARCINOMA

The term *minimal papillary carcinoma* refers to a small papillary tumor, usually <5 mm in diameter, that demonstrates no local invasiveness through the thyroid capsule, is not associated with lymph node metastases, and is often found in a young person as an occult lesion when thyroidectomy has been performed for another benign condition.[13] In such instances, lobectomy is sufficient and repeated surgeries are unnecessary; thyroid hormone is given to suppress serum thyroid-stimulating hormone (TSH) levels, and the patient is followed at regular intervals.

### STANDARD TREATMENT FOR MOST PAPILLARY CARCINOMAS

Most papillary carcinomas are neither minimal nor occult. Papillary cancers are known to be microscopically multicentric in up to 80% of cases, occasionally to invade locally into the trachea or esophagus,[14] to metastasize commonly to lymph nodes and later to the lungs and other tissues, and to recur clinically in the other thyroid lobe in 7% to 18% of patients if treated by only thyroid lobectomy.[15,16]

In the United States, ~1200 deaths occur each year from thyroid cancer and half of these deaths occur in patients with anaplastic thyroid carcinoma. Importantly, most patients with papillary thyroid cancer have a very good prognosis, particularly those who are young. Although the best treatment for most papillary cancers is near-total or total thyroidectomy, with appropriate central and lateral neck dissections when nodes are involved, the surgeon with limited experience should not perform total thyroidectomy unless capable of achieving a low incidence of recurrent laryngeal nerve injuries and permanent hypoparathyroidism. Otherwise, referral of these patients to a major medical center where such expertise is available may be advisable. Often, patients are treated with radioactive iodine postoperatively[17] (see Chap. 40). External irradiation and chemotherapy[17] are sometimes used for those special cases of severe, extensive disease that do not accumulate radioiodine.[18] In some studies,[19] patients receiving total or near-total thyroidectomy with radioiodine therapy for papillary cancers of 1 cm or larger had decreased mortality and recurrence of disease compared with those receiving lesser operations and no radioactive iodine therapy.

Studies have attempted to predict the potential aggressiveness of a given papillary carcinoma by determination of nuclear DNA measurement[20] as well as by formulations of a set of risk factors, including the age of the patient, the size of the tumor, presence or absence of local invasion or distant metastases, the tumor grade, and whether or not all tumor could be resected.[16,21,22] Clearly, young patients with small tumors that can be totally resected and that exhibit no local invasion or distant metastases have an excellent prognosis (approximately a 2% mortality from their papillary cancer). Older age, larger tumor size, local tumor invasiveness, presence of distant metastases, and nonresectable tumor are factors that portend a much greater cancer mortality. Approximately 80% of all papillary cancers fall in the low-risk category by these criteria, but 20% are much more aggressive.

## FOLLICULAR CARCINOMA

The prevalence of true follicular cancers has greatly diminished in recent years, perhaps due to an increase in iodine in the diet. Multicentricity of follicular carcinoma within the thyroid and lymph node metastases is less common than with papillary cancer. Metastatic spread occurs to the lungs, bones, and other peripheral tissues by hematogenous dissemination.

The ideal operation for follicular carcinoma is similar to that for papillary cancer, but the rationale differs. Small lesions with only minimal capsular invasion and no vascular invasion have a very good prognosis and require only lobectomy. Near-total or total thyroidectomy should be performed not for multicentricity but to make possible a later total body scan with radioiodine. If peripheral metastases are detected, they should be treated with high-dose radioiodine therapy.[17] In patients with either papillary or follicular cancer, if lymph node metastases are present in the lateral neck, a modified radical neck dissection should be performed (see Chap. 40). Prophylactic modified radical neck dissections, in the absence of clinical disease, should not be performed for differentiated thyroid cancers.

## ANAPLASTIC CARCINOMA

Anaplastic thyroid carcinoma remains one of the most virulent of all malignancies. Survival for most of these patients is measured in months. The type previously termed "small cell" is now considered to be a lymphoma by most pathologists and is treated by a combination of surgery, external radiation, and chemotherapy.[23] In treating lymphoma of the thyroid, major surgical resection has not been shown to be of therapeutic benefit. Therefore, operative management is usually limited to obtaining an adequate biopsy. The large cell type may present as a solitary thyroid nodule early in its clinical course and, if surgery is undertaken at that time, a near-total or total thyroidectomy should be performed, with appropriate central and lateral neck dissections. However, most commonly, the carcinoma is advanced when the patient is first evaluated. In these patients, surgical cure is unlikely, no matter how aggressive; in particularly advanced cases, diagnosis by needle biopsy or by small open biopsy may be all that is appropriate. Sometimes, the isthmus can be divided to relieve tracheal compression, or a tracheostomy might be beneficial. Most treatment, however, is by external radiotherapy or chemotherapy or both.[24] Hyperfractionation external radiation therapy that uses several treatments per day has some enthusiasts. Radioiodine treatment is ineffective because tumor uptake is absent. Although some success has been observed with doxorubicin, prolonged remissions are rarely achieved and multidrug regimens and combinations of chemotherapy with radiotherapy are being tried.[18] Currently, the author's protocol involves preoperative treatment with a chemotherapy regimen of cisplatin, hydroxyurea, and Taxol with external radiation therapy of 7500 rads. Total thyroidectomy follows if no distant metastases are present.[25] (Also see Chap. 41.)

## MEDULLARY THYROID CARCINOMA

Medullary thyroid carcinoma is a C-cell, calcitonin-producing tumor that contains amyloid or an amyloid-like substance, may secrete other peptides and amines, and may be transmitted in a familial pattern (see Chaps. 40 and 188). This tumor, or its precursor, C-cell hyperplasia, occurs as a part of the multiple endocrine neoplasia type 2 syndromes (MEN2A and MEN2B), as well as the less common familial medullary thyroid cancer syndrome.[26,26a,26b] Hence, patients with medullary thyroid carcinoma should be screened for hyperparathyroidism and pheochromocytoma. If a pheochromocytoma or adrenal medullary hyperplasia is present, this should be operated on first, because it represents the greatest immediate risk.

Medullary thyroid carcinoma is unilateral in sporadic cases and bilateral (often with C-cell hyperplasia when familial). It spreads to lymph nodes of the neck and mediastinum and later disseminates to the lungs, bone, liver, and elsewhere. The tumor is relatively radioresistant, it does not take up radioiodine, and it is not responsive to thyroid hormone suppression. Hence, an aggressive surgical approach is mandatory. The operation of choice for medullary thyroid carcinoma is total thyroidectomy with an extensive central compartment dissection down into the mediastinum. Lateral nodes are sampled. If central or lateral lymph nodes contain tumor, then appropriate unilateral or bilateral modified radical neck dissections are required. Repeated surgeries for metastatic tumor based on catheterization studies with blood sampling and calcitonin determinations alone have been proposed by some groups.[27] Others believe that surgery should be repeated only after localization of metastatic disease, usually by magnetic resonance imaging or computed tomographic scanning.[28] Octreotide or thallium scanning and positron emission tomography are useful in localizing metastatic diseases.[29,30] Extensive reoperations of the central and lateral neck compartments have rendered 25% to 30% of patients eucalcitonemic.[27,31] Some surgeons recommend laparoscopic evaluation of the liver to rule out metastatic disease before repeat operations in the neck are performed.[31]

Cure has been shown to be most frequent in young patients with familial disease whose disease was found by calcitonin screening[26] or by screening of the RET oncogene.[32,33] Prophylactic thyroidectomy is now being practiced at age 5 in patients with MEN2A who exhibit a mutated RET oncogene. Children of families with MEN2B who exhibit a mutated RET oncogene are given prophylactic surgery at an earlier age. Patients with MEN2A have a better prognosis than those with sporadic tumor, but patients with MEN2B have very aggressive tumors and often do not survive past age 40 years. In some patients, postoperative radiotherapy has been used, but most clinicians reserve this treatment for disease that cannot be resected.

In MEN2 syndromes, bilateral adrenalectomy is thought to be appropriate by some investigators if a pheochromocytoma or adrenal medullary hyperplasia is diagnosed, because each is likely to be a bilateral condition (see Chap. 188). Others believe that, especially in young children with an apparent unilateral pheochromocytoma, only the affected gland should be removed first, with the knowledge that the other gland may have to be removed in the future. This method has the advantage of permitting the child to grow with normal adrenal cortical function for a period of time. One report[34] supports unilateral adrenalectomy, because 48% of patients did not develop a pheochromocytoma in the other gland at 5.2 years of follow-up and no hypertensive crises occurred in these individuals. Furthermore, 23% of patients had an addisonian crisis after bilateral adrenalectomy with the occurrence of one death. Subtotal parathyroidectomy is necessary if primary hyperparathyroidism is diagnosed in MEN2A patients, because parathyroid hyperplasia is almost always present (see Chaps. 58 and 62).

## OPERATIVE TECHNIQUE FOR THYROIDECTOMY[35-37]

While under general endotracheal anesthesia, the patient is placed in a supine position with the neck extended. A low collar incision is made and is carried down through the subcutaneous tissue and platysma muscle. Superior and inferior flaps are developed, and the strap muscles are divided vertically in the midline and retracted laterally.

The thyroid lobe is bluntly dissected free from its investing fascia and rotated medially. The thyroid isthmus is often divided early in the dissection. The middle thyroid vein is ligated. The superior pole of the thyroid is dissected free, and care is taken to identify and preserve the external branch of the superior laryngeal nerve (Fig. 44-1). The superior pole vessels are ligated adjacent to the thyroid lobe, rather than ceph-

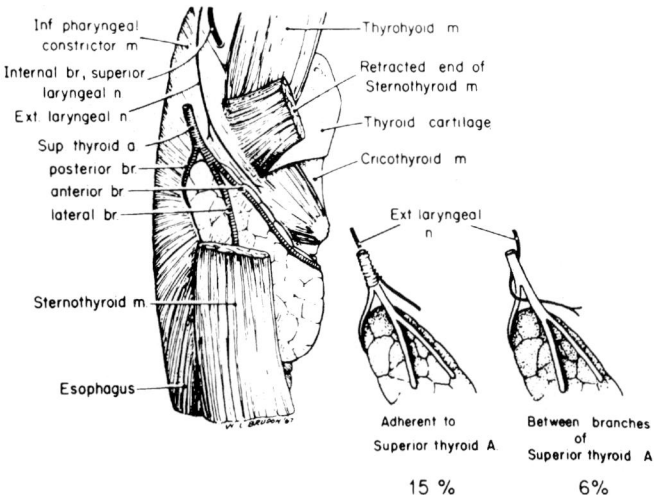

**FIGURE 44-1.** Proximity of the external branch of the superior laryngeal nerve to the superior thyroid vessels is clearly shown. (*Inf.*, inferior; *m.*, muscle; *br.*, branch; *n.*, nerve; *ext.*, external; *Sup.*, superior; *a.*, artery.) (From Moosman DA, DeWeese MS. The external laryngeal nerve as related to thyroidectomy. Surg Gynecol Obstet 1968; 127:1011. By permission of Surgery, Gynecology, & Obstetrics, now known as the Journal of the American College of Surgeons.)

alad to it, to prevent damage to this nerve. The inferior thyroid artery and recurrent laryngeal nerve are identified. To preserve the blood supply to the parathyroid glands, the inferior thyroid artery should not be ligated laterally; rather, its branches should be ligated individually on the capsule of the lobe after they have supplied the parathyroid glands (Fig. 44-2). The parathyroid glands are identified and an attempt is made to leave each with an adequate blood supply. Any parathyroid gland that appears to be devascularized can be minced and implanted into the sternocleidomastoid muscle after its identification by frozen section. Care is taken to identify the recurrent laryngeal nerve along its entire course if a

total lobectomy is to be done. The nerve is gently unroofed from surrounding tissue so that trauma to it is avoided. The nerve is in greatest danger near the junction of the trachea with the larynx, because here it is adjacent to the thyroid gland. Once the nerve and parathyroid glands have been identified and preserved, the thyroid lobe can be removed from its tracheal attachments (ligament of Berry). The contralateral thyroid lobe is removed in a similar manner when a *total thyroidectomy* is performed. A near-total thyroidectomy means that a small amount of thyroid tissue is left on the contralateral side to protect the parathyroid glands and recurrent nerve.[38,39] Careful hemostasis and visualization of all important anatomic structures are mandatory for success. The strap muscles are approximated in the midline with only one suture to decrease the possibility of a hematoma in this deep space, which could result in tracheal compression. Several deep dermal sutures of 4-0 absorbable sutures are used. The dermis is approximated by a subcuticular stitch of interrupted 5-0 synthetic absorbable sutures, and the skin edges are approximated with sterile paper tapes. A small suction catheter is often inserted through a stab wound and is usually removed by the following morning.

A *lateral neck dissection* is not done prophylactically for papillary or follicular cancer but, rather, only when metastatic disease is identified in the lateral triangle. "Cherry-picking operations" are not appropriate, but true modified radical lymph node dissections (Fig. 44-3), which leave the spinal accessory nerve, sternocleidomastoid muscle, and, in most cases, the jugular vein intact, are effective and provide a very satisfactory functional and cosmetic result.

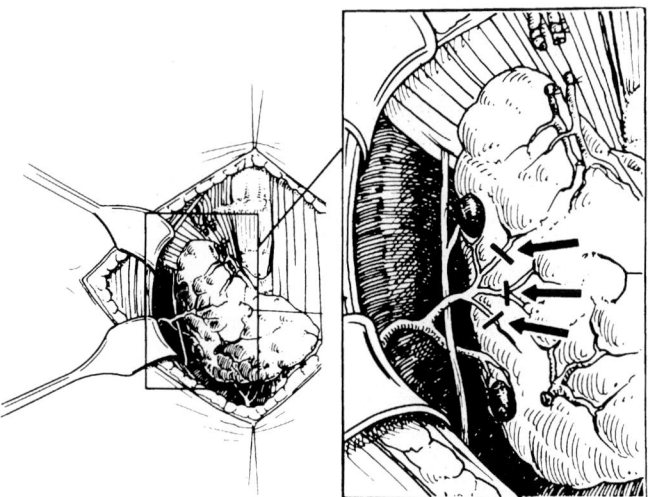

**FIGURE 44-2.** The thyroid lobe is retracted medially and, by careful blunt dissection, the recurrent laryngeal nerve, the inferior thyroid artery, and the parathyroid glands are identified. The inferior thyroid artery is not ligated laterally as a single trunk. Rather, each small branch is ligated and divided at a point distal to the parathyroid glands (*arrows*) to preserve their blood supply. Then, the thyroid lobe can be removed from its tracheal attachments if a lobectomy is to be performed. (From Kaplan EL. Surgery of the thyroid gland. In: De Groot LS, Larsen PR, Refetoff S, Stanbury JB, eds. The thyroid and its diseases. New York: John Wiley and Sons, 1984:851.)

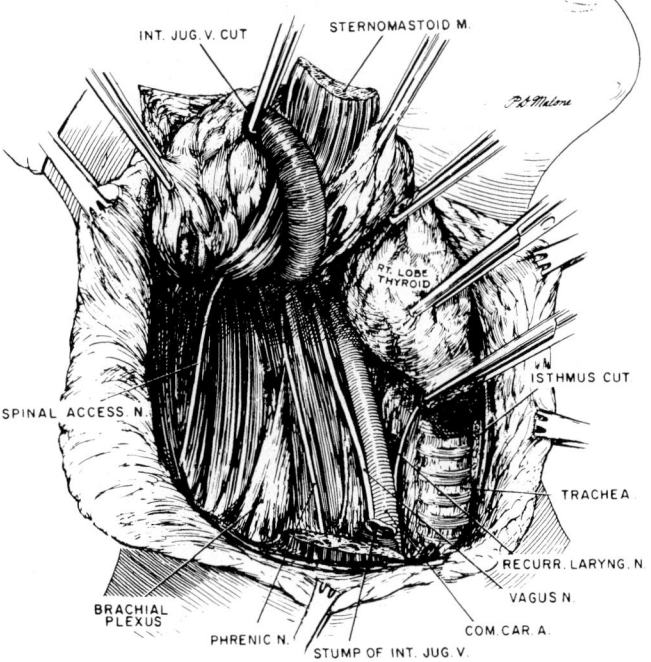

**FIGURE 44-3.** Modified radical neck dissection. The sternocleidomastoid muscle and internal jugular vein have been divided inferiorly and the dissection performed along the carotid sheath from below upward, exposing underlying structures. The thyroid gland is dissected free from the trachea, sparing the recurrent laryngeal nerve and leaving the parathyroid glands with a good blood supply. The vagus, phrenic, and spinal accessory nerves as well as the brachial plexus are left intact. At the end of the procedure, the divided sternocleidomastoid muscle can be reattached. In most instances, this muscle does not need to be divided, and the jugular vein can be left in situ if nodes are not fixed to it. (*Int. jug. v.*, internal jugular vein; *m.*, muscle; *Spinal access n.*, spinal accessory nerve; *Recurr. laryng. n.*, recurrent laryngeal nerve; *Com. car. a.*, common carotid artery.) (From Cady B, Rossi R. In: Surgery of the thyroid and parathyroid glands. Philadelphia: WB Saunders, 1991:204.)

*Subtotal thyroidectomy* is used for the surgical treatment of Graves disease. Two to 4 g of thyroid tissue should be left to attain satisfactory postoperative thyroid function without a high incidence of recurrent thyrotoxicosis. Less thyroid is left in young patients. When operations are performed for ophthalmopathy, a near-total or total thyroidectomy should be performed. Once more, the parathyroid glands and recurrent nerves should be identified and preserved in an intact state.

After a thyroidectomy, even with a modified radical neck dissection, the patient is almost always discharged on the first postoperative morning. Some surgeons currently discharge patients several hours after thyroidectomy, but the author thinks this is unsafe because late bleeding may occur. The skin tapes are removed at the time of the first outpatient visit, 8 to 10 days postoperatively.

Video-assisted thyroidectomy or *endoscopic resection of thyroid tumors* is being pioneered in several centers.[40–42] Its aim is to minimize the length of incisions in the neck or to hide the incisions by placing them below the clavicle or far lateral in the neck. In the hands of very skilled operators, the recurrent laryngeal nerve and parathyroid glands can be seen and a lobectomy performed. Other groups have performed mainly nodulectomy. Although this method may have merit for small lesions, the results and complications must be carefully assessed. Is the proper thyroid resection still being performed? Will there be a learning curve (as occurs with most new procedures) with increased rates of bleeding, nerve injuries, or hypoparathyroidism? Finally, do the improved cosmetic results warrant the possibility of greater morbidity? A careful assessment of the new procedures seems warranted.

# POSTOPERATIVE COMPLICATIONS

Many authors have reported large series of thyroidectomies with no deaths. In other reports, mortality does not differ greatly from that due to anesthesia alone. Four major complications are associated with thyroid surgery: thyroid storm, wound hemorrhage, recurrent laryngeal nerve injury, and hypoparathyroidism.

## THYROID STORM

Thyroid storm reflects an exacerbation of a thyrotoxic state and is seen most often in Graves disease, but it can occur rarely in patients with toxic adenoma or toxic multinodular goiter. Clinical manifestations and management of thyroid storm are discussed in Chapter 42.

## WOUND HEMORRHAGE

Wound hemorrhage with hematoma is an uncommon complication, reported in 0.3% to 1.0% of patients in most large series. However, it is a well recognized and potentially lethal complication. A small amount of hematoma deep to the strap muscles can compress the trachea. A suction closed-drainage system placed in the wound is not adequate for decompression if bleeding is from a major vessel. Swelling of the neck and bulging of the wound can be followed shortly thereafter by respiratory impairment. Treatment consists of immediately opening the wound and evacuating the clot, even at the bedside. Later, the bleeding vessel can be ligated in a careful and leisurely manner in the operating room. The urgency of treating this condition when it occurs cannot be overemphasized.

## INJURY TO THE RECURRENT LARYNGEAL NERVE

Recurrent laryngeal nerve injuries[43] occur in 1% to 2% or more of thyroid operations, especially when performed for malignant disease. The injuries can be unilateral or bilateral, temporary or permanent. Loss of function can be caused by transection, ligation, or handling of the nerve. In *unilateral recurrent nerve injuries*, the voice becomes husky because the vocal cords do not approximate one another. Usually vocal function returns within 6 to 9 months. If improvement is insufficient, injection of the paralyzed vocal cord with collagen may help.[44] One surgery involves insertion of a plug of silicone rubber, fashioned to the correct size to push the paralyzed vocal cord to the midline and thus improve vocal function.

*Bilateral recurrent laryngeal nerve damage* is much more serious because both vocal cords may assume a median or paramedian position, which results in airway obstruction and difficulty with respiratory toilet. Often, tracheostomy is required. Recurrent nerve injury is best avoided by always attempting to identify each nerve along its course. Accidental transection occurs most often at the level of the upper two tracheal rings, where the nerve is closely approximated to the thyroid lobe in the area of the ligament of Berry. If the transection is recognized, the transected nerve should be reapproximated by microsurgical techniques. A number of procedures to reinnervate the laryngeal muscles have been attempted with limited success.[45]

Injury to the *external branch of the superior laryngeal nerve* occurs when the upper pole vessels are divided (see Fig. 44-1) and results in an inability to forcefully project one's voice or to sing high notes. Often, this disability improves during the first 3 months after surgery.

## HYPOPARATHYROIDISM

The incidence of permanent hypoparathyroidism has been reported to be as high as 20% when a total thyroidectomy and radical neck dissection are performed and as low as 0.9% for subtotal thyroidectomy.[46] However, many surgeons can perform total or near-total thyroidectomy with a very low incidence of this complication. Postoperative hypoparathyroidism is rarely the result of inadvertent removal of all parathyroid glands but, more commonly, is due to disruption of their blood supply. Devascularization can be minimized by carefully ligating the branches of the inferior thyroid artery on the thyroid capsule distal to their supply of the parathyroid glands and by treating the parathyroids with great care (see Fig. 44-2). If a parathyroid gland is recognized to be nonviable during surgery, after identification by frozen section, it can be minced into 1- to 2-mm cubes and placed into pockets in the sternocleidomastoid muscle or elsewhere.[47]

Postoperative hypoparathyroidism results in hypocalcemia and hyperphosphatemia and is manifested by circumoral numbness, tingling, and intense anxiety during the first few days after operation. Chvostek sign appears early, and carpopedal spasm can occur. Most patients develop symptoms when the serum calcium level is <8 mg/dL.[48]

Routinely, the author measures the serum calcium level on the postoperative evening, on the following morning, and every 12 hours thereafter if the patient remains in the hospital. Oral calcium as calcium carbonate is used liberally, especially because most patients now leave on the first postoperative morning. Symptomatic patients should not be discharged and should be given 1 g (10 mL) of 10% calcium gluconate intravenously over 10 minutes. Then 2 to 5 g of this calcium solution should be mixed in a 500-mL bottle to run intravenously during each subsequent 6- to 8-hour period. On this treatment regimen of oral and intravenous calcium, most patients become asymptomatic, and intravenous therapy usually can be stopped. The patient can be discharged if asymptomatic on oral calcium therapy. If more severe hypocalcemia is present, more calcium gluconate may be needed intravenously, and 1,25-dihydroxyvitamin D should be given orally to promote the absorption of oral calcium. The management of more persistent hypocalcemia is discussed in Chapter 60.

# REFERENCES

1. Billroth T. Chirurgische Klinik Zurich, 1860–1867. Berlin, 1867.
2. Kocher T. Zur pathologie und therapie des propfes. Deutsch Z Chir 1874; 4.
3. Halsted WS. The operative story of goitre. Johns Hopkins Hosp Rep 1920; 19:71.
4. Becker C. Hypothyroidism and atherosclerotic heart disease: pathogenesis, medical management, and the role of coronary artery bypass surgery. Endocr Rev 1985; 6:432.
5. Sridama V, Reilly M, Kaplan EL, et al. Long term follow-up study of compensated low dose $^{131}$I therapy for Graves' disease. N Engl J Med 1984; 311:426.
6. Mitchie W, Hamer-Hodges DW, Pegg CAS, et al. Beta-blockade and partial thyroidectomy for thyrotoxicosis. Lancet 1974; 1:1009.
7. Lennquist S, Jortso E, Anderberg B, Smeds S. Beta-blockers compared with antithyroid drugs as preoperative treatment of hyperthyroidism: drug tolerance, complications and postoperative thyroid function. Surgery 1985; 98:1141.
8. Eriksson M, Rubenfeld S, Garber AJ, Kohler PO. Propranolol does not prevent thyroid storm. N Engl J Med 1977; 296:263.
9. Heppe H, Armin A, Calandra DB, et al. Hürthle cell tumors of the thyroid gland. Surgery 1985; 98:1162.
10. Brooks JR, Starnes HF, Brooks DC, Pelkey JN. Surgical therapy for thyroid carcinoma: a review of 1249 solitary thyroid nodules. Surgery 1988; 104:940.
11. Kaplan EL. An operative approach to the irradiated thyroid gland with possible carcinoma: criteria technique and results. In: DeGroot LJ, Frohman LA, Kaplan EL, Refetoff S, eds. Radiation associated carcinoma of the thyroid. New York: Grune & Stratton, 1977:371.
12. DeGroot LJ. Clinical features and management of radiation-associated thyroid carcinoma. In: Kaplan EL, ed. Surgery of the thyroid and parathyroid glands. Edinburgh: Churchill-Livingstone, 1983:40.
13. Sampson RJ. Prevalence and significance of occult thyroid cancer. In: DeGroot LJ, Frohman LA, Kaplan EL, Refetoff S, eds. Radiation associated thyroid carcinoma. New York: Grune & Stratton, 1977:137.
14. McCaffrey TV, Bergstralh EJ, Hay ID. Locally invasive papillary thyroid carcinoma: 1940–1990. Head Neck 1994; 16:165.
15. Clark OH. Total thyroidectomy: the treatment of choice for patients with differentiated thyroid cancer. Ann Surg 1982; 196:361.
16. Grant CS, Hay ID, Gough IR, Bergstralh EJ. Local recurrence in papillary thyroid carcinoma: is extent of surgical resection important? Surgery 1988; 104:954.
17. Beierwaltes WH. Treatment of metastatic thyroid cancer with radioiodine and external radiation therapy. In: Kaplan EL, ed. Surgery of the thyroid and parathyroid glands. Clinical surgery international, vol 4. Edinburgh: Churchill-Livingstone, 1983:103.
18. Hill SC Jr. Chemotherapy of thyroid cancer. In: Kaplan EL, ed. Surgery of the thyroid and parathyroid glands. Clinical surgery international, vol 4. Edinburgh: Churchill-Livingstone, 1983:120.
19. DeGroot LJ, Kaplan EL, Straus FH Jr, Shukla MS. Does the method of management of papillary thyroid carcinoma make a difference in outcome? World J Surg 1994; 18:123.
20. Bäckdahl M, Wallin G, Löwhagen T, et al. Fine needle biopsy cytology and DNA analysis. Surg Clin North Am 1987; 67:197.
21. Hay ID, Grant CS, Taylor WF, et al. Ipsilateral lobectomy versus bilateral lobar resection in papillary thyroid carcinoma: a retrospective analysis of surgical outcome using a novel prognostic scoring system. Surgery 1987; 102:1088.
22. Cady B, Rossi R. An expanded view of risk-group definition in differentiated thyroid carcinoma. Surgery 1988; 104:947.
23. Rasbach DA, Mondschein MS, Harris NL, et al. Malignant lymphoma of the thyroid gland: a clinical and pathological study of twenty cases. Surgery 1985; 98:1166.
24. Kim JH, Leeper RD. Treatment of anaplastic and spindle cell carcinoma of the thyroid with combination Adriamycin and radiation therapy. Cancer 1983; 52:954.
25. Sweeney PJ, Haraf DJ, Recant W, et al. Clinical case: anaplastic carcinoma of the thyroid. Ann Oncol 1996; 7:739.
26. Sizemore GW, van Heerden JA, Carney JA. Medullary carcinoma of the thyroid gland and the multiple endocrine neoplasia type 2 syndrome. In: Kaplan EL, ed. Surgery of the thyroid and parathyroid glands. Clinical surgery international, vol 4. Edinburgh: Churchill-Livingstone, 1983:75.
26a. Kebrew E, Ituarte PH, Siperstein AE, et al. Medullary thyroid carcinoma: clinical characteristics, treatment, prognostic factors, and a comparison of staging systems. Cancer 2000; 88:1139.
26b. Cohen R, Campos JM, Salaun C, et al. Preoperative calcitonin levels are predictive of tumor size and postoperative calcitonin normalization in medullary thyroid carcinoma. Group d'Etude d'Tumeurs a Calcitonine (GETC). J Clin Endocrinol Metab 2000; 85:919.
27. Tisell LE, Hansson G, Jansson S, Salander H. Reoperation in the treatment of asymptomatic metastasizing medullary thyroid carcinoma. Surgery 1986; 99:60.
28. van Heerden JA, Grant CS, Gharib H, et al. Long-term course of patients with persistent hypercalcitoninemia after apparent curative primary surgery for medullary thyroid carcinoma. Ann Surg 1990; 212:395.
29. Dorr U, Wurstlin S, Frank-Raue K, et al. Somatostatin receptor scintigraphy and magnetic resonance imaging in recurrent medullary thyroid carcinoma: a comparative study. Horm Metab Res Suppl 1993; 27:48.
30. Waddington WA, Kettle AG, Heddle RM, Coakley AJ. Intraoperative localization of recurrent medullary carcinoma of the thyroid using indium-111 pentetreotide and a nuclear surgical probe. Eur J Nucl Med 1994; 2:363.
31. Moley JF, Wells SA, Dilley WG, Tisell LE. Reoperation for recurrent or persistent medullary thyroid cancer. Surgery 1993; 114:1090.
32. Donis-Keller H, Dou S, Chi D, et al. Mutations in the RET proto-oncogene are associated with MEN 2A and FMTC. Hum Mol Genet 1993; 2:851.
33. Wells SA Jr, Donis-Keller H. Current perspectives on the diagnosis and management of patients with multiple endocrine neoplasia type 2 syndromes. Endocrinol Metab Clin North Am 1994; 23:215.
34. Lairmore TC, Ball DW, Baylin SB, Wells SA Jr. Management of pheochromocytomas in patients with multiple endocrine neoplasia type 2 syndromes. Ann Surg 1993; 217:595.
35. Moosman DA, DeWeese JS. The external laryngeal nerve as related to thyroidectomy. Surg Gynecol Obstet 1968; 127:1011.
36. Kaplan EL. Surgery of the thyroid gland. In: DeGroot LJ, Larsen PR, Refetoff S, eds. The thyroid and its diseases. New York: John Wiley and Sons, 1984:851.
37. Sedgwick CE, Cady B. Surgery of the thyroid and parathyroid glands. Philadelphia: WB Saunders, 1980:180.
38. Sarda AK, Bai S, Kapur MM. Near-total thyroidectomy for carcinoma of the thyroid. Br J Surg 1989; 76:90.
39. Lumsden AB, McGarity WC. A technique for subtotal thyroidectomy. Surg Gynecol Obstet 1989; 168:177.
40. Iacconi P, Bendinelli C, Miccoli P. Endoscopic thyroid and parathyroid surgery. Surg Endosc 1999; 13(3):314.
41. Shimizu K, Akira S, Tanaka S. Video-assisted neck surgery: endoscopic resection of benign thyroid tumor aiming at scarless surgery of the neck. J Surg Oncol 1998; 69(3):178.
42. Yeung GH. Endoscopic surgery of the neck: a new frontier. Surg Laparosc Endosc 1998; 8(3):227.
43. Lennquist S, Cahlin C, Smeds S. The superior laryngeal nerve in thyroid surgery. Surgery 1987; 102:999.
44. Ford CN, Martin DW, Warner TF. Injectable collagen in laryngeal rehabilitation. Laryngoscope 1984; 94:513.
45. May M, Beery P. Muscle-nerve pedicle laryngeal reinnervation. Laryngoscope 1986; 96:1196.
46. Mazzaferri EL. Papillary and follicular cancer: a selective approach to diagnosis and treatment. Annu Rev Med 1981; 32:73.
47. Wells SA, Farndon JR, Dale JK, et al. Long-term evaluation of patients with primary parathyroid hyperplasia managed by total parathyroidectomy and heterotopic autotransplantation. Ann Surg 1980; 192:451.
48. Kaplan EL, Sugimoto J, Yang H, Fredland A. Postoperative hypoparathyroidism: diagnosis and management. In: Kaplan EL, ed. Surgery of the thyroid and parathyroid glands. Clinical surgery international, vol 4. Edinburgh: Churchill-Livingstone, 1983:262.

---

# CHAPTER 45

# HYPOTHYROIDISM

LAWRENCE E. SHAPIRO AND MARTIN I. SURKS

*Hypothyroidism* is the appellation for any degree of thyroid hormone deficiency. The term *myxedema* is often used to indicate the result of a thyroid hormone deficiency that is of sufficient severity and chronicity to cause characteristic changes in the physical examination.

## HISTORY AND EPIDEMIOLOGY

By the end of the nineteenth century, the syndrome of acquired thyroid hormone deficiency in adults was described as a "cretinoid" state by Gull.[1] Ord proposed the term *myxoedema* to be applied to this condition, which he observed in middle-aged women.[2] Kocher[3] described its occurrence after thyroidectomy, and by 1894, Raven[4] had described the use of oral thyroid medication in the treatment of this disease.

Although most physicians appreciate that thyroid disorders are relatively common in the general population, the true incidence is less certain. Undoubtedly, there is a significant population of patients with undiagnosed thyroid disease who still function relatively normally. The Whickham survey, performed in a rural area of England, specifically sought to determine the incidence of thyroid disease in the general population.[5] Hypothyroidism, diagnosed by history and blood analysis, was

**TABLE 45-1.**
**Causes of Transient or Permanent Hypothyroidism**

**DESTRUCTIVE**
  Postoperative
  Radioactive iodine
  External radiation to neck
  Infiltrative disease (e.g., sarcoidosis, amyloidosis, lymphoma, metastatic
    carcinoma)
**AUTOIMMUNE**
  Hashimoto disease
  After Graves disease
**THYROIDITIS**
  Subacute (e.g., viral)
  Silent
  Postpartum
**DRUG-INDUCED**
  Iodides
  Lithium
  Thionamides
**HEREDITARY OR CONGENITAL**
  Enzyme deficiency affecting thyroid hormone biosynthesis
  Agenesis
  Hormone resistance
  Endemic cretinism
**HYPOTHALAMIC-PITUITARY DISORDERS**
  Thyrotropin-releasing hormone deficiency
  Thyroid-stimulating hormone deficiency
**IDIOPATHIC**
  No cause determined

found in more than 2% of 2800 persons tested. The mean age of diagnosis was 57 years, and the disease was ten-fold more common in women than in men. The disease is particularly prevalent in women older than 40 years of age. The disease is prevalent in debilitated geriatric patients of both sexes.[6]

## ETIOLOGY

Hypothyroidism may develop from any one of a number of acquired thyroid diseases or their treatments, from hereditary abnormalities, or secondarily from hypothalamic-pituitary disease (Table 45-1). Usually, hypothyroidism develops as a consequence of Hashimoto disease or of prior radioactive iodine or surgical management of Graves disease. In 20% of patients treated for Graves disease, the hypothyroidism that develops after radioactive iodine therapy occurs within the first 12 months of treatment. The initial incidence is locally influenced by the dosage of radiation used. A slower but relentlessly progressive increase in incidence of hypothyroidism continues at a rate of 2% to 4% of the population at risk each year.[7]

Hypothyroidism may also develop as a late consequence of Graves disease in patients who previously were not treated with radioactive iodine or surgery.[8] Studies suggest that thyrotropin-binding inhibitor immunoglobulins circulate in some of these patients.[9] The hyperthyroidism of Graves disease may be supplanted by hypothyroidism, because the autoimmune production of thyrotropin receptor-blocking antibodies has resulted in inhibition of thyroid-stimulating hormone (TSH) receptor function.

*Idiopathic hypothyroidism* implies that an appropriate clinical and laboratory evaluation has failed to reveal a specific etiologic factor for this disorder. This is a common occurrence in patients with acquired hypothyroidism. Because many of these patients have low titers of antithyroid antibodies, and because some may have associated autoimmune disorders,

such as pernicious anemia, most investigators believe that the hypothyroidism represents the end stage of autoimmune thyroid disease. The progressive development of hypothyroidism is readily apparent in many patients with Hashimoto thyroiditis. In this disease, there is continual replacement of normal thyroid tissue with lymphocytic and fibrous tissue, until insufficient thyroid tissue remains to maintain normal hormone production.

Temporary hypothyroidism may also develop during other forms of *thyroiditis,* such as viral (i.e., subacute) thyroiditis, silent thyroiditis, or postpartum thyroiditis (see Chap. 46). Although the causes of these forms of thyroiditis probably are distinct, some aspects of their clinical presentation and course can be similar. These patients often present with hyperthyroidism that is associated with decreased thyroid gland function, as determined by a very low uptake of radioactive iodine. The hyperthyroidism probably results from disruption of follicular structure, with the release of hormone systemically. This stage may last from a few weeks to several months. It is generally followed by a euthyroid stage, then often by a hypothyroid stage that may persist for several months. The hypothyroid stage of the disease is characterized by a healing and partially functioning thyroid gland that is not yet producing sufficient thyroid hormone to maintain the euthyroid state. Hypothyroidism in these settings usually is transient and does not require lifelong thyroid hormone replacement.

Several *pharmacologic* agents may influence thyroid function, but only thionamides and iodides are commonly associated with hypothyroidism. Good clinical management dictates that hypothyroidism should not occur during management of Graves disease with thionamides. As thyrotoxicosis is controlled, the physician should decrease the dosage of thionamides to a level that allows sufficient hormone production to maintain the euthyroid state or, alternatively, supplement thionamides with a daily replacement dose of thyroid hormone. If these modifications are not made, hypothyroidism may occur, often associated with an enlarging thyroid gland.

Iodide-induced hypothyroidism may be more difficult to document because the source of excessive iodide ingestion may be obscure. Common sources are iodine-containing pharmaceuticals, such as amiodarone, radiopaque contrast agents, expectorants, and topical antiseptics. Although failure to adapt to the acute Wolff-Chaikoff effect (see Chap. 37) is unusual in individuals without thyroid disease, iodide-induced hypothyroidism by this mechanism occurs readily in patients with preexisting thyroid diseases, such as Hashimoto disease or Graves disease, previously treated with radioactive iodine.[10] Iodide-induced hypothyroidism in these settings may be treated by reducing the excessive iodide intake or by the administration of thyroid hormone.

Hypothyroidism may also be caused by several *hereditary disorders,* particularly of the enzymatic pathways that are responsible for iodothyronine synthesis. Although an occasional adult may present with hypothyroidism and goiter because of hormone dysgenesis, most of these patients are diagnosed and treated during childhood. Defects in the genes coding for the β form of the thyroid hormone nuclear receptor have been reported to occur in familial forms of generalized thyroid hormone resistance.[11] Patients with thyroid hormone resistance manifest a spectrum of syndromes, ranging from cases of mental retardation and abnormal somatic development to clinically euthyroid patients diagnosed only because of elevated levels of TSH and thyroid hormones (see Chap. 32). Familial syndromes of thyroid gland agenesis have been shown to be caused by an inactivating mutation of the TSH receptor.[12]

In a small fraction of hypothyroid patients, the disorder results from decreased stimulation of the thyroid by TSH. The hypothalamic or pituitary disorders that are responsible for decreased TSH production are discussed in Chapter 15. Clinically, attention is focused on secondary or hypothalamic-pituitary–induced hypothyroidism by the finding of a normal or decreased serum TSH concentration concomitant with hypothyroidism.

## SYSTEMIC EFFECTS OF THYROID HORMONE DEFICIENCY

The clinical spectrum of thyroid hormone deficiency ranges from the asymptomatic person without abnormal physical findings to the classic myxedematous patient in whom the diagnosis can readily be made on physical examination. Physical findings are most striking in young, otherwise healthy patients. Advanced age or nonthyroidal disease can commonly produce symptoms or physical findings that suggest thyroid disease and require thyroid function tests to aid in a diagnosis.

Thyroid hormone deficiency causes generally decreased oxygen consumption and defects specific to individual organs. The common symptoms of thyroid hormone deficiency include lethargy and decreased physical ability. The decrease in tissue calorigenesis results in cold intolerance.

### SKIN AND CUTANEOUS APPENDAGES

In myxedema, the epidermis demonstrates an atrophied cellular layer with hyperkeratosis of traumatized areas. The dermis is infiltrated with mucopolysaccharides, hyaluronic acid, and chondroitin sulfate, resulting in increased fluid retention and nonpitting edema. Acinar gland secretion is decreased. On physical examination, decreases in surface temperature and pallor, resulting from cutaneous vasoconstriction, are observed. These changes produce the cool, dry roughness of the skin of the myxedematous patient (see Chap. 218). The hair and nails are brittle. Hair loss is common, but it usually is reversible with treatment.

### GASTROINTESTINAL SYSTEM

The usually modest weight gain in hypothyroidism probably is the result of a decreased metabolic rate. Marked obesity does not result from thyroid hormone deficiency. The sense of taste is decreased. Gastric atrophy and decreased gastric acid production are common. Antiparietal cell antibodies are present in approximately one-third of patients, and pernicious anemia has been reported in 10%.[13] Constipation is a common symptom, but ileus is seen only in patients with severe myxedema. Ascites is rarely evident, although it may exist in the markedly myxedematous patient who may also have pericardial and pleural effusions (see Chap. 204).

### CARDIOVASCULAR SYSTEM

Cardiac function is affected by hypothyroidism; however, this is significant only in patients with coexistent cardiac disease. There is decreased contractility, decreased cardiac output, and diminished cardiac oxygen consumption in hypothyroid patients.[14] In hypothyroid patients without coexisting heart disease, low exercise tolerance and shortness of breath on exertion may be partially caused by decreased cardiac function, but symptoms and signs specific for congestive heart failure usually are absent. In the patient with an already compromised heart, hypothyroidism may cause significant further deterioration. However, the lower tissue demands for cardiac output and tissue oxygenation may compensate for poor cardiac function (see Chap. 203). Unless ventricular function is compromised by a large myxedematous pericardial effusion, the authors believe that clinically significant cardiac dysfunction very rarely results from hypothyroidism. Occasionally, severe congestive heart failure coexists in patients with hypothyroidism. Such patients should be given thyroxine ($T_4$) with caution. The potential benefit of $T_4$ would be to increase contractility

and cardiac output. The potential harm would be that increased myocardial oxygen requirements might further compromise a failing heart.

The diagnosis of autoimmune thyroid disease per se did not increase the risk of ischemic heart disease after a 20-year follow-up.[15] However, elevations of serum lipids in hypothyroid patients are likely risk factors for coronary artery disease. The component of the hyperlipidemia that is due to thyroid hormone deficiency is variable, and it resolves after normalization of thyroid hormone levels. Because myocardial oxygen consumption is augmented by thyroid hormone, a hypothyroid patient with a deficient coronary artery circulation may not tolerate full replacement doses.

### RESPIRATORY SYSTEM

In the absence of primary respiratory disease, the diminution of respiratory function in the hypothyroid patient is not significant. These patients have measurably decreased responses to hypoxia and hypercapnea, but usually this lack of response is of little clinical importance. However, respiratory muscle function may be seriously affected in the severely myxedematous patient, in whom hypoventilation may occur. Hypothyroidism may be a reversible component in rare patients with clinically significant sleep apnea syndrome.[16] Myxedematous patients experiencing sleep apnea syndrome often have pharyngeal obstruction due to macroglossia. In the patients requiring prolonged mechanical ventilation, aggressive $T_4$ replacement may facilitate weaning from the respirator. However, coexisting heart disease may limit the dosage of $T_4$ that may be given safely (see also Chap. 202).

### BLOOD

Patients with myxedema commonly have a mild normochromic, normocytic anemia coexisting with a decreased red cell mass (see Chap. 212). In the childbearing years, hypothyroid women are often iron deficient because of an associated menorrhagia. Macrocytosis can occur in hypothyroidism because of folic acid or vitamin $B_{12}$ deficiency.[13] Pernicious anemia occurs in 10% of hypothyroid patients. In general, hypothyroid patients do not report abnormal bleeding. However, a clinically evident bleeding tendency may be caused by a defect in clotting factors VIII and IX, increased capillary fragility, or abnormal platelet function.

### NEUROMUSCULAR SYSTEM

Unlike many other tissues, oxygen consumption in the adult cerebrum does not depend on thyroid hormone. However, the hypothyroid patient may have diminished cerebral blood flow that is due to decreased cardiac output. Although this situation is usually clinically insignificant, it may play a role in the psychiatric[17] and neurologic disorders occasionally seen in severe hypothyroidism[18] (see Chap. 200).

Patients with severe myxedema may have general depression of central nervous system function, characterized by sluggish responses to questions and sleepiness. Rarely, in extreme cases, agitated psychosis may be seen, and seizures can occur. Myxedema coma often occurs in the complicated setting of severe trauma or systemic illness, and the diagnosis should be suspected in cases of depression, hypothermia, hypoventilation, hyponatremia, and an exaggerated response to sedatives or narcotics.

Nerve compression by myxedematous fluid may cause the carpal tunnel syndrome. Diminished hearing and poor night vision have been described. Cerebellar dysfunction may occur in severe cases of hypothyroidism; posterior column symptomatology probably indicates coexisting pernicious anemia. Deep tendon reflexes have a characteristic delayed relaxation phase that is relatively specific for hypothyroidism. Muscle cramps are common, but muscle weakness is not prominent. Persistent elevation of serum creatine phosphokinase is commonly seen and is not indicative of active muscle inflammation (see Chap. 210).

## RENAL FUNCTION

The decrease in cardiac output diminishes renal blood flow, which rarely has clinical implications (see Chap. 208). Decreased free water clearance may be encountered in severe hypothyroidism, causing hyponatremia that is similar to the syndrome of inappropriate secretion of antidiuretic hormone (see Chap. 27). However, abnormalities in antidiuretic hormone regulation have not been documented.[19]

## BONE

The effects of hypothyroidism on bone and calcium metabolism in adults are rarely significant. Serum calcium is usually normal, and there is no characteristic bone disease.

## ADRENOCORTICAL SYSTEM

Patients with hypothyroidism exhibit a decrease in the rates of cortisol secretion and cortisol metabolism.[20] Nevertheless, patients with primary hypothyroidism, in the absence of coexisting adrenal or pituitary disease, have normal plasma cortisol levels and a normal cortisol response to corticotropin.

However, hypothyroidism can coexist with primary adrenal deficiency resulting from autoimmune disease[21] or can be associated with a secondary adrenal insufficiency caused by an underlying hypothalamic-pituitary disease. If deficiencies of thyroid and adrenocortical hormones do occur, symptoms of the latter disease may be masked by the decreased requirement for glucocorticoids in the unstressed hypothyroid patient. In such a case, manifestations of adrenal failure may occur if thyroid hormone alone is prescribed.

## REPRODUCTIVE SYSTEM

In adult women of childbearing age, excessive menstrual bleeding is common. Fertility decreases, and there is an increased incidence of early abortions.[22] Libido is diminished in both sexes.

Hypothyroidism alters the metabolism of sex hormones and the concentrations of sex hormone–binding proteins. To avoid confusing results, it is prudent to postpone a nonemergency evaluation of sex hormone function until the hypothyroidism is corrected. Serum prolactin levels can be elevated in women with hypothyroidism, and it resolves with treatment.[23]

## PREGNANCY

High levels of estrogens, as occur in pregnancy, result in the elevation of serum $T_4$–binding globulin and an ~30% to 50% increase in serum total $T_4$. Consequently, determination of serum total $T_4$ yields an inaccurate assessment of thyroid function in pregnancy, and measurements of serum free $T_4$ ($FT_4$) and TSH should be obtained (see Chap. 110).

The thyroid status of the mother affects both fetal and childhood health.[23b] If the pregnant patient is newly diagnosed as hypothyroid and has no coexisting medical disease, the rapid replacement of thyroid hormone should be prescribed.[23b] Treatment should begin with a dose of $T_4$ estimated to result in full replacement. The adequacy of this dose can be assessed by determination of TSH and $FT_4$ after 4 weeks.[24]

A patient who is euthyroid while taking $T_4$ therapy for hypothyroidism should contact her endocrinologist when pregnancy occurs to determine whether the current dose of $T_4$ still results in normal levels of serum TSH. An increase in $T_4$

dose may be required in some pregnant patients.[25] All $T_4$-treated hypothyroid patients require reassessment of $FT_4$ and TSH by the end of the first trimester of pregnancy. Any adjustment of $T_4$ dosage requires reevaluation by assessing $FT_4$ and TSH after 4 weeks.

If the pregnant patient has hypothyroidism as a result of previous treatment for Graves disease, further attention is required. Although the continued presence of thyroid-stimulating immunoglobulin may be clinically occult in the mother, the passive transfer of maternal immunoglobulins place the fetus and newborn at risk for Graves disease. The presence of high levels of thyroid-stimulating immunoglobulin in late pregnancy may predict the presence of fetal Graves disease.

Postpartum thyroid dysfunction may occur 2 to 8 months after delivery in a patient not previously known to have thyroid disease. The reported incidence of postpartum dysfunction is 2% to 20%.[26] The usual course is reminiscent of "silent thyroiditis." Patients first develop hyperthyroidism, with a nontender, firm goiter that has decreased ability to concentrate radioactive iodine. Subsequently, thyroid hormone levels fall, and hypothyroidism occurs. The full-time course of the illness is usually several months before recovery occurs. However, patients with postpartum thyroiditis have serum antithyroid antibodies, often have recurrences after each pregnancy, and may eventually develop permanent hypothyroidism.

## INTERMEDIARY METABOLISM

Some evidence of the general slowing of metabolism may be clinically apparent. An associated diabetes mellitus often is ameliorated in the presence of hypothyroidism with a decreased requirement for insulin or oral hypoglycemic drugs. Hyperlipidemia, caused by reduced clearance, can increase levels of low-density lipoprotein, total cholesterol, and triglycerides. Another risk factor for coronary heart disease, plasma total homocysteine levels, which are elevated in hypothyroidism, is corrected by thyroxine treatment.[27,27b]

## DRUG METABOLISM

Thyroid hormone regulates the metabolism of drugs by the hepatic cytochrome p450 enzymes. Examples of drugs with a metabolism that decreases in hypothyroidism are antiseizure medications, digoxin, and narcotics. In addition, the effect of warfarin therapy may change because of alteration of the turnover of serum clotting factors. Thus, the dose requirements of these medications may change as a result of $T_4$ treatment.

## CLINICAL DIAGNOSIS

### HISTORY

Adult-onset hypothyroidism usually causes an insidious progression of multiple symptoms and signs, the exact onset of which often cannot be specified by the patient, close family members, or even the personal physician who is seeing the patient on a regular basis (Fig. 45-1 and Table 45-2). This usually is the result of the gradual decline of thyroid hormone levels that occurs in most cases. The physician should seek any history of prior thyroid disease or of therapy directed at the thyroid gland. A history of external irradiation of the head or neck could result in pituitary or thyroid failure. Any history of the use of compounds containing iodine or lithium should be elicited. Iodine deficiency is not a tenable cause of hypothyroidism in the United States because of the commercial practice of supplementing salt and bread with iodine. There may be a family history of thyroid disorders such as Graves or Hashimoto diseases or, more rarely, congenital thyroid disease or dyshormonogenetic goiter. If secondary hypothyroidism is suspected,

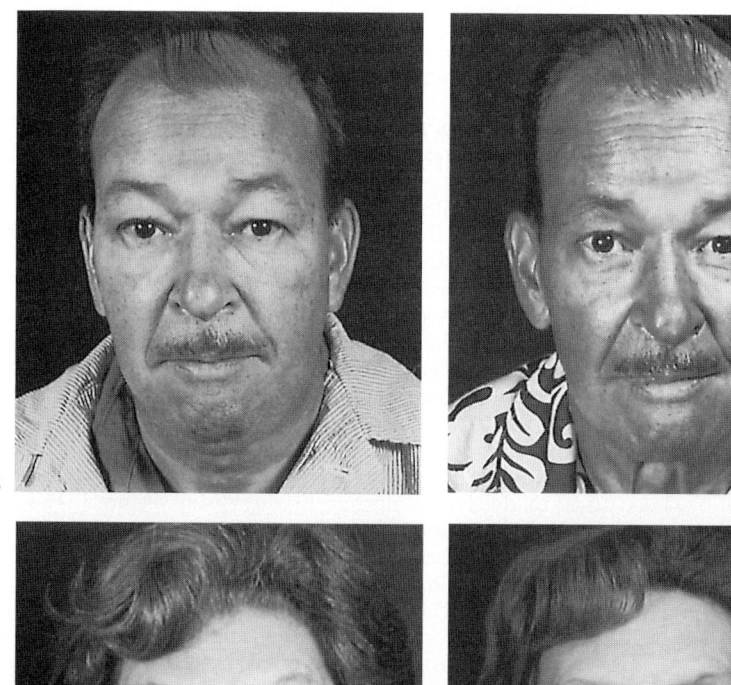

A,B

C,D

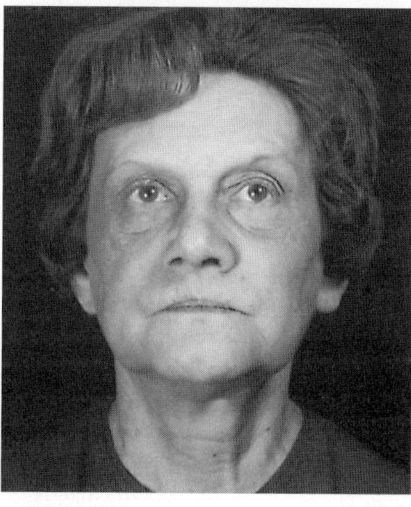

**FIGURE 45-1.** Two hypothyroid patients before (**A,** **C**) and after (**B, D**) full replacement with thyroid hormone. **A,** Notice the loss of eyelashes, the areas of vitiligo around the mouth, the region around the eyes, and the scalp. **C,** Notice the lethargic expression and the periorbital puffiness that disappear with therapy (**D**).

symptoms pertinent to other pituitary hormonal deficits should be elicited. A personal and family history of autoimmune processes should be explored in cases of "idiopathic" thyroid failure. Thoracic obstructive symptoms—such as dysphagia, dyspnea, and lightheadedness on raising the arms—may be present because of a large retroclavicular goiter.

The unusual occurrence of rapidly progressive symptoms of hypothyroidism should suggest one of a few relatively rare diseases. Some forms of thyroiditis are associated with a hyperthyroid and a subsequent hypothyroid phase. These include subacute thyroiditis, silent thyroiditis, and postpartum thyroid disorders (see Chaps. 42 and 46). Occasionally, the physician encounters a demented patient without the ability to give an accurate history who was previously euthyroid on thyroid replacement before the unintentional cessation of treatment. The exposure to iodine or lithium in a patient with an occult thyroid disorder may precipitate an abrupt onset of hypothyroidism.

The most common symptoms of hypothyroidism are listed in Table 45-2. There may be a slight weight gain or an inability to lose weight by dieting, but morbid obesity does not occur. Respiratory and cardiovascular symptoms are usually limited to shortness of breath on exertion, with no symptoms at rest or when lying flat in bed. The skin, hair, nail, and voice changes are most obvious in young patients; in the older population, they may erroneously be attributed to aging.

### PHYSICAL EXAMINATION

The features typical of the physical examination are listed in Table 45-2. In myxedema, there may be a typical facies that is "puffy," with loss of eyebrows and coarse skin (see Fig. 45-1).

The voice may have a unique, deep croaking quality. The tongue may be enlarged. If thyroid failure has resulted from treatment of Graves disease, orbitopathy may be present. Examination of the neck may reveal a scar from prior thyroid surgery. A goiter may be present, although often there is no palpable thyroid tissue. In hypothyroidism, the areolae are normally pigmented, unless there is coexistent adrenal disease, for which there may be decreased pigment (i.e., in pituitary failure) or increased pigment (i.e., in primary adrenal failure). Axillary and pubic hair are present, unless other endocrine failure coexists. Percussion of the chest may reveal basal dullness that is due to the bilateral pleural effusions seen occasionally in advanced cases of myxedema. The breath sounds should be normal.

Examination of the heart may reveal remarkable enlargement if myxedematous pericardial effusion exists. In this case, the cardiac impulse is not palpable, and heart sounds are distant. Signs of pericardial constriction should be sought. The abdomen often is mildly obese, without organomegaly. In severe myxedema, the examiner may encounter an ileus. Examination of the extremities may demonstrate a thickened, nonpitting puffiness. The neurologic examination reveals a delay in the relaxation phase of deep tendon reflexes.

### LABORATORY DIAGNOSIS

### THYROID HORMONE MEASUREMENTS

In patients with typical symptoms and signs, the diagnosis of hypothyroidism generally can be confirmed by measurement of the $FT_4$ level. Hypothyroidism is characterized by a decrease

**TABLE 45-2.**
**Clinical Presentation of Thyroid Hormone Deficiency**

| Affected Areas | Symptoms | Signs |
|---|---|---|
| GENERAL | Cold intolerance | Hypothermia |
| | Fatigue | |
| | Mild weight gain | |
| NERVOUS SYS-TEM | Lethargy | Somnolence |
| | Memory defects | Slow speech |
| | Poor attention span | Myxedema wit |
| | Personality change | Psychopathology: myxedema madness |
| | | Diminished hearing and taste |
| | | Cerebellar ataxia |
| NEUROMUSCU-LAR SYSTEM | Weakness | Delayed relaxation of deep tendon reflexes |
| | Muscle cramps | |
| | Joint pain | Carpal tunnel syndrome |
| GASTROINTESTI-NAL SYSTEM | Nausea | Large tongue |
| | Constipation | Ascites |
| CARDIORESPIRA-TORY SYSTEM | Decreased exercise tolerance | Hoarse voice |
| | | Bradycardia |
| | | Mild hypertension |
| | | Pericardial effusion |
| | | Pleural effusion |
| REPRODUCTIVE SYSTEM | Decreased libido | |
| | Decreased fertility | |
| | Menstrual disorders | |
| SKIN AND APPENDAGES | Dry, rough skin | Nonpitting edema of hands, face, and ankles |
| | Puffy facies | Periorbital swelling |
| | Hair loss | Pallor |
| | Brittle nails | Yellowish skin (i.e., carotenemia) |
| | | Coarse hair |
| | | Dry axillae |

of $T_4$ secretion and a decrease of the serum $FT_4$ levels; measurement of total $T_4$ levels in serum usually correlate with levels of $FT_4$. However, alterations of plasma thyroid hormone–binding proteins can result in decreased serum total $T_4$ values in the absence of hypothyroidism or in normal total $T_4$ values in the presence of hypothyroidism. A decrease in serum-binding proteins and serum total $T_4$ levels occurs most commonly in chronic nonthyroidal illness, but it also occurs during androgen treatment and in patients with a hereditary decrease in serum $T_4$–binding globulin. Alternatively, an increase in serum $T_4$–binding may occur because of estrogen-containing medications, pregnancy, acute liver dysfunction, human immunodeficiency virus infection, or several familial syndromes. Because thyroid regulation is not affected by abnormalities of thyroid hormone binding, the levels of serum $FT_4$ and TSH are in the normal ranges. In nonthyroidal disease, serum $FT_4$ may be in the normal range or increased. This contrasts with the findings in a patient with hypothyroidism in whom the serum $FT_4$ is decreased.[28] Thus, the measurement of serum $FT_4$ may be helpful.

Although triiodothyronine ($T_3$) is the most biologically active of the thyroid hormones, a decrease in serum $T_3$ concentration is not a sufficiently specific marker of hypothyroidism to be useful diagnostically. As with $T_4$, the serum $T_3$ value may be affected by alterations in serum iodothyronine–binding proteins; it also may be low in elderly patients. Nonetheless, in the absence of significant nonthyroidal disease, $FT_4$ levels are normal in patients as old as 110 years of age.[29] Serum $T_3$ levels frequently are decreased in euthyroid patients with nonthyroidal disease and during fasting or food restriction because of a diminished extrathyroidal conversion of $T_4$ to $T_3$. Because of the common occurrence of low serum $T_3$ values in euthyroid patients, serum levels of this hormone should not be used to confirm hypothyroidism.[30]

## THYROID-STIMULATING HORMONE MEASUREMENT AND THYROTROPIN-RELEASING HORMONE TESTS

In patients with hypothyroidism caused by disease of the thyroid gland, decreased iodothyronine production is always associated with an increase in serum TSH. A low serum $FT_4$ concomitant with an increased serum TSH confirms the diagnosis of hypothyroidism and signifies that the hypothyroidism is caused by failure of the thyroid gland. In the few patients who have hypothyroidism because of hypothalamic or pituitary disease, the serum TSH level is decreased or within normal limits. In the past, inadequate sensitivity of TSH measurements in many laboratories generally precluded differentiating normal from low values. Ultrasensitive immunoassays for TSH have been used to determine normal or decreased serum TSH in patients with secondary hypothyroidism.[31] The surprising detection of normal serum levels of TSH in some patients with secondary hypothyroidism may be the result of the presence of biologically inactive TSH in these patients.[32]

The use of thyrotropic-releasing hormone (TRH) is not recommended to diagnose or to determine the cause of hypothyroidism. In patients with hypothalamic or pituitary disease, the TSH response to TRH may be depressed or normal. Moreover, the TSH response to TRH is not sufficiently specific to determine whether the lesion is in the pituitary or hypothalamus.[32] However, the TSH response to TRH is always increased in patients with primary hypothyroidism. Because an elevation in the baseline serum TSH value confirms the diagnosis of primary hypothyroidism, testing with TRH does not play a role in the diagnosis of this disorder.

The negative-feedback regulation of TSH secretion by thyroid hormones is sensitive to changes of 10% to 20% in serum $T_4$ and $T_3$.[33] Even a small decrease in iodothyronine production that results in a decrease in serum $T_4$ to a value that may still be within the normal range may result in a TSH elevation (Fig. 45-2, *time A*). The finding of a normal serum $T_4$ value associated with an elevation in the serum TSH level is probably the first indication of failure of the thyroid gland and subclinical hypothyroidism. Because an elevation of the serum TSH concentration is the most sensitive indication of early primary hypothyroidism, TSH levels should be monitored, particularly in patients who are at high risk for developing this condition, including those who have had thyroid surgery or radioiodine treatment, patients with Hashimoto disease or Graves disease in remission, patients with malignancies of the head or neck who have undergone radiation therapy, and patients with multinodular goiter or with a strong family history of thyroid dysfunction (see Chap. 15).

## OTHER TESTS

Before radioimmunoassay measurements of serum $FT_4$, $T_4$, and TSH were available, tests using radioactive iodine were a mainstay in the diagnosis of hypothyroidism. A decrease in thyroidal uptake of radioiodine does occur in patients with hypothyroidism, but an increasing iodide intake in the United States has resulted in a lower normal range for thyroidal radioiodine uptake, which now significantly overlaps with the range for hypothyroid patients.[34] Although radioiodine testing may occasionally be useful to elucidate the abnormal iodine kinetics of certain forms of hypothyroidism, the inconvenience, expense, and radiation exposure of this test have markedly reduced its use to substantiate hypothyroidism.

Other tests that reflect, in part, the biologic activity of thyroid hormones were extensively used. These procedures included determination of oxygen consumption, serum cholesterol, and

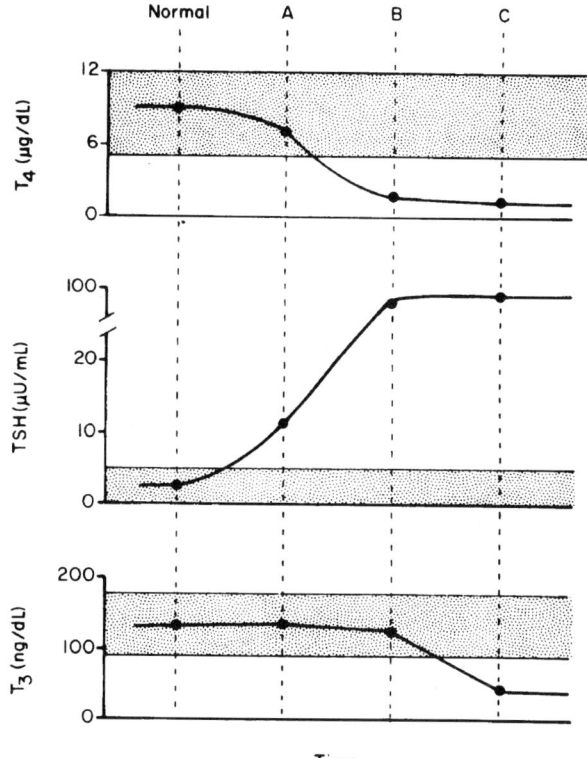

**FIGURE 45-2.** Progressive changes in serum thyroxine ($T_4$), triiodothyronine ($T_3$), and thyroid-stimulating hormone (*TSH*) concentrations during the development of hypothyroidism. The shaded areas represent the normal ranges for the three hormones. The time points may be months or years apart. At time A, the minimal decrease in serum $T_4$ to a value that is still within the normal range results in a rise in serum TSH. At time B, serum $T_4$ has decreased to a very low value, and serum TSH is markedly elevated. The patient may have few symptoms, because serum $T_3$ is still relatively normal. At time C, all patients have symptomatic hypothyroidism.

Achilles tendon reflex relaxation time. Later, tests such as cardiac systolic ejection intervals and serum levels of sex hormone–binding globulin were used (see Chap. 33). All these tests suffered from deficient sensitivity and have been supplanted by the specific and sensitive measurements of serum $FT_4$ and TSH concentrations. Several additional manifestations of the hypothyroid state include an increase in the activity of serum creatinine phosphokinase, serum oxaloacetic transaminase, and lactate dehydrogenase, but these changes are not sufficiently specific to be useful in routine diagnosis.

# THERAPY

## GUIDELINES FOR STANDARD THERAPY

Several pharmaceutical preparations are available for the treatment of hypothyroidism. The careful use of any of these preparations can reverse the hypothyroidism and restore the euthyroid state. Before commencing therapy, it is important to define whether hypothyroidism is caused by thyroid failure or by the much less common failure of TSH secretion because of hypothalamic or pituitary disease. In the latter case, coexisting impairment of adrenocorticotropic hormone secretion may precipitate an adrenal failure that had been satisfactorily tolerated during hypothyroidism. Even when TSH elevation demonstrates hypothyroidism that is due to thyroid failure, it is important to consider coexisting autoimmune disease of the adrenal gland. Treatment of the hypothyroidism alone raises

the metabolic rate and the rate of cortisol metabolism and may then "unmask" adrenocortical hormone deficiency. In these settings, cortisol should be administered with the thyroid hormone replacement.

Animal products, such as desiccated thyroid and thyroglobulin, were standard replacement therapy for several decades. These products are being replaced with synthetic preparations of L-thyroxine (L-$T_4$), L-triiodothyronine (L-$T_3$), or medications that combine synthetic $T_4$ and $T_3$. The use of synthetic preparations is recommended because of their stability and because their standardization is by hormone content rather than by iodine content. Among the synthetic products, only L-$T_4$ produces relatively unchanged serum $T_4$ and $T_3$ levels throughout the 24-hour day.[35] Because of its small distribution pool in blood, $T_3$ as well as synthetic combinations of $T_4$ and $T_3$ result in a postabsorptive increase in serum $T_3$ to hyperthyroid values. The consequent instability of serum $T_3$ levels in patients treated with $T_3$ does not allow assessment of the thyroidal state by measurement of serum levels of iodothyronine. Thyroid hormone receptors in some tissues (e.g., brain) are occupied by the $T_3$ that is produced within the target tissue from deiodination of $T_4$.[36] Because oral $T_3$ would not deliver thyroid hormone to such tissues in a physiologic manner, it is recommended that synthetic L-$T_4$ be used for replacement therapy. One of the well-standardized brands (e.g., Synthroid, Levothroid, Levoxyl) is recommended, because variations in potency have been reported for some generic preparations.[37]

The initial dosage of L-$T_4$ depends on the severity of the hypothyroid disorder, the age of the patient, and the presence of associated or underlying medical conditions. The half-life of L-$T_4$, which is ~6 days in euthyroid individuals, may be significantly prolonged in hypothyroid patients. A full replacement dose has been considered to be between 1.5 and 2.0 µg $T_4$/kg of body weight.[33] Most patients' deficiencies are fully replaced with a daily dosage of 0.075 to 0.15 mg per day. In young, otherwise healthy patients with mild hypothyroidism, a full daily replacement dose of L-$T_4$ (usually 0.075 to 0.10 mg) may be given at the beginning of therapy. The initial dose of L-$T_4$ in patients with severe hypothyroidism or in patients with clinically apparent or probable underlying atherosclerotic heart disease or in elderly patients is generally 0.0125 to 0.025 mg per day. This low dose is recommended because an abrupt increase in metabolic rate and demand for increased cardiac output may precipitate angina pectoris, myocardial infarction, congestive heart failure, or arrhythmias.[38] After this low initial daily dosage of L-$T_4$ is fully equilibrated (4 to 6 weeks), and if the patient has no symptoms or signs of cardiac decompensation, the daily dosage may be cautiously increased.

Doses are assessed at monthly intervals until the clinical syndrome is relieved or until laboratory tests demonstrate that full replacement has been achieved. The therapeutic goal for lifelong replacement therapy should be alleviation of the clinical syndrome and the normalization of serum TSH. It is essential to use a TSH assay of sufficient sensitivity to detect serum TSH levels that fall below the normal range in response to excess $T_4$. Appropriate practice requires that $T_4$ dosage be adjusted to normalize serum TSH to prevent possible adverse effects of chronic excess $T_4$ therapy on bone mineral density[39] or cardiac function.[40] These therapeutic goals may be modified in elderly patients with cardiovascular disease. In such individuals, optimal therapy may be a daily dosage of L-$T_4$ that relieves most of the symptoms of hypothyroidism without causing myocardial decompensation. Such a dose may not fully normalize serum $T_4$ and TSH.

After the desired dose of $T_4$ is established, patients are reevaluated annually to assess changing requirements or altered absorption of L-$T_4$ and their reliability in ingestion of medication. The dosage of L-$T_4$ should be evaluated when the patient's status changes. Pregnancy may increase the dosage needed to normalize serum TSH. The prescription of some medications may alter the absorption (bile acid binders, iron supplements, or aluminum-containing antacids), or metabolism (antiseizure medications or rifampin), of L-$T_4$. If the patient develops symptoms of thyroid dysfunction or heart disease, a dosage adjustment may be required.

# SPECIAL CLINICAL PROBLEMS

## DIAGNOSIS AND MANAGEMENT OF PATIENTS WITH NONTHYROIDAL DISEASE

Nonthyroidal disease complicates the evaluation of thyroid function. Differentiating hypothyroidism from the effects of nonthyroidal disease is a common reason to request endocrine consultation in hospitalized patients. Although patients who have nonthyroidal disease are not clinically hypothyroid, their clinical state may have some features in common with hypothyroidism, such as lethargy, hypothermia, and constipation. Moreover, the effects of nonthyroidal disease on binding proteins and iodothyronine metabolism may result in changes that suggest associated hypothyroidism.[30] Most clinical investigators think that the decreased conversion of $T_4$ to $T_3$ that occurs in illness facilitates the conservation of body protein stores and does not indicate hypothyroidism (see Chaps. 30, 36, and 232).

Although patients with primary hypothyroidism have decreased serum $T_4$ and increased serum TSH levels, patients with nonthyroidal disease may have decreased levels of serum $T_3$ and normal or reduced levels of serum $T_4$.[28] Decreased serum $T_3$ levels are encountered so frequently in these sick patients that this determination is of little value.[41] When the serum $T_4$ level remains normal in patients with nonthyroidal disease, there is no difficulty in excluding hypothyroidism.[28] However, when patients with severe nonthyroidal disease have decreased serum $T_4$ levels, the serum $FT_4$ concentration often remains normal, a finding that also would exclude hypothyroidism. Nevertheless, because of the presence of circulating inhibitors of thyroid hormone binding to plasma-binding proteins, and depending on the technique used to determine $FT_4$, even this value may be decreased in very sick patients.[42] A diagnosis of primary hypothyroidism usually can be excluded in such patients by finding a normal level of serum TSH, but studies have shown that the magnitude of the TSH secretory response to TRH after an experimentally produced decrease in serum $T_4$ and $T_3$ levels may be reduced in approximately one-half of older individuals and in patients with nonthyroidal disease.[43] These findings suggest that TSH may fail to rise in some in whom nonthyroidal disease coexists with primary hypothyroidism. Experience and clinical judgment are essential to complement laboratory values in evaluating thyroid status in some sick patients with low serum $T_4$ and TSH concentrations.

The finding of TSH elevation in an intensive care unit (ICU) patient usually indicates primary hypothyroidism. In a study of 86 patients who were hospitalized in an ICU, only two patients had hypothyroidism, and both had elevated serum levels of TSH.[44] There is a caveat to the interpretation of an elevated TSH in an ICU patient recovering from a recent, severe illness: TSH levels are elevated during the *recovery* of patients without endocrine disease whose serum $T_4$ levels were diminished during severe nonthyroidal illness. In such patients, the TSH elevation is transient and resolves after normalization of the serum $T_4$ level.[45]

Because the concentration of reverse $T_3$ is normal or increased in nonthyroidal disease and is decreased in hypothyroidism, the measurement of reverse $T_3$ may be helpful in differentiating patients with low TSH and secondary hypothyroidism caused by hypopituitarism from patients with nonthyroidal illness.[42] Serum $T_4$ and TSH concentrations may be decreased in both clinical settings. The finding of low serum levels of $T_4$ without elevations of serum TSH in a severely ill ICU patient most often occurs in the absence of endocrine disease. However, these laboratory data are also consistent with TSH deficiency. Because pituitary failure may coexist in an ICU patient, assessment of this life-threatening possibility is an important part of the endocrine evaluation of these patients.

## EFFECTS OF NONTHYROIDAL DISEASE ON PATIENTS WITH HYPOTHYROIDISM

Patients who have hypothyroidism and nonthyroidal disease represent special management problems, because the treatment of either disorder may adversely affect the other. For example, the use of iodine-rich radiopaque contrast agents for diagnostic procedures may acutely worsen subclinical or established hypothyroidism. The treatment of hypothyroidism may precipitate angina pectoris, myocardial infarction, arrhythmia, or congestive heart failure in patients with underlying heart disease.

The coexistence of hypothyroidism with a severe nonthyroidal disease represents a challenge to the clinician. Hypothyroid patients frequently have substantial anemia, a decrease in free water clearance, and a decrease in the rate of drug metabolism. These factors must be carefully considered in the management of the associated nonthyroidal disease. These issues are heightened when surgical management of the nonthyroidal disease is required. Hypothyroidism significantly increases the risk of anesthesia and surgery because of delayed metabolism of anesthetic agents and drugs, abnormal fluid balance, alveolar hypoventilation, reduced cardiac output, and other factors. Because of these potentially serious problems, a decision for surgery should be made only after extensive discussions among the surgeon, anesthesiologist, and the clinicians responsible for medical management. Evidence suggests that optimal combined management results in an excellent outcome for hypothyroid patients who undergo coronary bypass surgery. In this instance, thyroid hormone replacement usually is delayed until after surgery has been performed.[38]

## TREATMENT OF ASYMPTOMATIC OR "CHEMICAL" HYPOTHYROIDISM

Because hypothyroidism may develop insidiously, over many years in some patients, abnormal serum $T_4$ and TSH concentrations may be found before the typical symptoms and signs of hypothyroidism become apparent. The increase in serum TSH, which accompanies a decreasing serum $T_4$ level as thyroid function fails, stimulates the thyroid to produce more $T_3$ relative to $T_4$. Patients in the early stages of thyroid failure may have relatively normal serum $T_3$ levels, despite a marked decrease in serum $T_4$ and increase in serum TSH concentration (see Fig. 45-2, *time B*). These patients may be clinically euthyroid.[46]

Because of the frequency of thyroid hormone tests as part of multiphasic screening, several individuals who are identified as having "chemical hypothyroidism" because of abnormal results do not appear to have a compatible clinical syndrome. Some clinicians do not think that treatment with thyroid hormone replacement should be started in such patients, because the rate of progression of the thyroid failure is uncertain. It is possible that clinically relevant hypothyroidism may never develop in some of these persons. However, the presence of elevated serum TSH "marks" the patient with exhausted thyroid reserve who is at the "edge" of worsening hypothyroidism.

The presence of antithyroid antibodies increases the risk of progressive thyroid failure, prompting L-$T_4$ treatment.[47,48] If the patient is not treated, the physician must plan to reevaluate thyroid function on a regular basis. Although there are no prospective studies to reference, the authors suggest that there are several reasons why most patients with subclinical hypothyroidism should be treated:

1. Symptoms of hypothyroidism may be subtle and not appreciated by the patient until full replacement therapy has resulted in beneficial changes.

2. Patients with underlying thyroid disease and subclinical hypothyroidism are at risk for rapid development of severe hypothyroidism after exposure to iodides, because in many instances, they fail to adapt to the acute Wolff-Chaikoff effect. In a similar manner, treatment with lithium can precipitate worsening thyroid hormone deficiency.

3. The $T_3$ content of some tissues in the body is derived from intracellular $T_4$ rather than the plasma $T_3$. The failure to restore $T_4$ levels to normal in patients with chemical hypothyroidism may theoretically result in low $T_3$ levels within these tissues.

4. The effects of potent drugs, such as warfarin and digoxin, and antiseizure medications may be inconstant.

5. $T_4$ therapy is safe, simple, and relatively inexpensive. The assays for TSH allow the physician to avoid subtle $T_4$ overdosage.

6. The need for routine follow-up is as great (or greater) for the patient who is observed without treatment than it is for the treated patient.

7. Treatment of subclinical hypothyroidism decreases serum cholesterol.[49]

## MYXEDEMA COMA

Coma, as an end stage of myxedema, was described by Ord in 1880.[2] Thereafter, it was accepted that severe myxedema with coma was usually lethal. Only within the last three decades has there been success in treatment. Two factors seem important for improved survivability: The first is successful specific treatment of the intercurrent nonthyroidal disease that often precipitates the comatose state, and the second is that newer methods of intensive care for general medical management have increased survival for critically ill patients in general. Hypothyroidism is compatible with life in the otherwise healthy individual. The patient with a history of years or even decades of hypothyroidism is not rare. However, such a person has dysfunction of many organs and is less able to tolerate life-threatening illness than the euthyroid person. Survival of the critically ill patient with severe hypothyroidism depends on vigorous treatment of nonthyroidal life-threatening processes and prompt therapy with thyroid hormones.

The presence of coma may be a marker of the patient's clinical deterioration more than a primary effect of hypothyroidism. Often, there is a critical insult in the form of infection, surgery, convulsive seizure, congestive heart failure, cerebral vascular accident, gastrointestinal bleeding, cold exposure, or the administration of sedatives that precipitates myxedema coma.[50] Generally, the patient has clinical features of hypothyroidism on physical examination, is hypothermic, and has laboratory evidence of primary hypothyroidism. Other frequent findings are hypoventilation and hyponatremia.

The rare occurrence of myxedema coma and the heterogeneity of coexisting nonthyroidal diseases make it difficult to evaluate modes of treatment. Therapy is based on the successful treatment of seven clinically myxedematous patients with various associated and severe nonthyroidal diseases.[51] These investigators administered 400 to 500 μg of L-$T_4$ intravenously. This dose is sufficient to restore normal $T_4$ levels. They also used pharmacologic doses of glucocorticoids in some of these patients, a practice commonly recommended to treat potential adrenal insufficiency. Vigorous therapeutic attention should be paid to coexisting problems, such as hypothermia, shock, and $CO_2$ retention. Some clinicians use high doses of intravenous $T_4$, although others prefer to use smaller doses of $T_4$ or to use $T_3$ because of its more rapid onset of effect.[52–54] However, in some reports in which relatively high doses of $T_3$ have been used, an increased incidence of cardiovascular complications was observed.[55]

The authors' approach is to consider each case individually, with a careful search for coexisting diseases and assessment of the integrity of the patient's coronary arteries. The patient should be in an ICU. Vigorous therapeutic attention should be paid to coexisting diseases and life-threatening manifestations, such as hypothermia, shock, and $CO_2$ retention.

$T_4$ should be given intravenously. At least 50 μg is given daily—this dosage is sufficient to initiate therapy and minimizes adverse effects on a potentially diseased cardiovascular system. Glucocorticoids are used if the setting suggests coexisting adrenal insufficiency. In the authors' experience, the principal determinant of the patient's outcome is the degree of success achieved in diagnosing and treating coexisting diseases while the appropriate hormone therapy is being applied.

## TREATMENT OF THYROID CANCER

Patients treated for thyroid epithelial cell cancer are often athyrotic after surgery and radioiodine treatment. In these patients, the goal of L-$T_4$ therapy is to just suppress serum TSH, thus creating minimal biochemical thyroid hormone excess. Current studies suggest that this goal can be accomplished without the occurrence of cardiac dysfunction[56] or diminished bone mineral density.[57]

## THE NONCOMPLIANT PATIENT

A common cause of failure to normalize serum TSH is patient noncompliance. Because of its long serum half-life, L-$T_4$ can be given at greater than daily intervals. The patient should double the daily dosage on the day after a missed dose. In the extreme, the single ingestion of a week's dosage of $T_4$ every 7 days has been reported to achieve a reasonable therapeutic result.[58]

## REFERENCES

1. Gull WW. On a cretinoid state supervening in adult life in women. Trans Clin Soc Lond 1874; 7:180.
2. Ord WM. Cases of myxoedema. Trans Clin Soc Lond 1879; 13:15.
3. Kocher TH. Uber kropfextirpation und ihre folgen. Langenbecks Arch Klin Chir 1883; 29:254.
4. Raven TF. Myxoedema treated with thyroid tablets. BMJ 1894; 1:12.
5. Tunbridge WM, Evered DC, Hall R, et al. Lipid profiles and cardiovascular disease in the Whickham area with particular reference to thyroid failure. Clin Endocrinol (Oxf) 1977; 7:481.
6. Helfand M, Crapo LM. Screening for thyroid disease. Ann Intern Med 1990; 112:840.
7. Cevallos JL, Hagen GA, Maloof F, et al. Low-dosage $^{131}$I therapy of thyrotoxicosis (diffuse goiters). A five-year follow-up study. N Engl J Med 1974; 290:141.
8. Tamai H, Kasagi K, Takaichi Y, et al. Development of spontaneous hypothyroidism in patients with Graves' disease treated with antithyroid drugs: clinical, immunological and histological findings in 26 patients. J Clin Endocrinol Metab 1989; 69:49.
9. Konishi J, Iida Y, Kasagi K, et al. Primary myxedema with thyrotrophin-binding inhibitor immunoglobulins. Clinical and laboratory findings in 15 patients. Ann Intern Med 1985; 103:26.
10. Wolff J. Iodide goiter and the pharmacologic effects of excess iodide. Am J Med 1969; 47:101.
11. Takeda K, Balzano S, Sakurai A, et al. Screening of nineteen unrelated families with generalized resistance to thyroid hormone for known point mutations in the thyroid hormone receptor gene and detection of a new mutation. J Clin Invest 1991; 87:496.
12. Gagne N, Parma J, Deal C, et al. Apparent congenital athyreosis contrasting with normal thyroglobulin levels and associated with inactivating mutations in the thyrotropin gene. J Clin Endocrinol Metab 1998; 83:1771.
13. Tudhope GR, Wilson GM. Anaemia in hypothyroidism. Q J Med 1960; 29:513.
14. Woeber KA. Thyrotoxicosis and the heart. N Engl J Med 1992; 232:94.
15. Vanderpump MP, Tunbridge WM, French JM et al. The development of ischemic heart disease in relation to autoimmune thyroid disease in a 20-year follow up study of an English community. Thyroid 1996; 6:155.
16. Skjodt NM, Atkar R, Easton PA. Screening for hypothyroidism in sleep apnea. Am J Respir Crit Care Med 1999; 160:732.
17. Jackson IM. The thyroid axis and depression. Thyroid 1998; 8:951.
18. Hall RCW. Psychiatric effects of thyroid hormone disturbance. Psychosomatics 1983; 24:7.
19. Iwasaki Y, Oiso Y, Yamauchi K, et al. Osmoregulation of plasma vasopressin in myxedema. J Clin Endocrinol Metab 1990; 70:534.

20. Gordon GG, Southren AL. Thyroid hormone effects on steroid hormone metabolism. Bull NY Acad Med 1977; 53:241.

21. Edmonds M, Lamki L, Killinger DW, Volpe R. Autoimmune thyroiditis, adrenalitis and oophoritis. Am J Med 1973; 54:782.

22. Stephenson MD. Frequency of factors associated with habitual abortion in 197 couples. Fertil Steril 1996; 66:24.

23. Honbo KS, Van Herle AJ, Kellett KA. Serum prolactin levels in untreated primary hypothyroidism. Am J Med 1978; 64:782.

23b. Haddow JE, Palomaki GE, Allan WC, et al. Maternal thyroid deficiency during pregnancy and subsequent neuropsychological development of the child. N Engl J Med 1999; 341:541.

24. Montoro, MN. Management of hypothyroidism during pregnancy. Clin Obstet Gynecol 1997; 40:65.

25. Mandel PJ, Larsen PR, Seely GW, et al. Increased need for thyroxine during pregnancy in women with primary hypothyroidism. N Engl J Med 1990; 323:126.

26. Gerstein HC. How common is postpartum thyroiditis? Arch Intern Med 1990; 150:1397.

27. Nedrebo BG, Ericsson U-B, Nygard O, et al. Plasma total homocysteine levels in hyperthyroid and hypothyroid patients. Metabolism 1998; 47:89.

27b. Hussein WI, Green R, Jacobsen DW, et al. Normalization of hyperhomocysteinemia with L-thyroxine in hypothyroidism. Ann Intern Med 1999; 131:348.

28. Surks MI, Hupart KH, Pan C, et al. Normal free thyroxine in critical nonthyroidal illnesses measured by ultrafiltration at undiluted serum and equilibrium dialysis. J Clin Endocrinol Metab 1988; 67:1031.

29. Mariotti S, Barbesino G, Caturegli P. Complex alteration of thyroid function in healthy centenarians. J Clin Endocrinol Metab 1993; 77:1130.

30. Tibaldi JM, Surks MI. Effects of nonthyroidal illness on thyroid function. Med Clin North Am 1985; 69:899.

31. Spencer CA. Clinical utility and cost effectiveness of sensitive thyrotropin assays in ambulatory and hospitalized patients. Mayo Clin Proc 1988; 63:1214.

32. Faglia G, Bitensky L, Pinchera A, et al. Thyrotropin secretion in patients with central hypothyroidism: evidence for reduced biological activity of immunoreactive thyrotropin. J Clin Endocrinol Metab 1979; 48:989.

33. Ordene KW, Pan C, Barzel US, et al. Variable thyrotropin response to thyrotropin releasing hormone after small decreases in plasma thyroid hormone concentrations in patients of advanced age. Metabolism 1983; 32:881.

34. Pittman JA, Dailey GE, Beschi RJ. Changing normal values for thyroidal radioiodine uptake. N Engl J Med 1969; 280:1431.

35. Surks MI, Schadlow AR, Oppenheimer JH. A new radioimmunoassay for plasma L-triiodothyronine: measurements in thyroid disease and in patients maintained on hormonal replacement. J Clin Invest 1972; 51:3104.

36. Larsen PR, Silva JE, Kaplan MM. Relationships between circulating and intracellular thyroid hormones: physiological and clinical implications. Endocr Rev 1981; 2:87.

36b. Toft AD (Editorial). Thyroid hormone replacement—one hormone or two? N Engl J Med 1999; 340:469.

37. Fish LH, Schwartz HL, Cavanaugh J, et al. Replacement dose metabolism and bioavailability of levothyroxine in treatment of hypothyroidism. N Engl J Med 1987; 37:764.

38. Becker C. Hypothyroidism and atherosclerotic heart disease: pathogenesis, medical management and the role of coronary bypass surgery. Endocr Rev 1985; 6:432.

39. Taelman P, Kaufman JM, Janssens X, et al. Reduced forearm bone mineral content and biochemical evidence of increased bone turnover in women with euthyroid goitre treated with thyroid hormone. Clin Endocrinol (Oxf) 1990; 33:107.

40. Biondi B, Fazio S, Carella C, et al. Cardiac effects of long term thyrotropin-suppressive therapy with levothyroxine. J Clin Endocrinol Metab 1993; 77:334.

41. Bermudez F, Surks MI, Oppenheimer JH. High incidence of decreased serum triiodothyronine concentration in patients with nonthyroidal disease. J Clin Endocrinol Metab 1975; 41:27.

42. Chopra IJ, Solomon DH, Hepner GW, et al. Misleading low free thyroxine index and usefulness of reverse triiodothyronine measurement in non-thyroidal disease. Ann Intern Med 1979; 90:905.

43. Maturlo SJ, Rosenbaum RL, Pan C, et al. Variable thyrotropin response to thyrotropin-releasing hormone following small decreases in plasma free thyroid hormone concentrations in patients with nonthyroidal diseases. J Clin Invest 1980; 66:451.

44. Slag MF, Morley JE, Elson MK, et al. Hypothyroxinemia in critically ill patients as a predictor of high mortality. JAMA 1981; 245:43.

45. Hamblin PS, Dyer SA, Mohr VS, et al. Relationship between thyrotropin and thyroxine changes during recovery from severe hypothyroxinemia of critical illness. J Clin Endocrinol Metab 1986; 62:717.

46. Zulewski H, Muller B, Exer P, et al. Estimation of tissue hypothyroidism by a new clinical score. J Clin Endocrinol Metab 1997; 82:771.

47. Rosenthal MJ, Hunt WC, Garry PJ. Thyroidal failure in the elderly: microsomal antibodies as a discriminant for therapy. JAMA 1987; 258:209.

48. Vanderpump MP, Turnbridge WM, French JM et al. The incidence of thyroid disorders in a community hospital: a twenty year follow up of the Whickham Survey. Clin Endocrinol (Oxf) 1995;43:55.

49. Tanis BC, Westendorp GJ, Smelt HM. Effect of thyroid substitution on hypercholesterolaemia in patients with subclinical hypothyroidism. Clin Endocrinol (Oxf) 1996; 44:643.

50. Wartofsky L. Myxedema coma. In: Braverman LE, Utiger RD, eds. The thyroid, 6th ed. Philadelphia: JB Lippincott, 1991:1084.

51. Holvey DN, Goodner CJ, Nicoloff JT, et al. Treatment of myxedema coma with intravenous thyroxine. Arch Intern Med 1964; 113:139.

52. McConahey WM. Diagnosing and treating myxedema and myxedema coma. Geriatrics 1978; 33:61.

53. Rosenberg IN. Hypothyroidism and coma. Surg Clin North Am 1968; 48:353.

54. Capiferri R, Evered D. Investigation and treatment of hypothyroidism. Clin Endocrinol Metab 1979; 8:39.

55. Hylander B, Rosenquist U. Treatment of myxoedema coma-induced factors associated with fatal outcome. Acta Endocrinol (Copenh) 1985; 108:65.

56. Shapiro LE, Sievert R, Ong L, et al. Minimal cardiac effects in asymptomatic athyreotic patients chronically treated with thyrotropin-suppressive doses of L-thyroxine. J Clin Endocrinol Metab 1997; 82:2592.

57. Rosen HN, Moses AC, Garber J, et al. Randomized trial of pamidronate in patients with thyroid cancer: bone density is not reduced by suppressive dose of thyroxine, but is increased by cyclic intravenous pamidronate. J Clin Endocrinol Metab 1998; 83:2324.

58. Grebe SK, Cooke RR, Ford HC, et al. Treatment of hypothyroidism with once weekly thyroxine. J Clin Endocrinol Metab 1997; 82:870.

# CHAPTER 46

# THYROIDITIS

IVOR M. D. JACKSON AND JAMES V. HENNESSEY

*Thyroiditis* is a term used for a wide variety of thyroid disorders or different etiologies. Patients may present with vastly different clinical features. The evaluation and therapy of thyroiditis and the relevant pathology and etiology are herein reviewed.

## SUPPURATIVE THYROIDITIS

### ETIOLOGY

Suppurative thyroiditis, an uncommon but potentially serious disorder, is an acute, subacute, or chronic infection of the thyroid caused by either a bacterial or fungal infection. The organisms most commonly involved in acute suppurative thyroiditis include *Staphylococcus aureus*, *Streptococcus hemolyticus*, *Escherichia coli*, pneumococcus, and *Salmonella* sp.[1] *Bacteroides* sp and other anaerobic bacteria may occasionally initiate this disorder.[2] Acute inflammatory changes in the thyroid usually occur by direct hematogenous spread, either from a nearby infected tissue or from a distant site. Conversely, tuberculous or syphilitic involvement and fungal infection typically lead to a more chronic indolent process (see Chap. 213). *Pneumocystis carinii* has been documented as a cause of thyroid infection in patients with acquired immunodeficiency syndrome. In addition, cases of *Coccidioides immitis* thyroiditis have been reported in immune-suppressed patients in the context of disseminated coccidioidal disease.[3] These findings suggest that patients infected with human immunodeficiency virus and other immune-compromised individuals may be predisposed to a variety of thyroid infections with more unusual, opportunistic organisms.

### CLINICAL FEATURES AND LABORATORY EVALUATION

Patients with acute bacterial suppurative thyroiditis usually present with severe pain, tenderness, and swelling of the thyroid. Systemic signs and symptoms such as fever, rigor, and malaise frequently occur. Although pain usually is localized to the thyroid, it may be referred to the occiput, ear, or mandible. Examination characteristically reveals a tender thyroid gland, with warmth and erythema over the site of a nodule, and cervical lymphadenopathy. Patients with tuberculous thyroiditis may

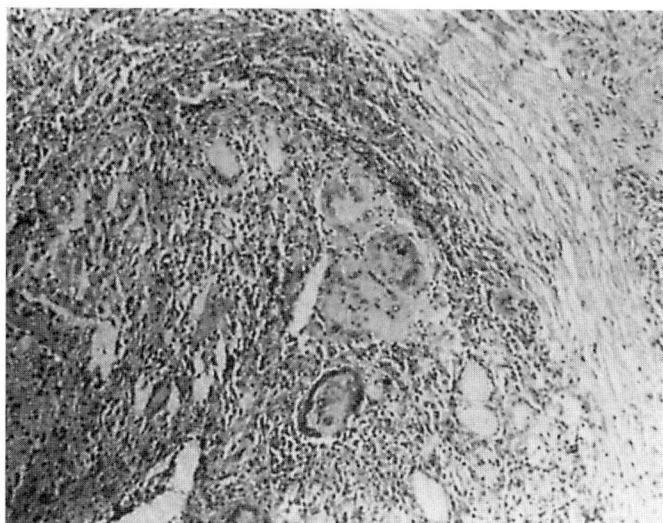

**FIGURE 46-1.** Subacute (granulomatous) thyroiditis. Note the numerous giant cells. ×125 (From LiVolsi VA, LoGerfo P, eds. Thyroiditis. Boca Raton, FL: CRC Press, 1981.)

have thyroid swelling but absence of pain and tenderness. Serum thyroid hormone levels in all types of suppurative thyroiditis are usually normal, but rare cases with thyrotoxicosis are reported that are due to tissue necrosis with release of a high concentration of thyroid hormone into the systemic circulation.[4] A specific diagnosis, with demonstration of the offending organism, usually can be made after aspiration of the infected area.

## TREATMENT

Treatment of suppurative thyroiditis necessitates surgical drainage of any abscess and administration of the appropriate antibiotics. Although some patients may respond to antibiotics alone, a failure to respond indicates the need to consider surgical measures.[5] Patients with a persistent thyroglossal duct or an internal fistula may require surgery for prevention of recurrence.[6] The prognosis in properly treated patients is good; normal residual thyroid function is the rule.

## SUBACUTE THYROIDITIS

### ETIOLOGY

Subacute thyroiditis is an inflammatory disorder of the thyroid thought to be viral in origin. Previously, this condition was termed *granulomatous thyroiditis, De Quervain thyroiditis, struma granulomatosa,* and *pseudotuberculous thyroiditis.* The pathologic hallmarks are granulomas and pseudo giant cells (Fig. 46-1). Evidence that suggests a viral infection includes the following:

1. Subacute thyroiditis often occurs after an upper respiratory tract infection or during a viral epidemic.
2. There is no associated polymorphonuclear leukocytosis.
3. Coxsackie virus antibody titers have been noted to rise.[7]
4. The mumps virus has been cultured from thyroid tissue of patients with subacute thyroiditis.[8]
5. The process is self-limited.

All current evidence suggests that subacute thyroiditis is not an autoimmune disease. Although low levels of antithyroid antibodies may appear transiently during the course of the disorder, the levels are not of the same magnitude seen in patients with other autoimmune thyroid disorders. Subjects with subacute thyroiditis, but not those with Hashimoto disease, have a higher frequency of a certain human leukocyte antigen (HLA) haplotype (HLA-B35)[7];

it is possible that this HLA association may reflect a genetic susceptibility to subacute thyroiditis after various viral infections.[9]

### CLINICAL FEATURES

These patients characteristically present with a painful, tender goiter that is firm, with pain radiating to the ears, mandible, or occiput. In some patients, however, these features may be minimal or even absent.[7] Cervical lymphadenopathy usually is not present, but many patients have prodromal symptoms of an upper respiratory tract infection, fever, myalgia, or arthralgia. Additionally, patients with subacute thyroiditis often experience a series of changes in thyroid function related to the inflammatory effects in the gland. Early in the course, symptomatic thyrotoxicosis may arise from the leakage of thyroid hormones from damaged follicular cells (see Chap. 42). Subsequently, patients may develop transient hypothyroidism after passing through a euthyroid phase. The hypothyroidism results from a depletion of thyroxine ($T_4$) and triiodothyronine ($T_3$) from the thyroid gland after the destructive, inflammatory process. However, patients usually experience a spontaneous recovery of normal thyroid function. Not all patients with subacute thyroiditis experience all phases of these alterations in thyroid function. The duration of the illness often is 6 weeks but may be 3 to 6 months. The inflammatory process may migrate from one area of the thyroid to another and often crosses between the two lobes ("creeping thyroiditis").

### LABORATORY EVALUATION

Laboratory evaluation usually reveals the following: elevated erythrocyte sedimentation rate (often >55 mm per hour); normal or near-normal leukocyte count; transient elevations of antithyroid antibodies in low titers; and serum $T_4$ and $T_3$ values that may be high, normal, or low, depending on the phase of the disease. In the thyrotoxic phase, the serum thyroid-stimulating hormone (TSH) value is suppressed but may be detectable in third-generation assays in nearly 80% of those evaluated.[10] TSH is normal during the euthyroid phase and elevated during the hypothyroid phase. A thyroid scan during an episode of subacute thyroiditis shows a cold region in the involved section of the thyroid. Additionally, during the thyrotoxic and euthyroid phases, the radioactive iodine (RAI) uptake is often <1%. This finding is of diagnostic importance in the evaluation of patients with suspected thyrotoxicosis, as a low uptake reflects the underlying etiology of destructive thyroiditis—not increased thyroid hormone production and secretion, as in Graves disease or toxic nodular goiter (in which the uptake is normal or high). Further, the serum thyroglobulin is frequently markedly elevated, a finding that is of value in the differential diagnosis of thyrotoxicosis that is due to surreptitious ingestion of thyroid hormone (thyrotoxicosis factitia). In the latter disorder, the RAI uptake and the serum thyroglobulin are low. Although the diagnosis of subacute thyroiditis usually is apparent in patients with typical clinical features, occasionally there is difficulty in establishing the diagnosis—such as with sudden enlargement of the thyroid gland—raising the possibility of anaplastic carcinoma. In this situation, a thyroid biopsy may be helpful. The usual microscopic features include degeneration of the follicular epithelium; infiltration of the tissue with leukocytes, lymphocytes, and histiocytes; and formation of granulomas composed of giant cells surrounding colloid. In approximately one-half of patients, microabscesses may be found.[11] In most patients with subacute thyroiditis, the diagnosis can be made clinically.

### TREATMENT

The management of patients with subacute thyroiditis is based on relief of symptoms, because no specific therapy is available. Two aspects of this therapy must be addressed in each patient:

the local symptoms and the effects of thyroid dysfunction. Frequently, pain and tenderness in the neck respond to treatment with salicylates, 0.65 g every 4 hours. If no benefit ensues within 48 hours, nonsteroidal antiinflammatory agents may be administered, although it is unclear whether these agents are superior to the salicylates. Approximately 5% of patients require corticosteroids for the relief of symptoms. Prednisone in doses of 30 to 40 mg per day usually results in prompt improvement; however, it may be difficult to reduce the dose without return of pain, so that treatment for 4 to 8 weeks may be necessary before a successful tapering is accomplished.[7] If the patient does not respond to prednisone within 24 to 48 hours, the diagnosis of subacute thyroiditis should be reevaluated. Thyroidectomy occasionally is used in patients with severe or recurrent pain that is unresponsive to other therapy, but this approach is required infrequently. If thyrotoxic symptoms are foremost, the patient should be managed with β-blockade (e.g., propranolol). The thyrotoxic phase in these patients is transient, and definitive therapy with RAI is neither indicated nor of value because the thyroid uptake is low. Likewise, the antithyroid drugs propylthiouracil or methimazole (Tapazole) should not be given because these medications are also ineffective. These drugs impair thyroid hormone synthesis, but the excess serum thyroid hormone levels in subacute thyroiditis result from leakage of $T_3$ and $T_4$ from the damaged follicles and not from enhanced synthesis and secretion. The hypothyroid phase of subacute thyroiditis is usually transient and is often asymptomatic; therefore, thyroid hormone replacement frequently is not necessary. Additionally, the increased TSH secretion at this time may be important in the recovery of thyroid gland function; consequently, there may be a relative contraindication to thyroid hormone treatment unless the patient is clearly symptomatic.

The long-term prognosis for patients with subacute thyroiditis is excellent. Recurrent episodes, although uncommon, do occur, in as many as 2% of affected patients yearly,[12] but eventual normal thyroid function is the rule. Discomfort in the thyroid area can, however, continue for many months. Rarely, patients with subacute thyroiditis may develop permanent hypothyroidism. Patients who have had prior thyroid surgery or who have coexistent autoimmune thyroiditis[13] may be especially prone to such an outcome.

# HASHIMOTO THYROIDITIS (AUTOIMMUNE THYROIDITIS)

Hashimoto thyroiditis, an autoimmune disorder, is the most common cause of hypothyroidism. It is also referred to as *chronic lymphocytic thyroiditis* and *autoimmune thyroiditis.* It occurs in all age groups, but it is most common in middle age.

## ETIOLOGY

Numerous features of Hashimoto thyroiditis indicate an autoimmune cause in which multiple genetic factors likely play an important role.[14] Because the disorder is much more common in women than in men, the possibility of a gene related to sex-steroid action has been considered.[14] Patients with Hashimoto thyroiditis are characterized by the presence of circulating antibodies to microsomal and thyroglobulin antigens, often present in high titer. The disorder occurs frequently in certain families, particularly among the female members.[15] Patients with Hashimoto thyroiditis and their relatives have an increased prevalence of other autoimmune disorders, such as Addison disease, diabetes mellitus, pernicious anemia, and myasthenia gravis—one or more of these may develop over time. The disease is characterized pathologically by infiltration of the thyroid by plasma cells and lymphocytes. Autoimmune thyroiditis resulting in hypothyroidism may represent a spec-

trum from Hashimoto disease (with a goiter) to atrophic lymphocytic thyroiditis (without a goiter, often called *primary myxedema*). The variability in these related disorders may reflect the production of different types of antithyroid antibodies. For example, patients with agoitrous autoimmune thyroiditis may have a blocking antibody that inhibits the growth of thyroid tissue induced by TSH.[16] This antibody most likely is absent in patients with Hashimoto thyroiditis and a goiter. The antimicrosomal antibodies found in patients with Hashimoto thyroiditis are primarily directed against the thyroid peroxidase (TPO) enzyme. Inhibition of this enzyme by the TPO antibody may be partly responsible for the hypothyroidism seen in these patients.[17] In addition, patients with Hashimoto thyroiditis may have antibodies that block TSH-dependent production of cyclic adenosine monophosphate, thus inhibiting thyroid hormone production. In one study,[18] it was shown that patients with overt hypothyroidism that is due to Hashimoto thyroiditis have a higher prevalence of TSH-blocking antibodies than patients with subclinical hypothyroidism.

The autoimmune thyroid diseases represent a wide spectrum of immune abnormalities, from Graves thyrotoxicosis, caused by antibodies that stimulate the TSH receptor, to Hashimoto thyroiditis, which results from a complex process of immunologic events leading to impaired thyroid function. Both these autoimmune thyroid diseases share a common pathophysiologic bond: the production of an abnormal thyroid state resulting from an immune process directed against the thyroid gland. Volpé[15] suggested that Hashimoto thyroiditis is predominantly a disorder of cell-mediated immunity that is manifested by a genetic defect in the suppressor T-cell function. This theory postulates that as a result of defective suppressor T cells, helper (CD4) T cells are not suppressed appropriately and, therefore, are able to activate and cooperate with certain B lymphocytes. Additionally, the helper T cells produce various cytokines, including interferon-γ, which induce thyrocytes to express major histocompatibility complex class II surface HLA-DR antigens and render them susceptible to immunologic attack. The activated B lymphocytes then produce antibodies that react with thyroid antigens. However, the antimicrosomal (anti-TPO) and antithyroglobulin antibodies used as serologic markers to identify patients with Hashimoto thyroiditis are likely not the direct cause of the thyroid destruction. There is evidence that cytotoxic T lymphocytes show variants in the promoter of antigen 4 (CTLA-4) and represent a risk factor for Hashimoto disease.[19] These cells act in concert with complement and killer (or K) lymphocytes to cause lymphocytic thyroiditis. In addition to autoimmune mechanisms of thyroid cell damage, various environmental factors may be involved in the pathogenesis of Hashimoto thyroiditis.[19a] For example, iodide ingestion may help trigger the development of autoimmune thyroiditis.[20] Further, the administration of granulocyte macrophage colony-stimulating factor or interleukin-2 may induce the temporary development of thyroid autoantibodies and reversible hypothyroidism in treated patients.[21,22] This finding suggests that patients receiving hematopoietic growth factors or cytokines should be monitored for the development of autoimmune thyroiditis and hypothyroidism.

Apoptosis (programmed cell death) may play a major role in the massive thyrocyte destruction in Hashimoto thyroiditis.[23] Cross-linking of the Fas receptor with its ligand (Fas L) induces apoptosis, whereas this process is inhibited by the protooncogene Bc1-2. Immunostaining of Hashimoto tissue shows enhanced expression of Fas and Fas L but diminished Bc1-2 protein in thyroid follicles, effects activated by the cytokine interleukin-1β (IL-1β), which is abundantly produced in a Hashimoto gland.[24]

Certain HLA tissue types, such as HLA-DR5, are more common in patients with Hashimoto thyroiditis than in the general population (see Chap. 194). Patients with primary myxedema (agoitrous hypothyroidism) have an increased prevalence of DR3 but not the DR5 antigen, suggesting that these autoim-

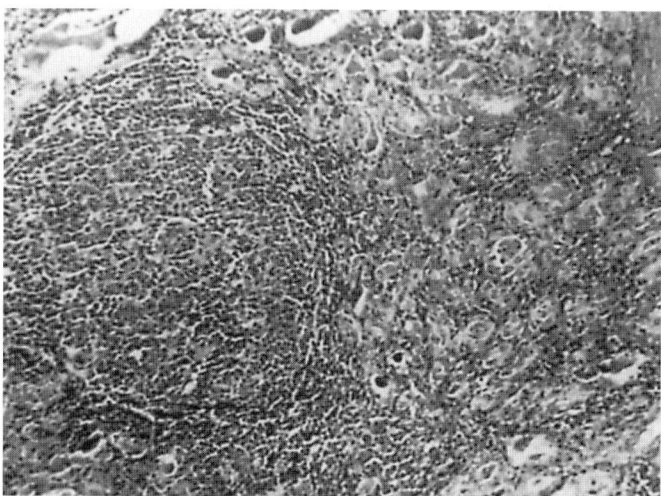

**FIGURE 46-2.** Histology of Hashimoto thyroiditis. ×125 (From LiVolsi VA, LoGerfo P, eds. Thyroiditis. Boca Raton, FL: CRC Press, 1981.)

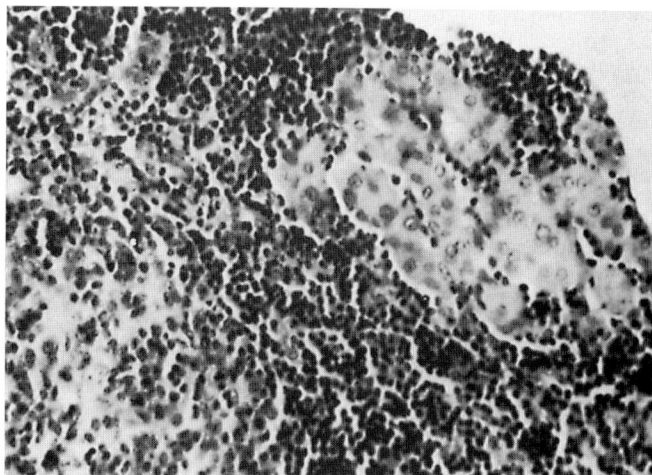

**FIGURE 46-3.** Histology of Hashimoto thyroiditis. Note the presence of lymphocytic and plasma cell infiltration, germinal centers, and eosinophilic Askanazy cells. ×200 (From LiVolsi VA, LoGerfo P, eds. Thyroiditis. Boca Raton, FL: CRC Press, 1981.)

mune thyroid disorders are separate genetic entities.[25] Because Graves disease and Hashimoto thyroiditis may coexist in the same patient, it is interesting that in both conditions there is an increased prevalence of HLA-AW30.[26] Graves disease, however, is associated with an excess of DR3 (as in primary myxedema) but not the DR5 antigen.[27] HLA-DR antigens are not normally expressed on thyroid cells. However, in Hashimoto disease the thyroid follicular cells present these antigens on their surface, which may trigger the autoimmune process.[28] There remains, however, considerable debate on the role that the HLA system plays in the pathogenesis of Hashimoto thyroiditis. It has been suggested that the tendency to develop thyroid autoantibodies is inherited as a mendelian dominant trait and not primarily through the HLA-related gene systems.[20] In addition, age, sex, and environmental factors (e.g., iodide or viral exposures) may play modifying roles in defining which genetically predisposed patients develop autoimmune thyroiditis.

## PATHOLOGY

Pathologically, Hashimoto thyroiditis is characterized by the infiltration of the gland with lymphocytes and plasma cells, follicular destruction and fibrosis, colloid depletion, and, at times, the presence of germinal centers (Figs. 46-2 and 46-3). In some patients, only isolated areas of lymphocytic infiltration are noted (termed *focal thyroiditis*). This may represent an early phase of Hashimoto thyroiditis, because there is a correlation between the degree of lymphocytic infiltration and the presence of antimicrosomal and antithyroglobulin antibodies in the serum of affected patients.[29] Also characteristically found in the glands of adults (but not children) with Hashimoto thyroiditis are eosinophilic epithelial cells called *Hürthle* or *Askanazy cells.*[16] In the juvenile form of Hashimoto thyroiditis, lymphoid follicles usually are not present.

## CLINICAL FEATURES

Patients may present in one of or a combination of the following three ways: with a goiter or thyroid nodule; with hypothyroidism; or with thyrotoxicosis, in which the condition is often referred to as *hashitoxicosis*. It appears likely that in most of the latter patients, the thyrotoxicosis represents the coexistence of Graves disease or silent thyroiditis with Hashimoto thyroiditis. The clinical features of the hyperthyroidism in patients with an apparent combination of Graves and Hashimoto disorders are essentially identical to the features of thyrotoxicosis in patients with only Graves disease. It is probable, however, that patients

with Graves disease and coexistent Hashimoto thyroiditis have an increased chance of spontaneous remission of the thyrotoxicosis and may be more prone to develop spontaneous hypothyroidism.

Goiter is a common presentation for patients with Hashimoto thyroiditis. In these patients, the gland is characteristically firm and bosselated, often with a palpable pyramidal lobe. Usually, patients have a diffusely enlarged gland; however, some patients may have a multinodular goiter or, more rarely, a single nodule. Although the goiter most often is asymptomatic, occasional patients develop pain and tenderness in the thyroid. In these patients, goiter growth may have been rapid, and the antithyroid antibody titers usually are high. The goiter also may cause local symptoms, such as pressure in the neck or dysphagia, but these symptoms are unusual. Hashimoto thyroiditis is not associated with cervical lymphadenopathy, and most patients (75–80%) presenting with a goiter are euthyroid when initially evaluated. Other patients have hypothyroidism that may be apparent clinically, or it may be subclinical and documented only by thyroid function testing. Commonly, patients present with hypothyroid symptoms, and a careful physical examination reveals a small goiter, the presence of which the patient may have been unaware. The diagnosis of Hashimoto thyroiditis should be strongly suspected in a euthyroid or hypothyroid patient who presents with a thyroid gland that has the "feel" of a Hashimoto gland. This determination is more easily made with extensive experience so that the typical firm and somewhat rubbery consistency of the thyroid tissue can be recognized. This disorder, which can occur in children, may be present as an acute confusional state with a gradual impairment of cognitive function, even mimicking stroke.[31a]

## OTHER ASSOCIATED CLINICAL DISORDERS

Patients with depression may have an increased prevalence of antithyroid antibodies, suggesting that autoimmune thyroiditis may predispose to this disorder.[30] Additionally, a rapidly progressive dementia may occur in patients with Hashimoto disease (Hashimoto encephalopathy), which often responds to treatment with high dose glucocorticoid therapy.[31]

## LABORATORY EVALUATION

A full laboratory evaluation of any patient suspected of having Hashimoto thyroiditis must include a determination of thyroid function. Rarely, patients may be thyrotoxic, in which case ele-

PART III: THE THYROID GLAND

vated serum $T_4$ and/or $T_3$ levels usually are found, along with a suppressed TSH. However, most patients are euthyroid or hypothyroid when first evaluated. In the hypothyroid patients, one may variably see reduced serum $T_4$ and $T_3$ levels and $T_3$ uptake with an elevated serum TSH. In patients with milder degrees of hypothyroidism, however, one may see only an elevated serum TSH concentration (or even a normal basal TSH value with an exaggerated TSH response to thyrotropin-releasing hormone). In these patients, the hypothyroidism probably is at an earlier stage, as manifested by the normal levels of serum $T_4$ and $T_3$. Without thyroid hormone replacement, many of these patients would eventually develop frank clinical hypothyroidism with low serum $T_4$ and $T_3$ levels. An immunologic diagnosis of Hashimoto thyroiditis can be made by the determination of antimicrosomal and antithyroglobulin antibodies in the serum using various methods.[32] The availability of recombinant TPO has led to the development of assays for anti-TPO, which have enhanced the sensitivity of the serologic diagnosis for Hashimoto thyroiditis. As a consequence, the antimicrosomal antibody determination is becoming obsolete. In biopsy-proven Hashimoto thyroiditis, the antimicrosomal levels are elevated more commonly than are the antithyroglobulin levels. Low titers of antithyroid antibodies may be found in patients with a wide variety of thyroid disorders and in apparently asymptomatic patients who have no evidence of thyroid disease. It is possible that the presence of low levels of antithyroid antibodies represents an early stage of Hashimoto thyroiditis, before the development of a goiter or thyroid function abnormalities. Furthermore, seronegative Hashimoto thyroiditis, presumably related to an organ-restricted form of this autoimmune disorder, has been reported.[33] Low titers of the antibodies also may represent a nonspecific response to thyroid tissue damage, as may be seen in patients with thyroid carcinoma.

In many patients who present with a diffuse goiter or hypothyroidism, a thyroid RAI uptake and scan are not crucial to the management. When a patient presents with a solitary nodule, a fine-needle aspiration biopsy is indicated to evaluate the possibility of malignancy (see Chap. 34). Of note is evidence that the presence of a cold nodule on nuclear scan in Hashimoto thyroiditis may reflect an even higher risk for malignancy than is normally found in such nodules.[34] If a thyroidal RAI uptake is done, one finds normal or low values in most patients, with rare patients showing an elevated uptake. Additionally, patients with Hashimoto thyroiditis may have a positive perchlorate discharge test (see Chap. 34), but this finding is also seen in patients with other thyroid disorders, such as in Graves disease after iodine-131 ($^{131}$I) therapy. The scan in patients with Hashimoto thyroiditis often is symmetric but with a patchy uptake evident.[35]

In summary, to establish a diagnosis of Hashimoto thyroiditis in patients presenting with a goiter or thyroid function abnormalities, the determination of the titer of the anti-TPO antibody is the most helpful laboratory test available. A thyroid fine-needle aspiration biopsy is not routinely necessary, but can be helpful in establishing the diagnosis in antibody negative subjects (~10%). In patients with a solitary nodule, it should be undertaken to rule out a thyroid malignancy. Ultrasonography demonstrates reduced thyroid echogenicity in both Hashimoto and Graves diseases.[35a] This finding on ultrasound may be a useful predictor of these autoimmune diseases.[35a]

## TREATMENT

Treatment usually involves the administration of physiologic doses of thyroid hormone, for example 0.1 to 0.15 mg per day of L-$T_4$. (In elderly hypothyroid patients or those with coronary disease, the initial dosage is lower, 0.0125–0.025 mg per day.) In patients with clinical or even subclinical hypothyroidism and Hashimoto thyroiditis, the therapy is directed at the hypothyroidism. In patients with a goiter but no hypothyroidism, the authors usually still consider the use of thyroid hormone replacement, for two reasons. First, the thyroid hormone administration may shrink the goiter, or at least limit growth. In patients with local symptoms (such as dysphagia), the thyroid hormone may lead to some improvement. The second reason relates to the natural history of the disease. In a number of patients with Hashimoto thyroiditis, hypothyroidism develops eventually.[36] Therefore, it seems reasonable to institute replacement in these patients early in the course of the disease rather than waiting until symptoms develop. This decision, however, is optional, and it would not be unreasonable to observe such patients carefully and to institute $T_4$ replacement when hypothyroidism actually occurs.

Previously, it was thought that hypothyroidism resulting from Hashimoto thyroiditis was likely permanent. However, more recent evidence has shown that some patients with hypothyroidism that is due to Hashimoto thyroiditis may have transient hypothyroidism. Approximately 20% of such patients have a spontaneous recovery of thyroid function while taking thyroid hormone replacement.[37] Another study[38] demonstrated that the mechanism of such recovery likely involves a disappearance of the TSH-blocking antibodies that previously were the apparent cause of the hypothyroidism. In the atypical, uncommon patient with rapid thyroid growth and pain, Hashimoto thyroiditis can be treated with corticosteroids, primarily to alleviate the local symptoms. An initial dosage of 60 to 80 mg per day of oral prednisone has been recommended, with a gradual tapering over a period of 3 to 4 weeks.

Surgery is rarely indicated in patients with Hashimoto thyroiditis; it usually is undertaken to relieve severe local effects (e.g., obstructive symptoms unresponsive to corticosteroids), to exclude the possible presence of a thyroid malignancy in a patient with a solitary thyroid nodule, or to treat a patient whose goiter continues to grow despite thyroid hormone administration.

The long-term prognosis of most patients with Hashimoto thyroiditis is good, because the hypothyroidism can be corrected by L-$T_4$, and the goiter usually is not large enough to cause serious problems. However, patients with Hashimoto thyroiditis may be at a significantly higher risk of developing a thyroid lymphoma[39] (see Chap. 40). Although this is uncommon, any increase in thyroid gland size during L-$T_4$ administration necessitates the exclusion of a malignant change.

## SILENT THYROIDITIS

### ETIOLOGY

During the past two decades, physicians increasingly have observed patients presenting with signs and symptoms of thyrotoxicosis; a small, painless, nontender goiter; and a low RAI uptake. Furthermore, the thyrotoxicosis has been transient. This syndrome, usually termed *silent thyroiditis* (absence of thyroid pain)[40] also has been termed *hyperthyroiditis*,[41] *painless subacute thyroiditis, atypical subacute thyroiditis*, and *lymphocytic thyroiditis with spontaneously resolving hyperthyroidism*. It is apparent from the range of the terms used to describe this disorder that the etiology and relation to several other forms of thyroiditis are somewhat unclear. Additionally, the reported frequency with which silent thyroiditis causes thyrotoxicosis ranges widely, from 4% to 23%.[42,43] The clinical course resembles that seen in subacute thyroiditis in regard to thyroid function. At biopsy, however, the thyroid tissue from patients with silent thyroiditis reveals findings more suggestive of Hashimoto disease (chronic lymphocytic thyroiditis), because extensive lymphocytic infiltration is observed. Often, severe disruption of the follicles is seen, Hürthle cell transformation is absent, and occasionally lymphoid follicles are present.[44] Despite these histologic changes that are compatible with Hashimoto thyroiditis, as many as 40% of patients with silent thyroiditis do not have significantly elevated titers of antimicrosomal or antithyroglobulin antibodies, the serologic hallmark of Hashimoto disease.[7]

Silent thyroiditis is associated with an excess of HLA-DR3.[45] This association links silent thyroiditis to autoimmune thyroiditis rather than to subacute thyroiditis.[46] Other observations that implicate an autoimmune etiology for this entity are the onset of silent thyroiditis (which has been observed after the resection of a thymoma)[47] and the appearance of a mixture of TSH-receptor antibodies that may mediate the various phases of thyroid function that are observed.[48] Silent thyroiditis has also been reported in conjunction with amiodarone[7] and lithium, and with the use of interferon-α in the treatment of hepatitis C patients.[49,50] The prevalence of antibodies before interferon treatment generally is low,[51] but treatment may induce antibodies in as many as 15% of patients, most of whom may experience thyrotoxicosis and/or hypothyroidism.[52] A report[53] was made of silent thyroiditis in a husband whose wife previously had subacute thyroiditis. Similar to subacute thyroiditis, the thyrotoxicosis[54] in silent thyroiditis results from damage to follicular cells by the inflammatory process, with the subsequent release of excessive amounts of thyroid hormone. This process also impairs the capacity of the thyroid to trap iodine—hence, the observed low RAI uptake. Because the damaged follicular cells temporarily cannot make additional thyroid hormone, patients experience a euthyroid phase and then become hypothyroid when the stored thyroid hormone is depleted; in most cases, they ultimately are restored to euthyroidism. The presence of high titers of anti-TPO (especially in the postpartum variety) may predispose to permanent hypothyroidism.

## CLINICAL FEATURES

Patients with silent thyroiditis present with the signs and symptoms of thyrotoxicosis, such as nervousness, weight loss, and often palpitations.[7] Thyroid examination, although variable, often reveals a slightly enlarged, firm, nontender gland. The thyroid, however, may be normal in size, but if enlarged, it usually is symmetric without nodules. These patients do not have the infiltrative eye signs or skin changes (pretibial myxedema) seen in Graves hyperthyroidism, a distinction that is helpful clinically. A history of a recent viral illness is not usually obtained. The differentiation from Graves hyperthyroidism is important as the prevalence of silent thyroiditis ranges from 1% of cases of thyrotoxicosis in Wales to 23% in some parts of the United States.[7] As in subacute thyroiditis, patients characteristically progress from a thyrotoxic state to euthyroid and hypothyroid phases before recovering normal thyroid function. The thyrotoxic phase of silent thyroiditis usually is transient, lasting ~2 to 4 months (rare patients may have thyrotoxicosis lasting 12 months[44]).

Occasional patients, however, may develop permanent, rather than transient, hypothyroidism, especially if the antimicrosomal (or anti-TPO) antibody titers are elevated. This, along with the HLA findings, suggests that silent thyroiditis in these patients represents a form of Hashimoto disease.

## LABORATORY EVALUATION AND TREATMENT

The diagnosis of silent thyroiditis is based on the finding of hyperthyroidism in the context of a low RAI uptake and a painless thyroid gland. These patients usually present in the thyrotoxic phase, and laboratory evaluation shows an elevated serum $T_4$, $T_3$, and $T_3$ uptake, and a suppressed TSH. TSH suppression is below the lower limit of detectability with a third-generation TSH assay in 90% of subjects with silent thyroiditis,[10] similar to Graves disease.[10] Anti-TPO or antithyroglobulin antibodies may only be present in relatively low titers (although some patients have raised titers), and the white blood cell count typically is normal. The erythrocyte sedimentation rate is normal or slightly elevated. An RAI uptake is low (often 1% to 2%) at 6 and 24 hours,[55] differentiating this form of thyrotoxicosis from Graves hyperthyroidism or Plummer disease (see Chap. 34). This is important because the management of thyrotoxic patients with silent thyroiditis is different from that for Graves hyperthyroidism or toxic nodular goiter. Because the hyperthyroxinemia in silent thyroiditis, as in subacute thyroiditis, results from the excessive release of thyroid hormone from damaged thyroid follicular cells and not from excess synthesis, antithyroid medication (propylthiouracil, methimazole) or $^{131}I$ therapy are inappropriate. The thyrotoxicosis should normally be treated symptomatically with β-adrenergic blockade, such as propranolol, 10 to 40 mg orally three or four times daily, if there are no contraindications to this form of therapy (i.e., congestive heart failure or asthma). Decreased $T_4$ to $T_3$ conversion may also be accomplished by administering sodium ipodate in doses of 500 mg per day. Ipodate has been demonstrated to be effective in rapidly decreasing $T_3$ levels and symptoms.[56] It may be continued for 2 to 6 weeks as the clinical syndrome resolves in individuals with severe destructive thyrotoxicosis. In occasional patients (10% to 20%) who do not respond to β-blockade, prednisone may be tried. Prednisone, started at 50 mg per day orally, then tapered over 4 weeks, has been used in patients with silent thyroiditis.

Rarely, surgery may be indicated in patients with recurrent episodes of severe thyrotoxic silent thyroiditis. Patients in the hypothyroid phase of silent thyroiditis often do not need thyroid hormone replacement because the hypothyroidism is usually transient and often symptomatically mild. Furthermore, as in subacute thyroiditis, the elevated serum TSH at this time may enhance the spontaneous return of normal thyroid function. In patients who are symptomatic and require treatment, it has been suggested that a lower-than-usual dose of thyroid hormone replacement be given to allow the TSH to remain slightly elevated. This may enhance the subsequent recovery of thyroid function.[57] Similarly, such patients may be treated with L-$T_4$ for ~9 months and then receive a tapering dose of thyroid hormone to determine if recovery of thyroid function has occurred.[58] In patients who appear to have developed permanent hypothyroidism (persistence of low serum $T_4$, elevated serum TSH levels, and hypothyroid symptoms for longer than 4 to 9 months), long-term thyroid hormone replacement is indicated.

Thyroid biopsy usually is not necessary to make the diagnosis. In many patients with this disorder, the thyroid gland is only barely enlarged; therefore, this procedure can be technically difficult. However, all nonpregnant patients with suspected hyperthyroidism, whose diagnosis appears to be other than Graves disease or a toxic nodular goiter by examination, should have an RAI uptake to establish the presence of this disorder. If the gland is painless and the uptake is low, a diagnosis of silent thyroiditis can usually be made. These patients can be reassured that the thyrotoxic phase is generally transient, and β-blockade is the treatment of choice if relief of thyrotoxic symptoms is necessary.

Studies of the natural history of silent thyroiditis suggest that a number of patients have recurrences (in one study, 11%[59]); patients with chronically elevated titers of antithyroid antibodies tend to develop permanent hypothyroidism. Because this disorder was recognized only relatively recently, however, additional studies are needed to document more clearly the long-term features of the disorder.

At least five conditions exist in which symptoms of thyrotoxicosis may be associated with a low RAI uptake: subacute thyroiditis; silent thyroiditis; recent iodide ingestion by patients with Graves disease, toxic multinodular goiter, or toxic adenoma; thyrotoxicosis factitia; and ectopic hyperthyroidism (struma ovarii or functioning metastatic thyroid carcinoma).

## POSTPARTUM THYROIDITIS

Like spontaneous lymphocytic thyroiditis, postpartum thyroiditis is associated with HLA-DR3, but an association with

DR5 also is observed.[45] This postpartum entity occurs in 5% to 9% of all pregnancies.[58,60–62] These observations are of particular interest for the probable autoimmune nature of this and the classic form of silent thyroiditis, as it is well established that many autoimmune diseases flare during the postpartum period after resolution of the immune suppression normally seen to occur during pregnancy. Higher ratios of helper (CD4+) to suppressor (CD8+) T cells seen in the postpregnancy state may play a critical role in the development of this postpartum dysfunction.[63] Patients with type 1 diabetes mellitus are especially prone to the development of postpartum thyroiditis; as many as 25% experience this disorder.[59,64]

## CLINICAL FEATURES AND LABORATORY EVALUATION

Fewer than 33% of affected women have a classic thyrotoxic, euthyroid, hypothyroid pattern followed by euthyroid recovery.[7] Many patients may present only as hypothyroidism when the thyrotoxic phase is mild or brief.[64] For those presenting with clear symptoms or laboratory evidence of thyrotoxicosis or hyperthyroxinemia and thyrotropin suppression, differentiation of a postpartum flare of Graves hyperthyroidism with an RAI uptake is essential to appropriately intervene. This diagnostic intervention may be problematic, because it interrupts the course of breast-feeding at a critical stage of bonding and necessitates discarding RAI-contaminated milk for 1 week after the ingestion of the diagnostic iodine dose. It is not enough to assume that thyrotoxicosis in the postpartum period is due to thyroiditis or even preexisting Graves disease; one study has demonstrated that 26 of 96 women with prior Graves disease who subsequently developed postpartum thyrotoxicosis actually had low uptake thyroiditis.[65]

Postpartum thyroiditis typically occurs with subsequent pregnancies among those who are HLA-DR5 positive[45] and may be partially predicted by the presence of thyroid autoantibodies which are seen in ~10% of affected women at 16 weeks of gestation.[58,66] Titers of antithyroid antibodies reach peak levels 3 to 7 months postpartum, corresponding to the thyrotoxic (~14 weeks) and hypothyroid (19 weeks) phases of the process.[58] Approximately 25% of patients with prior episodes of postpartum thyroiditis subsequently develop permanent hypothyroidism.[62] The majority, therefore, should be expected to recover from their postpartum episode and maintain euthyroidism.[7,58]

## TREATMENT

Treatment of the thyrotoxic phase with a β-blocker may be necessary for symptomatic individuals. L-$T_4$ may be indicated for symptoms during the hypothyroid phase. As most patients do recover normal thyroid function, $T_4$ should be withdrawn after 6 to 9 months of replacement.

## RIEDEL THYROIDITIS

Riedel thyroiditis is a most unusual and rare form of thyroid disease, which is characterized by extensive fibrosis of the thyroid gland. In these patients, the gland is hard, woody in consistency, and often fixed to the adjacent tissues. Occasionally, the gland may be asymmetric, presenting as a unilateral mass. In many patients with Riedel thyroiditis, local symptoms, including hoarseness (recurrent laryngeal nerve involvement) or dysphagia, are present. Pathologically, the gland shows an inflammatory fibrous process consisting of activated T lymphocytes, macrophages, aggregates of B lymphocytes, eosinophilia, and deposition of eosinophilic products, which may stimulate fibrosis[67] both within and outside the thyroid capsule (Fig. 46-4). Because invasion of local tissues typically occurs, the pathologic appearance initially may resemble invasive anaplastic car-

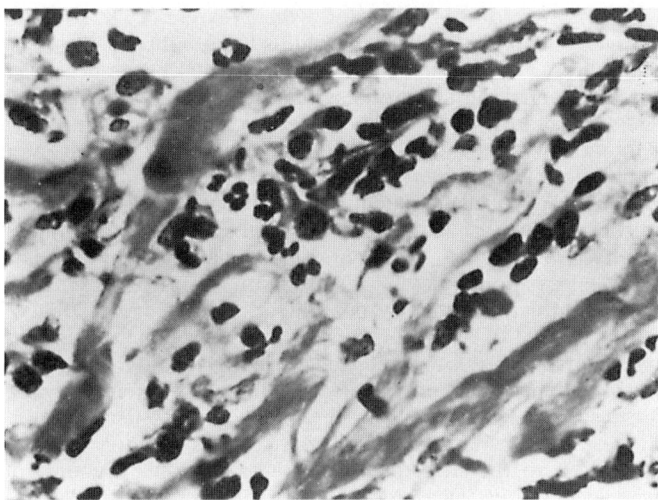

**FIGURE 46-4.** Riedel thyroiditis. Note fibrous tissue proliferation with cellular exudate consisting of lymphocytes, plasma cells, and polymorphonuclear leukocytes. ×650 (From Thomson JA, Jackson IMD, Duguid WP. The effect of steroid therapy on Riedel's thyroiditis. Scott Med J 1968; 13:13.)

cinoma.[68] The etiology is unclear, but it may represent a variant of Hashimoto thyroiditis, as evidenced by the mononuclear infiltrate, the detection of thyroid-specific autoantibodies in many patients, and the response to glucocorticoid treatment.[67] Riedel thyroiditis may represent the extension into the thyroid of a more generalized, invasive fibrosis syndrome, such as retroperitoneal fibrosis. Indeed, patients have been described with both Riedel thyroiditis and retroperitoneal fibrosis. This diagnosis should be considered in patients who present with a woody, hard thyroid gland that is fixed in position and associated with local symptoms. Laboratory evaluation—including thyroid function tests, erythrocyte sedimentation rate, and thyroid antibodies—may be normal, but a thyroid scan may reveal a nonspecific reduction in uptake in the affected areas. The diagnosis can be best established by a biopsy; however, specimens from patients with other thyroid disorders (e.g., Hashimoto thyroiditis) also may contain notable fibrotic tissue. Surgical treatment may be required if there are significant local symptoms or evidence of tracheal compression. Corticosteroids occasionally have been helpful in reducing the goiter size and alleviating local symptoms.[69]

## RADIATION THYROIDITIS

Radiation injury to the thyroid gland may affect it in several ways, depending on the dose and type of radiation. Pathologically, the thyroid changes seen after acute radiation injury (radiation thyroiditis) include cellular necrosis, follicular disruption, infiltration by neutrophils, and local edema.[70] Soon thereafter, vascular damage is evident in the form of hemorrhage and thrombosis. The more long-term changes of radiation thyroiditis (years after the injury) include fibrosis, atrophy of the follicles, nuclear abnormalities, lymphocytic infiltration, oxyphilic changes, and arteriolar hyalinization.

### RADIOISOTOPE THERAPY-INDUCED INJURY

Internal irradiation (e.g., [131]I or [125]I) for the treatment of hyperthyroidism or thyroid cancer can induce a radiation thyroiditis that may abruptly present clinically as pain and tenderness in the thyroid, swelling in the neck, and transient thyrotoxicosis. Indeed, thyroid storm occasionally has occurred after [131]I treatment of thyrotoxicosis.[71] These acute changes usually occur within 1 week of the RAI treatment and subside within

3 to 4 weeks.[70] As a consequence of [131]I or [125]I therapy for hyperthyroidism, the most common long-term clinical abnormality relates to the development of hypothyroidism. Therefore, after RAI therapy, patients need to be monitored indefinitely for the occurrence of hypothyroidism. However, there does not appear to be any increased incidence of thyroid cancer in patients receiving RAI therapeutically. This absence of an increased incidence of thyroid cancer after [131]I or [125]I therapy or *high-dose* external irradiation for head and neck cancer may relate to the fact that very high levels of intrathyroidal radiation are achieved, thereby destroying thyroid cells and obviating the potential for the later development of thyroid cell carcinoma.

## EXTERNAL RADIATION-INDUCED INJURY

Three effects may be seen on the thyroid gland after external irradiation of the thyroid: goitrous formation caused by thyroiditis, the induction of thyroid tumors, and the development of hypothyroidism. An increased incidence of goiter and of thyroid carcinoma has been observed in patients who previously received external irradiation to the head and neck in infancy or childhood for the treatment of such conditions as enlarged thymus or tonsils or for acne vulgaris (radiation dose usually <10 Gy [<1000 rads]; see Chap. 40). The development of thyroid cancer 10 to 40 years later after this type of *low-dose* external irradiation may occur. The effects are dose related from 0.5 to 10 Gy (50–1000 rads). Hypothyroidism does not occur at this dose range.

The radiation doses used for treatment of head or neck cancers or lymphomas (40–50 Gy) may lead to the development of thyrotoxic thyroiditis with subsequent hypothyroidism months to years after the radiation exposure.[72] Experience indicates that thyroid cancer is not a risk from this treatment.

## OTHER FORMS OF THYROIDITIS

### PERINEOPLASTIC THYROIDITIS

*Perineoplastic thyroiditis* is a term used to describe thyroiditis in a gland containing a thyroid neoplasm. Most commonly, this refers to lymphocytic thyroiditis in the tissue surrounding a thyroid neoplasm, most often a papillary thyroid carcinoma (PTC), but this finding has also been reported in medullary thyroid cancer. The frequency with which perineoplastic lymphocytic infiltration in PTC occurs varies with race and sex. It has been suggested that the lymphocytic thyroiditis represents an autoimmune reaction to the thyroid neoplasm and that it may be beneficial in reducing the spread of the tumor. Lymphocytes derived from tissue containing PTC are unusual, because they express both CD4 and CD8 markers and may display intense cytolytic activity in vitro. Significantly improved outcomes occur in PTC and medullary thyroid cancer patients who have lymphocytic infiltration when compared with patients with these tumors and no lymphocytic tissue response.[73] This finding may, if confirmed, be useful in treatment planning for patients with thyroid cancer.[74] Despite the increased incidence of thyroid lymphoma in patients with Hashimoto thyroiditis, clinical lymphocytic thyroiditis generally is not regarded as a significant premalignant lesion and was found in only ~1% of PTC cases in one series.[73] Therefore, the removal of thyroid glands containing chronic lymphocytic thyroiditis, which might be aimed at preventing the development of a thyroid neoplasm, does not seem justified. The coexistence of thyroiditis and a neoplasm in the same gland indicates that caution must be exercised in the interpretation of a thyroid biopsy that demonstrates thyroiditis. Because the lymphocytic changes are often noted near or mixed with the tumor, a biopsy of a tumor may show only thyroiditis. Multiple biopsy samples should allow sampling of actual tumor tissue and prevent the cancer from being missed.

## PALPATION THYROIDITIS

Palpation of the thyroid gland also can lead to a type of thyroiditis referred to as *palpation thyroiditis*. Most thyroid glands removed from patients who had recent thyroid physical examinations may reveal this form of inflammation.[75] Histologic examination demonstrates infiltration of lymphocytes, plasma cells, and occasionally giant cells. Hemorrhage also may be present. The clinical significance of palpation thyroiditis is unclear; however, few adverse effects are expected in most patients. Transient thyroiditis causing thyrotoxicosis may occur after throat trauma, thyroid biopsy, parathyroid surgery, and after surgical resection of hypopharyngeal cancer. These patients most likely develop a form of palpation thyroiditis because of trauma to the thyroid at the time of surgery. The possibility of such thyroiditis should be considered in postoperative patients who develop signs or symptoms suggestive of hyperthyroidism.

## GRANULOMATOUS DISORDERS

Infiltrative disorders, such as sarcoidosis or eosinophilic granuloma, may involve the thyroid gland and result in a lymphocytic thyroiditis, probably occurring as a reaction to the induced damage in the gland. Noncaseating granulomas have been noted occasionally in the thyroid glands of patients with sarcoidosis and usually are found between the thyroid follicles. If such granulomas are noted in a biopsy or surgical specimen from the thyroid, the patient should be evaluated for the systemic presence of sarcoidosis.

## REFERENCES

1. Volpé R. Acute and subacute thyroiditis. Pharmacol Ther 1976; 1:171.
2. Abe K, Taguchi T, Ohumo A, et al. Recurrent acute suppurative thyroiditis. Am J Dis Child 1978; 132:990.
3. Smilack JD, Rodolfo A. Coccidioidal infection of the thyroid. Arch Intern Med 1998; 158:89.
4. Golshan MM, McHenry CR, deVente J, et al. Acute suppurative thyroiditis and necrosis of the thyroid gland: a rare endocrine manifestation of acquired immunodeficiency syndrome. Surgery 1997; 233:593.
5. Dolgin C, LoGerfo P. Surgical management of thyroiditis. In: LiVolsi VA, LoGerfo P, eds. Thyroiditis. Boca Raton, FL: CRC Press, 1981:174.
6. Takai S, Matsuzaka F, Miyauchi A, et al. Internal fistula as a route of infection in acute suppurative thyroiditis. Lancet 1979; 1:751.
7. Ross DS. Syndromes of thyrotoxicosis with low radioactive iodine uptake. Endocrinol Metab Clin North Am 1998; 27:169.
8. Eylan E, Zmucky R, Sheba C. Mumps virus and subacute thyroiditis: evidence of a causal association. Lancet 1957; 1:1062.
9. Bech K, Nerup J, Thomsen M, et al. Subacute thyroiditis de Quervain: a disease associated with a HLA-B antigen. Acta Endocrinol (Copenh) 1977; 86:504.
10. Ito M, Takamatsu J, Yoshida S, et al. Incomplete thyrotroph suppression determined by third generation thyrotropin assay in subacute thyroiditis compared to silent thyroiditis or hyperthyroid Graves' disease. J Clin Endocrinol Metab 1997; 82:616.
11. Hannibal E, LiVolsi V. Subacute thyroiditis. In: LiVolsi VA, LoGerfo P, eds. Thyroiditis. Boca Raton, FL: CRC Press, 1981:31.
12. Iitaka M, Momotani N, Ishii J. Incidence of subacute thyroiditis recurrences after a prolonged latency: 24-year survey. J Clin Endocrinol Metab 1996; 81:466.
13. Tikkanen M, Lamberg BA. Hypothyroidism following subacute thyroiditis. Acta Endocrinol (Copenh) 1982; 101:348.
14. Barbesino G, Tomer Y, Concepcion ES, et al. International Consortium for the Genetics of Autoimmune Thyroid Disease. Linkage analysis of candidate genes in autoimmune thyroid disease II. Selected gender-related genes and the X-chromosome. J Clin Endocrinol Metab 1998; 83:3290.
15. Volpé R. Autoimmune thyroiditis. In: Braverman LE, Utiger RD, eds. Werner and Ingbar's the thyroid, 5th ed. Philadelphia: JB Lippincott, 1991:921.
16. Drexhage H, Bottazzo G, Bitensky L, et al. Thyroid growth-blocking antibodies in primary myxedema. Nature 1981; 289:594.
17. Okamoto Y, Hamada N, Saito H, et al. Thyroid peroxidase activity-inhibiting immunoglobulins in patients with autoimmune thyroid disease. J Clin Endocrinol Metab 1989; 68:730.
18. Chiovato L, Vitti P, Santini F, et al. Incidence of antibodies blocking thyrotropin effect in vitro in patients with euthyroid or hypothyroid autoimmune thyroiditis. J Clin Endocrinol Metab 1990; 71:40.

19. Braun J, Donner H, Siegmund T, et al. CTLA-4 promoter variants in patients with Graves' disease and Hashimoto's thyroiditis. Tissue Antigens 1998; 51:563.

19a. Tomer Y, Barberino G, Greenberg DA, et al. Mapping the major susceptibility loci for familial Graves' and Hashimoto's diseases: evidence for genetic heterogeneity and gene interaction. J Clin Endocrinol Metab 1999; 84:4656.

20. Weetman A, McGregor AM. Autoimmune thyroid disease: further developments in our understanding. Endocr Rev 1994; 15:788.

21. Hoekmank K, von Blomberg-van Der Flier BME, Wagstaff J, et al. Reversible thyroid dysfunction during treatment with GM-CSF. Lancet 1991; 338:541.

22. Atkins MB, Mier JW, Parkinson DR, et al. Hypothyroidism after treatment with interleukin-2 and lymphokine-activated killer cells. N Engl J Med 1988; 318:1557.

23. Mitsiades N, Poulaki V, Kotoula V, et al. Fas/Fas ligand up-regulation and Bcl-2 down-regulation may be significant in the pathogenesis of Hashimoto's thyroiditis. J Clin Endocrinol Metab 1998; 83:199.

24. Giordano C, Stassi G, De Maria R, et al. Potential involvement of FAS and its ligand in the pathogenesis of Hashimoto's thyroiditis. Science 1997; 275:960.

25. Doniach D. Hashimoto's thyroiditis and primary myxedema viewed as separate entities. Eur J Clin Invest 1981; 11:245.

26. Brown J, Solomon DH, Beall GN, et al. Autoimmune thyroid disease: Graves' and Hashimoto's. Ann Intern Med 1978; 88:379.

27. Strakosch C, Wenzel B, Row V, Volpé R. Immunology of autoimmune thyroid diseases. N Engl J Med 1982; 307:1499.

28. Botazzo G, Pujol-Borrell R, Hanafusa T. Role of HLA-DR expression and antigen presentation in induction of endocrine autoimmunity. Lancet 1983; 2:1115.

29. Yoshida H, Amino N, Yagawa K, et al. Association of serum antithyroid antibodies and lymphocytic infiltration of the thyroid gland: studies of 70 autopsied cases. J Clin Endocrinol Metab 1978; 46:859.

30. Nemeroff CB, Simon JS, Haggerty JJ, Evans DL. Antithyroid antibodies in depressed patients. Am J Psychiatry 1983; 14:840.

31. Wilhelm-Gossling C, Weckbecker K, Brabant EG, Dengler R. Autoimmune encephalopathy in Hashimoto's thyroiditis. A differential diagnosis in progressive dementia syndrome. Deutsche Medizinische Wochenschrift 1998; 123:279.

31a. Watemberg N, Willis D, Pollock JM. Encephalopathy as the presenting symptom of Hashimoto's thyroiditis. J Child Neurol 2000; 15:66.

32. Engler H, Staub J-J, Althaus B, et al. Assessment of antithyroglobulin and antimicrosomal autoantibodies in patients with autoimmune thyroid disease: comparison of haemagglutination assay, enzyme-linked immunoassay and radio-ligand assay. Clin Chim Acta 1989; 179:251.

33. Baker JR Jr, Saunders NB, Wartofsky L, et al. Seronegative Hashimoto thyroiditis with thyroid autoantibody production localized to the thyroid. Ann Intern Med 1988; 108:26.

34. Ott RA, Calandra DB, McCall A, et al. The incidence of thyroid carcinoma in patients with Hashimoto's thyroiditis and solitary cold nodules. Surgery 1985; 98:1203.

35. Yarman S, Mudun A, Alagol F, et al. Scintigraphic varieties in Hashimoto's thyroiditis and comparison with ultrasonography. Nucl Med Commun 1997; 18:951.

35a. Pederson OM, Aordal NP, Larssen TB, et al. The value of ultrasonography in predicting autoimmune thyroid disease. Thyroid 2000; 10:251.

36. Gordin A, Lamberg BA. Natural course of symptomless autoimmune thyroiditis. Lancet 1975; 2:1234.

37. Takasu N, Komiya I, Asawa T, et al. Test for recovery from hypothyroidism during thyroxine therapy in Hashimoto's thyroiditis. Lancet 1990; 336:1084.

38. Takasu N, Yamada T, Takasu M, et al. Disappearance of thyrotropin-blocking antibodies and spontaneous recovery from hypothyroidism in autoimmune thyroiditis. N Engl J Med 1992; 326:513.

39. Holm L, Blomgren H, Löwhagen T. Cancer risks in patients with chronic lymphocytic thyroiditis. N Engl J Med 1985; 312:601.

40. Papapetrou P, Jackson IMD. Thyrotoxicosis due to "silent" thyroiditis. Lancet 1975; 1:36.

41. Jackson IMD. "Hyper-thyroiditis": a diagnostic pitfall. N Engl J Med 1975; 293:661.

42. Vitug A, Goldman J. Silent (painless) thyroiditis: evidence of a geographic variation in frequency. Arch Intern Med 1985; 145:473.

43. Nikolai TF, Brosseau J, Kettrick MA, et al. Lymphocytic thyroiditis with spontaneously resolving hyperthyroidism (silent thyroiditis). Arch Intern Med 1980; 140:478.

44. Woolf P. Transient painless thyroiditis with hyperthyroidism: a variant of lymphocytic thyroiditis? Endocr Rev 1980; 1:411.

45. Farid NR, Hawe B, Walfish PG. Association of HLA-DR3 and HLA-DR5 to antigens in the painless thyroiditis with transient thyrotoxicosis syndrome. Clin Endocrinol Metab 1983; 19:699.

46. Volpé R. Is silent thyroiditis an autoimmune disease? [Editorial]. Arch Intern Med 1988; 148:1907.

47. Murao Y, Yoshinouchi T, Sato M, et al. Silent thyroiditis after excision of a thymoma. Intern Med 1998; 37:604.

48. Sarlis NJ, Brucker-Davis F, Swift JP, et al. Graves' disease following thyrotoxic painless thyroiditis: analysis of antibody activities against the thyrotropin receptor in two cases. Thyroid 1997; 7:829.

49. Wada M, Shimoyama T, Hamada A, Fukuchi M. Antithyroid peroxidase antibody and development of silent thyroiditis during interferon-$\alpha_{2a}$ treatment of chronic hepatitis C. Am J Gastroenterol 1995; 90:1366.

50. Roti E, Minelli R, Giuberti T, et al. Multiple changes in thyroid function in patients with chronic HCV hepatitis treated with recombinant interferon-α. Am J Med 1996; 101:482.

51. Boardas J, Rodriguez-Espinosa J, Enriquez J, et al. Prevalence of thyroid autoantibodies is not increased in blood donors with hepatitis C virus infection. J Hepatol 1995; 22:611.

52. Custro N, Montalto G, Scafidi V, et al. Prospective study on thyroid autoimmunity and dysfunction related to chronic hepatitis C and interferon therapy. J Endocrinol Invest 1997; 20:374.

53. Morrison J, Caplan RH. Typical and atypical ("silent") subacute thyroiditis in a wife and husband. Arch Intern Med 1978; 138:45.

54. Barclay ML, Brownlie BE, Turner JG, Wells JE. Lithium associated thyrotoxicosis: a report of 14 cases with statistical analysis of incidence. Clin Endocrinol (Oxf) 1994; 40:759.

55. Hennessey JV, Berg LA, Ibrahim M, Markert RJ. Evaluation of the early (5-6 hour) iodine-123 uptake for diagnosis and treatment planning in Graves' disease. Arch Intern Med 1995; 155:621.

56. Aren R, Munipalli B. Ipodate therapy in patients with severe destruction-induced thyrotoxicosis. Arch Intern Med 1996; 156:1752.

57. Nikolai TF, Coombs GJ, McKenzie AK, et al. Treatment of lymphocytic thyroiditis with spontaneously resolving hyperthyroidism (silent thyroiditis). Arch Intern Med 1982; 142:2281.

58. Lazarus JH. Prediction of postpartum thyroiditis. Eur J Endocrinol 1998; 139:12.

59. Alvarez-Marfany M, Roman SH, Drexler AJ, et al. Long-term prospective study of postpartum thyroid dysfunction in women with insulin-dependent diabetes mellitus. J Clin Endocrinol Metab 1994; 79:10.

60. Davies TF. The thyroid immunology of the postpartum period. Thyroid 1999; 9:675.

61. Hayslip CC, Fein HG, O'Donnell VM, et al. The value of serum antimicrosomal antibody testing in screening for symptomatic postpartum thyroid dysfunction. Am J Obstet Gynecol 1988; 159(1):203.

62. Amino N, Miyai K, Kuro R, et al. Transient post-partum hypothyroidism: fourteen cases with autoimmune thyroiditis. Ann Intern Med 1977; 87:155.

63. Stagnaro-Green A, Roman S, Cobin R, et al. A prospective study of lymphocyte-initiated immunosuppression in normal pregnancy: evidence of a T-cell etiology for postpartum thyroid dysfunction. J Clin Endocrinol Metab 1992; 74:645.

64. Stagnaro-Green A. Postpartum thyroiditis: prevalence, etiology and clinical implications. Thyroid Today 1993; 16:1.

65. Momotani N, Noh J, Ishikawa N, et al. Relationship between silent thyroiditis and recurrent Graves' disease in the postpartum period. J Clin Endocrinol Metab 1994; 79:285.

66. Roti E, Emerson C. Postpartum thyroiditis. J Clin Endocrinol Metab 1992; 74:3.

67. Heufelder AE, Goellmer JR, Bahn RS, et al. Tissue eosinophilia and eosinophil degranulation in Riedel's invasive fibrous thyroiditis. J Clin Endocrinol Metab 1996; 81:977.

68. Wan SK, Chan JK, Tang SK. Paucicellular variant of anaplastic thyroid carcinoma: a mimic of Riedel's thyroiditis. Am J Clin Pathol 1996; 105:388.

69. Bagnasco M, Passalacqua G, Pronzato C, et al. Fibrous invasive (Riedel's) thyroiditis with critical response to steroid treatment. J Endocrinol Invest 1995; 18:305.

70. LiVolsi VA. Radiation-associated thyroiditis. In: LiVolsi VA, LoGerfo P, eds. Thyroiditis. Boca Raton, FL: CRC Press, 1981:113.

71. McDermott MT, Kidd GS, Dodson LE, Hofeldt FD. Radioiodine-induced thyroid storm: case report and literature review. Am J Med 1983; 75:353.

72. Aizawa T, Watanabe T, Suzuki N, et al. Radiation-induced painless thyrotoxic thyroiditis followed by hypothyroidism: a case report and review of the literature. Thyroid 1998; 8:273.

73. Matsubayashi S, Kawai K, Matsumoto Y, et al. The correlation between papillary thyroid carcinoma and lymphocytic infiltration in the thyroid gland. J Clin Endocrinol Metab 1995; 80:3421.

74. Baker JR. The immune response to papillary thyroid carcinoma. J Clin Endocrinol Metab 1995; 80:3419.

75. LiVolsi VA. Palpation thyroiditis. In: LiVolsi VA, LoGerfo P, eds. Thyroiditis. Boca Raton, FL: CRC Press, 1981:43.

CHAPTER 47

# THYROID DISORDERS OF INFANCY AND CHILDHOOD

WELLINGTON HUNG

Thyroid hormones are important for the general growth and development of the infant and child, particularly in the differentiation and function of the nervous system. They are essential elements in the maturational events involved in the transition of the neonate to the adult.

**TABLE 47-1.**
**Age-Related Levels for Serum Parameters of Thyroid Function**

| Parameter | Age | Value |
|---|---|---|
| Total T$_4$ (µg/dL) | Preterm infants, age 28–36 weeks, first week of life | 4.0–17.4 |
| | Cord blood, >37 weeks | 5.9–15.0 |
| | 1–4 days | 14.0–28.4 |
| | 1–11 months | 7.2–15.7 |
| | 1–9 years | 6.0–14.2 |
| | 10–19 years | 4.7–12.4 |
| Free T$_4$* (ng/dL) | Preterm infants, 28–36 weeks, first week of life | 1.0–4.1 |
| | Cord blood, >37 weeks | 1.2–2.2 |
| | Birth–4 days | 2.2–5.3 |
| | 2 weeks–20 years | 0.8–2.0 |
| Total T$_3$ (ng/dL) | Cord blood, >37 weeks | 43–99 |
| | 1–3 days | 100–740 |
| | 1–11 months | 105–245 |
| | 1–4 years | 105–269 |
| | 5–9 years | 94–241 |
| | 10–14 years | 82–213 |
| | 15–19 years | 80–210 |
| TSH† (mIU/L) | Preterm infants, age 28–36 weeks, first week of life | 0.7–27.0 |
| | Cord blood, >37 weeks | 2.3–13.2 |
| | Birth–4 days | 1.0–38.9 |
| | 2–20 weeks | 1.7–9.1 |
| | 5 months–20 years | 0.7–6.4 |
| T$_4$-binding globulin (mg/dL) | Cord blood, >37 weeks | 2.1–3.7 |
| | 1–5 days | 2.2–4.2 boys; 2.2–4.2 girls |
| | 1–11 months | 1.6–3.6 boys; 1.7–3.7 girls |
| | 1–9 years | 1.4–2.6 boys; 1.5–2.7 girls |
| | 10–19 years | 1.4–2.6 boys; 1.4–3.0 girls |
| Thyroglobulin (ng/dL) | Cord blood | 14.7–101.1 |
| | Birth–35 months | 10.6–92.0 |
| | 3–11 years | 5.6–41.9 |
| | 12–17 years | 2.7–21.9 |
| | 18 years | ≥25 |
| T$_3$ reverse (ng/dL) | Cord blood, >37 weeks | 102–342 |
| | 1 month–20 years | 10–35 |
| T$_3$ uptake (units) | 1–9 years | 0.61–1.13 boys; 0.96–1.68 girls |
| | 10–19 years | 0.67–1.09 boys; 0.64—1.00 girls |

*Direct dialysis.
†Third generation, immunochemiluminometric assay.
T$_3$, triiodothyronine; T$_4$, thyroxine; TSH, thyroid-stimulating hormone.
(From Fisher DA. Pediatric endocrine testing. San Juan Capistrano, CA: Nichols Institute Reference Laboratories, 1993.)

## HYPOTHALAMIC–PITUITARY–THYROID INTERRELATIONSHIPS

In the human fetus, the period of maturation of thyroid function extends throughout gestation and into the neonatal period.[1,2] Thyrotropin-releasing hormone has been detected in the human fetal hypothalamus at 10 to 12 weeks of gestation, and levels increase to term. Pituitary thyroid stimulating hormone (TSH) is detectable at 8 to 10 weeks of gestation, remains low until 16 to 18 weeks, and then increases to a plateau level by 28 weeks of gestation. Human fetal serum TSH is detectable by 10 weeks of gestation and increases to a mean level of ~15 µU/mL between 20 and 30 weeks. Fetal serum total thyroxine (T$_4$) levels are low before 16 to 18 weeks of gestation and, thereafter, progressively increase to levels of 10 to 12 µg/dL at 34 to 36 weeks of gestation. By 40 weeks, the mean serum fetal TSH

**TABLE 47-2.**
**Newborn Screening Serum T$_4$ Values by Birth Weight**

| Weight (g) | T$_4$ (µg/dL), mean ± SD |
|---|---|
| <1000 | 5.6 ± 3.0 |
| 1000–1500 | 7.7 ± 2.7 |
| 1500–2000 | 9.6 ± 2.7 |
| 2000–2500 | 11.2 ± 2.4 |
| >2500 | 12.0 ± 2.0 |

SD, standard deviation; T$_4$, thyroxine.
(Modified from Frank FE, Faix JE, Hermos RJ, et al. Thyroid function in very low birth weight infants: effects on neonatal hypothyroidism screening. J Pediatr 1996; 128:548.)

decreases to a mean value of ~10 µU/mL, indicating maturation of the feedback mechanism.

Normal children and adults show a diurnal variation of TSH secretion with lower values at 11 a.m. and peak values around 11 p.m. No diurnal rhythm is detectable in preterm and full-term infants younger than 4 weeks of age.[3] Development of TSH circadian rhythm begins after the first month of life.

## PHYSIOLOGIC CHANGES IN THYROID FUNCTION TESTS

The proper interpretation of serum TSH, T$_4$, triiodothyronine (T$_3$), reverse T$_3$, T$_3$ uptake, and thyroglobulin (Tg) concentrations in pediatric patients requires a knowledge of the age dependency of these hormones. Normal values relative to age are shown in Table 47-1. Importantly, preterm and small-for-gestational-age neonates have serum thyroid hormone values different from those of normal-term infants. In preterm infants, the cord serum T$_4$ is decreased in proportion to gestational age and birth weight. Newborn screening serum T$_4$ concentrations obtained from filter paper blood specimens in very-low-birth-weight infants (<1500 g) and in low-birth-weight infants (1500–2499 g) are presented in Table 47-2.[4]

## HYPOTHYROIDISM IN THE NEONATE AND CHILD

### ETIOLOGY

The causes of pediatric hypothyroidism are listed in Table 47-3. Because most of the congenital and acquired causes are similar, they are discussed together. The terms *cretinism* and *congenital hypothyroidism* are used for hypothyroidism present before or at birth.

Endemic iodine deficiency may cause congenital hypothyroidism (cretinism) (Fig. 47-1). *Thyroid dysgenesis* is the most common cause of congenital hypothyroidism in nonendemic areas. The term includes aplasia, ectopy, and hypoplasia of the thyroid gland. It is twice as frequent among women as men. Interestingly, circulating antithyroid antibodies are found in a higher percentage of sera from mothers of nongoitrous cretins than in control mothers. Although these antibodies can cross the placenta, they probably do not destroy the fetal thyroid gland. Thus, the possible role, if any, of circulating or cellular antithyroid antibodies in the causation of congenital athyrosis is not clear. In mothers with Graves disease with or without thyrotoxicosis, TSH receptor-blocking antibodies may cross the placenta and cause transient neonatal hypothyroidism (see Chap. 42).[5]

Ectopy of the thyroid gland is an important cause of hypothyroidism. Approximately 75% of patients with lingual thyroid glands do not have any normally located thyroid tissue

**TABLE 47-3.**
**Causes of Hypothyroidism**

**CONGENITAL**

Thyroid dysgenesis

Partial or complete athyrosis

Ectopic thyroid gland

Inborn errors of thyroid hormone synthesis

Hypothalamic–pituitary–thyroid axis abnormalities

TRH deficiency or insensitivity

TSH deficiency

Thyroid gland unresponsiveness to TSH

Iodide deficiency

Transplacental passage of antithyroid drugs, chemicals, or agents

Peripheral resistance to thyroid hormone

**ACQUIRED**

Ectopic thyroid gland

TRH or TSH deficiency, or both

Inborn errors of thyroid hormone synthesis

Postthyroidectomy

Post–radioactive iodine therapy

Goitrogenic induced: iodide excess, propylthiouracil, methimazole, cobalt

Postsuppurative or -nonsuppurative thyroiditis

Chronic lymphocytic thyroiditis

Infiltrative diseases of the thyroid: cystinosis, histocytosis X

*TRH,* thyroid-releasing hormone; *TSH,* thyroid-stimulating hormone.
(From Hung W, August GP, Glasgow AM. Pediatric endocrinology. New Hyde Park, NY: Medical Examination Publishing, 1983:130.)

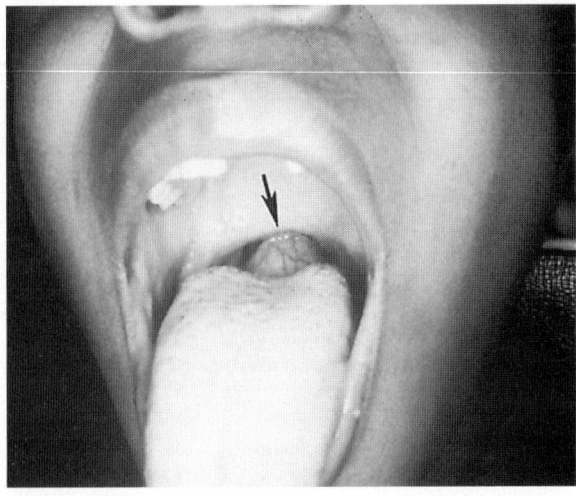

**FIGURE 47-2.** Eight-year-old child with lingual thyroid gland (*arrow*).

(Figs. 47-2 and 47-3). Usually, the amount of ectopic thyroid tissue is insufficient to prevent hypothyroidism, although it can respond to TSH stimulation. Ectopic thyroid glands must be included in the differential diagnosis of midline lingual and sublingual masses. All children with ectopic thyroid glands should have a trial of full replacement thyroid hormone therapy before surgical excision is contemplated. Thyroid hormone therapy prevents further hypertrophy and hyperplasia. There is no evidence that lingual or sublingual thyroid glands are malignant in the pediatric patient. In infants, the combination of elevated serum TSH and normal or low-normal $T_4$ levels suggests the presence of thyroid ectopy.[6] Infants with aplasia or hypoplasia of the thyroid gland also have high serum TSH and low $T_4$ levels.

Hypothyroidism may occur because of a hereditary enzymatic deficiency that prevents synthesis of $T_4$ and $T_3$. Hereditary enzymatic defects of thyroid hormone synthesis are the second most common cause of congenital hypothyroidism

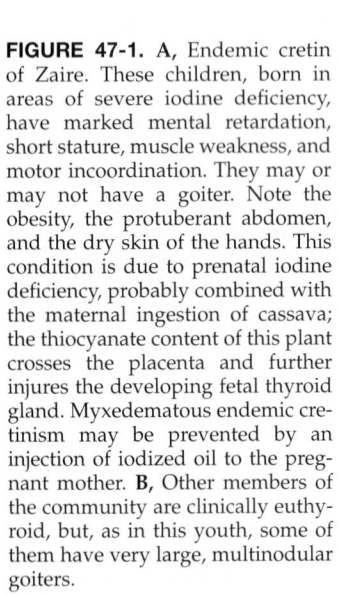

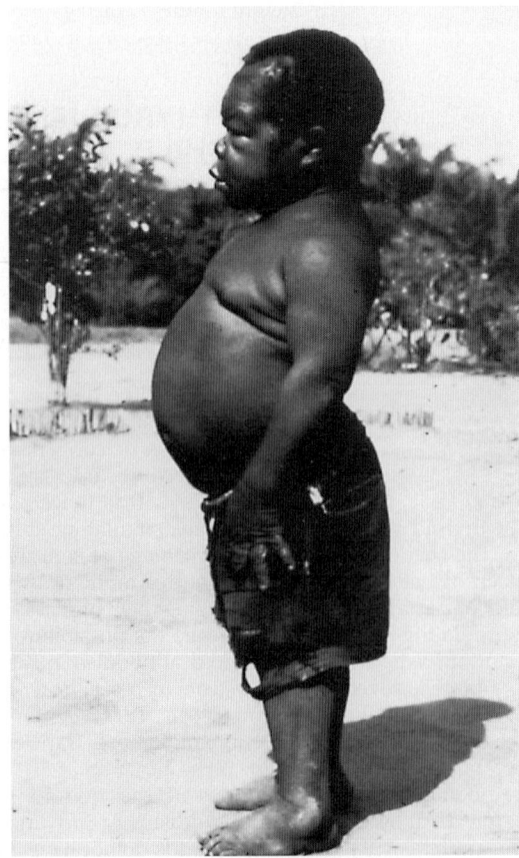

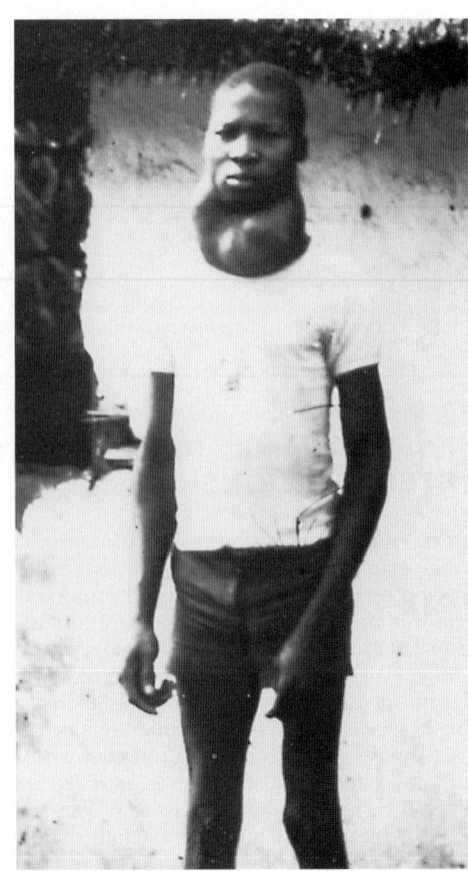

**FIGURE 47-1. A,** Endemic cretin of Zaire. These children, born in areas of severe iodine deficiency, have marked mental retardation, short stature, muscle weakness, and motor incoordination. They may or may not have a goiter. Note the obesity, the protuberant abdomen, and the dry skin of the hands. This condition is due to prenatal iodine deficiency, probably combined with the maternal ingestion of cassava; the thiocyanate content of this plant crosses the placenta and further injures the developing fetal thyroid gland. Myxedematous endemic cretinism may be prevented by an injection of iodized oil to the pregnant mother. **B,** Other members of the community are clinically euthyroid, but, as in this youth, some of them have very large, multinodular goiters.

A,B

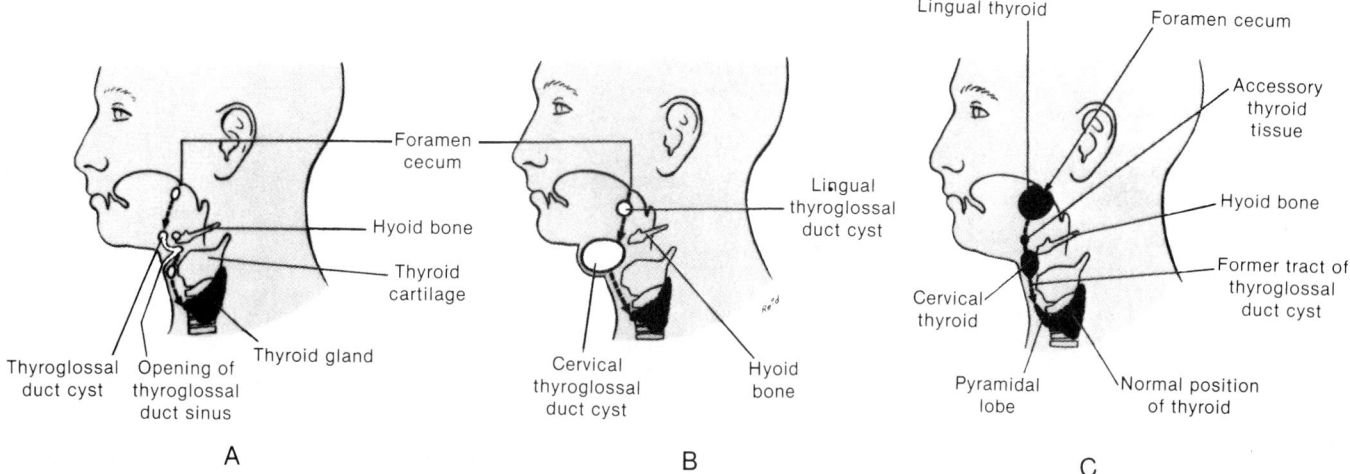

**FIGURE 47-3.** Diagrammatic representation of development and migration of thyroid, indicating locations of thyroid-related anomalies and of ectopic thyroid tissue. The thyroid gland develops from a midline endodermal thickening in the pharyngeal floor. The descending thyroid is connected to the tongue by the thyroglossal duct; its lingual opening is termed the *foramen cecum*. By the seventh week, the thyroglossal duct usually has disappeared. **A** and **B** show possible locations of thyroglossal duct cysts, as well as a thyroglossal duct sinus (opening at the skin surface). The broken line illustrates the normal course of the descending thyroglossal duct and thyroid gland. **C** shows the most common locations of ectopic thyroid tissue. (The commonly present pyramidal lobe of the thyroid is formed from a persistent remnant of the lower end of the thyroglossal duct.) Although accessory thyroid tissue is often functional, it frequently fails to maintain the euthyroid state if the thyroid gland is removed. (From Moore KL. The developing human, 5th ed. Philadelphia: WB Saunders, 1993:202.)

(Table 47-4).[7] Patients with enzymatic defects may present with hypothyroidism with or without goiter or euthyroidism with goiter. Because the thyroid gland is not always palpable in infants, infants with congenital hypothyroidism caused by an enzymatic defect cannot always be differentiated by physical examination from those with athyrotic hypothyroidism. The diagnosis depends on specific tests of the various steps in thyroid hormone synthesis and release. Pendred syndrome is an autosomal recessive disorder characterized by a goiter resulting from a peroxidase defect, with euthyroidism or mild hypothyroidism and congenital sensorineural hearing loss. The Pendred syndrome gene is mapped to chromosome 7q31 and has been found to encode a putative sulfate transporter.[8,9] Mutations have been found in the Pendred syndrome gene.[8,9] Congenital hypothyroidism caused by mutations in the thyrotropin-receptor gene has been reported.[10] The inherited disorders of thyroid hormone transport, $T_4$-binding globulin deficiency must also be considered in the differential

**TABLE 47-4.**
**Hereditary Defects in Thyroid Hormone Synthesis or Action Causing Hypothyroidism**

| Defect | Inheritance | Goiter | Plasma $T_4$ | Plasma TSH | Radioactive Iodine Uptake | Other Features |
|---|---|---|---|---|---|---|
| Iodide transport defect | Autosomal recessive | + | ↓ | N or ↑* | ↓ | No salivary radioactive iodine concentration; no TSH response |
| Organification defect | Autosomal recessive | + | N or ↓ | N or ↓* | ↑ | Positive perchlorate discharge of radioactive iodine from thyroid; mental retardation likely |
| Pendred syndrome | Autosomal recessive | + | N or ↓ | N | — | Milder form of organification defect; sensorineural deafness may be present at birth or develop shortly thereafter; goiter develops before puberty but may be present at birth |
| Deiodinase (iodotyrosine dehalogenase) defect | Autosomal recessive | + | N or ↓ | N or ↑* | ↑ | Injected [131I]DIT or [131I]MIT excreted unchanged in urine; increased incidence of thyroid carcinoma |
| Coupling defect | Autosomal recessive(?) | + | N or ↓ | N or ↑* | ↑ | Diagnosis made by exclusion of other defects |
| Thyroglobulin defect | Autosomal recessive(?) | + | N or ↓ | N or ↑* | ↑ | Serum protein-bound iodine level much greater than $T_4$ iodine level and difference is not caused by iodide-containing medications or contrast medium |
| Unresponsiveness to TSH | Autosomal recessive(?) | No | ↓ | ↑ | ↓ | Absence of thyroidal response to exogenous TSH; mental retardation |
| Resistance to thyroid hormone | Autosomal recessive(?) | + | ↑ | N | ↑ | Resistance may be partial and variable and be inhibited in three ways: generalized tissue unresponsiveness, selective pituitary unresponsiveness, and peripheral tissue, but not pituitary resistance; elevated serum $T_4$ and $T_3$ and inappropriately elevated TSH |

↓, decreased; ↑, increased; *DIT*, diiodotyrosine; *MIT*, monoiodotyrosine; *N*, normal; $T_3$, triiodothyronine; $T_4$, thyroxine; *TSH*, thyroid-stimulating hormone.
*Depends on age of patient and degree of defect.

**TABLE 47-5.**
**Inherited Defects in Thyroid Hormone Transport**

| Defect | Inheritance | T$_4$ | T$_3$ | Free T$_4$, T$_3$ | T$_3$ Uptake | Free T$_4$ Index |
|---|---|---|---|---|---|---|
| T$_4$-binding globulin deficiency (may be partial or complete) | X-linked | ↓ | ↓ | N | ↑ | N |
| T$_4$-binding globulin excess | X-linked | ↑ | ↑ | N | ↓ | N |
| T$_4$-binding prealbumin excess | Unknown | ↑ | N | N | N | ↑ |
| Familial dysalbuminemic hyperthyroxinemia | Autosomal dominant | ↑ | N | N | N | ↑ |

↓, decreased; ↑, increased; N, normal; T$_3$, triiodothyronine; T$_4$, thyroxine.

diagnosis of hypothyroidism (Table 47-5). However, in this condition, the patient is clinically euthyroid.

Chronic lymphocytic thyroiditis is the most common cause of acquired hypothyroidism in pediatric practice.

## TRANSIENT DISORDERS OF THYROID FUNCTION

Several transient disorders of thyroid function may occur in pediatric patients. These include transient hypothyroxinemia, transient hyperthyrotropinemia, and the euthyroid sick syndrome.

## CLINICAL FINDINGS IN HYPOTHYROIDISM

Patients with hypothyroidism differ in appearance depending on the age at which the deficiency occurs and its duration and severity before therapy is instituted. In complete athyrosis, symptoms may be present at birth but, more commonly, they occur during the first 2 months of life. Features in the neonate that should suggest the possible presence of hypothyroidism include prolonged gestation with large size at birth, large posterior fontanelle, respiratory distress, hypothermia, peripheral cyanosis, hypoactivity, feeding difficulties, constipation, abdominal distention with vomiting, prolonged jaundice, and dry skin. The skin may be dry and cool, and circulatory mottling may be present.

As the neonate ages, the facial features become coarse and puffy, and the tongue becomes broad and thick (Fig. 47-4). Linear growth may decline during the first month of life. Mental retardation occurs if the diagnosis is not made and therapy is not instituted. Diminished physical activity is a prominent finding. Any infant who must be awakened for feedings and who rarely cries must be suspected of having hypothyroidism.

Patients who develop hypothyroidism in early childhood have clinical manifestations different from neonates. Symptoms may appear gradually over several years. Delayed dentition and decelerated linear growth occurs. Mental sluggishness develops, but mental retardation usually does not occur if hypothyroidism develops after 2 years of age. If hypothyroidism has been present since infancy, infantile body proportions persist. Cold intolerance, dry skin, constipation, and muscle weakness are common findings.

An infrequently recognized syndrome in hypothyroid children is the Kocher-Debré-Sémelaigne syndrome (see Chap. 210), which consists of generalized muscular hypertrophy involving particularly the muscles of the extremities. The pathogenesis of the muscle hypertrophy is not known; it disappears with thyroid hormone therapy.

In the older child and adolescent, growth retardation is a common finding. Hypothyroidism affects the circulatory and neuromuscular systems, as it does in the younger patient. Significant delay in sexual maturation is characteristic. Multicystic ovaries occur frequently in girls with hypothyroidism.

A rare syndrome in children consists of severe hypothyroidism and isosexual precocity. The etiology is not entirely resolved. Studies suggest that there is some binding of the elevated circulating TSH to the follicle-stimulating hormone receptor, with follicle-stimulating hormone activity producing sexual precocity.[11] The signs of hypothyroidism and sexual precocity regress with therapy, and complete sexual maturation occurs at a normal age.

## LABORATORY FINDINGS

In primary hypothyroidism, serum TSH levels are elevated, whereas in secondary and tertiary hypothyroidism, serum TSH levels are low or undetectable. Serum T$_4$, T$_3$, and T$_3$ uptake values all are low. Plasma Tg levels are very low or undetectable in congenital hypothyroidism that is due to athyrosis. However, it is possible that low levels may be present in a patient with a defect in Tg synthesis or secretion. Thyroid scintiscan or ultrasonography may provide important information concerning the etiology of hypothyroidism in the neonate. Plasma somatomedin C concentrations are low in hypothyroidism, as is the serum alkaline phosphatase.

The bone age is retarded. Epiphyseal dysgenesis or stippling of the epiphyses can be present (Fig. 47-5). Enlargement of the sella turcica occasionally can be seen in primary hypothyroidism.[6] With thyroid hormone therapy, the bone age returns to normal, the epiphyseal dysgenesis regresses, and the radiographic appearance normalizes.

## THERAPY

The treatment goal is to restore euthyroidism as rapidly as is safe for the patient. In the neonate and very young infant, therapy is essential to protect the brain from damage. However, caution is necessary in the therapy for markedly hypothyroid neonates and infants because of the possible presence of a myxedematous myocardium. Vigorous therapy may cause cardiac failure or serious arrhythmias.

The initial single daily oral dose of L-T$_4$ in full-term neonates is 10 to 15 μg/kg per day.[12] In preterm neonates, the starting

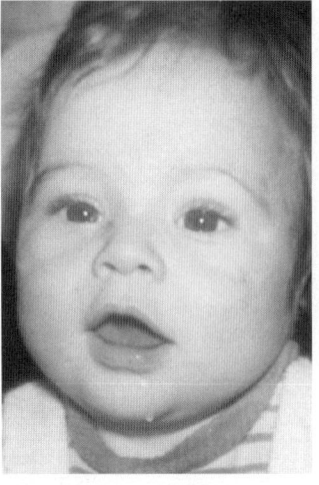

**A,B**

**FIGURE 47-4. A,** Hypothyroid neonate. Note typical cretinoid facies with dull appearance and myxedema of the face, eyelids, lips, and tongue. **B,** The same patient after therapy and disappearance of myxedema.

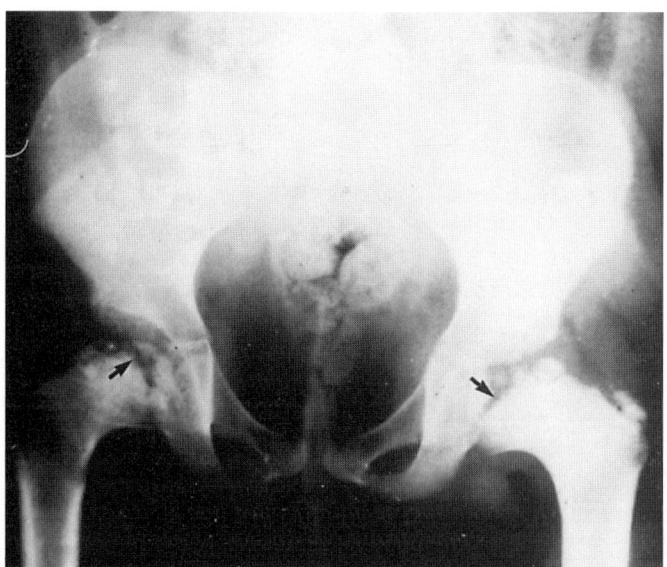

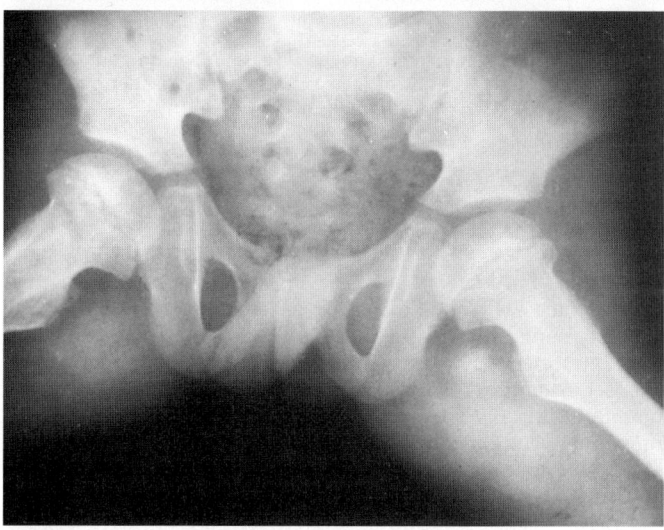

**FIGURE 47-5. A,** Radiograph of 13-year-old hypothyroid child with epiphyseal dysgenesis. There is fragmentation of the femoral heads and widening of the epiphyseal lines (*arrows*). **B,** At 6 months after commencement of thyroid hormone treatment, the femoral heads are now well formed and the epiphyseal lines appear relatively normal.

dosage is 10 µg/kg per day; usually the dose can be increased to 15 µg/kg per day in 4 to 6 weeks. In infants, children, and adolescents, the initial oral dose of L-T$_4$ is ~100 µg/m$^2$ per day.[13]

In children, suppression of serum TSH to normal levels is the best index of adequate therapy in primary hypothyroidism. However, neonates and infants with congenital hypothyroidism may have an abnormal "threshold" for the inhibition of TSH secretion; the feedback set-point seems to be increased, so that excessive serum levels of T$_4$ are required to suppress the TSH.[14] Serum TSH values may remain elevated for as long as 2 years, despite normal T$_4$ and T$_3$ levels produced by replacement therapy. Therefore, normal serum TSH levels must not be used as the only criterion of adequacy of therapy. Other indicators of adequate therapy include normal growth and development and normal skeletal maturation; however, children with long-standing acquired hypothyroidism appear to sustain a permanent height deficit at maturity, despite treatment.[15] Pseudotumor cerebri may occur after the initiation of L-T$_4$ therapy. Excessive thyroid hormone therapy may delay neurologic development.[16]

## NEONATAL SCREENING FOR HYPOTHYROIDISM

The clinical diagnosis of congenital hypothyroidism during the neonatal period can be difficult and is frequently missed. Thus, neonatal screening programs for congenital hypothyroidism have been established. Most screening programs measure T$_4$ and TSH in blood collected on filter paper before the neonate is discharged from the hospital. A supplemental TSH determination is performed on the lowest 3% to 5% of T$_4$ results. This provides the most comprehensive screening, identifying infants with primary hypothyroidism and those at risk for secondary hypothyroidism and Tg deficiency. Positive results should be confirmed by serum determinations. Screening programs throughout the world have shown an incidence of 1:3500 to 1:4500 births.[17]

The preliminary results of follow-up psychometric studies of neonates detected by screening programs have been encouraging. Studies indicate that the earlier the diagnosis of congenital hypothyroidism is made and therapy started, the better the prognosis for intelligence.[18] The prognosis also appears to be related to the etiology of the congenital hypothyroidism.

## HUMAN BREAST MILK AND NEONATAL SCREENING

Both T$_4$ and T$_3$ are present in human milk, but levels of T$_4$ and T$_3$ in various reports differ widely, probably because sampling methods were different. Also, in some studies, extracted milk was analyzed, whereas in other studies, nonextracted milk was used. It has been suggested that there is sufficient thyroid hormone in human milk to mitigate the effect of congenital hypothyroidism. Nevertheless, breast-feeding does not impair the detection of congenital hypothyroidism in neonatal screening programs.[19]

# HYPERTHYROIDISM IN THE CHILD

The various types of hyperthyroidism seen in pediatric patients are *congenital* (neonatal Graves disease and transitory Graves disease caused by transplacental passage of thyroid-stimulating immunoglobulins [TSIs]); and *acquired* (autoimmune thyroid disease, Graves disease, chronic lymphocytic thyroiditis, nodular toxic goiter [Plummer disease], thyroid carcinoma, exogenous iodide-induced hyperthyroidism [jod-basedow phenomenon], TSH-producing pituitary tumor, inappropriate secretion of TSH, and factitious hyperthyroidism). Graves disease is the most common type of hyperthyroidism. TSIs are responsible for causing Graves disease (see Chap. 42).

## CLINICAL FINDINGS

Graves disease in the child and adolescent is much like the disease in adults. Its course is characterized by variable severity and a tendency for spontaneous remissions and exacerbations. The disease may appear at any age and occurs approximately five times as frequently among girls as among boys. The frequency increases with age after the first year of life, peaking during adolescence.

Nervousness, irritability, emotional lability, excessive sweating, increased bowel movements, and increased appetite with or without weight loss are the most commonly noted symptoms. Occasionally, obesity may occur. Mild exophthalmos, lid retraction and stare, goiter, tachycardia, increased systolic blood pressure with wide pulse pressure, and tremors almost always are present on physical examination. Usually, the onset of symptoms and signs is gradual. Deterioration in school performance is not an uncommon symptom.

Mild ophthalmopathy, including proptosis, stare, and lid retraction, is present. However, severe ophthalmopathy, such as might be seen in adults, is very rare in pediatric patients. Accelerated growth may occur, but this is not followed by a significant increase in maximal attained adult height. Thyroid storm is very rare in children and adolescents.

## LABORATORY FINDINGS

Serum $T_4$, $T_3$, free $T_4$, free $T_3$, and $T_3$ uptake values are elevated in most patients; $T_3$ toxicosis and $T_4$ toxicosis can occur in pediatric patients.

## TREATMENT

There is controversy over the therapy of Graves disease in children and adolescents because no available therapy is ideal; each has distinct advantages and disadvantages.[20,21] Antithyroid drugs, surgery, and radioactive iodine have been used. The selection of treatment depends on many factors, including the age and sex of the patient, severity and duration of the disease, size of the thyroid gland, presence of other complicating medical conditions, availability of experienced surgeons, ability of the patient and family to cooperate, and fear of ionizing irradiation and its potential genetic effects.

Antithyroid drugs probably are the most common therapy for Graves disease in pediatric patients. The usual initial daily dosage of propylthiouracil is 300 mg and that of methimazole is 30 mg. The daily dosage of each drug should be divided into three equal doses and given approximately every 8 hours. Some physicians prescribe methimazole once daily. On the other hand, propylthiouracil may be less effective when given as a single daily dose. The recommended duration of therapy ranges from 1 to 3 years. Children and adolescents experience the same potential adverse effects of antithyroid drugs as do adults. The contraindications to medical therapy are drug toxicity and patient noncompliance. The main disadvantages are the relatively long period of therapy required and the difficulty of obtaining the continued cooperation of the patient.

Surgery usually offers the advantage of rapid and permanent control of hyperthyroidism. Potential disadvantages include mortality; hypoparathyroidism; hypothyroidism; injury to the recurrent laryngeal nerves; and laryngotracheal edema, sometimes requiring tracheotomy. The indications for surgery include (a) toxicity to antithyroid drugs, (b) failure of cure after an adequate course of antithyroid drug therapy, (c) lack of patient compliance, and (d) failure of antithyroid drug therapy to shrink a large, conspicuous goiter.

The use of $^{131}I$ in the treatment of Graves disease in pediatric patients has been controversial.[20,21] The advantages of such therapy are that it is easily administered and is effective. The disadvantages include a high incidence of hypothyroidism, the fact that complete control requires weeks to months, the unknown long-term effects on the induction of neoplasia, and the unknown genetic effects.

## NEONATAL GRAVES DISEASE AND FETAL THYROTOXICOSIS

Neonatal Graves disease is a rare condition in neonates born to mothers with active or previously active Graves disease. Neonatal Graves disease occurs in ~1 in 25,000 pregnancies, and almost all cases are caused by transplacental passage of TSI from mother to fetus.[22] In some neonates, the disease lasts for months or years, much longer than could be explained by persistence of passively transferred TSI in utero. The disease can be severe. There have been reports of neonatal Graves disease caused by a mutation in the thyrotopin-receptor gene.[23]

Fetal thyrotoxicosis is rarely diagnosed but is important because of the potential for significant morbidity and mortality.[24,25] It is caused by transplacental passage of TSI.

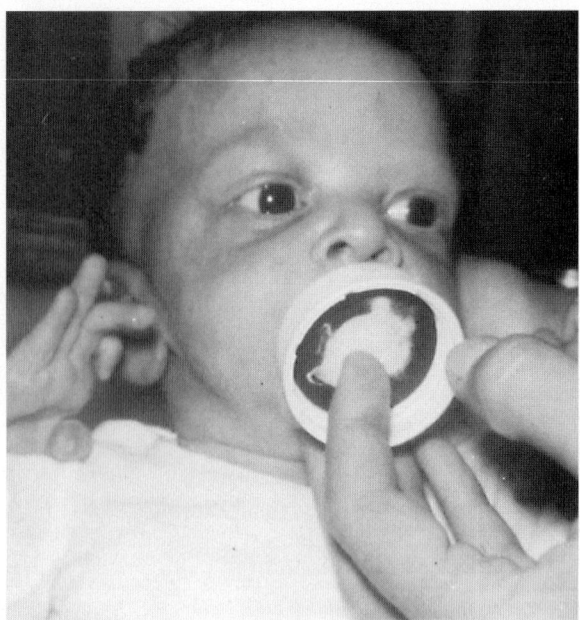

**FIGURE 47-6.** Neonate with Graves disease. Note prominent eyes, stare, and wet hair, a result of increased sweating. Pacifier had to be used to decrease constant movement of hands and arms.

## CLINICAL FINDINGS

The clinical findings of neonatal Graves disease include prematurity, goiter, exophthalmos, tachycardia, hypertension, hyperirritability, congestive heart failure, jaundice, hepatosplenomegaly, and thrombocytopenia (Fig. 47-6). If the neonate has been exposed to antithyroid medication in utero, the illness may not manifest clinically for 5 to 10 days after birth. The mortality ranges between 15% and 20%, and sequelae include craniosynostosis and intellectual impairment.

Clinical findings in fetal thyrotoxicosis include tachycardia (>160 beats per minute), goiter, congestive heart failure, and intrauterine growth retardation. The goiter can be detected by ultrasound examination. If there is evidence of fetal thyrotoxicosis, cordocentesis should be performed to monitor fetal thyroid function and the effects of maternal antithyroid therapy. However, the need for accurate assessment of fetal thyroid function must be weighed against the risk of cordocentesis.

## TREATMENT

The diagnosis of neonatal Graves disease should be followed immediately by therapy with propylthiouracil, 5 to 10 mg/kg per day, or methimazole, 0.5 to 1.0 mg/kg per day, in divided doses every 8 hours by gavage. This, then, should be followed by the administration of iodides, either orally (1 drop of supersaturated potassium iodide daily) or intravenously (as sodium iodide). Propranolol may be necessary if marked tachycardia and other catecholamine-mediated signs and symptoms are present. The dose of propranolol is 2 mg/kg per day in divided doses. Propranolol should never be used alone because of the associated complications and hazards of this drug in the neonate. In life-threatening situations, vigorous supportive therapies—including the use of glucocorticoids (prednisone, 2 mg/kg per day), intravenous fluids, sedation, oxygen, and a cooling blanket—may be necessary. Assuming that the Graves disease is self-limited, therapy should be gradually discontinued at 2 months. If there is a recurrence, antithyroid drugs should be restarted.

# GOITERS

Goiter in the pediatric patient is not rare. The incidence in school-age children and adolescents is between 3.9% and 6%.[26] The most common cause is chronic lymphocytic thyroiditis (autoimmune or Hashimoto thyroiditis).[27] Chronic lymphocytic thyroiditis (see Chap. 46) is the single most frequent thyroid disorder seen in pediatric patients and is the most common cause of acquired hypothyroidism. Colloid or simple goiter is the second most common cause of euthyroid goiter.

## CHRONIC LYMPHOCYTIC THYROIDITIS

### CLINICAL FINDINGS

Usually, the goiter is completely asymptomatic and the patient is clinically euthyroid. However, symptoms and signs of hypothyroidism or hyperthyroidism may be present. The goiter may be firm and smooth, lobulated, or nodular and is non-tender. If asymmetry of the thyroid gland is present, the right lobe is usually larger.

### LABORATORY FINDINGS

The presence of antibodies (anti-Tg and antithyroid peroxidase) against thyroid gland components is consistent with the diagnosis of chronic lymphocytic thyroiditis. However, antithyroid antibodies may not be detectable even in histologically proven cases of this disease. Serum levels of $T_4$ and $T_3$ may be normal, low, or elevated. Serum TSH levels may be normal, but they are frequently elevated despite normal serum $T_4$ concentrations. Thyroid scintiscan may show thyromegaly, with asymmetric or patchy areas of radioisotope uptake. Defective binding of inorganic iodide may occur in chronic lymphocytic thyroiditis, with substantial accumulation of iodide; significant discharge follows the inhibition of iodide transport. One test of the integrity of the organic-binding mechanism is the iodide-perchlorate discharge test (see Chap. 34).

A definite diagnosis of chronic lymphocytic thyroiditis may require a biopsy. However, the diagnosis may be made with reasonable certainty by the clinical picture and appropriate laboratory studies.

### TREATMENT

There is no general agreement about the treatment of chronic lymphocytic thyroiditis in pediatric patients, except for those with hypothyroidism for whom thyroid hormone therapy is essential. Some authors believe that the condition ultimately leads to hypothyroidism if untreated; therefore, they place all patients on full replacement doses of L-$T_4$ indefinitely to prevent either continued enlargement of the thyroid gland or hypothyroidism. Other physicians wait until there is biochemical evidence of hypothyroidism before instituting thyroid hormone therapy.

Other autoimmune disorders occur in increased frequency in pediatric patients with chronic lymphocytic thyroiditis and include Graves disease, type 1 diabetes mellitus, Addison disease, idiopathic hypoparathyroidism, and pernicious anemia. Therefore, periodic evaluation for these disorders is recommended.

## COLLOID OR SIMPLE GOITER

Colloid or simple goiter constitutes the second most common cause of euthyroid goiter in pediatric patients.[28] Almost all patients have no symptoms suggestive of hypothyroidism or hyperthyroidism. The physical examination and laboratory studies frequently do not differentiate between a colloid goiter and chronic lymphocytic thyroiditis.

The course of a colloid goiter is unpredictable. It has been postulated that simple diffuse enlargement of the thyroid gland in a young patient can lead to a large multinodular goiter in the older individual. This is the rationale for prescribing thyroid hormone therapy in a young patient with a large colloid goiter.

# EVALUATION OF THE THYROID NODULE

Single or multiple nodules of the thyroid gland are an uncommon finding in pediatric patients. Patients with nontoxic goiters may present with either solitary or multiple discrete nodules. Multinodular goiter may appear in childhood, particularly in areas in which there is chronic dietary iodine deficiency. The differential diagnosis of solitary nodules of the thyroid gland include chronic lymphocytic thyroiditis, cyst, adenoma, carcinoma, hyperplasia, toxic nodule, and embryonic defects such as intrathyroidal thyroglossal duct cysts.[29] The causes of multiple thyroid nodules include toxic goiter, toxic goiter after [131]I therapy, chronic lymphocytic thyroiditis, and adenomatous goiter.

Nodules of the thyroid gland in children and adolescents usually are asymptomatic and are noted incidentally by the patient or parents or detected during a routine physical examination. The primary challenge is to rule out the presence of a malignancy. The appropriate evaluation and therapy for solitary or multiple nodules in pediatric patients, particularly for solitary thyroid nodules, are controversial because the diagnostic techniques used to distinguish a benign from a malignant lesion vary in reliability.

## CLINICAL FINDINGS

In evaluation, the history is important and should include questions about previous irradiation of the head, neck, or upper thorax. External therapeutic irradiation of the head and neck is associated with the subsequent development of neoplastic changes in the thyroid gland.[30] Also, extensive *diagnostic* irradiation of the head and neck of children may be a causative factor in inducing subsequent thyroid neoplasia.[31] The family history should be explored for evidence of thyroid disease, pheochromocytoma, or hyperparathyroidism. Medullary thyroid carcinoma can occur sporadically or be transmitted as an autosomal dominant trait and may be associated with pheochromocytomas and hyperparathyroidism (multiple endocrine neoplasia type 2A) or can occur in association with pheochromocytoma and mucosal neuromas (multiple endocrine neoplasia type 2B) (see Chap. 188).

Information on the rate of growth of the mass, the presence of local or systemic symptoms, and hoarseness or dysphagia should be obtained. The painless, rapid growth of a nodule suggests anaplastic thyroid cancer. Pain in the thyroid gland is an uncommon symptom with malignancy. Pain is associated more commonly with a rapidly enlarging nodule caused by hemorrhage into a cyst or a benign degenerating nodule.

Careful palpation of a thyroid nodule may help define its nature. A soft, compressible, circumscribed nodule is probably not malignant; it is more likely to be a colloid or adenomatous cyst. Tenderness in a nodule suggests hemorrhage or an inflammatory process. Thyroid malignancy should be suspected if the nodule is hard or firm, if there is fixation to surrounding structures, or if there is vocal cord paralysis. Enlarged cervical lymph nodes, particularly low in the neck, increase the likelihood that a thyroid nodule is malignant. In most patients with malignant nodules, the surrounding thyroid tissue feels normal and the gland is of normal size.

Medullary thyroid carcinoma is implicated in a patient who presents with multiple mucosal neuromas, which appear as whitish nodules on the tongue, lips, and the palpebral conjunctiva; such patients may also manifest a marfanoid habitus and various skeletal defects (multiple endocrine neoplasia type 2B).

## LABORATORY FINDINGS

Serum $T_4$, $T_3$, and TSH determinations are helpful in determining the functional status of the thyroid gland. Importantly, the degree of hyperthyroidism resulting from a toxic nodule may not be sufficiently severe to allow diagnosis on clinical grounds alone. Serum antithyroid antibody studies may be helpful if one suspects chronic lymphocytic thyroiditis. Serum Tg lacks specificity as a marker of thyroid cancer when used preoperatively but has been useful in detecting postoperative recurrences of differentiated thyroid carcinomas. The measurement of serum calcitonin is essential if one suspects medullary thyroid carcinoma. Patients with this tumor may have elevated basal levels of serum calcitonin that increase further after the infusion of calcium or pentagastrin or both (see Chaps. 40 and 188).

Thyroid scintiscan is not particularly helpful in distinguishing between benign and malignant lesions (see Chaps. 34 and 40). Nevertheless, it should be performed preoperatively to preclude a nodule being an ectopic thyroid gland and perhaps being the sole functioning thyroid tissue. Furthermore, the scan might identify other nodules that are not detected by physical examination as well as an autonomous nodule. Ultrasonography is useful in defining accurately the size of a nodule, the anatomic relationship to other structures, and whether a cold nodule is cystic, solid, or mixed. Roentgenography of the neck may be helpful because medullary thyroid carcinoma may be associated with calcification in the region of the thyroid gland or in the cervical lymph nodes. Pulmonary metastases of thyroid cancer may be detected on a chest radiograph.

Fine-needle aspiration biopsy is used routinely in the evaluation of thyroid nodules in adults (see Chap. 39) and is being used more frequently in pediatric patients.

## TREATMENT

The primary challenge in the management of a multinodular thyroid gland or a solitary nodule of the thyroid is to exclude malignancy. The risk of malignancy is lower for a thyroid with multiple nodules than for a thyroid with a solitary nodule. Some clinicians recommend excision of all thyroid nodules in pediatric patients.[29] Others recommend thyroid suppression for a 4- to 6-month period in all patients who have no findings that suggest that their solitary nodule might be malignant.[32] If the nodule grows during this period, or if the nodule does not decrease in size by 50% over a 1-year period, surgery is recommended. More widespread application of needle aspiration biopsy (see Chap. 39) in the future should direct management choices more specifically.

A hyperfunctional or "hot" nodule may represent a follicular adenoma, focal hyperplasia, chronic lymphocytic thyroiditis, or, very rarely, a carcinoma. A hot nodule can be mimicked in patients with agenesis of the contralateral lobe of the thyroid. This particular anomaly must be differentiated from a hot nodule because excision is contraindicated. Repeat thyroid scanning after TSH stimulation excludes the functioning tissue as being the only thyroid tissue present.

Solitary hot nodules may be autonomous and may be toxic or nontoxic. A toxic, hot nodule should be removed surgically after proper preparation with antithyroid drugs. Hot nodules that do not produce hyperthyroidism initially may occasionally increase their secretion of thyroid hormones gradually and insidiously until the patient becomes hyperthyroid; therefore, prolonged observation of the pediatric patient is necessary. The surgical excision of nontoxic, autonomous, solitary thyroid nodules is recommended to avoid lifelong observation.

A hypofunctional or "cold" nodule presents the greatest clinical problem in differentiating malignant from benign lesions. Cold nodules may be found in chronic lymphocytic thyroiditis or may represent cysts, follicular adenomas, abscesses, carcinomas, or embryonic defects such as intrathyroidal thyroglossal duct cysts.[29] In one series of surgically removed solitary nodules of the thyroid, 5 of 27 patients (18.5%) with a cold nodule had carcinoma, whereas no patients with either a warm or hot nodule had a malignancy.[29]

In the few reports concerning the histopathology of solitary thyroid nodules in children and adolescents, the incidence of carcinomas has been from 16% to 24%.[29]

# THYROID CANCER

Carcinoma of the thyroid gland in pediatric patients is rare.[33] Its incidence has increased since 1951, when Winship was able to find 93 cases in the world's literature, to which he added 99 cases in 1970.[34] Since 1970, the incidence may be decreasing.

## ETIOLOGY

There is a significant association between thyroid carcinoma in children and adolescents and irradiation to the head and neck (see Chaps. 39 and 40). Also, there is some evidence that an increased serum TSH level may be implicated in thyroid cancer. Several retrospective studies have indicated that the recurrence of cancer can be minimized and survival improved with thyroid hormone therapy. Differentiated thyroid cancers have TSH receptors, and in vitro these tumors respond metabolically to TSH stimulation.

## PATHOLOGY

All of the histologic types of thyroid cancer that occur in adults are found in children and adolescents but, fortunately, with a slightly higher proportion of differentiated carcinomas. Papillary adenocarcinoma is the most common histologic type. Papillary cancers often contain follicular elements and may be designated mixed papillary and follicular carcinomas. Papillary carcinomas spread to the normal surrounding thyroid parenchyma and regional lymph nodes as they invade lymphatics. These carcinomas characteristically grow slowly. Follicular carcinomas have a marked tendency for vascular invasion and spread to bone and lung. Medullary thyroid cancer arises from the C cells of the thyroid and secretes calcitonin and other substances. Early spread is typically through the lymphatics. Undifferentiated carcinoma (anaplastic) is uncommon in children and causes early death because of extensive local and disseminated disease (see Chap. 40).

## CLINICAL FINDINGS

Thyroid cancer is approximately twice as common in women as in men. In children it usually presents as one or more firm, painless nodules in the neck. These nodules may be a metastatic lesion to the cervical lymph nodes without any detectable thyroid nodule, the primary thyroid tumor being occult. Usually, these lymph nodes are movable, smooth, nontender, and discrete. Carcinoma localized only to the thyroid gland is unusual.

## DIAGNOSIS

The diagnostic investigation for suspected thyroid cancer is identical with that discussed for the evaluation of thyroid nodules. Almost all pediatric patients with thyroid cancer are euthyroid. A definitive diagnosis of malignancy can be made only by histopathologic examination.

## TREATMENT

The therapy for thyroid cancer in children and adolescents is primarily surgical. However, there is controversy because of differences in criteria for diagnosis, a variable and usually prolonged course of the disease, and the lack of controlled studies of surgical and adjuvant types of therapy. The main controversy relates to the extent of surgery; recommendations vary from none, if the cancer has extended beyond the capsule or to the regional lymph nodes, to total thyroidectomy and prophylactic node dissection in all cases.[35,36] There is seldom an indication for radical surgery in children. Most forms of undifferentiated thyroid cancer are unresectable at the time of surgery; therefore, the goal is to obtain tissue for histologic examination so that radiation therapy can be initiated.

A total-body [131]I scan should be obtained after surgery to determine if there is any [131]I-concentrating tissue anywhere in the body. Remnants of normal thyroid tissue are usually present after surgery is performed for thyroid cancer. Most differentiated thyroid cancers do not concentrate [131]I in the presence of significant amounts of normal thyroid tissue. This necessitates ablation of the normal thyroid remnants with low doses of [131]I before the administration of therapeutic doses of radioactive iodine.

Thyroid hormone should be prescribed after the surgery and radioactive iodine therapy to suppress TSH release. Thyroid hormone therapy seems to be more effective in papillary and mixed papillary-follicular carcinomas than in follicular carcinomas.

The serum Tg concentration is a useful marker for metastatic differentiated thyroid cancer. However, for reliability, residual normal thyroid tissue must have been ablated.

Chemotherapy is indicated for a patient with thyroid cancer that is unresponsive to surgery, thyroid hormone therapy, or radiation therapy. The effectiveness of available chemotherapeutic agents has not, however, been evaluated extensively in pediatric patients.

Patients with medullary thyroid cancer who have undergone thyroidectomy should be evaluated for residual tumor or metastases by basal and provocative tests using calcium or pentagastrin to stimulate the release of calcitonin. If residual medullary thyroid cancer is present, serum and urine calcitonin levels increase in response to stimulation. External-beam irradiation should be considered in locally advanced, incompletely resected, recurrent, or metastatic disease.

## FOLLOW-UP

Children or adolescents with differentiated thyroid carcinoma should be observed for the rest of their lives. The course of these tumors is extremely slow and unpredictable.[37] The tumor may remain quiescent for a long period and then produce metastases. Follow-up evaluation should include a clinical examination for evidence of lung metastases, measurement of serum thyroid hormone and TSH levels to ensure an adequate suppressive dose of exogenous thyroid hormone, determination of serum Tg in patients with differentiated thyroid cancer, and measurement of serum or urine calcitonin in patients with medullary thyroid cancer.

## REFERENCES

1. Burrow GN, Fisher DA, Larsen PR. Maternal and fetal thyroid function. N Engl J Med 1994; 331:1072.
2. Fisher DA, Nelson JC, Carlton EI, Wilcox RB. Maturation of human hypothalamic-pituitary-thyroid function and control. Thyroid 2000; 10:229.
3. Mantagos S, Koulouris A, Makai M, Vegenakis AG. Development of thyrotropin circadian rhythm in infancy. J Clin Endocrinol Metab 1992; 74:71.
4. Frank FE, Faix JE, Hermos RJ, et al. Thyroid function in very low birth weight infants: effects on neonatal hypothyroidism screening. J Pediatr 1996; 128:548.
5. Usala AL, Wexler I, Poech A, Gupta MK. Elimination kinetics of maternally derived thyrotropin receptor-blocking antibodies in a newborn with significant thyrotropin elevation. Am J Dis Child 1992; 146:1074.
6. Hung W, Fitz CR, Lee EDH. Pituitary enlargement due to lingual thyroid gland and primary hypothyroidism. Pediatr Neurol 1990; 6:60.
7. Medeiros-Neto G. Clinical and molecular advances in inherited disorders of the thyroid system. Thyroid Today 1996; 19:1.
8. Everett LA, Glaser B, Beck JC, et al. Pendred syndrome is caused by mutations in a putative sulphate transporter gene (PDS). Nat Genet 1997; 17:411.
9. Coyle B, Reardon W, Herbrick JA, et al. Molecular analysis of the PDS gene in Pendred syndrome. Hum Mol Genet 1998; 7:1105.
10. Biebermann H, Schoeneberg T, Gudermann T. Congenital hypothyroidism caused by mutations in the thyrotropin-receptor gene. N Engl J Med 1997; 336:1390.
11. Anasti JN, Flack MR, Froehlich J, et al. A potential novel mechanism for precocious puberty in juvenile hypothyroidism. J Clin Endocrinol Metab 1995; 80:276.
12. Fisher DA. Management of congenital hypothyroidism. J Clin Endocrinol Metab 1991; 72:523.
13. Hodges S, O'Malley BP, Northover BN, et al. Reappraisal of thyroxine treatment in primary hypothyroidism. Arch Dis Child 1990; 65:1129.
14. Redmond GP, Soyka LF. Abnormal TSH secretory dynamics in congenital hypothyroidism. J Pediatr 1981; 98:83.
15. Rivkees SA, Bode HH, Crawford JD. Long-term growth in juvenile acquired hypothyroidism: the failure to achieve normal adult stature. N Engl J Med 1988; 318:599.
16. Weichsel ME. Thyroid hormone replacement therapy in the perinatal period: neurologic considerations. J Pediatr 1978; 92:1035.
17. Fisher DA. Hypothyroidism. Pediatr Rev 1994; 15:227.
18. Dubuis JM, Glorieux J, Richer F, et al. Outcome of severe congenital hypothyroidism: closing the developmental gap with early high dose levothyroxine treatment. J Clin Endocrinol Metab 1996; 81:222.
19. Hahn HB, Spiekerman AM, Otto WR, Hossalla DE. Thyroid function tests in neonates fed human milk. Am J Dis Child 1983; 137:220.
20. Zimmerman D, Lteif AN. Thyrotoxicosis in children. Endocrinol Metab Clin North Am 1998; 27:109.
21. Rivkees SA, Sklar C, Freemark M. The management of Graves' disease in children, with special emphasis on radioiodine treatment. J Clin Endocrinol Metab 1998; 83:3767.
22. Zimmerman D. Fetal and neonatal hyperthyroidism. Thyroid 1999; 9:727.
23. de Roux N, Polak M, Couet J, et al. A neomutation of the thyroid-stimulating hormone receptor in a severe neonatal hyperthyroidism. J Clin Endocrinol Metab 1996; 81:2023.
24. Wilace C, Couch R, Ginsberg J. Fetal thyrotoxicosis: a case report and recommendations for prediction, diagnosis and treatment. Thyroid 1995; 5:125.
25. Bowman ML, Bergmann M, Smith JF. Intrapartum labetalol for the treatment of maternal and fetal thyrotoxicosis. Thyroid 1998; 8:795.
26. Rallison ML, Dobyns BM, Meikle AW, et al. Natural history of thyroid abnormalities: prevalence, incidence, and regression of thyroid disease in adolescents and young adults. Am J Med 1991; 91:363.
27. Moore DC. Natural course of "subclinical" hypothyroidism in childhood and adolescence. Arch Pediatr Adolesc Med 1996; 150:293.
28. Hung W, Chandra R, August GP, Altman RP. Clinical, laboratory and histologic observations in euthyroid children and adolescents with goiter. J Pediatr 1973; 82:10.
29. Hung W. Solitary thyroid nodules in 93 children and adolescents. Horm Res 1999; 52:15.
30. Hempelman LH, Hall WL, Phillips M, et al. Neoplasms in persons treated with x-ray in infancy: fourth survey in 20 years. J Natl Cancer Inst 1975; 55:519.
31. Pillay R, Graham-Pole J, Miraldi F, et al. Diagnostic irradiation as a possible etiologic agent in thyroid neoplasms of childhood. J Pediatr 1982; 101:566.
32. Fisher DA. Thyroid nodules in childhood and their management. J Pediatr 1976; 89:866.
33. Hung W. Well-differentiated thyroid carcinoma in children and adolescents: a review. Endocrinologist 1994; 4:117.
34. Winship T, Rosvoll RF. Thyroid carcinoma in children: final report on a 20-year study. Clin Proc Child Hosp DC 1970; 26:327.
35. Robie DK, Dinauer CW, Tuttle RM, et al. The impact of initial surgical management on outcome in young patients with differentiated thyroid cancer. J Pediatr Surg 1998; 33:1134.
36. Millman B, Pellitteri PK. Thyroid carcinoma in children and adolescents. Arch Otolaryngol Head Neck Surg 1995; 121:1261.
37. Farahati J, Bucsky P, Parlowsky T, et al. Characteristics of differentiated thyroid carcinoma in children and adolescents with respect to age, gender, and histology. Cancer 1997; 80:2156.

# PART IV

# CALCIUM AND BONE METABOLISM

JOHN P. BILEZIKIAN, EDITOR

# CHAPTER 48

# MORPHOLOGY OF THE PARATHYROID GLANDS

VIRGINIA A. LIVOLSI

## EMBRYOLOGY

The parathyroid glands develop from the third and fourth pharyngeal (branchial) pouches (see Chap. 53, Fig. 53-4). The *third* pharyngeal pouch, containing the thymus and parathyroid tissue, migrates downward until the embryo is 18 mm in size, at which time the two *inferior* parathyroids attain their normal location at the lower poles of the thyroid.[1] The *fourth* pharyngeal pouch is the source of the two *upper* parathyroid glands, which remain attached to the upper poles of the thyroid.[1]

## ANATOMY

Anatomic studies have attempted to enumerate and localize the parathyroid glands in normal human cadavers.[1–3] Although 80% of normal adults have four parathyroid glands, from 1 to 12 may be observed.[1–3]

The location of the four parathyroid glands also varies. The superior glands may be found embedded in the capsule of the thyroid or in the pharynx, behind the esophagus, or lateral to the larynx.[1,3] The inferior glands, which normally rest near the lower pole of the thyroid, may be found near the bifurcation of the common carotid arteries, behind any part of the thyroid, paratracheally, in the thorax, or within the thymus. Despite this variable location, the parathyroid glands tend to be bilaterally symmetric.[1]

## GROSS ANATOMY

In normal adults, the total weight (mean ± standard deviation) of all parathyroid tissue is 120 ± 3.5 mg in men and 142 ± 5.2 mg in women.[4] (If both the parenchyma and fat are included in total gland weight, the weights are more variable.) Densitometry measurements show that parenchymal cell mass accounts for 74% of parathyroid gland weight.[1,5] Variations in parathyroid gland weights are found between males and females and between blacks and whites.[6] The size of the parathyroid glands ranges from 2 to 7 mm in length, 2 to 4 mm in width, and 0.5 to 2.0 mm in thickness. The glands are kidney bean shaped, soft, and brown to rust colored—although color varies with fat content, degree of vascular congestion, and the number of oxyphil cells present.[1,4]

## HISTOLOGY

The parathyroid glands are each surrounded by a thin connective tissue capsule that extends into the parenchyma, where fibrous septa divide the gland into lobules.[1,4] The parenchymal cells of the parathyroid glands are arranged in cords, nests, or sheets around capillaries.[1,4] Small clusters or spheres of cells are interspersed with foci of adipose tissue.

The adult parathyroid is composed of chief and oxyphil cells, a fibrous stroma, and variable amounts of fat (Fig. 48-1). The ratio of parenchymal to fat cells varies and probably is age dependent. Studies indicate that the formerly designated fat/cells ratio (50:50) may not reflect the normal state; in truth, normal parathyroid glands have only 17% fat.[1,6–9]

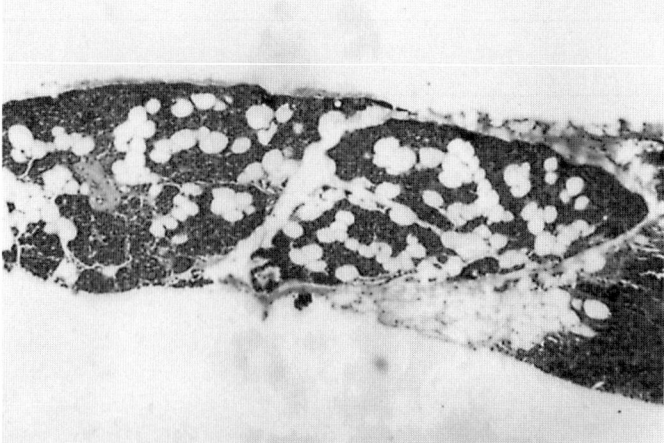

**FIGURE 48-1.** Normal parathyroid gland from a 40-year-old woman who had surgery for a thyroid nodule. Note 70:30 cell/fat ratio. Lymphoid tissue is at right. ×20

Normal parathyroid glands contain *chief cells, oxyphil cells,* and *clear cells.* These distinguishable cells probably represent different morphologic expressions of the same basic parenchymal element.

The chief cell is polyhedral and measures 6 to 8 nm in diameter.[4] It has amphophilic or slightly eosinophilic cytoplasm, a sharply outlined nuclear membrane, and abundant nuclear chromatin. Intracellular fat is found in most normal chief cells. After puberty, oxyphils appear,[4] and these increase in number with age (Fig. 48-2). The oxyphil measures 8 to 12 nm in diameter and has a well-demarcated cell membrane, abundant eosinophilic granular cytoplasm, and a pyknotic nucleus. Clear cells represent chief cells with an excessive amount of cytoplasmic glycogen.[4] The presence of follicles is a normal finding, but these may mimic thyroid histology and cause concern during intraoperative frozen section analysis.[10]

## ULTRASTRUCTURE

Electron microscopic studies of parathyroid cells have shown that the chief cells undergo morphologic change caused by the synthesis of parathyroid hormone. The Golgi apparatus increases in

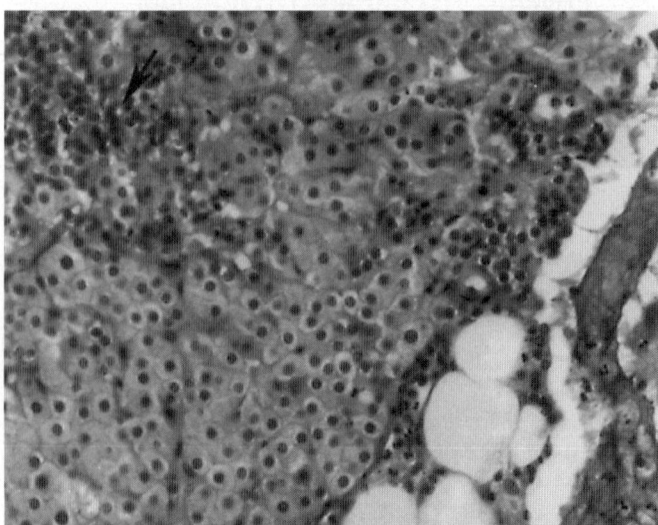

**FIGURE 48-2.** Oxyphil nodule, which abuts fat on right, and smaller chief cells on left (*arrow*). Cells are larger than chief cells with more abundant cytoplasm; the latter is distinctly eosinophilic and granular. Nodules such as this are common in adult glands. ×100

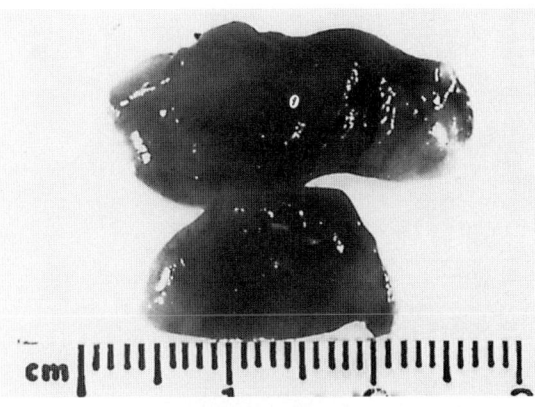

**FIGURE 48-3.** Transected parathyroid adenoma is shown. It weighed 1.1 g and had a brown, homogeneous surface. No rim is visible.

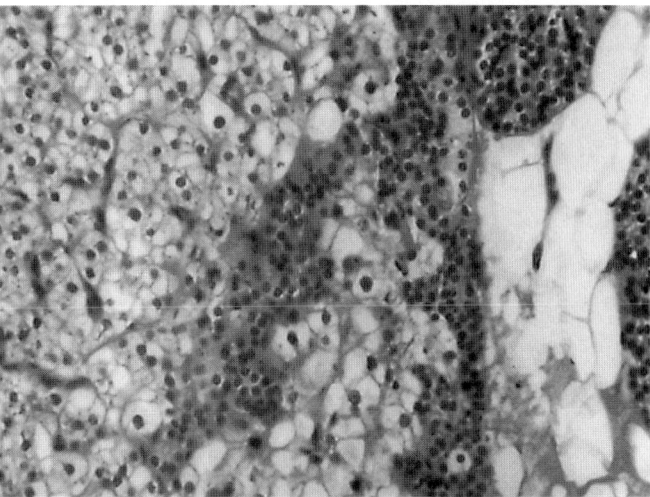

**FIGURE 48-4.** Portion of parathyroid adenoma (*left*) abutting "normal" rim. In this example, the adenoma cells have clear to slightly foamy cytoplasm. Cords of chief cells also are seen. On the *right* is fat and a group of normal chief cells. ×100

size; vesicles are prominent. In active parathyroid cells, little lipid is present.[11] In the involuting and resting phase, the cytoplasm of the chief cells contains glycogen and lipid. In the euparathyroid normal adult, only ~20% of the chief cells appears to be producing hormone at any one time.[4,11] Ultrastructurally, oxyphil cells contain numerous tightly packed mitochondria, some glycogen, and few free ribosomes. Evidence at the ultrastructural level for parathyroid hormone secretion is rarely observed in oxyphils.[4,11]

## PATHOLOGY

Most patients with primary hyperparathyroidism harbor a parathyroid adenoma (see Chap. 58); usually, a single adenoma occurs in ~80% of patients.[1,4,12,13] Occasionally, multiple adenomas are found either at surgery or after the "single" adenoma is removed. These cases most likely represent asynchronous parathyroid hyperplasia.

## PARATHYROID ADENOMA

The parathyroid adenoma is more frequently located among the lower glands than among the upper ones. Grossly, a parathyroid adenoma is oval, reddish-brown, and smooth, circumscribed, or encapsulated (Fig. 48-3). It may show areas of hemorrhage and, if large, cystic degeneration. In small adenomas, a grossly visible rim of yellow-brown normal parathyroid tissue occasionally may be seen. Weights vary from 300 mg to several grams. The overall size ranges from smaller than 1 cm to larger than 3 cm.[4]

Histologically, parathyroid adenomas are composed of sheets of parathyroid chief cells interspersed with a delicate capillary network. If not very large, most adenomas—consonant with their gross appearance—reveal a rim of normal or atrophic parathyroid tissue beyond the adenoma capsule[1,4,12,13] (Fig. 48-4). The extraadenomatous, normal cells tend to be smaller and more uniform than those in the adenoma. Stromal and cytoplasmic fat is frequently abundant here but absent in the adenoma.[13,14] The absence of a rim of normal tissue does not preclude the diagnosis of an adenoma, because large tumors may have overgrown the preexisting normal gland; alternatively, the rim may be lost when the tissue is sectioned.[15] Zones of fibrosis with hemorrhage, cholesterol clefts, and calcification may be found in larger tumors.[3,5]

Adenoma cells range in configuration from regular to severely atypical (Figs. 48-5 and 48-6). Focally, bizarre multinucleated cells with dark crinkled nuclei are occasionally seen; only rarely do these cells occur in large areas of the tumor. Nuclear

DNA measurements in such multinucleate lesions show polyploid, not aneuploid,[16] values, reflecting degenerative changes. Mitoses are only rarely found in a parathyroid adenoma. The belief was long held that mitotic figures are virtually never found in a benign parathyroid adenoma and that their presence should raise the suspicion of malignancy. This has been called into question, and parathyroid tumors with mitotic activity may, in fact, be benign.[17–19] However, long-term follow-up in the reported series is brief, and parathyroid carcinoma has a long natural history, so the issue remains controversial. Not infrequently, in a predominantly chief cell adenoma, scattered small foci of oxyphil cells may be found.[1,4] Ultrastructurally, adenoma cells have features of secretory activity, with prominent Golgi, rough endoplasmic reticulum, and secretory granules.[11]

When a single adenoma is present, the three nonadenomatous glands often show normal to increased fat content, and examination of biopsy tissue from the normal glands shows hypercellularity. Whether this observation reflects a real increase in cell number, difficulty in defining normal appearance, or sampling error is uncertain. Furthermore, some glands that contain a normal cell/fat ratio may have parenchyma that is unevenly dispersed throughout the gland, which makes a biopsy nonrepresentative.

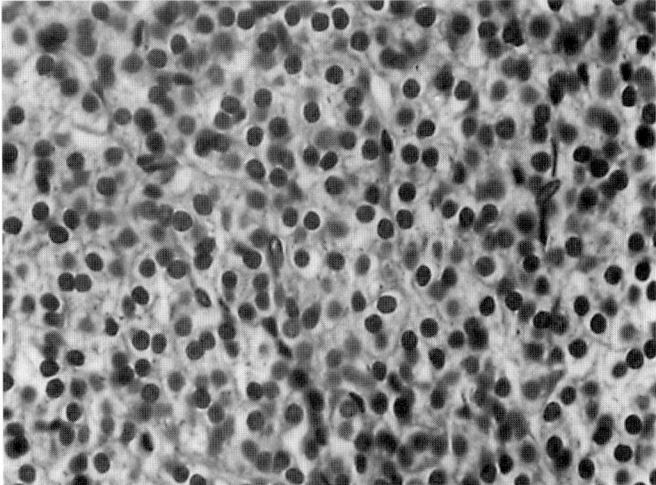

**FIGURE 48-5.** Center of chief cell adenoma. Note vascularity of the lesion; in this area, cells are nearly uniform. ×250

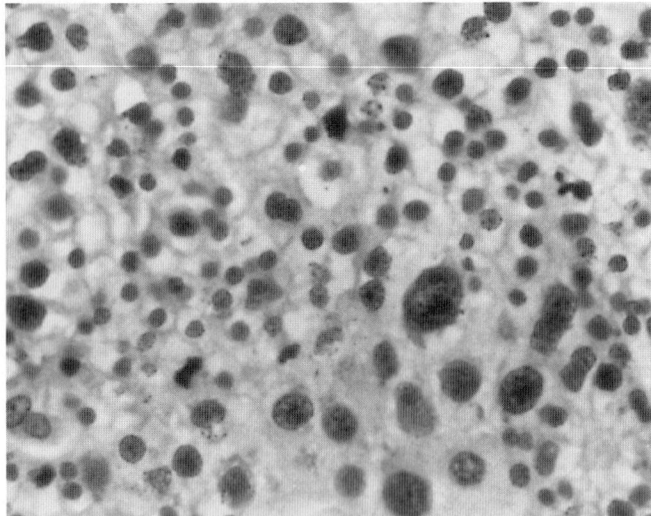

**FIGURE 48-6.** Another adenoma is shown. Bizarre nuclear shapes and large size of nuclei characterize this area of the lesion. No mitoses were found. Bizarre cells are considered a degeneration phenomenon; the cells are polyploid, not aneuploid, by microspectrophotometric measurements. ×250

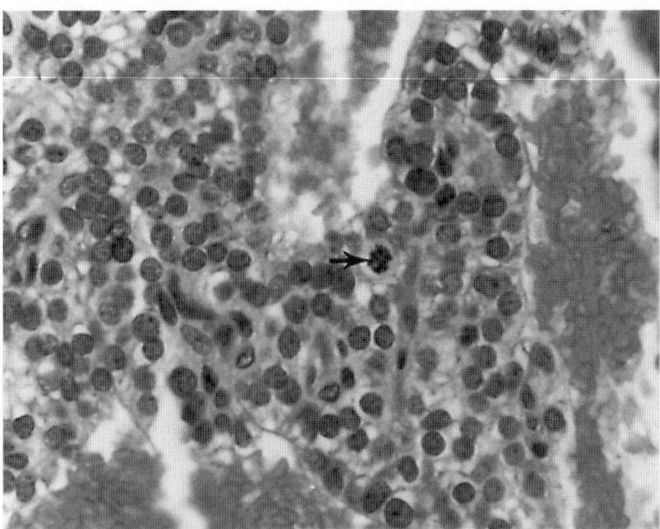

**FIGURE 48-7.** Parathyroid carcinoma from a 42-year-old patient with hyperparathyroidism. At surgery, the gland stuck to the esophagus and thyroid. The *arrow* points to mitotic figure in the parathyroid tumor. Such a finding is common in parathyroid malignancy. ×250

Rarely, oxyphil or oncocytic adenomas occur as functional lesions.[4] Such tumors tend to be large and are associated clinically with mild degrees of hypercalcemia. Ultrastructurally, large numbers of mitochondria are found.

In light of the embryology of the parathyroids, the finding of parathyroid tissue in nonclassic locations is not unexpected. Hence, adenomas are found in the superior mediastinum, behind the esophagus, or in an intrathyroidal location.[2–4]

## PRIMARY PARATHYROID HYPERPLASIA

### CHIEF CELL HYPERPLASIA

Chief cell hyperplasia accounts for ~15% of patients with primary hyperparathyroidism.[1,4] Significantly, 25% to 35% of individuals with chief cell hyperplasia have a history of familial hyperparathyroidism or multiple endocrine neoplasia[1,4] (see Chap. 188).

In chief cell hyperplasia, all four glands are enlarged.[4] If the glands are of unequal size, it is usually the lower glands that are larger.[5] Occasionally, the finding of one gland that is much larger than the others may erroneously suggest an adenoma. The combined weight of all four hyperplastic glands may range from 150 mg to >20 g, but usually it is 1 to 3 g.[4] Lobulation, a red-brown color, and a homogeneous appearance are characteristic. Microscopically, two major patterns are found. In diffuse chief cell hyperplasia, solid masses of cells are present with minimal or absent stromal fat. Usually, these sheets comprise chief cells with rare oxyphil elements. Nodular (adenomatous or pseudoadenomatous) hyperplasia consists of circumscribed nodules of chief or oxyphil cells. Each nodule is devoid of fat, and little fat is found in the intervening stroma.[1,4] Usually, no rim of normal parathyroid can be found; however, in nodular glands, relatively parvicellular zones may encompass totally cellular nodules, mimicking an adenoma.[4] Bizarre nuclei are rare in primary hyperplasia; mitoses are found occasionally.[19]

Electron microscopy reveals active-appearing chief cells, with large Golgi complexes, secretory vacuoles, and prominent endoplasmic reticulum virtually identical with chief cell adenomas.[11] Usually, intracellular fat is decreased or absent at the ultrastructural level and by fat stain.[13,15,20]

## CLEAR CELL (WATER CLEAR CELL) HYPERPLASIA

Clear cell (water clear cell) hyperplasia,[21] a rare cause of primary hyperparathyroidism, occurs as a sporadic, nonfamilial disorder. Grossly, unlike other hyperplasias, the superior glands are larger than the lower. Total weight of such parathyroids always exceeds 1 g, and weights of 5 to 10 g may occur.[1,4] The glands are irregular and exhibit cysts. No nodules are seen. The color is distinctly mahogany.

Histologically, the glands are composed of diffuse sheets of water clear cells without the admixture of other cell types. No rim of normal tissue is present. The clear cell is large, 10 to 15 mm in diameter, with sharp cell borders that occasionally fuse. The nuclei are located basally. Nuclear pleomorphism is absent, although multinucleation may be observed. Acini, papillae, or follicles may form and may be interspersed with solid sheets of clear cells.[1,4] Ultrastructurally, the cytoplasm is not empty but contains numerous membrane-bound vacuoles, secretion granules, Golgi apparatus, and endoplasmic reticulum.[11]

## PARATHYROID CARCINOMA

Parathyroid carcinoma is responsible for <1% of cases of primary hyperparathyroidism.[1,4,17,22,23] Often, the tumors are larger than adenomas, with an average weight of 12 g. Microscopically, parathyroid carcinoma is characterized by a trabecular arrangement of tumor cells (the latter divided by thick, fibrous bands), capsular and blood vessel invasion, and the presence of mitotic figures.[17,22,23] The mitotic figures must be found in tumor cells, not in stromal or endothelial elements[22] (Fig. 48-7). Cellular atypia, frequently found in benign parathyroid tumors, is uncommon in parathyroid carcinoma.[17,22] The mere presence of capsular invasion cannot be equated with malignancy in a parathyroid tumor because large parathyroid adenomas may have undergone prior hemorrhage, with subsequent fibrosis and trapping of tumor cells within the capsule. Similarly, vascular invasion is difficult to determine, except if seen outside the vicinity of the neoplasm. Grossly, the surgeon often notes that the gland is adherent to or invasive into neighboring tissues (e.g., nerve, esophagus). Metastases at the time of presentation are unusual, but they may be found in local or regional lymph nodes. Indeed, in some patients, the diagnosis of parathyroid carcinoma may not be made until metastases appear. The loss of the retinoblastoma (Rb) tumor-suppressor gene formerly was considered to be a marker for parathyroid carcinoma.[24] However, its loss in some adenomas and its retention in some carcinomas have diminished the diagnostic usefulness of testing for loss of Rb in parathyroid tumors.[23]

A group of solitary parathyroid tumors demonstrate some of the features of parathyroid carcinoma. These lesions appear to represent a pathologic spectrum of tumors that deserve careful clinicopathologic study and long-term follow-up. Such atypical lesions include (a) large parathyroid tumors with fibrous bands and uniform cytology but no mitoses (atypical adenoma), (b) parathyroid tumors of uniform pattern with easily identifiable mitoses but no other features of malignancy (atypical adenoma), and (c) circumscribed parathyroid adenomas within which are found one or more nodules of uniform histologic pattern with easily discernible mitoses (possibly, carcinoma in situ).

In rare instances of hyperparathyroidism due to primary hyperplasia, nests of hyperplastic parathyroid cells can be found in the neck outside of hyperplastic glands. This pathology is referred to as *parathyromatosis*. In some individuals, these nests of parathyroid cells are discovered at the first neck exploration. During embryologic development, nests of pharyngeal tissue containing parathyroid cells are assumed to be scattered throughout the adipose tissue of the neck and mediastinum. Normally, these nests are inconspicuous, but in the process of diffuse hyperplasia of the parathyroids, all functioning tissue becomes hyperplastic and appears as separate fragments on histologic evaluation. More commonly, a similar lesion may occur after surgery due to spillage and implantation of hyperplastic parathyroid tissue in the neck[25–27]; this may occur in the setting of either primary or secondary hyperparathyroidism.

## INTRAOPERATIVE ASSESSMENT OF PARATHYROID PATHOLOGY

### FAT STAINS

Because prominent, large fat droplets are found in the cytoplasm of normal chief cells and are absent in abnormal ones, the use of a sudan IV fat stain intraoperatively, at the time of frozen section, may conveniently and rapidly distinguish pathologic parathyroid tissue from normal tissue. In normal parathyroid glands, 80% of the cells are in a nonsecretory phase and contain cytoplasmic fat.[10] The potential usefulness of the fat stain is illustrated as follows. A biopsy specimen of an enlarged parathyroid gland is sent for frozen section, and, by routine hematoxylin and eosin stain, is shown to be hypercellular with little or no stromal fat. Thus, it appears to represent an adenoma or hyperplastic gland. A biopsy specimen of the second parathyroid gland is normocellular or minimally hypercellular. The fat stain shows abundant cytoplasmic fat; hence, this second gland is normal. The enlarged gland, therefore, represents an adenoma. However, these clear-cut distinctions are not supported by some authors, who indicate that the use of the fat stain is helpful only in distinguishing normal from abnormal in ~80% of cases. Complicating this issue is the fact that normal glands may show decreased fat.[8,13,20] Thus, fat stains should serve as an adjunctive technique and should be considered in the light of gross findings, gland weight, and size.[1,13,14,20,28]

### DENSITY GRADIENTS

Another rapid technique that may prove useful for the intraoperative assessment of parathyroid pathology is density gradient measurements of tissue. The gland is weighed, small pieces are removed from the center and from the rim, and their densities are determined in a 25% mannitol solution.[1,5] Abnormal parathyroid tissue sinks because of decreased fat and high parenchymal mass. One study reported >90% accuracy in distinguishing abnormal from normal parathyroid glands with this technique performed intraoperatively.[29]

## OTHER TYPES OF PARATHYROID PATHOLOGY

### SECONDARY HYPERPARATHYROIDISM

Grossly, in secondary hyperparathyroidism, all four glands are enlarged. Without clinical data, however, primary hyperplasia cannot be distinguished from secondary parathyroid hyperplasia microscopically.[4]

The anatomic variations of the parathyroid gland locations makes the surgical treatment of secondary hyperparathyroidism a challenge.[30]

### FAMILIAL HYPOCALCIURIC HYPERCALCEMIA

In familial hypocalciuric hypercalcemia (see Chap. 58) the parathyroid glands are described as normal or as showing minimal hyperplasia.[31]

### HUMORAL HYPERCALCEMIA OF MALIGNANCY

In patients with hypercalcemia caused by a nonparathyroid malignancy that is secreting a humoral substance, the parathyroids would be expected to demonstrate a normal histologic appearance[32] or atrophy, because they would be suppressed by the systemic hypercalcemia. Although uncommon, hyperplastic parathyroid tissue in such patients has been described by some authors.[5]

## REFERENCES

1. Grimelius L, Akerström G, Johansson H, Bergstrüm R. Anatomy and histopathology of human parathyroid glands. Pathol Annu 1981; 16(Part II):1.
2. Akerström G, Malmaeus J, Bergström S. Surgical anatomy of human parathyroid glands. Surgery 1984; 95:14.
3. Wang CA. The anatomic basis of parathyroid surgery. Ann Surg 1976; 183:271.
4. Castleman B, Roth SI. Tumors of the parathyroid glands, series II, fasc 14. Washington: Armed Forces Institute of Pathology, 1978.
5. Akerström G, Grimelius L, Johansson H, et al. Estimation of parathyroid parenchymal cell mass by density gradients. Am J Pathol 1980; 99:685.
6. Dufour DR, Wilkerson SY. Factors related to parathyroid weight in normal persons. Arch Pathol Lab Med 1983; 107:167.
7. Dufour DR, Wilkerson SY. The normal parathyroid revisited: percent of stromal fat. Hum Pathol 1982; 13:717.
8. Dekker A, Dunsford HA, Geyer SJ. The normal parathyroid gland at autopsy: the significance of stromal fat in adult patients. J Pathol 1979; 128:127.
9. Saffos RO, Rhatigan RM, Urgulu S. The normal parathyroid and the borderline with early hyperplasia: a light microscopic study. Histopathology 1984; 8:407.
10. Cinti S, Balercia G, Zingaretti MC, et al. The normal human parathyroid gland. Submicrosc Cytol 1983; 15:661.
11. Johannessen JV. Parathyroid glands. In: Johannessen JV, ed. Electron microscopy in human medicine, vol 10. New York: McGraw-Hill, 1981:111.
12. LiVolsi VA. Pathology of the parathyroid glands. In: Barnes L, ed. Surgical pathology of the head and neck. New York: Marcel Dekker, 1985:1487.
13. Grimelius L, Johansson H. Pathology of parathyroid tumors. Semin Surg Oncol 1997; 13:142.
14. Dekker A, Watson CG, Barnes EL. The pathologic assessment of primary hyperparathyroidism and its major impact on therapy: a prospective evaluation of 50 cases with oil-red-O stain. Ann Surg 1979; 190:671.
15. Ghandur-Mnaymneh L, Kimura N. The parathyroid adenoma. Am J Pathol 1984; 115:70.
16. Bowiby LS, DeBault LE, Abraham SR. Flow cytometric DNA analysis of parathyroid glands. Am J Pathol 1987; 128:338.
17. Bondeson L, Sandelin K, Grimelius L. Histopathological variables and DNA cytometry in parathyroid carcinoma. Am J Surg Pathol 1993; 17:820.

18. Chaitin BA, Goldman RL. Mitotic activity in benign parathyroid disease. (Letter). Am J Clin Pathol 1981; 76:363.
19. Snover DC, Foucar K. Mitotic activity in benign parathyroid disease. Am J Clin Pathol 1981; 75:345.
20. Dufour DR, Durkowski C. Sudan IV staining: its limitations in evaluating parathyroid functional status. Arch Pathol Lab Med 1982; 106:224.
21. Hedback G, Oden A. Parathyroid water clear cell hyperplasia, an O-allele associated condition. Hum Genet 1994; 94:195.
22. Schantz A, Castleman B. Parathyroid carcinoma: a study of 70 cases. Cancer 1973; 31:600.
23. Favia G, Lumachi F, Polistina F, D'Amico DF. Parathyroid carcinoma: sixteen new cases and suggestions for correct management. World J Surg 1998; 22:1225.
24. Cryns VL, Thor A, Hu HJ, et al. Loss of the retinoblastoma tumor suppressor gene in parathyroid carcinoma. N Engl J Med 1994; 330:757.
25. Reddick RL, Costa JC, Marx SJ. Parathyroid hyperplasia and parathyromatosis. Lancet 1977; 1:549.
26. Fitko R, Roth SI, Hines JR, et al. Parathyromatosis in hyperparathyroidism. Hum Pathol 1990; 21:234.
27. Sokol MS, Kavolius J, Schaaf M, et al. Recurrent hyperparathyroidism from benign neoplastic seeding: a review with recommendations for management. Surgery 1993; 113:456.
28. Bondeson AG, Bondeson L, Ljungberg O, Tibblin S. Fat staining in parathyroid disease: diagnostic value and impact on surgical strategy. Clinicopathologic analysis of 191 cases. Hum Pathol 1985; 16:1255.
29. Wang CA, Rieder SV. A density test for the intraoperative differentiation of parathyroid hyperplasia from neoplasia. Ann Surg 1978; 187:63.
30. Butterworth PC, Nicholson MI. Surgical anatomy of the parathyroid glands in secondary hyperparathyroidism. J R Coll Surg Edinb 1998; 43:271.
31. Thorgiersson U, Costa J, Marx SJ. The parathyroid glands in familial hypocalciuric hypercalcemia. Hum Pathol 1981; 12:229.
32. Dufour DR, Marx SJ, Spiegel AM. Parathyroid gland morphology in nonparathyroid hormone-mediated hypercalcemia. Am J Surg Pathol 1985; 9:43.

# CHAPTER 49

# PHYSIOLOGY OF CALCIUM METABOLISM

EDWARD M. BROWN

## ROLE OF CALCIUM

Calcium ions ($Ca^{2+}$) play numerous critical roles in both intracellular and extracellular physiology (Table 49-1). Intracellular $Ca^{2+}$ is an important regulator of a variety of cellular functions, including processes as diverse as muscle contraction, hormonal secretion, glycogen metabolism, and cell division.[1–3] Many of these functions are accomplished through the interaction of $Ca^{2+}$ with intracellular binding proteins, such as *calmodulin*, which then activate enzymes and other intracellular effectors.[2,3] The *cytosolic free calcium concentration* in resting cells is ~100 nmol/L. It is regulated by channels, pumps, and other transport mechanisms that control the movements of $Ca^{2+}$ into and out of cells and between various intracellular compartments.[1–3] Consonant with its role as a key intracellular second messenger, the cytosolic free $Ca^{2+}$ concentration ($Ca_i$) can rise by as much as 100-fold (i.e., to 1–10 μmol/L) during cellular activation. Such increases in $Ca_i$ are the result of uptake of extracellular $Ca^{2+}$ through $Ca^{2+}$-permeable channels in the plasma membrane, release of $Ca^{2+}$ from its intracellular stores, such as the endoplasmic reticulum, or both factors. Despite the importance of intracellular $Ca^{2+}$ in cellular metabolism, this compartment comprises only 1% of total body calcium.[4]

In contrast to intracellular $Ca^{2+}$ concentration, the *extracellular free $Ca^{2+}$ concentration ($Ca^{2+}_o$)* is ~1 mmol/L. It is closely regulated by a complex homeostatic system involving the parathyroid hormone (PTH)–secreting parathyroid glands and calcitonin-secreting thyroidal C cells as well as specialized $Ca^{2+}$-transporting cells in the intestine, skeleton, and kidney.[4–7] This system regulates the flow of $Ca^{2+}$ into and out of the body as well as between various bodily compartments, particularly between the skeleton and extracellular fluid. The rigid control of $Ca^{2+}_o$ ensures a steady supply of $Ca^{2+}$ for vital intracellular functions. $Ca^{2+}_o$ has other important roles, such as maintaining intercellular adhesion, promoting the integrity of the plasma membrane, and ensuring the clotting of blood, which further emphasizes the importance of maintaining near constancy of $Ca^{2+}_o$. The total amount of soluble extracellular calcium, however, like intracellular $Ca^{2+}$, constitutes only a minute fraction of total bodily $Ca^{2+}$ (~0.1%; see Table 49-1). Most of the $Ca^{2+}$ within the body (>99%) resides as calcium phosphate salts within the skeleton, where it serves two important functions. First, it protects vital internal organs and acts as a rigid framework that facilitates locomotion and other bodily movements. Second, it provides a nearly inexhaustible reservoir of calcium and phosphate ions for times of need when intestinal absorption and renal conservation are insufficient to maintain adequate levels of these ions within the extracellular fluid.

Thus, although $Ca^{2+}$ within all bodily compartments plays essential roles, the fraction that is most closely regulated by the homeostatic system and, in turn, affects all other compartments is $Ca^{2+}_o$. An understanding of overall extracellular calcium homeostasis requires knowledge of the various forms of $Ca^{2+}$ in the circulation and extracellular fluid as well as the movements of $Ca^{2+}$ between the organism and the environment and among various bodily compartments (i.e., overall $Ca^{2+}$ balance). Finally, $Ca^{2+}$ homeostasis depends critically on a recognition system for $Ca^{2+}_o$ and the effector systems by which changes in the circulating levels of calciotropic hormones (i.e., PTH; 1,25-dihydroxyvitamin $D_3$ [$1,25(OH)_2D_3$]; and calcitonin) restore $Ca^{2+}$ homeostasis. The form of Vitamin D produced by the body is vitamin $D_3$, which is then metabolized to 25-hydroxyvitamin $D_3$ and 1,25-dihydroxyvitamin $D_3$ as described later in this chapter. Thus, vitamin $D_3$ and its respective metabolites are referred to throughout this chapter. The reader should recognize, however, that some dietary forms of vitamin D and medications contain vitamin $D_2$. Vitamin $D_2$ is metabolized to 25-hydroxyvitamin $D_2$ and 1,25-dihydroxyvitamin $D_2$, which in humans are equivalent in their potencies to the same metabolites of vitamin $D_3$. As is described in more detail later, mineral ions themselves (i.e., extracellular calcium and phosphate ions) can also function in a calciotropic hormone-like manner, directly regulating the functions of many, if not all, of the tissues involved in maintaining $Ca^{2+}$ homeostasis.[7]

### FORMS OF CALCIUM IN BLOOD

Although the extracellular ionized $Ca^{2+}$ concentration within the interstitial fluid that bathes the various tissues of the body is perhaps most relevant to the $Ca^{2+}$ homeostatic system, it is not readily measurable. Generally, the total or ionized serum $Ca^{2+}$ concentration is determined. Of the serum total $Ca^{2+}$ concentration, some 47% is *ionized* or free $Ca^{2+}$, an equivalent amount (~46%) is *protein-bound*, and the remainder (5–10%) is complexed to small anions, including phosphate, citrate, bicarbonate, and others.[8] Ultrafilterable $Ca^{2+}$ comprises both free and complexed $Ca^{2+}$, but only the former is metabolically active (i.e., available for binding to extracellular $Ca^{2+}$ binding sites or for uptake into cells). Albumin is the principal protein that binds $Ca^{2+}$ in the circulation, and ~75% of bound serum calcium resides on albumin. The remainder is bound to various globulins.

Several factors alter the amount of $Ca^{2+}$ bound to proteins. Hypoalbuminemia and hyperalbuminemia reduce and increase, respectively, the amount of $Ca^{2+}$ in the blood that is bound to albumin (and, therefore, the total $Ca^{2+}$ concentration) without altering the level of ionized $Ca^{2+}$ (see Chap. 60). A simple way to correct the total $Ca^{2+}$ concentration for changes in serum albumin is to add or subtract 0.8 mg/dL of total $Ca^{2+}$ for each 1 g/dL decrease or increase, respectively, in serum albumin concentration. Rarely, patients with multiple myeloma present with an increase in total $Ca^{2+}$ concentration despite a normal serum ionized $Ca^{2+}$ concentration because of a $Ca^{2+}$-binding paraprotein in the circulation.[9]

**TABLE 49-1.**
**Some Properties of Calcium in Humans**

| Form | Location | Mass (% of total) | Functions |
|---|---|---|---|
| **INTRACELLULAR** | | | |
| Soluble | Cytosol, nucleus | 0.2 mg | Action potentials |
| | | | Contraction and motility |
| | | | Metabolic regulation |
| | | | Cytoskeletal function |
| | | | Cell division |
| | | | Secretion |
| Insoluble | Plasma membrane | 9 g (0.9%) | Structural integrity |
| | | | Storage |
| | Endoplasmic reticulum | | |
| | Mitochondria | | |
| | Other organelles | | |
| **EXTRACELLULAR** | | | |
| Soluble | Extracellular fluid | 1 g (0.1%) | Blood clotting |
| | | | Kinin generation |
| | | | Regulation of plasma membrane potential |
| | | | Exocytosis* |
| | | | Contraction* |
| Insoluble | Bones and teeth | 1–2 kg (99%) | Protection |
| | | | Locomotion |
| | | | Ingestion of minerals and other nutrients |
| | | | Mineral storage |

*The activation of exocytosis and muscle contraction depends, in part, on cellular uptake of extracellular calcium.

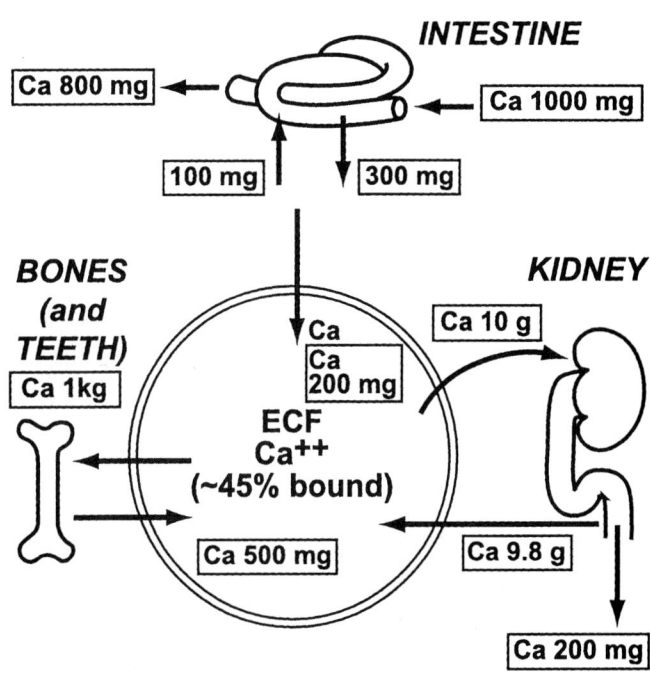

**FIGURE 49-1.** Overall $Ca^{2+}$ balance in a normal individual. Of the 1 g of elemental $Ca^{2+}$ ingested, net absorption is 200 mg (300 mg true absorption, 100 mg endogenous fecal secretion). Balance is achieved by renal excretion of 200 mg of $Ca^{2+}$ because equivalent amounts of $Ca^{2+}$ are laid down and removed from the skeleton on a daily basis in this individual. (*ECF*, extracellular fluid.) (Adapted from Brown EM, LeBoff MS. Pathophysiology of hyperparathyroidism. In: Rothmund M, Wells SA Jr, eds. Progress in surgery, vol 18. Parathyroid surgery. Basel: Karger, 1986:13.)

The binding of $Ca^{2+}$ to serum proteins is also pH dependent; acidosis reduces binding and alkalosis increases it, thereby producing reciprocal changes in serum ionized $Ca^{2+}$ concentration. The carpal spasm encountered in some patients during hyperventilation is, in part, due to a concomitant reduction in serum ionized $Ca^{2+}$ concentration caused by alkalosis. For each increase in pH of 0.1 unit, the serum ionized $Ca^{2+}$ concentration decreases by ~0.1 mEq/L, and vice versa.

## OVERALL CALCIUM BALANCE

During skeletal and somatic growth in childhood, more $Ca^{2+}$ enters the body through the gastrointestinal (GI) tract than leaves it through the kidneys, GI tract, and perspiration (generally, loss of $Ca^{2+}$ in sweat is insignificant). That is, the organism is in positive $Ca^{2+}$ balance. Conversely, in the elderly (see Chap. 64), total body $Ca^{2+}$ decreases, principally because of loss from the skeleton (i.e., $Ca^{2+}$ balance is negative). During several decades of adult life, however, the $Ca^{2+}$ homeostatic system precisely balances intake and output of $Ca^{2+}$ to maintain a constant total body level (Fig. 49-1) while at the same time maintaining near constancy of $Ca^{2+}_o$. Of the 1000 mg of elemental $Ca^{2+}$ ingested daily by this hypothetical individual, ~30% or 300 mg is actually absorbed by the intestine. Some 100 mg of $Ca^{2+}$ is lost into the gut lumen by intestinal secretion daily, so that net absorption is 200 mg. Approximately 500 mg of $Ca^{2+}$ enters and leaves the skeleton daily through the processes of bone formation and resorption, respectively. To maintain $Ca^{2+}$ balance, 200 mg of $Ca^{2+}$ are lost in the urine. The latter comprises only 2% of the daily filtered load of $Ca^{2+}$ (10 g), illustrating the remarkable efficiency of the kidney in reabsorbing $Ca^{2+}$ and its potential for modifying $Ca^{2+}$ balance via changes in net $Ca^{2+}$ reabsorption.

Because of the increasing recognition of osteoporosis as a major public health problem for individuals in later life, a great deal of interest has been shown in $Ca^{2+}$ nutrition as a function of

age, hormonal status, and other factors (see Chap. 64). The recommended daily allowance (RDA) in the United States had been 800 mg. However, although this level of intake may be sufficient to maintain some young adults in zero or positive balance, it may be insufficient for growing children and can lead to a negative balance in older people. In particular, a mean calcium intake of ~1000 mg prevents negative balance in perimenopausal, estrogen-replete women, whereas nearly 1500 mg is necessary to achieve zero balance in estrogen-deficient women of this age.[10] Indeed, the RDAs for various groups of individuals have been modified to the following values: *800 mg until age 10; 1200 mg in adolescence; and 1000 mg thereafter, increasing to 1200 mg during pregnancy and lactation and to 1500 mg if at increased risk of osteoporosis or >65 years of age.*[11] Intake of calcium in these quantities should not be considered as a supplementation but rather as a nutritional requirement for skeletal health. Interestingly, the RDA for humans is nearly five-fold lower than that for other species of animals ranging in size from 1 to 800 kg.[10]

The form of calcium ingested has some impact on the efficiency with which it is absorbed. A high phosphate/calcium ratio may have deleterious skeletal consequences, because increases in serum phosphate can lower $Ca^{2+}_o$ concentration and promote secondary hyperparathyroidism. Nevertheless, the relatively high content of phosphorus in dairy products does not appear to reduce substantially the absorption of $Ca^{2+}$ from this source. Calcium carbonate is a commonly used dietary $Ca^{2+}$ supplement. A pH below ~5 is required for solubilization of calcium carbonate in the stomach.[12] Therefore, in the presence of achlorhydria—a common condition in the aging population—absorption of the carbonate salt of calcium can be reduced. In this situation, more soluble forms of $Ca^{2+}$, such as calcium citrate, are preferable.[13] Certain dietary sugars, such as lactose, enhance the absorption of ingested $Ca^{2+}$ by a mechanism that is independent of vitamin D. This potential beneficial effect of lactose is often offset by lactose intolerance in older

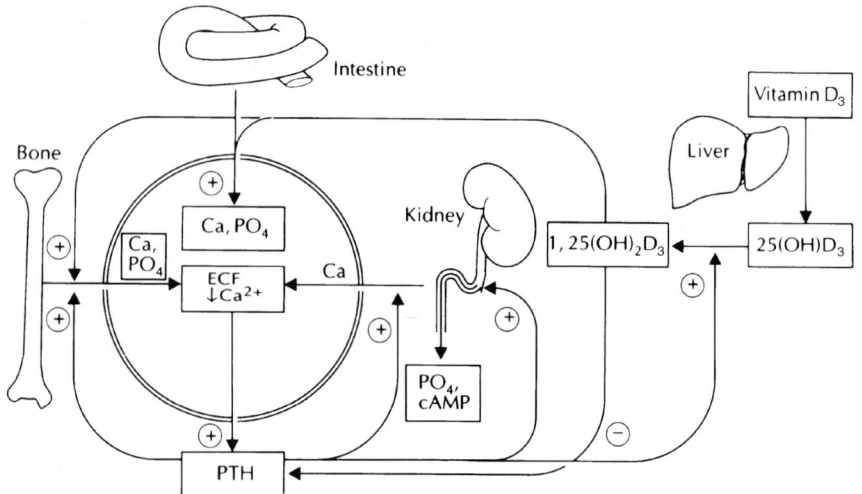

**FIGURE 49-2.** The hormonal control of calcium and phosphate homeostasis by parathyroid hormone (PTH) and vitamin D (*solid lines and arrows*). $Ca^{2+}$ regulates PTH secretion in an inverse fashion. In turn, PTH affects renal handling of calcium and phosphate as well as renal synthesis of $1,25(OH)_2D_3$. PTH and $1,25(OH)_2D_3$ synergistically mobilize calcium and phosphate from bone, whereas the latter increases intestinal absorption of both ions. Also shown are direct actions of calcium and phosphate ions on tissues involved in maintaining mineral ion homeostasis (*lines and arrows*), illustrating the role of these ions as extracellular, first messengers. For example, elevated $Ca^{2+}_o$ directly suppresses renal synthesis of $1,25(OH)_2D_3$, tubular reabsorption of $Ca^{2+}$ in the thick ascending limb, and the resorptive activities of osteoclasts. Thus, calcium ions modulate their own homeostasis not only through direct actions on the secretion of calciotropic hormones but also by exerting direct effects on target tissues that tend to lower $Ca^{2+}_o$. In effect, calcium and phosphate ions act as $Ca^{2+}_o$-regulating factors or "hormones" because they transmit information about the state of mineral ion metabolism from one part of the homeostatic system to other parts. For additional details, see text. (Reproduced from Brown EM, Pollak M, Hebert SC. Cloning and characterization of extracellular $Ca^{2+}$-sensing receptors from parathyroid and kidney. Molecular physiology and pathophysiology of $Ca^{2+}$-sensing. The Endocrinologist 1994; 4:419.)

patients. The treatment of milk with lactase largely overcomes this problem in the lactose-intolerant patient. Conversely, phytate, which is present in some cereal grains, can bind $Ca^{2+}$ in the intestinal lumen and impair absorption.

## HORMONAL CONTROL OF CALCIUM HOMEOSTASIS

A complex homeostatic system has evolved that is designed to maintain near constancy of $Ca^{2+}_o$ through calciotropic hormone, and direct, $Ca^{2+}_o$-induced alterations in the GI, renal, and/or skeletal handling of $Ca^{2+}$ (Fig. 49-2).[4–7] Usually, this is accomplished in such a way that extracellular (including skeletal) and cellular $Ca^{2+}$ homeostasis and balance are maintained simultaneously. Conditions of gross $Ca^{2+}$ excess, however, may induce positive $Ca^{2+}$ balance (e.g., deposition of $Ca^{2+}$ in bone and soft tissues) to maintain a normal or near-normal level of $Ca^{2+}_o$. Conversely, severe $Ca^{2+}$ deficiency leads to mobilization of skeletal $Ca^{2+}$ to preserve normocalcemia. Overall $Ca^{2+}_o$ homeostasis may be understood in terms of the following general principles: (a) The first priority of the homeostatic system is to maintain a normal level of $Ca^{2+}_o$; (b) with moderate stresses on the system, intestinal and renal adaptations are usually sufficient to sustain $Ca^{2+}_o$ homeostasis without changes in net bone mass; and (c) with severe hypocalcemic stresses, skeletal stores of $Ca^{2+}$ are mobilized to maintain $Ca^{2+}_o$ homeostasis, potentially compromising the structural integrity of the skeleton.

The homeostatic system comprises two essential components. The first is several cell types that sense changes in $Ca^{2+}_o$ and respond with appropriate alterations in their output of $Ca^{2+}_o$-regulating hormones (PTH, calcitonin, and $1,25[OH]_2D_3$). The parathyroid glands are key sensors of variations in $Ca^{2+}_o$, responding with alterations in PTH secretion that are inversely related to ambient levels of $Ca^{2+}_o$.[7] Parathyroid cells recognize changes in $Ca^{2+}_o$

through a cell-surface $Ca^{2+}_o$-sensing receptor[14]—described in more detail later—that is a member of the superfamily of G protein–coupled receptors that includes the receptors for PTH and calcitonin. The C cells of the thyroid gland also respond to changes in $Ca^{2+}_o$ with alterations in calcitonin secretion—with high $Ca^{2+}_o$ stimulating calcitonin secretion—through the same $Ca^{2+}_o$-sensing receptor. The physiologic relevance of changes in circulating levels of calcitonin in adult humans, however, remains uncertain (see Chap. 53). Finally, the production of $1,25(OH)_2D_3$ is likewise directly regulated by $Ca^{2+}_o$, with hypocalcemia stimulating its synthesis in the renal proximal tubule and hypercalcemia inhibiting it.[15] The second key component of the homeostatic system is the effector cells that control the renal, intestinal, and skeletal handling of $Ca^{2+}$. The translocation of calcium and phosphate ions into or out of the extracellular fluid by these tissues is regulated by PTH, calcitonin, and $1,25(OH)_2D_3$ as well as by mineral ions themselves.

The overall operation of the homeostatic system is as follows (see Fig. 49-2). In response to slight decrements in the $Ca^{2+}_o$, for example, a prompt increase occurs in the secretory rate for PTH. This hormone has several important effects on the kidney, which include inducing phosphaturia, enhancing distal tubular reabsorption of $Ca^{2+}$, and increasing generation of $1,25(OH)_2D_3$ from 25-hydroxyvitamin $D_3$, or $25(OH)D_3$.[16] The increased circulating levels of this potent metabolite of vitamin $D_3$ directly stimulate absorption of calcium and phosphate by the intestine through independent transport systems.[4–6,17] PTH and $1,25(OH)_2D_3$ also synergistically enhance the net release of calcium and phosphate from bone. The increased movement of $Ca^{2+}$ into the extracellular fluid from intestine and bone, coupled with PTH-induced renal retention of this ion, normalize circulating levels of $Ca^{2+}_o$, thereby inhibiting PTH release and closing the negative-feedback loop. In addition, $1,25(OH)_2D_3$, formed in response to the action of PTH on the kidney, directly inhibits the synthesis and secretion of PTH,[7] contributing to the negative feedback control of parathyroid function by the homeostatic system. Excess phosphate mobilized from bone and intestine is excreted in the urine via the phosphaturic action of PTH.

Both calcium and phosphate ions can exert direct effects on various cells and tissues involved in mineral ion metabolism (see Fig. 49-2). For instance, calcium ions not only reduce PTH secretion but also directly inhibit proximal tubular synthesis of $1,25(OH)_2D_3$,[15] stimulate the function of osteoblasts,[18] and inhibit the function of osteoclasts.[19] Phosphate ions reduce $1\alpha$-hydroxylation of vitamin D, stimulate bone formation, inhibit bone resorption,[4-7] and stimulate various aspects of parathyroid function,[20] as described in more detail in the next section. These actions play important roles in mineral ion homeostasis by enabling both the hormone-secreting and effector elements of the homeostatic system to sense changes in the ambient concentrations of mineral ions and to respond in a physiologically appropriate manner. Indeed, by virtue of their direct actions on cells involved in mineral ion metabolism, calcium and phosphate ions can be viewed as serving a hormone-like role as extracellular first messengers.[7] Although the cloning of the $Ca^{2+}_o$-sensing receptor that mediates direct actions of $Ca^{2+}_o$ on parathyroid and renal function has clarified substantially how cells sense $Ca^{2+}_o$,[21] the mechanism underlying phosphate sensing remains obscure.

## REGULATION OF PARATHYROID HORMONE SECRETION BY CALCIUM AND OTHER FACTORS

A steep, inverse sigmoidal relationship exists between PTH secretion and $Ca^{2+}_o$ (Fig. 49-3)—hence, the exquisite sensitivity of the parathyroid gland to $Ca^{2+}_o$ that is critical to maintaining stable normocalcemia.[7] This sigmoidal function can be described in terms of maximal and minimal secretory rates, midpoint or setpoint, and slope at the midpoint (see Fig. 49-3). The maximal secretory rate provides a measure of the acute secretory reserve of the gland in response to a maximal hypocalcemic stress. Maximal secretory capacity increases with parathyroid cellular hyperplasia, as in primary or secondary hyperparathyroidism.[4-7,21] The secretion of PTH from the parathyroid cell apparently is incapable of being totally suppressed, even at very high levels of $Ca^{2+}_o$ (see Fig. 49-3). Importantly, this implies that a sufficient mass of even normal parathyroid tissue could cause hypersecretion of PTH with resultant hypercalcemia. This has, in fact, been documented in rats by transplanting sufficient numbers of normal rat parathyroid glands to cause hypercalcemia in the recipient animals.[22] This may, in part, contribute to the hypersecretion of PTH in hypercalcemic hyperparathyroidism The setpoint of normal human parathyroid cells in vitro is ~1.0 mmol/L of ionized $Ca^{2+}$ and is close to the ambient level of $Ca^{2+}_o$ in humans (1.1–1.3 mmol/L).[7] This parameter is important in determining the level at which the $Ca^{2+}_o$ is set by the homeostatic system (the setpoint for $Ca^{2+}_o$ is slightly higher than that for the parathyroid cell per se, also being a function of the tissues that are targets for the actions of PTH). In primary hyperparathyroidism, the setpoint of pathologic parathyroid cells is increased to 1.2 to 1.4 mmol/L $Ca^{2+}$, or sometimes higher, and the serum $Ca^{2+}$ concentration is correspondingly reset to an elevated level[7,21] (see Chap. 58). The steep slope of the relationship between PTH release and $Ca^{2+}_o$ ensures a large change in secretory rate for a small change in $Ca^{2+}_o$ and is important in maintaining the serum $Ca^{2+}$ concentration within a narrow range. In addition to its sensitivity to $Ca^{2+}_o$, the parathyroid cell alters its secretory rate within seconds to a perturbation in $Ca^{2+}_o$ and may also be responsive to other variables, such as the rate and direction of the change.[23,24]

The technique of expression cloning in *Xenopus laevis* oocytes enabled isolation of a phosphoinositide-coupled, $Ca^{2+}_o$-sensing receptor from bovine parathyroid gland through which parathyroid, kidney, and other cells sense $Ca^{2+}_o$.[14] This receptor has a large amino-terminal extracellular domain that is involved in binding $Ca^{2+}_o$, followed by seven membrane-spanning segments characteristic of the superfamily of G protein–coupled receptors, and a cytoplasmic carboxy terminus (Fig. 49-4). In addition to rec-

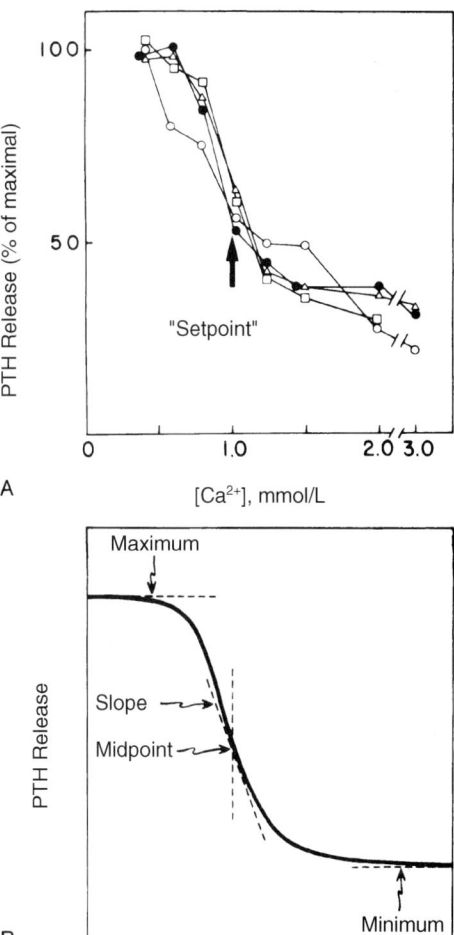

**FIGURE 49-3. A,** Relationship between parathyroid hormone (*PTH*) secretion and extracellular $Ca^{2+}$ concentration in normal human parathyroid cells. Dispersed parathyroid cells were prepared and incubated with the indicated ionized $Ca^{2+}$ concentrations. The PTH released was determined using a radioimmunoassay that recognizes the intact hormone and the COOH-terminal fragments of the molecule. **B,** The four parameters that can be used to describe the relationship between PTH secretion and the extracellular ionized $Ca^{2+}$ concentration: maximal and minimal secretory rates at low and high $Ca^{2+}$ concentrations, respectively; slope of the curve at its midpoint; and setpoint (the level of $Ca^{2+}$ producing half of the maximal inhibition of PTH release). (**A** from Brown EM. Regulation of the synthesis, metabolism and actions of parathyroid hormones. In: Brenner BM, Stein H, eds. Contemporary issues in nephrology, vol 2. Divalent ion homeostasis. New York: Churchill-Livingstone, 1983.)

ognizing $Ca^{2+}_o$, the receptor responds to other polyvalent cations as well, including $Mg^{2+}$, trivalent cations, and neomycin.[14] The possibility exists, therefore, that the $Ca^{2+}_o$-sensing receptor can function as a $Mg^{2+}_o$-sensing receptor, and that some of the direct effects of $Ca^{2+}_o$ as well as the toxic actions of aminoglycosides on the kidney are mediated through it.[21] The receptor plays a key role in $Ca^{2+}_o$ sensing by the parathyroid and kidney because the human homolog of the receptor harbors inactivating or activating mutations in several human genetic diseases that manifest abnormal $Ca^{2+}_o$ sensing.[21] In *familial hypocalciuric hypercalcemia (FHH)*,[25] individuals with heterozygous inactivating mutations of the $Ca^{2+}_o$-sensing receptor have mild to moderate hypercalcemia with inappropriately normal (e.g., nonsuppressed) circulating levels of PTH and normal or even frankly low levels of urinary calcium excretion. In contrast, persons with homozygous FHH, which presents clinically as *neonatal severe hyperparathyroidism (NSHPT)*, have severe hypercalcemia with marked hyperparathyroidism.[25] (NSHPT can also be caused by compound heterozygous inactivating mutations of the $Ca^{2+}_o$-sensing receptor [i.e.,

**FIGURE 49-4.** Proposed structural model of the predicted bovine parathyroid $Ca^{2+}$-sensing receptor protein. The large amino-terminal domain is located extracellularly and contains nine consensus *N*-glycosylation sites that are shown as branched chains. Amino acids of the deduced protein are shown at intervals of 50 in the amino-terminal domain. The amino-acid segments that comprise each of the seven predicted membrane-spanning helices are numbered (M1–M7). Potential protein kinase C (*PKC*) phosphorylation sites are also shown. Each symbol (*circle* or *triangle*) represents an individual amino acid; those that are conserved with the metabotropic glutamate receptors are shown as solid symbols, of which acidic residues are indicated by solid triangles and all others by solid circles. Also indicated are multiple cysteine residues conserved with the metabotropic glutamate receptors (which may be involved in stabilizing the large extracellular domain) as well as clusters of acidic residues in the extracellular domain (*open and solid triangles*) that could be involved in binding of $Ca^{2+}$ and other polyvalent cations. (*SP*, signal peptide; *HS*, hydrophobic segment.) (From Brown EM, Gamba G, Riccardi D, et al. Cloning and characterization of an extracellular $Ca^{2+}$-sensing receptor from bovine parathyroid. Nature 1993; 366:575.)

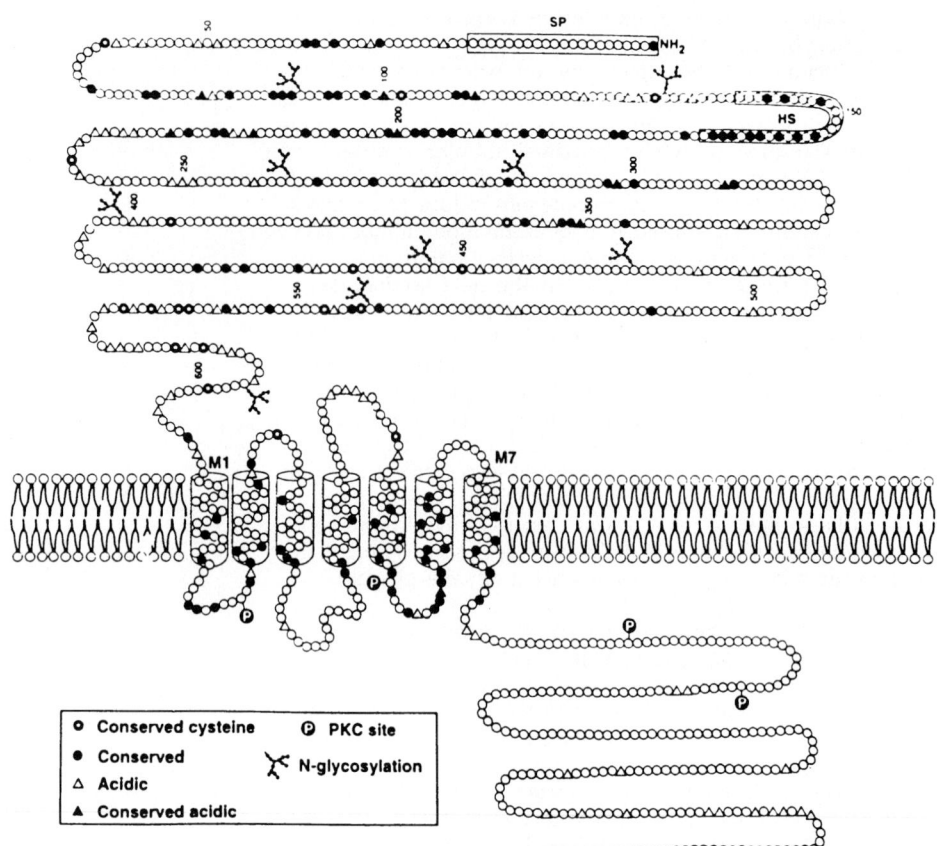

patients harbor a different mutation in each allele of the receptor[26]] or by the presence of heterozygous inactivating mutations that exert a dominant negative effect on the wild-type receptor.[27]) Finally, some families with an autosomal dominant or, occasionally, a sporadic form of hypocalcemia accompanied by relative hypercalciuria (e.g., inappropriately high for the serum calcium concentration) harbor activating mutations in this receptor, a finding that provides further evidence of its importance in $Ca^{2+}_o$ sensing in the parathyroid and kidney.[28]

In addition to being present in parathyroid, the $Ca^{2+}_o$-sensing receptor is also present along much of the renal tubule[29]; it is present at the highest levels in the cortical thick ascending limb of the nephron (a segment that is likely responsible for the abnormal renal handling of $Ca^{2+}$ in FHH).[25] Receptor transcripts are also found in thyroid, brain, and several other tissues, including intestine and bone, as described later.[30] The presence of the receptor in kidney probably accounts for several of the long-recognized but poorly understood direct effects of $Ca^{2+}_o$ on renal function (such as the reduced urinary concentrating ability encountered in some hypercalcemic patients).[31] In the thyroid, the $Ca^{2+}_o$-sensing receptor resides almost exclusively in the C cells and is thought to mediate the stimulatory effect of elevated $Ca^{2+}_o$ on calcitonin secretion. $Ca^{2+}_o$-sensing receptors in the brain might mediate as yet unknown actions of $Ca^{2+}_o$ on neuronal function.[30] Interestingly, among the G protein–coupled receptors, the $Ca^{2+}_o$-sensing receptor exhibits only limited homology with three subclasses of receptors sharing its overall topology, particularly the presence of a very large amino-terminal extracellular domain. These are the *metabotropic glutamate receptors (mGluRs)*, targets for glutamate, the major excitatory neurotransmitter in the brain; the $GABA_B$ *receptor*, which is activated by γ-aminobutyric acid (GABA), the major inhibitory neurotransmitter in the brain; and a family of putative *pheromone receptors*.[30] All three classes of receptor presumably arose from a common ancestral gene. Further understanding of their struc-

tural similarities may clarify previously unknown relationships between $Ca^{2+}_o$ homeostasis or other functions of $Ca^{2+}$ in the nervous system and in systemic $Ca^{2+}_o$ homeostasis.

As with $Ca^{2+}$, high concentrations of $Mg^{2+}_o$ inhibit PTH release via the $Ca^{2+}_o$-sensing receptor, although, on a molar basis, $Mg^{2+}_o$ is two to three times less potent than $Ca^{2+}_o$.[32] Levels of $Mg^{2+}_o$ in the blood sufficiently high to modulate PTH secretion are generally achieved only during pharmacologic interventions, such as the intravenous infusion of $Mg^{2+}$ for the treatment of preeclampsia. Because of the reabsorption of more NaCl, water, and $Ca^{2+}$ than of $Mg^{2+}$ in the proximal tubule, however, the level of $Mg^{2+}$ in the thick ascending limb can rise to approximately 1.6-fold higher than that initially filtered at the glomerulus.[33] Therefore, locally higher $Mg^{2+}$ concentrations could interact with $Ca^{2+}_o$-sensing receptors in the thick ascending limb, a major site of hormonally regulated (i.e., PTH-regulated) $Mg^{2+}$ and $Ca^{2+}$ reabsorption. Abnormally low $Mg^{2+}_o$ is also associated with a reduced rate of PTH release due to an unknown mechanism, which can cause hypocalcemia.[34] This biphasic secretory response to $Mg^{2+}_o$ differs from that to $Ca^{2+}_o$ because near-maximal rates of PTH release can be maintained at very low levels of $Ca^{2+}_o$.

Various other factors, including metabolites of vitamin D, a variety of catecholamines and other biogenic amines, prostaglandins and peptide hormones, phosphate, and monovalent cations such as potassium and lithium also modify PTH release.[7,35] Of these, the most physiologically relevant are the active vitamin D metabolite $1,25(OH)_2D_3$ and changes in the serum phosphate concentration. Studies have documented that $1,25(OH)_2D_3$ plays an important role in the longer-term (over days or longer) regulation of parathyroid function, tonically inhibiting PTH secretion,[36,37] PTH gene expression,[38,39] and probably parathyroid cellular proliferation.[40] Therefore, the actions of PTH on its target tissues produce negative feedback regulation of parathyroid cellular function not only by increasing the serum $Ca^{2+}$ concentration but also by stimulating the formation of $1,25(OH)_2D_3$, which exerts direct negative feedback actions on the parathyroid. Elevations and reductions in serum phosphate concentrations increase and decrease, respectively, PTH gene expression, PTH secretion (perhaps indirectly through changes in the expression of its gene), and parathyroid cellular proliferation.[20]

The use of lithium in the treatment of manic-depressive illness may induce hypercalcemia and hypersecretion of PTH.[41] These findings can mimic the biochemical abnormalities of primary hyperparathyroidism or FHH (e.g., lithium treatment can also be accompanied by hypocalciuria and a tendency toward hypermagnesemia). Indeed, of patients being treated long term with lithium, some 10% to 15% develop overt hyperparathyroidism, although whether this results from a direct action of lithium to induce the disorder or from unmasking of preexistent mild primary hyperparathyroidism is not entirely clear. In vitro, lithium produces a rightward shift in the setpoint of bovine parathyroid cells for $Ca^{2+}_o$[42] (e.g., a change similar to that seen in parathyroid adenomas), possibly due to interference with the process of $Ca^{2+}_o$ sensing.

## INTRACELLULAR MECHANISMS REGULATING PARATHYROID HORMONE RELEASE

After its biosynthesis as preproPTH, its subsequent metabolism to proPTH, and then its metabolism to PTH, the hormone is stored in secretory granules before its release into the circulation[43] (see Chap. 51). The regulation of hormonal secretion involves the transduction of information about changes in $Ca^{2+}_o$ by the $Ca^{2+}_o$-sensing receptor into alterations in the levels of one or more intracellular mediators that ultimately modify the secretory process.[7,14,43] The definitive identification of the relevant mediators, however, remains elusive. Although cyclic adenosine monophosphate (cAMP) mediates the actions of potent secretagogues, such as β-adrenergic catecholamines, on PTH release, it cannot account quantitatively for the effects of $Ca^{2+}_o$ on hormonal secretion.[7] Increases in $Ca^{2+}_o$ produce an initial transient rise in $Ca_i$,[44] most likely because of $Ca^{2+}$-receptor–mediated hydrolysis of polyphosphoinositides (PIs). The resultant production of inositol 1,4,5-trisphosphate[14,45] stimulates the release of $Ca^{2+}$ from intracellular stores. A more sustained increase in $Ca_i$ then ensues,[44] owing to uptake of extracellular $Ca^{2+}$ through plasma membrane channels for which the properties and mode of regulation remain to be fully defined. Activation of phospholipase C and the resultant hydrolysis of polyphosphoinositides in response to elevations in $Ca^{2+}_o$, likely plays a key role in the concomitant inhibition of PTH secretion and of parathyroid cellular proliferation. However, the identification of the most relevant downstream mediator(s) of these inhibitory effects on parathyroid function remain elusive. Patients with homozygous FHH have dramatic hypersecretion of PTH due to severe primary hyperparathyroidism with a substantial shift to the right in setpoint as well as marked glandular enlargement and parathyroid cellular hyperplasia.[46] This experiment in nature shows, therefore, that the $Ca^{2+}_o$-sensing receptor contributes to the tonic inhibition of parathyroid cellular proliferation under normal circumstances.

## EFFECTS OF PARATHYROID HORMONE ON CALCIUM-REGULATING TISSUES

### CONTROL OF GASTROINTESTINAL CALCIUM ABSORPTION

The net amount of $Ca^{2+}$ absorbed from the GI tract is the difference between the total mass of $Ca^{2+}$ moving from lumen to plasma (absorption) and plasma to lumen.[47] The latter, termed *endogenous fecal calcium*, results from the secretion by the intestinal mucosa of ~100 mg per day of $Ca^{2+}$; it varies little in different states of $Ca^{2+}$ balance. $Ca^{2+}$ absorption results from both passive diffusion across the intestinal mucosa and active trans-

port. The passive diffusion of $Ca^{2+}$ is a concentration-dependent, nonsaturable process that accounts for absorption of 10% to 15% of the $Ca^{2+}$ in the normal diet (i.e., 100–150 mg per day of ingested $Ca^{2+}$). The active component of $Ca^{2+}$ absorption is a saturable, carrier-mediated mechanism[46a,46b] regulated by $1,25(OH)_2D_3$. The highest density of sites of active $Ca^{2+}$ absorption is in the duodenum.[47,48] Clearly, however, vitamin D–responsive $Ca^{2+}$ absorption occurs in more distal portions of the bowel as well, including the small intestine (ileum more than jejunum) and portions of the colon. Because these segments of the GI tract are anatomically much longer than the duodenum, they may contribute significantly to overall $Ca^{2+}$ absorption.

After $1,25(OH)_2D_3$ is administered to vitamin D–deficient animals, an increase occurs in the GI absorption of $Ca^{2+}$ over several hours, which generally is paralleled by the induction in intestinal mucosal cells of several vitamin D–dependent proteins, including a *$Ca^{2+}$-binding protein (calbindin $D_{9K}$)*, alkaline phosphatase, and $Ca^{2+}$-$Mg^{2+}$-adenosine triphosphatase.[47,48] These proteins may be involved in the mechanism by which vitamin D enhances $Ca^{2+}$ absorption. Probably, $Ca^{2+}$ ions in the intestinal lumen move down their electrochemical gradient across the brush border of the epithelium via an uptake channel[46a,46b] and are pumped out of the basolateral aspect of the cell on their way to the extracellular fluid. The metabolite $1,25(OH)_2D_3$ appears to stimulate both the influx and the egress of $Ca^{2+}$ from the intestinal epithelial cells.[49,50]

Most phosphate absorption from the intestine occurs in the small bowel through a vitamin D–responsive mechanism distinct from the $Ca^{2+}$ mechanism.[4–6,47] Even in vitamin D deficiency, however, approximately half of dietary phosphorus is absorbed. The less stringent regulation of phosphate absorption in the gut is consonant with the ubiquity of this ion in the diet and the looser control of the serum phosphate concentration.

An important aspect of the $Ca^{2+}_o$ homeostatic system is its capacity to adapt the efficiency of $Ca^{2+}$ absorption to dietary intake. When patients are placed on a low $Ca^{2+}$ diet, serum levels of $1,25(OH)_2D_3$ increase by 50% within 24 to 48 hours, whereas when they are exposed to a high $Ca^{2+}$ diet this metabolite decreases by 50% over this period.[51] In experimental animals, the increase in $1,25(OH)_2D_3$ levels on a low $Ca^{2+}$ diet is largely abolished by prior parathyroidectomy,[52] a finding which suggests that dietary $Ca^{2+}$-induced changes in $1,25(OH)_2D_3$ concentration arise from changes in serum $Ca^{2+}$ concentration that alter vitamin D metabolism through alterations in the rate of PTH secretion. Nevertheless, lowering and raising the level of $Ca^{2+}_o$ also directly stimulate or inhibit, respectively, the 1-hydroxylation of $25(OH)D_3$.[15] The latter effects of $Ca^{2+}_o$ could potentially be mediated by the $Ca^{2+}_o$-sensing receptor present in the renal proximal tubular cells (see later).[29] The $Ca^{2+}_o$-sensing receptor is also expressed along the entire GI tract, but whether it directly regulates the absorption of mineral ions is not known.[30] Because of the $Ca^{2+}_o$- and PTH-evoked, $1,25(OH)_2D_3$-mediated adaptation in the efficiency of the absorption of $Ca^{2+}$ by the intestine, the absorption of this ion varies less than its content in the diet. Absorption of supplemental $Ca^{2+}$ may be predominantly through the vitamin D–independent route.[53] Phosphate intake also modulates the production of $1,25(OH)_2D_3$, with hypophosphatemia stimulating and hyperphosphatemia inhibiting its renal synthesis.[4–6]

### CONTROL OF RENAL CALCIUM EXCRETION

PTH- and direct $Ca^{2+}_o$-induced changes in renal $Ca^{2+}$ handling play an important role in overall fine-tuning of $Ca^{2+}$ balance[54,55,55b] (see Chap. 206). Conversely, vitamin D and its metabolites have only minor direct effects. Of the approximately 10 g of $Ca^{2+}$ filtered daily by the kidney, 65% is reabsorbed in the proximal tubule.[55] $Ca^{2+}$ reabsorption in this site is closely linked to bulk solute and water transport. PTH has little effect on $Ca^{2+}$ transport in this nephron segment. In fact,

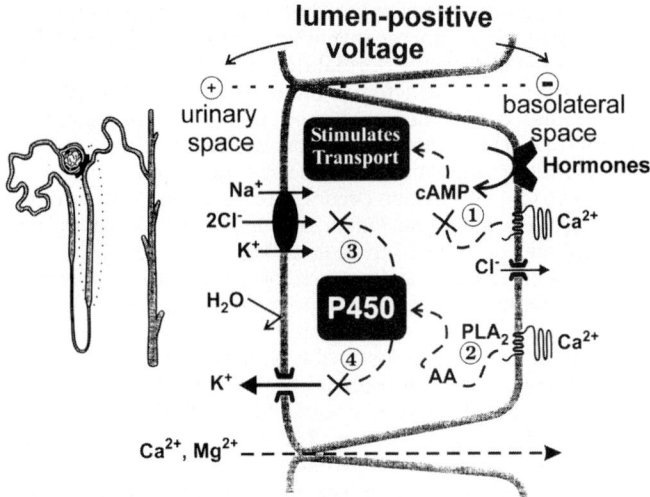

**FIGURE 49-5.** Diagram showing how the $Ca^{2+}_o$-sensing receptor (*CaR*) may regulate intracellular second messengers and, in turn, transport of NaCl, $K^+$, $Mg^{2+}$, and $Ca^{2+}$ in the cortical thick ascending limb. Hormones stimulating cyclic adenosine monophosphate (*cAMP*) accumulation, such as parathyroid hormone, increase the reabsorption of $Ca^{2+}$ and $Mg^{2+}$ through the paracellular pathway by elevating the lumen-positive transepithelial potential, $V_{te}$, via stimulation of the activity of the Na/K/2Cl cotransporter and an apical $K^+$ channel. The CaR, also present on the basolateral membrane, increases arachidonic acid (*AA*) formation by activating phospholipase $A_2$ ($PLA_2$) (2). AA is metabolized via the P450 pathway to produce an active metabolite, probably 20-hydroxyeicosatetraenoic acid, which inhibits the apical $K^+$ channel (4) and, perhaps, the Na/K/2Cl cotransporter (3). Both actions reduce overall cotransporter activity, thereby diminishing $V_{te}$ and, in turn, paracellular transport of $Ca^{2+}$ and $Mg^{2+}$. The CaR probably also inhibits adenylate cyclase (1), thereby decreasing hormone- and cAMP-stimulated divalent cation transport. (Reproduced with permission from Brown EM, Hebert SC. Calcium-receptor regulated parathyroid and renal function. Bone 1997; 20:303.)

in some studies, PTH inhibits the proximal tubular reabsorption of $Ca^{2+}$, perhaps because the hormone reduces sodium reabsorption.[55]

Of the more distal portions of the renal tubule, the descending and ascending thin limbs of Henle loop transport little $Ca^{2+}$.[55] Conversely, the thick ascending limb (TAL) of the loop and the distal convoluted tubule (DCT) reabsorb ~20% and 10%, respectively, of the filtered load of $Ca^{2+}$. In experimental animals, PTH rapidly increases the reabsorption of $Ca^{2+}$ in both segments of the nephron by increasing transport of the ion from lumen to plasma.[5,6,55] It exerts this effect, like its other actions in the kidney and in other tissues, by interacting with a G protein–coupled cell-surface receptor linked to activation of both adenylate cyclase and phospholipase C.[56] Several lines of evidence support a primary role for cAMP in mediating PTH-induced changes in renal $Ca^{2+}$ handling. In microdissected portions of the mammalian renal tubule, PTH-sensitive adenylate cyclase is present in the proximal tubule, cortical portion of the TAL, and portions of the distal tubule (e.g., DCT).[57] The location of the enzyme in the proximal tubule is thought to be linked to the well-known PTH-induced phosphaturia. The PTH-activated adenylate cyclase activity in the latter two locations correlates well with the sites of action of the hormone in promoting $Ca^{2+}$ reabsorption. Moreover, the exposure of renal tubules to analogs of cAMP mimics the effects of PTH on $Ca^{2+}$ transport, further supporting the mediatory role of cAMP. In the cortical thick ascending limb (CTAL), PTH is thought to increase the overall activity of the Na/K/2Cl cotransporter that drives transcellular reabsorption of NaCl in this nephron segment (Fig. 49-5).[31,33,55] This increase in transcellular transport is associated with an increase in the lumen-positive, transepithelial potential difference that is responsible for driving ~50% of the reabsorp-

tion of NaCl and most of the reabsorption of $Ca^{2+}$ and $Mg^{2+}$ in the CTAL. In contrast, raising $Ca^{2+}_o$ by activating the $Ca^{2+}_o$-sensing receptor present in the same epithelial cells of the CTAL reduces overall cotransporter activity, probably by inhibiting both the cotransporter itself as well as the apical potassium channel that recycles potassium ions back into the tubular lumen.[31] The transepithelial potential gradient is consequently reduced (see Fig. 49-5), leading to diminished paracellular reabsorption of both $Ca^{2+}$ and $Mg^{2+}$. In effect, $Ca^{2+}_o$, acting in a fashion analogous to that of "loop" diuretics (e.g., furosemide), regulates its own reabsorption (and that of $Mg^{2+}$) by a direct renal action that antagonizes the action of PTH.[31]

Although the detailed cellular mechanism by which PTH regulates $Ca^{2+}$ transport in the DCT remains incompletely understood, it likely involves a PTH-stimulated increase in the apical uptake of $Ca^{2+}$ through a channel.[46a,55,55a] The ensuing transcellular transport of $Ca^{2+}$ is facilitated by a vitamin D–dependent $Ca^{2+}$-binding protein, *calbindin $D_{28K}$*, which is expressed in this nephron segment and is distinct from that participating in vitamin D–mediated GI absorption of $Ca^{2+}$.[58] Another small amount of $Ca^{2+}$ (~5% of the filtered load) is reabsorbed in the collecting ducts, but transport at this site is not PTH regulated. Although the $Ca^{2+}_o$-sensing receptor is present in the DCT,[29] its role, if any, in regulating tubular reabsorption of $Ca^{2+}$ is not known.

The net action of PTH on renal $Ca^{2+}$ handling is to reduce the amount of $Ca^{2+}$ excreted at any given level of serum $Ca^{2+}$.[54] This has been demonstrated by examining renal $Ca^{2+}$ excretion as a function of serum $Ca^{2+}$ concentration in subjects with underactive, normal, or overactive parathyroid function (Fig. 49-6).[54] In patients with primary hyperparathyroidism, although the total amount of $Ca^{2+}$ excreted over 24 hours in the urine may be elevated, less $Ca^{2+}$ is excreted than in a normal person whose serum $Ca^{2+}$ concentration is equally elevated. Conversely, hypoparathyroid patients have a renal $Ca^{2+}$ leak, excreting more calcium than normal at a given serum $Ca^{2+}$ concentration. Therefore, during therapy with vitamin D, the total serum $Ca^{2+}$ concentration of patients with hypoparathyroidism should be maintained in the range of 8 to 9 mg/dL to avoid hypercalciuria (see Chap. 60). The data in Figure 49-6 also illustrate the steep positive relationship between serum and urine $Ca^{2+}$, which is likely mediated by the $Ca^{2+}_o$-sensing receptor.[31] This relation-

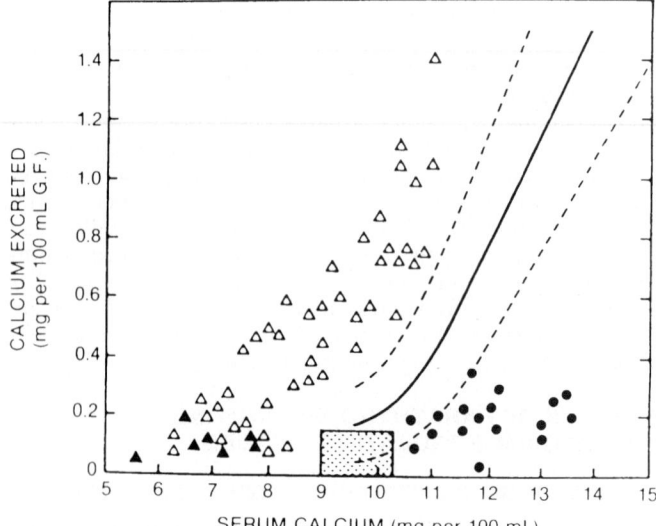

**FIGURE 49-6.** Urinary excretion of $Ca^{2+}$ expressed as a function of serum $Ca^{2+}$ in normal individuals (*area enclosed by the dotted lines*, which shows mean ± 2 standard deviations) as well as in hypoparathyroid subjects (*open* and *solid triangles*; *solid triangles* represent basal values) and hyperparathyroid subjects (*solid circles*). The *shaded area* is the normal physiologic situation. (*GF*, glomerular filtrate.) (From Nordin BEC, Peacock M. Role of the kidney in regulation of plasma calcium. Lancet 1969; 2:1280.)

ship is reset as a function of the prevailing state of parathyroid function, shifting rightward and leftward with chronic increases and decreases, respectively, in the circulating levels of PTH.[54]

Along with its effects on renal $Ca^{2+}$ handling in the distal nephron (i.e., CTAL and DCT), PTH also inhibits phosphate reabsorption in both proximal and distal sites and enhances the synthesis of $1,25(OH)_2D_3$ in the proximal tubule.[5,6] The first of these effects, like the actions of the hormone on $Ca^{2+}$ reabsorption, appears to be mediated by cAMP. PTH also activates PI turnover,[56] and evidence has implicated this pathway in the PTH-mediated stimulation of the synthesis of $1,25(OH)_2D_3$.[59]

In addition to regulating renal handling of $Ca^{2+}$ and $Mg^{2+}$, the $Ca^{2+}_o$-sensing receptor probably mediates the known action of hypercalcemia to reduce urinary concentrating ability.[31] It is thought to do so by two actions: First, by inhibiting NaCl reabsorption in the TAL, it reduces the medullary hypertonicity needed for passive, vasopressin-stimulated reabsorption of water in the collecting ducts. Second, in the inner medullary collecting duct, raising $Ca^{2+}_o$ directly reduces vasopressin-stimulated water flow, probably by an action mediated by the $Ca^{2+}_o$-sensing receptor on the apical membrane of these cells.[60] The resultant excretion of $Ca^{2+}$ in a more dilute urine may reduce the risk of renal stone formation when a $Ca^{2+}$ load requires disposal during times of antidiuresis.[31] In this way, the $Ca^{2+}_o$-sensing receptor may serve to coordinate the homeostatic mechanisms governing $Ca^{2+}_o$ and water metabolism.

## ROLE OF THE SKELETON IN CALCIUM HOMEOSTASIS

During the constant remodeling of the skeleton, osteoclastic bone breakdown is closely coupled to osteoblastic bone formation.[4–6,61] The formation of osteoblasts is coupled to the generation of osteoclasts from their precursors. Osteoclastic resorption of bone, in turn, is tightly linked to the ensuing replacement of the resorbed bone by osteoblasts. This constant turnover and renewal of bone (see Chap. 50) plays an important role in maintaining the structural integrity of this tissue. The precision of the coupling between resorption and formation is dramatically illustrated in Paget disease of bone, in which up to 10-fold increases in the rate of skeletal turnover are often unassociated with any alterations in the serum calcium concentration or overall calcium balance (see Chap. 65). Key mechanisms that link the differentiation and function of osteoblasts and osteoclasts are described briefly below and are discussed in more detail in Chap. 50.

PTH and other agents stimulating bone resorption (e.g., interleukin-11, prostaglandin $E_2$, and $1,25[OH]_2D_3$) activate osteoclast maturation and function only indirectly by enhancing the expression of *osteoclast differentiating factor (ODF)* (also sometimes called *TRANCE, RANKL,* or *osteoprotegerin-ligand*).[62] ODF is expressed on the cell surface of osteoblasts and stromal cells. It activates osteoclast development and increases the activity of mature osteoclasts by interacting with the ODF receptor (a protein called *RANK* or a closely related protein) on preosteoclasts, which then differentiate into mature osteoclasts if macrophage colony-stimulating factor (M-CSF) is also present.[62] Osteoclastic bone resorption, in turn, is coupled to subsequent osteoblastic formation of bone, at least in part through the release of skeletal growth factors, such as transforming growth factor-β and insulin-like growth factor-I, which stimulate osteoblastic differentiation and activity.[63]

The skeleton also serves as a nearly inexhaustible reservoir for calcium and phosphate ions.[5–7] Because the skeletal content of $Ca^{2+}$ is 1000-fold higher than that of the extracellular fluid, this function can be subserved by the net movement of relatively small amounts of $Ca^{2+}$ into or out of bone. After administration of PTH to animals, the structure of osteoclasts, osteoblasts, and osteocytes (those bone cells trapped within the calcified matrix) is altered within minutes.[5] Those morphologic changes are accompanied by increased activity of osteoclasts and inhibition

of osteoblastic function, leading to an increase in net skeletal calcium release within 2 to 3 hours. The PTH-induced increase in the size of the periosteocytic lacunae also has been considered presumptive evidence for a role for this cell type in skeletal calcium release. Continued exposure to PTH causes an increase in the number and activity of osteoclasts that is ultimately accompanied by an increase in osteoblastic activity through the coupling of bone resorption to formation, as noted previously. The mechanisms by which PTH modulates bone cell function remain to be fully elucidated. The hormone raises skeletal levels of cAMP[64] but may also act through other second messenger systems, including the activation of phospholipase C.[56]

In addition to modulating bone turnover indirectly, by altering the rate of PTH secretion and/or $1,25(OH)_2D_3$ production, changes in $Ca^{2+}_o$ also directly regulate bone cell function in vitro in ways that probably contribute to the control of bone turnover in vivo. Raising $Ca^{2+}_o$ stimulates several aspects of the functions of osteoblasts and preosteoblasts, such as enhancing their proliferation and chemotaxis.[18] These actions could contribute to the coupling of osteoclastic bone resorption to the subsequent replacement of the missing bone by osteoblasts. Conversely, elevated levels of $Ca^{2+}_o$ directly inhibit osteoclastic function,[19] possibly providing a way for osteoclasts to autoregulate their activity as a function of the amount of calcium that they have resorbed. Pharmacologic evidence has implicated distinct mechanisms for $Ca^{2+}_o$ sensing in osteoblasts and osteoclasts,[18,19] which differ in turn from the $Ca^{2+}_o$-sensing receptor that regulates various aspects of parathyroid and renal function.[7,14] The latter receptor, however, can be expressed by both osteoblastic[65] and osteoclastic cells,[66] and further studies are needed to establish with certainty the molecular mechanisms through which bone cells sense $Ca^{2+}_o$. Changes in the level of extracellular phosphate also modulate bone turnover as noted previously. Elevations in phosphate stimulate bone formation and inhibit bone resorption, whereas hypophosphatemia produces the converse effects.[7] As with the known direct actions of phosphate on parathyroid function, the mechanisms underlying the sensing of extracellular phosphate ions by bone cells remain obscure.

## REGULATION OF CIRCULATING CALCIUM CONCENTRATION

The information in Figure 49-2 does not delineate the temporal sequence of how the homeostatic system reacts to perturbations in $Ca^{2+}_o$. Actually, there is a hierarchy of responses by both the parathyroid gland and the effector systems that regulate calcium transport in the skeleton, kidney, and intestine.[7] The initial alteration in the secretory rate of PTH (release of preformed stores of hormone) occurs within seconds of the change in $Ca^{2+}_o$. Within 15 to 30 minutes, an increase occurs in the net synthesis of PTH, without any change in the levels of messenger RNA (mRNA), because of reduced intracellular degradation of PTH. If the hypocalcemic stimulus persists, the levels of PTH mRNA increase over the ensuing 12 to 24 hours or more.[38,39] Eventually, chronic hypocalcemia is associated with enhanced parathyroid cellular proliferation over days to weeks,[67] which further increases the secretory rate of the hormone. Reduced levels of $1,25(OH)_2D_3$ are also a likely stimulus for parathyroid cellular proliferation and contribute to the severe hyperparathyroidism that can be encountered in chronic renal insufficiency.

The most rapid changes in the handling of calcium by the effector organs of the homeostatic system occur in the skeleton and kidney. Alterations in distal tubular calcium reabsorption take place within minutes in vitro,[55] whereas the skeletal release of calcium occurs within 2 to 3 hours.[68] If these two functional changes are insufficient to restore normocalcemia, the continued hypersecretion of PTH stimulates increased synthesis of $1,25(OH)_2D_3$ within 1 to 2 days,[51] enhances the activity of existing osteoclasts, and promotes the appearance of new osteoclasts within days to weeks. Only rarely (e.g., in severe

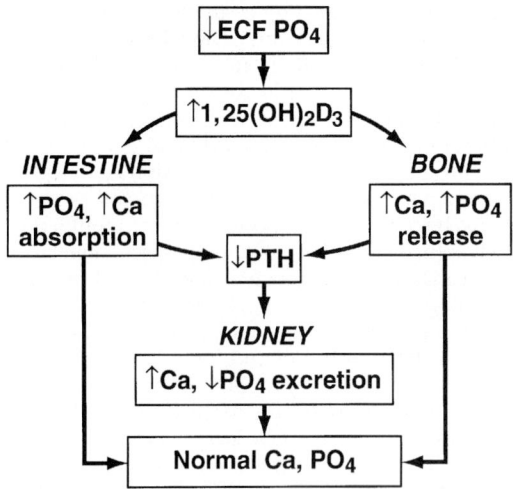

**FIGURE 49-7.** Response of the homeostatic system to hypophosphatemia. Hypophosphatemia per se stimulates synthesis of $1,25(OH)_2D_3$. Excess $Ca^{2+}$ mobilized with phosphate from bone and intestine suppresses parathyroid hormone (*PTH*) release, facilitating calciuresis. Decreased renal phosphate clearance resulting from reduced circulating levels of PTH retains phosphate available from intestine and bone. Low phosphate also may directly inhibit PTH release, increase bone resorption, and enhance renal phosphate reabsorption. (*ECF*, extracellular fluid.)

vitamin D deficiency) is the full complement of homeostatic responses insufficient to restore normocalcemia.

Exposure of the homeostatic system to a calcium load produces responses that are largely the opposite of those seen with hypocalcemia. The suppression of parathyroid function induces a renal leak of $Ca^{2+}$, reduces the release of skeletal $Ca^{2+}$, and ultimately suppresses GI absorption of $Ca^{2+}$ by inhibiting the synthesis of $1,25(OH)_2D_3$. The remarkable sensitivity of the system is illustrated by its response to the ingestion of the $Ca^{2+}$ present in a glass of milk. A minute rise in serum $Ca^{2+}$ causes approximately a 30% reduction in PTH secretion, which leads to prompt excretion of much of the extra $Ca^{2+}$ in the urine.[5] In response to severe loads of $Ca^{2+}$, the skeleton can buffer substantial quantities of $Ca^{2+}$, and the kidney can excrete up to 1 g of $Ca^{2+}$ over 24 hours; however, hypercalcemia may ensue, particularly if renal impairment develops.

One of the most elegant features of the homeostatic system for $Ca^{2+}$ is that it simultaneously contributes to the regulation of the serum phosphate concentration. With $Ca^{2+}$ deficiency sufficient to produce secondary hyperparathyroidism, the excess phosphate mobilized into the extracellular fluid from intestine and bone is excreted in the urine (mild hypophosphatemia may ensue). Conversely, with oral $Ca^{2+}$ loading, reduced GI and skeletal availability of phosphate are managed by decreased renal phosphate clearance because of reduced PTH secretion.

Primary abnormalities in phosphate metabolism also elicit changes in the $Ca^{2+}_o$ homeostatic system that tend to correct both serum phosphate and calcium concentrations. Hypophosphatemia, for example, enhances the synthesis of $1,25(OH)_2D_3$, which then increases intestinal absorption and skeletal release of phosphate and calcium[52] (Fig. 49-7). The increased movement of $Ca^{2+}$ into the extracellular fluid suppresses PTH release, thereby enhancing the excretion of the excess $Ca^{2+}$ as well as retaining the phosphate mobilized from intestine and bone. The net result of these adaptations is some normalization of serum phosphate without any change in the serum $Ca^{2+}$ concentration. Through poorly defined mechanisms, the kidney also retains phosphate more avidly in states of phosphate depletion, independent of alterations in PTH secretion. Clearly, as with the actions of phosphate on parathyroid and bone cells, some mechanism must exist through which these alterations in extracellular phosphate

availability and/or levels are recognized by the kidney and transduced into alterations in $1,25(OH)_2D_3$ synthesis and tubular phosphate reabsorption. Moreover, additional hormones regulating phosphate homeostasis likely will be discovered that are involved in the pathogenesis of inherited and acquired disorders of the regulation of the serum phosphate concentration.[69]

# CLINICAL ASSESSMENT OF CALCIUM HOMEOSTASIS

The clinical evaluation of normal and abnormal calcium homeostasis requires an accurate assessment of serum calcium and phosphate concentrations as well as the functions of the parathyroid glands and the effector systems regulating calcium homeostasis. Total serum calcium and phosphate measurements are usually reliable. Both dip-type and flow-through electrodes of improved quality are widely available for measuring serum ionized calcium and may be useful when changes in serum protein levels make the accurate estimation of ionized from total calcium levels difficult. Measurement of the serum ionized calcium concentration may also be helpful in cases of mild primary hyperparathyroidism, in which an elevation of serum ionized calcium is sometimes more readily detectable than one of serum total calcium concentration.

## DIRECT ASSAYS OF CALCIUM-REGULATING HORMONES IN BLOOD

### PARATHYROID HORMONE

Most of the immunoreactive PTH in the circulation represents inactive fragments of the hormone comprising the mid-molecule and carboxy-terminal portions of the molecule[70] (see Chap. 51). The amount of biologically active PTH (1-84) in the blood represents <10% of the total immunoreactivity. The advent of specific and sensitive double-antibody (e.g., immunoradiometric or immunochemiluminescent) assays specific for intact PTH has largely supplanted the previously used mid-molecule and carboxy-terminal assays.[71] Although these double-antibody assays were originally thought to recognize only the intact form of PTH, later studies have shown that they also detect variable amounts (10–25% or more) of additional forms of immunoreactive PTH.[72] Nevertheless, these intact PTH assays permit reliable diagnosis of primary and secondary hyperparathyroidism when interpreted in the context of the simultaneously measured serum calcium concentration. Furthermore, in hypercalcemia due to nonparathyroid causes, intact PTH levels are generally frankly suppressed, greatly facilitating the differential diagnosis of hypercalcemia. The need seldom arises, therefore, to measure PTH by the older immunoassays or more cumbersome bioassays. Because high-quality assays for parathyroid hormone–related protein are also routinely available,[73] measurement of urinary cAMP excretion is usually not required to diagnose parathyroid hormone–related, protein-mediated hypercalcemia of malignancy. An assay that appears to be specific for PTH (1-84) per se is under development.

### CALCITONIN

The determination of the immunoreactive calcitonin level is most useful in screening patients suspected of harboring medullary thyroid carcinoma (MTC).[74] In this setting, the calcitonin level is determined both before and after the administration of a secretagogue, such as calcium or pentagastrin. An abnormally large increase in the circulating level of calcitonin after pentagastrin administration generally indicates that the patient harbors a C-cell neoplasm. The identification of the gene (the *ret* oncogene) causing familial MTC and multiple endocrine neoplasia type 2 (MEN2)[75] now permits the clinician to identify obligate gene carriers by genetic means rather than relying solely on pentagastrin testing. How or to what extent serum calcitonin influences calcium homeostasis in normal humans is uncertain (see Chap. 53).

### VITAMIN D METABOLITES

Assays are available for measuring $25(OH)D_3$ and $1,25(OH)_2D_3$.[4-6] The former is measured to assess circulating stores of the vitamin. Serum is extracted and purified chromatographically; $25(OH)D_3$ is then measured either directly by its absorption of ultraviolet light, by a radioligand-binding assay that uses endogenous binding proteins, or by radioimmunoassay. Because of the low levels of $1,25(OH)_2D_3$ in blood (~30 pg/mL), this metabolite generally must be extensively purified before assay and then measured using the naturally occurring cellular receptor in radioligand assays or by radioimmunoassay. The clinical settings in which the measurement of this metabolite is useful are discussed in Chapters 63, 70, and 219.

## ASSESSMENT OF THE FUNCTION OF TARGET ORGANS FOR CALCIUM-REGULATING HORMONES

### KIDNEY

Along with measurement of urinary cAMP excretion, determination of the tubular reabsorption of phosphate (TRP) is another indirect assessment of PTH action on the kidney that is seldom required now that high-quality assays for intact PTH are widely available (see previous section on PTH assays). This parameter is calculated from the equation TRP = $1 - [U_p \times S_{cr}/U_{cr} \times S_p]$, where $U_p$ = urinary phosphate excretion, $U_{cr}$ = urinary creatinine excretion, and $S_p$ and $S_{cr}$ = serum phosphate and creatinine excretion, respectively. A particularly useful expression of renal phosphate handling is the tubular maximum for phosphate corrected for glomerular filtration rate, which can be calculated using an appropriate nomogram.[76] This parameter is particularly useful in assessing the contribution of renal leak of phosphate to hypophosphatemic, osteomalacic disorders (see Chaps. 63 and 70). The measurement of the relationship between serum calcium and urine calcium excretion provides some indirect information about the PTH-calciferol axis (see Fig. 49-6). Calcium excretion is often expressed in terms of the calcium/creatinine excretion ratio. A more rigorous parameter of renal calcium handling is the *ratio of calcium to creatinine clearance*, which is characteristically lower in patients with FHH (usually <0.01) than in those with primary hyperparathyroidism.[25]

### INTESTINE

The direct measurement of calcium absorption provides an indication of the intestinal response to circulating levels of $1,25(OH)_2D_3$ and, indirectly, PTH. Calcium absorption may be assessed by determining the difference between oral calcium intake and fecal calcium excretion or by using isotopic techniques.[77] The former is laborious and requires equilibration of mineral homeostasis to a constant diet over weeks. The latter is accomplished by administering a tracer dose of calcium-47 ($^{47}$Ca) or other isotopes of calcium with a fixed amount of stable calcium ($^{40}$Ca, usually 100 mg) and measuring the appearance of the isotope in blood samples during the following 0.5 to 6 hours. Unfortunately, neither technique is widely available.

### BONE

Alkaline phosphatase in serum originates from many sources, of which bone and liver are the two principal ones in adult humans.[78] Circulating alkaline phosphatase of skeletal origin derives primarily from osteoblasts; measurement of its activity in serum can be a useful, albeit indirect, indicator of osteoblastic activity. A crude way of distinguishing the activity of skeletal alkaline phosphatase from that arising from liver is the greater lability of the former to heat. Immunoassays specific for the skeletal isoenzyme of alkaline phosphatase are available; their utility will become clearer as greater experience with them accumulates.[78] A bone-derived serum protein, osteocalcin (sometimes called bone Gla protein), can be a marker of osteoblast function. This protein contains γ-carboxyglutamic acid (Gla) synthesized through a vitamin K–dependent carboxylation of glutamate, and it may be measured by radioimmunoassay.[79] When bone resorption and formation are coupled, it is a marker of bone turnover. If they are not well coupled (i.e., during therapy with glucocorticoids), it is a marker of bone formation.[78] Assays of bone formation are available that measure the serum levels of the amino-terminal and carboxy-terminal propeptides of type I collagen,[78] which are cleaved off during the maturation of bone collagen. Additional experience is needed to evaluate further their clinical utility, but as with other bone markers, they are a rather indirect measure of bone cell activity.

Several clinically useful markers of bone resorption arise from products of the degradation of bone collagen.[78] Because ~60% of total body collagen resides in bone, the determination of urine, or in some case serum, levels of these markers provides information about the turnover of bone matrix. The assay of urinary hydroxyproline as a measure of bone turnover has been supplanted by the developments of methods for measuring various breakdown products of the amino acids that crosslink collagen molecules in bone (hydroxylysyl pyridinolines = pyridinolines [Pyr]; or lysyl pyridinolines = deoxypyridinolines [d-Pyr]).[78] Approximately two-thirds of the Pyr and d-Pyr in urine are in the form of small peptides, and the remainder are the free amino acids. Pyr and d-Pyr are generally measured after acid hydrolysis to convert Pyr- and d-Pyr–containing peptides to the free amino acids. Two additional markers of bone resorption that are currently being evaluated are pyridinoline-containing peptides arising from the amino- and carboxy-termini of bone collagen (cross-linked N-telopeptides [NTx] and C-telopeptides [ICTP], respectively). As clinical experience accumulates, the indication is that assays based on cross-links of bone collagen will be useful, relatively specific urine (and perhaps serum) markers of bone resorption (see Chap. 56).

## REFERENCES

1. Rasmussen H. Calcium messenger system. N Engl J Med 1986; 314:1089.
2. Meldolesi J, Pozzan T. The endoplasmic reticulum $Ca^{2+}$ store: a view from the lumen. Trends Biochem Sci 1998; 23:10.
3. Nathanson MH. Cellular and subcellular calcium signaling in gastrointestinal epithelium. Gastroenterology 1994; 106:1349.
4. Parfitt AM, Kleerkoper M. The divalent ion homeostatic system: physiology and metabolism of calcium, phosphorous, magnesium, and bone. In: Maxwell MH, Kleeman CR, eds. Clinical disorders of fluid and electrolyte metabolism, 3rd ed. New York: McGraw-Hill, 1980:269.
5. Stewart AF, Broadus AE. Mineral metabolism. In: Felig P, Baxter JD, Broadus AE, Frohman LA, eds. Endocrinology and metabolism. New York: McGraw-Hill, 1987:1317.
6. Bringhurst FR. Calcium and phosphate distribution, turnover and metabolic actions. In: DeGroot LJ, ed. Endocrinology, 3rd ed. Philadelphia, WB Saunders, 1995:1015.
7. Brown EM. Extracellular $Ca^{2+}$-sensing, regulation of parathyroid cell function, and role of calcium and other ions as extracellular (first) messengers. Physiol Rev 1991; 71:371.
8. Walser M. Ion association. VI. Interactions between calcium, magnesium, inorganic phosphate, citrate, and protein in normal human plasma. J Clin Invest 1961; 40:723.
9. Lindgarde F, Zettervall O. Hypercalcemia and normal ionized serum calcium in a case of myelomatosis. Ann Intern Med 1973; 78:396.
10. Heaney RP, Gallagher JC, Johnston CC, et al. Calcium nutrition and bone health in the elderly. Am J Clin Nutr 1982; 36:986.
11. Miller GD, Groziak SM, DiRienzo D. Age considerations in nutrient needs for bone health. J Am Coll Nutr 1996; 15:553.
12. Bo-Linn GW, Davis GR, Buddru DJ, et al. An evaluation of the importance of gastric acid secretion in the absorption of dietary calcium. J Clin Invest 1984; 73:640.
13. Nicar MJ, Pak CY. Calcium bioavailability from calcium carbonate and calcium citrate. J Clin Endocrinol Metab 1985; 61:391.

14. Brown EM, Gamba G, Riccardi D, et al. Cloning and characterization of an extracellular $Ca^{2+}$-sensing receptor from bovine parathyroid. Nature 1993; 366:575.

15. Weisinger JR, Favus MJ, Langman CB, Bushinsky DA. Regulation of 1,25-dihydroxyvitamin $D_3$ by calcium in the parathyroidectomized, parathyroid hormone-replete rat. J Bone Miner Res 1989; 4:929.

16. Fraser DR, Kodicek E. Regulation of 25-hydroxy-cholecalciferol-hydroxylase activity in kidney by parathyroid hormone. Nature New Biol 1973; 241:163.

17. Holick MF. Vitamin D: photobiology, metabolism, and clinical applications. In: DeGroot L, Besser, H, Burger HG, et al., eds. Endocrinology, 3rd ed. Philadelphia, WB Saunders, 1995:990.

18. Quarles LD. Cation-sensing receptors in bone: a novel paradigm for regulating bone remodeling? J Bone Miner Res 1997; 12:1971.

19. Zaidi M, Adebanjo OA, Moonga BS, Sun L, Huang CL. Emerging insights into the role of calcium ions in osteoclast regulation. J Bone Miner Res 1999; 14:669.

20. Slatopolsky E, Finch J, Denda M, et al. Phosphorus restriction prevents parathyroid gland growth. High phosphorus directly stimulates PTH secretion in vitro. J Clin Invest 1996; 97:2534.

21. Brown EM, Vassilev PM, Quinn S, Hebert SC. G protein-coupled, extracellular $Ca^{2+}$-sensing receptor: a versatile regulator of diverse cellular functions. Vitamins and Hormones 1999; 55:1.

22. Gittes RF, Radde JC. Experimental model for hyperparathyroidism: effect of excessive numbers of transplanted isologous parathyroid glands. J Urol 1966; 95:595.

23. Adami S, Muirhead N, Manning RM, et al. Control of secretion of parathyroid hormone in secondary hyperparathyroidism. Clin Endocrinol 1982; 16:463.

24. Grant FD, Conlin PR, Brown EM. Rate and concentration dependence of parathyroid hormone dynamics during stepwise changes in serum ionized calcium in normal humans. J Clin Endocrinol Metab 1990; 71:370.

25. Brown EM, Kifor O, Bai M. Decreased Responsiveness to Extracellular $Ca^{2+}$ due to abnormalities in the $Ca^{2+}_o$-sensing receptor. In: Jameson U, ed. Contemporary Endocrinology: hormone resistance syndromes. Totowa, NJ: Humana Press 1999:87.

26. Kobayashi M, Tanaka H, Tsuzuki K, et al. Two novel missense mutations in calcium-sensing receptor gene associated with neonatal severe hyperparathyroidism. J Clin Endocrinol Metab 1997; 82:2716.

27. Bai M, Pearce SH, Kifor O, et al. In vivo and in vitro characterization of neonatal hyperparathyroidism resulting from a de novo, heterozygous mutation in the $Ca^{2+}$-sensing receptor gene: normal maternal calcium homeostasis as a cause of secondary hyperparathyroidism in familial benign hypocalciuric hypercalcemia. J Clin Invest 1997; 99:88.

28. Pollak MR, Brown EM, Estep HL, et al. Autosomal dominant hypocalcemia caused by a $Ca^{2+}$-sensing receptor gene mutation. Nat Genet 1994; 8:303.

29. Riccardi D, Hall AE, Chattopadhyay N, et al. Localization of the extracellular $Ca^{2+}$/polyvalent cation-sensing protein in rat kidney. Am J Physiol 1998; 274:F611.

30. Chattopadhyay N, Brown EM. Calcium-sensing receptor: roles in and beyond systemic calcium homeostasis. Biol Chem 1997; 378:759.

31. Hebert SC, Brown EM, Harris HW. Role of the $Ca^{2+}$-sensing receptor in divalent mineral ion homeostasis. J Exp Biol 1997; 200:295.

32. Habener JT, Potts JT Jr. Relative effectiveness of calcium and magnesium on the secretion and biosynthesis of parathyroid hormone in vitro. Endocrinology 1976; 98:197.

33. De Rouffignac C, Quamme GA. Renal magnesium handling and its hormonal control. Physiol Rev 1994; 74:305.

34. Anast CS, Mohs JM, Kaplan SL, Burns TW. Evidence for parathyroid failure in magnesium deficiency. Science 1972; 177:606.

35. Brown EM. Parathyroid secretion in vivo and in vitro: regulation by calcium and other secretagogues. Miner Electrolyte Metab 1982; 8:130.

36. Russell J, Silver J, Sherwood LM. The effects of calcium and vitamin D metabolites on cytoplasmic mRNA coding for preproparathyroid hormone in isolated parathyroid cells. Trans Assoc Am Physicians 1984; 97:269.

37. Chan YK, McKay C, Dye E, Slatopolsky E. The effect of 1,25 dihydroxycholecalciferol on parathyroid hormone secretion by monolayer cultures of bovine parathyroid cells. Calcif Tissue Int 1986; 38:27.

38. Yamamoto M, Igarishi T, Muramatsu M, et al. Hypocalcemia increases and hypercalcemia decreases the steady-state level of parathyroid hormone messenger RNA in the rat. J Clin Invest 1989; 83:1053.

39. Silver J, Naveh-Many T, Mayer H, et al. Regulation by vitamin D metabolites of parathyroid hormone gene transcription in vivo in the rat. J Clin Invest 1986; 78:1296.

40. Kremer R, Bolivar I, Goltzman D, Hendy GN. Influence of calcium and 1,25-dihydroxycholecalciferol on proliferation and proto-oncogene expression in primary cultures of bovine parathyroid cells. Endocrinology 1989; 125:935.

41. Mallette LE, Khouri K, Zengolita H, et al. Lithium treatment increases midregion parathyroid hormone and parathyroid volume. J Clin Endocrinol Metab 1989; 68:654.

42. Brown EM. Lithium induces abnormal calcium-regulated PTH release in dispersed bovine parathyroid cells. J Clin Endocrinol Metab 1981; 52:1046.

43. Silver J, Moallem E, Kilav R, et al. New insights into the regulation of parathyroid hormone synthesis and secretion in chronic renal failure. Nephrol Dial Transplant 1996; 11:2.

44. Nemeth EF, Scarpa A. Cytosolic $Ca^{++}$ and the regulation of secretion in parathyroid cells. FEBS Lett 1986; 213:15.

45. Kifor O, Kifor I, Brown EM. Effects of high extracellular calcium concentrations on phosphoinositide turnover and inositol phosphate in dispersed bovine parathyroid cells. J Bone Miner Metab 1992; 7:1327.

46. Marx SJ, Lasker R, Brown E, et al. Secretory dysfunction in parathyroid cells from a neonate with severe primary hyperparathyroidism. J Clin Endocrinol Metab 1986; 62:445.

46a. Hoenderop JGJ, Van de Graf AWCM, Hartog A, et al. Molecular identification of the apical $Ca^{2+}$ channel in 1,25-dihydroxyvitamin $D_3$-responsive epithelia. J Biol Chem 1999; 274:22739

46b. Peng JB, Chen XZ, Berger UV, et al. Molecular cloning and characterization of a channel-like transporter mediating intestinal absorption. J Biol Chem 1999; 274:22739.

47. Favus MJ. Intestinal absorption of calcium, magnesium and phosphorus. In: Coe FL, Favus MJ, eds. Disorders of bone and mineral metabolism. New York: Raven Press, 1992:57.

48. DeLuca HF. The Vitamin D story: a collaborative effort of basic science and clinical medicine. Fed Proc Am Soc Exper Biol 1988; 2:2124.

49. Rasmussen H, Fontaine O, Max EE, Goodman DBP. The effect of 1,alpha-hydroxyvitamin $D_3$ administration on calcium transport in chick intestine brush border membrane vesicles. J Biol Chem 1979; 25:2993.

50. Bikle DD. Regulation of intestinal calcium transport by vitamin D: role of membrane structure. In: Aloia RC, Curtain KC, Gordon LM, eds. Membrane transport and information storage. New York: Wiley Ross, 1990:191.

51. Adams ND, Gray RW, Lemann J. The effect of oral $CaCO_3$ loading and dietary calcium deprivation on plasma 1,25-dihydroxyvitamin D concentrations in healthy adults. J Clin Endocrinol Metab 1979; 48:1008.

52. Hughes MR, Brumbaugh PF, Haussler MR, et al. Regulation of serum 1,alpha-25-dihydroxyvitamin $D_3$ by calcium and phosphate in the rat. Science 1975; 190:578.

53. Sheikh MS, Ramirez A, Emmett M, et al. Role of vitamin D-independent mechanisms in absorption of food calcium. J Clin Invest 1988; 81:126.

54. Nordin BEC, Peacock M. Role of the kidney in regulation of plasma calcium. Lancet 1969; 2:1280.

55. Friedman PA, Gesek FA. Cellular calcium transport in renal epithelia: measurement, mechanisms. and regulation. Physiol Rev 1995; 75:429.

55a. Hoenderop JG, Willems PH, Bindels RJ. Toward a comprehensive molecular model of active calcium reabsorption. Am J Physiol 2000; 278:F352.

56. Abou-Samra A, Juppner H, Force T, et al. Expression cloning of a common receptor for parathyroid hormone and parathyroid hormone-related peptide from rat osteoblast-like cells: a single receptor stimulates intracellular accumulation of both cAMP and inositol phosphates and increases intracellular free calcium. Proc Natl Acad Sci U S A 1992; 89:2732.

57. Morel F, Chabardes D, Imbert-Teboul M, et al. Multiple hormonal control of adenylate cyclase in distal segments of the rat kidney. Kidney Int 1982; 11(Suppl):555.

58. Sonnenberg J, Pansini AR, Christakos S. Vitamin D-dependent rat renal calcium-binding proteins: development of a radioimmunoassay, tissue distribution, and immunologic identification. Endocrinology 1984; 115:640.

59. Ro HK, Tembe V, Favus MS. Evidence that activation of protein kinase C can stimulate 1,25-dihydroxyvitamin $D_3$ secretion by rat proximal tubules. Endocrinology 1992; 131:1424.

60. Sands JM, Naruse M, Baum M, et al. Apical extracellular calcium/polyvalent cation-sensing receptor regulates vasopressin-elicited water permeability in rat kidney inner medullary collecting duct. J Clin Invest 1997; 99:1399.

61. Rodan GA, Martin TJ. Role of osteoblasts in hormonal control of bone resorption: a hypothesis. Calcif Tissue Int 1981; 33:349.

62. Yasuda H, Shima N, Nakagawa N, et al. Osteoclast differentiation factor is a ligand for osteoprotegerin/osteoclastogenesis-inhibitory factor and is identical to TRANCE/RANKL. Proc Natl Acad Sci U S A 1998; 95:3597.

63. Canalis E, Pash J, Varghese S. Skeletal growth factors. Crit Rev Eukaryot Gene Expr 1993; 3:155.

64. Chase LR, Fedak SA, Aurbach GD. Activation of skeletal adenyl cyclase by parathyroid hormone in vitro. Endocrinology 1969; 84:761.

65. Yamaguchi T, Chattopadhyay N, Kifor O, et al. Mouse osteoblastic cell line (MC3T3-E1) expresses extracellular calcium ($Ca^{2+}_o$)-sensing receptor and its agonists stimulate chemotaxis and proliferation of MC3T3-E1 cells. J Bone Miner Res 1998; 13:1530.

66. Kameda T, Mano H, Yamada Y, et al. Calcium-sensing receptor in mature osteoclasts, which are bone resorbing cells. Biochem Biophys Res Commun 1998; 245:419.

67. Lee MJ, Roth SI. Effect of calcium and magnesium on deoxyribonucleic acid synthesis in rat parathyroid glands in vitro. Lab Invest 1975; 33:72.

68. Robertson WG, Peacock M, Alkins D. The effect of parathyroid hormone on the uptake and release of calcium by bone in tissue culture. Clin Sci 1972; 43:715.

69. Rowe PS, Oudet CL, Francis F, et al. Distribution of mutations in the PEX gene in families with X-linked hypophosphataemic rickets (HYP). Hum Mol Genet 1997; 6:539.

70. Martin KJ, Hruska KA, Freitag JJ, Slatopolsky E. The peripheral metabolism of parathyroid hormone. N Engl J Med 1979; 301:1092.

71. Nussbaum SR, Zahradnik RJ, Lavigne JR. Highly sensitive two-site immunoradiometric assay of parathyrin, and its clinical utility in evaluating patients with hypercalcemia. Clin Chem 1987; 33:1364.

72. Lepage R, Roy L, Brossard JH, et al. A non-(1-84) circulating parathyroid hormone (PTH) fragment interferes significantly with intact PTH commercial assay measurements in uremic samples. Clin Chem 1998; 44:805.

73. Burtis WJ, Brady TG, Orloff JJ, et al. Immunochemical characterization of hypercalcemia of malignancy. N Engl J Med 1990; 322:1106.

73a. John MR, Goodman WG, Gao P, et al. A novel immunoradiometric assay detects full-length human PTH but not amino-terminally truncated fragments: implications for PTH measurements in renal failure. J Clin Endocrinol Metab 1999; 84:4287.

74. Deftos LJ. Calcitonin and medullary thyroid carcinoma. In: Bennett JC, Plum F, eds. Cecil textbook of medicine, 20th ed. Philadelphia: WB Saunders, 1996:1372.

75. Gagel RF. Multiple endocrine neoplasia type II and familial medullary thyroid carcinoma. Impact of genetic screening on management. Cancer Treat Res 1997; 89:421.

76. Walton RJ, Bijvoet OLM. Nomogram for determination of renal threshold phosphate concentration. Lancet 1975; 2:309.

77. Heaney RP, Recker RR, Hinders SM. Variability of calcium absorption. Am J Clin Nutr 1988; 47:262.

78. Garnero P, Delmas PD. Biochemical markers of bone turnover. Applications for osteoporosis. Endocrinol Metab Clin North Am 1998; 27:303.

79. Price PA, Baukol SA. 1,25-Dihydroxyvitamin D₃ increases synthesis of the vitamin K-dependent bone protein by osteosarcoma cells. J Biol Chem 1980; 255:11660.

# CHAPTER 50

# PHYSIOLOGY OF BONE

LAWRENCE G. RAISZ

Understanding of the physiology of skeletal tissue has advanced remarkably during the past few decades. Studies of the various cell types in bone and their interactions have led to the concept of a system involving not only systemic hormones but also local factors that regulate bone turnover. Also, molecular biology techniques are now being applied to bone cells and have provided rapid advances.

Structurally, bone must provide a framework for locomotion, must protect internal organs and marrow, and must be able to adapt to changing physical stress. Metabolically, the skeleton functions as a storehouse and as a homeostatic buffer system. Presumably, bone evolved to fulfill both its structural and metabolic roles as our ancestors moved from the calcium-rich, buoyant ocean to fresh water, and then to dry land. Although the major reservoir function of bone is to supply calcium and phosphorus, the skeleton also serves as a reservoir and source of other ions, such as magnesium and sodium, and as a buffer to deal with hydrogen ion excess. Also, the ability of the skeleton to take up a variety of trace elements may serve as an important safeguard against their toxicity. To achieve its mechanical functions, the skeleton needs to be selectively responsive to different kinds of strain, light, of high tensile strength, and rigid but not brittle.[1,2] This is achieved by an orderly, slightly deformable, mineralized collagen structure distributed as a combination of *dense cortical bone* and *spongy trabecular bone*.

## EMBRYOLOGY AND ANATOMY OF BONE

The formation of the skeleton begins with condensation and differentiation of mesenchymal cells into cartilage. These provide the template for subsequent bone formation in two ways. Bone may begin to form by differentiation of osteoblasts adjacent to the cartilage rudiments. This occurs in the *membranous* bones, such as the skull and the periosteum of long bones. Here, the mesenchyme condenses, and osteoblasts differentiate on the surface of the cartilaginous template, which then degenerates. *Endochondral* bone formation occurs at the cartilage growth plate (Fig. 50-1). Here, the osteoblasts differentiate directly on calcified cartilage and form spicules of bone with a cartilaginous core. In either case, the first bone formed is of a loose, woven structure, and it is then replaced by lamellar bone.[3]

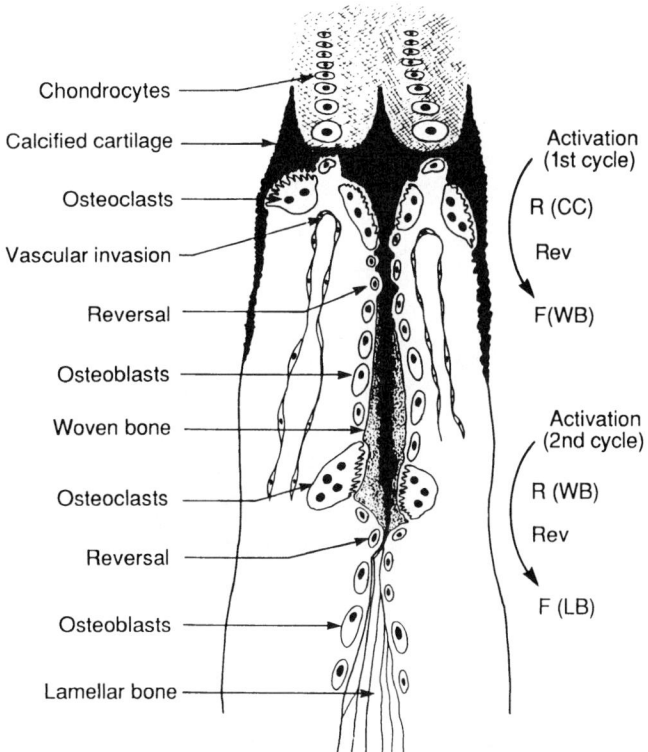

**FIGURE 50-1.** Bone remodeling and bone growth at the epiphyseal plate. (*R*, resorption; *CC*, calcified cartilage; *Rev*, reversal; *F*, formation; *WB*, woven bone; *LB*, lamellar bone.) (From Baron R. Anatomy and ultrastructure of bone. In: Primer on the metabolic bone diseases and disorders of bone metabolism, 3rd ed. New York: Raven Press, 1996.)

Long bones lengthen by the proliferation of cartilage cells. The cartilage undergoes an orderly change, in which the columns of cells in the proliferative zone become hypertrophied and the matrix between these columns becomes mineralized. This probably involves both breakdown of the highly hydrated high-molecular-weight proteoglycans of cartilage matrix and the release of matrix vesicles from hypertrophic chondrocytes. After the cartilage is mineralized, new bone formation by osteoblasts begins on the surface of the calcified cartilage spicules; this is called the *primary spongiosa*. Subsequently, the spicules are resorbed and replaced by bone, termed the *secondary spongiosa*. Early in fetal bone formation, collagen is laid down in a woven and irregular pattern, but soon the osteoblasts deposit an orderly lamellar arrangement of collagen.

The combination of a smooth, dense outer layer of *cortical* (*compact*) bone and *spongy trabecular* (*cancellous*) bone provides both the necessary strength without excessive weight and an extended surface on which rapid changes in formation or resorption can respond to changing metabolic needs. The metabolic responses of the skeleton occur mainly on the trabecular bone surfaces and the *endosteal* (inner) surface of the cortex. However, even the *periosteal* (outer) surface of the cortex can be affected by calcium-regulating hormones, as evidenced by the development of subperiosteal bone resorption in severe hyperparathyroidism.

## MODELING AND REMODELING

The term *modeling* refers to the process by which bone grows and alters its shape through resorption and formation at different sites. For example, the long bones enlarge by periosteal formation and endosteal resorption. As they lengthen, the large amount of bone formed at the growth plate is resorbed to maintain a hollow cylindrical structure (Fig. 50-2). The flat bones of

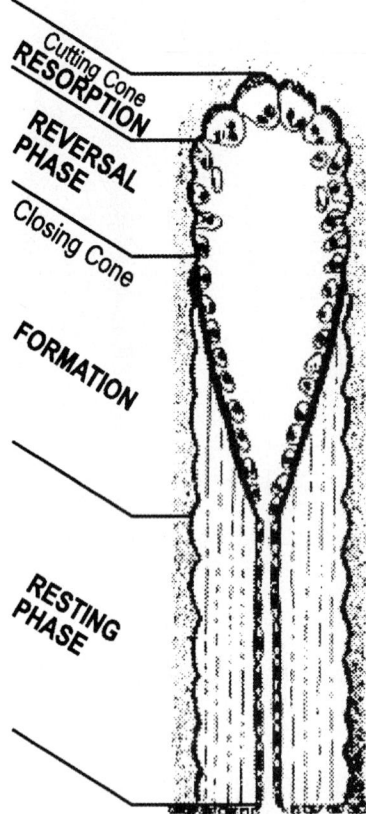

**FIGURE 50-2.** Modeling during the longitudinal growth of long bones. As the growth plate moves upward (see Fig. 50-1), the wider parts of the bone must be reshaped into a tubular diaphysis. (From Baron R. Anatomy and ultrastructure of bone. In: Primer on the metabolic bone diseases and disorders of bone metabolism, 3rd ed. New York: Raven Press, 1996.)

the skull and pelvis grow and change their shape by this process of formation at one site and resorption at another. Modeling can be influenced by mechanical stress. For example, bone mass increases in the most used long bones of athletes by both periosteal and endosteal apposition. Bone formation on one surface and resorption on the other permit teeth to be moved by mechanical forces. Even pressure from soft tissues can produce modeling changes. For example, increased endosteal resorption and periosteal apposition can occur in response to bone marrow hyperplasia.

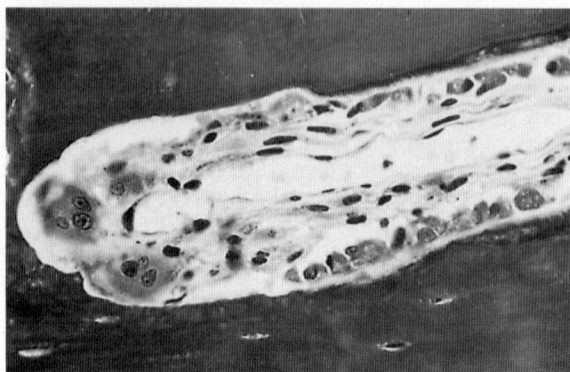

**FIGURE 50-3.** Haversian remodeling. This is a longitudinal section through a cortical bone remodeling unit (×400). The haversian canal is formed by an osteoclast-cutting cone. After the canal reaches maximal diameter, mesenchymal cells differentiate into osteoblasts and begin to form an osteon made of concentric lamellae of new matrix. (Courtesy of Dr. Robert Schenk.)

The term *remodeling* refers to the process in which *resorption* is followed by formation at the same site; hence, the two processes are "coupled."[4] This process is important for the overall growth and functional integrity of skeletal tissues as well as for the metabolic responses of the bone mineral reservoir. In large mammals, the cortical bone is remodeled by the development of a haversian system of osteons (Fig. 50-3). These structures are formed by osteoclastic removal of a cylinder of bone. Behind these osteoclasts are a vascular loop and mesenchymal cells that differentiate into osteoblasts and form concentric lamellae of new bone around the central vascular canal. The major importance of this system of osteons may be that it enables the cortex to participate in the metabolic functions of the skeleton without excessive loss of strength. Haversian remodeling may also be important in the repair of fatigue damage in bone.[5] Remodeling also occurs on the trabecular bone surface. This begins with the formation of the primary spongiosa. Osteoclasts excavate scalloped areas (called *Howship lacunae)* on mature trabecular bone, which are then replaced by packets of new lamellar bone laid down by osteoblasts. Although much is known about the anatomic sequence and time course of cycles of cortical and trabecular remodeling (Fig. 50-4), the cellular mechanisms are poorly understood. The initial activation involves a change in the lining cells or resting osteoblasts on the surface of bone, which may normally protect it from attack by osteoclasts. These may not only change shape but also release factors that stimulate osteoclastic activity. The development of osteoclasts requires an interaction between precursor cells of the osteoblastic and osteoclastic lineages; some of the proteins involved in this interaction are known (see later). Once osteoclasts have removed the bulk of bone mineral and matrix, a reversal phase occurs that involves the removal of additional elements of bone matrix by macrophages and the preparation of the bone surface for new osteoblastic formation. In the formation phase, successive generations of osteoblasts synthesize lamellar bone and replace the resorbed bone with a packet of new bone, called a *bone structural unit (BSU).*

## NATURAL HISTORY OF THE SKELETON

In humans, the skeleton continues to grow until 25 to 35 years of age. Before puberty, the bones grow by periosteal apposition and

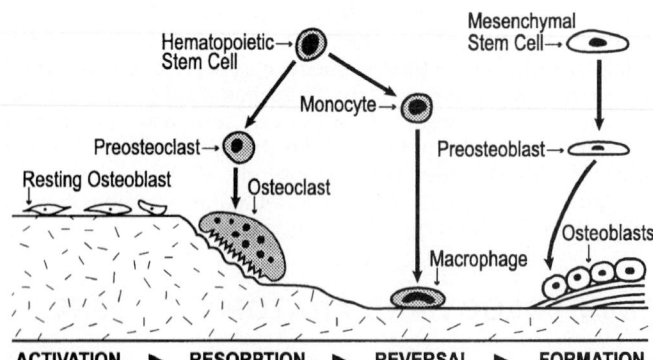

**FIGURE 50-4.** Bone remodeling cycle. Activation of this cycle begins with a change in the resting osteoblasts (also called *lining cells*) on the bone surface, which permits osteoclastic bone resorption, and a signal from cells of the osteoblastic lineage, which make contact with osteoclast precursors. Osteoclasts and macrophages are probably derived from different immediate precursors, but both originate from hematopoietic stem cells. During the reversal phase in trabecular bone remodeling, macrophages are seen on the bone surface, but their role is not established. Osteoblasts come from a separate mesenchymal stem cell population, probably related to stromal stem cells in the marrow, which differentiate into mature osteoblasts that replace the bone lost during the resorption phase. (From Raisz LG. Local and systemic factors in the pathogenesis of osteoporosis. N Engl J Med 1988; 318:818.)

endosteal resorption. During puberty and adolescence, a period of endosteal apposition and thickening of the trabeculae occurs, so that bone mass increases by 10% to 20% even after linear growth has ceased.[6] During the years from 20 to 50, bone mass is stable, because rates of formation and resorption are equal or coupled. The formation of new BSUs both in the cortex and on the surface of trabecular bone continues throughout life. Later in life, bone mass begins to decrease due to uncoupled remodeling. Age-related bone loss is greater for trabecular than for cortical bone, and more rapid in women than in men, largely because of the acceleration of remodeling at menopause. Bone mass can decrease simply because more BSUs are formed (increased turnover), because a time gap exists between resorption and formation even when the processes are coupled. This deficit is theoretically reversible if the rate of turnover decreases and the formation phase is allowed to proceed to complete replacement. Uncoupled remodeling can occur because so much endosteal or trabecular bone is removed that a template for osteoblastic replacement no longer exists. Thus, areas may appear in which trabecular plates develop holes or are converted to attenuated rods. Finally, the ability of successive populations of osteoblasts to complete the formation process is impaired with age, so that haversian canals remain enlarged and trabecular surfaces show only partial replacement of resorbed bone with small BSUs, that is, thinner packets of new bone.

## BONE CHEMISTRY AND MINERALIZATION

Bone mineral consists largely of *hydroxyapatite* [$Ca_{10}(PO_4)_6(OH)_2$] together with transition forms and other minerals absorbed on the surface. The hydroxyapatite crystals are small and often have lattice defects, although these crystals become more complete as bone matures. The major absorbed minerals are carbonate, magnesium, and sodium. Ninety-nine percent of body calcium, 90% of phosphorus, 80% of carbonate, 80% of citrate, 60% of magnesium, and 35% of sodium are in the skeleton.

All these ions may be accessed when deficits exist and stored when excesses occur. Hydrogen ion is generated when hydroxyapatite is formed from circulating calcium and hydrogen phosphate. When a hydrogen ion excess occurs in the extracellular fluid, it can be buffered by demineralization, in which carbonate and phosphate are released from bone. Many bone-seeking elements exist, such as aluminum, fluoride, lead, and strontium. Deposition of these elements in the skeleton can prevent soft-tissue damage but is likely to alter bone cell function.

The organic matrix of bone is made up largely of *type I collagen,* which consists of tightly coiled, long, triple helical molecules containing two $\alpha_1$ chains and one $\alpha_2$ chain. The collagen molecules are strengthened by covalent intramolecular and intermolecular cross-links and are assembled in ordered fibers. The other collagen types, such as types III, IV, and V, are not deposited in the matrix but are present in interstitial and vascular structures. Type II collagen predominates in cartilage.

Although 95% of the matrix is collagen, the noncollagenous components that constitute the remaining 5% are important in providing bone with some of its physical and chemical properties.[7] The *proteoglycan* of bone is of lower molecular weight and is more compact than that in cartilage. Small amounts of *proteolipid,* which can form complexes with calcium phosphate, are also found. Noncollagen proteins include a calcium-binding, $\gamma$-carboxyglutamic acid–containing protein (BGP or *osteocalcin*) and *osteonectin,* a highly phosphorylated glycoprotein that binds to collagen and calcium. *Osteopontin* and *bone sialoprotein* are highly acidic, have a high affinity for calcium, and have binding sites for integrin receptors. All these proteins are probably important in regulating mineralization, and their distribution may account for the delay between matrix deposition and mineralization. These proteins may also be involved in bone resorption. Osteocalcin is chemotactic for osteoclasts and their

precursors; and osteopontin, as well as other proteins, may be involved in the adhesion of osteoclasts to mineralized matrix.

Mineralization may also be controlled by cellular elements.[8] Matrix vesicles have been identified in calcifying cartilage and fetal bone. They contain cell membrane elements, are rich in alkaline phosphatase, and may initiate mineralization by increasing the local phosphate concentration or providing membrane proteolipids. The concept that *phosphatase* activity is essential for mineralization has been with us for >50 years, but the precise role of phosphatase is uncertain. Such enzymes may increase the local inorganic phosphate concentration by acting on organic phosphates, or they may cleave pyrophosphate, a potent inhibitor of calcification.

The delay between the deposition of matrix by osteoblasts and its mineralization is probably essential for extracellular modifications of matrix, such as collagen cross-linking, formation of large collagen fibers, and deposition of noncollagen proteins, all of which may increase the strength of mineralized tissues. Little evidence exists for direct hormonal control of these steps, but adequate supplies of calcium and phosphate are essential. Thus, animals lacking a vitamin D receptor, given enough calcium and phosphate, show normal mineralization.[9] Moreover, little evidence exists that parathyroid hormone (PTH) or calcitonin is essential for mineralization. The more important direct effects of the calcium-regulating hormones appear to be on matrix formation and bone resorption.

## CELL BIOLOGY OF BONE

The lineages of bone-forming cells (*osteoblasts*) and bone-resorbing cells (*osteoclasts*) probably become separate early in development. Their function is controlled by a complex system of intercellular signals that involve not only systemic calcium-regulating and growth-regulating hormones but also local factors. Bone disease occurs when an imbalance exists between the functions of forming and resorbing cells. Thus, accelerated resorption and diminished formation exacerbate decreases in bone mass in osteoporosis. Excessive bone mass can occur because bone resorption is impaired, as in congenital osteopetrosis, or because formation is excessive and disorderly, as in virally induced avian osteopetrosis and Paget disease.

### OSTEOBLASTS

The osteoblast, a highly specialized bone matrix–synthesizing cell, is derived from precursor cells in the periosteum or the stroma of the bone marrow called *determined osteoprogenitor cells.*[10] Bone can also form in ectopic sites from undifferentiated mesenchymal cells in response to certain inducing agents, particularly demineralized bone matrix. This may be due to the effects of specific proteins produced by bone cells and deposited in matrix.[11] Under these conditions, the sequence of endochondral bone formation is recapitulated; that is, cartilage is formed, mineralized, and then replaced by bone.

The mature osteoblast is a plump polygonal cell that has an eccentric nucleus, a prominent Golgi apparatus, and abundant rough endoplasmic reticulum (Fig. 50-5). These cells deposit a collagenous matrix and extend cytoplasmic processes into this matrix. As they complete their synthetic activity, they become buried in their own matrix and are called *osteocytes*. Osteoblasts may also stop producing matrix but remain on the bone surface; these *lining cells* or *resting osteoblasts* can be the sites for new remodeling cycles of activation, resorption, and formation. Lining cells may also be reactivated to functional osteoblasts in response to mechanical loading.

Osteoblasts produce most of the constituents of bone matrix; however, many proteins are taken up by matrix from the circulation, including $\alpha_2$-HS-glycoprotein and albumin.[12] Osteoblasts produce alkaline phosphatase and release it systemically. Hence,

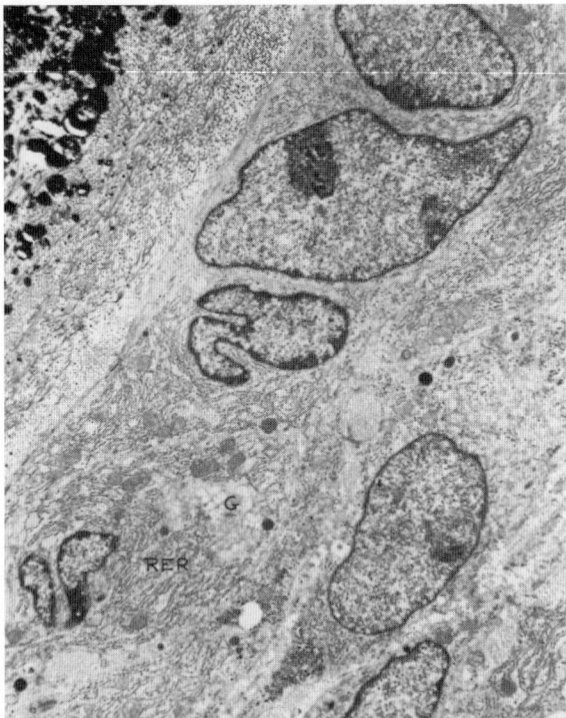

**FIGURE 50-5.** Osteoblasts shown on electron micrograph. A layer of plump cells rich in rough endoplasmic reticulum (*RER*) and with a large Golgi apparatus (*G*) is seen forming an osteoid seam consisting of a collagenous matrix that subsequently mineralizes. ~8000× (Courtesy of Dr. Marijke E. Holtrop.)

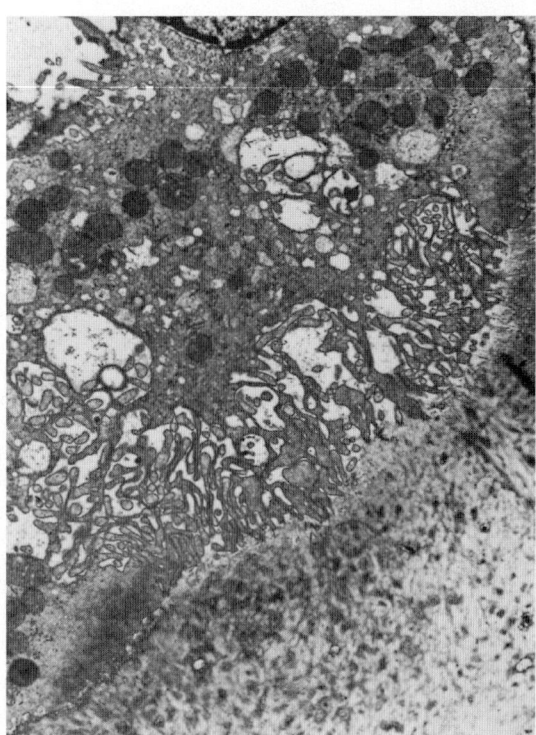

**FIGURE 50-6.** Resorbing apparatus of osteoclasts shown on electron micrograph. A section of an osteoclast with a highly infolded ruffled border is seen between two areas relatively devoid of subcellular particles, termed the *clear* or *sealing zone*. Large vacuoles are present in the osteoclast cytoplasm, and mitochondria are abundant. ~8000× (Courtesy of Dr. Marijke E. Holtrop.)

serum alkaline phosphatase activity correlates with osteoblastic activity. BGP is also released into the circulation from osteoblasts and provides another marker of their activity.[13] When procollagen is converted to collagen, large N- and C-terminal peptides are released. These can be measured in the circulation and reflect the overall rate of collagen synthesis in the body.

Osteoblasts have receptors for PTH and 1,25-dihydroxyvitamin $D_3$ [1,25(OH)$_2D_3$] and for systemic growth regulators.[14] They apparently are the major source of the autocrine factors that regulate local bone turnover, including cytokines, prostaglandins, and bone-derived growth factors. Osteoblasts may trigger bone resorption in the remodeling process. This activation step may involve shape changes or secretion of collagenase and related metalloproteinases as well as other proteolytic enzymes, such as plasminogen activator.[15] These changes may enhance the access of osteoclasts to the mineralized bone surface.

The concept that cells of the osteoblast lineage are critical in activating the resorption phase of the bone remodeling cycle has long been recognized, and some of the specific proteins involved in this interaction are known.[16–18] The ligands that regulate the osteoblast-osteoclast interaction are not specific for these cells but are also involved in lymphoid activation and may be produced by many other cells types. The activator protein, which is probably expressed in stromal precursor cells in the marrow, has been termed *osteoclast differentiating factor (ODF)* or *osteoprotegerin ligand (OPGL)* and is identical to the protein in the lymphoid series termed *TRANCE*. Its receptor on preosteoclasts is identical with another membrane protein on lymphoid cells called *RANK*. This interaction can be blocked by *osteoprotegerin (OPG)*, which binds to OPGL. The importance of this regulatory system has been demonstrated experimentally. The addition of synthetic ODF to cultures of preosteoclasts can replace cells of the osteoblast lineage in promoting differentiation and osteoclast formation. Animals in whom OPG has been knocked out show severe osteoporosis, due to increased bone resorption.[19]

Once the osteoblasts have completed their allotted portion of matrix synthesis, they can undergo one of three fates. Some cells become buried as *osteocytes*. These cells remain connected to the overlying osteoblast and to each other by cell processes enclosed in canaliculi within the mineralized bone. This syncytium of osteocytes and osteoblasts is probably critical for the signaling of the response to mechanical forces. One mechanism is the fluid shear-stress produced by small strains on the bone in the canaliculi and osteocyte lacunae, which can generate cellular responses, such as increased nitric oxide and prostaglandin production. A few osteoblasts remain on the inactive cell surface and spread out as thin *lining cells*. Finally, osteoblasts can undergo programmed cell death or *apoptosis*.[20] This process may be regulated by systemic hormones and local factors. A fourth possibility exists, namely, that osteoblasts can dedifferentiate and return to the marrow stoma as precursor cells, but this has not been demonstrated experimentally.

## OSTEOCLASTS

Osteoclasts resorb bone and calcified cartilage. These large multinucleated cells are formed by the fusion of mononuclear precursors. Osteoclasts presumably are derived from a hematopoietic stem cell rather than from the mesenchymal precursor of the osteoblast. The osteoclast cell line is related to the monocyte-macrophage lineage, but many of the surface markers for macrophages are missing from osteoclasts, and the osteoclast and monocyte precursor cell lines probably separate early in differentiation.[21] The stimulation of osteoclast precursor replication may be an important mechanism for increasing bone resorption. Once fusion has occurred, however, the nuclei in an osteoclast do not undergo further cell division.

The osteoclast cytoplasm contains abundant mitochondria, many lysosomes, and relatively little rough endoplasmic reticulum. The unique feature of the osteoclast is the ruffled border, which is the site of active resorption (Fig. 50-6). This is surrounded by a clear or sealing zone, which functions to attach the osteoclast to bone and isolate the ruffled border from extracellular fluid so that a high local concentration of hydrogen ions and lysosomal enzymes can be maintained. Osteoclasts are rich in acid phosphatase as well as other lysosomal enzymes, and in carbonic anhydrase, which facilitates hydrogen ion secretion. Osteoclasts also produce large amounts of *cathepsin K*, a relatively selective lysosomal enzyme that can degrade all components of bone matrix, including collagen, at a low pH.[22] Thus, the ruffled border area simulates a giant exteriorized phagolysosome in which hydrogen ions are important not only in mobilizing mineral but also in activating lysosomal enzymes.

The proton pump that transports hydrogen ions into the ruffled border area is similar but not identical to the vacuolar proton pump found in lysosomes and kidney cells. Other important features of the osteoclast are the cell attachment apparatus, which involves vitronectin receptors that can bind a wide variety of proteins containing Arg-Gly-Asp sequences.[23] The osteoclast may also have calcium-sensing receptors that mediate the inhibition of osteoclastic activity by high calcium concentrations. Osteoclast precursors express RANK; fully differentiated osteoclasts have not been shown to express RANK, but do respond to OPG, perhaps through some other binding protein.[24] Another critical factor for the formation of osteoclasts is colony-stimulating factor-1 (CSF-1) or macrophage colony-stimulating factor (M-CSF), which may play a role in the replication and differentiation of precursors.[25] Animals lacking CSF-1 have osteopetrosis.

## OTHER CELL TYPES IN BONE

*Macrophages* may be found at resorption sites after the initial removal of bone osteoclasts. Their function is uncertain, but they may remove residual matrix that has not been completely digested, because macrophages can secrete collagenase as well as lysosomal enzymes. Macrophages may also be a source of interleukin-1 (IL-1) and prostaglandin $E_2$ ($PGE_2$), which not only are potent stimulators of bone resorption but also can stimulate the replication of osteoblast precursors and may be involved in initiating the formation phase of the remodeling cycle. *Lymphocytes* may also play a role by secreting bone-resorbing factors.[26] Moreover, calcium-regulating hormones can act on these hematopoietic cells. For example, $1,25(OH)_2D_3$ increases the differentiation of monocyte precursors into macrophages.

*Fibroblastic cells* may also play a role by secreting local regulators. Insulin-like growth factor-I (IGF-I), which can be produced by fibroblasts, is a potent stimulator of bone growth. *Mast cells* are found adjacent to resorbing bone and can produce heparin, which enhances bone resorption in some culture systems[27] (see Chap. 181). Finally, *endothelial cells* and *nerve endings* may play a role by producing neuropeptides and growth factors.[28] Endothelial cells are also a major source of prostaglandins and nitric oxide, which can influence bone resorption and formation as well as affect bone blood flow.[29]

## EFFECTS OF HORMONES ON BONE CELLS

Despite many studies of the direct effects of hormones on bone, the complex regulation of bone resorption and formation still is inadequately explained. The effects of systemic agents are probably modulated by interactions with local intercellular mediators. For example, PTH is clearly a potent stimulator of bone resorption both in vivo and in vitro but has not been shown to act on isolated osteoclasts in the absence of other bone cells. Prostaglandins are also potent stimulators of bone resorption, but they decrease motility and resorptive activity of isolated osteoclasts, as does calcitonin. The major factors that influence bone metabolism and their most important direct effects are listed in Table 50-1.

**TABLE 50-1.**
**Systemic and Local Regulation of Bone Metabolism**

| Agent | Direct Effects on | |
| --- | --- | --- |
| | *Bone Resorption* | *Bone Formation* |
| **CALCIUM-REGULATING HORMONES** | | |
| Parathyroid hormone | ↑ | ↓ |
| 1,25-dihydroxyvitamin D | ↑ | ↓ |
| Calcitonin | ↓ | — |
| **SYSTEMIC HORMONES** | | |
| Glucocorticoids | ↓ | ↓ |
| Insulin | — | ↑ |
| Thyroxine | ↑ | ↑ |
| Sex hormones | ↓ | ↓↑* |
| Growth hormone | — | ↑ |
| **GROWTH FACTORS** | | |
| Insulin-like growth factors | — | ↑ |
| Epidermal growth factor + TGF-α† | ↑ | ↓ |
| Fibroblast growth factor† | ↑ | ↓ |
| Platelet-derived growth factor† | ↑ | ↑ |
| TGF-β† | ↑↓ | ↑↓ |
| **LOCAL FACTORS** | | |
| Prostaglandin $E_2$ | ↑ | ↑↓‡ |
| Interleukin-1† | ↑ | ↑↓‡ |
| Tumor necrosis factor | ↑ | ↑↓ |
| Bone-derived growth factors (BMP) | — | ↑↓ |

*TGF*, transforming growth factor; *BMP*, bone morphogenetic protein.
Direct effects are listed as increased (↑), decreased (↓), or unchanged (—) bone resorption or formation.
*Effects depend on age and concentration.
†Increase may be mediated by endogenous prostaglandin synthesis.
‡Depends on concentration and presence of glucocorticoids.

## PARATHYROID HORMONE

Although PTH was first shown to act directly on bone as a stimulator of resorption, much more is now known about its effects on osteoblasts at the cellular and molecular levels.[14,30–35] Much of this information has been derived from investigations of isolated bone cells or cloned osteosarcoma cells that have an osteoblastic phenotype, as well as from in vivo studies. The first effect of PTH on osteoblast-like cells is an activation of adenylate cyclase and protein kinase A. PTH can also accelerate phosphatidylinositol turnover, which leads to increased intracellular calcium and activation of protein kinase C. PTH causes rapid changes in osteoblast cell shape associated with polymerization of actin. A subsequent decrease in collagen synthesis is associated with a diminution of procollagen messenger RNA (mRNA) levels in the cell. Release of metalloproteinases from osteoblasts is also increased in response to PTH. Plasminogen activator activity is increased, in part by decreased production of an inhibitor, and this may result in the activation of latent collagenase. Alkaline phosphatase levels are usually decreased. PTH may also decrease BGP synthesis. PTH can increase prostaglandin synthesis and cell replication in bone cell and organ cultures.[36]

Most of these effects of PTH on bone can be considered catabolic; but prolonged, intermittent administration of low doses of PTH can elicit an anabolic effect, with increased bone mass.[37] This is the basis for the use of intermittent PTH administration to treat osteoporosis. The anabolic response may be due to stimulation of precursor cell replication by PTH or release of growth factors from bone cells or matrix.

Although the ability of PTH to stimulate bone resorption has been recognized for many years, the mechanism is poorly understood. In vivo, PTH rapidly increases the number and activity of osteoclasts as measured by the extent of ruffled border area. Increased release of calcium and matrix constituents of bone can be measured within a few hours, but increases in lysosomal enzyme release can be detected within minutes.

PTH stimulation of bone resorption presumably is receptor mediated. The role of cyclic adenosine monophosphate (cAMP) in mediating this response is controversial.[32,34] Stimulators of adenylate cyclase activity and phosphodiesterase inhibitors can enhance bone resorption, but their effect is generally smaller than that of PTH. Moreover, under certain conditions, these agents inhibit bone resorption, mimicking the action of calcitonin. Possibly, the stimulation of bone resorption involves multiple pathways, including activation of phospholipase C to release phosphatidylinositol and diacylglycerol. This results in increased cell calcium and activation of protein kinase C.

The major PTH receptor has been cloned. It is present in osteoblasts and their precursors but has not been demonstrated in mammalian osteoclasts. This single receptor can mediate increases in cAMP, phosphatidylinositol breakdown, and intracellular calcium. The receptor can be activated either by 1-34 PTH or by 1-34 PTH–related protein (PTHrP).[31] PTH and PTHrP, like other stimulators of bone resorption, can increase the expression of ODF and may also decrease the expression of OPG in osteoblastic cells.[38] Another PTH receptor has been identified with greater affinity for PTH than for PTHrP,[39,40] but its physiologic role is not known.

## 1,25-DIHYDROXYVITAMIN D₃

The major physiologic role of the hormonal form of vitamin D, $1,25(OH)_2D_3$ or calcitriol, is to promote intestinal absorption of calcium and phosphorus. It is also one of the most potent hormones acting on bone. Although the effects of $1,25(OH)_2D_3$ on the intestine promote skeletal growth and mineralization, the effects of high concentrations on bone appear to be catabolic, stimulating resorption and inhibiting formation. As with PTH, receptors for $1,25(OH)_2D_3$ have been demonstrated in osteoblastic cells. The hormone resembles PTH in inhibiting collagen synthesis but differs from PTH in its selective ability to increase osteocalcin production. Moreover, $1,25 (OH)_2D_3$ does not show the same marked anabolic effect as PTH, although it may prevent bone loss after ovariectomy in rats.[41]

Presumably $1,25(OH)_2D_3$ acts largely by a classic steroid hormone pathway, through a nuclear receptor that binds to chromatin.[42] This receptor has been demonstrated in osteoblasts and cells and can mediate such transcriptional effects as the increase in mRNA for BGP and the decrease in mRNA for collagen. A nongenomic effect of $1,25(OH)_2D_3$ may also be present, based on the finding of a binding protein for the hormone in plasma membrane and matrix vesicles, which appears to activate protein kinase C in intestinal cells and chondrocytes.[43]

Although $1,25(OH)_2D_3$ stimulates bone resorption, receptors have not been demonstrated in isolated osteoclasts, and the effect is likely to be mediated through osteoblasts as it is for other bone resorbers. The $1,25(OH)_2D_3$ also stimulates the production of multinucleated cells with an osteoclastic phenotype in bone marrow and spleen cell cultures when cells of the osteoblastic lineage are present. Resorption occurs at such low concentrations in organ culture that this effect can be used as a serum bioassay.[44] However, this assay requires extraction of the serum and, therefore, measures $1,25(OH)_2D_3$ that would normally circulate bound to vitamin D–binding protein. Hence, the concentrations that stimulate bone resorption in organ culture are probably at least 10-fold higher than the normal concentration of free hormone in the blood and extracellular fluid. When calcium and phosphate deprivation is severe, such high concentrations of $1,25(OH)_2D_3$ may be achieved that vitamin D is unable to maintain calcium and phosphorus levels by increasing intestinal absorption but must draw on the skeletal reservoir.

Although substantial evidence exists that $1,25(OH)_2D_3$ is the bioactive form of vitamin D, some evidence is found for effects of other metabolites on skeletal tissue. The metabolite 25-hydroxy-

vitamin D can stimulate bone resorption and inhibit bone formation at high concentrations, which may occur in vivo when toxic doses are given. The metabolite 24,25-dihydroxyvitamin D is formed by an alternative hydroxylation pathway in the kidney. This probably represents an inactivation process, but evidence exists that 24,25-dihydroxyvitamin D has anabolic effects, particularly on cartilage.

Not only does $1,25(OH)_2D_3$ have important direct effects on bone cells but it also may act on bone indirectly through its function as an immunomodulator.[45] The physiologic importance of these actions remains uncertain (see Chap. 195).

## CALCITONIN

Calcitonin is a potent direct inhibitor of osteoclastic activity (see Chap. 53). In contrast to PTH and $1,25(OH)_2D_3$, receptors for calcitonin have been identified on osteoclasts.[39] Moreover, isolated osteoclasts show a decrease in motility and resorptive activity when treated with this hormone. Calcitonin rapidly decreases the amount of active ruffled border of osteoclasts in organ cultures, although the cells may remain attached to the bone surfaces by their clear zones. In vivo, the number of osteoclasts decreases as the cells appear to migrate away from the bone surface. Calcitonin increases cAMP content in cell populations enriched with osteoclasts. Cyclic AMP is the mediator of inhibition of bone resorption, because agents that increase the cAMP concentration can mimic the action of calcitonin both in organ culture and in isolated osteoclasts. However, evidence also exists for an inhibitory pathway mediated by protein kinase C.[46]

The direct inhibition of osteoclastic activity by calcitonin is transient in isolated cell systems, in organ cultures, and in patients with hyperparathyroidism or hypercalcemia of malignancy. This "escape phenomenon" may be due to down-regulation of the calcitonin receptors.[39] Although calcitonin has been used clinically as an inhibitor of bone resorption, its physiologic role is probably limited. Patients with medullary carcinoma of the thyroid who have extremely high blood levels of calcitonin have normal bone turnover.

A number of peptides with homology to calcitonin may also affect bone metabolism. These include calcitonin gene-related peptide, amylin, and adrenomedullin.[47] The importance of these peptides in bone physiology is unknown; however, they have been shown to affect both bone resorption and bone formation in animal and in vitro models.[48]

## SYSTEMIC HORMONES THAT AFFECT BONE METABOLISM

Many hormones that regulate somatic growth act directly or indirectly on the skeleton. These hormones not only modulate physiologic skeletal growth and development but also are important in the pathogenesis of metabolic bone disease.

## GLUCOCORTICOIDS

Glucocorticoids have complex direct and indirect effects on skeletal tissue. The major indirect effect is the inhibition of calcium absorption in the intestine. This may lead to secondary hyperparathyroidism, which could explain the clinical observation that bone resorption is increased in some patients treated with glucocorticoids. Nevertheless, the major direct effect on bone is a dose-related decrease in formation.[49] This is probably mediated by a decrease in the replication and differentiation of osteoblast precursors. However, glucocorticoids can also have a positive effect on osteoblast function. In some cell and organ cultures, physiologic concentrations of glucocorticoids can increase collagen synthesis, increase alkaline phosphatase levels, and enhance the response to other hormones. These effects may be due to an increase in osteoblast differentiation.[14]

Glucocorticoids can have both stimulatory and inhibitory effects on bone resorption. Stimulation may be due to enhanced osteoclast differentiation as well as secondary hyperparathyroidism. Inhibition of resorption may be due to decreased replication of osteoclast precursors or decreased production of bone-resorbing factors by osteoblasts, such as prostaglandins and interleukins. Whatever the mechanisms, hypercalcemia has been observed in adrenal insufficiency, and decreased bone mass is an important adverse effect of glucocorticoid excess (see Chaps. 59 and 64).

## GROWTH HORMONE AND INSULIN-LIKE GROWTH FACTORS

Excesses and deficiencies of growth hormone are associated with increases and decreases in skeletal growth. This effect is probably mediated by IGF-I (see Chaps. 12 and 173).[50] A major source of IGF is the liver, but many other tissues, including skeletal tissue, can produce IGF-I and also IGF-II, which is not under growth hormone control. Moreover, growth hormone can stimulate IGF-I production by bone cells. IGF-I and IGF-II have pleiotropic effects, stimulating bone cell replication as well as collagen and noncollagen protein synthesis. The relative importance of IGF-I and IGF-II in regulating bone growth and in metabolic bone disease is uncertain. Possibly, the decrease in bone mass seen in malnutrition and gastrointestinal disorders is related to decreased production of these factors. An age-related decrease in growth hormone and IGF-I secretion may play a role in bone loss. Bone tissue produces not only IGF-I and IGF-II but also a number of IGF-binding proteins that can be both inhibitory and stimulatory. The regulation of these binding proteins may be as important as the regulation of IGFs themselves in the local control of bone formation.[51]

## INSULIN

Insulin is an important regulator of somatic growth. At physiologic concentrations, insulin appears to stimulate osteoblast function, selectively increasing collagen synthesis without affecting cell replication or protein synthesis in the periosteum.[14] At higher concentrations, insulin can produce a pleiotropic effect, perhaps by acting on the IGF-I receptor. Insulin may be important in skeletal development. Bone mass may be increased by hyperinsulinism in the infants of diabetic mothers and decreased in diabetic children with insulin deficiency.

## THYROID HORMONES

Thyroid hormones (thyroxine and triiodothyronine) are essential for maintaining skeletal growth and remodeling. They not only increase cartilage growth directly but also probably have a positive interaction with IGF-I. Thyroid hormones can increase bone turnover, an effect apparently due to direct stimulation of both bone resorption and formation.[52,53a] Decreased bone mass has been observed in hyperthyroid patients, including those who received large doses of exogenous thyroid hormones for long periods.[53]

## SEX HORMONES

Perhaps the greatest limitation in our understanding of skeletal physiology is that we do not know precisely how sex hormones act on bone. Androgens and estrogens are involved in the pubertal growth spurt and the maintenance of bone mass. Some of this may be due to changes in muscle mass, which then influence bone. The accelerated bone loss that occurs with estrogen withdrawal at menopause can be attributed to an increase in bone resorption. This has led to the concept that

estrogens oppose the resorptive activity of PTH or other stimulators of osteoclastic activity. Both estrogen and androgen receptors have been identified in bone cells, particularly those of the osteoblastic lineage. The sex hormones change the production of cytokines, prostaglandins, and growth factors by bone cells.[36,54,55] In rodent models, inhibition of IL-1 or tumor necrosis factor-α (TNF-α) can reverse the bone loss that follows ovariectomy. Moreover, ovariectomy does not cause bone loss in animals in whom the IL-1 receptor has been knocked out by homologous recombination. However, the relative importance of these effects in mediating the changes seen with sex hormone deficiency in humans remains to be determined.

Experiments of nature have helped us to understand the relative importance of estrogen and androgen.[56,56a] An abnormal skeletal phenotype has been defined in a man with loss of function due to a mutation in the estrogen receptor and in two men with aromatase deficiency who cannot convert testosterone to estrogen. These individuals showed failure of epiphyseal closure, high bone turnover, and decreased bone mass. In the aromatase-deficient men, treatment with estrogen could reverse these abnormalities. Because androgens are a source for estrogens, defining their specific role in bone is difficult. In women with androgen insensitivity, skeletal development is normal, although bone mineral density may be low.[57] However, estrogen may also play a role here, either because replacement has been inadequate or because a critical role is played by estrogen produced locally in bone by aromatase, which is expressed in human bone cells.

## OTHER SYSTEMIC HORMONES

In view of the many hormonal influences on the skeleton identified in the past few decades, additional effects of systemic hormones on skeletal function are likely to be discovered. Among the hormones that have been considered as possible skeletal regulators are progesterone,[58] prolactin,[59] and neuropeptides.[60,61]

## LOCAL REGULATORS

The ability of the skeleton to respond to local forces must depend on the existence of local regulators; moreover, these regulators are probably important in mediating the responses of systemic hormones as previously noted.

### PROSTAGLANDINS

Prostaglandins are ubiquitous local modulators of cell function (see Chap. 172). Their role in skeletal physiology was first suggested by the observations that $PGE_2$ can raise the cAMP concentration and stimulate bone resorption in vitro. Locally, prostaglandin production in bone can be stimulated by mechanical stress, by cytokines associated with inflammation and injury, and by growth factors. Systemically, PTH can stimulate and glucocorticoids can inhibit prostaglandin production in bone.

The effects of $PGE_2$ on bone metabolism are complex and biphasic.[36] $PGE_2$ can stimulate bone cell replication and differentiation and increase bone formation in vivo. At high concentrations in vitro, inhibition of osteoblastic collagen synthesis occurs. The ability of bone to respond to mechanical forces may be prostaglandin dependent.[62]

Stimulation of bone resorption by $PGE_2$ is important in mediating bone loss in inflammation and immobilization, and might play a role in osteoporosis.

### BONE-DERIVED GROWTH FACTORS

Two major families of growth factors are produced in bone and deposited in bone matrix: (a) the IGFs, including the IGF-binding proteins,[50] and (b) the transforming growth factor-β and bone morphogenetic protein family.[63,64] The latter group contains at least 10 different proteins that are related to other regulatory peptides, including the activin-inhibins and invertebrate growth factors.

## OTHER GROWTH FACTORS

Epidermal, fibroblast, and platelet-derived growth factors can all act on skeletal tissue (see Chap. 173). These factors can be derived from bone cells or from adjacent hematopoietic or vascular tissue. They can stimulate bone resorption by either prostaglandin-dependent or prostaglandin-independent mechanisms.[65] Their mitogenic effects may be associated with decreased collagen synthesis in acute experiments in vitro, but prolonged treatment may increase bone formation in vivo.

## CYTOKINES

Both bone cells and adjacent hematopoietic cells can produce cytokines, which profoundly influence bone metabolism[54] (see Chaps. 173 and 212). Cytokine-mediated bone resorption was first identified as being due to *osteoclast-activating factor*, produced by mitogen- or antigen-stimulated human leukocyte cultures. Subsequently, IL-1 was found to be the major bone-resorbing factor from macrophages. TNF is also produced by leukocytes and is an active bone resorber. These cytokines can stimulate bone resorption by both prostaglandin-dependent and prostaglandin-independent mechanisms and can inhibit collagen synthesis in osteoblasts. IL-6 is less potent as a direct stimulator of resorption but can synergize with IL-1 to increase bone resorption and prostaglandin production.[66] Some cytokines, such as IL-4, may inhibit bone resorption.[67]

Both IL-1 and IL-6 have been implicated as mediators of the increased bone resorption that occurs at menopause based largely on findings from rodent models.[54,68] Cytokines may mediate inflammatory bone loss and the hypercalcemia of multiple myeloma and other lymphoproliferative disorders.[69,70]

## IONS AS REGULATORS

Calcium, phosphate, and other ions important in bone metabolism not only are involved in feedback control of calcium-regulating hormone secretion but also can act as direct regulators. In addition to the critical role played by the supply of calcium and phosphorus in mineralization, organ culture studies suggest that both calcium and phosphate can influence the rate of matrix formation.[14] The effect of calcium is nonspecific in that this ion is required for cell growth generally. High serum phosphate concentrations are associated with rapid rates of bone growth. For example, in humans, phosphate concentrations are higher in the first year of life and at puberty, when the relative rates of skeletal growth are fastest. PTH secretion is inhibited and calcitonin secretion stimulated by calcium, whereas phosphate loading can lower ionized calcium and, thus, stimulate PTH secretion. Both calcium and phosphate have direct inhibitory effects on $1\alpha$-hydroxylase in the kidney and decrease $1,25(OH)_2D_3$ levels. High local concentrations of calcium, which develop during resorption in the ruffled border area, can cause loss of activity and detachment of osteoclasts. Phosphate may inhibit bone resorption directly by a physicochemical effect on mineral dissolution.

Magnesium has complex effects on skeletal metabolism (see Chap. 68). High concentrations can inhibit mineralization and PTH secretion, whereas severe magnesium depletion also is associated with decreased PTH secretion and decreased hormone responsiveness. Changes in hydrogen ion concentration can affect bone mineralization and demineralization. The increased hydrogen ion concentration in the ruffled border area is necessary not only for removal of mineral but also for maximal activity of the lysosomal enzymes that resorb matrix. Decreasing the hydrogen ion supply by inhibiting the proton pump, blocking carbonic anhydrase, or interfering with chloride-bicarbonate exchange all can inhibit bone resorption.

## REFERENCES

1. Turner CH. Three rules for bone adaptation to mechanical stimuli. Bone 1998; 23:339.
2. McLeod KJ, Rubin CT, Otter MW, Qin YX. Skeletal cell stresses and bone adaptation. Am J Med Sci 1998; 316:176.
3. Gorski JP. Is all bone the same? Distinctive distributions and properties of non-collagenous matrix proteins in lamellar vs. woven bone imply the existence of different underlying osteogenic mechanisms. Crit Rev Oral Biol Med 1998; 9:201.
4. Eriksen EF. Normal and pathological remodeling of human trabecular bone: three dimensional reconstruction of the remodeling sequence in normals and in metabolic bone disease. Endocrinol Rev 1986; 7:379.
5. Burr DB, Turner CH, Niack P, et al. Does microdamage accumulation affect the mechanical properties of bone? J Biomech 1998; 31:337.
6. Hui SL, Johnston CC Jr, Mazess RB. Bone mass in normal children and young adults. Growth 1985; 49:34.
7. Robey PG. Vertebrate mineralized matrix proteins: structure and function. Connect Tissue Res 1996; 35:131.
8. Hsu HHT, Anderson HC. Evidence of the presence of a specific ATPase responsible for ATP-initiated calcification by matrix vesicles isolated from cartilage and bone. J Biol Chem 1996; 271:26383.
9. Li YC, Amling M, Pirro AE, et al. Normalization of mineral ion homeostasis by dietary means prevents hyperparathyroidism, rickets, and osteomalacia, but not alopecia in vitamin D receptor-ablated mice. Endocrinology 1998; 139:4391.
10. Friedenstein AJ, Latzinik NV, Gorskaya YF, et al. Bone marrow stromal colony formation requires stimulation by haemopoietic cells. Bone Miner 1992; 18:199.
11. Raval P, Hsu HH, Schneider DJ, et al. Expression of bone morphogenetic proteins by osteoinductive and non-osteoinductive human osteosarcoma cells. J Dent Res 1996; 75:1518.
12. Delmas PD, Tracy RP, et al. Identification of the noncollagenous proteins of bovine bone by two-dimensional gel electrophoresis. Calcif Tissue Int 1984; 36:308.
13. Garnero P, Delmas PD. Biochemical markers of bone turnover—applications for osteoporosis. Endocrinol Metab Clin North Am 1998; 27:303.
14. Raisz LG, Kream BE. Medical progress: regulation of bone formation. N Engl J Med 1983; 309:29.
15. Allan EF, Martin TJ. The plasminogen activator inhibitor system in bone cell function. Clin Orthop 1995; 313:54.
16. Yasuda H, Shima N, Nakagawa N, et al. Osteoclast differentiation factor is a ligand for osteoprotegerin/osteoclastogenesis-inhibitory factor and is identical to TRANCE/RANKL. Proc Natl Acad Sci U S A 1998; 95:3597.
17. Quinn JMW, Elliott J, Gillespie MT, Martin TJ. A combination of osteoclast differentiation factor and macrophage-colony stimulating factor is sufficient for both human and mouse osteoclast formation in vitro. Endocrinology 1998; 139:4424.
18. Fuller K, Wong B, Fox S, et al. TRANCE is necessary and sufficient for osteoblast-mediated activation of bone resorption in osteoclasts. J Exp Med 1998; 188:997.
19. Mizuno A, Amizuka N, Irie K, et al. Severe osteoporosis in mice lacking osteoclastogenesis inhibitory factor/osteoprotegerin. Biochem Biophys Res Commun 1998; 147:610.
20. Jilka RL, Weinstein RS, Bellido T, et al. Osteoblast programmed cell death (apoptosis): modulation by growth factors and cytokines. J Bone Miner Res 1998; 13:793.
21. Teitelbaum SL, Tondravi MM, Ross FP. Osteoclasts, macrophages, and the molecular mechanisms of bone resorption. J Leukoc Biol 1997; 61:381.
22. Garnero P, Borel O, Byrjalsen I, et al. The collagenolytic activity of cathepsin K is unique among mammalian proteinases. J Biol Chem 1998; 48:32347.
23. Engleman VW, Nickols GA, Ross FP, et al. A peptidomimetic antagonist of the alpha (v) beta3 integrin inhibits bone resorption in vitro and prevents osteoporosis in vivo. J Clin Invest 1997; 99:2284.
24. Hakeda Y, Kobayashi Y, Yamaguchi K, et al. Osteoclastogenesis inhibitory factor (OCIF) directly inhibits bone-resorbing activity of isolated mature osteoclasts. Biochem Biophys Res Commun 1998; 251:796.
25. Flanagan AM, Lader CS. Update on the biologic effects of macrophage colony-stimulating factor. Curr Opin Hematol 1998; 5:181.
26. Miyaura C, Onoe Y, Inada M, et al. Increased B-lymphopoiesis by interleukin 7 induces bone loss in mice with intact ovarian function: similarity to estrogen deficiency. Proc Natl Acad Sci U S A 1997; 94:9360.
27. Nakamura M, Kuroda H, Narita K, Endo Y. Parathyroid hormone induces a rapid increase in the number of active osteoclasts by releasing histamine from mast cells. Life Sci 1996; 58:1861.
28. Konttinen Y, Imai S, Suda A. Neuropeptides and the puzzle of bone remodeling. State of the art. Acta Orthop Scand 1996; 67:632.
29. Chow JWM, Fox SW, Lean JM, Chambers TJ. Role of nitric oxide and prostaglandins in mechanically induced bone formation. J Bone Miner Res 1998; 13:1039.
30. Tetradis S, Nervina JM, Nemoto K, Kream BE. Parathyroid hormone induces expression of the inducible cAMP early repressor in osteoblastic MC3T3-E1 cells and mouse calvariae. J Bone Miner Res 1998; 13:1846.
31. Lanske B, Divieti P, Kovacs CS, et al. The parathyroid hormone (PTH)/PTH-related peptide receptor mediates actions of both ligands in murine bone. Endocrinology 1998; 139:5194.
32. Takasu H, Bringhurst FR. Type-1 parathyroid hormone (PTH) PTH-related peptide (PTHrP) receptors activate phospholipase C in response to carboxyl-truncated analogs of PTH (1-34). Endocrinology 1998; 139:4293.

33. Huang YF, Harrison JR, Lorenzo JA, Kream BE. Parathyroid hormone induces interleukin-6 heterogeneous nuclear and messenger RNA expression in murine calvarial organ cultures. Bone 1998; 23:327.

34. Schwindinger WF, Fredericks J, Watkins L, et al. Coupling of the PTH/PTHrP receptor to multiple G-proteins—Direct demonstration of receptor activation of $G_s$, $G_q$11, and $G_i(1)$ by {alpha-P-32} GTP-gamma-azidoanilide photoaffinity labeling. Endocrine 1998; 201.

35. Torrungruang K, Feister H, Swartz D, et al. Parathyroid hormone regulates the expression of the nuclear mitotic apparatus protein in the osteoblast-like cells, ROS 17/2.8. Bone 1998; 22:317.

36. Kawaguchi H, Pilbeam CC, Harrison JR, Raisz LG. The role of prostaglandins in the regulation of bone metabolism. Clin Orthop 1995; 313:36.

37. Dempster DW, Cosman F, Parisien M, et al. Anabolic actions of parathyroid hormone on bone. Endocr Rev 1993; 14:690.

38. Horwood NJ, Elliott J, Martin TJ, Gillespie MT. Osteotropic agents regulate the expression of osteoclast differentiation factor and osteoprotegerin in osteoblastic stromal cells. Endocrinology 1998; 139:4743.

39. Findlay DM, Martin TJ. Receptors of calciotropic hormones. Horm Metab Res 1997; 29128.

40. Turner PR, Mefford S, Bambino T, Nissenson RA. Transmembrane residues together with the amino terminus limit the response of the parathyroid hormone (PTH) 2 receptor to PTH-related peptide. J Biol Chem 1998; 273:3830.

41. Erben RG, Bromm S, Stangassinger M. Therapeutic efficacy of $1\alpha$, 25-dihydroxyvitamin $D_3$ and calcium in osteopenic ovariectomized rats: evidence for direct anabolic effect of $1\alpha$, 25-dihydroxyvitamin $D_3$ on bone. Endocrinology 1998; 139:4319.

42. Haussler MR, Whitfield GK, Haussler CA. The nuclear vitamin D receptor: biological and molecular regulatory properties revealed. J Bone Miner Res 1998; 13:325.

43. Nemere I, Schwatz Z, Pedroszo H, et al. Identification of a membrane receptor for 1,25-dihydroxyvitamin $D_3$ which mediates rapid activation of protein kinase C. J Bone Miner Res 1998; 13:1353.

44. Stern PH, Phillips TE, Mavreas T. Bioassay of 1,25-dihydroxyvitamin D in human plasma purified by partition, alkaline extraction, and high-pressure chromatography. Anal Biochem 1980; 102:22.

45. Morgan JW, Sliney DJ, Morgan DM, Maizel AL. Differential regulation of gene transcription in subpopulations of human B lymphocytes by vitamin D-3. Endocrinology 1999; 140:381.

46. Moonga BS, Dempster DW. Effects of peptide fragments of protein kinase C on isolated rat osteoclasts. Exp Physiol 1998; 83:717.

47. Cooper GJS. Amylin compared with calcitonin gene-related peptide—structure, biology, and relevance to metabolic disease. Endocrin Rev 1994; 15:163.

48. Cornish J, Callon KE, King AR. Systemic administration of amylin increases bone mass, linear growth, and adiposity in adult male mice. Am J Physiol 1998; 38:E694.

49. Advani S, LaFrancis D, Bogdanovic E, et al. Dexamethasone suppresses in vivo levels of bone collagen synthesis in neonatal mice. Bone 1997; 20:41.

50. Rosen CJ, Donahue LR. Insulin-like growth factors and bone—the osteoporosis connection revisited. Proc Soc Exp Biol Med 1998; 219:1.

51. Hakeda Y, Kawaguchi H, Hurley M, et al. Intact insulin-like growth factor binding protein-5 (IGFBP-5) associates with bone matrix and the soluble fragments of IGFBP-5 accumulated in culture medium of neonatal mouse calvariae by parathyroid hormone and prostaglandin E2-treatment. J Cell Physiol 1996; 166:370.

52. Kawaguchi H, Pilbeam CC, Raisz LG. Anabolic effects of 3,3',5-triiodothyronine and triiodothyroacetic acid in cultured neonatal mouse parietal bones. Endocrinology 1994; 135:971.

53. Derosa G, Testa A, Giacomini D, et al. Prospective study of bone loss in pre- and post-menopausal women on L-thyroxine therapy for non-toxic goitre. Clin Endocrinol 1997; 47:529.

53a. Pantazi H, Papapetrou PD. Changes in parameters of bone and mineral metabolism during therapy for hyperthyroidism. J Clin Endocrinal Metab 2000; 85:1099.

54. Pacifici R, Cytokines, estrogen, and postmenopausal osteoporosis—the second decade. Endocrinology 1998; 139:2659.

55. Srivastava S, Weitzmann MN, Kimble RB, et al. Estrogen blocks M-CSF gene expression and osteoclast formation by regulating phosphorylation of Egr-1 and its interaction with Sp-1. J Clin Invest 1998; 102:1850.

56. Bilezikian JP, Morishima A, Bell J, Grumbach MM. Increased bone mass as a result of estrogen therapy in a man with aromatase deficiency. N Engl J Med 1998; 339:599.

56a. Takagi M, Miyashita Y, Koga M, et al. Estrogen deficiency is a potential case for osteopenia in adult male patients with Noonan's syndrome. Calcif Tissue Int 2000; 66:200.

57. Mizunuma H, Soda M, Okano H, et al. Changes in bone mineral density after orchidectomy and hormone replacement therapy in individuals with androgen insensitivity syndrome. Hum Reprod 1998; 13:2816.

58. Manzi DL, Pilbeam CC, Raisz LG. The anabolic effects of progesterone on fetal rat calvaria in tissue culture. J Soc Gynecol Invest 1994; 1:302.

59. Clement-Lacroix P, Ormandy C, Lepescheux L, et al. Osteoblasts are a new target for prolactin: analysis of bone formation in prolactin receptor knockout mice. Endocrinology 1999; 140:96.

60. Konttinsen Y, Imai S, Suda A. Neuropeptides and the puzzle of bone remodeling. State of the art. Acta Orthop Scand 1996; 67:632.

61. Togari A, Arai M, Mizutani S, et al. Expression of MRNAs for neuropeptide receptors and beta-adrenergic receptors in human osteoblasts and human osteogenic sarcoma cells. Neurosci Lett 1997; 233:125.

62. Klein-Nulend J, Berger EH, Semeins CM, et al. Pulsating fluid flow stimulates prostaglandin release and inducible prostaglandin G/H synthase mRNA expression in primary mouse bone cells. J Bone Miner Res 1997; 12:45.

63. Bonewald LF, Dallas SL. Role of active and latent transforming growth factor beta in bone formation. J Cell Biochem 1994; 55:350.

64. Sakou T. Bone morphogenetic proteins: from basic studies to clinical approaches. Bone 1998; 22:591.

65. Zhang ZM, Chen JT, Jin D. Platelet-derived growth factor (PDGF)–BB stimulates osteoclastic bone resorption directly: the role of receptor beta. Biochem Biophys Res Commun 1998; 251:190.

66. Tai H, Miyaura C, Pilbeam CC, et al. Transcriptional induction of cyclooxygenase in osteoblasts is involved in interleukin-6-induced osteoclast formation. Endocrinology 1997; 138:2372.

67. Kawaguchi H, Nemoto K, Raisz LG, et al. Interleukin-4 inhibits prostaglandin G/H synthase-2 and cytosolic phospholipase A2 induction in neonatal mouse parietal bone cultures. J Bone Miner Res 1996; 11:358.

68. Papanicolaou DA, Wilder RL, Manolagas SC, Chrousos GP. The pathophysiologic roles of interleukin-6 in human disease. Ann Intern Med 1998; 128:127.

69. Daroszewska D, Bucknall RC, Chu P, Frazier WD. Severe hylpercalcemia in B-cell lymphoma: combined effects of PTH-RP, IL-6 and TNF. Postgrad Med J 1999; 75:672.

70. Trico G. New insights into role of microenvironment in multiple myeloma. Lancet 2000; 355:248.

# CHAPTER 51

# PARATHYROID HORMONE

DAVID GOLTZMAN AND GEOFFREY N. HENDY

Parathyroid hormone (PTH) is essential for the physiologic maintenance of calcium homeostasis, and a marked excess or deficiency can cause severe and potentially fatal illness. Because of its essential role in metabolism, skeletal function, and renal function, considerable effort has been expended and substantial advances have been made in understanding the biosynthesis, molecular biology, secretion, metabolism, and action of this hormone. Improved quantitation methods have enhanced our appreciation of its complex physiology and pathophysiology. The molecular biology approach has contributed valuable information about the structure and synthesis of this molecule and has led to the identification and characterization of a parathyroid hormone–like molecule, parathyroid hormone–related protein (PTHrP); a receptor that mediates the actions of PTH and PTHrP, the PTH/PTHrP receptor; and a parathyroid calcium-sensing receptor.

This chapter examines the production, metabolism, function, and measurement of PTH as a foundation for understanding the cause, pathogenesis, and diagnosis of disorders of the parathyroid glands.

## BIOSYNTHESIS OF PARATHYROID HORMONE

Parathyroid hormone follows a pattern of biosynthesis and of vectorial transport through organelles of the cell that now is well established for many peptide hormones (Fig. 51-1).[1,2] The major glandular form of the hormone, an 84-amino-acid, straight-chain peptide, PTH 1–84, is biosynthesized on the polyribosomes of the rough endoplasmic reticulum of the parathyroid gland. The gene for PTH encodes a precursor, prepro-PTH, that is extended at the amino-terminus of PTH 1–84 by 31 residues. The $NH_2$-terminal, 25-residue portion, characterized by its hydrophobicity, is called the *signal*, *leader*, or *pre* sequence, and it facilitates entry of the nascent hormone into the cisternae of the endoplasmic reticulum.

As the signal sequence of the synthesized hormone emerges from the ribosome, it binds to a *signal recognition particle* that stops further synthesis of the nascent protein. The signal recog-

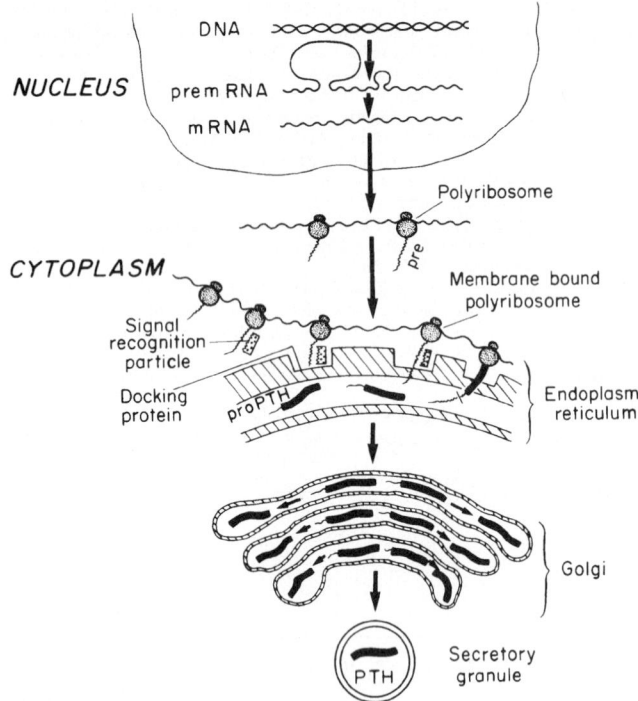

**FIGURE 51-1.** The biosynthesis of precursor and secretory forms of parathyroid hormone (*PTH*). Within the nucleus, transcription of the gene encoding PTH is followed by processing of the pre-mRNA through removal of intervening sequences. The mature mRNA leaves the nucleus and attaches to polyribosomes in the cytoplasm. The signal or pre-sequence of the hormone then binds to a signal recognition particle that interacts with a docking protein on the membrane of the endoplasmic reticulum, facilitating entry of the nascent peptide into the cisternae. The signal sequence is removed, leaving the precursor proPTH. The NH$_2$-terminal hexapeptide of this molecule is then removed in the Golgi apparatus, and the mature hormone, PTH 1–84, is packaged into secretory granules.

nition particle carrying the ribosome then binds to an integral membrane protein of the endoplasmic reticulum, called the *docking protein* or *signal recognition particle receptor*.[3] This protein releases the block in protein synthesis, and the nascent peptide is transported across the membrane into the cisternae of the endoplasmic reticulum. The signal sequence is simultaneously removed at the inner surface of the endoplasmic reticulum, enzymatically at a glycyl-lysyl bond. The resultant precursor molecule, proPTH, is extended at the NH$_2$-terminus of PTH 1–84 by only six amino acids. The *pro* sequence is necessary for efficient translocation and cleavage of the signal peptide. Once formed, proPTH is transported to the Golgi apparatus.

The prohormone hexapeptide has several basic residues that serve as a recognition sequence to yield the mature hormone. Unlike many other prohormones, proPTH does not contain another sequence at the COOH terminus and has not been detected within the circulation in states of parathyroid gland hyperfunction. ProPTH has little intrinsic biologic activity until cleaved to create the hormonal form.[1,4]

The translocation of proPTH from the rough endoplasmic reticulum to the Golgi apparatus is a process that requires energy.[2] The conversion of proPTH to PTH appears to occur within the Golgi apparatus through the action of endopeptidases with trypsin-like specificity.[1,4] The enzymes likely to be involved are furin and PC7, mammalian proprotein convertases that are related to bacterial subtilisins.[5,6] Little proPTH is stored within the gland.

The resultant mature 84-amino-acid form of the hormone is packaged in secretory granules and transported to the region of the plasma membrane. This appears to occur by a process involving vesicular budding and fusion that is driven by low-molecular-weight guanine nucleotide–binding proteins. The

hormone is released by exocytosis in response to the principal stimulus to secretion, *hypocalcemia*. The calcium ion has not been shown to influence the enzymatic cleavages involved in the processing of preproPTH or proPTH.

Little information is available concerning the posttranslational modification of the amino acid sequence of the hormone. Glycosylation does not appear to occur. Phosphorylation of proPTH and PTH occurs in vitro, where 10% to 20% of the hormone is phosphorylated at serine residues within the NH$_2$-terminal region of the molecule.[7] However, the influence of this process on intraglandular processing of the molecule or on bioactivity remains undefined.

## MOLECULAR BIOLOGY OF PARATHYROID HORMONE

### CHARACTERISTICS OF THE NORMAL PARATHYROID HORMONE GENE

The structural characterization of messenger RNAs (mRNAs) and genes encoding preproPTH from several mammalian species (i.e., humans, cattle, pigs, dogs, and both rats and mice) and one avian species (i.e., chicken) has been accomplished using the techniques of molecular biology.[8–12] In mammals, mature PTH has 84 amino acids, but the chicken form has 88 amino acids. The preproPTH gene is organized into three exons: exon I encoding the 5' untranslated region, exon II encoding the prepropeptide coding region and part of the prohormone cleavage site recognition sequence, and exon III encoding the Lys 2-Arg 1 of the prohormone cleavage site, the 84 amino acids of the mature hormone, and the 3' untranslated region.

Some of these organizational features are shared with the PTHrP gene, in which the same functional domains—the 5' untranslated region, prepro region of the precursor peptide, and the prohormone cleavage site and most or all of the mature peptide—are encoded by single exons[13–16] (Fig. 51-2; see Chap. 52). For PTHrP, exons encoding alternative 5' untranslated regions, carboxyl-terminal peptides, and 3' untranslated regions may also exist, depending on the species.

The PTH and PTHrP genes are both single-copy genes and have been mapped to the short arms of chromosomes 11 and 12, respectively.[17,18] These two human chromosomes are thought to have been derived by an ancient duplication of a single chromosome, and the PTH and PTHrP genes and their respective gene

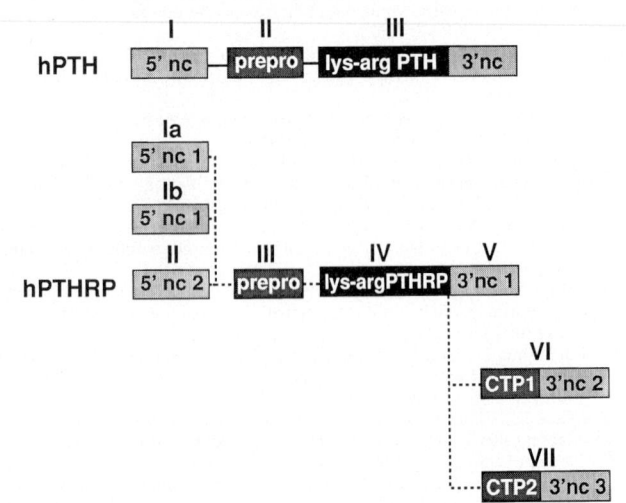

**FIGURE 51-2.** Comparison of the structural organization of the human parathyroid hormone (*PTH*) and parathyroid hormone–related protein (*PTHrP*) genes. (*Nc,* noncoding region; *CTP,* carboxyl-terminal peptide.) Roman numerals denote exons.

clusters have been maintained as syntenic groups in the human, rat, and mouse genomes.[18] Overall, because of the similarity in $NH_2$-terminal sequence of their mature peptides, their gene organization, and chromosomal location, it is likely that the PTH and PTHrP genes evolved from a single ancestral gene and form part of a single gene family.

Two common restriction-fragment-length polymorphisms for the restriction enzymes *Pst*I and *Taq*I have been detected at the human PTH gene locus, and a variable number of tandem repeat polymorphisms that occur with high frequency in the general population have been described within the human PTHrP gene.[19] These DNA markers are useful for testing for linkage of inherited disease genes to these loci in family studies.

## ALTERATIONS IN THE PARATHYROID HORMONE GENE STRUCTURE

The human PTH produced by patients with hyperparathyroidism is structurally normal.[8,20] In a small number of parathyroid tumors examined, the PTH gene sequence is rearranged, and the 5' flanking region of the PTH gene is placed upstream of the cyclin D gene located on the long arm of chromosome 11.[21] This is thought to lead to deregulated expression of the cyclin gene that contributes to tumor development. However, this type of gene rearrangement occurs infrequently in parathyroid tumors. A more common event involves the loss or inactivation of the multiple endocrine neoplasia type 1 gene, also on the long arm of chromosome 11. The protein encoded by the MEN1 gene,[22,23] called *menin*, is a 610-amino-acid nuclear protein;[24] its tumor suppressor function is thought to involve its binding to the transcription factor JunD and inhibition of JunD-activated transcription.[25] Germline mutations in the MEN1 gene cause familial and sporadic MEN1 and are found in 20% of non-MEN1 parathyroid adenomas. Loss of heterozygosity at 11q13 is found in MEN1 tumors and sporadic parathyroid adenomas, which is consistent with MEN1 being a tumor-suppressor gene.[26,27]

Mutations have been identified in the PTH gene in some cases of familial isolated hypoparathyroidism. One patient with autosomal-dominant hypoparathyroidism had a mutation within the protein-coding region of the PTH gene in which there was a single base substitution (T > C) in exon II, resulting in the substitution of arginine (CGT) for cysteine (TGT) in the signal peptide.[28] This places a charged amino acid in the hydrophobic core of the signal peptide, leading to inefficient processing of the mutant preproPTH to PTH. In a family with autosomal-recessive isolated hypoparathyroidism, a donor splice mutation was identified in the PTH gene of affected individuals at the exon II-intron II boundary that resulted in the loss of exon II, which encodes the initiation codon and signal peptide.[29]

A search for evidence of ectopic PTH synthesis (i.e., synthesis outside of parathyroid tissue) indicates that it occurs only rarely in malignancies associated with hypercalcemia.[30] However, with the advent of highly specific PTH immunoassays and mRNA analysis, a few cases of true ectopic PTH production have been documented. In one case of an ovarian carcinoma, the 5' PTH gene regulatory region that normally silences gene transcription in nonparathyroid cells was replaced by a foreign sequence that allowed inappropriate transcription to take place.[31]

## HORMONE SECRETION

### GENERAL FEATURES OF HORMONAL SECRETION

Relatively little PTH is stored in secretory granules within the parathyroid glands. In the absence of a stimulus for release, intraglandular metabolism occurs, causing complete degradation of the hormone to its constituent amino acids or partial degradation to fragments through a calcium-regulated enzymatic

mechanism.[32] In cases of hypercalcemia, the predominant hormonal entities released from parathyroid glands appear to be fragments composed of midregion or COOH-terminal sequences or both, containing little or no bioactivity.[33,34] In cases of hypocalcemia, degradation of PTH within the parathyroid cell is minimized, and the major hormonal entity released appears similar to or identical with the bioactive PTH 1–84 molecule.[35] Consequently, in the presence of hypocalcemia, increased amounts of bioactive PTH are secreted, even in the absence of additional synthesis of hormone. With a brief hypocalcemic stimulus, a biphasic secretory response often occurs. Hormone, presumably newly synthesized and derived from "immature" Golgi vesicles, is initially released in a large burst over a few minutes.[2] This is followed by a lower response sustained for a longer period, presumably representing hormone stored in secretory granules. However, hormone stores are insufficient to maintain secretion for more than a few hours in the presence of a sustained severe hypocalcemic stimulus; although other mechanisms—transcriptional and posttranscriptional—increase PTH synthesis to some extent, additional PTH secretion ultimately depends on an increase in the number of parathyroid cells. Such an increase appears to be modulated by the reductions in circulating 1,25-dihydroxyvitamin D that often accompany hypocalcemia.

A second protein, identical to chromogranin A from the adrenal medulla, is cosecreted with PTH in most conditions leading to the release of PTH.[36,37] This 50-kilodalton (kDa) protein is synthesized within the parathyroid gland and stored with PTH within secretory granules. This molecule, which can be glycosylated and phosphorylated, is a member of the chromogranin-secretogranin (granin) family of proteins that occurs in virtually all neuroendocrine cells.[38–40] The family of proteins plays several roles in the process of regulated secretion, including targeting peptide hormones and neurotransmitters to secretory granules of the regulated secretory pathway. Chromogranin A also functions as a precursor of biologically active peptides that modulate neuroendocrine cell secretion in an autocrine or paracrine fashion (see Chap. 175).

## MODULATORS OF PARATHYROID GLAND SECRETION

The calcium ion is the main regulator of parathyroid gland activity, although several other agents influence the release of PTH from parathyroid glands. These include various ions, agents altering the activity of the parathyroid cell adenylate cyclase system (e.g., β-adrenergic catecholamines, histamine), peptides derived from chromogranin A, and vitamin D metabolites.

A circadian rhythm has been reported for PTH secretion, with increased blood levels occurring at night and small amplitude pulses of PTH secretion occurring at much shorter intervals.[41,42] These studies may suggest neural or central nervous system influences on PTH secretion, or they could reflect circadian alterations in the levels of extracellular fluid calcium.

### IONS

**Cations.** The most potent of the cations modulating PTH release and the secretagogue that is most important in altering PTH release under physiologic and pathophysiologic circumstances is the calcium ion (Fig. 51-3). Although there is an inverse relationship between ambient calcium levels and PTH release, this is a curvilinear rather than proportional relationship.[43] From in vivo studies of cattle, maximal rates of PTH secretion of ~16 ng/kg per minute appear to be rapidly achieved at calcium levels below 7.5–8.0 mg/dL (1.88–2.00 mmol/L). When calcium levels are reduced from 10.0 to 9.5 mg/dL (2.50–2.38 mmol/L), a small and gradual increase in PTH secretion occurs that does exhibit a proportional relationship to the ambient calcium level. Half-maximal secretion rates normally occur at calcium levels of ~8.5 mg/dL (2.12 mmol/L), which is the *set-point* for PTH secretion. Basal secretion rates result after ambient calcium levels have risen above 11 mg/dL

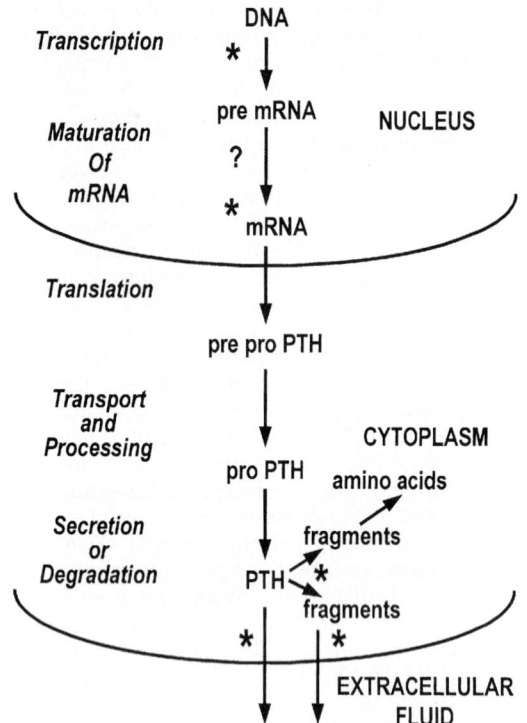

**FIGURE 51-3.** The sites of calcium regulation for parathyroid hormone (*PTH*) biosynthesis, intraglandular metabolism, and secretion. Sites known to be influenced by calcium (\*) include reversible reduction of preproPTH mRNA levels by elevated extracellular fluid calcium levels acting on preproPTH gene transcription and mRNA stability, increase in the production and release of COOH-terminal fragments by elevated calcium levels, and increase in secretion of the mature form of PTH by reduction in extracellular fluid calcium concentration. Whether calcium acts to alter the splicing of the pre-mRNA is unclear (?).

(2.75 mmol/L) and appear to persist despite further increases in calcium concentration, even up to 16–18 mg/dL (4.00–4.50 mmol/L). Similar results have been observed in studies with human parathyroid tissue in vitro. The nonsuppressible (more correctly, non–calcium suppressible) component of constitutive PTH secretion appears to comprise mainly bioinactive midregion and COOH-terminal fragments. However, direct determination of the activity of hormonal material released when calcium levels are markedly elevated also demonstrates some bioactivity.

This inverse relationship between PTH and extracellular calcium contrasts with the influence of the calcium ion as a secretagogue in most other secretory systems in which elevations in this ion enhance release of the secretory product. This distinction between the parathyroid cell and other secretory cells is maintained intracellularly, where elevations rather than decreases in cytosol calcium correlate with decreased PTH release.[44] Alterations in extracellular fluid calcium levels are transmitted through a parathyroid plasma membrane calcium sensing receptor that couples through a G-protein complex to phospholipase C. Increases in extracellular calcium lead to increases in inositol 1,4,5-trisphosphate ($IP_3$) and mobilization of intracellular calcium stores. The manner in which this inhibits hormone secretion is not understood. Although it would be anticipated that increases in diacylglycerol would accompany $IP_3$ increases caused by hydrolysis of phosphoinositides, activate protein kinase C, and result in reduced PTH secretion, this does not appear to occur in the parathyroid cell.[45] Paradoxically, agents that do stimulate protein kinase C, such as phorbol esters, stimulate rather than inhibit hormone secretion. This may be a result of phosphorylation of amino acids in the COOH-terminus of the CaSR, leading to its desensitization by blocking interaction of the receptor with its G protein.

The precise steps in the pathway from changes in extracellular calcium levels to hormone release remain to be elucidated.

The parathyroid cell $Ca^{2+}$-sensing receptor cDNA was identified by expression cloning in *Xenopus laevis* oocytes.[46] The mRNA of the human receptor encodes a polypeptide of 1078 amino acids that is predicted to contain a very large extracellular domain of ~600 amino acids and a seven transmembrane-spanning region characteristic of G-protein–coupled cell-surface receptors. Compared with the other known G-protein–coupled receptor family members, the $Ca^{2+}$-sensing receptor shows some homology with the metabotropic glutamate, γ-aminobutyric acid-B, and vomeronasal odorant receptors, sharing conserved cysteine residues and a hydrophobic sequence in the $NH_2$-terminal region. The $Ca^{2+}$-sensing receptor has a low affinity for $Ca^{2+}$, and consistent with this, the receptor sequence does not contain any of the $Ca^{2+}$ binding motifs found in high-affinity calcium-binding proteins. Highly acidic regions in the extracellular $NH_2$-terminal domain and the second extracellular loop may bind calcium as they do in other known low-affinity $Ca^{2+}$ binding proteins. Besides the parathyroid, the $Ca^{2+}$-sensing receptor is also expressed in other cells having $Ca^{2+}$-sensing functions, such as those of the kidney tubule, the calcitonin-secreting thyroid C-cells; and in diverse other organs and tissues such as brain, keratinocytes, gastrointestinal tract, and retina. Neomycin binds the receptor, possibly accounting for the toxic renal effects of aminoglycoside antibiotics.

The human $Ca^{2+}$-sensing receptor gene has been partially characterized and shown to consist of seven exons spanning more than 20 kb of genomic DNA.[47] The long extracellular domain is encoded by the first two to six exons, and the remainder of the molecule is encoded by exon seven. Exons 1A and 1B encode two alternative 5' untranslated regions of the CaSR mRNA. Inherited abnormalities of the CaSR gene, located on chromosome 3p13.3-21, can lead either to hypercalcemia or to hypocalcemia depending on whether they are inactivating or activating, respectively. Heterozygous loss-of-function mutations give rise to familial (benign) hypocalciuric hypercalcemia (FHH), in which the lifelong hypercalcemia is asymptomatic.[47–49] The homozygous condition manifests itself as *neonatal severe hyperparathyroidism* (NSHPT), which is a rare disorder characterized by extreme hypercalcemia and the bony changes of hyperparathyroidism that occur in infancy.[50,51] In several cases of NSHPT the parents are normocalcemic, and the cases seem to be sporadic. Autosomal-dominant hypocalcemia (ADH) is caused by gain-of-function mutations in the CaSR gene.[52] Autosomal-dominant hypocalcemia may be asymptomatic or present with neonatal or childhood seizures. Because of the overactive CaSR in the nephron, these patients are at greater risk of developing renal complications during vitamin D therapy than are patients with idiopathic hypoparathyroidism. A common polymorphism in the intracellular tail of the CaSR, Ala to Ser at position 986, has a modest effect on the serum calcium concentration in healthy individuals.[53] CaSR polymorphisms might also affect urinary calcium excretion and bone mass; therefore, the CaSR is a candidate gene for involvement in disorders such as idiopathic hypercalciuria and osteoporosis.

The CaSR is a target for phenylalkylamine compounds—so-called *calcimimetics*—that are allosteric stimulators of the affinity for cations by CaSR.[54] These orally active compounds have been evaluated for treatment of primary and secondary hyperparathyroidism and parathyroid carcinoma.[55]

The CaSR expressed in the developing parathyroid glands and in the placenta plays an important role in regulating fetal calcium concentrations. Normally, the fetal blood calcium level is elevated above the maternal level. This depends on the action of PTHrP (released from the fetal parathyroids and placenta) on placental calcium transport. Disruption of the CaSR, as shown by studies in CaSR-deficient mice, causes fetal hyperparathyroidism and hypercalcemia as a result of fetal bone resorption.[56] The transfer of calcium across the placenta is reduced, and renal calcium excretion is increased.

In vitro reductions in extracellular fluid calcium do not appear capable of enhancing specific PTH biosynthesis, which seems to occur at a maximal or near-maximal rate per cell; however, in vivo the reverse is the case, with biosynthesis of PTH normally being set at a low level. In vivo, PTH mRNA levels are markedly stimulated by decreased circulating calcium concentrations. It is thought that the relative insensitivity of parathyroid cell cultures to extracellular calcium is the result of reduced expression of the CaSR.[57,58] In vitro and in vivo studies have reported that elevated calcium levels reversibly and specifically reduce PTH mRNA.[59] This occurs, in part, by a direct effect on transcription of the pre-proPTH gene[60] and, in part, by a posttranscriptional mechanism, whereby hypocalcemia stabilizes and hypercalcemia destabilizes the PTH mRNA.[61] Although the results of in vitro studies are conflicting, prolonged hypocalcemia in vivo may stimulate DNA replication, cell division, and the production of increased numbers of parathyroid cells or parathyroid hyperplasia. This would increase the synthesis of proteins, including PTH, within the hypercellular parathyroid gland and ultimately would increase PTH release. In primary parathyroid gland hyperfunction resulting in hyperparathyroidism, alterations in the calcium-sensing mechanism may manifest as a setpoint error, producing a shift to the right of the curve relating PTH secretion to extracellular calcium levels.[62] Consequently, elevated concentrations of extracellular fluid calcium may be required to reduce PTH secretion, resulting in an adenomatous or hyperplastic parathyroid gland that is incompletely suppressed by calcium. Such a mechanism may underlie the observation that an increase in the mass of parathyroid tissue, such as that produced by transplantation, can be associated with hypercalcemia. The parathyroid glands of patients with primary and severe uremia secondary to hyperparathyroidism have reduced CaSR expression as assessed by immunostaining.[63] Loss of a functional CaSR, as in humans with NSHPT or in mice in which the CaSR gene has been ablated, leads to severe parathyroid hyperplasia.[64] If basal secretion per cell produces a significant amount of bioactive PTH, the cumulative increase in this basal or non–calcium-suppressible secretion arising from an increase in parathyroid cells also could be responsible for the hypercalcemia. The precise mechanistic relationship of extracellular calcium to parathyroid cell growth remains to be determined.

In studies in vitro, magnesium appears to parallel the effects of calcium on PTH release, although with reduced efficacy.[65,66] This is consistent with the known affinity of the parathyroid calcium-sensing receptor for magnesium that is lower than that for calcium itself. Mild hypomagnesemia or hypermagnesemia stimulates or suppresses, respectively, PTH secretion.[67] A special situation exists in clinical disorders associated with severe hypomagnesemia in which PTH secretion is impaired[67] (see Chap. 68). With the discovery of the syndrome of aluminum toxicity in uremia, characterized by osteomalacia, low circulating PTH levels, and a tendency toward hypercalcemia during treatment with vitamin D, the effects of aluminum on PTH secretion were assessed in vitro. Such studies, performed with rather high ambient aluminum concentrations, have shown suppression of PTH release by this cation,[68] whereas PTH mRNA expression is unaffected. A direct effect of aluminum on inhibition of PTH secretion in vivo therefore could contribute to the low circulating PTH levels seen in the presence of aluminum intoxication. It is unlikely that aluminum plays any physiologic role in the normal regulation of PTH secretion (see Chaps. 131 and 61).

**Anions.** The phosphate ion is of most interest clinically as a potential modulator of PTH release. Hyperphosphatemia induced by intravenous or oral administration of phosphate is associated with increased circulating levels of PTH. The effects have been thought to be indirect and a result of the hypocalcemia that accompanies the rise in serum phosphate.[69] However, it has been suggested that the anion can have a direct action on PTH secretion although the mechanism is unknown.[70,71] A parathyroid "phosphate sensor" analogous to the CaSR has yet to be identified. The physiologic role of other anions, such as chloride, that have been associated with alterations of PTH levels in vitro remains unclear.

## MODULATORS OF ADENYLATE CYCLASE ACTIVITY IN THE PARATHYROID CELL

A group of adenylate cyclase–stimulating agonists, such as catecholamines, prostaglandins of the E series, calcitonin, gut hormones of the secretin family, and histamine, influences PTH release in vitro.[72–74] β-Adrenergic agonists (e.g., epinephrine, isoproterenol) also enhance PTH release in animals, and some decreases in circulating PTH levels in humans have been reported with β-blockers. Despite the ability of the β-adrenergic catecholamines and histamine to induce PTH secretion, it is uncertain what physiologic or pathophysiologic role these biogenic amines may have in humans.[74,75]

Agents that may lower cyclic adenosine monophosphate (cAMP) levels within the parathyroid gland, such as $\alpha_2$-adrenergic agonists, prostaglandin $F_2$, and somatostatin, have been associated with decreased PTH secretion, mainly in vitro.

## CHROMOGRANIN A–DERIVED PEPTIDES

Peptides derived from chromogranin A (CgA), such as β-granin (i.e., CgA 1–113), synthetic βCgA 1–40, pancreastatin (i.e., porcine CgA 240–288), and parastatin (i.e., porcine CgA 347–419), have been reported to inhibit low-calcium–stimulated PTH release from parathyroid cells in culture.[76,77] The physiologic significance of these observations remains unclear. Within the parathyroid gland, processing of CgA to peptides occurs to a lesser extent than in some other endocrine tissues, such as the B cells of the pancreas, and the parathyroid cells could respond in a paracrine or endocrine fashion to CgA-derived peptides generated elsewhere.

## STEROLS AND STEROIDS

Various studies have demonstrated a role for vitamin D metabolites in the modulation of PTH release. A feedback loop between PTH-induced increase of vitamin D metabolite levels and vitamin D metabolite–induced decrease of PTH levels has been postulated. A high-affinity 1,25-dihydroxyvitamin D receptor (a member of the nuclear/steroid hormone receptor superfamily of transcriptional regulators) exists in parathyroid cells, and with the localization of injected 1,25-[³H]-dihydroxyvitamin D within the parathyroid cell, interest in this metabolite as a potential regulator of PTH synthesis or secretion has arisen. Efforts that focused on the role of 1,25-dihydroxyvitamin D in the biosynthesis of PTH provided evidence, in vitro and in vivo, that the sterol reversibly reduces levels of mRNA responsible for PTH synthesis.[78,79] This is effected by the action of the sterol on preproPTH gene transcription.

A vitamin D response element has been identified in the human PTH gene promoter, although the binding of the vitamin D receptor (VDR) to this element apparently does not require the retinoid X receptor, the normal heterodimerization partner of the VDR.[80] The precise mechanism of the down-regulation of PTH gene transcription by 1,25-dihydroxyvitamin D remains to be elucidated. Although 1,25-dihydroxyvitamin D is of uncertain importance in influencing immediate hormone release, it plays a role in modulating hormone synthesis within the gland, altering the quantities of hormone available for immediate release by secretagogues. Moreover, an early in vivo effect of reduction in 1,25-dihydroxyvitamin D appears to be an increase in maximal releasable PTH as a result of stimulation of glandular proliferation.[79] In vitro studies show that this effect of the sterol on cell proliferation is mediated by its action on early immediate response gene expression such as the *C-MYC* protooncogene.[81]

The role of other metabolites of vitamin D in modulating PTH biosynthesis or secretion remains unclear. However, "nonhypercalcemic" analogs of 1,25-dihydroxyvitamin D have been developed that do diminish PTH secretion in vitro and in vivo and that may serve in the future as therapeutics for hyperparathyroidism.

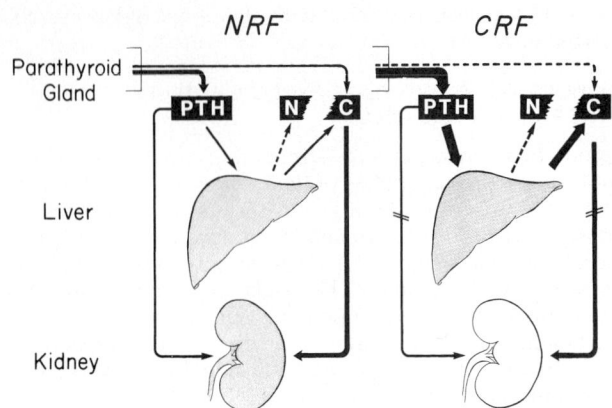

**FIGURE 51-4.** Model of parathyroid hormone (*PTH*) metabolism in the presence of normal renal function (*NRF*) and chronic renal failure (*CRF*). In the presence of NRF, PTH 1–84 released from the parathyroid gland is cleared by the kidney or metabolized in the liver, where amino (*N*; $NH_2$) and carboxyl (*C; COOH*) fragments are generated. Carboxyl, but generally not $NH_2$, fragments, are released into the circulation; these COOH fragments enter a pool, which also includes a contribution from the parathyroid gland, and are cleared by the kidney. In chronic renal failure, PTH secretion can be increased by a tendency toward hypocalcemia, and fewer COOH fragments are released from the parathyroid glands. Failure of the nonfunctioning kidneys to clear PTH results in hepatic metabolism of this moiety, with increased production of $NH_2$- and COOH fragments. Under these conditions, COOH-terminal fragments reach high circulating concentrations because of increased production and reduced renal clearance.

Cortisol, in some studies, has been reported to elevate extracellular levels of PTH in vivo and in vitro.[82] It is unclear, however, whether this effect is a direct effect on synthesis, on alteration of hormonal release, or on an alteration of the levels of enzymes metabolizing PTH within the parathyroid cell.[82] Although these findings could help explain the mild secondary hyperparathyroidism occasionally reported with glucocorticoid therapy, their overall significance remains unknown.

### PERIPHERAL METABOLISM

Besides metabolism within the parathyroid cell, PTH 1–84 undergoes extensive peripheral metabolism after release into the general circulation (Fig. 51-4). Although PTH 1–84 can be cleared from the circulation by the kidney and hormonal fragments may be generated in the kidney, such fragments probably do not reenter the circulation. Studies using sequence-specific radioimmunoassays coupled with gel filtration of serum or plasma have shown that the major circulating forms of PTH are the midregion and COOH-terminal fragments.[83–88] Such fragments may be released from the parathyroid gland in the presence of hypercalcemia.

Another major site of origin of PTH fragments appears to be the liver. Studies using [125]I-labeled PTH 1–84 injected intravenously into animals have demonstrated that initial cleavage occurs between residues 33 and 34 and at sites COOH-terminal to this. These and other studies have indicated that the hepatic Kupffer cell is the most likely site of peripheral hormonal cleavage.[89] The midregion and COOH-terminal fragments thus generated can enter the general circulation and subsequently be metabolized in the kidney.

In view of structure-function studies that have localized the bioactivity of PTH 1–84 to the $NH_2$-terminal third of the molecule, such midregion and COOH-terminal fragments should be biologically inert, at least with respect to calcium homeostatic actions mediated through the PTH/PTHrP receptor. Because of their long half-life in the circulation relative to intact PTH 1–84, such inert moieties generally comprise most circulating PTH-related entities.[90] Conversely, the corresponding $NH_2$-terminal

fragments generated during hepatic cleavage of PTH 1–84 would be expected to be bioactive, but such fragments seem to be completely degraded in the liver and do not reenter the circulation. The major circulating bioactive moiety is similar to or identical with the intact molecule PTH 1–84. Clearance of midregion and COOH-terminal fragments of PTH apparently depends almost solely on renal mechanisms. In cases of renal insufficiency, concentrations of midregion and COOH fragments may increase considerably (see Chaps. 58 and 61).

By using a sensitive renal cytochemical bioassay for PTH in association with gel filtration fractionation of plasma, it was possible to confirm that the major circulating bioactive moiety in hyperparathyroidism is similar to or identical with PTH 1–84.[91] These observations have been confirmed with the development of sensitive immunoradiometric assays that simultaneously recognize $NH_2$ and COOH epitopes on the PTH molecule and therefore detect only intact PTH 1–84. In secondary hyperparathyroidism associated with severe chronic renal failure, additional low-molecular-weight bioactive forms may occasionally be detected.[4]

The finding of a half-life of disappearance of intact bioactive PTH in end-stage renal disease that cannot be differentiated from normal kinetics indicates that, with the gradual evolution of renal insufficiency, extrarenal sites of degradation assume increasing importance in the clearance of the hormone.[4] This conclusion agrees with the finding that the clearance of $NH_2$-terminal immunoreactivity is not decreased in patients with renal failure.[90]

## ACTIONS OF PARATHYROID HORMONE

### PARATHYROID HORMONE FUNCTIONS

The major function of PTH appears to be the maintenance of a normal level of extracellular fluid calcium. The hormone exerts important effects on bone and kidney and indirectly influences the gastrointestinal tract. In response to a fall in the extracellular fluid ionized calcium concentration, PTH is released from the parathyroid cell and acts directly on the kidney to enhance renal calcium reabsorption and promote the conversion of 25-hydroxyvitamin D to 1,25-dihydroxyvitamin D.[92] This latter metabolite increases gastrointestinal absorption of calcium and, with PTH, induces skeletal resorption, causing the restoration of extracellular fluid calcium and the neutralization of the signal initiating PTH release. The opposite series of homeostatic events occurs in response to a rise in extracellular fluid calcium levels.

Although this scheme outlines the overall events that occur after a fall in calcium levels, aspects of the response may vary with the extent of the fall in calcium concentration and the consequent rise in PTH. There is some evidence that the actions of PTH on target tissues may depend on its prevailing concentration.[93] Consequently, certain actions of PTH, such as renal calcium retention and even skeletal anabolic actions, may predominate at relatively low circulating concentrations of PTH, but skeletal lysis may become evident only at higher levels of circulating PTH.

In addition to regulating calcium homeostasis, PTH elicits various other responses. Whether these other functions evolved independently or to complement the role of the hormone in maintaining calcium homeostasis is unclear. Among these other responses are perturbations of other ions, the most marked of which are those involving phosphate. As a consequence of PTH-enhanced 1,25-dihydroxyvitamin D production, the gastrointestinal absorption of phosphate is facilitated to some extent, and with PTH-induced skeletal lysis, phosphate and calcium are released. These effects increase the extracellular fluid phosphate levels, but the predominant effect of PTH on phosphate homeostasis is to inhibit renal phosphate reabsorption and produce phosphaturia. Consequently, a net decrease in

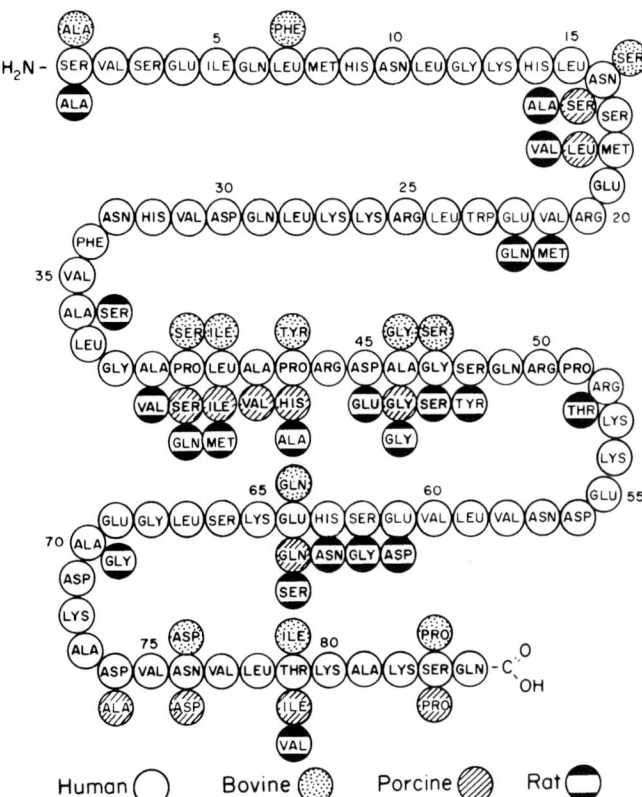

**FIGURE 51-5.** Amino acid sequence of mammalian parathyroid hormone 1–84. The backbone is that of the human sequence, and substitutions in each of the bovine, porcine, and rat hormones are shown at the specific sites.

extracellular fluid phosphate concentration occurs, and this may be viewed as adjunctive to the role of PTH in raising calcium levels.

In common with other peptide hormones, PTH interacts through a receptor on the outer surface of the plasma membrane of target cells. In these target tissues, the result of this interaction of PTH with the membrane receptor has classically been appreciated to be the stimulation of the enzyme adenylate cyclase on the inner surface of the plasma membrane, although the same receptor can couple to phosphatidylinositol turnover as well. The product of this adenylate cyclase activity, cellular cAMP, and the products of phospholipase activity, IP$_3$, diacylglycerol, and intracellular Ca$^{2+}$, initiate a cascade of events leading to the final cellular response to the hormone. The PTH receptor may activate both these intracellular signaling pathways in some target tissues and act preferentially by means of one or another pathway in other cells, but these issues are still under study.

## STRUCTURE OF PARATHYROID HORMONE CORRELATED WITH FUNCTION

The amino acid sequences of the major glandular form of mammalian PTH, PTH 1–84, have now been determined in humans, cattle, pigs, dogs, and rats (Fig. 51-5).[11,20] The corresponding amino acid sequence of the chicken peptide has also been determined and contains 88 rather than 84 amino acids. Studies correlating hormonal structure and function have emphasized the importance of the NH$_2$-terminal region to bioactivity. Considerable deletion of the middle and COOH-terminal region of the intact peptide can be tolerated without apparent loss of biologic activity. A peptide composed of the NH$_2$-terminal 34 residues,

PTH 1–34, appears to contain all of the conventional bioactivity of the intact hormone when tested in various bioassay systems.[94] Synthetic NH$_2$-terminal fragments of PTHrP, which share a high degree of homology with PTH within the NH$_2$-terminal 13 residues, have been shown to mimic PTH actions in many bioassay systems.[95–97]

Considerable effort has been expended to define the regions of the NH$_2$-terminal domain of the PTH molecule (and more recently of the PTHrP molecule) that are required to interact with the PTHR and stimulate downstream signaling. These studies examined full agonist, partial agonist, and antagonist activities of a variety of synthetic analogs of PTH (1-34), generally using in vitro adenylate cyclase–stimulating activity as an index of bioresponse. Early studies demonstrated that either deletion or extension of the NH$_2$ terminus of PTH markedly inhibited the capacity of this hormone to increase cAMP in target tissues.[94,98] Subsequently, the NH$_2$ terminus of PTHrP was shown to manifest similar sensitivity.[96] This work suggested that the NH$_2$-terminal domain of these hormones is a critical site for activation of the adenylate cyclase signaling system. Other work focused on the role of the COOH-terminal domain of PTH (1-34) in receptor binding, attempting to dissect a COOH-terminal "binding" domain in this entity from the NH$_2$-terminal "activation" domain. Stimulated by the initial observation that poorly active NH$_2$-terminal deleted analogs of PTH could still function as antagonists,[98] this work ultimately suggested that the 14-34 portion of PTH contains the predominant binding domain.[99] A number of studies have now been reported in which the structural basis of PTHrP function has also been analyzed, generally in comparison with PTH. For example, although PTH and PTHrP lack significant amino acid sequence homology in the 14-34 domains, these domains bind to osteoblastic cells with similar avidity, suggesting that these regions retain similar molecular topologies.[100,101] Despite many additional studies, however, it remains premature to assign exact functional equivalence to most of the different domains and residues in these two hormones.

Both PTH and PTHrP assume only a modestly ordered structural configuration in aqueous solution. Several nuclear magnetic resonance spectroscopy studies of PTH (1-34) and of PTHrP (1-34) in nonaqueous solutions (which are intended to mimic the membrane-bound receptor milieu) have disclosed some elements of secondary structure and have assigned two α-helical domains to these molecules, one less stable, extending for 7–11 amino acids in the NH$_2$-terminal region, and another more stable, of 9–15 residues in the COOH domain.[102–107] Some, but not all, studies have suggested interaction between the helices via a hydrophobic interface. In addition, the linker between the two helices is believed to be a turn or flexible hinge region. Cyclization of PTH and PTHrP analogs by a specific lactam apparently promotes α-helical conformation, and the stabilization of the α-helix in the putative COOH-terminal receptor-binding domain of PTH and PTHrP[108,109] has been correlated with enhanced bioactivity of these hormones. To date, however, determination of the three-dimensional x-ray structure of PTH or PTHrP has not been feasible because of the difficulty in obtaining high-quality crystals.

Although most in vitro studies correlating PTH structure and function have examined adenylate cyclase stimulating activity, several studies have been performed in which other in vitro activities have been assessed. Such studies have indicated that the NH$_2$ residues of PTH 1–34 may not be essential to induce effects on phosphoinositide metabolism and on the augmentation of intracellular calcium levels; rather that the PTH 23–34 sequence mediates this response. In vitro studies have described the mitogenic effects of the 25–47 region of PTH in osseous cells (not dependent on cAMP accumulation) and alkaline phosphatase–stimulating activity of the 53–84 sequence of PTH in osseous cells. The clinical significance of these in vitro observations remains to be determined.

# PARATHYROID HORMONE RECEPTORS

The PTH/PTHrP receptor is a member of the G-protein–linked receptor superfamily. These glycoproteins have hydrophobic sequences that are thought to span the plasma membrane seven times. These receptors couple to intracellular effectors through guanine nucleotide binding regulatory proteins or G proteins, which are heterotrimeric, consisting of alpha, beta, and gamma subunits. In the inactive state, the alpha subunit binds GDP; however, when the receptor is occupied by ligand, the G protein is activated by exchange of GTP for GDP and dissociates into $\alpha$ and $\beta$-$\gamma$ subunits. The alpha subunit, with GTP bound, can then stimulate ($G_s\alpha$) or inhibit ($G_i\alpha$), the activity of effector molecules such as adenylate cyclase or phospholipase C. The $\alpha$ subunit also has an intrinsic GTPase activity that hydrolyzes GTP to GDP, terminating the effector activation.

The PTH/PTHrP receptor belongs to a subgroup of the G-protein coupled receptor superfamily (group II GPCR) that, by virtue of their structural similarities, also includes the receptors binding secretin, calcitonin, vasoactive intestinal peptide, glucagon, glucagon-like peptide I, and growth hormone–releasing hormone. These receptors show no significant sequence identity with other known G-protein–linked receptors. All of these receptors couple to the adenylate cyclase effector by means of $G_s\alpha$. The activated PTH/PTHrP receptor couples to at least two effectors: adenylate cyclase and phospholipase C. Other members of this subgroup—including the receptors for calcitonin, glucagon, and glucagon-like peptide I—also couple to multiple signaling pathways.

PTH/PTHrP receptor cDNAs have been cloned and characterized from several species and tissues, including opossum kidney, rat bone, and human kidney and bone.[110–113] The amino acid sequences of the receptors are highly homologous, demonstrating a marked conservation across species. The opossum and rat PTH/PTHrP receptors bind $NH_2$-terminal analogs of PTH and PTHrP with similar affinity, while the human receptor appears to bind PTH somewhat preferentially. This is consistent with the study results of relative bioactivities of PTH and PTHrP in vivo in humans, that showed PTHrP 1–34 to be less potent than PTH 1–34.[114,114a]

The gene for the PTH/PTHrP receptor contains multiple introns (Fig. 51-6). For example, the mouse gene has at least 15 exons—14 of which encode the receptor protein—that span more than 32 kb of genomic DNA.[115] There are eight exons containing predicted membrane-spanning domains. These exons are heterogeneous in length, and three of the exon-intron boundaries fall within putative transmembrane sequences, suggesting that these exons did not arise from duplication events. The exon-intron organization of the PTH/PTHrP gene is similar to that of the growth hormone–releasing hormone gene, especially in the transmembrane regions, suggesting that the two genes evolved from a common precursor. PTH/PTHrP receptor gene transcription in mice is controlled by two promoters; P1, which is selectively active in kidney, and P2, which functions in a variety of tissues. Although P1 and P2 are conserved in the human PTH/PTHrP receptor gene, P1 activity in the kidney is weak, and a third promoter, P3, accounts for the majority of renal PTH/PTHrP receptor transcripts in humans.[116] During development, only P2 is active at midgestation in many human tissues, including calvaria and long bone. Thus, factors regulating the well-conserved P2 promoter control PTH/PTHrP receptor gene expression during skeletal development. Later in development, receptor gene expression is up-regulated with the induction of both P1 and P3 promoter activities.[116a]

The PTH/PTHrP receptor gene promoters lack consensus TATA elements, and the downstream promoter P2 and P3 promoters are GC-rich, which would be consistent with the widespread expression of the receptor mRNA. Although the receptor mRNA is highly expressed in kidney and bone, which are the primary target tissues of PTH, it is also expressed in nonclassic target tissues such as liver, brain, smooth muscle, spleen, testis, and skin.[112,117] In most of these tissues, the receptor probably mediates the local action of PTHrP. Although the predominant transcript is 2.5 kb, some tissues also express smaller or larger transcripts that probably are the result of alternative splicing of the primary transcript. The functional significance of these different forms of the receptor is unknown.

A second related receptor, PTHR2, which is the product of a distinct gene and binds PTH but not PTHrP, has been identified.[118] Its expression is limited to brain, pancreas, testis, and placenta; its function is unknown. Ligand-binding specificity of the PTH/PTHrP and the PTH2 receptors resides predominantly, but not exclusively, in its $NH_2$-terminal extracellular domain, whereas activation and generation of the cAMP signal is generated in the membrane-associated domain and involves specific amino acids in transmembrane domain (TM) 3 and extracellular loop 2. This suggests a two-step interaction of PTH and receptor, whereby the ligand first complexes with the $NH_2$-terminal domain of the receptor, after which the complex interacts with the membrane-associated part of the receptor to generate the signal.

Extensive analysis of the PTHR has also been performed in an attempt to delineate the structural basis of its function. Such studies using mutant and chimeric PTHR have indicated that the $NH_2$-terminal extracellular domain of the PTHR in particular is important for ligand binding and appears to interact with the COOH region of PTH or PTHrP.[119] Nevertheless, amino acid residues elsewhere in the PTHR, such as in the third extracellular loop, may also contribute to this binding.[120] Residues in the membrane-spanning helices of the PTHR may be required for binding residues in the $NH_2$-terminal domain of the ligand. Amino acids in the extracellular loops and the transmembrane regions are involved in signaling by PTH analogs, and residues in several intracellular loops and the COOH terminal intracellular tail are implicated in linkage to both $Gs\alpha$ and $Gq\alpha$. Residues in the second intracellular loop appear to be especially critical for interaction with $Gq\alpha$.[121] Other studies have identified sites in the COOH tail of the PTHR that may be important for receptor internalization and phosphorylation.[122] Consequently, a great deal of important information has been gleaned and continues to be generated on specific sites in the PTHR that may be necessary for hormone binding, for hormone signaling,

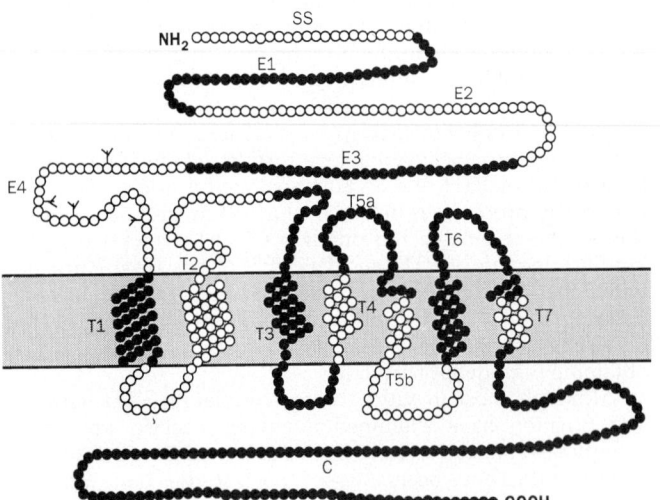

**FIGURE 51-6.** Schematic representation of the parathyroid hormone (*PTH*) and parathyroid hormone–related protein receptor. The gene contains at least 15 exons. Exon I encodes the 5′ untranslated region of the mRNA. The portions of the receptor encoded by the remaining 14 exons are schematically depicted by the alternate blocks of *unfilled* and *filled circles*. Exons are depicted as follows: *SS*; putative signal sequence; *E1–E4*; extracellular sequences; *T1–T7*; transmembrane sequences; *C*; cytoplasmic sequence. The mouse PTH/PTHrP receptor of 591 amino acids is shown.

and for PTHR regulation. Nevertheless, a comprehensive understanding of the detailed interaction of PTH and of PTHrP with the PTHR will have to await the determination of the three-dimensional structure of the bimolecular complex.

High circulating levels of PTH in hyperparathyroid states have been associated with hormonal desensitization in target tissues, apparently caused by diminished receptor capacity and a postreceptor reduction in functional levels of $G_s$.[123,124] PTH receptors, similar to many peptide hormone receptors, appear to be subject to down-regulation. The renal resistance to PTH often seen in hyperparathyroid states may be the partial result of this kind of regulatory mechanism.[125] More widespread reductions in $G_s$ are associated with hormone resistance in the disorder pseudohypoparathyroidism type 1a.

The human PTH/PTHrP receptor gene has been localized to chromosome 3p21.1-22[112] (and the PTHR2 gene to chromosome 2q33). A search for PTH/PTHrP receptor defects in patients with apparent resistance to endogenous PTH, such as in patients with pseudohypoparathyroidism type 1b, has produced negative results.[126,127] These patients have end-organ resistance to PTH without typical features of Albright hereditary osteodystrophy and therefore are thought likely to manifest a defect in PTH/PTHrP receptor expression or function. Because no mutations were identified in the receptor gene in such patients, it was indicated that mutations in genes for other proteins involved in the PTH/PTHrP signaling pathway are most likely responsible for the defects. Linkage to chromosome 20q13.3, which includes the GNAS1 locus encoding $G_s\alpha$ has been established in kindreds with PHP-1b.[128] In addition, the genetic defect is imprinted paternally and is therefore inherited in the same fashion as the PTH resistance in kindreds with PHP-1a and/or pseudopseudo-hypoparathyroidism and in a mouse model heterozygous for ablation of the Gnas gene.[129] Although the precise nature of mutations causing PHP-1b remains to be elucidated, an understanding of how mutations at a single chromosomal locus cause overlapping and/or distinct phenotypes is likely to be related to (a) the appreciation of the complex nature of the GNAS1 gene that because of its bidirectional imprinting encodes maternally, paternally, and biallelically derived proteins,[130] and (b) the subtle cell-specific imprinting of the $G_s\alpha$ transcript. Newly discovered exons upstream of the $G_s\alpha$ exons encode two different proteins, XLαs and NESP55, which are expressed in neuroendocrine cells and are probably important for secretory vesicle formation and function. It therefore is possible that a structural or regulatory mutation within the complex GNAS1 locus could account for PHP-1b, although this remains to be demonstrated.

Direct evidence that the PTH/PTHrP receptor mediates the calcium homeostatic actions of PTH and the growth plate actions of PTHrP in humans has come from the study of rare genetic disorders. *Jansen metaphyseal chondrodysplasia* (JMC) is inherited in an autosomal-dominant fashion although most reported cases are sporadic.[131] The disorder comprises short-limbed dwarfism secondary to severe growth plate abnormalities, asymptomatic hypercalcemia, and hypophosphatemia. There is increased bone resorption similar to that in primary hyperparathyroidism and urinary cAMP levels are elevated, but circulating PTH and PTHrP levels are low or undetectable. Although the PTH/PTHrP receptor is widely expressed in fetal and adult tissues, it is most abundant in three major organs, the kidney, bone, and metaphyseal or cartilaginous growth plate. It was hypothesized that the changes in mineral ion homeostasis and the growth plate in JMC are caused by constitutively active PTH/PTHrP receptors. Indeed, heterozygous PTH/PTHrP receptor gene mutations have now been identified in JMC patients. Two recurrent mutations have been described: one changes His to Arg at position 223 at the cytoplasmic end of the second transmembrane domain and the other is a Thr-to-Pro conversion at position 410 toward the cytoplasmic end of the sixth transmembrane domain.[132] Current theory holds that in the absence of agonist, G protein-coupled receptors are constrained in an inactive conformation by interactions between select amino acids in the transmembrane domains. Both His-223 and Thr-410 are highly conserved in members of the group II GPCRs, attesting to their functional importance for these receptors. Mutation of position 223 to any positively charged amino acid results in constitutive activity. Possibly, in the wild-type receptor, agonist binding leads to protonation of His-223 and results in activation. In the case of Thr-410 substitution with any other amino acid leads to constitutive activity indicating the key role Thr-410 plays in maintaining the receptor in an inactive state.

Inactivating or loss-of-function mutations in the PTH/PTHrP receptor have been implicated in the molecular pathogenesis of *Blomstrand lethal chondrodysplasia* (which was first described as a disease entity in 1985).[133] This rare disease is characterized by advanced endochondral bone maturation, short-limbed dwarfism, and fetal death, thus mimicking the phenotype of PTH/PTHrP receptor-less mice. The majority of patients with Blomstrand lethal chondrodysplasia were born to phenotypically normal, consanguineous parents, suggesting an autosomal-recessive mode of inheritance. In one such fetus, a homozygous missense mutation converting Pro-132 to Leu in the extracellular domain of the PTH/PTHrP receptor was identified.[134] Although the mutated receptor is expressed on the plasma membrane, it demonstrates reduced ligand binding and adenylate cyclase signaling. In another patient born to nonconsanguineous parents, a heterozygous deletion of 11 amino acids in the fifth transmembrane domain of the receptor was found.[135] This was the result of a G→A substitution in exon M5, which created a novel splice acceptor site in the maternal allele. The paternal allele is not expressed, although the reasons for this are not known. As in the other example, whereas the mutant receptor is well expressed in cells, it fails to bind ligand or stimulate cAMP or inositol phosphate production.

Evidence has accumulated for the possible existence of other receptors in the PTH/PTHrP system in addition to the two receptors already characterized. A receptor responsive to $NH_2$-terminal PTH and PTHrP, which signals through changes in intracellular free calcium rather than cAMP, has been found to exist in keratinocytes and other cells but has not yet been characterized. A receptor that signals in a similar manner but is only responsive to PTHrP-(1-34) mediates the release of arginine-vasopressin from the supraoptic nucleus. Unique biologic roles are predicted for the mid-region of PTHrP (transplacental calcium transport), the basic region of PTHrP (nuclear import and inhibition of apoptosis), the carboxyl-terminal region of PTHrP (inhibition of bone resorption), and the mid/carboxyl-terminal part of PTH (binding to osteoblast-like cells and modulation of their activity), each of which may act via discrete receptors.

Finally, discovery of the PTHR2 suggested the presence of an additional ligand in the PTH family. Thus, the PTHR2, responsive only to PTH and not PTHrP, is expressed mainly in brain, placenta, testis, and pancreas. A novel PTH-like ligand for the PTHR2 has been isolated from the hypothalamus.[135a]

## PARATHYROID HORMONE–INDUCED SIGNAL TRANSDUCTION ADENYLATE CYCLASE

Adenylate cyclase stimulation and the subsequent generation of cAMP are believed to be important events in the actions of PTH in the kidney and in the skeleton. Cyclic adenosine monophosphate mimics phosphaturic and calcium-retaining effects of PTH in the kidney in vivo and in vitro and mediates PTH-stimulated renal 1α-hydroxylase activity.[136] Cyclic adenosine monophosphate has also been implicated in the hypercalcemic action of PTH and may simulate PTH-induced bone resorption in vitro. Furthermore, the bone anabolic effect of PTH appears dependent on the capacity to stimulate cAMP.

Cyclic AMP produced in target cells for PTH is believed to stimulate cAMP-dependent *protein kinase isoenzymes*; types I and

II have different biochemical characteristics and may serve different functions. The isoenzymes are tetramers consisting of two regulatory and two catalytic subunits that have similar catalytic but different regulatory components, termed RI and RII, respectively. With binding of cAMP to the regulatory component, the holoenzyme dissociates, releasing the catalytic component that facilitates the transfer of a terminal phosphate group from a nucleotide donor, usually ATP, to an amino acid residue (i.e., serine, threonine, or tyrosine) of the substrate protein. PTH-induced stimulation of the two types of protein kinase has been demonstrated in normal osteoblasts and in a malignant osteoblast line.[137] One of the substrates of PKA is the widely expressed *cAMP response element binding protein* (CREB).[40] The phosphorylated CREB bound to the cAMP response element (CRE) in the promoters of responsive genes couples to the basal transcriptional machinery via cointegrators such as CREB-binding protein (CBP). PTH activates several osteoblastic genes, including c-fos,[138] by this mechanism.

### OTHER SECOND MESSENGERS OF PARATHYROID HORMONE ACTION

In addition to cAMP, other second messengers, such as the calcium ion, have been implicated as being potentially important in PTH action. In some species, transient hypocalcemia, presumably caused by calcium entry into bone cells, is the earliest event in the action of PTH on the skeleton in vivo. In vitro studies have shown that PTH promotes the uptake of calcium into isolated bone cells, that elevated calcium mimics or potentiates the effects of PTH on the enzymatic activities of isolated bone cells, and that calcium antagonists inhibit and calcium ionophores stimulate bone resorption.

PTH stimulates phosphatidylinositol turnover in certain cell types and in renal membranes.[139,140] In response to PTH-induced augmentation of phospholipase C action, presumably via Gq stimulation after occupancy of the PTH/PTHrP receptor, increased production of IP$_3$ and diacylglycerol occurs. Increases in cytoplasmic calcium, presumably induced by IP$_3$, have also been demonstrated, as has increased protein kinase C activity.

The cellular response to PTH may therefore involve multiple mechanisms of cell signaling, and modulation of one message by another ("cross talk") may affect the final response to the hormone. The relative contributions of adenylate cyclase versus phospholipase C stimulation to the pleiotropic effects of PTH in bone and kidney still remains to be clarified.

### EFFECTS OF PARATHYROID HORMONE IN TARGET TISSUES

#### BONE

Consistent with its prime function of raising the extracellular fluid calcium concentration, the most appreciated effect of PTH is a catabolic one in bone.[141,142] The end result is the breakdown of mineral constituents and bone matrix, as manifested in vivo by the release of calcium and phosphate, by increases in plasma and urinary hydroxyproline, and by other indices of bone resorption. This process appears to be mediated by *osteoclastic osteolysis*, but the mechanism by which PTH causes *osteoclastic stimulation* is indirect. Unlike calcitonin, PTH, when administered in vivo, does not bind directly to multinucleated osteoclasts.

In vivo studies using autoradiography have revealed PTH binding to mature osteoblasts and to skeletal mononuclear cells in the intertrabecular region of the metaphysis (apparently to preosteoblastic stromal cells).[143,144] Consequently, PTH-mediated increases in the number and function of osteoclasts (which are of hematogenous origin) appear to occur indirectly, through effects on cells of the osteoblast series (which are of mesenchymal origin).[145] The results of these studies have been confirmed in exper-

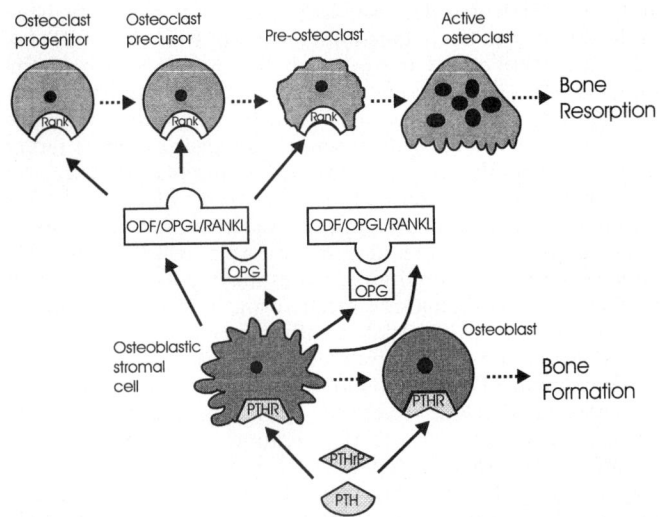

**FIGURE 51-7.** Model of the activation of bone resorption and formation by parathyroid hormone (*PTH*) or parathyroid hormone–related protein (*PTHrP*). PTH of PTHrP bind via their NH$_2$ terminus to the PTH/PTHrP receptor (*PTHR*) of osteoblastic stromal cells or osteoblasts. Osteoblastic stimulation may lead to bone formation. PTH/PTHrP binding to the PTHR, most likely on the osteoblastic stromal cell, can also lead to the binding of ODF/OPGL/RANKL to receptors (*RANK*) on cells of the osteoclast series. This cytokine can then enhance commitment, proliferation, differentiation, and fusion of osteoclast precursors to form active bone-resorbing osteoclasts. Alternatively, ODF/OPGL/RANKL may be bound by OPG, preventing osteoclastic bone resorption.

iments with the cloned PTH/PTHrP receptor; these have confirmed expression of the receptor in osteoblastic cells but not osteoclasts.[146] PTH-induced stimulation of multinucleated osteoclasts occurs through the action of PTH-stimulated osteoblastic activity.[147] This osteoblastic activity is characterized by release of intermediary factors such as cytokines.

One of the most important of these intermediary factors is *osteoclast differentiation factor* (ODF), also known as *osteoprotegerin ligand* (OPGL).[148] This protein is expressed in bone-lining cells or in osteoblast precursors that support osteoclast recruitment. ODF/OPGL, which is a member of the tumor necrosis factor (TNF) family, is identical to the molecule TRANCE/RANKL, which is expressed in T cells and previously was identified as a dendritic cell survival factor in vitro. Several bone resorbing factors, such as PTH, PTHrP, PGE$_2$, some of the interleukins, and 1,25(OH)$_2$D$_3$, up-regulate ODF/OPGL gene expression in osteoblasts and bone stromal cells (Fig. 51-7). Interaction of ODF/OPGL with its receptor on osteoclast progenitors and osteoclasts then stimulates their recruitment and activation and delays their degradation. The ablation of the ODF/OPGL gene in mice has confirmed it to be a key regulator of osteoclastogenesis as well as of lymphocyte development and lymph-node organogenesis.[149] *Osteoprotegerin* (OPG)/*osteoclastogenesis inhibitory factor* (OCIF)[150] is a soluble receptor for ODF/OPGL that inhibits recruitment, activation, and survival of osteoclasts and therefore inhibits osteoclastic bone resorption. OPG/OCIF acts as a natural decoy receptor to disrupt the interaction between ODF/OPGL, which is released by osteoblast-related cells, and the ODF/OPGL receptor on osteoclast progenitors.

Early and late phases of calcium mobilization have been described after in vivo administration of PTH.[151] The early hypercalcemic response occurs from 10 minutes to 3 hours after hormone exposure. This response may be a consequence of increased metabolic activity of preexisting osteoclasts or of other cell types that enhance the transfer to bone of calcium in bone that is already in solution.

A more sustained hypercalcemic response to PTH administration, occurring over approximately 24 hours, appears to depend on new protein synthesis and to involve a quantitative increase in osteoclasts, a change in the structure of the osteoclasts (i.e., increased ruffled borders, which is a zone of the cell believed to be involved in skeletal resorption); an increase in the secretion of lysosomal enzymes, including collagenase and acid hydrolases such as acid phosphatase; and acidification of the extracellular milieu of the osteoclast.

In contrast to sustained administration of PTH, which causes bone resorption and hypercalcemia, low and intermittent doses of PTH-(1-34)—and PTHrP-(1-34) and related analogs—promote bone formation.[152] Furthermore, in clinical studies, daily injections of PTH-(1-34) have been reported to increase hip and spine bone mineral density (BMD).

The consequences of the effects of PTH on osteoblast activity are therefore complex. Thus, in addition to using osteoblastic cells to relay signals to the osteoclast lineage to resorb bone, PTH also appears to stimulate osteoblastic cells to enhance new bone formation. This might occur as a result of the ability of PTH to stimulate the production of growth factors, such as IGF-I, by osteoblasts. However, the bone-forming activity of PTH may depend more on promoting differentiation of precursor cells into secretory osteoblasts than on an action on mature osteoblasts.[153] The precise mechanisms of the anabolic effect of PTH still remain to be clarified, however.

The anabolic and catabolic effects of PTH on osteoblasts may therefore represent a combination of direct and indirect effects; effects of different domains of the PTH molecule that signal differently; discrete functions of morphologically similar but functionally distinct osteoblastic cells; or differences in hormonal effects based on different times of exposure or different hormone concentrations.

## KIDNEY

One of the first-described effects of the administration of PTH intravenously was phosphaturia (see Chap. 206). Renal tubular reabsorption of phosphate is an active process, with a limited transport capacity resulting in a maximum rate of tubular reabsorption ($Tm\ PO_4$).[154] Because the absolute values of $Tm\ PO_4$ vary considerably among individuals and most of this variation can be explained by differences in glomerular filtration rate (GFR), the $Tm\ PO_4$/GFR ratio has been suggested as a more accurate index of phosphate reabsorption. This index, which represents the sum of the heterogeneous maximum reabsorption rates of all individual nephrons, is reduced by increased concentrations of PTH and increased in its absence.

The molecular basis of the inhibition of $Na^+$-dependent phosphate transport by PTH was clarified by the cloning of the $Na^+$-phosphate co-transporter, NPT-2.[155] Thus, inhibition of phosphate reabsorption by PTH in the renal proximal tubule appears to involve PTH-induced endocytosis of NPT-2 and its subsequent intracellular degradation.

Another relatively immediate effect of PTH that contributes to its role in calcium homeostasis is enhanced fractional reabsorption of calcium from the glomerular fluid. However, excessive circulating concentrations of PTH ultimately are associated with a rise in urinary calcium because of increases in extracellular calcium levels and therefore in the filtered load of calcium. The capacity of PTH to produce a mild renal tubular acidosis appears linked to its ability to inhibit the activation of the type 3 $Na^+$-$H^+$ exchanger (NHE3).[156]

Augmentation of urinary cAMP excretion in response to PTH administration is one of the earliest renal responses and is consistent with its postulated role as a second messenger for many or most renal responses. Nevertheless, evidence for an important role for inositol phosphates, protein kinase C, and intracellular calcium in the renal actions of PTH is also available; the relative in vivo contributions of the two pathways to the multiple effects of PTH in the kidney still requires clarification. The renal actions of PTH to increase urinary phosphate and cAMP excretion form the basis for the modified Ellsworth-Howard test that is used clinically to establish renal PTH responsiveness (see Chap. 60).

PTH alters renal function because of its interactions with multiple regions of the nephron. Evidence for PTH binding to the primary foot processes of podocytes of renal corpuscles and for the stimulation of adenylate cyclase activity in rat glomeruli can be correlated with reduction of the GFR in rats by PTH as a result of decreasing the ultrafiltration coefficient.[144] Evidence for the expression of the cloned PTH/PTHrP receptor in renal glomeruli confirms the previous findings.

PTH appears to reach the luminal surface of polar tubular cells by glomerular filtration and the basolateral surface through the peritubular capillary plexus. High-capacity binding sites have been described on the periluminal portion of the earliest part of the proximal tubule, at which, related to the microvillar surface, PTH degradative events appear to occur. Saturable, specific, low-capacity binding sites for PTH have been localized after injection in rats to the basolateral surface of the proximal convoluted tubule and pars recta, the thick ascending limb of the loop of Henle, and the distal convoluted tubule and pars arcuata of the collecting duct.[144] This pattern of PTH binding and activity correlates well with the expression of the cloned PTH/PTHrP receptor and with the localization of PTH-stimulated adenylate cyclase activity in rat nephrons, which was demonstrated in studies using microdissection of tubules.[156] These observations emphasize the diversity of PTH actions on the renal tubule, most of which can be mimicked by the infusion of cAMP onto the luminal aspect of tubular cells.[157,158]

The use of various techniques, including micropuncture and microperfusion, has localized PTH-induced inhibition of phosphate reabsorption to the proximal convoluted tubule and to the pars recta.[158] Inhibition of phosphate reabsorption in the proximal convoluted tubule appears to be accompanied by inhibition of sodium and fluid reabsorption. However, sodium is also reabsorbed more distally. Inhibition of phosphate reabsorption also may occur, although perhaps to a lesser extent, in the distal tubule. The proximal tubule appears to be the major site of action of PTH in stimulating the 1α-hydroxylase and increasing the production of 1,25-dihydroxyvitamin D. The PTH-induced inhibition of bicarbonate transport occurs in the proximal tubule and the pars recta, and the effect of PTH on this nephron segment may explain the rise in urinary bicarbonate produced by PTH infusion.[158] The important site of PTH action to increase calcium and probably magnesium transport appears to be in the thick ascending limb of the loop of Henle and in the distal convoluted tubule and earliest portion of the cortical collecting tubule.

Despite the demonstration of the dual role of PTH in increasing extracellular fluid calcium concentrations through renal and skeletal routes, the relative importance of each is unclear.[159] However, contributions of the kidney and skeleton to calcium homeostasis may depend on the concentration of circulating PTH and the duration of elevated hormonal levels.

## OTHER TARGET TISSUES

Although the administration of PTH in vivo can enhance intestinal calcium absorption, this effect appears to be indirect and mediated by the increased production of 1,25-dihydroxyvitamin D.[92] Among other reported effects of PTH are direct effects on vascular tone, stimulation or inhibition of mitosis of various cells in vitro, increased concentrations of calcium in mammary and in salivary glands, enhanced hepatic gluconeogenesis, and enhanced lipolysis in isolated fat cells. The demonstration of the widespread expression of the PTHrP gene and the equally disseminated expression of the PTH/PTHrP receptor gene suggests that many of the "noncalcemic" actions of PTH may be carried out by PTHrP acting in an autocrine or paracrine manner.[160]

# MEASUREMENT

## RADIOIMMUNOASSAYS

Radioimmunoassays (RIAs) developed for human PTH generally do not use human PTH (hPTH) 1–84 as a tracer because of its scarcity and because it lacks a tyrosine residue for convenient radioiodination. Instead, bovine PTH (bPTH) 1–84 is used, possibly contributing to the reduced sensitivity for hPTH. The antisera used in PTH RIAs are generally polyclonal and have been raised against bPTH 1–84 or hPTH 1–84. Nevertheless, populations of antibodies within polyclonal antisera directed against specific epitopes contained in the 1–84 molecule may predominate. Antibody populations recognizing the COOH-terminal region of PTH 1–84 usually are readily obtained after immunization with bPTH 1–84; antibodies recognizing the midregion also occur with high frequency.[161] Sufficiently sensitive antisera containing antibodies predominantly interacting with the NH$_2$-terminal region are more unusual but have been successfully raised.[162]

Attempts to direct antibody specificity have used several strategies. Although the development of monoclonal antibodies to PTH or PTH fragments would seem to be the most direct route to achieve specificity, this approach has not been successful for various technical and biochemical reasons. Instead, specificity has been achieved by using polyclonal antisera with predominant specificity for selected regions, as determined by their reactivity toward synthetic fragments of discrete regions of the molecule or by enhancing the specificity of such antisera by using synthetic fragments of the midregion or COOH-terminal end of PTH as tracers.

An important advance in the measurement of PTH is the development of immunoradiometric assays (IRMAs) that use antisera directed against the NH$_2$-terminal and midregion or COOH region of the molecule. These assays (i.e., "intact" assays) detect mainly intact PTH 1–84 and appear to be the most sensitive and specific.[163]

Defining the specificity of an RIA is important because of the complex metabolism of PTH, which results in a multiplicity of circulating molecular forms. The most abundant circulating forms are midregion and COOH fragments because of their longer half-life in the circulation; these become even more predominant in renal failure when clearance is further impaired.[89,90] The presumed bioactive forms, intact PTH 1–84 and the NH$_2$-terminal fragment, are cleared more readily and circulate at lower levels. Midregion and COOH-directed RIAs detect long-lived fragments and intact bioactive hormone. These RIAs generally do not require the high sensitivity of NH$_2$-directed assays to be useful, because they measure higher absolute levels of PTH.

Most material measured by these RIAs is thought to be inactive, but this has not greatly restricted their clinical usefulness in the diagnosis of primary or secondary hyperparathyroidism. For primary hyperparathyroidism, the midregion and COOH-directed RIAs may be especially useful in providing an index of integrated secretory function of the parathyroid glands.[85] However, first it should be established that a given midregion or COOH-terminal RIA is clinically useful. Amino-terminal RIAs, which determine the level of short-lived PTH forms, can also be used to detect hypersecretion in primary hyperparathyroidism but may be especially useful in assessing acute changes in PTH secretion in physiologic studies. Two-site IRMAs, which also measure bioactive hormone, are generally more sensitive and can substitute for NH$_2$-directed assays.

For cases of hyperparathyroidism associated with renal failure, NH$_2$-directed assays have the theoretical advantage of providing a better estimate of circulating bioactive PTH forms and differentiating decreased PTH clearance from hypersecretion. From a practical point of view, two-site IRMAs are preferred to NH$_2$-directed assays. If PTH levels are determined serially during the progression of renal failure, COOH-directed assays also may provide useful estimates of the severity of the hyperparathyroidism, and hormone levels determined by COOH-directed assays in renal failure have correlated well with the extent of skeletal resorption.[85] It has been suggested that midregion assays may detect intact PTH more readily than COOH-directed assays and may have a somewhat greater ability to measure a variety of PTH forms than the COOH-directed assays. However, midregion assays are subject to restrictions and advantages similar to those of the COOH-directed assays.

Few RIAs, no matter the degree of specificity, completely discriminate between concentrations of immunoreactive PTH found in healthy persons and those detected in hyperparathyroidism, although best results appear to be obtained with two-site IRMAs. It has been suggested that PTH levels should be interpreted in conjunction with prevailing levels of blood calcium. This assists in the assay analysis; if a given PTH level is measured in a normocalcemic individual and that same PTH level is found in a patient with hypercalcemia, the level in the latter case can be considered inappropriately elevated.

Another limitation of most RIAs is the inability to measure values in all healthy individuals. A lower limit of normality generally cannot be established, which makes it difficult to ascertain reduced PTH levels. Sensitive two-site IRMAs often approach a lower limit of normality. PTH RIAs are useful in differentiating hypocalcemia resulting from PTH deficiency (i.e., hypoparathyroidism) from hypocalcemia resulting from other causes. In the former situation, PTH is undetectable or is found in very low concentrations, but in the latter situation, the hypocalcemic stimulus is associated with increased PTH secretion and elevated levels of PTH (see Chaps. 58 and 61).

## BIOASSAYS

With the unraveling of the complex metabolism of PTH and the resulting heterogeneity of circulating hormone, the care that must be exercised in interpreting the results of PTH RIAs became apparent, and the possibility of using PTH bioassays to supplement the information obtained from RIAs arose. Some PTH bioassays estimate the biologic effects of the hormone in vivo, and some estimate levels of the hormone based on biologic effects in vitro. It has been estimated that the normal circulating levels of bioactive PTH are ~1 pmol/L.

### IN VIVO BIOASSAYS

Measurements of in vivo phosphaturic effects (e.g., determination of $Tm$ PO$_4$/GFR) and renal calcium retention (e.g., fractional excretion of calcium) provide estimates of PTH effects in vivo and have been useful as adjunctive studies of PTH. Partly because of their lack of specificity, these assays have not achieved widespread popularity as indices of PTH concentrations in most clinical situations. Conversely, estimates of urinary cAMP excretion (measured by RIA) have been fairly widely used.[164]

Several hormones in addition to PTH (e.g., vasopressin) contribute to urinary cAMP levels, although the PTH-produced component is the major fraction. Greater specificity of urinary cAMP for PTH can be achieved by measuring the fraction of urinary cAMP that is of renal origin. This nephrogenous component can be determined from the clearance of cAMP relative to the GFR, an estimate requiring plasma cAMP measurements, or it can be determined by relating the urinary cAMP to 100 mL of glomerular filtrate. Nephrogenous cAMP is a specific and rather sensitive in vivo bioassay for PTH.[164] Nephrogenous cAMP is often elevated in primary hyperparathyroidism and decreased in hypoparathyroidism. There is, however, overlap with the normal range. Most nephrogenous cAMP determinations accurately reflect circulating PTH levels as determined by RIA, but they do not have the sensitivity or specificity of the best two-site IRMAs.

## IN VITRO BIOASSAYS

Several attempts have been made to develop clinically useful in vitro bioassays for the measurement of active PTH. The capacity of PTH to stimulate adenylate cyclase, with the addition of guanyl nucleotides, in purified renal membrane preparations or tumor cell lines and the availability of synthetic antagonistic PTH fragments have imparted useful specificity to such renal membrane bioassay preparations.[165,166] Unfortunately, the relative insensitivity of this approach has precluded its use for anything other than experimental purposes.

Another approach is the cytochemical PTH bioassay. The most widely used has been a renal cytochemical bioassay (CBA) performed in guinea pig kidney segments maintained in nonproliferative organ culture.[4,91,167] The major drawbacks of the method are its technical difficulty and low throughput, which have precluded its use for routine clinical assay purposes.

## CONCLUSIONS

Considerable progress has been made in examining the biosynthesis of PTH, the regulation of PTH secretion, and the mechanism of PTH action. These advances include elucidation of the molecular genetics of PTH, discovery of the parathyroid calcium "sensor," and determination of the structure of the PTH/PTHrP receptor. Discovery of the ODF/OPGL/RANKL system and the cloning of NPT-2 have greatly contributed to the understanding of the mechanism of PTH action in bone and kidney. The identification of PTHrP has disclosed a new member of the PTH gene family and provided possibilities for understanding the biologic effects of both molecules. This improved comprehension of the biochemistry and physiology of PTH should translate into exciting insights into the pathophysiology of disease states in which PTH is implicated.

## REFERENCES

1. Kronenberg HM, Igarashi T, Freeman MW, et al. Structure and expression of the human parathyroid hormone gene. Recent Prog Horm Res 1986; 42:641.
2. Cohn DV, Elting J. Biosynthesis, processing and secretion of parathormone and secretory protein-I. Recent Prog Horm Res 1983; 39:181.
3. Walter P, Ibrahimi I, Blobel G. Translocation of proteins across the endoplasmic reticulum. 1. Signal recognition protein (SRP) binds to in vitro–assembled polysomes synthesizing secretory protein. J Cell Biol 1981; 91:545.
4. Goltzman D, Bennett HPJ, Koutsilieris M, et al. Studies of the multiple forms of bioactive parathyroid hormone and parathyroid hormone-like substances. Recent Prog Horm Res 1986; 42:665.
5. Hendy GN, Bennett HPJ, Lazure C, et al. Proparathyroid hormone (ProPTH) is preferentially cleaved to parathyroid hormone (PTH) by the prohormone convertase furin: a mass spectrometric study. J Biol Chem 1995; 270:9517.
6. Canaff L, Bennett HPJ, Hou Y, et al. Proparathyroid hormone processing by the proprotein convertase PC7: comparison with furin and assessment of modulation of parathyroid convertase mRNA levels by calcium and 1,25-dihydroxy vitamin D$_3$. Endocrinology 1999; 140:3633.
7. Rabbani SA, Kremer R, Bennett HPJ, Goltzman D. Phosphorylation of parathyroid hormone by human and bovine parathyroid glands. J Biol Chem 1984; 259:2949.
8. Hendy GN, Kronenberg HM, Potts JT Jr, Rich A. Nucleotide sequence of cloned DNAs encoding human preproparathyroid hormone. Proc Natl Acad Sci U S A 1981; 78:7365.
9. Vasicek TJ, McDevitt BE, Freeman MW, et al. Nucleotide sequence of genomic DNA encoding human parathyroid hormone. Proc Natl Acad Sci U S A 1983; 80:2127.
10. Weaver CA, Gordon DF, Kissil MS, et al. Isolation and complete nucleotide sequence of the gene for bovine parathyroid hormone. Gene 1984; 28:319.
11. Heinrich G, Kronenberg HM, Potts JT Jr, Habener JF. Gene encoding parathyroid hormone. Nucleotide sequence of the rat gene and deduced amino acid sequence of rat preproparathyroid hormone. J Biol Chem 1984; 259:3320.
12. Russell J, Sherwood LM. Nucleotide sequence of the DNA complementary to avian (chicken) preproparathyroid hormone mRNA and the deduced sequence of the hormone precursor. Mol Endocrinol 1989; 3:325.
13. Yasuda T, Banville D, Hendy GN, Goltzman D. Characterization of the human parathyroid hormone–like peptide gene: functional and evolutionary aspects. J Biol Chem 1989; 264:7720.
14. Mangin M, Ikeda K, Dreyer BE, Broadus AE. Isolation and characterization of the human parathyroid hormone–like peptide gene. Proc Natl Acad Sci U S A 1989; 86:2408.
15. Suva LJ, Mather KA, Gillespie MT, et al. Structure of the 5′ flanking region of the gene encoding human parathyroid hormone–related protein (PTHrP). Gene 1989; 77:95.
16. Karaplis AC, Yasuda T, Hendy GN, et al. Gene encoding parathyroid hormone–like peptide: nucleotide sequence of the rat gene and comparison with the human homologue. Mol Endocrinol 1990; 4:441.
17. Naylor SL, Sakaguchi AY, Shows TB, et al. Human parathyroid hormone gene (PTH) is on the short arm of chromosome 11. Somatic Cell Mol Genet 1983; 9:609.
18. Seldin MF, Mattei M-G, Hendy GN. Localization of mouse parathyroid hormone-like peptide gene (Pthlh) to distal chromosome 6 using interspecific backcross mice and in situ hybridization. Cytogenet Cell Genet 1992; 60:252.
19. Pausova Z, Morgan K, Fujiwara TM, et al. Molecular characterization of an intragenic minisatellite (VNTR) polymorphism in the human parathyroid hormone–related peptide gene in chromosome region 12p12.1–p11.2. Genomics 1993; 17:243.
20. Keutmann HT, Sauer MM, Hendy GN, et al. Complete amino acid sequence of human parathyroid hormone. Biochemistry 1978; 17:5723.
21. Motokura T, Bloom T, Kim HG, et al. A novel cyclin encoded by bcl1-linked candidate oncogene. Nature 1991; 350:512.
22. Chandrasekharappa SC, Guru SC, Manickam P, et al. Positional cloning of the gene for multiple endocrine neoplasia-type 1. Science 1997; 276:404.
23. European Consortium on MEN1. Identification of the multiple endocrine neoplasia type 1 (MEN1) gene. Hum Mol Genet 1997; 6:1177.
24. Guru SC, Goldsmith PK, Burns AL, et al. MENIN, the product of the MEN1 gene, is a nuclear protein. Proc Natl Acad Sci U S A 1998; 95:1630.
25. Agarwal SK, Guru SC, Heppner C, et al. Menin interacts with the AP1 transcription factor JunD and represses JunD-activated transcription. Cell 1999; 96:143.
26. Friedman E, Sakaguchi K, Bale AE, et al. Clonality of parathyroid tumors in familial multiple endocrine neoplasia type 1. N Engl J Med 1989; 321:213.
27. Thakker RV, Bouloux P, Wooding C, et al. Association of parathyroid tumors in multiple endocrine neoplasia type 1 with loss of alleles on chromosome 11. N Engl J Med 1989; 321:218.
28. Arnold A, Horst SA, Gardella TJ, et al. Mutation of the signal peptide-encoding region of the preproparathyroid hormone gene in familial isolated hypoparathyroidism. J Clin Invest 1990; 86:1084.
29. Parkinson DB, Thakker RV. A donor splice site mutation in the parathyroid hormone gene is associated with autosomal recessive hypoparathyroidism. Nature Genet 1992; 1:149.
30. Simpson EL, Mundy GR, D'Souza SM, et al. Absence of parathyroid hormone messenger RNA in nonparathyroid tumors associated with hypercalcemia. N Engl J Med 1983; 309:325.
31. Nussbaum SR, Gaz RD, Arnold A. Hypercalcemia and ectopic secretion of parathyroid hormone by an ovarian carcinoma with rearrangement of the gene for parathyroid hormone. N Engl J Med 1990; 323:1324.
32. Fischer JA, Oldham SB, Sizemore GW, Arnaud CD. Calcium-regulated parathyroid hormone peptidase. Proc Natl Acad Sci U S A 1972; 69:2341.
33. Flueck JA, DiBella FP, Edis AJ, et al. Immunoheterogeneity of parathyroid hormone in venous effluent serum from hyperfunctioning parathyroid glands. J Clin Invest 1977; 60:1367.
34. Hanley DA, Takatsuki K, Sultan JM, et al. Direct release of parathyroid hormone fragments from functioning bovine parathyroid glands in vitro. J Clin Invest 1978; 62:1247.
35. Mayer GP, Keaton JA, Hurst JG, Habener JF. Effect of plasma calcium concentrations on the relative proportion of hormone and carboxyl fragments in parathyroid venous blood. Endocrinology 1979; 104:1778.
36. Kemper B, Habener JF, Rich A, Potts JT Jr. Parathyroid secretion: discovery of a major calcium-dependent protein. Science 1974; 184:167.
37. Cohn DV, Zangerle R, Fischer-Colbrie R, et al. Similarity of secretory protein-I from parathyroid gland to chromogranin A from adrenal medulla. Proc Natl Acad Sci U S A 1982; 79:6056.
38. Bhargava G, Russell J, Sherwood LM. Phosphorylation of parathyroid secretory protein. Proc Natl Acad Sci U S A 1983; 80:878.
39. Mouland AJ, Bevan S, White JH, Hendy GN. Human chromogranin A gene; molecular cloning, structural analysis and neuroendocrine cell-specific expression. J Biol Chem 1994; 269:6918.
40. Canaff L, Bevan S, Wheeler D, et al. Analysis of molecular mechanisms controlling neuroendocrine cell specific transcription of the chromogranin A gene. Endocrinology 1998; 139:1184.
41. el-Hajj Fuleihan G, Klerman EB, Brown EN, et al. The parathyroid hormone circadian rhythm is truly endogenous—a general clinical research center study. J. Clin Endocrinol Metab 1997; 82:281.
42. Samuels MH, Veldhuis JD, Kramer P, et al. Episodic secretion of parathyroid hormone in postmenopausal women: assessment by deconvolution analysis and approximate entropy. J Bone Miner Res 1977; 12:616.
43. Mayer GP, Hurst JG. Sigmoidal relationship between parathyroid hormone secretion rate and plasma calcium in calves. Endocrinology 1978; 102:1036.
44. Shoback DM, Thatcher J, Leombruno R, Brown EM. Relationship between parathyroid hormone secretion and cytosolic calcium concentration in dispersed bovine parathyroid cells. Proc Natl Acad Sci U S A 1984; 81:3113.
45. Brown EM, Redgrave J, Thatcher J. Effect of the phorbol ester TPA on PTH secretion. Evidence for a role for protein kinase C in the control of PTH release. FEBS Lett 1984; 175:72.

46. Brown EM, Gambda G, Riccardi D, et al. Cloning and characterization of an extracellular $Ca^{2+}$-sensing receptor from bovine parathyroid. Nature 1993; 366:575.

47. Pollak MR, Brown EM, Chou Y-HW, et al. Mutations in the human $Ca^{2+}$-sensing receptor gene cause familial hypocalciuric hypercalcemia and neonatal severe hyperparathyroidism. Cell 1993; 75:1237.

48. Heath H III, Odelberg S, Jackson CE, et al. Clustered inactivating mutations and benign polymorphisms of the calcium receptor gene in familial benign hypocalciuric hypercalcemia suggest receptor functional domains. J Clin Endocrinol Metab 1996; 81:1312.

49. Cole DEC, Janicic N, Salisbury SR, Hendy, GN. Neonatal severe hyperparathyroidism, secondary hyperparathyroidism, and familial hypercalciuric hypercalcemia: multiple different phenotypes associated with an inactivating Alu insertion mutation of the calcium-sensing receptor gene. Am J Med Genet 1997; 71:202.

50. Pollak MR, Chou Y-HW, Marx SJ, et al. Familial hypocalciuric hypercalcemia and neonatal severe hyperparathyroidism. Effects of mutant gene dosage on phenotype. J Clin Invest 1994; 93:1108.

51. Bai M, Pearce SHS, Kifor O, et al. In vivo and in vitro characterization of neonatal hyperparathyroidism resulting from a de novo, heterozygous mutation in the $Ca^{2+}$-sensing receptor gene: normal maternal calcium homeostasis as a cause of secondary hyperparathyroidism in familial benign hypocalciuric hypercalcemia. J Clin Invest 1997; 99:88.

52. Pearce SHS, Williamson C, Kifor O, et al. A familial syndrome of hypocalcemia with hypercalciuria due to mutations in the calcium-sensing receptor. N Engl J Med 1996; 335:1115.

53. Cole DEC, Peltekova VD, Rubin LA, et al. A986S polymorphism of the calcium-sensing receptor and circulating calcium concentrations. Lancet 1999; 353:112.

54. Nemeth EF, Steffey ME, Hammerland LG, et al. Calcimimetics with potent and selective activity on the parathyroid calcium receptor. Proc Natl Acad Sci U S A 1998; 95:4040.

55. Silverberg SJ, Bone GH III, Marriott TB, et al. Short-term inhibition of parathyroid hormone secretion by a calcium-receptor agonist in patients with primary hyperparathyroidism. N Engl J Med 1997; 337:1506.

56. Kovacs CS, Ho-Pao CL, Hunzelman JL, et al. Regulation of murine fetal-placental calcium metabolism by the calcium-sensing receptor. J Clin Invest 1998; 101:2812.

57. Brown AJ, Zhong M, Ritter C, et al. Loss of calcium responsiveness in cultured bovine parathyroid cells is associated with decreased calcium receptor expression. Biochem Biophys Res Comm 1995; 212:861.

58. Mithal A, Kifor O, Kifor I, et al. The reduced responsiveness of cultured bovine parathyroid cells to extracellular $Ca^{2+}$ is associated with marked reduction in the expression of extracellular $Ca(^{2+})$-sensing receptor messenger ribonucleic acid and protein. Endocrinology 1995; 136:3087.

59. Russell J, Lettieri D, Sherwood LM. Direct regulation by calcium of cytoplasmic messenger ribonucleic acid coding for pre-proparathyroid hormone in isolated bovine parathyroid cells. J Clin Invest 1983; 72:1851.

60. Russell J, Sherwood LM. The effects of $1,25(OH)_2D_3$ and high calcium on transcription of the pre-proparathyroid hormone gene are direct. Trans Assoc Am Physicians 1987; 100:256.

61. Moallem E, Kilav R, Silver J, Naveh-Many T. RNA-protein binding and post-transcriptional regulation of parathyroid hormone gene expression by calcium and phosphate. J Biol Chem 1998; 273:5253.

62. Brown EM. Four-parameter model of the sigmoidal relationship between parathyroid hormone release and extracellular calcium concentration in normal and abnormal parathyroid tissue. Endocrinology 1983; 56:572.

63. Kifor O, Moore FD, Wang P, et al. Reduced immunostaining for the extracellular $Ca^{2+}$-sensing receptor in primary and secondary hyperparathyroidism. J Clin Endocrinol Metab 1996; 81:1598.

64. Ho C, Conner DA, Pollack MR, et al. A mouse model of human familial hypocalciuric hypercalcemia and neonatal severe hyperparathyroidism. Nature Genet 1995; 11:389.

65. Habener JF, Potts JT Jr. Relative effectiveness of magnesium and calcium on the secretion and biosynthesis of parathyroid hormone in vitro. Endocrinology 1976; 98:197.

66. Rude RK, Oldham SB, Sharp CF Jr, Singer FR. Parathyroid hormone secretion in magnesium deficiency. J Clin Endocrinol Metab 1978; 47:800.

67. Cholst IN, Steinberg SF, Tropper PJ, et al. The influence of hypermagnesemia on serum calcium and parathyroid hormone levels in human subjects. N Engl J Med 1984; 310:1221.

68. Morrissey J, Rothstein M, Mayer G, Slatopolsky E. Suppression of parathyroid hormone by aluminum. Kidney Int 1983; 23:699.

69. Sherwood LM, Mayer GP, Ramberg DF, et al. Regulation of parathyroid hormone secretion: proportional control by calcium, lack of effect of phosphate. Endocrinology 1968; 83:1043.

70. Almaden Y, Canelejo A, Hernandez A, et al. Direct effect of phosphorous on PTH secretion from whole rat parathyroid glands in vitro. J Bone Miner Res 1996; 11:970.

71. Slatopolsky E, Finch J, Denda M, et al. Phosphorous restriction prevents parathyroid gland growth: high phosphorous directly stimulates PTH secretion in vitro. J Clin Invest 1996; 97:2534.

72. Abe M, Sherwood LM. Regulation of parathyroid hormone secretion by adenylate cyclase. Biochem Biophys Res Commun 1972; 48:396.

73. Brown EM, Gardner DG, Windek RA, Aurbach GD. Relationship of intracellular 3',5'-adenosine monophosphate accumulation to parathyroid hormone release from dispersed bovine parathyroid cells. Endocrinology 1978; 103:2323.

74. Heath H III. Biogenic amines and the secretion of parathyroid hormone and calcitonin. Endocr Rev 1980; 1:319.

75. Epstein S, Heath H III, Bell NH. Lack of influence of isoproterenol, propranolol and dopamine on immunoreactive parathyroid hormone and calcitonin in normal man. Calcif Tissue Int 1983; 35:32.

76. Fasciotto BH, Gorr S-U, De Franco DJ, et al. Pancreastatin, a presumed product of chromogranin-A (secretory protein-1) processing, inhibits secretion from porcine parathyroid cells in culture. Endocrinology 1989; 125:1617.

77. Drees BM, Rouse J, Johnson J, Hamilton JW. Bovine parathyroid glands secrete a 26-kDa N-terminal fragment of chromogranin-A which inhibits parathyroid cell secretion. Endocrinology 1991; 129:3381.

78. Silver J, Russell J, Sherwood LM. Regulation by vitamin D metabolites of messenger ribonucleic acid for preproparathyroid hormone in isolated bovine parathyroid cells. Proc Natl Acad Sci U S A 1985; 82:4270.

79. Hendy GN, Stotland MS, Grunbaum D, et al. Characteristics of secondary hyperparathyroidism in vitamin D deficient dogs. Am J Physiol 1989; 256:E765.

80. Mackey SL, Heymont JL, Kronenberg HM, Demay MB. Vitamin D receptor binding to the negative human parathyroid hormone vitamin D response element does not require the retinoid x receptor. Molec Endocrinol 1996; 10:298.

81. Kremer R, Bolivar I, Goltzman D, Hendy GN. Influence of calcium and 1,25-dihdroxycholecalciferol on proliferation and proto-oncogene expression in primary cultures of bovine parathyroid cells. Endocrinology 1989; 125:935.

82. Fucik RF, Krukeja SC, Hargis GK, et al. Effect of glucocorticoids on function of the parathyroid glands in man. J Clin Endocrinol Metab 1975; 40:152.

83. Silverman R, Yalow RS. Heterogeneity of parathyroid hormone: clinical and physiologic studies. J Clin Invest 1973; 52:1958.

84. Segre GV, Niall HD, Habener JF, Potts JT Jr. Metabolism of parathyroid hormone: physiological and clinical significance. Am J Med 1974; 56:774.

85. Arnaud CD, Goldsmith RS, Bordier PJ, et al. Influence of immunoheterogeneity of circulating parathyroid hormone on radioimmunoassays of serum in man. Am J Med 1974; 56:785.

86. Reiss E, Canterbury JM. Emerging concepts of the nature of circulating parathyroid hormones: implications for clinical research. Recent Prog Horm Res 1974; 30:391.

87. Neuman WF, Neuman MW, Lane K, et al. The metabolism of labeled parathyroid hormone V. Collected biological studies. Calcif Tissue Res 1975; 18:271.

88. Martin KJ, Hruska KA, Freitag JJ, et al. The peripheral metabolism of parathyroid hormone. N Engl J Med 1979; 301:1092.

89. Segre GV, D'Amour P, Hultman A, Potts JT Jr. Effects of hepatectomy, nephrectomy, and nephrectomy/uremia on the metabolism of parathyroid hormone in the rat. J Clin Invest 1981; 67:439.

90. Papapoulos SE, Hendy GN, Tomlinson S, et al. Clearance of exogenous parathyroid hormone in normal and uraemic man. Clin Endocrinol 1977; 7:211.

91. Goltzman D, Henderson B, Loveridge N. Cytochemical bioassay of parathyroid hormone: characteristics of the assay and analysis of circulating hormonal forms. J Clin Invest 1980; 65:1309.

92. DeLuca HF. Recent advances in the metabolism of vitamin D. Ann Rev Physiol 1981; 43:199.

93. Parsons JA, Rafferty B, Gray D, et al. Pharmacology of parathyroid hormone and some of its fragments and analogues. In: Talmage RV, Owen M, Parsons JA, eds. Calcium-regulating hormones. Amsterdam: Excerpta Medica, 1975:33.

94. Tregear GW, van Rietschoten J, Greene E, et al. Bovine parathyroid hormone: minimum chain length of synthetic peptide required for biological activity. Endocrinology 1973; 93:1349.

95. Kemp BE, Moseley JM, Rodda CP, et al. Parathyroid hormone–related protein of malignancy: active synthetic fragments. Science 1987; 23:1568.

96. Horiuchi N, Caulfield MP, Fisher JE, et al. Similarity of synthetic peptide from human tumor to parathyroid hormone in vivo and in vitro. Science 1987; 23:1566.

97. Rabbani SA, Mitchell J, Roy DR, et al. Influence of the amino-terminus on in vitro and in vivo biological activity of synthetic parathyroid hormone–like peptides of malignancy. Endocrinology 1988; 123:2709.

98. Goltzman D, Peytremann A, Callahan E, et al. Analysis of the requirements for parathyroid hormone action in renal membranes with the use of inhibiting analogues. J Biol Chem 1975; 250:3199.

99. Nussbaum SR, Rosenblatt M, Potts JT Jr. Parathyroid hormone renal receptor interactions: demonstration of two receptor binding domains. J Biol Chem 1980; 255:10183.

100. Abou-Samra A-B, Uneno S, Jüppner H, et al. Non-homologous sequences of parathyroid hormone and the parathyroid hormone related peptide bind to a common receptor on ROS 17/2.8 cells. Endocrinology 1989; 125:2215.

101. Caulfield MP, McKee RL, Goldman ME, et al. The bovine renal parathyroid hormone (PTH) receptor has equal affinity for two different amino acid sequences: The receptor binding domains of PTH and PTH-related protein are located within the 14-34 region. Endocrinology 1990; 127: 83.

102. Klaus W, Dieckmann T, Wray V, et al. Investigation of the solution structure of the human parathyroid hormone fragment (1-34) by [1]H NMR spectros-

103. Cohen FE, Strewler GJ, Bradley MS, et al. Analogues of parathyroid hormone modified at positions 3 and 6: Effects on receptor binding and activation of adenylyl cyclase in kidney and bone. J Biol Chem 1991; 266:1997.

104. Barden JA, Kemp BE. Stabilized NMR structure of the hypercalcemia of malignancy peptide PTHrP [Ala-26](1-34) amide. Biochim Biophys Acta 1994; 1208:256.

105. Wray V, Federau T, Gronwald W, et al. The structure of human parathyroid hormone from a study of fragments in solution using 1H NMR spectroscopy and its biological implications. Biochemistry 1994; 33:1684.

106. Neugebauer W, Barbier J-R, Sung WL, et al. Solution structure and adenylyl cyclase stimulating activities of C-terminal truncated human parathyroid hormone analogues. Biochemistry 1995; 34:8835.

107. Maretto S, Mammi S, Bissacco E, et al. Mono- and bicyclic analogs of parathyroid hormone-related protein. 2. Conformational analysis of antagonists by CD, NMR, and distance geometry calculations. Biochemistry 1997; 36:3300.

108. Barbier J-R, Neugebauer W, Morley P, et al. Bioactivities and secondary stuctures of constrained analogues of human parathyroid hormone: cyclic lactams of the receptor binding region. J Medicinal Chem 1997; 40:1373.

109. Vickery BH, Avnur Z, Cheng Y, et al. RS-66271, a C-terminally substituted analog of human parathyroid hormone-related protein (1-34), increases trabecular and cortical bone in ovariectomized, osteopenic rats. J Bone Miner Res 1996; 11:1943.

110. Juppner H, Abou-Samra AB, Freeman MW, et al. A G protein–linked receptor for parathyroid hormone and parathyroid hormone–related peptide. Science 1991; 254:1024.

111. Abou-Samra AB, Jüppner H, Force T, et al. Expression cloning of a parathyroid hormone/parathyroid hormone-related peptide receptor from rat osteoblast-like cells: a single receptor stimulates intracellular accumulation of both cAMP and inositol triphosphate and increases intracellular free calcium. Proc Natl Acad Sci U S A 1992; 89:2732.

112. Pausova Z, Bourdon J, Clayton D, et al. Cloning of a parathyroid hormone/parathyroid hormone-related peptide receptor (PTHR) cDNA from a rat osteosarcoma (UMR 106) cell line: chromosomal assignment of the gene in the human, mouse, and rat genomes. Genomics 1994; 20:20.

113. Schipani E, Harga H, Karaplis AC, et al. Identical complementary deoxyribonucleic acids encode a human renal and bone parathyroid hormone (PTH)/PTH-related peptide receptor. Endocrinology 1993; 132:2157.

114. Fraher LJ, Hodsman AB, Jonas K, et al. A comparison of the in vivo biochemical responses to exogenous parathyroid hormone-(1–34) [PTH-(1–34)] and PTH-related peptide-(1–34) in man. J Clin Endocrinol Metab 1992; 75:417.

114a. Fraher LJ, Avram R, Watson PH, et al. Comparison of the biochemical responses to human parathyroid hormone-(1-31)NH₂ and hPTH-(1-34) in healthy humans. J Clin Endocrinol Metab 1999; 84:2739.

115. McCuaig KA, Clarke JC, White JH. Molecular cloning of the gene encoding the mouse parathyroid hormone/parathyroid hormone related peptide receptor. Proc Natl Acad Sci U S A 1994; 91:5051.

116. Bettoun JD, Minagawa M, Hendy GN, et al. Developmental upregulation of human parathyroid hormone (PTH)/PTH-related peptide receptor gene expression from conserved and human-specific promoters. J Clin Invest 1998; 102:958.

116a. Bettoun JD, Kwan MY, Minagawa M, et al. Methylation patterns of human parathyroid hormone (PTH)/PTH-related peptide receptor gene promoters are established several weeks prior to onset of their function. Biochem Biophys Res Commun 2000; 267:482.

117. Urena P, Kong X-F, Abou-Samra A-B, et al. Parathyroid hormone (PTH)/PTH-related peptide receptor messenger ribonucleic acids are widely distributed in rat tissues. Endocrinology 1993; 133:617.

118. Usdin TB, Gruber C, Bonner TI. Identification and functional expression of a receptor selectively recognizing parathyroid hormone, the PTH2 receptor. J Biol Chem 1995; 270:15455.

119. Lee CW, Gardella TJ, Abou-Samra AB, et al. Role of the extracellular regions of the PTH/PTHrP receptor in hormone-binding. Endocrinology 1994; 135:1488.

120. Lee CW, Luck MD, Jüppner H, et al. Homolog-scanning mutagenesis of the parathyroid hormone (PTH) receptor reveals PTH-(1-34) binding determinants in the third extracellular loop. Mol Endocrinol 1995; 9:1269.

121. Iida KA, Guo J, Takemura M, et al. Mutations in the second cytoplasmic loop of the rat parathyroid hormone (PTH)/PTH-related protein receptor result in selective loss of PTH-stimulated phospholipase C activity. J Biol Chem 1997; 272:6882.

122. Huang Z, Chen Y, Nissenson RA. The cytoplasmic tail of the G protein-coupled receptor for parathyroid hormone and parathyroid hormone-related protein contains positive and negative signals for endocytosis. J Biol Chem 1996; 270:151.

123. Mahoney CA, Nissenson RA. Canine renal receptors for parathyroid hormone: down-regulation in vivo by exogenous parathyroid hormone. J Clin Invest 1983; 72:411.

124. Forte LR, Langeluttig SG, Poelling RE, Thomas ML. Renal parathyroid hormone receptors in the chick: downregulation in secondary hyperparathyroid animal models. Am J Physiol 1982; 242:E154.

125. Tomlinson S, Hendy GN, Pemberton DM, O'Riordan JLH. Reversible resistance to the renal action of parathyroid hormone in man. Clin Sci Mol Med 1976; 51:59.

126. Schipani E, Weinstein LS, Bergwitz C, et al. Pseudohypoparathyroidism type 1b is not caused by a defect in the coding exons of the human parathyroid hormone (PTH)/PTH-related peptide gene. J Clin Endocrinol Metab 1995; 80:1611.

127. Bettoun JD, Minagawa M, Kwan MY, et al. Cloning and characterization of the promoter regions of the human parathyroid hormone (PTH)/PTH-related peptide receptor gene: analysis of deoxyribonucleic acid from normal subjects and patients with pseudohypoparathyroidism type 1b. J Clin Endocrinol Metab 1997; 82:1031.

128. Jüppner H, Schipani E, Bastepe M, et al. The gene responsible for pseudohypoparathyroidism type 1b is paternally imprinted and maps in four unrelated kindreds to chromosome 20q13.3. Proc Natl Acad Sci U S A 1998; 95:11798.

129. Yu S, Yu D, Lee E, et al. Variable and tissue-specific hormone resistance in heterotrimeric Gₛ protein α-subunit (Gₛα) knockout mice is due to tissue-specific imprinting of the Gₛα gene. Proc Natl Acad Sci U S A 1998; 95:8715.

130. Hayward BE, Moran V, Strain L, Bonthron DT. Bidirectional imprinting of a single gene: GNAS1 encodes maternally, paternally, and biallelically derived proteins. Proc Natl Acad Sci U S A 1998; 95:15475.

131. Jansen M. Über atypische Chondrodystrophie (Achondroplasie) und über eine noch nicht beschriebene angeborene Wachstumsstörung des Knochensystems: Metaphysäre Dysostosis. Orthop Chir 1934; 61:253.

132. Schipani E, Langman CB, Parfitt AM, et al. Constitutively activated receptors for parathyroid hormone-related peptide in Jansen's metaphyseal chondrodysplasia. N Engl J Med 1996; 335:708.

133. Blomstrand S, Claesson I, Save-Soderbergh J. A case of lethal congenital dwarfism with accelerated skeletal maturation. Pediatr Radiol 1985; 15:141.

134. Zhang P, Jobert A-S, Couvineau A, Silve C. A homozygous inactivating mutation in the parathyroid hormone/parathyroid hormone-related peptide receptor causing Blomstrand chondrodysplasia. J Clin Endocrinol Metab 1998; 83:3365.

135. Jobert A-S, Zhang P, Couvineau A, et al. Absence of functional receptors for parathyroid hormone and parathyroid hormone-related peptide in Blomstrand chondrodysplasia. J Clin Invest 1998; 102:34.

135a. Usdin TB, Hoare SR, Wang T, et al. TIP39: a new neuropeptide and PTH2-receptor agonist from hypothalamus. Nature Neuroscience 1999; 2:941.

136. Brenza HL, Kimmel-Jehan C, Jehan F, et al. Parathyroid hormone activation of the 25-hydroxyvitamin D₃-1 alpha-hydroxylase gene promoter. Proc Natl Acad Sci U S A 1998; 95:1387.

137. Livesey SA, Kemp BE, Re CA, et al. Selective hormonal activation of cyclic AMP-dependent protein-kinase isoenzymes in normal and malignant osteoblasts. J Biol Chem 1982; 257:14983.

138. Pearman AT, Chou WY, Bergman KD, et al. Parathyroid hormone induces c-fos promoter activity in osteoblastic cells through phosphorylated cAMP response element (CRE)-binding protein to the major CRE. J Biol Chem 1996; 271:25715.

139. Stern PH. Cationic agonists and antagonists of bone resorption. In: Cohn DV, Fujita T, Potts JT Jr, Talmage RV, eds. Endocrine control of bone and calcium metabolism. Amsterdam: Excerpta Medica, 1984:109.

140. Hruska KA, Moskowitz D, Esbrit P, et al. Stimulation of inositol triphosphate and diacylglycerol production in renal tubular cells by parathyroid hormone. J Clin Invest 1987; 79:230.

141. Bingham P, Brazell I, Owen M. The effect of parathyroid extract on cellular activity and plasma calcium levels in vivo. J Endocrinol 1969; 45:387.

142. Holtrop ME, Raisz LG, Simmons HA. The effect of parathyroid hormone, colchicine and calcitonin on the ultrastructure and activity of osteoblasts in organ culture. J Cell Biol 1974; 60:346.

143. Rouleau MF, Mitchell J, Goltzman D. In vivo distribution of parathyroid hormone receptors in bone. Evidence that a predominant osseous target cell is not the mature osteoblast. Endocrinology 1988; 123:187.

144. Rouleau MF, Warshawsky H, Goltzman D. Parathyroid hormone binding in vivo to renal, hepatic and skeletal tissues of the rat using a radioautographic approach. Endocrinology 1986; 118:919.

145. Rizzoli RE, Somerman M, Murray TM, Aurbach GD. Binding of radioiodinated parathyroid hormone to cloned bone cells. Endocrinology 1983; 113:1832.

146. Amizuka N, Karaplis AC, Henderson JE, et al. Haploinsufficiency of parathyroid hormone-related peptide (PTHrP) results in abnormal postnatal bone development. Dev Biol 1996; 175:166.

147. Takahashi N, Akatsu T, Udagawa N, et al. Osteoblastic cells are involved in osteoclast formation. Endocrinology 1988; 123:2600.

148. Lacey DL, Timms E, Tan HL, et al. Osteoprotegerin ligand is a cytokine that regulates osteoclast differentiation and activation. Cell 1998; 93:165.

149. Kong Y-Y, Yoshida H, Sarosi I, et al. OPGL is a key regulator of osteoclastogenesis, lymphocyte development and lymph-node organogenesis. Nature 1999; 397:315.

150. Simonet WS, Lacey DL, Dunstan CR, et al. Osteoprotegerin: A novel secreted protein involved in the regulation of bone density. Cell 1997; 89:309.

151. Parsons JA, Potts JT Jr. Physiology and chemistry of parathyroid hormone. In: MacIntyre I, ed. Clinics in endocrinology and metabolism, vol 1. Calcium metabolism and bone disease. London: WB Saunders, 1972:33.

152. Tam CS, Heersche JNM, Murray TM, Parsons JA. Parathyroid hormone stimulates the bone apposition rate independently of its resorptive action: differential effects of intermittent and continual administration. Endocrinology 1982; 110:506.

153. Corral DA, Amling M, Priemel M, et al. Dissociation between bone resorption and bone formation in osteopenic transgenic mice. Proc Natl Acad Sci U S A 1998; 95:13835.

154. Bijvoet OLM. Kidney function in calcium and phosphate metabolism. In: Avioli LV, Krane SM, eds. Metabolic bone disease, vol 1. New York: Academic Press, 1977:48.

155. Hartmann CM, Hewson AS, Kos CH, et al. Structure of murine and human renal type II Na⁺-phosphate cotransporter genes (Npt2 and NPT2). Proc Natl Acad Sci U S A 1996; 93:7409.

156. Azarani A, Goltzman D, Orlowski J. Structurally diverse N-terminal peptides of parathyroid hormone (PTH) and PTH-related peptide (PTHRP) inhibit the Na⁺/H⁺ exchanger NHE3 isoform by binding to the PTH/PTHRP receptor type I and activating distinct signalling pathways. J Biol Chem 1996; 271:14931.

157. Morel F. Regulation of kidney functions by hormones: a new approach. Recent Prog Horm Res 1983; 39:271.

158. Agus ZS, Wasserstein A, Goldfarb S. PTH, calcitonin, cyclic nucleotides and the kidney. Annu Rev Physiol 1981; 43:583.

159. Nordin BEC, Peacock M. Role of the kidney in regulation of plasma calcium. Lancet 1969; 2:1280.

160. Amizuka N, Warshawsky H, Henderson JE, et al. Parathyroid hormone-related peptide–depleted mice show abnormal epiphyseal cartilage development and altered endochondral bone formation J Cell Biol 1994; 126:1611.

161. Marx SJ, Sharp ME, Krudy A, et al. Radioimmunoassay for the middle region of human parathyroid hormone: studies with a radioiodinated synthetic peptide. J Clin Endocrinol Metab 1981; 53:76.

162. Papapoulos SE, Manning RM, Hendy GN, et al. Studies of circulating parathyroid hormone in man using a homologous amino-terminal specific immunoradiometric assay. Clin Endocrinol 1980; 13:57.

163. Nussbaum SR, Zahradnik RJ, Labigne JR, et al. A highly sensitive two-site immunoradiometric assay of parathyrin (PTH) and its clinical utility in evaluating patients with hypercalcemia. Clin Chem 1987; 33:1364.

164. Broadus AE. Nephrogenous cyclic AMP. Recent Prog Horm Res 1981; 37:667.

165. Nissenson RA, Abbott SR, Teitelbaum AP, et al. Endogenous biologically active human parathyroid hormone: measurement by a guanyl nucleotide-amplified renal adenylate cyclase assay. J Clin Endocrinol Metab 1981; 52:840.

166. Sato K, Han DC, Ozawa M, et al. A highly sensitive bioassay for PTH using ROS 17/2.8 subclonal cells. Acta Endocrinol (Copenh) 1987; 116:113.

167. Chambers DJ, Dunham J, Zanelli JM, et al. A sensitive bioassay of parathyroid hormone in plasma. Clin Endocrinol 1978; 9:375.

# CHAPTER 52

# PARATHYROID HORMONE–RELATED PROTEIN

GORDON J. STREWLER

Parathyroid hormone–related protein (PTHrP), sometimes referred to as *parathyroid hormone–like protein*, is the sister of PTH. Originally identified as the cause of humoral hypercalcemia in malignancy, PTHrP has a distinct set of physiologic functions that are unrelated to the regulation of systemic calcium homeostasis but rival the actions of PTH in their importance.

It has been recognized since Fuller Albright's time that in some ways patients with malignant tumors causing hypercalcemia resemble patients with primary hyperparathyroidism (pHPT). Malignancy-associated hypercalcemia is characterized not only by humorally mediated bone resorption but also by diminished tubule resorption of phosphate with consequent phosphaturia and hypophosphatemia. When it was recognized that the disorder also produced an increase in nephrogenous cyclic adenosine monophosphate (cAMP), which is the component of urinary cAMP secreted into the urine from the renal tubule,[1] it became clear that a humoral factor in patients with malignancy-associated hypercalcemia was mimicking PTH at the kidney. Increased nephrogenous cAMP was previously thought to be unique to hyperparathyroidism, reflecting increased secretion of cAMP from the renal tubule, where cAMP is the intracellular second messenger for PTH. Once it was understood that increased cAMP concentrations in kidney or bone cells could be used as a bioassay to detect the humoral factor secreted by malignant tumors, the substance responsible

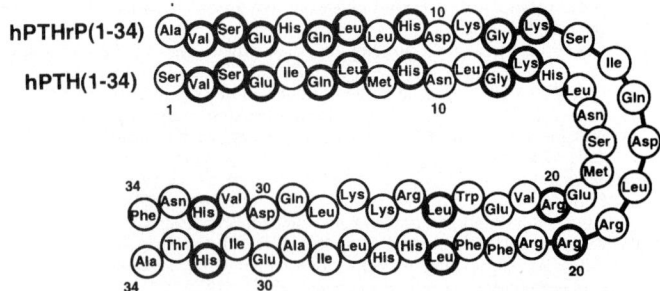

**FIGURE 52-1.** Primary structures of the aminoterminal part of parathyroid hormone–related protein and of parathyroid hormone. Compared are the human sequences 1–34. Identical amino acids are highlighted.

for malignancy-associated hypercalcemia was purified and shown to be a protein that was structurally related to PTH.[2–4]

## STRUCTURE AND BIOLOGIC PROPERTIES

### STRUCTURE AND PROCESSING OF PARATHYROID HORMONE–RELATED PROTEIN AND ITS GENE

PTHrP is a protein of 139 to 173 amino acids.[5–7] It resembles PTH in primary sequence only at the aminoterminus, where 8 of the first 13 amino acids in the two peptides are identical (Fig. 52-1). Although this is a limited region of homology, it is a critical region of both peptides; it is not required for binding but it is necessary for receptors occupied by either hormone to activate adenylate cyclase and hence to produce cAMP as a second messenger. Thus, the homology of PTH and PTHrP at the aminoterminal end is responsible for their shared biologic properties (see later in this chapter).

The gene for PTHrP is located on human chromosome 12. It is considerably more complex than the *PTH* gene, which is located on chromosome 11, with three promoters and four alternatively spliced exons upstream of the coding sequence.[8] The complexity of the promoter region allows for considerable flexibility in the regulation of *PTHrP* gene transcription. There is evidence that the promoters are used differentially in different tissues[8] and by the viral transactivating protein tax.[9]

Most of the prepro sequence of PTHrP is encoded on one exon, with the last 2 amino acids of the prepro sequence and 139 amino acids of the mature peptide encoded on a second exon. The splice junction between these two coding exons is precisely conserved between PTHrP and PTH. Downstream of the main coding sequence are two additional exons, which are alternatively spliced to contribute distinct carboxyterminal ends to the isoforms of PTHrP and distinct 3' noncoding sequences. The protein isoforms encoded by these exons are identical through amino acid 139 but comprise 139, 141, or 173 amino acids in toto. This downstream complexity of the *PTHrP* gene may also be used for regulation. The three transcript families with different 3' untranslated sequences have markedly different half-lives, ranging from 20 minutes to ~7 hours. In addition, their stability is differentially regulated. Exposure of cells to transforming growth factor-β specifically increases the half-life of the most unstable transcript, which encodes the 139 amino acid form of the protein.

It is clear from conservation of sequence, gene structure, and chromosomal localization that PTHrP and PTH arose from a common ancestral gene. In addition to the striking resemblance of their aminoterminal sequence and the conservation of the intron–exon boundaries between the two major coding exons, each gene is flanked by duplicated genes for lactate dehydrogenase. It is believed that chromosome 12, on which the *PTHrP* gene is located, and chromosome 11, where the *PTH* gene

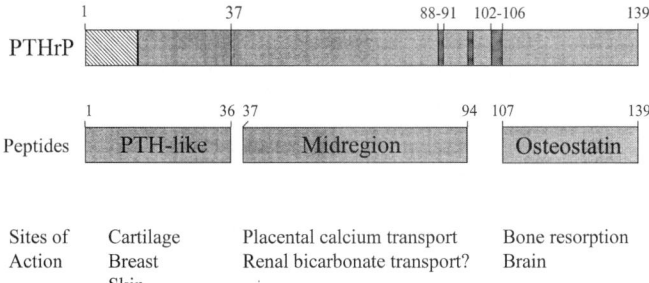

FIGURE 52-2. *Top,* Structural features of PTHrP. The PTH-homologous domain PTHrP(1–13) is delineated by hatched lines (▨), and potential cleavage sites are shown as vertical lines or crosshatched regions (▬). *Middle,* Peptides known or postulated to be derived from PTHrP. *Bottom,* Proven or postulated sites of action of individual PTHrP peptides are shown beneath each peptide.

resides, arose by an ancient duplication in which the ancestral *PTH/PTHrP* gene was evidently copied along with its neighbors.

## SECRETED FORMS: PEPTIDE HETEROGENEITY

The three mature PTHrP peptides predicted by cDNA are 139, 141, and 173 amino acids long. It is not clear whether any of them are secreted as intact proteins, although it seems likely they are.

### AMINOTERMINAL FRAGMENTS

The molecular size of PTHrP containing the bioactive aminoterminal part found in plasma and in tumor extracts ranges anywhere from 6 to 18 kDa,[2–4,10] and, apparently, several different aminoterminal fragments of PTHrP are secreted.[11] Three different cell types (renal carcinoma cells, PTHrP-transfected RIN-141 cells, and normal keratinocytes) use prohormone convertases to cleave PTHrP after arginine-37 to produce an aminoterminal fragment that is probably processed to PTHrP(1–36)[12] (Fig. 52-2). This aminoterminal PTHrP fragment contains the PTH-like region and could account completely for the PTH-like effects of PTHrP, as discussed later.

### MIDREGIONAL FRAGMENTS

The intracellular cleavage step at arginine-37 also produces midregional PTHrP fragments of ~50 to 70 amino acids beginning with alanine-38[12] (see Fig. 52-2). The carboxytermini of these fragments are located at amino acids 94, 95, and 101 in the highly basic region PTHrP(88–106).[13] Midregional fragments of PTHrP generated intracellularly can apparently enter the regulated pathway of peptide secretion and become packaged in dense neurosecretory granules, suggesting that they may be under separate secretory control from aminoterminal fragments.[12] Midregional PTHrP fragments of similar size are the predominant circulating forms in the plasma of patients with humoral hypercalcemia of malignancy.[14] These midregional PTHrPs play a physiologic role in transplacental calcium transport (see later), and synthetic midregion peptides also appear to have bioactivities in squamous carcinoma cells.

### CARBOXYTERMINAL FRAGMENTS

The size of the midregional fragments suggests the existence of additional carboxyterminal PTHrP fragments resulting from cleavage at the multibasic amino acid clusters at amino acids 88–106. Because the most carboxyterminal cleavage site is at amino acid 101, which precedes the lysine-arginine cluster at PTHrP(102–106), it is likely that carboxyterminal peptides such as PTHrP(107-139) are produced and secreted. Peptides with PTHrP(109–138) but not PTHrP(1–36) immunoreactivity have been found in sera of patients with humoral hypercalcemia of malignancy, and a peptide with PTHrP(109–138) immunoreac-

tivity circulates as a separate peptide that accumulates in patients with chronic renal failure.[10,15,16] The high degree of conservation between human, rat, and chicken PTHrP in the portion up to amino acid 111 suggests some biologic relevance of such peptides. The very carboxyterminal part of the conserved region, PTHrP(107–111), was found in several studies to be a potent inhibitor of osteoclastic bone resorption in vitro,[17,18] and has been given the name *osteostatin,* although this result has not been confirmed in all bone resorption assays.[19] The corresponding synthetic peptides (PTHrP[107–111] and PTHrP[107–139]) induce calcium transients in hippocampal neurons.[20]

PTHrP is posttranslationally modified in additional ways[21]; for example, PTHrP secreted by keratinocytes is glycosylated posttranslationally.[22] Whether this is also the case with other cell types and with PTHrP forms circulating in plasma is unknown.

The findings that cells process PTHrP to multiple peptide fragments, that some of these fragments may be under separate secretory control, and that one or more (in addition to its PTH-like aminoterminus) has its own bioactivity indicate that PTHrP is, like the adrenocorticotropic hormone-melanocyte-stimulating hormone–endorphin precursor pro-opiomelanocortin, a polyprotein precursor for multiple bioactive peptides.[23] The pattern of posttranslational modification may be tissue-specific, and this would add another dimension of specificity to the secreted forms of PTHrP.

## IMMUNOASSAYS

Because the known PTH-like bioactivity of PTHrP is located within the first 34 amino acids, most immunoassays have been directed against the aminoterminal sequence 1–34 to 1–40 of PTHrP in radioimmunoassays (RIAs)[24–26] or against larger fragments containing aminoterminal PTHrP in immunoradiometric assays.[16,27] Because the amounts of aminoterminal PTHrP extractable from normal serum are very low (<2.5 pmol/L),[26] prior extraction steps are often required to obtain clinically useful results with RIAs for aminoterminal PTHrP.[25,26] Typically, aminoterminal PTHrP is elevated in 60% to 80% of patients with hypercalcemia of malignancy and is undetectable in most healthy subjects (normal range, <2.5 pmol/L; Fig. 52-3).

As previously mentioned, a midregional PTHrP peptide is generated intracellularly and secreted. A RIA directed against a midregional epitope within the 53–84 region of PTHrP detects elevated PTHrP concentrations in the sera of ~80% of patients with hypercalcemia of malignancy.[28] The mean concentration of midregional PTHrP in these patients is ~50 pmol/L (see Fig. 52-3); this is ~10-fold higher than aminoterminal PTHrP concentrations.[25,26] Results with RIAs against this portion of PTHrP appear to be variable.[29,30] A RIA directed against a PTHrP epitope for the carboxyterminal (109–138) detected elevated levels in humoral hypercalcemia of malignancy but also revealed highly elevated levels in patients without malignancy who had chronic renal failure.[16] The 109–138 immunoreactive species appears to circulate as a separate carboxyterminal peptide.[10,15,16]

Assays with increased sensitivity and specificity have been developed by applying the two-site immunoradiometric assay technique to detect larger fragments containing aminoterminal and midregional PTHrP epitopes using PTHrP(1–74) to (1–86) standards.[16,27] Such two-site assays are now the preferred method for determining levels of circulating PTHrP. In patients with humoral hypercalcemia of malignancy, two-site assays usually detect elevated PTHrP serum concentrations in at least 80% of cases, with an average PTHrP concentration of 21 pmol/L (normal range, <5 pmol/L) in a typical assay (see Fig. 52-3), which is a range of concentrations similar to that detected by aminoterminal RIAs. Although such assays would fail to detect some bioactive aminoterminal fragments of PTHrP (e.g., PTHrP[1–36]), their performance in comparison to aminotermi-

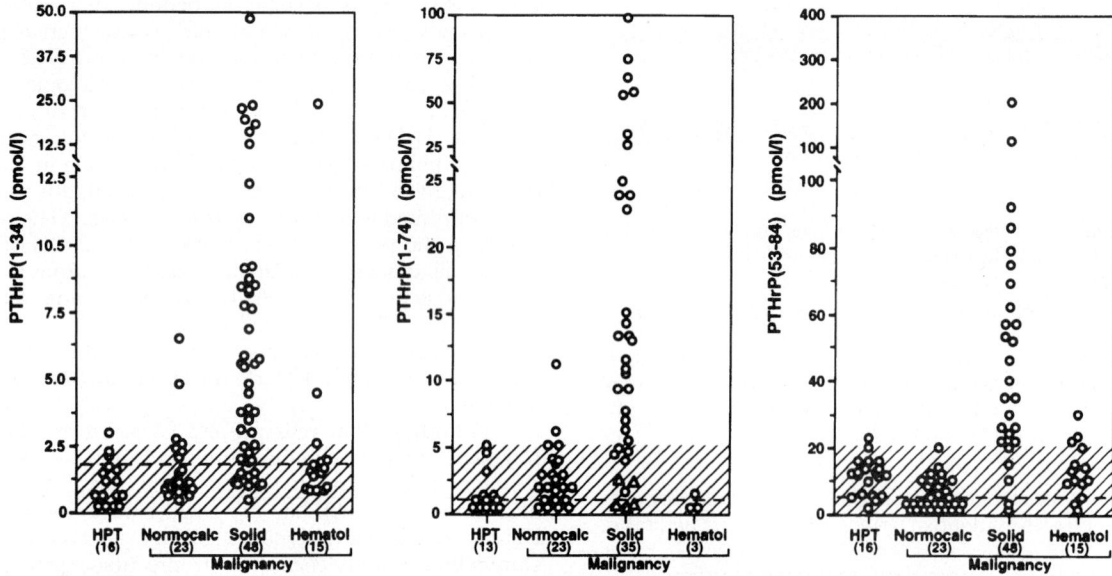

**FIGURE 52-3.** Plasma concentrations of parathyroid hormone–related protein (*PTHrP*) in patients with hyperparathyroidism (*HPT*), normocalcemic patients with malignancy (*Normocalc*), and patients with hypercalcemia of malignancy resulting from a solid tumor (*Solid*) or a hematologic malignancy (*Hematol*). Radioimmunoassay (*RIA*) for aminoterminal PTHrP(1–34) (*left panel*), an immunoradiometric assay (*IRMA*) for PTHrP(1–74) (*middle panel*), and an RIA for midregion PTHrP(53–84) (*right panel*). The hatched area represents the normal ranges, the dotted line the limits of detection, the numbers attached to each group indicate the number of patients. In the PTHrP(1–74) assay, the group *Solid* includes five patients classified as local osteolytic type of hypercalcemia (Δ) and two patients with lymphoma. Note the different scales of the Y-axes. (Modified from Budayr AA, Nissenson RA, Klein RF, et al. Increased serum levels of a parathyroid hormone-like protein in malignancy-associated hypercalcemia. Ann Intern Med 1989; 111:807; Burtis WJ, Brady TJ, Orloff JJ, et al. Immunochemical characterization of circulating parathyroid hormone-related protein in patients with humoral hypercalcemia of cancer. N Engl J Med 1990; 322:1106; and Blind E, Raue F, Götzmann J, et al. Circulating levels of midregional parathyroid hormone-related protein in hypercalcaemia of malignancy. Clin Endocrinol [Oxf] 1992; 37:290.)

nal RIAs in detecting PTHrP in patients with humoral hypercalcemia suggests that such fragments rarely predominate in tumor patients. Even the most sensitive assays of this type (reporting a lower limit of detection of 0.2 pmol/L) fail to detect PTHrP in at least half of normal people,[27,31] in contrast to the much higher normal range found for intact PTH in serum (1–6 pmol/L).

Direct comparison of PTHrP levels in different immunoassays shows heterogeneity of circulating forms secreted by individual tumors, which is consistent with the peptide's heterogeneity. Whether there are secretion patterns typical for certain tumors remains to be seen. Assay samples require the addition of proteinase inhibitors and rapid handling to avoid proteolysis after collection.[24,31] These assays are helpful in diagnosing humoral hypercalcemia of malignancy but not yet sufficiently sensitive to allow firm conclusions to be drawn about the presence or absence of PTHrP in the circulation of people under physiologic conditions.

## PARATHYROID HORMONE–RELATED PROTEIN RECEPTORS

Humoral hypercalcemia of malignancy shares several biochemical features with primary hyperparathyroidism (pHPT), closely reflecting the similarities of PTH and PTHrP action on bone and kidney. PTH and PTHrP bind with similar affinities to a shared receptor on osteoblast-like cells,[32–34] canine renal membranes,[33,35] and other tissues, owing to their homology in the aminoterminal portion (see Fig. 52-1). This adenylate cyclase-coupled receptor is a member of the family of G-protein coupled receptors[36] and is required for the developmentally crucial actions of PTHrP on the development of cartilage and bone, because ablation of the PTH/PTHrP receptor by homologous recombination produces a similar phenotype to ablation of the

PTHrP gene itself,[37] and expression of a constitutively active receptor produces a phenotype similar to overexpression of PTHrP.[38,39] In the brain,[40] in insulinoma cells,[41] and in skin,[42] there is evidence for receptors that are specific for aminoterminal PTHrP and do not recognize PTH. A receptor that is specific for PTH and does not recognize native PTHrP has been identified in brain by molecular cloning,[43] and the basis for its ligand specificity has been partially clarified.[44,45]

The observations that midregion PTHrP peptides have their own unique bioeffects (e.g., in the placenta,[46,47] as discussed later) clearly indicate that a separate receptor for midregion PTHrP must also exist. There is also evidence of a carboxyterminal PTHrP receptor in brain[20] and putatively in bone, where the carboxyterminal fragment of PTHrP (sometimes called *osteostatin*) appears to inhibit bone resorption.[18,48] Finally, as discussed later, some effects of PTHrP may result from direct intracrine actions in the nucleus of cells that secrete PTHrP,[49,50] and thus are possibly not mediated by a cell-surface receptor at all.

## BIOLOGIC PROPERTIES: ACTION ON BONE AND KIDNEY

Aminoterminal PTHrP is able to elicit the classic effects of PTH on target cells of calcium homeostasis. A number of studies have shown nearly identical effects with similar doses of aminoterminal fragments of PTH and PTHrP(1–34 to 1–40 region) on bone cells, such as stimulation of adenylate cyclase,[51–53] inhibition of alkaline phosphatase and growth, and activation of the intracellular calcium second messenger system.[54,55] In animals and in humans, aminoterminal PTHrP peptides reproduce the phosphaturic, hypocalciuric effects of PTH and activate the synthesis of 1,25-dihydroxyvitamin D.[51,53,56,57]

# ROLE OF PARATHYROID HORMONE–RELATED PROTEIN IN HYPERCALCEMIA

## TUMORS SECRETING PARATHYROID HORMONE–RELATED PROTEIN

The clinical manifestations of hypercalcemia in malignancy are discussed in Chapter 59. Here, evidence is presented on the involvement and the pathogenetic role of PTHrP.

### SOLID TUMORS

Elevated serum levels of PTHrP are found in ~80% of patients with solid tumors and hypercalcemia.[16,24–28,30,30a] PTHrP levels are almost always elevated in patients with hypercalcemia in the absence of bone metastasis (humoral hypercalcemia) and in solid tumors with squamous histologic features.[16,58] PTHrP secretion by tumor tissue should precede the development of hypercalcemia. Indeed, PTHrP elevations can be detected in a small percentage of cancer patients when they are still normocalcemic.[16,59]

### HUMORAL COMPONENT OF HYPERCALCEMIA

It was long assumed that in patients with radiologic evidence of extensive skeletal destruction by malignancy (especially in breast cancer), local osteolytic hypercalcemia was the mechanism responsible for hypercalcemia. A humoral form of the syndrome (humoral hypercalcemia of malignancy) was defined as hypercalcemia without bone metastasis. However, PTHrP levels are elevated with similar frequency in hypercalcemic patients with and without bone metastasis. In addition, the propensity of a given tumor type (e.g., lung cancer) to metastasize to bone is poorly correlated with the frequency of hypercalcemia; for example, tumors with small-cell histologic characteristics have the highest frequency of bone metastasis but rarely cause hypercalcemia. Thus, PTHrP can produce humoral hypercalcemia even in patients with bone metastases, and the diagnosis of humoral hypercalcemia in malignancy rests largely on the demonstration of elevated plasma PTHrP levels.

### BREAST CANCER

Hypercalcemia in breast cancer is most often seen in patients with extensive bone metastasis, but in 50% to 90%[16,24,26] of these patients, the serum PTHrP level is also elevated.[59] The finding that in breast cancer, hypercalcemia can occur in patients with or without increased circulating PTHrP levels suggests that hypercalcemia in breast carcinoma can have either a humoral or a local osteolytic cause. Fifty percent to 60% of breast cancer tissue is immunocytochemically positive for PTHrP,[59,60] but metastases in bone have been found to be PTHrP-positive (92%) more often than at other sites (17%).[61] This suggests that PTHrP may cause either local osteolytic hypercalcemia, when secreted at low levels from bone metastases, or humoral hypercalcemia, when secreted systemically at higher levels. Moreover, PTHrP-positive tumors may be more likely to metastasize to bone, possibly because of a survival advantage that results from the local osteolytic action of PTHrP. This possibility has been confirmed in an animal model of local osteolysis, in which introduction of PTHrP cDNA into breast cancer cells markedly increases the prevalence of lytic bone metastases.[62] This may have therapeutic consequences, because such a subgroup of patients could be treated prophylactically with bisphosphonates.[63] In addition, secretion of PTHrP may be activated in bone metastases by the local effects of bone matrix growth factors, such as transforming growth factor β, as shown in an animal model.[64] Approximately a century ago, Sir James Paget proposed that both seed and soil are important in bone metastasis, and the recent findings with regard to PTHrP illustrate this adage.

### HEMATOLOGIC MALIGNANCIES

PTHrP is rarely involved in the pathogenesis of hypercalcemia in hematologic malignancies. Multiple myeloma and lymphoma generally cause hypercalcemia by a local osteolytic mechanism, but humoral secretion of PTHrP is evident in a small fraction of hypercalcemic patients.[24,26,65] However, in the adult T-cell leukemia/lymphoma syndrome, which is caused by infection with the retrovirus human T-cell leukemia virus type 1 (HTLV-1), PTHrP-related hypercalcemia occurs in more than one-half of patients.[66–70] The tax protein encoded in the HTLV-1 genome can directly activate the PTHrP promoter,[9,71] and PTHrP expression in T lymphocytes may also be activated indirectly by HTLV-induced cytokines.[72,73]

## PATHOGENETIC ROLE OF PARATHYROID HORMONE–RELATED PROTEIN

Patients with humoral hypercalcemia of malignancy as well as normal persons infused with aminoterminal fragments of PTHrP[57,74] and animals treated with synthetic PTHrP show many of the hallmark effects of excess PTH, such as hypercalcemia, hypophosphatemia, hyperphosphaturia, elevated nephrogenous cAMP levels, and stimulation of osteoclastic bone resorption. PTHrP levels and calcium in plasma are positively correlated in patients with humoral hypercalcemia of malignancy, as are PTHrP levels and urinary cAMP concentrations.[16] Furthermore, the infusion of antibodies against PTHrP is able to reverse hypercalcemia and other manifestations in experimental humoral hypercalcemia of malignancy, including models in which human tumor cells produce hypercalcemia in nude mice.[75,76] Therefore, not only is PTHrP capable of producing hypercalcemia, but also secretion of PTHrP is necessary to develop hypercalcemia in such models.

To produce hypercalcemia in patients with hypercalcemia of malignancy, PTHrP may act in concert with bone-resorbing cytokines. Evidence from animal studies suggests that bone-resorbing factors such as tumor necrosis factor α may modulate hypercalcemia in humoral hypercalcemia of malignancy,[77] although there is little evidence that such factors by themselves cause humoral hypercalcemia of malignancy.

Some discrepancies exist between the clinical pictures of humoral hypercalcemia of malignancy and the PTH excess in pHPT with regard to bone and kidney. Although PTH and PTHrP act similarly on osteoblast-like cells in vitro, bone formation appears to be relatively lower in humoral hypercalcemia of malignancy than in pHPT,[78] although bone resorption is increased in both cases. Depressed bone formation in humoral hypercalcemia of malignancy may be caused by differences of action of PTHrP compared with PTH; but it may also result from the release of additional substances from tumors, such as cytokines, or it may be more indirectly caused by less specific effects of severe malignant disease.

Another discrepancy is the level of 1,25-dihydroxyvitamin D in the circulation: 1,25-dihydroxyvitamin D levels are often elevated in patients with pHPT but tend to be close to or below the lower limit of normal in hypercalcemia of malignancy.[1] Suppressed levels of 1,25-dihydroxyvitamin D in humoral hypercalcemia of malignancy (despite the presence of high PTHrP levels) rebound during calcium-lowering therapy, suggesting a dominance of inhibition of the renal 1α-hydroxylase by high serum calcium levels over the stimulatory effect of PTHrP.[79,80] As an underlying pathophysiologic mechanism, the existence of factors inhibiting the renal 1α-hydroxylase released by tumors has been suggested.[67]

Hypercalcemia of malignancy usually responds well to potent inhibitors of bone resorption, such as bisphosphonates, but some studies have shown that these substances are less effective in patients with increased serum PTHrP levels than in those with local osteolytic hypercalcemia.[81,82] Humoral hypercalcemia may be caused not only by bone resorption but also by increased calcium reabsorption by the kidney, owing to the hypocalciuric effect of PTHrP. The weaker response of patients with high PTHrP to bisphosphonates may be attributable to the effect of PTHrP-mediated renal calcium reabsorption on hypercalcemia in these patients, an effect that is not influenced by bisphosphonates. Additionally, high PTHrP levels may result in a more powerful stimulation of bone resorption, requiring higher doses of bisphosphonates.[82]

## USE OF PARATHYROID HORMONE–RELATED PROTEIN ASSAYS IN THE DIFFERENTIAL DIAGNOSIS OF HYPERCALCEMIA

PTHrP, as measured in immunoassays available today, is elevated in most patients with hypercalcemia caused by a solid tumor (see Fig. 52-3); an elevated PTHrP level can make a positive diagnosis of hypercalcemia of malignancy in ~80% of these patients. PTHrP levels are normal in almost all other causes of hypercalcemia, with rare exceptions, such as mammary hyperplasia (see later). However, to discriminate between pHPT and hypercalcemia of malignancy, the measurement of serum intact PTH is the variable of first choice. Although hypercalcemia is usually a complication of advanced malignancies that are obvious, a determination of intact PTH should be obtained on all patients because pHPT, which is a prevalent disorder, can present as an intercurrent illness in patients with malignancies. The demonstration of a suppressed or low-normal intact PTH level (<20 pg/mL) can exclude this possibility.

## ROLE OF PARATHYROID HORMONE–RELATED PROTEIN IN PHYSIOLOGY

Unlike PTH, whose expression is highly specific to the parathyroid glands, PTHrP is expressed in many tissues of fetuses and adults. These tissues include cartilage, bone, breast, skin, skeletal, heart and smooth muscle, uterus, and placenta. In addition, several endocrine organs—such as the fetal[83,84] and adult parathyroid,[85] fetal thyroid,[83] and pancreatic islets[86]—contain PTHrP transcripts or protein. In the central nervous system, PTHrP is expressed in neurons of the hippocampus, cerebral cortex, and cerebellar cortex.[87] Using the polymerase chain reaction, it has been shown that PTHrP expression is even more widespread.[88] This, together with the finding that the circulating level of PTHrP is significantly lower than that of PTH, suggests that PTHrP has protean tissue-specific functions, some of which are described here.

### CARTILAGE

The best understood action of PTHrP in normal physiology is as a regulator of cartilage growth and differentiation during the process of endochondral bone formation. The abolition of *PTHrP* gene expression by a targeted mutation of both PTHrP alleles produces embryonic lethality as the result of a severe disorder of cartilage development.[89] The limb bones are short, and there is a marked reduction in the width of the zone of proliferation of the growth plate, suggesting that the proliferation of growth plate chondrocytes is grossly impaired. In addition, endochondral bones in the skull base are heavily mineralized at birth, and the cranial vault is misshapen. The ribs are also prematurely mineralized, with a resultant decrease in the circumference of the chest cavity. Thus, the absence of PTHrP is associated with defective proliferation of chondrocytes and accelerated maturation to the hypertrophic stage, in which

chondrocytes mineralize their matrix. The converse phenotype is obtained when PTHrP is overexpressed in cartilage from a transgene driven by the cartilage-specific type II collagen promoter:[90] chondrocyte maturation is impaired, the growth plate is widened, and immature chondrocytes may be found within trabecular bone.

To carry out its actions in cartilage, PTHrP uses the shared PTH/PTHrP receptor, as evidenced by the similarity of phenotypes when PTHrP and the PTH/PTHrP receptor are ablated in mice[37] or in a rare human *chondrodysplasia*, the *Blomstrand type*.[91,92] Conversely, mutations that constitutively activate the PTH/PTHrP receptor inhibit chondrocyte maturation[38] and also induce life-long hypercalcemia, as reported in the human disorder *Jansen-type metaphysial chondrodysplasia*.[39]

As predicted from the sharing of a common receptor, PTH has most of the cartilage effects of PTHrP. PTH is a powerful mitogen for proliferating growth plate chondrocytes,[93,94] and it inhibits the mineralization of cartilage.[95] Yet PTH cannot substitute for the absence of PTHrP in PTHrP knockout mice. The common receptor in avascular cartilage may be relatively inaccessible to circulating PTH, compared with higher levels of PTHrP produced locally, and there may also be fewer PTH/PTHrP receptors in cartilage than in the primary target tissues of PTH, bone, and kidney.

PTHrP functions in endochondral bone formation as part of a feedback loop. Chondrocytes, which have just exited from the proliferative phase and begun to hypertrophy and terminally differentiate, produce the morphogen Indian hedgehog, a member of the hedgehog family of morphogens that regulate many important steps in vertebrate morphogenesis. Via its own receptor in the perichondrial layer surrounding the developing bone, Indian hedgehog signals for the secretion of PTHrP from proliferating chondrocytes, thus up-regulating the proliferation of cartilage cells and keeping them out of the terminal differentiation program.[37,96] The effect of the Indian hedgehog-PTHrP system is to relay a signal from mature cells back to the zone of decision. This feedback loop regulates the rate of entry into the differentiation pathway and thereby ensures that proliferation and maturation of chondrocytes is balanced and that cells are synchronized as they enter the last phase of their life, so that the linear growth of bone is orderly. This conclusion is supported by studies of chimeric mice in which clones of PTH/PTHrP receptor (−/−) cells are present in developing cartilage. These cells differentiate prematurely, activate the PTHrP-Indian hedgehog axis, and slow the differentiation of surrounding normal chondrocytes.[97]

To make available for study PTHrP knockout mice, they have been rescued from lethality by crossing heterozygotes for the PTHrP null genotype with transgenic mice in which expression either of PTHrP[98] or of a constitutively active PTH/PTHrP receptor[38] has been directed to cartilage. This produces some offspring, which express PTHrP or its constitutively active receptor in cartilage only, thus rescuing them from the fatal chondrodysplasia, while allowing study of the PTHrP null phenotype in other tissues.

### BREAST

Breast development in the PTHrP knockout mouse does not progress beyond the earliest stages of ingrowth of the mammary epithelial rudiment, which normally expresses PTHrP, into the underlying mesenchyme, which normally expresses its receptor[98] (see Fig. 52-2). This suggests that PTHrP is one of the signals in the complex interactions of epithelium and mesenchyme that underlie breast development. Restoration of PTHrP to mammary epithelium can be accomplished by a strategy similar to the rescue of PTHrP knockout mice, by crossing rescued PTHrP knockout mice with mice that express PTHrP constitutively in the mammary epithelium,[99] thus resulting in a mouse that produces PTHrP only in cartilage (thus, ensuring its survival) and the ingrowing mammary rudiment. This strategy restores the ingrowth of the breast bud, but the nipple still does not develop normally.[98] It should be possible to analyze the role of PTHrP in epithelial-mesenchymal signaling in detail by reconstituting explants of epithelium and mesenchyme from animals with differing genetic backgrounds.

The role of PTHrP in the breast is not confined to the developmental period. Glandular epithelial cells of the lactating breast as well as myoepithelial cells produce large amounts of PTHrP. This has led to the proposal that PTHrP may be the long-postulated signal that is responsible for the adaptation of maternal calcium metabolism to the stress of lactation. A nursing mother secretes gram quantities of calcium into milk to mineralize the skeleton of her offspring; in multiparous animals, lactation presents a particular challenge to calcium homeostasis. Yet the adaptation to this challenge does not seem to require any of the hormones of calcium homeostasis: a mother can successfully suckle her offspring in the face of calcium deficiency, hypoparathyroidism, or vitamin D deficiency, sacrificing a large portion of her skeletal mineral to do so.[100] Hypoparathyroid mothers can even maintain normocalcemia during lactation, but thereafter must return to vitamin D supplementation.[101] Some workers have reported detectable levels of PTHrP in the serum of nursing mothers.[102,103] However, even when detected, the levels of PTHrP are very low, and the level of PTH is not suppressed in lactation, as expected in the face of PTHrP-induced bone resorption. It remains to be shown conclusively that PTHrP is the long-sought lactational signal. Nonetheless, mammary PTHrP can probably produce systemic effects, because PTHrP levels are increased in rare syndromes of hypercalcemia associated with lactation[104] and massive mammary hypertrophy.[105]

In all mammalian and marsupial species that have been tested, PTHrP is found in milk at enormous levels—~10,000 times higher than the serum level.[58,106] The production of PTHrP during lactation is under the control of prolactin,[107] and the protein is secreted into milk by the glandular epithelial cells of the lactating mammary gland. This recapitulates for the nursing newborn the environment of its developing gut in utero, because amniotic fluid swallowed by the fetus also contains high levels of PTHrP.[108] It is possible that PTHrP plays a physiologic role in the developing alimentary tract or is absorbed to fulfill other functions. Receptors for PTHrP are present in the intestinal epithelium.[109] However, infants raised on soy-based formulas that do not contain PTHrP are healthy. It therefore appears that PTHrP in milk is dispensable.

## SKIN

One prominent site of normal production of PTHrP is the epidermis. The activation of the gene in epidermal keratinocytes probably accounts for the frequency of PTHrP-induced hypercalcemia in squamous carcinomas, which arise from this cell type. Expression of PTHrP seems to control the size of the proliferative pool of basal keratinocytes, from which keratinocytes exit to undergo terminal differentiation, keratinization, and programmed cell death. This pool is increased when PTHrP is overexpressed in the skin, but is diminished in rescued PTHrP knockout mice, with a reciprocal increase in granular cells that have entered the differentiation pathway, suggesting that in postnatal mice PTHrP regulates epidermal cell traffic in much the same way that it does in endochondral ossification prenatally.[110] PTHrP is also produced by cells of the inner root sheath of the hair follicle. The PTH/PTHrP receptor is present in the underlying dermis. Treatment with a PTHrP antagonist enhances entry of hair follicles into anagen, the active phase of hair growth.[111] This is another example of epithelial-mesenchymal interactions in which PTHrP serves as the messenger.

## TEETH

Rescue of PTHrP knockout mice, as previously described, discloses a failure of tooth eruption, which can be attributed to the absence of another epithelial-mesenchymal interaction. The formation of the teeth appears normal, but PTHrP is absent from the enamel epithelium, which caps the tooth rudiment as it pushes its way through the overlying alveolar bone to erupt. Restoration of PTHrP expression to enamel epithelium, using a strategy similar to those previously described, in which PTHrP is directed to this cell layer by a tissue-specific promoter, restores tooth eruption.[112] This implies that PTHrP secreted by the epithelial layer is normally targeted to receptors in the overlying bone, where it activates resorption of alveolar bone by osteoclasts to allow passage of the tooth. The signaling circuit in alveolar bone is distinctive, because there is no general defect in osteoclast function in transgenic mice. If present, impaired osteoclast function would produce generalized osteopetrosis.

## SMOOTH MUSCLE

PTHrP is a vasodilator[113,114] and also relaxes bladder, gastric, duodenal, and uterine smooth muscle beds.[115–117] The expression of PTHrP is increased in several types of smooth muscle by mechanical stretch[115] or by treatment with vasoconstrictors, such as angiotensin II.[118] Together, these findings raise the possibility that PTHrP released in response to increased smooth muscle tone acts locally to relax smooth muscle in a short-loop negative feedback system.[119,120] In keeping with this hypothesis, transgenic mice that overexpress PTHrP in vascular smooth muscle manifest a reduction in blood pressure.[121] This circuitry could be operative in the heart, in which PTHrP is released by atrial and ventricular myocytes[122] and has a positive chronotropic effect as well as a positive inotropic effect that probably results from coronary vasodilation.[123,124] PTHrP is also released from stromal cells of the spleen and other organs in response to endotoxic shock[125]; neutralization of PTHrP effects with antibodies prolongs survival after administration of lethal doses of endotoxin.[126]

In the arterial wall, PTHrP is expressed in proliferating vascular smooth muscle cells in culture[118] and after balloon angioplasty in vivo.[127] The level of PTHrP is increased in atherosclerotic coronary arteries.[128] Exposure of rat vascular smooth muscle cells to PTHrP has an antimitotic effect, suggesting that locally released PTHrP might act to throttle the response to a proliferative stimulus.[118] In contrast, when transfected into A10 rat vascular smooth muscle cells, PTHrP markedly induces proliferation.[49] The proliferative response does not occur with transfection of mutant forms of PTHrP from which polybasic amino acid sequences between residues 88 and 106 have been deleted. These sequences have been shown to function as nuclear localization sequences in other cells[50,129]; wild-type PTHrP, but not the deletion mutants, is targeted to the nucleus of A10 cells. It thus appears possible that in addition to binding to cell-surface receptors, PTHrP can have direct nuclear actions, termed *intracrine* actions. Because secreted fragments of PTHrP and its intracrine actions appear to have opposing effects on proliferation, PTHrP could interplay in a complex fashion with other proliferative factors in determining the response of the vascular wall to injury or atherosclerosis.

## UTERUS AND PLACENTA

In the human uteroplacental unit, PTHrP is expressed at high levels in the amniotic sac (as well as chorion, placenta, and decidua) and is secreted into the amniotic fluid.[108] The expression of PTHrP in amnion as well as rat myometrium[115] appears to be sensitive to stretch, and PTHrP in turn could modulate smooth muscle tone. Both fetal skin and the fetal gastrointestinal tract are exposed to high concentrations of PTHrP through at least the last half of pregnancy; thus, PTHrP could have a developmental function in these tissues.

The placenta maintains a calcium gradient by actively pumping calcium into the fetal circulation.[130] This gradient is abolished by fetal parathyroidectomy and in PTHrP knockout mice.[131] The transport of calcium can be restored by infusion of midregional fragments of PTHrP (e.g., PTHrP[46–68]), but not by aminoterminal PTHrP or by PTH.[46,47,131] As discussed in a previous section, this provides strong evidence for a distinct receptor for the midregion domain and establishes that PTHrP is a polyhormone. The fetus uses a midregion peptide from PTHrP for the regulation of systemic calcium economy, rather than the PTH-like aminoterminal domain. In so doing the fetus makes use of midregion PTHrP, perhaps secreted from the parathyroid gland (which expresses PTHrP[83,84]) in much the same way that PTH is used in the postnatal state.

# REFERENCES

1. Stewart AF, Horst R, Deftos LJ, et al. Biochemical evaluation of patients with cancer-associated hypercalcemia: evidence for humoral and non-humoral groups. N Engl J Med 1980; 303:1377.
2. Moseley JM, Kubota M, Diefenbach-Jagger H. Parathyroid hormone-related protein purified from a human lung cancer cell line. Proc Natl Acad Sci U S A 1987; 84:5048.
3. Strewler GJ, Stern PH, Jacobs JW. Parathyroid hormone-like protein from human renal carcinoma cells: structural and functional homology with parathyroid hormone. J Clin Invest 1987; 80:1803.
4. Stewart AF, Wu T, Goumas D, et al. N-terminal amino acid sequence of two novel tumor-derived adenylate cyclase-stimulating proteins: identification of parathyroid hormone-like and parathyroid hormone-unlike domains. Biochem Biophys Res Commun 1987; 146:672.
5. Thiede MA, Strewler GJ, Nissenson RA, et al. Human renal carcinoma expresses two messages encoding a parathyroid hormone-like peptide: evidence for the alternative splicing of a single-copy gene. Proc Natl Acad Sci U S A 1988; 85:4605.
6. Suva LJ, Winslow GA, Wettenhall RE, et al. A parathyroid hormone-related protein implicated in malignant hypercalcemia: cloning and expression. Science 1987; 237:893.
7. Mangin M, Webb AC, Dreyer BE, et al. Identification of a cDNA encoding a parathyroid hormone-like peptide from a human tumor associated with humoral hypercalcemia of malignancy. Proc Natl Acad Sci U S A 1988; 85:597.
8. Broadus A, Stewart A. Parathyroid hormone-related protein: structure, processing, and physiological actions. In: Bilezikian J, Levine M, Marcus R, eds. The parathyroids. New York: Raven Press, 1994:259.
9. Dittmer J, Gitlin SD, Reid RL, Brady JN. Transactivation of the P2 promoter of parathyroid hormone-related protein by human T-cell lymphotropic virus type I Tax1: evidence for the involvement of transcription factor Ets1. J Virol 1993; 67:6087.
10. Burtis WJ, Fodero JP, Gaich G, et al. Preliminary characterization of circulating amino- and carboxy-terminal fragments of parathyroid hormone-related peptide in humoral hypercalcemia of malignancy. J Clin Endocrinol Metab 1992; 75:1110.
11. Soifer NE, Stewart AF. Measurement of PTH-related protein and the role of PTH-related protein in malignancy-associated hypercalcemia. In: Halloran BP, Nissenson RA, eds. Parathyroid hormone-related protein: normal physiology and its role in cancer. Boca Raton: CRC Press, 1992.
12. Soifer NE, Stewart AF. Measurement of PTH-related protein and the role of PTH-related protein in malignancy-associated hypercalcemia. In: Halloran BP, Nissenson RA, eds. Parathyroid hormone-related protein: normal physiology and its role in cancer. Boca Raton: CRC Press, 1992:93.
13. Wu TL, Vasavada RC, Yang K, et al. Structural and physiologic characterization of the mid-region secretory species of parathyroid hormone-related protein. J Biol Chem 1996; 271:24371.
14. Burtis WJ, Dann P, Gaich GA, Soifer NE. A high abundance midregion species of parathyroid hormone-related protein: immunological and chromatographic characterization in plasma. J Clin Endocrinol Metab 1994; 78:317.
15. Orloff JJ, Soifer NE, Fodero JP, et al. Accumulation of carboxy-terminal fragments of parathyroid hormone-related protein in renal failure. Kidney Int 1993; 43:1371.
16. Burtis WJ, Brady TG, Orloff JJ, et al. Immunochemical characterization of circulating parathyroid hormone-related protein in patients with humoral hypercalcemia of cancer. N Engl J Med 1990; 322:1106.
17. Fenton AJ, Kemp BE, Hammonds RG Jr, et al. A potent inhibitor of osteoclastic bone resorption within a highly conserved pentapeptide region of parathyroid hormone-related protein; PTHrP[107-111]. Endocrinology 1991; 129:3424.
18. Cornish J, Callon KE, Nicholson GC, et al. Parathyroid hormone-related protein-(107-139) inhibits bone resorption in vivo. Endocrinology 1997; 138:1299.
19. Sone T, Kohno H, Kikuchi H, et al. Human parathyroid hormone-related peptide-(107-111) does not inhibit bone resorption in neonatal mouse calvariae. Endocrinology 1992; 131:2742.
20. Fukayama S, Tashjian AH Jr, Davis JN, et al. Signaling by N- and C-terminal sequences of parathyroid hormone-related protein in hippocampal neurons. Proc Natl Acad Sci U S A 1995; 92:10182.
21. Orloff JJ, Reddy D, de Papp AE, et al. Parathyroid hormone-related protein as a prohormone: posttranslational processing and receptor interactions. Endocr Rev 1994; 15:40.
22. Wu TL, Soifer NE, Burtis WJ, et al. Glycosylation of parathyroid hormone-related peptide secreted by human epidermal keratinocytes. J Clin Endocrinol Metab 1991; 73:1002.
23. Wysolmerski JJ, Stewart AF. The physiology of parathyroid hormone-related protein—an emerging role as a developmental factor. Annu Rev Physiol 1998; 60:431.
24. Grill V, Ho P, Body JJ, et al. Parathyroid hormone-related protein: elevated levels in both humoral hypercalcemia of malignancy and hypercalcemia complicating metastatic breast cancer. J Clin Endocrinol Metab 1991; 73:1309.
25. Kao PC, Klee GG, Taylor RL, Heath H III. Parathyroid hormone-related peptide in plasma of patients with hypercalcemia and malignant lesions. Mayo Clin Proc 1990; 65:1399.
26. Budayr AA, Nissenson RA, Klein RF, et al. Increased serum levels of a parathyroid hormone-like protein in malignancy-associated hypercalcemia. Ann Intern Med 1989; 111:807.
27. Ratcliffe WA, Norbury S, Heath DA, Ratcliffe JG. Development and validation of an immunoradiometric assay of parathyrin-related protein in unextracted plasma. Clin Chem 1991; 37:678.
28. Blind E, Raue F, Götzmann J, et al. Circulating levels of midregional parathyroid hormone-related protein in hypercalcaemia of malignancy. Clin Endocrinol (Oxf) 1992; 37:290.
29. Bucht E, Eklund A, Toss G, et al. Parathyroid hormone-related peptide, measured by a midmolecule radioimmunoassay, in various hypercalcaemic and normocalcaemic conditions. Acta Endocrinol (Copenh) 1992; 127:294.
30. Ratcliffe WA, Norbury S, Stott RA, et al. Immunoreactivity of plasma parathyrin-related peptide: three region-specific radioimmunoassays and a two-site immunoradiometric assay compared. Clin Chem 1991; 37:1781.
30a. Motellon JL, Javort Jiminez JF, deMiguel F, et al. Parathyroid hormone-related protein, parathyroid hormone, and vitamin D in hypercalcemia of malignancy. Clin Chim Acta 2000; 290:189.
31. Pandian MR, Morgan CH, Carlton E, Segre GV. Modified immunoradiometric assay of parathyroid hormone-related protein: clinical application in the differential diagnosis of hypercalcemia. Clin Chem 1992; 38:282.
32. Shigeno C, Yamamoto I, Kitamura N, et al. Interaction of human parathyroid hormone-related peptide with parathyroid hormone receptors in clonal rat osteosarcoma cells. J Biol Chem 1988; 263:18369.
33. Nissenson RA, Diep D, Strewler GJ. Synthetic peptides comprising the amino-terminal sequence of a parathyroid hormone-like protein from human malignancies: binding to parathyroid hormone receptors and activation of adenylate cyclase in bone cells and kidney. J Biol Chem 1988; 263:12866.
34. Jüppner H, Abou-Samra A, Uneno S, et al. The parathyroid hormone-like peptide associated with humoral hypercalcemia of malignancy and parathyroid hormone bind to the same receptor on the plasma membrane of ROS 17/2.8 cells. J Biol Chem 1988; 263:8557.
35. Orloff JJ, Wu TL, Heath HW, et al. Characterization of canine renal receptors for the parathyroid hormone-like protein associated with humoral hypercalcemia of malignancy. J Biol Chem 1989; 264:6097.
36. Lanske B, Kronenberg HM. Parathyroid hormone-related peptide (PTHrP) and parathyroid hormone (PTH)/PTHrP receptor. Crit Rev Eukaryot Gene Expr 1998; 8:297.
37. Lanske B, Karaplis AC, Lee K, et al. PTH/PTHrP receptor in early development and Indian hedgehog-regulated bone growth. Science 1996; 273:663.
38. Schipani E, Lanske B, Hunzelman J, et al. Targeted expression of constitutively active receptors for parathyroid hormone and parathyroid hormone-related peptide delays endochondral bone formation and rescues mice that lack parathyroid hormone-related peptide. Proc Natl Acad Sci U S A 1997; 94:13689.
39. Schipani E, Langman CB, Parfitt AM, et al. Constitutively activated receptors for parathyroid hormone and parathyroid hormone-related peptide in Jansen's metaphyseal chondrodysplasia. N Engl J Med 1996; 335:708.
40. Yamamoto S, Morimoto I, Yanagihara N, et al. Parathyroid hormone-related peptide-(1-34) [PTHrP-(1-34)] induces vasopressin release from the rat supraoptic nucleus in vitro through a novel receptor distinct from a type I or type II PTH/PTHrP receptor. Endocrinology 1997; 138:2066.
41. Gaich G, Orloff JJ, Atillasoy EJ, et al. Amino-terminal parathyroid hormone-related protein: Specific binding and cytosolic calcium responses in rat insulinoma cells. Endocrinology 1993; 132:1402.
42. Orloff JJ, Ganz MB, Ribaudo AE, et al. Analysis of PTHrP binding and signal transduction mechanisms in benign and malignant squamous cells. Am J Physiol 1992; 262:E599–E607.
43. Usdin TB, Gruber C, Bonner TI. Identification and functional expression of a receptor selectively recognizing parathyroid hormone, the PTH2 receptor. J Biol Chem 1995; 270:15455.
44. Behar V, Nakamoto C, Greenberg Z, et al. Histidine at position 5 is the specificity "switch" between two parathyroid hormone receptor subtypes. Endocrinology 1996; 137:4217.

45. Gardella TJ, Luck MD, Jensen GS, et al. Converting parathyroid hormone-related peptide (PTHrP) into a potent PTH-2 receptor agonist. J Biol Chem 1996; 271:19888.

46. Abbas SK, Pickard DW, Rodda CP, et al. Stimulation of ovine placental calcium transport by purified natural and recombinant parathyroid hormone-related protein (PTHrP) preparations. Q J Exp Physiol 1989; 74:549.

47. Care AD, Abbas SK, Pickard DW, et al. Stimulation of ovine placental transport of calcium and magnesium by mid-molecule fragments of human parathyroid hormone-related protein. Exp Physiol 1990; 75:605.

48. Fenton AJ, Kemp BE, Kent GN, et al. A carboxyl-terminal peptide from the parathyroid hormone-related protein inhibits bone resorption by osteoclasts. Endocrinology 1991; 129:1762.

49. Massfelder T, Dann P, Wu TL, et al. Opposing mitogenic and anti-mitogenic actions of parathyroid hormone-related protein in vascular smooth muscle cells—a critical role for nuclear targeting. Proc Natl Acad Sci U S A 1997; 94:13630.

50. Henderson JE, Amizuka N, Warshawsky H, et al. Nucleolar localization of parathyroid hormone-related peptide enhances survival of chondrocytes under conditions that promote apoptotic cell death. Mol Cell Biol 1995; 15:4064.

51. Horiochi N, Caulfield MP, Fisher JE, et al. Similarity of synthetic peptide from human tumor to PTH in vivo and in vitro. Science 1987; 238:1566.

52. Kemp BE, Moseley JM, Rodda CP, et al. Parathyroid hormone-related protein of malignancy: active synthetic fragments. Science 1987; 238:1568.

53. Stewart AF, Mangin M, Wu T, et al. A synthetic human parathyroid hormone-like protein stimulates bone resorption and causes hypercalcemia in rats. J Clin Invest 1988; 81:596.

54. Civitelli R, Martin TJ, Fausto A, et al. Parathyroid hormone-related peptide transiently increases cytosolic calcium in osteoblast-like cells: comparison with parathyroid hormone. Endocrinology 1989; 125:1204.

55. Yamada H, Tsutsumi M, Fukase M, et al. Effects of human PTH-related peptide and human PTH on cyclic AMP production and cytosolic free calcium in an osteoblastic cell clone. Bone Miner 1989; 6:45.

56. Yates AJ, Gutierrez GE, Smolens P, et al. Effects of a synthetic peptide of a parathyroid hormone-related protein on calcium homeostasis, renal tubular calcium reabsorption, and bone metabolism in vivo and in vitro in rodents. J Clin Invest 1988; 81:932.

57. Fraher LJ, Hodsman AB, Jonas K, et al. A comparison of the in vivo biochemical responses to exogenous parathyroid hormone-(1-34) [PTH-(1-34)] and PTH-related peptide-(1-34) in man. J Clin Endocrinol Metab 1992; 75:417.

58. Budayr AA, Halloran BP, King JC, et al. High levels of a parathyroid hormone-like protein in milk. Proc Natl Acad Sci U S A 1989; 86:7183.

59. Bundred NJ, Ratcliffe WA, Walker RA, et al. Parathyroid hormone related protein and hypercalcemia in breast cancer. BMJ 1991; 303:1506.

60. Southby J, Kissin MW, Danks JA, et al. Immunohistochemical localization of parathyroid hormone-related protein in human breast cancer. Cancer Res 1990; 50:7710.

61. Powell GJ, Southby J, Danks JA, et al. Localization of parathyroid hormone-related protein in breast cancer metastases: increased incidence in bone compared with other sites. Cancer Res 1991; 51:3059.

62. Guise TA, Yin JJ, Taylor SD, et al. Evidence for a causal role of parathyroid hormone-related protein in the pathogenesis of human breast cancer-mediated osteolysis. J Clin Invest 1996; 98:1544.

63. Heath DA. Parathyroid hormone related protein. Clin Endocrinol (Oxf ) 1993; 38:135.

64. Yin JJ, Selander K, Chirgwin JM, et al. TGF-β signaling blockade inhibits PTHrP secretion by breast cancer cells and bone metastases development. J Clin Invest 1999; 103:197.

65. Firkin F, Seymour JF, Watson AM, et al. Parathyroid hormone-related protein in hypercalcaemia associated with haematological malignancy. Br J Haematol 1996; 94:486.

66. Fukumoto S, Matsumoto T, Ikeda K, et al. Clinical evaluation of calcium metabolism in adult T-cell leukemia/lymphoma. Arch Intern Med 1988; 148:921.

67. Fukumoto S, Matsumoto T, Yamoto H, et al. Suppression of serum 1,25-dihydroxyvitamin D is caused by elaboration of a factor that inhibits renal 1,25-dihydroxyvitamin $D_3$ production. Endocrinology 1989; 124:2057.

68. Motokura T, Fukumoto S, Takahashi S, et al. Expression of parathyroid hormone-related protein in a human T cell lymphotrophic virus type I-infected T cell line. Biochem Biophys Res Commun 1988; 154:1182.

69. Motokura T, Fukumoto S, Matsumoto T, et al. Parathyroid hormone-related protein in adult T-cell leukemia-lymphoma. Ann Intern Med 1989; 111:484.

70. Ikeda K, Ohno H, Hane M, et al. Development of a sensitive two-site immunoradiometric assay for parathyroid hormone-related peptide: evidence for elevated levels in plasma from patients with adult T-cell leukemia/lymphoma and B-cell lymphoma. J Clin Endocrinol Metab 1994; 79:1322.

71. Watanabe T, Yamaguchi K, Takatsuki K, et al. Constitutive expression of parathyroid hormone-related protein gene in human T cell leukemia virus type 1 (HTLV-1) carriers and adult T cell leukemia patients that can be trans-activated by HTLV-1 tax gene. J Exp Med 1990; 172:759.

72. Ikeda K, Okazaki R, Inoue D, et al. Interleukin-2 increases production and secretion of parathyroid hormone-related peptide by human T cell leukemia virus type I-infected T cells: possible role in hypercalcemia associated with adult T cell leukemia. Endocrinology 1993; 132:2551.

73. Ikeda K, Okazaki R, Inoue D, et al. Transcription of the gene for parathyroid hormone-related peptide from the human is activated through a cAMP-dependent pathway by prostaglandin E1 in HTLV-I-infected T cells. J Biol Chem 1993; 268:1174.

74. Henry JG, Mitnick M, Dann PR, et al. Parathyroid hormone-related protein-(1-36) is biologically active when administered subcutaneously to humans. J Clin Endocrinol Metab 1997; 82:900.

75. Kukreja SC, Shevrin DH, Wimbiscus SA, et al. Antibodies to parathyroid hormone-related protein lower serum calcium in athymic mouse models of malignancy-associated hypercalcemia due to human tumors. J Clin Invest 1988; 82:1798.

76. Kukreja SC, Rosol TJ, Wimbiscus SA, et al. Tumor resection and antibodies to parathyroid hormone-related protein cause similar changes on bone histomorphometry in hypercalcemia of cancer. Endocrinology 1990; 127:305.

77. Guise TA, Yoneda T, Yates AJ, Mundy GR. The combined effect of tumor-produced parathyroid hormone-related protein and transforming growth factor-alpha enhance hypercalcemia in vivo and bone resorption in vitro. J Clin Endocrinol Metab 1993; 77:40.

78. Stewart A, Vignery A, Silverglate A, et al. Quantitative bone histomorphometry in humoral hypercalcemia of malignancy: uncoupling of bone cell activity. J Clin Endocrinol Metab 1982; 55:219.

79. Budayr AA, Zysset E, Jenzer A, et al. Effects of treatment of malignancy-associated hypercalcemia on serum parathyroid hormone-related protein. J Bone Miner Res 1994; 9:521.

80. Schilling T, Pecherstorfer M, Blind E, et al. Parathyroid hormone-related protein (PTHrP) does not regulate 1,25-dihydroxyvitamin D serum levels in hypercalcemia of malignancy. J Clin Endocrinol Metab 1993; 76:801.

81. Blind E, Raue F, Meinel T, et al. Levels of parathyroid hormone-related protein (PTHrP) in hypercalcemia of malignancy are not lowered by treatment with the biphosphonate BM 21.0955. Horm Metab Res 1993; 25:40.

82. Dodwell DJ, Abbas SK, Morton AR, Howell A. Parathyroid hormone-related protein[50-69] and response to pamidronate therapy for tumour-induced hypercalcemia. Eur J Cancer 1991; 27:1629.

83. Moseley JM, Hayman JA, Danks JA, et al. Immunohistochemical detection of parathyroid hormone-related protein in human fetal epithelia. J Clin Endocrinol Metab 1991; 73:478.

84. Rodda CP, Kubota M, Heath JA, et al. Evidence for a novel parathyroid hormone-related protein in fetal lamb parathyroid glands and sheep placenta: comparisons with a similar protein implicated in humoral hypercalcaemia of malignancy. J Endocrinol 1988; 117:261.

85. Ikeda K, Arnold A, Mangin M, et al. Expression of transcripts encoding a parathyroid hormone-related peptide in abnormal human parathyroid tissues. J Clin Endocrinol Metab 1989; 69:1240.

86. Drucker DJ, Asa SL, Henderson J, Goltzman D. The parathyroid hormone-like peptide gene is expressed in the normal and neoplastic human endocrine pancreas. Mol Endocrinol 1989; 3:1589.

87. Weir EC, Brines ML, Ikeda K, et al. Parathyroid hormone-related peptide gene is expressed in the mammalian central nervous system. Proc Natl Acad Sci U S A 1990; 87:108.

88. Selvanayagam P, Graves K, Cooper C, Rajaraman S. Expression of the parathyroid hormone-related peptide gene in rat tissues. Lab Invest 1991; 64:713.

89. Karaplis AC, Luz A, Glowacki J, et al. Lethal skeletal dysplasia from targeted disruption of the parathyroid hormone-related peptide gene. Genes Dev 1994; 8:277.

90. Weir EC, Philbrick WM, Amling M, et al. Targeted overexpression of parathyroid hormone-related peptide in chondrocytes causes chondrodysplasia and delayed endochondral bone formation. Proc Natl Acad Sci U S A 1996; 93:10240.

91. Jobert AS, Zhang P, Couvineau A, et al. Absence of functional receptors for parathyroid hormone and parathyroid hormone-related peptide in Blomstrand chondrodysplasia. J Clin Invest 1998; 102:34.

92. Zhang P, Jobert AS, Couvineau A, et al. A homozygous inactivating mutation in the parathyroid hormone/parathyroid hormone-related peptide receptor causing Blomstrand chondrodysplasia. J Clin Endocrinol Metab 1998; 83:3365.

93. Crabb ID, O'Keefe RJ, Puzas JE, Rosier RN. Differential effects of parathyroid hormone on chicken growth plate and articular chondrocytes. Calcif Tissue Int 1992; 50:61.

94. Koike T, Iwamoto M, Shimazu A, et al. Potent mitogenic effects of parathyroid hormone (PTH) on embryonic chick and rabbit chondrocytes: differential effects of age on growth, proteoglycan, and cyclic AMP responses of chondrocytes to PTH. J Clin Invest 1990; 85:626.

95. Kato Y, Shimazu A, Nakashima K, et al. Effects of parathyroid hormone and calcitonin on alkaline phosphatase activity and matrix calcification in rabbit growth-plate chondrocyte cultures. Endocrinology 1990; 127:114.

96. Vortkamp A, Lee K, Lanske B, et al. Regulation of rate of cartilage differentiation by Indian hedgehog and PTH-related protein. Science 1996; 273:613.

97. Chung UI, Lanske B, Lee K, et al. The parathyroid hormone/parathyroid hormone-related peptide receptor coordinates endochondral bone development by directly controlling chondrocyte differentiation. Proc Natl Acad Sci U S A 1998; 95:13030.

98. Wysolmerski JJ, Philbrick WM, Dunbar ME, et al. Rescue of the parathyroid hormone-related protein knockout mouse demonstrates that parathyroid hormone-related protein is essential for mammary gland development. Development 1998; 125:1285.

99. Wysolmerski JJ, McCaughern-Carucci, Daifotis AG, et al. Overexpression of parathyroid hormone-related protein or parathyroid hormone in trans-

genic mice impairs branching morphogenesis during mammary gland development. Development 1995; 121:3539.

100. Kovacs CS, Kronenberg HM. Maternal-fetal calcium and bone metabolism during pregnancy, puerperium, and lactation. Endocr Rev 1997; 18:832.

101. Mather KJ, Chik CL, Corenblum B. Maintenance of serum calcium by parathyroid hormone-related peptide during lactation in a hypoparathyroid patient. J Clin Endocrinol Metab 1999; 84:424.

102. Grill V, Hillary J, Ho PMW, et al. Parathyroid hormone-related protein; a possible endocrine function in lactation. Clin Endocrinol (Oxf ) 1992; 37:405.

103. Sowers MF, Hollis BW, Shapiro B, et al. Elevated parathyroid hormone-related peptide associated with lactation and bone density loss. JAMA 1996; 276:549.

104. Lepre F, Grill V, Ho PW, et al. Hypercalcemia in pregnancy and lactation associated with parathyroid hormone-related protein. N Engl J Med 1993; 328:666.

105. Braude S, Graham A, Mitchell D. Lymphoedema/hypercalcaemia syndrome mediated by parathyroid-hormone-related protein. Lancet 1991; 337:140.

106. Thurston AW, Cole JA, Hillman LS, et al. Purification and properties of parathyroid hormone-related peptide isolated from milk. Endocrinology 1990; 126:1183.

107. Thiede MA. The mRNA encoding a parathyroid hormone-like peptide is produced in mammary tissue in response to elevations in serum prolactin. Mol Endocrinol 1989; 3:1443.

108. Ferguson JE II, Gorman JV, Bruns DE, et al. Abundant expression of parathyroid hormone-related protein in human amnion and its association with labor. Proc Natl Acad Sci U S A 1992; 89:8384.

109. Li H, Seitz PK, Thomas ML, et al. Widespread expression of the parathyroid hormone-related peptide and PTH/PTHrP receptor genes in intestinal epithelial cells. Lab Invest 1995; 73:864.

110. Foley J, Longely BJ, Wysolmerski JJ, et al. PTHrP regulates epidermal differentiation in adult mice. J Invest Dermatol 1998; 111:1122.

111. Holick MF, Ray S, Chen TC, et al. A parathyroid hormone antagonist stimulates epidermal proliferation and hair growth in mice. Proc Natl Acad Sci U S A 1994; 91:8014.

112. Philbrick WM, Dreyer BE, Nakchbandi IA, et al. Parathyroid hormone-related protein is required for tooth eruption. Proc Natl Acad Sci U S A 1998; 95:11846.

113. Roca-Cusachs A, DiPette DJ, Nickols GA. Regional and systemic hemodynamic effects of parathyroid hormone-related protein: preservation of cardiac function and coronary and renal flow with reduced blood pressure. J Pharmacol Exp Ther 1991; 256:110.

114. Winquist RJ, Baskin EP, Vlasuk GP. Synthetic tumor-derived human hypercalcemic factor exhibits parathyroid hormone-like vasorelaxation in renal arteries. Biochem Biophys Res Commun 1987; 149:227.

115. Thiede MA, Daifotis AG, Weir EC, et al. Intrauterine occupancy controls expression of the parathyroid hormone-related peptide gene in preterm rat myometrium. Proc Natl Acad Sci U S A 1990; 87:6969.

116. Mok LL, Ajiwe E, Martin TJ, et al. Parathyroid hormone-related protein relaxes rat gastric smooth muscle and shows cross-desensitization with parathyroid hormone. J Bone Miner Res 1989; 4:433.

117. Mok LL, Cooper CW, Thompson JC. Parathyroid hormone and parathyroid hormone-related peptide inhibit phasic contraction of pig duodenal smooth muscle. Proc Soc Exp Biol Med 1989; 191:337.

118. Pirola CJ, Wang HM, Kamyar A, et al. Angiotensin II regulates parathyroid hormone-related protein expression in cultured rat aortic smooth muscle cells through transcriptional and post-transcriptional mechanisms. J Biol Chem 1993; 268:1987.

119. Massfelder T, Helwig JJ, Stewart AF. Parathyroid hormone-related protein as a cardiovascular regulatory peptide. Endocrinology 1996; 137:3151.

120. Massfelder T, Fiaschitaesch N, Stewart AF, et al. Parathyroid hormone-related peptide-a smooth muscle tone and proliferation regulatory protein. [Review.] Curr Opin Nephrol Hyperten 1998; 7:27.

121. Maeda S, Sutliff RL, Qian J, et al. Targeted overexpression of parathyroid hormone-related protein (PTHrP) to vascular smooth muscle in transgenic mice lowers blood pressure and alters vascular contractility. Endocrinology 1999; 140:1815.

122. Deftos LJ, Burton DW, Brandt DW. Parathyroid hormone-like protein is a secretory product of atrial myocytes. J Clin Invest 1993; 92:727.

123. Ogino K, Burkhoff D, Bilezikian JP. The hemodynamic basis for the cardiac effects of parathyroid hormone (PTH) and PTH-related protein. Endocrinology 1995; 136:3024.

124. Hara M, Liu YM, Zhen LC, et al. Positive chronotropic actions of parathyroid hormone and parathyroid hormone-related peptide are associated with increases in the current, I-F, and the slope of the pacemaker potential. Circulation 1997; 96:3704.

125. Funk JL, Krul EJ, Moser AH, et al. Endotoxin increases parathyroid hormone-related protein mRNA levels in mouse spleen. Mediation by tumor necrosis factor. J Clin Invest 1993; 92:2546.

126. Funk JL, Moser AH, Strewler GJ, et al. Parathyroid hormone-related protein is induced during lethal endotoxemia and contributes to endotoxin-induced mortality in rodents. Molecular Medicine 1996; 2:204.

127. Ozeki S, Ohtsuru A, Seto S, et al. Evidence that implicates the parathyroid hormone-related peptide in vascular stenosis-increased gene expression in the intima of injured rat carotid arteries and human restenotic coronary lesions. Arterioscler Thromb Vascul Biol 1996; 16:565.

128. Nakayama T, Ohtsuru A, Enomoto H, et al. Coronary atherosclerotic smooth muscle cells overexpress human parathyroid hormone-related peptides. Biochem Biophys Res Commun 1994; 200:1028.

129. Aarts MM, Levy D, He B, et al. Parathyroid hormone-related protein interacts with RNA. J Biol Chem 1999; 274:4832.

130. Strenler GJ. The philosophy of parathyroid hormone-related protein. N Engl J Med 2000; 342:177.

131. Kovacs CS, Lanske B, Hunzelman JL, et al. Parathyroid hormone-related peptide (PTHrP) regulates fetal-placental calcium transport through a receptor distinct from the PTH/PTHrP receptor. Proc Natl Acad Sci U S A 1996; 93:15233.

# CHAPTER 53

# CALCITONIN GENE FAMILY OF PEPTIDES

KENNETH L. BECKER, BEAT MÜLLER, ERIC S. NYLÉN, RÉGIS COHEN, OMEGA L. SILVA, JON C. WHITE, AND RICHARD H. SNIDER, JR.

The calcitonin gene family consists of five genes (*CALC-I* to *CALC-V*) that are located on chromosome 11 (*CALC-I*, *CALC-II*, *CALC-III*, and *CALC-V*) and on chromosome 12 (*CALC-IV*). In humans, the mRNAs arising from these genes generate multiple peptides, including calcitonin (CT), calcitonin gene–related peptide (CGRP), amylin, adrenomedullin (ADM), and various circulating precursor and derivative peptides, some of which may have biologic functions (Fig. 53-1).[1–5]

Several common features characterize the calcitonin gene family of peptides (Fig. 53-2). CT, the CGRPs, amylin, and ADM all contain two N-terminal cysteines that form a disulfide bridge resulting in a ring structure at the amino terminus. In addition, the carboxy-terminal amino acid of *all* these peptides is amidated. When the sequences of CT, CGRP, and amylin are aligned with a gap introduced in the CT sequence to maximize homology, the 12 identical matches and five conservative amino-acid substitutions suggest gene duplication of a common ancestral gene. Furthermore, the midregions of CGRP, CT, amylin, and ADM form an α-helical structure. Finally, the CT gene family peptides exert their overlapping bioeffects by *binding to the same family of receptors.*

## CALCITONIN

For reasons that are elucidated later, the following discussion distinguishes between CT and its precursor peptides (CTpr), which have been found to have important clinical and biologic functions. CT is initially biosynthesized as a larger precursor, procalcitonin (ProCT; Fig. 53-3), which is enzymatically cleaved into aminoprocalcitonin (NProCT) and the conjoined calcitonin:calcitonin carboxypeptide-I (CT:CCP-I), some of which, in turn, is further enzymatically processed to yield free immature CT and CCP-I. Immature CT is then amidated to yield the mature CT. (Procalcitonin and its subsequent posttranslational processing are discussed later.)

In this chapter, unless otherwise stated, the term *CT, without further qualification, refers to the mature amidated hormone* (molecular mass 3.42 kDa). The term *immunoreactive calcitonin (iCT)* is used to indicate either that the material being detected immunologically is not the mature hormone (i.e., it is incompletely processed CT or prohormone) or that in the particular referenced study, its precise molecular structure has not been determined or clarified. One should keep in mind that nearly all studies have used methodologies that do *not* distinguish mature CT from immature CT or CTpr and were performed before the distinct biologic functions of the various CT peptides were known. This important limitation should be kept in mind when scientific data of tissue distribution, control of secretion, and bioeffects are interpreted.

*Immature CT* is a 33-amino-acid glycine-terminated peptide contained initially within the procalcitonin molecule. In the peripheral blood of normal persons, however, immature CT is found within the procalcitonin molecule as a separate peptide in which it is conjoined to the calcitonin carboxy-terminal peptide (CCP-I), and also as the free 33-amino-acid peptide.

*Mature CT* is a free 32-amino-acid peptide terminating in an amidated proline. As with many other peptides, this amidation is important to the bioactivity of the hormone (see Chap. 167).

CT, in evolutionary terms, is a very conserved ancestral hormone that is found in primitive protochordate marine animals. Although the midportion of the hormone varies considerably among different species, common characteristics include the disulfide bond between the cysteine residues at the amino-terminal positions 1 and 7 and a carboxy-terminal proline amide. Of the known CTs, hamster and rat CT are the closest to the human form, differing by only two amino acids. Despite species differences, all of the CTs are bioactive in laboratory animals, although their potency and time curve of action vary with the receptor affinity and the rate of degradation.

## DISTRIBUTION OF CALCITONIN

The principal source of the iCT found in mammalian serum is probably the C cells. In submammals (e.g., birds, fish, amphibians, reptiles), the thyroidal C cells occur within a discrete, separate ultimobranchial gland. During early embryogenesis, CT-containing cells migrate from the neural crest to this gland. In humans and other mammals, however, the ultimobranchial gland subsequently fuses with the thyroid gland (Fig. 53-4). In the human, the C cells (also called parafollicular cells) are found in the central portion of each lateral lobe (see Chap. 29). Within the mammalian thyroid gland, these cells constitute an endocrine system that is quite separate from the thyroid follicular cells.

In addition to the thyroid gland, iCT is found in many other tissues, such as the lungs, adrenal medulla, hypothalamus, pituitary gland, thymus, parathyroid glands, and the gastrointestinal and genitourinary tracts.[6] In part, these tissue levels reflect the production of the hormone by their constituent neuroendocrine cells (see Chap. 175). However, nonneuroendocrine cells may contain low levels of iCT. Immunoreactive CT is found in the blood, urine, bile, gastric juice, and seminal fluid, and the concentration is particularly high in milk.

The wide distribution of iCT is similar to that of several other peptides of the diffuse neuroendocrine system (see Chap. 175) (e.g., somatostatin, cholecystokinin, mammalian bombesin, neurotensin) that were originally thought to emanate from a single tissue. In mammals, a large contribution to serum iCT is made by the C cells of the thyroid gland, and the responsivity of the mature CT to induced hypercalcemia appears to reside mostly within these cells.

The highest concentration of CT in the body is found within the C-cell region of the thyroid gland. Within the lung, iCT is found in the pulmonary neuroendocrine (PNE) cells, and in humans, more iCT is found within the lungs than in the thyroid gland[7]; however, the extent to which extrathyroidal neuroendocrine production of CT contributes to circulating levels of the hormone is uncertain. Although the thyroid C cells originate from the neural crest, the iCT-containing cells of the gut and respiratory tract probably arise embryologically from a different source. (For a discussion of iCT in extrathyroidal tissues, see later in section Calcitonin Precursors and Derivative Peptides.)

## CONTROL OF CALCITONIN SECRETION

The secretory control of CT is poorly understood. The physiologic secretagogues probably *vary with the location of the hormone*. Because of the hypocalcemic effects of pharmacologic doses of the hormone, early experiments searching for a possible feedback mechanism had focused on the stimulatory influence of increased serum calcium on iCT secretion.[8] The relationship between serum calcium and iCT secretion is not consistent, however, and small, sudden changes of endogenous circulating calcium do not influence the serum hormone levels in humans.

Hypermagnesemia but not hyperphosphatemia induces iCT release from the thyroid gland.[9] Various hormones are known to release thyroidal iCT, some of them involving cyclic AMP (cAMP); usually, these effects are induced by pharmacologic concentrations, and whether these responses are physiologically relevant in humans is unknown. These substances include cholecystokinin, cerulein, secretin, glucagon, and gastrin. Physiologically, modulation by the sympathetic nervous system may be important because β-adrenergic agonists may induce secretion, and β-adrenergic antagonists and α-adrenergic agonists may diminish iCT secretion. Within the lung, the iCT of the pulmonary neuroendocrine cells is released by a nicotinic-cholinergic mechanism.[10,11]

Factors that decrease iCT secretion include dopamine, somatostatin, and the $H_2$-receptor blocker, cimetidine.

## EFFECTS OF CALCITONIN

Despite hundreds of studies, the physiologic role of CT remains unclear. Many of the investigations used pharmacologic doses of the hormone. The studies used different in vivo and in vitro models that employed different species of the hormone and different species of animals. The full bioeffects of CT require the presence of the disulfide bridge and an intact $NH_2$-terminal end, and the majority of pharmacologic studies have used the "mature" (processed and amidated) forms of CT.

Although multiple target tissues have been identified, bones, the gastrointestinal tract, the kidneys, and the central nervous system appear to be particularly important.

### BONE EFFECTS

The osseous effect of CT is related to its *inhibition of osteoclast function*, which causes diminished bone resorption (Fig. 53-5).[12] In addition, some data suggest that CT may also exert stimulatory effects on osteoblasts.[13] In vivo, in most animals, the administration of large amounts of CT induces hypocalcemia and hypophosphatemia, an effect that is attributed to the decreased bone resorption. In vitro, CT protects against the bone-resorbing effects of parathyroid hormone, prostaglandins, and vitamin A. In humans, however, CT does not appear to play a role in the fine regulation of serum calcium. Thus, although the hormone may prevent a postprandial increase in serum calcium in some animals, this is not true in the human adult.

An effect of CT that may indirectly impact bone metabolism is its apparent influence on vitamin D metabolism; in some species, the hormone stimulates formation of 1,25-dihydroxyvitamin D, which increases intestinal absorption of calcium.[14]

In humans, neither endogenous hypercalcitonemia (e.g., in medullary thyroid cancer [MTC]) nor diminished CT (e.g., in total thyroidectomy) is associated with alterations of serum calcium, nor are any marked effects seen on osseous metabolism. Accordingly, some researchers have postulated that the main function of CT in relation to calcium metabolism is to protect the skeleton during times of increased need, such as during growth, pregnancy, or lactation. The hormone may also combat postprandial hypercalcemia in the newborn.[15]

# A. Human *CALC-I* Gene

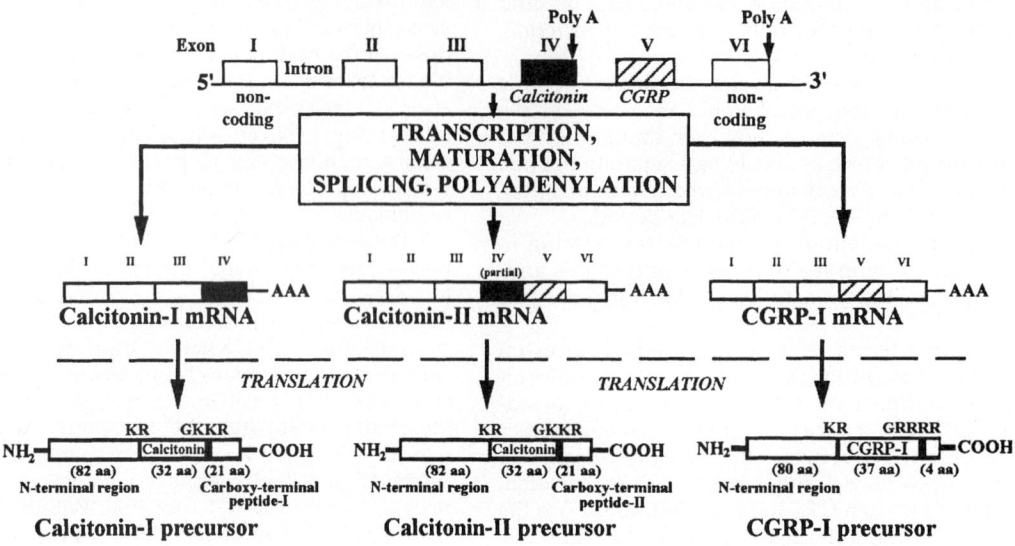

# B. Human *CALC-II* Gene

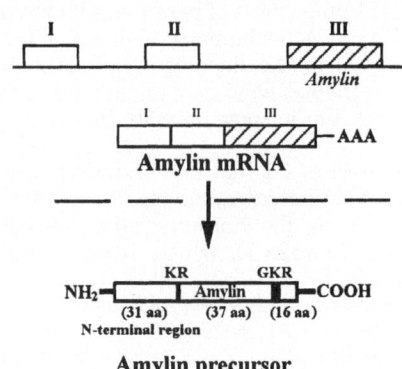

# C. Human *CALC-III* Gene

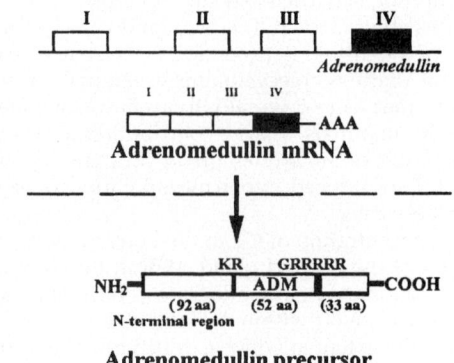

# D. Human *CALC-IV* Gene

# E. Human *CALC-V* Gene

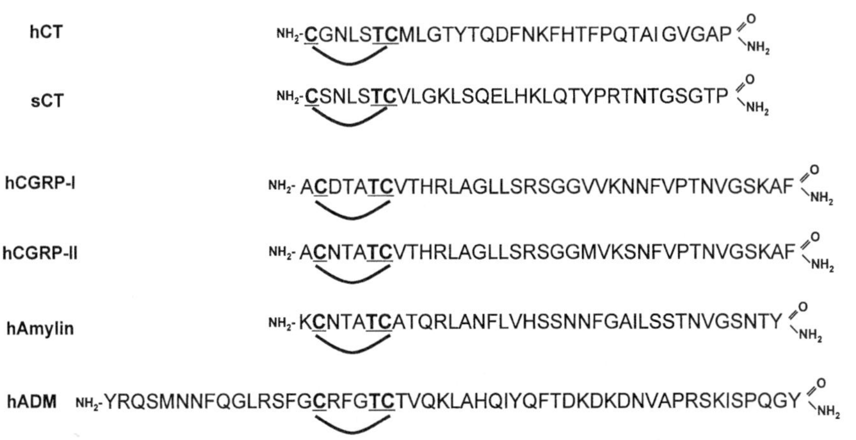

hCT    NH₂-<u>C</u>GNLS<u>TC</u>MLGTYTQDFNKFHTFPQTAI GVGAP〈°,NH₂

sCT    NH₂-<u>C</u>SNLS<u>TC</u>VLGKLSQELHKLQTYPRTNTGSGTP〈°,NH₂

hCGRP-I    NH₂-A<u>C</u>DTA<u>TC</u>VTHRLAGLLSRSGGVVKNNFVPTNVGSKAF〈°,NH₂

hCGRP-II    NH₂-A<u>C</u>NTA<u>TC</u>VTHRLAGLLSRSGGMVKSNFVPTNVGSKAF〈°,NH₂

hAmylin    NH₂-K<u>C</u>NTA<u>TC</u>ATQRLANFLVHSSNNFGAILSSTNVGSNTY〈°,NH₂

hADM    NH₂-YRQSMNNFQGLRSFG<u>C</u>RFG<u>TC</u>TVQKLAHQIYQFTDKDKDNVAPRSKISPQGY〈°,NH₂

**FIGURE 53-2.** Amino-acid sequences of human calcitonin (*hCT*), salmon CT (*sCT*), human calcitonin gene–related peptide-I (*hCGRP-I*), human calcitonin gene–related peptide-II (*hCGRP-II*), human amylin (*hAmylin*), and human adrenomedullin (*hADM*).

## GASTROINTESTINAL EFFECTS

Pharmacologically, CT decreases the secretion of pancreatic enzymes, gastrin, gastric acid, pancreatic glucagon, motilin, pancreatic polypeptide, gastric inhibitory peptide, and glucose-stimulated insulin; it also decreases the small intestinal secretion of potassium, chloride, sodium, and water. The gastrointestinal secretion of somatostatin is increased. Because some hormones that are found within the gastrointestinal tract stimulate the release of iCT, the existence of a food-related gut hormone–CT axis has been proposed.[16,17]

## RENAL EFFECTS

Renal cell membranes have receptors to CT, and this hormone decreases the tubular reabsorption of calcium and phosphate. Often this results in hypercalciuria and phosphaturia (see Chap. 206). In humans, CT increases the excretion of sodium, chloride, potassium, and magnesium.

## PULMONARY EFFECTS

For a discussion of pulmonary effects, see the section Neuroendocrine Tumors Other Than Medullary Thyroid Cancer.

## CENTRAL NERVOUS SYSTEM EFFECTS

The intracerebral administration of CT induces analgesia, decreases the intake of food and water, decreases gastric acid secretion, diminishes intestinal motility, and augments the glucose-stimulated release of insulin.[18]

## EFFECTS IN THE REPRODUCTIVE SYSTEM

Patients with ovarian failure have been reported to have decreased circulating iCT concentrations and a decreased iCT reserve in the thyroidal C cells.[19,20] Whether exogenous administration of estrogen increases the production of iCT by C cells is controversial.[21,22] Interestingly, iCT is secreted by the pregnant uterus.[23] This secretion is tightly regulated by the ovarian

◀ **FIGURE 53-1.** The human calcitonin (CT) gene family: organization of genes, mRNAs, and their hormone precursors. Based on their nucleotide sequence homologies, five genes belong to this family: *CALC-I* (CT/calcitonin gene–related peptide-I [*CGRP-I*]), *CALC-II* (*CGRP-II*), *CALC-III*, *CALC-IV* (amylin), and the *CALC-V* (adrenomedullin [*ADM*]) genes. Two structural features that are essential for full functional activity are conserved between the peptides: They contain two N-terminal cysteines that form a disulfide bridge resulting in an N-terminal loop and a C-terminal amide. **A,** The *CALC-I* primary transcript is processed into three different mRNAs: CT, CT-II, and CGRP-I mRNAs. The different products are generated by the inclusion or exclusion of exons by a mechanism termed *splicing*. Exons I–III are common for all mRNAs. Exon IV codes for CT, and exon V codes for CGRP-I. CT mRNA includes exons I + II + III + IV. CT-II mRNA includes exons I + II + III + IV (partial) + V + VI. CGRP-I mRNA is composed of exons I + II + III + V + VI. Each mRNA codes for a specific precursor. CT mRNA codes mainly for an N-terminal region, mature CT, and a specific C-terminal peptide (i.e., katacalcin, PDN-21, or calcitonin carboxy-terminal peptide-I [*CCP-I*]) that consists of 21 amino acids (*aa*). The N-terminal region includes a signal peptide of 25 amino acids and an N-terminal peptide of 57 amino acids (i.e., aminoprocalcitonin [*NProCT*] or PAS-57). The CT-II precursor differs from the CT-I precursor by its specific C-terminal peptide, CCP-II. CCP-I differs from CCP-II by its last eight amino acids. CGRP-I mRNA codes for an N-terminal region, mature CGRP-I, and a cryptic peptide. The commitment of primary transcript in the different splicing pathways is determined, in part, by a tissue specificity. Although some overlap is seen, the CGRP-I mRNA is expressed mainly in nervous tissue, and CT mRNA is the major mRNA product in thyroid tissue and other tissues, whereas CT-II was found to be expressed in liver. **B,** The *CALC-II* gene codes only for a CGRP-II precursor. Its organization is similar to that of the *CALC-I* gene, containing 6 exons. Sequence homologies are important. Examination of the exon IV–like region of *CALC-II* indicates that CT mRNA is unlikely. Splicing at the site equivalent to the exon III–exon IV junction in human CT mRNA would result in a stop codon within the reading frame of the precursor polypeptide. Although *CALC-II* appears to be a pseudogene for CT, it is a structural gene for CGRP-II. The CGRP-II hormone differs from CGRP-I by three amino acids. **C,** The *CALC-III* gene contains only two exons. Their sequences have homologies with exon II and III of the *CALC-I* and *CALC-II* genes. The *CALC-III* gene does not seem to encode a CT- or CGRP-related peptide hormone and is probably a pseudogene that is not translated into a protein. **D,** The *CALC-IV* gene codes for a precursor containing the amylin peptide. This gene contains only three exons. The third exon codes for amylin. This 37-amino-acid peptide has marked homology with the CGRP peptides. The suggestion has been made that the CT and CGRP exons are derived from a primordial gene and that the different CT/CGRP/ADM/amylin genes have arisen by duplication and sequence-divergent events. **E,** The *CALC-V* gene is translated into ADM. This gene contains four exons. ADM is coded by the fourth exon. The amino-terminal peptides, encoded by exons II and III, also have some bioactivity.

```
 -84  -83  -82  -81  -80  -79  -78  -77  -76  -75  -74  -73  -72  -71  -70  -69  -68  -67
Met-Gly-Phe-Gln-Lys-Phe-Ser-Pro-Phe-Leu-Ala-Leu-Ser-Ile-Leu-Val-Leu-Leu-

 -66  -65  -64  -63  -62  -61  -60     -59  -58  -57  -56  -55  -54  -53  -52  -51  -50  -49
Gln-Ala-Gly-Ser-Leu-His-Ala- Ala-Pro-Phe-Arg-Ser-Ala-Leu-Glu-Ser-Ser-Pro-

 -48  -47  -46  -45  -44  -43  -42  -41  -40  -39  -38  -37  -36  -35  -34  -33  -32  -31
Ala-Asp-Pro-Ala-Thr-Leu-Ser-Glu-Asp-Glu-Ala-Arg-Leu-Leu-Leu-Ala-Ala-Leu-

 -30  -29  -28  -27  -26  -25  -24  -23  -22  -21  -20  -19  -18  -17  -16  -15  -14  -13
Val-Gln-Asp-Tyr-Val-Gln-Met-Lys-Ala-Ser-Glu-Leu-Glu-Gln-Glu-Gln-Glu-Arg-

 -12  -11  -10   -9   -8   -7   -6   -5   -4   -3     -2   -1     1    2    3    4    5
Glu-Gly-Ser-Ser-Leu-Asp-Ser-Pro-Arg-Ser- -Lys-Arg- Cys-Gly-Asn-Leu-Ser-

   6    7    8    9   10   11   12   13   14   15   16   17   18   19   20   21   22   23
Thr-Cys-Met-Leu-Gly-Thr-Tyr-Thr-Gln-Asp-Phe-Asn-Lys-Phe-His-Thr-Phe-Pro-

  24   25   26   27   28   29   30   31   32                        1    2    3    4
Gln-Thr-Ala-Ile-Gly-Val-Gly-Ala-Pro-Gly- -Lys-Lys-Arg- Asp-Met-Ser-Ser-

   5    6    7    8    9   10   11   12   13   14   15   16   17   18   19   20   21
Asp-Leu-Glu-Arg-Asp-His-Arg-Pro-His-Val-Ser-Met-Pro-Gln-Asn-Ala-Asn
```

**FIGURE 53-3.** Amino-acid sequence of procalcitonin. This prohormone consists of 116 amino acids. At the amino terminus is a 57-amino-acid peptide, aminoprocalcitonin. The midportion consists of the 33-amino-acid immature calcitonin. The final 21 amino acids comprise calcitonin carboxy-terminal peptide-I (*CCP-I*). (Smaller amounts of another flanking peptide [CCP-II] are found in nervous tissue.)

hormones estrogen and progesterone, which limit its expression to a brief period during the time of blastocyst implantation. CT is expressed in the preimplantation embryo, as shown in a mouse model.[24] The binding of CT to its receptor activates adenylate cyclase and elevates cytosolic calcium levels, accelerating the development of the preimplantation embryo. Thus, CT might play a role in pregnancy during the implantation of the embryo.

### METABOLIC EFFECTS

Experimentally, CT increases plasma lactate and glucose concentrations, inhibits insulin secretion, and, in the rat model, causes peripheral insulin resistance by inhibiting insulin-stimulated incorporation of glucose in glycogen.[5]

### SERUM LEVELS OF IMMUNOREACTIVE CALCITONIN

Serum iCT has been measured by bioassay, radioreceptor assay, and immunoassay. Bioassay studies (e.g., induced hypocalcemia in laboratory animals, in vitro generation of adenylate cyclase from renal cell membranes, inhibition of calcium-45 release from prelabeled mouse calvaria) have demonstrated that not all of the immunologically detectable CT is bioactive.

Because of differences in the structure of CT, often little or no immunologic cross-reaction occurs among species, except among some rodents. In humans, after total thyroidectomy some immunoassays still detect serum iCT, but at low levels. Nevertheless, the serum iCT of the thyroidectomized human does not respond to an intravenous calcium challenge.

When serum iCT levels are being evaluated, only well-characterized assays should be used, and the assay conditions should not vary. In the past, most physiologic studies involving serum determinations have used techniques and antibodies that detect the immature CT (whether free or as part of precursor molecules), as well as mature CT. Mature CT assays (usually double-antibody techniques) use an antibody that specifically recognizes the carboxy terminus of CT. Previously, many investigators have reported that serum iCT levels are higher in men than in women.[25] Some have reported that iCT

levels are higher in children than in adults, and that the premature infant has higher levels than the full-term newborn, who has higher levels than the young child.[26]

Serum iCT levels do not change appreciably after meals. The existence of a circadian variation in serum levels is controversial. Values do not vary significantly during the menstrual cycle. Serum iCT is higher during pregnancy and may be increased during lactation. These findings have not been adequately verified using assays specific for mature CT.

The basal levels of CT, when measured using a sensitive and specific immunoassay are <10 pg/mL (<3 fmol/mL).

The endogenous secretion rate of iCT is 100 to 200 µg per day. In humans, the half-life of intravenously administered CT is ~10 minutes, and the hormone is degraded predominantly by the kidney.[27] Immunoreactive CT appears in the urine in a molecular form that is larger than the mature hormone. The specific chemical structure of this iCT is unknown. Values in the urine are also higher in the young than in the adult, and higher in men than in women when carboxy terminal–recognizing antisera are used.[28]

### THERAPEUTIC USES OF CALCITONIN

The CT preparation available in the United States for therapeutic purposes is synthetic salmon CT; the human peptide is no longer available for this purpose. Salmon CT differs from human CT by 16 of its 32-amino-acid sites (see Fig. 53-2). It is thought to have greater hypocalcemic potency in humans than does the human hormone (on a weight basis), greater binding affinity to target tissues, and slower degradation and clearance. When injected subcutaneously, local itching and redness at the site of injection are common but progressively diminish. Other side effects may include flushing, nausea, vomiting, and anorexia. Usually, these effects are mild and disappear or diminish with time; therefore, initial therapy should be at bedtime. A slight natriuretic effect may cause mild urinary frequency. In an occasional patient, the nausea is sufficiently bothersome to require cessation of therapy. The nasal preparation causes fewer systemic symptoms.

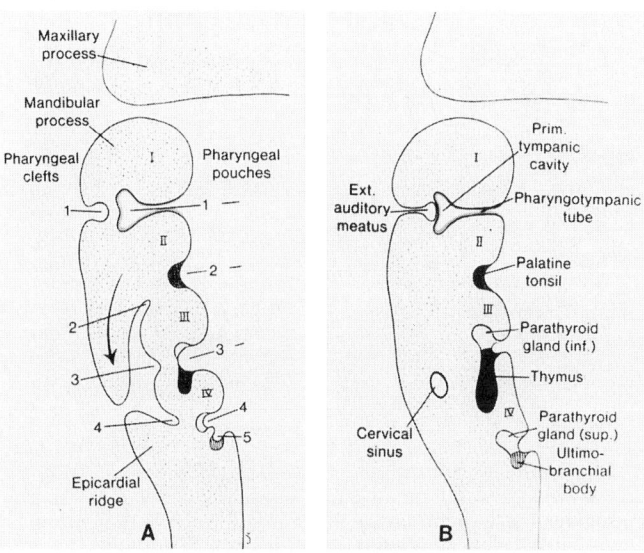

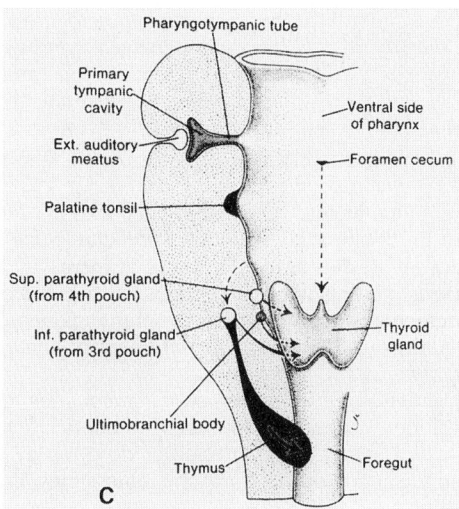

**FIGURE 53-4.** Embryology of the endocrine structures of the human neck, showing the progressive development and migration of the ultimobranchial body. **A,** In the fifth week, *pharyngeal arches* appear (I, II, III, IV). They are separated and demarcated by *pharyngeal clefts* (1, 2, 3, 4). Simultaneously, along the lateral walls of the primitive pharynx, the *pharyngeal pouches* form (1, 2, 3, 4, 5). The pharyngeal arches (i.e., brachial arches) participate in the formation of structures of the face, head, and neck. **B,** The third pharyngeal pouches develop into the inferior parathyroid glands and the thymus; the fourth pouches develop into the superior parathyroid glands. The fifth pouches, which some consider to be part of the fourth, develop into the ultimobranchial bodies. **C,** Notice the migration of the ultimobranchial bodies into the thyroid gland after the latter organ has descended from the level of the foramen cecum. The caudally migrating thymus pulls down the inferior parathyroid glands, and even though these glands have originated from the third pouches, their eventual location is below the superior parathyroid glands, which had originated from the fourth pouches. (*inf.,* inferior; *sup.,* superior; *Ext.,* exterior.) (From Sadler TW. Langman's medical embryology. Baltimore: Williams & Wilkins, 1985.)

## PAGET DISEASE

The most widespread and efficacious use of synthetic CT is for treatment of *Paget disease* (see Chap. 65). Usually, subcutaneous CT therapy (100 IU daily) results in a decrease of serum alkaline phosphatase, osteocalcin, and urinary hydroxyproline. Pain often is improved, the overlying warm skin may become cooler, the progress of the disease may be halted, and neurologic compressive symptoms may regress dramatically. Radiologically, an arrest of the lytic front and some remineralization of lytic lesions may be apparent. Moreover, CT has an analgesic effect in Paget disease that partially, but not entirely, depends on its effect on decreasing bone turnover. The progression of hearing loss, if present, may be halted.[29] Another use of CT in Paget disease is to decrease hyperemia of involved bones before surgical procedures, such as hip replacement. To minimize nausea, the patient should start at half-dose levels for the first week. The nasal preparation, which has a markedly diminished effect in Paget disease, is not approved for the treatment of this condition.

## HYPERCALCEMIA

Salmon CT has a role in the treatment of *acute hypercalcemia*.[30,31] The drug is particularly useful for short-term therapy. It lowers the increased serum calcium by 0.5 to 1.5 mg/dL in ~75% of patients regardless of the cause (Fig. 53-6). It can be used in association with any other therapy (e.g., intravenous fluids, intravenous pamidronate). Salmon CT is extremely well tolerated in this setting and can be used safely in patients with congestive heart failure, renal disease, liver disease, or bone marrow deficiency. The principal value of CT is to "take the top off" the hypercalcemia—an obtunded patient may become more alert, diagnostic studies may proceed, and the physician need have no concern about possible contraindications. One of the most effective drug therapies for acute hypercalcemia, intravenous pamidronate, requires 48 to 72 hours to exert its hypocalcemic effect; consequently, salmon CT has a very useful role before this time. Occasionally a patient with mild hypercalcemia can be treated with long-term use of salmon CT, although resistance ("CT escape") usually eventuates fairly rapidly; the cause of this early resistance, which also occurs when using human CT, is not known. Corticosteroid therapy has been alleged to nullify this escape phenomenon, but this has not been adequately documented, and such treatment adds the effects of harmful exogenous hypercortisolism to the clinical condition. Thus, intravenous pamidronate, repeated as needed, is a more appropriate therapy for the long-term control of hypercalcemia. Salmon CT is administered subcutaneously at a dosage of 4 IU/kg every 12 hours; in the authors' experience, a further increase of the dosage or the use of intravenous therapy seldom provides any additional benefit. Whether the nasal route of administration would be effective for hypercalcemia is not known, and it is not approved for this purpose.

## OSTEOPOROSIS

The use of CT in *osteoporosis* seems logical because many forms of this illness are caused by excessive bone resorption. The proposal has been made, based on no direct evidence, that a relative endogenous CT deficiency contributes to the development of osteoporosis. In this regard, many investigators found that serum iCT is lower in normal women than in men and responds less to a calcium infusion.[32] Some investigators found that serum iCT is higher in blacks (who have greater bone density than whites). Some found that estrogen therapy increases basal levels of serum iCT in postmenopausal women and may augment the CT responsivity to intravenous calcium challenge. In addition, a decreased iCT reserve in response to stimulation testing has been reported in the elderly of both sexes. Osteoporotic women, in particular, have been reported to have poor iCT reserves, although this latter finding is disputed. (None of these aforementioned studies used assays specific for mature CT.)

Nevertheless, in the patient undergoing thyroid hormone replacement, total thyroidectomy does *not* cause osteoporosis. Furthermore, patients with extremely high CT levels, such as those with MTC, do *not* have increased bone mass, *nor* does the uninvolved bone of elderly patients with Paget disease who have received long-term CT therapy appear to be influenced markedly.

Several studies have evaluated the use of CT as therapy for established osteoporosis or for the control of its progression. In

## Control                    Calcitonin, 10 min                    Calcitonin, 40 min

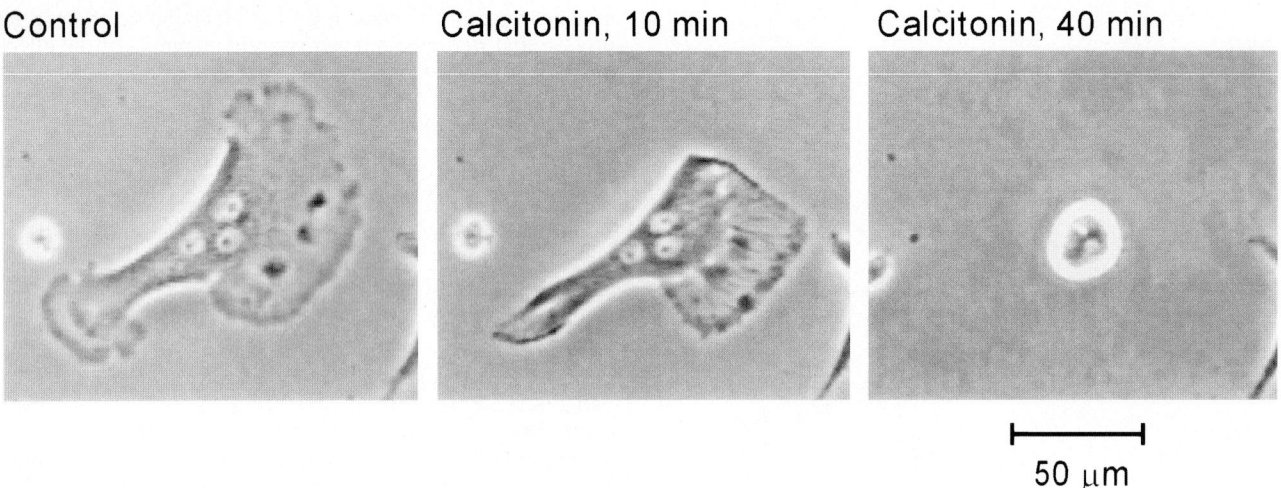

50 μm

**FIGURE 53-5.** Effect of calcitonin on the osteoclast. Series of video micrographs taken with phase-contrast microscopy shows a single osteoclast. Frame at left was taken immediately before addition of calcitonin (100 ng/mL final concentration). Middle frame shows osteoclast 10 minutes after addition of calcitonin, by which time the retraction of peripheral pseudopods was initiated. Frame at right shows the same osteoclast 40 minutes after treatment with calcitonin, with complete retraction of pseudopods. (Courtesy of S. Jeffrey Dixon and Stephen M. Sims, University of Western Ontario, London, Canada.)

cases of postmenopausal osteoporosis, some investigators observed a reduction of bone loss, and others reported increased bone mineral calcium and decreased urinary total hydroxyproline.[33-35] CT treatment of postmenopausal osteoporosis appears to be most effective in patients with increased bone turnover.[36] The increase of bone mass in patients with postmenopausal osteoporosis appear to be less for CT than for alendronate.[37]

After several months to 1 to 2 years, the beneficial effects of CT therapy may become limited by a subsequent decline in bone formation. The intermittent use of CT (e.g., 2 or 3 months on, and 2 or 3 months off) may prolong the beneficial effects on bone.[38]

Both the subcutaneous and nasal preparations have been reported to increase axial and appendicular bone density, although not all studies agree. Evidence is increasing that the fracture rate is diminished,[39-41] perhaps with greater efficacy than the augmentation of bone density might suggest. The dosage of subcutaneous salmon CT is 100 IU daily; the dosage of the nasal spray is 200 IU daily.

The administration of either subcutaneous or nasal CT induces antibody formation in many patients after several months of use. Usually, these antibodies do not play a role in resistance to the action of this hormone, unless they are present in very high titer.

Patient compliance is greatly increased when the nasal spray is used.[42] Few studies are available concerning the efficiency of the nasal route in other conditions, and this route is approved only for osteoporosis. When treating osteoporosis, both the subcutaneous and nasal preparations should be supplemented with daily oral doses of 1000 mg of elemental calcium and 400 IU of vitamin D. Further studies are needed to systematically compare the effects of nasal CT with those of subcutaneous CT.

CT has been used to treat the osteoporosis of immobilization as well as that caused by corticosteroid usage with rather disappointing results. In patients with temporal arteritis and polymyalgia rheumatica who were starting high-dose, long-term corticosteroids, salmon CT with calcium and vitamin D provided no greater bone preservation than that observed with calcium and vitamin D alone.[43] Therapy using this hormone has been tried in osteogenesis imperfecta with variable, but not dramatic, results. In treatment of the regional osteoporosis of Sudeck atrophy (reflex sympathetic dystrophy), CT has been alleged to diminish the pain, edema, and osteolytic process.

### OTHER USES

In acute pancreatitis, the diminution of pancreatic enzyme secretion caused by the administration of CT has been reported to produce a quicker clinical and biochemical recovery. CT also has been used as therapy for pain of various types with variable results.[44]

Receptors for CT have been identified in some human cancer cells, including those of lung, breast, bone, prostate, and MTC, suggesting that an imaging agent for the receptors might

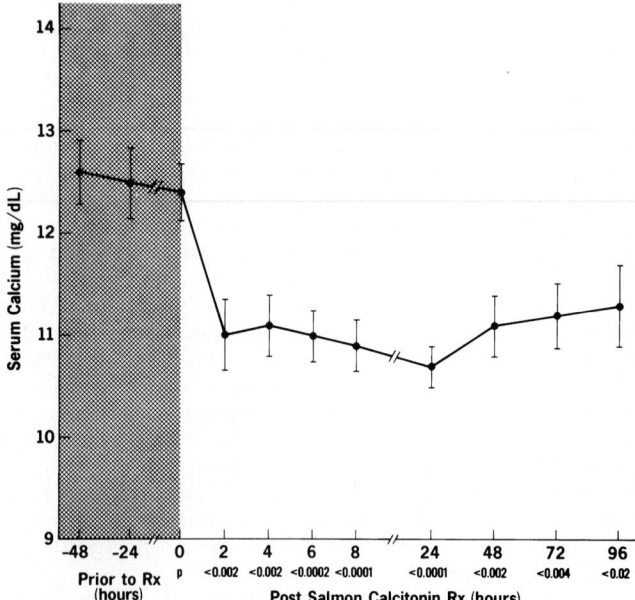

**FIGURE 53-6.** Salmon calcitonin treatment of hypercalcemia of various etiologies. Mean serum calcium (± standard error of the mean) for 24 hypercalcemic patients (0-, 24-, 48-, 72-, and 96-hour determinations are before first morning injection); $p$ value indicates statistical significance of difference from initial pretherapy serum calcium value. (From Wisneski LA, Croom WP, Silva OL, et al. Salmon calcitonin in hypercalcemia. Clin Pharmacol Ther 1978; 24:219.)

be useful in nuclear oncology. Radiolabeled mature CT is not optimal for nuclear imaging, however, because of rapid breakdown and clearance from target tissues.[45]

## PROCALCITONIN AND ITS DERIVATIVE PEPTIDES

The *CALC-I* gene encodes the information for the structure of the polypeptide precursor of CT, *preprocalcitonin (Pre-ProCT)*. Early in posttranslational processing, the leader sequence is cleaved from this precursor molecule by a signal peptidase. The resultant prohormone, procalcitonin (ProCT, also termed PAN116), consists of 116 amino-acid residues (molecular mass 12.79 kDa) (see Fig. 53-3). The function of ProCT, which is present at low levels in normal human serum (<5 pg/mL; <0.4 fmol/mL),[46] is unknown; an immunomodulatory role has been postulated.

At the amino-terminus portion of ProCT is found a 57-amino-acid peptide, *NProCT* (also termed PAS-57), which has a molecular mass of 6.22 kDa. NProCT, which is readily detectable in normal human serum (10–70 pg/mL; 1.6–12 fmol/mL), has no known definite function, although it has been reported to be a mitogen for osteoclasts.[46,47] The *immature CT* is centrally placed within the ProCT molecule. This peptide, which also is present in normal serum, has no known function other than as a precursor of mature CT. The final 21-amino-acid residues comprise *CCP-I* (also termed PDN-21 and previously called katacalcin). As shown in Figure 53-1, the *CALC-I* gene can also produce a *CCP-II* peptide arising from a different form of CT mRNA. CCP-I, which differs from CCP-II in its eight terminal amino acids, occurs predominantly in thyroidal C cells and neuroendocrine malignancies such as MTC tissue, and also in the serum of normal persons, whereas CCP-II, which has been insufficiently studied, is found mostly in the pituitary and in neurologic tissues.[48] Although these peptides may have a biologic function, none has yet been proven. Lastly, as part of the processing of the ProCT molecule, a peptide consisting of the *conjoined immature CT and CCP-I peptide (CT:CCP-I)* occurs in normal serum, where its function, if any, is unknown.[46]

All of the peptides that contain the CT molecule in its immature form (i.e., ProCT, CT:CCP-I, and immature CT) cross-react with antisera specific for the midportion of the immature CT molecule and, along with NProCT, have been termed CT precursors (CTpr), precalcitonin peptides, or large-molecular-weight CT.

**Regulated versus Constitutive Secretion.** The extent of posttranslational processing of ProCT largely depends on whether the prohormone is secreted mainly by a *regulated pathway*, as in the thyroidal C cells, or a *constitutive pathway*.[49] In regulated secretion, the Golgi apparatus identifies and selects ProCT to be routed to newly formed secretory vesicles, where the mature CT is produced and progressively concentrated. Subsequently, these electron-dense vesicles serve as storage repositories for later secretion. On the appropriate signal at the plasma membrane, a brief increased concentration of cytosolic free $Ca^{2+}$ induces secretion (i.e., migration to the cell periphery, fusion with the apical portion of the cell membrane, and discharge of hormone contents in a quantal release). In regulated secretion, in addition to CT, these vesicles also contain and extrude variable concentrations of the other processed products of ProCT (i.e., NProCT and CCP-I). ProCT and CT:CCP-I are largely absent from the storage vesicles.

In contrast, under certain conditions, constitutive secretion occurs, in which less-dense vesicles receive CT precursors, bud off from the trans-Golgi, and migrate rapidly to the cell surface. This nonstoring, continuous secretion of newly synthesized peptide(s) is a bulk-flow system by which hor-

monal material is rapidly secreted. Because of the lack of processing machinery within these different, rapidly transported and rapidly extruded vesicles, the relative proportion of CT in relation to precursor peptides is considerably diminished. In the case of the ProCT molecule, this form of secretion may occur to a small extent in normal persons, whereas in some pathophysiologic conditions, it is greatly increased (see later). It is uncertain why some tumors (e.g., MTC, small cell lung cancer [SCLC], bronchial carcinoid) secrete relatively small amounts of CT in comparison with large amounts of CTpr despite their abundant number of dense-core secretion vesicles, which are characteristic of regulated secretion.

## DISORDERS ASSOCIATED WITH ABERRANT PRODUCTION AND SECRETION OF CALCITONIN PRECURSORS AND DERIVATIVE PEPTIDES

### MEDULLARY THYROID CARCINOMA

Although the assay for CT has become the standard marker for the clinical detection and follow-up of MTC, CT precursors and other derivative peptides are also increased in the sera of these patients, frequently to a greater extent than is the CT.[50] Furthermore, some of these lesions secrete CGRP and precursor CGRP peptides as well. Nevertheless, the time-honored marker remains mature CT, and care should be taken to use the most specific assay.[51]

Nearly all MTC patients have increased basal serum CT (see Chaps. 40 and 188), and nearly all patients with MTC respond markedly to a calcium and/or pentagastrin challenge, even when in a "subclinical" stage (i.e., C-cell hyperplasia).

A patient with a thyroid mass and increased basal CT probably has MTC, and this usually can be readily confirmed by a fine-needle aspiration biopsy and immunocytochemical staining. In most sporadic cases of MTC, the basal serum CT level usually has not been obtained preoperatively, and the diagnosis most often is made by examination of the surgical specimen. In this respect, some clinicians believe that a screening basal serum CT level should be measured preoperatively for all nodular thyroid disease.[52] Furthermore, preoperative basal CT levels are predictive of the tumor size and offer information concerning the probability of postoperative normalization of the hormone level.[53] In those patients proven to have MTC, follow-up CT testing after surgery is essential to detect persistent local disease or to document the presence of metastases; later, long-term follow-up is essential to detect a subsequent recurrence or further tumor growth. In the past, the major use of provocative testing had been for the initial screening of the family members of a patient with MTC to help determine whether the patient had the sporadic or the familial variety of the disease, and also for the screening and follow-up of relatives of known familial cases. Currently, genetic studies (i.e., *Ret* protooncogene) have largely replaced the use of provocative testing of family members of an index case with known disease for the purpose of determining whether any specific relative is affected. In the future, provocative testing will probably become limited to the follow-up examination of individual nonhypercalcitonemic family members previously shown to possess the genetic abnormality and for whom prophylactic thyroidectomy is not selected (see Chap. 188). The authors' preference had been to perform a combined calcium and pentagastrin stimulation, because the effect of the latter hormone is additive with that of induced hypercalcemia. Pentagastrin often causes marked epigastric and chest pain, however, and is not an approved drug in the United States. Intravenous stimulation testing of family members is onerous and, for children, frightening. For family members and for patients with diagnosed C-cell hyperplasia whose serum CT has normalized after surgery, the measurement of iCT in a single urine specimen has proved to be more sensitive than serum measurements. The urine assay readily detects early disease in a family member or recurrent disease in the index case and often obviates the need for stimulation testing.[54]

## NEUROENDOCRINE HYPERPLASIAS

The study of some chronic nonneoplastic pulmonary conditions has demonstrated a slight to moderate increase of CTpr. Usually, levels of serum CT remain within the normal range. These conditions include chronic bronchitis, chronic obstructive pulmonary disease, chronic pulmonary tuberculosis, and cystic fibrosis. PNE cells (see later) are hyperplastic in some chronic lung conditions and may be the cause of this phenomenon.[55] A similar occurrence may be encountered in inflammatory bowel disease (e.g., regional enteritis), in which iCT-producing enteric neuroendocrine cells may undergo hyperplasia. In the case of the PNE cells, one of the exogenous stimuli to PNE cell hyperplasia may be cigarette smoke. In hamsters and in humans, cigarette smoke immediately increases serum iCT, probably due to the nicotine content of this smoke. Cholinergic-nicotinic receptors are found on the PNE cell, and nicotine stimulates the growth of these cells. A similar phenomenon occurs after exposure to the carcinogen diethylnitrosamine, which has nicotinic characteristics.[56]

## NEUROENDOCRINE TUMORS OTHER THAN MEDULLARY THYROID CANCER

The PNE cells, which have electron-dense vesicles containing iCT as well as other peptides, are situated near the basement membrane of the human trachea, larynx, and bronchial tree.[57] They are particularly common within the lungs of the newborn, where they often are strategically located in clusters called *neuroepithelial bodies*. In both the newborn and adults, the PNE cells secrete their contents into the bronchial lumen and also communicate with other types of pulmonary cells in a paracrine manner. Functionally, PNE cells appear to play a role in pulmonary maturation, transcellular and intracellular movements of calcium, and chondrogenesis of the bronchial tree; also, perhaps they locally modulate pulmonary blood flow (see Chap. 177). The iCT that is secreted in the short term by these cells is mostly the mature CT hormone.

SCLC, the third most common form of lung cancer, is a very virulent tumor. It is nearly always associated with cigarette smoking. Electron microscopy reveals that these cells are strikingly similar to PNE cells; they contain similar secretion granules, and contain and secrete iCT. This cancer as well as the more benign pulmonary carcinoid tumor are believed to arise from PNE cells or their progenitors.[58] Although these tumor cells contain mostly CT intracellularly, in contrast to PNE cells, they secrete predominantly CTpr. The carcinoid tumor, which occurs in extrapulmonary locations (e.g., small intestine), and extrapulmonary SCLC behave in a similar fashion.

Occasionally, other neuroendocrine tumors may contain and secrete iCT (e.g., pancreatic islet cell cancer, pheochromocytoma, thymoma). Furthermore, pulmonary neoplasms other than SCLC or carcinoid tumor may be associated with high levels of iCT in the serum (e.g., pulmonary epidermoid cancer, adenocarcinoma, or large cell cancer). This may be due to an admixture of SCLC cells within the tumor, hyperplasia of PNE cells in the vicinity of the cancer, or the smoking-related PNE cell hyperplasia that occurs in some of these affected patients.[59]

In the case of SCLC and pulmonary and extrapulmonary carcinoid tumors, as well as some of the above-mentioned iCT-secreting neoplasms, the sequential measurement of serum iCT may be a very useful marker for the presence of these lesions and their response to therapeutic measures (i.e., surgery, irradiation, and/or chemotherapy).[60] In such cases, the measurement of serum CTpr, which are always present in considerably higher concentrations than is CT, is preferable.

## INFLAMMATION, INFECTION, AND SEPSIS

Potent stimuli (e.g., trauma, extensive surgery, burns, pancreatitis, stroke, or bacterial infection) often initiate a marked augmentation of proinflammatory cytokines and other humoral substances that may result in inflammation. Locally, among other phenomena, inflammation is characterized by vasodilation and a concomitantly increased blood supply, attraction of leukocytes and lymphocytes, activation of macrophages, alteration of capillary function, and transudation into the tissues of serum along with its protein, peptide, and electrolyte constituents. Inflammation may be systemic, in which case the patient may note malaise, loss of appetite, or muscle aching. Fever or hypothermia, leukocytosis, or leukopenia, tachycardia, and/or tachypnea may be present. Systemic inflammation may be self-limited or may progress to multiple organ dysfunction, which is characterized by varying degrees of hypoxemia, myocardial insufficiency, hypoperfusion, diminished mental status, and circulatory dysfunction. Further complications include coagulopathy, acute respiratory distress syndrome, cardiac failure, shock, renal failure, and/or coma (see Chaps. 227 and 228). The term "sepsis" has been used to describe a condition in which a patient's cytokine and humoral response to an infection leads to some of these marked symptoms, signs, and complications. In sepsis, the patient is ill, not primarily because of the initial injury or infection, but because of the harmful pathophysiologic overreaction by the host.

**Calcitonin Precursors as a Marker for Inflammation, Infection, and Sepsis.** Although the serum levels of several humoral substances may be increased in the patient with systemic inflammation, infection, or sepsis, very few are reliable markers for the presence of the conditions, their clinical course, the response to therapy, or the prognosis. Data that have been accumulating since the 1980s indicate that large-molecular-weight CT-containing peptides (i.e., CTpr) as well as ProCT itself are dramatically increased in these conditions, attaining levels ranging from moderate elevations to thousands of times higher than normal.[7,61–63] In all of these illnesses, although the relative proportions of the different peptides may vary, serum levels of CT remain normal or only modestly increased because of incomplete processing and/or more rapid degradation.

Several techniques have been used to quantitate the CTpr of patients with inflammation, infection, and sepsis (e.g., gel filtration or high-performance liquid chromatography with associated immunoassay, and single-site assay, or two-site immunoassays). When selecting an assay, measuring more than one of the CTpr may be best, because of the varying degrees of increases in the serum of any individual patient. The two current assays include a single-site NProCT assay, which detects NProCT, ProCT, and procalcitonin gene–related peptide, and a two-site assay, which detects ProCT and CT:CCP-I.[63,64] When these assays are used, most patients with marked illness are found to have increased serum CTpr, and values tend to correlate with the severity of the condition and with the prognosis. Indeed, serum CTpr levels have now become the best markers, and one can follow the day-to-day course of the patient with considerable reliability.[65]

**Stimulus to Increased Serum Calcitonin Precursor Levels in Systemic Inflammation, Infection, and Sepsis.** The injection of endotoxin into normal human volunteers provokes an early increase of tumor necrosis factor-$\alpha$ (TNF-$\alpha$) and interleukin-1$\beta$ (IL-1$\beta$). Injection of TNF-$\alpha$ into normal hamsters provokes a marked increase of CTpr, reaching levels comparable to those observed in septic animals.[66] Various injuries (e.g., burns or trauma) are known to induce translocation across the bowel wall of endotoxin that normally is contained within the cell walls of the *Escherichia coli* flora of the gut. Endotoxin arising endogenously from the gut or exogenously from an acquired infection likely is the initial triggering factor that precipitates the cytokine cascade leading to increased CTpr. Bacterial exotoxins, other known precipitants of a cytokine cascade, may constitute additional offenders.

**Calcitonin Precursors as a Toxic Factor in Sepsis.**    In experimental systemic sepsis, CTpr have been found to contribute to the severity and mortality of the condition. In hamsters with induced sepsis due to peritonitis, the mortality is doubled by the addition of human ProCT but not by the addition of CT. Furthermore, in these septic animals, immunoneutralization of ProCT using an antiserum to the CT portion of ProCT improves outcome and reduces mortality.[67] In a similar model of sepsis in pigs, the preventive immunoneutralization of ProCT using an antiserum to the N-ProCT portion of ProCT markedly mitigates the onset and symptomatology of sepsis and prolongs life.[68]

**Origin of the High Serum Calcitonin Precursor Levels in Systemic Inflammation, Infection, and Sepsis.**    The levels of CTpr in septic tissues (e.g., kidney, liver, lung) are significantly increased compared with levels in tissues from healthy controls. Reverse transcriptase polymerase chain reaction studies in septic hamsters and pigs reveal detectable CT mRNA, not only in the thyroid gland, but also in *all* extrathyroidal tissues studied (e.g., kidney, liver, lung, brain, fat, muscle, spleen, testes, etc.). In contrast, in control hamsters, CT mRNA is detectable only in the thyroid and lung. Furthermore, in situ hybridization studies reveal that multiple cell types within these organs and tissues are involved. In this respect, during the marked host response, the whole organism is transformed into an endocrine gland.[69] Presumably, the increase of *CALC* gene transcription is mediated by one or several stimulus-specific sepsis-response elements in the gene promotor.

**Cause of Calcitonin Precursor Toxicity in Sepsis.**    In preliminary and limited experiments in healthy hamsters, the injection of human ProCT did not cause mortality. A mild hyperglycemia and a slight decrease of serum calcium were noted. In vitro, the addition of human ProCT to human endotoxin–stimulated mononuclear cells of peripheral blood markedly increased the ambient levels of proinflammatory cytokines (i.e., TNF-α, IL-1β, and interleukin 8)[70]; presumably this would be a harmful occurrence in sepsis. Furthermore, the administration of human ProCT to normal hamsters blocks the marked hypocalcemic effect of administered CT, suggesting that ProCT blocks tissue receptors for CT.[71] In this respect, previous studies have shown that ProCT does indeed bind to CT receptors. Such a blockage becomes potentially even more significant when one considers the extremely long half-life of serum ProCT (probably because of prolonged stimulus to secretion and the resistance to degradation) that occurs after endotoxin injection in humans. Thus, one could speculate that the toxicity of ProCT, may, in part, be related to receptor blockade, which prevents the various peptides of the CT gene family (e.g., CT, CGRP, amylin, and ADM) from exerting an otherwise beneficial effect in sepsis.

# CALCITONIN GENE–RELATED PEPTIDES

## ALTERNATIVE GENE EXPRESSION

The *CALC-I* gene gives rise to more than one bioactive peptide: CT and CGRP. This occurs because of alternative processing of the primary RNA transcript[72] (see Chap. 3; see Fig. 53-1).

Two very similar human CGRPs are found: CGRP-I (or α) from the *CALC-I* gene and CGRP-II (or β) from the *CALC-II* gene. CGRP-I is a 37-amino-acid hormone; in humans, CGRP-II differs from CGRP-I by only three amino acids (see Fig. 53-2).[73] The CGRPs have only a modest homology with CT. As is the case for CT, however, the CGRPs have an $NH_2$-terminal disulfide bridge and a COOH-terminal amide. The *CALC-II* gene does not seem to be alternatively expressed. The *CALC-I* and *CALC-II* genes, plus a pseudogene, *CALC-III*, probably arose by local duplication of a common ancestral gene.[74] Unlike with CT, the structure of the CGRPs is highly conserved in different animal species.

CT and CGRP-I can be coexpressed by a single cell, and several tissues contain both of them.[75] However, usually a prefer-

ence is seen for synthesis of either CT or CGRP-I according to the cellular type and localization. In the C cell, CT is preferentially produced; in the nervous system, CGRP-I predominates. The decision concerning the prevailing mode of synthesis is not immutable; for example, it can be modified by dexamethasone and by the naturally occurring fatty acid butyrate. Whether the expression of *CALC-I* and *CALC-II* genes is independently regulated is uncertain.

CGRP-I and CGRP-II occur in tissues of the normal human.[76] They are also found in some tumors, such as SCLC.[77] In the rat, in situ hybridization demonstrates a similar tissue distribution of the CGRP-I and CGRP-II mRNAs. Most immunohistochemical studies of specific tissue localization have used antisera that probably *cannot differentiate* the very similar CGRP-I and CGRP-II; consequently, when location and action are discussed, the more noncommital term CGRP is used.

CGRP is predominantly a neuropeptide, found mostly in various regions of the brain, cranial nerves, ganglia, and spinal cord. In peripheral nerves, CGRP is often costored and released with other neurotransmitters. Within the gastrointestinal tract, it is found in the myenteric plexus and in neuroendocrine cells. It also is found in the pituitary gland, the adrenal medulla, the pancreatic islets, the pulmonary nerves, and the PNE cells. The peptide circulates in a heterogeneous form in the blood. Serum levels of immunoreactive CGRP are higher in females than in males, and oral contraceptive use further increases these levels. Levels are normal in as many as 50% of patients with MTC, and its measurement does not improve detection of this tumor.

## EFFECTS

Many receptor sites react to CGRP in the nervous system and peripheral tissues; most, but not all, of these are not linked to adenylate cyclase (see the section Receptors of the Calcitonin Gene Family of Peptides).

As with CT, induced hypercalcemia can stimulate the release of CGRP, but in the case of this latter peptide, this probably is a nonphysiologic phenomenon. CGRP acts directly on rat osteoclasts to inhibit bone resorption.[78] Although administration of this hormone in some laboratory animals has a hypocalcemic effect, however, this does not occur in humans.

CGRP functions as a peptidergic messenger and is involved in neurocrine modulation. Capsaicin, the sensory nerve neurotoxin that is found in hot peppers, depletes CGRP, suggesting that this peptide is involved in sensory function. Intracerebrally, the hormone decreases food intake and gastric acid secretion. Commonly, CGRP is colocalized with substance P and sometimes is found with somatostatin, galanin, vasoactive intestinal peptide, or cholecystokinin.[79] This association with other peptides may have functional consequences. For example, the synergistic action of CGRP with substance P and the other neurokinins may induce plasma protein leakage from the vasculature and promote the inflammatory response.

Experimentally, the administration of CGRP has many effects, most of which may have no physiologic relevance but some of which may reflect a physiologic neurosensory influence. Using various experimental models, some have reported pharmacologic effects including flushing of skin (related to peripheral arteriolar vasodilatation), hypotension, chronotropic and inotropic cardiac effects, contraction of smooth muscle of the gut, and inhibition of contraction of smooth muscle of the uterus and vas deferens. The extremely potent vasorelaxant actions of CGRP are mediated partly by cAMP-dependent mechanisms. The release of this hormone from vascular nerve endings may be of importance in the physiologic control of blood pressure. Although blood levels of CGRP are only slightly increased in sepsis, an increase in paracrine secretion of CGRP may play an important role in sepsis-induced vasodilation and shock. In vitro studies suggest that CGRP may be implicated in the regulation of B-lymphocyte development and T-lymphocyte function.[80] The hormone exerts positive inotropic and chronotropic effects.

The CGRPs may have a role in pulmonary pathophysiology. CGRP-containing pulmonary neuroendocrine cells are increased in infants with chronic lung disease associated with bronchodysplasia. CGRP and other sensory peptides are potentially capable of producing many of the characteristic features of asthma, including bronchoconstriction and edema.[81] CGRP also induces a dose-dependent relaxation of the spontaneously contracting myometrium of pregnant women.

Infusion of pharmacologic doses of CGRP has metabolic effects similar to those of amylin (i.e., it also induces insulin resistance, decreases peripheral glucose clearance, and increases hepatic glucose output).[82]

CGRP, similarly to CT, may also have central effects: These include alteration of food intake and release of growth hormone and prolactin from the pituitary.[83] Interestingly, increased serum levels of CGRP are found in patients with migraine, even between attacks, suggesting a possible role in this disorder.[84]

## AMYLIN

Amylin was first isolated from amyloid deposits in an insulinoma, but it is also found in the amyloid of pancreatic islets of patients with type 2 diabetes, as well as in normal islets. Pancreatic amyloid is formed by the aggregation of amylin. Consequently, the hormone is also known as *islet amyloid polypeptide*.

This 37-amino-acid peptide originates from the *CALC-IV* gene (see Fig. 53-1). It has 43% sequence homology with CGRP-I and 49% homology with CGRP-II, as well as overlapping bioactivity.[85]

### EFFECTS

Amylin is packaged within B-cell granules and is cosecreted with insulin in response to hyperglycemia. In the human fetal pancreas, amylin is colocalized within the pancreatic neuroendocrine cells, along with insulin and glucagon. Intraislet somatostatin appears to be an inhibitory regulator of both of these peptide hormones.[86] In obese insulin-resistant patients, amylin values increase ten-fold after meals or glucose, whereas in patients with type 1 diabetes, serum values remain low or absent.

Various metabolic actions of amylin are related to the regulation of fuel metabolism, but whether they are physiologic or pharmacologic is uncertain. Thus, in muscle, the hormone opposes glycogen synthesis and activates glycogenolysis and glycolysis. The resultant increased lactate output provides substrate for hepatic gluconeogenesis and glycogen synthesis (Cori cycle). Presumably, the increased serum glucose reflects the gluconeogenesis. Intracerebrally, amylin exhibits an anorectic action. In experimental models, amylin causes insulin resistance by inhibiting glycogen synthesis in muscle, but whether serum amylin levels are increased in humans with insulin resistance is controversial. In the kidney, amylin stimulates the secretion of renin.

Because of its restraining effect on gastric emptying,[87] the insulin agonist pramlintide has been suggested as a potential therapy to mitigate hypoglycemia in insulin-treated patients with type 1 diabetes. After a long period of therapy with this agent, however, a potential risk of inducing systemic amyloidosis may be present. In this respect, pancreatic amyloid may be pathogenic[88]; amyloid fibrils, which accumulate in the islets of patients with type 2 diabetes, are cytotoxic to pancreatic cell lines and may be directly associated with the development or the worsening of type 2 diabetes. Furthermore, amylin fibrils, found in Alzheimer disease, promote the production of proinflammatory cytokines such as TNF-α, IL-1β, and IL-6, and may contribute to the pathology of this disease.[89]

In the rat, amylin appears to act centrally to elevate blood pressure, perhaps through activation of the renin-angiotensin system. However, pramlintide does not alter blood pressure in humans.

Amylin has weak osteoclast-inhibitory and hypocalcemic actions and, like CT and CGRP, has an antiinflammatory action. Amylin activates CGRP receptors and thereby induces vasodilation. Like CT, amylin has a gastroprotective action in some models of gastric ulcer.

## ADRENOMEDULLIN

ADM, originating from the *CALC-V* gene (see Figs. 53-1 and 53-2), is a 52-amino-acid peptide originally isolated from human adrenal pheochromocytoma.[90,91] As is the case for iCT, a significant fraction of circulating immunoreactive ADM (iADM) consists of one or more precursor peptides with potential bioactivity.

ADM is produced by and secreted from vascular endothelium, smooth muscle cells, fibroblasts, monocytes/macrophages, and many other cell types.[92,93] Immunoreactive ADM has been detected in many tissues throughout the body (e.g., kidney, lung, skin). ADM is cleared by the kidneys. High levels of the hormone are found in the urine, and serum levels increase with renal failure.[94]

### EFFECTS

Endothelial cells produce ADM and express specific receptors linked to the cAMP second messenger system.[95] ADM is a potent vasodilator, apparently via the generation of nitric oxide. Alternative cleavage products of the ADM prohormone, *adrenotensin*, have been reported to have an opposite effect on vascular tone. Hence, ADM may function not only as a circulating vasodilating hormone but also as a local regulating agent for vascular tone. It exerts positive inotropic and chronotropic effects.

Other effects of ADM include stimulation of insulin secretion, inhibition of adrenocorticotropic hormone (ACTH) secretion, inhibition of angiotensin II–induced aldosterone secretion, bronchodilation, natriuresis and diuresis, delay of gastric emptying, immunomodulation, stimulation of the growth of osteoblasts, and an antiinflammatory activity.[96–99]

### PATHOPHYSIOLOGY

Lipopolysaccharide and inflammatory cytokines (e.g., IL-1 and TNF) are potent stimulants of ADM production.[100] In patients with septic shock, serum ADM concentrations are increased compared with controls, and the levels correlate with hemodynamic disturbances (i.e., high cardiac output and low vascular resistance).[101] Serum ADM is elevated in patients with essential hypertension, congestive heart failure, myocardial infarction, and chronic obstructive pulmonary disease.

The *N-terminal peptide of proadrenomedullin* appears to function presynaptically to inhibit adrenergic nerves that innervate blood vessels. This latter peptide is increased in patients with essential hypertension. Its vasodilating effect is considerably weaker than that of ADM.

## RECEPTORS OF THE CALCITONIN GENE FAMILY OF PEPTIDES

The peptides of the CT-gene family exert their bioeffects through binding to characteristic receptors with seven transmembrane hydrophobic domains. The receptors belong to the G protein–coupled receptors, in which the guanidine nucleotide guanosine triphosphate mediates receptor function by binding to specific mediator proteins.[5] The receptors are categorized into two major subgroups, *CT receptors (CRs)* and *CT receptor–like receptors (CRLRs)*. The different members of the CT family of peptides bind with different affinity to CRs and to CRLRs.[5] Therefore, their bioeffects are in part overlapping.

## CALCITONIN RECEPTORS

Several isoforms of the CR are found. They are derived from a single gene by alternative splicing of mRNA, which results in variable amino-acid sequence, length, and functional properties of the receptor domains.[102] The CRs consist of a single glycosylated polypeptide of 70 to 90 kDa, equivalent to 450 to 500 amino acids. CRs are related to receptors of parathyroid hormone and parathyroid hormone–related protein, secretin, vasoactive intestinal peptide, pituitary adenylate cyclase–activating peptide, growth hormone–releasing hormone, glucagon-like peptide-1, and glucagon. This suggests that these receptors may comprise a distinct subfamily of G protein–coupled receptors.[103]

The CRs are widely distributed and are particularly numerous in osteoclasts of the bone, in cells of the distal nephron of the kidney, and in the central nervous system.[104] CRs are also expressed in preimplantation embryos in mice. As mentioned earlier, CT is thought to be involved in blastocyst differentiation and implantation. Human T lymphocytes have high–affinity CRs on their surfaces. Thus, the markedly increased CTpr levels seen in infection and sepsis might be immunoregulatory.[105]

The bioactivity of CR is coupled to several signal-transduction pathways. Stimulation of the CR involves binding of a guanine nucleotide–coupled regulatory protein. This binding is coupled with the activation of adenylate cyclase with cAMP formation and activation of protein kinase A.[106] The same receptor is also coupled to activation of phosphoinositol-dependent phospholipase C, which results in calcium mobilization, and protein kinase C activation.[107] The two signal-transduction pathways require the presence of mediator proteins (namely, the cholera toxin–sensitive $G_s$ and the pertussis toxin–sensitive $G_i$). Coupling of the CT-CR complex to these distinct G proteins leads to opposite bioeffects. For example, the $Na^+$ pump is stimulated by protein kinase A and inhibited by protein kinase C. Furthermore, selective activation of the pathways can occur in a cell cycle–dependent manner because $G_s$ is activated in $G_2$ phase and no longer stimulated in S phase. Conversely, CRs couple to $G_i$ in S phase, but not in $G_2$ phase.[108]

The expression and activity of the CR is strongly regulated. CRs exhibit constitutive signaling activity (i.e., they cause elevation of intracellular cAMP even in the absence of CT agonist). This may be a mechanism to adapt their signaling properties in the absence of agonist, so that the cell is more sensitive to the hormone.[109] Conversely, treatment of mature osteoclasts with CT causes a rapid and prolonged decrease in CR mRNA levels, which is reflected in a loss of cell-surface CRs. Because these cells regain resorption competence, the data support the concept that the clinical phenomenon of "escape" from the hypocalcemic action of CT results from a loss of sensitivity of osteoclasts to the hormone.[110]

## CALCITONIN RECEPTOR–LIKE RECEPTORS

The classic ligands for the CRLRs had been considered to be CGRP-I and CGRP-II. At least two isoforms of the receptor were postulated, according to the presence or absence of antagonistic activity of the 8-37 fragment of CGRP-I. The molecular sequence of a CGRP receptor type 1 has been cloned. This receptor has a significant peptide sequence homology with the CR and shares similarities with this receptor in general structure and length.[111]

The CRLRs are expressed in a variety of tissues. They are most prevalent in various brain areas, where the regional distri-

bution is well conserved among different species. In addition, they are expressed in high densities in the cardiovascular system, especially within the intima and media layers of blood vessels. In the heart, CGRP binds in highest densities in coronary arteries, heart valves, and the right atrium. CRLRs are also expressed in the adrenal and pituitary glands, exocrine pancreas, kidney, and bone.

## RECEPTOR-ACTIVITY–MODIFYING PROTEIN AND THE PLASTICITY OF THE RECEPTORS FOR THE HORMONES OF THE CALCITONIN GENE FAMILY OF PEPTIDES

The search for the "specific" receptors for the peptides of the calcitonin gene family has been arduous and elusive. Identifying a specific and unique receptor for any one of these peptides has been difficult or impossible. Rather, a complex and fascinating overlapping of receptivity by the candidate receptors appears to exist. This phenomenon is related to the *multipotentiality of the two principal receptors* (or classes of receptors): CRs and CRLRs. These receptors manifest alternative physiologic profiles, which are conferred on them by the actions of certain accessory proteins; these allow a response to CT, to CGRP, to amylin, and/or to ADM in a dynamic and varying manner.

*RAMPs, or receptor-activity–modifying proteins*, are single-transmembrane-domain proteins that alter the phenotype of both CRs and CRLRs.[112] Three RAMPs are known: RAMP-1, RAMP-2, and RAMP-3. RAMPs act on CRs, probably by modifying the receptor gene. They act on the CRLRs, however, by influencing their transport to the plasma membrane. *The specific cellular phenotype of the receptors that is ultimately expressed on the cell surface is determined by the presence, concentration, and/or timing of one or more of the three known RAMPs.*

**Action of Receptor-Activity–Modifying Proteins on Calcitonin Receptors.** RAMP-1 induces a high-affinity amylin receptor, which also responds well to CGRP but poorly to CT (Table 53-1). RAMP-2 induces receptors with a high affinity for CT, a lower affinity for CGRP, and a weak binding to amylin. RAMP-3 induces a high-affinity amylin receptor with poor affinity for CGRP.

**Action of Receptor-Activity–Modifying Proteins on Calcitonin Receptor–Like Receptors.** RAMP-1 induces a CRLR with a strong affinity for CGRP. RAMP-2 or RAMP-3 induces a receptor with strong affinity for ADM (see Table 53-1).

**Impact of the Receptor-Activity–Modifying Proteins.** RAMPs, the expression of which is subject to humoral influences,[113] effect an astonishingly elegant regulation and diversi-

**TABLE 53-1.**

**RAMP-Induced Heterogeneity of Receptor Affinity to the Calcitonin Gene Family of Peptides and the Postulated Effects**

| Receptor RAMP Combination | Effect |
|---|---|
| **CR + RAMP-1** | High affinity for amylin and CGRP; low affinity for CT |
| **CR + RAMP-2** | High affinity for CT; low affinity for CGRP and amylin |
| **CR + RAMP-3** | High affinity for amylin; low affinity for CGRP |
| **CRLR + RAMP-1** | High affinity for CGRP |
| **CRLR + RAMP-2** | High affinity for adrenomedullin |
| **CRLR + RAMP-3** | High affinity for adrenomedullin |

*RAMP*, receptor-activity–modifying protein; *CR*, calcitonin receptor; *CGRP*, calcitonin gene–related peptide; *CT*, calcitonin; *CRLR*, calcitonin receptor–like receptor.
    See references 114–117.

fication of receptor function. They induce alternative profiles in the receptors for the peptides of the calcitonin gene family and presumably modulate hormonal responsivity according to ambient needs.

## CONCLUSION

Although much remains to be elucidated, knowledge concerning CT has increased enormously. The role of the peptide, first thought to be an important regulator of serum calcium, is still elusive. In spite of its as yet imperfectly defined functions, CT has become an important therapeutic agent. Furthermore, appreciable amounts of CTpr are now known to circulate in normal persons, and their potential hormonal roles require elucidation. Several common and often life-threatening conditions are associated with dramatic increases of these peptides. One of these peptides, ProCT, may contribute markedly to the morbidity and mortality of some of these conditions, and its immunoneutralization offers considerable therapeutic promise. Importantly, other related peptides have been discovered that comprise a calcitonin gene family. This family includes the CGRPs, amylin, and ADM. These latter peptides have some overlapping effects, as well as some very unique functions. Thus, that which conceptually began as a single hormone has broadened to include a great panoply of known or potential hormones.

## REFERENCES

1. Le Moullec JM, Jullienne A, Chenais J, et al. The complete sequence of human preprocalcitonin. FEBS Lett 1984; 167:93.
2. Steenbergh PH, Hoppener JW, Zandberg J, et al. Structure and expression of the human calcitonin/CGRP genes. FEBS Lett 1986; 209:97.
3. Nishi M, Sanke T, Seino S, et al. Human islet amyloid polypeptide gene: complete nucleotide sequence, chromosomal localization, and evolutionary history. Mol Endocrinol 1989; 3:1775.
4. Yeakley JM, Hedjran F, Morfin JP, et al. Control of calcitonin/calcitonin gene-related peptide pre-mRNA processing by constitutive intron and exon elements. Mol Cell Biol 1993; 13:5999.
5. Wimalawansa SJ. Amylin, calcitonin gene-related peptide, calcitonin, and adrenomedullin: a peptide superfamily. Crit Rev Neurobiol 1997; 11:167.
6. Becker KL, Snider RH, Moore CF, et al. Calcitonin in extrathyroidal tissues of man. Acta Endocrinol (Copenh) 1979; 92:746.
7. Becker KL, Silva OL, Snider RH, et al. The pathophysiology of pulmonary calcitonin. In: Becker KL, Gazdar AF, eds. The endocrine lung in health and disease. Philadelphia: WB Saunders, 1984:chap 16,277.
8. Copp DH, Cameron EC, Cheney BA, et al. Evidence for calcitonin—a new hormone from the parathyroid that lowers blood calcium. Endocrinology 1962; 70:638.
9. Suzuki K, Kono N, Onishi T, Tarin S. The effect of hypermagnesemia on serum immunoreactive calcitonin levels in normal human subjects. Acta Endocrinol (Copenh) 1987; 116:282.
10. Tabassian AR, Nylén ES, Giron AE, et al. Evidence for cigarette smoke-induced calcitonin secretion from lungs of man and hamster. Life Sci 1988; 42:2323.
11. Nylén ES, Becker KL, Snider RH Jr., et al. Cholinergic-nicotinic control of growth and secretion of cultured pulmonary neuroendocrine cells. Anat Rec 1993; 236:129.
12. Chambers TJ, Chambers JC, Symonds J, Darby JA. The effect of human calcitonin on the cytoplasmic spreading of rat osteoclasts. J Clin Endocrinol Metab 1986; 63:1080.
13. Wergedal J. The bone anabolic effect of antiresorptive drugs. In: Christiansen C, ed. Postmenopausal osteoporosis. State of the art 1994. Rodovre, Denmark: Osteopress ApS, 1994:20.
14. Jaeger P, Jones W, Clemens TL, Hayslett JP. Evidence that calcitonin stimulates 1,25-dihydroxyvitamin D production and intestinal absorption of calcium in vivo. J Clin Invest 1986; 78:456.
15. Stevenson JC, Hillyard CJ, MacIntyre I, et al. A physiological role for calcitonin: protection of the maternal skeleton. Lancet 1979; 2:769.
16. Care AD, Bruce JB, Boelkins J, et al. Role of pancreozymin-cholecystokinin and structurally related compounds as calcitonin secretogogues. Endocrinology 1971; 89:262.
17. Cooper CW, Schwesinger WH, Ontjes DA, et al. Stimulation of secretion of pig thyrocalcitonin by gastrin and related hormonal peptides. Endocrinology 1972; 91:1079.
18. Greeley GH Jr, Cooper CW, Jeng YJ, et al. Intracerebroventricular administration of calcitonin enhances glucose-stimulated release of insulin. Regul Pept 1989; 24:259.
19. Taggart HM, Chesnut CH, Ivey JL, et al. Deficient calcitonin response to calcium stimulation in postmenopausal osteoporosis? Lancet 1982; 1:475.
20. Stevenson JC, Whitehead MI. Calcitonin secretion and postmenopausal osteoporosis. [Letter]. Lancet 1982; 1:804.
21. Hurley DL, Tiegs RD, Barta J, et al. Effects of oral contraceptive and estrogen administration on plasma calcitonin in pre- and postmenopausal women. J Bone Miner Res 1989; 4:89.
22. Dick IM, Prince RL. Transdermal estrogen replacement does not increase calcitonin secretory reserve in postmenopausal women. Acta Endocrinol (Copenh) 1991; 125:241.
23. Kumar S, Zhu LJ, Polihronis M, Armant DR. Progesterone induces calcitonin gene expression in human endometrium within the putative window of implantation. J Clin Endocrinol Metab 1998; 83:4443.
24. Wang J, Rout UK, Bagchi IC, et al. Expression of calcitonin receptors in mouse preimplantation embryos and their function in the regulation of blastocyst differentiation by calcitonin. Development 1998; 125:4293.
25. Heath HD, Sizemore GW. Plasma calcitonin in normal man. Differences between men and women. J Clin Invest 1977; 60:1135.
26. Samaan NA, Anderson GD, Adam-Mayne ME. Immunoreactive calcitonin in the mother, neonate, child and adult. Am J Obstet Gynecol 1975; 121:622.
27. Simmons RE, Hjelle JT, Mahoney C, et al. Renal metabolism of calcitonin. Am J Physiol 1988; 254:F593.
28. Snider RH, Moore CF, Silva OL, Becker KL. Radioimmunoassay of calcitonin in normal human urine. Anal Chem 1978; 50:449.
29. Nylén ES, O'Neill W, Jordan MH, et al. Serum procalcitonin as an index of inhalation injury in burns. Horm Metab Res 1992; 24:439.
30. Silva OL, Becker KL. Salmon calcitonin in the treatment of hypercalcemia. Arch Intern Med 1973; 132:337.
31. Wisneski LA, Croom WP, Silva OL, et al. Salmon calcitonin in hypercalcemia. Clin Pharmacol Ther 1978; 24:219.
32. Garcia-Ameijeiras A, De La Torre W, Rodriguez-Espinosa J, et al. Does testosterone influence the post-stimulatory levels of calcitonin in normal men? Clin Endocrinol (Oxf) 1987; 27:545.
33. Mazzuoli GF, Passeri M, Gennari C, et al. Effects of salmon calcitonin in postmenopausal osteoporosis: a controlled double-blind clinical study. Calcif Tissue Int 1986; 38:3.
34. Gnudi S, Mongiorgi R, Moroni A, Bertocchi G. Densitometric analysis in in vivo evaluation of synthetic salmon calcitonin activity. J Clin Pharmacol Ther 1988; 13:125.
35. Peichl P, Rintelen B, Kumpan W, Broll H. Increase of axial and appendicular trabecular and cortical bone density in established osteoporosis with intermittent nasal salmon calcitonin therapy. Gynecol Endocrinol 1999; 13:7.
36. Civitelli R, Gonnelli S, Zacchei F, et al. Bone turnover in postmenopausal osteoporosis. Effect of calcitonin treatment. J Clin Invest 1988; 82:1268.
37. Downs RW Jr, Bell NH, Ettinger MP, et al. Comparison of alendronate and intranasal calcitonin for treatment of osteoporosis in postmenopausal women. J Clin Endocrinol Metab 2000; 85:1783.
38. Gennari C, Agnusdei D, Camporeale A. Long-term treatment with calcitonin in osteoporosis. Horm Metab Res 1993; 25:484.
39. Chesnut C, Baylink D, Doyle D, et al. Salmon calcitonin nasal spray prevents vertebral fractures in established osteoporosis. Osteoporosis Int 1998; 8:13.
40. Hizmetli S, Elden H, Kaptanoglu E, et al. The effect of different doses of calcitonin on bone mineral density and fracture risk in postmenopausal osteoporosis. Int J Clin Pract 1998; 52:453.
41. Kanis JA, McCloskey EV. Effect of calcitonin on vertebral and other fractures. QJM 1999; 92:143.
42. Reginster JY, Denis D, Deroisy R, et al. Long-term (3 years) prevention of trabecular postmenopausal bone loss with low-dose intermittent nasal salmon calcitonin. J Bone Miner Res 1994; 9:69.
43. Healey JH, Paget SA, Williams-Russo P, et al. A randomized controlled trial of salmon calcitonin to prevent bone loss in corticosteroid-treated temporal arteritis and polymyalgia rheumatica. Calcif Tissue Int 1996; 58:73.
44. Roth A, Kolaric K. Analgesic activity of calcitonin in patients with painful osteolytic metastases of breast cancer. Results of a controlled randomized study. Oncology 1986; 43:283.
45. Blower PJ, Puncher MRB, Kettle AG, et al. Iodine-123 salmon calcitonin, an imaging agent for calcitonin receptors: synthesis, biodistribution, metabolism and dosimetry in humans. Eur J Nucl Med 1998; 25:101.
46. Snider RH Jr, Nylén ES, Becker KL. Procalcitonin and its component peptides in systemic inflammation: immunochemical characterization. J Investig Med 1997; 45:552.
47. Born W, Beglinger C, Fischer JA. Diagnostic relevance of the amino-terminal cleavage peptide of procalcitonin (PAS-57), calcitonin and calcitonin gene-related peptide in medullary thyroid carcinoma patients. Regul Pept 1991; 32:311.
48. Cohen R, Giscard-Darteville S, Bracq S, et al. Calcitonin genes (I and II) expression in human nervous and medullary thyroid carcinoma tissues. Neuropeptides 1994; 26:215.
49. Burgess TL, Kelly RB. Constitutive and regulated secretion of proteins. Annu Rev Cell Biol 1987; 3:243.
50. Snider RH, Silva OL, Moore CF, Becker KL. Immunochemical heterogeneity of calcitonin in man: effect on radioimmunoassay. Clin Chim Acta 1977; 76:1.
51. Engelbach M, Gorges R, Forst T, et al. Improved diagnostic methods in the follow-up of medullary thyroid carcinoma by highly specific calcitonin measurements. J Clin Endocrinol Metab 2000; 85:1890.

52. Pacini F, Fontanelli M, Fugazzola L, et al. Routine measurement of serum calcitonin in nodular thyroid diseases allows the preoperative diagnosis of unsuspected sporadic medullary thyroid carcinoma. J Clin Endocrinol Metab 1994; 78:826.

53. Cohen R, Campos JM, Salaun C, et al. Preoperative calcitonin levels are predictive of tumor size and postoperative calcitonin normalization in medullary thyroid carcinoma. Groupe d'Etudes des Tumeurs à calcitonine (GETC). J Clin Endocrinol Metab 2000; 85:919.

54. Silva OL, Snider RH Jr, Moore CF, Becker KL. Urine calcitonin as a test for medullary thyroid cancer: a new screening procedure. Ann Surg 1979; 189:269.

55. Becker KL, Nash D, Silva OL, et al. Increased serum and urinary calcitonin levels in patients with pulmonary disease. Chest 1981; 79:211.

56. Linnoila RI, Becker KL, Snider RH, Moore CF. Calcitonin as a marker for diethylnitrosamine induced pulmonary endocrine cell hyperplasia in hamsters. Lab Invest 1984; 51:39.

57. Becker KL. The coming of age of a bronchial epithelial cell. Am Rev Respir Dis 1993; 148:1166.

58. Becker KL, Gazdar AF. What can the biology of small cell cancer teach us about the endocrine lung? Biochem Pharmacol 1985; 34:155.

59. Kelley MJ, Becker KL, Rushin JM, et al. Calcitonin elevation in small cell lung cancer without ectopic production. Am J Respir Crit Care Med 1994; 149:183.

60. Silva OL, Broder LE, Doppman JL, et al. Calcitonin as a marker for bronchogenic cancer: a prospective study. Cancer 1979; 44:680.

61. Mallet E, Lanse X, Devaux AM, et al. Hypercalcitoninaemia in fulminant meningococcaemia in children. Lancet 1983; 1:294.

62. Chesney RW, McCarron DM, Haddad JG, et al. Pathogenic mechanisms of the hypocalcemia of the staphylococcal toxic-shock syndrome. J Lab Clin Med 1983; 101:576.

63. Assicot M, Gendrel D, Carsin H, et al. High serum calcitonin concentrations in patients with sepsis and infection. Lancet 1993; 34:515.

64. Whang K, Steinwald PM, White JC, et al. Serum calcitonin precursors in sepsis and systemic infection. J Clin Endocrinol Metab 1998; 83:3296.

65. Müller B, Becker KL, Schächinger H, et al. Calcitonin precursors are reliable markers of sepsis in a medical intensive care unit. Crit Care Med 2000; 28:977.

66. Whang KT, Vath SD, Becker KL, et al. Procalcitonin and pro-inflammatory cytokine interactions in sepsis. Shock 2000; 14:73.

67. Nylén ES, Whang KT, Snider RH Jr, et al. Mortality is increased by procalcitonin and decreased by an antiserum reactive to procalcitonin in experimental sepsis. Crit Care Med 1998; 26:1001.

68. Wagner KE, Vath SD, Snider RH, et al. Immunoneutralization of elevated calcitonin precursors markedly attenuates the harmful physiologic response to sepsis. Paper presented at: 40th Interscience Conference on Antimicrobial Agents and Chemotherapy; September 17–20, 2000; Toronto, Canada.

69. Müller B, White JC, Nylén ES, et al. Ubiquitous expression of the calcitonin-1 gene in multiple tissues in response to sepsis. J Clin Endocrinol Metab 2001; 86:396.

70. Müller B, Becker KL, Snider RH, et al. Procalcitonin induces the synthesis of inflammatory cytokines by human peripheral blood mononuclear cells. Paper presented at: 39th Interscience Conference on Antimicrobial Agents and Chemotherapy; September 26–29, 1999; San Diego, CA.

71. Whang KT, Snider RH, White JC, et al. Impact of precalcitonin peptides on calcium in experimental sepsis. Paper presented at: Endocrine Society; June 24, 1998; New Orleans, LA.

72. Amara SG, Jonas V, Rosenfeld MG, et al. Alternative RNA processing in calcitonin gene expression generates mRNAs encoding different polypeptide products. Nature 1982; 298:240.

73. Steenbergh PH, Hoppener JW, Zandberg J, et al. A second human calcitonin/CGRP gene. FEBS Lett 1985; 183:403.

74. Hoppener JW, Steenbergh PH, Zandberg J, et al. A third human CALC (pseudo)gene on chromosome 11. FEBS Lett 1988; 233:57.

75. Williams ED, Ponder BJ, Craig RK. Immunohistochemical study of calcitonin gene-related peptide in human medullary carcinoma and C cell hyperplasia. Clin Endocrinol (Oxf) 1987; 27:107.

76. Petermann JB, Born W, Chang JY, Fischer JA. Identification in the human central nervous system, pituitary, and thyroid of a novel calcitonin gene-related peptide, and partial amino acid sequence in the spinal cord. J Biol Chem 1987; 262:542.

77. Kelley MJ, Snider RH, Becker KL, Johson BE. Small cell lung carcinoma cell lines express mRNA for calcitonin and α- and β-calcitonin gene related peptides. Cancer Lett 1994; 81:19.

78. Zaidi M, Chambers TJ, Gaines DR, et al. A direct action of human calcitonin gene-related peptide on isolated osteoclasts. J Endocrinol 1987; 115:511.

79. Donnerer J, Schuligoi R, Stein C, Amann R. Upregulation, release and axonal transport of substance P and calcitonin gene-related peptide in adjuvant inflammation and regulatory function of nerve growth factor. Regul Pept 1993; 46:150.

80. Fernandez S, Knopf MA, McGillis JP. Calcitonin-gene related peptide (CGRP) inhibits interleukin-7-induced pre-B cell colony formation. J Leukoc Biol 2000; 67:669.

81. Palmer JB, Cuss FM, Mulderry PK, et al. Calcitonin gene-related peptide is localized to human airway nerves and potently constricts human airway smooth muscle. Br J Pharmacol 1987; 91:95.

82. Molina JM, Cooper GJ, Leighton B, Olefsky JM. Induction of insulin resistance in vivo by amylin and calcitonin gene-related peptide. Diabetes 1990; 39:260.

83. Fahim A, Rettori V, McCann SM. The role of calcitonin gene-related peptide in the control of growth hormone and prolactin release. Neuroendocrinology 1990; 51:688.

84. Ashina M, Bendsten L, Jensen R, et al. Evidence for increased plasma levels of calcitonin gene-related peptide in migraine outside of attacks. Pain 2000; 86:133.

85. Benvenga S, Trimarchi F, Facchiano A. Homology of calcitonin with the amyloid-related proteins. J Endocrinol Invest 1994; 17:119.

86. Kleinman RM, Fagan SP, Ray MK, et al. Differential inhibition of insulin and islet amyloid polypeptide secretion by intraislet somatostatin in the isolated perfused human pancreas. Pancreas 1999; 19:346.

87. Samsom M, Szarka LA, Camilleri M, et al. Pramlintide, an amylin analog selectively delays gastric emptying: potential role of vagal inhibition. Am J Physiol Gastrointest Liver Physiol 2000; 278:G946.

88. Tenidis K, Waldner M, Bernhagen J, et al. Identification of a penta- and hexapeptide of islet amyloid polypeptide (IAPP) with amyloidogenic and cytotoxic properties. J Mol Biol 2000; 295:1055.

89. Yates SL, Burgess LH, Kocsis-Angle J, et al. Amyloid beta and amylin fibrils induce increases in proinflammatory cytokine and chemokine production by THP-1 cells and murine microglia. J Neurochem 2000; 74:1017.

90. Kitamura K, Kangawa K, Kawamoto M, et al. Adrenomedullin: a novel hypotensive peptide isolated from human pheochromocytoma. Biochem Biophys Res Commun 1993; 192:553.

91. Hinson JP, Kapas S, Smith DM. Adrenomedullin, a multifunctional regulatory peptide. Endocr Rev 2000; 21:138.

92. Ishihara T, Kato J, Kitamura K, et al. Production of adrenomedullin in human vascular endothelial cells. Life Sci 1997; 60:1763.

93. Kubo A, Minamino N, Isumi Y, et al. Adrenomedullin production is correlated with differentiation in human leukemia cell lines and peripheral blood monocytes. FEBS Lett 1998; 426:233.

94. Sato K, Hirata Y, Imai T, et al. Characterization of immunoreactive adrenomedullin in human plasma and urine. Life Sci 1995; 57:189.

95. Kato J, Kitamura K, Kangawa K, Eto T. Receptors for adrenomedullin in human vascular endothelial cells. Eur J Pharmacol 1995; 289:383.

96. Kanazawa H, Kurihara N, Hirata K, et al. Adrenomedullin, a newly discovered hypotensive peptide, is a potent bronchodilator. Biochem Biophys Res Commun 1994; 205:251.

97. Petrie MC, Hillier C, Morton JJ, McMurray JJ. Adrenomedullin selectively inhibits angiotensin II-induced aldosterone secretion in humans. J Hypertens 2000; 18:61.

98. Kamoi H, Kanazawa H, Hirata K, et al. Adrenomedullin inhibits the secretion of cytokine-induced neutrophil chemoattractant, a member of the interleukin-8 family, from rat alveolar macrophages. Biochem Biophys Res Commun 1995; 211:1031.

99. Yamaguchi T, Baba K, Doi Y, et al. Inhibition of aldosterone production by adrenomedullin, a hypotensive peptide, in the rat. Hypertension 1996; 28:308.

100. Sugo S, Minamino N, Shoji H, et al. Interleukin-1, tumor necrosis factor and lipopolysaccharide additively stimulate production of adrenomedullin in vascular smooth muscle cells. Biochem Biophys Res Commun 1995; 207:25.

101. Nishio K, Akai Y, Murao Y, et al. Increased plasma concentrations of adrenomedullin correlate with relaxation of vascular tone in patients with septic shock. Crit Care Med 1997; 25:953.

102. Moore EE, Kuestner RE, Stroop SD, et al. Functionally different isoforms of the human calcitonin receptor result from alternative splicing of the gene transcript. Mol Endocrinol 1995; 9:959.

103. Goldring SR. The structure and molecular biology of calcitonin receptor. In: Bilezikian JP, Raisz LG, Rodan GA, eds. Principles of bone biology. New York: Academic Press, 1996:461.

104. Marx SJ, Woodward CJ, Aurbach GD. Calcitonin receptors of kidney and bone. Science 1972; 178:999.

105. Body JJ, Fernandez G, Lacroix M, et al. Regulation of lymphocyte calcitonin receptors by interleukin-1 and interleukin-2. Calcif Tissue Int 1994; 55:109.

106. Barsony J, Marx SJ. Dual effects of calcitonin and calcitonin gene-related peptide on intracellular cyclic 3',5'-monophosphate in a human breast cancer cell line. Endocrinology 1988; 122:1218.

107. Teti A, Paniccia R, Goldring SR. Calcitonin increases cytosolic free calcium concentration via capacitative calcium influx. J Biol Chem 1995; 270:16666.

108. Chakraborty M, Chatterjee D, Kellokumpu S, et al. Cell cycle-dependent coupling of the calcitonin receptor to different G proteins. Science 1991; 251:1078.

109. Cohen DP, Thaw CN, Varma A, et al. Human calcitonin receptors exhibit agonist-independent (constitutive) signaling activity. Endocrinology 1997; 138:1400.

110. Findlay DM, Martin TJ. Receptors of calciotropic hormones. Horm Metab Res 1997; 29:128.

111. Aiyar N, Rand K, Elshourbagy NA, et al. A cDNA encoding the calcitonin gene-related peptide type 1 receptor. J Biol Chem 1996; 271:11325.

112. McLatchie LM, Fraser NJ, Main MJ, et al. RAMPs regulate the transport and ligand specificity of the calcitonin-receptor-like receptor. Nature 1998; 393:333.

113. Frayon S, Cueille C, Gnidehou S, et al. Dexamethasone increases RAMP1 and CRLR mRNA expressions in human vascular smooth muscle cells. Biochem Biophys Res Commun 2000; 270:1063.

114. Muff R, Bühlmann N, Fischer JA, Born W. An amylin receptor is revealed following co-transfection of a calcitonin receptor with receptor activity modifying proteins-1 or -3. Endocrinology 1999; 140:2924.
115. Christopoulos G, Perrk J, Morfis M, et al. Multiple amylin receptors arise from receptor activity-modifying protein interaction with the calcitonin receptor gene product. Mol Pharmacol 1999; 56:235.
116. Sumpe ET, Tilakaratne N, Fraser NJ, et al. Multiple ramp domains are required for generation of amylin receptor phenotype from the calcitonin receptor gene product. Biochem Biophys Res Commun 2000; 267:368.
117. Martínez A, Kapas S, Miller M-J, et al. Coexpression of receptors for adrenomedullin, calcitonin gene-related peptide, and amylin in pancreatic β cells. Endocrinology 2000; 141:406.

# CHAPTER 54

# VITAMIN D

THOMAS L. CLEMENS AND JEFFREY L. H. O'RIORDAN

## CHEMISTRY

Vitamin D and its analogs form a group of fat-soluble secosterols with antirachitic properties.[1] The two parent forms of vitamin D are *ergocalciferol (vitamin $D_2$)* and *cholecalciferol (vitamin $D_3$)*. Ergocalciferol derives its name from its immediate precursor, ergosterol, the plant sterol from which it was originally prepared. Cholecalciferol is the natural form of the vitamin and is produced by irradiation of the precursor, 7-dehydrocholesterol. The D vitamins are structurally related to C-21 steroids but differ by having an opened B ring that forms a conjugated triene structure (Fig. 54-1). Vitamin $D_2$ differs structurally from vitamin $D_3$ by having a double bond between the carbon positions 22 and 23 and a methyl group at C-24. Both vitamin $D_2$ and vitamin $D_3$ are metabolized along the same pathways, producing active metabolites with equivalent biologic effects (Fig. 54-2). When written without the subscript, the term *vitamin D* may refer to either compound.

## PRODUCTION AND METABOLISM OF VITAMIN D

### PHOTOPRODUCTION

Technically, vitamin $D_3$ is not a true vitamin because it can be produced in the body. Its synthesis in skin can provide the body's entire requirement unless exposure to sunlight is restricted (see Chap. 185). The reaction proceeds by nonenzy-

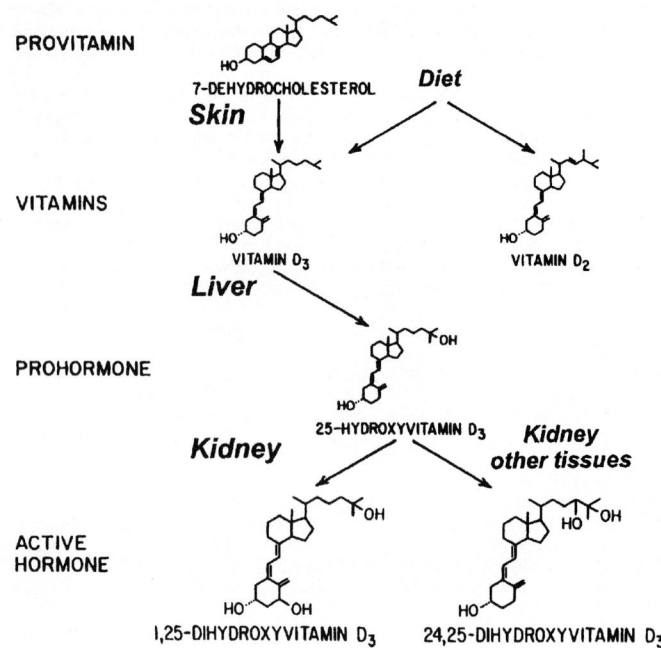

**FIGURE 54-2.** The main metabolic pathways of vitamin $D_3$ production and activation. Vitamin $D_2$ from the diet is metabolized along the same pathways, yielding the corresponding vitamin $D_2$ metabolites (not shown).

matic photolysis of 7-dehydrocholesterol (provitamin D) in the epidermis.[2] Near-ultraviolet (UV) light (wavelengths 290–315 nm) penetrates to the basal layer and cleaves the bond between carbon atoms 9 and 10 of 7-dehydrocholesterol, forming previtamin $D_3$ (see Fig. 54-2). Previtamin $D_3$ and vitamin $D_3$ are in thermal equilibrium; production of the latter is favored at body temperature. The time-dependent thermal isomerization of previtamin $D_3$ to vitamin $D_3$ allows the continuous release of vitamin $D_3$ into the circulation for several days after exposure to sunlight. Previtamin $D_3$ is subject to further photolysis, yielding the biologically inert photoproducts, lumisterol and tachysterol. Studies measuring circulating vitamin $D_3$ in subjects who have been given graded amounts of UV light have estimated that exposure to one minimal erythema dose results in the formation of at least 30 μg of vitamin $D_3$ per square meter of body surface. The skin pigment melanin, when present in large amounts, competes with 7-dehydrocholesterol for absorption of UV energy. Thus, heavily pigmented black persons make less vitamin $D_3$ in response to UV exposure than do lightly pigmented white persons.

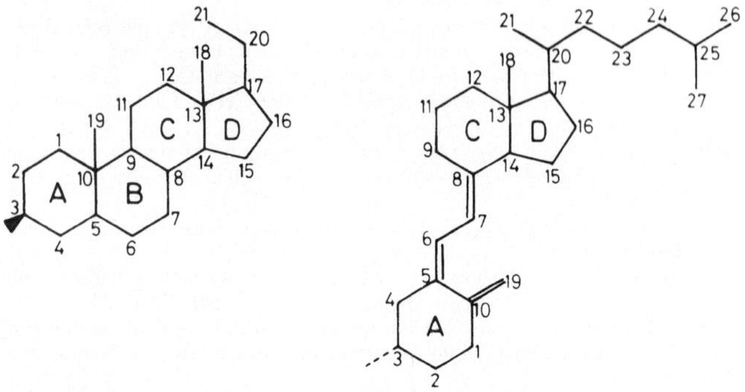

### DIETARY SOURCES

Few foods naturally contain appreciable amounts of vitamin D. The livers of fatty fish are a relatively rich source,[2a] which accounts for the efficacy of cod-liver oil as a cure for rickets. Insignificant amounts of vitamin D exist naturally in dairy products. The limited dietary availability of vitamin D led to its use as a supplement in certain foods. In the United States, federal regulation stipulates that 10 μg (400 IU) of vitamin D be added to every quart of milk. (In the United Kingdom, milk is not fortified with vitamin D, which may partly explain the lower vitamin D stores of its residents.) Multivitamin preparations typically contain 10 μg, which is twice the recommended dietary allowance of vitamin D as noted by the National Academy of Sciences. It has been estimated that the true vitamin D requirement in the absence of sunlight exposure could be as much as 600 IU or 15 μg per day.[3] Previously, the exclusive use of vitamin $D_2$ as a food additive made it the source of the circulating metabolites. Today,

**FIGURE 54-1.** The structure of vitamin $D_3$: A 9–10 secosterol (*right*), and a C-21 steroid (*left*).

however, either vitamin $D_2$ or vitamin $D_3$ is added to foods, so that vitamin $D_3$ metabolites in the circulation may have originated from endogenous or from dietary sources.

## METABOLIC ACTIVATION OF VITAMIN D

Vitamin D has little, if any, intrinsic bioactivity. Sequential hydroxylation reactions, which occur first in the liver and then in the kidney, are required for the production of the biologically active form, 1,25-dihydroxyvitamin D (1,25[OH]$_2$D).[1] The addition of the two hydroxyl groups enables 1,25(OH)$_2$D to bind to intracellular receptors in target tissues with high affinity. The metabolism and mode of action of vitamin D, therefore, are similar to those of other steroid hormones.

## 25-HYDROXYLATION IN THE LIVER

The first step in the activation of vitamin D is 25-hydroxylation, which occurs in the liver and is obligatory for further metabolism of the vitamin. Although other tissues can metabolize [$^3$H]vitamin $D_3$ to [$^3$H]25(OH)$D_3$ in vitro, the liver is the principal site of production; total hepatectomy causes the virtual disappearance of 25-hydroxyvitamin $D_3$ (25[OH]$D_3$) from the circulation. Hepatic 25-hydroxylase enzyme activity is associated with both mitochondrial and microsomal fractions. The mitochondrial enzyme, a cytochrome P-450 protein designated CYP27,[4,5] has been cloned and also has been shown to hydroxylate cholesterol and sterols involved in bile acid synthesis. Normally, 25(OH)D circulates at 5 to 65 ng/mL and has a circulating half-life of ~15 days. It is not considered bioactive at physiologic concentrations in vivo, but appears to be active at high concentrations when assessed in vitro. Its order of potency in calcium transport bioassay systems is similar to its 1,25(OH)$_2$D intestinal receptor binding activity, suggesting that, at high serum concentrations in vivo, it has agonist activity.[6] Accordingly, the hypercalcemia produced by vitamin D intoxication is almost certainly mediated by 25(OH)D.

## 1α-HYDROXYLATION IN THE KIDNEY

The final step in the activation of vitamin D occurs in the kidney, in which 25(OH)D is converted to 1,25(OH)$_2$D, the biologically active and most potent metabolite.[6a] The major site of 1α-hydroxylation is the renal proximal tubule.[7] Although other tissues and cultured cells produce 1,25(OH)$_2$D$_3$ in vitro, 1,25-(OH)$_2$D$_3$ is absent from the serum of anephric animals and humans, suggesting that extrarenal sources do not contribute significantly to circulating 1,25(OH)$_2$D concentrations under normal physiologic conditions. However, in pregnancy, the placenta synthesizes 1,25(OH)$_2$D and supplies additional hormone to the circulation.[8] Extrarenal synthesis of the metabolite also occurs in patients with sarcoidosis, in whom hypercalcemia and elevated 1,25(OH)$_2$D levels have been demonstrated, even in the anephric state[9] (Fig. 54-3). The synthesis of [$^3$H]1,25(OH)$_2$D$_3$ by pulmonary alveolar macrophages from patients with sarcoidosis has been demonstrated in vitro, suggesting that these cells are the source of the ectopic production.[10] It is likely that the hypercalcemia associated with other granulomatous diseases, such as tuberculosis, and with certain lymphomas also is attributable to extrarenal production of 1,25(OH)$_2$D (see Chap. 59).

The enzyme responsible for the conversion of 25(OH)D to 1,25(OH)$_2$D, vitamin D-25 1α-hydroxylase (CYP1), has been cloned[11] and is a mixed-function cytochrome P450 protein.[11a] The enzyme requires NADPH generated in the inner mitochondrial membrane of the renal proximal convoluted tubule cell by an energy-dependent trans-hydrogenase. Thus, inhibitors of oxidative phosphorylation or electron transport will inhibit 1α-hydroxylation in vitro.[12] Along with 25(OH)D, 24,25(OH)$_2$D and 25,26(OH)$_2$D also can serve as substrates to yield 1,24,25(OH)$_3$D and 1,25,26(OH)$_3$D, respectively. Under normal

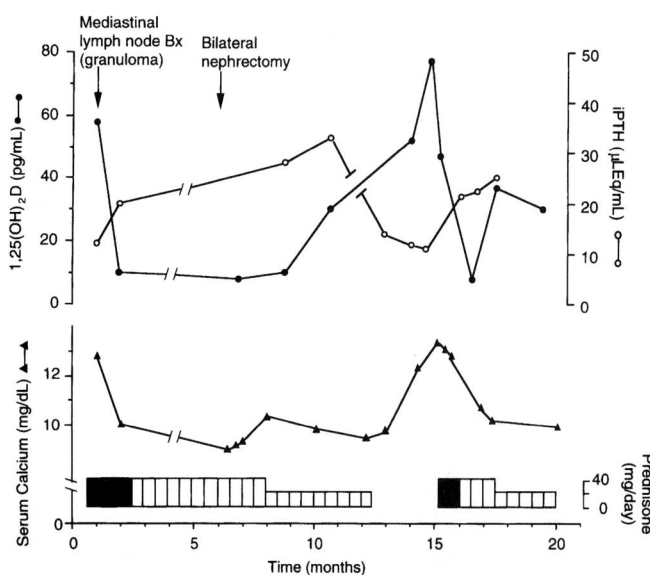

**FIGURE 54-3.** Extrarenal production of 1,25(OH)$_2$D in an anephric patient with sarcoidosis. The patient had progressive hypercalcemia in the face of renal failure that was associated with elevated serum 1,25(OH)$_2$D levels and suppressed immunoreactive parathyroid hormone (*iPTH*) concentrations. Bilateral nephrectomy and reduction of the prednisone dosage resulted in marked elevations in serum 1,25(OH)$_2$D levels and worsening of the hypercalcemia, implicating an extrarenal source of the 1,25(OH)$_2$D production. (From Barbour GL, Coburn JW, Slatopolsky E, et al. Hypercalcemia in a anephric patient with sarcoidosis: evidence for extrarenal generation of 1,25-dihydroxyvitamin D. N Engl J Med 1981; 305:440.)

physiologic conditions, the circulating concentration of 1,25(OH)$_2$D is 500 to 1000 times lower than that of 25(OH)D. In humans, 1 μg of 1,25(OH)$_2$D is produced each day; its circulating half-life is ~4 to 6 hours.[13]

## 24-HYDROXYLATION

25-Hydroxyvitamin D also is subject to hydroxylation at C-24, producing 24,25(OH)$_2$D, which is the second most abundant circulating metabolite of vitamin D. Most circulating 24,25(OH)$_2$D is made in the kidney. Other tissues, most notably cartilage and intestine, also can produce 24,25(OH)$_2$D$_3$ in vitro. The renal 24-hydroxylase (CYP24) also has been cloned,[14] and like the vitamin D-25 1-hydroxylase is a mixed function P450-dependent enzyme. It is expressed in mitochondria of renal tubular cells, but is distinct from the vitamin D-25 1α-hydroxylase and demonstrates a broader tissue distribution.[14,15] The main substrate is 25(OH)D, but under certain conditions, the enzyme also will hydroxylate 1,25(OH)$_2$D to form 1,24,25(OH)$_3$D. Normally, 24,25(OH)$_2$D circulates at concentrations that are ten-fold lower than those of 25(OH)D. Compared with 1,25(OH)$_2$D$_3$, 24,25(OH)$_2$D$_3$ is far less active when bioassayed in the systems that are responsive to vitamin D. No clear role can be ascribed to 24,25(OH)$_2$D; however, it may simply be a product of the further metabolism and inactivation of vitamin $D_3$, because 24-hydroxylation renders the molecule susceptible to side-chain cleavage and oxidation.

## OTHER PATHWAYS OF VITAMIN D METABOLISM

Other circulating forms of vitamin D have been isolated and identified.[16] 25,26-Dihydroxyvitamin D is produced in the kidney and probably in the liver. Its serum concentration usually is slightly lower than that of 24,25(OH)$_2$D. The 25(OH)D$_3$26,23-lactone has been identified in the plasma of animals and humans. Studies of the metabolism of 1,25(OH)$_2$D have identified a major oxidative cleavage product as the C-23 carboxylic acid. Other side-chain metabolites of vitamin D have been iso-lated from animals given large doses of the vitamin or from tis-sues incubated with 25(OH)D$_3$ in vitro. The physiologic significance of these metabolites, aside from being intermedi-ates in the vitamin D catabolic pathway, is unknown.

## REGULATION OF VITAMIN D METABOLISM

The metabolic activation of vitamin D is subject to both coarse- and fine-control mechanisms operating at the principal enzy-matic steps.[17] Hepatic 25-hydroxylation is more efficient at low levels of substrate, and the absolute amount of 25(OH)D in the circulation declines when the supply of vitamin D increases. Nevertheless, the degree of regulation of 25(OH)D synthesis is not sufficient to prevent vitamin D intoxication after the inges-tion of large amounts of vitamin D.[18]

In contrast to the relatively coarse control of hepatic 25-hydroxylation, renal 1α-hydroxylation is regulated strictly and represents the most important regulatory mechanism in the metabolism of vitamin D. In normal adults, serum concentrations of 1,25(OH)$_2$D change little in response to repeated dosing with vitamin D, and remain normal or even decline in vitamin D intox-ication. The three major factors that regulate the enzyme's activity are blood parathyroid hormone (PTH), calcium, and phosphorus.

### PARATHYROID HORMONE

Parathyroid hormone is the main hormonal stimulus for 1α-hydroxylation, increasing systemic 1,25(OH)$_2$D levels after administration to human research subjects.[19] Hypocalcemia also stimulates 1α-hydroxylation, but this effect is achieved largely through a feedback loop (see Chap. 58) involving the parathyroid glands[17]; hypocalcemia stimulates PTH secretion, which raises serum 1,25(OH)$_2$D concentrations. 1,25(OH)$_2$D enhances calcium absorption, and the increased serum calcium concentration then inhibits PTH secretion (Fig. 54-4). Some experimental studies suggest that the extracellular calcium con-centration can directly influence the renal 1α-hydroxylase.

### PHOSPHORUS

The blood phosphorus concentration is the third major control factor. In rats and in humans, hypophosphatemia stimulates 1α-hydroxylase activity and increases the 1,25(OH)$_2$D concentration in serum, whereas hyperphosphatemia inhibits formation of the metabolite (see Fig. 54-4). This adaptive effect does not depend on PTH, but it may require insulin-like growth factor-I.[20]

### OTHER REGULATORS

Other factors may directly or indirectly affect the activity of the renal 1α-hydroxylase enzyme. 1,25(OH)$_2$D$_3$ inhibits its own pro-duction in cultured kidney cells.[21] In rats, calcitonin stimulates the production of 1,25(OH)$_2$D, apparently through a mechanism different from PTH stimulation.[22] Prolactin, insulin, and growth hormone all stimulate 1α-hydroxylase in mammals. In birds, enhanced estrogen and progesterone secretion during ovulation stimulates 1α-hydroxylation and increases serum 1,25(OH)$_2$D concentrations. Therefore, these hormones appear to stimulate 1,25(OH)$_2$D$_3$ production to accommodate the increased mineral ion requirement during growth and reproduction.

### CONTROL OF 24-HYDROXYLATION

When blood calcium, phosphorus, and PTH levels are normal, 25(OH)D is converted mainly to 24,25(OH)$_2$D, whereas in the vitamin D–deficient state, the production of 1,25(OH)$_2$D$_3$ is induced and the synthesis of 24,25(OH)$_2$D$_3$ is suppressed. This reciprocal relationship between the production of these metab-

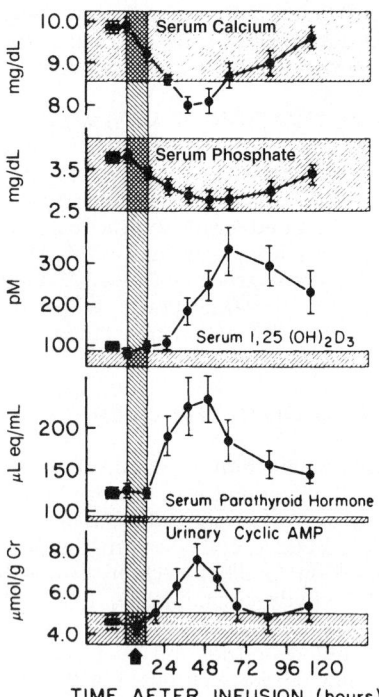

**FIGURE 54-4.** Effect of a decline in plasma calcium on circulating para-thyroid hormone and 1,25(OH)$_2$D concentrations in humans. Eight patients with Paget disease received plicamycin (25 μg/kg) by infusion. This resulted in a sudden reduction of plasma calcium levels followed by an increase in parathyroid hormone and 1,25(OH)$_2$D$_3$ concentra-tions. (*AMP*, adenosine monophosphate.) (Modified from Bilezikian JP, Canfield RE, Jacobs JP. Response of 1α-dihydroxyvitamin D$_3$ to hypo-calcemia in human subjects. N Engl J Med 1978; 299:437.)

olites has been demonstrated elegantly in cultured kidney cells.[21] The 24-hydroxylase enzyme activity and expression of its mRNA are acutely induced by 1,25(OH)$_2$D$_3$ in kidney and in other vitamin D–responsive cells.[23] As mentioned earlier, this appears to represent a mechanism by which activity of 1,25(OH)$_2$D$_3$ is limited.

### MATERNAL-FETAL METABOLISM

During human fetal development, ~30 g of calcium is trans-ferred from mother to fetus. Adaptations in maternal vitamin D metabolism during pregnancy are important in supplying this extra calcium to the fetus.[24] The increase in intestinal calcium absorption that persists throughout pregnancy is sufficient to sustain a positive calcium balance.[25] The circulating concentra-tions of 1,25(OH)$_2$D and its transporting protein (vitamin D–binding protein) increase in parallel during the first two trimes-ters. During the third trimester, however, total serum 1,25(OH)$_2$D levels continue to increase, whereas vitamin D–binding protein concentrations fall slightly.[26] This finding sug-gests that elevation in the biologically important, free 1,25(OH)$_2$D concentration stimulates maternal intestinal cal-cium absorption. The placental 1α-hydroxylase enzyme sup-plies additional 1,25(OH)$_2$D to the mother and child during pregnancy. The assayed concentrations of 1,25(OH)$_2$D in mater-nal and cord blood are positively correlated, suggesting placen-tal transfer of the metabolite, or stimulation of both fetal and maternal 1α-hydroxylase by common hormonal factors. Con-versely, maternal and fetal 24,25(OH)$_2$D concentrations decrease during this period. Enhanced hepatic synthesis of vitamin D–binding protein, which would cause a transient decrease in free 1,25(OH)$_2$D levels, may be the initial stimulus for the subsequent increase in 1,25(OH)$_2$D concentrations. PTH and prolactin also probably play a role in the adaptation of vitamin D metabolism during pregnancy.

## ABSORPTION, TRANSPORT, AND EXCRETION

Dietary vitamin D is absorbed with fats in the small intestine and is incorporated into chylomicrons. The efficiency of absorption normally is 60% to 90%, and interruptions of this process, such as in steatorrhea, can lead to vitamin D malabsorption (see Chap. 63). In the vitamin D–replete state, as much as 50% of the absorbed vitamin may be stored in body fats. Thus, high tissue concentrations of 25(OH)D may persist in patients long after treatment with pharmacologic doses of vitamin D has been discontinued.

### VITAMIN D–BINDING PROTEIN

Vitamin D entering the circulation from either dietary or epidermal sources is bound by vitamin D–binding protein (DBP), an α-globulin of 55,000 daltons that is identical with a serum protein originally described as the group-specific component.[27] This protein has a single, high-affinity binding site that will bind vitamin D and all its metabolites, although it has higher affinity for 25(OH)$D_3$, 24,25(OH)$_2D_3$, and 25,26(OH)$_2D_3$ than for vitamin $D_3$ or 1,25(OH)$_2D_3$.[28] This order of selectivity may facilitate the partitioning of vitamin D in lipid stores and favors entry of biologically active 1,25(OH)$_2D_3$ into target cells. Mice null for the DBP gene develop normally, but demonstrate an increased rate of clearance of 25(OH)D compared with controls,[29] which is consistent with the notion that DBP functions primarily as a vitamin D metabolite carrier protein. The serum concentration of DBP greatly exceeds the concentration of all the known metabolites of the vitamin, so that only 3% to 5% of available binding sites are occupied. Hepatic synthesis of the protein is increased during pregnancy and there is appreciable urinary loss in patients with hypoproteinemia. Nevertheless, its serum concentration is largely unaltered in other disorders of mineral or skeletal homeostasis.[30]

### EXCRETION

The pathways for excretion of vitamin D and its metabolites are still poorly understood. Bile appears to be a principal route; the biliary excretion of vitamin D metabolites increases when anticonvulsant drugs are administered.[31] There is little urinary excretion of vitamin D. Sulfate conjugates of vitamin $D_3$, with no related biologic activity, have been identified in urine and in breast milk.[32]

## BIOLOGIC ACTIONS OF VITAMIN D

### INTESTINE

#### CALCIUM TRANSPORT

The most important bioeffect of 1,25(OH)$_2D_3$ is to increase the intestinal absorption of calcium. Although the details of the mechanisms underlying this process remain sketchy, several key steps have been characterized.[33] In the absence of vitamin D, $Ca^{2+}$ is able to enter the cell, but little is absorbed as a result of its sequestration in the brush border terminal web. When 1,25(OH)$_2D_3$ is given to a vitamin D–deficient animal, there is a rapid increase in $Ca^{2+}$ entry over ~30 minutes. A second phase of calcium transport peaks several hours after administration of 1,25(OH)$_2D_3$, and termination of the entire transcellular $Ca^{2+}$ absorption process is not complete for several more hours. During this lag period, calbindin (see later) and other vitamin D–induced proteins are synthesized and are believed to participate in the delivery of $Ca^{2+}$ to the basolateral membrane, where

the ion is extruded by the action of the $Na^+/Ca^{2+}$ exchanger. The number of functional $Na^+/Ca^{2+}$ exchangers is increased by vitamin-D treatment.

The best characterized vitamin D–induced protein is a cytoplasmic, 28,000-dalton calcium-binding protein (calbindin 28K) that was first identified in chick intestine.[34] This protein has four high-affinity calcium-binding sites, and its dependence on vitamin D distinguishes it from calmodulin and other intracellular calcium-binding proteins. A separate 9000-dalton vitamin D–dependent calcium-binding protein (calbindin 9K), with 2 $Ca^{2+}$ binding sites, is expressed in mammalian intestine. In vitamin D–deficient chickens given 1,25(OH)$_2D$ orally, both the induction of calcium transport and the appearance of calbindin in villus enterocytes are demonstrable within a few hours after dosing. As indicated earlier, calbindin is thought to play a direct role in calcium transport but it may also mediate specific calcium-dependent processes within the enterocyte. The vitamin D–dependent calbindin 28K also is expressed in kidney,[35] brain,[36] bone, and other tissues.[34] Although the calbindins were initially viewed as vitamin D–dependent proteins, it is now clear that they are expressed in a wide array of tissues in a vitamin D–independent fashion. It has been suggested that the calbindins might serve as a buffer to guard against large fluctuations in intracellular calcium.

### PHOSPHATE TRANSPORT

The impact of vitamin D on phosphate transport was described in the 1960s by Harrison and Harrison using an everted gut sac method. Phosphate, like calcium, is transferred across the intestinal epithelium via a multi-step process.[37] An energy-dependent step is required for entry of the negatively charged phosphate ion into the cell, whereas the extrusion step occurs primarily by diffusional processes. Studies in vitamin D–deficient chicks administered $^{32}P$-phosphate suggest that vitamin D exerts effects on both the phosphate entry and exit mechanisms. The phosphate-entry step is $Na^+$-dependent, which is reminiscent of the absorption of a number of nonelectrolytes, such as glucose and amino acids. Several isoforms of the renal $Na^+$/phosphate co-transporters have been identified in intestinal mucosa. In addition, vitamin D induces the synthesis of a $Na^+$/phosphate co-transporter on the basolateral membrane. A $Na^+$/phosphate co-transporter is expressed on the basolateral membrane; however, it is unclear whether vitamin D affects the synthesis of this protein.

### EFFECT ON MEMBRANE LIPID

1,25-Dihydroxyvitamin D affects the lipid composition of intestinal brush border epithelial cells. 1,25(OH)$_2D$-induced synthesis of phosphatidylcholine occurs over a time course similar to the 1,25(OH)$_2D$-stimulated uptake of calcium into brush border membrane vesicles.[38] These observations gave rise to the concept that 1,25(OH)$_2D_3$ may exert some of its actions through nongenomic mechanisms. Consistent with this notion are studies that show rapid influxes in intracellular calcium in several cell types in vitro and acute increases in intestinal calcium uptake in ex vivo preparations of chicken intestine.[39] Presumably, these activities would require 1,25(OH)$_2D_3$ binding to a membrane receptor. Such a receptor has been proposed but has not yet been identified.

### SKELETON

The most familiar property of the D vitamins is their ability to cure rickets. However, normalization of blood calcium and phosphorus levels by intravenous infusion of calcium into vitamin D–deficient rats can cure rickets in the absence of circulating 1,25(OH)$_2D$.[40] Hence, the main antirachitogenic effects of 1,25(OH)$_2D_3$ rely more on its mobilization of calcium and phosphorus at the level of the intestine than on any direct effect it has on bone formation. Nonetheless, treatment of osteoblast cells with 1,25(OH)$_2D$ in vitro is associated with marked

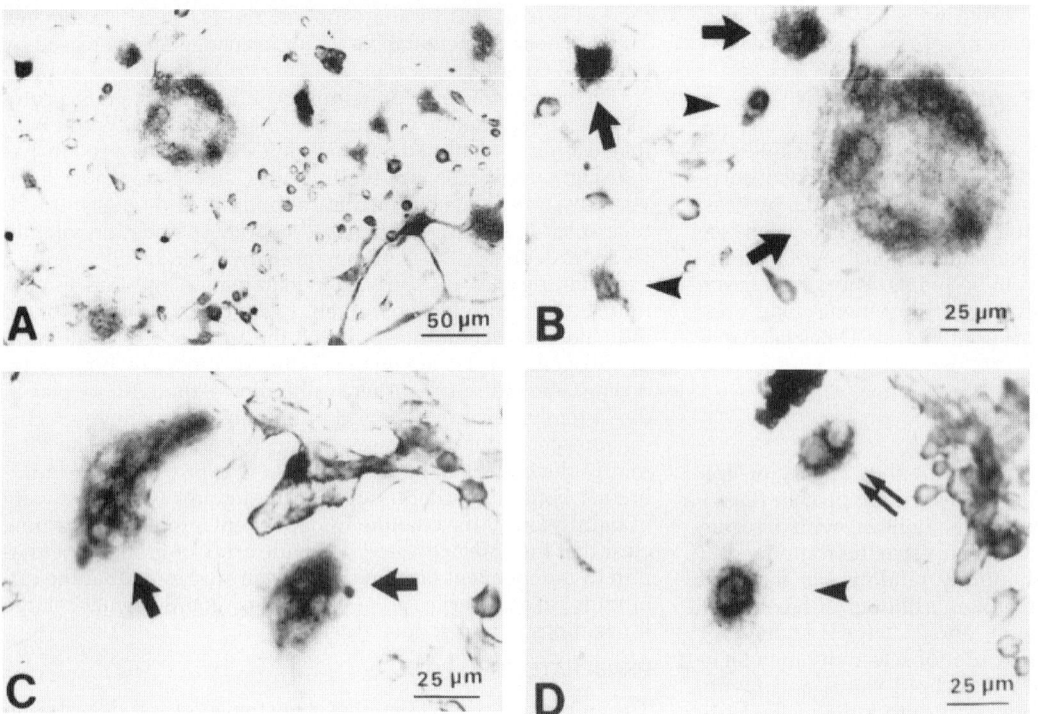

**FIGURE 54-5.** Induction of osteoclast-like cells by 1,25-(OH)$_2$D$_3$ in vitro. Autoradiographs of [$^{125}$I] calcitonin binding in mouse bone marrow cultures exposed to 1,25-(OH)$_2$D$_3$ for 8 days (**A** through **C**) or 3 days (**D**). Arrows are pointing to binding of [$^{125}$I] calcitonin to calcitonin receptors. Panel **B** shows a high-power micrograph of multinucleate cells staining positive for tartrate-resistant acid phosphatase (*TRAP*) and demonstrating calcitonin binding (indicated by the dense silver grains), two markers for osteoclasts. (From Takahashi N, Akatsu T, Sakasi T, et al. Induction of calcitonin receptors by 1,25-dihydroxyvitamin D$_3$ in osteoclast-like multinucleated cells formed in mouse bone marrow cells. Endocrinology 1988; 123:1504.)

changes in expression of osteoblast-specific genes.[41] 1,25(OH)$_2$D$_3$ decreases the rate of synthesis of collagen and citrate decarboxylase and increases alkaline phosphatase activity and the synthesis of the noncollagenous proteins, osteocalcin, and osteopontin. The precise role of 1,25(OH)$_2$D$_3$ in osteoblast function remains controversial, in part because of the differences in the experimental osteoblast cell models. By contrast, the ability of 1,25(OH)$_2$D to cause bone mineral resorption is uncontested. Studies in vitro, using neonatal calvaria or long bones prelabeled with $^{45}$Ca, have readily demonstrated increases in cell-mediated resorption.[42] 1,25(OH)$_2$D$_3$ increases the activity of existing osteoclasts and the rate of recruitment from mononuclear cell precursors.[43] Each of these activities appears to occur indirectly, after stimulation of an osteoblast factor called osteoprotegerin, which is a soluble member of the tumor necrosis factor (TNF) receptor family (see Chap. 61).

## ACTIONS ON OTHER TISSUES

In addition to the classic actions of vitamin D on mineral ion homeostasis, many other biologic processes are affected by 1,25(OH)$_2$D$_3$. As mentioned earlier, 1,25(OH)$_2$D$_3$ induces the 24-hydroxylase enzyme activity in kidney and other tissues. An inhibitory effect of 1,25(OH)$_2$D$_3$ on PTH secretion has been demonstrated, thus documenting a feedback loop in the control of 1,25(OH)$_2$D$_3$ synthesis.[44] This observation has led to the use of intravenous 1,25(OH)$_2$D$_3$ in the treatment of secondary hyperparathyroidism of chronic renal failure.[45] Vitamin D–deficient animals have reduced insulin secretion and impaired glucose tolerance that can be corrected by the administration of 1,25(OH)$_2$D$_3$.[46]

An increasingly appreciated action of 1,25(OH)$_2$D$_3$ is its ability to alter the developmental program of a diverse array of cell types. Exposure to near-physiologic concentrations of 1,25(OH)$_2$D$_3$ induces maturation of basal epidermal skin cells into keratinocytes and stimulates mouse myeloid leukemic cells to differentiate into macrophage-like cells.[47–49] As previously mentioned, 1,25(OH)$_2$D$_3$ stimulates the formation of multinucleated osteoclast-like cells in bone marrow cultures[50] (Fig. 54-5). These activities are accompanied by alterations in

biochemical markers and morphologic changes consistent with the differentiated phenotype. Such pleiotropic actions of 1,25(OH)$_2$D$_3$, together with the multiple-tissue distribution of the vitamin D receptor, suggest that the hormone functions during development and organogenesis.

## NONHYPERCALCEMIC VITAMIN D ANALOGS

Synthetic vitamin D analogs have been prepared that retain the ability to bind and activate the vitamin D receptor but are less calcemic than 1,25(OH)$_2$D$_3$ when administered to animals. These so-called *nonhypercalcemic analogs* (which is not a strictly accurate term because they cause hypercalcemia when administered at large doses) have a chemically modified side chain that reduces affinity for the serum vitamin D–binding protein and accelerates their metabolic degradation.[51] This property apparently accounts in part for their selective action on certain tissues (e.g., the parathyroid gland). It is likely that these analogs eventually will be used therapeutically in the treatment of such conditions as secondary hyperparathyroidism of chronic renal failure and hyperproliferative disorders such as psoriasis.

## BIOCHEMICAL MECHANISM OF ACTION

### INTRACELLULAR RECEPTORS

Tissues that are responsive to vitamin D express a specific intracellular receptor for 1,25(OH)$_2$D.[52] The fraction of circulating 1,25(OH)$_2$D that is not bound to serum vitamin D–binding protein diffuses across the target cell membrane and binds to an intracellular receptor protein. The protein from chick intestine has a molecular mass of 60,000 daltons and appears to be located predominantly within the nucleus, although a separate cytoplasmic component may serve to translocate the 1,25(OH)$_2$D ligand to the nuclear compartment. The rank order of receptor binding for a series of vitamin D metabolites correlates well with their order of biologic activities. Biochemical characterization of the vitamin D receptor (VDR) and its molecular cloning has revealed that it is closely related to the thyroid hormone and retinoic acid

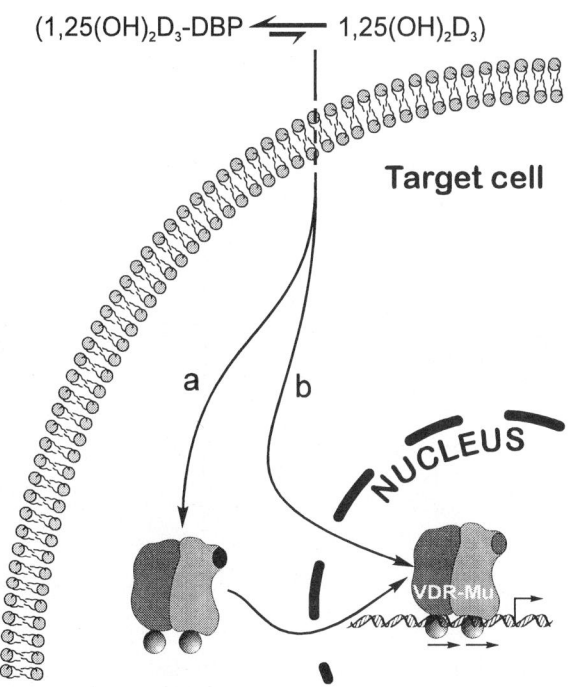

$$(1,25(OH)_2D_3\text{-}DBP) \rightleftharpoons 1,25(OH)_2D_3)$$

**Target cell**

a        b

NUCLEUS

VDR-Mu

**FIGURE 54-6.** The molecular mechanism of action of $1,25(OH)_2D_3$. The hormone dissociates from serum vitamin D binding protein (*DBP*), enters the cell, and interacts with the vitamin D receptor (*VDR*). Activation by the ligand leads to interaction of the VDR with responsive gene and modulation of gene expression. VDR-Mu, or VDR modulatory unit, comprises one VDR molecule and an associated protein, which is exemplified by but not restricted to a retinoid X receptor isoform. (a) An early model wherein the VDR, shown located in the cytoplasm, undergoes cytoplasmic to nuclear translocation on ligand activation and eventually binds to the regulatory region of a modulated gene. (b) Modern view of the location of the VDR, wherein the receptor is located in the nucleus and following ligand activation binds to the regulatory region of a vitamin D modulated gene. (From Pike JW. The vitamin D receptor and its gene. In: Feldman D, Glorieux FH, Pike JW, eds. Vitamin D. San Diego: Academic Press, 1997:105.)

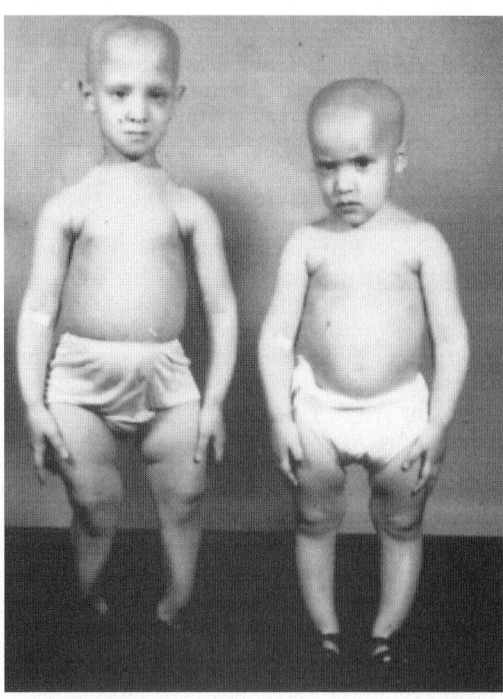

**FIGURE 54-7.** Two siblings with vitamin D–dependent rickets type II and alopecia. (From Rosen JF, Fleischman AR, Finberg L, et al. Rickets with alopecia: an inborn error of Vitamin D metabolism. J Pediatrics 1979; 94:729.)

receptors, which, like the vitamin D receptor, function as ligand-activated transcription factors. Each receptor exhibits functional domains for ligand binding and a highly conserved zinc finger region that mediates DNA binding. All three receptors bind to response elements consisting of the consensus hexamer AGGTCA, organized into combinations of direct and inverted repeat motifs. The specificity of each receptor for a particular target gene, therefore, would depend on the numbers and spacing of these elements, as well as on the presence and abundance of other coregulatory proteins; the retinoic acid X receptor functions as one such coregulator, but there are likely to be others. This complex interplay between the receptors, their cis-acting response elements, and the presence and abundance of specific transacting nuclear proteins would apparently constitute the means for tissue-specific and developmental actions for each hormone. The vitamin D response element has been identified in several $1,25(OH)_2D_3$-responsive genes, including osteocalcin, PTH, osteopontin, and the 25-hydroxy, 24-hydroxylase genes. A molecular model for $1,25(OH)_2D_3$ transcriptional activation of responsive genes is shown in Figure 54-6.

### RECEPTOR DEFECTS

Knowledge of the various components of the $1,25(OH)_2D$ receptor has been helpful in establishing the pathogenesis of vitamin D–dependent rickets type II (see Chaps. 63 and 70). In this rare, autosomal-recessive disorder, severe hypocalcemia and rickets develop early in childhood and are unresponsive to all forms of

vitamin D (Fig. 54-7). Affected persons demonstrate reduced receptor-binding capacity or defective nuclear internalization of hormone in skin fibroblasts.[53] Some also exhibit alopecia totalis. The genetic basis for dysfunctional vitamin D receptors has been identified in several affected kindreds by analysis of the chromosomal gene. Point mutations in nucleotides encoding amino acids in both ligand binding and zinc finger DNA binding domains have been demonstrated.[54] Mice lacking the vitamin D receptor (VDR) develop severe hypocalcemia, defective bone mineralization, and secondary hyperparathyroidism and alopecia, a phenotype that closely resembles that seen in patients with vitamin D–dependent rickets type II.[55]

Another consequence of altered vitamin D receptor expression may manifest itself at the level of bone mass. Studies have shown that a common allelic variation in the vitamin D receptor locus is a "predictor" for bone mass.[56,57] For example, bone mineral density was similar in dizygotic twin pairs with the same VDR genotype and much more variable in twin pairs with different VDR genotypes. Thus, the VDR (or a closely linked gene) appears to contribute to the development of peak bone mass, but the mechanism or mechanisms underlying this association remain obscure. However, conflicting results have been obtained by others[58]; therefore, the exact significance of the VDR locus to the development of peak bone mass remains to be established.

## MEASUREMENT OF VITAMIN D METABOLITES

### METHODS

The measurement of vitamin D in biologic fluids was pioneered with bioassays that measured either the linear calcification rate (line test) or a rise in blood calcium concentration (calcemic assay) in rats after the administration of vitamin D or its 25(OH)D analog. Modern assays, which are less tedious and more specific, use radioligand-binding techniques, physicochemical methods, or a combination of these.[59]

## 25-HYDROXYVITAMIN D

In the early 1970s, the first competitive protein-binding assays for 25(OH)D were developed.[60,61] This method uses the vitamin D transport protein as a specific binder. Extraction and chromatographic purification of 25(OH)D generally are required before the binding assay can be conducted. It also is possible to measure 25(OH)D by high-pressure liquid chromatography and UV absorbance spectroscopy.

The circulating concentration of 25(OH)D generally reflects the amount of vitamin D transmitted to the liver from dietary or epidermal sources, and therefore serves as the best index of overall vitamin D status. There is a seasonal fluctuation in serum 25(OH)D concentrations, with the highest values occurring in late summer and the lowest seen in late winter.[62] The normal range for 25(OH)D varies among laboratories, but generally is accepted to be 5 to 65 ng/mL. Frankly low values are found in patients with nutritional vitamin D deficiency and those with intestinal malabsorption syndromes.[63] Conversely, serum concentrations as high as 600 ng/mL are found in persons with vitamin D toxicity.

## 24,25-DIHYDROXYVITAMIN D AND 25,26-DIHYDROXYVITAMIN D

Because 24,25-dihydroxyvitamin D and 25,26-dihydroxyvitamin D also have strong affinity for vitamin D–binding protein, they can be measured using the competitive protein-binding technique if they first are separated individually by chromatography. The normal range for 24,25-dihydroxyvitamin D is 1 to 4 ng/mL; for 25,26-dihydroxyvitamin D, it is slightly lower. In the absence of renal disease, the serum concentrations of these two dihydroxy metabolites reflect the amount of substrate 25(OH)D.

## 1,25-DIHYDROXYVITAMIN D

The development of an assay for 1,25(OH)$_2$D has relied mainly on the use of its native receptor protein in radioreceptor assays, or on the technique of radioimmunoassay.[64,65] The prior separation of 1,25(OH)$_2$D from other metabolites is achieved by chromatography. The normal range varies somewhat depending on the method used, but is generally accepted to be from 18 to 65 pg/mL. The physiologic status of the individual must be considered carefully when interpreting the serum level. For example, during growth, pregnancy, or lactation, renal 1,25(OH)$_2$D synthesis may be appropriately increased. Hypocalcemia associated with vitamin D deficiency also is accompanied by augmented 1α-hydroxylase activity. Therefore, it is common to find elevated serum 1,25(OH)$_2$D concentrations in patients undergoing repletion of vitamin D.

# ASSESSMENT OF VITAMIN D STATUS

Because of the wide anatomic distribution of the sites of synthesis, metabolism, and action of vitamin D, clinical deficiency can result from disturbances at many levels (Fig. 54-8). Insufficient intake or production of vitamin D can lead to inadequate substrate concentrations for the conversion to 1,25(OH)$_2$D. Disturbances in the metabolism of vitamin D at the level of the liver or kidney can cause deficient production of 1,25(OH)$_2$D. In renal disease, a decline in the functional renal mass combined with increased phosphate retention eventually reduces or entirely eliminates 1,25(OH)$_2$D production. The loss or failure of parathyroid function in hypoparathyroidism or pseudohypoparathyroidism also is associated with low 1,25(OH)$_2$D levels. Serum concentrations are low in vitamin D–dependent rickets type I because of an inherited defect in the renal 1α-hydroxylase enzyme. End-organ resistance in patients with vitamin D–dependent rickets type II also can result from inherited defects in the receptor mechanism for 1,25(OH)$_2$D. In this disorder, serum 1,25(OH)$_2$D levels are grossly elevated in response to hypocalcemia.

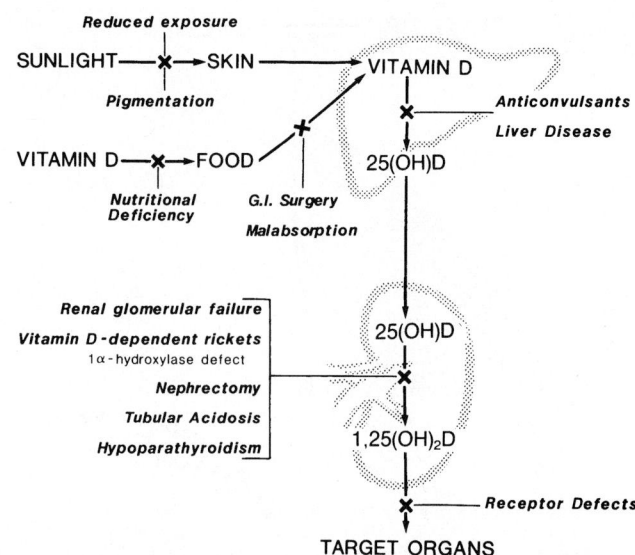

**FIGURE 54-8.** Potential clinical disturbances in intake, metabolism, and action of vitamin D. (*G.I.*, gastrointestinal.)

For accurate assessment of vitamin D status, it often is essential to consider both 25(OH)D and 1,25(OH)$_2$D concentrations. For example, a low 1,25(OH)$_2$D level need not indicate defective renal production of the metabolite. Instead, it could result from insufficient vitamin D intake (nutritional vitamin D deficiency), indicated by the finding of a low serum 25(OH)D concentration. If, however, 1,25(OH)$_2$D levels are low in the face of a normal concentration of 25(OH)D, then a disturbance in the renal synthesis of 1,25(OH)$_2$D$_3$ is likely. Further aspects of clinical disturbances in vitamin D metabolism are discussed in Chapters 61, 63, and 70.

# REFERENCES

1. DeLuca HF. Historical overview. In: Feldman D, Glorieux FH, Pike JW, eds. Vitamin D. San Diego: Academic Press, 1997:3.
2. Holick MF. Vitamin D: new horizons for the 21st century. Am J Clin Nutr 1994; 60:619.
2a. Nakamura K, Nashimoto M, Hori Y, Yamamoto M. Serum 25-hydroxyvitamin B concentrations and related dietary factors in peri- and postmenopausal Japanese women. Am J Clin Nutr 2000; 71:1161.
3. Chapuy M-C, Meunier PJ. Vitamin D insufficiency in adults and the elderly. In: Feldman D, Glorieux FH, Pike JW, eds. Vitamin D. San Diego: Academic Press, 1997:679.
4. Usui E, Noshiro M, Okuda K. Molecular cloning of cDNA for vitamin D$_3$ 25-hydroxylase from rat liver mitochondria. FEBS Lett 1990; 262(Mar 12;1):135.
5. Okuda K, Usui E, Ohyama Y. Recent progress in enzymology and molecular biology of enzymes involved in vitamin D metabolism. J Lipid Res 1995; 36:1641.
6. Bouillon R, Okamura WH, Norman AW. Structure-function relationships in the vitamin D endocrine system. Endocr Rev 1995; 16:200.
6a. Bland R, Zehnder P, Hewison M. Expression of 25-hydroxyvitamin D$_3$–1 alpha-hydroxylase along the nephron: new insights into renal vitamin D metabolism. Curr Opin Nephrol Hypertens 2000; 9:17.
7. Kawashima H, Jorika S, Kurokawa K. Localization of 25-hydroxyvitamin D$_3$-1α-hydroxylase and 24-hydroxylase along the rat nephron. Proc Natl Acad Sci U S A 1981; 78:1199.
8. Halloran BP. Cellular growth and differentiation during embryogenesis and fetal development. The role of vitamin D. Adv Exp Med Biol 1994; 352:227.
9. Barbour GL, Coburn JW, Slatopolsky E, et al. Hypercalcemia in an anephric patient with sarcoidosis: evidence for extrarenal generation of 1,25-dihydroxyvitamin D. N Engl J Med 1981; 305:440.
10. Adams TS, Sharma DP, Gacad MA, Singer FR. Metabolism of 25-hydroxyvitamin D$_3$ by cultured pulmonary alveolar macrophages in sarcoidosis. J Clin Invest 1983; 72:1856.
11. Takeyama K, Kitanaka S, Sato T, et al. 25-Hydroxyvitamin D$_3$ 1α-hydroxylase and vitamin D synthesis. Science 1997; 277:1827.
11a. Hewison M, Zehnder D, Bland R, Stewart PM. 1 alpha-hydroxylase and the action of vitamin D. J Mol Endocrinol 2000; 25:141.
12. Yoon PS, DeLuca HF. Purification and properties of chick renal mitochondrial ferredoxin. Biochemistry 1980; 19:2165.
13. Halloran BP, Portale AA, Lonergan ET, Morris RC Jr. Production and metabolic clearance of 1,25-dihydroxyvitamin D in men: effect of advancing age. J Clin Endocrinol Metab 1990; 70:318.

14. Ohyama Y, Noshiro M, Okuda K. Cloning and expression of cDNA encoding 25-hydroxyvitamin $D_3$ 24-hydroxylase. FEBS Lett 1991; 28;278:195.

15. Omdahl J, May B. The 25-hydroxyvitamin D 24-hydroxylase. In: Feldman D, Glorieux FH, Pike JW, eds. Vitamin D. San Diego: Academic Press, 1997:69.

16. Horst RL, Reinhardt TA. Vitamin D metabolism In: Feldman D, Glorieux FH, Pike JW, eds. Vitamin D. San Diego: Academic Press, 1997:13.

17. Fraser DR. Regulation of the metabolism of vitamin D. Physiol Rev 1980; 60:551.

18. Selby PL, Davies M, Marks JS, Mawer EB. Vitamin D intoxication causes hypercalcaemia by increased bone resorption which responds to pamidronate. Clin Endocrinol (Oxf) 1995; 43:531.

19. Slovik DM, Daly MA, Potts JT Jr, Neer RM. Renal 1,25-dihydroxyvitamin D, phosphaturic, and cyclic-AMP responses to intravenous synthetic human parathyroid hormone-(1-34) administration in normal subjects. Clin Endocrinol (Oxf) 1984; 20:369.

20. Gray RW. Evidence that somatomedins mediate the effect of hypophosphatemia to increase serum 1,25-dihydroxyvitamin $D_3$ levels in rats. Endocrinology 1987; 121(2):504.

21. Henry HL, Norman AW. Vitamin D: metabolism and biological actions. Annu Rev Nutr 1984; 4:493.

22. Horiuchi N, Takahashi H, Matsumoto T, et al. Salmon calcitonin-induced stimulation of 1,25-dihydroxycholecalciferol synthesis in rats involving mechanism independent of adenosine 3,5-cyclic monophosphate. Biochem J 1979; 184:269.

23. Chen ML, Boltz MA, Armbrecht HJ. Effects of 1,25-dihydroxyvitamin $D_3$ and phorbol ester on 25-hydroxyvitamin $D_3$ 24-hydroxylase cytochrome P450 messenger ribonucleic acid levels in primary cultures of rat renal cells. Endocrinology 1993; 132:1782.

24. Care AD. Vitamin D in pregnancy, the fetoplacental unit and lactation. In: Feldman D, Glorieux FH, Pike JW, eds. Vitamin D. San Diego: Academic Press, 1997:437.

25. Heaney RP, Skillman JG. Calcium metabolism in normal pregnancy. J Clin Endocrinol Metab 1971; 24:661.

26. Bouillon R, Van Assche FA, Van Baelen H, et al. Influence of the vitamin D–binding protein on the serum concentration of 1,25-dihydroxyvitamin D. J Clin Invest 1981; 67:689.

27. Daiger SP, Shanfield MS, Calli-Sforza LL. Group-specific components (GC) proteins bind vitamin D and 25-hydroxyvitamin D. Proc Natl Acad Sci U S A 1975; 72:2076.

28. Belsey R, Clark MB, Bernat M, et al. The physiologic significance of plasma transport of vitamin D and metabolites. Am J Med 1974; 57:50.

29. Safadi FF, Thornton P, Magiera H, et al. Osteopathy and resistance to vitamin D toxicity in mice null for vitamin D binding protein. J Clin Invest 1999; 103:239.

30. Cooke NE, Haddad JG. Vitamin D binding proteins. In: Feldman D, Glorieux FH, Pike JW, eds. Vitamin D. San Diego: Academic Press, 1997:87.

31. Hahn JT, Birge SJ, Scharp CK, Avioli LV. Phenobarbital-induced alterations in vitamin D metabolism. J Clin Invest 1972; 51:741.

32. Hollis BW, Lambert PW, Horst RL. Factors affecting the antirachitic sterol content of native milk. In: Holick MF, Anast CS, Gray TK, eds. Calcium, phosphate and vitamin D metabolism in pregnancy and neonate. Amsterdam: Elsevier, 1983:157.

33. Wasserman R. Vitamin D and intestinal absorption of calcium and phosphorus. In: Feldman D, Glorieux FH, Pike JW, eds. Vitamin D. San Diego: Academic Press, 1997:259.

34. Christakos S, Gabrielides C, Rhoten WB. Vitamin D–dependent calcium binding proteins: chemistry, distribution, functional considerations, and molecular biology. Endocr Rev 1989; 10:3.

35. Craviso GL, Garrett KP, Clemens TL. 1,25-Dihydroxyvitamin $D_3$ induces synthesis of vitamin D–dependent calcium-binding protein in cultured chick kidney cells. Endocrinology 1987; 120:894.

36. DelValle ME, Vazquez E, Represa J, et al. Immunohistochemical localization of calcium-binding proteins in the human cutaneous sensory corpuscles. Neurosci Lett 1994; 168:247.

37. Lee DB. Mechanisms and regulation of intestinal phosphate transport. Adv Exp Med Biol 1986; 208:207.

38. Matsumota T, Fontain OP, Rasmussen H. Effect of 1,25-dihydroxyvitamin $D_3$ on phospholipid metabolism in chick duodenal mucosa cell. J Biol Chem 1981; 256:3354.

39. Norman AW. Rapid biological actions mediated by 1α,25-dihydroxyvitamin $D_3$: a case study of transcaltachia (rapid hormonal stimulation of intestinal calcium transport). In: Feldman D, Glorieux FH, Pike JW, eds. Vitamin D. San Diego: Academic Press, 1997:233.

40. Underwood J, DeLuca HF. Vitamin D is not directly necessary for bone growth and mineralization. Am J Physiol 1984; 246:E493.

41. Raisz LG, Kream BE. Regulation of bone formation (parts I and II). N Engl J Med 1983; 309:29.

42. Aubin JE, Heershe JNM. Vitamin D and osteoblasts. In: Feldman D, Glorieux FH, Pike JW, eds. Vitamin D. San Diego: Academic Press, 1997:313.

43. Takahashi N, Yamana H, Yoshiki S, et al. Osteoclast-like cell formation by osteotropic hormones in mouse bone marrow cultures. Endocrinology 1988; 122:1373.

44. Russell J, Letteriere D, Sherwood LM. Suppression by 1,25-$(OH)_2D_3$ of transcription of the preproparathyroid hormone gene. Endocrinology 1986; 119:2864.

45. Slatopolsky E, Weerts C, Thielan J, et al. Marked suppression of secondary hyperparathyroidism by intravenous administration of 1,25-dihydroxycholecalciferol in uremic patients. J Clin Invest 1984; 74:2136.

46. Kadowski S, Norman AW. Dietary vitamin D is essential for normal insulin secretion from the perfused rat pancreas. J Clin Invest 1984; 73:759.

47. Abe E, Mayaura C, Sakagami H, et al. Differentiation of mouse myeloid leukemia cells induced by 1,25-dihydroxyvitamin $D_3$. Proc Natl Acad Sci U S A 1981; 78:4990.

48. Hosomi J, Hosoi J, Abe E, et al. Regulation of terminal differentiation of cultured mouse epidermal cells by 1,25-dihydroxyvitamin $D_3$. Endocrinology 1983; 113:1950.

49. Amento EP. Vitamin D and the immune system. Steroids 1987; 49:55.

50. Takahashi N, Akatsu T, Sakasi T, et al. Induction of calcitonin receptors by 1,25-dihydroxyvitamin $D_3$ in osteoclast-like multinucleated cells formed in mouse bone marrow cells. Endocrinology 1988; 123:1504.

51. Boiullon R, Allewaert K, Xiang DZ, et al. Vitamin D analogs with low affinity for the vitamin D binding protein: enhanced in vitro and decreased in vivo activity. J Bone Miner Res 1993; 6:1051.

52. Pike JW. The vitamin D receptor and its gene. In: Feldman D, Glorieux FH, Pike JW, eds. Vitamin D. San Diego: Academic Press, 1997:105.

53. Lieberman UA, Eil C, Marx SJ. Resistance to 1,25-$(OH)_2$-D: association with heterogeneous defects in cultured skin fibroblasts. J Clin Invest 1983; 71:192.

54. Hewison M, Rut AR, Kristjansson K, et al. Tissue resistance to vitamin D without a mutation of the vitamin D receptor gene. Clin Endocrinol (Oxf) 1993; 39:663.

55. Li YC, Pirro AE, Amling M, et al. Targeted ablation of the vitamin D receptor: an animal model of vitamin D–dependent rickets type II with alopecia. Proc Natl Acad Sci U S A 1997; 94:9831.

56. Morrison NA, Yeoman R, Kelly PJ, Eisman JA. Contribution of trans-acting factor alleles to the normal physiological variability: vitamin D receptor gene polymorphism and circulating osteocalcin. Proc Natl Acad Sci U S A 1992; 89:6665.

57. Morrison NA, Qi JC, Tolita A, et al. Prediction of bone density from vitamin D receptor alleles. Nature 1994; 367:284.

58. Cooper GS, Umbach DM. Are vitamin D receptor polymorphisms associated with bone mineral density? A meta-analysis. J Bone Miner Res 1996; 11:1841.

59. Hollis BW. Detection of vitamin D and its major metabolites. In: Feldman D, Glorieux FH, Pike JW, eds. Vitamin D. San Diego: Academic Press, 1997:587.

60. Belsey R, DeLuca HF, Potts JT Jr. Competitive protein-binding assay for vitamin D and 25-OH-vitamin D. J Clin Endocrinol Metab 1971; 33:554.

61. Haddad JG, Chyu KJ. Competitive protein-binding radioassay for 25-hydroxycholecalciferol. J Clin Endocrinol Metab 1971; 32:992.

62. Stamp TCB, Round JM. Seasonal changes in human plasma levels of 25-hydroxyvitamin D. Nature 1974; 247:1563.

63. Preece MA, Tomlinson S, Ribot CA, et al. Studies of vitamin D deficiency in man. Q J Med 1975; 44:575.

64. Brumbaugh PF, Haussler DH, Bursac KM, Haussler MR. Filter assay for 1,25-dihydroxyvitamin $D_3$: utilization of the hormone's target tissue chromatin receptor. Biochemistry 1974; 13:4091.

65. Clemens TL, Hendy GN, Papapoulos SE, et al. Measurement of 1,25-dihydroxycholecalciferol in man by radioimmunoassay. Clin Endocrinol (Oxf) 1979; 11:325.

# CHAPTER 55

# BONE QUANTIFICATION AND DYNAMICS OF TURNOVER

DAVID W. DEMPSTER AND ELIZABETH SHANE

The period since the 1970s has produced tremendous growth in the understanding of the pathophysiology of bone. This has resulted largely from an increased comprehension of normal and abnormal bone structure and from a much clearer grasp of the dynamic cellular processes involved in bone remodeling. Three major advances have greatly facilitated the accumulation of this information. First, the advent of plastic embedding media has made it possible to obtain, routinely, good quality histologic sections of fully mineralized bone. Previously, it was necessary to decalcify all bone specimens before histologic evaluation, and fundamental structural information was literally washed down the sink with the decalcifying fluid. The second important advance was the discovery that the tetracycline antibiotics are permanently incorporated at sites of bone formation, allowing these regions to be visualized and quantitatively analyzed in histologic sections. Finally, a simple, safe, and relatively atraumatic surgical technique for obtaining well-preserved and adequately sized biopsy samples with the patient under local anesthesia was perfected.

Consequently, the iliac crest biopsy has become one of the most powerful clinical and research tools available for the study of metabolic bone disease. This chapter describes the surgical procedure for obtaining the specimen, the methods by which the bone sample is prepared and analyzed, the variables that are measured and their clinical relevance, and the indications for biopsy.

## TECHNIQUE OF ILIAC CREST BIOPSY

### PRETREATMENT OF THE PATIENT WITH TETRACYCLINE

The information obtainable from an iliac crest biopsy is significantly increased by the use of in vivo markers of bone formation, such as the tetracycline antibiotics.[1] Approximately 3 weeks before the scheduled biopsy, tetracycline is administered for 2 days. This is followed by an interval of 12 drug-free days and then a 4-day course of tetracycline (2:12:4 sequence). The tetracycline is incorporated into bone at sites of new bone formation, binding irreversibly to hydroxyapatite at the mineralization front. When thin biopsy sections are subsequently viewed under violet or blue light, the tetracycline fluoresces so that bright lines ("labels") are visible at the formation sites (Fig. 55-1). At sites where bone formation was ongoing during the entire labeling sequence, two tetracycline labels are present, corresponding to the two discrete periods of tetracycline exposure. At sites where formation either commenced or ended in the interval with no tetracycline administration, only single fluorescent labels are visible. At least 5 days should elapse between the last day of tetracycline administration and the date of the biopsy to prevent the last label from diffusing out.

Demeclocycline, tetracycline, and oxytetracycline all are effective labeling agents, although demeclocycline appears to produce more intense fluorescent bands. Demeclocycline, 600

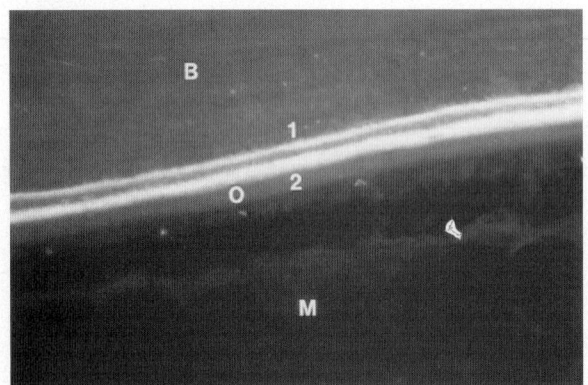

**FIGURE 55-1.** Double tetracycline labels at a site of active bone formation in an iliac crest biopsy specimen. The labeling sequence was 2:12:4. The first and second labels are indicated. Note that the second label, which was deposited over 4 days, is broader than the first. This may be helpful in distinguishing the labels that have been administered for bone biopsy purposes from those deposited during previous treatment with tetracyclines as antibiotic agents. (*B*, mineralized bone; *O*, osteoid; *M*, marrow.) Epifluorescence microscopy with a mercury light source and a violet excitation filter. Field width = 0.45 mm.

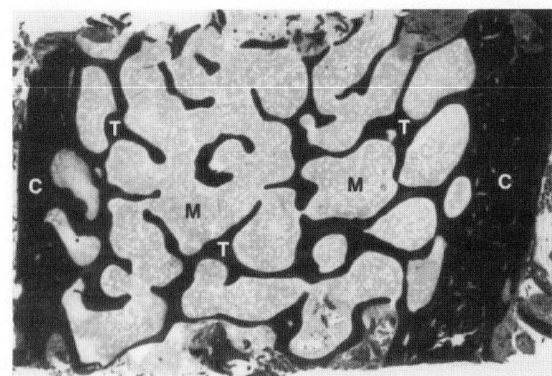

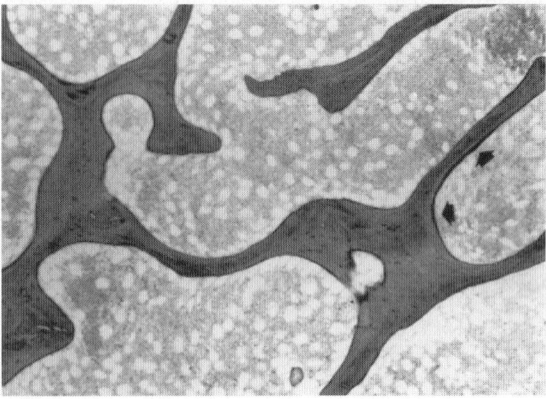

**FIGURE 55-2. A,** Iliac crest biopsy specimen from a 33-year-old normal man. Note the inner and outer cortices (*C*) and intervening trabecular bone (*T*). Goldner trichrome stain. (*M,* marrow.) Field width = 9.6 mm. **B,** Higher-power view of normal trabecular architecture. Arrows indicate normal osteoid seam. Field width = 2.3 mm.

mg per day (4 × 150-mg tablets), is taken on an empty stomach; dairy products and antacids containing aluminum, calcium, or magnesium impair absorption. Tetracyclines should not be given to children younger than 8 years of age or to pregnant women because it is incorporated into growing teeth and causes discoloration. Although tetracycline is generally well tolerated, some patients react adversely to these drugs with nausea, vomiting, or diarrhea. All patients should avoid direct exposure to sunlight or ultraviolet light during the time of administration because of potential skin phototoxicity.

### THE SITE AND THE SURGICAL PROCEDURE

The anterior iliac crest is the preferred site for several reasons: (a) it is easily accessible, making the surgical procedure simple and safe; (b) the bone sample obtained consists of both trabecular and cortical bone (Fig. 55-2A); (c) the amount of trabecular bone correlates with that of the axial skeleton (vertebral bodies); and (d) a large body of histomorphometric data has been accumulated at this site in both normal persons and patients with a wide variety of bone diseases.[2–5]

The biopsy generally is performed with a standard trephine of the type designed by Bordier. The internal diameter of the trephine should be 8 mm to obtain sufficient tissue, minimize compression of the sample, and reduce sampling error.[3,4]

The patient should be sedated, usually with intravenous meperidine hydrochloride (Demerol) and diazepam (Valium), immediately before the procedure. It is important to provide thorough local anesthesia of the skin, subcutaneous tissue, muscle, and, particularly, the periosteum covering both the lateral and the medial aspects of the ilium. The specimen is obtained through an incision 2–3 cm long made at a point 2 cm posterior and 2 cm inferior to the anterior superior iliac spine

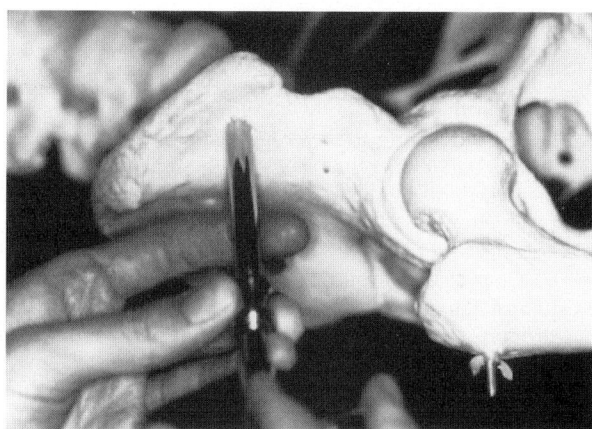

**FIGURE 55-3.** Demonstration of anterior iliac crest for Meunier trephine biopsy (2 cm posterior and 2 cm inferior to the anterior superior iliac spine).

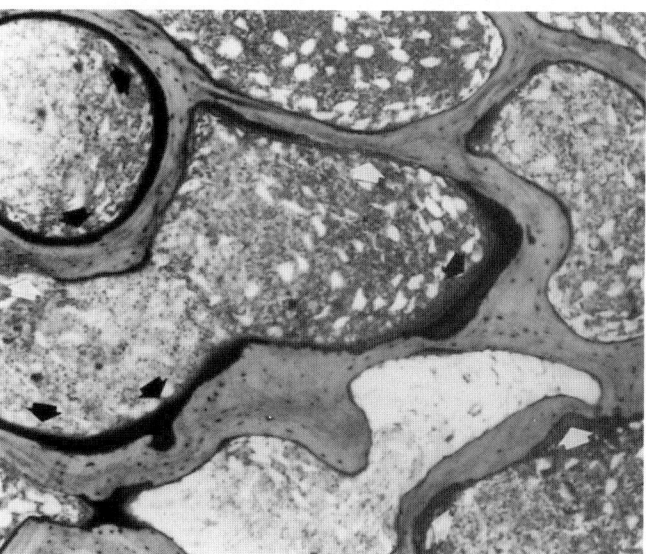

**FIGURE 55-4.** Iliac crest biopsy specimen from a patient with primary hyperparathyroidism caused by parathyroid carcinoma. Note extended resorption surface (*white arrows*) with associated marrow fibrosis and increased osteoid surface (*black arrows*). Goldner trichrome stain. Field width = 2.3 mm.

(Fig. 55-3). Proper positioning of the trephine is essential for accurate interpretation of the biopsy. The needle should be rotated back and forth with gentle but firm pressure so that it cuts rather than pushes through the ilium. Excessive force may yield a damaged and uninterpretable biopsy specimen. After the procedure, the patient should refrain from excessive activity for 24 hours; a mild analgesic may be necessary.

When a transiliac crest bone biopsy is performed with adequate sedation and with careful local anesthesia of the skin and periosteum, there is minimal discomfort, and patient acceptance is generally excellent. Significant complications from transiliac bone biopsy are unusual. In an international multicenter study involving 9131 transiliac biopsies, complications were recorded in 64 patients (0.7%).[3] The most common complications were pain at the biopsy site that persisted for more than 7 days after the procedure and hematoma; rarer complications included wound infection, fracture through the iliac crest, and osteomyelitis.

## PREPARATION AND ANALYSIS OF THE BIOPSY SPECIMEN

The biopsy should be fixed in 70% ethanol because more aqueous fixatives may leach the tetracycline from the bone. After a fixation period of 4–7 days, the biopsy is dehydrated in ethanol, cleared in toluene, and embedded in methyl methacrylate. No decalcification steps are performed. Once polymerized, the methyl methacrylate provides a sufficiently hard but flexible supporting matrix to allow good quality undecalcified sections to be cut with a heavy-duty microtome, usually equipped with a tungsten carbide-edged knife. The 5- to 10-μm sections are then stained with a variety of dyes to allow good discrimination between calcified bone matrix and noncalcified "osteoid" (Figs. 55-4 and 55-5A) and clear visualization of the cellular components of bone and marrow (Fig. 55-5B). Unstained sections also are prepared to allow observation of the tetracycline labels by fluorescence microscopy (see Fig. 55-1).[6,7]

The sections are analyzed morphometrically, according to standard stereologic principles, using either simple "point-counting" techniques or the less time-consuming method of computer-aided planimetry.[8–10]

## VARIABLES ROUTINELY MEASURED IN THE ANALYSIS OF THE BIOPSY SPECIMEN

An abundance of quantitative information may be obtained from the biopsy. Because the morphometric analysis is a labor-intensive process, the number of variables evaluated depends on whether the biopsy specimen is being analyzed for diagnostic or research purposes. Listed below are eight indices of trabecular bone that are of particular clinical relevance. A detailed account of the complete analysis of bone biopsy specimens is found in more specialized texts.[2,11]

The histomorphometric parameters are generally divided into two categories. *Static variables* provide information on the amount of bone present and the proportion of bone surface engaged in a particular phase of remodeling activity. *Dynamic variables* yield information on the rate of cell-mediated processes involved in remodeling. This category can be evaluated only in biopsy specimens that have been appropriately labeled with tetracycline. Importantly, inferences about the rate of cellular activities can be made only from an analysis of the dynamic variables. An increase in resorption surface, a static variable, does not necessarily indicate an increase in resorption rate. The bone formation rate may be calculated directly from selected dynamic variables measured in an appropriately labeled biopsy specimen. Resorption rate, on the other hand, can be computed only indirectly, using certain indices of bone formation, in a single biopsy specimen or from two sequential biopsy specimens.[11,12]

## STATIC VARIABLES

The following variables are categorized as static. The terms and abbreviations used are consistent with the recommendation of the Bone Histomorphometry Nomenclature Committee of the American Society for Bone and Mineral Research.[13]

    Cancellous bone volume (Cn-BV/TV, %). This is the fraction of a given volume of whole cancellous bone tissue (i.e., bone + marrow) that consists of mineralized and nonmineralized bone.
    Osteoid volume (OV/BV, %). This is the fraction of a given volume of bone tissue (mineralized bone + osteoid) that is osteoid (i.e., unmineralized matrix).
    Osteoid surface (OS/BS, %). This is the fraction of the entire trabecular surface that is covered by osteoid seams.
    Osteoid thickness (O.Th, μm). This is the average width of the osteoid seams.

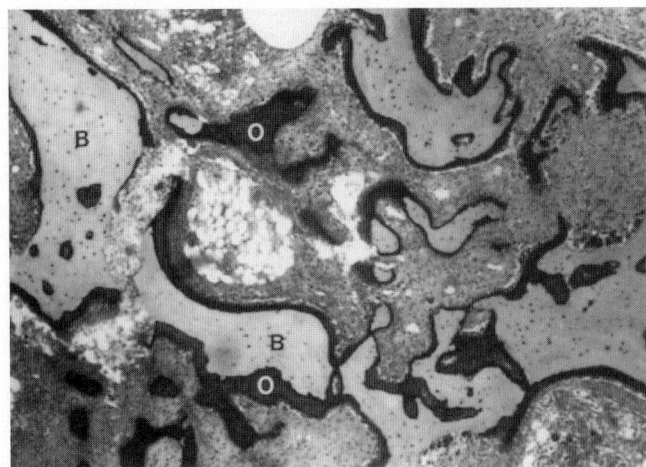

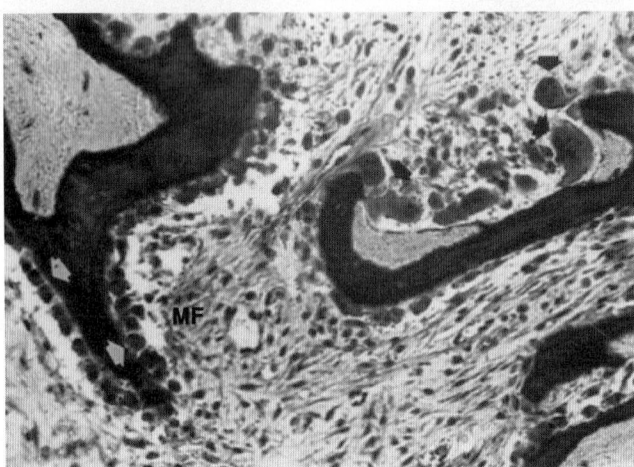

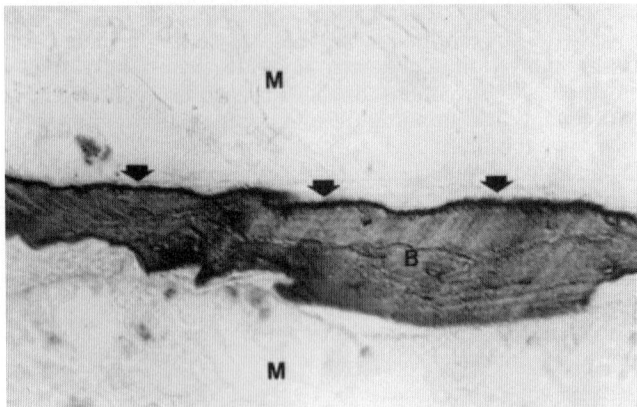

**FIGURE 55-5. A,** Iliac crest biopsy specimen from a patient with renal osteodystrophy. This is an example of "mixed" bone disease with evidence of secondary hyperparathyroidism (extended resorption and osteoid surface) and osteomalacia (increased width of osteoid seams). (*O,* osteoid; *B,* mineralized bone.) Goldner trichrome stain. Field width = 2.3 mm. **B,** Higher-power view of the area indicated in **A** to show osteoclasts (*black arrows*), osteoblasts (*white arrows*), and extensive marrow fibrosis (*MF*). Goldner trichrome stain. Field width = 0.47 mm. **C,** Histochemical staining procedure reveals the presence of aluminum (*arrows*) at the junction of an osteoid seam and mineralized bone in a patient with renal osteodystrophy who is receiving long-term hemodialysis. (*B,* mineralized bone; *M,* marrow.) Field width = 0.52 mm.

Eroded surface (ES/BS, %). This is the fraction of the entire trabecular surface that is occupied by resorption bays (Howship lacunae), including both those with and without osteoclasts.

## DYNAMIC VARIABLES

The following variables are categorized as dynamic.

> Mineral apposition rate (MAR, μm per day). This is calculated by dividing the average distance between the first and second tetracycline labels by the time interval (e.g., 12 days) separating them. It is a measure of the linear rate of production of calcified bone matrix by the osteoblasts.
>
> Mineralizing surface (MS/BS, %). This is the fraction of trabecular surface bearing double tetracycline labels plus one-half of the singly labeled surface. It is a measure of the proportion of bone surface on which new mineralized bone was being deposited at the time of tetracycline labeling.
>
> Bone Formation Rate (BFR/BS, $\mu m^3/\mu m^2$ per day). This is the volume of mineralized bone made per unit surface of trabecular bone per year. It is calculated by multiplying the mineralizing surface by the mineral apposition rate.

Table 55-1 indicates how each of these variables is altered in different disease states.

## NORMAL BONE REMODELING

Bone is remodeled continuously throughout life—old, worn-out bone is replaced by new bone. Approximately 25% of trabecular bone and 3% of cortical bone is replaced annually. The remodeling process is a quantum phenomenon because it occurs in discrete units or "packets." Osteoclasts resorb a preprogrammed volume of old bone. Shortly thereafter, the osteoclasts are replaced by osteoblasts, which refill the resorption cavity with a new packet of bone. The group of cells (osteoclasts and osteoblasts) that creates one new packet of bone is called a *bone remodeling unit.* In normal trabecular bone, ~900 bone remodeling units are activated each day. In cortical bone, the activation frequency is ~180 per day.[2,14–16]

## HYPERPARATHYROIDISM

Elevated circulating levels of parathyroid hormone (PTH) stimulate the activation frequency of bone remodeling units, resulting in increased numbers of osteoclasts in bone and, because of the coupling process, increased numbers of osteoblasts. Consequently, quantitative analysis of a biopsy specimen from a patient with either primary or secondary hyperparathyroidism reveals increases in *eroded surface, osteoid surface,* and *mineralizing surface* (see Fig. 55-4).[10,17–19] The extension of surface double labeled by tetracycline has allowed precise determination of the *mineral apposition rate,* which has been shown to be reduced. Because the *osteoid thickness* is normal in this disorder, the reduction in *mineral apposition rate* indicates a decreased rate of organic matrix production by the osteoblasts, rather than a defect in calcification. However, the extension of *mineralizing surface* overcompensates for the decrease in *mineral apposition rate,* so that the overall *bone formation rate,* the product of these two variables, is still increased. Thus, in hyperparathyroidism, bone resorption and formation rates are increased, which is a situation commonly referred to as a "high turnover" state. Bone turnover is higher in hyperthyroid patients with vitamin D insufficiency.[18a] Despite the rapid remodeling that occurs in primary hyperparathyroidism, the balance between resorption and formation is generally conserved because *cancellous bone volume* is normal or may even be increased, and trabecular connectivity is preserved.[19] Often accompanying the increased bone turnover rate are increased deposition of immature (woven) bone and marrow fibrosis. These features are particularly prominent in severe secondary hyperparathyroidism.

**TABLE 55-1.**
**Bone Biopsy Variables in a Variety of Disease States**

| Disease State | Cancellous Bone Volume | Osteoid Volume | Osteoid Surface | Osteoid Thickness | Eroded Surface | Mineral Apposition Rate | Mineralizing Surface | Bone Formation Rate |
|---|---|---|---|---|---|---|---|---|
| Hyperparathyroidism[10,17-19] | N or ↑ | ↑ | ↑ | N | ↑ | ↓ | ↑ | ↑ |
| Osteomalacia[10,20-22] | N | ↑ | ↑ | ↑ | ↑ | ↓ | ↓ | ↓ |
| Renal osteodystrophy/dialysis[23-35] | ↓ or ↑ | ↓ or ↑ | ↓ or ↑ | ↓ or ↑ | ↑ | ↑ or ↓ | ↑ or ↓ | ↑ or ↓ |
| Postmenopausal or senile osteoporosis[36-45] | ↓ or N | N or ↑ | N or ↑ | N or ↓ | N or ↑ | N or ↓ | N, ↑ or ↓ | N, ↑ or ↓ |
| Cushing syndrome and corticosteroid-induced osteoporosis[46,47] | ↓ or N | N | ↑ | ↓ | ↑ | ↓ | — | — |
| Paget disease[48] | ↑ | ↑ | ↑ | ↓ | ↑ | ↑ | ↑ | ↑ |
| Thyrotoxicosis[17] | ↓ | ↑ | ↑ | ↓ | ↑ | ↑ | ↑ | ↑ |
| Hypothyroidism[17] | N | ↓ | N | ↓ | N | ↓ | ↓ | ↓ |
| Medullary thyroid carcinoma[17] | N | ↑ | ↑ | N | ↑ | ↓ | ↑ | N |
| Multiple myeloma[49] | N, ↑ or ↓ | ↑ | ↑ | ↓ | ↑ | ↓ | ↑ | — |
| Osteogenesis imperfecta tarda[50,51] | ↓ | N | ↑ | ↓ | ↑ or N | ↓ | N | ↓ |

*N*, normal; ↑, increased; ↓, decreased.

Because the hallmarks of excessive remodeling activity (e.g., increased *eroded surface*) accumulate in bone over time, the biopsy can be a sensitive indicator of parathyroid gland hyperactivity, especially when this is mild or intermittent. However, the biopsy alone does not distinguish between primary and secondary hyperparathyroidism.

## OSTEOMALACIA

Numerous causative mechanisms underlie osteomalacia (see Chaps. 63 and 70). Most of the mechanisms involve processes that decrease the circulating calcium × phosphate product below the levels required for bone mineralization. Although calcification of the organic matrix is inhibited, the osteoblasts continue to synthesize and secrete the matrix. An accumulation of unmineralized matrix ("osteoid") results (Fig. 55-6). The *cancellous bone volume* is normal in osteomalacia, but as the *osteoid volume* is increased, the amount of mineralized bone is actually reduced.

Analysis of the dynamic variables is particularly important in osteomalacia. At some formation sites, mineral is still deposited, but less rapidly than normal, resulting in reduced separation between the double tetracycline labels and, consequently, low values for *mineral apposition rate*. At other formation sites, calcification may be completely inhibited, decreasing the extent of tetracycline uptake and therefore the *mineralizing surface*. The fall in both these variables markedly reduces *bone formation rate*. As regards the static variables, the accumulation of unmineralized matrix is reflected by increased *osteoid thickness, osteoid surface,* and *osteoid volume*. If PTH secretion is elevated, the activation frequency of bone remodeling units is enhanced and the biopsy reveals an increase in *eroded surface*. The elevated remodeling rate, along with the mineralization failure, accentuates the increased deposition of osteoid.[10,20-22]

## RENAL OSTEODYSTROPHY

Chronic renal failure is generally accompanied by phosphate retention and hyperphosphatemia, which lead to a reciprocal decrease in serum ionized calcium concentration and a consequent increase in secretion of PTH. Moreover, as functional renal mass decreases, the plasma 1,25-dihydroxyvitamin D level falls (see Chaps. 54 and 209), leading to impaired intestinal calcium absorption, which contributes to the tendency for hypocalcemia and ultimately may result in reduced bone mineralization. Consequent to these marked changes in calcium and phosphate metabolism, the bone biopsy specimen in renal osteodystrophy may display a heterogeneous picture; bone biopsy has contrib-

uted significantly to the current classification of renal bone disease.[23-35] Thus, renal osteodystrophy has been subdivided into two broad categories, primarily on the basis of histomorphomet-

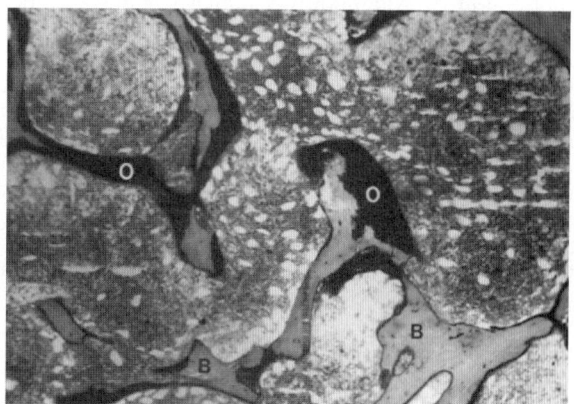

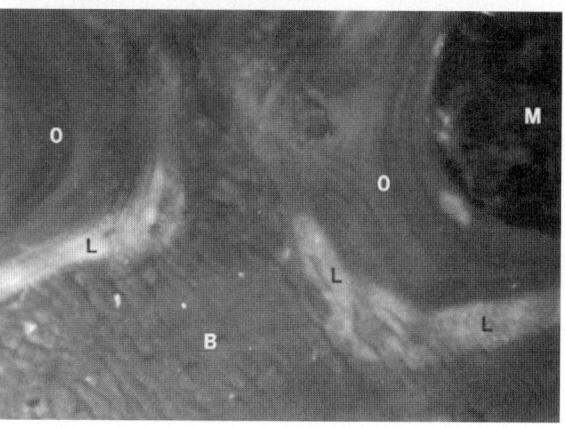

**FIGURE 55-6. A,** Iliac crest biopsy specimen from a patient with osteomalacia (tumor-induced).[22] There is a marked increase in the osteoid volume as a result of increased extent and thickness of osteoid seams. (*O*, osteoid; *B*, mineralized bone.) Goldner trichrome stain. Field width = 2.3 mm. **B,** Abnormal tetracycline deposition in the same patient. Compared with normal double labels seen in Figure 55-1, the labels (*L*) are broad, dull, and diffused. This pattern of tetracycline uptake is typical of osteomalacia and is thought to result from the presence of increased amounts of immature mineral that is capable of binding tetracycline.[20] (*B*, mineralized bone; *O*, osteoid; *M*, marrow.) Epifluorescence microscopy with a mercury light source and a violet excitation filter. Field width = 0.45 mm.

ric features: one characterized by normal or high bone turnover and a second characterized by low bone turnover.

In patients with end-stage renal disease, the most frequently observed biopsy changes arise from the effects of chronic excess PTH secretion on the skeleton, are classified as normal/high turnover, and include (a) osteitis fibrosa, (b) mild hyperparathyroidism, and (c) mixed bone disease. As a group, these forms are characterized histologically by increases in *eroded surface, osteoid surface,* and *mineralizing surface.* With osteitis fibrosa, however, there is deposition of woven osteoid and variable amounts of peritrabecular marrow fibrosis, in contrast to the minimal or absent fibrosis observed in mild hyperparathyroidism. States of low bone turnover also are frequently observed in patients undergoing dialysis, albeit less often than high turnover disease. The low turnover states are classified as (d) osteomalacia and (e) aplastic or adynamic bone disease. Patients with osteomalacia have evidence of reduced values for dynamic variables associated with the accumulation of excess unmineralized osteoid, whereas those with aplastic or adynamic disease have reduced bone formation as measured by tetracycline labeling, but normal or reduced *osteoid volume.* Most symptomatic patients with osteomalacia or aplastic bone disease have a significant extent (>25%) of surfaces covered with stainable aluminum and are considered to have aluminum-related bone disease.[24–27] The major sources of this aluminum are the aluminum-containing phosphate binders used to control hyperphosphatemia and dialysate solutions contaminated with aluminum (see Chaps. 61 and 131). Aluminum accumulates at sites of bone formation (see Fig. 55-5C), where it may directly inhibit mineralization, leading to an increase in *osteoid thickness* and *osteoid surface.* However, aluminum also is toxic to osteoblasts and may impair their ability both to synthesize and to mineralize bone matrix. These two effects of aluminum reduce both the *mineral apposition rate* and the *mineralizing surface.* However, if matrix production also is inhibited, osteoid thickness is not increased. With greater recognition of the potential sources of aluminum and the substitution of phosphate binders containing calcium for those containing aluminum, aluminum-related bone disease is becoming less of a clinical problem.

Another form of low-turnover bone disease has been described that is termed *idiopathic aplastic* or *adynamic bone disease* and is not characterized by significant aluminum accumulation or staining. Its pathogenesis is unclear but may be related to various therapeutic maneuvers designed to prevent or treat hyperparathyroidism in patients undergoing dialysis, including the use of dialysates with higher calcium concentrations (3.0–3.5 mEq/L), large doses of calcium-containing phosphate binders, and calcitriol therapy. In general, these patients tend to have few or no symptoms of bone disease, and this "disease" ultimately may prove to be a histologic rather than a clinically relevant form of bone disorder. It is unknown whether patients with aplastic bone disease are at increased risk for the development of clinical problems in the future.

The form of renal bone disease that is classified as mixed disease is characterized histologically by features of both osteitis fibrosa and osteomalacia. Such lesions are observed most commonly in patients who are in transition between osteitis fibrosa and aluminum-related bone disease.

## OSTEOPOROSIS

The most striking feature of bone biopsy specimens from patients with osteoporosis is the reduction in *cancellous bone volume* (see Chap. 64). Approximately 80% of patients with vertebral crush fractures have values that are lower than normal. The reduction in *cancellous bone volume* results primarily from progressive loss of entire trabeculae and, to a lesser degree, from thinning of those that remain (Fig. 55-7).[36–39,39a]

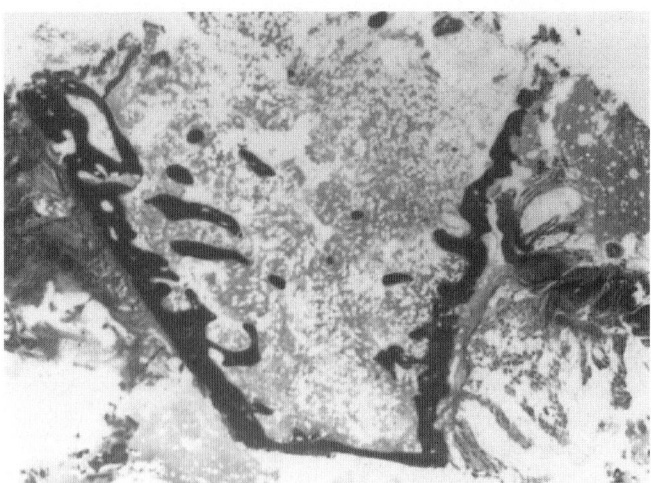

**FIGURE 55-7.** Iliac crest biopsy specimen from a patient with postmenopausal osteoporosis. Note the marked reduction in cancellous bone volume and in the thickness of the cortices compared with the normal biopsy specimen shown in Figure 55-2A. Goldner trichrome stain. Field width = 9.6 mm.

Concerning the changes in the other static and dynamic variables in osteoporosis, there is still considerable debate over whether patients can be stratified into high, normal, or low turnover groups. Even if they can, the pathogenetic and clinical significance of this so-called "histologic heterogeneity" in patients with osteoporosis is unclear. In a study of 50 postmenopausal women with untreated osteoporosis, the investigators identified two subsets of patients, one with normal turnover and one with high turnover, the latter representing 30% of the cases.[40] However, this conclusion was based on the finding of a bimodal distribution in *osteoid surface.* The tetracycline-based *bone formation rate,* a more reliable measure of turnover rate, showed a normal distribution. Based on the interval between the 10th percentile and the 90th percentile for calculated *bone resorption rate* in a large group (*n* = 32) of normal postmenopausal women, another study classified 30% of women with untreated postmenopausal osteoporosis as having high turnover, whereas 64% and 6% had normal and low turnover, respectively.[41] When *bone formation rate* was used as the discriminant variable, 19% were classified as having high turnover, 72% as having normal turnover, and 9% as having low turnover. Alternatively, in two studies of postmenopausal women with osteoporosis and their normal counterparts, the same wide variation in turnover indices was found in both groups, leading to the conclusion that there were no important subsets of patients with osteoporosis.[42,43] These studies, however, confirmed the earlier observations of others that, as a group, women with osteoporosis display a decrease in *bone formation rate,* and that some patients show profoundly depressed formation with little or no tetracycline uptake.[38]

From a clinical perspective, the impetus for classifying patients with osteoporosis according to their turnover status stems from the notion that the turnover rate may influence the response to particular therapeutic agents. For example, patients with high turnover rates may respond better to antiresorptive treatments. There is evidence that this is true for calcitonin.[44] However, in clinical practice, the biopsy is an impractical way to determine turnover status, and it is likely that biochemical markers of bone resorption and formation will be used increasingly for this purpose.

It is important to note that, in most cases, bone biopsy is performed when the disease is in an advanced stage, with multiple fractures already having occurred. It is probable that, in many cases, the disturbances in bone metabolism that led to the reduction in bone mass took place several years before the time of the biopsy and are no longer evident.[45] Another confounding factor is that most patients who undergo biopsy for osteoporosis already have been treated with one or more pharmaceutical agents.

## INDICATIONS FOR BIOPSY

Generally, biopsy of the iliac crest is useful only in diffuse diseases of the skeleton. A major use of the bone biopsy is as a diagnostic tool in patients with skeletal disease manifested by bone pain, fractures, or osteopenia of unclear cause or pathogenesis. In such cases, a biopsy specimen can provide important information about a pathologic process. There are only exceptional indications for performing this procedure in patients with localized skeletal disease such as Paget disease of bone, primary bone tumors, or bone metastases involving the iliac crest.

The indications for bone biopsy in women with postmenopausal osteoporosis are controversial. It would be difficult to perform biopsies on the many women who have this disease. However, bone biopsy can provide useful information in groups of patients less commonly affected by osteoporosis, such as young men and premenopausal women. Patients with osteopenia or women with postmenopausal osteoporosis should not undergo biopsy merely to measure *cancellous bone volume* to confirm the diagnosis of osteoporosis. The intraindividual and interindividual variability in *cancellous bone volume* is too great, and there is too much overlap between *cancellous bone volumes* in patients with clinical osteoporosis and normal persons to make it useful. However, bone biopsy is useful to exclude subclinical osteomalacia. In one study, 5% of patients with typical crush fracture syndrome had clear-cut histologic evidence of osteomalacia despite normal biochemical and radiologic variables.[52] Moreover, the biopsy can be useful in defining, more precisely, the probable mechanisms of bone loss in individual patients with osteoporosis, and may aid in choosing the most appropriate course of action. For example, if the biopsy reveals or confirms a high bone turnover rate, it is important to carefully rule out endocrine disorders, such as hyperthyroidism and hyperparathyroidism. Finally, the biopsy is the best available way to evaluate the effect of various therapeutic maneuvers on bone cell function.[53,54]

Persons with renal osteodystrophy represent another group of patients in whom a transiliac crest bone biopsy may be extremely helpful. Once again, however, the large number of patients with renal disease precludes the use of this procedure in every case. Generally, if a symptomatic patient has biochemical evidence of secondary hyperparathyroidism (hyperphosphatemia, hypocalcemia, and markedly elevated intact PTH levels), biopsy is unnecessary because it almost certainly will reveal osteitis fibrosa. However, patients with renal disease who have bone pain and fractures but who do not have the biochemical hallmarks typical of secondary hyperparathyroidism should undergo biopsy to determine whether they have osteomalacia or idiopathic aplastic bone disease, and whether aluminum accumulation appears to be the primary etiologic factor. Although biopsy can be useful in the clinical management of certain patients with bone disease, its primary use today is as a powerful research tool.

## REFERENCES

1. Frost HM. Bone histomorphometry: choice of marking agent and labeling schedule. In: Recker RR, ed. Bone histomorphometry: techniques and interpretation. Boca Raton, FL: CRC Press, 1983:37.
2. Parfitt AM. The physiological and clinical significance of bone histomorphometric data. In: Recker RR, ed. Bone histomorphometry: techniques and interpretation. Boca Raton, FL: CRC Press, 1983:143.
3. Rao DS. Practical approach to bone biopsy. In: Recker RR, ed. Bone histomorphometry: techniques and interpretation. Boca Raton, FL: CRC Press, 1983:3.
4. Bordier P, Matrajt H, Miravet B, Hioco D. Mesure histologique de la masse et de la résorption des través osseuse. Pathol Biol (Paris) 1964; 12:1238.
5. Dempster DW. The relationship between the iliac crest bone biopsy and other skeletal sites. In: Kleerekoper M, Krane S, eds. Clinical disorders of bone and mineral metabolism. New York: Mary Ann Liebert, Inc, 1988:247.
6. Baron R, Vignery A, Neff L, et al. Processing of undecalcified bone specimens for bone histomorphometry. In: Recker RR, ed. Bone histomorphometry: techniques and interpretation. Boca Raton, FL: CRC Press, 1983:13.
7. Weinstein RS. Clinical use of bone biopsy. In: Coe FL, Favus MJ, eds. Disorders of bone and mineral metabolism. New York: Raven Press, 1992:455.
8. Parfitt AM. Stereological basis of bone histomorphometry; theory of quantitative microscopy and reconstruction of the third dimension. In: Recker RR, ed. Bone histomorphometry: techniques and interpretation. Boca Raton, FL: CRC Press, 1983:53.
9. Compston J. Bone histomorphometry. In: Arnett TR, Henderson B, eds. Methods in bone biology. London: Chapman and Hall, 1997:177.
10. Malluche HH, Faugere M-C. Atlas of mineralized bone histology. Basel: Karger, 1987.
11. Frost HM. Bone histomorphometry: analysis of trabecular bone dynamics. In: Recker RR, ed. Bone histomorphometry: techniques and interpretation. Boca Raton, FL: CRC Press, 1983:109.
12. Eriksen EF. Normal and pathological remodeling of human trabecular bone: three dimensional reconstruction of the remodeling sequence in normals and in metabolic bone disease. Endocr Rev 1986; 7:379.
13. Parfitt AM, Drezner MK, Glorieux FH, et al. Bone histomorphometry: standardization of nomenclature, symbols, and units. J Bone Miner Res 1987; 2:595.
14. Frost HM. Bone remodeling and its relationship to metabolic bone diseases. Springfield, IL: Charles C Thomas Publisher, 1973.
15. Parfitt AM. Bone remodeling: relationship to the amount and structure of bone, and the pathogenesis and prevention of fractures. In: Riggs BL, Melton LJ III, eds. Osteoporosis: etiology, diagnosis, and management. New York: Raven Press, 1988:45.
16. Dempster DW. Bone remodeling. In: Coe FL, Favus MJ, eds. Disorders of bone and mineral metabolism. New York: Raven Press, 1992:355.
17. Melsen F, Mosekilde L, Kragstrup J. Metabolic bone diseases as evaluated by bone histomorphometry. In: Recker RR, ed. Bone histomorphometry: techniques and interpretation. Boca Raton, FL: CRC Press, 1983:265.
18. Parisien M, Silverberg SJ, Shane E, et al. The histomorphometry of bone in primary hyperparathyroidism: preservation of cancellous bone structure. J Clin Endocrinol Metab 1990; 70:930.
18a. Silverberg SJ, Shane E, Dempster DW, Bilezikian JP. The effects of vitamin D insufficiency in patients with primary hyperparathyroidism. Am J Med 1999; 107:561.
19. Parisien MV, Mellish RWE, Silverberg SJ, et al. Maintenance of cancellous bone connectivity in primary hyperparathyroidism: trabecular strut analysis. J Bone Miner Res 1992; 7:913.
20. Teitelbaum SL. Pathological manifestations of osteomalacia and rickets. J Clin Endocrinol Metab 1980; 9:43.
21. Jaworksi ZFG. Histomorphometric characteristics of metabolic bone disease. In: Recker RR, ed. Bone histomorphometry: techniques and interpretation. Boca Raton, FL: CRC Press, 1983:241.
22. Siris ES, Clemens TL, Dempster DW, et al. Tumor-induced osteomalacia. Kinetics of calcium, phosphorus, and vitamin D metabolism and characteristics of bone histomorphometry. Am J Med 1987; 82:307.
23. Malluche HH, Ritz E, Lange HP, et al. Bone histology in incipient and advanced renal failure. Kidney Int 1976; 9:355.
24. Hodsman AB, Sherrard DJ, Alfrey AC, et al. Bone aluminum and histomorphometric features of renal osteodystrophy. J Clin Endocrinol Metab 1982; 54:539.
25. Boyce BF, Fell GS, Elder HY, et al. Hypercalcemic osteomalacia due to aluminum toxicity. Lancet 1982; 2:1009.
26. Dunstan CR, Hills E, Norman AW, et al. The pathogenesis of renal osteodystrophy: role of vitamin D, aluminum, parathyroid hormone, calcium and phosphorus. Q J Med 1985; 55:127.
27. Parisien M, Charhon SA, Mainetti E, et al. Evidence for a toxic effect of aluminum on osteoblasts: a histomorphometric study in hemodialysis patients with adynamic bone disease. J Bone Miner Res 1988; 3:259.
28. Charhon SA, Berland YF, Olmer MJ, et al. Effects of parathyroidectomy on bone formation and mineralization in hemodialized patients. Kidney Int 1985; 27:426.
29. Sherrard DJ, Hercz G, Pei Y, et al. The spectrum of bone disease in end-stage renal failure—an evolving disorder. Kidney Int 1993; 43:435.
30. Coburn JW, Salusky IB. Hyperparathyroidism in renal failure: clinical features, diagnosis, and management. In: Bilezikian JP, Levine MA, Marcuo R, eds. The parathyroids. New York: Raven Press, 1994:721.
31. Slatopolsky E, Delmaz J. Bone disease in chronic renal failure and after renal transplantation. In: Coe FL, Favus MF, eds. Disorders of bone and mineral metabolism. New York: Raven Press, 1992:905.
32. Felsenfeld AJ, Rodriguez M, Dunlay R, Llach F. A comparison of parathyroid gland function in haemodialysis patients with different forms of renal osteodystrophy. Nephrol Dial Transplant 1991; 6:244.
33. Salusky IB, Coburn JW, Brill J, et al. Bone disease in pediatric patients undergoing dialysis with CAPD or CCPD. Kidney Int 1988; 33:975.
34. Moriniere P, Cohen-Solal M, Belbrik S, et al. Disappearance of aluminic bone disease in a long-term asymptomatic dialysis population restricting Al(OH)$_3$ intake: emergence of an idiopathic adynamic bone disease not related to aluminum. Nephron 1989; 53:93.
35. Hercz F, Pei Y, Greenwood C, et al. Low turnover osteodystrophy without aluminum: the role of "suppressed" parathyroid function. Kidney Int 1993; 44:860.
36. Meunier PJ, Sellami S, Briancon D, Edouard C. Histological heterogeneity

of apparently idiopathic osteoporosis. In: Deluca HF, Frost HM, Jee WSS, et al, eds. Osteoporosis, recent advances in pathogenesis and treatment. Baltimore: University Park Press, 1981:293.

37. Parfitt AM, Matthews CHE, Villanueva AR, et al. Relationships between surface, volume and thickness of iliac trabecular bone in aging and in osteoporosis. Implications for the microanatomic and cellular mechanisms of bone loss. J Clin Invest 1983; 72:1396.

38. Whyte MP, Bergfeld MA, Murphy WA, et al. Postmenopausal osteoporosis; a heterogeneous disorder as assessed by histomorphometric analysis of iliac crest bone from untreated patients. Am J Med 1982; 72:193.

39. Meunier PJ. Assessment of bone turnover by histomorphometry in osteoporosis. In: Riggs BL, Melton LJ III, eds. Osteoporosis: etiology, diagnosis, and management. New York: Raven Press, 1988:317.

39a. Dempster DW. The contribution of trabecular architecture to cancellous bone quality. J Bone Miner Res 2000; 15:20.

40. Arlot ME, Delmas PD, Chappard D, Meunier PJ. Trabecular and endocortical bone remodeling in postmenopausal osteoporosis: comparison with normal postmenopausal women. Osteoporos Int 1990; 1:41.

41. Eriksen EF, Hodgson SF, Eastell R, et al. Cancellous bone remodeling in type I (postmenopausal) osteoporosis: quantitative assessment of rates of formation, resorption, and bone loss at tissue and cellular levels. J Bone Miner Res 1990; 5:311.

42. Kimmel DB, Recker RR, Gallagher JC, et al. A comparison of iliac bone histomorphometric data in post-menopausal osteoporotic and normal subjects. Bone Miner 1990; 11:217.

43. Garcia Carasco M, de Vernejoul MC, Sterkers Y, et al. Decreased bone formation in osteoporotic patients compared with age-matched controls. Calcif Tissue Int 1989; 44:173.

44. Civitelli R, Gonnelli S, Zacchei F, et al. Bone turnover in postmenopausal osteoporosis. Effect of calcitonin treatment. J Clin Invest 1988; 82:1268.

45. Steiniche T, Christiansen P, Vesterby A, et al. Marked changes in iliac crest bone structure in postmenopausal women without any signs of disturbed bone remodeling or balance. Bone 1994; 15:73.

46. Bressot C, Meunier PJ, Chapuy MC, et al. Histomorphometric profile, pathophysiology and reversibility of corticosteroid-induced osteoporosis. Metab Bone Dis Relat Res 1979; 1:303.

47. Dempster DW. Bone histomorphometry in glucocorticoid-induced osteoporosis. J Bone Miner Res 1989; 4:137.

48. Meunier PJ, Coindre JM, Edouard CM, Arlot ME. Bone histomorphometry in Paget's disease; quantitative and dynamic analysis of Pagetic and non-pagetic bone tissue. Arthritis Rheum 1980; 23:1095.

49. Valentin-Opran A, Charhon SA, Meunier PJ, et al. Quantitative histology of myeloma-induced bone changes. Br J Haematol 1982; 52:601.

50. Baron R, Gertner JM, Lang R, Vignery A. Increased bone turnover with decreased bone formation by osteoblasts in children with osteogenesis imperfecta tarda. Pediatr Res 1983; 17:204.

51. Ste-Marie LG, Charhon SA, Edouard C, et al. Iliac bone histomorphometry in adults and children with osteogenesis imperfecta. J Clin Pathol 1984; 37:1081.

52. Meunier PJ. Bone biopsy in diagnosis of metabolic bone disease. In: Cohn DV, Talmage R, Matthews JL, eds. Hormonal control of calcium metabolism. Proceedings of the Seventh International Conference on Calcium Regulating Hormones. Amsterdam: Excerpta Medica, 1981:109.

53. Holland EFN, Chow JWM, Studd JWW, et al. Histomorphometric changes in the skeleton of postmenopausal women with low bone mineral density treated with percutaneous estradiol implants. Obstet Gynecol 1994; 83:387.

54. Marcus R, Leary D, Schneider DL, et al. The contribution of testosterone to skeletal development and maintenance: lessons from the androgen insensitivity syndrome. J Clin Endocrinol Metab 2000; 85:1032.

# CHAPTER 56

# MARKERS OF BONE METABOLISM

MARKUS J. SEIBEL, SIMON P. ROBINS, AND JOHN P. BILEZIKIAN

Bone is a metabolically active tissue that throughout life undergoes constant remodeling. Skeletal turnover is achieved by two counteracting processes: bone formation and bone resorption. Whereas bone formation is a function of *osteoblast* activity, bone resorption is attributed to *osteoclast* activity. The metabolic and cellular events in the skeleton are regulated by a large number of systemic and local modulators, such as parathyroid hormone, vitamin D, sex hormones, glucocorticoids, calcitonin, prostaglandins, growth factors, and cytokines (see Chaps. 49–51, 54, 55, and 173).

Under normal conditions, bone formation and resorption are closely coupled to each other, and this balance maintains a stable bone mass. Metabolic bone diseases, in contrast, are characterized by more or less pronounced imbalances in bone turnover (often referred to as "uncoupling"). The long-term result of such imbalances in bone turnover often is changes in bone mass and structure, which either become clinically symptomatic (e.g., fracture), or may be detected by means of radiographic or densitometric techniques. In addition to these static measures, markers of bone turnover can be used to detect the dynamics of the metabolic imbalance itself. Bone mass and bone turnover are, therefore, complementary parameters in the assessment of skeletal homeostasis.

This chapter reviews the basic biochemistry, methodology, and clinical application of the currently known markers of bone turnover (Tables 56-1 and 56-2). The endocrine regulation of calcium homeostasis and bone metabolism is discussed in Chapters 49 and 50.

## BIOCHEMISTRY OF BONE

Bone is composed of ~70% mineral and 30% organic matter. The mineral, primarily in the form of *hydroxyapatite* [$Ca_{10}(PO_4)_6(OH)_2$] crystals, is embedded in and aligned with the collagen fibrils, which play an important role in crystal formation. This calcium-collagen composite ensures the two main functions of bone: providing a structural framework and acting as a reservoir for mineral ions.

The organic phase of bone is made of cells and a protein matrix, of which ~90% is collagen type I. Bone also contains a large number of different proteins, glycoproteins, and proteoglycans, many of which are negatively charged (Table 56-3). Although their precise functions are not established, these noncollagenous proteins are probably associated with the organization and mineralization of the skeletal matrix.

*Collagen* is synthesized by osteoblasts as a larger precursor molecule. This *"procollagen"* molecule contains the triple helix portion, which bears several hydroxyproline residues, and globular extensions at the N- and the C-terminal ends (i.e., N- and C-terminal propeptides). After secretion of the collagen molecule, these propeptides are removed en bloc by specific proteases at the cell surface. The *C-terminal propeptide* remains intact and appears as a 100-kDa protein in the blood. The helical collagen molecules spontaneously assemble into fibrils, which are then covalently cross-linked to impart the necessary tensile strength. This process is initiated extracellularly through the action of a single enzyme, lysyl oxidase. Thereafter, reactions of the lysine-derived aldehydes occur spontaneously and culminate in the formation of trifunctional *pyridinium cross-links* (Fig. 56-1). Unlike hydroxyproline, which is already present in the newly synthesized protein, the pyridinium cross-links are found exclusively in mature collagens of the established extracellular matrix. Of the two cross-link analogs produced, deoxypyridinoline is located primarily in bone collagen. Pyridinoline occurs in cartilage and other soft tissues as well as in bone (see Chap. 189).

Of the noncollagenous proteins in bone, osteocalcin, or bone Gla protein, is one of the most abundant (~15%). The protein contains 49 amino-acid residues, three of which are γ-carboxyglutamic acid (GLA). Whereas the latter are formed in a posttranslational vitamin K–dependent process, transcription of the OC gene itself is controlled by 1,25-dihydroxyvitamin $D_3$. A small proportion of the newly synthesized protein is transported directly into the blood, from which it is eliminated mainly through the kidneys.

Other noncollagenous proteins in the extracellular matrix of bone are summarized in Table 56-3. Because many of these components are produced by osteoblasts and by a variety of other cell types, they may be found in nonskeletal tissues as well. This distribution is explained by the fact that most of

**TABLE 56-1.**
**Biomarkers of Bone Formation**

| Marker (Abbreviation) | Tissue of Origin | Specimen | Method | Specificity |
|---|---|---|---|---|
| Total alkaline phosphatase (AP, TAP) | Bone, liver, intestine, kidney, placenta | Serum | Colorimetric | In healthy adults, 1:1 ratio between liver or biliary and bone-derived enzyme. |
| Bone-specific alkaline phosphatase (BAP) | Bone | Serum | Colorimetric, electrophoretic, precipitation, IRMA, EIA | Specific product of osteoblasts; in some assays, cross-reactivity with liver isoenzyme. |
| Osteocalcin (OC, BGP) | Bone, platelets | Serum | RIA, ELISA | Specific product of osteoblasts; many immunoreactive forms in blood; some may be derived from bone resorption. |
| Carboxyterminal propeptide of type I procollagen (PICP) | Bone, soft tissue, skin | Serum | RIA, ELISA | Specific product of proliferating osteoblasts and fibroblasts. |
| Amino-terminal propeptide of type I procollagen (PINP) | Bone, soft tissue, skin | Serum | RIA, ELISA | Specific product of proliferating osteoblast and fibroblasts; partly incorporated into bone extracellular matrix. |

*IRMA*, immunoradiometric assay; *EIA*, enzyme immunoassay; *RIA*, radioimmunoassay; *ELISA*, enzyme-linked immunosorbent assay.

these proteins play an important role in the general organization of the extracellular matrix, mediating basic processes such as cell attachment and migration, growth, development, and fibril formation. Thus, both *osteopontin* and *bone sialoprotein* are found predominantly in mineralizing tissues, where they serve as cell-attachment proteins by means of their intrinsic RGD amino-acid sequences. In bone, the proteins are synthesized by osteoblasts and mediate the attachment of osteoclasts to the mineralized matrix.

Approximately 25% of the noncollagenous proteins found in the extracellular matrix of bone are actually derived from the serum and are not osteogenic products (see Table 56-3).

Besides the collagenous and noncollagenous proteins of bone, several specific enzymes play an important role in skeletal metabolism. Alkaline phosphatase is a characteristic product of active osteoblasts and young osteocytes. Although the function of this enzyme in bone metabolism is not clear, a close asso-

ciation with bone formation processes (i.e., maturation and mineralization of osteoid) has been established.

The main bone-resorbing cell is the osteoclast. Interactions of specific cell-surface components form a secondary, extracellular lysosome with a ruffled border through which hydrogen ions are pumped to produce a low-pH local environment. This process is necessary to demineralize the bone, after which the matrix is removed by a series of acidic proteases that are released by the osteoclasts. One of these enzymes is tartrate-resistant acid phosphatase, which also is found in blood and is considered to be an osteoclast-specific product.

## MARKERS OF BONE METABOLISM

Assays of biochemical markers of bone turnover are noninvasive and, when the results are applied and interpreted cor-

**TABLE 56-2.**
**Biomarkers of Bone Resorption**

| Marker (Abbreviation) | Tissue of Origin | Specimen | Method | Specificity |
|---|---|---|---|---|
| Hydroxyproline, total and dialyzable (OH-Pro, OHP) | Bone, cartilage, soft tissue, skin, blood | Urine | Colorimetric, HPLC | All fibrillar collagens and partly collagenous proteins, including C1q and elastin; present in newly synthesized and mature collagen. |
| Pyridinoline (PYD; Pyr) | Bone, cartilage, tendon, blood vessels | Urine Serum | HPLC, ELISA, RIA | Collagens, with highest concentrations in cartilage and bone; absent from skin; present in mature collagen only. |
| Deoxypyridinoline (DPD, d-Pyr) | Bone, dentin | Urine Serum | HPLC, ELISA, RIA | Collagens, with highest concentration in bone; absent from cartilage or skin; present in mature collagen only. |
| Carboxy-terminal cross-linked telopeptide of type I collagen (ICTP) | Bone, skin | Serum | RIA | Collagen type I, with highest contribution probably from bone; may be derived from newly synthesized collagen. |
| Carboxy-terminal cross-linked telopeptide of type I collagen (CTx) | All tissues containing type I collagen | Urine Serum | ELISA, RIA | Collagen type I, with highest contribution probably from bone. |
| Amino-terminal cross-linked telopeptide of type I collagen (INTP, NTx) | All tissues containing type I collagen | Urine Serum | ELISA RIA | Collagen type I, with highest contribution probably from bone. |
| Hydroxylysine glycosides | Bone, soft tissue, skin, serum complement | Urine | HPLC | Collagens and collagenous proteins; glycosylgalactosyl-OHLys in high proportion in collagens of soft tissues, and C1q; galactosyl-OHLys in high proportion in skeletal collagens. |
| Bone sialoprotein (BSP) | Mineralized tissues, such as bone, dentin, hypertrophic cartilage | Serum | RIA, ELISA | Synthesized by active osteoblasts and laid down in bone extracellular matrix. Appears to reflect osteoclast activity. |
| Tartrate-resistant acid phosphatase (TRAP) (TRAP5b) | Bone, blood | Plasma, serum | Colorimetric, RIA, ELISA | Osteoclasts, platelets, erythrocytes. |
| Free γ-carboxyglutamic acid (GLA) | Bone, blood | Serum, urine | HPLC | Derived from bone proteins (e.g., osteocalcin, matrix Gla protein) and from blood-clotting factors. |

*HPLC*, high-performance liquid chromatography; *ELISA*, enzyme-linked immunosorbent assay; *RIA*, radioimmunoassay.

**TABLE 56-3.**
**Biochemical Components of Bone**

| Components | Origin | Percentage of NCP | Average Size (kDa) | Function |
|---|---|---|---|---|
| Collagen type I | Osteoblast | | 300 | Framework, stability |
| Osteocalcin | Osteoblast | <1–15 | 5–6 | Unknown, mineralization (?) |
| Matrix Gla protein | Osteoblast | 1–2 | 9–15 | Unknown, growth (?) |
| Osteonectin | Osteoblast | 10–15 | 35–50 | Unknown, mineralization (?) |
| Osteopontin | Osteoblast | 5–10 | 60–80 | Cell attachment (e.g., osteoclast) |
| Bone sialoprotein | Osteoblast | 5–10 | 75–80 | Cell attachment |
| Fibronectin | Osteoblast | <1 | 450–500 | Cell attachment and migration |
| Thrombospondin | Osteoblast | <1 | 450–500 | Cell attachment |
| PG-I (biglycan) | Osteoblast | 2–5 | 100–200 | Unknown, matrix organization (?) |
| PG-II (decorin) | Osteoblast | 2–5 | 120–200 | Collagen fibrillogenesis |
| Alkaline phosphatase | Osteoblast | | 50–200 | Unknown, matrix biosynthesis |
| Acid phosphatase | Osteoclast | | 11–140 | Matrix degradation |
| Albumin | Liver | <1–3 | 60 | |
| $\alpha_2$-HS-glycoprotein | Liver | <1–20 | 50 | |

*NCP*, noncollagenous proteins; *PG*, proteoglycan.

rectly, are very helpful tools in the assessment of metabolic bone disease.

The various serum and urinary components used as markers of bone turnover include *enzymes* released by bone cells and *peptides* derived from the skeletal matrix during bone formation or bone resorption. For clinical purposes, bone biomarkers are usually classified according to the metabolic process they are considered to reflect; that is, bone formation or bone resorption (see Tables 56-1 and 56-2). Some components, such as the serum amino-terminal procollagen type I propeptide and urinary hydroxyproline, are derived from anabolic and catabolic processes and are, therefore, influenced by the rate of bone formation *and* bone resorption. Other markers, such as the bone isoenzyme of alkaline phosphatase or the pyridinium cross-links of collagen, are more specific to individual metabolic processes.

Most of the compounds that are used as markers of skeletal metabolism are *not* unique to bone, as they also occur in other tissues (see Tables 56-1 and 56-2). Few or perhaps none of the available markers is absolutely specific for bone. Moreover, most serum and urinary indices are *influenced by nonskeletal diseases*, such as inflammatory conditions, malignancies, and

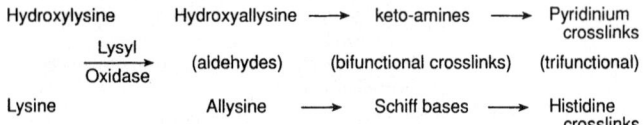

**FIGURE 56-1.** Lysyl-oxidase–derived cross-links. Scheme illustrating the tissue-specific differences in the trifunctional, mature cross-links formed, depending on whether lysine or hydroxylysine residues in the telopeptides are oxidized.

chronic renal or hepatic failure. Changes in biochemical markers of bone metabolism are, therefore, *not* disease specific; abnormal results should always be interpreted within the context of the clinical picture. With these notions in mind, one may use bone markers for the following purposes:

1. To evaluate bone turnover in individual patients and disorders
2. To predict future bone loss and hip fractures in larger cohorts
3. To select therapy for individual patients
4. To predict therapeutic response in individual patients
5. To monitor therapeutic response and efficacy in individual patients

## MARKERS OF BONE FORMATION

All bone formation markers are products or enzymes released by active osteoblasts and are generally measured in serum or plasma. The most commonly used markers of bone formation are alkaline phosphatase, OC, and the propeptides of type I collagen.

### ALKALINE PHOSPHATASE

The alkaline phosphatases form a family of isoenzymes that are found in a multitude of tissues, including bone (e.g., in osteoblasts), liver, intestines, kidney, and placenta.[1] The various isoforms can be differentiated by their carbohydrate content. Several methods have been established to determine specifically the enzyme fraction derived from osteoblasts, including selective denaturation, inhibition or activation, electrophoretic separation, and immunologic quantification.[2]

In healthy adults, ~50% of the *total serum alkaline phosphatase (TAP) activity* is derived from osteoblasts, whereas the other half is usually of biliary-hepatic origin. Particularly in elderly patients, elevated serum TAP activities are more often the result of hepatic afflictions than of skeletal diseases (Table 56-4). Therefore, serum TAP levels should be used as an index of bone formation only if an impairment of liver and biliary function can be excluded. In contrast, the *bone-specific isoenzyme of alkaline phosphatase (BAP)* is located exclusively in the osteoblast membrane, from which it is released into the circulation on osteoblast activation. Compared to the total enzyme pool, serum BAP levels are clearly less affected by nonskeletal disorders and therefore more specific for changes in bone formation. In the clinical setting, however, the diagnostic sensitivity of serum BAP is not superior to that of serum TAP.[2]

Total alkaline phosphatase is the classic laboratory marker of skeletal activity in Paget disease of bone. Serum levels of the total and bone-specific enzymes are markedly increased when the disease is active, but are normal or only slightly elevated when patients have monostotic, mild polyostotic, or inactive disease. In certain cases, determination of serum BAP instead of TAP may help identify patients with very mild disease. Rather high levels of serum TAP or BAP are typically seen in patients with involvement of the skull, and sometimes in cases with sarcomatous degeneration of pagetic bone. Serial measurements of serum TAP are helpful to monitor a therapeutic response and to detect a recrudescence of disease activity.

Primary hyperparathyroidism was previously often associated with significantly elevated levels of serum alkaline phosphatase, indicating gross bone involvement. However, as the clinical profile of the disorder has evolved toward a predominance of cases with asymptomatic hypercalcemia, marked elevations in serum alkaline phosphatase are rarely seen (see Chap. 58).[3] The expectation that serum BAP may be a more sensitive parameter of bone involvement in asymptomatic primary hyperparathyroidism has not yet been met.[2]

For the use of serum TAP and/or BAP measurements in osteoporosis, see last section of this chapter.

**TABLE 56-4.**
**Factors Affecting the Serum Levels of Total Alkaline Phosphatase**

| Increase | Decrease | Increase or Decrease |
|---|---|---|
| Somatic growth | Growth hormone deficiency | Race |
| Paget disease of bone | | Diurnal rhythms |
| Rickets and osteomalacia | Hypoparathyroid- ism | Seasonal rhythms |
| Renal osteodystrophy | Hypothyroidism | |
| Hyperparathyroidism (severe) | Familial or sporadic hypophos- phatasemia | Rheum- atoid arthritis |
| Thyrotoxicosis | | |
| Acromegaly (active) | | |
| Skeletal malignancies (e.g., osteosar- coma) | Achondroplasia | |
| Multiple myeloma | Anemia (severe) | |
| Metastatic bone disease (e.g., osteo- blastic) | | |
| Osteogenesis imperfecta | | |
| Fibrous dysplasia | | |
| Familial hyperphosphatasemia | | |
| Idiopathic hyperphosphatasemia | | |
| Hyperostosis frontalis interna | | |
| Recent fractures | | |
| Age | | |
| Hepatic and biliary disease, includ- ing hepatotoxicity and malignan- cies | | |
| Other malignancies (i.e., production of ectopic AP, such as Regan-, Nagao-AP) | | |
| Late pregnancy (e.g., placental AP) | | |

| *Treatment with* | *Treatment with* |
|---|---|
| Corticosteroids | Bisphosphonates |
| Anticonvulsants | Calcitonin |
| Fluorides | Estrogen |
| Growth hormones | |
| Vitamin $D_3$ | |

*AP, alkaline phosphatase.*

In osteomalacia, total and bone-specific enzyme activities are markedly elevated; the determination of serum alkaline phosphatase is often a clue to the diagnosis of this disorder. In renal osteodystrophy, elevated levels of serum alkaline phosphatase may be indicative of progressive skeletal involvement and, particularly in patients on chronic hemodialysis, should prompt appropriate diagnostic and therapeutic measures.

Serum levels of TAP and BAP may be elevated in primary and secondary skeletal malignancies. High serum activities are often found in osteoblastic bone metastases and after multiple fractures. In contrast, the alkaline phosphatase level is usually low in multiple myeloma. Because of its rather low sensitivity and specificity, serum alkaline phosphatase is not recom- mended as a tumor marker for clinical use.

## OSTEOCALCIN

*Osteocalcin (OC, or bone Gla protein)*, a small, GLA–rich peptide syn- thesized by osteoblasts, is one of the major noncollagenous pro- teins of the bone matrix.[4,5] The molecule is found exclusively in mineralized tissues, and although its precise function is unknown, one obviously important property of OC is its high affinity for hydroxyapatite. Interestingly, OC-deficient knock-out mice have increased cortical and trabecular bone thickness, and mechanically more stable bones than wild-type mice.[6] Therefore, during miner- alization, OC may act via a negative feedback mechanism.

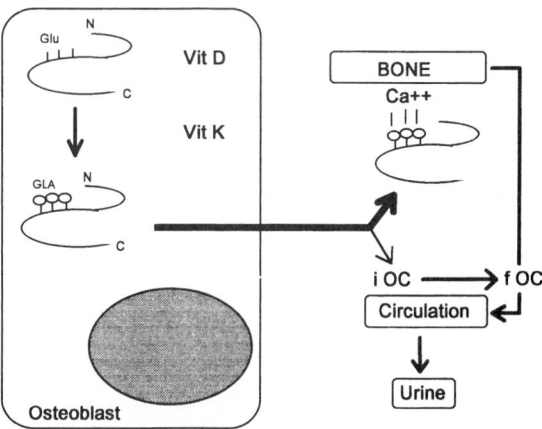

**FIGURE 56-2.** Synthesis and metabolism of osteocalcin. Although the synthesis of osteocalcin is stimulated by vitamin D, γ-carboxylation of glutamic acid (*Glu*) residues depends on vitamin K. Because of the affinity of γ-carboxyglutamic acid (*GLA*) residues to hydroxylapatite, 70% to 80% of the newly synthesized peptide is bound to the mineraliz- ing matrix of bone, and 20% to 30% enters the circulation as intact osteocalcin (*iOC*). Circulating osteocalcin is rapidly degraded into smaller fragments (*fOC*), some of which may also be derived from bone resorption. (*Vit*, Vitamin; *N*, amino terminus; *C*, carboxyl terminus.)

After its secretion by activated osteoblasts, the major frac- tion of OC is incorporated into the extracellular matrix. How- ever, 15% to 30% of the newly synthesized peptide is released into the general circulation, where it may be detected and quan- tified by immunoassay (Fig. 56-2). Although serum levels of cir- culating OC correlate well with the rate of bone formation,[7] significant drawbacks are encountered in the practical use of this marker. Serum OC levels are strongly affected by the pro- nounced thermal instability of the molecule, the specificity of the antibodies, and factors such as hormonal status, renal func- tion, age, and sex [4,4a] (Tables 56-5 and 56-6).

With the exception of Paget disease of bone, in which serum OC levels are often normal, *most conditions with increased bone and mineral formation are characterized by elevated serum concentra- tions of OC.* This is the case in primary hyperparathyroidism and hyperthyroidism, in which serum OC levels correlate with the extent of bone involvement.[8] In healthy women, a transient, two-fold increase of serum OC is seen during early menopause, and individual values appear to correlate with the rate of bone loss in this population.[9,10] In contrast, a wide range of values is observed in overt postmenopausal osteoporosis, which may be caused in part by the heterogeneity of the disease.

A different situation may be present in the elderly and in patients with senile osteoporosis. In this population, the effect of aging and possibly a deficiency of vitamins K and D may lead to an impairment in the γ-carboxylation of OC and ulti- mately to an increase in the proportion of partially undercar- boxylated circulating OC. Several studies now indicate that the proportion of undercarboxylated OC in serum may be an important determinant of femoral bone mineral density in elderly women, because high serum levels of undercarboxy- lated OC are associated with a low bone density at the hip and an increased risk of hip fractures.[11] (See also the last section of this chapter.)

Serum OC levels are often elevated in untreated osteomala- cia, in which they correlate with histomorphometric indices of osteoid formation.[12] However, serum OC levels are usually much less elevated than the corresponding serum TAP or BAP levels.

In advanced renal failure (i.e., glomerular filtration rate of <20–30 mL/minute/1.73 m²), the accumulation of intact OC

**TABLE 56-5.**
**Factors Affecting the Serum Levels of Osteocalcin**

| Increase | Decrease | Increase or Decrease |
|---|---|---|
| Somatic growth | Growth hormone | Metastatic bone disease |
| Acromegaly | deficiency | Hypercalcemia of |
| Hyperparathyroidism | Hypoparathyroid- | malignancy |
| Hyperthyroidism | ism | Osteomalacia |
| Malignancies | Hypothyroidism | Paget disease of bone |
| Renal osteodystrophy | Senile osteoporosis | Postmenopausal |
| Osteogenesis imperfecta | (i.e., intact OC) | osteoporosis |
| Recent fractures | Alcoholism | Race |
| Senile osteoporosis (i.e., | Anorexia nervosa | Diurnal rhythms |
| undercarboxylated OC) | Liver disease | Menstrual cycle |
| Age older than 50 years | Microprolactinoma | Seasonal rhythms |
| Female gender | Pregnancy | Osteoarthritis |
| Chronic renal failure | | Rheumatoid arthritis |
| Exercise | | |
| Lactation | | |
| Obesity | | |

| Treatment with | Treatment with |
|---|---|
| Fluorides | Bisphosphonates |
| Growth hormones | Calcitonin |
| Thyroid hormones (TSH | Corticosteroids |
| suppressive) | Estrogen |
| Vitamin $D_3$ | |
| Anticonvulsants | |

*OC*, osteocalcin; *TSH*, thyroid-stimulating hormone.

and its various immunoreactive fragments may lead to very high serum levels, even in the absence of significant skeletal disease (see Table 56-6). OC levels are not affected by hemodialysis. Because of impaired renal clearance and increased bone turnover, serum OC usually is elevated in patients with renal osteodystrophy.

Serum OC levels may be elevated in patients with metastatic bone disease, for whom it has been shown to be a useful marker of therapeutic responsiveness. Compared to the pyridinium cross-links, however, the diagnostic validity of serum OC for metastatic bone disease is low.[13,14]

Unlike in states of high bone turnover, serum OC levels are reduced in patients with glucocorticosteroid excess, such as Cushing disease or corticosteroid-induced osteoporosis. Also, low levels of serum OC have been correlated with poor survival in patients with stage III multiple myeloma.

Serum free and urinary GLA are in part derived from the breakdown of OC and matrix Gla protein. However, many other components, such as certain clotting factors and plasma proteins, contain considerable amounts of GLA. Although increased levels have been found in Paget disease and osteoporosis, neither serum nor urinary GLA has achieved clinical relevance.

## PROCOLLAGEN TYPE I PROPEPTIDES

During the process of collagen synthesis and before fibril formation, the N- and C-terminal procollagen propeptides are cleaved from the newly formed molecule and are released into the circulation. Because collagen and procollagen propeptides are generated stoichiometrically, levels of circulating procollagen propeptides are considered to reflect collagen neosynthesis (Fig. 56-3). Despite significant correlations between bone formation rates and the serum levels of procollagen type I propeptide, tissues other than bone contribute to the serum concentrations of these components[15,16] (see Table 56-1). As the procollagen propeptides are cleared from the circulation, mainly through uptake by endothelial cells of the liver, their serum and urinary concentrations are strongly influenced by hepatic function (see Table 56-6).

Several polyclonal immunoassays have been developed to determine specifically the *N- and C-terminal propeptides of procollagen type I* (*PINP* and *PICP*, respectively) in body fluids.[17,18] A number of different studies have shown good correlations between serum procollagen type I propeptide levels and the rate of bone formation or serum TAP activity.[13,16] Increased serum levels of both procollagen propeptides are generally seen in conditions involving somatic growth or enhanced bone turnover. Serum levels of both propeptides are much higher in prepubertal children and adolescents than in healthy adults. In children with somatic growth disorders, serum PICP levels correlate with linear growth velocity before and during growth

**TABLE 56-6.**
**Technical Characteristics of Bone Biomarkers**

| Marker (Abbreviation) | Stability and Recommended Storage | Concentrations Influenced by | Diurnal Rhythms |
|---|---|---|---|
| Total alkaline phosphatase (AP, TAP) | Stable < –20°C | Liver function* | Negligible |
| Bone-specific alkaline phosphatase (BAP) | Stable < –20°C | Liver function* | Negligible |
| Osteocalcin (OC, BGP) | Unstable < –80°C | Renal function† | Significant |
| Carboxy-terminal propeptide of type I procollagen (PICP) | Stable < –20°C | Liver function | Significant |
| Amino-terminal propeptide of type I procollagen (PINP) | Stable < –20°C | Liver function | Significant |
| Hydroxyproline, total and dialyzable (OH-Pro; OHP) | Stable < –20°C | Liver function, diet, inflammation (e.g., C1q) | Significant |
| Pyridinoline (PYD; Pyr) | Stable < –20°C | Liver function, active arthritis | Significant |
| Deoxypyridinoline (DPD; d-Pyr) | Stable < –20°C | Liver function | Significant |
| Carboxy-terminal cross-linked telopeptide of type I collagen (ICTP) | Stable < –20°C | Renal function, liver function | Significant |
| Carboxy-terminal cross-linked telopeptide of type I collagen (CTx) | Stable < –20°C | Renal function, liver function | Significant |
| Amino-terminal cross-linked telopeptide of type I collagen (INTP, NTx) | Stable < –20°C | Liver function | Significant |
| Hydroxylysine glycosides (Hyl-Glyc) | Stable < –20°C | Liver function | Significant |
| Bone sialoprotein (BSP) | Stable < –20°C | Renal function, liver function | Significant |
| Tartrate-resistant acid phosphatase (TRAP) | Unstable < –80°C | Hemolysis, blood clotting | Negligible |
| Free γ-carboxyglutamic acid (GLA) | | Diet (e.g., vitamin K), blood clotting | Negligible |

*See also Table 56-4.
†See also Table 56-5.

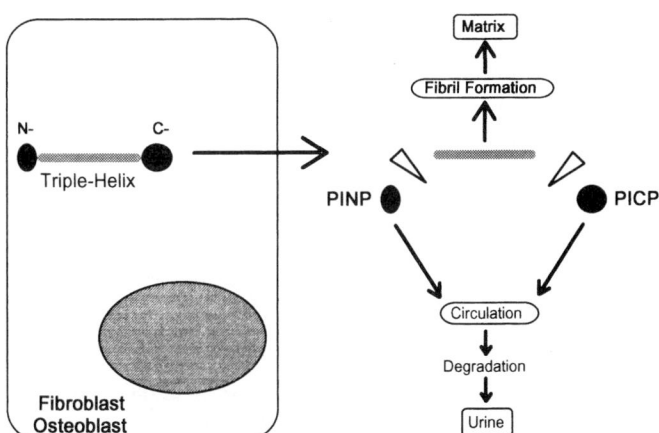

**FIGURE 56-3.** Synthesis and metabolism of procollagen propeptides. After the synthesis and secretion of the procollagen molecule by osteoblasts, the amino- (N-) and carboxy-terminal (C-) propeptides of type I collagen (e.g., PINP, PICP) are cleaved extracellularly from the procollagen molecule by specific proteases. The propeptides are considered to enter the circulation in an equimolar ratio to newly synthesized collagen and are regarded as specific markers of collagen biosynthesis. Similar mechanisms exist for other fibrillar collagens, such as type III collagen (e.g., PIIINP, PIIICP), which is typically found in soft tissues and mainly produced by fibroblasts.

hormone treatment.[19] Like most other biochemical markers of bone metabolism, serum propeptide levels are elevated in patients with Paget disease of bone; declining levels are seen after effective treatment. Normal menopause induces only slight changes in serum PICP and somewhat more pronounced elevations in PINP levels. Hormone-replacement therapy may be monitored by serum PICP or PINP, although the effect is usually less pronounced than with other markers of bone metabolism.

## MARKERS OF BONE RESORPTION

Markers of bone resorption are either enzymes released by active osteoclasts (i.e., tartrate-resistant acid phosphatase), or degradation products of the extracellular bone matrix. The latter are mainly collagen-related compounds such as the pyridinium cross-links. Also, noncollagenous proteins such as bone sialoprotein are being investigated as markers of bone resorption.

Unlike the formation markers, most resorption markers are routinely measured in urine, a medium that for several reasons is associated with a relatively high degree of imprecision. During the past few years, therefore, immunoassays for the measurement of type I collagen telopeptides have been developed (see later). The data so far are promising, and these new serum assays most likely will replace the urine-based techniques in the near future.

### HYDROXYPYRIDINIUM CROSS-LINKS OF TYPE I COLLAGEN AND RELATED STRUCTURES

The 3-hydroxypyridinium cross-links, pyridinoline (PYD) and deoxypyridinoline (DPD), are formed during extracellular maturation and are located in the telopeptide region of skeletal (type I) collagens. When mature collagen is broken down, both compounds and parts of the telopeptide region are released into the circulation and are ultimately excreted in the urine (Fig. 56-4). The pyridinium cross-links and the related telopeptides of type I collagen are currently considered *the most specific and sensitive markers of bone resorption.*[20]

The pattern of collagen cross-linking is tissue-specific in regard to cross-link type and concentration. Although PYD is found in cartilage, bone, tendons, and vascular tissues, DPD is

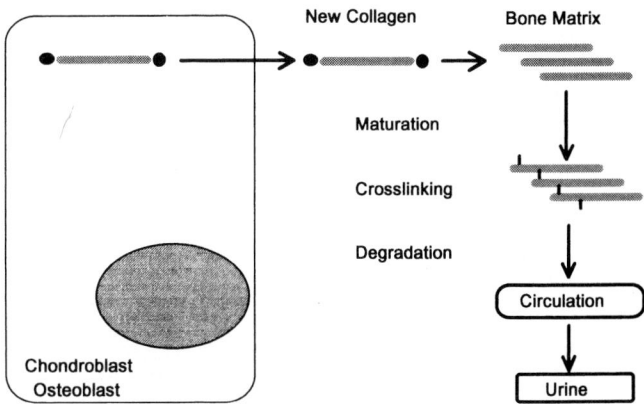

**FIGURE 56-4.** Synthesis and metabolism of pyridinium cross-links of collagen. After their extracellular aggregation, the collagen molecules are covalently cross-linked by type- and tissue-specific compounds derived from lysine (see Fig. 56-1). These components are released from the extracellular matrix during bone resorption and are ultimately excreted in the urine.

found almost exclusively in bone and dentin.[21,22] Moreover, because the formation of collagen cross-links is a time-dependent, posttranslational process, the source of the pyridinium components is restricted to mature collagens that have already been formed in the extracellular tissue matrix. Unlike urinary hydroxyproline, which may also be derived from the degradation of immature collagens (see later), the urinary excretion of PYD and DPD is not influenced by the breakdown of newly synthesized protein but instead reflects exclusively the degradation of mature collagens, as in bone resorption (Fig. 56-5).

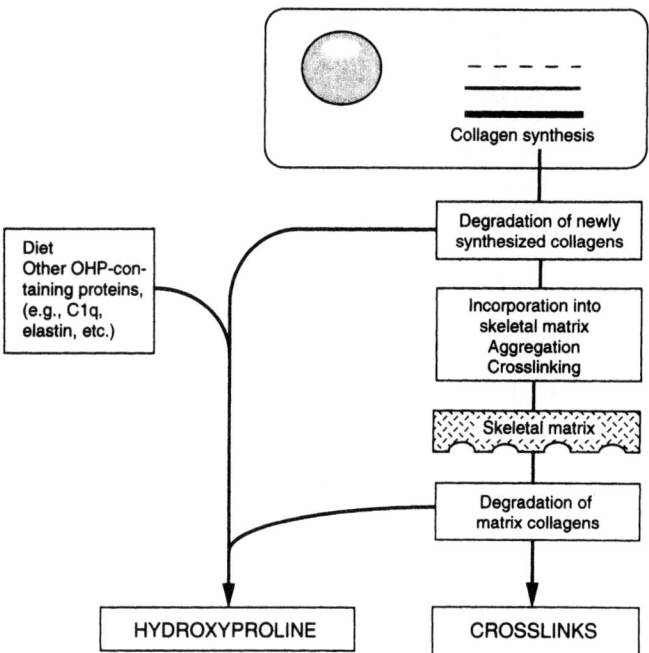

**FIGURE 56-5.** Comparison of hydroxyproline (*OHP*) and hydroxypyridinium cross-links in urine. Urinary hydroxyproline is derived from the degradation of mature *and* newly synthesized collagens. Additional sources of hydroxyproline are dietary intake and partly collagenous proteins, such as elastin and the complement component, C1q. The hydroxypyridinium cross-links are formed later in the process of collagen maturation and are exclusively derived from the breakdown of mature matrix collagens.

Approximately 50% to 60% of the total urinary cross-link pool is peptide-bound, with the cross-link incorporated into collagen peptides of various lengths. The remaining fraction is present in (peptide) free form. Several assays have been developed for the determination of pyridinium cross-link compounds in urine, including high-performance liquid chromatography (HPLC) and immunoassay techniques. The HPLC method makes use of the natural fluorescence of free cross-link compounds and, after complete acid hydrolysis of the urine, measures the total amount of urinary cross-link components.[23,24] In contrast, the various antibodies used in the commercially available immunoassays detect either the free cross-link components per se,[25–27] or small collagen peptides containing a cross-linking structure.[28,29]

The direct immunoassays for free PYD and DPD in urine are based on the fact that the proportion of free to peptide-bound cross-links in urine remains stable over a wide spectrum of bone pathologies. Measurement of the free cross-link fraction, therefore, provides similar information about bone resorption as does the determination of the total cross-link pool. This assumption has been confirmed in a number of clinical studies,[25–27] and assays for free pyridinium cross-links are currently a standard technique in many clinical laboratories throughout the world.

Parallel developments have resulted in several immunoassays for the measurement of collagen type I telopeptides in urine and in serum (Fig. 56-6). These assays are based on the fact that the cross-linking of collagen always involves a specific region of the molecule, the amino-terminal (N-) or carboxy-terminal (C-) telopeptide. The various types of assays currently available or under investigation are characterized as follows:

*C-terminal type I collagen telopeptide (ICTP) in serum*[29]: Antigenic determinant requires a trivalent cross-link; assay is not as sensitive to normal bone turnover as urinary cross-link assays but is more sensitive to abnormal bone resorption as in multiple myeloma or metastatic bone disease.

*C-terminal telopeptide of type I collagen (CTx) in urine or serum*[30–33]: Antigenic determinant is a synthetic octapeptide (EKAHDGGR) containing the cross-linking site of the C-terminal type I collagen telopeptide. Because of protein aging, the aspartyl may be present as isoaspartyl (βD),[31] which is also the form recognized in the serum assay.[33]

*N-terminal telopeptide of type I collagen (NTx) in urine and serum*[28]: Antigenic determinant requires the α-2 chain of type I collagen (QYDGKGVG); antibody reacts with several cross-linking components and is identical for urine- and serum-based assays.[34]

In healthy individuals, the excretion of PYD and DPD varies within a relatively narrow range, although a significant diurnal rhythm is observed, with highest values in the early morning hours and lowest values at night.[35] Menopause is associated with a two- to three-fold increase.[36] As these changes occur in healthy, nonosteoporotic women, they are likely to reflect the increase in bone turnover associated with estrogen withdrawal. Very similar results are seen with the immunoassays for either free DPD or the N- and C-terminal telopeptides (CTx, NTx).

In active Paget disease of bone, all collagen-related resorption markers are greatly elevated; a rapid decrease in urine or serum concentrations is seen after treatment with bisphosphonates, known inhibitors of osteoclast function.[34,37]

Approximately 60% of patients with mild primary hyperparathyroidism have elevated urinary cross-link concentrations, revealing subclinical bone involvement. After successful parathyroidectomy, urinary levels of DPD fall quickly, preceding the changes in urinary hydroxyproline and serum alkaline phosphatase by ~6 months.[38]

Overt metastatic bone disease and multiple myeloma are generally associated with marked changes in collagen-related resorption markers.[38a] In fact, these markers may be used to diagnose and/or monitor the therapeutic response in individ-

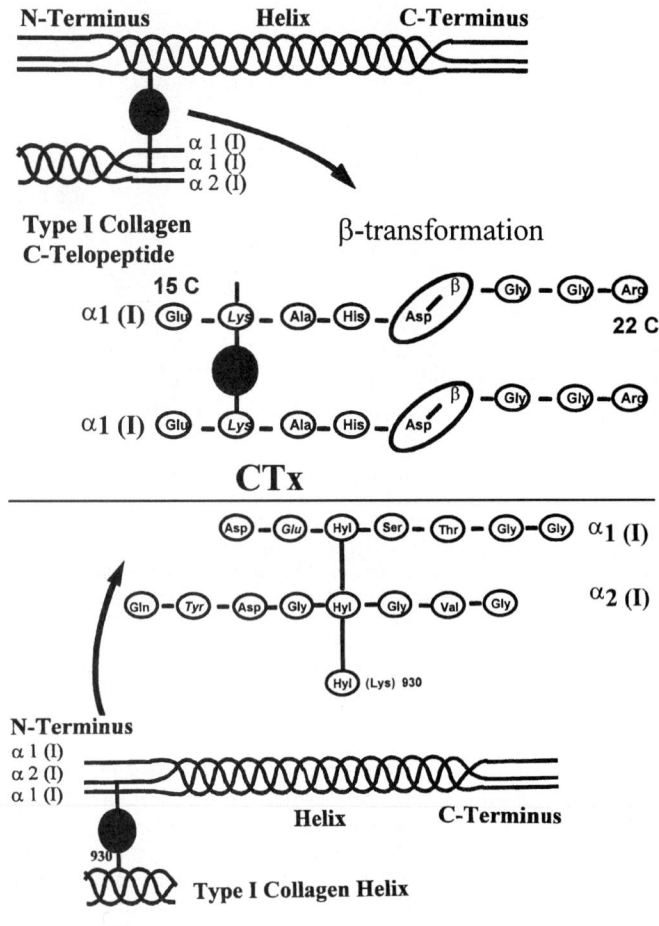

**FIGURE 56-6.** Structure and proposed epitopes of the carboxy-terminal (*CTx; upper panel*) and amino-terminal (NTx; *lower panel*) cross-linked telopeptides of type I collagen. The C-terminal telopeptide of type I collagen (β-CTx) excreted in urine requires only one strand of the octapeptide Glu-Lys-Ala-His-βAsp-Gly-Gly-Arg (EKAH-βD-GGR), which contains the cross-linking site of the C-terminal type I collagen telopeptide (K). The transformation of aspartyl to isoaspartyl (*βAsp*) results from protein aging. In serum, the epitope is thought to be a cross-linked β-isomerized dipeptide of the C-terminal telopeptide region (*oval insert*). The N-terminal telopeptide of type I collagen (*NTx*) excreted in urine and serum requires the α-2 chain of type I collagen. The sequence is Gln-Tyr-Asp-Gly-Hyl-Gly-Val-Gly (QYDGKGVG), and is identical for both the urine- and serum-based assay.

ual patients[13,14] (Fig. 56-7). Serum ICTP is a sensitive marker of osteolytic bone destruction in multiple myeloma and appears to predict disease progression independently from immunoglobulin production.[39]

For the use of cross-link compounds and related markers in osteoporosis, see the last section of this chapter.

## HYDROXYPROLINE AND HYDROXYLYSINE GLYCOSIDES

Fibrillar collagens are rich in the amino acids *hydroxyproline (OHP)* and *hydroxylysine (OHL)*, both of which are excreted in the urine after collagen degradation and are considered to be markers of bone resorption. Urinary OHP is a rather nonspecific and insensitive index of total body collagen turnover. First, OHP is formed intracellularly as one of the earliest posttranslational modifications of the collagen molecule. The amino acid is already present in newly synthesized collagens, and ~10% of the total OHP excreted in urine is likely to be derived from the degradation of immature collagens. Second, 90% to 95% of

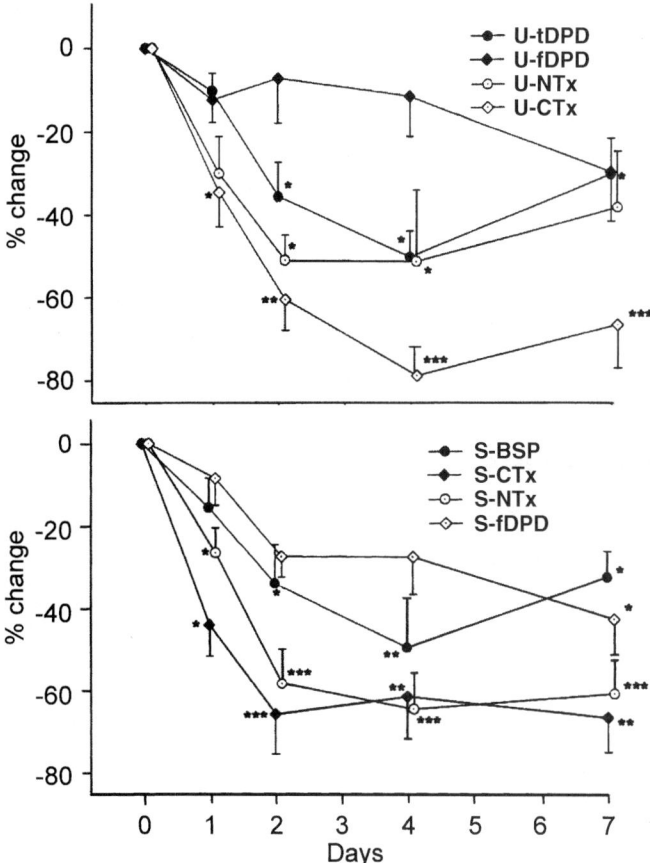

**FIGURE 56-7.** Changes in urinary (*upper panel*) and serum (*lower panel*) levels of bone resorption markers in patients with hypercalcemia of malignancy after a single dose of intravenous pamidronate. Note that the magnitude of change is similar for both urinary and serum markers. (*U-*, urinary; *S-*, serum; *tDPD*, total deoxypyridinoline; *fDPD*, free immunoreactive deoxypyridinoline; *NTx*, amino-terminal telopeptide of type I collagen; *CTx*, carboxy-terminal telopeptide of type I collagen; *BSP*, bone sialoprotein.) (From Woitge HW, Oberwittler H, Farahmand I, et al. New serum markers of bone resorption. J Bone Miner Res 1999; 14: 792.)

OHP released from various tissues is metabolized in the liver, and only a small fraction of the total circulating pool is actually excreted and measured in the urine. Third, urinary OHP levels are considerably influenced by dietary protein intake (especially meat) and by the metabolism of other collagenous proteins such as elastin and the complement component C1q (see Fig. 56-5). The amino acid is present in all fibrillar collagens and therefore in other soft tissues, especially in the skin[40] (see Table 56-2).

The urinary excretion of OHP is increased in states of physiologically high turnover, such as somatic growth and during early menopause, and in high-turnover osteopathies, such as Paget disease of bone, osteomalacia, renal osteodystrophy, hyperthyroidism, multiple myeloma, and metastatic bone disease. Because of its low sensitivity and specificity, urinary OHP is often normal in cases of asymptomatic or mild hyperparathyroidism and in patients with postmenopausal osteoporosis.

OHL may be present in two glycosylated forms: β-1-galactosyl-OHL and β-1,2-glucosyl-galactosyl-OHL. The type and concentration of OHL-glycoside vary among tissues, but the β-1-galactosyl-OHL appears to be a specific component of bone collagen. Unlike OHP, the lysine glycosides are not metabolized and may be more sensitive markers of collagen metabolism than OHP. The urinary levels of glycosylated OHL are not influenced by diet. The use of glycosylated OHL was long ham-

pered by the lack of appropriate methods. With the development of an HPLC technique, this marker is now applicable to clinical studies.[41] Data suggest that the determination of urinary OHL glycosides may be a helpful index of bone metabolism in women with postmenopausal osteoporosis and in growth-deficient children.[42,43]

### TARTRATE-RESISTANT ACID PHOSPHATASE

Human acid phosphatases form a heterogeneous group of at least five electrophoretically different isoenzymes that are found in prostate, various bloods cells, and osteoclasts. All acid phosphatases are inhibited by (+)-tartrate, except for the band 5 isoenzymes, of which the subtype 5b appears to be found in and secreted by osteoclasts. Serum or plasma *tartrate-resistant acid phosphatase (TRAP)* activity has been suggested as a marker of osteoclast activity in bone resorption. Circulating levels of TRAP may be determined by electrophoretic, spectrophotometric, and immunoassay procedures.[44] Although most assays are easily performed, the pronounced thermal instability of the enzyme has so far precluded use of this marker in routine clinical application. Artificially high values are often seen in hemolytic samples, due to the release of erythrocytic TRAP (see Table 56-6). Serum TRAP activity is elevated in healthy children, during somatic growth, and in a variety of metabolic bone diseases associated with increased bone resorption, such as Paget disease of bone, hyperparathyroidism, multiple myeloma, and metastatic bone disease.[45,46] Serum TRAP activity may be elevated in postmenopausal healthy and osteoporotic women, in whom TRAP activity is inversely correlated with bone mineral density.[47] In patients on long-term maintenance hemodialysis, serum TRAP levels have been shown to reflect osteoclast activity.

### BONE SIALOPROTEIN

*Bone sialoprotein (BSP)*, a major synthetic product of active osteoblasts and odontoblasts, accounts for ≤10% of the noncollagenous matrix of bone. The expression of BSP is restricted to mineralized tissue (e.g., bone and dentin), and to the interface of calcifying cartilage. The intact molecule contains an Arg-Gly-Asp (RGD) integrin-recognition sequence, and plays an important role in the supramolecular organization of the extracellular matrix of mineralized tissues.

Immunoassays have been developed for the determination of immunoreactive BSP in serum.[48,49] Elevated levels of serum BSP were found in children and adolescents as well as in patients with high turnover osteopathies such as Paget disease of bone, primary hyperparathyroidism, active rheumatoid arthritis, metastatic bone disease, and multiple myeloma.[50,50a] In patients with the latter, high baseline serum BSP levels appear to predict poor survival. Furthermore, in patients with newly diagnosed primary breast cancer, baseline levels of serum BSP above 24 ng/mL are associated with a high risk of early bone metastases.[51]

Based on clinical data and the rapid reduction of serum BSP levels after intravenous bisphosphonate treatment (see Fig. 56-7), serum BSP levels are currently considered to reflect processes related to bone resorption or osteoclast activity.

## USE OF BIOCHEMICAL MARKERS OF BONE TURNOVER IN OSTEOPOROSIS

Since the previous edition of this textbook, major advances have been made with regard to the application of biomarkers of bone turnover in osteoporosis. In particular, a number of studies have shown that bone turnover, as assessed by markers of bone formation or of bone resorption, are predictive of future bone loss and fracture risk. Thus, individuals with high rates of bone turnover have been shown to lose bone at a much faster rate than subjects with normal or low bone turnover[52,53] (Fig. 56-8). Furthermore, vertebral fracture rates seem to increase as a direct

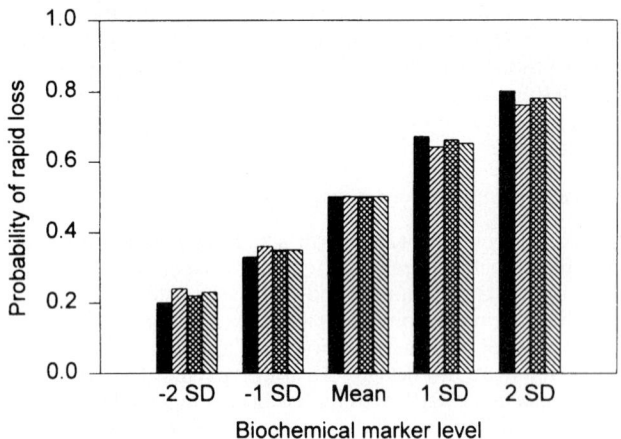

**FIGURE 56-8.** Probability of rapid bone loss as a function of biochemical marker levels as determined in a retrospective study over 14 years. The odds of rapid bone loss increased by 1.8 to 2.0 times for each 1.0 standard deviation (*SD*) increase of the marker. For example, for serum bone-specific alkaline phosphatase (*BAP*) (*filled bars*), the probability of rapid bone loss was 80% when the marker level was 2 SD above the group mean, but only 20% when the level was 2 SD below the mean (*n* = 200). Note that all markers yielded similar results. (2nd bar from left, osteocalcin [OC]; 3rd bar from left, pyridinoline [PYD]; 4th bar from left, deoxypyridinoline [DPD].) (From Ross PD, Knowlton W. Rapid bone loss is associated with increased levels of biochemical markers. J Bone Miner Res 1998; 13:297.)

function of either increased bone turnover or decreased vertebral bone mineral density (BMD).[54] A prospective, population-based study of elderly women (older than 75 years) demonstrated that an increase in the urinary excretion of total or free DPD was associated with an increased risk of hip fracture.[55] Later analyses of data from the same study revealed that *low* serum intact OC levels were also associated with an increased risk of hip fracture. Similar results have been reported for the urinary telopeptide markers (β-CTx).[56] Importantly, not only were the relative risks similar (as defined by either BMD or marker measurements), but also the combined measurement of hip bone density and of bone markers predicted future hip fractures better than the determination of either bone density or markers alone. This means that in older postmenopausal women, the statistical risk of future hip fracture is highest in subjects with a combination of low bone mass *and* high rates of bone turnover.

In contrast, markers of bone turnover are less useful in the primary diagnosis of vertebral osteoporosis. Usually, a broad overlap in marker levels is seen between osteoporotic and healthy populations, and most markers have insufficient diagnostic power to distinguish between vertebral osteopenia and osteoporosis.[36] Markers of bone turnover are, therefore, *not* useful in the *diagnosis* of osteoporosis.

An emerging application of biochemical bone markers is their use in therapeutic decision making. This is based on the observation that osteoporotic patients with high bone turnover benefit more from antiresorptive treatment than do patients with low bone turnover.[52,57,58] Depending on the baseline rate of bone turnover, both an increase in vertebral BMD and a decrease in bone turnover are equally effective in reducing vertebral fractures in osteoporotic women.[54] These results may provide a rationale for the use of bone markers in the selection of therapy and in the prediction of therapeutic response. So far, however, this relationship has been shown only for estrogen or calcitonin treatments, not for treatment with other antiresorptives such as the bisphosphonates or vitamin D.

The clinically most relevant application of bone biomarkers is their use in the *monitoring of ongoing therapy.* Although the efficacy of therapy is assessed primarily by a reduction in incidence of fracture, and secondarily by an increase in bone density, these effects usually occur slowly and within several years

of treatment. In contrast, some markers of bone metabolism change as early as 72 hours after intravenous bisphosphonate therapy. Most other interventions result in significant changes within 6 weeks of implementation[50,59–61] (see Fig. 56-7). One should bear in mind, however, that most biochemical markers are characterized by a high degree of variability, and that, depending on the type of marker used, posttherapeutic changes of 30% to 60% are required to reach significance.[62]

Newer studies indicate that the magnitude of the change in bone marker levels at 3, 4, or 6 months of treatment with hormone-replacement therapy or bisphosphonates correlates with the increase in BMD after 12 or 24 months of treatment.[52] Serial measurements of bone markers soon after implementation of therapy may therefore be helpful in deciding whether a patient has responded to a specific treatment regimen.

# REFERENCES

1. Harri, H. The human alkaline phosphatases: what we know and what we don't know. Clin Chim Acta 1989; 186:133.
2. Woitge HW, Seibel MJ, Ziegler R. Comparison of total and bone specific alkaline phosphatase in skeletal and non-skeletal diseases. Clin Chem 1996; 42:1796.
3. Silverberg SJ, Shane E, DeLaCruz L, et al. Skeletal disease in primary hyperparathyroidism. J Bone Miner Res 1989; 4:283.
4. Lian JB, Gundberg CM. Osteocalcin. Biochemical considerations and clinical applications. Clin Orthop Rel Res 1988; 226:267.
4a. Kakonen SM, Hellman J, Karp M, et al. Development and evaluation of three immunofluorometric assays that measure different forms of osteocalcin in serum. Clin Chem 2000; 46:332.
5. Power MJ, Fottrell PF. Osteocalcin: diagnostic methods and clinical applications. Crit Rev Clin Lab Sci 1991; 28:287.
6. Ducy P, Desbois C, Boycem B, et al. Increased bone formation in osteocalcin-deficient mice. Nature 1996; 382:448.
7. Malluche HH, Faugere MC, Fant P, Price PA. Plasma levels of bone Gla-protein reflect bone formation in patients on chronic maintenance dialysis. Kidney Int 1984; 26:869.
8. Charles P, Mosekilde L, Jensen FT. Primary hyperparathyroidism: evaluated by 47 calcium kinetics, calcium balance, and serum bone–Gla-protein. Eur J Clin Invest 1986; 16:277.
9. Epstein S, Poser J, McClintock R, et al. Differences in serum bone Gla protein with age and sex. Lancet 1984; 1:307.
10. Chen JT, Hosoda K, Hasumi K, et al. Serum N-terminal osteocalcin is a good indicator for estimating responders to hormone replacement therapy in postmenopausal women. J Bone Miner Res 1996; 11:1784.
11. Vergnaud P, Garnero P, Meunier P, et al. Undercarboxylated osteocalcin measured with a specific immunoassay predicts hip fracture in elderly women. The EPIDOS study. J Clin Endocrinol Metab 1998; 82:719.
12. Demiaux B, Arlot ME, Chapuy MC, et al. Serum osteocalcin is increased in patients with osteomalacia: correlations with biochemical and histomorphometric findings. J Clin Endocrinol Metab 1992; 74:1146.
13. Pecherstorfer M, Zimmer-Roth I, Schilling T, et al. The diagnostic value of urinary pyridinium cross-links of collagen, serum total alkaline phosphatase, and urinary calcium excretion in neoplastic bone disease. J Clin Endocrinol Metab 1995; 80:97.
14. Pecherstorfer M, Seibel MJ, Woitge H, et al. Urinary pyridinium crosslinks in multiple myeloma, MGUS and osteoporosis. Blood 1997; 90:3743.
15. Parfitt AM, Simon LS, Villanueva AR, Krane SM. Procollagen type I carboxyterminal extension propeptide in serum as a marker of collagen biosynthesis in bone. J Bone Miner Res 1987; 5:427.
16. Eriksen EF, Charles P, Meisen F, et al. Serum markers of type 1 collagen formation and degradation in metabolic bone disease: correlation with bone histomorphometry. J Bone Miner Res 1993; 8:127.
17. Melkko J, Niemi S, Risteli L, Risteli J. Radioimmunoassay of the carboxyterminal propeptide of human type I procollagen. Clin Chem 1990; 36:1328.
18. Pedersen BJ, Bonde M. Purification of human procollagen type I carboxylterminal propeptide cleaved as in vivo from procollagen and used to calibrate a radioimmunoassay of the propeptide. Clin Chem 1994; 40:811.
19. Trivedi P, Risteli J, Risteli L, et al. Serum concentrations of the type I and III procollagen propeptides as biochemical markers of growth velocity in healthy infants and children with growth disorders. Pediatr Res 1991; 30:276.
20. Seibel MJ, Baylink F, Farley H, et al. Basic science and clinical application of bone biomarkers. Exp Clin Endocrinol Diabetes 1997; 105:125.
21. Robins SP, Duncan A. Pyridinium crosslinks of bone collagen and their location in peptides isolated from rat femur. Biochim Biophys Acta 1987; 914:233.
22. Eyre D, Dickson IR, Van Ness K. Collagen crosslinking in human bone and articular cartilage. Biochem J 1988; 252:495.
23. Black D, Duncan A, Robins SP. Quantitative analysis of the pyridinium crosslinks of collagen in urine using ion-paired reverse-phase high-performance liquid chromatography. Anal Biochem 1988; 169:197.
24. Pratt DA, Daniloff Y, Duncan A, Robins SP. Automated analysis of the pyridinium crosslinks of collagen in tissue and urine using solid-phase extrac-

tion and reversed-phase high-performance liquid chromatography. Ann Biochem 1992; 207:168.

25. Seyedin S, Kung VT, Daniloff YN, et al. Immunoassay for urinary pyridino-line: the new marker of bone resorption. J Bone Miner Res 1993; 8:635.

26. Seibel MJ, Woitge HW, Scheidt-Nave C, et al. Urinary hydroxypyridinium crosslinks of collagen in population-based screening for overt vertebral osteoporosis: results of a pilot study. J Bone Miner Res 1994; 9:1433.

27. Robins SP, Woitge H, Hesley R, et al. A direct enzyme-linked immunoassay for urinary deoxypyridinoline as a specific marker for measuring bone resorption. J Bone Miner Res 1994; 9:1643.

28. Hansen DA, Weis MA, Bollen AM, et al. A specific immunoassay for moni-toring human bone resorption: quantitation of type I collagen cross-linked N-telopeptides in urine. J Bone Miner Res 1992; 7:1251.

29. Risteli J, Elomaa I, Niemi S, Novamo A, Risteli L. Radioimmunoassay for the pyridinoline crosslinked carboxyterminal telopeptide of type I collagen: a new serum marker of bone collagen degradation. Clin Chem 1993; 39:655.

30. Bonde MQP, Fledelius C, Riis BJ, Christiansen C. Immunoassay for quantify-ing type I degradation products in urine evaluated. Clin Chem 1994; 40:2022.

31. Fledelius C, Johnsen AH, Cloos PAC, et al. Characterization of urinary deg-radation products derived from type I collagen. Identification of a beta-isomerized Asp-Gly sequence within the C-terminal telopeptide (alpha1) region. J Biol Chem 1997; 272:9755.

32. Bonde M, Fledelius C, Qvist P, Christiansen C. Coated-tube radioimmu-noassay for C-telopeptides of type I collagen to assess bone resorption. Clin Chem 1996; 42:1639.

33. Bonde M, Garnero P, Fledelius C, et al. Measurement of bone degradation products in serum using antibodies reactive with an isomerized form of an 8 amino acid sequence of the C-telopeptide of type I collagen. J Bone Miner Res 1997; 12:1028.

34. Woitge HW, Oberwittler H, Farahmand I, et al. New serum markers of bone resorption. J Bone Miner Res 1999; 14:792.

35. Seibel MJ, Duncan A, Robins SP. Urinary pyridinium crosslinks of collagen provide indices of cartilage and bone involvement in arthritic diseases. J Rheumatol 1989; 16:970.

36. Seibel MJ, Cosman V, Shen V, et al. Urinary hydroxypyridinium crosslinks of collagen as markers of bone resorption and estrogen efficacy in post-menopausal osteoporosis. J Bone Miner Res 1993; 8:881.

37. Robins SP, Black D, Paterson RD, et al. Evaluation of urinary hydroxypyri-dinium crosslink measurement as resorption markers in metabolic bone disease. Eur J Clin Invest 1991; 21:310.

38. Seibel MJ, Gartenberg F, Silverberg S, et al. Urinary hydroxypyridinium crosslinks of collagen in primary hyperparathyroidism. J Clin Endocrinol Metab 1992; 74:481.

38a. Demers LM, Costa L, Lipton A. Biochemical markers and skeletal metastases. Cancer 2000; 88(2 Suppl):2919.

39. Elomaa I, Virkkunen P, Risteli L, Risteli J. Serum concentrations of the crosslinked carboxyterminal telopeptide of type I collagen (ICTP) is a use-ful prognostic indicator in multiple myeloma. Br J Cancer 1992; 66:337.

40. Kivirikko KI. Urinary excretion of hydroxyproline in health and disease. Int Rev Connect Tissue Res 1970; 5:93.

41. Moro L, Modricky C, Stagni N, et al. High performance liquid chromato-graphic analysis of urinary hydroxylysine glycosides as indicators of col-lagen turnover. Analyst 1984; 109:1621.

42. Moro L, Mucelli RS, Gazzarrini C, et al. Urinary β-1-galactosyl-O-hydroxylysine (GH) as a marker of collagen turnover in bone. Calcif Tissue Int 1988; 42:87.

43. Rauch F, Schonau E, Woitge E, et al. Urinary excretion of hydroxypyridin-ium cross-links of collagen reflects skeletal growth velocity in normal chil-dren. Exp Clin Endocrinol 1994; 102:104.

44. Lau KH, Onishi T, Wergedal JE, et al. Characterization and assay of tar-trate-resistant acid phosphatase activity in serum: potential use to assess bone resorption. Clin Chem 1987; 33:458.

45. Stepan JJ, Silinkova E, Havranek T, et al. Relationship of plasma tartrate-resistant acid phosphatase to the bone isoenzyme of serum alkaline phos-phatase in hyperparathyroidism. Clin Chim Acta 1983; 133:189.

46. Colson F, Berny C, Tebib J, et al. Assessment of bone resorption by measuring tartrate-resistant acid phosphatase (TAcP) activity in serum. In: Christiansen C, Overgaard K, eds. Osteoporosis. Copenhagen: Osteopress, 1990:621.

47. De la Piedra C, Torres R, Rapado A, et al. Serum tartrate-resistant acid phosphatase and bone mineral content in postmenopausal osteoporosis. Calcif Tissue Int 1989; 45:58.

48. Saxne T, Zunino L, Heinegard D. Increased release of bone sialoprotein into synovial fluid reflects tissue destruction in rheumatoid arthritis. Arthritis Rheum 1995; 38:82.

49. Karmatschek M, Woitge HW, Armbruster FP, et al. Improved purification of human bone sialoprotein and development of a homologous radioim-munoassay. Clin Chem 1997; 43:2076.

50. Seibel MJ, Woitge HW, Pecherstorfer M, et al. Serum immunoreactive bone sialoprotein as a new marker of bone turnover in metabolic and malignant bone disease. J Clin Endocrinol Metab 1996; 81:3289.

50a. Ogata Y, Nakao S, Kim RH, et al. Parathyroid hormone regulation of bone sialoprotein (BSP) gene transcription is mediated through a pituitary-specific transcription factor-1 (Pit-1) motif in the rat BSP gene promoter. Matrix Biol 2000; 19:395.

51. Diel IJ, Solomayer EF, Siebel MJ, et al. Serum bone sialoprotein in patients with primary breast cancer is a prognostic marker for subsequent bone metastases. Clin Cancer Res 1999; 5:3914.

52. Chesnut CH III, Bell NH, Clark GS, et al. Hormone replacement therapy in postmenopausal woman: urinary N-telopeptide of type I collagen moni-tors therapeutic effect and predicts response of bone mineral density. Am J Med 1997; 102:29.

53. Ross PD, Knowlton W. Rapid bone loss is associated with increased levels of biochemical markers. J Bone Miner Res 1998; 13:297.

54. Riggs BL, Melton LJ III, O'Fallon WM. Drug therapy for vertebral fractures in osteoporosis: evidence that decreases in bone turnover and increases in bone mass both determine antifracture efficacy. Bone 1996; 18:197S.

55. Van Daele PL, Seibel MJ, Burger H, et al. Case control analysis of bone resorption markers, disability and hip fracture risk: the Rotterdam study. BMJ 1996; 312:482.

56. Garnero P, Hausherr E, Chapuy MC, et al. Markers of bone resorption pre-dict hip fractures in elderly women. The EPIDOS study. J Bone Mineral Res 1996; 11(10):1531.

57. Civitelli R, Gonnelli S, Zacchei F, et al. Bone turnover in postmenopausal osteoporosis. J Clin Invest 1988; 82:1268.

58. Nielsen NM, Von der Recke P, Hansen MA, et al. Estimation of the effect of salmon calcitonin in established osteoporosis by biochemical bone mark-ers. Calcif Tissue Int 1994; 55:8.

59. Kraenzlin ME, Seibel MJ, Trechsel U, et al. The effect of intranasal salmon calcitonin on postmenopausal bone turnover: evidence for maximal effect after 8 weeks of continuous treatment. Calcif Tissue Int 1996; 58:216.

60. Raisz LG, Wiita B, Artis A, et al. Comparison of the effects of estrogen alone and estrogen plus androgen on biochemical markers of bone formation and resorption in postmenopausal women. J Clin Endocrinol Metab 1996; 81:37.

61. Heikkinen AM, Parvianen M, Niskanen L, et al. Biochemical bone markers and bone mineral density during postmenopausal hormone replacement therapy with and without vitamin $D_3$: a prospective, controlled, random-ized study. J Clin Endocrinol Metab 1997; 82:2476.

62. Hannon R, Blumsohn A, Naylor K, Eastell R. Response of biochemical markers of bone turnover to hormone replacement therapy: impact of bio-logical variability. J Bone Miner Res 1998; 13:1124.

# CHAPTER 57

# CLINICAL APPLICATION OF BONE MINERAL DENSITY MEASUREMENTS

PAUL D. MILLER, ABBY ERICKSON, AND CAROL ZAPALOWSKI

Bone densitometry is accepted as a useful quantitative measure-ment for assessing skeletal status and predicting the risk of fragil-ity fractures.[1] Low bone mineral density (BMD) is the most important risk factor for fracture. BMD testing is an objective mea-surement, and extensive data demonstrate that bone mass and future fracture risk are inversely correlated. Low bone mass pre-dicts fracture in the same way that high cholesterol and high blood pressure predict myocardial infarction and stroke, respectively.[2]

Historical risk factors cannot identify individual patients with low bone mass with adequate certainty.[3] This does not discount the importance of assessing risk factors other than BMD for frac-ture. These risk factors add valuable information required for individual patient management decisions. Also, some risk fac-tors can be modified to help reduce fracture risk.[4] This is particu-larly true in the perimenopausal population and in patients with secondary conditions associated with bone loss.

Measurement techniques for quantitating BMD that use radio-isotopes as their photon energy source have been replaced by tech-niques that use dual-energy x-ray sources.

Another technique, currently under evaluation, is quantitative ultrasound.[4a] *Dual-energy x-ray absorptiometry (DXA)* can be per-formed at several skeletal sites (e.g., hip, spine, finger, wrist, or heel) and does not require a water bath for the equalization of the soft tissue surrounding bone. DXA uses a dual-energy x-ray sys-tem to separate bone from soft tissue.

The radiologic and technical aspects for quantitating bone mass and the principles of bone mass measurement physics are

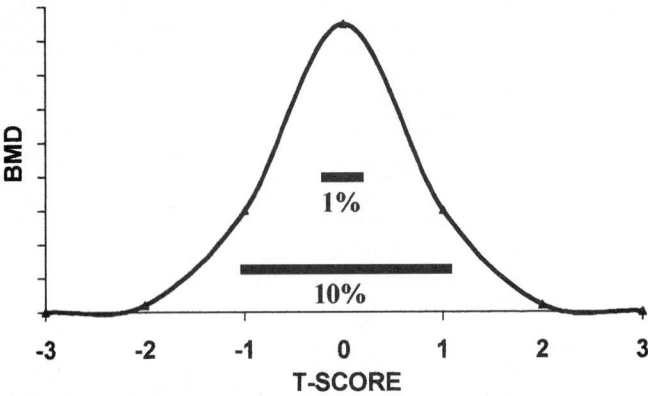

**FIGURE 57-1.** The effect of accuracy error on the distribution of T score. A 1% accuracy error has little effect on diagnosis, whereas a 10% accuracy error can change the T score in an individual patient from +1 to –1 SD. (*BMD,* bone minderal density.)

well documented.[5,6] Two technical terms, *accuracy* and *precision,* are important for the understanding of bone mass measurements.

Accuracy relates to the ability of a bone mass measurement device to measure the actual amount of bone tissue per unit volume present. It is determined using in situ and/or cadaveric bone samples that are measured—using the device being tested—in grams per centimeter (g/cm), with comparison of these values to the ashed-weight in grams per centimeter of the identical area of bone. Accuracy studies have been performed on most technical methods, and the accuracy ranges from 90% to 99%. Therefore, the accuracy error is 1% to 10%. The lower the accuracy error, the greater the accuracy of the measurement. The greater the accuracy of the device, the closer the measurement is to the actual bone mineral content per unit volume of the bone. Accuracy errors of 1% have very little effect on patient diagnosis if the number of standard deviations from a young normal mean is used for diagnostic criteria. Accuracy errors of 10%, on the other hand, may profoundly affect patient diagnosis (Fig. 57-1). Fortunately, the accuracy errors of the central DXA machines are ~6% and those of peripheral devices are ~3%. Accuracy errors are generally lower in peripheral devices because of decreased soft tissue at peripheral sites.

Precision, or reproducibility, pertains to the measurement error introduced by repetitive or serial tests. The precision error of the BMD testing devices is very low (1% to 2%). The lower the precision error, the better the precision of a device. The more precise the device, the shorter period of time required for a significant change in BMD to be detected. The metabolic bone community suggests that a serial measurement fall within the 95% confidence interval to be significant, and, therefore, represents a BMD change rather than a change caused by simply measurement error. Hence, for a serial BMD change to be significant, it must be at least 2.8 times the precision error of the bone mass measurement technique. Each densitometry facility should perform *daily quality control* (in vitro) using a phantom as well as an in vivo precision study for each skeletal site in normal subjects and in subjects with low bone mass to determine the precision error of their individual machine and technologist.

## DIAGNOSIS OF OSTEOPOROSIS USING BONE DENSITOMETRY: THE WORLD HEALTH ORGANIZATION CRITERIA

To allow bone densitometry to be used for the identification of asymptomatic individuals at risk for fracture, a paradigm shift in the definition of osteoporosis had to occur. The accepted def-

inition of osteoporosis is "a systemic skeletal disease characterized by low bone mass and microarchitectural deterioration of bone tissue, with a consequent increase in bone fragility and susceptibility to fracture risk"[7] (see Chap. 64). Although this accepted definition includes the terms low BMD, systemic disease, microarchitectural deterioration, and increased bone fragility, only BMD can presently be *objectively* measured in clinical practice. Before this consensus statement defined osteoporosis, a diagnosis was made on the basis of the presence of a fragility fracture, which usually occurs only in the advanced osteoporotic state. Recently, osteoporosis has been defined on the basis of a reduced level of BMD. This new definition was implemented by the World Health Organization (WHO) Consensus Development Conference on Osteoporosis.[2] The goal of the WHO Working Group was to establish a relationship between bone mineral content (BMC) per centimeter measured, at that time, predominantly at the radius and hip, and the prevalence of fractures in elderly postmenopausal white women. It was determined that those women in the lowest quintile of BMD had the greatest prevalence of global fractures. The lowest BMD quintile, when corrected for different instrument calibrations, corresponded to 2.5 standard deviations (SD) below the mean of the reference population. Therefore, the new definition of *osteoporosis* became a *bone mass that is at least 2.5 SD below the mean of a young normal reference population.* One major clinical justification for changing the diagnostic criteria for osteoporosis from one of prevalent fragility fractures to one of low BMD are data that established a higher risk for a second fracture once a first fracture has occurred.[8] In addition, the combination of low bone mass and a vertebral fracture increased the risk of a hip fracture. This risk is far greater than the risk of a first fracture in elderly individuals who have low bone mass alone.[8] The logical corollary of these data is the need to identify individuals with low bone mass *before* the first fracture.

The WHO criteria for the diagnosis of osteopenia and osteoporosis (Table 57-1) are based on a patient's comparison to *peak adult bone mass (PABM)* and use standardized scores (T score). The WHO Working Group chose to categorize individuals using the number of SD a patient's bone mass is below the mean bone mass of a young normal reference population. Because fracture risk is a gradient, increasing with declining levels of bone mass,[9] the WHO created a second diagnostic category of *osteopenia* (low bone mass, T score >–2.5 but <–1.0 SD) to alert the clinician that individuals with smaller reductions in bone mass merit attention, particularly if they are postmenopausal or have secondary conditions associated with bone loss. Data suggest that postmenopausal women who are not receiving hormone-replacement therapy (HRT) will predictably lose bone.[10,11] As the emphasis on skeletal health shifts from treatment to prevention, the diagnostic category of osteopenia may become increasingly important. Postmenopausal women not receiving therapy to prevent bone loss may unknowingly continue to lose bone, thereby progressively increasing their fracture risk as they age. Hence, postmenopausal women identified as osteopenic may be targeted for prevention strategies to preserve their skeletal mass. Individuals with osteopenia may also experience fragility fractures, particularly when risk factors for fracture are present.[12] Such factors include increased rates of bone turnover, advancing age, increased likelihood of falling, etc. It, therefore, is not surprising that some patients with small

**TABLE 57-1.**

**World Health Organization Criteria for the Diagnosis of Osteopenia and Osteoporosis**

| |
|---|
| Osteopenia = T score <–1.0 and >–2.5 |
| Osteoporosis = T score <–2.5 |

**TABLE 57-2.**
**World Health Organization Criteria for the Diagnosis
of Osteopenia/Osteoporosis: Pros and Cons**

**TABLE 57-2.**
**World Health Organization Criteria for the Diagnosis
of Osteopenia/Osteoporosis: Pros and Cons**

**PRO**

Provides a simple objective diagnostic number for use by practitioners.

Recognizes that osteoporosis should be diagnosed before the first fragility fracture.

**CON**

Limited data relating World Health Organization criteria to fracture risk in nonwhite races or in men.

Dependent on peak adult bone mass reference databases.

Not all low bone mass is osteoporosis.

Fracture risk is a gradient, not a threshold, and –2.5 SD may be used as a threshold cutoff.

Application to healthy premenopausal, estrogen-replete women and young men is inappropriate.

reductions in BMD and the presence of other risk factors may have fragility fractures. For this reason, the National Osteoporosis Foundation (NOF) clinical guidelines recommend treating all postmenopausal women with T scores <–2.0 SD without risk factors and <–1.5 SD with one or more risk factors.[13]

Like all diagnostic criteria, there are strengths and limitations to the WHO criteria for the diagnosis of osteoporosis. These are listed in Table 57-2. The WHO criteria provide a practitioner with objective values to be used for the diagnosis of low bone mass, akin to blood pressure for the diagnosis of hypertension. Practitioners have objective criteria that initiate the cognitive process of assessment of low bone mass, leading to intervention. In addition, the WHO criteria stress the importance of making a diagnosis of low bone mass (osteopenia) or osteoporosis *before* the first fracture occurs.

The limitations presented in Table 57-2 appear to outnumber the strengths. However, this belies the beneficial impact the WHO criteria have had on the prevention and management of osteoporosis. The WHO criteria have facilitated the widespread measurement of bone mass for the identification of individuals at risk for fracture.

One of the limitations of the WHO criteria is its restricted data for its application to nonwhite women. The WHO criteria are based on BMD and prevalence of low bone mass and fracture prevalence in *postmenopausal white women*. Similar data in men and women of other racial groups are *not* well established. However, some studies have shown that fracture rates in white men per standard deviation (SD) reduction in BMD may parallel that seen in white women[14–16]; however, one study suggests that this relationship may not be the same for men.[17] Nonetheless, it may be reasonable to use the WHO criteria to approximate fracture rates in elderly white men as well. As prospective fracture data are obtained for other races, the applicability of the WHO criteria can be judged more accurately. The WHO criteria were never intended to be applied to healthy premenopausal women of any race.

BMD data for the total hip and femoral neck have been analyzed in men and women of different races with T scores derived from a common database for the hip (NHANES III).[18] These data have helped determine the prevalence of osteoporosis at the hip in men and women of different races, using the WHO criteria.[18,19] The incorporation of the common hip reference database (NHANES III) into the central dual-energy x-ray absorptiometry (DXA) equipment produced by the three major manufacturers has eliminated the potential for machine-specific misdiagnoses of osteoporosis or osteopenia at the hip.[20] Regardless of the database issues as they relate to WHO classifications, low bone mass (g/cm) in any elderly individual is still the most important factor in the determination of fragility fracture risk.

Manufacturers' devices that measure skeletal sites other than the hip still use nonuniform young normal reference databases. This is a serious issue in the field of bone densitometry, because one of the basic principles of statistics is that each sample derived from a given population yields a different mean and potentially a different SD. The young normal mean and SD from that mean form the basis of the calculation of the T score (T score = [measured BMD in g/cm² – PABM mean in g/cm²] / PABM SD in g/cm²) or for ultrasound devices (T score = [mean young normal broadband ultrasound attenuation (BUA) or speed of sound (SOS) – measured BUA or SOS] / young normal SD of BUA or SOS). Therefore, an individual may be classified quite differently if different young normal sample populations are used to create the reference database to which the patient is being compared.[21,22]

Dissimilar T scores in the same patient, measured on different devices, is also in part a result of different accuracy errors of various technologies and differing age-dependent rates of bone loss from different skeletal sites.[23] These present clinical dilemmas, because the same patient may be classified differently by various bone mass measurement devices. The T score dissimilarities related to the young normal database could be resolved by the creation of a universal reference database for each skeletal site and technique used. In support of this proposal, data have shown that bone mass measured by various heel devices (ultrasound and DXA) and hip DXA result in similar T scores in postmenopausal women when calculated using a universal young normal reference population.[24] A universal database represents, at least in part, the long-term solution to this clinical dilemma.

A short-term solution has been suggested by a committee of the National Osteoporosis Foundation (NOF) and the International Society for Clinical Densitometry (ISCD). A "T score equivalent" for different manufacturers' devices can be calculated, based on the prevalence of low bone mass as determined by each device or risk if device-specific fracture data are available. A 50% prevalence in 60- to 69-year-old women is set by any device equal to the established 50% prevalence at the femoral neck established by NHANES III, which occurs at a T score of –1.5 SD. This 50% prevalence cutoff of –1.5 SD seems reasonable, because it captures 60% of the women who will ultimately have a hip or spine fracture; it corresponds to the NOF treatment threshold for postmenopausal women with one or more risk factors (–1.5 SD); and it equals global fracture risk prediction by all devices (RR 1.5/SD reduction).[25] Thus, the equivalent T score might be –0.8 SD for one device and –1.2 SD for another device. This short-term (T-score equivalent) solution would reduce the number of patient misclassifications resulting from the use of different devices, until a universal database is completed. The NOF/ISCD Committee is also examining the potential of calculating the T-score equivalence of different devices based on risk rather than prevalence. Both methods may be incorporated into the final T-score equivalence calculations, because prevalence approaches allow the clinician to make a diagnosis, and risk approaches assist with the prediction of the disease outcome of fragility fracture. Equating a level of risk to a level of prevalence may also be appealing.

A final solution to patient misclassification is to abandon the T score as a diagnostic or intervention tool and instead use the absolute BMD value as it relates to absolute fracture prediction for patient classification. This would require comparing a patient's BMD to instrument-specific fracture data for the calculation of fracture risk. This could also minimize discrepancies observed in individual patients measured on different equipment. Absolute fracture risk may be similar regardless of the technique used.[26]

The WHO-defined criteria for osteoporosis are made on the basis of the T score (*based on young normal bone mass*), rather than the Z score (*based on age-matched bone mass*). Although bone mass declines with advancing age,[27] it is no longer logical to assume that bone loss is inevitable. If only those individuals who lose more bone than predicted for their age are termed "diseased," then many individuals with increased risk of fracture will be

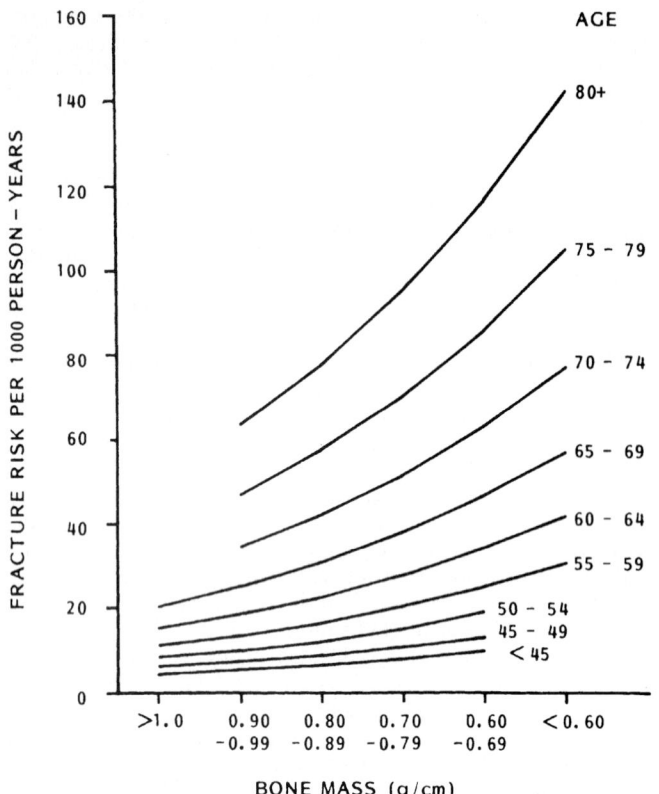

**FIGURE 57-2.** Increasing age increases fracture risk at equivalent levels of bone mass.

classified as "normal" and remain untreated. If the prevalence of osteoporosis were defined using age-matched BMD data, there would be no increase in prevalence with advancing age. This is illogical, because the number of fragility fractures increase with age and fragility fracture is the result of osteoporosis. The use of age-matched Z scores would result in the underdiagnosis of osteoporosis.[2] This would damage the credibility of bone densitometry by incorrectly describing elderly patients with fragile skeletons or possibly prevalent fragility fractures as "normal for age." Even if 70% of white women older than age 80 years are osteoporotic using the WHO criteria, this may not be an overestimate, because 50% of these women will experience a fragility fracture if untreated.[28] Use of the T score for diagnosis recognizes the true magnitude of the osteoporotic problem.

Age-matched data are appropriate, however, for comparisons in the adolescent population, before peak adult bone mass is achieved.[29] Once peak bone mass is achieved, the goal is to maintain that level of bone mass for the remainder of the patient's life. After peak adult bone mass has been achieved, age-matched Z scores that are < –2.0 SD may indicate the presence of a metabolic process causing bone loss or impeding bone acquisition in addition to aging and/or estrogen deficiency in the elderly population. Aging bone has *altered quality and microarchitectural deterioration* that cannot presently be clinically measured and may increase fracture risk in the elderly. These unmeasurable bone quality changes in the elderly explain higher fracture risks at equal BMD levels as age increases.

As mentioned previously, the WHO criteria were not meant to be applied to healthy, estrogen-replete premenopausal women. Peak adult bone mass is normally distributed. Hence, a healthy, estrogen-replete premenopausal woman with a T score of –1.8 SD may not have lost bone. Because her level falls within the normal bell-shaped curve, this T score could simply represent a low peak adult bone mass. Furthermore, *healthy premenopausal women with low peak adult bone mass may not have any greater risk of fragility fracture than age-matched women with normal bone mass.* There are scant

data in younger women that relate fracture risk to BMD, because premenopausal women rarely fracture and early postmenopausal women fracture only infrequently. Cross-sectional[29] and prospective fracture studies in premenopausal women have small numbers with wide confidence intervals.[30] Additionally, whereas there are some data to suggest that a subset of healthy, estrogen-replete premenopausal women may lose bone mass before the menopause, the majority of prospective longitudinal studies indicate that premenopausal women *do not* lose bone mass until the perimenopausal period.[31,32] Fracture risk has been shown to be much less for a 55-year-old woman than for a 75-year-old woman at equivalent levels of BMD (Fig. 57-2).[33] The inappropriate use of the WHO diagnostic criteria may cause undue fear regarding fracture risk and the inappropriate initiation of pharmacologic therapy in premenopausal women in the absence of data on efficacy and safety. The majority of longitudinal data suggest that healthy, estrogen-replete premenopausal women are not losing bone mass.[31] Healthy, estrogen-replete premenopausal women who seek advice after the discovery of low bone mass require a basic assessment to exclude secondary causes of *potential* bone loss, possibly a biomarker of bone turnover, conservative prevention advice, and a repeat bone mass measurement in 2 years to ensure that bone loss is not occurring. Most importantly, they need prompt protection of their skeleton at the menopause.[32] There are firm data that after the age of 50 years, postmenopausal women who are losing bone mass have fracture rates that are higher than those for age-matched postmenopausal women who have the same baseline BMD that, however, remains stable.[34]

## WHY ARE BONE MASS MEASUREMENTS PERFORMED?

There are three clinical applications for bone mass measurement. Each has a distinct value in clinical decision making. The three applications are

1. Diagnosis of osteopenia or osteoporosis (see Chap. 64).
2. Fracture risk prediction.
3. Serial monitoring to measure response to interventions, diseases, or medications that affect bone.

Clinicians have at their disposal various devices that measure bone mineral density. These devices are characterized as *central* or *peripheral*. Central devices measure the spine or the hip and peripheral devices measure the wrist, heel, finger, or tibia. These devices are listed in Table 57-3.

For each of the three applications of bone density measurements previously listed, the central and peripheral devices have advantages and disadvantages.[35,36]

### THE DIAGNOSIS OF OSTEOPENIA AND OSTEOPOROSIS

The diagnosis of osteopenia (T score of <–1.0 but >–2.5) is clinically important, independent of fracture-risk assessment, for

**TABLE 57-3.**
**Techniques for Bone Mass Measurement**

**CENTRAL SKELETON**
  DXA—spine (AP or lateral), or hip
  QCT—spine or hip
**PERIPHERAL SKELETON**
  QCT—wrist
  DXA—wrist, heel, finger
  Ultrasound—calcaneus, finger, tibia

*AP,* anteroposterior; *DXA,* dual energy x-ray absorptiometry; *QCT,* quantitative computerized tomography.

the initiation of early postmenopausal prevention strategies. This diagnostic category represents the range of bone density for which prevention strategies were designed. It has been shown that the recognition of low bone mass in early post-menopausal women facilitates the acceptance of hormone-replacement therapy (HRT).[37,38] This observation will most likely be the same for other preventive interventions in early postmenopausal women.

The utility of central or peripheral devices for the detection of osteopenia is dependent on the age of the patient and the particular skeletal site measured. In early menopausal patients, it is more likely that a diagnosis of osteopenia or osteoporosis will be missed if only one skeletal site is measured. In the elderly, bone mass may be more concordant at various skeletal sites. This reduces, but does not abolish, the likelihood of missing a diagnosis of osteopenia or osteoporosis if only one skeletal site is measured. The exception to the ability to use a single measurement in the elderly is the anteroposterior (AP) spine study by DXA. The AP spine measurement by DXA is frequently *falsely elevated by osteophytes and/or facet sclerosis of the posterior elements;* this may lead to underdiagnosis in this population.[39] In the elderly, all peripheral and central measurements, with the exception of the AP spine measurement by DXA, have nearly equivalent value for diagnosing osteopenia or osteoporosis.[27,40,41] There are fewer prospective fracture data for lateral spine DXA measurements. However, there is a strong correlation between lateral spine DXA BMD and spine quantitative computerized tomography (QCT) BMD, the latter of which has adequate fracture data. This suggests that *low* lateral spine DXA values should predict increased fracture risk in the elderly.[42,43]

BMD is more discordant throughout the skeleton in the early menopausal population than in the elderly (older than 65 years) population.[27,40,44] There are at least four potential explanations for this discordance:

1. Differences in development of PABM at various sites.[45]
2. Differences in rates of age-dependent bone loss between cancellous bone and cortical bone after the menopause.
3. Differences in the accuracy of measuring BMD using various techniques.
4. T scores being derived from different young normal databases.

Data suggest that in early menopausal women, if one skeletal site is osteoporotic (T score <–2.5 SD), there is a <10% chance that another skeletal site will be normal (T score >–1.0 SD).[27,46] Studies have not yet clarified how many early postmenopausal women have normal BMD at one site and osteopenia at another. These numbers may not be insignificant. Bone mass measurements can be used to "rule in" a diagnosis of low bone mass, but cannot be used to "rule out" a diagnosis (i.e., if they are normal). Hence, many early menopausal women will need additional BMD testing if a single skeletal site is normal to avoid missing an abnormal measurement at another skeletal site. This is particularly true in women with additional risk factors for low BMD or when a diagnosis of osteopenia would change the pharmacologic intervention. Patients with a normal single skeletal site BMD who may need additional testing are described in Table 57-4. These guidelines will minimize the potential for misdiagnosis.[47]

There are other patient populations in which a diagnosis of osteopenia may change intervention strategies. The prevention of bone loss associated with glucocorticoid therapy is recommended in patients with T scores <–1.0.[48] It may also be appropriate to intervene in other medical conditions associated with bone loss (i.e., hyperthyroidism [see Chap. 42], hyperparathyroidism [see Chap. 58], posttransplantation, etc.) based on a finding of osteopenia.

## THE PREDICTION OF FRACTURE RISK

It has been established that low bone mass is the most important predictor of fragility fracture. Approximately 80% of the variance in bone strength and resistance to fracture can be explained by bone mineral content per unit volume of bone in animal models.[49] Other risk factors are predictive of fracture, only some of which can be modified.[50] Risk factors such as increased height (>5 feet 7 inches), low body weight (<127 pounds), smoking, or maternal history of hip fracture are strong predictors of hip fracture. BMD is an objective, quantifiable measurement that offers clinical value akin to measuring a patient's blood pressure or cholesterol level.

The relationship between fracture risk and bone density is a gradient rather than a single threshold value. The diagnostic category of osteopenia is valuable clinically because it may facilitate the acceptance of preventive interventions in early menopausal women to reduce their lifetime fracture risk. The measurement of low bone mass may also be used to determine current fracture risk, within 5 years, in elderly women. A 1.0 SD reduction in BMD is associated with an average 1.5-fold relative risk (RR) increase in global fracture risk in postmenopausal women and elderly men. The RR is greater with the same reduction in BMD as age increases.[51] Because bone loss is an asymptomatic process, identifying small reductions in bone mass in the early menopausal patients is important to allow early intervention to halt this process. Patients may fracture with minimally reduced BMD (osteopenia), because of the effects of other factors that lead to bone fragility. The rate of bone turnover or the nature of a fall may lead to fracture with only a minimal reduction in BMD.[12,52,53]

Fracture prediction can be expressed as *current fracture risk* or *lifetime fracture risk.* Current risk is the risk of fracture within 3 to 5 years of the bone mass measurement. Current fracture risk can be expressed as RR, absolute risk or incidence, or annual risk. Relative risk, the ratio of two absolute risks, is increased 1.5 to 3 times for each 1.0 SD reduction in BMD.[8,54] All the data available in the *elderly* suggests that fracture risk is not dependent on the skeletal site measured or the technique (central or peripheral) used.[25,54,55] This observation is probably related to the concordance of bone mass measurements at different skeletal sites in the elderly population. Thus, in the elderly, low BMD measured at any skeletal site is more likely to represent increased fracture risk at other sites because of a global reduction in BMD and therefore increased fracture risk. The one exception is the prediction of hip fracture risk, which appears to be slightly better if the BMD is measured at the proximal femoral sites.[54] This observation does not, however, diminish the strong predictive value of peripheral bone mass for hip fracture.

**TABLE 57-4.**
**Patients with a Normal Single Skeletal Site Bone Mass Who May Need Additional Bone Mass Testing**

1. Postmenopausal patients concerned about osteoporosis, not receiving hormone-replacement therapy (HRT), but would accept HRT, bisphosphonates or SERMs if BMD were found to be low.
2. Patients at high risk for hip fracture, who have a maternal history of hip fracture, who are >5' 7" tall, who weigh <127 pounds, or who smoke.
3. Patients receiving medications associated with bone loss (e.g., glucocorticoids, antiseizure medications, chronic heparin, etc.).
4. Patients with secondary conditions associated with low bone mass or bone loss (e.g., hyperparathyroidism, malabsorption, hemigastrectomy, hyperthyroidism, etc.).
5. Patients found to have high urinary collagen cross-links (>1.0 SD above the upper limit for premenopausal women), where more rapid bone loss may be present.
6. Patients with a history of fragility fractures.

SERMs, selective estrogen receptor modulators; BMD, bone mineral density.
From Miller PD, Bonnick SL, Johnston CC Jr, et al. The challenges of peripheral bone density testing. J Clin Densitometry 1998; 1:1.

Data on current fracture risk have been obtained only in the elderly because younger women fracture only infrequently and bone mass technology has not existed long enough to follow a sufficient number of younger women for an adequate period of time.[8,16,19,54,56] Current fracture risk data should not be applied to younger perimenopausal women or premenopausal women with low peak adult bone mass for the age-related reasons previously stated.

After 60 years, advancing age is an independent predictor of fracture. In counseling patients, it is correct to state that the current fracture risk of a 50-year-old woman at a given level of BMD is substantially lower than the current fracture risk of a 70-year-old woman with the same BMD.[51] However, the 50-year-old woman with low BMD may have a greater lifetime fracture risk than her 50-year-old counterpart with a normal BMD[57-59] if no measures are taken to preserve skeletal mass. No direct data exist to validate these lifetime risk statistical models.[57-60] Certainly if the 50-year-old woman with low bone mass is postmenopausal, she should be counseled about preventive therapeutic options. She should be advised to continue with her usual life activities without excessive fear of fracture.

## SERIAL ASSESSMENTS OF BONE MASS

Bone densitometry is also valuable for serial monitoring of the natural progression of disease processes (such as primary hyperparathyroidism) or for monitoring the response of bone to pharmacologic interventions.[60a] There is currently a clear advantage of using the central skeleton instead of the peripheral skeleton for serial monitoring. The axial skeleton measured by DXA or QCT consistently demonstrates a greater magnitude of change over time to allow monitoring of the bone response to pharmacologic therapy.[11,61-65] The femur demonstrates smaller changes in response to pharmacologic interventions, and little or no change is observed at the wrist, finger, or heel. The reason for these discrepancies is unclear.[66] It is not the result of any limitations of the technology, because the precision of the peripheral techniques is excellent (1.0%). Several hypotheses have been suggested to explain this observation. There may be differences in the bone marrow environment of the peripheral skeleton versus the central skeleton, the surface area of the bone may be different, or differences in blood flow may exist between the cortical and cancellous bone compartments. No matter which hypothesis is correct, the bone mass of the spine and hip is more responsive to pharmacologic intervention. There are some limited data suggesting that forearm bone mass measurements may be valuable for monitoring the bone response to hormone-replacement therapy in some patients.[67] This study needs to be repeated and confirmed. The heel site is not recommended for this purpose for the reasons previously mentioned.

To summarize, the issue is not one of precision using peripheral measurements, but instead is related to the slow, small response to pharmacologic interventions seen at peripheral sites. Nevertheless, peripheral measurements have been approved by the Health Care Finance Administration (HCFA) for both diagnosis and longitudinal monitoring. Bone mass measurements using both central and peripheral technologies may be appropriate within the same year if the intent of the two measurements is different (e.g., peripheral for diagnosis and central for monitoring). Guidelines regarding which patients may not need central skeletal testing once they are diagnosed with low bone mass by a peripheral device have been published.[68] These latter guidelines are intended to preclude overuse of both technologies yet provide some assurance that a treated patient is being effectively monitored.

Biochemical markers of bone turnover can also be used to assess pharmacologic effects and help to guide management decisions. They can also be used to limit the number of patients

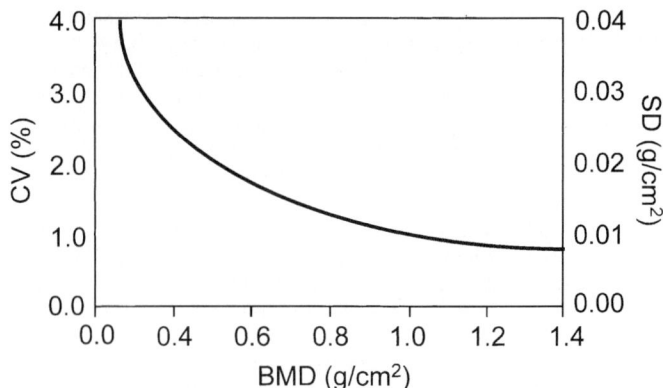

**FIGURE 57-3.** Precision error (CV%) of serial bone mass measurements deteriorates at lower level of bone mass. (*BMD*, bone mineral density.)

who receive both peripheral and central testing in the same year.[69]

In contrast to pharmacologic therapies, the forearm appears to be the best skeletal site for monitoring the effects of excess parathyroid hormone.[70] It may also be valuable in decisions regarding the timing of surgical parathyroidectomy.

No matter which BMD technique is used, serial changes can be expressed as the percentage of change (% change)(1st BMD – 2nd BMD/1st BMD × 100) or absolute change (g/cm²) between the two measurements. Either format is acceptable, providing that the precision of the device and the skeletal site is known. Individual manufacturers report precision errors of 1% to 2% at the AP spine. However, their precision error may be higher (3% to 4%) in the elderly population with low BMD values.[71] This is the result of an increased coefficient of variation (precision error) as BMD declines at each skeletal site (Fig. 57-3). In addition, different operators may introduce variability based on their training and skill during positioning or analysis. Therefore, each bone densitometry facility should calculate their individual precision error for each bone densitometry device used. Once the precision error is known, the significance of a serial BMD change can be determined. At the 95% confidence level, a significant BMD change needs to be at least 2.8 times the precision error. For example, if the precision error is 1.5%, then a 4.16% change would be necessary for significance at the 95% confidence level. In contrast, if the precision error is 3%, an 8.3% change would be necessary for significance.[6] Misleading conclusions may be drawn based on nonsignificant serial changes, with attendant inappropriate alterations in treatments, if serial measurements are interpreted incorrectly.

In contrast, absolute change has a small margin of error because the SD of absolute BMD is reasonably constant over a wide range. Any change in BMD that is > 0.04 g/cm² at the AP spine or 0.05 g/cm² at the femoral neck is significant at the 95% confidence level. Absolute change is calculated by subtracting the second BMD measurement from the baseline measurement. In most of the medical literature, serial BMD change is expressed as a percentage; however, either method is valid. BMD testing for serial monitoring is generally performed every 12 to 24 months, depending on the disease process or therapeutic intervention. In patients who have a documented response to pharmacologic intervention—which may be defined as either a gain or no loss in BMD—annual BMD measurements may not be necessary after the first year. In patients with a documented response to HRT, repeat BMD measurements every 3 to 5 years may improve the long-term compliance to therapy. Even in elderly women who have previously been documented as estrogen responders, bone mass measurements at 3- to 5-year intervals may document continued response and compliance to therapy. In this elderly population, age-related bone loss may overcome estrogen therapy causing further bone loss.[72] Thus, the NOF recommends BMD testing in women older than 65 years of age even if they have no risk factors and are receiving hormone-replacement therapy.[13] The frequency of serial monitoring may differ for non-estrogen therapy (e.g., bisphosphonates and calcitonin).

It is very difficult to compare serial changes if the measurements are performed on machines from different manufacturers. It even is sometimes difficult to compare values obtained from different machines made by the same manufacturer. It would be ideal if patients had serial measurements performed on the same machine by the same technician. However, this is unrealistic. The International Bone Densitometry Standards Committee has established a standardized BMD (sBMD), which allows for comparisons to be made between BMD values obtained from different manufacturers' equipment.[73] Using the calculated sBMD of the spine and hip for serial comparison reduces but does not eliminate the variance in measurements. As a general rule, the precision error should be increased by 1% for the calculation of percentage change if sBMD is used.

## CONCLUSIONS

Bone densitometry has revolutionized the clinical approach to osteoporosis. This technology provides a direct measurement of bone mineral density by which fracture risk can be estimated. If the results of testing are used responsibly and competently, patient care will be enhanced. The measurement of bone mineral density enables physicians and their patients to make informed decisions regarding preventive and therapeutic strategies. It also allows the physician to monitor the longitudinal efficacy of these interventions.

## REFERENCES

1. Miller PD, Bonnick SL, Rosen CJ, et al. Clinical utility of bone mass measurements in adults: consensus of an international panel. Semin Arthritis Rheum 1996; 25:361.
2. The WHO Study Group. Assessment of fracture risk and its application to screening for postmenopausal osteoporosis. Geneva: World Health Organization, 1994.
3. Hui SL, Slemenda CW, Carey MA, Johnston CC Jr. Choosing between predictors of fracture. J Bone Miner Res 1995; 10:186.
4. Cummings SR. Treatable and untreatable risk factors for hip fracture. Bone 1996; 18:165S.
4a. Peretz A, Penaloza A, Mesquita M, et al. Quantitative ultrasound and dual x-ray absorptiometry measurements of the calcaneus in patients on maintenance hemodialysis. Bone 2000; 27:287.
5. Genant HK, Engelke K, Fuerst T, et al. Noninvasive assessment of bone mineral and structure: state of the art. J Bone Miner Res 1996; 11:707.
6. Faulkner KG, von Stetten E, Miller P. Discordance in patient classification using T-scores. J Clin Densitom 1999; 2(3):343.
7. Anonymous. Consensus development conference: diagnosis, prophylaxis and treatment of osteoporosis. Am J Med 1993; 94:646.
8. Ross PD, Davis JW, Epstein RS, Wasnich RD. Pre-existing fractures and bone mass predict vertebral fracture incidence in women. Ann Intern Med 1991; 114:919.
9. Huang C, Ross PD, Wasnich RD. Short-term and long-term fracture prediction by bone mass measurements: a prospective study. J Bone Miner Res 1998; 13:107.
10. Ravn P, Overgaard K, Huang C, et al. Comparison of bone density of the phalanges, distal forearm and axial skeleton in early postmenopausal women participating in the EPIC study. Osteoporosis Int 1996; 6:308.
11. Writing Group for PEPI trial. Effects of hormone therapy on bone mineral density. JAMA 1996; 276:1389.
12. Riis BJ, Hansen MA, Jensen AM, et al. Low bone mass and fast rate of bone loss at menopause: equal risk factors for future fracture: a 15-year follow-up study. Bone 1996; 19:9.
13. Lindsay R. Risk assessment using bone mineral density determination. Osteoporosis Int 1998; 8(S1):28.
14. Lunt M, Felsenberg D, Reeve J, et al. Bone density variation and its effect on risk of vertebral deformity in men and women studied in thirteen European centers: the EVOS study. J Bone Miner Res 1997; 12:1883.
15. Mussolino ME, Looker AC, Madans JH, et al. Risk factors for hip fracture in white men: the NHANES I epidemiological follow-up study. J Bone Miner Res 1998; 13:918.
16. De Laet CEDH, Van Hout BA, Burger H, et al. Hip fracture prediction in the elderly men and women: validation in the Rotterdam study. J Bone Miner Res 1998; 13:1587.
17. Melton LJ III, Atkinson EJ, O'Connor MK, et al. Bone density and fracture risk in men. J Bone Miner Res 1998; 13:1915.
18. Looker AC, Wahner HW, Dunn WL, et al. Proximal femur bone mineral levels of US adults. Osteoporosis Int 1995; 5:389.
19. Melton LJ III. How many women have osteoporosis now? J Bone Miner Res 1995; 10:175.
20. Faulkner KG, Roberts LA, McClung MR. Discrepancies in normative data between Lunar and Hologic DXA system. Osteoporosis Int 1996; 6:432.
21. Ahmed AIH, Blake GM, Rymer JM, Fogelman I. Screening for osteopenia and osteoporosis: do the accepted normal ranges lead to overdiagnosis? Osteoporosis Int 1997; 7:432.
22. Simmons A, Simpson DE, O'Doherty MJ, et al. The effects of standardization and reference values on patient classification for spine and femur dual-energy x-ray absorptiometry. Osteoporosis Int 1997; 7:200.
23. Faulkner K, von Stetten E, Miller P. Discordance in patient classification using T-scores. J Clin Densitometry 1999; 2(3):343.
24. Greenspan SL, Bouxein ML, Melton ME, et al. Precision and discriminatory ability of calcaneal bone assessment technologies. J Bone Miner Res 1997; 12:1303.
25. Marshall D, Johnell O, Wedel H. Meta-analysis of how well measures of bone mineral density predict occurrence of osteoporotic fractures. BMJ 1996; 312:1254.
26. Grampp S, Genant HK, Mathur A, et al. Comparisons of noninvasive bone mineral measurements is assessing age-related loss, fracture discrimination, and diagnostic classification. J Bone Miner Res 1997; 12:697.
27. Arlot ME, Sornay-Rendu E, Garnero P, et al. Apparent pre- and postmenopausal bone loss evaluated by DXA at different skeletal sites in women: the OLEFY cohort. J Bone Miner Res 1997; 12:683.
28. Cummings SR, Black DM, Rubin SM. Lifetime risks of hip, Colles' or vertebral fracture and coronary heart disease among white postmenopausal women. Arch Intern Med 1989; 149:2556.
29. Goulding A, Cannan R, Williams SM, et al. Bone mineral density in girls with forearm fractures. J Bone Miner Res 1998; 13:143.
30. Duppe H, Gardsell P, Nilsson B, Johnell O. A single bone density measurement can predict fractures over 25 years. Calcif Tissue Int 1997; 60:171.
31. Riis BJ. Premenopausal bone loss: fact or artifact? Osteoporosis Int 1994; S1:S35.
32. Recker RR, Lappe JM, Davies KM, Kimmel DB. Change in bone mass immediately before menopause. J Bone Miner Res 1992; 7:857.
33. Hui SL, Slemenda CW, Johnston CC Jr. Age and bone mass as predictors of fracture in a prospective study. J Clin Invest 1988; 81:1804.
34. Melton LJ III, Khosla S, Atkinson EJ, et al. Relationship of bone turnover to bone density and fractures. J Bone Miner Res 1997; 12:1083.
35. Miller PD, McClung M. Prediction of fracture risk I: bone density. Am J Med Sci 1996; 312:257.
36. Baran DT, Faulkner KG, Genant HK, et al. Diagnosis and management of osteoporosis: guidelines for the utilization of bone densitometry. Calcif Tissue Int 1997; 61:433.
37. Rubin SM, Cummings SR. Results of bone densitometry affect women's decisions about taking measures to prevent fractures. Ann Intern Med 1992; 116:990.
38. Silverman SL, Greenwald M, Klein RA, Drinkwater BL. Effect of bone density information on decisions about hormone replacement therapy: a randomized trial. Obstet Gynecol 1997; 89:321.
39. Greenspan SL, Maitland-Ramsey L, Myers E. Classification of osteoporosis in the elderly is dependent on site-specific analysis. Calcif Tissue Int 1995; 58:409.
40. Melton LJ III, Chrischilles EA, Cooper C, et al. How many women have osteoporosis? J Bone Miner Res 1992; 7:1005.
41. Mazess RB. Advances in bone densitometry. Ital J Miner Electrolyte Metab 1997; 11:73.
42. Finkelstein JS, Cleary RL, Butler JP, et al. A comparison of lateral versus anterior-posterior spine dual energy x-ray absorptiometry for the diagnosis of osteopenia. J Clin Endocrinol Metab 1994; 78:724.
43. Ross PD, Genant HK, Davis JW, et al. Predicting vertebral fracture incidence from prevalent fractures and bone density among non-black osteoporotic women. Osteoporosis Int 1993; 3:120.
44. Pouilles JM, Tremollieres F, Ribot C. Spine and femur densitometry at the menopause: are both sites necessary in the assessment of the risk of osteoporosis? Calcif Tissue Int 1993; 52:344.
45. Bonnick SL, Nichols DL, Sanborn CF, et al. Dissimilar spine and femoral Z-scores in premenopausal women. Calcif Tissue Int 1997; 61:263.
46. Nelson DA, Molloy R, Kleerekoper M. Prevalence of osteoporosis in women referred for bone density testing: utility of multiple skeletal sites. J Clin Densitometry 1998; 1:5.
47. Miller PD, Bonnick SL, Johnston CC Jr, et al. The challenges of peripheral bone density testing. J Clin Densitometry 1998; 1:1.
48. Reid I. Glucocorticoid-induced osteoporosis: assessment and treatment. J Clin Densitometry 1998; 1:55.
49. Yang R-S, Wang S-S, Lin H-J, et al. Differential effects of bone mineral content and bone area on vertebral strength in a swine model. Calcif Tissue Int 1998; 63:86.
50. Cummings SR, Nevitt MC, Browner WS, et al. Risk factors for hip fracture in white women. N Engl J Med 1995; 332:767.

51. Hui SL, Slemenda CW, Johnston CC Jr. Age and bone mass as predictors of fracture in a prospective study. J Clin Invest 1988; 81:1804.
52. Garnero P, Hausherr E, Chapuy M-C, et al. Markers of bone resorption predict hip fracture in elderly women: the EPIDOS prospective study. J Bone Miner Res 1996; 11:1531.
53. Greenspan SL, Myers ER, Maitland LA, et al. Fall severity and bone mineral density as risk factors for hip fracture in ambulatory elderly. JAMA 1994; 271:128.
54. Cummings SR, Black DM, Nevitt MC, et al. Bone density at various sites for prediction of hip fracture. Lancet 1993; 341:72.
55. Yates AJ, Ross PD, Lydick E, Epstein RS. Radiographic absorptiometry in the diagnosis of osteoporosis. Am J Med 1995; 98(S2A):41S.
56. Hans D, Dargent-Molina P, Scott AM, et al. Ultrasonographic heel measurements to predict hip fracture in elderly women. The EPIDOS prospective study. Lancet 1996; 348:511.
57. Kanis JA. Diagnosis of osteoporosis. Osteoporosis Int 1997; 7(S3):S108.
58. Black DM, Cummings SR, Melton LJ III. Appendicular bone mineral and a woman's lifetime risk of hip fracture. J Bone Miner Res 1992; 7:639.
59. Melton LJ III, Atkinson EJ, O'Fallon WM, et al. Long-term fracture prediction by bone mineral assessed at different skeletal sites. J Bone Miner Res 1993; 8:1227.
60. Huang C, Ross PD, Wasnich RD. Short-term and long-term fracture prediction by bone mass measurements: a prospective study. J Bone Miner Res 1998; 13:107.
60a. Orwoll E, Ettinger M, Weiss S, et al. Alendronate for the treatment of osteoporosis in men. N Engl J Med 2000; 343:604.
61. Lufkin EG, Wahner HW, O'Fallon WM, et al. Treatment of postmenopausal osteoporosis with transdermal estrogen. Ann Intern Med 1992; 117:1.
62. Watts NB, Harris ST, Genant HK, et al. Intermittent cyclic etidronate treatment of postmenopausal osteoporosis. N Engl J Med 1990; 323:73.
63. Liberman UA, Weiss SR, Broll J, et al. Effect of oral alendronate on bone mineral density and the incidence of fractures in postmenopausal osteoporosis. N Engl J Med 1995; 333:1437.
64. Black DM, Cummings SR, Karpf DB, et al. Randomized trial of effect of alendronate on risk of fracture in women with existing vertebral fractures. Lancet 1996; 348:1535.
65. McClung M, Clemmesen B, Daifotis A, et al. Alendronate prevents postmenopausal bone loss in women without osteoporosis. Ann Intern Med 1998; 128:253.
66. Rosenthall L, Caminis J, Tenehouse A. Calcaneal ultrasonometry: response to treatment in comparison with dual x-ray absorptiometry measurements of the lumbar spine and femur. Calcif Tissue Int 1999; 64:200.
67. Christiansen C, Lindsay R. Estrogens, bone loss and preservation. Osteoporosis Int 1990; 1:7.
68. Miller PD, Bonnick SL, Johnston CC Jr, et al. The challenges of peripheral bone density testing. Which patients need additional central density skeletal measurement. J Clin Densitometry 1998; 1:211.
69. Greenspan SL, Parker RA, Ferguson L, et al. Early changes in biochemical markers of bone turnover predict the long-term response to alendronate therapy in representative elderly women: a randomized clinical trial. J Bone Miner Res 1998; 13:1431.
70. Silverberg SJ, Shane E, de la Cruz L, et al. Skeletal disease in primary hyperparathyroidism. J Bone Miner Res 1989; 4:283.
71. Faulkner KG, McClung MR. Quality control of DXA instruments in multicenter trials. Osteoporosis Int 1995; 5:218.
72. Cauley JA, Seeley DG, Ensrud K, et al. Estrogen replacement therapy and fracture in older women. Ann Intern Med 1995; 122:9.
73. Steiger P, for the International Committee for Standards in Bone Measurement. Letter to the editor: standardization of spine BMD measurements. J Bone Miner Res 1995; 10:1602.

# C H A P T E R   5 8

# PRIMARY HYPERPARATHYROIDISM

SHONNI J. SILVERBERG AND JOHN P. BILEZIKIAN

Primary hyperparathyroidism is caused by excessive, abnormally regulated secretion of parathyroid hormone (PTH) from the parathyroid glands. Chronic exposure of its two principal target organs, *bone* and *kidney*, to PTH causes hypercalcemia, a major hallmark of the disease. The incidence, pathophysiology, cause, clinical manifestations, diagnostic evaluation, and therapy of primary hyperparathyroidism are discussed in this chapter. Pathology and surgical therapy are covered separately in Chapters 48 and 62, respectively.

## INCIDENCE

The widespread clinical use of the multichannel screening test coincided with a dramatic increase in the incidence of primary hyperparathyroidism.[1,2] Before routine determinations of serum calcium were initiated in the early 1970s, primary hyperparathyroidism was an infrequent diagnosis; in the 1990s, it was diagnosed in as many as 1 person of every 1000 members of the general population. The dramatic four- to five-fold increase in apparent incidence that occurred within 10 years of introduction of the multichannel screening test has returned to a relatively stable rate. The incidence of the disease (i.e., recognized cases) now closely approximates the prevalence (i.e., disease detected and undetected) in the population. One study, as yet unconfirmed, suggests a declining incidence of primary hyperparathyroidism.[3]

Primary hyperparathyroidism occurs at all ages but remains distinctly unusual in children. The peak incidence of primary hyperparathyroidism is in the fifth to sixth decade of life, with a female to male ratio of 3:1.

Primary hyperparathyroidism results from a *single parathyroid adenoma* in 80% of individuals with surgically proven disease. Involvement of more than one parathyroid gland in a different pathologic process, *hyperplasia*, occurs in most of the remaining individuals. Primary hyperparathyroidism associated with four-gland parathyroid hyperplasia occurs commonly in conjunction with the syndromes of multiple endocrine neoplasia types 1 and 2A (MEN1 and MEN2A) (see Chap. 188). Rarely, patients with primary hyperparathyroidism harbor *multiple adenomas*. Even less commonly (<1%), pathologic analysis reveals *parathyroid carcinoma*. The histologic features that differentiate parathyroid adenoma, hyperplasia, and carcinoma are discussed in Chapter 48.

## PATHOPHYSIOLOGY

The functional abnormality of primary hyperparathyroidism is incompletely understood. Normally, PTH secretion is tightly regulated by the serum ionized calcium concentration; it is stimulated when the ionized calcium concentration decreases and suppressed when this concentration increases. In primary hyperparathyroidism, this sensitive regulatory control is lost, and the parathyroid glands continue to secrete PTH despite an elevated ionized calcium level. The cellular basis for altered control could be an altered setpoint, so that the parathyroid cell can be suppressed only if the ionized calcium concentration is raised to a level that is higher than normal. Alternatively, the excessive secretion of PTH could result from an increased number of parathyroid cells without a change in the setpoint for calcium. In primary hyperparathyroidism caused by adenoma, both mechanisms are likely to be operative. Conversely, in primary hyperparathyroidism with hyperplasia, the setpoint appears to be closer to normal.[4,5] The abnormal secretion of PTH probably arises from the increased number of parathyroid cells (see Chap. 49).

Evidence suggests that circulating growth factors may be related to the hyperparathyroidism associated with MEN1.[6] Although other regulators of PTH secretion, such as β-adrenergic catecholamines, histamine, and ions other than calcium, may possibly be important factors in the pathogenesis of primary hyperparathyroidism, the evidence suggests that these secretagogues are not important pathophysiologic factors in the establishment or maintenance of the hyperparathyroid state.[7]

Abnormal regulation of PTH by calcium is found in primary hyperparathyroidism, but the glands are not completely autonomous. The abnormal parathyroid gland is suppressible by some level of calcium; otherwise, all patients with the disorder would have uncontrolled hypercalcemia instead of relatively

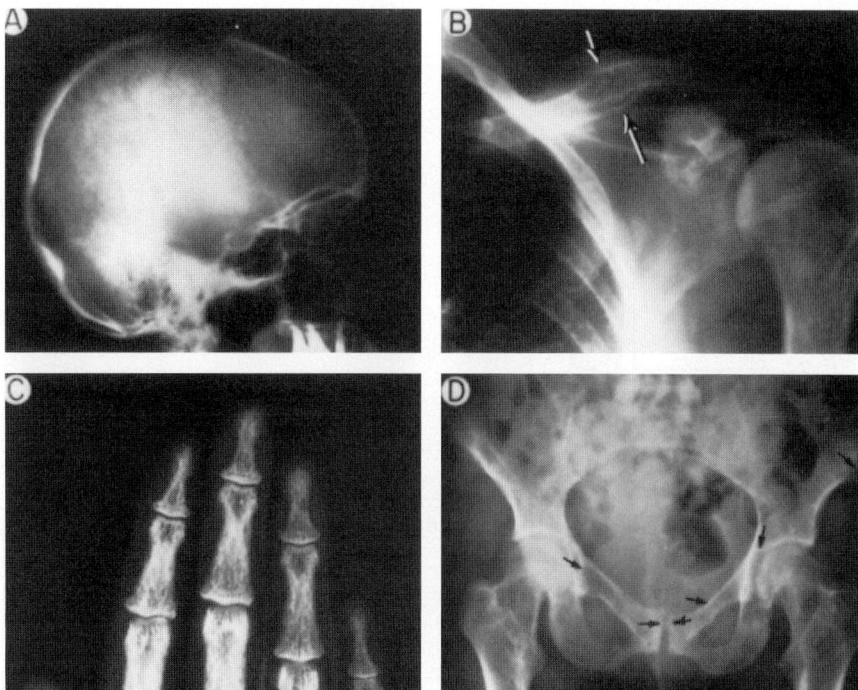

**FIGURE 58-1.** Radiographic representations of osteitis fibrosa cystica in primary hyperparathyroidism. **A,** Salt-and-pepper erosions of the skull. **B,** Cystic bone disease in the clavicle (*arrows*). **C,** Subperiosteal bone resorption of the digits. **D,** Cortical erosions (*arrows*).

stable, albeit abnormal levels. Patients with primary hyperparathyroidism who have a relatively high calcium intake (1 g daily) have PTH levels that are lower than patients whose calcium intake is less (400 mg daily).[8]

## ETIOLOGY

The cause of primary hyperparathyroidism is known only for a small subset of patients. Patients who had prior irradiation to the neck region may be at risk years later for the development of primary hyperparathyroidism.[9–10] The forms of primary hyperparathyroidism associated with familial syndromes have a genetic origin.[6,11–15] However, most patients with primary hyperparathyroidism do not have a family history of primary hyperparathyroidism or of its associated familial syndromes.

Genetic abnormalities that could be linked to sporadic parathyroid tumors have generated great interest; the first to be described is a rearrangement of the cyclin D1/(PRAD 1) oncogene. The gene defect for abnormal parathyroid tissue from some patients with primary hyperparathyroidism has been shown to be repositioned close to the strong tissue-specific enhancer elements of the PTH gene.[16] This realignment of DNA associates a growth promoter (*cyclin D1*) with a regulatory element that normally controls only a hormonal function, namely synthesis of PTH. Under these circumstances, whenever PTH is stimulated, cellular growth is also stimulated. Despite the attractiveness of this concept of a molecular mechanism of monoclonal parathyroid gland growth, only a few parathyroid tumors have been demonstrated to harbor this defect. Nevertheless, cyclin D1 protein levels are increased in as many as 20% of parathyroid adenomas.[17]

Another attractive molecular mechanism postulated to account for abnormal parathyroid secretion in primary hyperparathyroidism is loss of tumor-suppressor gene function. Abnormalities in the MEN1 gene have been shown to cause the MEN1 syndrome[18,19] (see Chap. 188). The view was long held that both copies of this tumor-suppressor gene might well be inactivated and, thus, contribute to the development of sporadic parathyroid adenomas. A somatic mutation in the MEN1 gene has been found to be associated with 15% to 25% of nonfamilial parathyroid adenomas.[20–22]

In addition to the MEN1 gene, other tumor-suppressor genes have been implicated in the pathogenesis of sporadic parathyroid tumors. Chromosomal regions of interest include 1p and 1q, 6q, 9p, and 15q.[23,24]

Mutations in the gene for the calcium-sensing receptor cause two well-known parathyroid disorders.[25,26] In *neonatal severe hyperparathyroidism, homozygous* mutations completely inactivate this gene; thus, uncontrolled hypercalcemia results. In the *heterozygous* counterpart, *familial hypocalciuric hypercalcemia (FHH)*, a point mutation in one allele leads to a condition that simulates primary hyperparathyroidism but is distinctly different. In sporadic primary hyperparathyroidism, no somatic mutations in the calcium-sensing receptor gene have been detected,[27] although in many adenomas, calcium-receptor protein and sometimes even its messenger RNA is reduced.[28,29]

## CLINICAL MANIFESTATIONS

The signs and symptoms of primary hyperparathyroidism result from the hypercalcemia (see Chap. 59) and the hyperparathyroid state. In primary hyperparathyroidism, the classic target organs are the bones and the kidneys.

### BONE DISEASE

In classic primary hyperparathyroidism, the skeleton is involved in a process known as *osteitis fibrosa cystica*.[30] Radiographically, subperiosteal bone resorption is seen in several typical sites (Fig. 58-1). The salt-and-pepper appearance of the skull, resorption of the distal phalanges, and tapering of the distal clavicles are classic features of the resorptive process in bone. Bone cysts and brown tumors also may be seen. Brown tumors are collections of osteoclasts intermixed with poorly mineralized woven bone. Another important radiologic feature of hyperparathyroid bone disease is demineralization caused by prolonged bone resorption. Osteopenia alone may be a radiographic characteristic of primary hyperparathyroidism. The differential diagnosis of osteoporosis should always include an evaluation for primary hyperparathyroidism.

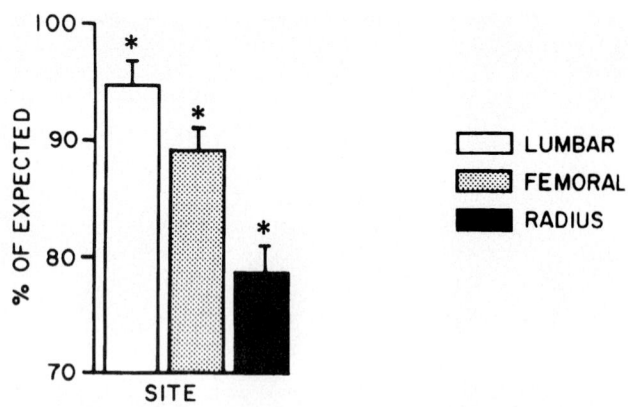

**FIGURE 58-2.** Bone densitometry can reveal mineral loss and bone thinning in patients with primary hyperparathyroidism. Patients' lumbar spine, femoral neck, and radius values are compared with the expected values from age- and sex-matched controls. The divergence from expected value is different at each site (*asterisk* indicates that the change is significant at the level of *p* <.0001).

Before the widespread use of the multichannel autoanalyzer in the early 1970s, the incidence of radiologically apparent bone disease in hyperparathyroidism was 10% to 15%. This figure is now much lower (<5%) because of the markedly higher detection of asymptomatic primary hyperparathyroidism in patients. Although grossly evident bone disease is no longer a frequent finding in primary hyperparathyroidism, more sophisticated diagnostic testing shows continued involvement of the skeleton in the hyperparathyroidism. Bone mineral densitometry and quantitative bone histomorphometry, for example, have detected evidence for hyperparathyroidism among patients without otherwise apparent hyperparathyroid bone disease.[30] The changes are seen at cortical bone, which is found predominantly in the appendicular skeleton. Thinning of cortical bone can be detected by bone mineral densitometry. Figure 58-2 demonstrates typical preferential loss of cortical bone in primary hyperparathyroidism. In contrast, excess PTH secretion appears to have a relative protective effect against bone loss at sites of cancellous bone, such as vertebral bone. Trabecular plates are typically maintained in number and in connectivity in primary hyperparathyroidism (Fig. 58-3; see Chap. 55).[31–33]

Awareness of the potential for bone involvement in patients with asymptomatic primary hyperparathyroidism has led to the routine use of bone mineral densitometry as part of the clinical evaluation of the disease. The results are used to help determine whether the patient should undergo parathyroid surgery.

## RENAL COMPLICATIONS

Nephrolithiasis was and still is the most frequent complication of primary hyperparathyroidism. In older studies, as many as 40% of patients had stone disease.[34] Just as the incidence of overt bone disease in primary hyperparathyroidism has decreased, the incidence of nephrolithiasis has also diminished with the changing clinical profile of the disease.[35] The incidence of nephrolithiasis is ~20%.

Other renal complications include nephrocalcinosis, a radiographic presentation of diffuse renal calcification, and hypercalciuria (see Chap. 208). Although PTH stimulates distal tubular reabsorption of calcium, the increased filtered load of calcium caused by hypercalcemia may lead to increased renal calcium excretion. As many as 35% to 40% of patients with primary hyperparathyroidism may have a urinary calcium excretion of >250 mg daily. Patients with primary hyperparathyroidism may show only a decrease in the creatinine clearance. However,

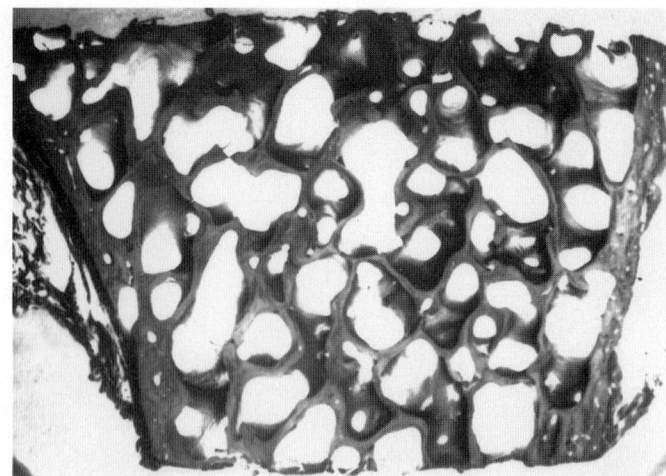

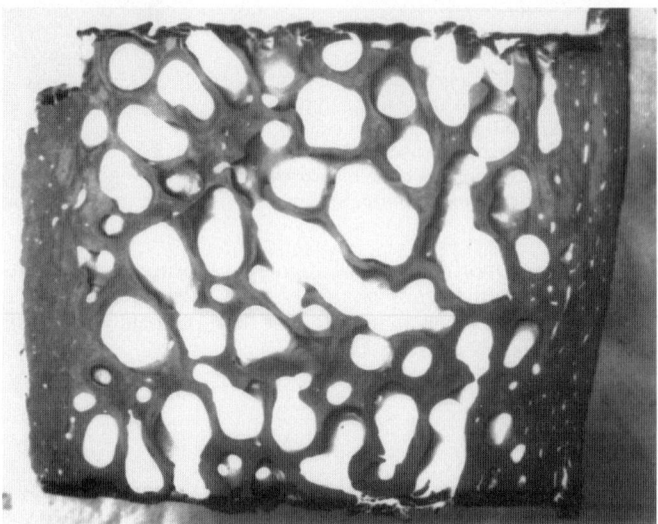

**FIGURE 58-3.** Primary hyperparathyroidism as seen by electron microscopy. **A,** Bone from a 45-year-old man is compared with (**B**) normal bone from an age- and sex-matched normal person. The trabecular plates are conserved in primary hyperparathyroidism, but the cortex is considerably thinner. (Courtesy of Dr. David Dempster.)

successful removal of the parathyroid adenoma does not predictably lead to an improvement in the creatinine clearance.

## OTHER SYSTEMIC EFFECTS

Organs other than skeleton and kidneys may be primary targets for complications of primary hyperparathyroidism. Muscle weakness and easy fatigability can occur. The underlying abnormality appears to be muscle atrophy directed toward, but not limited to, type II muscle fibers.[36] Atrophy of these fibers can explain the clinical finding of proximal muscle weakness. However, patients with primary hyperparathyroidism no longer demonstrate the classic neuromuscular signs of the disease, probably because so many patients are diagnosed with mild hypercalcemia.[37] Nevertheless, the presentation of weakness and easy fatigability may be considered a nonspecific manifestation of primary hyperparathyroidism.

The gastrointestinal tract is a focus for symptoms of hypercalcemia and a potential site of complications of primary hyperparathyroidism. Peptic ulcer disease and acute pancreatitis are classically associated with primary hyperparathyroidism. Whether these gastrointestinal disorders reflect a tendency for common diseases to appear coincidentally in some patients or whether an abnormal functional association exists between primary hyperparathyroidism and gastrointestinal disease is uncertain[38] (see Chap. 204). Similarly, the increased prevalence of hypertension in patients with primary hyperparathyroidism may not have a pathophysiologic basis. Successful removal of a parathyroid adenoma does not usually change the degree of hypertension, nor does it improve antihypertensive management.[39]

Gout and pseudogout have occurred in patients with primary hyperparathyroidism, particularly during the postoperative period[40] (see Chap. 211). Normocytic, normochromic anemia is observed only in patients with advanced parathyroid disease and corrects itself after cure of the hyperparathyroid state.[41]

Among the psychiatric manifestations of primary hyperparathyroidism, depression may be prominent. Less serious, but nevertheless important, is a set of cognitive complaints that patients may bring to the physician's attention. A general decrease in attentiveness and a sense of intellectual weariness have been observed among middle-aged individuals with primary hyperparathyroidism (see Chap. 200). This is another area in which associating a causal role for the hyperparathyroid state is difficult.[42] Reports of improvement in this area after successful parathyroidectomy are difficult to evaluate because of the paucity of accurate quantitative tools for assessing these features and the lack of adequately controlled clinical trials.[43,44]

In very rare cases, primary hyperparathyroidism has been described in association with several unusual nonendocrine manifestations. In some cases of *familial isolated primary hyperparathyroidism (FIPH)*, coexisting ossifying jaw tumors have been described.[13,15] Parathyroid adenomata in association with *Cowden disease* has also been reported.[45] This is a rare, but well described, syndrome characterized by diffuse gastrointestinal polyposis and oral and cutaneous hamartomas.

## HYPERCALCEMIC MANIFESTATIONS

Other signs and symptoms of primary hyperparathyroidism are not specific features of the disorder but reflect the hypercalcemia itself (see Chap. 59). They are not unique to primary hyperparathyroidism and may be associated with any hypercalcemic state. The extent to which patients demonstrate signs of hypercalcemia (e.g., shortened QT interval on the electrocardiogram) or symptoms of hypercalcemia (e.g., anorexia, nausea, vomiting, constipation, polyuria) depends on the actual level of the serum calcium and its rate of rise.

## CLINICAL PRESENTATION

Patients with primary hyperparathyroidism may present with one of several clinical pictures: asymptomatic hypercalcemia; bone or stone disease; other recognized complications, such as neuromuscular, gastrointestinal, articular, hematologic, or central nervous system features; "normocalcemic" hyperparathyroidism; acute primary hyperparathyroidism; parathyroid carcinoma; MEN1 or MEN2A; FIPH; familial cystic parathyroid adenomatosis; or neonatal hyperparathyroidism.[46] The most common form is mild hypercalcemia without any specific signs or symptoms.

The increased incidence of primary hyperparathyroidism reflects recognition of a population brought to the physician's attention by the incidental determination of calcium levels. Usually, these asymptomatic patients have serum calcium levels that are not more than 1 mg/dL above the upper limits of normal.[47] Other test results, such as those for serum phosphorus and the alkaline phosphatase, are usually normal. In marked contrast to this presentation is an unusual and life-threatening form, *acute primary hyperparathyroidism*. Patients with this disorder are symptomatic and present with extremely high serum calcium values (>15 mg/dL).[48] Approximately 25% of patients reported with this form of primary hyperparathyroidism have a previous history of mild hypercalcemia. Patients with acute primary hyperparathyroidism have extremely high serum PTH levels. In one review, the serum calcium value for 43 patients was 17.5 ± 2.1 mg/dL (mean ± standard deviation). In marked contrast to patients with asymptomatic primary hyperparathyroidism, virtually all patients were symptomatic. Unlike primary hyperparathyroidism, acute primary hyperparathyroidism involved both bone and kidney in one-half of the patients. More than two-thirds of patients had nephrolithiasis or nephrocalcinosis. The clinician must recognize that life-threatening hypercalcemia may be the result of acute primary hyperparathyroidism, because this is a curable disease.

Another clinical presentation of primary hyperparathyroidism is that associated with a limited set of complications. As expected, the skeleton, kidneys, or neuromuscular system is most commonly involved. Primary hyperparathyroidism may also occur in a hereditary syndrome in association with MEN1 or MEN2A or simply as FIPH. Patients with FIPH do not have any manifestations of MEN. Patients from these kindreds often present at a younger age than the typical individual with sporadic primary hyperparathyroidism. Their disease generally affects more than one gland and is often recurrent. Because of the high recurrence rate after removal of a single adenoma, subtotal parathyroidectomy is the preferred approach in such individuals.[49,50] Neonatal primary hyperparathyroidism also occurs (see Chap. 70).

Another familial form of primary hyperparathyroidism is characterized by distinctive cystic pathologic features.[51] Patients from these kindreds typically develop recurrent primary hyperparathyroidism resulting from another cystic adenoma years after successful removal of the first adenoma. No other endocrine tumors have been described in this syndrome, but several fibrous maxillary or mandibular tumors have been seen.

Results of the physical examination of patients with primary hyperparathyroidism are not noteworthy. The clinical sign of calcium deposition in the cornea, band keratopathy, is rarely seen (see Chap. 215). Similarly, palpation of an enlarged parathyroid gland is unusual unless parathyroid carcinoma is present.

## LABORATORY EVALUATION

The diagnosis of primary hyperparathyroidism depends on laboratory tests. The serum calcium concentration is virtually always elevated. The serum phosphorus value may be decreased, but it is usually normal, although typically in the lower range of normal.

Newer markers of bone metabolism are useful to evaluate the presence of underlying bone involvement in cases of primary hyperparathyroidism. Markers of bone formation and resorption tend to be elevated, even in asymptomatic primary hyperparathyroidism. Whether quantification of these markers is useful to predict the extent of PTH-dependent skeletal tumors or whether they are useful predictors of the course of the skeletal involvement is not yet certain, however.

The bone formation marker, total alkaline phosphatase activity, which is readily available on routine multichannel panels, continues to be a useful marker in primary hyperparathyroidism,[52] and its bone-specific isoenzyme is often clearly elevated in patients with mild primary hyperparathyroidism.[53,54] Osteocalcin is also generally increased in patients with primary hyperparathyroidism.[54–56]

Bone resorption is reflected in a product of osteoclast activity, tartrate-resistant acid phosphatase (TRAP), and collagen breakdown products such as hydroxyproline, hydroxypyridin-

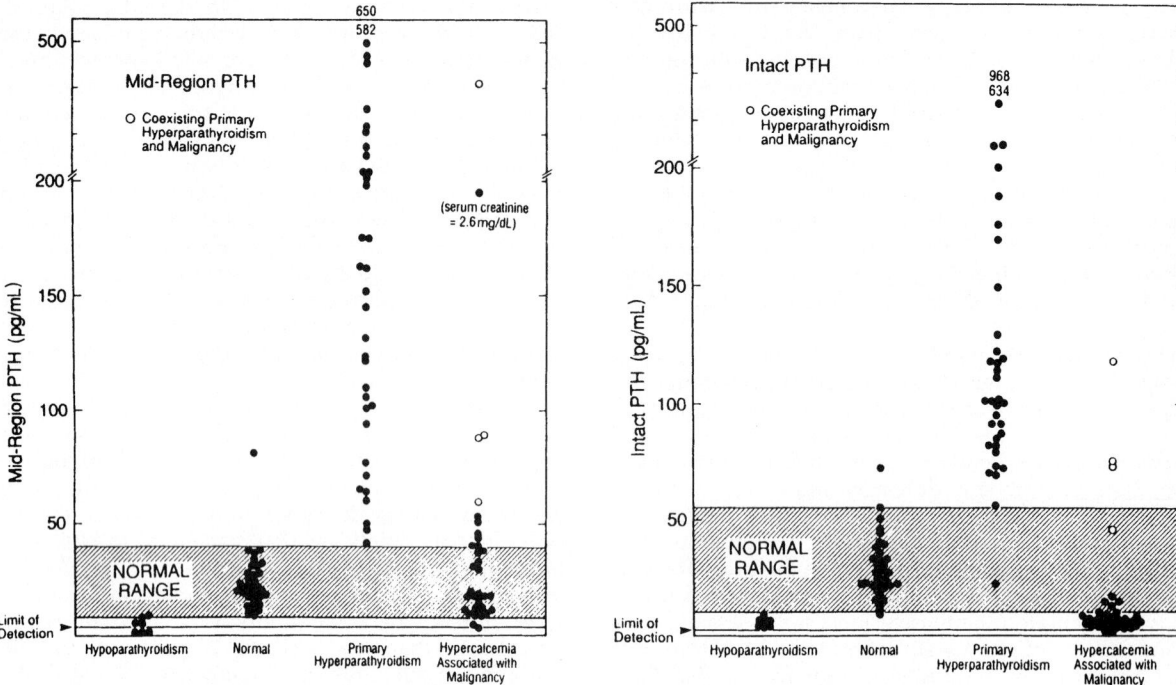

**FIGURE 58-4.** Comparison of midregion radioimmunoassay and immunoradiometric assay for parathyroid hormone (*PTH*) in primary hyperparathyroidism and hypercalcemia associated with malignancy. (From Nussbaum SR, Zahradnik RJ, Lavigne JR, et al. Highly sensitive two-site immunoradiometric assay of parathyrin and its clinical utility in evaluating patients with hypercalcemia. Clin Chem 1987; 33:1364.)

ium cross-links of collagen, and the small N- and C-telopeptides of collagen metabolism. The oldest known marker of bone resorption,[57,58] urinary hydroxyproline excretion, is frankly elevated in patients with *osteitis fibrosa cystica*. However, in patients with mild, asymptomatic primary hyperparathyroidism, values are often entirely normal. The hydroxypyridinium cross-links of collagen have replaced hydroxyproline excretion as markers of bone resorption used in evaluating primary hyperparathyroidism (see Chap. 56). These cross-links of collagen (pyridinoline and deoxypyridinoline) are mildly elevated.[59] Studies of TRAP levels in primary hyperparathyroidism are limited, although levels have been shown to be elevated.[60] Bone sialoprotein is a phosphorylated glycoprotein that makes up ~5% to 10% of the noncollagenous protein of bone. It is elevated in high-turnover states and reflects, in part, bone resorption. In primary hyperparathyroidism, bone sialoprotein levels are elevated and correlate with urinary pyridinoline and deoxypyridinoline.[61] Although their measurement is not mandatory for the evaluation of the patient with primary hyperparathyroidism, bone marker levels can provide useful information about the extent to which the skeleton is involved in the hyperparathyroid process.

## PARATHYROID HORMONE MEASUREMENT

The diagnosis of primary hyperparathyroidism is substantiated by measurement of the concentration of PTH. For most patients with primary hyperparathyroidism, assays show frankly elevated levels of PTH associated with the sine qua non of the disease, hypercalcemia. Fragment assays for circulating midregion or COOH-terminal forms of PTH reliably show elevations by radioimmunoassay. Circulating intact PTH can be measured by immunoradiometric or immunochemiluminometric assays (Fig. 58-4; see Chap. 51).[62,63] Elevated levels of circulating, intact PTH occur in ~90% of patients with primary hyperparathyroidism. The remaining 10% of patients have levels that are in the upper range of normal, concentrations that are inappropriately

high in the face of hypercalcemia. If these patients with "normal" levels of PTH are monitored over time, they invariably show elevated levels.

In addition to helping to establish the diagnosis of primary hyperparathyroidism, the assays for PTH help to differentiate it from the other most common cause of hypercalcemia, malignancy-associated hypercalcemia. In malignancy-associated hypercalcemia, even that associated with the production of parathyroid hormone–related protein (PTHrP), PTH levels are suppressed. This is because PTHrP is not recognized in assays for PTH (see Chap. 52).

In virtually all other hypercalcemic states, the parathyroid glands are normally suppressed, and levels of PTH are not detected in the circulation.

## OTHER TESTS

As a reflection of the increased concentration of biologically active PTH in the circulation of patients with primary hyperparathyroidism, total and nephrogenous urinary cyclic adenosine monophosphate (cAMP) levels are elevated.[64] However, with clinically proven assays for PTH, urinary cAMP measurement does not offer any additional information. Urinary calcium excretion is not useful for diagnostic purposes but does help in the overall assessment of the patient and in the process of decision making for surgery.

Serum 1,25-dihydroxyvitamin D [1,25(OH)$_2$D] may be elevated in primary hyperparathyroidism, reflecting an action of PTH to stimulate the conversion of 25-hydroxyvitamin D [25(OH)D] to 1,25(OH)$_2$D. Further insight into the functional abnormality of primary hyperparathyroidism derives from the observation that patients with this disorder convert more 25(OH)D to 1,25(OH)$_2$D than do normal people.[65] The level of 1,25(OH)$_2$D in primary hyperparathyroidism may reflect the actions of PTH on the renal 1$\alpha$-hydroxylase enzyme. However, the elevated 1,25(OH)$_2$D level in primary hyperparathyroidism is not specific. Many patients with primary hyperparathyroidism do not show elevations in this vitamin D metabolite, and other disorders associated with hypercalcemia (e.g., certain granulomatous diseases, lymphomas, sarcoidosis, vitamin D toxicity) may be associated with elevations in the $1,25(OH)_2D$ concentration.

Patients with primary hyperparathyroidism demonstrate characteristic histopathologic changes of the hyperparathyroid state on bone biopsy (see Chap. 55). Presently, bone biopsy has little clinical utility in management of this disease.

## DIAGNOSIS

The diagnostic hallmarks of primary hyperparathyroidism are hypercalcemia and an elevated level of PTH. Just as a normal circulating PTH concentration is a relatively unusual finding in primary hyperparathyroidism, a normal level of serum calcium is also most unusual in primary hyperparathyroidism. When this occurs, the circulating serum proteins may be low, and the "normal" serum calcium value may be associated with an elevated ionized calcium concentration (see Chap. 49). Only in this unusual situation of suspected primary hyperparathyroidism—elevated PTH and normal serum calcium—may ionized serum calcium values be a valuable adjunct to other diagnostic tests. Nonetheless, primary hyperparathyroidism is seen occasionally with a truly normal serum calcium concentration. The name *normocalcemic primary hyperparathyroidism* was given to this clinical presentation; over time, however, the serum calcium level does become elevated.[66] Presumably, this situation reflects increased parathyroid glandular activity that has not yet caused frank hypercalcemia. Rarely can primary hyperparathyroidism be shown to be present in an individual for whom serum calcium determinations are always normal.

In a small number of patients with primary hyperparathyroidism, the circulating PTH concentration is *not* frankly elevated. Values are instead in the upper range of normal. The PTH level is, however, inappropriately high given the patient's hypercalcemia. Any patient with hypercalcemia should have *suppressed* levels of PTH unless primary hyperparathyroidism is present. *Exceptions* to this rule include patients with FHH and those who are taking *thiazide diuretics* or *lithium*. Some data also suggest that *younger* individuals (i.e., younger than 45 years of age) may normally have lower levels of PTH than their older counterparts.[67] Thus, a value at the upper end of the normal range in a 40-year-old patient with hypercalcemia is probably indicative of hyperparathyroidism.

If the serum calcium level is consistently normal when the PTH concentration is elevated, the physician must consider a *secondary* cause for the hyperparathyroid state. The distinction between primary and secondary hyperparathyroidism is made readily. Parathyroid glandular overactivity in secondary hyperparathyroidism has a nonparathyroid cause, a condition associated with a depressed serum calcium level. Parathyroid tissues respond to this hypocalcemic stimulus with an increased secretory rate. The increased PTH concentration returns the serum calcium level toward normal. Secondary hyperparathyroidism has many causes (see Chaps. 61 and 63), but usually it is related to renal insufficiency or to gastrointestinal tract disorders in which malabsorption of vitamin D, calcium, or both occurs. All four parathyroid glands respond to hypocalcemia with the development of hyperplasia. In renal disease, if the hypocalcemic signal is uncontrolled and prolonged, the parathyroid tissue may become relatively autonomous, a condition called *tertiary hyperparathyroidism*, in which extreme elevations of PTH, sometimes >10 times normal, occur with hypercalcemia.

Before determination of PTH became the most useful test in the differential diagnosis of hypercalcemia, several other tests and measurements were used that now have only historic interest. These tests include the decreased basal tubular reabsorption of phosphate, the lack of effect of exogenous PTH on the tubular reabsorption of phosphate, an increased chloride/

bicarbonate ratio, and the failure to suppress serum calcium with prednisone. None of these maneuvers is of diagnostic value and they are not used to establish the diagnosis of primary hyperparathyroidism.

## DIFFERENTIAL DIAGNOSIS

The differential diagnosis of hypercalcemia is covered in Chapter 59, but several points are particularly relevant to the discussion of primary hyperparathyroidism. If previous medical records are available, the patient may be found to have had serum calcium levels at the upper limits of normal before frank hypercalcemia became evident.

### LITHIUM USE

Lithium administration has been associated with hypercalcemia and an apparent hyperparathyroid state. In vitro studies suggest that lithium may alter the calcium setpoint for calcium-mediated inhibition of PTH secretion.[68] Anecdotal clinical reports describe reversible hyperparathyroidism in patients treated with lithium. Confounding variables, such as diuretic therapy or renal failure, preclude definite conclusions in many of these case reports. Lithium treatment has been associated with hypercalcemia, hypermagnesemia, and reduced urinary calcium.[69] A controlled study involving normal volunteers assessed lithium effects on PTH secretion. No significant difference was found in serum calcium, plasma PTH, or nephrogenous cAMP measurements after calcium infusion in normal volunteers, off or on lithium therapy.[70] These data suggest that clinically relevant lithium levels do not alter the calcium setpoint of PTH release, but evidence suggests that the setpoint for calcium may be altered short term and that PTH levels may rise over time.[71] Practically, the diagnosis of primary hyperparathyroidism is on firmer grounds if lithium can be withdrawn and the patient shown to have persistent hypercalcemia over the ensuing several months.

### THIAZIDE USE

Another medication in common use, thiazide diuretics, may be associated with hypercalcemia.[72] The mechanism for hypercalcemia is related to several factors: reduced plasma volume, increased proximal tubular reabsorption of calcium, and perhaps activity at the level of the parathyroid glands themselves. Some patients who develop hypercalcemia in association with thiazide diuretic therapy are ultimately shown to have primary hyperparathyroidism. In these patients, the hypercalcemia persists after thiazides are withdrawn. Other patients who develop hypercalcemia during thiazide therapy show a return to normal of the serum calcium and serum PTH levels. The diagnosis of primary hyperparathyroidism cannot be made with confidence in hypercalcemic patients receiving thiazides unless the calcium and parathyroid levels are still elevated 2 to 3 months after the diuretic is discontinued.

### COEXISTENCE OF TWO CAUSES OF HYPERCALCEMIA

Because primary hyperparathyroidism is a relatively common disorder, it may coexist with another disorder associated with hypercalcemia, such as malignancy.

## THERAPY

### SURGERY

In view of the modern clinical profile of primary hyperparathyroidism, not all patients have features that would prompt a recommendation for surgery. The existence of asymptomatic

**TABLE 58-1.**
**Criteria for Surgery in Primary Hyperparathyroidism**

1. Serum calcium >12 mg/dL
2. Marked hypercalciuria (>400 mg/day)
3. Any overt manifestation of primary hyperparathyroidism (e.g., nephrolithiasis, osteitis fibrosa cystica, classic neuromuscular disease)
4. Markedly reduced cortical bone density (radius $z$ score < –2)
5. Reduced creatinine clearance in the absence of other cause
6. Age younger than 50 years

patients with primary hyperparathyroidism has engendered controversy about the need for parathyroidectomy and surgical guidelines.

At the Consensus Development Conference on the Diagnosis and Management of Asymptomatic Primary Hyperparathyroidism, a set of surgical guidelines was endorsed[73] (Table 58-1). The criteria for surgery include serum calcium concentration >12 mg/dL; any complication of primary hyperparathyroidism (e.g., overt bone disease, nephrolithiasis, nephrocalcinosis, classic neuromuscular disease); marked hypercalciuria (>400 mg per day); reduction in bone density more than two standard deviations below normal at the site of cortical bone, as in the forearm; an episode of acute hyperparathyroidism; and age younger than 50 years (see Table 58-1). Approximately 50% of patients with primary hyperparathyroidism meet one or more of these criteria. This is a significantly greater percentage of patients that have symptomatic primary hyperparathyroidism (20–30%). Some patients with asymptomatic primary hyperparathyroidism do meet surgical criteria and are candidates for parathyroid surgery, and in individual cases, surgical guidelines may be altered according to clinical judgment.

Parathyroidectomy leads to the rapid resolution of the biochemical abnormalities of primary hyperparathyroidism.[74] Surgery has also been documented to be of clear benefit in reducing the incidence of recurrent nephrolithiasis[75,76] and in leading to an improvement in bone mineral density.[74] Parathyroidectomy leads to a 12% rise in bone density mainly at the cancellous lumbar spine and femoral neck (Fig. 58-5). This increase is sustained over at least four years after surgery.

A few patients show a densitometric profile that is unusual for patients with asymptomatic primary hyperparathyroidism. These individuals do not show the usual sparing of cancellous bone; rather, they have low bone density at the spine. In these patients, the postoperative increase in vertebral bone density is even more dramatic than that seen in the average patient; this has led to the recommendation that patients with low vertebral bone density also should be considered for parathyroidectomy.[77]

Special mention should be made of surgery in postmenopausal women with primary hyperparathyroidism.[78] Many postmenopausal women with primary hyperparathyroidism have bone mass of the lumbar spine that is not below normal. Bone loss in the cancellous spine, typical of the postmenopausal state, may not be apparent. In these patients, the hyperparathyroid state could conceivably afford a relative protection, and the physician could use this information to proceed with a more conservative approach to management, especially if other guidelines for surgery are not met. On the other hand, the increase in bone density after surgery (at the spine and hip) is also seen in postmenopausal women.[74]

Issues related to parathyroid surgery and to preoperative localization of parathyroid tissue are also covered in Chapter 62.[79]

## NONSURGICAL MEDICAL APPROACHES

In patients who are not candidates for surgery at the time primary hyperparathyroidism is recognized, the course over the next 10 years often is stable (see Fig. 58-5).[74,80] Serum calcium

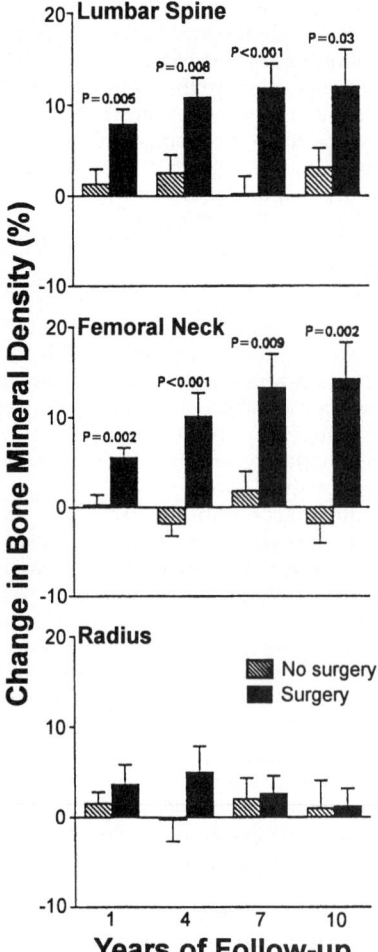

**FIGURE 58-5.** Mean (±SE) bone mineral density at three sites in two groups of patients with primary hyperthyroidism. Cumulative percentage change (mean ±SEM) from baseline by site at year 1, year 4, year 7, and year 10 of follow-up, reported in patients followed with no intervention (*hatched bars*) and after parathyroidectomy (*solid bars*). Differences between parathyroidectomy and no intervention groups are shown. (From Silverberg SJ, Gartenberg F, Jacobs TP, et al. Increased bone mineral density following parathyroidectomy in primary hyperparathyroidism. J Clin Endocrinol Metab 1995; 80:729.

and PTH levels, urinary calcium excretion, and other biochemical indices do not appear to show any changes or trends over time. Bone mineral densitometry at all three sites (i.e., forearm, hip, lumbar spine) does not appear to show any unusual changes or trends over time.[81,82] Fractures might be expected to be increased in patients followed conservatively, because of the reduction in bone mineral density typically seen in this disease. In fact, an increased incidence of distal radial fractures would be consistent with the known selective effects of PTH to reduce cortical bone mass. Despite publication of a few reports, no conclusion can be drawn as to whether fracture incidence is increased in primary hyperparathyroidism or whether these potential adverse events show site or time dependence.[83,84]

Relatively little is known about survival in patients who develop primary hyperparathyroidism. The indolent nature of the disease, as well as the difficulty in long-term follow-up, account, in part, for lack of pertinent information about mortality in this disease. However, the Mayo Clinic's review of the records of >400 patients with primary hyperparathyroidism for ~30 years indicates that survival, on average, is indistinguishable from the expected longevity from life tables.[85] Patients with hypercalcemia in the highest quartile ($Ca^{2+}$ of 11.2–16.0

mg/dL) may have had higher mortality; however, this becomes apparent only after 15 years. These findings are different from those of earlier studies in which an increased risk of death from cancer and cardiovascular events was reported.[86,87] These differences may be attributed to the apparently much milder disease observed in the Mayo Clinic population, very much like that usually seen in the United States today.

Although knowledge of the natural history of primary hyperparathyroidism managed without parathyroid surgery is still incomplete, medical approaches to the management of primary hyperparathyroidism should be considered in nonsurgical patients. Patients with acute primary hyperparathyroidism should be treated the same as any patient with severe hypercalcemia[88,89] (see Chap. 59). Long-term management of chronically elevated, mild hypercalcemia centers on adequate hydration and ambulation. If possible, diuretics should be avoided; in particular, thiazide diuretics may worsen the hypercalcemia in some patients. Other diuretics, such as furosemide, may place the patient at risk for dehydration and electrolyte imbalances. General recommendations for diet are not yet certain, and rationales exist for both low- and high-calcium diets in patients with hyperparathyroidism. Diets high in calcium may suppress levels of endogenous PTH. However, high-calcium diets may lead to greater absorption of calcium because of the elevated levels of $1,25(OH)_2D$ in some patients.[90,91] The recommendation for a low-calcium diet is based on the notion that less calcium is available for absorption. However, low-calcium diets may predispose patients to further stimulation of endogenous PTH levels. One study showed no effect of dietary calcium on biochemical indices or bone densitometry in patients with primary hyperparathyroidism.[92] A *normal* calcium intake can be followed without adverse effects, except in those patients with elevated 1,25-dihydroxyvitamin D levels. Such patients are advised to be more moderate in their calcium intake to prevent hypercalciuria.

Other approaches to the medical management of primary hyperparathyroidism have been considered. Attempts to block PTH secretion with β-adrenergic inhibitors or $H_2$-receptor antagonists have not been successful.[7] Oral phosphate, which has been used for many years in primary hyperparathyroidism, lowers serum calcium by 0.5 to 1.0 mg/dL in most patients. The average dosage is 1 to 2 g daily in divided doses. Phosphate appears to have several mechanisms of action. It may inhibit calcium absorption from the gastrointestinal tract; it prevents calcium mobilization from bone; and it may also impair the production of $1,25(OH)_2D$. The risks of the long-term use of phosphate in the management of patients with primary hyperparathyroidism are unknown. One concern is the possibility of ectopic calcification in soft tissues when the normal solubility product of $Ca^{2+} \times PO_4^{3-}$ is exceeded (normally ~40). Phosphate therapy is contraindicated when renal insufficiency or hyperphosphatemia is present. If phosphate is to be used, the serum levels of calcium and phosphate should be monitored at regular intervals. Moreover, the long-term use of phosphate in patients with primary hyperparathyroidism promotes a further increase in PTH.[93] The possibility that some of the symptoms and signs of primary hyperparathyroidism are caused by PTH itself and not by hypercalcemia raises questions about further increasing PTH levels in conjunction with phosphate therapy. If sufficient concern exists about lowering the serum calcium level in patients with asymptomatic primary hyperparathyroidism, parathyroid surgery remains the treatment of choice.

Estrogen therapy has been proposed as a means of lowering serum calcium, especially because prevalence of primary hyperparathyroidism among women is increased in the postmenopausal years. Estrogens have well-known but not clearly understood antagonist actions on PTH-induced bone resorption. The serum calcium does tend to fall by ~0.5 to 1.0 mg/dL in women receiving estrogens.[94–96] However, PTH and phosphorus levels do not change. More studies are required to better delineate the role of estrogen therapy.

To date, no available data exist on the role of selective estrogen-receptor modulators (SERMs) in the treatment of primary hyperparathyroidism. Because the antiresorptive actions of these drugs are similar to those of estrogens, SERMs might be predicted to lower serum calcium levels in postmenopausal women with primary hyperparathyroidism in a fashion similar to that seen with estrogen. This hypothesis remains to be tested.

Calcitonin may have a potential use in treating primary hyperparathyroidism, but no controlled trial has been conducted to test the efficacy of calcitonin for management of this condition. Data from the use of calcitonin in other states of increased bone turnover indicate that it may never become a useful long-term therapy for primary hyperparathyroidism.

The bisphosphonates represent a class of important antiresorbing agents that may emerge as a useful approach to the medical management of primary hyperparathyroidism. Oral etidronate is not useful, and the effect of oral clodronate and alendronate is limited in duration of effect.[97] Of the third-generation bisphosphonates, risedronate has been shown to have some efficacy in preliminary studies of patients with primary hyperparathyroidism.[98]

Finally, specifically targeted medical therapy for primary hyperparathyroidism is under active investigation. Calcimimetic agents that target the calcium-sensing receptor on the parathyroid cell[99] have shown early promise in animal and in vitro studies.[100,101] Data from human investigations are also encouraging. In early studies, one such calcimimetic has been shown to lower serum calcium and PTH levels both in a patient with parathyroid carcinoma and in a group of postmenopausal women with mild primary hyperparathyroidism.[102,103]

## PRIMARY HYPERPARATHYROIDISM DURING PREGNANCY

Rarely, primary hyperparathyroidism becomes evident during pregnancy.[104] Hyperparathyroidism during pregnancy used to be associated with an increased incidence of fetal death. Perinatal and neonatal complications were also thought to be increased in the hypocalcemic infant whose endogenous PTH production is suppressed by maternal hypercalcemia. Neonatal hypocalcemia and tetany can be the first sign of primary hyperparathyroidism in the mother.

Although systematically collected and controlled data are unavailable, experience has indicated that primary hyperparathyroidism during pregnancy can be managed successfully without resorting to surgery.[105,106] The management of primary hyperparathyroidism during pregnancy is controversial.[107] Some clinicians advocate surgery during the second trimester to reduce fetal risk of chronic hypercalcemia during the gestational period. Others advocate a much more conservative approach.

## PARATHYROID CARCINOMA

Parathyroid carcinoma is a rare form of primary hyperparathyroidism.[108,109] These patients often have hypercalcemia that is more severe than that usually seen in primary hyperparathyroidism. Serum calcium values >14 mg/dL may suggest a parathyroid malignancy. However, parathyroid carcinoma is uncommon, occurring in <0.5% of patients with primary hyperparathyroidism. Making the clinical diagnosis of parathyroid carcinoma before surgery is often difficult. Along with the high serum calcium level, the PTH level tends to be markedly elevated. Patients with parathyroid carcinoma often have coexistent complications related to the skeleton and the kidney. This combination is unusual in benign primary hyperparathyroidism. Another striking feature may be a palpable neck mass. The clinical features of palpable neck mass, marked hypercalcemia, high concentrations of PTH, and coexistent skeletal resorption and kidney stones should alert the clinician to the possibility of parathyroid carcinoma.[110] The diagnosis of parathyroid carcinoma may not be made until the time of surgery. The gross appearance of the parathyroid tissue may indicate the diagnosis. At times, the histologic features of parathyroid carcinoma may be typical (see Chap. 48), or it may be difficult to diagnose. Surgery is the mainstay of therapy for parathyroid carcinoma.

With the clinical presentation of benign disease changing, the case may well be that parathyroid cancer also will be diagnosed much earlier in its natural history. Patients with parathyroid carcinoma might be expected to show biochemical evidence for somewhat more active disease than seen usually in the benign disorder, but not like the older classical descriptions. The diagnosis would rest primarily with the histologic examination of the parathyroid tissue removed at the time of surgery.[111]

The management of parathyroid carcinoma that has metastasized to local structures or to more distant sites, such as liver or lung, is difficult. Because this malignancy causes symptoms and signs resulting from the hypercalcemia and not necessarily from enlargement of the tumor, surgery has a role in the management of metastatic disease. Removal of local metastases or nodules in the lung has been associated with prolonged survival. Because parathyroid carcinoma tissue is not responsive to feedback of ambient hypercalcemia, debulking the tumor with removal of functional tissue is helpful in controlling hypercalcemia. When the disease is no longer amenable to surgical intervention, management becomes limited to the control of hypercalcemia. In the long run, hypercalcemia is responsible for the morbidity and mortality of the disease. However, parathyroid carcinoma is an indolent malignancy, and patients often survive for years after the diagnosis is made. The probability of 5-year survival in two series approached 60%.[110]

As mentioned earlier (see Nonsurgical Medical Approaches), calcimimetic agents may hold some promise for the future in the treatment of this disease. One patient was treated with such an agent to control life-threatening hypercalcemia with good results.[103] Whether calcimimetic agents would have any efficacy in treating the tumor per se, or only in controlling its manifestations (hypercalcemia), is unknown. Finally, one report describes immunotherapy in the treatment of parathyroid carcinoma.[112] One patient was treated with autoantibodies raised against PTH, with a resulting decrease in hypercalcemia.

# FAMILIAL HYPOCALCIURIC HYPERCALCEMIA

FHH is a benign disorder associated with hypercalcemia.[113] Differentiating individuals with FHH from those with primary hyperparathyroidism is extremely difficult. This disorder is a familial disease that has an autosomal dominant pattern of transmission. Penetrance is high, and the hypercalcemia often manifests in affected individuals in childhood. The disease is characterized by hypercalcemia and relative hypocalciuria. The hypocalciuria may be marked, but it is not absolutely discriminatory when compared with urinary calcium levels in patients with primary hyperparathyroidism. Subtotal parathyroidectomy does not cure the hypercalcemia. Laboratory findings for patients with FHH include mild hypercalcemia but normal serum levels of phosphate and 1,25(OH)$_2$D. The PTH concentration is usually normal, although in several cases, it has been elevated. The serum magnesium concentration is normal to moderately elevated. Typically, the renal calcium clearance/creatinine clearance ratio is <0.01. Family screening is often necessary to differentiate FHH from primary hyperparathyroidism.

## PATHOPHYSIOLOGY

The pathophysiologic basis of FHH is not clear. The normal serum PTH level and urinary cAMP level suggest that this is not a disorder of parathyroid hyperactivity. Provocative tests to raise the calcium further lead to responses that suggest a set-point error.[5] In this respect, patients with FHH are different from patients with primary hyperparathyroidism.

Mutations in the calcium-sensing receptor (CaR) have clearly been shown to be the cause of FHH in almost all cases. Many families with FHH have now been identified who have inactivating mutations in the CaR.[114–116] The kindreds generally harbor unique heterozygous mutations, most of which are missense. These mutations can be found in any region of the receptor. When there are two mutations, the disorder presents in infancy as neonatal severe hypercalcemia. Although most patients with FHH express a defect in the CaR, which is located on 3q13-q21,[117] two other genes for FHH have been described. In one family, the disorder was traced to the short arm of chromosome 19.[118] In another kindred, the disorder is characterized by progressive elevations in PTH, hypophosphatemia, and osteomalacia without assignment to either chromosome 3 or 19.[119]

## MANIFESTATIONS AND THERAPY

Familial hypocalciuric hypercalcemia is not associated with signs and symptoms of primary hyperparathyroidism. Nephrolithiasis and evidence for hyperparathyroid bone disease are not found, nor do other potential complications of primary hyperparathyroidism occur. The disorder usually appears to be relatively benign. It may be associated with pancreatitis, hypertension, gallstones, and chondrocalcinosis, but the pathophysiologic bases of these relationships are unclear. Because of the benign natural history of FHH and because subtotal parathyroidectomy does not cure the disorder, these patients should not undergo neck exploration. After the diagnosis is made, the wise course is to observe these patients but not to engage in any aggressive intervention. Family screening is also recommended.

## REFERENCES

1. Heath H III, Hodgson SF, Kennedy MA. Primary hyperparathyroidism: incidence, morbidity, and potential economic impact in a community. N Engl J Med 1980; 302:189.
2. Mundy GR, Cove DH, Fisken R. Primary hyperparathyroidism: changes in the pattern of clinical presentation. Lancet 1980; 1:1317.
3. Wermers RA, Khosla S, Atkinson EJ, et al. The rise and fall of primary hyperparathyroidism in Rochester, Minnesota; a population based study. Ann Intern Med 1997; 126:433.
4. Brown EM, Broadus AE, Brennan MF, et al. Direct comparison in vivo and in vitro of suppressibility of parathyroid function by calcium in primary hyperparathyroidism. J Clin Endocrinol Metab 1979; 48:604.
5. Khosla S, Ebeling PR, Firek AF, et al. Calcium infusion suggests a "set-point" abnormality of parathyroid gland function in familial benign hypercalcemia and more complex disturbances in primary hyperparathyroidism. J Clin Endocrinol Metab 1993; 76:715.
6. Friedman E, Larsson C, Amorosi A, et al. Multiple endocrine neoplasia type I: pathology, pathophysiology, molecular genetics, and differential diagnosis. In: Bilezikian JP, Levine MA, Marcus R, eds. The parathyroids. New York: Raven Press, 1994:647.
7. Heath H III. Biogenic amines and the secretion of parathyroid hormone and calcitonin. Endocr Rev 1980; 1:319.
8. Insogna KL, Mitnick ME, Stewart AS, et al. Sensitivity of the parathyroid hormone–1,25-dihydroxyvitamin D axis to variations in calcium intake in patients with primary hyperparathyroidism. N Engl J Med 1985; 313:1126.
9. Melton LJ. Therapeutic radiation and hyperparathyroidism. A case-control study in Rochester, Minn. Arch Intern Med 1989; 149:1887.
10. Parfitt AM, Braunstein GD, Katz A. Radiation-associated hyperparathyroidism: comparison of adenoma growth rates, inferred from weight and duration of latency, with prevalence of mitosis. J Clin Endocrinol Metab 1993; 77:1318.
11. Wassif WS, Moniz CF, Friedman E, et al. Familial isolated hyperparathyroidism: a distinct genetic entity with an increased risk of parathyroid cancer. J Clin Endocrinol Metab 1993; 77:1485.

12. Metz DC, Jensen RT, Bale AE, et al. Multiple endocrine neoplasia type I: clinical features and management. In: Bilezikian JP, Levine MA, Marcus R, eds. The parathyroids. New York: Raven Press, 1994:591.

13. Teh BT, Farnebo F, Kristoffersson U, et al. Autosomal dominant primary hyperparathyroidism and jaw tumor syndrome associated with renal hamartomas: linkage to 1q21-q32 and loss of the wild-type allele in renal hamartomas. J Clin Endocrinol Metab 1996; 81:4204.

14. Teh BT, Kytola S, Farnebo F, et al. Mutation analysis of the MEN1 gene in MEN1, familial acromegaly and familial isolated hyperparathyroidism. J Clin Endocrinol Metab 1998; 83:2621.

15. Teh BT, Farnebo F, Twigg S, et al. Familial isolated hyperparathyroidism maps to 1q21-q32 in a subset of families. J Clin Endocrinol Metab 1998; 83:2114.

16. Rosenberg CL, Motokura T, Kronenberg HM, Arnold A. Coding sequence of the overexpressed transcript of the putative oncogene PRAD1/cyclin D1 in two primary human tumors. Oncogene 1993; 8:519.

17. Hsi ED, Zukerberg LR, Yang W-I, Arnold A. Cyclin D1/PRAD 1 expression in parathyroid adenomas: an immunohistochemical study. J Clin Endocrinol Metab 1996; 81:1736.

18. Chandrasekharappa SC, Guru SC, Manickam P, et al. Position cloning of the gene for multiple endocrine neoplasia type 1. Science 1997; 276:404.

19. European Consortium on MEN I Gene. Hum Mol Genet 1997; 6:1177.

20. Heppner C, Kester MB, Agarwal SK, et al. Somatic mutations of the MEN 1 gene in parathyroid tumors. Nat Genet 1997; 16:375.

21. Farnebo F, Teh BT, Kytola S, et al. Alterations of the MEN1 gene in sporadic parathyroid tumors. J Clin Endocrinol Metab 1998; 83:2627.

22. Carling T, Correa P, Hessman O, et al. Parathyroid MEN 1 gene mutations in relation to clinical characteristics of nonfamilial primary hyperparathyroidism. J Clin Endocrinol Metab 1998; 83:2960.

23. Tahara H, Smith AP, Gaz RD, et al. Genomic localization of novel candidate tumor suppressor gene loci in human parathyroid adenomas. Cancer Res 1996; 56:599.

24. Tahara H, Smith AP, Gaz RD, Arnold A. Loss of chromosome arm 9p DNA and analysis of the p16 and p15 cyclin-dependent kinase inhibitor genes in human parathyroid adenomas. J Clin Endocrinol Metab 1996; 81:3663.

25. Brown EM, Steinham B. In vivo and in vitro characterization of neonatal hyperparathyroidism resulting from a de novo, heterozygous mutation in the CaSR gene: normal maternal calcium as a cause of hyperparathyroidism in familial hypocalciuric hypercalcemia. J Clin Invest 1997; 99:88.

26. Pollack MR, Seidman CE, Brown EM. Three inherited disorders of calcium sensing. Medicine 1996; 75:115.

27. Hosokawa Y, Pollak MR, Brown EM, Arnold A. Mutational analysis of the extracellular Ca$^{2+}$-sensing receptor gene in human parathyroid tumors. J Clin Endocrinol Metab 1997; 80:3107.

28. Kifor O, Moore FD Jr, Wang P, et al. Reduced immunostaining for the extracellular Ca$^{2+}$-sensing receptor in primary and uremic secondary hyperparathyroidism. J Clin Endocrinol Metab 1996; 81:1598.

29. Gogusev J, Duchambon P, Hory B, et al. Depressed expression of calcium receptor in parathyroid gland tissue of patients with primary hyperparathyroidism. Kidney Int 1997; 51:328.

30. Bilezikian JP, Silverberg SJ, Gartenberg F, et al. Clinical presentation of primary hyperparathyroidism. In: Bilezikian JP, Marcus R, Levine MA, eds. The parathyroids. New York: Raven Press, 1994:457.

31. Parisien M, Silverberg SJ, Shane E, et al. The histomorphometry of bone in primary hyperparathyroidism: preservation of cancellous bone. J Clin Endocrinol Metab 1990; 70:930.

32. Parisien M, Mellish RW, Silverberg SJ, et al. Maintenance of cancellous bone connectivity in primary hyperparathyroidism: trabecular and strut analysis. J Bone Miner Res 1992; 7:913.

33. Parisien M, Cosman F, Mellish RWE, et al. Bone structure in postmenopausal hyperparathyroid, osteoporotic and normal women. J Bone Min Res 1995; 10:1393.

34. Mallette LE, Bilezikian JP, Heath DA, Aurbach GD. Hyperparathyroidism: a review of 52 cases. Medicine (Baltimore) 1974; 53:127.

35. Silverberg SJ, Shane E, Jacobs TP, et al. Nephrolithiasis and bone involvement in primary hyperparathyroidism. Am J Med 1990; 89:327.

36. Patten BM, Bilezikian JP, Mallette LE, et al. The neuromuscular disease of hyperparathyroidism. Ann Intern Med 1974; 80:182.

37. Turken SA, Cafferty M, Silverberg SJ, et al. Neuromuscular involvement in mild, asymptomatic primary hyperparathyroidism. Am J Med 1989; 87:553.

38. Linos DA, Van Heerden JA, Abboad CF, Edis AJ. Primary hyperparathyroidism and peptic ulcer disease. Arch Surg 1978; 113:384.

39. Scholz DA. Hypertension and hyperparathyroidism. Arch Intern Med 1977; 137:1123.

40. Bilezikian JP, Aurbach GD, Connor TB, et al. Pseudogout following parathyroidectomy. Lancet 1973; 1:445.

41. Mallette LE. Anemia in hypercalcemic hyperparathyroidism: renewed interest in an old observation. Arch Intern Med 1977; 137:572.

42. Ljunghall S, Jakobsson S, Joborn C, et al. Longitudinal studies of mild primary hyperparathyroidism. J Bone Miner Res 1991; 6(Suppl 2):S111.

43. Solomon BL, Schaaf M, Smallridge RC. Psychologic symptoms before and after parathyroid surgery. Am J Med 1994; 96:101.

44. Kleerekoper M, Bilezikian JP. Parathyroidectomy for non-traditional features of primary hyperparathyroidism. Am J Med 1994; 96:99.

45. Hamby LS, Lee EY, Schwartz RW. Parathyroid adenoma and gastric carcinoma as manifestations of Cowden's disease. Surgery 1995; 118:115.

46. Mallette LE. The functional and pathologic spectrum of parathyroid abnormalities in hyperparathyroidism. In: Bilezikian JP, Levine MA, Marcus R, eds. The parathyroids. New York: Raven Press, 1994:423.

47. Potts JT. Proceedings of the NIH Consensus Development Conference on Diagnosis and Management of Asymptomatic Primary Hyperparathyroidism. J Bone Miner Res 1991; 6(Suppl 2):S1.

48. Fitzpatrick LA, Bilezikian JP. Acute primary hyperparathyroidism: a review of 48 patients. Am J Med 1987; 82:275.

49. Huang SM, Duh QY, Shaver J, et al. Familial hyperparathyroidism without MEN. World J Surg 1997; 21:22.

50. Barry MK, van Heerdon JA, Grant CS, et al. Is familial hyperparathyroidism a unique disease? Surgery 1997; 122:1028.

51. Mallette LE, Malini S, Rappaport MP, Kirkland JL. Familial cystic parathyroid adenomatosis. Ann Intern Med 1987; 107:54.

52. Moss DW. Perspectives in alkaline phosphatase research. Clin Chem 1992; 38:2486.

53. Silverberg SJ, Deftos LJ, Kim T, Hill CS. Bone alkaline phosphatase in primary hyperparathyroidism. J Bone Mineral Res 1991; 6:A624.

54. Duda RJ, O'Brien JF, Katzman JA, et al. Concurrent assays of circulating bone Gla-protein and bone alkaline phosphatase: effects of sex, age, and metabolic bone disease. J Clin Endocrinol Metab 1988; 5:1.

55. Price PA, Parthemore JG, Deftos LJ. New biochemical marker for bone metabolism. Measurement by radioimmunoassay of bone Gla-protein in the plasma of normal subjects and patients with bone disease. J Clin Invest 1980; 66:878.

56. Deftos LJ, Parthemore JG, Price PA. Changes in plasma bone Gla-protein during treatment of bone disease. Calcif Tissue Int 1982; 34:121.

57. Deftos LJ. Bone protein and peptide assays in the diagnosis and management of skeletal disease. Clin Chem 1991; 37:1143.

58. Delmas PH. Biochemical markers of bone turnover: methodology and clinical use in osteoporosis. Am J Med 1991; 91:169.

59. Seibel MJ, Gartenberg F, Silverberg SJ, et al. Urinary hydroxypyridinium cross-links of collagen in primary hyperparathyroidism. J Clin Endocrinol Metab 1992; 74:481.

60. Kraenzlin ME, Lau KHW, Liang L, et al. Development of an immunoassay for human serum osteoclastic tartrate-resistant acid phosphatase. J Clin Endocrinol Metab 1990; 71:442.

61. Seibel MJ, Woigte HW, Pecherstorfer M, et al. Serum immunoreactive bone sialoprotein as a new marker of bone turnover in metabolic and malignant diseases. J Clin Endocrinol Metab 1996; 81:3289.

62. Kao PC, van Heerden JA, Grant CS, et al. Clinical performance of parathyroid hormone immunometric assays. Mayo Clin Proc 1992; 67:637.

63. Nussbaum SR, Potts JT Jr. Advances in immunoassays for parathyroid hormone: clinical applications to skeletal disorders of bone and mineral metabolism. In: Bilezikian JP, Levine MA, Marcus R, eds. The parathyroids. New York: Raven Press, 1994:157.

64. Broadus AE. Nephrogenous cyclic AMP as a parathyroid function test. Nephron 1979; 23:136.

65. Locascio V, Adami S, Galvanini G, et al. Substrate-product relation of 1-hydroxylase activity in primary hyperparathyroidism. N Engl J Med 1985; 313:1123.

66. Wills MR, Pak CYC, Hammond WG, Bartter FC. Normocalcemic primary hyperparathyroidism. Am J Med 1969; 47:384.

67. Segre GV. Personal communication.

68. Brown E. Lithium induces abnormal calcium-regulated PTH release in dispersed bovine parathyroid cells. J Clin Endocrinol Metab 1981; 52:1046.

69. Christiansen C, Baastrup P, Transbol I. Development of "primary" hyperparathyroidism during lithium therapy: longitudinal study. Neuropsychobiology 1980; 6:280.

70. Spiegel A, Rudorfer M, Marx S, Linnoila M. The effect of short term lithium administration on suppressibility of parathyroid hormone secretion by calcium in vivo. J Clin Endocrinol Metab 1984; 59:354.

71. Mallette LE, Khouri K, Zengotita H, et al. Lithium treatment increases intact and midregion parathyroid hormone and parathyroid volume. J Clin Endocrinol Metab 1989; 68:654.

72. Middler S, Pak CY, Murad F, Bartter F. Thiazide diuretics and calcium metabolism. Metabolism 1973; 22:1438.

73. National Institutes of Health Consensus Development Conference statement on primary hyperparathyroidism. J Bone Miner Res 1991; 6(Suppl 2):S9.

74. Silverberg SJ, Gartenberg F, Jacobs TP, et al. Increased bone mineral density following parathyroidectomy in primary hyperparathyroidism. J Clin Endocrinol Metab 1995; 80:729.

75. Klugman VA, Favus M, Pak CYC. Nephrolithiasis in primary hyperparathyroidism. In: Bilezikian JP, Levine MA, Marcus R, eds. The parathyroids. New York: Raven Press, 1994:505.

76. Deaconson TF, Wilson SD, Lemann J. The effect of parathyroidectomy on the recurrence of nephrolithiasis. Surgery 1987; 215:241.

77. Silverberg SJ, Locker FG, Bilezikian JP. Vertebral osteopenia: a new indication for surgery in primary hyperparathyroidism. J Clin Endocrinol Metab 1996; 81:4007.

78. Bilezikian JP. Primary hyperparathyroidism: another important metabolic bone disease of women. J Women Health 1994; 3:21.

79. Thule P, Thakore K, Vansant J, et al. Preoperative localization of parathyroid tissue with technetium-99m Sestamibi $^{123}$I subtraction scanning. J Clin Endocrinol Metab 1994; 78:77.

80. Parfitt AM, Rao DS, Kleerekoper M. Asymptomatic primary hyperparathyroidism discovered by multichannel biochemical screening: clinical course

and considerations bearing on the need for surgical intervention. J Bone Miner Res 1991; 6(Suppl 2):S97.

81. Sudhaker RD, Wilson RJ, Kleerekoper M, Parfitt AM. Lack of biochemical progression or continuation of accelerated bone loss in mild asymptomatic primary hyperparathyroidism. J Clin Endocrinol Metab 1988; 67:1294.

82. Silverberg SJ, Gartenberg F, Jacobs TP, et al. Longitudinal bone density measurements in untreated primary hyperparathyroidism. J Clin Endocrinol Metab 1995; 90:723.

83. Melton U III, Atkinson EJ, O'Fallon WM, Heath H. Risk of age-related fractures in patients with primary hyperparathyroidism. Arch Intern Med 1992; 152:2269.

84. Wilson RJ, Rao DS, Ellis B, Kleerekoper M, Parfitt AM. Mild asymptomatic primary hyperparathyroidism is not a risk factor for vertebral fractures. Ann Intern Med 1988; 109:959.

85. Wermers RA, Khosla S, Atkinson EJ, et al. Survival after the diagnosis of primary hyperparathyroidism. Am J Med 1998; 104:115.

86. Hedback G, Tisell LE, Bengtsson BA, et al. Premature death in patients operated on for primary hyperparathyroidism. World J Surgery 1990; 14:829.

87. Palmer M, Adami HO, Krusemo UB, Ljunghall S. Increased risk of malignant diseases after surgery for primary hyperparathyroidism: a nationwide cohort study. Am J Epidemiol 1988; 127:1031.

88. Bilezikian JP. Management of acute hypercalcemia. N Engl J Med 1992; 326:1196.

89. Bilezikian JP. Management of hypercalcemia. J Clin Endocrinol Metab 1993; 77:1445.

90. Kaplan RA, Haussler MR, Deftos LJ, et al. The role of 1,25-dihydroxyvitamin D in the mediation of intestinal hyperabsorption of calcium in primary hyperparathyroidism and absorptive hypercalciuria. J Clin Invest 1977; 59:756.

91. Broadus AE, Horst RL, Lang R, et al. The importance of circulating 1,25-dihydroxyvitamin D in the pathogenesis of hypercalciuria and renal-stone formation in primary hyperparathyroidism. N Engl J Med 1980; 302:421.

92. Locker FG, Silverberg SJ, Bilezikian JP. Optimal dietary calcium intake in primary hyperparathyroidism. Am J Med 1997; 102:543.

93. Broadus AE, Magee JS, Mallette LE, et al. A detailed evaluation of oral phosphate therapy in selected patients with primary hyperparathyroidism. J Clin Endocrinol Metab 1983; 56:953.

94. Marcus R, Madvig P, Crim M, et al. Conjugated estrogens in the treatment of postmenopausal women with hyperparathyroidism. Ann Intern Med 1984; 100:633.

95. Selby PL, Peacock M. Ethinyl estradiol and norethindrone in the treatment of primary hyperparathyroidism in post menopausal women. N Engl J Med 1986; 314:1481.

96. Stock JL. Medical management of primary hyperparathyroidism. In: Bilezikian JP, Levine MA, Marcus R, eds. The parathyroids. New York: Raven Press, 1994:519.

97. Hamdy NAT, Gray E, McCloskey E, et al. Clodronate in the medical management of hyperparathyroidism. Bone 1987; 8(Suppl 1):569.

98. Reisner CA, Stone MD, Hoshiy DJ, et al. Acute changes in calcium homeostasis during treatment of primary hyperparathyroidism with risedronate. J Clin Endocrinol Metab 1993; 77:1067.

99. Brown EM, Gamba G, Riccardi D, et al. Cloning and characterization of an extracellular calcium-sensing receptor from bovine parathyroid. Nature 1993; 366:575.

100. Rogers KV, Fox J, Nemeth EF. The calcimimetic compound NPS467 reduces plasma calcium in a dose-dependent and stereospecific manner. J Bone Miner Res 1993; 8(Suppl 1):S180.

101. Steffey ME, Fox J, Van Wagenen BC, et al. Calcimimetics: structurally and mechanistically novel compounds that inhibit hormone secretion from parathyroid cells. J Bone Miner Res 1993; 8(Suppl 1):S175.

102. Silverberg SJ, Bone HG 3rd, Marriott TB, et al. Short term inhibition of parathyroid hormone secretion by a calcium receptor agonist in primary hyperparathyroidism. N Engl J Med 1997; 337(21):1506.

103. Collins MT, Skarulis MC, Bilezikian JP, et al. Treatment of hypercalcemia secondary to parathyroid carcinoma with a novel calcimimetic agent. J Clin Endocrinol Metab 1998; 83:1083.

104. Kristofferson A, Dahlgren S, Lithner F, Jarhult J. Primary hyperparathyroidism in pregnancy. Surgery 1985; 97:326.

105. Kelly TR. Primary hyperparathyroidism during pregnancy. Surgery 1991; 110:1028.

106. Haenel LC IV, Mayfield RK. Primary hyperparathyroidism in a twin pregnancy and review of fetal/maternal calcium homeostasis. Am J Med Sci 2000; 319:191.

107. Ficinski ML, Mestman JH. Primary hyperparathyroidism during pregnancy. Endocr Pract 1996; 2:362.

108. Wynne AG, van Heerden J, Carney JA, Fitzpatrick LA. Parathyroid carcinoma: clinical and pathologic features in 43 patients. Medicine (Baltimore) 1992; 71:197.

109. Kytola S, Farnebo F, Obara T, et al. Patterns of chromosomal imbalances in parathyroid carcinomas. Am J Pathol 2000; 157:579.

110. Shane E, Bilezikian JP. Parathyroid carcinoma. In: Williams CJ, Krikorian JC, Green MR, Raghavan D, eds. Textbook of uncommon cancer. New York: John Wiley and Sons, 1988:763.

111. Silverberg SJ, Lowenfeld A, Perzin K, et al. Parathyroid cancer presents with a new phenotype in the 1990's. J Bone Mineral Res 1997; 12(Suppl 1):S522.

112. Bradwell AR, Harvey TC. Control of hypercalcaemia of parathyroid carcinoma by immunisation. Lancet 1999; 353:370.

113. Heath H III. Familial benign (hypocalciuric) hypercalcemia. A troublesome mimic of mild primary hyperparathyroidism. Endocrinol Metab Clin North Am 1989; 18:723.

114. Pollak MR, Brown EM, Chou YHW, et al. Mutations in the human $Ca^{2+}$-sensing receptor gene cause familial hypocalciuric hypercalcemia and neonatal severe hyperparathyroidism. Cell 1993; 75:1297.

115. Thakker RV. Molecular genetics of parathyroid disease. Curr Opin Endocrinol Diabetes 1996; 3:521.

116. Hendy GN, D'Souza-Li L, Yang B, et al. Mutations of the calcium-sensing receptor (CASR) in familial hypocalciuric hypercalcemia, neonatal severe hyperparathyroidism, and autosomal dominant hypocalcemia. Hum Mutat 2000; 16:281.

117. Chou YHW, Brown EM, Levi T, et al. The gene responsible for familial hypocalciuric hypercalcemia maps to chromosome 3q in four unrelated families. Nat Genet 1992; 1:295.

118. Heath H III, Jackson CE, Otterud B, Leppert MF. Genetic linkage analysis in familial benign (hypocalciuric) hypercalcemia: evidence for locus heterogeneity. Am J Hum Genet 1993; 53:193.

119. Trump D, Whyte M, Wooding C, et al. Linkage studies in a kindred from Oklahoma, with familial benign (hypocalciuric) hypercalcemia (FBH) and developmental elevations in serum parathyroid hormone levels, indicate a third locus for FBH. Hum Genet 1995; 96:183.

# CHAPTER 59

# NONPARATHYROID HYPERCALCEMIA

ANDREW F. STEWART

Primary hyperparathyroidism is the most common cause of hypercalcemia among nonhospitalized patients (see Chap. 58). This chapter focuses on nonparathyroid causes of hypercalcemia, the most common of which is malignancy.

Ionized extracellular fluid calcium has quantitatively important interfaces with four physiologic compartments: *serum proteins* (predominantly albumin), the *skeleton*, the *gastrointestinal tract*, and the *kidneys*. A disorder at the level of any one of these compartments may cause hypercalcemia. For example, a malignancy that is metastatic to the skeleton may cause hypercalcemia primarily through skeletal resorption (*resorptive hypercalcemia*). Alternatively, sarcoidosis appears to lead to hypercalcemia largely because of intestinal calcium hyperabsorption (*absorptive hypercalcemia*). Use of thiazide diuretics results in hypercalcemia mainly because of excessive renal calcium reabsorption (*renal hypercalcemia*). Finally, serum protein abnormalities may lead to elevations in total, but not ionized, serum calcium (*factitious hypercalcemia*). Combinations of renal, absorptive, resorptive, and protein-binding components all may contribute to a given patient's hypercalcemia. For example, hypercalcemia in a dehydrated patient with sarcoidosis may include all four components. Nevertheless, the grouping and conceptualization of the types of hypercalcemia into this pathophysiologic framework aids in both diagnosing and treating individual cases of hypercalcemia.

## SIGNS AND SYMPTOMS OF HYPERCALCEMIA

Hypercalcemia, through its effect on cellular sodium-potassium adenosine triphosphatase, leads to hyperpolarization of cell membranes. This hyperpolarization or refractoriness of cell membranes is particularly apparent in nervous and muscle tissue. Neurologic manifestations of hypercalcemia include the spectrum of *metabolic central nervous system dysfunction*, which involves apathy, drowsiness, and depression, progressing to obtundation and coma (see Chap. 200). Skeletal muscle and neurologic dysfunction may present as weakness (see Chap. 210). Smooth-muscle hyperpolarization may be manifest as bowel hypomotility and constipation. The most reproducible cardiac conduction abnormality is a shortening of the $QT_c$ interval.

Hypercalcemia interferes with vasopressin-induced urinary concentrating ability (see Chaps. 206 and 208). Thus, a clinical syndrome of nephrogenic diabetes insipidus is common in patients with hypercalcemia; it is manifested by polyuria, polydipsia, and dehydration. A reduced glomerular filtration rate is particularly common in patients with hypercalcemia. The azotemia is multifactorial, reflecting reductions in renal blood flow caused by nephrogenic diabetes insipidus–induced dehydration and hypercalcemia-induced afferent arteriolar vasoconstriction, as well as by nephrocalcinosis and, in some cases, obstructive uropathy resulting from nephrolithiasis. Nephrocalcinosis is particularly likely to occur in patients with nonparathyroid hypercalcemia, perhaps because their serum phosphate concentrations are normal to elevated in comparison to those of patients with primary hyperparathyroidism. Calcium phosphate salts are insoluble at alkaline pH values. Nephrocalcinosis is believed to result from calcium phosphate precipitation in the alkaline renal medulla. Calcium phosphate precipitation may occur in other alkaline environments, including the cornea (rarely observed on physical examination as band keratopathy), gastric mucosal cells, and the pancreas (leading to pancreatitis).

Gastrointestinal complaints such as nausea, anorexia, vomiting, abdominal pain, and constipation are common in patients with hypercalcemia (see Chap. 204). In the older literature, hypercalcemia was reported to be associated with peptic ulcer disease, particularly when primary hyperparathyroidism was present. This apparent correlation may relate to the coexistence of gastrin-secreting islet cell tumors with parathyroid adenomas or hyperplasia (multiple endocrine neoplasia type 1 [MEN1]), to related development of the milk-alkali syndrome, or to the simple coincidence of two common syndromes. The suggestion has been made that peptic ulcer disease may result from calcium-induced gastrin secretion or gastric acid hypersecretion.

# DIFFERENTIAL DIAGNOSIS OF HYPERCALCEMIA

Nonparathyroid disorders that may lead to hypercalcemia are listed in Table 59-1. The most common of these is malignancy, which is second in frequency only to primary hyperparathyroidism among ambulatory patients with hypercalcemia and is considerably more common than hyperparathyroidism among hospitalized patients with hypercalcemia.

## MALIGNANCY-ASSOCIATED HYPERCALCEMIA

Malignancy-associated hypercalcemia may arise through four general mechanisms: local osteolysis, humoral hypercalcemia of malignancy (HHM), excessive production of 1,25-dihydroxyvitamin D [$1,25(OH)_2D$], and paraneoplastic secretion of parathyroid hormone (PTH).

### LOCAL OSTEOLYTIC HYPERCALCEMIA

The first type of hypercalcemia to be well described clinically was that which accompanies multiple myeloma and breast cancer.[1] Most cases of lymphoma-induced hypercalcemia probably also belong in this group. This category comprises ~20% of patients with malignancy-associated hypercalcemia. Typically, affected patients display widespread skeletal tumor involvement as evidenced by radiographs, bone radionuclide scans, bone marrow biopsies, and postmortem examinations (Fig. 59-1). Histologically, the bone marrow space is infiltrated by tumor cells, and bone surfaces are lined by numerous active osteoclasts. Because of this histologic picture, tumor cells within the marrow space are widely believed to secrete local factors that stimulate osteoclastic bone resorption. With this apparent local mechanism in mind, these patients may be referred to as having local osteolytic hypercalcemia

**TABLE 59-1.**
**Nonparathyroid Causes of Hypercalcemia**

| Cause | Reference |
|---|---|
| **MALIGNANCY** | |
| Local osteolytic hypercalcemia | 1–21 |
| Humoral hypercalcemia of malignancy | 1–21 |
| 1,25-dihydroxyvitamin D–mediated hypercalcemia | 32–34 |
| Ectopic parathyroid hormone secretion | 35,36 |
| Unusual variants | 9,37 |
| **ENDOCRINOPATHIES** | |
| Thyrotoxicosis | 38–40 |
| Pheochromocytoma | 41–43 |
| Addisonian crisis | 44, 45 |
| VIPoma syndrome | 46 |
| **MEDICATIONS** | |
| Vitamins D and A (intoxication) | 47–54 |
| Lithium | 55–57 |
| Thiazide diuretics | 58,59 |
| Estrogens/antiestrogens | 60,61 |
| Growth hormone | 62,63 |
| Theophylline | 64 |
| Foscarnet | 65 |
| **GRANULOMATOUS DISORDERS** | |
| Sarcoidosis | 69,70,113 |
| Berylliosis | |
| Wegener granulomatosis | 114 |
| Tuberculosis | 68 |
| Histoplasmosis | 71 |
| Coccidioidomycosis | 115 |
| Nocardiasis | 116 |
| Candidiasis | 117 |
| Cat scratch fever | 118 |
| Eosinophilic granuloma | 119 |
| Crohn disease | 120 |
| Silicone implants, paraffin injection | 72,121 |
| **IMMOBILIZATION PLUS** | |
| Juvenile skeleton | 76,77 |
| Malignancy | |
| Paget disease | |
| Primary hyperparathyroidism | |
| Renal failure | |
| **MILK-ALKALI SYNDROME** | 80 |
| **PARENTERAL NUTRITION** | 81,83 |
| **FAMILIAL HYPOCALCIURIC HYPERCALCEMIA** | Chap. 58 |
| **HYPOPHOSPHATEMIA** | |
| **RENAL FAILURE** | 84 |
| **IDIOPATHIC HYPERCALCEMIA OF INFANCY** | Chap. 70 |
| **HYPERPROTEINEMIA** | 85,86 |
| **MANGANESE INTOXICATION** | 87,88 |
| **ADVANCED CHRONIC LIVER DISEASE** | 89 |

(LOH). The nature of the bone-resorbing or osteoclast-activating factors secreted by the tumor cells remains incompletely defined. Several factors have been proposed, including tumor necrosis factor α,[2] lymphotoxin,[3] interleukin-1,[4] PTH-related protein (PTHrP),[5–7] interleukin-6,[8] and prostaglandin $E_2$,[9] all of which stimulate osteoclastic bone resorption in in vitro systems. Direct bone resorption of devitalized bone in vitro also has been demonstrated by breast cancer cells.[10] Possibly, in some instances, tumors may directly phagocytose bone. Biochemical studies of patients with LOH characteristically reveal increases in fractional calcium excretion, normal or near-normal serum phosphate concentrations and renal phosphate threshold values, decreases in circulating immunoreactive PTH and $1,25(OH)_2D$ concentrations, and reductions in nephrogenous cyclic adenosine monophosphate (cAMP)

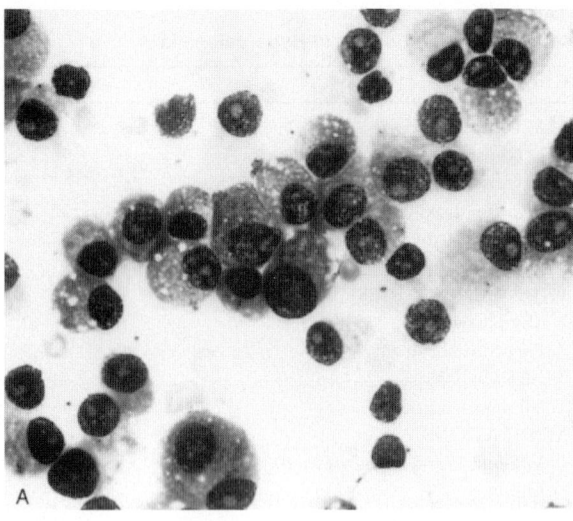

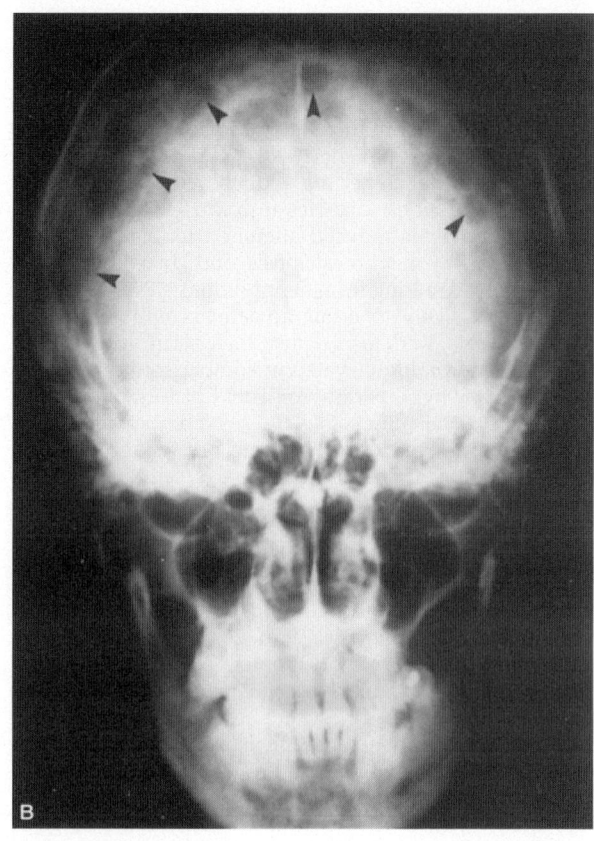

**FIGURE 59-1.** Multiple myeloma. **A,** Bone marrow aspirate showing extensive infiltration with myeloma cells. The cells and nuclei are of varying sizes. The nuclei are eccentrically placed, and the nucleoli are prominent. **B,** Skull radiograph of a hypercalcemic patient with multiple myeloma, showing multiple lytic lesions (*arrowheads*). (**A,** Courtesy of Dr. Geraldine P. Schecter.)

excretion[11,12] (Figs. 59-2 and 59-3). Bone resorption markers, such as hydroxyproline cross-links and N-telopeptide, are increased.[13]

### HUMORAL HYPERCALCEMIA OF MALIGNANCY

A second group of patients with malignancy-associated hypercalcemia includes those with HHM. This group comprises ~80% of patients with malignancy-associated hypercalcemia in unselected series.[11–15] The syndrome was first described in 1941. In contrast to the tumors encountered in patients with LOH,

those with HHM typically have squamous carcinomas of any site (including the head and neck, lung, esophagus, cervix, vulva, and skin); renal carcinomas; transitional carcinomas of the bladder; ovarian carcinomas; and human T-cell lymphoma/leukemia.[11–16] In addition, although skeletal metastases are the cause of hypercalcemia in most women with breast cancer, a significant minority (perhaps as many as 30%) have a humoral form of hypercalcemia.[17,18] The evidence that hypercalcemia is humoral in origin includes the observations that (a) these

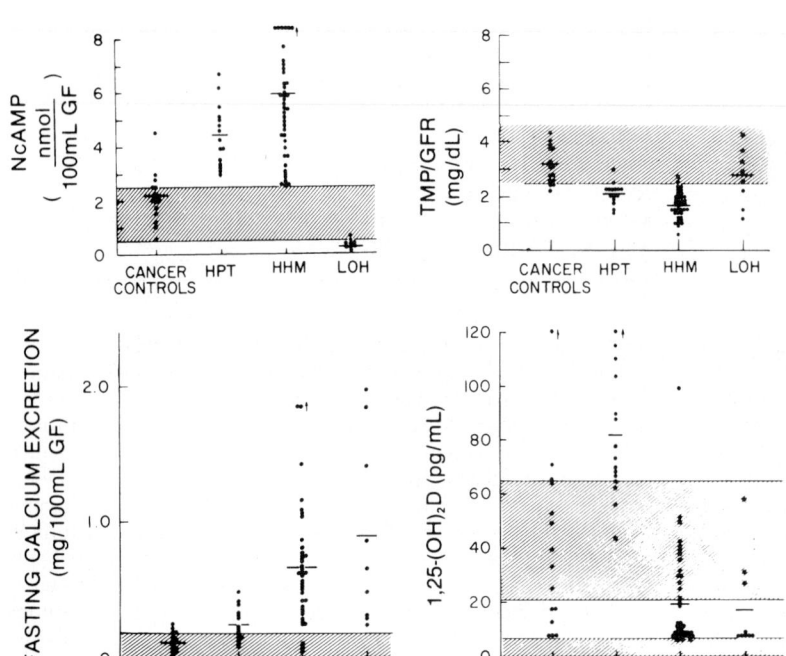

**FIGURE 59-2.** Biochemical profiles in patients with cancer and normal calcium values (cancer controls), patients with primary hyperparathyroidism (*HPT*), patients with humoral hypercalcemia of malignancy (*HHM*), and patients with local osteolytic hypercalcemia (*LOH*). (*NcAMP*, nephrogenous cyclic adenosine monophosphate excretion; *GF*, glomerular filtration; *TMP/GFR*, renal phosphorus threshold; *1,25(OH)₂D*, 1,25-dihydroxyvitamin D.) (Adapted from Stewart AF, Horst R, Deftos LJ, et al. Biochemical evaluation of patients with cancer-associated hypercalcemia: evidence for humoral and nonhumoral groups. N Engl J Med 1980; 303:1377.)

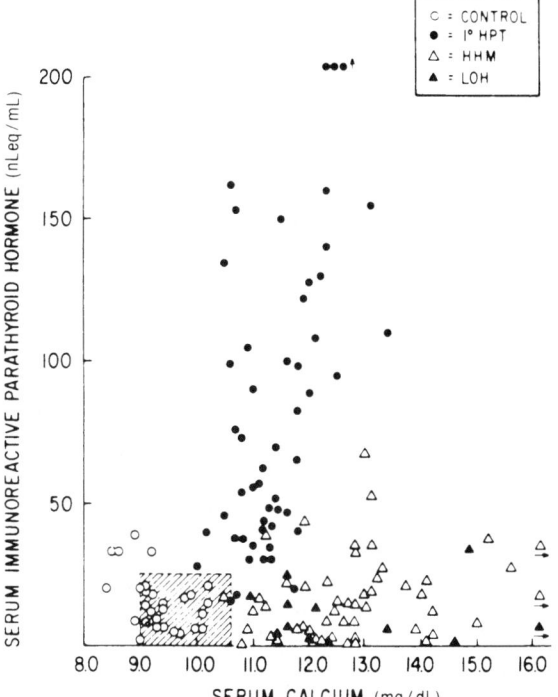

of phosphorus/glomerular filtration rate), accelerated osteoclastic bone resorption, and increases in nephrogenous (i.e., renal tubule–derived) cAMP excretion (see Figs. 59-2 and 59-3).[11,13,20] Unlike patients with primary hyperparathyroidism, however, patients with HHM display reductions in circulating concentrations of $1,25(OH)_2D$, reductions in immunoreactive PTH, and reductions of osteoblastic bone formation.[11,13,20] Markers of bone resorption (hydroxyproline, pyridinoline cross-links, N-telopeptide) are increased, whereas markers of bone formation (alkaline phosphatase, osteocalcin) are reduced.[13] Immunoreactive PTHrP concentrations in the circulation are elevated in HHM.[11,15,18] Although this point is controversial, patients with HHM appear to have a higher fractional excretion of calcium than do patients with primary hyperparathyroidism.[11,30] From a pathophysiologic standpoint, hypercalcemia results primarily from accelerated net bone resorption. Intestinal calcium absorption is reduced,[31] as would be predicted by the reduced plasma $1,25(OH)_2D$ concentrations.[11,13] Hypercalcemia occurs when the rate of calcium mobilization from the skeleton exceeds the ability of the kidney to clear this calcium load.

Although enormous progress has been made during the past decade in understanding the pathophysiology underlying HHM, three unanswered questions remain. First, why is osteoblastic activity uncoupled from the increase in osteoclastic activity in patients with HHM,[20] and why does this differ from the situation observed in patients with primary hyperparathyroidism, in whom a coupled increase occurs in both osteoblastic and osteoclastic activity?[20] Second, why are plasma $1,25(OH)_2D$ concentrations elevated in primary hyperparathyroidism but reduced in HHM?[11,13] Third, do differences truly exist in fractional calcium excretion and distal tubular calcium handling in patients with HHM and primary hyperparathyroidism,[11,30] and if so, why?

### EXCESSIVE PRODUCTION OF 1,25-DIHYDROXYVITAMIN D

A third subtype of malignancy-associated hypercalcemia has been defined in patients with lymphoma. Approximately 30 such patients have been described.[32–34] No clear unifying pattern of tumor histology is found. Circulating $1,25(OH)_2D$ concentrations in these patients are dramatically elevated (Fig. 59-4). The belief is that the serum $1,25(OH)_2D$ elevations result from excessive and unregulated conversion of circulating 25-hydroxyvitamin D [25(OH)D] to $1,25(OH)_2D$ by the lymphomatous tissue, and that the $1,25(OH)_2D$ elevations lead to hypercalcemia through intestinal calcium hyperabsorption and bone resorption. Nephrogenous cAMP excretion and serum PTH values are reduced.[32–34]

### PARANEOPLASTIC (ECTOPIC) SECRETION OF PARATHYROID HORMONE

As noted earlier, HHM was once thought to result almost exclusively from the ectopic secretion of PTH. With the advent of second-generation and third-generation PTH immunoassays and of molecular techniques for the measurement of PTH mRNA, it became apparent in the 1980s that HHM was not caused by ectopic secretion of PTH. The discovery of PTHrP and the development of sensitive and specific PTHrP immunoassays have now demonstrated that HHM results from systemic secretion of PTHrP by tumors. The concept of hyperparathyroidism due to ectopic secretion of PTH was abandoned.

Interestingly, however, seven cases of true ectopic secretion of PTH have been documented.[35,36] The tumors in these cases contained actual PTH mRNA and secreted authentic PTH. The tumors responsible were a small cell carcinoma of the lung, a small cell carcinoma of the ovary, a thymoma, a primitive neuroendocrine tumor, squamous carcinomas of the lung, and a clear cell carcinoma of the ovary. PTH levels declined with resection of the responsible tumors. In one case, the ectopic production of PTH was found to result from a gene rearrangement in tumor DNA that placed the coding region of the PTH gene under the control of a promoter for an ovarian gene product.[35]

**FIGURE 59-3.** Serum immunoreactive parathyroid hormone (*PTH*) levels obtained using a midregion PTH immunoassay in the patient groups described in Figure 59-2. Note that PTH concentrations correlate with the serum calcium concentration in patients with primary hyperparathyroidism (*HPT*) but not in patients with humoral hypercalcemia of malignancy (*HHM*) or local osteolytic hypercalcemia (*LOH*); also, although PTH values are "normal" in the two cancer hypercalcemia groups, they are indistinguishable, suggesting that the normal PTH values are related to immunoassay methodology and not physiology. (From Godsall JW, Burtis WJ, Insogna KL, et al. Nephrogenous cyclic AMP, adenylate cyclase-stimulating activity, and the humoral hypercalcemia of malignancy. Recent Prog Horm Res 1986; 42:705.)

patients typically display hypercalcemia in the setting of few or no skeletal metastases,[11,12] (b) hypercalcemia reverses with the resection of primary tumors (e.g., of the lung or kidney) that do not involve the skeleton,[19] and (c) skeletal biopsies from these patients reveal striking osteoclastic activation in the absence of tumor invasion of marrow.[20] From the initial description of this syndrome in 1941 through the early 1980s, the humoral factor responsible for this syndrome was variously believed to be PTH (causing "ectopic hyperparathyroidism" or "pseudohyperparathyroidism"), vitamin D–related phytosterols, or prostaglandins of the E series. It is now clear that the majority of cases of HHM result from overproduction of PTHrP by the tumor (see Chap. 52).[20a] The evidence that PTHrP causes HHM can be summarized as follows. First, PTHrP is produced by and has been purified from tumors associated with HHM.[21–24] Second, PTHrP is structurally homologous with PTH, binds to PTH receptors, and mimics the effects of PTH in bone and kidney.[21,25] Third, infusion of PTHrP into laboratory animals and humans reproduces the major features of the syndrome.[21,26,27] Fourth, PTHrP concentrations in the circulation are elevated in patients with HHM but not in patients with other types of hypercalcemia or in patients with cancer who do not have hypercalcemia.[14,15] Finally, the infusion of anti-PTHrP antisera into animals with HHM reverses the syndrome.[28,29]

Similar to patients with primary hyperparathyroidism, patients with HHM display hypercalcemia, a reduction in the renal phosphorus threshold (maximal rate of tubular resorption

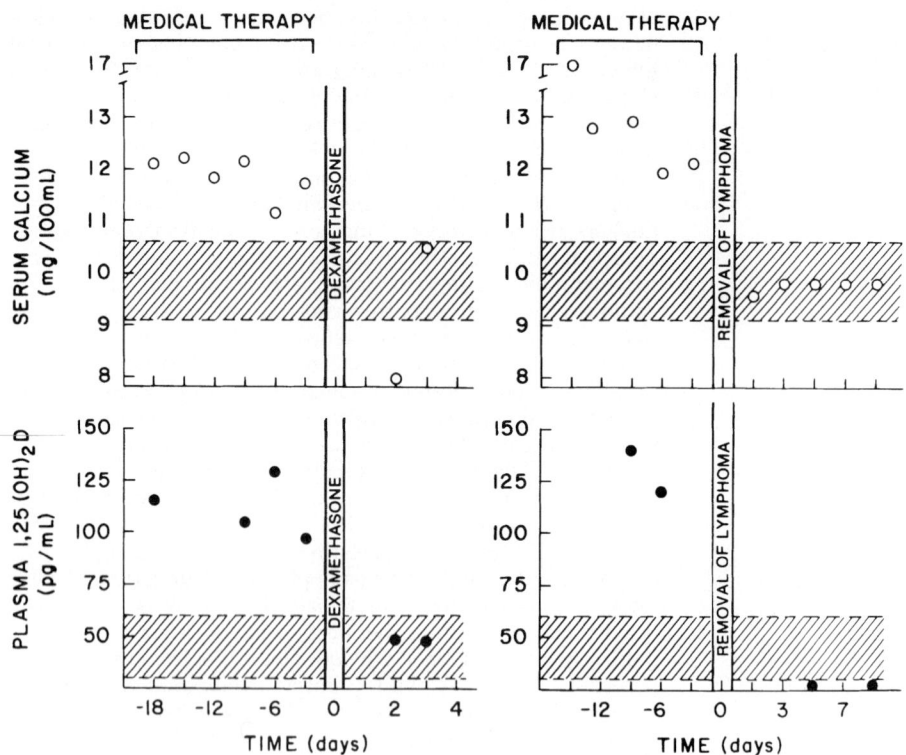

**FIGURE 59-4.** Serum calcium and plasma 1,25-dihydroxyvitamin D [*1,25(OH)₂D*] concentrations in two patients with lymphoma. Note that in contrast to patients with humoral hypercalcemia of malignancy and local osteolytic hypercalcemia (see Fig. 59-2), plasma 1,25(OH)₂D concentrations are strikingly elevated. These values reversed after glucocorticoid therapy in one patient (*left panel*) and resection of a solitary splenic lymphoma in the other patient (*right panel*). (From Rosenthal ND, Insogna KL, Godsall JW, et al. 1,25 dihydroxyvitamin D–mediated humoral hypercalcemia in malignant lymphoma. J Clin Endocrinol Metab 1985; 60:29.)

From a clinical standpoint, these observations have three implications. First, ectopic secretion of PTH, although extremely rare, does occur. Second, affected patients display elevations in circulating authentic PTH, even when measured by modern, highly specific PTH immunoassays. Third, this diagnosis should be considered before surgery in all patients with otherwise typical primary hyperparathyroidism and should be actively excluded in patients with primary hyperparathyroidism who have failed to respond to parathyroidectomy.

## MISCELLANEOUS CAUSES OF MALIGNANCY-ASSOCIATED HYPERCALCEMIA

In some cases of malignancy-associated hypercalcemia, the mechanism cannot be easily categorized. For example, the author has described a young woman with an ovarian dysgerminoma who had low nephrogenous cAMP values but who clearly had a humoral form of hypercalcemia of malignancy, because no bone metastases were apparent and her hypercalcemia reversed with resection of her tumor.[37]

Certain common tumors are rarely associated with hypercalcemia. Examples include adenocarcinomas of the prostate, colon, and stomach, and small cell carcinomas of the lung. The discovery of hypercalcemia in these patients should alert the physician to causes other than malignancy, to the presence of a second primary neoplasm, or to an incorrect histologic diagnosis.

Finally, hyperparathyroidism caused by a parathyroid adenoma or hyperplasia may coexist in a patient with cancer. Some authors have suggested that primary hyperparathyroidism actually is more common in patients with cancer than in the general population. In a study of 133 patients with malignancy and hypercalcemia, 8 proved to have primary hyperparathyroidism as the cause.[12]

## ENDOCRINOPATHIES ASSOCIATED WITH HYPERCALCEMIA

### THYROTOXICOSIS

Mild hypercalcemia, as assessed by ionized serum calcium measurement, occurs in as many as 47% of patients with thyrotoxicosis,[38,39] but total serum calcium values exceeding 11.0 mg/dL are rare. Commonly, the serum alkaline phosphatase level is increased. In a few cases, the patients have coexisting Graves disease and primary hyperparathyroidism, but usually thyrotoxicosis is believed to be the cause of the hypercalcemia. The circulating 1,25(OH)₂D level falls in thyrotoxicosis.[40] Because intestinal calcium absorption is reduced and osteoclastic activity is increased in hyperthyroidism, high circulating levels of thyroxine and triiodothyronine are believed to produce hypercalcemia through excessive osteoclastic activity. In these patients, β-adrenergic blockade may reduce the hypercalcemia. The diagnosis is established when the hypercalcemia reverses with successful treatment of the hyperthyroidism.

### PHEOCHROMOCYTOMA

Patients with pheochromocytoma may have mild to severe hypercalcemia.[41–43] The mechanisms responsible for this hypercalcemia may theoretically include (a) hyperparathyroidism occurring as part of the MEN2A syndrome, (b) hyperparathyroidism occurring as a result of catecholamine-mediated PTH secretion from the parathyroid glands, (c) ectopic PTH secretion from the pheochromocytoma, (d) catecholamine-induced bone resorption, and (e) secretion by the pheochromocytoma of PTHrP. Among these possibilities, strong evidence exists to support only the first and the last. In pheochromocytoma, hypercalcemia caused by primary hyperparathyroidism in the context of the MEN2A syndrome has been reported most commonly. In these patients, as expected, hypercalcemia persists after the resection of the adrenal tumor; however, a few patients with pheochromocytoma have been described whose hypercalcemia reversed after surgery.

From a clinical standpoint, patients discovered to have hypercalcemia and a pheochromocytoma should have the pheochromocytoma resected before consideration of parathyroidectomy, because the hypercalcemia rarely reverses after adrenalectomy, and performance of a parathyroidectomy in a patient with a pheochromocytoma may result in hypertensive crisis. As a corollary, patients with hypertension who have well-documented primary hyperparathyroidism should be screened for a pheochromocytoma before parathyroidectomy for these same reasons (see Chaps. 86 and 188).

## ADDISONIAN CRISIS

Mild hypercalcemia has been described rarely in patients with addisonian crisis.[44,45] Their hypercalcemia usually is mild (11.0–12.0 mg/dL) and could be the result of hemoconcentration and hyperalbuminemia. Rehydration and glucocorticoid therapy readily normalize the serum calcium level. In some patients, excessive renal calcium resorption, caused by dehydration and enhanced skeletal mobilization, may be present.[45] Most of these patients were described several decades ago when tuberculosis was the predominant cause of adrenal insufficiency; this raises the interesting, but undocumented, possibility that the glucocorticoid-reversible hypercalcemia was related not to adrenal insufficiency but to tuberculosis.

## VASOACTIVE INTESTINAL PEPTIDE–SECRETING TUMORS

Benign and malignant islet cell tumors that secrete vasoactive intestinal peptide (VIP) present with a characteristic clinical picture including watery diarrhea, hypokalemia, and achlorhydria (VIPoma syndrome, pancreatic cholera, or WDHA syndrome; see Chap. 220). Approximately 50% of these patients have hypercalcemia, which occasionally is severe.[46] Although the hypercalcemia may result from primary hyperparathyroidism occurring as part of the MEN1 syndrome, the fact that it sometimes reverses with surgical resection of the VIPoma suggests that VIP or another islet cell product is responsible.

## MEDICATIONS

### VITAMIN D

Vitamin D intoxication is an unusual but frequently overlooked cause of hypercalcemia.[47,48] The dosage of vitamin D required to produce hypercalcemia is large, usually at least 50,000 U three times weekly. This dose is available only by prescription (most multivitamins contain 400 U per tablet); thus, vitamin D intoxication usually occurs inadvertently in the setting of vitamin D therapy for osteoporosis, hypoparathyroidism, or renal osteodystrophy. It also may occur in patients taking self-administered megavitamin therapy. Moreover, vitamin D intoxication may occur in patients receiving any of the available analogs of vitamin D, such as $1,25(OH)_2D$ (see Chap. 54). Vitamin D intoxication resulting from excessive addition of vitamin D to milk also may occur.[49,50] Frequently, hypercalcemia in patients with vitamin D intoxication goes unrecognized, with the symptoms of nausea, vomiting, lethargy, and weakness being attributed to a viral syndrome. Hence, patients being treated with pharmacologic dosages of vitamin D should be warned of the possibility of hypercalcemia should flu-like symptoms develop.

In vitamin D toxicity, hypercalcemia develops largely because of excessive intestinal calcium absorption; however, accelerated bone resorption also plays a role, because patients with vitamin D intoxication are in negative calcium balance, and vitamin D is known to resorb bone in vitro. Decreased renal clearance of calcium also is important in most patients with vitamin D intoxication because of hypercalcemia-induced reduction in the glomerular filtration rate.

The diagnosis of vitamin D intoxication is made on clinical grounds. Because dosages of vitamin D sufficient to cause hypercalcemia can be obtained only by prescription, most patients who are vitamin D intoxicated are taking their vitamin D for osteoporosis, hypoparathyroidism, or chronic renal failure in excessive dosages or at too frequent dosing intervals. In all patients taking pharmacologic dosages of vitamin D, plasma concentrations of $25(OH)D$ are markedly elevated, regardless of the serum calcium value, and thus may not be diagnostic. Plasma $1,25(OH)_2D$ concentrations are not markedly elevated in patients with vitamin D intoxication and often are normal or low, as would be expected in the setting of reduced circulating

PTH concentrations. Azotemia may be present, and the serum phosphate value may be normal or increased. The serum alkaline phosphatase level is normal. A diagnosis of vitamin D intoxication is secured when hypercalcemia reverses with hydration, a low-calcium diet, and glucocorticoid therapy, and does not recur after dosage reduction or discontinuation of therapy with the offending vitamin D compound. Hypercalcemia usually reverses rapidly (within days) in patients intoxicated with $1,25(OH)_2D$ after use of the medication is discontinued, reflecting its short biologic half-life. Conversely, hypercalcemia may persist for weeks after the discontinuation of vitamin D use, reflecting accumulation in, and prolonged release from, adipose tissue.

### VITAMIN A

Hypercalcemia has been described in rare patients with vitamin A intoxication.[51,52] Usually, these persons have ingested vitamin A at a dosage of 50,000 IU per day for weeks to months. The recommended daily allowance is 5000 IU per day. The serum alkaline phosphatase concentration may be elevated. Although this syndrome has been reported only rarely in the past, the current widespread use of vitamin A from health food stores and of vitamin A congeners such as *cis*-retinoic acid in dermatologic disorders[53] and chemotherapy[54] suggests that it may be encountered more frequently in the future. Vitamin A is presumed to cause hypercalcemia through excessive bone resorption; *cis*-retinoic acid causes bone resorption in vitro. The diagnosis is made on clinical grounds, with heavy reliance on a history of excessive vitamin A intake, associated findings (alopecia, dermatitis, hepatic dysfunction), and reversal of hypercalcemia after cessation of vitamin intake. Measurements of circulating vitamin A and retinyl ester are useful to establish the diagnosis.

### LITHIUM

Lithium therapy has been associated with hypercalcemia.[55–57] In one study from Denmark, 12 of 96 patients taking lithium were noted to have hypercalcemia. In vitro and in vivo evidence suggests that lithium may alter the parathyroid cell setpoint for PTH secretion. Cessation of lithium therapy completely reverses the hypercalcemia in many patients. The hypercalcemia persists in other patients, however, and primary hyperparathyroidism eventually is diagnosed. Although the hypercalcemia encountered in these patients is mild (10.5–11.5 mg/dL), the question usually arises as to whether this mild hypercalcemia is contributing to, or perpetuating, the psychiatric symptoms and findings that originally required the lithium therapy. This can be resolved only by discontinuing or reducing the dosage of lithium.

### THIAZIDE DIURETICS

Use of thiazide diuretics (but not loop diuretics) has been associated with mild hypercalcemia.[58] Cessation of thiazide therapy reverses the hypercalcemia in many cases, although it persists in some patients. Thiazide diuretics stimulate renal tubular calcium reabsorption, a finding that has led to their use in the treatment of "renal leak" hypercalciuria and hypoparathyroidism. However, the kidney is not likely to be the only organ involved in thiazide-mediated hypercalcemia, because hypercalcemia may develop in anephric patients treated with chlorthalidone.[59] As with lithium-induced hypercalcemia, the diagnosis is confirmed by the reversal of hypercalcemia after the cessation of thiazide therapy.

### ESTROGENS AND ANTIESTROGENS

Estrogen and antiestrogen therapy causes hypercalcemia in as many as one-third of patients with breast cancer.[60,61] This "estrogen flare" hypercalcemia apparently occurs only in the setting of extensive skeletal metastases. Interestingly, if the hypercalcemia can be controlled with hydration and other measures, and administration of the estrogen/antiestrogen can be continued, a hypercalcemic response to estrogen/antiestrogen therapy may be a favorable predictor of response to hormonal therapy. The mechanism of the estrogen/antiestrogen flare remains obscure, but it usually responds to hydration, diuresis, and administration of glucocorticoids and agents that inhibit bone resorption.

### GROWTH HORMONE

Growth hormone anabolic therapy used in the setting of the intensive care unit (in treatment of burns, respiratory failure, poor wound healing) or in the treatment of acquired immuno-deficiency syndrome (AIDS) has been associated with hypercalcemia in the 11 to 12 mg/dL range.[62,63]

### THEOPHYLLINE

Large doses of theophylline, used in the treatment of asthma, have caused hypercalcemia. The specific mechanism is unknown.[64]

### FOSCARNET

Foscarnet is an antiviral agent used in the AIDS setting. It has been reported to cause hypercalcemia.[65]

### GRANULOMATOUS DISORDERS

Each of the granulomatous diseases listed in Table 59-1 has been associated with hypercalcemia. Other granulomatous diseases (e.g., chronic granulomatous disease of the young, Crohn disease), however, have not. Clearly $1,25(OH)_2D$ not only is involved in mineral metabolism but also is a lympho-kine produced by, and acting on, subsets of T cells, B cells, and macrophages.[66,67] Although the normal immunologic role of $1,25(OH)_2D$ has been only partially characterized, excessive systemic production of $1,25(OH)_2D$ is clearly a feature of tuberculosis,[68] sarcoidosis[69,70] (Fig. 59-5), histoplasmosis,[71] the granulomatous reaction to silicone implants,[72] and other granulomatous disorders (see Table 59-1). In contrast to the normal situation, in which the renal conversion of circulating $25(OH)D$ to $1,25(OH)_2D$ is tightly regulated, in patients with these granulomatous disorders, $1,25(OH)_2D$ production appears to be largely, and perhaps exclusively, substrate dependent. Thus, exposure to even small amounts of dietary vitamin D or to solar or other ultraviolet radiation leads to the expected physiologic increase in circulating $25(OH)D$, which is then converted in an unregulated fashion to $1,25(OH)_2D$. Although in most of the examples cited, evidence for this extrarenal conversion is inferential, direct conversion of $25(OH)D$ to $1,25(OH)_2D$ has been demonstrated by sarcoidosis-derived pulmonary alveolar macrophages[73] and by lymph node homogenates.[74] Hypercalcemia appears to result from $1,25(OH)_2D$-mediated intestinal calcium hyperabsorption, $1,25(OH)_2D$-mediated bone resorption (patients may remain hypercalcemic and hypercalciuric on very-low-calcium diets), and hypercalcemia-induced reductions in the glomerular filtration rate.

Because of the increases in $1\alpha$-hydroxylase activity [the enzyme that converts $25(OH)D$ to $1,25(OH)D$], patients with these disorders may be exquisitely sensitive to small increases in dietary vitamin D intake, to sunlight or other forms of ultraviolet radiation, and to dietary calcium intake. Patients with granuloma-induced $1,25(OH)_2D$ elevations appear to be, from a physiologic standpoint, the benign equivalent of those with $1,25(OH)_2D$-secreting malignant lymphomas. Generally, patients with these disorders have widespread pulmonary and extra-pulmonary disease, and the diagnosis is obvious at presentation. Exceptions do exist, however. The author's practice is to measure circulating $1,25(OH)_2D$ values in patients with unexplained hypercalcemia. If the values are elevated, and if other causes for $1,25(OH)_2D$ elevation (lymphoma, primary hyperparathyroidism, pregnancy, absorptive hypercalciuria) are not apparent, then a systematic search for pulmonary, renal, hepatic, ocular, and bone marrow granulomas is made. Occasionally, a glucocorticoid suppression test is warranted to exclude primary hyperparathyroidism (i.e., failure of the calcium to be suppressed to normal levels in patients with hyperparathyroidism).[75] If this is done, care should be taken to establish a stable baseline; that is, serum calcium values should be monitored and should be stable for 3 to 4 days before glucocorticoid administration is begun. In this test, hydrocortisone is administered orally, 40 mg every 8 hours for 10 days, and a serum calcium evaluation is performed each morning.

### IMMOBILIZATION

Weightlessness (as occurs in space flight) and complete immobilization (as occurs in spinal cord injury and other neuromuscular disorders, extensive casting for skeletal fractures, or prolonged bed rest associated with a chronic debilitating illness) regularly lead to calcium mobilization from the skeleton. Hypercalcemia rarely occurs in patients whose underlying bone turnover rate is normal or low. However, in persons with elevated bone turnover rates, such as young adults, adolescents, and children[76–78]; rare patients with Paget disease (who have focal increases in bone turnover); patients with malignancy with or without bone metastases; and patients with primary or secondary hyperparathyroidism, immobilization can produce or aggravate hypercalcemia. An example of the latter would be an elderly woman with mild primary hyperparathyroidism (serum calcium value, 10.6 mg/dL) who becomes bedridden and develops further hypercalcemia (serum calcium value, 12 or 13 mg/dL).

As with hypercalcemia occurring in other settings, hypercalcemia associated with immobilization may present as lethargy and depression. In a young adult with quadriplegia, the depression may be misinterpreted as an appropriate psychologic response to a devastating injury, and the hypercalcemia may go undetected and untreated. In particular, abdominal pain syndromes caused by hypercalcemia may be difficult to evaluate in patients with spinal cord injury and have led to unnecessary laparotomy.

Immobilization leads to rapid demineralization of the skeleton. In young adults who are completely immobilized, as much as 30% of the skeleton may be lost in the first few weeks to

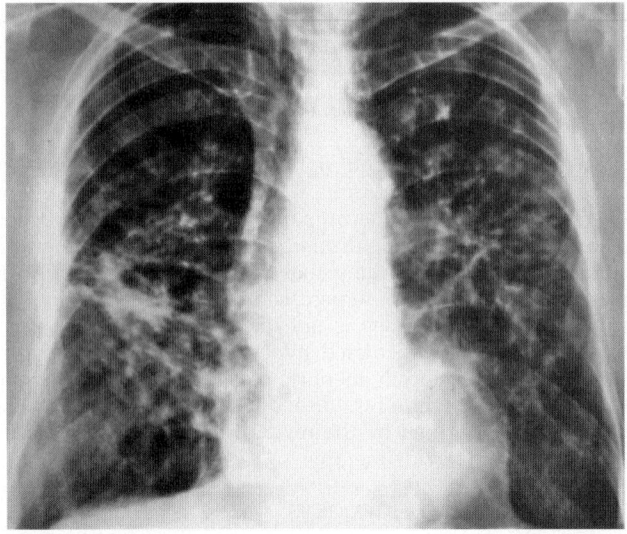

**FIGURE 59-5.** Radiograph of a patient with sarcoidosis and hypercalcemia. A typical-appearing, diffuse, bilateral, reticulonodular infiltrate is seen, predominantly in the midlung regions.

months. Although the mechanism by which immobilization leads to accelerated bone resorption remains unclear, bone histologic studies have shown that it is associated with an increase in osteoclastic activity and a decrease in osteoblastic activity.[79] This uncoupling of bone cell activity is reminiscent of that encountered in malignancy-associated hypercalcemia, and explains the hypercalcemia, hypercalciuria, increased urinary hydroxyproline excretion, and normal circulating alkaline phosphatase values typically encountered in these patients. Interestingly, previous parathyroidectomy appears to prevent skeletal mineral loss in animal models of immobilization, suggesting that the skeleton must be primed by PTH for immobilization to be followed by increases in osteoclastic activity. Bone resorption continues for as long as 12 to 18 months and then ceases spontaneously, despite continued immobilization.

Nephrolithiasis (infection or triple phosphate stones) is a frequent finding in patients with spinal cord injury. This occurs in part because of urinary tract infections resulting from stasis and long-term or intermittent bladder catheterization, regardless of whether hypercalcemia is present. The incidence of nephrolithiasis among patients with spinal cord injuries, both for infection stones and for calcium oxalate stones, is higher in those who have hypercalciuria than in those who do not.[78]

In immobilization-induced hypercalcemia, parathyroid function is suppressed, as indicated by measurement of low circulating immunoreactive PTH and $1,25(OH)_2D$ concentrations and by low nephrogenous cAMP excretion.[76] The diagnosis is made in the presence of the biochemical findings just described, together with a clinical picture of complete immobilization.

## MILK-ALKALI SYNDROME

Hypercalcemia was described in the 1920s as a result of peptic ulcer treatment regimens that included excessive amounts of milk or cream (gallons per day) and absorbable antacids such as sodium bicarbonate.[80,81] The original milk-alkali syndrome presented as moderate to severe hypercalcemia associated with advanced renal failure, hyperphosphatemia, and a systemic alkalosis. This variety of milk-alkali syndrome has largely disappeared, as this form of antiulcer regimen has disappeared. In more modern times, hypercalcemia has occurred principally in people taking large quantities of absorbable calcium-containing antacids for the treatment of esophagitis or peptic symptoms. Typically, patients report having taken > 4 g of elemental calcium per day in the form of calcium carbonate tablets (e.g., 200-mg tablets) or liquid calcium carbonate antacids. In contrast to the $1,25(OH)_2D$–regulated intestinal absorption of calcium that occurs when dietary calcium intake is normal (~1000 mg per day), ingestion of large amounts of dietary calcium can lead to passive, unregulated, and inappropriate calcium absorption.

This latter variety of milk-alkali syndrome is frequently overlooked by physicians for two reasons. First, patients often fail to volunteer the fact that they are using large amounts of calcium carbonate, because they do not consider it a medication. Second, physicians fail to specifically ask patients with hypercalcemia if they are using antacids.

Hypercalcemia leads to polyuria, polydipsia, mental status changes, dehydration, prerenal reductions in the glomerular filtration rate; if hypercalcemia, hyperphosphatemia, and dehydration persist, nephrocalcinosis and permanent renal impairment may occur. The diagnosis is made by excluding other causes of hypercalcemia and documenting calcium intakes in excess of 4 g per day of elemental calcium. Treatment includes the discontinuation of the calcium antacid, hydration, and education regarding the large amounts of calcium that can be ingested unintentionally.

## PARENTERAL NUTRITION

Hypercalcemia may develop in two groups of patients receiving parenteral hyperalimentation. The first group includes patients in whom hypercalcemia develops while they are receiving large amounts (>300 mg per day) of intravenous calcium, particularly when renal compromise is present. In this group, a reduction in parenteral calcium administration reverses the hypercalcemia and hypercalciuria. In the second group of patients, hypercalcemia may develop after long-term parenteral hyperalimentation, despite only modest parenteral calcium administration, and hypercalcemia and hypercalciuria may persist after the cessation of parenteral calcium administration.[81–83] Affected patients may have symptomatic bone disease, and most have a histologic picture on bone biopsy that is suggestive of osteomalacia. Osteomalacia in these patients may result in part from aluminum intoxication. Aluminum has been delivered to these patients in the past through antacids and as a component of the amino-acid hydrolysates used in parenteral nutrition preparations. With the recognition of aluminum intoxication in these patients and the elimination of aluminum from hyperalimentation solutions, this syndrome appears to be disappearing.

## FAMILIAL HYPOCALCIURIC HYPERCALCEMIA

The hypercalcemia that occurs in patients with familial hypocalciuric hypercalcemia, also known as *familial benign hypercalcemia* (see Chap. 58), has been attributed to diminished renal calcium clearance (excessive tubular reabsorption of calcium) as well as failure of parathyroid gland calcium sensing, both occurring most commonly as a result of inactivating mutations in the calcium-sensing receptor.[83a]

## HYPOPHOSPHATEMIA

In animals, hypophosphatemia leads to osteoclast stimulation, inhibition of mineralization, hypercalciuria, and hypercalcemia. This is true even when animals have been rendered vitamin D deficient and surgically hypoparathyroid. In humans, severe hypophosphatemia leads to hypercalciuria, presumably reflecting both increases in osteoclastic activity and hypophosphatemia-induced increases in renal $1,25(OH)_2D$ production, with consequent enhanced intestinal calcium absorption. Although hypercalcemia resulting exclusively from hypophosphatemia has *not* been described in humans, it seems likely that when hypophosphatemia complicates hypercalcemia of any cause, it exacerbates the hypercalcemia. Hypophosphatemia is particularly common among patients with hypercalcemia, regardless of the underlying cause, for the following reasons: Food intake may be reduced due to vomiting or anorexia; dietary phosphorus absorption may be limited by the use of phosphate-binding antacids; hypercalcemia per se is phosphaturic; PTH and PTHrP reduce the renal phosphate threshold; and agents that are used to treat hypercalcemia (calcitonin, loop diuretics, saline infusion) induce phosphaturia.

## RENAL FAILURE

Hypercalcemia has been described occasionally in patients with acute tubular necrosis, especially during the polyuric phase. In one careful study of patients with acute tubular necrosis resulting from rhabdomyolysis, patients initially were hypocalcemic because of severe hyperphosphatemia but later became hypercalcemic with the reversal of oliguria and hyperphosphatemia.[84] The hypercalcemia was transient and may have resulted from (a) mobilization of soft-tissue calcium phosphate salts deposited during the early hyperphosphatemic period, and (b) rebound hypercalcemia from the transiently elevated PTH and $1,25(OH)_2D$ values that occurred during the early hypocalcemic period.

Hypercalcemia often develops in patients with chronic renal failure who are receiving hemodialysis. Hypercalcemia is difficult to evaluate in such patients because the usual biochemical values [renal phosphate and calcium excretion, serum PTH, serum $1,25(OH)_2D$, and nephrogenous cAMP] are difficult to interpret in this setting. Nevertheless, reductions in dietary calcium intake and vitamin D supplements may correct the hypercalcemia, a result which suggests that increased intestinal calcium absorption in the face of diminished renal clearance may account for hypercalcemia in some patients. Immobilization of patients receiving hemodialysis may lead to hypercalcemia, presumably through acceleration of the underlying high rates of bone turnover. Tertiary hyperparathyroidism (the evolution of autonomous parathyroid-dependent hypercalcemia in patients with renal failure and chronic secondary hyperparathyroidism) may occur. Dialysis against a high-calcium bath also may lead to hypercalcemia. Finally, hypercalcemia may occur as part of the aluminum bone disease that forms an important aspect of renal osteodystrophy.

## IDIOPATHIC HYPERCALCEMIA OF INFANCY

The complex of disorders known as *idiopathic hypercalcemia of infancy* is discussed in Chapter 70.

## HYPERPROTEINEMIA

Hyperalbuminemia may lead to hypercalcemia because albumin is the major circulating calcium-binding protein. The hypercalcemia is usually mild, and patients in whom the diagnosis is suspected generally are severely dehydrated. Rapid rehydration often corrects the hypercalcemia before careful biochemical evaluation can be performed. In practice, this form of hypercalcemia can be diagnosed by the determination of a normal ionized calcium value in a patient with mildly elevated total serum calcium values, markedly elevated serum albumin levels, and none of the other causes for hypercalcemia listed in Table 59-1.

Rarely, patients with multiple myeloma have been described who display elevations in the total serum calcium concentration (sometimes striking elevations) but normal ionized calcium values.[85,86] This factitious hypercalcemia is caused by unusual immunoglobulins with an extremely high binding capacity for calcium. Hypercalciuria, electrocardiographic changes, and symptoms of hypercalcemia are absent in these unusual patients. Although hypercalcemia caused by a myeloma calcium-binding protein is unusual, it should be considered before attributing hypercalcemia in patients with multiple myeloma to the more common cause, osteolytic bone disease.

## MANGANESE INTOXICATION

Hypercalcemia has been reported to occur in patients with manganese intoxication.[87,88] Exposure to manganese in doses sufficient to cause intoxication has been reported in miners, in welders, and in people drinking water from manganese-contaminated wells. The mechanisms responsible for the development of hypercalcemia are uncertain. The hypercalcemia may be mild (e.g., 11.5 mg/dL) or severe (e.g., 20 mg/dL).

## ADVANCED CHRONIC LIVER DISEASE

Mild to severe hypercalcemia has been described in one series of 11 patients with advanced chronic liver disease awaiting liver transplantation.[89] All the patients had severe jaundice (the mean serum bilirubin value was 28.7 mg/dL), and most had hypoalbuminemia and prolonged prothrombin times and were in mild renal failure (the mean serum creatinine level was 2.8 mg/dL). Hypercalcemia was associated with normal to reduced plasma $1,25(OH)_2D$, $25(OH)D$, and PTH concentrations. Ionized serum calcium values were elevated. The cause of the syndrome appeared to be multifactorial, reflecting contri-

butions from renal failure, immobilization, total parenteral nutrition, and vitamin D supplementation.

## TREATMENT OF HYPERCALCEMIA

Principles of therapy for hypercalcemia should be based on an understanding of its cause, knowledge of its pathophysiology, and careful assessment of the symptom complex in individual patients. The treatment of mild hypercalcemia in a patient with asymptomatic primary hyperparathyroidism (i.e., without nephrolithiasis or apparent skeletal disease) is controversial (see Chap. 58). Similarly, mild hypercalcemia associated with thyrotoxicosis requires no treatment because it resolves spontaneously with treatment of the hyperthyroidism. The hypercalcemia in patients with familial hypocalciuric hypercalcemia almost always is asymptomatic and requires no therapy. Some may argue that severe hypercalcemia in a comatose patient with terminal cancer is best left untreated.

The treatment of hypercalcemia in a patient with significant symptomatology may be an urgent problem. The severity of symptoms of hypercalcemia can be related to the absolute calcium concentration; the rate of development of hypercalcemia (the faster the increase, the greater the symptoms); and the duration of the hypercalcemia. These points, as well as the patient's overall status and prognosis, should be considered before commencing therapy.

Therapy is best determined with an understanding of the pathophysiology of a given patient's hypercalcemia. For example, the absorptive hypercalcemia of sarcoidosis is best treated with dietary calcium restriction, whereas the resorptive hypercalcemia of immobilization and malignancy is most appropriately treated with measures aimed at diminishing osteoclastic activity.

Specific treatment of most of the disorders listed in Table 59-1 is self-evident. Therapy for the hypercalcemia associated with primary hyperparathyroidism, renal osteodystrophy, and neonatal disorders is discussed in Chapters 58, 61, and 70, respectively. Treatment of the underlying disorder responsible for hypercalcemia is an obvious, but frequently overlooked, goal, particularly in patients with malignancy-associated hypercalcemia. In these patients, antitumor therapy should be planned and initiated early in the hospital course, because other measures are effective only transiently and may be associated with toxicity. Usually, long-term control of malignancy-associated hypercalcemia can be accomplished only by successful antitumor therapy.

## SALINE INFUSION

Renal calcium excretion is enhanced by saline infusion, because of both the increase in glomerular filtration rate and the role of the filtered load of sodium in blocking proximal tubular calcium reabsorption.[90] The rate of infusion should be adjusted to the clinical situation. The uncertain cardiovascular status of these patients, many of whom are elderly, dictates caution. Infusion rates of 200 to 400 mL per hour of 0.9% saline are commonly used. The status of hydration should be checked frequently by physical signs (rales, skin turgor, mucous membrane hydration, blood pressure) and by hemodynamic monitoring when appropriate. Aggressive saline infusion may lead to hypokalemia, hypophosphatemia, and hypomagnesemia. These ions should be measured and replaced as necessary.

## LOOP DIURETICS

Loop diuretics appear to inhibit calcium reabsorption at the level of the thick ascending limb of the Henle loop.[90] In theory, use of agents such as *furosemide* should enhance the calciuresis of a saline infusion. Furosemide in dosages of 40 mg or more, given intravenously or orally, is widely used for this purpose. This drug should not be administered to dehydrated patients until rehydration is complete, because it may further reduce the glomerular filtration rate and, thereby, reduce the filtered load of calcium, decreasing renal calcium clearance even more. The drug is particularly useful if the patient has coexistent congestive heart failure. Again, careful surveillance of a patient's fluid, electrolyte, and renal status during therapy is critical.

## RESTRICTION OF CALCIUM AND VITAMIN D INTAKE

Dietary calcium and vitamin D restriction and avoidance of exposure to sunlight and other ultraviolet light sources is appropriate in patients with absorptive causes of hypercalcemia, such as sarcoidosis and other granulomatous diseases during their active stages.[90] Dietary calcium intake should be kept at <400 mg per day, the use of vitamin D supplements should be discontinued, and the patient should be advised to limit sun exposure as much as possible. These same guidelines probably apply to the occasional patient with 1,25(OH)$_2$D-mediated hypercalcemia associated with lymphoma.[32–34] Similarly, vitamin D intoxication and the milk-alkali syndrome should be treated with dietary calcium restriction.

Conversely, dietary calcium intake should not be reduced in patients with primarily resorptive, that is, malignancy-associated, hypercalcemia. Plasma 1,25(OH)$_2$D values are reduced in these patients, and dietary calcium absorption is inefficient. Unpalatable calcium-restricted diets are unnecessary and may further the nutritional deterioration and general misery of these patients.

## CALCITONIN

Most causes of acute hypercalcemia requiring aggressive treatment are related to accelerated bone resorption. Therefore, agents that inhibit osteoclastic function are important aspects of therapy. Bone resorption in vivo and in vitro can be inhibited by calcitonin. Calcitonin use has been disappointing in treating moderate to severe hypercalcemia because it does not work in all patients. The decrease in serum calcium is generally small, and most patients escape from the osteoclast-inhibiting effects of calcitonin in several days. Furthermore, the treatment is extremely expensive.[90,91] Nevertheless, given its low incidence of side effects and the rapidity with which the serum calcium level falls after administration of the hormone (2 to 4 hours), it is useful in some clinical settings. The dosage of salmon calcitonin suggested by the manufacturer is 4 IU/kg every 12 hours given subcutaneously or intramuscularly. Patients should undergo skin testing for hypersensitivity before use, as described in the package insert. Although interest has been shown in, and an argument made for, the synergistic effects of calcitonin and glucocorticoids, evidence supporting the efficacy of a combined regimen is not compelling (see Chap. 53).

## PLICAMYCIN

Plicamycin (Mithramycin) was once a staple of hypercalcemia management, but it has now largely been replaced by the bisphosphonates. It inhibits osteoclastic bone resorption in a predictable and impressive fashion.[90,92] Its mechanism of action on bone cells is unknown. The nadir in serum calcium after a dose of plicamycin occurs at ~48 hours. The usual dosage is 25 µg/kg given intravenously over 4 to 6 hours, repeated as necessary every 2 to 7 days. Despite the reliability and efficacy of plicamycin, its use may be limited by the associated toxicity in the form of transaminase elevations, proteinuria, azotemia, bone marrow suppression, or a failure of platelet aggregation. These side effects were more commonly reported in the older literature describing the use of larger dosages of plicamycin.[93] They occur rarely when the lower dosage is used for a limited duration. Patients without liver, bone marrow, or renal problems generally tolerate the agent well. In patients with preexisting disease of the marrow, kidney, or liver, if the agent is used at all, the dosage should be decreased to 12.5 µg/kg and the number of repeated infusions should be minimized. Plicamycin is best reserved for patients with moderate to severe hypercalcemia that threatens the central nervous system or renal function and for whom bisphosphonates are not an option. Most often, it is used in patients with malignancy-associated hypercalcemia. It also has been used in patients with acute primary hyperparathyroidism, patients with parathyroid carcinoma, and patients with severe Paget disease who have normal or elevated calcium levels, to limit bone resorption.

## GLUCOCORTICOIDS

Glucocorticoids have classically been used in the treatment of hypercalcemia associated with multiple myeloma, lymphoma, breast cancer, Addison disease, granulomatous disorders, and vitamin D intoxication.[75,90,94] The oral dosages used have been ~25 mg of cortisone acetate to as high as 20 mg of prednisone, or their parenteral equivalents, given 3 to 4 times per day. The hypocalcemic response may take 7 to 10 days to become apparent. The mechanism of response to glucocorticoids includes "tumorlytic" (or "granulomalytic") effects, inhibition of 1α-hydroxylase activity (in granulomatous disorders and lymphomas), direct inhibition of intestinal calcium transport (independent of corticosteroid effects on vitamin D metabolism), and inhibition of osteoclastic activity. Side effects of glucocorticoids (demineralization, generalized catabolic effects, immunosuppression), the slow response time, and interference with chemotherapeutic regimens have made these agents only moderately useful in treating patients with malignancy-associated hypercalcemia. Glucocorticoids do not reverse PTH-mediated hypercalcemia. Whether they are effective in treating HHM, mediated by PTHrP, remains an open question.[75]

## PHOSPHORUS

Phosphorus depletion exacerbates the hypercalcemia associated with most of the disorders described in Table 59-1. For this reason, if hypophosphatemia occurs, it should be corrected in patients with hypercalcemia using oral phosphorus. Detailed guidelines for phosphorus repletion have been reported.[95] Generally, in hospitalized patients with malignancy-associated hypercalcemia, 250 mg (8 mmol) of phosphorus is given orally four times a day if the serum phosphate value is <3.0 mg/dL. The use of phosphate-binding antacids should be discontinued if possible. Meticulous care should be taken in following up serum calcium, phosphate, and creatinine values in patients with hypercalcemia who are treated with phosphorus preparations, because renal failure resulting from calcium phosphate precipitation (nephrocalcinosis) may occur abruptly. The use of phosphorus should be discontinued at the first sign of a rise in creatinine values or when serum phosphate values exceed 4.0 mg/dL. Oral phosphorus should be used with similar caution in the treatment of outpatients with hypercalcemia caused by primary hyperparathyroidism (see Chap. 58).

Intravenous phosphorus has been used in patients with malignancy-associated hypercalcemia, usually with dramatic decreases in serum calcium levels but frequently with the abrupt onset of renal failure.[96] Intravenous phosphorus administration is potentially dangerous and should be reserved for the rare patients with life-threatening hypercalcemia who cannot be treated using any other approach. Again, great care should be taken in following up serum calcium, phosphate, and creatinine values, and the minimum dose required to normalize the serum phosphate level should be administered.

## BISPHOSPHONATES

The treatment of HHM, LOH, and parathyroid carcinoma has been facilitated by the advent of bisphosphonate therapy.[90,97–99] Originally used as industrial detergents, bisphosphonates were found to inhibit osteoclastic bone resorption, the predominant or sole pathophysiologic mechanism underlying hypercalcemia of malignancy. The cellular mechanism responsible for this inhibition is not clear. The bisphosphonates are pyrophosphate analogs with a P-C-P bond that is resistant to hydrolysis by alkaline phosphatase. They bind to hydroxyapatite in bone. Bisphosphonates are poorly absorbed from the gastrointestinal tract (only 1–2% of an oral dose is absorbed) and, thus, are more effective when given intravenously. In the United States, two bisphosphonates, etidronate (1-hydroxy-ethylidene bisphosphonic acid) and pamidronate (3-amino-1-hydroxypropylidene bisphosphonic acid), are available for intravenous administration for malignancy-associated hypercalcemia. Pamidronate enjoys wider usage because of its single-day dosing and its greater potency.

Unlike etidronate, pamidronate,[100–103] a second-generation bisphosphonate, does not inhibit bone mineralization or increase phosphate levels at dosages in the therapeutic range. It is 100-fold more potent than etidronate and can be given intravenously in 250 mL of saline or 5% dextrose over the course of 4 to 24 hours in doses of 60 or 90 mg. The serum calcium concentration begins to decline 1 to 2 days after the infusion, with the nadir occurring 3 to 6 days later. Normocalcemia may last for 1 to 8 weeks.[91] The most common side effect is a transient fever (1°C to 2°C above normal) beginning 24 to 48 hours after the infusion and lasting up to 3 days. This effect is usually observed only after the first dose. Rarely, first-dose effects of leukopenia and lymphopenia may occur. Hypophosphatemia, hypomagnesemia, and mild hypocalcemia may occur.

Several newer, more potent bisphosphonates are under development and will become available for clinical use in the next several years. Their relative lack of side effects, together with their reliability and effectiveness, make the bisphosphonates the therapeutic agents of choice in most patients with malignancy-associated hypercalcemia.

## GALLIUM NITRATE

Gallium nitrate, originally used as an antineoplastic agent, was found incidentally to cause hypocalcemia in previously normocalcemic patients.[104–106] Although the drug appears to be effective, the need for continuous intravenous infusion and the potential for nephrotoxicity limit its use.

## OTHER MEASURES

To the extent that an immobilized patient can perform *active weight-bearing exercise*, this is desirable. The response to mobilization in such patients may be rapid (within days) and dramatic.

If parenteral calcium is being administered to patients with hypercalcemia, it should be withdrawn; in this regard, the presence of calcium supplements in parenteral hyperalimentation solutions is frequently overlooked.

*Hemodialysis* and *peritoneal dialysis* may cause dramatic reductions in serum calcium levels in patients with hypercalcemia who are in renal failure, particularly when low-calcium or zero-calcium dialysate is used.[107–109] Although most patients with malignancy-associated hypercalcemia are not candidates for dialysis, a few are. Dialysis also has been used to treat patients in hypercalcemic crisis, including patients with severe primary hyperparathyroidism.[109]

*Prostaglandin synthetase inhibitors* (aspirin and indomethacin) have been used to treat malignancy-associated hypercalcemia. Although prostaglandins clearly are important in bone metabolism, the use of the inhibiting agents in hypercalcemia has been disappointing.[110]

Several *experimental therapies for hypercalcemia* are being examined. Ethiophos (WR-2721) is a chemoprotective agent that has inhibitory effects on bone resorption and on PTH secretion.[111] Thionaphthene-2-carboxylic acid and related compounds, which also appear to inhibit bone resorption, have been shown to reverse hypercalcemia in a rat model of HHM.[112]

## REFERENCES

1. Gutman AB, Tyson TL, Gutman EB. Serum calcium, inorganic phosphatase activity in hyperparathyroidism, Paget's disease, multiple myeloma and neoplastic disease of the bones. Arch Intern Med 1936; 57:379.
2. Thompson BM, Mundy GR, Chambers TJ. Tumor necrosis factors alpha and beta induce osteoblastic cells to stimulate osteoclastic bone resorption. J Immunol 1987; 138:775.
3. Garrett RI, Durie BGM, Nedwin GE, et al. Production of the bone resorbing cytokine lymphotoxin by cultured human myeloma cells. N Engl J Med 1987; 317:526.
4. Cozzolino F, Torcia M, Aldinucci D, et al. Production of interleukin-1 by bone marrow myeloma cells. Blood 1989; 74:387.
5. Firkin F, Seymour JF, Watson AM, et al. Parathyroid hormone-related protein in hypercalcemia associated with hematological malignancy. Br J Hematol 1996; 94:486.
6. Horiuchi T, Miyachi T, Arai T, et al. Raised plasma concentrations of parathyroid hormone–related protein in hypercalcemic multiple myeloma. Horm Metab Res 1997; 29:469.
7. Guise TA, Yin JJ, Taylor SD, et al. Evidence for a causal role of parathyroid hormone-related protein in the pathogenesis of human breast cancer-mediated osteolysis. J Clin Invest 1996; 98:1544.
8. Bataille R, Jourdan M, Zhang X-G, Klein B. Serum levels of interleukin-6, a potent myeloma cell growth factor, as a reflection of disease in plasma cell dyscrasias. J Clin Invest 1989; 84:2008.
9. Metz SA, McRae JR, Robertson RP. Prostaglandins as mediators of paraneoplastic syndromes. Metabolism 1981; 30:299.
10. Eilon G, Mundy GR. Direct resorption of bone by human breast cancer cells in vitro. Nature 1978; 276:726.
11. Stewart AF, Horst R, Deftos LJ, et al. Biochemical evaluation of patients with cancer-associated hypercalcemia: evidence for humoral and non-humoral groups. N Engl J Med 1980; 303:1377.
12. Godsall JW, Burtis WJ, Insogna KL, et al. Nephrogenous cyclic AMP, adenylate cyclase-stimulating activity, and the humoral hypercalcemia of malignancy. Recent Prog Horm Res 1986; 40:705.
13. Nakayama K, Fukumoto S, Takeda S, et al. Differences in bone and vitamin D metabolism between primary hyperparathyroidism and malignancy-associated hypercalcemia. J Clin Endocrinol Metab 1996; 81:607.
14. Burtis WJ, Brady TG, Orloff JJ, et al. Immunochemical characterization of circulating parathyroid hormone-related protein in patients with humoral hypercalcemia of malignancy. N Engl J Med 1990; 322:1106.
15. Budayr AA, Nissenson RA, Klein RF, et al. Increased serum levels of a parathyroid hormone–like protein in malignancy-associated hypercalcemia. Ann Intern Med 1989; 111:807.
16. Motokura T, Fukumoto S, Matsumoto T, et al. Parathyroid hormone–related protein in adult T-cell leukemia-lymphoma. Ann Intern Med 1989; 111:484.
17. Isales C, Carcangiu ML, Stewart AF. Hypercalcemia in breast cancer: a reassessment of the mechanism. Am J Med 1987; 82:1143.
18. Grill V, Ho P, Body JJ, et al. Parathyroid hormone-related protein: elevated levels in both humoral hypercalcemia of malignancy and hypercalcemia complicating metastatic breast cancer. J Clin Endocrinol Metab 1991; 73:1309.
19. Plimpton CH, Gellhorn A. Hypercalcemia in malignant disease without evidence of bone destruction. Am J Med 1956; 21:750.
20. Stewart AF, Vignery A, Silvergate A, et al. Quantitative bone histomorphometry in humoral hypercalcemia of malignancy: uncoupling of bone cell activity. J Clin Endocrinol Metab 1982; 55:219.
20a. Rabbani SA. Molecular mechanism of action of parathyroid hormone related peptide in hypercalcemia of malignancy: therapeutic strategies. Int J Oncol 2000; 16:197.
21. Halloran BD, Nissenson BP. Parathyroid hormone-related protein: normal physiology and its role in cancer. Boca Raton, FL: CRC Press, 1992.
22. Burtis WJ, Wu T, Bunch C, et al. Identification of a novel 17,000 dalton PTH-like adenylate cyclase stimulating protein from a tumor associated with humoral hypercalcemia of malignancy. J Biol Chem 1987; 262:7151.
23. Moseley JM, Kubota M, Diefenbach-Jagger H, et al. Parathyroid hormone-related protein purified from a human lung cancer cell line. Proc Natl Acad Sci U S A 1987; 84:5048.
24. Strewler GJ, Stern PH, Jacobs JW, et al. Parathyroid hormone-related protein from human renal carcinoma cells. J Clin Invest 1987; 80:1803.
25. Orloff JJ, Reddy DR, dePapp AE, et al. Parathyroid hormone-related protein as a prohormone: posttranslational processing and receptor interactions. Endocr Rev 1994; 15:40.

26. Stewart A, Mangin M, Wu T, et al. A synthetic human parathyroid hormone-like protein stimulates bone resorption and causes hypercalcemia in rats. J Clin Invest 1988; 81:596.
27. Everhart-Caye M, Inzucchi SE, Guinness-Henry J, Mitnick MA, Stewart AF. Parathyroid hormone-related protein(1-36) is equipotent with parathyroid hormone(1-34) in humans. J Clin Endocrinol Metab 1996; 81:199
28. Kukreja SC, Shevrin DH, Wimbiscus SA, et al. Antibodies to PTH-related protein lower serum calcium in athymic mouse models of malignancy-associated hypercalcemia due to human tumors. J Clin Invest 1988; 82:1798.
29. Henderson J, Bernier S, D'Amour, et al. Effect of passive immunization against PTH-like peptide and PTH in hypercalcemia tumor-bearing rats and normocalcemic controls. Endocrinology 1990; 127:1310.
30. Bonjour J-P, Phillipe J, Guelpa G. Bone and renal components in hypercalcemia of malignancy and response to a single infusion of clodronate. Bone 1988; 9:123.
31. Coombes RC, Ward MK, Greenberg PB, et al. Calcium metabolism in cancer. Cancer 1976; 38:211.
32. Breslau NA, McGuire JL, Zerwekh JR, et al. Hypercalcemia associated with increased serum calcitriol levels in three patients with lymphoma. Ann Intern Med 1984; 100:1.
33. Rosenthal NR, Insogna KL, Godsall JW, et al. 1,25 dihydroxyvitamin D-mediated humoral hypercalcemia in malignant lymphoma. J Clin Endocrinol Metab 1985; 60:29.
34. Adams JS, Fernandez M, Gacad MA, et al. Vitamin D metabolite–mediated hypercalcemia and hypercalcemia in patients with AIDS- and non-AIDS-associated lymphoma. Blood 1989; 73:235.
35. Nussbaum SR, Gaz RD, Arnold A. Hypercalcemia and ectopic secretion of parathyroid hormone by an ovarian carcinoma with rearrangement of the gene for PTH. N Engl J Med 1990; 323:1324.
36. Nielsen PK, Rasmussen AK, Feldt-Rasmussen U, et al. Ectopic production of intact parathyroid hormone by a squamous cell lung carcinoma in vivo and in vitro. J Clin Endocrinol Metab 1996; 81:3793.
37. Stewart AF, Broadus AE, Schwartz PE, et al. Hypercalcemia in gynecologic neoplasms. Cancer 1982; 49:2389.
38. Burman KD, Monchik JM, Earll JM, Wartofsky L. Ionized and total serum calcium and parathyroid hormone in hyperthyroidism. Ann Intern Med 1976; 84:668.
39. Ross DS, Nussbaum SR. Reciprocal changes in parathyroid hormone and thyroid function after radioiodine treatment of hyperthyroidism. J Clin Endocrinol Metab 1989; 68:1216.
40. Peerenboom H, Keck E, Kruskeniper HL, Strohmeyer G. The defect in intestinal calcium transport in hyperthyroidism and its response to therapy. J Clin Endocrinol Metab 1984; 59:936.
41. Stewart AF, Hoecker J, Segre GV, et al. Hypercalcemia in pheochromocytoma: evidence for a novel mechanism. Ann Intern Med 1985; 102:276.
42. Miller SS, Sizemore GW, Sheps SG, Tyce GM. Parathyroid function in patients with pheochromocytoma. Ann Intern Med 1975; 82:372.
43. Mune T, Katakami H, Kato Y. Production and secretion of PTH-related protein in pheochromocytoma. J Clin Endocrinol Metab 1993; 76:757.
44. Pederson KO. Hypercalcemia in Addison's disease. Acta Med Scand 1967; 181:691.
45. Muls E, Bouillon R, Boelart J, et al. Etiology of hypercalcemia in a patient with Addison's disease. Calcif Tissue Int 1982; 34:523.
46. Verner JV, Morrison AB. Endocrine pancreatic islet disease with diarrhea. Arch Intern Med 1974; 133:492.
47. Haussler MR, McCain TA. Basic and clinical concepts related to vitamin D metabolism and action. N Engl J Med 1977; 297:974.
48. Markowitz ME, Rosen JF, Smith C, DeLuca HF. 1,25-Dihydroxyvitamin $D_3$-treated hypoparathyroidism: 35 patient years in 10 children. J Clin Endocrinol Metab 1982; 55:727.
49. Jacobus CH, Holick MF, Shao Q. Hypervitaminosis D associated with drinking milk. N Engl J Med 1992; 326:1173.
50. Holick MF, Shau Q, Liu WW, Chen TC. The vitamin D content of fortified milk and infant formula. N Engl J Med 1992; 326:1178.
51. Hofman KJ, Milne FJ, Schmidt C. Acne, hypervitaminosis A, and hypercalcemia. S Afr Med J 1978; 54:579.
52. Ragavan W, Smith JE, Bilezikian JP. Vitamin A toxicity and hypercalcemia. Am J Med Sci 1982; 283:161.
53. Valente JP, Elias AN, Weinstein GD. Hypercalcemia associated with oral isotretinoin in the treatment of severe acne. JAMA 1983; 250:1899.
54. Villablanca JG, Khan AA, Avramis VI, et al. Phase I trial of *cis*-retinoic acid in children with neuroblastoma following bone marrow transplantation. J Clin Oncol 1995; 13:894.
55. Christiansen C, Baastrup PC, Lindgreen P, Transbol I. Endocrine effects of lithium. Acta Endocrinol (Copenh) 1978; 88:528.
56. Spiegel AM, Rudorfer MV, Marx SJ, Linnoila M. The effect of short-term lithium administration on suppressibility of parathyroid hormone secretion by calcium in vivo. J Clin Endocrinol Metab 1984; 59:354.
57. Haden ST, Stoll AL, McCormick S, et al. Alterations in parathyroid dynamics in lithium-treated subjects. J Clin Endocrinol Metab 1997; 82:2844.
58. Porter RH, Cox BG, Heaney D, et al. Treatment of hypoparathyroid patients with chlorthalidone. N Engl J Med 1978; 298:577.
59. Koppel MH, Massry SG, Shinaberger JH, et al. Thiazide-induced rise in serum calcium and magnesium in patients on maintenance hemodialysis. Ann Intern Med 1970; 72:895.
60. Legha SS, Powell K, Buzdar AU, Blumenachein GR. Tamoxifen-induced hypercalcemia in breast cancer. Cancer 1981; 47:2803.
61. Valentin-Opran A, Eilon G, Saez S, Mundy GR. Estrogens and antiestrogens stimulate release of bone resorbing activity in cultured human breast cancer cells. J Clin Invest 1985; 75:726.
62. Knox JB, Demling RH, Wilmore DW, Sarraf P, Santos AA, Hypercalcemia associated with the use of growth hormone in an adult surgical intensive care unit. Arch Surg 1995; 130:442.
63. Sakoulas G, Tritos NA, Lally M, et al. Hypercalcemia in an AIDS patient treated with growth hormone. AIDS 1997; 11:1353.
64. McPherson SR, Prince SR, Atamer ER, et al. Theophylline-induced hypercalcemia. Ann Intern Med 1986; 105:52.
65. Gayet S, Ville E, Durand JM, et al. Foscarnet-induced hypercalcemia in AIDS. AIDS 1997; 11:1068.
66. Tsoukas CD, Provvedini DM, Manolagas SC. 1,25-Dihydroxyvitamin $D_3$: a novel immunoregulatory hormone. Science 1984; 224:1438.
67. Amento EP. Vitamin D and the immune system. Steroids 1987; 49:55.
68. Gkonos PJ, London R, Hendler ED. Hypercalcemia and elevated 1,25$(OH)_2$D levels in a patient with end stage renal disease and active tuberculosis. N Engl J Med 1984; 311:1683.
69. Adams JS, Singer FR, Gacad MA, et al. Isolation and structural identification of 1,25-dihydroxyvitamin D produced by cultured alveolar macrophages in sarcoidosis. J Clin Endocrinol Metab 1985; 60:960.
70. Peris P, Font J, Grau JM, et al. Calcitriol-mediated hypercalcemia and increased interleukins in a patient with sarcoid myopathy. Clin Rheumatol 1999; 18:488.
71. Murray JJ, Helm CR. Hypercalcemia in disseminated histoplasmosis. Am J Med 1985; 78:881.
72. Kozemy GA, Barbato AL, Bansal VK, et al. Hypercalcemia associated with silicone-induced granulomas. N Engl J Med 1984; 311:1103.
73. Adams JS, Sharma OP, Gacad MA, Singer FR. Metabolism of 25-hydroxyvitamin $D_3$ by cultured pulmonary alveolar macrophages in sarcoidosis. J Clin Invest 1983; 72:1856.
74. Mason RS, Frankel TI, Chan YL, et al. Vitamin D conversion by sarcoid lymph node homogenate. Ann Intern Med 1984; 100:59.
75. Watson L, Moxham J, Fraser P. Hydrocortisone suppression test and discriminant analysis in differential diagnosis of hypercalcemia. Lancet 1980; 1:1320.
76. Stewart AF, Alder M, Byers CM, et al. Calcium homeostasis in immobilization: an example of resorptive hypercalciuria. N Engl J Med 1982; 306:1136.
77. Bergstrom WH. Hypercalciuria and hypercalcemia complicating immobilization. Am J Dis Child 1978; 132:553.
78. Tori JA, Kewalramani LS. Urolithiasis in children with spinal cord injury. Paraplegia 1979; 16:357.
79. Minaine P, Meunier P, Edouard C, et al. Quantitative histological data on disuse osteoporosis. Calcif Tissue Res 1974; 17:57.
80. Beall DP, Scofield H. Milk-alkali syndrome associated with calcium carbonate consumption. Medicine 1995; 74-89.
81. Klein GL, Horst RL, Norman AW, et al. Reduced serum 1,25-dihydroxyvitamin D during long-term total parenteral nutrition. Ann Intern Med 1981; 94:638.
82. Shike M, Sturtridge WC, Tam CS, et al. A possible role of vitamin D in the genesis of parenteral nutrition-induced metabolic bone disease. Ann Intern Med 1981; 95:560.
83. Ott SM, Maloney NA, Klein GL, et al. Aluminum is associated with low bone formation in patients receiving chronic parenteral nutrition. Ann Intern Med 1983; 98:910.
83a. Schwarz P, Larsen NE, Lonborg Friis IM, et al. Familial hypocalciuric hypercalcemia and neonatal severe hyperparathyroidism associated with mutations in the human $Ca^{2+}$-sensing receptor gene in three Danish families. Scand J Clin Lab Invest 2000; 60:221.
84. Llach F, Felsenfeld AJ, Haussler MR. The pathophysiology of altered calcium metabolism in rhabdomyolysis-induced acute renal failure. N Engl J Med 1981; 305:117.
85. Merlini G, Fitzpatrick IA, Siris ES, et al. A human myeloma immunoglobulin G binding four moles of calcium associated with asymptomatic hypercalcemia. J Clin Immunol 1984; 4:185.
86. John R, Oleesky D, Issa B, et al. Pseudohypercalcemia in two patients with IgM paraproteinemia. Ann Clin Biochem 1997; 34:694.
87. Chandra SV, Seth PK, Mankeshu JK. Manganese poisoning: clinical and biochemical observations. Environ Res 1974; 7:374.
88. Chandra SV, Shukla GS, Srivastava RS. An exploratory study of manganese exposure to welders. Clin Toxicol 1981; 18:407.
89. Gerhardt A, Greenberg A, Reilly JJ, Van Theil DH. Hypercalcemia: a complication of advanced chronic liver disease. Arch Intern Med 1987; 147:274.
90. Yang KH, Stewart AF. Treatment of hypercalcemia. In: Mazzaferri EL, Bar RS, Kreisberg RA, eds. Advances in endocrinology and metabolism, vol 4. St. Louis: Mosby, 1993:305.
91. Binstock ML, Mundy GR. Effect of calcitonin and glucocorticoids in combination on the hypercalcemia of malignancy. Ann Intern Med 1980; 93:269.
92. Perlia CP, Gubisch NJ, Cootter J, et al. Mithramycin treatment of hypercalcemia. Cancer 1970; 25:389.
93. Kennedy BJ. Metabolic and toxic effects of mithramycin during tumor therapy. Am J Med 1970; 49:494.
94. Zerwekh JE, Pak CYC, Kaplan RA, et al. Pathogenic role of 1,25 dihydroxyvitamin D in sarcoidosis and absorptive hypercalciuria: different response to prednisolone therapy. J Clin Endocrinol Metab 1980; 51:381.
95. Lentz RD, Brown DM. Treatment of severe hypophosphatemia. Ann Intern Med 1978; 89:941.
96. Goldsmith RS, Ingbar SH. Inorganic phosphorus in the treatment of hypercalcemia of diverse etiologies. N Engl J Med 1966; 274:1.
97. Bilezikian JP. Management of hypercalcemia. J Clin Endocrinol Metab 1993; 77:1445.

98. Bilezikian JP. Management of acute hypercalcemia. N Engl J Med 1992; 326:1196.

99. Body JJ. Current and future directions in medical therapy: hypercalcemia. Cancer 2000; 88(12 Suppl):3054.

100. Fitton A, McTavish D. Pamidronate: a review of its pharmacological properties and therapeutic efficacy in resorptive bone disease. Drugs 1991; 41:289.

101. Thiebaud D, Jaeger PH, Jacquet AF, et al. Dose-response in the treatment of hypercalcemia of malignancy by a single infusion of the bisphosphonate AHPrBP. J Clin Oncol 1988; 6:762.

102. Nussbaum SR, Younger J, VandePol CJ, et al. Single-dose intravenous therapy with pamidronate for the treatment of hypercalcemia of malignancy: comparison of 30-, 60-, and 90-mg dosages. Am J Med 1993; 95:297.

103. Gucalp R, Ritch P, Wiernik PH, et al. Comparative study of pamidronate disodium and etidronate disodium in the treatment of cancer-related hypercalcemia. J Clin Oncol 1992; 10:134.

104. Todd PA, Fitton A. Gallium nitrate: a review of its pharmacological properties and therapeutic potential in cancer-related hypercalcemia. Drugs 1991; 42:261.

105. Warrell RP, Isreal R, Frisone M, et al. Gallium nitrate for acute treatment of cancer-related hypercalcemia. A randomized, double blind comparison to calcitonin. Ann Intern Med 1988; 108:669.

106. Warrell RP, Murphy WK, Schulman P, et al. A randomized double-blind study of gallium nitrate compared with etidronate for acute control of cancer-related hypercalcemia. J Clin Oncol 1991; 9:1467.

107. Hegbrun PJ, Selby PL, Peacock M, et al. Peritoneal dialysis in the management of severe hypercalcemia. Mayo Clin Proc 1980; 280:525.

108. Bayat-Moktari F, Palmieri GMA, Momuddin M, Pourmand R. Parathyroid storm. Arch Intern Med 1980; 140:1092.

109. Kaiser W, Biesenbach G, Kramar R, Zazgornik J. Kalziumfreie hamodialyse-stellenwert in der therapie der hyperkalzamischen krise. Klin Wochenschr 1989; 67:86.

110. Brenner DE, Harvey HA, Lipton A, Demers L. A study of prostaglandin E₂, parathormone and response to indomethacin in patients with hypercalcemia of malignancy. Cancer 1982; 49:556.

111. Glover DJ, Shaw L, Glick JH, et al. Treatment of hypercalcemia in parathyroid cancer with WR-2721, S-2(3-aminopropylamino)ethyl-phosphorothiotic acid. Ann Intern Med 1985; 103:55.

112. Johannssen AJ, Onkelinx C, Rodan GA, Raisz LR. Thionaphthene-2-carboxylic acid: a new antihypercalcemic agent. Endocrinology 1985; 117:1508.

113. Zeimer HJ, Greenaway TM, Slavin J, et al. Parathyroid hormone–related protein in sarcoidosis. Am J Pathol 1998; 152:17.

114. Bosch X, Lopez-Soto A, Morello A, et al. Vitamin D metabolite–mediated hypercalcemia in Wegener's granulomatosis. Mayo Clin Proc 1997; 72:440.

115. Lee JC, Catanzaro A, Parthemore JG, et al. Hypercalcemia in disseminated coccidiomycosis. N Engl J Med 1977; 297:431.

116. Dockrell D, Poland G. Hypercalcemia in a patient with hypoparathyroidism and *Nocardia asteroides* infection. Mayo Clin Proc 1997; 72:757.

117. Kantarjian HM, Saad MR, Estey EH, et al. Hypercalcemia in disseminated candidiasis. Am J Med 1983; 74:721.

118. Bosch X. Hypercalcemia due to endogenous overproduction of active vitamin D in identical twins with cat-scratch disease. JAMA 1998; 279:532.

119. Jurney TH. Hypercalcemia in a patient with eosinophilic granuloma. Am J Med 1984; 76:527.

120. Bosch X. Hypercalcemia due to endogenous overproduction of 1,25-dihydroxyvitamin D in Crohn's disease. Gastroenterology 1998; 114:1061.

121. Albitar S, Genin R, Fen-Chong M, et al. Multisystem granulomatous injuries 28 years after paraffin injections. Nephrol Dial Transplant 1997; 12:1974.

## HYPOALBUMINEMIA

Albumin is the major calcium-binding serum protein, and hypoalbuminemia, rather than a decrease in the concentration of ionized calcium, accounts for most cases of low total serum calcium in hospitalized patients. Because reliable direct measurement of ionized serum calcium is not always readily available, a number of algorithms based on albumin or total protein concentrations[2,3] have been proposed for the "correction" of total serum calcium. None of these correction factors should be regarded as absolutely accurate, but they are useful as general indicators of the concentration of ionized calcium in serum. One widely used algorithm estimates that total serum calcium declines by ~0.8 mg/dL for each 1-g/dL decrease in albumin concentration, without a change in ionized calcium.

## IONIZED AND BOUND FRACTIONS

Sudden changes in the distribution of calcium between ionized and bound fractions may cause symptoms of hypocalcemia, even in patients who have normal hormonal mechanisms for the regulation of the ionized calcium concentration. Increases in the extracellular fluid concentration of anions such as phosphate, citrate, bicarbonate, or edetic acid increase the proportion of bound calcium and decrease ionized calcium until intact regulatory mechanisms normalize ionized calcium. Extracellular fluid pH also affects the distribution of calcium between ionized and bound fractions. Acidosis increases the ionized calcium, whereas alkalosis decreases it.[1]

## EFFECTS OF PARATHYROID HORMONE AND VITAMIN D

The concentration of extracellular ionized calcium is tightly regulated by parathyroid hormone (PTH) and 1,25-dihydroxyvitamin D [1,25(OH)₂D; calcitriol]. PTH has direct effects on bone to regulate calcium exchange at osteocytic sites and to enhance osteoclast-mediated bone resorption. In the kidney, PTH directly enhances distal tubular reabsorption of calcium, decreases the proximal tubular reabsorption of phosphate, and stimulates the metabolic conversion of 25-hydroxyvitamin D [25(OH)D] to 1,25(OH)₂D, the active vitamin D metabolite (Fig. 60-1). The 1,25(OH)₂D acts on bone to enhance bone resorption and on the gastrointestinal mucosa to increase absorption of dietary calcium (see Chaps. 49 and 54). Clinical disorders causing hypocalcemia

# CHAPTER 60

# HYPOPARATHYROIDISM AND OTHER CAUSES OF HYPOCALCEMIA

SUZANNE M. JAN DE BEUR, ELIZABETH A. STREETEN, AND MICHAEL A. LEVINE

## MECHANISMS OF HYPOCALCEMIA

Calcium is present in serum in three forms: *bound* to serum protein (40–45%), *complexed* to inorganic anions (5–10%), and *ionized* (~45–50%).[1] Although total serum calcium is most commonly measured, the ionized fraction is most important physiologically.

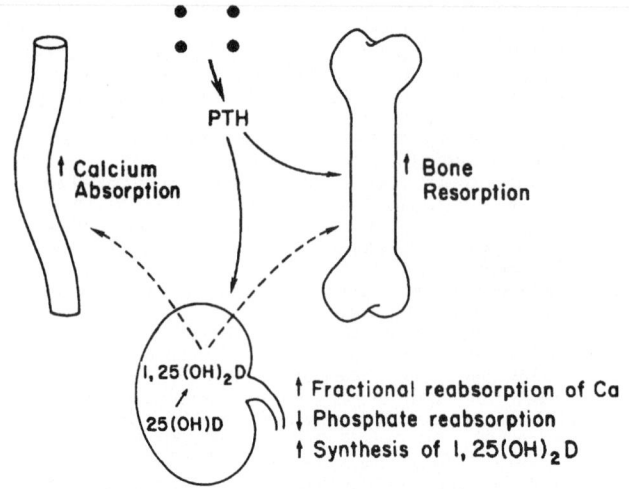

**FIGURE 60-1.** Schema for effects of parathyroid hormone (*PTH*). Secondary hyperparathyroidism develops in response to the hypocalcemia of vitamin D deficiency. (*1,25(OH)₂D*, 1,25-dihydroxyvitamin D; *25(OH)D*, 25-hydroxyvitamin D.)

**TABLE 60-1.**
**Biochemical Characteristics of Hypocalcemic Disorders**

| Disorder | Serum PO$_4$ | PTH | 25(OH)D | 1,25(OH)$_2$D | PTH Infusion $U_{cAMP}$ | PTH Infusion $U_{PO4}$ | Multiple Endocrine Defects |
|---|---|---|---|---|---|---|---|
| Hypoparathyroidism | ↑ | ↓ | Normal | ↓ | Normal | Normal | Occasionally* |
| Pseudohypoparathyroidism | | | | | | | |
|   Type 1a (low G$_s$) | ↑ | ↑ | Normal | ↓ | ↓ | ↓ | Characteristic |
|   Type 1b | ↑ | ↑ | Normal | ↓ | ↓ | ↓ | No |
|   Type 1c | ↑ | ↑ | Normal | ↓ | ↓ | ↓ | Yes |
|   Type 2 | ↑ | ↑ | Normal | ↓ | Normal | ↓ | No |
| Vitamin D deficiency | ↓ | ↑ | ↓ | Low normal | | | |
| 1α-Hydroxylase deficiency | ↓ | ↑ | Normal | ↓ | | | |
| 1,25(OH)$_2$D resistance | ↓ | ↑ | Normal | ↑ | | | |

*PTH*, parathyroid hormone; *25(OH)D*, 25-hydroxyvitamin D; *1,25(OH)$_2$D*, 1,25-dihydroxyvitamin D; $U_{cAMP}$, urinary cyclic AMP; $U_{PO4}$, uninary phosphorus; ↑, increased; ↓, decreased.
*Depending on the cause of hypoparathyroidism.

occur if the production of biologically active PTH or 1,25(OH)$_2$D is impaired or if target organ responses to these hormones are abnormal, either because of a specific biochemical defect or because of generalized target organ damage (Table 60-1).

In the hypoparathyroid states in which PTH secretion or action is deficient, the normal effects of PTH on bone and kidney are absent; the efflux of calcium from bone is diminished, and distal renal tubular calcium reabsorption is impaired. In the absence of PTH action, the proximal tubular reabsorption of phosphate is enhanced and hyperphosphatemia is common. The deficiency of PTH action and the hyperphosphatemia result in decreased renal production of 1,25(OH)$_2$D and impaired intestinal calcium absorption. Hypoparathyroidism, therefore, is characterized by a decreased entry of calcium into the extracellular fluid compartment from bone, kidney, and intestine, and is associated with hypocalcemia and hyperphosphatemia.

In states of vitamin D deficiency or vitamin D insensitivity, hypocalcemia is caused by decreases in intestinal calcium absorption. The 1,25(OH)$_2$D is a potent stimulator of bone resorption, and its absence may also decrease the availability of calcium from bone. Because the parathyroid glands are intact in the vitamin D–deficient states, hypocalcemia induces secondary hyperparathyroidism, and renal phosphate clearance is enhanced. Thus, hypocalcemia in vitamin D deficiency results from decreased calcium absorption and a limited availability of calcium from bone despite secondary hyperparathyroidism; characteristically, it is accompanied by hypophosphatemia.

## SIGNS AND SYMPTOMS OF HYPOCALCEMIA

Ionized calcium, rather than total calcium, is the primary determinant of symptoms in patients with hypocalcemia. A low extracellular fluid ionized calcium concentration enhances neuromuscular excitability, an effect that is potentiated by hyperkalemia and hypomagnesemia.

Substantial variation is seen among patients in the severity of symptoms. Those with chronic hypocalcemia sometimes have few, if any, symptoms of neuromuscular irritability despite quite low total serum calcium concentrations. Patients with acute hypocalcemia often do have symptoms, although no absolute level of serum calcium exists at which symptoms predictably occur. Most patients have at least mild symptoms of circumoral numbness, paresthesias of the distal extremities, or muscle cramping. Symptoms of fatigue, hyperirritability, anxiety, and depression are common. Severe manifestations of hypocalcemia include carpopedal spasm, laryngospasm, and focal or sometimes life-threatening generalized seizures (which

must be distinguished from the generalized tonic muscle contractions that occur in severe tetany).

Clinical signs of the neuromuscular irritability associated with latent tetany include *Chvostek sign* and *Trousseau sign*. Chvostek sign is elicited by tapping the facial nerve just anterior to the ear to produce ipsilateral contraction of the facial muscles. Slightly positive reactions occur in 10% to 30% of normal adults[4]; thus, this sign cannot be considered diagnostic of hypocalcemia unless one knows that it previously was absent. Trousseau sign is present if carpal spasm is induced by pressure ischemia of nerves in the upper arm during the inflation of a sphygmomanometer above systolic blood pressure for 3 to 5 minutes.[5] Both of these signs can be absent even in patients with definite hypocalcemia.

Hypocalcemia is also associated with nonspecific electroencephalographic changes, increases in intracranial pressure, and papilledema. Prolongation of the corrected QT interval on the electrocardiogram is a useful sign of significant hypocalcemia (Fig. 60-2), but other causes of QT prolongation exist. Cardiac dysfunction that reversed with treatment of the hypocalcemia has been reported. This may range from subclinical impairment of cardiac performance that is noted only with exercise[6] to life-threatening cardiac failure.[7,8] The somatosensory-evoked potential recovery period may be a tool for assessing the effects of and recovery from hypocalcemia.[9]

## SIGNS OF CHRONIC HYPOCALCEMIA

Chronic hypocalcemia is associated with other signs. Ectodermal findings such as dry skin, coarse hair, and brittle nails are common, but they are frequently overlooked. Dental and enamel hypoplasia and absence of adult teeth indicate that hypocalcemia has been present since childhood[10] (see Chap. 217). The pattern of dental abnormality may help date the onset of hypocalcemia. Calcification of the frontal lobes and basal ganglia can occur in all forms of hypoparathyroidism and are now detected with computed tomographic scanning even when routine skull radiographs do not demonstrate intracerebral calcification.[11] Occasionally, the calcification of the basal ganglia is associated with parkinsonism or chorea, and the prevalence of dystonic reactions to phenothiazines is reported to be high in hypoparathyroid patients.[12] Subcapsular cataracts are common in untreated hypoparathyroidism and are best seen with slit-lamp examination (see Chap. 215). Treatment may reverse or decrease the progression of the cataracts. Rickets and osteomalacia, although not characteristic, do occur occasionally in hypoparathyroidism after prolonged hypocalcemia.[13,14] Patients with longstanding hypoparathyroidism have been reported to have significantly increased bone mineral density whether they are treated[15,16] or untreated.[17]

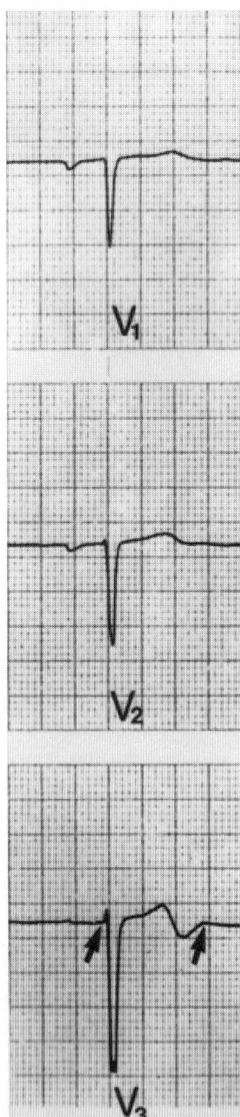

**FIGURE 60-2.** Electrocardiogram of patient with hypocalcemia, demonstrating a long QT interval. The QT interval, which comprises the duration of ventricular depolarization and repolarization, is measured from the beginning of the QRS complex to the end of the T wave (*arrows*). The interval increases with a decreasing heart rate and may be corrected (QTc) by measuring the RR interval and using the following formula: QTc = QT/(R − R). Alternatively, one may consult a nomogram. Serum calcium affects the second or plateau phase (ST segment) of the ventricular action potential; hypocalcemia results in a prolonged QTc interval. In this patient, the QT interval is ~600 msec and the QTc is ~525 msec. The upper limit of normal is 440 msec. (Because the exact end of the T wave may be difficult to determine, some clinicians use the $Q_aT_c$ interval, which comprises the onset of the QRS complex to the apex of the T wave.) (Courtesy of Dr. Steven Singh.)

Other features exist that are characteristic for the particular disorders which cause hypocalcemia. Recognition of these specific features can be helpful in the differential diagnosis of hypocalcemic states.

# SPECIFIC CAUSES OF HYPOCALCEMIA

## HYPOPARATHYROIDISM

A biochemical state of functional hypoparathyroidism occurs either because of failure of secretion of PTH or, less commonly, failure of PTH action at its target tissues. The clinical forms and

**TABLE 60-2.**
**Causes of Hypocalcemia**

**HYPOPROTEINEMIA ("PSEUDOHYPOCALCEMIA")**
**HYPOPARATHYROIDISM**
Decreased secretion of parathyroid hormone
  Postsurgical
  Idiopathic (autoimmune, genetic, sporadic)
  Developmental disorders of the parathyroid gland
  Infiltration (hemochromatosis, Wilson disease, metastatic tumor)
  Postirradiation
  Burns transient hypoparathyroidism (neonatal, postsuppression)
  Reversible hypoparathyroidism (hypomagnesemia, hypermagnesemia)
**RESISTANCE TO PARATHYROID HORMONE ACTION**
Pseudohypoparathyroidism
  Type 1a, deficient adenylate cyclase–coupling protein ($G_s\alpha$)
  Type 1b, possible deficient adenylate cyclase–coupling protein ($G_s\alpha$)
  Type 1c, abnormal cyclase catalytic unit
  Type 2, abnormal renal cyclic adenosine monophosphate action
Hypomagnesemia
**ALTERED BOUND CALCIUM**
Hyperphosphatemia
  Rhabdomyolysis
  Tumor lysis
  Phosphate infusion/enema
Citrate
  Massive blood transfusion
  Dialysis with citrate anticoagulation
Respiratory alkalosis
Acute severe illness (pancreatitis, sepsis, burns)
**DECREASED BONE RESORPTION (CALCITONIN, PLICAMYCIN [MITHRAMYCIN], BISPHOSPHONATE TREATMENT)**
**INCREASED OSTEOBLASTIC ACTIVITY**
Postparathyroidectomy hungry bones syndrome
Osteoblastic tumor metastasis
**DISORDERS OF VITAMIN D METABOLISM**
Decreased precursors
Dietary deficiency
Malabsorption
Nephrotic syndrome (urinary losses)
Liver disease
Disrupted enterohepatic circulation
**DECREASED CONVERSION TO ACTIVE METABOLITES**
1α-hydroxylase deficiency (vitamin D–dependent rickets, type I)
**RESISTANCE TO 1,25(OH)₂D ACTION**
$1,25(OH)_2D$ resistance (vitamin D-dependent rickets type II)

*$1,25(OH)_2D$, 1,25-dihydroxyvitamin D.*

characteristics of hypoparathyroidism are described below and in Table 60-2.

## SURGICAL HYPOPARATHYROIDISM

Hypoparathyroidism occurs most commonly as a result of parathyroid or thyroid surgery or after radical surgery for laryngeal or esophageal carcinoma. The resulting hypoparathyroidism can be transient or permanent and sometimes may not develop for many years. In some patients, a chronic state of "decreased parathyroid reserve" may exist[18] in which hypocalcemia becomes apparent only when mineral homeostasis is stressed further by other factors such as pregnancy, lactation, or illness.

**Transient Hypocalcemia after Parathyroid Surgery.** Hypocalcemia frequently occurs after removal of a hyperfunctioning parathyroid adenoma because of deficient secretion of PTH by the remaining previously suppressed parathyroid tissue. Hypoparathyroidism is usually transient, because the normal parathyroid glands recover function quickly (generally within 1 week), even after long-term suppression. Transient postoperative hypocalcemia may be exaggerated or prolonged in those patients who have significant preexisting hyperparathyroid bone disease. In these patients the surgically induced reduction of previously elevated plasma PTH results in an increased movement of plasma calcium (and phosphorus) into remineralizing "hungry bones."[19] Treatment with calcium and a short-acting vitamin D metabolite may be required until the bones heal.

**Permanent Hypoparathyroidism after Parathyroid Surgery.** Permanent hypoparathyroidism after an initial neck exploration for primary hyperparathyroidism is rare and develops in ~1% of patients. The incidence is greatly increased with repeated neck surgery for recurrent or persistent hyperparathyroidism, after subtotal parathyroidectomy for parathyroid hyperplasia, or when surgery is performed by an inexperienced surgeon.

**Hypocalcemia after Thyroid Surgery.** After thyroid surgery, the incidence of permanent hypoparathyroidism varies widely, depending on the underlying thyroid lesion and the extent of the procedure, as well as on the experience of the surgeon. Hypoparathyroidism may result from direct injury, inadvertent removal, or devascularization of the parathyroid glands. Permanent hypoparathyroidism is distinctly unusual after a hemithyroidectomy and should be relatively uncommon even after total thyroidectomy.[20,21] However, up to 33% of patients who undergo a total thyroidectomy for cancer may develop transient postoperative parathyroid insufficiency.[22]

Transient hypocalcemia occurs in approximately one-third of patients who undergo a subtotal thyroidectomy for thyrotoxicosis. The fall in plasma calcium level generally occurs within 24 to 48 hours after surgery and can be sufficient to produce symptoms of tetany. The mechanism of this hypocalcemia is not well understood. Frequently, hyperthyroidism is associated with increased bone turnover and resorption, elevated plasma ionized calcium levels, and suppressed parathyroid function. Although the proposal has been made that hypocalcemia occurs as calcium moves into remineralizing hungry bones after reduction of thyroid hormone levels,[23] the early development of hypocalcemia appears to be inconsistent with this abnormality. Some patients may have unappreciated damage to the parathyroid glands[18]; whether thyroidectomy causes hypocalcemia by producing hypercalcitonemia is disputed.[24,25] Clearly, whatever the initiating cause, the secretory response of the suppressed parathyroid glands is inadequate to maintain a normal plasma calcium.[24,25]

## IDIOPATHIC HYPOPARATHYROIDISM

The term *idiopathic hypoparathyroidism* describes a heterogeneous group of rare disorders that share in common the deficient secretion of PTH. Although most cases are sporadic, the familial occurrence of idiopathic hypoparathyroidism has been reported. Within these families hypoparathyroidism may occur as part of a complex autoimmune disorder (see Chap. 197) associated with multiple endocrine deficiencies (i.e., type 1 polyglandular syndrome)[26] or in association with diverse developmental abnormalities (e.g., nephropathy, lymphedema, nerve deafness, or tetralogy of Fallot).[27–42] The pleiotropic nature of many of these various syndromes suggests that the genetic basis of PTH deficiency is not related to a specific defect intrinsic to the parathyroid gland.

**Type 1 Polyglandular Syndrome.** Type 1 polyglandular syndrome may be sporadic or familial with an autosomal recessive inheritance pattern. The classic triad of this syndrome is *h*ypoparathyroidism, *a*drenal insufficiency, and *m*ucocutaneous candidiasis (HAM). The recognition that affected patients may have additional components has led to the suggestion that a more inclusive term be used to describe the syndrome: *a*utoimmune *p*oly*e*ndocrinopathy–*c*andidiasis–*e*ctodermal *d*ystrophy (APECED).[43] The syndrome is first recognized in early child-

hood, although a few individuals have developed the condition after the first decade of life. The clinical onset of the three principal components of the syndrome typically follows a predictable pattern, in which mucocutaneous candidiasis first appears at a mean age of 5 years, followed by hypoparathyroidism at a mean age of 9 years and adrenal insufficiency at a mean age of 14 years.[43] Patients may not manifest all three elements of the triad. Alopecia, keratoconjunctivitis, malabsorption and steatorrhea, gonadal failure, pernicious anemia, chronic active hepatitis, thyroid disease, and insulin-requiring diabetes mellitus occur in some patients.[26] Antibodies directed against the parathyroid, thyroid, and adrenal glands are demonstrable in many patients,[44] and a T-cell abnormality has been described.[45,46] The presence of antibodies may not correlate well with the clinical findings. In those cases that have been examined pathologically, complete parathyroid atrophy or destruction has been demonstrated. In some patients, treatment of hypoparathyroidism has been complicated by apparent vitamin D "resistance," possibly related to coexistent hepatic disease or steatorrhea, or both. Mutations in the gene *AIRE* (*autoimmune regulator gene*) have been identified in patients with APECED. *AIRE*, located on chromosome 21 (21q22.3), encodes a nuclear protein containing zinc-finger motifs; this suggests that it may play a role as a transcriptional regulator.[47,48] *AIRE* is expressed in tissues important in the development and regulation of the immune system (e.g., the thymus and lymph nodes). Although many different mutations have been reported throughout the world,[48a] the majority of patients harbor either the R257X mutation or a 13-base-pair deletion in exon 8, each resulting in a truncated AIRE protein.[49,50] The function of the AIRE protein remains unknown. The hypothesis has been made that the AIRE protein may regulate the immune response via B- and T-cell stimuli.[47] Functional analysis of the AIRE protein and further molecular analysis of the *AIRE* gene will elucidate the molecular pathogenesis of APECED.

**Isolated Hypoparathyroidism.** Isolated idiopathic hypoparathyroidism, in which PTH deficiency is unassociated with other endocrine disorders or developmental defects, is usually sporadic, but it may occur on a familial basis. Most commonly, the onset of isolated hypoparathyroidism is between the ages of 2 and 10 years, although it may first be recognized in adult life, and the onset may be at any age up to the eighth decade. Females are affected twice as often as males.

A high incidence of parathyroid antibodies is seen in patients with isolated idiopathic hypoparathyroidism, and some cases may be examples of incomplete expression of the type 1 polyglandular syndrome (APECED, see earlier). Some patients may possess antibodies that inhibit the secretion of PTH,[51] rather than cause parathyroid gland destruction.[52] In other cases that have been examined pathologically, fatty replacement[53] or atrophy with fatty infiltration and fibrosis[54] has been described.

**Familial Isolated Hypoparathyroidism.** In rare instances, isolated hypoparathyroidism may be familial, with the PTH deficiency being inherited by autosomal dominant, autosomal recessive, or X-linked modes of transmission.[55] The age at onset covers a broad range (1 month to 30 years), and the condition is often recognized first in the child, rather than in the parent. Parathyroid antibodies are absent.

As the preproPTH gene is located on the short arm of chromosome 11, molecular genetic studies of familial isolated hypoparathyroidism have focused first on kindreds in which inheritance of hypoparathyroidism is consistent with an autosomal mode of transmission. In one pedigree in which hypoparathyroidism was inherited in an autosomal dominant manner, DNA sequencing revealed a point mutation (T→C) in exon 2 that resulted in the substitution of arginine (CGT) for cysteine (TGT) in the leader sequence of preproPTH.[56] The substitution of a charged amino acid in the hydrophobic core of the leader sequence inhibits processing of the mutant preproPTH molecule by signal peptidase[56] and is presumed to impair translocation of the mutant and normal proteins across the plasma membrane of the endoplasmic reticulum. An abnormality of the preproPTH gene has also been found in a consanguineous family with autosomal recessive hypoparathyroidism.[57] Affected members of this family are homozygous for a single base transversion (G→C) at the exon 2–intron 2 boundary. This mutation leads to abnormal processing of the nascent prepro-PTH mRNA and results in mature transcripts in which exon 1 is spliced to exon 3 (i.e., exon skipping).[57] Although the molecular pathophysiology of hypoparathyroidism has been defined in these two families, detailed analyses of the preproPTH gene have failed to disclose defects in affected members of other autosomal recessive and dominant kindreds.[57]

Familial hypoparathyroidism is also inherited as an X-linked disorder that is, of course, unrelated to the preproPTH gene. Using a battery of X chromosome gene markers, linkage studies of two large multigenerational families with X-linked hypoparathyroidism have localized the defective gene to the region Xq26-27.[58,59] The defective gene or genes in this syndrome appear to be important for parathyroid cell development or function.[58] The early onset of hypocalcemia and the absence of parathyroid tissue at autopsy in individuals with this disorder are consistent with an important role for this genetic locus in the embryologic development of the parathyroid glands.[60]

## AUTOSOMAL DOMINANT HYPOCALCEMIA: A MODEL OF HUMAN DISEASE DUE TO DEFECTIVE G PROTEIN–COUPLED RECEPTOR SIGNALING

New insights into the molecular pathology of hypoparathyroidism have come from the cloning and characterization of the *calcium-sensing receptor (CaR)*, a cell surface protein that binds extracellular calcium.[61] The CaR is a member of the superfamily of heptahelical receptor proteins that are coupled via signal-transducing G proteins to a variety of intracellular signal effectors (e.g., enzymes such as adenylate cyclase and phospholipase C). *G protein–coupled receptors (GPCRs)* detect extracellular signals as diverse as light, odorants, hormones, growth factors, neurotransmitters, and ions, and interact with heterotrimeric *guanine nucleotide–binding proteins* (G proteins), which couple the extracellular receptors to intracellular effector enzymes and ion channels. *GPCR mutations* may be activating or inactivating.

The CaR is present in a variety of tissues, but its expression on parathyroid and renal tubular cells is the basis for its role in regulating serum and urinary calcium levels. Expression of the CaR on the surface of parathyroid cells is required for calcium-sensitive regulation of PTH secretion, and changes in the number or activity of CaRs can alter the calcium setpoint for PTH secretion.[62] Although the precise molecular basis for calcium-dependent regulation of PTH secretion remains unknown, the cloning of the CaR has led to the identification of the initial steps in the signaling pathway. Binding of extracellular calcium to CaRs on the surface of the parathyroid cell leads to activation of $G_q$, a G protein that stimulates phospholipase C activity. Phospholipase C hydrolyzes phosphoinositides, leading to the generation of inositol 1,4,5-triphosphate, which releases intracellular calcium from storage in the endoplasmic reticulum, and diacylglycerol, which activates protein kinase C.[63] The calcium-dependent activation of these second messenger pathways ultimately inhibits secretion of PTH (see Chap. 50). Heterozygous mutations in the CaR gene that lead to constitutive (ligand-independent) activation of CaRs (i.e., gain of function mutations) have been identified in several kindreds with autosomal dominant hypocalcemia, a syndrome associated with low serum PTH and relative hypercalciuria.[64] In other cases, linkage of hypocalcemia to the chromosomal locus for the CaR gene (3q13.3-21) has indirectly implicated this gene in familial hypoparathyroidism.[65] Preliminary studies have identified similar activating mutations of the CaR in cases of sporadic hypoparathyroidism. In both familial and sporadic cases, each proband has a unique mutation. These observations suggest that mutation

of the CaR gene may be the most common cause of genetic hypoparathyroidism. Further confirmation of the important role that the CaR plays in regulating PTH secretion derives from studies of patients with the contrasting syndrome of *familial* (benign) *hypocalciuric hypercalcemia (FHH)*, an autosomal dominant disorder associated with excessive secretion of PTH due to reduced sensitivity of the parathyroid glands to extracellular calcium.[66–68] Heterozygous mutations that result in loss of function of the CaR are present in most patients with FHH. Although FHH is typically a benign condition, in unusual cases, an affected subject may develop severe neonatal hyperparathyroidism, a life-threatening hypercalcemic disorder that is generally associated with inheritance of defective CaR genes from both parents.[69,70]

Defects in other GPCRs have been identified as the bases for a variety of human diseases. Several syndromes of inherited hormonal resistance result from germline loss of function mutations in GPCR, including the PTH/parathyroid hormone–related protein (PTHrP),[71,72] thyroid-stimulating hormone (TSH),[73,74] luteinizing hormone (LH),[75,76] growth hormone–releasing hormone (GHRH),[77–80] adrenocorticotropic hormone (ACTH),[81,82] V2 vasopressin,[83] follicle-stimulating hormone (FSH),[84] and gonadotropin-releasing hormone (GnRH)[85] receptors (Table 60-3). With the exception of the CaR, inheritance of these resistance syndromes is recessive. Gain of function mutations may be either germline or sporadic and are typically heterozygous. Somatic activating mutations in the TSH receptor result in ligand-independent stimulation and formation of hyperfunctioning thyroid nodules.[86] When similar TSH receptor–activating mutations occur in the germline, *familial nonautoimmune hyperthyroidism* results.[87,88] Activating mutations of PTH/PTHrP[89] and LH receptors,[90,91] which also have been identified (see Table 60-3), result in ligand-independent activation of hormone-sensitive signaling pathways. As previously noted for the CaR, many GPCRs have been associated with

## TABLE 60-3.
### G Protein–Coupled Receptor Mutations and Related Endocrine Disorders

| Disease | Receptor | Mutation |
|---|---|---|
| Jansen metaphyseal chondrodysplasia | PTH/PTHrP | Gain of function |
| Blomstrand chondrodysplasia | PTH/PTHrP | Loss of function |
| Familial hypocalciuric hypercalcemia and neonatal severe primary hyperparathyroidism | CaR | Loss of function |
| Autosomal dominant hypocalcemia and familial hypocalcemia with hypercalciuria | CaR | Gain of function |
| Familial hypothyroidism | TSH | Loss of function |
| Sporadic hyperfunctioning thyroid nodules | TSH | Gain of function |
| Familial nonautoimmune hyperthyroidism | TSH | Gain of function |
| Male pseudohermaphroditism | LH | Loss of function |
| Female Leydig cell hypoplasia | LH | Loss of function |
| Familial precocious puberty (male) | LH | Gain of function |
| Familial growth hormone deficiency | GHRH | Loss of function |
| Familial ACTH resistance | ACTH | Loss of function |
| Nephrogenic diabetes insipidus | V2 vasopressin | Loss of function |
| Hypergonadotropic ovarian dysgenesis | FSH | Loss of function |
| Isolated central hypothyroidism | TRH | Loss of function |
| Hypogonadotropic hypogonadism | GnRH | Loss of function |
| Dwarfism with GH deficiency | GHRH | Loss of function |

*PTH*, parathyroid hormone; *PTHrP*, parathyroid hormone–related protein; *CaR*, calcium-sensing receptor; *TSH*, thyroid-stimulating hormone; *LH*, luteinizing hormone; *GHRH*, growth hormone–releasing hormone; *ACTH*, adrenocorticotropic hormone; *FSH*, follicle-stimulating hormone; *TRH*, thyrotropin-releasing hormone; *GnRH*, gonadotropin-releasing hormone; *GH*, growth hormone; *GHRH*, GH-releasing hormone.

both gain of function and loss of function mutations, with generation of contrasting clinical syndromes. Another relevant example is the PTH/PTHrP receptor. Heterozygous activating mutations result in *Jansen metaphyseal chondrodysplasia*, a rare form of dwarfism with PTH-independent hypercalcemia and abnormal endochondral bone formation secondary to constitutive activity of the PTH/PTHrP receptor.[89] Homozygous inactivating mutations in the PTH/PTHrP receptor cause a rare lethal disorder of accelerated endochondral bone maturation known as *Blomstrand chondrodysplasia*.[71,72]

## DEVELOPMENTAL DISORDERS OF THE PARATHYROID GLAND

Hypoparathyroidism may result from agenesis or dysgenesis of the parathyroid glands. The most well-described example of parathyroid gland dysembryogenesis is the *DiGeorge syndrome* (DGS), in which maldevelopment of the third and fourth branchial pouches is frequently associated with congenital absence of not only the parathyroids but also the thymus. Because of thymic aplasia, T-cell–mediated immunity is impaired, and affected infants have an increased susceptibility to recurrent viral and fungal infections. Maldevelopment of the first and fifth branchial pouches occurs frequently as well, producing characteristic facial anomalies (Fig. 60-3), including hypertelorism, antimongoloid slant of the eyes, low-set and notched ears, short philtrum of the lip, and micrognathia (first branchial pouch) or aortic arch abnormalities, such as right-sided arch, truncus arteriosus, or tetralogy of Fallot. Most cases of branchial pouch dysembryogenesis are sporadic, but familial occurrence with apparent autosomal dominant inheritance has been described.[30,31] Although most children with DGS die of infections or cardiac failure by the age of 6 years, survival into adolescence or adulthood is possible when the syndrome is only partially expressed. Molecular mapping studies have demonstrated an association between the syndrome and deletions involving 22q11[32–34] or 10p.[35,36] Large deletions of genetic material at 22q11 result in hemizygosity for genes located

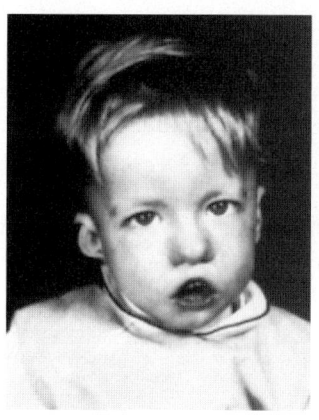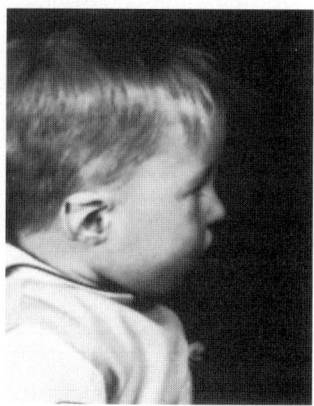

**FIGURE 60-3.** An 18-month-old boy with DiGeorge syndrome. Initially, he presented on the third day of life with a seizure that did not respond to phenobarbital. On examination, mild hypertelorism (increased interpupillary distance); slight antimongoloid slant of the eyes (outer canthus lower than inner canthus); asymmetric, malformed ears that were low set; and a short philtrum (infranasal groove) were noted. The serum calcium level was 6.8 mg/dL, the serum phosphate level was 6.8 mg/dL, and the chest radiograph revealed a right-sided aortic arch. No thymus shadow was present. The seizures responded to calcium gluconate therapy. The subsequent course was characterized by upper respiratory tract infections and episodes of otitis media. When the patient was seen again at the time of the photograph, retardation of growth and mental development were observed. Note the broad nose, cupid bow mouth, and mandibular hypoplasia. The serum calcium concentration was 8.2 mg/dL, and the serum phosphate level was 7.8 mg/dL. Calcium gluconate therapy was discontinued without a further drop in serum calcium levels or a recurrence of seizures. (From Kretschmer R, Say B, Brown D, Rosen F. Congenital aplasia of the thymus gland [DiGeorge's syndrome]. N Engl J Med 1968; 279:1295.)

in this region, and they are associated with contiguous gene deletion syndromes, which include not only the DGS but also the overlapping conotruncal anomaly and velocardiofacial syndromes. More than 20 candidate genes from the deleted region in DGS have been identified, and none has been shown to cause DGS.[92] Evidence both from the *hand2* knock-out mouse, which has characteristics that resemble DGS,[93] and from a DGS patient with a small deletion in the region of the ubiquitin fusion degradation 1 (*UFD1L*) gene has implicated heterozygous loss of function of this gene as the basis for the DGS phenotype.[93,94] Underexpression of *UFD1L* may lead to cell death in the pharyngeal arches in embryonic development. *UFD1L* regulates the accumulation of protein substrates via finely tuned protein degradation. Accumulation of excess protein may be toxic and lead to aberrant cell signaling, abnormal cellular proliferation, or apoptosis of the pharyngeal arches where *UFD1L* is expressed.[92] Further investigation demonstrating mutations in the *UFD1L* gene alone in patients with DGS are needed to validate *UFD1L* as the DGS gene.

Hypoparathyroidism is also associated with several other less well understood developmental syndromes, including the autosomal dominant hypoparathyroidism-deafness-renal dysplasia (HDR) syndrome associated with *sensorineural deafness and renal dysplasia*, which has been linked to deletions on 10p 13-14[27,95,95a] that result in loss of the GATA3 gene.[95b] Mutations in the GATA3 gene, which encodes a zinc-finger transcription factor, are also a cause of HDR.[95] The syndrome of lymphedema, prolapsing mitral valve, brachydactyly, and nephropathy[29]; and severe growth failure and dysmorphic features that include microcephaly, beaked nose, and micrognathia[40,42] as well as the *Kenney-Caffey syndrome* (short stature, osteosclerosis, basal ganglion calcifications, ophthalmic defects) are also associated with hypoparathyroidism.[60] Studies in mice show that loss of the *GCMB* gene, which encodes a transcription factor, results in hypoparathyroidism.[95c] Thus, this gene is the first specific regulator of parathyroid embryogenesis. Similar inactivating mutations in the *GCMB* gene have been described in patients with neonatal isolated hypoparathyroidism.[95d]

## TRANSIENT HYPOPARATHYROIDISM OF THE NEONATE

Shortly after birth, a physiologic fall occurs in the serum calcium concentration, and many normal infants may have serum calcium levels <8 mg/dL during the first 3 weeks of life. Hypocalcemia in the neonate can be divided into *early hypocalcemia*, starting within the first 24 to 72 hours of life before feedings have been given, and *late hypocalcemia*, usually appearing after several days to weeks of feeding.

**Early Neonatal Hypocalcemia.** Early neonatal hypocalcemia represents an exaggeration of the normal fall in serum calcium concentration and theoretically is due to deficient release of PTH by immature parathyroid glands. Prematurity, low birth weight, hypoglycemia, maternal diabetes, difficult delivery, and respiratory distress syndrome are frequently associated findings. Symptoms may be absent, or irritability, muscular twitching, or convulsive seizures may occur. Although the course is self-limited, symptomatic infants should be treated with oral or intravenous calcium. Transient congenital hypoparathyroidism can also occur in infants with DGS.[95e] A more severe form of transient neonatal hypoparathyroidism and tetany may also occur in children born to mothers with hyperparathyroidism or hypercalcemia. In these infants, parathyroid activity has been more profoundly suppressed in utero by maternal hypercalcemia.

**Late Neonatal Hypocalcemia.** Late neonatal hypocalcemia may develop 4 to 6 days (or later) after birth and may be considered a transient form of relative immaturity of renal phosphorus handling or of the renal adenylate cyclase system. Hypocalcemia may be precipitated by a high-phosphate diet and appears to occur particularly in those infants who are fed with artificial foods such as cow's milk–based formulas.[96] In these infants, the renal response to PTH is inadequate and hypocalcemia results. The reduction of serum calcium ion concentration is probably secondary to elevated serum phosphate levels and should stimulate para-thyroid gland activity. This form of hypocalcemia is the most common cause of seizures in the newborn period. A spontaneous recovery of normal mineral homeostasis typically occurs after a few weeks, but the serum calcium levels of symptomatic infants can be increased within 1 to 2 days by feeding a supplemented milk mixture with a high (3:1 to 4:1) calcium/phosphorus ratio.

## OTHER FORMS OF PARATHYROID GLAND DYSFUNCTION

**Irradiation and Drugs.** The parathyroid glands appear remarkably resistant to damage by a great many toxic agents and processes. Transient hypoparathyroidism has been associated with ingestion of large quantities of alcohol.[97] The administration of iodine-131 for the treatment of benign or malignant thyroid disease or for the deliberate induction of hypoparathyroidism has only rarely caused permanent, symptomatic hypoparathyroidism. Similarly, parathyroid gland function is altered only occasionally by most chemotherapeutic or cytotoxic agents. Notable exceptions include asparaginase, which causes parathyroid necrosis in rabbits, and ethiofos, a radio- and chemoprotector that causes a dose-dependent and reversible inhibition of PTH secretion.[98,99] Along with its effects on the parathyroid gland, ethiofos blocks the ability of osteoclasts to respond to hormonal stimuli. Thus, a significant component of its calcium-reducing effect derives from the ability of this agent to inhibit osteoclast-directed bone resorption and calcium release from bone.

**Infiltrative Disease of the Parathyroids.** Parathyroid gland function may also be impaired by infiltrative processes. Iron overload caused by hemochromatosis (see Chap. 131) or trans-fusion therapy is frequently associated with significant para-thyroid gland iron deposition and, occasionally, clinical hypoparathyroidism. Moreover, a similar pathologic picture has been described in one patient with Wilson disease and increased copper storage who developed symptomatic hypo-parathyroidism.[100] Pathologic involvement of the parathyroid glands can also occur in metastatic neoplasia, miliary tuberculosis, amyloidosis, and syphilis, but clinical hypoparathyroidism rarely occurs in these conditions.

**Magnesium Deficiency.** Reversible alterations of parathyroid gland function and PTH secretion are associated with magnesium depletion. Modest declines in magnesium slightly increase PTH secretion. However, as magnesium deficiency becomes more severe, PTH secretion becomes inappropriately low,[101,102] and hypocalcemia with tetany may ensue. With even more severe magnesium depletion, resistance to the action of PTH occurs, which is reversible with magnesium repletion (see Chap. 68).[103] By contrast, magnesium replacement does not appear to reverse the hypoparathyroidism associated with burns and hypomagnesemia.[103a]

**Hypermagnesemia.** Hypermagnesemia also may cause hypocalcemia.[104] This situation is commonly encountered in obstetric practice when high-dose magnesium infusions are used for the treatment of toxemia or premature labor. Because the hypocalcemia is accompanied by significant hyper-magnesemia, neuromuscular irritability should be less than that expected when similar calcium concentrations occur with normal magnesium; clinical tetany usually does not occur.

# PARATHYROID HORMONE RESISTANCE

## PSEUDOHYPOPARATHYROIDISM TYPE 1

The term *pseudohypoparathyroidism (PHP)* describes a heterogeneous syndrome characterized by biochemical hypoparathyroidism (i.e., hypocalcemia and hyperphosphatemia), increased plasma levels of PTH, and peripheral unresponsiveness to the biologic actions of PTH. Thus PHP differs substantially from true hypoparathyroidism; in contrast with the latter condition, PTH secretion is excessive and the parathyroid glands are hyperplastic.[105]

PHP was the first recognized human disease to be ascribed to diminished responsiveness to a hormone by otherwise normal target organs (subsequently, many others have been described) (see below).[106] Albright's initial description of the blunted calcemic and phosphaturic response to PTH administration in patients with PHP provided the basis for his original hypothesis that the disorder is due to target organ resistance.[107]

## MOLECULAR BASIS FOR PSEUDOHYPOPARATHYROIDISM: A MODEL FOR HUMAN G PROTEIN DISEASE

Characterization of the molecular basis for PHP commenced when research showed that cyclic adenosine monophosphate (cAMP) mediates the actions of PTH on kidney and bone and that PTH infusion in humans leads to a significant increase in urinary excretion of cAMP.[108,109] When these observations were applied to the study of PHP, affected persons were found to have a blunted urinary response of nephrogenous cAMP to PTH infusion in comparison with normal persons and patients with other forms of hypoparathyroidism (Fig. 60-4).[109] These findings formed the basis for the most reliable test presently available for the diagnosis of PHP type 1. Moreover, these results suggested that PTH resistance is caused by a defect in the plasma membrane–bound PTH receptor–adenylate cyclase complex that produces cAMP. Evi-

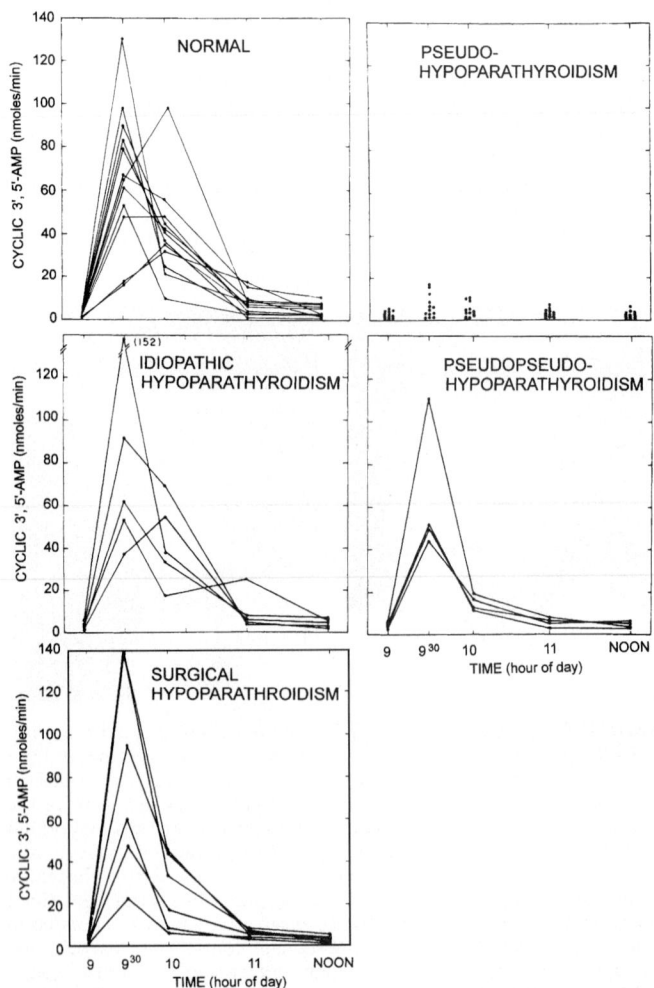

**FIGURE 60-4.** Cyclic adenosine monophosphate (*AMP*) excretion in urine in response to the injection of parathyroid hormone (300 USP units of bovine parathyroid extract infused from 9:00 to 9:15 a.m.). (Reproduced from Chase LR, Melson GL, Aurbach GD. Pseudohypoparathyroidism: defective excretion of 3'5'-AMP in response to parathyroid hormone. J Clin Invest 1969; 48:1836, by permission of the authors and the American Society for Clinical Investigation.)

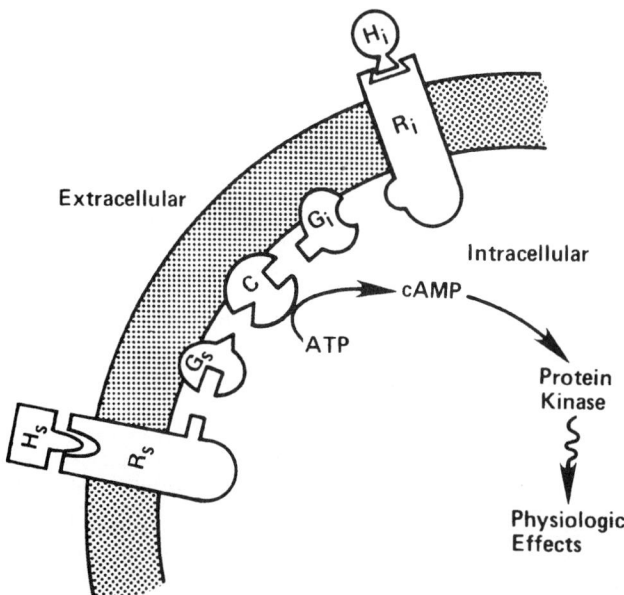

**FIGURE 60-5.** Schematic outline of the adenylate cyclase–cyclic adenosine monophosphate (*cAMP*) system. $H_s$ and $H_i$ denote stimulatory and inhibitory agents, respectively; $R_s$ and $R_i$ stimulatory and inhibitory receptors; and $G_s$ and $G_i$ the stimulatory and inhibitory guanine nucleotide–binding regulatory proteins. The rate of conversion of substrate adenosine triphosphate (*ATP*) to product cAMP by the catalytic (*C*) unit of adenylate cyclase is regulated by the interactions of $G_s$ and $G_i$. Details of the interactions are described in the text.

dence is accumulating that some actions of PTH may be cAMP independent, with signal transduction through inositol phospholipids, intracellular calcium mobilization, and protein kinase C activation (Fig. 60-5).[110–113] This may explain why some patients with PHP who have blunted urinary cAMP responses after PTH infusion still have evidence for PTH-mediated effects on renal tubular calcium handling[114,115] and skeletal remodeling (see later).

The adenylate cyclase system is far more complex than originally suspected, consisting of at least three types of proteins embedded in the plasma membrane (i.e., receptors, G proteins, and adenylate cyclase [Fig. 60-6; see Chap. 4]).[116] The signal-transducing G proteins are comprised of three subunits (αβγ) that are

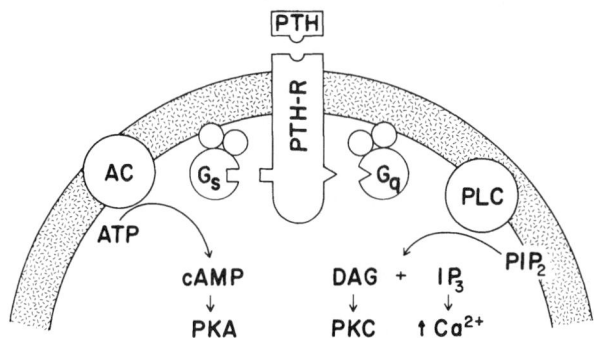

**FIGURE 60-6.** Cell surface receptors for parathyroid hormone (*PTH*) appear to be coupled to two classes of G proteins. $G_s$ mediates stimulation of adenylate cyclase (*AC*) and the production of cyclic adenosine monophosphate (*cAMP*), which in turn activates protein kinase A (*PKA*). $G_q$ stimulates phospholipase C (*PLC*) to form the second messengers inositol 1,4,5-trisphosphate (*IP₃*) and diacylglycerol (*DAG*) from membrane-bound phosphatidylinositol 4,5-bisphosphate (*PIP₂*). IP₃ increases intracellular calcium (*Ca²⁺*) and DAG stimulates protein kinase C (*PKC*) activity. Each G protein consists of a unique α chain and a βγ dimer. (*ATP*, adenosine triphosphate; *PTH-R*, parathyroid hormone receptor.) (From Bilezikian JP, Levine MA, Marcus R, eds. The parathyroids: basic and clinical concepts. New York: Raven Press, 1994:782.)

encoded by 16α, 6β, and 12γ genes. The α subunits are loosely associated with tightly coupled βγ dimers; this facilitates great combinatorial variability and allows G proteins to interact with as many as 1000 different GPCRs and effector proteins.[117] G proteins have been divided into four subfamilies: $G_s$, $G_i$, $G_q$, and $G_{12}$, based on structural and functional similarities. Members of the $G_s$ family activate adenylate cyclase and members of the $G_q$ family activate phospholipase C; members of the $G_i$ subfamily inhibit adenylate cyclase ($G_i$) or participate in visual ($G_{t1}$ and $G_{t2}$) or gustatory ($G_{gust}$) neurosensory processes. $G_{13}$ stimulates the exchange of sodium and hydrogen ions and cytoskeletal rearrangements.[117–119] The activity of the heterotrimeric protein is regulated by the binding and hydrolysis of guanosine triphosphate (GTP) by the Gα subunit. When Gβγ is bound to GDP, it is inactive and loosely associates with the βγ dimer. Receptor activation results in release of GDP by the heterotrimeric αβγ complex, binding of GTP to Gα, and dissociation of the Gα-GTP complex from the βγ dimer and receptor. Both the Gα-GTP chain and free βγ dimer can regulate downstream effectors. Termination of receptor signaling results from the hydrolysis of GTP to guanosine diphosphate (GDP), allowing the βγ dimer to reassociate with Gα-GDP.[117]

Mutations in G proteins tend to affect a variety of tissues, as demonstrated by the occurrence of multihormonal resistance in PHP type 1a. By contrast, receptor mutations are generally limited to one or a few tissues in which the defective receptor is expressed (e.g., defects in the CaR produce a disturbance in calcium sensing that appears limited to parathyroid and kidney cells). The determinants of phenotypic expression of the G protein and GPCR disease are the range of expression of the gene (*tissue distribution*), the developmental timing of the mutation (*germline vs. somatic*), and the nature of the mutation (*loss or gain of function*).

## PSEUDOHYPOPARATHYROIDISM TYPE 1A

Albright's original description of PHP focused on PTH resistance in this disorder. Resistance to PTH alone would be consistent with a defect in the cell surface receptor specific for PTH. However, some patients with PHP type 1 are resistant to multiple hormones whose effects are mediated by cAMP and have additional abnormalities, such as hypothyroidism and hypogonadism,[120] mental retardation,[121] and defective olfaction.[122] These patients, whose disorder is referred to as PHP type 1a, have ~ 50% reduction in the activity of $G_s$ (Fig. 60-7). This reduction occurs in all tissues that have been examined (including erythrocytes, platelets, fibroblasts, transformed lymphocytes, and, in one case, renal cortex).[123–125] A generalized deficiency of $G_s$ activity apparently results in a reduced ability of hormones and neurotransmitters to activate adenylate cyclase in diverse tissues and thereby leads to widespread hormone resistance (Fig. 60-8).

Patients with PHP type 1a show a unique phenotype characterized by round facies, short stature, obesity, brachydactyly (short metacarpal and metatarsal bones), heterotopic subcutaneous ossification, and bony exostoses (Fig. 60-9). Mental retardation may be present. In 1942, Albright and co-workers[107] first observed these unusual developmental defects, subsequently termed *Albright hereditary osteodystrophy* (*AHO*), in three patients during the initial description of PHP.

Ten years after the description of PHP, Albright and colleagues[126] described a patient with a habitus typical of AHO but who lacked biochemical evidence of target organ resistance to PTH. This normocalcemic variant of AHO was termed *pseudopseudohypoparathyroidism* (pseudoPHP) to call attention to the physical similarity with AHO yet indicate the metabolic dissimilarity (PTH responsiveness) of this disorder.

PseudoPHP is genetically related to PHP. Early clinical observations of AHO kindreds in which several affected members had only AHO (i.e., pseudoPHP), whereas others had PTH resistance as well (i.e., PHP) first suggested that the two disorders might reflect variability in expression of a single genetic lesion. Further support for this hypothesis derives from bio-

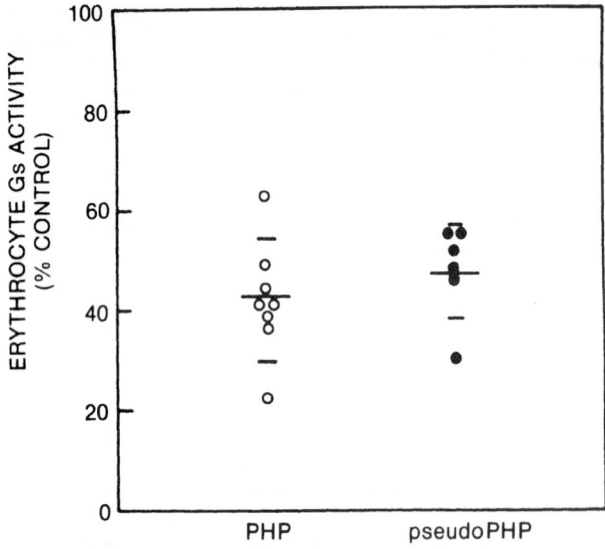

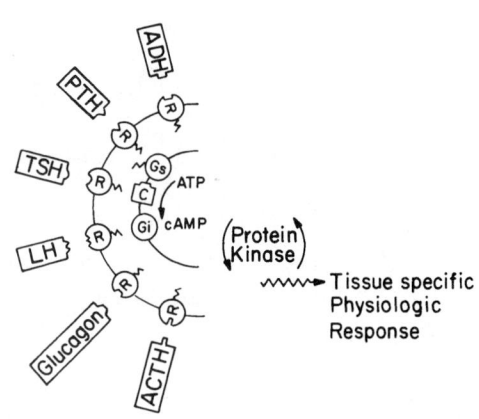

**FIGURE 60-7.** $G_s$ activity in pseudohypoparathyroidism (*PHP*) type 1a and in pseudopseudohypoparathyroidism (*pseudoPHP*). $G_s$ activity was measured in erythrocyte membrane extracts by complementation with $G_s$-deficient membranes from S49 cyc cells. The resultant adenylate cyclase activity is expressed as a percentage of a pooled normal human erythrocyte membrane standard. (From Levine MA, Jap T, Mauseth RS, et al. Activity of the stimulatory guanine nucleotide–binding protein is reduced in erythrocytes from patients with pseudohypoparathyroidism and pseudopseudohypoparathyroidism: biochemical, endocrine, and genetic analysis of Albrights hereditary osteodystrophy in six kindreds. J Clin Endocrinol Metab 1986; 62:497.)

**FIGURE 60-8.** Model showing some of the multiple receptors that are coupled by means of $G_s$ to activation of adenylate cyclase. Gene mutations that reduce $G_s\alpha$ activity commonly impair transmembrane signal transduction processes and result in hormone resistance. By contrast, activating mutations of $G_s\alpha$ produce constitutive signal transduction in the absence of hormone or neurotransmitters and can result in autonomous cell function and proliferation. (*ADH*, antidiuretic hormone; *PTH*, parathyroid hormone; *TSH*, thyroid-stimulating hormone; *LH*, luteinizing hormone; *ACTH*, adrenocorticotropic hormone; *R*, receptor; *C*, catalytic unit of adenylate cyclase; *ATP*, adenosine triphosphate; *cAMP*, cyclic adenosine monophosphate.)

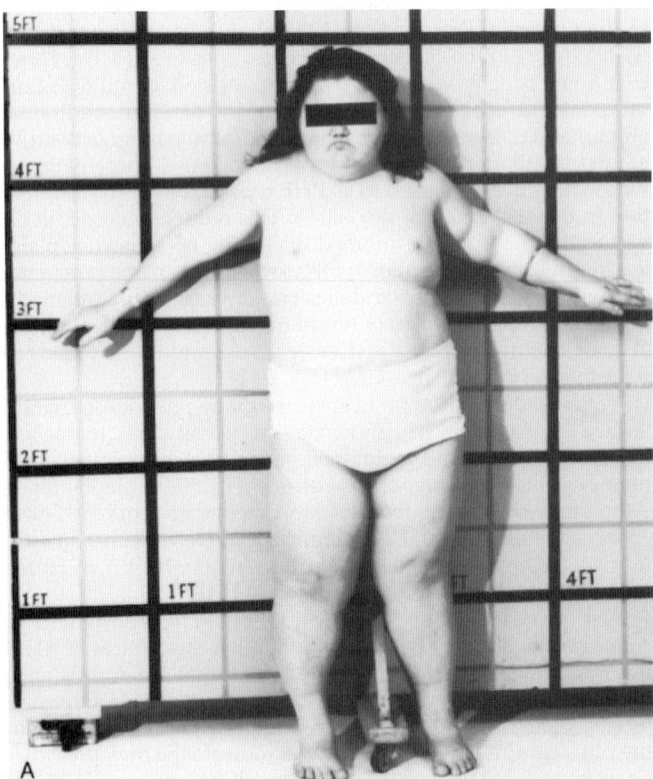

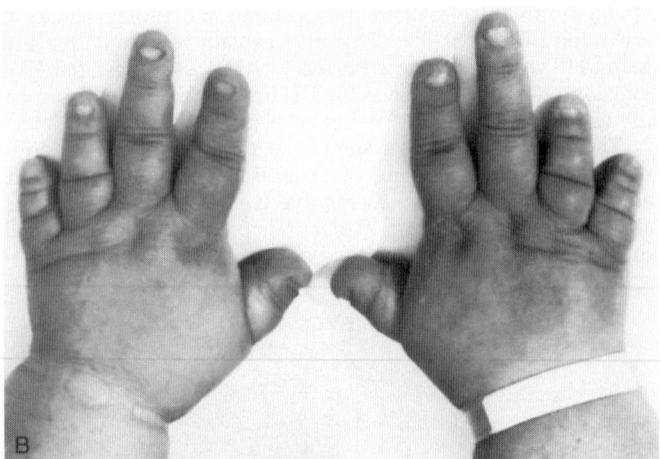

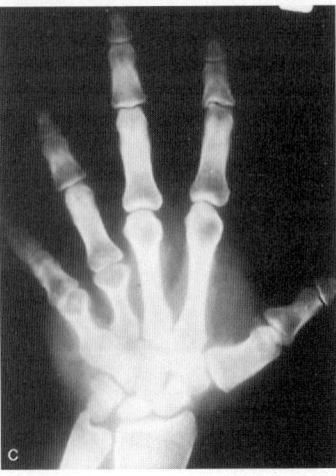

**FIGURE 60-9. A,** Young woman with Albright hereditary osteodystrophy. Note the short stature and rounded facies. **B,** Brachydactyly, particularly manifest in many patients as shortened fourth fingers. A "dimpling" of the fourth and fifth knuckle region may be seen when a fist is made. **C,** The radiograph reveals characteristic shortening of the fourth metacarpal, as well as shortening of the fifth metacarpal.

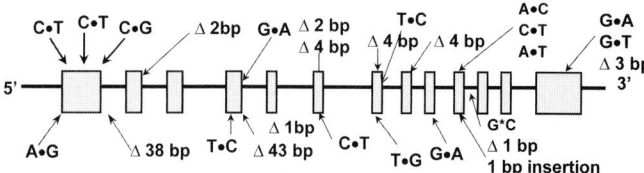

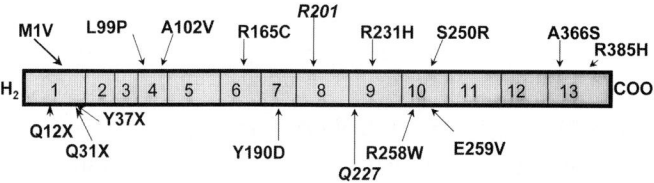

**FIGURE 60-10.** Mutations in the $G_s\alpha$ gene in Albright hereditary osteodystrophy. The upper diagram depicts the human $G_s\alpha$ gene, which spans over 20-kilobase pairs and contains 13 exons and 12 introns. Deletions (denoted by $\Delta$), missense (denoted by *asterisk*), nonsense, and splice-site mutations are noted in the appropriate location in the *GNAS1* gene. The lower panel depicts the amino acid changes in the protein as a result of the missense mutations in the gene. (*bp*, base pairs.)

chemical studies which indicate that patients with pseudoPHP who are related to patients with PHP type 1a have equivalent functional $G_s\alpha$ deficiency (see Fig. 60-7)[127] and identical gene defects (see later). Therefore, it seems reasonable to use the term *Albright hereditary osteodystrophy* to simplify description of this syndrome and to acknowledge the common clinical and biochemical characteristics that patients with PHP type 1a and pseudoPHP share.

The inheritance of $G_s\alpha$ deficiency in patients with AHO[127,128] first led to the speculation that the primary defect in this disorder involves the $G_s\alpha$ gene. The primary structure of the human $G_s\alpha$ protein has been deduced from characterization of complementary[129] and genomic[130] DNA clones. $G_s\alpha$ is encoded by exons 1 to 13 of the *GNAS1* gene (Fig. 60-10),[131–135] a complex gene that has been mapped to chromosome 20q13.2→q13.3 in humans.[136] The observation that patients with AHO have reduced[137,138] or normal[137] levels of $G_s\alpha$ mRNA has suggested that $G_s\alpha$ deficiency might arise from a variety of genetic mutations. Distinct heterozygous mutations in the *GNAS1* gene, including missense mutations,[131,133,134,139–141] point mutations in sequences required for efficient splicing,[132] insertions,[142] and small deletions[132–135,143–147] have been found in most kindreds studied (see Fig. 60-10); these findings imply that new mutations sustain this disorder in the population. A four-base-pair deletion in exon 7, which has been identified in several unrelated kindreds, appears to be a mutational hot spot.[135,146–149] Most patients with AHO have genetic defects that impair the synthesis of $G_s\alpha$ protein and, therefore, have $G_s\alpha$ deficiency. In other patients, mutations in the *GNAS1* gene lead to synthesis of dysfunctional proteins. These studies provide a molecular basis for $G_s\alpha$ deficiency and confirm that transmission of *GNAS1* gene defects accounts for the autosomal dominant inheritance of AHO (see Fig. 60-10). The delineation of these defects does not explain the often striking variability in expression of the biochemical or clinical phenotype, however. For example, despite a generalized $G_s\alpha$ deficiency, only some $G_s\alpha$-coupled pathways show reduced hormone responsiveness (e.g., to PTH, TSH, gonadotropins), whereas other pathways are apparently unaffected (those for ACTH in the adrenal and vasopressin in the renal medulla) (see Fig. 60-8).

One possible interpretation of variable hormonal responsiveness is that haploinsufficiency of $G_s\alpha$ is tissue specific; that is, in some tissues a 50% reduction in $G_s\alpha$ is still sufficient to facilitate normal signal transduction. However, this explanation leaves unanswered the even more intriguing question of

why some subjects with $G_s\alpha$ deficiency have hormone resistance (PHP type 1a), whereas others lack hormone resistance (pseudoPHP). Analysis of published pedigrees has indicated that in most cases maternal transmission of $G_s\alpha$ deficiency leads to PHP type 1a, whereas paternal transmission of the defect leads to pseudoPHP,[150–152] findings that have implicated genomic imprinting of the *GNAS1* gene as a possible regulatory mechanism.[151] Studies have indeed confirmed that the *GNAS1* gene is imprinted, but in a far more complex manner than had been anticipated. Two upstream promoters, each associated with a large coding exon, lie 35 kilobases (kb) upstream of *GNAS1* exon 1. These promoters are only 11 kb apart, yet show opposite patterns of allele-specific methylation and monoallelic transcription. The more 5' of these exons encodes *NESP55*, which is expressed exclusively from the maternal allele. By contrast, the XLαs exon is paternally expressed.[153,154] Despite the simultaneous imprinting in both the paternal and maternal directions of the *GNAS1* gene, expression of $G_s\alpha$ appears to be biallelic in all human tissues examined.[153–155] The lack of access to relevant tissues in patients with PHP type 1a has hindered studies of $G_s\alpha$ expression and stimulated attempts to develop suitable animal models. Two groups have succeeded in developing mice in which one *gnas* gene is disrupted, thereby generating murine models of PHP type 1a.[156,157] Although these mice have reduced levels of $G_s\alpha$ protein, they lack many of the features of the human disorder. Biochemical analyses of these heterozygous *gnas* knock-out mice indicate that $G_s\alpha$ expression is similarly reduced in most tissues, regardless of whether maternal or paternal transmission of the defective allele has occurred. In some tissues (e.g., renal cortex), however, $G_s\alpha$ expression is less in mice with maternal inheritance of the defective allele than in mice with paternal inheritance of the defective allele. Accordingly, mice that inherit the defective *gnas* gene maternally express too little $G_s\alpha$ protein in the renal proximal tubular cells to facilitate normal PTH stimulation of adenylate cyclase. By contrast, the 50% reduction in $G_s\alpha$ expression that occurs in other tissues may account for more variable and moderate hormone resistance in these sites (e.g., the thyroid). Further studies are necessary to confirm that tissue-specific imprinting is the basis for these differences in $G_s\alpha$ expression.

## OTHER G PROTEIN DISEASES

G protein defects are responsible for a number of other human diseases, most of which are rare endocrine disorders[158,159] (Table 60-4). The *McCune-Albright syndrome* is characterized by the clinical triad of autonomous hyperfunction of one or more

**TABLE 60-4.**
**G Protein Mutations in Human Disease**

| Disease | Defective G Protein | Molecular Mechanism |
|---|---|---|
| Pseudohypoparathyroidism 1a | $G_s\alpha$ | Loss of function mutations |
| Pseudohypoparathyroidism 1b | Possibly $G_s\alpha$ | Imprinting defect |
| McCune-Albright syndrome | $G_s\alpha$ | Gain of function mutations |
| Pseudohypoparathyroidism with testotoxicosis | $G_s\alpha$ | Loss/gain of function mutations |
| Hyperfunctioning thyroid adenomas | $G_s\alpha$ | Gain of function mutations |
| Pituitary adenomas (GH and ACTH) | $G_s\alpha$ | Gain of function mutations |
| Adrenocortical adenomas | $G_{i2}\alpha$ | Gain of function mutations |
| Endocrine ovarian neoplasms | $G_s\alpha$ | Gain of function mutations |
| Essential hypertension | $\beta 3$ | Gain of function mutations |
| Night blindness | $G_t\alpha$ | Loss of function mutations |

*GH*, growth hormone; *ACTH*, adrenocorticotropic hormone.

endocrine glands, irregularly bordered café-au-lait lesions, and fibrous dysplasia. The variable expression of these features in different tissues results from the mosaic distribution of cells containing a postzygotic somatic mutation in the *GNAS1* gene that activates $G_s\alpha$ protein. These mutations replace arginine[201], the site of modification by cholera toxin, by either cysteine or histidine and thereby impair the ability of $G_s\alpha$ to hydrolyze GTP. As occurs in cholera, the modified $G_s\alpha$ protein has enhanced activity[160,161] and is able to activate adenylate cyclase in the absence of hormonal stimulation. In McCune-Albright syndrome, the presence of the activated $G_s\alpha$ protein in tissues in which cAMP is trophic leads to cellular proliferation and autonomous hyperfunction (see Fig. 60-8) and can result in hyperthyroidism, precocious puberty, and growth hormone excess.[159] The characterization of a unique missense mutation in the *GNAS1* gene in two unrelated males with AHO and precocious puberty provides an unusual mechanism by which one mutation may cause both hormone resistance and constitutive signaling.[134] An Arg[366] to Ser missense mutation in the G5 region of the protein, which is important for guanyl nucleotide exchange, results in a temperature-sensitive form of $G_s\alpha$ that is rapidly degraded at 37°C, thereby leading to hormone resistance in many target tissues. However, the abnormal $G_s\alpha$ chain is stable at 32°C, and therefore accumulates in the testes, where the Arg[366] to Ser substitution leads to constitutive activation of adenylate cyclase and precocious puberty.

Activating mutations in $G_s\alpha$ have been identified in up to 40% of sporadic somatotropic tumors in acromegaly. As in the McCune-Albright syndrome, mutations in $G_s\alpha$ arginine[201] and glutamine[227] impair the ability of $G_s\alpha$ to hydrolyze GTP and result in persistent stimulation of adenylate cyclase.[162] This constitutively active mutant $G_s\alpha$ has been termed the *gsp oncogene*; it mimics the intracellular signaling triggered by GHRH and stimulates release of growth hormone and proliferation of somatotropes. A few autonomously hyperfunctioning thyroid adenomas harbor similar activating $G_s\alpha$ mutations,[163] and gain of function mutations in $G_{i2}$ have been identified in adrenal cortical adenomas and the endocrine tumors of the ovary.[164]

## PSEUDOHYPOPARATHYROIDISM TYPE 1B

Some subjects with PHP type 1 lack features of AHO. These patients typically show hormone resistance that is limited to PTH target organs (see Fig. 60-8) and have normal $G_s\alpha$ activity.[123,124] This variant is termed *PHP type 1b*.[165] Although patients with PHP type 1b fail to show a nephrogenous cAMP response to PTH, they often manifest skeletal lesions similar to those that occur in patients with hyperparathyroidism. These observations have suggested that at least one intracellular signaling pathway coupled to the PTH receptor may be intact in patients with PHP type 1b (see Fig. 60-6).

The molecular basis for PTH resistance in PHP type 1b has not been clearly defined. Specific resistance to PTH and normal activity of $G_s\alpha$ in available cells have implicated decreased expression or function of the PTH/PTHrP receptor as the cause of the hormone resistance. Despite extensive analysis of the complementary DNA,[166,167] coding exons and exon/intron boundaries,[168] and the promoter regions of the PTH/PTHrP receptor gene,[169,170] no mutations have been identified in PHP type 1b patients, and linkage analysis studies have excluded unsequenced regions of the gene.[170a] Additional evidence against the notion that the defects in the PTH/PTHrP receptor cause PHP type 1b come from studies of mice[171] and humans[71,72] who are heterozygous for inactivation of the gene encoding the PTH/PTHrP receptor. Remarkably, loss of one PTH/PTHrP receptor gene does not cause PTH resistance or hypocalcemia. Finally, inheritance of two defective type PTH/PTHrP receptor genes results in *Blomstrand chondrodysplasia*, a lethal genetic disorder characterized by

advanced endochondral bone maturation.[71,72] Thus, the molecular defect in PHP type 1b is likely to reside in another gene or genes that regulate expression or activity of the PTH/PTHrP receptor. A linkage analysis of four unrelated PHP type 1b kindreds established linkage to 20q13.3, the region that includes the $G_s\alpha$ gene (*GNAS1*).[172] The chromosomal region most tightly linked to the phenotype in these kindreds is not *GNAS1* itself but an area centromeric to the $G_s\alpha$ gene. Although these data are consistent with the existence of a second gene involved in mineral ion homeostasis in close proximity to *GNAS1*, defects in *GNAS1* or the promoter region that might limit $G_s\alpha$ deficiency to the kidney cannot be excluded.

## PSEUDOHYPOPARATHYROIDISM TYPE 1C

In a few patients with PHP type 1, resistance to multiple hormones occurs in the absence of a demonstrable defect in $G_s$ or $G_i$[120] (see Fig. 60-8). The nature of the lesion in such patients is unclear, but it could be related to some other general component of the receptor-adenylate cyclase system, such as the catalytic unit.[173] Alternatively, these patients could have functional defects of $G_s$ (or $G_i$) that do not become apparent in the assays presently available.

## GENETICS

Genetic studies of AHO and other forms of PTH resistance have been hampered by incomplete clinical descriptions of affected patients and inadequate characterization of their biochemical defects. The inheritance of AHO has been controversial. X-linked, autosomal dominant, and autosomal recessive inheritance of AHO has been proposed[128]; however, the description of father-to-son transmission of AHO with $G_s\alpha$ deficiency provided strong evidence against an X-linked mode of inheritance.[174] The identification of defects in the *GNAS1* gene in subjects with AHO has provided compelling evidence for autosomal dominant inheritance of AHO, including PHP type 1a and pseudoPHP.

A striking feature of AHO is the occurrence of individuals with PHP type 1a and pseudoPHP in the same family who have identical mutations in the *GNAS1* gene and show similar reductions in function or expression of $G_s\alpha$. Perhaps even more remarkable is the observation that pseudoPHP and PHP type 1a do not occur in the same generation. Furthermore, the phenotypic expression of $G_s\alpha$ deficiency appears to become more severe with each successive generation.[175] This pattern had originally been attributed to genomic imprinting,[150,151] as reviews of published reports of AHO kindreds had indicated that maternal transmission of $G_s\alpha$ deficiency led to PHP type 1a, whereas paternal transmission led to pseudoPHP.[150,151] Although the *GNAS1* locus is within an imprinted region of the genome, several lines of evidence argue against a model of simple imprinting as the mechanism for variable phenotype (see earlier). First, analysis of cells from patients with PHP type 1a and pseudoPHP have shown that these cells contain equivalent amounts of $G_s\alpha$ protein.[127] Second, the description of both maternal and paternal transmission of PHP type 1a[176] in a single multiplex family with $G_s\alpha$ deficiency[177] has suggested that the parental origin of the *GNAS1* mutation may be unrelated to phenotype. Third, although transcripts encoding *NESP55* and XL$\alpha$s are derived from only the maternal or the paternal allele, respectively (see earlier), $G_s\alpha$ transcripts are actively transcribed from both *GNAS1* genes in all fetal[177] and adult human tissues analyzed,[153,154] indicating that both $G_s\alpha$ alleles are expressed in a wide variety of tissues. This suggests that either tissue-specific imprinting or other mechanisms may be responsible for the variable expression of *GNAS1* gene defects observed within members of the same kindred.

The inheritance of other forms of PHP is less well characterized. Inheritance of PHP type 1b is most consistent with an autosomal dominant pattern.[172]

## PSEUDOHYPOPARATHYROIDISM TYPE 2

A few patients have been described in whom renal resistance to PTH is manifested by a reduced phosphaturic response to exogenous PTH, despite a normal increase in urinary cAMP excretion.[178] These observations suggest that the PTH receptor–adenylate cyclase complex is functionally normal but that PTH resistance arises from an inability of intracellular cAMP to initiate the chain of metabolic events that results in the ultimate expression of PTH action. Although no supportive data are yet available, a defective cAMP-dependent protein kinase A has been postulated.[178]

Pseudohypoparathyroidism type 2 is a clinically heterogeneous disorder without a clear genetic or familial basis. Fewer than 25 patients with the disorder have been reported, and biochemical characterization in many cases has been incomplete. The frequent observation that normalization of the serum calcium concentration can correct the defective phosphaturic response to PTH has suggested that the metabolic defect in this disorder may be a failure of PTH to activate a calcium-dependent second messenger system. In addition, apparent PTH resistance in some of these cases could be the result of severe hypocalcemia caused by an unrecognized acquired deficiency of vitamin D or its metabolites.[179]

## PSEUDOHYPOPARATHYROIDISM WITH SKELETAL RESPONSIVENESS

Although, generally, the assumption has been that PTH resistance extends to the skeleton, this remains unproved. Evidence that bone cells are unresponsive to PTH in patients with PHP has been inferred from the attendant hypocalcemia in the disorder that is not corrected with the administration of PTH. However, bone demineralization occurs frequently in patients with PHP types 1a and 1b,[180] although clinically significant hyperparathyroid bone disease with radiologic or histologic features of severe osteitis fibrosa cystica is rare. Whether these latter patients represent the extreme end of a spectrum of bone demineralization or a qualitatively different disease mechanism is unclear. In PHP, a deficiency of 1,25(OH)$_2$D may underlie the presence of the hypocalcemia and the apparent PTH unresponsiveness of the bone homeostatic mechanism in PHP; this conflicts with the premise that bone cells are intrinsically resistant to the actions of PTH.

## BIOINEFFECTIVE PARATHYROID HORMONE

The secretion of an abnormal, biologically inactive PTH molecule is a theoretical cause of functional hypoparathyroidism. Individuals with such a disorder might be expected to have elevated levels of circulating immunoreactive PTH and should respond normally to exogenous PTH, thus distinguishing them from patients with PHP. To date, a few cases have been reported in which the biochemical data were supportive of such a mechanism. In one previously reported case of bioineffective PTH, repeat study revealed clearly reduced or absent plasma levels of PTH in radioimmunoassays that were midmolecule specific or carboxy-terminal specific, despite symptomatic hypocalcemia.[55]

A second form of bioineffective PTH has been proposed as a mechanism to explain resistance to PTH in some patients with PHP.[181–183] In these patients an "inhibitor" is presumed to be secreted by the parathyroid gland with the characteristics of a PTH antagonist. Thus, subjects show elevated circulating levels of PTH by radioimmunoassay, absent or reduced levels of PTH by a sensitive cytochemical bioassay, and a defective urinary cAMP response to exogenous PTH. The nature of this putative inhibitor remains elusive. Whether such an inhibitor is an abnormal form of PTH or even a product of the parathyroid gland is not clear from available data. Conceivably this inhibitor may provide the

pathophysiologic basis for PTH resistance for some patients with PHP; however, the possibility that a circulating PTH inhibitor arises because of the primary biochemical defect is equally likely.

## OTHER CAUSES OF HYPOCALCEMIA

### HYPERPHOSPHATEMIA

Hypocalcemia may also occur because of acute or chronic hyperphosphatemia. Plasma phosphate, when elevated, complexes with calcium to cause subsequent extraskeletal calcifications; if chronically maintained, this elevation depresses renal 1α-hydroxylase activity and leads to reduced production of 1,25(OH)$_2$D. Hyperphosphatemia may result from iatrogenic administration of phosphate (either parenterally, orally, or rectally) or release from cells (e.g., after rapid tumor lysis during chemotherapy for Burkitt lymphoma or acute lymphoblastic leukemia).

### RHABDOMYOLYSIS

Hypocalcemia also occurs in rhabdomyolysis and in acute severe illnesses (pancreatitis, sepsis, burns).[103a,184] In these disorders, the cause of hypocalcemia is unclear, but it may be related to cell lysis with hyperphosphatemia or to movement of calcium into soft tissues with an inadequate acute response of the PTH–vitamin D homeostatic system.

### CANCER

Hypocalcemia frequently occurs in patients with cancer, but it usually represents a reduction in total, rather than ionized, calcium because of the effect of hypoproteinemia. Conversely, true reductions in ionized calcium occur in patients with cancer, particularly of breast and prostate, who have osteoblastic metastases.[185,186] Hypocalcemia in these patients has been attributed to increased calcium flux into the osteoblastic lesions.

Hypocalcemia of unknown cause is commonly associated with acute illness and carries a poor prognosis. Frequently, these patients are experiencing stress related to sepsis.[187]

### DISORDERS OF VITAMIN D METABOLISM

Abnormalities in vitamin D metabolism cause reduced intestinal calcium absorption; moreover, PTH-induced mobilization of calcium from bone to blood is impaired. Both of these factors may produce hypocalcemia if compensatory actions of PTH or 1,25(OH)$_2$D are inadequate.

#### ACQUIRED VITAMIN D DEFICIENCIES

Deficiencies of vitamin D or its active metabolite, 1,25(OH)$_2$D, are accompanied by hypocalcemia and secondary (adaptive) hyperparathyroidism. Deficiency of vitamin D may arise because of inadequate sunlight exposure, dietary deficiency, or malabsorption. A specific deficiency of 25(OH)D may develop in some patients with severe hepatobiliary disease. The principal example of an acquired deficiency of 1,25(OH)$_2$D is chronic renal insufficiency (see Chap. 61). Several drugs, most notably corticosteroids, barbiturates, and phenytoin, can interfere with vitamin D metabolism or action, and occasionally they can cause clinical hypocalcemia and secondary hyperparathyroidism.

#### HEREDITARY DISORDERS OF VITAMIN D METABOLISM

Hypocalcemia and secondary hyperparathyroidism can be biochemical manifestations of hereditary disorders of vitamin D function. Deficient 1,25(OH)$_2$D formation and action are causes of hypocalcemia and osteomalacia in patients who have either 1α-hydroxylase deficiency (vitamin D–dependent rickets type I)[188] or hereditary resistance to 1,25(OH)$_2$D (vitamin D–dependent rickets type II), respectively[189] (see Chap. 63).

# DIFFERENTIAL DIAGNOSIS OF HYPOCALCEMIA

The history and physical examination are quite important in the evaluation of hypocalcemia. The goal of the bedside examination is to characterize the severity of symptoms and the duration of hypocalcemia, to detect underlying medical conditions, and to search for specific features of the various states of hypoparathyroidism and other disorders of mineral metabolism. Often, the clinical evaluation provides a tentative diagnosis that can be confirmed by appropriate laboratory tests.

An understanding of the causes of hypocalcemia (see Table 60-2) provides the basis for the clinical evaluation. If the patient is asymptomatic and the hypocalcemia has been detected by blood tests performed for other reasons, one should first estimate the likelihood of true ionized hypocalcemia by examining the concentrations of serum proteins. Occasionally, the measurement of ionized calcium by a reliable laboratory is helpful. Acute changes in the distribution of calcium between ionized and bound fractions may be indicated by a history of hyperventilation (respiratory alkalosis), recent massive blood transfusion (citrate), trauma with rhabdomyolysis, tumor lysis after chemotherapy, or phosphate administration by enema or intravenous infusion.

Transient hypoparathyroidism can often be anticipated (in neonates and in patients with parathyroid suppression after treatment of hypercalcemia); therefore, it is usually not a diagnostic problem. Reversible hypoparathyroidism associated with hypomagnesemia may be suggested by a history of alcoholism, gastrointestinal disease, or treatment with drugs that cause renal magnesium wasting. Chronic genetic or acquired hypoparathyroidism often is associated with characteristic features, such as family history, abnormal habitus, other endocrine disturbances, or a history of damage to the parathyroid glands. Steatorrhea, liver disease, or renal insufficiency may suggest a deficiency of vitamin D metabolites (see Chap. 63).

One occasionally may be confronted with a patient in tetany for whom no previous medical history is available. Even if urgent therapy is deemed necessary, a blood sample should be obtained quickly, before the administration of calcium, for the determination of levels of calcium, phosphorus, blood urea nitrogen or creatinine, albumin, electrolytes, and magnesium, and for PTH radioimmunoassay. The results of these determinations can direct the subsequent evaluation.

In the absence of renal insufficiency, and if no history of an acute phosphate load is present, hyperphosphatemia is often an indication of deficient PTH secretion or abnormal PTH action. If the patient's nutritional status is normal, then hypophosphatemia may be suspected of being associated with secondary hyperparathyroidism in states of abnormal vitamin D action.

## SERUM PARATHYROID HORMONE LEVELS

Specific endocrine tests often are helpful in the evaluation. Because normally hypocalcemia is a potent stimulus for the secretion of PTH, patients with intact parathyroid gland function should be expected to have high circulating levels of PTH during hypocalcemic episodes. Low levels of serum PTH, and, with some assays, even inappropriately "normal" levels despite hypocalcemia, should prompt consideration of the various forms of hypoparathyroidism (see Table 60-2). Given the clinical history, duration of hypocalcemia, and physical findings, the cause of deficient parathyroid gland function can usually be determined. Because a number of different PTH assays are available (see Chaps. 51, 58, and 61), correct interpretation depends on familiarity with the results to be expected in the

particular assay. Caution should be exercised in the interpretation of the PTH assay if the patient has renal insufficiency.

If PTH levels are appropriately elevated in a hypocalcemic patient, then pseudohypoparathyroidism, disorders of vitamin D metabolism or action, and a variety of other conditions (see Table 60-2) need to be considered.

## PARATHYROID HORMONE INFUSION

Pseudohypoparathyroidism can sometimes be suggested by the characteristic habitus or the finding of hyperphosphatemia. The confirmation of the diagnosis depends on the demonstration of a deficient target organ response to PTH. This is usually accomplished by demonstrating a lack of the normal brisk increase in urinary excretion of cAMP and phosphate after an infusion of PTH.[190] Deficient activity of the adenylate cyclase coupling protein (G$_s$) in cell membranes from those patients with pseudohypoparathyroidism type 1a can also be demonstrated with specialized techniques available in some centers. Under some circumstances, analyzing the response of plasma cAMP to an intravenous infusion of synthetic human PTH (1-34) is more convenient, particularly in patients in whom collection of urine is not possible or practical. Although this testing protocol can differentiate patients with PHP type 1a from normal subjects and patients with pseudoPHP or hypoparathyroidism,[191,192] normal changes in plasma cAMP are less dramatic than the changes in urinary cAMP. The observation of an apparently normal plasma cAMP response to PTH in a 3-month-old child who later developed clinical and biochemical evidence of PHP type 1a, including an abnormal plasma cAMP response to PTH, suggests that testing be delayed until after 6 months of age.[193]

## MEASUREMENT OF SERUM VITAMIN D METABOLITES

The measurement of vitamin D metabolites can be helpful in documenting abnormalities of vitamin D metabolism or action as causes of hypocalcemia. Low serum 25(OH)D levels suggest nutritional deficiency, malabsorption, or liver disease. Low serum 1,25(OH)$_2$D levels may be seen in patients who have a specific defect of renal 1α-hydroxylase and in patients with renal failure. Low serum levels of 1,25(OH)$_2$D are also found in patients with hypoparathyroidism and pseudohypoparathyroidism, so results must be interpreted in the light of other tests of PTH secretion and action. Very high levels of 1,25(OH)$_2$D in patients with hypocalcemia may indicate resistance to the action of calcitriol.

Other causes of hypocalcemia with appropriate elevations of PTH are numerous (see Table 60-2) but are often acute in onset, with a definite precipitating event that can be determined by a careful history.

# THERAPY FOR HYPOCALCEMIA

Before treating hypocalcemia, one should recall that hypoalbuminemia is the most common cause of low total serum calcium concentration; it often occurs in patients with malnutrition or other debilitating diseases. In such patients, nutritional support, rather than treatment of hypocalcemia, is appropriate. If hypoalbuminemia cannot account for the observed decrease in total calcium, or if the ionized calcium level is found to be low, an evaluation and treatment of the hypocalcemia are indicated. Underlying disorders, such as hypomagnesemia or malabsorption, should be sought and corrected whenever possible.

## EMERGENCY THERAPY

Urgent therapy with intravenous calcium is required for patients who have acute hypocalcemic crisis manifested by severe tetany, laryngospasm, or convulsions. In adults, 10 to 20 mL of 10% calcium gluconate (93 mg elemental calcium per 10 mL, 4.65 mEq/10 mL) may be infused over 10 minutes. For children, 2 mg of elemental calcium per kilogram of body weight (~0.2 mL/kg of 10% calcium gluconate) may be used. Patients who require immediate treatment for tetany and patients who have symptoms of hypocalcemia without tetany are often candidates for intravenous calcium infusion over a longer period. Elemental calcium (10–15 mg/kg) may be infused over 6 to 8 hours while serum calcium levels are monitored to assess the adequacy of the administered dose. Calcium salts are extremely irritating; therefore, care should be taken to avoid extravasation of the dose, and dilution of the calcium in at least 50 to 100 mL of electrolyte solution is recommended. Certain anions, such as bicarbonate and phosphate, cause the precipitation of calcium.

## LONG-TERM THERAPY

Maintenance therapy for hypoparathyroidism consists of supplemental administration of oral calcium or vitamin D, or both. Because patients with hypoparathyroidism lack the renal effects of PTH, they usually have hypercalciuria at serum calcium concentrations within the normal range.[194] Therefore, the serum calcium concentration should be maintained in the range of 8 to 9 mg/dL. This is sufficiently high to prevent most symptoms of hypocalcemia and to retard the progression of cataracts, but low enough that hypercalciuria is uncommon. Nevertheless, episodes of hypercalciuria and hypercalcemia can occur even in patients who have taken stable doses of calcium and vitamin D for years. By contrast, hypercalciuria is unusual in patients with pseudohypoparathyroidism.

## TREATMENT WITH CALCIUM SALTS

A relatively high dose of a calcium salt (1500–2500 mg elemental calcium as a daily supplement) is recommended to provide a level of ingested calcium that is adequate to minimize fluctuations caused by variable dietary calcium intake. Patients can also be educated to consume a consistent quantity of calcium from dietary sources each day. Calcium content differs considerably among the available oral preparations[195] (see Chap. 236). Because therapy for hypoparathyroidism must be individualized to obtain a desired serum calcium level, few absolute guidelines exist for choosing one calcium salt over another. However, the patient may have a preference, and compliance can be maximized by suggesting the most tolerable dosage form. Calcium carbonate and calcium phosphate are poorly absorbed by patients with achlorhydria; optimal absorption requires that these salts be taken with meals.[196]

## THERAPY WITH VITAMIN D OR ITS METABOLITES

In some patients with decreased parathyroid reserve, oral calcium supplementation may be sufficient to alleviate symptoms of hypocalcemia. In most patients, however, treatment with vitamin D or one of its metabolites is required. In patients with some disorders of vitamin D metabolism, treating with a precursor metabolite is reasonable, so that the ability of PTH to regulate conversion of precursors to $1,25(OH)_2D$ can be preserved as a defense against drug toxicity. In hypoparathyroidism, PTH action is absent and regulated conversion of precursors to $1,25(OH)_2D$ does not occur. Therefore, the choice of vitamin D or another metabolite may be based on other considerations. Vitamin $D_2$ (ergocalciferol) is effective in treating patients with all forms of hypoparathyroidism and is the least expensive of the available preparations. The dosage required for the treatment of hypoparathyroidism is usually 50,000 to 100,000 U per day (1.25–2.5 mg per day), but dosage must be

individualized. During treatment with vitamin $D_2$, serum levels of 25(OH)D can be measured, if necessary, to assess compliance and drug absorption.[197] Vitamin $D_2$ is lipophilic, and a period of several weeks is required for its full effect to be established on beginning therapy. Likewise, if it must be discontinued, a prolonged period will be required for its effect to decrease. More active metabolites, such as calcitriol and 1α-OH-cholecalciferol (available outside the United States), have a more rapid onset of action, and a shorter period of time is required for their effects to decrease after discontinuation. However, these metabolites are more expensive, and frequent monitoring is necessary to avoid toxicity. Dihydrotachysterol is also active in patients who lack PTH action, and its moderate (1- to 4-week) duration of action and low cost offer a satisfactory compromise to vitamin $D_2$ and calcitriol. A disadvantage is that plasma levels of dihydrotachysterol cannot be monitored. The assessment of compliance may be more difficult when the patient is receiving a short-acting drug.

## VITAMIN D TOXICITY

Drug toxicity is a major concern whenever vitamin D or one of its metabolites is prescribed. For all of the agents, the therapeutic dose is close to the dose at which toxicity occurs; hence, therapy must be individualized and closely monitored. Frequent testing should include a determination of the serum calcium concentration, the urinary calcium excretion, and the serum creatinine level. Early toxicity can be recognized as asymptomatic hypercalciuria; more severe vitamin D intoxication is associated with asymptomatic or symptomatic hypercalcemia. Renal function can deteriorate during episodes of toxicity, and repeated episodes of vitamin D toxicity can lead to progressive renal insufficiency. If hypercalcemia occurs, both vitamin D and supplemental calcium should be discontinued and the patient should be treated, if necessary, for vitamin D intoxication (see Chap. 59). Those patients taking short-acting vitamin D metabolites can be rapidly switched to another dose form; patients taking vitamin $D_2$ may need to limit calcium intake for a prolonged period, until body stores of vitamin D decrease.

## INFLUENCE OF OTHER DRUGS

A number of commonly used drugs have important effects in patients who are treated with vitamin D and calcium. Thiazide diuretics enhance renal calcium reabsorption and may precipitate hypercalcemia in a patient taking vitamin D and calcium.[198] Treatment of patients who have mild hypoparathyroidism with sodium restriction and a long-acting thiazide diuretic has been reported to increase total and ionized serum calcium levels, even in patients not treated with vitamin D supplements[199]; however, the effect of thiazides to decrease renal calcium excretion is modest compared with the effect of vitamin D to increase intestinal calcium absorption.[200] Patients with hypoparathyroidism are markedly sensitive to the calciuric effects of loop diuretics and may become hypocalcemic after treatment with such drugs.[201] Glucocorticosteroids antagonize the actions of vitamin D metabolites. Anticonvulsants and other inducers of hepatic microsomal oxidases may increase the clearance of vitamin D metabolites.

Treatment with phosphate-binding antacids to decrease the level of serum phosphate is rarely necessary in patients with hypoparathyroidism, because renal phosphate clearance increases as serum calcium rises.[202]

Parathyroid allotransplantation has been attempted in some patients who have complicated hypoparathyroidism, with occasional success.[203] Long-term immunosuppression is required to maintain a functional graft, however, so that most patients with hypoparathyroidism are not candidates for such therapy.

## THERAPY DURING PREGNANCY

Neonatal hyperparathyroidism has been reported in the infants of hypocalcemic mothers; therefore, women with hypocalcemia should be appropriately treated during pregnancy. Because the mineral demands of the fetus change significantly during the course of pregnancy, patients should be monitored closely and treatment with a short-acting metabolite of vitamin D should be begun, so that dosage adjustments are immediately effective.

## REFERENCES

1. Moore EW. Ionized calcium in normal serum, ultrafiltrates, and whole blood determined by ion-exchange electrodes. J Clin Invest 1970; 49:318.
2. Ladenson JH, Lewis JW, Boyd JC. Failure of total calcium corrected for protein, albumin, and pH to correctly assess free calcium status. J Clin Endocrinol Metab 1978; 46:986.
3. Berry EM, Gupta MM, Turner SJ, Burns RR. Variations in plasma calcium with induced changes in plasma specific gravity, total protein, and albumin. BMJ 1973; 4:640.
4. Hoffman E. The Chvostek sign: a clinical study. Am J Surg 1958; 96:33.
5. Simpson JA. The neurologic manifestations of idiopathic hypoparathyroidism. Brain 1952; 75:76.
6. Wong CK, Lau CP, Cheng CH, et al. Hypocalcemic myocardial dysfunction: short and long-term improvement with calcium replacement. Am Heart J 1990; 120:381.
7. Levine SN, Rheams CN. Hypocalcemic heart failure. Am J Med 1975; 78:1022.
8. Rimailho A, Bouchard P, Schaison G, et al. Improvement of hypocalcemic cardiomyopathy by correction of serum calcium level. Am Heart J 1985; 109:611.
9. Kanda F, Jinnai I, Fujita T. Somatosensory evoked potentials in patients with hypocalcaemia after parathyroidectomy. J Neurol 1988; 235:136.
10. Nikiforuk G, Fraser D. Chemical determinants of enamel hypoplasia in children with disorders of calcium and phosphate homeostasis. J Dent Res 1979; 58(B):1014.
11. Illum F, Dupont E. Prevalence of CT-detected calcification in the basal ganglia in idiopathic hypoparathyroidism and pseudohypoparathyroidism. Neuroradiology 1985; 27:32.
12. Schaaf M, Payne C. Dystonic reactions to prochlorperazine in hypoparathyroidism. N Engl J Med 1966; 275:991.
13. Drezner ML, Neelan FA, Haussler M, et al. 1,25-Dihydroxycholecalciferol deficiency: the probable cause of hypocalcemia and metabolic bone disease in pseudohypoparathyroidism. J Clin Endocrinol Metab 1976; 42:621.
14. Schutt-Aine JC, Young MA, Pescovitz DH, et al. Hypoparathyroidism: a possible cause of rickets. J Pediatr 1985; 106:255.
15. Abugassa S, Nordenstrom J, Eriksson S, Sjoden G. Bone mineral density in patients with chronic hypoparathyroidism. J Clin Endocrinol Metab 1993; 76:1617.
16. Shukla S, Gillespy T III, Thomas WC Jr. The effect of hypoparathyroidism on the aging skeleton. J Am Geriatr Soc 1990; 38:884.
17. Orr-Walker B, Harris R, Holdaway IM, et al. High peripheral and axial bone densities in a postmenopausal woman with untreated hypoparathyroidism. Postgrad Med J 1990; 66:1061.
18. Wade JSH, Fourman P, Deane L. Recovery of parathyroid function in patients with "transient" hypoparathyroidism after thyroidectomy. Br J Surg 1965; 52:493.
19. Dent CE. Some problems of hyperparathyroidism. BMJ 1962; 2:1419.
20. Edis AJ. Prevention and management of complications associated with thyroid and parathyroid surgery. Surg Clin North Am 1979; 59:83.
21. Loré JM Jr. Complications in management of thyroid cancer. Semin Surg Oncol 1991; 7:120.
22. Gann DS, Paone JF. Delayed hypocalcemia after thyroidectomy for Graves' disease is prevented by parathyroid autotransplantation. Ann Surg 1979; 190:508.
23. Michie W, Stowers JM, Duncan T, et al. Mechanism of hypocalcemia after thyroidectomy for thyrotoxicosis. Lancet 1971; 1:508.
24. Watson CG, Steed DL, Robinson AG, Deftos LJ. The role of calcitonin and parathyroid hormone in the pathogenesis of post-thyroidectomy hypocalcemia. Metabolism 1981; 30:588.
25. Percival RC, Hargreaves AW, Kanis JA. The mechanism of hypocalcemia following thyroidectomy. Acta Endocrinol (Copenh) 1985; 109:220.
26. Neufield RB, Maclaren N, Blizzard R. Two types of autoimmune Addison's disease associated with different polyglandular autoimmune syndromes. Medicine (Baltimore) 1981; 60:355.
27. Barakat AY, D'Albora JB, Martin MM, Jose PA. Familial nephrosis, nerve deafness, and hypoparathyroidism. J Pediatr 1977; 91:61.
28. Benson PF, Parsons V. Hereditary hypoparathyroidism presenting with oedema in the neonatal period. QJM 1964; 130:197.
29. Dahlberg PJ, Borer WZ, Newcomer KL, Yutac WR. Autosomal or X-linked recessive syndrome of congenital lymphedema, hypoparathyroidism, nephropathy, prolapsing mitral valve, and brachytelephalangy. Am J Med Genet 1983; 16:99.
30. Raatikka M, Ropola J, Tuteri L, et al. Familial third and fourth pharyngeal pouch syndrome with truncus arteriosus: DiGeorge syndrome. Pediatrics 1981; 67:173.
31. Rohn RD, Leffell MS, Leadem P, et al. Familial third-fourth pharyngeal pouch syndrome with apparent autosomal dominant transmission. J Pediatr 1984; 105:47.
32. de la Chapelle A, Herra R, Kiovisto M, Aula P. A deletion in chromosome 22 can cause DiGeorge syndrome. Hum Genet 1981; 57:253.
33. Kelley RI, Zackai FH, Emanuel BS, et al. The association of the DiGeorge anomalad with partial monosomy of chromosome 22. J Pediatr 1982; 101:197.
34. Driscoll DA, Budarf ML, Emanuel BS. A genetic etiology for DiGeorge syndrome: consistent deletions and microdeletions of 22q11. Am J Hum Genet 1991; 50:924.
35. Monaco G, Pignata C, Rossi E, et al. DiGeorge anomaly associated with 10p deletion. Am J Med Genet 1991; 19:215.
36. Lai MMR, Scriven PN, Ball C, Berry AC. Simultaneous partial monosomy 10p and trisomy 5q in a case of hypoparathyroidism. J Med Genet 1992; 29:586.
37. Spinner MW, Blizzard RM, Childs B. Clinical and genetic heterogeneity in idiopathic Addison's disease and hypoparathyroidism. J Clin Endocrinol Metab 1968; 28:795.
38. Winter WE, Silverstein JH, Barrett DJ, Kiel E. Familial DiGeorge syndrome with tetralogy of Fallot and prolonged survival. Eur J Pediatr 1984; 141:171
39. Shaw NJ, Haigh D, Lealmann GT, et al. Autosomal recessive hypoparathyroidism with renal insufficiency and developmental delay. Arch Dis Child 1991; 66:1191.
40. Sanjad SA, Sakati NA, Abu-Osba YK, et al. A new syndrome of congenital hypoparathyroidism, severe growth failure, and dysmorphic features. Arch Dis Child 1991; 66:193.
41. Billous RW, Murty G, Parkinson DB, et al. Brief report: autosomal dominant familial hypoparathyroidism, sensorineural deafness, and renal dysplasia. N Engl J Med 1992; 327:1069.
42. Richardson RJ, Kirk JM. Short stature, mental retardation, and hypoparathyroidism: a new syndrome. Arch Dis Child 1990; 65:1113.
43. Ahonen P, Myllarniemi S, Sipila I, Perheentupa J. Clinical variation of autoimmune polyendocrinopathy–candidiasis–ectodermal dystrophy (APECED) in a series of 68 patients. N Engl J Med 1990; 322:1829.
44. Blizzard RM, Chee D, Davis W. The incidence of parathyroid and other antibodies in the sera of patients with idiopathic hypoparathyroidism. Clin Exp Immunol 1966; 1:119.
45. Verghese MW, Ward FE, Eisenbarth GS. Lymphocyte suppressor activity in patients with polyglandular failure. Hum Immunol 1981; 3:173.
46. Jackson RA, Haynes BF, Burch WM, et al. 1a+ T cells in new onset Graves' disease. J Clin Endocrinol Metab 1984; 59:187.
47. Nagamine K, Peterson P, Scott HS, et al. Positional cloning of the APECED gene. Nat Genet 1997; 17:393.
48. The Finnish-German APECED Consortium. An autoimmune disease, APECED, caused by mutations in a novel gene featuring two PHD-type zinc-finger domains. Nat Genet 1997; 17:399.
48a. Ishii T, Suzuki Y, Ando N, et al. Novel mutations of the autoimmune regulator gene in two siblings with autoimmune polyendocrinopathy-candidiasis-ectodermal dystrophy. J Clin Endocrinol Metab 2000; 85(8):2922.
49. Wang CY, Davoodi-Semiromi A, Huang W, et al. Characterization of mutations in patients with autoimmune polyglandular syndrome type 1 (APS1). Hum Genet 1998; 103:681.
50. Ward L, Paquette J, Seidman E, et al. Severe autoimmune polyendocrinopathy candidiasis-ectodermal dystrophy in an adolescent girl with a novel AIRE mutation: response to immunosuppressive therapy. J Clin Endocrinol Metab 1999; 84:844.
51. Posillico JT, Wortsman J, Srikanta S, et al. Parathyroid cell surface autoantibodies that inhibit parathyroid hormone secretion from dispersed human parathyroid cells. J Bone Miner Res 1986; 1:475.
52. Brandi ML, Aurbach GD, Fattorossi A, et al. Antibodies cytotoxic to bovine parathyroid cells in autoimmune hypoparathyroidism. Proc Natl Acad Sci U S A 1986; 83:8366.
53. Drake TG, Albright F, Bauer W. Chronic idiopathic hypoparathyroidism: report of 6 cases with autopsy findings in one. Ann Intern Med 1934; 12:1751.
54. Treusch JV. Idiopathic hypoparathyroidism: follow-up study including autopsy findings of a case previously reported. Ann Intern Med 1962; 56:484.
55. Ahn TG, Antonarakis SE, Kronenberg HM, et al. Familial isolated hypoparathyroidism: a molecular genetic analysis of 8 families with 23 affected persons. Medicine (Baltimore) 1986; 65:73.
56. Arnold A, Horst SA, Gardella TJ, et al. Mutation of the signal peptide–encoding region of the preproparathyroid hormone gene in familial isolated hypoparathyroidism. J Clin Invest 1990; 86:1084.
57. Parkinson DB, Shaw NJ, Himsworth RL, Thakker RV. Parathyroid hormone gene analysis in autosomal hypoparathyroidism using an intragenic tetranucleotide (AAAT)n polymorphism. Hum Genet 1993; 91:281.
58. Thakker RV, Davies KE, Whyte MP, et al. Mapping the gene causing X-linked recessive idiopathic hypoparathyroidism to Xq26-Xq27 by linkage studies. J Clin Invest 1990; 86:40.
59. Trump D, Dixon PH, Mumm S, et al. Localization of X-linked recessive idiopathic hypoparathyroidism to a 1.5 Mb region on Xq26-q27. J Med Genet 1998; 35:905.
60. Thakker RV. Molecular basis of PTH underexpression. In: Bilezikian JP, Raisz LG, Rodan GA, eds. Principles of bone biology. San Diego: Academic Press, 1996:837.
61. Brown EM, Gamba G, Riccardi D, et al. Cloning and characterization of an extracellular $Ca^{2+}$-sensing receptor from bovine parathyroid. Nature 1993; 366:575.
62. Brown EM. Physiology and pathophysiology of the extracellular calcium-sensing receptor. Am J Med 1999; 106:238.

63. Arthur JM, Collinsworth GP, Gettys TW, et al. Specific coupling of a cation-sensing receptor to G protein alpha-subunits in MDCK cells. Am J Physiol 1997; 273: F129.

64. Pearce SH, Williamson C, Kifor O, et al. A familial syndrome of hypocalcemia with hypercalciuria due to mutations in the calcium-sensing receptor [see comments]. N Engl J Med 1996; 335:1115.

65. Finegold DN, Armitage MM, Galiani M, et al. Preliminary localization of a gene for autosomal dominant hypoparathyroidism to chromosome 3q13. Pediatr Res 1994; 36:414.

66. Pollak MR, Brown EM, Chou YW, et al. Mutations in the human Ca$^{2+}$-sensing receptor gene cause familial hypocalciuric hypercalcemia and neonatal severe hyperparathyroidism. Cell 1993; 75:1297.

67. Pearce SH, Bai M, Quinn SJ, et al. Functional characterization of calcium-sensing receptor mutations expressed in human embryonic kidney cells. J Clin Invest 1996; 98:1860.

68. Pollak MR, Seidman CE, Brown EM. Three inherited disorders of calcium sensing. Medicine (Baltimore) 1996; 75:115.

69. Pollak MR, Brown EM, Estep HL, et al. Autosomal dominant hypocalcemia caused by a Ca$^{2+}$-sensing receptor gene mutation. Nat Genet 1994; 8:303.

70. Bai M, Quinn S, Trivedi S, et al. Expression and characterization of inactivating and activating mutations in the human Ca$^{2+}_o$-sensing receptor. J Biol Chem 1996; 271:19537.

71. Zhang P, Jobert AS, Couvinea A, Silve C. A homozygous inactivating mutation in the parathyroid hormone/parathyroid hormone related peptide receptor causing Blomstrand chondrodysplasia. J Clin Endocrinol Metab 1998; 83:3365.

72. Jobert AS, Zhang P, Couvineau A, et al. Absence of functional receptors for parathyroid hormone and parathyroid hormone-related peptide in Blomstrand chondrodysplasia. J Clin Invest 1998; 102:34.

73. Abramowicz MJ, Duprez L, Parma J, et al. Familial congenital hypothyroidism due to inactivating mutation of the thyrotropin receptor causing profound hypoplasia of the thyroid gland. J Clin Invest 1997; 99:3018.

74. Sunthornthepvarakul T, Gottschalk ME, Hayashi Y, Refetoff, S. Brief report: resistance to thyrotropin caused by mutations in the thyrotropin-receptor gene [see comments]. N Engl J Med 1995; 332:155.

75. Kremer H, Kraaij R, Toledo SPA, et al. Male pseudohermaphroditism due to homozygous missense mutation of the luteinizing hormone receptor gene. Nat Genet 1995; 9:160.

76. Latronico AC, Anasti J, Arnhold IJP, et al. Testicular and ovarian resistance to luteinizing hormone caused by inactivating mutations of the luteinizing hormone receptor gene. N Engl J Med 1996; 507.

77. Wajnrajch MP, Gertner JM, Harbison MD, et al. Nonsense mutation in the human growth hormone-releasing hormone receptor causes growth failure analogous to the little (lit) mouse. Nat Genet 1996; 12:88.

78. Netchine I, Talon P, Dastot F, Vitaux F, Goossens M, Amselem S. Extensive phenotypic analysis of a family with growth hormone (GH) deficiency caused by a mutation in the GH-releasing hormone receptor gene. J Clin Endocrinol Metab 1998; 83:432.

79. Salvatori R, Hayashida CY, Aguiar-Oliveira MH, et al. Familial dwarfism due to a novel mutation of the growth hormone-releasing hormone receptor gene. J Clin Endocrinol Metab 1999; 84:917.

80. Maheshwari HG, Silverman BL, Dupuis J, Baumann G. Phenotype and genetic analysis of a syndrome caused by an inactivating mutation in the growth hormone-releasing hormone receptor: dwarfism of Sindh. J Clin Endocrinol Metab 1998; 83:4065.

81. Weber A, Toppari J, Harvey RD, et al. Adrenocorticotropin receptor gene mutations in familial glucocorticoid deficiency: relationships with clinical features in four families. J Clin Endocrinol Metab 1995; 80:65.

82. Tsigos C, Arai K, Hung W, Chrousos GP. Hereditary isolated glucocorticoid deficiency is associated with abnormalities of the adrenocorticotropin receptor gene. J Clin Invest 1993; 92:2458.

83. Rosenthal W, Antaramian A, Gilbert S, Birnbaumer M. Nephrogenic diabetes insipidus. A V2 vasopressin receptor unable to stimulate adenylyl cyclase. J Biol Chem 1993; 268:13030.

84. Aittomaki K, Lucena JLD, Pakarinen P, et al. Mutation in the follicle-stimulating hormone receptor gene causes hereditary hypergonadotrophic ovarian failure. Cell 1995; 82:959.

85. De Roux N, Young J, Misrahi M, et al. A family with hypogonadotrophic hypogonadism and mutations in the gonadotrophin releasing hormone receptor. N Engl J Med 1997; 337:1597.

86. Parma J, Duprez L, Van Sande J, et al. Somatic mutations in the thyrotropin receptor gene cause hyperfunctioning thyroid adenomas. Nature 1993; 365:649.

87. Refetoff S, Sunthornthepvarakul T, Gottschalk ME, Hayashi, Y. Resistance to thyrotropin and other abnormalities of the thyrotropin receptor. Recent Prog Horm Res 1996; 51:97.

88. Duprez L, Parma J, Van Sande J, et al. Germline mutations in the thyrotropin receptor gene cause non-autoimmune autosomal dominant hyperthyroidism. Nat Genet 1994; 7:396.

89. Schipani E, Parfitt AM, Jensen GS, et al. Constitutively activated receptors for parathyroid hormone and parathyroid hormone related peptide in Jansen's metaphyseal chondrodysplasia. N Engl J Med 1996; 335:708.

90. Shenker A, Laue L, Kosugi S, et al. A constitutively activating mutation of the luteinizing hormone receptor in familial male precocious puberty. Nature 1993; 365:652.

91. Yano K, Hidaka A, Saji M, et al. A sporadic case of male-limited precocious puberty has the same constitutively activating point mutation in the luteinizing hormone/choriogonadotropin receptor gene as familial cases. J Clin Endocrinol Metab 1994; 79:1818.

92. Baldini A. Is the genetic basis of DiGeorge syndrome in HAND? Nat Genet 1999; 21:246.

93. Yamagishi H, Garg V, Matsuoka R, et al. A molecular pathway revealing a genetic basis for human cardiac and craniofacial defects. Science 1999; 283:1158.

94. Pizzuti A, Novelli G, Rattie A, et al. UFD1L, a developmentally expressed ubiquitination gene, is deleted in CATCH 22 syndrome. Hum Mol Genet 1997; 6:259.

95. Watanabe, Mochizuki H, Kohda N, et al. Autosomal dominant familial hypoparathyroidism and sensorineural deafness without renal dysplasia. Eur J Endocrinol 1998; 139:631.

95a. Lichtner P, Konig R, Hasegawa T, et al. An HDR (hypoparathyroidism, deafness, renal dysplasia) syndrome locus maps distal to the DiGeorge syndrome region on 10p13/14. J Med Genet 2000; 37(1):33.

95b. Van Esch H, Groenen P, Nesbit MA, et al. GATA3 haplo-insufficiency causes human HDR syndrome. Nature 2000; 406(6794):419.

95c. Gunther T, Chen ZF, Kim J, et al. Genetic ablation of parathyroid glands reveals another source of parathyroid hormone. Nature 2000; 406(6792):199.

95d. Ding C, Buckingham B, Levine MA. Neonatal hypoparathyroidism attributable to homozygous partial deletion of the human glial cell missing gene-B. Proceedings of the annual meeting of the Endocrine Society Toronto, 2000:CA409 (Abstr).

95e. Garcia-Garcia E, Camacho-Alonso J, Gomez-Rodriguez MJ, et al. Transient congenital hypoparathyroidism and 22q11 deletion. J Pediatr Endocrinol Metab 2000; 13(6):659.

96. Baltrop D. Neonatal hypocalcemia. Postgrad Med 1975; 51(Suppl 3):18.

97. Laitinen K, Tahtela R, Valimanki M. The dose-dependency of alcohol-induced hypoparathyroidism, hypercalciuria, and hypermagnesuria. Bone Miner 1992; 19:75.

98. Attie MF, Fallon MD, Spar B, et al. Bone and parathyroid inhibitory effects of S-2(3-aminopropylamino) ethylphosphorothioic acid. J Clin Invest 1985; 75:1191.

99. Hirschel-Scholz S, Caverzasio J, Bonjour J-P. Inhibition of parathyroid hormone secretion and parathyroid hormone–independent diminution of tubular calcium reabsorption by WR-2721, a unique hypocalcemic agent. J Clin Invest 1985; 76:1851.

100. Carpenter TO, Carnes DL Jr, Anast CS. Hypoparathyroidism in Wilson's disease. N Engl J Med 1983; 309:873.

101. Duran MJ, Borst GC, Osburne RC, Eil C. Concurrent renal hypomagnesemia and hypoparathyroidism with normal parathormone responsiveness. Am J Med 1984; 76:151.

102. Anast CS, Mohs JM, Kaplan SL, Burns TW. Evidence for parathyroid failure in magnesium deficiency. Science 1972; 177:606.

103. Estep H, Shaw WA, Watlington C, et al. Hypocalcemia due to hypomagnesemia and reversible parathyroid hormone unresponsiveness. J Clin Endocrinol Metab 1969; 29:842.

103a. Klein GL, Langman CB, Herndon DN. Persistent hypoparathyroidism following magnesium repletion in burn-injured children. Pediatr Nephrol 2000; 14(4):301.

104. Cholst IN, Steinberg SF, Tropper PJ, et al. The influence of hypermagnesemia on serum calcium and parathyroid hormone levels in human subjects. N Engl J Med 1984; 310:1221.

105. Kerr D, Hosking DJ. Pseudohypoparathyroidism: clinical expression of PTH resistance. QJM 1987; 247:889.

106. Verhoeven GFM, Wilson JD. The syndromes of primary hormone resistance. Metabolism 1979; 28:253.

107. Albright F, Burnett CH, Smith PH, Parson W. Pseudohypoparathyroidism—an example of "Seabright-Bantam syndrome." Endocrinology 1942; 3:922.

108. Chase LR, Aurbach GD. Parathyroid function and the renal excretion of 3'5'-adenylic acid. Proc Natl Acad Sci U S A 1967; 55:518.

109. Chase LR, Melson GL, Aurbach GD. Pseudohypoparathyroidism: defective excretion of 3'5'-AMP in response to parathyroid hormone. J Clin Invest 1969; 48:1832.

110. Hruska KA, Moskowitz D, Esbrit P, et al. Stimulation of inositol triphosphate and diacylglycerol production in renal tubular cells by parathyroid hormone. J Clin Invest 1987; 79:230.

111. Reid IR, Civitelli R, Halstead LR, et al. Parathyroid hormone acutely elevates intracellular calcium in osteoblast-like cells. Am J Physiol 1987; 252:E45.

112. Cole JA, Eber SL, Poelling RE, et al. A dual mechanism for regulation of kidney phosphate transport by parathyroid hormone. Am J Physiol 1987; 253:E221.

113. Yamaguchi DT, Hahn TJ, Iida-Klein A, et al. Parathyroid hormone-activated calcium channels in an osteoblast-like clonal osteosarcoma cell line: cAMP-dependent and cAMP-independent calcium channels. J Biol Chem 1987; 262:7711.

114. Yamamoto M, Takuwa Y, Masuko S, Ogata E. Effects of endogenous and exogenous parathyroid hormone on tubular reabsorption of calcium in pseudohypoparathyroidism. J Clin Endocrinol Metab 1988; 66:618.

115. Stone MD, Hosking DJ, Garcia-Himmelstine C, et al. The renal response to exogenous parathyroid hormone in treated pseudohypoparathyroidism. Bone 1993; 14:727.

116. Gilman AG. G proteins and dual control of adenylate cyclase. Cell 1984; 36:577.

117. Farfel Z, Bourne H, Iiri T. The expanding spectrum of G protein diseases. N Engl J Med 1999; 340:1012.

118. Hamm H. The many faces of G protein signalling. J Biol Chem 1998; 273:669.

119. Sprang SR. G protein mechanisms: insights from structural analysis. Annu Rev Biochem 1997; 66:639.

120. Levine MA, Downs RW Jr, Moses AM, et al. Resistance to multiple hormones in patients with pseudohypoparathyroidism: association with deficient activity of the guanine nucleotide regulatory protein. Am J Med 1983; 74:545.

121. Farfel Z, Friedman E. Mental deficiency in pseudohypoparathyroidism type 1 is associated with Ns-protein deficiency. Ann Intern Med 1986; 105:197.

122. Weinstock RS, Wright HN, Spiegel AM, et al. Olfactory dysfunction in humans with deficient guanine nucleotide-binding protein. Nature 1986; 322:635.

123. Levine MA, Downs RW Jr, Singer MJ, et al. Deficient activity of guanine nucleotide regulatory protein in erythrocytes from patients with pseudohypoparathyroidism. Biochem Biophys Res Commun 1980; 94:1319.

124. Farfel Z, Brickman AS, Kaslow HR, et al. Deficiency of receptor-cyclase coupling protein in pseudohypoparathyroidism. N Engl J Med 1980; 303:237.

125. Downs RW, Levine MA, Drezner MK, et al. Deficient adenylate cyclase regulatory protein in renal membranes from a patient with pseudohypoparathyroidism. J Clin Invest 1983; 71:231.

126. Albright F, Forbes AP, Henneman PH. Pseudopseudohypoparathyroidism. Trans Assoc Am Physicians 1952; 65:337.

127. Levine MA, Jap T, Mauseth RS, et al. Activity of the stimulatory guanine nucleotide-binding protein is reduced in erythrocytes from patients with pseudohypoparathyroidism and pseudopseudohypoparathyroidism: biochemical, endocrine, and genetic analysis of Albright's hereditary osteodystrophy in six kindreds. J Clin Endocrinol Metab 1986; 62:497.

128. Fitch N. The identification and inheritance of Albright's hereditary osteodystrophy. Am J Med Genet 1982; 11:11.

129. Bray P, Carter A, Simons C, et al. Human cDNA clones for four species of Gsα signal transduction protein. Proc Natl Acad Sci U S A 1986; 83:8893.

130. Kozasa T, Itoh H, Tsukamoto T, Kaziro Y. Isolation and characterization of the human Gsα gene. Proc Natl Acad Sci U S A 1988; 85:2081.

131. Patten JL, Johns DR, Valle D, et al. Mutation in the gene encoding the stimulatory G protein of adenylate cyclase in Albright's hereditary osteodystrophy. N Engl J Med 1990; 322:1412.

132. Weinstein LS, Gejman PV, Friedman E, et al. Mutations of the Gs alpha-subunit gene in Albright hereditary osteodystrophy detected by denaturing gradient gel electrophoresis. Proc Natl Acad Sci U S A 1990; 87:8287.

133. Miric A, Vechio JD, Levine MA. Heterogeneous mutations in the gene encoding the alpha subunit of the stimulatory G protein of adenylyl cyclase in Albright hereditary osteodystrophy. J Clin Endocrinol Metab 1993; 76:1560.

134. Iiri T, Herzmark P, Nakamoto JM, et al. Rapid GDP release from Gsα in patients with gain and loss of function. Nature 1994; 371:164.

135. Weinstein LS, Gejman PV, de Mazancourt P, et al. A heterozygous 4-bp deletion mutation in the Gsα gene (GNAS1) in a patient with Albright hereditary osteodystrophy. Genomics 1992; 13:1319.

136. Levine MA, Modi WS, O'Brien SJ. Mapping of the gene encoding the alpha subunit of the stimulatory G protein of adenylyl cyclase (GNAS1) to 20q13.2-q13.3 in human by in situ hybridization. Genomics 1991; 11:478.

137. Levine MA, Ahn TG, Kaufman K, et al. Genetic deficiency of the alpha-subunit of Gs as the molecular basis for Albright's hereditary osteodystrophy. Proc Natl Acad Sci U S A 1988; 85:617.

138. Carter A, Bardin C, Collins R, et al. Reduced expression of multiple forms of the alpha subunit of the stimulatory GTP-binding protein in pseudohypoparathyroidism type 1a. Proc Natl Acad Sci U S A 1987; 84:7266.

139. Jan de Beur SM, Deng ZC, Ding CL, Levine MA. Amplification of GC rich exon 1 of GNAS1 and identification of three novel missense mutations. (Abstract). Endocrine Soc Abstracts 1998; Abs. OR7-6:62.

140. Warner DR, Gejman PV, Collins RM, Weinstein LS. A novel mutation adjacent of switch III domain of G_sα in a patient with pseudohypoparathyroidism. Mol Endocrinol 1997; 11:1718.

141. Warner DR, Weng G, Yu S, et al. A novel mutation in the Switch 3 region of Gsα in a patient with Albright hereditary osteodystrophy impairs GDP binding and receptor activation. J Biol Chem 1998; 273:23976.

142. Farfel Z, Iiri T, Shapira H, et al. Pseudohypoparathyroidism, a novel mutation in the βγ contact region of Gsα impairs receptor stimulation. J Biol Chem 1996; 271:19653.

143. Shapira H, Mouallem M, Shapiro MS, Weisman Y, Farfel Z. Pseudohypoparathyroidism type 1a: two new heterozygous frameshift mutations in exon 5 and 10 of the Gsα gene. Hum Genet 1996; 97:73.

144. Fischer JA, Egert F, Werder E, Born W. An inherited mutation associated with functional deficiency of the alpha subunit of the guanine nucleotide-binding protein Gs in pseudo- and pseudopseudohypoparathyroidism. J Clin Endocrinol Metab 1999; 83:935.

145. Luttikhuis ME, Wilson LC, Leonard JV, Trembath RC. Characterization of a de novo 43-bp deletion of the Gs alpha gene (GNAS1) in Albright hereditary osteodystrophy. Genomics 1994; 21:455.

146. Yu S, Yu D, Hainline BE, et al. A deletion hot-spot in exon 7 of the Gs alpha gene (GNAS1) in patients with Albright hereditary osteodystrophy. Hum Mol Genet 1995; 4:2001.

147. Walden U, Weissortel R, Corria Z, et al. Stimulatory guanine nucleotide binding protein subunit 1 mutation in two sibling with pseudohypoparathyroidism type 1a and mother with pseudopseudohypoparathyroidism. Eur J Pediatr 1999; 158:200.

148. Ahmed SF, Dixon PH, Bonthron DT, et al. GNAS1 mutational analysis in pseudohypoparathyroidism. Clin Endocrinol 1998; 49:525.

149. Yokoyama M, Takeda K, Iyota K, et al. A 4 base pair deletion mutation of the Gsα gene in a Japanese patient with pseudohypoparathyroidism. J Endocrinol Invest 1996; 19:236.

150. Wilson LC, Oude Luttikhuis ME, Clayton PT, et al. Parental origin of Gs alpha gene mutations in Albright's hereditary osteodystrophy. J Med Genet 1994; 31:835.

151. Davies SJ, Hughes HE. Imprinting in Albright's hereditary osteodystrophy. J Med Genet 1993; 30:101.

152. Nakamoto JM, Sandstrom AT, Brickman AS, et al. Pseudohypoparathyroidism type 1a from maternal but not paternal transmission of a Gsa gene mutation. Am J Med Genet 1998; 77:261.

153. Hayward BE, Kamiya M, Strain L, et al. The human GNAS1 gene is imprinted and encodes distinct paternally and biallelically expressed G proteins. Proc Natl Acad Sci U S A 1998; 95:10038.

154. Hayward BE, Moran V, Strain L, Bonthron DT. Bidirectional imprinting of a single gene: GNAS1 encodes maternally, paternally, and biallelically derived proteins. Proc Natl Acad Sci U S A 1998; 95:15475.

155. Campbell R, Gosden CM, Bonthron DT. Parental origin of transcription from the human GNAS1 gene. J Med Genet 1994; 31:607.

156. Yu S, Yu D, Lee E, et al. Variable and tissue-specific hormone resistance in heterotrimeric Gs protein alpha-subunit (Gsalpha) knockout mice is due to tissue-specific imprinting of the Gsα gene. Proc Natl Acad Sci U S A 1998; 95:8715.

157. Schwindinger WF, Earnest KA, McCarthy EF, Levine MA. Mice with deficiency of Gas demonstrate a renal but not a skeletal phenotype. American Society for Bone and Mineral Research 1998:S115(Abstr).

158. Speigel A. Mutations in G proteins and G protein-coupled receptors in endocrine disease. J Clin Endocrinol Metab 1996; 81:2434.

159. Ringel MD, Schwindinger WF, Levine MA. Clinical implications of genetic defects in G proteins. Medicine 1996; 171.

160. Schwindinger WF, Francomano CA, Levine MA. Identification of a mutation in the gene encoding the alpha subunit of the stimulatory G protein of adenylyl cyclase in McCune-Albright syndrome. Proc Natl Acad Sci U S A 1992; 89:5152.

161. Weinstein LS, Shenker A, Gejman PV, et al. Activating mutations of the stimulatory G protein in the McCune-Albright syndrome. N Engl J Med 1991; 325:1688.

162. Landis CA, Masters SB, Spada A, et al. GTPase inhibiting mutations activate the alpha chain of Gs and stimulate adenylyl cyclase in human pituitary tumours. Nature 1989; 340:692.

163. Russo D, Arturi F, Wicker R, et al. Genetic alterations in thyroid hyperfunctioning adenomas. J Clin Endocrinol Metab 1995; 80:1347.

164. Lyons J, Landis CA, Griffith H, et al. Two G protein oncogenes in human endocrine tumors. Science 1990; 249:655.

165. Silve C, Santora A, Breslau N, et al. Selective resistance to parathyroid hormone in cultured skin fibroblasts from patients with pseudohypoparathyroidism type 1b. J Clin Endocrinol Metab 1986; 62:640.

166. Fukumoto S, Suzawa M, Takeuchi Y, et al. Absence of mutations in parathyroid hormone (PTH)/PTH-related protein receptor complementary deoxyribonucleic acid in patients with pseudohypoparathyroidism type 1b. J Clin Endocrinol Metab 1996; 81:2554.

167. Ding CL, Usdin TB, LaBuda MC, Levine MA. Molecular genetic analysis of pseudohypoparathyroidism 1B: exclusion of the genes encoding the type 1 and type 2 PTH receptors. (Abstract). J Bone Miner Res 1996; 11: S302.

168. Schipani E, Weinstein LS, Bergwitz C, et al. Pseudohypoparathyroidism type 1b is not caused by mutations in the coding exons of the human parathyroid hormone (PTH)/PTH-related peptide receptor gene. J Clin Endocrinol Metab 1995; 80:1611.

169. Bettoun JD, Minagawa M, Kwan MY, et al. Cloning and characterization of the promoter regions of the human parathyroid hormone (PTH)/PTH-related peptide receptor gene: analysis of deoxyribonucleic acid from normal subjects and patients with pseudohypoparathyroidism type 1b. J Clin Endocrinol Metab 1997; 82:1031.

170. Minagawa M, Watanabe T, Minamitani K, et al. Analysis of P3 promoter of human PTH/PTHrp receptor gene in pseudohypoparathyroidism type 1b. Bone 1998; 23, S462.

170a. Jan de Beur SM, Ding CL, LaBuda MC, et al. Pseudohypoparathyroidism 1b: exclusion of parathyroid hormone and its receptors as candidate disease genes. J Clin Endocrinol Metab 2000; 85:2239.

171. Lanske B, Karapalis AC, Lee K, et al. PTH/PTHrP receptor in early development and Indian hedgehog-regulated bone growth. Science 1996; 273:663.

172. Juppner H, Schipani E, Bastepe M, et al. The gene responsible for pseudohypoparathyroidism type 1b is paternally imprinted and maps in four unrelated kindreds to chromosome 20q13.3. Proc Natl Acad Sci U S A 1998; 95:11798.

173. Barrett D, Breslau NA, Wax MB, et al. A new form of pseudohypoparathyroidism with abnormal catalytic adenylate cyclase. Am J Physiol 1989; 257:E277.

174. Van Dop C, Bourne HR, Neer RM. Father to son transmission of decreased Ns activity in pseudohypoparathyroidism type 1a. J Clin Endocrinol Metab 1984; 59:825.

175. Levine MA. Pseudohypoparathyroidism. In: Avioli LV, Krane SM, eds. Metabolic bone disease and clinically related disorders, 3rd ed. San Diego: Academic Press, 1998:507.

176. Schuster V, Kress W, Kruse K. Paternal and maternal transmission of pseudohypoparathyroidism type 1a in a family with Albright hereditary osteodystrophy: no evidence of genomic imprinting. (Letter). J Med Genet 1994; 31:84.

177. Schuster V, Eschenhagen T, Kruse K, et al. Endocrine and molecular biological studies in a German family with Albright hereditary osteodystrophy. Eur J Pediatr 1993; 152:185.

178. Drezner MK, Neelon FA, Lebovitz HE. Pseudohypoparathyroidism type II: a possible defect in the reception of the cyclic AMP signal. N Engl J Med 1973; 280:1056.

179. Gascon-Barre M, Haddad P, Provencher SJ, et al. Chronic hypocalcemia of vitamin D deficiency leads to lower intracellular calcium concentrations in rat hepatocytes. J Clin Invest 1994; 93:2159.

180. Breslau NA, Moses AM, Pak CYC. Evidence for bone remodeling but lack of calcium mobilization in response to parathyroid hormone in pseudohypoparathyroidism. J Clin Endocrinol Metab 1983; 57:638.

181. Nagant de Deuxchaines C, Fischer JA, Dambacher MA, et al. Dissociation

of parathyroid hormone bioactivity and immunoreactivity in pseudohypoparathyroidism type 1. J Clin Endocrinol Metab 1981; 53:1105.

182. Loveridge N, Fischer JA, Nagant de Deuxchaines C, et al. Inhibition of cytochemical bioactivity of parathyroid hormone by plasma in pseudohypoparathyroidism type 1. J Clin Endocrinol Metab 1982; 54:1274.

183. Mitchell J, Goltzman D. Examination of circulating parathyroid hormone in pseudohypoparathyroidism. J Clin Endocrinol Metab 1985; 61:328.

184. Chernow B, Zaloga G, McFadden E, et al. Hypocalcemia in critically ill patients. Crit Care Med 1982; 10:848.

185. Raskin P, McClain CJ, Medsger TA. Hypocalcemia associated with metastatic bone disease: a retrospective study. Arch Intern Med 1973; 132:539.

186. Smallridge RC, Wray HL, Schaaf M. Hypocalcemia with osteoblastic metastases in a patient with prostatic carcinoma: a cause of secondary hyperparathyroidism. Am J Med 1981; 71:184.

187. Desai TK, Carlson RW, Geheb MA. Prevalence and clinical implications of hypocalcemia in acutely ill patients in a medical intensive care setting. Am J Med 1988; 84:209.

188. Kitanaka S, Takeyama KI, Murayama A, et al. Inactivating mutations in the 25 hydroxyvitamin $D_3$ 1$\alpha$-hydroxylase gene in patients with pseudovitamin D-deficiency rickets. N Engl J Med 1998; 338:653.

189. Malloy PJ, Wesley Pike J, Feldman D. The vitamin D receptor and the syndrome of hereditary 1,25-dihydroxyvitamin D resistant rickets. Endocr Rev 1999; 20:156.

190. Mallette LE, Kirkland JL, Gagel RF, et al. Synthetic human parathyroid hormone-(1-34) for the study of pseudohypoparathyroidism. J Clin Endocrinol Metab 1988; 67:964.

191. Sohn HE, Furukawa Y, Yumita S, et al. Effect of synthetic 1-34 fragment of human parathyroid hormone on plasma adenosine 3',5'-monophosphate (cAMP) concentrations and the diagnostic criteria based on the plasma cAMP response in Ellsworth-Howard test. Endocrinol Jpn 1984; 31:33.

192. Stirling HF, Darling JA, Barr DG. Plasma cyclic AMP response to intravenous parathyroid hormone in pseudohypoparathyroidism. Acta Paediatr Scand 1991; 80:333.

193. Barr DG, Stirling HF, Darling JA. Evolution of pseudohypoparathyroidism: an informative family study. Arch Dis Child 1994; 70:337.

194. Peacock M, Robertson WG, Nordin BEC. Relation between serum and urinary calcium with particular reference to parathyroid activity. Lancet 1969; 1:384.

195. Nicar NJ, Pak CYC. Calcium bioavailability from calcium carbonate and calcium citrate. J Clin Endocrinol Metab 1985; 61:391.

196. Recker R. Calcium absorption and achlorhydria. N Engl J Med 1985; 313:70.

197. Mason RS, Posen S. The relevance of 25-hydroxycalciferol measurements in the treatment of hypoparathyroidism. Clin Endocrinol (Oxf ) 1979; 10:265.

198. Parfitt AM. Thiazide-induced hypercalcemia in vitamin D–treated hypoparathyroidism. Ann Intern Med 1972; 77:557.

199. Porter RH, Cox BG, Heaney D, et al. Treatment of hypoparathyroid patients with chlorthalidone. N Engl J Med 1978; 298:577.

200. Newman GH, Wade M, Hosking DJ. Effect of bendrofluazide on calcium reabsorption in hypoparathyroidism. Eur J Clin Pharm 1984; 27:41.

201. Gabow PA, Hanson TJ, Popovitzer MM, Schrier RW. Furosemide-induced reduction in ionized calcium in hypoparathyroid patients. Ann Intern Med 1977; 86:579.

202. Eisenberg E. Effects of serum calcium level and parathyroid extracts on phosphate and calcium excretion in hypoparathyroid patients. J Clin Invest 1965; 44:942.

203. Duarte B, Mozes MF, John E, et al. Parathyroid allotransplantation in the treatment of complicated primary hypoparathyroidism. Surgery 1985; 98:1072.

# CHAPTER 61

# RENAL OSTEODYSTROPHY

KEVIN J. MARTIN, ESTHER A. GONZALEZ, AND EDUARDO SLATOPOLSKY

The association of skeletal disease with renal failure has been recognized for many years. The term *renal osteodystrophy* is used to encompass the many complex disorders of the skeleton that occur in patients with chronic renal disease and includes disorders with high bone turnover such as *osteitis fibrosa* as well as disorders with abnormally low bone turnover such as adynamic bone and *osteomalacia;* in addition, *osteoporosis* and, in children, *growth retardation* may be seen. Areas of *osteosclerosis* as well as *cystic bone lesions* may be present. These disorders may occur together to variable degrees in any given patient. Thus, to prevent and treat bone disease in patients with renal failure, an

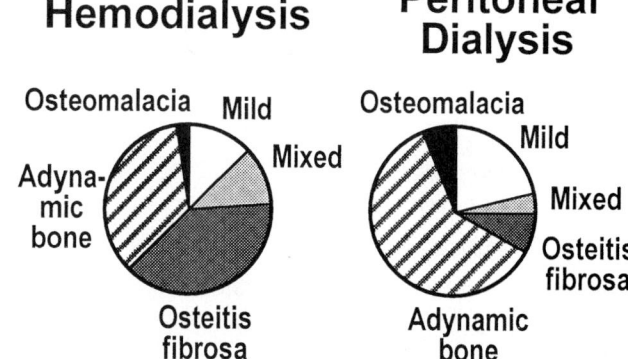

**FIGURE 61-1.** The spectrum of histologic abnormalities of bone in patients with end-stage renal disease on hemodialysis or peritoneal dialysis. (Adapted from Sherrard DJ, Hercz G, Pei Y, et al. The spectrum of bone disease in end-stage renal failure: an evolving disorder. Kidney Int 1993; 43:436.)

understanding of the pathogenesis, diagnosis, and treatment of the various types of bone disease is essential. The prevalence of the various types of bone disease encountered in patients with end-stage renal disease differs somewhat according to the modality of dialysis used, as illustrated in Figure 61-1.

## PATHOGENESIS

### OSTEITIS FIBROSA

Osteitis fibrosa results from high circulating levels of biologically active parathyroid hormone (PTH). Elevated levels of immunoreactive PTH (iPTH) and hyperplasia of the parathyroid glands are among the most consistent abnormalities of mineral metabolism in patients with chronic renal disease.[1,2] The elevation of serum PTH occurs in patients with only mild (~20%) reductions in renal function.

The principal factors involved in the pathogenesis of the secondary hyperparathyroidism of chronic renal disease include (a) retention of serum phosphorus because of a reduced glomerular filtration rate (GFR), (b) altered production of [1,25(OH)$_2$D], (c) abnormal parathyroid growth and function, and (d) resistance to the calcemic effect of PTH.

### RETENTION OF PHOSPHORUS

Considerable evidence supports the importance of phosphorus retention in the genesis of secondary hyperparathyroidism.[3-5] In normal subjects, the oral administration of elemental phosphorus (1 g) causes an increase in serum phosphorus, a fall in serum ionized calcium levels, and an increase in serum iPTH. Moreover, the long-term administration of a high-phosphorus diet can result in parathyroid hyperplasia and increased levels of iPTH. In experimentally induced renal disease, if dietary phosphorus is restricted in proportion to the decrease in renal function, secondary hyperparathyroidism can be prevented or markedly attenuated for at least 2 years[6] (Fig. 61-2). These findings have been confirmed in patients with mild to moderate renal insufficiency. Even in more advanced renal insufficiency, phosphorus restriction has resulted in substantial reductions in serum iPTH, although the levels remain above normal.

Studies have begun to refine our understanding of the mechanisms by which phosphorus retention alters parathyroid activity, as illustrated in Figure 61-3. Phosphorus directly increases the secretion of PTH[7,8] and also appears to influence the growth of the parathyroid cells[9] as well as to indirectly affect parathy-

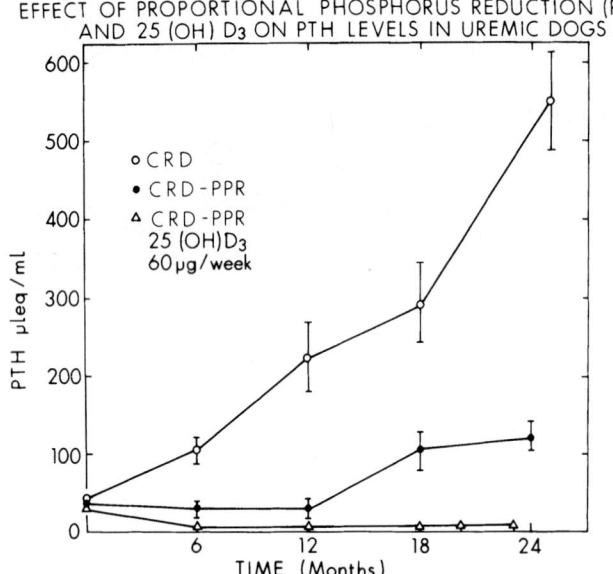

EFFECT OF PROPORTIONAL PHOSPHORUS REDUCTION (PPR)
AND 25 (OH) D₃ ON PTH LEVELS IN UREMIC DOGS

**FIGURE 61-2.** Serial determinations of parathyroid hormone (*PTH*) in dogs with chronic renal disease (*CRD*). The animals received a normal diet (O—O), a diet with phosphorus content reduced in proportion to the decrement in glomerular filtration rate (●—●), or this latter diet plus 25-hydroxyvitamin D₃ [*25(OH)D₃*], 20 µg three times per week for 2 years (△—△). (Modified from Rutherford WE, Bordier P, Marie P. Phosphate control and 25-hydroxycholecalciferol administration in preventing experimental renal osteodystrophy in the dog. J Clin Invest 1977; 60:332.)

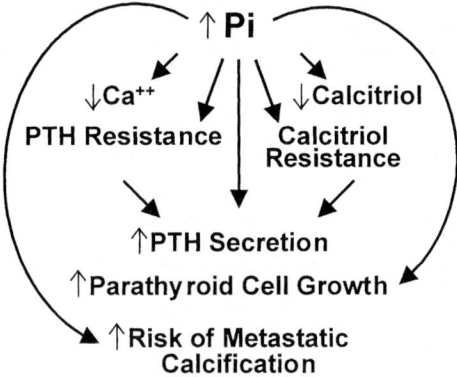

**FIGURE 61-3.** The consequences of hyperphosphatemia (for full description see text). (*Pi*, inorganic phosphate; *PTH*, parathyroid hormone.)

roid function. Furthermore, the effects of phosphorus on parathyroid cell growth have been shown to occur early in the course of experimentally induced renal insufficiency.[10]

The phosphorus retention that decreases the levels of ionized calcium (either by causing the formation of complexes with calcium that precipitate in soft tissues or, alternatively, by decreasing the production of calcitriol) also contributes to the genesis of hyperparathyroidism.[11] Thus, the decreased production of calcitriol may lead to hypocalcemia by decreasing intestinal absorption of calcium or by altering PTH secretion (see later). Hyperphosphatemia also leads to resistance to the actions of PTH, as manifested by decreased release of calcium from bone, as well as to resistance to the actions of calcitriol. However, neither hypocalcemia nor hyperphosphatemia is a universal finding in patients with early renal insufficiency,[12] and experimental studies have shown that hyperparathyroidism may occur without any hypocalcemia.[13] Support for the role of decreased levels of calcitriol is provided by the observation that hyperparathyroidism can be prevented by the administration of calcitriol immediately after the induction of renal insufficiency.[14]

## ALTERED PRODUCTION OF CALCITRIOL

Because the kidney is the major site of production of calcitriol[14] (see Chap. 54), low levels of calcitriol may accentuate the abnormalities of mineral metabolism seen in patients with chronic renal disease. Thus, the fact that intestinal absorption of calcium is decreased in patients with far-advanced renal insufficiency is explained by the concomitant low levels of serum calcitriol. Considerable evidence exists that abnormal vitamin D metabolism contributes to the altered mineral metabolism in patients with advanced renal insufficiency. Plasma levels of calcitriol in adult patients with mild to moderate decreases in GFR (e.g., 40–60 mL per minute) are relatively normal, whereas patients with more advanced renal insufficiency have low levels of this hormone.[15,16] These observations agree with studies that show that intestinal absorption of calcium is not decreased

in patients with renal insufficiency until the GFR is <30% of normal.[17,18] Because PTH increases the production of calcitriol, however, even normal levels of calcitriol may be inappropriately low for the prevailing metabolic state. An additional important role of low levels of calcitriol in the genesis of secondary hyperparathyroidism may be its influence on the regulation of PTH secretion at the level of the parathyroid gland.

## ALTERED PARATHYROID FUNCTION

Several lines of evidence suggest the presence of intrinsic abnormalities in the parathyroid glands resected from patients with renal insufficiency and severe hyperparathyroidism. Membranes prepared from hyperplastic parathyroid glands obtained from patients with chronic renal insufficiency are less susceptible to the inhibition of adenylate cyclase activity by calcium.[19] Thus, the setpoint for calcium (i.e., the calcium concentration required to inhibit enzyme activity by 50%) may be elevated in the hyperfunctioning parathyroid glands. Similar findings were obtained for calcium-regulated PTH secretion from isolated parathyroid cells from hyperfunctioning human parathyroid glands.[20] These in vitro data show that a higher concentration of calcium is required to inhibit PTH secretion in cells from the hyperplastic glands. This abnormal regulation of PTH secretion by calcium can potentially represent the consequences of low levels of calcitriol, which can have several important effects on parathyroid function, as illustrated in Figure 61-4. The finding that the parathyroid glands express vitamin D receptors was followed by the demonstration that calcitriol directly decreases PTH secretion in vitro.[21–27] Clinical studies confirmed the effects of calcitriol on the parathyroid by demonstrating that intravenous administration of calcitriol markedly suppresses PTH secretion in uremic patients on hemodialysis.[28] Furthermore, the effect of calcitriol may extend to restoring the abnormal calcium setpoint to normal.[29] This latter effect, however, is not seen in all studies, perhaps due to differences in the relative degree of hyperparathyroidism.[30] The consequences of low levels of calcitriol on the parathyroid may become amplified because calcitriol receptors are decreased in the parathyroid glands of hyperparathyroid patients[31] and animals.[32,33] The low levels of calcitriol may lead to decreased expression of calcitriol receptors in the parathyroid, because research has shown that calcitriol receptors can be up-regulated by the administration of calcitriol.[34] Calcitriol also regulates the growth of parathyroid cells associated with the altered expression of replication-associated oncogenes.[35] Thus, decreased levels of calcitriol may potentially lead to enhanced parathyroid cell growth. These observations are consistent with the findings of altered distribution of calcitriol receptors in the parathyroid glands from uremic subjects, in whom disordered regulation of PTH secretion and nodular hyperplasia occur.[36] In some

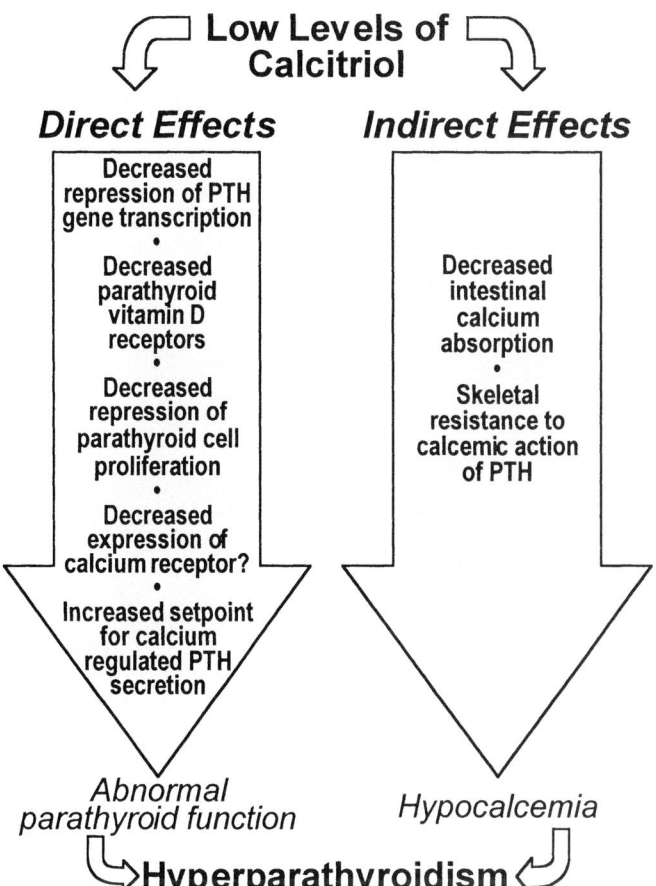

## Low Levels of Calcitriol

### Direct Effects

- Decreased repression of PTH gene transcription
- Decreased parathyroid vitamin D receptors
- Decreased repression of parathyroid cell proliferation
- Decreased expression of calcium receptor?
- Increased setpoint for calcium regulated PTH secretion

### Indirect Effects

- Decreased intestinal calcium absorption
- Skeletal resistance to calcemic action of PTH

*Abnormal parathyroid function*

*Hypocalcemia*

## Hyperparathyroidism

**FIGURE 61-4.** The direct and indirect effects of low levels of calcitriol on parathyroid gland activity and function. (*PTH*, parathyroid hormone.)

patients, the nodular hyperplasia has been shown to be due to monoclonal expansion of parathyroid cells.[37] Parathyroid glands from patients with severe hyperparathyroidism also have decreased expression of the calcium-sensing receptor; this likely contributes to the abnormal regulation of PTH secretion and, possibly, parathyroid cell growth.[38,39]

### SKELETAL RESISTANCE TO THE CALCEMIC EFFECT OF PARATHYROID HORMONE

That the calcemic response to PTH is less than normal in patients with renal insufficiency indicates that this phenomenon may be another cause of hypocalcemia and a further stimulus to PTH secretion in azotemic patients. This has been demonstrated not only by the administration of exogenous PTH but also by the studies showing a delayed recovery from induced hypocalcemia in patients with renal insufficiency, despite a greater augmentation in serum PTH levels. The pathogenesis of the apparent skeletal resistance to the calcemic effect of PTH remains unclear. The suggestion has been made that this abnormality is due to lower levels of calcitriol.[40,41] However, other evidence suggests that this phenomenon also may be due to desensitization of the skeletal response to PTH because of the high levels of circulating PTH.[42,43] Moreover, hyperphosphatemia may limit the release of calcium from bone.

### IMPAIRED RENAL METABOLISM OF CIRCULATING PARATHYROID HORMONE

In patients with chronic renal disease, an increased rate of PTH secretion is the major factor responsible for high plasma PTH levels. Nonetheless, the kidney is important for the peripheral

metabolism of PTH.[44,45] The metabolic clearance rate for PTH is prolonged in renal insufficiency; thus, decreased removal of this hormone from the circulation may accentuate the hyperparathyroidism of renal failure.

### OSTEOMALACIA AND ADYNAMIC BONE

Osteomalacia, manifested by increased osteoid seams and an abnormal or decreased mineralization front in bone, has not been frequently encountered since the realization that the major factor in its pathogenesis was the accumulation of aluminum in patients with chronic renal failure.[46,47] Initially, the source of this metal was thought to be the dialysate, because in geographic areas where the aluminum content of water was high, the incidence of osteomalacia decreased when the aluminum was removed[46]; however, the most important source of aluminum was found to be the ingestion of aluminum-containing antacids, which were used to complex dietary phosphorus. These are now used infrequently because other phosphate binders have become available to complement dietary phosphorus restriction. Accumulation of iron at the mineralization front has also been described and may also give rise to osteomalacia on bone histology.[48]

A disorder of bone characterized by extremely low bone turnover in the absence of aluminum, known as *adynamic bone*, is being increasingly recognized in patients on long-term dialysis and is now a major type of abnormal bone histology in patients with renal disease (see Fig. 61-1).[49] Symptoms referable to the skeletal system, such as bone pain or fractures, are relatively uncommon with this type of bone histology.[49] The pathogenesis of this abnormality is not well understood. Possibly it represents physiologic suppression of bone turnover as a consequence of the increased use of calcitriol and calcium salts as phosphorus binders, together with dialysate calcium concentrations that result in a positive calcium transfer to the patient. This would account for the increased incidence of this type of bone histology in patients on continuous ambulatory peritoneal dialysis (CAPD) and the associated suppression of the blood levels of PTH. Other patients with this syndrome—low bone turnover without demonstrable aluminum—include patients with diabetes mellitus and elderly patients.

### $\beta_2$-MICROGLOBULIN AND BONE

Patients on long-term dialysis may develop juxtaarticular radiolucent cysts in bone, destructive arthropathies, and carpal tunnel syndrome. These abnormalities appear to be due to deposition of $\beta_2$-microglobulin in tissues in the form of amyloid fibrils.[50] (See also refs. 50a and 50b.) The factors responsible for its deposition are not known. The increase of plasma $\beta_2$-microglobulin in dialysis patients reflects the increased production rates and decreased removal by dialysis.

### CLINICAL FEATURES

Symptoms of renal osteodystrophy usually appear only in patients with advanced renal failure, although the abnormalities in mineral metabolism occur early in renal insufficiency. Numerous signs and symptoms may appear. The classic symptom of renal osteodystrophy is *bone pain*, which may be so severe that the patient becomes bedridden. This may occur whether the major abnormality of bone is osteomalacia or osteitis fibrosa. More commonly, the bone pain is vague and localized to the lower back, hips, or legs. Low back pain may arise from collapse of a vertebral body. Chest pain may arise from spontaneous rib fractures. *Muscle weakness* is often a major associated symptom. The muscle enzymes are normal, and electromyographic findings are nonspecific. In severe cases, electron microscopy of muscle shows local disorganization of myofibrils and dispersion of Z bands.[51] *Itching* is common in patients with renal osteodystrophy, especially in those with severe hyperparathyroidism. This has been attributed to the deposition of calcium in the skin. Peripheral ischemic necrosis and vascular calcifications may also be found. Acute joint pain and periarthritis, owing to the deposition of hydroxyapatite crystals, may also occur concomitantly with severe hyperparathyroidism. Tendon rupture may ensue from the abnormal collagen metabolism of uremia and has been associated with $\beta_2$-microglobulin accumulation. In children, skeletal deformities, bowing of the tibia and femur, and slipped epiphysis are not uncommon. Growth retardation is usual and is due to the combination of malnutrition, acidosis, and osteomalacia. The correction of these abnormalities may improve growth.

## ABNORMALITIES OF LABORATORY TESTS

One of the earliest changes in patients with chronic renal failure is increased plasma levels of PTH. As the disease progresses, hypocalcemia may occur. Although hyperphosphatemia is not seen until the GFR is <25 mL per minute, one should remember that serum phosphorus remains normal as a consequence of the development of hyperparathyroidism, which occurs early in the course of renal insufficiency. The magnitude of the hyperphosphatemia depends on the amount of phosphorus ingested, the intestinal absorption, and the excretion of phosphorus by the diseased kidney. Hypermagnesemia occurs with a GFR of <15 mL per minute; the administration of magnesium-containing antacids must be monitored closely. Serum alkaline phosphatase levels are often increased with osteitis fibrosa, osteomalacia, or mixed lesions. Metabolic acidosis commonly is present when the GFR is <25 mL per minute.[52]

### ASSAYS FOR PARATHYROID HORMONE

Because hyperparathyroidism plays a major role in renal osteodystrophy, serum PTH must be measured to monitor the degree of hyperparathyroidism and the effects of treatment. Specific two-site immunoassays for intact PTH have become the most widely used and are readily available.[53] The desired range for levels of intact PTH that are associated with normal bone turnover in patients with end-stage renal disease appears to be 150 to 300 pg/mL, or 2.5- to 5-fold greater than the upper limit of normal for the intact PTH assays; this higher range presumably represents the need for higher levels of the hormone to overcome the skeletal resistance to PTH discussed previously.[54,55]

### BONE HISTOLOGY

An examination of undecalcified sections of bone is required for the precise diagnosis of renal osteodystrophy. *Osteitis fibrosa* is a manifestation of secondary hyperparathyroidism. This condition manifests with increased osteoclast number and increased resorption surface. Double tetracycline labeling shows an increase in bone turnover and an increased quantity of woven osteoid (see Chap. 55). The deposition of calcium phosphate may explain the osteosclerosis in some uremic patients. Double tetracycline labeling is mandatory for the diagnosis of osteomalacia, characterized by an increase in osteoid and an abnormal or decreased mineralization front. Bone turnover is decreased in osteomalacia as well as in the adynamic bone lesions of renal osteodystrophy. The lesions of osteitis fibrosa and osteomalacia can occur alone or in combination. Special stains may directly indicate the presence of aluminum.

### RADIOLOGIC ABNORMALITIES

The main radiographic feature of hyperparathyroidism is increased bone resorption, most commonly seen in the subperi-

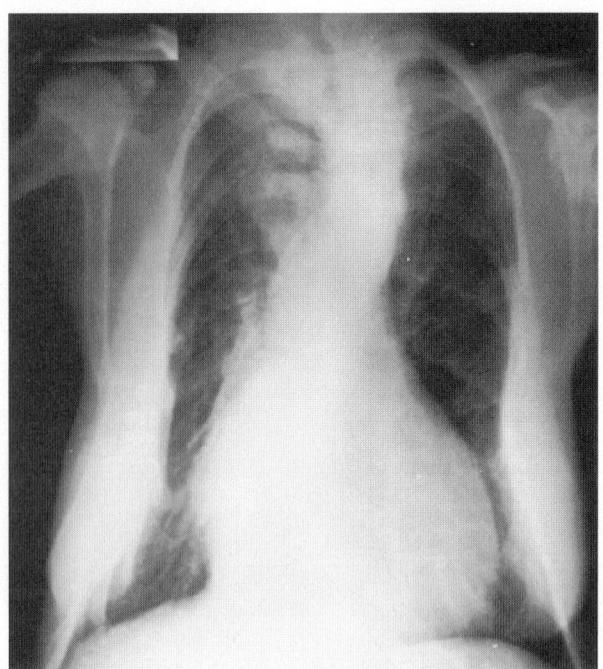

**FIGURE 61-5.** Chest radiograph of a patient with severe renal osteodystrophy secondary to chronic renal disease as a child. Note the deformity of the rib cage. The inset (*top left*) demonstrates severe osteitis fibrosa cystica.

osteal surfaces of the hands, neck of femur, and clavicle (Fig. 61-5). These radiologic features correlate well with serum PTH levels and evidence of osteitis fibrosa by bone histology.[56,57] Skull radiographs show a granular mottled appearance (Fig. 61-6). Osteosclerosis, owing to increased thickness and increased number of trabeculae, accounts for the classic radiographic appearance of the spine, called *"rugger-jersey" spine* (Fig. 61-7). Looser zones or pseudofractures may be seen in osteomalacia (see Chap. 63). Although radiographs are useful for the diagnosis of severe hyper-

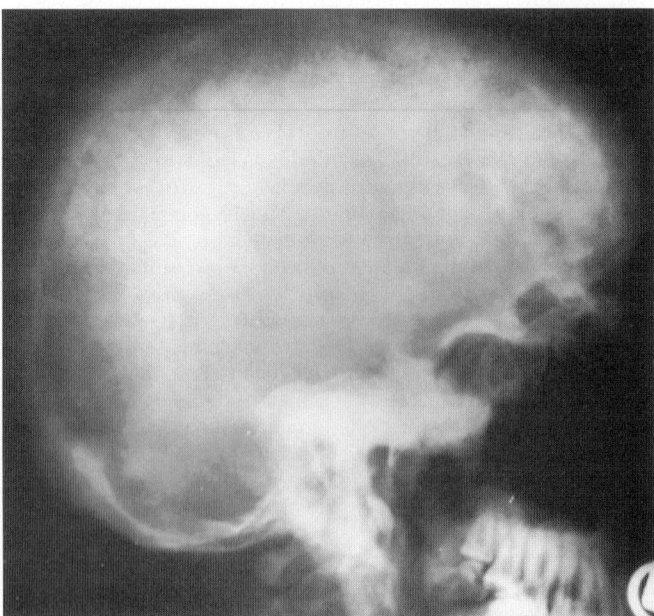

**FIGURE 61-6.** Abnormalities of skull radiograph in a patient with secondary hyperparathyroidism noted on bone biopsy. The skull has a diffuse granular appearance with focal areas of sclerosis.

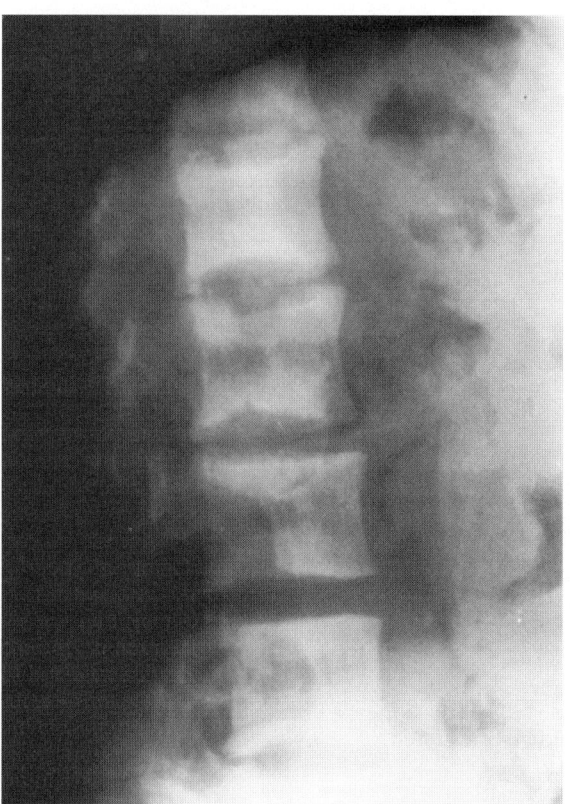

**FIGURE 61-7.** Radiograph of lateral lumbar spine of a patient with chronic renal failure and secondary hyperparathyroidism showing a "rugger-jersey" spine.

parathyroidism, the less distinct changes of osteomalacia or adynamic bone may require bone biopsy for definitive diagnosis. Extraskeletal calcifications may also be found by these radiologic studies (Fig. 61-8). Juxtaarticular radiolucent cysts are suggestive of $\beta_2$-microglobulin amyloid deposition.

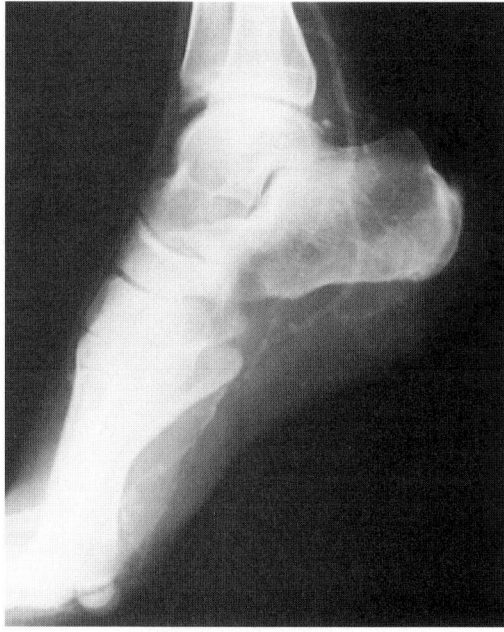

**FIGURE 61-8.** Radiograph of a foot of a patient with chronic renal failure and persistent hyperphosphatemia. The "auto-arteriogram" is the result of extensive vascular calcification.

# PREVENTION, DIAGNOSIS, AND MANAGEMENT

An understanding of the pathogenesis of renal osteodystrophy leads to a number of maneuvers that are effective in its prevention and treatment; these are summarized in Table 61-1.

## DIETARY PHOSPHORUS RESTRICTION

The cornerstone for the prevention and treatment of renal osteodystrophy is the restriction of phosphorus and the prevention of hyperphosphatemia. The usual phosphorus intake by normal adults is 1 to 1.6 g per day, from meat and dairy products. The dietary restriction of these foods is useful, but as renal failure becomes advanced, additional strategies to limit phosphate absorption are required. This is achieved by the use of calcium salts, calcium carbonate or calcium acetate, or sevelamer, a non–calcium-containing phosphate-binding polymer, taken with meals, which bind the ingested phosphorus in the gastrointestinal tract and prevent its absorption.[58–62] The goal of this treatment is to reduce the serum phosphate level to ~5 mg/dL. Serum phosphate levels should be closely monitored to avoid hypophosphatemia. Although aluminum-containing antacids are extremely effective in controlling serum phosphorus levels, these agents are not often used except for short-term administration because of the toxicity of aluminum in causing dialysis dementia and osteomalacia.[46,63] The administration of antacids such as calcium carbonate, calcium acetate, or sevelamer must be adjusted according to the approximate phosphorus content of the meal. Thus, a small breakfast (50–75 mg of phosphorus) may require small amounts of a phosphate binder, whereas a larger meal (600 mg of phosphorus) may require increased amounts. Calcium citrate should not be used, because aluminum absorption may be increased.

## CALCIUM SUPPLEMENTATION

Because intestinal calcium absorption is decreased in patients with advanced renal failure, and because their diets are usually low in calcium, the supplementation of calcium intake is required.[64,65] The minimum requirement is 1.5 g per day of elemental calcium; larger doses may be given, especially if hypocalcemia persists. As discussed previously, large doses of calcium carbonate or calcium acetate are also useful as phosphate binders for the control of hyperphosphatemia and prevention of hyperparathyroidism; if such doses of calcium are given, the levels of serum calcium and phosphate must be monitored frequently to avoid hypercalcemia and an elevation of the calcium-phosphorus product.

## USE OF VITAMIN D STEROLS

Because low levels of calcitriol play a major role in the pathogenesis of hyperparathyroidism in chronic renal disease, the administration of calcitriol has an important role in its treatment. In some countries, 1α-hydroxycholecalciferol, which is metabolized to calcitriol, is used. The administration of calcitriol is effective in achieving suppression of PTH levels with significant improvements in skeletal histology.[66] The use of calcitriol may vary according to the degree of renal insufficiency and the degree of hyperparathyroidism. In early renal failure, the oral administration of calcitriol, 0.25 to 0.5 μg per day, may be effective in minimizing hyperparathyroidism. However, that therapy should be monitored closely so that hypercalcemia and hypercalciuria do not occur, because a risk exists that renal function may be compromised. In end-stage renal disease, larger doses of calcitriol may be required. In patients on hemodialysis, the intravenous administration of calcitriol is associated with marked suppression of elevated PTH values and improvement in renal osteodystrophy. The

**TABLE 61–1.**
**Treatment of Renal Osteodystrophy at Various Stages of Renal Insufficiency**

| Mild GFR 50–80 mL/mm | Moderate GFR 25–50 mL/min | Severe and ESRD GFR<25mL/min |
|---|---|---|
| Monitor PTH ———————————————————————————————————→ | | |
| Phosphorus restriction ————————————————————————————→ | | |
| Calcium carbonate or acetate —————————————————————→ | | |
| Sevelamer ————————————————————————————————————→ | | |
| | Treat acidosis ———————————————————————→ | |
| | Avoid aluminum ——————————————————————→ | |
| | (Calcitriol) ———————————————————————————→ | |
| | | Calcitriol po or iv |
| | | Vitamin D analogs |
| | | Parathyroidectomy* |
| | | Bone biopsy† |
| | | Treat Al overloads‡ |
| | | Adjust dialysate calcium |
| | | Choice of dialyzer? |

GFR, glomerular filtration rate; ESRD, end-stage renal disease; PTH, parathyroid hormone; po, by mouth; iv, intravenously; Al, aluminum.
*Indications: severe hyperparathyroidism, osteitis fibrosa, very high PTH, hypercalcemia, extravascular calcifications, and calciphylaxis.
†Indications: symptomatic bone disease with hypercalcemia, high serum aluminum, positive deferoxamine test, and normal or slightly elevated PTH.
‡Indications: osteomalacia, myopathy, encephalopathy, positive bone biopsy, and high serum aluminum.

doses required are 1 to 3 µg given intravenously with each dialysis. As before, levels of calcium and phosphorus and their products must be monitored closely to avoid severe hypercalcemia, an elevated calcium × phosphate product, and metastatic calcification. The intermittent administration of large doses of calcitriol orally (2–5 µg twice per week) has also been shown to be effective, and this *pulse dosing* can achieve a significant reduction in PTH levels, comparable to that achieved with intravenous administration.[67–69] This mode of administration is also applicable to patients on CAPD.[70] The increased efficacy of intermittent administration, whether by intravenous or oral routes, may be due to the high levels achieved in serum, which allow increased delivery to peripheral tissues, including the parathyroid glands.[71] In the parathyroid, the induction of the vitamin D receptor by calcitriol may allow the glands to become more responsive to the prevailing levels of calcitriol and calcium. If the degree of hyperparathyroidism is severe (e.g., intact PTH of >2000 pg/mL), suppression of PTH by calcitriol may prove difficult. This may be explained by the relative lack of vitamin D receptor and calcium-sensing receptor in nodular hyperplastic parathyroid glands; thus, the administered calcitriol or elevations in serum calcium would be less effective in suppressing PTH biosynthesis. Such large glands may require excision. An analog of calcitriol with less calcemic effects, 19-nor-1α-25-dihydroxyvitamin $D_2$ (paricalcitol) is available for the treatment of hyperparathyroidism in renal failure.[72] Other analogs, 22-oxacalcitriol, falecalcitriol, and 1α-hydroxyvitamin $D_2$, are in clinical trials for the same purpose.[73–75]

## USE OF CALCIUM AND VITAMIN D STEROLS IN ALUMINUM-ASSOCIATED OSTEOMALACIA

Although serum calcium should be monitored in all patients treated with large doses of calcium or calcitriol, patients with aluminum-associated bone disease or low bone turnover, such as adynamic bone, are particularly prone to develop hypercalcemia. Presumably, this tendency to hypercalcemia arises because the increased calcium absorbed in the intestine cannot be deposited in bone in which normal mineralization is defective. Thus, patients who show mild hypercalcemia and markedly lower levels of iPTH than are found in those with severe osteitis fibrosa should be treated with caution; if severe hypercalcemia occurs at relatively low dosages of calcium or calcitriol, adynamic bone or aluminum-associated osteomalacia should be considered.

## PARATHYROIDECTOMY

Although the treatment regimens outlined earlier are often effective in improving mineral homeostasis, reversing the symptoms of bone disease, and reducing the serum levels of PTH, occasionally these measures are not totally effective, and parathyroidectomy may be indicated. When parathyroidectomy is considered, substantial evidence of severe hyperparathyroidism should be present, such as very high serum levels of PTH (as are found with severe osteitis fibrosa) or severe osteitis fibrosa on bone biopsy. Aluminum-associated osteomalacia should be excluded. Other features that are an indication for parathyroidectomy include a high PTH and (a) severe hypercalcemia, especially if symptomatic; (b) intractable pruritus; (c) progressive extraskeletal calcification with elevated calcium-phosphate product; (d) progressive skeletal pain and fractures; and (e) *calciphylaxis* (ischemic lesions of the skin and soft tissue and vascular calcifications).[76–78] Importantly, hypercalcemia may occur in patients who lack evidence of secondary hyperparathyroidism, such as in aluminum intoxication, or those with adynamic bone. Parathyroidectomy should not be undertaken unless firm evidence of hyperparathyroidism is found. Prior to surgery, parathyroid imaging is helpful.[79] The most common surgical procedure is to identify all four parathyroid glands and to remove three totally plus a portion of the remaining gland, leaving 80 to 100 mg of parathyroid tissue. Alternatively, total parathyroidectomy is performed, coupled with autotransplantation of parathyroid tissue to the forearm.[80] When the latter procedure is performed, the availability of cryopreservation facilities to store the remaining tissue is desirable so that further implants may be performed if the initial graft fails or is insufficient.

Because hypocalcemia may occur postoperatively, beginning treatment with calcitriol before surgery usually is desirable. Postoperative hypocalcemia is controlled with intravenous and oral administration of calcium supplements and calcitriol. Serum phosphorus may also decrease after surgery, so that temporary discontinuance of phosphorus binders is required. Although alkaline phosphatase may rise postoperatively, a fall toward normal may indicate that skeletal remineralization is slowing and that calcium and vitamin D therapy may be reduced.

## ALUMINUM ACCUMULATION

The main sources of aluminum for patients with renal failure are the dialysis water and aluminum-containing antacids. Appropriate water purification should be routine and a dialysis fluid aluminum concentration of <10 µg/L should be maintained. Deferoxamine has been found to be useful both for diagnosing and treating aluminum accumulation.[81–83] A rise in serum aluminum of >150 µg/L in response to administration of deferoxamine together with a PTH level of <200 pg/mL suggests that the patient is at risk for bone disease secondary to aluminum accumulation.[84] The definitive diagnosis is made by bone biopsy with special aluminum staining. If the diagnosis is confirmed, all sources of aluminum must be sought and removed. Deferoxamine therapy may be used to remove large amounts of aluminum (also see Chap. 131).

## RENAL TRANSPLANTATION

Many of the factors responsible for the altered divalent cation metabolism of chronic renal failure are corrected by successful renal transplantation. However, new problems may arise. Hyperparathyroidism gradually decreases after transplantation; PTH levels generally approach normal within 4 to 6 months if renal function is adequate. Sometimes, hyperparathyroidism may persist and hypercalcemia may occur, especially if the hyperparathyroidism was severe and of long duration. Hypophosphatemia may occur after transplantation because of this persistent hyperparathyroidism, because of antacid therapy, or because of an acquired renal tubular defect independent of PTH. The management of mild hypercalcemia and hypophosphatemia usually is conservative, with oral phosphate therapy and careful follow-up. If hypercalcemia persists or is associated with decreasing renal function, and PTH levels remain elevated, parathyroidectomy may be required. Long-term therapy with corticosteroids in renal transplant recipients has been associated with aseptic necrosis of bone and corticosteroid-induced osteopenia (see Chaps. 64 and 211).

## REFERENCES

1. Reiss E, Canterbury JM, Egdahl RH. Measurement of serum parathyroid hormone in renal insufficiency. Trans Assoc Am Physicians 1968; 81:104.
2. Arnaud CD. Hyperparathyroidism and renal failure. Kidney Int 1973; 4:89.
3. Slatopolsky E, Caglar S, Pennell IP, et al. On the pathogenesis of hyperparathyroidism in chronic experimental insufficiency in the dog. J Clin Invest 1971; 50:492.
4. Slatopolsky E, Delmez JA. Pathogenesis of secondary hyperparathyroidism. Am J Kidney Dis 1994; 23:229.
5. Slatopolsky E, Bricker NS. The role of phosphorus restriction in the prevention of secondary hyperparathyroidism in chronic renal disease. Kidney Int 1973; 4:141.
6. Rutherford WE, Bordier P, Marie P. Phosphate control and 25-hydroxy-cholecalciferol administration in preventing experimental renal osteodystrophy in the dog. J Clin Invest 1977; 60:332.
7. Slatopolsky E, Finch J, Denda M, et al. Phosphorus restriction prevents parathyroid gland growth. High phosphorus directly stimulates PTH secretion in vitro. J Clin Invest 1996; 97:2534.
8. Almaden Y, Canalejo A, Hernandez A, et al. Direct effect of phosphorus on PTH secretion from whole rat parathyroid glands in vitro. J Bone Miner Res 1996; 11:970.
9. Naveh-Many T, Rahamimov R, Livni N, Silver J. Parathyroid cell proliferation in normal and chronic renal failure rats. The effects of calcium, phosphate, and vitamin D. J Clin Invest 1995; 96:1786.
10. Denda M, Finch J, Slatopolsky E. Phosphorus accelerates the development of parathyroid hyperplasia and secondary hyperparathyroidism in rats with renal failure. Am J Kidney Dis 1996; 28:596.
11. Tanaka Y, DeLuca HF. The control of 25-hydroxyvitamin D metabolism by inorganic phosphorus. Arch Biochem Biophys 1973; 159:566.
12. Portale AA, Booth BE, Halloran BP, Morris RC Jr. Effect of dietary phosphorus on circulating concentrations of 1,25-dihydroxyvitamin $D_3$ and immunoreactive parathyroid hormone in children with moderate renal insufficiency. J Clin Invest 1984; 73:1580.
13. Lopez-Hilker S, Gelceram T, Chen Y, et al. Hypocalcemia may not be essential for the development of secondary hyperparathyroidism in chronic renal failure. J Clin Invest 1986; 78:1079.
14. Lopez-Hilker S, Dusso AS, Rapp NS, et al. Phosphorus restriction reverses hyperparathyroidism in uremia independent of changes in calcium and calcitriol. Am J Physiol 1990; 259:F432.
15. Slatopolsky E, Gray R, Adams ND, et al. The pathogenesis of secondary hyperparathyroidism in early renal failure. In: Norman A, ed. Fourth International Workshop on Vitamin D. Berlin: deGruyter, 1979:1209.
16. Cheung AK, Manolagas SC, Catherwood BD, et al. Determination of serum 1,25(OH)$_2$D$_3$ levels in renal disease. Kidney Int 1983; 24:104.
17. Coburn JW, Koppel MH, Brickman AS, Massry SG. Study of intestinal absorption of calcium in patients with renal failure. Kidney Int 1973; 3:264.
18. Malluche HH, Werner E, Ritz E. Intestinal absorption of calcium and whole-body calcium retention in incipient and advanced renal failure. Miner Electrolyte Metab 1978; 1:263.
19. Bellorin-Font E, Martin KJ, Freitag JJ, et al. Altered adenylate cyclase kinetics in hyperfunctioning human parathyroid glands. J Clin Endocrinol Metab 1981; 52:499.
20. Brown EM, Wilson RE, Eastman RC, et al. Abnormal regulation of parathyroid hormone release by calcium in secondary hyperparathyroidism due to chronic renal failure. J Clin Endocrinol Metab 1982; 54:172.
21. Brumbaugh PF, Hughes MR, Haussler MR. Cytoplasmic and nuclear binding components for 1,25-dihydroxyvitamin $D_3$ in chick parathyroid glands. Proc Natl Acad Sci U S A 1975; 72:4871.
22. Chertow BS, Baylink DJ, Wergedal MH, et al. Decrease in serum immunoreactive parathyroid hormone in rats and in parathyroid hormone secretion in vivo by 1,25-dihydroxycholecalciferol. J Clin Invest 1975; 56:668.
23. Au WYW, Bukowsky A. Inhibition of PTH secretion by vitamin D metabolites in organ cultures of rat parathyroids. Fed Proc 1976; 35:530.
24. Dietel M, Dorn G, Montz R, Altenahr E. Influence of vitamin $D_3$, 1,25-dihydroxyvitamin $D_3$ and 24,25-dihydroxyvitamin $D_3$ on parathyroid hormone secretion, adenosine 3',5'-monophosphate release, and ultrastructure of parathyroid glands in organ culture. Endocrinology 1979; 105:237.
25. Silver J, Russell J, Sherwood LM. Regulation by vitamin-D metabolites of messenger ribonucleic-acid for preproparathyroid hormone in isolated bovine parathyroid cells. Proc Natl Acad Sci U S A 1985; 82:4270.
26. Silver J, Navey-Many T, Mayer H, et al. Regulation by vitamin D metabolites of parathyroid hormone gene transcription in vivo in the rat. J Clin Invest 1986; 78:1296.
27. Russell J, Lettieri D, Sherwood LM. Suppression by 1,25-(OH)$_2$D$_3$ of transcription of the parathyroid hormone gene. Endocrinology 1986; 119:2864.
28. Slatopolsky E, Weerts C, Thielan J, et al. Marked suppression of secondary hyperparathyroidism in intravenous administration of 1,25-dihydroxycholecalciferol in uremic patients. J Clin Invest 1984; 74:2136.
29. Delmez AJ, Tindira C, Grooms P, et al. Parathyroid hormone suppression by intravenous 1,25-dihydroxyvitamin D: a role for increased sensitivity to calcium. J Clin Invest 1989; 83:1349.
30. Ramirez JA, Goodman WG, Gornbein J, et al. Direct in vivo comparison of calcium-regulated parathyroid hormone secretion in normal volunteers and patients with secondary hyperparathyroidism. J Clin Endocrinol Metab 1993; 76:1489.
31. Korkor AB. Reduced binding of [3H] 1,25-dihydroxyvitamin $D_3$ in the parathyroid glands of patients with renal failure. N Engl J Med 1987; 316:1573.
32. Brown AJ, Dusso A, Lopez-Hilker S, et al. 1,25-(OH)$_2$D receptors are decreased in parathyroid glands from chronically uremic dogs. Kidney Int 1989; 35:19.
33. Menke J, Hugel U, Zlotkowski A, et al. Diminished parathyroid 1,25(OH)$_2$D$_3$ receptors in experimental uremia. Kidney Int 1987; 32:350.
34. Naveh-Many T, Marx R, Keshet E, et al. Regulation of 1,25-dihydroxyvitamin $D_3$ receptor gene expression by 1,25-dihydroxyvitamin $D_3$ in the parathyroid in vivo. J Clin Invest 1990; 86:1968.
35. Kremer R, Bolivar I, Goltzman D, Hendy GN. Influence of calcium and 1,25-dihydroxycholecalciferol on proliferation and proto-oncogene expression in primary cultures of bovine parathyroid cells. Endocrinology 1989; 125:935.
36. Fukada N, Tanaka H, Tominaga Y, et al. Decreased 1,25-dihydroxyvitamin $D_3$ receptor density is associated with a more severe form of parathyroid hyperplasia in chronic uremic patients. J Clin Invest 1993; 92:1436.
37. Arnold A, Brown MF, Urena P, et al. Monoclonality of parathyroid tumors in chronic renal failure and in primary parathyroid hyperplasia. J Clin Invest 1995; 95:2047.
38. Kifor O, Moore FD Jr, Wang P, et al. Reduced immunostaining for the extracellular Ca$^{2+}$-sensing receptor in primary and uremic secondary hyperparathyroidism [see comments]. J Clin Endocrinol Metab 1996; 81:1598.
39. Gogusev J, Duchambon P, Hory B, et al. Depressed expression of calcium receptor in parathyroid gland tissue of patients with hyperparathyroidism. Kidney Int 1997; 51:328.
40. Somerville PJ, Kaye M. Resistance to parathyroid hormone in renal failure: role of vitamin D metabolites. Kidney Int 1978; 14:245.
41. Massry SG, Stein R, Garty J, et al. Skeletal resistance to the calcemic action of parathyroid hormone in uremia: role of 1,25(OH)$_2$D$_3$. Kidney Int 1976; 9:467.
42. Galceran T, Martin KJ, Morrissey JJ, Slatopolsky E. Role of 1,25-dihydroxy-vitamin D on the skeletal resistance to parathyroid hormone. Kidney Int 1987; 32:801.
43. Rodruigez M, Felsenfeld AJ, Llach F. Calcemic response to parathyroid hormone in renal failure: role of calcitriol and the effect of parathyroidectomy. Kidney Int 1991; 40:1063.
44. Hruska KA, Kopelman R, Rutherford WE, et al. Metabolism of immunoreactive parathyroid hormone in the dog: the role of the kidney and the effects of chronic renal disease. J Clin Invest 1975; 56:39.
45. Martin KJ, Hruska KA, Lewis J, et al. The renal handling of parathyroid

hormone: role of peritubular uptake and glomerular filtration. J Clin Invest 1977; 60:808.

46. Ward MK, Feest TG, Ellis HA, et al. Osteomalacic dialysis osteodystrophy: evidence for a water borne aetiological agent, probably aluminum. Lancet 1978; 1:841.

47. González EA, Martin KJ. Aluminum and renal osteodystrophy: a diminishing clinical problem. Trends Endocrinol Metab 1992; 3:371.

48. Phelps KR, Vigorita VJ, Bansal M, Einhorn TA. Histochemical demonstration of iron but not aluminum in a case of dialysis-associated osteomalacia. Am J Med 1988; 84:775.

49. Pei Y, Hercz G, Greenwood C, et al. Non-invasive prediction of aluminum bone disease in hemo- and peritoneal dialysis patients. Kidney Int 1992; 41:1374.

50. Gejyo F, Yamada T, Odani S, et al. A new form of amyloid protein associated with chronic hemodialysis was identified as β-2 microglobulin. Biochem Biophys Res Commun 1985; 129:701.

50a. Moe SM, Singh GK, Bailey AM. Beta-2 microglobulin induces MMP-1 but not TIMP–1 expression in human synovial fibroblasts. Kidney Int 2000; 57:2023.

50b. Lornoy W, Becaus I, Billiouw JM, et al. On-line haemodiafiltration. Remarkable removal of beta2-microglobulin. Long-term clinical observations. Nephrol Dial Transplant 2000; 15(Suppl 1):49.

51. Schoenfeld PJ, Martin JA, Barnes B, Teitelbaum SL. Amelioration of myopathy with 25-dihydroxyvitamin $D_3$ therapy (25 OH $D_3$) in patients on chronic hemodialysis. Abstract Book. Third Workshop on Vitamin D. Asilomar, California, 1977:160.

52. Hakim RM, Lazarus JM. Biochemical parameters in chronic renal failure. Am J Kidney Dis 1988; 11:238.

53. Nussbaum SR, Zahradnik RJ, Lavigne JR, et al. Highly sensitive two-site immunoradiometric assay of parathyrin, and its clinical utility in evaluating patients with hypercalcemia. Clin Chem 1987; 33:1364.

54. Wang M, Hercz G, Sherrard DJ, et al. Relationship between intact 1-84 parathyroid hormone and bone histomorphometric parameters in dialysis patients without aluminum toxicity. Am J Kidney Dis 1995; 26:836.

55. Quarles LD, Lobaugh B, Murphy G. Intact parathyroid hormone overestimates the presence and severity of parathyroid-mediated osseous abnormalities in uremia. J Clin Endocrinol Metab 1992; 75:145.

56. Hruska KA, Teitelbaum SL, Kopelman R, et al. The predictability of the histologic features of uremic bone disease by non-invasive techniques. Metab Bone Dis Relat Res 1978; 1:39.

57. Ritz E, Malluche HH, Bommar J, et al. Metabolic bone disease in patients on maintenance hemodialysis. Nephron 1974; 12:393.

58. Morniere PH, Roussel A, Tahiri Y, et al. Substitution of aluminum hydroxide by high doses of calcium carbonate in patients on chronic hemodialysis: disappearance of hyperaluminemia and equal control of hyperparathyroidism. Proc Eur Dial Transplant Assoc 1982; 19:784.

59. Slatopolsky E, Weerts C, Lopez-Hilker S, et al. Calcium carbonate is an effective phosphate binder in dialysis patients. N Engl J Med 1986; 315:157.

60. Salusky IB, Coburn JW, Foley J, et al. Calcium carbonate as a phosphate binder in children on dialysis. Kidney Int 1985; 27:185A.

61. Sheikh MS, Maquire JA, Emmett M, et al. Reduction of dietary phosphorus absorption by phosphorus binders. J Clin Invest 1989; 83:66.

62. Slatopolsky EA, Burke SK, Dillon MA, and the RenaGel Study Group. RenaGel, a non-absorbed calcium- and aluminum free phosphate binder, lowers serum phosphorus and parathyroid hormone. Kidney Int 1999; 55:299.

63. Fournier AE, Johnson WJ, Taves DR, et al. Etiology of hyperparathyroidism and bone disease during chronic hemodialysis. I. Association of bone disease with potentially etiologic factors. J Clin Invest 1971; 50:592.

64. Kopple JD, Coburn JW. Metabolic studies of low protein diets in uremia. II. Calcium, phosphorus and magnesium. Medicine 1973; 52:597.

65. Clarkson EM, Eastwood JB, Koutsaimanis KG, de Wardener HE. Net intestinal absorption of calcium in patients with chronic renal failure. Kidney Int 1973; 3:258.

66. Cannella G, Bonucci E, Rolla D, et al. Evidence of healing of secondary hyperparathyroidism in chronically hemodialyzed uremic patients treated with long-term intravenous calcitriol. Kidney Int 1994; 46:1124.

67. Indridason OS, Quarles LD. Oral versus intravenous calcitriol: is the route of administration really important? Curr Opin Nephrol Hypertens 1995; 4:307.

68. Tsukamoto Y, Nomura M, Maurmo F. Pharmacological parathyroidectomy by oral 1,25(OH)$_2$D$_3$ pulse therapy. Nephron 1989; 51:130.

69. Tsukamoto Y, Nomura M, Takahashi Y, et al. The "oral 1,25(OH)$_2$D$_3$ pulse therapy" in hemodialysis patients with severe secondary hyperparathyroidism. Nephron 1991; 57:23.

70. Martin KJ, Ballal HS, Domoto DT, et al. Pulse oral calcitriol for the treatment of hyperparathyroidism in patients on continuous ambulatory peritoneal dialysis: preliminary observations. Am J Kidney Dis 1992; 19:540.

71. Reichel H, Szabo A, Uhl J, et al. Intermittent versus continuous administration of 1,25-dihydroxyvitamin D$_3$ in experimental renal hyperparathyroidism. Kidney Int 1993; 44:1259.

72. Martin KJ, González EA, Gellens M, et al. 19-Nor-1-α-25-dihydroxyvitamin D$_2$ (paricalcitol) safely and effectively reduces the levels of intact PTH in patients on hemodialysis. J Am Soc of Nephrol 1998; 10:1427.

73. Kurokawa K, Akizawa T, Suzuki M, et al. Effect of 22-oxacalcitriol on hyperparathyroidism of dialysis patients: results of a preliminary study. Nephrol Dial Transplant 1996; 11:121.

74. Tan AU Jr, Levine BS, Mazess RB, et al. Effective suppression of parathyroid hormone by 1 alpha-hydroxy-vitamin D2 in hemodialysis patients with moderate to severe secondary hyperparathyroidism. Kidney Int 1997; 51:317.

75. Akiba T, Marumo F, Owada A, et al. Controlled trial of falecalcitriol versus

76. alfacalcidol in suppression of parathyroid hormone in hemodialysis patients with secondary hyperparathyroidism. Am J Kidney Dis 1998; 32:238.

76. Bleyer AJ, Choi M, Igwemezie B, et al. A case control study of proximal calciphylaxis. Am J Kidney Dis 1998; 32:376.

77. Coates T, Kirkland GS, Dymock RB, et al. Cutaneous necrosis from calcific uremic arteriolopathy. Am J Kidney Dis 1998; 32:384.

78. Llach F. Calcific uremic arteriolopathy (calciphylaxis): an evolving entity? Am J Kidney Dis 1998; 32:514.

79. Ambrosoni P, Olaizola I, Heuguerot C, et al. The role of imaging techniques in the study of renal osteodystrophy. Am J Med Sci 2000; 320:90.

80. Wells SA Jr, Gumells JC, Shelburne JD, et al. Transplantation of the parathyroid glands in man: clinical indications and results. Surgery 1975; 78:34.

81. Milliner DS, Nebeker HG, Ott SM, et al. Use of the desferrioxamine infusion test in the diagnosis of aluminum-related osteodystrophy. Ann Intern Med 1984; 101:775.

82. Ackrill P, Day JP, Gargstang FM, et al. Treatment of fracturing renal osteodystrophy by desferrioxamine. Proc Eur Dial Transplant Assoc 1982; 19:203.

83. Malluche HH, Smith AL, Abreo K, Faugere M-C. The use of desferrioxamine in the management of aluminum accumulation in bone in patients with renal failure. N Engl J Med 1984; 311:140.

84. Pei Y, Hercz G, Greenwood C, et al. Non-invasive prediction of aluminum bone disease in hemo- and peritoneal dialysis patients. Kidney Int 1992; 41:1374.

# CHAPTER 62

# SURGERY OF THE PARATHYROID GLANDS

GERARD M. DOHERTY AND SAMUEL A. WELLS, JR.

Hyperparathyroidism occurs in ~1 in 1000 persons in the United States. Successful parathyroid surgery requires an understanding of the anatomy of the head and neck area as well as the embryology and pathology of the parathyroid glands (see Chap. 48).

## STANDARD INITIAL OPERATIVE MANAGEMENT

Under general anesthesia, the patient is positioned supine with arms at the sides and the neck extended to maximally expose the anterior cervical region. A curvilinear incision is made low in the neck and extended through the platysma muscle. The strap muscles are separated in the midline to expose the underlying thyroid gland. After mobilization and medial retraction of the respective thyroid lobe, the recurrent laryngeal nerve and inferior thyroid artery are identified, and the search for the parathyroid glands begins.

The goal of the initial neck exploration for hyperparathyroidism is first to identify all four parathyroid glands and then to remove those that are enlarged. This requires exploration of both sides of the neck to identify all parathyroid glands. Stopping the exploration after finding one normal gland and one abnormal gland on one side of the neck leads to an increased incidence of missed tumors.[1] The size of the parathyroid gland should be the factor that determines resection, because the pathologists' interpretations of "adenoma" or "hyperplasia" are misleading. In most patients, only one parathyroid gland is enlarged. The large parathyroid glands should be excised, and the normal-appearing parathyroid glands should be left in situ. The surgical decision should not be based only on the histologic interpretation. In addition, tests of gland density (water immersion test) and histochemical staining for cytoplasmic lipid content are unreliable indicators of parathyroid gland behavior.

In most patients with *single-gland disease*, removal of the enlarged parathyroid gland is curative.[2] Infrequently, patients with hyperparathyroidism harbor *two or three enlarged parathyroid glands,* all of which should be removed. In one study, 76 patients with hyperparathyroidism caused by two or three enlarged parathyroid glands were evaluated from 12 to 140 months after resection of only the large parathyroids.[3] Persistent or recurrent postoperative hypercalcemia developed in eight patients (10.5%) from 1 to 133 months postoperatively. Thus, these patients appear to have an increased incidence of persistent or recurrent hypercalcemia compared with patients with hyperparathyroidism caused by single-gland disease.

A difficult management problem occurs in patients with hyperparathyroidism caused by *four-gland enlargement (parathyroid hyperplasia).*[4] This entity occurs in 10% to 15% of cases. Primary hyperplasia includes the rare *water clear cell hyperplasia* and the more common *chief cell hyperplasia,* which may occur alone or in association with certain familial endocrinopathies, including multiple endocrine neoplasia types 1 (MEN1) and 2A (MEN2A) (see Chap. 188). These patients are especially difficult to manage, and the postoperative results are less satisfactory than for patients undergoing surgery for one-, two-, or three-gland enlargement. Patients with parathyroid hyperplasia may be managed by subtotal parathyroidectomy (removal of three and one-half glands) or, alternatively, total parathyroidectomy and heterotopic autotransplantation of parathyroid tissue to the forearm. The former approach is more commonly used and leaves the remaining parathyroid tissue with its native blood supply. The latter approach has the advantage of removing all known parathyroid tissue from the neck and grafting it to a heterotopic site to simplify reoperation in case of recurrent hyperparathyroidism. Both operations are dependent on a meticulous initial neck exploration to identify all parathyroid glands. After subtotal parathyroidectomy for nonfamilial parathyroid hyperplasia, the incidence of recurrent hypercalcemia is 0% to 16%, and the incidence of permanent hypoparathyroidism is 4% to 5%.[5–8] In patients with MEN1, however, subtotal parathyroidectomy has led to recurrent hypercalcemia in 26% to 66% of patients at long-term follow-up (mean time to recurrence, >5 years).[9–11] Total parathyroidectomy is associated with a significant incidence of permanent hypoparathyroidism (5–36%) and possibly a higher incidence of graft-dependent recurrent hyperparathyroidism (familial, 20–64%; nonfamilial, 20%).[11,12] However, reoperation for recurrent hypercalcemia is simpler if the parathyroid tissue is in the forearm rather than in the neck. For patients with nonfamilial parathyroid hyperplasia, either approach is acceptable; however, patients with MEN1 or MEN2A should have total parathyroidectomy with autotransplantation.

Occasionally, only three parathyroid glands are found or, if four glands are seen, none is enlarged. The surgeon then must explore the "thyrothymic ligament" and superior mediastinum through the cervical incision, even removing a portion of the thymus if a lower parathyroid gland is missing. The lateral neck, from the thymus to the pharynx, should be explored for an undescended "parathymus." Rarely, an enlarged parathyroid gland is located within a crevice in the thyroid, between nodules, or it may be embedded within the thyroid parenchyma. Intraoperative ultrasonography may be useful to identify ectopic parathyroid tissue either within the thyroid or elsewhere in the neck. As a last resort, the surgeon should consider resecting the thyroid lobe on the side of the missing parathyroid gland. The superior parathyroid glands are more constant in location but are far posterior and may be overlooked. The upper glands, when enlarged, may descend into the tracheoesophageal groove or into the posterior mediastinum, where they may be extracted by the examining finger. Confirming all abnormal parathyroid tissue by biopsy, and confirming each parathyroid gland in patients with more than one abnormal gland, is wise. However, one should not completely resect a normal parathyroid gland.

If no enlarged parathyroid gland is identified after a thorough examination of the neck, the operation should be terminated. Postoperatively, the biochemical diagnosis of primary hyperpara-thyroidism should be confirmed. Localization studies should then be performed before repeat neck exploration. Localization procedures are not generally indicated in patients undergoing initial full neck exploration for hyperparathyroidism because the experienced endocrine surgeon identifies four parathyroid glands and successfully performs corrective surgery in nearly all cases.[13]

# PROMISING TECHNIQUES FOR INITIAL PARATHYROID EXPLORATION

Three technological advancements have made selective exploration strategies viable in the initial exploration of the neck. These advances are (a) the ability to rapidly (in 10–15 minutes) and accurately measure the serum level of PTH; (b) the improved ability to localize abnormal parathyroid tissue with technetium Tc 99m sestamibi ($^{99m}$Tc sestamibi) scanning, using either preoperative imaging or intraoperative handheld gamma probe localization; and (c) the improvement of videoscopic surgical instruments. A variety of strategies have been described that use combinations of these technologies to treat primary hyperparathyroidism. As the standard full neck exploration cures ~95% of patients, these newer strategies are designed to match those outcome results, with less surgical trauma. The long-term evaluations of these approaches remain to be accomplished; however, the early results are very promising.

## CONCISE PARATHYROIDECTOMY

The term "concise parathyroidectomy" was first used to describe a unilateral exploration approach.[14] This approach uses preoperative $^{99m}$Tc sestamibi imaging to select one side of the neck for exploration. During the operation, parathyroid hormone (PTH) levels are measured before and after the removal of the localized abnormal parathyroid tissue. If the PTH level falls sufficiently after the resection, then the exploration is terminated. If the PTH level does not fall, then the neck is explored further.[15] This approach avoids bilateral neck exploration in a significant number of patients, and may shorten both operative time and the risk of recurrent laryngeal nerve injury on the side contralateral to the abnormal parathyroid tissue. The more limited exploration may also facilitate the use of local or regional anesthesia with sedation, avoiding the morbidity of general anesthesia.

## RADIOGUIDED PARATHYROIDECTOMY

An alternative strategy depends on the ability to localize the abnormal parathyroid tissue using $^{99m}$Tc sestamibi scanning and a handheld gamma probe for intraoperative localization.[16] This technique can be performed with or without concurrent intraoperative PTH monitoring. Because the handheld probe can be used to localize the abnormal parathyroid gland in many cases, very small incisions and local anesthesia can be used to identify and remove the localized parathyroid gland. Prospective trials are currently under way at several institutions to evaluate this technique as well as the utility of combining the radioguided approach with intraoperative PTH monitoring to avoid persistent hyperparathyroidism in patients with multiple gland disease.

## VIDEOSCOPIC PARATHYROIDECTOMY

A minimally invasive approach to the removal of the parathyroid glands has been reported using videoscopic surgical techniques. This approach is currently applied in selected centers, and always in combination with preoperative $^{99m}$Tc sestamibi scanning and intraoperative PTH monitoring.[17] The technique has been performed from a variety of anatomic approaches, but to date includes visualization of just one parathyroid gland and resection using small (2–5 mm) videoscopic instruments, through an operative space created by a balloon expander. The value of this technique awaits the results of further experience.

## TECHNIQUES FOR LOCALIZATION OF ABNORMAL PARATHYROID TISSUE IN PATIENTS WITH PERSISTENT OR RECURRENT HYPERPARATHYROIDISM

Several noninvasive techniques have been developed for localizing hyperfunctioning parathyroid tissue. Barium swallow, cineesophagography, and thyroid scanning are rarely helpful, whereas other procedures such as computed tomographic (CT) scans, magnetic resonance imaging, [99m]Tc sestamibi scanning, and high-resolution real-time ultrasonography identify enlarged parathyroid glands in 40% to 60% of patients studied.[18–20] CT scans, [99m]Tc sestamibi scans, and sestamibi/iodine subtraction single photon emission computed tomography (SPECT)[20a] are most useful for identifying lesions in the neck and mediastinum (Fig. 62-1). Sometimes, these techniques are coupled with needle aspiration of an identified mass followed by assay of the aspirate for PTH. Markedly increased PTH values, compared with an aspirate from muscle, document the presence of parathyroid tissue.

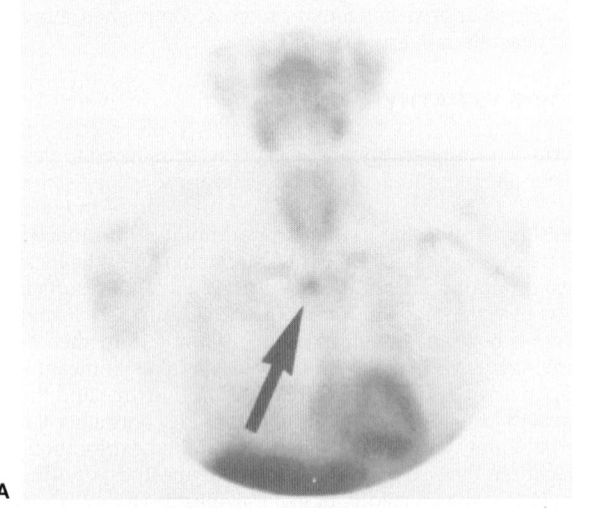

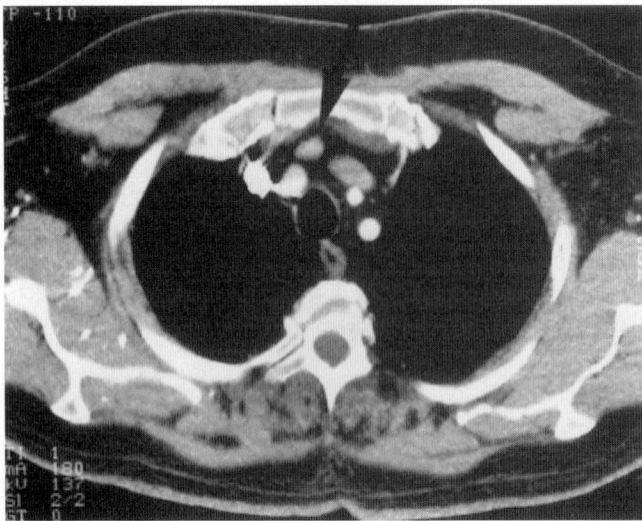

**FIGURE 62-1. A,** Sestamibi scan. The technetium-99m sestamibi scintigram shows concentration of the nuclide in ectopic parathyroid tissue in the anterior mediastinum (*arrow*). **B,** Computed tomographic scan of the mediastinum in the same patient as shown in **A** reveals a soft-tissue mass anterior to the brachiocephalic artery consistent with parathyroid adenoma (*arrow*).

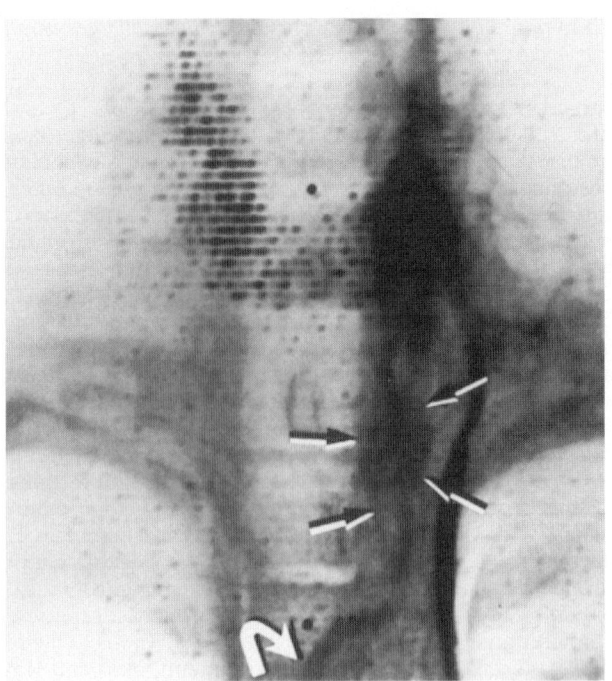

**FIGURE 62-2.** Selective arteriography. Late phase of an inferior thyroid arteriogram. A left lower parathyroid adenoma stain is indicated by the *four small arrows.* The normal thyroid gland blush is superior and is identified as such by superimposition of the thyroid scan. The *curved arrow* denotes the draining inferior thyroid vein. (From Wells SA Jr. The parathyroid glands. In: Sabiston DC Jr, ed. Textbook of surgery. Philadelphia: WB Saunders, 1972:656.)

Invasive localization techniques include selective thyroid arteriography and selective venous sampling with assay of plasma levels of PTH.[19,21] Selective arteriography (Fig. 62-2) identifies hyperfunctioning parathyroid tissue in 50% to 70% of cases. Arteriography should be performed only by an experienced angiographer, because the technique may have significant morbidity. In rare patients for whom there are significant reasons to avoid reoperation, angiographic ablation of hyperfunctioning parathyroid tissue may be appropriate.[22] Selective thyroid venous sampling with PTH assay is useful in lateralizing the side of the neck in which hyperfunctioning parathyroid tissue resides (Fig. 62-3).

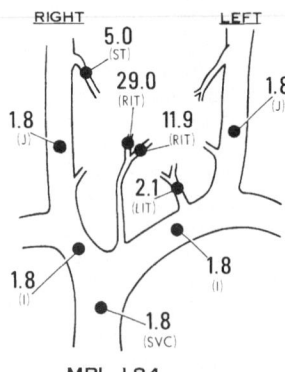

**FIGURE 62-3.** Selective thyroid venous sampling in a patient with a retained hyperfunctioning right inferior parathyroid gland. Plasma parathyroid hormone concentrations in samples obtained at different points in the venous circulation. Veins are jugular (*J*), innominate (*I*), superior vena cava (*SVC*), superior thyroid (*ST*), left inferior thyroid (*LIT*), and right inferior thyroid (*RIT*). *MBL* is mean background level; sites of sampling indicated by •; adjacent numbers indicate plasma PTH concentration in ng/mL. (Adapted from Potts J, et al. Parathyroid re-exploration sequence, synthesis, immunoassay studies. Am J Med 1971; 50:639.)

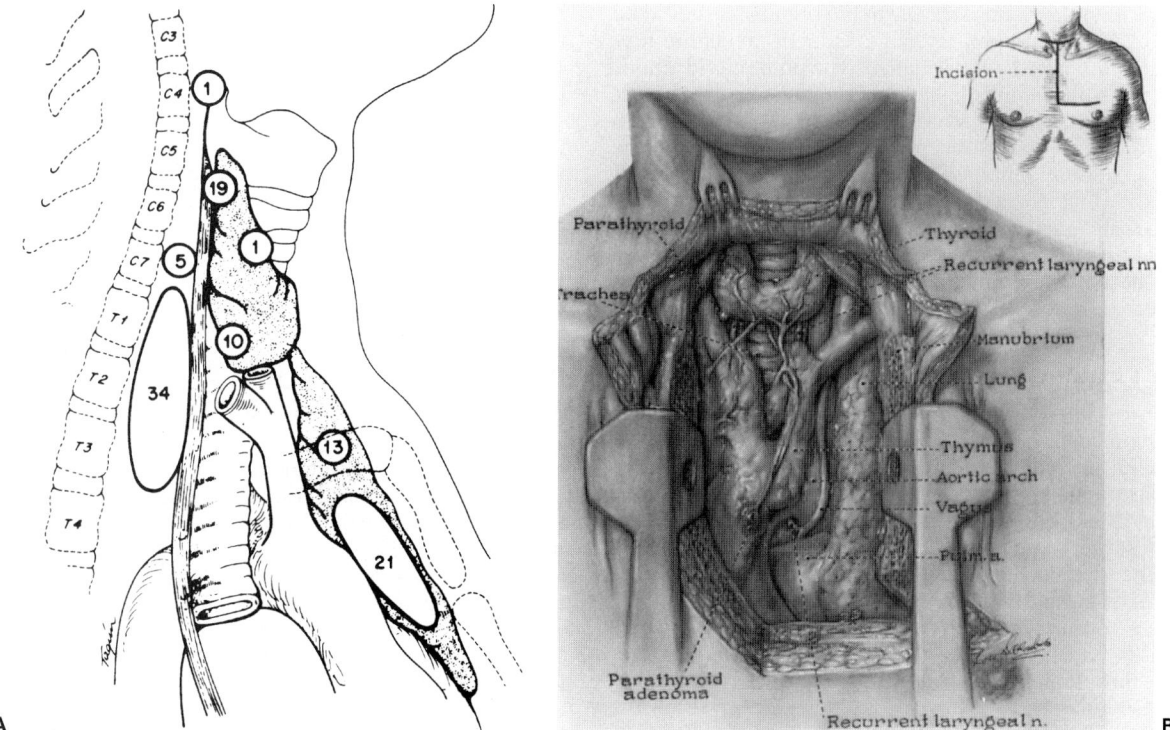

**FIGURE 62-4.** **A,** Schematic representation of location, at reexploration, of 104 missing parathyroid glands. The sites in which the missing parathyroid glands were most frequently located were the superior posterior mediastinum, the mediastinal thymus, the superior thyroid pole, the thymic tongue, and the inferior portion of the thyroid gland. Thus, 81% of the missing glands were reached by way of the neck and 19% by way of the mediastinum. **B,** Surgical technique of median sternotomy to reach an enlarged parathyroid gland in the thymus. (**A** from Wang CA. Parathyroid re-exploration: a clinical and pathological study of 112 cases. Ann Surg 1977; 186:140.)

The combined techniques of arteriography and selective venous catheterization can accurately localize hyperfunctioning tissue in 70% to 85% of reoperative cases. For patients who have previously undergone exploration by an experienced endocrine surgeon, most clinicians would use noninvasive and then (if no two studies concur) invasive localization studies.

## STRATEGY AT REOPERATION FOR RECURRENT OR PERSISTENT HYPERPARATHYROIDISM

Parathyroid reoperation may be necessary in cases of persistent or recurrent primary hyperparathyroidism. Persistent primary hyperparathyroidism is the more common cause of postoperative hypercalcemia and represents a continuation of an elevated serum calcium level through the immediate postoperative period or its development within 6 months of operation. This usually is the result of a missed hyperfunctioning parathyroid gland or of inadequate resection of hyperfunctioning parathyroid tissue in a patient with multiglandular hyperparathyroidism. Presumably, recurrent primary hyperparathyroidism results from hyperfunction of a previously normal parathyroid gland, incomplete resection of a parathyroid, incomplete resection of hyperfunctional parathyroid tissue, or hypertrophy of autotransplanted abnormal parathyroid tissue.

The severity of the parathyroid disease should be carefully assessed to justify the increased risk of parathyroid reoperation. Reexploration is usually limited to patients with a serum calcium concentration of >12 mg/dL or patients who have renal stones and in whom deteriorating renal function, skeletal fractures, peptic ulcer disease, hypertension, neuromuscular dysfunction, or other complications of primary hyperparathyroidism are present, regardless of the degree of hypercalcemia. In a totally

asymptomatic patient with a serum calcium level of <11 mg/dL and no evidence of skeletal or renal disease, a nonoperative course should be considered.

Before repeat neck exploration, the surgeon should review previous surgical notes, pathology reports, and histologic sections of all resected tissue. Reoperation is generally deferred until localization tests can be performed. If initially generalized parathyroid gland enlargement was found and either a three-gland or a three-and-one-half-gland parathyroidectomy was performed and confirmed histologically, one may undertake repeat neck exploration without performing localization procedures, on the assumption that the remaining gland or gland remnant is the cause of hypercalcemia. The same course may be undertaken if the previous neck exploration has been performed by an inexperienced parathyroid surgeon.

In 75% to 90% of patients undergoing repeat surgery for primary hyperparathyroidism, the hyperfunctioning tissue can be reached through a cervical incision (Fig. 62-4A). Therefore, the neck should be explored first. Even if a parathyroid tumor is identified in the mediastinum by localization techniques, it may be possible to extract it through a cervical incision. The use of a thymectomy retractor can facilitate this mediastinal exploration.[23]

Repeat neck exploration is technically more difficult than the initial surgery and has a greater risk of recurrent laryngeal nerve damage and permanent hypoparathyroidism. Hypoparathyroidism can be prevented by cryopreserving a portion of abnormal parathyroid tissue. The reported success rate in repeat parathyroid surgery varies from 60% to 91%.

## MEDIASTINAL EXPLORATION

The mediastinum is explored through either a cervical incision[23] or a median sternotomy (see Fig. 62-4B). If the enlarged parathyroid gland is visible in the thymus, it should be selectively excised. If no parathyroid is evident, the entire thymus should be removed and sectioned. The parathyroid tumor may not be identified until the pathologist reviews the permanent sections of the submitted tissue. The surgeon should also explore the entire mediastinum around the great vessels and the pericardium. After an enlarged parathyroid gland is identified, if doubt exists that normal parathyroid tissue remains in the neck, the resected parathyroid gland should be sliced into 1-mm × 3-mm pieces and cryopreserved in liquid nitrogen.[24] If the patient has been rendered hypoparathyroid, then the viably frozen tissue can be autotransplanted into a forearm muscle.

## PARATHYROID AUTOTRANSPLANTATION

Clinical circumstances in which parathyroid autotransplantation is useful include radical thyroid surgery with either unavoidable or inadvertent devascularization of parathyroid tissue, renal osteodystrophy, primary parathyroid hyperplasia, and repeat surgery for recurrent or persistent hyperparathyroidism. The decision to autotransplant parathyroid tissue depends on the individual patient.

In the case of inadvertent devascularization of normal parathyroid tissue, such as during radical thyroid surgery, immediate autotransplantation is indicated. The devascularized gland is removed and placed in cold saline. A frozen section is obtained to confirm that the tissue is parathyroid. After thyroidectomy, the parathyroid tissue is sliced into 1-mm × 3-mm slivers and immediately implanted into the sternocleidomastoid muscle. Each implantation site contains one or two parathyroid fragments and is marked with a silk suture. Some investigators question the need to perform this technique if other in situ parathyroid glands appear viable. However, assessing viability by macroscopic appearance is difficult. If any question exists regarding adequacy of the blood supply to a parathyroid, the gland should be removed and transplanted.

Reduction of the hyperplastic parathyroid tissue mass is indicated in patients with renal osteodystrophy who are refractory to medical management and who have fractures or severe bone pain, extraosseous soft tissue or vascular calcification, or intractable pruritus (see Chap. 61). The role of parathyroid surgery in the management of secondary hyperparathyroidism has been complicated by the recognition of aluminum-related osteodystrophy (see Chaps. 61 and 131). All patients with severe secondary hyperparathyroidism (tertiary hyperparathyroidism) should be evaluated for the presence of this entity. Evidence suggests that, for these patients, parathyroid surgery is not the treatment of choice and actually may further predispose to aluminum bone disease. However, in patients with severe renal osteodystrophy that is not related to aluminum and in whom the control of secondary hyperparathyroidism is impossible by an aggressive medical approach, surgery may be necessary. In this setting, subtotal parathyroidectomy is generally indicated.[25] Total parathyroidectomy with heterotopic autografting[4,26–28] is an equivalent or superior option because cervical reexploration for recurrent disease, with the risk of hypoparathyroidism and recurrent laryngeal nerve injury, is precluded, and the bone symptom improvements may be more durable.[29] A thorough neck exploration is undertaken, with removal of all parathyroid glands. Each gland should have a small portion removed for frozen-section examination. These glands are then placed in cold sterile tissue culture medium and sliced into 1-mm × 3-mm pieces. After closure of the cervical incision, ~20 pieces of tissue are implanted into the brachioradialis muscle of the nondominant forearm. In cases in which fewer than four parathyroid glands are identified despite a thorough neck exploration, the harvested parathyroid tissue is cryopreserved, and parathyroid grafting is delayed. The patient should then be monitored postoperatively for evidence of parathyroid hyperfunction or hypofunction. If prolonged

hypocalcemia develops, forearm engraftment under local anesthesia can be carried out at a convenient time. Persistent hypercalcemia indicates that an inadequate amount of parathyroid tissue was resected.

A 10% to 40% incidence of persistent or recurrent hyperparathyroidism is reported in patients managed by subtotal parathyroidectomy for renal osteodystrophy.[30] Cervical reexploration results in postoperative hypoparathyroidism in approximately one-third of these patients. With immediate or delayed autografting, graft failure is reported to occur in 5% of patients; hyperfunction of the heterotopic autograft is readily managed by partial graft resection under local anesthesia.

## IMMEDIATE VERSUS DELAYED AUTOGRAFTING

The decision to use immediate versus delayed autografting depends on the potential risk of graft loss during the freezing and thawing process, versus the risk of graft-dependent hypercalcemia. The incidence of graft-dependent hypercalcemia is 30% within 3 months to 2 years after the autografting of fresh hyperfunctioning parathyroid tissue.[12] Also, cases of recalcitrant or recurrent graft-dependent hypercalcemia have been reported.[31] Whether persistent parathyroid hyperfunction is caused by pathologic tissue left in situ or by the hyperfunctioning graft may be unclear. Assay for forearm PTH levels may aid in this differentiation. For these reasons, some have advocated delayed autografting using in vitro–tested cryopreserved parathyroid tissue.

If delayed transplantation is the decided course, fresh tissue removed at the time of operation is divided into 1-mm × 3-mm fragments and cryopreserved.[24] Long-term tissue viability has been demonstrated by successful engraftment after 9 to 48 months of storage. During subsequent transplantation, the tissue is thawed, and fragments are implanted into the forearm muscle pockets as a heterotopic autograft. A single sliver of parathyroid tissue is implanted into an individual muscle pocket. The musculature and fascia above the graft are then enclosed with a single 5-0 nonabsorbable suture, which provides a marker of the graft site. Implantation must be carried out without hemorrhage into the muscle pocket, and care must be taken not to impale the graft tissue—either will result in graft failure.

## PARATHYROID CARCINOMA

Hyperparathyroidism caused by parathyroid carcinoma is rare; the reported incidence is from 0.5% to 4% (see Chaps. 48 and 58). This diagnosis should be suspected when (a) a palpable neck mass is present, (b) the serum calcium level exceeds 14 mg/dL, (c) the serum PTH level is markedly elevated, and (d) a previously unoperated patient is hoarse from a recurrent laryngeal nerve invasion. At surgery, parathyroid carcinomas appear white and very firm, unlike adenomas, which are reddish brown and soft. The initial operation must be aggressive yet meticulous, with en bloc resection of the parathyroid tumor and all adjacent invaded tissues, including the ipsilateral thyroid lobe. Care must be taken not to rupture the capsule and spill the tumor. Radical neck dissection is reserved for patients with clinically overt cervical node metastases. Distinguishing early parathyroid carcinoma from atypical parathyroid adenoma by histologic and clinical criteria may be difficult. In these cases, DNA cytometry can be helpful, because an aneuploid pattern and higher nuclear DNA content are typical of carcinomas but not of adenomas. For recurrent disease, repeated resection of local cervical implants and distant metastases is important in palliative management. Tumor recurrence is generally apparent within 6 months to 3 years of surgery and may denote an incurable process. However, select patients appear to benefit greatly from re-resection of locally recurrent tumors.

# REFERENCES

1. Duh Q-Y, Uden P, Clark OH. Unilateral neck exploration for primary hyperparathyroidism: analysis of a controversy using a mathematical model. World J Surg 1992; 16:654.
2. Brasier A, Wang C-A, Nussbaum S. Recovery of parathyroid hormone secretion after parathyroid adenectomy. J Clin Endocrinol Metab 1988; 66:495.
3. Wells SA, Leight GS, Hensley M, Dilley WG. Hyperparathyroidism associated with the enlargement of two or three parathyroid glands. Ann Surg 1985; 202:533.
4. Cope O, Keynes WM, Roth SI, Castleman B. Primary chief cell hyperplasia of the parathyroid glands: a new entity in the surgery of hyperparathyroidism. Ann Surg 1958; 148:375.
5. Rudberg C, Akerström G, Palmer M, et al. Late results of operation for primary hyperparathyroidism in 441 patients. Surgery 1986; 99:643.
6. Edis AJ, van Heerden JA, Scholz DA. Results of subtotal parathyroidectomy for primary chief cell hyperplasia. Surgery 1979; 86:462.
7. Bonjer HJ, Bruining HA, Birkenhager JC, et al. Single and multigland disease in primary hyperparathyroidism: clinical follow-up, histopathology, and flow cytometric DNA analysis. World J Surg 1992; 16:737.
8. Proye C, Carnaille B, Quievreux J-L, et al. Late outcome of 304 consecutive patients with multiple gland enlargement in primary hyperparathyroidism treated by conservative surgery. World J Surg 1998; 22:526.
9. Rizzoli R, Green J III, Marx SJ. Primary hyperparathyroidism in familial multiple endocrine neoplasia type I: long-term follow-up of serum calcium levels after parathyroidectomy. Am J Med 1985; 78:467.
10. Kraimps J, Duh Q-Y, Demeure M, Clark O. Hyperparathyroidism in multiple endocrine neoplasia syndrome. Surgery 1992; 112:1080.
11. Hellman P, Skogseid B, Oberg K, et al. Primary and reoperative parathyroid operations in hyperparathyroidism of multiple endocrine neoplasia type 1. Surgery 1998; 124:993.
12. Wells SA Jr, Farndon JR, Dale JK, et al. Long-term evaluation of patients with primary parathyroid hyperplasia managed by total parathyroidectomy and heterotopic autotransplantation. Ann Surg 1980; 192:451.
13. Consensus Development Conference Panel. Diagnosis and management of asymptomatic primary hyperparathyroidism: Consensus Development Conference statement. Ann Intern Med 1991; 114:593.
14. Carty S, Worsey M, Virji M, et al. Concise parathyroidectomy: the impact of preoperative SPECT $^{99m}$Tc sestamibi scanning and intraoperative quick parathormone assay. Surgery 1997; 122:1107.
15. Boggs JE, Irvin GL 3rd, Molinari AS, Deriso GT. Intraoperative parathyroid hormone monitoring as an adjunct to parathyroidectomy. Surgery 1996; 120:954.
16. Norman J, Chheda H, Farrell C. Minimally invasive parathyroidectomy for primary hyperparathyroidism: decreasing operative time and potential complications while improving cosmetic results. Ann Surg 1998; 64:391.
17. Miccoli P, Bendinelli C, Vignali E, et al. Endoscopic parathyroidectomy: report of an initial experience. Surgery 1998; 124:1077.
18. Miller DL, Doppman JL, Shawker TH, et al. Localization of parathyroid adenomas in patients who have undergone surgery. Part I. Noninvasive imaging methods. Radiology 1987; 162:133.
19. Levin KE, Gooding GAW, Okerlund M, et al. Localizing studies in patients with persistent or recurrent hyperparathyroidism. Surgery 1987; 102:917.
20. Wei J, Burke G, Munsberger A. Prospective evaluation of the efficacy of technetium 99m sestamibi and iodine 123 radionuclide imaging of abnormal parathyroid glands. Surgery 1992; 112:1111.
20a. Neumann DR, Esselstyn CB Jr, Madera AM. Sestamibi/iodine subtraction single photon emission computed tomography in reoperative secondary hyperparathyroidism. Surgery 2000; 128:22.
21. Miller DL, Doppman JL, Krudy AG, et al. Localization of parathyroid adenomas in patients who have undergone surgery. Part II. Invasive procedures. Radiology 1987; 162:138.
22. Doherty GM, Doppman JL, Miller DL, et al. Results of a multidisciplinary strategy for management of mediastinal parathyroid adenoma as a cause of persistent primary hyperparathyroidism. Ann Surg 1992; 215:101.
23. Wells SA Jr, Cooper JD. Closed mediastinal exploration in patients with persistent hyperparathyroidism. Ann Surg 1991; 214:555.
24. Wells SA, Gunnells JC, Gutman RA, et al. The successful transplantation of frozen parathyroid tissue in man. Surgery 1977; 81:86.
25. Stanbury S, Lumb G, Nicholson W. Selective subtotal parathyroidectomy for renal hyperparathyroidism. Lancet 1960; 1:793.
26. Cordell LJ, Maxwell JG, Warden GD. Parathyroidectomy in chronic renal failure. Am J Surg 1979; 138:951.
27. Dubost C, Drueke T, Jeaneau P, et al. Hyperparathyroidie secondaire: parathyroidectomie subtotale ou totale avec autotransplantation parathyroidienne. Nouvelle Presse Médicale 1980; 9:2709.
28. Niederle B, Roka R, Brennan MF. The transplantation of parathyroid tissue in man: development, indications, techniques, and results. Endocr Rev 1982; 3:345.
29. Rothmund M, Wagner PK, Schark C. Subtotal parathyroidectomy versus total parathyroidectomy and autotransplantation in secondary hyperparathyroidism: a randomized trial. World J Surg 1991; 15:745.
30. Rothmund M, Wagner P. Reoperations for persistent and recurrent secondary hyperparathyroidism. Ann Surg 1988; 207:310.
31. D'Avanzo A, Parangi S, Morita E, et al. Hyperparathyroidism after thyroid surgery and autotransplantation of histologically normal parathyroid glands. J Am Coll Surg 2000; 190:546.

# CHAPTER 63

# OSTEOMALACIA AND RICKETS

NORMAN H. BELL

## DEFINITION

Osteomalacia is a disorder of mineralization of newly formed organic matrix that occurs in adults. Rickets is a disease of children in which abnormal calcification of matrix also occurs. Further, defective mineralization of cartilage takes place in the epiphyseal cartilage growth plate so that disorganization of cellular development ensues, which leads to widening of the ends of long bones and, possibly, retardation of growth and skeletal deformities.

## PATHOGENESIS

For mineralization to take place normally, newly formed osteoid must be normal both qualitatively and quantitatively, the concentrations of calcium and phosphate in extracellular fluid must be sufficient, the activity of alkaline phosphatase must be adequate, the pH at the site of calcification must be optimal, and excess concentration of inhibitors of calcification must be prevented. Bone formation takes place in two steps. The organic matrix or osteoid derived from osteoblasts, or bone-forming cells, is laid down and then undergoes a process of maturation that requires 10 to 15 days before mineralization takes place.[1] Whereas osteomalacia could result from abnormal structure of organic matrix so that calcification cannot take place normally, it much more frequently is caused by alterations in mineral metabolism in which reduced serum concentrations of calcium or phosphate, or both, occur.[2]

Normal mineralization is incompletely understood (see Chap. 50). Calcium and phosphate in extracellular fluid are supersaturated, and metastatic calcification is prevented by pyrophosphate and possibly other substances that include peptides. Bone mineral is first deposited as amorphous calcium phosphate that eventually undergoes conversion to hydroxyapatite $[Ca_{10}(PO_4)_6(OH)_2]$. Calcium in extracellular fluid space is taken up by mitochondria in osteoblasts and transported to matrix vesicles for mineralization. The phosphate that is used in mineralization is made available by alkaline phosphatase that is present in the matrix vesicles. Deposition and eventual conversion of amorphous calcium phosphate to hydroxyapatite occur at gaps, "hole zones," between the distal ends of two molecules of collagen.

The rate of bone formation and calcification can be measured accurately by histomorphometric techniques, which require double tetracycline labeling (see Chap. 55). Tetracyclines are deposited in the skeleton at the mineralization front in a band-like pattern. They fluoresce and are easily visualized on histologic sections under a fluorescence microscope. After two brief courses of administration, with an intervening interval, the appositional growth rate of the skeleton can be estimated in biopsy samples of the iliac crest by determining the distance between the two fluorescent bands. In normal adults, this distance averages ~1 μm per day.[3] In osteomalacia, the distance is reduced. In some patients with osteomalacia, mineralization of the skeleton is so abnormal that only a single ill-defined band of fluorescence can be discerned. Newly synthesized matrix that is abnormally mineralized appears as a wide osteoid seam. The two cardinal histomorphometric features of osteomalacia are the wide osteoid seam and the reduced calcification rate; these two findings are essential for the diagnosis, because wide osteoid seams occur without abnormal mineralization in bone disease associated with hyperthyroidism, Paget disease, and primary hyperparathyroidism.[4]

## CLINICAL PRESENTATION

Sometimes patients with osteomalacia have no symptoms, so that the diagnosis is not readily apparent early in the course of the disease. When present, symptoms include diffuse skeletal pain and muscle weakness. The pain often is described as dull and aching and is worsened by activity. It is present in the lower back and hips or at sites where fractures have taken place. Bone tenderness may be present on palpation. Fractures most commonly occur in the ribs, vertebrae, and long bones, and may lead to skeletal deformities. Muscle weakness, often present in patients with osteomalacia, may be severe and associated with wasting.[5] Because weakness usually involves the proximal muscle groups, particularly of the lower extremities, it may contribute to the characteristic waddling gait.

Numerous factors appear to play a role in the development of the muscle weakness associated with osteomalacia. Whereas myopathic muscle changes sometimes are evident by electromyography, denervation rarely is seen on muscle biopsy.[6] However, neurogenic atrophy or type II muscle fiber atrophy occasionally is observed.[7] Hypophosphatemia itself can cause muscle weakness; therefore, the weakness can be improved simply by correction of the hypophosphatemia. Secondary hyperparathyroidism may be important in the pathogenesis of the neuromuscular disease in osteomalacia, because clinical and laboratory findings similar to those that occur in patients with osteomalacia occasionally are found in patients with primary hyperparathyroidism.

## RADIOGRAPHIC FINDINGS

The most common radiographic change in osteomalacia is reduced skeletal density, a nonspecific finding with little diagnostic value. More helpful are the less frequently occurring coarsening of trabecular pattern and the *Looser zones* or *pseudofractures*.[8,9] The loss of distinctness of trabeculae in vertebral bodies is attributed to the loss of secondary trabeculae and to inadequate mineralization of osteoid. Because of softening, the vertebral bodies in more advanced disease may become concave, termed "codfish" vertebrae. Conversely, the vertebral disks are large and biconvex. Compression fractures of the spine occur but are less common than in osteoporosis.

Looser zones are narrow lines of radiolucency that usually transect and lie either at right angles or obliquely to the cortical margins of bones. They typically are bilateral and symmetric. Common sites include the axillary margins of the scapulae, the lower ribs, the superior and inferior pubic rami, the inner margins and neck of the proximal femora, and the posterior margins of the proximal ulnae. Multiple, bilateral, and symmetric pseudofractures in a patient with osteomalacia are called *Milkman syndrome*.[10,11] The pathogenesis of Looser zones is thought by some to be stress fractures that are repaired by the laying down of inadequately mineralized osteoid. Because the pseudofractures often lie adjacent to arteries, others attribute the lesions to mechanical erosion caused by arterial pulsations, a concept that is supported by the arteriographic demonstra-

tion that arteries frequently overlie sites of the pseudofractures.[8,12] True fractures can occur at these weakened areas.

Deformities of the skeleton often occur with rickets during childhood, some of which may persist into adulthood.[13] Skeletal abnormalities occur at sites of rapid growth. Because the rate of growth of different bones varies with age, the skeletal changes of rickets vary with age and may indicate the age of onset of the disease. Because of rapid growth, the skull is particularly affected in neonates. Softening of the cranium, or *craniotabes*, may be associated with parietal flattening, frontal bossing, and widened sutures. Rapid growth of the arms and rib cage in early childhood is reflected in the widening of the forearm at the wrist, and the thickening of the costochondral junctions that produces the *rachitic rosary* (see Chap. 70). Indentations of the lower ribs at the site of attachment of the diaphragm are called *Harrison grooves*. With increased growth of long bones, bowing of the lower extremities may result as a consequence of weight-bearing. Deformities of the pelvis occur and can produce major problems at the time of weight-bearing.

Because of secondary hyperparathyroidism, skeletal changes resulting from increases in circulating parathyroid hormone (PTH) may be present. These include subperiosteal resorption of the phalanges and resorption of the distal ends of long bones such as the clavicle and humerus.

In patients with osteomalacia, bone mass, determined by single- and dual-photon absorptiometry, is reduced,[14] and bone scans show increased uptake of technetium 99m pyrophosphate by long bones and wrists, and prominence of the calvaria and mandible.[15] Less prominent is beading of the costochondral junctions and marked uptake of the tracer by the sternum and its margins, the "tie sternum." Moreover, pseudofractures appear as hot spots.[15] Sometimes pseudofractures may be evident only on radiographs and other times only on bone scan. Hot spots may be erroneously diagnosed as metastatic lesions.

## TYPES OF OSTEOMALACIA

Osteomalacia can result from abnormalities in vitamin D metabolism, phosphate deficiency, various mineralization defects, and states of rapid bone formation (Table 63-1; see Chap. 70).

### NUTRITIONAL DEFICIENCY

Normally, vitamin $D_3$ derived by dermal production from 7-dehydrocholesterol is the major source of the vitamin (see Chap. 54). Because exposure to sunlight is adequate and dairy products are fortified with vitamin D, osteomalacia resulting from nutritional deficiency is rarely seen in the United States. When it does occur, lack of exposure to sunlight usually is responsible. Conversely, nutritional deficiency of vitamin D is more common in other parts of the world. In the United Kingdom, osteomalacia occurs in immigrant Indians and Pakistanis.[16–18] Ethnic traditions and dietary patterns contribute to the development of osteomalacia in the Asian population in England. Endogenous production of vitamin $D_3$ is limited in women who remain indoors and wear traditional clothing, because of diminished exposure to the sun. Chupatti flour, a dietary staple of these population groups, has a high phytate content in the wheat and binds calcium, causing increased fecal excretion. Lignin, a component of wheat fiber, binds to bile acids, preventing their absorption.[19] Vitamin D, which normally forms micelles with bile acids, a requirement for its absorption by the intestine, may be bound by the lignin-bile acid complex instead and not be absorbed. Removal of the chupatti flour from the diet corrects abnormal vitamin D and mineral metabolism. In addition, fortification of the diet with vitamin D can correct the deficiency.

In the United States and other countries, rickets occurs in newborns who are breast-fed because the content of vitamin D

**TABLE 63-1.**
**Etiology of Osteomalacia**

I. **ABNORMALITIES IN VITAMIN D METABOLISM**
  A. Vitamin D deficiency
    1. Nutritional deficiency
    2. Lack of exposure to sunlight
    3. Malabsorption syndromes
      a. Postgastrectomy, partial or total
      b. Small bowel disease
      c. Pancreatic insufficiency
  B. Defective dermal production of vitamin D
    1. Chronic renal disease
    2. Aging
  C. Defective hepatic 25-hydroxylation of vitamin D
    1. Deficiency of hepatic D-25 hydroxylase
    2. Primary biliary cirrhosis
    3. Biliary atresia
    4. Biliary fistula
  D. Defective renal 1α-hydroxylation of 25-hydroxyvitamin D
    1. Hypoparathyroidism
    2. Pseudohypoparathyroidism
    3. Chronic renal insufficiency
    4. Vitamin D–dependent rickets type I
    5. Hypophosphatemic rickets
    6. Tumor-induced osteomalacia
    7. Age-related osteomalacia
  E. Defective target organ response to 1,25-dihydroxyvitamin D
    1. Vitamin D–dependent rickets type II
    2. Anticonvulsant therapy
  F. Renal loss of vitamin D–binding protein
    1. Nephrotic syndrome
II. **PHOSPHATE DEFICIENCY**
  A. Diminished intake
    1. Neonatal rickets
    2. Excess aluminum hydroxide ingestion
  B. Impaired renal tubular phosphate reabsorption

    1. Primary renal tubular defects
      a. X-linked hypophosphatemic osteomalacia
      b. Adult-onset hypophosphatemic osteomalacia
      c. Sporadic acquired hypophosphatemic osteomalacia
      d. Fanconi syndromes
        i. Wilson disease
        ii. Lowe disease
        iii. Tyrosinemia
        iv. Glycogen storage disease
        v. Cystinosis
    2. Secondary renal tubular "defects"
      a. Primary hyperparathyroidism
      b. Secondary hyperparathyroidism
      c. Renal tubular acidosis
      d. Tumor-induced osteomalacia
III. **MINERALIZATION DEFECTS**
  A. Enzyme deficiency
    1. Hypophosphatasia
  B. Circulating inhibitor(s) of calcification
    1. Chronic renal failure
    2. Hypophosphatasia (increased pyrophosphate)
  C. Drugs and ions
    1. Bisphosphonates
    2. Fluoride
    3. Aluminum intoxication
  D. Abnormal bone collagen or matrix
    1. Chronic renal failure
    2. Osteogenesis imperfecta
    3. Fibrogenesis imperfecta ossium
IV. **STATES OF RAPID BONE FORMATION**
  A. Postoperative primary hyperparathyroidism with osteitis fibrosa cystica
  B. Osteopetrosis
V. **MISCELLANEOUS**
  A. Parenteral alimentation

---

and 25-hydroxyvitamin D [25(OH)D] in human milk is not adequate.[20] In the northern hemisphere, blacks, Pakistanis, and Asian Indian infants are particularly at risk for rickets because maternal serum vitamin D and 25(OH)D values are low as a consequence of increased skin pigmentation and diminished dermal synthesis of vitamin D. Asian Indians and Pakistanis, but not blacks, are at risk for vitamin D deficiency and osteomalacia in later life.[21] However, osteomalacia caused by nutritional vitamin D deficiency does not occur in blacks. In developed countries, osteomalacia occurs in the elderly, who appear to be the population at greatest risk for this disorder. This is especially true for individuals who are housebound or institutionalized. An age-related decline in the dermal synthesis of 7-dehydrocholesterol,[22] inadequate intake of vitamin D, and impaired production of 25(OH)D in the liver and 1,25-dihydroxyvitamin D [1,25(OH)$_2$D] in the kidney[23] also may be contributing factors.

## VITAMIN D-25-HYDROXYLASE DEFICIENCY

Rarely, rickets occurs as a consequence of deficiency of vitamin D-25-hydroxylase.[24,25] The disease apparently is transmitted genetically as an autosomal recessive trait. Affected children show evidence of rickets during early childhood. Clinical findings include irritability, seizures, growth retardation, and poor motor development. Hypocalcemia of variable degree, hypophosphatemia, elevated serum alkaline phosphatase and serum immunoreactive PTH (iPTH) values, low serum 25(OH)D values, and normal or elevated serum levels of 1,25 dihydroxyvita-

min D [1,25(OH)$_2$D] are found. The diagnosis is made as follows: demonstration of a low serum 25(OH)D value; poor response to physiologic doses of vitamin D; correction of biochemical, clinical, and radiographic changes of rickets after treatment with physiologic doses of 25(OH)D; the lack of hepatic, gastrointestinal, or renal disease; and no history of consumption of anticonvulsants.

## GASTROINTESTINAL AND HEPATIC DISEASES

Intestinal malabsorption associated with diseases of the small intestine, hepatobiliary tree, and pancreas is the most common cause of vitamin D deficiency in the United States.[26] Disorders of the small intestine that may cause malabsorption and osteomalacia include celiac disease or sprue, regional enteritis, scleroderma, multiple jejunal diverticula, and the blind loop syndrome. In some cases, the bone disease is more evident than the gastrointestinal disease. Impaired absorption of calcium as well as vitamin D may contribute to the development of osteomalacia. Although vitamin D undergoes an enterohepatic circulation, intestinal loss of endogenous vitamin D has not been demonstrated to be important in the pathogenesis of osteomalacia in enteric diseases.

In adults, osteomalacia is a common complication of intestinal bypass surgery for the treatment of morbid obesity. In these patients, histologic changes of osteomalacia are more common than are radiographic changes.[27]

Osteomalacia is a complication of partial gastrectomy, especially in association with the Billroth II operation, which excludes the duodenum.[28] Deficient intake of vitamin D, postgastrectomy steatorrhea, and diminished exposure to sunlight and calcium absorption are contributing factors. The incidence of postgastrectomy osteomalacia will probably decline with the advent of more effective medical treatment of peptic ulcer disease.

Osteomalacia occurs as a complication of hepatocellular biliary disorders[29] but is infrequent in pancreatic disorders. Biliary obstruction or parenchymal disease of the liver can diminish the synthesis of 25(OH)D and interfere with the intestinal absorption of vitamin D and calcium. In some patients, the defect in vitamin D-25-hydroxylation may be so great that vitamin D is an ineffective means of treatment and 25(OH)D must be administered.

## HYPOPARATHYROIDISM

Osteomalacia only rarely occurs in patients with hypoparathyroidism (see Chap. 60). Bone pain suggests the diagnosis, and in some instances, because radiographs of the skeleton may be unremarkable, the diagnosis can be made only by histomorphometric analysis of bone biopsy material.[30] Hypocalcemia and low or low-normal serum $1,25(OH)_2D$ usually are present and appear to be important in the pathogenesis of the bone disease. Because PTH is the major regulator of the renal synthesis of $1,25(OH)_2D$, the low serum $1,25(OH)_2D$ value and hypocalcemia result from its deficiency. Some patients can be treated effectively with vitamin D, whereas others require treatment with $1,25(OH)_2D$.[30]

## PSEUDOHYPOPARATHYROIDISM

In pseudohypoparathyroidism (see Chap. 60), resistance to PTH results in hypocalcemia, retention of phosphate, and low serum $1,25(OH)_2D$ values.[30-32] Patients with pseudohypoparathyroidism rarely have osteomalacia.[30] Hypocalcemia and a low serum $1,25(OH)_2D$ value are important factors in the pathogenesis of the bone disease.[30] As in hypoparathyroidism, some patients can be treated with vitamin D and others with $1,25(OH)D$.[30]

## CHRONIC RENAL INSUFFICIENCY

Sometimes osteomalacia occurs in patients with chronic renal failure (see Chap. 61). Several factors may contribute. These include low serum $1,25(OH)_2D$ value resulting from loss of renal tissue and the enzyme 25(OH)D–1α-hydroxylase,[33] retention of inhibitors of calcification, metabolic acidosis, and formation of abnormal collagen matrix. More commonly, skeletal changes of osteitis fibrosa cystica occur as a consequence of secondary hyperparathyroidism, sometimes in association with osteomalacia.[34] Subperiosteal resorption may be present on the medial aspect of the middle phalanges. Resorption also may be evident at other sites, including the medial margins of the femoral necks and the inner aspects of the proximal tibiae. Osteomalacia may develop as a consequence of excessive intake of aluminum-containing phosphate binders,[35] as a result of dialysis-induced phosphate depletion[36] or renal phosphate wasting after renal transplantation.[37]

Osteomalacia may be caused by aluminum derived from water that is used for hemodialysis or from aluminum hydroxide gels that are used to bind phosphate (see Chaps. 61 and 131). Aluminum is deposited in bone at the mineralization front and may impair calcification and cause osteomalacia.[38] In aluminum-induced osteomalacia, serum iPTH is normal or minimally elevated, and the bone disease does not respond to treatment with vitamin D or its analogs. Long-term treatment with the chelating agent deferoxamine is effective in removing aluminum from bone.[39] The osteomalacia can then be treated by calcium together with either 25(OH)D or $1,25(OH)_2D$.

## VITAMIN D–1α-HYDROXYLASE DEFICIENCY

Vitamin D–1α-hydroxylase deficiency, or vitamin D–dependent rickets type I, is an inborn error of vitamin D metabolism that is transmitted genetically as an autosomal recessive trait.[40,41] Affected children appear to be normal at birth and show evidence of the clinical and biochemical changes of rickets during the first year of life. Hypocalcemia is a consistent finding, together with hypophosphatemia and elevated serum iPTH and alkaline phosphatase values. The diagnosis is made by demonstration of a normal or elevated serum 25(OH)D level and normal or low serum $1,25(OH)_2D$ level in association with a low serum calcium level. Some patients are treated successfully with large doses of vitamin D or 25(OH)D but readily respond to physiologic doses of $1,25(OH)_2D$.[40,41]

When 25(OH)D–1α-hydroxylase, which had been cloned from human keratinocytes, was sequenced, it was found to consist of 508 amino acids with an N-terminal mitochondrial signal sequence and a heme-binding region.[42] One patient had deletion/frameshift mutations at codons 211 and 231 that produced a stop codon after amino acid 233; this resulted in a severely truncated protein, which would not bind heme or express 25(OH)D–1α-hydroxylase activity. More recent studies have demonstrated mutations at amino acids 65, 189, 212, 241, 389, 409, 429, 438, 453, 497, 958, 1921, and 1984 (the latter three outside the coding region), which are associated with diminished bioactivity (Fig. 63-1).[43] The gene contains duplicated 7 base-pair (bp) sequences encoding residues 438 and 442. In a number of patients, a third 7 bp copy was found that altered the downstream reading frame and created a premature TGA stop signal.[43] Deletion of glycine 958 is the most common mutation. The disease in these patients is attributed to two autosomal recessive mutations, each inherited from one of the parents.[42,43]

## HYPOPHOSPHATEMIC RICKETS

Hypophosphatemic rickets or osteomalacia is characterized by hypophosphatemia and renal wasting of phosphate.[44,45] The primary defect is one of impaired reabsorption of filtered phosphate by the proximal renal tubule. Two separate mechanisms exist for phosphate transport in the renal tubule: a PTH-dependent component that is responsible for two-thirds of the net tubular reabsorption, and a PTH-independent component that is regulated by the serum calcium and is responsible for the remaining one-third of the net reabsorption.[46] The PTH-dependent component is lacking in men and is partially deficient in women with hypophosphatemic osteomalacia. Defective phosphate transport also

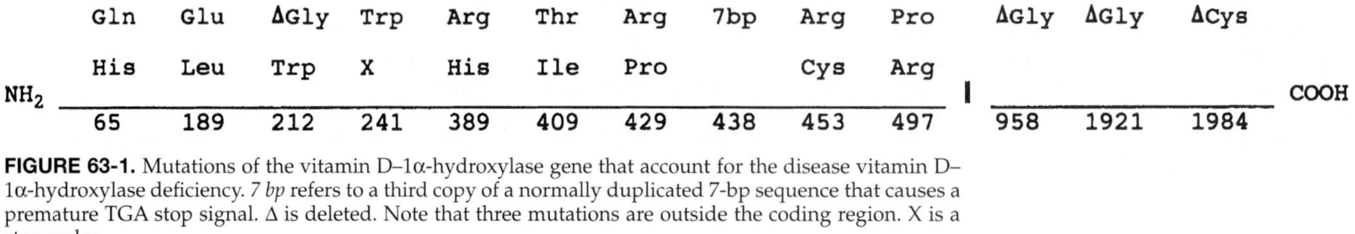

| | Gln | Glu | ΔGly | Trp | Arg | Thr | Arg | 7bp | Arg | Pro | | ΔGly | ΔGly | ΔCys | |
|---|-----|-----|------|-----|-----|-----|-----|-----|-----|-----|---|------|------|------|---|
| | His | Leu | Trp | X | His | Ile | Pro | | Cys | Arg | | | | | |
| NH₂ | 65 | 189 | 212 | 241 | 389 | 409 | 429 | 438 | 453 | 497 | | 958 | 1921 | 1984 | COOH |

**FIGURE 63-1.** Mutations of the vitamin D–1α-hydroxylase gene that account for the disease vitamin D–1α-hydroxylase deficiency. *7 bp* refers to a third copy of a normally duplicated 7-bp sequence that causes a premature TGA stop signal. Δ is deleted. Note that three mutations are outside the coding region. X is a stop codon.

is present in the intestinal mucosa, suggesting that the deficit is generalized and not restricted to the kidney.[47]

Hypophosphatemic rickets usually is familial, but occasionally is sporadic. It is transmitted as an X-linked dominant trait. Onset occurs between 1 and 1.5 years of age and is associated with delayed or abnormal dentition. Screening studies in families indicate that *fasting* hypophosphatemia is the most common manifestation of the disorder. Serum calcium and serum iPTH levels usually are normal. The clinical spectrum is broad, varying from patients who have hypophosphatemia and no apparent bone disease (usually girls) to patients who have symptoms and severe bone disease.[39,40] Patients with the disorder are short and stocky and have bowed legs, particularly when treatment has been inadequate.[47a] The degree of hypophosphatemia and the severity of the bone disease are not correlated. However, diminished growth rate is attributed to hypophosphatemia.

Defective phosphate transport by the kidney and intestine and the production of a phosphaturic substance have been implicated in the pathophysiology of the disorder. However, cross-transplantation experiments in the X-linked hypophosphatemic (*Hyp*) mouse, a model for the human disease, demonstrated that the *Hyp*-mouse phenotype is not corrected or transferred by renal transplantation.[48] These findings support the likelihood of a humoral factor rather than an intrinsic renal or intestinal abnormality in the etiology of hypophosphatemic rickets.

A type II sodium/phosphate cotransporter in the brush border membranes is the rate-limiting, physiologic mediator of proximal renal tubular phosphate reabsorption. Expression of sodium/phosphate cotransporter mRNA and protein is reduced in proximal renal tubular brush border membranes of *Hyp* mice with impaired renal tubular reabsorption of phosphate.[49]

The renal production of $1,25(OH)_2D$ is impaired in patients with hypophosphatemic osteomalacia. Serum values are inappropriately low for the degree of hypophosphatemia and respond poorly to administration of PTH.[50] The defect appears to be coupled to the abnormality in renal phosphate transport. Plasma $1,25(OH)_2D$ values vary directly with the renal tubular maximum of phosphate glomerular filtration rate (TmP/GFR) in patients with X-linked hypophosphatemia, normal individuals, and patients with other defects in phosphate transport, including tumor-induced osteomalacia (Fig. 63-2).[51] Although the renal production of $1,25(OH)_2D$ and the renal tubular reabsorption of phosphate probably are linked, treatment with $1,25(OH)_2D$ does not reverse the renal phosphate wasting, and normalization of the serum phosphate value does not enhance the renal production of $1,25(OH)_2D$. Interestingly, serum $1,25(OH)_2D$ and TmP/GFR are elevated in patients with tumoral calcinosis, a disease that appears to be the mirror image of X-linked hypophosphatemia and tumor-induced osteomalacia in which the renal tubular reabsorption of phosphate is abnormally increased.

Mutations in the *PEX* gene, a phosphate-regulating endopeptidase, have been shown to be the cause of X-linked phosphatemic rickets in patients and in the *Hyp* mouse.[52] It has been proposed that the *PEX* gene product acts to increase a phosphaturic factor, phosphatonin, that inhibits the renal tubular reabsorption of phosphate. Preliminary studies with cultured osteoblasts from normal and *Hyp* mice have shown that PEX and phosphatonin production are maturationally dependent and that aberrant degradation of phosphatonin by PEX may be involved in the pathogenesis of the disease.[53]

The treatment of hypophosphatemic osteomalacia is lifelong administration of phosphate and $1,25(OH)_2D$. The bone disease can be completely reversed with adequate therapy.[52] However, sometimes hypercalcemia and nephrocalcinosis are complications.

## TUMOR-INDUCED OSTEOMALACIA

In tumor-induced osteomalacia (oncogenous osteomalacia), renal phosphate wasting and osteomalacia occur in association with a variety of benign or malignant neoplasms and disappear

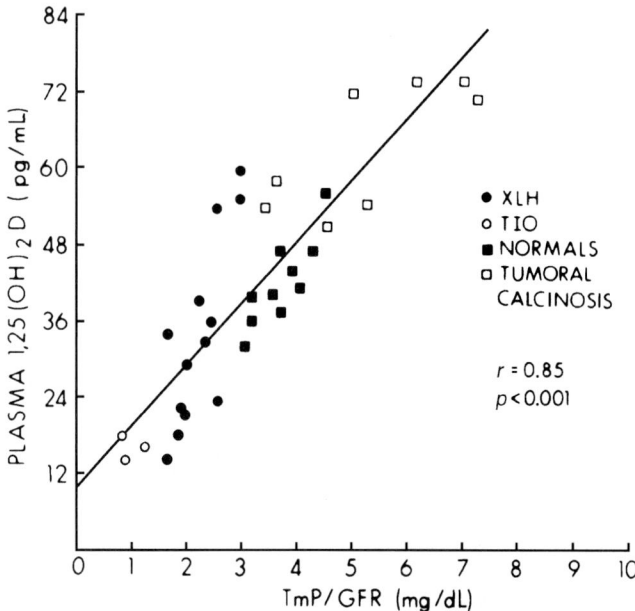

**FIGURE 63-2.** Relation between plasma 1,25 dihydroxyvitamin D [*1,25(OH)₂D*] and renal tubular maximum of phosphate glomerular filtration rate (*TmP/GFR*) in normal subjects and in patients with hypophosphatemic rickets (*XLH*), tumor-induced osteomalacia (*TIO*), and tumoral calcinosis. Note that values tend to be low in XLH and TIO, and high in tumoral calcinosis. Also note the highly significant positive correlation between plasma 1,25(OH)₂D and renal TmP/GFR. These results point to the possibility that renal tubular reabsorption of phosphate may be a major determinant of the renal production of 1,25(OH)₂D. (From Drezner MK. Understanding the pathogenesis of X-linked hypophosphatemic rickets: a requisite for successful therapy. In: Zackson DA, ed. A CPC series: cases in metabolic bone disease. New York: Triclinica Publishing, 1987:1.)

with removal or irradiation of the tumors.[54] Lesions responsible for the disease often are of mesenchymal origin, are vascular, show foci of new bone formation, and include sarcomas, hemangiomas, and giant cell tumors of bone as well as carcinoma of the breast and prostate. Osteomalacia associated with fibrous dysplasia of bone, neurofibromatosis,[55] and linear nevus sebaceous syndrome may be associated with tumors as well.[54] The clinical and biochemical features are typical of osteomalacia; patients often have generalized muscle weakness and bone pain. Serum calcium values usually are normal to slightly reduced, serum phosphate values are low, and serum alkaline phosphatase and urinary calcium values are elevated. Serum $1,25(OH)_2D$ values and calcium absorption may be low, and contribute to the pathogenesis of the bone disease.

The hypophosphatemia probably results from one or more factors produced by the tumors that alter the renal tubular reabsorption of phosphate in the proximal tubule and interfere with the renal production of $1,25(OH)_2D$.[55a] Evidence for this is the demonstration of phosphaturic activity in tumor extracts, the occurrence of renal phosphate wasting and diminished 25(OH)D–1α-hydroxylase activity in tumor-bearing athymic nude mice, and reduced activity of the enzyme in kidney cell cultures exposed to extracts of tumors.[52,54] The pathophysiology of the disease may be similar to that of X-linked hypophosphatemic osteomalacia.[54] Increased expression of normal *PEX* mRNA and protein were found in tumors of two patients with tumor-induced osteomalacia.[56] Thus, mutations of the *PEX* gene did not account for the disease in these two patients. These findings illustrate the complexity of the relationship between *PEX* and hypophosphatemia.

Treatment of tumor-induced osteomalacia is resection or irradiation of the lesion. If this is not possible, treatment with phosphate and $1,25(OH)_2D$ may be used (see Chap. 219).

## HEREDITARY HYPOPHOSPHATEMIC RICKETS WITH HYPERCALCIURIA

Hereditary hypophosphatemic rickets with hypercalciuria is a rare autosomal recessive disorder characterized by hypophosphatemic rickets, increased serum $1,25(OH)_2D$, normocalcemia, suppression of serum PTH and urinary cyclic adenosine 3',5'-monophosphate, and hypercalciuria.[57] Onset occurs during infancy and childhood. Clinical findings include muscle weakness, short stature, disproportionately short lower limbs, genu varum or valgum, anterior external bowing of the femur, coxa vara, radiologic signs of rickets, and diminished bone density. Relatives with mild hypophosphatemia and no bone disease are considered to have a milder form of the disease.[58]

The disorder is attributed to a primary defect in the renal tubular reabsorption of phosphate that results in hypophosphatemia and stimulation of renal $25(OH)D–1\alpha$-hydroxylase, increases in serum $1,25(OH)_2D$, intestinal absorption of calcium, inhibition of secretion of PTH, and hypercalciuria.

## VITAMIN D–DEPENDENT RICKETS TYPE II

Vitamin D–dependent rickets type II results from resistance of target organs to $1,25(OH)_2D$[59,60] and is usually caused by mutations of the vitamin D receptor. The development of the bone disease can occur at any time from infancy to adolescence. It is rare, and the occurrence is sporadic or familial. Sometimes it results from a consanguineous marriage and is transmitted as an autosomal recessive trait. Infants with the familial disease may have permanent alopecia, which usually is a sign of increased severity. In these patients, serum $1,25(OH)_2D$ values may be as high as 700 pg/mL. Studies of cultured skin fibroblasts from patients with the disorder demonstrate a wide variety of abnormalities in the uptake and nuclear binding of $^3$H-labeled $1,25(OH)_2D$. These findings indicate considerable genetic heterogeneity in the disorder.[60]

Five different types of intracellular defects have been identified: (a) hormone-binding negative, (b) defect in hormone-binding capacity, (c) defect in hormone-binding affinity, (d) deficient nuclear localization, and (e) normal or near-normal binding of $1,25(OH)_2D$ to the vitamin D receptor but diminished binding of the hormone receptor to DNA.[60] As noted later, subsequent studies indicate that the heterogeneity is caused by genetic mutations at different sites of the vitamin D receptor.[61,62]

The $1,25(OH)_2D$ binds to specific intracellular receptors in target cells, and the receptor–hormone complex acts in *trans* by binding to specific *cis*-acting DNA sequences in the promoter region of hormone-responsive genes to modulate transcription. The gene for the human vitamin D receptor has been cloned and sequenced.[63] The receptor consists of a hydrophilic DNA-binding domain that includes two "zinc fingers," a hinge, and a hydrophobic hormone-binding domain. As shown in Figure 63-3, 19 sites of mutations in the receptor have been described to date: nine in the DNA-binding domain, nine in the hormone-binding domain, and one in the hinge region. Single-point mutations at sites 30, 33, 35, 70, and 73 that include one of the two zinc fingers, or at sites 44, 45, 46, 50, and 80 lying between or near the two zinc fingers in the DNA-binding domain, result in a vitamin D receptor of normal size with normal binding to $1,25(OH)_2D$ and diminished binding of the $1,25(OH)_2D$ receptor complex to DNA (type V). Stop codons

at sites 30, 73, 152, 259, and 295 result in a truncated vitamin D receptor that is unable to bind $1,25(OH)_2D$ or promote gene expression (type I). Finally, vitamin D–dependent rickets type II can occur in patients with a normal vitamin D receptor, which has been found to be caused by inadequate calcium intake.[64,64a]

In general, patients with type III (deficient affinity) and type IV (deficient nuclear localization) defects respond to high doses of vitamin D or its metabolites with complete remission, whereas patients with the type II (low-capacity) defect and most patients with type I (receptor-negative) and type V (receptor-positive) defects respond either poorly or not at all to such treatment.[60] However, these patients can be treated with prolonged administration of intravenous calcium.[65]

## ANTICONVULSANT-INDUCED OSTEOMALACIA

Osteomalacia occasionally occurs in patients with epilepsy who are receiving anticonvulsant therapy, especially phenobarbital and phenytoin.[66,67] Other anticonvulsants also are implicated.[67a] Whereas the incidence of bone disease is low, hypocalcemia, diminished intestinal absorption of calcium, and increased serum alkaline phosphatase are more common. The clinical spectrum ranges from patients with reduced bone mass who have no symptoms to patients with hypocalcemia, clinically apparent bone disease, fractures, and pseudofractures. The administration of more than one anticonvulsant drug increases the incidence of bone disease.

Anticonvulsant drugs alter vitamin D metabolism. This alteration includes increased hepatic conversion of vitamin D to $25(OH)D$ and increased hepatic conversion of vitamin D and $25(OH)D$ to more polar biologically inactive metabolites.[68] As a consequence, serum $25(OH)D$ values are reduced. Serum $1,25(OH)_2D$ values are normal; however, the bone disease may not be caused by abnormal vitamin D metabolism. In animals, phenytoin inhibits the intestinal absorption of calcium, and both phenytoin and phenobarbital inhibit the mobilization of calcium from bone in vitro. Thus, the drugs may cause bone disease by blocking the actions of $1,25(OH)_2D$ in target organs.

The administration of vitamin D corrects and prevents the biochemical and radiographic abnormalities of osteomalacia and decreases the incidence of fractures.[69]

## RENAL TUBULAR ACIDOSIS

Osteomalacia occurs in renal tubular acidosis[70] and in the acidosis that occurs after ureterosigmoidoscopy.[71] Chronic acidosis may cause bone disease by decreasing the conversion of amorphous calcium phosphate to hydroxyapatite at the mineralization front and by causing renal phosphate wasting. Systemic acidosis enhances the dissolution of bone and results in hypercalciuria.[11] Acidosis enhances the response of bone to PTH in vitro and may contribute to skeletal loss of calcium. In humans, systemic acidosis does not compromise the metabolism of vitamin D, that is, the renal production of $1,25(OH)_2D$.

In patients with renal tubular acidosis and osteomalacia, serum calcium values are normal, serum phosphate values are normal or reduced, and serum alkaline phosphatase values are elevated. Because of hypercalciuria, nephrocalcinosis and renal lithiasis occur. Some patients have salt wasting, so that second-

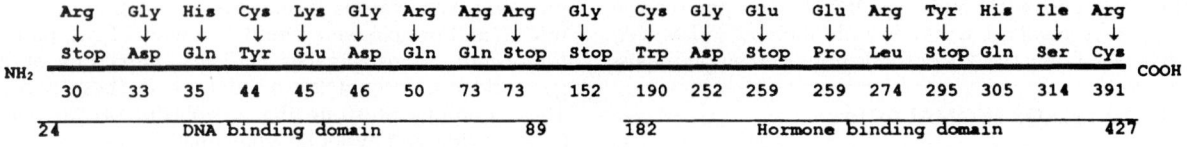

| | Arg | Gly | His | Cys | Lys | Gly | Arg | Arg | Arg | Gly | Cys | Gly | Glu | Glu | Arg | Tyr | His | Ile | Arg | |
|---|---|---|---|---|---|---|---|---|---|---|---|---|---|---|---|---|---|---|---|---|
| | ↓ | ↓ | ↓ | ↓ | ↓ | ↓ | ↓ | ↓ | ↓ | ↓ | ↓ | ↓ | ↓ | ↓ | ↓ | ↓ | ↓ | ↓ | ↓ | |
| | Stop | Asp | Gln | Tyr | Glu | Asp | Gln | Gln | Stop | Stop | Trp | Asp | Stop | Pro | Leu | Stop | Gln | Ser | Cys | |
| NH₂ | | | | | | | | | | | | | | | | | | | | COOH |
| | 30 | 33 | 35 | 44 | 45 | 46 | 50 | 73 | 73 | 152 | 190 | 252 | 259 | 259 | 274 | 295 | 305 | 314 | 391 | |

| 24 | DNA binding domain | 89 | 182 | Hormone binding domain | 427 |
|---|---|---|---|---|---|

**FIGURE 63-3.** Sites of mutations reported for the vitamin D receptor gene in patients with vitamin D–dependent rickets type II.

ary aldosteronism and hypokalemia develop. Under these circumstances, muscle weakness is profound, and an erroneous diagnosis of poliomyelitis may be made.

Osteomalacia from chronic acidosis can be treated successfully with bicarbonate.[70] Patients with hypokalemia can be treated with potassium. Vitamin D and calcium may be given at the outset to hasten healing of the bone disease but usually are not required for long-term treatment.

## MINERALIZATION DEFECTS

Bisphosphonates are compounds that have the structure P-C-P and are analogs of pyrophosphate P-O-P. The drugs are taken up selectively by skeletal tissue. In the case of etidronate, when it is administered in high doses, it may inhibit mineralization, causing osteomalacia.[72,73]

Aluminum has been implicated in the development of the osteomalacia and fractures that occur in patients who are receiving total parenteral nutrition and amino acids in the form of casein hydrolysate.[74] Aluminum occurs in high concentrations in casein hydrolysate and also in the osseous tissue of these patients. In patients who have osteomalacia while receiving treatment with total parenteral nutrition, serum iPTH values are either abnormally low or in the lower range of normal, and the rate of bone formation is reduced. The pathogenesis apparently is similar to that of the aluminum-related osteomalacia that occurs in patients with chronic renal failure. The bone disease improves when the use of aluminum-containing preparations is avoided in patients who are receiving total parenteral nutrition.[75]

## HYPOPHOSPHATASIA

Hypophosphatasia is a rare disease characterized by abnormally low alkaline phosphatase values in the serum and skeleton, abnormal mineralization of the skeleton with rickets and osteomalacia, increased phosphoethanolamine and pyrophosphate values in the blood and urine, and premature loss of deciduous teeth. It is transmitted as an autosomal recessive trait and is prevalent in inbred populations. The disorder is usually caused by missense mutations of the tissue nonspecific alkaline phosphatase gene, particularly in severe forms of the disease.[76] Mutations that have been reported are outlined in Figure 63-4. Many patients are compound heterozygotes and inherit one or more mutations from each parent. Mutations occur along almost the entire length of the alkaline phosphatase gene.

Three types of hypophosphatasia occur: *infantile, childhood,* and *adult.*[77] Whereas in most patients the disorder is diagnosed in infancy or childhood, in others it is not recognized until adulthood. Neonatal or infantile hypophosphatasia is most common, and the diagnosis is evident before the age of 6 months and sometimes even in utero. Impaired mineralization of the skeleton, increased intracranial pressure, hypercalcemia, hypercalciuria, and nephrocalcinosis generally are present. The skeletal disease is so severe that <50% of infants survive.

Childhood hypophosphatasia is associated with premature loss of deciduous teeth, increased susceptibility to infection, and retarded growth. A generalized deossification with a coarse trabecular pattern is present on radiographs, together with bowing deformities and fractures. Craniosynostosis is common. Irregu-

lar epiphyses and islands of radiolucency are present in the shafts of bones. Spontaneous healing usually occurs.

Adult hypophosphatasia is rare, and patients may have fractures that are delayed in healing. They also may have histories of rickets and loss of deciduous teeth in childhood, and loss of density of the skeleton. Radiographs show a coarse trabecular pattern, Looser zones and subperiosteal bone formation.

The diagnosis is established by the findings of low serum alkaline phosphatase values and elevated serum and urine phosphoethanolamine values.

No effective treatment exists. Vitamin D administration produces improvement in some patients, but the treatment may cause vitamin D intoxication. Treatment with phosphate improves mineralization of the skeleton in some instances when given in daily doses of 1.25 to 3.0 g as neutral phosphate.

## TREATMENT

In patients with osteomalacia, the goals of treatment are (a) to correct hypocalcemia and the related symptoms and to prevent the consequences of hypocalcemia, including seizures and cataracts; (b) to correct and prevent skeletal deformities and changes resulting from secondary hyperparathyroidism; and (c) to prevent hypercalcemia, hypercalciuria, and renal complications, including stone formation, nephrocalcinosis, and renal damage.

Vitamin $D_2$ and several of its derivatives are available in the United States. Vitamin D is marketed in 50,000-IU (1.25-mg) capsules for oral administration, in sesame oil (500,000 IU or 12.5 mg/mL) for injection, and in propylene glycol (250 IU or 6.25 µg/drop; 8000 IU/mL) for oral administration. The advantages of vitamin D are that the cost is modest and it often is effective even in patients with abnormal vitamin D metabolism. The disadvantages of vitamin D are that several weeks may be required before optimal therapeutic effectiveness is achieved, the therapeutic dose is near the toxic dose, and the bioactivity persists after its administration is discontinued.

The metabolite $25(OH)D_3$ is available in capsules of 20 and 50 µg. The drug may be particularly useful in patients with hepatic disease and impaired synthesis of $25(OH)D_3$. Its onset of action is more rapid than that of vitamin D, and it has similar disadvantages. However, the half-life of $25(OH)D_3$, 2 to 3 weeks, may be shorter than that of vitamin $D_2$, which is stored in fat, so that the biologic effects after cessation of administration may not be as long-lasting as those of vitamin $D_2$.

The metabolite $1,25(OH)_2D_3$ is marketed as capsules of 0.25 and 0.50 µg. The advantages of the drug are its rapid onset of action and rapid disappearance of its biologic effects after discontinuation. Its half-life is <6 hours. One disadvantage is that hypercalcemia may occur after long-term treatment during which the abnormal calcium metabolism has been stabilized.[78] The hypercalcemia can be treated by discontinuing administration of the drug and is prevented by decreasing the dose. Hypercalcemia occurs fairly frequently, so patients must be followed up closely. Treatment with $1,25(OH)_2D_3$ is most useful in diseases in which its synthesis by the kidney is impaired. Sometimes it is of value in disorders that have resistance to its effects at the cellular level. In these cases, higher doses are required.

| NH$_2$ | Ala | Arg | Arg | Gln | Tyr | Ala | Asp | Asp | Arg | Arg | Tyr | Ala | Glu | Gln | None | Asp | Asp | Tyr | |
|---|---|---|---|---|---|---|---|---|---|---|---|---|---|---|---|---|---|---|---|
| | Val | Cys | Pro | Pro | His | Val | Ala | Val | Cys | Pro | His | Thr | Lys | Pro | | Ala | Val | His | COOH |
| | 16 | 54 | 174 | 190 | 246 | 274 | 277 | 361 | 387 | 388 | 419 | 711 | 747 | 796 | 1052 | 1057 | 1309 | 1482 | |

**FIGURE 63-4.** Mutations of tissue nonspecific alkaline phosphate that account for abnormal bone and mineral metabolim in hypophosphatasia.

Dihydrotachysterol is available as tablets of 0.125, 0.2, and 0.4 mg. The drug has a rapid onset of action and a relatively short duration of biologic action after cessation of administration. The 180-degree rotation of the A ring permits the hydroxyl group in the 3 position to act as a pseudohydroxyl group. The drug becomes bioactive after it undergoes 25-hydroxylation in the liver. Because it does not need to be hydroxylated in the 1α position, dihydrotachysterol is of potential value in treating the same diseases for which $1,25(OH)_2D_3$ is used.

Calcium supplements should be administered in divided doses, because calcium absorption is abnormally low in most patients with osteomalacia. The administration of calcium decreases the amount of vitamin D or its analogs that is required for treatment. The content of elemental calcium varies among preparations, so the amount that provides 1 g of elemental calcium also varies (calcium carbonate = 40% elemental calcium; calcium chloride = 36%; calcium lactate = 13%; and calcium gluconate = 9%). From 1 to 2 g per day of elemental calcium should be administered to adults in divided doses. The dosage should be modified depending on the severity of disease.

Deficiency of vitamin D is treated by the administration of 5000 IU (125 μg) to 10,000 IU (250 μg) per day of vitamin $D_2$ until healing of the bone disease occurs. The dosage then is decreased to 400 IU (10 μg) per day, the recommended daily requirement. Larger doses of 50,000 to 100,000 IU (1250 to 2500 μg) per day may be required in patients with gastrointestinal or hepatic disease. Treatment with $25(OH)D_3$ is indicated when the hepatic vitamin D-25-hydroxylase is markedly impaired.

Vitamin $D_2$, 50,000 to 100,000 IU (1250 to 2500 μg) per day or more, is often effective in treating osteomalacia resulting from diseases that are associated with renal insufficiency, hypoparathyroidism, and pseudohypoparathyroidism, but it may not be effective in the treatment of bone disease associated with vitamin D–dependent rickets type I, hypophosphatemic rickets, and tumor-induced osteomalacia. In these disorders, $1,25(OH)_2D_3$, 0.5 to 3.0 μg per day, usually is effective. The requirements of vitamin D, $25(OH)D_3$, and $1,25(OH)_2D_3$ vary from patient to patient, so that the dosage for a given individual must be determined by trial and error. Phosphate supplements, 2 to 4 g per day in divided oral doses, are essential for the treatment of hypophosphatemic rickets to heal the bone disease, along with as much as 4 μg per day of $1,25(OH)_2D_3$. Lifelong treatment is required. Removal or irradiation of the tumor is necessary to treat tumor-induced osteomalacia.

Sometimes osteomalacia associated with vitamin D–dependent rickets type II responds to treatment with vitamin D.[60] However, in instances of a more profound target-organ defect, administration of $1,25(OH)_2D_3$ is necessary. Dosages as high as 15 to 20 μg per day may be required, and even these may not be effective. Under these circumstances, long-term parenteral administration of calcium can be used to heal the bone disease.[65]

Osteomalacia associated with renal tubular acidosis is treated initially with 5000 to 10,000 IU (125 to 250 μg) per day of vitamin $D_3$. The acidosis is corrected by treatment with sodium bicarbonate. Once the bone disease heals, however, vitamin D is not required.

Sometimes hypercalcemia and hypercalciuria occur during treatment with vitamin D and its metabolites. Patients may have no symptoms, or they may have anorexia, nausea, vomiting, weight loss, headache, constipation, polyuria, polydipsia, and altered mental status. The abnormal calcium metabolism is characterized by increased intestinal absorption and enhanced release of calcium from skeletal tissue. A decline in renal function, nephrocalcinosis, nephrolithiasis, urinary tract infections, and even death may ensue. Patients who are receiving long-term treatment with vitamin D and its analogs require careful follow-up at intervals of 4 to 6 weeks with measurement of serum and urinary calcium and serum creatinine. Careful evaluation of patients is important, because no means exist to predict when or in whom vitamin D intoxication will develop (see Chap. 59). The most effective means of treating these side effects and complica-

tions is prevention. When intoxication does occur, administration of the drug and of calcium supplements should be discontinued, and fluids, 3 to 4 L per day, should be given. When intoxication is severe, the use of prednisone or salmon calcitonin may be necessary. The dosage of either vitamin D or its derivatives should be reduced, or another drug should be substituted.

# REFERENCES

1. Frost HM. Tetracycline-based histological analysis of bone remodeling. Calcif Tissue Res 1969; 3:211.
2. Frame B, Parfitt AM. Osteomalacia: current concepts. Ann Intern Med 1978; 89:966.
3. Lee WR. Bone formation in Paget's disease. A quantitative microscopic study using tetracycline markers. J Bone Joint Surg 1967; 49B:146.
4. Parfitt AM. The physiologic and clinical significance of bone histomorphometric data. In: Recker RR, ed. Bone histomorphometry: techniques and interpretation. Boca Raton, FL: CRC Press, 1983:143.
5. Schott GD, Wills MR. Muscle weakness in osteomalacia. Lancet 1976; 1:626.
6. Prineas JW, Stuart AM, Henson RA. Myopathy in metabolic bone disease. BMJ 1965; 1:1034.
7. Mallette LE, Patten BM, King WE. Neuromuscular disease in secondary hyperparathyroidism. Ann Intern Med 1975; 82:474.
8. Steinbach HL, Kolb FO, Crane JT. Unusual roentgen manifestations of osteomalacia. AJR Am J Roentgenol 1959; 82:875.
9. Steinbach HL, Noetzli M. Roentgen appearance of the skeleton in osteomalacia and rickets. AJR Am J Roentgenol 1964; 91:955.
10. Milkman LA. Multiple spontaneous idiopathic symmetrical fractures. AJR Am J Roentgenol 1934; 32:622.
11. Albright F, Reifenstein EC Jr. The parathyroid glands and metabolic bone disease. Baltimore: Williams & Wilkins, 1948:1.
12. Goldring SR, Krane SM. Disorders of calcification: osteomalacia and rickets. In: DeGroot LJ, ed. Endocrinology. New York: Grune & Stratton, 1979; 2:853.
13. Park EA. The Blackader lecture on some aspects of rickets. Can Med Assoc J 1932; 26:3.
14. Wahner HA. Single- and dual-photon absorptiometry in osteoporosis and osteomalacia. Semin Nucl Med 1987; 27:305.
15. Fogelman I, McKillop JA, Bessent RG, et al. The role of bone scanning in osteomalacia. J Nucl Med 1978; 19:245.
16. Stamp TCB, Exton-Smith AN, Richens A. Classical rickets and osteomalacia in Britain. Lancet 1976; 2:308.
17. Holmes AM, Enoch BA, Taylor JL, Jones ME. Occult rickets and osteomalacia amongst the Asian immigrant population. QJM 1973; 42:125.
18. Pietrek J, Preece MA, Windo J, et al. Prevention of vitamin-D deficiency in Asians. Lancet 1976; 1:1145.
19. Eastwood MA, Girdwood RH. Lignin: a bile-salt sequestrating agent. Lancet 1968; 2:1170.
20. Mitra D, Bell NH. Racial, geographic, genetic, and body habitus effects on vitamin D metabolism. In: Feldman D, Glorieux FH, Pike JW, eds. Vitamin D. San Diego: Academic Press, 1997:521.
21. Awumey EMK, Mitra DA, Hollis BW, et al. Vitamin D metabolism is altered in Asian Indians in the Southern United States: a Clinical Research Center study. J Clin Endocrinol Metab 1998; 83:169.
22. MacLaughlin J, Holick MF. Aging decreases the capacity of human skin to produce vitamin $D_3$. J Clin Invest 1985; 76:1536.
23. Gallagher JC, Riggs BL, Esiman JA, et al. Intestinal calcium absorption and serum vitamin D metabolites in normal subjects and osteoporotic patients. J Clin Invest 1979; 64:729.
24. Casella SJ, Reiner BJ, Chen TC, et al. A possible genetic defect in 25-hydroxylation as a cause of rickets. J Pediatr 1994; 124:929.
25. Walter Nützenadel W, Mehis O, Klaus G. A new defect in vitamin D metabolism. J Pediatr 1995; 126:76.
26. Coburn JW, Brickman AS, Hartenblower DL. Clinical disorders. In: Norman AW, Schaeffer P, eds. Vitamin D and problems related to uremic bone disease. New York: de Gruyter, 1975:219.
27. Parfitt AM, Podenphant J, Villanueva AR, Frame B. Metabolic bone disease with and without osteomalacia after intestinal bypass surgery. Bone 1985; 6:211.
28. Eddy RL. Metabolic bone disease after gastrectomy. Am J Med 1971; 50:442.
29. Compston JE. Hepatic osteodystrophy: vitamin D metabolism in patients with liver disease. Gut 1986; 27:1073.
30. Epstein S, Meunier PJ, Lambert PW, et al. 1α,25-Dihydroxyvitamin $D_3$ corrects osteomalacia in hypoparathyroidism and pseudohypoparathyroidism. Acta Endocrinol (Copenh) 1983; 103:241.
31. Chase LR, Melson GL, Aurbach GD. Pseudohypoparathyroidism: defective excretion of 3',5'cAMP in response to parathyroid hormone. J Clin Invest 1969; 48:1832.
32. Levine MA, Downs RW Jr, Moses AM, et al. Resistance to multiple hormones in patients with pseudohypoparathyroidism: association with deficient activity of guanine nucleotide regulating protein. Am J Med 1983; 74:545.
33. Haussler MR, Baylink DJ, Hughes MR, et al. The assay of 1α,25-dihydroxyvitamin $D_3$: physiologic and pathologic modulation of circulating hormone levels. Clin Endocrinol (Oxf) 1976; 5:151S.
34. Coburn JW, Sherrard DJ, Ott SM, et al. Bone disease in uremia: a reap-

praisal. In: Norman AW, Schaefer K, Herrath DV, Grigoleit H-G, eds. Vitamin D: chemical, biochemical and clinical endocrinology of calcium metabolism. New York: de Gruyter, 1982:835.

35. Ravid M, Robson M. Proximal myopathy caused by iatrogenic depletion. JAMA 1976; 236:1380.
36. Pierdes AM, Ellis HA, Kerr DNS. Phosphate-deficiency during regular haemodialysis. Lancet 1976; 2:746.
37. Moorhead JF, Wills MR, Ahmet KY, et al. Hypophosphataemic osteomalacia after cadaveric renal transplantation. Lancet 1974; 1:694.
38. Hodsman AB, Sherrard DJ, Alfrey AC, et al. Bone aluminum and histomorphometric features of renal osteodystrophy. J Clin Endocrinol Metab 1982; 54:539.
39. Brown DJ, Dawborn JK, Ham KN, Xipell JM. Treatment of dialysis osteomalacia with desferrioxamine. Lancet 1982; 2:343.
40. Fraser D, Kooh SW, Kind HP, et al. Pathogenesis of hereditary vitamin D-dependent rickets (an inborn error of vitamin D metabolism involving defective conversion of 25-hydroxyvitamin D to 1,25-dihydroxyvitamin D). N Engl J Med 1973; 289:817.
41. Scriver CR, Reade TM, DeLuca HF, Hamstra AJ. Serum 1,25-dihydroxyvitamin D levels in normal subjects and in patients with hereditary rickets or bone disease. N Engl J Med 1978; 299:976.
42. Fu GK, Lin D, Ahang MYH, et al. Cloning of human 25-hydrovitamin D–1α-hydroxylase and mutations causing vitamin D–dependent rickets type I. Mol Endocrinol 1997; 11:1961.
43. Wang JT, Lin C-J, Burridge SM, et al. Genetics of vitamin D 1α-hydroxylase deficiency in 17 families. Am J Hum Genet 1998; 63:1694.
44. Graham JB, McFalls VW, Winters RW. Familial hypophosphatemia with vitamin D resistant rickets. III. Three additional kindreds of sex-linked dominant type with a genetic analysis of four such families. Am J Hum Genet 1959; 11:311.
45. Lobaugh B, Burch WM Jr, Drezner MK. Abnormalities of vitamin D metabolism and action in the vitamin D resistant rachitic and osteomalacic diseases. In: Kumar R, ed. Vitamin D basic and clinical aspects. Boston: Martinus Nijhoff, 1984:665.
46. Glorieux FH, Scriver CR. Loss of a parathyroid hormone-sensitive component of phosphate transport in X-linked hypophosphatemia. Science 1972; 175:997.
47. Short EM, Binder HJ, Rosenberg LE. Familial hypophosphatemic rickets: defective transport of inorganic phosphate by intestinal mucosa. Science 1973; 179:700.
47a. Miyamoto J, Koto S, Hasegawa Y. Final height of Japanese patients with x-linked hypophosphatemic rickets: effect of vitamin D and phosphate therapy. Endocr J 2000; 47:163.
48. Nesbitt T, Coffman TM, Griffiths R, Drezner MK. Crosstransplantation of kidneys in normal and *Hyp* mice: evidence that the *Hyp* mouse phenotype is unrelated to an intrinsic renal defect. J Clin Invest 1992; 89:1453.
49. Collins JF, Scheving LA, Ghishan FK. Decreased transcription of the sodium-phosphate transporter gene in the hypophosphatemic mouse. Am J Physiol 1995; 269:F439.
50. Lyles KW, Drezner MK. Parathyroid hormone effects on serum 1,25-dihydroxy-vitamin D levels in patients with X-linked hypophosphatemic rickets: evidence for abnormal 25-hydroxyvitamin D-1-hydroxylase activity. J Clin Endocrinol Metab 1982; 54:638.
51. Drezner MK. Understanding the pathogenesis of X-linked hypophosphatemic rickets: a requisite for successful therapy. In: Zackson DA, ed. A CPC series: cases in metabolic bone disease. New York: Triclinica Publications, 1987:1.
52. Drezner MK. Clinical disorders of phosphate homeostasis. In: Feldman D, Glorieux FH, Pike JW, eds. Vitamin D. San Diego: Academic Press, 1997:733.
53. Nesbitt T, Hamrick JL, Quarles LD, Drezner MK. Coordinated developmental regulation of PEX and phosphatonin: evidence for the pathophysiological role of PEX in XLH. J Bone Miner Res 1997; 12:S113.
54. Drezner MK. Tumor associated rickets and osteomalacia. In: Favus M, Christakos S, Gagel RF, et al., eds. Primer on the metabolic bone diseases and disorders of mineral metabolism, 3rd ed. Philadelphia: Lippincott–Raven Publishers, 1996:319.
55. Konishi K, Nakamura M, Yamakawa H, et al. Case report: hypophosphatemic osteomalacia in von Recklinghausen neurofibromatosis. Am J Med Sci 1991; 301:322.
55a. Kumar R. Tumor-induced osteomalacia and the regulation of phosphate homeostasis. Bone 2000; 27:333.
56. Panda D, Lipman ML, Henderson JE, et al. Cloning of human PEX cDNA from tumors causing hypophosphatemic osteomalacia. J Bone Miner Res 1997; 12:S113.
57. Tieder M, Modai D, Samuel R, et al. Hereditary hypophosphatemic rickets with hypercalciuria. N Engl J Med 1985; 312:611.
58. Tieder M, Modai D, Shaked U, et al. "Idiopathic" hypercalciuria and hereditary hypophosphatemic rickets; two phenotypical expressions of a common genetic defect. N Engl J Med 1987; 316:125.
59. Brooks MH, Bell NH, Love L, Stern PH, et al. Vitamin D–dependent rickets type II: resistance of target organs to 1,25-dihydroxyvitamin D. N Engl J Med 1978; 298:996.
60. Liberman UA, Marx SJ. Vitamin D dependent rickets. In: Favus M, Christakos S, Gagel RF, et al., eds. Primer on the metabolic bone diseases and disorders of mineral metabolism, 2nd ed. New York: Raven Press, 1993; 274.
61. Whitfield GK, Selznick SH, Haussler CA, et al. Vitamin D receptors from patients with resistance to 1,25-dihydroxyvitamin $D_3$: point mutations confer reduced transactivation in response to ligand and impaired interaction with the retinoid X receptor heterodimeric partner. Mol Endocrinol 1996; 10:1617.
62. Malloy PJ, Pike JW, Feldman D. Hereditary 1,25-dihydroxyvitamin D resistant rickets. In Feldman D, Glorieux D, Pike JW, eds. Vitamin D. San Diego: Academic Press, 1997:765.
63. Baker AR, McDonnell DP, Hughes M, et al. Cloning and expression of full-length cDNA encoding human vitamin D receptor. Proc Natl Acad Sci U S A 1988; 85:3294.
64. Giraldo A, Pino W, Garcia-Ramirez LF, et al. Vitamin D dependent rickets type II and normal vitamin D receptor cDNA sequence. A cluster in a rural area of Cauca, Colombia, with more than 200 affected children. Clin Gen 1995; 48:57.
64a. Sierra OL, Alarcon Y, Penaloza LN, et al. Fractional intestinal calcium absorption in children with rickets and controls from Cauca, Columbia. J Bone Miner Res 2000; Su105(abstract).
65. Balsan S, Barabédian M, Larchet M, et al. Long-term nocturnal calcium infusions can cure rickets and promote normal mineralization in hereditary resistance to 1,25-dihydroxyvitamin D. J Clin Invest 1986; 77:1661.
66. Sotaniemi EA, Hakkarainen HK, Puranen JA, Lahti RO. Radiologic bone changes and hypocalcemia with anticonvulsant therapy in epilepsy. Ann Intern Med 1972; 77:389.
67. Winnacker JL, Yeager H, Saunders JA, et al. Rickets in children receiving anticonvulsant drugs. Am J Dis Child 1977; 131:286.
67a. Karaaslan Y, Haznedaroglu S, Ozturk M. Osteomalacia associated with carbamazepine/valproate. Ann Pharmacother 2000; 34:264.
68. Hahn JT. Drug-induced disorders of vitamin D and mineral metabolism. Clin Endocrinol Metab 1980; 9:107.
69. Sherk HH, Cruz M, Stambaugh J. Vitamin D prophylaxis and the lowered incidence of fractures in anticonvulsant rickets and osteomalacia. Clin Orthop Rel Res 1977; 129:251.
70. Richards P, Chamberlain MJ, Wrong OM. Treatment of osteomalacia of renal tubular acidosis by sodium bicarbonate alone. Lancet 1972; 2:994.
71. Cunningham J, Fraher LJ, Clemens TL, et al. Chronic acidosis with metabolic bone disease. Am J Med 1982; 73:199.
72. Russell RGG, Smith R, Preston C, et al. Diphosphonates in Paget's disease. Lancet 1974; 1:894.
73. Khairi MRA, Altman RD, DeRosa GP, et al. Sodium etidronate in the treatment of Paget's disease of bone. Ann Intern Med 1977; 87:656.
74. Ott SM, Maloney NA, Klein GL, et al. Aluminum is associated with low bone formation in patients receiving chronic parenteral nutrition. Ann Intern Med 1983; 98:910.
75. Vargas JH, Klein GL, Ament ME, et al. Metabolic bone disease of total parenteral nutrition: course after changing from casein to amino acids in parenteral solutions with reduced aluminum content. Am J Clin Nutr 1988; 48:1070.
76. Henthorn PS, Raducha M, Fedde KN, et al. Different missense mutations at the tissue-nonspecific alkaline phosphatase gene locus in autosomal recessively inherited forms of mild and severe hypophosphatasia. Proc Natl Acad Sci U S A 1992; 89:9924.
77. Whyte MP. Hypophosphatasia. In: Scriver CR, Beaudet AL, Sly WS, Valle D, eds. The metabolic and molecular bases of inherited disease, 7th ed. New York: McGraw-Hill, 1995:4095.
78. Bell NH, Stern PH. Hypercalcemia and increases in serum hormone value during prolonged administration of 1α,25-dihydroxyvitamin D. N Engl J Med 1978; 298:1241.

# CHAPTER 64

# OSTEOPOROSIS

ROBERT LINDSAY AND FELICIA COSMAN

Osteoporosis, the most common bone disease in clinical practice, is a skeletal disorder characterized by a reduction in bone mass with accompanying microarchitectural damage that increases bone fragility and the risk of fracture.[1,2] Histologically, the cortices are thinned and porous, and the trabeculae are fewer, thinner, and less connected. Clinically the disease is important because of the fractures that occur as a consequence.

## EPIDEMIOLOGY

The incidence of osteoporosis increases with age. It becomes widely prevalent in the elderly, in whom it is a major public health problem, causing >1.3 million fractures annually and costing more than $13 billion per year in the United States.[1,3]

Peak bone mass occurs at ~18 to 30 years of age, after which bone is progressively lost. This phenomenon is seen in all populations, regardless of race, sex, economic development, or geographic location.[4] Fracture rates vary in different groups; they are

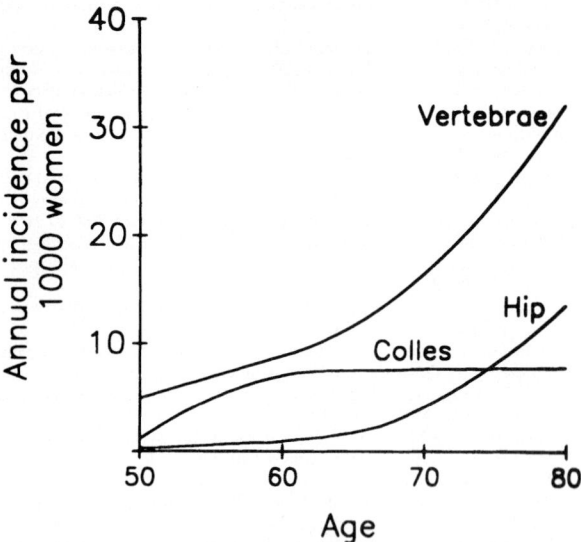

FIGURE 64-1. Incidence rates for vertebral, Colles, and hip fractures in women. (From Wasnich RD. In: Favus MJ, et al. Primer on the metabolic bone diseases and disorders of mineral metabolism. Philadelphia: Lippincott-Raven Publishers, 1996:249.)

higher in whites and Asians than in blacks, and usually are higher among women than among men. The incidence of limb fractures doubles approximately every 5 to 8 years after the fifth decade among women but does not increase substantially until after the seventh decade among men. The most common fracture sites are in the *thoracic* and *lumbar vertebral bodies* (i.e., crush or wedge fractures), the *neck* and *intertrochanteric regions of the femur* (i.e., hip fractures), and the *distal radius* (i.e., Colles fractures); however, in osteoporosis, fracture of any bone is possible (Fig. 64-1).

The prevalence of hip fractures in the United States reaches 15% by age 80 and exceeds 25% by age 90, with a female/male predominance of ~2:1 among whites.[4] In other populations, however, such as those of Singapore and Hong Kong, and the South African Bantu, the incidence of hip fractures in men may equal or exceed that in women.[5] Approximately 300,000 hip fractures occur in the United States every year. The incidence has been rising, with a 40% increase reported between 1970 and 1980. However, data suggest that this rise has plateaued.[6] The mortality rate associated with hip fracture and its complications is 12% to 20% within the first year, and a large proportion of patients are mildly or severely disabled permanently.[1,2]

The true prevalence of vertebral fracture is unknown because of the variable definitions of vertebral fracture and variable clinical expressions. More than 25% of all women older than 65 years of age may have sustained a crush fracture, many of which are asymptomatic. The female/male predominance of vertebral fracture is estimated to be between 2:1 and 8:1.[7,8]

Like hypertension, osteoporosis has many causes and pathogenetic mechanisms. The *primary* form of the disease is the most common and can be further classified into several types. *Secondary osteoporosis* is seen in many endocrine, genetic, and other illnesses (Table 64-1), but the most common form is that associated with the therapeutic use of corticosteroids.

## POSTMENOPAUSAL AND AGE-RELATED PRIMARY OSTEOPOROSIS

### PATHOPHYSIOLOGY AND ETIOLOGIC CONSIDERATIONS

More than 80% of osteoporosis cases occur among postmenopausal and aging populations. Although some differences in pathogenetic mechanisms have been described,[9,10] the overlap

**TABLE 64-1.**
**Classification of Osteoporosis**

I. PRIMARY OSTEOPOROSIS
  1. *Postmenopausal osteoporosis (type I)*
  2. *Age-related osteoporosis (type II)*
  3. *Juvenile osteoporosis*
  4. *Idiopathic osteoporosis (of young adults)*
  5. *Regional osteoporosis*
     A. Immobilization osteoporosis
     B. Reflex sympathetic dystrophy
     C. Transient osteoporosis of the hip
     D. Regional migratory osteoporosis
     E. Osteolysis syndromes
II. SECONDARY OSTEOPOROSIS
  1. *Endocrine etiology*
     A. Cushing syndrome
     B. Hypogonadism
     C. Hyperthyroidism
     D. Hyperparathyroidism
     E. Diabetes mellitus
     F. Acromegaly
     G. Hyperprolactinemia
  2. *Genetic diseases*
     A. Osteogenesis imperfecta
     B. Homocystinuria
     C. Ehlers-Danlos syndrome
     D. Marfan syndrome
     E. Menkes steely hair disease
     F. Riley-Day syndrome (familial dysautonomia)
     G. Gaucher disease and other glycogen storage diseases
     H. Sickle cell anemia
     I. Thalassemia
     J. Hypophosphatasia
  3. *Iatrogenic causes*
     A. Glucocorticoid therapy
     B. Heparin therapy
     C. Chemotherapy
     D. Thyroxine therapy
     E. Therapy with gonadotropin-releasing hormone agonists
     F. Anticonvulsant therapy
  4. *Miscellaneous*
     A. Alcohol abuse
     B. Multiple myeloma
     C. Gastrointestinal diseases
     D. Chronic liver disease
     E. Pregnancy-related osteoporosis
     F. Chronic obstructive pulmonary disease
     G. Rheumatoid arthritis
     H. Malnutrition
     I. Diffuse cancer
     J. Systemic mastocytosis
     K. Amyloidosis
     L. Hemochromatosis

between populations seen clinically is sufficient for them to be considered together. Fracture risk at any age is determined primarily by skeletal mass,[11,12] which depends on the *maximal mass achieved at maturity* and on the *subsequent rate and duration of bone loss*. Various interrelated factors are thought to control the two processes.[13] The frequency of falling and factors predisposing to falls are also determinants of fracture risk, particularly for limb fractures.[14] Thus, the frail elderly are more likely to sustain fractures than those who maintain their health, coordination, and strength. Reduced bone elasticity and decreased dissipation of force over bone by weaker and less coordinated muscle contractions also add to fracture risk. The presence of vertebral fractures has been found to be an independent predictor of further vertebral fracture risk,[15] and also increases the risk of fractures at other sites, notably the hip.[16] The occurrence of any fracture after the age of 40 doubles the risk of further osteoporotic fractures in later life.[17]

## DETERMINANTS OF MAXIMUM BONE MASS

Maximum bone mass is achieved some time after puberty (age 18–30) and is primarily determined genetically.[18,19] Race, gender, and body size are the principal genetic determinants; consequently, maximum bone mass probably is under polygenic control. The inequality between the sexes is probably not evident prepubertally,[20] but is clear after transition through puberty, with total bone mass becoming significantly greater among males.[21–23] The positive correlation between body size and bone mass is well established.[23] Bone density is also a function of skeletal size, because the usual two-dimensional techniques employed do not adequately correct for the size of the bone. Gender differences in true density are less than those in bone mass in young adults, and in some studies are found to be insignificant.[23] Racial differences in both mass and density are apparent in young adults, with black populations generally having a 5% to 10% greater bone mass.[24] In cross-sectional studies these racial differences are maintained with increased age, whereas gender differences become yet greater.

Investigations into the genetic control of bone mass and density have focused on several candidate genes that, by virtue of the known function of their products, have some biologic credibility.[19] Thus, investigators have evaluated polymorphisms in the vitamin D receptor; the estrogen receptor (ER-α); the gene for type I collagen, osteocalcin, and the interleukins; and receptors and receptor antagonists. Although all have provided some promising data, each contributes only a small amount to the variability seen in bone density or bone turnover.

Although multiple genetic factors clearly play an important role in determining peak bone mass, other influences are also important. Adequate nutrition, health, and exercise in childhood can modify the likelihood that any individual will reach his or her genetic potential.[25,26] Nutritional factors include not only calcium but calories and protein. Furthermore, a normal progression through puberty and the associated growth spurt as well as normal menstrual function are critical to adult skeletal health. Osteoporosis has been dubbed *a disease that presents in the geriatric population but often has its roots in the pediatric population*.

## DETERMINANTS AND PATHOGENESIS OF BONE LOSS

In women, bone loss begins between 20 to 30 years of age, at least in the hip. Bone mass may be more stable in the spine.[27] This premenopausal loss of bone in the hip may be related to marginal estrogen deficiency or decreased physical activity.[28] Bone loss in the spine probably does not occur until after the fifth decade of life and is more dependent on the decreasing production of estrogen as women approach the menopause.[28,29] Bone loss in the spine in men also may begin at this age but occurs at a slower rate and without the accelerated loss that is typically seen in menopausal women.

Net loss of bone may be a universal phenomenon with increasing age, at least in humans.[30] Whether such bone loss with increasing age occurs in other animal species is unclear. This is an important issue, because unique facets of human life may have consequences for skeletal health. The rate of bone loss is determined by endocrine, environmental, and various local factors, and probably also by genetic influences. Eskimos, for example, have rapid age-related bone loss and a high frequency of fracture.[31] Those traits probably have both environmental and genetic causes.

The adult skeleton undergoes a process of remodeling by which old bone is removed and replaced by new, young bone.[32] Before menopause, the bone that is removed is replaced by an equal amount of new bone tissue, and the frequency with which bone remodeling units are initiated is constant. With estrogen deficiency in women, and with increasing age in both sexes, changes occur in the remodeling process.[33] Across menopause, an increase is seen in the number of new bone remodeling units initiated per unit time. This creates a transient loss of bone mass. For continued loss to occur, however, an imbalance must exist between formation and resorption within each remodeling unit.[34] This can occur for one of several reasons: (a) more bone may be removed by more aggressive osteoclasts, (b) insufficient new bone may be laid down by new osteoblasts, (c) a combination of these two may occur, or (d) aggressive osteoclasts may penetrate trabeculae, removing the template on which new bone may be laid down. Variable combinations of these effects probably occur.

In postmenopausal women, the rate at which new remodeling sites are initiated increases. The suggestion has been made that the osteoclast population is hyperactive, leading to excessive bone resorption.[35] A combination of these effects results in a net bone loss within each remodeling site and a stochastic probability of increased trabecular penetration. In glucocorticoid-induced osteoporosis, the same effects occur but are exacerbated by impaired osteoblast activity.[36] This remodeling process takes place on the surface of cancellous bone at the endocortical junction and within the cortex of bone where the completed remodeling process is seen as Haversian systems. The fact that the majority of the activity occurs on the surface means that, when situations of imbalance occur, the loss of tissue is greatest at high surface areas and, within sites of equal surface, is highest at sites within red marrow in juxtaposition.[37] Consequently, in any situation in which excessive bone loss occurs, bone loss occurs first and most markedly in cancellous bone, which contributes 80% of the surface area of the skeleton but only 20% of the skeletal mass.

In healthy individuals, the process of bone loss is insidious, occurring over many years in an asymptomatic fashion. The average negative calcium balance of 30 to 50 mg per day after three decades can cause as much as 30% to 50% loss of skeletal mass. Superimposed on these slow changes are the endocrine changes at menopause, in which a loss of estrogen produces increased bone remodeling.[33–38] After spontaneous or surgical menopause, vertebral bone loss rates of 3% to 5% per year have been recorded for the first 5 to 10 years. Thereafter, the process of bone loss becomes slower, but it continues in many people until old age. Some indications are found that bone loss may accelerate in the very old individual.[39] Menopause-related changes in bone remodeling are clearly triggered by the declining estrogen level.[40] The mechanisms by which estrogen deficiency induces bone loss are only now beginning to be understood. Estrogen receptors, both ER-α and ER-β, have been detected in a variety of cells within marrow and on cells of osteoblast and osteoclast lineage.[41–43] However, whether the estrogen effects are mediated through ER-α or ER-β in the skeleton is unknown. Multiple target cells for estrogens probably exist within the skeleton, including macrophages, monocytes, lymphocytes, and other cells within marrow, as well as osteoblasts, preosteoclasts, and osteoclasts. In addition, osteocytes may be target cells for estrogen. Consequently, the fact that estrogen actions depend on a variety of cell-cell interactions, and a release of a variety of local cytokines and growth factors, is not surprising.[44] Thus, implicated in the estrogen actions on the skeleton are interleukins 1, 6, and 11, prostaglandin E₂, tumor necrosis factor-α (TNF-α), transforming growth factor-β (TGF-β), insulin-like growth factor-I (IGF-I), and perhaps also IGF-II.[45–57] Moreover, direct effects of estrogen may include control of cell life span for osteoblasts, osteoclasts, and/or osteocytes, and control of the synthesis of new osteoclasts via osteoclast differentiation factor (or RANK ligand), which could be the final effectors of estrogen action in the recruitment process of new osteoclasts.[58–60] Effects on other estrogen-responsive genes (e.g., *c-phos* and *c-jun*) have not been integrated into these processes.[61]

The consequence of the changes in the bone turnover with estrogen deficiency can be detected by the increased mean and median levels of bone biochemical markers in serum and urine.[62–74] The ranges of these marker levels are also increased; many individuals still have levels of biochemical markers within the expected premenopausal range, whereas others have levels that are distinctly elevated. Thus, the suggestion has been made that measurement of biochemical marker levels may provide a useful test for determining the rates of bone loss. However, although several studies have examined the relationship between baseline biochemical marker values and changes in bone mineral density (BMD) in untreated postmenopausal women, in general, the relationships are modest; biochemical marker levels are inadequate for clinical use in determining whether individual patients will lose bone rapidly.[70–72] Although increased levels of biochemical markers do indicate the increased remodeling activity within the skeleton, the inherent intraindividual variability of marker levels probably limits their usefulness.[73]

The consequence of this increased skeletal remodeling is loss of bone mass. As noted, loss of bone occurs earliest and most rapidly in areas of cancellous bone, which can be seen in the vertebral body. The risk of fracture increases with declining bone mass.[74–81] That women who lose bone at the greatest rate will have the greatest deterioration in skeletal architecture,[82] and subsequently be at even higher risk of fracture regardless of bone density, seems logical. This suggests that biochemical markers should correlate with the risk of fracture. Several studies have now indicated that biochemical marker levels do predict the risk of fracture in several populations.[83–86] In addition, the suggestion has been made that biochemical markers of bone resorption predict the risk of fracture independently of bone mass and that the two effects are additive.[83,87] However, this combination of tests has yet to be applied clinically.

Bone loss continues among postmenopausal women and becomes more apparent in men older than age 60 years.[39,88] Some have argued that this process of bone loss in older individuals is related to features other than estrogen deficiency.[89,90] Data have shown, however, that rates of bone loss in this population are dependent on endogenous estrogen production and that estrogen intervention prevents bone loss in the elderly, just as it does in women in the early years after the menopause.[91] Thus, these findings suggest that at least part of the process of bone loss in elderly individuals is estrogen sensitive.

The report of a man with estrogen resistance due to absence of the estrogen receptor who presented with osteoporosis and continued growth because of failure of the epiphyses to fuse suggests that, in men, estrogen is responsible for control of skeletal homeostasis and may also be important in determining rates of bone loss.[92] Declining ability to aromatize androgens to estrogen may also contribute to bone loss in aging men.[93]

One alternative hypothesis regarding bone loss after menopause is that a primary renal leak of calcium occurs, with increased obligatory loss of calcium that is offset by an increased skeletal remodeling required to maintain serum calcium.[94] This hypothesis has some biologic plausibility, because hypercalciuria is a known risk factor for osteoporosis,[95] particularly among men.[96] Some studies have suggested that the increased renal loss of calcium may be estrogen dependent in women and, thus, a feature of postmenopausal bone loss.[94] Thus estrogen deficiency may affect mineral metabolism. The net effect is to increase the likelihood that bone will be resorbed more easily by any stimulus to remodeling.[97] Bone is less resistant to the resorbing effects of parathyroid hormone (PTH) infusion in the estrogen-deficient state, confirming this hypothesis.[98]

## OTHER RISK FACTORS

A large number of risk factors have been implicated in postmenopausal osteoporosis (Table 64-2).[99] Some of these affect bone mass and its loss, thereby altering fracture risk, whereas others modify the risk of fracture independently of bone mass.

**TABLE 64-2.**
**Risk Factors, Diseases, and Drugs Associated with an Increased Risk of Osteoporosis in Adults**

**RISK FACTORS FOR OSTEOPOROSIS-RELATED FRACTURES AMONG POSTMENOPAUSAL WOMEN**

*Among White Women Used in These Analyses*
  Personal history of fracture as an adult
  History of fracture in a first-degree relative
  Low body weight (<127 lb)
  Current cigarette smoking
*Additional Risk Factors*
  Ovariectomy at early age* (younger than 45 yrs)
  Dementia
  Poor health/frailty§
  Recent falls
  Low calcium intake
  Inadequate physical activity
  Imperfect eyesight despite adequate correction

**INCREASED RISK OF GENERALIZED OSTEOPOROSIS IN ADULTS**

*Diseases*

| | |
|---|---|
| Acromegaly | Lymphoma and leukemia |
| Amyloidosis | Malabsorption syndromes |
| Ankylosing spondylitis | Mastocytosis |
| Celiac disease | Multiple myeloma |
| Chronic obstructive pulmonary disease | Multiple sclerosis |
| | Organ transplantation |
| Congenital porphyria | Osteogenesis imperfecta |
| Cushing syndrome | Pernicious anemia |
| Endometriosis | Rheumatoid arthritis |
| Gastrectomy | Severe liver disease, especially primary biliary cirrhosis |
| Gaucher disease | |
| Gonadal insufficiency (primary and secondary) | Spinal cord transsection |
| | Stroke |
| Hemochromatosis | Thalassemia |
| Hyperparathyroidism | Thyrotoxicosis |
| Inflammatory bowel disease | Type 1 diabetes mellitus |
| Immobilization | |

*Drugs*

| | |
|---|---|
| Anticonvulsants | Gonadotropin-releasing hormone agonists |
| Cigarette smoking | |
| Coumadin | Long-term use of heparin |
| Cytotoxic drugs | Immunosuppressants |
| Excessive thyroxine | Tamoxifen use in premenopausal women |
| Glucocorticoids and adrenocorticotropin | |
| | Total parenteral nutrition |

*Without hormone replacement therapy. Premature ovarian failure (<45 yrs) may also be a risk factor, but is less well documented.
§May be self-reported.

Some risk factors may have effects on both bone mass and fracture risk. One example is cigarette use, which may affect bone turnover and the age of menopause, and, through its harmful effects on general health, may independently raise fracture risk.[100] More conveniently, from the clinician's viewpoint, risk factors are usually categorized conceptually into those that are modifiable and those that are not. Although all are important in determining an individual's likelihood of fracture, it is the former that must be addressed when making treatment decisions.

**Nonmodifiable Risk Factors.** Of the factors that influence risk and *cannot be changed*, age is the single most important.[101–103] In addition, gender, a family history of osteoporosis, and a past history of fracture affect risk.[101–105] In most societies, fractures occur more commonly in women, and in white and Asian groups in most Western countries, female gender doubles fracture risk. The same appears true for the black population, although the absolute risk is significantly lower for blacks than for those of other races.[106] In the United States, the risk of fracture among black women is roughly equal to that among white males. Not surprisingly, persons with a family history of hip fracture in a parent are at approximately twice the risk of others for hip fracture.[101] Data suggest that those with a family history of osteoporosis have lower peak bone mass, and parental bone mass is correlated with bone mass in offspring.[107–110]

The clinical experience that patients who present with fractures are more likely to fracture in the future has been confirmed by several formal studies.[101,111] The view is now generally accepted that those who present with a history of fracture are at approximately twice the risk of future fracture, an increase in risk that is independent of bone mass. The occurrence of vertebral fractures dramatically increases the risk of subsequent vertebral fractures by five-fold for one fracture and by 12-fold for two or more fractures, while doubling the risk for other osteoporotic fractures.[111]

**Modifiable Risk Factors.** Although the results of studies evaluating those factors that might be *modifiable* in any individual patient have varied, some broad agreement exists regarding evaluations for fracture risk. Furthermore, a large number of chronic diseases and medications have been associated with an increased risk of osteoporosis (see Table 64-2).

NUTRITION. Good nutrition is as important for skeletal health as it is for general health.[112] During growth, an adequate supply of calories, protein, and minerals is a prerequisite for the attainment of peak skeletal mass.[18,26,27,112,113] Although the effect has not been proven by long-term studies, undernutrition in childhood leads to a skeletal deficit that cannot be repaired during adult life and presumably, therefore, would lead to an increase in the risk of osteoporotic fracture in later life. During adult life, an adequate intake of calcium is required to ensure that serum calcium can be maintained within the normal range (Table 64-3). Inadequate intake necessitates the use of calcium from the skeleton to maintain levels of serum calcium and leads to a consequent increase in bone turnover that results in a loss of skeletal mass.[38] The effects of inadequate calcium intake are likely to be less among premenopausal women with adequate ovarian function than among women in an estrogen-deficient state.[114–116] In the early postmenopausal years, the effects of estrogen deficiency are sufficiently potent that calcium supplementation has only modest effects.[117] As individuals age, however, the role of calcium appears to become more important.[118] Thus, studies of calcium supplementation conducted among older individuals show significant beneficial effects on bone mass and the incidence of fractures.[119–127] The message to patients must be that calcium intake is important at all ages.

The role of vitamin D in the pathogenesis of osteoporosis has been debated for some time.[128] Although clearly vitamin D deficiency leads to osteomalacia in adults, whether lesser degrees of vitamin D deprivation can lead to osteoporosis is unclear. Certain populations frequently have circulating levels of 25-dihydroxyvitamin D [25(OH)D] that are considered to be in the borderline range (5 to 20 ng/mL).[129–131] Because costs and risks are minimal, recommending supplementation to these groups seems prudent. These populations include the elderly, the institutionalized, and those who are chronically ill, especially those with malabsorption and diseases causing diminished ambulation, such as multiple sclerosis.[132–136] For these groups, ingestion of 400 to 800 U per day of cholecalciferol is safe and cost effective.

The suggestion has also been made that the reduced intestinal calcium absorption seen in osteoporosis is the primary defect and part of a more general resistance to the actions of 1,25-hydroxyvitamin D [1,25(OH)$_2$D], which, in turn, could be related to a reduced receptor density.[9] Evidence also exists of a reduced supply of the active metabolite, 1,25(OH)$_2$D, perhaps related to an age-dependent decline in renal function.[13] Superimposed on these metabolic features is the decline in physical activity with age, which may play an important role in determining rates and duration of bone loss, especially in the hip. The hypothesis argues that the skeleton has an inbuilt "mechanostat," which sets bone mass according to the degree of stress placed on the skeleton. This is most obvious in the increase of bone mass during growth and in the loss of bone that occurs after disuse. A smaller loss could be precipitated by the gradually reduced stress of lessening physical activity, as is often seen in the elderly. In any individual some combination of these events may conspire to produce a negative skeletal balance. Superimposed on these age-related changes are secondary causes of bone loss and, in women, the effects of estrogen deficiency at menopause.

An often underrecognized nutritional factor in the pathogenesis of osteoporosis is sodium intake.[137] A high intake of sodium results in an obligatory loss of calcium in the urine in excess of the normal urinary losses. This phenomenon, continued over years (especially if not compensated for by an adequate calcium intake), would be expected to exacerbate other risk factors for osteoporosis. Whether limitation of sodium intake can reduce bone loss has not been determined.

Other nutritional factors that have been implicated in the pathogenesis of osteoporosis include excessive intake of protein, especially animal protein.[138] The suspicion is that this is the effect of the acid load of such diets. Excess caffeine intake has also been implicated, either because it increases urinary calcium excretion or because it leads to a minor diminution of calcium absorption. However, demonstrating a relationship between caffeine intake and fracture is difficult, partly because of the difficulty of determining the level of caffeine intake, partly because of the confounding effects of other risk factors,[138,139] and partly because caffeine appears to have such a minor effect on skeletal metabolism. Phosphorus intake, such as in cola drinks, also has been implicated, but has a very minor effect on bone metabolism. The major importance of this latter nutrient is that phosphorus-containing drinks often substitute for calcium-containing ones, such as milk. Perhaps the most controversial nutritional risk factor is alcohol. No doubt exists that excess alcohol intake is detrimental to the skeleton[140,141]; a high intake is a risk factor for osteoporosis among men. The role of moderate intakes is less clear, however. Some data suggest that consumption of one to two alcoholic drinks per day may have a positive effect on bone mass, but because those data are from epidemiologic studies, other biases cannot be excluded.[142]

The current calcium recommendations should be adequate to offset effects for patients with even moderately high intakes of protein, caffeine, and salt, as are often seen in the U.S. population.

LIFESTYLE. Data from several studies suggest that cigarette use is a significant risk factor for osteoporotic fracture[101,142] (Fig. 64-2). Several mechanisms exist by which this effect might be mediated. Cigarette use results in a menopause that is earlier by as much as 2 years and lowers estradiol levels in both pre- and postmenopausal women.[143] In some animal models of osteoporosis, exposure to cigarette tobacco has direct toxic effects on

**TABLE 64-3.**
**Adequate Intake Levels for Calcium and Vitamin D**

| Age (Years) | Calcium* (mg) | Vitamin D[†] [IU (μg)] |
|---|---|---|
| 4–8 | 800 | 200 (5) |
| 9–18 | 1300 | 200 (5) |
| 19–50 | 1000 | 200 (5) |
| 51–65 | 1200 | 400 (10) |
| >65 | 1200 | 600–800 (15–20) |

*Calcium needs may increase in the presence of malabsorption, achlorhydria, and other chronic conditions that decrease calcium absorption or increase calcium excretion.

[†]Vitamin D requirement in the absence of adequate exposure to sunlight. Those at greatest risk of vitamin D deficiency include strict vegetarians without adequate exposure to sunlight, the elderly, and housebound, institutionalized, and/or chronically ill individuals. Adults of all ages at greatest risk of deficiency may need 600–800 IU per day. Individuals should not consume >800 IU per day except under the guidance of a physician.

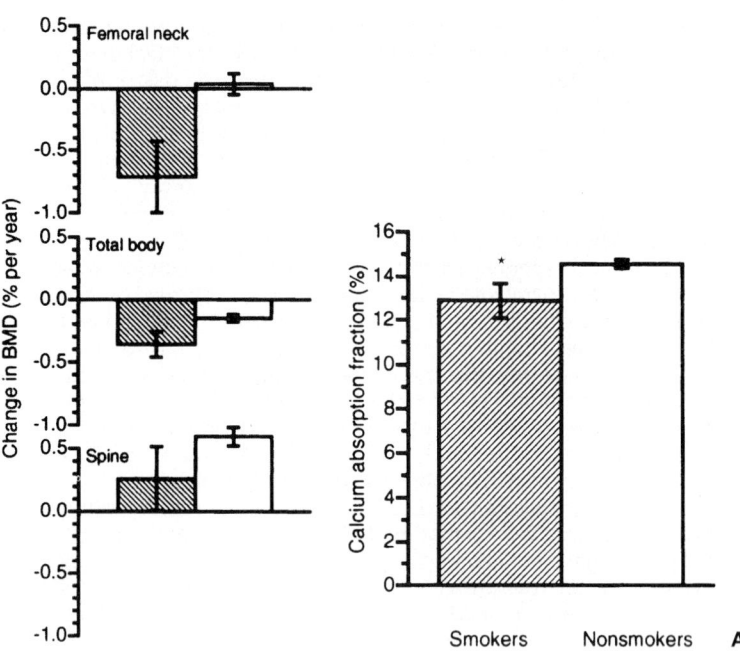

**FIGURE 64-2.** **A,** Mean (± standard error of the mean) adjusted annual rates of bone mineral density (*BMD*) change of the femoral neck, total body, and lumbar spine in smokers (*hatched bars*) and nonsmokers (*white bars*). Rates are adjusted for baseline BMD, weight, age, gender, supplementation status (calcium plus vitamin D or placebos), and dietary calcium intake. Values at the femoral neck are −0.714 ± 0.285% per year for 31 smokers versus +0.038 ± 0.084% per year for 355 nonsmokers, $p$ <.02; for the total body, −0.360 ± 0.101% per year for 354 nonsmokers, $p$ <.05; and at the spine, +0.260 ± 0.252% per year for 29 smokers versus +0.593 ± 0.074% per year for 339 nonsmokers, $p$ = .21. **B,** Mean (± standard error of the mean) adjusted fractional calcium absorption in smokers (*hatched bar*) and nonsmokers (*white bar*). Means are adjusted for gender, age, supplementation status (placebo or calcium plus vitamin D), and dietary calcium and vitamin D intakes. Values are 12.9 ± 0.8% for 23 smokers and 14.6 ± 0.2% for 310 nonsmokers, $p$ <.05. (From Krall EA, Dawson-Hughes B. Smoking increases bone loss and decreases intestinal calcium absorption. J Bone Miner Res 1999; 14:215.)

the skeleton. Cigarette use may also be associated with decreased physical activity. Finally, the effects of cigarettes on general health may result in frail individuals who are more at risk for falls and subsequent injury.[144] Consequently, some of the risk conferred by cigarette use is independent of its effects on bone.[101] Among the elderly, current cigarette use doubles the risk of hip fracture.[101]

PHYSICAL ACTIVITY.   The popular belief exists that physical activity is important for good skeletal health. Cross-sectional data clearly show dramatic effects on the skeleton at the extremes of activity.[145–148] Complete loss of activity causes loss of bone mass, just as muscle mass is lost. Highly active individuals have greater skeletal mass than average; this may be specific to the underlying bone used in the activity (e.g., forearm bone in tennis players).[148] Within the average range of physical activity in the general population, however, demonstrating marked effects of changing activity on bone mass has been difficult. Most studies do suggest modest effects, with the changes in activity producing bone mass differences of 1% to 2%. Metaanalyses confirm decreased bone loss in exercisers compared with sedentary individuals. Most would agree that activity has an important role to play in the prevention of osteoporotic fracture. Among the elderly, this may be related to the effects of maintaining activity on the risk of falls and subsequent injury.[149–152] Thus, patients with or at risk of osteoporosis should incorporate exercise into their therapy.

## CLINICAL FEATURES

In general, osteoporosis has no symptoms, and the clinical features with which it presents are those of its complications, that is, fractures. Vertebral fracture is the most common clinical manifestation of osteoporosis. It is often asymptomatic and identified incidentally on a chest radiograph; only 10% to 30% of vertebral fractures present with acute pain. Multiple vertebral fractures ("crush fractures") lead to increased dorsal kyphosis, loss of height, and dowager's hump (Fig. 64-3). When fractures are symptomatic, acute pain may develop suddenly after minimal force or strain from routine activities such as bending, reaching, or lifting. This pain subsides within a few weeks, but may be followed by a period of chronic, dull, diffuse pain, which may last for months to years. In part, this chronic pain is related to the changing biomechanical competence of the spine. Progressive vertebral body collapse, with loss of thoracolumbar height, may cause the lower ribs to rest on the iliac crest, which may produce some relief of back pain but may result in lower rib and flank

pain. This altered body configuration compresses pulmonary and abdominal organs and may be associated with exertional dyspnea and gastrointestinal distress, including early satiety, bloating, and constipation.[153–159] Psychosocial consequences (fear, depression, irritability, and loneliness) often follow multiple vertebral fractures. Neurologic signs and symptoms of nerve root or spinal cord compression are seldom caused by osteoporotic vertebral fractures and should prompt a search for other causes of fracture.

Hip fractures (e.g., subcapital femoral neck, intertrochanteric, and subtrochanteric) occur in 15% of women and 5% of men by age 80 years[4] (Fig. 64-4). Surgical intervention is almost always necessary if patients are expected to return to an ambulatory status. Hip fracture is a common cause of nursing home admission. Because of the surgery and postsurgical complications, hip fractures are associated with a 5% to 20% excess mortality in the first

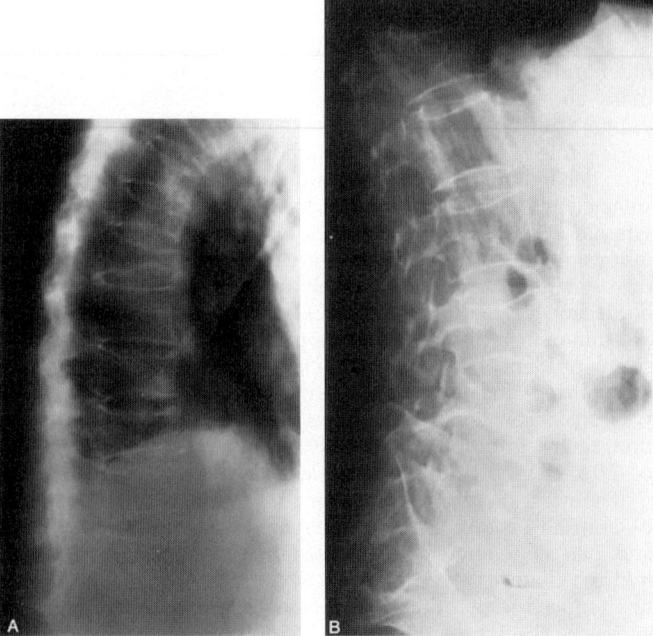

**FIGURE 64-3.** Radiographic appearance of the dorsal spine (**A**) and the lumbar spine (**B**) showing anterior wedging and vertebral lapse, radiolucency, and biconcavities.

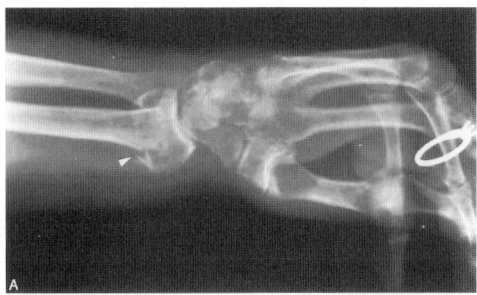

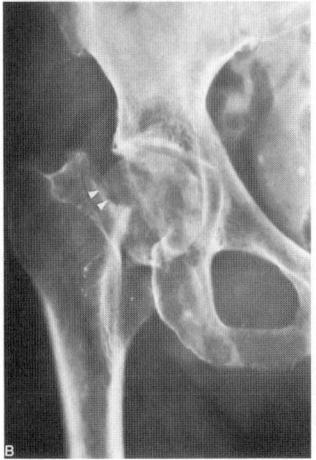 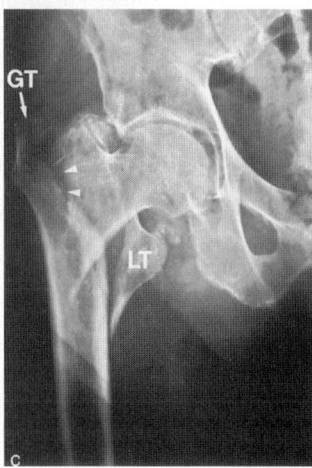

**FIGURE 64-4. A,** A 54-year-old osteoporotic woman with typical Colles fracture caused by a fall on the outstretched hand. There is a fracture of the distal end of the radius (*arrowhead*), with angulation and impaction of the distal fragment. **B,** A 75-year-old osteoporotic man with a subcapital femoral fracture (*arrowheads*). Notice that the broken-off head of the femur is completely displaced from the neck. The usual treatment of a fracture with this degree of displacement is surgical excision of the femoral head and replacement with a metallic prosthesis. **C,** A 77-year-old man with intertrochanteric femoral fracture. The fracture line (*arrowheads*) extends from the center of the greater trochanter (*GT*) to the lesser trochanter (*LT*). In this instance, the LT has broken off as a separate fragment. The treatment of this fracture is by internal fixation with a metallic device. (Courtesy of Dr. Bahman Sadr, Washington, DC.)

year after fracture.[4,14,160–166] Approximately 30% to 50% of patients with hip fracture never return to their level of activity before the fracture. Distal radius fractures (i.e., Colles fractures) cause less morbidity than hip or vertebral fracture (see Fig. 64-4). However, wrist fractures increase in frequency at an earlier age than do fractures of the hip or spine.[4,167–170] Any individual who fractures a wrist should be considered possibly at risk for osteoporosis and should be considered for evaluation. Because osteoporosis is a systemic disease, fractures of any bone can occur, and fracture of any bone after the age of 40 should raise a suspicion of osteoporosis in any individual.

### HISTORY AND PHYSICAL EXAMINATION

Postmenopausal osteoporosis is a diagnosis of exclusion. Clinical evaluation is specifically directed toward determining if secondary causes of the disease are present. Evaluation of all prior fractures, current or past renal stone or other renal disease, thyroid disease, glucocorticoid use, Cushing syndrome, diabetes, hypogonadism, immobilization, liver disease, intestinal disease, and gastric or intestinal surgery should be made. Back pain should be evaluated, as it might be the presenting symptom of vertebral osteoporosis. The consideration of possible systemic symptoms of malignancy, especially of multiple myeloma, is essential in any patient. In women, the age of menopause, menarche, and reproductive history are important. A history of excessive alcohol or caffeine consumption and of

cigarette smoking should be elicited. Lifelong calcium intake and exercise history should be determined. Nutritional calcium status is easily estimated. The family's medical history should be ascertained, particularly with respect to hip and wrist fractures and significant height loss or change in thoracic shape. Physical evaluation should include a general physical examination with measurement of height, weight, and arm span (which gives an estimate of original height) and with a search for signs of secondary diseases. Suspicion of secondary disease should be particularly high in patients who are neither postmenopausal women nor elderly.

### LABORATORY TESTS

All laboratory values, including indices of mineral metabolism, are usually normal in patients with primary or postmenopausal osteoporosis, except in those with recent fractures, who may show elevations in serum alkaline phosphatase related to fracture healing. Laboratory evaluation could include measurement of serum calcium, phosphorus, alkaline phosphatase, and thyroid-stimulating hormone levels, complete blood count, erythrocyte sedimentation rate, tests of renal and hepatic function, and serum protein electrophoresis, depending on clinical suspicion. If adrenocortical hyperfunction is suspected, a urinary free cortisol test or an overnight dexamethasone suppression test should be performed.

When serum calcium is high, the serum PTH level should be obtained. If questions exist regarding the nutritional status in elderly patients, patients with other chronic diseases, or patients on antiepileptic drugs, the measurement of the 25(OH)D level may be helpful. Some recommend supplementation with cholecalciferol in these circumstances without necessarily obtaining a biochemical measurement.

### BONE MASS MEASUREMENT

Osteoporosis is defined as a disease of bone mass in which bone mass or density has fallen below the expected range for young adults. The analogy is the upper limits of normal for blood pressure or cholesterol, which are taken as indicators of hypertension or hypercholesterolemia. These risk factors for the clinical catastrophes of stroke or myocardial infarction are in common use in clinical practice. Bone mass measurement, which is at least as good a predictor of the clinical outcome, merits similar use.[74–81]

Two sensitive and noninvasive tests are available for measuring bone density in clinical practice. The first, dual-energy x-ray absorptiometry (DXA), which is used to measure appendicular and axial sites and can be used to measure total body bone mass, is the most precise method available, produces minimal radiation exposure, and has become widely available. The second, quantitative computed tomography (QCT), has the advantage of measuring only trabecular bone and may be the most sensitive indicator of cancellous bone loss after menopause; however, this advantage is outweighed by poor precision in comparison to other techniques and much greater radiation exposure (see Chap. 57).

Several techniques that measure peripheral bone have the advantage of small size, which allows them to be easily housed in an office. These techniques include peripheral CT, peripheral dual-energy x-ray absorptiometry, single-energy x-ray absorptiometry, and ultrasonography. (The advantage of ultrasonography is the lack of x-ray exposure and the possibility that it might measure structural characteristics of the bone that contribute to skeletal fragility, although this remains to be proven.)

Bone densitometry is used to determine the risk of fracture. An inverse relationship is seen between density and the likelihood that a patient will experience fracture.[74–81] The risk of hip fracture increases 2.5-fold for every one standard deviation decline in bone density when measured at the hip. Measurements of bone density at the *hip* allow estimation of risk of fractures at other sites, for which the relative risk is ~1.5 for every standard deviation change in bone density. Measurements of bone density at other sites are less effective in identifying those patients most likely to experience hip fracture, and because hip fracture is the most serious consequence of osteoporosis, measurements of the hip are generally preferred in predicting risk. However, for the early postmenopausal woman whose major concern may be vertebral fractures, measurements of the *spine* may be more appropriate. Measurements of the spine are often uninterpretable in the elderly because of facet joint disease and extraosseous calcification, so that measurements of the hip are preferable. When measurements of the hip and spine are not available, *peripheral bone* measurements may be substituted. However, although guidelines exist for intervention based on bone density measurements of the central skeleton, such guidelines do not exist for measurements of the peripheral skeleton.

Bone density measurement has become an almost routine clinical tool in evaluation of patients for risk of osteoporosis and evaluation of those who have already had fractures. For asymptomatic individuals, bone densitometry should be offered to every woman by the age of 65. For women who are postmenopausal but younger than age 65 years, if risk factors other than menopause exist, bone densitometry should be recommended. All persons who present with fracture at >40 years should be considered for bone densitometry. Medicare guidelines allow repeat bone densitometry at intervals of ~2 years after the progression of the disease or 1 year after a new treatment is initiated. Bone density measurements must change by at least 3% to 4% in the spine and at least 5% to 6% in the hip to be considered significant in individual patients.

### TESTS OF BONE TURNOVER

Several tests are available to measure either breakdown products from the skeleton or specific enzymes or proteins synthesized by osteoblasts. Levels of these *markers of bone turnover* have several possible uses in the management of patients with osteoporosis. First, they may provide some information on the baseline status of bone remodeling, which, when increased as occurs in postmenopausal women, adds to the risk of osteoporotic fracture. Second, these tests can be used to monitor the response to treatment. The tests available in the United States are listed in Table 64-4. These tests should be used only in selected patients, because the results may be difficult to interpret due to significant inter- and intraindividual variability.

In unusual situations, when osteoporosis presents in young individuals, a bone biopsy may be used to evaluate cellular activity on the surface of the skeleton. Such situations are, however, increasingly unusual.

### RADIOLOGIC FEATURES

Greater than 30% loss of bone mass has to occur before detectable changes can be seen on plain radiograph. In the spine, individual trabeculae are thinned and, because the horizontal trabeculae are preferentially lost, vertical trabeculae appear more prominent. The vertebral bodies eventually appear as empty shells, and changes in shape begin to occur. Schmorl nodes, caused by the indentation of the disk into the vertebral body, are not pathognomonic of osteoporosis but certainly raise clinical suspicion.[171] The classic wedge-shaped deformity is characterized by reduced anterior vertebral height (see Fig. 64-3). This decrement is thought to be significant when the anterior height becomes >15% lower than that of the immediate craniad vertebra, or alternatively, more than three standard deviations below the expected mean for the anterior height of the vertebrae itself. Biconcavity or "codfish vertebra" indicates the collapse of the central vertebral body and is particularly common in the lumbar spine. Posterior wedging is less common and may suggest a destructive lesion, especially if posterior extrusion of a fragment toward the cord is seen. A true crush fracture is a decrease in all aspects of vertebral height (anterior, central, and posterior). Vertebral fractures seldom occur above the level of T4 and their frequency is maximal between T8 and L3. Single vertebral fractures are often asymptomatic; however, single severe wedge fractures at the level of T7 can be particularly symptomatic because they produce an especially prominent kyphotic angulation. Radiographs can also be useful to rule out other bone diseases, such as Paget disease, in patients with bone pain and/or fractures.

Radiographs taken after wrist or hip injury show the typical changes of fractures at those sites (see Fig. 64-4).[171] Radionuclide scans may be used to make the diagnosis of fracture at any site for which the routine radiograph is not definitive. Radionuclide scans and magnetic resonance images can also be used in certain clinical settings to rule out diseases that produce hip pain, such as avascular necrosis of the femoral head.

## INTERVENTION IN POSTMENOPAUSAL OSTEOPOROSIS

The first approach to the prevention or treatment of osteoporosis is *risk reduction*.[172] Improving calcium intake and increasing physical activity are the most frequently adopted strategies. Indeed, for their general effects on health and their modest cost and low risk, these are strategies that should be recommended to all. In addition, elimination of cigarette use and moderation of alcohol intake are valuable. Limiting doses of drugs that adversely affect the skeleton and reviewing environmental safety concepts to reduce falling risk, particularly for elderly individuals, are also important.

### CALCIUM INTAKE

All individuals should be advised of the recommended intake of calcium. The recommendations of the National Academy of Sciences (see Table 64-3) are somewhat lower than those previously suggested by the National Institutes of Health but are probably more easily achieved for those with average intakes (~50% of recommended intake).[173] The improvement in intake should be obtained by improving diet. In the United States, this primarily means increasing consumption of dairy products, a move that is resisted by many on the grounds that it will result in increased fat or calorie intake. Opting for nonfat or low-fat products helps avoid this problem. Lactose intolerance is a problem that increases in frequency with age, although not all who claim lactose intolerance have true lactase deficiency. Those who cannot increase dietary calcium sufficiently in this way can consume calcium-fortified foods such as fruit juices, which have as much calcium per ounce as milk. Furthermore, many calcium supplement preparations are available. When advising about supplements, the clinician must remember that the aim is to increase intake to the recommended levels. A simple assessment of basal intake can be made easily and supplements can be added as required. For most individuals, an extra intake of 500 to 750 mg per day of elemental calcium is sufficient. When supplements are used, the least expensive is usually a calcium carbonate preparation with a USP label (which

**TABLE 64-4.**
**Biochemical Markers of Bone Turnover**

**BONE FORMATION**
  Serum osteocalcin (OC)
  Propeptide of type I procollagen (PICP)
  Bone-specific alkaline phosphatase
**BONE RESORPTION**
  Urine pyridinoline and deoxypyridinoline
  Urine and serum cross-linked N-telopeptide
  Urine and serum cross-linked C-telopeptide
  Serum tartrate-resistant acid phosphatase

ensures solubility). Calcium supplements should be taken in divided doses. Calcium carbonate should be taken at the end of a meal when the acid load of the meal will assist the availability of the calcium (this is not required when calcium citrate is used). Although some suggest that calcium should be taken at bedtime to reduce the nocturnal increase in bone remodeling, no available data indicate a greater beneficial effect.

Such increases in calcium intake are important at all ages and may improve peak bone mass and slow premenopausal loss. Although this strategy by itself does not prevent the loss of bone that is driven by estrogen deficiency, improving calcium intake among the elderly clearly reduces the risk of fracture significantly, perhaps by as much as 50%.[112–126]

## PHYSICAL ACTIVITY

The general belief that increased physical activity improves bone mass is based mainly on cross-sectional data.[148–152] Longitudinal data suggest that in adults the effects of physical activity on bone density are modest, although most studies show some increase.[173–182] Whether the effects of physical activity on bone modify fracture risk is not known and cannot easily be tested. Exercise has other effects on the organism that are likely to yield positive effects on fracture risk (e.g., effects on the neuromuscular system). Improved reaction time and strength might be expected to reduce the risk of falls and, thereby, the risk of injury.

Physical activity is a habit. To obtain the maximum benefit from any activity program, the earlier in life that it is begun and the longer in life it is continued, the better. Exercise has many health benefits beyond its effects on the skeleton; thus, the argument for increased activity at all ages is only enhanced by the skeletal effects that might accrue directly or indirectly. No specific exercise prescription for osteoporosis exists, and components of strength training as well as activities that improve cardiovascular performance are required. The authors recommend a pragmatic approach, recognizing that adherence to a program is more important than the program itself. The activities that the individual enjoys are recorded as part of the history-taking, and the patient is encouraged to increase their use. In addition, use of the buddy system is stressed, because participation with a friend makes adherence more likely.

## PHARMACOLOGIC INTERVENTION

Agents available in the United States include bone-specific drugs (*bisphosphonates, calcitonin*) and agents that have more general effects (e.g., *estrogens* and *tissue-selective estrogens*).[183,184] Each has different advantages and disadvantages, but their availability allows treatment to be tailored to individual needs.

**Estrogen.** Hormone-replacement therapy (HRT; the terms "hormone-replacement therapy" and "estrogen-replacement therapy" are generally used interchangeably) has been available for >50 years and is considered to be the gold standard for the prevention and treatment of osteoporosis.[183,184] Most available data support the conclusion that HRT is an effective intervention for osteoporosis prevention and treatment.[185–192] In terms of prevention of *vertebral fracture*, one long-term primary prevention study has reported an ~75% protection rate over 10 years.[185] Small secondary prevention studies, in which patients with osteoporosis were treated with hormones indicate an ~50% reduction in fracture risk.[193]

Epidemiologic data indicate an ~50% reduction in overall risk of hip fractures.[194–203] One study suggested that the effect may be even greater among older women (older than 65 years) who have taken estrogen for >10 years.[203] A 75% reduction in the risk of hip fracture was evident only among those women with a long history of estrogen therapy who were currently taking treatment.

In a clinical trial evaluating the effects of estrogen on myocardial infarction in patients with established heart disease, no evidence was found of an effect of estrogen use on *nonspinal* fractures.[204] Because the study was not specifically designed as

an osteoporosis study, its importance is uncertain. However, it does suggest that some of the findings regarding estrogen effects on fractures may be related to the "healthy user" phenomenon[205]—that is, *women who receive HRT are healthier and are more likely to have healthy lifestyles* (i.e., no tobacco use, higher exercise activity, better diets). One study of 460 early menopausal women suggested that HRT did reduce the risk of non-spine fractures by ~60% compared to placebo.[199] Further controlled studies are necessary to determine the effect of HRT on nonspinal osteoporosis-related fractures.

Considerable clinical trial data indicate that estrogen intervention in women after menopause (surgical or natural) reduces the rate of bone remodeling to premenopausal levels and prevents the loss of bone mass.[184–192,206–215] Most studies have followed patients for 2 to 3 years.[185,208] HRT appears to be effective for as long as it is given, although some bone loss may occur in older individuals, in whom bone remodeling is being influenced by factors other than estrogen deficiency. Some data indicate that even in such aged individuals bone loss is partially sensitive to estrogen status and may be influenced by the low level of endogenous estrogen production.[216,217] Thus, even in those older than 70 years of age, HRT can produce positive effects on the skeleton. Intervention with HRT is effective only while estrogen is being taken.[203] Many individuals may not fill their prescriptions, and, of those that do, many (probably ~50%) fail to complete one year of treatment; thus, many fail to take estrogen for sufficiently long to derive the health benefits.[218]

For women who have passed a natural menopause, HRT is generally prescribed as a combination of estrogen and a progestin.[219] The progestin may be given cyclically (younger women) or continuously (older women). The cyclic regimens are associated with more regular menstrual-type vaginal bleeding, whereas the continuous regimens induce amenorrhea. While continuous regimens are often associated with irregular bleeding during the early months of treatment, most women cease bleeding within 6 to 12 months. This bleeding pattern needs to be explained to the patient, because it can result in serious patient concerns about the safety of the medicine. Several different preparations of estrogen are available, and combined preparations are available that obviate the need for two separate medications. Progestins need not be taken by women who do not have a uterus.

Controversy continues about the dosage of estrogen required to achieve a bone-sparing effect.[191,220,221] Available data suggest that 0.625 mg per day conjugated equine estrogen (CEE) or its equivalent is >90% effective. In a metaanalysis of the estrogen studies performed with and without calcium supplementation, the effect of estrogen on bone density was found to be enhanced by adequate calcium intake.[222] A controlled clinical trial evaluating the effect of 0.3 mg per day CEE (with adequate calcium and vitamin D intake) confirmed that, in the presence of good nutrition, this lower dosage of estrogen is sufficient. Similar results have been obtained with other estrogen products at equivalent dosages.[220,223]

Estrogens can be administered by oral, transdermal, buccal, vaginal, percutaneous, or subcutaneous routes. Provided that enough estrogen is supplied, an effect on bone remodeling and bone density occurs, although no studies on fractures have been published other than for oral or transdermal administration. No cross-comparison studies have been undertaken; thus, equivalency is based on studies of each compound in *different* populations, with *differing* trial designs.

Estrogens have multiple tissue effects in the body and are still prescribed principally for the relief of menopausal symptoms.[219,224] Consequently, much of the use is relatively short-term and insufficient to prevent osteoporosis. Although the hypothesis has been put forward that estrogen use is associated with reductions in the risk of myocardial infarction among postmenopausal women,[224] the data are epidemiologic.[205] In fact, one secondary prevention study (a controlled clinical trial) undertaken in women with established heart disease showed a transient *increase* in cardiac events during the early treatment and no favorable effect until 4 to 5 years had passed.[204] This study has caused some reexamination of the data supporting estrogen use for heart disease. Estrogen also may have a protective effect against Alzheimer disease.[225–227] Controlled clinical trial data do suggest that use of estrogens may improve cognitive function among postmenopausal women; however, the data regarding dementia are *very preliminary*.[228] Estrogen use has been associated with an increased risk of breast cancer in some epidemiologic studies, findings that potentially limit long-term use of estrogens for prevention of osteoporosis.[229] As might be expected, the prescription of estrogens for postmenopausal women is complicated, and often patients refuse this pharmacologic intervention.

**Bisphosphonates.** Bisphosphonates are analogs of pyrophosphate in which the oxygen is replaced by a carbon atom,[230] yielding a stable compound that resists metabolism and allows two side chains to be added to the carbon atom. These agents have varied affinities for bone and differing activities for inhibition of bone resorption. Controlled clinical trials with *etidronate* demonstrated increased bone density but failed to provide definitive fracture data.[230a] Thus, etidronate is marketed in the United States for Paget disease, hypercalcemia, and myositis ossificans but *not* for use in treatment of osteoporosis.

Alendronate was the first of the bisphosphonates approved in the United States for osteoporosis treatment and prevention. Clinical trials demonstrated marked reductions in bone remodeling and increases in BMD of spine and hip[231–233] (Fig. 64-5). These remodeling modifications were accompanied by reductions in the risk of fractures. In a large multicenter study, patients with prevalent vertebral fractures experienced reductions in the risk of vertebral fractures (~50%) and a reduction in hip and forearm fractures of ~50%.[232] Patients with low bone density but without prevalent fractures experienced no overall reduction of clinical fractures (although *radiographically* demonstrated vertebral fractures were reduced by 44%)[233]; however, when the analysis was limited to those who had osteoporosis by bone density criteria, a significant reduction in clinical fractures was seen. This suggests that alendronate is best used for either those who have fractures at presentation or those who have osteoporosis.

For osteoporosis, the dose of alendronate approved for *prevention is 5 mg* and for *treatment is 10 mg*. A modest but significantly greater effect on BMD is seen with 10 mg, but either dose is probably equally effective[232] (based on the fracture intervention trials in which the 5-mg dose was used for the first two years, with a change to 10 mg only for the latter portion of the study[232–233]). In the United States, both doses cost the same; therefore, the 10-mg dose is often preferred as the initial dose.

Bisphosphonates are poorly absorbed (<1% of the ingested dose absorbed on an empty stomach).[230] Food interferes with absorption. Consequently, alendronate must be taken in the morning on an empty stomach with water (6–8 ounces) ≥30 minutes before any food is consumed. The patient must also remain in the upright position (standing or sitting) to avoid reflux of the tablet into the esophagus. For some patients this rigid schedule is difficult, although most seem to manage once the rationale is explained.

Esophagitis has been reported, particularly with the 10-mg dose.[234,235] Amino-containing bisphosphonates are irritating (although little evidence of this was observed in the alendronate clinical trials).[231–233] The incidence of such problems may be as much as 15% to 40%, but most cases are minor and can be resolved by temporarily discontinuing the drug for a week before resuming treatment. If symptoms recur, treatment should be stopped, and the patient should be changed to an alternative drug or the dose should be lowered to 5 mg. Rarely, a more serious esophageal erosion with ulceration can occur. This may lead to perforation (incidence ≤1%). Usually, esophageal side effects occur in the early months of treatment. Use of

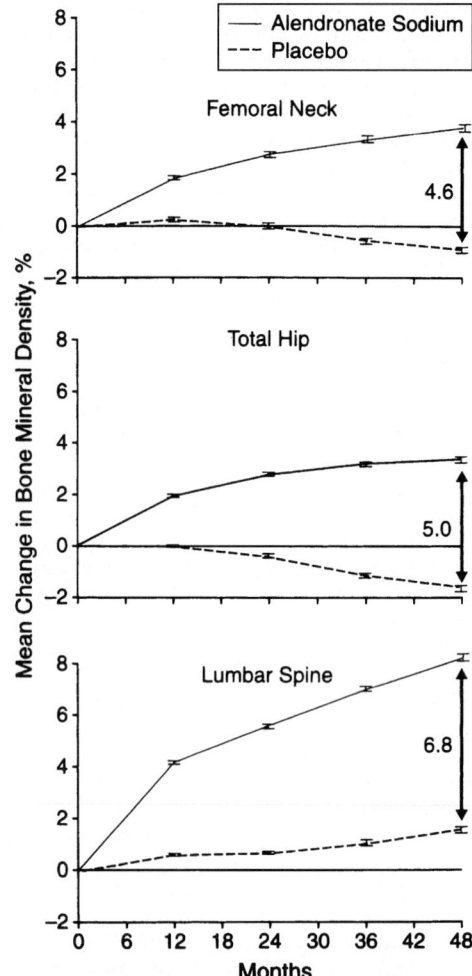

**FIGURE 64-5.** Mean (± standard deviation) percentage changes in bone mineral density from baseline to 48 months in patients receiving alendronate therapy and in those receiving a placebo. (From Cummings SR, Black DM, Thompson DE, et al. Effect of alendronate on risk of fracture in women with low bone density but without vertebral fractures: results from the Fracture Intervention Trial. JAMA 1998; 280:2077.)

alendronate should be avoided in those with active upper gastrointestinal disease.

Occasionally, patients report some general aches and pains during the early months of alendronate treatment. The cause is unclear and the symptoms usually are minor and self-limiting.

Risedronate is approved for treatment and prevention of osteoporosis and corticosteroid-induced osteoporosis. Risedronate has a potent effect on bone mass, and turnover. Data show a rapid and sustained reduction in vertebral fracture occurrence and a reduction in all non-spine fractures, including those of the hip in patients with osteoporosis.[236,237] Other bisphosphonates include tiludronate and, intravenously, pamidronate.

The major clinical problem with bisphosphonates, as with other therapeutic agents used in the treatment of largely asymptomatic conditions (e.g., hypertension, hypercholesterolemia), is obtaining long-term compliance. The median duration of bisphosphonate use in the United States is ~6 months,[238] which clearly seems inadequate to obtain long-term protection against fractures. This is similar to the median duration of use of HRT and calcitonin, again not providing long-term protection. Thus, a major advance in patient management would be to lengthen adherence to treatment.

**Calcitonin.** Salmon calcitonin (SCT), originally given in the form of a subcutaneous injection, currently is most frequently used as an intranasal spray. Intranasal administration of

SCT (200 units per day in a single spray, given to alternate nostrils on successive days) is approved for treatment of osteoporosis in the United States. Controlled clinical trials have confirmed that this dosage reduces bone turnover, although less than do the bisphosphonates. The effect on bone mass is also less. However, administration of this dosage for 5 years reduces vertebral fractures by 36%, a result that more closely matches the reduction in fracture risk with bisphosphonates than would be predicted from calcitonin's effects on bone mass or turnover.[239]

The major advantage to calcitonin is safety. No long-term safety concerns have arisen, either in clinical trials or from long experience with subcutaneous therapy. Only nasal irritation may occur, and this is usually mild. The major disadvantage is related to the modest effects on surrogate markers of efficacy, because the changes in bone mass or turnover are insufficient in most individuals to detect whether the treatment is having an effect. No data indicate that this agent significantly reduces the risk of fractures other than those of the vertebrae.

**Selective Estrogen-Receptor Modulators.** Most data concerning efficacy of estrogens at reducing fracture risk are observational.

Furthermore, even if all of the alleged beneficial effects of estrogen are confirmed (prevention of spine and other osteoporotic fractures, reduction of heart disease, and blunting of the cognitive decline in Alzheimer disease), concern still exists about breast cancer in many women. Agents are needed that can achieve some of the possible benefits of estrogen without the adverse side effects. Selective estrogen-receptor modulators (SERMs) bind to the estrogen receptor but have tissue-selective effects (estrogenic action in some tissues and estrogen antagonist action in others). Different SERMs have their own specific phenotypic profiles with differential potency and effect on different organ systems.[240] The two most important SERMs currently available for postmenopausal women are tamoxifen and raloxifene. Only raloxifene has been approved for prevention of osteoporosis and is currently being evaluated for treatment of osteoporosis. Tamoxifen has beneficial effects on bone density and bone turnover in postmenopausal women. A breast cancer prevention trial involving 13,388 pre- and postmenopausal women showed a reduction in the risk of classic osteoporotic fractures in the tamoxifen group, although the reductions in hip and Colles fracture was not quite significant.[241] Overall, the trend toward reduced clinical fracture was ~21% in women older than 50 years. Tamoxifen *reduces* bone density in premenopausal women and increases it in postmenopausal women.[242] The use of tamoxifen is indicated in breast cancer and in women at "increased risk for breast cancer." Postmenopausal women taking this agent can probably be considered to be on a bone-active drug. In such circumstances, monitoring with tests of BMD and/or bone turnover markers might be useful. Tamoxifen clearly reduces the risk of breast cancer in high-risk women, but the effects on heart and cerebrovascular disease are unclear, and tamoxifen use is associated with a number of benign uterine conditions as well as uterine malignancy. Unfortunately, as is the case for raloxifene and estrogens, the risk of venous thromboembolic disease is also increased (approximately three-fold relative risk).[240]

Raloxifene has been studied in several osteoporosis prevention trials as well as an osteoporosis treatment trial called "MORE" (Multiple Outcomes of Raloxifene Evaluation). In both the prevention and treatment cohorts, raloxifene was associated with small increments of bone density at all skeletal sites and reductions in bone turnover (as measured by both bone formation and bone resorption variables). Data from the 3-year point showed that the drug reduced the risk of vertebral fracture by 40% to 50%.[243] However, no reduction in the risk of nonspinal fractures was observed. Raloxifene apparently has beneficial effects on serum lipoproteins (similar to those of tamoxifen[240]); however, the ultimate outcomes for heart and cerebrovascular disease are unknown. Raloxifene's

reduction of the risk of invasive breast cancer by 76% over 3.5 years is quite compelling but needs to be confirmed in ongoing clinical trials. The drug does not increase the risk of uterine cancer.[244]

Both tamoxifen and raloxifene can increase the prevalence of hot flashes in postmenopausal women. However, absolute risk is still quite low in the normal ambulatory population.[240]

**Experimental Therapies.** Fluoride (sodium fluoride), originally used at dosages of 40 to 60 mg per day, has been in clinical development for a number of years; marked increases occurred in bone mass, most obvious in the spine. However, little evidence was seen for a reduction in fracture risk, even in the spine.[245,246] In addition, uncontrolled clinical data indicated that fluoride therapy is associated with an increase in the risk of hip fracture. Use of lower-dose fluoride (slow-release fluoride), investigated in clinical trials, has led to increased bone mass that is more controlled, with a concomitant reduction in the risk of vertebral fractures.[247] Currently, fluoride is not approved as therapy for osteoporosis in the United States.

PTH increases vertebral bone mass when delivered by daily subcutaneous injection, either as the intact hormone or as the 1–34 amino-acid peptide.[248] In studies in which PTH alone was used during 1 year of therapy, little if any effect was seen on bone mass in the hip. Indeed, total body bone mass declined by ~2%. These changes are probably related to activation of bone remodeling. PTH has also been administered in combination with antiresorptive therapy: Long-term studies in combination with HRT showed marked (15–30%) increases in spinal BMD with accompanying, although smaller, increases in BMD of the hip and in total body bone mass (Fig. 64-6). In two studies, the risk of vertebral fractures appeared to be reduced.[249,249a] Furthermore, a substantial effect of PTH on all non-spine fractures was seen in the larger of these two studies.[249a]

# OTHER FORMS OF PRIMARY OSTEOPOROSIS

## OSTEOPOROSIS IN MEN

Although osteoporosis is more common in women, it is not unusual in men. One-fifth of all hip fractures and approximately one-seventh of all vertebral fractures are seen in men. One in six men has a hip fracture by the age of 90.[7,8] The lower incidence of osteoporosis in men may be attributed to the higher peak bone mass attained (~10% higher) and to the absence of a menopause equivalent in men. Adult men with a history of constitutional delay in puberty have lower radial and spinal bone mineral densities.[250] Overall, when osteoporosis is encountered in a nonelderly man, the two most frequent causes are alcohol abuse and hypogonadism.[43,44,134,135,251] Heavy smoking also is common in young men with osteoporosis. Preliminary data suggest that alendronate therapy might improve bone mass in osteoporotic men.

## JUVENILE OSTEOPOROSIS

Juvenile osteoporosis is a rare, self-limiting disease of prepubertal children.[252] These patients commonly present between the ages of 8 and 14 with the acute onset of back pain secondary to vertebral compression fractures. Spontaneous remission usually occurs after 2 to 6 years. Juvenile osteoporosis must be differentiated from osteogenesis imperfecta, Cushing syndrome, leukemia, and other disorders of bone marrow. Laboratory values are generally normal, as in the adult with osteoporosis. Although the temporal relation of juvenile osteoporosis to puberty implies an endocrine cause, the primary defect is unknown. Biopsy data suggest a relatively uncontrolled activity of metaphyseal osteoclasts.

Analgesic therapy, early mobilization, supportive physical therapy, and preventive measures against further bone loss are used. Currently no treatment approved by the Food and Drug

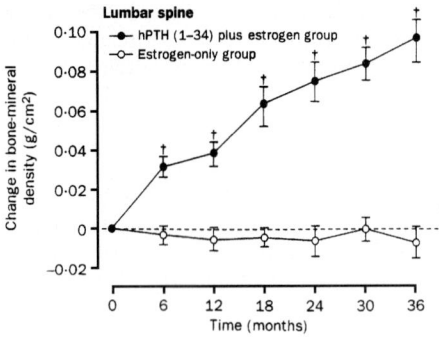

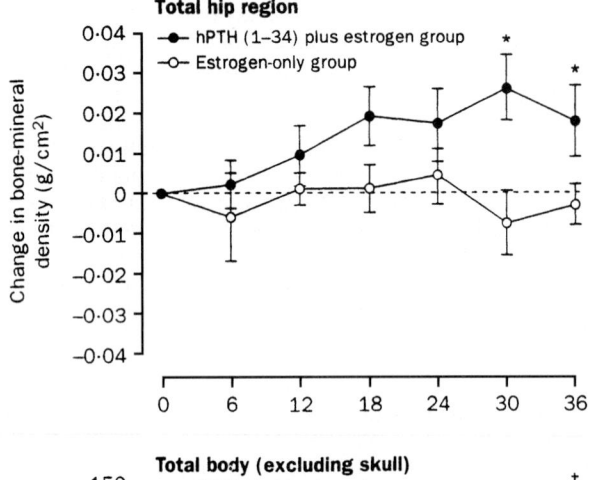

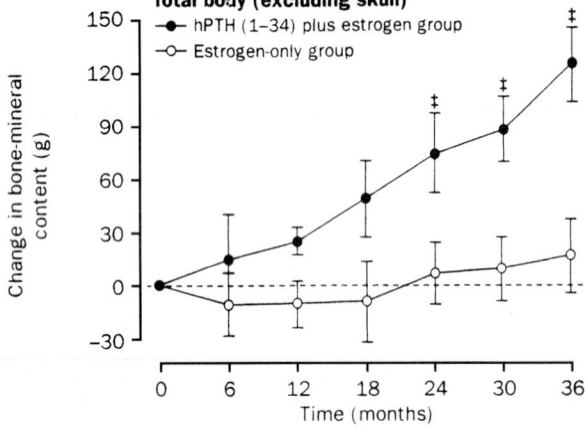

**FIGURE 64-6.** Changes in bone mass during 3 years of therapy for group receiving parathyroid hormone (*hPTH*) plus estrogen and group receiving estrogen only. Level of statistical significance of differences between groups is indicated as follows: †, $p < .02$; *, $p < .001$; ‡, $p < .02$. (Lindsay R, Nieves J, Formica C, et al. Randomized controlled study of effect of parathyroid hormone on vertebral-bone mass and fracture incidence among postmenopausal women on oestrogen with osteoporosis. Lancet 1997; 350:550.)

Administration exists for osteoporosis in children. Sex hormone therapy is not effective (and not advisable), and the use of bisphosphonates[253] should not be recommended because of their long skeletal half-lives.

## IDIOPATHIC OSTEOPOROSIS IN YOUNG ADULTS

Idiopathic osteoporosis, an uncommon condition, occurs between the ages of 30 and 50 and is more frequent in men than in women. The axial skeleton is most severely affected, and vertebral fractures are common. Serum laboratory values are normal, but hypercalciuria and consequent nephrolithiasis are

often seen. The high urinary calcium losses may be associated with mild secondary hyperparathyroidism. The bone histology often shows active remodeling with excessive osteoclast activity or decreased bone formation.[254] Exclusion of a late-onset form of osteogenesis imperfecta, even by biopsy, may be difficult. The treatment of this condition is the same as for other forms of osteoporosis, although it may be more rapidly progressive and disabling.[254,255]

## REGIONAL OSTEOPOROSIS

The classic example of regional osteoporosis is that following disuse or immobilization of a limb. Total immobilization in patients with fractures, motor paralysis, or chronic disabling ailments is associated with rapid and generalized loss of bone. Immobilization is linked to a rapid and significant increase in bone resorption and a slight increase in bone formation followed after a few weeks by a marked reduction in formation. The result is a high-turnover form of osteoporosis characterized by hypercalciuria and hyperphosphaturia.[145–147] Occasionally, especially in the first few weeks, mild hypercalcemia and hyperphosphatemia may develop. The process may be self-limited, and a new steady state may be reached. However, severe bone loss of ~50% of skeletal mass sometimes occurs. Weight-bearing and positive-stress maneuvers may help to decrease the rate of bone loss, but additional vascular, neurogenic, and humoral factors certainly play a role in the process. Radiologic evidence of osteoporosis may appear within 2 months of the immobilization, and a regional distribution over the areas immobilized is characteristic. If the immobilization time is not so prolonged as to result in permanent loss of bone, remineralization can occur on mobilization. Rheumatoid arthritis and infectious arthritis also may produce a localized osteoporosis adjacent to the affected joints (Fig. 64-7). Sometimes, regional osteoporosis occurs without a history of immobilization (Fig. 64-8).

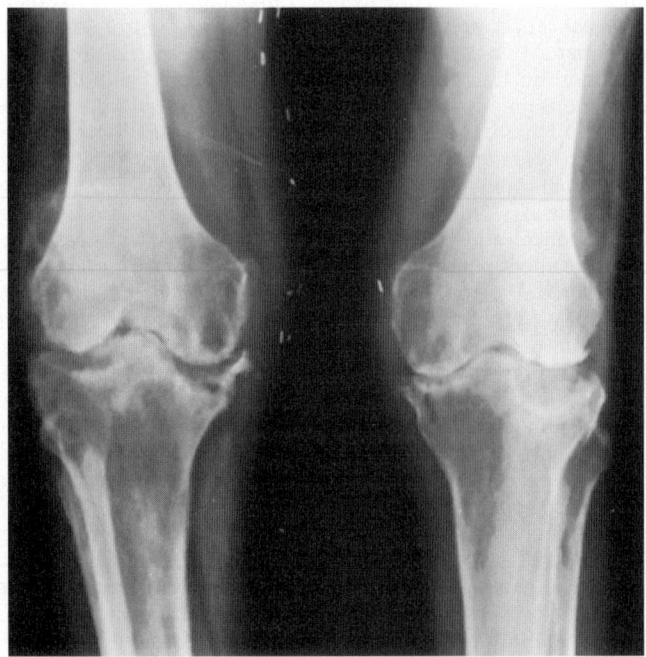

**FIGURE 64-7.** Regional osteoporosis in a 64-year-old man with relative immobilization caused by severe rheumatoid arthritis. Bilateral, symmetric loss of the joint spaces of the knees is seen, with large subcortical bone cysts. Marked juxta-articular osteoporosis is present. The patient had a generalized diminution of bone density on radiography. In such cases, the hypothesis has been that the inflammatory process produces bone-resorbing growth factors. (The patient had saphenous vein surgery related to a coronary artery bypass graft procedure.)

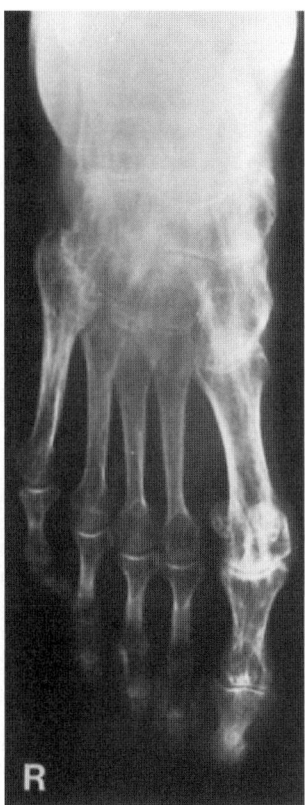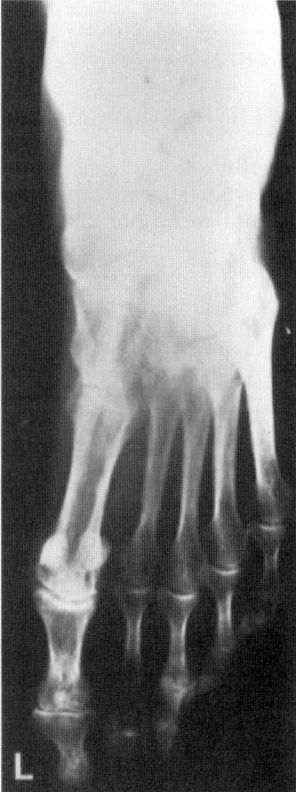

**FIGURE 64-8.** Regional osteoporosis of the right foot of a 57-year-old white woman. The patient had no history of trauma or immobilization of the involved limb, and the cause was obscure. (*R*, right; *L*, left.)

## REFLEX SYMPATHETIC DYSTROPHY

Reflex sympathetic dystrophy (RSD) is a distinct entity that is also called Sudeck atrophy, osteodystrophy, causalgia, acute bony atrophy, posttraumatic osteoporosis, and shoulder-hand syndrome.[256] It follows conditions such as myocardial infarction, trauma, limb surgery, neoplasms, calcific tendinitis, vasculitis, and degenerative disease of the cervical spine. Overactivity of the sympathetic nervous system, with secondarily increased blood flow and activation of sensory fibers, has been suggested as the pathogenetic mechanism.

The clinical picture is variable, although it commonly involves the shoulder and the hand with swelling, vasomotor changes (i.e., spasm or dilatation), and hyperesthesia. The symptoms are usually unilateral, but bilateral involvement can occur. The resolution of swelling and vasomotor changes occurs within several months, with the appearance of skin pigmentation, hyperhidrosis, hypertrichosis, skin and nail atrophic changes, and contracture. These phenomena may persist for years or gradually disappear.

Radiographs and bone density measurements reveal localized osteoporosis, and soft-tissue swelling is evident in RSD patients. Bone resorption is characteristically seen. Radionuclide imaging reveals increased uptake, which is probably related to increased vascularity. Magnetic resonance imaging tests are normal or nonspecific.[257]

Histologic examination reveals accelerated bone resorption with excessive osteoclast activity, and intense synovitis is often evident. Treatment is supportive, although corticosteroids have been useful in alleviating pain and decreasing radionuclide uptake in bones and joints. Calcitonin has been used with good symptomatic response, and attempts have been made to attenuate the sympathetic tone with variable success.[258]

## TRANSIENT OSTEOPOROSIS OF THE HIP

Transient osteoporosis of the hip, first described in patients in the third trimester of pregnancy, was subsequently reported in young and middle-aged men and nonpregnant women.[259] The hip pain begins spontaneously, without an antecedent history of trauma or infection. Radiographic films show osteoporosis of the periarticular bones of the hip joint, especially in the femoral head. No diminution of the joint space occurs. Bone density measurement of the hip may show some localized bone loss. Magnetic resonance imaging and radionuclide bone scan may be valuable in establishing the diagnosis and in follow-up care.[260] The clinical course is self-limited, with complete regression of the radiographic and clinical signs and symptoms within months to 1 year. The cause is unknown, and the treatment is supportive and aimed at symptomatic relief.

## REGIONAL MIGRATORY OSTEOPOROSIS

In the syndrome of regional migratory osteoporosis, local pain and swelling rapidly develop in the ankle, foot, or knee and are accompanied by the radiographic appearance of localized osteoporosis in those areas.[261] Spontaneous recovery occurs after weeks or months, but with recurrence in other regions of the same or opposite extremity. These events may be repeated over a few years. Radionuclide bone scanning reveals increased activity in involved areas. The cause is unknown. The differential diagnosis includes rheumatoid arthritis, but involvement of the joint space is lacking, as is symmetric involvement of multiple joints. Other monoarticular syndromes, such as septic arthritis, pigmented villonodular synovitis, and idiopathic synovial osteochondromatosis, must be considered in the differential diagnosis; however, these conditions follow a course characterized by rapid joint destruction with only minimal secondary osteoporosis.

The treatment of regional migratory osteoporosis is supportive, and includes use of antiinflammatory agents and occasional short courses of glucocorticoids. Calcitonin therapy has been associated with some clinical improvement.

# OTHER OSTEOLYTIC SYNDROMES

A number of rare syndromes can lead to some degree of bone lysis. These osteolytic syndromes can result from infectious, neoplastic, traumatic, metabolic, vascular, congenital, and genetic causes. Hyperparathyroidism and Paget disease can cause significant osteolysis as well.

The most common form of secondary osteoporosis is corticosteroid-induced osteoporosis[262]; however, many other drugs, other endocrinopathies, and genetic diseases produce osteoporotic-like syndromes in which bone mass is reduced sufficiently to increase the risk of fracture. Frequently, secondary forms of osteoporosis coexist with the primary form of the disease. Recognition of the secondary form is important because treatment of the primary condition or elimination of the drug providing the insult to the skeleton can improve the patient's outcome.

## CORTICOSTEROID-INDUCED OSTEOPOROSIS

Corticosteroid-induced osteoporosis is the most common form of secondary osteoporosis. It may also be the presenting sign of Cushing syndrome. In such situations, the clinical onset may be heralded by a cluster of vertebral and rib fractures. Usually, the patient has overt signs of Cushing syndrome. The more common form of corticosteroid-induced osteoporosis occurs in individuals who require long-term pharmacologic doses of steroid.[263] The higher incidence in women of rheumatic diseases that may require corticosteroid therapy (e.g., rheumatoid arthritis, systemic lupus erythematosus [SLE], temporal arteritis, multiple sclerosis), coupled with the relatively compromised skeletal status of the aging female, explains why corticosteroid-induced osteoporosis is more common among women. Nonetheless, corticosteroid-induced osteoporosis can occur in both sexes and in connection with any disorder (e.g., chronic lung disease requiring long-term corticosteroid therapy).

Prospective studies have revealed that bone loss can be rapid, with significant loss occurring within the first 3 to 6 months of therapy. Surprisingly, however, in some individuals bone loss does not occur, even on very high dosages of corticosteroid. In other individuals, bone mass may be lost on prednisone regimens as low as 5 mg per day. Bone loss also occurs in patients with Addison disease on standard corticosteroid-replacement therapy. Corticosteroid-induced bone loss occurs throughout the skeleton but is generally greater in trabecular than in cortical bone. One-third or more of corticosteroid-treated patients have vertebral fractures, and the risk of hip fracture is 50% greater than in controls.

Glucocorticoid excess causes bone loss by several mechanisms. These drugs inhibit the synthesis of bone matrix by the osteoblast and slow down the recruitment of newer osteoblasts. Histomorphometric studies have shown decreased mineral apposition and decreased width of trabecular packets. Osteocalcin levels in the blood are reduced within 1 day of initiation of glucocorticoid therapy and generally remain suppressed for as long as the therapy continues.[264] In addition, bone resorption may be increased. Secondary hyperparathyroidism may be present, for which several potential causes exist: (a) glucocorticoids reduce the efficiency of calcium absorption by a direct effect on the intestinal cells, (b) glucocorticoids may increase obligatory urinary calcium loss, and (c) density of the $1,25(OH)_2D$ receptor in the cell may be reduced. The compensatory secondary hyperparathyroidism that follows is thought to be responsible for accelerating bone loss. In addition, glucocorticoid therapy may reduce circulating levels of estradiol or testosterone through inhibitory effects on the adrenal gland and perhaps also direct effects on the ovary and intestine, exacerbating sex hormone deficiency.

The principles of treatment for glucocorticoid-induced osteoporosis are similar to those for postmenopausal osteoporosis. Limitation of dosage and duration of corticosteroid therapy are important. Alternate-day regimens may be beneficial. Patients on corticosteroids should receive calcium supplementation (1.2 g per day) and vitamin D (800 U per day). Physical activity should be encouraged, if possible, because the adverse effects of immobilization may exacerbate the situation. Whether administration of calcitriol is beneficial remains inconclusive.[265] Controlled clinical trials have demonstrated preservation of bone mass using bisphosphonate therapy. Furthermore, two separate clinical trials (one using daily doses of alendronate and the other, intermittent cyclical therapy with etidronate) showed a decreased risk of vertebral compression deformity in postmenopausal women. Risedronate also increases bone mass and reduces vertebral fracture occurence in women with steroid-induced osteoporosis. HRT therapy may be appropriate for postmenopausal women, provided it is not contraindicated by the primary diagnosis (e.g., SLE).

Patients with corticosteroid-induced osteoporosis perhaps might benefit most from use of an anabolic agent capable of stimulating osteoblast synthesis of new bone. Controlled clinical trials of PTH therapy demonstrated marked increments in bone mass in patients with a variety of rheumatologic disorders who were on baseline treatment with HRT. However, PTH is not currently marketed for use in the United States.

## PRIMARY HYPERPARATHYROIDISM

Although the classic bone disease of primary hyperparathyroidism is osteitis fibrosa cystica, generalized skeletal demineralization without osteitis may be seen. Bone densitometry has uncovered a higher prevalence of subclinical skeletal involvement, usually a preferential loss of cortical bone, in patients with primary hyperparathyroidism[151] (see Chap. 58). Indeed, spinal BMD might be specifically preserved in mild forms of the disorder.

## HYPERTHYROIDISM

Hyperthyroidism consistently increases bone turnover, and mild hypercalcemia occurs in ~10% of cases. Both bone formation and resorption are usually increased. A mild and prolonged hyperthyroid state may aggravate an underlying process of bone loss, and the correction of hyperthyroidism may lead to some restoration of bone mass. Hypothyroidism is prevalent in the elderly, and overreplacement with thyroid hormone may accelerate bone loss and uncover clinical osteoporosis.[266] Because the daily requirements for thyroid hormone may decrease with age, a periodic reassessment of the replacement dose is appropriate in this age group.

## AMENORRHEA AND ANOREXIA NERVOSA

Hypogonadal states are associated with osteoporosis.[267,268] These include primary gonadal disorders, such as in Turner and Klinefelter syndromes, and secondary gonadal failure, as in patients with pituitary tumors and hypothalamic pituitary insufficiency. The latter may be associated with exercise-induced or stress-induced amenorrhea.

Many studies have shown that rapid and profound bone loss occurs with estrogen deficiency in younger women. For example, a 5% to 10% loss in spinal and femoral bone density occurs within 6 months of gonadotropin-releasing hormone agonist therapy.[269] Similarly, rapid bone loss is seen with exercise-induced amenorrhea.[270,271] In patients with anorexia nervosa, bone loss is related to the accompanying amenorrhea but is not fully corrected with estrogen treatment alone, a finding that indicates the importance of nutritional and perhaps genetic factors.[272]

## HYPERPROLACTINEMIA

When hyperprolactinemia is associated with infertility, aggressive management is the rule, and in women, an attempt should be made to restore menses. When fertility is not important, any decision to withhold bromocriptine therapy for a microadenoma should include consideration of the concomitant hypogonadism and the subsequent increased risk of osteoporosis. Moreover, some studies have suggested a direct negative effect of prolactin on bone, independent of the presence of hypogonadism.[273] An oral contraceptive containing estrogen should be given to patients with untreated microadenomas associated with amenorrhea or oligomenorrhea.

## TYPE 1 (INSULIN-DEPENDENT) DIABETES

A reduction in bone mass is seen in patients with type 1 (insulin-dependent) diabetes mellitus.[274] This may become detectable as early as 2 to 3 years after the onset of clinical diabetes. A similar reduction in bone mass is not usually seen in diabetes mellitus type 2. Hypercalciuria is common in type 1 diabetics, but plasma levels of PTH and vitamin D metabolites are generally normal. Subtle changes have been reported in some patients, however, suggesting a relative deficiency of vitamin D metabolites and possibly calcium malabsorption. Insulin deficiency may reduce bone formation by means of diminished synthesis of collagen by the osteoblasts. In patients with type 1 diabetes, hypercalciuria and reduced tubular reabsorption of phosphate are improved by strict glucose control.

## ACROMEGALY

Osteoporosis in patients with acromegaly is related in part to a concomitant hypogonadal state. Nevertheless, a unique form of high-turnover bone disease, which predominantly affects cortical bone, appears to be connected to the increased serum levels of growth hormone (presumably mediated through insulin-like growth factors).[275] Radiographically, new periosteal bone formation and a characteristic increased anteroposterior diameter of the vertebral bodies, with significant osteophyte formation, are noted. In the absence of hypogonadism, trabecular bone involvement is uncommon. Hyperphosphatemia, a well-known feature of acromegaly, probably results from growth hormone–induced stimulation of renal tubular reabsorption of phosphate. Growth hormone also stimulates the production of $1,25(OH)_2D$ and directly stimulates calcium absorption, both of which may lead to hypercalciuria.[276]

## OSTEOGENESIS IMPERFECTA

Osteogenesis imperfecta is a common heritable disorder of bone, found in 1 of 20,000 live births. This disease can be diagnosed by a skin biopsy followed by fibroblast culture and collagen analysis. A blood test for certain genotypes is also available. There may be forms of the disease (tarda) that do not manifest abnormalities until later in life. Other phenotypic features can include blue sclerae, arcus senilis, and dental and hearing disorders. The disappearance of sex hormone protection with the menopause may cause a second rise in fracture incidence among women with the disorder; these women may benefit from HRT.[277]

## OTHER GENETIC DISORDERS

Other genetic disorders involving defective collagen synthesis or collagen cross-linking may be associated with osteoporosis. These include *homocystinuria, Ehlers-Danlos syndrome, Marfan syndrome,* and *Menkes syndrome* (Fig. 64-9). Congenital anemias that cause bone marrow hyperplasia, such as *thalassemia* and *sickle cell anemia,* frequently are accompanied by osteoporosis. *Glycogen storage diseases, hypophosphatasia, hemochromatosis,* and *familial dysautonomia* (i.e., Riley-Day syndrome) are associated with osteoporosis (see Chap. 66).

## ALCOHOLISM

An association is seen between marked alcohol consumption and the development of osteoporosis. Whether mild or moderate alcohol consumption is associated with a negative effect on

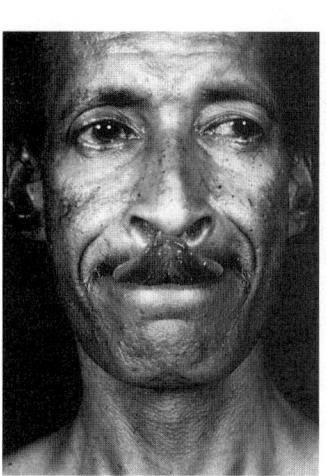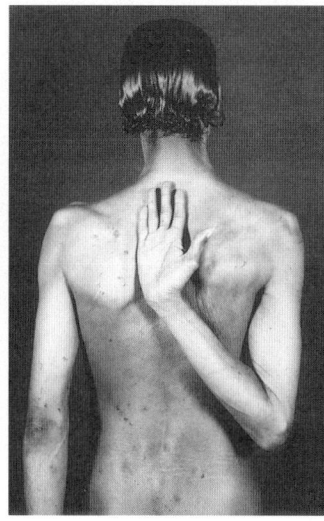

**FIGURE 64-9.** A 46-year-old man with Ehlers-Danlos syndrome, a heritable connective tissue disorder. The patient had marked osteoporosis. The patient had soft and atrophic skin that was hyperextensible and marked hypermobility of the joints.

the skeleton is unknown; one large study suggested that such an intake is not detrimental.[277a] Alcohol abuse can cause calcium and vitamin D malabsorption secondary to pancreatic or liver disease and may inhibit calcium absorption directly. It may also result in hypercalciuria through a direct renal effect. The poor nutritional habits of alcoholics frequently result in low calcium intake. Alterations in liver function may produce abnormalities in vitamin D metabolism, with reduced 25(OH)D and $1,25(OH)_2D$ levels. PTH secretion or function may be impaired directly by ethanol or indirectly by concomitant hypomagnesemia. Moreover, gonadal function is often impaired in alcoholics, with deficient testosterone production in men.

Alcohol appears to exert a direct, toxic depressant effect on osteoblast function. Several studies have demonstrated a reduction in skeletal mass (mostly in trabecular bone) in alcoholics. Some histologic studies have found evidence of osteomalacia, although this usually occurs in the presence of gross malnutrition. In "healthier" alcohol abusers, bone histology shows a profound reduction in bone formation and resorption, which strongly suggests a direct effect of alcohol on bone cells.

## MULTIPLE MYELOMA AND OTHER MALIGNANCIES

Multiple myeloma is often associated with generalized osteoporosis. Spinal crush fractures, back pain, and diffuse skeletal demineralization seen on radiographic films are often the initial clinical features of the illness. The production of osteoclast-activating factors (or humoral hypercalcemic factors) by plasma cells may mediate the demineralization. Diffuse osteoporosis may also occur as a result of bone marrow infiltration by carcinoma cells from other malignancies. Moreover, the use of chemotherapeutic agents such as methotrexate and other antimetabolites has been associated with the development of osteoporosis.[278]

## PREGNANCY AND LACTATION

A specific and rare syndrome of osteoporosis has been associated with pregnancy and lactation, during which fractures may occur.[279] Pregnancy and lactation are generally periods during which calcium is passed from the mother to the fetus and infant. The skeleton of the newborn infant contains almost 30 g of calcium; another 40 g are passed on through the milk of the mother over 3 months of lactation. However, pregnancy is accompanied by regulatory defense mechanisms, including increased calcium absorption and possibly increased calcitonin secretion. Whether similar mechanisms occur during lactation is unknown, but maternal skeletal mass may increase during pregnancy in preparation for the calcium demands of lactation.[280] Nulliparity and prolonged lactation are often cited as risk factors for osteoporosis. In the osteoporosis syndrome that develops during pregnancy and lactation, a deficiency of $1,25(OH)_2D$ has been suggested. Bone histology studies have not revealed evidence for osteomalacia or an increase of bone turnover. The syndrome is self-limiting, and fractures may not occur over prolonged periods of follow-up despite subsequent pregnancies.

## GASTROINTESTINAL DISEASE

A variety of gastrointestinal diseases are associated with osteoporosis and osteomalacia due to malabsorption of calcium or vitamin D. Whether osteoporosis or osteomalacia dominates depends on the severity of the malabsorption process. Subtotal gastrectomy, particularly of the Billroth II type, is associated with the development of osteomalacia and osteoporosis in 5% to 10% of cases many years after the surgery. The mechanism may be that of calcium malabsorption, similar to that which occurs with achlorhydria and old age. The role of *lactase deficiency* with milk intolerance and resultant calcium deficiency may also be important in the development of osteoporosis.

## OBSTRUCTIVE LIVER DISEASE

Chronic obstructive liver disease may interfere with the enterohepatic circulation of vitamin D metabolites and predispose the patient to osteomalacia.[281] Osteoporosis, more often than osteomalacia, is associated with primary biliary cirrhosis, and histomorphometric studies reveal inactive remodeling with depressed bone formation.

## HEPARIN-INDUCED OSTEOPOROSIS

Chronic heparin administration (15,000 U or more daily) for 6 months or longer has been associated with the development of osteoporosis and increased fractures.[282] The changes may be reversible with cessation of therapy. Heparin activates lysosomal bone resorption as shown in vitro. It may also inhibit bone formation. Moreover, *systemic mastocytosis* has been associated with generalized demineralization in this disorder. Abnormally proliferating mast cells are thought to produce heparin, although a role for histamine and other mediators has not been excluded.[283]

## ANTICONVULSANT THERAPY

Diphenylhydantoin has been associated with a syndrome of osteomalacia that is thought to be related to abnormal vitamin D metabolism in the liver.[284] A smaller effect has also been reported with phenobarbital. Phenytoin and carbamazepine may also have more subtle direct effects on bone cells, resulting in osteopenia, particularly in the hip region. Increases in the markers of bone formation and resorption have been seen.[285]

## REFERENCES

1. Consensus development conference: prophylaxis and treatment of osteoporosis. Osteoporos Int 1991; 1:114.
2. Peck WA. Consensus development conference: diagnosis, prophylaxis, and treatment of osteoporosis. Am J Med 1993; 94:646.
3. Melton LJ III. How many women have osteoporosis now? J Bone Miner Res 1995; 10:175.
4. Melton LJ III, Riggs BL. Epidemiology of age-related fractures. In: Avioli LV, ed. The osteoporotic syndrome. New York: Grune & Stratton, 1987:1.
5. Chalmers J, Ho KC. Geographical variations in senile osteoporosis. The association with physical activity. J Bone Miner Res 1970; 52B:667.
6. Wallace WA. The increasing incidence of fractures of the proximal femur: an orthopedic epidemic. Lancet 1983; 1:1413.
7. Cooper C, Melton LJ. Epidemiology of osteoporosis. Trends Endocrinol Metab 1992; 3:224.
8. Kanis JA, McCloskey EV. Epidemiology of vertebral osteoporosis. Bone 1992; 13(Suppl 2):S1.
9. Riggs BL, Melton LJ III. Medical progress: involutional osteoporosis. N Engl J Med 1986; 314:1676.
10. Richelson LS, Wahner HW, Melton LJ III, Riggs BL. Relative contribution of aging and estrogen deficiency to postmenopausal bone loss. N Engl J Med 1985; 311:1273.
11. Cummings SR, Black DM, Nevitt MC, et al. Bone density at various sites for prediction of hip fractures. Lancet 1993; 341:72.
12. Ross PD, Davis JW, Vogel JM, Wasnich RD. A critical review of bone mass and the risk of fractures in osteoporosis. Calcif Tissue Int 1990; 46:149.
13. Dempster DW, Lindsay R. Pathogenesis of osteoporosis. Lancet 1993; 341:797.
14. Kelsey JL, Browner WS, Seeley DG, et al. Risk factors for fractures of the distal forearm and proximal humerus. Am J Epidemiol 1992; 135:477.
15. Ross PD, Davis JW, Epstein RS, Wasnich RD. Pre-existing fractures and bone mass predict vertebral fracture incidence in women. Ann Intern Med 1991; 114:919.
16. Cummings SR. Treatable and untreatable risk factors for hip fracture. Bone 1996; 18(Suppl 3):165S.
17. Ross PD, Genant HK, Davis J, et al. Predicting vertebral fracture incidence from prevalent fractures and bone density in older women. Osteoporos Int 1993; 3:120.
18. Sowers MR, Galuska DA. Epidemiology of bone mass in premenopausal women. Epidemiol Rev 1993; 15:374.
19. Sambrook N, Kelly PJ, White CP, et al. Genetic determinants of bone mass. In: Marcus R, Feldman D, Kelsey J, eds. Osteoporosis. San Diego: Academic Press, 1996:477.
20. Southard R, Morris J, Mahan J, et al. Bone mass in healthy children measurement with quantitative DXA. Radiology 1991; 179:735.
21. Katzman DK, Bachrach LK, Carter DR, Marcus R. Clinical and anthropometric correlates of bone mineral acquisition in healthy adolescent girls. J Clin Endocrinol Metab 1991; 73:1332.
22. Bonjour JP, Theintz G, Buchs B, et al. Critical years and stages of puberty for spinal and femoral bone mass accumulation during adolescence. J Clin Endocrinol Metab 1991; 73:555.
23. Gilsanz V, Boechat I, Roe TF, et al. Gender differences in vertebral body sizes in children and adolescents. Radiology 190; 1994:673.
24. Gilsanz V, Roe TF, Mora S, et al. Changes in vertebral bone density in black girls and white girls during childhood and puberty. N Engl J Med 1991; 325:1597.
25. Matkovic V, Fontana D, Tominac C, et al. Factors that influence peak bone mass formation: a study of calcium balance and the inheritance of bone mass in adolescent females. Am J Clin Nutr 1990; 52:878.
26. Bonjour JP, Rizzoli R. Bone acquisition in adolescence In: Marcus R, Feldman D, Kelsey J, eds. Osteoporosis. San Diego: Academic Press, 1996:477.
27. Steinberg KK, Frein-Titulaer LW, DePuey EG, et al. Sex steroids and bone density in premenopausal and perimenopausal women. J Clin Endocrinol Metab 1989; 69:533.
28. Sowers MF. Premenopausal reproductive and hormonal characteristics and the risk for osteoporosis. In: Marcus R, Feldman D, Kelsey J, eds. Osteoporosis. San Diego: Academic Press, 1996:477.
29. Sowers M, Crutchfield M, Bandekar R, et al. Bone mineral density and its change in pre- and perimenopausal white women: the Michigan bone health study. J Bone Miner Res 1998; 13(7):1134.
30. Meema HE. Cortical bone atrophy and osteoporosis as a manifestation of aging. AJR Am J Roentgenol 1963; 89:1287.
31. Mazess RB, Mather W. Bone mineral content of North Alaskan Eskimos. Am J Clin Nutr 1974; 27:916.
32. Parfitt AM. Skeletal heterogeneity and the purposes of bone remodeling: implications for the understanding of osteoporosis. In: Marcus R, Feldman D, Kelsey J, eds. Osteoporosis. San Diego: Academic Press, 1996:477.
33. Heaney RP, Recker RR, Saville PD. Menopausal changes in bone remodeling. J Lab Clin Med 1978; 92:964.
34. Eriksen EF. Normal and pathological remodeling of human trabecular bone: three dimensional reconstruction of the remodeling sequence in normals and in metabolic disease. Endocr Rev 1986; 4:379.
35. Parfitt AM. Age-related structural changes in trabecular and cortical bone: cellular mechanism and biomechanical response. Calcif Tissue 1984; 36:8123.
36. Chiodini I, Carnevale V, Torlontano M, et al. Alterations of bone turnover and bone mass at different skeletal sites due to pure glucocorticoid excess: study in eumenorrheic patients with Cushing's syndrome. J Clin Endocrinol Metab 1998; 83(6):1863.
37. Krempien B, Lemminger FM, Ritz E, Weber E. The reaction of different skeletal sites to metabolic bone disease—a micromorphometric study. Klin Wochenschr 1978; 56:755.
38. Heaney RP, Recker RR, Saville PD. Menopausal changes in calcium balance. J Lab Clin Med 1978; 92:953.
39. Hui SL, Zhou L, Evans R, et al. Rates of growth and loss of bone mineral in the spine and femoral neck in white females. Osteoporos Int 1999; 9:200.
40. Johnston CC Jr, Hui SL, Witt RM, et al. Early menopausal changes in bone mass and sex steroids. J Clin Endocrinol Metab 1985; 61:905.
41. Kusec V, Virdi AS, Prince R, Triffitt JT. Localization of estrogen receptor-α in human and rabbit skeletal tissues. J Clin Endocrinol Metab 1998; 83(7):2421.
42. Onoe Y, Miyaura C, Ohta H, Nozawa S, Suda T. Expression of estrogen receptor β in rat bone. Endocrinology 1997; 138:4509.
43. Arts J, Kuiper GGJM, Janssen JMMF, et al. Differential expression of estrogen receptors α and β mRNA during differentiation of human osteoblast SV-HFO cells. Endocrinology 1997; 138:5067.
44. Mundy GR, Boyce BF, Yoneda T, et al. Cytokines and bone remodeling. In: Marcus R, Feldman D, Kelsey J, eds. Osteoporosis. San Diego: Academic Press, 1996:477.
45. Horowitz MC. Cytokines and estrogens in bone: anti-osteoporotic effects. Science 1993; 260:626.
46. Girasole G, Jilka RL, Passeri G, et al. 17β-estradiol inhibits interleukin-6 production by bone marrow derived stromal cells and osteoblasts in vitro: a potential mechanism for the antiosteoporotic effect of estrogens. J Clin Invest 1992; 89:883.
47. Cheleuitte D, Mizuno S, Glowacki J. In vitro secretion of cytokines by human bone marrow: effects of age and estrogen status. J Clin Endocrinol Metab 1998; 83:2043.
48. Cohen-Solal ME, Boitte F, Bernard-Poenaru O, et al. Increased bone resorbing activity of peripheral monocyte culture supernatants in elderly women. J Clin Endocrinol Metab 1998; 83:1687.
49. Chen MM, Yeh JK, Aloia JF. Anabolic effect of prostaglandin E$_2$ in bone is not dependent on pituitary hormones in rats. Calcif Tissue Int 1998; 63:236.
50. Kodama Y, Takeuchi Y, Suzawa M, et al. Reduced expression of interleukin-11 in bone marrow stroma cells of senescence-accelerated mice (SAMP6): relationship to osteopenia with enhanced adipogenesis. J Bone Miner Res 1998; 13:1370.
51. Shimizu T, Mehdi R, Yoshimura Y, et al. Sequential expression of bone morphogenetic protein, tumor necrosis factor, and their receptors in bone-forming reaction after mouse femoral marrow ablation. Bone 1998; 23:127.
52. Raisz LG. Local and systemic factors in the pathogenesis of osteoporosis. N Engl J Med 1988; 318:818.

53. Pacifici R, Rifas L, Teitelbaum S, et al. Spontaneous release of interleukin-1 from human blood monocytes reflects bone formation in idiopathic osteoporosis. Proc Natl Acad Sci U S A 1987; 84:4616.

54. Pacifici R, Brown C, Puscheck E, et al. Effect of surgical menopause and estrogen replacement on cytokine release from human blood mononuclear cells. Proc Natl Acad Sci U S A 1991; 88:514.

55. Gowen M, Wood DD, Ihrie EJ, et al. An interleukin-1 like factor stimulates bone resorption in vitro. Nature 1989; 306:378.

56. Stock JL, Coderre JA, MacDonald B, Rosenwasser LJ. Effects of estrogen in vivo and in vitro on spontaneous interleukin-1 release by monocytes from postmenopausal women. J Clin Endocrinol Metab 1989; 68:364.

57. Jilka RL, Hangoe G, Girasole G. Increased osteoclast development after estrogen loss: mediation by interleukin-6. Science 1992; 257:88.

58. Matsuzaki K, Udagawa N, Takahashi N, et al. Osteoclast differentiation factor (ODF) induces osteoclast-like cell formation in human peripheral blood mononuclear cell cultures. Biochem Biophys Res Commun 1998; 246:199.

59. Mizuno A, Amizuka N, Irie K, et al. Severe osteoporosis in mice lacking osteoclastogenesis inhibitory factor/osteoprotegerin. Biochem Biophys Res Commun 1998; 247:610.

60. Yasuda H, Shima N, Nakagawa N, et al. Osteoclast differentiation factor is a ligand for osteoprotegerin/osteoclastogenesis-inhibitory factor and is identical to TRANCE/RANKL. Proc Natl Acad Sci U S A 1998; 95:3597.

61. Turner RT, Riggs BL, Spelsberg TC. Skeletal effects of estrogen. Endocr Rev 1994; 15:275.

62. Uebelhart D, Schlemmer A, Johansen JS, et al. Effect of menopause and hormone replacement therapy on the urinary excretion of pyridinium crosslinks. J Clin Endocrinol Metab 1991; 72:367.

63. Hassager C, Fabbri-Mabelli G, Christiansen C. The effect of the menopause and hormone replacement therapy on serum carboxyterminal propeptide of type I collagen. Osteoporos Int 1993; 3:50.

64. Calvo MS, Eyre DR, Gundberg CM. Molecular basis and clinical application of biological markers of bone turnover. Endocr Rev 1996; 17(4):333.

65. Hansen M. Assessment of age and risk factors on bone density and bone turnover in healthy premenopausal women. Osteoporos Int 1994; 4:123.

66. Mazzuoli G, Minisola S, Valtorta C, et al. Changes in mineral content and biochemical bone markers at the menopause. Isr J Med Sci 1985; 21:875.

67. Stepan JJ, Pospichal J, Presl J, Pacovsky V. Bone loss and biochemical indices of bone remodeling in surgically induced postmenopausal women. Bone 1987; 8:279.

68. Seibel MJ, Cosman F, Shen V, et al. Urinary hydroxypyridinium crosslinks of collagen as markers of bone resorption and estrogen efficacy in postmenopausal osteoporosis. J Bone Miner Res 1993; 8:881.

69. Garnero P, Sornay-Rendu E, Chapuy MC, Delmas PD. Increased bone turnover in late postmenopausal women is a major determinant of osteoporosis. J Bone Miner Res 1996; 11(3):337.

70. Cosman F, Nieves J, Wilkinson C, et al. Bone density change and biochemical indices of skeletal turnover. Calcif Tissue Int 1996; 58:236.

71. Blumsohn A, Eastell R. The performance and utility of biochemical markers of bone turnover: do we know enough to use them in clinical practice? Ann Clin Biochem 1997; 34:449.

72. Rosen CJ, Chesnut III CH, Mallinak NJS. The predictive value of biochemical markers of bone turnover for bone mineral density in early postmenopausal women treated with hormone replacement or calcium supplementation. J Clin Endocrinol Metab 1997; 82(6):1904.

73. Hannon R, Blumsohn A, Naylor K, Eastell R. Response of biochemical markers of bone turnover to hormone replacement therapy: impact of biological variability. J Bone Miner Res 1998; 13(7):1124.

74. Schott AM, Cormier C, Hans D, et al. How hip and whole-body bone mineral density predict hip fracture in elderly women: the EPIDOS prospective study. Osteoporos Int 1998; 8:247.

75. Cummings SR, Black DM, Nevitt MC, et al. Bone density at various sites for prediction of hip fractures. Lancet 1993; 341:72.

76. Wasnich RD, Ross PD, Heilburn LK, et al. Prediction of postmenopausal fracture risk with use of bone mineral measurements. Am J Obstet Gynecol 1985; 153:745.

77. Melton LJ III, Atkinson EJ, O'Fallon WM, et al. Long-term fracture prediction of bone mineral assessed at different sites. J Bone Miner Res 1993; 10:1227.

78. Wasnich RD, Ross PD, Heilbrun LK, Vogel JM. Prediction of postmenopausal fracture risk with use of bone mineral measurements. Am J Obstet Gynecol 1985; 153:745.

79. Nevitt MC, Johnell O, Black DM, et al. For the Study of Osteoporotic Fractures Research Group. Bone mineral density predicts non-spine fractures in very elderly women. Osteoporos Int 1994; 4:325.

80. Gardsell P, Johnell O, Nilsson BE. Predicting fractures in women by using forearm bone densitometry. Calcif Tissue Int 1989; 44:235.

81. Hui SL, Slemenda CW, Johnston CC. Baseline measurements of bone mass predict fracture in white women. Ann Intern Med 1989; 111:355.

82. Dempster DW, Shane E, Horbett W, Linday R. A simple method for correlative light and scanning electron microscopy of human iliac crest bone biopsies: qualitative observations in normal and osteoporotic subjects. J Bone Miner Res 1986; 1:15.

83. Garnero P, Hausherr E, Chapuy MC, et al. Markers of bone resorption predict hip fracture in elderly women: the EPIDOS prospective study. J Bone Miner Res 1996; 11:1531.

84. Van Daele PLA, Seibel MJ, Burger H, et al. Case-control analysis of bone resorption markers, disability, and hip fracture risk: The Rotterdam Study. BMJ 1996; 312:482.

85. Akesson K, Ljunghall S, Jonsson B, et al. Assessment of biochemical markers of bone metabolism in relation to the occurrence of fracture: a retrospective and prospective population-based study of women. J Bone Miner Res 1995; 10:1823.

86. Ross PD, Wasnich RD, Knowlton WK. Skeletal alkaline phosphatase (Tandem©-R Ostase©) measurements predict vertebral fractures: a prospective study. (Abstract). J Bone Miner Res 1997; 12(Suppl 1):S150.

87. Delmas PD. The role of markers of bone turnover in the assessment of fracture risk in postmenopausal women. Osteoporos Int 1998; 8(Suppl 1):S32.

88. Looker AC, Wahner HW, Dunn WL, et al. Updated data on proximal femur bone mineral levels of US adults. Osteoporos Int 1998; 8:468.

89. Riggs BL, Melton LJ III. Evidence for two distinct syndromes of involutional osteoporosis. Am J Med 1983; 75:899.

90. Cummings SR, Browner WS, Bauer D, et al. For the Study of Osteoporotic Fractures Research Group. Endogenous hormones and the risk of hip and vertebral fractures among older women. N Engl J Med 1998; 339:733.

91. Ettinger B, Pressman A, Sklarin P, et al. Associations between low levels of serum estradiol, bone density, and fractures among elderly women: the Study of Osteoporotic Fractures. J Clin Endocrinol Metab 1998; 83:2239.

92. Smith EP, Boyd J, Frank GR, et al. Estrogen resistance caused by a mutation in the estrogen-receptor gene in a man. N Engl J Med 1994; 331:1056.

93. Center JR, Nguyen TV, White CP, Eisman JA. Male osteoporosis predictors: sex hormones and calcitropic hormones. J Bone Miner Res 1997; 12(S1):S368.

94. Nordin BEC, Need AG, Morris HA, et al. Evidence for a renal calcium leak in postmenopausal women. J Clin Endocrinol Metab 1991; 72(2):401.

95. Sakhaee K, Nicar MJ, Glass K, Pak CYC. Postmenopausal osteoporosis as a manifestation of renal hypercalciuria with secondary hyperparathyroidism. J Clin Endocrinol Metab 1985; 61:368.

96. Coe FL, Canterbury JM, Firpo JJ, Reiss E. Evidence for secondary hyperparathyroidism in idiopathic hypercalciuria. J Clin Invest 1973; 52:134.

97. Heaney RP. A unified concept of osteoporosis. Am J Med 1965; 39:377.

98. Cosman F, Shen V, Xie F, Seibel M, et al. Estrogen protection against bone resorbing effects of parathyroid hormone infusion: assessment by use of biochemical markers. Ann Intern Med 1993; 118:337.

99. Kanis JK, ed. Osteoporosis. London: Blackwell Healthcare Communications, 1997.

100. Eddy DM, Johnston CC Jr, Cummings SR, et al. Osteoporosis: review of the evidence for prevention, diagnosis, and treatment and cost-effectiveness analysis. Osteoporos Int 1998; 8(Suppl 4):S1.

101. Cummings SR, Nevitt MC, Browner WS, et al. For the Study of Osteoporotic Fractures Research Group. Risk factors for hip fracture in white women. N Engl J Med 1995; 332:767.

102. Johnell O, Gullberg B, Kanis JA, et al. Risk factors for hip fracture in European women—the MEDOS study. J Bone Miner Res 1995; 10(11):1802.

103. Dargent-Molina P, Favier F, Grandjean H, et al. For the EPIDOS Study Group. Fall-related factors and risk of hip fracture: the EPIDOS prospective study. Lancet 1996; 348:145.

104. Cummings SR, Kelsey JL, Nevitt MC, O'Dowd KJ. Epidemiology of osteoporosis and osteoporotic fractures. Epidemiol Rev 1985; 7:178.

105. Lindsay R. Estrogen deficiency. In: Riggs BL, Melton III LJ, eds. Osteoporosis. Philadelphia: Lippincott–Raven Publishers, 1995:133.

106. Farmer ME, White LR, Brody JA. Race and sex differences in hip fracture incidence. Am J Public Health 1984; 74:1374.

107. Garn SM. Population differences and family line differences in cortical thickness. In: The earlier gain and the later loss of cortical bone, in nutritional perspective. Springfield, IL: Charles C Thomas, 1970.

108. Seeman E, Hopper JL, Bach LA, et al. Reduced bone mass in daughters of women with osteoporosis. N Engl J Med 1989; 320:554.

109. Lutz J. Bone mineral, serum calcium and dietary intakes of mother/daughter pairs. Am J Clin Nutr 1986; 44:99.

110. Tylavsky FA, Bortz AD, Hancock R, Anderson JJB. Familial resemblance of radial bone mass between premenopausal mothers and their college-age daughters. Calcif Tissue Int 1989; 45:265.

111. Ross PD, Davis JW, Epstein RS, Wasnich RD. Pre-existing fractures and bone mass predict vertebral fracture incidence in women. Ann Intern Med 1991; 114:919.

112. Lloyd T, Andon MD, Rollings N, et al. Calcium supplementation and bone mineral density in adolescent girls. JAMA 1993; 270:841.

113. Johnston CC Jr, Miller JZ, Slemenda CW, et al. Calcium supplementation and increases in bone mineral density in children. N Engl J Med 1992; 327:82.

114. Matkovic V, Fontana D, Tominac C, et al. Factors which influence peak bone mass formation: a study of calcium balance and the inheritance of bone mass in adolescent females. Am J Clin Nutr 1990; 52:878.

115. Kanders B, Dempster DW, Lindsay R. Interaction of calcium, nutrition, and physical activity on bone mass in young women. J Bone Miner Res 1988; 3:145.

116. Baran D, Sorensen A, Grimes J, et al. Dietary modification with dairy products for preventing vertebral bone loss in premenopausal women: a three year prospective study. J Clin Endocrinol Metab 1989; 70:264.

117. Elders PJM, Netelendo JC, Lips P, et al. Calcium supplementation reduces vertebral bone loss in postmenopausal women: a controlled trial in 248

women between 46 and 55 years of age. J Clin Endocrinol Metab 1991; 73:533.

118. Heaney RP. Calcium intake requirement and bone mass in the elderly. J Lab Clin Med 1982; 100:309.

119. Holbrook TL, Barrett-Connor E, Wingard DL. Dietary calcium and risk of hip fracture: 14 year prospective population study. Lancet 1988; 2:1046.

120. Dawson-Hughes B, Dallal GE, Krall EA, et al. A controlled trial of the effect of calcium supplementation on bone density in postmenopausal women. N Engl J Med 1990; 323:878.

121. Tillyard MW, Spears GFS, Thomson J, Dovey S. Treatment of postmenopausal osteoporosis with calcitriol or calcium. N Engl J Med 1992; 326.

122. Recker RR, Hinders S, Davies KM, et al. Correcting calcium nutritional deficiency prevents spine fractures in elderly women. J Bone Miner Res 1996; 11:1961.

123. Aloia JF, Vaswani A, Yeh JK, et al. Calcium supplementation with and without hormone replacement therapy to prevent postmenopausal bone loss. Ann Intern Med 1994; 120:97.

124. Reid IR, Ames RW, Evans MC, et al. Long-term effects of calcium supplementation on bone loss and fractures in postmenopausal women. A randomized controlled trial. Am J Med 1995; 98:331.

125. Chapuy MC, Arlot ME, Duboeuf F, et al. Vitamin D$_3$ and calcium to prevent hip fractures in elderly women. N Engl J Med 1992; 327:1637.

126. Kanis JA, Johnell O, Gullberg B, et al. Evidence for efficacy of drugs affecting bone metabolism in preventing hip fracture. BMJ 1992; 305:1124.

127. Dawson-Hughes B, Dallal GE, Krall EA, et al. A controlled trial of the effect of calcium supplementation on bone density in postmenopausal women. N Engl J Med 1990; 323:878.

128. Parfitt AM, Gallagher JC, Heaney RP, et al. Vitamin D and bone health in the elderly. Am J Clin Nutr 1982; 36:1014.

129. O'Dowd KJ, Clemens TL, Kelsey JL, Lindsay R. Exogenous calciferol (vitamin D) and vitamin D endocrine status among elderly nursing home residents in the New York City area. J Am Geriatr Soc 1993; 41:414.

130. Nieves J, Cosman F, Herbert J, et al. High prevalence of vitamin D deficiency and reduced bone mass in multiple sclerosis. Neurology 1994; 44:1687.

131. Thomas MK, Lloyd-Jones DM, Thadhani RI, et al. Hypovitaminosis D in medical inpatients. N Engl J Med 1998; 338:777.

132. Komar L, Nieves J, Cosman F, et al. Calcium homeostasis of an elderly population upon admission to a nursing home. J Am Geriatr Soc 1993; 41:1057.

133. Tsai KS, Heath HH III, Kumar R, Riggs BL. Impaired vitamin D metabolism with aging in women: possible role in pathogenesis of senile osteoporosis. J Clin Invest 1984; 73:1668.

134. Silverberg SJ, Shane E, de la Cruz L, et al. Abnormalities in parathyroid hormone secretion and 1,25-dihydroxyvitamin D formation in women with osteoporosis. N Engl J Med 1989; 320(5):277.

135. Villareal DT, Civitelli R, Chines A, Avioli LV. Subclinical vitamin D deficiency in postmenopausal women with low vertebral bone mass. J Clin Endocrinol Metab 1991; 72:628.

136. Khaw K, Sneyd M, Compston J. Bone density, parathyroid hormone and 25-hydroxyvitamin D concentrations in middle aged women. BMJ 1992; 305:273.

137. Nordin BEC, Need AG, Morris HA, Horowitz M. The nature and significance of the relationship between urinary sodium and urinary calcium in women. J Nutr 1993; 123:1615.

138. Heaney RP, Recker RR. Effects of nitrogen, phosphorus and caffeine on calcium balance in women. J Lab Clin Med 1982; 99:46.

139. Barrett-Connor E, Chang JC, Edelstein SL, et al. Coffee-associated osteoporosis offset by daily milk consumption: the Rancho Bernardo study. JAMA 1994; 271:280.

140. Bikle DD, Genant HK, Cann C, et al. Bone disease in alcohol abuse. Ann Intern Med 1985; 103:42.

141. Peris P, Pares A, Guanabens N, et al. Reduced spinal and femoral bone mass and deranged bone mineral metabolism in chronic alcoholics. Alcohol Alcohol 1992; 27:619.

142. Seeman E. The effects of tobacco and alcohol use on bone. In: Marcus R, Feldman D, Kelsey J, eds. Osteoporosis. San Diego: Academic Press, 1996:477.

143. Hopper JL, Seeman E. Bone density in twins discordant for tobacco use. N Engl J Med 1994; 330:387.

144. Hirota Y, Hirohata T, Fukuda K. Association of intake, cigarette smoking and occupational status with the risk of idiopathic osteonecrosis of the femoral head. Am J Epidemiol 1993; 137:530.

145. Krolner B, Toft B. Vertebral bone loss: an unheeded side-effect of therapeutic bed rest. Clin Sci 1983; 64:537.

146. Mazess RB, Whedon JD. Immobilization and bone. Calcif Tissue Int 1983; 35:265.

147. Vogel JM, Whittle MW. Bone mineral changes; the second manned Skylab mission. Aviat Space Environ Med 1976; 47:396.

148. Huddleson AL, Rockwell D, Kurland DN, Harrison B. Bone mass in lifetime tennis athletes. JAMA 1980; 244:1107.

149. Krolner B, Toft B, Nielsen SP, Tondevold E. Physical exercise as prophylaxis against involutional vertebral bone loss: a controlled trial. Clin Sci 1983; 64:541.

150. Smith EL, Reddan W, Smith PE. Physical activity and calcium modalities for bone mineral increase in aged women. Med Sci Sports Exerc 1981; 13:60.

151. Gutin B, Kasper MJ. Can vigorous exercise play a role in osteoporosis prevention? A review. Osteoporos Int 1992; 2:55.

152. Krall EA, Dawson-Hughes B. Walking is related to bone density and rates of bone loss. Am J Med 1994; 96:20.

153. Greendale GA, Barrett-Connor E. Outcomes of osteoporotic fractures. In: Marcus R, Freedman D, Kelsey J, eds. Osteoporosis. San Diego: Academic Press, 1996.

154. Ensrud KE, Black DM, Harris F, et al. Correlates of kyphosis in older women. The fracture intervention trial research group. J Am Geriatr Soc 1997; 45(6):682.

155. Finsen V. Osteoporosis and back pain among the elderly. Acta Med Scand 1998; 223:443.

156. Bergenudd H, Nilson B, Uden A, Wilner S. Bone mineral content, gender, body posture, and build in relation to back pain in middle age. Spine 1989; 14:577.

157. Nicholson PT, Haddaway MW, Davie MWJ, Evans SF. Vertebral deformity, bone mineral density, back pain, and height loss in unscreened women over 50 years. Osteoporos Int 1993; 3:300.

158. Leidig G, Minne HW, Sauer P, et al. A study of complaints and their relation to vertebral destruction in patients with osteoporosis. Bone Miner 1990; 8:217.

159. Lyles KW, Gold DT, Shipp KM, et al. Association of osteoporotic vertebral compression fractures with impaired functional status. Am J Med 1993; 94:595.

160. Mossey JM, Mutran E, Knott K, Craik R. Determinants of recovery 12 months after hip fracture: the importance of psychosocial factors. Am J Public Health 1989; 79(3):279.

161. US Congress, Office of Technology Assessment. Hip fracture outcomes in people age 50 and over—background paper OTA-BP-H-120. Washington: US Government Printing Office, 1994.

162. Miller CW. Survival and ambulation following hip fracture. J Bone Joint Surg 1978; 60-A:930.

163. Marottoli RA, Berkman LF, Cooney LM. Decline in physical function following hip fracture. J Am Geriatr Soc 1992; 40:861.

164. Greendale GA, Barrett-Connor E. Outcomes of osteoporotic fractures. In: Marcus R, Freedman D, Kelsey J, eds. Osteoporosis. San Diego: Academic Press, 1996.

165. White BL, Fisher WD, Laurin CA. Rate of mortality for elderly patients after fracture of the hip in the 1980s. J Bone Joint Surg 1987; 69-A:1335.

166. Poor G, Atkinson EJ, O'Fallon WM, Melton LJ III. Determinants of reduced survival following hip fractures in men. Clin Orthop 1995; 319:260.

167. Kaukonen JP, Karaharju EO, Porras M, et al. Functional recovery after fracture of the distal forearm. Ann Chir Gynaecol 1988; 77:27.

168. Gartland JJ, Werley CW. Evaluation of healed Colles fractures. J Bone Joint Surg 1951; 33A:895.

169. Field J, Warwick D, Bannister GC, et al. Long-term prognosis of displaced Colles fracture: a 10 year prospective review. Injury 1992; 23:529.

170. Altissimi M, Antenucci R, Fiacca C, et al. Long-term results of conservative treatment of fractures of the distal radius. Clin Orthop Relat Res 1986; 206:202.

171. Stevenson JC, Marsh MS, Lindsay R. An atlas of osteoporosis, 2nd ed. London: Parthenon Publishing Group, 1999.

172. National Osteoporosis Foundation. Physician's guide to prevention and treatment of osteoporosis. Belle Mead, New Jersey: Excerpta Medica, 1998.

173. Chow R, Harrison JE, Notarius C. Effect of two randomized exercise programs on bone mass of healthy postmenopausal women. BMJ 1987; 295:1441.

174. Friedlander AL, Genant HK, Sadowsky S, et al. A two-year program of aerobics and weight training enhances bone mineral density of young women. J Bone Miner Res 1995; 10:574.

175. Grove KA, Londeree BR. Bone density in postmenopausal women: high impact vs. low impact exercise. Med Sci Sports Exerc 1992; 24:1190.

176. Hatori M, Hasegawa A, Adachi H, et al. The effects of walking at the anaerobic threshold level on vertebral bone loss in postmenopausal women. Calcif Tissue Int 1993; 52:411.

177. Nelson ME, Fiatarone MA, Morganti CM, et al. Effects of high-intensity strength training on multiple risk factors for osteoporotic fractures. A randomized controlled trial. JAMA 1994; 272:1909.

178. Simkin A, Ayalon J, Leichter I. Increased trabecular bone density due to bone-loading exercises in postmenopausal osteoporotic women. Calcif Tissue Int 1987; 40:59.

179. Snow-Harter C, Bouxsein ML, Lewis BT, et al. Effects of resistance and endurance exercise on bone mineral status of young women: a randomized exercise intervention trial. J Bone Miner Res 1992; 7:761.

180. Bassey EJ, Ramsdale SJ. Weight-bearing exercise and ground reaction forces: a 12-month randomized controlled trial of effects on bone mineral density in healthy postmenopausal women. Bone 1995; 16:469.

181. Sinaki M, Wahner HW, Offord DP, Hodgson SF. Efficacy of nonloading exercises in prevention of vertebral bone loss in postmenopausal women: a controlled trial. Mayo Clin Proc 1989; 64:762.

182. Dalsky GP, Stocke KS, Ehsani AA, et al. Weight-bearing exercise training and lumbar bone mineral content in postmenopausal women. Ann Intern Med 1998; 108:824.

183. Eastell R. Drug therapy: treatment of postmenopausal osteoporosis. N Engl J Med 1998; 338:736.

184. Lindsay R. Prevention and treatment of osteoporosis. Lancet 1993; 341:801.

185. Lindsay R, Hart DM, Forrest C, Baird C. Prevention of spinal osteoporosis in oophorectomized women. Lancet 1980; 2:1151.

186. Albright F. The effect of hormones on osteogenesis in man. Recent Prog Horm Res 1947; 1:293.

187. Lindsay R, Aitken JM, Anderson JB, et al. Long-term prevention of postmenopausal osteoporosis by estrogen. Lancet 1976; 1(7968):1038.

188. Lindsay R, Hart DM, Purdie P, et al. Comparative effects of estrogen and a progestogen on bone loss in postmenopausal women. Clin Sci Mol Med 1978; 54:193.

189. Christiansen C, Rodbro P. Does postmenopausal bone loss respond to estrogen replacement therapy independent of bone loss rate? Calcif Tissue 1983; 35:720.

190. Christiansen C, Christiansen MS, McNair P. Prevention of early postmenopausal bone loss: conducted 2 years study in 315 normal females. Eur J Clin Invest 1980; 10:273.

191. Davis ME, Lanzl LH, Cos AB. Detection, prevention and retardation of postmenopausal osteoporosis. Obstet Gynecol 1970; 36:187.

192. Robert R, Recker K, Davies M, et al. The effect of low-dose continuous estrogen and progesterone therapy with calcium and vitamin D on bone in elderly women. Ann Intern Med 1999; 130:897.

193. Lufkin EG, Wahner HW, O'Fallon WM, et al. Treatment of postmenopausal osteoporosis with transdermal estrogen. Ann Intern Med 1992; 117:1.

194. Paganini-Hill A, Ross RK, Gerkins VR, et al. Menopausal estrogen therapy and hip fractures. Ann Intern Med 1981; 95:28.

195. Hutchinson TA, Polansky JM, Fienstein AR. Postmenopausal oestrogens protect against fracture of hip and distal radius. Lancet 1979; 2(8145):705.

196. Kreiger N, Kelsey JL, Holford TR. An epidemiological study of hip fracture in postmenopausal women. Am J Epidemiol 1982; 116:141.

197. Weiss NS, Szekely DR, Dallas R, et al. Endometrial cancer in relation to patterns of menopausal estrogen use. JAMA 1979; 242:261.

198. Ettinger B, Genant HK, Cann CE. Long-term estrogen therapy prevents bone loss and fracture. Ann Intern Med 1985; 102:319.

199. Komulainen MH, Kroger H, Tuppurainen MT, et al. HRT and vitamin D in prevention of non-vertebral fractures in postmenopausal women; a 5 year randomized trial. Maturitas 1998; 13:45.

200. Burch JC, Byrd BF, Vaughn WK. The effects of long-term estrogen on hysterectomized women. Am J Obstet Gynecol 1974; 118:778.

201. Kiel DP, Felson DT, Anderson JJ. Hip fracture and the use of estrogens in postmenopausal women. N Engl J Med 1987; 317:1169.

202. Williams AR, Weiss NS, Ure C, et al. Effect of weight, smoking, and estrogen use on the risk of hip and forearm fractures in postmenopausal women. Obstet Gynecol 1982; 60:695.

203. Cauley JA, Seeley DG, Ensrud K, et al. For the Study of Osteoporotic Fractures Research Group. Estrogen replacement therapy and fractures in older women. Ann Intern Med 1995; 122:9.

204. Hulley S, Grady D, Bush T, et al. Randomized trial of estrogen plus progestin for secondary prevention of coronary heart disease in postmenopausal women. Heart and Estrogen/progestin Replacement Study (HERS) Research Group. JAMA 1998; 280:605.

205. Barrett-Connor E. Postmenopausal estrogen and prevention bias. Ann Intern Med 1991; 115:455.

206. Horsman A, Gallagher JC, Simpson M, Nordin BEC. Prospective trial of estrogen and calcium in postmenopausal women. BMJ 1977; 2:789.

207. Lindsay R, Hart DM, Clark DM. The minimum effective dose of estrogen for prevention of postmenopausal bone loss. Obstet Gynecol 1984; 63:759.

208. Nachtigall LE, Nachtigall RH, Nachtigall RD. Estrogen replacement therapy I: a 10-year prospective study in the relationship to osteoporosis. Obstet Gynecol 1979; 53:277.

209. Quigley MET, Martin PL, Burnier AM, Brooks P. Estrogen therapy arrests bone loss in elderly women. Am J Obstet Gynecol 1987; 156:1516.

210. Recker RR, Saville PD, Heaney RP. The effect of estrogens and calcium carbonate on bone loss in postmenopausal women. Ann Intern Med 1977; 87:649.

211. Riggs BL, Jowsey J, Kelly PJ, et al. Effect of sex hormones on bone in primary osteoporosis. J Clin Invest 1969; 48:1065.

212. Meema S, Bunker ML, Meema HE. Preventive effect of estrogen on postmenopausal bone loss. Arch Intern Med 1975; 135:1436.

213. Riis B, Thomsen K, Strom V, Christiansen C. The effect of percutaneous estradiol and natural progesterone on postmenopausal bone loss. Am J Obstet Gynecol 1987; 156:61.

214. Jensen GF, Christiansen C, Transbol I. Treatment of postmenopausal osteoporosis: a controlled therapeutic trial comparing estrogen/gestagen, 1,25-dihydroxy-vitamin $D_3$ and calcium. Clin Endocrinol 1982; 16:515.

215. Ettinger B, Genant HK, Cann CE. Postmenopausal bone loss is prevented by treatment with low-dosage estrogen and calcium. Ann Intern Med 1978; 106:40.

216. Khosla S, Melton LJ 3rd, Atkinson EJ, et al. Relationship of serum sex steroid levels and bone turnover markers with bone mineral density in men and women: a key role for bioavailable estrogen. J Clin Endocrinol Metab 1998; 83(7):2266.

217. Cummings SR, Browner WS, Bauer D, et al. Endogenous hormones and the risk of hip and vertebral fractures among older women. N Engl J Med 1998; 339(11):733.

218. Ravnikar VA. Compliance with hormone replacement therapy: are women receiving the full impact of hormone replacement therapy preventive health benefits? Women's Health Issues 1992; 2:75.

219. Ettinger B. Overview of estrogen replacement therapy: a historical perspective. Proc Soc Exp Biol Med 1998; 217:2.

220. Genant HK, Lucas J, Weiss S, et al. Low-dose esterified estrogen therapy: effects on bone, plasma estradiol concentrations, endometrium, and lipid levels. Estratab Osteoporosis Study Group. Arch Intern Med 1997; 157:2609.

221. Arnold JS, Bartley MH, Tont SA, Jenkins DP. Effects of hormone therapy on bone mineral density: results from the Postmenopausal Estrogen/Progestin Interventions (PEPI) trial. The Writing Group for the PEPI Trial. JAMA 1996; 276:1389.

222. Nieves JW, Komar L, Cosman F, Lindsay R. Interaction between antiresorptive therapy and calcium intake: review and analysis. Am J Clin Nutr 1998; 67:18.

223. Speroff L, Rowan J, Symons J, et al. The comparative effect on bone density, endometrium, and lipids of continuous hormones as replacement therapy (CHART Study). A randomized controlled trial. JAMA 1996; 276:1397.

224. Santoro NF, Nananda F, Eckman MH, et al. Therapeutic controversy. Hormone replacement therapy—where are we going? J Clin Endocrinol Metab 1999; 84:1798.

225. Henderson VW. The epidemiology of estrogen replacement therapy and Alzheimer's disease. Neurology 1997; 48:S27.

226. Yaffe K, Sawaya G, Lieberburg I, Grady D. Estrogen therapy in postmenopausal women: effects on cognitive function and dementia. JAMA 1998; 279:688.

227. Paganini-Hill A. Does estrogen replacement therapy protect against Alzheimer's disease? Osteoporos Int 1997; 7(Suppl 1):S12.

228. Haskell SG, Richardson ED, Horwitz RI. The effect of estrogen replacement therapy on cognitive function in women: a critical review of the literature. J Clin Epidemiol 1997; 50:1249.

229. Collaborative Group on Hormonal Factors in Breast Cancer. Breast cancer and hormone replacement therapy: collaborative re-analysis of data from 51 epidemiological studies of 52,705 women with breast cancer and 108,411 women without breast cancer. Lancet 1997; 350:1047.

230. Papapoulos S. Bisphosphonates. Pharmacology and use in the treatment of osteoporosis. In: Marcus R, Freedman D, Kelsey J, eds. Osteoporosis. San Diego: Academic Press, 1996:1209.

230a. Harris SJ, Watts NB, Jackson RD, et al. Four year study of intermittent cyclic etidronate treatment of postmenopausal osteoporosis: three years of blinded treatment followed by one year of open treatment. Am J Med 1993; 95:557.

231. Liberman UA, Weiss SR, Broll J. Effect of oral alendronate on bone mineral density and the incidence of fractures in postmenopausal osteoporosis. N Engl J Med 1995; 333:1437.

232. Black DM, Cummings SR, Karpf DB. Randomised trial of effect of alendronate on risk of fracture in women with existing vertebral fractures. Lancet 1996; 348:1535.

233. Cummings SR, Black DM, Thompson DE, et al. Effect of alendronate on risk fracture in women with low bone density but without vertebral fractures. JAMA 1998; 280:2077.

234. Peter CP, Handt LK, Smity SM. Esophageal irritation due to alendronate sodium tablets: possible mechanisms. Dig Dis Sci 1998; 43:1998.

235. De Grouen PC, Lubbe DF, Hirsch LJ, et al. Esophagitis associated with the use of alendronate. N Engl J Med 1996; 35:1016.

236. Harris ST, Watts NB, Genant HK, et al. Effects of risedronate treatment on vertebral and nonvertebral fractures in women with postmenopausal osteoporosis. A randomized controlled trial. JAMA 1999; 282:14.

237. Miller P, Roux C, McClung M, et al. Risedronate reduces hip fractures in patients with low femoral neck bone mineral density. Arthritis & Rheumatism 1999; 42:2.

238. Ettinger B, Pressman A, Schein J, et al. Alendronate use among 812 women: prevalence of gastrointestinal complaints, noncompliance with patient instructions, and discontinuation. J Managed Care Pharm 1998:488.

239. Chestnut CH III, Silverman S, Andriano K, et al., for the PROOF Study Group. A randomized trial of nasal spray salmon calcitonin in postmenopausal women with established osteoporosis: the prevent recurrence of osteoporotic fractures study. Am J Med 2000; 109:267.

240. Cosman F, Lindsay R. Selective estrogen receptor modulators: clinical spectrum. Endocr Rev 1999; 20:418.

241. Fisher B, Costantino JP, Wickerham DL, et al. Tamoxifen for prevention of breast cancer: report of the National Surgical Adjuvant Breast and Bowel Project P-1 Study. J Natl Cancer Inst 1998; 90:1371.

242. Powles TJ, Hickish T, Kanis JA, et al. Effect of tamoxifen on bone mineral density measured by dual energy x-ray absorptiometry in healthy premenopausal and postmenopausal women. J Clin Oncol 1996; 14:78.

243. Delmas PD, Ensrud KE, Harris S, et al. Raloxifene therapy for 3 years reduces the risk of incident vertebral fractures in postmenopausal women. Paper presented at: 26th European Symposium on Calcified Tissues; 1999; The Netherlands.

244. Cummings SR, Eckert S, Krueger KA, et al. The effect of raloxifene on risk of breast cancer in postmenopausal women. Results from the MORE randomized trial. JAMA 1999; 281:2189.

245. Riggs BL, O'Fallon WM, Lane A, et al. Clinical trial of fluoride therapy in postmenopausal osteoporotic women: extended observations and additional analysis. J Bone Miner Res 1994; 9:265.

246. Kleerekoper M, Mendlovic DB. Sodium fluoride therapy of postmenopausal osteoporosis. Endocr Rev 1993; 14:312.

247. Pak CYC, Sakhaee K, Piziak V, et al. Slow-release sodium fluoride in the management of postmenopausal osteoporosis. A randomized clinical trial. Ann Intern Med 1994; 120:625.

248. Cosman F, Lindsay R. Is parathyroid hormone a therapeutic option for osteoporosis? Calcif Tissue 1998; 62:475.

249. Lindsay R, Nieves JW, Formica C, et al. Randomized controlled study of effect of parathyroid hormone on vertebral bone mass and fracture incidence among postmenopausal women on estrogen with osteoporosis. Lancet 1997; 350:550.

249a. Neer R. Recombinant human PTH reduces the risk of spine and non-spine fractures in psotmenopausal osteoporosis. Toronto, Canada: Endocrine Society 2000.

250. Finklestein JS, Neer RM, Biller BMK, et al. Osteopenia in men with history of delayed puberty. N Engl J Med 1992; 326:600.

251. Jackson JA, Kleerekoper M. Osteoporosis in men: diagnosis, pathophysiology and prevention. Medicine (Baltimore) 1990; 69:137.

252. Teotia M, Teotia SPS, Singh RK. Idiopathic juvenile osteoporosis. Am J Dis Child 1979; 133:894.

253. Hoekman J, Papapoulos SE, Peters ACB, Bijvoet OLM. Characteristics and bisphosphonate treatment of a patient with juvenile osteoporosis. J Clin Endocrinol Metab 1985; 61:952.

254. Zerwekh JE, Sakhaee K, Breslau NA, et al. Impaired bone formation in male idiopathic osteoporosis: further reduction in the presence of concomitant hypercalciuria. Osteoporos Int 1992; 2:128.

255. Ljunghalls S, Johansson AG, Burmen P, et al. Low levels of insulin-like growth factor I (IGF-I) in male patients with idiopathic osteoporosis. J Intern Med 1992; 232:59.

256. Kozin F, McCarty DJ, Simms J, Genant H. The reflex sympathetic dystrophy syndrome. I. Clinical and histologic studies: evidence for bilaterality, response to corticosteroid and articular movement. Am J Med 1976; 60:321.

257. Koch E, Hofer HO, Sialer G, et al. Failure of MR imaging to detect reflex sympathetic dystrophy of the extremities. AJR Am J Roentgenol 1991; 56(1):113.

258. Ford SR, Forrest WH Jr, Eltherington L. The treatment of reflex sympathetic dystrophy with intravenous regional bretylium. Anesthesiology 1988; 66:137.

259. Schils J, Piraino D, Richmond BJ, et al. Transient osteoporosis of the hip: clinical and imaging features. Cleve Clin J Med 1992; 59:483.

260. Potter H, Moran M, Schneider R, et al. Magnetic resonance imaging in the diagnosis of transient osteoporosis of the hip. Clin Orthop 1992; 280:223.

261. Kim SM, Desai AG, Krakovitz M, et al. Scintigraphic evaluation of regional migratory osteoporosis. Clin Nucl Med 1989; 14:36.

262. Lukert BP, Raisz LG. Glucocorticoid-induced osteoporosis: pathogenesis and management. Ann Intern Med 1990; 112:352.

263. Meunier PJ. Is steroid induced osteoporosis preventable? N Engl J Med 1993; 323:1781.

264. Cosman F, Nieves J, Herbert J, et al. High dose glucocorticoids in multiple sclerosis patients exert direct effects on the kidney and skeleton. J Bone Miner Res 1994; 9:1097.

265. Tillyard MW, Spears GFS, Thomson J, Dovey S. Treatment of postmenopausal osteoporosis with calcitriol or calcium. N Engl J Med 1992; 326.

266. Greenspan SL, Greenspan FS. The effect of thyroid hormone on skeletal integrity. Ann Intern Med 1999; 130:750.

267. Shore RM, Chesney RW, Mazess RB, et al. Skeletal demineralization in Turner syndrome. Calcif Tissue Int 1982; 34:519.

268. Smith DAS, Walker MS. Changes in plasma steroids in bone density in Klinefelter syndrome. Calcif Tissue Int 1977; 22(Suppl):225.

269. Rico H, Arnanz F, Revilla M. Total and regional bone mineral content in women treated with GnRH agonists. Calcif Tissue Int 1993; 52:354.

270. Warren MP. Amenorrhea in endurance runners. J Clin Endocrinol Metab 1992; 75:393.

271. Slemenda CW, Johnson CC. High intensity activities in young women: site-specific bone mass effects among female figure skaters. Bone Miner 1993; 20:125.

272. Rigotti NA, Neer RM, Skates SJ, et al. The clinical course of osteoporosis in anorexia nervosa: a longitudinal study of cortical bone mass. JAMA 1991; 265:1133.

273. Schlechte JA, Sherman B, Martin R. Bone density in amenorrheic women with and without hyperprolactinemia. J Clin Endocrinol Metab 1983; 56:1120.

274. Soejima K, Landing BH. Osteoporosis in juvenile-onset diabetes mellitus: morphometric and comparative studies. Pediatr Pathol 1986; 6:289.

275. Riggs BL, Randall RV, Wahner HW, et al. The nature of the metabolic bone disorder in acromegaly. J Clin Endocrinol Metab 1972; 34:911.

276. Gray RW, Garthwaite TL. Activation of renal 1,25-dihydroxyvitamin D synthesis by phosphate deprivation: evidence for a role of growth hormone. Endocrinology 1983; 116:1989.

277. Paterson CR, McAllion S, Stellman JL. Osteogenesis imperfecta after the menopause. N Engl J Med 1984; 310:1694.

277a. Ganry O, Baudoin C, Fardellone P. Effect of alcohol intake on bone mineral density in elderly women: The EPIDOS study. Am J Epidemiol 2000; 151:773.

278. Schwartz AM, Leonides JC. Methotrexate osteopathy. Skeletal Radiol 1984; 11:13.

279. Smith R, Stevenson JC, Winearls CJ, et al. Osteoporosis of pregnancy. Lancet 1985; 1:1178.

280. Hillman L, Sateesna S, Haussler M, et al. Control of mineral homeostasis during lactation: interrelationships of 25-hydroxyvitamin D, 24,25-dihydroxy D, 1,25-dihydroxy D, parathyroid hormone, calcitonin, prolactin, and estradiol. Am J Obstet Gynecol 1981; 139:471.

281. Long RG, Meinhard E, Skinner RK, et al. Clinical, biochemical, and histological studies of osteomalacia, osteoporosis, and parathyroid function in chronic liver disease. Gut 1978; 19:85.

282. Avioli LV. Heparin-induced osteopenia: an appraisal. Adv Exp Med Biol 1975; 52:375.

283. Chines A, Pacifici R, Avioli LV, et al. Systemic mastocytosis presenting as osteoporosis: a clinical and histomorphologic study. J Clin Endocrinol Metab 1991; 72:140.

284. Hahn TJ, Hendin BA, Scharp CR, et al. Serum 25-hydroxycalciferol levels and bone mass in children on chronic anticonvulsant therapy. N Engl J Med 1975; 292:550.

285. Valimaki MJ, Tiihone M, Laitinen K, et al. Bone mineral density measured by dual energy x-ray absorptiometry and novel markers of bone formation and resorption in patients on antiepileptic drugs. J Bone Miner Res 1994; 9:631.

# CHAPTER 65

# PAGET DISEASE OF BONE

ETHEL S. SIRIS

Paget disease of bone is a localized disorder of skeletal remodeling in which abnormally increased rates of both bone resorption and new bone formation change bone architecture. Typically, pagetic bone shows a characteristic radiographic appearance (Fig. 65-1). The affected bone is often larger, generally less compact, more vascular, and more susceptible to deformity and fracture than normal bone. Paget disease occurs predominantly in persons older than 40 years, affecting men slightly more often than women. In the United States, up to 2% to 3% of the population in their 50s and 60s have this bone disease, and the frequency rises in the ensuing decades.[1a] Most patients are asymptomatic, although a significant minority do experience signs and symptoms related to the area of involved bone, the degree of increased bone turnover, and the structural changes that result at affected sites.

## ETIOLOGY

The precise etiology of Paget disease remains unknown; genetic and environmental—specifically viral—factors play a role. Geographic and ethnic epidemiologic data document the common occurrence of Paget disease in some parts of the world and its rarity in others. Earlier studies had indicated that Paget disease was present in 4% to 5% of older Britons.[1] A focus of the disorder occurred in the Lancashire area, where as many as 8% of the older population showed radiographic evidence of this condition.[2] Interestingly, more recent epidemiologic studies from the United Kingdom and New Zealand suggest both a decreasing frequency and decreasing severity of the disease.[2a,2b] Nonetheless, it is relatively common in those countries, as well as in Australia and throughout western Europe (with the exception of Scandinavia, where it is infrequently seen).[3] The disorder is uncommon in both southern Asia (i.e., the Indian subcontinent), eastern Asia (i.e., China, Japan), and sub-Saharan Africa. In the United States, it occurs primarily in people of Anglo-Saxon or European descent but is seen in blacks, although apparently to a smaller degree than in whites.[4]

Paget disease is often present in more than one member of a family; this is noted in up to 40% of cases.[5–7] This value may be an underestimate, because many patients with the condition never know they have it. Early studies analyzing pedigrees of several affected kindreds suggest autosomal dominant inheritance.[8] Familial aggregation studies in the United States indicate that first-degree relatives of patients with Paget disease have seven times the risk of developing it than do persons without such a family history. The risk increases if the affected relative had deforming disease or was younger than 50 years old when the disease was diagnosed.[9] Linkage of Paget disease to HLA is not conclusive.[10–13] Specific susceptibility loci for Paget disease may occur on chromosome 18q, the apparent site of the gene responsible for a similar but rare bone dysplasia called *familial expansile osteolysis*.[14] Studies have reported some families with

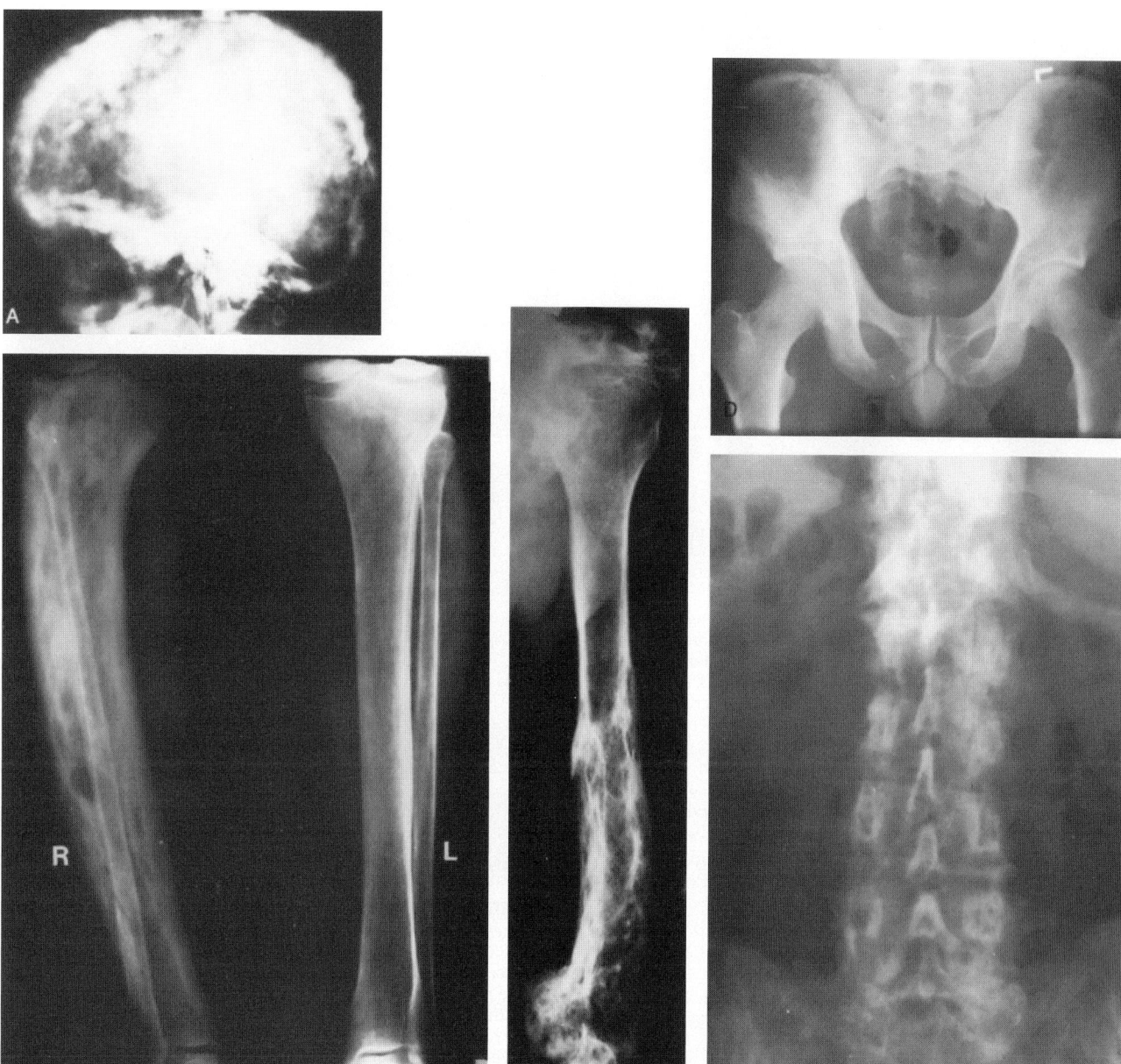

**FIGURE 65-1.** Radiographic findings in pagetic bone. **A,** Typical "cotton wool" appearance of the skull. Areas of extensive blastic change are present, and the cortex of the bone is markedly thickened. **B,** A normal left tibia and fibula contrasted with a pagetic, bowed right tibia. The affected tibia is larger, has areas of increased density as well as localized hyperlucent foci, and is bowed. **C,** Evidence of the localized nature of Paget disease, showing a normal proximal half of the humerus with pagetic involvement in the entire distal half. A sharp line of demarcation exists between normal and involved bone at the midshaft point. This radiograph also demonstrates the poor architectural quality of the pagetic bone. **D,** Relatively early changes of Paget disease in the right hemipelvis include thickening of the ilioischial and iliopectineal lines as well as sclerosis in the ilium and ischium, in contrast to the normal findings in the left hemipelvis. **E,** Extensive Paget disease involving the entire lumbosacral spine (and visible pelvis), with marked coarsening of trabecular markings. Secondary degenerative changes with loss of disc spaces are seen as well. (*R*, right; *L*, left.) (**A** through **C** from Siris ES, Canfield RE, Jacobs TP. Paget's disease of bone. Bull N Y Acad Med 1980; 56:285.)

Paget disease that display genetic linkage to this site,[15,16] but such linkage has not been found in others.[16] Genetic heterogeneity is very likely.

Another area of research to elucidate the etiology of Paget disease involves the possible role of one or more viral agents. At sites of active Paget disease, osteoclasts are abnormally increased in both number and size, containing up to 20 times the usual number of nuclei per cell.[17] Initial studies described viral nucleocapsid–like structures in both the nuclei and cytoplasm of pagetic osteoclasts[18,19] (Fig. 65-2). Such virus-like inclusions are not found in osteoclasts in normal bone, although they have been reported in other bone diseases such as osteopetrosis.[20] Some subsequent studies using immunofluorescence techniques detected nucleocapsid protein antigens of both measles and respiratory syncytial

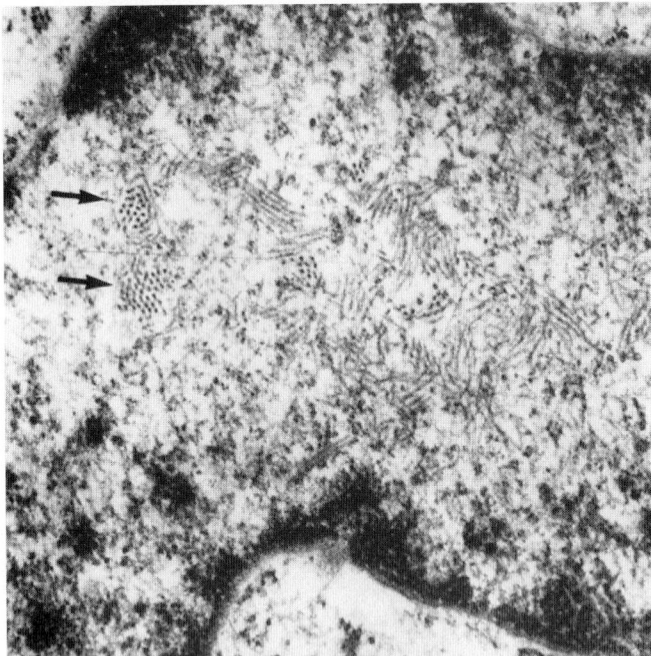

**FIGURE 65-2.** Electron micrograph showing the characteristic inclusions seen in an osteoclast nucleus from pagetic bone. A paracrystalline arrangement of ~12.5-nm filaments is noted (*arrows*). Scattered, nonoriented filaments throughout the karyoplasm are also seen. The filaments are not membrane bound or attached to any nuclear structure. ×80,000 (Courtesy of Dr. Barbara Mills.)

virus antigens in these cells,[21,22] whereas others implicated canine distemper virus.[23] Each of these is one of the paramyxoviruses, a group of viruses for which the members promote the fusion of infected cells and the formation of multinucleated giant cells.[24] Conflicting results have emerged, however, when RNA extraction and polymerase chain reaction techniques have been used to search for viral identification in tissue from pagetic patients.[25–29] Thus, a role for a viral cause as at least part of the etiology of Paget disease is suggested, but clearly not proven.

Measles virus transcripts have been detected in both bone marrow mononuclear cells[28] and in peripheral blood cells,[29] including both osteoclast precursors and more primitive hematopoietic stem cells. Because Paget disease is a localized process, the ubiquitous finding of osteoclast precursors bearing evidence of measles virus throughout the circulation is puzzling. One possible approach to explaining this comes from the observation that increased concentrations of interleukin-6 are produced by pagetic osteoclasts and that they express high levels of interleukin-6 receptor on their surfaces.[30,31] This suggests that interleukin-6 is an autocrine/paracrine factor that influences and enhances osteoclast activity. Perhaps such cytokines in the marrow microenvironment may influence the differentiation of osteoclast precursors, limiting the extent of pagetic involvement to localized sites once the initial lesion occurs. However, how that initial lesion is established is unknown.

## PATHOLOGY

The initial abnormality in Paget disease is a marked increase in the rate of bone resorption at localized sites, mediated by large and numerous pagetic osteoclasts. In response to the increased bone resorption, large numbers of osteoblasts are recruited to these sites and promote a compensatory increase in new bone formation. The osteoblasts probably are inherently normal, although a possible pathologic role for these cells in the initiation of the pagetic process has not been completely excluded.

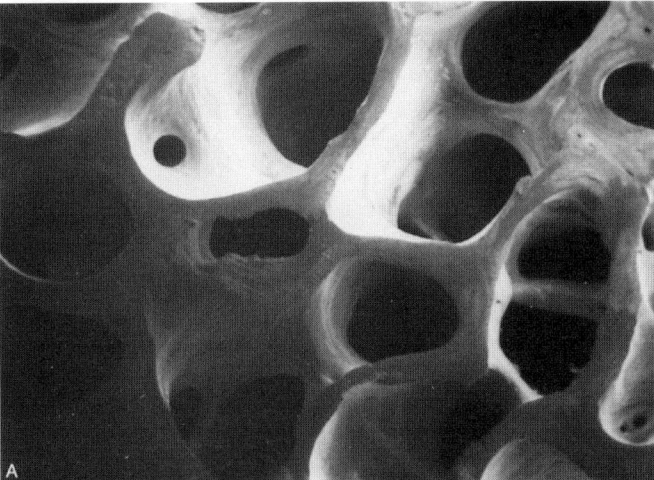

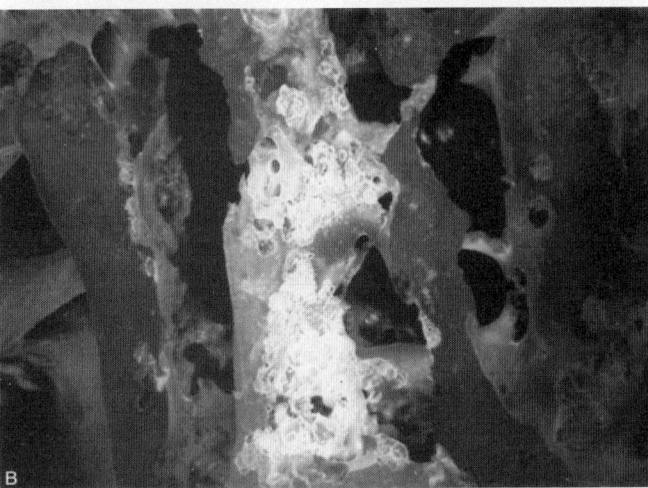

**FIGURE 65-3.** Scanning electron micrographs of trabecular bone from iliac crest biopsies taken from a normal person (**A**) and from a patient with Paget disease (**B**). The normal biopsy specimen consists of a honeycomb-like network of trabecular plates and cylinders surrounding the marrow cavities. This architecture is lost in the specimen from the patient with Paget disease, in which the trabeculae are coarse and the architecture is disorganized. Note the extensive imprints of osteoclastic bone resorption in the center portion of the specimen of pagetic bone. (Courtesy of Dr. David Dempster.)

The earliest phase of Paget disease is represented radiographically by an advancing lytic wedge or "blade of grass" lesion in a long bone, or by *osteoporosis circumscripta*, as seen in the skull. The next phase is a mixture of the initial abnormality, increased bone resorption, and a compensatory increase of new bone formation. Both osteoclasts and osteoblasts are found at active sites in this stage. Presumably because of the rapidity of the process, newly deposited collagen fibers are laid down in a haphazard, rather than a linear, fashion, creating a mosaic pattern in bone—a more primitive *woven bone*—instead of the normal *lamellar* pattern. The bone marrow becomes infiltrated by an excess of fibrous connective tissue, and a marked increase in blood vessels is seen, which causes the bone to become hypervascular. Usually, the bone matrix is normally mineralized, although areas of reduced mineralization (widened osteoid seams) can be found in isolated areas of some bone biopsy specimens.[5] Eventually, the hypercellularity at a given locus may decrease, leaving only the sclerotic mosaic bone ("burned out" disease) without evidence of active bone turnover. Usually, all different phases are seen concomitantly in different areas of pagetic involvement in a given patient. Figure 65-3 compares the appearance of normal and pagetic bone by scanning elec-

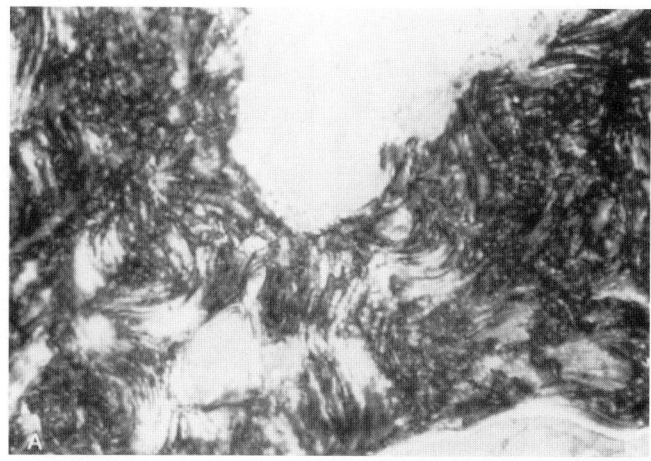

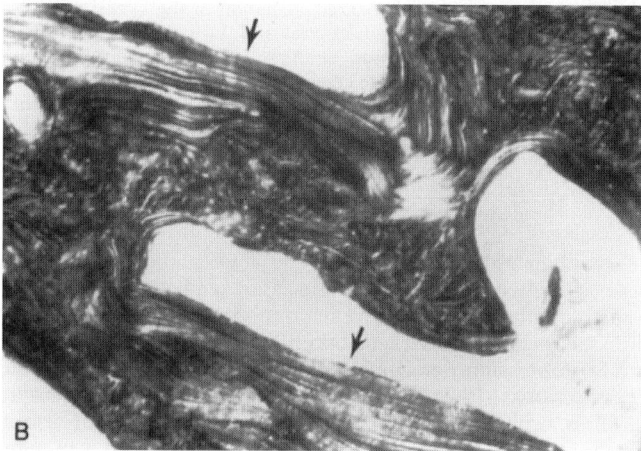

**FIGURE 65-4.** These photomicrographs, using polarized light, demonstrate the typical pattern of woven bone in a biopsy from a pagetic iliac crest before treatment (**A**) and after bisphosphonate therapy (**B**). The first biopsy specimen demonstrates the chaotic and more primitive pattern of collagen deposition that is characteristic of Paget disease. The posttreatment specimen shows areas in which a restoration toward a more lamellar pattern has occurred (*arrows*). (Courtesy of Dr. Pierre Meunier.)

tron microscopy, and Figure 65-4*A* shows the pattern of woven bone in Paget disease.

The increased bone resorption increases the urinary excretion of products of the degradation of bone collagen, including total hydroxyproline and more specific bone markers such as pyridinoline, deoxypyridinoline, and both the N- and C-telopeptides of collagen. The increased osteoblastic activity is associated with a rise in the serum alkaline phosphatase level. Because overall bone resorption and bone formation in most patients are coupled, these values rise in proportion to each other and are useful markers of metabolic activity. Moreover, as specific treatment is instituted, decreases in these indices serve as evidence of a therapeutic response.

Serum calcium is typically normal in Paget disease. However, when a patient with extensive and active disease is immobilized and loses the weight-bearing stimulus to new bone formation, hypercalcemia or clinically significant hypercalciuria may occur. In an ambulatory, otherwise healthy patient with Paget disease, the discovery of an elevated serum calcium level usually leads to a diagnosis of coexisting primary hyperparathyroidism. No data exist to support the idea that the two conditions are causally linked in such people, and the presence of both disorders in the same person is considered a clinical coincidence.[32] Some studies have suggested, however, that secondary hyperparathyroidism may emerge in a

subset of patients with active Paget disease because of markedly increased calcium requirements during periods of intensive new bone formation.[33,34] In patients with either primary or secondary hyperparathyroidism, increased levels of parathyroid hormone stimulate pagetic osteoclasts to even higher levels of activity and may cause a worsening of the underlying bone remodeling abnormality. When primary hyperparathyroidism coexists, surgical removal of the parathyroid adenoma is often associated with an improvement of the Paget disease. The treatment of coexisting secondary hyperparathyroidism involves maintaining an adequate intake of calcium and vitamin D.

## CLINICAL PRESENTATION

The localized nature of Paget disease leads to a variable clinical presentation. Frequently, only one or two bones are involved; alternatively, many bones may be affected. The most commonly involved sites include the pelvis, spine, skull, femur, and tibia. The bones of the upper extremities, the clavicles, scapulae, and ribs are somewhat less commonly involved, and the hands and feet are seldom affected. Clinical symptoms and complications of Paget disease depend greatly on the sites of involvement, the relation of pagetic bone to adjacent structures, and the extent of ongoing metabolic activity.

Most patients with Paget disease are asymptomatic, and the diagnosis is an incidental finding, made when either an elevated serum alkaline phosphatase level is discovered or a radiograph showing classic pagetic changes is obtained for some unrelated reason. Other patients have symptoms referable to the skeleton, but these may reflect a range of causes, including problems with the bone itself, joint dysfunction adjacent to pagetic bone, neurologic abnormalities, and changes associated with increased blood flow. Depending on the site of involvement and the nature of the skeletal alterations that are occurring, a simple complaint such as bone pain may be difficult to characterize. For example, patients with skull involvement may describe headaches or tightness across the scalp, or they may note a sensation of warmth, presumably reflecting the increased blood flow through pagetic bone and surrounding soft tissues. A symptom of pain in the back in the setting of one or more enlarged pagetic vertebrae may come from the bone itself, but is probably due to degenerative changes of the joints that are exacerbated by the presence of Paget disease, with or without spinal nerve impingement and muscle spasm. Pagetic involvement of the pelvis or proximal femur may include the hip joint, leading to pain in the groin or in the thigh, often radiating to the knee. This common pattern is a major source of discomfort in patients with Paget disease at this site.

Bone deformity may be the patient's presenting problem. Enlargement or bowing of the femur or tibia is a readily apparent finding, as are skull enlargement with classic frontal bossing, asymmetry of the pelvic or shoulder girdle areas, and kyphosis (Fig. 65-5). When the femur or tibia on one side of the body has a bowing deformity caused by Paget disease, adjacent joints are subjected to mechanical stresses from the curvature; in addition, the bowed limb is typically shortened, increasing the likelihood of back pain or contralateral joint dysfunction and pain resulting from the abnormal gait. These symptoms are among the most common. As with the skull, a sensation of increased heat in a bowed extremity is a frequently stated complaint. Often this increased warmth is felt by the examiner's hand.

Fracture through pagetic bone is a more serious complication. Pagetic fractures may be either traumatic or pathologic, especially, but not exclusively, involving long bones with active areas of advancing lytic disease. Usually these fractures heal normally, but the rate of nonunion may be as high as 10%.[35] The

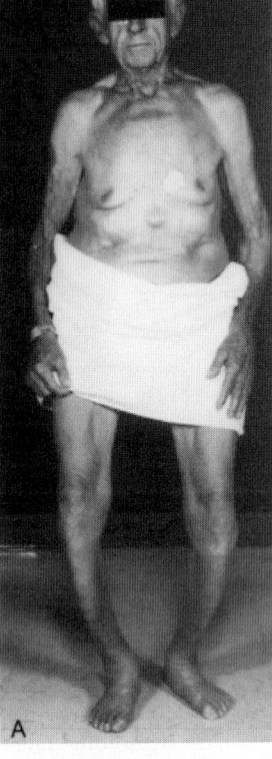

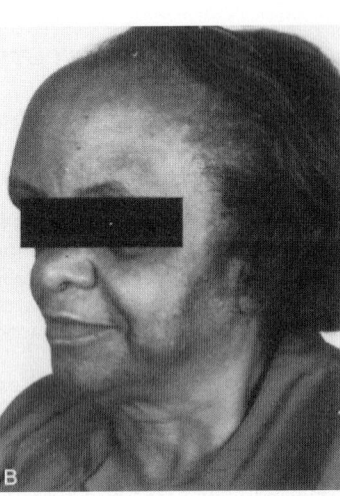

**FIGURE 65-5.** **A,** Extensive Paget disease in an elderly man, showing considerable deformity of the lower extremities. Outward bowing of the femoral, tibial, and fibular bones and anterior bowing of the shins (saber shins) are seen. The patient also has thoracic kyphosis. Considerable secondary degenerative arthritis of the knees and hips is present. (The nodule on the abdomen is a sebaceous cyst.) **B,** Severe pagetic involvement of the skull, showing deformity and enlargement of the frontal bone. The patient complained of a throbbing discomfort of the head, and the overlying skin was very warm.

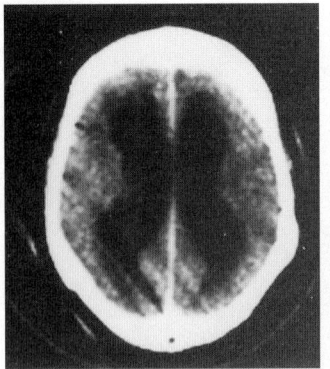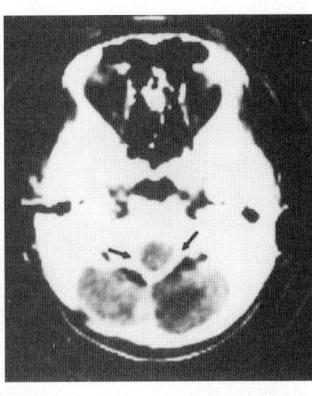

A,B

**FIGURE 65-6.** These two photographs are sections of a computed tomographic scan of a pagetic skull, obtained from a patient with radiographic evidence of basilar invagination in whom coma and a unilateral dilated pupil had developed acutely. **A,** The thickened cortex of the skull is demonstrated, and marked dilatation of the lateral ventricles reveals evidence of severe hydrocephalus. **B,** Virtual encasement of the brainstem region by increased amounts of pagetic bone is shown (*arrows*). Chronic obstruction to cerebrospinal fluid flow had developed in this patient as a result of pagetic bone encroachment. A ventricular shunt was performed immediately, with rapid resolution of her acute, central nervous system decompensation. (From Siris ES, Canfield RE, Jacobs TP. Paget's disease of bone. Bull N Y Acad Med 1980; 56:285.)

most serious and probably most common fractures involve the femoral shaft or subtrochanteric area.[5,35] Some of these fractures are the result of progression from small cortical "fissure" fractures. Rarely, a fracture occurs in association with an area of malignant degeneration (i.e., through an osteogenic sarcoma in pagetic bone).

When Paget disease affects the axial skeleton, it may be associated with neurologic complications. Patients with skull involvement may experience hearing loss of either a sensorineural or a conductive type, or both. Typically, cochlear dysfunction is present and, less commonly, direct eighth nerve compression occurs.[36] Vertigo, Bell palsy, and other cranial nerve abnormalities are seen less often. Extensive skull involvement may lead to a softening of the base of the skull, causing platybasia or frank basilar impression. The slow sinking of the skull onto the odontoid process may lead to narrowing of the foraminal space and potentially to an obstructive hydrocephalus. Radiographic criteria for basilar invagination are often met in cases with massive skull involvement, but neurologic sequelae from this are relatively uncommon. When they do occur, however, these sequelae are serious and life-threatening. Brainstem or cerebellar compression or obstruction of cerebrospinal fluid flow from blockage of the fourth ventricle or the foramina of Magendie and Luschka may lead to fairly rapid and progressive neurologic decompensation. The use of computed tomographic scanning and magnetic resonance imaging has made the prompt diagnosis of ventricular enlargement much easier and allows rapid and appropriate neurosurgical intervention. Figure 65-6 shows an example of this complication.

Involvement of one or more vertebral bodies also may be associated with neurologic signs and symptoms. Sometimes radiculopathy from nerve root compression, particularly in the lumbar region, is observed. Lumbar spinal stenosis and vertebral compression deformities may be seen. Less common, but more serious, is the occurrence of spinal cord compression syndromes, especially at the narrowed thoracic region but also in the lumbar region. Occasionally, the injury to the cord is thought to result not from direct compression by bone, but rather from ischemia of the neural structures, owing to a diversion of blood to the extremely vascular pagetic bone (i.e., a "steal" syndrome).[37] Progressive development of sensory changes and motor weakness below the affected level may be slow or relatively rapid, and always requires immediate attention.

The cardiovascular complications of Paget disease include increased cardiac output related to increased blood flow in the thickened and vascular bone. These patients also are prone to the development of vascular calcifications. The aortic valve, in particular, has been shown to develop calcification in parallel with advancing stages of the disease.[38]

Malignant degeneration in pagetic bone occurs with an incidence of <1%.[3] The development of increasing pain at a pagetic site may be the first evidence of this rare but extremely grave complication. In 50 years of experience at the Mayo Clinic, the site of malignant change most commonly was the pelvis, with the femur and humerus next in frequency.[39] Most of the tumors were osteosarcomas, although fibrosarcomas and chondrosarcomas also occurred. Death resulting from local extension of tumor or from pulmonary metastases occurs in most cases within 1 to 3 years, because no effective treatment regimens are available.

Benign giant cell tumors also may arise in pagetic bone, typically presenting as localized protuberances at the involved site that may show lytic changes on radiography. These tumors often initially are thought to represent osteosarcomas, but after biopsy they prove to be clusters of large osteoclasts, which may represent reparative granulomas.[40] Many of these giant cell tumors are extremely sensitive to corticosteroids and may literally melt away after a course of dexamethasone.[41] An interesting geographic or familial clustering of giant cell tumor cases among patients with Paget disease from the region of Avellino, Italy, has been described.[41]

# DIAGNOSIS

The diagnosis of Paget disease is based on a combination of the medical history and physical examination (particularly when increased heat or bone deformity is present), laboratory tests (measurement of serum alkaline phosphatase, and in some instances, a urinary marker of bone resorption), and radiographic studies (bone scans and conventional radiographs). Bone biopsy is indicated only occasionally in this disorder, primarily as a means of distinguishing between Paget disease and malignant conditions.

Perhaps the most specific and straightforward diagnostic test in the evaluation of Paget disease is a radiograph of an involved site, because the changes in the appearance of bone are characteristic (see Fig. 65-1). These include enlargement or expansion of bone, coarsening of trabecular markings, and pathognomonic patterns of lytic and sclerotic change. A bone scan is not a specific diagnostic test for Paget disease but is extremely useful, primarily for its sensitivity in identifying active sites of involvement. Radiographs of these areas then can be obtained to confirm the diagnosis and to provide information on the appearance of the process. For example, radiographs of an involved femur will reveal the extent of sclerotic versus lytic change, provide data on the status of the hip joint, identify areas of fissure fractures if present, and demonstrate bowing.

The serum alkaline phosphatase level is probably the most useful blood test in the diagnostic evaluation. A markedly elevated serum alkaline phosphatase level in a healthy older patient with no evidence of liver disease and a normal serum calcium level probably is due to Paget disease. The degree of elevation of the alkaline phosphatase level is generally a measure of metabolic activity. For reasons not well understood, the highest levels usually are seen in patients whose involved sites include the skull. Minimally elevated levels of alkaline phosphatase in patients with a single site of pagetic change (e.g., a tibia or a single vertebra) may represent progressive disease at that site. Conversely, extensive skeletal involvement identified radiographically and a minimal alkaline phosphatase increase denote relatively inactive or burned out disease in most instances. In patients with coexistent liver disease, serum bone-specific alkaline phosphatase is the most helpful marker. Although a urinary marker of bone resorption reflects more directly the initiating bone-resorptive lesion, its measurement is not usually required for diagnosis. Occasionally, however, a patient may present with radiographic evidence of Paget disease and a *normal* serum alkaline phosphatase level but an elevated level of urinary resorption marker, presumably indicating ongoing lytic pagetic change. Measurement of serum osteocalcin is not helpful in Paget disease.

Problems with differential diagnosis occur infrequently because of the characteristic radiographic appearance in established Paget disease. Occasionally, however, a patient may have bone pain, elevated levels of serum alkaline phosphatase and a urinary resorption marker, a positive bone scan result, and less than typical osteolytic or sclerotic changes on radiography. In this situation, uncertainty may exist as to whether the disorder is Paget disease or metastatic cancer to bone. Old radiographic films and laboratory reports may be helpful in such cases; if the serum alkaline phosphatase level and radiograph of the involved bone were normal a year earlier, Paget disease is much less likely, particularly in a 60- or 70-year-old person. Occasionally, someone with long-standing Paget disease develops nonspecific radiographic changes in a new area. Because the spread of Paget disease to new sites years after its initial appearance is distinctly unusual, the clinical suspicion of another process should be high. When this type of diagnostic problem is encountered, bone biopsy may be indicated.

# TREATMENT

Issues regarding therapy for Paget disease include questions about the indications for specific medical treatment, anticipated benefits from these treatments, choices among the antipagetic agents, and the utility of nonspecific therapies (e.g., analgesics, nonsteroidal antiinflammatory drugs). In patients with a range of signs and symptoms, the localized nature of this disorder makes highly individualized treatment decisions necessary.

The goals of treatment are to relieve symptoms and to attempt to prevent future complications. The currently available therapies for Paget disease in the United States include the bisphosphonate agents etidronate, pamidronate, alendronate, tiludronate, and risedronate, as well as salmon calcitonin and plicamycin. All appear to act by decreasing osteoclastic bone resorption. The first-choice therapy is a potent bisphosphonate, but parenteral salmon calcitonin may be an alternative for patients who are not candidates for bisphosphonate therapy. Plicamycin has largely been replaced by the potent newer bisphosphonates, especially intravenous pamidronate. Initial and early reductions in the levels of urinary resorption markers, followed by decreases in serum alkaline phosphatase (reflecting a subsequent slowing of new bone formation) nearly always result from appropriate treatment with these agents. Consequently, a variety of pagetic symptoms may be ameliorated. Moreover, bone biopsies taken before and after courses of treatment provide evidence for normalization of bone morphology (see Fig. 65-4*B*). Thus, the goal of relieving symptoms is one that often can be met. Some data suggest that the prevention of future complications through an arrest or slowing of active pagetic bone turnover may be possible in some patients, especially with the newer bisphosphonates that have the capacity to achieve a biochemical remission for extended periods of time in most patients.[42]

Therefore, the indications for treatment include (a) symptoms referable to Paget disease and (b) asymptomatic but active involvement (i.e., associated with elevated bone turnover markers) in areas of the skeleton where future serious complications might arise. Examples of this second indication include marked skull or vertebral involvement, which carries the threat of future neurologic problems; involvement of bones adjacent to major joints, such as the hip, knee, or ankle, with the potential for disabling joint problems; or pagetic change in a long bone, particularly in the lower extremity, so that a future bowing deformity is possible with disease progression over time. These issues are especially important in younger patients who may live with the disorder for many years. On the other hand, a small area of pagetic change in the calvarium or asymptomatic disease in the pelvis not involving the hip joint may be observed without treatment, particularly in elderly patients.

The kinds of symptoms that are likely to respond to treatment also must be considered. The early clinical trials with bisphosphonates made it clear that a substantial placebo effect occurs from virtually any therapy. However, when the experience with treatment is analyzed carefully, several points become apparent. The reduction in the activity of Paget disease often decreases bone pain, pagetic headache, excessive warmth, some arthritic complaints, and, in some instances, the signs and symptoms associated with neurologic compression syndromes. In the relatively rare patient with high-output cardiac failure associated with extensive Paget disease (usually a person with underlying heart disease), treatment of the Paget disease may lead to some amelioration of cardiac symptoms. Hearing loss would not be expected to reverse itself (although progression might be slowed), bowed limbs may continue to bow with weight-bearing, and severely narrowed joint spaces will remain arthritic, although perhaps become less painful.

## BISPHOSPHONATES

Five bisphosphonate compounds are used to treat Paget disease in the United States, including the first oral agent used for the disorder, etidronate; the only intravenous preparation, pamidronate; and three newer oral agents, tiludronate, alendronate, and risedronate. These are discussed in the order in which they became available.

**Etidronate.** *Etidronate* became available at approximately the same time as salmon calcitonin.[43,44] Indeed, these two agents were the mainstays of therapy for this disorder for nearly 20 years, after which the newer and more potent bisphosphonates emerged. Etidronate is given orally at a dose of 5 mg/kg per day (400 mg in most patients), taken with a small amount of water or clear juice at a point midway through a 4-hour fast (e.g., between two meals at least 4 hours apart or at bedtime at least 2 hours after any food has been ingested). It is given for a treatment course of 6 months' duration, typically achieving ~50% reduction in elevated indices of pagetic bone turnover in most patients, as well as a relief of those symptoms likely to respond to decreased turnover as previously noted. Thus, in patients with mild disease, indices may return to normal and remain that way with continued symptom relief for several years after a single 6-month course.[45] However, individuals with initial elevations of serum alkaline phosphatase more than three to four times the upper limit of normal typically continue to have biochemically elevated turnover indices despite the 50% or so reduction, even if symptoms improve. Such patients are typically retreated at the same dose in repeated cycles of 6 months on, 6 months off therapy, a program that has maintained a reduced level of turnover for up to 10 years in some patients,[45] although others have experienced a loss of effectiveness with repeated cycles.[46]

The *failure of indices to return to normal or near normal* in most of the more severely affected patients has been suggested as one explanation for the finding of *disease progression* in many patients treated with etidronate.[47] Interestingly, higher dosages of etidronate for longer treatment intervals produce greater degrees of biochemical suppression than the recommended regimen, but clearly such therapy often leads to clinically significant *osteomalacia*.[43] This is the basis for the recommendation that the 400-mg dose be given for no longer than 6 months, followed by at least a 6-month etidronate-free interval, an approach that is generally quite safe. All bisphosphonates have the capacity to impair mineralization of newly forming bone if enough is given for a long enough time period (the process reverses itself once the agent is stopped), but, of the currently available bisphosphonates, only etidronate at excessive dosages is likely to do so. Etidronate has also been shown to be associated with progression of lytic disease in some patients with this manifestation of the disorder[48]; thus, the drug should not be used in individuals with advancing lytic disease in weight-bearing bone or in patients with healing fractures. As is noted later, the newer bisphosphonates do *not* appear to impair mineralization at the therapeutic doses that are highly effective in treating this disease.

**Pamidronate.** The first of the more potent bisphosphonates to become available in the United States is intravenously administered *pamidronate*. This agent has been extensively studied using a variety of different regimens for its administration,[49–53] all of which are effective. Overall, pamidronate use clearly is associated with reduction in symptoms, improvement in lytic disease, and normalization of serum alkaline phosphatase for a year or more after a given number of infusions (dose and frequency may be individualized to the characteristics of the given patient). The package insert for the use of pamidronate in Paget disease calls for a dose of 30 mg daily for 3 days, each given in 500 mL of 5% dextrose in water over 4 hours, because this was the protocol used in the clinical trial that led to Food and Drug Administration clearance. This regimen actually resulted in an ~50% reduction in elevated indices. However, clinical experience suggests that this approach is cumbersome and not at all optimal for achieving the substantial benefits of this agent. In patients with relatively mild or monostotic disease, a single infusion of 60 or 90 mg infused over 2 to 3 hours (volume must be adequate to avoid superficial phlebitis at the infusion site, so the rapidity of the treatment depends on how quickly the patient can receive 400 to 500 mL of fluid) usually produces a normal serum alkaline phosphatase level with a prolonged biochemical remission before indices again rise above normal and retreatment is required.[53] In persons with more severe disease (i.e., serum alkaline phosphatase values 5 to 10 times normal or higher) who rarely achieved normal values with etidronate or calcitonin, 60 to 90 mg can be given weekly or biweekly (depending on doctor and patient convenience) for three or four doses, with a reassessment of the indices 6 to 8 weeks after the final dose. After this, additional infusions can be given if needed (i.e., if the chemistries are still significantly elevated) to attempt to bring the alkaline phosphatase into the normal range over the next few weeks to months. Although some patients do not achieve normal indices even after use of very high doses,[54] *most do or at least come much closer to normal than was possible with the older agents.* Typically, the remission lasts a year or more before indices rise above normal; this means that the patient can be followed with an alkaline phosphatase measurement every 6 months. Because retreatment will be given when values rise slightly above normal, the total dose for retreatment may be a fraction of what was initially required. Asymptomatic localized mineralization defects have been reported with as little as 180 mg of pamidronate,[55] but this is a rare finding in the literature. More significant, perhaps, has been the suggestive evidence that some degree of secondary resistance to pamidronate may occur with repeat treatment courses, requiring the use of higher dosages or a change to another, more potent bisphosphonate.[56] The main side effect of pamidronate is a transient acute-phase reaction with fever and myalgias a day after the first-ever infusion.

**Tiludronate.** Three oral bisphosphonates are available that are *more potent* than etidronate and that do *not* appear to be associated with mineralization defects at clinically effective doses. *Tiludronate* is somewhat more potent than etidronate and is given at a dosage of 400 mg per day for 3 months, with a follow-up observation period off therapy of 3 months, during which the serum alkaline phosphatase level continues to decline to its posttreatment nadir. This approach has reduced the serum alkaline phosphatase level by 50% to 60% in ~60% of patients after 3 months and resulted in a normal serum alkaline phosphatase in 24% to 35% of subjects in clinical trials.[57,58] The agent is given in the form of two 200-mg tablets (ingested at the same time) taken with 6 to 8 oz of water at least 2 hours before or after consumption of food. Calcium supplements must not be taken for at least 2 hours after tiludronate is taken. Generally, the drug is well tolerated, with only mild upper gastrointestinal tract upset observed in a minority of patients. Patients should be followed with measurement of serum alkaline phosphatase every 3 to 6 months and should be retreated once indices rise above the prior nadir.

**Alendronate.** *Alendronate* is several hundred times more potent than etidronate and substantially more potent than pamidronate. It is given in a dosage of 40 mg daily for 6 months. The agent must be taken on arising, on an empty stomach, with 8 oz of plain (not mineral) water. The patient should remain upright and should not eat or drink anything but water (including no other medications) for the next 30 minutes. This regimen has produced a normal serum alkaline phosphatase in 48% to 63% of patients with moderately severe disease[59,60]; among patients whose serum alkaline phosphatase normalized, in approximately half, levels were still within normal limits 24 months after the end of the initial 6-month course of treatment. Analysis of bone biopsy specimens in these studies indicated no evidence of mineralization impairment and revealed normal bone deposition at sites of newly forming bone after successful treatment. Healing of lytic fronts is also seen with alendronate. In the clinical trials, up to 17% of patients had generally mild upper gastrointestinal tract side effects with rare esophageal erosions. Serum alkaline phosphatase can be measured every 4 to 6 months or so, with retreatment once levels rise above normal or above the posttreatment nadir.

**Risedronate.** *Risedronate*, which is more potent than alendronate and pamidronate, is given at a dosage of 30 mg per day for 2 months as the basic regimen. It is taken in a manner identical to that for alendronate (see earlier). Its use for 2 to 3 months in clinical trials by patients with moderate to severe disease resulted in a normal serum alkaline phosphatase level in 50% to 70% of patients; most of those who attained normal values maintained these values for up to 16 months after the end of the 2-month course.[61,62] Like alendronate, risedronate causes no impairment of mineralization at therapeutic doses and promotes normal bone deposition. Approximately 15% of patients have mild upper gastrointestinal tract side effects. Both pamidronate and risedronate have been associated with iritis in rare instances.

Because normalization of biochemical indices and a prolonged remission is a major goal of treatment, the choice of bisphosphonate should take into account each agent's likelihood of achieving that goal.

With any potent bisphosphonate (e.g., pamidronate, alendronate, risedronate), confirming that the patient is *vitamin D replete* and is receiving *adequate oral calcium* is important; to this end, a wise course is to offer 500 mg of calcium twice daily and 400 to 800 U of vitamin D each day to avoid hypocalcemia and transient secondary hyperparathyroidism.

## CALCITONIN

The biochemistry and physiology of calcitonin secretion are discussed elsewhere (see Chap. 53). The form of calcitonin that is clinically available is *synthetic salmon calcitonin*. Because calcitonin is a peptide hormone, it cannot be taken orally. The form approved for the treatment of Paget disease in the United States is administered parenterally. Use of the nasal spray form of salmon calcitonin in Paget disease has been studied,[63] but its utility for most patients has not been determined.

Salmon calcitonin therapy is ordinarily initiated at a dose of 100 U injected subcutaneously by the patient each day. As early as 2 to 3 weeks later, symptomatic benefit may be appreciated, and any benefit that is likely to occur should be apparent by the end of 3 months. Therapeutic responses to calcitonin include the reduction of both bone pain and excessive warmth. Radiographic improvement with healing of lytic areas and improvement of neurologic complications has been reported. Serum alkaline phosphatase and urinary hydroxyproline values generally decline to ~50% of pretreatment levels by the end of the first 6 months of treatment,[64] after which the calcitonin dosage often may be reduced to 50 to 100 U three times a week, with maintenance of symptomatic and biochemical benefit. The discontinuation of treatment after an initial 1- to 2-year course may be followed by another year or more of persistent disease suppression, but a return of the biochemical indices to pretreatment values usually occurs after this.[65] Thus, depending on the patient's age, extent of disease, and symptoms, an indefinite course of treatment at the lowest effective dosage (e.g., typically recommended to be 50 U three times a week) may be indicated.

After a prolonged period of treatment with salmon calcitonin, biochemical indices may begin to rise again in some patients, often back to pretreatment levels. In some cases, this escape from effectiveness reflects the development of high titers of neutralizing antibodies to the salmon hormone.[66] However, in other instances titers are not increased, and the suggestion has been made that a down-regulation of calcitonin receptors at target cells may occur, with a resulting decreased therapeutic response.

Treatment with salmon calcitonin at full dosages is expensive, and sometimes the need for parenteral administration elicits problems with continued patient compliance. Side effects, which occur in 10% to 20% of patients, consist of nausea, less commonly vomiting or diarrhea, and occasionally marked cutaneous flushing. For this reason, treatment may be initiated using only 50% of the desired dose each day for the first week, with an increase to the full dose if the agent is well tolerated; side effects may be less troublesome if the agent is given at bedtime; in many patients, they diminish substantially as treatment continues. Calcitonin causes a mild and usually asymptomatic decrease (~1 mg/dL) of serum calcium 4 to 6 hours after injection in patients with active Paget disease, but this change in the serum calcium level diminishes as the pagetic process responds to therapy.

## PLICAMYCIN (MITHRAMYCIN)

Plicamycin is a cytotoxic compound that binds to DNA and inhibits RNA synthesis. It is an effective therapy for the hypercalcemia of malignancy by virtue of its inhibition of osteoclast-mediated bone resorption. For this same reason, it is an effective means of treating Paget disease.[67] However, its significant systemic toxicity (nausea, vomiting, elevation of hepatocellular enzymes, and, less commonly, reversible nephrotoxicity, as well as thrombocytopenia and a hemorrhagic diathesis) markedly limits its use. It is rarely needed today because of the availability of potent bisphosphonates such as pamidronate, alendronate, and risedronate. Nevertheless, in the rare patient who needs treatment and who fails to respond to such agents, a course of plicamycin (12.5 to 20 µg/kg given intravenously over 4 to 8 hours every second to third day for five to ten total doses) may be of significant value.

## NONSTEROIDAL ANTIINFLAMMATORY DRUGS

Many of the most troublesome symptoms for patients with Paget disease result from a *secondary arthritis* involving the hip, knee, ankle, or spine. Analgesics such as aspirin or acetaminophen may provide pain relief, and the use of nonsteroidal antiinflammatory compounds or COX-2 inhibitors can be extremely effective in alleviating symptoms caused by arthritic complications of Paget disease. In patients with metabolically inactive Paget disease (i.e., normal serum alkaline phosphatase levels) but with significant joint symptoms, one of these agents may be the only required therapy. In cases in which Paget disease is active, these compounds may serve as useful adjuncts to either a bisphosphonate or calcitonin.

## SURGICAL INTERVENTION

Several of the mechanical complications of Paget disease can best be managed surgically.[68] Joint replacement may be the only means of eliminating severe pain, particularly in the hip, but should be undertaken only by an orthopedic surgeon who has had experience in operating on vascular, pagetic bone.[69] Other elective orthopedic procedures include internal stabilization of an impending fracture, particularly when the lytic changes are progressive and pain develops, and, occasionally, osteotomy of a severely bowed limb when a serious gait disturbance or pain unrelieved by medical therapy is interfering with daily function. In general, elective surgery should be delayed until disease activity—manifested by the level of serum alkaline phosphatase—is reduced to the lowest possible level through the use of a course of intravenous pamidronate or, if time permits, oral alendronate or risedronate. If the alkaline phosphatase level is reduced to normal or at least to under two to three times the upper limit of normal, hypervascularity of the pagetic bone should be substantially decreased, limiting the potential for excessive bleeding at surgery.

Sometimes neurosurgical intervention is necessary as therapy for rapidly progressive spinal cord compression or for neurologic decompensation caused by obstructive hydrocephalus. In acute situations, high doses of dexamethasone (up to 16 mg per day in divided doses) in the hours before surgery also may decrease vascularity and provide some initial degree of decompression.

## REFERENCES

1. Barker DJP. The epidemiology of Paget's disease. Br Med Bull 1984; 40:396.
1a. Altman RD, Block DA, Hochberg MC, Murphy WA. Prevalence of pelvic Paget's disease of bone in the United States. J Bone Miner Res 2000; 15:461.
2. Barker DJP, Chamberlain AT, Guyer PB, Gardner MJ. Paget's disease of bone: the Lancashire focus. BMJ 1980; 280:1105.
2a. Cooper C, Shafheutle K, Dennison E, et al. The epidemiology of Paget's disease in Britain: is the prevalence decreasing? J Bone Miner Res 1999; 14:192.
2b. Cundy T, McAnulty K, Wattie D, et al. Evidence for secular changes in Paget's disease. Bone 1997; 20:69.
3. Barry HC. Paget's disease of bone. Edinburgh: E & S Livingstone, 1969.
4. Guyer PB, Chamberlain AT. Paget's disease of bone in two American cities. BMJ 1980; 280:985.
5. Singer FR. Paget's disease of bone. New York: Plenum Publishing, 1977.
6. Siris ES, Canfield RE, Jacobs TP. Paget's disease of bone. Bull N Y Acad Med 1980; 56:285.
7. Morales-Piga AA, Rey-Rey JS, Corres-Gonzalez J, et al. Frequency and characteristics of familial aggregation of Paget's disease of bone. J Bone Miner Res 1995; 10:663.
8. McKusick VA. Heritable disorders of connective tissue. St. Louis: CV Mosby, 1972:718.
9. Siris ES, Ottman R, Flaster E, Kelsey JL. Familial aggregation of Paget's disease of bone. J Bone Miner Res 1991; 6:495
10. Singer FR, Mills BG, Park MS, et al. Increased HLA-DQw1 antigen frequency in Paget's disease of bone. Proceedings of the 7th Annual Meeting of the American Society for Bone and Mineral Research. Washington, DC: 1985:128.
11. Tilyard MW, Gardner RJM, Milligan L, et al. A probable linkage between familial Paget's disease and the HLA foci. Aust N Z J Med 1982; 12:498.
12. Foldes J, Shamir S, Brautbar C, et al. HLA-D antigens and Paget's disease of bone. Clin Orthop 1991; 266:301.
13. Singer FR, Siris ES, Knieriem A, et al. The HLA DRB1*1104 gene frequency is increased in Ashkenazi Jews with Paget's disease of bone. J Bone Miner Res 1996; 11:S369.
14. Hughes AE, Shearmen AM, Weber JL, et al. Genetic linkage of familial expansile osteolysis to chromosome 18q. Hum Mol Genet 1994; 3:359.
15. Cody JD, Singer FR, Roodman GD, et al. Genetic linkage of Paget disease of the bone to chromosome 18q. Am J Hum Genet 1997; 61:1117.
16. Haslam SI, Van Hul W, Morales-Piga A, et al. Paget's disease of bone: evidence for a susceptibility locus on chromosome 18q and for genetic heterogeneity. J Bone Miner Res 1998; 13:911.
17. Rasmussen H, Bordier P. The physiological and cellular basis of metabolic bone disease. Baltimore: Williams & Wilkins, 1974:293.
18. Mills BG, Singer FR. Nuclear inclusions in Paget's disease of bone. Science 1976; 194:201.
19. Rebel A, Malkani K, Basle M, Bregeon C. Nuclear inclusions in osteoclasts in Paget's bone disease. Calcif Tissue Res 1976; 21(Suppl):113.
20. Mills BG, Yabe H, Singer FR. Osteoclasts in human osteopetrosis contain viral-nucleocapsid-like nuclear inclusions. J Bone Miner Res 1988; 3:101.
21. Rebel A, Basle M, Pouplard A, et al. Viral antigens in osteoclasts from Paget's disease of bone. Lancet 1980; 2:344.
22. Mills BG, Singer FR, Weiner LP, et al. Evidence for both respiratory syncytial virus and measles virus antigens in the osteoclasts of patients with Paget's disease of bone. Clin Orthop 1984; 183:303.
23. Gordon MT, Anderson DC, Sharpe PT. Canine distemper virus localized in bone cells of patients with Paget's disease. Bone 1991; 12:195.
24. Fraser KB, Martin SJ. Measles virus and its biology. New York: Academic Press, 1978.
25. Gordon MT, Mee AP, Anderson DC, Sharpe PT. Canine distemper virus transcripts sequenced from pagetic bone. Bone Miner 1992; 19:159.
26. Ralston SH, Digiovine FFS, Gallacher SJ, et al. Failure to detect paramyxovirus sequences in Paget's disease of bone using the polymerase chain reaction. J Bone Miner Res 1991; 6:1243.
27. Birch MA, Taylor W, Fraser WD, et al. Absence of paramyxovirus RNA in cultures of pagetic bone cells and in pagetic bone. J Bone Miner Res 1994; 9:11.
28. Reddy SV, Singer FR, Roodman GD. Bone marrow mononuclear cells from patients with Paget's disease contain measles virus nucleocapsid messenger ribonucleic acid that has mutations in a specific region of the sequence. J Clin Endocrinol Metab 1995; 80:2108.
29. Reddy SV, Singer FR, Mallette L, Roodman GD. Detection of measles virus nucleocapsid transcripts in circulating blood cells from patients with Paget's disease. J Bone Miner Res 1996; 11:1603.
30. Roodman GD, Kurihara N, Oksaki Y, et al. IL-6. A potential autocrine/paracrine factor in Paget's disease of bone. J Clin Invest 1992; 89:46.
31. Hoyland JA, Freemont AJ, Sharpe PT. Interleukin-6, IL-6 receptor, and IL-6 nuclear factor gene expression in Paget's disease. J Bone Miner Res 1993; 9:75.
32. Posen S, Clifton-Bligh P, Wilkinson W. Paget's disease of bone and hyperparathyroidism: coincidence or causal relationship? Calcif Tissue Res 1978; 26:107.
33. Meunier PJ, Coindre JM, Edouard CM, Arlot ME. Bone histomorphometry in Paget's disease: quantitative and dynamic analysis of pagetic and nonpagetic bone tissue. Arthritis Rheum 1980; 23:1095.
34. Siris ES, Clemens TP, McMahon D, et al. Parathyroid function in Paget's disease of bone. J Bone Miner Res 1989; 4:75.
35. Barry HC. Orthopedic aspects of Paget's disease of bone. Arthritis Rheum 1980; 23:1128.
36. Monsell EM, Bone HG, Cody DD, et al. Hearing loss in Paget's disease of bone: evidence of auditory nerve integrity. Am J Otol 1995; 16:27.
37. Herzberg L, Bayliss E. Spinal cord syndrome due to non-compressive Paget's disease of bone: a spinal artery steal phenomenon reversible with calcitonin. Lancet 1980; 2:13.
38. Strickberger SA, Schulman SP, Hutchins GM. Association of Paget's disease of bone with calcific aortic valve disease. Am J Med 1987; 82:953.
39. Wick MR, Siegal GP, Unni KK, et al. Sarcomas of bone complicating osteitis deformans (Paget's disease). Am J Surg Pathol 1981; 5:47.
40. Upchurch KS, Simon LS, Schiller AL, et al. Giant cell reparative granuloma of Paget's disease of bone: a unique clinical entity. Ann Intern Med 1983; 98:35.
41. Jacobs TP, Michelsen J, Polay JS, et al. Giant cell tumor in Paget's disease of bone. Familial and geographic clustering. Cancer 1979; 44:742.
42. Siris ES. Clinical review. Paget's disease of bone. J Bone Miner Res 1998; 13:1061.
43. Canfield R, Rosner W, Skinner J, et al. Diphosphonate therapy of Paget's disease of bone. J Clin Endocrinol Metab 1977; 44:96.
44. Khairi MRA, Altman RD, DeRosa GP, et al. Sodium etidronate in the treatment of Paget's disease of bone. Ann Intern Med 1977; 87:656.
45. Siris ES, Canfield RE, Jacobs TP, et al. Clinical and biochemical effects of EHDP in Paget's disease of bone: patterns of response to initial treatment and to long-term therapy. Metab Bone Dis Relat Res 1981; 3:301.
46. Altman R. Long-term follow-up of therapy with intermittent etidronate disodium in Paget's disease of bone. Am J Med 1985; 79:583.
47. Meunier PJ, Vignot E. Therapeutic strategy in Paget's disease of bone. Bone 1995; 17:489S.
48. Nagant de Deuxchaisnes C, Rombouts-Lindeman C, Huaux JP, et al. Roentgenologic evaluation of the action of the diphosphonate EHDP and of combined therapy (EHDP and calcitonin) in Paget's disease of bone. In: MacIntyre I, Szelke M, eds. Molecular endocrinology. Amsterdam: Elsevier, 1979:405.
49. Cantrill JA, Buckler HM, Anderson DC. Low dose intravenous 3-amino-1-hydroxypropylidene-1,1-bisphosphonate (APD) for the treatment of Paget's disease of the bone. Ann Rheum Dis 1986; 45:1012.
50. Gallacher SJ, Boyce BF, Patel U, et al. Clinical experience with pamidronate in the treatment of Paget's disease of bone. Ann Rheum Dis 1991; 50:930.
51. Harinck HI, Papapoulos SE, Blanksma HJ, et al. Paget's disease of bone: early and late responses to three different modes of treatment with aminohydroxypropylidene biphosphonate (APD). BMJ 1987; 295:1301.
52. Patel S, Stone MD, Coupland C, Hosking DJ. Determinants of remission in Paget's disease of bone. J Bone Miner Res 1993; 8:1467.
53. Thiebaud D, Jaeger P, Gobelet C, et al. A single infusion of AHPrBP (APD) as treatment of Paget's disease of bone. Am J Med 1988; 85:207.
54. Cundy T, Wattie D, King AR. High dose pamidronate in the management of Paget's disease of bone. Calcif Tissue Res 1996; 58:6.
55. Adamson BB, Gallacher SJ, Byars J, et al. Mineralisation defects with pamidronate therapy for Paget's disease. Lancet 1993; 342:1459.
56. Gutteridge DH, Ward LC, Stewart GO, et al. Paget's disease: acquired resistance to one aminobisphosphonate with retained response to another. J Bone Miner Res 1999; 14:79.
57. Roux C, Gennari C, Farrerons J, et al. Comparative prospective, double-blind, multicenter study of the efficacy of tiludronate and etidronate in the treatment of Paget's disease. Arthritis Rheum 1995; 38:851.
58. McClung M, Tou CPK, Goldstein NH, Picot C. Tiludronate therapy for Paget's disease of bone. Bone 1995; 17:493S.
59. Siris E, Weinstein RS, Altman R, et al. Comparative study of alendronate versus etidronate for the treatment of Paget's disease of bone. J Clin Endocrinol Metab 1996; 81:961.
60. Reid IR, Nicholson GC, Weinstein RS, et al. Biochemical and radiologic improvement in Paget's disease of bone treated with alendronate: a randomized, placebo-controlled trial. Am J Med 1996; 171:341.
61. Siris ES, Chines AA, Altman RD, et al. Risedronate in the treatment of Paget's disease: an open-label, multicenter study. J Bone Miner Res 1998; 13:103.
62. Miller PD, Brown JP, Siris ES, et al. A prospective, multicenter, randomized, double-blind comparison of risedronate and etidronate in the treatment of Paget's disease of bone. Am J Med 1999; 106:513.
63. Nagant de Deuxchaisnes C, Devogelaer JP, Huaux JP, et al. Effect of a nasal spray of salmon calcitonin in normal subjects and in patients with Paget's disease. Proceedings of the 7th Annual Meeting of the American Society for Bone and Mineral Research. Washington, DC: 1985:369.
64. DeRose J, Singer FR, Avramides A, et al. Response of Paget's disease to porcine and salmon calcitonins. Am J Med 1974; 56:858.
65. Avramides A, Flores A, DeRose J, Wallach S. Paget's disease of bone: observations after cessation of long-term synthetic salmon calcitonin treatment. J Clin Endocrinol Metab 1976; 42:459.
66. Haddad J, Caldwell JG. Calcitonin resistance: clinical and immunological studies in subjects with Paget's disease of bone treated with porcine and salmon calcitonins. J Clin Invest 1972; 51:3133.
67. Ryan WG, Schwartz TB, Perlia CP. Effects of Mithramycin on Paget's disease of bone. Ann Intern Med 1969; 70:549.
68. Sochart DH, Porter ML. Charnley low-friction arthroplasty for Paget's disease of the hip. J Arthroplasty 2000; 15:210.
69. McDonald DJ, Sim FH. Total hip arthroplasty in Paget's disease. A follow-up note. J Bone Joint Surg Am 1987; 69:766.

# CHAPTER 66

# RARE DISORDERS OF SKELETAL FORMATION AND HOMEOSTASIS

MICHAEL P. WHYTE

Although they are individually rare, many unusual disorders of skeletal formation and homeostasis exist.[1–7] Some entities are mere radiographic curiosities; others are lethal. Some are associated with well-defined endocrine or metabolic abnormalities, and the endocrinologist may be consulted for his or her expertise, especially regarding metabolic bone disease. Cumulatively, the number of affected individuals is significant. Accordingly, this chapter provides a review of several of these conditions.

## OSTEOPETROSIS

Osteopetrosis (marble bone disease) is one of many disorders that cause high bone mass (Table 66-1).[6] Two principal forms are well characterized: an *autosomal dominant (benign) type* with few or no symptoms, and an *autosomal recessive (malignant) type* that is typically fatal during the first decade of life if untreated.[8,9] Both of these forms of osteopetrosis have been genetically mapped,[10,11] but the gene defects are partly known. An *intermediate form* of osteopetrosis also exists; it is inherited as an autosomal recessive trait and presents during childhood with some of the clinical manifestations of the malignant type, but its impact on life expectancy is unclear.[12] Also, an autosomal recessive syndrome of *osteopetrosis with renal tubular acidosis and cerebral calcification* is seen; this form is due to an inborn error of metabolism characterized by deficiency of the *carbonic anhydrase II (CA II) isoenzyme.*[13] At least *nine forms* of osteopetrosis are found in humans; most have a genetic basis.[8,9,14]

All forms of osteopetrosis in humans result from a *failure of osteoclasts to resorb skeletal tissue,* including the cartilage deposited during endochondral bone formation (primary spongiosa).[15] The precise cause of osteoclast malfunction is understood only for CA II deficiency, for which several mutations in the CA II gene have been characterized,[13] and for a subset of patients with malignant osteopetrosis who have defects in a gene that encodes a vacuolar proton pump.[13a] A considerable variety of defects in osteoclast formation and function will likely be found to explain these clinically and genetically heterogeneous conditions,[8,9,15,16] for which animal models increasingly provide insight concerning potential etiology and pathogenesis.[17,18]

In the malignant form of osteopetrosis, symptoms begin during infancy.[19] Often, an early observation is nasal stuffiness attributable to malformation of paranasal and mastoid sinuses. Subsequently, patients fail to thrive and often develop palsies of the facial, optic, or oculomotor nerves from compression by narrow cranial foramina; delayed dentition; bone fragility; and infection with spontaneous bruising and bleeding secondary to myelophthisic anemia with extramedullary hematopoiesis.[8,9] Some develop hydrocephalus.[20] Short stature, a large head, frontal bossing, nystagmus, "adenoid" appearance, hepatosplenomegaly, and genu valgum may be apparent. Death results from bronchopneumonia, sepsis, hemorrhage, or severe anemia.[8,9]

Children with intermediate osteopetrosis are of short stature and may have macrocephaly, ankylosed teeth that predispose them to osteomyelitis of the jaw, and recurrent fractures.[12] Cranial nerve deficits can occur. Some develop progressive myelophthisic anemia.

**TABLE 66-1.**
**Disorders That Cause High Bone Mass**

**DYSPLASIAS AND DYSOSTOSES**
  Autosomal dominant osteosclerosis
  Central osteosclerosis with ectodermal dysplasia
  Craniodiaphyseal dysplasia
  Craniometaphyseal dysplasia
  Dysosteosclerosis
  Endosteal hyperostosis
    Sclerosteosis
    Van Buchem disease
  Frontometaphyseal dysplasia
  Infantile cortical hyperostosis (Caffey disease)
  Lenz-Majewski syndrome
  Melorheostosis
  Metaphyseal dysplasia (Pyle disease)
  Mixed sclerosing bone dystrophy
  Oculodento-osseous dysplasia
  Osteodysplasia of Melnick and Needles
  Osteoectasia with hyperphosphatasia (hyperostosis corticalis)
  Osteomesopyknosis
  Osteopathia striata
  Osteopetrosis
  Osteopoikilosis
  Pachydermoperiostosis
  Progressive diaphyseal dysplasia (Engelmann disease)
  Pycnodysostosis
  Tubular stenosis (Kenny-Caffey syndrome)
**METABOLIC DISORDERS**
  Carbonic anhydrase II deficiency
  Fluorosis
  Heavy metal poisoning
  Hepatitis C–associated osteosclerosis
  Hypervitaminosis A, D
  Hyper-, hypo-, and pseudohypoparathyroidism
  Hypophosphatemic osteomalacia
  Milk-alkali syndrome
  Renal osteodystrophy
  X-linked hypophosphatemia
**OTHER**
  Axial osteomalacia
  Diffuse idiopathic skeletal hyperostosis (DISH)
  Fibrogenesis imperfecta ossium
  Hypertrophic osteoarthropathy
  Exposure to ionizing radiation
  Leukemia
  Lymphoma
  Mastocytosis
  Multiple myeloma
  Myelofibrosis
  Osteomyelitis
  Osteonecrosis
  Paget disease
  Polycythemia vera
  Sarcoidosis
  Sickle cell disease
  Skeletal metastases
  Sterno-costo-clavicular hypertosis
  Tuberous sclerosis

(Reproduced from Whyte MP. Skeletal disorders characterized by osteosclerosis or hyperostosis. In: Avioli LV, Krane SM, eds. Metabolic bone disease and clinically related disorders, 2nd ed. San Diego: Academic Press, 1997.)

In the benign form of osteopetrosis, increased bone density can appear during childhood, but reportedly in two radiographic patterns.[21] Although many affected individuals are asymptomatic, the long bones are brittle, and occasionally pathologic

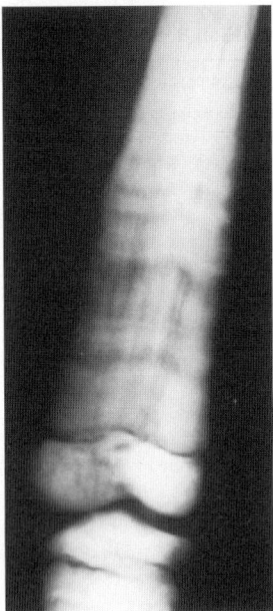

**FIGURE 66-1.** Osteopetrosis. The classic radiographic changes in the long bones are shown here in a distal femur and proximal tibia. They include increased radiodensity, loss of distinction between cortex and medullary space, modeling defects that result in flask-shaped tubular bones (especially in children), and radiodense transverse striations and longitudinal bands in the metaphyses.

fractures occur. Osteomyelitis of the jaw, osteoarthritis, and in rare cases deafness and facial palsy are potential complications.[22]

CA II deficiency typically manifests in infancy or early childhood with fracture or failure to thrive; short stature, psychomotor delay, and visual or auditory impairment may be present.[13] Hematologic abnormalities are usually absent. Most patients have a mixed renal tubular acidosis; hypokalemic paralysis has occurred in several affected individuals. The disorder seems compatible with a long life.

Other, even rarer, types of osteopetrosis may have devastating or benign outcomes.[8,9]

Routine biochemical parameters of mineral homeostasis are usually normal in osteopetrosis. In some severely affected infants or children, hypocalcemia with secondary hyperparathyroidism and elevated serum 1,25-dihydroxyvitamin D levels can occur. Although the cause is poorly understood, acid phosphatase and creatine kinase ("brain" isoenzyme) are often aberrantly increased or detectable, respectively, in patient sera.[8] In the malignant form, dysfunction of circulating monocytes and granulocytes is seen.[23]

Defective osteoclast action manifests radiographically as abnormalities in skeletal growth, modeling, and remodeling causing a generalized symmetrical increase in bone mass.[5] In the axial skeleton, sclerosis of the base of the skull, underpneumatization of the paranasal and mastoid sinuses, and a "mask sign" on anteroposterior view of the skull (especially prominent in children) are present. On lateral view of the spine, *endobones* (bone-within-bone) or a "rugger-jersey" appearance is seen. In the appendicular skeleton, erosion of the distal phalanges may be present. The classic change in the distal femur, an Erlenmeyer flask deformity, is shown in Figure 66-1. Skeletal scintigraphy may disclose fractures or osteomyelitis.

Although the radiographic features can be diagnostic, the principal pathogenetic disturbance provides a histologic finding that is characteristic for all forms of osteopetrosis. Persistence of primary spongiosa is reflected by the presence of unresorbed "islands" or "bars" of cartilage encased within bone (Fig. 66-2). In the malignant form, osteoclasts are generally numerous, and the marrow space is crowded with fibrous tissue (see Fig. 66-2). In other forms of osteopetrosis, osteoclasts are present in increased, normal, or decreased numbers.[8]

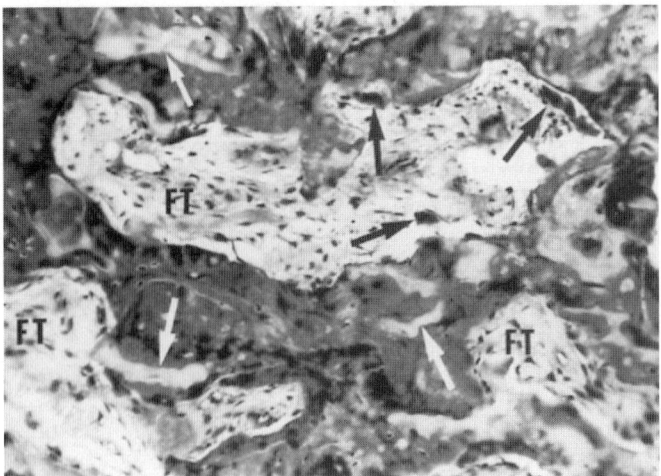

**FIGURE 66-2.** Osteopetrosis. The characteristic histopathologic change in all forms of osteopetrosis reflects the failure of osteoclasts to resorb primary spongiosa; that is, lightly stained cartilage bars (*white arrows*) remain within darkly stained (well-mineralized) trabecular bone. As shown here in the malignant form, numerous osteoclasts (*black arrows*) and marked accumulation of fibrous tissue (*FT*) in the medullary space are also present. (Masson trichrome stain, ×160)

Because intensive treatment is necessary for malignant osteopetrosis, whereas the prognosis for the intermediate form and for CA II deficiency is more benign,[13,24–26] correct diagnosis is crucial.[19] Infants or young children with CA II deficiency can have radiographic changes consistent with the malignant form of osteopetrosis, yet sequential studies may reveal gradual spontaneous resolution of their high bone mass and its complications.[27]

Bone marrow transplantation from HLA-identical normal donors to patients with malignant osteopetrosis has been followed by marked clinical improvement (including the reversal of hematologic, radiographic, histologic, and sometimes neurologic abnormalities).[24–26,28] Demonstration after transplantation that osteoclasts, but not osteoblasts, are of donor origin is consistent with defective osteoclast-mediated bone resorption in osteopetrosis and development of these polykaryons from fusion of cells of monocyte/macrophage lineage produced by marrow hematopoietic stem cells.[15,18]

Although the responses have not been as dramatic or as well documented compared with those of the bone marrow recipients, favorable biochemical changes have been reported in a few patients with malignant osteopetrosis treated with large oral doses of 1,25-dihydroxyvitamin $D_3$ (calcitriol) together with a low-calcium diet.[9,18,26] Calcitriol potentiates osteoclast activity. Long-term trials, however, are needed. Interferon-γ-1b is effective for malignant osteopetrosis and is especially appropriate for patients who are not good candidates for transplantation.[29] Glucocorticoid treatment helps the hematologic problems.[30] Transfusion of CA II–replete erythrocytes to one woman with CA II deficiency did not correct her systemic acidosis.[31] Hyperbaric oxygenation has been used for osteomyelitis. Surgical decompression of the facial and optic nerves has been described.[20]

Prenatal diagnosis of the malignant form of osteopetrosis may be possible by conventional radiographs late in the pregnancy.[32] Successful diagnosis using ultrasonography is occasionally reported.[33] CA II deficiency can be detected in utero by mutation analysis.[34]

## PYCNODYSOSTOSIS

Pycnodysostosis, an autosomal recessive disorder, perhaps affected the French impressionist painter Henri de Toulouse-

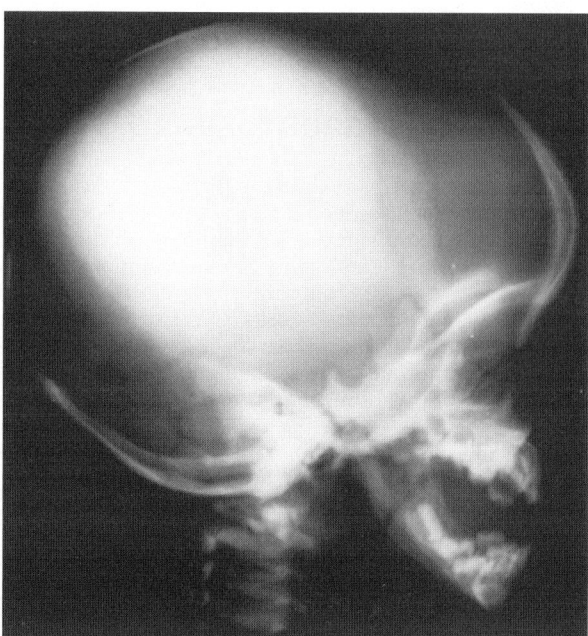

**FIGURE 66-3.** Pycnodysostosis. The skull of this 7-year-old child shows characteristic markedly widened cranial sutures, a flattened mandibular angle, several wormian bones at the occiput, and increased radiodensity at the base.

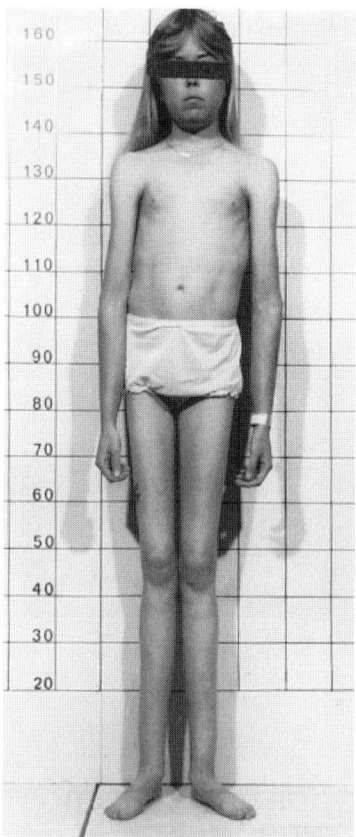

**FIGURE 66-4.** Progressive diaphyseal dysplasia. This 17-year-old girl has the typical appearance of severe disease. She is of normal height yet is prepubescent, has marked thickening of the long bones, and has a paucity of muscle mass and subcutaneous tissue in the extremities.

Lautrec.[2,6] Patients present in childhood with disproportionate short stature, a relatively large cranium, frontooccipital prominence, small facies, obtuse mandibular angle, small chin, dental malocclusion, high palate, exophthalmos, blue-tinged sclerae, a pointed and beaked nose, and short, clubbed fingers with hypoplastic nails. Recurrent fractures, with deformity, scoliosis, kyphosis, and genu valgum, may occur. Generalized uniform osteosclerosis increases with age but is not accompanied by the modeling defects of osteopetrosis.[5] Unlike in osteopetrosis, the fontanelles remain open (especially the anterior; Fig. 66-3), radiodense striations and endobones do not occur, wormian bones may be present near the parietal sutures, the mandibular angle is obtuse, and hypoplasia of the facial bones, clavicles, and terminal phalanges is present.

*Defects in the cathepsin K gene* have been found to cause Pycnodysostosis.[35] Treatment for associated growth hormone deficiency seems helpful.[36] Fractures of the long bones generally heal well.

## PROGRESSIVE DIAPHYSEAL DYSPLASIA (CAMURATI-ENGELMANN DISEASE)

Progressive diaphyseal dysplasia is a sclerosing bone disorder that is inherited in an autosomal dominant pattern, but with variable penetrance.[1,6,37] Patients have defects in the gene that encodes transforming growth factor B.[37a] New bone formation occurs progressively along both the periosteal and endosteal surfaces of major tubular bones and is associated with pain and gait disturbance.

During childhood, the patient experiences leg pains and often has a limp.[38,39] Muscle wasting and a paucity of subcutaneous fat in the extremities is common, and the gait may be waddling and broad-based. In severe cases, the axial skeleton (including the cranium) is affected. Patients may have an enlarged head, prominent forehead, proptosis, cranial nerve palsies, and a characteristic body habitus (Fig. 66-4). Sometimes puberty is delayed due to hypothalamic hypogonadotropic hypogonadism. Skeletal symptoms may remit during adolescence. Especially rare, mild, sporadic cases have been referred to as *Ribbing disease.*[37] Such patients seem to represent new, relatively benign expressions of the disorder.

Routine studies of bone and mineral metabolism are typically normal. With severe disease, a modest hypocalcemia and hypocalciuria can be present—findings that appear to reflect markedly positive calcium balance.[39] Serum alkaline phosphatase activity and the erythrocyte sedimentation rate may be increased.

Radiographic changes feature gradual, generally symmetrical, diaphyseal and metaphyseal sclerosis; the epiphyses are spared.[5] Periosteal and endosteal new bone formation increase the outer diameter and cause medullary stenosis, respectively, of affected long bones (Fig. 66-5). The tibiae and femora are most frequently involved. When the skull is affected, progressive diaphyseal dysplasia may be difficult to distinguish from mild forms of craniodiaphyseal dysplasia.[5] Although bone scintigraphy and radiographic findings are usually concordant, in some patients bone scanning may be unremarkable, whereas radiographic study shows distinct abnormalities.[40] Here, the disease process may be quiescent. The converse situation also occurs and probably reflects active but early disease. Biopsy of affected skeletal tissue reveals periosteal and endosteal new bone that is disorganized (woven) peripherally but undergoing maturation and cancellous compaction toward the cortex.[37]

Glucocorticoid therapy—generally low-dose, alternate-day treatment with prednisone—usually relieves bone pain; histologic improvement has been described.[41] Courses of pamidronate may also be effective.[42] Surgical removal of especially painful areas of cortical bone can be helpful (personal observation).[37]

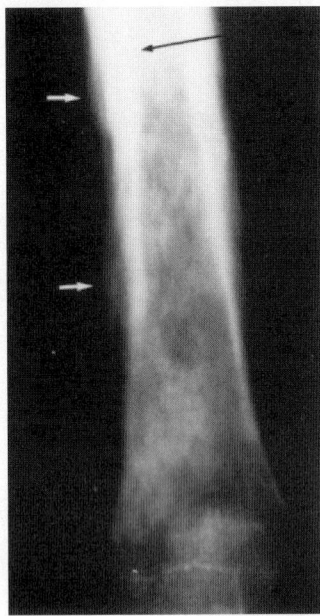

**FIGURE 66-5.** Progressive diaphyseal dysplasia. There is marked cortical thickening of the tibial diaphysis from both periosteal (*white arrows*) and endosteal (*black arrow*) new bone formation.

## INFANTILE CORTICAL HYPEROSTOSIS (CAFFEY SYNDROME)

Infantile cortical hyperostosis is a self-limited, focal skeletal disorder in which exuberant periosteal new bone causes transient swellings that involve adjacent musculature, fascia, and connective tissues. The swellings slowly resolve but often recur and can cause deformity.[5,7] Autosomal dominant transmission with variable expression and incomplete penetrance can occur.[43]

Symptoms generally begin abruptly before 5 months of age. Fever, irritability, anorexia, pallor, and pleurisy may be present. Soft-tissue swellings—precursors of the periosteal new bone formation—are tender and hard but generally not warm. Some infants appear to have pseudoparalysis, as they "splint" affected bones. Erb palsy may be diagnosed erroneously before radiographic changes are noted.[44] The clinical course is variable; manifestations may subside gradually over months, but occasionally the disease remains intermittently active for years. Patients may develop limb-length inequality or synostosis; some die of secondary infection.

Caffey syndrome is diagnosed radiologically.[5] The erythrocyte sedimentation rate, serum alkaline phosphatase activity, and leukocyte count may be elevated during episodes of swelling. Some patients have mild anemia. Skeletal involvement can be unifocal or may follow a sequential pattern of multifocal disease.[5] The mandible, clavicles, and ribs are involved most frequently—sometimes symmetrically. The skull, scapulae, and long bones may also be affected. Characteristically, diaphyseal cortical hyperostosis begins as new bone within the soft-tissue mass. The swelling then joins with the subjacent osseous tissue, causing bone enlargement, with dense thickening of the cortex secondary to periosteal elevation. Histologically, the periosteum is inflamed and thickened. Immature lamellar bone is present initially but undergoes maturation. Marrow spaces may be filled with vascular fibrous tissue. Dystrophic calcification can occur. Destructive lesions can involve the skull.

Infantile cortical hyperostosis generally resolves by 1 year of age. No specific medical or surgical treatment exists, although glucocorticoid therapy can cause prompt improvement. Patients should be observed and managed for symptoms. Sedation for irritability may be necessary.

## ENDOSTEAL HYPEROSTOSIS

Endosteal hyperostosis is inherited either as a clinically severe autosomal recessive disorder (*sclerosteosis* or *van Buchem disease*) or as a relatively benign autosomal dominant condition (*Worth type*).[6] The clinical and radiographic manifestations, however, are similar.[1,6,45] During puberty, progressive asymmetric enlargement of the mandible occurs. Occasionally, facial palsy or deafness is caused by cranial nerve entrapment, but the head circumference is normal. Serum alkaline phosphatase activity may be increased in van Buchem disease. Radiographic abnormalities include sclerosis of the axial skeleton and the skull (where the table may be wide), mandibular enlargement, and thickening of the diaphyses of long bones due to selective endosteal hyperostosis (bones remain properly shaped).[5] Some cases reported as van Buchem disease have features suggesting sclerostenosis or craniodiaphyseal dysplasia.[46] Previously, sclerostenosis had been differentiated from van Buchem disease because patients with the former condition were of excessive height and had syndactyly; however, both conditions map to chromosome 17q12-q21; thus, they may be allelic disorders.[47] No effective medical treatment exists.

## FLUOROSIS

Chronic ingestion or inhalation of large amounts of fluoride causes fluorosis.[48] In the United States, prolonged administration of sodium fluoride as a therapy for postmenopausal osteoporosis represents an increasingly unlikely cause. Mottled discoloration of the teeth, diffuse bone pain reflecting an underlying osteomalacia, and a plantar fascia syndrome characterized by painful feet may be presenting features. Biochemical diagnosis by assay of the fluoride ion in 24-hour urine collections can be obtained through commercial laboratories. Early radiographic signs include irregularity at the point of attachment of muscles to the iliac spine and calcification of ligaments in the pelvis, vertebrae, and interosseous membranes.[5] Later, generalized osteosclerosis can occur. Histopathologic studies may reveal osteomalacia (fluoride stimulates osteoid synthesis by osteoblasts, yet mineral deposition is impaired). Treatment consists of protection from fluoride exposure and, if osteomalacia is present, calcium supplementation to mineralize the excess osteoid (see Chaps. 63 and 131).

## OSTEOPOIKILOSIS

Osteopoikilosis (spotted bones) is a radiographic curiosity.[5,6] If unrecognized, however, it may lead to investigation for metastatic disease, mastocytosis, tuberous sclerosis, or other disorders. It is inherited as an autosomal dominant trait and manifests as numerous well-defined, small, homogeneous, symmetric, round or oval, periarticular foci of osteosclerosis (Fig. 66-6). Bone scanning, however, is unremarkable.[49] In some kindreds focal, asymptomatic accumulation of dermal elastin (dermatofibrosis lenticularis disseminata) is found, and the disorder is called *Buschke-Ollendorff syndrome*.[50]

## OSTEOPATHIA STRIATA

Osteopathia striata is characterized radiographically by symmetric, regular, dense bony striations in the metaphyseal regions of tubular bones (Fig. 66-7) and by fan-like linear pro-

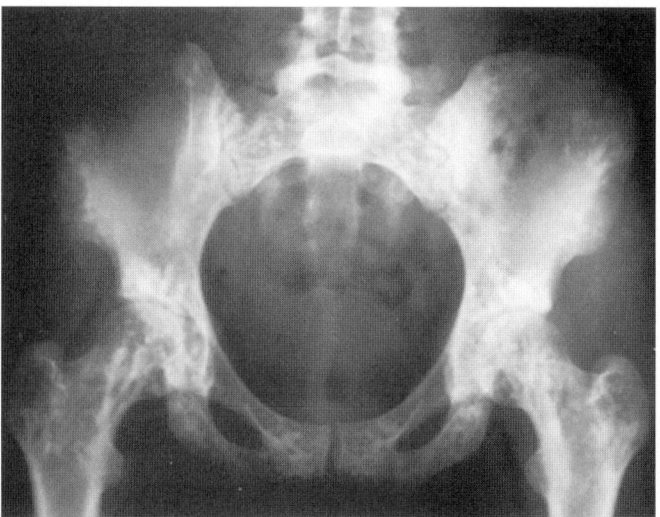

**FIGURE 66-6.** Osteopoikilosis. Characteristic features shown here include the spotted appearance of the pelvis and meta-epiphyseal regions of the femora.

jections in the iliac wings.[5] It is inherited as an autosomal dominant trait and is a radiographic curiosity unless associated with ectodermal manifestations (i.e., focal dermal hypoplasia, *Goltz syndrome*) or with additional skeletal lesions. Bone scanning is unremarkable.[49]

## MELORHEOSTOSIS

Melorheostosis, a sporadic, asymmetric hyperostosis that usually affects the long bones, can cause pain and intermittent swelling of joints and limit mobility. Deformity and limb-length discrepancy may result from shortening of muscles, ligaments, and tendons.[51] Often, cutaneous changes are present over subsequently involved skeletal areas. No sex preference is seen;

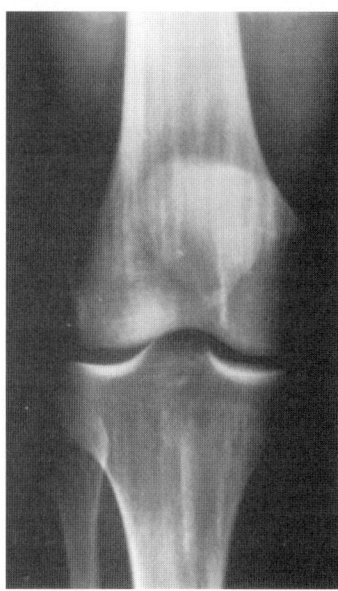

**FIGURE 66-7.** Osteopathia striata. Typical longitudinal striations are present in the metaphyseal regions of the femur, tibia, and fibula. (From Whyte MP, Murphy WA. Osteopathia striata associated with familial dermopathy and white forelock: evidence for postnatal development of osteopathia striata. Am J Med Genet 1980; 5:227.)

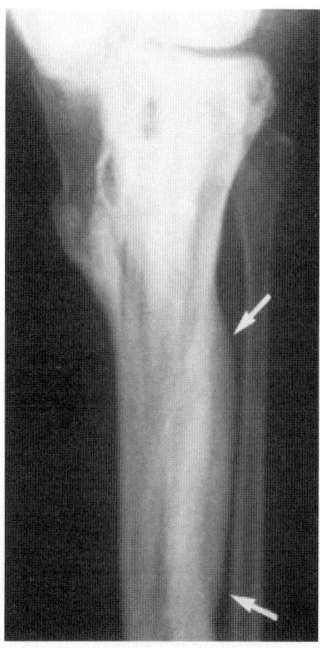

**FIGURE 66-8.** Melorheostosis. Characteristic patchy cortical sclerosis, which gives a "dripping-candle-wax" appearance to the cortex (*arrows*), is present in most of the proximal tibia.

symptoms usually begin before 20 years of age. The disorder may progress, but it is commonly present in only one limb, generally a lower extremity, of which one or several bones are affected. Radiographic examination reveals a "dripping-candle-wax" appearance to the cortex (Fig. 66-8). Bone scanning shows increased radionuclide uptake in involved areas.[49] No effective medical treatment exists. Some patients require surgery to relieve symptoms from contractions or neurovascular entrapment.

## MIXED SCLEROSING BONE DYSTROPHY

Rarely, a patient may have various combinations of osteopathia striata, melorheostosis, osteopoikilosis, cranial sclerosis, diaphyseal dysplasia, or other defects in bone formation.[52] Individuals with melorheostotic features or cranial sclerosis can have symptoms from compression of neurovascular tissue.[53] This is a sporadic condition. No known medical treatment exists.

## FIBRODYSPLASIA (MYOSITIS) OSSIFICANS PROGRESSIVA

Fibrodysplasia (myositis) ossificans progressiva (FOP) features accumulation of true bone in the fibrous connective tissue of striated muscle, ligaments, tendons, and fascia; however, smooth muscle is spared.[2,4–6] Patients have congenital anomalies of the digits (75% incidence of bilateral microdactyly of the great toe with synostosis and hypoplasia of the phalanges), allowing a presumptive diagnosis at birth.[5] The pathogenesis involves endochondral bone formation in soft tissues.[54] Most cases appear to represent new mutations for this autosomal dominant disorder (advanced paternal age seems to be a causal factor).

The severity of FOP can be quite variable.[55] Ectopic bone formation generally begins during the first decade of life as a painful, warm swelling (commonly in the sternocleidomastoid muscle) that regresses over 1 to 2 months, leaving a bony residuum. Trauma can provoke the appearance of lesions. Episodes

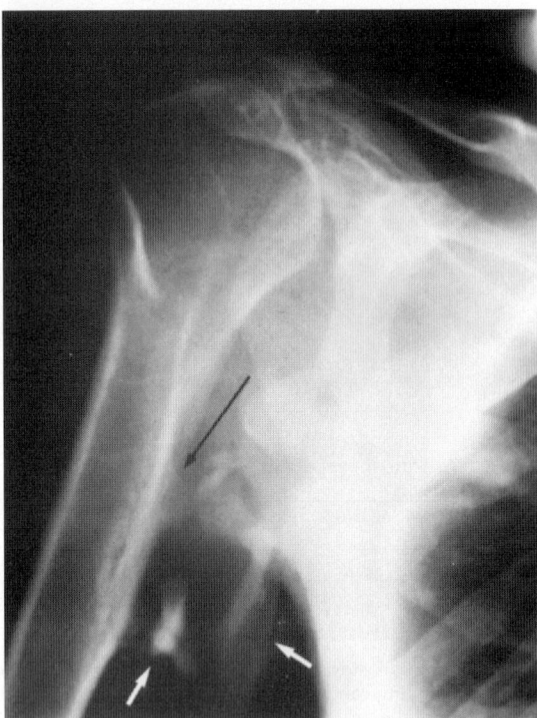

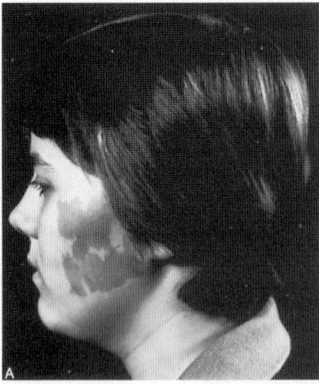 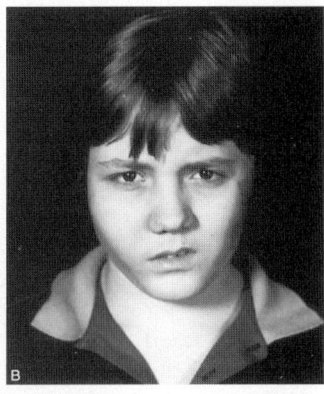

**FIGURE 66-10. A,** Fibrous dysplasia. Café-au-lait spots are typically ipsilateral to and near the skeletal lesions. These café-au-lait macules have irregular ("coast of Maine") margins unlike in neurofibromatosis, in which they have smooth ("coast of California") borders. **B,** This 13-year-old boy, however, has bilateral skeletal disease that resulted in characteristic deformity of the face on the contralateral side.

**FIGURE 66-9.** Fibrodysplasia ossificans progressiva. Typical struts of ectopic bone (*white arrows*) are seen in the periarticular soft tissues of the shoulder of this 17-year-old boy. Exostoses (*black arrow*) are common.

occur with considerable irregularity, which makes assessment of attempted therapies or prognosis difficult. The shoulder girdle, upper arms, spine, and pelvis may be affected—generally in that sequence. Accumulation of ectopic bone eventually limits range of motion, especially in the neck and shoulders; thoracic deformity, due to involvement of the intercostal and paravertebral muscles, causes constriction of the chest. Restrictive pulmonary disease and recurrent pneumonia can follow. Patients may die from adolescence onward from restrictive lung disease, infection, or inanition owing to masseter muscle disease, although a long life is possible.[4]

Routine biochemical studies are generally normal. Radiographic features include ossification of an entire muscle or the appearance of a plate of ectopic bone that outlines a fascial plane.[5] Metaphyseal exostoses may be present (Fig. 66-9). In the spine, fusion of the apophyseal joints is followed by fusion of the vertebrae. Radiographically, the differential diagnosis includes calcinosis universalis, dermatomyositis, tumoral calcinosis, and other disorders of mineral homeostasis that produce ectopic calcification. Histologic examination reveals true bone (i.e., mature bone with trabeculae and haversian systems, sometimes including marrow).

No medical therapy is established for FOP.[56] Administration of disodium etidronate, a bisphosphonate that in large doses inhibits bone formation, produces equivocal results. Warfarin treatment to disrupt γ-carboxylation of skeletal calcium-binding protein reportedly decreases urinary γ-carboxyglutamic acid levels but does not limit the ectopic calcification.[57] Treatment of FOP is supportive. Physical therapy to maintain joint mobility may exacerbate the condition or provoke new lesions. Trauma to muscle (e.g., surgery, intramuscular injections) should be avoided whenever possible. Sometimes, surgical release of the jaw is successful and may be essential to improve nutrition. Dental procedures should be completed early in life.

FOP lesions are a form of ectopic endochondral bone formation.[54] The temporal-spatial appearance of the lesions is reminiscent of the distribution of the decapentaplegia mutation in

*Drosophila* species. In FOP, a disturbance in circulating levels of bone morphogenetic protein (BMP) has been reported.[58] One patient has been shown to have a defect in the gene that encodes noggin, a BMP inhibitor.[58a]

# FIBROUS DYSPLASIA

Fibrous dysplasia, a sporadic unifocal or multifocal developmental skeletal disorder, affects either sex and often causes fractures and deformities.[59] The pathogenetic abnormality is an expanding fibrous lesion of bone-forming mesenchyme.[4] Monostotic disease typically presents during the second or third decade of life; polyostotic disease manifests before 10 years of age.[60] Long bones or the skull are usually affected. Before adolescence, expansile skeletal lesions may fracture, cause deformity, and sometimes entrap nerves. Affected bones occasionally become sarcomatous (incidence of <1%), especially with involvement of the facial bones or the femur.[61] Pregnancy may reactivate previously quiescent lesions. Some patients have characteristic hyperpigmented skin macules called *café-au-lait spots* (Fig. 66-10) and endocrine hyperfunction (i.e., *McCune-Albright syndrome*).[59] The endocrinopathy is usually pseudoprecocious puberty in girls and less commonly thyrotoxicosis, Cushing syndrome, acromegaly, hyperprolactinemia, or hyperparathyroidism.[62] Rarely, patients with McCune-Albright syndrome also have renal phosphate wasting and hypophosphatemic bone disease that may represent a form of "oncogenic" rickets or osteomalacia[63] (see Chaps. 63, 67, 70, and 219).

Although serum alkaline phosphatase activity can be increased in fibrous dysplasia, blood calcium and phosphate levels are usually normal. Monostotic disease is more common than polyostotic involvement, but any bone can be affected.[5] The femur, tibia, ribs, and facial bones are most frequently involved. Small bones are affected in 50% of the patients with polyostotic disease. Lesions in the long bones occur in the metaphyses and diaphyses. They are generally discrete, sometimes lobulated or trabeculated, areas of radiolucency characteristically with thin cortices and a ground-glass appearance (Fig. 66-11).

Monostotic and polyostotic lesions have similar histologic findings. They are well defined but not encapsulated. Characteristically, spindle-shaped fibroblasts form a swirl in marrow spaces with haphazardly arranged trabeculae consisting of immature woven bone (Fig. 66-12). Cartilage tissue is present especially in polyostotic disease. Cystic areas, which are lined by multinucleated giant cells, may also be found. The lesion is reminiscent of the changes seen in hyperparathyroidism, but unlike in osteitis fibrosa cystica, mature osteoblasts are absent.

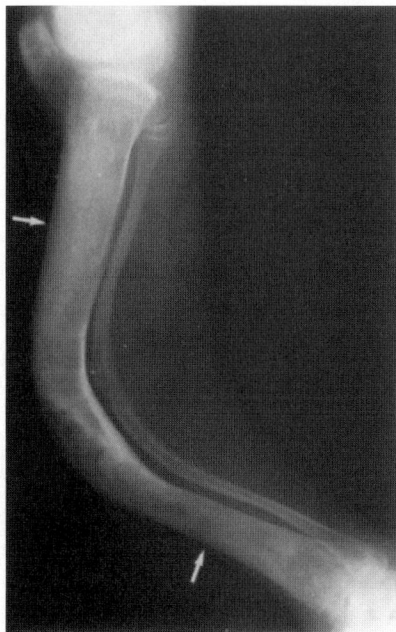

**FIGURE 66-11.** Fibrous dysplasia. Classic features in long bones include an expansile lesion in the diaphysis associated with thin but intact cortices (*arrows*) and an overall ground-glass appearance—changes present in the tibia of this 16-year-old boy with polyostotic disease who also developed hypophosphatemic osteomalacia.

The cause of McCune-Albright syndrome and fibrous dysplasia is somatic mosaicism for activating mutations in the gene encoding the $G_s\alpha$ subunit of the G protein that couples hormone receptors to adenylate cyclase.[64] Endocrine abnormalities in McCune-Albright syndrome are due to end-organ hyperactivity rather than premature hypothalamic maturation with secretion of releasing hormones.[62] No established medical treatment exists for the skeletal disease; however, promising responses have been reported with intravenous administration of pamidronate.[65] Spontaneous improvement does not occur. Skeletal lesions may progress, and new ones may appear; however, in most patients with mild disease, lesions are quiescent. Girls with precocious puberty have responded favorably to the

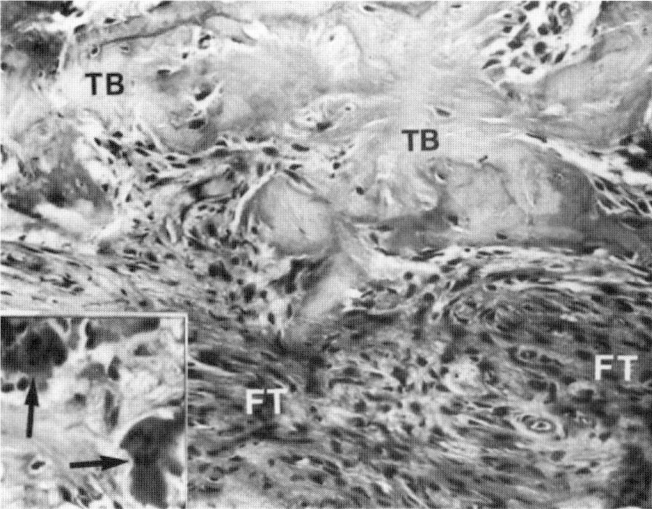

**FIGURE 66-12.** Fibrous dysplasia. Characteristic histopathologic findings include whorls of abundant fibrous tissue (*FT*) in the medullary space, trabecular bone (*TB*) composed of woven collagen, and, as shown in the inset, osteoclastosis (*arrows*) yet *absence* of osteoblasts.

aromatase inhibitor testolactone.[66] Although painful stress or fissure fractures may be difficult to detect, generally fractures heal well. The potential for development of endocrinopathies or skeletal sarcomas should be remembered. Calcitriol and inorganic phosphate supplementation may be helpful for associated hypophosphatemic bone disease.

## OSTEOGENESIS IMPERFECTA

Osteogenesis imperfecta (OI; brittle-bone disease) is characterized by osteopenia with recurrent fractures and deformity, dental disease, and premature hearing loss[67] (see Chaps. 70 and 189). Clinical severity is extremely variable, ranging from stillbirth to deafness or fracture late in adult life. The pathogenesis involves quantitative and often qualitative abnormalities in the biosynthesis of type I collagen, the most abundant protein in bone. Connective tissue in ligaments, skin, sclerae, and dentin is also affected, because type I collagen is normally present in these structures as well. Classification into several clinical types has been useful, but the understanding of OI has been greatly improved by the identification of > 250 distinct mutations in the genes that encode the $\alpha_1$ and $\alpha_2$ procollagen chains which intertwine to form the type I collagen heterotrimer[2,3,68] (see Chap. 189).

Patients with OI may also be troubled by ligamentous laxity causing joint hypermobility, excessive diaphoresis, and bruising. They are predisposed to pulmonary infections if they have severe thoracic deformity from vertebral collapses and kyphoscoliosis. Mitral valve clicks are common, but significant cardiac disease is unusual. Hearing loss affects approximately half of patients younger than 30 years of age and nearly all who are older. Deafness may be conductive, sensorineural, or of mixed pathogenesis. The differential diagnosis of multiple fractures in the pediatric population includes the "battered baby" syndrome and congenital indifference to pain. Generalized osteopenia in children may be due to idiopathic juvenile osteoporosis, Cushing disease, or many other disorders.[4]

The classification scheme of Silence, which emphasizes the apparent mode of inheritance and severity of the skeletal manifestations of OI, is referenced frequently[68] (see Chap. 189); however, essentially all forms of OI are inherited as autosomal dominant disorders.[68] Type I OI is associated with blue sclerae (especially obvious in childhood), osteopenia with recurrent fracture but often normal stature, and deafness during early adulthood (30% of cases). Dentinogenesis imperfecta may be absent or present in different kindreds (types IA and IB, respectively). Joint laxity or hernias can also occur. Affected women, who may first present with fractures late in adult life, can be mistakenly thought to have postmenopausal or involutional osteoporosis, and radiographic findings may not distinguish the disorders. Approximately one-third of OI patients represent new mutations.[68] Histomorphometric assessment of undecalcified specimens of bone reveal an increased number of cortical osteocytes in some patients.[68a]

Patients with Silence types II, III, or IV OI are affected more severely. Phenotypic features include a triangle-shaped face, high-pitched voice, deformities of the long bones of the extremities (yet normal-appearing hands and feet), pectus excavatum or carinatum, joint hyperextensibility, excessive sweating, and hernias. Even patients with the most severe skeletal manifestations are generally of normal intelligence.[67,68]

Routine biochemical studies are usually unremarkable; elevated serum alkaline phosphatase activity and urine hydroxyproline levels occur in some patients. Hypercalciuria is common in severely affected children.[69] This finding may be explained by poor skeletal growth despite effective absorption of dietary calcium.

Characteristic radiographic changes occur in severely affected patients.[5] Generalized osteopenia and deformity of long bones

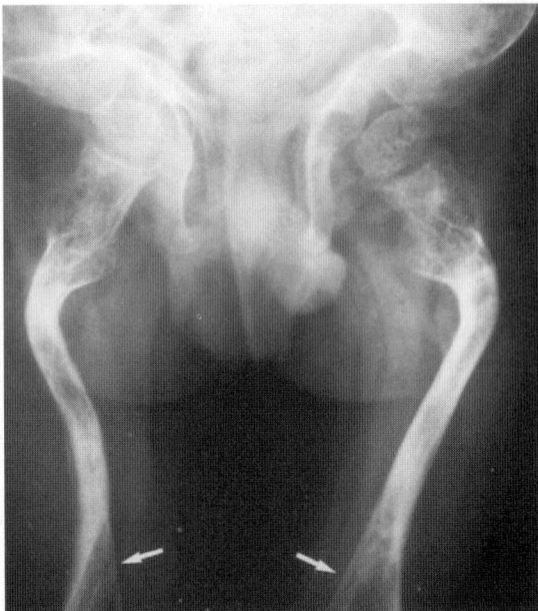

**FIGURE 66-13.** Osteogenesis imperfecta. In the more severely affected patients (here a 4.5-year-old boy), long bones are characteristically gracile (narrow diameter) with thin cortices (*arrows*); they fracture easily, resulting in bowing deformity.

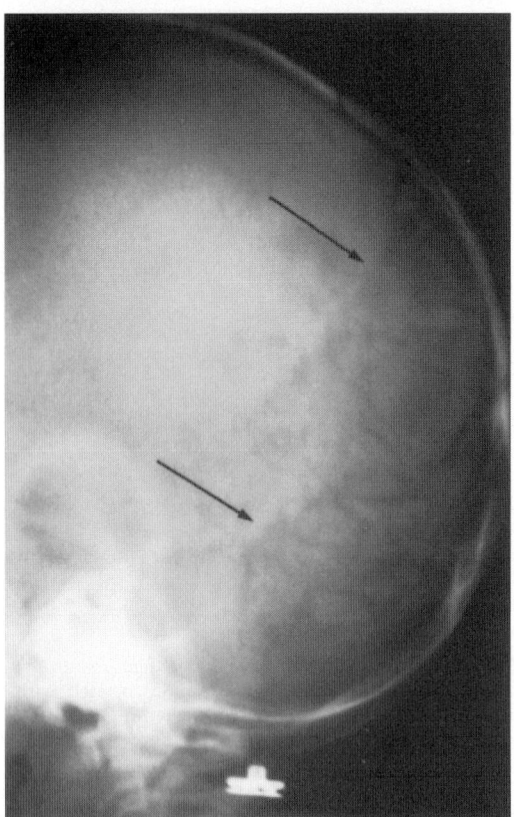

**FIGURE 66-14.** Osteogenesis imperfecta. Wormian bones (*arrows*), although not pathognomonic of this disorder, are often found in the lambdoidal suture of the posterior occiput.

from recurrent fractures are present, and vertebrae may be collapsed. Periosteal bone formation is defective, which retards the circumferential growth of bone and causes a gracile appearance in ribs and long bones in the limbs (Fig. 66-13). In some severely affected infants with an especially poor prognosis, severe micromelia (major long bones appear short but thick in their external diameter) and marked bowing deformities are present. Wormian bones may be noted (Fig. 66-14), and the pelvis can be triradiate shaped. Radiographic abnormalities may change considerably during growth.[5] *Popcorn calcifications* are rare developmental lesions in the epiphyses and metaphyses of major long bones (predominantly at the knees and ankles) that may be due to traumatic fragmentation of growth plate cartilage. They are observed during childhood, appear to resolve at adolescence, and may severely limit skeletal growth. Understandably, patients are predisposed to osteoarthritis. Fractures are often transverse, yet they heal at normal rates—sometimes with exuberant callus formation if motion persists at the fracture site. Platybasia can also occur, occasionally with basilar impression.[67,68]

Undecalcified specimens of bone may reveal abnormal skeletal matrix, especially in more severely affected patients. Disorganized, "woven" bone can be abundant. Polarized-light microscopy may demonstrate thin collagen bundles in areas of lamellar bone. The number of osteocytes in cortical bone can be increased, a finding that perhaps reflects decreased activity of individual osteoblasts, although the overall rate of bone turnover is rapid. Histomorphometric studies after in vivo tetracycline labeling support this hypothesis.[4,68a]

The perinatal form of OI (type II) can result from large rearrangements or even point mutations within the genes encoding the pro-$\alpha_1$ or pro-$\alpha_2$ chains of type I procollagen.[2,3,68] The nascent collagen molecule undergoes excessive posttranslational modification that, in turn, results in diminished secretion of unstable bone matrix (see Chap. 189). In the milder forms (e.g., type I), the amount of type I procollagen synthesized is decreased, but a variety of secondary quantitative defects in noncollagenous bone proteins occur as well, reflecting a more profound defect in the development of hard tissues.

Although remarkable progress has been made in our understanding of the heterogeneous genetic defects in OI, no established medical therapy exists.[68] Intravenous infusions of pamidronate seem promising in uncontrolled trials.[70,70a] Treatment is supportive and often requires expert dental care with orthopedic and rehabilitation therapy for the recurrent fractures and limb deformities, kyphosis, and scoliosis. Support groups (e.g., Osteogenesis Imperfecta Foundation, Inc.) are an important source of comfort and current information for patients and their families.

Genetic counseling should be offered and periodically updated, because progress in this area has been important.[68] Although very rarely some cases represent an autosomal recessive condition, gonadal mosaicism can account for new-onset OI in affected siblings. Prenatal diagnosis by a variety of techniques, including ultrasonography in severe cases and molecular testing, has been successful.[71]

## HYPOPHOSPHATASIA

Hypophosphatasia is an inborn error of metabolism characterized clinically by premature tooth loss and rickets or osteomalacia, and biochemically by subnormal serum alkaline phosphatase activity.[72] Delineation of this condition has shown that alkaline phosphatase functions importantly as an ectoenzyme in skeletal mineralization. Four clinical forms, classified according to the patient's age when skeletal disease is first noted (perinatal, infantile, childhood, adult), are generally reported. Actually, the severity of hypophosphatasia is a continuum that ranges from stillbirth to hypophosphatasemia in asymptomatic adults with unremarkable radiologic and histopathologic studies of bone.[73,74] When hypophosphatasia manifests at birth, it may be confused with a severe form of OI because of profound hypomineralization of the skeleton, or with cleidocranial dysplasia because of wide cranial sutures.[5] If the onset is within the first 6 months of life (infantile form), only hypotonia may be noted perinatally, but subsequently failure to thrive may occur as patients develop clinically apparent rickets and hypercalcemia, recurrent pneumonias, and sometimes seizures or periodic apnea. Onset later in infancy or during childhood may cause short stature, rachitic deformity, early loss of deciduous teeth, and premature cranial synostosis.[72,73] In the adult form, a history of dental disease often precedes painful recurrent stress fractures in the feet and pseudofractures (Looser zones) in the proximal femora.[74] The severe forms are inherited as autosomal recessive traits.[72] The adult form can be transmitted as an autosomal dominant trait, but with variable penetrance.[74] *Odontohypophosphatasia* refers to the disorder in patients (primarily children) who have only dental manifestations. More than 58 different mutations in the gene that encodes the isoenzyme form of alkaline phosphatase found in bone have been detected in individuals with hypophosphatasia.[75]

The diagnosis requires a finding of subnormal serum alkaline phosphatase activity for the patient's age. (Note: Several clinical situations cause hypophosphatasemia, e.g., glucocorticoid therapy, starvation, vitamin D intoxication, scurvy, hypothyroidism, milk-alkali syndrome, magnesium deficiency, massive transfusion, severe anemia, or improper collection of blood.) Sometimes, clinical laboratories neglect to report a lower limit of serum alkaline phosphatase activity or fail to provide age-appropriate normal ranges. Increased levels of *plasma pyridoxal 5'-phosphate* or *urinary phosphoethanolamine* (natural substrates for alkaline phosphatase) give supportive biochemical evidence.[76] *Inorganic pyrophosphate* (an endogenous inhibitor of bone mineralization) is increased in blood and urine, but the assay is a research procedure.

Radiographic findings in children often provide more information than merely the suggestion of some form of rickets. Along with rachitic changes, characteristic focal "tongues" of metaphyseal radiolucency are seen (Fig. 66-15). Adults can be osteopenic and have unhealed stress fractures of the feet or elsewhere. Looser zones may be present in the femora and, although unexplained, are often situated laterally rather than medially as in other forms of osteomalacia. Chondrocalcinosis and additional changes consistent with pyrophosphate arthropathy result from articular accumulation of calcium pyrophosphate.[77] As in all forms of rickets and osteomalacia, a generalized

defect in skeletal mineralization is present in hypophosphatasia. However, *no* pathognomonic histopathologic changes in bone are seen. Histochemical studies demonstrate deficient alkaline phosphatase activity.[73] Evidence of secondary hyperparathyroidism is generally absent. Conversely, *histologic examination of teeth* can be an excellent aid for diagnosis and characteristically shows absence or hypoplasia of cementum.

No established medical therapy is available for hypophosphatasia. Hypercalcemia in infants may be improved by dietary calcium restriction (glucocorticoid or calcitonin treatment has also been used). Nevertheless, progressive skeletal demineralization often follows. Calcium supplementation or administration of vitamin D or one of its bioactive metabolites may cause hypercalcemia and hypercalciuria. Inorganic phosphate supplementation to enhance urinary excretion of inorganic pyrophosphate and enzyme-replacement therapy using intravenous infusion of alkaline phosphatases have been disappointing.[72] Infusion of pooled normal plasma was followed by remarkable transient skeletal remineralization in a boy with the infantile form.[78] Bone marrow transplantation seemed beneficial for another infant.[79] A trial of vitamin B$_6$ should be given for unexplained seizures.[76] Optimal orthopedic management of femoral fractures and pseudofractures in adults may require insertion of intramedullary rods.[80] Craniotomy may be necessary to correct premature synostosis. Prenatal diagnosis of the severe perinatal (lethal) form is possible with ultrasonography and by assay of alkaline phosphatase activity in chorionic villus samples.[81] Molecular diagnosis is becoming feasible.

## AXIAL OSTEOMALACIA

Axial osteomalacia features defective bone mineralization despite normal serum levels of calcium and phosphate and increased alkaline phosphatase activity. Men seem to be affected more frequently than women; in one study,[82] this disorder was found to be familial. The condition may be discovered incidentally; occasionally, patients present with a vague, chronic axial skeletal pain. Radiographic studies reveal osteosclerosis of the axial skeleton in which the trabecular pattern is coarse, as in other forms of osteomalacia.[5] The appendicular skeleton appears unaffected, and Looser zones have not been reported. Features of ankylosing spondylitis may be present. Histopathologic studies of bone reveal osteoidosis and failure of tetracycline deposition but no evidence of secondary hyperparathyroidism. Osteoblasts are inactive-appearing (flat) lining cells.[82] Because the disorder seems to reflect a defect in the bone tissue, use of vitamin D and mineral supplementation is not recommended. No effective medical therapy exists.

## FIBROGENESIS IMPERFECTA OSSIUM

Fibrogenesis imperfecta ossium is a sporadic, idiopathic disorder in which pathologic changes seem to affect collagen within the skeleton only. Symptoms begin in adult life. There is progressive pain, recurrent fractures, and then weakness, muscle atrophy, and contractures. Patients become immobilized and debilitated. Marked bone tenderness is elicited by palpation. Serum calcium and phosphate levels are unremarkable, although alkaline phosphatase activity may be increased. Radiographic abnormalities occur throughout the skeleton, except the skull.[5] Although generalized osteopenia (most marked in the axial skeleton and periarticular regions) with a paucity of spongy bone is present, trabeculae appear coarse and dense. An abnormal trabecular pattern replaces cortical bone. Deformity secondary to fracture may be present, but bony contours are usually normal. Vertebral end plates can appear sclerotic and mimic a *"rugger-jersey"* spine. The radiographic differential diagnosis includes advanced osteitis fibrosa

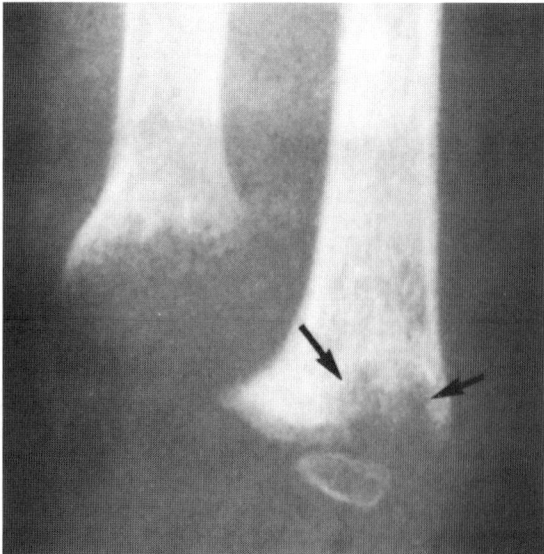

**FIGURE 66-15.** Hypophosphatasia. Projections ("tongues") of radiolucency from a widened growth plate into the metaphysis (*arrows*) are a characteristic feature of the rickets of hypophosphatasia, demonstrated here in the forearm of a 2-year-old boy.

cystica, Paget bone disease, and axial osteomalacia.[5] Histopathologic studies are important and show that the birefringent pattern normally formed by collagen fibrils is absent in lamellar bone. Electron microscopy reveals a random, tangled pattern of thin collagen fibrils.[83] Increased numbers of osteoid seams do not take up tetracycline labels. The pathogenesis seems to involve a defect in bone matrix rather than in mineral metabolism. No effective medical therapy is known.

## METAPHYSEAL AND SPONDYLOMETAPHYSEAL DYSPLASIAS

Not all disorders in children that result in widened growth plates and metaphyseal irregularity are forms of rickets (i.e., generalized disturbance of mineralization of skeletal matrix).[5] Metaphyseal or spondylometaphyseal dysplasias may mimic rickets radiographically[5]; however, the biochemical aberrations associated with rachitic disorders are absent.[84] Serum levels of calcium, phosphate, and alkaline phosphatase activity are normal, and biopsy of skeletal tissue away from the metaphyses (after in vivo tetracycline labeling) confirms that bone remodeling is unremarkable. Instead, these disorders involve dysplastic processes occurring in growth plates. They are heritable with various patterns of genetic transmission.[1,4,7,84] Mutations in the genes that encode types II, IX, and X collagen have been discovered.

The most common metaphyseal dysplasia, the Schmid type, is a form of short-limb dwarfism. Patients present with short stature and occasionally with rachitic-like deformities of the legs. They grow steadily, but height is generally below the fifth percentile. An especially severe (Jensen) type, which is associated with hypercalcemia and marked short stature, is caused by activating mutations in the parathyroid hormone/parathyroid hormone–related protein receptor.[85] Patients with spondylometaphyseal dysplasia have vertebral abnormalities as well as metaphyseal defects. Accordingly, thoracic deformity often occurs in these individuals.

The medical history, physical findings, and unremarkable screening biochemical studies are usually sufficient to exclude rickets. Experienced radiologists generally provide a correct diagnosis.[5] In milder or more unclear cases, histologic examination of nondecalcified bone sections (obtained after in vivo tetracycline administration) helps to exclude rickets or osteomalacia.

Orthopedic management may include bracing of bowing deformities. Occasionally, osteotomy is necessary to prevent osteoarthritis or premature closure of growth plates.[84] When the spine is involved, instability may occur from dysplastic changes of the vertebrae. If such abnormalities affect the cervical region, odontoid hypoplasia can be an important problem that may require neurosurgical intervention.

## IDIOPATHIC JUVENILE OSTEOPOROSIS

Idiopathic juvenile osteoporosis is a poorly characterized, heterogeneous condition that almost certainly has a variety of causes.[4] A few case reports and small clinical series indicate that the disorder typically presents during late childhood with fracture—especially in the lower limbs and with vertebral collapse—but afterwards improves spontaneously.[86] Distinction from OI requires a careful physical examination and family history. Idiopathic juvenile osteoporosis is generally a diagnosis of exclusion; secondary causes of osteopenia in children must always be considered (see Chap. 70).[4] No established therapy exists, but dietary deficiencies (e.g., suboptimal calcium intake) should be corrected, and patients should be cautioned against stooping to lift heavy objects or participating in potentially traumatic physical activity. Bisphosphonate therapy is being evaluated.

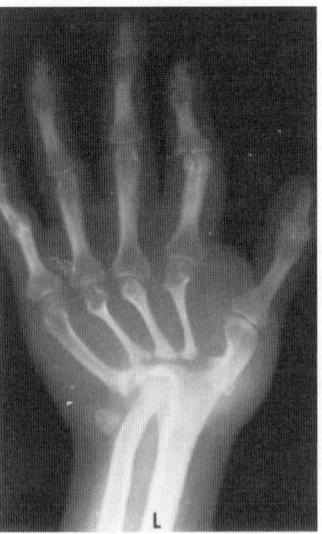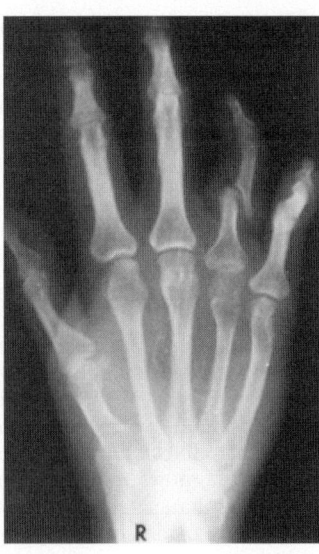

**FIGURE 66-16.** Carpotarsal osteolysis. Classic radiographic features include gradual disappearance of carpal and tarsal bones during childhood, leaving just a residual tapered ("sucked candy") appearance to the metacarpals. In this 40-year-old man, the radiographic changes of the disease are early in the right hand, yet advanced in the left hand. (*L*, left; *R*, right.) (From Whyte MP, Murphy WA, Kleerekoper M, et al. Idiopathic multicentric osteolysis: report of an affected father and son. Arthritis Rheum 1978; 21:367.)

## IDIOPATHIC OSTEOLYSIS

Unifocal or multifocal osteolytic lesions manifest in a variety of sporadic idiopathic or hereditary disorders.[87] Acro-osteolysis occurs with polyvinyl chloride poisoning, hand trauma (e.g., use of vibrating instruments), systemic lupus erythematosus, and other conditions.[87,88] Carpotarsal osteolysis (Fig. 66-16) is characterized by episodes of pain and swelling in the wrists and ankles during childhood that accompany osteolysis of predominantly the carpal and tarsal bones.[89] The disorder occurs as an isolated problem when transmitted as an autosomal dominant trait; nephropathy occurs in some sporadic or autosomal recessive cases. In Gorham massive osteolysis, unifocal areas of osteolysis can cause considerable bone destruction.[90]

## ECTOPIC CALCIFICATION

Many conditions are associated with extraskeletal deposition of calcium and phosphate.[4] In some, the pathogenesis is an elevation in the circulating calcium-phosphate product (i.e., metastatic calcification).[91] In others, the precise mechanism is unknown, and either amorphous calcium (dystrophic calcification) or true bone is deposited.[91] Metastatic calcification occurs with hypercalcemia of any cause (e.g., milk-alkali syndrome, hypervitaminosis D, tumoral calcinosis, sarcoidosis, hyperparathyroidism, and renal osteodystrophy). Typically, deposits occur in the kidneys, lungs, media of large arteries, fundus of the stomach, and periarticular regions. Hyperphosphatemia is also associated with ectopic calcification (e.g., hypoparathyroidism and pseudohypoparathyroidism), renal insufficiency, and massive cell destruction with liberation of inorganic phosphate (e.g., chemotherapy for leukemia). Dystrophic calcification, in which the calcium-phosphate product is normal, occurs in necrotic tissue in the calcinosis universalis and calcinosis circumscripta that accompany scleroderma, dermatomyositis, systemic lupus erythematosus, trauma, and metastatic malignancy, and as a primary cutaneous disease.[4] Fasciitis is associated with ectopic bone formation (e.g., myositis ossificans progressiva), although other soft tissues can ossify, as in neurologic injury, burns, and trauma. Progressive osseous heteroplasia, an autosomal dominant disorder featuring extraskeletal ossification in subcutaneous and deep tissues, is caused by mutation in the GNASI gene that encodes the $G_s\alpha$ stimulatory protein.[91a]

## ISCHEMIC NECROSIS

Ischemic (avascular) necrosis is common[92] (see Chap. 211). The condition has multiple causes: endocrine or metabolic (e.g., glucocorticoid therapy, Cushing disease, alcohol abuse, gout, osteomalacia, hyperparathyroidism, hypothyroidism), storage diseases (e.g., Gaucher disease), hemoglobinopathies, trauma, dysbaric disorders, irradiation, and pancreatitis.[93] Some cases are idiopathic, and some are familial. The most common causes are prolonged exposure to glucocorticoids and alcohol abuse. Patients present with deep aching pain in the diseased region. Often, the head of the femur is affected. Microfracture of dead trabecular bone destroys the support for overlying cortical bone and articular cartilage. Radiographic studies typically reveal sclerosis of subcortical bone.[5] Nuclear magnetic resonance imaging provides the greatest sensitivity and specificity to aid in early diagnosis.[94] Treatment may require core decompression or joint arthroplasty or replacement with a prosthesis.

## REFERENCES

1. Beighton P. Inherited disorders of the skeleton, 2nd ed. New York: Churchill Livingstone, 1988.
2. Royce PM, Steinmann BU, eds. Connective tissue and its heritable disorders, 2nd ed. New York: Wiley-Liss, 2001; in press.
3. Beighton P, ed. Heritable disorders of connective tissue, 5th ed. St. Louis: Mosby–Year Book, 1993.
4. Favus MJ, ed. Primer on the metabolic bone diseases and disorders of mineral metabolism, 4th ed. Philadelphia: Lippincott Williams & Wilkins, 1999.
5. Resnick D. Diagnosis of bone and joint disorders, 3rd ed. Philadelphia: WB Saunders, 1995.
6. Whyte MP. Skeletal disorders characterized by osteosclerosis or hyperostosis. In: Avioli LV, Krane SM, eds. Metabolic bone disease and clinically related disorders, 2nd ed. San Diego: Academic Press, 1997.
7. Taybi H, Lachman RS. Radiology of syndromes, metabolic disorders, and skeletal dysplasias, 4th ed. St. Louis: Mosby, 1996.
8. Whyte MP. Osteopetrosis. In: Royce PM, Steinmann BU, eds. Connective tissue and its heritable disorders, 2nd ed. New York: Wiley-Liss, 2001; in press.
9. Key LL Jr, Ries WL. Osteopetrosis. In: Bilezikian JP, Raisz LG, Rodan GA, eds. Principles of bone biology. San Diego: Academic Press, 1996.
10. Heaney C, Shalev H, Elbedour K, et al. Human autosomal recessive osteopetrosis maps to 11q13, a position predicted by comparative mapping of the murine osteosclerosis (oc) mutation. Hum Mol Genet 1998; 7:1407.
11. Van Hul W, Bollerslev J, Gram J, et al. Localization of a gene for autosomal dominant osteopetrosis (Albers-Schönberg disease) to chromosome 1p21. Am J Hum Genet 1997; 61:363.
12. Kahler SG, Burns JA, Aylsworth AS. A mild autosomal recessive form of osteopetrosis. Am J Med Genet 1984; 17:451.
13. Whyte MP. Carbonic anhydrase II deficiency. Clin Orthop 1993; 294:52.
13a. Frattini A, Orchard PJ, Sobacchi C, et al. Defects in TCIRG1 subunit of the vacuolar proton pump are responsible for a subset of human autosomal recessive osteopetrosis. Nat Genet 2000; 25:343.
14. Whyte MP. Recent advances in osteopetrosis. In: Cohn DV, Gennari C, Tashjian AH Jr, eds. Calcium regulating hormones and bone metabolism. New York: Elsevier Science, 1992.
15. Athanasou NA, Sabokbar A. Human osteoclast ontogeny and pathological bone resorption. Histol Histopathol 1999; 14:635.
16. Marks SC Jr. Osteopetrosis: multiple pathways for the interruption of osteoclast function. Appl Pathol 1987; 5:172.
17. Marks SC Jr. Osteoclast biology: lessons from mammalian mutations. Am J Med Genet 1989; 34:43.
18. Schneider GB, Key LL, Popoff SN. Osteopetrosis: therapeutic strategies. Endocrinologist 1998; 8:409.
19. Gerritsen EJ, Vossen JM, van Loo IH, et al. Autosomal recessive osteopetrosis. Pediatrics 1994; 93:247.
20. Lehman RA, Reeves JD, Wilson, WB, Wesenberg RL. Neurological complications of infantile osteopetrosis. Ann Neurol 1977; 2:378.
21. Bollerslev J. Autosomal dominant osteopetrosis: bone metabolism and epidemiological, clinical, and hormonal aspects. Endocr Rev 1989; 10:45.
22. Johnston CC Jr, Lavy N, Lord T, et al. Osteopetrosis: a clinical, genetic, metabolic, and morphologic study of the dominantly inherited, benign form. Medicine (Baltimore) 1968; 47:149.
23. Reeves JD, August CS, Humbert JR, Weston WL. Host defense in infantile osteopetrosis. Pediatrics 1979; 64:202.
24. Eapen M, Davies SM, Ramsay NK, Orchard PJ. Hematopoietic stem cell transplantation for osteopetrosis. Bone Marrow Transplant 1998; 22:941.
25. Locatelli F, Beluffi G, Giorgiani G, et al. Transplantation of cord blood progenitor cells can promote bone resorption in autosomal recessive osteopetrosis. Bone Marrow Transplant 1997; 20:701.
26. Kubo T, Tanaka H, Ono H, et al. Malignant osteopetrosis treated with high doses of 1α-hydroxyvitamin $D_3$ and interferon gamma. J Pediatr 1993; 123:264.
27. Whyte MP, Murphy WA, Fallon MD, et al. Osteopetrosis, renal tubular acidosis, and basal ganglia calcification in three sisters. Am J Med 1980; 69:64.
28. Orchard PJ, Dickerman JD, Mathews CHE, et al. Haploidentical bone marrow transplantation for osteopetrosis. Am J Pediatr Hematol Oncol 1987; 9:335.
29. Key LL Jr, Ries WL, Rodriguiz RM, Hatcher HC. Recombinant human interferon gamma therapy for osteopetrosis. J Pediatr 1992; 121:119.
30. Ozsoylu S. High dose intravenous methylprednisolone in treatment of recessive osteopetrosis. (Letter). Arch Dis Child 1987; 62:214.
31. Whyte MP, Hamm LL 3rd, Sly WS. Transfusion of carbonic anhydrase-replete erythrocytes fails to correct the acidification defect in the syndrome of osteopetrosis, renal tubular acidosis, and cerebral calcification (carbonic anhydrase-II deficiency). J Bone Miner Res 1988; 3:385.
32. Ogur G, Ogur E, Celasun B, et al. Prenatal diagnosis of autosomal recessive osteopetrosis, infantile type, by X-ray evaluation. Prenat Diagn 1995; 15:477.
33. Sen C, Madazli R, Aksoy F, Ocak V. Antenatal diagnosis of lethal osteopetrosis. Ultrasound Obstet Gynecol 1995; 5:278.
34. Strisciuglio P, Hu PY, Lim EJ, et al. Clinical and molecular heterogeneity in carbonic anhydrase II deficiency and prenatal diagnosis in an Italian family. J Pediatr 1998; 132:717.
35. Gelb BD, Shi GP, Chapman HA, Desnick RJ. Pycnodysostosis, a lysosomal disease caused by cathepsin K deficiency. Science 1996; 273:1236.
36. Soliman AT, Rajab A, AlSalmi I, et al. Defective growth hormone secretion in children with pycnodysostosis and improved linear growth after growth hormone treatment. Arch Dis Child 1996; 75:242.
37. Fallon MD, Whyte MP, Murphy WA. Progressive diaphyseal dysplasia (Engelmann's disease). J Bone Joint Surg Am 1980; 62:465.
37a. Kinoshita A, Saito T, Tomita H, et al. Domain-specific mutations in TGFB1 result in Camurati-Engelmann disease. Nat Genet 2000; 26:19.
38. Hundley JD, Wilson FC. Progressive diaphyseal dysplasia. Review of the literature and report of seven cases in one family. J Bone Joint Surg Am 1973; 55:461.
39. Smith R, Walton RJ, Corner BD, Gordon IR. Clinical and biochemical studies in Engelmann's disease (progressive diaphyseal dysplasia). QJM 1977; 46:273.
40. Kumar B, Murphy WA, Whyte MP. Progressive diaphyseal dysplasia (Engelmann disease): scintigraphic-radiographic-clinical correlations. Radiology 1981; 140:87.
41. Naveh Y, Alon U, Kaftori JK, Berant M. Progressive diaphyseal dysplasia: evaluation of corticosteroid therapy. Pediatrics 1985; 75:321.
42. De Rubin ZS, Ghiringhello G, Mansur JL. Clinical, humoral and scintigraphic assessment of a bisphosphonate as potential treatment of diaphyseal dysplasia: Ribbing and Camurati-Engelmann diseases. Medicina 1997; 57(Suppl 1):56.
43. Saul RA, Lee WH, Stevenson RE. Caffey's disease revisited: further evidence for autosomal dominant inheritance with incomplete penetrance. Am J Dis Child 1982; 136:55.
44. Holtzman D. Infantile cortical hyperostosis of the scapula presenting as an ipsilateral Erb's palsy. J Pediatr 1972; 81:785.
45. Van Buchem FSP, Prick JJG, Jasper HHJ. Hyperostosis corticalis generalisata familiaris (van Buchem's disease). Amsterdam: Excerpta, 1976.
46. Eastman JR, Bixler D. Generalized cortical hyperostosis (van Buchem disease): nosologic considerations. Radiology 1977; 125:297.
47. Balemans W, Van Den Ende J, Paes-Alves AF, et al. Localization of the gene for sclerosteosis to the van Buchem Disease-gene region on chromosome 17q12-q21. Am J Hum Genet 1999; 64:1661.
48. Krishnamachari KA. Skeletal fluorosis in humans: a review of recent progress in the understanding of the disease. Prog Food Nutr Sci 1986; 10:279.
49. Whyte MP, Murphy WA, Siegel BA. 99mTc-pyrophosphate bone imaging in osteopoikilosis, osteopathia striata, and melorheostosis. Radiology 1978; 127:439.
50. Uitto J, Starcher BC, Santa-Cruz DJ, et al. Biochemical and ultrastructural demonstration of elastin accumulation in the skin lesions of the Buschke-Ollendorff syndrome. J Invest Dermatol 1981; 76:284.
51. Beauvais P, Faure C, Montagne J, et al. Leri's melorheostosis: three pediatric cases and a review of the literature. Pediatr Radiol 1977; 6:153.
52. Whyte MP, Murphy WA, Fallon MD, Hahn TJ. Mixed-sclerosing-bone-dystrophy: report of a case and review of the literature. Skeletal Radiol 1981; 6:95.
53. Pacifici R, Murphy WA, Teitelbaum SL, Whyte MP. Mixed-sclerosing-bone-dystrophy: 42-year follow-up of a case reported as osteopetrosis. Calcif Tissue Int 1986; 38:175.
54. Kaplan FS, Tabas JA, Gannon FH, et al. The histopathology of fibrodysplasia ossificans progressiva: an endochondral process. J Bone Joint Surg Am 1993; 75:220.
55. Connor JM, Evans DA. Fibrodysplasia ossificans progressiva. The clinical features and natural history of 34 patients. J Bone Joint Surg Br 1982; 64:76.
56. Smith R, Russell RG, Woods CG. Myositis ossificans progressiva. Clinical features of eight patients. J Bone Joint Surg A 1976; 58:48.

57. Moore SE, Jump AA, Smiley JD. Effect of warfarin sodium therapy on excretion of 4-carboxy-L-glutamic acid in scleroderma, dermatomyositis, and myositis ossificans progressiva. Arthritis Rheum 1986; 29:344.
58. Shafritz AB, Shore EM, Gannon FH, et al. Overexpression of an osteogenic morphogen in fibrodysplasia ossificans progressiva. N Engl J Med 1996; 335:555.
58a. Lucotte G, Semonin O, Lutz P. A de novo heterozygous deletion of 42 base-pairs in the noggin gene of a fibrodysplasia ossificans progressiva patient (Letter). Clin Genet 1999; 56:469.
59. Whyte MP. Hereditary metabolic and dysplastic skeletal disorders. In: Coe FL, Favus MJ, eds. Disorders of bone and mineral metabolism. New York: Raven Press 1992:977.
60. Harris WH, Dudley HR Jr, Barry RJ. The natural history of fibrosis dysplasia. J Bone Joint Surg Am 1962; 44:207.
61. Johnson CB, Gilbert EF, Gottlieb LI. Malignant transformation of polyostotic fibrous dysplasia. South Med J 1979; 72:353.
62. Harris RI. Polyostotic fibrous dysplasia with acromegaly. Am J Med 1985; 78:539.
63. Lever EG, Pettingale KW. Albright's syndrome associated with a soft-tissue myxoma and hypophosphataemic osteomalacia: report of a case and review of the literature. J Bone Joint Surg Br 1983; 65:621.
64. Shenker A, Weinstein LS, Moran A, et al. Severe endocrine and nonendocrine manifestations of the McCune-Albright syndrome associated with activating mutations of stimulatory G-protein GS. J Pediatr 1993; 123:509.
65. Chapurlat RD, Meunier PJ. Fibrous dysplasia of bone. Bailliére's Clin Rheumatol 2000; 14:385.
66. Feuillan PP, Foster CM, Pescovitz OH, et al. Treatment of precocious puberty in the McCune-Albright syndrome with the aromatase inhibitor testolactone. N Engl J Med 1986; 315:1115.
67. Albright JA, Millar EA. Osteogenesis imperfecta (symposium). Clin Orthop 1981; 159:1.
68. Byers PH. Disorders of collagen biosynthesis and structure. In: Scriver CR, Beaudet AL, Sly WS, Valle D, eds. The metabolic and molecular basis of inherited disease, 7th ed. New York: McGraw-Hill, 1995:4029.
68a. Rauch F, Travers R, Parfitt AM, Glorieux FH. Static and dynamic bone histomorphometry in children with osteogenesis imperfecta. Bone 2000; 26:581.
69. Chines A, Petersen DJ, Schranck FW, Whyte MP. Hypercalciuria in children severely affected with osteogenesis imperfecta. J Pediatr 1991; 119:51.
70. Glorieux FH, Bishop NJ, Plotkin H, et al. Cyclic administration of pamidronate in children with severe osteogenesis imperfecta. N Engl J Med 1998; 339:947.
70a. Plotkin H, Rauch F, Bishop NJ, et al. Pamidronate treatment of severe osteogenesis imperfecta in children under 3 years of age. J Clin Endocrinol Metab 2000; 85:1846.
71. Brons JT, van der Harten HJ, Wladimiroff JW, et al. Prenatal ultrasonographic diagnosis of osteogenesis imperfecta. Am J Obstet Gynecol 1988; 159:176.
72. Whyte MP. Hypophosphatasia. In: Scriver CR, Beaudet AL, Sly WS, Valle D, eds. The metabolic and molecular bases of inherited disease, 7th ed. New York: McGraw-Hill, 1995:4095.
73. Fallon MD, Teitelbaum SL, Weinstein RS, et al. Hypophosphatasia: clinico-pathologic comparison of the infantile, childhood, and adult forms. Medicine (Baltimore) 1984; 63:12.
74. Whyte MP, Teitelbaum SL, Murphy WA, et al. Adult hypophosphatasia: clinical, laboratory, and genetic investigation of a large kindred with review of the literature. Medicine (Baltimore) 1979; 58:329.
75. Whyte MP. Hypophosphatasia. In: Econs MJ, ed. The genetics of osteoporosis and metabolic bone disease. Totowa, NJ: Humana Press, 1999; in press.
76. Whyte MP, Mahuren JD, Vrabel LA, Coburn SP. Markedly increased circulating pyridoxal-5′-phosphate levels in hypophosphatasia: alkaline phosphatase acts in vitamin B6 metabolism. J Clin Invest 1985; 76:752.
77. Whyte MP, Murphy WA, Fallon MD. Adult hypophosphatasia with chondrocalcinosis and arthropathy: variable penetrance of hypophosphatasemia in a large Oklahoma kindred. Am J Med 1982; 72:631.
78. Whyte MP, Magill HL, Fallon MD, Herrod HG. Infantile hypophosphatasia: normalization of circulating bone alkaline phosphatase activity followed by skeletal remineralization (evidence for an intact structural gene for tissue nonspecific alkaline phosphatase). J Pediatr 1986; 108:82.
79. Fedde KN, Blair L, Terzic F, et al. Amelioration of the skeletal disease in hypophosphatasia by bone marrow transplantation using the alkaline phosphatase-knockout mouse model. (Abstract). Am J Hum Genet 1996; 59:A.
80. Coe JD, Murphy WA, Whyte MP. Management of femoral fractures and pseudofractures in hypophosphatasia. J Bone Joint Surg Am 1986; 68:981.
81. Brock DJ, Barron L. First-trimester prenatal diagnosis of hypophosphatasia: experience with 16 cases. Prenat Diagn 1991; 11:387.
82. Whyte MP, Fallon MD, Murphy WA, Teitelbaum SL. Axial osteomalacia: clinical, laboratory and genetic investigation of an affected mother and son. Am J Med 1981; 71:1041.
83. Lang R, Vignery AM, Jensen PS. Fibrogenesis imperfecta ossium with early onset: observations after 20 years of illness. Bone 1986; 7:237.
84. Patel AC, McAlister WH, Whyte MP. Spondyloepimetaphyseal dysplasia: clinical and radiologic investigation of a large kindred manifesting autosomal dominant inheritance. Medicine 1993; 72:326.
85. Kruse K, Schutz C. Calcium metabolism in the Jansen type of metaphyseal dysplasia. Eur J Pediatr 1993; 152:912.
86. Evans RA, Dunstan CR, Hills E. Bone metabolism in idiopathic juvenile osteoporosis: a case report. Calcif Tissue Int 1983; 35:5.
87. Whyte MP, Eddy MC, Podgornik MN, McAlister WH. Polycystic bone disease: a new, autosomal dominant disorder. J Bone Miner Res 1999; 14:1261.
88. Destouet JM, Murphy WA. Acquired acroosteolysis and acronecrosis. Arthritis Rheum 1983; 26:1150.
89. Whyte MP, Murphy WA, Kleerekoper M, et al. Idiopathic multicentric osteolysis. Arthritis Rheum 1978; 21:367.
90. Bullough PG. Massive osteolysis. N Y State J Med 1971; 71:2267.
91. Anderson HC. Calcific diseases: a concept. Arch Pathol Lab Med 1983; 107:341.
91a. Eddy MC, Jan de Beur SM, Yandow SM, et al. Deficiency of the α-subunit of the stimulatory G protein and severe extraskeletal ossification. J Bone Miner Res 2000; 15:2074.
92. Anonymous. Symposium on idiopathic osteonecrosis. Orthop Clin North Am 1985; 16:593.
93. Chang CC, Greenspan A, Gershwin ME. Osteonecrosis: current perspectives on pathogenesis and treatment. Semin Arthritis Rheum 1993; 23:47.
94. Totty WG, Murphy WA, Ganz WI, et al. Magnetic resonance imaging of the normal and ischemic femoral head. AJR Am J Roentgenol 1984; 143:1273.

# CHAPTER 67

# DISEASES OF ABNORMAL PHOSPHATE METABOLISM

MARC K. DREZNER

Phosphorus is one of the most abundant constituents of all tissues, and disturbances in phosphate homeostasis can affect almost any organ system. Most phosphorus within the body is in bone (600–700 g), whereas much of the remainder is distributed in soft tissue (100–200 g). Less than 1% is in extracellular fluids. As the major intracellular anion, phosphorus plays a critical role in many aspects of cell function. These include (a) serving as a source of the high-energy phosphate in adenosine triphosphate (ATP); (b) providing an essential element of phospholipid in cell membranes; and (c) directly influencing a variety of enzymatic reactions (e.g., glycolysis) and protein functions (e.g., the oxygen-carrying capacity of hemoglobin by regulation of 2,3-diphosphoglycerate [2,3-DPG] synthesis). The plasma contains ~14 mg/dL phosphorus, of which 8 to 9 mg is lipid phosphorus, a trace is an anion of pyrophosphoric acid, and the remainder is inorganic phosphate (Pi). The Pi is present in the circulation as monohydrogen phosphate, which is divalent, and as dihydrogen phosphate, which is monovalent. At pH 7.4, the relative concentrations of monohydrogen to dihydrogen phosphate are 4:1. Although phosphorus is present as phosphate in biologic fluids, the concentration of elemental phosphorus is measured in routine serum assays and averages 2.5 to 4.5 mg/dL in normal adults. In children, normal levels are higher. The mechanism for this difference is not established but may be related to the higher levels of circulating growth hormone in growing children and the associated increases in the tubular reabsorption of phosphate.

## REGULATION OF PHOSPHATE METABOLISM

The critical role that phosphorus plays in cell physiology has resulted in the development of elaborate mechanisms for extracting phosphates from the diet and the conservation of phosphate absorbed by the intestine. Such regulation maintains the plasma and extracellular fluid phosphorus within a relatively narrow range and centers on the intestine and kidney as the major organs of regulation.

### PHOSPHATE HOMEOSTASIS: INTESTINE

The average dietary phosphate intake in humans, derived largely from dairy products, meat, and cereals, is 1200 to 1500 mg per day, two-fold to three-fold greater than the estimated minimum requirement. Approximately 60% to 70% of phosphate in the diet is absorbed, so that net absorption is proportional to intake. Absorption probably occurs throughout the small intestine; transport is greatest in the jejunum, less in the duodenum, and minimal in the ileum.[1] The movement of phosphorus from the intestinal lumen to the blood requires (1) transport across the luminal brush border membrane; (2) movement transcellularly; and (3) transport across the basolateral plasma membrane of the epithelium.

Phosphate transport at the luminal brush border membrane occurs by way of a saturable process against a lumen/intracellular electrochemical gradient at lumen phosphate concentrations below 2 mmol/L; above this concentration, transport predominantly proceeds by passive diffusion. The active transport of phosphate occurs by way of two independent carrier-mediated processes, a high-affinity and a low-affinity system. Both processes are dependent on sodium and potassium; however, the high-affinity transport system is enhanced by acid pH, whereas both alkaline pH and calcium stimulate the low-affinity system. The molecular basis for the sodium-dependent phosphate transport remains unknown.

Likewise, little is known about the cellular events that mediate the movement of phosphorus from the luminal to the basolateral membrane. Nevertheless, available evidence suggests a role for the microtubule system in conveying phosphorus transcellularly and in extrusion of phosphorus at the basolateral membrane.

Extrusion of phosphorus at the basolateral membrane of intestinal epithelial cells is passive, occurring via an anion-exchange mechanism, because the electrochemical gradient favors such movement. However, there have been reports of an ATP- and Na$^+$-dependent transport process at this locus.

Calcitriol [1,25(OH)$_2$D$_3$] is the principal hormonal factor that influences gastrointestinal phosphate absorption.[2,3] Facilitation of transport occurs by way of a calcium-dependent duodenal process and a calcium-independent jejunal system. The latter activity is modulated by calcitriol-induced transcription of messenger RNA. A major cause of defective phosphate absorption is calcitriol deficiency (secondary to a nutritional deficiency or caused by malabsorption). Alternatively, genetic and acquired disorders of vitamin D metabolism may decrease the availability of vitamin D (see Chaps. 54, 63, and 70).

Besides calcitriol deficiency, a number of additional factors may adversely influence the intestinal absorption of phosphate. Principal among these is the formation of nonabsorbable calcium, aluminum, or magnesium phosphate salts in the intestine. Moreover, phosphate absorption is reduced by more than one-half with advancing age in laboratory animals and probably in humans.

## PHOSPHATE HOMEOSTASIS: KIDNEYS

The kidney is immediately responsive to changes in serum levels or dietary intake of phosphate.[4,5] Altering either the filtered load or the tubular reabsorption of phosphate controls renal adaptation.

The concentration of phosphate in the glomerular ultrafiltrate is essentially identical to that in plasma. Thus, the product of the serum phosphorus concentration and the glomerular filtration rate (GFR) is equal to the filtered load of phosphate. A change in the GFR may influence phosphate homeostasis if uncompensated by commensurate changes in tubular reabsorption.

Normally, 80% to 90% of the filtered phosphate load is reabsorbed, predominantly in the proximal portions of the nephron.[6-8] Sixty to seventy percent is reabsorbed in the proximal convoluted tubule and a smaller but significant fraction is reabsorbed in the pars recta. Along the proximal convoluted tubule, the transport is heterogeneous. In the most proximal portion, the S1 segment, phosphate reabsorption exceeds that of sodium and water, whereas, more distally, phosphate reabsorption parallels that of fluid and sodium. Ample evidence also supports the existence of one or more distal tubular reabsorptive sites for phosphorus. However, conclusive proof for tubular secretion of phosphate in humans is lacking.

In the proximal convoluted tubule, transepithelial phosphate transport is essentially unidirectional and involves uptake across the brush border membrane (BBM), translocation across the cell, and efflux at the basolateral membrane. The phosphate uptake at the apical cell surface proceeds by way of an active rate-limiting step in the reabsorptive process and is mediated by Na$^+$-dependent Pi transporters. The transporters are located in the BBM and depend on the basolateral membrane-associated Na$^+$,K$^+$-ATPase to maintain the Na$^+$ gradient that drives the transport process. Recently, cDNAs encoding two classes of Na$^+$-Pi cotransporters have been identified and designated NPT1 and NPT2. Although both transporters mediate high-affinity Na$^+$-Pi cotransport, the pH profile and documented hormonal modulation of NPT2 indicate that the NPT2 transporter is the primary functional protein that regulates phosphate transport.[9] In contrast to this regulated process, the exit of phosphate across the contraluminal membrane into the peritubular fluid is passive, going down a concentration gradient. The monovalent ion (H$_2$PO$_4^-$) is preferentially transported, and reabsorptive capacity is saturated at a physiologic tubular fluid phosphate concentration of 2 mmol/L. Little is known regarding the mechanisms of transport in the distal nephron.

A transport maximum (TmP) or threshold that, when exceeded, results in quantitative excretion of filtered phosphate characterizes renal phosphate reabsorption in humans. In the fasting state, the phosphate concentration in the renal ultrafiltrate is generally less than the TmP; however, some of the filtered phosphate is excreted in the urine secondary to nephron heterogeneity with regard to GFR and reabsorption.

The TmP can be determined in patients by phosphate infusions, but this method is cumbersome and nonphysiologic. Alternatively, a simplified method to accurately estimate the TmP has been developed.[4] Using a nomogram, TmP is determined by measurements of serum and urine phosphorus (PO$_4$) and creatinine (Cr) and calculation of the tubular reabsorption of phosphate (TRP):

$$TRP(\%) = (1 - C_{PO_4}/C_{Cr}) \times 100$$

Several factors modulate the renal TmP (Table 67-1). The best known and most important regulator is parathyroid hormone (PTH). PTH administration decreases renal phosphate reabsorption, causing major increases of urinary phosphate.[10] Conversely, parathyroidectomy increases renal phosphate reabsorption and decreases phosphate excretion. The PTH-dependent changes result primarily from alteration of ion transport in the proximal convoluted tubule. Calcium-mediated, 1,25(OH)$_2$D$_3$-mediated, calcitonin-mediated, and estrogen-mediated changes in renal TmP have also been reported (see Chap. 206). In addition, dietary Pi intake is a major regulator of renal Pi handling. Pi deprivation elicits an increase, and Pi loading a decrease, in TmP/GFR, changes that are caused by an adaptive increase or decrease in BBM Na$^+$-Pi cotransport. In any case, a change in phosphate reabsorption and the TmP generally yields a comparable change in the serum phosphorus and eventually in the total phosphorus balance.

## DIFFERENTIAL DIAGNOSIS OF AN ABNORMAL SERUM PHOSPHORUS LEVEL

Frequently, a careful history and physical examination reveal the apparent cause of an abnormal serum phosphorus concentration. However, the variety of diseases, therapeutic agents, and physiologic states that affect phosphate homeostasis are numerous, and clinicians should make every effort to determine the mechanism underlying changes in the serum phos-

**TABLE 67-1.**
**Control of Renal Phosphate Reabsorption**

| DECREASED TRANSPORT MAXIMUM | INCREASED TRANSPORT MAXIMUM |
|---|---|
| *Hormones* | *Hormones* |
| Parathyroid hormone | Insulin |
| Calcitonin | Growth hormone |
| Glucocorticoids | Thyroid hormone |
| Antidiuretic hormone | Angiotensin II |
| Estrogen | Calcitriol |
| *Drugs/Metabolic Alterations* | *Drugs/Metabolic Alterations* |
| Alcohol ingestion | Hypercalcemia |
| Extracellular fluid excess | Hypermagnesemia |
| Diuretics | Decreased dietary phosphorus intake |
| Metabolic acidosis or alkalosis | Bisphosphonates |
| Acute respiratory acidosis | Prostaglandin |
| Increased dietary phosphorus intake | |
| Luminal glucose | |
| Acetazolamide | |

phorus level in each patient. Determining the cause for the abnormality permits a rational choice of appropriate therapy.

## HYPERPHOSPHATEMIA

Two mechanisms generally underlie the genesis of hyperphosphatemia in humans. First and most commonly, reduced renal excretion of phosphate may cause phosphate retention. The reduction reflects either a reduced GFR or increased renal tubular reabsorption of phosphate (see Table 67-1). Second, hyperphosphatemia rarely ensues after an increase in phosphate intake or an acute increment of endogenous phosphate released into the extracellular fluid.

### REDUCED RENAL PHOSPHATE EXCRETION

**Renal Failure.** The most common cause of hyperphosphatemia is chronic renal failure. The increased serum phosphate concentration results from a decline of the GFR.[11] However, in early stages of renal failure, compensatory changes in the renal tubular reabsorption of phosphate, in part because of elevated circulating levels of PTH, limit expression of this abnormality. Indeed, only at a GFR of ~25 mL/min/l.73 m² or less is hyperphosphatemia commonly seen. With advanced renal failure, however, serum phosphorus levels may increase up to a level of 11 or 12 mg/dL if dietary phosphate is high and phosphorus is freely mobilized from the skeleton by severe secondary hyperparathyroidism. Retention of phosphate in this disorder leads to the development of renal osteodystrophy, ectopic calcification (see later), depression of renal calcitriol synthesis, and impaired intestinal absorption of calcium. Hyperphosphatemia also lowers the serum ionized calcium and stimulates hypertrophy of the parathyroid glands and secretion of PTH.

**Hypoparathyroidism.** Hyperphosphatemia characteristically complicates the hypoparathyroid states (idiopathic or postsurgical, or pseudohypoparathyroidism).[12] The increased serum phosphate levels are secondary to enhanced renal reabsorption of phosphate. In idiopathic and postsurgical hypoparathyroidism, deficient PTH causes a loss of the hormonal effect to decrease the TmP. Conversely, the increased renal reabsorption of phosphate in the pseudohypoparathyroid disorders arises from renal resistance to PTH.

The concurrence of clinically significant hypocalcemia and hyperphosphatemia usually leads to the diagnosis of hypoparathyroidism. Some studies have revealed that the causes of idiopathic hypoparathyroidism in some affected patients include (a) gain-of-function calcium-receptor mutations that result in autosomal-dominant and sporadic disease[13]; (b) an autoimmune polyglandular syndrome caused by a genetic

abnormality at 21q22.3[14]; (c) an X-linked recessive inherited form of the disorder[15]; and (d) autoimmune-targeting of the calcium-sensing receptor.[13] In contrast, investigations of the familial parathyroid hormone-resistance syndromes indicate that (a) pseudohypoparathyroidism type 1a occurs because of paternally imprinted mutations of GNAS1 on chromosome 20q13.11, resulting in abnormalities of the α subunit of the G protein, which couples receptor binding to activation of adenylate cyclase[16]; and (b) pseudohypoparathyroidism type 1b similarly manifests secondarily to a paternally imprinted mutation of the stimulatory G protein that maps to 20q13.3.[17] In all of these disorders, treatment of the hypocalcemia with oral calcium supplements and vitamin D preparations may reduce but not necessarily normalize the serum phosphate levels and the renal TmP. This effect may be the result of the elevation of the serum calcium concentration, or perhaps it is the result of a direct effect of 1,25(OH)$_2$D$_3$ on renal tubular phosphate handling. Thus, patients with hypoparathyroidism who are successfully treated may have normal calcium and phosphate levels.

**Tumoral Calcinosis.** Tumoral calcinosis is a rare genetic disease characterized by periarticular cystic and solid tumorous calcifications (Fig. 67-1). Specific biochemical markers of the

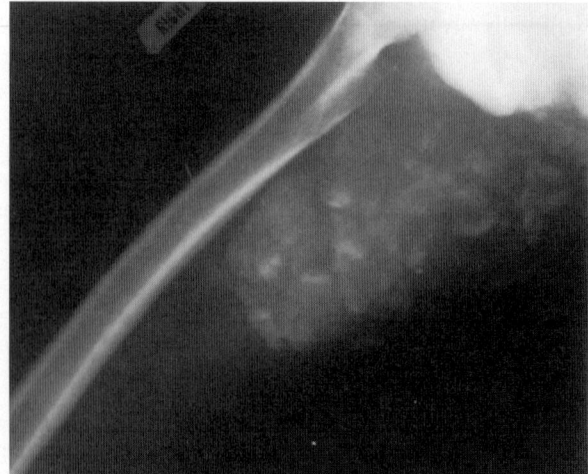

**FIGURE 67-1.** Tumoral calcinosis. Radiograph of right femur and pelvis of a 9-year-old boy with hyperphosphatemic tumoral calcinosis. This tumor was his fourth, and it had to be removed surgically. Serum phosphate level was 7.92 mg/dL (normal, 4.5–6.5 mg/dL); 1,25 dihydroxyvitamin D was 80 pg/mL (normal, 19–50 pg/mL).

disorder include hyperphosphatemia and an elevated serum $1,25(OH)_2D_3$ concentration. Using these criteria, evidence has been presented for autosomal-recessive inheritance of this syndrome. However, an abnormality of dentition, marked by short bulbous roots, pulp stones, and radicular dentin deposited in swirls, is a phenotypic marker of the disease that is variably expressed. Thus, this disorder may have multiple formes frustes that could complicate genetic analysis. Indeed, using the dental lesion as well as the more classic biochemical and clinical hallmarks of the disease, an autosomal-dominant pattern of transmission for tumoral calcinosis has been documented.[18]

An increase in capacity of renal tubular phosphate reabsorption causes the hyperphosphatemia that is typical in affected subjects. Hypocalcemia is not a consequence of this abnormality, however, and the serum PTH concentration is normal. Moreover, the phosphaturic and urinary cyclic adenosine monophosphate (cAMP) responses to PTH are not disturbed. Thus, the defect does not represent renal insensitivity to PTH, or hypoparathyroidism. Rather, the basis of the disease is probably a primary abnormality of the renal tubule that enhances phosphate reabsorption. Undoubtedly, the calcific tumors result from the elevated calcium-phosphorus product. The observation that long-term phosphorus depletion alone or in association with administration of acetazolamide, a phosphaturic agent, leads to resolution of the tumor masses supports this possibility.[19,20]

An acquired form of this disease is rarely seen in patients with end-stage renal failure. Affected patients manifest hyperphosphatemia in association with either (a) an inappropriately elevated calcitriol level for the degree of renal failure, hyperparathyroidism, or hyperphosphatemia[21,22]; or (b) long-term treatment with calcium carbonate, calcitriol, or high calcium-content dialysates. Calcific tumors again likely result from an elevated calcium–phosphorus product. Indeed, complete remission of the tumors occurs on treatment with low-calcium dialysate[23] or with vinpocetine, a mineral scavenger drug.[24]

**Hyperthyroidism.** Up to one-third of patients with thyrotoxicosis may have hyperphosphatemia. The elevation of the serum phosphorus is caused by increased bone resorption and calcium mobilization, consequent PTH suppression, and an increase in renal tubular reabsorption of phosphate. The frequent concurrence of an elevated serum osteocalcin and alkaline phosphatase activity, as well as increased urinary calcium and hydroxyproline, indicates that thyroid hormone effects on bone cause the hyperphosphatemia.[25,26] The increased TmP has been confirmed by direct measurements and by reports of elevated tubular reabsorption of phosphate in hyperthyroidism that reverts to normal after successful treatment. Secondary hypoparathyroidism, which is a response to thyroid hormone–associated hypercalcemia (see Chap. 42), is probably not the only explanation for the abnormal phosphate transport. Several studies suggest that thyroxine and triiodothyronine directly influence renal tubular phosphate reabsorption, but both enhanced and diminished phosphate transport have been reported. In any case, the hyperphosphatemia, when present, has no discernible effect on the clinical expression of the signs and symptoms of thyrotoxicosis.

**Acromegaly.** Approximately two-thirds of patients with acromegaly have an elevated serum phosphate concentration that is secondary to the chronic effects of growth hormone on renal tubular reabsorption of phosphate[27] (see Chap. 206). The serum phosphate level in affected subjects seldom exceeds 5.5 mg/dL but does correlate with disease activity. The mechanism underlying the increased phosphate reabsorption remains unknown. Although the administration of growth hormone to laboratory animals yields increased renal tubular phosphate reabsorption independent of alterations in the PTH concentration,[28] somatotropin does not influence renal phosphate transport in a variety of in vitro systems. The widely distributed presence of insulin-like growth factor-I receptors in the kidney[29]

suggests that insulin-like growth factor-I probably mediates the effect of growth hormone on renal TmP (see Chap. 12).

**Bisphosphonate Therapy.** The administration of disodium etidronate, a pyrophosphate analog, in doses generally higher than 5 mg/kg per day, can induce an increase in the serum phosphate concentration.[30] The drug, which is used in the treatment of Paget disease and osteoporosis, causes a time-dependent and dose-dependent increment of the renal TmP and consequent phosphate retention that is largely responsible for the hyperphosphatemia. However, an inhibition of the normal intracellular translocation of phosphorus also contributes to the elevated serum levels. Although an elevation in serum phosphate levels occurs soon after the initiation of therapy, the maximum elevation of the phosphate concentration does not occur until after several days of treatment. The mechanism by which disodium etidronate alters the renal tubular reabsorption of phosphate is unclear. Drug therapy does not alter the serum PTH concentration. Moreover, the drug does not inhibit the urinary cAMP and phosphaturic response to infused PTH. A direct effect on renal phosphate transport, therefore, appears likely.

## INCREASED PHOSPHATE LOAD

**Vitamin D Intoxication.** An increase of the Pi load from exogenous sources generally does not cause hyperphosphatemia because the kidney excretes the excessive phosphorus. However, an increased serum phosphate concentration may occur in vitamin D intoxication when the gastrointestinal absorption of phosphate is markedly enhanced. Increased phosphate mobilization from bone and a reduction of GFR, secondary to hypercalcemia or nephrocalcinosis, may also contribute to the evolution of the hyperphosphatemia.

The chronic ingestion of large doses of vitamin D, in excess of 100,000 U per day, is generally required to cause intoxication. Suspected hypervitaminosis D may be investigated through competitive binding protein assays, which can document excessive amounts of vitamin D and its metabolites in the circulation (see Chaps. 54 and 59).

**Rhabdomyolysis.** Because muscle contains a large amount of phosphate, necrosis of muscle tissue may acutely increase the endogenous phosphate load and result in hyperphosphatemia. Such muscle necrosis (rhabdomyolysis) may complicate heatstroke, acute arterial occlusion, hyperosmolar nonketotic coma, trauma, toxic agents such as ethanol and heroin, and idiopathic paroxysmal myoglobinuria.[31,32] Muscle biopsy often reveals myolytic denervation, and, as a consequence, acute renal failure caused by myoglobin excretion frequently complicates the clinical presentation and contributes to the hyperphosphatemia. However, an elevated serum phosphate concentration may precede evidence of renal failure or may occur in its complete absence when rhabdomyolysis is present. The diagnosis is confirmed by elevated serum creatine phosphokinase, uric acid, and lactate dehydrogenase concentrations and by the demonstration of heme-positive urine in the absence of red blood cells. Therapy is directed at the underlying disorder, with maintenance of the extracellular volume to avoid volume depletion and alkalinization of the urine to prevent uric acid accumulation and consequent acute tubular necrosis.

**Cytotoxic Therapy.** Cytotoxic therapy often causes cell destruction and liberation of phosphorus into the circulation.[33] The lysis of tumor cells begins within 1 to 2 days after treatment is initiated and is followed quickly by an elevation of the serum phosphate concentration. Hyperphosphatemia supervenes, however, only when the treated malignancies have a large tumor burden, rapid cell turnover, and substantial intracellular phosphorus content. Such malignancies include lymphoblastic leukemia, various types of lymphoma, and acute myeloproliferative syndromes, as well as solid tumors (e.g., small cell carcinoma, breast cancer, and neuroblastoma). Common risk factors for this syndrome include pretreatment renal insufficiency, elevated serum lactate dehydrogenase (LDH) concentration, and hyperuricemia. Additional biochemical abnormalities observed in affected patients include hyperkalemia and hypocalcemia.

**Malignant Hyperthermia.** Malignant hyperthermia is a rare familial syndrome that is characterized by an abrupt rise in body temperature during the course of anesthesia.[34] The disease appears to be autosomal dominant in transmission; an elevated serum creatine phosphokinase concentration is found in otherwise normal family members. Hyperphosphatemia results from shifts of phosphate from muscle cells to the extracellular pool. A high mortality rate accompanies the syndrome.

## HYPOPHOSPHATEMIA

Routine measurement of the serum phosphate concentration in hospitalized patients frequently reveals hypophosphatemia (<2.5 mg/dL). The hypophosphatemia may be of no clinical significance or may reflect significant disease and phosphate depletion.[35]

Hypophosphatemia in humans may result from any one or a combination of three factors: (a) a decrease in either dietary intake or gastrointestinal absorption of Pi; (b) renal phosphate loss, owing to a decrease in the TmP (see Table 67-1); or (c) the transcellular shift of Pi from the extracellular to the intracellular space. The pathologic consequences of hypophosphatemia are variable and depend on the rapidity with which the serum phosphate concentration declines and the concurrence of such related abnormalities as defective vitamin D metabolism or inappropriate PTH secretion.

### DISTURBANCE OF PHOSPHATE INTAKE/GASTROINTESTINAL ABSORPTION

**Phosphate Deprivation.** Hypophosphatemia and Pi depletion resulting from inadequate dietary intake are rare. With a decline in ingested phosphate, the renal TmP increases and urinary phosphate excretion decreases.[36] In addition, gastrointestinal phosphate secretion gradually lessens. However, severe dietary deprivation (<100 mg/d) leads to a prolonged period of negative phosphate balance and total body depletion. Affected female patients may display hypophosphatemia (1.5–2.5 mg/dL); in interesting contrast, male patients generally do not manifest a decreased serum phosphate concentration in response to the deprivation. The reasons underlying this sex difference are not clear. Nevertheless, attempts to maintain phosphate homeostasis in both sexes include suppression of the serum PTH concentration and increased $1,25(OH)_2D_3$ production.

Such a phosphate deprivation syndrome occurs frequently in children with kwashiorkor. Affected subjects manifest severe hypophosphatemia (<1.0 mg/dL) that is often life threatening.

Total starvation does not cause hypophosphatemia. The catabolic effects of total food deprivation result in the release of phosphate from intracellular stores, which compensates for the negative phosphorus balance. However, refeeding of the starved person results in hypophosphatemia when phosphate deprivation is maintained. Hypophosphatemia also occurs in response to prolonged vomiting and gastric suction and is worsened by an associated hypochloremic alkalosis, which results in a urinary phosphate loss.

**Gastrointestinal Malabsorption.** Gastrointestinal absorption of phosphorus may be decreased with the use of antacids that contain aluminum or magnesium; prolonged use of these drugs in large amounts has been associated with hypophosphatemia and a negative phosphorus balance.[37] Actually, long-term reduction of the serum phosphorus concentration, owing to chronic, excessive use of antacids, leads to frank osteomalacia and myopathy.

Mild to moderate hypophosphatemia may also occur secondary to gastrointestinal diseases that cause steatorrhea or rapid transit time (e.g., Crohn disease, postgastrectomy states, and intestinal fistulas). The decreased serum phosphate concentration is caused by vitamin D malabsorption or deficiency and by resultant secondary hyperparathyroidism and renal phosphate wasting. Affected patients variably manifest osteomalacia.[38] However, the relationship between the metabolic bone disease, vitamin D deficiency, and hypophosphatemia is complex. Indeed, osteomalacia may occur in the absence of hypophosphatemia.

### RENAL PHOSPHATE LOSS

**Hyperparathyroidism.** Approximately 30% of patients with hyperparathyroidism have hypophosphatemia. The decreased serum phosphate concentration results from a PTH-directed decrement of the renal TmP.[39] The effects of PTH on the kidney are mediated by cAMP and the dual second messengers inositol triphosphate and diacylglycerol. Thus, nephrogenous cAMP is often elevated. The almost universal concurrence of hypercalcemia in primary hyperparathyroidism distinguishes hypophosphatemia caused by this disorder from virtually all other causes of hypophosphatemia. The presence and extent of hypophosphatemia reflects the extent of the hyperparathyroidism. Other factors, however, are important. The absence of a decreased serum phosphate level in more than one-half of the affected population, for example, may be the result of the effects of phosphate depletion, which in turn limits urinary phosphate excretion.

**X-linked Hypophosphatemic Rickets/Osteomalacia.** The X-linked hypophosphatemic rickets/osteomalacia (XLH) syndrome is an X-linked dominant disorder characterized by hypophosphatemia, a low TmP, growth retardation, osteomalacia, and rickets in growing children (Fig. 67-2). This disease represents the prototypic genetic disorder, causing phosphopenic rickets/osteomalacia (Table 67-2; see Chaps. 63 and 70). Studies

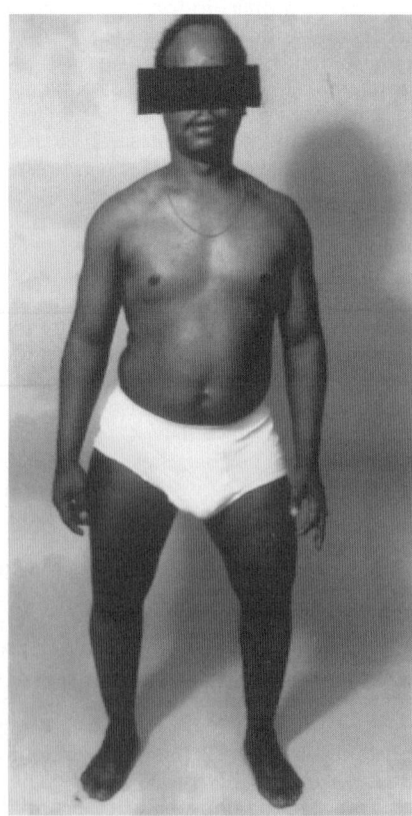

**FIGURE 67-2.** X-linked hypophosphatemic rickets. This patient has X-linked hypophosphatemic rickets. Note that the skull has frontal bossing that has occurred from premature closure of the sutures. The legs are bowed despite previous tibial osteotomies to correct the bowing. The patient also has hypertrophy of the quadriceps muscles secondary to the bowing.

**TABLE 67-2.**
Abnormalities Characteristic of the Rachitic/Osteomalacic Disorders

| | Phosphopenic | | | | | Calciopenic | |
|---|---|---|---|---|---|---|---|
| | *XLH* | *AHR* | *ADHR* | *TIO* | *HHRH* | *VDDR I* | *VDDR II* |
| **SERUM BIOCHEMISTRY** | | | | | | | |
| Calcium | N | N | N | N | N | ↓ | ↓ |
| Phosphorus | ↓ | ↓ | ↓ | ↓ | ↓ | ↓ | ↓ |
| Alkaline phosphatase | ↑ | ↑ | ↑ | ↑ | ↑ | ↑ | ↑ |
| Parathyroid hormone | N | N | N | N | N | ↑ | ↑ |
| 25(OH)D | N | N | N | N | N | N/↑ | N |
| 1,25(OH)$_2$D$_3$ | N/↓ | N/↓ | N | ↓ | ↑ | ↓ | ↑ |
| **GASTROINTESTINAL FUNCTION** | | | | | | | |
| Calcium absorption | ↓ | ↓ | ? | ↓ | ↑ | ↓ | ↓ |
| Phosphorus absorption | ↓ | ↓ | ? | ↓ | ↑ | ↓ | ↓ |
| **RENAL FUNCTION** | | | | | | | |
| Urinary calcium | ↓ | ↓ | ? | ↓ | ↑ | ↓ | ↓ |
| Urinary phosphorus | ↑ | ↑ | ↑ | ↑ | ↑ | ↑ | ↑ |

*25(OH)D*, 25-hydroxyvitamin D; *1,25(OH)$_2$D$_3$*, 1,25 dihydroxyvitamin D$_3$; *XLH*, X-linked hypophosphatemic rickets/osteomalacia; *AHR*, adult hypophosphatemic rickets; *ADHR*, autosomal-dominant hypophosphatemic rickets/osteomalacia; *TIO*, tumor-induced osteomalacia; *HHRH*, hereditary hypophosphatemic rickets with hypercalciuria; *VDDR I*, vitamin D–dependent rickets type I; *VDDR II*, vitamin D–dependent rickets type II; *N*, normal; ↑, increased; ↓, decreased.

that localized the gene locus for this disorder to the chromosome Xp22.1 led to construction of a *YAC* contig spanning the *HYP* gene region and ultimately made possible the cloning and identification of the disease gene as PHEX—phosphate-regulating gene with homologies to endopeptidases located on the X chromosome.[40] More recent investigations suggest that inactivating mutations of PHEX produce inadequate amounts of the endopeptidase, resulting in (a) ineffective or inadequate degradation/inactivation of a phosphate-transport inhibitory protein (phosphatonin); (b) circulation of excessive amounts of this protein; (c) consequent repressed expression of the sodium-dependent phosphate cotransporter; and (d) renal phosphate wasting and hypophosphatemia. In any case, the clinical expression of the disease is widely variable, ranging from an apparent asymptomatic defect to severe bone disease.[41] The mildest abnormality is hypophosphatemia without clinically evident bone disease, and the most common clinical manifestation is short stature. Strikingly absent are any abnormalities in the calcium concentration and muscle weakness, both of which are common features of vitamin D–deficiency osteomalacia.

Several factors undoubtedly contribute to the short stature that commonly affects patients with XLH. Refractory hypophosphatemia is most likely a contributing cause. This view is supported by the normal growth realized during infancy in most affected children, in whom the onset of hypophosphatemia does not occur until 6 to 12 months of age. Moreover, the improved growth rate observed in many children when treated adequately (phosphorus and calcitriol) to normalize the serum phosphate level further supports the role of hypophosphatemia in the genesis of the growth abnormality.[42] Likewise, the beneficial effects of growth hormone on the short stature of affected youths is associated with an increase in the serum phosphorus concentration secondary to the influence of this hormone on renal phosphate excretion (see earlier).

The hypophosphatemia in XLH is associated with increased urinary phosphate excretion that arises from a decrease of the renal TmP. Until recently, whether this renal abnormality is primary or secondary to the elaboration of a humoral factor has been controversial. In this regard, the presence of a primary renal abnormality is supported by the observation that primary cultures of renal tubule cells from *hyp*-mice exhibit a persistent defect in renal Pi transport, which is probably caused by decreased expression of the Na$^+$-phosphate co-transporter (NPT-2) mRNA and immunoreactive protein.[43] In contrast, transfer of the defect in renal Pi transport to normal and/or

parathyroidectomized normal mice parabiosed to *hyp*-mice has implicated a humoral factor in the pathogenesis of the disease.[44] Current studies have provided compelling evidence that the defect in renal Pi transport in XLH is secondary to the effects of a circulating hormone or metabolic factor. Thus, immortalized cell cultures from the renal tubules of *hyp*- and *gy*-mice exhibit normal Na$^+$-phosphate transport, suggesting that the paradoxical effects observed in primary cultures may represent the effects of impressed memory and not an intrinsic abnormality.[45] Moreover, the report that cross-transplantation of kidneys in normal and *hyp*-mice results in neither transfer of the mutant phenotype nor its correction unequivocally established the humoral basis for XLH.[46] Subsequent efforts that resulted in localization of the gene encoding the Na$^+$-phosphate co-transporter to chromosome 5 further substantiated the conclusion that the renal defect in brush border membrane phosphate transport is not intrinsic to the kidney in XLH. Although these data establish the presence of a humoral abnormality in XLH, the identity of the putative factor, the spectrum of its activity, and the mechanism by which it functions have not been definitively elucidated. Regardless, preliminary reports suggest the production of a phosphaturic factor by *hyp*-mouse osteoblasts and marrow mesenchymal cells maintained in culture. These studies argue that a circulating factor, phosphatonin, may play an important role in the pathophysiologic cascade responsible for XLH.

An ancillary abnormality in patients with XLH that affects the phenotypic expression of the disease is defective vitamin D metabolism.[41] Several investigators have observed that untreated youths and adults have normal serum 1,25(OH)$_2$D$_3$ levels. However, an elevation of this active vitamin D metabolite would be anticipated in the setting of hypophosphatemia and phosphate depletion, factors that increase 1,25(OH)$_2$D$_3$ production in humans. The paradoxical occurrence of hypophosphatemia and normal serum 1,25(OH)$_2$D$_3$ levels is the result of abnormal regulation of renal 25(OH)D-1α-hydroxylase activity. Indeed, studies in *hyp*-mice have established that defective regulation is confined to the enzyme localized in the proximal convoluted tubule, which is the site of the abnormal phosphate transport.[47,48] Thus, the aberrant vitamin D metabolism would appear to be an acquired defect secondary to changes in the intracellular milieu that depend on the abnormal phosphate transport. Moreover, evidence indicates that increased renal catabolism of calcitriol may also contribute to the aberrant regulation of vitamin D metabolism.[49]

In any case, data indicate that the collective effects of hypophosphatemia and abnormal vitamin D metabolism underlie the phenotypic expression of XLH. Included in these data is the observation that differences in the manifestations of XLH and the syndrome of hereditary hypophosphatemic rickets with hypercalciuria (HHRH),[50] two diseases marked by renal phosphate wasting, can be attributed to the normal vitamin D metabolism maintained in the latter disease (see Table 67-2). Thus, the elevated serum 1,25(OH)$_2$D$_3$ levels in patients with HHRH induce increased gastrointestinal absorption of calcium and phosphorus. Conversely, the defective vitamin D metabolism in patients with XLH abrogates the normal homeostatic response to phosphate depletion (increased gastrointestinal absorption) and alters the therapy required for healing of the bone disease. Successful treatment of XLH requires pharmacologic amounts of calcitriol as well as phosphate supplementation (Fig. 67-3). In fact, some studies indicate that the interplay between hypophosphatemia and vitamin D metabolism may be more complex, because decreased serum phosphate levels may impair binding of 1,25(OH)$_2$D$_3$ receptor complexes to nuclei and thereby promote vitamin D resistance.[51]

**Fanconi Syndrome.** The Fanconi syndrome represents a group of diseases, both genetic and acquired, in which hypophosphatemia, owing to a reduced renal TmP, is associated with additional renal tubular defects, causing loss of glucose, bicarbonate, and amino acids. Additional features of the disorder include rickets, osteomalacia, short stature, and hypokalemia. Among the genetic diseases that cause the syndrome are cystinosis, tyrosinemia, galactosemia, Wilson disease, and fructose intolerance. Acquired forms of the disease have been described in association with heavy metal poisoning, hematologic malignancies, connective tissue diseases, and the use of outdated tetracycline. The disease is primary or idiopathic when the cause is unknown or when only the mode of inheritance is evident. The idiopathic disorder may be sporadic, autosomal-dominant, autosomal-recessive, or X-linked. The clinical presentation of the disease is variable, depending on the cause. However, rickets and osteomalacia are invariable consequences of the hypophosphatemia. In most patients, a decreased or inappropriately normal serum 1,25(OH)$_2$D$_3$ level contributes to the bone disease. In contrast, a small subgroup of affected subjects with inherited disease exhibits an appropriately elevated 1,25(OH)$_2$D$_3$ level. Phenotypic expression of the disorder in these patients is modified in a fashion similar to that in subjects with HHRH[52] (see earlier). In any case, regardless of the underlying cause, osteomalacia associated with Fanconi syndrome appears to respond well to treatment with phosphate and vitamin D replacement. In fact, these patients do not necessarily appear to require 1,25(OH)$_3$D$_3$.

**Vitamin D–Dependent Rickets.** Vitamin D–dependent rickets is an autosomal-recessive disorder that resembles vitamin D deficiency clinically and is often referred to as *pseudo–vitamin D deficiency rickets*[53] (VDDR; see Chaps. 63 and 70). Affected patients demonstrate, within the first 3 months of life, muscle weakness, hypocalcemia, and evidence of secondary hyperparathyroidism, including aminoaciduria, phosphaturia, and hypophosphatemia (see Table 67-2). With progression, patients develop classic signs of rickets and osteomalacia. Although a decreased serum phosphate concentration is common, this VDDR syndrome is generally considered a calciopenic form of rickets/osteomalacia because of the marked hypocalcemia. The type I disorder results from missense and null mutations in the 1α-hydroxylase gene, localized to chromosome 12q13.3, that abolish enzyme activity and limit production of the active vitamin D metabolite, 1,25(OH)$_2$D.[54] A physiologic dose of calcitriol (1 μg per day) generally promotes complete healing of the bone disease and resolution of the biochemical abnormalities, whereas a pharmacologic dose of vitamin D or 25(OH)D is required to achieve similar effects. In the majority of affected patients, therapy with vitamin D or its metabolites must be con-

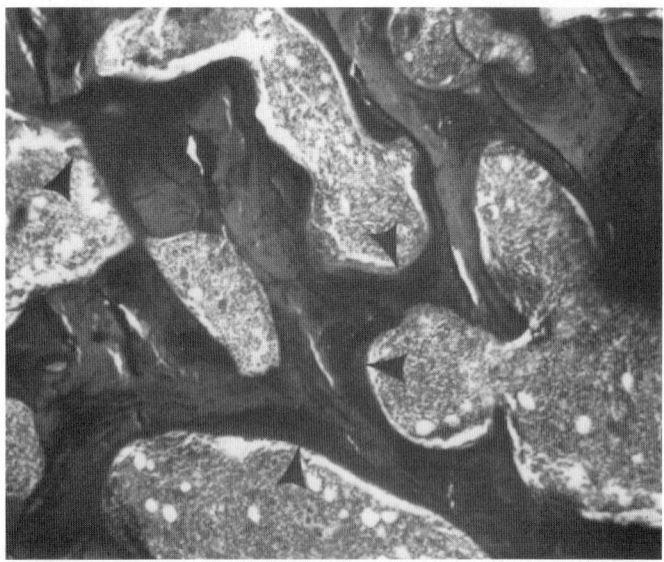
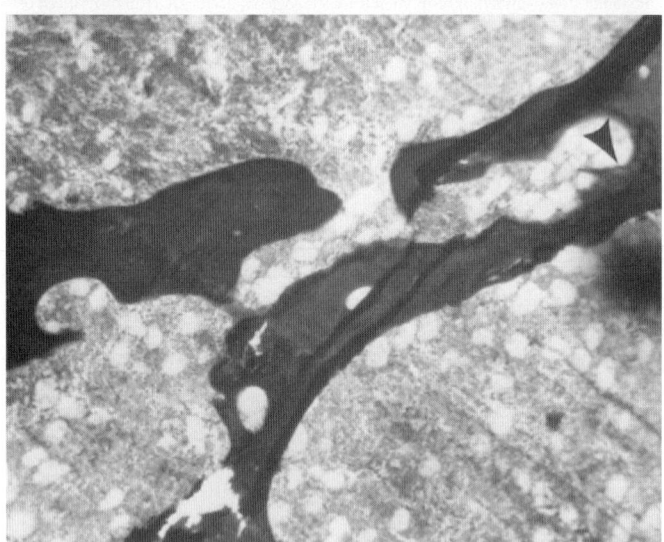

**FIGURE 67-3. A,** Bone biopsy specimen (Goldner stained) from an untreated patient with X-linked hypophosphatemic rickets viewed under high-power microscope. Characteristically, an excess of osteoid appears along mineralized trabecular bone surfaces. The thick osteoid seams are highlighted by the black arrowheads. **B,** Bone biopsy specimen (Goldner stained) from a patient with XLH after 9 months of treatment with calcitriol (1.5 μg, bid) and oral phosphate supplements (2 g per day; 8 phosphorus supplement [K-Phos Neutral] tablets per day). There is notable resolution of the excess osteoid, and only normal amounts remain (*arrowhead*). Indeed, quantitative histomorphologic analysis of the specimen confirms complete healing of the osteomalacia, an event unprecedented when other forms of treatment are used.

tinued lifelong to prevent relapse. Another group of patients with similar features of VDDR but elevated serum 1,25(OH)$_2$D$_3$ levels has been described[53] (see Table 67-2). These patients, with calciopenic rickets/osteomalacia, have variably associated abnormalities, including alopecia, ectodermal anomalies (e.g., multiple milia, epidermal cysts, and oligodontia), and immune dysfunction. This autosomal-recessive form of VDDR (type II) results from mutations in the DNA- and ligand-binding domains of the vitamin D receptor that cause decreased target-organ responsiveness to 1,25(OH)$_2$D$_3$ (Fig. 67-4). The role of the vitamin D receptor in the pathogenesis of this disorder has been confirmed in mice by targeted ablation of the DNA-binding domain of the receptor that causes hypocalcemia, hyperparathyroidism, and alopecia within the first month of life. Effective treatment of this disease likely depends on the nature of the

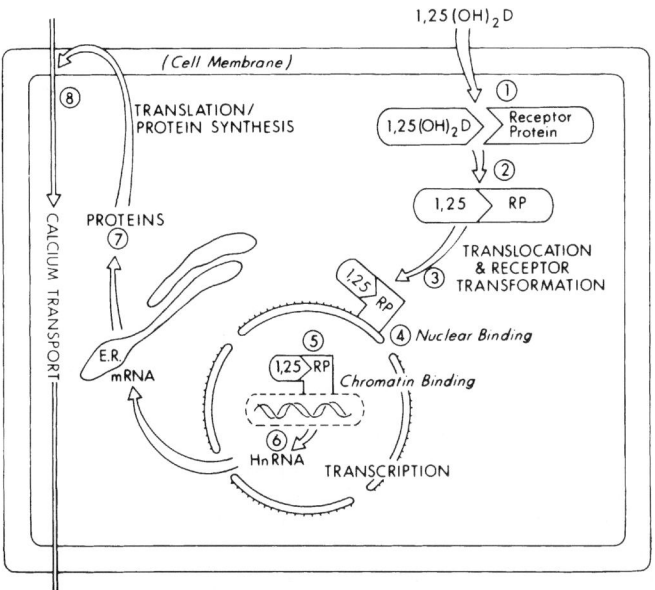

**FIGURE 67-4.** Model for potential cellular defects underlying vitamin D–dependent rickets type II. Sites of potential abnormalities underlying vitamin D–dependent rickets type II are indicated by the circled numbers. These defects include (1) a decreased number of cytosolic receptors for $1,25(OH)_2D_3$; (2) altered affinity or stability of the cytosolic receptor; (3) abnormal translocation and/or transformation of the $1,25(OH)_2D_3$ receptor; (4, 5) an altered nuclear and/or chromatin binding site; (6) abnormal transcription; and/or (7, 8) defective protein synthesis or action, thereby precluding expression of $1,25(OH)_2D_3$-specific effects such as calcium transport. [*1,25*, $1,25(OH)_2D_3$; *RP*, receptor protein; *HnRNA*, heterogeneous RNA; *ER*, endoplasmic reticulum.]

underlying abnormality. Thus, patients with deficient affinity of $1,25(OH)_2D_3$ to receptor and inadequate nuclear translocation respond to high-dose vitamin D or $1,25(OH)_2D$ with complete clinical and biochemical remission. In contrast, patients with other forms of the disease generally remain refractory to treatment with vitamin D or its analogs. However, every patient should receive a 6-month trial of therapy with supplemental calcium (1–3 g per day) and vitamin D or its analogs [25(OH)D or $1,25(OH)_2D$], often in massive doses in severe cases. If the abnormalities of the syndrome do not normalize in response to this treatment, clinical remission may be achieved by administering high-dose oral calcium or long-term intracaval infusion of calcium.[55]

**Autosomal-Dominant Hypophosphatemic Rickets.** The existence of autosomal-dominant hypophosphatemic rickets was first reported in 1979,[56] and the autosomal-dominant transmission of this disease has since been confirmed. Affected patients exhibit hypophosphatemia as a result of renal phosphate wasting (without a diffuse tubular abnormality), lower-extremity bowing, rickets, and osteomalacia. Subgroups of these patients demonstrate delayed penetrance of clinically apparent disease and an increased tendency to fracture or apparent resolution of the disease postadolescence. Regardless, all patients with the disorder manifest aberrant regulation of vitamin D metabolism, similar to that found in other phosphopenic rachitic diseases, and normal serum parathyroid hormone levels. The gene locus for this disorder has been identified as chromosome 12p13 in the 18-cM interval between the flanking markers D12S100 and D12S397.[57]

**Tumor-Induced Osteomalacia.** The tumor-induced osteomalacia syndrome is characterized by the remission of unexplained osteomalacia and rickets after resection of a coexisting tumor. The cases of ~100 patients with this disorder have been reported.[41,58] Tumors associated with the syndrome have gener-

ally been of mesenchymal origin (e.g., giant cell tumors of bone, sarcomas, and hemangiomas).[58a] However, the frequent occurrence of Looser zones in the radiographs of moribund patients with carcinomas of epidermal and endodermal derivation indicates that the disease may be more widespread and prevalent than previously recognized. The observation of tumor-induced osteomalacia in association with breast carcinoma and prostate carcinoma supports this conclusion (see Chaps. 63 and 219).

Hypophosphatemia is the primary biochemical abnormality in affected patients, and it results from a decreased renal TmP. Moreover, affected subjects invariably exhibit a decreased serum $1,25(OH)_2D_3$ concentration that apparently results from inhibition of renal 25(OH)D-1α-hydroxylase activity (see Table 67-2). These abnormalities result from the adverse effects of a tumor-secreted product on normal biochemical processes. Although a heat-sensitive protein of 8000 to 25,000 daltons has been isolated from a sclerosing hemangioma and is a likely tumor-secreted product,[59] other studies, which document the presence in various disease states of additional phosphate-transport inhibitors, indicate that the tumor-secreted factors are heterogeneous.

In affected patients, if tumor resection is possible, the hypophosphatemia [and abnormal serum $1,25(OH)_2D_3$ levels] quickly normalize. If tumor resection is precluded by the size of the primary lesion or metastases, treatment with $1,25(OH)_2D_3$ alone or with phosphate supplements restores the serum phosphate and often effects healing of the bone disease.

**Hereditary Hypophosphatemic Rickets with Hypercalciuria.** Hereditary hypophosphatemic rickets with hypercalciuria is a rare, genetic disease marked by hypophosphatemia (secondary to a decreased renal TmP) and hypercalciuria.[50] In contrast to the other diseases in which renal phosphate transport is abnormal, serum $1,25(OH)_2D_3$ levels are elevated. The increased bioactive vitamin D causes enhanced gastrointestinal absorption of calcium and consequent hypercalciuria. In affected subjects, hypophosphatemia (and bone disease) often respond to phosphate supplements alone.

## TRANSCELLULAR SHIFT OF PHOSPHORUS

In a large proportion of clinically important cases of hypophosphatemia, a sudden shift of phosphorus from the extracellular to the intracellular compartment is responsible for the decline of the serum phosphate concentration. This ion movement occurs in response to naturally occurring disturbances and after the administration of certain compounds.

**Alkalosis.** Alkalosis secondary to intense hyperventilation may depress serum phosphate levels to < 1 mg/dL.[60] A similar degree of alkalemia, owing to excess bicarbonate, also causes hypophosphatemia, but of a much lesser magnitude (2.5–3.5 mg/dL). The disparity between the effects of a respiratory and metabolic alkalosis is related to the more pronounced intracellular alkalosis that occurs during hyperventilation. The phosphate shift to the intracellular compartment results from its use for glucose phosphorylation, which is a process stimulated by a pH-dependent activation of phosphofructokinase.

**Glucose Administration.** The administration of glucose and insulin often results in moderate hypophosphatemia.[61] Endogenous or exogenous insulin increases the cellular uptake not only of glucose but also of phosphorus. The most responsive cells are those of the liver and skeletal muscle. The decline of the serum phosphate concentration generally does not exceed 0.5 mg/dL. A lesser decrease is manifest in patients with type 2 diabetes mellitus and insulin resistance or those with a disease causing a diminished skeletal mass. The administration of fructose and glycerol similarly reduces the serum phosphate concentration. In contrast to glucose, fructose administration may be associated with more pronounced hypophosphatemia; the more striking effect is caused by unregulated uptake by the liver.

## COMBINED MECHANISMS

Special clinical situations occur in which more than one mechanism contributes to the development of hypophosphatemia. These disorders represent some of the more common and profound causes of a decreased serum phosphorus concentration.

**Alcoholism.** Alcoholic patients frequently enter the hospital with hypophosphatemia. However, many do not exhibit a decreased serum phosphate concentration until several days have elapsed and refeeding has begun. The multiple factors that underlie the hypophosphatemia include poor dietary intake, use of phosphate binders to treat gastritis, excessive urinary loss of phosphorus, and shift of phosphorus from the extracellular to the intracellular compartment resulting from glucose administration or hyperventilation, which occurs in patients with cirrhosis or during alcohol withdrawal.[61] Moreover, many alcoholic patients are hypomagnesemic, which potentiates renal-phosphate wasting by an unclear mechanism.

**Burns.** Within several days after sustaining an extensive burn, patients often manifest severe hypophosphatemia. The initial insult induces a transient retention of salt and water. When the fluid is mobilized, significant urinary phosphorus loss ensues. Coupled with the shift of phosphorus to the intracellular compartment (which occurs secondary to hyperventilation), phosphate loss in cutaneous exudates, and the anabolic state, profound hypophosphatemia may result.

**Nutritional Recovery Syndrome.** Refeeding of starved patients or maintaining nutritional support by parenteral nutrition or by tube feeding without adequate phosphorus supplementation may also cause hypophosphatemia.[62] A prerequisite for the decreased serum phosphate concentration in affected patients is that their cells must be capable of an anabolic response. As new proteins are synthesized and glucose is transported intracellularly, phosphate demand depletes reserves. Several days are generally required after the initiation of refeeding to establish an anabolic condition. In patients receiving total parenteral nutrition, serum phosphate levels may be further depressed if sepsis supervenes and a respiratory alkalosis develops.

**Diabetic Ketoacidosis.** Poor control of blood glucose levels and consequent glycosuria, polyuria, and ketoacidosis invariably cause renal phosphate wasting.[61] The concomitant volume contraction may yield a normal serum phosphate concentration. However, with insulin therapy, the administration of fluids, and correction of the acidosis, serum and urine phosphate levels fall precipitously. The resultant hypophosphatemia may contribute to insulin resistance and slow the resolution of the ketoacidosis. Hence, the administration of phosphate may improve the capacity to metabolize glucose and facilitate recovery.

**Acute Phase Response Syndrome.** Hypophosphatemia is common (11.4%) in acutely ill patients who have experienced severe trauma or infection and manifest fever with leukopenia or leukocytosis. Affected patients often have an associated hyperglycemia secondary to tissue injury and/or infection. Thus, the hypophosphatemia is most likely caused by shifts of the extracellular phosphate into cells. Alternatively, the high levels of inflammatory cytokines, which characterize early sepsis, may play a role in the genesis of the hypophosphatemia. With resolution of the acute phase of illness, the hypophosphatemia resolves.

## CLINICAL SIGNS AND SYMPTOMS OF ABNORMAL SERUM PHOSPHATE LEVELS

A wide variety of diseases and syndromes with varying clinical manifestations have the characteristic biochemical abnormalities of hyperphosphatemia or hypophosphatemia. Furthermore, a unique complex of disturbances often is directly related to the abnormal phosphate homeostasis. The recognition of these signs and symptoms may lead to appropriate biochemical testing, the diagnosis of an unsuspected disease, and initiation of lifesaving or curative treatment.

## HYPERPHOSPHATEMIA

Hypocalcemia and consequent tetany are the most serious clinical sequelae of hyperphosphatemia.[63] The decreased serum calcium concentration results from the deposition of calcium–phosphate salts in soft tissue, a process that may lead to symptomatic ectopic calcification. The dystrophic calcification is frequently seen in acute and chronic renal failure, hypoparathyroidism, pseudohypoparathyroidism, and tumoral calcinosis. Indeed, deposition of calcium–phosphate complexes in the kidney may predispose a patient to acute renal failure. When the calcium–phosphate product exceeds 70, the probability that soft-tissue calcification will occur increases sharply. In addition, local factors, such as tissue pH and injury (e.g., necrotic or hypoxic tissue), may predispose the patient to precipitation of the calcium–phosphate salts. In chronic renal failure, calcification occurs in arteries, muscle tissue, periarticular spaces, myocardial conduction system, lungs, and kidney. Affected patients may also have ocular calcification, causing the "red eye" syndrome of uremia, and subcutaneous calcification, which also plays a role in uremic pruritus. Alternatively, a predisposition to calcification of periarticular surfaces of the hips, elbows, shoulders, and other large joints occurs in tumoral calcinosis.

In some disease states, hyperphosphatemia may also play an important role in the development of secondary hyperparathyroidism.[27] A decrement in the serum calcium concentration secondary to hyperphosphatemia stimulates the release of PTH. Furthermore, hyperphosphatemia decreases the activity of renal $25(OH)D-1\alpha$-hydroxylase. The consequent diminished production of $1,25(OH)_2D_3$ impairs the gastrointestinal absorption of calcium and induces skeletal resistance to PTH, which are influences that augment the development of hyperparathyroidism.

Thus, hyperphosphatemia triggers a cascade of events that have an impact on calcium homeostasis at multiple sites. The prevention of secondary hyperparathyroidism, metabolic bone disease, and soft-tissue and vascular calcification in affected patients, therefore, depends on ultimately controlling the serum phosphate concentration.

## HYPOPHOSPHATEMIA

A low serum phosphorus level is associated with symptoms only if there is concomitant phosphate depletion. The presence of phosphate deficiency, however, may cause widespread disturbances. This is not surprising, because severe hypophosphatemia causes two critical abnormalities that have an impact on virtually all organ systems. First, a deficiency of 2,3-diphosphoglycerate (2,3-DPG) occurs in red cells, which is associated with an increased affinity of hemoglobin for oxygen and, therefore, tissue hypoxia. Second, there is a decline of tissue ATP content and a concomitant decrease in the availability of energy-rich phosphate compounds that are essential for cell function.[64,65] The major clinical syndromes resulting from these abnormalities include nervous system dysfunction, anorexia, nausea, vomiting, ileus, muscle weakness, cardiomyopathy, respiratory insufficiency, hemolytic anemia, and impaired leukocyte and platelet function. Additionally, phosphate deficiency causes osteomalacia and bone pain, which are clinical sequelae that are probably independent of the aforementioned abnormalities.

Central nervous system dysfunction has been well characterized in severe hypophosphatemia, especially in patients receiving total parenteral nutrition for diseases causing severe weight loss. A sequence of symptoms compatible with a metabolic encephalopathy usually begins one or more weeks after the initiation of therapy with solutions that contain glucose and amino acids but lack adequate phosphorus supplementation to prevent hypophosphatemia. Irritability, muscle weakness, numbness, and paresthesia mark the onset of dysfunction, with progression to dysarthria, confusion, obtundation, coma, and death.[66] These patients have a profoundly diminished red-cell 2,3-DPG content. Both biochemical abnormalities and clinical symptoms improve as patients receive phosphorus supplementation. Peripheral neuropathies, Guillain-Barré–like paralysis, hyporeflexia, intention tremor, and ballismus have also been described with hypophosphatemia and phosphate depletion.

The effects of hypophosphatemia on muscle depend on the severity and chronicity of the deficiency. Chronic phosphorus deficiency results in a proximal myopathy with striking atrophy and weakness. Osteomalacia frequently accompanies the myopathy, so patients complain of pain in weight-bearing bones. Normal values for serum creatine phosphokinase and aldolase activities are characteristically present. Rhabdomyolysis does not occur with chronic phosphate depletion.

In contrast, acute hypophosphatemia can lead to rhabdomyolysis with muscle weakness and pain. Most cases occur in chronic alcoholics or patients receiving total parenteral nutrition. In both groups of patients, muscle pain, swelling, and stiffness occur 3 to 8 days after the initiation of therapies that do not contain adequate amounts of phosphorus. Muscle paralysis and diaphragmatic failure may occur. Studies of muscle tissue from chronically phosphate-depleted dogs made acutely hypophosphatemic showed a decrement in cellular content of phosphorus, ATP, and adenosine diphosphate. Rhabdomyolysis occurred in these muscle fibers. The laboratory findings in patients with hypophosphatemic myopathy and with rhabdomyolysis include elevated serum creatine phosphokinase levels; however, serum phosphate levels may become normal if enough necrosis has occurred with subsequent phosphorus release. Also, renal failure and hypocalcemia can be associated with the syndrome.

Myocardial performance can be abnormal at serum phosphate levels of 0.7 to 1.4 mg/dL. This occurs when ATP depletion causes impairment of the actin–myosin interaction, the calcium pump of the sarcoplasma, and the sodium–potassium pump of the cell membrane.[67] The net result is reduced stroke work and cardiac output, which may progress to congestive heart failure. These problems are reversible with phosphate replacement.

Respiratory failure can occur as a result of failure of diaphragmatic contraction in hypophosphatemic patients. When serum phosphate levels are raised, diaphragmatic contractility improves. The postulated mechanism for the respiratory failure is muscle weakness secondary to inadequate levels of ATP and decreased glycolysis as the result of phosphate depletion.[68]

Two disturbances of red-cell function may occur secondary to phosphorus deficiency. First, as intraerythrocyte ATP production is decreased, the erythrocyte cell membrane becomes rigid, which can cause hemolysis.[69] This is rare and is usually seen in septic, uremic, acidotic, or alcoholic patients when serum phosphate levels are <0.5 mg/dL. Second, the limited production of 2,3-DPG causes a leftward shift of the oxyhemoglobin curve and impairs the release of oxygen to peripheral tissues.

Leukocyte dysfunction, which complicates phosphate deficiency, includes decreased chemotaxis, phagocytosis, and bactericidal activity.[70] These abnormalities increase the host susceptibility to infection. The mechanism by which hypophosphatemia impairs the various activities of the leukocyte probably is related to impairment of ATP synthesis. Decreased availability of energy impairs microtubules that regulate the mechanical properties of leukocytes and limit the rate of synthesis of organic phosphate compounds that are necessary for endocytosis.

Abnormal platelet survival, causing profuse gastrointestinal bleeding and cutaneous bleeding, has also been described in association with phosphate depletion in animal studies. Despite these abnormalities, there is little evidence that hypophosphatemia is a primary cause of hemorrhage in humans.

Perhaps the most consistent abnormalities associated with phosphate depletion are those on bone. Acute phosphate deple-

tion induces dissolution of apatite crystal from the osseous matrix. This effect may be a result of the 1,25(OH)$_2$D$_3$ level, which is increased in response to phosphate depletion in both animals and humans. More prolonged hypophosphatemia leads to rickets and osteomalacia. This complication is a common feature of phosphate depletion. However, the ultimate cause is variable. Although simple phosphate depletion alone may underlie the genesis of the abnormal mineralization, in many disorders, the defect is secondary to phosphate depletion and commensurate 1,25(OH)$_2$D$_3$ deficiency. Thus, treatment of this complication may often require combination therapy, including phosphate supplements and calcitriol.

## TREATMENT OF ABNORMAL SERUM PHOSPHATE LEVELS

Treatment of the myriad of diseases that characteristically display hyperphosphatemia or hypophosphatemia depends on determining the mechanism underlying their pathogenesis. The cause can almost always be ascertained by assessment of the clinical setting, determination of renal function, measurement of urinary phosphate excretion, and analysis of arterial carbon dioxide tension and pH. Therapy is aimed at correcting both the serum phosphate concentration and the associated complications.

Theoretically, elevated serum phosphate levels may be reduced by decreasing the TmP, increasing the GFR, or diminishing the phosphate load (exogenous or endogenous). There are no generally available pharmacologic means of acutely altering the GFR or reducing the TmP. However, chronic use of drugs, such as acetazolamide, which decreases TmP and induces phosphaturia, is effective as ancillary treatment of disorders such as tumoral calcinosis. Nevertheless, regulation of hyperphosphatemia is most often achieved by reducing the renal phosphate load. In tumoral calcinosis and chronic renal failure, such an effect is obtained by restricting the dietary phosphate intake or by administering calcium carbonate or aluminum hydroxide. Alternative strategies for management of load-dependent hyperphosphatemia include the administration of intravenous calcium or intravenous glucose and insulin. The consequence of such intervention is sequestration of phosphate in bone or soft tissues. Dialysis can also be used for the acute management of load-dependent disorders or for the chronic maintenance of phosphate overload, such as that which complicates chronic renal failure. In the latter condition, phosphate binders are essential.[71,72]

The treatment of phosphate depletion depends on replacing body phosphorus stores. Preventive measures, however, preclude the onset of phosphate depletion. Thus, appropriate monitoring of patients taking large doses of antacids that contain aluminum and provision of phosphorus intravenously to patients with diabetic ketoacidosis preserves phosphate stores. Alternatively, the treatment of established phosphate depletion may require 2.5 to 4.0 g per day of phosphate, preferably administered orally in four equally divided doses. This can be done by giving phosphorus supplement tablets (K-Phos Neutral), which contain 250 mg elemental phosphorus per tablet. If oral therapy is not tolerated and the serum phosphate level shows a downward trend, approaching dangerous levels (<1.2 mg/dL), intravenous phosphate supplementation at a dose of 10 mg/kg per day may be administered. Such therapy should be discontinued when the serum phosphate concentration reaches values > 2 mg/dL. However, therapy is not required for many of the conditions resulting in phosphate depletion. Only when the consequences of severe depletion are manifest does treatment need to be initiated.

In many of the chronic causes of hypophosphatemia, marked by a reduction in the TmP, correction of the hypophosphatemia is difficult. In these diseases, chronic phosphate supplementation with K-Phos Neutral alone or in combination with vitamin D or its metabolites increases the serum phosphorus (not always to normal) and improves the complications associated with hypophosphatemia.

# REFERENCES

1. Wilkinson R. Absorption of calcium, phosphorus and magnesium. In: Nordin BEC, ed. Calcium, phosphate and magnesium metabolism. New York: Longman, 1976:218.
2. Gennari C, Bernini M, Nordi P, Fusi L. Dissociation of absorptions of calcium and phosphate in different pathophysiological states in man. In: Massry SG, Maschio G, Ritz E, eds. Phosphate and mineral metabolism. New York: Plenum Press, 1984:195.
3. Walling MW. Intestinal calcium and phosphate transport: differential responses to vitamin D3 metabolites. Am J Physiol 1977; 233:E488.
4. Bijvoet OLM. Kidney function in calcium and phosphate metabolism. In: Avioli LV, Krane SM, eds. Metabolic bone disease, vol 1. New York: Academic Press, 1977:49.
5. Trohler U, Bonjour J-P, Fleisch H. Inorganic: phosphate homeostasis: renal adaptation to the dietary intake in intact and thyroparathyroidectomized rats. J Clin Invest 1976; 57:264.
6. Agus ZS. Renal handling of phosphate. In: Massry SG, Glassock RJ, eds. Textbook of nephrology. Baltimore: Williams & Wilkins, 1983:389.
7. Cheng L, Jacktor B. Sodium gradient-dependent phosphate transport in renal brush border membrane vesicles. J Biol Chem 1981; 256:1556.
8. Donsa TP, Kempson SA. Regulation of renal brush border membrane transport of phosphate. Miner Electrolyte Metab 1982; 7:113.
9. Tenenhous HS. Cellular and molecular mechanisms of renal phosphate transport. J Bone Miner Res 1997; 12:159.
10. Dennis VW, Stead WW, Myers JL. Renal handling of phosphate and calcium. Annu Rev Physiol 1979; 41:257.
11. Slatopolsky E, Robson AM, Elkan I, Bricker NS. Control of phosphate excretion in uremic man. J Clin Invest 1968; 47:1865.
12. Nagant De Deuxchaisnes C, Krane SM. Hypoparathyroidism. In: Avioli LV, Krane SM, eds. Metabolic bone diseases, vol 11. New York: Academic Press, 1978:183.
13. De Luca F, Baron J. Molecular biology and clinical importance of the $Ca^{2+}$-sensing receptor. Curr Opin Pediatr 1998; 10:435.
14. Pearce SH, Cheetham T, Imrie H, et al. A common and recurrent 1 3-bp deletion in the autoimmune regulator gene in British kindreds with autoimmune polyendocrinopathy type 1. Am J Hum Gen 1998; 63:1675.
15. Trump D, Dixon PH, Mumm S, et al. Localisation of X linked recessive idiopathic hypoparathyroidism to a 1.5 Mb region on Xq26-q27. J Med Gen 1998; 35:905.
16. Ahmed SF, Dixon PH, Bonthron DT, et al. GNAS 1 mutational analysis in pseudohypoparathyroidism. Clin Endocrinol (Oxf) 1998; 49:525.
17. Jüppner H, Schipani E, Bastepe M, et al. The gene responsible for pseudohypoparathyroidism type 1b is paternally imprinted and maps in four unrelated kindreds to chromosome 20q13.3. Proc Natl Acad Sci U S A 1998; 95:11798.
18. Lyles KW, Burkes EJ, Ellis GJ, et al. Genetic transmission of tumoral calcinosis: autosomal dominant, with variable clinical impressivity. J Clin Endocrinol Metab 1985; 60:1093.
19. Mozaffanan G, Lafferty FW, Pearson OH. Treatment of tumoral calcinosis with phosphorus deprivation. Ann Intern Med 1972; 77:741.
20. Sinah TK, Allen DO, Queener SF, et al. Effects of acetazolamide on the renal excretion of phosphate in hyperparathyroidism and pseudohypoparathyroidism. J Lab Clin Med 1977; 89:1188.
21. Quarles LD, Murphy G, Econs MJ, et al. Uremic tumoral calcinosis: preliminary observations suggesting an association with aberrant vitamin D homeostasis. Am J Kidney Dis 1991; 18:706.
22. Tezelman S, Siperstein AE, Duh QV, et al. Tumoral calcinosis: controversies in the etiology and alternatives in the treatment. Arch Surg 1993; 128:737.
23. Kuriyama S, Tomonari H, Nakayama M, et al. Successful treatment of tumoral calcinosis using CAPD combined with hemodialysis with low-calcium dialysate. Blood Purif 1998; 16:43.
24. Ueyoshi A, Ota K. Clinical appraisal of vinpocetine for the removal of intractable tumoral calcinosis in hemodialysis patients with renal failure. J Int Med Res 1992; 20:435.
25. Simionesciu L, Dumitriu L, Dumitriu V, et al. The serum osteocalcin levels in patients with thyroid disease. Endocrinologie 1988; 26:27.
26. DeMenis E, DaRin G, Roiter I, et al. Bone turnover in overt and subclinical hyperthyroidism due to autonomous thyroid adenoma. Horm Res 1992; 37:217.
27. Slatopolsky E, Rutherford WE, Rosenbaum R, et al. Hyperphosphatemia. Clin Nephrol 1977; 7:138.
28. Corvilain J, Abramov M, Bergaus A. Effect of growth hormone on tubular transport of phosphate in normal and parathyroidectomized dogs. J Clin Invest 1964; 43:1608.
29. Ohashi H, Rosen KM, Smith FE, et al. Characterization of type 1 IGF receptor and IGF 1 mRNA expression in cultured human and bovine glomerular cells. Regul Pept 1993; 48:9.
30. Walton RJ, Russell RGG, Smith R. Changes in the renal and extra-renal handling of phosphate induced by disodium etidronate (EHDP) in man. Clin Sci Mol Med 1975; 49:45.
31. Grossman RA, Hamilton RW, Morse BM, et al. Nontraumatic rhabdomyolysis and acute renal failure. N Engl J Med 1974; 291:807.
32. Koffler A, Fnedler RM, Massry SG. Acute renal failure due to nontraumatic rhabdomyolysis. Ann Intern Med 1976; 85:25.
33. Zusman J, Brown DM, Nesbitt ME. Hyperphosphatemia, hyperphosphaturia and hypocalcemia in acute lymphoblastic leukemia. N Engl J Med 1973; 289:1335.
34. Denborough MA, Forster JFA, Hudson MC, et al. Biochemical changes in malignant hyperpyrexia. Lancet 1970; 1:1137.
35. Halevy J, Bulvik S. Severe hypophosphatemia in hospitalized patients. Arch Intern Med 1988; 148:153.
36. Levine BS, Cooks PW, Katz JA, et al. Early events during renal adaptation to low dietary phosphorus. Kidney Int 1984; 25:148.
37. Latz M, Zisman E, Bartter FC. Evidence for a phosphorus-depletion syndrome in man. N Engl J Med 1968; 278:409.
38. Baker LRI, Acknll P, Cattell WR, et al. Iatrogenic osteomalacia and myopathy due to phosphate depletion. BMJ 1974; 3:150.
39. Haas HG, Dambacher MA, Buncaga J, Lauffenburger T. Renal effects of calcitonin and parathyroid extract in man. J Clin Invest 1971; 50:2689.
40. Francis F, Henning S, Korn B, et al. A gene (PEX) with homologies to endopeptidases is mutated in patients with X-linked hypophosphatemic rickets. Nat Gen 1995; 11:130.
41. Lobaugh B, Burch WM Jr, Drezner MK. Abnormalities of vitamin D metabolism and action in the vitamin D resistant rachitic and osteomalacic diseases. In: Kumar R, ed. Vitamin D: basic and clinical aspects. Boston: Martinus Nijhoff, 1984:665.
42. Friedman NE, Lobaugh B, Drezner MK. Effects of calcitriol and phosphorus therapy on the growth of patients with X-linked hypophosphatemia. J Clin Endocrinol Metab 1993; 76:839.
43. Bell CL, Tennenhouse HS, Scriver CR. Primary cultures of renal epithelial cells from X-linked hypophosphatemic (Hyp) mice express defects in phosphate transport and vitamin D metabolism. Am J Hum Genet 1988; 43:293.
44. Meyer RA Jr, Meyer MH, Gray RW. Parabiosis suggests a humoral factor is involved in X-linked hypophosphatemia in mice. J Bone Miner Res 1989; 4:493.
45. Nesbitt T, Econs MJ, Byun JK, et al. Phosphate transport in immortalized cell cultures from the renal proximal tubule of normal and hyp mice. Evidence that the Hyp gene locus product is an extrarenal factor. J Bone Miner Res 1995; 10:1327.
46. Nesbitt T, Coffman TM, Griffiths R, et al. Crosstransplantation of kidneys in normal and hyp-mice: evidence that the hyp-mouse phenotype is unrelated to an intrinsic renal defect. J Clin Invest 1992; 89:1453.
47. Nesbitt T, Drezner MK, Lobaugh B. Abnormal parathyroid hormone stimulation of 25-hydroxyvitamin D-1α-hydroxylase activity in the hypophosphatemic mouse: evidence for a generalized defect of vitamin D metabolism. J Clin Invest 1986; 77:181.
48. Nesbitt T, Lobaugh B, Drezner MK. Calcitonin stimulation of renal 25 hydroxyvitamin D-1α hydroxylase activity in Hyp-mice: evidence that the regulation of calcitriol production is not universally abnormal in X-linked hypophosphatemia. J Clin Invest 1987; 79:15.
49. Tenenhouse HS, Yip A, Jones G. Increased renal catabolism of 1,25-dihydroxyvitamin $D_3$ in murine X-linked hypophosphatemic rickets. J Clin Invest 1988; 81:461.
50. Tieder M, Modai D, Samuel R, et al. Hereditary hypophosphatemic rickets with hypercalciuria (HHRH): a new syndrome. In: Norman AW, Schaefer K, Grigoleit H-G, Herrath DV, eds. Vitamin D: a chemical, biochemical and clinical update. Berlin: Walter de Gruyter, 1985:1107.
51. Yamamoto T, Seino Y, Tanaka H, et al. Effects of the administration of phosphate on nuclear 1,25-dihydroxyvitamin D3 uptake by duodenal mucosal cells of Hyp-mice. Endocrinology 1988; 122:576.
52. Tieder M, Arie R, Modai D, et al. Elevated serum 1 ,25-dihydroxyvitamin D concentrations in siblings with primary Fanconi's syndrome. N Engl J Med 1988; 319:845.
53. Lieberman UA, Eil C, Marx SJ. Hereditary hypocalcemic vitamin D resistant rickets (HHDR). In: Frame B, Potts JT, eds. Clinical disorders of bone and mineral metabolism. Amsterdam: Excerpta Medica, 1983:441.
54. Fu GK, Lin D, Zhang MY, et al. Cloning of human 25-hydroxyvitamin D-1α-hydroxylase and mutations causing vitamin D-dependent rickets type 1. Mol Endocrinol 1997; 11:1961.
55. Bliziotes M, Yergey AJ, Nanes MS, et al. Absent intestinal response to calciferols in hereditary resistance to 1 ,25-dihydroxyvitamin D: documentation and effective therapy with high dose intravenous calcium infusions. J Clin Endocrinol Metab 1988; 66:294.
56. Harrison HE, Harrison HC. Rickets and osteomalacia. In: Harrison HE, Harrison HC. Disorders of calcium and phosphate metabolism. Philadelphia: WB Saunders, 1979;141.
57. Econs MJ, McEnery PT, Lennon F, et al. Autosomal dominant hypophosphatemic rickets is linked to chromosome 12p13. J Clin Invest 1997; 100:2653.
58. Drezner MK. Tumor-associated rickets and osteomalacia.. In: Favus MJ, ed. Primer on the metabolic bone diseases and disorders of mineral metabolism, ed 2. New York: Raven Press, 1993:282.
58a. Sandhu FA, Martuza RL. Craniofacial hemangiopericytoma associated with oncogenic osteomalacia. J Neurooncol 2000; 46:241.
59. Cai Q, Hodgson MD, Kao PC, et al. Inhibition of renal phosphate transport by a tumor product in a patient with oncogenic osteomalacia. N Engl J Med 1994; 330:1645.
60. Mostellar ME, Tuttle EP. Effects of alkalosis on plasma concentration and urinary excretion of inorganic phosphate in man. J Clin Invest 1964; 43:138.

61. Knochel JP. The pathophysiology and clinical characteristics of severe hypophosphatemia. Arch Intern Med 1977; 137:203.
62. Sheldon GF, Grzyb S. Phosphate depletion and repletion: relation to parenteral nutrition and oxygen transport. Ann Surg 1975; 182:683.
63. Herbert LA, Lemann J, Peterson JR, Lennon EJ. Studies of the mechanism by which phosphate infusion lowers serum calcium concentration. J Clin Invest 1966; 45:1886.
64. Duhm J. 2,3-DPG-induced displacements of the oxyhemoglobin dissociation curve of blood: mechanisms and consequences. Adv Exp Biol Med 1971; 37A:179.
65. Travis SF, Sugerman HJ, Ruberg RL, et al. Alterations of red cell glycolytic intermediates and oxygen transport as a consequence of hypophosphatemia in patients receiving intravenous hyperalimentation. N Engl J Med 1977; 297:901.
66. Parfitt AM, Kleerekoper M. Clinical disorders of calcium, phosphorus and magnesium metabolism. In: Maxwell MH, Kleeman CR, eds. Clinical disorders of fluid and electrolyte metabolism. New York: McGraw-Hill, 1980:947.
67. O'Connor LR, Wheeler WS, Bethune JE. Effect of hypophosphatemia on myocardial performance in man. N Engl J Med 1977; 297:901.
68. Newman JH, Neff TA, Ziporen P. Acute respiratory failure associated with hypophosphatemia. N Engl J Med 1977; 296:1101.
69. Klock JC, Williams HE, Mentzer WK. Hemolytic anemia and somatic cell dysfunction in severe hypophosphatemia. Arch Intern Med 1974; 134:360.
70. Craddock PR, Yawota Y, Van Santen L, et al. Acquired phagocyte dysfunction: a complication of the hypophosphatemia of parenteral hyperalimentation. N Engl J Med 1974; 290:1403.
71. Block GA, Port FK. Re-evaluation of risks associated with hyperphosphatemia and hyperparathyroidism in dialysis patients: recommendations for a change in management. Am J Kidn Dis 2000; 35:1226.
72. Chertow GM, Dillon MA, Amin N, Burke SK. Sevelamer with and without calcium and vitamin D: observations from a long-term open-label clinical trial. J Ren Nutr 2000; 10:125.

# CHAPTER 68

# MAGNESIUM METABOLISM

ROBERT K. RUDE

Magnesium is the fourth most abundant cation in the body and the major intracellular divalent cation. The amount of magnesium in an adult human is ~2000 mEq (24 g), of which 60% is in the skeleton and 40% is intracellular. Less than 1% is found in the extracellular fluid compartment.[1–3] Magnesium is essential for the function of many enzyme systems, including those that use adenosine triphosphate.[4,5] Magnesium can be absorbed along the entire gastrointestinal tract, including both the small and large intestine, but it is absorbed most efficiently in the jejunum and ileum, through both a saturable transport system and passive diffusion.[6,7] Fractional intestinal magnesium absorption appears to depend on the amount of magnesium in the diet; with an average magnesium intake, ~40% is absorbed.[6,7] The major dietary sources of magnesium include vegetables and meats, but magnesium is ubiquitous in food. Some studies have suggested that 1,25-dihydroxyvitamin D [1,25(OH)$_2$D] enhances intestinal magnesium absorption,[8] although this may be secondary to the effect of this vitamin on calcium transport.[9] The regulation of magnesium homeostasis occurs primarily in the kidney.[10] Micropuncture studies have demonstrated that magnesium is absorbed along the proximal convoluted tubule (5% to 15%), the thick ascending limb of the loop of Henle (50% to 60%), and the distal tubule (10%).[11] Although a true tubular maximum for magnesium has not been demonstrated in isolated micropuncture studies of the nephron, the whole kidney does demonstrate a maximal capacity to reabsorb magnesium.[12,13] When the filtered magnesium load exceeds that amount filtered under normal circumstances (serum ultrafilterable magnesium concentration of ~1.3 mEq/L), the excess is excreted. Under conditions of magnesium deprivation, however, when the filtered load is below 1.3 mEq/L, magnesium is virtually completely reabsorbed.

Despite efficient regulation of magnesium metabolism, no factor or hormone has yet been described that primarily regulates this system.

## MAGNESIUM DEFICIENCY

### ETIOLOGY OF MAGNESIUM DEFICIENCY

Although magnesium is avidly conserved by the body, magnesium deficiency is a common occurrence. Up to 10% of the patients admitted to large city hospitals are hypomagnesemic.[14] In one hospital, 65% of the patients in a medical intensive care unit were hypomagnesemic.[15] Because magnesium is found in virtually all foods, dietary deprivation is a most unusual cause of hypomagnesemia in persons with normal caloric intake. Much more commonly, magnesium deficiency is caused by excessive losses from either the gastrointestinal tract or the kidney.[16] Table 68-1 outlines causes of magnesium deficiency.

**TABLE 68-1.**
**Differential Diagnosis of Magnesium Deficiency**

**GASTROINTESTINAL DISORDERS**
  Malabsorption syndromes
  Extensive bowel resection
  Acute and chronic diarrhea
  Intestinal and biliary fistulas
  Protein–calorie malnutrition
  Acute hemorrhagic pancreatitis
  Primary hypomagnesemia (neonatal)
**RENAL LOSS**
  Chronic parenteral fluid therapy
  Hypercalcemia
  Osmotic diuresis
    Glucose (diabetes mellitus)
    Mannitol
    Urea
  Alcohol
  Acidosis (e.g., starvation, diabetes)
  Drugs
    Diuretics (furosemide, ethacrynic acid)
    Aminoglycosides
    Cisplatin
    Cyclosporine
    Amphotericin B
    Pentamidine
    Cardiac glycosides (possible)
  Renal diseases
    Chronic pyelonephritis and glomerulonephritis
    Diuretic phase of acute tubular necrosis
    Post–obstructive nephropathy
    Renal tubular acidosis
    Post–renal transplant
  Primary hypomagnesemia
**ENDOCRINE AND METABOLIC**
  Phosphate depletion
  Primary hyperparathyroidism
  Hypoparathyroidism
  Hyperthyroidism
  Hypothyroidism
  Primary aldosteronism
  Hungry bone syndrome
  Excessive lactation
  Massive transfusion with citrated blood

## GASTROINTESTINAL DISORDERS

Magnesium may be lost via the gastrointestinal tract, either by excessive loss of secreted fluids or impaired absorption of both dietary and endogenous magnesium.[2,7] The magnesium concentration of upper intestinal tract fluids is ~0.5 mmol/L, and vomiting or nasogastric suction may contribute to magnesium depletion because of loss of these fluids. Disorders of the small bowel are frequently associated with magnesium deficiency.[2,7] Intestinal mucosal damage from nontropical sprue, radiation injury from the treatment for Whipple disease, and intestinal lymphectasia may cause magnesium deficiency. Steatorrhea also may cause or potentiate magnesium malabsorption through formation of nonabsorbable magnesium-lipid salts. The resection or bypass of the ileum for obesity, enteritis, or vascular infarction often results in magnesium deficiency. The magnesium content of intestinal fluids can be as high as 15 mEq/L.[17] Thus, excessive magnesium loss may occur in acute or chronic diarrheal states, including regional enteritis and ulcerative colitis, or in patients with intestinal or biliary fistulas. The diarrhea encountered in protein–calorie malnutrition may be one mechanism for magnesium depletion. Acute hemorrhagic or edematous pancreatitis can also produce hypomagnesemia. The reason is unclear, but it may be the result of saponification of magnesium in the necrotic peripancreatic fat, which is a mechanism similar to that proposed for the hypocalcemia of acute pancreatitis. A selective defect in intestinal magnesium absorption (primary intestinal hypomagnesemia) is thought to be one cause of neonatal hypomagnesemia.

## RENAL LOSS

Urinary loss of magnesium is a common contributing cause of magnesium deficiency.[2,13,18] The renal magnesium transport is influenced by the filtered sodium and calcium load. Thus, excess urinary excretion of sodium and calcium will increase magnesium clearance and lead to urinary magnesium losses. The administration of excessive sodium in parenteral fluids is a common factor in the pathogenesis of hypomagnesemia in hospitalized patients. Most disorders causing an increase in the serum calcium concentration will also lead to renal magnesium wasting, presumably because of activation of the $Ca^{2+}$-sensing receptor in the thick ascending limb of Henle, resulting in a decrease in the transepithelial voltage and a subsequent decrease in calcium and magnesium reabsorption.[11,19] An exception is familial hypocalciuric hypercalcemia caused by an inactivating mutation of the $Ca^{2+}$-sensing receptor, and lithium ingestion, in which urinary magnesium excretion is decreased.

Commonly, diabetes mellitus is associated with magnesium deficiency and exemplifies osmotic-induced magnesium deficiency.[20] The acidosis resulting from diabetic ketoacidosis, starvation, or alcoholism may also lead to renal magnesium wasting.[2] The association of alcoholism with magnesium depletion is well known. Although the reason for magnesium deficiency is usually multifactorial in these patients, a rising blood alcohol level has been shown to cause renal magnesium loss.

A wide spectrum of therapeutic agents may be associated with renal magnesium wasting.[21] Hypomagnesemia is observed with the use of loop diuretics, such as furosemide and ethacrynic acid, and with therapy with the aminoglycosides, cisplatin, cyclosporine, amphotericin B, and pentamidine.[22] Cardiac glycosides increase renal magnesium loss in dogs, but the pathophysiologic role they play in human magnesium depletion is unclear.

Many renal glomerular and tubular diseases are associated with renal magnesium wasting.[2] There may be other accompanying tubular abnormalities, and a reduced glomerular filtration rate (GFR) may or may not be present. A rare form of hypomagnesemia (primary renal hypomagnesemia) is characterized by renal magnesium wasting in the absence of any other renal abnormality. This disorder may occur in children or in adults and may be familial.

## ENDOCRINE AND METABOLIC CAUSES

Other disorders may also be associated with a disturbance in magnesium metabolism.[2,23] Phosphate depletion, which is a common problem in hospitalized patients, causes renal magnesium wasting. An increase in urinary magnesium excretion and occasional hypomagnesemia is seen also in primary hyperparathyroidism, treated hypoparathyroidism, and hyperthyroidism.[2,24] In these situations, hypercalciuria probably promotes the renal magnesium losses. In hypothyroidism, low intracellular magnesium content is found in association with high serum magnesium levels. A tendency to low serum magnesium concentrations in primary aldosteronism may be related to renal magnesium wasting resulting from volume expansion. Marked hypomagnesemia may occasionally accompany the "hungry bone syndrome," which is a phase of rapid bone mineral accretion most commonly seen in patients with preexisting hyperparathyroid bone disease who undergo successful neck surgery for hyperparathyroidism. Hypomagnesemia caused by excessive lactation is a rare occurrence. Massive transfusion with citrated blood may result in hypomagnesemia as well as hypocalcemia.

## MANIFESTATIONS OF MAGNESIUM DEFICIENCY

### SIGNS AND SYMPTOMS

Pure magnesium deficiency in the absence of hormonal, gastrointestinal, or other metabolic disorders is uncommon. Signs and symptoms of magnesium deficiency are shown in Table 68-2. Because magnesium deficiency is usually associated with other disease states, the signs and symptoms of the primary disease process may mask those of magnesium deficiency.[25] Neuromuscular hyperirritability may be the most common presenting problem in magnesium-depleted patients.[2,23,26] Latent tetany may be present and may be elicited by positive Chvostek and Trousseau signs. Some patients may have spontaneous carpopedal spasm. Generalized seizures have also been reported. These neurologic signs in part may be caused by coexisting hypocalcemia. However, tetany has also been documented in magnesium-deficient patients with normal serum calcium levels.[27] Other neurologic findings in hypomagnesemia include

**TABLE 68-2.**
**Common Clinical Manifestations of Magnesium Deficiency**

**NEUROMUSCULAR**
Positive Chvostek and Trousseau signs
Spontaneous carpal-pedal spasm
Vertigo, ataxia, nystagmus, athetoid and choreiform movements
Muscular weakness, tremor, fasciculation, and wasting
Psychiatric: depression, psychosis
**CARDIAC ARRHYTHMIA**
Junctional arrhythmias
Ventricular premature contractions, tachycardia, fibrillation
Sensitivity to digitalis intoxication
Torsades de pointes
**BIOCHEMICAL**
Hypocalcemia
Impaired parathyroid hormone secretion
Renal and skeletal resistance to parathyroid hormone
Resistance to vitamin D
Hypokalemia
Renal potassium wasting
Decreased intracellular potassium

athetoid and choreiform movements, nystagmus, ataxia, and vertigo. Psychiatric abnormalities have been reported. Muscular complaints, such as tremors, fasciculations, muscle wasting, and weakness, may also occur.

Cardiac arrhythmias are a serious complication of magnesium depletion.[2,28–30] Atrial and ventricular arrhythmias, including premature ventricular contractions, ventricular tachycardia, torsades de pointes, and ventricular fibrillation have been reported. Arrhythmias after myocardial infarction have also been associated with hypomagnesemia, and magnesium therapy has been demonstrated to decrease arrhythmias and improve survival in patients with acute myocardial infarction in some,[31,32] but not all studies.[33] Other electrocardiographic abnormalities include prolonged PR interval, U waves, and an increased QT interval. Associated hypokalemia and intracellular potassium depletion may contribute to these electrocardiographic abnormalities. Arrhythmias in magnesium-deficient patients may be resistant to the usual antiarrhythmic therapy and may respond only to magnesium therapy.[29,34] An increased susceptibility of magnesium-deficient patients to digitalis intoxication has also been observed.[28] Evidence also suggests that magnesium modulates vascular tone and may play a role in essential hypertension.[34a,35] Other less recognized complaints include dysphagia caused by esophageal spasm.[2] Also, anemia, characterized by short red blood cell survival, reticulocytosis, spherocytosis, microcytosis, and erythroid hyperplasia, has been described.[2] Platelet-dependent thrombosis may occur.[35a]

Magnesium therapy has been suggested as a beneficial form of therapy in renal calcium stone formation.[36,37] In vitro studies have demonstrated that magnesium can prevent the precipitation and growth of calcium oxalate and calcium phosphate crystals.[36] Experimental magnesium deficiency in rats results in nephrocalcinosis, and some patients with idiopathic renal magnesium wasting also have nephrocalcinosis.[38] Assessment of magnesium status in renal stone formers, however, has demonstrated normal serum magnesium concentrations, muscle magnesium contents, and magnesium tolerance testing results.[38] Gastrointestinal magnesium absorption was also found to be normal. Because of the influence of magnesium on crystal formation, alterations in renal magnesium excretion may be a potential cause of renal stone formation. Stone formers, however, have been found to have urinary magnesium excretion that is similar to a control population in most but not all studies.[38,39] The ratio of urinary magnesium to urinary calcium has also been used as an index of the propensity to form stones. Magnesium excretion for corresponding calcium is lower in stone-forming patients, and a reduced ratio has been reported to be associated with an increased frequency of stones.[36,40]

Studies have assessed the benefit of magnesium supplementation in stone disease. One study of 56 patients who received 400 mg magnesium per day for 2 years noted a decrease in the rate of stone episodes from 0.8 stones per year to 0.003 stones per year.[36] A control group also had a decrease in stone episodes of 0.5 to 0.22 stones per year. This was ascribed to the expected interval-free period after a stone episode. Another study suggested that oral magnesium supplements decrease intestinal calcium absorption in patients with hyperabsorptive hypercalciuric stone disease.[37] Magnesium therapy, therefore, may be of benefit in reducing the recurrence rate in renal calcium stone disease.

## HYPOCALCEMIA

An important clinical complication of magnesium deficiency is hypocalcemia.[2] The hypocalcemia is caused in part by the suppressive effect of magnesium depletion on parathyroid hormone (PTH) secretion. Under normal circumstances, an abrupt decrease in magnesium causes an increase in PTH secretion, similar to that induced by a decrease in the serum calcium concentration. Magnesium affects PTH secretion by binding to the calcium-sensing

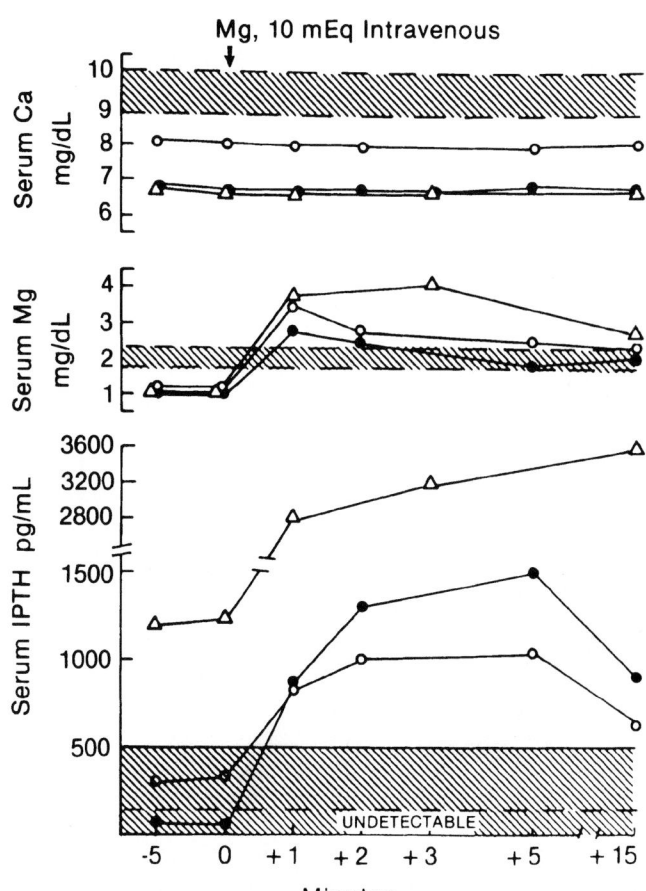

**FIGURE 68-1.** The effect of an intravenous injection of 10 mEq magnesium on the serum concentrations of calcium, magnesium, and immunoreactive parathyroid hormone (*IPTH*) in hypocalcemic magnesium-deficient patients with undetectable (●—●), normal (○—○), or elevated (Δ—Δ) levels of IPTH. Shaded areas represent the range of normal for each assay. The broken line for the IPTH assay represents the level of detectability. The magnesium injection resulted in a marked rise in parathyroid hormone secretion within 1 minute in all three patients.

receptor.[20] Chronic severe hypomagnesemia, however, impairs the secretion of PTH. Serum immunoreactive PTH (IPTH) concentrations are undetectable or inappropriately low in most hypocalcemic patients with magnesium depletion, although some patients will have IPTH concentrations that are higher than normal.[41,42] The ability of low magnesium concentrations to impair PTH secretion—as opposed to PTH synthesis—is well illustrated by the rapid increase in serum PTH levels after an intravenous injection of magnesium.[41] An example of the acute response to magnesium administration in three magnesium-deficient patients with varying basal serum IPTH concentrations is shown in Figure 68-1.

Along with impaired PTH secretion in hypomagnesemia, patients may demonstrate end-organ resistance to PTH. Both skeletal and renal resistance to PTH have been demonstrated in magnesium-deficient patients by decreased rises in the serum calcium concentration and in urinary cyclic adenosine monophosphate (cAMP) excretion in response to exogenously administered PTH.[42] Although the defect in PTH secretion is restored within minutes of magnesium administration, the skeletal resistance is not reversed as quickly. Figure 68-2 shows a 5-day course of magnesium therapy in a typical patient with hypocalcemia and magnesium depletion. In this patient, the serum calcium concentration does not rise appreciably until after ~2 days and is normalized only after 5 days of therapy. Serum PTH concentrations remain high until the serum calcium concentration returns to normal. The degree of PTH resistance seems to depend on the

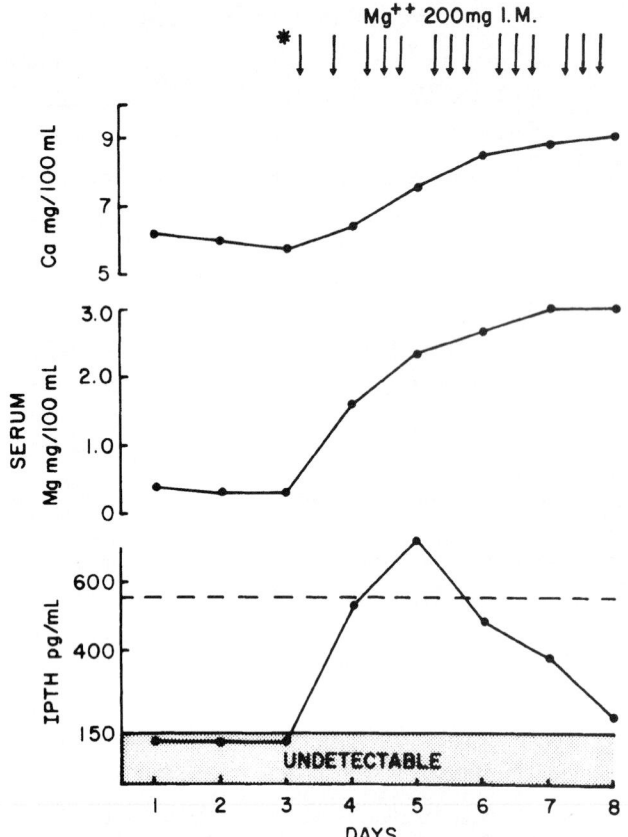

**FIGURE 68-2.** Changes in the serum calcium, magnesium, and immunoreactive parathyroid hormone (*IPTH*) concentrations during 5 days of magnesium therapy in a patient with magnesium deficiency. The horizontal *dashed* line indicates the upper limit of normal for the serum IPTH concentration. *Arrows* indicate times of intramuscular injection of 200 mg elemental magnesium. *Asterisk* indicates an initial intravenous injection of 300 mg elemental magnesium. Magnesium therapy resulted in a rise in the serum calcium, magnesium, and IPTH. The serum calcium concentration had returned to normal by the fourth or fifth day of therapy. (From Rude RK, Oldham SB, Singer FR. Functional hypoparathyroidism and parathyroid hormone end-organ resistance in human magnesium deficiency. Clin Endocrinol 1976; 5:209.)

severity of the magnesium depletion. The fall in serum PTH in normal subjects experimentally depleted of magnesium correlated with the fall in red blood cell free magnesium.[43]

The serum concentration of 1,25-dihydroxyvitamin D [1,25(OH)$_2$D] has been found to be low in most hypocalcemic magnesium-deficient patients.[44] The 1,25(OH)$_2$D level remains low for several days after initiation of magnesium therapy, during which time the serum calcium concentration returns to normal. The reason for the low 1,25(OH)$_2$D level is unclear, but it does not appear to be related to either the amount of vitamin D–binding protein in the plasma or the affinity of 1,25(OH)$_2$D for the binding protein. Magnesium-deficient patients with hypocalcemia are also resistant to the effects of pharmacologic doses of vitamin D as high as 50,000 units per day.[45] The overall effect of magnesium deficiency on calcium metabolism is illustrated in Figure 68-3.

### HYPOKALEMIA

Hypokalemia is a frequent and important complication of magnesium deficiency.[2,46–48] In one study, hypomagnesemia was present in 42% of patients with hypokalemia.[47] Such patients also have a marked reduction in intracellular potassium content. Experimental human magnesium deficiency has demonstrated that the abnormalities in potassium metabolism are caused by a reduction in the ability of the kidney to conserve potassium.[49] Potassium therapy alone will neither increase the

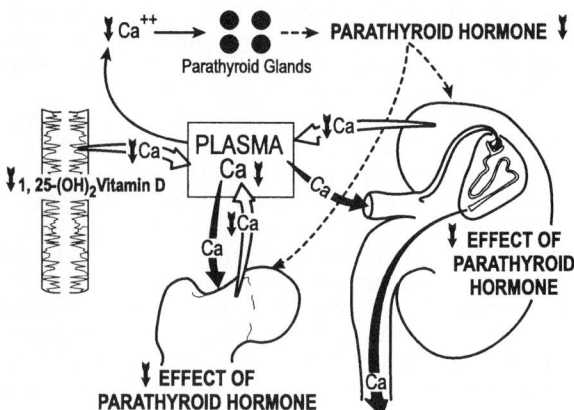

**FIGURE 68-3.** Disturbance of calcium metabolism during magnesium deficiency. Hypocalcemia is caused by a decrease in parathyroid hormone secretion as well as renal and skeletal resistance to the action of this hormone. Low serum concentrations of 1,25-dihydroxyvitamin D [*1,25(OH)$_2$D*] result in reduced intestinal calcium absorption.

intracellular potassium stores nor correct the renal potassium leak. Only simultaneous magnesium therapy will reverse the renal defect and normalize both the serum potassium concentration and the intracellular potassium content.[50]

### DIAGNOSIS

The serum magnesium concentration is the most commonly available index for assessing the presence of magnesium deficiency. The concentration of magnesium in the serum is commonly expressed in milliequivalents per liter or milligrams per deciliter. Milliequivalents of magnesium may be converted to milligrams by using the formula

$$mEq = \frac{[mg \times 2 \text{ (valence)}]}{24(MW)}$$

A low serum concentration (<1.5 mEq/L) usually indicates magnesium deficiency. However, the magnesium concentration in the extracellular fluid compartment does not always accurately represent total body magnesium stores, because only ~1% of body magnesium is in the extracellular fluid. Magnesium deficiency with clinical manifestations may exist in the presence of a normal serum magnesium concentration.[2,15,28,42,51] Ion-specific electrodes have become available for determining ionized magnesium in serum or plasma.[52] Results suggest that these may provide a better index of magnesium status than the total serum magnesium concentration. Differences between ionized-magnesium analyzers must be resolved, however, before they are used in routine patient care.[53] The mean intracellular peripheral lymphocyte magnesium content is reduced in patients with hypomagnesemia and in normomagnesemic patients at high risk for magnesium deficiency and, therefore, may be more precise in reflecting total body magnesium stores.[51,54] Clinically, however, considerable overlap with normal values limits the usefulness of this index in an individual patient. Perhaps the most accurate assessment of magnesium deficiency in use is a magnesium tolerance test that is based on the amount of magnesium retained after a dose is administered parenterally[55] (Table 68-3). In one study, the retention of a low dose of magnesium (0.2 mEq/kg or 2.4 mg/kg lean body weight) given intravenously over 4 hours was determined in hypomagnesemic patients, normomagnesemic patients at high risk for having magnesium deficiency, and normal controls by measuring the 24-hour urine magnesium excretion. Hypomagnesemic patients retained a mean of 78% ± 7% of the magnesium load. Normomagnesemic patients at risk for magnesium depletion retained 43% ± 5% of the magnesium load, whereas normal controls retained only 15% ± 5% of the administered magnesium. A

**TABLE 68-3.**
**Suggested Protocol for Clinical Use of Magnesium Tolerance Test**

1. Collect baseline urine (spot or timed) for magnesium/creatinine ratio.
2. Infuse 0.2 mEq (2.4 mg)/kg lean body weight of elemental magnesium in 50 mL 5% dextrose over 4 hours.
3. Collect 24-hour urine (starting with infusion) for magnesium and creatinine.
4. Calculate percentage magnesium retained using the formula:

$$\% \text{ Magnesium retained } = \left[ 1 - \left( \frac{\text{postinfusion 24-h urine magnesium} - \text{preinfusion urine magnesium/creatinine} \times \text{postinfusion urine creatinine}}{\text{Total elemental magnesium infused}} \right) \right] \times 100$$

5. Criteria for magnesium deficiency:
   >50% retention at 24 h = definite deficiency
   >25% retention at 24 h = probable deficiency

(From Ryzen E, Elbaum N, Singer FR, Rude RK. Parenteral magnesium tolerance testing in the evaluation of magnesium deficiency. Magnesium 1985; 4:137.)

suggested protocol for this magnesium tolerance test is outlined in Table 68-2. For example, a 70-kg patient underwent the magnesium tolerance test. The urinary magnesium/creatinine ratio was 0.02 before the start of the magnesium infusion. The patient was given 168 mg magnesium (2.4 mg/kg) intravenously over 4 hours. A 24-hour urine collection beginning with the infusion contained 120 mg magnesium and 1200 mg creatinine:

% magnesium retained

$$= \left[ 1 - \left( \frac{120 \text{ mg Mg} - [0.02 \text{ Mg/creat} \times 1200 \text{ mg creat}]}{168 \text{ mg Mg}} \right) \right] \times 100$$

$$= 43\%$$

The retention of 43% of the intravenous magnesium load supports the diagnosis of magnesium deficiency.

## THERAPY

Patients with symptoms or complications of magnesium deficiency should be treated with magnesium salts.[2,56] Mild degrees of depletion may be corrected with oral magnesium supplementation, or even diet alone, if the process that caused the magnesium deficiency has resolved. Importantly, the hypocalcemia, hypokalemia, and other aspects of magnesium deficiency require treatment with magnesium. Treatment with vitamin D, calcium, or potassium alone usually is ineffective.

Moderate to severe magnesium depletion is usually treated by the parenteral administration of magnesium, especially if there are continuing magnesium losses from the intestine or kidney. An effective treatment regimen is the intramuscular administration of 2 g $MgSO_4 \cdot 7H_2O$ (16.2 mEq magnesium) as a 50% solution every 8 hours. Because these injections may be painful, a continuous intravenous infusion (48 mEq/24 h) may be better tolerated. This treatment usually yields a serum magnesium concentration of 1.7 to 2.1 mEq/L. Therapy should be continued for at least 5 days, or until the hypocalcemia and hypokalemia are corrected. Note that in the patient whose treatment course is shown in Figure 68-2, the serum calcium concentration did not become normal until the fifth day of therapy. Continuing magnesium losses may require longer therapy to maintain magnesium stores. If the patient is unable to eat, a maintenance dose of ~8 mEq should be added daily to the intravenous fluids once repletion is accomplished. If the patient has a reduced GFR, the dose of magnesium given should be reduced (one-half) to avoid magnesium intoxication. Serum magnesium concentrations should be determined daily when a patient with azotemia is given magnesium-replacement therapy.

Occasionally, some patients may require long-term oral magnesium supplementation. Oral magnesium salts in the form of oxide, sulfate, lactate, hydroxide, chloride, or glycerophosphate can be used. An initial dose of ~300 mg elemental magnesium usually is well tolerated. The dose may be increased to the desired amount until side effects such as diarrhea occur. If the magnesium is given in small doses, three to four times a day, the cathartic effect of magnesium can be minimized.

## MAGNESIUM EXCESS

Magnesium intoxication is an uncommon clinical problem, although mild to moderate elevations in the serum magnesium concentration are not unusual. In acute care hospitals, up to 12% of admissions have been found to have hypermagnesemia, usually in association with chronic renal failure.[14]

### ETIOLOGY OF HYPERMAGNESEMIA

Orally administered magnesium has rarely been reported to result in hypermagnesemia because excess magnesium is normally excreted rapidly in the urine. However, enemas and cathartics that contain magnesium[57] have been reported to cause hypermagnesemia in patients with apparently normal renal function.

A reduction in the GFR is the most common factor related to elevation in the serum magnesium concentration.[2,13] As the GFR falls, so does the clearance of magnesium. Hypermagnesemia is commonly seen when the GFR is <30 mL per minute. The presence of frank magnesium intoxication in these patients is usually associated with the administration of antacids, enemas, or parenterally administered fluids that contain magnesium. Dialysates high in magnesium content have also been reported to result in hypermagnesemia. Hypermagnesemia may be seen in acute renal failure. Contributing factors may include azotemia, rhabdomyolysis, acidosis, and magnesium administration.

The parenteral administration of magnesium in patients with normal renal function is uncommonly associated with magnesium intoxication. The treatment of pregnancy-induced hypertension (toxemia of pregnancy) with magnesium salts results in serum magnesium concentrations of 4 to 7 mEq/L as a therapeutic end point. Excessive magnesium administration in these patients could lead to symptomatic magnesium intoxication. Hypermagnesemia also has been reported to occur in the neonates of mothers treated with parenteral magnesium.

Other uncommon diseases associated with an increase in the serum concentration of magnesium include familial hypocalciuric hypercalcemia, lithium ingestion, hypothyroidism, milk-alkali syndrome, viral hepatitis, and Addison disease.

### MANIFESTATIONS

Symptoms of magnesium intoxication are usually not apparent until the serum magnesium concentration exceeds at least 4 mEq/L.[2,58] One biochemical clue may be the presence of unexplained hypocalcemia, because hypermagnesemia causes a fall in the serum calcium concentration. This may be the result of decreased PTH secretion[59]; however, a fall in the serum calcium concentration also occurs in treated hypoparathyroid patients, suggesting a peripheral effect of magnesium.[60] Hypermagnesemia may directly decrease the biologic effect of PTH on its end-organ.[61] Hypermagnesemia has been reported to increase serum calcitonin levels despite the associated decrease in serum calcium levels.

Neuromuscular symptoms are the most common presenting problem of magnesium intoxication.[2,62] Disappearance of the deep tendon reflexes occurs when the serum magnesium concentration reaches 4 to 6 mEq/L. Somnolence may be observed at concentrations of 4 to 7 mEq/L or above. Impaired respiration and apnea caused by paralysis of the voluntary muscles occurs at serum magnesium levels of 10 mEq/L or higher. Excessive magnesium decreases impulse transmission across the neuromuscular junction and, therefore, has a curare-like effect.[63]

A moderate elevation in the serum magnesium concentration to 4 to 5 mEq/L may result in bradycardia and mild supine and orthostatic hypotension. Higher concentrations (5–10 mEq/L) are associated with electrocardiographic changes including an increase in the PR interval and an increase in the QRS and QT intervals. Complete heart block as well as cardiac arrest in systole may occur at levels higher than 15 mEq/L.[63]

Other nonspecific manifestations of magnesium intoxication include nausea, vomiting, and cutaneous flushing at serum magnesium concentrations of 3 to 9 mEq/L.

## THERAPY

Most cases of magnesium intoxication can be prevented.[2] It should be anticipated in any patient receiving parenteral magnesium, and, especially if there is a reduction in renal function, monitoring of the serum magnesium should be performed daily. Magnesium therapy should be discontinued in patients with mild to moderate elevations of the serum magnesium level. Excess magnesium will be excreted by the kidney, and any symptoms or signs of magnesium intoxication will resolve. Patients with severe magnesium intoxication may be treated with intravenous calcium; calcium antagonizes the toxic effects.[58,62] The usual dose is an infusion of 100 to 200 mg elemental calcium over 5 to 10 minutes. If the patient is in renal failure, peritoneal dialysis or hemodialysis will rapidly and effectively lower the serum magnesium concentration.

## REFERENCES

1. Elin R. Assessment of magnesium status. Clin Chem 1987; 33:1965.
2. Rude RK. Magnesium disorders. In: Kokko JP, Tannen RL, eds. Fluids and electrolytes, 3rd ed. Philadelphia: WB Saunders, 1996:421.
3. Teuboi S, Nakagaki H, Ishiguro K, et al. Magnesium distribution in human bone. Calcif Tissue Int 1994; 54:34.
4. Frausto da Silva JJR, Williams RJP. The biological chemistry of magnesium:phosphate metabolism. In: Fraústo Da Silva JR, Williams RJP. The biological chemistry of the elements. Oxford: Oxford University Press, 1991:241.
5. Birch NJ. Magnesium and the cell. New York: Academic Press, 1993.
6. Fine KD, Santa Ana CA, Porter JL, et al. Intestinal absorption of magnesium from food and supplements. J Clin Invest 1991; 88:396.
7. Kayne LH, Lee DBN. Intestinal magnesium absorption. Miner Electrolyte Metab 1993; 19:210.
8. Krejs GJ, Nicar MJ, Zerwekh JE, et al. Effect of 1,25-dihydroxyvitamin D$_3$ on calcium and magnesium absorption in the healthy human jejunum and ileum. Am J Med 1983; 75:973.
9. Hodgkinson A, Marshall DH, Nordin BEC. Vitamin D and magnesium absorption in man. Clin Sci 1979; 57:121.
10. Quamme GH. Magnesium homeostasis and renal magnesium handling. Miner Electrolyte Metab 1993; 19:218.
11. Quamme GA. Renal magnesium handling: new insights in understanding old problems. Kidney Int 1997; 52:1180.
12. Rude RK, Bethune JE, Singer FR. Renal tubular maximum for magnesium in normal, hypoparathyroid, and hyperthyroid man. J Clin Endocrinol Metab 1980; 51:1425.
13. Massry SG. Pharmacology of magnesium. Ann Rev Pharmacol Toxicol 1977; 17:67.
14. Wong ET, Rude RK, Singer FR. A high prevalence of hypomagnesemia in hospitalized patients. Am J Clin Pathol 1983; 79:348.
15. Ryzen E, Wagers PW, Singer FR, Rude RK. Magnesium deficiency in a medical ICU population. Crit Care Med 1985; 13:19.
16. Dorup I. Magnesium and potassium deficiency. Acta Physiol Scand 1994; 150(Suppl 618):2.
17. Thoren L. Magnesium deficiency in gastrointestinal fluid loss. Acta Chir Scand Suppl 1963; 306:5.
18. Sutton RAL, Domrongkitchaiporn S. Abnormal renal magnesium handling. Miner Electrolyte Metab 1993; 19:232.
19. Brown EM, Hebert SC. A cloned Ca$^{2+}$-sensing receptor: a mediator of direct effects of extracellular Ca$^{2+}$ on renal function. J Am Soc Nephrol 1995; 6:1530.
20. Tosiello L. Hypomagnesemia and diabetes mellitus. A review of clinical implications. Arch Intern Med 1996; 156:1143.
21. Shah GM, Kirschenbaum MA. Renal magnesium wasting associated with therapeutic agents. Miner Electrolyte Metab 1991; 17:58.
22. Shah GM, Alvarado P, Kirschenbaum MA. Symptomatic hypocalcemia and hypomagnesemia with renal magnesium wasting associated with pentamidine therapy in a patient with AIDS. Am J Med 1990; 89:380.
23. Flink E. Magnesium deficiency: etiology and clinical spectrum. Acta Med Scand 1981; 647:125.
24. Disashi T, Iwaoka T, Inoue J, et al. Magnesium metabolism in hyperthyroidism. Endocrinol J 1996; 43:97.
25. Kingston ME, Al-Sibai MB, Skooge WC. Clinical manifestations of hypomagnesemia. Crit Care Med 1986; 14:950.
26. Whang R, Hampton EM, Whang DD. Magnesium homeostasis and clinical disorders of magnesium deficiency. Ann Pharmacol 1994; 28:220.
27. Wacker WEC, Moore FD, Ulmer DD, Vallee BL. Normocalcemic magnesium deficiency tetany. JAMA 1962; 180:161.
28. Cohen L, Kitzes R. Magnesium sulfate and digitalis—toxic arrhythmias. JAMA 1983; 249:2808.
29. Ebel H. Role of magnesium in cardiac disease. J Clin Chem Clin Biochem 1983; 21:249.
30. Hollifield JW. Magnesium depletion, diuretics, and arrythmias. Am J Med 1987; 82(Suppl 3A):30.
31. Rasmussen HS, McNair P, Norregard P, et al. Intravenous magnesium in acute myocardial infarction. Lancet 1986; 1:234.
32. Woods KL, Fletcher S. Long-term intravenous magnesium sulfate in suspected acute myocardial infarction: the second Leicester Intravenous Intervention TRIAL (LIMIT-2). Lancet 1994; 343:816.
33. ISIS-4. A randomized factorial trial assessing early oral captopril, oral mononitrate, and intravenous magnesium sulphate in 58,050 patients with suspected acute myocardial infarction. Lancet 1995; 345:669.
34. Boriss MN, Papa L. Magnesium: a discussion of its role in the treatment of ventricular dysrhythmia. Crit Care Med 1988; 16:292.
34a. Yang ZW, Wang J, Zheng T, et al. Low Mg$^{2+}$ induces contraction of cerebral arteries: roles of cytokine and mitogen-activated protein kinases. Am J Physiol Heart Circ Physiol 2000; 279:H185.
35. Nadler JL, Goodsow S, Rude RK. Evidence that prostacyclin mediates the vascular action of magnesium in man. Hypertension 1987; 9:379.
35a. Shechter M, Merz CN, Rude RK, et al. Low intracellular magnesium levels promote platelet-dependent thrombosis in patients with coronary artery disease. Am Heart J 2000; 140:212.
36. Johansson G, Backman U, Danielson BG, et al. Biochemical and clinical effects of the prophylactic treatment of renal calcium stones with magnesium hydroxide. J Urol 1980; 124:770.
37. De Swart PMJR, Sokole EB, Wilmink JM. The interrelationship of calcium and magnesium absorption in idiopathic hypercalciuria and renal calcium stone disease. J Urol 1998; 159:669.
38. Johansson G, Backman U, Danielson BG, et al. Magnesium metabolism in renal stone disease. Invest Urol 1980; 18:93.
39. Evans RA, Forbes MA, Sutton RAL, Watson L. Urinary excretion of calcium and magnesium in patients with calcium-containing renal stones. Lancet 1967; 2:958.
40. Oreopoulos DG, Soyannwo MA, McGeown MG. Magnesium-calcium ratio in urine of patients with renal stones. Lancet 1968; 2:420.
41. Rude RK, Oldham SB, Sharp CF, Singer FR. Parathyroid hormone secretion in magnesium deficiency. J Clin Endocrinol Metab 1978; 47:800.
42. Rude RK, Oldham SB, Singer FR. Functional hypoparathyroidism and parathyroid hormone end-organ resistance in human magnesium deficiency. Clin Endocrinol (Oxf) 1976; 5:209.
43. Fatemi S, Ryzen E, Flores JF, et al. Effect of experimental human magnesium depletion on PTH secretion and 1,25(OH)$_2$ vitamin D metabolism. J Clin Endocrinol Metab 1991; 72:1067.
44. Rude RK, Adams JS, Ryzen E, et al. Low serum concentrations of 1,25-dihydroxyvitamin D in human magnesium deficiency. J Clin Endocrinol Metab 1985; 61:933.
45. Medalle R, Waterhouse C, Hahn TJ. Vitamin D resistance in magnesium deficiency. Am J Clin Nutr 1976; 29:854.
46. Ryan MP. Interrelationships of magnesium and potassium homeostasis. 1993; 19:290.
47. Whang R, Oei TO, Arkawa JK, et al. Predictors of clinical hypomagnesemia. Arch Intern Med 1984; 144:1794.
48. Chernow B, Bamberger S, Stoiko M, et al. Hypomagnesemia in patients in postoperative intensive care. Chest 1989; 95:391.
49. Shils ME. Experimental human magnesium depletion. Medicine 1969; 48:61.
50. Cronin RE, Knockel JP. Magnesium deficiency. Adv Intern Med 1983; 28:509.
51. Ryzen E, Elkayam U, Rude RK. Low blood mononuclear cell magnesium in intensive cardiac care unit patients. Am Heart J 1986; 111:475.
52. Altura BT, Shirey TL, Young CC, et al. A new method for the rapid determination of ionized Mg in whole blood, serum and plasma. Methods Find Exp Clin Pharmacol 1992; 14:297.
53. Cecco SA, Hristova EN, Rehak NN, Elin RJ. Clinically important intermethod differences for physiologically abnormal ionized magnesium results. Clin J Clin Pathol 1997; 108:564.
54. Ryzen E, Nelson TA, Rude RK. Low blood mononuclear cell magnesium content and hypocalcemia in normomagnesemic patients. West J Med 1987; 147:549.

55. Hebert P, Mehta N, Wang J, et al. Functional magnesium deficiency in critically ill patients identified using a magnesium-loading test. Crit Care Med 1997; 25:749.
56. McLean RM. Magnesium and its therapeutic uses: a review. Am J Med 1994; 96:63.
57. Weber CA, Santiago RM. Hypermagnesemia: a potential complication during treatment of theophylline intoxication with oral activated charcoal and magnesium-containing cathartics. Chest 1989; 95:56.
58. Mordes JP, Wacker WEC. Excess magnesium. Pharmacol Rev 1978; 29:273.
59. Cholst IN, Steinberg SF, Tropper PJ, et al. The influence of hypermagnesemia on serum calcium and parathyroid hormone levels in human subjects. N Engl J Med 1984; 310:1221.
60. Jones KH, Fourman P. Effects of infusions of magnesium and of calcium in parathyroid insufficiency. Clin Sci 1966; 30:139.
61. Slatopolsky E, Mercado A, Morrison A, et al. Inhibitory effects of hypermagnesemia on the renal action of parathyroid hormone. J Clin Invest 1976; 58:1273.
62. Fishman RA. Neurological aspects of magnesium metabolism. Arch Neurol 1965; 12:562.
63. Morisaki H, Yamamoto S, Morita Y, et al. Hypermagnesemia-induced cardiopulmonary arrest before induction of anesthesia for emergency cesarean section. J Clin Anesth 2000; 12:224.

# CHAPTER 69

# NEPHROLITHIASIS

MURRAY J. FAVUS AND FREDRIC L. COE

## CLINICAL FEATURES OF STONE DISEASE

### TYPES OF KIDNEY STONES

Kidney stones usually consist of *calcium salts, uric acid, cystine,* or *struvite* (magnesium ammonium phosphate). Each of the four types of stones has its own natural history, pathogenesis, and forms of treatment, but all stones share a set of general clinical features. Kidney stones are formed on the surfaces of the renal papillae and represent a form of pathologic soft-tissue mineralization. The stones are composed of crystals embedded in a protein matrix; often they contain several types of crystals. When the stones escape the renal surface, they act as foreign bodies in the urinary tract, causing obstruction, pain, bleeding, and a tendency to infection.

### CALCIUM STONES

Calcium forms salts with oxalic acid and with phosphate. Because these salts are extremely insoluble, they frequently crystallize to form renal stones. The most common stone, accounting for 66% to 70% of the total stones in unselected series,[1] consists of mainly *calcium oxalate* monohydrate or dihydrate crystals. These common stones are usually small, 1 mm to 1 cm in their maximal dimension, black, radiodense, and hard. Approximately 5% to 15% of the crystals in a calcium oxalate stone are *calcium phosphate* in the form of apatite. Less commonly, in 1% to 5% of patients, the stones are mainly calcium phosphate, either apatite or brushite (calcium hydrogen phosphate). The formation of these stones is favored when the urine pH is abnormally elevated. Approximately 10% of calcium oxalate stones contain uric acid, and patients who form such stones pose special treatment problems.

### URIC ACID STONES

Uric acid contains two dissociable protons; the undissociated uric acid is sparingly soluble in human urine at 37° C (98 ± 2 mg/L).[2] When the urine is unduly acidic, or when uric acid excretion is abnormally high, stones can be produced. Uric acid stones are radiolucent and often so large that they fill the renal pelvis and even extend out into the branches of the calyces to form a branching *staghorn* stone. They are white or red because of adsorption of the pigment urochrome from urine.

### CYSTINE STONES

Cystine, an essential sulfur-containing amino acid, is poorly soluble (e.g., urine at 37° C dissolves only 300 mg/L). Patients with a hereditary tubular defect for the reabsorption of filtered cystine excrete so much that stones form.[2a] Cystine stones are moderately radiopaque because of the sulfur, and, like uric acid stones, they often grow to be large. The stones are lemon-yellow, hard, and covered with sparkling, shiny crystals that resemble crystallized sugar.

### STRUVITE STONES

Magnesium, ammonium, and phosphate ions spontaneously combine to form an insoluble triple salt called *struvite*. This occurs in urine only because of infection with bacteria, usually *Proteus* sp,[3] that possess the enzyme urease. This enzyme hydrolyzes urea to ammonia and carbon dioxide, and these stones are often called *infection stones*. Struvite stones grow to be extremely large and frequently form staghorns. They are gray to yellow, friable, and radiopaque. Because of their size and their intimate association with urinary tract infection, struvite stones are frequently damaging to the kidneys.

## EPIDEMIOLOGY OF STONES

Calcium stones occur more frequently in men than in women and in the wealthy than in the poor. Overall, the incidence in the United States is ~0.5%, and these patients are clustered geographically in warm regions. Uric acid stones develop mainly in men, especially in those predisposed to gout. Cystine stones occur equally among men and women. Struvite stones occur mainly in women. There are no obvious geographic or socioeconomic predictors of cystine or struvite stones.

## SYMPTOMS AND SIGNS OF STONES

### ATTACKS OF COLIC

As long as they are firmly attached to the renal papillae, stones are painless; but once they break loose, they tend to pass into the renal pelvis and urinary tract, obstructing the flow of urine and causing an acute attack of pain, called *renal colic*. The pain is the result of sudden dilation of the urinary tract from increased pressure. Typically, the pain begins suddenly on one side. It may start in the flank, lower back, or lower anterior abdomen. Although it is called colic, it increases steadily in intensity over about an hour and remains constant as long as the stone remains in one place. As the stone moves downward, the pain shifts with it. Stones at the junction of the ureter and the bladder cause urinary frequency and dysuria, often incorrectly ascribed to urinary tract infection. Pain from low-lying stones radiates to the ipsilateral testicle or vulva, mimicking genital disease. If the stone passes, the pain ends rapidly. Colic causes nausea and vomiting, and diarrhea is common. These latter symptoms may falsely suggest intestinal obstruction, biliary colic, or acute diverticulitis.

Renal colic is thought to be among the worst pains that can be encountered, and its management usually requires analgesic medications, including narcotics. Hydration with intravenous fluid is needed if vomiting is protracted. Once an attack ends, by stone removal or passage, little or no further treatment is needed.

### SILENT OBSTRUCTION

Large stones, even staghorn stones, may occlude the ureteropelvic junction so slowly that no pain occurs, even though hydronephrosis may damage or destroy the kidney. A mass in the flank from a hydronephrotic kidney, recurrent infection, unexplained azotemia (when obstruction is bilateral or involves a solitary functioning kidney), or the passage of stone fragments may call the problem to attention. Frequently, however, the stone is found in the course of an unrelated radiographic procedure.

### CRYSTALLURIA

Calcium oxalate or phosphate crystalluria, or uric acid crystals, commonly cause episodes of colic that are unassociated with a stone but resemble a stone attack. Hematuria is common, although transient. The urine contains large amounts of crystals, but only briefly after the attack.

### HEMATURIA

Crystals and stones are common causes of isolated hematuria, abnormal proteinuria, or infection. The other main causes are malignant or benign tumors of the kidneys and urinary tract, infections such as tuberculosis, cysts of the kidneys, and bleeding from the prostatic bed. Hematuria even occurs from stones that are anchored to the renal papillae and otherwise are asymptomatic.

### NEPHROCALCINOSIS

Numerous small papillary stones that are seen on an abdominal radiograph are termed *nephrocalcinosis*. A better term is *papillary nephrocalcinosis*, which distinguishes this localized condition from generalized renal calcification caused by hypercalcemic states. Because of its dramatic radiographic appearance, nephrocalcinosis suggests unusual diseases but usually is a result of the routine causes of calcium stone disease and requires no special evaluation.[4] Medullary sponge kidneys, a hereditary cystic renal disease, is associated with nephrocalcinosis,[5] probably because the ectasia of terminal collecting ducts causes stasis and favors the deposition of small crystals in the renal papillary areas.

## SURGICAL TREATMENT OF STONES

Stones need surgical intervention if they cause severe pain, bleeding, obstruction, or serious infection. Most attacks of colic can be managed medically for a few days to determine if an obstructing stone is gradually moving downward. Based on stone size alone, the likelihood of spontaneous passage for stones >6 mm is ~25%; for stones from 4 to 6 mm it is ~60%, and for stones <4 mm it is ~90%. Many stones in the kidneys do not cause symptoms and are not obstructing. Also, most episodes of colic terminate by spontaneous stone passage. When intervention is required, cystoscopy, surgery, or shock-wave lithotripsy are used. The frequency of these procedures varies with the cause of the calcium oxalate stone. Patients with hyperuricosuria and calcium oxalate stones are more likely to require stone-removal procedures or nephrectomy.

### CYSTOSCOPY

The indication for cystoscopy is removal of a stone that is close to or at the ureterovesical junction. Another reason for cystoscopy is to perform retrograde pyelography to assess the patency of the urinary tract. Sometimes, a stone is in the bladder but cannot pass because of a narrow bladder outlet or because it gradually has grown too large. In these locations, the stone can be fragmented and removed.

### OPERATIVE PROCEDURES

Stones lodged in the ureter may be removed by ureterolithotomy. Stones in the renal pelvis have been removed by pyelolithotomy, which is a major surgical procedure involving a flank incision and prolonged recovery. Most of these stones are now removed by lithotripsy.

### LITHOTRIPSY

A form of stone therapy that has revolutionized the treatment of many stones is shock-wave lithotripsy. Shock waves reduce the stones to small fragments that are then passed with relative ease. In one form of treatment, the patient is lowered into a tank of water, either under general anesthesia or spinal anesthesia, and positioned so that the stone is centered at the secondary focus of a parabolic reflector. An electric spark generator is positioned such that the shock wave it produces in the water is at the primary focus of the reflector, and electrical discharges are produced. The mechanism is synchronized with the standard electrocardiogram so that the shock waves occur immediately after the QRS complex. The shock waves pass through the stone and disrupt it. Anywhere from 500 to 1500 or more discharges are needed to fragment stones of moderate size. The stone fragments move into the ureter and are subsequently passed. The procedure works well with stones in the renal pelvis or calyces. Kidney stones smaller than 2 cm but larger than 0.5 cm in diameter are best treated with lithotripsy. Stones greater than 2 cm or those larger than 1 cm in the lower poles of the kidney are best treated with percutaneous nephrolithotomy. Ureterolithotomy is used for removal of stones of any size located in the lower ureter below the pelvic brim. Transurethral ureterolithotripsy (TUL) and laser technology disintegrate ureteral stones and have largely supplanted the open surgical procedures. Most stones (80% to 90%) subjected to lithotripsy are passed, and there is only limited information on the fate of retention of small fragments or the recurrence of new stones.[6] Infrequent but serious complications include bleeding into the renal parenchyma, spinal cord damage, and paraplegia.[7]

## MEDICAL TREATMENT OF STONES

### PREVENTION

The main goals of the internist are to identify the metabolic disturbance that causes stone formation in a given patient and, through specific treatment, to prevent the development of new stones. The search may involve considerable effort because most of the abnormalities are found in the chemical analysis of the urine; however, such studies are not widely available in hospital clinical chemistry laboratories.

### ATTEMPTS AT DISSOLUTION

Uric acid stones and some cystine stones may be dissolved by altering the urine chemistry. Calcium stones and struvite stones are rarely dissolved, despite vigorous treatment.

## CALCIUM STONES

### PATHOGENETIC FACTORS

The factors critical to calcium stone formation are *supersaturation* and *nucleation*. Supersaturation of a solution occurs when a solution contains a salt (e.g., calcium oxalate) at a concentration that exceeds its solubility.[1,8] When such a solution comes into contact with a precipitated salt with which it is already supersaturated, the solid phase serves as a nucleation center for the aggregation and precipitation of the excess salt in solution. Supersaturation is defined and measured in terms of the particular salts present in concentrations exceeding their solubilities. A solution may be supersaturated with several salts, each to a different extent. The magnitude of the supersaturation provides the driving force for crystallization of the solid phase (e.g., stone formation from urine).

The supersaturation of urine with calcium oxalate and calcium phosphate phases, such as brushite or apatite, is determined by (1) the concentrations of calcium, oxalate, and phosphate; (2) the concentrations of calcium ligands such as citrate (which chelates calcium, preventing the precipitation of calcium oxalate or phosphate salts); and (3) the pH (determines relative concentrations of hydrogen phosphate and phosphates, which form brushite and apatite, respectively). The actual measurement of supersaturation is difficult but useful, because the elevation of supersaturation corresponds to stone composition.[9] Clinically, the excretion rates and concentrations of calcium and oxalate and the urine pH are measured to detect patients with hypercalciuria, hyperoxaluria, or abnormally alkaline urine. These measurements frequently represent the diagnostic end points of patient evaluation for supersaturation.

Important to the formation of renal stones is a surface (nucleation center) within the supersaturated solution that can promote aggregation of ions to form crystals. Given a foreign surface to which ions can adhere to form clusters, stones can be formed, even if supersaturation is mild; therefore, the probability of stone formation can be increased simply by a foreign nucleation surface. Clinical examples of foreign, or "heterogeneous," nucleation include stone crystallization on an injured urothelial surface and calcium oxalate stones grown on a crystal of uric acid induced by low urine pH and increased uric acid excretion. The uric acid crystals offer a nucleation surface on which calcium oxalate overgrowth is likely to occur.[10] When the foreign surface strongly resembles the one to be formed, the ions aggregate on the surface in a strongly oriented manner, reflecting the alignment of the overgrowing and preformed crystals. This process is called *epitaxial* growth, and although it has been proposed as a mechanism for uric acid nucleation of calcium oxalate,[10,11] it is unlikely to be a common occurrence.

Urine contains substances that inhibit the growth and formation of calcium oxalate and phosphate stones. Citrate, which lowers the supersaturation of calcium salts by chelating calcium, can also reduce the growth of calcium oxalate and phosphate crystals.[12,13] An anionic glycoprotein inhibitor, glycoprotein crystal growth-inhibitor (GCI) protein,[14,15] which is in urine, dramatically inhibits calcium oxalate growth. Patients with stones often have low citrate levels and excrete an abnormal form of GCI.[14] Urinary inorganic pyrophosphate inhibits calcium phosphate crystal growth.[12,16] Magnesium may inhibit calcium oxalate crystal growth because it forms a soluble complex with oxalate.

## DISORDERS OF CALCIUM STONE FORMATION

### BENIGN FAMILIAL "IDIOPATHIC" HYPERCALCIURIA

The abnormality that is found in 50% to 75% of patients with calcium stones is a *normocalcemic hypercalciuria* that is unexplained by any known systemic disease, such as sarcoidosis, hyperthyroidism, rapidly progressive bone disease, vitamin D intoxication, immobilization, Paget disease, malignancy, or glucocorticoid excess.[1,17] Called *idiopathic hypercalciuria*, it is more appropriately named *benign familial hypercalciuria* because it is found in the families of affected patients in a pattern that is compatible with an autosomal-dominant inheritance[18,19,19a] (Fig. 69-1). Familial hypercalciuria affects 2% to 4% of normal adults and accounts for ~40% of stone formers. In ~80% to 90% of patients, hypercalciuria is silent. The distribution of values for calcium excretion in the population is not bimodal, as expected for an inherited disorder, but non-Gaussian, with a long tail of high values. Therefore, the upper limit of normal for calcium excretion and the diagnosis of idiopathic hypercalciuria are arbitrary. An outpatient 24-hour urine collection is obtained; the patient eats ad libitum, including dairy products. Many investigators have determined calcium excretion under various dietary conditions that are important for studies of the pathogenesis of the disease. However, because changes in dietary calcium intake or the use of artificial diets change the urine chemistry, the authors believe that a free-choice diet is preferable when the diagnosis is in doubt. Hypercalciuria is determined by a 24-hour calcium excretion of above 300 mg for men and 250 mg for women, or either 4 mg/kg of body weight or 140 mg/g of urinary creati-

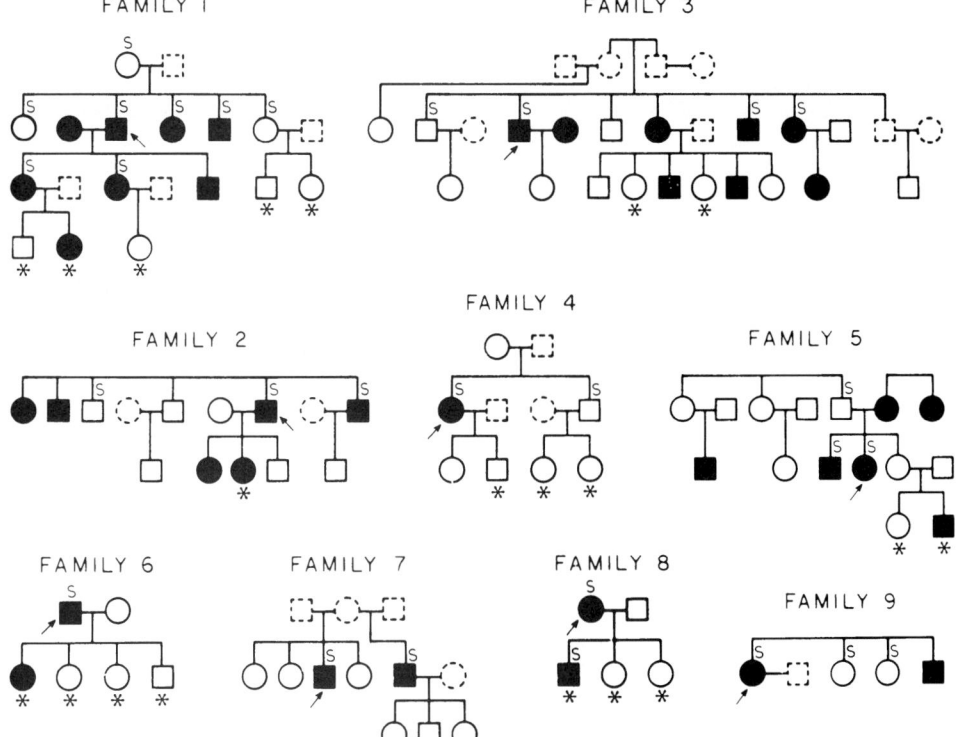

**FIGURE 69-1.** Family pedigrees of nine probands with idiopathic hypercalciuria. Marginal hypercalciuria was present in four siblings, one each in families 1, 2, 3, and 5; in the mother of proband 4; in two aunts and one niece in family 5; and in one nephew in family 3. Altogether, hypercalciuria occurred in 11 of 24 siblings, 7 of 16 offspring, and 1 of 3 parents of the probands. (*Squares* indicate males; *circles* indicate females; *solid circles* and *squares,* family members with hypercalciuria; *S,* stone disease; *\*,* children younger than 20 years of age; *arrows,* probands; *interrupted circles* and *squares,* relatives who were not studied but who were included to complete the pedigree.) (From Coe FL, Parks JH, Moore ES. Familial idiopathic hypercalciuria. N Engl J Med 1979; 300:337.)

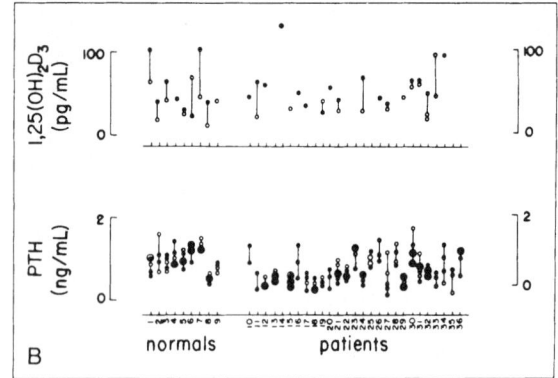

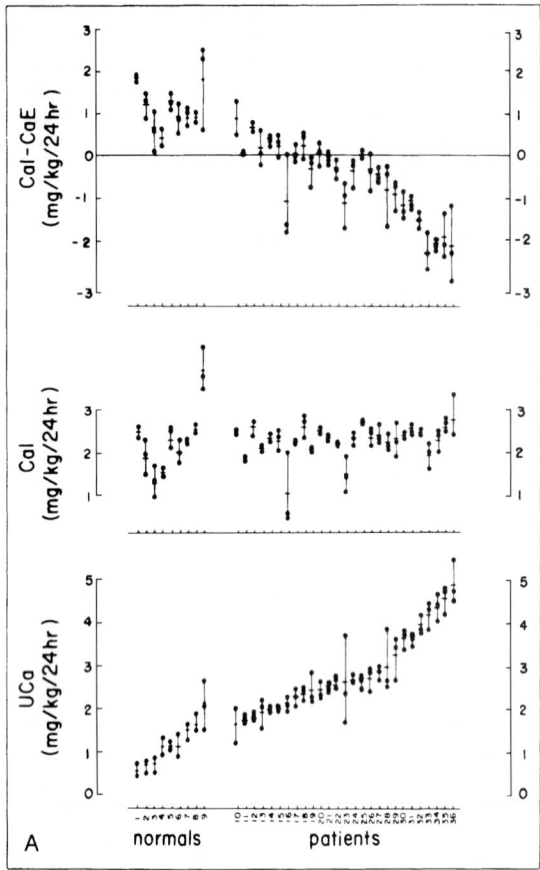

**FIGURE 69-2.** Calcium intake and excretion (*CaE*) (**A**) and serum parathyroid hormone (*PTH*) and 1,25(OH)$_2$D$_3$ (**B**) values in patients and normal subjects. Urine calcium excretion (*UCa*) and intake (*CaI*) are during low calcium diet. Serum values for 1,25(OH)$_2$D$_3$ and PTH during low calcium diet (Ca intake of 2 mg/kg body weight [*BW*] per day for 10 days, *solid circles*) and free-choice diet (*open circles*) are both shown. Mean calcium intake of normal subjects (2.29 ± 0.15 SEM in mg/kg BW of calcium in 24 hours) and patients (2.31 ± 0.05) did not differ. Mean excretion rates during low calcium diet (1.18 ± 0.11 vs. 2.87 ± 0.11, *p* <.001) for normal subjects and patients, respectively, and values of intake minus excretion (CaI – CaE, 1.14 ± 0.12 vs. –0.58 ± 0.11, *p* <.001) differed significantly from each other. Calcium excretion in normal subjects (1.78 ± 0.16) and patients (4.38 ± 0.15) during free-choice diet (not shown) differed from each other (*p* <.001) and from values during low calcium diet (*p* <.01, both normal subjects and patients). Normal subjects and patients are shown in order of ascending mean calcium excretion; numbers are for identification of individual normals and patients. [From Coe FL, Favus MJ, Crockett T, et al. Effects of low-calcium diet on urine calcium excretion, parathyroid function, and serum 1,25(OH)$_2$D levels in patients with idiopathic hypercalciuria and normal patients. Am J Med 1982; 72:25.]

nine in either sex. Hypercalciuria increases urine supersaturation with calcium oxalate or brushite.[20,21]

The excessive urinary calcium excretion arises from increased intestinal calcium absorption.[1] The pathogenesis of benign familial hypercalciuria is probably heterogeneous, with some patients overproducing 1,25-dihydroxyvitamin D$_3$ [1,25(OH)$_2$D$_3$], the biologically active form of vitamin D that stimulates intestinal calcium absorption.[22] Target organ hyperresponsiveness to 1,25(OH)$_2$D$_3$ may also be present, and elevated and normal serum 1,25(OH)$_2$D$_3$ levels have been reported.[1] The apparent discrepancies of 1,25(OH)$_2$D$_3$ measurements among familial hypercalciuric patients may reflect their sensitivity to dietary calcium intake.[23] The stimulus for increased 1,25(OH)$_2$D$_3$ production remains unknown, but low serum phosphorus or excess parathyroid hormone is unlikely. If dietary calcium is reduced severely, calcium balance becomes more negative than in normal people given an equivalent diet[1]; urine calcium excretion remains high in many of these patients[24] (Fig. 69-2). This observation suggests that, under these conditions, calcium is being mobilized from bone. Because of this adverse response to a low calcium diet, which also occurs in normal people who are made hypercalciuric but not hypercalcemic by exogenous 1,25(OH)$_2$D$_3$, a low calcium diet is not advisable for these patients.[25]

Therapies to prevent stone recurrence focus on the importance of the urine chemistry, specifically, the level of supersaturation with calcium oxalate and calcium phosphate (Table 69-1). Urine calcium is the major predictor of supersaturation and stone recurrence. Thiazide diuretic agents lower calcium excretion, diminish supersaturation with calcium oxalate monohydrate, and decrease new stone formation.[17] These results have been documented in a placebo-controlled trial.[26] When pretreatment and posttreatment stone formation rates are compared, thiazide may reduce new stone formation by 90%.[17] Thiazide reduces urine calcium by increasing distal tubular cal-

cium reabsorption. The higher the pretreatment urine calcium level, the greater is the reduction of the urine calcium concentration with thiazide. Urine calcium values may decline by 200 mg per day in patients with idiopathic hypercalciuria. The maximally effective dose is determined by the fall in urine calcium. Although the dose of thiazide varies with the specific agent, a starting dose can be equivalent to the usual dose for the treatment of edema or hypertension. The effect of thiazide on calcium excretion should be evaluated after 6 weeks of treatment by analysis of calcium in a 24-hour urine collection. Possible adverse effects of thiazides include hypokalemia, increased serum cholesterol levels, and reduced glucose tolerance. Interestingly, thiazides may increase bone mass.[27] Amiloride can reduce the potassium wasting, and it may increase the hypocalciuric effect.

Other treatments include orthophosphate, which increases the urine concentration of the crystal growth inhibitor, pyrophosphate. Magnesium therapy may reduce urine supersaturation of calcium oxalate, but this requires further study. Cellulose phosphate is a nonabsorbable substance that binds dietary calcium in the lumen of the intestinal tract, preventing absorption. Like dietary calcium restriction, cellulose phosphate may not be suitable for patients with idiopathic hypercalciuria who mobilize calcium from bone during low calcium intake.[25]

### PRIMARY HYPERPARATHYROIDISM

Approximately 5% of patients with calcium stones have primary hyperparathyroidism[1,17] (see Chap. 58). The mechanism for stone production appears to be hypercalciuria, which is presumed to arise from a high filtered load of calcium because of the hypercalcemia. The increased urinary calcium excretion is associated with increased intestinal calcium absorption caused by increased serum 1,25(OH)$_2$D$_3$ levels.[28] However, patients with primary hyperparathyroidism and stones have 1,25(OH)$_2$D$_3$ levels that

**TABLE 69-1.**
Urine Uric Acid Saturation in Calcium Oxalate Renal Stone Formers

| 24-Hour Urine Values | Metabolic Group | | | | |
|---|---|---|---|---|---|
| | *Normal (20)* | *IH (24)* | *HU (12)* | *Both (14)* | *Neither (17)* |
| Number of samples | 24 | 69 | 36 | 42 | 51 |
| Total uric acid (mg/L) | 503 ± 32 | 421 ± 23 | 575 ± 28 | 616 ± 27** | 462 ± 32 |
| Urine volume (mL) | 1268 ± 65 | 1717 ± 133 | 1501 ± 79* | 1397 ± 70 | 1387 ± 90 |
| Urine pH | 6.22 | 5.92 | 5.62** | 5.74** | 5.67*** |
| Undissociated uric acid (mg/L)‡ | 57 ± 8 | 84 ± 11 | 155 ± 21*** | 150 ± 15**** | 128 ± 18** |
| CPR, monosodium hydrogen urate | 2.8 ± 0.3† | 2.2 ± 0.2 | 2.7 ± 0.2 | 3.1 ± 0.2 | 2.2 ± 0.2 |
| [Na]·[Urate] (mol² × 10⁻⁵), initial§ | 37 ± 4 | 27 ± 3 | 35 ± 4 | 42 ± 3ǁ | 29 ± 3 |
| Sodium concentration (mEq/L) | 131 ± 8 | 118 ± 7 | 130 ± 7 | 149 ± 7 | 132 ± 7 |

All values except the numbers of samples and the numbers of people in each metabolic group (in parentheses) are means ± SEM.
*IH*, idiopathic hypercalciuria; *HU*, hyperuricosuria; *CPR*, concentration product ratio; *[Na]*, sodium concentration (mEq/L); *[Urate]*, urate concentration (mmol/L).
*Differs from control, $p < .05$; ** $p < .02$; *** $p < .01$; **** $p < .001$.
†Based on the study of 16 of the 20 normal subjects who had CPR measurements.
‡The mean equilibrium value, determined in 26 urine samples of pH below 5.6, after 48 hours of incubation with crystals of uric acid, was 90 ± 5 (SEM) mg/L. Values were calculated using a pKa of 5.345.
§Before incubation with crystals of sodium hydrogen urate.
ǁMen differed from women, $p < .05$.
(Reprinted from Coe FL, Strauss AL, Tembe V, Dun SL. Uric acid saturation in calcium nephrolithiasis. Kidney Int 1980; 17:662.)

are no different from those of patients without stones. The treatment for patients with stone disease and primary hyperparathyroidism is parathyroidectomy.

## HYPOCALCEMIA AND HYPERCALCIURIA

A phenotype of familial hypocalcemia with hypercalciuria has been described in six kindred.[29] Treatment of the hypocalcemia with vitamin D and calcium resulted in nephrocalcinosis and renal impairment. Mutations of the calcium-sensing receptor gene lead to a gain of function in which lower levels of serum calcium are required to reduce parathyroid hormone secretion.

## HYPEROXALURIA

Excessive urinary oxalate excretion may increase supersaturation, thereby increasing the risk for stone formation. The pathogenesis of hyperoxaluria is diverse and may be genetic or acquired.[29a,29b] It may be separated into two categories: *metabolic overproduction of oxalate* (hereditary, types I and II; ethylene glycol ingestion; methoxyflurane excess; and pyridoxine deficiency, which occurs in the experimental animal but perhaps not in humans), and *gastrointestinal overabsorption of oxalate* (oxalate overingestion; ileal resection as in Crohn disease; malabsorption syndromes such as celiac sprue or pancreatic insufficiency; small-bowel bypass surgery; and cellulose phosphate ingestion).

**Enteric Hyperoxaluria.** Patients with malabsorption syndrome and a functioning colon are prone to increased absorption and urine excretion of oxalate and to severe stone disease.[30] Usual clinical settings for enteric hyperoxaluria are intestinal bypass surgery for obesity, Crohn disease, ileal resection for any cause, and other forms of malabsorption.[30] Steatorrhea is almost invariably present.[31] The hyperabsorption of oxalate occurs in the colon; hence, patients with an ileostomy do not develop enteric hyperoxaluria. Urine oxalate excretion, normally 20 to 40 mg per day, frequently is 60 to 80 mg per day or more.

The mechanism of oxalate overabsorption appears to be increased colon permeability to oxalate, resulting from delivery of undigested medium-chain fatty acids and bile salts to this site.[32] The colon appears to possess a size- and charge-selective barrier to neutral sugars that reduces the permeability of oxalate below that predicted from the molecule's molecular radii. Ricinoleate, a medium-chain fatty acid normally absorbed in the small bowel, increases the absorption of oxalate and other small molecules by increasing the epithelial permeability of the colon.

Hyperoxaluria greatly raises urine calcium oxalate supersaturation,[33] causing stones. Tubulointerstitial nephropathy also is produced by the crystals; hence, progressive azotemia and defects of tubule function, such as renal tubular acidosis (RTA), may occur.[34] The effects of hyperoxaluria are exaggerated by the loss of urine citrate that occurs in small-bowel malabsorption states; by low urine volumes caused by fluid loss from diarrhea; and by an acid urine pH from intestinal bicarbonate loss, which promotes uric acid crystallization and the formation of both uric acid and calcium oxalate stones.

The treatment of enteric hyperoxaluria is directed mainly at reducing intestinal oxalate absorption. If intestinal bypass surgery has been performed, reanastomosis is indicated. A low oxalate diet is practical and useful to the extent that variety in the diet and good nutrition can be maintained. A low-fat diet helps by reducing the colonic delivery of undigested fatty acids; the dietary fat content should be as low as is consistent with good nutrition. Because these patients often have marginally adequate nutrition, each patient requires an individual assessment of the role of dietary modification. An additional therapeutic approach is oral calcium, which can reduce oxalate absorption, probably by precipitating calcium oxalate in the intestinal lumen.[35] The dose of calcium preparation should be commenced at 1 g elemental calcium in four divided doses and gradually increased to 2 to 4 g in four divided doses as needed, depending on the urine oxalate excretion rate. Finally, the ion-exchange resin, cholestyramine, can be used in a dosage of 4 to 16 g in four daily divided doses. This resin binds oxalate, preventing its absorption, and also binds bile salts so they cannot injure the colonic epithelial surface.[36] The doses of calcium and cholestyramine depend on patient tolerance. Calcium may cause constipation and abdominal discomfort, which may limit its usefulness. Cholestyramine has an unpleasant taste and causes abdominal pain and diarrhea in some patients.

Urine calcium and oxalate levels must be monitored during treatment because calcium loading may raise urine calcium without lowering urine oxalate, thus increasing the risk of stones. Cholestyramine may interfere with the absorption of drugs, and it often causes a vitamin K depletion that must be offset by monthly supplements. Low urine citrate and pH are best treated, if present, with oral citrate or bicarbonate, 2 to 4 mEq/kg, in four divided doses daily.

**Primary Hyperoxaluria.** Rarely, stone formers have hyperoxaluria caused by one of several hereditary diseases.[1,34,37] The urinary oxalate excretion is frequently above 100 mg per day, leading to supersaturation. Consequently, stones are numerous, tubulointerstitial nephropathy is progressive, and chronic renal failure may develop. Stones usually begin in childhood, and in most people, renal failure develops by 20 to 30 years of age. Unfortunately, the treatment is highly unsatisfactory. Pyridoxine, 400 mg per day, may reduce oxalate production. High fluid intake, above 3 L per day, reduces supersaturation. Orthophosphate, in a dosage of 1 to 2 g phosphate in four divided doses daily, may lower urine calcium and reduce crystallization.[34] Despite treatment, stone disease and renal failure are frequently progressive. The missing enzyme in type I disease can be restored by liver transplantation.[38]

**Dietary Hyperoxaluria.** Some patients excrete excessive amounts of oxalate, in the range of 50 to 70 mg per day, because of dietary excesses of foods high in oxalate, such as spinach, rhubarb, nuts, chocolate, pepper, and tea.[1] The extent of oxaluria reflects the dietary load, which is usually variable. Renal damage usually does not occur. The treatment is dietary modification.

## RENAL TUBULAR ACIDOSIS

Few patients with calcium stones, perhaps 1%, develop stones as a result of disordered renal acidification. The stones are composed mainly of calcium phosphate, such as brushite or apatite. Many patients who have RTA acquired it from previous stone disease or other renal disease. A few patients have the hereditary form of RTA. Whether acquired or hereditary, the mechanisms of stone formation are the same.

Renal tubular acidosis conventionally is divided into five types: *type 1*, gradient; *type 2*, proximal; *type 3*, mixed 1 and 2; *type 4*, acquired, associated with hyperkalemia and an acid urine; and *type 5*, resulting from chronic renal failure.[39] Of these, it is type 1 that is associated with stones. In type 1 RTA, the renal tubules lose their capacity to lower urine pH normally, causing inadequate net acid excretion and systemic metabolic acidosis. The acidosis causes hypercalciuria and reduces urine citrate excretion.[39,40] The alkaline urine pH increases the concentration of phosphate ion and of monohydrogen phosphate; consequently, apatite and brushite become further supersaturated.[41] The result is calcium phosphate crystalluria, nephrocalcinosis, and stones. The stones frequently are large and numerous.

The diagnosis of RTA is suggested in any patient who repeatedly forms calcium phosphate stones. The pH of the 24-hour urine is elevated above the normal mean of 6.1. It does not fall below 5.5 in the 6 hours after administration of oral ammonium chloride, 1.9 mEq/kg, given as a single dose in the morning in the postabsorptive state (available as 500-mg tablets; 1 g ammonium chloride = 18.7 mEq chloride). The presence or absence of metabolic acidosis does not critically affect the diagnosis because some stone formers who cannot lower urine pH properly nevertheless can excrete acid in the form of ammonium at a rate sufficient to prevent systemic acidosis. These patients have *incomplete RTA*. Because hereditary RTA is a dominant trait, family members should be screened for stone disease or metabolic acidosis (serum bicarbonate <24 mEq/L).

The chronic metabolic acidosis of hereditary RTA may cause stunted growth and bone disease.[42] The reduced growth rate can be restored by alkali treatment. Bone disease is not common, but when it occurs, it takes the form of rickets in children and osteomalacia in adults. In children, the acidosis is markedly worsened by intercurrent illness; they may develop severe dyspnea as a respiratory compensation to the systemic acidosis. The presentation may resemble pneumonia.

The treatment of RTA is with alkali, 2 to 4 mEq/kg in four daily divided doses, in the form of bicarbonate or citrate. The alkali raises urine citrate levels and lowers those of urine calcium; the results of its use are excellent.[43] Patients with incomplete RTA may have acquired RTA as well as benign familial hypercalciuria. Along with alkali, thiazides may be required to further lower urinary calcium excretion.

## HYPERURICOSURIA AND LOW URINE PH

**Calcium Oxalate Uric Acid Stones.** Approximately 10% of patients form stones that contain variable amounts of uric acid admixed with calcium oxalate.[1] The urine of such patients most often is abnormally supersaturated with calcium oxalate and with undissociated uric acid. In contrast, urine from patients with calcium oxalate stones is not supersaturated with uric acid, and urine from patients with pure uric acid stones is not overly supersaturated with calcium oxalate. The supposedly dual supersaturation with calcium oxalate and uric acid leads to crystallization from both phases and the development of mixed stones. Because the urine is supersaturated with calcium oxalate monohydrate, uric acid crystals become a favorable surface for promoting calcium oxalate nucleation. Whenever the uric acid forms crystals, calcium oxalate formation is fostered. The actual stones show calcium oxalate and uric acid aligned along one dimension compatible with heterogeneous nucleation.

The treatment of this type of mixed stone is directed both at the hyperuricosuria (above 800 mg for men or 750 mg for women) and at the urine pH that is below normal. Both the uricosuria and the low pH are caused by excessive dietary intake of meat, fish, and poultry[44] and often can be corrected by dietary counseling. When dietary treatment is unsuccessful, allopurinol is an alternative.[17]

**Calcium Oxalate Stones.** The pattern of uric acid supersaturation combined with modest calcium oxalate supersaturation is also encountered in some patients whose stones predominantly are calcium oxalate. Uric acid may play a critical role in nucleation, but quantitatively it may be only a trivial component of the eventual mass of the stone. It appears that uric acid supersaturation fosters uric acid crystallization, which in turn promotes heterogeneous nucleation of calcium oxalate monohydrate.[1] As in patients with mixed stones, the hyperuricosuria and mildly acidic urine pH found in patients with calcium oxalate stones can be treated by either changes in diet or allopurinol. Only the latter has been studied clinically.[17]

## HYPOCITRICURIA

**Secondary Hypocitricuria.** Low excretion of urinary citrate occurs whenever there is systemic acidosis. RTA and malabsorption have already been mentioned in connection with hypocitricuria. Other causes are ileostomy, chronic colitis with loss of bicarbonate, and potassium depletion. In all these conditions, the replacement of alkali, either as bicarbonate or citrate, increases urinary citrate and lowers the urine calcium ion concentration. Angiotensin II converting-enzyme inhibitors decrease urine citrate, but the doses commonly used have not been associated with calcium nephrolithiasis.[45]

**Primary Hypocitricuria.** In the absence of systemic disease, some patients with stones excrete less citrate than normal.[46] The term *primary hypocitricuria* is not yet used routinely for this condition, but it seems appropriate. Generally, women excrete more citrate than men. Stone formers excrete less citrate than normal people of the same sex. The disparity in urinary citrate excretion between normal people and stone formers is more dramatic in women than in men. The mechanism of low citrate excretion appears to be enhanced reabsorption by the renal tubules.

Reasonable limits for normal urine citrate excretion for both sexes are given in Table 69-2. The normal range depends on local populations and must be determined by each laboratory. Low urinary citrate levels may occur in isolation or in association with hypercalciuria, hyperuricosuria, hyperoxaluria, or bowel disease. Whatever the cause, it should be treated by either potassium citrate or by potassium bicarbonate. Potassium lowers urine calcium and increases calcium balance.[47] The initial dosage of alkali, in any form, should be 1 to 2 mEq/kg per day, in two or three divided doses, and adjusted as needed, according to the response of urine citrate excretion.

**TABLE 69-2.**
**Selected Urinary Measurements**

| Measurement | Men | | Women | |
|---|---|---|---|---|
| | *Normal* | *Stones* | *Normal* | *Stones* |
| Volume (mL/24 h) | 1293 ± 84 | 1626 ± 40[†§] | 1372 ± 136 | 1370 ± 72 |
| Weight (kg) | 77 ± 2 | 81 ± 1 | 62 ± 2 | 66 ± 2* |
| Calcium (mg/24 h) | 181 ± 14 | 254 ± 7[‡] | 125 ± 12 | 206 ± 9[‡] |
| Oxalate (mg/24 h) | 33 ± 2 | 39 ± 1[†] | 25 ± 1 | 29 ± 1* |
| Citrate (mg/24 h) | 547 ± 31 | 516 ± 15 | 729 ± 47 | 551 ± 24[†] |
| Uric acid (mg/24 h) | 699 ± 33 | 740 ± 11 | 520 ± 21 | 557 ± 13* |

*Differs from normal, same sex, $p < .05$; [†]$p < .02$; [‡]$p < .002$. All values are means ± SEM.

[§]Differs from women, same group, $p < .02$. Excretion rates of calcium, oxalate, uric acid, sodium, magnesium, and phosphorus by men exceeded those of corresponding women, $p < .01$ for all comparisons. Urine calcium and citrate excretion of women and men patients exceeded normal ($p < .01$) when expressed per kilogram body weight, grams of creatinine, or liters of creatinine clearance (not shown).

(Reprinted from Parks JH, Coe FL. Urine citrate and calcium in calcium nephrolithiasis. In: Massry S, ed. Proceedings of the 7th International Workshop on Phosphate Metabolism. Sept 1–4, 1985: New York: Plenum Press, 1986.)

## ABNORMALITIES OF GLYCOPROTEIN CRYSTAL GROWTH-INHIBITOR PROTEIN

Gross measurements of the degree to which urine inhibits the growth of calcium oxalate monohydrate have repeatedly shown less inhibition by the urine of patients with stones.[48] Whether the reduction was caused by fewer inhibitor molecules or by abnormal molecules of poor inhibitory activity could not be determined, because the actual molecules were unknown. Now, one such inhibitor substance, the GCI protein, has been purified from urine and from a human renal cell line[49]; its properties in normal people and stone formers have been partly determined. Normal GCI contains γ-carboxyglutamic acid (GLA), two to three residues per mole.[14] It forms strong films at the air–water interface and has an apparent affinity for the calcium oxalate crystal surface of 100 nmol/L.[14] It also exhibits microheterogeneity, as shown in four distinct peaks eluting from ion-exchange columns. All four peaks have the same molecular mass of 14,000 daltons and the same affinity, but they have decreasing amounts of GLA and decreasing air–water interfacial stability.[14]

When compared with that of normal people, the GCI from patients with calcium oxalate stones lacks GLA altogether and forms weak films at the air–water interface.[14] More important, the third and fourth peaks of GCI, which comprise half of the total GCI in urine, have a much lower affinity for the crystal surface (1 μmol/L), making it weaker as an inhibitor. The obvious implication of these results is that some inherited or acquired defect of GCI may diminish its effectiveness and expose some people to a greater than normal risk of calcium oxalate crystal formation. In principle, defective GCI permits stone formation to occur even with normal supersaturation, so that specific disorders of urine minerals need not occur in such patients. The validity of this hypothesis remains to be tested.

## RENAL STONES IN PATIENTS WITHOUT ANY KNOWN ABNORMALITIES

Every stone program reports that some patients (~20%) have no disorder explaining their stones. The recent recognition of low urinary citrate and the new discovery of abnormal GCI proteins inevitably will decrease the number of these patients. The conventional criterion for hypercalciuria is the top fifth percentile of a normal population. However, lower urinary calcium excretion than these rates may confer a risk of stones. The use of more refined criteria and these newer measurements should decrease the percentage of patients in whom stone disease is not associated with any recognized abnormalities.

Thiazide treatment of patients with calcium oxalate stones who have no discernible metabolic disorder reduces the rate of new stone formation by reducing urine calcium excretion and calcium oxalate supersaturation. Like patients with idiopathic hypercalciuria, normocalciuric stone formers may lose bone

mass when fed a diet severely restricted in calcium. Neutral orthophosphate may also reduce the rate of calcium oxalate stone formation, but this regimen has not been adequately tested.

# URIC ACID STONES

## PATHOGENESIS

### LOW URINE PH

The main cause of increases in uric acid supersaturation is a low urine pH (Fig. 69-3). The concentration of undissociated uric acid, which is the only form that crystallizes under most circumstances, is controlled by pH.[2] Two other factors, low urine volume and hyperuricosuria, are less important. Reasons for a low urine pH include a hereditary predisposition (as in patients with clinical gout and familial uric acid nephrolithia-

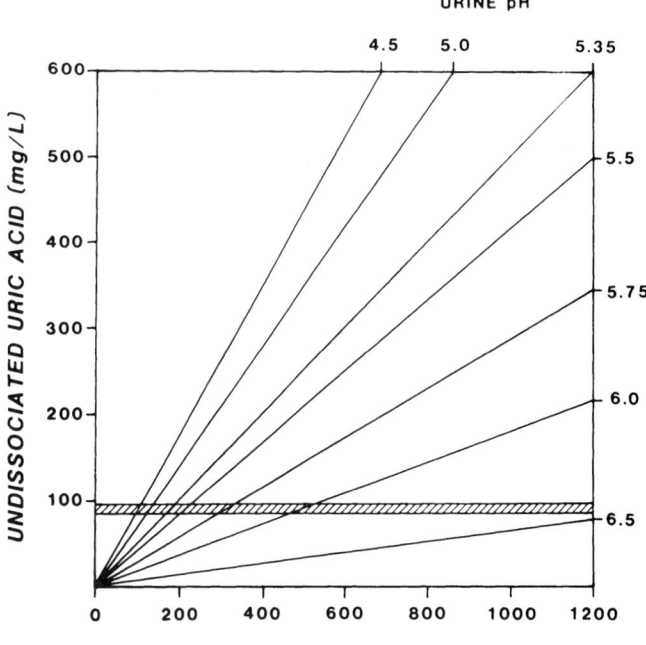

**FIGURE 69-3.** Nomogram showing the undissociated uric acid concentration at values of urine pH and total uric acid concentration. The solubility limit for uric acid is shown by crosshatched bars (96 ± 2 mg/L). (From Coe FL. Uric acid and calcium oxalate nephrolithiasis. Kidney Int 1983; 24:392.)

sis), ileostomy, small-bowel malabsorption, colitis, chronic renal insufficiency, and diets with a high methionine content (so-called *acid ash diets*).[50] The latter is common in calcium stone formers who eat large amounts of meat. Dehydration, from any cause, increases the urine uric acid concentration and increases supersaturation at any given pH.

### HYPERURICOSURIA

The main causes of hyperuricosuria are diets high in purines and primary overproduction of uric acid. The latter occurs in gout and in rare hereditary disorders of purine metabolism (see Chap. 192). Figure 69-3 illustrates that rises in the urine pH and the urine volume easily prevent excessive supersaturation of uric acid up to excretion levels of 1000 mg per day. Thus, hyperuricosuria is a much less important risk factor for uric acid stone disease than is the urine pH.

Before hyperuricosuria is implicated, the urine should be studied on at least three occasions. All drugs that could produce a falsely high measurement of urine uric acid must be discontinued. The colorimetric method, which is not completely specific, yields falsely high values in the presence of ascorbic acid, salicylates, caffeine, theophylline, high concentrations of glucose, and certain chromogens retained in renal failure. The uricase method is much more specific and does not give falsely high readings, but it is not generally available.

### TREATMENT

#### ALKALI

The goal of treatment is to raise the average urine pH to ~6, as determined by a 24-hour collection. The urine pH should be kept above 6 throughout the day, as determined by monitoring the patient at each voiding. Generally, 2 to 4 mEq/kg alkali is needed in four divided doses. Sodium bicarbonate has a rapid rate of absorption and excretion in the urine, giving rise to sharp increases and decreases in pH. Citrate produces a more sustained increase of urine pH. The potassium salt of citrate may be preferable to sodium bicarbonate because it is more palatable. It is important to avoid alkaline pH values above 6.5, which foster crystallization of brushite and apatite.

#### ALLOPURINOL

Reduction of the uric acid excretion rate is advisable only when total uric acid excretion is above 1000 mg per day; allopurinol, 100 mg twice daily, usually is sufficient. The twice-daily dosage is helpful in achieving continuous control of the urine uric acid level.

## CYSTINE STONES

### PATHOGENESIS

The only known cause of cystine stones is a hereditary defect of renal tubule transport that permits large amounts of cystine to pass into the urine. The defects, which include three separate varieties,[51] involve not only cystine but also the other dibasic amino acids—ornithine, lysine, and arginine. Only the cystinuria has consequences that are clinically important. One might think that cystine loss would cause an amino-acid deficiency state, but this is not a recognized problem. Stone formation primarily is caused by the low solubility of cystine: 300 mg/L urine. Normal people excrete < 60 mg per day of cystine, a level below supersaturation. Heterozygotes for the so-called type 1 form of cystinuria excrete normal amounts of cystine; heterozygotes for types 2 and 3 excrete abnormal amounts, in the range of 80 to 300 mg per day, along with an excess of the other three dibasic amino acids. However, heterozygotes do not form stones. Homozygous cystinurics, of all three types, excrete more than 400 mg per day of cystine. Patients with cystinuria may have other causes of stones as well, including those associated with calcium salts.

### TREATMENT

Treatment is based on high fluid intake to produce at least 3 L per day of urine. Urine output should be distributed evenly between the day and night. The amount of urine to be excreted can be calculated by dividing the total cystine excretion by the solubility of cystine. Any period of dehydration can cause fresh crystallization; hence, these patients should never be allowed to develop the sensation of thirst or symptoms of dehydration. Moreover, hydration is important because preformed stones can be dissolved by high fluid intake.

Another therapeutic approach is to increase urine pH. Above pH 7.5, cystine solubility increases dramatically.[1] Treatment with alkali is controversial. It often is used at a dosage of 2 mEq/kg per day, when fluids alone are insufficient. With a bedtime dose of acetazolamide, 250 to 500 mg, a high urine pH can be maintained and excessive sodium alkali salts excreted. The danger of alkali administration is calcium phosphate stone formation, especially in patients who also are hypercalciuric.

When fluids are insufficient, D-penicillamine can be tried. This drug forms a soluble disulfide with cysteine that is in equilibrium with cystine. Cystine dissociates to cysteine as cysteine binds to the penicillamine, so the concentration of cystine falls. Cysteine–penicillamine is significantly more soluble than cystine. The drug is effective in doses of 1 to 2 g per day in four divided doses, but it has many potential side effects: skin eruptions, fever, lymphadenopathy, arthritis, leukopenia, thrombocytopenia, a form of pseudothrombocytopenia caused by clumping of platelets in vitro (that deceives cell-counting machines), loss of the senses of smell and taste, proteinuria with focal glomerulitis, cutaneous lupus, and, rarely, Goodpasture syndrome with pulmonary hemorrhage and hemorrhagic acute renal failure.[51]

## STRUVITE STONES

### PATHOGENESIS

Some bacteria, especially *Proteus, Pseudomonas, Klebsiella,* and *Aerobacter* sp, possess urease, which is an enzyme that catalyzes the hydrolysis of urea to $CO_2$ and ammonia. By accepting protons to become $NH_4^+$, the pH of the urine is raised. Therefore, the concentration of $PO_4^{3-}$ increases, and the ion associates with $NH_4^+$ and magnesium ion to form the crystalline struvite stone.[1,52] Because the amounts of urea, phosphate, and magnesium generally are large, struvite stones grow rapidly to form staghorns. The other product of urea hydrolysis, $CO_2$, is readily converted to $HCO_3^-$ in the tubules. The $HCO_3^-$, in turn, becomes carbonate ($CO_3^{2-}$) as it loses a proton to $NH_3$. The $CO_3^{2-}$ ion crystallizes with calcium to form calcium carbonate, which helps to increase the mass of stone material, and accounts for the almost universal finding of calcium salts in struvite stones.[53]

Many patients with struvite stone disease initially are metabolic stone formers with calcium or uric acid stones. Presumably, infection from stone passage or from instrumentation leads to treatment that selects for resistant, urease-possessing organisms that are responsible for struvite stone formation. Struvite stone formers should also be evaluated for metabolic causes of stone formation.

### TREATMENT

#### ROLE OF ANTIBIOTICS

Virtually all struvite stones, when cultured, are infected, even when the urine from the patient contains so few bacteria that cultures are sterile. Antibacterial treatment is directed against an infected foreign body as well as infected tissue. Although antibiotics are not successful in preventing stone growth, they may sterilize the urine and the stone surface. At best, the prolonged use of antibiotics may slow the growth of stones. Their principal use is to treat acute infections, which presumably represent an invasion of bacteria into the renal tissue or the urinary tract wall. Another use of antibiotics is after the removal or disruption of a stone, to sterilize the kidneys and urinary tract and any tiny stone fragments that are left behind. For both purposes, bactericidal agents should be used in full dose, for a full time-course, and selected to correspond to the sensitivity pattern of the infecting bacteria.

## SURGERY

The indications for surgery or lithotripsy are, in order of frequency, pain, obstruction, and serious infection. Bleeding is rarely of sufficient magnitude to require treatment.

## LITHOTRIPSY

Lithotripsy is not always effective for large stones, such as are common when struvite stones are present. The number of shock waves needed to disrupt a stone increases with its mass; after several thousand shocks, there is a risk of renal damage. Furthermore, the volume of debris from a large stone may obstruct the ureter, requiring antegrade or retrograde instrumentation. Percutaneous removal, or pyelolithotomy, may be preferable for large stones despite the known hazards of major surgery.[54–56]

## EVALUATION PROTOCOL FOR PATIENTS WITH NEPHROLITHIASIS

A protocol for patient evaluation is presented in Table 69-3. Three 24-hour urine collections are obtained from outpatients eating their own ad libitum diets. Three corresponding blood samples are drawn between 8:00 and 9:00 a.m., in the postabsorptive state. Hypercalcemia, hypercalciuria, hyperoxaluria, hyperuricosuria, low pH, and hypocitricuria all are specifically investigated. This information, along with a complete history, physical examination, and review of available radiographs,

allows reasonably good classification into a particular type of stone disease. Appropriate treatment is then instituted.

## REFERENCES

1. Coe FL, Favus MJ. Disorders of stone formation. In: Brenner BM, Rector FC Jr, eds. The kidney. Philadelphia: WB Saunders, 1986:1403.
2. Coe FL, Strauss AL, Tembe V, Dun SL. Uric acid saturation in calcium nephrolithiasis. Kidney Int 1980; 17:662.
2a. Guillen M, Corella D, Cabello ML, et al. Association between M467T and 114 C-->A gene and some phenotypical variants within the SLC3A1 traits in cystinuria patients from Spain. Hum Genet 2000; 106:314.
3. Griffith DP, Gibson JR, Clinton C, Musher DM. Acetohydroxamic acid: clinical studies of a urease inhibitor in patients with staghorn calculi. J Urol 1978; 119:9.
4. Cotran RS, Rubin RH, Tolkoff-Rubin NE. Tubulointerstitial diseases. In: Brenner BM, Rector FC Jr, eds. The kidney. Philadelphia: WB Saunders, 1986:1143.
5. Kuiper JJ. Medullary sponge kidney. In: Gardner KD Jr, ed. Cystic diseases of the kidney. New York: John Wiley & Sons, 1976:1168.
6. Miles SG, Kaude JV, Newman RC, et al. Extracorporeal shock-wave lithotripsy: prevalence of renal stones 3–21 months after treatment. AJR Am J Roentgenol 1988; 150:307.
7. Williams CM, Kaude JV, Newman RC, et al. Extracorporeal shock-wave lithotripsy: long term complications. AJR Am J Roentgenol 1988; 150:311.
8. Coe FL, Parks JH. New insights into the pathophysiology and treatment of nephrolithiasis: new research venues. J Bone Miner Res 1997; 12:522.
9. Parks JH, Coward M, Coe FL. Correspondence between stone composition and urine supersaturation in nephrolithiasis. Kidney Int 1997; 51:894.
10. Coe FL, Lawton RB, Goldstein RB, Tembe V. Sodium urate accelerates precipitation of calcium oxalate in vitro. Proc Soc Exp Biol Med 1975; 149:926.
11. Nielson AE. Kinetics of precipitation. New York: Pergamon Press, 1964.
12. Bisaz S, Felix R, Neuman WF, Fleisch H. Quantitative determination of inhibitors of calcium phosphate precipitation in whole urine. Miner Electrolyte Metab 1978; 1:74.
13. Meyer JL, Smith LH. Growth of calcium oxalate crystal. Invest Urol 1975; 13:36.
14. Nakagawa Y, Abram V, Parks JH, et al. Urine glycoprotein crystal growth inhibitors: evidence for a molecular abnormality in calcium oxalate nephrolithiasis. J Clin Invest 1985; 76:1455.
15. Nakagawa Y, Ahmed M, Hall SL, et al. Isolation from human calcium oxalate renal stones of nephrocalcin, a glycoprotein inhibitor of calcium oxalate growth. J Clin Invest 1987; 79:1782.
16. Fleisch H, Bisaz S. Isolation from urine of pyrophosphate, a calcification inhibitor. Am J Physiol 1962; 203:671.
17. Coe FL. Treated and untreated recurrent calcium nephrolithiasis in patients with idiopathic hypercalciuria, hyperuricosuria, or no metabolic disorder. Ann Intern Med 1977; 87:404.
18. Coe FL, Parks JH, Moore ES. Familial idiopathic hypercalciuria. N Engl J Med 1979; 300:337.
19. Favus MJ. Familial forms of hypercalciuria. J Urol 1989; 141:719.
19a. Alon US, Berenbom A. Idiopathic hypercalciuria of childhood: 4- to 11-year outcome. Pediatr Nephrol 2000; 14:1011.
20. Pak CYC, Holt K. Nucleation and growth of brushite and calcium oxalate in urine of stone formers. Metabolism 1976; 25:665.
21. Marshall RW, Cochran M, Robertson WG, et al. The relationship between the concentration of calcium salts in the urine and renal stone composition in patients with calcium containing stones. Clin Sci 1972; 43:433.
22. Insogna KL, Broadus AE, Dryer BE, et al. Elevated production rate for 1,25-dihydroxyvitamin D in patients with absorptive hypercalciuria. J Clin Endocrinol Metab 1985; 61:490.
23. Broadus AE, Insogna KL, Lang RAS, et al. Evidence for disordered control of 1,25-dihydroxyvitamin D in absorptive hypercalciuria. N Engl J Med 1984; 31:73.
24. Coe FL, Favus MJ, Crockett T, et al. Effects of low-calcium diet on urine calcium excretion, parathyroid function and serum 1,25(OH)$_2$D levels in patients with idiopathic hypercalciuria and normal patients. Am J Med 1982; 72:25.
25. Coe FL, Parks JH, Favus MJ. Diet and calcium: the end of an era? Ann Intern Med 1997; 126:553.
26. Laerum E, Larsen S. Thiazide prophylaxis of urolithiasis: a double-blind study in general practice. Acta Med Scand 1984; 215:383.
27. Coe FL, Parks JH, Bushinsky DA, et al. Chlorothalidone promotes mineral retention in patients with idiopathic hypercalciuria. Kidney Int 1988; 33:1140.
28. Kaplan RA, Haussler MR, Deftos LJ, et al. The role of 1,25-dihydroxyvitamin D in the mediation of hyperabsorption of calcium in primary hyperparathyroidism and absorptive hypercalciuria. J Clin Invest 1977; 59:756.
29. Pearce SH, Williamson C, Kifor O, et al. A familial syndrome of hypocalcemia with hypercalciuria due to mutations in the calcium-sensing receptor. N Engl J Med 1996; 335:1115.
29a. Basmaison O, Rolland MO, Cochat P, Bozon D. Identification of 5 novel mutations in the AGXT gene. Hum Mutat 2000; 15:577.
29b. Mashour S, Turner JF Jr, Merrell R. Acute renal failure, oxalosis, and vitamin C supplementation. Chest 2000; 118:561.
30. Smith LH, Fromm H, Hofman AF. Acquired hyperoxaluria, nephrolithiasis and intestinal disease. N Engl J Med 1972; 286:1371.
31. Dobbins JW, Binder HJ. Importance of colon in enteric hyperoxaluria. N Engl J Med 1977; 296:298.

**TABLE 69-3.**
**Protocol for Evaluation of Urine and Serum Chemistry Profiles in Kidney Stone Formers**

| Measurement | Day 1 | Day 2 | Day 3 |
|---|---|---|---|
| **SERUM** | | | |
| Calcium | × | × | × |
| Magnesium | × | × | × |
| Phosphorus | × | × | × |
| Creatinine | × | × | × |
| Uric acid | × | × | × |
| Sodium | × | | |
| Potassium | × | | |
| Bicarbonate | × | | |
| **24-HOUR URINE** | | | |
| pH | × | × | × |
| Calcium | × | × | × |
| Magnesium | × | × | × |
| Phosphorus | × | × | × |
| Creatinine | × | × | × |
| Uric acid | × | × | × |
| Sodium | × | × | × |
| Oxalate | × | × | × |
| CPR | × | × | × |
| Citrate | × | × | × |
| Cystine screen | × | | |

*CPR*, concentration product ratio: an estimate of the state of supersaturation of calcium oxalate.

32. Kathpalia SC, Favus MJ, Coe FL. Evidence for size and charge permeability of rat ascending colon: effects of ricinoleate and bile salts on oxalic acid and neutral sugar transport. J Clin Invest 1984; 74:805.

33. Robertson WG, Peacock M, Nordin BEC. Calcium oxalate crystalluria and urine saturation in recurrent renal stone formers. Clin Sci 1971; 40:365.

34. Smith LH. Enteric hyperoxaluria and other hyperoxaluric states. In: Coe FL, Brenner BM, Stein JH, eds. Contemporary issues in nephrology, vol 4. New York: Churchill Livingstone, 1980:136.

35. Barilla DE, Notz C, Kennedy D, Pak CYC. Renal oxalate excretion following oral oxalate loads in patients with ileal disease and with renal and absorptive hypercalciurias: effect of calcium and magnesium. Am J Med 1978; 64:579.

36. Chadwick VS, Modha K, Dowling RH. Mechanism for hyperoxaluria in patients with ileal dysfunction. N Engl J Med 1973; 289:172.

37. Chlebeck PT, Milliner DS, Smith LH. Long-term prognosis in primary hyperoxaluria type II (L-glyceric aciduria.) Am J Kidney Dis 1994; 23:255.

38. Watts RWE, Morgan SH, Danpure CL, et al. Combined hepatic and renal transplantation in primary hyperoxaluria type I: clinical report of nine cases. Am J Med 1991; 90:179.

39. Alpern RJ, Warnock DG, Rector FC Jr. Renal acidification mechanisms. In: Brenner BM, Rector FC Jr, eds. The kidney. Philadelphia: WB Saunders, 1986:206.

40. Lemann J Jr, Lennon EJ, Goodman AD, et al. The net balance of acid in subjects given large loads of acid or alkali. J Clin Invest 1965; 44:507.

41. Robertson WG, Peacock M, Nordin BEC. Activity products in stone-forming and non-stone-forming urine. Clin Sci 1968; 34:579.

42. McSherry E, Morris RC Jr. Attainment and maintenance of normal stature with alkali therapy in infants and children with classic renal tubular acidosis. J Clin Invest 1978; 61:509.

43. Coe FL, Parks JH. Stone disease in hereditary distal renal tubular acidosis. Ann Intern Med 1980; 93:60.

44. Coe FL, Moran E, Kavalach AG. Dietary purine consumption by hyperuricosuric calcium oxalate kidney stone formers and normal subjects. J Chronic Dis 1976; 29:793.

45. Melnick JZ, Preisig PA, Haynes S, et al. Converting enzyme inhibition causes hypocitraturia independent of acidosis or hypokalemia. Kidney Int 1998; 54:1670.

46. Parks JH, Coe FL. Pathogenesis and treatment of calcium stones. Semin Nephrol 1996; 16:398.

47. Lemann J Jr, Gray RW, Pleuss JA. Potassium bicarbonate, but not sodium bicarbonate, reduces urinary calcium excretion and improves calcium balance in healthy men. Kidney Int 1989; 35:688.

48. Fleisch H. Inhibitors and promoters of stone formation. Kidney Int 1978; 13:361.

49. Nakagawa Y, Margolis HC, Yokoyama S, et al. Purification and characterization of a calcium oxalate monohydrate crystal growth inhibitor from human kidney tissue culture medium. J Biol Chem 1981; 256:3936.

50. Hall AP, Berry PE, Dawber TR, et al. Epidemiology of gout and hyperuricosuria: a long term population study. Am J Med 1967; 42:27.

51. Geeson MJ, Kobashi K, Griffith DP. Noncalcium nephrolithiasis. In: Coe FL, Favus MJ, eds. Disorders of bone and mineral metabolism. New York: Raven Press, 1992:801.

52. Elliot JS, Sharp RF, Lewis L. The solubility of struvite in urine. J Urol 1959; 80:169.

53. Kristensen C, Parks JH, Lindheimer M, Coe FL. Reduced glomerular filtration rate and hypercalciuria in primary struvite nephrolithiasis. Kidney Int 1987; 32:749.

54. Chaussy CG, Fuchs GJ. Current state and future developments of noninvasive treatment of human urinary stones with extracorporeal shock wave lithotripsy. J Urol 1989; 141:782.

55. Lingeman JE, Woods J, Toth PD, et al. Role of lithotripsy and its side effects. J Urol 1989; 141:793.

56. Lingeman JE, Siegel YI, Steele B. Management of lower pole nephrolithiasis: a critical analysis. J Urol 1994; 151:663.

# CHAPTER 70

# DISORDERS OF CALCIUM AND BONE METABOLISM IN INFANCY AND CHILDHOOD

THOMAS O. CARPENTER

## ABNORMAL SERUM CALCIUM

Hypocalcemia is the most common disorder of mineral metabolism in the neonatal period and is observed frequently in premature infants. Although less common, hypercalcemia may also occur in the neonatal period and, if severe, may be life threatening.

## NEONATAL HYPOCALCEMIA

Except for the unusual cases of congenital hypoparathyroidism, neonatal hypocalcemia is usually transient, persisting for a few days to a few weeks.[1,2] Neonatal hypocalcemia is categorized according to the time of its onset: early neonatal hypocalcemia and late neonatal hypocalcemia.

### EARLY NEONATAL HYPOCALCEMIA

Early neonatal hypocalcemia occurs in the first 24 to 48 hours of life and is observed most frequently in premature infants, sick infants, and infants born of an abnormal labor or pregnancy. The condition can be explained as an exaggeration of the normal postnatal decrease in serum calcium; the fall in serum calcium is inversely proportional to the gestational age of the infant. The serum calcium remains low for a few to several days and then gradually increases, usually reaching normal levels by 1 to 2 weeks of age. The serum inorganic phosphate concentration is usually normal, although it may be elevated in asphyxiated infants and in infants born of diabetic mothers.

It has been suggested that inappropriate parathyroid secretion, parathyroid hormone (PTH) resistance, and/or vitamin D metabolic abnormalities may contribute to the development of this condition, but no single conclusive mechanism has been confirmed. Many premature infants with early neonatal hypocalcemia are asymptomatic, but in others, tetany or convulsions may be present. Symptomatic infants obviously require calcium therapy, but there is no unanimity regarding treatment of hypocalcemic infants who are asymptomatic. The emergency treatment of neonatal hypocalcemia consists of the intravenous administration of 1 mL per minute 10% calcium gluconate, which should not exceed 2.0 mL/kg. This may be repeated three to four times in 24 hours to control the acute symptoms. After the acute symptoms have been controlled, 5.0 mL/kg 10% calcium gluconate may be given with intravenous fluids over a 24-hour period, or calcium supplements may be given orally if feedings are tolerated. Occasionally, hypomagnesemia is concomitantly identified; this can be treated with 0.1 to 0.2 mL/kg of a 50% solution of magnesium sulfate ($MgSO_4 \bullet 7H_2O$).

### LATE NEONATAL HYPOCALCEMIA

Late neonatal hypocalcemia appears at the end of the first week of life or later, often in full-term infants who have received a high phosphate load, such as that formerly encountered with feedings of evaporated cow's milk formula or from a phosphate enema.[2a] Infants with late neonatal hypocalcemia usually have clinical manifestations of tetany or convulsions. Hyperphosphatemia is a prominent feature, and the serum PTH level may be low, reflecting a state of functional hypoparathyroidism in the presence of hypocalcemia. This form of hypocalcemia is seen in infants born to hyperparathyroid mothers and in children with congenital heart disease in the postoperative period.

The emergency treatment of acute tetany or convulsions secondary to hypocalcemia is the same as for early neonatal hypocalcemia. Dietary factors are of importance in the management of late neonatal hypocalcemia; the phosphate load should be diminished, with an increase of the calcium/phosphate ratio of milk feedings to 4:1. The author often uses Similac PM 60/40 (Ross Laboratories, Columbus, Ohio) in this setting. The serum calcium level usually increases when the infants are given such milk feedings; and, after several days to weeks, the serum PTH level gradually rises and the infants can tolerate higher phosphate loads. The pathogenesis of the transient hypoparathyroidism in these infants is unknown.

## NEONATAL HYPERCALCEMIA

Neonatal hypercalcemia is found in association with several disorders of calcium metabolism.[3] In the presence of mild to

**TABLE 70-1.**
**Clinical Disorders Associated with Hypercalcemia in the Neonatal Period**

| Disorder | Comments |
|---|---|
| Neonatal primary hyperparathyroidism | Association with familial hypocalciuric hypercalcemia |
| Neonatal hyperparathyroidism associated with maternal hypoparathyroidism and pseudohypoparathyroidism | Fetal hypocalemia results in secondary hyperparathyroidism |
| Idiopathic infantile hypercalcemia, including Williams syndrome | Defect in vitamin D metabolism(?) |
| Subcutaneous fat necrosis | Increased 1,25(OH)$_2$ vitamin D |
| Blue diaper syndrome | Defect in intestinal transport of tryptophan |
| Hyperabsorption of calcium by very-low-birth-weight infants receiving human milk fortifier | — |
| Phosphate depletion | Most common in premature infants who receive human milk |

(Modified from Anast CS. Disorders of mineral and bone metabolism. In: Avery ME, Taeusch WH, eds. Schaffer's diseases of the newborn. Philadelphia: WB Saunders, 1984:464.)

moderate hypercalcemia (11.0–13.0 mg/dL) the infant is often asymptomatic. Infants with more severe hypercalcemia have various clinical findings, including failure to thrive, poor feeding, hypotonia, vomiting, seizures, lethargy, polyuria, and hypertension. The medical management of acute symptomatic hypercalcemia consists of the administration of intravenous saline. Additionally, furosemide, in a dose of 1 mg/kg, is frequently given intravenously at 6- to 8-hour intervals. Intravenous infusion of pamidronate has also been useful in this setting. Specific long-term therapy depends on the specific hypercalcemic disorder. Disorders associated with neonatal hypercalcemia are listed in Table 70-1.

### PRIMARY HYPERPARATHYROIDISM IN THE NEONATAL PERIOD

In infants with neonatal primary hyperparathyroidism, the symptoms of hypercalcemia usually develop during the early days of life. Severe hypercalcemia is usually present, with serum calcium levels that range between 15 and 30 mg/dL. Occasionally, however, the hypercalcemia is mild, with serum calcium values between 11 and 13 mg/dL. The serum inorganic phosphate level is often depressed, whereas the serum PTH level is elevated (see Chap. 58). Radiographic studies of bone are characteristic of primary hyperparathyroidism. Moreover, renal calcinosis may be present.

Primary hyperparathyroidism may be sporadic, or it may be inherited in an autosomal-recessive fashion. An interesting association between neonatal severe primary hyperparathyroidism and familial hypocalciuric hypercalcemia (FHH) occurs[4] (see Chap. 58). FHH, an autosomal-dominant trait, is manifest by modest asymptomatic hypercalcemia with relative hypocalciuria and either normal or somewhat elevated serum PTH levels. An inactivating mutation in the gene for the extracellular calcium-sensing receptor, which is present on parathyroid cells, acts in a dominant negative manner in FHH. A greater level of serum ionized calcium is required to suppress PTH secretion than would normally be necessary; thus, modest increases in serum calcium are maintained. Individuals who are homozygous for such a mutation effectively fail to suppress PTH secretion and manifest severe neonatal hyperparathyroidism.[5]

Severe neonatal primary hyperparathyroidism is considered a surgical emergency. The serum calcium levels often range between 15 and 30 mg/dL. Total parathyroidectomy may be necessary because of recurrence after subtotal parathyroidectomy.[6] Parathyroidectomy and heterotopic autotransplantation have also been suggested; however, a current common practice

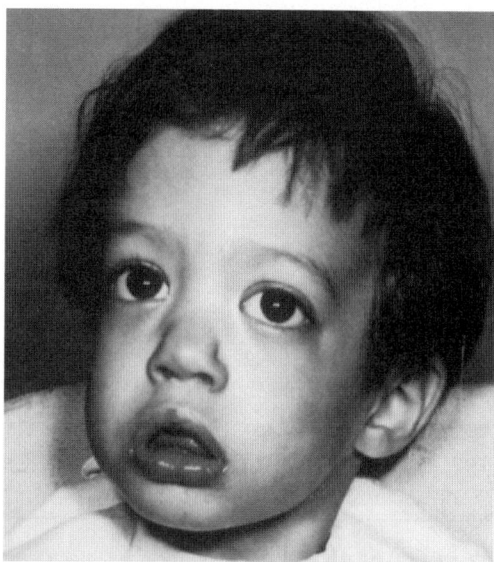

**FIGURE 70-1.** Idiopathic hypercalcemia (Williams syndrome) in a 3-year-old boy. Note the typical broad forehead, depressed bridge of the nose, anteverted nares, long philtrum (the vertical median groove extending from beneath the nose to the upper lip), the slight strabismus, the wide mouth with large lips, the drooping of the lower lip, and the large ears. The cheeks are full and dependent, and there is mandibular hypoplasia.

is to leave a small portion of one gland in the neck, marked with a surgical clip for ease in identification should reexploration be necessary. In some infants, the disorder is milder, with low serum calcium concentrations (i.e., 11–13 mg/dL). These infants may not require surgical intervention; their bony lesions may heal spontaneously, they may be asymptomatic in the presence of modest hypercalcemia in association with relative hypocalciuria, and the disorder may be self-limited.[7]

### IDIOPATHIC HYPERCALCEMIA

There are mild and severe forms of idiopathic infantile hypercalcemia. In the mild form, symptoms associated with hypercalcemia usually appear between 2 and 9 months of age. The infants may fail to thrive and, in a few, a cardiac murmur may be apparent. The facies frequently appears normal, and the prognosis for physical and mental development is usually good.

In the severe form, the symptoms may date from birth; however, this is frequently difficult to document. Prenatal and postnatal growth failure are common, and a number of the phenotypic features of Williams syndrome (Fig. 70-1) are observed in some patients with the severe disorder. These features, in addition to hypercalcemia, include cardiovascular abnormalities (usually supravalvular aortic stenosis or peripheral pulmonic stenosis), late psychomotor development, selective mental deficiency, a characteristic unusual facies, and short stature. A deletion of the elastin gene is found in many cases of Williams syndrome.[8]

The serum calcium levels range between 12 and 19 mg/dL. The hypercalcemia usually subsides spontaneously by the age of 4 years. The prognosis for patients with the severe form is poor, and the mortality may be as high as 25% during the first 4 years of life.

The pathogenesis of idiopathic hypercalcemia is uncertain. In one study, an exaggerated 25-hydroxyvitamin D [25(OH)D] response to vitamin D administration was observed, suggesting that the regulation of this metabolite may be abnormal.[9] There are conflicting reports on the circulating levels of 1,25-dihydroxyvitamin D [1,25(OH)$_2$D] in the severe form of idiopathic hypercalcemia.[10,11]

Treatment consists of placing the child on a low calcium, vitamin D–free diet. In some resistant cases, short-term therapy with

**TABLE 70-2.**
**Causes of Rickets**

| Type | Calciopenic Causes | Phosphopenic Causes |
|---|---|---|
| **NUTRITIONAL** **TRANSPORT** | Vitamin D deprivation; calcium deprivation<br>Impaired absorption; bile salt depletion (effect on vitamin D absorption)<br>Sprue, celiac disease, etc. (effect on calcium and vitamin D absorption) | Phosphate deprivation/antacid abuse<br>Hypophosphatemic rickets secondary to renal phosphate tubulopathies<br>X-linked,* autosomal-recessive or autosomal-dominant transmission<br>Acquired, late-onset<br>Fanconi syndrome (ifosfamide)<br>Oncogenic*<br>Hypophosphatemic rickets associated with hypercalciuria† |
| **METABOLISM** | Defective synthesis of 25(OH)D; hepatocellular disease<br>Defective synthesis of 1,25(OH)$_2$D; renal parenchymal disease; mutations of 1α-hydroxylase (vitamin D–dependent rickets, type I)<br>Hereditary resistance to 1,25(OH)$_2$D; mutations of the vitamin D receptor (vitamin D–dependent rickets type II) | |

*Impaired generation of 1,25-dihydroxyvitamin D [*1,25(OH)$_2$D*].
†Elevated serum 1,25-dihydroxyvitamin D levels.

corticosteroids may be necessary. The author has used intravenous pamidronate to correct hypercalcemia in Williams syndrome.

Although rare in the neonatal period, intoxication with vitamin D or vitamin A should be excluded in older infants with hypercalcemia. Another rare condition in this differential diagnosis includes subcutaneous fat necrosis, a self-limited disorder of infancy for which increased production of 1,25(OH)$_2$D has been described.[12]

# RICKETS

*Rickets* may be defined as a disorder in which there is a lag in the rate of mineralization of the matrix of bone and growth cartilage. Growth plate cartilage typically hypertrophies in an unorganized fashion, producing the characteristic widened ends of the long bones seen in this disorder. The formation of hydroxyapatite depends on adequate concentrations of extracellular calcium and phosphate; therefore, a deficiency of either or both of these minerals may cause rickets.

There are more than 30 causes of rickets: One classification scheme that categorizes the various forms of rickets is shown in Table 70-2 (see Chap. 63).

## VITAMIN D–DEPRIVATION AND CALCIUM DEFICIENCY

There has been a resurgence of vitamin D–deprivation rickets associated with breast-feeding and special dietary practices, including macrobiotic and other vegetarian diets. Human breast milk may provide as little as 10 to 20 IU of vitamin D per day, and macrobiotic diets may provide comparable amounts of vitamin D. Marginal vitamin D stores are often present in the breast-feeding mother of a rachitic infant. Thus, infants who receive only human milk and children who receive macrobiotic diets are at high risk for developing rickets in the early months and years of life.

The physical findings at the time of the rickets diagnosis may include flaring of the wrists and ankles, frontal bossing, rachitic rosary, Harrison grooves (a groove extending laterally from the xiphoid process that corresponds to the diaphragmatic attachment), long-bone fractures, bowed legs, leg tenderness, and large fontanelles (Figs. 70-2 to 70-4). The biochemical findings include a low serum calcium or phosphate level, or both, and elevated serum alkaline phosphatase activity. In the presence of hypocalcemia, the circulating PTH level is increased, which, in turn, leads to generalized aminoaciduria. The serum 25(OH)D concentrations are depressed, whereas the serum 1,25(OH)$_2$D levels may be either low, normal, or modestly elevated. Radiographic

findings include widening of the space between the calcified plate at the end of the metaphysis and the center of ossification. Other changes at the cartilage-shaft junction include cupping, spreading, spur formation, fringing, and stippling.

The author usually prescribes 1000 to 2000 IU vitamin D per day as treatment for vitamin D–deficient rickets. Others may prefer the administration of intermediate amounts of oral vitamin D (i.e., 8000–16,000 IU per day). After radiographic evidence of healing, the dosage is usually reduced to prophylactic amounts of 400 IU per day. Where compliance is an issue, the so-called *stoss* form of therapy is used, which consists of the administration of a single oral or intramuscular dose of 600,000 IU vitamin D. (Some prefer to divide the large oral dose into two or more doses given several hours apart on the same day.)

Often, these children are referred to specialty clinics after the diagnosis is suspected and supplementation with some form of

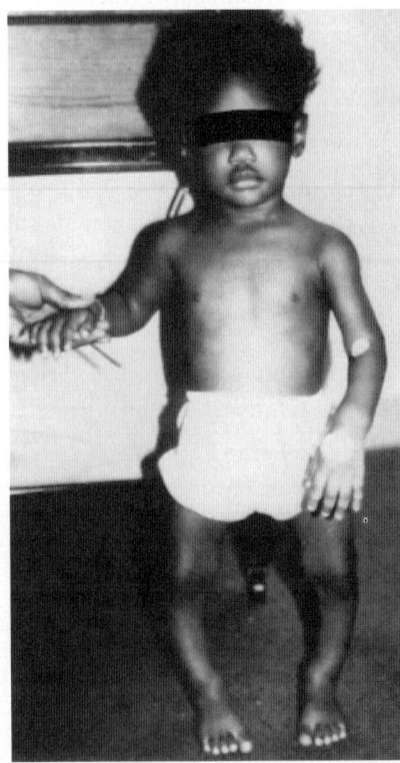

**FIGURE 70-2.** Nutritional rickets (vitamin D deficiency) in a 3-year-old boy. Note the severe bowing of the lower extremities and the widened wrists and ankles.

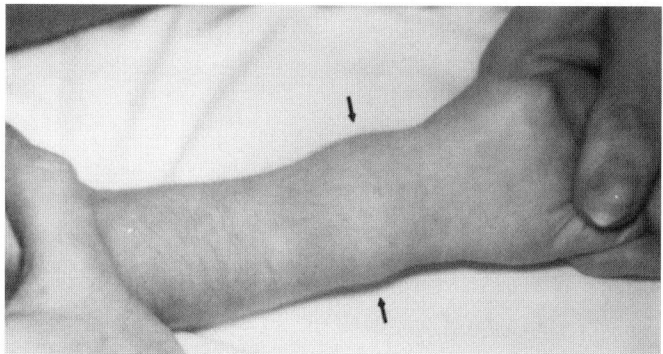

**FIGURE 70-3.** Flaring of the wrists (*arrows*) of a 2-year-old boy with rickets.

vitamin D has been initiated. These children often have low normal levels of 25(OH)D. The radiographic hallmark of partially treated vitamin D–resistant rickets is a thin dense line of opacity at the metaphyses of long bones, representing recent rapid mineralization at the edge of the growth plate.

It is not infrequent for children with vitamin D deficiency to require supplemental calcium. Some of these children apparently have a low dietary intake of calcium, and others may manifest the hungry bone syndrome, in which mineralization is sufficiently rapid to effect a decrease in the serum calcium levels. For this reason, supplemental calcium (such as calcium glubionate or calcium carbonate) should be included in the therapy, so that the child receives a total daily intake of 30 to 50 mg/kg elemental calcium. Indeed, stores of vitamin D are subject to relatively rapid turnover in the setting of concomitant low dietary intake of calcium.[13]

## INHERITED DISORDERS OF VITAMIN D METABOLISM AND ACTIVITY

*Autosomal recessive 1α-hydroxylase deficiency* (also known as *hereditary pseudovitamin D deficiency rickets* or *vitamin D–dependent rickets type I*) is an autosomal-recessive disorder in which the renal 25(OH)D 1α-hydroxylase that converts 25(OH)D to

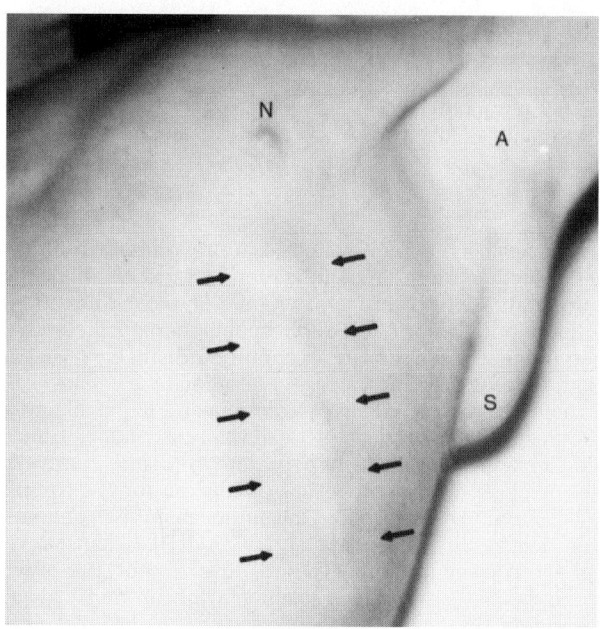

**FIGURE 70-4.** Rachitic rosary (*arrows*) in a 5-year-old boy. This condition is caused by enlargement of the costochondral junctions. (*N*, nipple; *A*, axilla; *S*, scapula.)

1,25(OH)$_2$D is dysfunctional. Individuals with this disorder have a mutation in the gene encoding a specific cytochrome P450 that donates electrons to the substrate, 25(OH)D.[14] Thus, this enzyme component is essential to the hydroxylation reaction. Onset of symptoms is usually within 4 to 12 months of age, and the clinical course and biochemical features are similar to those of severe vitamin D–deficiency rickets. In contrast to vitamin D–deficient rickets, there is a history of adequate dietary intake of vitamin D or of sunlight exposure. In untreated patients, the serum 25(OH)D level is normal. The serum 1,25(OH)$_2$D is low to low-normal and remains so in patients treated with pharmacologic doses of vitamin D or 25(OH)D. Patients with 1α-hydroxylase deficiency may respond to high dosages of vitamin D or 25(OH)D; however, treatment with 1,25(OH)$_2$D is optimal, using initial dosages from 0.5 to 3.0 μg per day and maintenance dosages ranging from 0.25 to 2.0 μg per day.

*Hereditary vitamin D resistance* (also known as *vitamin D–dependent rickets type II*) is a rare inherited disorder transmitted as an autosomal-recessive trait. The clinical, radiologic, and most of the biochemical features are similar to those observed in 1α-hydroxylase deficiency (Fig. 70-5). The major biochemical distinction is that circulating 1,25(OH)$_2$D levels are high in patients with hereditary vitamin D resistance and low in patients with 1α-hydroxylase deficiency. A unique clinical feature in some kindreds with hereditary vitamin D resistance is total body and scalp alopecia. Other patients may demonstrate oligodontia (Fig. 70-6). Studies in affected individuals of several kindreds have revealed defects in the 1,25(OH)$_2$D receptor, which is one of a large superfamily of hormone receptors, including glucocorticoid, mineralocorticoid, and thyroid hormone receptors. Mutations, which have been identified in the gene encoding this receptor, result in altered DNA binding, altered ligand binding, or interruption of complete synthesis of the receptor (see Chap. 54). In some families, no genetic defect has been identified.

Patients with hereditary vitamin D resistance have been treated with megadoses of vitamin D or vitamin D metabolites with variable responses to such therapy. Parenteral administration of calcium has been shown to completely correct the skeletal abnormalities in severe forms of this disorder.[15]

## X-LINKED HYPOPHOSPHATEMIC RICKETS

X-Linked hypophosphatemic rickets[16] (XLH) is inherited as an X-linked dominant trait and is characterized by hypophosphatemia and decreased renal tubular phosphate reabsorption. The inherited disorder may vary in degree, from severe to mild bone disease associated with hypophosphatemia, to hypophosphatemia alone without evidence of active or former rickets. The severity of bone disease does not correlate with the degree of hypophosphatemia. Children with XLH are usually seen in the second or third year of life with bowed legs and short stature. Controversy exists whether the mineralized tissue abnormalities are more severe in affected males compared with females.[17,18] Hallmark laboratory findings include hypophosphatemia, normocalcemia, and elevated serum alkaline phosphatase activity. The tubular reabsorption rate and the maximum reabsorption rate of phosphate are decreased. The serum PTH level is usually normal but can be elevated in the untreated state. Hyperparathyroidism is not infrequently seen as a complication of therapy. In the untreated state, the serum 25(OH)D levels are normal. The serum 1,25(OH)$_2$D levels are either normal or somewhat decreased. The "normal" circulating levels of this metabolite are inappropriately low in the presence of hypophosphatemia.

Pathophysiologic features of XLH include a defect in renal tubular transport of phosphate and impaired generation of 1,25(OH)$_2$D in response to both phosphate deprivation and PTH. The mutated gene[19] (PHEX) encodes a protein with

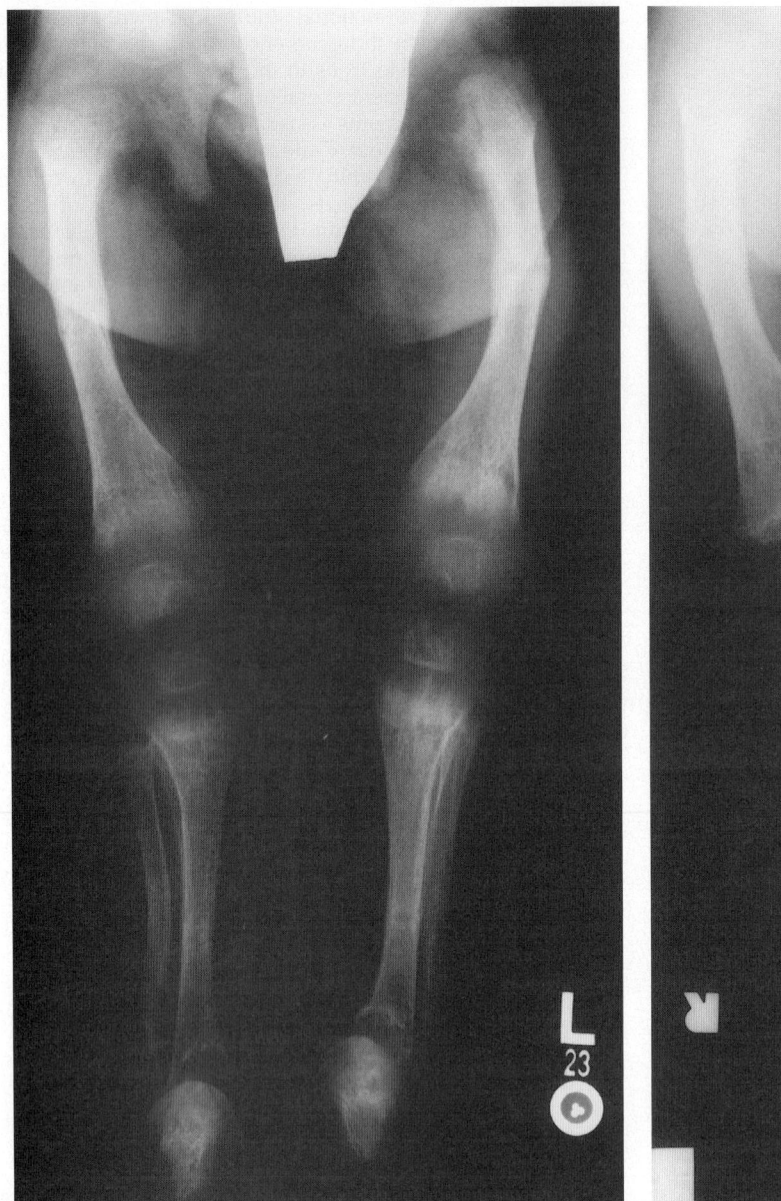
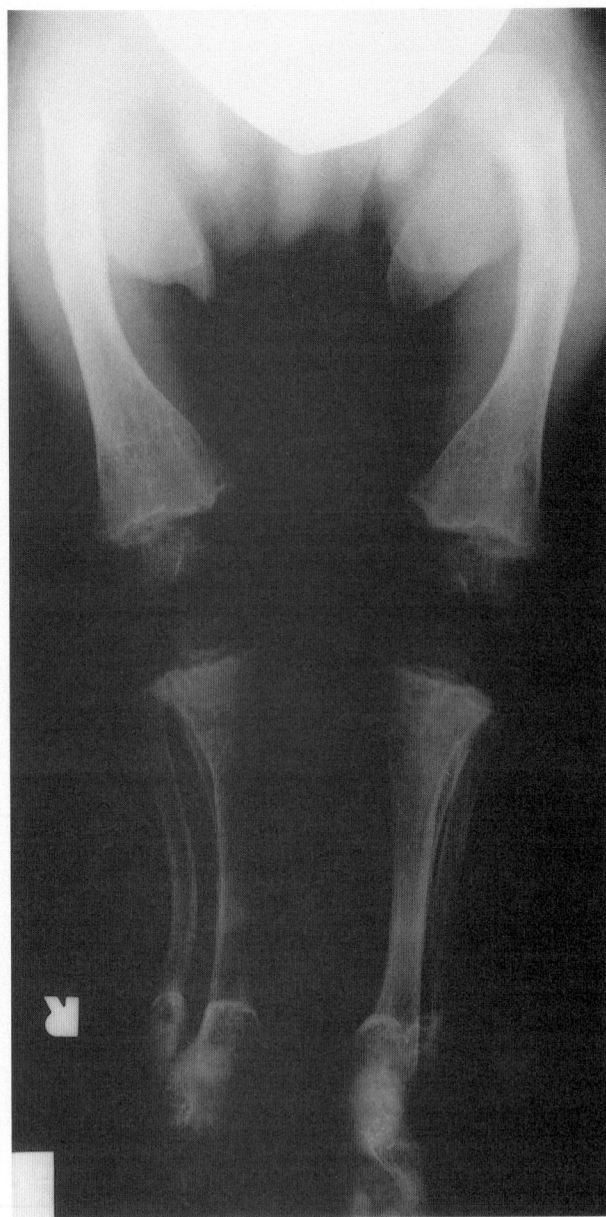

**FIGURE 70-5.** Rachitic changes in the lower extremities of a 2½-year-old girl with hereditary resistance to vitamin D. At presentation (**A**) severely deformed epiphyses, demineralization, and bilateral fractures of the femora and tibiae are evident. After 4 months of therapy with high-dose calcitriol (**B**), dramatic remodeling of the metaphyseal edges has occurred.

homology to known metallo-endopeptidases (including nephrolysin and endothelin-converting enzyme-1), although the role of such an enzyme in the pathophysiology of the disease has not been clearly established. Studies in an animal model, the *hyp* mouse, indicate that a circulating factor influences the renal phosphate transport.[20,21] Whether the mutation directly affects the skeleton independent of serum phosphate levels is not entirely clear, but has been suggested by other experiments in *hyp* mice.[22,23]

Treatment consists of the administration of phosphate plus vitamin D or a vitamin D metabolite. Phosphate treatment alone, or in conjunction with vitamin D, induces healing of the rachitic lesions at the growth plate, but has little effect on the mineralization defect in trabecular bone. Furthermore, hyperparathyroidism is likely to result from solitary phosphate therapy. In practice, treatment of XLH has employed relatively large amounts of phosphorus (1–4 g per day) in conjunction with $1,25(OH)_2D$ (0.5–2.0 µg per day or 10–40 ng/kg per day). This regimen has been demonstrated to improve the rachitic lesion at the growth plate and mineralization in trabecular bone.[24] The administration of vitamin D or vitamin D metabolites counteracts the hypocalcemic effect of phosphate therapy, thereby serving to prevent secondary hyperparathyroidism. Complications of higher dosages of $1,25(OH)_2D$ (averaging 68.2 ± 10 ng/kg per day in one study) include hypercalcemia and hypercalciuria.[25]

Because of the propensity to develop secondary[26] and, in some instances, tertiary hyperparathyroidism[27] with large doses of phosphate, and because of concern for the complication of vitamin D intoxication, the author maintains patients on lower dosages of phosphate and $1,25(OH)_2D$ than previous reports recommend. The average dose in our pre-pubertal patients is 0.75 g per day of elemental phosphorus, given in three to four divided doses; rarely does the author recommend more than 1.5 g per day of phosphorus. The average dose of $1,25(OH)_2D$ used is 0.75 µg per day, which is usually given in two divided doses. Furthermore, the author has found that

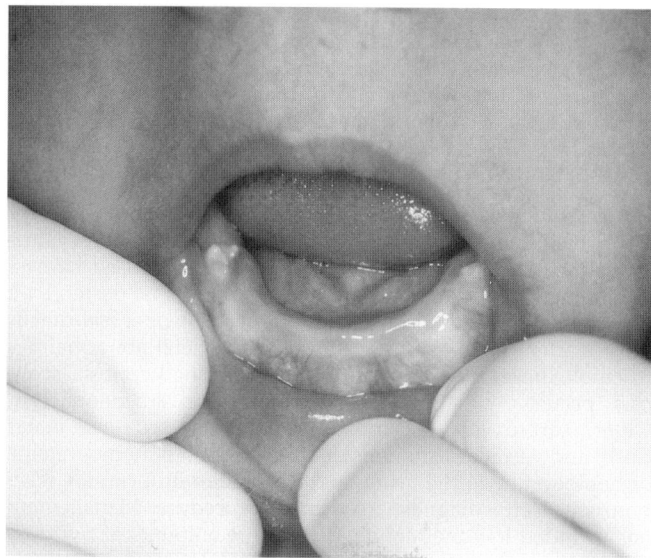

**FIGURE 70-6.** The limited eruption of teeth (oligodontia), as shown here, is characteristic of certain kindreds with hereditary resistance to vitamin D.

supplementation of this regimen with 24,25(OH)$_2$D at a dose of 10 μg per day can aid in the correction of mild secondary hyperparathyroidism.[28] The rachitic disease is exacerbated by the adolescent growth spurt; doses of 1,25(OH)$_2$D may be transiently increased to as high as 2.0 μg per day, but such high-dose therapy is rarely used for longer than a year and should be carefully monitored. Likewise, oral phosphorus during this phase may be transiently increased to 2 g per day, but careful monitoring is important. In the past, treatment has been limited to affected children and stopped after achievement of ultimate height. It now appears likely, however, that symptomatic adults may benefit from therapy.[29]

Nephrocalcinosis is common in treated patients with X-linked hypophosphatemia. Ultrasound examinations of the kidney should be performed occasionally to monitor this complication. Data suggest that the clinical significance of this lesion is very limited.[30]

In addition to X-linked transmission, both autosomal-recessive and autosomal-dominant transmission patterns of hypophosphatemic rickets have been reported. The gene associated with the autosomal-dominant form has been mapped to the short arm of chromosome 12.[31] Acquired, sporadic forms of hypophosphatemic rickets occur later in childhood or in adulthood. Hypophosphatemic rickets, with a low serum 1,25(OH)$_2$D concentration in some patients, is found in association with skeletal and soft tissue mesenchymal tumors; the term *oncogenic rickets* has been applied to these cases. It is possible that a mesenchymal tumor may be a pathogenetic factor in many cases of acquired hypophosphatemic rickets, but because the tumors are often benign and small, they may not be discovered (see Chaps. 63 and 219).

Phosphate-wasting rickets also occurs in linear sebaceous nevus syndrome,[32] neurofibromatosis,[33] and in the McCune-Albright syndrome. In this disorder, a somatic mutation of the membrane guanyl nucleotide stimulatory protein results in constitutive stimulation of adenylate cyclase. The somatic nature of the mutation results in a random pattern of affected tissues (see Chap. 60).[34] Should the renal tubule possess the mutation, a PTH-like inhibition of phosphate transport and renal phosphate wasting may result.

Hereditary hypophosphatemic rickets with hypercalciuria is yet another form of phosphate-wasting rickets, which is distinguished from X-linked hypophosphatemia by an autosomal-recessive mode of transmission and a normal hypo-

phosphatemia–1α-hydroxylase axis.[35] Such patients, therefore, have an appropriately elevated circulating 1,25(OH)$_2$D level, which results in increased intestinal calcium absorption, a propensity to hypercalcemia, hypercalciuria, and reduced circulating PTH levels. Patients generally respond well to treatment with phosphate salts alone, and vitamin D supplementation provokes frank hypercalcemia. Urinary calcium excretion should be determined in children with phosphate-wasting rickets to correctly identify this disease variant.

## OSTEOPENIA IN CHILDHOOD

Children occasionally come to the physician's attention because of osteopenia (radiographic evidence of reduced bone mass). Abnormalities in serum calcium, phosphorus, or alkaline phosphatase may confirm the suspicion of rickets. In less clear cases, however, differentiation between osteomalacia (defective mineralization of osteoid) and osteoporosis (decreased organic and calcified bone mass) must be sought (see Chaps. 55 and 64). This discussion is concerned primarily with disorders in which osteopenia is a presenting feature (Table 70-3). There are several conditions in which osteopenia may be an associated finding and not the primary manifestation of the disease (e.g., thyrotoxicosis, acromegaly, hypogonadism [Klinefelter syndrome, Noonan syndrome, hyperprolactinemia], hyperparathyroidism, diabetes mellitus, the lactating adolescent, heparin therapy, mastocytosis, increased erythropoiesis, Down syndrome, Wilson disease, cystic fibrosis, familial dysautonomia, anorexia nervosa, and other severe chronic diseases).

It appears that racial differences in bone mass begin at an early age. Adequate but not excess calcium intake in children may have positive effects on bone mineral status in adulthood.

### MAJOR CHILDHOOD OSTEOPENIA

#### IMMOBILIZATION

Severe trauma, myelodysplasia, and juvenile rheumatoid arthritis are predisposing conditions for immobilization-related osteoporosis in children.

#### OSTEOGENESIS IMPERFECTA

Osteogenesis imperfecta, a heterogeneous group of diseases, has an estimated incidence of 1 per 15,000 live births. The osteopenia results from abnormal production of bone matrix secondary to defective collagen synthesis or assembly.[36] Other tissues that

**TABLE 70-3.**
**Osteoporotic Disorders with Osteopenia as Presenting Feature**

| Disorder | Mechanism |
|---|---|
| Immobilization | (?) |
| Osteogenesis imperfecta | Abnormal synthesis or assembly of collagen |
| Idiopathic juvenile osteoporosis | (?) |
| Turner syndrome | Hypogonadism vs. associated chromosomal aberration (?); controversial existence |
| Homocystinuria | Defective cross-linking of collagen |
| Lysinuric protein intolerance | Generalized protein malnutrition → poor matrix formation |
| Menkes syndrome | Defective cross-linking of collagen |
| Malnutrition | — |
| Protein | Poor matrix formation |
| Copper deficiency | Defective cross-linking of collagen |
| Hypercortisolism | Generalized decrease in body protein synthesis |
| Leukemia | (?) |

contain collagen may be affected, as evidenced by joint laxity and thin skin. The sclerae may appear blue because of thinning, allowing the blue pigment of the choroid to be transmitted. Improper formation of dentin may occur, and teeth may be yellow or opalescent and chip easily. Sensorineural or conductive hearing loss may be present. The skeleton is variably affected. Wormian bones (islands of bone with a rich vascular supply) are frequently observed on skull radiographs. Biochemical findings are nonspecific; however, mild hypercalcemia and hypercalciuria may be present in younger patients. Markers of bone turnover—such as serum alkaline phosphatase activity and osteocalcin as well as urinary excretion of resorptive markers—may also have higher than average values. Serum PTH and vitamin D metabolites are nearly always normal.

Numerous mutations in genes encoding the $\alpha_1$ and $\alpha_2$ chains of type I collagen (bone collagen) have been described.[36a] Most kindreds are affected with unique mutations, and sporadic mutations are not uncommonly reported. Studies note variable severity associated with the mutations, being dependent on the region of the gene in which the mutation occurs; thus a "regional model" for site of mutation/severity has been proposed.[37] Mutations in introns resulting in abnormal mRNA processing have been described; these result in abnormal ratios of chain production, not abnormal chains, per se.

Prenatal diagnosis of osteogenesis imperfecta has been possible through genetic studies of chorionic villous samples or through high-resolution fetal ultrasound studies in severe cases.

After years of disappointing results with various experimental therapies of the disease, trials with intravenous pamidronate have shown dramatic changes in the bone density and fracture rate over the short term.[38] The bisphosphonate preparation is given intravenously in 3- to 4-hour daily infusions that are repeated for 3 successive days per cycle. The cycle is repeated at 4-month intervals. Therapy is sufficiently new that long-term effects on the skeleton have not yet been clearly established. Nevertheless, serious consideration for therapy should be undertaken in patients with severe disease. It is less clear whether mild forms of the disease warrant such an intervention.

Finally, it seems likely that a number of unidentified mutations in the collagen gene could be responsible for disorders of childhood osteoporosis that have not classically been diagnosed as osteogenesis imperfecta. Related connective tissue disorders, particularly the Ehlers-Danlos syndrome and, rarely, Marfan syndrome, may also manifest osteopenia (see Chaps. 66 and 189).

### IDIOPATHIC JUVENILE OSTEOPOROSIS

In contrast to osteogenesis imperfecta, idiopathic juvenile osteoporosis usually becomes evident just before puberty. Such individuals may have pain in the weight-bearing skeleton, refusal to walk, or gait abnormalities. Radiographs can show generalized osteopenia, compression fractures of the thoracolumbar vertebrae, and metaphyseal compression fractures. Marked osteopenia in the metaphyseal region of new bone formation is characteristic.

There are no consistent biochemical changes in this disorder. Increased hydroxyproline excretion and negative calcium balance may occur. The circulating PTH level has been reported as elevated relative to the serum calcium level. Serum $1,25(OH)_2D$ levels may be decreased, normal, or increased. The active disease is almost always transient, but residual deformity is not uncommon. Rarely, patients have persistence of active osteoporosis through adolescence and into adulthood (see Chap. 64). Some patients have been shown to respond to bisphosphonate therapy.[39]

### TURNER SYNDROME

A number of skeletal abnormalities have been reported in Turner syndrome, including osteopenia. However, recent stud-

ies of bone density in girls with Turner syndrome have indicated that when bone mineral density is normalized to height or body mass rather than age, bone mass may actually be normal. Girls or older women with Turner syndrome may have an increased incidence of fractures.

### HOMOCYSTINURIA

*Homocystinuria* refers to several disorders of methionine metabolism resulting in increased blood and urinary homocystine levels (see Chap 191). The prototype disorder, caused by cystathionine β-synthase deficiency, is commonly manifested by a dislocated lens and a consistent, marked osteoporosis that is most evident in the spine. Some of the skeletal abnormalities resemble those of Marfan syndrome, including kyphosis, scoliosis, pectus excavatum and carinatum, and arachnodactyly. Other features include mental retardation, seizures, malar flush, and vascular thromboses. The detection of homocysteine or homocystine in the urine by the cyanide-nitroprusside reaction is a useful diagnostic screening procedure. Management has included low methionine diets, large amounts of pyridoxine, and supportive management of complications.

### LYSINURIC PROTEIN INTOLERANCE

Osteopenia is an almost constant feature of lysinuric protein intolerance, which is an autosomal-recessive disorder of amino-acid transport. Episodic vomiting, anorexia, variable hepatomegaly, protein aversion, or unexplained osteopenia may bring the child to the physician's attention. Defective renal, intestinal, and hepatocellular transport of dibasic amino acids (ornithine, lysine, and arginine) cause limited urea cycle activity and episodic hyperammonemia. Characteristically, decreased levels of circulating dibasic amino acids and massive urinary excretion of lysine occur. Generalized aminoaciduria also may be present. Very marked elevations in serum lactate dehydrogenase may occur, as well as elevations in serum transaminases. Histomorphometric analysis of bone in one patient confirmed an osteoporotic process. Restricted protein intake probably accounts for the osteoporosis. Citrulline therapy has improved general well-being as well as the osteoporosis.

### MENKES KINKY HAIR SYNDROME

Menkes kinky hair syndrome is an X-linked disorder characterized by defective intestinal absorption and tissue accumulation of copper. Deficient copper-dependent enzymes result in abnormal hair, neuronal degeneration, and hypothermia. The osteoporosis is caused by defective collagen synthesis, resulting from the defective copper-dependent enzyme lysyl oxidase, which is required for normal cross-linking (also see Chap. 131).

### MALNUTRITION

Celiac disease, protein–calorie malnutrition, and copper deficiency may result in osteoporosis. Copper deficiency is thought to cause osteoporosis secondary to defective cross-linking of collagen.

### HYPERCORTISOLISM

Cushing syndrome, which is caused by an excess of endogenous glucocorticoids, may present as osteopenia, although other features of hypercortisolism are usually evident. The vitamin D metabolites 25-OHD and $1,25(OH)_2D$ have been proposed as therapeutic agents for steroid-induced osteoporosis, although use of the latter in adults resulted in a significant incidence of hypercalcemia. Biphosphate therapy may prove to be useful in this setting.

### LEUKEMIA

Leukemia may produce osteoporosis before abnormal cellular forms are evident in the peripheral circulation.

## OSTEOPENIA OF PREMATURITY

Osteopenia of prematurity is common in low-birth-weight infants, in whom it is difficult to provide, ex utero, the mineral requirements necessary for the rapidly growing and developing skeleton. Rickets or osteomalacia may be a significant factor in the bone disease of these patients. Human milk fortifiers have been developed to provide adequate mineral to counter this problem but are not without complications (see section on hypercalcemia).

## TOWARD A DEFINITIVE DIAGNOSIS

In the absence of evidence of primary osteomalacia or other systemic disease, determinations of serum copper, bicarbonate, uric acid, and serum and urine amino-acid levels and, occasionally, chromosomal analysis should be performed. A search for evidence of hyperadrenalism is undertaken if subtle cushingoid manifestations are present. If the child is severely affected or systemically ill, yet with no features of a specific disorder, a bone marrow aspiration may be necessary and could be performed during a bone biopsy procedure. Usually, no definitive diagnosis is evident, and one is left to distinguish between idiopathic juvenile osteoporosis and mild osteogenesis imperfecta. Analysis of collagen produced in skin samples obtained at biopsy may confirm a diagnosis of osteogenesis imperfecta. A definitive diagnosis is important in view of the potentially effective therapy with bisphosphonates described earlier.

## REFERENCES

1. Hillman LS, Haddad JG. Hypocalcemia and other abnormalities of mineral homeostasis during the neonatal period. In: Heath DA, Marx SJ, eds. Calcium disorders. Clinical endocrinology, Butterworths international medical reviews. London: Butterworths, 1982; 248.
2. Cole DEC, Carpenter TO, Goltzman D. Calcium homeostasis and disorders of bone and mineral metabolism. In: Collu R, ed. Pediatric endocrinology, comprehensive endocrinology series. New York: Raven Press, 1988; 509.
2a. Walton DM, Thomas DC, Aly HZ, Short BL. Morbid hypocalcemia associated with phosphate enema in a six-week-old infant. Pediatrics 2000; 106:E37.
3. Anast CS, David L. Human neonatal hypercalcemia. In: Holick MF, Anast CS, Gray TK, eds. Perinatal calcium and phosphorus metabolism. Amsterdam: Elsevier 1983; 363.
4. Marx SJ, Attie MF, Spiegel AM, et al. An association between severe primary hyperparathyroidism and familial hypocalciuric hypercalcemia in three kindreds. N Engl J Med 1982; 306:257.
5. Pollack MR, Chou Y-HW, Marx SJ, et al. Familial hypocalciuric hypocalcemia and neonatal severe hyperparathyroidism: effects of mutant gene dosage on phenotype. J Clin Invest 1994; 93:1108.
6. Cooper L, Wertheimer J, Levy R, et al. Severe primary hyperparathyroidism in a neonate who was the product of two related hypercalcemic parents managed by a parathyroidectomy and heterotopic autotransplantation. Pediatrics 1986; 78:263.
7. Harris SS, D'Ercole J. Neonatal hyperparathyroidism: the natural course in the absence of surgical intervention. Pediatrics 1989; 83:53.
8. Ewart AK, Morris CA, Atkinson D, et al. Hemizygosity at the elastin locus in a developmental disorder, Williams syndrome. Nat Genet 1993; 5:11.
9. Taylor AB, Stern PH, Bell NH. Abnormal regulation of circulating 25-hydroxyvitamin D in the Williams syndrome. N Engl J Med 1982; 306:972.
10. Goodyer PR, Frank A, Kaplan BS. Observations on the evolution and treatment of idiopathic infantile hypercalcemia. J Pediatr 1984; 105:771.
11. Garabedian M, Jacqz E, Guillozo H, et al. Elevated plasma 1,25-dihydroxyvitamin D concentrations in infants with hypercalcemia and an elfin facies. N Engl J Med 1985; 312:948.
12. Kruse K, Irle U, Uhlig R. Elevated 1,25-dihydroxyvitamin D serum concentrations in infants with subcutaneous fat necrosis. J Pediatr 1993; 122:460.
13. Clements MR, Johnson L, Fraser DR. A new mechanism for induced vitamin D deficiency in children. Nature 1987; 325:62.
14. Fu GK, Lin D, Zhang MY, et al. Cloning of human 25-hydroxyvitamin D-1α-hydroxylase and mutations causing vitamin D–dependent rickets type 1. Mol Endocrinol 1997; 11:1961.
15. Balsan S, Garabedian M, Larchet M, et al. Long-term nocturnal calcium infusions can cure rickets and promote normal mineralization in hereditary resistance to 1,25-dihydroxyvitamin D. J Clin Invest 1986; 77:1661.
16. Carpenter TO. New perspectives on the biology and treatment of X-linked hypophosphatemic rickets. Pediatr Clin North Am 1997; 44:443.
17. Whyte MP, Schranck FW, Armamento-Villareal R. X-linked hypophosphatemia: a search for gender, race, anticipation, or parent of origin effects on disease expression in children. J Clin Endocrinol Metab 1996; 81:4075.
18. Winters RW, Graham JB, Williams TF, et al. A genetic study of familial hypophosphatemia and vitamin D resistant rickets with a review of the literature. Medicine 1958; 37:97.
19. The HYP Consortium. A gene (PEX) with homologies to endopeptidases is mutated in patients with X-linked hypophosphatemia. Nat Genet 1995; 11:130.
20. Nesbitt T, Coffman TM, Griffiths R, et al. Cross transplantation of kidneys in normal and *Hyp* mice: evidence that the *Hyp* mouse phenotype is unrelated to an intrinsic renal defect. J Clin Invest 1992; 89:1453.
21. Meyer RA Jr, Meyer MH, Gray RW. Parabiosis suggests a humoral factor is involved in X-linked hypophosphatemia in mice. J Bone Miner Res 1989; 4:493.
22. Ecarot B, Glorieux FH, Desbarats M, et al. Effect of 1,25-dihydroxyvitamin D₃ treatment on bone formation by transplanted cells from normal and X-linked hypophosphatemic mice. J Bone Miner Res 1995; 10:424.
23. Carpenter TO, Gundberg CM. Osteocalcin abnormalities in *Hyp* mice reflect altered genetic expression and are not due to altered clearance, affinity for mineral, or ambient phosphorus levels. Endocrinology 1996; 137:5213.
24. Glorieux FH, Pierre JM, Pettifor JM, Delvin EE. Bone response to phosphate salts, ergocalciferol, and calcitriol in hypophosphatemic vitamin D–resistant rickets. N Engl J Med 1980; 303:1023.
25. Harrell RM, Lyles KW, Harrelson JM, et al. Healing of bone disease in X-linked hypophosphatemic rickets/osteomalacia. J Clin Invest 1985; 75:1858.
26. Carpenter TO, Mitnick MA, Ellison A, et al. Nocturnal hyperparathyroidism: a frequent feature of X-linked hypophosphatemia. J Clin Endocrinol Metab 1994; 78:1383.
27. Rivkees SA, El-Hajj-Fuleihan G, Brown EM, Crawford JD. Tertiary hyperparathyroidism during high phosphate therapy of familial hypophosphatemic rickets. J Clin Endocrinol Metab 1992; 75:1514.
28. Carpenter TO, Keller M, Schwartz D, et al. 24,25 Dihydroxyvitamin D supplementation corrects hyperparathyroidism and improves skeletal abnormalities in X-linked hypophosphatemic rickets—a clinical research center study. J Clin Endocrinol Metab 1996; 81:2381.
29. Sullivan W, Carpenter TO, Glorieux F, et al. A prospective trial of phosphate and 1,25 dihydroxyvitamin D₃ therapy in symptomatic adults with X-linked hypophosphatemic rickets. J Clin Endocrinol Metab 1992; 75:879.
30. Eddy MC, McAlister WH, Whyte MP. X-linked hypophosphatemia: normal renal function despite medullary nephrocalcinosis 25 years after transient vitamin D₂-induced renal azotemia. Bone 1997; 21:515.
31. Econs MJ, McEnery PT, Lennon F, Speer MC. Autosomal dominant hypophosphatemic rickets is linked to chromosome 12p13. J Clin Invest 1997; 100:2653.
32. O'Neill EM. Linear sebaceous naevus syndrome with oncogenic rickets and diffuse pulmonary angiomatosis. J R Soc Med 1993; 86:177.
33. Konishi K, Nakamura M, Yamakawa H, et al. Case report: hypophosphatemic osteomalacia in von Recklinghausen neurofibromatosis. Am J Med Sci 1991; 301(5):322.
34. Hahn SB, Lee SB, Kim DH. Albright's syndrome with hypophosphatemic rickets and hyperthyroidism: a case report. Yonsei Med J 1991; 32(2):179.
35. Chen C, Carpenter TO, Steg N, et al. Hypercalciuric hypophosphatemic rickets: mineral balance, bone histomorphometry, and therapeutic implications of hypercalciuria. Pediatrics 1989; 84:276.
36. Prockop DJ, Kivirikko KI. Collagens: molecular biology, diseases, and potentials for therapy. Ann Rev Biochem 1995; 64:403.
36a. Nuytinck L, Tutel T, Kayserili H, et al. Glycine to tryptophan substitution in type I collagen in a patient with OI type III: a unique collagen mutation. J Med Genet 2000; 37:371.
37. Wang Q, Orrison BM, Marini JC. Two additional cases of osteogenesis imperfecta with substitutions for glycine in the alpha 2(I) collagen chain. A regional model relating mutation location in phenotype. J Biol Chem 1993; 268(33):25162.
38. Glorieux F, Bishop NJ, Plotkin H, et al. Cyclic administration of pamidronate in children with severe osteogenesis imperfecta. N Engl J Med 1998; 349:947.
39. Shaw NJ, Boivin CM, Crabtree NJ. Intravenous pamidronate in juvenile osteoporosis. Arch Dis Child 2000; 83:143.

# PART V

# THE ADRENAL GLANDS

D. LYNN LORIAUX, EDITOR

# CHAPTER 71

# MORPHOLOGY OF THE ADRENAL CORTEX AND MEDULLA

## DONNA M. ARAB O'BRIEN

The adrenal glands are paired organs adjacent to the kidneys, containing a cortex and a medulla. These two divisions are best understood as functionally separate endocrine organs. This chapter reviews the embryology, anatomy, and histopathology of the adrenal cortex and medulla, emphasizing those aspects most relevant to clinical endocrinologists.[1-5]

## EMBRYOLOGY

The adrenal cortex and medulla arise from separate embryologic tissues (Fig. 71-1). Beginning in the fourth week of gestation, cells destined to form the adrenal cortex develop from primitive mesoderm just medial to the urogenital ridge. These cells penetrate the overlying retroperitoneal mesenchyme and, over the next several weeks, form a gradually enlarging adrenal cortex. During the sixth week of gestation, the developing cortex is penetrated by nerve fibers, along which primitive medullary cells will eventually migrate. By the eighth week, the cortex has formed two distinct zones: a relatively large and centrally located *fetal zone* and a thin rim of definitive cortex, which will later form the *adult adrenal cortex*. Throughout this period, proliferation is largely confined to the outer definitive cortex, suggesting that the same cells give rise to both the fetal and definitive zones. About this time, the fetal adrenal circulation is established, with several adrenal arteries arising from the descending aorta, and a central vein draining each adrenal gland. Between the second and third month of gestation, the adrenal glands increase in weight from about 5 to 80 mg, are much larger than the adjacent kidney, and reach their greatest size relative to total fetal weight. Growth of the adrenal cortex after the 20th week of gestation is dependent on pituitary stimulation (anencephalic fetuses are born with an atrophic adrenal fetal zone). After birth, the fetal zone involutes and the definitive cortex evolves into the three zones of the adult adrenal cortex (Fig. 71-2).

During fetal development, primitive adrenocortical cells may migrate widely. *Accessory adrenocortical rests* have been found adjacent to the celiac plexus, in the broad ligament, adjacent to ovarian or spermatic vessels, and around the kidney or uterus. Less common sites include the abdominal organs and, even more rarely, the lung, spinal nerves, or brain. These rests may be responsible for recurrent Cushing disease (see Chap. 75) after bilateral adrenalectomy and, rarely, for neoplastic transformation. Intratesticular or intraovarian adrenal rests represent a special problem because they may be difficult to distinguish from normal gonadal tissue. Such rests are rarely recognized in normal persons, but they may appear as gonadal enlargement in patients with Nelson syndrome or untreated congenital adrenal hyperplasia (CAH).

The adrenal medulla arises from primitive sympathetic nervous system cells (sympathogonia) derived from the neuroectoderm. These cells differentiate into neuroblasts, which migrate ventrally from the neural crest to form paravertebral and preaortic sympathetic ganglia, and into pheochromoblasts, which form catecholamine-secreting (chromaffin) cells (see Fig. 71-1). In the fetus, chromaffin cells are found not only in the adrenal medulla but also throughout the sympathetic chain. Similarly, neuroblast cell clusters often are present in the fetal adrenal medulla and involute after birth. A rudimentary adrenal medulla may be seen after the sixth week of gestation, but chromaffin cells continue to migrate to this location throughout the third month. After birth, extraadrenal chromaffin tissue generally involutes, although it may persist near the origin of the celiac and mesenteric arteries. The paired *organs of Zuckerkandl*, located near the inferior mesenteric artery and prominent in the first year of life, represent such extraadrenal catecholamine–secreting tissue. The widespread prenatal occurrence of extraadrenal chromaffin cells accounts for the location of extraadrenal pheochromocytomas later in life.

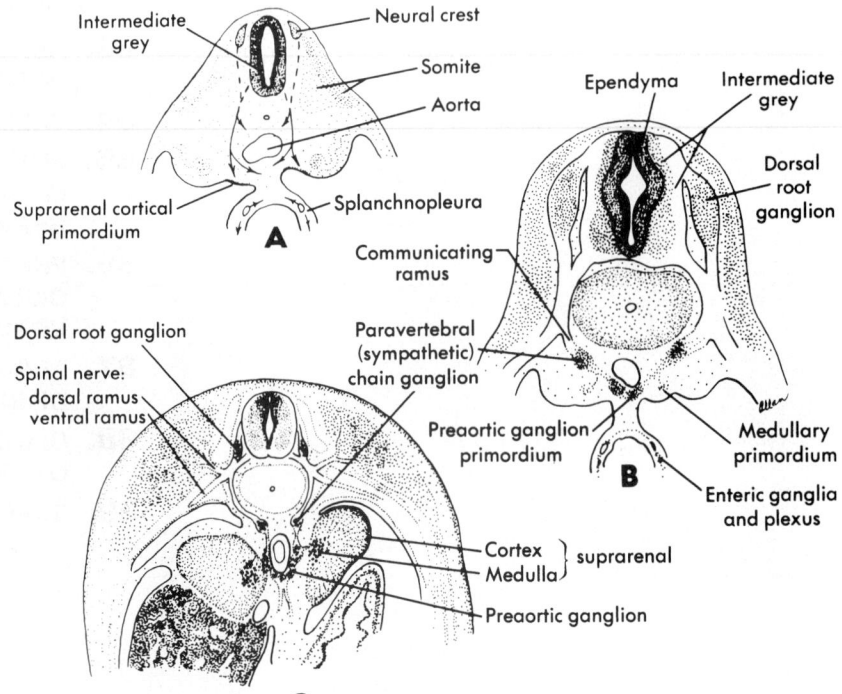

**FIGURE 71-1.** Formation of the human adrenal (suprarenal) gland and sympathetic ganglia. **A,** Migration of sympathetic ganglion and chromaffin cells from the neural crest and neural tube. **B,** The formation of the sympathetic ganglia. **C,** The chromaffin cells of the future suprarenal medulla reaching the provisional cortex. (From Allan FD. Essentials of human embryology, 2nd ed. New York: Oxford University Press, 1969.)

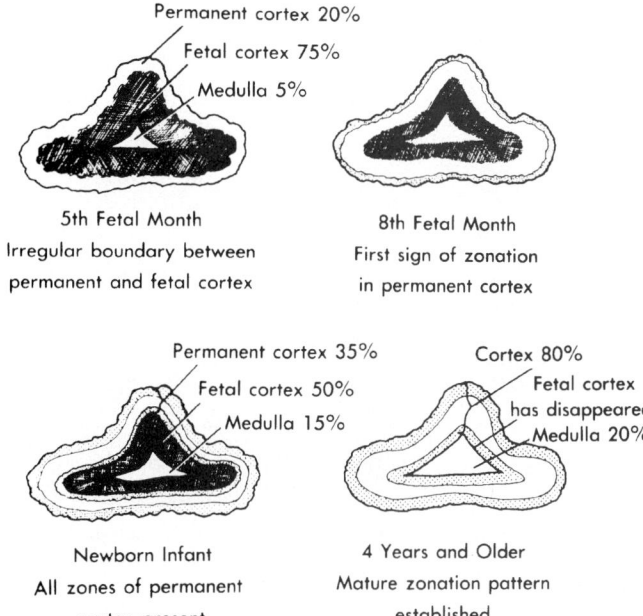

FIGURE 71-2. Internal development of the human suprarenal gland. The fetal cortex (*cross-hatched*) decreases in volume from the fifth fetal month to its complete disappearance in the first year of postnatal life. Zonation of the permanent cortex begins with the zona glomerulosa, indicated in the eighth fetal month; complete zonation is established by the fourth year of life. (From Gray SW. Embryology for surgeons. Philadelphia: WB Saunders, 1972:555; based on data from Sucheston ME, Cannon MS. Development of zonular patterns in the human adrenal gland. J Morphol 1968; 126:477.)

## ANATOMY

The adrenal glands are paired structures in the retroperitoneal space, lying anteromedial to the upper pole of the kidneys between the level of the 11th thoracic and the first lumbar vertebrae (Fig. 71-3). Although often abutting the kidneys, the adrenals in obese patients can be widely separated from the kidneys and other retroperitoneal organs by fat.

Normal adult adrenal glands average about 5.0 × 2.5 cm in length and width and are, at most, only about 0.6 cm thick. In cross-section, as seen with computerized imaging (see Chap. 88), the right gland is thickest centrally with two wings of tissue extending at each side, whereas the left gland often has a semilunar appearance. Each gland has a head, body, and tail. The head lies inferiorly, is the largest portion, and contains most of the medulla. The average weight of each gland is between 3 and 5 g, but this may increase by more than 50% during stress.

The adrenals are supplied by numerous small arteries arising from the celiac, superior mesenteric, inferior phrenic, renal, and iliac arteries and from the aorta. These arteries anastomose over the surface of the glands, with numerous smaller unbranched arteries descending through the capsule (Fig. 71-4). Blood supplying the adrenal medulla first traverses the cortex through capillary sinusoids. Adrenal blood flow is differentially regulated in the cortex and the medulla.[6] Nitric oxide is important for maintaining high basal levels of blood flow in both zones. Blood flow in the medulla is neurally regulated and correlates with catecholamine secretion. In the cortex, blood flow is not as closely linked to cortical secretory activity, although in many models, increased cortical blood flow is associated with increased adrenal steroid secretion.

The adrenal blood empties through a single central vein, which is surrounded by a cuff of normal adrenocortical tissue as it passes through the medulla. The adrenal vein enters the infe-

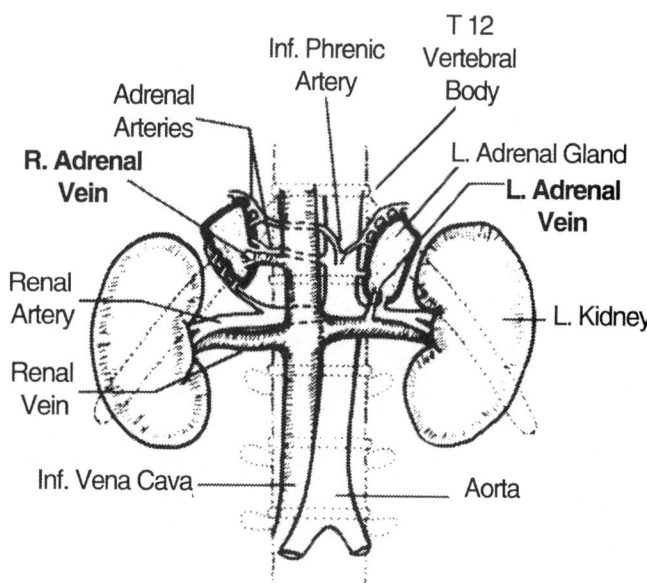

FIGURE 71-3. Normal adrenal anatomy. Both adrenal glands are supplied by multiple small arteries. The right adrenal vein empties directly into the vena cava, whereas the left adrenal vein enters the left renal vein.

rior vena cava on the right and the renal vein on the left. The acute angle between the right adrenal vein and the vena cava often makes catheterization of this vessel technically difficult.

## HISTOPATHOLOGY OF THE ADRENAL CORTEX

### NORMAL HISTOLOGY

The adult adrenal cortex includes the outer 80% of the adrenal glands and a cuff of cortex surrounding the central vein. Three

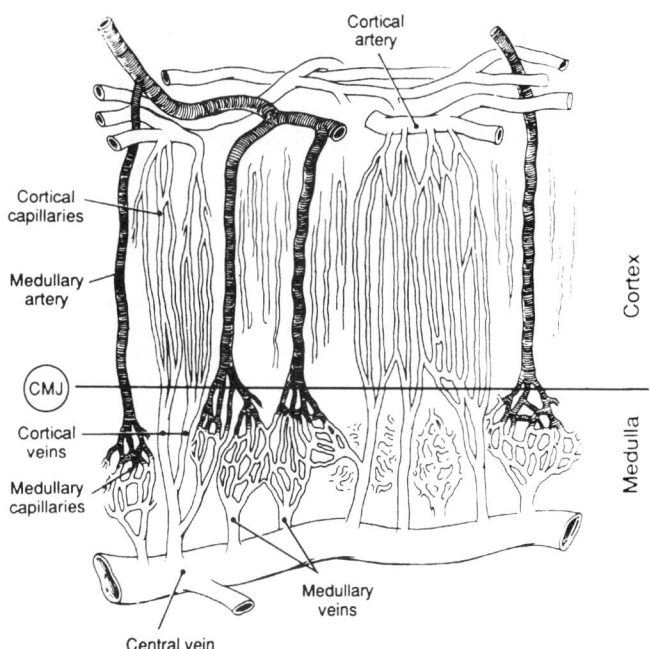

FIGURE 71-4. The adrenal vasculature showing distinct arteries supplying medulla and cortex. Note transition of cortical capillaries into veins at the corticomedullary junction (*CMJ*). (From Breslow MJ. Regulation of adrenal medullary and cortical blood flow. Am J Physiol 1992; 262:H1317.)

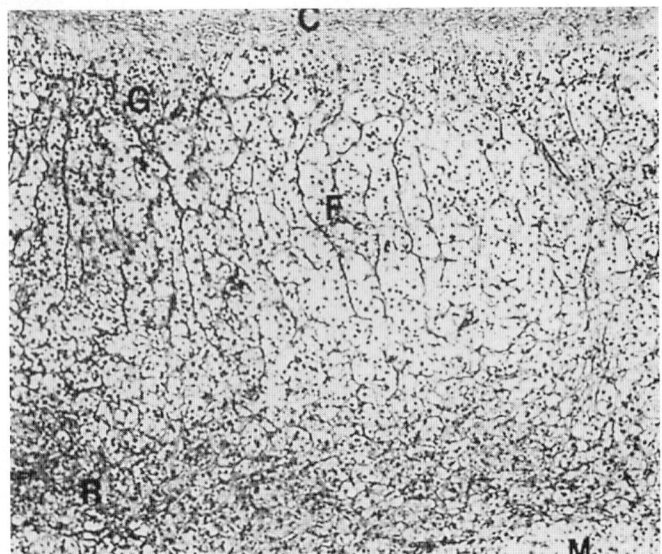

**FIGURE 71-5.** Histologic features of the normal adrenal cortex. Zona glomerulosa cells (*G*) are distributed focally beneath the capsule (*C*). Clear cells of the zona fasciculata (*F*) are arranged in columns between the cortex (or glomerulosa) and the inner compact cells of the zona reticularis (*R*). A small area of adrenal medulla can be seen at the lower right (*M*). (From Neville AM, O'Hare MJ. The human adrenal cortex. Pathology and biology—an integrated approach. New York: Springer-Verlag, 1982:20.)

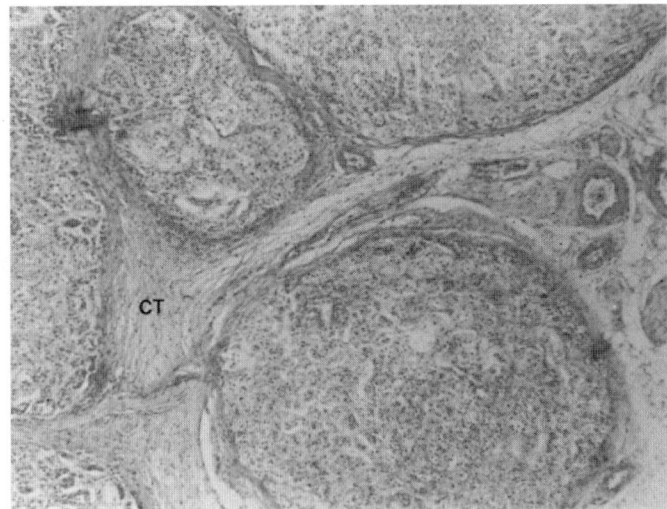

**FIGURE 71-6.** Adrenal nodules. Multiple nodules are shown, separated by fibrovascular connective tissue (*CT*). Normal cortical architecture is totally disrupted. (Courtesy of Dr. Stephen Boudreau.)

functional zones are present: glomerulosa, fasciculata, and reticularis (Fig. 71-5). The zona glomerulosa is responsible for aldosterone secretion and constitutes about 5% of the cortex. It is a discontinuous layer of nests of cells beneath the adrenal capsule. These cells are small, with a dense nucleus, a high nuclear/cytoplasmic ratio, and relatively low cytoplasmic lipid content. On electron microscopic examination, there are elongate mitochondria with abundant tubular cristae, a small amount of smooth endoplasmic reticulum (SER), and few lysosomes and microvilli.

Functionally, the zonae fasciculata and reticularis form a unit, with both cell types having the capacity to secrete cortisol and androgens. Histologically, however, they are distinct. The zona fasciculata makes up about 70% of the adrenal cortex and consists of columns of cells extending from the inner reticularis zone to the glomerulosa (or to the capsule where the glomerulosa is absent). The cells are large, with a low nuclear/cytoplasmic ratio and abundant cytoplasmic lipid. During fixation, the lipid is removed, giving the cells a vacuolated appearance and hence the name *clear cells*. On electron microscopic examination, the cells form a continuum: from the outer zone, in which the cells have ovoid mitochondria with few internal vesicles, little SER, and few lysosomes, to the inner zone, in which the cells contain spherical mitochondria with numerous internal vesicles, more SER, and more lysosomes.

The zona reticularis comprises the inner 25% of the adrenal cortex. It consists of anastomosing columns of cells that vary widely in size and contain densely granular cytoplasm and sparse lipid (hence, the name *compact cells*). The nuclear/cytoplasmic ratio is intermediate to that between cells of the glomerulosa and cells of the fasciculata. Electron microscopic examination reveals ovoid to elongate mitochondria with tubular to vesicular cristae, abundant SER, and numerous lysosomes. In older persons, an increasing amount of lipofuscin may be seen, which imparts a darker color to these cells.

The reason for functional zonation of the adrenal cortex has been a matter of considerable debate. Embryologic evidence

suggests that all cortical cells arise from the same precursor. Although cells from each of the three zones initially have distinct steroid secretory patterns in vitro, long-term cultures demonstrate that the histologic and functional distinctions between these cells disappear.[2] The blood supply to the adrenal glands flows inwardly from the capsule. This creates a gradient of increasing steroid hormone concentration from the outer to the inner cortex. Intraadrenal steroid concentrations may modulate the relative activities of the steroidogenic enzymes.[7-9] Such hormone gradients, which likely increase with increasing adrenal size, may explain not only the functional zonation of the adrenal cortex but also the development of the reticularis zone during adrenarche.

Electron microscopy has been useful in differentiating among cortical cell types, demonstrating transitional cells between the three zones of the adrenal cortex. It has not been useful, however, in elucidating pathologic changes in the adrenal cortex or in making the difficult distinction between benign and malignant neoplasms.

## PATHOLOGY

### ADRENAL NODULES: THE ADRENAL RESPONSE TO AGING

With advancing age, the adrenal glands of most persons begin to show microscopic nodular changes within the cortex. These changes begin as nests of clear cells located peripherally in the cortex or in cortical tissue surrounding the central vein. Larger nodules compress the adjacent cortex and eventually distort the adrenal capsule. They may contain foci of compact cells and areas of fibrosis, hemorrhage, and cyst formation (Fig. 71-6). These "yellow nodules" have been recognized in 3% of normotensive research subjects and may reach 2 to 3 cm in diameter. Their incidence appears to increase not only with age but also with the presence of vascular damage, as is seen with hypertension and diabetes. Pigmented ("black") nodules seen at autopsy appear to represent a variant of yellow nodules and contain compact (zona reticularis–like) cells with increased amounts of lipofuscin.

These nodules are not neoplasms and, although they produce steroids in vitro, are not associated with adrenocortical hyperfunction. The unaffected cortex remains normal in appearance. Their main significance lies in their incidental detection on radiologic imaging. In the absence of clinical or biochemical evidence of hormonal hypersecretion, small asymptomatic adrenal nodules seen incidentally during abdominal imaging procedures are unlikely to represent clinically significant pathologic entities.[10]

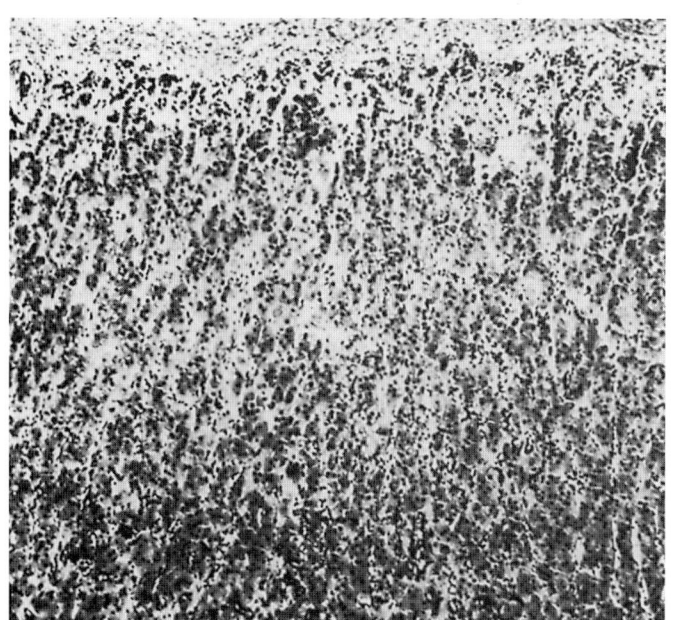

**FIGURE 71-7.** Effect of stress on the adrenal cortex. Columns of compact cells have totally replaced the clear cells of the normal zona fasciculata. (From Neville AM, O'Hare MJ. Histopathology of the adrenal cortex. J Clin Endocrinol Metab 1985; 14:791.)

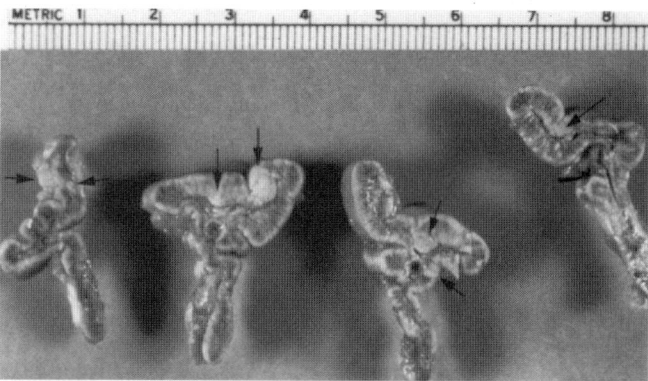

**FIGURE 71-8.** Bilateral nodular hyperplasia with cortical nodules. The adrenal glands from this patient with Cushing disease demonstrate a hyperplastic cortex (dark areas beneath the light-colored capsule) containing multiple small light-colored nodules (*arrows*). (Courtesy of Dr. Stephen Boudreau.)

## ADRENOCORTICAL HYPERFUNCTION

**Response to Stress.** Adrenal glands examined at autopsies after prolonged illnesses have mean weights of about 6 g and may weigh as much as 9 g. This appears to be the result of prolonged corticotropin (ACTH) stimulation. Histologically, within several hours of ACTH stimulation, clear (fasciculata) cells at the fasciculata-reticularis junction begin to lose their lipid content and take on the light-microscopic and ultrastructural appearance of compact (reticularis) cells (Fig. 71-7). Eventually, this "lipid depletion" may involve the entire fasciculata, and compact cells may extend from the medulla to the glomerulosa or adrenal capsule.

**Corticotropin-Dependent Cushing Syndrome.** Corticotropin-dependent Cushing syndrome includes both pituitary hypersecretion of ACTH (Cushing disease) and paraneoplastic (ectopic) ACTH secretion from a benign or malignant neoplasm. The pathologic changes in the adrenal glands form a continuum from the mild stress-induced changes to the extreme changes resulting from severe, prolonged ACTH hypersecretion commonly seen with the paraneoplastic ACTH syndrome. Cushing disease accounts for about 60% of endogenous (noniatrogenic) Cushing syndrome in adults and ~35% in children (see Chaps. 14, 75, and 83). The ACTH hypersecretion is generally mild but often prolonged. The adrenal glands are usually enlarged, each weighing 6 to 12 g. The cortex is widened, with a broadened zone of compact cells, suggesting a hyperplastic zona reticularis. Some of the reticularis may be replaced by lipid. The clear cells often are larger than normal, with increased lipid content. The zona glomerulosa is normal. Cortical micronodules, consisting of clusters of clear cells, also may be seen in the periphery or around the central vein (Fig. 71-8). The only difference between these micronodules and those seen with aging is that the remainder of the cortex is hyperplastic.

With prolonged ACTH stimulation, macronodular hyperplasia may occur. Clinically, this is seen as unilateral or bilateral nodules in bilaterally hyperplastic adrenal glands in patients with long-standing Cushing disease.[11] Each nodule-containing gland usually weighs between 12 and 20 g, although much larger glands are possible. The nodules have macroscopic and microscopic features similar to those of the nodules seen with aging. The remainder of the cortex is hyperplastic. Although adrenal glands with macronodular hyperplasia are not capable of prolonged cortisol secretion without ACTH, there is evidence that such glands have limited autonomy compared with glands with bilateral hyperplasia that do not have nodules (see Chap. 75).

Paraneoplastic ACTH secretion accounts for ~15% of endogenous Cushing syndrome in adults. The ACTH levels range from normal to greatly increased. Because of the natural history of the underlying tumor, the duration of disease is often brief (see Chap. 219). The adrenal glands frequently are markedly enlarged, weighing from 12 g to more than 20 g, but nodules usually are not present. Microscopically, columns of hypertrophic compact cells extend from the medulla to the glomerulosa or capsule. Foci of clear cells may be seen capping the compact cell columns.

**Corticotropin-Independent Cushing Syndrome.** The category of ACTH-independent Cushing syndrome includes cortisol-secreting adrenocortical neoplasms, micronodular adrenal disease (which is seen in children and young adults), and drug-induced Cushing syndrome (which induces adrenocortical atrophy; see Chap. 75). Benign cortisol-secreting adenomas account for 10% to 15% of cases of endogenous Cushing syndrome. These tumors usually are small (<50 g). Functionally, they tend to present a pure picture of glucocorticoid excess, with little or no androgen production. Gross and microscopic appearances resemble adrenal nodules, with the important exception that the noninvolved adrenal cortex is atrophic with cortisol-secreting tumors. Most adenomas contain both clear and compact cells in various proportions, although clear cells generally predominate. Necrosis is uncommon in adrenal adenomas, presumably because of their small size.

Cortisol-secreting adrenal carcinomas account for ~10% of cases of endogenous Cushing syndrome in adults but represent nearly 50% of these cases in children. Adrenocortical carcinomas are inefficient hormone producers, usually weigh more than 100 g, and may exceed 1000 g by the time they become clinically apparent. Adrenal carcinomas produce multiple hormones, and the mixed clinical presentation of Cushing syndrome and virilization, with markedly elevated serum levels of testosterone and dehydroepiandrosterone sulfate, is common. These characteristics often suggest to the clinician the malignant nature of an adrenal neoplasm, even when metastases are absent. Nevertheless, benign and malignant adrenocortical neoplasms may be difficult to distinguish. On gross examination, areas of necrosis, hemorrhage, or calcification are common with adrenal carcinoma, but these features appear to be related more to the size of the tumor than to its malignant potential.

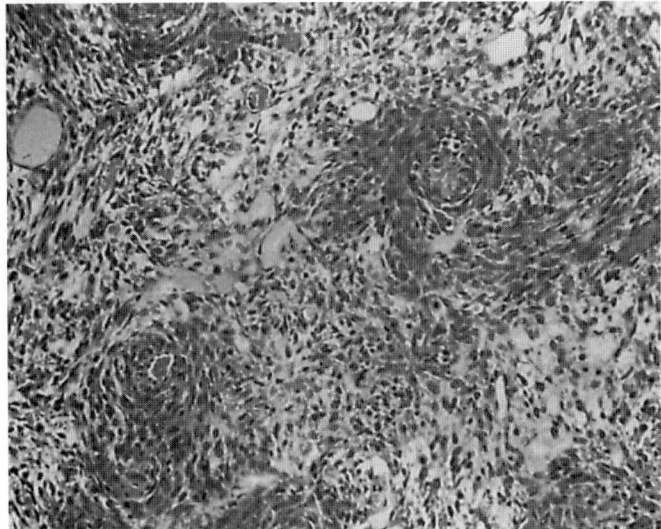

**FIGURE 71-9.** Adrenal carcinoma. Marked cellular pleomorphism and atypia are seen in this clearly malignant neoplasm. (Courtesy of Dr. Stephen Boudreau.)

When satellite lesions, metastases, capsular penetration, or vascular invasion are present, the malignant nature of these lesions is confirmed. Often, however, none of these features is evident. Similarly, whereas compact cells often predominate in carcinomas, the cellular morphology and the degree of cellular atypia overlaps with benign tumors (Fig. 71-9). Electron microscopy also is not useful in making the distinction between benign and malignant lesions. Adrenal carcinomas metastasize most commonly to local lymph nodes, peritoneum, lung, and liver, and less commonly to bone, pleura, mediastinum, brain, and kidney.

Micronodular adrenal disease is a rare form of Cushing syndrome seen almost exclusively in children and young adults. It occurs either as an isolated entity or in combination with other abnormalities, such as cardiac and cutaneous myxomas and a variety of pigmented skin lesions.[12] The adrenal glands range from small to slightly enlarged for age. Although they have a diffusely nodular appearance on gross examination, the nodules are usually too small (<3 mm) to be apparent on radiographs. In infancy, nodular hyperplasia of the definitive and fetal zones may be seen, whereas in later childhood, the intracortical nodules consist largely of compact cells. The nonnodular adrenal cortex has been described as atrophic[12,13] or normal[1]; however, ACTH levels are undetectable and the hypercortisolism is not suppressed by dexamethasone. Although the cause is unknown, these characteristics suggest that micronodular adrenal disease represents a primary adrenal disorder.

**Virilizing and Feminizing Adrenal Syndromes.** The virilizing and feminizing adrenal syndromes include sex hormone–producing adrenal neoplasms and CAH (see Chaps. 75 and 77). Virilizing and feminizing adrenal tumors are rare. They are recognized most frequently in children and young adults, although they can occur at any age. They also may present with signs of hypercortisolism or hyperaldosteronism. As with cortisol-producing neoplasms, the larger tumors (>200 g) are more likely to be malignant, whereas those weighing <70 g usually are benign. Considerable overlap exists, however. The cells of small sex hormone–secreting neoplasms consist almost exclusively of compact cells, resembling those of normal zona reticularis. With increasing size, greater cellular atypia occurs, as well as a higher frequency of hemorrhage, necrosis, and calcification. Although certain tumors can be classified as benign or malignant based on extremes of cellular morphology, the degree of cellular and nuclear pleomorphism overlaps in benign and malignant sex hormone–producing neoplasms.

The pattern of androgen secretion by an adrenal neoplasm depends on the relative enzyme activities within the tumor. Adenomas often are relatively deficient in 17,20-lyase (desmolase) activity, resulting in diminished androgen secretion relative to cortisol. Adrenal carcinomas frequently have diminished 3β-hydroxysteroid dehydrogenase activity, resulting in diminished cortisol and mineralocorticoid secretion and enhanced secretion of androgen precursors. These patterns of enzyme activity explain the association of virilization with adrenal carcinomas.[14]

The CAHs are all characterized by defects in cortisol synthesis, causing ACTH hypersecretion. In untreated patients, the adrenal glands are variably enlarged, depending on the degree of enzyme deficiency and the age of the patient. In adults with 21-hydroxylase deficiency, individual glands weighing more than 30 g have been found. The adrenal glands are multinodular with diffuse cortical hyperplasia. The cortex is widened and convoluted, consisting almost entirely of compact cells. Hyperplasia of the zona glomerulosa usually is present in patients with coexistent mineralocorticoid deficiency. The adrenal abnormalities in some of the rarer, nonlethal forms of CAH (such as 17-hydroxylase deficiency) have not been described but are likely to be similar. Adrenal glands from patients with a deficiency of the cholesterol side chain cleavage enzyme, however, demonstrate cortical hyperplasia with exclusively clear, lipid-laden cells (*congenital lipoid hyperplasia*). This feature is consistent with the inability of the adrenal glands to mobilize cholesterol for the synthesis of steroid hormones.

**Primary Hyperaldosteronism.** Although primary hyperaldosteronism includes several syndromes, pathologically these patients can be divided into those who harbor solitary adenomas (or, rarely, carcinoma) and those who have only diffuse hyperplasia. Complicating the pathologic presentation is that hypertension alone is associated with an increased frequency of nonfunctional adrenal nodule formation and that true functional adenomas also may be associated with diffuse (nodular or nonnodular) hyperplasia of the zona glomerulosa. Because patients without an adenoma do not benefit from surgical therapy, it is crucial that the differential diagnosis of hyperaldosteronism be made on biochemical grounds.

Twenty percent to 50% of patients with primary hyperaldosteronism have bilateral hyperplasia as the cause of their mineralocorticoid excess (the variation in incidence depends, in part, on the criteria used to differentiate bilateral hyperplasia from low-renin essential hypertension; see Chap. 80). Most of the remaining patients have solitary adenomas. Multiple adenomas have been reported, but most of these cases, in retrospect, represented nodules. Malignant aldosterone-secreting neoplasms are rare and do not differ in size or behavior from other adrenocortical carcinomas.

Aldosterone-secreting adenomas usually weigh <10 g, and fewer than 10% weigh >20 g. They have a characteristic golden yellow cut surface, which allows them to be differentiated macroscopically from other hormone-secreting adenomas. The cellular morphology of these adenomas also is distinct, with large and small clear cells, compact cells, and glomerulosa cells being present to varying degrees in the same adenoma (Fig. 71-10). Some investigators feel that this variability may be related to the influence of local microvasculature and corticosteroid concentrations on cellular structure, analogous to that which occurs in the normal adrenal cortex.[1] Surprisingly, the uninvolved cortex in patients with aldosterone-secreting adenomas demonstrates hyperplasia of the zona glomerulosa. The glomerulosa may surround the entire cortex and is increased in width. Moreover, clear-cell nodules as large as 3 cm in diameter, similar to those generally seen in patients with hypertension, may be present throughout the cortex. Removal of the adenoma results in correction of the hyperaldosteronism, which suggests that the morphologically hyperplastic zona glomerulosa does not contribute to the pathologic condition.

The adrenal morphology in patients with hyperaldosteronism and bilateral hyperplasia (without an adenoma) does not

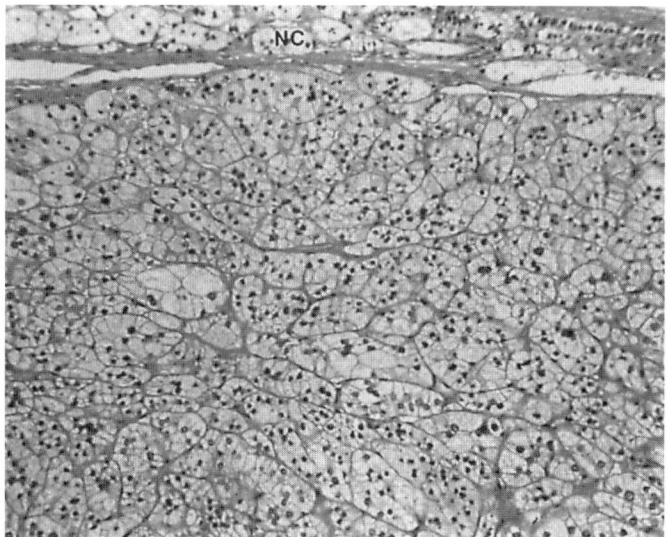

**FIGURE 71-10.** Aldosterone-secreting adenoma. Lipid-laden clear cells are arranged in nests and cords. A compressed rim of normal cortex (*NC*) can be seen at the top of the photograph. (Courtesy of Dr. Stephen Boudreau.)

differ from that described in patients with adenomas, except that the aldosterone-secreting tumor is not present. The adrenals usually are normal to moderately increased in size. Often, the cortex appears micronodular, although macronodules may be present and may cause confusion radiologically with aldosterone-secreting adenomas. Similar findings are noted in patients with secondary hyperaldosteronism. Hypertension generally is not corrected by bilateral adrenalectomy in these patients, which suggests that the morphologic changes are related to the hypertension.

## NONSECRETORY ADRENAL TUMORS

*Nonsecretory adrenal adenomas* produce no symptoms and have the same clinical relevance as adrenal nodules. *Nonfunctioning adrenal carcinomas* are similar to hormone-producing adrenocortical carcinomas except that they are often detected even later. They usually secrete inactive steroid hormone precursors and thus are not truly "nonfunctioning." They have a poor prognosis, similar to that of the cortisol-secreting adrenal carcinomas.

*Myelolipomas* are uncommon benign adrenocortical tumors that usually occur in older persons.[15] They generally are <2 cm in diameter but have been reported as large as 34 cm in diameter. Myelolipomas contain varying amounts of adipose and bone marrow cells. They present mainly in the differential diagnosis of incidental, nonsecretory adrenal masses, although larger ones may be associated with pain, abdominal fullness, or hematuria.

## ADRENOCORTICAL HYPOFUNCTION

**Secondary Adrenal Insufficiency (Corticotropin Deficiency).** Secondary adrenal insufficiency includes hypopituitarism and drug-induced (iatrogenic) Cushing syndrome. Both conditions result in adrenal atrophy, the extent of which is dependent on the degree of ACTH deficiency. The adrenal glands are decreased in size. The cortex is thinned and consists of a normal zona glomerulosa; a decreased, but otherwise normal-appearing zona fasciculata; and an absent zona reticularis. When this condition is present at birth, the definitive zone is relatively normal but the fetal zone is greatly diminished in width.

**Primary Adrenal Insufficiency.** The two principal causes of Addison disease are autoimmune adrenalitis and adrenal tuberculosis (see Chap. 76). Adrenal hemorrhage, acquired immunodeficiency syndrome, and metastatic cancer uncommonly cause sufficient adrenocortical damage to result in adrenal insufficiency. Systemic fungal infections, sarcoidosis, amyloidosis, neonatal and sex-linked adrenoleukodystrophy, and congenital adrenal hypoplasia are much less common causes.[16,17]

The adrenal glands in autoimmune adrenalitis are mildly to markedly reduced in size. The cortex is thinned and may be absent. The remaining cortical cells usually resemble those of the zona reticularis. Hypertrophied cells and micronodules also may be found. Often, a diffuse mononuclear cell infiltrate is present. The medulla is histologically normal.

The adrenal glands in tuberculous adrenalitis are as much as fourfold enlarged. The adrenals may be adherent to surrounding tissues and, in acute cases, are replaced by a caseous semisolid exudate. The normal cellular architecture is destroyed, and caseous necrosis is present throughout the glands. A lymphocytic and giant-cell infiltrate usually is present in the acute stage. Tuberculous bacilli can be seen in about half the acute cases. Fibrosis and calcium deposition are present in varying amounts, depending on the duration of the destructive process (see Chap. 213).

Clinically significant adrenal hemorrhage generally occurs in the setting of hypotension, severe illness, or systemic anticoagulation.[18–20] Although adrenal hemorrhage is present in about 1% of subjects at autopsy, this is often microscopic and not associated with adrenal insufficiency. At the other extreme, extensive retroperitoneal bleeding may result from adrenal hemorrhage. Pathologically, the hemorrhage often appears to start in the medulla, with the hematoma extending outward into the cortex. Large hematomas cause capsular rupture and a retroperitoneal mass. Although areas of necrosis usually accompany the bleeding, extensive cortical destruction must occur before adrenal insufficiency results. Areas of calcification within the adrenal glands may be seen in patients who survive.

Adrenal insufficiency has been described but is uncommon in patients with human immunodeficiency virus infection.[21] Despite higher than normal plasma ACTH levels, basal and stimulated cortisol and aldosterone concentrations and plasma renin activity are normal in most patients with the acquired immunodeficiency syndrome.[22] At autopsy, a necrotizing adrenalitis has been found to be associated with cytomegalovirus infection. The hemorrhage and necrosis are most prominent in the medulla, although the cortex also may be involved.

# HISTOPATHOLOGY OF THE ADRENAL MEDULLA

## NORMAL HISTOLOGY

The medulla is located primarily in the head of the adrenal glands and accounts for ~10% of their normal adult weight. The chromaffin cell is the major cell type, named for the yellow-brown color imparted to its epinephrine-containing granules by chromatic salts. Chromaffin cells are rounded or polygonal, with a finely granular cytoplasm and an eccentric nucleus with prominent nucleoli. The cells are arranged in nests or cords. They are surrounded and directly innervated by preganglionic sympathetic nerve fibers and hence are analogous to norepinephrine-secreting postganglionic fibers in the remainder of the sympathetic nervous system. When specific immunostains are used, chromaffin cells have been found in the human adrenal cortex and cortical cells have been found in the adrenal medulla, which provides a cellular basis for potential intraadrenal interactions.[23] The medullary blood supply is derived mainly from the capillary plexus draining the cortex. The resulting high intramedullary cortisol levels are thought to be important in inducing the enzyme that converts norepinephrine to epinephrine in the chromaffin cells.

## ADRENAL MEDULLARY HYPERFUNCTION

Adrenal medullary hyperfunctional states include adrenal medullary hyperplasia, neuroblastoma, and pheochromocytoma.

There is a close relationship between neural cells of the sympathetic ganglia and chromaffin cells. Small numbers of ganglion cells can be found in the adrenal medulla, and chromaffin cells occur in the sympathetic ganglia. Hence, neoplastic disorders affecting either cell type can arise throughout this system.

The diagnosis of adrenal medullary hyperplasia depends on an increased volume of adrenal medulla in relation to the cortex. There is a diffuse nodular proliferation of normal medullary elements. This condition is seen mainly in families with multiple endocrine neoplasia type 2A and is considered a preneoplastic condition (see Chap. 188).

Neuroblastomas, ganglioneuroblastomas, and ganglioneuromas arise from neuroblasts. These tumors form a continuum from least to most differentiated and from malignant to benign. Neuroblastoma usually is a tumor of infancy and childhood, with a median incidence at the age of 2 years. It originates in the paraganglia of the sympathetic nervous system or the adrenal medulla, and 60% arise in the abdomen. Grossly, it is a multinodular tumor with areas of hemorrhage, necrosis, and cystic degeneration.[24] The cells are arranged in nests and contain small, dark-staining nuclei with little cytoplasm. Although the light-microscopic features are not necessarily distinct from those of other childhood tumors, electron microscopic examination shows characteristic cytoplasmic neurosecretory granules. Neuroblastomas usually secrete catecholamines, their metabolites, or both. Characteristically, these tumors grow rapidly and metastasize early to local lymph nodes, the liver and other abdominal organs, and bone. Although spontaneous regression or differentiation into a more benign tumor may occur, mortality is high and treatment often includes combinations of palliative surgery, radiation, and chemotherapy.[25] Ganglioneuroblastomas contain some mature ganglion cells and have a better prognosis. Ganglioneuromas are benign tumors arising from mature neuronal elements.[26,27]

Pheochromocytomas arise from chromaffin cells. As expected from their cellular origin, 95% or more are in the abdomen, with most being in the adrenal glands.[28] Similar to chromaffin cells, however, they occasionally can be found anywhere along the sympathetic chain of ganglia from the base of the skull to the neck of the urinary bladder. Ten percent of patients with sporadic pheochromocytomas and 50% of those with familial pheochromocytomas have bilateral tumors. The pheochromocytoma that may occur in von Hippel-Lindau disease commonly is bilateral.[29,30] Although only 5% to 10% are malignant, it is often impossible to distinguish benign from malignant neoplasms histologically. Pheochromocytomas are highly vascular tumors with local hemorrhage and cystic degeneration. Microscopically, they often have a chaotic pattern of pleomorphic elongated cells with prominent cytoplasmic granules (see Chap. 86). Although the light-microscopic features may not be diagnostic, electron microscopic examination demonstrates characteristic dense catecholamine secretory granules.

## ADRENAL MEDULLARY HYPOFUNCTION

The adrenal medulla is affected by the same systemic diseases (tubercular and fungal infections, sarcoidosis, amyloidosis) as is the cortex and also is often the initial site of hemorrhage. Isolated adrenal medullary hypofunction is uncommon and usually occurs in the setting of diffuse autonomic insufficiency. Sparse amounts of medullary tissue may be found in some elderly persons, but no specific abnormality has been described.

## REFERENCES

1. Neville AM, O'Hare MJ. Histopathology of the adrenal cortex. J Clin Endocrinol Metab 1985; 14:791.
2. Neville AM, O'Hare MJ. The human adrenal cortex. Pathology and biology—an integrated approach. New York: Springer-Verlag, 1982.
3. Symington T. The adrenal cortex. In: Bloodworth JMB Jr, ed. Endocrine pathology. General and surgical. Baltimore: Williams & Wilkins, 1982:419.
4. Gould VE, Sommers SC. Adrenal medulla and paraganglia. In: Bloodworth JMB Jr, ed. Endocrine pathology. General and surgical. Baltimore: Williams & Wilkins, 1982:473.
5. Francis IR, Gross MD, Shapiro B, et al. Integrated imaging of adrenal disease. Radiology 1992; 184:1.
6. Breslow MJ. Regulation of adrenal medullary and cortical blood flow. Am J Physiol 1992; 262:H1317.
7. Hornsby PJ. Regulation of adrenocortical function by control of growth and structure. In: Anderson DC, Winter JSD, eds. Adrenal cortex: BIMR clinical endocrinology. Boston: Butterworth, 1985:1.
8. Hyatt PJ. Functional significance of the adrenal zones. In: D'Agata R, Chrousos GP, eds. Recent advances in adrenal regulation and function. New York: Raven Press, 1987:35.
9. Winter JSD. Functional changes in the adrenal gland during life. In: D'Agata R, Chrousos GP, eds. Recent advances in adrenal regulation and function. New York: Raven Press, 1987:51.
10. Copeland PM. The incidentally discovered adrenal mass. Ann Intern Med 1983; 98:940.
11. Doppman JL, Miller DL, Dryer AJ, et al. Macronodular adrenal hyperplasia in Cushing's disease. Radiology 1988; 166:347.
12. Carney JA, Young WF Jr. Primary pigmented nodular adrenocortical disease and its associated conditions. The Endocrinologist 1992; 2:6.
13. Ruder HJ, Loriaux DL, Lipsett MB. Severe osteopenia in young adults associated with Cushing's syndrome due to micronodular adrenal disease. J Clin Endocrinol Metab 1974; 39:1138.
14. Sakai Y, Yanase T, Hara T, et al. Mechanism of abnormal production of adrenal androgens in patients with adrenocortical adenomas and carcinomas. J Clin Endocrinol Metab 1994; 78:36.
15. Del Gaudio A, Solidoro G. Myelolipoma of the adrenal gland: report of two cases with a review of the literature. Surgery 1986; 90:293.
16. Kelley RI, Datta NS, Dobyns WB, et al. Neonatal adrenoleukodystrophy: new cases, biochemical studies, and differentiation from Zellweger and related peroxisomal polydystrophy syndromes. Am J Med Genet 1986; 23:869.
17. Schwartz RE, Stayer SA, Pasquariello CA, et al. Anesthesia for the patient with neonatal adrenoleukodystrophy. Can J Anaesth 1994; 41:56.
18. Xarli VP, Steele AA, Davis PJ, et al. Adrenal hemorrhage in the adult. Medicine (Baltimore) 1978; 57:211.
19. Rao RH, Vagnucci AH, Amico JA. Bilateral massive adrenal hemorrhage: early recognition and treatment. Ann Intern Med 1989; 110:227.
20. Caron P, Chabanier MH, Cambus JP, et al. Definitive adrenal insufficiency due to bilateral adrenal hemorrhage and primary antiphospholipid syndrome. J Clin Endocrinol Metab 1998; 83:1437.
21. Stolarczykk, Ruio SI, Smolyar D, et al. Twenty-four-hour urinary free cortisol in patients with acquired immunodeficiency syndrome. Metabolism 1998; 47:690.
22. Verges B, Chavanet P, Degres J, et al. Adrenal function in HIV infected patients. Acta Endocrinol (Copenh) 1989; 121:633.
23. Bornstein SR, Gonzalez-Hernandez JA, Erhart-Bornstein M, et al. Intimate contact of chromaffin and cortical cells within the human adrenal gland forms the basis for important intraadrenal interactions. J Clin Endocrinol Metab 1994; 78:225.
24. Askin FB, Perlman EJ. Neuroblastoma and peripheral neuroectodermal tumors. Am J Clin Pathol 1998; 109(4 Suppl 1):S23.
25. Katzenstein HM, Cohn SL. Advances in the diagnosis and treatment of neuroblastoma. Curr Opin Oncol 1998; 10:43.
26. Schulman H, Laufer L, Barki Y, et al. Ganglioneuroma: an 'incidentaloma' of childhood. Eur Radiol 1998; 8:582.
27. Fujiwara T, Kawamura M, Sasou S, Hiramori K. Results of surgery for a compound tumor consisting of pheochromocytoma and ganglioneuroblastoma in an adult; 5-year follow-up. Intern Med 2000; 39:58.
28. Meideiros LJ, Wolf BC, Balogh K, Federman M. Adrenal pheochromocytoma: a clinicopathologic review of 60 cases. Hum Pathol 1985; 16:580.
29. Chew SL, Dacie JE, Reznik RH, et al. Bilateral pheochromocytomas in von Hippel-Lindau disease. Q J Med 1994; 87:49.
30. Couch V, Lindor HM, Karnes PS, Michels VV. von Hippel-Lindau disease. Mayo Clin Proc 2000; 75:265.

# CHAPTER 72

# SYNTHESIS AND METABOLISM OF CORTICOSTEROIDS

PERRIN C. WHITE

The adrenal glands are endocrinologically complex organs that are composed of two distinct endocrine tissues derived from different embryologic sources[1] (see Chap. 71). The adrenal cortex (outer layer) constitutes 80% to 90% of the gland and is the

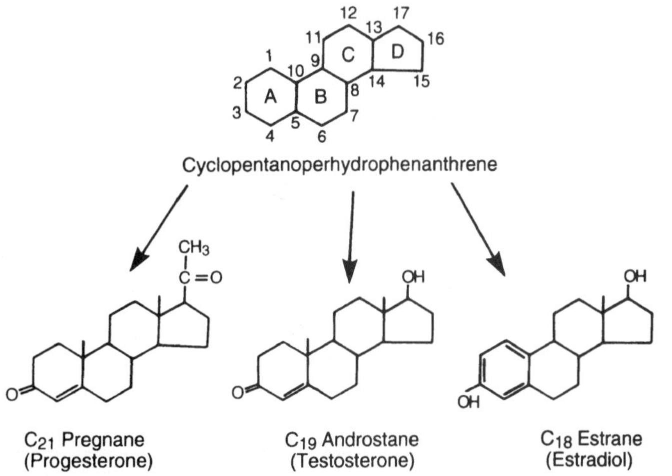

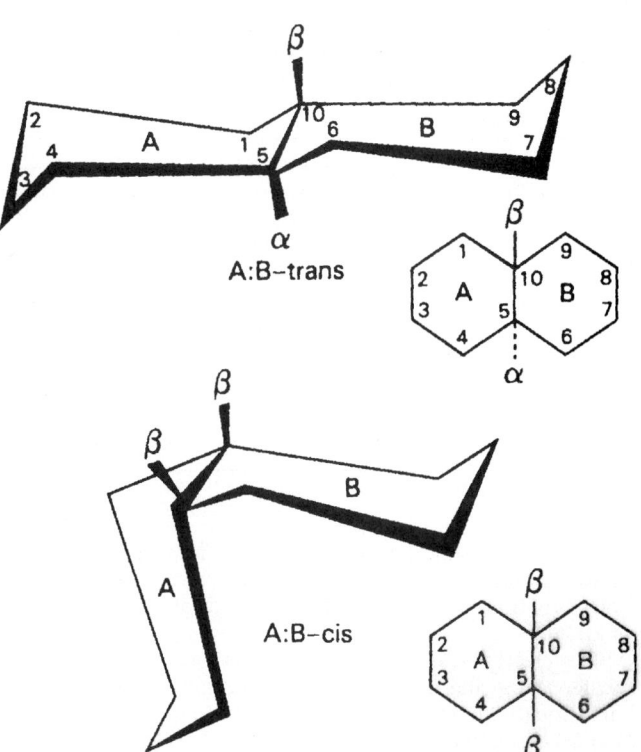

**FIGURE 72-1.** The steroid nucleus. The four rings are labeled *A, B, C, D,* and the carbons are numbered as shown. Examples are shown of steroids from each of the three structural categories of steroid hormones: the 21-carbon pregnane derivatives, the 19-carbon androstane derivatives, and the 18-carbon estrane derivatives. The names of the individual steroids shown are indicated in parentheses.

**FIGURE 72-2.** *Cis-trans* orientation of the steroid nucleus and location of the α- and β-substituents.

source of the steroid hormones, whereas the adrenal medulla is the source of catecholamines. Although the adrenal cortex and medulla are in close proximity, they function independently. This chapter describes the biosynthesis, metabolism, mechanisms of action, and regulation of the steroid products of the adrenal cortex.

Three major groups of hormones are produced by the adrenal cortex: *mineralocorticoids, glucocorticoids,* and *sex steroids.* Mineralocorticoids are produced primarily by the zona glomerulosa; glucocorticoids are produced by the zona fasciculata; and sex steroids originate primarily from the zona reticularis. The hormonal products of the adrenal cortex share cholesterol as a common precursor. Cholesterol is also the precursor for the gonadal steroids, vitamin D and derivatives, and the bile acids.

## STRUCTURE AND NOMENCLATURE

Steroids have a common structure with 17-carbon atoms arranged in three six-membered rings and a fourth five-membered ring labeled A, B, C, and D, respectively (Fig. 72-1). Each of the 17 carbons is numbered in a standard way. Two additional carbons, numbered 18 and 19, may be attached at carbons 13 and 10, respectively. Carbon atoms 20 and 21 may be attached at the 17 position. These various additions yield three steroid families: the $C_{18}$ *estranes* with an aromatic ring (estrogens); the $C_{19}$ *androstanes* (androgens); and the $C_{21}$ *pregnanes* (corticoids and progestins) (see Fig. 72-1). The steroid nucleus lies in a plane that can be modified by the addition of substituents either above or below (Fig. 72-2). The α-*substituents occur below the plane* (indicated by dotted lines in Fig. 72-2) and the β-*substituents lie above the plane* (indicated by solid lines). The A and B rings may be attached so that the substituents at positions 5 and 10 are in either the *cis* or *trans* orientations (see Fig. 72-2).

A multiplicity of *trivial* and *systematic* or *biochemical* names exist for each steroid (Table 72-1). Between 1930 and 1950, two groups under the direction of Reichstein and of Kendall isolated most of the naturally occurring steroids. Each group labeled steroids alphabetically in the order in which they were discovered, with the result that the same compound was sometimes given two different alphabetical designations. Thus, Kendall's compound A is not the same as Reichstein's compound A.

## BIOSYNTHESIS

### IMPORTATION INTO MITOCHONDRIA

The rate-limiting step in steroid biosynthesis is importation of cholesterol from cellular stores to the matrix side of the mitochondria inner membrane where the cholesterol side-chain cleavage system (CYP11A, adrenodoxin, adrenodoxin reductase) is located. This is controlled by the *steroidogenic acute regulatory protein (StAR),*[2,2a] the synthesis of which is increased within minutes by trophic stimuli such as adrenocorticotropic hormone (ACTH) or, in the zona glomerulosa, by increased intracellular calcium. StAR is synthesized as a 37-kDa phosphoprotein that contains a mitochondrial importation signal peptide. However, importation into mitochondria is not necessary for StAR to stimulate steroidogenesis; to the contrary, the likeli-

**TABLE 72-1.**
**Adrenal Steroidogenesis: Nomenclature**

| Nomenclature of the Major Naturally Occurring Steroid Hormones | | |
|---|---|---|
| *Common Name* | *Biochemical Name* | *Letter* |
| Aldosterone | Pregn-4-en-11β,21-diol-18-al-3,20-dione | |
| Corticosterone | Pregn-4-en-11β,21-diol-3,20-dione | B |
| Cortisol (hydrocortisone) | Pregn-4-en-11β,17α,21-triol-3,20-dione | F |
| Cortisone | Pregn-4-en-17α,21-diol-3,11,20-trione | E |
| Dehydroepiandrosterone (DHA, DHEA) | Androst-5-en-3β-ol-17-one | |
| Deoxycorticosterone (DOC) | Pregn-4-en-21-ol-3,20-dione | |
| Deoxycortisol | Pregn-4-en-17α,21-diol-3,20-dione | S |
| Estradiol | Estra-1,3,4(10)-trien-3,17β-diol | |
| Progesterone | Pregn-4-en-3,20-dione | |
| Testosterone | Androst-4-en-17β-ol-3-one | |

**TABLE 72-2.**
**Characteristics of Enzymes Involved in Adrenal Steroid Biosynthesis**

| Gene | Alias | Enzyme | Chromosome | Gene Size (kb) | Number Exons | Number Amino Acids* | Subcellular Location |
|------|-------|--------|-----------|---------------|-------------|--------------------|--------------------|
| CYP11A | P450scc | Cholesterol desmolase | 15q23-24 | 20 | 9 | 521/482 | Mitochondria |
| CYP17 | P450c17 | 17α-Hydroxylase/17,20-lyase | 10q24.3 | 6.7 | 8 | 508 | ER |
| HSD3B2 | 3β-HSD | 3β-Hydroxysteroid dehydrogenase/$\Delta^5$-$\Delta^4$-isomerase | 1p11-13 | 8 | 4 | 371 | ER |
| CYP21 | P450c21 | 21-Hydroxylase | 6p21.3 | 3.1 | 10 | 494 | ER |
| CYP11B1 | P450c11 | 11β-Hydroxylase | 8q22 | 7 | 9 | 503/479 | Mitochondria |
| CYP11B2 | P450aldo | Aldosterone synthase | 8q22 | 7 | 9 | 503/479 | Mitochondria |
| CYP19 | P450arom | Aromatase | 15q21.1 | 70 | 9 | 503 | ER |
| HSD11B2 | 11-HSD2 | 11β-Hydroxysteroid dehydrogenase | 16q22 | 7 | 5 | 405 | ER |

*ER*, endoplasmic reticulum.
*Mitochondrial enzymes are synthesized as prohormones that are cleaved in mitochondria to the mature proteins; both sizes are given.

hood now appears that mitochondrial importation rapidly inactivates StAR.[3] The mechanism by which StAR mediates cholesterol transport across the mitochondrial membrane is not yet known.

StAR clearly is not the only protein that mediates cholesterol transfer across the mitochondrial membrane. Another protein that appears necessary (but not sufficient, at least in the adrenals and gonads) for this process is the *peripheral benzodiazepine receptor*, an 18-kDa protein in the mitochondrial outer membrane that is complexed with the mitochondrial voltage-dependent anion carrier in contact sites between the outer and inner mitochondrial membranes.[4] This protein does not appear to be directly regulated by typical trophic stimuli but is stimulated by *endozepines*, peptide hormones also called *diazepam-binding inhibitors*. *Endozepines* may be regulated by ACTH to some extent, but not with a rapid time course. Thus far, whether or not a direct physical interaction exists between StAR and the peripheral benzodiazepine receptor is not clear.

## ENZYMES

The enzymes required for adrenal steroid biosynthesis comprise two classes: *cytochrome P450 enzymes* and *short chain dehydrogenases* (Table 72-2).[5] These enzymes are located in either the lipophilic membranes of the smooth endoplasmic reticulum or the mitochondrial inner membrane. As the successive biosynthetic reactions involved in steroidogenesis occur, the adrenal steroids shuttle between the mitochondria and the smooth endoplasmic reticulum (Fig. 72-3).

### CYTOCHROME P450 ENZYMES

*Cytochrome P450 (CYP) enzymes* are responsible for most of the enzymatic conversions from cholesterol to biologically active steroid hormones.[5,6] Five P450 enzymes are involved in cortisol and aldosterone synthesis (see Table 72-2). Three—CYP11A (cholesterol desmolase, P450scc; the "scc" stands for "side chain cleavage"), CYP11B1 (11β-hydroxylase, P450c11), and CYP11B2 (aldosterone synthase, P450aldo)—have been localized in mitochondria; two—CYP17 (17α-hydroxylase/17,20-lyase, P450c17) and CYP21 (21-hydroxylase, P450c21)—are located in the endoplasmic reticulum (see Fig. 72-3).

*P450 enzymes* are membrane-bound hemoproteins with molecular masses of ~50 kDa. Their name arises from their property of absorbing light at a peak wavelength of 450 nm. These enzymes are located in the membranes of the smooth endoplasmic reticulum and the mitochondrial inner membrane and are encoded by a large superfamily of genes.[7]

P450s are *mixed function oxidases*. They use molecular oxygen and reducing equivalents (i.e., electrons) provided by reduced nicotinamide-adenine dinucleotide phosphate (NADPH) to cat-

alyze oxidative conversions of an extremely wide variety of mostly lipophilic substrates.

The reducing equivalents are not accepted directly from NADPH but instead from accessory electron transport proteins. These accessory proteins are necessary because NADPH donates electrons in pairs, whereas P450s can only accept single electrons.[8] Microsomal P450s use a single accessory protein, NADPH-dependent cytochrome P450 reductase. Mitochondrial P450s require two proteins; NADPH-dependent adrenodoxin reductase donates electrons to adrenodoxin, which in turn transfers them to the P450.[9] Adrenodoxin (or ferredoxin) reductase, like cytochrome P450 reductase, is a flavoprotein. Adrenodoxin (or ferredoxin) contains nonheme iron complexed with sulfur. One gene encodes each accessory protein in mammals.

The heart of the P450 catalytic site is a heme group that interacts with a highly conserved peptide of the P450. A completely conserved cysteine near the C terminus[10] is the fifth

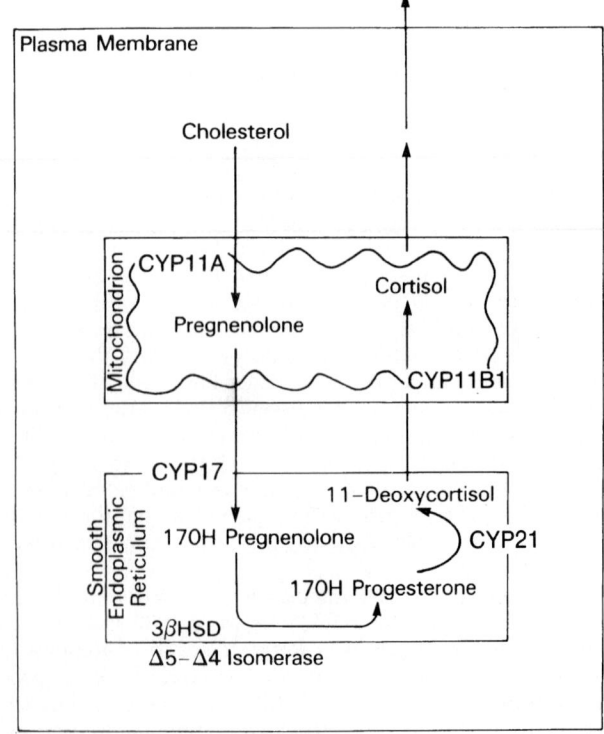

**FIGURE 72-3.** Biosynthesis of cortisol from cholesterol. The functional names of the steroidogenic enzymes are listed in Table 72-2 and Figure 72-4.

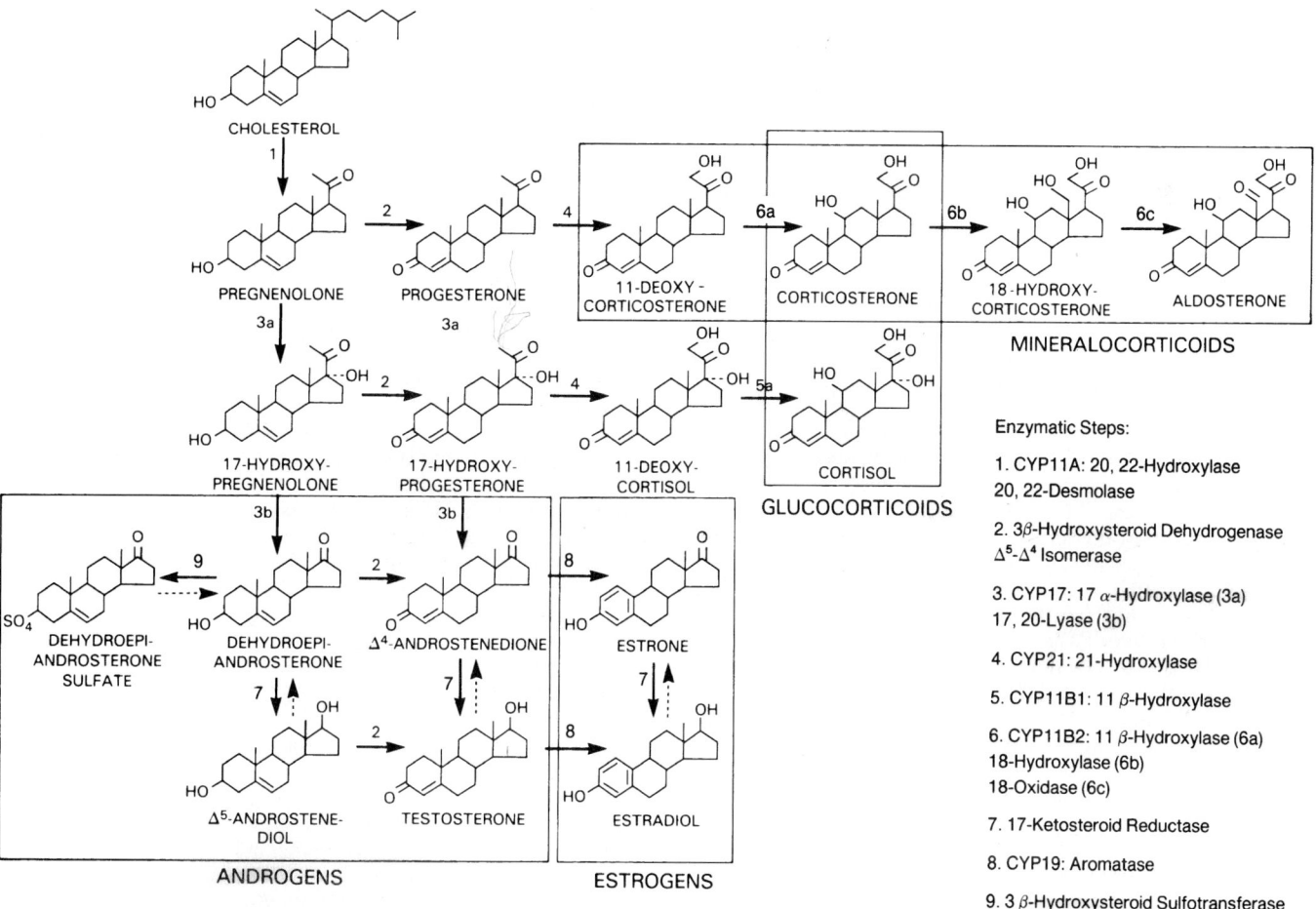

**FIGURE 72-4.** The steroidogenic pathway and enzymatic steps.

ligand of the heme iron atom. The other axial ligand is either water or molecular oxygen. When oxygen is bound, the long axis of the oxygen molecule is parallel with the axis of the heme iron. According to one of the several proposed models of catalysis,[11] the first step of the reaction is binding of substrate to oxidized (ferric, $Fe^{3+}$) enzyme. One electron is donated from the accessory electron transport protein to the enzyme so that the iron is in the reduced (ferrous, $Fe^{2+}$) state. This complex binds molecular oxygen and then accepts a second electron from the accessory protein, leaving the bound oxygen molecule with a negative charge. The distal oxygen atom accepts two protons from a conserved threonine residue, possibly via a bound water molecule.[12] The distal oxygen atom is then released as a water molecule, leaving the iron in the $Fe^{3+}$ state. The remaining oxygen atom is highly reactive (the iron-oxygen complex is a "ferryl" moiety) and attacks the substrate, resulting in an hydroxylation.

**Cholesterol Desmolase (CYP11A, P450scc).**    The first enzymatic step in all steroid hormone biosynthesis is the conversion of cholesterol to pregnenolone by CYP11A (Fig. 72-4; see also Fig. 72-3). This enzyme catalyzes 20α- and 22R-hydroxylation followed by oxidative cleavage of the $C_{20-22}$ carbon bond of cholesterol to release the $C_{22-27}$ side chain.[13] These reactions require a total of three oxygen molecules and six electrons. Like other mitochondrial cytochrome P450 enzymes, CYP11A receives these electrons from NADPH through the accessory proteins, adrenodoxin reductase and adrenodoxin. The three oxidations are normally performed in succession without release of hydroxylated intermediates from the enzyme.

CYP11A is structurally related to the CYP11B (11β-hydroxylase) isozymes (see later). It is synthesized as a precursor protein. As is the case with other mitochondrial proteins encoded by nuclear genes, an amino-terminal peptide is required for transport to the mitochondrial inner membrane. This peptide of 39 residues is removed in the mitochondria to yield the mature protein.

**17α-Hydroxylase/17,20-Lyase (CYP17, P450c17).**    CYP17 catalyzes conversion of pregnenolone to 17-hydroxypregnenolone. In rats, this enzyme also converts progesterone to 17-hydroxyprogesterone, but progesterone is not a good substrate for the human enzyme. CYP17 also catalyzes an oxidative cleavage of the 17,20 carbon-carbon bond, converting 17-hydroxypregnenolone and 17-hydroxyprogesterone to dehydroepiandrosterone (DHEA) and androstenedione, respectively.[14] A pair of electrons and a molecule of oxygen are required for each hydroxylation or lyase reaction. CYP17 is a microsomal cytochrome P450 and accepts these electrons from NADPH-dependent cytochrome P450 reductase.

In the human adrenal cortex, 17α-hydroxylase activity is required for the synthesis of cortisol. The human enzyme preferentially uses pregnenolone rather than progesterone, and 3β-hydroxysteroid dehydrogenase then converts 17-hydroxypregnenolone to 17-hydroxyprogesterone. Because most rodents do not express CYP17 in the adrenal cortex, they secrete corticosterone as their primary glucocorticoid. Both 17α-hydroxylase and 17,20-lyase activities are required for androgen and estrogen biosynthesis.

Because the same enzyme catalyzes production of cortisol in the adrenal cortex and androgens in the gonads, the relative level of 17,20-lyase activity must be independently regulated by a mechanism other than gene expression, or else excessive amounts of androgens would be synthesized in the adrenal cortex. Cytochrome b5 levels are likely to be one such mechanism, because interactions with cytochrome b5 increase 17,20-lyase activity, and mutations in cytochrome b5 interfere with androgen biosynthesis. Phosphorylation of specific serines and threonines in CYP17 may also be important.[15]

**21-Hydroxylase (CYP21, P450c21).** The enzyme 21-hydroxylase resides in the endoplasmic reticulum and is responsible for hydroxylating 17-hydroxyprogesterone to 11-deoxycortisol and progesterone to 11-deoxycorticosterone. The preferred substrate for the human enzyme is 17-hydroxyprogesterone. The structural gene encoding human CYP21 (*CYP21*, *CYP21A2*, or *CYP21B*) and a pseudogene (CYP21P, CYP21A1P, or CYP21A) are located in the HLA major histocompatibility complex on chromosome 6p21.3 ~30 kilobases (kb) apart, adjacent to and alternating with the *C4B* and *C4A* genes encoding the fourth component of serum complement. Both the *CYP21* and C4 genes are transcribed in the same direction. CYP21 and CYP21P each contain 10 exons spaced over 3.1 kb. Their nucleotide sequences are 98% identical in exons and ~96% identical in introns. This tandem duplication is genetically unstable and frequent recombinations occur between *CYP21* and CYP21P, causing congenital adrenal hyperplasia due to 21-hydroxylase deficiency[16] (see Chap. 77).

The two microsomal enzymes, CYP21 and CYP17, are 36% identical in amino-acid sequence and their genes have a similar intron-exon organization, a finding which suggests that both genes evolved from a common ancestor.[17]

**11β-Hydroxylase (CYP11B1, P450c11) and Aldosterone Synthase (CYP11B2, P450aldo).** Humans have distinct 11β-hydroxylase isozymes, CYP11B1 and CYP11B2, that are responsible for cortisol and aldosterone biosynthesis, respectively. In vitro, both isozymes can convert 11β-hydroxylate 11-deoxycorticosterone to corticosterone and 11-deoxycortisol to cortisol. CYP11B2 also has 18-hydroxylase and 18-oxidase activities, so that it can convert deoxycorticosterone to aldosterone. In contrast, the CYP11B1 isozyme does not synthesize detectable amounts of aldosterone from corticosterone or 18-hydroxycorticosterone.[18]

These isozymes are mitochondrial cytochrome P450 enzymes and are synthesized with a signal peptide that is cleaved in mitochondria. The sequences of the proteins are 93% identical. CYP11B1 and CYP11B2 are encoded by two genes on chromosome 8q21-q22. CYP11B2 is located to the left of CYP11B1 if the genes are pictured as being transcribed from left to right; the genes are located approximately 40 kb apart. The location of introns in each gene is identical to that seen in the CYP11A gene encoding cholesterol desmolase, and the predicted protein sequences of the CYP11B isozymes are each ~36% identical to that of CYP11A.

CYP11B1 is expressed at high levels in normal adrenal glands. CYP11B2 is normally expressed at low levels, but its expression is dramatically increased in aldosterone-secreting tumors. Transcription of CYP11B1 is regulated mainly by ACTH, whereas CYP11B2 is regulated by angiotensin II and potassium levels (see later). Recombinations between these two genes can lead to abnormal regulation of CYP11B2 and cause hypertension, a condition termed *glucocorticoid suppressible hyperaldosteronism* (see Chap. 80).

### SHORT CHAIN DEHYDROGENASES

Most short chain dehydrogenases catalyze reversible reactions.[19] In the dehydrogenase direction, a hydride (i.e., a proton plus two electrons) is removed from the substrate and transferred to an electron acceptor that, depending on the enzyme, is oxidized nicotinamide-adenine dinucleotide (NAD+) or oxidized nicotinamide-adenine dinucleotide phosphate (NADP+). If, for example, the reaction involves a hydroxylated substrate, the reaction converts the hydroxyl to a keto group; NADH or NADPH and a proton are also produced. Oxoreductase reactions reverse this process. Unlike oxidations mediated by cytochrome P450 enzymes, no accessory protein is required for these reactions.

Most short chain dehydrogenases contain 250 to 300 amino-acid residues. Some enzymes are found in cytosol, whereas others are located mainly in the endoplasmic reticulum. These enzymes have a conserved cofactor-binding domain near the N terminus and all have tyrosine and lysine residues near the C terminus that are crucial for catalysis.[20] The lysine residue lowers the apparent $pK_a$ of the phenolic hydroxyl of tyrosine from 10.0, its value in solution, into the physiologic range. The deprotonated hydroxyl is then able to remove a proton from the hydroxyl group of the substrate, which facilitates transfer of a hydride from the substrate to the oxidized cofactor.

The most important enzyme of this type in the adrenal cortex is 3β-hydroxysteroid dehydrogenase. This enzyme is only ~15% identical to most other short chain dehydrogenases, although it retains the essential structural features of this class of enzymes. Other enzymes of this type that are important in steroid metabolism include 11β-hydroxysteroid dehydrogenase, which interconverts cortisol and cortisone, and 17-ketosteroid reductase, which converts androstenedione and estrone to testosterone and estradiol, respectively.

**3β-Hydroxysteroid Dehydrogenase/Δ⁵-Δ⁴-Isomerase.** Conversion of $\Delta^5$-3β-hydroxysteroids (pregnenolone, 17-hydroxypregnenolone, DHEA) to $\Delta^4$-3-ketosteroids (progesterone, 17-hydroxyprogesterone, androstenedione) is mediated by 3β-hydroxysteroid dehydrogenase (3β-HSD) in the endoplasmic reticulum. This enzyme uses NAD+ as an electron acceptor. In addition to 3β-hydroxysteroid dehydrogenase activity, the enzyme mediates a $\Delta^5$-$\Delta^4$-ene isomerase reaction that transfers a double bond from the B ring to the A ring of the steroid so that it is conjugated with the 3-keto group. Certain isozymes are also able to mediate 3-ketosteroid reduction of several substrates using NADH as an electron donor. Genomic blot analysis suggests that as many as six closely linked *HSD3B* genes exist in humans, but only two isozymes have actually been identified. *HSD3B1* encodes the type I isozyme expressed in placenta, skin, and adipose tissue,[21] whereas *HSD3B2* encodes the type II isozyme expressed in the adrenals and gonads.[22] The remaining genes apparently do not encode active enzymes.

Any of the enzymatic conversions required for cortisol biosynthesis may be defective.[5] Inherited disorders of cortisol biosynthesis are collectively termed *congenital adrenal hyperplasia*. These disorders are discussed in Chapter 77.

**11β-Hydroxysteroid Dehydrogenase.** The interconversion of cortisol and cortisone is mediated by two isozymes of 11β-hydroxysteroid dehydrogenase (11-HSD).[23] The "liver" or 11-HSD1 isozyme is expressed at the highest levels in liver. In vivo, it acts primarily as a reductase and uses NADPH as an electron donor. It may act to "buffer" circulating levels of cortisol. This enzyme is responsible for the bioactivity of intrinsically inactive steroids like cortisone and prednisone when they are administered systemically. The "kidney" or 11-HSD2 isozyme is expressed mainly in mineralocorticoid target tissues, such as the kidney, colon and salivary glands, and also in placenta. It acts almost exclusively as a dehydrogenase, uses NAD+ as an electron acceptor, and has a much higher affinity for steroids than 11-HSD1 (10–100 nmol/L versus 1 μmol/L). The two isozymes are only 20% identical in amino-acid sequence. The 11-HSD2 isozyme plays a critical role in maintaining ligand specificity of the mineralocorticoid receptor, which can otherwise be activated by cortisol. Deficiency of this isozyme leads to a severe form of hypertension termed *apparent mineralocorticoid excess*. This is discussed in more detail in Chapter 82.

## PATHWAYS

### ORIGIN OF CHOLESTEROL

Cholesterol, the common precursor of all adrenal steroids, is a 27-carbon compound that originates from three sources (Fig. 72-5). Most cholesterol used in steroidogenesis is derived from the lysosomal degradation of circulating low-density lipoproteins. Cholesterol-rich low-density lipoprotein binds to specific

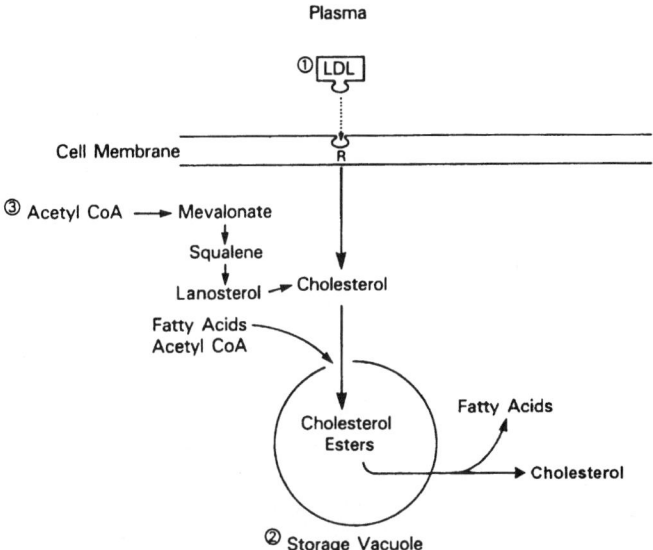

**FIGURE 72-5.** Sources of the cholesterol used in adrenal steroidogenesis: (1) low-density lipoprotein (*LDL*) cholesterol, (2) release from storage vacuoles, and (3) de novo synthesis from acetate. (*R*, LDL receptor; *CoA*, coenzyme A.)

plasma membrane receptors on adrenocortical cells, is internalized by endocytosis, and is degraded to liberate free cholesterol. The cholesterol that is not used in steroidogenesis is esterified and stored within cytoplasmic vacuoles in the cortical cells. When additional steroid production is needed, the stored cholesterol esters are hydrolyzed by cytoplasmic enzymes to

generate free cholesterol. Finally, adrenocortical cells produce some of their cholesterol by de novo synthesis from acetate.

## SECRETORY PRODUCTS

The relative activities of the steroidogenic enzymes within a given steroid-secreting cell determine which secretory products that cell produces. For example, $17\alpha$-hydroxylase activity exists only in the zona fasciculata and reticularis. Therefore, cortisol and adrenal androgens cannot be synthesized by the zona glomerulosa.

All of the precursors to the major adrenal biosynthetic products are measurable in the peripheral circulation. Because steroid hormones cannot be stored in steroidogenic cells, they are secreted immediately after their biosynthesis. Cortisol, 11-deoxycortisol, aldosterone, corticosterone, and 11-deoxycorticosterone are derived almost exclusively from adrenal secretion, whereas most other steroids are derived from a combination of adrenal and gonadal sources. Table 72-3 gives representative values for the production rates, basal plasma concentrations, and relative adrenal contribution to the blood production rate for the principal steroids of adrenal origin.

### GLUCOCORTICOIDS

Cortisol is the principal glucocorticoid in humans. It is synthesized primarily in the zona fasciculata with a small contribution from the zona reticularis. In humans, the five necessary transformations proceed predominantly as follows (see Fig. 72-3). Cholesterol is imported into mitochondria and converted to pregnenolone by cholesterol desmolase (CYP11A). Pregnenolone is transferred to the endoplasmic reticulum, where $17\alpha$-hydroxylase (CYP17) converts it to 17-hydroxypregnenolone. This is converted to 17-hydroxyprogesterone by $3\beta$-hydroxysteroid dehydrogenase/$\Delta^5$-$\Delta^4$ isomerase in the

**TABLE 72-3.**
**Mean Blood Production Rate, Adrenal Contribution, and Normal Plasma Concentration of the Major Steroids in the Circulation**

| Steroid | Mean Blood Production Rate (BPR, mg/24 h) | | Adrenal Contribution to BPR (%) | | Normal a.m. Plasma Concentration | | |
|---|---|---|---|---|---|---|---|
| | *Male* | *Female* | *Male* | *Female* | *Male* | *Female* | *Unit* |
| **Cortisol** | 20 | 16 | 100 | 100 | 6–25 | 6–25 | μg/dL |
| **11-Deoxycortisol** | 0.4 | 0.4 | 100 | 100 | 25–300 | 25–300 | ng/dL |
| **Aldosterone** | 0.1* | 0.1* | 100 | 100 | 4–12[†] | 4–12[†] | ng/dL |
| | | | | | 4–28[‡] | 4–28[‡] | ng/dL |
| **18-Hydroxycorticosterone** | NA | NA | 100 | 100 | 10–35 | 10–35 | ng/dL |
| **Corticosterone** | 4 | 4 | 100 | 100 | 150–1500 | 150–1500 | ng/dL |
| **11-Deoxycorticosterone (DOC)** | 0.1 | 0.1 | 100 | 100 | 4–12 | 4–12 | ng/dL |
| **18-Hydroxy-DOC** | NA | NA | 100 | 100 | <10 | <10 | ng/dL |
| **Pregnenolone** | 1.2 | | 70 | 40 | 30–100 | 30–200[¶] | ng/dL |
| **17-Hydroxypregnenolone** | 7 | 5 | 70 | 90 | 40–400 | 30–300 | ng/dL |
| **Progesterone** | 0.3 | 0.5[§] | | 60[§] | 10–40 | 10–80[§] | ng/dL |
| **17-Hydroxyprogesterone** | 1.6 | 1[§] | 10 | 10 | <200 | <200 | ng/dL |
| **DHEA** | 16 | 16 | >90 | >90 | 200–1000[#] | 200–1000[#] | ng/dL |
| **DHEAS** | 10 | 8 | >90 | >90 | 90–400[#] | 80–350[#] | μg/dL |
| **$\Delta^5$-Androstenediol** | 1.4 | 1 | 50 | 80 | 60–200 | 60–200 | ng/dL |
| **$\Delta^4$-Androstenedione** | 2 | 3.4 | 70 | 50 | 80–200 | 80–350 | ng/dL |
| **Testosterone** | 7 | 0.2 | 1.5 | 50 | 250–1200 | 20–60 | ng/dL |
| **Estrone** | 0.1 | 0.1[§] | 40 | 40[§] | <10–70 | 30–110[§] | pg/mL |
| **Estradiol** | 0.03 | 0.1[§] | 10 | 4[§] | <10–58 | 10–100[§] | pg/mL |

*NA*, not available; *DHEA*, dehydroepiandrosterone; *DHEAS*, dehydroepiandrosterone sulfate.
*Normal salt intake.
[†]Supine.
[‡]Erect.
[§]Follicular phase.
[¶]Premenopausal.
[#]Young adults; normal range declines with age.
(Modified from Loriaux DL, Cutler GB Jr. Diseases of the adrenal glands. In: Kohler PO, ed. The human adrenal cortex. New York: John Wiley and Sons, 1986:167.)

endoplasmic reticulum. A further hydroxylation in the smooth endoplasmic reticulum by 21-hydroxylase (CYP21) converts 17-hydroxyprogesterone to 11-deoxycortisol. The latter is transferred back to the mitochondria and is converted to cortisol by 11β-hydroxylase (CYP11B1). This step is highly efficient, resulting in 98% conversion of 11-deoxycortisol to cortisol. The end product, cortisol, diffuses rapidly into the circulation without significant storage in adrenal cortex.

## MINERALOCORTICOIDS

Aldosterone is the major mineralocorticoid. It is normally produced solely by the zona glomerulosa. The biosynthetic pathway of aldosterone initially parallels that of cortisol, except that 17-hydroxylation does not occur because of absent CYP17 in the zona glomerulosa. Thus, 11-deoxycorticosterone is produced in the endoplasmic reticulum rather than 11-deoxycortisol. The 11-deoxycorticosterone is transferred to the mitochondria, where a zone-specific 11β-hydroxylase isozyme (CYP11B2, aldosterone synthase) converts 11-deoxycorticosterone to corticosterone (and, to a lesser degree, 18-hydroxy, 11-deoxycorticosterone) and progressively oxidizes it to 18-hydroxycorticosterone and aldosterone. The secretion of 18-hydroxycorticosterone closely parallels that of aldosterone, and normally it is derived almost entirely from the zona glomerulosa. However, circulating levels of 11-deoxycorticosterone, 18-hydroxydeoxycorticosterone, and corticosterone originate primarily in the zona fasciculata due to the presence of a "17-deoxy" pathway in that zone.

Although aldosterone is the most potent endogenous mineralocorticoid, many steroids, including 11-deoxycorticosterone, 18-hydroxydeoxycorticosterone, corticosterone, and cortisol, possess a lesser degree of mineralocorticoid activity. Their metabolites, such as 19-nordeoxycorticosterone, also act as mineralocorticoids. Any of these steroids may contribute significant mineralocorticoid activity in pathologic states, such as adrenal tumor or congenital adrenal hyperplasia. However, only cortisol is thought to exert appreciable mineralocorticoid activity under normal circumstances.

## ANDROGENS

The adrenal sex steroids are produced primarily in the zona reticularis, although the fasciculata is also capable of their production. The key enzyme in their production is CYP17, which has both 17α-hydroxylase and 17,20-lyase (oxidative cleavage of the $C_{17-20}$ bond) activities. This enzyme is not necessary for mineralocorticoid synthesis and is absent in the zona glomerulosa. DHEA is the principal $\Delta^5$ steroid produced by the adrenal glands. It may also undergo sulfation by a sulfokinase to form DHEA sulfate (DHEAS).[24] These two steroids have no intrinsic androgenic activity but can be converted to the potent androgen, testosterone. This conversion requires the enzymes 3β-hydroxysteroid dehydrogenase/$\Delta^5$-$\Delta^4$ isomerase and 17-ketosteroid reductase. Depending on the sequence of these reactions, conversion of DHEA to testosterone proceeds through either androstenedione or $\Delta^5$-androstenediol as an intermediate (see Fig. 72-4; see Chap. 114). In men, the testis produces such a large quantity of testosterone (~7000 µg per day) that the contribution of the adrenal glands (~100 µg per day) is insignificant. In women, however, the adrenal glands contribute ~50% of total circulating androgens, either directly or through the secretion of precursors such as DHEA and androstenedione that are converted peripherally to testosterone.

## ESTROGENS

In both men and women, estrogens are derived either from the adrenal gland or the gonad. The aromatase enzyme converts androgens to estrogens: testosterone is converted to estradiol, and androstenedione to estrone.[25] Aromatase activity is present both in the adrenal gland and in peripheral tissues such as fat.

Therefore, circulating estrogens are produced by both adrenal and gonadal aromatization and by peripheral aromatization of adrenal and gonadal precursors. In the normal woman with intact ovarian function, the adrenal contribution to the circulating estrogens is relatively insignificant. However, in the absence of normal ovarian function, such as in postmenopausal or agonadal women, the adrenal gland may be the principal or only source of endogenous estrogen.

# REGULATION OF ADRENAL CORTICOSTEROID PRODUCTION

## CORTISOL SECRETION

### ADRENOCORTICOTROPIC HORMONE

ACTH is a 39-amino-acid peptide that is produced in the anterior pituitary. It is synthesized as part of a larger molecular weight precursor peptide known as *proopiomelanocortin (POMC)*. This precursor peptide is also the source of β-lipotropin (β-LPH). In addition, ACTH and β-LPH are cleaved further to yield`α- and β-melanocyte-stimulating hormone (α-MSH and β-MSH, respectively), corticotropin-like intermediate lobe peptide (CLIP), γ-LPH, β- and γ-endorphin, and enkephalin (see Chap. 14). The POMC precursor peptide is found in a variety of extrahypothalamic tissues, including the gastrointestinal tract, numerous tumors, and the testis. It is secreted in small amounts from the anterior pituitary gland and does not bind significantly to the ACTH receptor.

ACTH is the primary regulator of adrenal cortisol secretion. ACTH acts through a specific G protein–coupled receptor to increase levels of cAMP (cyclic or 3',5'-adenosine monophosphate).[26] The cAMP has short-term effects (minutes to hours) on cholesterol transport into mitochondria[2] but longer term effects (hours to days) on transcription of genes encoding the enzymes required to synthesize cortisol.[27] The transcriptional effects occur, at least in part, through increased activity of protein kinase A, which phosphorylates transcriptional regulatory factors, not all of which have been identified. ACTH also influences the remainder of the steps in steroidogenesis as well as the uptake of cholesterol from the plasma lipoproteins and the maintenance of the size of the adrenal glands. In addition to these effects on the adrenal gland, it also stimulates melanocytes and results in hyperpigmentation when secreted in excess (see Chap. 14).

### CORTICOTROPIN-RELEASING HORMONE

Corticotropin-releasing hormone (CRH) is the principal hypothalamic factor that stimulates the pituitary production of ACTH.[28,29] Vasopressin also stimulates ACTH release, synergizes with CRH, and is an important physiologic regulator of ACTH.[30] CRH is produced in the paraventricular nuclei of the hypothalamus and is also found in other parts of the central nervous system (CNS) as well as in extra-CNS locations such as the peripheral leukocytes. Hypothalamic CRH is transported to the anterior pituitary cells by the hypophysial portal vessels. CRH activates ACTH secretion through a cAMP-dependent mechanism. CRH is secreted in a pulsatile fashion that results in the episodic secretion of ACTH and the diurnal variation of cortisol secretion. The diurnal variation of cortisol secretion also is discussed in Chapters 6 and 14. Numerous factors, such as metabolic, physical, or emotional stress, result in increased glucocorticoid secretion, which is mediated by hypothalamic secretion of CRH and vasopressin.

### HYPOTHALAMIC–PITUITARY–ADRENAL AXIS

Cortisol is the primary regulator of resting activity of the hypothalamic–pituitary–adrenal (HPA) axis by its negative feedback

**TABLE 72-4.**
**Steroid-Binding Proteins and Factors Affecting Their Circulating Levels**

| Steroid-Binding Proteins | | | Factors Affecting Circulating Levels of Steroid-Binding Proteins | |
| --- | --- | --- | --- | --- |
| *Characteristic* | *CBG* | *Albumin* | *Factor* | *Effect on Binding Protein* |
| Molecular weight | 52,000 | 69,000 | Estrogen | Increases CBG and TeBG |
| Concentration ($\mu$mol/L) | 0.71 | 550 | Pregnancy | Increases CBG and TeBG |
| $K_d$ for cortisol (37°C) (mol/L) | $3 \times 10^{-8}$ | $2 \times 10^{-4}$ | Oral contraceptive use | Increases CBG and TeBG |
| Cortisol-binding capacity ($\mu$g/dL) | 25 | >20,000 | Diabetes mellitus | Increases CBG and TeBG |
| % Cortisol bound | ~85 | ~7 | Thyroid hormone | Increases CBG and TeBG |
| % Aldosterone bound | ~17 | ~47 | Hypoproteinemia (nephrotic syndrome) | Decreases CBG |
| % Deoxycorticosterone bound | ~36 | ~60 | Obesity | Decreases CBG and TeBG |
| | | | Genetic excess of CBG | Increases CBG |
| | | | Mitotane (*o,p'*-DDD) | Increases CBG |
| | | | Genetic deficiency of CBG | Decreases CBG |
| | | | Cirrhosis | Increases TeBG |
| | | | Testosterone | Decreases TeBG |
| | | | Age | Decreases TeBG |

CBG, corticosteroid-binding globulin; *TeBG*, testosterone-binding globulin; $K_d$, dissociation constant.

effects on ACTH and CRH (see Chap. 14). Furthermore, it may inhibit some of the higher cortical activities that lead to CRH stimulation. The negative feedback effects of cortisol are exerted at the level of both the hypothalamus and the pituitary. The magnitude of the cortisol response to each ACTH burst remains relatively constant, whereas the number of secretory bursts may vary. Therefore, it is the number of secretory periods of CRH and ACTH that determines the total daily cortisol secretion. The increased cortisol secretion observed during the early morning hours, and the increased secretion in response to stress, result primarily from increased CNS activity, possibly mediated by vasopressin, rather than by decreased sensitivity to the negative feedback effects of cortisol. For example, the diurnal variation in cortisol secretion is not abolished in the addisonian patient in whom little cortisol is present to suppress CRH and ACTH secretion. In addition, in major stress situations, the negative feedback effects of cortisol are overridden by increased CRH and ACTH activity, which results in an increase in cortisol secretion.

## ALDOSTERONE SECRETION

The rate of aldosterone synthesis, which is normally 100- to 1000-fold less than that of cortisol synthesis, is regulated mainly by angiotensin II and potassium levels, with ACTH having only a short-term effect.[31] Angiotensin II occupies a G protein–coupled receptor,[32] activating phospholipase C. The latter protein hydrolyzes phosphatidylinositol bisphosphate to produce inositol triphosphate and diacylglycerol, which raise intracellular calcium levels and activate protein kinase C and CaM kinases. Similarly, increased levels of extracellular potassium depolarize the cell membrane and increase calcium influx through voltage-gated L-type calcium channels.[33] Phosphorylation of as yet unidentified factors by CaM kinases increases transcription of the aldosterone synthase (CYP11B2) enzyme required for aldosterone synthesis.[31]

## ANDROGEN SECRETION

The mechanisms by which the adrenal steroids, DHEAS and androstenedione, are regulated are not completely understood. The compounds themselves have only weak androgenic activity, but because they serve as precursors for more active androgens, testosterone and dihydrotestosterone, they are often referred to as the adrenal androgens. *Adrenarche* is a matura-

tional process in the adrenal gland that results in increased adrenal androgen secretion between the ages of 5 and 20 years.[34] The process begins before the earliest signs of puberty and continues throughout the years when puberty is occurring. Histologically, it is associated with the appearance of the zona reticularis. Whereas ACTH stimulates adrenal androgen production acutely and clearly is the primary stimulus for cortisol release (see earlier), additional factors have been implicated in the stimulation of the adrenal androgens. These include a relative decrease in expression of 3-hydroxysteroid dehydrogenase in the zona reticularis,[35] and possibly increases in 17,20-lyase activity due to phosphorylation or increased cytochrome b5 expression.[15]

## DISTRIBUTION IN THE CIRCULATION

Substantial variability exists in the production rate of the various steroids by males and females (see Table 72-3). Steroid products are secreted into the circulation as free hormones, where they bind to plasma proteins[36,37] (Table 72-4). Only the free hormone is biologically active. However, the amount of hormone that is potentially available to tissues is determined by the equilibrium of the free and bound fractions. Bound hormone may be freed from the binding protein as the free hormone is metabolized or taken up into tissues. Thus, binding to plasma proteins increases the amount of hormone that can circulate in the blood and serves as a mechanism for transport of steroids in an inactive form. Binding makes the hormones more resistant to metabolism, thereby increasing the plasma half-life ($t_{1/2}$).

### GLUCOCORTICOIDS

Only 3% to 10% of circulating cortisol is in the free state. Approximately 80% to 90% is bound to a specific $\alpha_2$-globulin, known as *corticosteroid-binding globulin* (CBG) or transcortin.[36,37] This 52-kDa glycoprotein binds cortisol with high affinity and specificity. It is produced primarily in the liver and has been found in all mammalian species. The association constant for a single molecule of cortisol is $3 \times 10^7$ L/mol. The CBG circulates in a concentration of ~3 mg/dL. The cortisol-binding capacity of CBG is ~20 $\mu$g/dL, and it is increased in patients receiving oral estrogen or the adrenolytic drug mitotane (*o,p'*-DDD). The CBG also has high affinity for cortisone, corticosterone, 11-deoxycorticosterone, progesterone, and 17-hydroxyprogesterone.

Between 5% and 10% of cortisol is bound to *albumin.* Albumin has a lower affinity for cortisol than CBG but a much higher capacity. The dissociation of cortisol from albumin is more rapid. Therefore, the steroid bound by albumin is more readily available to the tissues than that bound by CBG.

A third binding protein, $\alpha_1$-*acid glycoprotein,* also binds cortisol, but it appears to be of minor importance. It binds principally to progesterone.

## ALDOSTERONE

Although aldosterone does not have a specific binding protein, ~64% of the total circulating aldosterone is in a bound form. Approximately 17% is weakly bound to CBG. Aldosterone also binds to red blood cells, albumin (47%), and other plasma proteins. It dissociates quickly from the plasma proteins to which it binds, so that it is readily available to its target tissues.

## ADRENAL SEX STEROIDS

The adrenal androgens DHEA and androstenedione are bound weakly to plasma proteins, predominantly albumin. DHEAS, however, is tightly bound to albumin, explaining its slow metabolic clearance rate and high, stable levels in plasma. The sex steroids testosterone and estradiol are bound by a distinct binding protein, known as sex hormone–binding globulin (SHBG) or testosterone-binding globulin (TeBG).[36,37] The relative binding affinity to TeBG, in order of decreasing affinity, is dihydrotestosterone, testosterone, androstenediol, androstanediol, estradiol, and estrone.

## ALTERATIONS IN BINDING PROTEINS

Generally, it is the total level of a hormone that is measured. Many factors can alter binding globulin concentrations in plasma[38] (see Table 72-4). Because the free hormone determines biologic activity, knowledge of the conditions affecting the binding proteins is important in assessing total serum steroid levels. Sex steroids—in particular, estrogen—increase CBG levels. Therefore, in pregnant women or women taking oral contraceptives, higher circulating serum cortisol levels are expected, although free cortisol and cortisol activity should be normal. Thyroid hormone also stimulates CBG synthesis. Some families appear to have inherited elevations in CBG levels; elevations may also be seen in diabetes mellitus. Subnormal levels are seen in states of decreased protein production, such as in liver disease, or in states of protein loss (e.g., the nephrotic syndrome). Some patients have heritable varients in their CBG, resulting in low cortisol-binding affinity.[38a] Hypothyroidism, multiple myeloma, and obesity have all been associated with low circulating CBG levels. The circulating concentration of TeBG is affected by age, body weight, and circulating estrogen, testosterone, and thyroid hormone levels.

## METABOLISM

The liver and the kidney are the principal organs involved in clearing the steroid hormones from the circulation. Although most tissues can metabolize steroids, the liver is the primary site of steroid hormone metabolism, and the kidney is the primary site of steroid hormone excretion. Unconjugated steroids that are filtered by the kidney are largely reabsorbed. Hepatic metabolism accomplishes two functions: a decrease in the biologic activity of the hormones; and an increase in their water solubility, because of conversion to a hydrophilic form that can

be excreted in urine. Additional metabolism and excretion may take place in the gut, although most of the metabolized products are reabsorbed.

Because plasma cortisol is bound with such high affinity, it is relatively protected from degradation. The plasma $t_{1/2}$ of cortisol is 60 to 100 minutes. This contrasts with many other steroids, such as aldosterone, DHEA, androstenedione, testosterone, and estradiol, that have metabolic clearance rates of ~2000 L per day, corresponding to a $t_{1/2}$ of under 20 minutes. Although these compounds also circulate in a bound form, they dissociate more rapidly from their binding proteins, making them more susceptible to degradation. The episodic secretion of these adrenal hormones, combined with this short $t_{1/2}$, results in wide fluctuations in plasma steroid concentrations. By contrast, the steroid sulfates, such as DHEAS, which bind with high affinity to albumin, are cleared slowly from the circulation and have high stable plasma concentrations.

The pathways involved in metabolism of the steroids yield more than 50 different metabolic products formed by approximately a dozen distinct enzymatic reactions.

## CORTISOL, CORTICOSTERONE, 11-DEOXYCORTICOSTERONE, AND 11-DEOXYCORTISOL

Metabolized products of cortisol can be measured in the urine (Fig. 72-6). Unmetabolized cortisol comprises only ~0.1% of the total urinary cortisol metabolites. At least 90% of the cortisol and cortisone metabolites are excreted as the sulfate or the glucuronide conjugates. The metabolism of corticosterone, 11-deoxycorticosterone, and 11-deoxycortisol resembles that of cortisol. The major reactions involved in the metabolism of cortisol include (a) *reduction of the $C_{4-5}$ double bond,* from either the α or β side of the A ring; this reaction is irreversible and produces dihydrocortisol, which is further rapidly metabolized by (b) *reduction of the $C_3$ ketone group;* this reaction yields tetrahydrocortisol, which is rapidly (c) *conjugated with glucuronic acid at the 3-hydroxyl position,* yielding a highly water soluble form; (d) tetrahydrocortisol also undergoes *reduction at the $C_{20}$ position* to yield cortol.[39] Another important pathway of cortisol metabolism includes *oxidation at the 11β-hydroxyl group* to yield cortisone (see Chap 73). Cortisone may then be metabolized by steps a, b, c, and d, as outlined for cortisol. The resulting products include tetrahydrocortisone, cortolone, and the conjugated products of each. In infants, *6β-hydroxylation* is an important metabolic pathway. Moreover, *16α-hydroxylation,* which is important for the conversion of estradiol to estriol, may be a minor pathway in the metabolism of cortisol. Finally, *cleavage of the $C_{17}$ side chain* may take place, producing $C_{19}$ metabolites that have a ketone group at the $C_{17}$ position, such as 11β-hydroxyandrostenedione and 11-ketoetiocholanolone, which are measured as 17-ketosteroids.

## ALDOSTERONE

Aldosterone has a plasma $t_{1/2}$ of <15 minutes. Less than 0.5% of the aldosterone is secreted into the urine in the free state. It is metabolized in a fashion similar to cortisol to yield tetrahydroaldosterone and its conjugate, tetrahydroaldosterone glucuronide. It also is conjugated in the $C_{18}$ position to yield aldosterone glucuronide.[40] Urinary assays for aldosterone usually measure this metabolite. Further metabolic pathways for aldosterone, such as oxidation at the 11β hydroxyl group, play a smaller role. When aldosterone is in aqueous solution, the 11β hydroxyl group is in a hemiketal conformation with the adjacent 18-aldehyde group and, thus, is protected from oxidation. This fact allows aldosterone to occupy the mineralocorticoid receptor in target tissues, whereas cortisol is oxidized to cortisone by 11β-hydroxysteroid dehydrogenase.

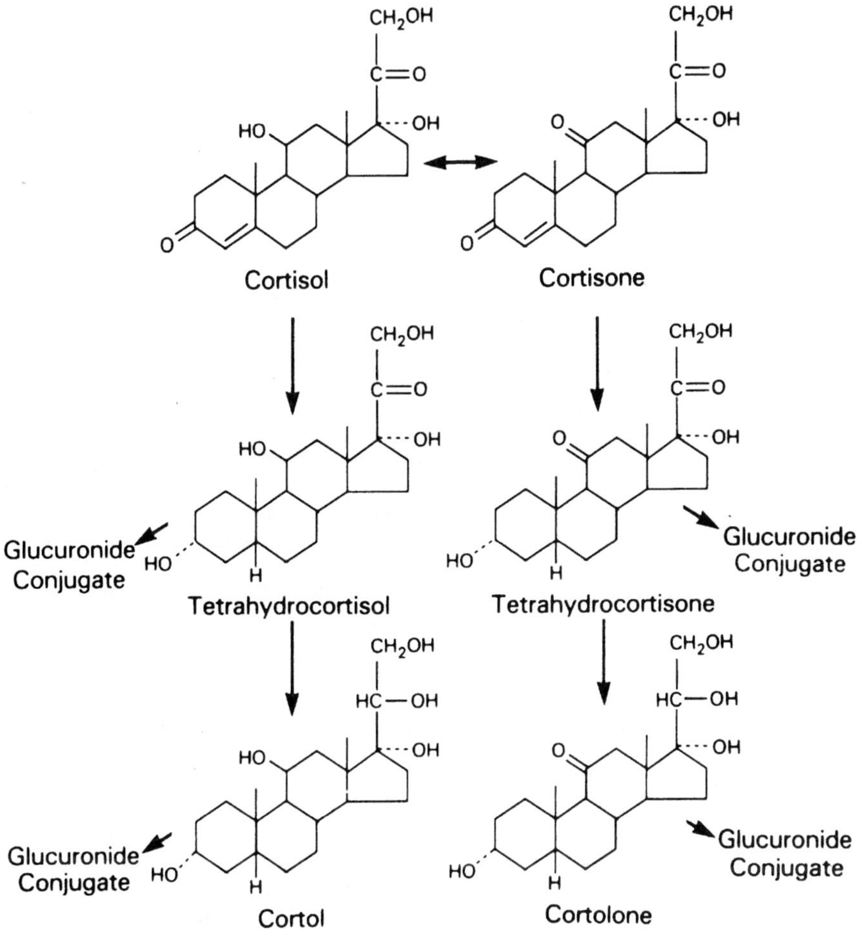

**FIGURE 72-6.** Major metabolic pathways for cortisol. Reduction of the double bond at $C_4$ produces urinary metabolites with both the 5β and 5α orientations.

# REFERENCES

1. Mesiano S, Jaffe RB. Developmental and functional biology of the primate fetal adrenal cortex. Endocr Rev 1997; 18:378.
2. Stocco DM, Clark BJ. Regulation of the acute production of steroids in steroidogenic cells. Endocr Rev 1996; 17:221.
2a. Stocco DM. The role of the STAR protein in steroidogenesis: challenges for the future. J Endocrinol 2000; 164:247.
3. Arakane F, Kallen CB, Watari H, et al. The mechanism of action of steroidogenic acute regulatory protein (StAR). StAR acts on the outside of mitochondria to stimulate steroidogenesis. J Biol Chem 1998; 273:16339.
4. Papadopoulos V. Structure and function of the peripheral-type benzodiazepine receptor in steroidogenic cells. Proc Soc Exp Biol Med 1998; 217:130.
5. White PC. Genetic diseases of steroid metabolism. Vitam Horm 1994; 49:131.
6. Nebert DW, Nelson DR, Coon MJ, et al. The P450 superfamily: update on new sequences, gene mapping, and recommended nomenclature [published erratum in DNA Cell Biol 1991 10(5):397]. DNA Cell Biol 1991; 10:1.
7. Schenkman JB, Greim H. Cytochrome P450. Berlin: Springer-Verlag, 1993.
8. Sevrioukova IF, Peterson JA. NADPH-P-450 reductase: structural and functional comparisons of the eukaryotic and prokaryotic isoforms. Biochimie 1995; 77:562.
9. Lambeth JD, Seybert DW, Lancaster JRJ, et al. Steroidogenic electron transport in adrenal cortex mitochondria. Mol Cell Biochem 1982; 45:13.
10. Nelson DR, Strobel HW. On the membrane topology of vertebrate cytochrome P-450 proteins. J Biol Chem 1988; 263:6038.
11. Rein H, Jung C. Metabolic reactions: mechanisms of substrate oxygenation. In: Schenkman JB, Greim H, eds. Cytochrome P450. Berlin: Springer-Verlag, 1993:105.
12. Ravichandran KG, Boddupalli SS, Hasemann CA, et al. Crystal structure of hemoprotein domain of P450BM-3, a prototype for microsomal P450's. Science 1993; 261:731.
13. Lambeth JD, Kitchen SE, Farooqui AA, et al. Cytochrome P450scc-substrate interactions. Studies of binding and catalytic activity using hydroxycholesterols. J Biol Chem 1982; 257:1876.
14. Yanase T, Simpson ER, Waterman MR. 17 alpha-hydroxylase/17,20-lyase deficiency: from clinical investigation to molecular definition. Endocr Rev 1991; 12:91.
15. Miller WL, Auchus RJ, Geller DH. The regulation of 17,20 lyase activity. Steroids 1997; 62:133.
16. Speiser PW, White PC. Congenital adrenal hyperplasia due to steroid 21-hydroxylase deficiency. Clin Endocrinol (Oxf) 1998; 49:411.
17. Picado-Leonard J, Miller WL. Cloning and sequence of the human gene for P450c17 (steroid 17 alpha-hydroxylase/17,20 lyase): similarity with the gene for P450c21. DNA 1987; 6:439.
18. White PC, Curnow KM, Pascoe L. Disorders of steroid 11 beta hydroxylase isozymes. Endocr Rev 1994; 15:421.
19. Persson B, Krook M, Jornvall H. Characteristics of short-chain alcohol dehydrogenases and related enzymes. Eur J Biochem 1991; 200:537.
20. Obeid J, White PC. Tyr-179 and Lys-183 are essential for enzymatic activity of 11 beta-hydroxysteroid dehydrogenase. Biochem Biophys Res Commun 1992; 188:222.
21. Lachance Y, Luu-The V, Labrie C, et al. Characterization of human 3beta-hydroxysteroid dehydrogenase/delta 5-delta 4-isomerase gene and its expression in mammalian cells [published erratum in J Biol Chem 1992; 267(5):3551]. J Biol Chem 1990; 265:20469.
22. Lachance Y, Luu-The V, Verreault H, et al. Structure of the human type II 3beta-hydroxysteroid dehydrogenase/delta 5-delta 4 isomerase (3 beta-HSD) gene: adrenal and gonadal specificity. DNA Cell Biol 1991; 10:701.
23. White PC, Mune T, Agarwal AK. 11β-hydroxysteroid dehydrogenase and the syndrome of apparent mineralocorticoid excess. Endocr Rev 1997; 18:135.
24. Longcope C. Dehydroepiandrosterone metabolism. J Endocrinol 1996; 150(Suppl):S125.
25. Simpson ER, Mahendroo MS, Means GD, et al. Aromatase cytochrome P450, the enzyme responsible for estrogen biosynthesis. Endocr Rev 1994; 15:342.
26. Mountjoy KG, Robbins LS, Mortrud MT, Cone RD. The cloning of a family of genes that encode the melanocortin receptors. Science 1992; 257:1248.
27. Waterman MR, Bischof LJ. Cytochromes P450 12: diversity of ACTH (cAMP)-dependent transcription of bovine steroid hydroxylase genes. FASEB J 1997; 11:419.
28. Orth DN. Cushing's syndrome [published erratum in N Engl J Med 1995; 332(22):1527]. N Engl J Med 1995; 332:791.
29. Itoi K, Seasholtz AF, Watson SJ. Cellular and extracellular regulatory mechanisms of hypothalamic corticotropin-releasing hormone neurons. Endocr J 1998; 45:13.
30. Scott LV, Dinan TG. Vasopressin and the regulation of hypothalamic-pituitary-adrenal axis function: implications for the pathophysiology of depression. Life Sci 1998; 62:1985.
31. Rainey WE, White PC. Functional adrenal zonation and regulation of aldosterone biosynthesis. Curr Opin Endocrinol Diabetes 1998; 5:175.
32. Matsusaka T, Ichikawa I. Biological functions of angiotensin and its receptors. Annu Rev Physiol 1997; 59:395.

33. Barrett PQ, Bollag WB, Isales CM, et al. Role of calcium in angiotensin II–mediated aldosterone secretion. Endocr Rev 1989; 10:496.

34. McKenna TJ, Fearon U, Clarke D, Cunningham SK. A critical review of the origin and control of adrenal androgens. Baillières Clin Obstet Gynaecol 1997; 11:229.

35. Gell JS, Carr BR, Sasano H, et al. Adrenarche results from development of a 3beta-hydroxysteroid dehydrogenase-deficient adrenal reticularis. J Clin Endocrinol Metab 1998; 83:3695.

36. Rosner W. The functions of corticosteroid-binding globulin and sex hormone–binding globulin: recent advances. Endocr Rev 1990; 11:80.

37. Hammond GL. Molecular properties of corticosteroid binding globulin and the sex-steroid binding proteins. Endocr Rev 1990; 11:65.

38. Hammond GL. Determinants of steroid hormone bioavailability. Biochem Soc Trans 1997; 25:577.

38a. Emptoz-Bonneton A, Cousin P, Seguehik, et al. Novel human corticosteroid-binding globulin variant with low cortisol-binding affinity. J Clin Endocrinol Metab 2000; 85:361.

39. Brownie AC. The metabolism of adrenal cortical steroids. In: James VH, ed. The adrenal gland, 2nd ed. New York: Raven Press, 1992:209.

40. Morris DJ, Brem AS. Metabolic derivatives of aldosterone. Am J Physiol 1987; 252:F365.

---

# CHAPTER 73

# CORTICOSTEROID ACTION

PERRIN C. WHITE

## GENERAL MECHANISMS OF ACTION

The steroid hormones, vitamin D, retinoic acid, and the thyroid hormones all share a similar mechanism of action.[1,2] These hormones diffuse through the target cell membrane and interact with a specific receptor protein for each hormone. The activated hormone-receptor complex binds to specific DNA sequences, the hormone-responsive elements (HREs), which are usually located in the 5' flanking region of each hormone-responsive gene. These complexes may also bind to other transcription factors. The binding of the hormone-receptor complex to these DNA sequences or transcription factors leads to selective increases or decreases in gene transcription. The altered protein levels that result from this change in transcription rate are responsible for the hormonal response seen in that particular tissue.[3]

At least six classes of *steroid receptors* exist, corresponding to the known bioactivities of the steroid hormones: glucocorticoid, mineralocorticoid, progestin, estrogen, androgen, and vitamin D. Additional "orphan" receptors of incompletely understood function are found that bind related compounds such as androstanes.[4] Steroid receptors belong to a larger superfamily of nuclear transcriptional factors that includes the thyroid hormone and retinoic acid receptors. All of these receptors share a common structure that includes *a carboxy-terminal ligand-binding domain and a midregion DNA-binding domain*. The latter domain contains two "zinc fingers," each of which consists of a loop of amino acids stabilized by four cysteine residues chelating a zinc ion.[5]

Unliganded steroid hormone receptors shuttle between the cytoplasm and the cell nucleus. Importation into the nucleus is an energy-dependent process. This process requires one or more nuclear localization signal sequences on the receptor, which consist of clusters of basic amino-acid residues located in or near the DNA-binding domain. When not occupied by ligand, the various hormone receptors differ in their propensity to be transported to the nucleus. For example, the estrogen receptor is predominantly located within the nucleus, whereas the unoccupied glucocorticoid and mineralocorticoid receptors are found mainly in the cytosol.[6]

The cytosolic glucocorticoid receptor, when not bound to its steroid ligand, forms a heterooligomer with two molecules of heat shock protein (HSP) 90 and one molecule each of HSP 70 and HSP 56 (immunophilin).[7] Binding of ligand changes the conformation of the receptor and, thus, has several effects. HSP 90 is associated with the unliganded glucocorticoid receptor at the ligand-binding domain and dissociates from the receptor complex after glucocorticoid binds to the receptor. A dimerization region that overlaps the steroid-binding domain is exposed, promoting dimerization of the occupied receptor. Finally, a hormone-dependent nuclear localization signal located in a "hinge" between the DNA and steroid-binding domains is activated, which leads to increased importation of occupied receptors into the nucleus. The occupied receptors are then able to bind DNA and/or other transcription factors and modulate transcription of various genes.[8,9]

Glucocorticoids affect transcription of a wide variety of genes through several different mechanisms.[8] First, the glucocorticoid-receptor complex can stimulate transcription by binding to specific glucocorticoid-responsive elements (GREs) in the 5' flanking region of glucocorticoid-responsive genes. GREs, like other specific hormone response elements, are often imperfect palindromes (in a palindrome, the two complementary strands of a DNA molecule, when "read" in opposite directions, have the identical sequence). Most often, GREs are variants of the sequence GGTACAnnnTGTTCT, where "n" is any nucleotide. The existence of two "half-sites" separated by three nucleotides suggests that glucocorticoid receptors interact with GREs as dimers, with one monomer binding to each half-site. However, many GREs consist of isolated half-sites or half-sites with variable spacing between them. Moreover, marked variations in sequence can be tolerated in one half-site. Thus, monomeric glucocorticoid receptors can also bind DNA, but the binding can apparently be stabilized by interactions with other bound receptor molecules or other transcription factors. Thus, binding of the monomeric receptor to one half-site markedly increases the ability of a second monomer to bind to the other half-site.

The interaction of the glucocorticoid receptor and DNA has been studied in detail by x-ray crystallography and nuclear magnetic resonance techniques.[5] The two zinc fingers form a single domain. Alpha helices adjacent to each finger on the carboxy-terminal side are oriented perpendicularly to each other; the first helix fits into the major groove of the DNA helix and makes direct contact with bases. The tips of both fingers contact the phosphate backbone, and the second finger also mediates DNA-dependent dimerization of the receptor.

GREs cannot constitute the only DNA sequences mediating the transcriptional effects of glucocorticoids. GREs are indistinguishable in sequence from the elements binding mineralocorticoid, progestin, and androgen receptors, and these receptors are >90% identical in amino-acid sequence in their DNA-binding domains. However, the amino-terminal domains of these receptors are <15% identical in amino-acid sequence, and at least some interactions with other transcriptional factors are mediated by this domain.[10]

As a second type of effect, glucocorticoid receptors can inhibit or activate transcription by interacting with other transcription factors.[8,9,11] In particular, they can regulate gene activity by repressing gene transcription mediated by "AP-1" or NF-κB elements in the regulatory regions of some genes. These AP-1 and NF-κB sites bind cFos-cJun or RelA-p50 heterodimers, respectively. The ligand-bound glucocorticoid receptor monomer and/or dimer interacts with AP-1 or NF-κB and prevents them from exerting their transactivational effects on the genes they normally regulate. AP-1 and NF-κB serve as intracellular messenger systems for many growth factors and inflammatory cytokines, respectively. The profound antigrowth and antiinflammatory effects of glucocorticoids are exerted to a great extent via transrepression of these transcription factors. In addition, glucocorticoid receptors may modulate effects of the Stat4, Stat5, NF-1, Oct-1, SP-1, C/EBP, HNF3, and HNF4 transcription factors.

Unlike glucocorticoids, mineralocorticoids do not appear to interfere with cFos-cJun or NF-κB binding. This functional difference may be localized to the amino-terminal domain of the receptor.[10]

Two new classes of nuclear proteins that influence the transactivational activity of nuclear receptors have been identified and collectively called *coregulators*.[12,13] According to their ability to potentiate or diminish the activity of nuclear receptors, they are respectively called *coactivators* and *corepressors*. Known coregulators are large proteins with many functional domains. One could think of coactivators as bridges between the DNA-bound nuclear receptor and components of the transcription machinery, such as ancillary factors of DNA polymerase II, that stabilize and hence stimulate the activity of the initiation complex. In addition, coactivators have enzymatic activities that promote transcription, such as histone acetyl-transferase activity, which loosens the DNA double helix from the nucleosome and allows the polymerase complex to exert its activity.[14] On the other hand, corepressors prevent the nuclear receptor from binding to DNA and/or transactivating their target genes and have enzymatic activities that impede transcription, such as histone deacetylase, which strengthens the interactions of the DNA with the nucleosome. Coregulators are expressed in a tissue-specific fashion and have varying degrees of specificity for particular nuclear receptors. Some of these proteins serve as coregulators of other transcription factors, such as AP-1, NF-κB, and the Stats, and hence serve as cross-points between different signal transduction systems in the cell.

Several factors regulate tissue-specific effects of steroids at several levels both before and after the receptor. Most obviously, hormone receptors are widely but not ubiquitously expressed, and a particular class of steroid fails to have effects on cells that do not express the corresponding receptor. Of physiologic importance, enzymes may increase or decrease the affinity of steroids for their receptors and thus modulate their activity. For example, the mineralocorticoid receptor has identical affinities in vitro for cortisol and aldosterone, yet cortisol is a weak mineralocorticoid in vivo. This discrepancy may result from the action of 11β-hydroxysteroid dehydrogenase, which converts cortisol to cortisone. Cortisone is not a ligand for the receptor, whereas aldosterone is not a substrate for the enzyme. Pharmacologic or genetic inhibition of this enzyme allows cortisol to occupy renal mineralocorticoid receptors and produce sodium retention and hypertension.[15]

Whereas different steroids may share bioactivities because of their ability to bind to the same receptor, a given steroid may exert diverse biologic effects in different tissues. The diversity of hormonal responses is determined by the different genes that are regulated by the hormone in different tissues. Glucocorticoids, for example, have primarily GRE-mediated metabolic effects in liver and mainly anti–NF-κB–mediated antiinflammatory properties in lymphoid tissue.[16]

In addition to the actions resulting from the binding of steroids to nuclear steroid receptors, some effects might be mediated through other mechanisms. Such effects often take place with extreme rapidity (milliseconds to minutes) and/or have been documented not to require protein synthesis, a sine qua non of the transcriptional effects mediated by nuclear-hormone receptors. These effects have been most extensively documented for 1,25-dihydroxyvitamin $D_3$, progesterone, and aldosterone; they appear to involve second messengers systems including protein kinase C, intracellular calcium levels, nitric oxide, and tyrosine kinases.[17] Thus far, however, no steroid-specific membrane receptors have been isolated or cloned. (Also see Chaps. 4 and 54.)

## ACTIONS OF THE GLUCOCORTICOIDS

Glucocorticoids are essential for survival. The term *glucocorticoid* refers to the glucose-regulating properties of these hormones. However, the glucocorticoids have multiple effects that

**TABLE 73-1.**
**Major Glucocorticoid Actions**

**METABOLIC EFFECTS**
*Carbohydrate*
  Increase blood sugar
  Increase gluconeogenesis in liver and kidney
  Increase hepatic glycogenesis
  Increase cellular resistance to insulin; decrease glucose uptake in tissues
*Lipid*
  Increase lipolysis
*Protein*
  Increase proteolysis
**IMMUNOLOGIC EFFECTS (PHARMACOLOGIC LEVELS)**
  Stabilize lysosomal membranes
  Block bradykinin, histamine, interleukin-1 and interleukin-2, plasminogen-activating factor
  Decrease vascular permeability
  Increase polymorphonuclear (PMN) cell release from bone marrow:neutrophilia
  Block PMN diapedesis, chemotaxis, and phagocytosis
  Deplete circulating lymphocytes:lymphocytopenia affecting T cells more than B cells
  Decrease antibody formation from B lymphocytes
  Deplete circulating monocytes:monocytopenia
  Deplete circulating eosinophils:eosinopenia
  Decrease thymic and lymphoid tissue mass
  Impair delayed hypersensitivity reaction
  Decrease resistance to bacterial, fungal, viral, and parasitic infections
**CONNECTIVE TISSUE EFFECTS**
  Decrease collagen formation
  Impair granulation tissue formation and wound healing
**CALCIUM AND BONE EFFECTS**
  Decrease serum calcium
  Accelerate osteoporosis
**CIRCULATORY EFFECTS**
  Increase cardiac output
  Increase response to catecholamines
**RENAL EFFECTS**
  Increase renal blood flow and glomerular filtration rate
  Increase free water clearance
  Inhibit vasopressin
**CENTRAL NERVOUS SYSTEM EFFECTS**
  Increase mood lability
  Cause euphoria
  Produce psychosis
  Decrease libido
  Blunt thyrotropin and gonadotropin activity
**EYE EFFECTS**
  May induce posterior subcapsular cataracts
**GROWTH AND DEVELOPMENTAL EFFECTS**
  Inhibit skeletal growth (pharmacologic doses)
  Mature surfactant, hepatic, and gastrointestinal systems

*PMN, polymorphonucleocytes; TSH, thyrotropin.*

include an important role in carbohydrate, lipid, and protein metabolism (Table 73-1). They also regulate immune, circulatory, and renal function. They influence growth, development, bone metabolism, and central nervous system (CNS) activity.

In stress situations, glucocorticoid secretion can increase up to almost 10-fold.[18,19] This increase is believed to enhance survival by increasing cardiac contractility, cardiac output, sensitivity to the pressor effects of the catecholamines and other pressor hormones, work capacity of the skeletal muscles, and capacity to mobilize energy through gluconeogenesis, proteolysis, and lipolysis. Persons with unrecognized adrenal insufficiency are at risk of life-threatening adrenal crisis if subjected to stress without glucocorticoid replacement.[20]

## CARBOHYDRATE METABOLISM

The daily secretion rate of cortisol varies little in the absence of stress. Cortisol interacts in a permissive fashion with many other hormones, including insulin, glucagon, catecholamines, and growth hormone, to achieve full homeostasis. For example, glucocorticoids are essential for normal epinephrine- or glucagon-stimulated lipolysis, gluconeogenesis, and glycogenolysis.[21,22] Excess cortisol increases hepatic glycogen and glucose production and decreases glucose uptake and utilization in the peripheral tissues. These effects combine to cause hyperglycemia. This may lead to overt diabetes in persons who have a decreased capacity to produce insulin. By contrast, glucocorticoid deficiency decreases glucose production and hepatic glycogen content and may cause hypoglycemia. However, serum glucose levels may be normal in the chronically ill patient with Addison disease because of a compensatory decrease in insulin secretion.

The primary action of the glucocorticoids on carbohydrate metabolism is to increase glucose production by increasing hepatic gluconeogenesis. Gluconeogenesis uses substrates derived from glycolysis, proteolysis, and lipolysis. Lactate is derived from glycolysis in muscle. Alanine is the primary substrate derived from proteolysis; fatty acids and glycerol are derived from lipolysis. In addition to inducing gluconeogenic enzymes, glucocorticoids stimulate glycolysis, proteolysis, and lipolysis, thus providing more substrate for gluconeogenesis. Glucocorticoids also increase cellular resistance to insulin, thereby decreasing entry of glucose into the cell. This inhibition of glucose uptake occurs in adipocytes, muscle cells, and fibroblasts. (Also see Chaps. 75 and 139.)

In addition to opposing insulin action, glucocorticoids may work in parallel with insulin to protect against long-term starvation by stimulating glycogen deposition and production in liver. Both hormones stimulate glycogen synthetase activity and decrease glycogen breakdown.

## LIPID METABOLISM

Glucocorticoids increase free fatty acid levels by enhancing lipolysis, decreasing cellular glucose uptake, and decreasing glycerol production, which is necessary for reesterification of fatty acids. This increase in lipolysis is also stimulated through the permissive enhancement of the lipolytic action of other factors such as epinephrine. This action affects adipocytes differently according to their anatomic locations. In the patient with glucocorticoid excess, fat is lost in the extremities, but it is increased in the trunk (centripetal obesity), neck, and face (moon facies).[23] This may involve effects on adipocyte differentiation.[24]

## PROTEIN METABOLISM

The glucocorticoids generally exert a catabolic/antianabolic effect on protein metabolism. This proteolysis in fat, skeletal muscle, bone, and lymphoid and connective tissue increases amino-acid substrates that can be used in gluconeogenesis. In muscle, the type II white glycolytic fibers are more affected than the type I fibers. Cardiac muscle and the diaphragm are almost entirely spared from this catabolic effect.

## IMMUNOLOGIC EFFECTS

Glucocorticoids play a profound role in immune regulation.[16,18] At high concentrations, they inhibit most immunologic and inflammatory responses. Although these effects may have beneficial aspects, they may also be detrimental to the host by inducing a state of immunosuppression that predisposes to infection. Glucocorticoids inhibit eicosanoid and glycolipid synthesis and the actions of bradykinin. They also block histamine and proinflammatory cytokine (tumor necrosis factor α, interleukin-1, and interleukin-6) secretion and effects.[25] These actions inhibit vasoactive agents and diminish the inflammatory process. Glucocorticoids may cause lymphocytopenia with a relative T-cell depletion, monocytopenia, and eosinopenia. They do so at least in part by inducing cell cycle arrest in the $G_1$ phase and by activating the apoptosis pathway through glucocorticoid receptor–mediated effects.[26]

In contrast, glucocorticoids increase circulating polymorphonuclear cell counts, mostly by preventing their egress from the circulation. Generally, glucocorticoids decrease diapedesis, chemotaxis, and phagocytosis of polymorphonuclear cells. Thus, the mobility of these cells is altered such that they do not arrive at the site of inflammation to mount an appropriate immune response. Some of these effects may be mediated by changes in levels of the cytokine migration inhibitory factor (MIF) from macrophages and T cells. Whereas physiologic levels of glucocorticoids promote release of MIF, pharmacologic doses inhibit MIF secretion.[27]

The suppressive effect of glucocorticoids is primarily exerted on T helper 1 cells and hence on cellular immunity, whereas the T helper 2 cells are spared, which effectively leads to a predominantly humoral immune response.[16,28] Indeed, glucocorticoids enhance secondary anamnestic antibody responses, whereas they inhibit primary antibody responses. Pharmacologic doses of glucocorticoids may also decrease the size of the immunologic tissues (i.e., the spleen, thymus, and lymph nodes).

In summary, high levels of glucocorticoids decrease inflammatory and cellular immune responses and increase susceptibility to certain bacterial, viral, fungal, and parasitic infections.

## EFFECTS ON SKIN

Glucocorticoids inhibit fibroblasts, which leads to increased bruising and poor wound healing through cutaneous atrophy. This effect explains the thinning of the skin that is seen in patients with Cushing syndrome[29] (see Chap. 75). Immunosuppressive effects of glucocorticoids makes them effective for skin conditions such as psoriasis.

## EFFECTS ON BONE AND CALCIUM

Glucocorticoids have the overall effect of decreasing serum calcium and have been used in emergency therapy for certain types of hypercalcemia (see Chap. 59). This hypocalcemic effect probably results from a decrease in the intestinal absorption of calcium and a decrease in the renal reabsorption of calcium and phosphorus. The serum calcium level, however, generally does not fall below normal because of the secondary increase in parathyroid hormone secretion.

The most significant effect of long-term glucocorticoid excess on calcium and bone metabolism is osteoporosis.[30] Glucocorticoids inhibit osteoblastic activity by decreasing the number and activity of osteoblasts.[31] Glucocorticoids also decrease osteoclastic activity, but to a lesser extent, leading to low bone turnover with an overall negative balance. The tendency of glucocorticoids to lower serum calcium and phosphate levels causes secondary hyperparathyroidism. Together, these actions decrease bone accretion and cause a net loss of bone mineral.

## CIRCULATORY AND RENAL EFFECTS

Glucocorticoids have a positive inotropic influence on the heart, increasing the left ventricular work index. Moreover, they have a permissive effect on the actions of epinephrine and norepinephrine on both the heart and the blood vessels. In the absence of glucocorticoids, decreased cardiac output and shock may develop; in states of glucocorticoid excess, hypertension is frequently observed. This may be due to activation of the mineralocorticoid receptor (see later) that occurs when renal 11β-hydroxysteroid dehydrogenase is saturated by excessive levels of glucocorticoids.

## CENTRAL NERVOUS SYSTEM EFFECTS

Glucocorticoids readily penetrate the blood–brain barrier and have direct effects on brain metabolism. They decrease CNS edema and are commonly used in therapy for increased intracranial pressure. Paradoxically, they also may contribute to the development of pseudotumor cerebri (increased intracranial pressure in the absence of a structural lesion). Their effects on mood and behavior are well recognized. They stimulate appetite and cause insomnia with a reduction in rapid eye movement sleep. An increase in irritability and emotional lability is seen, with an impairment of memory and ability to concentrate. Libido is decreased—an effect that may be secondary to both a direct glucocorticoid effect on behavior and glucocorticoid-induced inhibition of the reproductive system.

Glucocorticoid excess and deficiency may both be associated with clinical depression. Furthermore, glucocorticoid excess may produce a psychosis in some patients. Mild to moderate glucocorticoid excess for a limited period of time often causes a feeling of euphoria or well-being. Therefore, patients may object to a decrease in glucocorticoid dosage. Patients who have primary psychiatric disorders, such as depression or anorexia nervosa, may have abolition of the normal circadian pattern of glucocorticoid secretion and an increase in glucocorticoid production. These abnormalities are reversible with remission of the psychiatric illness and have been referred to as states of pseudo-Cushing syndrome (see Chap. 201).

Glucocorticoid effects in brain are mediated largely through interactions with two closely related receptors, sometimes referred to as type I and type II receptors. The type II receptor is the conventional glucocorticoid receptor. The type I receptor is identical to the mineralocorticoid receptor, but it has identical affinities for both glucocorticoids and mineralocorticoids in most areas of the brain in which it is expressed because of lack of concomitant expression of 11β-hydroxysteroid dehydrogenase[15] (see later and Chap. 72); this enzyme oxidizes glucocorticoids to inactive compounds in mineralocorticoid target tissues. The type I receptor, which is expressed at highest levels in the limbic system (i.e., the hippocampus),[32] has a 10-fold higher affinity for glucocorticoids than the type II receptor. Thus, glucocorticoid effects in the limbic system may be mediated predominantly through the type I receptor at normal levels and may activate the type II receptor mainly at elevated levels as seen under stress conditions.[32,33] These receptors have divergent and in some cases opposing effects. For example, activation of the type I receptors reduces sensitivity of hippocampal neurons to the neurotransmitter serotonin whereas activation of the type II receptors increases it.[34] Increased sensitivity of the hippocampus to serotonin may help explain the euphoria associated with high doses of glucocorticoids. In an analogous manner, glucocorticoids suppress release of corticotropin-releasing hormone (CRH) in the anterior hypothalamus but stimulate it in the central nucleus of the amygdala and lateral bed nucleus of the stria terminalis, where it may mediate fear and anxiety states.[35]

In addition, glucocorticoids and other steroids may have nongenomic effects by modulating activities of both γ-amino butyric acid (GABA) and N-methyl-D-aspartate (NMDA) receptors.[36]

## GROWTH

In excess, glucocorticoids inhibit linear growth and skeletal maturation in children.[37] This results primarily from the direct inhibitory effect of glucocorticoids on the epiphyses. This effect may in part be mediated by decreasing levels of insulin-like growth factor-I (IGF-I)[31] and by increasing levels of IGF-binding protein-1 (IGFBP-1), which inhibits somatic growth by decreasing circulating levels of free IGF-I.[38] Also, chronic glucocorticoid excess has been associated with inhibition of growth hormone secretion.[39]

Although excess glucocorticoids clearly impair growth, glucocorticoids are necessary for normal growth and development. In the fetus and neonate, they accelerate the differentiation and development of various tissues. Their actions include promoting the development of the hepatic and gastrointestinal systems as well as the production of surfactant in the fetal lung (see Chap. 202). Glucocorticoids are routinely given to pregnant women at risk for delivery of premature infants in an effort to accelerate these maturational processes.

## EFFECTS ON OTHER HORMONES

Glucocorticoids have several effects on pituitary function.[19,40] They primarily regulate adrenocorticotropic hormone (ACTH) secretion through glucocorticoid (type II) receptor–mediated effects at the hypothalamic and pituitary levels (see Chap. 72). In addition, they affect both thyroid and reproductive function.

**Thyroid Function.**    Glucocorticoids blunt the thyroid-stimulating hormone response to thyrotropin-releasing hormone stimulation. They decrease the peripheral conversion of thyroxine ($T_4$) to triiodothyronine ($T_3$) with a concomitant increase in reverse $T_3$. A decrease in both thyroid-binding globulin and thyroid-binding prealbumin is seen. The sum of these effects is usually a low-normal total $T_4$ and free $T_4$ level, without clinical manifestations of hypothyroidism.

**Gonadal Function.**    The glucocorticoids inhibit gonadotropin secretion both in the basal state and in response to gonadotropin-releasing hormone. These actions cause a decrease in gonadal sex steroid production.[41] The glucocorticoids also have direct inhibitory effects on the gonad, and they lead to a decrease in libido.[42] Together, these actions impair reproductive function.

## ACTIONS OF THE MINERALOCORTICOIDS

In order of decreasing potency, the mineralocorticoids include aldosterone, 11-deoxycorticosterone, 18-oxocortisol, corticosterone, and cortisol. As a class of hormones, they have more specific actions than the glucocorticoids. Their major function is to maintain intravascular volume by conserving sodium and eliminating potassium and hydrogen ions. They exert these actions in kidney, gut, and salivary and sweat glands. In addition, aldosterone may have distinct effects in other tissues. Mineralocorticoid receptors are found in the heart and vascular endothelium,[43] and aldosterone increases myocardial fibrosis.[44] Such receptors are also found in the brain (see earlier); although they are occupied predominantly by glucocorticoids in some regions of the brain, aldosterone has distinct effects in increasing salt hunger and blood pressure when administered into the cerebral ventricles.[45]

The distal convoluted tubules and collecting ducts of the kidney are the major sites of action of the mineralocorticoids.[46] In the cortical collecting duct, mineralocorticoids induce reabsorption of sodium and secretion of potassium. In the medullary collecting duct, they act in a permissive fashion to allow vasopressin to increase osmotic water flux.

Patients with mineralocorticoid deficiency may develop weight loss, hypotension, hyponatremia, and hyperkalemia, whereas patients with mineralocorticoid excess may develop hypertension, hypokalemia, and metabolic alkalosis[47] (see Chaps. 79 through 81).

The mechanisms by which aldosterone affects sodium excretion are incompletely understood. Most effects of aldosterone are presumably due to changes in gene expression mediated by the mineralocorticoid receptor; indeed, levels of subunits of both the $Na^+/K^+$–adenosine triphosphatase and the epithelial sodium channel (ENaC) increase in response to aldosterone. However, the mineralocorticoid receptor has not been shown to bind to hormone-response elements or to influence the transcription of these or any other genes. Moreover, the effects of aldosterone on the activity of the ENaC are considerably more rapid than these effects on gene expression, suggesting that aldosterone also (or perhaps mainly) affects translocation of channels to the apical cell membrane or the percentage of time the channels stay open. Such effects might be mediated by post-translational modifications to the regulatory subunits of ENaC, including proteolysis, phosphorylation, or carboxymethylation.[48] These changes might be mediated by the mineralocorticoid receptor or they might represent nongenomic effects, which have also been implicated in effects of aldosterone on cardiovascular function and leukocyte cell volume.[17]

Because the mineralocorticoid receptor actually has comparable affinities for cortisol and aldosterone, yet circulating levels of aldosterone are normally much lower than those of cortisol, aldosterone is able to have discrete bioeffects only because the 11β-hydroxysteroid dehydrogenase enzyme is able to oxidize glucocorticoids, but not aldosterone, to inactive steroids.[15]

## ACTIONS OF THE ADRENAL ANDROGENS

Many actions of adrenal androgens are exerted through their conversion to active androgens or estrogens such as testosterone, dihydrotestosterone, estrone, and estradiol. In men, <2% of the biologically important androgens are derived from adrenal production, whereas in women ~50% of androgens are of adrenal origin. The adrenal contribution to circulating estrogen levels is mainly important in pathologic conditions, such as feminizing adrenal tumors. Adrenal androgens contribute to the physiologic development of pubic and axillary hair during normal puberty. They also play an important role in the pathophysiology of congenital adrenal hyperplasia, premature adrenarche, adrenal tumors, and Cushing syndrome (see Chaps. 75, 77, and 83).

In humans, circulating levels of dehydroepiandrosterone (DHEA) and dehydroepiandrosterone sulfate (DHEAS), the chief adrenal androgens, reach a peak in early adulthood and then decline.[49] This has led to speculation that age-related physiologic changes might be reversed by DHEA administration, and beneficial effects have been proposed for insulin sensitivity, bone mineral density, muscle mass, cardiovascular risk, obesity, cancer risk, autoimmunity, and the central nervous system.[50] Many of these effects have been observed in rodents, which normally do not synthesize significant amounts of these steroids, but the extent to which they exist in humans is controversial at this time.

## REFERENCES

1. Mangelsdorf DJ, Thummel C, Beato M, et al. The nuclear receptor superfamily: the second decade. Cell 1995; 83:835.
2. Luisi BF, Schwabe JW, Freedman LP. The steroid/nuclear receptors: from three-dimensional structure to complex function. Vitam Horm 1994; 49:1.
3. Katzenellenbogen JA, O'Malley BW, Katzenellenbogen BS. Tripartite steroid hormone receptor pharmacology: interaction with multiple effector sites as a basis for the cell- and promoter-specific action of these hormones. Mol Endocrinol 1996; 10:119.
4. Forman BM, Tzameli I, Choi HS, et al. Androstane metabolites bind to and deactivate the nuclear receptor CAR-beta. Nature 1998; 395:612.
5. Freedman LP. Anatomy of the steroid receptor zinc finger region. Endocr Rev 1992; 13:129.
6. Akner G, Wikstrom AC, Gustafsson JA. Subcellular distribution of the glucocorticoid receptor and evidence for its association with microtubules. J Steroid Biochem Mol Biol 1995; 52:1.
7. Pratt WB, Toft DO. Steroid receptor interactions with heat shock protein and immunophilin chaperones. Endocr Rev 1997; 18:306.
8. Bamberger CM, Schulte HM, Chrousos GP. Molecular determinants of glucocorticoid receptor function and tissue sensitivity to glucocorticoids. Endocr Rev 1996; 17:245.
9. Truss M, Beato M. Steroid hormone receptors: interaction with deoxyribonucleic acid and transcription factors. Endocr Rev 1993; 14:459.
10. Pearce D, Yamamoto KR. Mineralocorticoid and glucocorticoid receptor activities distinguished by nonreceptor factors at a composite response element. Science 1993; 259:1161.
11. McEwan IJ, Wright AP, Gustafsson JA. Mechanism of gene expression by the glucocorticoid receptor: role of protein-protein interactions. Bioessays 1997; 19:153.
12. Shibata H, Spencer TE, Onate SA, et al. Role of co-activators and co-repressors in the mechanism of steroid/thyroid receptor action. Recent Prog Horm Res 1997; 52:141.
13. Horwitz KB, Jackson TA, Bain DL, et al. Nuclear receptor coactivators and corepressors. Mol Endocrinol 1996; 10:1167.
14. Spencer TE, Jenster G, Burcin MM, Allis CD, Zhou J, Mizzen CA, et al. Steroid receptor coactivator-1 is a histone acetyltransferase. Nature 1997; 389:194.
15. White PC, Mune T, Agarwal AK. 11β-hydroxysteroid dehydrogenase and the syndrome of apparent mineralocorticoid excess. Endocr Rev 1997; 18:135.
16. Chrousos GP. The hypothalamic-pituitary-adrenal axis and immune-mediated inflammation. N Engl J Med 1995; 332:1351.
17. Wehling M. Specific, nongenomic actions of steroid hormones. Annu Rev Physiol 1997; 59:365.
18. McEwen BS, Biron CA, Brunson KW, et al. The role of adrenocorticoids as modulators of immune function in health and disease: neural, endocrine and immune interactions. Brain Res Brain Res Rev 1997; 23:79.
19. Chrousos GP. Stressors, stress, and neuroendocrine integration of the adaptive response. The 1997 Hans Selye Memorial Lecture. Ann N Y Acad Sci 1998; 851:311.
20. Lamberts SW, Bruining HA, de Jong FH. Corticosteroid therapy in severe illness. N Engl J Med 1997; 337:1285.
21. McMahon M, Gerich J, Rizza R. Effects of glucocorticoids on carbohydrate metabolism. Diabetes Metab Rev 1988; 4:17.
22. Pilkis SJ, Granner DK. Molecular physiology of the regulation of hepatic gluconeogenesis and glycolysis. Annu Rev Physiol 1992; 54:885.
23. Bjorntorp P. Body fat distribution, insulin resistance, and metabolic diseases. Nutrition 1997; 13:795.
24. MacDougald OA, Lane MD. Transcriptional regulation of gene expression during adipocyte differentiation. Annu Rev Biochem 1995; 64:345.
25. Almawi WY, Beyhum HN, Rahme AA, Rieder MJ. Regulation of cytokine and cytokine receptor expression by glucocorticoids. J Leukoc Biol 1996; 60:563.
26. Cidlowski JA, King KL, Evans-Storms RB, et al. The biochemistry and molecular biology of glucocorticoid-induced apoptosis in the immune system. Recent Prog Horm Res 1996; 51:457.
27. Bucala R. MIF rediscovered: cytokine, pituitary hormone, and glucocorticoid-induced regulator of the immune response. FASEB J 1996; 10:1607.
28. Norbiato G, Bevilacqua M, Vago T, Clerici M. Glucocorticoids and Th-1, Th-2 type cytokines in rheumatoid arthritis, osteoarthritis, asthma, atopic dermatitis and AIDS. Clin Exp Rheumatol 1997; 15:315.
29. Yanovski JA, Cutler GBJ. Glucocorticoid action and the clinical features of Cushing's syndrome. Endocrinol Metab Clin North Am 1994; 23:487.
30. Lane NE, Lukert B. The science and therapy of glucocorticoid-induced bone loss. Endocrinol Metab Clin North Am 1998; 27:465.
31. Delany AM, Dong Y, Canalis E. Mechanisms of glucocorticoid action in bone cells. J Cell Biochem 1994; 56:295.
32. de Kloet ER, Vreugdenhil E, Oitzl MS, Joels M. Brain corticosteroid receptor balance in health and disease. Endocr Rev 1998; 19:269.
33. Lupien SJ, McEwen BS. The acute effects of corticosteroids on cognition: integration of animal and human model studies. Brain Res Brain Res Rev 1997; 24:1.
34. Meijer OC, de Kloet ER. Corticosterone and serotonergic neurotransmission in the hippocampus: functional implications of central corticosteroid receptor diversity. Crit Rev Neurobiol 1998; 12:1.
35. Schulkin J, Gold PW, McEwen BS. Induction of corticotropin-releasing hormone gene expression by glucocorticoids: implication for understanding the states of fear and anxiety and allostatic load. Psychoneuroendocrinology 1998; 23:219.
36. Revelli A, Tesarik J, Massobrio M. Nongenomic effects of neurosteroids. Gynecol Endocrinol 1998; 12:61.
37. Allen DB. Growth suppression by glucocorticoid therapy. Endocrinol Metab Clin North Am 1996; 25:699.
38. Lee PD, Giudice LC, Conover CA, Powell DR. Insulin-like growth factor binding protein-1: recent findings and new directions. Proc Soc Exp Biol Med 1997; 216:319.
39. Bertherat J, Bluet-Pajot MT, Epelbaum J. Neuroendocrine regulation of growth hormone. Eur J Endocrinol 1995; 132:12.
40. Kononen J, Honkaniemi J, Gustafsson JA, Pelto-Huikko M. Glucocorticoid receptor colocalization with pituitary hormones in the rat pituitary gland. Mol Cell Endocrinol 1993; 93:97.
41. Chrousos GP, Torpy DJ, Gold PW. Interactions between the hypothalamic-pituitary-adrenal axis and the female reproductive system: clinical implications. Ann Intern Med 1998; 129:229.
42. Michael AE, Cooke BA. A working hypothesis for the regulation of steroidogenesis and germ cell development in the gonads by glucocorticoids

and 11β-hydroxysteroid dehydrogenase (11β–HSD). Mol Cell Endocrinol 1994; 100:55.

43. Lombes M, Alfaidy N, Eugene E, et al. Prerequisite for cardiac aldosterone action. Mineralocorticoid receptor and 11β-hydroxysteroid dehydrogenase in the human heart. Circulation 1995; 92:175.

44. Young M, Fullerton MJ, Dilley R, Funder JW. Mineralocorticoids, hypertension, and cardiac fibrosis. J Clin Invest 1994; 93:2578.

45. Gomez-Sanchez EP. Central hypertensive effects of aldosterone. Front Neuroendocrinol 1997; 18:440.

46. Rogerson FM, Fuller PJ. Mineralocorticoid action. Steroids 2000; 65:61.

47. White PC. Disorders of aldosterone biosynthesis and action. N Engl J Med 1994; 331:250.

48. Garty H, Palmer LG. Epithelial sodium channels: function, structure, and regulation. Physiol Rev 1997; 77:359.

49. Lamberts SW, van den Beld AW, van der Lely AJ. The endocrinology of aging. Science 1997; 278:419.

50. Baulieu EE, Robel P. Dehydroepiandrosterone (DHEA) and dehydroepiandrosterone sulfate (DHEAS) as neuroactive neurosteroids. Proc Natl Acad Sci U S A 1998; 95:4089.

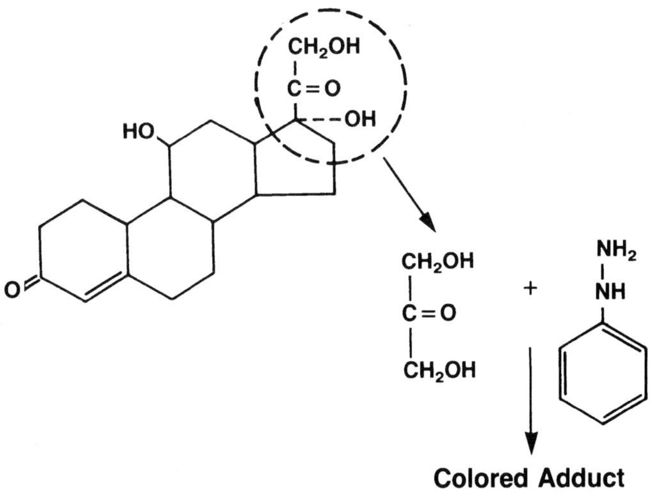

**FIGURE 74-1.** Principle of measurement of Porter-Silber chromogens.

# CHAPTER 74

# TESTS OF ADRENOCORTICAL FUNCTION

D. LYNN LORIAUX

The diagnosis of adrenocortical disease depends on accurate and precise laboratory measurements. The optimal application of the available tests is an evolving process. This chapter concentrates on those tests that the author believes are most useful. The discussion focuses on three categories of test: *tests used to document hypercortisolism or hypocortisolism; tests used for the differential diagnosis of hypercortisolism or hypocortisolism;* and *tests used to localize disease.* Further details concerning the rationale and interpretation of adrenal function tests are found in Chapters 14, 17, 75 through 83, 237, and 241.

## TESTS FOR DOCUMENTING HYPERCORTISOLISM

### URINARY FREE CORTISOL

Urinary free cortisol is cortisol in urine that is not conjugated to amino acids or glucuronic acid and, hence, is "free." Urinary free cortisol retains its preferential solubility in organic solvents and can be extracted from urine with diethyl ether or dichloromethane. After extraction, the organic solvent is evaporated and the residual cortisol is measured by one of several techniques. The most popular is radioimmunoassay (RIA).[1]

The advantage of the measurement of urinary free cortisol over other techniques used to document hypercortisolism is sensitivity. Patients with hypercortisolism rarely fall into the normal range.[2–4] The ranges of urinary free cortisol excretion for normal persons and persons subsequently proved to have hypercortisolism overlap by only 1% to 2%. This overlap is considerably greater with other methods. The physiologic mechanism underlying this high degree of specificity is probably the relationship between corticosteroid-binding globulin (CBG) binding capacity and the normal cortisol production rate. The binding capacity of CBG is nearly saturated at normal rates of cortisol production. At greater than normal rates of cortisol secretion, the unbound fraction of plasma cortisol increases disproportionately. Because urinary free cortisol is derived from the unbound or bioactive cortisol by glomerular filtration, the free cortisol concentration in the urine rises rapidly as the bind-ing capacity of CBG is exceeded. Thus, the urinary free cortisol level directly reflects the bioactive plasma cortisol concentration. The most important variable affecting the excretion of urinary free cortisol is its reabsorption by the nephron. Because >95% of filtered cortisol is reabsorbed, small changes in the reabsorbed fraction can make large differences in the quantitative urinary excretion of the hormone. Fortunately, this is not a complicating variable in most cases of hypercortisolism. The normal values for urinary free cortisol, as with all tests, vary with the individual laboratory, but the normal basal excretion of urinary free cortisol typically is <100 µg/d.

## PORTER-SILBER CHROMOGENS

Porter-Silber chromogen measurement often is termed the *17-hydroxycorticosteroids* test. Measurement of Porter-Silber chromogens and 17-hydroxycorticosteroids, however, are different tests. In the United States, the available test virtually always is the Porter-Silber chromogens test.[5] In this procedure, the side chain of cortisol (carbons 17, 20, and 21) is measured. This side chain can be thought of as dihydroxyacetone. Dihydroxyacetone forms a colored adduct with phenylhydrazine that has an absorption maximum at 410 nm, which allows the concentration to be measured using spectrophotometry (Fig. 74-1). The measurement involves, first, a hydrolysis step to free the steroid of its conjugate and render it lipid soluble; second, an extraction with an organic solvent; and, third, a color reaction followed by spectrophotometric measurement. The main steroids measured by this test are metabolites of cortisol, not cortisol itself (Fig. 74-2).

The complexity of the test offers several opportunities for artifact. Examples include drug-induced interference with the hydrolysis step (e.g., by aspirin)[6]; decreased efficiency of organic extraction subsequent to increased polarity of the metabolites of cortisol, resulting from a drug-induced alteration in hepatic metabolism (e.g., by phenytoin, phenobarbital)[7,8]; and interference with the color reaction by medications and their metabolites (e.g., some of the minor tranquilizers). Many other unrecognized hazards can render the test unreliable. Because most of these hazards can be attributed to medications, the test always should be performed with the patient in a drug-free state.

The normal range for Porter-Silber chromogens remains constant throughout life, at 4.5 ± 2.5 mg/g creatinine per day.[9] Approximately one-third of the daily production of cortisol finds its way into the Porter-Silber chromogen pool. A note of caution: Porter-Silber chromogen excretion has a diurnal variation, whereas creatinine excretion does not. Thus, inadequate

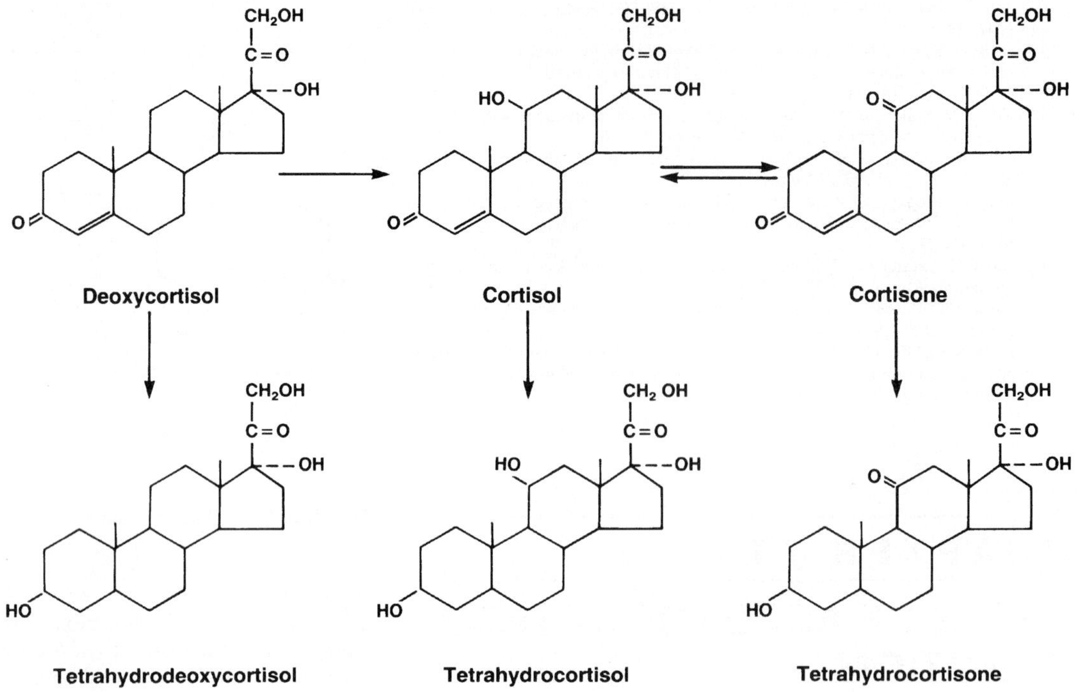

FIGURE 74-2. Urinary corticosteroids measured by Porter-Silber chromogen technique.

**Deoxycortisol**    **Cortisol**    **Cortisone**

**Tetrahydrodeoxycortisol**    **Tetrahydrocortisol**    **Tetrahydrocortisone**

urine collections *cannot* be corrected on the basis of the creatinine measurement. Collections that are deficient early in the day give artificially low values when corrected in this assay, and collections that are deficient late in the day give artificially high values.

## PLASMA CORTISOL

Cortisol is secreted episodically. Normally, 8 to 10 bursts of cortisol are secreted each day. These bursts tend to cluster in the morning hours, which leads to a diurnal pattern in the concentration of plasma cortisol.[10] This feature of cortisol secretion makes the interpretation of a single plasma cortisol value hazardous. An additional confounding factor is that cortisol circulates bound to CBG. The concentration of this α-globulin modulates the concentration of plasma cortisol at any given production rate. Thus, factors that change plasma CBG concentration (e.g., estrogens) ultimately are reflected in the plasma concentration of cortisol.[11]

Plasma cortisol is measured almost exclusively by RIA. This technique involves the extraction of cortisol from plasma with an organic solvent and subsequent measurement based on a competition with radiolabeled cortisol for binding sites on antibodies with high affinity and specificity for cortisol. The technique is fast, inexpensive, and reliable. The physician should be aware, however, that, depending on the antibody used, molecules other than cortisol can compete for binding sites. The most important of these are 11-deoxycortisol (especially during the administration of metyrapone) and synthetic glucocorticoids such as prednisone and dexamethasone.[1]

## TESTS FOR THE DIFFERENTIAL DIAGNOSIS OF HYPERCORTISOLISM

The traditional differential diagnostic tests for adrenal hyperfunction, which focus on establishing the presence or absence of an intact feedback loop, are the dexamethasone suppression test and the metyrapone test. These tests are difficult to interpret and are quickly becoming obsolete. Because metyrapone is

now hard to obtain, this test is included here mainly for historical interest.

## DEXAMETHASONE SUPPRESSION TEST

As developed by Liddle and colleagues, the dexamethasone suppression test measures the response of the Porter-Silber chromogens to the exogenous administration of dexamethasone.[12] Urine collections are made for 6 days. Basal, or control, collections are made on days 1 and 2 of the test. Dexamethasone is given at a dose of 2 mg per day on days 3 and 4, and 8 mg per day on days 5 and 6. At some point during the test, the excretion of Porter-Silber chromogens is reduced by half in 95% of patients with Cushing disease (Fig. 74-3). It is reduced by less

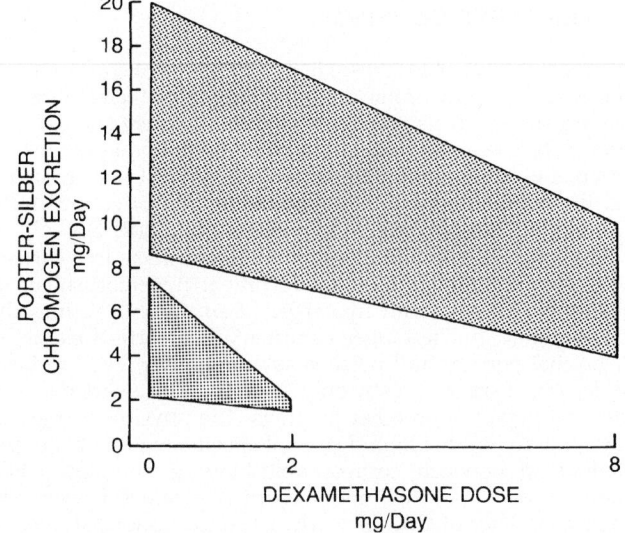

FIGURE 74-3. The pattern of Porter-Silber chromogen excretion in normal humans (*lower area*) and in patients with Cushing disease (*upper area*) in response to the administration of dexamethasone. Porter-Silber chromogens are reduced in both groups, but considerably less so in patients with Cushing disease.

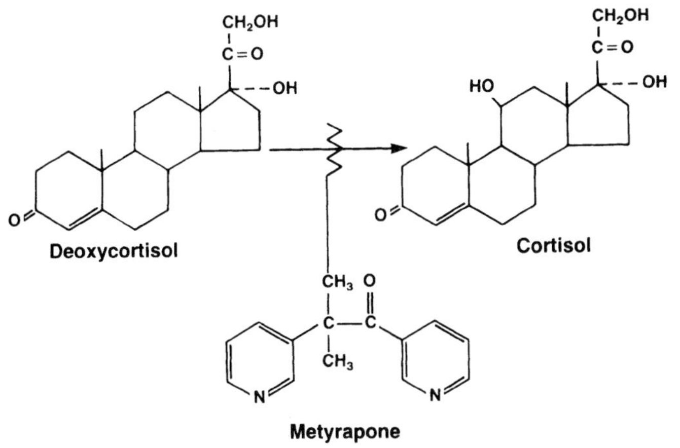

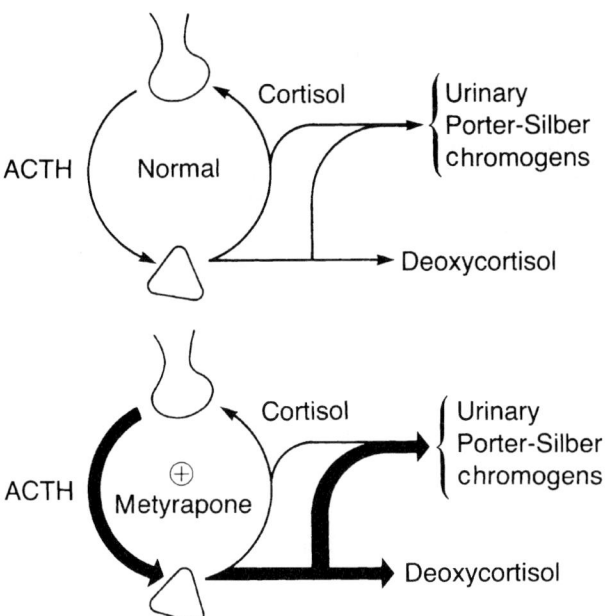

**FIGURE 74-4.** Metyrapone blockade of biosynthesis of cortisol.

than half in patients with other causes of Cushing syndrome. The urine free cortisol also can be used as an end point, but must decrease by 80% or more to indicate that suppression has occurred[13] (see Chap. 75).

## METYRAPONE TEST

Metyrapone is a competitive inhibitor of the 11-hydroxylase enzyme (Fig. 74-4). It blocks the biosynthesis of cortisol. This leads to a reduced plasma cortisol concentration. If the feedback axis is intact, adrenocorticotropic hormone (ACTH) secretion increases in an attempt to reestablish normal plasma cortisol concentrations. Because large amounts of 11-deoxycortisol are produced, 11-deoxycortisol and its metabolites raise the urinary concentration of Porter-Silber chromogens (Fig. 74-5). The traditional rule of thumb is that a doubling of the basal level of Porter-Silber chromogens indicates an intact feedback axis.[14]

A similar pattern of changes can be seen in the plasma concentrations of cortisol and 11-deoxycortisol. During effective blockade with metyrapone, plasma cortisol concentrations fall to <5 µg/dL. Plasma 11-deoxycortisol concentrations rise to over 50% of the baseline cortisol concentrations (always >7 µg/dL) if the feedback axis is intact. Before the metyrapone test can be interpreted, it must be shown that a blocking dose of metyrapone has been delivered. Plasma cortisol concentrations at the detection limit of the cortisol assay are the most reliable guide for this.[15]

The two main variations of the metyrapone test are the standard 2-day test and the overnight test. The standard 2-day test is performed by giving 750 mg of metyrapone orally every 4 hours for 1 day. The urinary concentration of Porter-Silber chromogens is measured that day and again the next day. A doubling of the level of Porter-Silber chromogens is a rough guide to the normal response. Plasma cortisol, measured 4 hours after the last metyrapone dose, should be <5 µg/dL, and plasma 11-deoxycortisol should range between 10 and 30 µg/dL. The overnight metyrapone test is performed by giving metyrapone, 30 mg/kg orally, at midnight. Plasma cortisol values at 8:00 a.m. should be lower than 5 µg/dL and 11-deoxycortisol levels should be >7 µg/dL.[16]

The response to metyrapone can be altered by abnormalities of thyroid function.[17] Several drugs, including estrogens and diphenylhydantoin, can invalidate the test.[18,19]

## CORTICOTROPIN-RELEASING HORMONE TEST

The corticotropin-releasing hormone (CRH) test is currently the test of choice for the differential diagnosis of Cushing syndrome.[20] CRH, a 41–amino-acid peptide of hypothalamic origin, plays an important role in the regulation of ACTH secretion (see Chap. 14). A single intravenous bolus of CRH stimulates the release of ACTH in normal persons (Fig. 74-6). Plasma cortisol concentrations >20 µg/dL, however, prevent the release of ACTH from the normal pituitary gland. Thus, CRH fails to stimulate the release of ACTH in patients with Cushing syndrome if the cause is anything other than a pituitary tumor that is secreting ACTH. Alternatively, ACTH-secreting pituitary tumors are resistant to the feedback effects of cortisol; they retain the ability to respond to CRH, even at high plasma cortisol concentrations. A plasma ACTH concentration of >10 pg/mL after CRH administration defines ACTH-dependent hypercortisolism. Values of <10 pg/mL are characteristic of ACTH-independent hypercortisolism.[21]

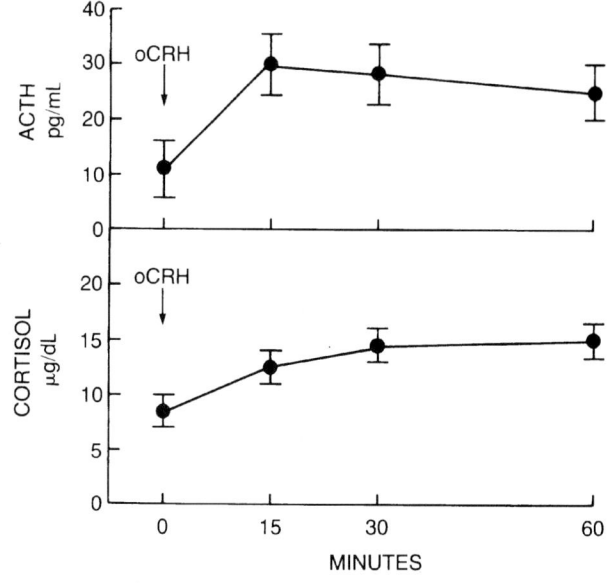

**FIGURE 74-5.** Principle of metyrapone testing. See text for explanation. (*ACTH*, adrenocorticotropic hormone.)

**FIGURE 74-6.** Effect of ovine corticotropin-releasing hormone (*oCRH*) on levels of plasma adrenocorticotropic hormone (*ACTH*) and cortisol in normal persons.

The test is performed by administering ovine CRH, 1 µg/kg, intravenously over 1 minute. Blood samples are drawn after 30, 45, and 60 minutes for the measurement of ACTH. A positive response is any value >10 pg/mL.

The untoward effects of CRH are limited to a facial flush and sense of warmth, which occur in ~10% of patients. Larger doses can induce hypotension and should not be used.

## TESTS FOR ADRENAL HYPOFUNCTION

The normal ranges of plasma cortisol and urinary free cortisol overlap the detection limit of most assays. In other words, a value of "zero" can be normal. Thus, reliable tests of adrenal insufficiency evaluate the ability of plasma cortisol to respond to an ACTH stimulus. The cosyntropin (Cortrosyn) test is the most convenient and reliable. This test is performed by administering an intravenous bolus of 250 µg of synthetic β1-24 ACTH and measuring the plasma cortisol concentration 45 and 60 minutes later.[22] A plasma cortisol concentration of 20 µg/dL is the lower limit of the normal response. Anything less than this suggests impaired adrenal function.[23] Localizing the cause of adrenal insufficiency to the adrenal gland itself or to the hypothalamic-pituitary unit can be accomplished efficiently by measuring plasma ACTH. High ACTH concentrations localize the defect to the adrenal gland; normal or low concentrations localize the defect to the hypothalamus or pituitary.[24] The RIA for ACTH has been notoriously unreliable, but the commercially available two-site immunoradiometric assay measurements are of high quality.[25]

## TESTS FOR CONGENITAL ADRENAL HYPERPLASIA

Diagnosis of the various syndromes of congenital adrenal hyperplasia depends on the measurement of the steroid biosynthetic intermediate before the blocked step (see Chap. 77). All the plasma marker steroids now can be measured by specific RIAs. The appropriate measurements include 17-hydroxyprogesterone (for 21-hydroxylase deficiency), 11-deoxycortisol (for 11-hydroxylase deficiency), 17-hydroxypregnenolone (for 3β-hydroxysteroid dehydrogenase deficiency), and progesterone or pregnenolone (for 17-hydroxylase deficiency).

## TESTS FOR LOCALIZATION

Four tests are useful in localizing the site of disease in disorders of adrenal function: petrosal sinus sampling, computed tomography (CT), magnetic resonance imaging, and the iodocholesterol scan.

### PETROSAL SINUS SAMPLING

The venous drainage of the pituitary gland can be sampled in the inferior petrosal sinuses (Fig. 74-7). The finding of an ACTH gradient between petrosal sinus blood and peripheral blood in a patient with hypercortisolism localizes the site of ACTH production to the sella or parasellar region.[26,26a] Because the venous drainage of the pituitary gland tends to lateralize (the right half drains into the right inferior petrosal sinus and the left half drains into the left sinus), the site of an ACTH-producing microadenoma usually can be localized within the pituitary gland. The usefulness of the test is increased by sampling during the administration of CRH: the central/peripheral ACTH gradients and the right/left gradient are enhanced by this addition. The average gradient in Cushing disease is ~15, with a lower limit of 1.7. The lower limit increases to 3 after CRH administra-

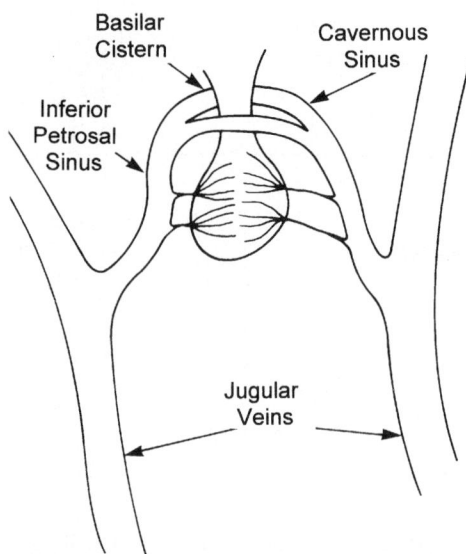

**FIGURE 74-7.** Anatomy of venous draining of the pituitary gland.

tion, which completely separates this population from those with nonpituitary causes of Cushing syndrome. Current data suggest that the test correctly identifies pituitary disease >95% of the time, which makes it the most powerful single test for differential diagnosis in Cushing syndrome.[27] In previously untreated patients, the procedure correctly lateralizes the disease ~85% of the time. Untoward effects are largely confined to the catheterization process. A few patients have had transient signs and symptoms of brainstem dysfunction or other neurological findings.[27a] These have not led to permanent disability. Other untoward effects include bleeding, bruising, and minor infections at the venipuncture site.

### COMPUTED TOMOGRAPHY

CT has become the procedure of choice in localizing adrenal disease (see Chap. 88). Most adrenal cancers are large, and CT, for practical purposes, identifies all these, as well as nearly all the smaller adrenal adenomas. Other useful findings revealed by CT include adrenal hyperplasia, usually bilateral and symmetric, and an abnormal intraabdominal fat distribution that supports the clinical diagnosis of Cushing syndrome.[28–31]

### MAGNETIC RESONANCE IMAGING

Magnetic resonance imaging offers only a single advantage over CT in the differential diagnosis of adrenal disease: the classification of adrenal masses into probably benign versus probably malignant categories on the basis of the T2-weighted image.[32] Normal adrenal glands are dark on T1-weighted magnetic resonance imaging scans. Benign adenomas remain dark when the scan is shifted to T2-weighting, but malignant lesions become bright. A hyperintense rim on fat-saturated spin-echo magnetic resonance imaging is often seen in adrenal adenomas and may aid in their differentiation from adrenal metastases.[33] Adrenal cysts and pheochromocytomas also are bright, but usually present no problem in diagnosis when viewed in the context of other endocrine tests and the ultrasound examination for cystic structure (see Chap. 88).

### IODOCHOLESTEROL SCAN

The iodocholesterol scan is an imaging procedure that depends on the *function* of the adrenal gland. It is rarely required in the differential diagnosis of hypercortisolism. Circulating cholesterol serves as the precursor for most of the steroids produced by the adrenal gland. Not surprisingly, therefore, circulating cholesterol is concentrated in the adrenal glands. Iodocholesterol, a γ-emitter, can be used to examine this physiologic process. Normal and hyperactive glands image bilaterally. Adenomas causing Cushing syndrome image, but the contralateral side does not, because the resultant hypercortisolism suppresses ACTH and diminishes the function of the normal gland. Adrenal carcinomas causing Cushing syndrome fail to produce an image because of an inefficient cholesterol-concentrating mechanism. The contralateral normal side also fails to image because ACTH secretion is suppressed. Thus, if both sides are visualized, an ACTH-dependent process is implied. If one side is visualized, an adrenal adenoma is implied. If neither side is seen, adrenal carcinoma or factitious disease is suggested.[34–36]

## REFERENCES

1. Ruder HJ, Guy RL, Lipsett MB. Radioimmunoassay for cortisol in plasma and urine. J Clin Endocrinol Metab 1972; 35:219.
2. Murphy BEP. Clinical evaluation of urinary cortisol determinations by competitive protein binding radioassay. J Clin Endocrinol Metab 1968; 28:343.
3. Hsu TH, Bledsoe T. Measurement of urinary free corticoids by competitive protein binding radioassay in hypoadrenal states. J Clin Endocrinol Metab 1970; 30:443.
4. Beardwell CG, Burke CW, Cope CL. Urinary free cortisol measured by competitive protein binding. J Endocrinol 1968; 42:79.
5. Silber RH, Porter CC. The determination of 17-21-dihydroxy, 20-ketosteroids in urine and plasma. J Biol Chem 1954; 210:923.
6. Borushek S, Gold JJ. Commonly used medications that interfere with routine endocrine laboratory procedures. Clin Chem 1964; 10:41.
7. Werk EE, MacBee T, Sholiton LJ. Effect of diphenylhydantoin on cortisol metabolism in man. J Clin Invest 1964; 43:1824.
8. Burstein S, Klaiber EL. Phenobarbital-induced increase in 6-hydroxycortisol excretion: clue to its significance in human urine. J Clin Endocrinol Metab 1965; 25:293.
9. Franks RC. Urinary 17-hydroxycorticosteroid and cortisol excretion in childhood. J Clin Endocrinol Metab 1973; 36:702.
10. Krieger DT, Allen W, Rizzo F, Krieger HP. Characterization of the normal temporal pattern of plasma corticosteroid levels. J Clin Endocrinol Metab 1971; 32:266.
11. Doe RP, Zimmerman HH, Flink EB. Significance of the concentration of nonprotein bound plasma cortisol in normal subjects, Cushing's syndrome, pregnancy, and during estrogen therapy. J Clin Endocrinol Metab 1960; 20:1484.
12. Liddle GW, Island DP, Meador CK. Normal and abnormal regulation of corticotropin secretion in man. Recent Prog Horm Res 1962; 18:125.
13. Flack MR, Loriaux DL, Nieman LK. Urinary free cortisol excretion: a better measure of response to the dexamethasone suppression test in Cushing's syndrome? (Abstract). New Orleans: Endocrine Society, 1988:1.
14. Liddle GW, Estep HL, Kendall TW. Clinical application of a new test of pituitary reserve. J Clin Endocrinol Metab 1959; 19:875.
15. Meikle AW, Jubiz W, Hutchings MD, et al. A simplified metyrapone test with determination of plasma 11-deoxycortisol (metyrapone test with plasma S). J Clin Endocrinol Metab 1969; 29:985.
16. Jubiz W, Meikle AW, West CD, Tyler FH. A single dose metyrapone test. Arch Intern Med 1970; 125:472.
17. Cushman P. Hypothalamic-pituitary-adrenal function in thyroid disorders: effects of metyrapone infusion on plasma corticosteroids. Metabolism 1968; 17:263.
18. Meikle AW, Jubiz W, Matsukura S, et al. Effect of estrogen on the metabolism of metyrapone and release of ACTH. J Clin Endocrinol Metab 1970; 30:259.
19. Jubiz W, Levinson RA, Meikle AW. Absorption and conjugation of metyrapone during diphenylhydantoin therapy: mechanism of abnormal response to oral metyrapone. Endocrinology 1970; 86:328.
20. Chrousos GP, Schulte HM, Oldfield EH, et al. The corticotropin releasing factor stimulation test: an aid in the evaluation of patients with Cushing's syndrome. N Engl J Med 1984; 310:622.
21. Nieman LK, Chrousos GP, Oldfield EH, et al. The corticotropin-releasing hormone stimulation test and the dexamethasone suppression test in the differential diagnosis of Cushing's syndrome. Ann Intern Med 1986; 105:862.
22. Kehlet H, Binder C. Value of an ACTH test in assessing hypothalamic-pituitary-adrenocortical function in glucocorticoid treated patients. BMJ 1973; 2:147.
23. Lindholm J, Kehlet H, Blichert-Toft M. Reliability of the 30-minute ACTH test in assessing hypothalamic-pituitary-adrenal function. J Clin Endocrinol Metab 1978; 47:272.
24. Schulte HM, Chrousos GP, Avgerinos P. The CRF test: a possible aid in the evaluation of adrenal insufficiency. J Clin Endocrinol Metab 1984; 58:1064.
25. Slyper AH, Findling JW. Use of a two-site immunoradiometric assay to resolve a factitious elevation of ACTH in primary pigmented nodular adrenocortical disease. J Pediatr Endocrinol 1994; 7:61.
26. Oldfield EH, Chrousos GP, Schulte HM, et al. Preoperative localization of ACTH secreting pituitary microadenomas by bilateral and simultaneous inferior petrosal sinus sampling. N Engl J Med 1985; 312:100.
27. Zovickian J, Oldfield EH, Doppman JL, et al. Usefulness of inferior petrosal sinus venous endocrine markers in Cushing's disease. J Neurosurg 1988; 68:205.
27a. Lefournier V, Gatta B, Martinie M, et al. One transient neurological complication (sixth nerve palsy) in 166 consecutive interior petrosal sinus samplings for the etiological diagnosis of Cushing's syndrome. J Clin Endocrinol Metab 1999; 84:3401.
28. Vincent JM, Morrison ID, Armstrong P, Reznek RH. The size of normal adrenal glands on computed tomography. Clin Radiol 1994; 49:453.
29. Ganguly A, Pratt JH, Yune HY, et al. Detection of adrenal tumors by computerized tomographic scan in endocrine hypertension. Arch Intern Med 1979; 139:590.
30. Kelestimur F, Unlu Y, Ozesmi M, Tolu I. A hormonal and radiological evaluation of adrenal gland in patients with acute or chronic pulmonary tuberculosis. Clin Radiol 1994; 49:453.
31. White FE, White MC, Drury PL, et al. Value of computed tomography of the abdomen and chest in investigation of Cushing's syndrome. BMJ 1982; 284:771.
32. Heinz-Peer G, Honigschabel S, Schneider B, et al. Characterization of adrenal masses using MR imaging with histopathologic correlation. AJR Am J Roentgenol 1999; 173:15.
33. Ichikawa T, Ohtamo K, Uchiyama G, et al. Adrenal adenomas: characteristic hyperintense rim sign on fat-saturated spin-echo MR images. Radiology 1994; 193:247.
34. Moses DC, Schteingart DS, Sturman MF, et al. Efficacy of radiocholesterol imaging of the adrenal glands in Cushing's syndrome. Surg Gynecol Obstet 1974; 139:201.
35. Chatal JR, Charbonnel B, Le Mevel BP, et al. Uptake of $^{131}$I-19-iodocholesterol by an adrenal cortical carcinoma and its metastases. J Clin Endocrinol Metab 1976; 43:248.
36. Beierwaltes WH, Sisson JC, Shapiro B. Diagnosis of adrenal tumors with radionuclide imaging. Spec Top Endocrinol Metab 1984; 6:1.

# CHAPTER 75

# CUSHING SYNDROME

DAVID E. SCHTEINGART

Cushing syndrome is the clinical expression of the metabolic effects of persistent, inappropriate hypercortisolism. Since the disorder was first described by Harvey Cushing in 1932, great progress has been made in understanding its pathophysiology and the spectrum of its clinical presentation. The diagnosis can now be precisely established by biochemical means, by noninvasive imaging of the pituitary and adrenal lesions, and by selective identification of the source of corticotropin (ACTH or adrenocorticotropic hormone) in the ACTH-dependent types.

The clinical manifestations of Cushing syndrome involve many organ systems and metabolic processes.[1] Hypertension, obesity, diabetes, androgen-type hirsutism, and acne are commonly seen in these patients and are prevalent in patients who do not have primary cortisol excess. When present, the following findings increase the suspicion of Cushing syndrome: symptoms and signs of protein catabolism (e.g., ecchymoses, myopathy, osteopenia); truncal obesity; lanugal hirsutism; cutaneous lesions (i.e., wide, purple striae; tinea versicolor; verruca vulgaris); hyperpigmentation; and psychiatric manifestations (i.e., impairment of affect, cognition, and vegetative functions).[2–6] In some instances, the diagnosis of Cushing syndrome can be strongly suspected on clinical grounds alone, but for most patients, the diagnosis is established by laboratory studies.[7]

## PATHOPHYSIOLOGY

Cushing syndrome can be *exogenous*, resulting from the administration of glucocorticoids or ACTH, or *endogenous*, resulting from a primary increased secretion of cortisol or ACTH. An etiologic classification of Cushing syndrome is given in Figure 75-1.

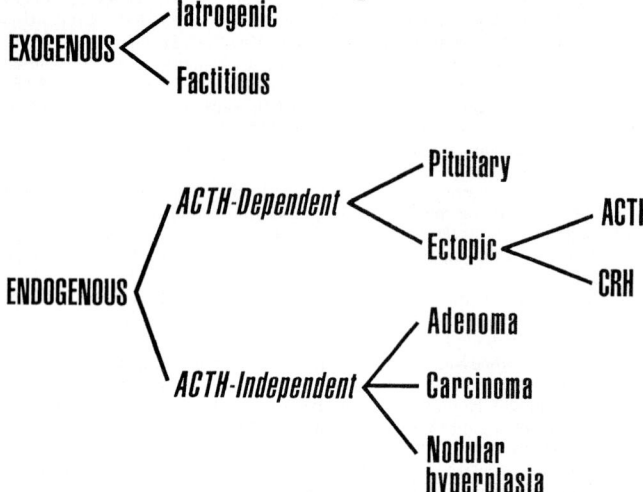

**FIGURE 75-1.** Classification of Cushing syndrome. (*ACTH*, corticotropin; *CRH*, corticotropin-releasing hormone.)

The changes in ACTH and cortisol secretion observed in patients with *ACTH-dependent* and *ACTH-independent* Cushing syndrome are illustrated in Figure 75-2. In the ACTH-dependent types, ACTH is secreted by the pituitary gland or by an extrapituitary neoplasm capable of producing peptide hormones, including ACTH and corticotropin-releasing hormone (CRH). In pituitary-dependent *Cushing disease*, the feedback relationship between the pituitary and the adrenal glands is maintained but is abnormal. In the *ectopic ACTH syndrome*, pituitary ACTH release is suppressed by excessive production of cortisol, which is stimulated by an unsuppressible overproduction of ACTH by the ectopic source. In *ectopic CRH syndrome*, tumor CRH stimulates ACTH secretion by the pituitary cortico-

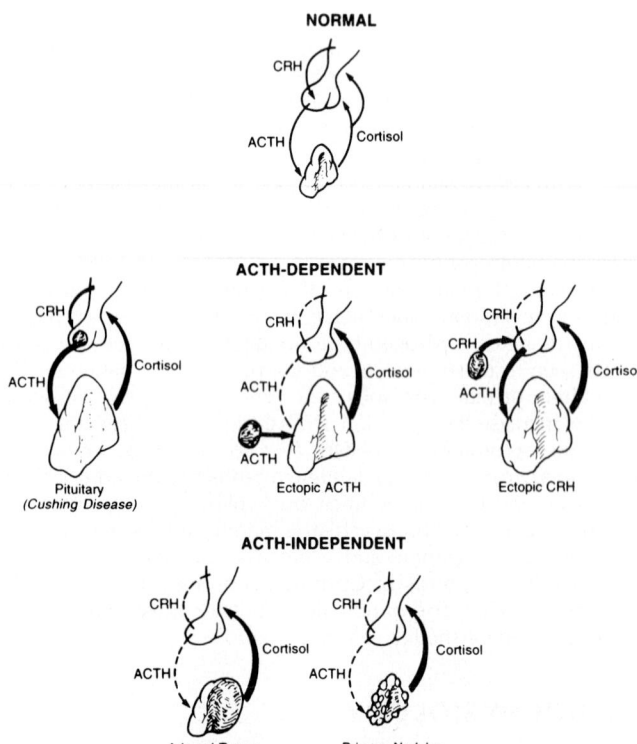

**FIGURE 75-2.** Corticotropin (*ACTH*) and cortisol levels in ACTH-dependent and ACTH-independent types of Cushing syndrome. (*CRH*, corticotropin-releasing hormone.)

tropes; this causes an excessive production of cortisol that is not sufficient to suppress ACTH secretion. In patients with ACTH-independent types of Cushing syndrome, pituitary ACTH secretion is suppressed by excessive cortisol production that originates in *adrenocortical tumors* (i.e., adenomas or carcinomas) or in *autonomous nodular hyperplastic glands*.

# CORTICOTROPIN-DEPENDENT CUSHING SYNDROME

## PITUITARY CORTICOTROPIN-DEPENDENT CUSHING SYNDROME

Approximately 85% of patients with pituitary ACTH-dependent Cushing syndrome, also called Cushing disease, have pituitary microadenomas. The origin, nature, and biochemical characteristics of these microadenomas are not clear.[8,9] In most cases, the microadenomas are located in the periphery of the gland and can be identified by imaging techniques or transsphenoidal pituitary exploration. Occasionally, they are located deep in the central wedge of the pituitary and can be missed on imaging or at surgery.[8] The suggestion has been made that excessive ACTH secretion may be caused by neurohypothalamic stimulation, which results in corticotrope hyperplasia.[10,11] However, fewer than 17% of cases of Cushing disease are associated with ACTH hypersecretion by nonneoplastic corticotrope cells.[12] Whether pituitary ACTH-dependent Cushing disease develops from a primary pituitary disorder or is the result of corticotrope stimulation by CRH has been unclear. In the case of a pituitary adenoma, the nonadenomatous corticotropes are usually suppressed, and removal of the adenoma is followed by ACTH and cortisol insufficiency. In the rare cases of corticotrope hyperplasia, the possibility exists that these corticotropes have been stimulated from a hypothalamic source. Clonal analysis of the pituitary tissue obtained from patients with Cushing disease shows that ACTH-secreting adenomas have a monoclonal pattern consistent with a monoclonal proliferation of a genetically altered cell. Thus, a spontaneous somatic mutation in pituitary corticotropes is the primary pathogenetic mechanism in this disorder. In contrast, the corticotrope hyperplasia seen in patients with CRH-secreting bronchial carcinoids is polyclonal.[13] Direct measurement of CRH levels in patients with Cushing disease secondary to a pituitary adenoma has not been performed. In the few patients in whom CRH levels have been measured in the spinal fluid, low levels have been found, suggesting suppressed CRH secretion.

The manifestations of abnormal ACTH secretion in Cushing disease are a loss of normal negative feedback and a blunted circadian rhythm of ACTH and cortisol secretion. Although the relative sensitivity of ACTH release to corticosteroid suppression remains in most of these patients, as many as 40% exhibit resistance to suppression and resemble patients with the ectopic ACTH syndrome. Unusual abnormal patterns of release of ACTH and cortisol have been described, and episodes of hypersecretion have persisted for hours or weeks and are interrupted by periods of normal secretion.[14,15] This *periodic hormonogenesis* has been found in patients with and without ACTH-secreting pituitary adenomas.

## ECTOPIC CORTICOTROPIN SYNDROME

The association of Cushing syndrome with nonadrenal neoplasms has been recognized for decades and is called the *ectopic ACTH syndrome*.[16] Typically, a rapidly developing malignancy causes the autonomous secretion of high levels of ACTH and cortisol, with clinical manifestations of Cushing syndrome and pigmentation. Approximately 50% of these ectopic ACTH-secreting tumors are in the lung, and the remainder occur in a variety of tissues. Table 75-1 describes the type and frequency of these tumors.

**TABLE 75-1.**
Tumors Causing Ectopic Corticotropin Syndrome

| Tumor | Percentage of Patients with Tumor | |
|---|---|---|
| | (25 *Patients**) | (16 *Patients†*) |
| Bronchial carcinoid | 28 | 37 |
| Small cell carcinoma of lung | 20 | 19 |
| Thymic carcinoid | 8 | 12 |
| Pancreatic carcinoma | 4 | |
| Islet cell pancreatic tumor | 16 | 12 |
| Pheochromocytoma | 12 | 6 |
| Ovarian tumor | 4 | |

*Data from Jex RK, Vanheerden JA, Carpenter PC, et al. Ectopic ACTH syndrome—diagnostic and therapeutic aspects. Am J Surg 1985; 149:276.

†Data from Howlett TA, Drury PL, Perry L, et al. Diagnosis and management of an ACTH-dependent Cushing's syndrome: comparison of the features of an ectopic and pituitary ACTH production. Clin Endocrinol 1986; 24:699.

Pancreatic islet cell tumors have been associated with Cushing syndrome in fewer than 5% of patients. In addition to ACTH, these tumors sometimes contain other hormones, such as insulin, gastrin, and glucagon, which are not produced in sufficient amounts to cause a metabolic syndrome. Less frequent causes of the ectopic ACTH syndrome include thymic carcinoids; gastric and appendicular carcinomas; pheochromocytomas; adrenal medullary paragangliomas; cystadenomas of the pancreas; epithelial carcinomas of the thymus; medullary thyroid carcinomas; prostatic carcinomas; carcinomas of the esophagus, ileum, and colon; ovarian tumors; squamous cell carcinoma of the lung, larynx, and cervix; and melanomas. Although the relationship between the more commonly occurring tumors and ectopic ACTH production has been well established, the production of ACTH by the less frequently occurring tumors has not been absolutely proved.[17]

Several mechanisms of ectopic elaboration of peptide hormones have been postulated. Neoplastic transformation of dormant stem cells results in expression by the tumor of a specific hormone gene that would not otherwise be expressed by the mature cells of that organ. An alternative hypothesis is that cells with endocrine potential migrate to various organs during embryogenesis, where they remain dormant. These cells have the capacity to initiate amine precursor uptake and decarboxylation (APUD) and synthesize a variety of peptides.[18] This hypothesis does not account for the large number of ectopic hormones elaborated by non-APUD cells. An enhanced expression of genes normally encoding for proopiomelanocortin (POMC) in extrapituitary tissues is a more likely explanation for the development of ectopic hormone syndromes. These tissues include stomach, adrenal medulla, pancreas, brain, and placenta.[19] The tumor cells in patients with the ectopic ACTH syndrome appear to have developed a more efficient mechanism for translation of messenger RNA (mRNA) to immunoreactive POMC-derived peptides or may have lost the mechanism for preventing the continuous expression of the POMC gene.[20] Unique transcription factors may be constitutively expressed in tumor cells and cause unregulated secretion of POMC-derived peptides.[21]

An unusual cause of ectopic ACTH production is an *ectopic pituitary adenoma.* In some cases, normal pituitary tissue occurs in an ectopic location and not in continuity with intrasellar pituitary tissue. Occasionally, adenomas may develop in this ectopic pituitary tissue, causing excessive ACTH production.[22] From the biochemical standpoint, these patients resemble those with pituitary ACTH-dependent or ectopic ACTH-dependent Cushing syndrome. The possibility of an ectopic pituitary adenoma in a patient presenting with an ACTH-dependent Cushing syndrome should be considered if the patient exhibits an atypical hormonal profile in the absence of an ectopic ACTH-secreting, extracranial neoplasm or in the absence of a pituitary abnormality at the time of transsphenoidal exploration. A computerized tomographic (CT) study of the parasellar region and the sphenoid sinus may help to identify such ectopically located pituitary adenomas.

## ECTOPIC CORTICOTROPIN-RELEASING HORMONE SYNDROME

Ectopic CRH production can cause Cushing syndrome.[23,24] Tumors with a capacity to secrete CRH ectopically include bronchial carcinoids, medullary thyroid carcinoma, and metastatic prostatic carcinoma. In patients with ectopic ACTH production, the pituitary ACTH content is low and only Crooke changes (i.e., hyaline degeneration) are observed in pituitary corticotropes. In contrast, patients with ectopic CRH secretion demonstrate corticotrope hyperplasia. The presence of an ectopic CRH-secreting tumor should be suspected in patients who have disease that behaves biochemically like pituitary ACTH-dependent disease but who have a clinical course of short duration and high plasma ACTH levels.

# CORTICOTROPIN-INDEPENDENT CUSHING SYNDROME

Primary nodular hyperplasia, adrenocortical adenomas, and carcinomas as well as rare cases of ectopic cortisol production by tumor are found in 30% of patients presenting with Cushing syndrome.[25]

## PRIMARY BILATERAL MICRONODULAR HYPERPLASIA

Primary bilateral micronodular hyperplasia is characterized by the presence in the adrenal cortex of one or more yellow nodules visible to the naked eye and 2 to 3 cm in diameter. Its pathogenesis is unknown. Whether this type of hyperplasia is of primary adrenal origin or the result of a combined mechanism by which the pituitary predominates initially but the adrenal eventually becomes autonomous, is not clear.[26] Increased adrenocortical cell sensitivity to ACTH has also been suggested.[27]

Histologically, the micronodules consist of clear cells arranged in acini and cords, and are occasionally encapsulated and surrounded by simple or micronodular cortical hyperplasia. The frequency of mitotic figures is low. In one form of ACTH-independent micronodular adrenal disease, darkly pigmented micronodules are seen in the presence of atrophy of the perinodular adrenal tissue, disorganization of normal zonation of the cortex, and small glands[28] (Fig. 75-3). Microscopically, the nodules are

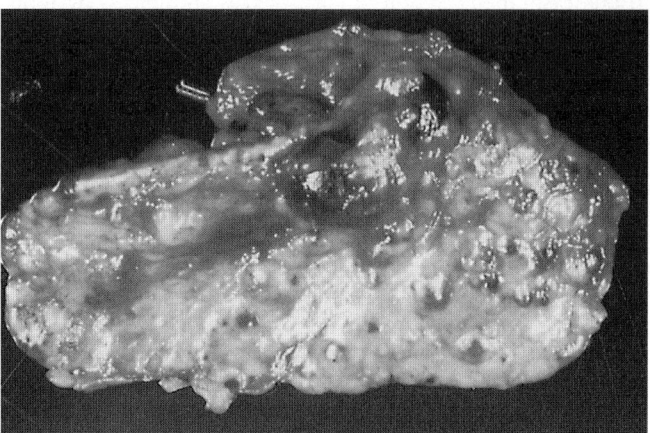

**FIGURE 75-3.** Appearance of an adrenal gland with pigmented micronodular hyperplasia removed from a patient with familial, corticotropin-independent Cushing syndrome. The patient was also found to have an atrial myxoma and a Sertoli cell testicular tumor.

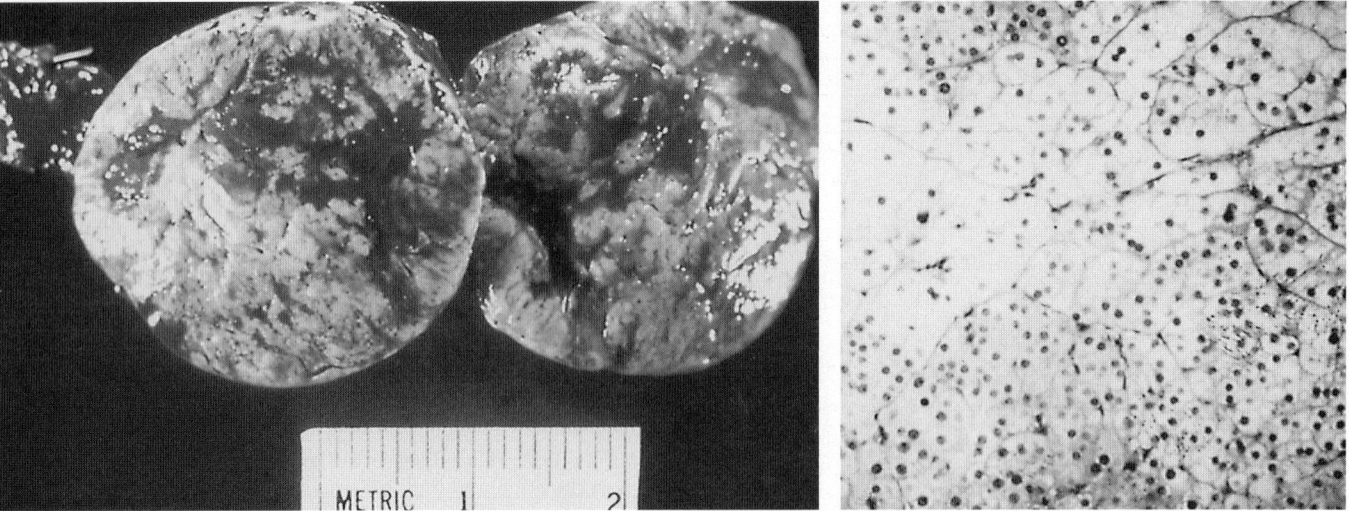

**FIGURE 75-4. A,** This well-encapsulated, adrenal cortical adenoma, 2.6 cm in diameter, with homogeneous appearance, was removed from a 35-year-old woman with a 3-year history of Cushing syndrome. **B,** The histologic pattern was consistent with a benign adrenal adenoma, with clear and compact cells arranged in cords.

composed predominantly of large globular cortical cells with granular eosinophilic cytoplasm that often contains lipofuscin.

A condition associated with pigmented micronodular hyperplasia is Carney complex, a form of multiple endocrine neoplasia. Patients with this condition have, in addition to the adrenal cortical disease, growth hormone–secreting pituitary tumors, Sertoli cell testicular tumors, atrial or ventricular myxomas, single or multiple mammary fibroadenomas, and cutaneous myxomas. A prominent feature in these patients is spotty skin pigmentation similar to that observed in several lentiginosis syndromes. The genetic defect(s) responsible for Carney complex map(s) to the short arm of chromosome 2 (2p16). This region has been found to exhibit cytogenic aberrations in atrial myxomas associated with the complex and has been characterized by microsatellite instability in human neoplasias.[29]

ACTH-independent macronodular adrenal cortical hyperplasia is a rare cause of Cushing syndrome in which the adrenal glands become very enlarged and occupied by multiple large cortical nodules. In some patients, the masses can be extremely large and weigh close to 100 g each. Histologically, the nodules are composed mostly of clear cells, and no cortical architecture has been observed in the internodular regions.[30] Several interesting pathogenic mechanisms have been described in patients with ACTH-independent nodular adrenal cortical hyperplasia. In one case, the secretion of cortisol was stimulated by food. The patient had elevated postprandial cortisol levels that could not be suppressed with dexamethasone. Cortisol increased in response to oral glucose, a lipid-rich meal, or a protein-rich meal but not to the intravenous administration of glucose. In response to test meals, plasma glucose-dependent insulinotropic polypeptide (GIP) increased in parallel to the plasma cortisol. The ability of GIP to stimulate adrenal cortisol production could be demonstrated in cell suspensions of adrenal tissue from the patient. Nodular adrenal cortical hyperplasia and Cushing syndrome were postulated to be food dependent and to result from abnormal responsiveness of adrenal cells to the physiologic secretion of GIP. The suggestion was made that ectopic expression of GIP receptors on the adrenal cells mediate this disorder.[31]

A case of Cushing syndrome secondary to ACTH-independent bilateral adrenal hyperplasia was also described in which cortisol secretion responded to catecholamines acting through ectopic adrenal β receptors. The increased cortisol secretion was inhibited by β-blockade with propranolol. High-affinity binding sites compatible with $\beta_1$ or $\beta_2$ receptors were detected in the adrenal tissue

from this patient but not from control subjects. The ectopic expression of β receptors in the adrenal cortex of this patient led to nodular hyperplasia, hypersecretion of cortisol and aldosterone, and feedback suppression of ACTH and angiotensin.[32]

## ADRENAL ADENOMA AND CARCINOMA

Adrenal adenomas are unilateral, well-circumscribed, brown to yellow tumors with a homogeneous appearance, weighing <30 g. Histologically, they have the characteristics of normal adrenal cortex, with compact and clear cells arranged in cords (Fig. 75-4). Adrenal carcinomas are large neoplasms with irregularly shaped nodules, exhibiting areas of necrosis or hemorrhage. Histologically, the cells are small, with nuclear pleomorphism and mitotic figures, and evidence of capsular and blood vessel invasion by tumor is found (Fig. 75-5).

Adrenal cortical carcinoma may develop in patients with hereditary cancer syndromes. The Li-Fraumeni syndrome is characterized by cancers derived from all three germinal cell lines, and include sarcomas, brain tumors, leukemia, lymphoma, and adrenal cortical carcinoma, in addition to early-onset breast cancer. These tumors tend to occur in family members under the age of 45. Mutations in the p53 tumor-suppressor gene have been identified in patients with cancer associated with Li-Fraumeni syndrome.[33,34]

## CLINICAL PRESENTATIONS

The clinical manifestations of Cushing syndrome are determined by the increased abnormal secretion of cortisol, ACTH, and other adrenocortical steroids under ACTH control. However, the clinical presentation varies among the different types.

### CORTICOTROPIN-DEPENDENT CUSHING DISEASE

Patients with pituitary ACTH-dependent disease (i.e., Cushing disease) usually have a history of disease that begins 2 to 3 years before a definitive diagnosis is made. In milder cases, symptoms may be present for 5 to 10 years. Earliest symptoms include weight gain, progressive changes in physical appearance, hypertension, and glucose intolerance. Patients may have been treated for these conditions with weight-reduction diets, antihypertensive drugs, and oral hypoglycemic agents. The

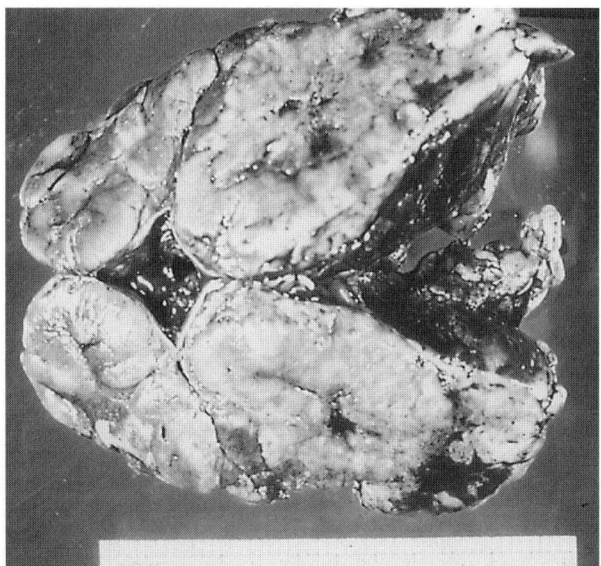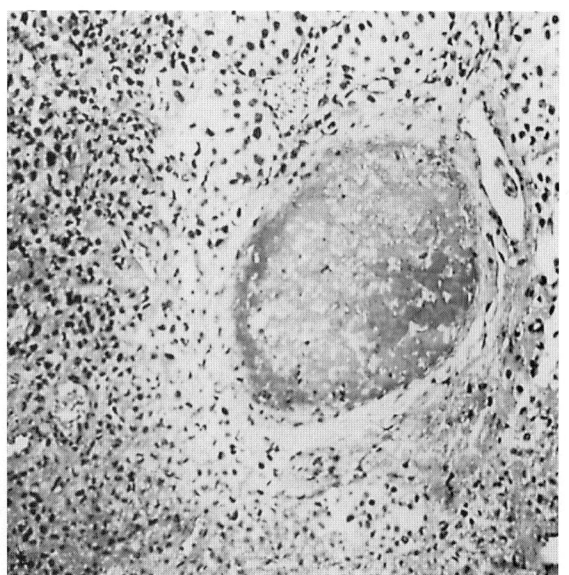

**FIGURE 75-5. A,** This 4.2 × 8.5 cm adrenal neoplasm with multiple, large nodules and evidence of capsular invasion was removed from a 50-year-old woman with a 9-month history of Cushing syndrome. **B,** Histologically, this tumor revealed angioinvasion and small cells with nuclear pleomorphism and numerous mitotic figures.

response to diet is frequently unsuccessful. Those who do not experience actual weight gain notice redistribution of adipose tissue resulting in changes in appearance, with facial rounding, increased central adiposity, and thinning of upper and lower extremities.

After 2 to 3 years of mild symptoms, additional symptoms or increased severity of the initial symptoms draw patients to the attention of the physician. Patients relate the appearance of striae, easy bruising, and increased body hair growth; irregular menses or amenorrhea may be present in women or gynecomastia in men. Proximal muscle weakness and atrophy are common, and some patients exhibit manifestations of a steroid myopathy. Other manifestations include peripheral edema, back pain, and loss of height if patients have developed severe osteoporosis and compression fractures of the vertebrae (Fig. 75-6A).

The physical examination reveals plethora, a round face with preauricular fullness, a prominent upper lip (i.e., the Cupid bow), supraclavicular fossa fullness, and a cervicodorsal fat pad (i.e., buffalo hump) disproportionate to the degree of obesity (see Fig. 75-6B). Patients exhibit truncal obesity, with large breasts or gynecomastia and a protuberant abdomen. This protuberance is the result of an increased abdominal panniculus and relaxed abdominal muscles. The extremities are thin, with decreased muscle mass and strength. Patients may show pretibial edema. The skin is thin, with wide, atrophic purple striae present over the abdomen, chest, and upper thighs (see Fig. 75-6C). Other skin lesions include keratosis pilaris seen over the upper trunk, tinea versicolor over the anterior chest and back (see Fig. 75-6D), and verruca vulgaris, which occasionally may be large and present in multiple locations (see Fig. 75-6E). Hirsutism is often present as a mixture of fine, lanugal-type hair growth over the face and trunk, together with coarse, terminal-type hair over the face, trunk, and extremities. This latter type of hair is associated with increased androgen secretion.

Increased skin pigmentation is infrequent in patients with pituitary ACTH-dependent Cushing disease, because ACTH levels are not sufficiently elevated to induce hyperpigmentation. When hyperpigmentation is present, it is associated with high ACTH levels and characterized by pigmentation of the hands, palmar creases, elbows and knees, gums, and oral mucosae. Another type of pigmentation is associated with insu-

lin resistance and hyperinsulinemia; this type is localized to the neck, elbows, and dorsum of the hands and has the characteristics of acanthosis nigricans. In individuals with dark skin, a history of further darkening is indicative of development of hyperpigmentation.

## ECTOPIC CORTICOTROPIN AND CORTICOTROPIN-RELEASING HORMONE SYNDROMES

The duration of symptoms is usually shorter in patients with the ectopic ACTH syndrome than in those with the pituitary ACTH-dependent type, because the source of ACTH is a malignant neoplasm, often one with a rapidly progressive course. Frequently, the symptoms and signs of Cushing syndrome appear 4 to 6 months before a diagnosis is made. Some patients exhibit minimal symptoms of Cushing syndrome because of the short duration of hypercortisolemia. In these patients, very high cortisol levels are often associated with manifestations of mineralocorticoid excess, including hypernatremia, hypokalemia, and metabolic alkalosis. Because the levels of ACTH in these patients are 5 to 10 times higher than in those with pituitary ACTH-dependent disease, hyperpigmentation of the skin and oral mucosa may be an early manifestation. Severe hypokalemia may also lead to significant muscle weakness. The manifestations of the underlying malignant neoplasm, including anorexia, weight loss, and focal symptoms of organ involvement, may occur with the manifestations of cortisol excess. Some patients with the ectopic ACTH syndrome have a more protracted disease course. These are patients with bronchial or mediastinal carcinoids that may be present for several years before detection and whose disease may share clinical and biochemical features with pituitary ACTH-dependent disease.

## CORTICOTROPIN-INDEPENDENT TYPES OF CUSHING SYNDROME

Patients with benign adrenocortical adenomas usually have a long history of manifestations of cortisol excess before a definitive diagnosis is made. Because adrenocortical adenomas are often monotropic and purely cortisol-secreting tumors, the predominant clinical manifestations are indicative of the protein catabolic effects of cortisol unopposed by androgen excess.

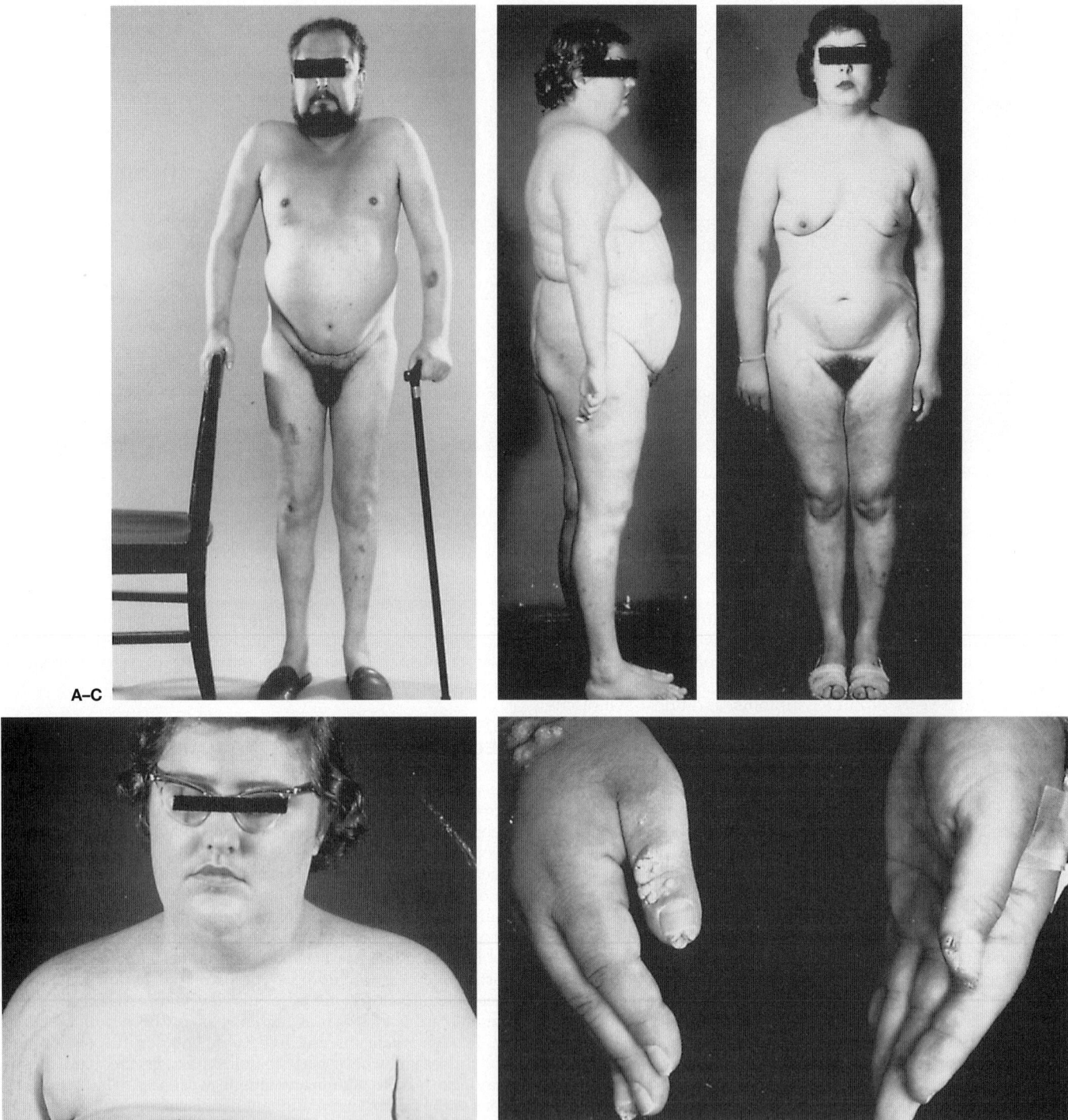

**FIGURE 75-6. A,** A 45-year-old man with a 2-year history of progressive muscle weakness and atrophy, truncal obesity, severe back pain, loss of height, and multiple ecchymoses. **B,** Truncal obesity with a very prominent cervicodorsal fat pad (i.e., buffalo hump) in a woman with Cushing syndrome. **C,** Atrophic striae over hips, breasts, and axillae in a 24-year-old woman with Cushing syndrome. **D,** A 28-year-old woman with Cushing syndrome. She had pigmented lesions of tinea versicolor over the anterior upper chest. **E,** Severe, intractable verruca vulgaris lesions over the fingers in a 32-year-old man with Cushing syndrome and a markedly depressed T-lymphocyte count.

These include skin and muscle atrophy, easy bruising, and osteopenia. The patients have the typical fat distribution associated with hypercortisolism, but acne and coarse, terminal-type hair growth are unusual.

Patients with adrenocortical carcinoma have a disease history of shorter duration, with symptoms appearing within 4 to 6 months of diagnosis. The severity of the clinical manifestations depends on the degree of hypercortisolemia. Patients with adrenocortical carcinoma may exhibit manifestations of androgen excess, including hirsutism, acne, scalp hair loss, and clitoromegaly. The androgen excess can moderate the severity of the catabolic effects of hypercortisolism. In particular, skin and muscle atrophy may not be as apparent. Because adrenocortical carcinomas are large, frequently >100 g, they may be palpable on the abdominal examination, and hepatomegaly may be noted if hepatic metastases are present.

**TABLE 75-2.**
**Outpatient Evaluation of Cushing Syndrome**

---

**Urinary Free Cortisol**
  Normal: 20–90 µg/day
  Cushing syndrome: >150 µg/day
**1.0-mg Dexamethasone Suppression**
  Cortisol
    Normal: <5 µg/dL
    Cushing: >10 µg/dL
  ACTH
    Normal: <9 pg/mL (IRMA)
    Cushing: >50 pg/mL
**8.0-mg Dexamethasone Suppression**
  Cortisol
    Pituitary ACTH dependent: <50% of baseline
    Ectopic ACTH or ACTH independent: >50% of baseline

---

*ACTH,* corticotropin; *IRMA,* immunoradiometric assay.

---

Although the discovery of an adrenocortical adenoma is usually made while a patient is being investigated for the possibility of Cushing syndrome, the adenoma occasionally is discovered incidentally during the investigation of abdominal complaints. Silent adrenal masses are found in 2% to 3% of patients who are undergoing CT scans for investigation of abdominal symptoms.[34a] Although these patients may not have obvious clinical manifestations of Cushing syndrome and their baseline urinary cortisol levels are normal, cortisol secretion is autonomous. Evidence of autonomous cortisol secretion includes a blunted circadian rhythm, suppressed ACTH levels, and a lack of response to dexamethasone. Adrenal scintigraphy with iodocholesterol shows increased uptake on the side of the tumor but suppression of uptake in the contralateral adrenal gland.

Although these patients may have minimal manifestations of Cushing syndrome, these manifestations improve after surgical removal of the lesion. Patients with primary nodular adrenocortical hyperplasia are clinically indistinguishable from patients with benign adrenocortical adenomas or pituitary ACTH-dependent disease.

# DIAGNOSIS

## STANDARD DIAGNOSTIC EVALUATION

A biochemical evaluation of Cushing syndrome is necessary for confirming the clinical diagnosis and for determining the presence of the syndrome in patients with an equivocal clinical presentation.[35] Preliminary testing includes the *measurement of urinary free cortisol* and of the *ability to suppress serum cortisol levels with a low dose of dexamethasone* (Table 75-2). In patients with Cushing syndrome, the urinary free cortisol usually exceeds 90 µg per day. Serum cortisol levels obtained 9 hours after the oral administration of 1 mg of dexamethasone at 23:00 hours fail to decrease below 10 µg/dL, and plasma ACTH levels (assessed by immunoradiometric assay) fail to decrease to <9 pg/mL.[36] In patients without Cushing syndrome, cortisol levels are suppressed below 5 µg/dL. In patients whose levels fall between these two values, additional studies are required for confirmation of the diagnosis. After the preliminary diagnosis has been determined, a definitive diagnosis may require more extensive testing (Table 75-3). This includes the measurement of serum cortisol and plasma ACTH levels at various times of the day to determine the absence of a *circadian rhythm.*

Patients with Cushing syndrome, regardless of cause or type, have high baseline urinary free cortisol and serum cortisol levels and lack normal circadian changes in level. Occasionally, the early morning cortisol levels may be indistinguishable from normal, but levels obtained between 22:00 hours and midnight are clearly higher than in normal persons. This testing, however, requires that the patient be hospitalized for blood drawing. A more convenient procedure is the measurement of salivary cortisol at 08:00 and 22:00 hours or midnight in a collection that can be obtained by the patient at home. Salivary cortisol testing measures free cortisol and results correlate well with plasma cortisol levels. Patients with Cushing syndrome have high evening salivary cortisol levels.[37] In borderline or confusing cases, loss of circadian rhythm may be key to establishing the differential diagnosis between Cushing syndrome and normal cortisol secretion. The pituitary response to dexamethasone is measured to detect abnormal feedback regulation of ACTH and cortisol secretion. Dexamethasone is given in doses of 0.5 mg every 6 hours for 8 doses, followed by 2 mg every 6 hours for 8 doses.

The response of plasma ACTH levels to dexamethasone depends on the type of Cushing syndrome. When an immunoradiometric assay is used (normal levels, 9–52 pg/mL), baseline levels are normal or high (50–100 pg/mL) in ACTH-dependent types and low (<9 pg/mL) in ACTH-independent types. Although ACTH levels are frequently at the upper limit of normal in patients with pituitary causes, they range from 200 to 1000 pg/mL in patients with the ectopic ACTH syndrome. The lack of normal suppression of cortisol with low doses of dexamethasone is found in all types of Cushing syndrome, but most patients with pituitary ACTH-dependent Cushing syndrome (i.e., Cushing disease) shown suppression with high doses of dexamethasone to values below 50% of the baseline levels (Table 75-4). Fewer than 10% of patients with ectopic ACTH syndrome respond in this manner. In patients with ACTH-dependent Cushing syndrome, high ACTH levels and lack of response to dexamethasone should strongly raise the possibility of ectopic ACTH syndrome.

The *high-dose dexamethasone suppression test* can be performed as a rapid *single oral dose test* and by *intravenous administration* in hospitalized patients unable to take oral medication.[38,39] A sin-

---

**TABLE 75-3.**
**Definitive Evaluation of Cushing Syndrome**

| Test | Days | Biochemical Measurements | | | | |
| --- | --- | --- | --- | --- | --- | --- |
| | | U 17-OHCS | UFC | S Cortisol | P ACTH | S 11-Deoxycortisol |
| **BASELINE** | 1 | √ | √ | √ | √ | |
| **METYRAPONE** | 2 | √ | | √ | √ | √ |
| **LOW-DOSE (2-mg) DEXAMETHASONE SUPPRESSION** | 2 | √ | √ | √ | √ | |
| **HIGH-DOSE (8-mg) DEXAMETHASONE SUPPRESSION** | 2 | √ | √ | √ | √ | |
| **CRH INFUSION** | 1 | | | √ | √ | |

√, indicates that the test should be obtained; *U,* urine; *P,* plasma; *S,* serum; *17-OHCS,* 17-hydroxycorticosteroids; *UFC,* urinary free cortisol; *ACTH,* corticotropin; *CRH,* corticotropin-releasing hormone.

**TABLE 75-4.**
**Differential Diagnosis of Pituitary and Ectopic Corticotropin (ACTH)-Dependent Cushing Syndrome**

| Test | Pituitary ACTH-Dependent Syndrome | Ectopic ACTH-Dependent Syndrome | | Ectopic CRH Syndrome |
| | | Rapidly Growing | Slow Growing | |
|---|---|---|---|---|
| **BASELINE** | | | | |
| *Cortisol* | ↑ | ↑↑ | ↑–↑↑ | ↑–↑↑ |
| *ACTH* | ↑ | ↑↑ | ↑–↑↑ | ↑–↑↑ |
| **RESPONSE TO** | | | | |
| *Dexamethasone (8.0 mg)* | ↓ >50% | → | ↓ >50% | ↓ or 50% |
| *CRH* | ↑↑ | → | → | ↑ |

*CRH*, corticotropin-releasing hormone; ↑, increased or positive; ↓, decreased or negative; →, no change.

gle dose of 8 mg of dexamethasone is given at 23:00 hours, and the serum cortisol level is measured at 08:00 hours the next morning. A suppression of plasma cortisol levels to <50% of baseline values suggests a pituitary cause, and a lack of suppression below that limit indicates the existence of an adrenal tumor or of ectopic ACTH syndrome. The diagnostic efficacy or predictive power of the overnight high-dose dexamethasone suppression test (defined as the ratio between the number of cases in which the diagnosis is correctly predicted and the total number of cases) is at least 82.4%, compared with 84.6% for the classic 8-mg Liddle test. Because the two tests are comparable, the shorter test has the obvious advantage of speed and lower cost.

The *ACTH response to the intravenous administration of CRH* is also a useful test in the differential diagnosis of pituitary and ectopic ACTH syndrome.[40,41] After the administration of ovine CRH (1 μg/kg), patients with Cushing disease usually show a further increase in the elevated levels of ACTH and cortisol. In contrast, most patients with the ectopic ACTH syndrome who also have high basal plasma concentrations of ACTH and cortisol fail to respond to CRH (see Chaps. 74 and 241).

Several tests have been suggested for establishing a diagnosis of Cushing disease in patients with borderline elevations of cortisol and negative pituitary imaging for a pituitary adenoma. These tests include the high-dose dexamethasone suppression test with revised criteria to improve sensitivity and specificity; the combined CRH stimulation/dexamethasone suppression test (CRH/DST), and a hydrocortisone suppression test in cases for which dexamethasone gives a false-negative result.[42]

In the CRH/DST, the CRH stimulation is performed 2 hours after completion of the low-dose dexamethasone suppression test. Normal individuals and patients with pseudo-Cushing states show a lower response to CRH than patients with pituitary ACTH-dependent Cushing syndrome. The separation appears to be valid even in patients with mild Cushing disease.[43] The combined CRH/DST could be a potentially useful modification of the dexamethasone suppression test and the CRH stimulation test to distinguish patients with pseudo-Cushing from those with pituitary ACTH-dependent Cushing syndrome.

Benign and malignant adrenocortical tumors can be differentiated biochemically. Malignant neoplasms often have partial enzymatic deficiencies in the steroid biosynthetic pathway. When this occurs, steroid biosynthetic intermediates or other metabolites are found in increased quantity in serum or urine. Impaired activities of 3β-hydroxysteroid dehydrogenase and 11β-hydroxylase are the most common. These deficiencies lead to increased serum levels of pregnenolone and 11-deoxycortisol.

## DIFFICULTIES IN INTERPRETATION OF THE DIAGNOSTIC TESTS

The tests described produce a small but significant percentage of false-positive and false-negative results that contribute to difficulties in establishing a clear biochemical diagnosis of the disease.[44] For example, the 08:00-hour plasma cortisol values are found to yield 9% false-positive and 60% false-negative results. A diurnal variation of cortisol occurs in 30% of patients with Cushing syndrome and is lacking in 18% of patients without Cushing syndrome. The overnight dexamethasone suppression test may be abnormal in 30% of hospitalized patients. In contrast, urinary free cortisol level has a very great sensitivity and specificity (uncorrected or corrected for creatinine) and is the most efficient screening method for Cushing syndrome in hospitalized patients.

Several factors can lower the sensitivity and specificity of these tests. First, cortisol secretion is episodic or pulsatile and can result in widely variable levels. A normal diurnal variation is a pattern in which plasma cortisol levels from 16:00 hours to midnight are <75% of the 08:00-hour values. Values at 16:00 hours can show considerable overlap in normal individuals and patients with Cushing syndrome. The *plasma cortisol value at 23:00 hours* is probably superior, because only ~3% of patients with Cushing syndrome have been shown to have normal plasma cortisol levels at that time. Frequent sampling for serum cortisol is useful but requires hospitalization and may be relatively expensive. Second, 30% to 50% of obese people, particularly those with abdominal obesity and without Cushing syndrome, have increased cortisol secretion rates, but urinary free cortisol values in patients with Cushing syndrome are separated by at least 60 μg per day from those in obese individuals. Third, a variety of drugs that cause induction of hepatic microsomal hydroxylating enzymes may increase the metabolism of dexamethasone and result in lower levels of these compounds than expected for the dose administered.[45] Under these circumstances, the response to dexamethasone may be abnormal without the presence of Cushing syndrome. Patients with Cushing disease who show normal suppression with the low-dose dexamethasone test usually show a decrease in the clearance of dexamethasone, which produces plasma dexamethasone levels that are higher than expected.[46]

The measurement of plasma dexamethasone together with cortisol can help exclude abnormalities in dexamethasone clearance. Rarely, patients with factitious Cushing syndrome, who have been taking pharmacologic doses of synthetic glucocorticoids, present with a paradoxical finding of the clinical manifestations of Cushing syndrome with suppressed ACTH and cortisol levels.

## ANATOMIC LOCALIZATION

### DETECTION OF PITUITARY LESIONS

After the diagnosis of Cushing disease has been established on clinical and biochemical grounds, the presence of pituitary lesions should be further determined by *magnetic resonance imaging (MRI) of the sella turcica*. Because of the small size of most pituitary tumors associated with Cushing disease, the results of plain radiographic studies are often normal or misleading. Large microadenomas secreting ACTH are extremely rare at the time the initial diagnosis of the disease is made. However, small (<10 mm) pituitary microadenomas can be identified by MRI of the pituitary gland with gadolinium contrast using coronal cuts in approximately 70% of patients with Cushing disease. On T1-weighted images, the lesion usually appears as a nonenhancing abnormality surrounded by an enhancing normal pituitary gland (Fig. 75-7).

*Petrosal sinus sampling with or without CRH stimulation* can be used for localization of pituitary tumors.[47] Through a percuta-

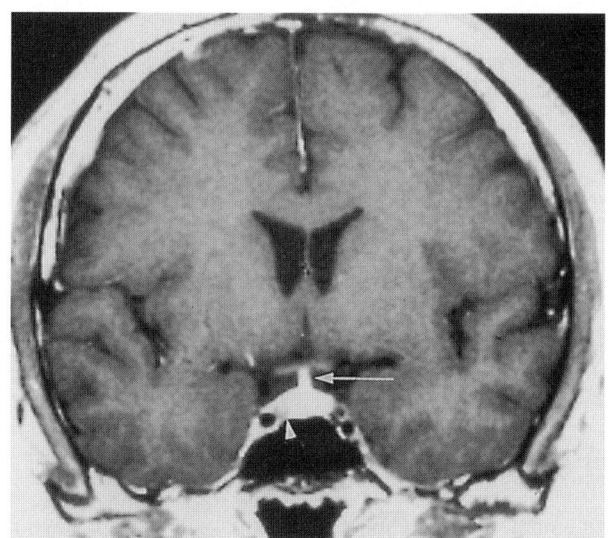

**FIGURE 75-7.** T1-weighted magnetic resonance image of the pituitary gland with gadolinium contrast in a patient with corticotropin-dependent Cushing syndrome (Cushing disease). The pituitary gland and the stalk (*arrow*) enhanced with contrast, and an area of decreased enhancement (*arrowhead*) consistent with an adenoma was outlined in the right side of the gland.

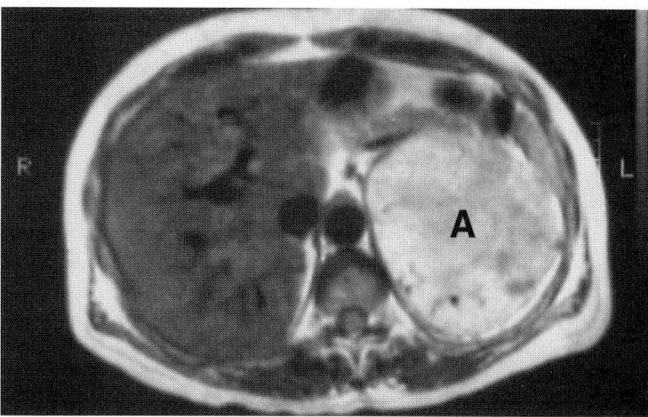

**FIGURE 75-8.** A 13-cm left adrenal mass (*A*) with areas of necrosis was detected by computed tomographic scanning in a 72-year-old woman with abdominal pain. She also had pulmonary nodules consistent with metastatic adrenal carcinoma.

neous bilateral femoral approach, catheters are placed in the left and right inferior petrosal sinuses, and blood for ACTH is withdrawn simultaneously from both catheters and from a peripheral vein. To account for fluctuations in levels caused by the pulsatile nature of ACTH secretion, sequential samples (i.e., four samples drawn on both sides over a 20-second period at 2- to 5-minute intervals) are obtained. A *plasma ACTH concentration gradient* (i.e., petrosal sinus/peripheral vein ACTH of ≥1.6) verifies the pituitary source of ACTH. A *right to left discrepancy* may also help to lateralize ACTH secretion and aids in the preoperative localization of the lesion. A lateralization of the source of ACTH by this procedure can help in cases in which a tumor is not found at the time of surgery. Partial resection of the side of the pituitary where the highest ACTH levels are recorded can be accompanied by remission of the disease. Failure to find the pituitary microadenoma or to induce cure after resection of the side of the pituitary with the highest concentration of ACTH may be due to failure to remove the involved part of the pituitary gland completely or to the fact that confluent pituitary veins do not invariably drain into the ipsilateral inferior petrosal sinus, so that a microadenoma may be present in the opposite side of the pituitary gland.[48]

Another possibility is the presence of multiple microadenomas. The administration of CRH at the time of catheterization may enhance differences between the two sides; however, a simultaneous response by the uninvolved gland may blur the differences.

To correct for unequal dilution by nonpituitary venous blood, other pituitary hormones, including prolactin, thyroid-stimulating hormone (TSH), human chorionic gonadotropin, and α subunit, have been measured simultaneously. The assumption was that an ACTH-secreting microadenoma would not cause unequal delivery of these hormones into the two inferior petrosal sinuses, but correction of the ACTH gradients by these hormones did not improve the discriminatory ability of the test.[49]

Catheterization of the inferior petrosal sinuses requires a great deal of technical expertise. To make this type of testing more accessible to neuroradiologists with limited experience in this procedure, the diagnostic accuracy of the less invasive sampling of the internal jugular veins has been compared with sampling of the inferior petrosal sinuses.[50] Jugular vein sam-

pling correctly identified ACTH-secreting adenomas in 80% of patients with proven Cushing disease. Administration of CRH was essential for diagnostic results in 65% of the patients. Negative results on jugular vein sampling should be confirmed by petrosal sinus sampling.

## DETECTION OF ADRENAL LESIONS

Techniques for the anatomic localization of adrenal lesions include *abdominal CT scans* and *MRI, ultrasonography,* and *adrenal scintigraphy* with 6-β-($^{131}$I)-iodomethyl-19-norcholesterol.[51] These techniques are noninvasive and provide good definition of structure and function of the adrenal glands.

Adrenocortical masses can be *anatomically defined* by CT scanning, MRI, or ultrasonography (Fig. 75-8). CT can identify adrenal lesions as small as 1 cm in diameter. This level of resolution can be important in patients with adrenal carcinoma to detect involved lymph nodes and hepatic and pulmonary metastases. Hepatic metastases are found in approximately 42% of patients, and pulmonary metastases are found in 45%.

MRI is also helpful. Adrenal carcinomas are *hypointense* compared with liver in *T1-weighted images.* They are *hyperintense* compared with liver in *T2-weighted images.* The superior blood vessel identification and the multiplanar capacity of MRI may make it the modality of choice in evaluating the extent of disease and in planning surgical excision.[52]

Ultrasonography can help define the benign or malignant character of a lesion. Malignant lesions are heterogeneous in appearance, with focal or scattered echopenic or echogenic zones representing areas of tumor necrosis, hemorrhage, or calcification.[53]

Scintigraphy with *iodocholesterol* provides an image reflective of the structure of the adrenal gland and information about its function. Patients with bilateral adrenocortical hyperplasia demonstrate bilateral increased adrenal uptake of iodocholesterol. Patients with cortisol-secreting adrenocortical adenomas, which suppress pituitary ACTH secretion and the function of the contralateral gland, demonstrate unilateral concentration of the tracer. Patients with Cushing syndrome secondary to an adrenocortical carcinoma fail to show tracer uptake on either side. Carcinomas have relatively low functional capacity per gram of tissue and fail to concentrate iodocholesterol in quantities sufficient to produce an image.[54] Occasionally, actively secreting carcinomas may image in a manner indistinguishable from that of a benign tumor.

Patients with primary macronodular hyperplasia may show asymmetric uptake, with greater activity on the side of the predominant nodules. This finding is important in determining the

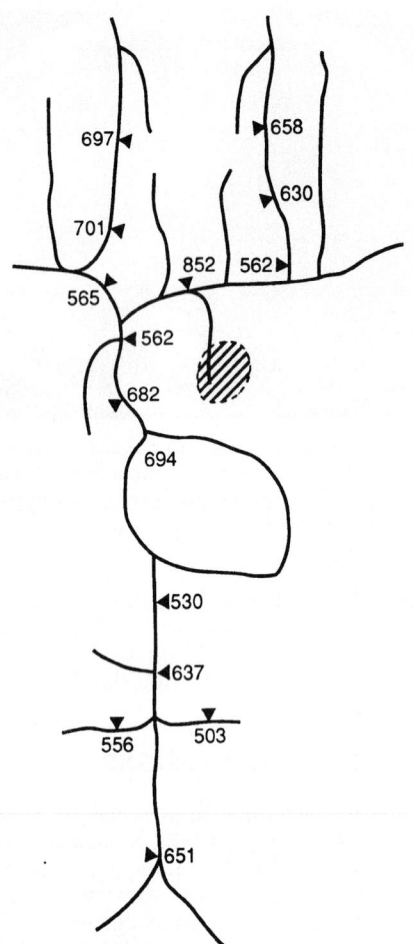

**FIGURE 75-9.** Results of selective venous catheterization and sampling in a 55-year-old man with ectopic corticotropin (*ACTH*)-dependent Cushing syndrome. ACTH levels (pg/mL) were measured in samples obtained throughout the venous system. A peak level in the left innominate vein led to the discovery of a malignant, ACTH-secreting thymoma.

presence of bilateral adrenocortical disease, because a CT scan or MRI may show a mass on one side, but surgical resection of that mass may not result in remission if the contralateral gland is also abnormal. Radiographic differences between patients with macronodular hyperplasia secondary to ACTH-secreting pituitary adenomas and primary micronodular hyperplasia of the adrenal glands have been described. In macronodular adrenocortical hyperplasia, the nodules are visible on CT or MRI, and in micronodular disease, the micronodules are seen microscopically, but the adrenal glands do not demonstrate focal masses.[55]

## LOCALIZATION OF ECTOPIC CORTICOTROPIN-SECRETING LESIONS

Ectopic sources of ACTH are localized using a variety of procedures, including CT of the chest, CT or MRI of the abdomen, thyroid scan, and selective venous catheterization and sampling in search of concentration gradients of ACTH (Fig. 75-9). Approximately 50% of these tumors are within the thorax (e.g., small cell carcinomas, bronchial carcinoids, thymomas), and thoracic CT scans usually can localize the lesion. Other ACTH-secreting tumors are found in the pancreas (islet cell tumors), the thyroid (medullary carcinoma), and the adrenal medulla (pheochromocytoma).

Ectopic ACTH-secreting carcinoids may be small and slow growing, and many years may elapse before they become radiographically apparent.[56] Carcinoid tumors that possess somatostatin receptors may take up the somatostatin analog octreotide. Use of indium-111 ($^{111}$In) pentetreotide has allowed these tumors to be detected as areas of increased uptake at the exact location of a suspected thoracic lesion seen on CT.[57] However, these scans are often negative when a lesion is not detected by CT.

The finding of a pulmonary lesion may lead to a percutaneous biopsy for confirmation and eventual surgical excision of the lesion. The biopsy tissue can be analyzed by immunocytochemistry to demonstrate POMC-derived peptide secretory granules in the tumor cells or by extraction and analysis of the ACTH content in the tumor. The presence of POMC mRNA may also be a way of confirming that the tumor has the ability to produce ACTH.[58–60]

## PSEUDO–CUSHING SYNDROME

Hypercortisolism may exist in patients who do not have true Cushing syndrome. These patients experience obesity, depression, alcoholism, anorexia nervosa, bulimia, or acute stress. Because their clinical presentation and biochemical findings overlap with those of patients with Cushing syndrome, the differential diagnosis can be challenging.

### OBESITY

Obese people, particularly those with abdominal or upper-body-segment obesity, share many of the metabolic, hormonal, and behavioral findings observed in Cushing syndrome. These include diabetes mellitus, hypertension, myocardial infarction, insomnia, and depression.[61] Obesity is associated with increased cortisol production, as indicated by high cortisol secretion rates and levels of urinary 17-hydroxycorticosteroids, but normal or slightly diminished serum cortisol levels; these findings suggest an increased metabolic clearance rate for cortisol.[62] Urinary free cortisol is increased in proportion to the waist-to-hip ratio; these individuals also exhibit increased cortisol responsiveness to ACTH stimulation and to physical and mental stress.[63]

Unlike in Cushing syndrome with its well-defined causes, in pseudo–Cushing syndrome the cause of the abnormality in adrenal function and its relationship to the complications of obesity have not been established. From the clinical standpoint, obese people do not usually exhibit signs of protein catabolism. Biochemically, they have a normal circadian rhythm of cortisol and ACTH secretion and show normal suppression with a low dose of dexamethasone.[62]

### MAJOR DEPRESSIVE DISORDER

Approximately 50% of patients with major depressive disorder (MDD) hypersecrete cortisol and show early escape from the normal feedback inhibition by dexamethasone. Conversely, neuropsychiatric symptoms such as irritability, decreased libido, insomnia, and depressed mood also are frequently seen in patients with Cushing syndrome. Deciding whether a patient with hypercortisolemia has primary depression or early Cushing syndrome may be difficult. Some patients who eventually show full-blown Cushing syndrome begin with only intermittent elevations of cortisol and symptoms of a major affective disorder.

Although similar in many respects to MDD, the depression seen in Cushing syndrome does have distinguishing clinical characteristics that may aid in the differential diagnosis. Irritability is a prominent and consistent feature, as are symptoms of autonomic activation such as shaking, palpitations, and sweating. Depressed affect is often intermittent, and Cushing patients feel their best, not their worst, in the morning. Psychomotor retardation is not so pronounced as to be clinically obvious, and most of these patients are not withdrawn, apathetic, or hopeless. Significant cognitive impairment, including disorder of memory, is a consistent and prominent clinical feature.[64] Biochemically, patients with Cushing syndrome exhibit higher cortisol levels than those with MDD, and these levels do not return to normal with administration of antidepressants. Assessment of the ACTH response to CRH may be helpful in the differential diagnosis. Although a substantial overlap exists between the two groups, patients with Cushing syndrome show a response, and those with MDD fail to respond to CRH.[65]

## ALCOHOL-INDUCED PSEUDO–CUSHING SYNDROME

As originally described in the literature, patients with alcohol-induced pseudo–Cushing syndrome present with moon facies, truncal obesity, easy bruising, and biochemical features consistent with hypercortisolism. They may fail to show normal suppression with the 1.0-mg overnight dexamethasone test but recover normal suppressibility within 3 weeks of alcohol withdrawal. Similarly, the initially elevated 24-hour urinary free cortisol level returns to normal within a few days.[66,67] Doubt exists, however, as to whether chronic alcohol use leads to stimulation of the hypothalamic–pituitary–adrenal axis. In cases in which cortisol levels have been found to be increased, patients had consumed large quantities of alcohol and appeared intoxicated, with nausea, vomiting, and considerable stress. Some of the phenotypic changes associated with chronic alcohol abuse—such as central adiposity, myopathy, skin atrophy, depression, and psychosis—may be the result of ethanol itself rather than of cortisol. Bruises and rib fractures may result from falls, and diabetes may result from pancreatitis. Thus, whether alcohol-induced pseudo–Cushing syndrome really exists is questionable.[68]

## DIFFERENTIAL DIAGNOSIS OF CUSHING-TYPE HYPERCORTISOLISM AND PSEUDO–CUSHING SYNDROME

The biochemical and phenotypic presentation of patients with mild hypercortisolism in Cushing syndrome is often indistinguishable from that seen in pseudo-Cushing states such as depression. These include elevated urine free cortisol and 17-hydroxycorticosteroid excretion and abnormalities in the normal suppression of plasma cortisol after the administration of a low (1-mg) dose of dexamethasone. In most cases of pseudo–Cushing syndrome, the history and physical examination provide important clues as to whether a given patient has Cushing syndrome or one of these other clinical states. This is particularly true with regard to obesity, in which comorbid conditions exist that overlap with those of Cushing syndrome. In these cases, biochemical studies are necessary to establish a differential diagnosis. Several of the tests used in this differential diagnosis vary in the level of diagnostic accuracy. The low-dose dexamethasone suppression test has 74% specificity, 69% sensitivity, and 71% diagnostic accuracy using the standard criterion of suppression of urinary 17-hydroxycorticoids to <2.5 mg per day on the second day of suppression. For urinary free cortisol, a value >36 µg per day (100 nmol per day) has 100% specificity, 56% sensitivity, and 71% diagnostic accuracy for Cushing syndrome. The CRH stimulation test without dexamethasone pretreatment has 100% specificity, 64% sensitivity, and 76% diagnostic accuracy. The diagnostic accuracy of the CRH/DST for the diagnosis of Cushing syndrome is greater than the accuracy of either the low-dose dexamethasone test or the CRH test alone.[69] A plasma cortisol concentration of >1.4 µg/dL (38 nmol/L) measured 15 min after the administration of CRH had 100% specificity, sensitivity, and diagnostic accuracy. The test has not been worked out for patients with severe melancholic depression, anorexia nervosa, cortisol resistance syndrome, or recent surgical stress. It also has not been defined for patients

with periodic hormonogenesis and intermittent Cushing syndrome. In these patients, measurement of repeated 24-hour urine free cortisol levels may help detect times when an upsurge of ACTH and cortisol secretion occurs. The hypothesis behind the test is that at a dexamethasone dose sufficient to suppress normal cortisol production, patients with pseudo-Cushing states exhibit low basal plasma cortisol and ACTH levels and a diminished response to exogenous CRH. By contrast, patients with Cushing disease have higher basal cortisol and ACTH levels after the administration of dexamethasone and a greater peak response after CRH.[69]

## CORTICOTROPIN-RELEASING HORMONE IN THE PATHOPHYSIOLOGY OF PSEUDO–CUSHING SYNDROME

CRH secretion may help to differentiate pseudo–Cushing syndrome and true Cushing syndrome. Although CRH secretion may be increased in patients with pseudo–Cushing syndrome, in most patients with ACTH-dependent or ACTH-independent Cushing syndrome, CRH secretion appears to be suppressed. When exogenous CRH is administered to patients with MDD, ambulatory alcoholics, and patients with anorexia nervosa, the ACTH response is diminished, whereas the response is increased in patients with pituitary ACTH-dependent disease. Unfortunately, a 25% overlap is found between the two groups.[65]

## TREATMENT OF CUSHING DISEASE

Optimal treatment of Cushing disease depends on an accurate diagnosis of the underlying pathology. Four approaches are used in the management of pituitary ACTH-dependent Cushing disease: *pituitary surgery, pituitary irradiation, adrenal surgery, and drug therapy.*[7,70–72]

### PITUITARY SURGERY

The treatment of choice for pituitary ACTH-dependent Cushing disease is the microsurgical removal of microadenomas or macroadenomas. If a pituitary adenoma or microadenoma can be demonstrated by radiographic techniques, a transsphenoidal operation of the pituitary gland should be the preferred treatment. If a tumor is not detected by imaging techniques, a transsphenoidal exploration of the pituitary gland is still in order, because the tumor can be found in ~90% of patients.[73–75] Even with considerable suprasellar extension, the tumor can be resected transsphenoidally. If a tumor invades the dura, total resection may be impossible, but good remission rates of 45% to 75% have been described for these cases. The microsurgical transsphenoidal selective resection of ACTH-secreting pituitary microadenomas is the most common treatment of Cushing syndrome and comes closest to the ideal form of treatment for this condition.[76–78] Several reports have described a high cure rate with transsphenoidal surgical treatment of Cushing disease.[73–75,79,80] The probability of finding pituitary pathology and of surgically correcting the disease is highest among patients with a typical endocrine testing pattern.[81] *Typical* diagnostic criteria for Cushing disease consist of elevated basal urinary 17-hydroxycorticosteroids and free cortisol levels, cortisol secretion rates, and mean basal serum cortisol levels; a positive response to metyrapone (i.e., elevated ACTH levels associated with a rise in urinary 17-hydroxycorticosteroids); and abnormal suppression with low-dose dexamethasone but >50% suppression with high-dose dexamethasone. Patients with *atypical* diagnostic criteria have elevated basal levels but do not respond as described to metyrapone or to low or high doses of dexamethasone. Pituitary disease was found in 18 of 19 patients with typical preoperative endocrine test results but in only 6 of 11 patients with atypical test results.

If a microadenoma can be identified and totally and discretely *resected*, then the remaining pituitary tissue remains functional, and patients can enjoy remission without loss of endocrine function.[82] If a specific adenoma cannot be identified during surgery, the decision must be made as to whether to perform a *partial* or *total hypophysectomy*. If preoperative inferior petrosal sinus sampling has been carried out and is clearly lateralizing, an appropriate hemiresection of the hypophysis should be performed. If the endocrine studies strongly indicate a pituitary origin but the petrosal sinus sampling is not lateralizing and the patient does not wish to have children, a total hypophysectomy should be considered, but only after a lengthy preoperative discussion with the patient regarding this possibility. If the patient wishes to have children, alternative forms of therapy, including medical treatment or a total adrenalectomy, must be considered. Transsphenoidal surgery for Cushing disease seems to be a reasonably safe procedure, with a mortality rate of <1%. Main complications in these patients are anterior pituitary insufficiency, which occurs in 19%, and diabetes insipidus, which occurs in 18%. Overall incidence of cerebrospinal fluid fistulas is 4%. Other complications, including meningitis, carotid artery injuries, loss of vision, and hypothalamic injuries, occur in from 1% to 2% of patients. An inverse relationship is found between the experience of the surgeon and the likelihood of complications. A statistically significant decreased incidence of morbidity and death has been reported after 200 and even 500 transsphenoidal operations have been performed.[83] With transsphenoidal surgery, permanent anterior or posterior pituitary hormone deficiencies are rare. Transient diabetes insipidus may occur during the early weeks after surgery. Permanent diabetes insipidus and cerebrospinal fluid rhinorrhea are uncommon complications with an initial procedure but may occur more commonly with repeated transsphenoidal surgery. Treatment failures are most common in patients with pituitary macroadenomas or in those in whom a distinct microadenoma has not been found.

### DELAYED RECURRENCE

A delayed recurrence of Cushing disease after removal of a pituitary adenoma may be the result of regrowth of adenoma cells left behind in the peritumoral tissue during the first operation. Attempts are usually made to prevent this cause of recurrence by peritumoral edge resection after selective adenomectomy.[74] The rates of disease recurrence vary among series, which may reflect the evaluation criteria and the technical ability of the pituitary neurosurgeons.[84]

After selective adenoma resection, patients commonly experience transient secondary adrenal insufficiency (of 6 months to 2 years) requiring maintenance hydrocortisone replacement. During this period, the ACTH response to CRH is subnormal.[85] If ACTH and cortisol do not fall to low levels, recurrence is more likely. Within 6 to 8 months after surgery, recovery of hypothalamic pituitary adrenal function and other tropic function usually takes place. The finding of transient deficiency of ACTH secretion after resection of a microadenoma favors the hypothesis of a pituitary origin of the disease. This contrasts with cases of CRH hypersecretion in which overstimulation of the residual corticotropes would be expected after the resection of the adenomatous tissue, leading to persistent or recurrent disease.

### SURGICAL RESULTS IN CHILDREN

Transsphenoidal microadenomectomy is also successful in children and adolescents with Cushing disease.[86] With successful treatment, growth retardation is replaced by catch-up growth or resumption of the growth rate; hypogonadism is followed by pubertal maturation and normal pubertal levels of gonadal steroids; and the blunted TSH response to thyroid-releasing hormone returns to normal. Effective treatment of Cushing disease must be instituted early to prevent early fusion of the epiphysis and permanent stunting of growth.

### PITUITARY IRRADIATION

When transsphenoidal surgery has failed or alternative forms of treatment are desired, pituitary irradiation is an option. The most widely used type of pituitary irradiation is high-voltage irradiation provided by cobalt-60 ($^{60}$Co). The total recommended dose is 40 to 50 Gy, and favorable results can be achieved in ~50% of patients.[70] The best responses are observed in patients with the juvenile form of the disease or in adults younger than 40 years.

When successful, $^{60}$Co irradiation has several advantages. Remission occurs with preservation of pituitary and adrenal function; panhypopituitarism seldom develops; normal reproductive function is restored when the patient is in remission; corticosteroid replacement therapy is not needed; recurrence is rare; and normal cortisol secretion may be restored (i.e., circadian rhythm, normal suppressibility on dexamethasone).[87] The major disadvantage is the slow therapeutic response to pituitary irradiation; 6 to 18 months may elapse before a clinical and biochemical remission is achieved.

Treatment with $^{60}$Co irradiation alone is not adequate in patients who have severe Cushing syndrome. Symptoms may progress if the patient waits for remission, and severe, perhaps irreversible, complications may result. Heavy particle beam irradiation and Bragg peak proton irradiation therapy, with a rate of improvement or remission as high as 80%, appears to be more effective than $^{60}$Co irradiation in the treatment of Cushing syndrome.[88,89] However, the prevalence of postirradiation panhypopituitarism is high. Implants of gold-198 or yttrium-90 yield complete or partial response in 77% of patients with Cushing disease, but the treatment is also complicated by hypopituitarism in 30% to 50% of the patients. Some reports suggest that significant disturbances of hypothalamic-pituitary function follow megavoltage therapy; these disturbances may progress to overt hypopituitarism.[90]

The side effects and the efficacy of therapy may be related to the dosage regimen, with the greatest responses being observed when the highest dose of irradiation is administered. A higher incidence of postirradiation side effects, including radiation necrosis of the brain, occurs with higher dosage.[91] Because this complication may occur from 2 to 20 years after completion of radiation therapy, its possibility should be entertained when local neurologic symptoms develop in patients with a history of radiation therapy for pituitary disease.

Another method of focally targeted radiation therapy is stereotactic radiosurgery or gamma knife therapy. These techniques have been applied to patients who experience recurrence of Cushing disease after transsphenoidal resection of pituitary adenomas and in whom residual tumor can be detected on MRI. Radiation doses of 20 to 35 Gy delivered to the center of the tumor have produced remission of Cushing syndrome and stabilization of tumor growth.[92,93]

### ADRENAL SURGERY

In patients with advanced Cushing disease in whom transsphenoidal surgery has failed, bilateral total adrenalectomy is the preferred treatment. The major disadvantage of adrenalectomy is that it fails to attack the cause underlying the hypersecretion of ACTH. A complication that may occur months or years later is *Nelson syndrome*, with hyperpigmentation and an ACTH-secreting pituitary macroadenoma becoming clinically apparent.[94] These ACTH-secreting tumors may become locally invasive and difficult to control by surgery or radiation therapy. Rarely, these tumors undergo distant metastases, and discrete hepatic metastatic nodules have been found. In a series of 79 consecutive patients with Cushing disease treated with bilateral adrenalectomy, three early postoperative deaths occurred, but most patients did not fare worse than the general population.[95] The most common cause of death among patients who had undergone adrenalectomy for Cushing disease was cardiovascular disease; in other cases, death was the result of the local effects of pituitary tumors. Laparoscopic adrenalectomy has become a common procedure for resection of benign adrenal cortical tumors. Bilateral adrenalectomy can also be performed by laparoscopic technique. The operating time is longer than with open adrenalectomy, but the duration of the procedure depends on the surgical instrumentation used and the experience of the surgeon. Laparoscopic surgery may take 3 to 4 hours to complete in contrast to 1 to 1.5 hours for the open procedure. Estimated blood losses are comparable. The main advantage of laparoscopic surgery is the short recovery time; most patients are able to resume oral intake and ambulation 1 to 4 days postoperatively and normal daily activities in 5 to 7 days.[96]

## DRUG THERAPY

### INHIBITORS OF ADRENAL FUNCTION

Various inhibitors of adrenal function have been used to suppress cortisol secretion in patients with Cushing syndrome. They include *aminoglutethimide, ketoconazole,* and *mitotane.*

**Aminoglutethimide.**    When initially used as an anticonvulsive drug, aminoglutethimide was observed to inhibit cortisol secretion. Subsequently, aminoglutethimide was shown to suppress cortisol secretion effectively in patients with adrenal cancer and ACTH-dependent Cushing disease.[97,98] The mechanism of action of aminoglutethimide is the inhibition of cholesterol side-chain cleavage and blocking of the conversion of cholesterol to $\Delta^5$-pregnenolone in the adrenal cortex. As a result, the synthesis of cortisol, aldosterone, and androgens is inhibited. Histologically, the adrenocortical cells appear loaded with cholesterol droplets as in the lipoidic form of congenital adrenal hyperplasia. Aminoglutethimide also inhibits the aromatization of androstenedione to estrone, an effect that has made it useful in the treatment of patients with carcinoma of the breast.

The drug has been used in adults and in children in doses of 0.5 to 2 g daily.[99,100] Cortisol levels fall gradually, and eventually patients may need glucocorticoid replacement. In persons with cortisol-secreting adrenocortical carcinoma, the effect of aminoglutethimide can be maintained for many months with regression of the clinical manifestations of Cushing syndrome.[97] The drug is only transiently effective in patients with ACTH-dependent Cushing syndrome. The inhibitory effect of the drug is overcome by the high levels of ACTH and cortisol levels, which return to pretreatment levels within days of instituting therapy.[98] The effect of aminoglutethimide is promptly reversed by interruption of therapy.

Aminoglutethimide causes gastrointestinal symptoms (i.e., anorexia, nausea, vomiting) and neurologic side effects (i.e., lethargy, sedation, blurred vision) and can cause hypothyroidism in 5% of patients. A skin rash is frequently observed during the first 10 days of treatment; this usually subsides despite continuation of treatment. Headaches have also been observed when the larger doses are given.

**Ketoconazole.**    Ketoconazole is an imidazole derivative that inhibits the synthesis of ergosterol in fungi and cholesterol in mammalian cells by blocking demethylation of lanosterol. In addition to the effect on cholesterol synthesis, ketoconazole inhibits mitochondrial cytochrome P450–dependent enzymes, such as 11β-hydroxylase and the enzymes needed for cholesterol side-chain cleavage. The drug was also found to inhibit H-dexamethasone binding to glucocorticoid receptors in hepatoma tissue culture cell cytosol and to block glucocorticoid action.

Used in clinical practice as an antifungal medication, ketoconazole has been found to be a potent inhibitor of gonadal and adrenal steroidogenesis in vivo.[101] In normal men, ketoconazole, administered in doses of 200 to 600 mg per day, is a potent inhibitor of testosterone production. Ketoconazole can also inhibit abnormal cortisol production in patients with adrenal adenoma and Cushing syndrome. These patients respond promptly, with disappearance of the clinical and metabolic manifestations of the disease within 4 to 6 weeks of treatment.[101] The effect of ketoconazole appears to be persistent, because no escape from its suppressive effect has been reported for patients who receive the drug for prolonged periods. When patients are treated with ketoconazole, adrenal insufficiency is avoided by decreasing the dose sufficiently to maintain normal cortisol levels.

The most frequent adverse reactions to this drug are nausea and vomiting, abdominal pain, and pruritus in 1% to 3% of patients. Hepatotoxicity, primarily of the hepatocellular type, has been associated with its use. The patient should be monitored for this side effect by performing liver function tests such as those for alkaline phosphatase, serum aspartate aminotransferase (AST), serum alanine aminotransferase (ALT), and bilirubin, which should be measured before starting treatment and at intervals during treatment. Transient minor elevations in liver enzymes have occurred during treatment, but the drug should be discontinued if even minor liver function test abnormalities persist, if the abnormalities worsen, or if they are accompanied by symptoms of possible liver injury.

**Mitotane.**    Of all the pharmacologic agents described, mitotane is the only one that inhibits biosynthesis of corticosteroids and destroys adrenocortical cells secreting cortisol, producing a long-lasting effect. Mitotane acts on adrenocortical cell mitochondria, where it inhibits 11β-hydroxylase and cholesterol side-chain cleavage enzymes. As a result of this inhibition, the production of cortisol, aldosterone, and dehydroepiandrosterone is suppressed. Mitotane appears to require metabolism for its action. Under the effect of mitochondrial P450 monooxygenases, the drug is probably transformed into an acylchloride, which covalently binds to important macromolecules in the cell mitochondria. The result is the destruction of the mitochondria with necrosis of the adrenal cortex. The zona reticularis of the adrenal cortex appears to be most sensitive to the action of mitotane, and the glomerulosa is the least sensitive.

A combination of $^{60}$Co irradiation of the pituitary gland and selective suppression of cortisol secretion with mitotane has been used in the treatment of Cushing disease.[102] Eighty percent of the patients treated with this drug plus pituitary irradiation had clinical and biochemical remission of their disease (Fig. 75-10). One-half of the patients treated by this combination of therapy had suppression of their elevated cortisol levels within 4 months of therapy. The initial decrease in cortisol secretion appeared to be a response to the administration of mitotane, because plasma ACTH levels were still high when

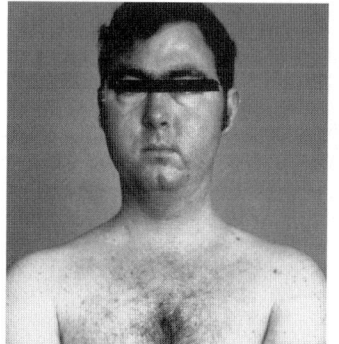 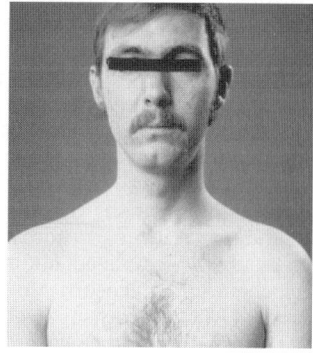

A,B

**FIGURE 75-10.** **A,** A 24-year-old man with severe Cushing disease failed to respond to $^{60}$Co pituitary irradiation. **B,** After mitotane therapy for 9 months, the features of Cushing syndrome disappeared.

indices of cortisol secretion returned to normal. In addition to suppressing cortisol secretion, this drug appears to have a partial suppressive effect on ACTH. After suppression of cortisol secretion, minimal feedback increase in ACTH production occurred, and in 70% of treated patients, an actual decrease in ACTH levels was observed. This response contrasts with the increase in ACTH levels in patients treated by adrenalectomy or with other adrenal inhibitors.

Mitotane is a selective inhibitor of the reticularis and fasciculata zones of the adrenal cortex. Aldosterone secretion is usually spared, and the patients do not require mineralocorticoid replacement when they develop adrenal insufficiency. The side effects of therapy include anorexia, nausea, diarrhea, somnolence, pruritus, hypercholesterolemia, and hypouricemia. Elevated alkaline phosphatase levels can also occur as a result of the hepatotoxic effects of mitotane. Hypouricemia, a consistent finding, appears to be caused by increased renal clearance of uric acid. Low thyroxine levels found in patients treated with mitotane are probably the result of interference with protein-binding for this hormone. Mitotane competitively binds to thyroxine-binding globulin in a manner similar to that of phenytoin, another diphenyl compound. Other indices of thyroid function are in the normal range. All of the side effects described can be reversed by reducing the dose or by interrupting therapy.

Mitotane also has well-known extraadrenal effects, derived from its effect as an inducer of microsomal hydroxylating enzymes. As such, it can alter cortisol metabolism and the metabolic degradation of synthetic substituted steroids, which are predominantly inactivated by hydroxylation. A consequence of this effect is an early fall in the urinary excretion of 17-hydroxycorticosteroids, which occurs independently of the suppressive effects on cortisol secretion. Because of this effect, measurement of urinary 17-hydroxycorticosteroid levels does not provide a reliable index of adrenal suppression by the drug. Assessment of changes in cortisol secretion rates, urinary free cortisol levels, and plasma cortisol levels is required to determine the biochemical response.

Combined therapy with pituitary irradiation and mitotane can be given as primary medical treatment of Cushing syndrome when surgery is contraindicated or as the next modality of therapy when transsphenoidal pituitary surgery fails to bring about remission of the disease. The dose used for the treatment of Cushing disease is 2 to 4 g daily. Therapy may be initiated with a dose of 500 mg twice daily and increased to 1 g four times daily, as needed to achieve adrenal-suppressive effects. The urinary free cortisol excretion should be monitored, and the dose should be titrated to maintain the urinary free cortisol excretion in the normal range. If adrenal insufficiency is suspected, hydrocortisone should be given orally. Because mitotane induces liver monooxygenases, which metabolize corticosteroids and other drugs, the adequate dosage of fludrocortisone or hydrocortisone may be higher than expected. As the effect of radiation therapy becomes apparent with suppression of ACTH secretion, treatment with the drug can be gradually discontinued.

A compound of a different class, mifepristone or RU-486 [17-β-hydroxy-11-β-(4-dimethyl amino)-17-α-(1-propynyl) estra-4,9-dien-3-one] is a glucocorticoid antagonist that has been shown to effectively antagonize hypercortisolism causing Cushing syndrome.[103] This compound is a 19-norsteroid with substitutions at positions $C_{11}$ and $C_{17}$; it antagonizes cortisol action competitively at the receptor level. With therapy, the somatic features of Cushing syndrome ameliorate, mean arterial blood pressure is normalized, and suicidal depression can resolve. All biochemical glucocorticoid-sensitive parameters normalize, and ACTH and cortisol levels, as expected, remain unchanged. Although this drug may be effective in patients with autonomous cortisol production, the blocking effect of the compound on cortisol receptors may increase the secretion of ACTH in patients with pituitary ACTH-dependent Cushing syndrome

**TABLE 75-5.**

**Staging of Adrenal Cortical Carcinoma Based on Size and Extent of Tumor Involvement**

| Stage | Size | Lymphade-nopathy | Local Invasion | Metastases |
|---|---|---|---|---|
| I | <5 cm | – | – | – |
| II | >5 cm | – | – | – |
| III | Any size | + | + | – |
| IV | Any size | + | + | + |

+, present; –, absent

and cause a further increase in cortisol production. This additional cortisol production may be sufficient to overcome the antiglucocorticoid effect of the drug.

Mifepristone is well tolerated and nontoxic in doses ranging between 10 and 20 mg/kg per day. It is still an investigational drug, and its use is limited to investigational protocols.

## TREATMENT OF ECTOPIC ADRENOCORTICOTROPIN SYNDROME

Treatment of the ectopic ACTH syndrome involves the surgical resection of the primary tumor, followed by radiation therapy or chemotherapy, depending on the type of neoplasm producing the illness. In patients whose neoplasms cannot be resected, the use of adrenal inhibitors such as aminoglutethimide, metyrapone, and ketoconazole may ameliorate the clinical manifestations of the Cushing syndrome. However, the very high ACTH levels may overcome the suppressive effect of these drugs. Bilateral adrenalectomy is an alternative approach but is not a practical one for patients who have rapidly progressive metastatic disease. Because the underlying tumors may occasionally be slow growing (e.g., metastatic carcinoid, bronchial carcinoids), an adrenalectomy followed by replacement therapy with normal amounts of hydrocortisone may improve considerably the metabolic consequence of the Cushing syndrome.

## TREATMENT OF CORTICOTROPIN-INDEPENDENT CUSHING SYNDROME

### ADRENOCORTICAL ADENOMA

Adrenocortical adenomas should be surgically removed.[104] Because of suppression of the hypothalamic–pituitary–adrenal axis in these patients, adrenal insufficiency occurs postoperatively. These patients require replacement therapy with physiologic doses of cortisol until recovery of the hypothalamic-pituitary–adrenal axis takes place. This recovery may require 6 to 16 months. Occasionally, recovery of pituitary-adrenal function never occurs and patients require lifelong replacement therapy with cortisol.

### ADRENAL CARCINOMA

Adrenal carcinomas causing Cushing syndrome are highly malignant neoplasms resulting in a shortened life expectancy.[105,105a] Their treatment has not been well standardized, and the prognosis has been poor regardless of therapy. Prognosis depends on the stage of the tumor at the time of diagnosis. Staging by size and extent (Table 75-5) is helpful in assessing the magnitude of the disease and probable life expectancy.[106] Patients with stage I or stage II tumors may experience cure or long disease-free periods. Patients with stage IV tumors have short life expectancy even with currently available chemotherapy.

Several approaches to therapy have been used. One method is surgical excision of the primary tumor and of large neoplastic abdominal masses. Although temporary remission of the disease frequently occurs with this approach, recurrence and eventual death from metastatic disease is the rule.[107] Another approach is radiation therapy and nonspecific chemotherapy.[108] These have been generally effective only for palliation of local disease, because this neoplasm is generally resistant to these types of therapy.

Agents that block corticosteroid hormone production by the tumor have also been used. Although effective in reversing the metabolic consequences of these tumors, these drugs do not alter the progression and eventual fatal outcome of the disease. Mitotane has been the only drug that has proven effective in patients with adrenocortical carcinoma.[109] Most of the experience with mitotane comes from its use in patients with obvious metastases, but its effectiveness under those conditions has been disputed in the literature.[107,110–112] Decreases in elevated urinary steroid levels, measurable disease response, and overall clinical response have been described.[111] However, mean survival is short (8 months) when the drug is used after the appearance of metastatic disease. Isolated case reports have described impressive remissions and even cures of adrenocortical carcinoma after therapy with this drug.[109,113,114] In general, survival appears to depend on the size of the primary lesion and the degree of local and distant extension of the neoplasm at the time of initial surgery. Criteria for staging adrenal cancer have been suggested. Patients with primary tumors <5 cm in diameter and without local or distant extension appear to have relatively good prognosis and longer survival.

If mitotane therapy is to be effective, it should be instituted early, as adjuvant therapy, after the resection of the primary tumor and before local extension or distant metastasis has occurred.[112,115] Adverse effects of mitotane therapy are found to be dose dependent; they are intolerable with doses higher than 6 g daily. Treatment is usually begun with doses of 1 g twice daily and gradually increased up to tolerance. The drug should be administered with fat-containing food, because its absorption and transport appear to be coupled to lipoproteins. The prominent early side effects of larger doses are anorexia and nausea. The discomfort with these side effects can be minimized by administering the largest dose at bedtime so that patients sleep through the most uncomfortable period. Side effects are usually reversed by interrupting therapy for several days and restarting the drug at a lower dose level. Because of possible teratogenic effects, patients on mitotane should be advised against pregnancy.

# REFERENCES

1. Gold EM. The Cushing's syndromes: changing views of diagnosis and treatment. Ann Intern Med 1979; 90:829.
2. Kathol RG, Delahunt JW, Hannah L. Transition from bipolar affective disorder to intermittent Cushing's syndrome: case report. J Clin Psychiatry 1985; 46:194.
3. Kelly WF, Checkley SA, Bender BA. Cushing's syndrome and depression—a prospective study of 26 patients. Br J Psychiatry 1983; 142:16.
4. Reed K, Watkins M, Dobson H. Mania in Cushing's syndrome: case report. J Clin Psychiatry 1983; 44:416.
5. Saad MF, Adams F, Mackay B, et al. Occult Cushing's disease presenting with acute psychosis. Am J Med 1984; 76:759.
6. Starkman MN, Schteingart DE. Neuropsychiatric manifestations of patients with Cushing's syndrome. Arch Intern Med 1981; 141:215.
7. Schteingart DE. The diagnosis and medical management of Cushing's syndrome. In: Thompson NW, Vinik AL, eds. Endocrine surgery update. New York: Grune & Stratton, 1983:87.
8. Daughaday, WH. Cushing's disease and basophilic microadenomas—editorial retrospective. N Engl J Med 1984; 310:919.
9. Lamberts SWJ, Delange SA, Stefanko SZ. Adrenocorticotropin-secreting pituitary adenomas originate from the anterior or intermediate lobe in Cushing's disease: differences in the regulation of hormone secretion. J Clin Endocrinol Metab 1982; 54:286.
10. Lamberts SWJ, Stefanko SA, deLange SA, et al. Failure of clinical remission after transsphenoidal removal of a microadenoma in a patient with Cushing's disease: multiple hyperplastic and adenomatous cell nests in surrounding pituitary tissue. J Clin Endocrinol Metab 1980; 50:793.
11. Young WF, Scheithauer BW, Gharib H, et al. Cushing's syndrome due to primary multinodular corticotrope hyperplasia. Mayo Clin Proc 1988; 63:256.
12. McKeever PE, Koppelman MCS, Metcalf D, et al. Refractory Cushing's disease caused by multinodular ACTH-cell hyperplasia. J Neuropathol Exp Neurol 1982; 41:490.
13. Biller BM, Alexander JM, Zervas NT, et al. Clonal origins of adrenocorticotropin-secreting pituitary tissue in Cushing's disease. J Clin Endocrinol Metab 1992; 75(5):1303.
14. Glass AR, Zabadil AP, Halberg F, et al. Circadian rhythm of serum cortisol in Cushing's disease. J Clin Endocrinol Metab 1984; 59:161.
15. Schteingart DE, McKenzie AK. Twelve hour cycles of ACTH and cortisol secretion in Cushing's disease. J Clin Endocrinol Metab 1980; 51:1195.
16. Liddle GW, Island DP, Ney RI. Cushing's syndrome caused by recurrent malignant bronchial carcinoid. Arch Intern Med 1963; 111:471.
17. Schteingart DE. Ectopic secretion of peptides of the proopiomelanocortin family. Endocrinol Metab Clin North Am 1991; 20:453.
18. Melmed S, Rushakoff RJ. Ectopic pituitary and hypothalamic hormone syndromes. Endocrinol Metab Clin North Am 1987; 16:805.
19. DeBold CR, Menefee JK, Nicholson WE, et al. Proopiomelanocortin gene is expressed in many normal tissues and in tumors not associated with ectopic adrenocorticotropin syndrome. Mol Endocrinol 1988; 2:862.
20. White A, Clark AJ, Stewart MF. The synthesis of ACTH and related peptides by tumors. Baillières Clin Endocrinol Metab 1990; 4:1.
21. Picon A, Leblond-Francillard M, Raffin-Sanson ML, et al. Functional analysis of the human pro-opiomelanocortin promoter in the small cell lung carcinoma cell line DMS-79. J Mol Endocrinol 1995; 15:187.
22. Schteingart DE, Chandler WF, Lloyd RV, et al. Cushing's syndrome caused by an ectopic pituitary adenoma. Neurosurgery 1987; 21:223.
23. Belsky JL, Cuello B, Swanson LW, et al. Cushing's syndrome due to ectopic production of corticotropin-releasing factor. J Clin Endocrinol Metab 1985; 60:496.
24. Schteingart DE, Lloyd RV, Akil H, et al. Cushing's syndrome secondary to ectopic CRH-ACTH secretion. J Clin Endocrinol Metab 1986; 63:770.
25. Marieb NJ, Spangler S, Kashgarian M, et al. Cushing's syndrome secondary to ectopic cortisol production by ovarian carcinoma. J Clin Endocrinol Metab 1983; 57:737.
26. Smalls AGH, Pieters GFFM, Van Haelst UJG, et al. Micronodular adrenocortical hyperplasia in long standing Cushing's disease. J Clin Endocrinol Metab 1983; 58:25.
27. Lamberts SWJ, Bons EG, Bruining HA. Different sensitivity to adrenocorticotropin of dispersed adrenocortical cells from patients with Cushing's disease with macronodular and diffuse adrenal hyperplasia. J Clin Endocrinol Metab 1984; 58:1106.
28. Shenoy BV, Carpenter PC, Carney JA. Bilateral primary pigmented nodular adrenal cortical disease—rare cause of Cushing's syndrome. Am J Surg Pathol 1984; 8:335.
29. Stratakis CA, Carney JA, Lin JP, et al. Carney complex. A familial multiple neoplasia and lentiginosis syndrome: analysis of 11 kindreds and linkage to the short arm of chromosome 2. J Clin Invest 1996; 97(3):699.
30. Terzolo M, Boccuzzi A, Ali A, et al. Cushing's syndrome due to ACTH-independent bilateral adrenocortical hyperplasia. J Endocrinol Invest 1997; 20 (5):270.
31. Lacroix A, Bolte E, Tremblay J, et al. Gastric inhibitory polypeptide-dependent cortisol hypersecretion—a new cause of Cushing's syndrome. N Engl J Med 1992; 327(14):974.
32. Lacroix A, Tremblay J, Russeau G, et al. Brief report: propranolol therapy for ectopic (beta)-adrenergic receptors in adrenal Cushing's syndrome. N Engl J Med 1997; 337(20):1429.
33. Lynch HT, Lynch J, Conway T, et al. Hereditary breast cancer and family cancer syndromes. World J Surg 1994; 18(1):21.
34. Tsunematsu Y, Watanabe S, Oka T. et al. Familiar aggregation of cancer from proband cases with childhood adrenal cortical carcinoma. Jap J Cancer Res 1991; 82(8):893.
34a. Schteingart DE. Management approaches to adrenal incidentalomas. A view from Ann Arbor, Michigan. Endocrinol Metab Clin North Am 2000; 29(1):127.
35. Crapo L. Cushing's syndrome: a review of diagnostic tests. Metabolism 1971; 28:955.
36. Kennedy L, Atkinson AB, Johnston H, et al. Serum cortisol concentrations during low dose dexamethasone suppression test to screen for Cushing's syndrome. BMJ 1984; 289:1188.
37. Raff H, Raff JL, Findling JW. Late-night salivary cortisol as a screening test for Cushing's syndrome. J Clin Endocrinol Metab 1998; 83(8):2681.
38. Bruno OD, Rossi MA, Contreras LN, et al. Nocturnal high dose dexamethasone suppression test in the etiological diagnosis of Cushing's syndrome. Acta Endocrinol 1985; 109:158.
39. Abou Samra AB, Dechaud H, Estour B, et al. Beta-lipotropin and cortisol responses to intravenous infusion dexamethasone suppression test in Cushing's syndrome and obesity. J Clin Endocrinol Metab 1985; 61:116.
40. Chrousos GP, Schulte HM, Oldfield EH, et al. A corticotropin-releasing factor stimulation test—an aid in the evaluation of patients with Cushing's syndrome. N Engl J Med 1984; 310:622.
41. Orth DN, DeBold CR, DeCherney GS, et al. Pituitary microadenomas causing Cushing's disease respond to corticotropin-releasing factor. J Clin Endocrinol Metab 1982; 55:1017.
42. Joebson RV, Hockings GI, Torpy PJ. New diagnostic tests for Cushing's syndrome. Clin Exp Physiol 1996; 23(6–7):579.
43. Yanovski JA, Cutler GB, Chrousos GP, Nieman LK. The dexamethasone-suppressed, corticotropin-releasing hormone stimulation test differentiates mild Cushing's disease from normal physiology. J Clin Endocrinol Metab 1998; 83(2):348.

44. Dunlap NE, Grizzle WE, Siegel AL. Cushing's—screening methods in hospitalized patients. Arch Pathol Lab Med 1985; 109:222.

45. Werk EE, MacGee J, Sholiton LJ. Effect of diphenylhydantoin on cortisol metabolism in man. J Clin Invest 1964; 43:1824.

46. Kapcala LP, Hamilton SM, Meikle AW. Cushing's disease with "normal suppression" due to decreased dexamethasone clearance. Arch Intern Med 1984; 144:636.

47. Oldfield EH, Chrousos GP, Schulte HM, et al. Preoperative lateralization of ACTH-secreting pituitary microadenomas by bilateral and simultaneous inferior petrosal venous sinus sampling. N Engl J Med 1985; 312:100.

48. Snow RB, Patterson RH, Howith M, et al. Usefulness of preoperative inferior petrosal vein sampling in Cushing's disease. Surg Neurol 1988; 29:17.

49. Zovickian J, Oldfield EH, Doppman JL, et al. Usefulness of inferior petrosal sinus venous endocrine markers in Cushing's disease. J Neurosurg 1988; 68:205.

50. Doppman JL, Oldfield EH, Nieman LK. Bilateral sampling of internal jugular vein to distinguish between mechanisms of adrenocorticotropic hormone-dependent-Cushing syndrome. Ann Intern Med 1998; 128(1):33.

51. Moses DC, Schteingart DE, Sturman MF, et al. Efficacy of radiocholesterol imaging of the adrenal glands in Cushing's syndrome. Surg Obstet Gynecol 1974; 139:1.

52. Smith SM, Patel SK, Turner DA, Matalon TA. Magnetic resonance imaging of adrenal cortical carcinoma. Urol Radiol 1989; 11:1.

53. Hamper UM, Fishman EK, Hartman DS, et al. Primary adrenocortical carcinoma: sonographic evaluation with clinical and pathological correlation in 26 patients. AJR Am J Roentgenol 1987; 148:915.

54. Schteingart DE, Seabold JE, Gross MD, et al. Iodocholesterol adrenal tissue uptake and imaging in adrenal neoplasms. J Clin Endocrinol Metab 1981; 52:1157.

55. Doppman JL, Miller DL, Dwyer AJ, et al. Macronodular adrenal hyperplasia in Cushing's disease. Radiology 1988; 166:347.

56. DeStefano D, Lloyd RV, Schteingart DE. Cushing's syndrome produced by a bronchial carcinoid tumor. Hum Pathol 1984; 15:890.

57. Philipponneau M, Nocaudie M, Epelbaum J, et al. Somatostatin analogs for the localization and preoperative treatment of adrenocorticotropin-secreting bronchial carcinoid tumor. J Clin Endocrinol Metab 1994; 78:20.

58. Barbareschi M, Mariscotti C, Frigo B, et al. Mediastinal malignant carcinoid with Cushing's syndrome: immunohistochemical and ultrastructural study. Appl Pathol 1989; 7:161.

59. Coates PJ, Doniach I, Howlett TA, et al. Immunocytochemical study of 18 tumors causing ectopic Cushing's syndrome. J Clin Pathol 1986; 39:955.

60. Doppman JL, Loughlin T, Miller DL, et al. Identification of ACTH producing intrathoracic tumors by measuring ACTH levels in aspirated specimens. Radiology 1987; 163:501.

61. Lapidus L, Bengtsson C, Höllström T, Björntorp P. Obesity, adipose tissue distribution and health in women. Results from a population study in Gothenburg, Sweden. Appetite 1989; 12:25.

62. Schteingart DE, Gregerman RI, Conn JW. A comparison of the characteristics of increased adrenocortical function in obesity and in Cushing's syndrome. Metabolism 1963; 12:484.

63. Marin P, Darin N, Aneniva T, et al. Cortisol secretion in relationship to body fat distribution in premenopausal women. Metabolism 1992; 41:882.

64. Starkman MN. The HPA axis and psychopathology. Cushing's syndrome. Psychiatr Ann 1993; 23:691.

65. Gold PW, Loriaux DL, Roy A, et al. Responses to corticotropin-releasing hormone in the hypercortisolism of depression and Cushing's disease. N Engl J Med 1986; 314:1329.

66. Rees LH, Besser GM, Jeffcoate WF, et al. Alcohol-induced pseudo-Cushing's syndrome. Lancet 1977; 1:726.

67. Lambert SW, Klijn JGM, deJong FH, Birkenhager JC. Hormone secretion in alcohol-induced pseudo-Cushing's syndrome: differential diagnosis with Cushing's disease. JAMA 1979; 242:1640.

68. Jeffcoate W. Alcohol-induced pseudo-Cushing's syndrome. Lancet 1993; 341(8846):676.

69. Yanovski JA, Cutler GB, Chrousos GP, Nieman LK. Corticotropin-releasing hormone stimulation following low-dose dexamethasone administration: a new test to distinguish Cushing's syndrome from pseudo-Cushing's states. JAMA 1993; 269(17):2232.

70. Aron DC. Cushing's syndrome: current concepts in diagnosis and treatment. Compr Ther 1987; 13:37.

71. Jeffcoate WJ. Treating Cushing's disease. BMJ 1988; 296:227.

72. Orth D, Liddle GW. Results of treatment in 108 patients with Cushing's syndrome. N Engl J Med 1971; 285:243.

73. Boggan JE, Tyrrell JB, Wilson CB. Transsphenoidal microsurgical management of Cushing's disease—report of 100 cases. J Neurosurg 1983; 59:195.

74. Nakane T, Kuwayama A, Watanabe M, et al. Long term results of transsphenoidal adenomectomy in patients with Cushing's disease. Neurosurgery 1987; 21:218.

75. Pelkonen R, Eistola P, Grahme B, et al. Treatment of pituitary Cushing's disease: results of adrenal and pituitary surgery. Acta Endocrinol Suppl 1983; 251:38.

76. Hardy J. Transsphenoidal surgery of hypersecreting pituitary tumors. In: Kohler PO, Ross GT, eds. Diagnosis and treatment of pituitary tumors. Amsterdam: Excerpta Medica, 1979:179.

77. Salassa RM, Laws ER Jr, Carpenter PC, et al. Transsphenoidal removal of pituitary microadenoma in Cushing's disease. Mayo Clin Proc 1978; 53:24.

78. Tyrrell JB, Brooks RM, Fitzgerald PA, et al. Cushing's disease: selective transsphenoidal resection of pituitary microadenomas. N Engl J Med 1978; 289:753.

79. Kuwayama A, Kageyama N. Current management of Cushing's disease. Part I. Contemp Neurosurg 1985; 7:1.

80. Swearingen B, Biller BM, Barker FG II, et al. Long-term mortality after transsphenoidal surgery for Cushing disease. Ann Intern Med 1999; 130 (10):821.

81. Chandler WF, Schteingart DE, Lloyd RV, et al. Surgical treatment of Cushing's disease. J Neurosurg 1987; 66:204.

82. Schnall AM, Brodkey JS, Kaufman B, et al. Pituitary function after removal of pituitary microadenomas in Cushing's disease. J Clin Endocrinol Metab 1978; 47:410.

83. Ciric I, Ragin A, Baumgartner C, Pierce D. Complications of transsphenoidal surgery: results of a national survey, review of the literature, and personal experience. Neurosurgery 1997; 40(2):225.

84. Burch WM. Diagnosis and treatment of Cushing's disease at Duke University (1977–1982). N C Med J 1983; 44:293.

85. Avgerinos PC, Chrousos GP, Nieman LK, et al. The corticotropin-releasing hormone test in the postoperative evaluation of patients with Cushing's syndrome. J Clin Endocrinol Metab 1987; 65:906.

86. Styne DM, Grumbach MM, Kaplan SL, et al. Treatment of Cushing's disease in childhood and adolescence by transphenoidal microadenomectomy. N Engl J Med 1984; 310:889.

87. Futterweit W, Krieger DT, Gabrilove JL. Adrenal cortical function studies in Cushing's syndrome due to nontumorous adrenocortical hyperfunction treated with pituitary irradiation. J Clin Endocrinol Metab 1962; 22:364.

88. Kjellberg RN, Kliman B. A system for therapy of pituitary tumors. In: Kohler PO, Ross GT, eds. Diagnosis and treatment of pituitary tumors. Amsterdam: Excerpta Medica, 1973:234.

89. Lawrence JH, Okerlund MD, Linfoot JE, et al. Heavy particle treatment of Cushing's disease. N Engl J Med 1971; 285:1263.

90. Sharpe GF, Kendall-Taylor P, Prescott RWG, et al. Pituitary function following megavoltage therapy for Cushing's disease: long-term follow-up. Clin Endocrinol 1985; 22:169.

91. Aristizabal S, Caldwell WL, Avila J, et al. Relationship of time/dose factors to tumor control and complications in the treatment of Cushing's disease by irradiation. Int J Radiat Oncol Biol Phys 1977; 2:47.

92. Seo Y, Fukuoka S, Takanashi M, et al. Gamma knife surgery for Cushing's disease. Surg Neurol 1995; 43(2):170.

93. Wolffenbuttel BH, Kitz K, Beuls EM. Beneficial gamma-knife radiosurgery in a patient with Nelson's syndrome. Clin Neurol Neurosurg 1998; 100(1):60.

94. Nelson DH, Meakin JW, Thorn GW. ACTH-producing pituitary tumors following adrenalectomy for Cushing's syndrome. Ann Intern Med 1970; 52:560.

95. Welbourn RB. Survival and cause of death after an adrenalectomy for Cushing's disease. Surgery 1985; 97:16.

96. Gagner M, Pomp A, Heniford BT, et al. Laparoscopic adrenalectomy: lessons learned from 100 consecutive procedures. Ann Surg 1997; 226(3):238.

97. Schteingart DE, Cash R, Conn JW. Aminoglutethimide and metastatic adrenal cancer. Maintained reversal (six months) of Cushing's syndrome. JAMA 1966; 198:1007.

98. Schteingart DE, Conn JW. Effects of aminoglutethimide upon adrenal function and cortisol metabolism in Cushing's syndrome. J Clin Endocrinol Metab 1967; 27:1657.

99. Misbin RI, Canary J, Willard D. Aminoglutethimide in the treatment of Cushing's syndrome. J Clin Pharmacol 1976; 16:645.

100. Zachman N, Gitzelmann RT, Zagalaka M, et al. Effect of aminoglutethimide on urinary cortisol and cortisol metabolites in adolescents with Cushing's syndrome. Clin Endocrinol 1977; 7:63.

101. Sonino N, Boscaro M, Merola G, et al. Prolonged treatment of Cushing's disease by ketoconazole. J Clin Endocrinol Metab 1985; 61:718.

102. Schteingart DE, Tsao HS, Taylor CI, et al. Sustained remission of Cushing's disease with mitotane and pituitary irradiation. Ann Intern Med 1980; 92:613.

103. Nieman LK, Chrousos GP, Kellner C, et al. Successful treatment of Cushing's syndrome with a glucocorticoid antagonist RU486. J Clin Endocrinol Metab 1985; 71:536.

104. Scott HW, Abumrad NN, Orth DN. Tumors of the adrenal cortex in Cushing's syndrome. Ann Surg 1985; 201:586.

105. Huvos AJ, Hajdu SI, Brosfield RD, et al. Adrenal cortical carcinoma: clinico-pathologic study of 34 cases. Cancer 1970; 25:354.

105a. Wajchenberg BL, Albegaria Pereira MA, Medonca BB, et al. Adrenocortical carcinoma : clinical and laboratory observations. Cancer 2000; 88:711.

106. Hogan T. A clinical and pathological study of adrenocortical carcinoma; therapeutic implications. Cancer 1980; 45:2880.

107. Hajjar RA, Hickey RC, Samaan NA. Adrenal cortical carcinoma: a study of 22 patients. Cancer 1975; 35:549.

108. Percarpio B, Knowlton AH. Radiation therapy of adrenal cortical carcinoma. Acta Radiol Oncol Radiat Phys Biol 1976; 15:288.

109. Becker D, Schumacher OP. o,p'-DDD therapy in invasive adrenocortical carcinoma. Ann Intern Med 1977; 82:677.

110. Hoffman DL, Mattox VL. Treatment of adrenocortical carcinoma with o,p'-DDD. Med Clin North Am 1972; 50:999.

111. Hutter AM Jr, Kayhoe DE. Adrenal cortical carcinoma: results of treatment with o,p'-DDD in 138 patients. Am J Med 1966; 41:581.

112. Lubitz JA, Freeman L, Okun R. Mitotane use in inoperable adrenal cortical carcinoma. JAMA 1973; 223:1109.

113. Downing V, Eule J, Huseby RA. Regression of an adrenal cortical carcinoma and its neovascular bed, following mitotane therapy: a case report. Cancer 1974; 34:1882.

114. Jarabak J, Rice K. Metastatic adrenocortical carcinoma: prolonged regression with mitotane therapy. JAMA 1981; 246:1706.

115. Schteingart DE, Motazedi A, Noonan RA, et al. The treatment of adrenal carcinoma. Arch Surg 1982; 117:1142.

# CHAPTER 76

# ADRENOCORTICAL INSUFFICIENCY

## D. LYNN LORIAUX

## SYNDROMES OF ADRENAL INSUFFICIENCY

The adrenal glands produce three classes of steroid hormone: *glucocorticoid, mineralocorticoid,* and *adrenal androgen* (actually, androgen precursor). The primary glucocorticoid in humans is hydrocortisone. This hormone is essential for life. The syndrome of adrenal insufficiency is the clinical manifestation of deficient production of this hormone. The central pathophysiologic alteration is cardiovascular: reduced cardiac output and decreased vascular tone with relative hypovolemia. This stimulates increased vasopressin secretion, which results in water retention and hyponatremia. If salt balance is not maintained, a situation that occurs if aldosterone also is deficient, hyponatremia is accompanied by hyperkalemia. Left untreated, this disorder leads to debility, prostration, coma, and death. The causes of adrenal insufficiency can be considered under two general headings: *primary adrenal insufficiency* (Addison disease), caused by destruction of the adrenal glands themselves, and *secondary adrenal insufficiency,* caused by disordered hypothalamic-pituitary function leading to a relative or complete deficiency of adrenocorticotropic hormone (ACTH).

## PRIMARY ADRENAL INSUFFICIENCY

The two main causes of primary adrenal disease are tuberculosis and autoimmune adrenal destruction.[1] The latter is a component of the polyendocrine deficiency syndrome[2] (see Chap. 197). The causes of primary adrenal insufficiency are listed in Table 76-1.

Estimates are that 70% of the cases of primary adrenal insufficiency in the industrialized world are associated with the

**TABLE 76-1.**
**Etiology of Adrenal Insufficiency**

| Cause | Occurrence |
|---|---|
| **PRIMARY ADRENAL INSUFFICIENCY** | |
| Autoimmune (polyendocrine deficiency syndrome) | 70% |
| Tuberculosis | 20% |
| *Other* | 10% |
| Fungal infections | |
| Adrenal hemorrhage | |
| Congenital adrenal hypoplasia | |
| Sarcoidosis | |
| Amyloidosis | |
| Acquired immunodeficiency syndrome | |
| Adrenoleukodystrophy | |
| Adrenomyeloneuropathy | |
| Metastatic neoplasia | |
| Congenital unresponsiveness to corticotropin | |
| **SECONDARY ADRENAL INSUFFICIENCY** | |
| After exogenous glucocorticoids or corticotropin | Very common |
| After the cure of Cushing syndrome (removal of endogenous glucocorticoids) | Common |
| Hypothalamic and pituitary lesions | Uncommon |

**TABLE 76-2.**
**Features of the Autoimmune Polyglandular Syndromes**

| Characteristic | Type 1 | Type 2 |
|---|---|---|
| Peak age of onset | 12 yr | 30 yr |
| HLA association | None | B8 |
| Hypoparathyroidism | ++ | 0 |
| Mucocutaneous candidiasis | ++ | 0 |
| Alopecia | + | 0 |
| Chronic active hepatitis | + | 0 |
| Pernicious anemia | + | 0 |
| Hypogonadism | + | 0 |
| Autoimmune thyroid disease | + | ++ |
| Diabetes mellitus, type 1 | 0 | + |

+, occasional association; ++, frequent association; 0, no association.
(From Neufeld M, MacLaren N, Blizzard R. Autoimmune polyglandular syndromes. Pediatr Ann 1980; 9:154.)

polyendocrine deficiency syndrome. This disorder is autoimmune. Findings that support this conclusion include a high prevalence of suppressor T-cell abnormalities, the presence of antibodies against endocrine organs, and an association with other disorders of known autoimmune etiology such as vitiligo, alopecia areata, celiac disease, autoimmune thyroiditis, and mucocutaneous candidiasis.[3,4] The histologic picture in the adrenal glands reveals lymphocytic infiltration, fibrosis, a loss of cortical cells, and an intact adrenal medulla.

The disorder has two recognizable subtypes (Table 76-2). Type 1 is an illness of childhood, with a mean age of onset of 12 years. Adrenal insufficiency, hypoparathyroidism, and mucocutaneous candidiasis are the most common manifestations. Associated conditions include hypogonadism, pernicious anemia, chronic active hepatitis, and alopecia. The disorder has a recessive pattern of inheritance, clustering across sibships without apparent vertical transmission (see Chap. 187).

Type 2 is a disorder of young adults. The mean age of onset is in the mid-20s. Adrenal insufficiency, autoimmune thyroid disease, and diabetes mellitus are the most common manifestations. Associated immune disorders are rare. Susceptibility to this disorder seems to be inherited as a dominant trait in linkage disequilibrium with the HLA-B region of chromosome 6 (see Chap. 194). This form of the disease exhibits a vertical pattern of transmission.[5]

Worldwide, tuberculosis still is the most common cause of primary adrenal insufficiency[6] (see Chap. 213). The adrenal glands can be replaced entirely by caseating granulomas. This phenomenon is virtually always accompanied by evidence of tuberculosis in other organ systems, especially the lungs and kidneys. Tuberculous adrenal glands are large and often contain calcium. This contrasts strikingly with the normal-sized or small, noncalcified glands found in patients with the polyendocrine deficiency syndrome.

Fungi can colonize and destroy the adrenal cortex. All the commonly occurring fungi, except *Candida,* can cause adrenal insufficiency.[7–10] Histoplasmosis is the most frequently occurring. The adrenal glands are involved in more than one-third of persons who die of histoplasmosis. This fungus is endemic in the Piedmont plateau of the Middle Atlantic states and in the Ohio and Tennessee Valley regions of the Mississippi watershed. The gross and microscopic anatomic findings in adrenal glands infected with fungi are similar to those seen in tuberculosis.

Rare causes of adrenal insufficiency include amyloidosis,[11] adrenal hemorrhage[12] (which is especially common during sepsis and anticoagulation), congenital adrenal hypoplasia,[13] and two demyelinating disorders—*adrenoleukodystrophy,* or Brown-Schilder disease, and *adrenomyeloneuropathy,* or sudanophilic leukodystrophy.[14–16] The demyelinating diseases are similar in that they have an X-linked inheritance pattern (and, hence, are diseases of males) and markedly increased plasma C-26 fatty acid concentrations that are thought to reflect the biochemical abnormality responsible for the disorders. Both disorders can be diagnosed by showing an increased plasma concentration of C-26 fatty acids and by demonstrating the pathognomonic, multilamellated inclusion bodies in the steroidogenic cells of the adrenal glands and testes. The two diseases differ in that adrenoleukodystrophy, a disorder of childhood, is dominated by a central neuropathy featuring cortical blindness and coma. Adrenomyeloneuropathy, a disorder of young adults, is dominated by an ascending mixed motor and sensory neuropathy culminating in spastic paraparesis.[16a] Two rare causes of primary adrenal insufficiency include heparin-induced thrombosis and adrenal insufficiency associated with the antiphospholipid antibody syndrome.[17,18]

Metastatic cancer often is cited as a cause of adrenal insufficiency. Although the adrenal glands are a common site of metastasis, these lesions uncommonly result in adrenal insufficiency.[19] When adrenal insufficiency does occur in association with malignancy, the malignancy usually is an infiltrative neoplasm, such as lymphoma or leukemia, although metastatic carcinoma of the lung or breast are occasional offenders.

Finally, the acquired immunodeficiency syndrome has an association with adrenal insufficiency (see Chap. 213). Whether this is the result of a direct effect of the virus on the adrenal glands or of a secondary superinfection (i.e., *Cryptococcus, Mycobacterium* sp., or cytomegalovirus) remains unresolved.[20–22]

## SECONDARY ADRENAL INSUFFICIENCY

Secondary adrenal insufficiency has three causes: adrenal suppression after exogenous glucocorticoid or ACTH administration, adrenal suppression after the correction of endogenous glucocorticoid hypersecretion, and abnormalities of the hypothalamus or pituitary gland leading to ACTH deficiency.

The histologic appearance of the adrenal glands in secondary adrenal insufficiency varies from normal-appearing to simple atrophy of the cortex with a normal medulla.

Adrenal suppression by exogenous glucocorticoids is the most common cause of secondary adrenal insufficiency.[23–25] The frequent use of glucocorticoids to treat inflammatory disorders, such as dermatitis, arthritis, and hepatitis, is the underlying reason. Supraphysiologic doses of glucocorticoids given long enough suppress hypothalamic corticotropin-releasing hormone production and the ability of the anterior pituitary gland to respond to this hormone. The degree of adrenal suppression depends on three variables: dosage, schedule of administration, and duration of administration. Significant adrenal suppression is rarely seen with dosages of hydrocortisone (or its equivalent) of $<15$ mg/m$^2$ per day. A divided dosage schedule is more suppressive than is a once-a-day or once-every-other-day schedule. Finally, the longer the duration of administration, the greater the likelihood of suppression. Treatment periods of $<14$ days, for example, rarely lead to clinically important adrenal suppression, whereas treatment periods long enough to allow the emergence of the signs of Cushing syndrome usually are associated with clinically significant suppression of adrenal function. Secondary adrenal insufficiency can become manifest shortly after the cessation of corticosteroid therapy or months later in a stressful setting such as after an injury or a surgical procedure. The duration of impairment can be as long as 1 year after the correction of hypercortisolism.[26] These findings have led to the conservative practice of replacing glucocorticoid before an anticipated stress in any patient who has received supraphysiologic dosages of glucocorticoids within the past year. An alternative, and more satisfactory, practice is to test the functional capacity of the adrenal glands directly with ACTH and to base the need for glucocorticoid supplementation on the results (see Chap. 78 for an extensive discussion of exogenous corticosteroid administration and its complications).[27]

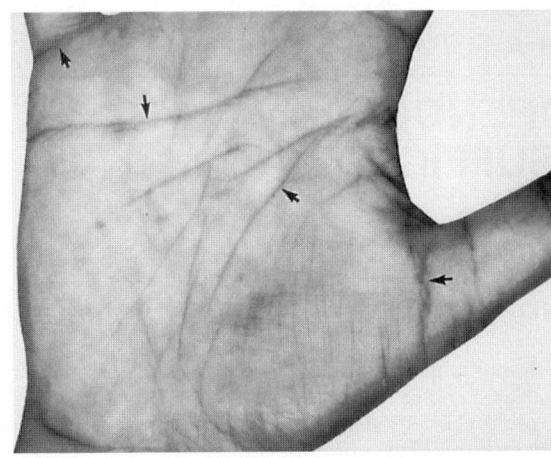

**FIGURE 76-1.** An example of the increased skin pigmentation most characteristic of chronic primary adrenal insufficiency, with accentuation in the creases of the fingers and palms (*arrows*).

Any lesion of the hypothalamus or pituitary gland can lead to secondary adrenal insufficiency; examples include space-occupying lesions such as craniopharyngioma,[28] pituitary adenoma,[29] metastases from distant malignancies,[30] sarcoidosis,[31] and infections with fungi (*Nocardia, Actinomyces*) or the tubercle bacillus.[32] Trauma to the stalk or its blood supply also can lead to adrenal insufficiency.[33] A deficiency of ACTH in the absence of any of these underlying causes is rare (see Chaps. 11 and 17).

## SYMPTOMS AND SIGNS

The symptoms and signs of primary and secondary adrenal insufficiency can be categorized as related to the *chronic* and *acute* syndromes.[34] Symptoms of the chronic syndrome include weakness, fatigue, anorexia, nausea, abdominal pain, and diarrhea. An occasional patient, particularly one with primary adrenal insufficiency, complains of orthostatic dizziness and, rarely, syncope. Signs include weight loss and, particularly in primary insufficiency, orthostatic hypotension. Symptoms and signs specific to primary adrenal insufficiency include salt craving and pigmentation of the skin and mucous membranes (Figs. 76-1 through 76-3). Vitiligo and alopecia also can occur in the autoimmune form of primary adrenal insufficiency.[35] Radiologic findings include large, often calcified, glands in patients with an infectious cause.[20]

The symptoms of the acute syndrome include muscle, joint, and abdominal pain, and postural hypotension. Associated signs include fever, hypotension, and clouded sensorium. The patient may appear dehydrated. No hyperpigmentation is seen in acute primary adrenal insufficiency, unless the acute insufficiency is superimposed on a prior chronic condition.

## LABORATORY FINDINGS

The complete blood count can show a normocytic, normochromic anemia; neutropenia and eosinophilia (rarely $>10\%$); and a relative lymphocytosis. Common chemical abnormalities include metabolic acidosis and prerenal azotemia. If the patient has not been eating, hypoglycemia can occur. Hyponatremia is found in 90% of patients with chronic primary adrenal insufficiency. Hyperkalemia occurs in 65%.[36] Hypercalcemia occurs, but is rare[37] (see Chap. 59).

The electrolyte abnormalities differ in primary and secondary adrenal insufficiency. The pattern of electrolyte alterations in primary adrenal insufficiency usually is dominated by deficient mineralocorticoid activity, leading to hyponatremia and hyperkalemia. The electrolyte abnormalities in secondary adre-

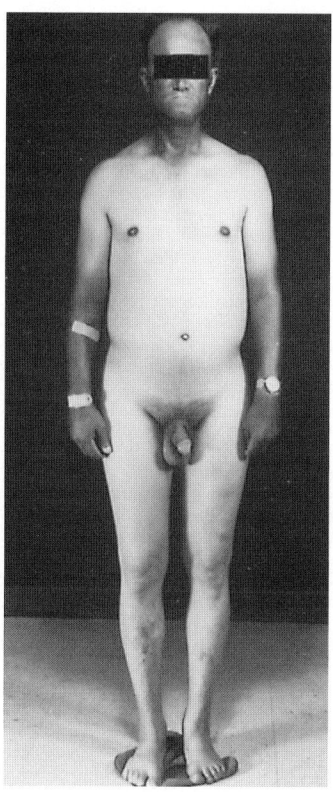

**FIGURE 76-2.** Patient with autoimmune adrenal insufficiency. Note the darkening of sun-exposed areas of the face, neck, and arms; the dark nipples; and the darkened scars of the pretibial region. Other common sites of pigmentation in this disease are areas of pressure or irritation, such as the elbows, knees, and knuckles.

nal insufficiency generally are dominated by water retention caused by increased vasopressin secretion, leading to a generalized hemodilution. Potassium concentrations are normal.[38]

## DIAGNOSIS

The diagnosis of adrenal insufficiency requires the presence of both clinical and chemical abnormalities compatible with the known manifestations of the disorder.

### ACUTE ADRENAL INSUFFICIENCY

Acute adrenal insufficiency should be suspected when hypotension occurs in a patient with chronic adrenal insufficiency or in association with any of the known causes of adre-

nal insufficiency (see Table 76-1). When it is suspected, a blood sample should be drawn immediately for the measurement of plasma cortisol. Because plasma cortisol concentrations range between 20 and 120 μg/dL during severe stress or shock in patients with normal adrenal function, a plasma cortisol concentration of <20 μg/dL favors a diagnosis of adrenal insufficiency. Treatment should not wait for the result but should be initiated as soon as the blood sample for cortisol has been obtained. Initial treatment should consist of the intravenous administration of 100 mg of hydrocortisone in association with steps to maintain blood pressure. Hydrocortisone, 100 mg every 6 hours, should be administered until the crisis is past or the diagnosis is excluded. Steps designed to establish a definitive diagnosis should be instituted immediately.

### CHRONIC ADRENAL INSUFFICIENCY

When chronic adrenal insufficiency is suspected, or when the diagnosis of acute adrenal insufficiency is being confirmed, ACTH should be given as a screening test. Synthetic ACTH (Cortrosyn), 250 μg, is given as an intravenous injection over 1 minute. Blood is drawn at 45 and 60 minutes for the measurement of cortisol.[39] The lower limit of the normal response range is 20 μg/dL. (Note that the results of this test may be normal in patients with adrenal insufficiency that immediately follows the removal of an exogenous or endogenous ACTH source[40]; see Chap. 74.)

Two tests are useful for the differential diagnosis of chronic adrenal insufficiency: the measurement of plasma ACTH[41] and computed tomography (CT) of the adrenal glands. High levels of plasma ACTH imply primary adrenal insufficiency; normal or low levels suggest secondary adrenal insufficiency.[42] A finding of large adrenal glands by CT implies primary disease.[43]

Aldosterone deficiency also points to primary adrenal disease. This can be diagnosed best by testing the ability of the patient to retain salt.[44] On a diet with 10 mEq of sodium, normal persons come into balance in 3 days. To the extent that a patient fails to achieve this balance, salt supplementation or fludrocortisone treatment is required (see Chap. 78). An elevated resting plasma renin level also is a rough guide to mineralocorticoid deficiency. Patients who appear to have secondary adrenal insufficiency without an obvious cause, such as exogenous glucocorticoid or ACTH administration, must undergo careful examination of the pituitary gland and hypothalamus by CT scanning or magnetic resonance imaging to exclude space-occupying lesions of these organs.

## TREATMENT

The treatment of adrenal insufficiency consists of replacing the missing hormones.[45] The treatment of an adrenal crisis theoretically would require administration of ~200 mg of hydrocorti-

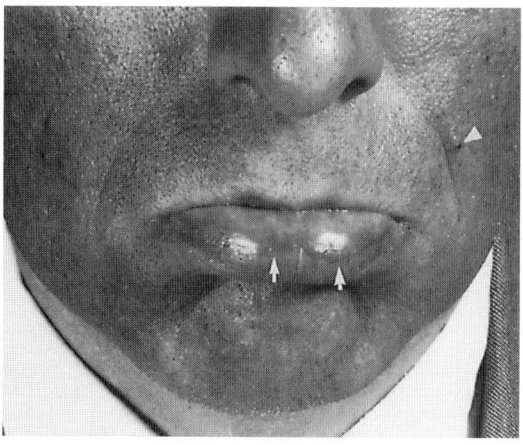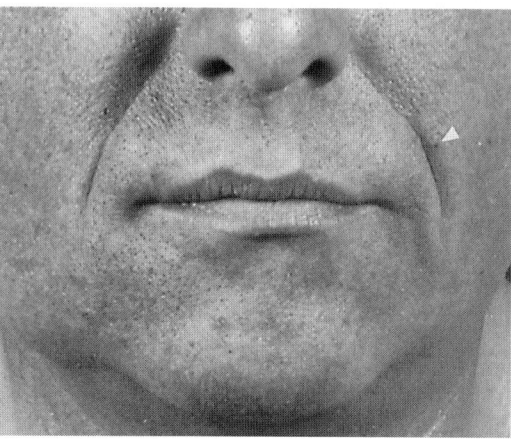

**FIGURE 76-3.** Patient with tuberculous Addison disease before (*left*) and 2 years after (*right*) commencement of cortisol therapy. The hyperpigmentation of the face and lips has disappeared. Note the lightening of the freckle (*arrowhead*).

sone daily. The standard regimen used in most centers provides 400 mg per day intravenously, approximately twice the amount calculated to be necessary. The basal production rate of cortisol has been thought to be 12 to 15 mg/m$^2$ per day. Some studies have challenged this, however, suggesting that the production rate of cortisol may be lower by as much as half. Nevertheless, replacement of cortisol at the rate of 12 to 15 mg/m$^2$ per day provides an adequate amount of bioactive cortisol at the cellular level. Although current practice favors a split dose of cortisol, the frequency of administration often can be reduced to once a day. In the author's experience, compliance is enhanced by a once-a-day regimen.

The current standard of practice also recommends an increase in the rate of cortisol administration during stress. The definition of *stress* is vague, but conservative criteria include fever >38°C (100°F), surgical procedures or injuries, and gastroenteritis with associated vomiting and diarrhea. Some studies question the need for increased cortisol during such periods; until this is firmly demonstrated in humans, however, current guidelines should be followed.[46] The generally accepted guideline is that the daily dose of glucocorticoid should be doubled during periods of *minor* stress such as low-grade fever, vomiting, and diarrhea. In such circumstances, if the patient is not eating, the corticosteroid must be given parenterally. During periods of *major* stress, such as intraabdominal surgical procedures or major trauma, the dosage of hydrocortisone should be increased to 200 mg per day. Once the stress has passed, usually by the second postoperative day, the dosage of glucocorticoid is reduced immediately and directly to the usual daily rate of 12 to 15 mg/m$^2$ (see Chap. 78). The measurement of serum cortisol, serum ACTH, or urinary free cortisol, or of Porter-Silber chromogens is not a reliable guide to the appropriate maintenance dosage of glucocorticoid. Normal serum electrolyte levels, a good appetite, and the patient's feeling of well-being are the best guides to adequate replacement. The appearance of the signs of Cushing syndrome, such as hypertension, weight gain, facial rounding, or supraclavicular puffiness, indicate overtreatment. Overtreatment also may result in diminished bone density.[47]

The production rate of aldosterone is ~100 µg per day at all stages of life in salt-replete humans.[48] Fludrocortisone is roughly equipotent with aldosterone but is available only as an oral preparation. In normal persons, mineralocorticoid activity is supplied by both aldosterone and cortisol in roughly equal proportions. Thus, if cortisol is used for replacement, fludrocortisone, 100 µg per day, will supply the remaining complement of mineralocorticoid activity. If the glucocorticoid preparation used does not have significant mineralocorticoid activity (i.e., prednisone or dexamethasone, which are not recommended for replacement therapy), the dosage of fludrocortisone should be doubled. The serum potassium level is the best guide to the adequacy of mineralocorticoid replacement.

## REFERENCES

1. O'Donnell WM. Changing pathogenesis of Addison's disease. Arch Intern Med 1950; 86:266.
2. Loriaux DL. The polyendocrine deficiency syndromes. N Engl J Med 1985; 312:1568.
3. Neufeld M, MacLaren N, Blizzard R. Autoimmune polyglandular syndromes. Pediatr Ann 1980; 9:154.
4. Vibo R, Aavik E, Peterson P, et al. Autoantibodies to cytochrome P450 enzymes P450 sec, P450 c17, and P450 c21 in autoimmune polyglandular disease types I and II and in isolated Addison's disease. J Clin Endocrinol Metab 1994; 78:323.
5. Eisenbarth G, Wilson P, Ward F, Lebovitz HE. HLA type and occurrence of disease in familial polyglandular failure. N Engl J Med 1978; 298:92.
6. Irvine WJ, Barnes EW. Adrenocortical insufficiency. J Clin Endocrinol Metab 1972; 1:549.
7. Crispell KR, Parson W, Hamlin J. Addison's disease associated with histoplasmosis. Am J Med 1956; 20:23.
8. Eberle DE, Evans RB, Johnson RH. Disseminated North American blastomycosis: occurrence with clinical manifestations of adrenal insufficiency. JAMA 1977; 238:2629.
9. Rawson AJ, Collins LH, Grant JL. Histoplasmosis and torulosis as causes of adrenal insufficiency. Am J Med Sci 1948; 215:363.
10. Forbus WD, Beilerbreurtje AM. Coccidioidomycosis: a study of 95 cases of the disseminated type with special reference to the pathogenesis of the disease. Mil Surg 1946; 99:653.
11. Irvine WJ, Toft AD, Feede CM. Addison's disease. In: James VHT, ed. The adrenal gland. New York: Raven Press, 1979:131.
12. O'Connell TX, Aston SJ. Acute adrenal hemorrhage complicating anticoagulant therapy. Surg Gynecol Obstet 1974; 139:355.
13. Sperling MW, Wolfsen AR, Fisher DA. Congenital adrenal hypoplasia: an isolated defect of organogenesis. J Pediatr 1973; 82:444.
14. Schaumberg H, Powers JW, Raine CS. Adrenoleukodystrophy: a clinical and pathological study of 17 cases. Arch Neurol 1975; 32:577.
15. Griffen JW, Goren E, Schaumberg H, et al. Adrenomyeloneuropathy: a probable variant of adrenoleucodystrophy. Neurology 1977; 27:1107.
16. Blevins LS Jr, Shankroff J, Moser HW, Ladanson PW. Elevated plasma adrenocorticotropin concentration as evidence of limited adrenocortical reserve in patients with adrenomyeloneuropathy. J Clin Endocrinol Metab 1994; 78:261.
16a. Powers JM, DeCiero DP, Ito M, et al. Adrenomyeloneuropathy: a neuropathologic review featuring its noninflammatory myelopathy. J Neuropathol Exp Neurol 2000; 59:89.
17. Bleasd JF, et al. Acute adrenal insufficiency secondary to heparin-induced thrombocytopenia-thrombosis syndrome. Med J Aust 1952; 157:192.
18. Caron P, Chabannier MH, Cambus JP, et al. Definitive adrenal insufficiency due to bilateral adrenal hemorrhage and primary anti-phospholipid syndrome. J Clin Endocrinol Metab 1998; 83:1437.
19. Sheeler LR, Myers JM, Eversham JJ, Taylor HC. Adrenal insufficiency secondary to carcinoma metastatic to the adrenal gland. Cancer 1983; 52:1312.
20. Tapper ML, Rotterdam HZ, Lerner CW, et al. Adrenal necrosis in the acquired immunodeficiency syndrome. Ann Intern Med 1984; 100:239.
21. Greene LW, Cole W, Green JB. Adrenal insufficiency as a complication of the acquired immunodeficiency syndrome. Ann Intern Med 1984; 101:497.
22. Aron DC. Endocrine complications of the acquired immunodeficiency syndrome. Arch Intern Med 1989; 149:330.
23. Danowski TS, Bonessi JV, Sabek G. Probabilities of pituitary-adrenal responsiveness after steroid therapy. Ann Intern Med 1964; 101:11.
24. Plager JE, Cushman P. Suppression of the pituitary ACTH response in man by administration of ACTH or cortisol. J Clin Endocrinol Metab 1962; 22:147.
25. Jasani MK, Boyle TA, Dick WC, et al. Corticosteroid-induced hypothalamo-pituitary-adrenal axis suppression: prospective study using two regimens of corticosteroid therapy. Ann Rheum Dis 1968; 27:352.
26. Graber AL, Ney RL, Nicholson WE. Natural history of pituitary-adrenal recovery following long term suppression with corticosteroids. J Clin Endocrinol Metab 1965; 25:11.
27. Kehlet H, Binder C. Value of an ACTH test in assessing hypothalamic-pituitary-adrenocortical function in glucocorticoid treated patients. BMJ 1973; 2:147.
28. Banna M. Craniopharyngioma: a review article based on 160 cases. Br J Radiol 1976; 49:206.
29. Hankinson T, Banna M. Pituitary and parapituitary tumors. London: WB Saunders, 1976:51.
30. Vita JA, Silverberg SJ, Goland RS, et al. Clinical clues to the cause of Addison's disease. Am J Med 1985; 78:461.
31. Stuart CA, Neelon FA, Lebovitz HE. Hypothalamic insufficiency: the cause of hypopituitarism in sarcoidosis. Ann Intern Med 1978; 88:589.
32. Tandon PN, Pathak SN. Tuberculosis of the central nervous system. In: Tropical neurology. London: Oxford University Press, 1973:37.
33. Ortega FJV, Longridge NS. Fracture of the sella turcica. Injury 1975; 6:335.
34. Thorn GW. Diagnosis and treatment of adrenal insufficiency. Springfield, IL: Charles C Thomas, 1951.
35. Hertz KC, Gazze LA, Kirkpatrick CH, Katz SI. Autoimmune vitiligo: detection of antibodies to melanin producing cells. N Engl J Med 1977; 297:634.
36. Lipsett MB, Pearson OH. Pathophysiology and treatment of adrenal crises. N Engl J Med 1956; 254:511.
37. Jorgensen H. Hypercalcemia in adrenocortical insufficiency. Acta Med Scand 1973; 193:175.
38. Pearson OH, Whitmore WF, West CD. Clinical and metabolic studies of bilateral adrenalectomy for advanced cancer in man. Surgery 1953; 34:543.
39. Lindholm J, Kehlet H, Blichert-Toft M. Reliability of the 30 minute ACTH test in assessing hypothalamic-pituitary-adrenal function. J Clin Endocrinol Metab 1978; 47:272.
40. Kehlet H, Lindholm J, Bjerre P. Value of the 30 min ACTH test in assessing hypothalamic-pituitary-adrenocortical function after pituitary surgery in Cushing's disease. Clin Endocrinol (Oxf) 1984; 20:349.
41. Oelkers W, Diederich S, Bahr V. Diagnosis and therapy surveillance in Addison's disease: rapid adrenocorticotropin (ACTH) test and measurement of plasma ACTH, renin activity and aldosterone. J Clin Endocrinol Metab 1992; 75:259.
42. Schulte HM, Chrousos GP, Avgerinos P. The corticotropin-releasing hormone stimulation test: a possible aid in the evaluation of patients with adrenal insufficiency. J Clin Endocrinol Metab 1984; 58:1064.
43. Schultz CL, Haaga JR, Fletcher BD. Magnetic resonance imaging of the adrenal glands: a comparison with computed tomography. Am J Radiol 1984; 143:1235.
44. Gill JR, Bell NH, Barrter FL. Impaired conservation of sodium and potassium in renal tubular acidosis. Clin Sci 1967; 33:577.
45. Thorn GW, Lauler DP. Clinical therapeutics of adrenal disorders. Am J Med 1977; 53:673.

46. Symreng T, Karlberg BE, Kagedal B, Schlidt B. Physiological cortisol substitution of long term steroid-treated patients undergoing major surgery. Br J Anaesth 1981; 53:949.

47. Zelissen PM, Croughs RJ, van Rijk PP, Raymakers JA. Effect of glucocorticoid replacement therapy on bone mineral density in patients with Addison's disease. Ann Intern Med 1994; 120:207.

48. New MI, Seaman MP, Peterson RE. A method for the simultaneous determination of the secretion rates of cortisol, 11-deoxycortisol, corticosterone, 11-deoxycorticosterone, and aldosterone. J Clin Endocrinol Metab 1969; 29:514.

# CHAPTER 77

# CONGENITAL ADRENAL HYPERPLASIA

PHYLLIS W. SPEISER

Congenital adrenal hyperplasia (CAH) is a group of inherited diseases caused by defective activity in one of five enzymes that contribute to the synthesis of cortisol from cholesterol in the adrenal cortex (Fig. 77-1). Details of normal adrenal steroidogenesis are discussed in detail in Chapter 72. The term *adrenal hyperplasia* derives from the tendency to glandular enlargement under the influence of adrenocorticotropic hormone (ACTH) in an effort to compensate for inadequate cortisol synthesis. The alternate term *adrenogenital syndrome* refers to the common associated finding of ambiguous external genitalia due to incidental deficiency or excess production of adrenal androgens. Each particular enzyme deficiency produces characteristic alterations in the ratio of precursor hormone to product hormones. These hormonal imbalances are accompanied by clinically evident abnormalities, including abnormal development of the genitalia and pseudohermaphroditism, disturbances in sodium and potassium homeostasis, blood pressure dysregulation, and abnormal somatic growth[1,2,2a] (Table 77-1). The molecular genetic basis for all but one of the enzymatic deficiencies is known; disease-causing mutations have been identified for the genes encoding the respective steroidogenic enzymes.

The most prevalent form of CAH is caused by deficiency of the cytochrome P450 enzyme, 21-hydroxylase (>90% of cases), followed by a deficiency of 11β-hydroxylase, 17α-hydroxylase/17,20-lyase, and 3β-hydroxysteroid dehydrogenase. No mutations have been identified in the gene encoding cholesterol desmolase (also termed *side-chain cleavage*); this apparent enzyme deficiency is instead explained by defective steroidogenic acute regulatory protein. Deficiency of the enzymes that do not impair cortisol synthesis do not come under the rubric of CAH and are therefore not discussed here. In addition to a classic form with onset in prenatal life, nonclassic forms of the enzyme deficiencies with onset in childhood or young adult life are also described.

## EMBRYOLOGY

The fetal gonads remain undifferentiated until about the seventh week of gestation (see Chap. 90). At that time, in normal 46,XY fetuses, the gene encoding the sex-determining factor of the Y chromosome (i.e., *SRY*) is transcribed and testicular differentiation begins. *SRY* initiates a complex cascade of events[3] in which other genes are inhibited (e.g., *DAX-1*, important in ovarian determination) or activated (e.g., *SOX9* and *SF-1*, important in Sertoli cell differentiation and indirectly involved in ovarian inhibition via antimüllerian hormone, AMH). Testosterone secretion begins by ~8 weeks of fetal life. In normal 46,XX fetuses, the absence of high local concentrations of AMH allows differentiation of the ovaries, beginning at ~10 weeks' gestation (see Chap. 90).

The internal genital duct structures are recognizable by 7 weeks. Müllerian ducts develop into the rostral third of the vagina, the uterus, and fallopian tubes. Wolffian ducts develop into epididymis, vas deferens, seminal vesicles, and ejaculatory ducts under the influence of adequate local quantities of androgen. Embryonal development of the gonads and internal ducts are generally unaffected by vagaries in sex steroid hormone synthesis.

In females, the development of the external genitals is passive. The urogenital sinus differentiates into separate urethral and vaginal orifices in normal females, and the labioscrotal folds remain separated by the labia minora, which hood the clitoris. In males, under the influence of high circulating levels of androgen, the urethral and genital orifices fuse to form an elongated penile urethra, and the labioscrotal folds fuse to form the scrotum. The latter changes may also occur in 46,XX fetuses exposed to high androgen levels from fetal adrenal or maternal sources. Conversely, male external genitals may be hypoplastic if a defect exists in testosterone synthesis or action.

At ~7 weeks of gestation, the adrenal cortex differentiates from mesodermal tissues. Soon after, two adrenal zones form: a small peripheral adult cortex and a large inner fetal cortex. Steroid production by the fetal cortex begins in the latter half of the first trimester. Adrenal mass increases markedly during this time, and peaks at 15 weeks.[4] General regulation of adrenal growth early in gestation is incompletely understood and is thought to be only partly attributable to ACTH. Other likely trophic hormones include transforming growth factor-β

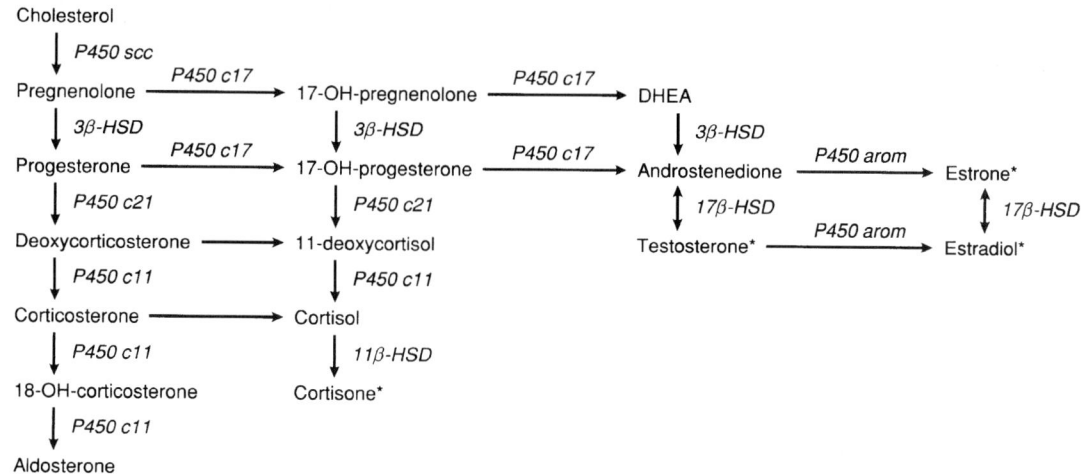

FIGURE 77-1. The pathways of corticosteroid synthesis are diagrammed. Cholesterol is converted in several steps to aldosterone, cortisol, or sex steroids. Hormones marked by an asterisk (*) are produced largely outside the adrenal cortex. Deficiency of a given enzyme causes accumulation of hormonal precursors and a deficiency of products. (*DHEA*, dehydroepiandrosterone; *HSD*, hydroxysteroid dehydrogenase.)

**TABLE 77-1.**
**Clinical, Biochemical, and Genetic Characteristics of Congenital Adrenal Hyperplasia**

| Characteristic | P450c21 Enzyme | P450c21 Enzyme | P450c11 Enzyme | P450c17 Enzyme | 3β-HSD Enzyme | 3β-HSD Enzyme | P450scc Enzyme |
|---|---|---|---|---|---|---|---|
| Deficient phenotype | Classic | Nonclassic | Classic | Classic | Classic | Nonclassic | Classic |
| Ambiguous genitalia | + in 46,XX | | + in 46,XX | + in 46,XY<br>− Puberty in ♀ | + in 46,XY<br>Mild in 46,XX | | + |
| Addisonian crisis | + in SW | | Rare | | + | | ++ (lethal) |
| Incidence (gen. pop.) | 1:14,000 | 1:100 | 1:100,000 | ~120 cases | ? | Common (?) | Rare |
| Hormones | | | | | | | |
|   Glucocorticoids | ↓ | nl | ↓ | ↓ | ↓ | nl | ↓ |
|   Mineralocorticoids | ↓ in SW | nl | ↑ | ↑ | ↓ often | nl | ↓ |
|   Androgens | ↑↑ prenatally | ↑ postnatally | ↑↑ prenatally | ↓ | ↓ in ♂<br>Weak androgens | ↑ in ♀ | ↓ |
|   Estrogens | Relative deficiency in ♀ | Relative deficiency in ♀ | Relative deficiency in ♀ | ↓ | ↓ | ↓ | ↓ |
| Physiology | | | | | | | |
|   Blood pressure | ↓ untreated | nl | ↑ often | ↑ often | ↓ | nl | ↓ |
|   Na balance | ↓ in SW | nl | ↑ | ↑ | ↓ often | nl | ↓ |
|   K balance | ↑ in SW | nl | ↓ | ↓ | ↑ often | nl | ↑ |
|   Acidosis | + in SW | | ± alkalosis | ± alkalosis | + if SW | | + |
| Diagnosis | | | | | | | |
|   Metabolite ↑ | ++++ 17OHP | + 17OHP | DOC, S | DOC, B | DHEA, 17Δ⁵Preg | | None |
|   Common mutations | SW: del; nt 656 A→G<br>SV: I172N | V281L | R448H, frame shifts | Term, frame shifts | Term, frame shifts | | StAR gene defect |

*P450c*, cytochrome P450; *HSD*, hydroxysteroid dehydrogenase; +, present; ?, unknown; ↓, diminished quantity; ↑, increased quantity; ♂, male; ♀, female; *SW*, salt-water; *nl*, normal; *17OHP*, 17-hydroxyprogesterone; *DOC*, deoxycorticosterone; *S*, 11-deoxycortisol; *B*, corticosterone; *DHEA*, dehydroepiandrosterone; *17D⁵Preg*, 17-D⁵-pregnenolone; *del*, deletion; *nt*, nucleotide number; *V281L*, mutation at valine 281 resulting in leucine substitution; *R448H*, mutation at arginine 448 resulting in histidine substitution; *Term*, termination mutation; *StAR*, steroidogenic acute regulatory protein; *SV*, simple virilizer; *I172N*, mutation at isoleucine 172 resulting in asparagine substitution.

(TGF-β), basic fibroblast growth factor (bFGF), and insulin-like growth factor-II (IGF-II).[5] Beyond 20 weeks of gestation, adrenal growth and steroidogenesis are almost exclusively responsive to ACTH. In utero administration of glucocorticoids suppresses fetal ACTH and, under most circumstances, inhibits adventitious adrenal steroid production in fetuses affected with a severe virilizing form of CAH (e.g., 21- or 11β-hydroxylase deficiency).

## CLINICAL FEATURES

### 21-HYDROXYLASE (P450C21) DEFICIENCY

Patients with this commonly diagnosed enzyme deficiency cannot adequately synthesize cortisol. Insufficient cortisol synthesis results in overproduction of adrenal androgens, which are synthesized independently of 21-hydroxylase. Androgens induce somatic growth with inappropriately rapid advancement of linear growth, early epiphyseal fusion of the long bones, and short stature. Other features include precocious development of sexual hair, apocrine body odor, and penile or clitoral enlargement. Reduced fertility may be observed in both sexes. Clinical features are outlined in Table 77-1.

Females affected with the severe classic form of 21-hydroxylase deficiency are exposed to excess androgens prenatally and are born with masculinized external genitalia (Fig. 77-2). If the disease goes undiagnosed and the infant is untreated, further virilization ensues (Fig. 77-3). Approximately 75% of patients with the classic form cannot synthesize aldosterone efficiently because of impaired 21-hydroxylation of progesterone; these *salt-wasting* individuals fail to conserve sodium normally and usually come to medical attention in the neonatal period with hyponatremia, hyperkalemia, and hypovolemic shock. These adrenal crises may prove fatal if proper medical care is not delivered. Patients with sufficient

aldosterone production and no salt wasting who have signs of prenatal virilization and markedly increased production of hormonal precursors of 21-hydroxylase (e.g., 17-hydroxyprogesterone) are referred to as *simple virilizers*. Earlier confusion regarding the origins of these two classic phenotypes has been resolved to a large extent by the understanding of the molecular genetics of the disease, and allelic variation in the gene encoding active 21-hydroxylase (*CYP21*) appears to be responsible for most phenotypic variation, as is discussed later.

Patients affected with the milder, nonclassic form of 21-hydroxylase deficiency may have signs of postnatal androgen excess.[6] Except for rare cases showing mild clitoromegaly,

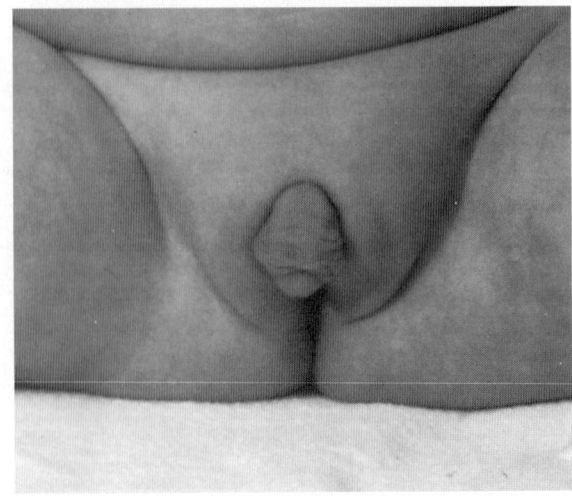

**FIGURE 77-2.** External genitalia of a 2-month-old female infant with 21-hydroxylase deficiency.

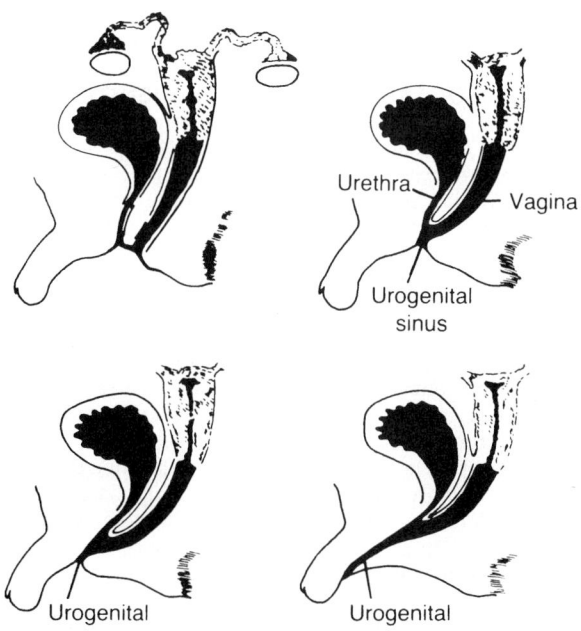

**FIGURE 77-3.** Variations in the differentiation of the external genitalia in congenital adrenal hyperplasia. In genetic females, adrenal androgen hypersecretion (enzymes 2, 4, and 5) is associated with various degrees of masculinization, leading to apparent male external genitalia. (From Grumbach MM, Ducharme J. The effects of androgens on fetal development: androgen-induced female pseudohermaphroditism. Fertil Steril 1960; 11:157.)

females with the nonclassic disorder are born with normal external genitalia. The syndrome of polycystic ovarian disease has often been confused with nonclassic CAH 21-hydroxylase deficiency in young women with hirsutism, oligomenorrhea, and diminished fertility. Precise clinical distinction between the classic simple virilizing disease and nonclassic disorder is sometimes difficult among males, because the hormonal reference standards for diagnosis represent a continuum. Moreover, because males do not manifest ambiguous genitalia as a sign of in utero androgen excess, the only other distinguishing clinical parameters are bone age and somatic growth pattern, which are nonpathognomonic. Phenotypic severity in nonclassic 21-hydroxylase deficiency varies greatly, and in some individuals the disease has been detected solely on the basis of hormonal or genetic testing in the course of family studies. Aldosterone synthesis is normal in patients with nonclassic 21-hydroxylase deficiency. Table 77-2 describes features distinguishing salt-wasting, simple virilizing, and nonclassic forms of 21-hydroxylase deficiency. Table 77-3 describes specific mutations.

Neonatal screening for 21-hydroxylase deficiency measuring 17-hydroxyprogesterone levels in heel-stick blood has been

**TABLE 77-2.**
**Phenotype in 21-Hydroxylase Deficiency**

| Characteristic | Salt Wasting | Simple Virilizing | Nonclassic Form |
|---|---|---|---|
| Age at diagnosis | Infancy | Infancy (females) or childhood (males) | Childhood or adulthood |
| Aldosterone | Low | Normal | Normal |
| Virilization | Severe to moderate | Moderate to severe | None to mild |
| Mutation | Severe | Moderate (severe + moderate) | Mild (mild to moderate, mild + severe) |

**TABLE 77-3.**
**Most Common Disease-Causing Mutations in *CYP21***

| Designation | Site | Percentage of Normal Enzyme Activity |
|---|---|---|
| **GROUP A: NO ENZYME ACTIVITY** | | |
| Deletion | Exons 1 to 8 | 0 |
| Deletion of 8 base pairs | Exon 3 | 0 |
| Cluster: Ile-236→Asn | Exon 6 | 0 |
| Val-237→Glu | | |
| Met-239→Lys | | |
| Insert T Phe-306 | Exon 7 | 0 |
| Gln-318→term | Exon 8 | 0 |
| Arg-356→Trp | Exon 8 | 0 |
| nt 656 A→G | Intron 2 | ? amount residual activity |
| **GROUP B: SEVERELY REDUCED ENZYME ACTIVITY** | | |
| Ile-172→Asn | Exon 4 | 2 |
| **GROUP C: MODERATELY REDUCED ENZYME ACTIVITY** | | |
| Pro-30→Leu | Exon 1 | 30–60 |
| Val-281→Leu | Exon 7 | 20–50 |

?, indeterminate amount of residual activity; *term*, termination mutation; *nt*, nucleotide number.

effective in reducing neonatal morbidity and mortality.[7] This has been particularly useful in males with salt-wasting disease in whom no obvious phenotypic clue to the diagnosis, such as ambiguous genitalia, is present. The radioimmunoassay of heel-stick blood on filter paper was first used on a wide scale among the Alaskan Yupik Eskimos, one of two geographically isolated and genetically homogeneous groups at high risk for 21-hydroxylase deficiency CAH.[8] Subsequently, many other newborn screening programs were developed for 21-hydroxylase deficiency CAH.[9,9a] The worldwide incidence of 21-hydroxylase deficiency CAH based on newborn screening is 1 in 14,554 live births; approximately 75% of infants in whom the disease is detected in these programs manifest the salt-wasting phenotype.[9] According to the Hardy-Weinberg law for populations at equilibrium, the heterozygote frequency for all classic 21-hydroxylase gene defects is 1 in 61 persons.

A high frequency of nonclassic 21-hydroxylase deficiency has also been discerned.[10] This disorder occurs most frequently among Ashkenazi Jews (1 in 27), but it is also common among other ethnic groups, such as Hispanics, residents of the former Yugoslavia, and Italians. Overall, in a mixed white population, the disease is estimated to occur in ~1 in 100 individuals. These disease frequencies were derived indirectly based on response to ACTH stimulation combined with HLA typing. Confirmation was obtained using the statistical method of commingling distributions.[11] Nonclassic 21-hydroxylase deficiency is among the most frequent autosomal recessive disorders in humans. Clinical investigation to diagnose nonclassic 21-hydroxylase deficiency is warranted in any patient showing the signs of androgen excess described previously; particularly high-risk groups include Ashkenazi Jews, children with precocious pubarche, and girls or women with hirsutism and oligomenorrhea.

## 11β-HYDROXYLASE (P450C11) DEFICIENCY

As in the case of 21-hydroxylase deficiency, in patients with 11β-hydroxylase deficiency accumulating precursor steroids are channeled into androgen pathways beginning in prenatal life, which causes genital ambiguity in affected newborn females. Male infants show no abnormality of external genitalia. Later signs of androgen excess are observed in both sexes affected with 11β-hydroxylase deficiency if the disease is not promptly recognized and treated.[12] Patients with 11β-hydroxylase deficiency account for approximately 5% of all CAH cases. Although in the general population this enzyme defect is found in ~1 in 100,000 live births, the disease frequency is ~1 in 5000 to 7000 among Jews of Moroccan descent.[13] No systematic screening programs have been initiated to detect forms of CAH other than 21-hydroxylase deficiency. Nonclassic variants of 11β-hydroxylase deficiency have also been described.[12]

Hormonal imbalances differentiate 21-hydroxylase from 11β-hydroxylase deficiency. In most cases, classic 21-hydroxylase deficiency is accompanied by deficient aldosterone synthesis and limited ability to conserve sodium. In contrast, in patients with 11β-hydroxylase deficiency, excessive production of the mineralocorticoid agonist deoxycorticosterone (DOC) or its metabolites results in sodium retention, hypokalemia, volume expansion, suppressed plasma renin activity (PRA), and hypertension. Hypertension, however, is not the sine qua non for diagnosis of 11β-hydroxylase deficiency and is often absent in young children. Nonclassic cases may show variable elevations of DOC and 11β-deoxycortisol (compound S) and have normal PRA levels.

## 17α-HYDROXYLASE/17,20-LYASE (P450C17) DEFICIENCY

In 17α-hydroxylase/17,20-lyase deficiency, impaired production of glucocorticoids and sex steroids ($C_{19}/C_{18}$ compounds) causes failure to develop estrogenic sexual characteristics at puberty in genetic females and incomplete development of the external genitals in genetic males.[14,15] Shunting of P450c17 precursor steroids into the 17-deoxy pathway produces mineralocorticoid excess, with hypokalemic alkalosis and hypertension similar to that in the 11β-hydroxylase deficiency. In rare cases, selective 17,20-lyase deficiency is detected. In such patients, cortisol and DOC levels are normal, but adrenal and gonadal $C_{21}$ to $C_{19}$ steroid conversion is impaired, so that normal sex steroid production is prevented.

More than 120 cases have been reported of severe or complete 17α-hydroxylase deficiency, mostly in combination with 17,20-lyase deficiency.[16] Patients from Canadian-Dutch Mennonite kindreds who share the same genotype have been reported.[17] Relatively few genetic females have been detected. Partial deficiency of this enzymatic activity may be found in males with ambiguous genitalia.[18]

## 3β-HYDROXYSTEROID DEHYDROGENASE DEFICIENCY

The enzyme 3β-hydroxysteroid dehydrogenase (3β-HSD) is responsible for conversion of $\Delta^5$ to $\Delta^4$ steroids. Deficiency of this enzyme results in inefficient cortisol synthesis; oversecretion of dehydroepiandrosterone (DHEA), which is only weakly androgenic; and oversecretion of pregnenolone, which is ineffective as a mineralocorticoid. Affected individuals typically have cortisol insufficiency and salt wasting. Genital ambiguity is also part of the syndrome. Although lack of potent androgens produces hypospadias in males, high levels of DHEA may cause clitoromegaly without urogenital sinus formation in females.[19] In 3β-HSD and 17α-hydroxylase/17,20-lyase deficiencies, potent androgens are deficient in prenatal life, which predisposes males to gynecomastia. The precise frequency of severe defects in the adrenal 3β-HSD gene is unknown.

A nonclassic form of 3β-HSD deficiency is diagnosed with variable frequency in children with precocious pubarche and females with hirsutism and oligomenorrhea,[20,21] but the hormonal profile with ACTH stimulation is less robust a diagnostic tool than that described for 21-hydroxylase deficiency. Some investigators have suggested that ovarian hyperandrogenism may be confused with 3β-HSD deficiency.[22] The physician must also exercise caution in the interpretation of ACTH stimulation tests performed in infants younger than 1 year of age, because 3β-HSD is normally deficient in fetal life and relatively inactive in early infancy. Molecular genetic investigation has not revealed mutations to explain cases of mild 3β-HSD deficiency. No marked vari-

ations in the ethnic incidence of this defect are known; several classic cases have been identified in consanguineous families.

## 20,22-DESMOLASE (P450SCC) DEFICIENCY

Deficiency of 20,22-desmolase is also called *lipoid adrenal hyperplasia* or *apparent cholesterol desmolase deficiency*. This enzyme catalyzes the initial reaction for all steroid production from cholesterol substrate. Apparent deficiency of side-chain cleavage or cholesterol desmolase is extremely rare, with only ~30 cases reported in the world's literature.[23,24] Complete cholesterol desmolase deficiency would be expected to produce global adrenocortical insufficiency and death because of marked cortisol deficiency and severe salt wasting. Partial apparent defects in this enzyme result in pseudohermaphroditism in genetic males; lack of secondary sexual characteristics can be expected in genetic females. A single case report describes long-term follow-up of a patient diagnosed in the newborn period and successfully treated for 18 years.[25] Apparent cholesterol desmolase deficiency seems to occur with less severity and somewhat more frequently among the Japanese. Lipoid adrenal hyperplasia is now known to result from genetic defects in the gene encoding steroidogenic acute regulatory protein, rather than from actual defects in cholesterol desmolase.[25a]

## DIAGNOSIS

### POSTNATAL DIAGNOSIS

The diagnosis of 21-hydroxylase deficiency may be confirmed by administering an intravenous bolus of ACTH and measuring the resultant elevation in blood levels of 17-hydroxyprogesterone.[26] Usually, a panel of adrenal hormones is assayed before and after ACTH administration, but the most specific available marker for which testing is commercially available is 17-hydroxyprogesterone. Clinicians should be aware that cortisol stimulation is suboptimal after ACTH infusion in patients with severe defects in adrenal steroid synthesis. If for any reason blood testing cannot be used or radioimmunoassays for 17-hydroxyprogesterone are unavailable, the examiner can measure 17-ketosteroids or pregnanetriol in a 24-hour urine collection. The latter steroid is the principal direct urinary metabolite of 17-hydroxyprogesterone.

Ancillary tests used in the initial evaluation of infants with ambiguous genitalia include karyotype analysis, pelvic and abdominal ultrasonography, and sonogram of the urogenital orifices using radiopaque dyes.

Patients with nonclassic 21-hydroxylase deficiency have 17-hydroxyprogesterone levels that exceed those seen in heterozygous carriers of an affected gene, but these levels are lower than those of patients with the classic form of the disorder.[26] In the nonstimulated state, these patients may have near-normal serum hormone levels. A serum 17-hydroxyprogesterone level below 200 ng/dL effectively excludes this diagnosis if the sample is obtained in the early morning (i.e., by 8:00 a.m.).

The diagnosis of 11β-hydroxylase deficiency is made by the measurement of elevated basal or ACTH-stimulated DOC and/or 11-deoxycortisol (i.e., compound S) in the serum or elevated levels of the tetrahydro-compounds (i.e., DOC and/or S) in a 24-hour urine collection.[27] Another marker useful in pediatric diagnosis is 6α-hydroxytetrahydro-11-deoxycortisol, which can be measured by gas chromatography and mass spectrometry of urine.[28] As in 21-hydroxylase deficiency, urinary 17-ketosteroids are usually elevated, reflecting increased shunting of 11β-hydroxylase hormonal precursors into the sex steroid pathway. PRA is usually low in older children and is accompanied by low levels of aldosterone.

The diagnosis of 17α-hydroxylase/17,20-lyase deficiency is made by a finding of marked elevations of serum DOC and corticosterone (i.e., compound B) and the metabolites of these two steroids.[14] Aldosterone is often low secondary to suppression of renin by excess DOC, as in the case of 11β-hydroxylase deficiency. The 17α-hydroxylase-deficient patients do not experience adrenal crisis despite inadequate cortisol synthesis. Overproduction of corticosterone provides adequate physiologic response to stress. Plasma ACTH levels are less elevated than in other conditions of impaired cortisol production. Gonadotropin production is extremely elevated in both sexes because of the absence of any sex steroid feedback; the gonads are atrophic.

A high ratio of $\Delta^5$ to $\Delta^4$ steroids characterizes the 3β-HSD deficiency.[29] Serum levels of 17-hydroxypregnenolone and DHEA are elevated before and after ACTH stimulation. Increased excretion of the $\Delta^5$ metabolites pregnanetriol and 16-pregnanetriol in the urine is also diagnostic for this enzyme disorder.

## PRENATAL DIAGNOSIS

Prenatal testing for 21-hydroxylase deficiency has been used for two decades in pregnancies known to be at risk.[30,31] Hormonal diagnosis is accomplished by finding elevated levels of 17-hydroxyprogesterone or 21-deoxycortisol in amniotic fluid.[32,33] Genetic diagnosis was first performed by identifying HLA markers on fetal cells cultured from the amniotic fluid; the genes encoding HLA antigens are closely linked to CYP21.[34,35] Problems encountered with these diagnostic techniques included false-negative 17-hydroxyprogesterone levels in non–salt-losing cases and intra-HLA recombination.[36] Early amniocentesis and chorionic villus sampling have permitted diagnostic studies to be performed at the end of the first trimester.[37,38] DNA obtained from such procedures may be analyzed by molecular genetic techniques, such as allele-specific hybridization with oligonucleotide probes for the normal and mutant alleles of CYP21.[39,40]

In pregnancies known to have a 25% risk for 21-hydroxylase deficiency, "blind" prenatal treatment of the fetus may be initiated by administering dexamethasone to the mother beginning in the first trimester.[41–43] Deferral of therapy until a molecular genetic diagnosis is known could hamper the ability to prevent genital ambiguity.[44] Although prenatal treatment usually ameliorates virilization of affected females, results of prenatal treatment have not been completely successful in this regard.[45,46] Failure to produce normal female genitalia in 20% to 25%[47] of affected girls through the use of prenatal dexamethasone therapy has been attributed to cessation of therapy in midgestation, to noncompliance, or to suboptimal dosing. Some treatment failures had no ready explanation.[48]

No fetus treated with low-dose dexamethasone has been born with a congenital malformation specifically attributable to dexamethasone therapy.[49] The incidence of fetal deaths in treated pregnancies does not exceed that for the general population. Complications observed in a rodent model of in utero exposure to high-dose glucocorticoids included cleft palate, placental degeneration, intrauterine growth retardation, and unexplained fetal death.[50] Other concerns for human fetal exposure have been raised based on observations of relatively late sequelae involving neurologic and vascular changes in lower mammals.[51] Although at present no data exist to suggest that such sequelae occur in humans, the oldest prenatally treated children from CAH studies are only now reaching adolescence, and more long-term follow-up is required.

The incidence of maternal complications has varied among investigations. Serious side effects, such as overt Cushing syndrome, massive weight gain, and hypertension, have been reported in ~1% of all treated pregnant women.

Caution must be exercised in recommending prenatal therapy with dexamethasone, and women must be fully informed of these potential risks and nonuniformity of beneficial outcome to the affected female fetus. Despite these caveats, many parents of affected girls still choose prenatal medical treatment because of the severe psychological impact of ambiguous genitalia.

A similar diagnostic and therapeutic approach is effective in cases of 11β-hydroxylase deficiency, in which affected female fetuses are also at risk for prenatal virilization.

## TREATMENT

Patients with simple virilizing or salt-wasting classic 21-hydroxylase deficiency or those with 11β-hydroxylase, 17α-hydroxylase/17,20-lyase, and 3β-HSD deficiencies, as well as select symptomatic patients with nonclassic forms of these diseases, are treated with daily oral hydrocortisone or similar drugs. Treatment with glucocorticoids suppresses excessive secretion of ACTH, correcting the adrenal hormone imbalance. Patients with the salt-wasting form of CAH require additional supplementation with mineralocorticoids (e.g., fludrocortisone acetate [Florinef], 50–200 µg per day) and sodium chloride supplements (1 to 2 g/10 kg body weight). Older children and adults with simple virilizing disease who are treated adequately with glucocorticoids usually do not have a clinically apparent deficiency of aldosterone, nor is renin markedly elevated. Many pediatric endocrinologists empirically treat all CAH patients with fludrocortisone and sodium chloride despite the lack of signs of salt wasting. Prudence dictates following PRA in all patients as an index of the need for mineralocorticoid and salt supplements. Caution is advised to avoid development of hypertension consequent to excessive or unnecessary treatment with the latter regimen.

Glucocorticoid treatment also leads to reduction of mineralocorticoid hormones in 11β-hydroxylase and 17α-hydroxylase deficiency, with amelioration of hypertension. In cases of long-standing hypertension, adjunctive antihypertensive drugs may be required to completely normalize blood pressure.

The usual mode of treatment for CAH in childhood is with two to three divided daily doses of hydrocortisone totaling 10 to 20 mg/m$^2$ per day (average dosage ~15 mg/m$^2$ per day). Even this relatively low dosage may be supraphysiologic, because healthy children and adolescents secrete an average of ~7 µg/m$^2$ of cortisol daily.[52,53] Experience indicates that once-daily doses of hydrocortisone, because of its relatively rapid metabolism, is therapeutically suboptimal over the long term.

Treatment efficacy should be monitored with frequent measurements of serum 17-hydroxyprogesterone (good control is indicated by a level of <1000 ng/dL), androstenedione, and testosterone, in addition to PRA in young children,[54] and assessment of growth, skeletal maturation, and pubertal status.

If the response to maintenance hydrocortisone at the standard dosage is poor despite good medical compliance, a 2- to 4-day trial of dexamethasone (in a dosage of ~20–30 µg/kg per day to a maximum of 2 mg per day) may be more effective in suppressing the adrenal. Maintenance hydrocortisone may then be resumed, and adrenal hormone levels are monitored. If epiphyses are fused and linear growth is not at risk, the maintenance regimen may be changed to one of the longer-acting glucocorticoids, prednisone or dexamethasone. The greater potency of these drugs means that slight dosing errors may result in iatrogenic Cushing syndrome and growth retardation in children. Life-threatening stress, severe illness, or surgery demand parenteral therapy with high doses of hydrocortisone in any patient who is undergoing chronic treatment with exogenous glucocorticoids.

Clinical trials have been initiated in classic CAH using androgen-receptor blockers and inhibitors of steroid synthesis in conjunction with glucocorticoids to ameliorate virilization and to prevent iatrogenic glucocorticoid-induced growth retardation.[55] Preliminary results appear promising, but more data are required.[56] Compliance with multidrug regimens may be difficult for many patients. Another potentially useful adjunct to standard therapy is the gonadotropin-releasing hormone analogs, which serve to delay the onset of gonadarche.

Adrenalectomy has been performed in a limited number of severely affected patients refractory to adrenocortical suppression with standard medical therapies.[57] This approach remains experimental, and such patients must obviously be treated with lifelong physiologic replacement dosages of glucocorticoid and mineralocorticoid.

The suggestion has been made that androgen-receptor blockade may be preferable to glucocorticoids as primary treatment of mild 21-hydroxylase deficiency.[58] Therapeutic trials of the latter treatment have been prompted by the observation that, although menses usually resume regularity within 2 to 6 months after initiation of glucocorticoid therapy in young women with nonclassic 21-hydroxylase deficiency, hirsutism is quite refractory to this mode of treatment.

Surgical therapy is recommended in cases of ambiguous genitalia. Most often, this involves clitoroplasty and vaginoplasty in virilized females. Improved surgical techniques now permit these procedures to be performed in a single-stage operation by experienced urologists.[59]

Given the recognition of disturbed gender identity and role among young women with CAH, providing early and continuing psychological counseling for them is extremely important.[60,61] With improved medical, surgical, and psychological treatments, an improved psychosexual outcome can be achieved.

# GENETICS

The autosomal recessive mode of inheritance of adrenal steroidogenic defects was recognized in the early 1950s.[62–64] The linkage of 21-hydroxylase deficiency to the HLA complex on chromosome arm 6p was discovered in the late 1970s,[65] and by the mid-1980s, further molecular genetic details had been unravelled.[66] Other human adrenal steroidogenic defects also have been successfully subjected to molecular genetic analysis.

## 21-HYDROXYLASE DEFICIENCY

The *CYP21* (*CYP21B*) structural gene encoding steroid 21-hydroxylase and a pseudogene (CYP21P or CYP21A) are located 30 kilobases (kb) apart in the HLA complex on chromosome band 6p21.3.[67,68] Although the two genes are 98% identical in nucleotide sequence, CYP21P has accumulated a number of mutations that render any gene product completely inactive. These include an 8-base-pair (bp) deletion in exon 3, a frame shift in exon 7, and a nonsense mutation in exon 8.

Most mutations causing 21-hydroxylase deficiency are caused by apparent recombinations between *CYP21* and CYP21P. Approximately 20% of these are unequal meiotic crossovers resulting in a deletion of a 30-kb DNA segment that includes the 3' end of the pseudogene and the greater portion of the active gene.[69] This deleted haplotype is incapable of producing any active enzyme. About 80% of mutations result from apparent gene conversions that transfer small segments containing one or more deleterious mutations from CYP21P to *CYP21*. The most common of these, accounting for an additional ~25% of mutant haplotypes, is a single A→G transition at nucleotide 656 that causes abnormal pre–messenger RNA (mRNA) splicing. Less commonly found are missense mutations, which cause changes in the protein's amino-acid sequence.

Several large studies have examined the prevalence of individual mutations in an attempt to correlate specific mutations with particular clinical manifestations of the disease.[70–74] These correlations are most reliably made in individuals who are homozygous or hemizygous (the other chromosome carries a deletion) for each mutation. Table 77-3 illustrates the mutations commonly found in classic and nonclassic forms of 21-hydroxylase deficiency, grouped into three categories according to the predicted level of enzymatic activity based on in vitro mutagenesis and expression.[75–78] Group A, with total ablation of enzyme activity, is most

often associated with salt-wasting disease; group B, with 2% normal activity, consists predominantly of patients with simple virilizing disease; and group C, with 20% to 60% of normal activity, is most often associated with the nonclassic disorder.

These studies suggest that mutant *CYP21* enzymes carrying discrete amino-acid substitutions identified in CAH patients exhibit in vivo activities that are generally consistent with in vitro predictions, and correlate with disease severity. Exceptions to this rule include patients with moderate or severe mutations and relatively mild disease. Because aldosterone is normally secreted at a rate 100 to 1000 times lower than that of cortisol, residual enzyme activity as low as 0.6% of normal activity, as seen in the Ile-172→Asn nonconservative substitution, allows enough aldosterone synthesis to prevent symptoms of salt wasting, resulting in the simple virilizing phenotype. Factors outside the *CYP21* locus may also influence development of the salt-wasting phenotype.

Another point of interest in phenotype-genotype analysis is the wide range of clinical manifestations in patients carrying the group C nonclassic mutations (e.g., Val-281→Leu and Pro-30→Leu). These mutations are expected to reduce enzyme activity to 20% to 60% of normal, with 17-hydroxyprogesterone being the preferred substrate. An individual heterozygous for a deletion of *CYP21* (i.e., ablation of all enzyme activity derived from one chromosome) is also expected to have ~50% of normal 21-hydroxylase activity, but such individuals have no signs of disease and have hormonal abnormalities detectable only with ACTH stimulation. This suggests that in vivo 21-hydroxylase activity in patients with nonclassic 21-hydroxylase deficiency is often <50% of normal. One plausible explanation for such differences in clinical manifestations of disease is fluctuating intraadrenal concentrations of progesterone, which at physiologic levels (2–4 μmol/L)[79] acts as a competitive inhibitor of the nonclassic mutant enzyme for its main substrate, 17-hydroxyprogesterone. Individuals carrying two nonclassic alleles may have closer to 20% net 21-hydroxylase activity as intraadrenal progesterone concentration increases. Other factors contributing to phenotypic variability might include pseudosubstrate inhibition of other steroidogenic enzymes by accumulated precursors of 21-hydroxylase. Study of naturally occurring mutations has also shed light on structure-function relationships for the 21-hydroxylase enzyme; for example, G291s is important for catalytic activity, and E196 deletion and R483P reduce enzyme half-life.[80]

## 11β-HYDROXYLASE DEFICIENCY

Two human genes on chromosome band 8q21-q22 encode 11-hydroxylase (CYP11B) isozymes with predicted amino-acid sequences that are 93% identical.[81,82] Each has 9 exons spaced over ~7 kb. *CYP11B1*, expressed at high levels in normal adrenal glands, is regulated by ACTH.[81,83] *CYP11B2*, not readily detectable in Northern blots using normal adrenal RNA, is regulated primarily by angiotensin II, rather than by ACTH.[81] Transcripts of *CYP11B2* have been detected by hybridization to RNA from an aldosterone-secreting tumor or in normal adrenal mRNA by the more sensitive technique of reverse transcription coupled with the polymerase chain reaction.[84,85]

Defects in the *CYP11B1* gene result in virilizing, hypertensive CAH, and defects in *CYP11B2* cause a rare salt-wasting disease known as corticosterone methyl oxidase II (CMO II) deficiency. A third disease, glucocorticoid-suppressible aldosteronism, ensues when the regulatory region of *CYP11B1* is transposed to a position at which it controls synthesis of *CYP11B2*, promoting glucocorticoid-suppressible and ACTH-stimulable aldosterone synthesis.[86]

Mutations in the *CYP11B1* gene tend to cluster in exons 6, 7, and 8.[87] The most common genetic alteration in Moroccan Jews with 11β-hydroxylase deficiency is Arg-448→His.[88] When introduced into *CYP11B1* complementary DNA and expressed in cultured cells, this mutation abolishes normal enzymatic activity and is therefore consistent with the classic, severe virilizing phenotype observed in these patients. Blood pressure was not uniformly elevated in all patients carrying this mutation, and as observed in 21-hydroxylase deficiency, apparently other factors exist that modify phenotype. Numerous other genetic defects in 11β-hydroxylase–deficient patients from other ethnic backgrounds have been described, including insertions and nonsense, missense, and splice mutations.[89–94] Mild missense mutations have been identified in some patients with nonclassic 11β-hydroxylase deficiency.[95]

## 17α-HYDROXYLASE/17,20-LYASE DEFICIENCY

The P450c17 structural gene (*CYP17*) spans 12.6 kb on chromosome 10,[96] with an intron-exon organization similar to that of *CYP21*. The same gene is expressed in both the adrenal and the testis.[97] Molecular characterization of specific mutations in *CYP17* have been reported in a number of patients.[16] In patients with classic, severe 17α-hydroxylase and 17,20-lyase deficiencies, these have included a point mutation creating a termination codon in the first exon, a 7-bp duplication in exon 2 that produces a frame shift, and a four-base duplication in exon 8. Homozygous deletion of 3 bp in exon 1 was detected in a patient with apparent selective compromise of 17,20-lyase activity, a phenotypic female with sexual infantilism. A genetic male with ambiguous genitalia was found to be a compound heterozygote with a termination codon introduced by a single base substitution in exon 4 on one chromosome and a nonconservative proline→threonine substitution in exon 6 on the second chromosome. Another patient with male pseudohermaphroditism was a compound heterozygote for two null mutations, including a splice mutation deleting exon 2.[98]

## 3β-HYDROXYSTEROID DEHYDROGENASE DEFICIENCY

Two homologous genes encoding 3β-HSD type I, expressed in placenta and skin, and type II, expressed in adrenal and gonads, have been identified on chromosome band 1p13.[99–102] This is the only enzyme discussed here that is not encoded by a gene in the cytochrome P450 superfamily. Type II gene mutations have been described in patients with classic 3β-HSD deficiency.[102a] These include two separate point mutations introducing termination codons in exon 4, insertion of a single base causing a frame shift, and two separate amino-acid substitutions in highly conserved portions of the protein.[103–105] Mutations have not been detected in either the type I or II gene to explain mild or nonclassic 3β-HSD deficiency.[106] Thus, the latter syndromes appear to be attributable to other causes, perhaps not genetic.

## CHOLESTEROL DESMOLASE DEFICIENCY

The *CYP11A* gene encoding cholesterol desmolase encompasses 20 kb on chromosome 15.[107] Mutations in this gene have not been identified in patients with lipoid adrenal hyperplasia,[108] although in vitro studies suggest that the 20α-hydroxylase function is deficient in at least one patient with the syndrome. Mutations affecting another cellular component fundamental to early steroidogenesis, steroidogenic acute regulatory proteins (StAR), are responsible for this syndrome.[109]

## OTHER GENETIC DISORDERS RELATED TO CONGENITAL ADRENAL HYPERPLASIA

Several other disorders involve adrenal steroid-synthesizing enzymes. Strictly speaking, the CMO deficiencies and other enzyme defects discussed below are not included among the adrenal hyperplasias, because they do not affect cortisol synthesis and cause no disturbance of the hypothalamic–pituitary–adrenal axis. A distal block in aldosterone synthesis results from defects in the *CYP11B2* gene encoding 18-hydroxylase (CMO I) and 18-oxidase (CMO II) and causes rare forms of recessively inherited salt wasting with hypotension and failure to thrive in infancy. The biochemical profile in cases of CMO II deficiency is notable for low levels of aldosterone, with high PRA, and high serum corticosterone and 18-hydroxycorticosterone. The latter steroid is found in low levels in cases of CMO I deficiency.[110] Affected individuals are often clinically asymptomatic in later life.

Defects in the *CYP19* gene encoding cytochrome P450 aromatase (P450arom) prevent the normal synthesis of estrogens and create a relative abundance of androgens. Such defects have been identified as a novel cause of ambiguous genitalia in 46,XX neonates, of primary amenorrhea with hypergonadotropic hypogonadism in adolescent girls, or of virilism in the setting of polycystic ovaries in young women.[111,112] In men the defect results in continued linear bone growth beyond puberty, delayed bone age, and failure of epiphyseal closure, findings which prove that estrogens are critical for epiphyseal fusion. These symptoms are alleviated by estrogen administration.[113]

Classic deficiency of 17-ketosteroid reductase (i.e., 17β-hydroxysteroid dehydrogenase) is a cause of ambiguous genitalia in 46,XY neonates, who have a tendency to virilize at puberty, probably by means of extragonadal 17β-HSD activity and enhanced 5α-reductase activity.[114,115] Mild forms of this enzyme deficiency exist in young men with gynecomastia and in women with hirsutism and polycystic ovaries.[116,117] Specific defects in the gene *HSD17B3* encoding gonadal 17β-HSD have been identified in subjects with classic deficiency of this enzyme.[118,119] The typical hormonal profile shows a markedly elevated ratio of androstenedione to testosterone.

Other rare inherited disorders of steroidogenesis, such as glucocorticoid-suppressible hyperaldosteronism (i.e., glucocorticoid-remediable aldosteronism or dexamethasone-suppressible hyperaldosteronism), a regulatory defect of the *CYP11B2* gene,[120] and apparent mineralocorticoid excess, a defect in the renal isozyme 11-hydroxysteroid dehydrogenase, are discussed in Chapter 80.

## CONCLUSION

The adrenal hyperplasias have been extensively studied from the clinical and molecular genetic perspectives. The molecular bases for the various forms of CAH have been identified. Severe mutations in the genes encoding steroidogenic enzymes, such as deletions, frame shifts, and nonsense codons, result in gene products with no enzymatic activity. In contrast, milder mutations, such as conservative or nonconservative substitutions, may cause a lesser degree of enzyme impairment. The catalytic activity of such gene products may be differently affected for each of two different substrates. Interindividual variation also may occur in individuals with similar genotypes. Two apparent enzyme deficiencies, nonclassic 3β-HSD deficiency and cholesterol desmolase/lipoid CAH, are not due to defects in the structural genes encoding these respective enzymes.

One practical result of molecular genetic characterization is the ability to perform accurate and early prenatal diagnosis. Current research efforts are focused on achieving regulation of these genes, understanding more about gene and enzyme structure-function relationships, identifying further clinical-genetic correlations, and optimizing treatment.

## REFERENCES

1. New MI, White PC, Pang S, et al. The adrenal hyperplasias. In: Scriver CR, Beaudet AL, Sly WS, Valle D, eds. The metabolic basis of inherited disease, 6th ed. New York: McGraw-Hill, 1989:1881.
2. White PC, New MI, Dupont B. Congenital adrenal hyperplasia. N Engl J Med 1987; 316:1519.
2a. Speiser PW, White PC. Congenital adrenal hyperplasia. Endocr Rev 2000; in press.

3. Swain A, Lovell-Badge R. A molecular approach to sex determination in mammals. Acta Paediatr Suppl 1997; 423:46.

4. Branchaud CL, Murphy BEP. Physiopathology of the fetal adrenal. In: Pasqualini JR, Scholler R, eds. Hormones and fetal pathophysiology. New York: Marcel Dekker, 1992:53.

5. Estivariz FE, Lowry PJ, Jackson S. Control of adrenal growth. In: James VHT, ed. The adrenal gland, 2nd ed. New York: Raven Press, 1992:43.

6. Kohn B, Levine LS, Pollack MS, et al. Late-onset steroid 21-hydroxylase deficiency: a variant of classical congenital adrenal hyperplasia. J Clin Endocrinol Metab 1982; 55:817.

7. Pang S, Hotchkiss J, Drash AL, Levine LS, New MI. Microfilter paper method for 17α-progesterone radioimmunoassay: its application for rapid screening for congenital adrenal hyperplasia. J Clin Endocrinol Metab 1977; 45:1003.

8. Pang S, Murphey W, Levine LS, et al. A pilot newborn screening for congenital adrenal hyperplasia (CAH) in Alaska. Pediatr Res 1981; 15:512.

9. Pang SP, Wallace MA, Hofman L, et al. Worldwide experience in newborn screening for classical congenital adrenal hyperplasia due to 21-hydroxylase deficiency. Pediatrics 1988; 81:866.

9a. Therrell BL Jr, Berenbaum SA, Manter-Kapanke V, et al. Results of screening 1.9 million Texas newborns for 21-hydroxylase-deficient congenital adrenal hyperplasia. Pediatrics 1998; 101(4 Pt 1):583.

10. Speiser PW, Dupont B, Rubinstein P, et al. High frequency of nonclassical steroid 21-hydroxylase deficiency. Am J Hum Genet 1985; 37:650.

11. Sherman SL, Aston CE, Morton NE, et al. A segregation and linkage study of classical and nonclassical 21-hydroxylase deficiency. Am J Hum Genet 1988; 42:830.

12. Zachmann M, Tassinari D, Prader A. Clinical and biochemical variability of congenital adrenal hyperplasia due to 11 beta-hydroxylase deficiency. A study of 25 patients. J Clin Endocrinol Metab 1983; 56:222.

13. Rosler A, Leiberman E, Cohen T. High frequency of congenital adrenal hyperplasia (classic 11 beta-hydroxylase deficiency) among Jews from Morocco. Am J Med Genet 1992; 42:827.

14. Biglieri EG, Herron MA, Brust M. 17-Hydroxylation deficiency in man. J Clin Invest 1966; 45:1946.

15. New MI. Male pseudohermaphroditism due to 17α-hydroxylase deficiency. J Clin Invest 1970; 49:1930.

16. Yanase T, Simpson ER, Waterman MR. 17α-Hydroxylase/17,20-lyase deficiency: from clinical investigation to molecular definition. Endocr Rev 1991; 12:91.

17. Imai T, Toshihiko T, Waterman MR, et al. Canadian Mennonites and individuals residing in the Friesland region of the Netherlands share the same molecular basis of 17α-hydroxylase deficiency. Hum Genet 1992; 89:95.

18. Ahlgren R, Yanase T, Simpson ER, et al. Compound heterozygous mutations (Arg239→stop, Pro342→Thr) in the CYP17 (P45017α) gene lead to ambiguous external genitalia in a male patient with partial combined 17α-hydroxylase deficiency. J Clin Endocrinol Metab 1992; 74:667.

19. Bongiovanni AM. The adrenogenital syndrome with deficiency of 3β-hydroxysteroid dehydrogenase. J Clin Invest 1962; 41:2086.

20. Bongiovanni AM. Acquired adrenal hyperplasia: with special reference to 3β-hydroxysteroid dehydrogenase. Fertil Steril 1981; 35:599.

21. Zerah M, Schram P, New MI. The diagnosis and treatment of nonclassical 3β-HSD deficiency. Endocrinologist 1991; 1:75.

22. Ehrmann DA, Rosenfield RL. Hirsutism—beyond the steroidogenic block. N Engl J Med 1990; 323:909.

23. Prader A, Gurtner HP. Das Syndrom des Pseudohermaphroditismus masculinus bei kongenitaler Nebennierenrinden-Hyperplasie ohne Androgenüberproduktion (adrenaler Pseudoherm masc). Helv Pediatr Acta 1955; 10:397.

24. Prader A, Siebenmann RE. Nebennereninsuffizienz bei kongenitaler Lipoid-hyperplasie der Nebennieren. Helv Pediatr Acta 1957; 12:569.

25. Hauffa BP, Miller WL, Grumbach MM, et al. Congenital adrenal hyperplasia due to deficient cholesterol side-chain cleavage activity (20,22-desmolase) in a patient treated for 18 years. Clin Endocrinol 1985; 23:481.

25a. Stocco DM. The role of the StAR protein in steroidogenesis: challenges for the future. J Endocrinol 2000; 164(3):247.

26. New MI, Lorenzen F, Lerner AJ, et al. Genotyping steroid 21-hydroxylase deficiency: hormonal reference data. J Clin Endocrinol Metab 1983; 57:320.

27. Eberlein WR, Bongiovanni AM. Plasma and urinary corticosteroids in the hypertensive form of congenital adrenal hyperplasia. J Biol Chem 1956; 223:85.

28. Hughes IA, Arisaka O, Perry LA, et al. Early diagnosis of 11-beta-hydroxylase deficiency in two siblings confirmed by analysis of a novel steroid metabolite in newborn urine. Acta Endocrinol (Copenh) 1986; 111:349.

29. Bongiovanni AM. Urinary excretion of pregnanetriol and pregnenetriol in two forms of congenital adrenal hyperplasia. J Clin Invest 1971; 60:2751.

30. Jeffcoate TNA, Fleigner JRH, Russell SH, et al. Diagnosis of the adrenogenital syndrome before birth. Lancet 1965; 2:553.

31. Merkatz IR, New MI, Seaman MP. Prenatal diagnosis of adrenogenital syndrome by amniocentesis. J Pediatr 1969; 75:977.

32. Frasier SD, Thorneycroft IH, Weiss BA, Horton R. Elevated amniotic fluid concentration of 17α-hydroxyprogesterone in congenital adrenal hyperplasia. J Pediatr 1975; 86:310.

33. Gueux B, Fiet J, Couillin P, et al. Prenatal diagnosis of 21-hydroxylase deficiency congenital adrenal hyperplasia by simultaneous radioimmunoassay of 21-deoxycortisol and 17-hydroxyprogesterone in amniotic fluid. J Clin Endocrinol Metab 1988; 66:534.

34. Couillin P, Nicolas H, Boue J, Boue A. HLA typing of amniotic-fluid cells applied to prenatal diagnosis of congenital adrenal hyperplasia. Lancet 1979; 1:1076.

35. Pollack MS, Levine LS, Pang S, et al. Prenatal diagnosis of congenital adrenal hyperplasia (21-hydroxylase deficiency) by HLA typing. Lancet 1979; 1:1107.

36. Pang S, Pollack MS, Loo M, et al. Pitfalls of prenatal diagnosis of 21-hydroxylase deficiency congenital adrenal hyperplasia. J Clin Endocrinol Metab 1985; 61:89.

37. Odink RJH, Boue A, Jansen M. The value of chorion villus sampling in early detection of 21-hydroxylase deficiency. Pediatr Res 1988; 23:131A.

38. Shulman DI, Mueller OT, Gallardo LA, et al. Treatment of congenital adrenal hyperplasia in utero. Pediatr Res 1989; 25:93A.

39. Owerbach D, Draznin MB, Carpenter RJ, Greenberg F. Prenatal diagnosis of 21-hydroxylase deficiency congenital adrenal hyperplasia using the polymerase chain reaction. Hum Genet 1992; 89:109.

40. Speiser PW, White PC, Dupont J, et al. Prenatal diagnosis of congenital adrenal hyperplasia due to 21-hydroxylase deficiency by allele-specific hybridization and Southern blot. Hum Genet 1994; 93:424.

41. David M, Forest MG. Prenatal treatment of congenital adrenal hyperplasia resulting from 21-hydroxylase deficiency. J Pediatr 1984; 105:799.

42. Evans MI, Chrousos GP, Mann DW, et al. Pharmacologic suppression of the fetal adrenal gland in utero. JAMA 1985; 253:1015.

43. Forest MG, Betuel H, David M. Prenatal treatment of congenital adrenal hyperplasia with 21-hydroxylase deficiency: a multicenter study. Ann Endocrinol (Paris) 1987; 48:31.

44. Speiser PW, LaForgia N, Kato K, et al. First trimester prenatal treatment and molecular genetic diagnosis of congenital adrenal hyperplasia (21-hydroxylase deficiency). J Clin Endocrinol Metab 1990; 70:838.

45. Migeon CJ. Comments about the need for prenatal treatment of congenital adrenal hyperplasia due to 21-hydroxylase deficiency. (Editorial). J Clin Endocrinol Metab 1990; 70:836.

46. Prenatal treatment of congenital adrenal hyperplasia. (Editorial). Lancet 1990; 510.

47. Forest MG, Morel Y, David M. Prenatal diagnosis and treatment of congenital adrenal hyperplasia. Horm Res 1997; 48(suppl 2): 22.

48. Pang S, Pollack MS, Marshall RN, Immken L. Prenatal treatment of congenital adrenal hyperplasia due to 21-hydroxylase deficiency. N Engl J Med 1990; 322:111.

49. Lajic S, Wedell A, Bui TH, Ritzen EM, Holst M. Long-term somatic follow-up of prenatally treated children with congenital adrenal hyperplasia. J Clin Endocrinol Metab 1998; 83:3872.

50. Goldman AS, Sharpior BH, Katsumata M. Human foetal palatal corticoid receptors and teratogens for cleft palate. Nature 1978; 272:464.

51. Seckl JR, Miller WL. How safe is long-term prenatal glucocorticoid treatment? JAMA 1997; 277:1077.

52. New MI, Seaman MP. Secretion rates of cortisol and aldosterone in various forms of congenital adrenal hyperplasia. J Clin Endocrinol Metab 1970; 30:361.

53. Linder BL, Esteban NV, Yergey AL, et al. Cortisol production rate in childhood and adolescence. J Pediatr 1990; 117:892.

54. Golden MP, Lippe BM, Kaplan SA, et al. Management of congenital adrenal hyperplasia using serum dehydroepiandrosterone sulfate and 17-hydroxyprogesterone concentrations. Pediatrics 1978; 61:867.

55. Cutler GB Jr, Laue L. Seminars in medicine of the Beth Israel Hospital, Boston: congenital adrenal hyperplasia due to 21-hydroxylase deficiency. N Engl J Med 1990; 323:1806.

56. Merke DP, Keil MF, Jones JV, et al. Flutamide, testolactone, and reduced hydrocortisone dose maintain normal growth velocity and bone maturation despite elevated androgen levels in children with congenital adrenal hyperplasia. J Clin Endocrinol Metab 2000; 85(3):1114.

57. Van Wyk JJ, Gunther DF, Ritzen EM, et al. The use of adrenalectomy as a treatment for congenital adrenal hyperplasia. J Clin Endocrinol Metab 1996; 81:3180.

58. Spritzer P, Billaud L, Thalabard J-C, et al. Cyproterone acetate versus hydrocortisone treatment in late-onset adrenal hyperplasia. J Clin Endocrinol Metab 1990; 70:642.

59. Donahoe PK, Gustafson ML. Early one-stage surgical reconstruction of the extremely high vagina in patients with congenital adrenal hyperplasia. J Pediatr Surg 1994; 29:352.

60. Mulaikal RM, Migeon CJ, Rock JA. Fertility rates in female patients with congenital adrenal hyperplasia due to 21-hydroxylase deficiency. N Engl J Med 1987; 316:178.

61. Kuhnle U, Bollinger M, Schwarz HP, Knorr D. Partnership and sexuality in adult female patients with congenital adrenal hyperplasia. First results of a cross-sectional quality-of-life evaluation. J Steroid Biochem Mol Biol 1993; 45:123.

62. Knudson AG Jr. Mixed adrenal disease of infancy. J Pediatr 1951; 39:408.

63. Bentinck RC, Hinman F Sr, Lisser H, et al. The familial congenital adrenal syndrome: report of two cases and review of the literature. Postgrad Med 1952; 11:301.

64. Childs B, Grumbach MM, Van Wyk JJ. Virilizing adrenal hyperplasia: a genetic and hormonal study. J Clin Invest 1956; 35:213.

65. Dupont B, Oberfield SE, Smithwick EM, et al. Close genetic linkage between HLA and congenital adrenal hyperplasia (21-hydroxylase deficiency). Lancet 1977; 2:1309.

66. White PC, New MI. Genetic basis of endocrine disease, 2: congenital adrenal hyperplasia due to 21-hydroxylase deficiency. J Clin Endocrinol Metab 1992; 74:6.

67. White PC, Grossberger D, Onufer BJ, et al. Two genes encoding steroid 21-hydroxylase are located near the genes encoding the fourth component of complement in man. Proc Natl Acad Sci U S A 1985; 82:1089.

68. Carroll MC, Campbell RD, Porter RR. The mapping of 21-hydroxylase genes adjacent to complement component C4 genes in HLA, the major histocompatibility complex in man. Proc Natl Acad Sci U S A 1985; 82:521.

69. White PC, Vitek A, Dupont B, New MI. Characterization of frequent dele-

tions causing steroid 21-hydroxylase deficiency. Proc Natl Acad Sci U S A 1988; 85:4436.

70. Owerbach D, Crawford YM, Draznin MB. Direct analysis of CYP21B genes in 21-hydroxylase deficiency using polymerase chain reaction amplification. Mol Endocrinol 1990; 4:125.

71. Mornet E, Crete P, Kuttenn F, et al. Distribution of deletions and seven point mutations on CYP21B genes in three clinical forms of steroid 21-hydroxylase deficiency. Am J Hum Genet 1991; 48:79.

72. Higashi Y, Hiromasa T, Tanae A, et al. Effects of individual mutations in the P-450(C21) pseudogene on the P-450(C21) activity and their distribution in the patient genomes of congenital steroid 21-hydroxylase deficiency. J Biochem 1991; 109:638.

73. Speiser PW, Dupont J, Zhu D, et al. Disease expression and molecular genotype in congenital adrenal hyperplasia due to 21-hydroxylase deficiency. J Clin Invest 1992; 90:584.

74. Wedell A, Thilén A, Ritzén EM, et al. Mutational spectrum of the steroid 21-hydroxylase gene in Sweden: implications for genetic diagnosis and association with disease manifestation. J Clin Endocrinol Metab 1994; 78:1145.

75. Higashi Y, Tanae A, Inoue H, et al. Aberrant splicing and missense mutations cause steroid 21-hydroxylase [P-450(C21)] deficiency in humans: possible gene conversion products. Proc Natl Acad Sci U S A 1988; 85:7486.

76. Tusie-Luna MT, Traktman P, White PC. Determination of functional effects of mutations in the steroid 21-hydroxylase gene (CYP21) using recombinant vaccinia virus. J Biol Chem 1990; 265:20916.

77. Tusie-Luna MT, Speiser PW, Dumic M, et al. A mutation (Pro-30 to Leu) in CYP21 represents a potential nonclassic steroid 21-hydroxylase deficiency allele. Mol Endocrinol 1991; 5:685.

78. Higashi Y, Hiromasa T, Tanae A, et al. Effects of individual mutations in the P-450(C21) pseudogene on the P-450(C21) activity and their distribution in the patient genomes of congenital steroid 21-hydroxylase deficiency. J Biochem (Tokyo) 1991; 109:638.

79. Dickerman Z, Grant DR, Faiman C, Winter JSD. Intraadrenal steroid concentrations in man: zonal differences and developmental changes. J Clin Endocrinol Metab 1984; 59:1031.

80. Nikoshkov A, Lajic S, Vlamis-Gardikas A, et al. Naturally occurring mutants of human steroid 21-hydroxylase (P450c21) pinpoint residues important for enzyme activity and stability. J Biol Chem 1998; 273:6163.

81. Mornet E, Dupont J, Vitek A, White PC. Characterization of two genes encoding human steroid 11β-hydroxylase (P-450 11β). J Biol Chem 1989; 264:20961.

82. Chua SC, Szabo P, Vitek A, et al. Cloning of cDNA encoding steroid 11β-hydroxylase (P450c11). Proc Natl Acad Sci U S A 1987; 84:7193.

83. Kawamoto T, Mitsuuchi Y, Toda K, et al. Cloning of cDNA and genomic DNA for human cytochrome P-450₁₁β . FEBS Lett 1990; 269:345.

84. Kawamoto T, Mitsuuchi Y, Ohnishi T, et al. Cloning and expression of a cDNA for human cytochrome P-450aldos as related to primary aldosteronism. Biochem Biophys Res Commun 1990; 173:309.

85. Curnow KM, Tusie-Luna MT, Pascoe L, et al. The product of the CYP11B2 gene is required for aldosterone biosynthesis in the human adrenal cortex. Mol Endocrinol 1991; 5:1513.

86. White PC, Pascoe L, Curnow KM, et al. Molecular biology of 11β-hydroxylase and 11β-hydroxysteroid dehydrogenase enzymes. J Steroid Biochem Mol Biol 1992; 43:827.

87. Curnow KM, Slutsker L, Vitek J, et al. Mutations in the CYP11B1 gene causing congenital adrenal hyperplasia and hypertension cluster in exons 6, 7, and 8. Proc Natl Acad Sci U S A 1993; 90:4552.

88. White PC, Dupont J, New MI, et al. A mutation in CYP11B1 (Arg-448→His) associated with steroid 11β-hydroxylase deficiency in Jews of Moroccan origin. J Clin Invest 1991; 87:1664.

89. Naiki Y, Kawamoto T, Mitsuuchi Y, et al. A nonsense mutation (TGG116TAG[Stop]) in CYP11B1 causes steroid 11β-hydroxylase deficiency. J Clin Endocrinol Metab 1993; 77:1677.

90. Helmberg A, Ausserer B, Kofler R. Frame shift by insertion of 2 basepairs in codon 394 of CYP11B1 causes congenital adrenal hyperplasia due to steroid 11 beta-hydroxylase deficiency. J Clin Endocrinol Metab 1992; 75:1278.

91. Nakagawa Y, Yamada M, Ogawa H, Igarashi Y. Missense mutation in CYP11B1 (CGA[Arg-384]→GGA[Gly]) causes steroid 11 beta-hydroxylase deficiency. Eur J Endocrinol 1995; 132:286.

92. Yang LX, Toda K, Miyahara K, et al. Classic steroid 11 beta-hydroxylase deficiency caused by a C→G transversion in exon 7 of CYP11B1. Biochem Biophys Res Commun 1995; 216:723.

93. Geley S, Kapelari K, Johrer K, et al. CYP11B1 mutations causing congenital adrenal hyperplasia due to 11 beta-hydroxylase deficiency. J Clin Endocrinol Metab 1996; 81:2896.

94. Merke DP, Tajima T, Chhabra A, et al. Novel CYP11B1 mutations in congenital adrenal hyperplasia due to steroid 11 beta-hydroxylase deficiency. J Clin Endocrinol Metab 1998; 83:270.

95. Joehrer K, Geley S, Strasser-Wozak EM, et al. CYP11B1 mutations causing non-classic adrenal hyperplasia due to 11 beta-hydroxylase deficiency. Hum Mol Genet 1997; 6:1829.

96. Matteson KJ, Picado-Leonard J, Chung B-C, et al. Assignment of the gene for adrenal P450c17 (steroid 17α-hydroxylase/17,20-lyase) to human chromosome 10. J Clin Endocrinol Metab 1986; 63:789.

97. Chung B-C, Picado-Leonard J, Haniu M, et al. Cytochrome P450c17 (steroid 17α-hydroxylase/17,20-lyase): cloning of human adrenal and testis cDNAs indicates the same gene is expressed in both tissues. Proc Natl Acad Sci U S A 1987; 84:407.

98. Suzuki Y, Nagashima T, Nomura Y, et al. A new compound heterozygous mutation (W17X, 436 + 5G→T) in the cytochrome P450c17 gene causes 17 alpha-hydroxylase/17,20-lyase deficiency. J Clin Endocrinol Metab 1998; 83:199.

99. Lachance Y, Luu-The V, Labrie C, et al. Characterization of human 3β-hydroxysteroid dehydrogenase/$\Delta^5$-$\Delta^4$ isomerase gene and its expression in mammalian cells. J Biol Chem 1990; 265:20469.

100. Lorence MC, Corbin CJ, Kamimura N, et al. Structural analysis of the gene encoding human 3β-hydroxysteroid dehydrogenase/$\Delta^{5\rightarrow4}$-isomerase. Mol Endocrinol 1990; 4:1850.

101. Lachance Y, Luu-The V, Verreault H, et al. Structure of the human type II 3β-hydroxysteroid dehydrogenase/$\Delta^5$-$\Delta^4$ isomerase (3β-HSD) gene: adrenal and gonadal specificity. DNA Cell Biol 1991; 10:701.

102. Berube D, Luu-The V, Lachance Y, et al. Assignment of the human 3β-HSD gene to the p13 band of chromosome 1. Cytogenet Cell Genet 1989; 52:199.

102a. McCartin S, Russell AJ, Fisher RA, et al. Phenotypic variability and origins of mutations, in the gene encoding 3β-hydroxysteroid dehydrogenase type II. Mol Endocrinol 2000; 24:75.

103. Rheaume E, Simard J, Morel Y, et al. Congenital adrenal hyperplasia due to point mutations in the type II 3β-hydroxysteroid dehydrogenase gene. Nature 1992; 1:239.

104. Chang YT, Kappy MS, Iwamoto K, et al. Mutations in the type II 3 beta-hydroxysteroid dehydrogenase (3 beta-HSD) gene in a patient with classic salt-wasting 3 beta-HSD deficiency congenital adrenal hyperplasia. Pediatr Res 1993; 34:698.

105. Simard J, Rheaume E, Sanchez R, et al. Molecular basis of congenital adrenal hyperplasia due to 3β-hydroxysteroid dehydrogenase deficiency. Mol Endocrinol 1993; 7:716.

106. Sakkal-Alkaddour H, Zhang L, Yang X, et al. Studies of 3 beta-hydroxy-steroid dehydrogenase genes in infants and children manifesting premature pubarche and increased adrenocorticotropin-stimulated delta 5-steroid levels. J Clin Endocrinol Metab 1996; 81:3961.

107. Chung BC, Matteson KJ, Voutilainen R, et al. Human cholesterol side-chain cleavage enzyme, P450scc: cDNA cloning, assignment of the gene to chromosome 15, and expression in the placenta. Proc Natl Acad Sci U S A 1986; 83:8962.

108. Lin D, Gitelman SE, Saenger P, Miller WL. Normal genes for the cholesterol side chain cleavage enzyme, P450ssc, in congenital lipoid adrenal hyperplasia. J Clin Invest 1991; 88:1955.

109. Miller WL. Congenital lipoid adrenal hyperplasia: the human gene knockout for the steroidogenic acute regulatory protein. J Mol Endocrinol 1997; 19:227.

110. Ulick S, Wang JZ, Morton DH. The biochemical phenotypes of two inborn errors in the biosynthesis of aldosterone. J Clin Endocrinol Metab 1992; 74:1415.

111. Harada N, Ogawa H, Shozu M, Yamada K. Genetic studies to characterize the origin of the mutation in placental aromatase deficiency. Am J Hum Genet 1992; 51:666.

112. Ito Y, Fisher CR, Conte FA, et al. Molecular basis of aromatase deficiency in an adult female with sexual infantilism and polycystic ovaries. Proc Natl Acad Sci U S A 1993; 90:11673.

113. Simpson ER, Zhao Y, Agarwal VR, et al. Aromatase expression in health and disease. Recent Prog Horm Res 1997; 52:185.

114. Eckstein B, Cohen S, Farkas A, Rosler A. The nature of the defect in familial male pseudohermaphroditism in Arabs of Gaza. J Clin Endocrinol Metab 1989; 68:477.

115. Rosler A, Belanger A, Labrie F. Mechanisms of androgen production in male pseudohermaphroditism due to 17 beta-hydroxysteroid dehydrogenase deficiency. J Clin Endocrinol Metab 1992; 75:773.

116. Castro-Magana M, Angulo M, Uy J. Male hypogonadism with gynecomastia caused by late-onset deficiency of testicular 17-ketosteroid reductase. N Engl J Med 1993; 328:1297.

117. Pang S, Softness B, Sweeney WJ, New MI. Hirsutism, polycystic ovarian disease, and ovarian 17-ketosteroid reductase deficiency. N Engl J Med 1987; 316:1295.

118. Andersson S, Moghrabi N. Physiology and molecular genetics of 17 beta-hydroxysteroid dehydrogenases. Steroids 1997; 62:143.

119. Moghrabi N, Hughes IA, Dunaif A, Andersson S. Deleterious missense mutations and silent polymorphism in the human 17beta-hydroxysteroid dehydrogenase 3 gene (HSD17B3). J Clin Endocrinol Metab 1998; 83:2855.

120. Nyckoff JA, Seely EW, Hurwitz S, et al. Glucocorticoid-remediable aldosteronism and pregnancy. Hypertension 2000; 35:668.

# CHAPTER 78

# CORTICOSTEROID THERAPY

LLOYD AXELROD

This chapter examines the risks associated with the use of glucocorticoids and of mineralocorticoids for various illnesses, and provides guidelines for the administration of these commonly prescribed substances.

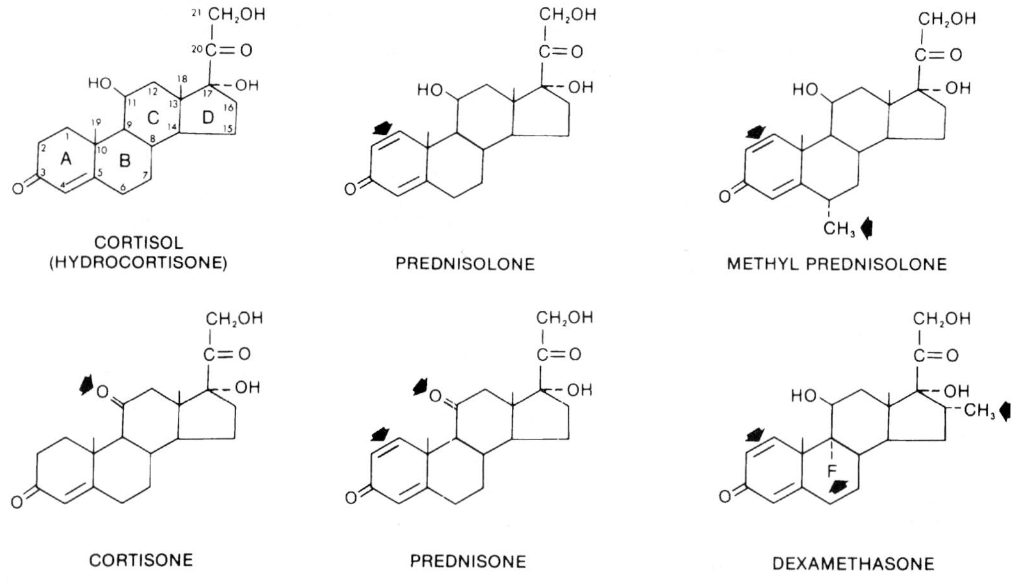

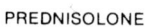

**FIGURE 78-1.** The structures of commonly used glucocorticoids. In the depiction of cortisol, the 21 carbon atoms of the glucocorticoid skeleton are indicated by numbers and the four rings are designated by letters. The *arrows* indicate the structural differences between cortisol and each of the other molecules. (From Axelrod L. Glucocorticoid therapy. Medicine [Baltimore] 1976; 55:39, and Axelrod L. Glucocorticoids. In: Kelley WN, Harris ED Jr, Ruddy S, Sledge CB, eds. Textbook of rheumatology, 4th ed. Philadelphia: WB Saunders, 1993:779.)

# GLUCOCORTICOIDS

## STRUCTURE OF COMMONLY USED GLUCOCORTICOIDS

Figure 78-1 indicates the structures of several commonly used glucocorticoids.[1,2] *Cortisol (hydrocortisone)* is the principal circulating glucocorticoid in humans.

Glucocorticoid activity requires a hydroxyl group at carbon 11 of the steroid molecule. Cortisone and prednisone are 11-keto compounds. Consequently, they lack glucocorticoid activity until they are converted in vivo to cortisol and prednisolone, the corresponding 11-hydroxyl compounds.[3,4] This conversion occurs predominantly in the liver. Thus, topical application of cortisone is ineffective in the treatment of dermatologic diseases that respond to topical application of cortisol.[4] Similarly, the antiinflammatory action of cortisone delivered by intraarticular injection is minimal compared with the effect of cortisol administered in the same manner.[3] Cortisone and prednisone are used only for systemic therapy. All glucocorticoid preparations marketed for topical or local use are 11-hydroxyl compounds, which obviates the need for biotransformation.

## PHARMACODYNAMICS

### HALF-LIFE, POTENCY, AND DURATION OF ACTION

The important differences among the systemically used glucocorticoid compounds are duration of action, relative glucocorticoid potency, and relative mineralocorticoid potency (Table 78-1).[1,2] The commonly used glucocorticoids are classified as *short-acting, intermediate-acting,* and *long-acting* on the basis of the duration of corticotropin (ACTH) suppression after a single dose, equivalent in antiinflammatory activity to 50 mg of prednisone (Table 78-1).[5] The relative potencies of the glucocorticoids correlate with their affinities for the intracellular glucocorticoid receptor.[6] The observed potency of a glucocorticoid, however, is determined not only by the intrinsic biologic potency, but also by the duration of action.[6,7] Consequently, the relative potency of two glucocorticoids varies as a function of the time interval between the administration of the two steroids and the determination of the potency. In particular, failure to account for the duration of action may lead to a marked underestimation of the potency of dexamethasone.[7]

The correlation between the *circulating half-life* ($T_{1/2}$) of a glucocorticoid and its *potency* is weak. The $T_{1/2}$ of cortisol in the circulation is in the range of 80 to 115 minutes.[1] The $T_{1/2}$s of other commonly used agents are cortisone, 0.5 hours; prednisone, 3.4 to 3.8 hours; prednisolone, 2.1 to 3.5 hours; methylprednisolone, 1.3 to 3.1 hours; and dexamethasone 1.8 to 4.7 hours.[1,7,8] Prednisolone and dexamethasone have comparable circulating $T_{1/2}$s, but dexamethasone is clearly more potent. Similarly, the correlation between the circulating $T_{1/2}$ of a glucocorticoid and its *duration of action* is poor. The many actions of glucocorticoids do not have an equal duration, and the duration of action may be a function of the dose.

The duration of ACTH suppression is not simply a function of the level of antiinflammatory activity, because variations in the duration of ACTH suppression are achieved by doses of glucocorticoids with comparable antiinflammatory activity. The duration of ACTH suppression produced by an individual glucocorticoid, however, probably is dose related.[5]

**TABLE 78-1.**
**Commonly Used Glucocorticoids**

| Duration of Action* | Gluco-corticoid Potency† | Equivalent Glucocorticoid Dose (mg) | Mineralo-corticoid Activity |
|---|---|---|---|
| **SHORT-ACTING** | | | |
| Cortisol (hydrocortisone) | 1 | 20 | Yes‡ |
| Cortisone | 0.8 | 25 | Yes‡ |
| Prednisone | 4 | 5 | No |
| Prednisolone | 4 | 5 | No |
| Methylprednisolone | 5 | 4 | No |
| **INTERMEDIATE-ACTING** | | | |
| Triamcinolone | 5 | 4 | No |
| **LONG-ACTING** | | | |
| Betamethasone | 25 | 0.60 | No |
| Dexamethasone | 30 | 0.75 | No |

*The classification by duration of action is based on Harter JG. Corticosteroids. NY State J Med 1966;66:827.

†The values given for glucocorticoid potency are relative. Cortisol is arbitrarily assigned a value of 1.

‡Mineralocorticoid effects are dose related. At doses close to or within the basal physiologic range for glucocorticoid activity, no such effect may be detectable.

(Data from Axelrod L. Glucocorticoid therapy. Medicine [Baltimore] 1976;55:39; Axelrod L. Adrenal corticosteroids. In: Miller RR, Greenblatt DJ, eds. Handbook of drug therapy. New York: Elsevier North-Holland, 1979:809; and Axelrod L. Glucocorticoids. In: Kelley WN, Harris ED Jr, Ruddy S, Sledge CB, eds. Textbook of rheumatology, 4th ed. Philadelphia: WB Saunders, 1993:779.)

In short, the slight differences in the circulating $T_{1/2}$s of the glucocorticoids contrast with their marked differences in potency and duration of ACTH suppression. Thus, the duration of action of a glucocorticoid is not determined by its presence in the circulation. This is consistent with the mechanism of action of steroid hormones. A steroid molecule binds to a specific intracellular receptor protein (see Chap. 4). This steroid-receptor complex modifies the process of transcription by which RNA is transcribed from the DNA template. This process alters the rate of synthesis of specific proteins. The steroid thereby modifies the phenotypic expression of the genetic information. Thus, the glucocorticoid *continues* to act inside the cell after it has disappeared from the circulation. Moreover, the events initiated by the glucocorticoid may continue to occur, or a product of these events (such as a specific protein) may be present after the disappearance of the glucocorticoid.

### BIOAVAILABILITY, ABSORPTION, AND BIOTRANSFORMATION

Normally, a person's plasma cortisol level is much lower after the oral administration of cortisone than after an equal dose of cortisol.[9] Consequently, although oral cortisone may be adequate replacement therapy in chronic adrenal insufficiency, the oral form of this agent should not be used when larger, pharmacologic effects are sought. Comparable plasma prednisolone levels are achieved in normal persons after equivalent oral doses of prednisone and prednisolone.[8,10] After the administration of either of these corticosteroids, however, there is wide variation in individual prednisolone concentrations, which may reflect variability in absorption.[8]

In contrast to the marked rises that follow the intramuscular injection of hydrocortisone, plasma cortisol levels rise little or not at all after an intramuscular injection of cortisone acetate. When it is given intramuscularly, cortisone acetate does not provide adequate plasma cortisol levels and offers no advantage over hydrocortisone delivered by the same route. The explanation for the failure of intramuscular cortisone acetate to provide adequate plasma cortisol levels is unknown. It may reflect poor absorption from the site of injection. Alternatively, intramuscular cortisone acetate, which reaches the liver through the systemic circulation, may be metabolically inactivated before it can be converted to cortisol in the liver, in contrast to oral cortisone acetate, which reaches the liver through the portal circulation.

### PLASMA TRANSPORT PROTEINS

In normal humans, circadian fluctuations occur in the capacity of corticosteroid-binding globulin (transcortin) to bind cortisol and prednisolone. Patients who have been treated with prednisone for a prolonged period have no diurnal variation in the binding capacity of corticosteroid-binding globulin for cortisol or prednisolone, and both capacities are reduced in comparison with normal persons. Thus, long-term glucocorticoid therapy not only alters the endogenous secretion of steroids, but also affects the transport of some glucocorticoids in the circulation. This may explain why the disappearance of prednisolone is more rapid in those persons who have previously received glucocorticoids.

### GLUCOCORTICOID THERAPY IN THE PRESENCE OF LIVER DISEASE

Plasma cortisol levels are normal in patients with hepatic disease. Although the clearance of cortisol is reduced in patients with cirrhosis, the hypothalamic-pituitary-adrenal (HPA) homeostatic mechanism remains intact. Consequently, the decreased rate of metabolism is accompanied by decreased synthesis of cortisol (see Chap. 205).

The conversion of prednisone to prednisolone is impaired in patients with active liver disease.[11] This is largely offset by a decreased rate of elimination of prednisolone from the plasma in these patients.[11] In patients with liver disease, the plasma availability of prednisolone is quite variable after oral doses of either prednisone or prednisolone.[12] This is further complicated by the lower percentage of plasma prednisolone that is bound to protein in patients with active liver disease; the unbound fraction is inversely related to the serum albumin concentration. An increased frequency of prednisone side effects is observed at low serum albumin levels.[12] Both these findings may reflect impaired hepatic function. Because the impairment of conversion of prednisone to prednisolone is quantitatively small in the presence of liver disease and is offset by a decreased rate of clearance of prednisolone, and because of the marked variability in plasma prednisolone levels after the administration of either corticosteroid, there is no clear mandate to use prednisolone rather than prednisone in patients with active liver disease or cirrhosis.[8] If prednisone or prednisolone is used, however, a somewhat lower than usual dose should be given if the serum albumin level is low.[8]

### GLUCOCORTICOID THERAPY AND THE NEPHROTIC SYNDROME

When hypoalbuminemia is caused by the nephrotic syndrome, the fraction of prednisolone that is protein bound is decreased. The unbound fraction is inversely related to the serum albumin concentration. The unbound prednisolone concentration remains normal, however.[13,14] Because the pharmacologic effect is determined by the unbound concentration, altered prednisolone kinetics do not explain the increased frequency of prednisolone-related side effects in these patients.

### GLUCOCORTICOID THERAPY AND HYPERTHYROIDISM

The bioavailability of prednisolone after an oral dose of prednisone is reduced in patients with hyperthyroidism because of decreased absorption of prednisone and increased hepatic clearance of prednisolone.[15]

### GLUCOCORTICOIDS DURING PREGNANCY

Glucocorticoid therapy is well tolerated in pregnancy.[16] Glucocorticoids cross the placenta, but there is no compelling evidence that this produces clinically significant HPA suppression or Cushing syndrome in neonates,[16] although subnormal responsiveness to exogenous ACTH may occur. Similarly, there is no evidence that glucocorticoids increase the incidence of congenital defects in humans.[16] Glucocorticoids do appear to decrease the birth weight of full-term infants; the long-term consequences of this are unknown. Because the concentrations of prednisone and prednisolone in breast milk are low, the administration of these drugs to the mother of a nursing infant is unlikely to produce deleterious effects in the infant.

### GLUCOCORTICOID THERAPY AND AGE

The clearance of prednisolone and methylprednisolone decreases with age.[17,18] Despite the higher prednisolone levels seen in elderly subjects compared with young subjects after comparable doses, endogenous plasma cortisol levels are suppressed to a lesser extent in the elderly.[17] These findings may be associated with an increased incidence of side effects and suggest the need to use smaller doses in the elderly than in young patients.

### DRUG INTERACTIONS

The concomitant use of medications can alter the effectiveness of glucocorticoids; the reverse also is true.[19]

#### EFFECTS OF OTHER MEDICATIONS ON GLUCOCORTICOIDS

The metabolism of glucocorticoids is accelerated by substances that induce hepatic microsomal enzyme activity, such as phenytoin, barbiturates, and rifampin. The administration of these medications can increase the corticosteroid requirements of patients with adrenal insufficiency or lead to deterioration in the conditions of patients whose underlying disorders are well controlled by glucocorticoid therapy. These substances should be avoided in patients receiving corticosteroids. Diazepam does not alter the metabolism of glucocorticoids and is preferable to barbiturates in this setting. If drugs that induce hepatic microsomal enzyme activity must be used in patients taking corticosteroids, an increase in the required dose of corticosteroids should be anticipated.

Conversely, ketoconazole increases the bioavailability of large doses of prednisolone (0.8 mg/kg) because of inhibition of hepatic microsomal enzyme activity.[20] Oral contraceptive use decreases the clearance of prednisone and increases its bioavailability.[21]

The bioavailability of prednisone is decreased by antacids in doses comparable to those used clinically.[22] The bioavailability of prednisolone is not impaired by sucralfate, $H_2$-receptor blockade, or cholestyramine.

### EFFECTS OF GLUCOCORTICOIDS ON OTHER MEDICATIONS

The concurrent administration of a glucocorticoid and a salicylate may reduce the serum salicylate level. Conversely, reduction of the corticosteroid dose during the administration of a fixed dose of salicylate may lead to a higher and possibly toxic serum salicylate level. This interaction may reflect the induction of salicylate metabolism by glucocorticoids.[23]

Glucocorticoids may increase the required dose of insulin or oral hypoglycemic agents, antihypertensive drugs, or glaucoma medications. They also may alter the required dose of sedative-hypnotic or antidepressant therapy. Digitalis toxicity can result from hypokalemia caused by glucocorticoids, as from hypokalemia of any cause. Glucocorticoids can reverse the neuromuscular blockade induced by pancuronium.

### CONSIDERATIONS BEFORE INITIATING THE USE OF GLUCOCORTICOIDS AS PHARMACOLOGIC AGENTS

Cushing syndrome (see Chap. 75) is a life-threatening disorder. The 5-year mortality was higher than 50% at the beginning of the era of glucocorticoid and ACTH therapy.[24] Infection and cardiovascular complications were frequent causes of death. High-dose exogenous glucocorticoid therapy is similarly hazardous.

Table 78-2 summarizes the important questions to consider before initiating glucocorticoid therapy.[25] These questions enable the physician to assess the potential risks that must be weighed against the possible benefits of treatment. The more severe the underlying disorder, the more readily can systemic glucocorticoid therapy be justified. Thus, corticosteroids are commonly used in patients with severe forms of systemic lupus erythematosus, sarcoidosis, active vasculitis, asthma, chronic active hepatitis, transplantation rejection, pemphigus, or diseases of comparable severity. Generally, systemic corticosteroids should not be administered to patients with mild rheumatoid arthritis or mild bronchial asthma; such patients should receive more conservative therapy first. Although these patients may experience symptomatic relief from glucocorticoids, it may prove difficult to withdraw the drugs. Consequently, they may unnecessarily experience Cushing syndrome and HPA suppression.

### DURATION OF THERAPY

The anticipated duration of glucocorticoid therapy is another critical issue. The use of glucocorticoids for 1 to 2 weeks for a condition such as poison ivy or allergic rhinitis is unlikely to be associated with serious side effects in the absence of a contraindication. An exception to this rule is a corticosteroid-induced psychosis. This complication may occur after only a few days of high-dose glucocorticoid therapy, even in patients with no previous history of psychiatric disease (see Chap. 201).[26,27] Because the risk of so many complications is related to the dose and duration

**TABLE 78-2.**
**Considerations before the Use of Glucocorticoids as Pharmacologic Agents**

1. How serious is the underlying disorder?
2. How long will therapy be required?
3. What is the anticipated effective corticosteroid dose?
4. Is the patient predisposed to any of the potential hazards of glucocorticoid therapy?
   Diabetes mellitus
   Osteoporosis
   Peptic ulcer, gastritis, or esophagitis
   Tuberculosis or other chronic infections
   Hypertension and cardiovascular disease
   Psychological difficulties
5. Which glucocorticoid preparation should be used?
6. Have other modes of therapy been used to minimize the glucocorticoid dosage and to minimize the side effects of glucocorticoid therapy?
7. Is an alternate-day regimen indicated?

(Modified from Thorn GW. Clinical considerations in the use of corticosteroids. N Engl J Med 1966; 274:775.)

of therapy, the smallest possible dose should be prescribed for the shortest possible period. If hypoalbuminemia is present, the dose should be reduced. If long-term treatment is indicated, the use of an alternate-day schedule should be considered.

### LOCAL USE

A local corticosteroid preparation should be used whenever possible because systemic effects are minimal when these substances are administered correctly. Examples include topical therapy in dermatologic disorders, corticosteroid aerosols in bronchial asthma and allergic rhinitis, and corticosteroid enemas in ulcerative proctitis. Systemic absorption of inhaled glucocorticoids leading to Cushing syndrome and HPA suppression is a rare occurrence when these agents are administered correctly at prescribed doses.[28,29] The intraarticular injection of corticosteroids may be of value in carefully selected patients if strict aseptic techniques are used and if frequent injections are avoided.

### SELECTING A SYSTEMIC PREPARATION

Agents with little or no mineralocorticoid activity should be used when a glucocorticoid is prescribed for pharmacologic purposes. If the dosage is to be tapered over a few days, a long-acting agent may be impractical. For alternate-day therapy, a short-acting agent that generally does not cause sodium retention (e.g., prednisone, prednisolone, or methylprednisolone) should be used. There is no indication for glucocorticoid conjugates designed to achieve a prolonged duration of action (several days or several weeks) after a single intramuscular injection. The bioavailability of such preparations cannot be regulated precisely, the duration of action cannot be estimated reliably, and it is not possible to taper the dosage rapidly in the event of an adverse reaction such as a corticosteroid-induced psychosis. The use of such preparations may cause HPA suppression more frequently than do comparable doses of the same glucocorticoid given orally. The use of supplemental medications to minimize the systemic corticosteroid dose and to reduce the side effects of systemic glucocorticoids should always be considered. In asthma, for example, treatment should include inhaled glucocorticoids and bronchodilators, such as β-adrenergic agonists and theophylline, and may include cromolyn.

### EFFECTS OF EXOGENOUS GLUCOCORTICOIDS

#### ANTIINFLAMMATORY AND IMMUNOSUPPRESSIVE EFFECTS

Endogenous glucocorticoids protect the organism from damage caused by its own defense reactions and the products of these reactions during stress.[30,30a] Consequently, the use of glucocorticoids as antiinflammatory and immunosuppressive agents represents an application of the physiologic effects of glucocorticoids to the treatment of disease.[30] Glucocorticoids have many effects on inflammatory and immune responses, which are described in this section.

Glucocorticoids inhibit synthesis of almost all known cytokines and of several cell surface molecules required for immune function.[31–33] When an immune stimulus such as tumor necrosis factor binds to its receptor, nuclear factor kappa B (NF-κB) moves to the nucleus, where it activates many immunoregulatory genes. This activation of NF-κB involves the degradation of its cytoplasmic inhibitor IκBα and the translocation of NF-κB to the nucleus. Glucocorticoids are potent inhibitors of NF-κB activation. This inhibition is mediated by the induction of the IκBα inhibitory protein, which traps activated NF-κB in inactive cytoplasmic complexes.[31–33] This reduction in NF-κB activity appears to explain the ability of glucocorticoids to inhibit the production of cytokines and cell surface molecules and to suppress the immune response.

**Influence on Blood Cells and on the Microvasculature.** Glucocorticoid effects on inflammatory and immune phenomena include effects on leukocyte movement, leukocyte function, and humoral factors (Table 78-3). In general, glucocorticoids have a greater effect on leukocyte traffic than on function, and more effect on cellular than on humoral processes.[34,35] Glucocorticoids alter the traffic of all the major leukocyte populations in the circulation (see Chap. 212).

Probably the most important antiinflammatory effect of glucocorticoids is the ability to inhibit the recruitment of neutrophils and monocyte-macrophages to an inflammatory site.[35] Corticosteroids modify the increased capillary and membrane permeability that occurs in an area of inflammation. By decreasing the dilation of the microvasculature and the increased capillary permeability that occur during an inflammatory response, the exudation of fluid and the formation of edema may be reduced, and the migration of leukocytes may be impaired.[2,35,36] The decrease in the accumulation of inflammatory cells is also related to decreased adherence of inflammatory cells to the vascular endothelium. It is not possible to determine the relative contributions of the direct vascular effect, the effect on inflammatory cell adherence to the vascular wall, and the effect on chemotaxis to the reduction in inflammation caused by glucocorticoids.

Glucocorticoids have multiple effects on leukocyte function.[35] Corticosteroids suppress cutaneous delayed hypersensitivity responses. Monocyte-macrophage traffic and function are sensitive to glucocorticoids (see Table 78-3). Glucocorticoids in divided daily doses depress the bactericidal activity of monocytes. The sensitivity of monocytes to glucocorticoids may explain the effectiveness of these agents in many granulomatous diseases because the monocyte is the principal cell involved in granuloma formation.[35] Although neutrophil traffic is sensitive to glucocorticoids, neutrophil function appears to be relatively resistant to these agents.[35] Whereas most in vivo studies of neutrophil phagocytosis have found no evidence for impairment of phagocytosis or bacterial killing,[35] other studies suggest that glucocorticoids induce a generalized phagocytic defect affecting both granulocytes and monocytes.

Glucocorticoid therapy retards the disappearance of sensitized erythrocytes, platelets, and artificial particles from the circulation.[35] This may account for the efficacy of glucocorticoids in the treatment of idiopathic thrombocytopenic purpura and autoimmune hemolytic anemia.

**Influence on Arachidonic Acid Derivatives.** Glucocorticoids inhibit prostaglandin (PG) and leukotriene synthesis by inhibiting the release of arachidonic acid from phospholipids.[37] This inhibition of arachidonic acid release appears to be mediated by the induction of lipocortins, a family of related proteins that inhibit phospholipase $A_2$, which is an enzyme that liberates arachidonic acid from phospholipids (see Chap. 172).[38,39] This mechanism is distinct from the mechanism of action of the nonsteroidal antiinflammatory agents, such as salicylates and indomethacin, which

inhibit the cyclooxygenase that converts arachidonic acid to the cyclic endoperoxide intermediates in the PG synthetic pathway; in some tissues, glucocorticoids inhibit cyclooxygenase activity. Thus, the glucocorticoids and the nonsteroidal antiinflammatory agents exert their antiinflammatory effects at two distinct but adjacent loci in the synthetic pathway of arachidonic acid metabolism. Glucocorticoids and nonsteroidal antiinflammatory agents have different spectra of antiinflammatory effects. Some of the therapeutic effects of corticosteroids that are not produced by the nonsteroidal agents may be related to the inhibition of leukotriene formation.[37]

**TABLE 78-3.**
**Effects of Glucocorticoids on Inflammatory and Immune Responses in Humans**

**EFFECTS ON LEUKOCYTE MOVEMENT**
*Lymphocytes*
  Circulating lymphocytopenia 4–6 hours after drug administration, secondary to redistribution of cells to other lymphoid compartments
  Depletion of recirculating lymphocytes
  Selective depletion of T lymphocytes more than B lymphocytes
*Monocyte-Macrophages*
  Circulating monocytopenia 4–6 hours after drug administration, probably secondary to redistribution
  Inhibition of accumulation of monocyte-macrophages at inflammatory sites
*Neutrophils*
  Circulating neutrophilia
  Accelerated release of neutrophils from the bone marrow
  Blockade of accumulation of neutrophils at inflammatory sites
*Eosinophils*
  Circulating eosinopenia, probably secondary to redistribution
  Decreased migration of eosinophils into immediate hypersensitivity skin test sites

**EFFECTS ON LEUKOCYTE FUNCTION**
*Lymphocytes*
  Suppression of delayed hypersensitivity skin testing by inhibition of recruitment of monocyte-macrophages
  Suppression of lymphocyte proliferation to antigens more easily than proliferation to mitogens
  Suppression of mixed leukocyte reaction proliferation
  Suppression of T lymphocyte–mediated cytotoxicity (at high concentrations in vitro)
  No effect on antibody-dependent cell-mediated cytotoxicity
  Suppression of spontaneous (natural) cytotoxicity
  Regulatory effects on helper and suppressor cell populations
*Monocyte-Macrophages*
  Suppression of cutaneous delayed hypersensitivity by inhibition of lymphokine effect on the macrophage
  Blockade of Fc receptor binding and function
  Depression of bactericidal activity
  Possible decrease in monocyte chemotaxis
*Neutrophils*
  Possibly no effect on phagocytic and bactericidal capability (controversial)
  Increase in antibody-dependent cellular cytotoxicity
  Probable decrease in lysosomal release but little effect on lysosomal membrane stabilization at pharmacologic concentrations
  Inhibition of chemotaxis only by suprapharmacologic concentrations

**EFFECTS ON HUMORAL FACTORS**
  Mild decrease in immunoglobulin levels
  Decreased reticuloendothelial clearance of antibody-coated cells
  Decreased synthesis of prostaglandins and leukotrienes
  Inhibition of plasminogen activator release
  Potentiation of the actions of catecholamines
  Antagonism of histamine-induced vasodilation

(Adapted from Parrillo JE, Fauci AS. Mechanisms of glucocorticoid action on immune processes. Annu Rev Pharmacol Toxicol 1979;19:179.)

**TABLE 78-4.**
**Adverse Reactions to Glucocorticoids**

**OPHTHALMIC**

Posterior subcapsular cataracts, increased intraocular pressure and glaucoma, exophthalmos

**CARDIOVASCULAR**

Hypertension

Congestive heart failure in predisposed patients

**GASTROINTESTINAL**

Peptic ulcer disease, pancreatitis

**ENDOCRINE-METABOLIC**

Truncal obesity, moon facies, supraclavicular fat deposition, posterior cervical fat deposition (buffalo hump), mediastinal widening (lipomatosis), hepatomegaly caused by fatty liver

Acne, hirsutism or virilism, erectile dysfunction, menstrual irregularities

Suppression of growth in children

Hyperglycemia; diabetic ketoacidosis; hyperosmolar, nonketotic diabetic coma; hyperlipoproteinemia

Negative balance of nitrogen, potassium, and calcium

Sodium retention, hypokalemia, metabolic alkalosis

Secondary adrenal insufficiency

**MUSCULOSKELETAL**

Myopathy

Osteoporosis, vertebral compression fractures, spontaneous fractures

Aseptic necrosis of femoral and humeral heads and other bones

**NEUROPSYCHIATRIC**

Convulsions

Benign intracranial hypertension (pseudotumor cerebri)

Alterations in mood or personality

Psychosis

**DERMATOLOGIC**

Facial erythema, thin fragile skin, petechiae and ecchymoses, violaceous striae, impaired wound healing

**IMMUNE, INFECTIOUS**

Suppression of delayed hypersensitivity

Neutrophilia, monocytopenia, lymphocytopenia, decreased inflammatory responses

Susceptibility to infections

(Data from Axelrod L. Adrenal corticosteroids. In: Miller RR, Greenblatt DJ, eds. Handbook of drug therapy. New York: Elsevier North-Holland, 1979:809; and Axelrod L. Glucocorticoids. In: Kelley WN, Harris ED Jr, Ruddy S, Sledge CB, eds. Textbook of rheumatology, 4th ed. Philadelphia: WB Saunders, 1993:779.)

## SIDE EFFECTS

The side effects of glucocorticoids include the diverse manifestations of Cushing syndrome and HPA suppression (Table 78-4).[40] Iatrogenic Cushing syndrome differs from endogenous Cushing syndrome in several respects: hypertension, acne, menstrual disturbances, male erectile dysfunction, hirsutism or virilism, striae, purpura, and plethora are more common in endogenous Cushing syndrome; benign intracranial hypertension, glaucoma, posterior subcapsular cataract, pancreatitis, and aseptic necrosis of bone are virtually unique to iatrogenic Cushing syndrome; and obesity, psychiatric symptoms, and poor wound healing have nearly equal frequency in both.[40,41] These differences may be explained as follows. When Cushing syndrome is caused by exogenous glucocorticoids, ACTH secretion is suppressed. In spontaneous, ACTH-dependent Cushing syndrome, the elevated ACTH output causes bilateral adrenal hyperplasia. In the former circumstance, the secretion of adrenocortical androgens and mineralocorticoids is not increased. Conversely, when ACTH output is elevated, the secretion of adrenal androgens and mineralocorticoids may be increased.[1] The augmented secretion of adrenal androgens may account for the higher prevalence of virilism, acne, and menstrual irregularities in the endogenous form of Cushing syndrome, and the enhanced production of mineralocorticoids may explain the higher prevalence of hypertension.[1]

Some of the complications that are virtually unique to iatrogenic Cushing syndrome arise after the prolonged use of large doses of glucocorticoids. Examples are benign intracranial hypertension, posterior subcapsular cataract, and aseptic necrosis of bone.[1]

Although the association of glucocorticoid therapy and peptic ulcer disease is controversial,[42–47] glucocorticoids appear to increase the risk of peptic ulcer disease and also gastrointestinal hemorrhage (see Chap. 204).[45,46] The magnitude of the association between glucocorticoid therapy and these complications is small and is related to the total dose and duration of therapy.[42,45] The risk of peptic ulcer disease and related gastrointestinal problems is increased by the concurrent use of glucocorticoids and nonsteroidal antiinflammatory drugs.[48,49]

Glucocorticoid therapy, especially daily therapy, may suppress the immune response to skin tests for tuberculosis. When possible, tuberculin skin testing is advisable before the initiation of glucocorticoid therapy. Routine isoniazid prophylaxis probably is not indicated for corticosteroid-treated patients, even for those with positive tuberculin skin test results.[50]

At similar doses, some patients respond to and experience side effects of glucocorticoids more readily than do others. Variations in responsiveness to glucocorticoids may be a consequence of drug interactions or of variations in the severity of the underlying disease. Alterations in bioavailability probably do not account for variations in the therapeutic response to glucocorticoids. In patients who experience side effects, the metabolic clearance rate of prednisolone and the volume of distribution are lower[10,51] and the circulating $T_{1/2}$ is longer[51] than in those who do not experience side effects. Impaired renal function may contribute to a decrease in the clearance of prednisolone and an increase in the prevalence of cushingoid features.[52] Patients who have a cushingoid habitus while taking prednisone have higher endogenous plasma cortisol levels than do those without this complication, perhaps because of resistance of the HPA axis to suppression by exogenous glucocorticoids.[53]

Variations in the effectiveness of corticosteroids may be the result of altered cellular responsiveness to the drugs.[54–57] In patients with primary open-angle glaucoma, exogenous glucocorticoids produce a more pronounced rise of intraocular pressure[54]; a greater suppression of the 8:00 a.m. plasma cortisol level when dexamethasone, 0.25 mg, is administered the previous evening at 11:00 p.m.[56]; and greater suppression of phytohemagglutinin-induced lymphocyte transformation[55,57] than in normal persons. Primary open-angle glaucoma is relatively common. These findings suggest that a distinct subpopulation of patients are hyperresponsive to glucocorticoids and that this sensitivity is genetically determined (see Chap. 215).

## PREVENTION OF SIDE EFFECTS

Increasingly, the issues of concern to physicians and patients with respect to glucocorticoid therapy are not only HPA suppression but long-term complications such as glucocorticoid-induced osteoporosis and *Pneumocystis carinii* pneumonia. Of course, the risk of many complications can be reduced by the use of the *lowest possible dose of a glucocorticoid for the shortest possible period*, by the use of *regional or topical* rather than systemic steroids, and by the use of *alternate-day corticosteroid therapy*. In addition, *pharmacologic interventions* to prevent specific complications such as bone disease and *P. carinii* pneumonia are now widely used.

**Osteoporosis.** The majority of patients who receive long-term glucocorticoid therapy will develop low bone mineral density. By some estimates, more than one-fourth of these patients will sustain osteoporotic fractures.[58] The prevalence of vertebral fractures in asthmatic patients on glucocorticoid therapy for at least a year is 11%.[58] Patients with rheumatoid arthritis who are treated with glucocorticoids have an increased incidence of fractures of the hips, ribs, spine, legs, ankles, and feet.[58] Skeletal wasting occurs most rapidly during the first year of therapy. Trabecular bone is affected more than cortical bone. The effects on the skeleton are related to the cumulative dose and duration of treatment.[58] Alternate-day glucocorticoid therapy does not reduce the risk of osteopenia. Inhaled steroids have been associated with bone loss.

The pathogenesis of glucocorticoid-induced osteoporosis involves several different mechanisms.[58] Glucocorticoids decrease intestinal absorption of calcium and phosphate by vitamin D-independent mechanisms. Urinary calcium excretion is increased, possibly as a result of direct effects on renal tubular calcium reabsorption. These changes may lead to secondary hyperparathyroidism in at least some patients. Glucocorticoids reduce sex hormone production. This may be a direct effect by decreasing gonadal hormone release. It may also be indirect by reducing ACTH secretion and adrenal androgen production. Also, inhibition of luteinizing hormone secretion can result in decreased estrogen and testosterone production by the gonads. Glucocorticoids also have an inhibitory effect on the proliferation of osteoblasts, attachment of osteoblasts to matrix, and the synthesis of type I collagen and noncollagenous proteins by osteoblasts.

The evaluation of a patient should emphasize medical risk factors for osteoporosis, including inadequate dietary calcium and vitamin D intake, alcohol consumption, smoking, menopause, and any history of infertility or impotence suggesting hypogonadism in males. Attention should also be devoted to the possible presence of thyrotoxicosis, overtreatment with thyroid medication, renal osteodystrophy, multiple myeloma, osteomalacia, or primary hyperparathyroidism. When appropriate, laboratory studies should be ordered for evaluation of these disorders. When glucocorticoid therapy will be administered for more than a few months, it is reasonable to obtain a baseline measurement of bone mineral density using dual energy x-ray absorptiometry.

In general, all patients should receive calcium and vitamin D supplementation to correct any nutritional deficiency. Calcium therapy alone is associated with rapid rates of spinal bone loss and offers only partial protection from this loss. There is no evidence that the combination of calcium and vitamin D completely prevents bone loss caused by glucocorticoids.[59] Calcitriol and bisphosphonates, specifically alendronate and etidronate, are effective in the prevention of bone loss.[60–63] If calcitriol is used, careful follow-up determinations of serum levels is necessary. Hypogonadotropic men should receive testosterone therapy; hormone replacement therapy should be considered for postmenopausal women. Patients should be educated about the risks and the consequences of osteoporosis and the factors in their own lives that may contribute. Because glucocorticoids also affect muscle mass and function, patients should be advised about exercises for maintaining muscle strength.

***Pneumocystis carinii* Pneumonia.** Glucocorticoids predispose patients to infections of many varieties. Until recently, prophylaxis against infections for patients treated with glucocorticoids was limited to patients receiving transplantation of organs, who also receive other forms of immunosuppression. Currently, prophylaxis for patients with other disorders who are treated with glucocorticoids is being used, particularly for *P. carinii* pneumonia.[64,65]

In a series of 116 patients without acquired immunodeficiency syndrome (AIDS) who experienced a first episode of *P. carinii* pneumonia between 1985 and 1991, 105 (90.5%) had received glucocorticoids within 1 month before the diagnosis of *P. carinii* pneumonia was established.[64] The median daily dose was equivalent to 30 mg prednisone; 25% of the patients had received as little as 16 mg daily. The median duration of glucocorticoid therapy was 12 weeks before the development of the pneumonia. In 25% of the patients, *P. carinii* pneumonia developed after 8 weeks or less of glucocorticoid therapy. However, the attack rate in patients with primary or metastatic central nervous system tumors who received glucocorticoid therapy

was 1.3% and may be lower in other conditions.[65] Also, prophylactic therapy may produce side effects.

Some physicians recommend prophylaxis (e.g., with trimethoprim-sulfa, one double-strength tablet a day) for patients with impaired immune competence conferred by chemotherapy, transplantation, or an inflammatory disorder who have received prednisone 20 mg or more per day for more than 1 month. No controlled studies with such prophylaxis in steroid-treated patients are available. Among patients undergoing bone marrow or organ transplantation at the Mayo Clinic from 1989 to 1995, no cases of *P. carinii* pneumonia were detected in those who received adequate chemoprophylaxis.

### WITHDRAWAL FROM GLUCOCORTICOIDS

The symptoms associated with glucocorticoid withdrawal include anorexia, myalgia, nausea, emesis, lethargy, headache, fever, desquamation, arthralgia, weight loss, and postural hypotension. Many of these symptoms can occur with normal plasma glucocorticoid levels and in patients with normal responsiveness to conventional tests of the HPA system.[66,67] These patients may have abnormal responses to a more sensitive test using 1 µg of α-1-24 ACTH rather than the conventional 250-µg dose.[68,69] Because glucocorticoids inhibit PG production and because many of the features of the corticosteroid withdrawal syndrome can be produced by PGs such as $PGE_2$ and $PGI_2$, this syndrome may be caused by a sudden increase in PG production after the withdrawal of exogenous corticosteroids. The corticosteroid withdrawal syndrome may contribute to psychologic dependence on glucocorticoid treatment and to difficulties in withdrawing such therapy.

### SUPPRESSION OF THE HYPOTHALAMIC-PITUITARY-ADRENAL SYSTEM

#### DEVELOPMENT OF HYPOTHALAMIC-PITUITARY-ADRENAL SUPPRESSION

Few well-documented cases of acute adrenocortical insufficiency have been reported after prolonged glucocorticoid therapy and none have been reported after ACTH therapy.[1] After the introduction of ACTH and glucocorticoids into clinical practice in the late 1940s, patients were described in whom shock was attributed to adrenocortical insufficiency induced by these agents, but biochemical evidence of adrenocortical insufficiency was not available to substantiate the diagnosis.[1] Prolonged hypotension, or even an apparent response of hypotension to intravenous hydrocortisone, is not a reliable means of assessing adrenocortical function. It must be demonstrated simultaneously that the plasma cortisol level is lower than the values found in normal persons experiencing a comparable degree of stress. When testing for plasma cortisol levels became available in the early 1960s, three cases were described in which these criteria were met. The paucity of reports may reflect the fact that acute adrenocortical insufficiency after glucocorticoid therapy is uncommon in properly treated patients, and that physicians may be reluctant to report such events.

The minimal duration of glucocorticoid therapy that can produce HPA suppression must be ascertained from studies of adrenocortical weight and adrenocortical responsiveness to provocative tests.[1,2] Any patient who has received a glucocorticoid in dosages equivalent to 20 to 30 mg per day of prednisone for more than 5 days should be suspected of having HPA suppression.[1,2] If the dosages are closer to but above the physiologic range, 1 month is probably the minimal interval.[1,2]

The stress of general anesthesia and surgery is not hazardous to patients who have received only replacement doses (no more than 25 mg hydrocortisone, 5 mg prednisone, 4 mg triamcinolone, or 0.75 mg dexamethasone), provided the corticosteroid is given early in the day. If doses of this size are given late in the day, suppression may occur as a result of inhibition of the diurnal surge of ACTH release.

**TABLE 78-5.**
**Assessment of Hypothalamic-Pituitary-Adrenal (HPA) Function in Patients Treated with Glucocorticoids**

**METHOD**

Withhold exogenous corticosteroids for 24 hr

Give cosyntropin [synthetic α1-24 ACTH] 250 μg as intravenous bolus or intramuscular injection

Obtain plasma cortisol level 30 or 60 min after administration of ACTH

Performance of the test in the morning is customary but not essential

**INTERPRETATION**

Normal response: Plasma cortisol level >18 μg/dL at 30 or 60 minutes after ACTH administration

Note: Traditional recommendations also specify an increment above baseline of 7 μg/dL at 30 minutes or 11 μg/dL at 60 minutes and a doubling of the baseline value at 60 minutes. These end-points are valid in normal, unstressed subjects but are frequently misleading in ill patients with a normal HPA axis, in whom stress may raise the baseline plasma cortisol level by an increase in *endogenous* ACTH levels.

(From Axelrod L. Glucocorticoids. In: Kelley WN, Harris ED Jr, Ruddy S, Sledge CB, eds. Textbook of rheumatology, 4th ed. Philadelphia: WB Saunders, 1993:779.)

## ASSESSMENT OF HYPOTHALAMIC-PITUITARY-ADRENAL FUNCTION

When HPA suppression is suspected, the physician may wish to assess the integrity of the HPA system. A test of HPA reserve is indicated only when the result will modify therapy. In practice, this applies to patients who may need an increase in the corticosteroid dosage to cover a stressful event (such as general anesthesia and surgery) and to patients in whom withdrawal of glucocorticoid therapy is contemplated. In the latter group, a test of the HPA axis usually is indicated only when the glucocorticoid dosage has been reduced to replacement levels, for example, 5 mg prednisone daily (or an equivalent dosage of another glucocorticoid). In stable patients receiving prolonged glucocorticoid therapeutic regimens, frequent tests of HPA reserve function are not indicated. For example, it is not necessary to test before each reduction in dosage during tapering of the steroid regimen. The responsiveness of the HPA system may change as corticosteroid therapy continues, and repeated testing is costly.

The short ACTH test is a useful guide to the presence or absence of HPA suppression in patients treated with glucocorticoids (Table 78-5). Although this test assesses directly only the adrenocortical response to ACTH, it is an effective measure of the integrity of the HPA axis. *Because hypothalamic-pituitary function returns before adrenocortical function during recovery from HPA suppression, a normal adrenocortical response to ACTH in this setting implies that hypothalamic-pituitary function also is normal.* This rationale is supported by direct observation. Thus, the maximal response of the plasma cortisol level to ACTH corresponds to the maximal plasma cortisol level observed during the induction of general anesthesia and surgery in patients who have received glucocorticoid therapy.[1,2] A normal response to ACTH before surgery is unlikely to be followed by markedly impaired secretion of cortisol during anesthesia and surgery in corticosteroid-treated patients. An abnormal response to ACTH is a necessary but not a sufficient condition for the diagnosis of adrenal insufficiency in glucocorticoid-treated patients who undergo surgery; some patients with an abnormal response to ACTH tolerate surgery without glucocorticoid treatment.[70] Moreover, hypotension in the operative or postoperative period in patients who have been treated previously with glucocorticoid therapy is often a result of other causes, such as volume depletion and reactions to anesthetic medication. The hypotension often responds to treatment of these factors.

Other tests of HPA function generally are not indicated. The *low-dose (1 μg) short ACTH test* is more sensitive than the conventional-dose ACTH test in patients who have been treated with glucocorticoids.[68,68a] The conventional dose of ACTH used in the short ACTH test (and other ACTH tests) produces circulating ACTH levels that are far above the physiologic range. These supraphysiologic levels may produce a normal plasma cortisol level in patients with partial adrenocortical insufficiency. Nevertheless, the low-dose short ACTH test has not yet replaced the conventional-dose short ACTH test. The *lower limit* of the normal range for the low-dose ACTH test has *not* yet been defined.[69] Also, there are *no* commercially available preparations of ACTH available for direct use in the low-dose short ACTH test. The injection for the low-dose short ACTH test must be prepared by dilution, which is a source of *inconvenience and possible error.* Insulin-induced hypoglycemia may be hazardous (especially in patients with cardiac or neurologic disease), and the symptoms may be uncomfortable. This procedure is more time-consuming and more costly than the ACTH test because more cortisol values must be determined. The measurement of plasma cortisol levels before and after the administration of corticotropin-releasing hormone also has been recommended.[71] This test also is longer and more expensive than the ACTH test and has not been compared to a physiologic stress such as anesthesia and surgery. It offers no clear advantage over the ACTH test.

## CORTICOTROPIN AND THE HYPOTHALAMIC-PITUITARY-ADRENAL SYSTEM

Pharmacologic doses of ACTH cause elevated cortisol secretory rates and increased plasma cortisol levels. The elevated plasma cortisol levels might be expected to suppress ACTH release. Actually, there is no evidence of clinically significant hypothalamic-pituitary suppression in patients who have received ACTH therapy.[1] The failure of ACTH to suppress HPA function is not explained by the dose of ACTH used, the frequency of injection, the time of administration, or the plasma cortisol pattern after ACTH administration. Alternatively, it is possible that the hyperplastic and overactive adrenal cortex that results from ACTH therapy compensates for hypothalamic or pituitary suppression. Although threshold adrenocortical sensitivity to ACTH is not changed in patients who have received daily ACTH therapy, there may be altered adrenocortical responsiveness to ACTH in the physiologic range. Moreover, the normal response of the plasma cortisol level in patients treated with ACTH may be preserved, at least in part, because ACTH treatment reduces the rate of ACTH secretion but not the total amount secreted, whereas glucocorticoids reduce both the rate of secretion and the total amount secreted.[72]

## RECOVERY FROM HYPOTHALAMIC-PITUITARY-ADRENAL SUPPRESSION

During the recovery from HPA suppression, hypothalamic-pituitary function returns before adrenocortical function.[1,2,73] Twelve months must elapse after the withdrawal of large doses of glucocorticoids given for a prolonged period before HPA function, including responsiveness to stress, returns to normal.[1,2,73] Conversely, recovery from HPA suppression that has been induced by a brief course of corticosteroids (i.e., 25 mg prednisone twice daily for 5 days) occurs within 5 days.[74] Patients with mild suppression of the HPA axis (i.e., normal basal plasma and urine corticosteroid levels but diminished responses to ACTH and insulin-induced hypoglycemia) resume normal HPA function more rapidly than do those with severe depression of the HPA axis (i.e., low basal plasma and urine corticosteroid levels and diminished responses to ACTH and insulin-induced hypoglycemia). The time course of recovery correlates with the total duration of previous glucocorticoid therapy and the total previous corticosteroid dose. Nevertheless, in an individual patient, it is not possible to predict the duration of recovery from a course of glucocorticoid therapy at supraphysiologic doses lasting more than a few weeks. Consequently, persistence of HPA suppression should be suspected for 12 months after such treatment. The recovery interval after suppression of the contralateral adrenal cortex by the products of an adrenocortical tumor may exceed 12 months. The recovery from HPA suppression that is induced by exogenous glucocorticoids may be more rapid in children than in adults.

## WITHDRAWAL OF PATIENTS FROM GLUCOCORTICOID THERAPY

### RISKS OF WITHDRAWAL

The decision to discontinue glucocorticoid therapy provokes apprehension among physicians. The deleterious consequences of such an action include precipitation of adrenocortical insufficiency, development of the corticosteroid withdrawal syndrome, or exacerbation of the underlying disease. Adrenocortical insufficiency after the withdrawal of glucocorticoids is justly feared. The likelihood of precipitating the underlying disease depends on the activity and natural history of the illness in question. When there is any possibility that the underlying illness will flare up, the glucocorticoid should be withdrawn gradually, over an interval of weeks to months, with frequent reassessment of the patient.

### TREATMENT OF PATIENTS WITH HYPOTHALAMIC-PITUITARY-ADRENAL SUPPRESSION

No proven means exists for hastening a return to normal HPA function once inhibition has resulted from glucocorticoid therapy. The use of ACTH does not prevent or reverse the development of glucocorticoid-induced adrenal insufficiency. Conversion to an alternate-day schedule permits but does not accelerate recovery. In children, alternate-day glucocorticoid therapy actually may delay recovery.

The recovery from corticosteroid-induced adrenal insufficiency is time dependent and spontaneous. The rate of recovery is determined not only by the doses given when the corticosteroids are being tapered, but also by the doses administered during the initial phase of treatment, before tapering is commenced. During the course of recovery, small doses of hydrocortisone (10–20 mg) or prednisone (2.5–5.0 mg) given in the morning may alleviate the withdrawal symptoms. Recovery of HPA function still occurs when small doses of glucocorticoids are administered in the morning. The possibility cannot be excluded, however, that small doses of glucocorticoids given in the morning retard the rate of recovery from HPA suppression.

## ALTERNATE-DAY GLUCOCORTICOID THERAPY

Alternate-day glucocorticoid therapy is defined as the administration of a short-acting glucocorticoid with no appreciable mineralocorticoid effect (i.e., prednisone, prednisolone, or methylprednisolone) once every 48 hours in the morning, at about 8:00 a.m. The purpose of this approach is to minimize the adverse effects of glucocorticoids while retaining the therapeutic benefits. The original basis for this schedule was the hypothesis that the antiinflammatory effects of glucocorticoids persist longer than do the undesirable metabolic effects.[75–77] This hypothesis is *not* supported by observations of the duration of corticosteroid effects. A second hypothesis emphasizes that intermittent rather than continuous administration produces a cyclic, although not diurnal, pattern of glucocorticoid levels in the circulation and within the target cells that simulates the normal diurnal cycle.[34] This may prevent the development of Cushing syndrome and HPA suppression while providing therapeutic benefit. Because the full expression of a disease frequently occurs only when the level of inflammatory activity is elevated over a protracted period, the intermittent administration of a glucocorticoid may be sufficient to shorten the interval during which the disorder develops without interruption and thereby to prevent the level of disease activity from becoming apparent clinically (Fig. 78-2).[34] The duration of action of the glucocorticoid is important here. The selection of prednisone, prednisolone, and methylprednisolone as the agents of choice

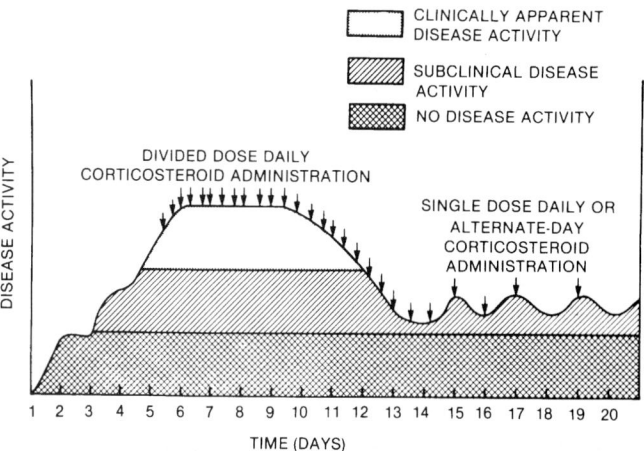

**FIGURE 78-2.** The effect of glucocorticoid administration on the activity of the underlying disease. A divided daily dosage schedule may be necessary initially in some disorders. When the disease is controlled, or from the start of therapy in certain diseases, alternate-day therapy may be effective. (From Fauci AS, Dale DC, Balow JE. Glucocorticosteroid therapy: mechanisms of action and clinical considerations. Ann Intern Med 1976; 84:304.)

for alternate-day therapy and of 48 hours as the appropriate interval between doses has an empiric basis. It has been found that intervals of 36, 24, and 12 hours were accompanied by adrenal suppression, and that an interval of 72 hours was therapeutically ineffective when prednisone (and, occasionally, triamcinolone) was used.[77] An interval of 48 hours is optimal.

### ALTERNATE-DAY GLUCOCORTICOID THERAPY AND MANIFESTATIONS OF CUSHING SYNDROME

An alternate-day regimen can prevent or ameliorate the manifestations of Cushing syndrome.[1,2] The susceptibility to infections that characterizes Cushing syndrome may be alleviated. Patients have been described in whom refractory infections appeared to clear after conversion from daily to alternate-day regimens. In addition, there is a low frequency of infections in patients receiving alternate-day therapy. Children treated with alternate-day steroid therapy regain or retain tonsillar and peripheral lymphoid tissue. The available information strongly suggests that alternate-day regimens are associated with a lower incidence of infections than are daily regimens, but it does not firmly establish this point.

Host defense mechanisms have been studied in patients receiving alternate-day therapy. Patients maintained on such schedules who have been studied on the days they do not take the medication have normal blood neutrophil and monocyte counts, normal cutaneous inflammatory responses, and normal neutrophil $T_{1/2}$s. Patients receiving daily therapy, however, demonstrate neutrophilia, monocytopenia, decreased cutaneous neutrophil and monocyte inflammatory responses, and prolongation of the neutrophil $T_{1/2}$. Patients studied on the days they do not receive treatment do not have the lymphocytopenia observed in patients who receive daily therapy. Monocyte cellular function is normal in patients receiving alternate-day treatment at 4 hours and at 24 hours after a dose. Intermittently normal leukocyte kinetics, preservation of delayed hypersensitivity, and preservation of monocyte cellular function may explain the apparently reduced susceptibility to infection of patients receiving alternate-day therapy.[78–80]

### EFFECTS OF ALTERNATE-DAY GLUCOCORTICOID THERAPY ON HYPOTHALAMIC-PITUITARY-ADRENAL RESPONSIVENESS

Patients receiving alternate-day glucocorticoid therapy may have some suppression of basal corticosteroid levels, but they have normal or nearly normal responsiveness to provocative tests such as the corticotropin-releasing hormone stimulation test, the ACTH stimulation test, insulin-induced hypoglycemia, and the metyrapone test.[1,2,81] They have less suppression of HPA function than do patients receiving daily therapy.

## EFFECTS OF ALTERNATE-DAY THERAPY ON THE UNDERLYING DISEASE

Alternate-day glucocorticoid therapy is as effective, or nearly as effective, in controlling diverse disorders as daily therapy in divided doses.[1,2] This approach has provided apparent benefit in patients with the following disorders: childhood nephrotic syndrome, adult nephrotic syndrome, membranous nephropathy, renal transplantation, mesangiocapillary glomerulonephritis, lupus nephritis, ulcerative colitis, rheumatoid arthritis, acute rheumatic fever, myasthenia gravis, Duchenne muscular dystrophy, dermatomyositis, idiopathic polyneuropathy, asthma, Sjögren syndrome, sarcoidosis, alopecia areata and other chronic dermatoses, and pemphigus vulgaris. Prospective, controlled studies demonstrate the efficacy of alternate-day therapy in membranous nephropathy and renal transplantation. The role of alternate-day therapy in giant cell arteritis is controversial.[82–84]

## USE OF ALTERNATE-DAY THERAPY

Because alternate-day therapy can *prevent or ameliorate the manifestations of Cushing syndrome, can avert or permit recovery from HPA suppression, and is as effective (or nearly as effective) as continuous therapy*, patients for whom long-term glucocorticoid administration is indicated should be placed on such programs whenever possible. Nevertheless, physicians sometimes are reluctant to use alternate-day schedules, often because of an unsuccessful experience. Many efforts fail because of lack of familiarity with the indications for and use of such therapy.

The benefits of alternate-day glucocorticoid therapy are demonstrable only when corticosteroids are used for a *prolonged* period. There is no reason to use an alternate-day schedule when the anticipated duration of therapy is less than several weeks.

Alternate-day therapy may not be necessary or appropriate during the initial stages of therapy or during exacerbation of the underlying disease. Nevertheless, patients with many chronic disorders have been treated with an alternate-day regimen as initial therapy with apparent benefit.[1,2] In patients with rheumatoid arthritis, it appears to be easier to establish treatment with alternate-day corticosteroids than to convert from daily therapy. Physicians treating recipients of renal transplants initially use daily therapy and then convert to an alternate-day schedule.

Alternate-day therapy may be hazardous in the presence of adrenocortical insufficiency of any cause because patients are unprotected against glucocorticoid insufficiency during the last 12 hours of the 48-hour cycle. In patients who have been taking glucocorticoids for more than a brief period, or in those who may have adrenal insufficiency on another basis, the adequacy of HPA function should be determined before the initiation of an alternate-day program. It may be possible to surmount this obstacle by giving a small dose of a short-acting glucocorticoid (i.e., 10 mg hydrocortisone) in the afternoon of the second day; this approach has not been studied systematically.

Alternate-day glucocorticoid therapy may fail to prevent or ameliorate the manifestations of Cushing syndrome or HPA suppression if a short-acting glucocorticoid is not used, or if it is used incorrectly. For example, the use of prednisone four times a day on alternate days may be less successful than the use of the same total dose once every 48 hours.

An abrupt alteration from daily to alternate-day therapy should be avoided. First, the prolonged use of daily-dose glucocorticoids may have caused HPA suppression. In addition, patients with normal HPA function may experience withdrawal symptoms and have an exacerbation of the underlying disease.

No program of conversion from continuous therapy to alternate-day therapy has been shown to be optimal. One approach is to reduce the frequency of drug administration until the total dose for each day is given in the morning, and then to increase the dosage gradually on the first day of each 2-day period and to decrease the dosage on the second day. Another approach is to double the dosage on the first day of each 2-day cycle, to give this as a single morning dose if possible, and then to taper the dosage gradually on the second day.[85] It is not clear how often changes in dosage should be made with any approach. This depends on many variables, including the underlying disease involved, the duration of previous glucocorticoid therapy, the personality of the patient, and the physician's ability to use adjunctive therapy. Nonetheless, the conversion should be made as quickly as the patient can tolerate it. If adrenal insufficiency, the corticosteroid withdrawal syndrome, or an exacerbation of the underlying disease develops, the previously effective regimen should be reinstituted and then tapered more gradually. Occasionally, it is necessary to resume full daily dosages temporarily. An absolute change of dosage represents a larger percentage change in dosage at small total daily doses than at large total daily doses. Changes in the dosage should be about 10 mg prednisone (or equivalent) at total daily doses of more than 30 mg, 5 mg at total doses of more than 20 mg, and 2.5 mg at lower doses. The interval between changes in the dosage may be as short as 1 day or as long as many weeks.

Optimal results from alternate-day glucocorticoid therapy may not be achieved because of failure to use supplemental therapy for the underlying disorder. Conservative (nonglucocorticoid) therapy often is used until a glucocorticoid is initiated, at which time these less toxic therapeutic measures are ignored. Adjunctive therapeutic measures may facilitate the use of the lowest possible corticosteroid dose. With alternate-day therapy, these measures especially should be used during the end of the second day, when symptoms may be prominent. Supplemental therapy may be especially helpful in disorders in which patients are likely to experience symptoms of the disease on the day off therapy, such as asthma and rheumatoid arthritis. In illnesses in which disabling symptoms are less likely to appear on the alternate day, such as the childhood nephrotic syndrome, less difficulty may be encountered.

Alternate-day therapy may fail because of failure to inform patients about the purposes of this regimen. Because glucocorticoids may induce euphoria, patients may be reluctant to accept modification of a schedule of frequent doses. A careful explanation about the risks of glucocorticoid excess, attuned to patients' intellectual and emotional ability to comprehend, enhances the prospects of success.

## DAILY SINGLE-DOSE GLUCOCORTICOID THERAPY

Sometimes, alternate-day therapy fails because patients experience symptoms of the underlying disease during the last few hours of the second day. In these situations, single-dose glucocorticoid therapy may be of value.[1,2] This regimen appears to be as effective as divided daily doses in controlling such underlying diseases as rheumatoid arthritis, systemic lupus erythematosus, polyarteritis, and proctocolitis. In giant cell arteritis, a daily dose in the morning is nearly as effective as daily therapy in divided doses.[82] Daily single-dose therapy reduces the likelihood that HPA suppression will develop. The manifestations of Cushing syndrome, however, probably are not prevented or ameliorated by a daily single-dose regimen.

## GLUCOCORTICOIDS OR CORTICOTROPIN?

Disorders that respond to glucocorticoid therapy also respond to ACTH therapy if the adrenal cortex is normal. There is no evidence, however, that ACTH is superior to glucocorticoids for the treatment of any disorder when comparable doses are used.[1,2,86] Hydrocortisone and ACTH, given intravenously in pharmacologically equivalent doses (determined by plasma cortisol levels and urinary corticosteroid excretion rates), are equally effective in the treatment of inflammatory bowel disease.[87] Similarly, there is no apparent difference in the effectiveness of prednisone and ACTH for the treatment of infantile spasms.[88] Because ACTH does not appear to offer any therapeutic advantage, glucocorticoids are preferable for therapeutic purposes: they can be administered orally, the dose can be regulated precisely, their effectiveness does not depend on adrenocortical responsiveness (an important consideration in patients who have been treated with glucocorticoids), and they produce a lower frequency of certain side effects such as acne, hypertension, and increased pigmentation.[1,2] If alternate-day therapy cannot be used, ACTH might appear to be preferable because it does not suppress the HPA axis. This benefit usually is outweighed by the advantages of glucocorticoids and by the fact that daily injections of ACTH are not superior to single daily doses of short-acting glucocorticoids; in both cases, HPA suppression is unlikely to result, but Cushing syndrome is not prevented. In life-threatening situations, glucocorticoids are indicated because maximal blood levels are obtained immediately after intravenous administration, whereas with ACTH infusion, the plasma cortisol level rises to a plateau over several hours. The principal indication for ACTH continues to be the assessment of adrenocortical function.

## DOSAGE

### ANTIINFLAMMATORY OR IMMUNOSUPPRESSIVE THERAPY

The glucocorticoid dosage required for antiinflammatory or immunosuppressive therapy is variable, and depends on the disease under treatment. In general, the dosage ranges from just above that needed for long-term replacement therapy up to 60 to 80 mg prednisone or its equivalent daily. Although much larger dosages sometimes are recommended for diseases such as asthma, systemic lupus erythematosus, and cerebral edema, controlled studies have not established the need for such large amounts of medication. The role of massive doses of corticosteroids in asthma is controversial.[89,90] Most studies report no advantage of high-dose therapy (e.g., more than 60–80 mg prednisone per day). Many physicians use intravenous pulse therapy (e.g., 1 g per day of methylprednisolone intravenously for 3 consecutive days) for severe manifestations of systemic lupus erythematosus, rapidly progressive glomerulonephritis, or other entities. There are no controlled studies that compare the results of pulse therapy with 60 to 80 mg per day of prednisone, however. Thus, the superiority of pulse therapy has not been demonstrated.[91,92]

When alternate-day therapy is used, the dosage is variable and depends on the disease under treatment. It may range from just above that needed for long-term replacement therapy to 150 mg prednisone every other day.

### PERIOPERATIVE MANAGEMENT

Traditional doses of glucocorticoids recommended for perioperative coverage in patients treated with steroids (e.g., 100 mg hydrocortisone intravenously every 8 hours or 20 mg methylprednisolone intravenously every 8 hours on the day of surgery, with a gradual taper over subsequent days) are arbitrary and have no empirical basis.[70] A study in cynomolgus monkeys explored the doses required to prevent postoperative hypotension.[93] Bilateral adrenalectomies were performed in the experimental animals, and replacement doses of glucocorticoids were given for 4 months. The animals were then divided into three groups, given normal, one-tenth normal, or 10 times the normal replacement doses of glucocorticoids. A cholecystectomy was performed on each animal under these conditions. The animals that received one-tenth normal replacement doses had an increased mortality rate, decreased peripheral vascular resistance, and hypotension. The group that received normal replacement doses of glucocorticoids had no more hypotension or postoperative complications than did the group receiving 10 times the replacement dose. A double-blind study in patients provided similar results.[94] The investigators studied patients who had taken at least 7.5 mg prednisone a day for several months and had an abnormal response to an ACTH test. All patients received their usual daily dose of prednisone on the day of surgery. One group of 12 patients received perioperative injections of saline. The other group of 6 patients received hydrocortisone in the saline. There was no significant difference in outcome between the groups in this small study. It appears that patients with secondary adrenal insufficiency resulting from glucocorticoid therapy do not experience hypotension or tachycardia when given only their usual daily dose of steroids for surgical procedures such as joint replacements and abdominal operations.

Based on an analysis of the literature, an interdisciplinary group suggests the use of variable doses, depending on the magnitude of the surgical stress.[70] For *minor surgical stress* (e.g., an inguinal herniorrhaphy), the glucocorticoid target dose would be 25 mg hydrocortisone or equivalent. For *moderate surgical stress* (e.g., a lower extremity revascularization or total joint replacement), the target would be 50 to 75 mg hydrocortisone or equivalent. This might constitute continuation of the patient's usual dose of prednisone (i.e., 10 mg a day) and 50 mg hydrocortisone intravenously intraoperatively. For *major surgical stress* (e.g., esophagogastrectomy or cardiopulmonary bypass), the patient might receive his or her usual steroid dose (e.g., 40 mg prednisone or the parental equivalent preoperatively within 2 hours of surgery) and 50 mg hydrocortisone intravenously every 8 hours after the initial dose for the first 48 to 72 hours. Corticosteroid therapy should not be tapered inadvertently to a dosage below that known to control the underlying disease.

In patients with primary adrenocortical insufficiency, hydrocortisone has the advantage of having mineralocorticoid as well as glucocorticoid activity at high dosages. At dosages less than 100 mg per day, it is necessary to use a mineralocorticoid agent in addition to hydrocortisone; fludrocortisone can be used when patients can take oral medications. Parenteral mineralocorticoid preparations such as desoxycorticosterone acetate are no longer available commercially in the United States.

### DRUG INTERACTIONS

If patients also must take a hepatic microsomal enzyme inducer, the metabolism of the glucocorticoid will be accelerated and larger daily dosages may be needed. The treatment of adrenocortical insufficiency is considered in Chapter 76.

## MINERALOCORTICOIDS

### PHARMACOLOGY

Mineralocorticoids are 21-carbon steroids characterized by their effects on fluid and electrolyte balance. They promote renal sodium reabsorption and potassium excretion (see Chap. 79). Mineralocorticoid deficiency (see Chap. 81) causes hyponatremia, volume depletion, hypotension, hyperkalemia, and a hyperchloremic metabolic acidosis. Mineralocorticoid excess (see Chap. 80) is associated with the retention of sodium and water, hypertension, potassium depletion, hypokalemia, and a metabolic alkalosis. The excessive secretion or administration of a mineralocorticoid causes sodium retention, with consequent fluid retention and weight gain. Patients retain several hundred milliequivalents of sodium and gain several kilograms of weight. If mineralocorticoid excess persists, *mineralocorticoid escape* occurs; further sodium retention and weight gain do not

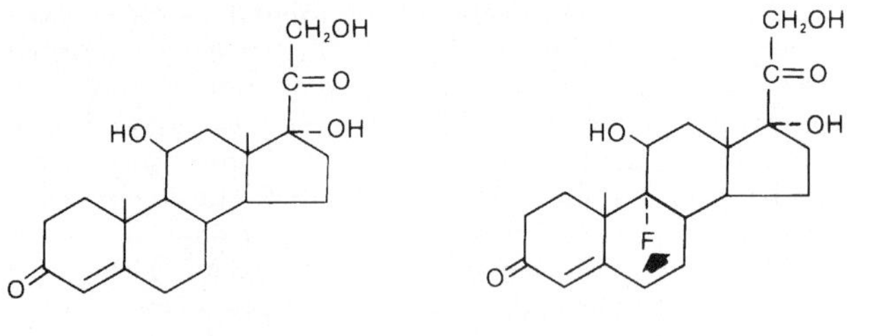

**FIGURE 78-3.** Structure of the mineralocorticoid fludrocortisone. The *arrow* indicates the structural difference between this synthetic steroid and cortisol.

occur. During this escape phenomenon, urinary sodium excretion increases until patients come into balance, and urinary sodium excretion again reflects sodium intake. Thus, patients with mineralocorticoid excess often do not retain sufficient fluid for peripheral edema to develop (although it occasionally does) unless there is another cause for edema such as hypoalbuminemia or right ventricular failure. Therefore, the absence of edema does not exclude the possibility of mineralocorticoid excess.

Aldosterone is the principal mineralocorticoid in humans. Desoxycorticosterone, corticosterone, and cortisol (hydrocortisone) also are secreted in amounts sufficient to cause salt retention in certain pathologic situations.

### AGENTS USED CLINICALLY

The agents with mineralocorticoid action that are used clinically are hydrocortisone and fludrocortisone (9α-fluorohydrocortisone, Florinef [Apothecon, a Bristol-Meyers Squibb Co., Princeton, NJ]; Fig. 78-3). When hydrocortisone is given in large dosages (e.g., 100 mg per day or more), a mineralocorticoid effect may be anticipated. Aldosterone is not used clinically, although it is a potent mineralocorticoid and is essentially devoid of glucocorticoid effect. It would be of limited value because of its brief duration of action.

Fludrocortisone is available only for oral therapy. The presence of the fluorine atom in the 9α position enhances the mineralocorticoid potency of hydrocortisone. The enhanced mineralocorticoid potency of 9α-fluorohydrocortisone is explained by impaired renal conversion of this molecule to 9α-fluorocortisone by 11-hydroxysteroid dehydrogenase, in contrast to the rapid conversion of cortisol to cortisone.[95] At recommended dosages, fludrocortisone is an effective mineralocorticoid, but it is essentially free of glucocorticoid activity. Its duration of action is ~12 to 24 hours.[96–99]

If patients also need large dosages of a glucocorticoid, hydrocortisone can be used alone. A dosage of 100 mg per day or more provides mineralocorticoid activity.[96–98] Experimentally, it was found that fludrocortisone, 1 mg per day orally, is equivalent in mineralocorticoid activity to aldosterone, 1 mg per day in four divided intramuscular doses.[98,99]

No mineralocorticoid by itself can increase the sodium stores of sodium-depleted patients. The effectiveness of a mineralocorticoid hormone depends on substrate availability; patients with mineralocorticoid deficiency not only need the hormone, they also need salt and water. Both hormonal therapy and proper fluid and electrolyte administration are necessary to achieve an optimal clinical response.

### DRUG INTERACTIONS

Mineralocorticoid activity is antagonized by spironolactone; the latter has no effect in patients with hypoaldosteronism. Amiloride (Midamor), a potassium-sparing diuretic agent that acts even in the absence of aldosterone, can reduce the effects of a mineralocorticoid on sodium and potassium balance.

Anything that promotes salt loss, such as a diuretic medication, impairs mineralocorticoid efficacy. For patients who ordinarily need a diuretic (e.g., for the treatment of hypertension or fluid retention), the desired effect may be achieved by modifying the dosage of mineralocorticoid, the intake of salt, or both. Medications that alter sweating or promote vomiting or diarrhea may affect salt balance and therefore change the effectiveness of a mineralocorticoid.

### INDICATIONS

Mineralocorticoid therapy is indicated for primary adrenocortical insufficiency; isolated hypoaldosteronism; salt-losing forms of congenital adrenal hyperplasia; and chronic orthostatic hypotension caused by autonomic insufficiency (multiple systems atrophy [e.g., the Shy-Drager syndrome], idiopathic orthostatic hypotension, and diabetic autonomic neuropathy).

### DOSAGE

The usual dosage of fludrocortisone is 0.1 mg daily, but may range from 0.1 mg on alternate days to 0.2 mg daily. Generally, the starting dosage is 0.1 mg daily, with adjustments made according to clinical response. Orthostatic vital signs are of great value in assessing the adequacy of mineralocorticoid replacement therapy. A marked rise in the heart rate or a fall in blood pressure on standing may precede other manifestations of mineralocorticoid deficiency.

## REFERENCES

1. Axelrod L. Glucocorticoid therapy. Medicine (Baltimore) 1976; 55:39.
2. Axelrod L. Glucocorticoids. In: Kelley WN, Harris ED Jr, Ruddy S, Sledge CB, eds. Textbook of rheumatology, 4th ed. Philadelphia: WB Saunders, 1993.
3. Hollander JL, Brown EM Jr, Jessar RA, Brown CY. Hydrocortisone and cortisone injected into arthritic joints. JAMA 1951; 147:1629.
4. Robinson RCV, Robinson HM Jr. Topical treatment of dermatoses with steroids. South Med J 1956; 49:260.
5. Harter JG. Corticosteroids: their physiologic use in allergic disease. NY State J Med 1966; 66:827.
6. Ballard PL, Carter JP, Graham BS, Baxter JD. A radioreceptor assay for evaluation of the plasma glucocorticoid activity of natural and synthetic steroids in man. J Clin Endocrinol Metab 1975; 41:290.
7. Meikle AW, Tyler FH. Potency and duration of action of glucocorticoids: effects of hydrocortisone, prednisone and dexamethasone on human pituitary-adrenal function. Am J Med 1977; 63:200.
8. Pickup ME. Clinical pharmacokinetics of prednisone and prednisolone. Clin Pharmacokinet 1979; 4:111.
9. Jenkins JS, Sampson PA. Conversion of cortisone to cortisol and prednisone to prednisolone. BMJ 1967; 2:205.
10. Gambertoglio JG, Amend WJC Jr, Benet LZ. Pharmacokinetics and bioavailability of prednisone and prednisolone in healthy volunteers and patients: a review. J Pharmacokinet Biopharm 1980; 8:1.
11. Davis M, Williams R, Chakraborty J, et al. Prednisone or prednisolone for the treatment of chronic active hepatitis? A comparison of plasma availability. Br J Clin Pharmacol 1978; 5:501.
12. Lewis GP, Jusko WJ, Burke CW, et al. Prednisone side effects and serum-protein levels, a collaborative study. Lancet 1971; 2:778.
13. Frey FJ, Frey BM. Altered prednisolone kinetics in patients with the nephrotic syndrome. Nephron 1982; 32:45.
14. Gatti G, Perucca E, Frigo GM, et al. Pharmacokinetics of prednisone and its metabolite prednisolone in children with nephrotic syndrome during the active phase and in remission. Br J Clin Pharmacol 1984; 17:423.
15. Frey FJ, Horber FF, Frey BM. Altered metabolism and decreased efficacy of prednisolone and prednisone in patients with hyperthyroidism. Clin Pharmacol Ther 1988; 44:510.
16. Schatz M, Patterson R, Zeitz S, et al. Corticosteroid therapy for the pregnant asthmatic patient. JAMA 1975; 233:804.
17. Stuck AE, Frey BM, Frey FJ. Kinetics of prednisolone and endogenous cortisol suppression in the elderly. Clin Pharmacol Ther 1988; 43:354.
18. Tornatore KM, Logue G, Venuto RC, Davis PJ. Pharmacokinetics of methylprednisolone in elderly and young healthy males. J Am Geriatr Soc 1994; 42:1118.
19. Jubiz W, Meikle AW. Alterations of glucocorticoid actions by other drugs and disease states. Drugs 1979; 18:113.
20. Zürcher RM, Frey BM, Frey FJ. Impact of ketoconazole on the metabolism of prednisolone. Clin Pharmacol Ther 1989; 45:366.

21. Legler UF, Benet LZ. Marked alterations in dose-dependent prednisolone kinetics in women taking oral contraceptives. Clin Pharmacol Ther 1986; 39:425.
22. Uribe M, Casian C, Rojas S, et al. Decreased bioavailability of prednisone due to antacids in patients with chronic active liver disease and in healthy volunteers. Gastroenterology 1981; 80:661.
23. Graham GG, Champion GD, Day RO, Paull PD. Patterns of plasma concentrations and urinary excretion of salicylate in rheumatoid arthritis. Clin Pharmacol Ther 1977; 22:410.
24. Plotz CM, Knowlton AI, Ragan C. The natural history of Cushing's syndrome. Am J Med 1952; 13:597.
25. Thorn GW. Clinical considerations in the use of corticosteroids. N Engl J Med 1966; 274:775.
26. Boston Collaborative Drug Surveillance Program. Acute adverse reactions to prednisone in relation to dosage. Clin Pharmacol Ther 1972; 13:694.
27. Perry PJ, Tsuang MT, Hwang MH. Prednisolone psychosis: clinical observations. Drug Intell Clin Pharm 1984; 18:603.
28. Hollman GA, Allen DB. Overt glucocorticoid excess due to inhaled corticosteroid therapy. Pediatrics 1988; 81:452.
29. Stead RJ, Cooke NJ. Adverse effects of inhaled corticosteroids. BMJ 1989; 298:403.
30. Munck A, Guyre PM. Glucocorticoid physiology and homeostasis in relation to anti-inflammatory actions. In: Schleimer RP, Claman HN, Oronsky A, eds. Anti-inflammatory steroid action: basic and clinical aspects. San Diego: Academic Press, 1989.
30a. Sapolsky RM, Romero LM, Munck AU. How do glucocorticoids influence stress responses? Integrating permissive, suppressive, stimulatory, and preparative actions. Endocr Rev 2000; 27:55.
31. Scheinman RI, Cogswell PC, Lofquist AK, Baldwin AS Jr. Role of transcriptional activation of IκBα in mediation of immunosuppression by glucocorticoids. Science 1995; 270:283.
32. Auphan N, DiDonato JA, Rosette C, et al. Immunosuppression by glucocorticoids: inhibition of NF-κB activity through induction of IκB synthesis. Science 1995; 270:286.
33. Marx J. How the glucocorticoids suppress immunity. Science 1995; 270:232.
34. Fauci AS, Dale DC, Balow JE. Glucocorticosteroid therapy: mechanisms of action and clinical considerations. Ann Intern Med 1976; 84:304.
35. Parrillo JE, Fauci AS. Mechanisms of glucocorticoid action on immune processes. Annu Rev Pharmacol Toxicol 1979; 19:179.
36. Cupps TR, Fauci AS. Corticosteroid-mediated immunoregulation in man. Immunol Rev 1982; 65:133.
37. Samuelsson B. Leukotrienes: mediators of immediate hypersensitivity reactions and inflammation. Science 1983; 220:568.
38. DiRosa M, Flower RJ, Hirata F, et al. Anti-phospholipase proteins. Prostaglandins 1984; 28:441.
39. Parente L, DiRosa M, Flower RJ, et al. Relationship between the anti-phospholipase and anti-inflammatory effects of glucocorticoid-induced proteins. Eur J Pharmacol 1984; 99:233.
40. Axelrod L. Side effects of glucocorticoid therapy. In: Schleimer RP, Claman H, Oronsky A, eds. Antiinflammatory steroid action: basic and clinical aspects. San Diego: Academic Press, 1989.
41. Ragan C. Corticotropin, cortisone and related steroids in clinical medicine: practical considerations. Bull NY Acad Med 1953; 29:355.
42. Conn HO, Blitzer BL. Nonassociation of adrenocorticosteroid therapy and peptic ulcer. N Engl J Med 1976; 294:473.
43. Langman MJS, Cooke AR. Gastric and duodenal ulcer and their associated diseases. Lancet 1976; 1:680.
44. Jick H, Porter J. Drug-induced gastrointestinal bleeding. Lancet 1978; 2:87.
45. Messer J, Reitman D, Sacks HS, et al. Association of adrenocorticosteroid therapy and peptic-ulcer disease. N Engl J Med 1983; 309:21.
46. Spiro HM. Is the steroid ulcer a myth? N Engl J Med 1983; 309:45.
47. Conn HO, Poynard T. Adrenocorticosteroid administration and peptic ulcer: a critical analysis. J Chronic Dis 1985; 38:457.
48. Piper JM, Ray WA, Daugherty JR, Griffin MR. Corticosteroid use and peptic ulcer disease: role of nonsteroidal anti-inflammatory drugs. Ann Intern Med 1991; 114:735.
49. Gabriel SE, Jaakkimainen L, Bombardier C. Risk for serious gastrointestinal complications related to use of nonsteroidal anti-inflammatory drugs. A meta-analysis. Ann Intern Med 1991; 115:787.
50. Schatz M, Patterson R, Kloner R, Falk J. The prevalence of tuberculosis and positive tuberculin skin tests in a steroid-treated asthmatic population. Ann Intern Med 1976; 84:261.
51. Kozower M, Veatch L, Kaplan MM. Decreased clearance of prednisolone, a factor in the development of corticosteroid side effects. J Clin Endocrinol Metab 1974; 38:407.
52. Bergrem H, Jervell J, Flatmark A. Prednisolone pharmacokinetics in cushingoid and non-cushingoid kidney transplant patients. Kidney Int 1985; 27:459.
53. Frey FJ, Amend WJC Jr, Lozada F, et al. Endogenous hydrocortisone, a possible factor contributing to the genesis of cushingoid habitus in patients on prednisone. J Clin Endocrinol Metab 1981; 53:1076.
54. Becker B. Intraocular pressure response to topical corticosteroids. Invest Ophthalmol 1965; 4:198.
55. Bigger JF, Palmberg PF, Becker B. Increased cellular sensitivity to glucocorticoids in primary open angle glaucoma. Invest Ophthalmol 1972; 11:832.
56. Becker B, Podos SM, Asseff CF, Cooper DG. Plasma cortisol suppression in glaucoma. Am J Ophthalmol 1973; 75:73.
57. Becker B, Shin DH, Palmberg PF, Waltman SR. HLA antigens and corticosteroid response. Science 1976; 194:1427.
58. American College of Rheumatology Task Force on Osteoporosis Guidelines. Recommendations for the prevention and treatment of glucocorticoid-induced osteoporosis. Arthritis Rheum 1996; 39:1791.
59. Sambrook PN. Calcium and vitamin D therapy in corticosteroid bone loss: what is the evidence? J Rheumatol 1996; 23:963.
60. Sambrook P, Birmingham J, Kelly P, et al. Prevention of corticosteroid osteoporosis. A comparison of calcium, calcitriol, and calcitonin. N Engl J Med 1993; 328:1747.
61. Adachi JD, Bensen WG, Brown J, et al. Intermittent etidronate therapy to prevent corticosteroid-induced osteoporosis. N Engl J Med 1997; 337:382.
62. Reid IR. Preventing glucocorticoid-induced osteoporosis. N Engl J Med 1997; 337:420.
63. Saag KG, Emkey R, Schnitzer TJ, et al. Alendronate for the prevention and treatment of glucocorticoid-induced osteoporosis. N Engl J Med 1998; 339:292.
64. Yale SH, Limper AH. *Pneumocystis carinii* pneumonia in patients without acquired immunodeficiency syndrome: associated illnesses and prior corticosteroid therapy. Mayo Clin Proc 1996; 71:5.
65. Sepkowitz KA. *Pneumocystis carinii* pneumonia without acquired immunodeficiency syndrome: who should receive prophylaxis? Mayo Clin Proc 1996;71:102.
66. Amatruda TT Jr, Hollingsworth DR, D'Esopo ND, et al. A study of the mechanism of the steroid withdrawal syndrome: evidence for integrity of the hypothalamic-pituitary-adrenal system. J Clin Endocrinol Metab 1960; 20:339.
67. Amatruda TT Jr, Hurst MM, D'Esopo ND. Certain endocrine and metabolic facets of the steroid withdrawal syndrome. J Clin Endocrinol Metab 1965; 25:1207.
68. Dickstein G, Shechner C, Nicholson WE, et al. Adrenocorticotropin stimulation test: effects of basal cortisol level, time of day, and suggested new sensitive low-dose test. J Clin Endocrinol Metab 1991; 72:773.
68a. Henzen C, Suter A, Lerch E, et al. Suppression and recovery of adrenal response after short-term, high-dose glucocorticoid treatment. Lancet 2000; 355:542.
69. Streeten DHP. Shortcomings in the low-dose (1 μg) ACTH test for the diagnosis of ACTH deficiency states. J Clin Endocrinol Metab 1999; 84:835.
70. Salem M, Tainsh RE Jr, Bromberg J, et al. Perioperative glucocorticoid coverage. A reassessment 42 years after emergence of a problem. Ann Surg 1994; 219:416.
71. Schlaghecke R, Kornely E, Santen RT, Ridderskamp P. The effect of long-term glucocorticoid therapy on pituitary-adrenal responses to exogenous corticotropin-releasing hormone. N Engl J Med 1992; 326:226.
72. Daly JR, Fletcher MR, Glass D, et al. Comparison of effects of long-term corticotrophin and corticosteroid treatment on responses of plasma growth hormone, ACTH, and corticosteroid to hypoglycaemia. BMJ 1974; 2:521.
73. Graber AL, Ney RL, Nicholson WE, et al. Natural history of pituitary-adrenal recovery following long-term suppression with corticosteroids. J Clin Endocrinol Metab 1965; 25:11.
74. Streck WF, Lockwood DH. Pituitary adrenal recovery following short-term suppression with corticosteroids. Am J Med 1979; 66:910.
75. Haugen HN, Reddy WJ, Harter JG. Intermittent steroid therapy in bronchial asthma. Nord Med 1960; 63:15.
76. Reichling GH, Kligman AM. Alternate-day corticosteroid therapy. Arch Dermatol 1961; 83:980.
77. Harter JG, Reddy WJ, Thorn GW. Studies on an intermittent corticosteroid dosage regimen. N Engl J Med 1963; 269:591.
78. MacGregor RR, Sheagren JN, Lipsett MB, Wolff SM. Alternate-day prednisone therapy: evaluation of delayed hypersensitivity responses, control of disease and steroid side effects. N Engl J Med 1969; 280:1427.
79. Dale DC, Fauci AS, Wolff SM. Alternate-day prednisone: leukocyte kinetics and susceptibility to infections. N Engl J Med 1974; 291:1154.
80. Fauci AS, Dale DC. Alternate-day therapy and human lymphocyte subpopulations. J Clin Invest 1975; 55:22.
81. Schürmeyer TH, Tsokos GC, Avgerinos PC, et al. Pituitary-adrenal responsiveness to corticotropin-releasing hormone in patients receiving chronic, alternate day glucocorticoid therapy. J Clin Endocrinol Metab 1985; 61:22.
82. Hunder GG, Sheps SG, Allen GL, Joyce JW. Daily and alternate day corticosteroid regimens in treatment of giant cell arteritis: comparison in a prospective study. Ann Intern Med 1975; 82:613.
83. Abruzzo JL. Alternate-day prednisone therapy. Ann Intern Med 1975; 82:714.
84. Bengtsson B-A, Malmvall B-E. An alternate-day corticosteroid regimen in maintenance therapy of giant cell arteritis. Acta Med Scand 1981; 209:347.
85. Fauci AS. Alternate-day corticosteroid therapy. Am J Med 1978; 64:729.
86. Allander E. ACTH or corticosteroids? A critical review of results and possibilities in the treatment of severe chronic disease. Acta Rheum Scand 1969; 15:277.
87. Kaplan HP, Portnoy B, Binder HJ, et al. A controlled evaluation of intravenous adrenocorticotropic hormone and hydrocortisone in the treatment of acute colitis. Gastroenterology 1975; 69:91.
88. Hrachovy RA, Frost JD Jr, Kellaway P, Zion TE. Double-blind study of ACTH vs prednisone therapy in infantile spasms. J Pediatr 1983; 103:641.
89. Editorial. Steroids in acute severe asthma. Lancet 1992; 340:1384.
90. McFadden ER Jr. Dosages of corticosteroids in asthma. Am Rev Respir Dis 1993; 147:1306.
91. Elenbaas J. Steroid pulse therapy in systemic lupus erythematosus. Drug Intell Clin Pharm 1983; 17:342.
92. Kurki P, ed. High dose intravenous corticosteroid therapy of systemic lupus erythematosus and primary crescenteric rapidly progressive glomerulonephritis. Proceedings of a symposium. Scand J Rheumatol 1984; Suppl 54:1.

93. Udelsman R, Ramp J, Gallucci WT, et al. Adaptation during surgical stress: a reevaluation of the role of glucocorticoids. J Clin Invest 1986; 77:1377.
94. Glowniak JV, Loriaux DL. A double-blind study of perioperative steroid requirements in secondary adrenal insufficiency. Surgery 1997; 121:123.
95. Oelkers W, Buchen S, Diederich S, et al. Impaired renal 11β-oxidation of 9α-fluorocortisol: an explanation for its mineralocorticoid potency. J Clin Endocrinol Metab 1994; 78:928.
96. Goldfein A, Laidlaw JC, Haydar NA, et al. Fluorohydrocortisone and chlorohydrocortisone, highly potent derivatives of compound F. N Engl J Med 1955; 252:415.
97. Renold AE, Haydar NA, Reddy WJ, et al. Biological effects of fluorinated derivatives of hydrocortisone and progesterone in man. Ann NY Acad Sci 1955; 61:582.
98. Thorn GW, Renold AE, Morse WI, et al. Highly potent adrenal cortical steroids; structure and biological activity. Ann Intern Med 1955; 43:979.
99. Thorn GW, Sheppard RH, Morse WI, et al. Comparative action of aldosterone and 9-alpha-fluorohydrocortisone in man. Ann NY Acad Sci 1955; 61:609.

# CHAPTER 79

# RENIN-ANGIOTENSIN SYSTEM AND ALDOSTERONE

DALILA B. CORRY AND MICHAEL L. TUCK

## THE RENIN-ANGIOTENSIN SYSTEM

### ANGIOTENSINOGEN

Angiotensinogen (AGT), also termed *renin substrate*, is the precursor for the angiotensin peptides, which include *angiotensin (A)-I, II, III, and IV, and A$_{1-7}$*. Levels of this peptide, which can be rate-limiting for the *renin-angiotensin system*, are produced mainly in the liver, where its precursor *preproangiotensinogen* is synthesized and glycosylated in the hepatocytes; nonetheless, there is evidence of production in other tissues as well (e.g., the heart, blood vessels, kidney, and adipocytes).

In the circulation, AGT, with a half-life of 16 hours, is cleaved by renin (~10%) and/or other enzymes to release A-I (Fig. 79-1). In many tissues not expressing renin, AGT can be cleaved by enzymes other than renin (e.g., cathepsin G, tonin, and chymase). The extent to which AGT is glycosylated may influence the kinetics of renin in the circulation. Indeed, this has been hypothesized in a proposed, separate, brain-AGT system.

There is one copy of the AGT gene in the mammalian genome, which is ~11,800 base pairs (bp) in length.[1,2] This gene

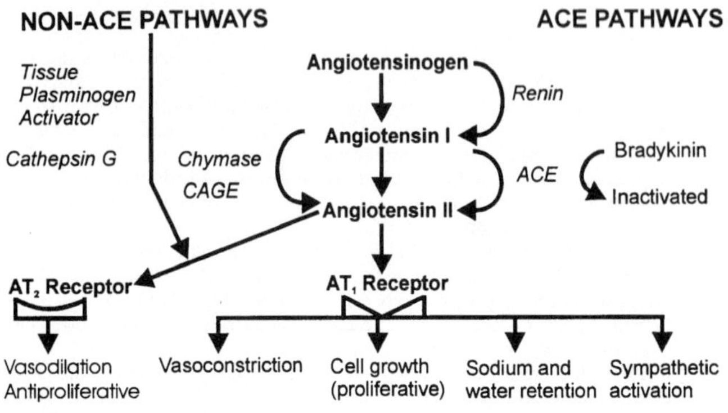

**FIGURE 79-1.** Angiotensinogen and angiotensin I and II pathways and their role in vascular and fluid homeostasis via angiotensin II receptors (*AT$_1$* and *AT$_2$*). (*CAGE*, chymotrypsin-like angiotensin-generating enzyme.)

has 5 exons that encode for the protein, separated by 4 introns. Exon 1 codes for the 5'-nontranslated region, whereas exon 2 contains the signal peptide and coding regions. AGT is secreted constitutively from hepatocytes; however, several factors (e.g., glucocorticoids, estrogens, thyroid hormone, insulin, and A-II) may exert a positive feedback.[3,4]

### RELATIONSHIP TO HYPERTENSION

A high molecular-weight form of AGT, which is released during pregnancy, may play a role in *pregnancy-induced hypertension*. In adipose tissue, there is a form of AGT that is increased by insulin and decreased by 3-adrenergic blockade and that possibly contributes to *obesity-related hypertension*. Moreover, AGT may play a role in certain other forms of hypertension, as observed in glucocorticoid excess states (e.g., Cushing syndrome) and thyroid disorders.[1-4] Interestingly, antisense nucleotide sequences that have been used to block AGT mRNA can reduce blood pressure. In spontaneously hypertensive rats, central nervous system (CNS) administration of antisense sequences against the mRNA encoding AGT lowers blood pressure.[5] Furthermore, rats made transgenic with human AGT develop hypertension because AGT is expressed in the blood vessel wall.[6,7] Thus, there is ample documentation for a role of AGT in experimental hypertension.

Further documentation for a role of AGT in hypertension is as follows: Epidemiologic studies have shown a relationship between plasma AGT and human hypertension.[8,9] Polymorphisms of the AGT gene have been linked to familial hypertension, renal disease, and cardiovascular risk factors.[9] Increased levels of AGT are associated with essential hypertension, and an M235T polymorphism in the AGT gene is associated with nephropathy in type 2 diabetics.[10] The AGT M235T molecular variant—threonine substituted for methionine at amino acid 235—is associated by linkage analysis with essential hypertension, especially in whites.[11,12] Subjects bearing the 235 allele have higher levels of AGT (i.e., a 20% increase in homozygous subjects [TT] and a 10% increase in heterozygous subjects [MT]) compared with homozygous (MM) individuals. This linkage of AGT variants to hypertension is population-dependent (i.e., strong in whites, weak in Mexican Americans[13] and the Chinese[14]). AGT mutations probably play a significant but modest role in blood pressure variation. All of these findings suggest that the renin-AGT reaction kinetics are increased by AGT variants, leading to more A-II production, which in turn may increase vascular resistance and growth. In turn, vascular injury induces AGT gene expression in the vascular media and neointima, suggesting that the renin-angiotensin system participates in myointimal proliferation.[15] Finally, gene knock-out mice for AGT develop hypotension with polyuria when challenged with a high-salt diet.[16]

### RENIN SYNTHESIS AND RELEASE

Renin, an aspartyl proteolytic enzyme, catalyzes the rate-limiting cleavage of AGT (between the leucine at position 10 and the valine at position 11) to form the *decapeptide A-I*, which is further converted by angiotensin-converting enzyme I (ACE-I) to the *octapeptide, A-II*. It is the plasma renin activity that is accepted as an index of the renin-angiotensin system, because it is difficult to measure other components (e.g., A-II).

Renin synthesis begins with the formation of *preprorenin* in the *juxtaglomerular (JG) cells* of the kidney.[17,18] This precursor is transported into the rough endoplasmic reticulum (Fig. 79-2), where it is cleaved to form a 23-amino-acid inactive form (*prorenin*), which is passed through the Golgi apparatus, glycosylated, and deposited in lysosomal granules.[18] Here it is cleaved by cathepsin B to form *renin*, which can be secreted in response to various stimuli.[18] Basally, there is a low rate of renin release, and this is increased several-fold in response to stimuli.

**Cytoplasm**

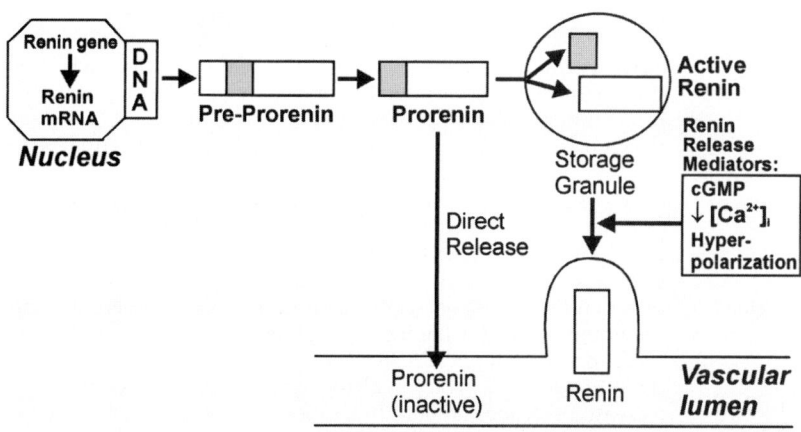

**FIGURE 79-2.** Renin synthesis, activation, and release.

Prorenin, which is not regulated by the factors that control renin release (i.e., pressure and volume changes), is released into the circulation at levels several-fold higher than those of bioactive renin.[19] Whereas the role of circulating prorenin is unknown, it is found in tissue sites such as the adrenal glands, pituitary, and submandibular glands as well as in the kidney, and in spontaneously hypertensive rats, which are stroke-prone, prorenin may raise blood pressure.[20]

Several local factors, which are under genetic control, also contribute to further enhance the renin response to salt restriction and to other stimuli. The vascular tissue-derived JG cells are situated in the afferent arteriole near the glomerulus and the *macula densa*. With salt depletion, there is a recruitment of new cells facilitating a continued renin release.[21] Additionally, the expression of the renin gene can be increased by sodium restriction.[22]

Regulation of renin release is multifactorial (i.e., by *renal baroreceptors, JG cells,* the *macula densa, renal nerves,* and *humoral factors*). The renal baroreceptor is an intrarenal vascular receptor in the afferent arteriole that stimulates renin secretion in response to reduced renal perfusion pressure. It is attenuated when renal perfusion is elevated (Fig. 79-3). This is the most powerful mechanism for renin release; it is exemplified in the Goldblatt models of hypertension, in which a unilateral stenotic lesion of the renal artery causes hypoperfusion. The hypoperfusion induces increases in renin, and, hence, results in a renin-dependent form of hypertension.

The macula densa is a modified group of cells in the distal tubules near the end of the loop of Henle and adjacent to the afferent arteriole and the JG cells. These cells sense distal tubular $Na^+$ delivery through $Cl^-$ and act through the $Na^+,K^+,Cl^-$ cotransporter pathway. Diuretics, which stimulate the cotransporter pathway, enhance renin release. Other factors (e.g., adenosine, prostaglandin $E_2$, nitric oxide, and the $\beta_1$-adrenergic system) also may mediate the macula densa renin-response pathway.[17,23]

The renal nerves (i.e., the $\beta_1$-adrenergic system) are stimulated through mechanoreceptors in the heart, pressor receptors in the aorta, and chemoreceptors in the vagal nerve. Central sympathetic stimulation increases renin secretion and is the major acute pathway for stress and posture; thus, upright posture increases plasma renin activity two- to four-fold.

Cyclic adenosine monophosphate (cAMP) is the main intracellular signal pathway for renin release, which is induced by $\beta_1$-adrenergic agonists and by prostaglandins.[24] Increased intracellular calcium provides another signal pathway; renin secretion is suppressed after rises in cytosolic calcium. Electrical depolarization of the JG cells (by increased A-II) opens calcium channels, and the high intracellular calcium inhibits renin release. Hyperpolarization of the JG cells with a resultant decrease of intracellular calcium has the opposite effect.[24] Other inhibitors of renin release include adenosine $A_1$, $\alpha$-adrenergic agonists, thromboxane, and endothelin.[24] Atrial natriuretic peptides (ANPs) and nitric oxide inhibit renin release through stimulation of cyclic guanosine monophosphate (cGMP) and guanylate cyclase. Phospholipase C-regulated changes in intracellular calcium also affect renin secretion.[24]

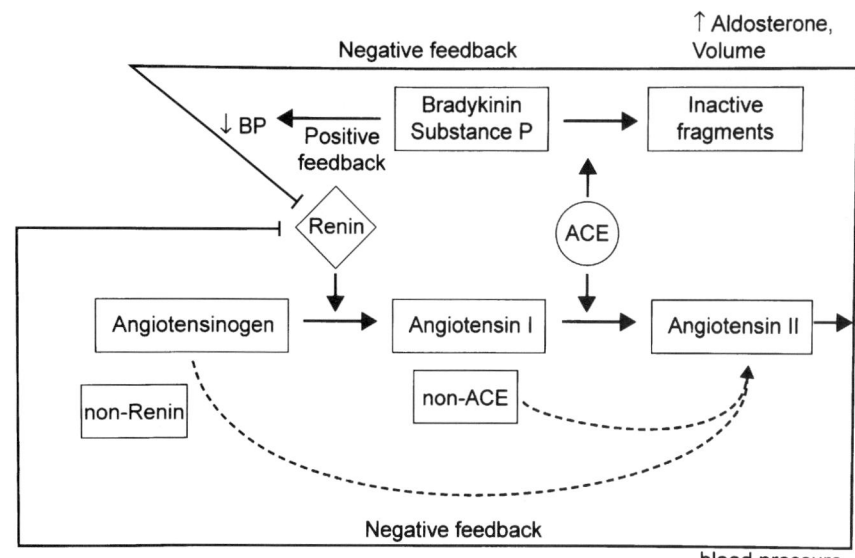

**FIGURE 79-3.** Control of renin release by negative feedback.

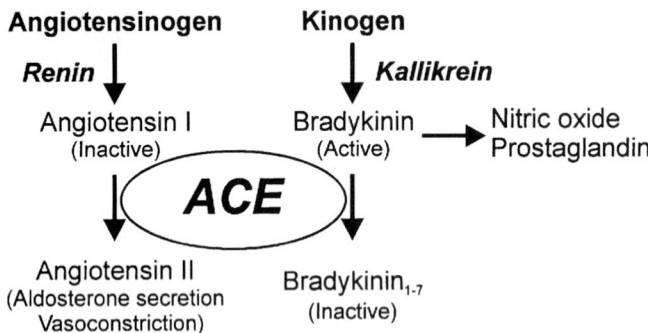

**FIGURE 79-4.** Metabolism of vasoactive peptides by angiotensin-I–converting enzyme (*ACE*).

Mice and rats that are transgenic for the renin message TGR(mREN2)27 (a model representing a precisely defined defect for the renin-angiotensin system) demonstrate that the renin gene is an important candidate gene for hypertension.[25] Thus, TGR(mREN2)27 rats, harboring the murine REN-2 gene, develop severe hypertension despite low levels of renin. The high expression of the transgene in several tissues should cause high tissue levels of renin and A-II. In this model, the high blood pressure and suppressed plasma renin activity in the face of an increased tissue renin expression suggests that an extrarenal renin-angiotensin system can mediate the hypertension.

## ANGIOTENSIN I-CONVERTING ENZYME

Angiotensin I-converting enzyme (ACE) converts the inactive decapeptide angiotensin I to the active octapeptide angiotensin II (Fig. 79-4). The enzyme is not specific for angiotensin because it cleaves bradykinin, luteinizing hormone-releasing hormone, the enkephalins, and substance P.[26,27] It is a more efficient kininase than it is a converting enzyme.[27] ACE activates the vasoconstrictor A-II and metabolizes the vasodilator bradykinin (see Fig. 79-4). ACE inhibitors block angiotensin formation and bradykinin degradation. The beneficial effects of ACE inhibitors in the heart and kidney may be a result of both A-II reduction and bradykinin accumulation.

ACE is a metalloenzyme that requires zinc as a cofactor and also needs chloride ions to cleave most substrates.[28] Human ACE has a molecular mass of 150 kDa to 180 kDa, of which 146.6 kDa is protein and the remainder is carbohydrate.[28] Most ACE is bound to plasma membranes of endothelial cells within vascular tissue. ACE is inserted into the membrane by a 17-amino acid hydrophobic region near the carboxyl terminus (*C-terminus hydrophobic anchor peptide*). ACE can be released from the plasma membrane by proteolytic cleavage; therefore, some soluble ACE can be detected in blood, urine, edema fluid, amniotic fluid, cerebrospinal fluid, lymph, seminal plasma, and prostate.[28,29]

The highest concentration of ACE is seen in the blood vessels of the lung, retina, and brain.[29] The human kidney also contains a very large amount of this enzyme.[28] The brush border of the proximal tubules (where A-II has major functions in electrolyte transport) is rich in ACE. It is also abundant in the choroid plexus, the placenta, and the epithelial lining of the small intestine, and seems to be highly concentrated in some areas of the brain (e.g., the subfornical organ, area postrema, substantia nigra, and locus coeruleus).

The primary structure of ACE consists of two active centers that are located within two homologous domains.[29,30] Most tissues have both domains, but testicular tissue has only one domain, perhaps representing an early form of the enzyme that has not been duplicated.[30] In endothelial cells, ACE contains two functional sites (requiring two zinc ions) and two inhibitor-binding sites.

ACE has in vitro activity for a broad range of substrates besides A-I (e.g., *N*-acetyl-seryl-aspartyl-lysyl-proline [Ac-SDKP], which is a regulatory factor for hematopoiesis).[26,27,31] In vivo, plasma levels of Ac-SDKP increase sharply after oral administration of an ACE inhibitor.[31] ACE inhibition, which is the treatment of choice for the erythrocytosis that occurs after renal transplantation, lowers the erythrocyte count independently of any effect on erythropoietin. Thus, ACE appears to have a role in the regulation of hematopoiesis.

The human ACE gene displays an insertion (I)/deletion (D) polymorphism, which accounts for at least half of the variability in serum ACE levels.[32] One such I/D polymorphism, which has been found in the noncoding region, corresponds to the presence or absence of a 287-bp sequence in intron 16.[32] Individuals who are homozygous for the insertion polymorphism (II) have lower levels of circulating ACE than do individuals with the deletion (DD) genotype.[33] The D allele may be associated with an increased risk for coronary heart disease and diabetic nephropathy. Individuals with diabetic nephropathy who are DD homozygous may respond less well to ACE inhibitors with respect to reducing blood pressure and proteinuria.[33] These individuals are also more salt sensitive, such that on a high salt diet, ACE inhibition is less effective. Furthermore, a deletion variant of the ACE D allele is associated with an increased risk of diabetic nephropathy and hastened progression of IgA nephropathy.[34] This deletion in ACE does not appear to affect outcome of renal transplants.[35] A link between the D allele and plasminogen activator inhibitor-l levels in diabetes and microangiopathy suggests that an adverse consequence of thrombotic mechanisms can be activated with ACE polymorphism.[36]

Other A-II–forming serine proteinases such as chymase have been identified in the human cardiac left ventricle and in vascular, renal, and other tissues.[37] These enzymes serve as alternative routes in the conversion of A-I to A-II.[37] These non-ACE enzymes may explain the incomplete blockade of A-II formation during ACE-inhibition therapy.

## ANGIOTENSIN METABOLISM

Of the several active angiotensins, A-II is the most important. The enzymes that are most active in degrading angiotensin are the aminopeptidases (Fig. 79-5). Glutamyl aminopeptidase cleaves A-II to form A-III ($A_{2-8}$), and arginyl aminopeptidase cleaves A-III to A-IV ($A_{3-8}$).[38] Although $A_{3-8}$ does not have major pressor activity, it does increase cGMP levels and may have central effects.[38] The amino-terminal heptapeptide, $A_{1-7}$ [des-phe8], which is formed directly from A-I by several tissue endopeptidases or by ACE,[39] can stimulate the release of arginine vasopressin (AVP), vasodilator prostaglandins, bradykinin, and nitric oxide.[39,40] Most angiotensins have a very short duration of action and undergo enzymatic degradation and endocytosis. The $AT_1$ receptor can mediate intracellular transport of A-II and the ligand-receptor can also be internalized. The acute inhibition of ACE decreases levels of A-II, but chronic inhibition therapy may not suppress A-II, although it does raise levels of $A_{1-7}$ (a competitive inhibitor of A-II); this phenomenon possibly explains the long-term antihypertensive effects of ACE-I.[39,40]

## TISSUE RENIN-ANGIOTENSIN SYSTEM

Local renin-angiotensin systems in multiple tissues can produce A-II independently of the circulating renin-angiotensin system (Table 79-1). Their function of these systems is probably to permit regional modulation of blood flow and also to assist in the action of growth factors. Most contractile cells (e.g., vascular smooth muscle, heart cells, mesangial cells, and sperm tails) have a well-defined local renin-angiotensin system. A-II is

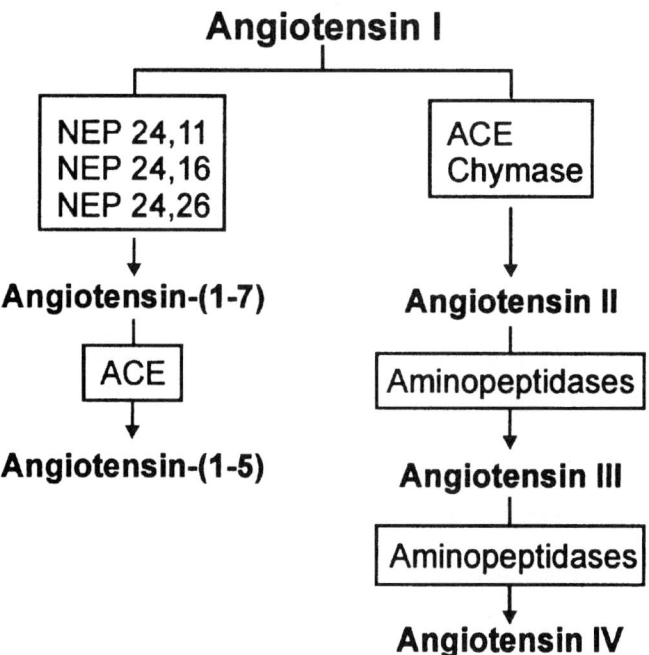

**FIGURE 79-5.** Enzymes that convert angiotensin I into other angiotensin peptide products.

**TABLE 79-1.**
Differences in Circulating and Tissue Renin-Angiotensin System Control and Action

|  | CIRCULATING | TISSUE |
|---|---|---|
| **Control** | Short-term effect due to rapid feedback | Long-term effects |
| **Kidney** | Na$^+$ and water reabsorption | Intraglomerular pressure |
| **Heart** | Chronotropic effect Arrythmogenic | Myocyte cell growth |
| **Vessels** | Vasoconstriction | Vascular cell growth |

formed in these cells either by renin or through other proteases such as chymase, cathepsin, or tonin.[41–43]

**Kidney Renin-Angiotensin System.** In addition to being the major site for release of systemic renin, the kidney has a local renin-angiotensin system that is involved in renal growth.[44] ACE-I administration during pregnancy causes severe fetal renal abnormalities. The tubular epithelial cells contain ACE, and local A-II is found in proximal tubules and mesangial cells.[45] The intrarenal A-II constricts afferent and efferent arterioles and directly increases Na$^+$ reabsorption. Locally, A-II is also involved in renal pathologic conditions (e.g., the development of nephrosclerosis).

**Cardiac Renin-Angiotensin System.** Evidence exists for a role for an intracardiac renin-angiotensin system in both normal and failing hearts.[41,42] There is a direct expression of AGT and the A-II receptor (AT$_1$) in cardiomyocytes. The exact source of the renin in cardiac tissue is controversial, because levels of mRNA are low.[43] The heart can also express A-I, which may be converted by intracardiac ACE to A-II.[43] Probably, cardiac renin-angiotensin system activity is regulated by the amount of AGT, ACE, or renin-binding protein in the cardiomyocytes. Consequently, local A-II can regulate vascular tone, contractility, growth, and cardiac hypertrophy.

**Vascular Renin-Angiotensin System.** Vascular tissue has an active tissue renin-angiotensin system. Both ACE mRNA and product are found in the endothelium, and also, to a lesser degree, in vascular smooth muscle cells.[43] AGT, which is also expressed in cultured vascular smooth muscle cells, is stimulated by insulin and insulin-like growth factor-I (IGF-I).[46] The specific origin of the renin in the vasculature is more controversial, because the mRNA is low. Nonetheless, in situ conversion of A-I to A-II does occur in the vasculature; thus, there is an active ACE, which probably has a regulatory role.[43] Insulin and IGF-I–induced vascular growth and hypertrophy are mediated in part by a local renin-angiotensin system and attenuated by ACE-I and AT$_1$-receptor blockers.[46]

**Ovarian Renin-Angiotensin System.** The ovarian cells produce high concentrations of both renin and prorenin, and all components of the renin-angiotensin system are found in follicular fluid.[47] The granulosa and theca cells also contain renin and angiotensin. Because prorenin is secreted throughout pregnancy,

it may have functional significance during this time. A possible role for A-II as a reproductive hormone is being investigated.[48]

**Testicular Renin-Angiotensin System.** A-I, -II, and -III are found in the testicular tissue, and AT$_1$ receptors are present in Leydig cells.[48,49] The structure of testicular ACE is unique; it has only one of the two binding domains. Perhaps, testicular ACE and A-II participate in spermatogenesis and may play a role in male fertility.[49]

**Adipose Renin-Angiotensin System.** Adipose tissue is a rich source for AGT.[50] Locally formed A-II from adipose tissue may cause vasoconstriction and hypertension, especially as body fat content increases.

**Skin Renin-Angiotensin System.** The human skin fibroblast expresses A-II and AGT mRNA. Local injury elevates local A-II concentrations, and it then participates in wound healing through growth factors.

**Adrenal Renin-Angiotensin System.** Some of the highest levels of A-II are found in the adrenal cortex, within the adrenal zona glomerulosa and fasciculata.[51] Local A-II is thought to play an important role in aldosterone and corticosteroid production. Renin is known to be produced in adrenal tissue and acts independently of plasma renin.

**Brain Renin-Angiotensin System.** The blood–brain barrier prevents any blood-borne components of the renin-angiotensin system from entering the brain; thus, this organ has a local renin-angiotensin system. The expression of renin mRNA is low in the brain, but some cells (e.g., glial cells) have marked expression of AGT.[52] However, the expression and production of ACE is widespread throughout the brain.[52] Moreover, AT$_1$ receptors are in the hypothalamus and AT$_2$ receptors are in the locus coeruleus and in the inferior olivary region. In addition, receptors for A-IV and A$_{1-7}$ are also found in the brain.[52] Direct injection of A-II into the brain causes changes in drinking behavior and elevations of blood pressure.

The anterior pituitary gland has high levels of renin and A-II (located mainly in the gonadotropes); thus, the renin-angiotensin system may contribute to the regulation of estrogen production in females and testosterone production in males. Interestingly, A-II inhibits prolactin release. Importantly, the human brain (especially the pineal gland) is rich in chymase, which can convert A-I to A-II.[53]

## ANGIOTENSIN RECEPTORS

A-II binds and acts on its receptors at the cell surface. Several receptor subtypes have been found, including the $AT_1$, $AT_2$, and $AT_4$.[54–56]

**AT$_1$ Receptor Subtype.** Almost all actions of A-II are mediated through the AT$_1$ receptor, including its effects on vasoconstriction and aldosterone production and cell growth (Fig. 79-6). The AT$_1$ receptor is part of the *superfamily* of peptide hormone receptors with seven membrane-spanning regions linked to G proteins (Fig. 79-7). AT$_1$ activates phospholipase C, which in turn hydrolyzes phosphoinositide to inositol triphosphate (IP$_3$) and diacylglycerol.[54] These changes increase the intracellular calcium levels that in turn activate protein kinases. Also, AT$_1$ receptors appear to lower levels of intracellular

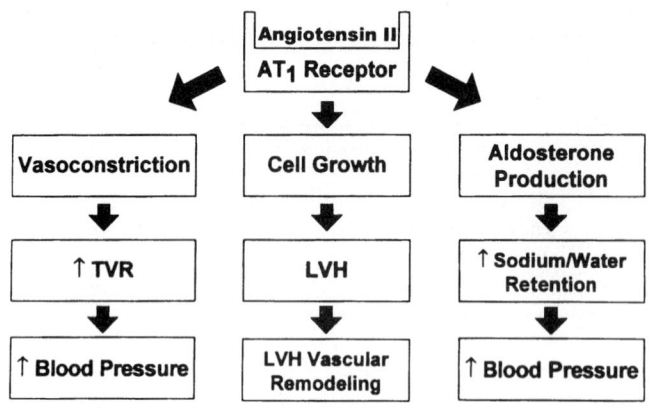

**FIGURE 79-6.** Three major pathways of the angiotensin II ($AT_1$) receptor.

cAMP, an effect that is most evident in the adrenal gland on the control of aldosterone secretion.[54]

Although the $AT_1$ receptor contains no intrinsic protein kinase activity, numerous studies indicate that A-II activates both nonreceptor-type and receptor-type tyrosine kinases.[56] Thus, A-II binding to the $AT_1$ receptor stimulates a large variety of regulated cellular events, including activation of phospholipases, second messenger generation, and protein phosphorylation. The enzymes that may be coupled to the $AT_1$ receptor include adenylate cyclase and phospholipases C, D, and A.[54]

**$AT_2$ Receptor Subtype.** Table 79-2 contrasts the actions of the A-II $AT_1$ and $AT_2$ receptor subtypes. Attention has been directed to the $AT_2$ receptor subtype, which is found in fetal tissue, where it is responsible for the growth and remodeling of organs.[57] It is likely that the actions of the $AT_2$ receptor may antagonize those of the $AT_1$ receptor (Table 79-2). Using the gene transfer approach, it has been shown that the $AT_2$ receptor participates in vascular smooth muscle growth through apoptosis.[57] $AT_2$ receptors have been identified in the adult brain, in the adre-

**TABLE 79-2.**
**Actions of the Angiotensin $AT_1$ and $AT_2$ Receptors**

| $AT_1$ RECEPTOR | $AT_2$ RECEPTOR |
|---|---|
| Vasoconstriction | Vasodilation |
| Growth | Growth inhibition |
| Anti-apoptotic | Pro-apoptotic |
| Pro-fibrotic | Fibrosis (?) |
| Pro-thrombotic | Thrombosis (?) |
| Pro-oxidant | Anti-oxidant (?) |

nal medulla, in the gastrointestinal tract, and in other tissues. $AT_2$ receptors also facilitate intestinal sodium reabsorption. It has been demonstrated that an A-II receptor antagonist can correct endothelial dysfunction in human essential hypertension.

## ACTIONS OF ANGIOTENSIN II

**Renal Sodium and Water Retention.** The best known function of A-II is *to support the circulation under conditions of reduced intravascular volume*. However, there are >50 known physiologic actions. These include vasoconstriction, salt retention through aldosterone, increased thirst and secretion of antidiuretic hormone resulting in retention of water, increased cardiac output, and stimulation of sympathetic nervous system activity (Table 79-3). Also, there are direct effects of A-II on early proximal tubule Na$^+$ reabsorption that are mediated in part through the Na$^+$, H$^+$ antiporter; this accounts for 40% to 50% of sodium and water reabsorption.[58] In AGT gene-null mutant mice, chronic volume depletion causes a sharp decrease in glomerular filtration rate (GFR) and a marked concentration defect, which is insensitive to AVP.[59] Furthermore, the renin-angiotensin system is essential for two fundamental homeostatic functions in the kidney, stabilizing the GFR and maintaining urine diluting and concentrating capacity.

**TABLE 79-3.**
**Angiotensin II Actions in Various Target Tissues**

| Action | Target Tissue |
|---|---|
| Vasoconstriction | Vascular smooth muscle |
| Hypertophy/hyperplasia | Vascular smooth muscle |
| Aldosterone secretion | Adrenal glomerulosa |
| Contractility, hypertrophy | Myocardium |
| Embryogenesis | Kidney |
| Sodium reabsorption | Proximal tubule of kidney |
| Contraction | Mesangium of kidney |
| Inhibition of renin release | Juxtaglomerular cells |
| Increased prostaglandins, nitric oxide, endothelin | Vascular endothelium |
| Extracellular matrix synthesis | Vascular connective tissue |
| Platelet aggregation | Platelets |
| Monocyte adhesion | Vessel wall |
| Prolactin inhibition | Anterior pituitary |
| ADH inhibition, thirst | Posterior pituitary |
| Norepinephrine release | Sympathetic neurons |
| Catecholamine release | Adrenal medulla |
| Pressor control | Brain |
| Baroreceptor control | Brain |
| ADH control | Brain |
| Salt/water absorption | Intestine ($AT_2$) |
| Angiotensinogen synthesis | Liver |
| Glycogenolysis | Liver |
| Decreased apoptosis | Tissues |

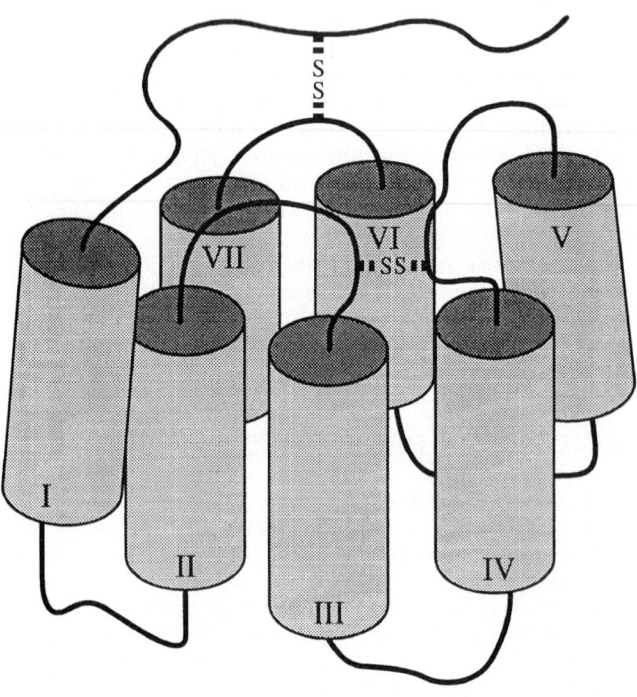

**FIGURE 79-7.** Model of angiotensin II ($AT_1$) receptor. (From Hunyady L, Balla T, Catt KJ. The ligand binding sites of the angiotensin AT1 receptor. Trends Pharmacol Sci 1996; 17:135.)

**Systemic Vasoconstriction.**    A-II produces arteriolar vaso-constriction and elevates vascular resistance and blood pressure. The signal transduction for this A-II–mediated vasoconstriction includes an increase of intracellular calcium and formation of protein kinase C.[60] The facilitated release of norepinephrine[61] and endothelin-I[62] may also contribute to the vasoconstriction that is induced by A-II. A-II stimulates the release of arachidonic acid products in the vasculature (e.g., lipoxygenase products and $P_{450}$ epoxides), which have vasoconstrictive properties.[63]

**Regulation of Gomerular Filtration Rate.**    A-II regulates the GFR and renal blood flow by constricting the efferent and afferent glomerular arterioles, and the interlobular artery.[64] A-II differentially increases efferent resistance to levels that are two to three times those of the afferent resistance; this elevates glomerular capillary pressure to maintain the single nephron GFR.

In AGT gene-null mutant mice, chronic volume depletion causes a sharp decrease in GFR and a marked concentration defect, which is insensitive to AVP.[59] These physiologic changes are paralleled by changes in renal structure at the glomerular level as well as at the renal papilla and underscore the key role of angiotensins in the development of the mammalian kidney. As mentioned previously, A-II can also stimulate prostaglandins (e.g., thromboxane) that mediate renal hemodynamics.[65] A-II controls the GFR by constricting the mesangium and altering tubuloglomerular feedback. In sodium-replete women, A-II infusion elicits a blunted renal microcirculatory response compared with the response in sodium-replete men; this demonstrates that sex steroids modulate the effects of A-II.[66] A-II also has nonhemodynamic effects on the kidney (e.g., stimulation of cytokines in diabetic nephropathy).[67]

**Cardiac Effects.**    The cardiac effects of the tissue angiotensin system are multiple.[68] A-II is involved in cardiac remodeling and, through the $AT_1$ receptor, promotes extracellular production of matrix as well as a fibrous tissue response and increasing collagen levels. In addition, the vasoconstriction caused by A-II and oxidative stress further contribute to ischemia and left ventricular hypertrophy with a resultant greater stiffness of the myocardial wall.[69] Elevations in plasma renin activity are associated with increased risk for myocardial infarction.[70] This risk may be related to renin-angiotensin-system–induced changes in the fibrinolytic system, because A-II inhibits fibrinolysis (thereby promoting clot formation) and stimulates excess production of plasminogen activator inhibitor.[71] Also, the ACE-induced breakdown of bradykinin leads to lower tissue type plasminogen activator levels and decreases nitric oxide concentrations. A low-salt diet increases plasminogen activator inhibitor activity by increasing the renin-angiotensin system and raising the aldosterone levels.[72] These findings help to explain why blockade of the renin-angiotensin system by ACE-I or by $AT_1$ receptor antagonists protect against thrombotic cardiac events and reduce the risk of recurrent myocardial infarctions.

**Brain Effects.**    There are several actions of the angiotensins in the brain, an organ in which all three receptor subtypes exist.[52] In addition, A-II exerts a central pressor activity and causes blunting of the baroreceptor; it also stimulates dipsogenic behavior and the synthesis of AVP.

**Other Effects.**    Other actions of A-II include platelet adhesion, glycogenolysis, and inhibition of prolactin release. A-II also has interactions with prostaglandins, nitric oxide, and endothelin. More diverse effects include contraction of the uterus, blockade of the effects of glucagon, stimulation of catecholamines, stimulation of endothelial cell growth, stimulation of ovulation, and regulation of steroidogenesis. Moreover, A-II selectively stimulates transforming growth factor-β and stimulates mRNA in the heart and kidneys (thereby contributing to cardiac and renal fibrosis), and it suppresses *clusterin*, a glycoprotein that is expressed in response to tissue injury.[73]

Functional analysis of A-II and other components of the renin-angiotensin system can now be achieved by transgenic and gene-targeting technology.[74,75] The direct transfection of the human renin gene using gene-transfer techniques in hepatocytes in vivo elevates blood pressure. In vivo transfection of antisense oligodeoxynucleotides for AGT decreases plasma AGT levels and blood pressure in spontaneously hypertensive rats.[74] Transfection of antisense to AGT or $AT_1$ receptors decreases blood pressure in spontaneously hypertensive rats.[76] Vascular injury is associated with abundant expression of AGT and ACE. This process of vascular hypertrophy can be duplicated by transfecting ACE vector locally into intact rat carotid arteries.[74] In vivo transfer of antisense ACE oligodeoxynucleotides inhibits neointimal formation in balloon-injured rat carotid arteries.[74]

Antisense technology has been used to examine the role of the renin-angiotensin system in the central nervous system (see earlier).[76] Conceivably, a gene therapy for hypertension could use an antisense inhibition with adeno-associated viral vector delivery to target the A-II type 1 receptor messenger ribonucleic acid.[76] Prolonged reductions in blood pressure in hypertension may be achieved with a single dose of adeno-associated viral vectors to deliver antisense oligodeoxynucleotides to inhibit $AT_1$ receptors.[76]

## ALDOSTERONE

Aldosterone is the most potent of several mineralocorticoid steroid hormones that act on the epithelium, especially in the kidney, to produce $Na^+$ reabsorption and $K^+$ excretion.[77] Other steroids that have weaker mineralocorticoid effects include deoxycorticosterone (DOC), 18-oxycortisol, 19-nor-deoxycorticosterone (19-nor-DOC), and 18-hydroxydeoxycorticosterone (18-OH-DOC).

### SYNTHESIS

The adrenal gland is partitioned into different zones, which contain specific enzymes that produce either glucocorticoids (i.e., cortisol), mineralocorticoids (i.e., aldosterone), or weak adrenal androgens.[78,79] Aldosterone is synthesized in the outer region of the adrenal gland (zona glomerulosa). Cortisol is synthesized in the inner regions in the zona fasciculata and reticularis. The same adrenal enzymes share most of the early synthetic steps of these steroids, but they differ markedly in their terminal enzymes. The zona glomerulosa is unique in lacking 17α-hydroxylase, the essential enzyme for cortisol formation. However, the zona glomerulosa is rich in the enzyme aldosterone synthase, which is required for the terminal steps in aldosterone synthesis.[78-80] Aldosterone synthase is a single multifunctional P450 enzyme on the inner mitochondrial membrane that converts corticosterone to aldosterone. It catalyzes three successive hydroxylation steps: (a) conversion of deoxycorticosterone to corticosterone; (b) addition of a hydroxyl group to corticosterone (18-OH-corticosterone); and (c) conversion of 18-OH-corticosterone to an aldehyde, with consequent formation of aldosterone. Two cytochrome P450 enzymes have been found, including 11β-hydroxylase and aldosterone synthase.[78] Their genes are located in close proximity (40 kb) on chromosome 8 (8q21-q22) and display 95% homology. In the familial disorder *glucocorticoid-remediable hyperaldosteronism*, there is hypertension and variable hypokalemia as a result of the formation of a chimeric gene that makes aldosterone synthesis ACTH-dependent[78] (see Chap. 80).

### MINERALOCORTICOID RECEPTORS

The mineralocorticoid receptor (*steroid receptor type 1 [SR1]*) binds both aldosterone and cortisol with equal affinity, whereas the cortisol receptor (*steroid receptor type 2 [SR2]*) binds only cortisol with high affinity.[81,82] Both receptors are part of the *steroid/vitamin D/retinoic acid superfamily of transcription regulators*. Both receptors have high amino acid homology and may overlap the actions of progesterone and androgen receptors. In humans, there are two isoforms of the SR1; the α and β isoforms.[83,84] The SR1s are found mainly on epithelial cells of the renal tubule, the parotid gland, and the colon. SR1s have been found in vascular smooth muscle, in the heart, and in areas of the brain. These receptors can undergo down-regulation, as seen with sodium loading in which the β isoform expression is decreased.[84] In contrast, SR2s are found in most cells of the body.

Glucocorticoids and mineralocorticoids bind to SR1 with equal affinity, and glucocorticoid levels are 1000-fold higher than those of mineralocorticoids; thus, one would expect the receptor to be saturated with cortisol. However, specificity is conferred by the enzyme 11β-*hydroxysteroid dehydrogenase (HSD)*,[78,79,85] which oxidizes cortisol to inactive corticosterone, thus allowing aldosterone to bind to its receptor. Thus, coexpression of 11β-HSD and SR1 in tissues appears to be a mechanism by which specificity is conferred to aldosterone action. There are multiple forms of this enzyme in the mammalian kidney,[86] including a high density form in the principal and intercalated cells.[87] In the *syndrome of apparent mineralocorticoid excess*, the renal isoform for 11β-HSD$_2$ is missing, thus allowing the normally high concentrations of cortisol in the kidney to bind to SR1.[78] This effect creates an excess Na$^+$ reabsorption with resultant hypertension and hypokalemia (see Chap. 80). The active ingredient of licorice, glycyrrhetinic acid, also inhibits 11β-HSD$_2$, causing an acquired syndrome of mineralocorticoid excess in humans. However, several questions remain regarding mineral corticoid receptors.[87a]

## ALDOSTERONE ACTION

The major site of aldosterone action is on the distal nephron, where it increases Na$^+$ reabsorption and K$^+$ and H$^+$ secretion. Aldosterone initiates its action by diffusing across the plasma membrane of the cell and binding avidly to specific receptors, which are located mostly in the cytoplasm.[82] In the nucleus, the aldosterone-receptor complex acts on chromatin to increase mRNA and ribosomal RNA transcription.[87,88] The binding of steroid to the carboxyl terminal of the receptor causes release of heat shock proteins, after which the receptor changes conformation to allow dimerization and binding to the regulatory end of specific target genes (*hormone-responsive elements*).[82]

Mineralocorticoids affect electrolyte balance by inducing and activating proteins in epithelial cells (e.g., *aldosterone-induced protein* may act as a regulatory unit for the luminal membrane Na$^+$ channel to allow luminal Na$^+$ to enter the cell).[89,90] Another aldosterone-induced protein may be a subunit of the Na$^+$, K$^+$ pump. This strengthens the argument that aldosterone not only has an indirect effect through ionic changes but also has a direct action on the Na$^+$, K$^+$ pump.[88]

The major sites for aldosterone action are in the connecting segment and in the collecting tubules.[78] Aldosterone promotes NaCl reabsorption and K$^+$ secretion in the connecting segments and in the principal cells in the cortical collecting tubules. In addition, it may act on Na$^+$ in the papillary (inner medullary) collecting tubule and is thought to increase ionic transport by increasing the number of open Na$^+$ and K$^+$ channels in the luminal membrane.[89,90] Aldosterone also stimulates the Na$^+$, K$^+$ pump in the basolateral membrane. Na$^+$ then diffuses into the tubular cells from which the Na$^+$ is removed by the Na$^+$, K$^+$ pump, thus creating an electrogenic negative potential difference within the lumen. K$^+$ is also secreted from the cell as Cl$^-$ moves in to maintain electroneutrality. Another mechanism for K$^+$ efflux is through the Na$^+$, K$^+$ pump. It is believed that aldosterone mediates Na$^+$ channel movement by the methylation of channel proteins that, in turn, activate silent or inoperative Na$^+$ channels.[90] Because amiloride blocks luminal Na$^+$ permeability, it is likely that increasing luminal permeability is one of the primary actions of aldosterone.[91] Intracellular calcium changes may serve as second messenger for this response by increasing the number of open Na$^+$ channels.[92]

The intercalated cells in the renal cortex and the tubular cells of the outer medullary region seem to be the sites for aldosterone action on H$^+$ secretion.[93] These cells do not activate Na$^+$ reabsorption; therefore, aldosterone-mediated H$^+$ secretion and Na$^+$ reabsorption occur in different regions of the kidney. However, there is a modest Na$^+$/H$^+$ exchange process mediated by aldosterone in the principal cells.

Although aldosterone acts almost exclusively on the kidney, there are other epithelial sites (e.g., the colon, sweat and salivary glands) where the hormone reduces the Na$^+$ and raises the K$^+$ content of secretions.[78] In very end-stage renal failure, the colonic secretion of K$^+$ can become an important route of elimination.

Aldosterone may be implicated in the fibrosis of left ventricular hypertrophy and congestive heart failure.[94-97] In fact, the heart could be capable of de novo synthesis. The hormone may have effects on vascular remodeling and collagen formation as well as modifying endothelial cell function, and the cardiac angiotensin AT$_1$ receptor may be one of its targets.[94-97] A local or tissue aldosterone, which has been found in vascular smooth muscle, may contribute to A-II–induced vascular hypertrophy.[96] Thus, hypertension, cardiac fibrosis, and hypertrophy by nonepithelial cells may, in part, be consequences of high aldosterone levels, in either the primary or the secondary forms of hyperaldosteronism.[95,96] Evidence suggests that many of the effects of aldosterone on blood pressure and the resultant pathologic changes could be mediated through specific mineralocorticoid receptors in the AV3V region of the brain and in the heart.[98] Some of these nonepithelial effects are blocked either by aldosterone-receptor antagonists (e.g., spironolactone) or by selective aldosterone-receptor agonists (e.g., eplerenone). In the Randomized Aldactone Evaluation Study (RALES) trial, the addition of low-dose spironolactone (25 mg) to standard therapy for congestive heart failure further reduced total mortality and/or the hospitalization rate for heart failure by 31%.[99] Hyperaldosteronism occurs in renal failure despite normal renin levels. Furthermore, aldosterone appears to contribute to the progression of renal disease by causing fibrosis and glomerular damage, as seen in the rat remnant kidney model.[100] More details of aldosterone action may be seen in a review.[100a]

## CONTROL OF ALDOSTERONE SECRETION

**The Renin-Angiotensin System.**   A-II is the major stimulator of aldosterone secretion. The proximal site of action of A-II is in enhancing the conversion of cholesterol to pregnenolone, but it also can modulate the distal regulatory site influencing the conversion of corticosterone to aldosterone by acting on aldosterone synthase.[80,101,102] In general, the renin-angiotensin system is the major mediator of the volume-induced changes in aldosterone. Thus, volume and/or salt depletion will stimulate renin release, producing more A-II to act on the adrenal gland. The resulting Na$^+$ retention then restores the volume to normal and shuts off renin release. The converse effect is seen with volume overload or with a high-salt diet, in which the renin-angiotensin system and aldosterone secretion are suppressed, allowing excess Na$^+$ to be excreted. With volume expansion, there also is release of the ANPs and of dopamine, which, as inhibitors of aldosterone secretion, may act in concert with a low A-II level to limit the release of this mineralocorticoid.

**Plasma Potassium Concentration.**   There is a direct relationship between increases in plasma K$^+$ and increases in aldosterone secretion.[103] Studies of K$^+$ infusion in humans show that a 0.1- to 0.2-mEq/L change in plasma K$^+$ can alter aldosterone levels, suggesting that the zona glomerulosa is exquisitely sensitive to K$^+$.[104] In the feedback cycle, an increasing plasma K$^+$ level stimulates aldosterone, which in turn increases K$^+$ secretion and restores it to normal. This mechanism protects against excessive K$^+$ in the body; it represents the single pathway for handling K$^+$ overload. K$^+$ has a direct effect on the zona glomerulosa cells to stimulate aldosterone synthesis, thereby activating the conversion of cholesterol to pregnenolone.[105] Although both A-II and K$^+$ act on the zona glomerulosa through different and independent effects, their cumulative action can be synergistic.[106] Thus, A-II is more effective in releasing aldosterone when the subject is on a high K$^+$ diet. This effect may be a result of adrenal renin, because in vitro studies show that K$^+$ enhances adrenal renin and adrenal A-II. Both young and elderly subjects have similar basal serum potassium levels and similar responses to a K$^+$ infusion; however, during a K$^+$ infusion, hyperkalemia is more pronounced in elderly subjects because of a blunted adrenal response.[107]

**Corticotropin.** As with cortisol release, ACTH, acting through adenylate cyclase, acutely stimulates aldosterone secretion in a dose-dependent manner; however, this effect is not sustained.[108] Thus, ACTH is not considered an important chronic regulator of aldosterone. ACTH initially stimulates and then suppresses the aldosterone-synthase gene.[108] ACTH also directs steroid biosynthesis through the enzyme 17α-hydroxylase, which diverts synthesis away from the mineralocorticoid pathway and into the glucocorticoid and androgen pathways.

**Other Factors.** The plasma Na$^+$ concentration is a weak regulator of aldosterone; hyponatremia increases aldosterone levels, and hypernatremia possibly has the opposite effect.[109] In humans, extreme changes in plasma Na$^+$ are required to alter aldosterone secretion independently from more powerful stimuli (e.g., A-II and K$^+$). Hyponatremia usually involves water retention, which (by suppression of A-II) overrides any direct action of Na$^+$ on adrenal gland aldosterone synthesis.[110] There is a modest effect of systemic acidosis on adrenal aldosterone release; this increases the excretion of acid and reduces systemic acidemia.[111] The effect of aldosterone is thought to be through the H$^+$-ATPase pumps on the luminal membrane of the collecting tubules.

*Aldosterone escape* occurs when, after several days of administration of this hormone, there is a loss of normal sodium- and fluid-retaining capacity, and a spontaneous diuresis occurs. This escape mechanism, which is caused by increases in ANPs and by a rise in renal perfusion pressure that limits Na$^+$ retention, is observed in primary hyperaldosteronism and perhaps in the inherited forms of mineralocorticoid hypertension, conditions in which edema is not seen, despite a volume retention state.[112]

# REFERENCES

1. Corvol P, Jeunemaitre X. Molecular genetics of human hypertension: role of angiotensinogen. Endocr Rev 1997; 18(5):662.
2. Kim HS, Krege JH, Kluckman KD, et al. Genetic control of blood pressure and the angiotensinogen locus. Proc Natl Acad Sci U S A 1995; 92:2735.
3. Brasier AR, Li J. Mechanisms for inducible control of angiotensinogen gene transcription. Hypertension 1996; 27:465.
4. Klett CP, Printz MP, Bader M, et al. Angiotensinogen messenger RNA stabilization by angiotensin II. J Hypertens 1996; 14(Suppl 1):S25.
5. Wielbo D, Sernia C, Gyurko R, Phillips MJ. Antisense inhibition of hypertension in the spontaneously hypertensive rat. Hypertension 1995; 25:314.
6. Naftilan AJ, Zuo WM, Ingelfinger J, et al. Localization and differential regulation of angiotensinogen mRNA expression in the vessel wall. J Clin Invest 1991; 88:1300.
7. Schunkert H, Ingelfinger JR, Hirsch AT, et al. Evidence for tissue specific activation of renal angiotensinogen mRNA expression in chronic stable experimental heart failure. J Clin Invest 1992; 90:1523.
8. Inoue I, Nakajima T, Williams CS, et al. A nucleotide substitution in the promoter of human angiotensinogen is associated with essential hypertension. J Clin Invest 1997; 99:1786.
9. Corvol P, Persu A, Gimenez-Roqueplo AP, Jeunemaitre X. Seven lessons from two candidate genes in human essential hypertension: angiotensinogen and epithelial sodium channel. Hypertension 1999; 33:1324.
10. Freire MBS, Ji L, Onuma T, et al. Gender-specific association of M235T polymorphism in angiotensinogen gene and diabetic nephropathy in NIDDM. Hypertension 1998; 31:896.
11. Kunz R, Kreutze R, Beige J, et al. Association between the angiotensinogen 235T variant and essential hypertension in whites: a systematic review and methodological appraisal. Hypertension 1997; 30:1331.
12. Staessen JA, Kuznetsova T, Wang JG, et al. M235T angiotensinogen polymorphism and cardiovascular renal risk. J Hypertens 1999; 17:9.
13. Atwood LD, Kammerer CM, Samollow PB. Linkage of essential hypertension to the angiotensinogen locus in Mexican Americans. Hypertension 1997; 30:326.
14. Niu T, Xu X, Rogus J, et al. Angiotensinogen gene and hypertension in Chinese. J Clin Invest 1998; 101:188.
15. Rakugi H, Jacob HJ, Krieger JE, et al. Vascular injury induces angiotensinogen gene expression in the media and neointima. Circulation 1993; 87:283.
16. Umemura S, Kihara M, Sumida Y, et al. Endocrinological abnormalities in angiotensinogen-gene knockout mice: studies of hormonal responses to dietary salt loading. J Hypertens 1998; 16:285.
17. Navar LG, Inscho EW, Majid SA, et al. Paracrine regulation of the renal microcirculation. Physiol Rev 1996; 76:425.
18. Skott O, Jensen BL. Cellular and intrarenal control of renin secretion. Clin Sci 1993; 84:1.
19. Toffelmire EB, Slater K, Corvol P, et al. Response of prorenin and active renin to chronic and acute alterations of renin secretion in normal humans. Studies using a direct immunoradiometric assay. J Clin Invest 1989; 83:679.
20. Hosoi M, Kim S, Takada T, et al. Effects of prorenin on blood pressure and plasma renin concentrations in stroke-prone spontaneously hypertensive rats. Am J Physiol 1992; 262:E234.
21. Gomez RA, Chevalier RL, Everett AD. Recruitment of renin gene-expressing cells in adult rat kidney. Am J Physiol 1990; 259:F660.
22. Sigmund CD, Gross KW. Structure, expression, and regulation of the murine ren genes. Hypertension 1991; 18:446.
23. Kopp U, DiBona GF. Interaction of renal β1-adrenoreceptors and prostaglandins in reflex renin release. Am J Physiol 1983; 244:F418.
24. Wagner C, Jensen BL, Kramer BK, Kurtz A. Control of the renal renin system by local factors. Kidney Int 1998; 54(Suppl 67):S78.
25. Lee MA, Bohm M, Paul M, et al. Physiologic characterization of the hypertensive transgenic rat TGR(mREN2)27. Am J Physiol 1996; 270(Endocrinol Metab 33):E919.
26. Erdos EG, Skidgel RA. Metabolism of bradykinin by peptidases in health and disease. In: Farmer SG, ed. The kinin system: handbook of immunopharmacology. London: Academic Press, 1997:112.
27. Linz W, Wiemer G, Gohlke P, et al. Contribution of the kinins to the cardiovascular actions of angiotensin-converting enzyme inhibitors. Pharmacol Rev 1995; 47:25.
28. Ramchandran R, Kasturi S, Douglas J, et al. Metalloprotease-mediated cleavage secretion of pulmonary ACE by vascular endothelial and kidney epithelial cells. Am J Physiol 1996; 271:H744.
29. Soubrier F, Wei L, Hubert C, et al. Molecular biology of the angiotensin I-converting enzyme, II: structure function: gene polymorphism and clinical implications. J Hypertens l993; 11:599.
30. Wei L, Clauser E, Athenc-Gelas F, Corval P. The two homologous domains of human angiotensin I-converting enzyme interact differently with competitive inhibitors. J Biol Chem 1992; 267:13398.
31. Azizi M, Rousseau A, Ezan E, et al. Acute angiotensin-converting enzyme inhibition increases the plasma level of the natural stem cell regulator N-acetylseryl-lysyl-proline. J Clin Invest 1996; 97:839.
32. Rigat B, Hubert C, Alhenc-Gelas F, et al. An insertion/deletion polymorphism in the angiotensin I-converting enzyme gene accounting for half the variance of serum enzyme levels. J Clin Invest 1990; 86:1343.
33. Van der Kliej FGH, Schmidt A, Navis GJ, et al. Angiotensin converting enzyme insertion/deletion polymorphism and short-term renal response to ACE inhibition: role of sodium status. Kidney Int 1998; 53(Suppl 63):S23.
34. Marre M, Bernadet P, Gallois Y, et al. Relationship between angiotensin I converting enzyme gene polymorphism, plasma levels, and diabetic retinal and renal complications. Diabetes 1994; 43:384.
35. Biege J, Scherer S, Weber A, et al. Angiotensin-converting enzyme genotype and renal allograft survival. J Am Soc Nephrol 1997; 8:1319.
36. Kimura H, Geiyo F, Suzuki S, et al. Polymorphisms of angiotensin converting enzyme and plasminogen activator inhibitor-1 genes in diabetes and microangiopathy. Kidney Int 1998; 54:1659.
37. Urata H, Nishimura H, Ganten D. Chymase-dependent angiotensin II forming system in humans. Am J Hypertens 1996; 9:277.
38. Harding JW, Wright JW, Swanson GN, et al. AT4 receptors: specificity and distribution. Kidney Int 1994; 46:1510.
39. Chappel MC, Pirro NT, Sykes A, Ferrario CM. Metabolism of angiotensin (1-7) by angiotensin converting enzyme. Hypertension 1998; 31:362.
40. Ferrario CM, Chappel MC, Tallant EA, et al. Counterregulatory actions of angiotensin (1-7). Hypertension 1997; 30:535.
41. Unger T, Gohlke P. Tissue renin-angiotensin systems in the heart and vasculature: possible involvement in the cardiovascular actions of converting enzyme inhibitors. Am J Cardiol 1990; 65:31.
42. Dostal DE, Baker KM. Evidence for a role of an intracardiac renin-angiotensin system in normal and failing hearts. Trends Cardiovasc Med 1993; 3:67.
43. Martin P, Wagner J, Dzau VJ. Gene expression of the renin-angiotensin system in human tissues: quantitative analysis by polymerase chain reaction. J Clin Invest 1993; 91:2058.
44. Wang DH, Du Y, Zhao H, et al. Regulation of angiotensin I receptor and its gene expression: role in renal growth. J Am Soc Nephrol 1997; 8:193.
45. Yanagawa N. Potential role of local luminal angiotensin II in proximal tubule sodium transport. Kidney Int Suppl 1991; 32:S33.
46. Kamide K, Hori M, Tuck ML, et al. Insulin-mediated growth in aortic smooth muscle and the vascular renin-angiotensin system. Hypertension 1998; 32:482.

47. Nemeth G, Pepperell JR, Yamada Y, et al. The basis and evidence of a role for the ovarian renin-angiotensin system in health and disease. J Soc Gynecol Investig 1994; 1:118.

48. Speth RC, Daubert DL, Grove KL. Angiotensin II: a reproductive hormone too? Regul Pept 1999; 79(l):25.

49. Hageman JR, Moyer JS, Bachman ES, et al. Angiotensin-converting enzyme and male fertility. Proc Natl Acad Sci U S A 1998; 95:2552.

50. Jones BH, Standbridge MK, Taylor JW, et al. Angiotensinogen gene expression in adipose tissue, analysis of obese models and hormonal and nutritional control. Am J Physiol 1997; 273(Regulatory Integrative Comp Physiol 42):236.

51. Kifor I, Moore TJ, Fallo F, et al. Potassium-stimulated angiotensin release from superfused adrenal capsules and enzymatically digested cells of the zona glomerulosa. Endocrinology 1991; 129:823.

52. Phillips MI, Speakman EA, Kimura B. Levels of angiotensin and molecular biology of the tissue renin angiotensin system. Regul Pept 1993; 43:1.

53. Baltatu O, Nishimura H, Hoffman S, et al. High levels of human chymase expression in the pineal and pituitary gland. Brain Res 1997; 759:269.

54. Griendling KK, Lassegue B, Alexander RW. The vascular angiotensin (AT1) receptor. Thromb Haemost 1993; 70(1):188.

55. Coffman TM. Gene targeting in physiological investigations: studies of the renin-angiotensin system. Am J Physiol 1998; 274 (Renal Physiol):F999.

56. Sadoshima J. Versatility of the angiotensin II type 1 receptor. Circ Res 1998; 82:1352.

56a. Schiffrin EL, Park JB, Intengan HD, Touyz RM. Correction of arterial structure and endothelial dysfunction in human essential hypertension by the angiotensin receptor antagonist losartan. Circulation 2000; 101(14):1653.

57. Horiuchi M, Akishita M, Dzau VJ. Recent progress in angiotensin II type 2 receptor research in the cardiovascular system. Hypertension 1999; 33:613.

58. Cogan MG. Angiotensin II: a powerful controller of sodium transport in the early proximal tubule. Hypertension 1990; 15:451.

59. Okubo S, Numura F, Matsusaka T, et al. Angiotensinogen gene null-mutant lacks homeostatic regulation of glomerular filtration and tubular reabsorption. Kidney Int 1998; 53:617.

60. Scholz H, Kurtz A. Role of protein kinase C in renal vasoconstriction caused by angiotensin II. Am J Physiol 1990; 259:C421.

61. Clemson B, Gaul L, Gubin SS, et al. Prejunctional angiotensin II receptors. Facilitation of norepinephrine release in the human forearm. J Clin Invest 1994; 93:684.

62. Moreau P, d'Uscio LV, Shaw S, et al. Angiotensin II increases tissue endothelin and induces vascular hypertrophy: reversal by ET(A)-receptor antagonist. Circulation 1997; 96:1593.

63. Golub MS, Hori MT, Tuck ML. Arachidonic acid metabolites in the vasculature. In: Sowers JR, ed. Endocrinology of the vasculature. Totowa, NJ: Humana Press, 1996:357.

64. Ichikawa I, Harris RC. Angiotensin actions in the kidney: renewed insight into the old hormone. Kidney Int 1991; 40:583.

65. Wilcox CS, Welch WJ, Snellen H. Thromboxane mediates renal hemodynamic response to infused angiotensin II. Kidney Int 1991; 40:1090.

66. Miller JA, Anacata LA, Cattran DC. Impact of gender on the response to angiotensin II. Kidney Int 1999; 55:278.

67. Wolf G, Ziyadeh FN. The role of angiotensin II in diabetic nephropathy: emphasis on nonhemodynamic mechanisms. Am J Kidney Dis 1997; 29:153.

68. Dzau VJ, Re R. Tissue angiotensin system in cardiovascular medicine: a paradigm shift. Circulation 1994; 89:493.

69. Gibbons GH. The pathophysiology of hypertension. The importance of angiotensin II in cardiovascular remodeling. Am J Hypertens 1998; 11:177S.

70. Alderman MH, Madhaven S, Ooi WL, et al. Association of renin-sodium profile with risk of myocardial infarction in patients with hypertension. N Engl J Med 1991; 324:1098.

71. Vaughan DE. The renin-angiotensin system and fibrinolysis. Am J Cardiol 1997; 79(5A):12.

72. Brown NJ, Agirbasli MA, Williams GH, et al. Effect of activation and inhibition of the renin-angiotensin system on plasma PAI-1. Hypertension 1998; 32:965.

73. Hwan K, Thornhill B, Wolstenholme T, Chevalier RL. Tissue-specific regulation of growth factors and clusterin by angiotensin II. Am J Hypertens 1998; 11:715.

74. Morishita R, Ogihara T. In vivo evaluation of in vitro hypothesis using "gain or loss" of function: functional analysis of the renin-angiotensin system. Am J Hypertens 1998; 11:507.

75. Tomita N, Morishita R, Higaki J, et al. Transient decrease in high blood pressure by in vitro transfer of antisense oligodeoxynucleotides against angiotensinogen. Hypertension 1995; 26:131.

76. Phillips MI. Antisense inhibition and adeno-associated viral vector delivery for reducing hypertension. Hypertension 1997; 29:177.

77. Marver D, Kokko JP. Renal target sites and the mechanism of action of aldosterone. Min Elect Metab 1983; 9:1.

78. White PC. Mechanisms of disease. Disorders of aldosterone biosynthesis and action. N Engl J Med 1994; 331:250.

79. Connell JM, Fraser R. Adrenal cortical synthesis and hypertension. J Hypertens 1991; 9:97.

80. Holland OB, Carr B. Modulation of aldosterone synthase messenger ribonucleic acid levels by dietary sodium and potassium and by adrenocorticotropin. Endocrinology 1993; 132:2666.

81. Arriza JL, Weinberger C, Cerelli C, et al. Cloning of human mineralocorticoid receptor complementary DNA: structural and functional kinship with the glucocorticoid receptor. Science 1987; 237:268.

82. Funder JW. Mineralocorticoids, glucocorticoids, receptors and response elements. Science 1993; 259:1132.

83. Bastl CP, Hayslett. The cellular action of aldosterone in target epithelia. Kidney Int 1992; 42:250.

84. Zennaro M-C, Farman N, Bonvalet J-P, et al. Tissue-specific expression of alpha and beta messenger ribonucleic acid isoforms of the human mineralocorticoid receptor in normal and pathological states. J Clin Endocrinol Metab 1997; 82:1345.

85. Funder JW. Enzymes and the regulation of sodium balance. Kidney Int 1992; 37(Suppl):S114.

86. Kenouch S, Coutry N, Farman N, Bonvalet J-P. Multiple patterns of 11β-hydroxysteroid dehydrogenase catalytic activity along the mammalian nephron. Kidney Int 1992; 42:56.

87. Naray-Fejes-Toth A, Rusvai E, Fejes-Toth G. Mineralocorticoid receptors and 11β-hydroxysteroid dehydrogenase activity in renal principal and intercalated cells. Am J Physiol 1994; 266:F76.

87a. Funder JW. Aldosterone and mineralocorticoid receptors: orphan questions. Kidney Int 2000; 57(4):1358.

88. Horisberger JD, Rossier BC. Aldosterone regulation of gene transcription leading to control of ion transport. Hypertension 1992; 19:221.

89. Szerlip H, Palevsky P, Cox M, Blazer-Yost B. Relationship of the aldosterone-induced protein GP70 to the conductive channel. J Am Soc Nephrol 1991; 2:1108.

90. Schafer JA, Hawk CT. Regulation of $Na^+$ channels in the cortical collecting duct by AVP and mineralocorticoids. Kidney Int 1992; 41:255.

91. Hayhurst RA, O'Neil RG. Time-dependent actions of aldosterone and amiloride-blockable sodium channels in A6 epithelia. Am J Physiol 1988; 254:F689.

92. Petzel D, Ganz MB, Nestler EJ, et al. Correlates of aldosterone-induced increases in $Ca_i^{2+}$ and Isc suggest that $Ca_i^{2+}$ is the second messenger for stimulation of apical membrane conductance. J Clin Invest 1992; 89:150.

93. Hays SR. Mineratocorticoid modulation of apical and basolateral membrane $H^+/OH^-/HCO_3^-$, transport processes in rabbit inner strip of outer medullary collecting duct. J Clin Invest 1992; 90:180.

94. Brilla CG, Weber KT. Mineralocorticoid excess, dietary medium and myocardial fibrosis. J Lab Clin Med 1992; 120:893.

95. Young M, Fullerton M, Dilley P, Funder J. Mineralocorticoids, hypertension and cardiac fibrosis. J Clin Invest 1994; 93:2578.

95a. Falkenstein E, Christ M, Feuring M, Wehling M. Specific nongenomic actions of aldosterone. Kidney Int 2000; 57(4):1390.

96. Hakeyama H, Miramuri I, Fujita T, et al. Vascular aldosterone, biosynthesis and a link to angiotensin II-induced hypertrophy of vascular smooth muscle. J Biol Chem 1994; 269:24316.

97. Robert V, Heymes C, Silvestre J-B, et al. Angiotensin AT1 receptor subtype as a cardiac target of aldosterone; role in aldosterone-salt-induced fibrosis. Hypertension 1999; 33:981.

98. Gomez Sanchez EP. What is the role of the central nervous system in mineralocorticoid hypertension? Am J Hypertension 1991; 4:374.

99. The RALES Investigators. Effectiveness of spironolactone added to an angiotensin converting enzyme inhibitor and a loop diuretic for severe chronic congestive heart failure (The Randomized Aldactone Evaluation Study [RALES]). Am J Cardiol 1996; 78:902.

100. Ibrahim HN, Rosenberg ME, Greene EL, et al. Aldosterone is a major factor in the progression of renal disease. Kidney Int 1997; 52(Suppl 63):S115.

100a. Farman N, Verrey F. Forefronts in nephrology news in aldosterone action. Kidney Int 2000; 57:1239.

101. Brann DW, Hendry LB, Mahesh VB. Emerging diversities in the mechanism of action of steroid hormones. J Steroid Biochem Molec Biol 1995; 52:113.

102. Adler GK, Chen R, Menachery AI, et al. Sodium restriction increases aldosterone synthesis by increased late pathway, not early pathway, messenger ribonucleic acid levels and enzyme activity in normal rats. Endocrinology 1993; 133:2235.

103. Young DB. Quantitative analysis of aldosterone's role in potassium regulation. Am J Physiol 1988; 255:F811.

104. Himathongan T, Dluhy R, Williams GH. Potassium-aldosterone-renin interrelationships. J Clin Endocrinol Metab 1975; 41:153.

105. Kifor I, Moore TJ, Fallo F, et al. Potassium-stimulated angiotensin release from superfused adrenal capsules and enzymatically digested cells of the zona glomerulosa. Endocrinology 1991; 129:823.

106. Young DB, Smith MJ Jr, Jackson TE, Scott RE. Multiplicative interaction between angiotensin II and K concentration in stimulation of aldosterone. Am J Physiol 1984; 247:E328.

107. Mulkerrin E, Epstein FH, Clark BA. Aldosterone responses to hyperkalemia in healthy elderly humans. J Am Soc Nephrol 1995; 6:1459.

108. Braley LM, Adler GK, Mortensen RM, et al. Dose effect of adrenocorticotropin on aldosterone and cortisol biosynthesis in cultured bovine adrenal glomerulosa cells. In vitro correlate of hyperreninemic hypoaldosterone. Endocrinology 1992; 131:187.

109. Merrill DC, Ebert TJ, Skelton MM, Cowley AW Jr. Effect of plasma sodium on aldosterone during angiotensin II stimulation in normal humans. Hypertension 1989; 14:164.

110. Taylor RE, Glass GT, Radke KJ, Schneider EG. Specificity of effect of osmolality on aldosterone secretion. Am J Physiol 1987; 252:E118.

111. Jones GV, Wall BM, Williams HH, et al. Modulation of plasma aldosterone by physiologic changes in hydrogen ion concentration. Am J Physiol 1992; 262:R269.

112. White PC. Inherited forms of mineralocorticoid hypertension. Hypertension 1996; 28:927.

# CHAPTER 80

# HYPERALDOSTERONISM

JOHN R. GILL, JR.

## DISORDERS OF MINERALOCORTICOID EXCESS

Mineralocorticoid excess, whether primary or secondary, and disorders that mimic it are commonly manifested clinically as hypokalemia, which usually but not always is accompanied by alkalosis. Thus, a useful strategy for diagnosing hypokalemia is to approach the evaluation as a differential diagnosis of disorders of mineralocorticoid excess. Clinical features that accompany hypokalemia and may be used to determine the specific disorders that need to be considered are illustrated in Table 80-1 and in the flow chart in Figure 80-1. This basic framework is expanded in the course of this review to include the disorders appropriate to each of the four listed patterns of abnormalities of renin and aldosterone. Ideally, evaluation of the renin and aldosterone systems should be done in the absence of medication during a standardized sodium intake (e.g., 100 mEq per day of sodium as sodium chloride). If this is not possible, then at least the use of medications that affect the production of renin and aldosterone (i.e., diuretics and angiotensin converting enzyme inhibitors) should be discontinued and the blood pressure should be controlled with a calcium channel blocking agent. The level of sodium intake immediately preceding the

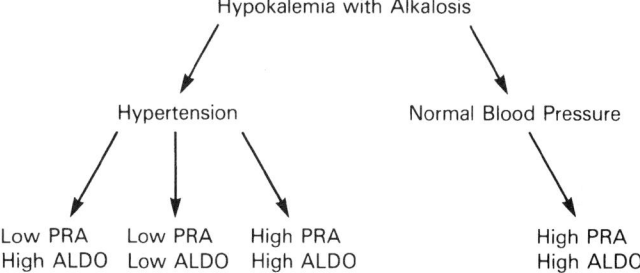

**FIGURE 80-1.** Flow chart for evaluation of patients with hypokalemic alkalosis. (*PRA,* plasma renin activity; *ALDO,* aldosterone.) (See Table 80-1 for continuation of evaluation.)

sampling of blood for plasma renin activity and plasma aldosterone should be estimated by collecting a 24-hour aliquot of urine for the determination of sodium excretion. The blood for the plasma renin activity and plasma aldosterone evaluations should be drawn after overnight bedrest (in the hospital) or after 30 minutes of bedrest (in the clinic), and then drawn again after 2 hours of standing and walking.

## PHYSIOLOGY OF ALDOSTERONE

### SYNTHESIS

The zona glomerulosa cells of the adrenal cortex synthesize aldosterone from *corticosterone* in a two-step, mixed function oxidation reaction that is catalyzed by the enzyme *corticosterone*

**TABLE 80-1.**
**Disorders Characterized by Hypokalemia and Alkalosis**

| | |
|---|---|
| **HYPERALDOSTERONISM (SO-CALLED "PRIMARY")** | Hypertension |
| *Clinical Features* | High plasma renin activity |
|   Hypokalemia | High aldosterone levels |
|   Alkalosis | *Disorders* |
|   Hypertension |   Renal artery stenosis |
|   Low plasma renin activity |   Renin-secreting tumor |
|   High aldosterone levels |   Malignant hypertension |
| *Disorders* |   Chronic renal disease |
|   Aldosterone-producing adenoma | **SECONDARY HYPERALDOSTERONISM AND NORMAL BLOOD PRESSURE** |
|   Idiopathic hyperaldosteronism | *Clinical Features* |
|   Primary adrenal hyperplasia |   Hypokalemia |
|   Dexamethasone-suppressible hyperaldosteronism |   Alkalosis |
|   Adrenocortical carcinoma |   Normal blood pressure |
| **SYNDROMES OF REAL OR APPARENT MINERALOCORTICOID EXCESS NOT CAUSED BY ALDOSTERONE** |   High plasma renin activity |
| *Clinical Features* |   High aldosterone levels |
|   Hypokalemia | *Disorders* |
|   Alkalosis |   Renal disorders |
|   Hypertension |     Renal tubular acidosis |
|   Low plasma renin activity |     Nephritis |
|   Low aldosterone levels |     Cystinosis |
| *Disorders* |     Bartter syndrome |
|   11β-Hydroxylase deficiency |     Magnesium-losing tubulopathy |
|   17-Hydroxylase deficiency |     Calcium-losing tubulopathy |
|   Liddle syndrome |   Hepatic cirrhosis |
|   11β-Hydroxysteroid dehydrogenase deficiency |   Cardiac failure |
|   Licorice ingestion |   Gastrointestinal disorders |
| **SECONDARY HYPERALDOSTERONISM AND HYPERTENSION** |     Covert vomiting |
| *Clinical Features* |     Covert laxative abuse |
|   Hypokalemia |     Familial chloride diarrhea |
|   Alkalosis |   Covert diuretic abuse |

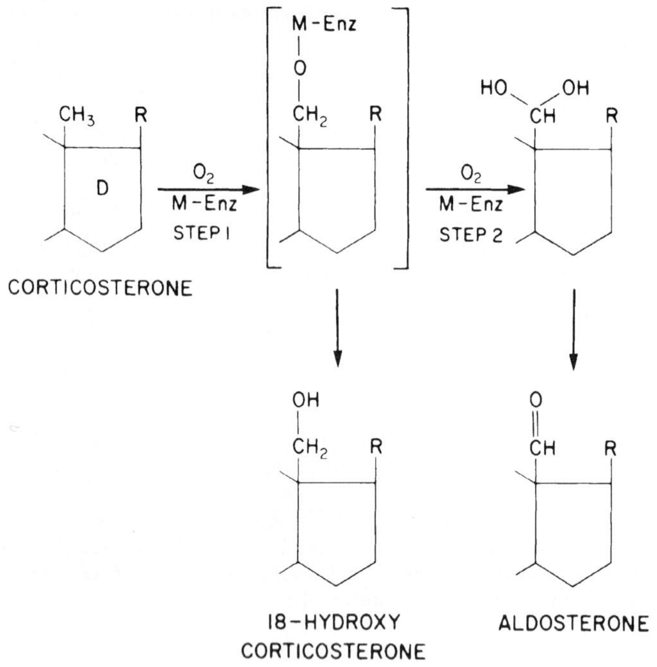

**FIGURE 80-2.** Proposed mechanism and structure of intermediates in the conversion of corticosterone to aldosterone. (From Ulick S. Diagnosis and nomenclature of the disorders of the terminal portion of the aldosterone biosynthetic pathway. J Clin Endocrinol Metab 1976; 43:92.)

*methyl oxidase*[1] (Fig. 80-2). Normally, the adrenal glands secrete 60 to 200 μg aldosterone each day, depending on the state of sodium chloride and water balance of the body; the steroid circulates in the blood either free or loosely bound to albumin. Although some of the circulating aldosterone may be excreted in the urine in the free form, most of it is metabolized by the liver to *tetrahydroaldosterone* and by the kidneys to *aldosterone-18-glucuronide*. Measurement of the excretion of the 18-glucuronide metabolite has been used as an index of aldosterone production; values obtained by this method range from 1 to 15 μg per day in normal persons receiving an unrestricted sodium chloride intake.

## SECRETION

Aldosterone biogenesis is regulated primarily by the *renin-angiotensin system*, with *potassium, atrial natriuretic hormone (ANH),* and *dopamine* also making important contributions. *Corticotropin* (ACTH) also may stimulate aldosterone production, but its effects are self-limited except in certain disease states. In addition, the factors that determine aldosterone secretion have direct effects on the kidney and vasculature and, along with aldosterone, contribute to the maintenance of the volume of extracellular fluid, the concentration of extracellular potassium, and, ultimately, blood pressure. Thus, when the intake of sodium chloride is restricted and blood volume is contracted, an increase in the formation of angiotensin II stimulates the secretion of aldosterone. Angiotensin II and aldosterone, in turn, both increase the reabsorption of sodium by the renal tubule to curtail sodium loss and restore extracellular volume. Conversely, when sodium chloride intake is increased and blood volume is expanded, the formation of angiotensin II decreases, ANH is secreted by the heart, and the formation of dopamine by the adrenal glands and kidneys increases. ANH and dopamine inhibit aldosterone biogenesis; they also increase sodium excretion through direct effects on the kidney. Potassium exerts differential effects on aldosterone biosynthesis. Hyperkalemia, secondary to potassium administration or retention, stimulates aldosterone secretion, whereas hypokalemia, secondary to potassium depletion, inhibits it. A more detailed discussion of the renin-angiotensin system and its control of aldosterone secretion is presented in Chapters 79 and 183; ANH is discussed in Chapter 178.

## ACTIONS

Aldosterone exerts its biologic actions by crossing the plasma membrane of target cells and binding to its receptor in the cytosol.[2] The aldosterone-receptor complex then migrates to the nucleus, where it binds, thereby initiating transcription, translation, and synthesis of proteins responsible for expression of the action of aldosterone on the functions of that target cell (see Chap. 4). Collecting tubule cells of the kidney and epithelial cells of other transporting tissues (i.e., sweat, salivary gland, and intestine) are target tissues in which the physiologic effects of aldosterone are most discernible, although effects on vascular[3] and other tissues may occur. In epithelial cells for which the physiologic actions of aldosterone have been extensively characterized, the steroid facilitates passage of sodium across the apical membrane into the cell and accelerates extrusion of sodium and uptake of potassium by $Na^+,K^+$-adenosine triphosphatase located in the basolateral membrane.[4] In the renal collecting tubule, these actions of aldosterone increase the reabsorption of sodium and the secretion of potassium, leading to retention of sodium by the body and loss of potassium (see Chap. 206).

As the foregoing discussion indicates, the renin-angiotensin-aldosterone systems regulate the volume of extracellular fluid and contribute to the maintenance of the extracellular potassium concentration. As a result of disease, the production of aldosterone may become supernormal and cease to be responsive to the physiologic stimuli that regulate it. The overproduction of aldosterone may result from overactivity of the renin-angiotensin system (*secondary hyperaldosteronism*) or from other abnormalities (*primary hyperaldosteronism*). The consequences of continual overproduction of aldosterone, or hyperaldosteronism, depend in part on the disorder with which it is associated, and may include excessive sodium chloride and water retention, potassium loss, alkalosis, and hypertension.

## "PRIMARY ALDOSTERONISM"

Autonomous overproduction of aldosterone occurs in ~2% of patients with hypertension and was recognized initially as being associated with either a unilateral adenoma (*aldosterone-producing adenoma,* or *APA*) or bilateral hyperplasia of the zona glomerulosa. Because patients with bilateral adrenal disease tended to have a clinical presentation similar to that of patients with an APA (hypertension and hypokalemia) and, like the patients with unilateral disease, they showed suppression of the renin-angiotensin system, they also were assumed to have a primary adrenal disorder. Subsequent observations have not proved this to be true; they suggest, instead, that bilateral hyperplasia of the zona glomerulosa probably is not a primary adrenal disorder in most cases and may have more than one cause. Unilateral adrenalectomy usually cures or ameliorates the hypertension in patients with an APA, whereas subtotal or total adrenalectomy, with few exceptions, has little effect on the blood pressure of patients with bilateral hyperplasia. In the case of those few patients who have primary adrenal hyperplasia, unilateral adrenalectomy may be curative.[5] In some patients with bilateral hyperplasia, the hyperaldosteronism was dependent on ACTH (so-called *glucocorticoid-remediable hyperaldosteronism*). The hypothesis that a trophic hormone, possibly of pituitary origin, may be responsible for bilateral hyperplasia not caused by ACTH has received considerable support, although it has not been definitively proved. As a result of advances in knowledge, the inclusive designation of "primary hyperaldosteronism" for those patients with hyperaldosteronism associated with both adenoma and bilateral hyperplasia has tended to be *replaced* by the more specific designations of *aldosterone-producing adenoma, idiopathic hyperaldosteronism,* primary adrenal hyperplasia, and *glucocorticoid-remediable hyperaldosteronism.* Rarely, *adrenocortical carcinoma* may overproduce aldosterone. These five disorders present as hypokalemic alkalosis, hypertension, low or suppressed plasma renin activity, and high aldosterone concentrations (see Table 80-1).

# ALDOSTERONE-PRODUCING ADENOMAS

## CLINICAL FEATURES AND PATHOPHYSIOLOGY

Aldosterone-producing adrenocortical adenomas usually are small (0.5–2.5 cm), unilateral, solitary, and associated with hypoplastic zona glomerulosa. Occasionally, however, these lesions may be multiple and associated with hyperplasia of the zona glomerulosa. This benign tumor of the adrenal cortex occurs most frequently in the third through the fifth decades of life but also has been observed in prepubertal children[6] and older persons (range, 13–66 years). Aldosterone-producing adenomas occur equally in men and women and do not appear to have a racial predisposition; they tend to develop more frequently in the left adrenal gland than in the right, but this difference is small.

(The occurrence of primary aldosteronism resulting from APA in two or more members of the same family has been reported,[7] as well as the familial occurrence of idiopathic aldosteronism. In one of the families, one member had bilateral nodular hyperplasia and another had APA. This familial form of primary aldosteronism was labeled *familial hyperaldosteronism type II* to distinguish it from glucocorticoid-remediable hyperaldosteronism. The clinical features of familial hyperaldosteronism type II do *not* differ from those of sporadic patients with APA or idiopathic hyperaldosteronism.)

The symptoms reported most frequently by patients with an APA are headache, easy fatigability, and weakness, although high blood pressure may be the only symptom in many cases. Hypokalemia, suppressed plasma renin activity, and high plasma and urinary aldosterone values are the findings usually associated with APA, but they may not always be demonstrable.[8]

Aldosterone production by an APA is autonomous and is affected only minimally by angiotensin II because of the decreased formation of this peptide as well as the decreased responsiveness of the adenoma. An APA is unresponsive to the infusion of dopamine, although endogenous dopamine may exert tonic inhibitory effects.[9] ANH, levels of which appear to be elevated in patients with this disorder,[10] does not inhibit aldosterone biogenesis by APA cells in vitro, as it does in normal glomerulosa cells.[11] Therefore, this hormone may have little effect on aldosterone secretion by an APA in vivo. In contrast, changes in serum potassium or ACTH levels may exert important regulatory effects on aldosterone secretion in patients with this tumor: aldosterone production may be blunted by the potassium loss and the hypokalemia that it induces. The circadian rhythm of aldosterone in patients with APA tends to mirror that of ACTH.

As a consequence of sustained overproduction of aldosterone, retention of sodium chloride and water occurs, but this usually is limited; "escape" occurs when extracellular fluid has been expanded by ~500 mL.[12] Initially, the renal excretion of potassium increases. As hypokalemia develops, potassium excretion decreases to reflect intake of this cation. Hydrogen ion excretion, which increases principally because of an increase in urinary ammonium, is responsible for the development and maintenance of metabolic alkalosis. Urinary calcium and magnesium levels are high; presumably, this is a reflection of the effects of expansion of extracellular fluid on the tubular reabsorption of these ions. The urinary concentrating ability is impaired because of potassium depletion. Although sodium

and water retention may contribute to the increase in blood pressure that occurs, the precise mechanisms responsible for an increase in peripheral resistance and the associated hypertension are unclear. Receptors for aldosterone have been found in blood vessels and in the brain, and the effects of aldosterone on ion transport in these tissues may be important mediators of the increase in blood pressure. Preliminary studies in dogs indicate that an amount of aldosterone that is too small to exert an effect when infused peripherally increases blood pressure when it is infused into the third ventricle of the brain.[13]

## DIAGNOSIS AND DIFFERENTIAL DIAGNOSIS

Patients with hypertension who have *borderline or low serum potassium* concentrations, *low stimulated plasma renin activity* (<2 ng/mL per hour), and *borderline or high plasma aldosterone* concentrations (>14 ng/dL) should be evaluated further for autonomous overproduction of aldosterone.

The evaluation should be done before antihypertensive treatment is instituted or after it has been discontinued for 2 weeks. *Determining aldosterone suppressibility,* by combining a high sodium intake and treatment with a mineralocorticoid such as 9-αfluorohydrocortisone for 3 or more days, or by intravenous saline infusion, is a useful first step. Of these two interventions, the infusion of 2 L normal saline over 4 hours with the measurement of plasma aldosterone levels before and at the conclusion of the infusion is simpler and may be readily adapted to the evaluation of outpatients.[14] At the conclusion of the infusion, the plasma aldosterone level normally is 5 ng/dL or less; in patients with hyperaldosteronism, it usually exceeds 10 ng/dL.

*Determination of the plasma aldosterone to plasma renin activity ratio* also has been used to detect aldosteronism. Single determinations of this ratio tend to be of limited use because values from patients with hyperaldosteronism frequently are the same as those from patients with normal adrenal function. A solution to the problem of overlap that appears to improve specificity considerably is to collect blood samples every 30 minutes for 6 hours, so that an *integrated plasma aldosterone/plasma renin activity ratio* can be determined.[15] A somewhat simpler but probably equally effective alternative is to collect blood 90 minutes after the administration of 25 to 50 mg *captopril,* which is a converting enzyme inhibitor, for determination of the plasma aldosterone/plasma renin activity ratio[16] (Fig. 80-3). Both procedures are safe and do not require dietary preparation or hospitalization. It has been suggested that all patients with hypertension undergo captopril screening tests,[17] because determination of the serum potassium concentration and plasma renin activity may be inadequate measures for screening the hypertensive population for hyperaldosteronism.[8] The normogram in Figure 80-3 indicates the degree of separation of patients with aldosterone excess from those with essential hypertension.[16] Subsequent evaluation of the captopril test indicates a false-negative rate of 6.3% and a false-positive rate of 0.6% in patients with primary hyperaldosteronism.[18] The problem of identifying those patients with hyperaldosteronism who harbor an adenoma has been greatly facilitated by technologic advances. *Computed tomography* (CT) appears to have the capacity to discern an adrenal mass in ~80% of patients with an aldosterone-producing adenoma.[19,20] *Magnetic resonance imaging* also has been used to evaluate the adrenal glands in patients with hyperaldosteronism; apart from confirming the findings of CT, however, it does not appear to offer any advantage over CT. These new techniques for imaging adrenal masses have replaced the more cumbersome and time-consuming procedure of [131I]iodocholesterol imaging in most centers (see Chap. 88). A limitation of all the imaging techniques, however, is that an adenoma may be poorly visualized or not detected at all. These problems result from the small size of some adenomas, which may be less than 1 cm in diameter. The problem

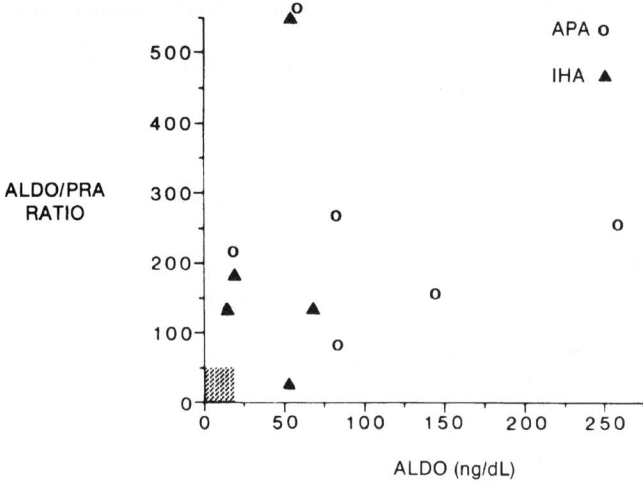

**FIGURE 80-3.** Values for the plasma aldosterone (*ALDO*)/plasma renin activity (*PRA*) ratio plotted as a function of plasma aldosterone for normal and hypertensive control subjects (*hatched area*), patients with aldosterone-producing adenoma (*APA*), and patients with idiopathic hyperaldosteronism (*IHA*) 2 hours after the administration of 25 mg captopril. The plasma aldosterone value decreased to <15 ng/dL in normal persons, but remained higher than this in most with IHA and in all with APA. The ALDO/PRA ratio was <50 in normal persons and >50 in most with IHA and all with APA. (From Lyons DF, Kem DC, Brown RD, et al. Single dose captopril as a diagnostic test for primary aldosteronism. J Clin Endocrinol Metab 1983; 57:892.)

of an inconclusive CT scan may be partially resolved by *determining the plasma 18-hydroxycorticosterone* level after overnight bedrest.[21] In a series of 50 patients with aldosteronism, all but 1 of the 24 patients with an adenoma had 18-hydroxycorticosterone values that exceeded 50 ng/dL.[8] Thus, a plasma 18-hydroxycorticosterone value >50 ng/dL in a patient with hyperaldosteronism suggests that the diagnosis is more likely to be an aldosterone-producing adenoma than bilateral hyperplasia, even though the adrenal glands may appear normal (Fig. 80-4). If the plasma aldosterone level were to show a "paradoxic" fall paralleling the circadian fall in plasma cortisol during 2 hours of ambulation after early morning sampling, this also would suggest that the diagnosis is more likely to be an aldosterone-producing adenoma than bilateral hyperplasia.[22] So many patients with an adenoma, like those with bilateral hyperplasia, show a rise rather than a fall in the plasma aldosterone level that *the usefulness of the procedure is limited*.[8]

The most reliable means of assessing adrenal glands in patients with hyperaldosteronism is *bilateral catheterization of adrenal veins* to sample for corticosteroids.[23] The aldosterone/cortisol ratio in samples of venous blood from both adrenal glands and a peripheral site, before and after ACTH stimulation, provides a good comparative characterization of adrenal function and an extremely reliable means of distinguishing between bilateral and unilateral overproduction of aldosterone. Table 80-2 shows the results of adrenal vein sampling in a patient with an aldosterone-producing adenoma. Determination of the cortisol level provides important confirmation of roentgenographic evidence that the site of sampling is actually an adrenal vein; it also is used to correct values of adrenal venous aldosterone for dilution by blood of extraadrenal origin. In the illustrated patient, the findings show the importance of stimulation with ACTH to ensure that an adenoma is functioning, rather than quiescent, at the time of sampling and also to demonstrate suppression of aldosterone production by the contralateral gland. Although adrenal vein sampling is an invasive procedure, it is associated with minimal morbidity. When used as just described, it has an accuracy >90% in the lateralization of an adenoma, making the distinction between an APA and those disorders associated with bilateral overproduction of

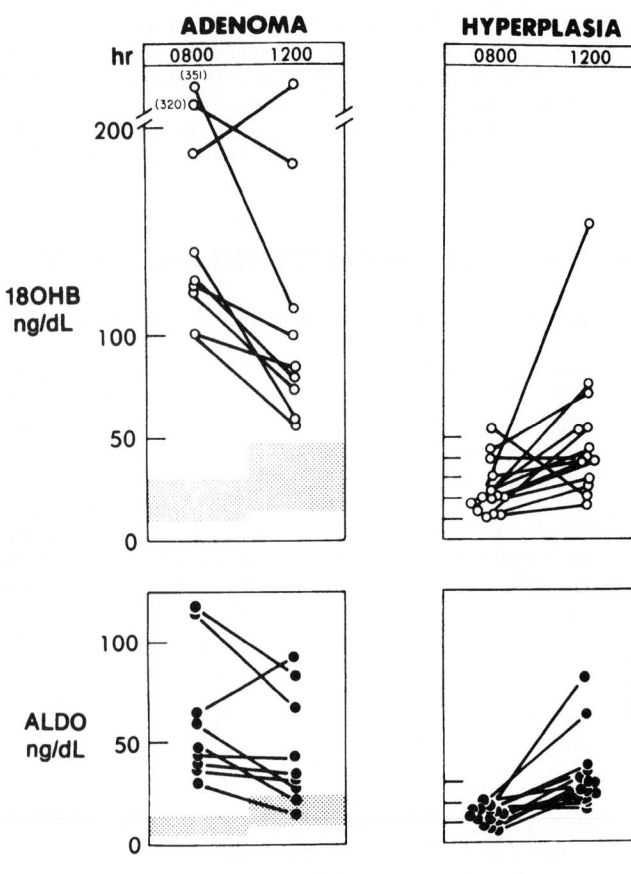

Normal Ranges

**FIGURE 80-4.** Plasma 18-hydroxycorticosterone (*18OHB*) and plasma aldosterone (*ALDO*) concentrations at bedrest and after 4 hours of ambulation in patients with aldosterone-producing adenomas (*adenoma*) or idiopathic hyperaldosteronism (*hyperplasia*). Note the wide separation in resting values for 18OHB between patients with adenoma and patients with hyperplasia and the different responses of the two groups to ambulation. (From Biglieri EG, Schambelan M. The significance of elevated levels of plasma 18-hydroxycorticosterone in patients with primary aldosteronism. J Clin Endocrinol Metab 1979; 49:87.)

**TABLE 80-2.**
**Adrenal Venous Sampling**

| Location | Aldosterone (ng/dL) | Cortisol (μg/dL) | Aldosterone/Cortisol Ratio |
|---|---|---|---|
| **PATIENT WITH ALDOSTERONE-PRODUCING ADENOMA** | | | |
| *Basal* | | | |
| Inferior vena cava | 17 | 13 | 1.3 |
| Left adrenal vein | 106 | 20 | 5.3 |
| Right adrenal vein | 110 | 571 | 0.2 |
| *After Corticotropin* | | | |
| Inferior vena cava | 91 | 25 | 3.6 |
| Left adrenal vein | 143,000 | 2230 | 64.1 |
| Right adrenal vein | 290 | 2440 | 0.1 |
| **PATIENT WITH IDIOPATHIC HYPERALDOSTERONISM** | | | |
| *Basal* | | | |
| Inferior vena cava | 18 | 9 | 2.0 |
| Left adrenal vein | 432 | 21 | 20.6 |
| Right adrenal vein | 300 | 18 | 16.7 |
| *After Corticotropin* | | | |
| Inferior vena cava | 36 | 14 | 2.6 |
| Left adrenal vein | 15,200 | 1700 | 8.9 |
| Right adrenal vein | 10,400 | 1230 | 8.6 |

aldosterone. The observations that APA may be associated with other abnormalities seen on CT scans such as ipsilateral and contralateral nonfunctioning nodules and thickening of an adrenal limb indicate the important role of adrenal vein sampling in reaching a correct diagnosis.[20] Only occasionally will a patient with idiopathic aldosteronism have a gradient between the two adrenal glands with an aldosterone/cortisol ratio that approaches 4 to 1, the lower limit of the range of the ratio of APA to normal adrenal.[24]

## TREATMENT

The preferred therapy for patients with an aldosterone-producing adenoma is operative removal of the adrenal gland containing the tumor.[25] Adenomectomy alone is not sufficient.[25a] This can be done laparoscopically with minimal morbidity[26] (see Chap. 89). The cure rate (correction of hypertension as well as aldosteronism) ranges from 60% to 75%. Because the prevalence of a family history of hypertension in patients with an aldosterone-producing adenoma may range from 40% to 60%, this, along with the duration of the hypertension, may account for the persistence of an elevated blood pressure despite the correction of hyperaldosteronism. Most of the patients who remain hypertensive after the correction of hyperaldosteronism become more responsive to antihypertensive medication.

Spironolactone is probably the single most effective drug for treating patients with an APA. It acts as a competitive inhibitor, competing with aldosterone for its cytosol receptor, thereby antagonizing the action of the mineralocorticoid in target tissue. Spironolactone also is both an antiandrogen and a progestagen, and this explains many of its distressing side effects; [2,4] decreased libido, mastodynia, and gynecomastia may occur in 50% or more of men, and menometrorrhagia and mastodynia may occur in an equally large number of women taking the drug.[27] The problem of side effects may preclude the long-term use of spironolactone, particularly in younger men and women, and is more likely to occur when the dosage exceeds 100 mg per day. The usual dosage of spironolactone ranges from 50 mg once daily to 100 mg twice daily.

Drugs such as amiloride and triamterene also may oppose the effect of aldosterone on the renal tubule, but these agents act by inhibiting sodium reabsorption and potassium secretion through a direct effect on the tubule cell, not by competing with aldosterone for its receptor. This may explain why triamterene and amiloride tend to be less effective than spironolactone as antihypertensive agents in patients with hyperaldosteronism.

Calcium channel blocking drugs, such as nifedipine, also may be useful therapeutic agents in patients with hyperaldosteronism. In addition to its antihypertensive action, nifedipine may decrease aldosterone production.[28] Thus, the combined use of nifedipine and a potassium-sparing diuretic may serve as an alternative to spironolactone in the medical treatment of patients with an APA.

# IDIOPATHIC HYPERALDOSTERONISM

## CLINICAL FEATURES AND PATHOPHYSIOLOGY

Idiopathic bilateral adrenocortical hyperplasia of the zona glomerulosa (idiopathic hyperaldosteronism) is characterized by features similar to those associated with APAs, although they are less pronounced in many patients.[29] The reported prevalence of idiopathic hyperaldosteronism has ranged from a high of 70% of those patients with primary hyperaldosteronism[14] to a low of 8%.[20] The true prevalence probably is somewhere between these two extremes and may be ~30%.

Although the etiology of idiopathic aldosteronism has not been established, the belief that a circulating stimulatory factor is responsible for hyperfunction of the zona glomerulosa is generally accepted. Extracts of urine from normal persons contain a protein fraction that selectively stimulates the production of aldosterone and produces hypertension when injected into rats.[30] Subsequent studies of one of these extracts have shown that (a) it is a peptide of pituitary origin, (b) it is increased in patients with idiopathic hyperaldosteronism but not in those with an APA, and (c) it is not suppressed by dexamethasone.[31] The specific peptide has not been identified. In other studies, plasma concentrations of γ-melanotropin[32] and of β-endorphin[33] were increased in patients with idiopathic hyperaldosteronism but not in those with an aldosterone-producing adenoma. These two peptides are fragments of a larger peptide, pro-opiomelanocortin, which is formed in the pituitary; they may stimulate the secretion of aldosterone or increase the sensitivity of the adrenal gland to angiotensin II, or both. The report of an enlargement of the intermediate lobe of the pituitary in a patient with idiopathic hyperaldosteronism,[34] together with the observations that central serotoninergic stimulation of aldosterone secretion may occur[35] and that cyproheptadine, which is an inhibitor of central serotonin release, may decrease plasma aldosterone in patients with idiopathic hyperaldosteronism,[36] is consistent with a possible role for the pituitary in the pathogenesis of idiopathic hyperaldosteronism. It should be noted, however, that a pathogenetic schema for idiopathic hyperaldosteronism has to account for the hypertension as well as the hyperaldosteronism because adrenalectomy rarely lowers blood pressure. Therefore, a putative aldosterone-stimulating factor of pituitary or other origin, or changes proximal to its release, must be responsible for the hypertension in idiopathic hyperaldosteronism, unless the hypertension is a separate process. The effects of the putative aldosterone-stimulating factors on blood pressure are not known. As in an APA, the overproduction of aldosterone in idiopathic hyperaldosteronism causes increased sodium reabsorption and potassium secretion by the renal tubule, expansion of the volume of extracellular fluid, suppression of plasma renin activity, and hypokalemia.

## DIAGNOSIS AND DIFFERENTIAL DIAGNOSIS

Although the features that characterize prolonged aldosterone excess may be as prominent in patients with idiopathic hyperaldosteronism as in patients with an APA, they usually are less pronounced and more subtle.[29] (It has been suggested that approximately half the patients with hypertension and suppressed plasma renin activity who show a decrease in plasma aldosterone to values between 5 and 10 ng/dL in response to saline infusion may have idiopathic hyperaldosteronism, even though baseline plasma aldosterone and serum potassium values may be normal.[14] When these diagnostic criteria are used, it may be difficult to distinguish between idiopathic hyperaldosteronism and low-renin essential hypertension. Such a sharp distinction between idiopathic hyperaldosteronism and low-renin essential hypertension may not be made with certainty until the pathogenesis of both disorders is more clearly delineated.) More important distinctions are those between idiopathic hyperaldosteronism and an APA, and between idiopathic hyperaldosteronism and primary bilateral adrenal hyperplasia, because therapy for these disorders is different. The *response to saline infusion* may be helpful because the aldosterone/cortisol ratio increases in an APA but remains unchanged or decreases, with a value of 2.2 or less, in idiopathic hyperaldosteronism[37] (Fig. 80-5). A value for plasma 18-hydroxycorticosterone less than 50 ng/dL at 8:00 a.m. after overnight bedrest is the usual finding in idiopathic hyperaldosteronism.[8,21] In patients with an APA, as well as in most patients with primary hyperplasia, values for 18-hydroxycorticosterone are >50 ng/dL and may exceed 100 ng/dL.[5,21,38] An increase in plasma aldosterone levels associated with a decrease in plasma cortisol levels after 2 hours of ambulation in the morning favors a diagnosis of idiopathic

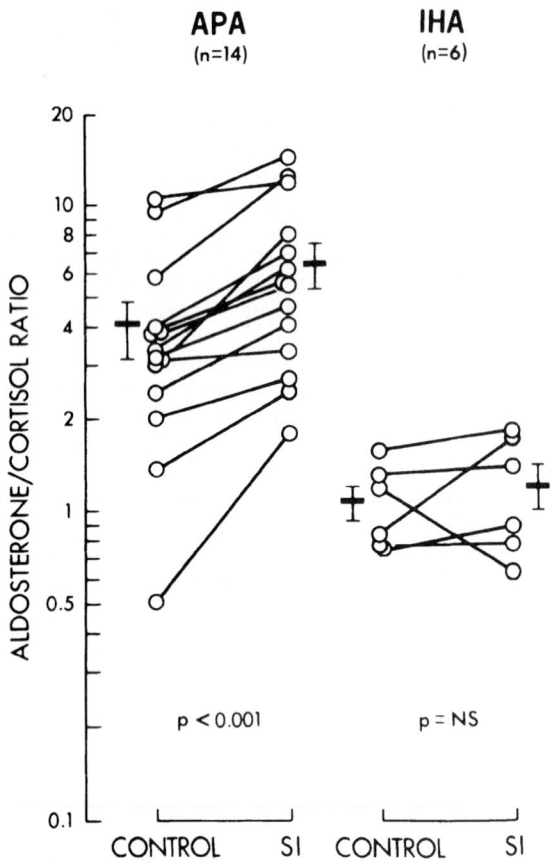

**FIGURE 80-5.** The plasma aldosterone/plasma cortisol ratio before (*control*) and after the administration of 1250 mL of a normal saline infusion (*SI*) over 2 hours from 8 a.m. to 10 a.m. Note consistent increases and higher values for the ratio in patients with aldosterone-producing adenoma (*APA*) than in those with idiopathic hyperaldosteronism (*IHA*). (From Arteaga E, Klein R, Biglieri EG. Use of the saline infusion test to diagnose the cause of primary aldosteronism. Am J Med 1985; 79:722.)

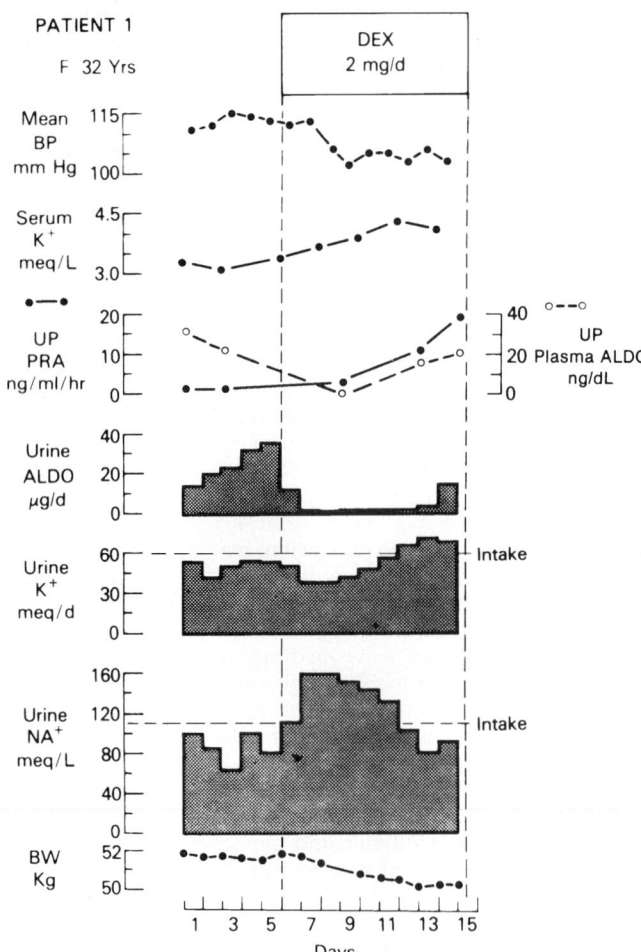

**FIGURE 80-6.** Response of mean blood pressure (*BP*), serum potassium (*K+*), ambulatory plasma renin activity (*UP PRA*), ambulatory plasma aldosterone concentration (*UP plasma ALDO*), urine ALDO, urine *K+*, urine sodium (*Na+*), and body weight (*BW*), to dexamethasone (*DEX*) in a patient with dexamethasone-suppressible hyperaldosteronism. Note the abrupt decrease in urine ALDO with DEX. (From Gill JR Jr, Bartter FC. Overproduction of sodium-retaining steroids by the zona glomerulosa is adrenocorticotropin-dependent and mediates hypertension in dexamethasone-suppressible aldosteronism. J Clin Endocrinol Metab 1981; 53:331.)

hyperaldosteronism but also may occur in association with an APA.[22] An increase in plasma aldosterone levels is more difficult to interpret than is a paradoxic decrease. Because of the number of false-positive and false-negative results, the test, as originally described, is not sufficiently dependable to be a reliable tool.[8] A refinement in the interpretation of the postural stimulation test (i.e., correction of the percentage increase in aldosterone by subtraction of the percentage increase in cortisol with standing) and acceptance of an increase in levels of plasma aldosterone with standing of <30% as a positive response for an adenoma has improved the predictive value of the test.[39] The response of plasma aldosterone to a single dose of a converting enzyme inhibitor, such as captopril, is more helpful in discriminating between hyperaldosteronism and low-renin essential hypertension than in separating patients with idiopathic hyperaldosteronism from those with an APA.[16] Interestingly, others have observed a decrease in aldosterone levels and blood pressure in patients with idiopathic hyperaldosteronism who are given larger doses of converting enzyme inhibitors for longer periods.[40] In contrast to the results obtained with a single dose of a converting enzyme inhibitor, testing with *saralasin*, which is an angiotensin II antagonist, correctly identified 15 patients with aldosteronism. After infusing saralasin, 10 μg/kg per minute for 30 minutes, plasma aldosterone levels increased in eight patients with idiopathic hyperaldosteronism but did not change in six patients with an adenoma.[41] Most important, these methods of evaluation assess adrenal function indirectly. Therefore, the more concordance there is among the results of several tests,

the more confidence one can have in the diagnosis. The best procedure for resolving uncertainty and making a more definitive diagnosis is adrenal vein catheterization. This procedure provides a direct assessment of adrenal biology; hence, bilateral supernormal secretion of aldosterone is readily distinguished from supernormal secretion of aldosterone by one adrenal gland with suppression of secretion from the contralateral gland. The results of adrenal vein catheterization in a representative patient with idiopathic hyperaldosteronism are shown in Table 80-2.

Once a tentative diagnosis of idiopathic hyperaldosteronism has been made, it is necessary to test for the less common disorder of dexamethasone-suppressible hyperaldosteronism, which also is characterized by bilateral adrenal hyperfunction. Because increased aldosterone production in dexamethasone-suppressible hyperaldosteronism is ACTH dependent, treatment with dexamethasone, 0.5 mg every 6 hours for 3 days, decreases plasma and urinary aldosterone activity to extremely low values[42] (<2.0 ng/dL and 2 μg per day, respectively; Fig. 80-6). Although treatment with glucocorticoids also decreases plasma and urinary aldosterone values in idiopathic hyperaldosteronism, the change occurs more slowly and is less pronounced (Fig. 80-7). If the results of dexamethasone suppression suggest that a patient

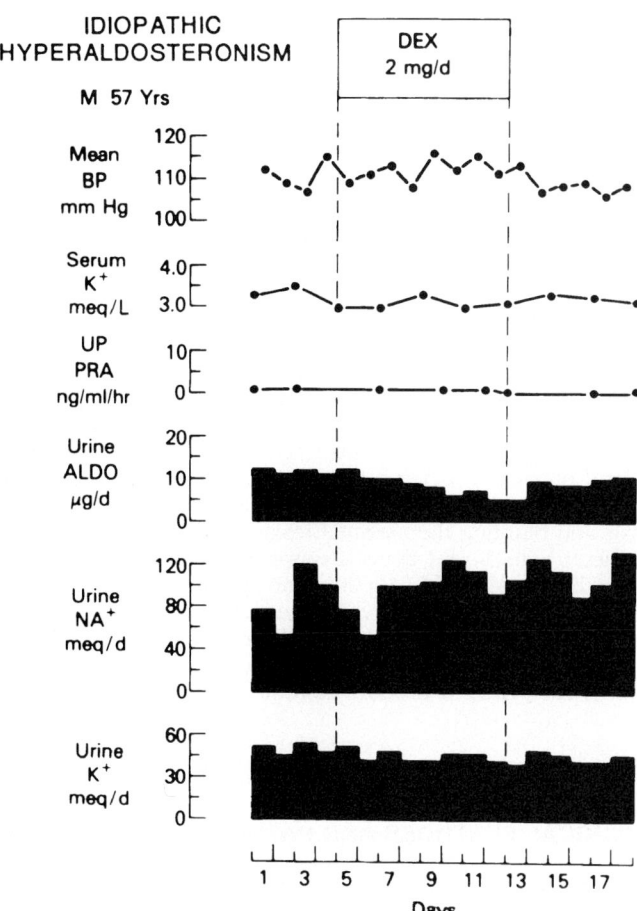

**FIGURE 80-7.** Response of mean blood pressure (*BP*), serum potassium (*K+*), ambulatory plasma renin activity (*UP PRA*), urine aldosterone (*ALDO*), urine sodium (*Na+*), and urine K+ to dexamethasone (*DEX*) in a patient with idiopathic hyperaldosteronism.

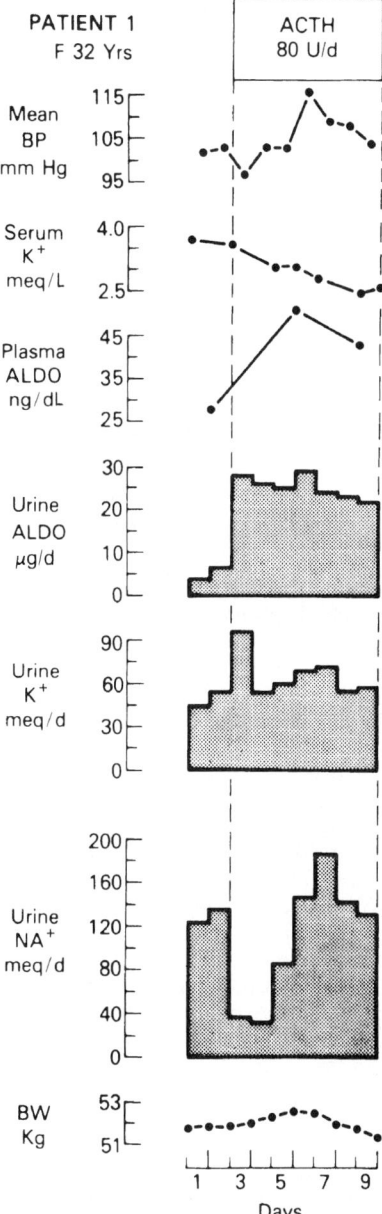

**FIGURE 80-8.** Response of mean blood pressure (*BP*), serum potassium (*K+*), plasma aldosterone (*plasma ALDO*), urine aldosterone (*urine ALDO*), urine K+, urine sodium (*Na+*), and body weight (*BW*) to adrenocorticotropin (*ACTH*) in a patient with dexamethasone-suppressible hyperaldosteronism. Note the sustained increase in ALDO during ACTH administration. (From Gill JR Jr, Bartter FC. Overproduction of sodium-retaining steroids by the zona glomerulosa is adrenocorticotropin-dependent and mediates hypertension in dexamethasone-suppressible aldosteronism. J Clin Endocrinol Metab 1981; 53:331.)

may have dexamethasone-suppressible hyperaldosteronism, determination of urinary 18-hydroxycortisol and 18-oxocortisol levels and of the response to ACTH should confirm the diagnosis. Identification of the gene mutations that cause dexamethasone-suppressible hyperaldosteronism makes it possible to screen for the disorder directly by genetic testing.[43]

## TREATMENT

Because adrenalectomy does not correct hypertension in idiopathic hyperaldosteronism,[44] except in rare patients with primary bilateral hyperplasia,[5,38] most patients must be treated medically. A calcium channel blocking drug, such as nifedipine, is a good antihypertensive agent in this condition because it decreases plasma aldosterone levels, presumably by inhibiting secretion, in addition to reducing blood pressure.[28] Enalapril, a converting enzyme inhibitor, also has been reported to decrease aldosterone production and to reduce blood pressure in a small series of patients with idiopathic hyperaldosteronism, and may prove to be a useful therapeutic agent.[40] If hypokalemia persists during treatment with nifedipine or enalapril, it usually can be managed by the addition of a potassium-sparing diuretic, such as triamterene or amiloride.

Unusual patients with bilateral hyperplasia who have high plasma aldosterone levels with positive postural stimulation test results and high 18-hydroxycorticosterone values should be given a trial of spironolactone.[5,38,40] If treatment with spironolactone produces a sustained decrease in blood pressure, then either unilateral or bilateral adrenalectomy may be curative.[5,38]

## DEXAMETHASONE-SUPPRESSIBLE HYPERALDOSTERONISM

### CLINICAL FEATURES AND PATHOPHYSIOLOGY

Dexamethasone-suppressible hyperaldosteronism (glucocorticoid-remediable aldosteronism) is a rare familial disorder inherited as an autosomal-dominant trait that exhibits the clinical features of hyperaldosteronism outlined previously.[45] As a result of an abnormality in the adrenal glands of patients with dexamethasone-suppressible hyperaldosteronism, ACTH causes a sustained overproduction of aldosterone (Fig. 80-8). This is in contrast to

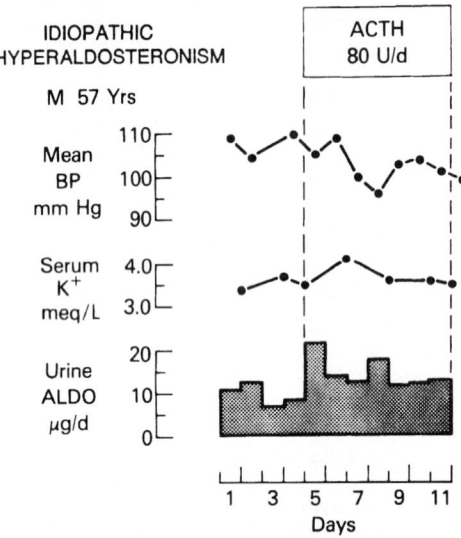

**FIGURE 80-9.** Response of mean blood pressure (*BP*), serum potassium (*K*+), and urine aldosterone (*ALDO*) to adrenocorticotropin (*ACTH*) in a patient with idiopathic hyperaldosteronism. Note transient response of ALDO to ACTH.

the usual response of aldosterone secretion to the prolonged administration of ACTH: after an initial rise, plasma aldosterone levels fall back to baseline values on the second day and show little change during the subsequent days of ACTH treatment (Fig. 80-9). Patients with dexamethasone-suppressible hyperaldosteronism exhibit gene duplication in which there is an unequal crossing over and fusion of the 5' regulatory region of 11β-hydroxylase with the coding region of aldosterone synthase to form a chimeric gene.[46] These chimeric gene formations probably have occurred because of the close proximity of the genes for 11β-hydroxylase and aldosterone synthase on chromosome 8 and their almost identical (95%) nucleotide sequences. These chimeric genes result in expression of aldosterone synthase under the regulatory control of ACTH in adrenal fasciculata cells. This explains why aldosterone is regulated by ACTH in these patients and why ACTH produces a sustained overproduction of aldosterone (see Fig. 80-8) instead of the normal transitory rise with a fall back to baseline values for the remainder of ACTH administration (see Fig. 80-9). The presence of an ACTH-regulated aldosterone synthase in adrenal fasciculata cells also explains why these patients form and excrete in their urine supernormal amounts of 18-hydroxycortisol and 18-oxocortisol[47] in addition to aldosterone. The production of aldosterone by fasciculata cells leads to suppression of the production of aldosterone by the zona glomerulosa. Because 18-oxocortisol has mineralocorticoid activity,[48] it may represent the mineralocorticoid activity seen in the radioreceptor assay that is not accounted for by summation of known mineralocorticoids.[49] An increase in 18-oxocortisol as well as in aldosterone during treatment with ACTH may explain the greater rise in blood pressure seen in patients with dexamethasone-suppressible hyperaldosteronism when ACTH is given than when high doses of aldosterone are given for a similar period.[50]

### DIAGNOSIS AND DIFFERENTIAL DIAGNOSIS

The unique clinical features of this subset of hyperaldosteronism are the rapid and complete suppression of plasma and urinary aldosterone levels in 24 to 48 hours by dexamethasone (see Fig. 80-6) and the sustained increase in aldosterone production that accompanies treatment with ACTH[42] (see Fig. 80-8). These features readily distinguish dexamethasone-suppressible hyperaldosteronism from idiopathic hyperaldosteronism, the disorder it most closely resembles. Improvement in hypertension

and in potassium wasting has been observed during pregnancy and may be a consequence of antagonism of overproduced mineralocorticoids by progesterone.[42] Once a diagnosis has been made, other members of the family should be screened by dexamethasone administration, by determination of urinary 18-hydroxycortisol and 18-oxocortisol levels, or by genetic testing. Although patients with dexamethasone-suppressible hyperaldosteronism usually have hypokalemia as well as hypertension, genetic screening has revealed that affected persons may have normal potassium levels with borderline elevation of the blood pressure.[42,51]

### TREATMENT

Dexamethasone, given in a dose that replaces the patient's output of glucocorticoids, corrects the overproduction of aldosterone, the hypokalemia, and the hyporeninemia, and reduces the blood pressure to normal levels (see Fig. 80-6). This treatment has the disadvantage of suppressing the hypothalamic-pituitary axis and blunting the maximal release of ACTH. Alternatively, patients with dexamethasone-suppressible hyperaldosteronism may be treated with a potassium-sparing diuretic, such as amiloride or triamterene, which is equally effective in correcting hypokalemia and decreasing blood pressure but does not affect the hypothalamic-pituitary axis. Spironolactone also is efficacious, but it tends to produce more side effects.

## ADRENOCORTICAL CARCINOMA

### CLINICAL FEATURES AND PATHOPHYSIOLOGY

Adrenocortical carcinoma is an extremely rare cause of hyperaldosteronism and accounts for fewer than 2% of aldosterone-producing tumors.[52,52a] Although aldosterone may be the only adrenal steroid overproduced early in the course of the disease, hypersecretion of cortisol usually occurs at some point. Occasionally, overproduction of adrenal androgens may occur. The circadian rhythm of plasma aldosterone levels, commonly seen in patients with an adenoma, is absent in patients with adrenal carcinoma, presumably because ACTH has little effect on aldosterone secretion by malignant tumor cells.

### DIAGNOSIS AND TREATMENT

The clinical presentation of adrenal carcinoma may be similar to that of adrenal adenoma, and the diagnosis may depend on the histologic demonstration of invasion of the capsule and blood vessels by tumor cells.[52] More commonly, the large size of the adrenal mass and its involvement of the kidney identifies it as a malignant tumor before surgery. Although metastases may not be demonstrable at the time the primary tumor is removed, they appear subsequently, with a course from diagnosis to death that may range from 2 to 13 years.[52] Treatment with mitotane (*o,p'*-DDD) appears to have little effect on the progression of the disease. Spironolactone may be variably effective in controlling renal potassium loss.

## SYNDROMES OF REAL OR APPARENT MINERALOCORTICOID EXCESS NOT CAUSED BY ALDOSTERONE

### CLINICAL FEATURES AND PATHOPHYSIOLOGY

Occasionally, patients may have features of mineralocorticoid excess (hypokalemic alkalosis, suppressed plasma renin activity, and hypertension) but plasma aldosterone concentrations that are low or undetectable (see Table 80-1). Some of these patients have increased production of other mineralocorticoids, such as deoxycorticosterone or corticosterone, as a result of 11β-hydroxylase deficiency or 17-hydroxylase deficiency, respectively (Table 80-3; see Chap. 77); others do not overproduce any of the known adrenal steroids. Still others accumulate an abnormal amount of cortisol in renal tubule cells because of 11β-hydroxysteroid dehydrogenase deficiency that leads to increased occupancy of mineralocorticoid receptors by cortisol.[53]

In *Liddle syndrome,* increased renal tubular reabsorption of sodium and secretion of potassium presumably are independent of stimulation by a mineralocorticoid because they are unaffected by treatment with spironolactone.[54] The cause of Liddle syndrome is mutations in the β subunit of the epithelial sodium channel.[55]

It now appears that most and possibly all of the described patients with apparent mineralocorticoid excess, some of them siblings, who were thought to be overproducing an unidentified steroid because they responded to spironolactone, have a deficiency of 11β-hydroxysteroid dehydrogenase.[56,57] As a result of this abnormality, those kidney and liver cells that lack the enzyme are unable to convert cortisol to cortisone. The manifestations of this block in cortisol metabolism are a prolonged half-life of plasma cortisol, suppression of ACTH, an accumulation of cortisol in renal tubule cells, and increased occupancy of mineralocorticoid receptors in those cells by cortisol. The last of these events is thought to mediate the changes of mineralocorticoid excess in these patients.[53] No defects have been found in the gene encoding for 11β-hydroxysteroid dehydrogenase.[58]

Studies suggest that the syndrome of apparent mineralocorticoid excess produced by the ingestion of *licorice* may be the result of inhibition of 11β-hydroxysteroid dehydrogenase by glycyrrhizic acid and its metabolite, glycyrrhetinic acid.[53,59] Normal volunteers fed glycyrrhetinic acid show a prolongation of the plasma cortisol half-life, with a tendency for the urinary metabolites of cortisol to increase and those of cortisone to decrease.[60] Because licorice compounds have no effect in adrenalectomized animals, they presumably induce sodium retention and potassium secretion by increasing the cortisol available to bind to mineralocorticoid receptors in renal tubule cells.

### DIAGNOSIS AND DIFFERENTIAL DIAGNOSIS

The syndrome of apparent mineralocorticoid excess caused by 11β-hydroxysteroid dehydrogenase deficiency can be readily diagnosed by determination of the urinary tetrahydrocortisol/tetrahydrocortisone ratio.[56,57] Because plasma cortisol levels are normal, and because deoxycorticosterone and corticosterone levels, similar to those of aldosterone, may be low or undetectable, these patients are readily distinguished from those with the adrenogenital syndromes, who have 11β-hydroxylase deficiency or 17-hydroxylase deficiency. In those patients with 11β-hydroxylase deficiency, boys also show precocious puberty and girls show virilization, and those with 17-hydroxylase deficiency are, for the most part, phenotypic females with sexual infantilism. Furthermore, hydrocortisone, which improves the adrenogenital syndromes, worsens the syndrome of 11β-hydroxysteroid dehydrogenase deficiency. Spironolactone produces improvement in patients with 11β-hydroxysteroid dehydrogenase deficiency as well as those with 11β-hydroxylase and 17-hydroxylase deficiency. This distinguishes these disorders from Liddle syndrome, which does not respond to the mineralocorticoid antagonist.

### TREATMENT

Treatment with spironolactone decreases the blood pressure and corrects other abnormal features of apparent mineralocorticoid excess resulting from 11β-hydroxysteroid dehydrogenase deficiency.[57] The effectiveness of dexamethasone, which has been reported to produce improvement in one patient but appeared to be ineffective in another, is uncertain.

**TABLE 80-3.**
**Hormonal Profile of Congenital Enzyme Deficiencies Causing Hypokalemia, Alkalosis, and Hypertension**

| ADRENAL STEROID PRODUCTION IN 11β-HYDROXYLASE DEFICIENCY | |
| --- | --- |
| *High* | *Low* |
| Progesterone | Cortisol |
| 17-Hydroxyprogesterone | Corticosterone |
| 11-Deoxycortisol | 18-Hydroxydeoxycorticosterone |
| Deoxycorticosterone | 18-Hydroxycorticosterone |
| | Aldosterone |

| ADRENAL STEROID PRODUCTION IN 17-HYDROXYLASE DEFICIENCY | |
| --- | --- |
| *High* | *Low* |
| Progestrone | 17-Hydroxyprogesterone |
| Deoxycorticosterone | Cortisol |
| Corticosterone | 18-Hydroxycorticosterone |
| 18-Hydroxydeoxycorticosterone | Aldosterone |

In patients with 11β-hydroxylase deficiency and 17-hydroxylase deficiency, treatment with hydrocortisone restores the overproduction of mineralocorticoids to normal levels. In Liddle syndrome, a potassium-sparing diuretic such as amiloride (5–10 mg daily) or triamterene (50–100 mg twice daily) is the drug of choice.[54] Infants or extremely young children may require smaller dosages.

## SECONDARY HYPERALDOSTERONISM

A variety of disorders of the kidney, heart, liver, and gastrointestinal tract may lead to hyperreninemia and, in turn, to hyperaldosteronism and hypokalemia. Because the blood pressure may be either normal or high, the disorders may be grouped on the basis of blood pressure.

Disorders that may give rise to hypertension with secondary hyperaldosteronism are renal artery stenosis (see Chap. 82), renin-secreting tumor (see Chap. 219), malignant hypertension, and chronic renal disease (see Table 80-1). Occasionally, the renal disorder may not be apparent clinically, and the hypertension and hypokalemia may be mistaken for primary aldosteronism. Determination of plasma renin activity after overnight bedrest and after ambulation for 2 hours should demonstrate whether this hormone is suppressed or stimulated and make the distinction between primary and secondary hyperaldosteronism. In chronic renal disease with renal insufficiency, plasma renin activity may be increased or suppressed. If it is suppressed, aldosterone also tends to be suppressed, except when the potassium concentration is high. Patients with hyperreninemia, hyperaldosteronism, and hypertension should be evaluated carefully for renal artery stenosis or renin-secreting tumor because these causes of hypertension may be curable.[61,62] Sampling of renal venous blood for the determination of plasma renin activity usually indicates whether the increase in renin release is bilateral or unilateral and, if it is unilateral, which kidney is the source.[61] Arteriography then can be performed to identify the nature of the disorder and confirm its location.

The development of percutaneous transluminal balloon dilation angioplasty for the treatment of renal artery stenosis has revolutionized the management of this disorder and stimulated a search for more effective ways to identify those patients with hypertension who have renal artery stenosis. The captopril test, in which the response of plasma renin activity and blood pressure to 50 mg captopril is determined over 60 minutes, reportedly has a high degree of sensitivity and specificity in untreated patients without renal parenchymal disease.[63]

Secondary hyperaldosteronism with normal blood pressure may occur in chronic renal disease, renal tubular acidosis, cardiac failure, cirrhosis of the liver, disorders of the gastrointesti-

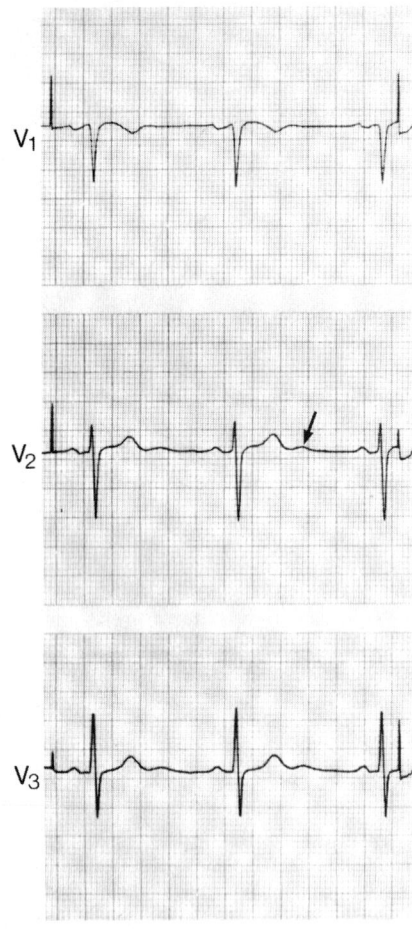

**FIGURE 80-10.** Severe potassium depletion caused by diuretics in a 58-year-old man. The serum potassium was 2.8 mEq/L. Note the prominent U waves (*arrow*), especially in lead $V_2$. Although all investigators are not in accord, most feel that severe hypokalemia may progress to potentially lethal ventricular arrhythmias. An electrocardiogram such as seen in this patient often is an initial clue to the presence of hypokalemia and may occur in many of the conditions discussed in this chapter. (Courtesy of Dr. Steven Singh.)

nal tract, and various renal tubulopathies (see Table 80-1). The mechanism that brings about an increase in renin release in each of these disorders is an alteration in cardiovascular function, which may be a decrease in either actual or effective circulating blood volume. Consideration of all these disorders in detail is beyond the scope of this review. The tubulopathies are discussed in some depth, but only those aspects of the other disorders that are responsible for secondary aldosteronism are noted.

Renal tubular acidosis and, at times, chronic renal disease are characterized by an impairment in the renal tubular secretion of hydrogen ions, with hypokalemia and acidosis. The defect in hydrogen ion secretion results in a loss of sodium and potassium, with contraction of the volume of extracellular fluid and stimulation of the renin-angiotensin-aldosterone system.[64] The increase in aldosterone secretion may intensify the renal potassium loss. In hepatic cirrhosis and cardiac failure, inadequate arterial filling appears to be the basis for increased renin release.[65]

The loss of potassium from the gastrointestinal tract or from the kidneys as a result of a disorder listed in Table 80-1 may cause severe potassium depletion (Fig. 80-10) and lead to hyperreninemia and hyperaldosteronism. Experimental evidence indicates that potassium depletion may decrease peripheral arterial resistance and increase pressor resistance of the arteries to angiotensin II, presumably by stimulating the synthesis of vasodilator prostaglandins, such as prostacyclin, in

vascular tissue, because treatment with a prostaglandin synthetase inhibitor corrects the abnormalities.[66,67] In hypokalemic animals, a dose of an angiotensin II antagonist that had no effect before the induction of potassium depletion produces a profound decrease in blood pressure.[66] This suggests that hyperreninemia is a compensatory adjustment that opposes vasodilator stimuli and helps to maintain blood pressure in the hypokalemic state. The overproduction of prostaglandins characterizes the severe potassium depletion that is produced by gastrointestinal disorders and renal tubulopathies,[68] and probably is the basis for the hyperreninemia, hyperaldosteronism, and pressor resistance associated with these disorders.

## BARTTER SYNDROME

### CLINICAL FEATURES AND PATHOPHYSIOLOGY

Bartter syndrome includes a number of disorders of tubular transport that may be familial or acquired as a result of a disease such as cystinosis.[69,70] The syndrome may present in childhood as a failure to thrive, weakness, salt craving, polyuria, and polydipsia, or in adulthood as an incidental finding with little associated symptomatology. In the latter instance, the syndrome may have been present since childhood in a mild form that was not detected. Serum chloride and potassium levels are low and serum carbon dioxide content is normal or increased. The serum magnesium concentration may be normal or low, and creatinine clearance may be normal or decreased.

Physiologic studies suggested that an impairment of chloride transport in the diluting segment of the nephron, presumably the thick ascending limb of the loop of Henle, was the cause of the syndrome in some patients.[71] The defect in chloride reabsorption would impair the ability of the tubule not only to dilute, but also to concentrate tubular fluid, because it results in a decrease in medullary hypertonicity. A defect in chloride transport by the thick ascending limb also would decrease potassium reabsorption in this segment and stimulate its secretion distally by increasing the volume of tubular fluid delivered to the distal nephron, in which potassium secretion is flow-dependent.[72] Molecular biology studies indicate that such patients may have a mutation in the gene encoding a renal chloride channel, CLCNKB.[73] This channel represents a major pathway through which chloride travels from cells of the thick ascending limb across their basolateral membrane into the interstitium. Hypercalciuria may or may not be an associated finding.

The $Na^+-K^+-2Cl^-$ cotransporter also mediates the reabsorption of chloride, in addition to sodium and potassium, in the thick ascending limb.[74] Mutations in the gene NKCC2 that encodes for this cotransporter produce a syndrome, apparent in the immediate postnatal period, characterized by failure to thrive, marked polyuria, and polydipsia.[75] The delivery is frequently premature and complicated by polyhydramnios. Hypercalciuria is present and usually complicated by nephrocalcinosis and, presumably, is the basis for the impairment in urinary concentrating ability. Diluting ability appears to remain intact.

Mutations in the gene ROMK that encodes for a potassium channel, which are also located in the luminal membrane of cells of the thick ascending limb, produce a syndrome clinically similar to that produced by mutations in NKCC2.[76] ROMK encodes for an ATP-sensitive potassium channel, which recycles potassium that has been reabsorbed from tubular fluid by thick ascending limb cells (from the cells back into the tubular lumen). This process of potassium recycling ensures sufficient luminal potassium for $Na^+-K^+-2Cl^-$ transporter to function. Thus, an impairment in function of this channel has physiologic consequences similar to those produced by mutations in NKCC2.

Mutations in the gene encoding for the thiazide-sensitive sodium-chloride cotransporter, TSC, located in the cells of the distal convoluted tubule produce a variant of Bartter syndrome also referred to as *Gitelman syndrome*.[77] These patients differ from those with mutations in CLCNKB, NKCC2, and ROMK in that they have hypocalciuria and hypermagnesiuria with hypomagnesemia. Urinary diluting and concentrating abilities are usually intact. The impaired function that results from mutations in TSC and its associated phenotype appears to account for the majority of patients diagnosed as Bartter syndrome.

The transport abnormalities previously discussed, by impairing sodium chloride reabsorption in the thick ascending limb or distal convoluted tubule, increase the delivery of these ions distally to the cortical collecting tubule, where increased sodium reabsorption leads to increased potassium secretion. Why impaired sodium chloride reabsorption in the thick ascending limb increases excretion of calcium but not that of magnesium, and why impaired sodium chloride reabsorption in the distal convoluted tubule decreases calcium excretion but increases that of magnesium is not yet understood.

Renal potassium loss and consequent potassium depletion stimulate prostaglandin overproduction and, in turn, the abnormalities that once were thought to be unique to Bartter syndrome but now are recognized as the pathophysiologic results of potassium depletion. Although it is not possible to demonstrate a decrease in peripheral resistance in Bartter syndrome, as was done in experimental potassium depletion in dogs, evidence for an increase in vasodilator stimuli may be inferred from the following observations:

1. A high level of urinary prostaglandins, especially 6-keto-PGF$_{1\alpha}$, which is a metabolite of prostacyclin, consistent with an increase in vasodilator prostaglandins in vascular tissue.[78]
2. Increased pressor resistance to angiotensin II that is corrected only partially when plasma angiotensin II is restored to normal by converting enzyme inhibition.[79]
3. Blood pressure that is normal despite hyperreninemia and increased sympathoadrenal activity and that decreases markedly when an antagonist of angiotensin II is given.[80,81]
4. Correction of prostaglandin overproduction by treatment with a prostaglandin synthetase inhibitor corrects the hyperreninemia, the increased sympathoadrenal activity, the pressor resistance to angiotensin II and to norepinephrine, and the hypotensive response to an angiotensin II inhibitor.[80–82]

The vasodilative stimuli of prostaglandins and the increase in plasma bradykinin associated with them are opposed by compensatory increases in activity of the renin-angiotensin and sympathoadrenal systems that stabilize blood pressure, as shown in Figure 80-11.

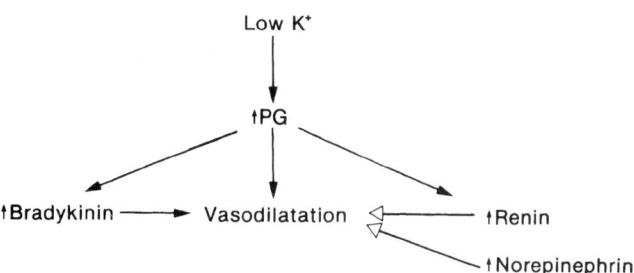

**FIGURE 80-11.** Bartter syndrome. Increased synthesis of prostaglandins (*PG*), presumably prostacyclin, by vascular tissue is stimulated by low body potassium levels (*K⁺*) and leads to vasodilatation and an increase in pressor resistance. An increase in bradykinin, associated with the increase in PGs, augments the vasodilatation. Increases in activity of the renin-angiotensin and sympathoadrenal systems oppose vasodilatation and maintain blood pressure. (From Gill JR Jr. The role of chloride transport in the thick ascending limb in the pathogenesis of Bartter syndrome. Klin Wochenschr 1982; 60:1212.)

**TABLE 80-4.**

**A Comparison of Phenotypic Findings Caused by Mutations in Genes That Encode for a Renal Tubular Cotransporter or Channel That Has Been Identified in Patients Diagnosed with Bartter Syndrome**

| MUTATED GENE: | NKCC2 | ROMK | CLCNKB | TSC |
|---|---|---|---|---|
| Serum magnesium | Normal | Normal | Normal | Low |
| Urinary magnesium | Normal | Normal | Normal | High |
| Urinary calcium | High | High | Normal or high | Low |
| Nephrocalcinosis | Present | Present | Absent | Absent |
| Urinary concentration | Decreased | Decreased | Decreased | Normal |

Gene and gene product: *NKCC2*, Na⁺-K⁺-2Cl⁻ cotransporter; *ROMK*, potassium channel; *CLCNKB*, chloride channel; *TSC*, thiazide sensitive Na-Cl cotransporter.

## DIAGNOSIS AND DIFFERENTIAL DIAGNOSIS

The clinical features of Bartter syndrome (hypokalemic alkalosis, hyperreninemia, and hyperaldosteronism with normal blood pressure) are not unique to this disorder because they may be caused by potassium loss from the gastrointestinal tract, as well as from the kidney. The clinical history may indicate the source of potassium loss when it is familial chloride diarrhea[83] or a similar problem, but when the loss is caused by covert vomiting or laxative abuse, the physician must resort to other strategies to make the diagnosis. The measurement of daily urinary sodium, chloride, and potassium levels while patients are consuming constant diets containing 100 mEq per day of sodium and chloride may be helpful. If the potassium loss is caused by a tubulopathy, genetic evaluation may indicate the specific autosomal-recessive genetic trait. The presence of such a trait is suggested by stable values for urinary sodium, chloride, and potassium that approximate oral intake. If potassium loss is from the gastrointestinal tract, the amount and pattern of urinary electrolytes will reflect this. Overall, excretion will be considerably lower than intake and, if vomiting is the cause, the excretion of chloride will be disproportionately lower than that of sodium. Although the urinary potassium level usually also is decreased, it may be inappropriately high if alkalosis and hypokalemia are severe enough to impair potassium reabsorption by the thick ascending limb of the loop of Henle.[84]

Distinguishing between covert diuretic abuse and Bartter syndrome can be difficult. In addition to the clinical features of potassium depletion, diuretics such as furosemide and thiazides also decrease sodium chloride reabsorption by the distal tubule, thereby mimicking the transport abnormalities of Bartter syndrome. Screening the urine for diuretics may be helpful in reaching the correct diagnosis.

To establish the diagnosis of the specific transport abnormality, the phenotype must be characterized by measurement of serum magnesium, urinary magnesium, and urinary calcium. Determination of maximal fractional free water clearance ($CH_2O/C_{IN}$) and concentrating ability provide additional information. The phenotypic patterns associated with the transport abnormalities demonstrated to date are shown in Table 80-4.

## TREATMENT

Supplementation with potassium chloride (120–160 mEq per day of potassium) and, if hypomagnesemia is present, magnesium chloride (30–50 mEq per day of magnesium) may be all that is required in some patients.[85] If symptoms persist, a potassium-sparing diuretic such as amiloride or triamterene may be added to the regimen. Although prostaglandin synthetase inhibition may correct the overproduction of prostaglandins and, in turn, the prostaglandin-dependent abnormalities, it does not prevent potassium loss. Generally, the side effects of prostaglandin synthetase inhibitors outweigh the benefits, except in those patients with hypercalciuria in whom they may ameliorate renal calcium loss in addition to correcting hyperreninemia and hyperaldosteronism.[85,86]

# REFERENCES

1. Ulick S. Diagnosis and nomenclature of the disorders of the terminal portion of the aldosterone biosynthetic pathway. J Clin Endocrinol Metab 1976; 43:92.
2. Fanestil DD, Kipnowski J. Molecular action of aldosterone. Klin Wochenschr 1982; 60:1180.
3. Kornel L, Kanamarlapudi N, Travers T, et al. Studies on high affinity binding of mineralo- and glucocorticoids in rabbit aorta cytosol. J Steroid Biochem 1982; 16:245.
4. Sweiry JH, Binder HJ. Characterization of aldosterone-induced potassium secretion in rat distal colon. J Clin Invest 1989; 83:844.
5. Irony I, Kater CE, Biglieri EG, Shackleton CHL. Correctable subsets of primary aldosteronism, primary adrenal hyperplasia and renin responsive adenoma. Am J Hypertens 1990; 3:576.
6. Etker S, Enger EA. Aldosterone-producing adrenal adenoma in children. Eur J Pediatr Surg 1992; 2:370.
7. Stowasser M, Gordon RD, Tunny TJ, et al. Familial hyperaldosteronism type II: five families with a new variety of primary aldosteronism. Clin Exp Pharmacol Physiol 1992; 19:319.
8. Bravo EL, Tarazi RC, Dunstan HP, et al. The changing clinical spectrum of primary aldosteronism. Am J Med 1983; 74:641.
9. Holland OB, Thomas C, Brown H, et al. Aldosterone suppression with dopamine infusion in low-renin hypertension. J Clin Invest 1983; 72:754.
10. Yamaji T, Ishibashi M, Sekihara H, et al. Plasma levels of atrial natriuretic peptide in primary aldosteronism and essential hypertension. J Clin Endocrinol Metab 1986; 63:815.
11. Higuchi K, Nawata H, Kato KI, et al. Lack of inhibitory effect of alpha-human atrial natriuretic polypeptide on aldosteronogenesis in aldosterone producing adenoma. J Clin Endocrinol Metab 1986; 63:192.
12. Biglieri EG, Forsham PH. Studies on the expanded extracellular fluid and the response to various stimuli in primary aldosteronism. Am J Med 1961; 30:564.
13. Kageyama Y, Bravo EL. Neurohumoral and hemodynamic responses to chronic intracerebroventricular infusion of aldosterone in conscious dogs. (Abstract.) Hypertension 1987; 10:373.
14. Holland OB, Brown H, Lavon K, et al. Further evaluation of saline infusion for the diagnosis of primary aldosteronism. Hypertension 1984; 6:717.
15. Zadik Z, Levin PA, Hamilton BP, Kowarski AA. Detection of primary aldosterone by the 6-hour integrated aldosterone-renin ratio. Hypertension 1986; 8:285.
16. Lyons DF, Kem DC, Brown RD, et al. Single dose captopril as a diagnostic test for primary aldosteronism. J Clin Endocrinol Metab 1983; 57:892.
17. Naomi S, Iwaoka T, Omeda T, et al. Clinical evaluation of the captopril screening test for primary aldosteronism. Jpn Heart J 1985; 26:549.
18. Iwaoka T, Umeda T, Naomi S, et al. The usefulness of the captopril test as a simultaneous screening for primary aldosteronism and renovascular hypertension. Am J Hypertens 1993; 6:899.
19. Vetter H, Fischer M, Galanski M, et al. Primary aldosteronism: diagnosis and noninvasive lateralization procedures. Cardiology 1985; 72(Suppl 1):57.
20. Doppman JL, Gill JR Jr, Miller DL, et al. Distinction between hyperaldosteronism due to bilateral hyperplasia and unilateral aldosteronoma: reliability of CT. Radiology 1992; 184:677.
21. Biglieri EG, Schambelan M. The significance of elevated levels of plasma 18-hydroxycorticosterone in patients with primary aldosteronism. J Clin Endocrinol Metab 1979; 49:87.
22. Ganguly A, Dowdy A, Luetscher JA, Melada GA. Anomalous postural response of plasma aldosterone concentration in patients with aldosterone producing adrenal adenoma. J Clin Endocrinol Metab 1973; 36:401.
23. Dunnick NR, Doppman JL, Gill JR Jr, et al. Localization of functional adrenal tumors by computed tomography and venous sampling. Radiology 1982; 142:429.
24. Young WF Jr, Stanson AW, Grant CS, et al. Primary aldosteronism: adrenal venous sampling. Surgery 1996; 120:913.
25. Bravo EL. Primary aldosteronism. Issues in diagnosis and management. Endocrinol Metab Clin North Am 1994; 23:271.
25a. Calvo-Romero JM, Ramos-Salado JL. Recurrence of adrenal aldosterone-producing adenoma. Postgrad Med J 2000; 76:160.
26. Walther MM. Laparoscopic surgery for adrenal disease. Updates Principles and Practice of Oncology 1997; 11:Number 12.
27. Loriaux DL, Menard R, Taylor A, et al. Spironolactone and endocrine dysfunction. Ann Intern Med 1976; 85:630.
28. Nadler JL, Hsueh W, Horton R. Therapeutic effect of calcium channel blockade in primary aldosteronism. J Clin Endocrinol Metab 1985; 60:896.
29. Ferris JR, Beavers DG, Brown JJ, et al. Clinical, biochemical and pathological features of low-renin ("primary") hyperaldosteronism. Am Heart J 1978; 95:375.
30. Sen S, Bravo EL, Bumpus FM. Isolation of a hypertension-producing compound from normal human urine. Circ Res 1977; 40(Suppl 1):1.
31. Carey RM, Sen S. Recent progress in the control of aldosterone secretion. Recent Prog Horm Res 1986; 42:251.
32. Griffing GT, Berelowitz B, Hudson M, et al. Plasma immunoreactive gamma-melanotropin in patients with idiopathic hyperaldosteronism,

aldosterone-producing adenomas, and essential hypertension. J Clin Invest 1985; 76:163.
33. Griffing GT, McIntosh T, Berelowitz B, et al. Plasma β-endorphin levels in primary aldosteronism. J Clin Endocrinol Metab 1985; 60:315.
34. Franco-Saenz R, Mulrow PJ, Kitai K. Idiopathic aldosteronism: a possible disease of the intermediate lobe of the pituitary. JAMA 1984; 251:2555.
35. Shenker Y, Gross MD, Grekin RJ. Central serotonergic stimulation of aldosterone secretion. J Clin Invest 1985; 76:1485.
36. Gross MD, Grekin RJ, Gniadek TC, Villareal JZ. Suppression of aldosterone by cyproheptadine in idiopathic aldosteronism. N Engl J Med 1981; 305:181.
37. Arteaga E, Klein R, Biglieri EG. Use of the saline infusion test to diagnose the cause of primary aldosteronism. Am J Med 1985; 79:722.
38. Banks WA, Kastin AJ, Biglieri EG, Ruiz AE. Primary adrenal hyperplasia: a new subset of primary hyperaldosteronism. J Clin Endocrinol Metab 1984; 58:783.
39. Fontes RG, Kater CE, Biglieri EG, Irony I. Reassessment of the predictive value of the postural stimulation test in primary aldosteronism. Am J Hypertens 1991; 4:786.
40. Griffing GT, Melby JC. The therapeutic effect of a new angiotensin-converting enzyme inhibitor, enalapril maleate, in idiopathic hyperaldosteronism. J Clin Hypertens 1985; 3:265.
41. Brown RD, Kem DC, Hogan MJ, Hegstad RL. Evaluation of a test using saralasin to differentiate primary aldosteronism due to an aldosterone-producing adenoma from idiopathic hyperaldosteronism. Metabolism 1984; 33:734.
42. Gill JR Jr, Bartter FC. Overproduction of sodium-retaining steroids by the zona glomerulosa is adrenocorticotropin-dependent and mediates hypertension in dexamethasone-suppressible aldosteronism. J Clin Endocrinol Metab 1981; 53:331.
43. Liddle GW, Bledsoe I, Coppage WS. A familial renal disorder simulating primary aldosteronism but with negligible aldosterone secretion. Trans Assoc Am Physicians 1963; 76:199.
44. George JM, Wright L, Bell NH, Bartter FC. The syndrome of primary aldosteronism. Am J Med 1970; 43:343.
45. Fallo F, Kuhnle Y, Bossaro M, Sonino N. Abnormality of aldosterone and cortisol late pathways in glucocorticoid-remediable aldosteronism. J Clin Endocrinol Metab 1994; 79:772.
46. Lifton RP, Dluhy RG, Powers M, et al. Hereditary hypertension caused by chimaeric gene duplications and ectopic expression of aldosterone synthase. Nature Genetics 1992; 2:66.
47. Ulick S, Chan CK, Gill JR Jr, et al. Defective fasciculata zone function as the mechanism of glucocorticoid-remediable aldosteronism. J Clin Endocrinol Metab 1990; 71:1151.
48. Ulick S, Land M, Chu MD. 18-Oxocortisol, a naturally occurring mineralocorticoid agonist. Endocrinology 1983; 113:2320.
49. Speiser PW, Martin KO, Kao-Lo G, New MI. Excess mineralocorticoid receptor activity in patients with dexamethasone-suppressible hyperaldosteronism is under adrenocorticotropin control. J Clin Endocrinol Metab 1985; 6:129.
50. New MI, Peterson RE, Saenger P, Levine LS. Evidence for an unidentified ACTH induced steroid hormone causing hypertension. J Clin Endocrinol Metab 1976; 43:1283.
51. Rich GM, Ulick S, Cook S, et al. Glucocorticoid-remediable aldosteronism in a large kindred: clinical spectrum and diagnosis using a characteristic biochemical phenotype. Ann Intern Med 1992; 116:813.
52. Arteaga E, Biglieri EG, Kater CE, et al. Aldosterone-producing adrenocortical carcinoma: preoperative recognition and course in three cases. Ann Intern Med 1984; 101:316.
52a. Yoshimoto T, Naruse M, Ito Y, et al. Adrenocortical carcinoma manifesting pure primary aldosteronism: a case report and analysis of steroidogenic enzymes. J Endocrinol Invest 2000; 23:112.
53. Edwards CR, Walker BR, Benediktsson R, Secki JR. Congenital and acquired syndromes of apparent mineralocorticoid excess. J Steroid Biochem Mol Biol 1993; 45:1.
54. Liddle GW, Bledsoe I, Coppage WS. A familial renal disorder simulating primary aldosteronism but with negligible aldosterone secretion. Trans Assoc Am Physicians 1963; 76:199.
55. Shimkets RA, Warnock DG, Bositis CM, et al. Liddles syndrome: Heritable human hypertension caused by mutations in the β subunits of the epithelial sodium channel. Cell 1994; 79:407.
56. Monder C, Shackleton CHL, Bradlow HC, et al. The syndrome of apparent mineralocorticoid excess: its association with 11β-dehydrogenase and 5β-reductase deficiency and some consequences for corticosteroid metabolism. J Clin Endocrinol Metab 1986; 63:550.
57. DiMartino-Nardi J, Stoner E, Martin K, et al. New findings in apparent mineralocorticoid excess. J Clin Endocrinol Metab 1987; 27:49.
58. Nikkila H, Tannin GM, New MI, et al. Defects in the HSD11 gene encoding 11 beta-hydroxysteroid dehydrogenase are not found in patients with apparent mineralocorticoid excess of 11-oxoreductase deficiency. J Clin Endocrinol Metab 1993; 77:687.
59. Walker BR, Edwards CR. Licorice-induced hypertension and syndromes of apparent mineralocorticoid excess. Endocrinol Metab Clin North Am 1994; 23:359.
60. Stewart PM, Valentino R, Wallace AM, et al. Mineralocorticoid activity of liquorice: 11-beta-hydroxysteroid dehydrogenase deficiency comes of age. Lancet 1987; 2:821.
61. Pickering TG, Sos TA, Vaughan ED Jr, Laragh JH. Differing patterns of renal vein renin in patients with renovascular hypertension and their role in predicting the response to angioplasty of one or both renal arteries. Nephron 1986; 44(Suppl 1):8.

62. Robertson JIS. Renin-secreting tumour. Contrib Nephrol 1984; 43:153.
63. Muller FB, Sealey JE, Case DB, et al. The captopril test for identifying renovascular disease in hypertensive patients. Am J Med 1986; 80:633.
64. Gill JR Jr, Bell NH, Bartter FC. Impaired conservation of sodium and potassium in renal tubular acidosis and its correction by buffer anions. Clin Sci 1967; 33:577.
65. Gill JR Jr. Edema. Annu Rev Med 1970; 21:269.
66. Galvez OG, Bay WH, Roberts BW, Ferris TF. The hemodynamic effects of potassium deficiency in the dog. Circ Res 1977; 40(Suppl 1):1.
67. Gullner H-G, Graf AK, Gill JR Jr, Mitchell MD. Hypokalemia stimulates prostacyclin synthesis in the rat. Clin Sci 1983; 65:43.
68. Gill JR Jr. Prostaglandins in Bartter's syndrome and in potassium-deficient disorders that mimic it. Miner Electrolyte Metab 1981; 6:76.
69. Godard C, Vallotton MD, Broyer M, Roger P. A study of the inhibition of the renin-angiotensin system in renal potassium wasting syndromes, including Bartter's syndrome. Helv Paediatr Acta 1972; 27:495.
70. Gitelman HJ. Unresolved issues in the pathogenesis of Bartter's syndrome and its variants. Curr Opin Nephrol Hypertens 1994; 3:471.
71. Gill JR Jr, Bartter FC. Evidence for a prostaglandin-independent defect in chloride reabsorption in the loop of Henle as a proximal cause of Bartter's syndrome. Am J Med 1978; 65:766.
72. Wright FC, Giebisch G. Renal potassium transport: contributions of individual nephron segments and populations. Am J Physiol 1978; 235:F515.
73. Simon DB, Bundra RS, Mansfield TA, et al. Mutations in the chloride channel gene, CLCNKB, cause Bartter's syndrome type III. Nature Genet 1997; 17:171.
74. Simon DB, Karet FE, Hamdan JM, et al. Bartter's syndrome, hypokalaemic alkalosis with hypercalciuria is caused by mutations in the Na-K-2Cl cotransporter NKCC2. Nature Genet 1996; 13:183.
75. Seyberth HW, Rascher W, Schweer H, et al. Congenital hypokalemia with hypercalciuria in preterm infants: a hyperprostaglandinuric tubular syndrome different from Bartter's syndrome. J Pediatr 1985; 107:694.
76. Simon DB, Karet FE, Rodriguez-Soriano J, et al. Genetic heterogeneity of Bartter's syndrome revealed by mutations in the K+ channel ROMK. Nature Genet 1996; 14:152.
77. Simon DB, Nelson-Williams C, Bia MJ, et al. Gitelman's variant of Bartter's syndrome, inherited hypokalemic alkalosis, is caused by mutations in the thiazide-sensitive Na-Cl cotransporter. Nature Genet 1996; 12:24.
78. Gullner H-G, Bartter FC, Cerletti C, et al. Prostacyclin overproduction in Bartter's syndrome. Lancet 1979; 2:767.
79. Fujita T, Ando K, Sato Y, et al. Independent roles of prostaglandins and the renin and angiotensin system in abnormal vascular reactivity in Bartter's syndrome. Am J Med 1982; 73:71.
80. Sasaki H, Okumura M, Asano T, et al. Responses to angiotensin II antagonist before and after treatment with indomethacin in Bartter's syndrome. BMJ 1977; 2:975.
81. Gullner H-G, Gill JR Jr, Bartter FC, et al. Correction of increased sympathoadrenal activity in Bartter's syndrome by inhibition of prostaglandin synthesis. J Clin Endocrinol Metab 1980; 50:857.
82. Bartter FC, Gill JR Jr, Frolich JL, et al. Prostaglandins are overproduced by the kidneys and mediate hyperreninemia in Bartter's syndrome. Trans Assoc Am Physicians 1976; 89:77.
83. Pearson AJG, Sladen GE, Edmonds CJ, et al. The pathophysiology of congenital chloridorrhoea. Q J Med 1973; 167:453.
84. Garella S, Chazan JA, Cohen JJ. Saline-resistant metabolic alkalosis or "chloride-wasting nephropathy." Ann Intern Med 1970; 73:31.
85. Gill JR Jr. Bartter's syndrome. In: Krieger DT, Bardin CW, eds. Current therapy in endocrinology and metabolism 1988–1989. St Louis: CV Mosby, 1988:153.
86. Mourani CC, Sanjad SA, Akatcherian CY. Bartter syndrome in a neonate: early treatment with indomethacin. Pediatr Nephrol 2000; 14:143.

# CHAPTER 81

# HYPOALDOSTERONISM

JAMES C. MELBY

## ISOLATED HYPOALDOSTERONISM

Isolated hypoaldosteronism, *a selective deficiency of aldosterone secretion without alteration in cortisol production*, results in a persistent hyperkalemia, which may be associated with profound muscle weakness and cardiac arrhythmias. Isolated hypoaldosteronism can result from inborn errors in aldosterone biosynthesis, failure of the zona glomerulosa owing to autoimmune adrenal disease in

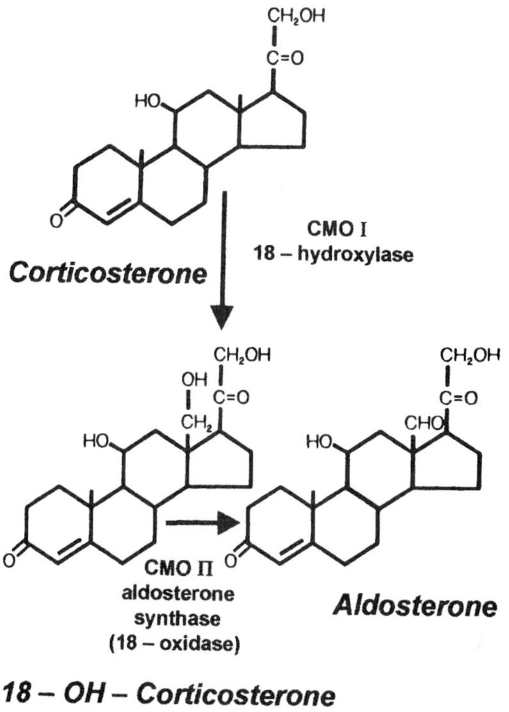

**FIGURE 81-1.** Terminal steps in the biosynthesis of aldosterone. Corticosterone methyl oxidase (*CMO*) type I and II deficiencies exhibit defects in the hydroxylase-oxidase reactions. In CMO type I deficiency, levels of the 18-hydroxylated product, 18-OH-corticosterone, are reduced. In CMO type II deficiency, 18-OH-corticosterone production is markedly increased. In both cases, aldosterone deficiency results.

association with critical illness, altered function of the renin-angiotensin system in the syndrome of hyporeninemic hypoaldosteronism, unilateral adrenalectomy for an aldosterone-producing adenoma, or pharmacologic inhibition of aldosterone. *Mineralocorticoid resistance* occurs when there is a lack of response to aldosterone despite the presence of this hormone.[1]

## PRIMARY DEFICIENCY

### INBORN ERRORS

Inborn errors in the oxidation of corticosterone to form aldosterone have been described as *corticosterone methyl oxidase type I deficiency* (CMO I) and *corticosterone methyl oxidase type II deficiency* (CMO II). Corticosterone is at first hydroxylated and oxidized at the 18th position to yield aldosterone. This sequence of enzymatic events is seen in Figure 81-1. CMO I is also referred to as *18-hydroxylase;* CMO II is also referred to as *aldosterone synthase* or *aldosterone oxidase*. CMO II deficiency is more common than CMO I deficiency. Some of the CMO I and CMO II enzymes have activity residing in the isozyme of steroid 11β-hydroxylase; this isozyme activity is limited to the zona glomerulosa. 18-Hydroxylase and 18-oxidase activities are required for the production of aldosterone. Mutations in the genes that encode the isozyme result in defective synthesis of aldosterone.

**Corticosterone Methyl Oxidase Type I Deficiency (18-Hydroxylase Deficiency).** CMO I deficiency is extremely rare. Biochemically, it is characterized by a marked overproduction of corticosterone by the zona glomerulosa without a corresponding increase in 18-hydroxycorticosterone and a virtual absence of aldosterone. Scrutiny of some case reports casts doubt on whether they represent type I or type II deficiency because 18-hydroxycorticosterone measurement was not available. However, clinical results for a North American kindred in Pennsylvania, although attributed to CMO II deficiency, probably represent the type I variant.[2,3]

**Corticosterone Methyl Oxidase Type II Deficiency (Aldosterone Synthase Deficiency).**  CMO II deficiency is inherited as an autosomal-recessive trait. This deficiency is rare but has been observed with an increased frequency among Jews of Iranian origin. The biomolecular studies have been extensive.[4]

In both CMO I and CMO II deficiencies, the severity of the clinical manifestations is inversely related to the age at diagnosis: it becomes less severe as the child ages. CMO II deficiency, if recognized clinically, has its onset between 1 week and 3 months of age and is characterized by severe dehydration, vomiting, and failure to grow. Hyponatremia, hyperkalemia, and metabolic acidosis are uniformly present. The plasma renin activity (PRA) is elevated, and plasma aldosterone levels are low. On the other hand, plasma 18-hydroxycorticosterone levels are markedly increased, and the 18-hydroxycorticosterone/aldosterone ratio in plasma exceeds 5. Also, the ratio of the urinary metabolite of 18-hydroxycorticosterone, 18-hydroxytetrahydroaldosterone, to the metabolite of aldosterone, tetrahydroaldosterone, also exceeds 5. In older children, adolescents, and adults, the abnormal steroid pattern described may be present and may persist throughout life without clinical manifestations.

Mineralocorticoid (fludrocortisone) is given during infancy and early childhood, but this therapy does not have to be continued in most cases. Moreover, spontaneous normalization of growth can occur in patients who are untreated. It is not understood why aldosterone deficiency is so much more threatening in infancy than in adult life. It is particularly puzzling that isolated hypoaldosteronism caused by low renin secretion in aging patients has clinical significance, whereas patients with asymptomatic inherited hypoaldosteronism, resulting from either CMO I or CMO II deficiency, exhibit none of the manifestations of hyporeninemic hypoaldosteronism. These same observations are true of patients with pseudohypoaldosteronism (PHA).

## FAILURE OF ADRENAL GLOMERULOSA FUNCTION

**Autoimmume Adrenal Failure.**  As autoimmune adrenal failure evolves, selective aldosterone deficiency may emerge in the presence of preservation of zona fasciculata cell function. Although glucocorticoid responsiveness to corticotropin (ACTH), metyrapone, or insulin-induced hypoglycemia may be normal, PRA is elevated in the presence of a low or undetectable plasma corticotropin level. This is accompanied by mild metabolic acidosis and, occasionally, hyponatremia. During late stages of the disease, progression to panadrenal insufficiency may occur. A period of up to 1 year may separate the onset of the mineralocorticoid and glucocorticoid deficiencies.[5]

In selective aldosterone deficiency caused by autoimmune disease, antiadrenal antibodies can be detected. Mucocutaneous candidiasis and hypoparathyroidism may occur concurrently,[6] a form of multiple autoimmune endocrinopathy.

A patient with idiopathic hemochromatosis, weakness, postural hypotension, and loss of libido was found to have mild glucose intolerance and low gonadotropins in addition to normokalemia, hyponatremia, and a modest elevation of urea. PRA was elevated, and aldosterone levels were suppressed. Cortisol response to ACTH and urinary 17-hydroxysteroid were normal. The patient failed to conserve sodium on a sodium-restricted diet. This suggests that isolated mineralocorticoid deficiency can occur secondary to glomerulosa cell failure caused by iron deposition.[7]

**Hypoaldosteronism in Ill Patients.**  Hyperreninemic hypoaldosteronism can occur in critically ill patients, such as those in septic states, or in hemodynamically compromised subjects. Most of these patients have prolonged illness and hypotension of long duration, with or without hyperkalemia. The cortisol secretion is elevated, commensurate with the level of the stressful state. Because aldosterone, corticosterone, and 18-hydroxycorticosterone (but not cortisol) secretions become suppressed within 48 to 96 hours of continuous ACTH stimulation of the

adrenal gland,[8] prolonged ACTH secretion secondary to stress may impair 11β-hydroxylase and 18β-hydroxylase enzymes and may be the underlying mechanism of this syndrome. However, these patients have an increased plasma 18-hydroxycorticosterone/aldosterone ratio, and their aldosterone response to angiotensin II (A-II) infusion is impaired; this suggests that a selective inhibition of CMO II may play a role in the development of this disease. Because hypoxia is associated with increased renin activity and cortisol secretion and diminished aldosterone secretion,[9] insufficiency of CMO II activity may be the result of hypoxia or other circulating factors affecting the zona glomerulosa. Autopsy studies in adrenal glands from patients with this syndrome have revealed atrophy or necrosis involving most of the layers of the adrenal gland, including the zona glomerulosa. However, an isolated necrosis of the zona glomerulosa has not been found; this is probably because blood flows from the outer cortex toward the medulla, and hypoperfusion would affect the inner corticomedullary region first.[10]

Hyperreninemic hypoaldosteronism may be caused by the release of various cytokines in chronic illness. Tumor necrosis factor (TNF) and interleukin-1 (IL-1), which act both pyrogenically and catabolically, have been found to be elevated in body fluids during severe infection, and TNF and IL-1 are known to inhibit the stimulatory actions of A-II and ACTH on aldosterone secretion. However, the action of potassium on aldosterone release is not altered. Although 12-hydroxyeicosanoic acid stimulates aldosterone and is a second messenger of A-II, TNF inhibits A-II stimulation of 12-hydroxyeicosanoic acid release.[11]

It is plausible that high circulating levels of atrial natriuretic hormone (ANH) during illness contribute to the aldosterone level in these patients. ANH is a powerful suppresser of aldosterone secretion both in vitro and in vivo. It suppresses aldosterone secretion in humans despite upright posture or A-II infusion.[12] In cultured adrenal cells, it also blunts the aldosterone secretion that ordinarily occurs after stimulation by potassium, A-II, and ACTH.[13] The ANH may be stimulated by subclinical volume expansion resulting from mildly reduced renal function, congestive heart failure, atrial arrhythmias, or other subclinical cardiac disease associated with atrial distension. In addition, many critically ill patients are on medications that may interfere with the renin-angiotensin-aldosterone axis (see later in this chapter) and consequently contribute to the reduced aldosterone production. Because no major clinical complications are reported with this form of hypoaldosteronism, it seldom requires treatment other than avoidance of drugs that may exacerbate the hypoaldosteronism.

## SECONDARY DEFICIENCY

### SYNDROME OF HYPORENINEMIC HYPOALDOSTERONISM

The syndrome of hyporeninemic hypoaldosteronism (SHH), also referred to as *distal renal tubular acidosis type 4*, is common; it usually occurs in middle-aged and elderly patients (median age, 68 years) and in men more often than women. Diabetes mellitus occurs in less than half the patients; chronic renal insufficiency is present in 80% of patients. The condition is frequent in patients with tubulointerstitial forms of renal disease, but it has been described in virtually every type of renal abnormality.[14] Fifty percent to 70% of patients with unexplained hyperkalemia and renal disease and a glomerular filtration rate that is sufficient to sustain normokalemia are found to have SHH.[15]

Most patients with this syndrome have low PRA and aldosterone that cannot be stimulated by appropriate maneuvers. Hyperchloremic metabolic acidosis occurs in less than 70% of cases, and mild to moderate hyponatremia is found in half of the patients. Importantly, hyperkalemia is observed in all subjects.[16] These patients exhibit decreased fractional excretion of potassium in relation to glomerular filtration rate and a reduced response to kaliuretic stimuli (including sodium bicarbonate, sodium sulfate, and diuretics) as well as to intravenous potassium chloride. The hyperkalemia is out of proportion to the degree of renal insufficiency. Proposed mechanisms include hyporeninemia caused by a damaged juxtaglomerular apparatus, sympathetic insufficiency, altered renal prostaglandin production, or impaired conversion of prorenin to renin.[17] Low renin production does not appear to be the sole factor because the PRA may be inappropriately normal in some patients. Certain cases may be explained by sodium retention leading to volume expansion and thus to a secondary suppression of renin and aldosterone.[18] The leading causes of interstitial nephritis, in which hyperkalemia can occur early and before chronic renal failure, are anatomic genitourinary abnormalities, analgesic abuse with aspirin or phenacetin, hyperuricemia, nephrocalcinosis, nephrolithiasis, and sickle cell disease.

Diabetic patients are predisposed to hyperkalemia because of insulin deficiency and hyperglycemia. Interestingly, both insulin deficiency and hyperglycemia can independently produce a maldistribution of total body potassium. Hyperglycemia results in extracellular hyperosmolality, producing an extracellular flux of potassium. Furthermore, insulin deficiency prevents the cellular uptake of potassium, presumably related to the metabolic actions of this hormone. Autonomic insufficiency, which can be a complication of diabetes, results in hyporeninemic hypoaldosteronism, and the degree of autonomic neuropathy correlates with the duration of hyperglycemia.[19]

Immunoglobulin M monoclonal gammopathy has been associated with nodular glomerulosclerosis, a concentrating defect, and hyporeninemic hypoaldosteronism. The hypoaldosteronism is associated with decreasing renal function, suggesting that κ light-chain nephropathy is a cause of this syndrome.[20]

Patients with the acquired immunodeficiency syndrome may have persistent hyperkalemia secondary to either adrenal insufficiency or, less frequently, hyporeninemic hypoaldosteronism. The hypoaldosterone patients usually have adequate aldosterone stimulation, suggesting that inadequate renin is the cause of the hypoaldosteronism.[21]

**Treatment.** No ideal medical therapy has been established for SHH. Most patients with mild selective hypoaldosteronism require no therapy. With preventive measures and education of patients, therapy may be avoided. The decision to treat SHH and the selection of specific therapeutic agents depend on a number of factors, including the degree of hyperkalemia, the extent of renal insufficiency, the presence of diabetes mellitus, the level of blood pressure, and the status of sodium balance. Once the diagnosis of SHH has been made, factors that precipitate or perpetuate suppression of renin biogenesis, aldosterone biogenesis, or both should be avoided (see Chaps. 79 and 183).

Reducing the extracellular potassium load can be the single most effective preventive measure in controlling hyperkalemia in SHH. Reducing dietary intake of potassium is helpful. Low sodium foods and use of salt substitutes, which often contain potassium as the alternative cation (such as low-salt milk, which contains 60 mEq/L potassium), should be avoided. Examples of foods high in potassium include dried fruits (30 mEq/cup), meat (60 mEq/lb), and decaffeinated coffee (4 mEq/cup). Other sources of potassium include transfusions of bank blood (30 mEq/L) and high-dose penicillin (1.7 mEq/10⁶ U).

The long-term control of glucose homeostasis in diabetes mellitus may reduce the risk of developing SHH. Perhaps autonomic insufficiency is avoidable in well-controlled diabetics. Because many medications can interfere at multiple points in the renin-aldosterone axis, avoidance of these drugs can be of major importance. β-Adrenergic receptor blockers, prostaglandin synthetase inhibitors, and potassium-sparing diuretics should be avoided in patients with known SHH and in diabetic patients with latent hypoaldosteronism. Calcium-channel blockers, antidopaminergic agents, and drugs that impair adrenal function should be used with caution. Patients on angio-

tensin-converting enzyme inhibitors should be carefully monitored for hyperkalemia. Prolonged administration of heparin should be avoided because it can worsen the hypoaldosteronism and it has been associated with lethal hyperkalemia.

In severe SHH, fludrocortisone acetate is used in dosages of 0.1 to 1.0 mg per day, which is equivalent to 200 to 2000 μg of aldosterone daily. Ninety percent of patients become normokalemic on fludrocortisone, which, however, carries the risk of salt retention and hypertension and edema.

Diuretics may be the cardinal therapy for patients with SHH and coexisting diseases associated with sodium retention. Older patients with hypertension, mild renal impairment, and congestive heart failure respond better to diuretic therapy than to mineralocorticoid replacement. Because kaliuresis is the goal of diuretic therapy, the choice of a potent kaliuretic drug is of the utmost importance. Chlorthalidone and hydrochlorothiazide, a slightly less kaliuretic agent, meet this requirement. The "loop" diuretics, such as furosemide and ethacrynic acid, are less potent kaliuretic agents and induce a greater degree of natriuresis. Another potential benefit of diuretic therapy is stimulation of residual renin release in patients with hyporeninism caused by autonomic insufficiency.

Sodium bicarbonate cannot be recommended as routine therapy in the treatment of hyporeninemic hypoaldosteronism because it is hazardous in elderly patients with coexisting renal impairment, congestive heart failure, and hypertension.

Sodium polystyrene sulfonate (Kayexalate), a cation exchange resin, removes ~1 mEq/g potassium by exchanging sodium for potassium in a ratio of 1.0 to 1.5. Thus, this drug increases sodium load and may be contraindicated in patients unable to tolerate an increase of this cation. Calcium-exchange resins are under investigation and may become available as an alternative therapy.

## HYPOALDOSTERONISM AFTER ADRENALECTOMY FOR ALDOSTERONOMA

Hypoaldosteronism from chronic volume expansion was reported in postadrenalectomy patients after surgical excision of an aldosterone-producing adenoma.[22] These patients develop severe hyperkalemia and hypotension lasting several days to several weeks after surgery. Similar forms of hypoaldosteronism due to volume expansion were also reported in patients chronically ingesting sodium bicarbonate (baking soda) for the treatment of gastrointestinal symptoms.

## PHARMACOLOGIC INHIBITION OF ALDOSTERONE

Pharmacologic agents such as cyclosporine, heparin sodium, and calcium-channel blockers specifically inhibit aldosterone biogenesis by the zona glomerulosa of the adrenal gland[23] (Table 81-1). Cyclosporine A produces hypoaldosteronism by dual effects on the adrenal cortex; first, an acute blockade of the A-II–induced aldosterone production, and second, an inhibition of growth and steroidogenic capacity of adrenocortical cells. The latter effect may be caused by an impairment of protein synthesis. Polysulfated glycosaminoglycans, such as heparin sodium, impair aldosterone biosynthesis from the zona glomerulosa. With prolonged administration, heparin sodium can produce significant hypoaldosteronism with severe hyperkalemia because of a direct toxic effect on the zona glomerulosa, evidenced by a hyperreninemic hypoaldosteronism and zona glomerulosa atrophy.[24] The least toxic dose of heparin sodium is unknown, but a dose of 20,000 U per day for 5 days has been observed to reduce aldosterone secretion. This is an uncommon cause of hypoaldosteronism, but it may result in fatal hyperkalemia. This effect appears to be caused by chlorbutanol, which is used as a preservative with heparin, rather than by the heparin itself. Heparin-induced aldosterone deficiency has been used therapeutically in some patients with chronic glomerulonephritis and initial hyperaldosteronism.[25] Calcium-channel

**TABLE 81-1.**

**Pharmacologic Agents That Induce Direct or Indirect Inhibition of Aldosterone or of Aldosterone Effects**

Heparin (via chlorbutanol)
Cyclosporine A
Calcium-channel blockers
β-Blockers
Prostaglandin synthetase inhibitors
Angiotensin-converting enzyme inhibitors
Spironolactone
Triamterene
Amiloride
Aminoglutethimide
Metyrapone
Trilostane
Bromocriptine (?)

blockers inhibit aldosterone biosynthesis and, under certain clinical conditions, may cause hypoaldosteronism by lowering aldosterone secretion through inhibition of calcium influx.

β-Blockers and prostaglandin synthetase inhibitors are frequent causes of hyporeninemic hypoaldosteronism. Juxtaglomerular cells, which synthesize and secrete renin, contain β-adrenergic receptors; either intrinsic neuronal or extrinsic adrenergic stimuli trigger these receptors, resulting in an immediate release of renin. As a result, β-blocking adrenergic drugs interfere with renin secretion and may cause hypoaldosteronism. Prostaglandin synthetase inhibitors, which specifically inhibit cyclooxygenase, block renin release and can result in severe hyperkalemia caused by hyporeninemic hypoaldosteronism. Prostaglandin $E_2$ ($PGE_2$) directly stimulates renin release, probably by a direct action on the juxtaglomerular apparatus. Furosemide-induced renin release is blunted by indomethacin and other prostaglandin synthetase inhibitors.[26]

Angiotensin-converting enzyme inhibitors and potassium-sparing diuretics may contribute to the hypoaldosteronism and hyperkalemia of various conditions. Angiotensin-converting enzyme inhibitors act by inactivating angiotensin-converting enzyme, which interrupts the renin-aldosterone axis and results in iatrogenic hypoaldosteronism.[27] Spironolactone has two effects: it is a mineralocorticoid receptor antagonist, and it inhibits aldosterone biosynthesis, presumably by competing with corticosteroid biogenesis.[28] Triamterene produces potassium retention by a direct action on non–aldosterone-mediated distal tubular exchange sites.[29] Amiloride acts on the luminal surfaces of epithelial membranes to block sodium channels, resulting in less sodium resorption but diminished potassium secretion.

Drugs that impair adrenal function are increasingly used for the hormonal treatment of breast cancer and medical management of Cushing syndrome; these agents can cause hypoaldosteronism. Aminoglutethimide, metyrapone, and trilostane block various enzymatic steps in the synthesis of mineralocorticoids, glucocorticoids, and adrenal sex steroids. Lower doses of these drugs may not be associated with hyperkalemia because secretion of aldosterone precursors, such as deoxycorticosterone, may confer significant mineralocorticoid activity.[27]

Drugs affecting the dopaminergic system produce significant alterations in aldosterone secretion. It is believed that aldosterone is under tonic dopamine inhibition; thus, the administration of dopaminergic agonists, such as bromocriptine, may impair aldosterone secretion in certain physiologic situations.[27]

# MINERALOCORTICOID RESISTANCE

Mineralocorticoid resistance implies a lack of response to aldosterone despite its presence. Aldosterone binds to intracellular mineralocorticoid receptors, which interact with DNA. To influence gene transcription and subsequent synthesis of protein such as $Na^+/K^+$-ATPase on the basolateral surface of renal epithelial cells and the amiloride-sensitive epithelial sodium channel (ENaC) on the apical membrane,[1] ENaC-mediated entry of sodium into the cell represents the rate-limiting step for the reabsorption of sodium.

## PSEUDOHYPOALDOSTERONISM TYPE I

*Pseudohypoaldosteronism type I (PHA I)* is a rare inherited salt-wasting disorder that was first described in 1958 as a defective renal-tubular response to mineralocorticoid in infancy.[30] Patients present in the neonatal period with *dehydration, hyponatremia, hypokalemia, metabolic acidosis, and failure to thrive despite normal glomerular filtration and normal renal and adrenal function.*[5] When patients fail to respond to mineralocorticoid therapy, PHA I should be considered the underlying disorder. Diagnosis includes an elevated plasma aldosterone level and increased plasma renin activity. PHA I can be inherited either as a recessive or dominant trait. Neonates affected with PHA I have a primary defect that affects the renal reabsorption of sodium.[30a]

Further analysis of PHA I has revealed that it can be divided into *two distinct disorders with unique physiologic and genetic characteristics—the renal form of PHA I and a multiorgan form of PHA I.* The renal form of PHA I follows mendelian inheritance and is transmitted in an autosomal-dominant manner. This disease is limited to a mineralocorticoid resistance only in the kidneys. Interestingly, the patient's condition spontaneously improves within the first several years of his or her life, thus allowing discontinuation of therapy.

The multiorgan or generalized form of PHA I also follows mendelian inheritance but is transmitted as an autosomal-recessive trait.[31] There is a high incidence of consanguinity in the families; the parents of these patients usually have physiologically normal levels of aldosterone and renin.[31] The two main characteristics that distinguish this form of PHA I from the renal form are (a) the patient has a multiorgan disorder such that mineralocorticoid resistance is not limited to the kidneys (it can be seen in the kidney, sweat and salivary glands, and the colonic mucosa), and (b) this condition does not spontaneously improve with age[31,31a]; hence, it is considered to be more severe. Because sodium reabsorption is coupled to potassium and hydrogen ion secretion, patients often exhibit decreased potassium- and hydrogen-ion secretion with decreased sodium reabsorption; hence, potassium and hydrogen ions accumulate in the body, ultimately causing hyperkalemia and metabolic acidosis. Moreover, a decrease in vascular volume is detected by vessels in the juxtaglomerular region, leading to increased secretion of renin. Elevated plasma renin levels will ultimately cause an increase in aldosterone secretion through the indirect impact of angiotensin II.

Originally, it had been thought that PHA I, analogous to a steroid-hormone resistance syndrome, might result from a defect in the mineralocorticoid receptor, either because of an absence or deficiency of receptors or because of an abnormality in the structure of the receptor (such as, perhaps, a defect in the aldosterone-binding domain). The mineralocorticoid-receptor gene was mapped to chromosome 4 by somatic cell hybridization and regionally localized to 4q31.1-31.2 by fluorescent in situ hybridization. Although evidence supporting a defect in the gene coding for the mineralocorticoid receptor was found in some studies, most studies have been inconsistent.[32]

Although the involvement of the mineralocorticoid receptor in PHA I was not completely ruled out, it has been hypothesized that PHA I may be a heterogeneous condition resulting from a disorder either at the prereceptor level or at the postreceptor level. At the prereceptor level, there may be some factor that competes for the aldosterone-binding site or causes the cleavage of the mineralocorticoid receptor. At the postreceptor level, it was hypothesized that PHA I might result from a defect in one or both of the aldosterone-induced proteins: the Na$^+$/K$^+$-ATPase and/or the ENaC.[31,31a]

## AMILORIDE-SENSITIVE EPITHELIAL SODIUM CHANNEL

The ENaC is a highly selective sodium channel found at the apical surface of salt-reabsorbing tight epithelia of tissues, including distal nephrons, the distal colon, salivary and sweat glands, lung, and taste buds.[33] As described earlier, it plays a critical role in the control of sodium balance, extracellular fluid volume, and blood pressure, because the ENaC-mediated entry of sodium into the cell in these epithelia represents the rate-limiting step for the movement of sodium from the mucosal side to the serosal side.[34] These channels allow the transport of sodium into the cell by diffusion without coupling to the flows of other solutes and without the direct input of metabolic energy.[33] ENaCs are often referred to as "amiloride-sensitive" because of their high sensitivity to the potassium-sparing diuretic amiloride and its analogs. These channels are directly stimulated by aldosterone and inhibited by amiloride.[33]

ENaCs are composed of three subunits: α, β, and γ, which are 35% homologous at the amino-acid level and are conserved throughout evolution.[35] Moreover, the three subunits are similar in structure and share the following characteristics: short intracellular amino-acid carboxyl termini, two transmembrane-spanning domains, and a large extracellular loop. The genetic locus of the gene coding for the α subunit of ENaC has been traced to chromosome 12, and the genes coding for the β and γ subunits have been traced to chromosome 16.[35] The α subunit has been regionally localized to 12p13.1–pter, and the α and γ subunits have been regionally localized to 16p12.2–13.11.[31] Of the three, the α subunit is thought to be the most important for the proper functioning of ENaC.

## LIDDLE SYNDROME (PSEUDOALDOSTERONISM)

(In 1994, evidence was found explaining the underlying cause of Liddle syndrome, a disorder for which the physiologic symptoms are *opposite* to those of PHA I.[36,37] This condition, also known as *pseudoaldosteronism*, is an autosomal-dominant form of hypertension characterized by *volume expansion*, *hypokalemia*, and *alkalosis*. Using genetic analysis, the illness was traced to two distinct mutations in the genes coding for the subunits of the ENaC. It was found that it is caused by mutations in the genes coding for the β and γ subunits of ENaC, which cause truncation of the cytoplasmic carboxyl termini that, in turn, lead to a constitutive activation of ENaC activity.[36] It is now believed that these mutations increase the number of sodium channels in the apical membrane by deleting a critical consensus motif.)

## PSEUDOHYPOALDOSTERONISM TYPE I—MULTIORGAN

Recognizing that PHA I may result from a loss of ENaC function, researchers have attempted to prove that mutations coding for the β, γ, and α subunits of ENaC (similar but *opposite* to those seen in Liddle syndrome) may render the ENaC nonfunctional and unresponsive to mineralocorticoids.

Three mutations have been found that result in a loss of ENaC function in neonates with the multiorgan type of PHA I.[31] These mutations better define the differences between the two forms of PHA I.

Two of the mutations involve the subunit, and one mutation involves the β subunit.[31] On the α subunit, a two base-pair deletion at codon 168 introduces a frameshift mutation and thus disrupts the protein before the first transmembrane domain. The other mutation of the α subunit is a single-base substitution at codon R508 that changes a cytosine base to thymine. This truncates the α subunit before the second transmembrane domain by introducing a premature termination codon in the extracellular domain. The result is normal production of the first transmembrane domain, but no production of a second

domain or of the intracytoplasmic carboxyl termini, and an incomplete production of the extracellular domain.

## THE TWO TYPES OF PSEUDOHYPOALDOSTERONISM TYPE I

The α subunit is the most important of the three subunits and is required for normal ENaC activity.[34] Thus, it is reasonable to assume that an α subunit not containing all its domains may lead to a nonfunctional channel protein. Both of these mutations lead to a loss of ENaC activity because both transmembrane domains are required for normal channel activity.

On the β subunit, a point mutation causes the substitution of serine for glycine at amino acid 37. The glycine at position 37 on the β subunit ENaC lies within a segment preceding the first transmembrane spanning region that is homologous among all members of the ENaC gene family. This mutation on the β subunit has been shown to diminish ENaC activity but does not lead to a complete loss of activity; after this mutation, ENaC activity is still higher than it would be in the absence of a β subunit.[36a]

The gating of ENaC involves a complex mechanism that remains poorly understood; however, it has been suggested that the highly conserved 20 amino-acid segment containing the conserved glycine may control the normal gating of ENaC such that the glycine-to-serine mutation on the β subunit would alter the open probability of ENaC.[34] The glycine-to-serine mutation may impair the normal functioning of the ENaC gating domain and shift the equilibrium between two different gating modes, thus favoring a mode with short open times and long closed times. Moreover, in addition to being involved in the gating of ENaC, glycine may be part of a functional domain of ENaC that is regulated directly or indirectly by aldosterone.[34] As stated previously, ENaC is stimulated by the presence of aldosterone; thus, the previous hypothesis would help to explain why a PHA I patient with this mutation on the β subunit fails to respond to the body's elevated levels of aldosterone and to exogenously administered mineralocorticoids.[8]

Two additional mutations on the γ subunit of ENaC further elucidate the cause of the autosomal-recessive form of PHA I.[36] One mutation involves a replacement of a highly conserved amino acid triplet Lys-Tyr-Ser by Asn in the extracellular loop immediately adjacent to the transmembrane domain. The other mutation is a 300-nucleotide deletion in the extracellular loop that introduces a stop codon before the second transmembrane domain; both of these mutations are thought to cause either a complete or a partial loss of ENaC activity.

## PSEUDOHYPOALDOSTERONISM TYPE I—RENAL

Once the genetic basis and pathophysiology of the autosomal-recessive or multiorgan form of PHA I had been defined, and studies had shown that ENaC was probably not involved in the pathophysiology of the autosomal-dominant or renal form of PHA I, attention turned to the mineralocorticoid receptor. Although some studies have found evidence supportive of a role for the mineralocorticoid receptor as a candidate for PHA I, other studies have failed to find functional mutations in the gene coding for the mineralocorticoid receptor. Retrospectively, it is noteworthy that *all but one of these studies investigated patients with the autosomal-recessive form* of PHA I, which has since been linked to the ENaC. Two frameshift mutations have been identified that may help to explain the underlying cause of the renal form of PHA I[37,38]; sequence analysis revealed two single base-pair deletions on exon 2, one at codon 335 and the other at codon 459. Both of these deletions result in frameshifts that lead to a gene product lacking the entire DNA- and hormone-binding domains, as well as the dimerization motif.[37]

**Improvement of Renal Pseudohypoaldosteronism Type I with Age.** A plausible hypothesis for the improvement of the renal form of PHA I with age is that the very important early role that aldosterone plays in salt homeostasis diminishes later in life because of a transition to a higher salt intake diet. Breast milk is very low in sodium, and aldosterone levels are elevated in infancy to increase sodium reabsorption. Only those infants in whom salt homeostasis is stressed by an intercurrent illness with volume depletion actually will manifest clinically recognizable PHA I.[38] Nevertheless, the phenomenon of improvement with age requires further study.

## TREATMENT

PHA I patients are *resistant to mineralocorticoid therapy*; therefore, standard treatment includes supplementation with sodium chloride (2–8 g per day) and cation exchange resins. This usually corrects the patient's biochemical imbalance. However, if a patient shows signs of severe hyperkalemia, peritoneal dialysis may be necessary. For those PHA I patients in whom *hypercalciuria* is found, the recommended course of treatment usually involves treatment either with indomethacin or with hydrochlorothiazide. Indomethacin is thought to act by causing a reduction in the glomerular filtration rate and/or an inhibition of the effect of prostaglandin $E_2$ on renal tubules.[39] Indomethacin reduces polyuria, sodium loss, and the hypercalciuria. (Hydrochlorothiazide, which is a potassium-losing diuretic that sometimes is administered to diminish hyperkalemia, also has been shown to reduce hypercalciuria in PHA I patients.[39])

In patients with the autosomal-dominant or *renal* form of PHA I, the signs and symptoms decrease with age; nevertheless, salt supplementation is required for the first 2 to 3 years of life.[14] In patients with the autosomal-recessive or *multi-organ* type of PHA I, however, resistance to therapy with sodium chloride or drugs that decrease serum potassium concentrations often occurs and may even lead to death in infancy of hyperkalemia.[40] These patients often require very high amounts of salt in their diet (as much as 45 g NaCl per day).[41]

Carbenoxolone (CBX), a derivative of glycyrrhetinic acid in licorice, is moderately successful in helping to reduce the high-salt requirement in the diets of renal PHA I patients (however, it is not useful in treating multiorgan PHA I patients).[41] CBX acts by inhibiting 11β-hydroxysteroid dehydrogenase (11β-HSD) activity. This enzyme, which is present at high levels in aldosterone-responsive target tissues, exerts a mineralocorticoid effect mainly in patients with the renal form of PHA I. Normally, 11β-HSD has an antimineralocorticoid effect, because it converts cortisol into its inactive form, cortisone. However, by inhibiting this enzyme, CBX allows unmetabolized cortisol to bind to and activate mineralocorticoid receptors in a manner similar to that of aldosterone.[41]

## PSEUDOHYPOALDOSTERONISM TYPE II

Pseudohypoaldosteronism type II (PHA II), also known as *familial hyperkalemia and hypertension* or *Gordon syndrome*, is a *non-salt-wasting disorder* characterized by *hyperkalemia despite normal renal glomerular filtration and hypertension*.[42] Hyperchloremia, metabolic acidosis, and suppressed plasma renin activity variably occur. Linkage analysis reveals autosomal-dominant transmission and locus heterogeneity of this trait to chromosomes 1q31-q42 and 17p11-q21.15. Although the pathogenesis has not been completely resolved, clinical studies suggest possible primary defects including (a) a recessive renal-sodium reabsorption proximal to the site of aldosterone action, (b) a generalized membrane defect impairing movement of potassium ions into cells, or (c) an increased renal-chloride reabsorption that in turn would impair potassium secretion. Treatment with a combination of furosemide, desmopressin (DDAVP), and sodium bicarbonate has been effective in controlling the hyperkalemia, hypertension, hyperchloremia, and hyperchloremic metabolic acidosis.[42]

## REFERENCES

1. White PC. Disorders of aldosterone biosynthesis and action. N Engl J Med 1994; 331:250.
2. Veldhuis JD, Kulin HE, Santen RJ, et al. Inborn error in the terminal step of aldosterone biosynthesis. N Engl J Med 1980; 303:117.
3. Ulick S, Wang J, Morton D. The biochemical phenotypes of two inborn errors in the biosynthesis of aldosterone. J Clin Endocrinol Metab 1992; 72:1415.
4. White PC, Pascoe L. Disorders of steroid 11β-hydroxylase isozymes. Trends Endocrinol Metab 1992; 3:229.
5. Kokko JP. Primary acquired hypoaldosteronism. Kidney Int 1985; 27:690.
6. Marieb NJ, Melby JC, Lyall SS. Isolated hypoaldosteronism associated with idiopathic hypoparathyroidism. Arch Intern Med 1974; 134:424.
7. Thomas JP. Aldosterone deficiency in a patient with idiopathic haemochromatosis. Clin Endocrinol (Oxf ) 1984; 21:271.
8. Aguilera G, Fujita K, Catt KJ. Mechanism of inhibition of aldosterone secretion by adrenocorticotropin. Endocrinology 1981; 108:522.
9. Slater JDH, Tuffey RE, Williams ES, et al. Control of aldosterone secretion during acclimatization to hypoxia in man. Clin Sci 1969; 37:327.
10. Davenport MW, Zipser RD. Association of hypotension with hyperreninemic hypoaldosteronism in critically ill patient. Arch Intern Med 1983; 143:735.
11. Antonipillai I, Wang Y, Horton R. Tumor necrosis factor and interleukin-1 may regulate renin secretion. Endocrinology 1990; 126:273.
12. Clark BA, Brown RS, Epstein FH. Effect of atrial natriuretic peptide on potassium-stimulated aldosterone secretion: potential relevance to hypoaldosteronism in man. J Clin Endocrinol Metab 1992; 75:399.
13. Rocco S, Opocher G, D'Agostino D, et al. Lack of aldosterone inhibition by atrial natriuretic factor in primary aldosteronism: in vitro studies. J Endocrinol Invest 1989; 12:13.
14. Schambelan M, Sebastian A, Biglieri EG. Prevalence, pathogenesis and functional significance of aldosterone deficiency in hyperkalemic patients with chronic renal insufficiency. Kidney Int 1980; 17:89.
15. DeFronzo RA. Hyperkalemia and hyporeninemic hypoaldosteronism. Kidney Int 1980; 17:118.
16. Batlle DC. Hyperkalemic hyperchloremic metabolic acidosis associated with selective aldosterone deficiency and distal renal tubular acidosis. Semin Nephrol 1981; 1:260.
17. Melby JC, Griffing GT. Isolated hypoaldosteronism. In, Kassier JP, ed: Current therapy in internal medicine. Philadelphia: BC Decker, 1991:1328.
18. Holland OB. Hypoaldosteronism: disease or normal response? N Engl J Med 1991; 324:488.
19. Jost-Vu E, Horton R, Antonipillai I. Altered regulation of renin secretion by insulin-like growth factors and angiotensin II in diabetic rats. Diabetes 1992; 41(9):1100.
20. Nakamoto Y, Imai H, Hamanaka S, et al. IgM monoclonal gammopathy accompanied by nodular glomerulosclerosis urine concentrating defect and hyporeninemic hypoaldosteronism. Am J Nephrol 1985; 5:53.
21. Kalin MF, Poretsky L, Seres DS, Zumoff B. Hyporeninemic hypoaldosteronism associated with acquired immune deficiency syndrome. Am J Med 1987; 82:1035.
22. Biglieri EG, Slaton PE Jr, Silen WS, et al. Post-operative studies of adrenal function in primary aldosteronism. J Clin Endocrinol Metab 1966; 26:553.
23. Sebastian A, Schambelan M, Lindenfeld S, Morris RC Jr. Amelioration of metabolic acidosis with fludrocortisone therapy in hyporeninemic hypoaldosteronism. N Engl J Med 1977; 297:576.
24. Rimmer JM, Horn JF, Gennari FJ. Hyperkalemia as a complication of drug therapy. Arch Intern Med 1987; 147:867.
25. Kutyrina IM, Nikshova TA, Tareyeva IE. Effects of heparin-induced aldosterone deficiency on renal function in patients with chronic glomerulonephritis. Nephrol Dial Transplant 1987; 2:219.
26. Kutyrina IM, Androsova SO, Tareyeva IE. Indomethacin-induced hyporeninaemic hypoaldosteronism. Lancet 1979; 1:785.
27. Ponce SP, Jennings AE, Madias NE, Harrington JT. Drug induced hyperkalemia. Medicine 1985; 64:357.
28. Corvol P, Claire M, Oblin ME, Greeving K, Rossier B. Mechanism of the antimineralocorticoid effects of spironolactones. Kidney Int 1981; 20:1.
29. Benos DJ. Amiloride: a molecular probe of sodium transport in tissues and cells. Am J Physiol 1982; 242:C131.
30. Corvol P. Editorial: The enigma of pseudohypoaldosteronism. J Clin Endocrinol Metab 1994; 79(1):25.
30a. Bonny O, Hummler E. Dysfunction of epithelial sodium transport: from human to mouse. Kidney Int 2000; 57:1313.
31. Chang SS, Grunder S, Hanukoglu A, et al. Mutations in subunits of the epithelial sodium channel cause salt wasting with hyberkalemic acidosis, pseudohypoaldosteronism type I. Nat Genet 1996; 12(3):248.
31a. Grunder S, Jaeger NF, Gautschi I, et al. Identification of a highly conserved segment at the N-terminus of the epithelial Nat channel alpha subunit involved in gating. Pflugers Arch 1999; 438:709.
32. Chung E, Hanukoglu A, Rees M, et al. Exclusion of the locus for autosomal recessive pseudohypoaldosteronism type I from the mineralocorticoid receptor gene region on human chromosome 4q by linkage analysis. J Clin Endocrinol Metab 1995; 80(11):3341.
33. Garty H, Palmer LG. Epithelial sodium channels: function, structure, and regulation. Physiol Rev 1997; 77(2):359.
34. Grunder S, Firsov D, Chang SS, et al. A mutation causing pseudohypoaldosteronism type I identifies a conserved glycine that is involved in the gating of the epithelial sodium channel. EMBO J 1997; 16(5):899.
35. Strautnieks SS, Thompson RJ, Gardiner RM, Chung E. A novel splice-site mutation in the subunit of the epithelial sodium channel gene in three pseudohypoaldosteronism type I families. Nat Genet 1996; 13(2):248.

36. Strautnieks SS, Thompson RJ, Hanukoglu A, et al. Localization of pseudo-hypoaldosteronism genes to chromosome 16p12.2-13.11 and 12p13.1-pter by homozygosity mapping. Hum Molec Genet 1996; 5(2):293.

36a. Bonny O, Chraibi A, Loffing J, et al. Functional expression of a pseudohy-poaldosteronism type I mutated epithelial Na+ channel lacking the pore-forming region of its alpha subunit. J Clin Invest 1999; 104(7):967.

37. Snyder PM. Liddle's syndrome mutations disrupt cAMP-mediated transloca-tions of the epithelial Na+ channel to the cell surface. J Clin Invest 2000; 105:45.

38. Geller DS, Rodriguez-Soriano J, Vallo Boado A, et al. Mutations in the min-eralocorticoid receptor gene cause autosomal dominant pseudohypoaldos-teronism type I. Nat Genet 1998; 19(3):279.

39. Stone RC, Vale P, Rosa FC. Effect of hydrochlorothiazide in pseudohypoal-dosteronism with hypercalciura and severe hyperkalemia. Pediatr Nephrol 1996; 10(4):501.

40. White PC: Mechanisms of disease: disorders of aldosterone biosynthesis and action. N Engl J Med 1994; 331(4):250.

41. Hanukoglu A, Joy O, Steinitz M, et al. Pseudohypoaldosteronism due to renal and multisystem resistance to mineralocorticoids respond differently to carbenoxolone. J Steroid Biochem Molec Biol 1997; 60(1-2):105.

42. Mansfield TA, Simon DB, Farfel Z, et al. Multilocus linkage of familial hyperkalemia and hypertension, pseudohypoaldosteronism type II, to chromosomes 1q31-42 and 17p11-q21. Nat Genet 1997; 16(2):202.

# CHAPTER 82

# ENDOCRINE ASPECTS OF HYPERTENSION

DALILA B. CORRY AND MICHAEL L. TUCK

## SPECTRUM OF HYPERTENSION

Hypertension is an extremely common disorder, affecting 15% to 20% of the population. More than 95% of hypertension is of unknown etiology, termed *primary* or *essential* hypertension. There are several causes of endocrine hypertension (Table 82-1), with the most common forms being renal artery stenosis, primary aldoster-onism, and pheochromocytoma. In the Hypertension Detection Follow-Up Program, 0.18% of 15,000 participants had secondary

**TABLE 82-1.**

**Endocrine Causes of Hypertension**

Essential hypertension (?)
Renovascular hypertension
Pheochromocytoma
Primary aldosteronism
Glucocorticoid-remediable aldosteronism
Apparent mineralocorticoid excess
Cushing syndrome
Cortisol resistance
Renal parenchymal disease (?)
Coarctation of the aorta (?)
Congenital adrenal hyperplasia
Exogenous agents (licorice)
Estrogen-induced hypertension
Diabetes mellitus
Obesity
Hyperparathyroidism
Pseudohypoparathyroidism
Hypothyroidism
Hyperthyroidism
Acromegaly
Liddle syndrome
Pregnancy-induced hypertension
Renin-secreting tumors

hypertension.[1] Because endocrine hypertension is rare, it is recom-mended by the Joint National Committee on Hypertension VI (JNC VI) that the new-onset hypertensive patient not have exten-sive testing for endocrine hypertension.[2] Thus, only if the history and physical examination suggest endocrine hypertension is it necessary to perform screening tests. Pheochromocytoma can be detected with high sensitivity and specificity using urine and plasma catecholamine measurements. Primary aldosteronism is suspected by low serum potassium and plasma renin activity (PRA); however, as screening tests, these measurements are not very sensitive or specific. The screening tests for renovascular hypertension are improving, but most testing procedures are either invasive or indirect and can be costly.

*Secondary hypertension* should be suspected in severe and resistant hypertension, new-onset hypertension in the young (<20 years) or the older patient (>55 years), hypertension with spontaneous hypokalemia, and episodic hypertension with sweating, tachycardia, and headaches. Important physical find-ings include the detection of an abdominal bruit (suggestive of renovascular hypertension); a radial-femoral pulse delay (sug-gestive of aortic coarctation); or central obesity, striae, and bruising (suggestive of Cushing syndrome). Other chapters deal in depth with aldosteronism, Cushing syndrome, congeni-tal adrenal hyperplasia, and pheochromocytoma (see Chaps. 75, 77, 80, and 86). This chapter deals with selected topics.

## RENOVASCULAR HYPERTENSION

Renovascular hypertension is the most common cause of sec-ondary hypertension (1% of cases of mild to moderate hyper-tension and up to 10% to 40% of subjects with acute, severe, or refractory hypertension).[3] There is still much debate over the method and extent of evaluation in such patients.[3-8]

Clinically, diffuse atherosclerosis with severe hypertension can be associated with a high incidence.[9,10] Acute elevation of serum creatinine is another presentation, either spontaneously or after initiation of an angiotensin-converting enzyme (ACE) inhibitor.[5] Asymmetric renal size is a clue, as are recurrent epi-sodes of acute ("flash") pulmonary edema and unexplained congestive heart failure.[11]

Hypertension results from obstructive lesions of the main renal artery or its segmental branches, but it takes ≥70% steno-sis to lead to hypoperfusion, reduced renal blood flow, and ischemia. Thus, the primary anatomic stenotic lesion may or may not be related to the blood pressure (BP), as it takes signifi-cant stenosis to activate the *renin-angiotensin system*, the main mediator of hypertension in renovascular hypertension.

Most renovascular hypertension results from either athero-sclerotic plaques or fibromuscular dysplasia. Of 2442 hyperten-sive patients included in the Renovascular Cooperative Study,[3] 63% had atherosclerotic lesions and 32% had fibromuscular dysplasia. Fibromuscular dysplasia occurs mostly in children and young adults, especially in women, whereas atheroscle-rotic plaques are seen in men over 45 who have a history of cig-arette smoking. The most common form of fibrous renal artery disease is medial fibroplasia; often it is bilateral (Fig. 82-1).

The syndrome of renovascular hypertension requires a broad definition (i.e., any secondary elevation of BP by any con-dition that interferes with the arterial circulation to kidney tis-sue).[12,13] Trauma and subcapsular hematoma can exert pressure on the kidney, causing renal ischemia without stenosis of the renal arteries. Other causes include renal transplantation, necrotizing vasculitis, intravenous drug abuse, malignant hypertension, renal artery emboli, coarctation or dissection of the aorta, and renal artery aneurysms.[13]

## PATHOGENESIS

The two main types of renovascular hypertension are *unilateral* and *bilateral renal artery stenosis*. The renin-angiotensin system is

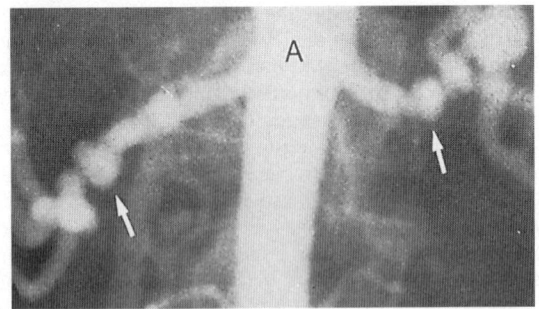

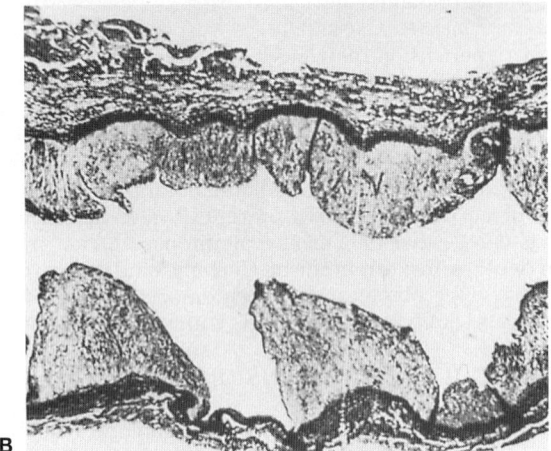

**FIGURE 82-1. A,** Angiographic picture of bilateral renal artery stenosis with multiple stenotic lesions. (*A*, aorta.) **B,** Anatomic cross section of renal artery from patient with fibromuscular dysplasia.

the major hormone system in the pathogenesis of renovascular hypertension, with the critical initiating event being reduced renal perfusion pressure[14–18] (see Chaps. 79 and 183). There is increased renin and angiotensin II (A-II) production by the stenotic kidney, although PRA levels often are normal to only moderately elevated, reflecting renin suppression in the nonstenotic kidney. In experimental one-kidney, one-clip renovascular hypertension, the renin levels increase for 6 to 10 days after renal artery clipping and then decline, yet the hypertension per-

sists. The long-term increase in BP is related to increases in vascular resistance; the early enhancement of the renin-angiotensin system triggers other factors, sustaining the hypertension. (Volume expansion may play a critical role in long-term BP elevations.) In contrast, in the two-kidney, one-clip model of renovascular hypertension, an elevated PRA persists throughout the chronic maintenance phase of hypertension.

In *unilateral renal artery stenosis*, the uninvolved kidney should protect against fluid and electrolyte imbalance and hypertension; the rise in BP should increase sodium excretion in the nonstenotic kidney. However, the nonstenotic kidney does not adapt appropriately; there is a paradoxical rise in local A-II, despite a suppressed PRA[15,16] (Fig. 82-2). This discordant response leads to mediation by A-II of vasoconstriction and sodium retention with a blunted pressure natriuresis response curve in the nonstenotic kidney.

In *bilateral renovascular hypertension*, the hormonal, neural, and volume responses are different from those in unilateral disease. There is an initial rise in the renin-angiotensin system, but with time, there is normalization of the renin-angiotensin system activity, and hypertension in the steady-state condition becomes more dependent on volume-mediated factors.

Other amplifying factors contribute to the maintenance of hypertension in renovascular hypertension; there may be a *neurogenic phase*, as enhanced sympathetic nervous system activity is found in the early stages.[19] Levels of several *vasoactive eicosanoids* are high in animals with renovascular hypertension.[14,16] A-II–induced activation of the lipoxygenase pathway of arachidonic acid has pressor functions and has been implicated in the sustained phase. Lipoxygenase inhibitors prevent the development of experimental renovascular hypertension.[19] A-II in the kidney is taken up and incorporated by renal cells through the A-II–AT$_1$ receptor[16]; this uptake might serve to prolong A-II action. Circulating levels of aldosterone are normal to high in renovascular disease, depending on the levels of renin. In marked renovascular hypertension, renin and aldosterone levels are high, and hypokalemia is found.[20]

## CLINICAL CLUES TO SCREEN FOR RENOVASCULAR HYPERTENSION

Abrupt onset of severe hypertension in a young (younger than 20 years) or older individual (older than 55 years).
Prepubertal hypertension .
Hypertension that is refractory to triple-drug therapy.

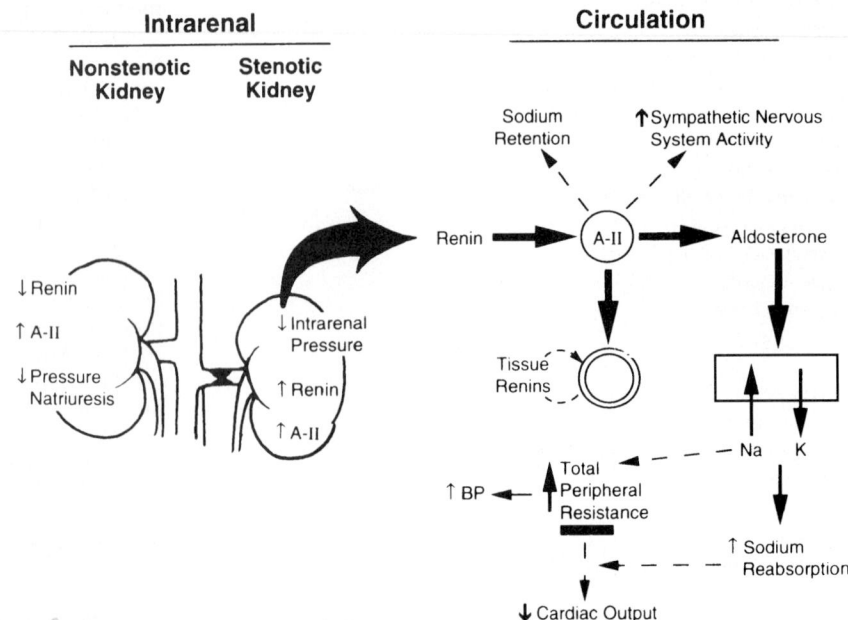

**FIGURE 82-2.** Changes in hemodynamics and the renin-angiotensin-aldosterone system in the kidneys and circulation in unilateral renal artery stenosis. Intrarenal changes begin in the stenotic kidney, with subsequent changes in the nonstenotic kidney. (*A-II*, angiotensin II; *BP*, blood pressure.)

Malignant or accelerated hypertension associated with grade III to IV retinopathy.

Sudden flank pain due to renal embolic infarction.

Unexplained azotemia.

Detection of an upper flank or abdominal bruit that radiates to the flanks. (The bruit may be systolic, systolic-diastolic, or continuous, and is high pitched and difficult to discern.) Bruit in a hypertensive young woman suggests fibromuscular disease.

Hypertension associated with diffuse atherosclerotic vascular disease, especially in a smoker.

Unexplained deterioration in renal function with the use of an ACE inhibitor.

Paradoxical worsening of hypertension with a diuretic.

Spontaneous hypokalemia.

Recurrent flash pulmonary edema.

Some patients have *no* such histories and are indistinguishable from those with essential hypertension.[3,4]

## LABORATORY EVALUATION

**Routine Laboratory Tests.**    Measurements of electrolytes, renal function tests, and urinalysis often give normal results in renovascular hypertension.[2] Hypokalemia is found in those cases in which secondary hyperaldosteronism is found. In unilateral stenosis of the renal artery, an impairment of renal function occurs infrequently, whereas in bilateral renal artery stenosis, serum creatinine and urea nitrogen may be increased. In embolic renovascular disease, hematuria may be detected.

## SCREENING TESTS

**Intravenous Pyelography.**    The findings on rapid-sequence pyelography that have the greatest significance are a unilateral decrease in renal size (>1.5 cm disparity in pole-to-pole diameter) and a unilateral delay in the appearance of contrast medium in the 1- to 5-minute exposures.[3] False-negative results often occur in cases of renovascular hypertension because of bilateral renal artery disease.[3,21] The hypertensive urogram has *low sensitivity* (a negative test does not exclude renovascular hypertension) *and specificity* and, importantly, has the *risk of nephrotoxicity* because of contrast agents.

**Plasma Renin Activity.**    Although hypoperfusion in the stenotic kidney activates the renin-angiotensin system, renin secretion in the nonstenotic kidney is often normal or low, so that the baseline or unstimulated circulating PRA levels are normal in most cases. Thus, when measured in peripheral venous samples, PRA is normal in 20% to 50% of cases of documented renovascular hypertension.[7,13,20] The interpretation is confounded by the fact that 16% to 20% of subjects with essential hypertension have PRA values that are moderately elevated.

However, in renovascular hypertension there are *exaggerated PRA responses* to procedures that *stimulate* the renin-angiotensin system, such as upright posture, sodium restriction, and the administration of angiotensin-converting enzyme inhibitors (ACEI).[22] ACEI interrupt the conversion of A-I to A-II; the negative feedback effect of A-II on renin release is diminished, resulting in an increase in secretion. The administration of the ACEI *captopril* to patients with renovascular hypertension produces a marked increase in PRA compared to responses in other forms of hypertension.[20,22–24] In the usual test procedure, captopril, 25 to 50 mg, is given orally, and PRA is obtained after 1 hour. The test has 75% to 100% sensitivity and 60% to 90% specificity.[22,24] Furthermore, it is safe and inexpensive, and can be done on an outpatient basis or simultaneously with captopril renography. The utility of the test is hampered by the need for strict standardization, the need to stop antihypertensive medications, its reduced accuracy in renal failure, and low sensitivity and poor predictive value compared to a renogram.

*Renal vein renin levels,* sampled by percutaneous catheterization, determine the functional significance of the stenotic lesion and predict the BP response to therapy.[3] Renin production is increased in the stenotic kidney and suppressed in the contralateral kidney; asymmetry of renin production yields a renal vein renin ratio of ≥1.5:1 in renovascular hypertension. This procedure has predictive value for surgical curability, but use has declined because it is invasive, and up to 60% of patients *do not lateralize* but are nevertheless improved by surgery.[25]

**Radionuclide Renography.**    The renogram relies on a disparity of renal function and of perfusion between the stenotic and nonstenotic kidneys. Isotopic compounds such as technetium-99m–diethylenetetraminepentaacetic acid (DTPA) accurately measure glomerular filtration rate, and compounds such as $^{99m}$Tc-mercapto acetyl triglycine ($^{99m}$Tc-MAG3) measure both glomerular filtration rate and tubular secretion and are good in renal insufficiency.[7] The addition of computer quantitation has improved their accuracy.[3–7,13,26] Patients with renovascular hypertension show decreased uptake, delayed peak values, and prolonged excretion of these agents. Because of the low-risk and noninvasive nature of renography, it has many advantages. However, renography used alone has a high incidence of false-negative and false-positive results.

Captopril administration during renography has improved its sensitivity and specificity.[5–7,22,24,26,27] Captopril (25–50 mg), which is given 1 hour before the isotope injection, reduces A-II–mediated vasoconstriction in the efferent arterioles and lowers glomerular pressure and filtration rate. In the stenotic kidney, captopril reduces renal perfusion more than in the nonstenotic kidney, thereby revealing the asymmetric reduction in renal function in renovascular hypertension. Scintiphotographs and time-activity curves are analyzed to assess renal perfusion, function, and size. In high-risk populations, sensitivity and specificity exceed 90% for high-grade stenosis. The predictive value of the ACE-inhibitor renogram is less in low-risk populations and in bilateral disease.

**Duplex Doppler Ultrasonography.**    Ultrasonography has been improved by the use of low-frequency transducers (B-mode imaging) for better visualization of the renal arteries, and Doppler for the measurement of differential blood flow velocities.[28–31] It has the advantage of determining *both the anatomic and the functional* significance of a stenotic lesion. A renal-aortic flow velocity ratio of ≥3.5 suggests renovascular hypertension. Duplex Doppler ultrasonography can detect unilateral and bilateral disease, can detect recurrent stenosis in previously treated patients, and can be enhanced with ACE inhibition[30] and color coding.[31] It has a 99% positive predictive value and a 97% negative predictive value.[29] (Disadvantages: time-consuming and highly operator-dependent.)

**Magnetic Resonance Angiography.**    Magnetic resonance (MR) angiography is promising and noninvasive, and may become the method of choice.[32–36] In comparison with arteriography, MR angiography showed 100% sensitivity and 96% specificity for finding stenosis of the main renal arteries.[32–36] A sensitivity of 100% and a specificity of 71% were found for lesions of the proximal renal arteries with 50% to 75% stenosis.[34]

Significant advances in techniques include breath-holding MR angiography and paramagnetic contrast material. Thus, the procedure may be able to visualize accessory arteries.[34] Phase-contrast MR angiography may enable determination of the hemodynamic significance of a stenotic lesion.[35] The procedure cannot be used in individuals with metallic implants such as a pacemaker or a clip for an aneurysm.

**Spiral (Helical) Computed Tomographic Scan and Computed Tomographic Angiography.**    This offers great promise as the best noninvasive screening test.[37] In a comparison of spiral computed tomography (CT) to arteriography in subjects investigated for renovascular hypertension, the sensitivity was 98% and the specificity 94%.[28] However, renal insufficiency reduces the accuracy of this procedure due to diminishing renal blood flow. It identifies lesions of the main renal arteries but has more difficulty in finding branch lesions. Although it is minimally invasive, the risk of radiocontrast-induced nephrotoxicity still exists.

**Angiography.** Despite the increase in types of procedures and technical advances in detecting renovascular hypertension, renal angiography by the percutaneous, transfemoral route remains the "gold standard" for detecting renal artery stenosis, as well as its location and pathology. Atherosclerotic lesions most often involve the proximal segment of the renal artery and have a circular configuration. By contrast, fibromuscular disease is in the more distal portions of the renal artery and is either localized or diffuse and bilateral. Angiography is costly and invasive and has the risk of nephrotoxicity. Because angiography does not always predict the functional significance of renal artery stenosis or its treatment outcome, many centers apply simultaneous angioplasty, with the BP response to percutaneous renal angioplasty or stenting serving as the indicator of functional significance.

Digital subtraction angiography avoids some of the complications of percutaneous catheterization, because computer enhancement of the renal area allows the injection of smaller amounts of contrast material.[3] Injection has been in a peripheral vein, but the specificity and sensitivity of the procedure are both 90% or less when compared to arterial procedures. Because 150 to 200 mL of dye is injected, there is still risk for nephrotoxicity. An intraaortic injection site provides better visualization. The procedure can be performed safely in azotemic patients, and it has been useful in hypertension after renal transplantation.[4]

Thus, the renal arteriogram best establishes the presence of renal artery stenosis but does not distinguish functional from nonfunctional lesions. Tests such as the intravenous pyelogram and radionucleotide renogram lack sensitivity for detecting renovascular hypertension and, if used alone, cannot consistently diagnose renovascular hypertension. The newer tests (e.g., captopril renography, MR angiography, duplex ultrasonography, and spiral CT) show great promise.

## TREATMENT OF RENOVASCULAR HYPERTENSION

The goals of therapy of renovascular hypertension are the control of BP and the preservation of renal function. The three therapies for treatment of renovascular hypertension are medical, percutaneous transluminal renal angioplasty, and surgery. Each approach has advantages and disadvantages, and the selection also depends on cause, severity, and age. Few trials have compared the three therapies. Often no single test can help in this decision, and experience and clinical judgment are paramount. There are several differences in the approach to unilateral versus bilateral renal artery stenosis.

### Unilateral Renal Artery Stenosis

SURGERY. Often, surgery is reserved for patients for whom hypertension cannot be controlled on medical therapy or for those who fail angioplasty and in whom renal function is deteriorating. However, some believe that surgery should be considered in patients <50 to 60 years of age, as the outcome is more definitive and spares the chronic use of medication.[38–41] Surgery is generally more effective than angioplasty, especially in patients with atherosclerosis. One indication for surgical revascularization is preservation of renal function, based on the emerging evidence of deteriorating renal function in atherosclerotic ischemic renal disease.[41–43] Revascularization procedures include bypass using natural or synthetic arteries; natural arteries provide a better outcome.[38–41] The surgical cure rate for hypertension due to unilateral atherosclerotic lesions may be up to 95%, especially if the disease is of short duration. Less favorable results are seen in older subjects with long-standing hypertension, probably due to either underlying essential hypertension or the onset of intrarenal disease. Mortality from surgery is ~2.5% in experienced centers; it is higher in older patients, especially those with diffuse atherosclerosis and heart failure.[40]

PERCUTANEOUS TRANSLUMINAL ANGIOPLASTY. The technical success and cure rate for percutaneous transluminal angioplasty are rapidly improving; this procedure and *stenting* are now treatments of choice.[44–50] Patients with fibromuscular dysplasia have the best outcome (<10% restenosis). Best results are obtained in lesions of the main renal artery that are only partly occluded.[44–47] In atherosclerotic lesions the results are not as good. Cure rates of only 10% to 20% are recorded; ~60% will improve but not be cured, and 15% incur no benefit. A failure can be predicted in the first 48 hours if BP fails to fall.[46] Technical complications include renal artery thrombosis and perforation. The main overall advantage of percutaneous transluminal angioplasty may be the ability to decrease the number of medications needed to control BP without the risks of surgery.[46,47] In transplant renal artery stenosis, angioplasty is first-line therapy, with a cure rate of 70% at 5 years; surgery is less successful because of extensive scar tissue.[3] *Ostial stenoses* are less likely to respond to angioplasty (recurrence rate as high as 47% for atherosclerotic lesions). Here, the outcome of angioplasty is better with intravascular stents.[48–50] Stents are placed most often after unsuccessful angioplasty and offset the effect of elastic recoil (success rate from 65% to 70%; restenosis in only 13%).[48,49]

MEDICAL THERAPY. In high-risk individuals with coexisting carotid or coronary artery disease in which surgical or angiographic risk is high, medical therapy is often the sole modality.[51–53] However, the natural course of renovascular hypertension, especially due to atherosclerotic disease, shows that many stenotic lesions progress over time and that renal damage can occur in untreated lesions.[52] Thus, it remains uncertain whether drug therapy—by only controlling BP—affects the progression of renovascular hypertension.

Because renovascular hypertension is a renin-dependent form of hypertension, ACEI and A-II–receptor blockers should show selective efficacy.[51] In unilateral renovascular hypertension, ACEI may be as effective as monotherapy.[51] However, ACE inhibitors can produce rapid loss of renal function especially in bilateral renovascular hypertension or in renovascular hypertension with a solitary kidney, owing to the almost complete dependency of renal function on A-II.[51] Usually, the use of ACEI in unilateral renovascular hypertension does not permanently reduce glomerular filtration and is safe and effective.[51] Some clinicians monitor serum creatinine, renal size, and periodic ultrasonography during such therapy.

Calcium antagonists are effective antihypertensive agents in renovascular hypertension and may induce less renal impairment than ACE inhibitors.[3] However, in critical, high-grade stenosis, any agent that lowers BP excessively can impair renal function. A-II–receptor blockers act by directly blocking the $AT_1$ receptor without affecting other peptides (e.g., bradykinin) as do the ACEI.

**Bilateral Renal Artery Stenosis.** Bilateral renal artery stenosis or unilateral stenosis in a solitary kidney usually involves more acute, severe, and difficult-to-treat hypertension, accompanied often by renal insufficiency. In bilateral renovascular hypertension, treatment should be guided toward lowering BP and preserving renal function. Patients who have bilateral disease with complete stenosis of one renal artery are at the greatest risk. Doppler ultrasound follow-up on bilateral renovascular hypertension shows that by 1 year, there often is a decrease in kidney size.[54] To preserve renal function, the use of surgery or angioplasty should be considered in bilateral disease.

Percutaneous transluminal angioplasty is generally less successful in bilateral renovascular hypertension and is associated with more complications (atheroemboli).[42,55] It is limited to people who are at high surgical risk or those who cannot be controlled by medication. Intravascular stents may expand the success of angioplasty in this disease.

Medical therapy in bilateral disease is best handled with ACEI or a calcium-channel blocker with the addition of a diuretic based on the volume expansion and volume-dependent

**TABLE 82-2.**
Biochemical Features of Hypertensive Syndromes Involving Mineralocorticoid and Glucocorticoid Excess

| | Blood Pressure | Serum Potassium | PRA | Aldosterone | Cortisol | DOC | ACTH |
|---|---|---|---|---|---|---|---|
| Primary aldosteronism | ↑ | ↓ | ↓ | ↑ | N | N | N |
| Cushing syndromes | | | | | | | |
| Pituitary or adrenal adenoma | ↑ | N | N/↑* | N | ↑ | N | ↑/N/↓ |
| Paraneoplastic ACTH | ↑ | ↓ | ↓ | ↓ | ↑ | ↑ | ↑ |
| 11β-Hydroxylase deficiency | ↑ | ↓ | ↓ | ↓ | ↓ | ↑ | ↑ |
| 17α-Hydroxylase deficiency | ↑ | ↓ | ↓ | ↓ | ↓ | ↑ | ↑ |
| Apparent mineralocorticoid excess | ↑ | ↓ | ↓ | ↓ | N† | N | N |
| Licorice ingestion | ↑ | ↓ | ↓ | ↓ | N† | N | N |
| Cortisol resistance | ↑ | ↓ | ↓ | ↓ | ↑ | ↑ | ↑ |

ACTH, corticotropin; DOC, deoxycorticosterone; PRA, plasma renin activity; N, not found.
*Increased renin substrate.
†Abnormal corticosteroid metabolism because of enzyme deficiency of 11β-hydroxysteroid dehydrogenase in the kidneys.

hypertension.[51] One can almost expect a hemodynamic decline in glomerular filtration rate following ACEI in bilateral renovascular hypertension, so careful monitoring is essential.

If possible, the surgical correction of bilateral renal artery stenosis should be pursued, because BP and renal function can improve after revascularization.[40,56] Optimal therapy for bilateral disease has not been established: Surgery is the treatment of choice in the young with bilateral severe stenosis. In older, high-risk subjects with atherosclerosis, medical therapy with either an ACEI or a calcium-channel blocker is indicated.

## RENIN-PRODUCING TUMORS

Renin-producing tumors, a rare form of endocrine hypertension that occurs in young persons, manifest *severe hypertension* and *hypokalemia*.[56,57] The PRA is among the highest recorded in hypertensive syndromes and can exceed 50 ng/mL/h.[56] The hypokalemia, often <2.0 mEq/L, is due to intense secondary hyperaldosteronism. The combined high PRA and aldosterone levels distinguish this disorder from primary aldosteronism. Two categories of renin-producing tumors cause this syndrome: *renal juxtaglomerular cell tumors* and a variety of *extrarenal tumors*, such as Wilms and ovarian tumors.[56,57] The renin originating from tumor production resembles that found in normal kidneys.[58] Extrarenal renin-secreting tumors have higher concentrations of *prorenin* than do tumors of renal origin.[57,59] Most cases of extrarenal renin-secreting tumors occur in women, and many are located in the reproductive tract.[59] In these patients, the high prorenin level serves as a marker for the tumor. One presentation is the *hyponatremic hypertensive syndrome and massive proteinuria* seen in patients with *renin-producing leiomyosarcomas*.[60] The ACEI captopril is effective in the control of BP due to renin tumors.[61]

In renal *renin-secreting tumors*, renal vein PRA measurements can localize the tumor. They are small, so that radiologic visualization, including urography, magnetic resonance imaging (MRI), ultrasonography, CT, and angiography may sometimes be unsuccessful[57,62]; even exploratory surgery may fail to find the lesion. In these patients, nephrectomy or selective tumor resection is curative, and ACEI are the medical treatment of choice.[28] An A-II–receptor blocker may be equally effective or superior by also blocking the antigensin type 2 (AT$_2$) receptor.[63]

## MINERALOCORTICOID HYPERTENSION

Several mineralocorticoids, such as aldosterone and deoxycorticosterone (DOC), produce hypertensive syndromes.[64–66] For more details of aldosterone function see review.[66a] Primary aldosteronism is the best example of mineralocorticoid hypertension. The mechanisms underlying hypertension include sodium retention, extracellular fluid expansion, high cardiac output,

increased sympathetic nervous system activity, and structural changes in blood vessels. Hyperaldosteronism is reviewed elsewhere (see Chap. 80), as is congenital adrenal hyperplasia (see Chap. 77).

Table 82-2 summarizes the levels of BP, serum potassium, PRA, aldosterone, cortisol, DOC, and corticotropin (ACTH) in several glucocorticoid and mineralocorticoid disorders associated with hypertension. *Glucocorticoid resistance* results in a mineralocorticoid form of hypertension accompanied by hypokalemia and suppressed renin and aldosterone (see Table 82-2). High levels of plasma cortisol and a paucity of stigmata of Cushing syndrome suggest the diagnosis.[67] The insensitivity to glucocorticoids is caused by inherited glucocorticoid receptor mutations.[67] An insensitivity to cortisol at the hypothalamic-pituitary feedback for ACTH increases ACTH production, which, in turn, stimulates DOC and corticosterone formation; the increased mineralocorticoid activity then causes volume expansion, hypertension, and the suppression of renin and aldosterone. An adrenal androgen excess can also be found, resulting in hirsutism in women and precocious pseudopuberty in children. The demonstration of a functionally abnormal glucocorticoid receptor in mononuclear cells confirms the diagnosis.[67] Mutations occur in the glucocorticoid receptor–ligand-binding domain and at a splice site.[67] High doses of dexamethasone reduce the ACTH, and thereby correct the BP and serum potassium abnormalities. A form of cortisol resistance has also been described in the acquired immunodeficiency syndrome.[67,68]

## HYPERTENSION IN OTHER ENDOCRINE DISORDERS

### CUSHING SYNDROME

Hypertension is common in endogenous Cushing syndrome (up to 80%) but occurs less frequently with exogenous glucocorticoid therapy.[69] The cardiovascular mortality and morbidity are much higher in Cushing syndrome,[70] attributed to the effects of cortisol on BP, on atherosclerosis, and on the heart. The hypertension is thought to directly result from cortisol excess through at least three mechanisms.[71] Glucocorticoid excess increases the hepatic synthesis of angiotensinogen, the substrate for the production of the vasoconstrictor A-II. This mechanism might suggest a renin-dependent form of hypertension, yet renin levels in Cushing syndrome often are normal to decreased. Glucocorticoid administration to normal subjects will enhance vascular reactivity to pressor hormones such as phenylephrine; indeed, many attribute its hypertensive action to this mechanism. Although cortisol in excess binds to mineralocorticoid receptors, most cases of Cushing syndrome resulting from pituitary or adrenal adenoma do not have strong evidence for mineralocorticoid excess such as hypokalemia and suppressed renin.

A more pronounced mineralocorticoid effect is seen in Cushing syndrome due to paraneoplastic ACTH production. In these disorders, the high levels of cortisol and DOC, but not aldosterone, cause a mineralocorticoid effect, leading to hypokalemia and hypertension[71] (see Chap. 219). High circulating ACTH levels in these ectopic syndromes preferentially stimulate adrenal secretion of DOC over aldosterone; the excess DOC causes volume expansion and the suppression of renin and aldosterone. One should be alerted to this scenario in an established or suspected cancer patient—with unexplained hypokalemia and metabolic alkalosis—who may or may not have hypertension.

Another mechanism for hypertension in paraneoplastic ACTH syndromes is one in which the renal form of the enzyme 11β-hydroxysteroid dehydrogenase (11β-HSD) is deficient or overwhelmed by the high circulating cortisol levels.[72] This defect leads to the accumulation of cortisol in the kidneys, where it binds in excess to the mineralocorticoid receptor. Diagnosis is made by demonstrating a high ratio of the urine metabolites of cortisol/cortisone. These findings are similar to those seen in the genetic or acquired (licorice) forms of *apparent mineralocorticoid excess*.[66] In some cases of adrenal carcinoma, there are partial enzyme blocks leading to the accumulation of steroid precursors (e.g., compound DOC), which can have mineralocorticoid effects.

## DIABETES MELLITUS AND HYPERTENSION

The frequency of hypertension in diabetes mellitus is high, reaching an incidence rate of about 50%.[73,74] Hypertension in the diabetic greatly enhances the risk of macrovascular atherosclerotic complications and the microvascular complications of nephropathy and retinopathy. It is also known that lowering BP slows the progression of diabetic nephropathy[75] and diabetic retinopathy.[76]

In *type 1 diabetes mellitus*, hypertension appears after several years and is seen almost uniquely in those 40% of type 1 diabetics who will develop diabetic nephropathy. The BP begins to rise at about 3 years after the onset of microalbuminuria, and hypertension is eventually seen in 85% of them. Thus, renal mechanisms explain most of the pathophysiology of hypertension in type 1 diabetes mellitus. In *type 2 diabetics*, 40% to 70% develop hypertension. Here, the hypertension is due to aging, obesity, insulin resistance, hyperinsulinemia, atherosclerosis, and renal disease; it may be present at the time of diagnosis or even have preceded the onset of diabetes mellitus. However, a significant number of type 2 diabetics have microalbuminuria, suggesting that renal disease can be a contributor. Nevertheless, obesity probably is the major cause of their hypertension; genetic factors also contribute, as there is an association between the $A_2$ allele of the glycogen synthase gene and insulin resistance.[77]

Unique mechanisms for the cause of hypertension in diabetes mellitus relate to the metabolic abnormalities; both type 1 and type 2 diabetics have increased vascular reactivity and sodium retention.[78,79] Norepinephrine, A-II, exercise, and mental stress in diabetic subjects lead to exaggerated BP responses.[78,79] Sodium retention and volume expansion in the diabetic are due to increased reabsorption through tubular glucose-sodium cotransport[80]; this causes a higher incidence of salt-sensitive hypertension.[81]

High levels of insulin in diabetes contribute to the hypertension. In type 2 diabetics, insulin resistance causes hyperinsulinemia; also, insulin excess may occur in type 1 diabetes due to exogenous therapy.[74] Insulin increases sodium reabsorption and sympathetic nervous system activity and has direct effects on vascular reactivity.[73,74] After starting insulin in type 2 diabetics, there is an increase in mean values of BP from 132/81 to 148/89 mm Hg.[82]

In human diabetes, as well as in experimental models, values for plasma renin activity often are reduced or completely suppressed,[83] whereas in certain tissues (e.g., the kidney) the expression of renin and its products is elevated.[84] Individuals with long-standing diabetes and renal impairment can have the *syndrome of hyporeninemic hypoaldosteronism*, which is detected by finding low PRA and aldosterone levels and hyperkalemia. The low PRA in diabetic patients is due to diabetic nephropathy, destruction of the juxtaglomerular apparatus, defective conversion of prorenin to active renin, chronic volume expansion, and decreased neural control of renin release.[83,84] The efficacy of ACEI in treatment of hypertension and target-organ protection in diabetes mellitus occurs despite low circulating levels of renin and is thought to be due to effects on the tissue renin-angiotensin system[84] and increases in bradykinin.[85] Endothelial dysfunction, which is common in diabetes, may further contribute to the hypertension[86]; in type 1 diabetics, ACEI therapy improves endothelial function.[87]

## INSULIN AND HYPERTENSION

There is a positive correlation between insulin resistance, hyperinsulinemia, and BP.[88–90] In high-risk patients with syndrome X, insulin resistance and hyperinsulinemia partly contribute to the hypertension as well as the dyslipidemia, atherosclerosis, and cardiovascular disease.[88–90] Insulin resistance and the clustering of other risk factors can be found in nondiabetic subjects who are obese or lean but often have impaired glucose tolerance. Approximately 50% of patients with essential hypertension have the insulin-resistance syndrome.[90] There has been disagreement over whether insulin resistance and hyperinsulinemia have the same risk impact on BP in African-Americans. A follow-up study demonstrated that in both African-Americans and whites, baseline insulin and the insulin/glucose ratio are associated with a higher risk of hypertension.[91] There also may be elevations of steroid hormones (e.g., androgens), since circulating androgen levels are directly related to the degree of abdominal fat.[92] Moreover, insulin resistance occurs with androgen excess in the polycystic ovary syndrome.[93] There is a genetic contribution to the insulin-resistance syndrome, as normotensive individuals from hypertensive families have higher insulin levels and more insulin resistance.[94,95] In a study to identify the genetic locus for diabetes and insulin resistance that might be linked to BP, linkage analysis was performed in 48 families with type 2 diabetes.[96] Although no linkage to genes for the components of the renin-angiotensin system were found, one region of the lipoprotein lipase gene correlated with systolic BP.

Insulin alters BP-regulating mechanisms, such as sympathetic nervous system activity, sodium handling, and vascular tone.[73,74,86] In normal persons, the infusion of insulin increases plasma norepinephrine levels, regional sympathetic neuronal burst activity, and sodium reabsorption.[73,74] Despite these changes, insulin infusion in normal subjects causes vasodilatation and increased blood flow, suggesting that insulin acts directly on blood vessels as a vasodilator—a finding that might not support its role in hypertension.[97] This vasodilatory effect is blunted in obese individuals and even more so in type 2 diabetics.[97] This implies that a resistance to insulin's normal vasodilating effect could lead to hypertension by shifting the vasomotor balance away from vasodilatation toward vasoconstriction. The decrease in forearm blood flow could also decrease glucose delivery to skeletal muscles, thus contributing to insulin resistance.[97] The vasodilatory effect of insulin is blocked by inhibitors of the nitric oxide pathway.[97,98] In insulin-resistance states, there may be simultaneous reductions in insulin-mediated glucose uptake and insulin-mediated vasodilatation through abnormal endothelial function and reduced nitric oxide accumulation.[97]

Insulin also has effects on the vascular renin-angiotensin system: There is an up-regulation of the A-II type 1 receptor through posttranscriptional changes[99] and increases in angiotensinogen levels.[100] Both insulin and insulin-like growth factor-I (IGF-I) increase vascular growth, an effect that is blocked by inhibitors of the renin-angiotensin system.[100] This suggests both a prohypertensive effect and a growth effect directly on blood vessels, mediated through the vascular renin-angiotensin system.

Not all studies show a positive effect of insulin on BP. In dogs, chronic insulin infusion has no effect on BP.[101] In essential hypertensive patients with insulin resistance, insulin administration for 2 weeks actually decreased BP by a small amount.[102] In addition, not all epidemiologic reports have found a correlation between insulin and BP.[89] Perhaps, in order for insulin to raise BP, other prohypertensive factors must be present.

## OBESITY AND HYPERTENSION

There is a positive relationship between body weight and BP; weight loss evokes a hypotensive effect that may be substantial.[103–106] Hypertensive individuals have a greater prevalence of obesity than do normotensives. Obesity carries a much greater risk of left ventricular hypertrophy that is partly independent of the BP.[107] The association of obesity with other risks, such as dyslipidemia and insulin resistance, further enhances total cardiovascular risk.

There is a major role of fat distribution in cardiovascular risk in obesity. Central obesity with intraabdominal fat excess represents a high-risk form of obesity.[103,104] Increased intraabdominal fat is associated with hypertension, insulin resistance, hyperinsulinemia, dyslipidemia, accelerated atherosclerosis, coagulation defects, and cardiovascular disease. There is an outpouring of free fatty acids that lead to increased Apo B and hepatic lipase, producing a typical lipid profile including increased triglycerides and small dense low-density lipoprotein (LDL) and reduced high-density lipoprotein (HDL).

Clinically, abdominal obesity is diagnosed by measuring the waist/hip circumference ratio (abnormal >0.95 in men and >0.85 in women). It is visceral or subcutaneous truncal fat rather than intraperitoneal fat that is high risk; this type of fat and its distribution are also predictors of a low $HDL_2$ cholesterol,[108] insulin resistance,[109] and diabetes.[110] Intraabdominal fat is detected more accurately by CT scan.

Obese hypertensive patients have a unique hemodynamic profile: Blood volume and cardiac output are increased, but systemic vascular resistance is normal to low.[107] There are differences between normotensive and hypertensive obese subjects: Normotensive obese subjects have high cardiac output but a systemic vascular resistance that is below the levels found in normotensive lean subjects. Hypertensive obese subjects have a higher systemic vascular resistance than do normotensive obese subjects.[107]

In obesity, norepinephrine and insulin levels are high.[105] Because insulin increases norepinephrine release, it is possible that the caloric excess causes hyperinsulinemia and stimulation of the sympathetic nervous system and BP.[111] Techniques to assess sympathetic nervous system activity in humans (plasma and urinary catecholamine levels, norepinephrine spillover, and microneurography) have provided important data on obesity and its relation to hypertension. Some studies have found that plasma norepinephrine levels are variably high in obesity. During weight loss there is an even more consistent relationship between reductions in norepinephrine and BP.[112] Regional norepinephrine spillover in obesity is high in the kidney and could lead to sodium retention.[113] Using microneurography techniques (which determine muscle sympathetic outflow), marked elevations were found in obese normotensive young men,[114] but it is unclear if sympathetic activity is higher in hypertensive obese subjects. Thus, human obesity is characterized by abnormalities in sympathetic cardiovascular control, but its role in hypertension is still undetermined.

Other variables may alter sympathetic nervous system activity and hypertension in obesity. Sleep apnea syndrome occurs in a substantial subgroup of obese patients, and activation of the sympathetic nervous system by repeated bouts of hypoxia could affect BP. The muscle sympathetic activity has been found to be high only in those obese subjects who have obstructive sleep apnea; when these patients are factored out, there are no demonstrable abnormalities in sympathetic nervous system activity in obesity.[115] Leptin produced in adipose tissue acts on central receptors to decrease appetite and increase energy expenditure. Like insulin, leptin has cardiovascular properties that include increasing sympathetic nervous system activity, altering sodium excretion, and possibly affecting BP.[116] Also, there is a reported association of a polymorphism in the $\beta_3$-adrenergic receptor gene with features of the insulin resistance syndrome.[117]

The hypotensive response to weight loss is accompanied by reductions in plasma volume, insulin, norepinephrine, and renin.[106,112] Often a successful BP response is attained before ideal body weight is achieved. Interestingly, sodium balance does not alter the effect of weight loss on BP.[106] Based on the results of multiple weight loss studies, it can be estimated that for every kilogram of weight loss there is a 0.5 to 1.0 mm Hg fall in mean BP. Reversal of obesity is difficult to achieve, and antihypertensive agents are often needed to control the hypertension.[118]

## HYPERCALCEMIA AND HYPERTENSION

Estimates of hypertension in primary hyperparathyroidism have ranged from 50% to 70%, and as many as 35% of patients with chronic hypercalcemia of other etiologies are hypertensive[119] (see Chaps. 58 and 59). Hypertension is also seen in the syndrome of parathyroid hormone (PTH) resistance (pseudohypoparathyroidism) and in secondary hyperparathyroidism due to severe renal failure. Hypertension in primary hyperparathyroidism is sometimes associated with renal insufficiency, but other factors, such as hypercalcemia; PTH and its analog, PTH-related protein; and phosphorus and magnesium deficiency contribute to the hypertension. Calcium is a major mediator of vascular contractility; calcium infusion can increase BP[120] and potentiate A-II and norepinephrine. The positive relationship between serum calcium and BP in hypertensive subjects suggests a cause-effect relationship.[120]

PTH may be involved in raising BP, but on acute administration it acts as a vasodilator and induces a fall in BP. However, more chronic exposure to PTH may raise BP. Approximately half of patients with pseudohypoparathyroidism have hypertension, but their serum calcium is low and their PTH is high.[121] Perhaps the high PTH sustains the hypertension, as normalization of calcium has no effect on BP.[121] 1,25-dihydroxycholecalciferol is high in primary hyperparathyroidism and can exert mild effects on calcium mobilization in blood vessels.

PRA is high in hyperparathyroidism, suggesting that the renin-angiotensin system participates in raising the BP[122]; in some, parathyroid surgery normalizes PRA, aldosterone, and the BP.[123] However, in renal insufficiency, hypertension persists or is only partially corrected.[123] Hypertension, per se, is not an indication for parathyroid surgery in patients with primary hyperparathyroidism. Despite the heightened renin-angiotensin system in primary hyperparathyroidism, the BP response to ACEI is limited, and there is no information on the best antihypertensive agent in this disorder.

Of note, hypocalcemia also can raise BP,[124] and, in such circumstances, calcium supplementation may show beneficial effects on systolic BP in patients with essential hypertension.[125] In studies of normocalcemic patients with essential hypertension, calcium supplementation produces a mild, but statistically significant, reduction in BP.[125] These studies have been disputed, but it appears that a subgroup of hypertensive patients do have BP sensitivity to calcium. An *ionic hypothesis of cardiovascular disease* is based on the findings of a negative correlation between ionic (free) calcium and magnesium, and BP.[126]

## ACROMEGALY AND HYPERTENSION

Hypertension is very common in acromegaly. In the largest published series, hypertension was found in up to 51% of 500 patients with acromegaly[127] (see Chap. 12). Human growth hormone promotes sodium reabsorption, and the extracellular fluid volume is increased in acromegaly; this is accompanied by suppressed renin levels.[128,129] Also, there is evidence for overactivity of the sympathetic nervous system in acromegaly. An increase of left ventricular mass is frequently found in active disease, accompanied by an increased stroke volume and a decreased afterload. Thus, increased cardiac output in acromegaly could be responsible for the rise in BP.[130] Moreover, some have postulated a specific cardiomyopathy of acromegaly that could accompany the hypertension. The successful treatment of acromegaly often normalizes or improves BP and is beneficial to the other cardiac abnormalities, especially if the disease is treated early.

## THYROID DISEASE AND HYPERTENSION

Thyroid hormone affects all regulatory aspects of the cardiovascular system.[131-134] Thyroid hormone excess increases heart rate, cardiac output, stroke volume, and systolic BP; however, it decreases peripheral vascular resistance and diastolic BP. Cardiovascular changes with thyroid hormone are attributed to increased adrenergic nervous system activity through the β-adrenergic receptor.[133,134] Because thyroid hormones are structurally related to catecholamines, they may be taken up and released at the neural synapse.[133,134] Thyroid hormone stimulates the renin-angiotensin system mainly through increasing the hepatic production of angiotensinogen (renin substrate).[134]

**Hypothyroidism and Hypertension.**    The hypertension, which occurs in some patients with hypothyroidism, mainly involves elevations in diastolic BP; the incidence of the hypertension is reported to be 15% to 30%, but reports have varied widely from 0% up to 50% of subjects.[135] Overall, hypothyroidism may account for 1% to 3% of patients who are diagnosed as having essential hypertension. Hypothyroidism is common in older individuals in whom the independent incidence of hypertension is high. However, comparison studies have shown an increased prevalence of hypertension in hypothyroid individuals even when age is accounted for.[135] Sympathetic nervous system activity is increased in hypothyroidism, as documented by high circulating levels of norepinephrine.[131-134] This enhanced sympathetic nervous system activity is predominantly α-adrenergic in origin and may raise total peripheral resistance and decrease cardiac output—hemodynamic findings that have been verified in hypertensive, hypothyroid patients. In general, PRA in hypertensive, hypothyroid patients is low.[135] In about 30% of these patients, thyroid hormone replacement alone will reduce BP, although most of the patients will require antihypertensive therapy.

**Hyperthyroidism and Hypertension.**    Approximately 30% of subjects with thyrotoxicosis will have elevated BP that is predominantly an elevation in systolic BP.[131,132,134] The high systolic pressure and pulse pressure are best explained by increased cardiac output. These cardiac adaptations to thyroid hormone excess are mediated through the adrenergic nervous system; β-adrenergic blockade reduces the cardiac output and pulse pressure.[133] Nevertheless, circulating catecholamine levels are normal to reduced in hyperthyroidism.[133] In hyperthyroid rats, there is an increased density of β-adrenergic receptors in the cardiovascular tissue, indicating that thyroid hormone may increase adrenergic activity through these receptors.[133] Although PRA levels are elevated in hyperthyroidism, the increased renin-angiotensin system activity is not thought to contribute to the hypertension.[131,132] Successful treatment of hyperthyroidism, especially in younger subjects, usually corrects the hemodynamic abnormalities and reduces the systolic BP (see Chap. 42).

## ENDOCRINE SYSTEMS IN ESSENTIAL HYPERTENSION

In essential hypertension, there is evidence for the participation of several hormone systems, e.g., the renin-angiotensin system, serum aldosterone, and the sympathetic nervous system. Also, natriuretic hormones (e.g., the atrial natriuretic peptides [ANPs]), ouabain-like factors, endogenous vasodilator substances (e.g., the eicosanoids [prostaglandins, lipoxygenases, P450 epoxides]), and the kallikrein-kinin system have been implicated in hypertension. Many of these systems act in an autocrine-paracrine fashion; new additions to this list include endothelial factors such as nitric oxide and endothelin. However, the clinical use of measurements of these systems in the evaluation of hypertensive subjects is limited to special study situations. On the other hand, therapy with agonists or antagonists of these systems may prove to be promising.

### RENIN-ANGIOTENSIN SYSTEM

In hypertension, the renin-angiotensin system activity, almost always measured as PRA, varies widely. There probably is a continuum of levels of PRA in hypertension; however, some authors, who believe that there are subsets, *profile* hypertensive subjects as having *low, normal,* and *high PRA.*[136,137] Procedures to test for the release of PRA include sodium restriction, upright posture, diuretic administration, or correlation of PRA with 24-hour sodium excretion. There is an inverse relationship between PRA and sodium excretion; the concept of renin profiling in hypertension may enable a more definitive classification of hypertension. In support of the renin-profiling procedure is the increased cardiovascular risk associated with high circulating levels of PRA.[137] There also may be differences in BP response in renin subgroups.

**Low-Renin Hypertension.**    Approximately 30% of subjects with essential hypertension have low PRA levels, and a higher incidence is found in certain ethnic groups such as African-Americans.[136] Normally, low PRA is also thought to be associated with older age, but PRA may not be suppressed in the hypertensive individuals who survive to an older age.[138] In patients with low-renin hypertension, there is an increased incidence of salt sensitivity, and these persons are at lower risk for myocardial infarction.[137] In addition, individuals with low-renin hypertension have a superior antihypertensive response to diuretics and calcium-channel blockers.[139] However, the magnitude of difference of BP response to thiazide diuretics between renin groups is small.[140] The mechanism for low renin in essential hypertension is probably multifactorial, including mineralocorticoid excess, alterations in the tissue renin-angiotensin system, disordered calcium metabolism, and/or low sympathetic function. The best example of low-renin hypertension is primary aldosteronism in which volume expansion suppresses PRA levels. Other genetic disorders of mineralocorticoid excess (including glucocorticoid remediable aldosteronism,[141] the apparent mineralocorticoid excess syndrome,[142] and Liddle syndrome[143]) exhibit a suppressed PRA accompanied by hypertension and hypokalemia. Initial studies of the mechanisms for low-renin hypertension focused on aldosterone and other mineralocorticoids. Several candidate steroids (18-hydroxycorticosterone, 18-hydroxy-DOC, DOC, and 19-norDOC) have turned out not to be the cause.[144] In addition, hypokalemia rarely occurs in low-renin essential hypertension, and aldosterone levels are normal. The exact cause of low-renin essential hypertension remains unknown; however, these subjects might have abnormal calcium and magnesium metabolism; they display a positive relationship between diastolic BP and cytosolic calcium and an inverse relationship between systolic and diastolic BP and intracellular free magnesium.[145]

**High-Renin Hypertension.**    Approximately 10% to 20% of patients with essential hypertension have elevated levels of PRA.[136] It is uncertain if these moderate increments represent a

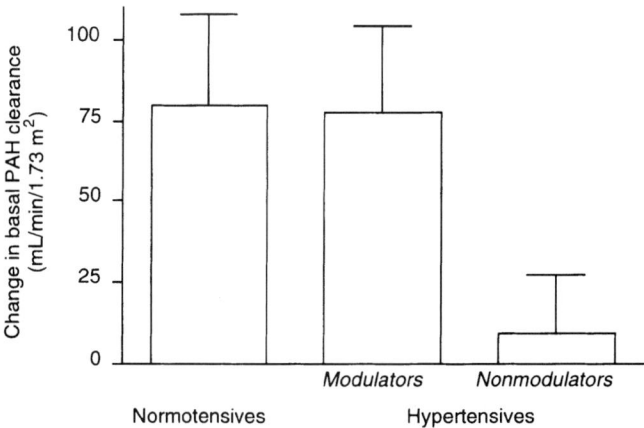

**FIGURE 82-3.** Changes in paraaminohippuric acid (*PAH*) clearance (renal blood flow) in normotensive and essential hypertensive subjects on high-sodium diet in response to angiotensin II. Nonmodulators fail to change renal blood flow with high salt and angiotensin II levels. (From Shoback D, Williams GH, Moore TJ, et al. Defect in the sodium-modulated tissue responsiveness to angiotensin II in essential hypertension. J Clin Invest 1983; 72:2115.)

distinct pathophysiologic abnormality, but these individuals are at greater risk for cardiovascular disease.[137] One explanation for elevated PRA in the hypertensive subject is nephron heterogeneity, with discordant renin secretion and sodium excretion; this causes a hypertensive vasoconstriction-volume relationship.[146] The renin dependency of the BP is supported by showing a greater hypotensive response to blockade of the renin-angiotensin system (ACEI, A-II–receptor blockers) in high-renin subjects. However, interpretation of these findings is difficult, as the antihypertensive responses related to ACEI correlate only minimally with baseline PRA.[147] Specific secondary causes of high-renin hypertension include renovascular hypertension, malignant hypertension, and renin-producing tumors.

**Normal-Renin Hypertension.** Normal PRA values are found in ~60% of subjects with hypertension.[136] An abnormal tissue response to A-II has been reported in subjects with normal-renin hypertension (termed *nonmodulating essential hypertension*).[148] The nonmodulation trait may be an intermediate phenotype that is inherited and is associated with a single nucleotide polymorphism (SNP) in the coding region of the angiotensinogen gene at codon 235.[149] The phenotype occurs twice as frequently in men.[149] Up to 85% of subjects have a family history of hypertension.[149] In these subjects, the aldosterone response to A-II infusion is subnormal on a low-sodium diet, and the renal blood flow response to A-II is subnormal on a high-sodium intake (Fig. 82-3). Thus, sodium fails to normally modulate the tissue response to A-II in both the adrenal glands and the kidneys. Because administration of an ACE inhibitor completely corrects the abnormal responses, tissue A-II defects may account for nonmodulation.[149] Nonmodulation could partially explain the impaired renal sodium handling and salt sensitivity that are found in hypertension. The diagnosis of nonmodulation is difficult, requiring sodium balance and A-II infusion. However, several tests, such as angiotensinogen gene expression and the red blood cell sodium, lithium ($Na^+,Li^+$) countertransport assay could be markers for nonmodulation.[149]

**Tissue Renin-Angiotensin System.** Many of the conclusions from profiling of circulating PRA must now be interpreted in light of the presence of a tissue (local) renin-angiotensin system in blood vessels, heart, kidney, adrenal glands, and other target organs.[150] *It is possible that much of the cause of essential hypertension resides in the tissue renin-angiotensin system.* For example, in the kidney, A-II levels can be 1000-fold higher than in the circulation, especially in certain areas such as

the glomerular and peritubular sites.[151] In transgenic rats in which a mouse renin gene is inserted, there is hypertension, but circulating levels of renin and A-II and renal renin content are low at the same time that vascular A-II is high.[152] Treatment with ACEI and removal of the adrenals corrects the BP, suggesting a tissue mediation of the hypertension in what was otherwise a low-renin state.[152]

**Genetics of the Renin-Angiotensin System.** Genetic aspects of the renin-angiotensin system in hypertension are being intensely studied. Polymorphisms of the angiotensinogen gene on chromosome 1 have been linked to essential hypertension, and there is a 33% excess of shared angiotensinogen alleles in male sibling pairs with diastolic hypertension.[153] This mutation might account for 6% of hypertension in young white subjects. One mutation, the T235 variant of the angiotensinogen gene, is associated with elevated levels of angiotensinogen. Another mutation, involving an A for G substitution in the 6 position of the promoter region, occurs on the angiotensinogen gene; in a large study, subjects with the AA genotype had better BP responses to sodium and weight reduction.[154] Thus, genotyping for angiotensinogen might potentially help to predict BP responses to therapy.

ACE gene polymorphism has also been noted in hypertension and vascular disease. The alleles found for ACE include insertion (I) and deletion (D); the DD genotype is associated with coronary heart disease,[155] carotid artery disease,[156] and atherosclerosis. These studies show that polymorphism of ACE is strongly associated with cardiovascular complications. Insulin resistance and angina pectoris also relate to converting-enzyme gene polymorphism.[157] Other studies have shown that the DD allele is associated with higher ACE levels and the II genotype with lower ACE levels in the renal disease of type 1 diabetic patients.[158] The diabetic group has less reduction in BP and proteinuria on treatment with an ACEI if the subjects are on a high-salt diet.[159]

## SYMPATHETIC NERVOUS SYSTEM IN HYPERTENSION

Increased sympathetic nervous system activity (see Chap. 85) occurs in essential hypertension.[160] In studies measuring plasma norepinephrine, young hypertensive subjects had higher values than did normotensive controls.[161] Hypertensive subjects also have increased renal and cardiac norepinephrine spillover, indicating regional sympathetic excess.[162] In studies using microneurography to measure regional sympathetic nerve activity, the recorded activity in skeletal muscle is high in essential hypertension.[163] Inhibitors of sympathetic activity lower BP proportionately to the baseline level of plasma norepinephrine. Stress, isometric exercise, and tilt table maneuvers all produce exaggerated norepinephrine responses in hypertension, and hyperactive BP responses occur with norepinephrine infusion. Thus, the combination of exaggerated BP responses and high norepinephrine levels could provide a substantial neurogenic stimulus for hypertension. Certain subgroups may be more prone to develop neurogenic hypertension, including young hypertensive subjects, very obese individuals, and those defined as having a hyperdynamic circulation.[160]

There may be two phases of sympathetic nervous system activity participation in the evolution of hypertension. In the early phase there is high cardiac output that is initiated by an increase in sympathetic nervous system activity.[160] This early hyperdynamic phase of hypertension then converts to a more long-term phase of chronic BP elevation in which cardiac output returns toward normal and systemic vascular resistance rises.[164] With time high sympathetic nervous system activity and BP also induce structural and hypertrophic changes in blood vessels that further sustain the hypertension.[165] In humans, there is support for the concept of an inappropriately high sympathetic nervous system activity, both early and late, in the course of essential hypertension, implying that factprs that would normally or physiologically suppress the sympathetic nervous system are not operative.[164] In studies to support this notion, drugs that lower BP cause an excessive response of norepinephrine, suggesting an unmasking of sympathetic nervous system responses. There may be a central disinhibition failure due to abnormal central function in the cells of the rostral ventricular medulla in neurogenic forms of hypertension.[166] Thus, values considered in the normal range in a person with established hypertension may be abnormal or inappropriately high. Much of the neurogenic contribution to hypertension may be at a regional or organ-specific level. Increased organ-specific radiotracer spillover has been demonstrated in the heart and kidneys of essential hypertensive subjects.[162] Similar regional increases in sympathetic burst activity or firing rates are found in borderline and established hypertensive individuals.[163] A mutually reinforcing effect of the sympathetic nervous system and renin-angiotensin system may sustain high BP, since adrenergic receptors mediate renin release and A-II can activate the sympathetic nervous system.[167] Both of these systems also have parallel growth-promoting properties that probably mediate the degenerative changes in chronic hypertension.

Dopamine is an indispensable catecholamine product that not only acts as a neurotransmitter in neuronal tissues but also has autocrine and paracrine functions in nonneuronal tissues. When stimulating specific receptors located in the blood vessels or along the nephron, dopamine can regulate renal hemodynamics as well as sodium and water transport, and in the adrenal gland inhibits aldosterone secretion. In humans with essential hypertension, the response to dopamine is impaired at the receptor level. Renal dopamine modulates sodium excretion during sodium loading, mediated through the renal dopamine $D_3$-receptor (as shown in mice with inactive $D_3$-receptors).[168] Both BP and the renin-angiotensin system are higher in these mice. The $D_3$-receptor may be an important regulator of renal renin release and BP.[168] A dopamine agonist (e.g., fenoldopam and the powerful dopamine $D_2$-receptor agonist carmoxirole) can lower BP in very severe hypertension and has been used in hypertensive crises.[169] Interestingly, a reduced urinary free dopamine response to salt loading is observed in essential hypertension, indicating a deficiency of renal dopamine that could blunt normal natriuretic mechanisms.[170]

## SODIUM AND HYPERTENSION

A positive relationship between sodium intake and hypertension is documented in epidemiologic studies,[171] but increased salt intake does not uniformly raise BP in all persons. There may be individual differences in BP sensitivity to salt.[171,172] Some hypertensive subjects may be *salt sensitive* (defined as an increase in mean BP of $\geq 10$ mm Hg in response to a high-salt diet). Salt-sensitive hypertension is more common in older subjects, in African-Americans, and in diabetic subjects.[171,172] Factors that control sodium (e.g., membrane transport systems, ANPs, and sodium pump inhibitors) are abnormal in hypertension. Other factors that regulate sodium (e.g., aldosterone, dopamine, prostaglandins, and bradykinin) also play a role in the relationship of salt to BP.

## MEMBRANE SODIUM TRANSPORT

A major function of most cells is to pump in an outward direction $Na^+$ in exchange for extracellular $K^+$ by the action of the $Na^+,K^+$-adenosine triphosphatase (ATPase) pump. The pump then establishes a gradient of sodium across cell membranes that can serve as energy for other passive ion transport systems. Red and white blood cells from subjects with essential hypertension show a high $Na^+$ content, a finding that matches the observations of high $Na^+$ content in blood vessels and other target tissue from hypertensive animal models.[173,174] Disturbances in several membrane ionic transport pathways are described in human hypertension.[173,174] Measurement of these transport systems in humans uses peripheral cells (erythrocytes, leukocytes, platelets). The transport pathways are discussed in the following sections.

**$Na^+,K^+$ Pump.**    The $Na^+,K^+$-ATPase or $Na^+,K^+$ pump mediates the active transport of $Na^+$ and $K^+$, and is central for acute and chronic regulation of cell ions. Factors such as insulin, catecholamines, and $\beta_2$-agonists increase intracellular uptake of $K^+$ through the pump. Compounds such as digitalis increase cell $Na^+$ by direct inhibition of the pump; the activity can be measured by ATPase enzyme activity, ion fluxes, ouabain binding, and so forth. In skeletal muscle, the activity of the pump is increased by training, thyroid hormones, and glucocorticoids. The pump is down-regulated in hypothyroidism, cardiac failure, muscle disease, $K^+$ deficiency, and some forms of hypertension. Insulin stimulates $K^+$ uptake through the pump in 3T3 fibroblasts by means of phosphatidylinositol 3-kinase and protein kinase C.[175]

Several studies found a defective pump activity in human and animal models of hypertension that could lead to a high intracellular $Na^+$.[176] This defect could produce hypertension by partial membrane depolarization and activation of voltage-dependent $Ca^{2+}$ channels (with increased influx of $Ca^{2+}$), thus promoting blood vessel contraction. Another proposal is that high intracellular $Na^+$ could activate the $Na^+,Ca^{2+}$ exchanger that would increase intracellular $Ca^{2+}$.[176] Other studies find high pump activity in blood vessels, especially in animal metabolic models such as the fructose-fed rat.[177]

**$Na^+,Li^+$ Countertransport.**    An elevated erythrocyte $Na^+,Li^+$ countertransport has been noted in numerous studies of subjects with essential hypertension.[173,174] The $Na^+,Li^+$-countertransport system is genetically transmitted by a single gene determinant and may be a candidate marker for genetic hypertension. $Na^+,Li^+$-countertransport kinetics are abnormal in relatives of hypertensive patients who have high countertransport.[178] One question has been the usefulness of this assay as a predictor of future hypertension. In a prospective study of normotensive middle-aged men, those who eventually developed hypertension had high $Na^+,Li^+$ countertransport, suggesting the assay as a predictor of subsequent hypertension.[179]

Enhanced erythrocyte $Na^+,Li^+$ countertransport is found in hypertensive patients who have hyperlipidemia.[180] High countertransport is also a marker for metabolic correlates [higher fasting blood glucose, greater glucose, and insulin responses to an oral glucose tolerance test (OGGT)] in hypertensive subjects.[181] In nonmodulating essential hypertension, in people who fail to change renal blood flow in response to high salt intake, countertransport is high, and the assay may be a marker for nonmodulation and salt-sensitive hypertension.[182]

The pathophysiologic consequences of an abnormal countertransport are more difficult to understand. The system is quantitatively a minor transport pathway, and its functional significance remains to be determined.

The $Na^+,Li^+$-countertransport system is also a risk marker for hypertension and renal complications in diabetes mellitus. A high countertransport appears to be an inherited-risk marker for diabetic nephropathy. The assay may identify those type 2 diabetics who will develop microalbuminuria.[183] The major kinetic abnormality of the $Na^+,Li^+$ countertransporter in diabetes with renal disease is a raised affinity for extracellular sodium.[184] Studies show a membrane defect in countertransport in diabetic nephropathy that explains the abnormal kinetics, including an increased $V_{max}$ and $V_{max}/K_m(So)$ ratio, which reflects higher ion association for the transport system.[185] The abnormal kinetic parameters can be completely corrected by thiol group alkylation with $N$-ethylmaleimide. Similar to the findings in essential hypertension, high countertransport values are correlated with insulin resistance and BP in patients with type 2 diabetes.[186]

**$Na^+,H^+$ Exchange.**    Elevated $Na^+,H^+$-exchanger activity is found in various cell types from patients with essential hypertension and is a recognized intermediate phenotype for this disorder.[187] The phenotype of an increased maximal transport capacity is preserved in Epstein-Barr virus immortalized lymphoblasts from hypertensive patients, suggesting strong genetic control.[188,189] Both lymphocytes[190] and erythrocytes[191] from patients with essential hypertension show an enhanced Na$^+$,H$^+$-exchanger activity. Higher Na$^+$,H$^+$ exchanger in peripheral cells is also noted in normotensive subjects with a family history of hypertension.[187] Very similar findings for elevated Na$^+$,H$^+$ exchanger are noted in vascular myocytes from the spontaneously hypertensive rat.[192,193] There is a family of Na$^+$,H$^+$-exchanger isoforms of which the most studied in hypertension is the NHE-1 isoform. The NHE-1 isoform and, in some tissues, the NHE-3 isoform have been reported to be elevated in human and experimental hypertension in several cells, including erythrocytes, platelets, and fibroblasts.[187] However, the gene for the NHE-1 isoform of the exchanger is not the cause of hypertension as shown in genetic linkage studies.[191] Although this transporter is involved in growth regulation, the enhanced proliferation pattern seen in vascular tissue in hypertension is mostly independent of ion transport.[194]

The mechanism of Na$^+$,H$^+$ abnormality in hypertension is unclear. The physiologic role of this transport system is to respond to intracellular acid loads, and intracellular pH does appear to be slightly lower in hypertension.[192] Exchanger abundance is identical in hypertensive versus normotensive subjects, indicating that the increased activity in the hypertensive group is due to elevated turnover of the exchanger.[188,195] Na$^+$,H$^+$ exchanger phosphorylation is elevated in quiescent cells.[188] Its dysfunction could represent a defect in signal transduction as it responds to several agonists including A-II.[188] It has been further noted that A-II stimulates p90rsk in vascular smooth muscle cells, leading to the hypothesis of a potential Na$^+$,H$^+$-exchanger kinase.[195] Metabolic acidosis, high salt intake, and circulating hormones (e.g., insulin) also regulate Na$^+$,H$^+$ exchange.[187] Although increased Na$^+$,H$^+$ exchange is high in the erythrocytes of patients with primary aldosteronism, aldosterone directly added to cells in vitro does not affect this system.[196]

ACEI corrects the Na$^+$,H$^+$-exchanger overactivity in essential hypertension.[197] The addition of chelerythrine, a blocker of protein kinase C, also reduces Na$^+$,H$^+$-exchanger activity in spontaneously hypertensive rats.[198] The addition of an amiloride derivative, which inhibits the Na$^+$,H$^+$ exchanger, increases BP in spontaneously hypertensive rats.[199]

The Na$^+$,H$^+$ exchanger also exhibits altered kinetics in diabetic nephropathy.[200,201] This phenotype persists in immortalized lymphoblasts[201] and in skin fibroblasts[202] from diabetic subjects with nephropathy. Similarly to hypertension, the mechanism in diabetes is due to posttranslational factors.[201,202]

**Na$^+$,K$^+$,(2Cl$^-$) Cotransport.** This transport pathway is inhibited by loop diuretics (furosemide, bumetanide). Initial studies found low erythrocyte cotransport in essential hypertension, but later reports noted high activity, probably representing a different hypertensive population.[203] Ethnic and geographic variations in cotransport may make it a poor marker for essential hypertension. In a metaanalysis from the literature, it was found that essential hypertension, family history of hypertension, gender, and antihypertensive medications were the main determinants of cotransport.[204] Indirect evidence has shown a circulating cotransport inhibitor of unknown nature.[205]

In summary, various membrane cation-transport defects are thought to contribute to the high cell sodium content and increased Na$^+$ reabsorption seen in hypertension. In addition, there is evidence for increased passive inward Na$^+$ leak in hypertension. These abnormal membrane ion transport pathways suggest a more complex picture for sodium handling than can be explained by a circulating pump inhibitor, natriuretic hormones, and many of the other factors that control sodium homeostasis.

### SODIUM PUMP INHIBITORS

Enhanced sodium excretion in response to volume expansion is associated with increased blood levels of a factor(s) that inhibits the Na$^+$,K$^+$-ATPase pump.[206] Reduced Na$^+$ excretion causes volume expansion and signals a circulating pump inhibitor to block sodium reabsorption and correct volume overload. This pump inhibitor, however, could act on other tissue Na$^+$,K$^+$-ATPase pump sites. For example, in the blood vessels, there would be an increase of intracellular Na$^+$ and Ca$^{2+}$ and a resetting of vascular tone.[206] Increased intracellular Na$^+$ and Ca$^{2+}$ and reduced Na$^+$,K$^+$-ATPase pump activity are found in experimental and human hypertension. The isolation and structural identification of a circulating compound that inhibits the Na$^+$,K$^+$-ATPase pump has been difficult. One group has identified and characterized a ouabain-like compound from human plasma and adrenal glands that inhibits Na$^+$,K$^+$-ATPase pump activity.[207] The physiologic effects of this endogenous ouabain include stimulation of vascular contraction and control of intracellular calcium stores.[207] The *endogenous ouabain* is a novel steroid counterpart that is isomeric with the plant glycoside ouabain.[207] The primary source of endogenous ouabain is in the adrenal zona glomerulosa where ACTH and A-II AT$_2$ receptors stimulate its release. The signal pathway for endogenous ouabain release is different than that for aldosterone. A binding site for endogenous ouabain has been found on the sodium pump. It mediates long-term BP control through neuronal pathways, yielding a slow pressor effect that could contribute to the induction of hypertension.

### ENDOGENOUS NATRIURETIC PEPTIDES

There is a family of endogenous natriuretic peptides, including ANP, brain natriuretic peptide (BNP), and C-type natriuretic peptide (CNP).[208,209] ANP, which was first isolated from the heart, has numerous actions, including stimulation of natriuresis and vasodilation, and inhibition of the renin-angiotensin system, aldosterone, the sympathetic nervous system, and the endothelin system.[208] ANP is synthesized in atrial myocytes, implying an endocrine function in the heart (see Chap. 178). ANP and BNP are released by atrial stretch (intravascular volume, atrial pressure). BNP has properties similar to those of ANP, but is synthesized and stored in the central nervous system and in atrial cells.[208] In hypertension, the levels of BNP may be greater than the levels of ANP; thus, it is debated which peptide is more important in guarding against BP elevations. CNP is produced in the endothelium and is a potent vasoactive peptide that dilates both veins and arteries, but it has no natriuretic properties. CNP is not a circulating peptide and acts in a paracrine fashion.

Much of the function of these ANPs is determined by their receptors. Two of these receptors, ANPR-A and ANPR-B, are linked to guanyl cyclases. ANP and BNP bind to A receptors in the endothelium of blood vessels, whereas CNP binds to B receptors.[208] The third is the ANPR-C receptor, which is a clearance receptor and plays an active role in determining availability of the peptides by controlling their rate of removal from the circulation.[208]

In essential hypertension, the levels of ANP and BNP are elevated, but it has been argued that these values are actually relatively low for the level of BP.[208] The concept of a natriuretic peptide deficiency state in essential hypertension is appealing, but unproved. The most promising therapeutic approach to raise natriuretic peptide levels and lower BP is through the regulation of the ANPR-C clearance receptors and use of neutral endopeptidase inhibition (ompatrilat) to potentiate their bioaction.[210] These agents also have ACE inhibitor properties and accumulate kinins.[210a] Cardiac natriuretic peptide levels may also be predictors of mortality in heart failure.[211]

### KININS IN HYPERTENSION

The products of the kallikrein-kinin system, the kinins, are natriuretic and diuretic and have vasodilating properties, through stimulation of nitric oxide and prostaglandins[212,213] (see Chap. 170). Kinins are produced from kininogens through cleavage by the enzyme kallikrein to form the two main kinins, bradykinin and lysyl-bradykinin (kallidin). Kinins act as paracrine and autocrine hormones through two receptors, the $B_1$- and $B_2$-receptors. The $B_2$-receptors, which belong to the family linked to G proteins, are the ones that mediate most known regulating effects on blood flow to meet metabolic demands. Renal kinins play a role in the regulation of the microcirculation and of water and sodium metabolism; the natriuretic effect is mediated in part by prostaglandins. Neutral endopeptidase inhibitors are natriuretic through the blocking of kinin hydrolysis leading to their accumulation. ACE is one of the main peptidases that hydrolyze kinins; ACE inhibitors block the breakdown of kinins. Tissue and urinary kinins increase with ACEI application. Although kinin accumulation potentiates the hypotensive action of ACE inhibitors, the administration of a kinin antagonist only blocks the acute but not chronic hypotensive effect of ACEI. Kinin release after ACEI may mediate the cardioprotection of ACEI during ischemic episodes and in the prevention of remodeling.[214,215]

A reduction in the kallikrein-kinin system has been found in animal models of genetic hypertension; in children, it is a good marker of genetic hypertension.[212,213] A restriction fragment length polymorphism for the kallikrein gene family is linked to BP in the spontaneously hypertensive rat.[212] The administration of kinin inhibitors raises BP, whereas in animals, which are transgenic for kinin expression, there is a prolonged hypotensive response. The bradykinin $B_2$-receptor gene knockout mouse also develops hypertension on a high-salt diet.

## NITRIC OXIDE IN HYPERTENSION

Nitric oxide (NO) is formed from endogenous arginine by nitric oxide synthase (NOS) or from exogenous nitrovasodilators such as nitroglycerin (see Chap. 179). Cells and tissues oxidize via a five-electron oxidation of the guanido nitrogen of arginine to form citrulline and NO.[216] This reaction is catalyzed by the enzyme NOS, which exists in three isoforms (neuronal NOS, inducible NOS, and endothelial eNOS).[216,217] Studies have found eNOS to be membrane associated in the Golgi apparatus, in plasmalemmal membranes, and in caveolae that contain several key signal-transduction complexes.[218] The enzymes are dependent on several cofactors, including reduced nicotinamide adenine dinucleotide phosphate (NADP), flavin, adenine dinucleotide, and tetrahydrobiopterin; they use heme as the prosthetic group. In addition, intracellular calcium and calmodulin can activate NOS and NO production, but there are also several calcium-independent pathways.[219] The actions of agents such as acetylcholine, histamine, thrombin, and insulin are mediated through NO. Certain cytokines and endotoxins also activate NO in vascular smooth muscle, liver, and peripheral cells. Shear stress induces NO production through activation of *heat-shock proteins* such as Hsp90.[220]

The major signal-transduction pathway for NO is through guanylate cyclase, forming cyclic guanosine monophosphate (GMP).[221] NO binds to the heme-containing enzyme guanylate cyclase to convert guanosine triphosphate (GTP) to cGMP. This reaction activates protein kinase G with phosphorylation of numerous proteins that mediate vascular relaxation and have antigrowth effects.

Numerous hormones and drugs regulate NO through effects on NOS activity and at other regulatory sites.[222] These factors can also act on the NO-cGMP complex to alter signal transduction. Several agents such as phosphodiesterase inhibitors, scavenger agents (hemoglobin), agents that alter cellular calcium, NOS-substrate inhibitors, and hormone and receptor antagonists will alter NO.

The NO-cGMP complex mediates smooth muscle vasodilatation in blood vessels and other hollow organs. The system is also operative in platelets, nerves, macrophages, and other target organs. NO contributes to the regulation of insulin secretion and action, platelet function, neurotransmission, memory, penile erection, cytotoxicity induced by macrophages, and

atherogenesis.[222] NO can operate through cGMP-independent pathways having molecular effects on iron-containing enzymes, free radicals, proteins, and DNA synthesis.

The role of NO in hypertensive vascular disease is complex.[223] With the preponderance of data showing that NO is crucial in vascular homeostasis, it should be a major contributor to hypertension. A logical hypothesis is that decreased eNOS expression should be seen in hypertension. There have been eNOS polymorphisms reported in essential hypertension such as a calcium repeat polymorphism in intron 13,[224] and a G to T substitution in exon 7 of the eNOS gene resulting in a Glu298Asp conversion.[225] However, these altered genes seem to have a weak effect on phenotype or cardiovascular risk. A depressed response of blood flow to acetylcholine, which is eNOS sensitive, is taken as an indicator of endothelial dysfunction and decreased bioactive NO. Attenuated vasodilator responses are seen in hypertension and coronary heart disease.[223] Paradoxically, NO responses can be increased in both genetic and primary hypertension, and the response may vary in different vascular beds.[226] In the spontaneous hypertensive rat, eNOS is up-regulated in the aorta but normal in other vascular beds. Oxidative stress may be another important determinant of endothelial function. Increased production of superoxide radicals ($O_2^-$) may account for the variable findings of NO activity in hypertension, as overproduction of the NO scavenger $O_2^-$ (rather than a change in eNOS production) may be important in endothelial dysfunction. An increased vascular $O_2^-$ has been associated with hypercholesterolemia and animal models of hypertension.[226]

In summary, reduced production or bioavailability of NO should promote cellular events in blood vessels that promote vasoconstriction, inhibit vasodilatation, and activate structural damage in vessels. Blockade of NO synthase with inhibitors will raise BP in humans and animal models.[223] Administration of arginine will cause a mild reduction in BP both in humans and in animal models.[223]

## ENDOTHELIN IN HYPERTENSION

Endothelin-1 (ET-1) is a potent 21-amino acid vasoconstrictor peptide produced by the endothelium. There are three mammalian endothelins (i.e., ET-1, ET-2, and ET-3), which were first found in the vascular endothelium but exist in many other cells.[227] They regulate cardiovascular function and other noncardiovascular actions such as airway smooth muscles, the digestive tract, endocrine glands, the renal system, and the nervous system.

Endothelial cells produce preproendothelin, from which is derived proendothelin, which is converted to big endothelin by endothelin-converting enzyme, a neutral endopeptidase.[227] Big endothelin (39 amino acids) then is processed into endothelin (22 amino acids). Vascular endothelial cells (VEC) release predominantly ET-1 in response to low shear stress, A-II, vasopressin, catecholamines, and transforming growth factor-β.

ET-1 acts on the $ET_A$ and $ET_B$ receptors to induce contraction, proliferation, and cell hypertrophy.[227] Through the $ET_B$ receptor, ET-1 may release NO and prostacyclin, thus having the capacity to be both a vasoconstrictor and a vasodilator. This dual activity depends on the receptor predominance in any vascular bed. Coronary arteries lack $ET_B$ receptors, so ET-1 is a vasoconstrictor, whereas in cardiomyocytes $ET_B$ receptors predominate. In the kidney, predominantly $ET_A$ receptors are found in blood vessels and mesangial cells. In the distal tubule, the $ET_A$ receptor regulates sodium excretion.

The endothelin system plays an important role in development. Several models of gene disruption produce malformations in the upper airways and aortic arch and abnormalities in pigment and megacolon. These models do not exhibit major changes in BP.

The endothelin system seems to be activated mostly in severe salt-dependent hypertension such as the deoxycorticosterone acetate, salt-sensitive rat and the Dahl salt-sensitive rat. These models overexpress ET-1 in blood vessels. Endothelin antagonist therapy reverses hypertrophic remodeling in small blood vessels.[228] In human hypertension, administration of endothelin-receptor antagonists has a mild BP-lowering effect, but the effect of a combined $ET_A/ET_B$ antagonist is equal to that of an ACE inhibitor.[229,230] Endothelins may be involved in renal failure–induced hypertension, in cyclosporine-induced hypertension, in erythropoietin-induced hypertension, in pheochromocytoma-induced hypertension, and in pregnancy-induced hypertension.[229] In general, although the exact role of endothelins in hypertension is not yet clear, the receptor antagonists may have a promising future in the control and prevention of cardiovascular disease.[229]

# REFERENCES

1. Hypertension Detection and Follow-Up Program Cooperative Group. The hypertension detection and follow-up program. Circ Res 1977; 40(Suppl 1):106.
2. The Sixth Report of the Joint National Committee on Detection, Evaluation and Treatment of High Blood Pressure (JNC VI). Arch Intern Med 1997; 157:2413.
3. Working Group on Renovascular Hypertension. Detection, evaluation and treatment. Arch Intern Med 1987; 147:820.
4. Mann SJ, Pickering TG. Detection of renovascular hypertension: state of the art. Ann Intern Med 1992; 117:845.
5. Connolly JO, Higgens RM, Walters HL, et al. Presentation, clinical features and outcome in different patterns of atherosclerotic renovascular disease. Q J Med 1994; 87:413.
6. Canzanello VJ, Textor SC. Noninvasive diagnosis of renovascular disease. Mayo Clin Proc 1994; 69:1172.
7. Ram CVS. Renovascular hypertension. Curr Opin Nephrol Hypertens 1997; 6:575.
8. McGrath BP, Clarke K. Renal artery stenosis: current diagnosis and treatment. Med J Aust 1993; 158:343.
9. Rimmer JM, Gennari FJ. Atherosclerotic renal vascular disease and progressive renal failure. Ann Intern Med 1993; 118:712.
10. Choudhri AH, Cleland JG, Rowlands PL. Unsuspected renal artery stenosis in peripheral vascular disease. Br Med J 1990; 301:1197.
11. Pickering TG, Devereux RB, James GD. Recurrent pulmonary edema in hypertension due to bilateral renal artery stenosis: treatment by angioplasty or surgical revascularization. Lancet 1988; 2:551.
12. Svetkey LP, Kadir S, Dunnick NR, et al. Similar prevalence of renovascular hypertension in selected blacks and whites. Hypertension 1991; 17:678.
13. Pohl MA. Renal artery stenosis, renal vascular hypertension and ischemic nephropathy. In: Schrier RW, Gottschalk CW, eds. Disease of the kidney, 6th ed. Boston: Little Brown and Company, 1997:1367.
14. Martinez-Maldonado M. Pathophysiology of renovascular hypertension. Hypertension 1991; 17:707.
15. Mitchell KD, Braam B, Navar LG. Hypertensinogenic mechanisms mediated by renal actions of renin-angiotensin system. Hypertension 1992; 19(Suppl 1):I-18-1.
16. Navar LG. The kidney in blood pressure regulation and development of hypertension. Med Clin North Am 1997; 8:1165.
17. Mitchell KD, Navar LG. Intrarenal actions of angiotensin II in pathogenesis of experimental hypertension. In: Laragh JH, Brenner BM, eds. Hypertension: pathophysiology, diagnosis, and management. New York: Raven Press, 1995:1437.
18. Guan S, Fox MJ, Mitchell KD, Navar LG. Angiotensin and angiotensin-converting enzyme tissue levels in two-kidney, one-clip hypertensive rats. Hypertension 1992; 20:763.
19. Romero JC, Feldstein AE, Rodriguez-Porcel MG, et al. New insights into the pathophysiology of renovascular hypertension. Mayo Clin Proc 1997 72:251.
20. Corry DB, Tuck ML. Secondary aldosteronism. Endocrinol Metab Clin North Am 1995; 24:511.
21. Thornbury JR, Stanley JC, Fryback DG. Hypertensive urogram: a nondiscriminatory test for renovascular hypertension. AJR 1982; 138:43.
22. Wilcox CS. Use of angiotensin-converting-enzyme inhibitors for diagnosing renovascular hypertension. Kidney Int 1993; 44:1379.
23. Elliot WJ, Martin WB, Murphy MB. Comparison of two noninvasive tests for renovascular hypertension. Arch Intern Med 1993; 153:755.
24. Postma CT, Van Der Steen PH, Hoefnagels WH, et al. The captopril test in the detection of renovascular disease in hypertensive patients. Arch Intern Med 1990; 150:625.
25. Roubidoux MA, Dunnick NR, Klotman PE, et al. Renal vein renins: inability to predict response to revascularization in patients with hypertension. Radiology 1991; 178:819.
26. Nally JV, Black HR. State of the art review: captopril renography pathophysiological considerations and clinical observations. Semin Nucl Med 1992; 22:85.
27. Mann SJ, Pickering TG, Sos TA, et al. Captopril renography in the diagnosis of renal artery stenosis: accuracy and limitations. Am J Med 1991; 90:30.
28. Halpern EJ, Deane CR, Needleman L, et al. Normal renal artery spectral Doppler wave form. A closer look. Radiology 1995; 196:667.
29. Olin JW, Piedmonte MR, Young JR, et al. The utility of duplex ultrasound scanning of the renal arteries for diagnosing significant renal artery stenosis. Ann Intern Med 1995; 196:667.
30. Rene PC, Oliva VL, Bui BT, et al. Renal artery stenosis: evaluation of Doppler US after inhibition of angiotensin converting enzyme with captopril. Radiology 1995; 196:675.
31. Riehl J, Schmitt H, Bongatz, et al. Renal artery stenosis: Evaluation with colour duplex ultrasonography. Nephrol Dial Transplant 1997; 12:1608.
32. Debatin JF, Spritzer CE, Grist TM, et al. Imaging of the renal arteries: value of MR angiography. AJR 1991; 157:981.
33. Postma CT, Joosten FB, Rosenbusch G, Thien T. Magnetic resonance angiography has a high reliability in the detection of renal artery stenosis. Am J Hypertens 1997; 10:957.
34. Rieumont MJ, Kaufman JA, Geller SC, et al. Evaluation of renal artery stenosis with dynamic gadolinium-enhanced MR angiography. AJR 1997; 169:39.
35. DeHaan MW, Kouwenhoven M, Thelissen GRP, et al. Renovascular disease in patients with hypertension: detection with systolic and diastolic gating in three-dimensional, phase-contrast MR angiography. Radiology 1996; 198:449.
36. Olbricht CJ, Arlet IP. Magnetic resonance angiography—the procedure of choice to diagnose renal artery stenosis? Nephrol Dial Transplant 1998; 13:1620.
37. Olbricht CJ, Paul K, Prokop M, et al. Minimally invasive diagnosis of renal artery stenosis by spiral computed tomography angiography. Kidney Int 1995; 48:1332.
38. Weibull H, Bergqvist D, Bergentz SE, et al. Percutaneous transluminal angioplasty versus reconstruction of atherosclerotic renal artery stenosis. Prospective randomized study. J Vasc Surg 1993; 18:841.
39. Lawrie GM, Morris GC, Glaeser DH, DeBakey MI. Renovascular reconstruction: factors affecting long-term prognosis in 919 patients followed up to 31 years. Am J Cardiol 1989; 63:1085.
40. Hansen KJ, Starr SM, Sands E, et al. Contemporary surgical management of renovascular disease. J Vasc Surg 1992; 16:310.
41. Textor SC. Revascularization in atherosclerotic renal artery disease. Kidney Dis 1998; 53:799.
42. Caps MT, Zierler RE, Polissar NL, et al. Risk of atrophy in kidneys with atherosclerotic renal artery stenosis. Kidney Int 1998; 53:735.
43. Greco BA, Breyer JA. Atherosclerotic ischemic renal disease. Am J Kidney Dis 1997; 29:167.
44. Derkx FH, Schalecamp MA. Renal artery stenosis and hypertension. Lancet 1994; 344:237.
45. Ramsey LE, Weller PC. Blood pressure response to percutaneous angioplasty. an overview of published series. Br Med J 1990; 300:569.
46. Bonelli FS, McKusick MA, Textor SC. Renal artery angioplasty: technical results and clinical outcome in 320 patients. Mayo Clin Proc 1995; 70:104.
47. Plouin PF, Chatellier G, Darne B, et al. Blood pressure outcome of angioplasty in atherosclerotic renal artery stenosis. A randomized trial. Hypertension 1998; 31:823.
48. Van de Ven PJ, Beutler JJ, Kaatee R. Transluminal vascular stent for ostial atherosclerotic renal artery stenosis. Lancet 1995; 346:672.
49. Blum U, Krumme B, Flugel P, et al. Treatment of ostial-artery stenosis with vascular endoprothesis after unsuccessful balloon angioplasty. N Engl J Med 1997; 336:459.
50. Shannon HM, Gillespie IN, Moss JG. Salvage of the solitary kidney by insertion of a renal artery stent. AJR 1998; 171:459.
51. Hollenberg NK. The treatment of renovascular hypertension: surgery, angioplasty, and medical therapy with converting enzyme inhibitors. Am J Kidney Dis 1987; 10(Suppl 1):52.
52. Pohl MA, Novick AC. Natural history of atherosclerotic and fibrous renal artery disease: clinical implications. Am J Kidney Dis 1985; 5(4):A120.
53. Dean RH. Comparison of medical and surgical treatment of renovascular hypertension. Nephron 1986; 44(Suppl 1):101.
54. Stradness DE Jr. Natural history of renal artery stenosis. Am J Kidney Dis 1994; 24:630.
55. Marshall FI, Hagen S, Mahaffy RG, et al. Percutaneous transluminal angioplasty for theromatous renal artery stenosis—blood pressure response and discriminant analysis of outcome predictors. Q J Med 1990; 75:483.
56. Corvol P, Pinet F, Galen FX, et al. Seven lessons from seven renin-secreting tumors. Kidney Int 1988; 34(Suppl 25):S38.
57. Mimran A. Renin-secreting tumors. In: Swales J, ed. Textbook of hypertension. Oxford, UK: Blackwell Science, 1994:858.
58. Bruneval P, Fournier JG, Soubrier F, et al. Detection and localization of renin messenger mRNA in human pathologic tissues using in situ hybridization. Am J Pathol 1988; 131:320.
59. Anderson PW, Macaulay L, Do YS, et al. Extrarenal renin-secreting tumors: insights into hypertension and ovarian renin production. Medicine 1990; 68:257.
60. Misiani R, Sonzogni A, Poletti EM, et al. Hyponatremic hypertensive syndrome and massive proteinuria in a patient with renin-producing leiomyosarcoma. Am J Kidney Dis 1994; 24:83.
61. Aurell M, Rudin A, Tisell LE, et al. Captopril effect on hypertension in patients with renin-producing tumor. Lancet 1979; 2:149.

62. Kawai M, Sahashi K, Yamase H, et al. Renin producing adrenal tumor: report of a case. Surg Today 1998; 28:974.
63. Carey RM, Wang ZQ, Siragy HM. Role of the angiotensin type 2 receptor in the regulation of blood pressure and renal function. Hypertension 2000; 35(1 Pt 2):155.
64. Lifton RP, Dluhy RG, Powers M, et al. Glucocorticoid remediable hyperaldosteronism: chimeric gene from cross-over between 11β-hydroxylase and aldosterone synthase genes. Nature 1992; 355:262.
65. Snyder PM, Price MP, McDonald FJ, et al. Mechanism by which Liddle's syndrome mutations increase activity of a human epithelial Na+ channel. Cell 1995; 83:969.
66. White PC, Speiser PW. Steroid 11β-hydroxylase deficiency and related disorders. Endocrinol Metab Clin North Am 1994; 23:325.
66a. Farman N, Verrey F. Forefronts in nephrology news in aldosterone action. Kidney Int 2000; 57:1239.
67. Malchoff DM, Brufsky A, Reardon G, et al. A mutation of the glucocorticoid receptor in primary cortisol resistance. J Clin Invest 1993; 91:1918.
68. Norbiato G, Bevilacqua M, Vago T, et al. Glucocorticoid resistance and the immune function in the immunodeficiency syndrome. Ann NY Acad Sci 1998; 840:835.
69. Gomez-Sanchez CE. Cushing's syndrome and hypertension. Hypertension 1986; 8:256.
70. Whitworth JA. Studies on the mechanisms of glucocorticoid hypertension in humans. Blood Pressure 1994; 3:24.
71. Danese RD, Aron DC. Cushing's syndrome and hypertension. In: Bravo EL, ed. Endocrine hypertension. Endocrinol Metab Clin North Am 1994; 23:299.
72. Parks LL, Turney MK, Gaitan D, Kovacs WJ. Expression of 11β-hydroxysteroid dehydrogenase type 2 in an ACTH-producing small cell lung cancer. J Steroid Biochem Mol Biol 1998; 67(4):341.
73. Sowers JR, Epstein M. Diabetes mellitus and associated hypertension, vascular disease and nephropathy. An update. Hypertension 1995; 26(Pt 1): 869.
74. Corry DB, Tuck ML. Insulin and glucoregulatory hormones: implications for antihypertensive therapy. In: Epstein M, ed. Calcium antagonists in clinical medicine. Philadelphia: Hanley and Belfus, 1998:217.
75. Mogensen CE. The kidney and hypertension. Boston: Kluwer Academic Publishers, 1998:1.
76. Chaturvedi N, Sjolie A-K, Stephenson JM, et al. Effect of lisinopril on progression of retinopathy in normotensive people with type 1 diabetes. Lancet 1998; 351:28.
77. Groop LC, Kankuri M, Schalin-Jantti, et al. Association between polymorphism of the glycogen synthase gene and non–insulin-dependent diabetes. Kidney Int 1993; 328:10.
78. Weidmann P, Boehlen LM, de Courten M. Pathogenesis and treatment of hypertension associated with diabetes mellitus. Am Heart J 1993; 125:1498.
79. Stern N, Tuck ML. Pathogenesis of hypertension in diabetes. In LeRoith D, Taylor S, Olefsky J, eds. Diabetes mellitus: a fundamental and clinical text. Philadelphia: Lippincott–Raven Publishers, 1996:780.
80. Nosandi R, Sambataro M, Thomaseth K, et al. Role of hyperglycemia and insulin resistance in determining sodium retention in non–insulin-dependent diabetes. Kidney Int 1993; 44:139.
81. Tuck ML, Corry DB, Trujillo A. Salt-sensitive blood pressure and exaggerated vascular reactivity in the hypertension of diabetes mellitus. Am J Med 1990; 88:210.
82. Randeree HA, Omar HA, Mortala AA, Seedat MA. Effect of insulin on blood pressure in NIDDM patients with secondary failure. Diabetes Care 1992; 15:1258.
83. Trujillo A, Egenna P, Barrett J, Tuck M. Renin regulation in type II diabetes mellitus: influence of dietary sodium. Hypertension 1989; 13:200.
84. Hseuh WA. Effect of renin-angiotensin system in the vascular disease of type II diabetes mellitus. Am J Med 1992; 92(Suppl):13S
85. Tomiyama H, Kushiro T, Abeta A, et al. Kinins contribute to the improvement of insulin sensitivity during treatment with angiotensin converting enzyme inhibitor. Hypertension 1994; 23:450.
86. Steinberg HO, Brechtel G, Johnson A, et al. Insulin-mediated skeletal muscle vasodilation is nitric oxide dependent. A novel mechanism for insulin resistance. J Clin Invest 1995; 96:786
87. O'Driscoll G, Green D, Rankin J, et al. Improvement in endothelial function by angiotensin converting enzyme in insulin-dependent diabetes mellitus. J Clin Invest 1997; 100:678.
88. Reaven GM, Lithell H, Landsberg L. Hypertension and associated metabolic abnormalities—the role of insulin resistance and the sympathoadrenal system. N Engl J Med 1996; 334:374.
89. Muller DC, Elahi D, Pratley RE, et al. An epidemiological test of the hyperinsulinemia-hypertension hypothesis. J Clin Endocrinol Metab 1993; 76:544.
90. Lithell HO. Hyperinsulinemia, insulin resistance and the treatment of hypertension. Am J Hypertens 1996; 9:154.
91. He J, Klag MJ, Caballero B, et al. Plasma insulin levels and incidence of hypertension in African Americans and whites. Arch Intern Med 1999; 159:498.
92. Tchernof A, Prud'homme D, Despres J-P, et al. Relation of steroid hormones to glucose tolerance and plasma insulin levels in men. Diabetes Care 1995; 18:292.
93. Mantzorose CS, Georgiadis EI, Young P, et al. Relative androgenicity, blood pressure levels, and cardiovascular risk factors in young healthy women. Am J Hypertens 1995; 8:606.
94. Masuo K, Mikami H, Ogihara T, Tuck ML. Differences in insulin and sympathetic responses to glucose ingestion due to family history of hypertension. Am J Hypertens 1996; 9:739.

95. Hausberg M, Sinkey CA, Mark AL, et al. Sympathetic nerve activity and insulin sensitivity in normotensive offspring of hypertensive parents. Am J Hypertens 1998; 11:1312.
96. Wu DA, Bu X, Warden CH, et al. Quantitative trait locus mapping of human blood pressure to a genetic region at or near the lipoprotein lipase gene locus on chromosome 8q22. J Clin Invest 1996; 97:2111.
97. Steinberg HO, Chaker H, Leaming R, et al. Obesity/insulin resistance is associated with endothelial dysfunction. Implications for the syndrome of insulin resistance. J Clin Invest 1996; 97:2601.
98. Zeng G, Quon MJ. Insulin-stimulated production of nitric oxide is inhibited by wotmannin. Direct measurement in vascular endothelial cells. J Clin Invest 1996; 98:894.
99. Nickenig G, Roling J, Strehlow K, et al. Insulin induces upregulation of vascular AT1 receptor gene expression by postranscriptional mechanisms. Circulation 1998; 98:2453.
100. Kamide K, Hori MT, Zhu J-H, Tuck ML. Insulin-mediated growth in aortic smooth muscle and the vascular renin-angiotensin system. Hypertension 1998; 32:482.
101. Hall JE, Coleman TG, Mizelle HL, Smith MJ. Chronic hyperinsulinemia and blood pressure regulation. Am J Physiol 1990; 258:F722.
102. Heise T, Magnusson K, Heinemann L, Sawicki PT. Insulin resistance and the effect of insulin on blood pressure in essential hypertension. Hypertension 1998; 32:243.
103. Kaplan NM. Obesity, insulin and hypertension. Cardiovasc Risk Factors 1994; 4:133.
104. Peiris AN, Sothman MS, Hoffman RG, et al. Adiposity, fat distribution and cardiovascular risk. Ann Intern Med 1989; 110:867.
105. Tuck ML. Obesity, the sympathetic nervous system, and essential hypertension. Hypertension 1992; 19(Suppl 1):I-67.
106. Reisin E. Sodium and obesity in the pathogenesis of hypertension. Am J Hypertens 1990; 3:164.
107. Schmieder RE, Messerli FH. Does obesity influence early target organ damage in hypertensive patients? Circulation 1993; 87:1482.
108. Ostlund RE, Staten M, Kohrt WM, et al. The ratio of waist-to-hip circumference, plasma insulin level, and glucose intolerance as independent predictors of the HDL2 cholesterol level in older adults. N Engl J Med 1990; 322:229.
109. Abate N, Garg A, Peshock RM, et al. Relationship of generalized and regional adiposity to insulin sensitivity in man. J Clin Invest 1995; 96:88.
110. Chan JM, Rimm EB, Colditz GA, et al. Obesity, fat distribution and weight gain as risk factors for clinical diabetes in men. Diabetes Care 1994; 17:961.
111. Landsberg L. Hyperinsulinemia: possible role in obesity-induced hypertension. Hypertension 1992; 19(Suppl 1):I-61.
112. Maxwell MH, Heber D, Waks AU, Tuck ML. Role of insulin and norepinephrine in the hypertension of obesity. Am J Hypertens 1994; 7:402.
113. Vaz M, Jennings G, Turner A, et al. Regional sympathetic and oxygen consumption in obese normotensive human subjects. Circulation 1997; 6:3423.
114. Grassi G, Seravalle G, Cattaneo BM, et al. Sympathetic activation in obese normotensive subjects. Hypertension 1995; 25[Pt I]:560.
115. Narkiewiez K, van de Borne PJ, Cooley RL, et al. Sympathetic activity in obese subjects with and without obstructive sleep apnea. Circulation 1998; 98:772.
116. Haynes WG, Morgan DA, Walsh SA, et al. Receptor-mediated regional sympathetic nerve activation by leptin. J Clin Invest 1997; 100:270
117. Wilden E, Lehto M, Kanninen T, et al. Association of a polymorphism in the β3-adrenergic receptor gene with features of the insulin resistance syndrome in Finns. N Engl J Med 1995; 333:348.
118. Reisin E, Mathew R, Falkner B, et al. Lisinopril versus hydrochlorothiazide in obese hypertensive patients. A multicenter placebo-controlled trial. Hypertension 1997; 30[Pt I]:140.
119. Lind L, Hvarfner A, Palmer M, et al. Hypertension in primary hyperparathyroidism in relation to histopathology. Eur J Surg 1991; 157:457.
120. Brickman AS, Nyby MD, vonHungen K, Tuck ML. Calciotropic hormones, platelet calcium and blood pressure in essential hypertension. Hypertension 1990; 16:515.
121. Brickman AS, Stern N, Sowers JR. Hypertension in pseudohypoparathyroidism. Am J Med 1988; 85:785.
122. Gennari C, Nami R, Gonelli A. Hypertension and primary hyperparathyroidism: the role of adrenergic and renin-angiotensin-aldosterone systems. Miner Electrolyte Metab 1995; 21:77.
123. Sancho JJ, Rouco J, Riera-Vidal R, Sitges-Serra A. Long-term effects of parathyroidectomy for primary hyperparathyroidism on arterial hypertension. World J Surg 1992; 16:732.
124. Zawada E Jr, Brickman AS, Maxwell MH, Tuck ML. Hypertension associated with hyperparathyroidism is not responsive to angiotensin blockade. J Clin Endocrinol Metab 1980; 50:912.
125. Sowers JR, Standley PR, Tuck ML, Ram JL. Calcium and calcium regulatory hormones in hypertension. In: Laragh JH, Brenner BM, eds. Hypertension: pathophysiology, diagnosis and management, 2nd ed. New York: Raven Press, 1995:1155.
126. Resnick L. The cellular ionic basis of hypertension and allied clinical conditions. Prog Cardiovasc Dis 1999; 42(1):1.
127. Ezzat S, Forster MJ, Berchtold P, et al. Acromegaly: clinical and biochemical features in 500 patients. Medicine 1994; 73:233.
128. Kratz C, Benker G, Weber F, et al. Acromegaly and hypertension: prevalence and relationship to the renin-angiotensin-aldosterone system. Klin Wochenschr 1990; 68:583.
129. Connell JMC, Davies DL. Endocrine hypertension: thyroid disease and

acromegaly. In: Swales JD, ed. Textbook of hypertension. Oxford, UK: Blackwell Science, 1994:959.

130. Lopez-Velasco R, Escobar-Morreale HF, Vega B, et al. Cardiac involvement in acromegaly: specific myocardiopathy or consequence of systemic hypertension? J Clin Endocrinol Metab 1997; 82:1047.

131. Akpununu BE, Mulrow PJ, Hoffman EA. Secondary hypertension: evaluation and treatment: thyrotoxicosis and hypertension. Dis Mon 1996; 42:689 and 42:696.

132. Saito I, Saruta T. Hypertension and thyroid disorders. Endocrinol Metab Clin North Am 1994; 23:379.

133. Levy GS, Klein I. Catecholamine-thyroid hormone interactions and cardiovascular manifestations of hyperthyroidism. Am J Med 1990; 88:642.

134. Klein I, Ojama K. Cardiovascular manifestations of endocrine disease. J Clin Endocrinol Metab 1992; 75:339.

135. Streeten DHP, Anderson GH, Howland T, et al. Effects of thyroid function on blood pressure: recognition of hypothyroid hypertension. Hypertension 1988; 11:78.

136. Laragh JH, Sealey JE. The renin-angiotensin-aldosterone system and the renal regulation of sodium and potassium and blood pressure homeostasis. In: Windhager EE, ed. Handbook of renal physiology. New York: Oxford University Press, 1992:1409.

137. Alderman MH, Madhavan S, Ooi WL, et al. Association of the renin-sodium profile with risk of myocardial infarction in patients with hypertension. N Engl J Med 1991; 324:1098.

138. Trenkwalder P, James GD, Laragh JH, Sealey JE. Plasma renin activity and plasma prorenin are not suppressed in hypertensives surviving to old age. Am J Hypertens 1996; 9:621.

139. Blaufox MD, Lee HB, Davis B, et al. Renin predicts the blood pressure response to nonpharmacologic and pharmacologic therapy. JAMA 1992; 267:1221.

140. Wyndham RN, Gimenez L, Walker WG, et al. Influence of renin levels on the treatment of essential hypertension with thiazide diuretics. Arch Intern Med 1987; 147:1021.

141. Rich GM, Ulick S, Cook S, et al. Glucocorticoid-remediable aldosteronism in a large kindred: clinical spectrum and diagnosis using a characteristic biochemical phenotype. Ann Intern Med 1992; 116:813.

142. Soro A, Ingram MC, Tonolo G, et al. Evidence of coexisting changes in 11β-dehydrogenase and 5β-reductase activity in subjects with untreated essential hypertension. Hypertension 1995; 25:67.

143. Snyder PM, Price MP, McDonald FJ, et al. Mechanism by which Liddle's syndrome mutations increase activity of a human epithelial Na+ channel. Cell 1995; 83:969.

144. Griffing GT, Dale SL, Holbrook MM, Melby JC. The regulation of urinary free 19-nordeoxycorticosterone and its relation to systemic arterial blood pressure in normotensive and hypertensive subjects. J Clin Endocrinol Metab 1983; 56:99.

145. Resnick LM, Muller FB, Laragh JH. Calcium-regulating hormones in essential hypertension. Relation to plasma renin activity and sodium metabolism. Ann Intern Med 1986; 105:649.

146. Sealey JE, Blumenfeld JD, Bell GM, et al. On the renal basis for essential hypertension: nephron heterogeneity with discordant renin secretion and sodium excretion causing a hypertensive vasoconstriction-volume relationship. J Hypertens 1988; 6:763.

147. Williams GH. Converting-enzyme inhibitors in the treatment of hypertension. N Engl J Med 1988; 319:1517.

148. Redgrave J, Rabinowe S, Hollenberg NK, Williams GH. Correction of abnormal renal blood flow response to angiotensin II by converting enzyme inhibitor. J Clin Invest 1985; 75:1285.

149. Williams GH, Fisher ND, Hunt SC, et al. Effects of gender and genotype on the phenotypic expression of nonmodulating essential hypertension. Kidney Int 2000; 57(4):1404.

150. Johnston CI, Franz Volhard Lecture. Renin-angiotensin system: a dual tissue and hormonal system for cardiovascular control. J Hypertens 1992; 10(Suppl 7):S13.

151. Seikaly MG, Arant BS, Seney FD. Endogenous angiotensin concentration in specific intrarenal fluid compartments of the rat. J Clin Invest 1990; 86:1352.

152. Bachman S, Peters J, Engler E, et al. Transgenic rats carrying the mouse renin gene-morphologic characterization of a low-renin hypertension model. Kidney Int 1992; 41:24.

153. Jeunemaitre X, Soubrier F, Kotelevtsev YV, et al. Molecular basis of human hypertension: role of angiotensinogen. Cell 1992; 71:169.

154. Hunt SC, Cook NR, Oberman A, et al. Angiotensinogen genotype, sodium retention, weight loss and prevention of hypertension: trials of hypertension prevention. Hypertension 1998; 32:393.

155. Lindpianter K, Pfeffer MA, Kreutz R, et al. A prospective evaluation of an angiotensin-converting enzyme gene polymorphism and the risk of ischemic heart disease. N Engl J Med 1995; 332:706.

156. Kauma H, Piavansalo M, Savolainen MJ, et al. Association between angiotensin converting enzyme gene polymorphism and carotid atherosclerosis. J Hypertens 1996; 14:1183.

157. Takezako T, Saku K, Zhang B, et al. Angiotensin I converting enzyme gene polymorphism and insulin resistance in patients with angina pectoris. Am J Hypertens 1999; 12:291.

158. Marre M, Bernadet P, Gallois Y, et al. Relationships between angiotensin I converting enzyme gene polymorphism, plasma levels, and diabetic retinal and renal complications. Diabetes 1994; 43:384.

159. Fujisawa T, Ikegami H, Kawaguchi Y, et al. Meta-analysis of association of insertion/deletion polymorphism of angiotensin I-converting gene with diabetic nephropathy and retinopathy. Diabetologia 1998; 41:47.

160. Julius S. Changing role of the autonomic nervous system in human hypertension. J Hypertens 1990; 9(Suppl 7):S59.

161. Goldstein DS, Kopin IJ. The autonomic nervous system and catecholamines in normal blood pressure control and in hypertension. In: Laragh JH, Brenner BM, eds. Hypertension: Pathophysiology, Diagnosis and Management. New York: Raven Press, 1990:711 .

162. Esler M, Jennings G, Lambert G, et al. Overflow of catecholamine neurotransmitters to the circulation: source, fate, and function. Physiol Rev 1990; 70:963.

163. Mark AL. The sympathetic nervous system in hypertension: a potential long-term regulator of arterial pressure. J Hypertens 1996; 14(Suppl):S159.

164. Izzo JL. Sympathoadrenal activity, catecholamines and the pathogenesis of vasculopathic hypertensive target-organ damage. Am J Hypertens 1989; 2:3055.

165. Brooks VL, Osborn JW. Hormonal-sympathetic interactions in the long-term of arterial pressure: an hypothesis. Am J Physiol 1995; 268:R1343.

166. McCarty R, Gold P. Catecholamine, stress and disease: a psychobiologic perspective. Psycosom Med 1996; 58:590.

167. Ichihara A, Inscho EW, Imig JD, et al. Role of renal nerves in afferent arteriolar reactivity in angiotensin-induced hypertension. Hypertension 1997; 29:442.

168. Ascio LP, Ladiness C, Fuchs S, et al. Distribution of the dopamine D3 receptor gene produces renin-dependent hypertension. J Clin Invest 1998; 102:493.

169. Pa J, Eisner GM. Renal dopamine receptors in health and hypertension. Pharmacol Ther 1998; 80:149.

170. Gill JR, Grossman E, Goldstein DS. High urinary dopa excretion and low urinary dopamine: dopa ratio in salt-sensitive hypertension. Hypertension 1991; 18:614.

171. Weinberger MH. Salt sensitivity of blood pressure in humans. Hypertension 1996; 27:481.

172. Lijnen P. Alterations in sodium metabolism as an etiological model for hypertension. Cardiovasc Drugs 1995; 9:377.

173. Corry DB, Tuck ML. Altered sodium and potassium metabolism in the pathogenesis of hypertension. In: Maxwell MH, Kleeman C, Narrins R, eds. Disorders of fluid and electrolyte metabolism, 5th ed. New York: McGraw-Hill, 1993:1245.

174. Bobick A, Neylon CB, Little PJ. Disturbances of vascular smooth muscle cation transport and the pathogenesis of hypertension. In: Swales JD, ed. Textbook of hypertension. Oxford, UK: Blackwell Science, 1994:175.

175. Sweeney G, Somwar R, Ramlal T, et al. Insulin stimulation of K+ uptake in 3T3-L1 fibroblasts involves phosphatidylinositol 3-kinase and protein kinase C-zeta. Diabetologia 1998; 41:1199.

176. Blaustein MP. Physiologic effects of endogenous ouabain: control of intracellular calcium stores and cell responsiveness. Am J Physiol 1993; 264:C1367.

177. Berger ME, Ormsby BL, Bunnag P, et al. Increased functional Na(+)-K(+) pump activity in the vasculature of fructose-fed hyperinsulinemic and hypertensive rats. Hypertens Rev 1998; 21(2):73.

178. Rutherford PA, Thomas TH, Wilkinson R. Na-Li countertransport kinetics in the relatives of hypertensive patients with abnormal Na-Li countertransport activity. Biochem Mol Med 1997; 62(1):106.

179. Strazzulo P, Siani A, Cappuccio FP, et al. Red blood cell sodium-lithium countertransport and risk of future hypertension: the Olivetti Prospective Heart Study. Hypertension 1998; 31(6):1284.

180. Van Norren K, Thien T, Berden JH, et al. Relevance of erythrocyte Na+/Li+ countertransport measurement in essential hypertension, hyperlipidemia and diabetic nephropathy: a critical review. Eur J Clin Invest 1998; 28(5):339.

181. Ragone E, Strazullo P, Siani A, et al. Ethnic differences in red blood cell sodium/lithium countertransport and metabolic correlates of hypertension: an international collaborative study. Am J Hypertens 1998; 11(8; Pt 1): 935.

182. Sanchez RA, Gimenez MI, Migliorini M, et al. Erythrocyte sodium-lithium countertransport in non-modulating offspring and essential hypertensive individuals: response to enalapril. Hypertension 1997; 30:99.

183. Monciotti CG, Semplicini A, Morocutti A, et al. Elevated sodium-lithium countertransport activity in erythrocytes is predictive of the development of microalbuminuria in IDDM. Diabetologia 1997; 40(6):654.

184. Carr SJ, Moore D, Sikand K, Norman RI. Raised affinity for extracellular sodium of the sodium-lithium countertransporter is associated with a family history of hypertension and uraemia in patients with renal disease. Clin Sci 1997; 92(5):497.

185. Jones SC, Thomas TH, Marshall SM. Thiol group modulation of sodium-lithium countertransport kinetics in diabetic nephropathy. Diabetologia 1997; 40:1079.

186. Giordano M, Castellino P, Solini A, et al. Na+/Li+ and Na+/H+ countertransport activity in hypertensive non–insulin-dependent diabetic patients: role of insulin resistance and antihypertensive treatment. Metabolism 1997; 46:1326.

187. Siffert W, Dusing R. Sodium-proton exchange and primary hypertension: an update. Hypertension 1995; 26:649.

188. Ng LL, Sweeney FP, Siczkowski M, Davies JE, et al. Na(+)-H(+) antiporter phenotype, abundance, and phosphorylation of immortalized lymphoblasts from humans with hypertension. Hypertension 1995; 25:971.

189. Rosskopf D, Schroder KJ, Siffert W. Role of sodium-hydrogen exchange in the proliferation of immortalized lymphoblasts from patients with essential hypertension and normotensive subjects. Cardiovasc Res 1995; 29:254.

190. Garciandia A, Lopez R, Tisaire J, et al. Enhanced Na$^{(+)}$-H$^{(+)}$ exchanger activity and NHE-1 mRNA expression in lymphocytes from patients with essential hypertension. Hypertension 1995; 25(3):356.

191. Diez J, Alonso A, Garciandia A, et al. Association of increased erythrocyte Na$^+$/H$^+$ exchanger with renal Na$^+$ retention in patients with essential hypertension. Am J Hypertens 1995; 8(2):124.

192. LaPointe MS, Ye M, Moe OW, et al. Na$^+$/H$^+$ antiporter (NHE-1 isoform) in cultured vascular smooth muscle from the spontaneously hypertensive rat. Kidney Int 1995; 47(1):78.

193. Siczkowski M, Davies JE, Ng LL. Na$^{(+)}$-H$^{(+)}$ exchanger isoform 1 phosphorylation in normal Wistar-Kyoto and spontaneously hypertensive rats. Circ Res 1995; 76:825.

194. Siffert W, Rosskopf D, Moritz A, et al. Enhanced G protein activation in immortalized lymphoblasts from patients with essential hypertension. J Clin Invest 1995; 96:759.

195. Takahashi E, Abe J, Berk BC. Angiotensin II stimulates p90rsk in vascular smooth muscle cells. A potential Na$^{(+)}$-K$^{(+)}$ exchanger kinase. Circ Res 1997; 81(2):268.

196. Koren W, Postnov IY, Postnov YV. Increased Na$^{(+)}$-H$^{(+)}$ exchange in red blood cells of patients with primary aldosteronism. Hypertension 1997; 29(2):587.

197. Fortuno A, Tisaire J, Lopez R, et al. Angiotensin converting enzyme inhibition corrects Na$^+$,H$^+$ exchanger overactivity in essential hypertension. Am J Hypertens 1997; 10(1):84.

198. Gende OA. Chelerythrine inhibits Na$^{(+)}$-H$^{(+)}$ exchange in platelets from spontaneously hypertensive rats. Hypertension 1996; 28(6):1013.

199. Chen YF, Yang RH, Meng QC, et al. Sodium-proton (Na$^+$/H$^+$) exchange inhibition increases blood pressure in spontaneously hypertensive rats. Am J Med Sci 1994; 308:145.

200. Trevisan R, Viberti G. Sodium-hydrogen antiporter: its possible role in the genesis of diabetic nephropathy. Nephrol Dialysis Transplant 1997; 12(4):643.

201. Ng LL, Davies JE, Siczkowski M, et al. Abnormal Na$^+$/H$^+$ antiporter phenotype and turnover of immortalized lymphoblasts from type 1 diabetic patients with nephropathy. J Clin Invest 1994; 93(6):2750.

202. Siczkowski M, Davies JE, Sweeney FP, et al. Na$^+$/K$^+$ exchanger isoform-1 abundance in skin fibroblasts of type I diabetic patients with nephropathy. Metabolism 1995; 44:791.

203. Tuck ML, Corry DB, Maxwell M, et al. Erythrocyte Na$^+$,K$^+$ cotransport and Na$^+$,K$^+$ pump in black and Caucasian hypertensive patients: a kinetic analysis. Hypertension 1987; 10:204.

204. Tepper T, Sluiter WJ, Huisman RM, deZeeuw D. Co-transport measurement in essential hypertension: useful diagnostic tool or failure? A meta-analysis of 17 years of literature.

205. Pares I, de la Sierra A, Coca MM, et al. Detection of a circulating inhibitor of the Na$^{(+)}$-K$^{(+)}$-Cl$^{(-)}$ cotransport system in plasma and urine after high salt intake. Am J Hypertens 1995; 8:965.

206. Blaustein MP. The physiological effects of endogenous ouabain: control of cell responsiveness. Am J Physiol 1993; 264:C1367.

207. Hamlyn JM, Hamilton BP, Manunta P. Endogenous ouabain, sodium balance and blood pressure: a review and an hypothesis. J Hypertens 1996; 14:151.

208. Wilkens MR, Redondo J, Brown LA. The natriuretic peptide family. Lancet 1997; 349:1307.

209. Koller KJ, Goeddel DV. Molecular biology of the natriuretic peptides and their receptors. Circulation 1992; 86:1081.

210. Burnett JC Jr. Vasopeptidase inhibition: a new concept in blood pressure management. J Hypertens 1999; 17(Suppl 1):S37.

210a. Schriger JA, Grantham JA, Kullo IJ, et al. Vascular actions of brain natriuretic peptide: modulation by atherosclerosis and neutral endopeptidase inhibition. J Am Coll Cardiol 2000; 35:796.

211. Lainchbury JG, Espinar EA, Frampton CM, et al. Cardiac natriuretic peptides as predictors of mortality. J Intern Med 1997; 241:257.

212. Bhoola KD, Figueroa CD, Worthy K. Bioregulation of kinins: kallikreins, kininogens, and kinases. Pharmacol Rev 1992; 44:1.

213. Carretero OA, Scili AG. The kallikrein-kinin system. In: Fozzard HA, ed. The heart and cardiovascular system. New York: Scientific Foundations, Raven Press, 1991:1851.

214. Liu LH, Yang XP, Sharov VG, et al. Effects of angiotensin-converting enzyme inhibitors and angiotensin II type 1 receptor antagonists in rats with heart failure: role of kinins and angiotensin type 2 receptor. J Clin Invest 1997; 99:1926.

215. Yang XP, Liu YH, Scili GM, et al. Role of kinins in the cardioprotective effect of preconditioning: study of myocardial ischemia/reperfusion injury in B$_2$ kinin receptor knockout mice and kininogen-deficient rats. Hypertension 1997; 30:735.

216. Dattilo JB, Makhoul RG. The role of nitric oxide in vascular biology and pathobiology. Ann Vasc Surg 1997; 11:307.

217. Ignarro L, Murad F. Nitric oxide biochemistry, molecular biology, and therapeutic implications. In: JT August, MW Anders, F Murad, ed. Advances in Pharmacology. New York: Academic Press, 1995.

218. Garcia-Cardena G, Martasek P, Masters BS, et al. Dissecting the interaction between nitric oxide synthase (NOS) and caveolin: functional significance of the NOS caveolin binding domain in vivo. J Biol Chem 1997; 272:25437.

219. Busse R, Fleming I. Nitric oxide, nitric oxide synthase and hypertensive vascular disease. Curr Hypertens Rep 1999; 1:88.

220. Garcia-Cardena G, Fan R, Shah V, et al. Dynamic activation of endothelial nitric oxide by Hsp90. Nature 1998; 292:821.

221. Murad F. The 1996 Albert Lasker Medical Research Awards. Signal transduction using nitric oxide and cyclic guanosine monophosphate. JAMA 1996; 276:1189.

222. Haller H. Endothelial function: general considerations. Drugs 1997; 53(Suppl 1):1.

223. Ferro CJ, Webb DJ. Endothelial dysfunction and hypertension. Drugs 1997; 53 (Suppl 1):30.

224. Nakayama T, Soma M, Takahashi Y, et al. Association analysis of CA repeat polymorphism of the endothelial nitric oxide synthase gene with essential hypertension in Japanese. Clin Genet 1997; 51:26.

225. Miyamoto Y, Saito Y, Kajiyama N, et al. Endothelial nitric oxide synthase gene expression is positively associated with essential hypertension. Hypertension 1998; 32:3.

226. Bauersachs J, Bouloumie A, Mulsch A, et al. Vasodilator dysfunction in aged spontaneously hypertensive rats; changes in NO synthase III and soluble guanylyl expression and in superoxide anion production. Cardiovasc Res 1998; 37:772.

227. Luscher TF, Oemar BS, Boulanger CM, Hahn AWA. Molecular and cellular biology of endothelin and its receptors, Pts 1 and 2. J Hypertens 1993; 11:7 and 11:121.

228. Schiffrin EL, Intengan HD, Thibault G, Touyz RM. Clinical significance of endothelin in cardiovascular disease. Curr Opin Cardiol 1997; 12:354.

229. Moreau P, Rabelink TJ. Endothelin and its antagonists in hypertension: can we foresee the future? Curr Hypertens Rep 1999; 1:69.

230. Krum H, Viskoper RV, Lacourciere Y, et al. The effects of an endothelin receptor antagonist, bosantin, on blood pressure in patients with essential hypertension. N Engl J Med 1998; 338:784.

# CHAPTER 83

# ADRENOCORTICAL DISORDERS IN INFANCY AND CHILDHOOD

ROBERT L. ROSENFIELD AND KE-NAN QIN

## GENERAL PRINCIPLES

Along with the well-known perturbations of fluid, electrolyte, and glucose homeostasis, adrenocortical diseases that occur in children also cause disturbed growth. The proper management of children with these disorders requires careful documentation of height and weight at regular intervals.

Physicians who are relatively unfamiliar with pediatric patients may assume that the fluid and electrolyte requirements of infants and children are similar to those of adults. Actually, infants are hypermetabolic, as compared to adults, because of the relatively large size of their high-energy-consuming organs (i.e., the brain, heart, liver, and kidneys) as compared to their somatic size. Water requirements change in proportion to caloric requirements. One milliliter of water is required for each kilocalorie of energy expenditure. Water and calorie requirements are approximately constant throughout life relative to surface area (1500 kcal/m$^2$ per day). Surface area can be calculated as the square root of (cm × kg/3600).

Normal daily sodium and potassium maintenance requirements are ~2 mEq/dL and 1 mEq/dL water, respectively. When calculating electrolyte replacement, it must be remembered that the exchangeable fluid compartment is relatively larger in children than in adults, ranging from 60% of body weight in small children to 40% in adults. Because of the rapid rate of turnover of children's body fluids, the electrolyte concentrations of parenteral fluids should be distributed evenly throughout the day to prevent shifts in the tonicity of body fluids.

Infants and children are intolerant of prolonged fasting because of their high metabolic rate and functionally immature gluconeogenic enzyme systems. When fasted, the normal young child will become hypoglycemic within as few as 20 hours. To prevent glycogenolysis, infants and young children need 6 to 8 mg/kg per minute of glucose.[1]

**TABLE 83-1.**
**Typical Normal Plasma Values in Infancy and Childhood for Renin-Aldosterone Axis**

| Age | PRA (ng/mL/h) Range | Aldosterone (ng/dL) Range |
|---|---|---|
| Term, <1 mo | <35 | 5–190 |
| 1–12 mo | <37 | 5–90 |
| 1–3 yr | <10 | 5–45 |
| 3–15 yr | <7 | 1–40 |
| >15 yr, ambulatory | 0.7–9 | 2–30 |
| >15 yr, supine | 0.2–3 | 1–15 |

*PRA,* plasma renin activity.
(Data from Endocrine Science Laboratories, Tarzana, CA; and Nichols Reference Laboratories, San Juan Capistrano, CA.)

The production of glucocorticoids and the excretion of their metabolites are essentially constant with respect to surface area and lean body mass throughout life. The daily secretion rate of cortisol approximates 6 to 8 mg/m$^2$.[2] Urinary cortisol excretion ranges from 15 to 70 μg/m$^2$ or μg/g creatinine. Urinary 17-hydroxycorticoid excretion (measured as Porter-Silber chromogens) is a poor index of cortisol secretion in the neonate due to deficient glucuronyl-transferase activity in the first month of life. Plasma cortisol concentrations vary from 4 to 25 μg/dL, as in adults. The circadian rhythm of adrenocortical secretion is established by 3 months of age.[3] The aldosterone secretion rate is constant throughout life at ~80 μg per day.[4] Thus, in infants it is several times more than that of adults in terms of surface area. Plasma aldosterone levels and plasma renin activity (PRA) are higher in infants than subsequently; the level of these two constituents gradually declines during childhood (Table 83-1), but absolute levels vary among laboratories.[5,6] Plasma dehydroepiandrosterone (DHEA) and DHEA sulfate (DHEAS) levels are at adult levels at birth as a consequence of the function of the fetal zone of the adrenal gland, fall during early infancy, and rise with adrenarche[7,8] (Table 83-2).

# ADRENOCORTICAL INSUFFICIENCY

## PRIMARY FORM

### ETIOLOGY

**Congenital Adrenal Hyperplasia and Hypoplasia.** The most prevalent cause of adrenocortical insufficiency in infancy is congenital adrenal hyperplasia (Fig. 83-1). This condition is dis-

cussed extensively in Chap. 77. Further details are emphasized in the sections Treatment and Precocious Pseudopuberty.

By contrast, congenital adrenal hypoplasia is a rare cause of adrenal insufficiency in infancy; it has been reported to occur as an apparently isolated defect, with or without a familial tendency.[9] The autosomal recessive form is associated with miniature, adult-type, adrenal architecture and may be secondary to isolated adrenocorticotropic hormone (ACTH) deficiency. The X-linked form is due to DAX-1 gene mutations and is associated with cytomegaly of fetal-like adrenocortical cells and congenital gonadotropin deficiency.[10] Mental retardation and other features may occur, depending on the extent of contiguous chromosomal deletion.

**Neonatal Adrenal Hemorrhage.** Neonatal adrenal hemorrhage usually presents with the symptoms of shock, severe jaundice, and an abdominal mass during the first week of life.[11] It is associated with birth trauma and is thought to result from severe hypoxemia. Ultrasonographic examination, repeated at 3- to 5-day intervals, may reveal a lesion that changes from solid to cystic as the hemorrhagic mass liquefies, and adrenal calcifications may be noted after 4 weeks of age. Children who survive should be tested for chronic adrenal insufficiency.

**Destruction of the Adrenal Cortex.** Beyond the newborn period, adrenal insufficiency usually is attributable to destruction of the adrenal cortex. Addison disease usually is caused by autoimmune endocrinopathy that may be associated with diseases affecting other glands (see Chaps. 76 and 197). The major autoantigens are the steroidogenic enzymes, particularly 21-hydroxylase (cytochrome P450c21),[12] but their presence does not necessarily predict adrenal failure.[13] There are two varieties of autoimmune polyglandular deficiency syndrome. Type I usually is seen in early life, with a mean age at onset of 12 years. Although Addison disease in this syndrome is commonly associated with hypoparathyroidism and mucocutaneous candidiasis, the incidence of associated type 1 diabetes mellitus and thyroid disease is low.[14] Pernicious anemia and other autoimmune disorders are seen occasionally. The disorder is an autosomal recessive disease due to mutation of an autoimmune regulator gene on chromosome 21q22.3.[15] Type II autoimmune polyglandular deficiency has a mean age at onset of 30 years. This form of the disease is associated with insulin-dependent diabetes mellitus, thyroid deficiency, or both, and has an autosomal dominant transmission pattern linked with the human leukocyte antigen (HLA)-B8 allele. Both type I and type II can be associated with vitiligo and primary gonadal failure.

Acute adrenal insufficiency can complicate septic shock. The classic association of acute adrenal hemorrhage and purpura with fulminating meningococcemia (Waterhouse-Friderichsen

**TABLE 83-2.**
**Basal Corticosteroids: Typical Plasma Values in Normal Infants, Children, and Adults**

| | DHEA (μg/dL) | DHEAS (ng/dL) | AD (ng/dL) | 17-Preg (ng/dL) | 17-Prog (ng/dL) | S (ng/dL) | F (μg/dL) | T (ng/dL) |
|---|---|---|---|---|---|---|---|---|
| **PREMATURE INFANTS (32 wk), 3 DAYS** | 122–710 | 80–3150 | 19–141 | 64–2380 | 26–568 | 48–579 | 3–9 | — |
| **TERM INFANTS, 3 DAYS** | 90–355 | 65–1250 | <140 | <830 | <80 | <145 | 2–14 | — |
| **PREADRENARCHAL (2–8 yr)** | <40 | <25–120 | <25–50 | <25–235 | <25–65 | <25–160 | 5–25 | <15 |
| **PREMATURE ADRENARCHAL** | 40–100 | 100–420 | 30–75 | <25–355 | <25–95 | <25–120 | 5–25 | 10–45 |
| **ADULT FEMALE** | 75–350 | 100–1000 | 45–175 | 40–400 | <25–65* | 30–220 | 5–25 | 20–70 |

*DHEAS,* dehydroepiandrosterone sulfate; *DHEA,* dehydroepiandrosterone; *AD,* androstenedione; *17-Preg,* 17-hydroxypregnenolone; *17-Prog,* 17-hydroxyprogesterone; *S,* 11-deoxycortisol; *F,* cortisol; *T,* testosterone.
*Early follicular phase (days 1–8 of cycle); 17-hydroxyprogesterone rises in the preovulatory phase and reaches a peak as high as 360 ng/dL in the luteal phase of the cycle.
(Data from Rosenfield RL, Rich BH, Lucky AW. Adrenarche as a cause of benign pseudopuberty in boys. J Pediatr 1982; 101:1005; Rosenfield RL, Helke J, Lucky AW. Dexamethasone preparation does not alter corticoid and androgen responses to adrenocorticotropin. J Clin Endocrinol Metab 1985; 60:585; Lucky AW, Rosenfield RL, McGuire J, et al. Adrenal androgen hyperresponsiveness to adrenocorticotropin in women with acne and/or hirsutism: adrenal enzyme defects and exaggerated adrenarche. J Clin Endocrinol Metab 1986; 62:840; Lee MM, Rajagopalan L, Berg GJ, Moshang T Jr. Serum adrenal steroid concentration in premature infants. J Clin Endocrinol Metab 1989; 69:1133; Lashansky G, Saenger P, Fishman K, et al. Normative data for adrenal steroidogenesis in a healthy pediatric population: age- and sex-related changes after adrenocorticotropin stimulation. J Clin Endocrinol Metab 1991; 73:674.)

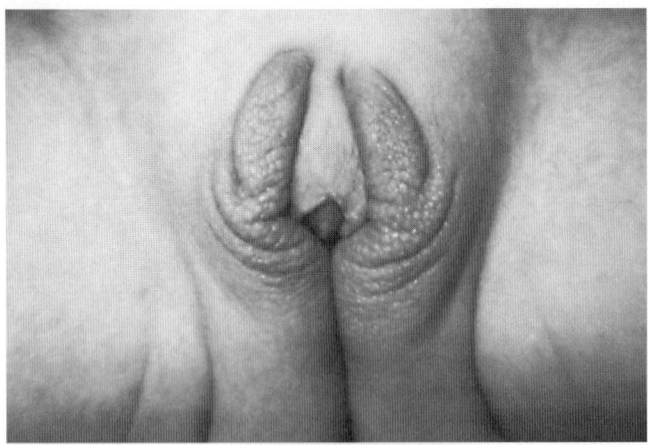

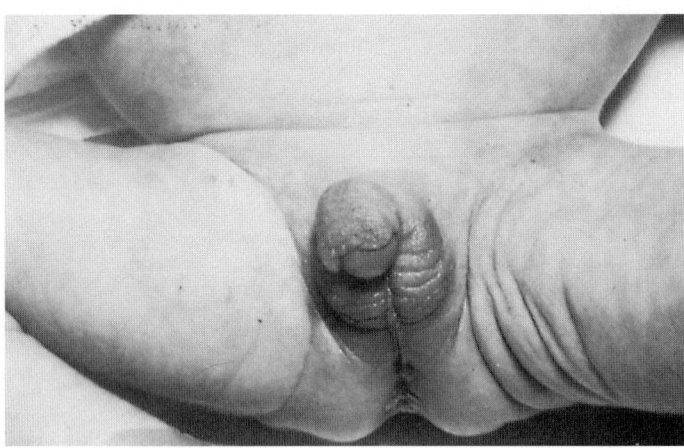

A

B

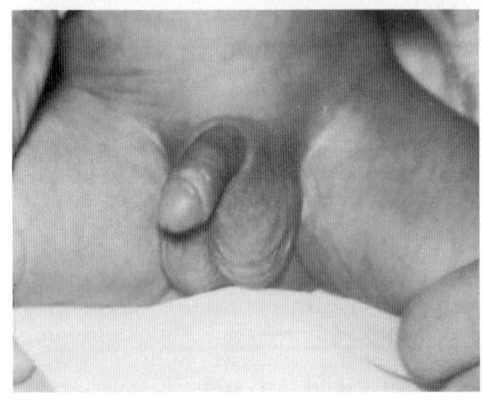

C

**FIGURE 83-1.** Congenital adrenal hyperplasia in three newborn infants, all with 21-hydroxylase deficiency. The female infants depicted in **A** and **B** have different degrees of ambiguity of the external genitalia. **A,** Clitoromegaly with labial enlargement. **B,** Severe clitoral hypertrophy and nearly complete labial fusion. Note the scrotal appearance of the labia. **C,** Male infant with precocious development of the external genitalia and rapid somatic growth (infant Hercules). (Courtesy of Dr. Wellington Hung.)

syndrome)[16] (Fig. 83-2; see Chap. 213). It resembles the generalized Shwartzman phenomenon.

Progressive degenerative or granulomatous diseases such as tuberculosis or histoplasmosis may involve the adrenal cortex and cause adrenal failure. Lysosomal acid lipase deficiency, or Wolman disease, is a disorder that occurs in infancy. It is caused by abnormal storage of triglycerides and cholesterol esters that cannot be degraded by the adrenals, spleen, liver, bone marrow, brain, or lymph nodes. The form of transmission is autosomal recessive.[17] Patients present in the early weeks of life with vomiting, diarrhea, failure to thrive, hepatosplenomegaly, and adrenal calcification. Invariably, the patient progresses to death by a few months of age despite corticosteroid treatment.

Adrenoleukodystrophy is a rare, fatal, or autosomal recessive demyelinating disorder of the brain that presents in childhood with blindness, quadriparesis, or dementia, typically before adrenal failure.[18,19] Adrenomyeloneuropathy, a more slowly progressive form, may present in boys as adrenal failure. These disorders result from accumulation of very long-chain fatty acids (C-24 and longer). Most forms are X-chromosome–linked, due to mutations of a gene encoding a peroxisomal integral membrane protein that is located on Xq28. Neonatal adrenoleukodystrophy is an autosomal recessive disease caused by defects in peroxisome assembly; it results from mutations of PEX genes.[19]

**Isolated Glucocorticoid Insufficiency.** Glucocorticoid deficiency in the presence of normal mineralocorticoid secretion can result from primary adrenal disease or be secondary to defects in the secretion or mode of action of ACTH. In the early stages of autoimmune Addison disease, aldosterone secretion is sometimes

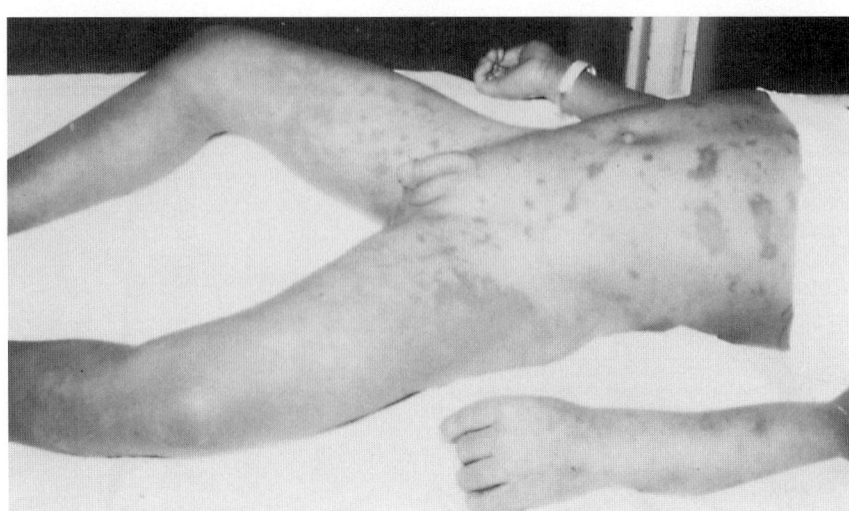

**FIGURE 83-2.** Seven-year-old boy with Waterhouse-Friderichsen syndrome secondary to severe meningococcemia. The child subsequently died. Note the massive hemorrhaging into the skin. (Courtesy of Dr. Wellington Hung.)

intact. This must be distinguished from ACTH deficiency, which has been reported in the polyglandular autoimmune syndrome.[20]

Familial isolated glucocorticoid deficiency appears to be caused by a heterogeneous group of autosomal recessive disorders. These include degenerative disorders of the zona fasciculata and defects in the ACTH receptor, or ACTH action.[21] ACTH resistance may result from degeneration of the zona fasciculata-reticularis in association with achalasia of the esophagus and alacrima (triple-A syndrome).[21] Approximately 15% of patients later develop mineralocorticoid deficiency. This disorder maps to a critical region on the chromosome 12q13 locus. Patients with isolated ACTH receptor defect average 2 standard deviations (SD) taller than average.

**Isolated Mineralocorticoid Deficiency.** Isolated aldosterone deficiency may result from defects in the terminal portion of the aldosterone biosynthetic pathway or from hyporeninemia.[22,23] Defective corticosterone 18-hydroxylation causes corticosterone overproduction. Defective 18-dehydrogenation (oxidation) of 18-hydroxycorticosterone is characterized biochemically by corticosterone and 18-hydroxycorticosterone overproduction (see Chap. 81). These enzyme activities, as well as 11β-hydroxylase, are all located on a single enzyme, cytochrome P450c11. Symptoms are reported to lessen as patients grow older. Isolated hypoaldosteronism resulting from defects in the renin-angiotensin system may be familial in infancy[23a] (also see Chap. 81). *Pseudohypoaldosteronism type I* is a syndrome of renal sodium chloride loss accompanied by hyperkalemia and metabolic acidosis that occurs as the result of an end-organ defect in the distal renal tubule that causes a failure of response to endogenous aldosterone. PRA, plasma aldosterone concentration, and urinary aldosterone excretion are usually elevated. The autosomal dominant form is a mild disease that remits with age and is usually due to mineralocorticoid receptor mutations.[24] The severe form that persists into adulthood is usually caused by autosomal recessive inactivating mutations in genes encoding subunits of the amiloride-sensitive epithelial sodium channel.[25] *Pseudohypoaldosteronism type II* is a very different form of aldosterone resistance. Hyperkalemia and hyperchloremic acidosis (type IV renal tubular acidosis) are accompanied by low or normal renin and aldosterone levels. It may result from a familial disorder in which hypertension is associated with an isolated increase in reabsorption of chloride by the renal tubule, a defect that can be corrected by hydrochlorothiazide.[26] This is an autosomal dominant disorder that has been mapped to two different loci, chromosomes 1q31–42 and 17p11–q21.[27] Either type of pseudohypoaldosteronism can also be acquired as the result of obstructive uropathy, sickle cell or lead nephropathy, amyloidosis or urinary tract infections.[28,29]

### CLINICAL CHARACTERISTICS

The characteristic, early symptoms of glucocorticoid deficiency—anorexia, weakness, and fatigue—may not be easy to elicit in the infant or young child. Abdominal pain, vomiting, and diarrhea are the nonspecific symptoms. In congenital forms, there may be a history of neonatal cholestatic jaundice due to "hepatitis."[21] Failure to thrive (particularly cachexia) may be the presenting complaint. Symptoms of hypoglycemia associated with ketosis often are the most prominent features (see Chap. 161). Anorexia, listlessness or irritability, tachypnea, tachycardia, emesis, and hypotonia may result from acute hypoglycemia. Hunger and excessive perspiration are unusual symptoms in young children. Hyperpigmentation indicates ACTH excess. Mineralocorticoid deficiency and related salt-wasting disorders cause sodium diuresis, which produces polyuria and enuresis, as well as hyponatremia, hyperkalemia, metabolic acidosis, aciduria, and dehydration. They can present as a salt-losing crisis or as failure to thrive.

### DIAGNOSIS

Plasma cortisol levels are seldom diagnostic of adrenal failure unless a low level is accompanied by a clearly elevated plasma ACTH level. Confirmation of primary adrenal insufficiency requires an ACTH test, which is usually performed with synthetic ACTH-(1-24) (cosyntropin), 0.15 mg/m², with sampling at 0 and 60 minutes. A peak plasma cortisol level ≥18 μg/dL, or an aldosterone increment ≥5 ng/dL above the control level, is indicative of normal adrenocortical reserve.[30,31]

Measurements of the 24-hour urine content of electrolytes and pH are useful in the assessment of hyponatremia and hyperkalemia.[28] A high urinary sodium level distinguishes aldosterone deficiency from prerenal sodium-losing states (e.g., cystic fibrosis, in which sodium may be lost through perspiration, or chronic sodium-losing diarrhea). Low urinary pH (<5.5) distinguishes aldosterone deficiency from renal tubular disorders that cause hyperkalemic acidosis. If aldosterone or PRA levels are indeterminate, measurements should be repeated either 3 hours after challenge with furosemide (30 mg/m² every 6 hours × 3) or after a low-salt diet (7 mEq/m² per day) for 5 days.

## SECONDARY FORM

### ETIOLOGY AND CLINICAL CHARACTERISTICS

The most frequent cause of isolated glucocorticoid deficiency is withdrawal from glucocorticoid excess (Cushing syndrome), the cause of which may be iatrogenic or spontaneous. The degree of hypothalamic-pituitary-adrenal (HPA) axis suppression is dependent on the dose, duration, and frequency of corticosteroid therapy. Recovery from high doses administered for long periods may be delayed for as long as 9 months after the discontinuation of therapy.[32] The data suggest successive recovery of the pituitary, adrenal, and hypothalamic portions of the axis, in that order.

The most common organic cause of hypothalamic corticotropin-releasing hormone (CRH) or ACTH insufficiency is intracranial tumor or its treatment, or both.

The sluggish HPA axis of extremely low birth weight newborns may predispose to transient glucocorticoid deficiency.[33] Neonatal ACTH deficit also occurs as part of the congenital hypopituitarism syndrome of hypoglycemia and cholestatic jaundice, with micropenis in boys.[34,35] Autoimmune hypophysitis involving corticotropes may occur as part of the polyglandular deficiency syndrome.[20]

Isolated ACTH deficiency may be congenital, or due to a proopiomelanocortin (POMC) mutation.[36,37] The POMC mutations yield a syndrome, resulting from the lack of POMC-derived ligands for the melanocortin receptors: ACTH deficiency (ACTH receptor, also termed *melanocortin 2 receptor*); red hair pigmentation due to α-melanocyte–stimulating hormone deficiency (*melanocortin 1 receptor*); and severe early-onset obesity due to α-melanocyte–stimulating hormone deficiency (*melanocortin 4 receptor*). However, most cases of isolated ACTH deficiency probably have an autoimmune basis.[36]

The clinical manifestations of ACTH deficiency are the same as those of isolated glucocorticoid deficiency, except for the absence of hyperpigmentation. Dilutional hyponatremia may occur due to an altered osmotic threshold for vasopressin release. Adrenal medullary insufficiency may complicate management of hypoglycemia.[38]

### DIAGNOSIS

Plasma DHEAS concentrations are useful in screening post-adrenarchal patients for adrenal failure.[39] The very low dose 1 μg/1.73 m² ACTH stimulation test should replace the standard 150 μg/m² ACTH stimulation test in screening the HPA axis for secondary hypocortisolism when the DHEAS level is indeterminate.[40,41] A cortisol level <18 mg/dL (500 nmol/L) after 30 minutes signifies impaired adrenocortical reserve. The technique of delivering the low dose of ACTH is critical. A definitive test should be performed if this test results in a borderline value and the diagnosis is questioned.[41]

The cortisol response to insulin-induced hypoglycemia has been the best single standard test for assessing the function of the entire HPA axis.[30] Insulin (0.05–0.15 U/kg) is administered by intravenous (iv) bolus under very close supervision to allow the study to be aborted instantaneously with iv administration of glucose should an emergency arise. Complications of hypoglycemia are unlikely in the absence of a history of syncope or seizures. A plasma cortisol level ≥18 μg/dL in response to a 40% reduction in blood glucose is considered to be indicative of normal HPA reserve. Insulin-induced hypoglycemia normally acts on the hypothalamus to trigger sequential ACTH and cortisol secretion through stimulation of CRH, vasopressin, and epinephrine.[42] It is not established, however, whether the outcome of this test corresponds with the capacity of the HPA axis to respond to stress in children with hypothalamic disease.

The metyrapone test specifically checks the integrity of the negative feedback system; therefore, the results do not necessarily correspond to those for insulin tolerance testing. Metyrapone is obtained from Novartis Pharmaceutical by special order. The dose is 15 mg/kg (maximum 0.5 g) orally every 4 hours for six doses, commencing at 8:00 a.m. Normally, plasma 11-deoxycortisol levels increase to 9.0 μg/dL or more 4 hours after the sixth dose.

The place for CRH testing in the diagnosis of secondary adrenal insufficiency remains to be established.[43] It is clear, however, that subnormal ACTH and cortisol responses indicate decreased ACTH secretion.

The adequacy of replacement doses of corticosteroids is hard to judge in patients on drugs that accelerate their metabolism, such as phenobarbital or phenytoin. Measurement of plasma cortisol levels 1 to 3 hours after the oral administration of 13 mg/m$^2$ may be helpful.[44]

## TREATMENT

In managing acute adrenal crisis, it is important to remember that affected children have incurred large losses of salt and water. Indeed, a newborn infant may excrete more than half a liter of isotonic urine daily, and will have accumulated a substantial salt deficit before the hyponatremic crisis occurs. Water, salt, and corticosteroids should be replaced intravenously. Intake and output should be strictly monitored, with special attention given to 24-hour sodium excretion. Fluid therapy should be initiated with 0.45% saline and 5% dextrose administered at twice the average maintenance rate (i.e., 200 mL/kg per day). Once serum electrolytes have been measured, an increase to 0.675% saline and 5% dextrose may be indicated to correct the calculated sodium deficit. Normal saline (20 mL/kg, administered by rapid iv infusion) or colloid may be required initially for the treatment of shock. Corticosteroid treatment may not have a perceptible effect on the patient's clinical course for several hours. Glucocorticoid therapy should be initiated with cortisol, 50 mg/m$^2$ iv immediately and 15 mg/m$^2$ iv every 6 hours intramuscularly (im).

When the crisis is past (within ~24–48 hours), oral feedings can begin, and iv hydrocortisone can be discontinued. Fludrocortisone (Florinef), 0.1 mg per day, should be started as soon as oral administration is possible. Feeding initially should include 1 g sodium chloride daily. This is administered as 15 mL saline with the first ounce of each of an infant's six feedings. After a few days, the sodium dosage should be individualized, keeping in mind that eyelid, presacral, or labioscrotal edema will be the first sign of overtreatment in an infant. With the typical uncomplicated clinical course, infants usually are thriving and have normal serum electrolyte levels by the sixth day of hospitalization.

Maintenance glucocorticoid therapy should be initiated with 15 (10–20) mg/m$^2$ per day oral hydrocortisone. This dose is twofold greater than the blood production rate to account for splanchnic metabolism. For infants, the dose of hydrocortisone

suspension (Cortef) should be measured accurately in a syringe after vigorous shaking. Three divided doses usually are required to maintain low plasma ACTH concentrations. This is especially important in patients with congenital adrenal hyperplasia, to minimize hyperandrogenemia.

In long-term therapy, the critical factor in avoiding glucocorticoid overdose is the careful monitoring of linear growth, since a subnormal growth rate is the earliest indicator of glucocorticoid excess. Patients with ACTH deficiency may require glucocorticoid replacement only during times of stressful illness; use of cortisol over 15 mg/m$^2$ for asymptomatic patients may increase the growth hormone requirement in hypopituitary patients. Patients should be monitored every 4 to 12 weeks during the period of rapid growth (birth to 1 year) to determine the lowest maintenance glucocorticoid dose that will normalize symptoms and the plasma ACTH concentration or, in the case of congenital adrenal hyperplasia, the appropriate plasma steroids. In older children, regular follow-up at 3- to 6-month intervals is advisable.

Occasionally, it is difficult to normalize some patients on standard therapeutic regimens.[45] Such patients are best treated with a longer-acting glucocorticoid, such as prednisone twice a day, or dexamethasone at bedtime. Prednisone causes fewer striae than does dexamethasone, and it is possible to adjust the dose of tablets more precisely. Prednisone is ~3 times and dexamethasone 80 times more potent in suppressing growth and ACTH than is cortisol.[46]

Because of associated adrenal medullary insufficiency, recovery from hypoglycemia may not be normalized by the usual replacement doses of cortisol. This is because of the lack of high local adrenomedullary concentrations of cortisol that seem to facilitate the N-methylation required for epinephrine synthesis.[38]

A dose of fludrocortisone acetate, 0.05 to 0.1 mg daily, is typically appropriate as mineralocorticoid replacement from infancy onward. The most sensitive index of the adequacy of salt and mineralocorticoid therapy is PRA (see Table 83-1). Underdose interferes with the control of androgens because angiotensin stimulates adrenal fasciculata-reticularis cells.[47] Overdosage is indicated by edema, hypertension, or hypokalemia. Spironolactone, a competitive antagonist of aldosterone, can be used as an adjunct to the treatment of mineralocorticoid excess forms of congenital adrenal hyperplasia.

Families should be given written instructions about emergency treatment, and the child should wear a bracelet (e.g., Medic Alert) that specifies the diagnosis in case of emergency.

## CORTICOSTEROID COVERAGE FOR STRESS

The goal of therapy during physiologic stress is to provide exogenous cortisol in a sufficient amount to mimic the known normal response. Excessive doses of corticosteroid are undesirable, since the drug may interfere with electrolyte homeostasis, retard healing, and increase the patient's susceptibility to infection. If surgery is required, the following treatment regimen is suggested. Cortisol, 15 mg/m$^2$, is administered orally on the evening before surgery, and cortisol, 15 mg/m$^2$, is administered iv immediately preoperatively, and parenterally every 6 hours thereafter until recovery from the acute effects of surgery has occurred.

During the course of any acute, stressful illness, such as diarrhea or an upper respiratory infection, the cortisol dose should be increased to two or three times maintenance. Such treatment is seldom required for more than 3 days. If medication cannot be taken orally or is vomited repeatedly, cortisol, 100 mg/m$^2$, should be administered im daily to prevent adrenocortical crisis.

Varicella is not dangerous to patients who are receiving replacement hydrocortisone therapy provided the dose of glucocorticoid does not exceed two-fold maintenance.[48]

# HYPERCORTISOLISM

## CLINICAL CHARACTERISTICS

Cushing syndrome is the clinical manifestation of excess gluco-corticoid. Along with the well-known manifestations in adults, affected children have attenuated linear growth.[49] Indeed, growth arrest may be the only clear clinical sign of Cushing syndrome. Interestingly, often these children tend to be highly responsible and obsessive about schoolwork, housework, and hobbies. Multiple factors[50–52] contribute to linear growth arrest. These range from direct inhibition of cell proliferation to inhibition of growth hormone release.

The abnormal glucose tolerance associated with hypercortisolism is attributable to increased gluconeogenesis. Ecchymosis secondary to increased capillary fragility, hypertrichosis resembling that seen in states of malnutrition, and muscle weakness and fatigue all appear to be related to increased protein catabolism. The hypertension is caused by increased vascular reactivity to vasoconstrictive factors,[53] increased plasma renin substrate,[53] cortisol overload,[54] and increased mineralocorticoid production.[55] Hyperpigmentation is seen in those patients with elevated plasma ACTH levels. Concomitant androgen excess is responsible for hirsutism or virilization, the latter of which suggests a tumor.

The most common cause of Cushing syndrome in children is pharmacologic glucocorticoid therapy. Attenuation of linear growth occurs at all doses that exceed the normal replacement range of 10 to 20 mg/m$^2$ per day cortisol, or the equivalent.[52] The syndrome can occur after use of topical corticoids, depending on the steroid and the dose. Some individuals are hyperreactive to glucocorticoids, and become cushingoid on normal replacement doses.[56] High doses of some synthetic progestins can cause cushingoid state.[56a]

Cushing disease is hyperadrenocorticolism secondary to excessive secretion of pituitary ACTH, which results in bilateral adrenal hyperplasia (see Chap. 75). In children, as in adults, it is usually caused by a pituitary microadenoma (Fig. 83-3). It may

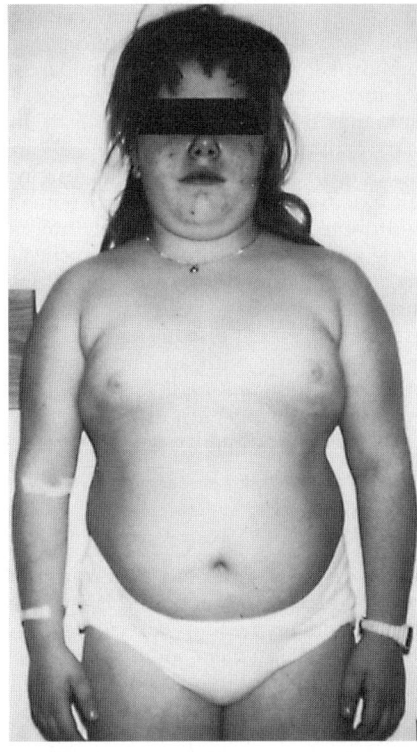

**FIGURE 83-3.** Nine-year-old girl with Cushing disease. Later, the condition was treated successfully by transsphenoidal adenectomy. (Courtesy of Dr. Wellington Hung.)

have an autoimmune basis.[57] Hyperfunctioning adrenocortical tumors occur three times more frequently in girls than in boys. Cushing syndrome secondary to ACTH production by nonendocrine tumors is very rare in the pediatric population. ACTH-independent, primary bilateral adrenal hyperplasia may be caused by McCune-Albright syndrome variants.[58] Adrenocortical micronodular dysplasia causing Cushing syndrome is primarily a disorder of young girls. It may be familial, associated with multiple endocrine neoplasia-type I,[59] or myxoid and other tumors,[60,61] or it can occur as an autoimmune disease.[49] In some cases, hormonogenesis is periodic, and in others it is estrogen-[61] or food-dependent.[62]

## DIAGNOSIS

The diagnostic criteria for Cushing syndrome in children are similar to those in adults. Generally, after determining that cortisol production is excessive, the next step in the workup is the two-step dexamethasone suppression test using successive 2-day courses of dexamethasone, 1 mg/m$^2$ and 2 mg/m$^2$ per day in four divided doses.[49] Plasma cortisol levels should decrease to <2 μg/dL, 24-hour urinary 17-hydroxycorticoids should fall to <2 mg/g creatinine, and urinary free cortisol should fall at least 90%. CRH testing shows promise in yielding the same information in less time. Imaging studies should be performed as in adults. The diagnosis in some cases may require petrosal sinus sampling during the CRH test. Periodic hormonogenesis may present a diagnostic dilemma.[63] The differential diagnosis of high cortisol levels includes familial cortisol resistance, which may be due to a defect in the receptor for glucocorticoids[64,65] or a receptor coactivator.[65a]

## TREATMENT

The potential for further growth and pubertal development is important to consider in reaching a decision about optimal therapy for children with Cushing disease. A trial of cyproheptadine hydrochloride may bring about remission.[66] However, in children and adolescents, transsphenoidal microadenomectomy, performed by an experienced surgeon, usually appears to be the treatment of choice.[67] Transsphenoidal surgery often corrects hypercortisolism, even if no adenoma is detected; cases of Cushing disease without definite pituitary adenoma have been reported in which removal of a portion of the central mucous zone of the pituitary gland was associated with remission. Following surgery, subsequent normal growth is expected, and few sequelae are reported. However, a few patients may require repeat transsphenoidal surgery. The presence of autoantibodies to corticotropes may be a marker indicating a poor prognosis.[57]

Pituitary irradiation of patients with Cushing disease, using ~4000 rad, has resulted in a 75% remission rate; however, this mode of treatment is also associated with a 50% incidence of growth hormone deficiency.[68] Bilateral adrenalectomy not only causes permanent hypoadrenalism, but also causes the development of Nelson syndrome in 27% of patients.[69]

In the postoperative period, patients must be treated to prevent secondary adrenal insufficiency. After cure of Cushing syndrome, catch-up growth often occurs.[70] Catch-up growth is poor in some cases with a long duration and high intensity of glucocorticoid exposure. The cause is unclear; perhaps, puberty causes chondrocytes to differentiate before recovery from inhibition of stem cell proliferation is completed. Catch-up growth is most likely to occur when glucocorticoid excess is relieved well before puberty.

## WITHDRAWAL FROM CORTICOSTEROID EXCESS IN CHILDREN

Children in whom long-term pharmacologic glucocorticoid therapy is being withdrawn or in whom the HPA axis has been

**TABLE 83-3.**
**ACTH-Stimulated Corticosteroids: Typical Normal Plasma Values in Children and Adults***

| | DHEAS (µg/dL) | DHEA (ng/dL) | AD (ng/dL) | 17-Preg (ng/dL) | 17-Prog (ng/dL) | S (ng/dL) | F (µg/dL) | T (ng/dL) |
|---|---|---|---|---|---|---|---|---|
| **PREADRENARCHAL (2–8 yr)** | <40 | 45–120 | <50 | 130–340 | 80–180 | <25–350 | 16–50 | <20 |
| **PREMATURE ADRENARCHAL** | 40–220 | 120–495 | 25–140 | 240–1100 | 40–190 | 40–300 | 16–50 | 15–45 |
| **ADULT FEMALE** | 75–350 | 225–1470 | 90–320 | 150–1085 | 40–130[†] | 40–275 | 17–45 | 20–70 |

*ACTH*, adrenocorticotropic hormone; *DHEAS*, dehydroepiandrosterone sulfate; *DHEA*, dehydroepiandrosterone; *AD*, androstenedione; *17-Preg*, 17-hydroxypregnenolone; *17-Prog*, 17-hydroxyprogesterone; *S*, 11-deoxycortisol; *F*, cortisol; *T*, testosterone.

*Thirty to 60 minutes after ACTH [1–24], 10 µg/m² to 250 µg as intravenous bolus.

†Early follicular phase (days 1–8 of cycle); 17-hydroxyprogesterone rises in the preovulatory phase and reaches a peak as high as 360 ng/dL in the luteal phase of the cycle.

(Data from Rosenfield RL, Rich BH, Lucky AW. Adrenarche as a cause of benign pseudopuberty in boys. J Pediatr 1982; 101:1005; Rosenfield RL, Helke J, Lucky AW. Dexamethasone preparation does not alter corticoid and androgen responses to adrenocorticotropin. J Clin Endocrinol Metab 1985; 60:585; Lucky AW, Rosenfield RL, McGuire J, et al. Adrenal androgen hyperresponsiveness to adrenocorticotropin in women with acne and/or hirsutism: adrenal enzyme defects and exaggerated adrenarche. J Clin Endocrinol Metab 1986; 62:840; Lashansky G, Saenger P, Fishman K, et al. Normative data for adrenal steroidogenesis in a healthy pediatric population: Age and sex related changes after adrenocorticotropin stimulation. J Clin Endocrinol Metab 1991;73:674.)

suppressed by Cushing syndrome require extended and gradually tapering therapeutic regimens. The dosage of corticosteroid can usually be lowered to a maintenance level (10–20 mg/m² per day of cortisol equivalents fairly rapidly; i.e., halving the dose at 1- to 2-week intervals over a few weeks). This will permit linear growth and prevent adrenal insufficiency. During this time, recrudescence of the underlying disease being treated, corticosteroid dependence,[71] or pseudotumor cerebri[72] may occur, necessitating a return to a higher corticosteroid dose followed by a slower taper. The use of alternate-morning administration of prednisone in such situations may minimize corticosteroid side effects and permit growth.[73,74]

After the patient is stabilized on maintenance glucocorticoids, it is appropriate to wean the patient from the corticosteroid over as long a period as the patient has been receiving therapy, up to 9 months.[32] The symptoms of too-rapid weaning are often vague, and are characteristic of isolated glucocorticoid deficiency. Of course, intercurrent, acute, stressful illness requires supplementation for a few days. The return of normal function of the HPA axis is indicated by an 8:00 a.m. plasma cortisol level of >10 µg/dL and a level >18 µg/dL in response to a very low dose ACTH challenge.[40,41]

# PRECOCIOUS PSEUDOPUBERTY

## ETIOLOGY AND CLINICAL CHARACTERISTICS

*Adrenarche* is an "adrenal puberty" during which the adrenal cortex acquires the ability to secrete 17-ketosteroids (see Table 83-2) and DHEA responsiveness to ACTH increases[75–77] (Table 83-3). It normally commences slowly in midchildhood, eventually accounting for most DHEAS production, and reaches a magnitude sufficient to bring about the growth of pubic hair at an average age of ~12 years.

Adrenarche is independent of true (gonadotropin-mediated) puberty. It is related to the development of the zona reticularis. DHEA synthesis increases because this zone has low 3β-hydroxysteroid dehydrogenase activity and seemingly high 17,20-lyase activity; DHEAS is formed from DHEA because of the high sulfokinase activity of this zone. The existence of a putative pituitary adrenocortical androgen-stimulating factor, which is responsible for adrenarche, has been argued. However, ACTH is necessary and sufficient to stimulate adrenal androgens and is the only hormone established to do so. The authors' concept is that an adrenarche factor need be responsible only for bringing about the development of the zona reticularis or a shift in its pattern of response to ACTH.

*Premature pubarche* (sexual pubic hair as an isolated phenomenon before 8.5 years of age in girls or 9.5 years in boys) usually is a benign condition. It has been termed "premature adrenarche" when the plasma DHEAS and testosterone levels are elevated for

age, but appropriate for the pubic hair stage. Premature adrenarche is more common in girls than boys. Neither a growth spurt nor clitoromegaly occurs. There are no signs of gonadal maturation, and the bone age is not advanced to an abnormal extent. It has been thought to be a normal phenomenon happening early. However, the androgen level, particularly that of androstenedione, in childhood correlates with the emergence of a polycystic ovary syndrome (PCOS)–like form of functional ovarian hyperandrogenism after menarche.[78] This suggests that some cases are due to dysregulation of androgen production, which seems to underlie the primary functional adrenal hyperandrogenism (formerly termed *exaggerated adrenarche*) that accounts for most cases of postmenarcheal adrenal androgen excess, as well as the frequently associated ovarian androgen excess.[77] Although such patients were originally thought to have a mild 3β-hydroxysteroid dehydrogenase deficiency, this is now known to be unlikely unless 17-hydroxypregnenolone responses to ACTH are 7 or more SD above average.[79]

Frankly virilizing adrenal disease is usually caused by congenital adrenal hyperplasia (see Chap. 77). Nonclassic congenital adrenal hyperplasia may closely resemble premature adrenarche; affected girls do not have the genital ambiguity of classic congenital adrenal hyperplasia. Rare causes of functional adrenal hyperandrogenism and premature pubarche are *congenitally excessive cortisol metabolism*[80] and *resistance to cortisol*.[65] Adrenal tumors may be responsible for virilism. In such cases, virilization is more often attributable to adrenal carcinoma than to adrenal adenoma. In patients with adrenal carcinoma, there is a high incidence of associated urinary tract anomalies, hemihypertrophy, neurofibromatosis, and familial tumors.[81,82] Tumor size and histologic grade are the major prognostic factors.[83]

Feminizing adrenal tumors are rare in children, but both adenomas and carcinomas have been reported.[84] These tumors cause abnormal advancement of bone age and sexual precocity in girls, and gynecomastia with advanced bone age in boys. Simultaneous feminization and androgenization occur in those tumors that produce androgens and estrogens. Urinary free cortisol and plasma DHEAS and estrogen levels typically are markedly elevated.

## DIAGNOSIS

Pseudopuberty is distinguished clinically from true puberty by the absence of gonadal development. This is indicated by the absence of breast enlargement in affected girls and by the absence of testicular enlargement in affected boys. Virilization is indicated by clitoromegaly in girls, an abnormally advanced bone age, and a plasma testosterone concentration greater than the adult female range.

Virilizing disorders can usually be distinguished from premature adrenarche (see Tables 83-2 and 83-3) and from one another by their characteristic plasma steroid patterns. Classic congenital

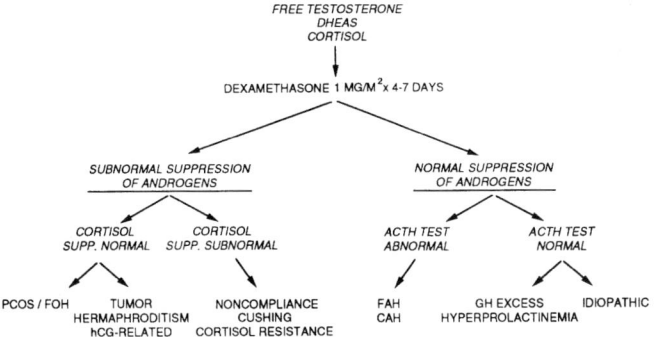

FREE TESTOSTERONE
DHEAS
CORTISOL

DEXAMETHASONE 1 MG/M²x 4-7 DAYS

SUBNORMAL SUPPRESSION
OF ANDROGENS

NORMAL SUPPRESSION
OF ANDROGENS

CORTISOL
SUPP. NORMAL

CORTISOL
SUPP. SUBNORMAL

ACTH TEST
ABNORMAL

ACTH TEST
NORMAL

PCOS / FOH

TUMOR
HERMAPHRODITISM
hCG-RELATED

NONCOMPLIANCE
CUSHING
CORTISOL RESISTANCE

FAH
CAH

GH EXCESS
HYPERPROLACTINEMIA

IDIOPATHIC

**FIGURE 83-4.** This algorithm illustrates the differential diagnosis of hyperandrogenemia. (*DHEAS,* dehydroepiandrosterone sulfate; *supp.,* suppression; *ACTH,* adrenocorticotropic hormone; *PCOS/FOH,* polycystic ovarian syndrome/functional ovarian hyperandrogenism; *hCG,* human chorionic gonadotropin; *FAH,* functional adrenal hyperandrogenism; *CAH,* congenital adrenal hyperplasia; *GH,* growth hormone.) (Modified from Rosenfield RL. The ovary and female maturation. In: Sperling M, ed. Pediatric endocrinology, 1st ed. Philadelphia: WB Saunders, 1996:329–385.)

adrenal hyperplasia (see Chap. 77) is characterized by very high levels of 17-hydroxyprogesterone (typically >2000 ng/dL), with only modest elevation of DHEAS. Nonclassic congenital adrenal hyperplasia may have plasma androgen levels in the adrenarchal range and normal baseline 17-hydroxyprogesterone levels. Adrenal tumors are associated with extremely high levels of DHEAS (>800 µg/dL) and very little elevation in plasma 17-hydroxyprogesterone. The differential diagnosis of extreme elevation of plasma DHEAS also includes the 3β-hydroxysteroid dehydrogenase deficiency form of congenital adrenal hyperplasia and steroid sulfatase deficiency. Gonadal tumors produce relatively large amounts of androstenedione, which causes a modest elevation in excretion of urinary 17-ketosteroids.

The dexamethasone suppression test is helpful in distinguishing among the causes of hyperandrogenemia (Fig. 83-4). Dexamethasone, 1 mg/m² (in three or four divided daily doses), is administered for 4 days (7 days if the patient weighs ≥100 kg). This will selectively suppress adrenal androgenic hyperfunction to normal levels in functional adrenal hyperandrogenism, including congenital adrenal hyperplasia. Normally, in prepubertal children, this regimen suppresses plasma androgens to preadrenarchal levels and suppresses cortisol levels to <2 µg/dL. An ACTH test is indicated to differentiate nonclassic congenital adrenal hyperplasia from other forms of functional adrenal hyperandrogenism, in which the bone age is abnormally advanced. Poor suppression of cortisol is most often due to noncompliance with the test regimen. The distinction between Cushing syndrome and cortisol resistance requires testing with graded doses of dexamethasone.[65] Subnormal suppression of androgens with normal suppression of cortisol indicates that the ovary or a tumor is the source of hyperandrogenism. In pubertal girls, functional ovarian hyperandrogenism, including PCOS, can usually be distinguished from tumor by the characteristic, gradual, perimenarcheal onset and modest elevation of plasma testosterone (<200 ng/dL). When a tumor is suspected, modern radiographic techniques should be used, as in adults, commencing with ultrasound.

## TREATMENT

Tumors that produce sex hormone require surgery. Adrenocortical carcinoma with metastases can be treated with mitotane (o,p′ DDD, Lysodren). In those conditions that cause precocious pseudopuberty that are amenable to therapy, sexual hair development typically regresses, although regression is incomplete in adrenarchal children, and improvement of growth potential

typically occurs following the early correction of virilizing disorders.[85] However, one must be alert to the complication of true sexual precocity in those children in whom the bone age has been advanced to a pubertal level.[86]

# SYNDROMES INVOLVING MINERALOCORTICOID EXCESS

## VARIETIES OF MINERALOCORTICOID EXCESS

A primary excess of any of the mineralocorticoids produced by the adrenals causes variable degrees of hypertension and, hypokalemic alkalosis. Blood pressure is lower in children than in adults. The upper limit of normal is 108/59 mm Hg at 1 year of age and gradually rises until puberty is complete.[87] Edema does not occur in uncomplicated cases because of escape from further sodium retention when blood volume has been expanded by only a few percentage points. The renal salt loss, which mediates this escape, may be due to atrial natriuretic hormone.[88]

### PRIMARY HYPERALDOSTERONISM

Bilateral adrenal hyperplasia, with or without nodule formation, is the most common cause of primary aldosteronism in childhood[89] (see Chap. 80). Boys have a greater incidence of bilateral hyperplasia than girls do. *Familial glucocorticoid-suppressible aldosteronism* (Sutherland syndrome) arises from a mutation that causes a chimeric gene for aldosterone synthase, which contains the ACTH promoter from the homologous 11β-hydroxylase gene.[22] Primary hyperaldosteronism may be due to familial hyperplasia or tumor.[89a] Solitary aldosteronoma or ectopic tumors are rare in children.

### EXCESS OF NON-ALDOSTERONE CORTICOIDS

Excessive secretion of deoxycorticosterone, corticosterone, or cortisol itself may account for mineralocorticoid excess in cases of Cushing syndrome, 17-hydroxylation deficiency, nonendocrine carcinomas, and hyperthyroidism.[54,55] *Primary cortisol resistance* is an autosomal disease in which coexistent elevations in deoxycorticosterone levels may cause a mineralocorticoid excess syndrome.[64,65] Resistance to multiple steroids may be found.[65a] The syndrome of *apparent mineralocorticoid excess* resembles pseudoaldosteronism. It appears to arise from heterogeneous defects in cortisol metabolism that allow filtered cortisol to escape inactivation by renal tubular 11β-hydroxysteroid dehydrogenase.[22,90] *Licorice abuse* produces the syndrome by competitively inhibiting this enzyme, thereby permitting filtered cortisol to reach renal mineralocorticoid receptors.[91]

### PSEUDOALDOSTERONISM

Type I pseudoaldosteronism (Liddle syndrome) is characterized by hypertension, hypokalemia, and low PRA, without overproduction of aldosterone. It is a rare, autosomal dominant, heritable cause of hypertension. This disorder is due to activating mutations in genes encoding subunits of the amiloride-sensitive epithelial sodium channel.[25] It responds to treatment with triamterene, but not spironolactone.[92] Renal transplant is curative. Type II pseudoaldosteronism is a disorder that apparently results from primary renal salt retention of unknown cause.[93]

### SECONDARY HYPERALDOSTERONISM

Secondary hyperaldosteronism is caused by the high PRA resulting from chronic intravascular volume depletion or renovascular disease. The manifestations of secondary hyperaldosteronism vary with the cause (Table 83-4). Metabolic alkalosis does not occur in the edematous forms of untreated secondary aldosteronism because too little sodium reaches the distal tubule for aldosterone to exert significant biologic effects. Uni-

**TABLE 83-4.**
**Differential Diagnosis of Hyperaldosteronism**

| Etiology | ↑ Blood Pressure | Edema | ↓ Serum K and ↑ Serum $CO_2$ | PRA |
|---|---|---|---|---|
| PRIMARY | + | – | + | ↓ |
| SECONDARY | | | | |
| Heart failure, nephrosis, cirrhosis | – | + | – | ↑ |
| Unilateral renal artery stenosis | + | – | + | ↑ |
| Renal salt-losing states | – | – | + | ↑ |

*PRA*, plasma renin activity; +, present; –, absent; ↑, high; ↓, low.

lateral renal artery stenosis may mimic primary aldosteronism clinically because hyperperfusion of the intact kidney delivers ample sodium for the excessive aldosterone to exchange for potassium and to increase blood volume. Malignant hypertension appears to cause secondary aldosteronism because of diffuse intrarenal arteriolar stenosis (see Table 83-4).

## BARTTER SYNDROME

Bartter syndrome is a form of secondary aldosteronism that is characterized by metabolic alkalosis and hypokalemia in the absence of edema or hypertension (see Chap. 80). The syndrome results from heterogeneous disorders causing defective sodium and potassium chloride reabsorption by the renal tubules.[94] Bartter syndrome occurs in neonatal and childhood forms. Affected neonates experience severe dehydration and frequently have hypercalciuria and very high prostaglandin E excretion; there is frequently a history of antenatal polyhydramnios. Autosomal recessive mutations in the furosemide-sensitive Na-K-2Cl cotransporter and other ion channels in the thick ascending loop of Henle have been described in some families. One patient, heterozygous for an angiotensin type 1 receptor mutation, has been described. *Gitelman syndrome* is a mild variant of Bartter syndrome that is characterized by delayed puberty, hypomagnesemic tetany, and hypocalciuria, but may be asymptomatic. It is an autosomal recessive disorder that is due to thiazide-sensitive sodium-chloride cotransporter gene mutation in the distal convoluted tubule. Diverse renal tubular disorders, congenital or acquired, may cause the syndrome.[95–97]

### DIFFERENTIAL DIAGNOSIS AND TREATMENT

The first step in the differential diagnosis of excessive aldosterone production is determination of the PRA (see Table 83-1). The ratio of plasma aldosterone to PRA in a random blood sample usually distinguishes primary from secondary hyperaldosteronism.[22,49] However, distinguishing normal from abnormal PRA may require dynamic testing. In renovascular hypertension, PRA hyperresponsiveness to challenge with captopril is found more often than is elevation of baseline PRA.[98] Suppression of PRA is indicated by the absence of a rise in response to an acute furosemide challenge or, more definitively, a low-salt diet (≤10 mEq NaCl) for 5 days. The differential diagnosis of hypertension and low PRA includes pseudoaldosteronism. The differential diagnosis of metabolic alkalosis includes hypertensive states, such as pseudoaldosteronism, excessive production of mineralocorticoids other than aldosterone, and licorice abuse. It also includes nonhypertensive states that are usually due to chloride depletion from chronic gastrointestinal or renal losses.[99] The determination of urinary electrolytes is useful for distinguishing between prerenal and renal sources of potassium loss and among the types of renal tubular disorders.[89] Potassium therapy may unmask hyperaldosteronism in hypokalemic patients with disordered renal tubular function.

Children with primary hyperaldosteronism require a search utilizing computed tomography (CT) or magnetic resonance imaging (MRI) for a surgically treatable lesion. In the absence of tumor, a 1-week therapeutic trial of dexamethasone to rule out glucocorticoid-suppressible aldosteronism is indicated. When hypermineralocorticoidism due to other steroids is suspected, a trial of spironolactone may be helpful.

The management of Bartter syndrome involves oral replacement of sodium, chloride, potassium, and other mineral deficits (e.g., magnesium), when indicated. The concomitant use of potassium-sparing diuretics, such as triamterene (~5–10 mg/m² per day) or spironolactone (~100 mg/m² per day) is often required to control the hypokalemic alkalosis. The use of prostaglandin synthetase inhibitors decreases PRA and ameliorates hypokalemia in some cases; it may be lifesaving in neonatal Bartter syndrome.

## REFERENCES

1. Cowett RM, Susa JB, Giletti B, et al. Glucose kinetics in infants of diabetic mothers. Am J Obstet Gynecol 1983; 146:781.
2. Metzger DL, Wright NM, Veldhuis JD, et al. Characterization of pulsatile secretion and clearance of plasma cortisol in premature and term neonates using deconvolution analysis. J Clin Endocrinol Metab 1993; 77:458.
3. Vermes I, Dohanics J, Toth G, Pongracz J. Maturation of the circadian rhythm of the adrenocortical functions in human neonates and infants. Horm Res 1980; 12:237.
4. Kowarski A, Katz H, Migeon CJ. Plasma aldosterone concentration in normal subjects from infancy to adulthood. J Clin Endocrinol Metab 1974; 38:489.
5. Pratt JH, Jones JJ, Miller JZ, et al. Racial differences in aldosterone excretion and plasma aldosterone concentrations in children. N Engl J Med 1989; 321:1152.
6. Harshfield GA, Alpert BS, Pulliam DA. Renin-angiotensin-aldosterone system in healthy subjects aged ten to eighteen years. J Pediatr 1993; 122:563.
7. Rosenfield RL, Lucky AW. Acne, hirsutism, and alopecia in adolescent girls. Clinical expressions of androgen excess. Endocrinol Metab Clin North Am 1993; 22:507.
8. Lee MM, Rajagopalan L, Berg GJ, Moshang T Jr. Serum adrenal steroid concentrations in premature infants. J Clin Endocrinol Metab 1989; 69:1133.
9. Blethen S, Wenick G, Hawkins L. Congenital adrenal hypoplasia in association with growth hormone deficiency, developmental delay, partial androgen resistance, unusual facies, and skeletal abnormalities. Dysmorphology Clin Genet 1990; 4:110.
10. Vilain E, Le Merrer M, Lecointre C, et al. IMAGe, a new clinical association of Intrauterine growth retardation, Metaphyseal dysplasia, Adrenal hypoplasia congenita, and Genital anomalies. J Clin Endocrinol Metab 1999; 84:4335.
11. Khuri FJ, Alton DJ, Hardy BE, et al. Adrenal hemorrhage in neonates: report of 5 cases and review of the literature. J Urol 1980; 124:684.
12. Chen S, Sawicka J, Betterle C, et al. Autoantibodies to steroidogenic enzymes in autoimmune polyglandular syndrome, Addison's disease, and premature ovarian failure. J Clin Endocrinol Metab 1996; 81:1871.
13. De Bellis A, Bizzarro A, Rossi R, et al. Remission of subclinical adrenocortical failure in subjects with adrenal autoantibodies. J Clin Endocrinol Metab 1993; 76:1002.
14. Betterle C, Greggio NA, Volpato M. Clinical review 93: autoimmune polyglandular syndrome type 1. J Clin Endocrinol Metab 1998; 83:1049.
15. Ward L, Paquette J, Seidman E, et al. Severe autoimmune polyendocrinopathy-candidiasis-ectodermal dystrophy in an adolescent girl with a novel AIRE mutation: response to immunosuppressive therapy. J Clin Endocrinol Metab 1999; 84:844.
16. Migeon CJ, Kenny FM, Hung W, et al. Study of adrenal function in children with meningitis. Pediatrics 1967; 40:163.
17. Pagani F, Pariyarath R, Garcia R, et al. New lysosomal acid lipase gene mutants explain the phenotype of Wolman disease and cholesteryl ester storage disease. J Lipid Res 1998; 39:1382.
18. Gartner J, Braun A, Holzinger A, et al. Clinical and genetic aspects of X-linked adrenoleukodystrophy. Neuropediatrics 1998; 29:3.
19. Geisbrecht BV, Collins CS, Reuber BE, et al. Disruption of a PEX1-PEX6 interaction is the most common cause of the neurologic disorders Zellweger syndrome, neonatal adrenoleukodystrophy, and infantile Refsum disease. Proc Natl Acad Sci U S A 1998; 95:8630.
20. Castells S, Inamdar S, Orti E. Familial moniliasis, defective delayed hypersensitivity, and adrenocorticotropic hormone deficiency. J Pediatr 1971; 79:72.
21. Clark A, Weber A. Adrenocorticotropin insensitivity syndromes. Endocr Rev 1998; 19:828.
22. White PC. Disorders of aldosterone biosynthesis and action. N Engl J Med 1994; 331:250.
23. Portrat-Doyen S, Tourniaire J, Richard O, et al. Isolated aldosterone synthase deficiency caused by simultaneous E198D and V386A mutations in the CYP11B2 gene. J Clin Endocrinol Metab 1998; 83:4156.
23a. Landier F, Guyenne TT, Boutignon H, et al. Hyporeninemic hypoaldosteronism in infancy: a familial disease. J Clin Endocrinol Metab 1984; 58:143.
24. Geller DS, Rodriguez-Soriano J, Vallo Boado A, et al. Mutations in the min-

eralocorticoid receptor gene cause autosomal dominant pseudohypoaldosteronism type I. Nat Genet 1998; 19:279.

25. Schaedel C, Marthinsen L, Kristoffersson A-C, et al. Lung symptoms in pseudohypoaldosteronism type 1 are associated with deficiency of the α-subunit of the epithelial sodium channel. J Pediatr 1999; 135:739.

26. Kuhnle U. Pseudohypoaldosteronism: mutation found, problem solved? Mol Cell Endocrinol 1997; 133:77.

27. Mansfield TA, Simon DB, Farfel Z, et al. Multilocus linkage of familial hyperkalaemia and hypertension, pseudohypoaldosteronism type II, to chromosomes 1q31–42 and 17p11–q21. Nat Genet 1997; 16:202.

28. Batlle DC, Kurtzman NA. Syndromes of aldosterone deficiency and excess. Med Clin North Am 1983; 67:879.

29. Gregory MJ, Schwartz GJ. Diagnosis and treatment of renal tubular disorders. Semin Nephrol 1998; 18:317.

30. Streeten DH, Anderson GH Jr, Dalakos TG, et al. Normal and abnormal function of the hypothalamic-pituitary-adrenocortical system in man. Endocr Rev 1984; 5:371.

31. Dluhy RG, Himathongkam T, Greenfield M. Rapid ACTH test with plasma aldosterone levels. Improved diagnostic discrimination. Ann Intern Med 1974; 80:693.

32. Graber A, Ney R, Nicholson W. Natural history of pituitary-adrenal recovery following long term suppression with corticoids. J Clin Endocrinol Metab 1965; 25:11.

33. Helbock HJ, Insoft RM, Conte FA. Glucocorticoid-responsive hypotension in extremely low birth weight newborns. Pediatrics 1993; 92:715.

34. Lanes R, Blanchette V, Edwin C, et al. Congenital hypopituitarism and conjugated hyperbilirubinemia in two infants. Am J Dis Child 1978; 132:926.

35. Choo-Kang LR, Sun CC, Counts DR. Cholestasis and hypoglycemia: manifestations of congenital anterior hypopituitarism. J Clin Endocrinol Metab 1996; 81:2786.

36. de Luis DA, Aller R, Romero E. Isolated ACTH deficiency. Horm Res 1998; 49:247.

37. Krude H, Biebermann H, Luck W, et al. Severe early-onset obesity, adrenal insufficiency and red hair pigmentation caused by POMC mutations in humans. Nat Genet 1998; 19:155.

38. Hung W, Migeon CJ. Hypoglycemia in a two-year-old boy with adrenocorticotropic hormone (ACTH) deficiency (probably isolated) and adrenal medullary unresponsiveness to insulin-induced hypoglycemia. J Clin Endocrinol Metab 1968; 28:146.

39. Korth-Schutz S, Levine LS, New MI. Dehydroepiandrosterone sulfate (DS) levels, a rapid test for abnormal adrenal androgen secretion. J Clin Endocrinol Metab 1976; 42:1005.

40. Henzen C, Suter A, Lerch E, et al. Suppression and recovery of adrenal response after short-term, high-dose glucocorticoid treatment. Lancet 2000; 355:542.

41. Streeten DHP. What test for hypothalamic-pituitary-adrenocortical insufficiency? Lancet 1999; 354:179.

42. Plotsky PM, Bruhn TO, Vale W. Central modulation of immunoreactive corticotropin-releasing factor secretion by arginine vasopressin. Endocrinology 1984; 115:1639.

43. Grinspoon SK, Biller BM. Clinical review 62: laboratory assessment of adrenal insufficiency. J Clin Endocrinol Metab 1994; 79:923.

44. Kyriazopoulou V, Parparousi O, Vagenakis AG. Rifampicin-induced adrenal crisis in addisonian patients receiving corticosteroid replacement therapy. J Clin Endocrinol Metab 1984; 59:1204.

45. Rosenfield RL, Bickel S, Razdan AK. Amenorrhea related to progestin excess in congenital adrenal hyperplasia. Obstet Gynecol 1980; 56:208.

46. Hansen JW, Loriaux DL. Variable efficacy of glucocorticoids in congenital adrenal hyperplasia. Pediatrics 1976; 57:942.

47. Lebrethon MC, Jaillard C, Defayes G, et al. Human cultured adrenal fasciculata-reticularis cells are targets for angiotensin-II: effects on cytochrome P450 cholesterol side-chain cleavage, cytochrome P450 17 alpha-hydroxylase, and 3 beta-hydroxysteroid-dehydrogenase messenger ribonucleic acid and proteins and on steroidogenic responsiveness to corticotropin and angiotensin-II. J Clin Endocrinol Metab 1994; 78:1212.

48. Dowell SF, Bresee JS. Severe varicella associated with steroid use. Pediatrics 1993; 92:223.

49. Magiakou MA, Mastorakos G, Oldfield EH, et al. Cushing's syndrome in children and adolescents. Presentation, diagnosis, and therapy. N Engl J Med 1994; 331:629.

50. Kilgore BS, McNatt ML, Meador S, et al. Alteration of cartilage glycosaminoglycan protein acceptor by somatomedin and cortisol. Pediatr Res 1979; 13:96.

51. Jonat C, Rahmsdorf HJ, Park KK, et al. Antitumor promotion and antiinflammation: down-modulation of AP-1 (Fos/Jun) activity by glucocorticoid hormone. Cell 1990; 62:1189.

52. Allen DB. Growth suppression by glucocorticoid therapy. Endocrinol Metab Clin North Am 1996; 25:699.

53. Saruta T, Suzuki H, Handa M, et al. Multiple factors contribute to the pathogenesis of hypertension in Cushing's syndrome. J Clin Endocrinol Metab 1986; 62:275.

54. Ulick S, Wang JZ, Blumenfeld JD, Pickering TG. Cortisol inactivation overload: a mechanism of mineralocorticoid hypertension in the ectopic adrenocorticotropin syndrome. J Clin Endocrinol Metab 1992; 74:963.

55. Biglieri EG, Slaton PE, Schambelan M, Kronfield SJ. Hypermineralocorticoidism. Am J Med 1968; 45:170.

56. Iida S, Nakamura Y, Fujii H, et al. A patient with hypocortisolism and Cushing's syndrome–like manifestations: cortisol hyperreactive syndrome. J Clin Endocrinol Metab 1990; 70:729.

56a. Stockheim JA, Daaboul JJ, Yogev R, et al. Adrenal suppression in children with the human immunodeficiency virus treated with megestrol acetate. J Pediatr 1999; 134:368.

57. Scherbaum WA, Schrell U, Gluck M, et al. Autoantibodies to pituitary corticotropin-producing cells: possible marker for unfavourable outcome after pituitary microsurgery for Cushing's disease. Lancet 1987; 1:1394.

58. Boston BA, Mandel S, LaFranchi S, et al. Activating mutation in the stimulatory guanine nucleotide-binding protein in an infant with Cushing's syndrome and nodular adrenal hyperplasia. J Clin Endocrinol Metab 1994; 79:890.

59. Gaitan D, Loosen PT, Orth DN. Two patients with Cushing's disease in a kindred with multiple endocrine neoplasia type I. J Clin Endocrinol Metab 1993; 76:1580.

60. Carney JA. Carney complex: the complex of myxomas, spotty pigmentation, endocrine overactivity, and schwannomas. Semin Dermatol 1995; 14:90.

61. Caticha O, Odell WD, Wilson DE, et al. Estradiol stimulates cortisol production by adrenal cells in estrogen-dependent primary adrenocortical nodular dysplasia. J Clin Endocrinol Metab 1993; 77:494.

62. N'Diaye N, Tremblay J, Hamet P, et al. Adrenocortical overexpression of gastric inhibitory polypeptide receptor underlies food-dependent Cushing's syndrome. J Clin Endocrinol Metab 1998; 83:2781.

63. Gomez Muguruza MT, Chrousos GP. Periodic Cushing syndrome in a short boy: usefulness of the ovine corticotropin releasing hormone test. J Pediatr 1989; 115:270.

64. Bamberger CM, Schulte HM, Chrousos GP. Molecular determinants of glucocorticoid receptor function and tissue sensitivity to glucocorticoids. Endocr Rev 1996; 17:245.

65. Malchoff CD, Javier EC, Malchoff DM, et al. Primary cortisol resistance presenting as isosexual precocity. J Clin Endocrinol Metab 1990; 70:503.

65a. New MI, Nimkarn S, Brandon DD, et al. Resistance to several steroids in two sisters. J Clin Endocrinol Metab 1999; 84:4454.

66. Couch RM, Smail PJ, Dean HJ, et al. Prolonged remission of Cushing disease after treatment with cyproheptadine. J Pediatr 1984; 104:906.

67. Devoe DJ, Miller WL, Conte FA, et al. Long-term outcome in children and adolescents after transsphenoidal surgery for Cushing's disease. J Clin Endocrinol Metab 1997; 82:3196.

68. Clayton PE, Shalet SM. Dose dependency of time of onset of radiation-induced growth hormone deficiency. J Pediatr 1991; 118:226.

69. Hopwood NJ, Kenny FM. Incidence of Nelson's syndrome after adrenalectomy for Cushing's disease in children: results of a nationwide survey. Am J Dis Child 1977; 131:1353.

70. Boersma B, Wit JM. Catch-up growth. Endocr Rev 1997; 18:646.

71. Dixon RB, Christy NP. On the various forms of corticosteroid withdrawal syndrome. Am J Med 1980; 68:224.

72. Weisberg LA, Chutorian AM. Pseudotumor cerebri of childhood. Am J Dis Child 1977; 131:1243.

73. Kaiser BA, Polinsky MS, Palmer JA, et al. Growth after conversion to alternate-day corticosteroids in children with renal transplants: a single-center study. Pediatr Nephrol 1994; 8:320.

74. Kamada AK, Szefler SJ. Glucocorticoids and growth in asthmatic children. Pediatr Allergy Immunol 1995; 6:145.

75. Rosenfeld RL. Normal and almost normal precocious variations in pubertal development premature pubarche and premature thelarche revisited. Horm Res 1994; 41:7.

76. Rosenfield R, Qin K. Normal adrenarche. In: Rose B, ed. UpToDate. Wellesley, MA: UpToDate, 1998.

77. Rosenfield RL. Ovarian and adrenal function in polycystic ovary syndrome. Endocrinol Metab Clin North Am 1999; 28:265.

78. Ibanez L, Potau N, Zampolli M, et al. Girls diagnosed with premature pubarche show an exaggerated ovarian androgen synthesis from the early stages of puberty: evidence from gonadotropin-releasing hormone agonist testing. Fertil Steril 1997; 67:849.

79. Pang S. Congenital adrenal hyperplasia. Clin Obstet Gynaecol 1997; 11:281.

80. Phillipov G, Palermo M, Shackleton C. Apparent cortisone reductase deficiency: a unique form of hypercortisolism. J Clin Endocrinol Metab 1996; 81:3855.

81. Lee PD, Winter RJ, Green OC. Virilizing adrenocortical tumors in childhood: eight cases and a review of the literature. Pediatrics 1985; 76:437.

82. Reincke M, Karl M, Travis WH, et al. p53 mutations in human adrenocortical neoplasms: immunohistochemical and molecular studies. J Clin Endocrinol Metab 1994; 78:790.

83. Mayer SK, Oligny LL, Deal C, et al. Childhood adrenocortical tumors: case series and reevaluation of prognosis—a 24-year experience. J Pediatr Surg 1997; 32:911.

84. Wohltmann H, Mathur RS, Williamson HO. Sexual precocity in a female infant due to feminizing adrenal carcinoma. J Clin Endocrinol Metab 1980; 50:186.

85. Bongiovanni AM, Moshang T Jr, Parks JS. Maturational deceleration after treatment of congenital adrenal hyperplasia. Helv Paediatr Acta 1973; 28:127.

86. Pescovitz OH, Comite F, Cassorla F, et al. True precocious puberty complicating congenital adrenal hyperplasia: treatment with a luteinizing hormone-releasing hormone analog. J Clin Endocrinol Metab 1984; 58:857.

87. Rosner B, Prineas RJ, Loggie JM, et al. Blood pressure nomograms for children and adolescents, by height, sex, and age, in the United States. J Pediatr 1993; 123:871.

88. Hunt PJ, Espiner EA, Richards AM, Daniels SR. Interactions of atrial and brain natriuretic peptides at pathophysiological levels in normal men. Am J Physiol 1995; 269:R1397.

89. New MI, Peterson RE. Disorders of aldosterone secretion in childhood. Pediatr Clin North Am 1966; 13:43.

89a. Gordon RD, Stowaasser M. Familial forms broaden the horizons for primary aldosteronism. Trends Endocrinol Metab 1998; 9:220.

90. Ulick S, Tedde R, Wang JZ. Defective ring A reduction of cortisol as the major metabolic error in the syndrome of apparent mineralocorticoid excess. J Clin Endocrinol Metab 1992; 74:593.

91. Edwards CR, Stewart PM, Burt D, et al. Localisation of 11 beta-hydroxysteroid dehydrogenase—tissue specific protector of the mineralocorticoid receptor. Lancet 1988; 2:986.

92. Vania A, Tucciarone L, Mazzeo D, et al. Liddle's syndrome: a 14-year follow-up of the youngest diagnosed case. Pediatr Nephrol 1997; 11:7.

93. Vallotton MB. Primary aldosteronism. Pt II. Differential diagnosis of primary hyperaldosteronism and pseudoaldosteronism. Clin Endocrinol (Oxf) 1996; 45:53.

94. Guay-Woodford LM. Bartter syndrome: unraveling the pathophysiologic enigma. Am J Med 1998; 105:151.

95. Goto Y, Itami N, Kajii N, et al. Renal tubular involvement mimicking Bartter syndrome in a patient with Kearns-Sayre syndrome. J Pediatr 1990; 116:904.

96. Walker SH, Firminger HI. Familial renal dysplasia with sodium wasting and hypokalemic alkalosis. Am J Dis Child 1974; 127:882.

97. Steiner RW, Omachi AS. A Bartter's-like syndrome from capreomycin, and a similar gentamicin tubulopathy. Am J Kidney Dis 1986; 7:245.

98. Hamed RM, Balfe JW, Ellis G. Use of the captopril test to assess renin responsiveness in children with hypertension and renal disease. Child Nephrol Urol 1991; 11:10.

99. Rosen RA, Julian BA, Dubovsky EV, et al. On the mechanism by which chloride corrects metabolic alkalosis in man. Am J Med 1988; 84:449.

---

# C H A P T E R   8 4

# THE INCIDENTAL ADRENAL MASS

D. LYNN LORIAUX

An unanticipated adrenal mass is found in ~4% of upper abdominal computed tomographic (CT) scans (see Chaps. 88 and 89). There are 100,000 such scans done annually. Thus, the consultation for an incidentally discovered adrenal mass is an important one for the endocrinologist. The primary questions posed in the consultation are two: What is the possibility that the mass is a primary adrenal cancer, and should the mass be surgically removed? The first question can be answered with some certainty. The one piece of "hard" data concerning this question is the known incidence of adrenocortical cancer, ~1 in 600,000 per year.[1] This number is taken from "pre-incidentaloma" registries and is based on criteria that ensure malignant behavior. If we assume a 3-year "preclinical" life, the prevalence of adrenocortical cancer can be estimated at 1 in 200,000. Let us assume, further, that all of these tumors will be found by the usual upper abdominal CT scan. Thus, if 200,000 people are scanned, 8000 nodules will be found, of which 1 will be a primary adrenal malignancy, a prevalence of 0.01%. In other words, the possibility that an "incidental" adrenal mass is a primary adrenal cancer is very small. Some series, however, report an incidence of adrenal cancer in incidental adrenal masses as high as 7%.[2,3] This means that 560 of the 8000 nodules would have the pathologic diagnosis of adrenal cancer, and only 1 would exhibit the clinical behavior of an adrenal cancer. Many of these nodules are removed by surgeons, are misdiagnosed by the pathologist as cancer, and, since they are in fact benign, do not recur—a cancer "pseudocure." It is this fact that introduces most of the confusion that bedevils the management of these patients.

The causes of an incidental adrenal mass are shown in Table 84-1. Three surprises emerge from a study of these data: the *high frequency of metastatic lesions to the adrenal gland that "present" as an incidental finding,* the *high percentage of pheochromocytomas* in this group of patients, and, as previously noted, the *extreme rarity of adrenocortical cancer.*

**TABLE 84-1.**
**Major Causes of Incidental Adrenal Masses**

| Cause | Percent |
| --- | --- |
| Benign adenoma or isolated hyperplasia | 50 |
| Cysts | 10 |
| Myelolipoma | 10 |
| Pheochromocytoma and ganglioneuroma | 10 |
| Metastasis in patients not known to have cancer | 6–30 |
| Adrenal cancer | 0.01 |

| **Of the nonfunctional incidental adrenal masses, the major causes are:** | |
| --- | --- |
| Benign adrenal adenoma | 70-90 |
| Metastasis | 5-20 |
| Cysts, myelolipoma, hemorrhage, etc. | 5-10 |

(Data taken from Kloos RT. Incidentally discovered adrenal masses. Endocr Rev 1995; 16:460; Cook DM, Loriaux DL. The incidental adrenal mass. Am J Med 1996; 101:88.)

Thus, the major challenge for the clinician managing these patients is to identify, with certainty, metastases to the adrenal gland and pheochromocytomas, and to develop a plan for following the remaining nodules of adrenal origin, including the identification of infectious causes of adrenal enlargement that need treatment, such as tuberculosis. A decision tree for the management of these patients is shown in Figure 84-1.

The *functional capacity* of the lesion should be assessed first; it should be assessed clinically and biochemically. Signs and symptoms of glucocorticoid and mineralocorticoid excess or deficiency, and symptoms of androgen excess in women and estrogen excess in men, should be sought out. The author's choices for supporting laboratory tests are shown in Table 84-2. There are many variations on this theme, and most can be defended. In the opinion of the author, all patients should have a standard *cosyntropin stimulation test* (250 µg) with measurements

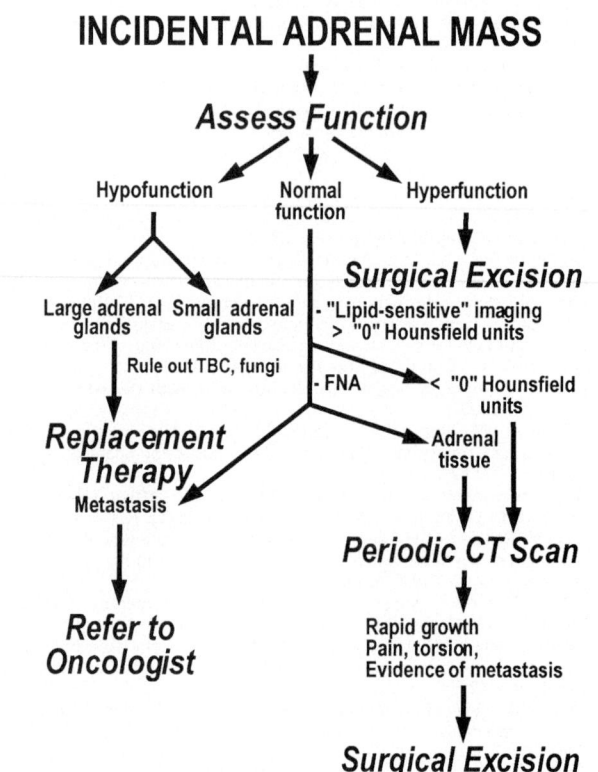

**FIGURE 84-1.** Decision tree for the management of patients with an incidentally discovered adrenal mass. (*TBC,* tuberculosis; *CT,* computed tomographic.)

**TABLE 84-2.**
**Tests of Endocrine Function**

| Disorder | Test |
| --- | --- |
| Glucocorticoid excess | Urine free cortisol |
| Glucocorticoid deficiency | 250 μg cosyntropin (Cortrosyn) stimulation test |
| Mineralocorticoid excess | Electrolytes and upright renin |
| Mineralocorticoid deficiency | Electrolytes and supine renin |
| Catecholamine excess | Fractionated urine catecholamines |
| Estrogen excess | Plasma estradiol |
| Androgen excess | Plasma testosterone |

of *cortisol, 17-hydroxyprogesterone,* and *fractionated urinary catecholamines.* The remaining tests should be used if the clinical picture is strong enough to warrant a corroboration.

Incidentally discovered adrenal masses associated with excess steroid hormone or catecholamine secretion should be surgically excised (see Chap. 89). Patients with glucocorticoid deficiency should receive replacement therapy with hydrocortisone and fludrocortisone, and infectious causes of adrenal insufficiency should be identified and treated. Nonclassical 21-hydroxylase deficiency should be treated with glucocorticoid replacement, in some cases, with the addition of a mineralocorticoid (fludrocortisone) and, in others, with the addition of an antiandrogen.

With dysfunctional lesions excluded, the primary differentiation now centers on *identifying metastases from an unknown primary neoplasm.* At this stage, the possibility of a metastasis is now enhanced, since masses with abnormal function have been excluded. The possibility that the mass is a metastasis in a patient with a known malignancy is high, in some series as high as 70%.[4]

These patients need no further evaluation by the endocrinologist and should be referred to an oncologist.

When it is explained to the patient that there is a strong possibility that the incidentally discovered lesion is the first manifestation of a nonadrenal malignancy, most patients will wish this possibility explored. The "gold standard" for this differentiation, in the opinion of the author, is a CT-guided *fine needle aspiration* (FNA) of the mass. Although pathologists cannot predict which lesions composed of adrenal tissue will metastasize, they can determine which lesions originate outside of the adrenal gland with an accuracy approaching 100%.[5] Recent advances in imaging have provided a methodology that may reduce the number of patients requiring FNA for this differentiation. For example, using a CT density cutoff of "0" Hounsfield units all adrenal lesions with a density below this level were found to be benign. Roughly half of the incidental adrenal masses fell below this cutoff. Thus, using the CT image as a screen, it is possible to reduce the theoretical number of FNAs by half. Chemical shift magnetic resonance imaging (MRI), in some hands, has differentiated metastasis from benign adenoma with an accuracy of 100%.[6] Together, these tools, as they become generally available, may obviate the need for FNA in most cases. However, currently, FNA remains a useful clinical tool.[7]

Once metastases are excluded, there are two treatment choices for the remaining adrenal nodules: *surgical removal versus watchful waiting.* At this point in the evaluation, the chance that any one of these masses is an adrenal cancer is ~1 in 2000 (0.05%).

Let us consider surgical intervention first. Assume that an operation will cure a cancer and that the associated surgical mortality is 1%. In this case, 20 people with benign lesions will die for every person "cured" of cancer. Clearly, these nodules, as a group, should *not* be surgically excised.

Could these odds be improved if only the largest lesions (>5 cm) are surgically removed? The prevalence of benign lesions of this size is difficult to determine, but in one series of 12,000 autopsies, four such lesions were found, giving an incidence of 1 in 3000.[7] The appropriate control population for this group would

be the incidence of adrenal cancer found at autopsy, which is ~1 in 600,000. Thus, if we assume that all cancers are >5 cm, the ratio of benign to malignant lesions in this group is 200:1. If the surgeon is operating to cure cancer, the operation should probably proceed by an anterior abdominal approach (see Chap. 89). This will have a higher mortality, perhaps 2%. In this analysis, four people with a benign lesion will die for every one cured of a cancer. If, on the other hand, the mortality is <0.5%, the operation could be defended, with the assumption that there will be a "cure" of the true cancer with high certainty. This, of course, is unknown; we currently have no way of predicting malignant behavior based on an examination of the tumor removed. This might be influenced by associated problems such as abdominal pain and the likelihood of torsion and necrosis of the tumor, all of which are compelling reasons to recommend surgery. It is in this context that the physician must make a recommendation. The prevailing standard of practice is to remove all lesions >5 to 6 cm in largest diameter. The opinion of the author is that the efficacy of "curative" surgery in this setting is equivocal, and that in the absence of pain, absences of torsion and necrosis, and absence of clear-cut signs of malignancy such as invasion of the renal vein, the kidney, or adjacent structures, surgery should be avoided.

On the other hand, it is quite clear that surgery prolongs life and improves the quality of life for patients with documented adrenocortical cancer (see Chap. 89). Studies have shown an average longevity of 48 months from diagnosis, and most of that gain can be attributed to surgical intervention; it is the only treatment known to be effective for adrenocortical cancer and should be applied with vigor at this stage of the disease.[9]

## REFERENCES

1. US Department of Health Services National Cancer Institute 1981 Surveillance, Epidemiology, and End Results; Incidence and Mortality Data, 1973–1977. NIH Publication No. 81-2330. Washington, DC: US Government Printing Office, 1981.
2. Terzolo M, Ali A, Osella G, Mazza E. The prevalence of adrenal carcinoma among incidentally discovered adrenal masses. Arch Surg 1997; 132:914.
3. Belldegrun A, Hussain S, Seltzer SE, et al. Incidentally discovered mass of the adrenal gland. Surg Gynecol Obstet 1986; 163:203.
4. Kloos RT. Incidentally discovered adrenal masses. Endocr Rev 1995; 16:460.
5. Cook DM, Loriaux DL. The incidental adrenal mass. Am J Med 1996; 101:88.
6. Bernardino ME, Walther MM, Phillips VM, et al. AJR 1985; 144:67.
7. Shin SJ, Hoda RS, Ying L, DeLellis RA. Diagnostic utility of the monoclonal antibody A103 in fine-needle aspiration biopsies of the adrenal. Am J Clin Pathol 2000; 113:295.
8. Mitchell DG, Crovello M, Matteucci T, et al. Benign adrenocortical masses: diagnosis with chemical shift MR imaging. Radiology. 1992; 185:345.
9. Vassilopoulou-Sellin R, Guinee VF, Klein MJ, et al. Impact of adjuvant mitotane on the clinical course of patients with adrenocortical cancer. Cancer 1993; 71:319.

# CHAPTER 85

# PHYSIOLOGY OF THE ADRENAL MEDULLA AND THE SYMPATHETIC NERVOUS SYSTEM

DAVID S. GOLDSTEIN

In responding to stressors, whether physical or psychological, trivial or mortal, the *autonomic nervous system* plays a crucial role. This system influences cardiovascular, metabolic, and visceral activity in the resting organism and determines the physiologic concomitants of virtually every motion and emotion.

According to Langley's conceptualization dating from approximately the turn of the twentieth century, the autonomic nervous system consists of the parasympathetic nervous system and the sympathetic nervous system. The former uses acetylcholine (ACh) as the main neurotransmitter, and the latter (with exceptions) uses the catecholamine norepinephrine (NE, noradrenaline). The adrenomedullary hormonal system uses the catecholamine epinephrine (EPI, adrenaline) as the main hormone secreted into the bloodstream.

Walter B. Cannon considered the adrenal gland to act in concert with the sympathetic nervous system to maintain homeostasis during emergencies, leading to the current use of the term *sympathoadrenal system*. As discussed in this chapter, however, recent evidence has indicated separate regulation of sympathoneural and adrenomedullary outflows during different forms of stress.[1] In addition, a third peripheral catecholaminergic system may use dopamine (DA) as an autocrine-paracrine substance.

## INTEGRATION AND ADAPTATION

An understanding of *sympathetic nervous and adrenomedullary hormonal* system activation may be facilitated by considering integrative actions in homeostasis and in adaptive responses during stress.[1] For instance, almost all the components of the *shock syndrome*—pallor, sweating, cutaneous vasoconstriction, piloerection, agitation, pupillary dilation, tachycardia, hyperventilation, increased total peripheral resistance, decreased gastrointestinal motility, hyperglycemia, and renal sodium retention—can be accounted for by increased activity of catecholaminergic systems in the ultimate attempt to preserve life. When these compensatory mechanisms are overwhelmed or give way, the organism dies.

Many principles of endocrinology and metabolism dealing with hormones, central and peripheral neurotransmission, receptors, and second messengers originated from classic investigations of the function of catecholamines. In addition, many effective therapies for clinical disorders, such as depression, myocardial ischemia, hypertension, and circulatory shock, have resulted directly from applications of these principles.

## EMBRYOLOGY

The *chromaffin tissue* of the adrenal medulla and that of the ganglia of the sympathetic nervous system share an embryonic origin from neural crest tissue. The term *chromaffin* refers to the histochemical identification of intracellular granules that turn brown when treated with oxidizing agents. In adult humans, chromaffin cells exist mainly in the adrenal medulla because sympathetic nerve terminals do not occur in a form concentrated enough to produce a detectable chromaffin reaction.

Precursors of sympathetic cells (sympathogonia) develop early in ontogeny in the area of the neural crest and tube. They migrate ventrally and differentiate into paravertebral and preaortic neuroblasts, the precursors of ganglion cells, and pheochromoblasts, the precursors of chromaffin cells. Thus, extraadrenal pheochromocytomas characteristically occur in paravertebral or preaortic regions.

Whereas adrenocortical tissue arises from coelomic epithelium, adrenomedullary tissue arises from pheochromoblasts that migrate from sympathetic ganglia and nest within adrenocortical tissue. The adrenomedullary cells differentiate into modified neuronal (gland) cells, not neurons. The separate origins of adrenocortical and adrenomedullary tissue are evident in amphibians and reptiles, in which the two types of glandular tissue are only loosely associated, and in fish, which have anatomically distinct glands. In humans, extraadrenal chromaffin tissue degenerates after birth, and adrenomedullary chromaffin tissue matures.

## FUNCTIONAL ANATOMY

Sympathetic *preganglionic* axons originate from cell bodies in the intermediolateral cell columns of the thoracolumbar spinal cord[2] (Fig. 85-1). A central neural site projecting to the intermediolateral cell columns has been identified in the rostral ventrolateral medulla,[3] and catecholaminergic neurons in this region appear to participate in regulation of blood pressure by more rostral structures and by baroreflexes; however, whether the rostral ventrolateral medulla cells that project to the sympathetic preganglionic neurons actually use catecholamines as the responsible transmitters now seems unlikely. After exiting the spinal cord, the preganglionic sympathetic axons synapse in the paravertebral chain of sympathetic ganglia and preaortic ganglia. Preganglionic fibers also pass through lower thoracic and lumbar ganglia to form the splanchnic neural innervation of the adrenal medulla. Adrenal nerve activity, therefore, at least partly reflects *preganglionic* outflow, whereas renal nerve sympathetic activity reflects *postganglionic* outflow. At the *ganglionic synapse* and at adrenomedullary cells, the neurotransmitter is ACh.

The postganglionic neurons end in nerve terminals throughout the body, especially in lattice-like networks in the adventitial and adventitial-medial layers of arterioles, where the terminals release NE into the synaptic clefts. Skeletal muscle beds, however, appear to possess both sympathetic noradrenergic and cholinergic innervation, and eccrine sweat glands, involved in thermoregulation, possess sympathetic cholinergic innervation.

The adrenal medulla secretes directly into the bloodstream. The cytoplasm of adrenomedullary cells contains large amounts of *phenylethanolamine N-methyltransferase* (PNMT), which catalyzes the conversion of NE to EPI. EPI constitutes ~85% of the catecholamine content of the adrenal medulla in humans and is the main catecholamine secreted by the gland.

Sympathetic nerve endings are not selectively coupled with single effector cells. Instead, they form plexuses, in which one axon innervates several effector cells and each effector cell receives innervation from several axons.

Fibers from the superior cervical ganglion innervate the head. Cardiac sympathetic innervation emanates from the three cervical sympathetic ganglia (the most caudal being the stellate ganglia) and from the upper thoracic ganglia, converging in the cardiac nerves. Gut organs receive innervation from preaortic plexuses, whereas the pelvic organs derive their innervation from the sacral spinal nerves and pelvic plexuses.

NE is not distributed uniformly in sympathetic nerve endings, but is localized in discrete areas called *varicosities*, ~25,000 of which may occur on a single axon.[4] Each varicosity contains ~1000 membrane-bound vesicles.[5] The electron-dense core found in a proportion of the vesicles is thought to represent ~15,000 molecules of stored NE. The vesicles also contain DA β-hydroxylase (DBH), adenosine triphosphate, and various peptides, including enkephalin, neuropeptide Y, and chromogranin A.

The blood supply to the adrenal medulla is derived from the inferior phrenic artery, the aorta, and the renal artery, and from a corticomedullary portal system originating in the zona reticularis. The last supply provides the anatomic substrate for the influence of adrenocortical steroids on catecholamine biosynthesis.

The parasympathetic nervous system, the other limb of the autonomic nervous system, is derived mainly from *cranial* (vagal) and *sacral* cholinergic efferents. The ganglionic synapses

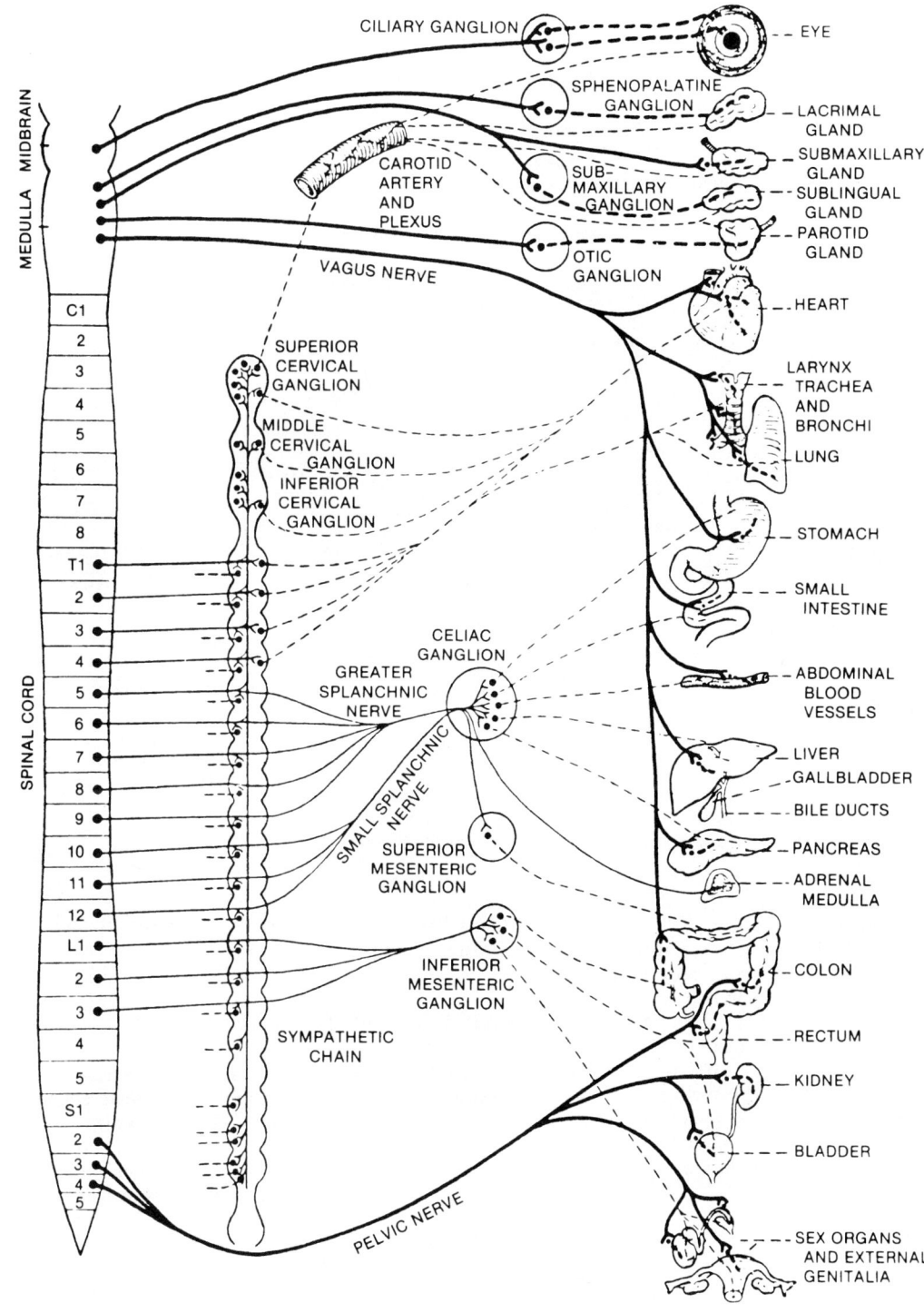

**FIGURE 85-1.** Diagram of efferent autonomic pathways. The *heavy lines* indicate parasympathetic pathways, and the *thin lines* represent sympathetic pathways. The *solid lines* represent preganglionic pathways, and the *dashed lines* postganglionic pathways. Note the emanation of sympathetic fibers predominantly from the thoracolumbar spinal cord, whereas the parasympathetic fibers originate predominantly from the brainstem and the sacral spinal cord. (From Youmans WB. Fundamentals of human physiology, 2nd ed. Chicago: Year Book Medical Publishers, 1962.)

usually are near or embedded in the parenchyma of the innervated organ.

## CATECHOLAMINE SYNTHESIS

The catecholamines contain a catechol (3,4-dihydroxyphenyl) nucleus (Fig. 85-2). Intracellular events in NE synthesis, turnover, and metabolism are depicted in Figure 85-3. The precursor of the catecholamines—the amino acid *tyrosine*—is a dietary constituent as well as a product of hepatic metabolism of dietary *phenylalanine*. Tyrosine is taken up by sympathetic neural tissue and is converted to *dihydroxyphenylalanine* (DOPA) by

the enzyme *tyrosine hydroxylase* (TH).[6,7] The specific enzymatic hydroxylation of tyrosine to DOPA is the rate-limiting step in catecholamine biosynthesis and is end product–inhibited by DOPA, DA, and NE. Although it is known that adrenomedullary chromaffin cells and tissues that possess sympathetic innervation contain TH, it is unknown whether, outside the brain, only sympathetic nerves and adrenomedullary cells contain TH. Current evidence suggests a nonneuronal synthesis of catecholamines.[8]

DOPA is converted to *DA* by *DOPA decarboxylase* (aromatic L-amino acid decarboxylase), which is found in many tissues. DA is taken up into vesicles containing DBH and converted to NE. DBH occurs only in the vesicles of NE- or EPI-synthesizing cells.

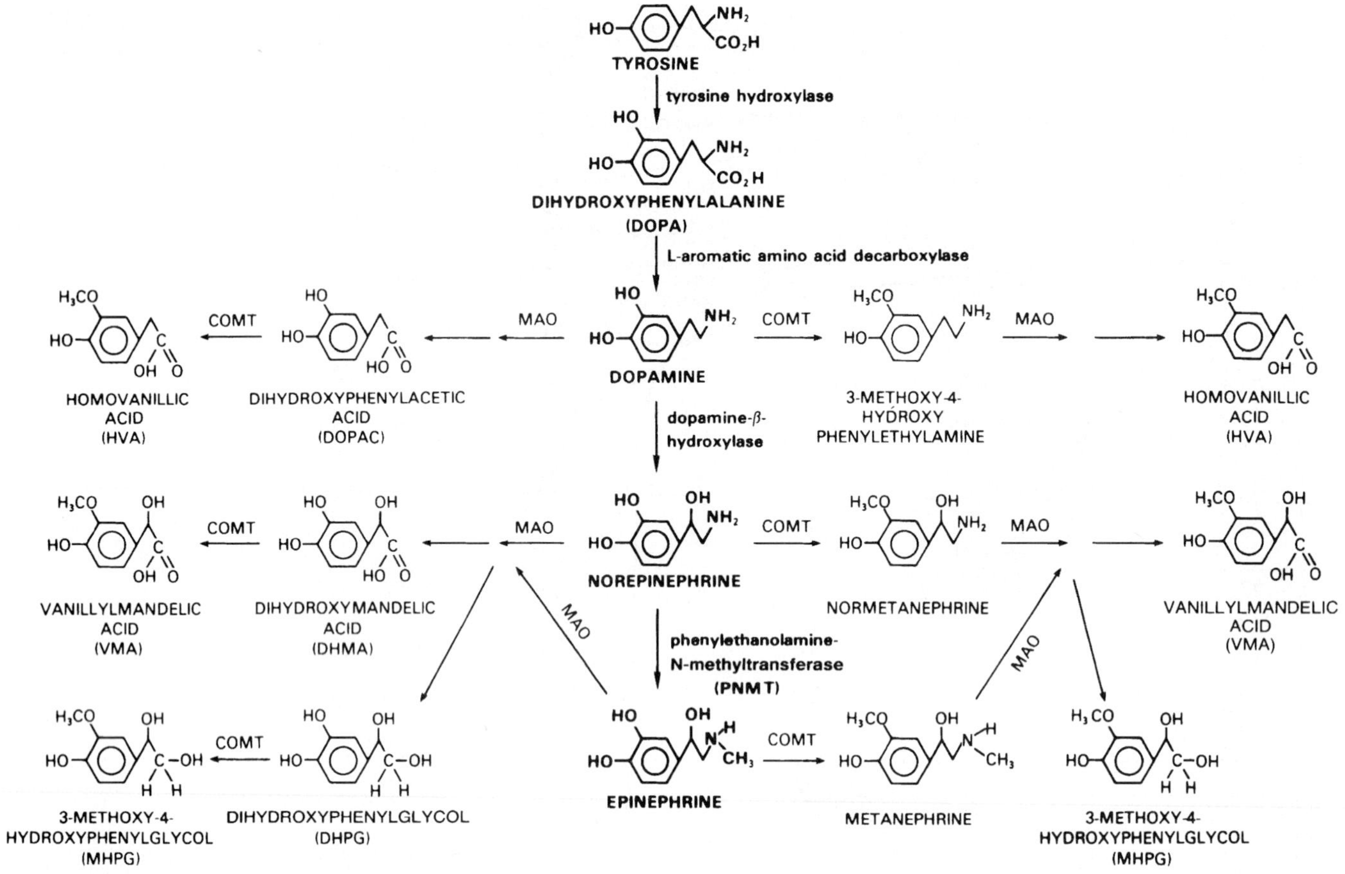

**FIGURE 85-2.** Structures of the endogenous catecholamines and major metabolites are illustrated. Substances in the main pathway of catecholamine biosynthesis appear in *boldface*. (*MAO,* monoamine oxidase; *COMT,* catechol-O-methyltransferase.)

In adrenomedullary tissue, NE is methylated to form EPI by the cytosolic, nonspecific enzyme PNMT.[9] Glucocorticoids, which occur at high concentrations in the adrenal medulla because of the corticomedullary portal system, induce PNMT activity.[10]

The catecholamine content of an organ changes little during sympathetic stimulation because of the small percent of the storage pool released, concurrent stimulation of catecholamine synthesis by induction of TH activity, and efficient recycling of the released NE. TH activity increases in response to loss of feedback inhibition during sympathetically mediated release of neurotransmitter and in response to cellular depolarization.

## CATECHOLAMINE RELEASE

ACh depolarizes chromaffin cells by increasing membrane permeability to sodium. Transmembrane influx of calcium directly or indirectly results from this increase in intracellular sodium; thus, cytoplasmic calcium levels increase. The latter process is thought to be part of an incompletely defined biomechanical final common pathway in cellular activation leading to exocytotic release of vesicular contents.

Indirect evidence suggests that neurosecretion occurs by actual exocytosis of the contents of the storage vesicles. Other soluble vesicular contents—adenosine triphosphate, enkephalins, chromogranins, neuropeptide Y, and DBH—are released during cellular activation, but cytoplasmic macromolecules are not.[11–13] Electron micrographs occasionally have demonstrated the so-called omega sign, as if a defect in the cell membrane were produced at the site of vesicle-plasmalemma fusion. Cytoplasmic NE does not appear to be released by nerve impulses. Sympathomimetic amines release NE by a nonexocytotic pro-

cess because DBH also is not released and because the release is not calcium-dependent.

## CATECHOLAMINE REMOVAL

The most prominent removal mechanism for released NE is reuptake into the presynaptic terminal by a nonstereospecific, energy-requiring process called *uptake-1.*[14,15] Cocaine, tricyclic antidepressants (e.g., desipramine hydrochloride), and ouabain inhibit uptake-1. The hypotensive effect of guanethidine and the hypertensive effect of tyramine depend on uptake of these drugs into presynaptic axons. Therefore, the administration of uptake-1 inhibitors attenuates these effects. Molecular genetic studies have confirmed the existence of a family of neurotransmitter transporters, including distinct transporters for DA and NE. Uptake-1 refers to the transporter for NE in sympathetic nerves.

NE in the axonal cytoplasm can be taken up into vesicles by a stereoselective process, or it can be oxidized by mitochondrial monoamine oxidase. Monoamine oxidase is present in both neural and nonneural tissue, and the deaminated metabolites are rapidly converted to dihydroxyphenylglycol (DHPG)[16] or dihydroxymandelic acid in the cell. Vesicular uptake is not specific for NE, and α-methyldopamine can be taken up into the vesicle, converted to α-methylnorepinephrine, and released during sympathetic stimulation.

NE also can be removed by extraneuronal uptake (uptake-2), a nonstereoselective, energy-requiring process that is inhibited by metanephrine and steroids. Extraneuronal tissues contain catechol-O-methyltransferase (COMT), which converts NE to normetanephrine and EPI to metanephrine. COMT exists pri-

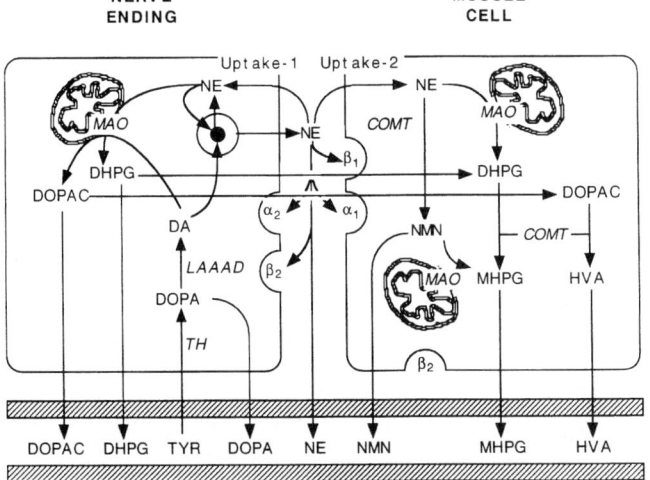

**FIGURE 85-3.** Mechanisms of norepinephrine (*NE*) synthesis, release, and metabolism. Tyrosine (*TYR*) is taken up into sympathetic nerves and converted to dihydroxyphenylalanine (*DOPA*) by tyrosine hydroxylase (*TH*). A small proportion of axoplasmic DOPA enters the bloodstream. DOPA is converted to dopamine (*DA*) by L-aromatic amino-acid decarboxylase (*LAAAD*), and DA is taken up into vesicles containing dopamine β-hydroxylase (*DBH*) and converted to NE, or is deaminated by monoamine oxidase (*MAO*) to form dihydroxyphenylacetic acid (*DOPAC*), the main neuronal metabolite of DA. Vesicular NE can leak into the axoplasm, undergoing deamination to form dihydroxyphenylglycol (*DHPG*), or it can be released by exocytosis. Most of the endogenously released NE is taken back up into the axoplasm by uptake-1. A small proportion of released NE enters the bloodstream or is taken up by extraneuronal uptake (*uptake-2*). NE in extraneuronal cells undergoes O-methylation by catechol-O-methyltransferase (*COMT*) to form normetanephrine (*NMN*), which enters the bloodstream or is deaminated to form methoxyhydroxyphenylglycol (*MHPG*) or (in the liver) to vanillylmandelic acid. DHPG and DOPAC in extraneuronal cells also undergo O-methylation to form MHPG and homovanillic acid (*HVA*), the latter being the main end product of DA metabolism.

marily in extraneuronal tissues, especially the liver and kidney. Adrenomedullary cells also contain COMT, and O-methylation of catecholamines in the adrenal gland constitutes the main determinant of circulating concentrations of metanephrines, both in healthy individuals and in patients harboring catecholamine-secreting adrenal tumors.[17] Products of combined actions of monoamine oxidase and COMT include vanillylmandelic acid and methoxyhydroxyphenylglycol, the former produced mainly in the liver and the latter produced in sympathetically innervated organs.

## PRESYNAPTIC MODULATION

NE can regulate its own release, by stimulating presynaptic, inhibitory $\alpha_2$-adrenergic receptors.[18,19] Other inhibitors of NE release that appear to act presynaptically include ACh,[20] DA, prostaglandins of the E series,[21] histamine, and purines. Stimulatory modulators include angiotensin II[22] and EPI, the latter of which appears to stimulate presynaptic $\beta_2$-adrenergic receptors. Substantial clinical evidence supports modulation of NE release by $\alpha_2$-adrenoceptors.[23] The roles of the other endogenous compounds remain less well established.

## ADRENERGIC RECEPTORS

Specific receptors for catecholamines exist in several tissues, including muscle (skeletal, myocardial, vascular, gastrointesti-

nal, ciliary, and bronchial) and glands (salivary, sweat, adrenocortical, and pancreatic).[24] These receptors mediate the effects of endogenously released as well as exogenously administered catecholamines (Table 85-1).

Ahlquist[25] introduced the concept of $\alpha$- and $\beta$-adrenergic receptors to explain contrasting cardiovascular responses to exogenous catecholamines. NE administration causes diffuse vasoconstriction and reflexive bradycardia, whereas EPI causes vasodilation of skeletal muscle beds, tachycardia, and increased myocardial contractility. According to this framework, the vasoconstrictor actions of NE and EPI result from stimulation of $\alpha$-adrenergic receptors, whereas the cardiotonic, tachycardiac, and vasodilator properties of EPI result from stimulation of $\beta$-adrenergic receptors.

Further subclassification to $\alpha_1$-, $\alpha_2$-, $\beta_1$-, and $\beta_2$-adrenergic receptors has been based on ligand-binding studies, on responses to synthetic agonists and antagonists, and on molecular genetic experiments.[26–28] *NE is an agonist at $\beta_1$-, $\alpha_1$-, and $\alpha_2$-adrenergic receptors, whereas EPI is an agonist at all four subtypes.* Stimulation of $\alpha_1$-receptors causes vasoconstriction. Phenylephrine is an example of a relatively specific $\alpha_1$-agonist, and prazosin is an example of an $\alpha_1$-antagonist. $\alpha_2$-Selective agonists, such as clonidine hydrochloride,[29] $\alpha$-methyldopa, and guanabenz,[30] exert more complex effects, because stimulation of $\alpha_2$-receptors on vascular smooth muscle cells elicits vasoconstriction and increased blood pressure, whereas stimulation of presynaptic $\alpha_2$-receptors inhibits NE release from sympathetic nerve endings, and stimulation of $\alpha_2$-receptors in the central nervous system causes decreases in sympathetic outflow and increases in vagal outflow. The latter effects predominate, and $\alpha_2$-agonists are used as antihypertensive medications. $\alpha_2$-Antagonists (e.g., yohimbine) cause increases in plasma NE, as well as a psychiatric pattern of heightened arousal and tremulousness, in contrast with the sedation induced by $\alpha_2$-agonists. Pharmacologic and molecular genetic studies have demonstrated the existence of several subtypes of $\alpha_2$-adrenoceptors. The structure of the subtype responsible for modulation of NE release from sympathetic nerves remains unknown.

$\beta_1$-Agonists increase heart rate, cardiac conduction velocity, and myocardial contractility, and produce lipolysis. In contrast, $\beta_2$-agonists (e.g., terbutaline sulfate and albuterol) predominantly cause skeletal muscle vasodilation, bronchial and gastrointestinal smooth muscle relaxation, increased renin secretion from the kidney, glycogenolysis, and enhanced release of NE from sympathetic nerve terminals. Because of the latter effect, $\beta_2$-agonists actually may elicit delayed constriction in some vascular beds. Relatively selective $\beta_1$-antagonists are being used with increasing frequency for cardiovascular disorders, such as angina pectoris, arrhythmias, and hypertension, because nonselective $\beta$-antagonists can aggravate bronchospastic responsiveness. Examples of $\beta_1$-adrenergic receptor-selective medications are atenolol and metoprolol. A third type of $\beta$-adrenoceptor has been described, $\beta_3$, which probably participates in catecholamine-induced lipolysis.

The intracellular mechanisms activated by $\alpha$-adrenergic receptor stimulation appear to be subtype-selective. Stimulation of $\alpha_1$-receptors releases ionized calcium into the cytoplasm from intracellular stores, by activation of the inositol triphosphate pathway[31] (see Chap. 4). Stimulation of $\alpha_2$-receptors appears to inhibit the adenylate cyclase–cyclic adenosine monophosphate (cAMP) system. Both $\beta_1$- and $\beta_2$-adrenergic receptor agonists stimulate the adenylate cyclase–cAMP system. The exact mechanism of inhibition of NE release by $\alpha_2$-adrenoceptor stimulation remains unknown.

The calculated number of adrenoceptors on cell surfaces can increase (up-regulate) or decrease (down-regulate) in response to changes in agonist concentrations at $\alpha$- or $\beta$-adrenergic receptors. Altered numbers of adrenergic receptors, altered affinity for catecholamines, or altered intracellular actions distal to receptor occupation provide explanations for tachyphylaxis

**TABLE 85-1.**
**Responses of Effector Organs to Autonomic Nerve Impulses**

| Effector Organs | Adrenergic Impulses | | Cholinergic Impulses |
|---|---|---|---|
| | Receptor Type | Responses* | Responses* |
| **EYE** | | | |
| Radial muscle, iris | $\alpha_1$ | Contraction (mydriasis)† | — |
| Sphincter muscle, iris | | — | Contraction (miosis)‡ |
| Ciliary muscle | $\beta$ | Relaxation for far vision§ | Contraction for near vision‡ |
| **HEART** | | | |
| Sinoatrial node | $\beta_1$ | Increase in heart rate† | Decrease in heart rate; vagal arrest‡ |
| Atria | $\beta_1$ | Increase in contractility and conduction velocity† | Decrease in contractility, and shortened action-potential duration† |
| Atrioventricular node | $\beta_1$ | Increase in automaticity and conduction velocity† | Decrease in conduction velocity; atrioventricular block‡ |
| His-Purkinje system | $\beta_1$ | Increase in automaticity and conduction velocity‡ | Little effect |
| Ventricles | $\beta_1$ | Increase in contractility, conduction velocity, automaticity, and rate of idioventricular pacemakers‡ | Slight decrease in contractility claimed by some |
| **ARTERIOLES** | | | |
| Coronary | $\alpha$; $\beta_2$ | Constriction§; dilatation‡†¶ | Dilatation‡ |
| Skin and mucosa | $\alpha$ | Constriction‡ | Dilatation¶ |
| Skeletal muscle | $\alpha$; $\beta_2$ | Constriction†; dilatation†¶# | Dilatation§** |
| Cerebral | $\alpha$ | Constriction (slight) | Dilatation¶ |
| Pulmonary | $\alpha$; $\beta_2$ | Constriction§; dilatation¶ | Dilatation¶ |
| Abdominal viscera | $\alpha$; $\beta_2$ | Constriction‡; dilatation§# | — |
| Salivary glands | $\alpha$ | Constriction‡ | Dilatation† |
| **RENAL** | $\alpha_1$; $\beta_1$; $\beta_2$ | Constriction‡; dilatation§# | — |
| **VEINS (SYSTEMIC)** | $\alpha$; $\beta_2$ | Constriction†; dilatation† | — |
| **LUNG** | | | |
| Tracheal and bronchial muscle | $\beta_2$ | Relaxation§ | Contraction† |
| Bronchial glands | $\alpha_1$; $\beta_2$ | Decreased secretion; increased secretion | Stimulation‡ |
| **STOMACH** | | | |
| Motility and tone | $\alpha_2$; $\beta_2$ | Decreased (usually)†§ | Increased‡ |
| Sphincters | $\alpha$ | Contraction (usually)§ | Relaxation (usually)§ |
| Secretion | | Inhibition (?) | Stimulation† |
| **INTESTINE** | | | |
| Motility and tone | $\alpha_1$; $\alpha_2$; $\beta_2$ | Decreased†§ | Increased† |
| Sphincters | $\alpha$ | Contraction (usually)§ | Relaxation (usually)§ |
| Secretion | | Inhibition (?) | Stimulation† |
| **GALLBLADDER AND DUCTS** | $\beta_2$ | Relaxation§ | Contraction§ |
| **KIDNEY** | $\beta_1$ | Renin secretion† | — |
| **URINARY BLADDER** | | | |
| Detrusor | $\beta$ | Relaxation (usually)§ | Contraction‡ |
| Trigone and sphincter | $\alpha$ | Contraction† | Relaxation† |
| **URETER** | | | |
| Motility and tone | $\alpha$ | Increased | Increased (?) |
| **UTERUS** | $\alpha$; $\beta_2$ | Pregnant: contraction ($\alpha$); relaxation ($\beta_2$). Nonpregnant: relaxation ($\beta_2$) | Variables†† |
| **SEX ORGANS, MALE** | $\alpha$ | Ejaculation‡ | Erection‡ |
| **SKIN** | | | |
| Pilomotor muscles | $\alpha$ | Contraction† | — |
| Sweat glands | $\alpha$ | Localized secretion§ §§ | Generalized secretion‡ |
| **SPLEEN CAPSULE** | $\alpha$; $\beta_2$ | Contraction‡; relaxation§ | — |
| **ADRENAL MEDULLA** | | — | Secretion of epinephrine and norepinephrine (nicotinic effect) |
| **SKELETAL MUSCLE** | $\beta_2$ | Increased contractility, glycogenolysis, K⁺ uptake | — |
| **LIVER** | $\alpha$; $\beta_2$ | Glycogenolysis and gluconeogenesis‡ | Glycogen synthesis§ |
| **PANCREAS** | | | |
| Acini | $\alpha$ | Decreased secretion§ | Secretion† |
| Islets (B cells) | $\alpha_2$ | Decreased secretion‡ | — |
| | $\beta_2$ | Increased secretion§ | — |
| **FAT CELLS** | $\alpha$; $\beta_1$ | Lipolysis‡ | — |
| **SALIVARY GLANDS** | $\alpha_1$ | Potassium and water secretion§ | Potassium and water secretion‡ |
| | $\beta$ | Amylase secretion§ | |
| **LACRIMAL GLANDS** | | — | Secretion‡ |
| **NASOPHARYNGEAL GLANDS** | | — | Secretion† |

(continued)

**TABLE 85-1. (continued)**

| Effector Organs | Adrenergic Impulses | | Cholinergic Impulses |
| | Receptor Type | Responses* | Responses* |
| --- | --- | --- | --- |
| PINEAL GLAND | β | Melatonin synthesis | — |
| POSTERIOR PITUITARY | β₁ | Antidiuretic hormone secretion | — |

*Responses are designated 1+ to 3+ to provide an approximate indication of the importance of adrenergic and cholinergic nerve activity in the control of the various organs and functions listed. A *long dash* signifies no known functional innervation.

†It has been proposed that adrenergic fibers terminate at inhibitory β-receptors on smooth muscle fibers, and at inhibitory α-receptors on parasympathetic cholinergic (excitatory) ganglion cells of Auerbach's plexus.

‡There is significant variation among species in the type of receptor that mediates certain metabolic responses; α and β responses have not been determined in humans.

§Dilatation predominates in situ because of metabolic autoregulatory phenomena.

¶Cholinergic vasodilatation at these sites is of questionable physiologic significance.

#Over the usual concentration range of physiologically released, circulating epinephrine, β-receptor response (vasodilatation) predominates in blood vessels of skeletal muscle and liver; α-receptor response (vasoconstriction) predominates in blood vessels of other abdominal viscera. The renal and mesenteric vessels also contain specific dopaminergic receptors, activation of which causes dilation.

**Sympathetic cholinergic system causes vasodilatation in skeletal muscle, but this is not involved in most physiologic responses.

††Depends on stage of menstrual cycle, amount of circulating estrogen and progesterone, and other factors.

§§Palms of hands and some other sites (adrenergic sweating).

(From Goodman LS, Gilman AG, eds. The pharmacologic basis of therapeutics, 7th ed. New York: Macmillan, 1985:72.)

(e.g., decreasing responsiveness to β-agonists after repeated administration to patients with asthma) and sensitization (e.g., increasing pressor responsiveness to administered NE in patients with idiopathic orthostatic hypotension).[32–35] Thyroid hormones and glucocorticoids can potentiate β-adrenergic receptor–mediated responses.[36] It has been proposed that decreased β-adrenergic receptor numbers in congestive heart failure may result from chronically increased release of endogenous NE.[35]

Although alterations in receptor numbers or in intracellular biomechanical events can affect responses to agonists, the main determinant of physiologic responses to sympathoadrenal activation is the amount of endogenous catecholamines released from the sympathetic nerve endings and the adrenal medulla, which reach adrenoceptors on effector cells.

## EFFECTS OF CATECHOLAMINES

### CIRCULATION

Cardiovascular function, both at rest and during stress, unquestionably depends on sympathetic neural activity. Interference with sympathetic outflow or inhibition of NE release from sympathetic nerve endings causes the blood pressure to decrease even in resting, healthy adults, and β-adrenergic receptor blockade causes a decrease in heart rate at rest, as well as attenuated heart rate responses to stress.

Circulatory responses during orthostasis, altered regional and total body metabolic demands imposed by exercise, changes in environmental temperature, hemorrhage, hypoglycemia, hypoxia, and emotion occur predominantly by patterned sympathoneural and adrenomedullary activation. Sympathetic stimulation causes tachycardia, increased cardiac inotropism, increasingly rapid cardiac conduction, acceleration of myocyte spontaneous depolarization, increased resistance to blood flow in most vascular beds, and venous constriction. Because of relatively scanty sympathetic innervation of the coronary and cerebral vessels, diffuse sympathetic stimulation generally preserves blood flow to these vital organs. Total peripheral resistance may remain unchanged or may decrease, depending on the extent of EPI-induced skeletal muscle vasodilation.

More indirect or longer-term effects of sympathoadrenal activation on circulatory function include (a) antidiuresis and stimulation of renal sodium retention by direct tubular effects, as well as by enhanced renin-angiotensin-aldosterone system activity, reduced intrarenal hydrostatic pressure, and increased vasopressin secretion, possibly shunting corticomedullary blood flow[37–46]; (b) stimulation of cell growth and division in cardiac and vascular smooth muscle tissue[42,43]; (c) α₂-adrenergic receptor–mediated promotion of platelet aggregation; (d) shunting of blood toward the cardiopulmonary region, which causes stimulation of low-pressure cardiac baroreceptors; and (e) adrenoceptor down-regulation.

### METABOLISM

Metabolic effects of pharmacologic doses of EPI include nonshivering thermogenesis, hyperglycemia, hyperlipidemia, hypokalemia, and increased oxygen consumption.[47–53] Most of these actions arise from β-receptor–mediated stimulation of adenylate cyclase in cell membranes, which catalyzes the conversion of adenosine triphosphate to cAMP in the cell. Mechanisms for the hyperglycemic response to EPI include stimulation of hepatic glycogen phosphorylase, the rate-limiting catalytic step in glycogenolysis; inhibition of glycogen synthase; stimulation of gluconeogenesis from amino acids and lactate; α-adrenergic receptor–mediated inhibition of insulin secretion; and stimulation of pancreatic secretion of glucagon.

### VISCERAL EFFECTS

Stimulation of α₁-adrenergic receptor causes smooth muscle contraction, and β₂-receptor stimulation of smooth muscle causes relaxation. Catecholamines also may produce indirect visceral effects by modifying ACh release at parasympathetic nerve terminals (see Table 85-1).

Catecholamines diffusely inhibit gut motility. They stimulate myoepithelial cells in the breast and ovary, affecting lactation and ovulation. Because DA inhibits prolactin secretion, the DA receptor agonist, bromocriptine, had been used to stop lactation in women after childbirth, but this indication was rescinded by the U.S. Food and Drug Administration.

Axillary sweating is stimulated by sympathetic noradrenergic innervation of apocrine glands. Eccrine glands, which participate importantly in thermoregulation, receive sympathetic cholinergic innervation.

In the eye, catecholamines stimulate secretion into the aqueous humor, and β-blockade is an established mode of therapy for some forms of glaucoma.[54] Stimulation of the sympathetic innervation of the iris from the superior cervical ganglia produces mydriasis, whereas interruption of this innervation produces Horner syndrome, characterized by ptosis, myosis, and facial anhidrosis.

Catecholamines affect the function of virtually all endocrine systems.[54] Generally, β-adrenergic receptor stimulation accentuates release of preformed hormone, whereas α-adrenergic receptor agonism attenuates the action of the physiologic stimulus for secretion of the hormone. In the kidneys, NE and EPI promote antinatriuresis by decreasing renal blood flow and increasing secretion of renin, whereas DA promotes natriuresis by increasing renal blood flow and inhibiting $Na^+/K^+$ adenosine triphosphatase in proximal tubular cells.

## CIRCULATING CATECHOLAMINES AND ACTIVITIES OF THE SYMPATHONEURAL AND ADRENOMEDULLARY SYSTEMS

Much of the catecholamine content of human plasma is sulfo-conjugated, especially DA, which is ~98% conjugated in peripheral blood. Most of DA sulfate production in humans occurs in the gastrointestinal tract.[55] Some of the free (i.e., non-conjugated) catecholamines circulate bound loosely to protein. The significance of this protein binding also is unclear.

NE and DA are not hemocrine hormones. That is, the cardiovascular and metabolic effects of these catecholamines require supraphysiologic plasma concentrations. In contrast, even within a physiologic range, circulating EPI can exert circulatory and metabolic effects. Therefore, EPI may be considered to be a hemocrine hormone.

Free and conjugated catecholamines and catecholamine metabolites are excreted in the urine. The renal mechanisms involved are poorly understood. By far the predominant free catecholamine in human urine is DA, and the main catechol is dihydroxyphenylacetic acid.[56] The prominence of DA and its metabolites in human urine, in contrast with NE, EPI, and their metabolites, remains unexplained. The measurement of total urinary catechol or catecholamine excretion, therefore, is not as useful a screening test for pheochromocytoma as is the measurement of the excretion of metabolites of NE and EPI.

The urinary excretion of DA in humans exceeds its renal clearance; a proportion of urinary DA must come from DA released by the kidney itself. In humans, most or all of urinary DA is derived from plasma levodopa (L-dopa).[56]

In the antecubital venous blood of resting, supine, healthy persons, plasma levels of NE average approximately 100 to 400 pg/mL, and those of EPI average ~5 to 50 pg/mL. Plasma levels of EPI can be less than 5 pg/mL, whereas plasma NE is detectable even in patients with sympathetic failure or those who are undergoing ganglion blockade. Plasma NE increases as a function of age among healthy persons,[57] but plasma EPI does not.

Catecholamine concentrations in antecubital venous blood are commonly used to indicate overall sympathetic "tone."[58,59] The validity of this application requires consideration of a few important principles. First, owing to the several removal mechanisms for NE, a large cleft-to-plasma concentration gradient exists, determined primarily by uptake-1.[60] Medications or pathologic states associated with inhibition of uptake-1 or overall NE removal may result in overestimation of sympathetic outflow. Second, the vasculature of the arm possesses extensive sympathetic innervation and contributes importantly to NE in the venous drainage. Third, any of several modulators can act presynaptically to enhance or attenuate NE release for a given amount of sympathetic nerve traffic. Last, sympathoneural responses are not always homogeneous among the several vascular beds, so that measuring antecubital venous plasma NE may not detect regional abnormalities in sympathetic outflow.

An effective blood–brain barrier exists for catecholamines. Because adrenalectomized patients have normal plasma NE levels, plasma NE in humans is thought to be derived mainly from peripheral sympathetic nerve endings.

The complex origin of plasma NE contrasts with the simple, single origin of plasma EPI from the adrenal medulla. The view that the level of plasma EPI provides the best measure of overall sympathetic outflow ignores differential changes in plasma NE and EPI during different forms of stress. The level of plasma EPI does provide a fairly direct assessment of adrenomedullary secretion.

The amount of regional release of NE into the venous drainage ("spillover") can be measured from the regional removal of NE, the arteriovenous increment in NE across the bed, and regional blood flow. The regional removal of NE can be assessed by determining the concentrations of radioactive and total NE in arterial and regional venous blood during the infusion of tracer-labeled NE.[61–63]

Combined measurements of catecholamines and their metabolites provide information about rates of uptake, turnover, and metabolism of NE. Plasma DHPG reflects intraneuronal metabolism of axoplasmic NE and, thereby, the turnover of vesicular NE, and plasma DOPA and dihydroxyphenylacetic acid partly reflect catecholamine biosynthesis. Because catecholamine synthesis normally balances turnover in sympathetic nerves, plasma DHPG levels correlate positively with plasma DOPA levels in humans.[64]

Many factors that are both common and difficult to control influence plasma levels of catecholamines. These include psychological stress, altered environmental temperature, posture (plasma NE doubles within 5 minutes of standing), exercise, hospitalization, medications, and sodium intake (salt restriction increases plasma NE[65]). Thus, the conditions of blood sampling must be monitored carefully.

One clinical method for sampling blood for catecholamine determinations includes testing at a consistent time of day at least 12 hours after the subject has discontinued smoking, alcohol ingestion, and ingestion of caffeine-containing foodstuffs, and after several days of a diet containing a normal amount of salt, as indicated by 24-hour urinary sodium excretion. Because even decaffeinated coffee contains caffeic acid, a catechol converted to dihydrocaffeic acid by gut bacteria, and because dihydrocaffeic acid can cause spuriously high levels of EPI or DA, even decaffeinated coffee should not be ingested for ~12 hours before testing.[66] Acetaminophen interferes with liquid chromatographic-electrochemical assays for normetanephrine.[67] For testing, the subject lies supine with an indwelling intravenous catheter or needle in place for at least 20 minutes before phlebotomy is performed without a tourniquet. The blood is drawn into a chilled, evacuated, heparinized glass tube; additives are unnecessary. The plasma is stored at –70°C or colder until the time of assay. Because virtually any medication can affect plasma catecholamine levels, it is advisable, if possible, to discontinue the use of all medications (particularly antihypertensive medications) for at least 2 weeks before testing.

Plasma catecholamines can be measured accurately by radioenzymatic assay[68] or liquid chromatography with electrochemical detection (LCED).[69] LCED has largely supplanted older radioenzymatic assay procedures, because it is less expensive, does not involve radionuclides, and can be used for simultaneous measurements of the catechols DOPA, dihydroxyphenylacetic acid, NE, EPI, DA, DHPG (the main intraneuronal metabolite of NE), and synthetic catecholamines used clinically as pressors.

## DIRECT MEASUREMENT OF SYMPATHETIC NEURAL ACTIVITY

Microneurography can measure sympathetic neural activity from the rate of pulse-synchronous bursts of directly recorded activity in a peripheral nerve, such as the peroneal nerve, supplying skeletal muscle.[70,71] This approach avoids many interpretational difficulties associated with catecholamine measurements, but the procedure requires extensive technical training and cannot measure sympathetic outflow in visceral vascular beds.

When skeletal muscle sympathetic activity has been compared with antecubital venous plasma NE, the agreement between these values has been surprisingly strong.[72,73] The agreement probably reflects concurrent changes in sympathetic outflows to several beds.

## OTHER METHODS

Power spectra of heart rate variability include a low-frequency component thought to reflect cardiac sympathetic tone. Parasympathetic activity also influences this component, however, and no studies have demonstrated the validity of analyses of heart rate variability in specifically indicating cardiac sympathetic activity in humans.

Nuclear scanning after the injection of radioactive sympathomimetic amines or catecholamines can visualize cardiac sympathetic innervation and may enable assessment of cardiac sympathetic function.[74,75]

## PATTERNS OF CATECHOLAMINERGIC ACTIVATION

Sympathoneural and adrenomedullary activation in response to physiologic or pharmacologic manipulations can be generalized or patterned. Consideration of the appropriateness of adjustments to a particular challenge can help to explain the observed patterns of responses.

Sympathetic neural outflow to most vascular beds increases in response to orthostasis, isometric exercise, exposure to cold, and extracellular volume depletion; thus, plasma NE increases.[76] Pharmacologic agents such as amphetamine, tyramine, clonidine, and isoproterenol also affect plasma NE levels preferentially. The pharmacologic findings imply that mechanisms of modulation of catecholamine release may differ between sympathetic nerve endings and adrenomedullary cells. The physiologic stimuli have in common a relatively minor influence on compensatory mechanisms for fuel production or utilization and seem mainly to elicit sympathetic neural responses leading to appropriate shifts in blood flow distribution or glandular secretion. Stimulation of arterial "high-pressure" baroreceptors appears to inhibit sympathetic outflow diffusely, although with quantitative differences among regional beds.[77]

Adrenomedullary activity increases markedly in response to hypoglycemia, hemorrhage, asphyxiation, circulatory collapse, and emotional distress; therefore, plasma EPI increases to a greater extent than does plasma NE in these situations.[77-79] Because of the potential threat to the organism's existence, even small decreases in levels of glucose trigger circulatory, metabolic, and visceral responses to maximize delivery of this vital fuel; adrenomedullary activation contributes importantly to these responses.

Many stimuli, when intense, elicit combined adrenomedullary and sympathetic neural discharge. The resulting syndrome—tachycardia, vasoconstriction, pallor, sweating, pupillary dilation, hyperglycemia, renal retention of sodium, ileus, hyperventilation, piloerection ("gooseflesh"), and agitation—defines the appearance of a patient in shock and has awed clinicians since ancient times.

The pattern of catecholaminergic responses to psychological stress in humans appears to be analogous to that associated with the defense reaction in animals preparing for fight-or-flight responses. Renal, gut, and cutaneous vasoconstriction occur, along with skeletal muscle vasodilation, tachycardia, and predominantly systolic hypertension. One theory about the pathogenesis of essential hypertension states that susceptible persons undergo many defense reactions daily in response to conditional stimuli, without the actual physical fight-or-flight behavior occurring. These chronically repeated pressor episodes eventually lead to more long-lasting structural adaptation of the arterioles. Because, in these situations, skeletal muscle sympathetic outflow increases little, or decreases, and because the arm contributes importantly to NE levels in its venous drainage, plasma NE levels in antecubital venous blood may change little.[80]

Vasodepressor responses involve skeletal vasodilation; cutaneous, renal, and gut vasoconstriction; EPI release; and vagally mediated bradycardia. Directly recorded skeletal sympathetic activity decreases markedly during these responses, and plasma NE fails to increase.[81,82]

Patterning of catecholaminergic responses to different stressors argues against the doctrine of nonspecificity,[83] a founding principle of the stress theory of Hans Selye, who introduced and popularized the notion of stress as a medical scientific idea. Alternatively, stress responses may contain a degree of primitive specificity, reflecting the evolution of adaptively advantageous patterns of responses involving several effector systems, including catecholaminergic systems.

Abel first deduced the chemical structure of a hormone; EPI. Elliott's hypothesis about the neuronal release of an "EPI-like substance" foreshadowed the theory of chemical neurotransmission. The discovery of cAMP, the first identified intracellular messenger, and of cellular activation by phosphorylation, depended on a knowledge of the hormonal effects of EPI. Ahlquist's explanation for the different effects of catecholamines, and Iversen's and Axelrod's findings about the disposition of catecholamines, led to the identification of the molecular structures of adrenoceptors and catecholamine transporters and to the discovery of pharmacologic agents now widely used in cardiology, neurology, and psychiatry. Thus, for a century, the study of catecholaminergic systems has proved to be a most fruitful endeavor. If the overall goal of physiologic research is to identify the "algorithms" that the body uses to maintain the internal environment, medical history predicts that catecholamine research will spearhead this quest.

## REFERENCES

1. Goldstein DS. Stress, catecholamines, and cardiovascular disease. New York: Oxford University Press, 1995.
2. Gabella G. Structure of the autonomic nervous system. London: Chapman & Hall, 1976.
3. Reis DJ, Granata AR, Joh TH, et al. Brain stem catecholamine mechanisms in tonic and reflex control of blood pressure. Hypertension 1984; 6:117.
4. Dahlström A, Haggendal J. Some quantitative studies on the noradrenaline content in the cell bodies and terminals of a sympathetic adrenergic neuron system. Acta Physiol Scand 1966; 67:271.
5. Geffen LB, Livett BG. Synaptic vesicles in sympathetic neurons. Physiol Rev 1971; 9:119.
6. Blaschko H. Catecholamine biosynthesis. Br Med Bull 1973; 29:105.
7. Udenfriend S. Tyrosine hydroxylase. Pharmacol Rev 1966; 18:43.
8. Kawamura M, Schwartz JP, Nomura T, et al. Differential effects of chemical sympathectomy on expression and activity of tyrosine hydroxylase and levels of catecholamines and DOPA in peripheral tissues of rats. Neurochem Res 1999; 24:25.
9. Axelrod J. Methylation reactions in the formation and metabolism of catecholamines and other biogenic amines. Pharmacol Rev 1966; 18:95.
10. Wurtman RJ, Axelrod J. Control of enzymatic synthesis of adrenaline in the adrenal medulla by adrenal cortical steroids. J Biol Chem 1966; 241:2301.
11. Slotkin TA, Kirshner N. All-or-none secretion of adrenal medullary storage vesicle contents in the rat. Biochem Pharmacol 1973; 22:205.
12. Smith AD. Mechanisms involved in the release of noradrenaline from sympathetic nerves. Br Med Bull 1973; 29:123.
13. Weinshilboum RM, Thoa NB, Johnson DG, et al. Proportional release of norepinephrine and dopamine-beta-hydroxylase from sympathetic nerves. Science 1971; 174:1349.
14. Iverson LL. Catecholamine uptake process. Br Med Bull 1973; 29:130.
15. Iverson LL. The uptake and storage of noradrenaline in sympathetic nerves. Cambridge: Cambridge University Press, 1967.
16. Eisenhofer G, Keiser HR, Friberg P, et al. Plasma metanephrines are markers of pheochromocytoma produced by catechol-O-methyltransferase within tumors. J Clin Endocrinol Metab 1998; 83:2175.

17. Goldstein DS, Eisenhofer G, Stull R, et al. Plasma dihydroxyphenylglycol and the intraneuronal disposition of norepinephrine in humans. J Clin Invest 1988; 81:213.
18. Goldstein DS, Golczynska A, Stuhlmuller J, et al. A test of the "epinephrine hypothesis" in humans. Hypertension 1999; 33:36.
19. Langer SZ. Presynaptic regulation of catecholamine release. Biochem Pharmacol 1974; 23:1793.
20. Levy MN, Blattberg B. Effect of vagal stimulation on the overflow of norepinephrine into the coronary sinus during cardiac sympathetic nerve stimulation in the dog. Circ Res 1976; 38:81.
21. Hedqvist P. Modulating effect of prostaglandin E-2 on noradrenaline release from the isolated cat spleen. Acta Physiol Scand 1969; 75:511.
22. Zimmerman BG. Adrenergic facilitation by angiotensin: does it serve a physiological function? Clin Sci 1976; 39:566.
23. Grossman E, Chang PC, Hoffman A, et al. Evidence for functional $\alpha_2$-adrenoceptors on vascular sympathetic nerve endings in the human forearm. Circ Res 1991; 69:887.
24. O'Dowd BF, Lefkowitz RJ, Caron MG. Structure of the adrenergic and related receptors. Annu Rev Neurosci 1989; 12:67.
25. Ahlquist RP. A study of the adrenotropic receptors. Am J Physiol 1948; 153:586.
26. Lefkowitz RJ. Direct binding studies of adrenergic receptors: biochemical, physiologic and clinical implications. Ann Intern Med 1979; 91:450.
27. Hoffman BB, Lefkowitz RJ. Alpha-adrenergic receptor subtypes. N Engl J Med 1980; 302:1390.
28. Motulsky HJ, Insel PA. Adrenergic receptors in man. Direct identification, physiologic regulation, and clinical alterations. N Engl J Med 1982; 307:18.
29. Jarrott B, Conway EL, Maccarrone C, Lewis SJ. Clonidine: understanding its disposition, sites and mechanism of action. Clin Exp Pharmacol Physiol 1987; 14:471.
30. Gehr M, MacCarthy EP, Goldberg M. Guanabenz: a centrally acting natriuretic antihypertensive drug. Kidney Int 1986; 29:1203.
31. Minneman KP. $\alpha_1$-Adrenergic receptor subtypes, inositol phosphates, and sources of cell $Ca^{2+}$. Pharmacol Rev 1988; 40:87.
32. Hollister AS, FitzGerald GA, Nadeau JHJ. Acute reduction in human platelet alpha-2-adrenoceptor affinity for agonist by endogenous and exogenous catecholamines. J Clin Invest 1983; 72:1498.
33. Fraser J, Nadeau J, Robertson D, Wood AJ. Regulation of human leukocyte beta receptors by endogenous catecholamines: relationship of leukocyte beta receptor density to the cardiac sensitivity to isoproterenol. J Clin Invest 1981; 67:1777.
34. Krall JF, Connelly M, Tuck ML. Acute regulation of beta adrenergic catecholamine sensitivity in human lymphocytes. J Pharmacol Exp Ther 1980; 214:554.
35. Bristow MR, Ginsburg R, Minobe W, et al. Decreased catecholamine sensitivity and beta-adrenergic-receptor density in failing human hearts. N Engl J Med 1982; 307:205.
36. Williams LT, Lefkowitz RJ, Watanabe AM, et al. Thyroid hormone regulation of beta-adrenergic receptor number. J Biol Chem 1977; 252:2787.
37. Gottshall RW, Itskovitz HD. Redistribution of renal cortical blood flow by renal nerve stimulation and norepinephrine infusion. Proc Soc Exp Biol Med 1977; 164:60.
38. Gottschalk CW. Renal nerves and sodium excretion. Annu Rev Physiol 1979; 41:229.
39. Prosnitz EH, DiBona GF. Effect of decreased renal sympathetic nerve activity on renal tubular sodium reabsorption. Am J Physiol 1978; 235:F557.
40. Bello-Reuss E, Trevino DL, Gottschalk CW. Effect of renal sympathetic nerve stimulation on proximal water and sodium reabsorption. J Clin Invest 1976; 57:1104.
41. Wagermark J, Ungerstedt U, Ljungqvist A. Sympathetic innervation of the juxtaglomerular cells of the kidney. Circ Res 1968; 22:149.
42. Bevan RS, Tsuru H. Functional and structural changes in the rabbit ear artery after sympathetic denervation. Circ Res 1981; 49:478.
43. Simpson P, McGrath A. Norepinephrine-stimulated hypertrophy of cultured rat myocardial cells is an alpha-1 adrenergic response. J Clin Invest 1983; 72:732.
44. Levi J, Coburn J, Kleeman CR. Mechanism of the antidiuretic effect of beta-adrenergic stimulation in man. Arch Intern Med 1976; 136:25.
45. Shimamoto K, Miyahara ML. Effect of norepinephrine infusion on plasma vasopressin levels in normal human subjects. J Clin Endocrinol Metab 1976; 43:201.
46. Berl T, Cadnapaphornchai P, Harbottle JA, Schrier RW. Mechanism of stimulation of vasopressin release during beta-adrenergic stimulation with isoproterenol. J Clin Invest 1974; 53:857.
47. Himms-Hagen J. Effects of catecholamines on metabolism. In: Blaschko H, Muscholl E, eds. Catecholamines: handbook of experimental pharmacology, vol 33. Berlin: Springer-Verlag, 1972:363.
48. Landsberg L, Saville ME, Young JB. The sympathoadrenal system and regulation of thermogenesis. Am J Physiol 1984; 247:E181.
49. Rosen SG, Clutter WE, Shah SD, Cryer PE. Direct alpha-adrenergic stimulation of hepatic glucose production in human subjects. Am J Physiol 1983; 245:E616.
50. Galster AD, Clutter WE, Cryer PE, et al. Epinephrine plasma thresholds for lipolytic effects in man: measurements of fatty acid transport with [1-13C] palmitic acid. J Clin Invest 1981; 67:1729.
51. Deibert DC, DeFronzo RA. Epinephrine-induced insulin resistance in man. J Clin Invest 1980; 65:717.
52. Smith U. Adrenergic control of lipid metabolism. Acta Med Scand 1983; 672(Suppl):41.
53. Brown MJ, Brown DC, Murphy MB. Hypokalemia from beta-2-receptor stimulation by circulating epinephrine. N Engl J Med 1983; 309:1414.
54. Potter DE. Adrenergic pharmacology of aqueous humor dynamics. Pharmacol Rev 1981; 33:133.
55. Goldstein DS, Swoboda KJ, Miles JM, et al. Sources and physiological significance of plasma dopamine sulfate. J Clin Endocrinol Metab 1999; 84:2523.
56. Wolfovitz E, Grossman E, Folio CJ, et al. Derivation of urinary dopamine from dihydroxyphenylalanine (DOPA) in humans. Clin Sci 1993; 84:549.
57. Ziegler MG, Lake CR, Kopin IJ. Plasma noradrenaline increases with age. Nature 1976; 261:333.
58. Lake CR, Ziegler MG, Kopin IJ. Use of plasma norepinephrine for evaluation of sympathetic neuronal function in man. Life Sci 1976; 18:1315.
59. Goldstein DS, McCarty R, Polinsky RJ, Kopin IJ. Relationship between plasma norepinephrine and sympathetic neural activity. Hypertension 1983; 5:552.
60. Kopin IJ, Zukowska-Grojec Z, Bayorh M, Goldstein DS. Estimation of intrasynaptic norepinephrine concentrations at vascular neuroeffector junctions in vivo. Naunyn Schmiedebergs Arch Pharmacol 1984; 325:298.
61. Esler M, Jennings G, Korner P, et al. Total, end organ–specific, noradrenaline plasma kinetics in essential hypertension. Clin Exp Hypertens 1984; 6:507.
62. Goldstein DS, Zimlichman R, Stull R, et al. Measurement of regional neuronal removal of norepinephrine in man. J Clin Invest 1985; 76:15.
63. Goldstein DS, Eisenhofer G, Sax FL, et al. Plasma norepinephrine pharmacokinetics during mental challenge. Psychosom Med 1987; 49:591.
64. Goldstein DS, Polinsky RJ, Garty M, et al. Patterns of plasma levels of catechols in neurogenic orthostatic hypotension. Ann Neurol 1989; 26:558.
65. Linares OA, Zech LA, Jacquez JA, et al. Effect of sodium-restricted diet and posture on norepinephrine kinetics in humans. Am J Physiol 1988; 254:E222.
66. Goldstein DS, Stull R, Markey SP, et al. Dihydrocaffeic acid: a common contaminant in the liquid chromatographic-electrochemical measurement of plasma catecholamines in man. J Chromatogr 1984; 311:148.
67. Lenders JWM, Eisenhofer G, Armando I, et al. Determination of metanephrines in plasma by liquid chromatography with electrochemical detection. Clin Chem 1993; 39:97.
68. Peuler JD, Johnson GA. Simultaneous single isotope radioenzymatic assay of plasma norepinephrine, epinephrine and dopamine. Life Sci 1977; 2:625.
69. Goldstein DS, Stull RW, Zimlichman R, et al. Simultaneous measurement of DOPA, DOPAC, and catecholamines in plasma by liquid chromatography with electrochemical detection. Clin Chem 1984; 30:815.
70. Sundlof G, Wallin BG. Human muscle nerve sympathetic activity at rest. Relationship to blood pressure and age. J Physiol (Lond) 1978; 274:621.
71. Wallin BG, Nerhed C. Relationship between spontaneous variations of muscle sympathetic activity and succeeding changes of blood pressure in man. J Auton Nerv Syst 1982; 6:293.
72. Morlin C, Wallin BG, Eriksson BM. Muscle sympathetic activity and plasma noradrenaline in normotensive and hypertensive man. Acta Physiol Scand 1983; 119:117.
73. Wallin BG, Sundlof G, Eriksson B-M, et al. Plasma noradrenaline correlates to sympathetic muscle nerve activity in normotensive man. Acta Physiol Scand 1981; 111:69.
74. Schwaiger M, Kalff V, Rosenspire K, et al. Noninvasive evaluation of sympathetic nervous system in human heart by positron emission tomography. Circulation 1990b; 82:457.
75. Goldstein DS, Holmes CS, Stuhlmuller JE, et al. 6-[$^{18}$F]Fluorodopamine PET scanning in the assessment of cardiac sympathoneural function. Clin Auton Res 1997; 7:17.
76. Robertson D, Johnson GA, Robertson RM, et al. Comparative assessment of stimuli that release neuronal and adrenomedullary catecholamines in man. Circulation 1979; 59:637.
77. Ninomiya I, Nisimaru N, Irisawa H. Sympathetic activity to the spleen, kidney, and heart in response to baroreceptor input. Am J Physiol 1971; 221:1346.
78. Chien S. Role of the sympathetic nervous system in hemorrhage. Physiol Rev 1967; 47:214.
79. Johnson TS, Young JB, Landsberg L. Sympathoadrenal responses to acute and chronic hypoxia in the rat. J Clin Invest 1983; 71:1263.
80. Goldstein DS, Dionne R, Sweet J, et al. Circulatory, plasma catecholamine, cortisol, lipid, and psychological responses to real-life stress (wisdom tooth extractions): effects of diazepam sedation and of inclusion of epinephrine with the local anesthetic. Psychosom Med 1982; 44:259.
81. Robertson RM, Medina E, Shah N, et al. Neurally mediated syncope: pathophysiology and implications for treatment. Am J Med Sci 1999; 317:102.
82. Wallin BG, Sundlof G. Sympathetic outflow to muscles during vasovagal syncope. J Auton Nerv Syst 1982; 6:287.
83. Pacak K, Palkovits M, Yadid G, et al. Heterogeneous neuroendocrine responses to various stressors: a test of Selye's doctrine of non-specificity. Am J Physiol 1998; 275:R1247.

# CHAPTER 86

# PHEOCHROMOCYTOMA AND OTHER DISEASES OF THE SYMPATHETIC NERVOUS SYSTEM

HARRY R. KEISER

## PHEOCHROMOCYTOMA

The most important disease of the adrenal medulla is pheochromocytoma.[1–7] Eighty-five percent to 90% of these tumors occur in the adrenal glands. They arise from cells of neural crest origin and can also be found in some extraadrenal locations (i.e., carotid body, aortic chemoreceptors, sympathetic ganglia, organ of Zuckerkandl). These extraadrenal tumors have been called *paragangliomas, chemodectomas,* and the like, depending on their anatomic location. Any tumor that makes, stores, and secretes catecholamines and produces symptoms of excessive catecholamine release should be considered a pheochromocytoma and treated as such, regardless of its location.

Pheochromocytomas are rare except in certain familial settings. They occur equally in both sexes and at any age, although they are most frequent between the ages of 30 and 50 years. They occur in all races, but less frequently in blacks. When they occur sporadically, 10% are bilateral. When they occur in families, ~50% are bilateral and they are usually intraadrenal. Pheochromocytomas may occur as a solitary entity or they may be familial, associated with other diseases, such as multiple endocrine neoplasia type 2A or type 2B, von Hippel-Lindau disease type 2, or neurofibromatosis type 1. In most familial disorders inheritance is autosomal dominant[8] (Table 86-1) (see Chap. 188). In one study, 23% of unselected patients with pheochromocytoma were found to be carriers of familial disorders—19% had von Hippel-Lindau disease and 4% had multiple endocrine neoplasia type 2.[9] In addition, 38% of carriers of von Hippel-Lindau disease and 24% of carriers of multiple endocrine neoplasia type 2 had pheochromocytoma as the only manifestation of their syndrome. Thus, all patients in families with multiple endocrine neoplasia type 2 or von Hippel-Lindau disease should be genetically screened to determine if they are carriers and require screening for specific phenotypic traits.[9a] Patients who are hypertensive or are scheduled to undergo surgery for another aspect of the disease should be screened for pheochromocytoma, even if they are asymptomatic. Although pheochromocytoma is not a normal part of multiple endocrine neoplasia type 1, it has been associated with pancreatic islet cell tumors in some families.[10] In all situations in which several different tumors have been discovered contemporaneously, the pheochromocytoma should be removed before any other surgery is performed. An adrenal gland should be removed only if it contains tumor. A normal-appearing adrenal gland should be left intact and carefully monitored. A pheochromocytoma may not develop in the remaining gland; in one study it appeared in 52% of patients after a mean of 11.87 years.[11]

Although ~5% of patients with pheochromocytoma have neurofibromatosis, only 1% of patients with neurofibromatosis have pheochromocytoma.[1] In children, 50% of pheochromocytomas are solitary and intraadrenal, 25% involve the adrenals bilaterally, and 25% are extraadrenal (see Chap. 87).

## CLINICAL MANIFESTATIONS

The hallmark of a pheochromocytoma is hypertension, either paroxysmal or sustained (both forms occur with equal frequency).

**TABLE 86-1.**
**Pathologic Conditions Associated with Pheochromocytoma**

| Disease or Disorder | Genetic Abnormality | Phenotypic Abnormalities |
|---|---|---|
| **MULTIPLE ENDOCRINE NEOPLASIA SYNDROMES** | | |
| Multiple Endocrine Neoplasia Type 2A (Sipple syndrome) | Chromosome 10 (10q11.2); *RET* protooncogene mutations affect tyrosine kinase ligand-binding domain | Medullary carcinoma of the thyroid, hyperparathyroidism |
| Multiple Endocrine Neoplasia Type 2B (or 3) | Chromosome 10 (10q11.2); *RET* protooncogene mutations affect tyrosine kinase catalytic site | Medullary carcinoma of the thyroid, mucosal neuromas, intestinal ganglioneuroma, megacolon, marfanoid habitus |
| **NEUROECTODERMAL SYNDROMES** | | |
| Neurofibromatosis (von Recklinghausen disease) Type 1 | Chromosome 17 (17q11); mutations affect *NF1*, tumor-suppressor gene | Peripheral neurofibromata |
| Cerebelloretinal hemangioblastomatosis (von Hippel-Lindau syndrome) Type 2 | Chromosome 3 (3p25-26); missense mutations affect *VHL*, tumor suppressor gene | Retinal angiomas; cerebellar and spinal cord hemangioblastomas; renal cell cancer; pancreatic, renal, epididymal, and endolymphatic cysts/tumors |

Usually, the hypertension is labile. A typical paroxysm is characterized by a sudden major increase in blood pressure, a severe, throbbing headache, profuse sweating over most of the body (especially the trunk), palpitations with or without tachycardia, anxiety, a sense of doom, skin pallor, nausea with or without emesis, and abdominal pain.[1,2] A study of 2585 hypertensive patients, including 11 with pheochromocytoma, noted that *headache, sweating,* and *palpitations* were reported by 71%, 65%, and 65%, respectively, of patients with pheochromocytoma.[12] When these three manifestations were present and associated with hypertension, they indicated the diagnosis of pheochromocytoma with a specificity of 93.8% and a sensitivity of 90.9%. In the absence of hypertension and this triad of symptoms, the diagnosis of pheochromocytoma could be excluded with a certainty of 99.9%. The hypertensive episode may appear to occur spontaneously, or it may follow acute physical (but not psychological) stress, an increase in abdominal pressure (induced, for example, by palpation of the tumor or defecation), a hypotensive episode, or any activation of the sympathetic nervous system. Hypertensive episodes are usually not caused by anxiety or psychological stress. They may last a few minutes to several hours, and they leave the patient feeling exhausted. These hypertensive episodes may occur in patients who are otherwise normotensive, or they may affect patients with sustained hypertension. Hypertensive episodes may be precipitated by drugs that lower blood pressure acutely (i.e., saralasin[13]), as well as by opiates, adrenocorticotropic hormone (ACTH), dopamine antagonists (i.e., metoclopramide[14] and droperidol), radiographic contrast media, indirect-acting amines (such as tyramine and amphetamine, which act by displacing the normal neurotransmitter), proprietary cold preparations, and drugs that block neuronal catecholamine reuptake (i.e., tricyclic antidepressants and cocaine). Other symptoms include dizziness and constipation. The patient may experience postural hypotension, hyperglycemia, hypermetabolism, weight loss, and even psychic changes. The hyperglycemia is generally mild, occurs with the hypertensive attacks, and usually does not require treatment. A few patients may say that they feel "flushed," but observation of an actual flush should bring into question the diagnosis of a pheochromocytoma.[3] The hypertensive crisis associated with pheochromocytoma may precipitate a myocardial infarction, even in the absence of coronary artery disease, or a cerebral hemorrhage. A prolonged excess of catecholamines may produce a cardiomyopathy that is manifested by congestive heart failure. Unexplained shock may also be the presenting feature of pheochromocytoma.[15]

A pheochromocytoma with all the classic signs and symptoms is easy to diagnose. However, the tumor may present with only part of the syndrome. Early in the course of a pheochromocytoma, symptoms may be very mild and infrequent, becoming progressively more severe and more frequent later. A patient may have symptoms for years before the diagnosis is made.

The extensive differential diagnosis of a pheochromocytoma includes anxiety and panic attacks, thyrotoxicosis, abrupt withdrawal of clonidine therapy, amphetamine use, cocaine use, ingestion of tyramine-containing foods or proprietary cold preparations (e.g., phenylephrine, pseudoephedrine, phenylpropanolamine) while taking monoamine oxidase inhibitors, hypoglycemia, insulin reaction, angina pectoris or myocardial infarction, brain tumor, subarachnoid hemorrhage, cardiovascular deconditioning, menopausal syndrome, neuroblastoma (in children), and toxemia of pregnancy, among others. A pseudopheochromocytoma has been reported in a patient with parkinsonism treated with selegiline, a monoamine oxidase type B inhibitor, and fluoxetine, an antidepressant that inhibits serotonin uptake.[16] Clozapine, a tricyclic dibenzodiazepine, has been reported to mimic pheochromocytoma with hypertension and increased urinary catecholamine levels, both of which revert to normal when the drug is stopped.[17] To make these diagnostic distinctions, the physician must obtain a detailed history and, if possible, observe and monitor a hypertensive episode. If this is done, the self-administration of various drugs, the abrupt withdrawal of clonidine (which causes a rebound in central sympathetic outflow resulting in the release of large amounts of epinephrine and norepinephrine), and other episodic disorders are evident. Two of the most difficult differential diagnoses are panic attacks and cardiovascular deconditioning, the latter of which indicates that a patient has been so sedentary that minimal physical activity causes marked tachycardia and sympathetic nervous system activity. These conditions present diagnostic difficulties because neither is characterized by specific symptoms, physical findings, or diagnostic tests. Thus, a pheochromocytoma must be excluded before either of these diagnoses may be established. Pheochromocytoma should be suspected in patients with hypertension that is refractory to therapy and in those who have a history of hypertensive episodes occurring during previous general anesthesia or abdominal surgery.

Pheochromocytomas may produce calcitonin, opioid peptides, somatostatin, ACTH, and vasoactive intestinal peptide.[4] The high serum calcitonin level may mistakenly suggest a medullary carcinoma of the thyroid until the pheochromocytoma is removed.[18] In some patients with pheochromocytoma, the ACTH production has been known to cause Cushing syndrome,[19] and production of vasoactive intestinal peptide has resulted in watery diarrhea.[6] Pheochromocytomas also produce and secrete into the blood neuron-specific enolase, chromogranin A (CGA), neuropeptide Y, and adrenomedullin.

## DIAGNOSIS

### URINE TESTS

The diagnosis of a pheochromocytoma must rest on biochemical determinations (i.e., the demonstration of elevated levels of catecholamines or their metabolites in blood or in urine). The traditional and easiest method is the measurement of epinephrine and norepinephrine, of metanephrines (methoxycatechola-

**TABLE 86-2.**
**Effects of Various Drugs on Results of Biochemical Urine Tests for Pheochromocytoma***

| | Catecholamines | Metanephrines | Vanillylmandelic acid |
|---|---|---|---|
| **NORMAL VALUES** | | | |
| Total catecholamines | <100 ng/24 hours | <1.3 mg/24 hours | <9.0 mg/24 hours |
| Epinephrine | <20 ng/24 hours | <300 µg/24 hours | |
| Norepinephrine | <80 ng/24 hours | <500 µg/24 hours | |
| **VALUES INCREASED BY** | Amphetamines | Amphetamines | Amphetamines |
| | Catecholamines | Catecholamines | Catecholamines |
| | Clonidine withdrawal | Clonidine withdrawal | Clonidine withdrawal |
| | Ethanol | Ethanol | Nalidixic acid |
| | Methyldopa | MAO inhibitors | |
| | L-Dopa | Chlorpromazine | |
| | Quinidine | | |
| | Theophylline | | |
| | Tetracycline | | |
| **VALUES DECREASED BY** | Metyrosine | Metyrosine | Metyrosine |
| | Reserpine | Reserpine | Reserpine |
| | Guanethidine | Guanethidine | Guanethidine |
| | | Methylglucamine from radiographic contrast media | MAO inhibitors |
| | | | Clofibrate |
| | | | Disulfiram |
| | | | Ethanol |

*MAO*, monoamine oxidase.
*Effect may be attributable to alterations in synthesis, release, or metabolism of catecholamines, or interference in the assay procedure.
(Adapted from Ram CV, Engleman K. Pheochromocytoma—recognition and management. Curr Probl Cardiol 1979; 4:1; and from Levine SN, McDonald JC. The evaluation and management of pheochromocytomas. Adv Surg 1984; 17:281.)

mines), or of vanillylmandelic acid in a 24-hour collection of urine (Table 86-2).[1-4] The urine must be collected in strong acid (i.e., 20 mL of 6N HCl or 25 mL of 50% acetic acid) in an easily sealed, leakproof container; it need not be refrigerated. The measurement of metanephrines in a single random urine sample, or of norepinephrine in a single overnight sample of urine, has been used successfully to diagnose pheochromocytoma.[20,21] However, such random specimens show greater variability and, therefore, have less diagnostic sensitivity than do 24-hour samples. Creatinine should be measured in all collections of urine to ensure adequacy of the collection and to serve as a denominator for timed or random samples. Simultaneous analysis of norepinephrine and its metabolite dihydroxyphenolglycol may improve specificity.[22] The amount of urinary total metanephrines and vanillylmandelic acid, when expressed in relation to creatinine, decreases with age in normal children.[23] Although an amine-free or "vanillylmandelic acid" diet is useful in metabolic studies, it is usually unnecessary in the diagnosis of a pheochromocytoma now that more specific analyses are used. The patient should cease taking all medications, if possible (see Table 86-2). If antihypertensive therapy must be continued, diuretics, vasodilators (hydralazine or minoxidil), calcium channel blockers, and angiotensin-converting enzyme inhibitors cause minimal interference. Although any one of the three urinary tests usually indicates the diagnosis, the determination of norepinephrine and epinephrine, or of normetanephrine and metanephrine, is preferred.[24,25] Specific assays for urinary epinephrine and norepinephrine are preferable to measurement of total catecholamines, because increased epinephrine may be the only abnormal finding in patients with multiple endocrine neoplasia.[26] A markedly elevated value for total catecholamines (i.e., 2000 µg per 24 hours) with normal values for metanephrines and vanillylmandelic acid suggests that the patient is taking methyldopa (metabolized to α-methylnorepinephrine and determined as a catecholamine) and does not have a pheochromocytoma. In most patients with a pheochromocytoma, the urine test results are abnormally elevated at all times. For the few patients with only infrequent episodes of hypertension, urine is best collected when the patient is hypertensive. This is accomplished most easily by giving the patient 5 mL of 6N HCl in a 1-L container with instructions to be followed when hypertensive symptoms occur. When symptoms are noted, the patient should void, discard the urine, and note the time. Then, 2 to 3 hours later, the patient should void again, now saving the urine in the container and again noting the time. This urine specimen should be assayed for epinephrine, norepinephrine, and creatinine. A greater than twofold increase in either catecholamine over levels obtained from testing a similar control collection is diagnostic.

### BLOOD TESTS

The blood sample to test for catecholamines[27] (see Chap. 85) must be drawn under controlled circumstances; the patient should be fasting and supine, and the needle should be in place in the vein for at least 20 minutes before the sample is drawn. The blood sample should immediately be placed on ice and centrifuged and the plasma drawn off and frozen within 1 hour. Normal values are generally <500 pg/mL for norepinephrine and <100 pg/mL for epinephrine; values >1500 pg/mL for norepinephrine and >300 pg/mL for epinephrine are diagnostic of a pheochromocytoma. Intermediate values may not represent a tumor but rather an exaggerated physiologic response. In this situation, a suppression test (see the following discussion) is indicated. The presence of dihydrocaffeic acid, a catecholamine metabolite of the caffeic acid that is present in all forms of coffee (decaffeinated, as well as regular) and many cola beverages may produce false-positive results.[28] Therefore, patients are best studied in the morning after an overnight fast. A report suggests that the plasma ratio of norepinephrine to dihydroxyphenolglycol (mainly from neuronally released norepinephrine) is >2.0 in patients with a pheochromocytoma and is <0.5 in normal and hypertensive subjects.[29] However, a normal plasma norepinephrine/dihydroxyphenolglycol ratio does not exclude the presence of a pheochromocytoma that produces predominantly epinephrine.[30]

Determination of the plasma metanephrines normetanephrine and metanephrine has been particularly useful in screening for pheochromocytoma because their sensitivity is 100% and their negative predictive value is 100%.[31,31a] Thus, normal plasma concentrations of metanephrines exclude the diagnosis of pheochromocytoma, because the adrenals serve as the major source of plasma free metanephrines; the increased metanephrines from pheochromocytoma arise from the production and metabolism of catecholamines within the tumor.[31,32] This assay is available in only a few laboratories, acetaminophen interferes, and levels are increased in renal failure.

Procedures that call for the measurement of plasma catecholamines before and after standing, exercise, and other activities generally confirm that a pheochromocytoma is not integrated into sympathetic nervous system responses but do not help in the diagnosis of a tumor. Most laboratories measure free catecholamines in plasma by means of high-pressure liquid chromatography with electrochemical detection. Radioimmunoassays that measured the sum of free and conjugated catecholamines have been replaced. Scant data are available to assess the usefulness of determinations of total catecholamines (i.e., free plus conjugated catecholamines). The plasma concentration of chromogranin A (see Chap. 175) is supranormal in some patients with a pheochromocytoma and is an excellent marker to follow in patients with any neuroendocrine tumor. It is not useful in the diagnosis of pheochromocytoma.[33–35]

### PHARMACOLOGIC TESTS

Phentolamine (Regitine), a short acting α-adrenergic antagonist, can be used as a diagnostic suppression test for pheochromocytoma. A reduction in blood pressure of >35 mm Hg systolic and 25 mm Hg diastolic after administration of 1 to 5 mg of the drug as an intravenous bolus is considered to be diagnostic. This reduction begins 2 minutes after the injection and lasts ~10 minutes. Because patients with a pheochromocytoma may become hypotensive after a large dose of phentolamine, the prudent course is to inject only 1.0 mg initially and to observe the response. If blood pressure is unaffected, the remaining 4.0 mg in the vial can then safely be administered. However, the test should be performed only when the patient is hypertensive and preferably when he or she is not receiving any other antihypertensive agents. The blood pressure and heart rate must be monitored every 30 to 60 seconds, and a patent intravenous line and vasopressors must be at hand. False-positive tests are common.

Clonidine (Catapres), a centrally acting, orally active, α₂-adrenergic agonist, can also be used as a diagnostic suppression test.[36] Blood is drawn to test for plasma catecholamines both before and 3 hours after the oral administration of clonidine (0.3 mg/70 kg). Blood pressure declines in most patients with hypertension of any cause. Plasma catecholamine levels decrease if they are under physiologic control, whereas in patients with pheochromocytoma, plasma catecholamines remain the same or increase. This test is very safe but is useful only if basal catecholamine values are abnormally high. Similarly, pentolinium, administered by the intravenous route, has been used in a suppression test. However, it has no unique advantages, and the intravenous form is no longer available in the United States.

Histamine,[37] tyramine, glucagon,[37,38] and metoclopramide[14] each has been used as a provocative test for pheochromocytoma. Such provocation is inherently dangerous, as indicated by the several deaths that have been reported during histamine tests. These tests should be used only if repeated assays of blood and urine are equivocal and if symptoms are classic, truly episodic, but too infrequent to permit prompt diagnosis. Although many physicians focus on the blood pressure response, it is only of value if the patient has discontinued all medications. Plasma catecholamines are best measured before and during the test (generally 2 minutes after injection of the drug) and only significant elevations of plasma catecholamines should be considered as diagnostic of a pheochromocytoma. If this is done, the provocation can provide useful diagnostic information, without any risk, in a patient who is receiving α- and β-adrenergic blockers. The usual dose of glucagon is 1.0 mg, delivered as an intravenous bolus. The usual dose for metoclopramide is 1 to 10 mg, also delivered as an intravenous bolus (the 1-mg dose is recommended initially; if the result is negative, then the 10-mg dose may be tried). Close monitoring of blood pressure is required, and phentolamine must be at hand for the treatment of any episodes of severe hypertension. Histamine and tyramine are rarely used anymore. A glucagon provocative test followed by a clonidine suppression test can be easily and safely performed on outpatients, and the combination yields increased sensitivity and specificity in the diagnosis of pheochromocytoma.[39] Even when glucagon is given to patients with known pheochromocytoma, only 18% have an elevation of systolic blood pressure over 200 mm Hg. The hypertension responds rapidly to bolus intravenous administration of phentolamine, 5 mg.

Urinary epinephrine and norepinephrine secretion is normally suppressed by sleep. In patients with pheochromocytoma, however, the catecholamine level may remain unregulated by sleep; this effect can be further accentuated with the addition of oral clonidine before bedtime.[40] The diagnostic utility and specificity of this procedure remain to be determined.

## LOCALIZATION

A computed tomographic (CT) scan of the abdomen is the best all-around technique for locating a pheochromocytoma. However, attempts to locate the tumor should *not* be made until biochemical studies have confirmed its presence. The demonstration of a mass in an adrenal gland does *not* prove that the mass is a pheochromocytoma, just as failure to find a mass in either adrenal gland does *not* prove that the patient does not have a pheochromocytoma. However, in certain familial settings (e.g., von Hippel-Lindau disease or multiple endocrine neoplasia type 2), a computed tomogram of the abdomen or a scan with radiolabeled metaiodobenzylguanidine (MIBG) may point to the need for further workup when the basal laboratory data have been equivocal and the patient is scheduled for surgery for another component of the syndrome.[9] A careful history and physical examination may yield important clues as to the location of a pheochromocytoma, as in the case of postmicturition hypertension secondary to a pheochromocytoma of the urinary bladder.[41] If epinephrine constitutes >15% of the total urinary catecholamines, then the tumor is almost always intraadrenal. Overall sensitivity of the studies in the localization of pheochromocytoma was 89% for CT, 98% for magnetic resonance imaging (MRI), and 81% for MIBG scan.[42]

MRI is a useful diagnostic tool because it provides sufficient histologic specificity to distinguish pheochromocytomas from other adrenal masses via T2 and spin echo sequences.[43,44]

The iodine-131 ([131]I)–labeled MIBG scan is accurate in revealing 80% to 95% of pheochromocytomas, but it may also visualize neuroblastoma and some other APUD (amine precursor uptake and decarboxylation) tumors (i.e., carcinoid and medullary carcinoma of the thyroid).[45,45a] Labetalol reduces tumor uptake of MIBG, and the drug should be stopped up to 1 week before an MIBG scan.[46] Other drugs known to reduce or suspected of reducing MIBG uptake include reserpine, cocaine, tricyclic antidepressants, sympathomimetics (including nonprescription compounds containing phenylpropanolamine), and calcium channel blockers.[46] MIBG scanning is most useful in detecting multiple tumors, tumor metastases, and tumors in unusual locations (e.g., cardiac tumors).[47] Both [123]I-MIBG and single photon emission CT have been used in place of planar imaging to provide improved resolution.[48] Use of a radiolabeled somatostatin analog, such as octreotide, is not as helpful as MIBG in locating a pheochromocytoma. In a comparative study of patients with known pheochromocytoma metastases, detection rates were 80% with MIBG and 44% with octreotide. However, octreotide imaging detected six metastases that were not detected by MIBG scanning. Thus, octreotide scanning may be used as a complementary method in detecting metastases when results from MIBG imaging are negative.[49]

The major role of ultrasonography has been to determine whether a mass seen on radiographic examination is attached to the kidney and whether it is solid or cystic. However, transesophageal echocardiography has proven to be valuable in the visualization of intrapericardial tumors.[50]

With the ready availability of CT and MRI, arteriography for the diagnosis of a pheochromocytoma is rarely indicated. An arteriogram imposes significant risk of a serious hypertensive crisis and offers little additional information. In the rare event that one is needed to clarify complicated vascular anatomy before surgery, the patient should be prepared and monitored as if he or she were undergoing surgery. A midstream injection into the abdominal aorta may yield all needed information and is much less likely to trigger a hypertensive crisis than is selective arterial injection.

The measurement of catecholamine levels in selected veins is a procedure that is also rarely needed, except when an extraadrenal tumor that escaped removal during previous surgery must be located. This procedure generally does not help to locate an intraadrenal tumor, because catecholamine levels in the adrenal veins normally vary tremendously over time, during stress, and from one side to the other. An excess of norepinephrine in the venous effluent of one adrenal would suggest a pheochromocytoma, because epinephrine normally predominates. Also, dilution effects are important, because the right adrenal vein is short and can be entered directly from the inferior vena cava, whereas the left adrenal vein is accessible only through the left renal vein. Simultaneous measurement of cortisol or aldosterone can provide the denominator necessary to control for the distance of the catheter from the tumor (see also Chap. 88).

## TREATMENT

Surgical removal of a pheochromocytoma is clearly the treatment of choice, because an unresected tumor represents a buried time bomb waiting to explode with a potentially fatal hypertensive crisis.[1–4] Safe surgical removal requires an integrated, cooperative, team effort by an internist, an anesthesiologist, and a surgeon, preferably one with prior experience in removal of pheochromocytoma (see Chap. 89). Preparation should start at least 7 days before surgery with the administration of the nonspecific α-adrenergic receptor blocker phenoxybenzamine (Dibenzyline). The initial dosage of 10 mg twice daily should be increased to an average dosage of 0.5 to 1.0 mg/kg daily, delivered in two to three divided doses. Prazosin (Minipress),[51] a specific $α_1$-antagonist (2–5 mg two to three times daily) or labetalol (Normodyne, Trandate), a drug with both α- and β-antagonist activity (200–600 mg orally, twice daily) may also be used. Large doses of these drugs may be necessary to control blood pressure and to restore the patient's diminished plasma volume. As normal blood volume is restored, the degree of postural hypotension decreases. However, if too much α-blocker is administered, the degree of postural hypotension increases and may cause symptoms, just as it does in normal subjects. A β-adrenergic blocker seldom is needed unless a significant tachycardia or catecholamine-induced arrhythmia occurs. Clearly, a β-blocker should never be used in the absence of an α-blocker, because the former would exacerbate epinephrine-induced vasoconstriction by blocking its vasodilator component.

The author has found that metyrosine (Demser, α-methyl-L-tyrosine) is very useful in treating patients with pheochromocytoma. The drug competitively inhibits tyrosine hydroxylation,[52] the rate-limiting step in catecholamine synthesis. It facilitates blood pressure control both before and during surgery, especially during the induction of anesthesia and manipulation of the tumor.[53] Treatment is customarily begun at a dosage of 250 mg every 6 hours; thereafter, the dosage is increased by 250 to 500 mg per day, as necessary, up to a total dose of 4 g per day. Because metyrosine is a substituted amino acid, it readily enters the brain. There, it inhibits catecholamine synthesis and may produce sedation (frequently) and extrapyramidal signs (rarely, parkinsonism in older patients). These symptoms disappear rapidly when the drug is discontinued. Adverse central nervous system symptoms are best handled by reducing the dosage if the patient reports unusually vivid or frightening dreams or if significant behavioral changes occur. Although the author prefers the more stable blood pressure produced by the combination of α-antagonists and metyrosine, physicians in some centers, such as the Cleveland Clinic and Mayo Clinic, report equally good results without metyrosine. The calcium channel blocker nifedipine (10 mg per administration, as necessary), which is absorbed quickly from the stomach, is useful in controlling infrequent spikes in blood pressure.[54,55] Nicardipine, another calcium channel blocker, has been used alone to control blood pressure both before and during surgical removal of pheochromocytoma.[56] Calcium channel blockers are potent vasodilators, and they also block the entry of calcium, which is needed for release of catecholamines from the tumor cell.

During surgery, phentolamine, nicardipine, or nitroprusside should be administered to control hypertensive episodes. The infusion of dilutions of the drug is preferable to bolus injections. Small amounts of β-blockers, such as propranolol, in intravenously administered doses of 0.1 to 1.0 mg can be used, if needed, to treat tachycardia or catecholamine-induced arrhythmias.

If hypotension occurs, either during surgery (especially after the tumor is removed) or after surgery, then volume replacement is the treatment of choice.[1,4] The use of pressor agents is ill-advised, especially if long-lasting α-blockers have been used, because of the difficulty with which patients are weaned from these agents. Control of postoperative hypotension is even more difficult if both metyrosine and phenoxybenzamine (Dibenzyline) are used preoperatively. This is because the former inhibits catecholamine synthesis by both the tumor and the sympathetic nervous system, whereas the latter blocks the action of any catecholamines that are synthesized. Thus, the vascular system is effectively paralyzed in a dilated state. The best way to control blood pressure is by careful attention to volume replacement. The volume of fluid required is frequently large (i.e., one-half to one and one-half times the patient's calculated blood volume) during the first 24 to 48 hours after removal of the tumor, because this long is required for the effects of both drugs to disappear and for the sympathetic nervous system to resume autoregulation. This return to autoregulation becomes apparent when the renal output suddenly begins to increase and the blood pressure and heart rate remain stable. At this time, replacement volumes can be decreased to standard amounts (i.e., 125 mL per hour).

Occurrence of postoperative hypertension may mean that some tumor tissue was not resected. However, during the first 24 hours after surgery, hypertension is most likely attributable to pain, volume overload, or autonomic instability.[52] Because major surgery causes large increases in both plasma and urinary catecholamine levels, a 5- to 7-day interval should precede any attempt to collect samples for biochemical evidence of residual tumor. A suppression test with phentolamine or clonidine may be very useful in clarifying the cause of persistent hypertension after the removal of a pheochromocytoma. In 25% of such cases, the hypertension is attributable to preexisting hypertension, usually the essential form.

## PHEOCHROMOCYTOMA IN PREGNANCY

A pheochromocytoma in a pregnant woman is a very dangerous condition.[1,5,57] The very high overall maternal and fetal mortality rates of 48% and 55%, respectively, as had been reported in 1980, can be reduced to 0% and 15%, respectively, only if the diagnosis of pheochromocytoma is made antenatally.[58,59] As soon as the diagnosis is made, α-adrenergic blockers should be administered; phenoxybenzamine is the drug of choice. Localization is best accomplished by ultrasonography or MRI. If a pheochromocytoma is discovered during the first or second trimester, the tumor should be removed as soon as the patient is prepared adequately with α-adrenergic blockers. This has been done laparoscopically.[60] The fetus can remain undisturbed, but spontaneous abortion is very likely. If a pheochromocytoma is discovered during the third trimester, the patient may be treated with α-adrenergic blockers and carefully monitored until the fetus matures to the point of viability. Then, cesarean section and removal of the tumor can be accomplished in one operation. If uncontrolled hypertension, hemorrhage, or other emergency occurs, the tumor should be removed at once.

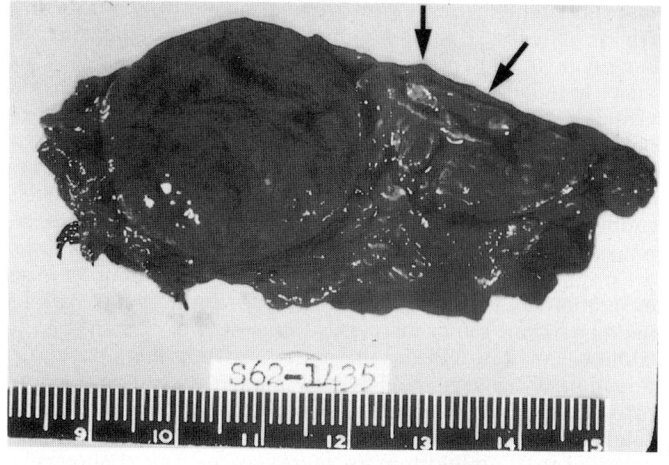

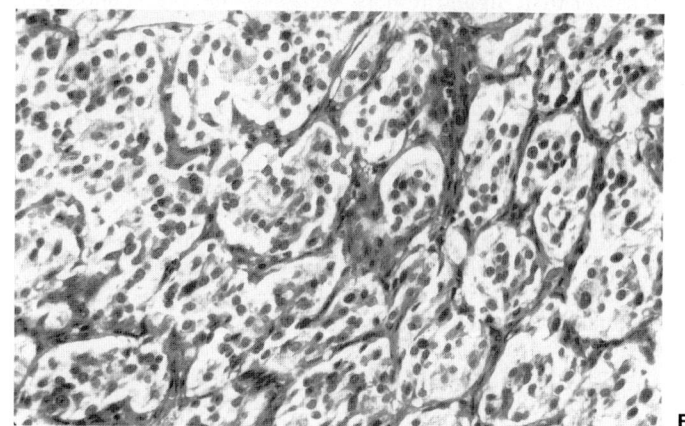

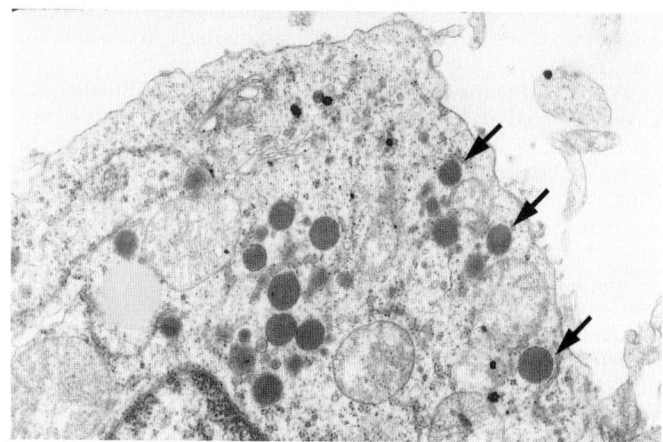

**FIGURE 86-1.** **A,** Cross-section of a well-demarcated intraadrenal pheochromocytoma with stippled areas of congestion. The normal adrenal cortex, which had a characteristic yellow-orange color when fresh, is marked with *arrows*. **B,** The typical histology of an adrenal pheochromocytoma is shown with cells in nests and trabeculae separated by a thin vascular stroma (hematoxylin and eosin; ×400). **C,** Electron microscopic view of an adrenal pheochromocytoma with many large, dense-core catecholamine-containing granules, some marked with *arrows*. These granules, with a thin uniform halo between the core and the investing membrane, are the epinephrine-containing type. Granules with a prominent eccentric lucent space between the core and the limiting membrane are the norepinephrine-containing type. ×13,500 (**B,** Courtesy of Dr. Ilona Linnoila.)

## MALIGNANT PHEOCHROMOCYTOMA

A pheochromocytoma is usually surrounded by a firm capsule or pseudocapsule. The cut surface shows many areas of hemorrhagic necrosis. Microscopic examination reveals that the tumor is composed of large, pleomorphic, chromaffin cells (Fig. 86-1) that contain many dense core granules on electron microscopy. For a pathologist to determine if a pheochromocytoma is benign or malignant is very difficult, if not impossible. The major criteria for differentiation are invasion of capsular blood vessels by tumor and metastatic invasion of other tissues. Without these findings, a pheochromocytoma may only appear to be benign. Thus, patients should have their blood pressure checked annually, and blood or urine catecholamine levels should be monitored annually for 5 years to detect any recurrence. A documented recurrence does not necessarily mean that the original tumor was malignant, but it should prompt a fresh evaluation of the patient.[61] Assessing the serum level of various neuroendocrine tumor markers, such as CGA or neuron-specific enolase,[62] may provide additional information that allows differentiation between benign and malignant tumors.[63] Flow cytometric DNA analyses of pheochromocytoma have indicated that nondiploid tumors are more prone to aggressive behavior than diploid tumors; therefore, the former should be monitored more carefully.[64]

Approximately 10% to 15% of pheochromocytomas are malignant. The larger number applies to extraadrenal tumors. Malignant pheochromocytomas grow larger, invade adjacent structures, and metastasize to bone, liver, lung, and lymph nodes. Aggressive surgical removal of all accessible tumor tissue is appropriate. Symptoms should be controlled with phenoxybenzamine or prazosin, metyrosine, and β-adrenergic blockers, as needed. Radiation therapy to bony metastases relieves pain and frequently kills tumor at that site. Originally, [131]I-labeled MIBG therapy held promise as a mode of treatment for malignant pheochromocytoma. However, current reports indicate that the treatment is only palliative.[65]

The rate of spread of malignant pheochromocytomas is highly variable; median survival is 5 years. A rapidly growing pheochromocytoma metastasis that produces impending compression of the spinal cord is a medical emergency that necessitates immediate high doses of corticosteroids and radiation therapy.

A chemotherapeutic regimen used for the treatment of the closely related neuroblastoma consists of intravenous cyclophosphamide, 750 mg/m², on day 1; vincristine, 1.4 mg/m², on day 1; and dacarbazine, 600 mg/m², on days 1 and 2. This regimen is then repeated every 21 days with adjustments being made in the dose of cyclophosphamide as hematologic parameters change and in the dose of vincristine if neurologic toxicity is noted. Fourteen patients with malignant pheochromocytoma were treated and followed for 6 to 35 months (median duration of 25 months). Two patients had complete remissions, 6 patients had >50% regression of all measurable tumor sites, and 3 patients had >25% regression (median duration of response was >17 months). In two patients, the disease stabilized after one course of therapy; one patient had progressive disease despite therapy.[66] All responding patients experienced improvement in performance status and hypertension, and a reduction in or elimination of antihypertensive therapy became possible. The excretion of catecholamines or their metabolites correlated with the tumor response in all cases. However, all treated patients eventually died of their disease. Therefore, this regimen of combination chemotherapy can produce a partial remission of significant duration in many patients with malignant pheochromocytoma; however, it cannot cure these patients, and it is effective for only a finite period. This regimen is recommended only after all other therapeutic modalities have been exhausted and the patient is documented as having progressive and measurable disease that is negatively affecting his or her quality of life.

## ADRENAL MEDULLARY HYPERPLASIA

Adrenal medullary hyperplasia has been reported in a few cases, most of which have been in the familial setting of multiple endocrine neoplasia type 2A or 2B.[67] The diagnosis is determined by analysis of an adrenal gland removed from a patient who appears to have a pheochromocytoma on the basis of signs, symptoms, and laboratory tests. Yet, on histologic examination, the adrenal gland does not contain a tumor but has diffuse, nonnodular, adrenal medullary hyperplasia, characterized by increased mitotic activity, decreased corticomedullary ratio, increased weight, and total catecholamine content. These cases suggest, but do not prove, that adrenal medullary hyperplasia may be a precursor of pheochromocytoma. In humans, no demonstrable physiologic consequences of the alternative state (i.e., adrenal medullary hypoplasia or aplasia) are seen.

## OTHER TUMORS THAT PRODUCE CATECHOLAMINES

Neuroblastoma, ganglioneuroblastoma, and ganglioneuroma are all solid tumors of neural crest origin that occur in sympathetic ganglia or the adrenal medulla. They all can synthesize and excrete the catecholamines and metabolites that are found in pheochromocytoma. Moreover, they also excrete increased amounts of the catecholamine precursors dihydroxyphenylalanine (DOPA) and dopamine, and of the metabolite homovanillic acid.[68] Only one in five patients with neuroblastoma is hypertensive, probably owing to the secretion of large amounts of inactive catecholamine precursors and only small amounts of active catecholamines.[69] The tumors form a wide spectrum of disease activity. Neuroblastomas occur mainly in children and are highly malignant. However, spontaneous regressions have been reported.[70] Ganglioneuromas occur in both adults and children and are benign, well-differentiated tumors. Ganglioneuroblastomas are intermediate in both their malignant nature and cellular differentiation. These tumors should be diagnosed and treated as if they were pheochromocytomas.

## ORTHOSTATIC HYPOTENSION

Orthostatic hypotension is defined as a critical and symptomatic reduction in blood pressure on the assumption of upright posture. It is caused by the failure of normal blood pressure homeostasis, and it reflects the loss of vasoconstrictor reflexes in both resistance and capacitance vessels. This loss is attributable to defects in either *peripheral (postganglionic) neurons* or *central (preganglionic) neurons*.[71] The first category, which is the largest, includes many diseases with associated peripheral neuropathies, such as diabetes mellitus, tabes dorsalis, alcoholism, amyloidosis, and the *Holmes-Adie syndrome* (unilateral, enlarged pupil, an absent or delayed response to light, a slow reaction on convergence, and a good response to miotics or mydriatics). In these diseases, the orthostatic hypotension is usually accompanied by dysfunctions in potency, sweating, and sphincter control.

A consensus statement has established the following categories of primary autonomic insufficiencies or dysautonomias: (a) pure autonomic failure that occurs without other neurologic features, (b) Parkinson's disease with autonomic failure, and (c) multiple system atrophy, a sporadic, progressive disorder of adults characterized by autonomic dysfunction, parkinsonism, and ataxia in any combination. The latter category is divided into three types: (a) striatonigral degeneration when parkinsonism predominates, (b) olivopontocerebellar atrophy when cerebellar features predominate, and (c) Shy-Drager syndrome when autonomic failure predominates.[71] Further differentiation of these disorders has been made on the basis of neurochemical analyses and positron emission tomography using 6-[18F]fluorodopamine.[72] A classification of dysautonomias has been proposed[72] in which sympathetic neurocirculatory failure results from peripheral sympathetic denervation or decreased or absent sympathoneural traffic, with or without signs of central neural degeneration, and in which both parkinsonism with sympathetic neurocirculatory failure and multiple system atrophy without sympathetic neurocirculatory failure differ from the Shy-Drager syndrome. Patients with the Shy-Drager syndrome have poor or no response to therapy with levodopa-carbidopa, intact cardiac sympathetic innervation, and a poor prognosis, whereas patients with parkinsonism, postural hypotension, and cardiac sympathetic denervation have a better prognosis.[72]

Treatment for orthostatic hypotension is mainly symptomatic once all treatable causes have been addressed. Certain nonpharmacologic measures should be implemented at once, including getting the patients on their feet for even short periods and having patients squat, bend over, and cross the legs. Support hose, fitted elastic stockings, and pressure suits have been used, but they correct only mild disorders. Fludrocortisone therapy plus a high-salt diet is the best treatment approach. Initial doses of 0.1 mg of fludrocortisone daily may be increased by 0.1 mg each week, as necessary, up to a maximum of 1 mg per day. This therapy should be combined with an increase in dietary salt to >150 mEq per day, either by consumption out of the salt shaker or by use of salt tablets. Serious complications occur that frequently limit this form of therapy. These include recumbent hypertension, congestive heart failure, edema, and hypokalemia. Recumbent hypertension is best treated by raising the head of the patient's bed.[73–75]

Various drugs that have been effective in the treatment of orthostatic hypotension include phenylpropanolamine, midodrine, yohimbine, and indomethacin. Ibuprofen, caffeine, and methylphenidate have been ineffective.[76] Generally, dosages have been difficult to control and must be individualized; many patients become hypertensive when recumbent and hypotensive when erect. One approach, which has been effective in some difficult cases, is to provide long-term administration of an oral monoamine oxidase inhibitor and to have the patient use phenylephrine nose drops before sitting or standing.[77] Such a regimen requires an intelligent, cooperative patient and some experimentation. Rapid atrial pacing on demand has been used successfully in one carefully selected patient with bradycardia and low cardiac output.[78] One research group has experimented with the use of a portable, servo-controlled, automated syringe, controlled by a microcomputer, to infuse a vasopressor for maintenance of the patient's blood pressure at a predetermined level.[79]

## FAMILIAL DYSAUTONOMIA (RILEY-DAY SYNDROME)

Familial dysautonomia, also known as Riley-Day syndrome, is characterized by autonomic instability. In neonates, the disease is manifested by dysphagia, difficulty in feeding, absence of fungiform papillae of the tongue, hyporeflexia, and slow movement.[80] Later, abnormalities in sweating, temperature control, and blood pressure regulation become evident, along with impairment in sensations of pain, temperature, and taste as well as lack of lacrimation. Hypersensitivity to both adrenergic and cholinergic agonists and loss of skin flare after the injection of histamine are noted. A loss of small-caliber neurons in peripheral nerves and in dorsal root and sympathetic ganglia also occurs. The disease is transmitted as an autosomal recessive trait and affects mainly Ashkenazi Jews. The gene responsible appears to reside at 9q31-33.[81] Only a few patients survive to adulthood. Usually, the diagnosis is self-evident. However, the labile blood pressure may lead to confusion with pheochromocytoma or neuroblastoma. Symptomatic postural hypotension has been treated with midodrine (see earlier). Basal supine plasma levels of norepinephrine are normal, but no increase occurs on assumption of upright posture. Urinary levels of dopamine and homovanillic acid are increased, whereas levels of vanillylmandelic acid and methoxyhydroxyphenylglycol are decreased.

## REFERENCES

1. Manger WM, Gifford RW Jr. Clinical and experimental pheochromocytoma, 2nd ed. Cambridge, MA: Blackwell Science, 1996.
2. Gifford RW Jr, Manger WM, Bravo EL. Pheochromocytoma. Endocrinol Metab Clin North Am 1994; 23:387.
3. Ram CV, Engelman K. Pheochromocytoma—recognition and management. Curr Probl Cardiol 1979; 4:1.
4. Kuchel O. Adrenal medulla: pheochromocytoma. In: Genest J, Kuchel O, Hamet P, Cantin M, eds. Hypertension, 2nd ed. New York: McGraw-Hill, 1983:947.
5. Young JB, Landsberg L. Catecholamines and the adrenal medulla: pheochromocytoma. In: Wilson JD, Foster DW, eds. William's textbook of endocrinology, 9th ed. Philadelphia: WB Saunders, 1998:chap 13, 665.
6. Hull CJ. Phaeochromocytoma: diagnosis, preoperative preparation and anaesthetic management. Br J Anaesthiol 1986; 58:1453.
7. Samaan NA, Hickey RC. Pheochromocytoma. Semin Oncol 1987; 14:297.
8. Sarosi G, Doe RP. Familial occurrence of parathyroid adenomas, pheochromocytoma and medullary carcinoma of the thyroid with amyloid stroma (Sipples syndrome). Ann Intern Med 1968; 68:1305.
9. Neumann HPH, Berger DP, Sigmund G, et al. Pheochromocytomas, multiple endocrine neoplasia type 2, and von Hippel-Lindau disease. N Engl J Med 1993; 329:1531.
9a. Sgambati MT, Stolle C, Choyke PL, et al. Mosaicism in von Hippel-Lindau disease: lessons from kindreds with germline mutations identified in offspring with mosaic parents. Am J Hum Genet 2000; 66:84.
10. Carney JA, Go VLW, Gordon H, et al. Familial pheochromocytoma and islet cell tumor of the pancreas. Am J Med 1980; 68:515.
11. Lairmore TC, Ball DW, Baylin SB, Wells SA Jr. Management of pheochromocytomas in patients with multiple endocrine neoplasia type 2 syndromes. Ann Surg 1993; 217:595.
12. Plouin PF, Degoulet P, Tugaye A, et al. Le dépistage du phéochromocytome: chez quels hypertendus?: Étude sémiologique chez 2585 hypertendus dont 11 ayant un phéochromocytome. Nouv Press Med 1981; 10:869.
13. Dunn FG, DeCarvalho JGR, Kem DC, et al. Pheochromocytoma crisis induced by saralasin: relation of angiotensin analogue to catecholamine release. N Engl J Med 1976; 295:605.
14. Plouin PF, Ménard J, Corvol P. Hypertensive crisis in patient with pheochromocytoma given metoclopramide. Lancet 1976; 2:1357.
15. Bergland BE. Pheochromocytoma presenting as shock. Am J Emerg Med 1989; 7:44.
16. Montastruc JL, Chamontin B, Senard JM, et al. Pseudopheochromocytoma in parkinsonian patient treated with fluoxetine plus selegiline. Lancet 1993; 341:555.
17. Li JKY, Yeung VTF, Leung CM, et al. Clozapine: a mimicry of phaeochromocytoma. Aust N Z J Psychiatry 1997; 31:889.
18. Heath H III, Edis AJ. Pheochromocytoma associated with hypercalcemia and ectopic secretion of calcitonin. Ann Intern Med 1979; 91:208.
19. Forman BH, Marban E, Kayne RD, et al. Ectopic ACTH syndrome due to pheochromocytoma: case report and review of the literature. Yale J Biol Med 1979; 52:181.
20. Kaplan NM, Kramer NJ, Holland OB, et al. Single-voided urine metanephrine assays in screening for pheochromocytoma. Arch Intern Med 1977; 137:190.
21. Ganguly A, Henry DP, Yune HY, et al. Diagnosis and localization of pheochromocytoma: detection by measurement of urinary norepinephrine excretion during sleep, plasma norepinephrine concentration and computerized axial tomography (CT scan). Am J Med 1979; 67:21.
22. Duncan MW, Compton P, Lazarus L, Smythe GA. Measurement of norepinephrine and 3,4-dihydroxyphenylglycol in urine and plasma for the diagnosis of pheochromocytoma. N Engl J Med 1988; 319:136.
23. Gitlow SE, Mendlowitz M, Wilk EK, et al. Excretion of catecholamine metabolites by normal children. J Lab Clin Med 1968; 72:612.
24. Stein PP, Black HR. A simplified diagnostic approach to pheochromocytoma: a review of the literature and report of one institution's experience. Medicine (Baltimore) 1991; 70:46.
25. Graham PE, Smythe GA, Edwards GA, Lazarus L. Laboratory diagnosis of pheochromocytoma: which analytes should we measure? Ann Clin Biochem 1993; 30:129.
26. Hamilton BP, Landsberg L, Levine RJ. Measurement of urinary epinephrine in screening for pheochromocytoma in multiple endocrine neoplasia type II. Am J Med 1978; 65:1027.
27. Shoup RE, Kissinger PT, Goldstein DS. Rapid liquid chromatographic methods for assay of norepinephrine, epinephrine, and dopamine in biological fluids and tissues. In: Ziegler MG, Lake CR, eds. Frontiers of clinical neuroscience, vol 2. Norepinephrine. Baltimore: Williams & Wilkins, 1984:38.
28. Goldstein DS, Stull R, Markey SP, et al. Dihydrocaffeic acid: a common contaminant in the liquid chromatographic electrochemical measurement of plasma catecholamines in man. J Chromatogr 1984; 311:148.
29. Brown MJ. Simultaneous assay of norepinephrine and its deaminated metabolite, dihydroxyphenylglycol, in plasma: a simplified approach to the exclusion of pheochromocytoma in patients with borderline elevation of plasma noradrenaline concentration. Eur J Clin Invest 1984; 14:67.
30. Lenders JWM, Willemsen JJ, Beissel T, et al. Value of the plasma norepinephrine/3,4-dihydroxyphenylglycol ratio for the diagnosis of pheochromocytoma. Am J Med 1992; 92:147.
31. Lenders JWM, Keiser HR, Goldstein DS, et al. Plasma metanephrines in the diagnosis of pheochromocytoma. Ann Intern Med 1995; 123:101.

31a. Eisenhofer G, Lenders JW, Linehan WM, et al. Plasma normetanephrine and metanephrine for detecting pheochromocytoma in von Hippel-Lindau disease and multiple endocrine neoplasia type 2. N Engl J Med 1999; 340:1872.

32. Eisenhofer G, Keiser H, Friberg P, et al. Plasma metanephrines are markers of pheochromocytoma produced by catechol-O-methyltransferase within tumors. J Clin Endocrinol Metab 1998; 83:2175.

33. O'Connor DT, Bernstein KN. Radioimmunoassay of chromogranin A in plasma as a measure of exocytotic sympathoadrenal activity in normal subjects and patients with pheochromocytoma. N Engl J Med 1984; 311:764.

34. Canale MP, Bravo EL. Diagnostic specificity of serum chromogranin-A for pheochromocytoma in patients with renal dysfunction. J Clin Endocrinol Metab 1994; 78:1139.

35. Baudin E, Gigliotti A, Ducreux M, et al. Neuron-specific enolase and chromogranin A as markers of neuroendocrine tumours. Br J Cancer 1998; 78:1102.

36. Bravo EL, Tarazi RC, Fouad FM, et al. Clonidine suppression test: a useful aid in the diagnosis of pheochromocytoma. N Engl J Med 1981; 305:623.

37. Sheps SG, Maher FT. Histamine and glucagon tests in diagnosis of pheochromocytoma. JAMA 1968; 205:895.

38. Levinson PD, Hamilton BP, Mersey JH, Kowarski AA. Plasma norepinephrine and epinephrine responses to glucagon in patients with suspected pheochromocytomas. Metabolism 1983; 32:998.

39. Grossman E, Goldstein DS, Hoffman A, Keiser HR. Glucagon and clonidine testing in the diagnosis of pheochromocytoma. Hypertension 1991; 17:733.

40. Macdougall IC, Isles CG, Stewart H, et al. Overnight clonidine suppression test in the diagnosis and exclusion of pheochromocytoma. Am J Med 1988; 84:993.

41. Raper AJ, Jessee EF, Texter JH Jr, et al. Pheochromocytoma of the urinary bladder: a broad clinical spectrum. Am J Cardiol 1977; 40:820.

42. Jalil ND, Pattou FN, Combemale F, et al. Effectiveness and limits of preoperative imaging studies for the localization of pheochromocytomas and paragangliomas: a review of 282 cases. French Association of Surgery (AFC), and The French Association of Endocrine Surgeons (AFCE). Eur J Surg 1998; 164:23.

43. Fink IJ, Reinig JW, Dwyer AJ, et al. MR imaging of pheochromocytomas. J Comput Assist Tomogr 1985; 9:454.

44. Doppman JL, Reinig JW, Dwyer AJ, et al. Differentiation of adrenal masses by magnetic resonance imaging. Surgery 1987; 102:1018.

45. Sisson JC, Frager MS, Valk TW, et al. Scintigraphic localization of pheochromocytoma. N Engl J Med 1981; 305:12.

45a. Rainis T, Ben-Haim S, Dickstein G. False positive metaiodobenzylguanidine scan in a patient with a huge adrenocortical carcinoma. J Clin Endocrinol Metab 2000; 85:5.

46. Khafagi FA, Shapiro B, Fig LM, et al. Labetolol reduces iodine-131 MIBG uptake by pheochromocytoma and normal tissues. J Nucl Med 1989; 30:481.

47. Jonsson A, Hallengren B, Manhem P, et al. Cardiac pheochromocytoma. J Intern Med 1994; 236:93.

48. Sinclair AJ, Bomanji J, Harris P, et al. Pre- and post-treatment distribution pattern of [123]I-MIBG in patients with phaeochromocytomas and paragangliomas. Nucl Med Commun 1989; 10:567.

49. Kopf D, Bockisch A, Steinert H, et al. Octreotide scintigraphy and catecholamine response to an octreotide challenge in malignant pheochromocytoma. Clin Endocrinol (Oxf) 1997; 46:39.

50. Rosamond TL, Hamburg MS, Vacek JL, Borkon AM. Intrapericardial pheochromocytoma. Am J Cardiol 1992; 70:700.

51. Cubeddu L, Zarate NA, Rosales CB, Zschaeck DW. Prazosin and propranolol in preoperative management of pheochromocytoma. Clin Pharmacol Ther 1982; 32:156.

52. Engelman K. Pheochromocytoma. Clin Endocrinol Metab 1977; 6:769.

53. Perry RR, Keiser HR, Norton JA, et al. Surgical management of pheochromocytoma with the use of metyrosine. Ann Surg 1990; 212:621.

54. Lenders JW, Sluiter HE, Thien T, Willemsen J. Treatment of a pheochromocytoma of the urinary bladder with nifedipine. BMJ 1985; 290:1624.

55. Chimori K, Miyazaki S, Nakajima T, Miura K. Preoperative management of pheochromocytoma with the calcium antagonist nifedipine. Clin Ther 1985; 7:372.

56. Proye C, Thevenin D, Cecat P, et al. Exclusive use of calcium channel blockers in preoperative and intraoperative control of pheochromocytomas: hemodynamics and free catecholamine assays in ten consecutive patients. Surgery 1989; 106:1149.

57. Schenker JG, Chowers I. Pheochromocytoma and pregnancy. Obstet Gynecol Surg 1971; 26:739.

58. Fudge TL, McKinnin WMP, Geary WL. Current surgical management of pheochromocytoma during pregnancy. Arch Surg 1980; 115:1224.

59. Harper MA, Murnaghan GA, Kennedy L, et al. Phaeochromocytoma in pregnancy: five cases and a review of the literature. Br J Obstet Gynaecol 1989; 96:594.

60. Demeure MJ, Carlsen B, Traul D, et al. Laparoscopic removal of a right adrenal pheochromocytoma in a pregnant woman. J Laparoendosc Adv Surg Tech A 1998; 8:315.

61. Brennan MF, Keiser HR. Persistent and recurrent pheochromocytoma: the role of surgery. World J Surg 1982; 6:397.

62. Oishi S, Sato T. Elevated serum neuron-specific enolase in patients with malignant pheochromocytoma. Cancer 1988; 61:1167.

63. Linnoila RI, Lack EE, Steinberg SM, Keiser HR. Decreased expression of neuropeptides in malignant paragangliomas. Hum Pathol 1988; 19:41.

64. Pang LC, Tsao KC. Flow cytometric DNA analysis for the determination of malignant potential in adrenal and extra-adrenal pheochromocytomas or paragangliomas. Arch Pathol Lab Med 1993; 117:1142.

65. Loh KC, Fitzgerald PA, Matthay KK, et al. The treatment of malignant pheochromocytoma with iodine-131 metaiodobenzylguanidine ([131]I-MIBG): a comprehensive review of 116 reported patients. J Endocrinol Invest 1997; 20:648.

66. Averbuch SD, Steakley CS, Young RC, et al. Malignant pheochromocytoma: effective treatment with a combination of cyclophosphamide, vincristine, and dacarbazine. Ann Intern Med 1988; 109:267.

67. DeLellis RA, Wolfe HJ, Gagel RF, et al. Adrenal medullary hyperplasia: a morphometric analysis in patients with familial medullary thyroid carcinoma. Am J Pathol 1976; 83:177.

68. Gitlow SE, Bertani LM, Rausen A, et al. Diagnosis of neuroblastoma by qualitative and quantitative determination of catecholamine metabolites in urine. Cancer 1970; 25:1377.

69. Weinblatt ME, Heisel MA, Siegal SE. Hypertension in children with neurogenic tumors. Pediatrics 1983; 71:947.

70. Conference on the biology of neuroblastoma. J Pediatr Surg 1968; 3:103.

71. Consensus statement on the definition of orthostatic hypotension, pure autonomic failure, and multiple system atrophy: the Consensus Committee of the American Autonomic Society and the American Academy of Neurology. Neurology 1996; 46:1470.

72. Goldstein DS, Holmes C, Cannon RO, et al. Sympathetic cardioneuropathy in dysautonomias. N Engl J Med 1997; 336:696.

73. Wieling W, van Lieshout JJ. Investigation and treatment of autonomic circulatory failure. Curr Opin Neurol Neurosurg 1993; 6:537.

74. Freeman R, Miyawaki E. The treatment of autonomic dysfunction. J Clin Neurophysiol 1993; 10:61.

75. Chobanian AV, Volicer L, Tifft CP, et al. Mineralocorticoid-induced hypertension in patients with orthostatic hypotension. N Engl J Med 1979; 301:68.

76. Jordan J, Shannon JR, Biaggioni I, et al. Contrasting actions of pressor agents in severe autonomic failure. Am J Med 1998; 105:166.

77. Itskovitz HD, Wartenburg A. Combined phenylephrine and tranylcypromine for postural hypotension. Am Heart J 1983; 106:598.

78. Moss AJ, Glaser W, Topol E. Atrial tachypacing in the treatment of a patient with primary orthostatic hypotension. N Engl J Med 1980; 302:1456.

79. Polinsky RJ, Samaras GM, Kopin IJ. Sympathetic neural prosthesis for managing orthostatic hypotension. Lancet 1983; 1:901.

80. Brant PW, McKusick VA. Familial dysautonomia: a report of genetic and clinical studies with a review of the literature. Medicine 1970; 49:343.

81. Eng CM, Slaughenhaupt SA, Blumenfeld A, et al. Prenatal diagnosis of familial dysautonomia by analysis of linked CA-repeat polymorphisms on chromosome 9q31-q33. Am J Med Genet 1995; 59:349.

# CHAPTER 87

# ADRENOMEDULLARY DISORDERS OF INFANCY AND CHILDHOOD

WELLINGTON HUNG

## CATECHOLAMINES IN THE INFANT AND CHILD

The physiology of the adrenal medulla has been discussed in Chapter 85. The normal values in pediatric patients for excretion of urinary catecholamines and their metabolites are shown in Tables 87-1 and 87-2. Values have been published according to age, body weight, and surface area, and in relation to milligrams of urinary creatinine.[1-6] In children, the daily urinary excretion of catecholamines and metabolites increases with age and is independent of the size of individuals.[1] No sex difference is found. The dietary content does not significantly alter the quantity of catecholamines, vanillylmandelic acid, homovanillic acid, or metanephrine excreted in the urine.[7]

Plasma epinephrine and metanephrine have been studied in normal infants and children using radioenzymatic assay. The concentrations fall rapidly during the first few minutes after birth, remain at this low level for the subsequent 3 hours, and then decline further by 12 to 48 hours of life.[8] At 48 hours of life and later, the plasma epinephrine level (mean, 26 pg/mL) and

**TABLE 87-1.**
Urinary Catecholamine Excretion in Full-Term and Premature Neonates on Day 1 of Age (Mean ± Standard Deviation)

| Catecholamine | Full-Term Infants | Premature Infants |
|---|---|---|
| Epinephrine (ng/mL) | 20.9 ± 18.4 | 5.7 ± 3.4 |
| Norepinephrine (ng/mL) | 21.2 ± 27.7 | 6.4 ± 2.8 |
| Dopamine (ng/mL) | 199 ± 177 | 47 ± 26 |
| Creatinine (mg/mL) | 0.31 ± 0.21 | 0.10 ± 0.05 |
| Epinephrine/creatinine (ng/mg) | 72.2 ± 44.7 | 69.2 ± 43.4 |
| Norepinephrine/creatinine (ng/mg) | 64.6 ± 50.3 | 76.7 ± 46.6 |
| Dopamine/creatinine (ng/mg) | 689 ± 417 | 576 ± 462 |

(From Maxwell GM, Crompton S, Davies A. Urinary catecholamine levels in the newborn infant. Eur J Pediatr 1985; 143:171.)

the norepinephrine level (mean, 283 pg/mL) are comparable to values in the resting adult.

# PHEOCHROMOCYTOMA

Less than 5% of all pheochromocytoma cases occur in childhood. Pheochromocytoma is approximately twice as common in boys as in girls. In children, most tumors occur in the adrenal medulla, but they may also be found in aberrant tissue along the sympathetic chain, the thorax, the paraaortic area, the aortic bifurcation, the retroperitoneum, and the bladder. In children with pheochromocytoma, the incidence of malignant adrenal tumors has been reported to be as high as 25%.[10]

## CLINICAL FEATURES

The symptoms and signs of pheochromocytoma in children are presented in Table 87-3. Pheochromocytomas in pediatric patients are extremely variable in clinical presentation, which can lead to delay in diagnosis.[11] In a large review of 100 children, 140 tumors were found.[12] Sixty-eight patients had single tumors, 19 of which were extraadrenal. Among the 32 patients with two or more tumors, 20 had bilateral adrenal tumors, 8 had both intraadrenal and extraadrenal tumors, and 4 had multiple extraadrenal tumors.

The association of pheochromocytoma with neurocutaneous syndromes is well known. These syndromes include mucosal neuromas (see Chap. 188) and neurofibromatosis. Bilateral pheochromocytoma may occur in patients with von Hippel-Lindau disease (a syndrome characterized by dominantly inherited angiomatosis of the retina, cerebellar angioma, and angiomas of other organs).[13] Extraadrenal pheochromocytoma may be found in patients with the triad of Carney (gastric epithelioid leiomyosarcoma, pulmonary chondroma, and functioning extraadrenal paraganglioma).[14]

**TABLE 87-3.**
Symptoms and Signs of Pheochromocytoma in Children

| Symptoms/Signs* | Hume[9] (85 Patients) | Stackpole et al.[12] (100 Patients) |
|---|---|---|
| Sustained hypertension | 92 | 88 |
| Headache | 81 | 75 |
| Sweating | 68 | 67 |
| Nausea and vomiting | 56 | 48 |
| Weight loss | 44 | 38 |
| Visual disturbances | 44 | 37 |
| Abdominal or chest pain | 35 | 32 |
| Palpitations, nervousness | 34 | Not given |
| Weakness, fatigue | 27 | Not given |
| Polydipsia and polyuria | 25 | 31 |
| Convulsions | 23 | 22 |
| Acrocyanosis | 11 | 22 |
| Intermittent hypertension | 8 | 12 |

Numbers given indicate approximate percentage of patients exhibiting a particular sign or symptom.
*Reversible catecholamine-induced dilated cardiomyopathy has also been reported.

## LABORATORY FINDINGS

As in adults, in children the definitive diagnosis of pheochromocytoma requires the detection of elevated urine or blood levels of catecholamines and their metabolites (Fig. 87-1). Generally, discontinuing all medications at least 2 weeks before obtaining urine collections is wise.

The most commonly used diagnostic tests in children are 24-hour urine determinations of free catecholamines, vanillylmandelic acid, and metanephrines.[15] Assays of urinary catecholamines and vanillylmandelic acid have been associated with an approximate 25% incidence of false-negative findings, whereas such results occur in only 4% of metanephrine determinations. Measurement of plasma catecholamines may be a useful adjunct to 24-hour urine studies.[15a] Patients must remain supine while blood samples are obtained; nevertheless, plasma determinations offer the major advantage of obviating 24-hour urine collections, which can be difficult in young children.

Routine laboratory findings may include an elevated hematocrit, which may be attributable to decreased plasma volume. Hyperglycemia may be present, resulting from decreased insulin release and increased gluconeogenesis. Elevated plasma renin activity (PRA) and aldosterone levels may also occur.[16]

Formerly, pharmacologic tests to aid in the diagnosis were used widely; however, they are rarely indicated at the present time.[17] Although the provocative tests are unnecessary and can be dangerous, the clonidine suppression test is a safe and accurate method for confirming the presence of a pheochromocytoma.[18]

**TABLE 87-2.**
24-Hour Urinary Excretion of Catecholamines and Metabolites in Normal Children by Age (Mean ± Standard Deviation)

| Catecholamine | 6 Months | 6–12 Months | 1–2 Years | 2–6 Years | 6–10 Years | 10–16 Years |
|---|---|---|---|---|---|---|
| Epinephrine (μg) | 1.2 ± 0.6 | 1.8 ± 1.4 | 2.1 ± 1.0 | 4.0 ± 3.1 | 5.7 ± 3.0 | 6.9 ± 3.7 |
| Norepinephrine (μg) | 9.1 ± 5.5 | 8.8 ± 3.8 | 8.1 ± 4.1 | 13.5 ± 5.1 | 22.3 ± 16.0 | 22.6 ± 10.7 |
| Normetanephrine (μg) | 12.1 ± 7.3 | 8.1 ± 5.7 | 10.9 ± 3.4 | 18.1 ± 12.7 | 26.5 ± 13.1 | 23.7 ± 11.0 |
| Metanephrine (μg) | 3.9 ± 2.6 | 4.8 ± 5.9 | 4.5 ± 2.6 | 5.3 ± 3.2 | 9.7 ± 5.6 | 8.4 ± 4.2 |
| Vanillylmandelic acid (mg) | 1.0 ± 0.5 | 1.3 ± 0.6 | 1.3 ± 0.5 | 1.4 ± 0.9 | 2.3 ± 1.2 | 2.6 ± 1.2 |
| Dihydroxyphenylalanine (μg) | 59.1 ± 27.7 | 71.0 ± 35.5 | 84.6 ± 39.1 | 82.6 ± 34.1 | 114.6 ± 45.6 | 112.4 ± 53.9 |
| Homovanillic acid (mg) | 0.9 ± 0.5 | 1.4 ± 0.7 | 1.2 ± 0.7 | 1.7 ± 1.1 | 2.1 ± 1.0 | 3.3 ± 1.5 |

(From De Schaepdryver AF, Hooft C, Delbeke MJ, Van Den Noortgaete M. Urinary catecholamines and metabolites in children. J Pediatr 1978; 93:266.)

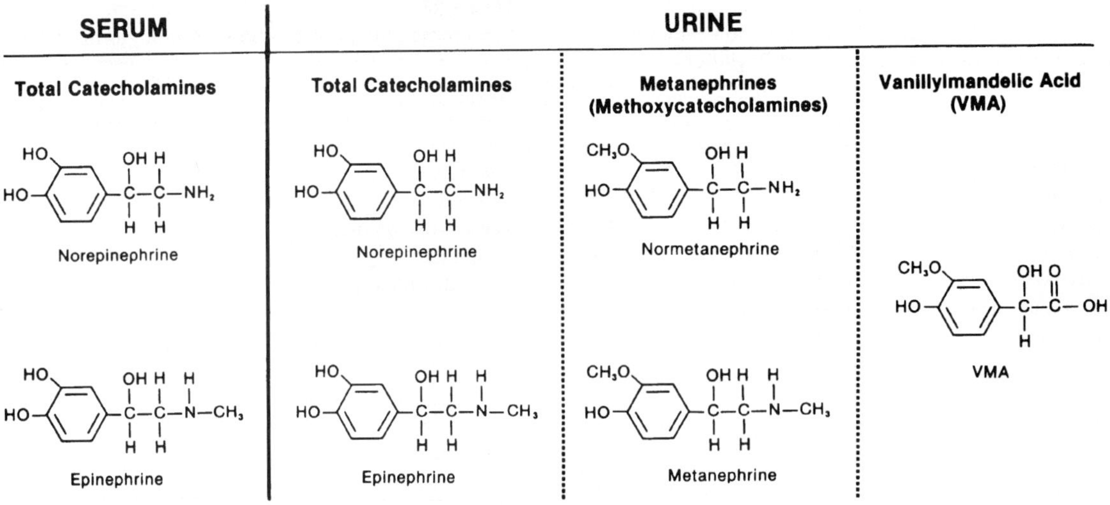

|     SERUM     |     | URINE |     |
|---|---|---|---|
| **Total Catecholamines** | **Total Catecholamines** | **Metanephrines (Methoxycatecholamines)** | **Vanillylmandelic Acid (VMA)** |

**FIGURE 87-1.** Serum and urinary constituents used for the diagnosis of pheochromocytoma. Norepinephrine and epinephrine are converted to normetanephrine and metanephrine, respectively, by the enzyme catechol-O-methyltransferase. Normetanephrine and metanephrine are then converted to vanillylmandelic acid by the enzyme monamine oxidase. (See Chap. 85 for details.)

## LOCALIZATION

Once the diagnosis of pheochromocytoma has been established, anatomic localization is essential. In children, the use of ultrasonography, computed tomography, and magnetic resonance imaging has essentially eliminated the need for preoperative localization of the tumor with arteriographic studies[19] (see Chap. 88). Selective caval sampling for catecholamine levels can be performed when an extraadrenal tumor is suspected but cannot be demonstrated by other techniques. Metaiodobenzylguanidine (MIBG) labeled with iodine-131 has been used routinely as a diagnostic imaging agent in children to localize pheochromocytomas.[20] Imaging cannot distinguish between benign and malignant tumors.[21] An occasional pheochromocytoma may not be revealed with MIBG imaging, and [18F]fluorodeoxyglucose positron emission tomography has been used successfully in detecting these tumors.[22]

## FAMILIAL PHEOCHROMOCYTOMA

Approximately 10% of pheochromocytomas in pediatric patients are familial, a frequency four times that in adults.[23] Testing all members of a family for pheochromocytomas is, therefore, important. Pheochromocytomas have also been associated with medullary thyroid carcinoma and multiple endocrine neoplasia types 2A and 2B. Therefore, all patients with pheochromocytomas should undergo careful palpation of the thyroid gland, and serum calcitonin levels should be determined. However, preoperatively, the serum calcitonin concentration can be elevated due to production of calcitonin by the pheochromocytoma (see Chaps. 53, 86, and 188).

## DIFFERENTIAL DIAGNOSIS

Particularly in children, pheochromocytoma is a difficult disease to detect by history and physical examination alone. Hyperthyroidism, cardiac disease, diabetes mellitus, and anxiety reaction may be considered initially in the differential diagnosis, but appropriate laboratory results exclude them.

## TREATMENT

Surgical removal of the pheochromocytoma should be undertaken after adequate preoperative preparation, which should include the administration of α-adrenergic and, sometimes, β-adrenergic

blocking agents.[24] The type and dosage of blockade vary from patient to patient and depend on the type of catecholamines produced by the tumor and on the response to the therapeutic agents.

For α-adrenergic blockade, phenoxybenzamine hydrochloride (Dibenzyline) or phentolamine mesylate (Regitine) can be used. Phenoxybenzamine is superior because it offers a longer duration of action and smoother control and has fewer side effects than phentolamine. In children, the usual dosage is 20 to 50 mg twice a day for 10 to 14 days preoperatively (or 1–2 mg/ kg per day divided, every 6–8 hours). The dosage of these and other α-adrenergic blocking drugs that is necessary to achieve the desired degree of blockade must be determined by careful titration while the patient is hospitalized.

Propranolol may be used for the control of β-adrenergic effects, but only after prior α-blockade. The appropriate oral dosage is 10 to 30 mg three to four times daily.

Drugs such as α-methyltyrosine that inhibit the synthesis of catecholamines have also been used in the treatment of pheochromocytoma. These agents block the conversion of tyrosine to dihydroxyphenylalanine (DOPA), thereby preventing the symptoms caused by an excess production of catecholamines.

Children with pheochromocytoma may have an increased red cell mass and chronic hypovolemia. Prolonged adrenergic activity and vasoconstriction are associated with the hypovolemia. The hypovolemia need not be manifested by a decreased hematocrit. Preoperative treatment with phenoxybenzamine for several days gradually causes expansion of the intravascular volume. Preoperative blood volume studies can be obtained, and blood can be administered in amounts calculated to expand the intravascular volume to 10% above normal.[25] Laparoscopic adrenalectomy has been used in adults but infrequently in pediatric patients.[25a] With greater experience this technique will probably be used more often in children.

In children, as in adults, the preoperative, operative, and postoperative management is of extreme importance.[26] If bilateral pheochromocytomas are diagnosed preoperatively, the child should receive intramuscular glucocorticoid therapy for 3 days before surgery in anticipation of bilateral adrenalectomy.

## POSTOPERATIVE CARE

Postoperative management should include monitoring the patient for the persistence of hypertension, which suggests residual pheochromocytoma or renovascular damage. The clinician should be alert for a contracted vascular volume, which may be present despite preoperative α-adrenergic blockade. Hypoglycemia may occur after removal of a pheochromocytoma; therefore, the plasma glucose concentration should also be monitored.

Urinary catecholamines and their metabolites should be measured during the first postoperative week. These should normalize within that time unless remaining tumor is present. Postoperatively, all patients diagnosed as having pheochromocytoma should undergo follow-up evaluations. At 6-month intervals, urinary or plasma catecholamine and metabolite studies are performed to detect any recurrence or, if the lesion was malignant, any active metastases. Rarely, a seemingly benign lesion may reveal its true nature by the subsequent finding of metastases years later; therefore, long-term follow-up is essential.[27]

## ADRENAL MEDULLARY HYPERPLASIA

Adrenal medullary hyperplasia is a rare disorder.[28] It has been described in children who were diagnosed clinically as having pheochromocytoma but in whom no tumor could be found on surgical exploration or at autopsy. The criteria that have been proposed for the diagnosis of adrenal medullary hyperplasia include (a) a clinical history of episodic hypertension with other symptoms and signs suggesting pheochromocytoma, generally associated with increased urinary catecholamine levels during attacks; (b) diffuse expansion of the adrenal medulla into the tail of the adrenal gland; (c) a medulla composed of enlarged cells with or without pleomorphism; and (d) an increased medulla/cortex ratio, together with an increased medullary weight. The suggestion has been made that diffuse adrenal medullary hyperplasia may be the initial pathologic change that subsequently leads to the development of nodular hyperplasia and a pheochromocytoma.[29]

## REFERENCES

1. De Schaepdryver AF, Hooft C, Delbeke MJ, Van Den Noortgaete M. Urinary catecholamines and metabolites in children. J Pediatr 1978; 93:266.
2. Voorhess ML. Urinary catecholamine excretion by healthy children. Pediatrics 1967; 39:252.
3. Gitlow SE, Mendlowitz M, Wilk EK, et al. Excretion of catecholamine catabolites by normal children. J Lab Clin Med 1968; 72:612.
4. Nakai T, Yamanda R. Urinary catecholamine excretion by various age groups with special reference to clinical value of measuring catecholamines in newborns. Pediatr Res 1983; 17:456.
5. Maxwell GM, Crompton S, Davies A. Urinary catecholamine levels in the newborn infant. Eur J Pediatr 1985; 143:171.
6. Tuchman M, Morris CL, Ramnaraine ML, et al. Value of random urinary homovanillic acid and vanillylmandelic acid levels in the diagnosis and management of patients with neuroblastoma: comparison with 234-hour urine collections. Pediatrics 1985; 75:324.
7. Weetman RM, Rider PS, Oei TO, et al. Effect of diet on urinary excretion of VMA, HVA, metanephrine and total free catecholamine in normal preschool children. J Pediatr 1976; 88:46.
8. Elito RJ, Lam R, Leake RD, et al. Plasma catecholamine concentration in infants at birth and during the first 48 hours of life. J Pediatr 1980; 96:311.
9. Hume DM. Pheochromocytoma in the adult and in the child. Am J Surg 1960; 99:458.
10. Perel Y, Schlumberger M, Marguerite G, et al. Pheochromocytoma and paraganglioma in children: a report of 24 cases of the French Society of Pediatric Oncology. Pediatr Hematol Oncol 1997; 14:413.
11. Januszewicz P, Wieteska-Klimczak A, Wyszka T. Pheochromocytoma in children: difficulties in diagnosis and localization. Clin Exp Hypertens 1990; 4:571.
12. Stackpole RH, Melicow MM, Uson AC. Pheochromocytoma in children: report of nine cases and review of the first 100 published cases with follow-up studies. J Pediatr 1963; 63:315.
13. Ritter MM, Frilling A, Crossey PA, et al. Isolated familial pheochromocytoma as a variant of von Hippel-Lindau disease. J Clin Endocrinol Metab 1996; 81:1035.
14. Carney JA. The triad of gastric epithelioid leiomyosarcoma, pulmonary chondroma, and functioning extra-adrenal paraganglioma. Medicine 1983; 62:159.
15. Fonkalsrud EW. Pheochromocytoma in childhood. Prog Pediatr Surg 1991; 26:103.
15a. Raber W, Raffesberg W, Kmen E, et al. Pheochromocytoma with normal urinary and plasma catecholamines but elevated plasma free metanephrines in a patient with adrenal incidentaloma. The Endocrinologist 2000; 10:65.
16. Hung W, August GP. Hyperreninemia and secondary hyperaldosteronism in pheochromocytoma. J Pediatr 1979; 94:215.
17. Young WF Jr. Pheochromocytoma and primary aldosteronism: diagnostic approaches. Endocrinol Metab Clinics North Am 1997; 26:801.
18. Bravo EL, Tarazi RC, Fouad FM, et al. Clonidine-suppression test: a useful aid in the diagnosis of pheochromocytoma. N Engl J Med 1981; 305:623.
19. Farrelly CA, Daneman A, Martin DJ, Chan HSL. Pheochromocytoma in childhood: the important role of computed tomography in tumor localization. Pediatr Radiol 1984; 13:210.
20. Gelfand MJ. Metaiodobenzylguanidine in children. Semin Nucl Med 1993; 23:231.
21. Abramson SJ. Adrenal neoplasms in children. Radiol Clin North Am 1997; 35:1415.
22. Arnold DR, Villemagne VL, Civelek AC, et al. FDG-PET: a sensitive tool for the localization of MIBG-negative pelvic pheochromocytomas. Endocrinologist 1998; 8:295.
23. Levine C, Skimming J, Levine E. Familial pheochromocytomas with unusual associations. J Pediatr Surg 1992; 27:447.
24. Brunjes A, Johns VJ, Crane MG. Pheochromocytoma. N Engl J Med 1960; 262:393.
25. Schwartz DL, Gann DS, Haller JA. Endocrine surgery in children. Surg Clin North Am 1974: 54:363.
25a. Clements RH, Goldstein RE, Holcomb III GW. Laparoscopic left adrenalectomy for pheochromocytoma in a child. J Pediatr Surg 1999; 34:1408.
26. Turner MC, Lieberman E, DeQuattro V. The perioperative management of pheochromocytomas in children. Clin Pediatr 1992; 31:583.
27. Em SH, Shandling B, Wesson D, Filler RM. Recurrent pheochromocytomas in children. J Pediatr Surg 1990; 10:1063.
28. Kurihara K, Mizuseki K, Kondo T, et al. Adrenal medullary hyperplasia. Hyperplasia-pheochromocytoma sequence. Acta Pathol Jpn 1990; 40:683.
29. Qupty G, Ishay A, Peretz H, et al. Pheochromocytoma due to unilateral adrenal medullary hyperplasia. Clin Endocrinol 1997; 47:613.

# CHAPTER 88

# DIAGNOSTIC IMAGING OF THE ADRENAL GLANDS

DONALD L. MILLER

Current imaging techniques permit the adrenal gland to be visualized with superb clarity and spatial resolution. Except in rare circumstances, other methods of adrenal imaging have been supplanted by computed tomography (CT) and magnetic resonance imaging (MRI).

CT should be the initial study for adrenal imaging in virtually all patients. It is capable of demonstrating the adrenal glands in virtually 100% of normal individuals. It provides greater spatial resolution than MRI and is less expensive. Ultrasonography costs less than CT, but it is operator dependent, has a high false-negative rate, and is often unable to permit imaging of the left adrenal gland. CT is more accurate than ultrasonography and can demonstrate both normal adrenal glands in virtually all patients (Fig. 88-1). MRI is more helpful for differential diagnosis of a known adrenal mass, but CT is a more appropriate screening technique. Oral and intravenous contrast materials are not normally required but can be helpful in some very thin patients.

The limbs of a normal adrenal gland vary considerably in length and width from individual to individual. The usual length is from 4 to 6 cm, and the usual width is from 2 to 3 mm. A good rule of thumb, when interpreting CT or MRI examinations, is that each limb should be no wider than the ipsilateral crus of the diaphragm.[1]

## ADRENAL ADENOMAS

*Incidentally discovered adrenal adenomas (incidentalomas)* are found in 1% to 4% of the population on CT scans.[1] Considerable effort has been devoted to the development of CT and MRI techniques for differentiating benign adrenal tumors from other adrenal masses.

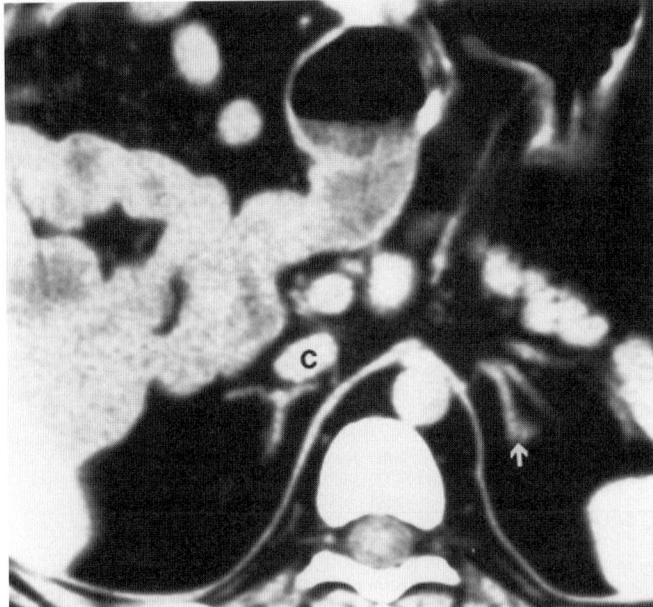

**FIGURE 88-1.** Normal adrenal glands in a patient with abundant retroperitoneal fat. The right gland lies directly behind the inferior vena cava (C) and consists of medial and lateral limbs. On the right, a small nodule (*arrow*) is seen on the tip of the medial limb, not an uncommon finding in middle-aged patients.

Adrenal adenomas are round or oval, homogeneous masses with a smooth, well-defined margin, and are usually <2 cm in diameter (Fig. 88-2).[2] In patients with known extraadrenal cancer, adrenal masses that are >3 cm in diameter or that have irregular margins have a high probability of malignancy.[3] Biopsy should be performed.

In patients who do not have a known malignancy, an incidentally discovered adrenal mass >5 cm may be an adrenal cancer. This size criterion had a sensitivity of 93% and a specificity of 64% for differentiating adenomas and carcinomas in a series of 210 patients with incidentally discovered adrenal masses.[4] Other features suggestive of adrenal carcinoma are central areas of decreased attenuation, calcification, and evidence of hepatic, venous, or nodal spread (Fig. 88-3).[5] Note, however, that large, degenerated adrenal adenomas often contain areas of calcification, hemorrhage, or necrosis.[5a] No universally reli-

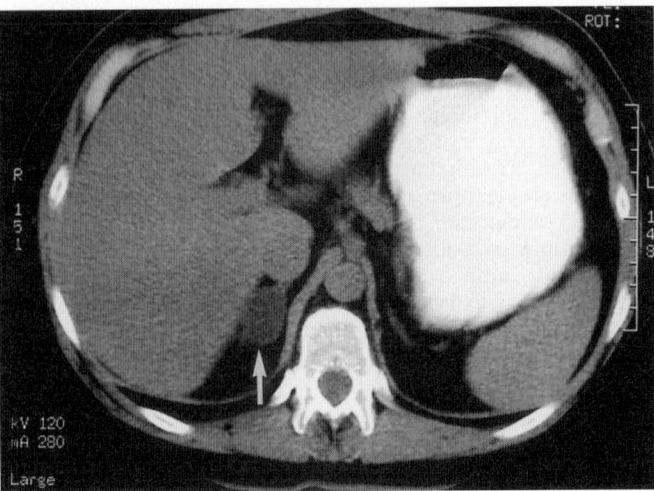

**FIGURE 88-2.** Adrenal adenoma. A homogeneous, oval, 2.5-cm mass with smooth margins is seen in the right adrenal gland (*arrow*). On this noncontrast CT scan, its attenuation is –3 Hounsfield units. It was an incidental finding in this 40-year-old woman.

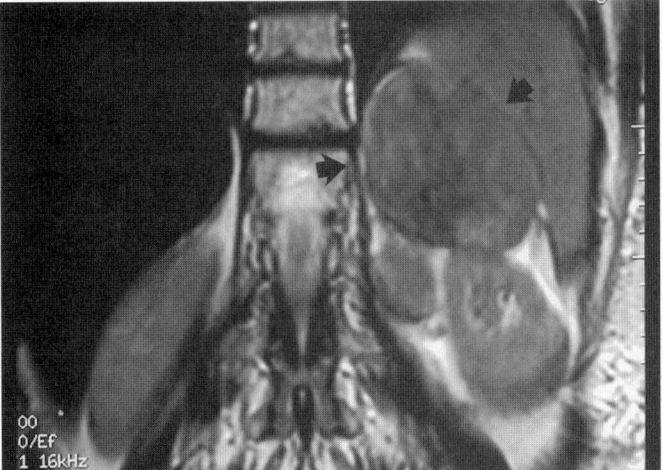

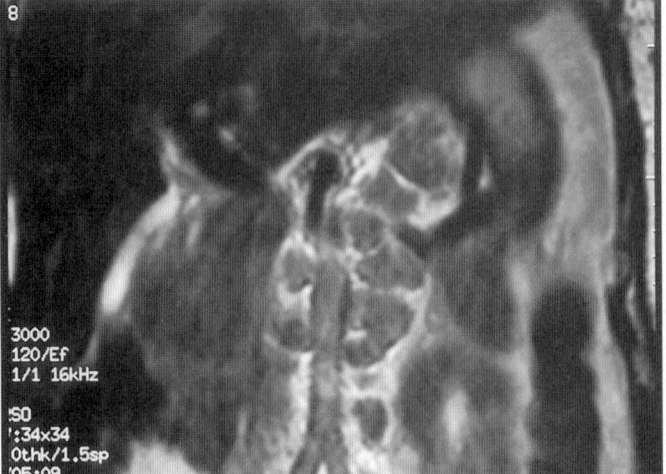

**FIGURE 88-3.** Adrenal carcinoma. **A,** The 9-cm mass in the left adrenal gland (*arrows*) has low signal intensity on this coronal T2-weighted magnetic resonance image and shows some central inhomogeneity. Whatever its imaging characteristics, the tumor's size alone suggests that adrenal carcinoma should be strongly considered. **B,** A more anterior coronal image demonstrates paraaortic adenopathy, which supports the diagnosis of adrenal carcinoma.

able imaging criteria, other than size, are available for differentiating adrenal adenoma from adrenal carcinoma on CT scans.

Adrenal adenomas, regardless of whether they demonstrate clinical endocrine function, usually contain an abundance of intracytoplasmic lipid; metastases do not.[6] Most CT and MRI maneuvers used to diagnose adrenal adenomas are designed to demonstrate or quantify this lipid content. The simplest method is measurement of adrenal attenuation on a CT scan obtained without intravenous contrast material. CT attenuation is measured in *Hounsfield units (HU)*, with water arbitrarily assigned a value of 0 HU. The greater the amount of lipid in an adrenal mass, the lower its attenuation. Some investigators have reported a mean attenuation of 2.5 HU for adrenal adenomas versus 32 HU for other adrenal lesions (see Fig. 88-2),[7] and others have found a mean attenuation of 4 HU for adenomas and 37 HU for other adrenal masses.[8] Unfortunately, substantial variability exists in the amount of lipid present from adenoma to adenoma; therefore, substantial variability is seen in attenuation as well. Threshold values from 20 HU to 2 HU have been used in the radiologic literature to distinguish between adenomas and other adrenal lesions. With a 20-HU threshold, sensitivity is 88%, but specificity is 84%. If a 2-HU threshold is used, specificity increases to 100%, but sensitivity is only 47%.[9] Many centers use a 10-HU cutoff value.[10]

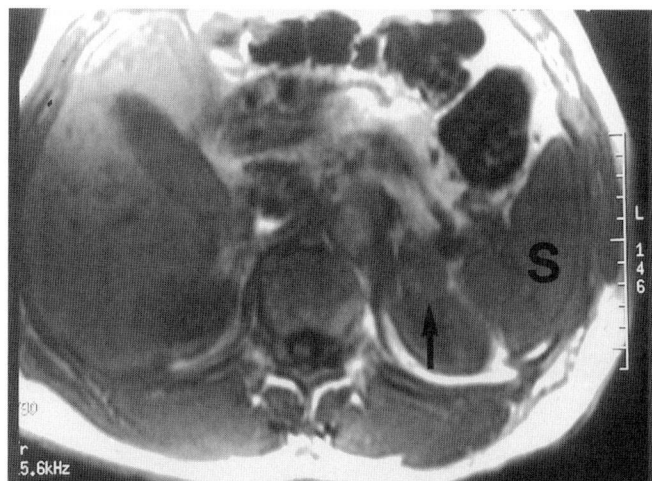

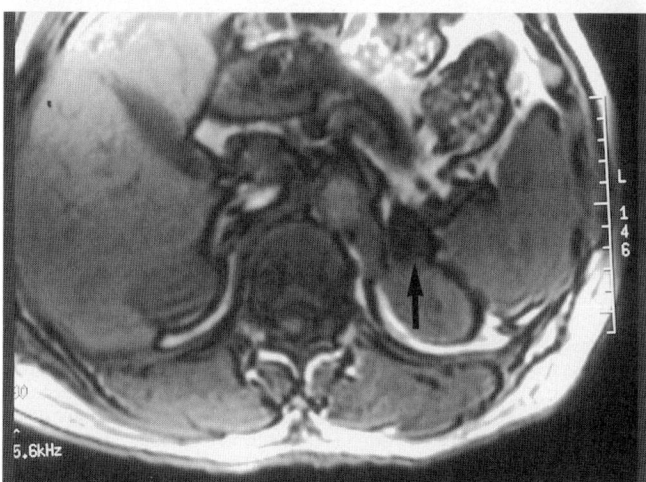

**FIGURE 88-4.** Magnetic resonance chemical-shift imaging in a patient with a left adrenal adenoma. **A,** An axial in-phase image demonstrates a left adrenal mass (*arrow*) of signal intensity approximately equal to that of the spleen (*S*). **B,** An opposed-phase image demonstrates markedly lower signal intensity in the same adrenal mass (*arrow*) as compared to the spleen, which indicates that the mass has a significant lipid content.

These threshold values cannot be used if the patient has been given intravenous contrast material for the CT scan, because this causes adrenal enhancement. Instead, attenuation may be measured at a specific time (≥3 min) after contrast material administration. The attenuation threshold depends on the delay between contrast material administration and scanning. A threshold of 39 HU at 30 minutes has been recommended.[8]

An alternative CT method for evaluation of adrenal lesions is the use of washout curves. After intravenous administration of contrast material, adrenal adenomas demonstrate contrast material washout (loss of enhancement) earlier and more rapidly than other adrenal masses.[11,12] The histopathologic and pathophysiologic correlates of this behavior are unclear. A similar phenomenon has been observed with MRI. Initial reports suggest that the sensitivity and specificity of this technique exceed 96%.[11,12]

MRI with chemical-shift imaging is another way to demonstrate adrenal lipid. This is generally done using opposed-phase images. T1-weighted gradient-echo MR images can be acquired so that water and lipid spins are either in phase or opposed. If lipid is present, comparison of in-phase and opposed-phase images will demonstrate that the signal intensity of the tissue is lower on the opposed-phase image (Fig. 88-4). Quantitative analysis may be performed by calculating the *chemical-shift ratio*—equal to the lesion-to-spleen intensity ratio in in-phase images

divided by the lesion-to-spleen ratio in opposed-phase images (see Fig. 88-4). Eighty percent sensitivity and nearly 100% specificity can be achieved with this technique, regardless of whether qualitative or quantitative methods are used.[5,13] In a study of 134 adrenal masses, the combination of MR chemical shift imaging and MR gadolinium washout techniques yielded a sensitivity of 91%, a specificity of 94%, and an accuracy of 93% for differentiating benign and malignant adrenal masses.[13a]

MR chemical–shift imaging and CT-attenuation techniques correlate well; a lesion that is considered indeterminate by one technique is likely to be indeterminate with the other technique.[14] This is not always true, however. A cost-effective algorithm uses CT attenuation as the first step, followed, if necessary, by MRI with chemical-shift imaging. If both of these studies are equivocal, biopsy should be performed.[15]

Clinically silent adrenal adenomas cannot be differentiated from functioning adrenal adenomas on the basis of any cross-sectional imaging method (i.e., CT, MRI, ultrasonography). This is an endocrine diagnosis, not a radiologic one, because imaging studies demonstrate morphology, not function. However, MRI signal intensity characteristics can usually aid in differentiating benign adrenal adenomas from otherwise morphologically identical pheochromocytomas, and often from small adrenal carcinomas.[16]

Adrenal scintigraphy with the cholesterol analog *NP-59* ([131]I-6β-iodomethylnorcholesterol), an investigational drug, has been used to differentiate adrenal adenomas from adrenal metastases. Advances in CT and MRI have essentially eliminated the need for this agent, which accumulates in, and irradiates, the adrenal glands, the gonads, and the thyroid.[1,17] [111]In-pentetreotide, an octreotide analog, may be helpful in problem cases because it is concentrated in most malignant adrenal lesions, but not in most benign lesions.[18] Uncommon nonfunctioning adrenal lesions identified on imaging studies include cystic lesions (hydatid cyst, endothelial cyst), solid lesions (hemangioma, ganglioneuroma, angiosarcoma, primary malignant melanoma), and solid fatty lesions (myelolipoma, collision tumor). Most of these lesions do not have specific imaging features.[18a]

## ADRENAL LESIONS WITH ENDOCRINE FUNCTION

The *cardinal rule of endocrine radiology* may be expressed in the phrase *diagnosis first, localization second.* When dealing with a patient with a suspected endocrine abnormality, the clinician must establish the diagnosis first, using endocrinologic methods. Only after the diagnosis is determined should radiologic methods be used in an attempt to locate an anatomic abnormality. Failure to heed this rule often results in a costly series of tests that produce only false-positive findings.

### PHEOCHROMOCYTOMA

*Adrenal pheochromocytomas* are almost always >2 cm in diameter and are readily identified by CT. Central necrosis and calcification may occur (Fig. 88-5).[2] Pheochromocytomas demonstrate very high signal intensities on T2-dependent spin-echo MRI images and are readily visible.[5] In a series of 282 patients with known pheochromocytomas, MRI had a sensitivity of 98%, CT had a sensitivity of 89%, and scanning with [131]I-metaiodobenzylguanidine (MIBG) had a sensitivity of 81%.[19] For this reason, MRI is the procedure of choice for the initial localization of pheochromocytomas.

Patients with elevated catecholamine levels and a unilateral adrenal mass on CT or MRI require no further localization studies. Bilateral tumors or adrenal medullary hyperplasia are common in multiple endocrine neoplasia syndrome (MEN) type 2A (Sipple syndrome) and type 2B.

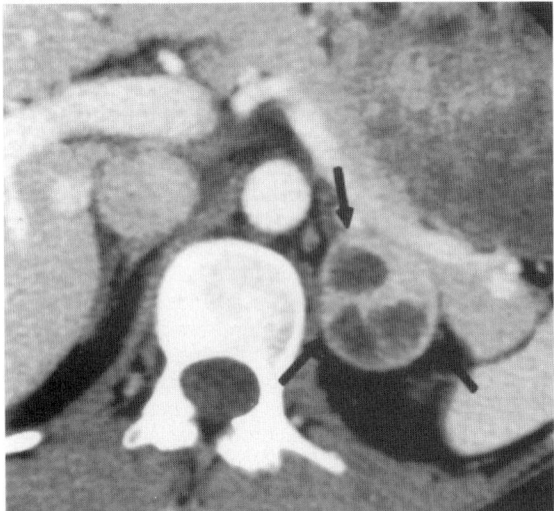

**A**

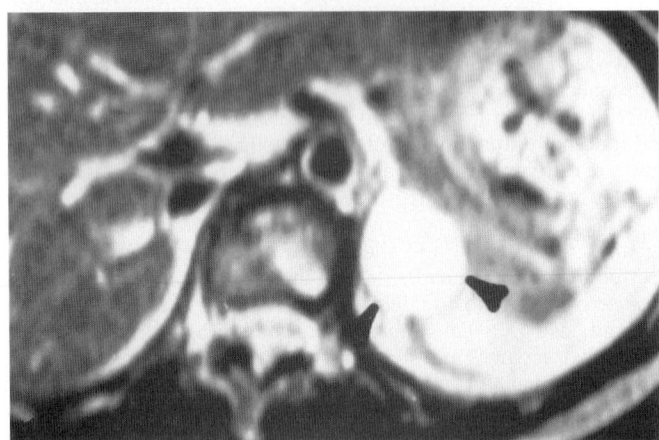

**B**

**FIGURE 88-5. A,** This contrast-enhanced computed tomographic scan shows a 3-cm pheochromocytoma in the left adrenal gland that contains focal areas of necrosis (*arrows*). **B,** A T2-weighted magnetic resonance imaging (*MRI*) scan shows very high signal intensity (*arrowheads*), typical for a pheochromocytoma. This characteristic high signal intensity on T2-weighted MRI scans makes MRI the preferred localization technique for ectopic pheochromocytomas.

When pheochromocytoma is suspected, MRI of the adrenal glands should be performed first, because 90% of these tumors are intraadrenal. If the adrenal glands are normal, MRI or CT of the entire abdomen and pelvis is appropriate, because 98% of all pheochromocytomas and 85% of all extraadrenal pheochromocytomas occur below the diaphragm.[20] Extraadrenal pheochromocytomas may occur in paravertebral locations, in the organ of Zuckerkandl, and anywhere from the base of the skull (e.g., glomus jugulare tumors) to the neck of the urinary bladder.

MIBG imaging has proven useful for the detection of ectopic pheochromocytomas. MIBG has a molecular structure that resembles norepinephrine. It is actively concentrated in chromaffin tissue and the adrenergic nervous system. Although MIBG imaging is less sensitive overall than MRI or CT, it is more specific than either.[21] For extraadrenal lesions, MIBG scanning has a sensitivity of 67% to 100%, and a specificity of 96%.[20] It is particularly helpful for the detection of metastases in patients with malignant pheochromocytomas (Fig. 88-6). MIBG scans alone may not provide sufficient anatomic detail to guide the surgeon, but they help to direct CT and MRI studies toward the ectopically located lesion.

In the rare patient in whom CT, MRI, and MIBG studies yield negative or equivocal results, *arteriography* or *venous sampling* may sometimes be helpful.[22] These procedures are safe in patients receiving adequate doses of blocking agents, such as

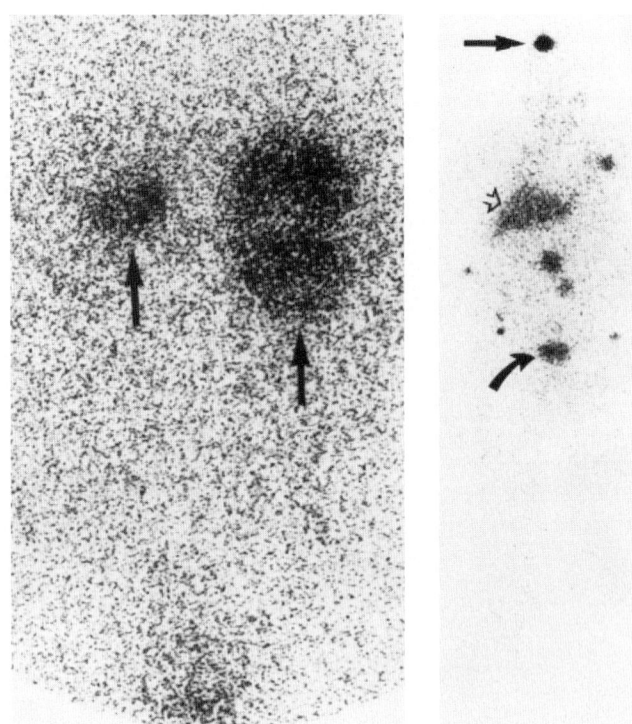

**A,B**

**FIGURE 88-6. A,** Iodine-131–labeled metaiodobenzylguanidine (*MIBG*) concentrates in pheochromocytomas, as demonstrated in the scan of this patient with bilateral adrenal tumors (*arrows*). This image was obtained 48 hours after injection of the radiopharmaceutical. The delay is a drawback of this method. **B,** In patients with malignant pheochromocytoma, a whole body scan may demonstrate metastases. A prominent lesion is seen in this patient's skull (*arrow*) and other metastases are noted elsewhere. Radioactivity is also evident in normal liver (*open arrow*) and the urinary bladder (*curved arrow*) on this anterior scan obtained 24 hours after administration of MIBG.

phenoxybenzamine. Nonionic contrast agents do not appear to affect circulating catecholamine levels.[23]

## HYPERALDOSTERONISM

*Hyperaldosteronism (Conn syndrome)* may be caused by a discrete, functioning aldosterone-producing adenoma (APA) or by bilateral hyperplasia. The decision between medical and surgi-

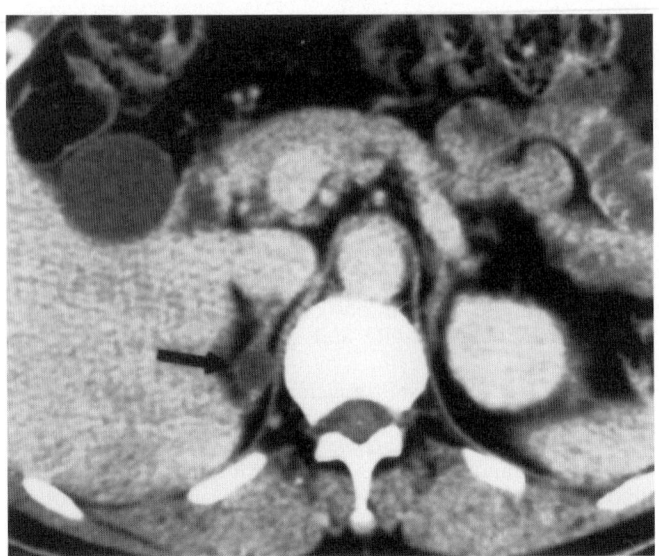

**FIGURE 88-7.** Aldosterone-producing adenomas are usually small and often contain relatively lucent focal areas of decreased attenuation (*arrow*).

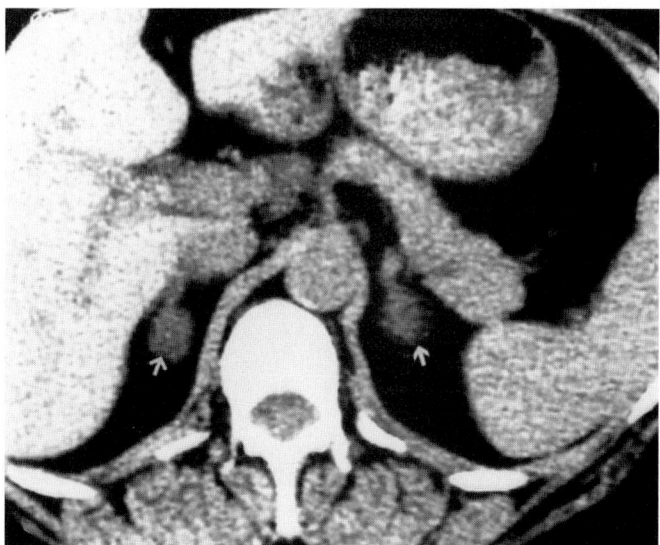

**FIGURE 88-8.** The bilateral adrenal masses (*arrows*) in this patient with hyperaldosteronism suggest the diagnosis of idiopathic hyperaldosteronism. Bilateral adrenal venous sampling revealed a right-sided aldosteronoma, confirmed by surgery. Aldosterone levels became normal after right adrenalectomy.

cal therapy hinges on the diagnosis of unilateral adrenal involvement (adenoma) or bilateral hyperplasia.[24] Because MRI is more expensive than CT and has a lower spatial resolution, CT is the preferred modality for initial evaluation of the adrenal glands in patients with hyperaldosteronism.[17]

Aldosterone-producing adenomas often appear on CT as relatively lucent, focal areas of decreased attenuation compared with the surrounding adrenal gland (Fig. 88-7).[2] This presumably reflects the high concentration of corticosteroids in the lesion. APAs are small: 50% are <1 cm in diameter. CT permits reliable detection of lesions >5 mm, but smaller APAs still may occasionally be missed. CT scans that demonstrate normal-appearing adrenal glands bilaterally are not diagnostic of hyperplasia, because a small, undetected adenoma may be present.[25] One should also remember that on rare occasions the aldosterone source may be a renal or ovarian tumor.[26]

A more common problem in differentiating adenoma from hyperplasia on CT and MRI is the presence of *bilateral adrenal nodules*. This finding is not diagnostic of idiopathic hyperplasia. In one series, 6 of 7 patients with bilateral adrenal nodules on CT had a unilateral aldosteronoma confirmed at surgery (Fig. 88-8).[27] The same difficulty arises when multiple nodules are identified in one gland, or when CT evidence of bilateral adrenal enlargement and a unilateral nodule is present. With current high-definition CT scanners, multiple small nodules or limb thickening are often observed in the adrenal glands of older adults.[28] Chemical-shift MRI can be used to define which, if any, of the nodules has a high lipid content and is therefore an APA.[29] In one series, chemical shift imaging was positive in 6 of 7 patients (86%) with APA and 8 of 9 patients (89%) with hyperplasia.[27]

Patients with primary hyperaldosteronism who have imaging findings of an obvious unilateral adrenal nodule and a normal contralateral gland on CT scans, and clinical findings that support a diagnosis of APA, may proceed directly to surgery.[1] Patients with CT evidence of bilateral adrenal nodules or bilateral normal-appearing adrenal glands should undergo bilateral adrenal vein sampling.[17,24,29] Scintigraphy with NP-59 has been used in patients with hyperaldosteronism, but it is relatively insensitive for APAs <15 mm; therefore, it is not helpful for the evaluation of small adrenal nodules.[17]

Imaging studies evaluate adrenal architecture, but *adrenal venous sampling* provides data on adrenal function. With proper

technique, venous sampling can correctly differentiate hyperplasia from APA in nearly 100% of patients; it can only lateralize in those patients who have APA.[27] Properly performed, venous sampling is the most reliable method available for this purpose.[24,30]

The purpose of adrenal venous sampling is not to demonstrate which adrenal is producing aldosterone but to demonstrate which gland is *not*.[31] A gland that is not producing aldosterone is physiologically suppressed and, therefore, normal. If both glands produce aldosterone, bilateral hyperplasia is present.

The technique of adrenal venous sampling has been described in detail.[27,31] Bilateral adrenal vein samples should be collected simultaneously before and after stimulation with adrenocorticotropic hormone (ACTH). Simultaneous peripheral vein samples are obtained as well. The right adrenal vein is short and difficult to catheterize, and dilution of right adrenal samples with blood from the inferior vena cava is a common problem. This can be corrected by calculating the aldosterone/cortisol ratio (A:C ratio) in each sample, because cortisol production should be uniform bilaterally.[32] Adrenal venography is not necessary to document sampling position; if cortisol levels are higher than those in the peripheral vein sample, the adrenal veins have been sampled.

When an APA is present, the A:C ratio in blood from the affected side is >1.5 times the A:C ratio of the peripheral sample, and the A:C ratios of blood from the normal (suppressed) adrenal and the peripheral vein are essentially the same. With adrenal hyperplasia, samples from both glands exhibit A:C ratios of >1.5 times the A:C ratio from the peripheral vein. Because catheterization of the right adrenal vein may be difficult, some patients have been evaluated using only left adrenal vein and peripheral samples. This method is accurate if an APA is present in the right adrenal gland, but bilateral adrenal hyperplasia and a left adrenal APA cannot be differentiated without a right adrenal vein sample.

## CUSHING SYNDROME

*Bilateral adrenal hyperplasia* secondary to ACTH-dependent Cushing disease can produce slightly enlarged glands; however, the adrenals may have a normal appearance. Paraneoplastic or

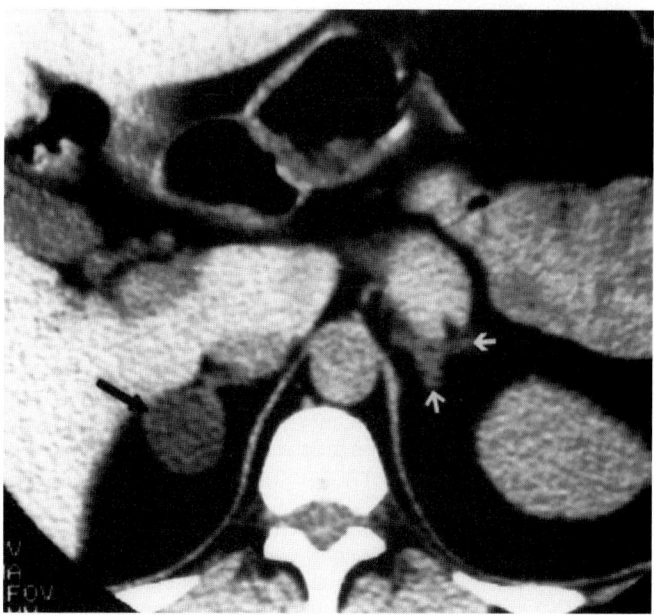

**FIGURE 88-9.** A 3-cm nodule (*black arrow*) in the right adrenal gland of a patient with Cushing syndrome. The presence of hyperplasia in the left adrenal gland (*white arrows*) identifies this as adrenocorticotropic hormone (*ACTH*)–dependent hypercortisolism with a unilateral nodule (i.e., asymmetric ACTH-dependent macronodular hyperplasia).

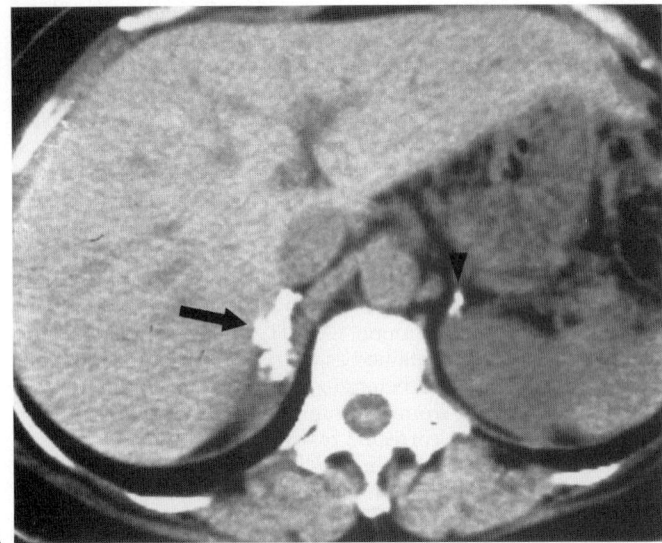

**A**

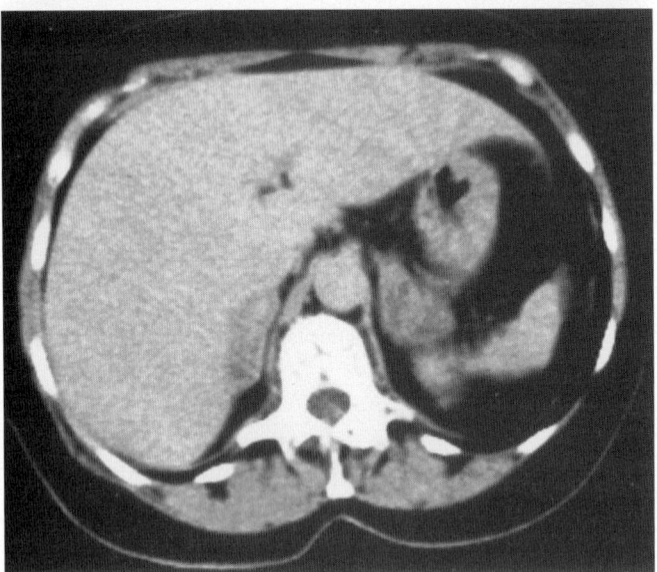

**B**

**FIGURE 88-10. A,** In chronic adrenal insufficiency due to granulomatous infection, bilateral calcification is often present (*arrow* and *arrowhead*). **B,** Acute adrenal insufficiency due to histoplasmosis presents as enlarged inhomogeneous adrenal glands that retain their adreniform shape.

ectopic production of ACTH may result in a greater degree of adrenal enlargement. Occasionally, unilateral macronodular hyperplasia may simulate the appearance of an adenoma (Fig. 88-9).[28] This may lead the unwary physician to recommend inappropriate unilateral adrenalectomy.

Two forms of bilateral adrenal involvement in ACTH-independent Cushing syndrome are found. *ACTH-independent macronodular adrenal hyperplasia*, also called *massive macronodular hyperplasia*, is a rare, distinct cause of Cushing syndrome.[33] Approximately 40 cases had been reported in a recent review.[33] Multiple adrenal nodules are present bilaterally, ranging in size from microscopic to 4 cm.[28] They obscure the normal adrenal contour, and the adrenal gland is recognizable as such only by its location. These patients require bilateral adrenalectomy, which is curative.[33]

*Primary pigmented nodular adrenocortical disease* may be a component of Carney complex, an autosomal dominant MEN syndrome that includes myxomas, spotty skin pigmentation, and tumors of the adrenal cortex, pituitary, thyroid, or gonads.[34,35] The pigmented nodules range from microscopic to 8 mm in diameter. Older patients may have larger nodules, up to 3 cm in diameter.[36] In individuals aged 14 years or older, CT scans obtained with 5-mm sections demonstrate tiny nodules in the adrenal limbs, with

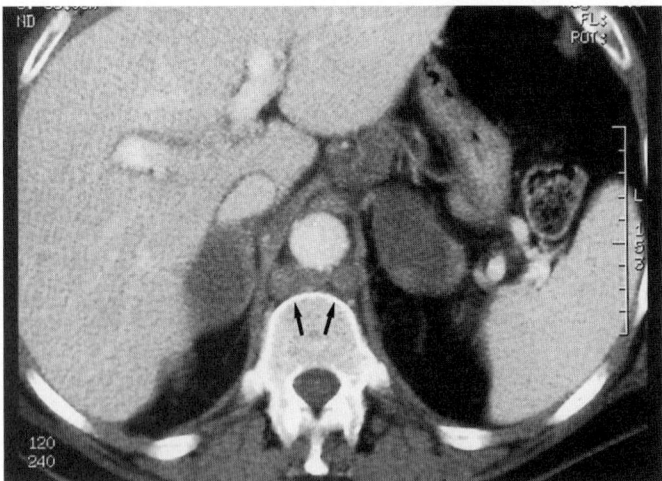

**FIGURE 88-11.** Bilateral adrenal lymphoma causing hypoadrenalism. In this 69-year-old man, both adrenal glands are enlarged, and paraaortic adenopathy (*arrows*) is also evident.

intervening areas of atrophy, which give rise to a characteristic "string-of-beads" appearance.[28,36] The lipofuscin pigment in the nodules does not affect their CT or MR appearance.

## ADRENAL HYPOFUNCTION

In *idiopathic Addison disease*, the size of the adrenal glands may be small or normal. Adrenal calcification or high attenuation of the adrenal glands can be seen in hypoadrenalism owing to certain specific causes, such as chronic tuberculosis, histoplasmosis, and hemochromatosis (Fig. 88-10). In hypoadrenalism of acute onset, the identification of enlarged glands with a normal contour should suggest acute granulomatous adrenalitis secondary to tuberculosis or histoplasmosis. Prompt treatment may restore adrenal function. Rarely, hypoadrenalism may be due to bilateral adrenal metastases (Fig. 88-11).

## REFERENCES

1. Cook DM. Adrenal mass. Endocrinol Metab Clin North Am 1997; 26:829.
2. Kawashima A, Sandler CM, Fishman EK, et al. Spectrum of CT findings in nonmalignant disease of the adrenal gland. Radiographics 1998; 18:393.
3. Candel AG, Gattuso P, Reyes CV, et al. Fine-needle aspiration biopsy of adrenal masses in patients with extraadrenal malignancy. Surgery 1993; 114:1132.
4. Terzolo M, Ali A, Osella G, Mazza E. Prevalence of adrenal carcinoma among incidentally discovered adrenal masses: a retrospective study from 1989 to 1994. Arch Surg 1997; 132:914.
5. Krebs TL, Wagner BJ. MR imaging of the adrenal gland: radiologic-pathologic correlation. Radiographics 1998; 18:1425.
5a. Newhouse JH, Heffess CS, Wagner BJ, et al. Large degenerated adrenal adenomas: radiologic-pathologic correlation. Radiology 1999; 210:385.
6. Korobkin M, Giordano TJ, Brodeur FJ, et al. Adrenal adenomas: relationship between histologic lipid and CT and MR findings. Radiology 1996; 200:743.
7. Korobkin M, Brodeur FJ, Yutzy GG, et al. Differentiation of adrenal adenomas from nonadenomas using CT attenuation values. AJR Am J Roentgenol 1996; 166:531.
8. Szolar DH, Kammerhuber F. Quantitative CT evaluation of adrenal gland masses: a step forward in the differentiation between adenomas and nonadenomas? Radiology 1997; 202:517.
9. Boland GWL, Lee MJ, Gazelle GS, et al. Characterization of adrenal masses using unenhanced CT: an analysis of the CT literature. AJR Am J Roentgenol 1998; 171:201.
10. Peppercorn PD, Grossman AB, Reznek RH. Imaging of incidentally discovered adrenal masses. Clin Endocrinol 1998; 48:379.
11. Szolar DH, Kammerhuber FH. Adrenal adenomas and nonadenomas: assessment of washout at delayed contrast-enhanced CT. Radiology 1998; 207:369.
12. Korobkin M, Brodeur FJ, Francis IR, et al. CT time-attenuation washout curves of adrenal adenomas and nonadenomas. AJR Am J Roentgenol 1998; 170:747.
13. Outwater EK, Blasbalg R, Siegelman ES, Vala M. Detection of lipid in

abdominal tissues with opposed-phase gradient-echo images at 1.5 T: techniques and diagnostic importance. Radiographics 1998; 18:1465.

13a. Heinz-Peer G, Hönigschnabl S, Schneider B, et al. Characterization of adrenal masses using MR imaging with histopathologic correlation. AJR Am J Roentgenol 1999; 173:15.

14. Outwater EK, Siegelman ES, Huang AB, Birnbaum BA. Adrenal masses: correlation between CT attenuation value and chemical shift ratio at MR imaging with in-phase and opposed-phase sequences. Radiology 1996; 200:749.

15. McNicholas MMJ, Lee MJ, Mayo-Smith WM, et al. An imaging algorithm for the differential diagnosis of adrenal adenomas and metastases. AJR Am J Roentgenol 1995; 165:1453.

16. Lee MJ, Mayo-Smith WW, Hahn PF, et al. State-of-the-art MR imaging of the adrenal gland. Radiographics 1994; 14:1015.

17. Young WF Jr. Pheochromocytoma and primary aldosteronism: diagnostic approaches. Endocrinol Metab Clin North Am 1997; 26:801.

18. Maurea S, Lastoria S, Salvatore M, et al. The role of radiolabeled somatostatin analogs in adrenal imaging. Nucl Med Biol 1996; 23:677.

18a. Otal P, Escourrou G, Mazerolles C, et al. Imaging features of uncommon adrenal masses with histopathologic correlation. Radiographics 1999; 19:589.

19. Jalil ND, Pattou FN, Combemale F, et al. Effectiveness and limits of preoperative imaging studies for the localisation of pheochromocytomas and paragangliomas: a review of 282 cases. Eur J Surg 1998; 164:23.

20. Whalen RK, Althausen AF, Daniels GH. Extra-adrenal pheochromocytoma. J Urol 1992; 147:1.

21. Maurea S, Cuocolo A, Reynolds JC, et al. Diagnostic imaging in patients with paragangliomas: computed tomography, magnetic resonance and MIBG scintigraphy comparison. Q J Nucl Med 1996; 40:365.

22. Walker IABL. Selective venous catheterization and plasma catecholamine analysis in the diagnosis of phaeochromocytoma. J R Soc Med 1996; 89:216P.

23. Mukherjee JJ, Peppercorn PD, Reznek RH, et al. Pheochromocytoma: effect of nonionic contrast medium in CT on circulating catecholamine levels. Radiology 1997; 202:227.

24. Ganguly A. Primary aldosteronism. N Engl J Med 1998; 339:1828.

25. Young WF Jr, Stanson AW, Grant CS, et al. Primary aldosteronism: adrenal venous sampling. Surgery 1996; 120:913.

26. Abdelhamid S, Müller-Lobeck H, Pahl S, et al. Prevalence of adrenal and extra-adrenal Conn syndrome in hypertensive patients. Arch Intern Med 1996; 156:1190.

27. Doppman JL, Gill JR Jr, Miller DL, et al. Distinction between hyperaldosteronism due to bilateral hyperplasia and unilateral aldosteronoma: reliability of CT. Radiology 1992; 184:677.

28. Doppman JL. The dilemma of bilateral adrenocortical nodularity in Conn's and Cushing's syndromes. Radiol Clin North Am 1993; 31:1039.

29. Doppman JL. Problems in endocrinologic imaging. Endocrinol Metab Clin North Am 1998; 26:973.

29a. Sohaib SA, Peppercorn PD, Allan C, et al. Primary hyperaldosteronism (Conn syndrome): MR imaging findings. Radiology 2000; 214:527.

30. Gleason PE, Weinberger MH, Pratt JH, et al. Evaluation of diagnostic tests in the differential diagnosis of primary aldosteronism: unilateral adenoma versus bilateral micronodular hyperplasia. J Urol 1993; 150:1365.

31. Doppman JL, Gill JR Jr. Hyperaldosteronism: sampling the adrenal veins. Radiology 1996; 198:309.

32. Tokunaga K, Nakamura H, Marukawa T, et al. Adrenal venous sampling analysis of primary aldosteronism: value of ACTH stimulation in the differentiation of adenoma and hyperplasia. Eur Radiol 1992; 2:223.

33. Swain JM, Grant CS, Schlinkert RT, et al. Corticotropin-independent macronodular adrenal hyperplasia: a clinicopathologic correlation. Arch Surg 1998; 133:541.

34. Stratakis CA, Kirschner LS. Clinical and genetic analysis of primary bilateral adrenal diseases (micro- and macronodular disease) leading to Cushing syndrome. Horm Metab Res 1998; 30:456.

35. Carney JA. The Carney complex (myxomas, spotty pigmentation, endocrine overactivity, and Schwannomas). Dermatol Clin 1995; 13:19.

36. Doppman JL, Travis WD, Nieman L, et al. Cushing syndrome due to primary pigmented nodular adrenocortical disease: findings at CT and MRI. Radiology 1989; 172:415.

# CHAPTER 89

# SURGERY OF THE ADRENAL GLANDS

GARY R. PEPLINSKI AND JEFFREY A. NORTON

Adrenalectomy is the most effective means available to eradicate localized cancers that arise within the adrenal glands, to eliminate adrenal sources of hormone overproduction, to relieve symptoms caused by mass effect, and to promptly establish definitive diagnoses for potentially malignant adrenal masses. *Minimally invasive laparoscopic approaches* for adrenalectomy have evolved dramatically and are now commonly practiced in high-volume endocrine surgery centers. Laparoscopic adrenalectomy can be safely performed by experienced surgeons, is effective treatment for selected adrenal conditions, and is consistently associated with prompt resumption of full patient activity. *Open adrenalectomy* remains the standard operation for resection of large adrenal tumors and adrenal cancers. In addition to surgical advances, success in treating patients with adrenal disorders is also due to improved understanding of endocrine pathophysiology, more sensitive and specific radiologic imaging and localization studies, and advances in anesthesia in perioperative patient care. This chapter presents the surgical perspective to assessing and treating the varied disorders of the adrenal glands.

## SURGICAL ANATOMY AND EMBRYOLOGY

Each adrenal gland lies high within the retroperitoneum in a central location within the body, near the midline and at the junction of the chest and abdomen. Careful dissection must be carried out near the inferior vena cava, kidneys, diaphragm, liver, aorta, splenic vessels, spleen, stomach, and pancreas.

The normal gland is identified resting on the superior aspect of the kidney and is usually 3 to 5 cm long, 2 to 3 cm wide, 0.5 cm thick, and 3 to 6 g in weight. The right adrenal is triangular in shape and abuts the posterolateral surface of the inferior vena cava. The left adrenal gland lies close to the aorta and is more crescentic in shape. Each gland is surrounded by a fibrous capsule and embedded within areolar perirenal fat. The normal adrenal cortex is bright yellow, and the medulla appears reddish brown. On palpation of the suprarenal area, the adrenal gland can be distinctly recognized by its firm consistency.

The adrenal glands are highly vascular. The *arterial blood supply* for each gland is variable and is derived from numerous sources. Several small arteries penetrate the perimeter of each gland along its superior, medial, and inferior aspects, arising from the phrenic artery superiorly, directly from the aorta medially, and from the renal arteries inferiorly.

*Venous drainage* of the adrenals is more constant; a single vein drains each gland. Knowledge of the specific location and course of each vein is crucial for successful surgery. Venous bleeding may result from damage to the fragile veins and may be difficult to localize and control. The *right adrenal vein* is wide and short, ~5 mm in length. This vein exits the right adrenal at its medial surface and drains directly into the inferior vena cava at its posterolateral aspect. Thus, this vessel may be difficult to control from an anterior exposure of the right adrenal, and the vein is easily torn when large right adrenal masses are retracted, which is a potentially fatal event. The *left adrenal vein* exits the left adrenal from its anterior surface and has a longer course medially to drain into the left renal vein, although aberrant venous drainage sometimes occurs.

Because intraoperative exploration is the definitive evaluation for the presence of disease, the common ectopic locations where adrenal tumors occur must be known. This requires an understanding of adrenal embryology. The adrenal cortex develops from coelomic mesoderm near the urogenital ridge. Accessory adrenal cortical tissue may be identified as yellow masses in tissues surrounding the adrenal glands, in the kidneys, ovaries, in broad ligaments, or in the testes. The incidence of *functioning extraadrenal cortical tissue* is very low; these tissues need not be excised.

The *adrenal medullae* arise from ectodermal neural crest cells in the thoracic region that migrate ventrolateral to the aorta and along adrenal vessels until contact is made with the primitive adrenocortical cells. Approximately 10% of sporadic pheochromocytomas arise in extraadrenal locations, most commonly in the *organ of Zuckerkandl* located to the left of the aortic bifurcation

**TABLE 89-1.**
**Adrenalectomy Procedures Indicated by Preoperative Diagnosis**

| Approach | Unilateral Adrenalectomy | Bilateral Adrenalectomy |
|---|---|---|
| **Open anterior** | Malignant or multifocal pheochromocytoma<br>Adrenocortical carcinoma<br>Virilizing or feminizing tumor<br>Incidental solid mass >6 cm | Pheochromocytoma involving both adrenal glands |
| **Open or laparoscopic** | Familial pheochromocytoma (MEN2A or MEN2B) involving one adrenal gland | Familial pheochromocytoma (MEN2A or MEN2B) involving both adrenal glands<br>Massive macronodular adrenal hyperplasia |
| **Laparoscopic** | Cortical adenoma causing Cushing syndrome<br>Aldosteronoma<br>Small pheochromocytoma (<5 cm) | Primary pigmented micronodular adrenal hyperplasia<br>Severe Cushing syndrome (due to an occult ACTH-producing tumor that is unresponsive to medical management) |

*MEN*, multiple endocrine neoplasia; *ACTH*, adrenocorticotropic hormone.

near the origin of the inferior mesenteric artery. Pheochromocytomas may arise anywhere in the periaortic sympathetic ganglia, however, as well as in the bladder, mediastinum, neck, anus, and vagina. Familial cases of pheochromocytomas have ~50% incidence of bilateral adrenal involvement. In contrast to ectopic adrenocortical tissue, extraadrenal pheochromocytomas frequently cause symptoms, and all gross tumor must be resected.

## INDICATIONS FOR ADRENALECTOMY

Surgical resection is the primary treatment for adrenal tumors that are functionally active or potentially malignant (Table 89-1). In general, adrenalectomy is indicated for functional cortical adenomas causing Cushing syndrome or primary aldosteronism, virilizing or feminizing tumors, adrenocortical carcinoma, pheochromocytoma, and incidental solid adrenal masses that are >6 cm in diameter on computed tomographic (CT) scan. Laparoscopic adrenalectomy has become the procedure of choice for solitary benign functional adenomas or pheochromocytomas that are small. Open resection is required for large masses (>5–6 cm in diameter) and cancers.

*Bilateral adrenalectomy* is indicated for conditions of primary bilateral adrenal gland hypersecretion, such as primary pigmented micronodular adrenal hyperplasia and massive macronodular adrenocortical hyperplasia (see Table 89-1).[1] Bilateral adrenalectomy is also an effective treatment for severe, debilitating Cushing syndrome caused by an ectopic adrenocorticotropic hormone (ACTH)–secreting tumor that is either occult and not identified on imaging studies or metastatic and unresectable. Bilateral adrenalectomy may also be indicated for those patients with Cushing disease in whom transsphenoidal surgery and medical management have not been successful.[2] Laparoscopy is the preferred surgical approach for these conditions because typical adrenal gland sizes are small enough to permit a minimally invasive procedure, and severely debilitated patients tolerate laparoscopic adrenalectomy better than open surgery. One exception is massive macronodular adrenocortical hyperplasia, which may require open resection because the adrenal glands may be quite large and tend to adhere to adjacent tissues.

Patients with multiple endocrine neoplasia (MEN) type 2A or type 2B have a high incidence of bilateral adrenal pheochromocytomas. Therefore, some surgeons recommend bilateral adrenalectomy at the time of detection of the initial pheochromocytoma, even if the contralateral gland appears free of disease. This is commonly performed laparoscopically. Others argue that the risk of acute adrenal insufficiency after bilateral adrenalectomy is unacceptably high and can be lethal if untreated. In addition, 12 years may elapse before a pheochromocytoma arises in the uninvolved contralateral adrenal gland.[3] Consequently, if the contralateral adrenal gland appears normal by preoperative studies and intraoperative examination, some recommend unilateral adrenalectomy to resect the identified pheochromocytoma and long-term follow-up with serial urinary screening tests for pheochromocytoma to detect the development of disease in the contralateral adrenal gland. Patient compliance with follow-up must be assured.

## ADRENAL INCIDENTALOMA

The more widespread availability and use of high-resolution CT scanners have resulted in the detection of asymptomatic adrenal masses, called adrenal "incidentalomas," which may have previously gone unrecognized. The dilemma for the surgeon is to identify and resect the *minority* of such tumors that are malignant or functional, and avoid risks of unnecessary operations for benign, nonfunctional adenomas, which occur commonly and do not require any treatment.

Initial evaluation of a solid incidentaloma consists of a careful history-taking and physical examination to detect signs or symptoms suggestive of hypercortisolism, primary aldosteronism, pheochromocytoma, primary adrenocortical cancer, or adrenal metastasis from an undiagnosed malignancy arising in another tissue (Fig. 89-1). Laboratory studies are obtained based on clinical suspicion of the presence of one of these disorders.[4] In addition, a 24-hour urinary free cortisol level should be obtained in each patient with an incidentaloma, because addisonian crisis may occur postoperatively in a few patients with clinically occult Cushing syndrome if stress doses of corticosteroids are not administered.[4a] Blood pressures and serum potassium level are also measured in each patient to help exclude an aldosteronoma.

Importantly, death may result from even a minor procedure that induces a surge of catecholamines from a pheochromocytoma in a patient who is either undiagnosed or inadequately prepared with α-blockade.[5] Therefore, the presence of a pheochromocytoma must be definitively excluded in every patient with a solid adrenal incidentaloma before any procedures are undertaken. Clinical evaluation alone is inadequate, because these tumors may produce only episodic symptoms and may be clinically occult. A finding of normal 24-hour urine levels of catecholamines, vanillylmandelic acid, and metanephrines excludes the presence of a pheochromocytoma. In addition, on T2-weighted magnetic resonance images (MRIs), a pheochromocytoma characteristically appears extremely bright (signal intensity is three times that of the liver). In contrast, primary adrenocortical cancer and cancer that is metastatic to the adrenal gland appear only slightly brighter than the liver on MRI T2-weighted images, and cortical adenomas appear darker than the liver.[6]

If an adrenal incidentaloma is a solid mass that is not functional based on the previously described evaluation, and the presence of a pheochromocytoma can be excluded, then the

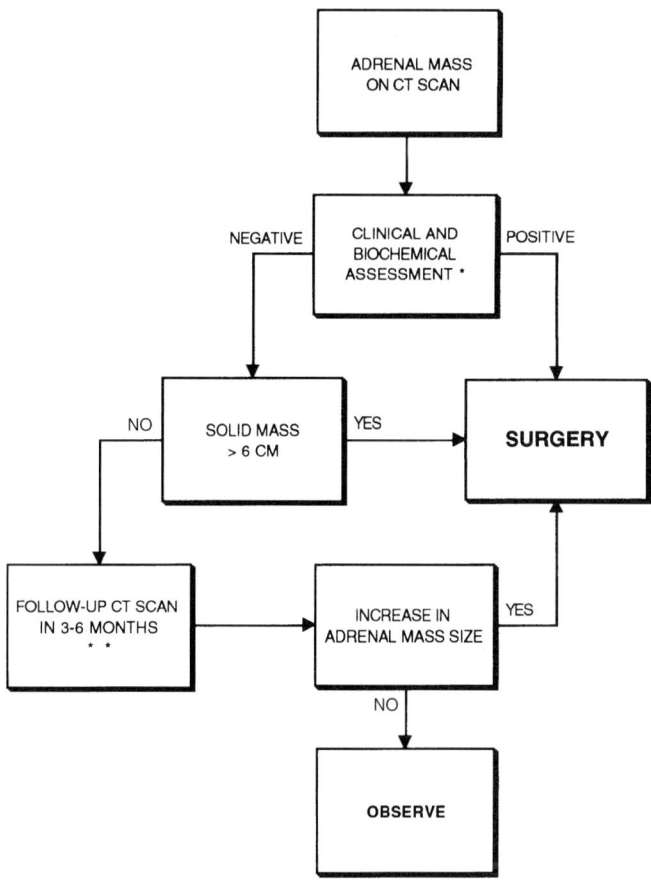

**FIGURE 89-1.** Management of an incidentally discovered adrenal mass. An asymptomatic solid adrenal mass may be identified on abdominal computed tomographic (*CT*) scans obtained to evaluate other intraabdominal processes. Functioning or potentially malignant adrenal lesions must be resected, whereas nonfunctioning, benign adrenocortical adenomas require no therapy. *, Clinical assessment consists of a careful history and physical examination for evidence of adrenal hyperfunction. Biochemical assessment includes measurement of the plasma potassium level and 24-hour urinary levels of catecholamines, vanillylmandelic acid, metanephrines, and free cortisol. **, If cancer metastatic to the adrenal gland is suspected, then CT-guided fine-needle aspiration may be attempted at this point for a confirmatory diagnosis.

final differentiation is a malignancy from a benign adrenal adenoma. Malignancy is most conclusively established or excluded by resecting each incidentaloma. However, this approach is not justified because primary adrenal carcinoma is rare, whereas benign adrenal adenomas occur frequently. If an adrenal mass is likely to be a metastasis from a malignancy arising in another tissue, then percutaneous biopsy for cytologic analysis, after a pheochromocytoma has been excluded, may be useful if a diagnosis of metastatic cancer can be established, and adrenalectomy can be avoided. However, if metastatic cancer is not likely, then percutaneous fine-needle biopsy of an adrenal incidentaloma is not indicated, because cytologic analysis cannot accurately differentiate primary adrenal cancers from benign adenomas. Laparoscopic adrenalectomy may be reasonable in healthy, young patients with moderate-sized nonfunctional adrenal incidentalomas (4–6 cm in diameter). The procedure must be performed safely with low risk by an experienced surgeon. In such cases, laparoscopic adrenalectomy provides a prompt, definitive diagnosis and peace of mind for the patient. Recovery to full preoperative activity occurs promptly, and repeated evaluations and testing are unnecessary if the mass is benign.

*The best radiologic factor to discriminate nonfunctioning benign and malignant adrenal tumors is the diameter of the mass on CT.*

**TABLE 89-2.**
**Patient Preparation before Adrenalectomy**

Assessment and optimization of the patient's general medical condition
Accurate preoperative diagnosis
Accurate localization of pathology
Radiologic imaging to define anatomy, the location of any mass and its size, and, for cancers, the extent of disease and involvement of adjacent structures
Correction of electrolyte and acid-base abnormalities
Cushing syndrome:
  Administration of stress doses of glucocorticoids
Pheochromocytoma:
  Stable α-adrenergic blockade to normalize blood pressure and symptoms
  β-Adrenergic blockade to control tachycardia and arrhythmias
  Adequate volume replacement
  Provision of central venous access
  Arterial catheterization for blood pressure monitoring

Most adrenocortical adenomas are <4 cm in diameter on CT, whereas the incidence of cancer in solid adrenal lesions of >6 cm is >35%. Therefore, every solid adrenal mass that is ≥6 cm in diameter should be resected (see Fig. 89-1). An adrenocortical carcinoma may be detected at an early stage, at <6 cm, and may be curable. Consequently, every patient with an adrenal incidentaloma that is not resected must have a repeat abdominal CT scan after 3 to 6 months to assess for growth of the lesion. Every tumor that increases in size must be resected after appropriate biochemical studies are obtained. Each of these patients should be reevaluated clinically for the development of new signs or symptoms of excessive adrenal function, which is also an indication for adrenalectomy after laboratory investigation. A well-circumscribed adrenal mass that is <6 cm in diameter, does not grow, and is not functional on repeat evaluation is virtually always benign. Resection is not indicated, and additional follow-up is *not* required.

## PREOPERATIVE PATIENT PREPARATION

Several factors must be considered to appropriately prepare a patient for adrenalectomy to obtain a successful outcome (Table 89-2) The patient's medical condition is carefully assessed and optimized to decrease operative risk. Patients with primary aldosteronism, for example, may have congestive heart failure, cardiac arrhythmias, or nephropathy. In addition, an accurate diagnosis is vital for appropriate surgical management. For pheochromocytoma, in particular, preoperative treatments and intraoperative monitoring are distinctly different from those used in other adrenal conditions.

Diagnostic biochemical tests and standard radiologic imaging may not definitively identify the cause of the endocrine disorder in some cases. Advances in imaging techniques and interventional radiologic procedures have greatly facilitated the diagnosis and localization of adrenal disorders. For example, for primary aldosteronism, adrenal vein sampling for aldosterone and cortisol is the definitive study if other radiologic imaging tests cannot differentiate an aldosteronoma from *idiopathic adrenocortical hyperplasia* as the cause. An aldosteronoma is effectively treated with adrenalectomy, while idiopathic adrenocortical hyperplasia is not improved after unilateral adrenalectomy and is managed medically.[7] Similarly, petrosal sinus sampling has facilitated the differentiation of pituitary-dependent and pituitary-independent Cushing syndrome in difficult cases. If biochemical tests suggest a primary adrenal cause of Cushing syndrome, but CT fails to show a discrete unilateral adrenal mass, then iodine-131 ([131]I)–labeled methylnorcholesterol imaging may be useful to image primary pigmented micronodular adrenal hyperplasia.[8] Bilateral adrenalectomy is curative for pri-

**TABLE 89-3.**
**Advantages and Limitations of Different Approaches for Adrenalectomy**

| Approach | Advantages | Limitations |
|---|---|---|
| **Open** | Excellent exposure | Postoperative ileus |
| | Large masses can be resected | Significant postoperative pain |
| | Allows potentially curative resections of cancers | Long recovery period |
| | Complete abdominal exploration possible | Adhesion formation and risk of subsequent bowel obstruction |
| | Extraadrenal masses can be resected | |
| **Laparoscopic** | No postoperative ileus | Large or invasive masses cannot be resected |
| | No adhesion formation | Scarring from prior surgery or trauma in the operative field inhibits use |
| | Less postoperative pain | Difficult to control hemorrhage |
| | Prompt return to full patient activity | Complete abdominal exploration more difficult |
| | Cosmetically acceptable incisions | Extraadrenal masses may not be resected |

mary pigmented micronodular adrenal hyperplasia and massive macronodular adrenal hyperplasia.[1]

Preoperative CT is useful for localizing pathology, defining anatomy, staging cancers, and showing involvement of extraadrenal tissues. MRI may provide additional information in localizing lesions and in predicting the pathology based on the T2-weighted mass signal intensity.[6] Scintigraphy using [[131]I]metaiodobenzylguanine may be used to localize pheochromocytomas that are not imaged by CT or MRI. This radiographic agent resembles norepinephrine and is concentrated in adrenergic tissues by amine uptake. The overall sensitivity of this test is ~87% and the specificity is virtually 100%. Preoperative venography and intraoperative ultrasonography are best to show tumor extension into the vena cava.

Correction of fluid, electrolyte, and acid-base abnormalities is important in the preoperative phase. Patients with primary aldosteronism uniformly have decreased potassium levels, and hypernatremia, metabolic alkalosis, or hypomagnesemia may be present. Use of spironolactone, an aldosterone antagonist, greatly facilitates preoperative electrolyte correction in these patients. Patients with pheochromocytomas typically have a lactic acidosis as a result of the metabolic effects of catecholamines and decreased perfusion from vasoconstriction. Arterial blood pH must be measured before inducing anesthesia. In addition, patients with pheochromocytomas have diminished intravascular volume and blunted sympathetic responses, important contributors to hypotension during surgery. Adequate hydration before induction of anesthesia is paramount. In patients with poor cardiac function, a Swan-Ganz catheter may need to be placed preoperatively to optimize hemodynamic status.

Stable α-adrenergic blockade must be achieved preoperatively in all patients with pheochromocytomas. Many medications may be used for this purpose, including prazosin, metyrosine, nifedipine, and nicardipine. Classically, the α-receptor antagonist, phenoxybenzamine, is given for at least 7 days before surgery at a starting dosage of 10 mg every 12 hours, which is increased until a therapeutic dosage is reached. At the therapeutic dosage, paroxysms should not occur, and blood pressure should be adequately controlled. Patients must be encouraged to drink fluids liberally and to use caution when sitting or standing, because almost all patients experience orthostatic hypotension. Patients who are symptomatic may require preoperative hospitalization. Preoperative normalization of blood pressure and symptoms is associated with fewer intraoperative and postoperative complications and has dramatically improved surgical management of these patients.[9] Once α-adrenergic blockade has been achieved, use of a β-blocker may then be initiated to control tachycardia and catecholamine-induced arrhythmias. Propranolol is commonly used at a dosage of 10 mg three to four times daily. A paradoxical increase in blood pressure may occur if β-blockade is started before successful α-blockade is achieved.

Patients with an adrenocortical adenoma causing Cushing syndrome usually have atrophied residual adrenocortical tissue. Stress corticosteroid doses are necessary in these patients perioperatively to avoid acute adrenocortical insufficiency. Some groups have reported using ketoconazole as an effective means to eliminate hypercortisolism before surgery. Ketoconazole therapy may be associated with addisonian crises and hepatotoxicity. In the experience of the authors, this treatment is not needed before resecting adrenal adenomas causing Cushing syndrome. However, preoperative ketoconazole therapy may be indicated when extremely severe symptoms of hypercortisolism are present, as observed in patients with paraneoplastic ACTH-secreting tumors.

## ADRENALECTOMY

The adrenal glands lie at a central, deep position within the body, and several different surgical approaches have been devised for their safe removal. Either adrenal gland may be resected using an open anterior transperitoneal approach or using minimally invasive laparoscopic methods. Laparoscopic adrenalectomy has essentially replaced the open posterior approach, which provided access to the adrenals through the back. General anesthesia is required for each operation. Several important factors are considered when choosing the surgical approach (Table 89-3). These include preoperative diagnosis, size and location of any adrenal mass, potential for malignancy, involvement of extraadrenal structures, the need to explore the entire abdomen, previous surgery in the planned operative area, and patient factors.

The trend has been increasingly in favor of using a laparoscopic approach for adrenalectomy whenever possible.[9a,9b] Data that have accrued with laparoscopic adrenalectomy have reproducibly demonstrated efficacy equivalent to that of open surgery in treating certain adrenal conditions and significantly reduced postoperative patient rehabilitation. In addition, ileus does not occur after laparoscopic surgery, and intraperitoneal adhesion formation is avoided, so that the associated risk of subsequent bowel obstruction is eliminated. For the surgeon, the magnification and clarity provided by modern videoscopic systems enable close visualization of deep regions and dissection with fine detail.

Requirements that must be satisfied for laparoscopic adrenalectomy include a benign condition, mass diameter <5 to 6 cm, noninvolvement of adjacent structures, no history of surgery or trauma resulting in scarring in the planned surgical field, surgeon experience in advanced laparoscopy and open adrenalectomy, and acceptable patient factors. Laparoscopic adrenalectomy is the procedure of choice for small functional adenomas causing aldosteronism or Cushing syndrome, small pheochromocytomas, small adrenal incidentalomas, and bilateral hyperfunctioning adrenal glands (e.g.,

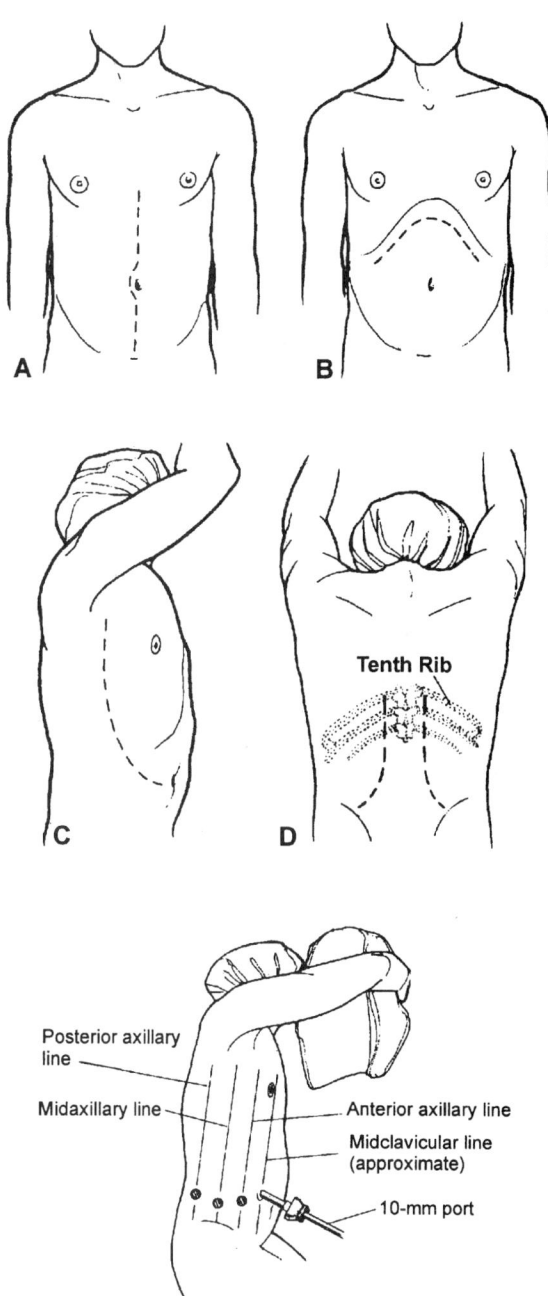

**FIGURE 89-2.** Patient positioning and skin incisions for adrenalectomy. Resection of either adrenal gland and any associated mass is accomplished using an open anterior transperitoneal approach or using laparoscopic techniques. **A,** Midline incision for open transperitoneal approach. **B,** Bilateral subcostal incision for open transperitoneal approach. **C,** Thoracoabdominal incision for large, invasive cancers. **D,** Posterior approach (not commonly used at present). **E,** Port entry sites for laparoscopic adrenalectomy. (From Peplinski GR, Norton JA. Adrenalectomy. Current Techniques in General Surgery 1994; 3[1]:1. Copyright 1994, Lawrence DellaCorte Publications, Inc. Artist: Molly Babich.)

of the entire abdomen, retroperitoneum, and contralateral adrenal gland is easily accomplished with an open anterior approach to accurately identify and resect all disease and to evaluate the extent of disease. Large sporadic pheochromocytomas and adrenocortical carcinomas should be resected with open surgery.

The inability to complete an adrenalectomy using laparoscopic methods also requires conversion to an open operation. Conditions that technically prevent a laparoscopic approach are large masses (generally >5–6 cm in diameter), involvement of extraadrenal structures, scarring that makes dissection difficult, significant bleeding, poor visualization, inconclusive anatomy, and equipment malfunction. Therefore, every surgeon performing laparoscopic adrenalectomy must be proficient in open abdominal and retroperitoneal surgery. The anatomic perspective with laparoscopic adrenalectomy may be unfamiliar to a surgeon inexperienced with this approach, and the added magnification provided by laparoscopy may lead to misidentification of important structures. Dissection of the vascular adrenal with inadequate hemostasis may cause bleeding that compromises visualization and the ultimate success of a laparoscopic approach. The adrenal glands themselves may be very difficult to locate with laparoscopy because only visualization and not palpation is possible, and the adrenals are embedded in retroperitoneal fat of similar color and consistency. The availability of *laparoscopic intraoperative ultrasonography* and familiarity with this advanced technique are necessary to locate the adrenal glands in difficult cases without converting to an open procedure. In addition, laparoscopic ultrasonography may be used to identify the location of important vascular structures so that injury is avoided.

For an open anterior approach,[9c] the patient is placed in the supine or lateral decubitus position, and either a midline, bilateral subcostal, or thoracoabdominal incision is made (Figs. 89-2A through 89-2C). For laparoscopic adrenalectomy, the patient is placed in the lateral decubitus position with the affected side superiorly. Four ports are placed transversely along the costal

primary pigmented micronodular adrenal hyperplasia). Large adrenal masses (>5–6 cm diameter) and those that are thought to be malignant should be resected using an open anterior transperitoneal approach. A thoracoabdominal incision with the patient in a partial lateral decubitus position may be used for open resection of localized large masses. Open surgery enables appropriate exposure for potentially curative cancer resections. In addition, thorough exploration

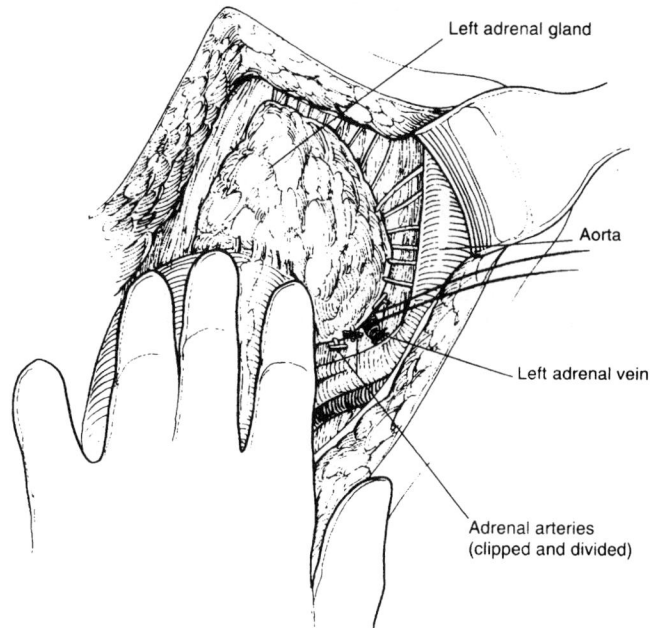

**FIGURE 89-3.** Posterior approach for left adrenalectomy. Removal of the 11th and 12th ribs and gentle inferior retraction on the kidney provides good exposure of the adrenal gland. The more superficial arteries are initially dissected, ligated, and divided until the adrenal vein is visualized. Gaining vascular control of the left adrenal vein is difficult from the posterior approach because it lies very deep, anterior to the adrenal gland. (From Peplinski GR, Norton JA. Adrenalectomy. Current Techniques in General Surgery 1994; 3:5. Copyright 1994, Lawrence DellaCorte Publications, Inc. Artist: Molly Babich.)

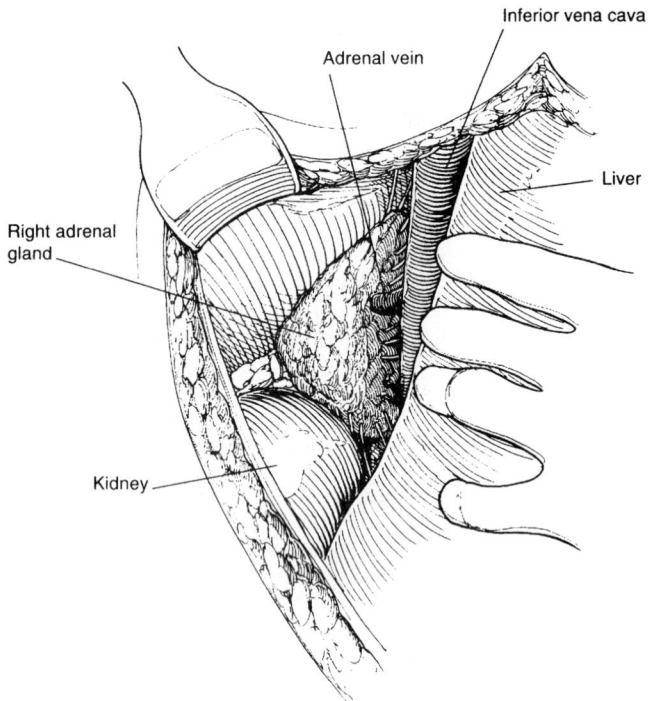

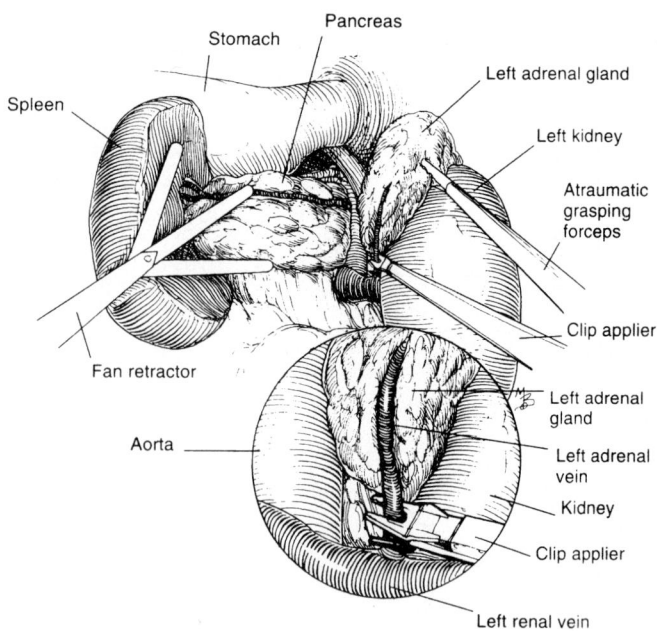

**FIGURE 89-4.** Open anterior, transperitoneal approach for right adrenalectomy. The right adrenal gland is exposed from within the abdomen by dividing the hepatic ligaments and mobilizing the right lobe of the liver medially. The adrenal gland is identified resting on the superior aspect of the kidney. The right adrenal vein is short and wide and drains directly into the posterolateral aspect of the inferior vena cava. (From Peplinski GR, Norton JA. Adrenalectomy. Current Techniques in General Surgery 1994; 3:3. Copyright 1994, Lawrence DellaCorte Publications, Inc. Artist: Molly Babich.)

**FIGURE 89-5.** Laparoscopic left adrenalectomy. The splenic flexure of the left colon and the splenic ligaments are dissected free to allow medial retraction of the spleen, stomach, and tail of the pancreas with a fan retractor, which exposes the left adrenal gland. The adrenal vein, which is identified on the anterior surface of the gland, is clipped and divided. Once dissected free, the adrenal gland is placed into a bag before removal to prevent spillage of tissue. (From Peplinski GR, Norton JA. Adrenalectomy. Current Techniques in General Surgery 1994; 3:7. Copyright 1994, Lawrence DellaCorte Publications, Inc. Artist: Molly Babich.)

margin from the midclavicular line to the posterior axillary line (see Fig. 89-2E). A videoscope is inserted through one port, and operating instruments—which include retractors, grasping forceps, dissecting forceps, irrigation, suction, and cautery—are manipulated through the other three ports. (Of historical interest, the posterior approach was performed by placing the patient in the prone jackknife position and making a curved incision that ran vertically from just lateral to the midline at the 10th rib to the superior aspect of the posterior iliac crest [see Fig. 89-2D]. Removal of the 11th and 12th ribs was common to improve access to the suprarenal area [Fig. 89-3].)

Laparoscopic and open adrenalectomy is performed with adherence to the same surgical principles. A thorough exploration of the abdomen is initially conducted to identify extra-adrenal or bilateral disease and to document other pathology. Laparoscopic exploration is limited to two-dimensional visualization, which may be obstructed by viscera, such as the bowel, that cannot be adequately mobilized away from the field. In contrast, open surgery enables a more thorough inspection and palpation of the entire abdomen and contralateral adrenal gland. The right adrenal gland is exposed by mobilizing the hepatic flexure of the right colon and the right lobe of the liver anteriorly and medially away from the right retroperitoneum (Fig. 89-4). The left adrenal gland is optimally exposed by reflecting the splenic flexure of the left colon, the spleen, and the tail of the pancreas medially away from the left retroperitoneum (Fig. 89-5). Considerably less dissection is required for laparoscopic resection than for open surgery. The adrenal gland is located by identifying normal anatomy, visualizing a mass, using intraoperative ultrasonography, and palpating.

Prompt identification, dissection, and ligation of the single adrenal vein is important to accomplish early in the operation.

Control of the vein decreases the risk of fatal hemorrhage from tearing it when a mass is present. In addition, venous occlusion prevents the systemic circulation of hormones produced by an adrenal tumor and its bioeffects. When a pheochromocytoma is resected, minimal handling of the involved adrenal gland until the vein is ligated causes less lability in intraoperative blood pressure due to catecholamine discharge. The right adrenal vein is most easily identified by dissecting along the posterolateral border of the inferior vena cava. This vein is very short and wide. The left adrenal vein is typically long and easily visualized on the anterior aspect of the left adrenal gland.

After the adrenal vein is controlled, the adrenal gland is then dissected free circumferentially. Multiple small arteries are encountered in this dissection, and each one must be securely clipped or ligated and divided. If an adrenal mass is present, it is included in the dissection. With laparoscopic resection, the specimen is placed into a bag before removal, to prevent spilling of tissue as it is negotiated through one of the port sites.

Potentially curative resections of cancers require complete removal of the malignant mass with margins of uninvolved tissue. Direct incision into the mass is avoided to prevent spillage and seeding of potentially cancerous cells. Invasion of adjacent organs, as may be encountered with adrenocortical carcinoma, requires en bloc resection of all the involved tissues. The best opportunity for potential cure of adrenocortical carcinoma is complete resection of all gross disease at the initial surgery. Cancers often exhibit a considerable degree of neovascularity, and hemostasis as dissection proceeds is critical.

Resection of a pheochromocytoma requires close cooperation between the anesthesiologist and surgeon. Continuous, close intraoperative monitoring of the patient's electrocardiogram, central venous pressure, and blood pressure by means of an arterial line has contributed to a reduction in operative mortality and morbidity for patients undergoing resections of pheochromocytomas.[9] For patients with significant cardiac disease, Swan-Ganz catheter-

**TABLE 89-4.**
**Outcomes and Follow-Up after Successful Adrenalectomy, by Diagnosis**

| Pathologic Diagnosis | Outcome | Follow-Up Issues |
|---|---|---|
| Benign adenoma | Excellent | None |
| Adenoma causing Cushing syndrome | Unilateral adrenalectomy is curative | Glucocorticoid replacement until pituitary-adrenal axis recovers |
| Aldosteronoma | Very good | Electrolytes normalize in all patients |
| | | Recurrent hypertension in 30% in 2–3 years |
| Bilateral adrenal hyperplasia (pigmented micronodular, massive macronodular) | Bilateral adrenalectomy is curative | Lifelong glucocorticoid and mineralocorticoid replacement |
| Sporadic pheochromocytoma | 5-year survival >95% after complete resection | Recurrent hypertension in 25% |
| | | Recurrent tumor (up to 50%) |
| | | Measurement of catecholamines; clonidine suppression tests; CT, MRI, MIBG imaging |
| | | Resection of recurrent tumor |
| Adrenocortical carcinoma | Overall 5-year survival is 10–20% | Recurrent cancer |
| | Stage I and II cancers may be cured after complete resection | Measurement of hormone levels; CT, MRI |
| | | Resection of slowly growing recurrences may prolong remissions |

*CT,* computed tomography; *MRI,* magnetic resonance imaging; *MIBG,* metaiodobenzylguanidine labeled with iodine-131.

ization is necessary. Acute episodes of intraoperative hypertension are treated with intravenous phentolamine or nitroprusside, which should be available for immediate use before the induction of anesthesia. Hypertensive episodes are most likely to occur during the induction of anesthesia, intubation, or manipulation of the tumor by the surgeon. An acute increase in blood pressure with intraoperative palpation of a mass strongly supports the diagnosis of pheochromocytoma. On removal of a pheochromocytoma, the patient's blood pressure should decrease. Hypotension is appropriately treated by the discontinuation of any vasodilatory agents and by volume resuscitation. Hypotension is potentiated by inadequate preoperative fluid administration. Tachycardia and ventricular ectopy usually respond to treatment with propranolol.

## POSTOPERATIVE CARE

After open surgery, a nasogastric tube that is placed at the time of operation may be continued and maintained on low suction until output is minimal. When bowel function returns, generally within 1 week, an oral feeding is instituted. Intravenous narcotic pain medication is required initially. The relief of pain is important to allow aggressive pulmonary physiotherapy and early ambulation after open surgery. After laparoscopic adrenalectomy, postoperative ileus does not typically occur, and oral feeding may be started the night of surgery or the following morning. Pain is often controlled adequately with oral pain medications and perhaps the administration of only a few doses of parenteral narcotics. As a result, patients resume independent activity quickly. Inpatient stay is reduced and the total hospital charges appear to be less for laparoscopic adrenalectomy.[10]

## OPERATIVE SEQUELAE

The morbidity after elective adrenalectomy performed by experienced surgeons is relatively low; the mortality rate is <1%. Improper operative technique may rapidly result in a potentially fatal situation. Massive intraoperative bleeding, for example, may occur if the adrenal vein is torn by a weighty adrenal mass that is momentarily unsupported, or if the inferior vena cava is injured. Unrecognized, inadvertent entry into the pleural cavity during the operation may result in a pneumothorax, which could lead to a potentially life-threatening tension pneumothorax. Wound infections, abscesses, and incisional hernias may also be encountered after adrenalectomy.

Acute adrenal insufficiency may occur after unilateral adrenalectomy if inadequate amounts of corticosteroids are provided to a patient who has a chronically suppressed pituitary-adrenal axis. Acute adrenal insufficiency is fatal if unsuspected but is easily treated once diagnosed. Weakness, fever, hypotension, nausea, vomiting, and abdominal pain suggest the diagnosis of acute adrenal insufficiency. In the postoperative setting, patients commonly exhibit at least some of these symptoms; thus, the diagnosis is not straightforward and a high index of suspicion must be maintained. The prompt administration of high-dose dexamethasone in a patient with acute adrenal insufficiency results in rapid improvement of symptoms and is lifesaving. The administration of mineralocorticoids is unnecessary. Dexamethasone does not interfere with subsequent tests that may be performed to confirm the diagnosis. A plasma free cortisol level of <15 µg/dL in the immediate postoperative period or a blunted rise in plasma cortisol levels after cosyntropin administration are consistent with adrenal insufficiency.

The administration of high-dose glucocorticoids perioperatively increases the risks of wound problems, due to their immunosuppressive and antiinflammatory effects. Fibroblast activity and collagen formation are decreased, resulting in connective tissue that is reduced in quantity and strength. Wound healing may be prolonged. The risk of postoperative wound infections and abscesses is greater in these immunosuppressed patients, and infections may not exhibit classic signs or symptoms. Aggressive treatment with drainage, debridement, and antibiotics is needed. Infections that are inappropriately treated may lead to sepsis or fascia dehiscence and evisceration, both life-threatening situations. Associated medical conditions, such as diabetes mellitus, may additionally impair healing and increase the risk of postoperative infections. Wound infection significantly increases the chances of a subsequent incisional hernia.

## POSTOPERATIVE FOLLOW-UP

For hypercortisolism caused by a hyperfunctional adrenal adenoma, successful adrenalectomy is curative, and the prognosis is excellent (Table 89-4). Due to atrophy of normal adrenal tissue from chronic suppression, the continued administration of glucocorticoids is necessary postoperatively for these patients. Hydrocortisone may be administered at a maintenance dosage of 12 to 15 mg/m² per day. Mineralocorticoid replacement is not required. Glucocorticoid replacement therapy is continued until the pituitary-adrenal axis recovers, which may take up to 2 years; recovery can be definitively evaluated with an ACTH stimulation test.[11] Postoperative hormone replacement therapy is generally unnecessary for patients who undergo unilateral adrenalectomy for other conditions.

Bilateral adrenalectomy for primary pigmented micronodular adrenal hyperplasia or massive macronodular adrenocortical hyperplasia is also curative. Lifelong glucocorticoid and mineralocorticoid replacement therapy is necessary for all patients who undergo bilateral adrenalectomy. Fludrocortisone at a dosage of 100 μg per day is added.

Up to 30% of patients who undergo unilateral adrenalectomy for an aldosteronoma develop recurrent hypertension within 2 to 3 years after surgery (see Table 89-4).[12] Serial blood pressure measurements should be taken, and antihypertensive medications should be added as needed. Electrolyte disturbances always resolve in these patients. In contrast, patients with idiopathic adrenocortical hyperplasia who undergo unilateral adrenalectomy for a misdiagnosed aldosteronoma experience no improvement in their abnormalities. These patients require medical treatment.

The complete resection of sporadic pheochromocytomas results in a 5-year survival rate of >95%. Hypertension is also cured in most patients after surgery, but it recurs in ~25% of patients. It is usually well controlled with standard antihypertensive medications. Studies have indicated that tumor recurrence or metastatic disease may approach 50%. The measurement of urinary catecholamines, the clonidine suppression test, and CT, MRI, and [$^{131}$I]metaiodobenzylguanine scans may be required on a yearly basis (see Table 89-4). Localized, solitary recurrences or metastases should be surgically resected, if possible.[13]

Patients with adrenocortical carcinoma need close follow-up after resection.[14] Patients with stage I or stage II disease may be cured if their cancers are completely resected with negative surgical margins. However, only ~30% of patients with adrenocortical carcinomas present with these early-stage cancers. A majority of patients have advanced disease, and the overall 5-year survival rate is only ~10% to 20%. The detection of recurrent disease and aggressive surgical resection of metastases in the liver, lungs, and brain may result in prolonged remissions, although no cures in such patients have been reported. Patients with slowly growing, functional metastases may benefit from surgical resection, even if complete resection is not possible.[15] Therefore, in an attempt to detect recurrent disease, hormone levels, especially of those hormones that were elevated preoperatively, are measured periodically after the resection of adrenocortical carcinoma. Plasma levels of 11-deoxycortisol,

dehydroepiandrosterone, and deoxycorticosterone are determined, as well as urinary levels of free cortisol and 17-ketosteroids. Local recurrences and metastases are identified using CT and MRI. Palliative radiation therapy may be administered for symptomatic bony lesions, and mitotane chemotherapy may be given in some cases, but survival is not significantly increased by these adjunctive treatments. The best opportunity for cure is the complete resection of cancer at the initial operation.

## REFERENCES

1. Zeiger MA, Nieman LK, Cutler GB, et al. Primary bilateral adrenocortical causes of Cushing syndrome. Surgery 1991; 110:1106.
2. Zeiger MA, Fraker DL, Pass HI, et al. Effective reversibility of the signs and symptoms of hypercortisolism by bilateral adrenalectomy. Surgery 1993; 114:1138.
3. Lairmore TC, Bail DW, Baylin SB, Wells SA Jr. Management of pheochromocytomas in patients with multiple endocrine neoplasia type 2 syndromes. Ann Surg 1993; 217:595.
4. Ross NS, Aron DC. Hormonal evaluation of the patient with an incidentally discovered adrenal mass. N Engl J Med 1990; 323:1401.
4a. Orth DN. Cushing's syndrome. N Engl J Med 1995; 332:791.
5. McCorkell SJ, Miles NL. Fine-needle aspiration of catecholamine-producing adrenal masses: a possibly fatal mistake. AJR Am J Roentgenol 1985; 145:113.
6. Doppman IL, Reinig JW, Dwyer AJ, et al. Differentiation of adrenal masses by magnetic resonance imaging. Surgery 1987; 102:1018.
7. Auda SP, Brennan MF, Gill JR. Evolution of the surgical management of primary aldosteronism. Ann Surg 1980; 191:1.
8. Perry RR, Nieman LK, Cutler GB, et al. Primary adrenal causes of Cushing syndrome: diagnosis and surgical management. Ann Surg 1989; 210:59.
9. Orchard T, Grant CS, van Heerden JA, Weaver A. Pheochromocytoma: continuing evolution of surgical therapy. Surgery 1993; 114:1153.
9a. Michel LA, de Canniere L, Hamoir E, et al. Asymptomatic adrenal tumors: criteria for endoscopic removal. Eur J Surg 1999; 165:767.
9b. Wells SA, Merke DP, Cutler GB Jr, et al. The role of laparoscopic surgery in adrenal disease. J Clin Endocrinol Metab 1998; 831:3041.
9c. Buell JF, Alexander HR, Norton JA, et al. Bilateral adrenalectomy for Cushing's syndrome: anterior versus posterior approach. Ann Surg 1997; 225:63.
10. Schell SR, Talamini MA, Udelsman R. Laparoscopic adrenalectomy for nonmalignant disease: improved safety, morbidity, and cost-effectiveness. Endoscopy 1999; 13:30.
11. Doherty GM, Nieman LK, Cutler GB Jr, et al. Time to recovery of the hypothalamic-pituitary-adrenal axis after curative resection of adrenal tumors in patients with Cushing syndrome. Surgery 1990; 108:1085.
12. Favia G, Lumachi F, Scarpa V, D'Amico DF. Adrenalectomy in primary aldosteronism: a long-term follow-up study in 52 patients. World J Surg 1992; 16:680.
13. Brennan MF, Keiser HR. Persistent and recurrent pheochromocytoma: the role of surgery. World J Surg 1982; 6:397.
14. Luton JP, Cerdas S, Billaud L, et al. Clinical features of adrenocortical carcinoma, prognostic factors and the effect of mitotane therapy. N Engl J Med 1990; 322:1195.
15. Jensen JC, Pass HI, Sindelar WF, Norton JA. Aggressive resection of recurrent or metastatic disease in select patients with adrenocortical carcinoma. Arch Surg 1991; 126:457.

# PART VI

# SEX DETERMINATION AND DEVELOPMENT

ROBERT W. REBAR AND
WILLIAM J. BREMNER, EDITORS

# CHAPTER 90

# NORMAL AND ABNORMAL SEXUAL DIFFERENTIATION AND DEVELOPMENT

JOE LEIGH SIMPSON AND ROBERT W. REBAR

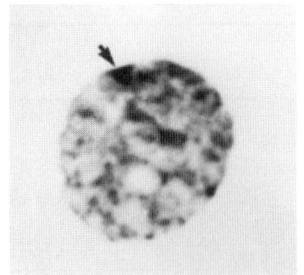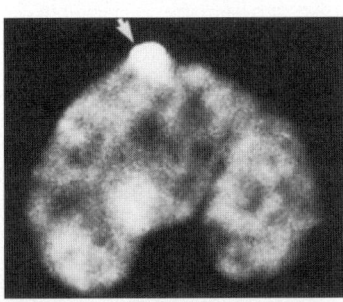

A,B

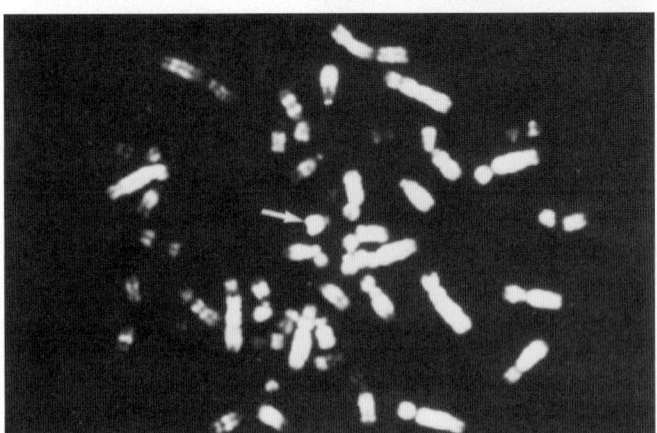

C

The purpose of this chapter is to describe briefly what is known about normal sexual differentiation and to consider the causes, diagnosis, and management of disorders in such differentiation. Abnormalities of embryonic development can be classified in several ways, and the disorders of sexual differentiation are no exception. The categorization presented here differs from that in most textbooks but is well suited to the clinician attempting to consider these disorders in a logical fashion. Disorders of the hypothalamic-pituitary axis sometimes included in such discussions are not considered in this chapter, because they are not truly errors of sexual differentiation and because they are discussed elsewhere in this book (see Chaps. 16, 18, 92, 93, 96, and 115). Some disorders dealt with briefly here are discussed in detail in other chapters.

## CYTOGENETIC PRINCIPLES

### NOMENCLATURE AND IDENTIFICATION OF CHROMOSOMES

Normal humans have 46 chromosomes—44 autosomes and two sex chromosomes. In females, the two sex chromosomes are X chromosomes; in males, one is an X and one a Y chromosome. By convention, chromosomes are numbered according to size and the position of the *centromere*, the primary constriction around which cell division occurs. As with other chromosomes, the centromere divides the X and the Y chromosomes into a *short arm*, designated p, and a *long arm*, designated q. Accepted nomenclature dictates that specific chromosome *bands* are designated by the chromosome, the arm (p or q), the region, and the specific band; bands are numbered consecutively from the centromere distally. Complements containing structurally abnormal X or Y chromosomes also require the symbol for the aberration present (e.g., i for isochromosome, del for deletion).[1,2]

Beginning in 1969, the development of banding techniques that produce horizontal "stripes" on the chromosome permitted the routine identification of individual chromosomes[1,2a] (Fig. 90-1D). Although the mechanism of chromosome banding is not completely understood, the various bands are known to reflect variations in DNA base sequences.

### CYTOLOGIC PROPERTIES OF THE X CHROMOSOME

One of the two X chromosomes in normal females is the last chromosome to complete DNA synthesis, a fact believed to reflect tighter condensation during interphase of this chromosome than of others. The late-replicating X is said to represent the heterochromatic X and appears as a planoconvex body, now called X-*chromatin* body and formerly known as sex chromatin or the Barr body, near the nuclear membrane[3] (see Fig. 90-1A). These bodies are observed in 30% or more of the cell nuclei from normal females. X-chromatin is the more nonfunctioning X chromosome and is present in the resting nuclei of somatic cells in mammals in which the cell has more than one X chromosome.[4] In interphase, only one X chromosome usually functions in a cell at a given time; all other X chromosomes are present in the form of X-chromatin bodies.

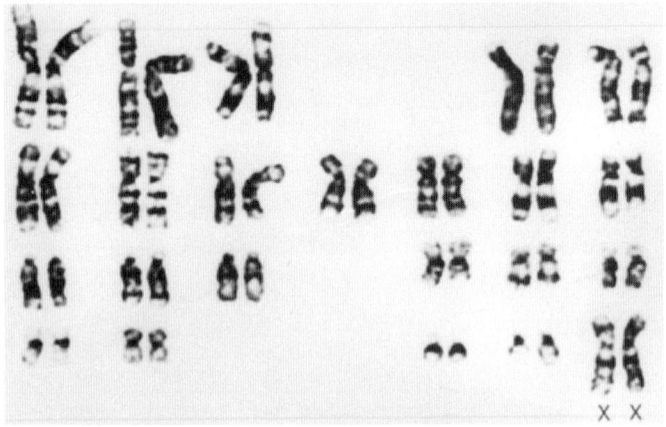

X  X    D

**FIGURE 90-1.** A, Nucleus of normal female cell from orcein-stained smear of buccal mucosa showing one X-chromatin mass, or Barr body (*arrow*). B, The nucleus of a peripheral leukocyte from a normal male, stained with quinacrine mustard and showing the fluorescent Y-chromatin (*arrow*). C, Quinacrine-stained metaphase chromosomes of a normal male from leukocyte culture: *arrow* indicates fluorescent Y chromosome. D, Giemsa-banded karyotype of normal female from leukocyte culture. Each human chromosome can be identified by its banding pattern. Giemsa banding (G-banding) is the most widely used procedure. The number of bands identified with this technique is ~500, which permits the detection of subtle chromosome alterations. Additional techniques include quinacrine banding (Q-banding), constitutive heterochromatin banding (C-banding), and reverse banding (R-banding). (Courtesy of Dr. Beverly White; reproduced from Rebar RW. Practical evaluation of hormonal status. In: Yen SSC, Jaffe RB, eds. Reproductive endocrinology: physiology, pathophysiology, and clinical management, 2nd ed. Philadelphia: WB Saunders, 1986:683.)

The time of X *inactivation* is uncertain but is probably around the time of implantation. The choice of which X chromosome (i.e., maternal or paternal) is inactivated in a given cell is random if both X chromosomes are normal. After a given X is inactivated, however, the descendants of that cell retain the identical pattern. Because X inactivation occurs only after the embryo contains hundreds of cells, normal females have two populations of cells: in one, the maternal X is active; in the other, the paternal X is active. The biochemical basis of X inactivation is not well understood, but the inactivated DNA appears to be more heavily methylated than in the active X. (See also ref. 4a.)

Although the heterochromatic X is considered inactive, in reality, some loci on this chromosome remain active.[5] For example, ovarian-maintenance determinants, which are located on the short and the long arms of the X chromosome, must remain active, because 45,X individuals would be normal if such were not the case. Both X chromosomes also remain active in oocytes.

Before chromosomal banding techniques became available, analysis of X-chromatin in buccal smears was used in evaluating individuals with gonadal failure. By itself, however, buccal smear analysis seldom is used diagnostically by cytogeneticists. The X-chromatin analysis is subject to technical problems even in experienced hands, and the analysis of buccal smears alone fails to differentiate 45,X from 46,XY cells. The precise number of X chromosomes can be more reliably determined by the number of signals made in interphase cells by X chromosome–specific DNA probes.

### CYTOLOGIC PROPERTIES OF THE Y CHROMOSOME

The normal Y chromosome differs in length from individual to individual because of polymorphism in the distal portion of the long arm, which fluoresces brilliantly[6] (see Fig. 90-1*B* and C). *Fluorescent Y-chromatin* can be identified in interphase cells and equals the number of Y chromosomes. Because the fluorescent portion can be absent in otherwise-normal males, however, and because regions of autosomal fluorescence may be mistaken for Y chromatin, sex determination should be made on the basis of complete cytogenetic analysis or use of Y-specific DNA probes.

### CELL DIVISION

#### MITOSIS

Mitosis is the process by which progeny cells receive identical copies of the parental genome (Fig. 90-2). Although mitosis has several distinct stages, the process occupies only a small portion of the cell cycle.

At the onset of *prophase*, the chromosomes are elongated. Although each chromosome appears to consist of only a single unit when viewed by light microscopy, DNA replication has occurred already, and each chromosome actually consists of two sister chromatids. Each chromosome subsequently becomes shorter, more compact, and more darkly staining. Toward the end of prophase, the centriole divides into two centrioles, and the new centrioles migrate to opposite poles of the nucleus.

*Metaphase* begins when the nuclear membrane disappears and the mitotic spindle forms between the centrioles. After division of the centromere along the longitudinal plane of each chromosome, the sister chromatids pass to opposite poles.

During *anaphase*, the chromosomes, actually again now each a single chromatid, move to opposite poles of the cell.

*Telophase* begins when the chromatids reach opposite poles. The mitotic spindle disappears, and new nuclear membranes form. With the division of the cytoplasm, two complete cells are formed.

#### MEIOSIS

The *diploid* number (2n = 46) of chromosomes in humans is derived from paternal and maternal sources. Because each parent contributes a *haploid* (n = 23) number to the zygote, the number of chromosomes in each *gamete* (oocyte or spermatozoon) must be reduced by one-half; otherwise, offspring would have twice the parental number of chromosomes. This reduction division, called *meiosis*, really involves two separate cell divisions, I and II (see Fig. 90-2). However, replication of DNA

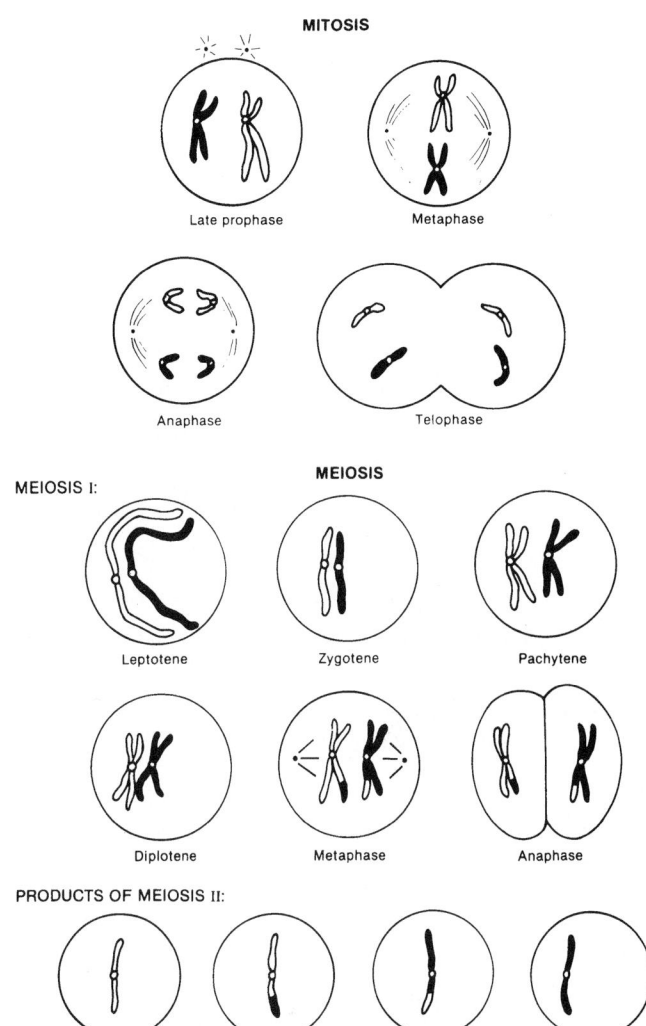

**FIGURE 90-2.** *Upper panel,* Stages of mitosis. Two chromosomes are represented. After DNA synthesis, each chromosome consists of two sister chromatids. After centromeric division in the longitudinal plane, each chromatid passes to different daughter cells. *Lower panel,* Stages of meiosis I and gametes present after meiosis II; the behavior of one pair of autosomes is shown. At zygotene, homologous chromosomes pair with each other along their longitudinal plane by a process known as synapsis. Synapsis occurs between the various alleles at a single locus. At some sites, segments are exchanged between nonsister chromatids (e.g., crossing over). During diplotene, chromosomes begin to separate. If crossing over occurs, no two of the four chromatids of a given chromosome pair are genetically identical. (From Simpson JL. Disorders of sexual differentiation: etiology and clinical delineation. New York: Academic Press, 1976.)

occurs only once. During *meiosis I*, the chromosome number is reduced from 2n to n; during *meiosis II*, each haploid germ cell divides into two other haploid cells. From a single diploid germ cell, as many as four haploid cells can be formed. In females, only one ovum results, with the remaining three cells becoming nonfunctional polar bodies.

### CHROMOSOMAL ABNORMALITIES

Certain disorders of sexual differentiation involve abnormalities in chromosomal number.[7] Most commonly, an additional chromosome is present (*trisomy,* 2n + 1), or one is lacking. Any deviation from the expected number of chromosomes (n or 2n) is called *aneuploidy.*

Trisomy may arise by several mechanisms, but in humans, it usually arises de novo after meiotic or mitotic nondisjunction.

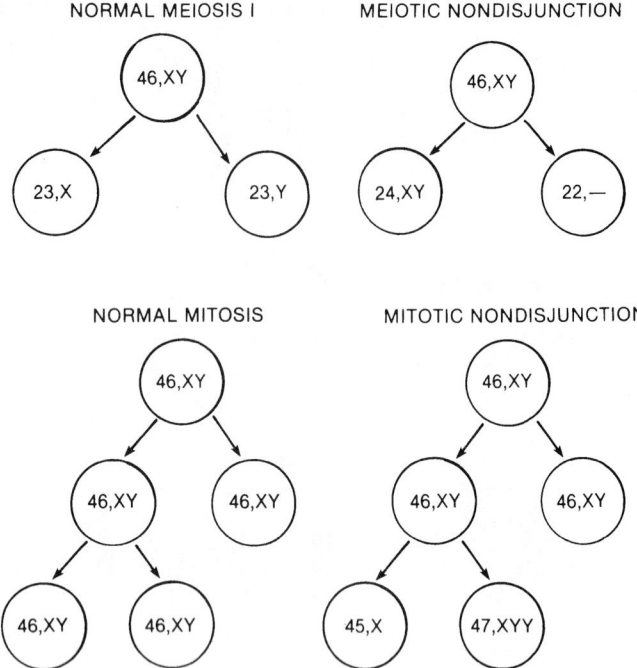

**FIGURE 90-3.** *Above,* Diagram of the products of normal meiosis and of meiosis in which nondisjunction produced two aneuploid gametes, 24,XY and 22. *Below,* Products of normal mitosis and of mitosis characterized by nondisjunction of a *Y chromosome.* If all daughter cells survived, the complement would be 45,X/46,XY/47,XYY. (From Simpson JL. Disorders of sexual differentiation: etiology and clinical delineation. New York: Academic Press, 1976.)

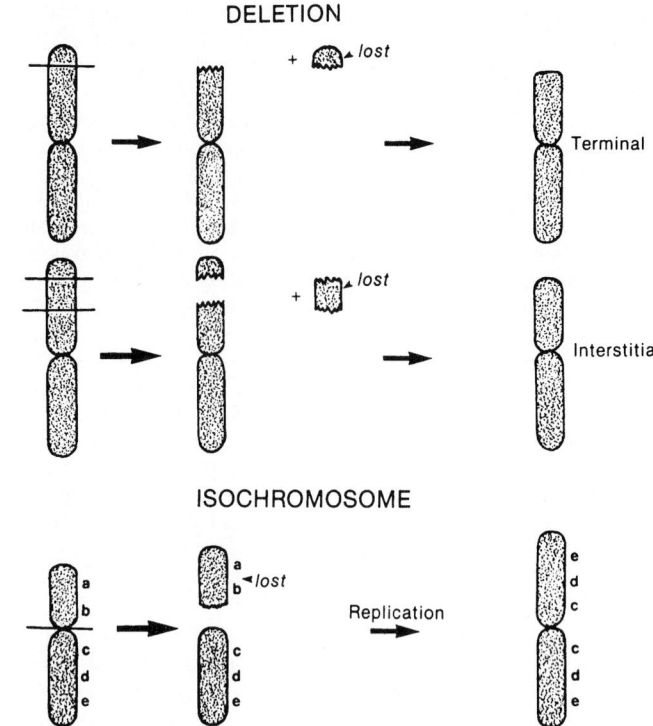

**FIGURE 90-4.** *Above,* Diagram of the origin of terminal and interstitial deletions. *Below,* Diagram of the origin of an isochromosome. An isochromosome has two identical arms. It arises from horizontal, rather than longitudinal, division of the centromere. One arm of the chromosome is completely absent, and, eventually, the two remaining arms are mirror images. (From Simpson JL. Disorders of sexual differentiation: etiology and clinical delineation. New York: Academic Press, 1976.)

Specifically, nondisjunction may follow failure of homologous chromosomes to disjoin in meiosis I or failure of sister chromatids to disjoin in meiosis II or mitosis. Cytologic factors predisposing to nondisjunction in meiosis I include failure of synapsis, absence of chiasmata, or premature terminalization. Nondisjunction during meiosis produces aneuploid gametes, and the resulting zygote has the identical chromosomal constitution in all cells (Fig. 90-3); however, nondisjunction during mitosis produces two or more cell lines (i.e., mosaicism). Another rare mechanism for trisomy involves normal meiotic segregation in a trisomic parent.

Although trisomies are presumed to result from nondisjunction, the biologic explanation for nondisjunction is unknown. Because various trisomies become more common with advancing maternal age, intrinsic aging of oocytes may predispose to nondisjunction. It is possible, but unlikely, that oocytes selected earlier for ovulation are more likely to be normal than those remaining in older women. Perhaps aneuploidy increases with advancing age because of accumulated exposure to various deleterious agents such as radiation.

Major structural alterations in chromosomes can lead to phenotypic abnormalities. Chromosomal *deletion* involves the loss of part of one chromosome, a terminal or an interstitial portion (Fig. 90-4). Deletions also may follow crossing over. Although deletions of even small portions of autosomes usually lead to embryonic death or malformations, deficiency in a sex chromosome is not necessarily so deleterious.

After chromosomal breakage, material may be exchanged between two or more chromosomes. *Translocation* is then said to have occurred. If the individual is phenotypically normal, no genetic material is presumed lost, and the translocation is said to be balanced.

*Isochromosomes* have identical arms. They arise if the centromere divides incorrectly, in a horizontal rather than in a longitudinal fashion, after duplication of the chromatids (see Fig. 90-4). One product contains no centromere and is lost at the next cell division, and the other contains the centromere and is capable of duplication. The isochromosome therefore consists of complete duplication of one arm, with complete deficiency of the other arm of the original chromosome. Both parts of the resulting chromosome are structurally and genetically identical. An isochromosome can be composed of identical long arms or identical short arms, depending on which arm retains the centromere. An isochromosome involving the X long arm (I[Xq]) is the most common structural abnormality associated with *gonadal dysgenesis.*

A *dicentric chromosome* has two centromeres. Its formation most commonly follows identical breaks in adjoining chromatids (Fig. 90-5). Fragments without centromeres are lost. The sister chromatids containing the centromere join. After longitudinal division of the centromere, the chromosome contains two centromeres and deficient and duplicated portions as well. Dicentric chromosomes are sometimes detected in 45,X/46,XY mosaicism, a form of gonadal dysgenesis predisposing to germ-cell neoplasia.

A *ring chromosome* arises after breaks in both of the long arms (see Fig. 90-5). The chromosomal regions contiguous with the centromere then fuse, and the portions without centromeres are lost. Ring chromosomes are inherently unstable, because the ring must open for each replication. The site of opening is not identical in every cell division, so that rings of various sizes may be present in neighboring cells.

## GENETIC CONTROL OF SEX DIFFERENTIATION

The X and Y sex chromosomes and the autosomes contain loci that must remain intact for normal sexual development. That

FORMATION OF DICENTRIC CHROMOSOME

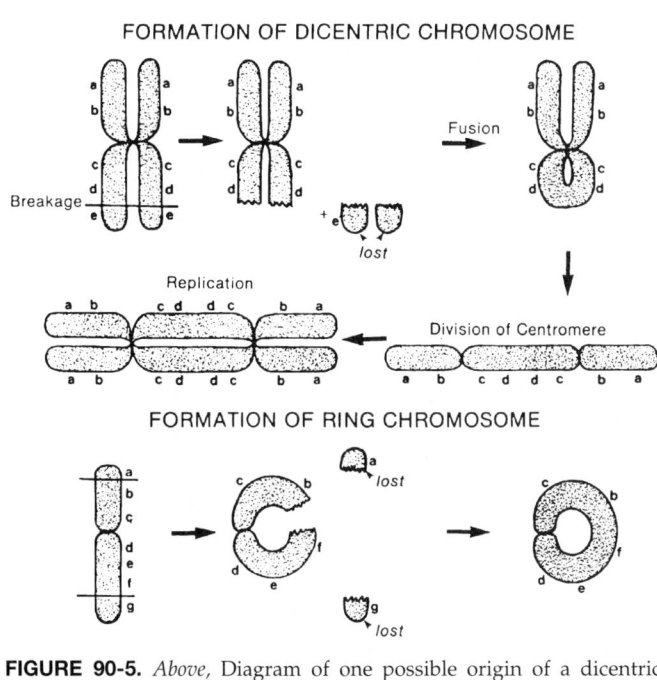

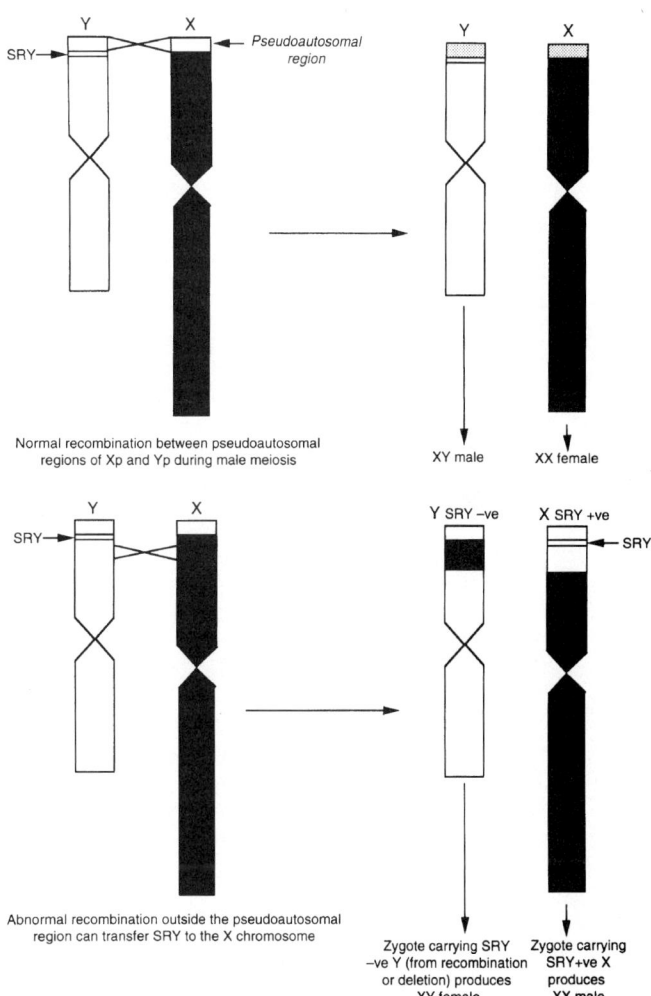

Normal recombination between pseudoautosomal regions of Xp and Yp during male meiosis

XY male    XX female

Abnormal recombination outside the pseudoautosomal region can transfer SRY to the X chromosome

Zygote carrying SRY –ve Y (from recombination or deletion) produces XY female    Zygote carrying SRY+ve X produces XX male

**FIGURE 90-5.** *Above,* Diagram of one possible origin of a dicentric chromosome. A dicentric chromosome also can arise after crossing over within a paracentric loop. *Below,* Diagram of the origin of a ring chromosome. (From Simpson JL. Disorders of sexual differentiation: etiology and clinical delineation. New York: Academic Press, 1976.)

**FIGURE 90-6.** The *SRY* gene has been localized to the short arm of the Y chromosome, immediately adjacent to the pseudoautosomal region that pairs with the pseudoautosomal region on the short arm of the X chromosome. Normal recombination between the pseudoautosomal regions of Xp and Yp occurs during male meiosis and results in normal XY males and XX females. If abnormal recombination outside the pseudoautosomal region occurs, the *SRY* gene can be transferred to the X chromosome, producing *SRY*-negative Y chromosomes, resulting in XY females, and *SRY*-positive X chromosomes, resulting in XX males. (Courtesy of Goodfellow PN, Department of Genetics, University of Cambridge, Cambridge, England.)

autosomal factors influence sexual development is potentially important for clinical management. For example, an autosomal translocation may result in genital abnormalities. Before the various disorders are formally considered, summarizing the genetic control of sex differentiation may be helpful.

## TESTICULAR DEVELOPMENT

Consideration of individuals with various abnormalities of the X and Y chromosomes led to the concept that the Y chromosome carries genetic information required for testis formation.[7] Such a hypothetical gene was named *testis-determining factor (TDF)* and was postulated to be present in males and absent in females. In that sense, *TDF* is the sex-determining gene, although many other genes are required for the formation of a testis, and these are distributed among the autosomes and the X chromosome. Several experiments have resulted in the identification and cloning of a gene located on the Y chromosome called the *sex-determining region Y (SRY)* gene that appears identical to the conceptual *TDF* gene.[8]

*SRY* was identified and cloned by constructing maps of the Y chromosome. The Y chromosome is composed of two parts with different functions. One part consists of the two pseudoautosomal regions that are found on the X and Y chromosomes and are required for correct pairing and segregation during meiosis.[9,10] The major pseudoautosomal region is located at the end of the short arm of each sex chromosome. During each male meiosis, a single recombination occurs between the X and Y chromosomes in this pseudoautosomal region (Fig. 90-6), allowing the construction of recombination maps of the terminal part of the short arms of the sex chromosomes.[11] (A second pseudoautosomal region exists at the ends of the long arm of the sex chromosomes.) The second part of the Y chromosome includes *TDF* and is not shared with the X chromosome. Because the Y-specific region does not normally recombine with the X chromosome, it is not amenable to classic genetic analysis. Study of the genomes of XX males, however, in which it was proposed that Y-derived sequences would be present on the X chromosome as a result of an abnormal recombination between the unique portions of the sex chromosomes

during male meiosis, has allowed the construction of maps of the short arm of the Y chromosome.[12,13] *TDF* was mapped to the most distal part (i.e., farthest from the centromere) of the unique portion of the short arm of the Y chromosome.

*SRY* is a single-copy gene located in the smallest Y chromosomal region capable of inducing sex reversal. It is expressed in the genital ridge only during the appropriate time of embryonic development when testicular cords form.[8] Moreover, it is deleted or mutated in cases of human XY females, and the presence of the equivalent gene in the mouse, called SRY, can sex-reverse XX mice into males.[8,14–17] The protein product of SRY contains an 80-amino-acid domain with a motif shared by a *high-mobility group* (HMG) of transcription factors that bind to DNA and are important in the regulation of gene transcription. Studies of the DNA-binding properties of the SRY HMG box of proteins in the promoter regions of the P450 aromatase gene (which converts testosterone to estradiol and is down-regulated in the male embryo) and of the antimüllerian hormone (AMH) gene (which is responsible for regression of the müllerian ducts) support the hypothesis that SRY directly regulates male development

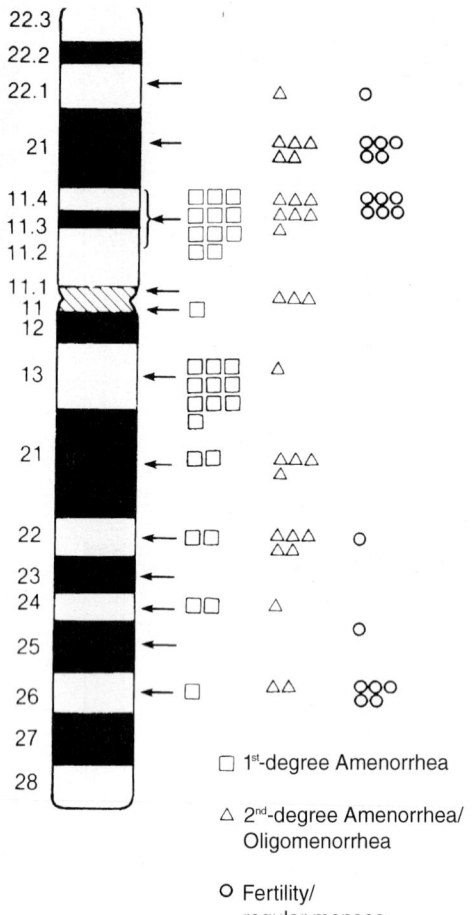

□ 1ˢᵗ-degree Amenorrhea

△ 2ⁿᵈ-degree Amenorrhea/
  Oligomenorrhea

○ Fertility/
  regular menses

**FIGURE 90-7.** Schematic diagram of gonadal function associated with terminal deletions of the X chromosome. The regions of both arms that are nearest to the centromere are those that are most necessary to maintenance of ovarian function. The schematized X chromosome has sharply drawn black and white bands; in actuality, a continuous transition occurs without sharp demarcation. (From Simpson JL. Phenotypic-karyotypic correlations of gonadal determinants: current status and relationship to molecular studies. In: Sperling K, Vogel F, eds. Proceedings of the Seventh International Congress on Human Genetics. Heidelberg: Springer-Verlag, 1987:224.)

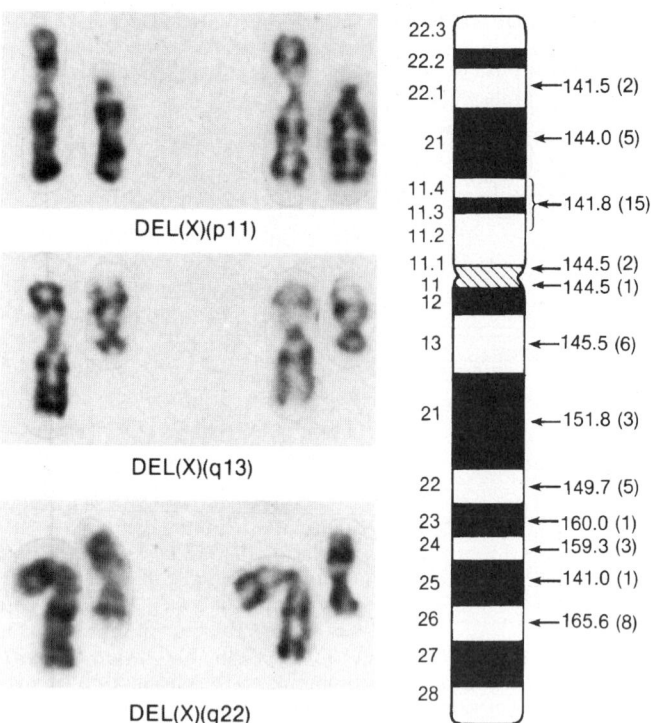

DEL(X)(p11)

DEL(X)(q13)

DEL(X)(q22)

**FIGURE 90-8.** *Left*, Pairs of X chromosomes from three individuals with terminal deletions. *Right*, Schematic diagram of mean heights (in cm) of adults (older than 15 years) reported to have terminal deletions at various regions of the X chromosome; number of patients is noted in parentheses. [*Left*, from Simpson JL, Le Beau MM. Gonadal and structural determinants on the X chromosome and their relationship to in-vitro studies showing prolonged cell cycles in 45,X; 46,X,del(X)(p11); 46,X,del(XXq13) and q(22) fibroblasts. Am J Obstet Gynecol 1981; 141:930; *Right*, from Simpson JL. Ovarian determinants through phenotypic-karyotypic deductions: progress and pitfalls. In: Rosenfield R, Grumbach M, eds. Turner syndrome. New York: Marcel Dekker, 1990:65.]

through sequence-specific regulation of target genes.[8,18,19] Other target genes remain to be identified.[19a] Active SRY participation in morphogenesis appears to be required for formation of a testis from the bipotential genital ridge.

In addition to regions on the Y chromosome, genes necessary for testicular differentiation exist on the X chromosome and on the autosomes. The importance of the genes on the X chromosome is evident from the existence of an X-linked recessive form of XY gonadal dysgenesis as well as the existence of a *(DDS) X chromosomal region* that, if duplicated, causes testicular repression.[19,20] Three chromosomal regions—9p, 10q, and 17q—have been implicated as sites of *autosomal testicular genes.* Moreover, autosomal locations for these genes can be deduced on the basis of various clinical syndromes. Agonadia has been reported in sibs, as has the rudimentary testes syndrome.[21,22] Autosomal factors are also responsible for germ-cell hypoplasia in genetic males (i.e., germinal cell aplasia) and genetic females (i.e., streak gonads).[23-27] (See also ref. 27a.)

## OVARIAN DEVELOPMENT

In the absence of a Y chromosome, the indifferent gonad develops into an ovary. Germ cells exist in cases of monosomy X (45,X) human fetuses, and 39,X mice.[28-30] The pathogenesis of

germ-cell failure in monosomy X involves accelerated germ-cell atresia. In the absence of two intact X chromosomes, as in the 45,X karyotype, ovarian follicles usually degenerate before birth. The second X chromosome is therefore responsible for *ovarian maintenance,* rather than ovarian differentiation. Further supporting constitutive ovarian differentiation are observations that oocyte development occurs in humans with XY gonadal dysgenesis and with the genitopalatocardiac syndrome.[31,32] Oocyte development in the presence of a Y chromosome also is well documented in mice.[33]

For years, efforts have been directed toward localizing the regions of the X chromosome important for ovarian maintenance. Research has made it clear that ovarian maintenance determinants exist on the X short arm and the X long arm[34-36] (Fig. 90-7). Each arm probably has at least two regions of importance for ovarian development. With respect to the short arm, 11 (45.8%) of 24 reported del(X)(p11.2→11.4) patients had primary amenorrhea.[34,35] The other 13 individuals developed secondary amenorrhea, but pregnancy was rare. A locus in regions Xp11.2→11.4 is important for ovarian maintenance. More telomeric deletions [del(X)(p21)] appear less deleterious; almost all women reported with these deletions menstruated. However, 5 of 10 del(X)(p21) women were infertile and manifested secondary amenorrhea. A second region exists on Xp that is important for ovarian maintenance, albeit less so than region Xp11.2→11.4.

Similar topography appears to exist on the X long arm (Xq). Deletions involving Xq11.3 or proximal Xq21 are usually (10 of 11 reported cases) associated with complete ovarian failure[34-36] (Fig. 90-8; see also Fig. 90-7). Region Xq25 or Xq26 also is neces-

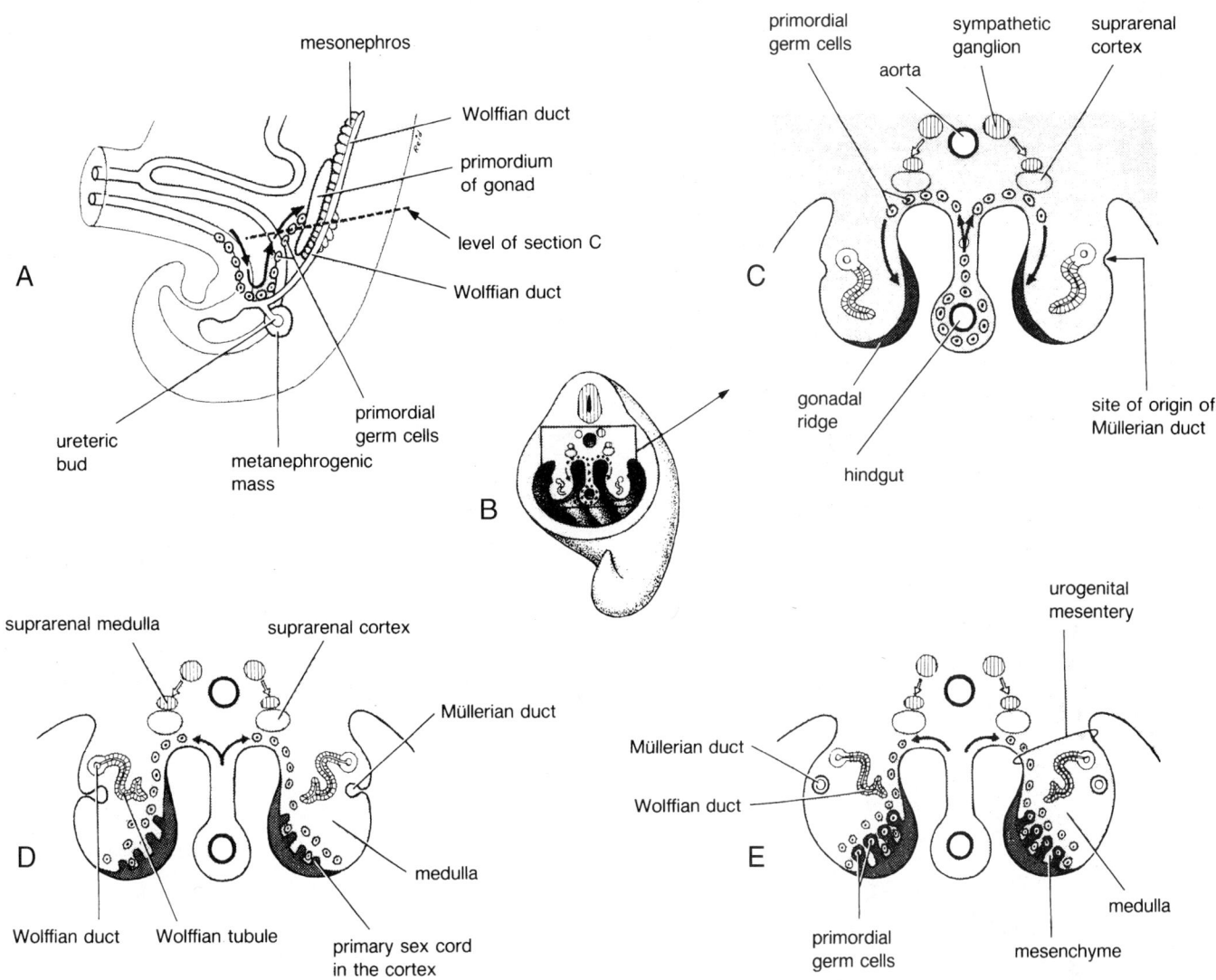

**FIGURE 90-9. A,** Drawing of 5-week embryo depicting migration of primordial germ cells. **B,** Three-dimensional sketch of caudal region of 5-week embryo, showing location and extent of the gonadal ridges on medial aspect of urogenital ridges. **C,** Transverse section, showing anlage of adrenal (suprarenal) glands, gonadal ridges, and migration of primordial germ cells. **D,** Transverse section through 6-week embryo, showing primary sex cords and developing müllerian (paramesonephric) ducts. **E,** Similar transverse section at later stage, showing the indifferent gonads and müllerian and wolffian (mesonephric) ducts. (From Moore KL. The developing human: clinically oriented embryology, 3rd ed. Philadelphia: WB Saunders, 1982:271.)

sary, however, because an interstitial deletion involving this region resulted in secondary amenorrhea in a mother and her daughters.[37] Familial terminal deletions of Xq25 and Xq26 yield similar phenotypes.[35,38] Two or more regions on Xq must play roles in ovarian maintenance, with the two regions differing in importance (see Fig. 90-7).

Certain autosomal loci also are essential for normal ovarian development. An autosomal recessive gene causes gonadal dysgenesis in XX individuals, and several distinct entities have been identified (i.e., genetic heterogeneity). Families exist in which autosomal genes are capable of causing germ-cell failure in males and females.

## REPRODUCTIVE EMBRYOLOGY

Early in ontogeny, the gonads of both sexes are *indifferent* and *bipotential*. Large *primordial germ cells* are visible in the fourth week among the endodermal cells of the wall of the yolk sac

near the origin of the allantois. In the fifth week, these germ cells migrate by ameboid movement along the dorsal mesentery of the hindgut to the gonadal ridges (Fig. 90-9). During the sixth week, the primordial germ cells migrate into the underlying mesenchyme and become incorporated in the primary sex cords (Fig. 90-10, see also Fig. 90-9).

Divergent development begins at ~40 days of gestation. With the development of the gonad, controlled by a gene or genes regulating testicular differentiation, the translation of gonadal sex into phenotypic sex follows predictably as a function of the type of gonad formed.

In males, gonaductal differentiation depends on at least two substances secreted by the fetal testes (Figs. 90-11 and 90-12). The first, *testosterone*, is produced by the Leydig cells. This hormone stabilizes the wolffian ducts to stimulate the growth and development of the epididymis, vasa deferentia, and seminal vesicles. The second, AMH, is a glycoprotein secreted by the Sertoli cells that acts locally to cause nearly complete regression of the müllerian ducts by 8 weeks of fetal age, before the secre-

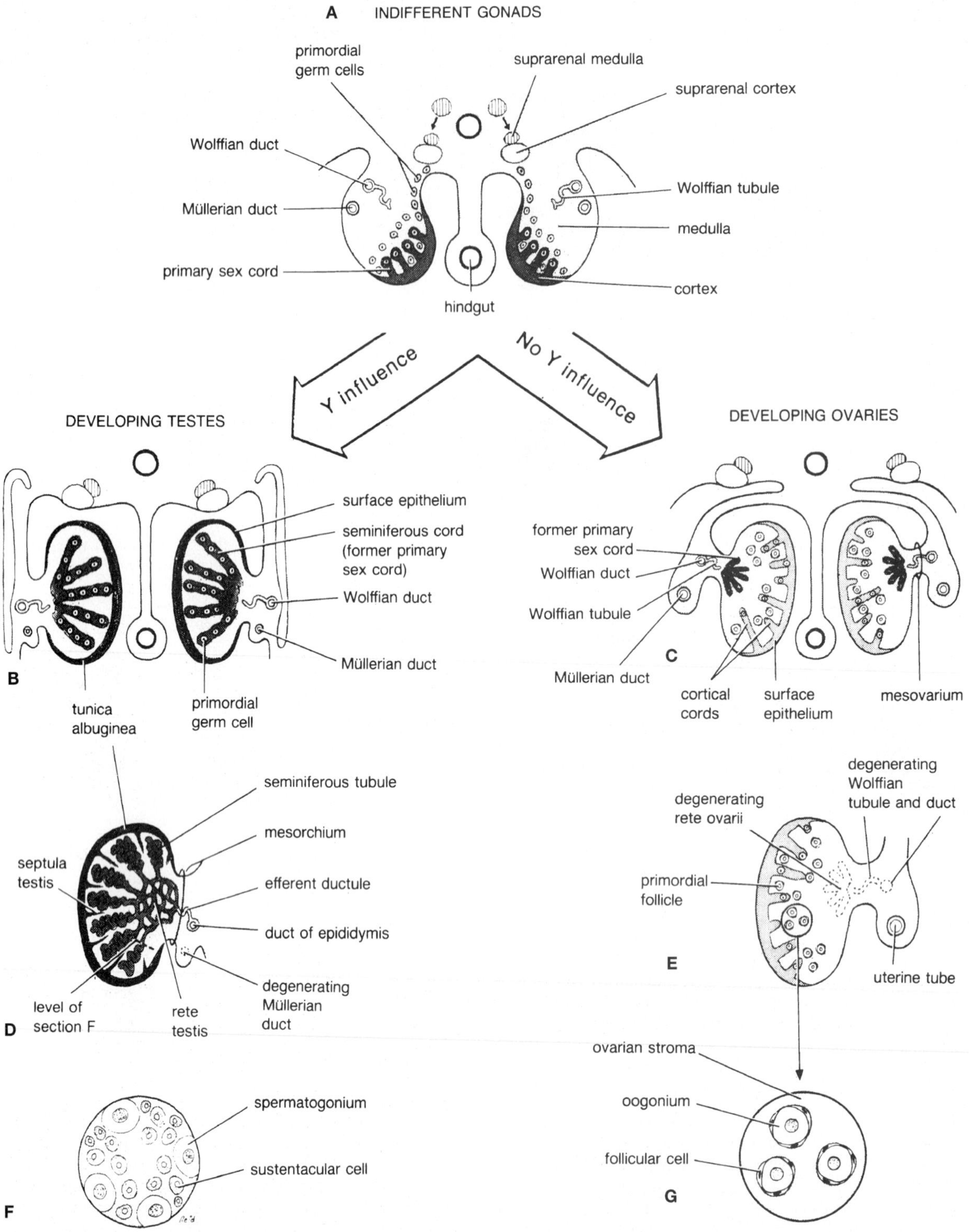

**A    INDIFFERENT GONADS**

primordial germ cells

suprarenal medulla

suprarenal cortex

Wolffian duct

Müllerian duct

primary sex cord

hindgut

Wolffian tubule

medulla

cortex

**DEVELOPING TESTES**

**Y influence**

**No Y influence**

**DEVELOPING OVARIES**

surface epithelium

seminiferous cord (former primary sex cord)

Wolffian duct

Müllerian duct

**B**

tunica albuginea

primordial germ cell

former primary sex cord

Wolffian duct

Wolffian tubule

Müllerian duct

**C**

cortical cords

surface epithelium

mesovarium

seminiferous tubule

mesorchium

efferent ductule

duct of epididymis

degenerating Müllerian duct

septula testis

level of section F

rete testis

**D**

degenerating rete ovarii

primordial follicle

degenerating Wolffian tubule and duct

uterine tube

**E**

spermatogonium

sustentacular cell

**F**

ovarian stroma

oogonium

follicular cell

**G**

**FIGURE 90-10.** Schematic sections illustrating differentiation of indifferent gonads into testes or ovaries. **A,** At 6 weeks, indifferent gonads are composed of outer cortex and inner medulla. **B,** By 7 weeks, testes begin to develop under the influence of the testes-determining factor on the Y chromosome. Primary sex cords have become seminiferous cords, and they are separated from the surface epithelium by the tunica albuginea. **C,** By 12 weeks, ovaries begin to develop in the absence of any influence from a Y chromosome. Cortical cords have extended from surface epithelium, displacing the primary sex cords centrally into the mesovarium, where they form rudimentary rete ovarii. **D,** Testis at 20 weeks has a well-developed rete testis and seminiferous tubules derived from the seminiferous cords. An efferent ductule has developed from a wolffian tubule, and the wolffian duct has become the duct of the epididymis. **E,** Ovary at 20 weeks contains primordial follicles formed from cortical cords. Rete ovarii derived from primary sex cords and wolffian tubule and duct are regressing. **F,** Section of seminiferous tubule from 20-week fetus. No lumen is present at this stage, and the seminiferous epithelium is composed of two kinds of cells. **G,** Section of ovarian cortex of 20-week fetus showing three primordial follicles. (From Moore KL. The developing human: clinically oriented embryology, 3rd ed. Philadelphia: WB Saunders, 1982:271.)

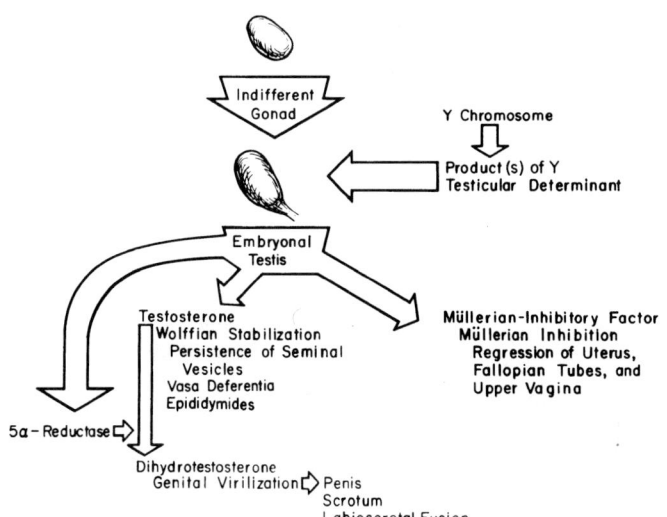

**FIGURE 90-11.** Diagram detailing embryonic development of male sex accessory organs and external genitalia. Central role of testis-determining factor (*TDF*) on Y chromosome is apparent. Needed also for complete sexual development are testosterone, dihydrotestosterone, and antimüllerian hormone (*AMH*), formerly known as müllerian inhibiting factor (*MIF*). (From Simpson JL. Disorders of gonads and internal ducts. In: Emery AEH, Rimoin DL, eds. Principles and practice of medical genetics, 2nd ed. Edinburgh: Churchill Livingstone, 1990.)

tion of testosterone and the stimulation of the wolffian ducts.[39] Studies have established that AMH is similar structurally to transforming growth factor-β (TGF-β) and to ovarian inhibin.[39–41] The structural locus has been localized to the short arm of chromosome 19.[42] The receptor for AMH, a serine-threonine kinase with a single transmembrane domain, is expressed in the region around the fetal müllerian duct and in Sertoli and granulosa cells.[43,44]

AMH may have extramüllerian functions. This hormone can exert an inhibitory effect on oocyte meiosis, play a role in the descent of the testes, and inhibit surfactant accumulation in the lungs.[45] Fragments of AMH, produced by proteolytic cleavage, can inhibit the growth of various neoplasms. Because AMH is detectable in the serum of males throughout life but is not measurable in females until the second decade of life, its measurement can serve as a sensitive *marker for the presence of testicular tissue in intersex anomalies.*[46]

Testosterone secreted by the fetal testes also is converted to *dihydrotestosterone* (DHT) by 5α-reductase, an enzyme in the primordia of the external genitalia. Acting locally, DHT stimulates differentiation of the glans penis and corpora cavernosa from the genital tubercle, the corpus spongiosum (which surrounds the penile urethra) from the urethral folds, and the scrotum from the labioscrotal swellings (Fig. 90-13). DHT also stimulates the formation of the prostate and Cowper glands.

Jost and colleagues have shown that the Sertoli cells have the function of organizing the gonad into a testis.[47] Consistent with this view are observations that Sertoli cells are the first identifiable cells to appear in differentiation. Moreover, Leydig and Sertoli cells are capable of functioning in isolation from the gonad.[9,48,49]

In the absence of testosterone, DHT, and AMH, the wolffian ducts regress; the müllerian ducts develop into the uterus, fallopian tubes, and upper vagina; and the external genitalia develop along female lines (see Figs. 90-12 and 90-13). The genital tubercle gives rise to a clitoris, the urethral folds to the labia minora, the labioscrotal swellings to the labia majora, and the urogenital sinus to the lower two-thirds of the vagina and the Bartholin and Skene glands (Table 90-1). Gonaductal and geni-

tal differentiation in females appears to be independent of fetal ovarian function. Such development occurs in 46,XX embryos and in castrated 46,XY embryos. Development along female lines also occurs in the absence of the Y chromosome. This occurs in 46,XX and in 45,X individuals.[29]

The combined observations illustrate the underlying principle that germ cells do not direct gonadal differentiation. Instead, germ cells take the form of the gonad in which they find themselves—oocytes in normal ovaries and spermatogonia in normal testes.

# DISORDERS OF SEXUAL DIFFERENTIATION

No classification scheme for the various disorders of sexual differentiation is ideal. The easiest approach is perhaps to consider such disorders on the basis of whether they affect primarily the gonads, the ductal structures involving the gonads, or the external genitalia (Table 90-2).

## ERRORS IN GONADAL DEVELOPMENT

### TRUE HERMAPHRODITISM

By definition, true hermaphrodites possess testicular and ovarian tissue, either separately or, more commonly, together as one or more ovotestes.[49a] Most true hermaphrodites (50–70%) have a 46,XX chromosomal complement; however, some have 46,XX/46,XY, 46,XX/47,XXY, 46,XY, or other complements.[50] Some evidence suggests that phenotype reflects karyotype, but this is unproved.[50]

**Phenotype.** Approximately two-thirds of true hermaphrodites are raised as males, although their external genitalia may be frankly ambiguous or predominantly female. Paradoxically, breast development usually occurs at puberty despite the presence of male external genitalia; virilization does not.

Gonadal tissue may be located in the ovarian, inguinal, or labioscrotal region. A testis or an ovotestis is more likely to be present on the right side than on the left. The greater the proportion of testicular tissue in an ovotestis, the greater the likelihood of gonadal descent. In 80% of ovotestes, the testicular and ovarian components exist immediately adjacent to each other in end-to-end fashion.[51,52] An ovotestes usually can be detected by inspection, or possibly by palpation, because testicular tissue is softer and darker than ovarian tissue. Spermatozoa are rarely present; however, apparently normal oocytes often are present, even in ovotestes.

Usually, a uterus is present, and commonly it is bicornuate or unicornuate. The absence of a uterine horn usually indicates the presence of an ipsilateral testis or ovotestis. The fimbriated end of the fallopian tube may be occluded ipsilateral to an ovotestis, and squamous metaplasia of the endocervix may occur. Most true hermaphrodites with a uterus menstruate. Five 46,XX true hermaphrodites have become pregnant—usually, but not always, after the removal of testicular tissue.[53,54]

Typically, the diagnosis of true hermaphroditism is made only after excluding the more common forms of male and female pseudohermaphroditism. A male sex-of-rearing is possible if genital status permits reconstruction and if the inappropriate (i.e., ovarian) tissue is extirpated.

All gonadal tissue should be biopsied, and tissue not compatible with the gender assignment removed. Despite the "dysgenetic" nature of the gonads in true hermaphrodites and the fact that a Y chromosome is sometimes present, gonadoblastomas have been reported far less frequently than in XY gonadal dysgenesis.[55,56] Carcinoma of the breast also has been reported.

**Etiology.** The cause of true hermaphroditism is uncertain but heterogeneous. Cases with 46,XX/46,XY karyotypes pre-

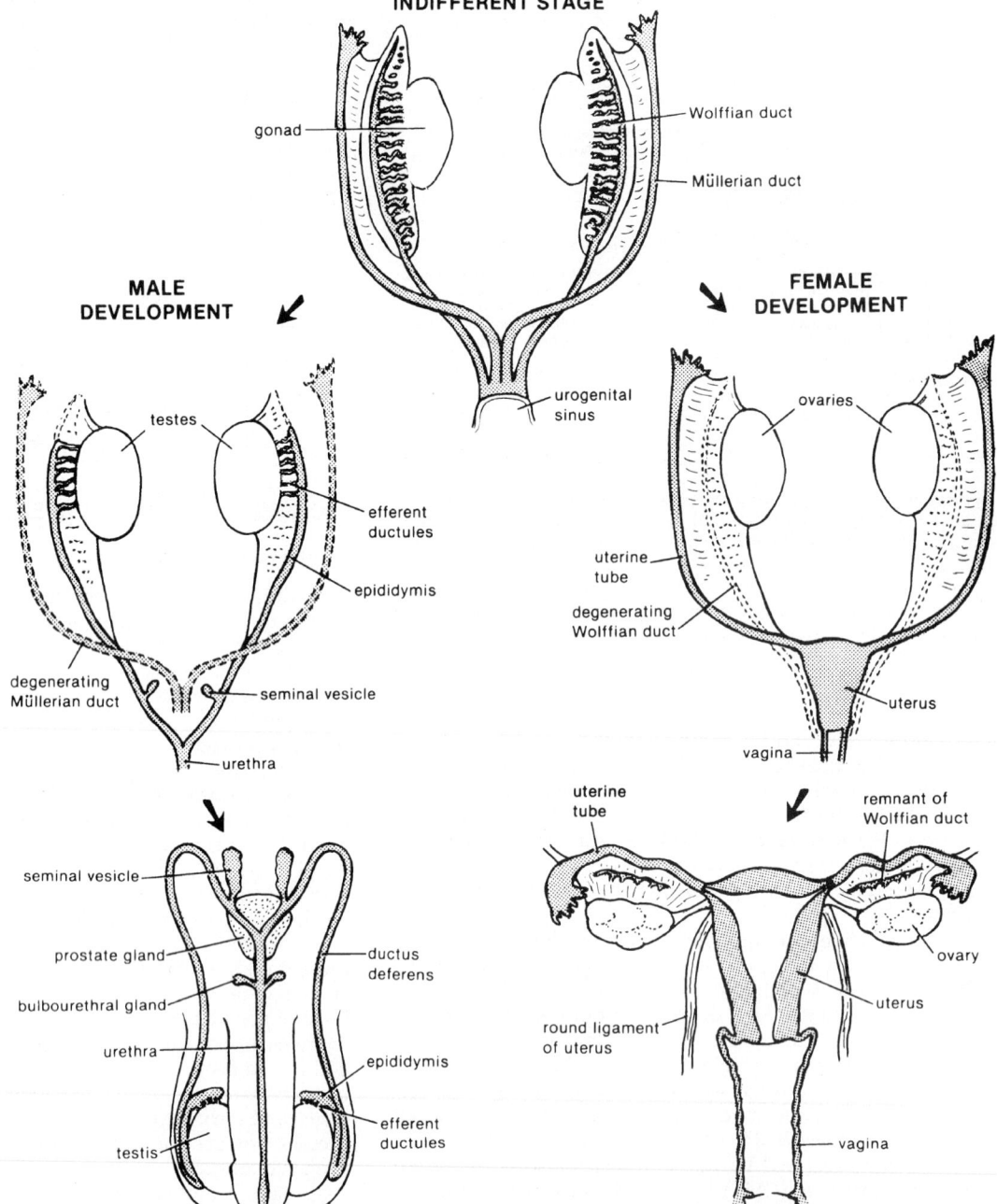

**FIGURE 90-12.** Embryonic development of male and female internal reproductive structures. The testes descend out of the abdominopelvic cavity into the scrotum, and the ovaries, which also descend, remain within pelvic cavity. (From Spence AP, Mason EB. Human anatomy and physiology, 3rd ed. Menlo Park, CA: Benjamin/Cummings Publishing, 1987:809.)

sumably result from *chimerism*, the presence of two or more cell lines, each derived from different zygotes, in a single individual. In one survey, 6 of 28 46,XX/46,XY cases were proved chimeras.[50] Experimental production of XX/XY mouse chimeras usually does not result in true hermaphroditism, however, nor do 46,XX/46,XY humans always have true hermaphroditism. The 46,XX/47,XXY cases may result from chimerism or mitotic nondisjunction.

A few 46,XX true hermaphrodites doubtless result from undetected chimerism; however, for various reasons, undetected chimerism cannot easily explain all 46,XX true hermaphrodites. The presence of testicular tissue in 46,XX individuals is perplexing, because the *TDF* is localized to the Y chromosome, specifically the short arm. Plausible explanations for the presence of testes in individuals who ostensibly lack a Y chromosome include translocation of *TDF* from the Y to an X, translocation of *TDF* from the Y to an autosome, undetected mosaicism or chimerism, and activation of sex-reversal genes, perhaps

located on autosomes. The first or second hypothesis is supported by the detection of H-Y antigen in almost all 46,XX true hermaphrodites.[19] Especially impressive are observations of H-Y antigen in each of two 46,XX true hermaphrodite sibs.[57] However, cloned DNA sequences known to be near *TDF* have not been detected in true hermaphrodites.[58] These observations contrast with those in 46,XX males, suggesting different pathogenetic mechanisms for the two sex-reversal states. Aggregates of sibs of 46,XX true hermaphrodites suggest that recessive genetic factors, perhaps activation of autosomal loci ordinarily suppressed in 46,XX individuals, are responsible.[59,60] That 46,XX males and 46,XX true hermaphrodites have occurred in multiple generations of the same kindreds may or may not be attributable to the same mechanism.[61,62] That XX males in some of these kindreds have not, in contrast to the usual male, shown *TDF* favors perturbation of an autosomal region as the cause of XX true hermaphroditism.[34,35,63,64] Indeed, *SRY* is almost always present.

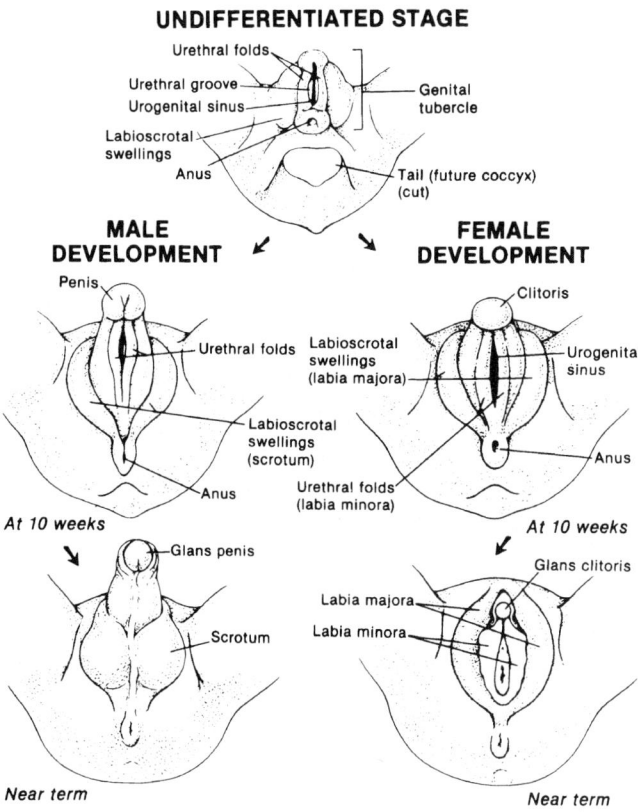

**FIGURE 90-13.** Embryonic development of male and female external reproductive structures from common anlagen. (From Spence AP, Mason EB. Human anatomy and physiology, 3rd ed. Menlo Park, CA: Benjamin/Cummings Publishing, 1987:809.)

**TABLE 90-1.**
**Adult Derivatives and Vestigial Remains of Embryonic Urogenital Structures**

| Male* | Embryonic Structure | Female* |
|---|---|---|
| *Testis* | Indifferent gonad | *Ovary* |
| *Seminiferous tubules* | Cortex | *Ovarian follicles* |
| *Rete testis* | Medulla | *Medulla* |
| | | Rete ovarii |
| Gubernaculum testis | Gubernaculum | *Ovarian ligament* |
| | | *Round ligament of uterus* |
| *Ductuli efferentes* | Mesonephric tubules | Epoophoron |
| Paradidymis | | Paroophoron |
| Appendix of epididymis | Wolffian (mesonephric) duct | Appendix vesiculosa |
| *Ductus epididymis* | | Duct of epoophoron |
| *Ductus deferens* | | Duct of Gartner |
| *Ureter, pelvis, calices, and collecting tubules* | | *Ureter, pelvis, calices, and collecting tubules* |
| *Ejaculatory duct and seminal vesicle* | | |
| Appendix testis | Müllerian (paramesonephric) duct | Hydatid (of Morgagni) |
| | | *Uterine tube* |
| | | *Uterus* |
| | | *Fibromuscular wall of vagina* |
| *Urinary bladder* | Urogenital sinus | *Urinary bladder* |
| Urethra (except *navicular fossa*) | | *Urethra* |
| Prostatic utricle | | *Vagina* |
| *Prostate gland* | | *Urethral and paraurethral glands* |
| *Bulbourethral glands* | | *Greater vestibular glands* |
| Seminal colliculus | Sinus Tubercle | Hymen |
| *Penis* | Phallus | *Clitoris* |
| *Glans penis* | | *Glans clitoridis* |
| *Corpora cavernosa penis* | | *Corpora cavernosa clitoridis* |
| *Corpus spongiosum penis* | | *Bulb of the vestibule* |
| *Ventral aspect of penis* | Urogenital folds | *Labia minora* |
| *Scrotum* | Labioscrotal swellings | *Labia majora* |

*Functional derivatives are in *italics*.
(From Moore KL. The developing human: clinically oriented embryology, 3rd ed. Philadelphia: WB Saunders, 1982:271.)

## GONADAL DYSGENESIS

In ovarian dysgenesis, the gonads traditionally are said to exist in the form of streak gonads (Fig. 90-14). The streaks are devoid of germ cells, accounting for the term *gonadal dysgenesis*. The streak is located in the position ordinarily occupied by the ovary. In the small percentage of individuals with gonadal dysgenesis who survive until adulthood, the normal gonad is usually replaced by a white fibrous streak 2 to 3 cm long and ~0.5 cm wide. This streak gonad is characterized histologically by interlacing waves of dense fibrous stroma, devoid of oocytes but otherwise indistinguishable from normal ovarian stroma. The karyotypes of affected individuals differ widely, with gonadal dysgenesis observed in a spectrum of karyotypes, including 45,X; 46,XX; 46,XY; various mosaics; and X or Y structural aberrations.

*Turner syndrome* is the term most frequently applied to the picture seen in individuals with gonadal dysgenesis. This designation is confusing, however, and application of the term *gonadal dysgenesis* in any instance of streak gonads is perhaps more appropriate. The term *Turner stigmata* is reserved for short stature and certain other somatic anomalies.[7]

**45,X Embryonic Lethality and Its Cellular Explanation.** Approximately 50% of spontaneous abortions occurring during the first 3 months of gestation are associated with a chromosomal abnormality. Twenty percent of chromosomally abnormal abortuses show monosomy X.[65] Of all pregnancies, 12% to 15% or more terminate in first-trimester spontaneous abortions, and 1% to 2% of all conceptions must be 45,X. Because the incidence of 45,X at birth is only ~1 per 10,000 females, >99% of all 45,X embryos can be assumed to be aborted. The high rate at which 45,X cell lines are spuriously detected in chorionic villi, however, raises the possibility that the frequency of 45,X in embryos is overestimated. Monosomy X may be relatively restricted to villi or membranes, those tissues most often available for cytogenetic studies, and the aborted embryo may have a different chromosomal complement. In any case, intrauterine growth restriction is characteristic of the rare surviving 45,X neonate.[66]

GONADAL DEVELOPMENT AND X-CHROMOSOME INACTIVATION.    The absence of oocytes in monosomy X is the result of increased oocyte atresia, not failure of germ-cell formation. The 45,X embryos and 45,X neonates have germ cells.[29,30] Inasmuch as germ cells are present in 45,X embryos, the fact that 3% to 5% of 45,X individuals menstruate spontaneously is not too surprising. Several fertile 45,X individuals have been reported.[67]

Because (according to the Lyon hypothesis) X chromosomes in excess of one are inactivated, why 45,X individuals should manifest developmental abnormalities is not so obvious. Relatively normal ovarian development occurs in 39,X mice and in most other monosomy X mammalian organisms. Data support several related explanations for these findings. First, some loci on the human heterochromatic (inactive) X are not inactivated. For example, the locus for steroid sulfatase, which is located on Xp, is not inactivated, and it would not be surprising if ovarian

**TABLE 90-2.**
**Classification of Disorders of Sexual Differentiation**

**ERRORS IN GONADAL DEVELOPMENT**
*True Hermaphroditism*
*Gonadal (Ovarian) Dysgenesis*
  With the stigmata of Turner syndrome
  Without any stigmata (i.e., 46,XX or 46,XY)
  Mixed gonadal dysgenesis
*Seminiferous Tubule Dysgenesis (Klinefelter syndrome) and Its Variants*
*Other Disorders Affecting Testes*
  Germinal cell aplasia (i.e., Sertoli-cell–only syndrome; del Castillo syndrome)
  Congenital anorchia (i.e., vanishing testis syndrome)
  Syndrome of rudimentary testes
  "Male Turner syndrome" (i.e., Ullrich-Noonan syndrome)
*Miscellaneous Disorders Affecting Germ Cells in Both Sexes*
**ERRORS IN DUCTAL DEVELOPMENT**
*Anomalies of the Distal Female Tract (see Table 90-4)*
  Imperforate hymen
  Vaginal septa
    Transverse
    Longitudinal
  Vaginal atresia
  Müllerian agenesis or hypoplasia
  Incomplete müllerian fusion
  Diethylstilbestrol-associated anomalies
*Anomalies of the Distal Male Tract*
  Wolffian aplasia
  Failure of fusion of epididymis and testis
  Persistence of müllerian derivatives in otherwise normal males (i.e., hernia uteri inguinale)
  Wolffian dysgenesis (e.g., cystic fibrosis)
**ERRORS IN GENITAL DIFFERENTIATION**
*Female Pseudohermaphroditism*
  Genetic forms (of congenital adrenal hyperplasia)
    21-hydroxylase deficiency
    11β-hydroxylase deficiency
    3β-hydroxysteroid dehydrogenase deficiency
  Teratogenic forms
  Idiopathic
*Male Pseudohermaphroditism*
  Defects in testicular activity
    Agonadia (i.e., testicular regression syndrome)
    Leydig cell agenesis
  Defects in androgen synthesis
    20,22-desmolase deficiency (i.e., congenital lipoid adrenal hyperplasia)
    3β-hydroxysteroid dehydrogenase deficiency
    17α-hydroxylase deficiency
    17,20-desmolase deficiency
    17-ketosteroid reductase deficiency
    Multiple enzyme defects
  Defects in androgen action
    Complete androgen insensitivity (i.e., testicular feminization)
    Incomplete androgen insensitivity and the Reifenstein syndrome
    5α-reductase deficiency (i.e., pseudovaginal perineoscrotal hypospadias)
    Infertile males with androgen resistance
  Unclassified disorders
    Hypospadias without other defects
    Genital ambiguity with multiple malformation patterns
    Microphallus

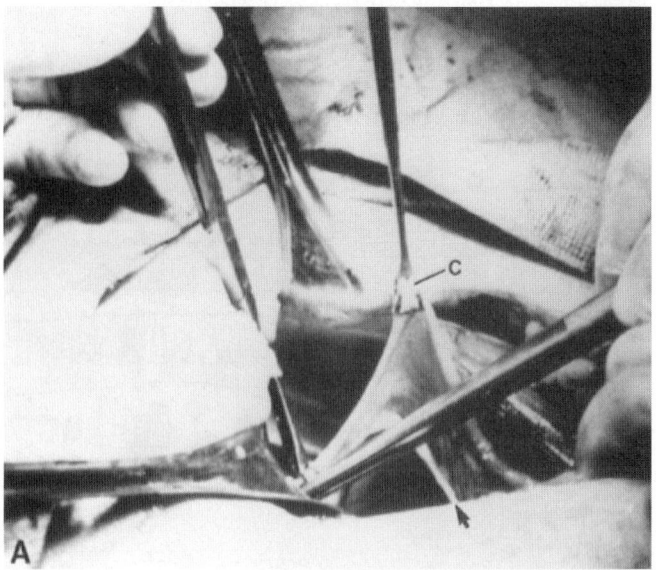

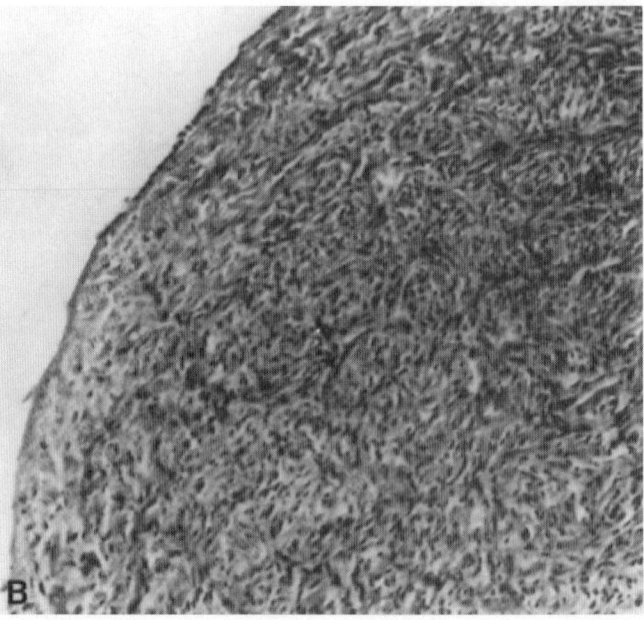

**FIGURE 90-14. A,** Streak gonad of patient with XY gonadal dysgenesis. Clamp (*C*) is elevating a fallopian tube. White streak perpendicular to forceps at lower right is the gonad (*arrow*). A streak gonad from a 45,X individual would look identical. **B,** Histologic appearance of streak gonad from an individual with 45,X gonadal dysgenesis. Only fibrous stroma is present; no oocytes are obvious. (From Simpson JL. Disorders of sexual differentiation: etiology and clinical delineation. New York: Academic Press, 1976.)

The parental origin of 45,X is of interest. In humans, 70% of live-born 45,X individuals have lost a *paternal* sex chromosome.[69] This helps explain why mean maternal age is not increased for 45,X abortuses or live borns.[70] Murine monosomy (39,X) also results from the loss of a paternal sex chromosome at the time of fertilization.[71]

Most commonly, individuals with gonadal dysgenesis have a 45,X karyotype and present with the Turner stigmata.[72] Secondary sexual development usually does not occur in 45,X individuals (Fig. 90-15). Pubic and axillary hair fail to develop in normal quantity. Although well differentiated, the external genitalia, the vagina, and the müllerian derivatives (e.g., uterus) remain small. As is true for virtually all individuals with gonadal dysgenesis, estrogen and androgen levels are decreased; levels of follicle-stimulating hormone (FSH) and luteinizing hormone (LH) are increased.

determinants likewise escaped X inactivation. Second, X inactivation never occurs in human oocytes, as evidenced by the fact that females who are heterozygous for the enzyme glucose-6-phosphate dehydrogenase synthesize both alleles in oocytes.[68]

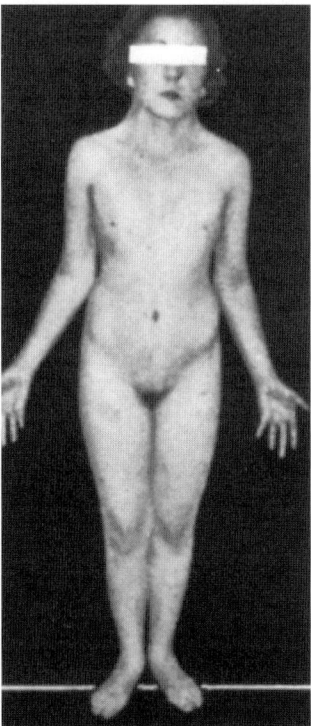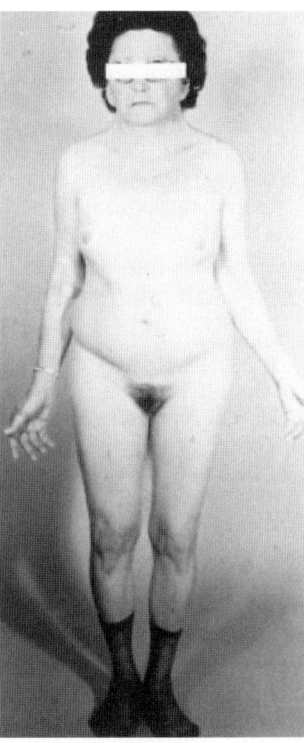

**A,B**

**FIGURE 90-15. A,** Appearance of one of original seven cases of Turner syndrome reported in 1938. **B,** Same patient, photographed in 1972, almost 35 years after publication of the original case report. The karyotype was documented to be 45,X. The patient had received little estrogen in intervening years and experienced severe osteoporosis. (Courtesy of Dr. R. Rebar and Dr. S. S. C. Yen, University of California, San Diego.)

NONGONADAL FEATURES OF TURNER SYNDROME. The common anomalies of Turner syndrome include epicanthal folds, high arched palate, low nuchal hairline, webbed neck, shield-like chest, coarctation of the aorta, ventricular septal defect, renal anomalies, pigmented nevi, lymphedema, hypoplastic nails, and cubitus valgus (Table 90-3). Inverted nipples and double eyelashes may be present as well. No feature is pathognomonic, but in aggregate, they form a spectrum of anomalies more likely to exist in 45,X individuals than in normal 46,XX individuals. These anomalies are the Turner stigmata, the presence of which suggests the coexistence of gonadal dysgenesis.

Individuals with a 45,X karyotype have low birth weights (adjusted mean, 2851.1 ± 65.1 g).[66] Total body length at birth is sometimes less than normal, but often it is normal. Height velocity before puberty generally lies in the 10th to the 15th percentile, and the mean heights of 45,X adults (16 years or older) range from 141 to 146 cm (55.5–57.5 in).[72–75] In untreated patients, the epiphyses remain open; additional growth occurs when sex steroids are administered. Despite the diminished final height of such patients, their adult stature tends to correlate with parental height.[75] (Also see ref. 75a.)

That not all patients with gonadal dysgenesis are short indicates that sex steroid deficiency is not the cause. For example, normal stature is characteristic of individuals with 46,XX gonadal dysgenesis. Growth hormone (GH) levels have long been considered essentially normal in individuals with gonadal dysgenesis.[76,77] Cellular resistance to GH, however, has been suggested. This relative resistance may be overcome by treatment with exogenous GH at higher doses than those used for classic GH deficiency.[78] Anti-GH antibodies have been detected, and GH reserve may be decreased.[79,80] More evidence suggests that abnormalities in GH or insulin-like growth factor-I (IGF-I), which fall below the normal range after 8 years of age, are secondary to the lack of gonadal activation and estrogen secretion.[81]

**TABLE 90-3.**
**Somatic Features Associated with 45,X Karyotype**

**GROWTH***
Decreased birth weight
Decreased adult height (mean, 141 ± 0.62 cm)
**INTELLECTUAL FUNCTION**
Verbal IQ > performance IQ
Cognitive deficits (e.g., space-form blindness)
Immature personality, probably secondary to short stature
**CRANIOFACIAL**
Premature fusion of spheno-occipital and other sutures, producing brachycephaly
Triangular facies
Low-set ears
Abnormal pinnae
Retruded mandible
Epicanthal folds (25%)[†]
Ptosis
High-arched palate (36%)
"Double" eyelashes
Abnormal dentition
Visual anomalies, usually strabismus (22%)
Auditory deficits: sensorineural or secondary to middle ear infections
"Wooly" hair
**NECK**
Pterygium coli (46%)
Short broad neck (74%)
Low nuchal hair line (71%)
**CHEST**
Rectangular contour (i.e., shield chest; 53%)
Apparent widely spaced nipples
Inverted nipples
Tapered lateral ends of clavicle
**CARDIOVASCULAR**
Coarctation of aorta or ventricular septal defect (10–16%)
Aortic stenosis
Pulmonic stenosis (rare)
**RENAL (38%)**
Horseshoe kidneys
Unilateral renal aplasia
Duplicated ureters
**GASTROINTESTINAL**
Telangiectasias
**SKIN AND LYMPHATICS**
Pigmented nevi (63%)
Capillary hemangiomas
Lymphedema (39%) secondary to hypoplasia of superficial vessels (especially neonatal)
**NAILS**
Hypoplasia or malformation (66%)
**SKELETAL**
Cubitus valgus (54%)
Radial tilt of articular surface of trochlear eminence of the humerus
Clinodactyly V
Short metacarpals, usually fourth finger (48%)
Decreased carpal arch (mean angle, 117 degrees)
Deformities of medial tibial condyle
Hypoplastic or fused (rarely) cervical vertebrae
Kyphosis
Scoliosis
Square lumbar vertebral bodies
**DERMATOGLYPHICS**
Increased total digital ridge count (mean, 166.1 ± 8.6)
Increased distance between palmar triradii a and b
Distal axial triradius in position t'
**PELVIC ALTERATIONS**
Android pelvic inlet
Small iliac wings
Narrow sacrosciatic notches
Narrow pubic arch

*A list of somatic anomalies frequently associated with a 45,X chromosomal complement. Many other anomalies have been reported in 45,X individuals.
†Frequencies are given in parentheses.
(Data from Simpson JL. Ovarian determinants through phenotypic-karyotypic deductions: progress and pitfalls. In: Rosenfield R, Grumbach M, eds. Turner syndrome. New York: Marcel Dekker, 1990:65; Simpson JL. Disorders of sexual differentiation: etiology and clinical delineation. New York: Academic Press, 1976; and Simpson JL. Gonadal dysgenesis and abnormalities of the human sex chromosomes: current status of phenotypic-karyotypic correlations. Birth Defects 1975; 11[4]:23.)

Short stature may be common in gonadal dysgenesis because the epiphyses are structurally abnormal. This hypothesis is compatible with observations that decreased growth occurs in the long bones, teeth, and skull.[82,83] One aspect of Turner syndrome may be a skeletal dysplasia.

Most 45,X patients have normal intelligence, but any given 45,X patient has a slightly higher probability of being retarded than a 46,XX individual. The frequency of overt retardation is 11% to 17%.[72] Biases of ascertainment dictate that this prevalence probably represents the maximum risk. Performance IQ is definitely lower than verbal IQ, however; 45,X individuals have an unusual cognitive defect characterized by an inability to appreciate the shapes and relations of objects with respect to one another (i.e., space-form blindness).[84–86] The patients usually appear socially immature, probably in part because they are short and sexually immature.[87]

METABOLIC ALTERATIONS.    Diabetes mellitus, thyroid disease, and essential hypertension often are present in individuals with 45,X karyotypes. Abnormal oral glucose-tolerance tests may occur in as many as 40% of these individuals.[88] Both autoimmune thyroiditis and Graves disease are observed with increased frequency in patients with Turner stigmata. Approximately one-third of adult 45,X patients have essential hypertension, which also may occur in young 45,X girls. Therapy for any metabolic alterations is not unique, although reduction or careful monitoring of exogenous estrogen therapy may be necessary.

**Abnormalities of the X Chromosome.**    Several different abnormalities of the X chromosome have been associated with gonadal dysgenesis. The cytologic origin of these defects was considered earlier.

DELETION OF THE SHORT ARM OF CHROMOSOME X.    A terminal deletion of the X short arm [del(Xp)] may or may not cause gonadal dysgenesis, short stature, and other features of the Turner stigmata. The phenotype depends on the amount of Xp that is deficient.

Spontaneous menstruation, albeit usually leading to secondary amenorrhea, has occurred in almost 40% of reported 46,X,del(X)(p11) individuals (see Fig. 90-7). Almost all 46,X,del(X)(p21) individuals menstruate, but only approximately one-half become pregnant.[7,34,89,90] These data indicate that ovarian tissue persists more often in del(Xp) individuals than in 45,X individuals and that complete ovarian failure (with primary amenorrhea) occurs only if the proximal and the terminal portions of Xp are deleted. However, the mean adult heights are 140 cm (55 in) for 46,X,del(X)(p11) and 146.5 cm (57.5 in) for 46,X,del(X)(p21) persons[89,91] (see Fig. 90-8). Inasmuch as 46,X,del(X)(p21) individuals are short but have normal ovarian function, determinants for ovarian maintenance and for stature must be located in different regions of Xp; statural determinants are more distal.[35,36,91] No evidence yet exists that any given X-specific probe bears a special relation to X-ovarian or X-structural determinants.

ISOCHROMOSOME FOR THE X LONG ARM (1[XQ]).    Almost all 46,X,i(Xq) patients have streak gonads, short stature, and features of the Turner stigmata. In addition to having a duplication of Xq,i(Xq), these individuals differ from del(X)(p11) persons because the terminal portion and almost all of Xp is deleted. The better gonadal function in del(X)(p11) than in i(Xq) individuals is consistent with the location of ovarian determinants at several different sites on Xp. A locus on Xp may be deleted in i(Xq) karyotype but be retained near the centromere in 46,X,del(X)(p11) cases. Because duplication of Xq (i.e., 46,X,i[Xq]) does not compensate for deficiency of Xp, the gonadal determinants on Xq and Xp must have different functions. Whether duplication of Xq per se produces abnormalities is unknown.

DELETION OF THE LONG ARM OF CHROMOSOME X (DEL[XQ]).    Most patients with a deletion of the X long arm have streak gonads and never menstruate. This is especially true of individuals with del(X)(q13). However, deletions of distal Xq are more likely to be associated with premature ovarian failure than with primary amenorrhea. The Xq appears to contain more than one region that is required for normal ovarian function. Perhaps several Xq loci can affect ovarian function in additive fashion. The only clue to the nature of any of these products is the suggestion that the diaphanous (*DIA*) gene, localized to Xq25, plays a role; however, other genes in distal Xq are also pivotal to ovarian development.

Originally, deletions of Xq were not thought to result in short stature, but later tabulations show a definitely decreased mean height of persons with del(X)(q13).[36,72,89,92] Whether the short stature reflects specific loci or vicissitudes of X-inactivation is unclear.[93]

**Mosaicism**

MOSAICISM INVOLVING ONLY X CHROMOSOMES.    The 45,X/46,XX individuals have fewer anomalies than 45,X individuals. In one survey, 12% of 45,X/46,XX individuals menstruated, compared with only 3% of 45,X individuals.[72] In that survey, the mean adult height was greater in 45,X/46,XX persons than in 45,X individuals. More mosaic patients (25%) than nonmosaic patients (5%) reach adult heights greater than 152 cm (60 in). Somatic anomalies are less likely to occur in 45,X/46,XX than in 45,X patients.

MOSAICISM WITH A Y CHROMOSOME.    Individuals with a 45,X cell line and at least one line containing a Y chromosome manifest a variety of phenotypes, ranging from almost normal males with cryptorchidism or penile hypospadias to females indistinguishable from those with the 45,X Turner syndrome. The different phenotypes presumably reflect different tissue distributions of the various cell lines, although this assumption remains unproven. At any rate, 45,X/46,XY individuals may show unambiguous female external genitalia, ambiguous external genitalia, or almost normal male external genitalia.

Some 45,X/46,XY individuals with female external genitalia have the Turner stigmata and are clinically indistinguishable from 45,X individuals. Others, however, are female but of normal stature and without somatic anomalies. As in other types of gonadal dysgenesis, the external genitalia, vagina, and müllerian derivatives remain unstimulated because of deficient sex steroids. Breasts fail to develop, and little pubic or axillary hair grows. In fact, breast development in a 45,X/46,XY individual should lead one to suspect an estrogen-secreting tumor, most commonly a gonadoblastoma or dysgerminoma.

The streak gonads of 45,X/46,XY individuals usually are indistinguishable histologically from the streak gonads of individuals with 45,X gonadal dysgenesis. However, gonadoblastomas or dysgerminomas develop in 15% to 20% of 45,X/46,XY individuals.[55,56,94] Such neoplasms may arise as early as the first two decades of life. Gonadoblastomas occur almost exclusively in 46,XY or 45,X/46,XY individuals and usually are benign. However, they may be associated with dysgerminomas or other germ-cell tumors that are malignant. The gonads of 45,X/46,XY individuals should be extirpated regardless of the patient's age. Because of the risk of neoplasia, 45,X/46,XY gonadal dysgenesis should be differentiated from forms of gonadal dysgenesis lacking a Y chromosome.

When the polymerase chain reaction for *SRY* was used, unrecognized Y-chromosome material was found in 1 of 40 patients with Turner syndrome.[95] Because the detection of *SRY* sequences in patients with gonadal dysgenesis is correlated with the presence of Y-chromosomal DNA and carries the risk of tumor development, the application of this technique in search of *SRY* may be justified in all individuals with this disorder.

Individuals may show one streak gonad and one dysgenetic testis. The terms *asymmetric gonadal dysgenesis* or *mixed gonadal dysgenesis* are often applied to such individuals. They usually have ambiguous external genitalia. Many investigators believe that the phenotype of asymmetric gonadal dysgenesis is almost always associated with 45,X/46,XY mosaicism, with ostensibly nonmosaic cases reflecting merely an inability to analyze appropriate tissues. Most 45,X/46,XY individuals with ambiguous

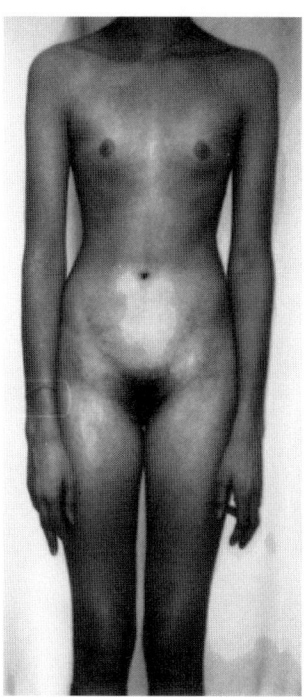

**FIGURE 90-16.** A case of 46,XX gonadal dysgenesis: a 19-year-old woman with primary amenorrhea. Notice the normal stature and diminished breast development. Circulating gonadotropin levels were markedly elevated.

external genitalia have müllerian derivatives (e.g., a uterus). The presence of a uterus is helpful diagnostically, because a uterus is absent in most genetic forms of male pseudohermaphroditism. If an individual has ambiguous external genitalia, bilateral testes, and a uterus, one may reasonably infer the presence of 45,X/46,XY mosaicism, whether or not both lines can be demonstrated cytogenetically. Occasionally, the uterus is rudimentary, or a fallopian tube fails to develop ipsilateral to a testis.

The 45,X/46,XY mosaicism has less commonly been detected in individuals with almost normal male external genitalia. In some individuals, hypospadias is present, but the sex-of-rearing is unequivocally male.

The 45,X/47,XXY and 45,X/46,XY/47,XXY complements exist, albeit much less often than 45,X/46,XY. These complements are associated with the same phenotypic spectrum as 45,X/46,XY. Of particular interest is one family in which two and possibly three sibs had 45,X/46,XY/47,XYY mosaicism.[96] The parents were second cousins, suggesting recessive factors.

**Gonadal Dysgenesis in 46,XX Individuals.**    The first individual with gonadal dysgenesis and an apparently normal female (46,XX) complement was reported in 1960.[12] By 1971, a survey of 61 such individuals led to the conclusion that the disorder was inherited in an autosomal recessive fashion.[12] A study of all XX gonadal dysgenesis cases in Finland confirmed this conclusion.[97]

The external genitalia and the streak gonads (see Fig. 90-14) in XX gonadal dysgenesis are indistinguishable from those in gonadal dysgenesis secondary to a sex chromosomal abnormality. Likewise, the endocrine profiles do not differ, but individuals with XX gonadal dysgenesis usually have normal stature (Fig. 90-16). Several pathogenic mechanisms can be postulated, but firm data have not been gathered. Phenocopies for XX gonadal dysgenesis also are well recognized (see Chap. 96).

Both XX gonadal dysgenesis and neurosensory deafness have occurred in multiple sibs in several families; the occurrence of deaf but fertile male sibs confirms autosomal inheritance.[98] The coexistence of gonadal and auditory anomalies probably indicates a syndrome distinct from XX gonadal dys-

genesis without deafness (i.e., genetic heterogeneity). Further evidence for genetic heterogeneity can be cited. In several other families, unique patterns of somatic anomalies indicate the existence of mutant genes distinct from those already discussed. These include: XX gonadal dysgenesis and myopathy; XX gonadal dysgenesis and cerebellar ataxia; XX gonadal dysgenesis and metabolic acidosis; XX gonadal dysgenesis, microcephaly, and arachnodactyly.[99–101]

**Follicle-Stimulating Hormone–Receptor Mutations.**    At least one form of XX gonadal dysgenesis is now known to be caused by a mutation of the FSH receptor (FSHR). Affected women present with primary or secondary amenorrhea and elevated serum FSH levels indicative of premature ovarian failure[97,102] (see Chap. 96). The mutation originally was identified in a large number of sporadic and familial cases in Finland. Most cases were found in north central Finland, a sparsely populated part of the country. The overall frequency of the disorder in Finland was 1 per 8300 females, a relatively high incidence attributed to a founder effect. The segregation ratio of 0.23 for female sibs was consistent with autosomal recessive inheritance, as was the consanguinity rate of 12%.

Sib-pair analysis using polymorphic DNA markers was used to localize the gene to a specific region of chromosome arm 2p, a region known to contain genes for both FSHR and the LH receptor (LHR). One specific mutation (C566T:alanine to valine) in exon 7 was observed in six multiplex families.[102,103] On transvaginal ultrasonography, most of these patients have demonstrable ovarian follicles, raising the possibility of residual receptor activity.[103]

The C566T mutation was not found in all Finnish XX gonadal dysgenesis patients and is rarely detected in 46,XX women with ovarian failure who reside outside Finland.[104,105]

**Gonadal Dysgenesis in 46,XY Individuals.**    Gonadal dysgenesis also can occur in 46,XY individuals. In XY gonadal dysgenesis, affected individuals are phenotypic females who show sexual infantilism and bilateral streak gonads (Fig. 90-17). The gonads may undergo neoplastic transformation (20–30% prevalence)[56] (Fig. 90-18). At least one form of XY gonadal dysgenesis results from an X-linked recessive or male-limited autosomal dominant gene.[106,107] Sporadic cases may result from deletion or point mutations within *SRY* on the Y short arm.[14,108,109]

Further evidence for genetic heterogeneity lies in the existence of at least three syndromes having *XY gonadal dysgenesis as one of their components: XY gonadal dysgenesis and long-limbed camptomelic dwarfism, XY gonadal dysgenesis and ectodermal defects,* and the *genitopalatocardiac syndrome.*[36,110–112]

**Rudimentary Ovary Syndrome and Unilateral Streak Gonad Syndrome.**    The rudimentary ovary syndrome is a poorly defined entity of unknown cause said to be characterized by decreased numbers of follicles. This "syndrome" is heterogeneous, not a single entity. Many cases have been associated with sex chromosomal abnormalities, particularly 45,X/46,XX mosaicism. Similar statements also apply to individuals with the unilateral streak ovary syndrome. For example, a unilateral streak gonad and a contralateral polycystic ovary have been observed in a 46,XX/46,X,i(Xq) individual who became pregnant.[113]

EVALUATION AND TREATMENT OF GONADAL DYSGENESIS. When Turner stigmata are present, the diagnosis of gonadal dysgenesis usually is made early in childhood. The index of suspicion should be high for any infant with lymphedema of the hands and feet at birth, especially because the somatic anomalies are not very obvious in neonates (see Fig. 90-9). Other children present for evaluation of sexual infantilism, and still others with a male sex-of-rearing may not virilize at the expected age of puberty. Short stature is another common reason that evaluation is sought.

The measurement of circulating gonadotropin concentrations and the determination of the karyotype can establish the

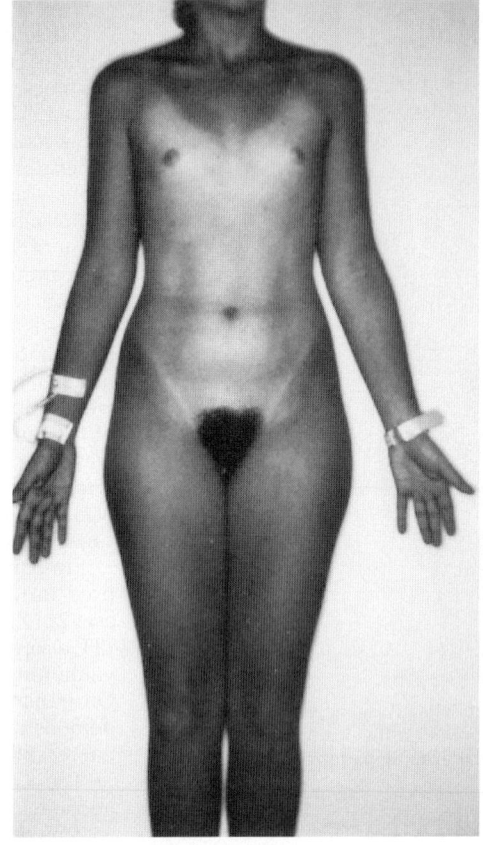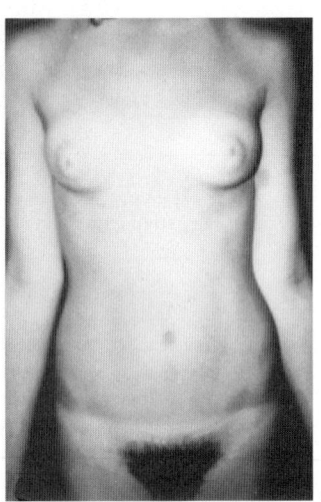

**A,B**

**FIGURE 90-17. A** and **B,** Two examples of 46,XY gonadal dysgenesis. Both 16-year-old individuals presented with primary amenorrhea and markedly elevated concentrations of circulating gonadotropins. Both patients had dysgerminoma of an ovary; the patient in **B** also had a large gonadoblastoma of the contralateral ovary. Breast development as in **B** is extremely rare and no doubt secondary to hormone production by the patient's gonadal neoplasm. (**B,** Photograph reproduced from Villanueva AL, Benirschke K, Campbell J, et al. Complete development of secondary sexual characteristics in a case of 46,XY gonadal dysgenesia. Obstet Gynecol 1984; 64:68S.)

diagnosis. Longitudinal studies have documented elevated gonadotropin levels at all ages in gonadal dysgenesis, indicating absence of appropriate feedback inhibition of the hypothalamic-pituitary unit by the dysgenetic gonads even in childhood.[114,115]

Chromosomal studies are indicated to eliminate the possibility of a Y chromosome. The use of the polymerase chain reaction to detect sequences of *SRY* may well be warranted. If the phenotype and karyotype are compatible, the only tissue needed is blood for lymphocyte culture. If the phenotype and karyotype are incompatible (e.g., tall "45,X" subjects), skin or gonadal fibroblasts also should be cultured to detect any mosaicism. If a Y chromosome is identified, surgical extirpation of the dysgenetic gonads is indicated to prevent neoplasms. Streak gonads usually can be removed by laparoscopy. In appropriate cases in which disseminated malignancies do not involve the gonads, the uterus may be left in situ for donor in vitro fertilization or embryo transfer. The evaluation of other commonly involved organ systems should include a careful physical examination, with special attention to the cardiovascular system, and should include thyroid function tests (including antibodies), fasting blood glucose level, renal function tests, and an intravenous urogram or a renal ultrasonographic scan.

The treatment of individuals with short stature has received significant attention. A multicenter, prospective, randomized trial of administration of GH, alone and in combination with oxandrolone, was initiated in 1983.[116,117] Data on 62 girls, who have received 3 to 6 years of treatment, have been published. Given an average height of 143 cm for untreated girls in the United States, the mean height of 151.9 cm in the 30 girls whose therapy was terminated represented a net increase of 8.1 cm (therapy was terminated because the subjects had met study criteria for cessation of treatment, including bone age >14 years and a growth velocity of <2.5 cm over 12 months, or because the subject was satisfied with her current height and elected to discontinue therapy).[117]

To increase the final height, administration of estrogens in very low doses and anabolic steroids (particularly oxandrolone) has been advocated.[117] The success in increasing the final adult height remains arguable, but increased growth in the first 2 or 3 years of therapy without undue acceleration of bone age has been verified.[116,118,119] Any increase in the final height appears to be no more than 6 to 8 cm. Although estrogens appear to act by increasing GH secretion, the mode of action of oxandrolone has not been determined. Oxandrolone does not appear to increase the secretion of GH or IGF-I, but it may act directly on growing cartilage. Long-term follow-up suggests that postprandial insulin levels are higher in patients treated with oxandrolone and GH than in patients treated with GH alone.

Treatment strategies that have exogenous GH as their key element are now commonly accepted. An adult height of >150 cm, the widely accepted lower limit of normal height for women in the United States, is now attainable by most girls with this disorder. What the exact dose of GH should be and what additional benefit oxandrolone may contribute are not known. GH administered in doses 25% above those recommended for GH deficiency is proving to be remarkably safe.

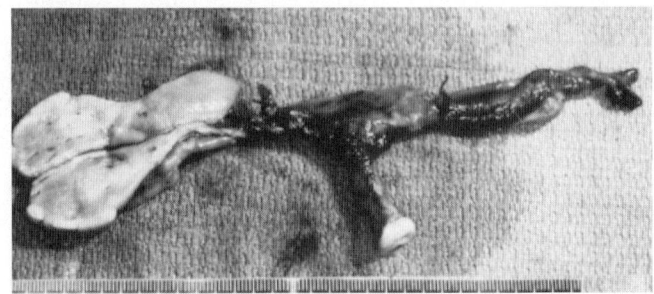

**FIGURE 90-18.** Gross appearance of the uterus, fallopian tubes, and gonads of 46,XY patient with gonadal dysgenesis. Right gonad (cut) contained dysgerminoma.

To enable the patient to achieve sexual maturation, estrogen therapy should be initiated when the patient is psychologically ready, perhaps at the age of 12 to 13 years, and after GH therapy is completed. Because the aim is to mimic normal pubertal development, therapy is initiated with low-dose estrogen alone (such as oral conjugated estrogens 0.3 mg daily) given continuously for the first several months. A progestogen (5–10 mg of oral medroxyprogesterone acetate or 200 mg of oral micronized progesterone daily for 14 days each month) is then added to prevent the development of endometrial hyperplasia, either when the patient notices vaginal bleeding or after 6 months of unopposed estrogen therapy. Thereafter, the dose of estrogen is increased slowly over 1 to 2 years to daily oral doses of 1.25 to 2.5 mg of conjugated estrogen, 1 to 2 mg of micronized 17β-estradiol, 1.25 to 2.5 mg of piperazine estrone sulfate orally, or 0.05 to 0.1 mg of estradiol transdermally, with the patch changed once or twice weekly depending on the specific preparation. Generally, continued breast tenderness is the first sign that the dose of estrogen is excessive. These patients must be observed especially closely for the development of hypertension with estrogen therapy. The patients and their parents should be informed of the emotional and physical changes that will occur with therapy. Additional principles for estrogen replacement may be found in Chapter 100 (also see ref. 119a).

Individuals with mosaic gonadal dysgenesis and other chromosomal aberrations such as del(X)(p11) or del(X)(q25 to q27) may develop normally at puberty. The decision whether to initiate estrogen therapy can be made on the basis of growth rates, bone age, uterine size determined by ultrasonography, and circulating gonadotropin concentrations. FSH levels in the normal range for age imply functional gonads.

Examination of individuals with sexual infantilism who have been treated with large doses of estrogen (especially conjugated estrogens) from the outset to effect maturation of secondary sexual characteristics often reveals abnormal and inappropriate breast development. The areola often becomes abnormally large, with minimal additional breast tissue. Whether breast contour can be improved in individuals subjected to such inappropriate therapy is not clear.

Pregnancies can now be achieved in these individuals, with success rates of >50%, by using donor oocytes.[120] Hormone-replacement regimens using transdermal estradiol-17β and intramuscular progesterone have generally been associated with the highest pregnancy rates among those regimens aimed at preparing the endometrium to receive an embryo.

TRIPLE-X SYNDROME (47,XXX). The existence of individuals with a 47,XXX karyotype was first reported in 1959, and an association with premature ovarian failure was noted.[121] Since then, study has shown that patients with the triple-X syndrome need not have any impairment in fertility nor any shortening of their reproductive lives.[122,123] Premature menopause occurs with increased frequency, however, compared with its incidence in karyotypically normal individuals.[124] Moreover, reports of patients with triple-X syndrome associated with immunoglobulin deficiency, together with the finding that the control of T-cell function may be related to the X chromosome, suggest an association between immunologic abnormalities and triple-X syndrome in females with premature ovarian failure.[125–127]

Because affected individuals are phenotypically normal, they usually are identified only after presenting with hypergonadotropic amenorrhea. Treatment for the premature ovarian failure is the same as it is for menopausal women and is discussed in Chapter 100.

ULLRICH-NOONAN SYNDROME. A syndrome now known as the Ullrich-Noonan or pseudo-Turner syndrome has been described in which phenotypic females present with many of the Turner stigmata and a normal 46,XX chromosomal complement.[128–131] Moreover, females have functioning ovaries, although the onset of puberty may be delayed. Males also may present with this disorder. The common stigmata include short stature, webbed neck, ptosis, and (unlike in gonadal dysgenesis) right-sided congenital heart disease. Pulmonic stenosis (occurring in perhaps 50% of individuals) and atrial septal defect are the most common cardiac anomalies, although ventricular septal defect, ventricular hypertrophy, patent ductus arteriosus, coarctation of the aorta, and aortic stenosis may be found. Mental retardation, pectus excavatum, cubitus valgus, and lymphedema also may occur (see Chap. 92).

The incidence of this syndrome has been estimated at ~1 in 8000, with >80% of cases arising from spontaneous mutations.[132] Familial clusters consistent with autosomal dominant inheritance have been described.

The existence of this syndrome reinforces the need to perform a karyotype study of individuals presenting with the Turner stigmata. Otherwise, individuals thought to have gonadal dysgenesis may develop normally at puberty and become fertile, much to the surprise of the physician.

### SEMINIFEROUS TUBULE DYSGENESIS AND ITS VARIANTS

**Klinefelter Syndrome.** Males with at least one Y chromosome and at least two X chromosomes have Klinefelter syndrome.[7] Most cases are 47,XXY, but the phenotype may also be associated with 46,XY/47,XXY; 48,XXYY; and 49,XXXXY complements.[133–135] The most characteristic features are seminiferous tubule dysgenesis and androgen deficiency. Somatic anomalies sometimes coexist.[133] The presence of a chromosomal abnormality and of elevated gonadotropin levels differentiates Klinefelter syndrome from hypogonadotropic hypogonadism. These conditions are discussed in Chapter 115.

**46,XX Sex-Reversed Males.** The 46,XX sex-reversed males are phenotypic males with bilateral testes.[7] Their chromosomal complement, however, appears to be that of a female (see Chap. 115). Affected patients have small testes and signs of androgen deficiency but otherwise have a normal male appearance. Facial and body hair are decreased, and pubic hair may be distributed in the pattern characteristic of females. Approximately one-third have gynecomastia. The penis and scrotum are small but usually well differentiated, and wolffian derivatives are normal. By definition, the sex-of-rearing is not in doubt.[136,137] Seminiferous tubules are decreased in number and in size, peritubular and interstitial fibrosis is present, Leydig cells are hyperplastic, and spermatogonia usually cannot be detected. Occasionally, immature spermatogonia are found, and sometimes the ejaculate contains spermatozoa.

In 46,XX males, as in 46,XX true hermaphrodites, testes develop, contrary to expectations that a Y chromosome is required for testicular differentiation. Translocation of the *TDF* from the Y to the X chromosome has been documented by molecular studies in most cases (80%).[63,138] Moreover, familial aggregates of 46,XX males alone or 46,XX males and 46,XX true hermaphrodites also have been reported.[61–64] Like XX true hermaphrodites, XX males in these kindreds may not show the Y-X translocation.[63,64] These observations support the possibility that autosomal sex-reversal genes exist or that mutation in an autosomal or X chromosomal gene that permits testicular differentiation in the absence of *TDF* has occurred.[34,35,64,138]

### OTHER DISORDERS AFFECTING THE TESTES

**Germinal Cell Aplasia.** Del Castillo and coworkers were the first to describe normally virilized yet sterile males with germinal cell aplasia (i.e., Sertoli cell–only syndrome or del Castillo syndrome).[139] Seminiferous tubules lack spermatogonia, and the testes are slightly smaller than average. Leydig cell function is normal, however, and secondary sexual development is normal. In germinal cell aplasia, FSH levels are elevated, but LH levels are normal.[139a] Tubular hyalinization and sclerosis usually do not occur. Occasionally, a few spermatozoa are present, but affected individuals usually are sterile. Despite infertility, androgen therapy is unnecessary because secondary sexual development is normal. In five families, a male with this condition has had a sister with streak gonads (see Chap. 115).

**Congenital Anorchia.** Males (46,XY) with anorchia (i.e., *vanishing testis syndrome*) have unambiguous male external genitalia, normal wolffian derivatives, no müllerian derivatives, and no detectable testes[7] (see Chap. 115). Unilateral anorchia is not extraordinarily rare, but bilateral anorchia is uncommon. Somatic abnormalities are rare. Despite the absence of testes, the phallus is well differentiated. The pathogenesis presumably involves atrophy of the fetal testes after 12 to 16 weeks of gestation, by which time genital virilization has occurred. The vasa deferentia terminate blindly, often in association with the spermatic vessels. The diagnosis should be applied only if testicular tissue is not detected in the scrotum, the inguinal canal, or the entire path along which the testes descend during embryogenesis. Splenic-gonadal fusion also can occur, mimicking the disorder.

Heritable tendencies exist, but the occurrence of monozygotic twins discordant for anorchia suggests that genetic factors are not paramount in all cases.[140,141] Perhaps a heritable tendency toward in utero torsion of the testicular artery exists, explaining occasional familial aggregates (see Chap. 115).

**Syndrome of Rudimentary Testes.** Men have also been reported who had well-formed but small testes (<1 cm in greatest diameter) and small penises.[142] These testes consisted of a few Leydig cells, small tubules containing Sertoli cells, and an occasional spermatogonium. Wolffian derivatives were present, but müllerian derivatives were absent. Relatively few individuals with the rudimentary testes syndrome have been described; however, five affected sibs have been reported.[22]

The pathogenesis is unclear, for it seems unlikely that such small testes could be responsible for normal male development. Perhaps the testes initially were normal during embryogenesis and only later decreased in size. The cause may be analogous to that of anorchia but with retention of some testicular tissue.

**Ullrich-Noonan Syndrome.** Phenotypic males with normal 46,XY chromosomal complements who present with the Turner stigmata often are said to have the "male Turner syndrome"[128–131] (see Chap. 115). Most have the Ullrich-Noonan syndrome (see earlier). In many such boys, the testes are undescended and hypoplastic. In contrast to girls with Ullrich-Noonan syndrome, in whom sexual development is normal, boys often require testosterone replacement at puberty.

## DISORDERS AFFECTING GERM CELLS IN BOTH SEXES

In five sibships, male sibs and female sibs have each had germinal cell failure. The females had streak gonads and the males had germ-cell aplasia (Sertoli cell–only syndrome or del Castillo phenotype). In two families, the parents were consanguineous; in neither family did affected offspring show somatic anomalies.[24,25] In three other families, distinctive patterns of somatic anomalies coexisted, suggesting distinct entities. In these kindreds, germ-cell abnormalities were associated with hypertension and deafness, alopecia, or microcephaly, short stature, and minor anomalies.[23,26,27]

These families demonstrate that several different autosomal genes are capable of affecting XX and XY germ cells, presumably acting at sites in early germ-cell development common to both sexes. The elucidation of such genes could have profound implications for the understanding of normal developmental processes.

## ERRORS IN DUCTAL DEVELOPMENT

### ANOMALIES OF THE DISTAL FEMALE REPRODUCTIVE TRACT

Anomalies of the distal female reproductive tract represent a heterogeneous group of malformations resulting from abnormal development of the müllerian ducts. Many of the less severe anomalies do not affect reproduction, but others may increase fetal wastage.[143] Fertility itself seems unaffected in

**TABLE 90-4.**
**Classification of Müllerian Anomalies**

**CLASS I. SEGMENTED MÜLLERIAN AGENESIS OR HYPOPLASIA**
  A. Vaginal
  B. Cervical
  C. Fundal
  D. Tubal
  E. Combined

**CLASS II. UNICORNUATE UTERUS**
  A. With a rudimentary horn
      1. With a communicating endometrial cavity
      2. With a noncommunicating cavity
      3. With no cavity
  B. Without any rudimentary horn

**CLASS III. UTERUS DIDELPHYS**

**CLASS IV. BICORNUATE UTERUS**
  A. Complete to the internal os
  B. Partial
  C. Arcuate

**CLASS V. SEPTATE UTERUS**
  A. With a complete septum
  B. With an incomplete septum

**CLASS VI. UTERUS WITH INTERNAL LUMINAL CHANGES**

(Adapted from Buttram VC Jr, Gibbons WE. Müllerian anomalies: a proposed classification [an analysis of 144 cases]. Fertil Steril 1979; 32:40.)

patients with uterine malformations only. The development of secondary sexual characteristics is virtually always normal, and ovulation generally occurs regularly.

The most logical classification that has been proposed appears in Table 90-4.[144] Although the incidence of these anomalies is unknown, initial estimates approximated 0.02% of the female population.[145] An apparent increase in the incidence may be valid, a result of maternal ingestion of diethylstilbestrol (DES) during pregnancy. Between the late 1940s and the early 1970s, an estimated 2 to 3 million women were given DES during their pregnancies, so that 1 to 1.5 million female progeny were exposed to the drug in utero. DES generally results in anomalies of the lumen of the uterus (class VI). Whether infertility and oligomenorrhea are increased in women with DES-related anomalies is not clear.[146,147]

Of the ductal anomalies unrelated to drugs, the septate uterus is most common. In some instances, abnormalities of the vagina or uterus are part of a syndrome of malformations including abnormalities of the skeleton (especially of the lumbosacral spine) and renal system (i.e., *Rokitansky-Küster-Hauser syndrome*).[7,148–150]

Regardless of the cause, uterine anomalies not involving segmental müllerian agenesis or hypoplasia (class I) are compatible with normal fertility. However, increased fetal wastage has been documented.[149] In addition to spontaneous abortion and premature labor, uterine malformations are associated with abnormal presentations (e.g., breech, transverse lie) and complications of labor (e.g., retained placenta) that may compromise maternal or fetal well-being and contribute to fetal wastage.

**Imperforate Hymen.** Although an imperforate hymen does not involve the genital ducts, it must be considered in the differential diagnosis of several anomalies of the müllerian system. Ordinarily, the central portion of the hymen is patent (perforate) and allows outflow of mucus and blood. If the hymen is imperforate, mucus and blood accumulate in the vagina or uterus (i.e., hydrocolpos or hydrometrocolpos). An imperforate hymen is not particularly rare. Fortunately, the anomaly is corrected easily by surgical incisions, preferably cruciform. An imperforate hymen may be suspected because a bulging membrane, often bluish, may be visible at the introitus. However, the differential diagnosis may not seem so simple on physical examination. Ultrasonography may be helpful in verifying the presence of a uterus.

**Transverse Vaginal Septa.** Transverse vaginal septa may occur at several locations and may be complete or incomplete. Usually, the septa are ~1 cm thick and located near the junction of the upper one-third and lower two-thirds of the vagina; however, they may be present in the middle or lower third of the vagina. If no perforation is present, mucus and menstrual fluid lack egress, and hydrocolpos or hydrometrocolpos may develop. Other pelvic organs are usually normal, although occasionally the uterus is bicornuate.

Transverse vaginal septa probably result from failure of the urogenital sinus derivatives and müllerian duct derivatives to fuse or to canalize. An autosomal recessive gene appears to be responsible for some cases, at least in people of Amish descent,[151] with the *TVS* gene (as yet unidentified) being localized to chromosome band 20p12.[22] Individuals with coexisting postaxial polydactyly and cardiac defects (the *McKusick-Kaufman syndrome*) may or may not be etiologically distinct.[152–154]

Before surgery, transverse vaginal septa may be indistinguishable from vaginal atresia or imperforate hymen. Resection of the septa with mucosal reanastomosis generally obviates future problems with conception. If a transverse vaginal septum or an imperforate hymen is not diagnosed for several menstrual cycles after menarche, endometriosis may arise secondarily and interfere with subsequent fertility.

**Longitudinal Vaginal Septa.** Although among the most common genital tract anomalies, with an estimated frequency of between 0.2 and 0.5 per 1000 live births, longitudinal vaginal septa (sagittal or coronal) rarely produce clinical problems.[149] These septa probably result from abnormal mesodermal proliferation or persisting epithelium. Occasionally, such septa impede the second stage of labor; rarely, they interfere with coitus. Surgical transection is then indicated. Heritable tendencies do not appear paramount factors in the cause. However, an autosomal dominant syndrome characterized by a longitudinal vaginal septum, hand anomalies, and a possible bladder neck anomaly has been reported.[155] A longitudinal septum may exist in müllerian fusion defects of the most extreme type.

**Vaginal Atresia.** In vaginal atresia, the urogenital sinus fails to contribute the caudal portion of the vagina. The lower 20% to 40% of the vagina is replaced by 2 to 3 cm of fibrous tissue, superior to which exist a well-differentiated upper vagina, cervix, uterine corpus, and fallopian tubes. Vaginal atresia is distinct from transverse vaginal septa and müllerian aplasia and is found in only 10% to 20% of patients who present clinically with "absence of the vagina."[7,149]

Familial aggregates of vaginal atresia have not been reported. However, an autosomal recessive syndrome characterized by vaginal atresia, renal hypoplasia or agenesis, and middle ear anomalies (e.g., malformed incus, fixation of the malleus and incus) has been described in three families.[156,157] Another malformation syndrome in which vaginal atresia occurs is the Fraser syndrome, characterized by cryptophthalmus with resulting blindness.[158] Agonadia, discussed subsequently, sometimes coexists in the Fraser syndrome.[159]

Surgical correction of true vaginal agenesis is facilitated by the existence of a rudimentary vagina and requires a normal cervix, uterus, and fallopian tubes.[149] A passageway to the uterus should not be created unless the cervix is normal; otherwise, the creation of a vagina may lead to recurrent pelvic infections. Hysterectomy should be performed if the cervix is abnormal or absent.[160,161] Even though vaginal stricture is a common postoperative problem, neovaginostomy frequently is successful.[162] In 28 cases of vaginal agenesis reported between 1927 and 1983, 20 pregnancies occurred among the 21 patients undergoing neovaginostomy.[149] Neovaginostomy obviously should be delayed until the woman is about to become sexually active or at least until she is mature enough to use vaginal dila-

tors to prevent stricture. Motivated individuals may be successful in creating a functional vagina with the use of dilators alone without any surgery (e.g., the Frank method).[163]

**Müllerian Agenesis or Hypoplasia.** Aplasia of the müllerian ducts leads to absence of the uterine corpus, uterine cervix, and upper portion of the vagina. A vagina only 1 to 2 cm in depth probably is derived exclusively from invagination of the urogenital sinus. Instances of cervical, uterine, and tubal agenesis are extremely rare in the absence of coexisting vaginal atresia.[149] Despite primary amenorrhea, secondary sexual development is normal. The differential diagnosis includes imperforate hymen, transverse vaginal septum, vaginal atresia, and the syndromes of androgen insensitivity.

Complete androgen insensitivity, also known as complete testicular feminization, is recognized easily because of the incomplete development of secondary sex characteristics, with the breasts developing to Tanner stage 3 and little or no pubic hair present. Affected individuals have a male (46,XY) chromosomal complement.

Renal anomalies are associated with müllerian aplasia more frequently than expected by chance. The most frequent of these anomalies are pelvic kidney, renal ectopia, and unilateral renal aplasia. Vertebral anomalies also are relatively common. Excretory urography and vertebral radiography are obligatory in the evaluation of patients with müllerian aplasia. Alternatively, ultrasonographic studies can be performed.

Genetic observations are most consistent with polygenic or multifactorial inheritance, although some controversy exists.[164–166]

**Incomplete Müllerian Fusion.** The müllerian ducts are paired structures early in embryogenesis. Subsequently, fusion and canalization produce the upper vagina, uterus, and fallopian tubes. Congenital uterine anomalies result from arrest or perturbation of the sequence of events that normally converts the bilateral müllerian ductal system into a single female reproductive tract. Possible anomalies include unicornuate, bicornuate, didelphic, and septate uteri (Fig. 90-19).

In unicornuate uteri, only a single normally differentiated müllerian horn exists, alone or together with a partially developed horn that in itself may or may not communicate externally. Ninety percent of rudimentary uterine horns are noncommunicating.[167] Women with a unicornuate uterus typically do not have problems with conception itself, but some have suggested that they have an incidence of first- and second-trimester abortions approaching 50%.[149] Because abortion rates in women referred for anomalies were 20% to 30% in one survey, this figure of 50% must be a maximum and reflects ascertainment bias.[168] If a pregnancy occurs in a rudimentary horn, the chances of a live-born infant are only ~1%.[167]

Surgical removal of a noncommunicating but functional uterine horn is indicated, because the associated hematometra and hematosalpinx may result in cyclic pelvic pain, secondary reflux endometriosis, and consequent irreversible infertility. The excision of a noncommunicating nonfunctional or a communicating horn does not appear indicated to improve fertility.

If the two müllerian ducts fuse incompletely, a bicornuate uterus may result. Hysterosalpingography, laparoscopy, and hysteroscopy have been used historically to differentiate a bicornuate from a septate uterus. Magnetic resonance imaging and endovaginal sonography (sometimes with sonohysterography) are as accurate as these invasive techniques in identifying the anomaly.[169] The prevalence of infertility in women with a bicornuate uterus is believed to be no greater than that in the general population. However, although the true incidence of spontaneous abortion in such individuals is unknown, the rate of abortion appears to be greater than in normal women.[149] As in women with a unicornuate uterus, those with a bicornuate uterus have an increased likelihood of premature labor and abnormal lies, with these problems occurring in ~25% of pregnancies. Estimates are that <60% of pregnancies of such women result in live births.[143,149] Various operative unification proce-

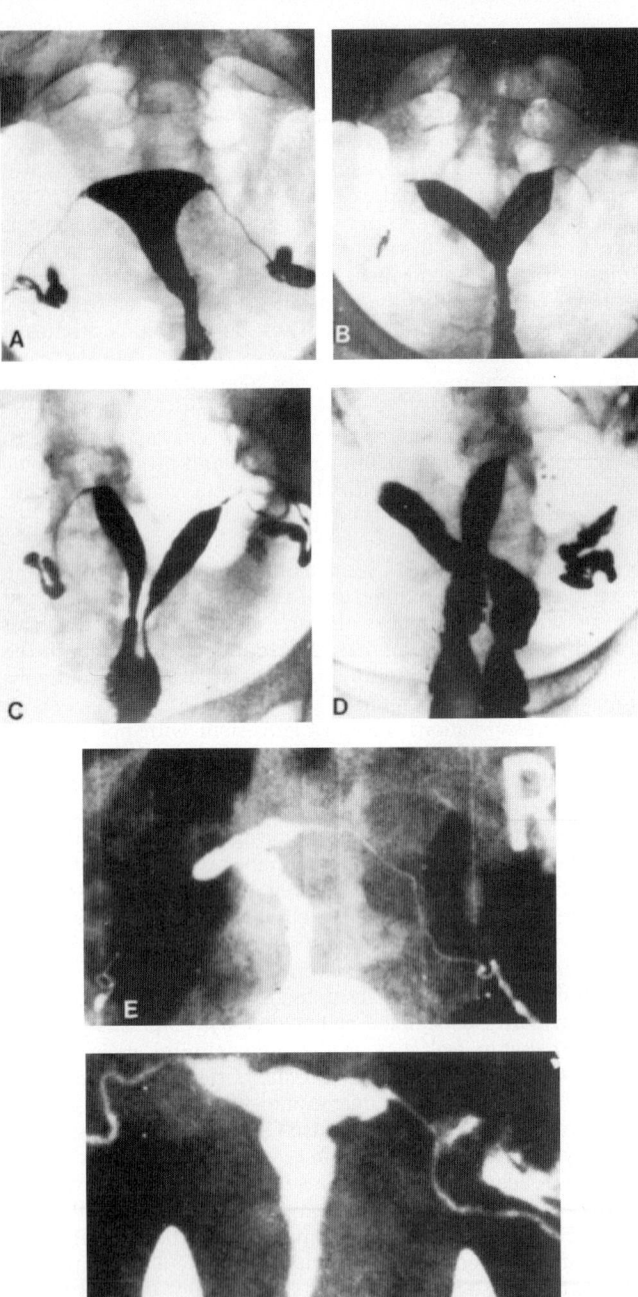

**FIGURE 90-19.** Hysterosalpingograms of normal and abnormal female genital tracts. **A,** Normal study with bilateral spill. **B,** Bicornuate uterus. **C,** Uterus didelphys. **D,** Uterus didelphys with double vagina. **E** and **F,** Typical appearance in women with in utero exposure to diethylstilbestrol; notice the T-shaped endometrial cavities, uterine constrictions, and bulbous dilatations. (Courtesy of Dr. A. Gerbie; reproduced with permission from Spitzer IB, Rebar RW. Counseling for women with medical problems: ovary and reproductive organs. In: Hollingsworth D, Resnik R, eds. Medical counseling before pregnancy. New York: Churchill Livingstone, 1988:213.)

dures can be performed in women with a bicornuate uterus and repeated pregnancy wastage[170,171] (Fig. 90-20). Women with a recognized bicornuate uterus may be permitted to conceive without surgery because many term pregnancies do result; however, such women should be counseled regarding the risk of pregnancy loss and the availability of surgical correction.

Complete lack of fusion of the müllerian ducts results in uterus didelphys. In the 75% of cases in which separate uteri and two cervical ostia are present, a longitudinal vaginal sep-

tum is also found (Fig. 90-21). By some estimates, almost 50% of the pregnancies in these women end in spontaneous abortion, and premature labor and abnormal lies also are markedly increased.[149] Surgical repair of uterine didelphys has been disappointing and now is rarely attempted. Although supporting data are lacking, many physicians perform cervical cerclage on these women during their pregnancies.

In cases of septate uterus, the uterine cavity is divided partially or completely by a longitudinal septum. Fetal wastage is high in this disorder, even though fertility is not affected.[149] Women with a septate uterus also manifest an increased frequency of postpartum hemorrhage and intrauterine adhesion formation, perhaps because the placenta attaches to a relatively avascular septum, leading to placenta accreta.[172] The excision of uterine septa is indicated in women with histories of repeated pregnancy loss. Surgery is accomplished most easily by hysteroscopy, after which the live birth rate is >90%.[173–175] Both the low recurrence risk of incomplete müllerian fusion observed in female siblings (3%) and the occasional reports of familial aggregates are consistent with polygenic or multifactorial inheritance.[176]

Incomplete müllerian fusion also may be one component of genetically determined malformation syndromes. One especially interesting syndrome is the hand-foot-uterus syndrome, an autosomal dominant disorder in which affected females have a bicornuate uterus and characteristic malformations of the hands and feet.[177] The frequency of this disorder, in which orthopedic management is needed, probably is underestimated.[178] A mutation in *HOXA13* was detected in a member of the originally described family.[179–181] In other families with this disorder, a *HOXA13* nonsense mutant has been detected.[180,182]

**Diethylstilbestrol-Associated Anomalies.** The teratogenic effects of DES are exerted only during the first 18 weeks of pregnancy.[147,183] Most anomalies are benign, with squamous metaplasia and vaginal adenosis occurring most commonly. Clear cell adenocarcinoma of the vagina and cervix in DES-exposed offspring is rare, estimated at 0.14 to 1.4 per 1000 of those exposed.[147] Strong evidence supports a müllerian origin for these tumors.

The reproductive consequences of DES exposure still are debated. The effect of DES-associated müllerian anomalies on fertility is not clear, but more agreement is found regarding the effect on obstetric outcomes. The frequencies of spontaneous abortion, premature labor, and even ectopic pregnancies are increased in affected women, but 70% to 80% of pregnancies end in live births.[184] DES exposure apparently has deleterious effects on uterine muscle development, resulting in a T-shaped endometrial cavity, an abnormally small uterine cavity, uterine constrictions, and bulbous dilation of the lower cervical segment[185] (see Fig. 90-19). Reproductive performance in DES-exposed women probably depends on the nature and extent of the resulting anomalies. DES-exposed women contemplating pregnancy and those who are infertile should be evaluated by hysterosalpingography to determine the extent of any anomaly.

After menarche, an initial examination consisting of cytology and colposcopy is recommended for DES-exposed women. In the absence of suspected malignancy or significant symptoms, routine examination every 6 to 12 months should suffice. No evidence exists that the use of oral contraceptives is contraindicated. Biopsy of any suspicious lesion is indicated, with appropriate staging and management of any adenocarcinoma by an oncologist.

## ANOMALIES OF THE MALE REPRODUCTIVE TRACT

**Wolffian Aplasia and Congenital Absence of the Vasa Deferentia.** Wolffian ducts differentiate into the *vasa deferentia*, *epididymides*, and *seminal vesicles*. Absence of wolffian derivatives (*wolffian aplasia*) may be an isolated defect, or it may be associated with absence of the upper urinary tract. Absence of

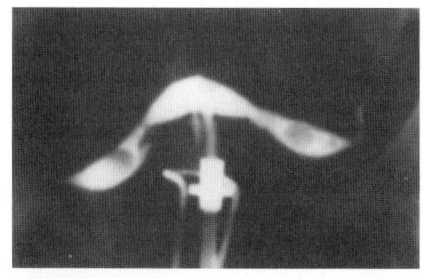
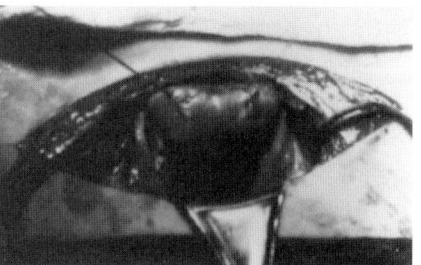

**A,B**

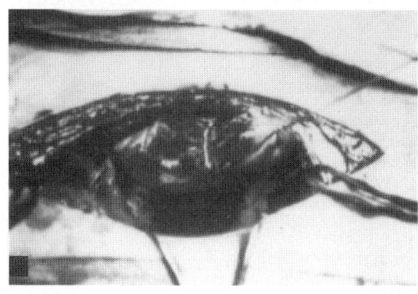
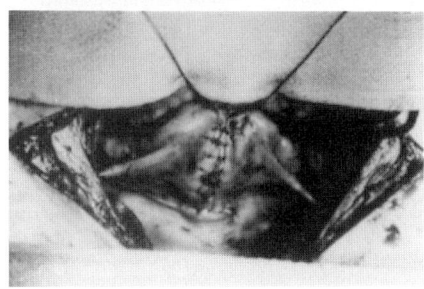

**C,D**

**FIGURE 90-20.** Surgical repair using Strassman procedure in 22-year-old woman with repeated pregnancy wastage. **A,** Hysterosalpingogram showing bicornuate uterus. **B,** Appearance of uterus at surgery. **C,** Incision into uterus. **D,** Appearance after repair. (From Spitzer IB, Rebar RW. Counseling for women with medical problems: ovary and reproductive organs. In: Hollingsworth D, Resnik R, eds. Medical counseling before pregnancy. New York: Churchill Livingstone, 1988:213.)

the upper urinary tract, as well, implies total failure of mesonephric development. By contrast, absence of wolffian derivatives without upper urinary tract anomalies implies resorption of wolffian elements after the wolffian duct reaches the cloaca. Irrespective of whether absence of wolffian derivatives is or is not accompanied by abnormalities of the upper urinary tract, the gonads are only rarely involved. More frequently, the upper urinary tract is normal in individuals who lack an epididymis, vas deferens, or seminal vesicle. If wolffian aplasia is bilateral, affected individuals are, of course, infertile due to azoospermia. If the defect is unilateral, patients are usually asymptomatic.

Cystic fibrosis is the result of a mutation in the cystic fibrosis transmembrane regulation (CFTR) gene on chromosome 7 that functions as a chloride channel. It has long been known that almost all cystic fibrosis homozygotes are infertile, usually because of *congenital absence of the vasa deferentia* (CAVD). More recently, a relationship has been shown to exist between cystic

fibrosis and absence of the vasa deferentia. Up to 70% of males with CAVD have cystic fibrosis,[186,187] usually in the form of compound heterozygosity. Thus, two mutant CFTR alleles should be assumed to be present, even if only one can be detected molecularly. The most common mutations are ΔF508 and R117H.

Several older reports have described affected sibs with congenital absence of the vas deferens.[188–190] These familial aggregates could reflect polygenic/multifactorial etiology, but, more likely, mutations in the CFTR locus explain familial aggregates of CAVD. If upper tract anomalies coexist, this explanation would not apply.

**Failure of Fusion of Epididymis and Testis.** Another relatively common urologic defect is failure of the testicular rete cords of the testis to fuse with the mesonephric tubules destined to form the ductule efferentia.[7] As a result, spermatozoa cannot exit the testes. If the defect is bilateral, infertility results. One or both testes may also fail to descend.

Fusion defects of this type occur in ~1% of cryptorchid and ~1% of azoospermic men. Familial aggregates have not been reported. Fertility is now achievable by aspirating sperm from the testes or epididymis and using assisted reproductive technologies such as *intracytoplasmic sperm injection* (ICSI).

**Persistence of Müllerian Derivatives in Otherwise Normal Males (Hernia Uteri Inguinale).** Occasionally, the uterus and fallopian tubes, which are müllerian derivatives, persist in ostensibly normal males. The external genitalia, wolffian (mesonephric) derivatives, and testes develop as expected; virilization occurs at puberty. However, the frequency of associated infertility is quite high, and ~5% of reported individuals have had a seminoma or other germ-cell tumor. The disorder is sometimes discovered because the uterus and fallopian tubes are found in inguinal hernias, hence the appellation *hernia uteri inguinale*. Failure of müllerian duct regression theoretically could result from end-organ (e.g., uterus) insensitivity to AMH (due to an abnormality in the AMH-receptor gene) or from failure of fetal Sertoli cells to synthesize or secrete AMH (due to a mutation of the gene transcribing AMH).

The AMH gene is located on chromosome arm 19p, is 2800 base pairs long, and consists of five exons.[191] Although AMH can be measured by enzyme-linked immunosorbent assay, AMH production is suppressed to undetectable levels after sexual maturation. In the absence of measurable AMH in boys with persistent müllerian derivatives (AMH-negative disorders), mutations in the structural gene often can be demonstrated.[191–193] The first three exons are most consistently involved.[192]

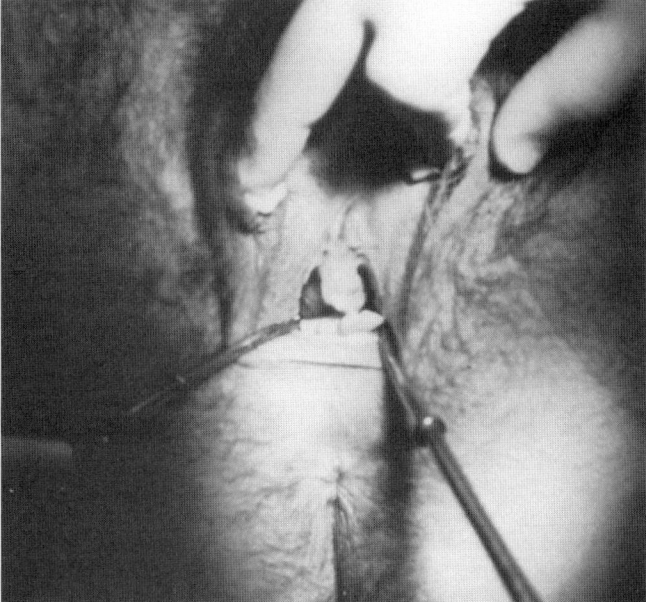

**FIGURE 90-21.** Introitus of teenaged girl with complete duplication of vagina, cervix, and uterus. (From Spitzer IB, Rebar RW. Counseling for women with medical problems: ovary and reproductive organs. In: Hollingsworth D, Resnik R, eds. Medical counseling before pregnancy. New York: Churchill Livingstone, 1988:213.)

**TABLE 90-5.**
**Types of Female Pseudohermaphroditism**

**GENETIC**
    Syndromes of congenital adrenal hyperplasia
        21-hydroxylase deficiency
        11β-hydroxylase deficiency
        3β-hydroxysteroid dehydrogenase deficiency
    Nonadrenal genetic forms associated with somatic anomalies
**TERATOGENIC**
    Maternal ingestion of substances with androgenic activity
    Androgen-producing neoplasia
**IDIOPATHIC**

---

**TABLE 90-6.**
**Female Pseudohermaphroditism: Androgens and Progestogens Potentially Capable of Virilizing Human Female Fetuses**

| Proven Virilization* | Not Associated with Virilization | Insufficient Data |
|---|---|---|
| Testosterone enanthate | Progesterone | Ethynodiol diacetate |
| Testosterone propionate | 17α-hydroxyprogester-one | Dimethisterone |
| Methylandrostenediol | Medroxyprogesterone | Norgestrel |
| 6α-methyltestosterone | Norethynodrel | |
| Ethisterone | | |
| Norethindrone | | |
| Danazol | | |

*Those that are considered proven to cause virilization do so only when administered in relatively high doses. Of those compounds for which insufficient data exist, norgestrel and dimethisterone are most worrisome. In low doses (e.g., in oral contraceptives), progestins, even including norethindrone, seem unlikely to virilize a female fetus.

The AMH-receptor gene is located on chromosome band 12q13 and consists of 11 exons. Mutations in the receptor have been found in some individuals with AMH-positive persistence of müllerian derivatives.[194] An informative animal model exists for AMH-receptor mutation in miniature Schnauzer dogs.[195]

## ERRORS IN GENITAL DIFFERENTIATION

In *pseudohermaphroditism*, the individual has sex chromosomes and gonads characteristic of one sex but some phenotypic features characteristic of each sex. In *female pseudohermaphroditism*, the individual's karyotype is typically 46,XX; in *male pseudohermaphroditism*, it is 46,XY or contains a 46,XY line.

Differentiation of the external genitalia begins ~7 weeks after the mother's last menstrual period, when the genital tubercle first becomes evident. The process is completed by 14 weeks in the female and by 16 weeks in the male. Pseudohermaphroditism indicates some abnormality in genital differentiation during this interval. In females, clitoral hypertrophy, labioscrotal fusion, and posterior displacement of the urethral orifice to create a urogenital sinus can occur. Clitoral hypertrophy is the only genital abnormality that can develop after 14 weeks of gestation. In males, hypospadias and undescended testicles occur, with nondescent the only abnormality that can develop after 16 weeks of gestation. Undescended testes are normal in infants born prematurely, with descent occurring in the first several weeks after birth.

The discussions of female and male pseudohermaphroditism that follow are limited to individuals with karyotypes and gonads characteristic of one sex but with incompletely developed external genitalia. However, the tables delineating the disorders have been expanded to include disorders of the external genitalia accompanied by abnormalities of the gonads or ducts or both. Such classification leads to some overlap of several entities already considered but allows comparison with schemata suggested by other researchers.

### FEMALE PSEUDOHERMAPHRODITISM

In female pseudohermaphroditism, genital differentiation is not that expected for 46,XX individuals; however, ovaries are present. Individuals generally present with genital ambiguity at birth, but sometimes the disorder is not detected for several years. A variety of distinct forms have been identified (Table 90-5).

**Genetic Forms of Adrenal Hyperplasia.**    The various syndromes of adrenal hyperplasia are the most frequent causes of female pseudohermaphroditism and are discussed in detail in Chapter 77. Nonclassic forms of adrenal hyperplasia are also discussed briefly in Chapters 96 and 101. Three adrenal enzyme defects—21-hydroxylase deficiency, 11β-hydroxylase deficiency, and 3β-hydroxysteroid dehydrogenase deficiency—result in increased androgen production in utero and consequent virilization of the external genitalia. These enzyme defects decrease cortisol secretion, causing increased pituitary adrenocorticotropic hormone (ACTH) secretion and consequent overproduction of adrenal androgens.

**Aromatase Mutations (*CYP19*).**    Conversion of androgens ($\Delta^4$-androstenedione) to estrogens (estrone) requires cytochrome P450 aromatase, an enzyme that is the gene product of a single 40-kilobase (kb) gene located on chromosome band 15q21.[196] The gene consists of 10 exons. A mutation in this *CYP19* (P450 arom) gene has been identified in an 18-year-old 46,XX woman with primary amenorrhea and cystic ovaries.[197] The patient was a compound heterozygote for two different point mutations in exon 10. The mutant protein had no activity.

**Teratogenic Forms.**    Rarely, ambiguous genitalia result from the maternal ingestion of various teratogens (Table 90-6). Exposure to the teratogen must occur during genital organogenesis. Moreover, not all fetuses exposed to a given teratogen manifest the same anomalies or even the presence of any anomaly; that is, fetuses demonstrate the principle of differing genetic susceptibility.

In general, synthetic steroids with androgenic properties can affect female genital differentiation. Extremely high levels of the naturally occurring androgens are required to masculinize a female fetus because of the tremendous capacity of the placenta to aromatize androgens to estrogens, but most synthetic androgens cannot be aromatized. Norethisterone in doses of 10 to 20 mg daily can cause virilization.[198,199] The same is true of danazol in doses of 800 mg daily.[200,201]

Most progestins are also weakly androgenic. Among the synthetic acetoxyprogesterones, medroxyprogesterone (6α-methyl-17-hydroxyprogesterone) has been reported to produce virilization in rats, albeit not consistently, but not in mice.[202,203] Medroxyprogesterone often has been administered to pregnant women in high doses in the hope of maintaining pregnancies and in lower doses for pregnancy diagnosis. Fortunately, virtually no evidence is found that medroxyprogesterone produces female virilization or even clitoral hypertrophy in humans. Only 1 of 82 female offspring of mothers who received 5 to 50 mg of medroxyprogesterone daily before the 12th week of pregnancy for a total dose of 50 to 7000 mg per patient had clitoral hypertrophy, and none was extensively virilized.[204] In another study, virilization was not observed among 72 female offspring, nor were deleterious effects observed in a report of empirically treated pregnancies.[205,206]

The naturally occurring progestins progesterone and 17α-hydroxyprogesterone exert weak androgenic effects and can be converted peripherally to androgens. The possibility of virilization exists if these progestogens are administered in very high doses during the critical stage of gestation. However, only a few cases have been reported in which female fetuses were masculinized after maternal progesterone or 17α-hydroxyprogesterone administration. In these cases, the hormones usually had been administered for a long interval in the hope of preventing abortion.

**TABLE 90-7.**
**Causes of Male Pseudohermaphroditism***

**DEFECTS IN TESTICULAR ACTIVITY**

Agonadia (testicular regression syndrome)

Leydig cell agenesis or hypoplasia

Defects in androgen synthesis

Deficiency before synthesis of pregnenolone (i.e., 20,22-desmolase deficiency)

3β-hydroxysteroid dehydrogenase deficiency

17α-hydroxylase deficiency

17,20-desmolase deficiency

17-ketosteroid reductase deficiency

Multiple enzyme defects

Defective antimüllerian hormone activity or receptors (i.e., hernia uteri inguinale)

**DEFECTS IN ANDROGEN ACTION**

Complete androgen insensitivity (i.e., testicular feminization)

Incomplete androgen insensitivity and the Reifenstein syndrome

5α-reductase deficiency (pseudovaginal perineoscrotal hypospadias)

Infertile males with androgen resistance

**UNCLASSIFIED DISORDERS**

Hypospadias without other defects

Genital ambiguity with multiple malformation patterns

Microphallus

**CYTOGENETIC ABNORMALITIES (e.g., 45,X/46,XY; MIXED GONADAL DYSGENESIS)**

**TERATOGENIC CAUSES (e.g., ESTROGENS, ANTIANDROGENS)**

*Based on an expanded definition of pseudohermaphroditism; see Chap. 115.

---

These cases may or may not indicate that progesterone and 17α-hydroxyprogesterone cause female virilization, especially because the hormones have been administered to so many pregnant women that the anomalies could have been coincidental. Several large studies have detected no increase in fetal anomalies. In one retrospective study, the rate of anomalies was no higher among infants of 837 pregnant women given 17α-hydroxyprogesterone caproate (250 to 500 mg by injection one to five times) than among infants of 110 controls.[207] Infants of women treated daily with 50-mg progesterone vaginal suppositories also do not have an increased incidence of anomalies.[208] Other investigators who routinely use large doses of these progestins have also observed no such deleterious effects.[209,210] These progestogens are unlikely to be teratogenic to the genital system.

The inadvertent ingestion of oral contraceptives, which contain relatively low doses of mestranol or ethinyl estradiol and a 19-norsteroid, rarely if ever results in virilization.[199]

## MALE PSEUDOHERMAPHRODITISM

In male pseudohermaphroditism, genital differentiation is not that expected for normal males, even though the chromosomal complement is 46,XY and testes are present. A variety of separate forms are distinguishable, but no unanimity exists regarding the classification of several of these disorders (Table 90-7).

**Defects in Testicular Activity.** The normal synthesis and secretion of testosterone by fetal Leydig cells are essential for male differentiation of the wolffian ducts and the external genitalia.

AGONADIA.    In agonadia (i.e., *testicular regression syndrome*), gonads are absent, the external genitalia are abnormal, and all but rudimentary müllerian or wolffian derivatives are absent. The external genitalia usually consist of a phallus about the size of a clitoris, underdeveloped labia majora, and near-complete fusion of the labioscrotal folds. Often, a persistent urogenital sinus is present. By definition, gonads cannot be detected. Neither normal müllerian derivatives nor normal wolffian derivatives are present, although rudimentary structures may be found along the lateral pelvic wall. Somatic anomalies are common, including craniofacial, vertebral, and dermatoglyphic anomalies, and, possibly, mental retardation.[211]

Any pathogenic explanation for agonadia must take into account the absence of gonads and the abnormal external genitalia and the lack of normal internal ducts. At least two explanations seem reasonable. The first postulates that the fetal testes functioned long enough to inhibit müllerian development but not long enough to complete male differentiation (i.e., testicular regression syndrome). The second theory posits that the entire gonadal, ductal, and genital systems developed abnormally as a result of defective anlage, defective connective tissue, or action of a teratogen. The frequent coexistence of somatic anomalies favors the existence of a teratogen or of defective connective tissue. In several kindreds, multiple affected sibs have been reported, and genetic factors should be considered.[212] The coexistence of anorchia and agonadia in a single sibship also has been observed.[213] In agonadia, the H-Y antigen is present, suggesting that pathogenesis need not involve an abnormality of this system.[214]

Although agonadia most often occurs in 46,XY individuals, 46,XX individuals may also show the phenotype.[215]

LEYDIG CELL AGENESIS.    Several individuals with 46,XY karyotypes presenting with male pseudohermaphroditism associated with Leydig cell unresponsiveness to human chorionic gonadotropin (hCG) or LH have been reported.[216–221] The presence of parental consanguinity in some families suggests autosomal recessive inheritance.

The external genitalia in reported cases have ranged from minimally masculinized genitalia with posterior labial fusion and a shortened vagina to hypoplastic male genitalia in individuals raised as males. The testes are typically small and undescended with an absent or decreased number of Leydig cells, normal Sertoli cells, and seminiferous tubules showing arrest of spermatogenesis. Müllerian duct regression is complete, presumably because the secretion of AMH (by Sertoli cells) is not impaired. Wolffian derivatives, including epididymides and vasa deferentia, invariably are present.

Virilization does not occur at puberty. After puberty, basal gonadotropin levels and responses to exogenous gonadotropin-releasing hormone (GnRH) are increased. Circulating levels of 17α-hydroxyprogesterone, androstenedione, and testosterone are very low, and no increase in testosterone levels can be elicited by hCG or LH. This decreased responsiveness of the Leydig cells to hCG and LH has been attributed to absent or abnormal gonadotropin receptors. Variations in the severity of the abnormality and in the quantity of testosterone produced apparently account for the variability in the clinical presentation.

Gonadotropin deficiency in utero, as may be observed in Kallmann syndrome, hypopituitarism, and anencephaly, is not associated with male pseudohermaphroditism, even though undescended testes and microphallus are common (see Chap. 115). Such observations implicate placental hCG as the important gonadotropin stimulating testosterone secretion by the fetal testis during the early critical period for differentiation of the external genitalia. Fetal pituitary LH and FSH are not necessary for differentiation of the fetal testis or the external genitalia.

Reports have suggested that the molecular basis of Leydig cell agenesis is a mutation in the luteinizing hormone (LH)–receptor gene, located on chromosome 2 near the FSHR gene. Two siblings of consanguineous parents, who were homozygous for a missense mutation (Ala$^{(593)}$→Pro), were reported.[222,223] In another case, a deletion in exon 11 was detected.[224] Leydig cells presumably fail to develop because luteinizing hormone cannot exert its effect during embryogenesis. This is reminiscent of ovarian failure due to FSH-receptor mutation.

In contrast to the Leydig cell agenesis produced by *inactivating* LHR mutations, *activating* mutations cause precocious puberty in males.[223] In the female, LHR activating–receptor mutations do not seem to exert the same effect.

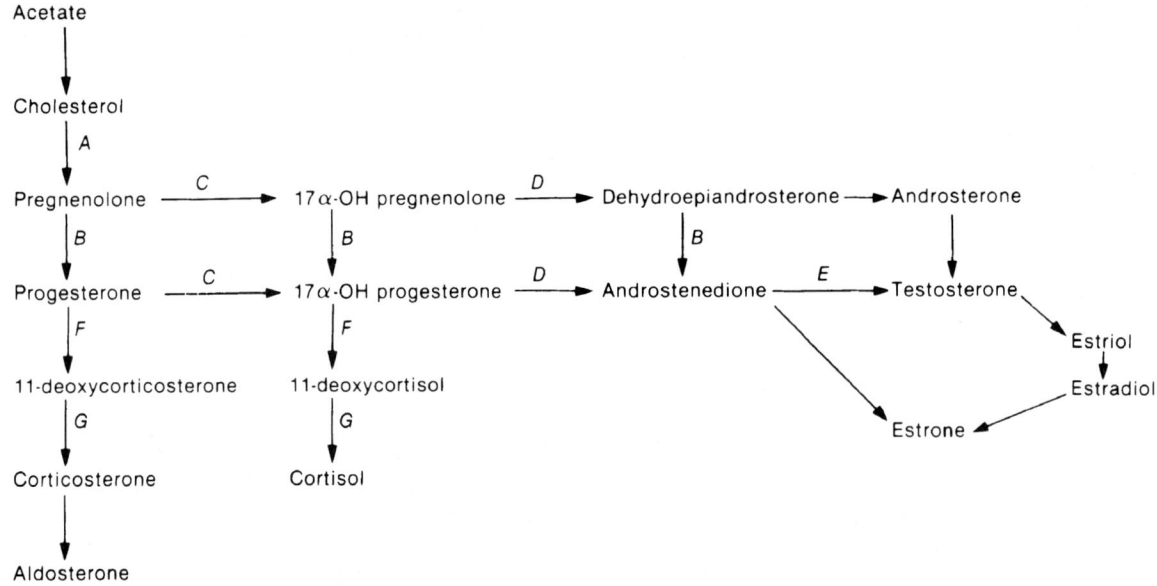

$A = 20\alpha\text{-}hydroxylase,\ 22\alpha\text{-}hydroxylase\ and\ 20,22\text{-}desmolase$
$B = 3\beta\text{-}hydroxysteroid\ dehydrogenase$
$C = 17\alpha\text{-}hydroxylase$
$D = 17,\ 20\text{-}desmolase$
$E = 17\text{-}ketosteroid\ reductase$
$F = 21\text{-}hydroxylase$
$G = 11\beta\text{-}hydroxylase$

**FIGURE 90-22.** Important adrenal and gonadal biosynthetic pathways and enzymes required for indicated conversions. (Modified from Simpson JL. Disorders of sexual differentiation etiology and clinical delineation. New York: Academic Press, 1976.)

**Defects in Androgen Synthesis.**    Five different enzyme defects in the synthesis of testosterone may result in male pseudohermaphroditism (Fig. 90-22; see Chaps. 77 and 115). Three defects (i.e., 20,22-desmolase, 3β-hydroxysteroid dehydrogenase, 17α-hydroxylase) involve enzymes required for the synthesis of cortisol and testosterone, and they are associated with compensatory increases in ACTH secretion and consequent congenital adrenal hyperplasia. The remaining two enzyme defects (i.e., 17,20-desmolase, 17-ketosteroid reductase) affect only gonadal steroidogenesis. The inheritance of 17,20-desmolase deficiency may be X-linked recessive, and only males have been found with 17-ketosteroid reductase deficiency. The other disorders are autosomal recessive.

An enzyme defect should be suspected in poorly masculinized individuals in whom the secretion of testosterone and its metabolites is diminished. Deficiencies in the 21-hydroxylase and 11β-hydroxylase enzymes, the most common causes of female pseudohermaphroditism (see Chap. 77), do not cause male pseudohermaphroditism. Males with 21-hydroxylase deficiency may lose sodium, however, and those with 11β-hydroxylase deficiency may retain sodium and develop hypervolemia and hypertension. Newborn male infants whose siblings had 21-hydroxylase or 11β-hydroxylase deficiency should be screened for electrolyte disturbances. These enzyme defects can be diagnosed by measuring 17α-hydroxyprogesterone in the serum or pregnanetriol in the urine.

CONGENITAL LIPOID ADRENAL HYPERPLASIA.    Male pseudohermaphrodites with lipoid adrenal hyperplasia have ambiguous or female-like external genitalia, abdominal or inguinal testes with wolffian differentiation, severe salt wasting, and adrenal glands characterized by foamy-appearing cells filled with cholesterol.[225] Approximately 30 cases have been reported.[226,227] Because males and females may be affected, autosomal recessive inheritance has been assumed. The gene is located on chromosome 15.[228] Most affected individuals have died during infancy in adrenal crisis.

The accumulation of cholesterol indicates that this compound cannot be converted to pregnenolone. Despite the appellation, the specific enzyme defect in this disorder is unknown, because any of the three enzymes required to convert cholesterol to pregnenolone (i.e., 20α-hydroxylase, 20,22-desmolase, 22α-hydroxylase) may be deficient (see Fig. 90-22). In any case, levels of all circulating steroids are low or immeasurable, and little if any urinary excretion of 17-ketosteroids, 17-hydroxysteroids, or aldosterone occurs.

Signs of adrenal insufficiency, with hyperkalemia and hyponatremia, generally occur within the first 2 weeks of life. In the phenotypic female infant or the infant with ambiguous genitalia and adrenal insufficiency, a 46,XY karyotype suggests the diagnosis of congenital adrenal hyperplasia. Low urinary 17-ketosteroid excretion and low circulating dehydroepiandrosterone levels differentiate this disorder from 3β-hydroxysteroid dehydrogenase deficiency. Immediate and continued glucocorticoid and mineralocorticoid replacement is required for survival. In males, sex hormone therapy must be initiated at the age of puberty and obviously should be consistent with the sex-of-rearing. In most males, the genital defects are so severe that a female sex-of-rearing is necessary.

The cytochrome P450 enzyme responsible for converting cholesterol to pregnenolone is called *P450scc* (*side chain cleavage*); the gene is *CYP11A*. P450scc converts cholesterol to pregnenolone via 20α-hydroxylase, 22α-hydroxylase, and 20,72-desmolase. *CYP11A* is a large gene, located on chromosome 15. Its length is 20 kb and it consists of 9 exons.

Surprisingly, perturbations of this gene have not been detected in congenital *adrenal lipoid hyperplasia*.[229] Rather, this disorder results from mutations of another gene, *steroidogenic acute regulatory (StAR) protein*. The StAR protein, ~30 kDa in size, delivers precursors for cholesterol side-chain cleavage and is very sensitive to trophic hormone action on the gonads and adrenals. The mutations reported in StAR result in nonfunctional protein consequent to deletions or truncated gene products.[230]

3β-HYDROXYSTEROID DEHYDROGENASE DEFICIENCY.    Complete deficiency of the 3β-hydroxysteroid dehydrogenase enzyme results in deficient cortisol, aldosterone, androgen, and estrogen secretion by the adrenal glands and gonads (see Fig. 90-22). Severely affected children present with adrenal insufficiency in infancy. Approximately 30 such cases have been reported.[231] In milder cases, sufficient cortisol and aldosterone are secreted to avert adrenal insufficiency in the newborn. Many older children with less severe defects have been identified.[232] A few mild cases have been reported that mimic the polycystic ovary syndrome (see Chap. 96). Heterogeneity is demonstrated by the existence of isoenzyme variants of this deficiency.[233] In most of those with a 46,XY karyotype, however, the genitalia are ambiguous at birth, and secondary sex characteristics fail to develop at puberty. Affected individuals with mutations in the type II 3β-hydroxysteroid dehydrogenase gene have been reported.[234,235]

The incompletely developed external genitalia of affected males are similar to the external genitalia of most other male pseudohermaphrodites: a small phallus, a urethra that opens proximally on the penis, and incomplete labioscrotal fusion. The testes and wolffian ducts differentiate normally.

The diagnosis is established by determining that plasma levels of pregnenolone, 17α-hydroxypregnenolone, and dehydroepiandrosterone are increased, and those of cortisol and aldosterone are reduced. Plasma $\Delta^4$-steroids (e.g., progesterone, 17α-hydroxyprogesterone, androstenedione, sometimes testosterone) may be normal or increased, suggesting intact hepatic and peripheral 3β-hydroxysteroid dehydrogenase:$\Delta^{4-5}$ isomerase activity. In contrast to the situation in the infant with 20,22-desmolase deficiency, urinary 17-ketosteroid excretion is normal or increased. As in 20,22-desmolase deficiency, treatment involves glucocorticoid and mineralocorticoid replacement, with sex steroids added as appropriate at puberty.

3β-Hydroxysteroid dehydrogenase is not a cytochrome P450 enzyme, but rather a microsomal enzyme. Two forms of the enzyme are found: type I is expressed in placenta, skin, and breasts, and type II, in adrenal cortex and gonads. The gene for the type II enzyme is located on chromosome band 1p 13.1. Point mutations resulting in male pseudohermaphroditism obviously involve type II 3β-hydroxysteroid dehydrogenase.[236]

17α-HYDROXYLASE/17,20-LYASE DEFICIENCY.    Males with deficiency of 17α-hydroxylase/17,20-lyase usually have ambiguous external genitalia, normal wolffian duct development, and normal testicular differentiation. Some severely affected males have entirely female external genitalia.[237] Gynecomastia can develop at puberty, with little or no virilization, making some affected males phenotypically similar to those with androgen insensitivity. Unlike females deficient in 17α-hydroxylase/17,20-lyase, males usually have normal blood pressure.

The enzyme 17α-hydroxylase/17,20-lyase is a single enzyme that converts pregnenolone and progesterone to 17α-hydroxypregnenolone and 17α-hydroxyprogesterone, respectively, and 17α-hydroxypregnenolone and 17α-hydroxyprogesterone to dehydroepiandrosterone and $\Delta^4$-androstenedione, respectively[238] (see Fig. 90-22). Because these enzyme conversions are needed to produce cortisol, corticotropin secretion is increased. As a result, secretion of the precursors pregnenolone, progesterone, deoxycorticosterone, corticosterone, and 18-hydroxycorticosterone is increased, and excretion of 17-hydroxysteroids and 17-ketosteroids is decreased. Generally, signs of glucocorticoid deficiency are not observed because of the glucocorticoid activity of corticosterone. The increased circulating deoxycorticosterone leads to increased sodium retention and increased plasma volume, hypertension, hypokalemia, and low plasma renin and aldosterone levels.

In affected adults, gonadotropin levels are elevated, and sex steroid concentrations are low. Glucocorticoid replacement therapy reverses the metabolic abnormalities and lowers the blood pressure in hypertensive individuals. Appropriate sex steroid therapy should begin at the age of puberty.

A family in which three members apparently had 17,20-desmolase deficiency was first reported in 1972.[239] This remains the only family in which multiple members have been affected. Unlike with other adrenal enzyme disorders, affected relatives were not confined to sibs. Two maternal first cousins had genital ambiguity, bilateral testes, and no müllerian derivatives; a maternal "aunt" was said to have abnormal external genitalia and bilateral testes. This disorder could be inherited in X-linked recessive fashion. Both cousins had low plasma testosterone and low dehydroepiandrosterone concentrations, but the normal urinary excretion of pregnanediol, pregnanetriol, and 17-hydroxycorticosteroids is characteristic of this disorder (see Fig. 90-22). In the initial cases, in vitro testicular tissue synthesized testosterone from androstenedione or dehydroepiandrosterone, excluding 17-ketosteroid reductase deficiency and suggesting 17,20-desmolase deficiency.[239] Testosterone secretion was not increased by the administration of corticotropin or hCG.

That a single gene/enzyme is responsible for both 17α-hydroxylase and 17,20-desmolase (or lyase) functions was a surprise, because enzyme studies had suggested two genetically distinct conditions involving two separate genes.[240] Mutations have been described in which only the 17,20-lyase function or both enzyme functions are affected, adding to the confusion.[241–243]

The single P450c17 enzyme is coded by a gene (*CYP17*) on chromosome band 10q24–25. This gene (*CYP17*) consists of 8 exons. It is structurally similar to its *CYP21* cousin, 21-hydroxylase, but no pseudogene coexists. Thus, deletions and gene conversions are uncommon; point mutations are the typical molecular perturbation.[244–247]

As with other disorders, the sex-of-rearing should be determined by the extent of ambiguity of the external genitalia. In more severe cases, patients should be raised as females, with gonadectomy performed before the age of puberty. Sex hormone therapy should begin at the age of puberty.

17-KETOSTEROID REDUCTASE DEFICIENCY.    Genetic males with 17-ketosteroid reductase deficiency generally have ambiguous external genitalia, bilateral testes, and no müllerian derivatives. Approximately 25 cases have been reported.[248] With few exceptions, the ambiguity has led to the children being raised as females. At puberty, breast development may or may not occur, apparently depending on the ratio of androgen to estrogen; however, virilization invariably occurs.[249]

The enzyme 17-ketosteroid reductase catalyzes the conversions of androstenedione to testosterone and of estrone to estradiol (see Fig. 90-22). In affected 46,XY individuals, circulating levels of androstenedione are increased, and testosterone levels are low to normal. Circulating LH levels are increased, and FSH levels are normal to increased.

Affected 46,XY children with female external genitalia should be raised as females, with gonadectomy performed during childhood to prevent pubertal virilization. Female sex hormone replacement therapy should be initiated at the age of puberty. In males with ambiguous genitalia that can be corrected surgically, male sex-of-rearing can be anticipated. Because one individual virilizing at puberty reportedly underwent a female-to-male sex role change, an attempt to make the correct diagnosis early in childhood is important.[249] Because the majority of reported cases involve 46,XY individuals, the inheritance pattern is unknown but is presumed to be autosomal recessive. Some 46,XX individuals with hirsutism, secondary amenorrhea, and polycystic ovaries have had biochemical evidence consistent with decreased 17-ketosteroid reductase[250,251] (see Chap. 115).

The 17β-hydroxysteroid dehydrogenase gene (*17HSD-3*) is located on chromosome 9 and consists of 11 exons.[252] Unlike

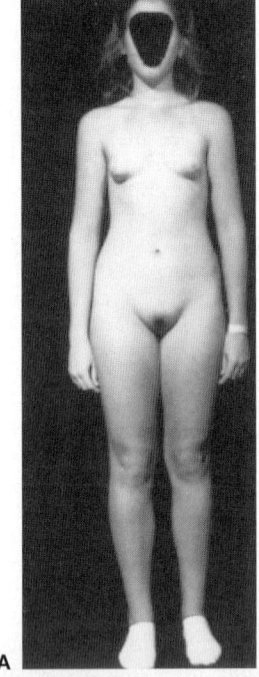

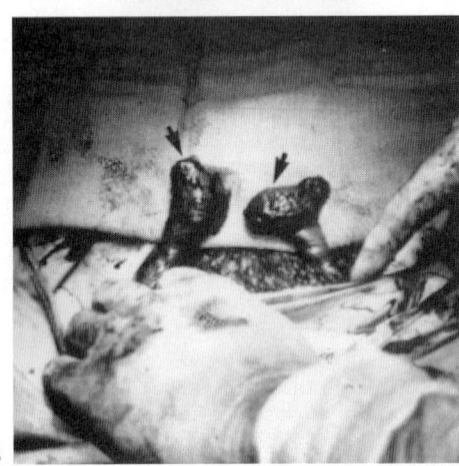

**FIGURE 90-23. A,** This 17-year-old individual had a 46,XY karyotype and complete androgen insensitivity; pubic hair was minimal and no axillary hair was present. Circulating testosterone concentrations were near upper limits of the range for normal men. **B,** Two inguinal testes (*arrows*) were found at surgery.

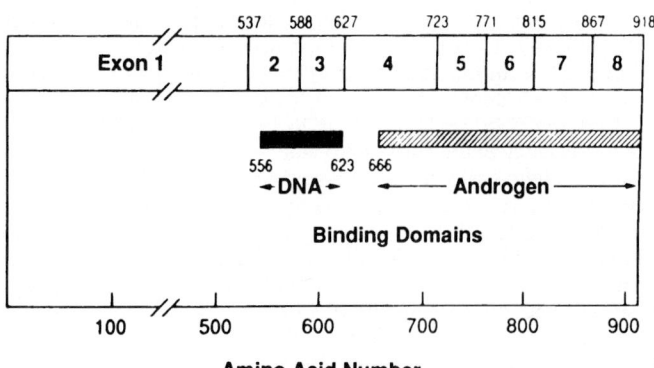

**FIGURE 90-24.** Diagram of the androgen-binding gene. Exons 2 through 4 relate to DNA binding, and exons 5 through 7 confer androgen binding. Sites of some reported mutations are noted. (Adapted from a diagram of Dr. Leonard Pinsky, Montreal, Quebec, Canada. From Simpson JL. Disorders of abnormal sexual differentiation. In: Sanfilippo JS, Muram D, Lee PA, Dewhurst J, eds. Pediatric and adolescent gynecology. Philadelphia: WB Saunders, 1994:77.)

many other steroid biosynthetic genes, this gene, just as 3β-hydroxysteroid dehydrogenase, is microsomal, reflecting action in the gonads rather than in the adrenals. Molecular perturbations typically involve single-amino-acid substitutions, but disruption of the splice junction involving intron 3 is not uncommon. Mutations may also occur in exons 2, 8, 9, 10, and 11. Missense mutations may result in secretion of negligible levels of testosterone due to complete impairment of the enzyme. No single predominant mutation is evident.

MULTIPLE ENZYME DEFECTS. A 46,XY infant with a female phenotype and ambiguous genitalia has been described who seemed to have defects differing from those previously associated with male pseudohermaphroditism.[253] The principal findings included high basal plasma levels of progesterone, pregnenolone, 17α-hydroxyprogesterone, 21-deoxycortisol, deoxycorticosterone, corticosterone, and 18-hydroxycorticosterone, and increased urinary levels of pregnanediol, pregnenediol, pregnanetriol, 17α-hydroxypregnanolone, pregnanetriolone, and the tetrahydro metabolites of corticosterone. These findings are compatible with

partial deficiencies of the microsomal mixed-function oxidases: 21-hydroxylase, 17α-hydroxylase, and 17,20-desmolase activities (see Fig. 90-22). Translocation of P450 into the endoplasmic reticulum of the adrenocortical microsomes may represent a single defect affecting the activities of all three oxidases.

A similar hormone profile has been found in two slightly virilized 46,XX teenage girls with ovaries and only mildly ambiguous external genitalia.[254] These findings are not in conflict, because in females with the combined disorder, despite reduced 17,20-desmolase activity, sufficient androgen may be produced from adrenal $C_{21}$ steroid precursors to permit mild masculinization.

### Defects in Androgen Action

COMPLETE ANDROGEN INSENSITIVITY. In androgen insensitivity (i.e., testicular feminization), 46,XY individuals have bilateral testes, female external genitalia, a blindly ending vagina, and no müllerian derivatives[255] (Fig. 90-23). Affected individuals undergo breast development and pubertal feminization. Some individuals with androgen insensitivity develop clitoral enlargement and labioscrotal fusion at puberty; to these cases, the term *incomplete androgen insensitivity* (i.e., incomplete testicular feminization) has been applied.

Complete and incomplete androgen insensitivity are inherited in X-linked recessive fashion.[256] The two disorders are genetically distinct, however, and heterogeneity exists in each. The androgen-receptor gene is localized to the Xq11-Xq12 region of the long arm of the X chromosome[257,258] (Fig. 90-24). This gene consists of eight exons. Exons 2 and 3 are the DNA-binding domains, whereas exons 4 through 8 are androgen-binding domains. No specific mutation has proved paramount. Deletions and insertions are rare; point mutations are more common. Usually these take the form of deletion of three nucleotides with preservation of an open-reading frame; single-nucleotide changes resulting in either substitution of an unscheduled amino acid or generation of a stop codon that would result in premature message termination; and production of a nonfunctional protein. Mutations are found throughout the gene, but particularly in exons 4–8 (androgen-binding domain). Mutations in exon 1 usually cause complete androgen insensitivity, but mutations in exons 2 and 3 produce either complete or partial androgen insensitivity, apparently randomly. In exons 5–8, the preponderance of mutations are missense.

Genetic heterogeneity with regard to the androgen receptor clearly exists among individuals with complete androgen insensitivity.[258a] In 60% to 70% of cases, androgen receptors are not present (i.e., the patient is receptor negative). In 30% to 40%, receptors are present (i.e., receptor positive), and in these, mutations in the DNA-binding domain have been documented or a defect at a more distal step in androgen action (i.e., postreceptor defect) must be postulated.[259–263] Receptor-positive and receptor-negative individuals are indistinguishable clinically.

The clinical features of individuals with complete androgen insensitivity are well known. These phenotypic females may be quite attractive and have advanced breast development, but most affected patients are similar in appearance to unaffected females. Breasts contain normal ductal and glandular tissue, but often the areolae are pale and poorly developed (Tanner stage 3). Statural growth and body proportions usually are normal, although occasionally the arms and legs are disproportionately long and the hands and feet disproportionately large. Pubic and axillary hair is sparse, but scalp hair is normal. The vagina terminates blindly and is shorter than usual, presumably because the müllerian ducts fail to contribute to the formation of the vagina. Occasionally, the vagina is only 1 to 2 cm long or represented merely by a dimple. Usually, neither a uterus nor fallopian tubes are present, although fibromuscular remnants or rudimentary fallopian tubes of presumptive müllerian origin sometimes can be detected.[264]

The absence of müllerian derivatives is not unexpected because the AMH secreted by the Sertoli cells of the fetal testes is not an androgen; therefore, müllerian regression occurs as in normal males. The testes usually are normal in size and may be located in the abdomen, inguinal canal, or labia—anywhere along the path of embryonic testicular descent. Testes in the inguinal canal may produce inguinal hernias, and one-half of all individuals with testicular feminization develop inguinal hernias. Determining the cytogenetic status of prepubertal girls with inguinal hernias is therefore desirable, although most are 46,XX.

The frequency of gonadal neoplasia is increased, but the precise extent is uncertain. In one frequently cited publication, 22% of reported patients had neoplasia.[265] Because of various biases, however, the actual risk probably is no greater than 5%.[55] Most investigators agree that the risk of neoplasia is low before the age of 25 to 30 years. The preferable course is to leave the testes in situ until after pubertal feminization, thereafter performing orchiectomy, because the risk of neoplasia increases with age. In postpubertal patients, benign tubular adenomas (i.e., Pick adenomas) are especially common, probably as a result of increased secretion of LH.

The diagnosis is suggested by the finding that normal male levels (or even somewhat elevated levels) of circulating testosterone are present in phenotypic females with blindly ending vaginas and little pubic and axillary hair. Levels of LH tend to be increased, but FSH levels tend to be normal because of inappropriate steroid feedback, as in the polycystic ovary syndrome. The finding of a 46,XY karyotype confirms the diagnosis.

Informing these phenotypic females with female gender of their karyotype may be inadvisable, because the psychological implications may be devastating. Family members should be informed that müllerian aplasia occurred and that the risk of neoplasia necessitates gonadectomy after puberty. Families also should undergo appropriate genetic counseling and screening because of the possibility that other family members are affected. Steroid replacement with estrogen is required after orchiectomy.

INCOMPLETE ANDROGEN INSENSITIVITY AND THE REIFENSTEIN SYNDROME.  At puberty, certain individuals feminize (e.g., show breast development) because of androgen insensitivity, but their external genitalia undergo phallic enlargement and partial labioscrotal fusion. Such individuals are said to have incomplete androgen insensitivity (i.e., incomplete testicular feminization). These individuals are otherwise identical to those with complete androgen insensitivity, and little or no other virilization occurs at puberty. An epididymis and one or both vasa deferentia usually are present.

The pathogenesis of incomplete androgen insensitivity appears to involve decreased numbers or qualitative defects of androgen receptors.[260,266–269] Molecular analysis has revealed several different mutations in the androgen-binding domains (exons, 5, 6, and 7) and in the DNA-binding domains (see Fig. 90-24). A poor correlation is found between receptor levels (and androgen-binding affinity) and the degree of masculinization. No simple correlation exists between the exon containing the mutation and the phenotype, whether complete or incomplete androgen insensitivity is present.

Incomplete (partial) androgen insensitivity appears to be an X-linked recessive condition encompassing several entities historically considered separate (i.e., *Lubs syndrome, Gilbert-Dreyfus syndrome, Reifenstein syndrome*). In 1974, Wilson and colleagues reported that individuals with the Reifenstein phenotype and the incomplete androgen insensitivity phenotype as traditionally defined were present in a single kindred.[270] In 1984, the same group confirmed partial androgen-receptor deficiency in two individuals with the Lubs syndrome phenotype.[271] These three disorders appear merely to represent *different manifestations of a single X-linked recessive disorder*, here called incomplete (partial) androgen insensitivity. Individuals characterized by female genitalia and failure of posterior labioscrotal fusion also may fit into this spectrum, although some disagree. Genetic heterogeneity may still exist, but its basis should not be considered to consist merely of differences in clinical appearance. (Also see ref. 271a.)

Traditionally, the appellation of Reifenstein syndrome was applied when a male had phallic development more nearly normal than in incomplete androgen insensitivity, no vagina-like perineal orifice, and lack of pubertal virilization.[272] Typically, the testes are small and undescended, and gynecomastia may occur at puberty. Logically, the decreased virilization in the Reifenstein syndrome would appear to result not from androgen insensitivity but from inadequate testosterone secretion; however, partial androgen insensitivity has been demonstrated.[273]

The clinical significance of the incomplete androgen insensitivity states is that they must be excluded before a male sex-of-rearing is assigned. The presence of androgen receptors and the demonstration of a response to exogenous androgen (regardless of receptor status) excludes these disorders. Individuals with moderate to severe defects in the external genitalia should be raised as females. If possible, orchiectomy should be performed before puberty to prevent virilization. Estrogen therapy should be initiated at the age of puberty. Individuals with mild hypospadias probably can be raised as males, but they will require surgery for repair of the hypospadias and for reduction of gynecomastia.

**Estrogen-Receptor Defects.**   The estrogen-receptor gene, consisting of eight exons, is coded on chromosome 6q24→27. As with the much better studied androgen-receptor gene (see earlier), DNA-binding (exons 2 and 3) and estrogen-binding domains (exons 4–8) are found.

Although it is not technically male pseudohermaphroditism, a mutation in the estrogen receptor has been reported in a 28-year-old genetic male with normal male sexual development.[274,275] Incomplete epiphyseal closure led to tall stature. Endogenous serum gonadotropin and estrogen levels were elevated, and neither decreased after exogenous estrogen administration. The molecular basis proved to be a homozygous transition in exon 2 that resulted in a premature stop codon.[274,275]

5α-REDUCTASE DEFICIENCY (PSEUDOVAGINAL PERINEOSCROTAL HYPOSPADIAS).   Some genetic males have ambiguous external genitalia at birth but otherwise develop like normal males. At puberty, they undergo virilization with phallic enlargement, increased facial hair, muscular hypertrophy, voice deepening, and no breast development (see Chap. 115). The external genitalia consist of a phallus that resembles a clitoris more than a penis, a perineal urethral orifice, and, usually, a

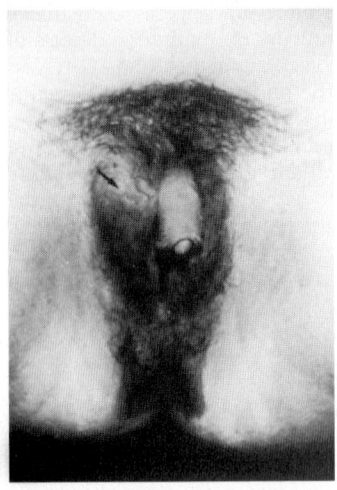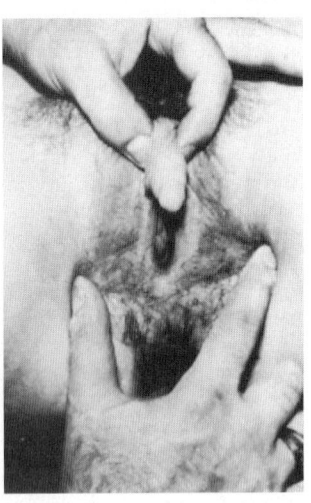

**A,B**

**FIGURE 90-25. A,** External genitalia of one of three 46,XY sibs with pseudovaginal perineoscrotal hypospadias (*PPSH*) phenotype who have deficiencies of 5α-reductase. The clitoris measures 5 to 6 cm long. Bilateral testes were present, one of which is visible (*arrow*). **B,** When phallus is elevated, the pseudovaginal opening is evident. (From Opitz JM, Simpson JL, Sarto CE, et al. Pseudovaginal perineoscrotal hypospadias. Clin Genet 1972; 3:1.)

separate blindly ending perineal orifice that resembles a vagina (i.e., pseudovagina; Fig. 90-25). The testes are relatively normal in size but may be undescended, and they secrete normal amounts of testosterone. Subjects have erections with ejaculation from the perineal urethra.

This abnormality, inherited in autosomal recessive fashion, results from a deficiency of 5α-reductase.[276–286] The enzyme 5α-reductase converts testosterone to DHT, the androgen active within cells. That intracellular 5α-reductase deficiency results in characteristic genital abnormalities is consistent with embryologic findings that virilization of the external genitalia during embryogenesis requires DHT, but wolffian differentiation requires only testosterone.

Two 5α-reductase (*SRD5*) genes exist. The type I gene (*SRD5A1*) is located on chromosome 5, and the type II gene (*SRD5A2*) on chromosome band 2p23. Only type II is expressed in gonads; thus, of the two isoforms, type II is deficient in male pseudohermaphroditism. Consisting of five exons,[283] the *SRD5A2* gene has been shown to have undergone deletions far less often[284] than point mutations.[285] Different ethnic groups have different mutations (*founder effect*), scattered among the five exons. The molecular etiology can be exploited for prenatal diagnosis and genetic counseling in kindreds, but usually only after one affected case has been identified.

In adolescent subjects, the diagnosis is made most easily by finding an elevated ratio of plasma testosterone to DHT after hCG stimulation. Circulating LH levels are increased despite the presence of normal to high levels of testosterone, suggesting a feedback role for DHT in the regulation of LH secretion. FSH levels also tend to be elevated, perhaps because of the testicular damage induced by cryptorchidism.

The deficiency in 5α-reductase also is present in cultured fibroblasts, in fibroblast homogenates, and in tissue homogenates. Because levels of 5α-reductase normally are highest in genital tissue, most investigators prefer to assay cells derived from genital tissue (e.g., foreskin). Unfortunately, a great variability exists in 5α-reductase activity, with near overlap between controls and patients clearly deficient for the enzyme.[287] Several hormonal studies may be needed to confirm the diagnosis. Measurement of 5α and 5β urinary metabolites constitutes one approach. The ratio of plasma testosterone to DHT can be measured after hCG stimulation or after testosterone stimulation.[287,288] The diagnosis can be made on the basis of

an elevated ratio of urinary tetrahydrocortisol to 5α-tetrahydrocortisol.[288]

Gender identity changes from female to male in untreated individuals have been reported, leading to the use of the descriptive term "penis at 12" ("guevedoces") syndrome to describe this disorder.[278] These changes in gender identity underscore the importance of androgens in affecting behavior and suggest that DHT is more important than testosterone in utero (see Chap. 115).

Two individuals with documented type II 5α-reductase deficiency had normal sperm concentrations, suggesting that dihydrotestosterone does not play a major role in spermatogenesis.[289] However, low levels of DHT may be sufficient for normal spermatogenesis.

INFERTILE MALES WITH ANDROGEN RESISTANCE.    Some phenotypic males with infertility have been said to have partial androgen resistance.[290] Gynecomastia may exist. The suggestion has been made that a significant proportion of male infertility may be due to this cause. This view is plausible, but whether the disorder constitutes one defect or several remains unclear. Affected males typically have azoospermia or oligospermia and normal or increased circulating levels of LH and testosterone. The family history is unremarkable, somewhat surprisingly in view of the inheritance patterns of other syndromes of androgen insensitivity and casts doubt on the primary role of androgen resistance as the cause of infertility. Histologically, the testes show maturation arrest of Sertoli cells only. Decreased or abnormal androgen receptors have been identified.

**Potential Teratogenic Forms.**    At least four potential teratogens have been identified, but fortunately none has been reported as causing a case of female pseudohermaphroditism in humans. Although not approved for this indication, the four drugs have been used to treat women with hirsutism. Cyproterone acts by blocking uptake of androgens by receptors and may have some effect on 5α-reductase as well[291]; thus, maternal ingestion of high doses during embryogenesis should result in female external genitalia in 46,XY fetuses. Spironolactone is an aldosterone antagonist that blocks androgen action by inhibiting cytochrome P450–linked enzymes involved in steroidogenesis and increases the clearance of testosterone.[292,293] Finasteride inhibits 5α-reductase, and thus should be capable of producing the form of pseudohermaphroditism bearing that designation (5α-reductase deficiency.)[294] Flutamide is a nonsteroidal compound that inhibits the androgen receptor[295] and may reduce the synthesis of androgens or increase their metabolism at high doses.[296]

**Other Disorders**

HYPOSPADIAS WITHOUT OTHER DEFECTS.    In hypospadias, the external urinary meatus terminates on the ventral aspect of the penis, proximal to its usual site at the tip of the glans penis. Hypospadias can be classified according to the site of the urethral meatus: along the glans penis, on the penile shaft, at the penoscrotal junction, or on the perineum (see Fig. 93-3). Sometimes, testicular hypoplasia coexists; however, more often testicular volume is normal (see Chap. 93).

Multiple affected sibs and affected individuals in several generations have been reported to have uncomplicated hypospadias.[7] After the birth of one affected child, the recurrence risk for subsequent male progeny is 6% to 10%.[297] These risks are higher than those usually associated with multifactorial or polygenic traits, suggesting genetic heterogeneity with the existence of unappreciated autosomal recessive forms. Hypospadias sometimes is only one of several components of multiple malformation patterns that are known to be inherited in this fashion. The presence of other anomalies should therefore be excluded before parents are quoted recurrence risks of 6% to 10%.

GENITAL AMBIGUITY WITH MULTIPLE MALFORMATION PATTERNS.    Genital ambiguity may occur in individuals with multiple malformation patterns, as tabulated elsewhere.[7] Previously unrecognized syndromes continue to be reported.[32,298]

MICROPHALLUS.    As measured from the pubic ramus to the tip of the glans, the mean stretched penile length in the term infant is 3.5 cm. The 3rd and 97th percentiles are 2.8 and 4.2 cm, respectively.[299] In premature infants, the mean stretched phallic length at 28 and 34 weeks is 2.2 and 2.8 cm, respectively. The mean width at term is 1.1 cm; the 3rd and 97th percentiles are 0.9 and 1.3 cm, respectively; and at 28 and 34 weeks the mean widths are 0.8 and 0.9 cm, respectively. If the phallus in a term infant is <1.5 by 0.7 cm, insufficient phallic growth may have occurred.

Microphallus (i.e., phallus of <2 cm long at birth) has heterogeneous causes, but fetal testosterone deficiency appears to be the most common cause in 46,XY males. In the human male fetus, placental hCG appears to stimulate testosterone synthesis during the critical period of male differentiation (8–12 weeks of gestation). Only after midgestation does fetal pituitary LH modulate testosterone synthesis and continued growth of the phallus. Because individuals with congenital hypopituitarism and isolated GH deficiency and those with isolated gonadotropin deficiency alone may present with microphallus, GH appears to be important in the growth of the phallus. Testicular failure beginning after genital differentiation can also present as microphallus at birth (see Chap. 93).

The infant with microphallus should undergo assessment of anterior pituitary function. An hCG stimulation test should be performed to determine if the testis can secrete testosterone. In individuals in whom fetal testosterone deficiency is a cause for the microphallus, intramuscular administration of testosterone enanthate (25–50 mg) monthly for 3 months should result in an increase in phallic length of 2 cm.[300] Failure of the phallus to increase in length in response to exogenous testosterone administration should lead to consideration of orchiectomy and assignment of female gender.

## CLINICAL APPROACH TO THE INFANT WITH GENITAL AMBIGUITY

### IMMEDIATE CONCERNS AND DIAGNOSTIC TESTS

Infants with genital ambiguity (Fig. 90-26) must be evaluated promptly and the correct diagnosis determined to prevent life-threatening complications and to assuage the concerns of the parents. Immediate management requires attention to medical and psychological factors. If a competent group of gynecologists, urologists, pediatricians, psychiatrists, geneticists, and endocrinologists is not available, the patient is best referred to a medical center having such a team.

Cytogenetic and endocrine studies should be initiated. To determine the genetic sex, the physician should rely on lymphocyte cultures and not solely on analysis of buccal epithelial cells (i.e., buccal smear) for the presence or absence of X-chromatin or Y-chromatin. Use of a chromosome-specific probe for the Y chromosome can provide a rapid diagnosis (fluorescent in situ hybridization) of interphase nuclei. A complete karyotype of chromosomes from peripheral leukocytes arrested in metaphase is now available within 48 hours. The X and Y chromosomes can be examined by high-resolution banding for deletions, rearrangements, nondisjunction, and other defects. The X and Y chromosomes can also be characterized by in situ hybridization using X chromosome–specific probes or Y chromosome–specific probes.

Increasingly, even more sophisticated genetic techniques are being used to identify specific gene defects in intersex disorders. Several genes important in sexual differentiation, including SRY and the genes for the androgen receptor, 5α-reductase, 21-hydroxylase, and antimüllerian hormone and its putative receptor, have all been cloned and are available as probes. Genomic DNA obtained from peripheral leukocytes

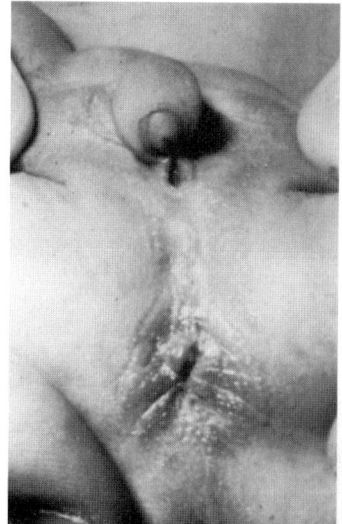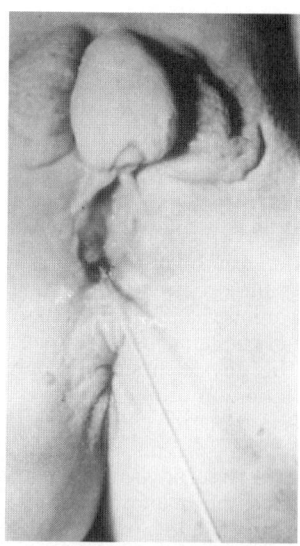

A,B

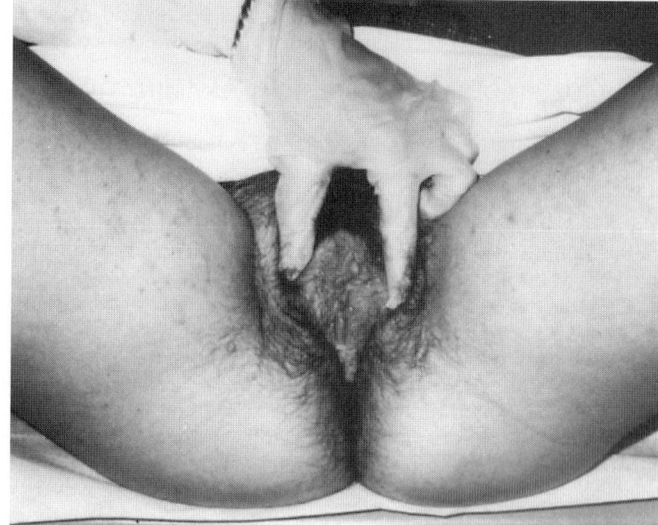

C

**FIGURE 90-26. A** and **B,** External genitalia of two 46,XX infants with ambiguous genitalia. Both infants had 21-hydroxylase deficiency. **B,** Probe identifies a cloacal opening. **C,** External genitalia of 22-year-old 46,XX individual who underwent clitorectomy at 2 years of age. This individual was found to have 21-hydroxylase deficiency as a young child and was treated with glucocorticoids. She subsequently conceived and vaginally delivered normal children.

and mRNA or complementary DNA from gonadal or genital skin biopsies can be used for these studies. Gene conversions, deletions, and insertions can be identified by northern and southern analysis. Restriction fragment length and other dinucleotide repeat polymorphisms have proved to be especially useful for studying segregation of 21-hydroxylase genes. DNA sequencing and polymerase chain reaction techniques can be used to detect single base mutations and microconversions in the genes that have been isolated. DNA diagnostic tests have proven disappointing in sporadic cases because of molecular heterogeneity. Once the molecular basis is known for an index case, however, a molecular basis exists for identifying other affected family members.

To exclude the syndromes of adrenal hyperplasia, the most common cause of genital ambiguity, levels of serum sodium, serum potassium, and serum 17α-hydroxyprogesterone, and the urinary excretion of 17-ketosteroids, pregnanetriol, and tetrahydrodeoxycortisol should be determined. Proper urine collection in infants requires that they be placed in metabolic beds designed to guarantee complete collection. Infants should be followed closely to prevent the development of dehydration, hyponatremia, and hyperkalemia, which may occur in some forms of congenital adrenal hyperplasia. It has also been recommended that AMH be measured as a sensitive indicator of testicular tissue, because it is elevated in males and undetectable in females in the first several years of life.[46,299]

During the 72 to 96 hours required for these tests, the emotional status of the parents must be considered. The preferable approach is to avoid any public indication that a special situation exists. The physician should attach no unusual significance to the occurrence of genital ambiguity and should inform the parents that their child has a "birth defect" involving the external genitalia, just as another birth defect may involve the heart. The physician should counsel the parents that the child will undergo normal psychosexual development, regardless of the sex-of-rearing chosen.

Some parents may be poorly equipped to cope with peer pressures. If so, advising them to withhold information concerning the sex of the infant from relatives may be preferable. Birth announcements should be deferred. If legally possible, the first name should be withheld from the birth certificate until the sex-of-rearing is chosen. Alternatively, a name suitable for a boy or girl may be selected. Occasionally, formal psychiatric consultation is necessary.

## HELPFUL FINDINGS ON PHYSICAL EXAMINATION

Although a careful physical examination should be performed on every infant with genital ambiguity, the diagnosis of a specific disorder usually cannot be made by physical examination alone. Nonetheless, some important generalizations are applicable. Potential penile function should be determined before arriving at the specific diagnosis.

That the external genitalia are rarely sufficiently distinctive to diagnose a particular condition is not surprising, because early in embryogenesis, male and female embryos have identical external genitalia. The genital tubercle and the genital folds can differentiate in the normal manner for embryos of a given sex, by incomplete masculinization of male embryos, or by unexpected virilization of female embryos. The size of the normal penis at birth has been detailed previously. The size of the phallus is less helpful diagnostically, however, than the location of the urethral opening. In normal males, the urethral orifice is located at the tip of the glans penis. In incomplete virilization, which results from decreased synthesis of fetal androgens or phallic unresponsiveness to androgens, the urethral orifice is located on the proximal glans penis, the shaft of the penis, or the perineum. Sometimes, the examiner can distinguish an underdeveloped penis from an overdeveloped clitoris by inspecting the frenulum on the ventral surface of the phallus. In normal males, only a single midline frenulum is present; in normal females, two frenula are found, each lateral to the midline. A female with clitoral hypertrophy has two paramedian frenula, and a male with hypospadias has a single midline frenulum or several irregularly spaced fibrous bands (chordee) that extend between the perineum and the penile shaft. A very large clitoris associated with normal urethral placement suggests exposure to androgens or progestins after genital differentiation in the first trimester.

Fusion of the labioscrotal folds results in formation of the scrotum and obliteration of the potential vagina. This process occurs in a posteroanterior direction, with the fusion site represented by the scrotal raphe. The processes that cause a hypoplastic penis also cause incomplete fusion of the labioscrotal folds. Likewise, processes that cause clitoral hypertrophy also cause unexpected fusion of the labioscrotal folds. If partial fusion occurs, the fused portion will be posterior.

An important point is determining whether müllerian derivatives (i.e., fallopian tubes, uterus, upper vagina) are present. If so, the infant has female pseudohermaphroditism, true hermaphroditism, or a cytogenetic form of male pseudohermaphroditism. A genetic form of male pseudohermaphroditism is unlikely to be associated with müllerian development. Frequently, a uterus can be palpated during the rectal examination; however, cystoscopic studies, ultrasonography, radiographic studies (e.g., vaginogram), or an examination with anesthesia may be necessary to verify the presence or absence of a uterus. Magnetic resonance imaging of the newborn pelvis can supplant these other diagnostic modalities.[301]

Sometimes, the composition of a gonad can be deduced by its location or consistency or by the surrounding organs based on several principles. First, a gonad located in the labial or inguinal regions almost invariably contains testicular tissue. In true hermaphroditism, the greater the amount of testicular tissue, the greater is the probability of gonadal descent. Second, a testis is softer than an ovary or a streak gonad and is more often surrounded by blood vessels that impart a reddish appearance. An ovary is white, convoluted, and of fibrous consistency. If various portions of a single gonad differ in consistency, the physician should consider the presence of an ovotestis or of a testis or streak gonad that has undergone neoplastic transformation. If a well-differentiated fallopian tube is absent on only one side, the ipsilateral gonad probably is a testis or ovotestis.

The presence of somatic anomalies comprising the Turner stigmata in association with genital ambiguity suggests 45,X/46,XY mosaicism, because the Turner stigmata presumably reflect the coexistence of 45,X cells.[36] Similarly, increased areolar and scrotal pigmentation may result from increased levels of ACTH, a hormone with melanocyte-stimulating properties.

Although genital ambiguity usually is recognized at birth, occasionally the problem is not recognized until later during infancy or even in childhood. The issue of changing the sex-of-rearing may arise. Traditionally, the belief has been that psychological problems do not develop if this change is accomplished before 2 years of age. Nevertheless, experience with individuals having 5α-reductase deficiency indicates that gender can be changed after age 2 in certain circumstances.[277] In any case, surgery to make the external genitalia as compatible with the sex-of-rearing as possible is indicated (see Fig. 90-26). Clitorectomy and clitoral recession are the most frequently performed surgical procedures.

## REFERENCES

1. Brown CJ, Goss SJ, Lubahn DB, et al. Androgen receptor locus on the human X chromosome: regional localization to Xq11→12 and description of a DNA polymorphism. Am J Hum Genet 1989; 44:264.
2. Standing Committee on Human Cytogenetic Nomenclature. An international system for human cytogenetic nomenclature (1978). Cytogenet Cell Genet 1978; 21:1.
2a. Sahin FI, Ergun MA, Tan E, Menvse A. The mechanism of G–banding detected by atomic force microscopy. Scanning 2000; 22:24.
3. Barr ML, Bertram EG. A morphological distinction between neurones of the male and female and the behavior of the nucleolar satellite during accelerated nucleoprotein synthesis. Nature 1949; 163:676.
4. Lyon MF. Gene action in the X-chromosome of the mouse (*Mus musculus* L.). Nature 1961; 190:372.
4a. Bailey JA, Carrel L, Chakravarti A, Eichler EE. Molecular evidence for a relationship between Line–1 elements and X chromosome inactivation: the Lyon repeat hypothesis. Proc Natl Acad Sci U S A 2000; 97:6634.
5. Polani PE, Angell R, Giannelli F, et al. Evidence that the Xg locus is inactivated in structurally abnormal X chromosomes. Nature 1970; 227:613.
6. Unnérus V, Fellman J, De La Chapelle A. The length of the human Y chromosome. Cytogenetics 1967; 6:213.
7. Simpson JL. Disorders of sexual differentiation: etiology and clinical delineation. New York: Academic Press, 1976.
8. Goodfellow PN, Lovell-Badge R. SRY and sex determination in mammals. Annu Rev Genet 1993; 27:71.
9. Ellis NA, Goodfellow PN. The mammalian pseudoautosomal region. Trends Genet 1989; 5:406.
10. Mohandas TK, Speed RM, Passage MB, et al. Role of the pseudoautosomal region in sex-chromosome pairing during male meiosis: meiotic studies in a man with a deletion of distal Xp. Am J Hum Genet 1992; 51:526.
11. Weissenbach J, Levilliers J, Petit C, et al. Normal and abnormal interchanges between the human X,Y chromosomes. Dev Suppl 1987; 101:67.
12. Ferguson-Smith MA. X-Y chromosomal interchange in the aetiology of true hermaphroditism and of XX Klinefelter's syndrome. Lancet 1966; 2:475.
13. Vergnaud G, Page DC, Simmler M-C, et al. A deletion map of the human Y chromosome based on DNA hybridization. Am J Hum Genet 1986; 38:109.

14. Jager RJ, Anvret M, Hall K, Scherer G. A human XY female with a frame shift mutation in the candidate testis-determining gene SRY. Nature 1990; 348:452.

15. Muller J, Schwartz M, Skakkebaek NE. Analysis of the sex-determining region of the Y chromosome (SRY) in sex reversed patients: point-mutation in SRY causing sex-reversion in a 46,XY female. J Clin Endocrinol Metab 1992; 75:331.

16. Koopman P, Gubbay J, Vivian N, et al. Male development of chromosomally female mice transgenic for SRY. Nature 1991; 351:117.

17. Haqq CM, King C-Y, Donahoe PK, Weiss MA. SRY recognizes conserved DNA sites in sex-specific promoters. Proc Natl Acad Sci U S A 1993; 90:1097.

18. McElreavey K, Vilain E, Cotinot C, et al. Control of sex determination in animals. Eur J Biochem 1993; 218:769.

19. Simpson JL, Christakos AC, Horwith M, et al. Gonadal dysgenesis associated with apparently normal chromosomal complements. Birth Defects 1971; 7(6):215.

19a. Sarafoglou K, Ostrer H. Clinical review 111: familial sex reversal: a review. J Clin Endocrinol Metab 2000; 85:483.

20. German J, Simpson JL, Chaganti RSK, et al. Genetically determined sex-reversal in 46,XY humans. Science 1978; 202:53.

21. De Grouchy J, Gompel A, Salmon-Bernard Y. Embryonic testicular regression syndrome and severe mental retardation in sibs. Ann Genet 1985; 28:154.

22. Najjar SS, Takla RJ, Nassar VH. The syndrome of rudimentary testes: occurrence in five siblings. J Pediatr 1974; 84:119.

23. Hamet P, Kuchel O, Nowacynski JM, et al. Hypertension with adrenal, genital, renal defects, and deafness. Arch Intern Med 1973; 131:563.

24. Smith A, Fraser IS, Noel M. Three siblings with premature gonadal failure. Fertil Steril 1979; 32:528.

25. Granat M, Amar A, Mor-Yosef S, et al. Familial gonadal germinative failure: endocrine and human leukocyte antigen studies. Fertil Steril 1983; 40:215.

26. Al-Alwadi SA, Farag TI, Teeb AS, et al. Primary hypergonadism and partial alopecia in three sibs with müllerian hypoplasia in the affected females. Am J Med Genet 1985; 22:619.

27. Mikati MA, Samir SN, Sahil IF. Microcephaly, hypergonadotropic hypogonadism, short stature and minor anomalies: a new syndrome. Am J Med Genet 1985; 22:599.

27a. Hiort O, Holterhus P-M. The molecular basis of male sexual differentiation. Eur J Endocrinol 2000; 142:101.

28. Jirasek J. Principles of reproductive embryology. In: Simpson JL, ed. Disorders of sexual differentiation. New York: Academic Press, 1976:51.

29. Singh RP, Carr DH. The anatomy and histology of XO human embryos and fetuses. Anat Rec 1966; 155:369.

30. Burgoyne PS, Baker TG. Perinatal oocyte loss in XO mice and its implication for the etiology of gonadal dysgenesis in XO women. J Reprod Fertil 1987; 175:633.

31. Cussen LK, McMahon R. Germ cells and ova in dysgenetic gonads of a 46,XY female dizygote twin. Arch Dis Child 1979; 133:373.

32. Greenberg F, Gresik MW, Carpenter RJ, et al. The Gardner-Silengo-Wachtel or genito-palato-cardiac syndrome: male pseudohermaphroditism with micrognathia, cleft palate, and conotruncal cardiac defects. Am J Med Genet 1987; 26:59.

33. Evans EP, Ford CE, Lyon MF. Direct evidence of the capacity of the XY germ cell in the mouse to become an oocyte. Nature 1977; 267:430.

34. Simpson JL. Phenotypic-karyotypic correlations of gonadal determinants: current status and relationship to molecular studies. In: Sperling K, Vogel F, eds. Proceedings of the Seventh International Congress on Human Genetics. Heidelberg: Springer-Verlag, 1987:224.

35. Simpson JL. Genetic control of sexual development. In: Ratnam SS, Teoh ES, eds. Proceedings of the 12th World Congress on Fertility and Sterility. Lancaster, UK: Parthenon Press, 1987:165.

36. Simpson JL. Ovarian determinants through phenotypic-karyotypic deductions: progress and pitfalls. In: Rosenfeld R, Grumbach M, eds. Turner syndrome. New York: Marcel Dekker, 1990:65.

37. Krauss CM, Turkray RN, Atkins L, et al. Familial premature ovarian failure due to interstitial deletion of the long arm of the X chromosome. N Engl J Med 1987; 317:125.

38. Fitch N, de Saint VJ, Richer CL, et al. Premature menopause due to small deletion in long arm of the X chromosome: a report of three cases and a review. Am J Obstet Gynecol 1982; 142:968.

39. Cate RL, Mattaliano RJ, Hession C, et al. Isolation of the bovine and human genes for Müllerian inhibiting substance and expression of the human gene in animal cells. Cell 1986; 45:686.

40. Derynck R, Jarrett JA, Chen EY, et al. Human transforming growth factor-β complementary DNA sequence and expression in normal and transformed cells. Nature 1985; 316:701.

41. Mason AJ, Hayflick JS, Ling N, et al. Complementary DNA sequences of ovarian follicular inhibin show precursor structure and homology with transforming growth factor-β. Nature 1985; 318:659.

42. Cohen-Haguenauer O, Picard JY, Mattei MG, et al. Mapping of the gene for anti-Müllerian hormone to the short arm of human chromosome 19. Cytogenet Cell Genet 1987; 44:2.

43. Visser JA, McLuskey A, van Beers T, et al. Structure and chromosomal localization of the human anti-müllerian hormone type II receptor gene. Biochem Biophys Res Commun 1995; 215:1029.

44. Josso N, di Clemente N. Serine/threonine kinase receptors and ligands. Curr Opin Genet Dev 1997; 7:371.

45. Lee MM, Donahoe PK. Müllerian inhibiting substance: a gonadal hormone with multiple functions. Endocr Rev 1993; 14:152.

46. Gustafson ML, Lee MM, Asmundson L, et al. Müllerian inhibiting substance in the diagnosis and management of intersex and gonadal abnormalities. J Pediatr Surg 1993; 28:439.

47. Jost A, Vigier B, Prepin J, et al. Studies on sex differentiation in mammals. Recent Prog Horm Res 1973; 29:1.

48. Patsavoudi E, Magre S, Castanier M, et al. Dissociation between testicular morphogenesis and functional differentiation of Leydig cells. J Endocrinol 1985; 105:235.

49. Magre S, Jost A. Dissociation between testicular morphogenesis and endocrine cytodifferentiation of Sertoli cells. Proc Natl Acad Sci U S A 1984; 81:7831.

49a. Walker AM, Walker JL, Adams S, et al. True hermaphroditism. J Paediatr Child Health 2000; 36:69.

50. Simpson JL. True hermaphroditism: etiology and phenotypic considerations. Birth Defects 1978; 14:9.

51. Van Niekerk WA, Retiel AE. The gonads of human true hermaphrodites. Hum Genet 1981; 58:117.

52. Van Niekerk WA. True hermaphroditism. New York: Harper & Row, 1974.

53. Tegenkemp TR, Brazzell JW, Tegenkamp I, et al. Pregnancy without benefit of reconstructive surgery in a bisexually active true hermaphrodite. Am J Obstet Gynecol 1979; 135:427.

54. Minowada S, Fukutani K, Hara M, et al. Childbirth in a true hermaphrodite. Eur Urol 1984; 10:414.

55. Simpson JL, Photopulos G. The relationship of neoplasia to disorders of abnormal sexual differentiation. Birth Defects 1976; 12(1):15.

56. Verp MS, Simpson JL. Abnormal sexual differentiation and neoplasia. Cancer Genet Cytogenet 1987; 25:191.

57. Fraccaro M, Tiepolo L, Zuffardio-Chiumello G, et al. Familial XX true hermaphroditism and H-Y antigen. Hum Genet 1979; 48:45.

58. Ramsey M, Bernstein R, Zwane F, et al. XX true hermaphroditism in southern African blacks: an enigma of primary sexual differentiation. Am J Hum Genet 1988; 43:4.

59. Armendares S, Salamanca F, Cantú JM, et al. Familial true hermaphroditism in three siblings. Hum Genet 1975; 29:99.

60. Mori V, Mitzutani S. Familial hermaphroditism in genetic families. Jpn J Urol 1968; 59:857.

61. Kasdan R, Nankin HP, Troen P, et al. Paternal transmissions of maleness in XX human beings. N Engl J Med 1987; 288:539.

62. Skordis NA, Stetka DG, MacGillivray MH, et al. Familial 46,XX coexisting with familial 46,XX true hermaphrodites in same pedigree. J Pediatr 1987; 110:244.

63. Page DC, de la Chapelle A, Wiessenbach J. Chromosome Y-specific DNA in related human XX males. J Pediatr 1987; 110:224.

64. De la Chapelle A. The complicated issue of human sex determination. Am J Hum Genet 1988; 43:1.

65. Simpson JL, Bombard AT. Chromosomal abnormalities in spontaneous abortions: frequency, pathology and genetic counselling. In: Edmonds K, Bennett MJ, eds. Spontaneous abortion. London: Blackwell, 1987:51.

66. Chen ATL, Chan Y-K, Falek A. The effects of chromosome abnormalities on birth weight in man. I: sex chromosome disorders. Hum Hered 1971; 21:543.

67. Simpson JL. Pregnancies in women with chromosomal abnormalities. In: Schulman JD, Simpson JL. Genetics in diseases in pregnancy. New York: Academic Press, 1981:439.

68. Gartler SM, Liskay RM, Campbell BK, et al. Evidence of two functional X chromosomes in human oocytes. Cell Differ 1972; 1:215.

69. Sanger R, Tippett P, Gavin J, et al. Xg groups and sex chromosome abnormalities in people of northern European ancestry: an addendum. J Med Genet 1977; 14:210.

70. Kajii T, Ohama K. Inverse maternal age effect in monosomy X. Hum Genet 1979; 51:147.

71. Russell LB. Chromosome aberrations in experimental mammals. Prog Med Genet 1962; 2:230.

72. Simpson JL. Gonadal dysgenesis and abnormalities of the human sex chromosomes: current status of phenotypic-karyotypic correlations. Birth Defects 1975; 11(4):23.

73. Ranke MB, Pfluger H, Rosendahl W, et al. Turner's syndrome: spontaneous growth in 150 cases and review of the literature. Eur J Pediatr 1983; 141:81.

74. Ranke MB, Preece MA, Grant DB. Growth curve for girls with Turner syndrome. Arch Dis Child 1985; 60:932.

75. Brook CGD, Murset G, Zachmann M, et al. Growth in children with 45,XO Turner's syndrome. Arch Dis Child 1974; 49:789.

75a. Binder G, Schwarze CP, Ranke MB. Identification of short stature caused by SHOX defects and therapeutic effect of recombinant human growth hormone. J Clin Endocrinol Metab 2000; 85:245.

76. Donaldson CL, Wegienko LC, Miller D, et al. Growth hormone studies in Turner's syndrome. J Clin Endocrinol Metab 1968; 28:383.

77. Ross JL, Long LM, Loriaux DL. Growth hormone secreting dynamics in Turner's syndrome. J Pediatr 1985; 106:202.

78. Saenger P. Clinical review 48: the current status of diagnosis and therapeutic intervention in Turner's syndrome. J Clin Endocrinol Metab 1993; 77:297.

79. Botazzo GF, McIntosh C, Stanford W, et al. Growth hormone cell antibodies and partial hormone deficiency in a girl with Turner's syndrome. Clin Endocrinol (Oxf) 1980; 12:1.

80. Laczi F, Julesz J, Janaky T, et al. Growth hormone reserve capacity in Turner's syndrome. Horm Metab Res 1979; 11:664.

81. Ranke MB, Blum WF, Hang F, et al. Growth hormone, somatomedin levels and growth regulation in Turner's syndrome. Acta Endocrinol (Copenh) 1987; 116:305.

82. Filipsson R, Lindstein J, Almqvist S. Time of eruption of the permanent teeth, cephalometric and tooth measurement and sulphation factor activity

in 45 patients with Turner's syndrome with different types of chromosome aberration. Acta Endocrinol (Copenh) 1965; 48:91.

83. Lindstein J, Fraccaro M. Turner's syndrome. In: Rashad MN, Morton WRM, eds. Genital anomalies. Springfield: Charles C Thomas, 1969:396.

84. Garron DC, Vander Stoep LR. Personality and intelligence in Turner's syndrome. Arch Gen Psychiatry 1969; 21:339.

85. Money J. Two cytogenetic syndromes: psychologic comparisons. I. Intelligence and specific-factor quotients. J Psychiatr Res 1964; 2:223.

86. Shaffer JW. A specific cognitive defect observed in gonadal aplasia (Turner's syndrome). J Clin Psychol 1962; 18:403.

87. McCauley E, Sybert V, Ehrhardt AA. Psychosocial adjustment of adult women with Turner syndrome. Clin Genet 1986; 29:284.

88. Polychronakos C, Letarte J, Collu R, et al. Carbohydrate intolerance in children and adolescents with Turner's syndrome. J Pediatr 1980; 96:1009.

89. Simpson JL, LeBeau MM. Gonadal and statural determinants on the X chromosome and their relationship to in vitro studies showing prolonged cell cycles in 45,X, 46,X, del(X)(p11); 46,X, del(X)(q13) and q(22) fibroblasts. Am J Obstet Gynecol 1981; 141:930.

90. Fraccaro M, Maraschio P, Pasquali F, et al. Women heterozygous for deficiency of the (p21→pter) region of the X chromosome are fertile. Hum Genet 1977; 39:283.

91. Simpson JL. Genetics of sex determination. In: Iizuka R, Semm K, eds. Human reproduction. Proceedings of the VIth World Congress on Human Reproduction. Amsterdam: Elsevier Science, 1988:19.

92. Ferguson-Smith MA. Karyotype-phenotype correlations in gonadal dysgenesis and their bearing on the pathogenesis of malformations. J Med Genet 1965; 2:142.

93. Geerkens C, Just W, Vogel W. Deletions of Xq and growth deficit: a review. Am J Med Genet 1994; 50:105.

94. Manuel M, Katayama KP, Jones HW Jr. The age of occurrence of gonadal tumors in intersex patients with a Y chromosome. Am J Obstet Gynecol 1976; 124:293.

95. Medlej R, Lobaccaro JM, Berta P, et al. Screening for Y-derived sex determining gene SRY in 40 patients with Turner syndrome. J Clin Endocrinol Metab 1992; 75:1289.

96. Hsu LYF, Hirschhorn K, Goldstein A, et al. Familial chromosomal mosaicism: genetic aspects. Ann Hum Genet 1970; 33:343.

97. Aittomäki K. The genetics of XX gonadal dysgenesis. Am J Hum Genet 1994; 58:844.

98. Pallister PD, Opitz JM. The Perrault syndrome: autosomal recessive ovarian dysgenesis with facultative, nonsex-limited sensorineural deafness. Am J Med Genet 1979; 4:239.

99. Lundgren PO. Hereditary myopathy, oliophrenia, cataract, skeletal abnormalities and hypergonadotrophic hypogonadism: a new syndrome. Eur J Neurol 1973; 10:261.

100. Skre H, Bassoe HH, Berg K, et al. Cerebellar ataxia and hypogonadism in the two kindreds: chance occurrence, pleiotropism or linkage? Clin Genet 1976; 9:234.

101. Maximilian C, Ionescu B, Bucur A. Two sisters with gonadal dysgenesis, short stature, microcephaly, and arachnodactyly, and 46,XX karyotype. J Genet Hum 1970; 18:365.

102. Aittomaki K, Luccena JL, Pakarinen P, et al. Mutation in the follicle-stimulating hormone receptor gene causes hereditary hypergonadotropic ovarian failure. Cell 1995; 82:959.

103. Aittomaki K, Herva R, Stenman UH, et al. Clinical features of primary ovarian failure caused by a point mutation in the follicle-stimulating hormone receptor gene. J Clin Endocrinol Metab 1996; 81:3722.

104. Layman LC, Amede S, Cohen DP, et al. The Finnish follicle-stimulating hormone receptor gene mutation is rare in North American women with 46,XX ovarian failure. Fertil Steril 1998; 69:300.

105. Liu JY, Gromoll J, Cedars MI. Identification of allelic variants in the follicle-stimulating hormone receptor genes of females with or without hypergonadotropic amenorrhea. Fertil Steril 1998; 70:326.

106. Simpson JL, Blagowidow N, Martin AO. XY gonadal dysgenesis: genetic heterogeneity based upon clinical observations: H-Y antigen status and segregation analysis. Hum Genet 1981; 58:91.

107. Sternberg WH, Barclay DL, Kloeper HW. Familial XY gonadal dysgenesis. N Engl J Med 1968; 278:695.

108. Page DC. Sex reversal: deletion mapping the male determining function of the Y chromosome. Cold Spring Harb Symp Quant Biol 1986; 51:229.

109. Pionick EK, Wachtel S, Woods D, et al. Mutations in the conserved domain of SRY are uncommon in XY gonadal dysgenesis. Hum Genet 1992; 90:308.

110. Mann JR, Corkery JJ, Fisher HJW, et al. The X-linked recessive form of XY gonadal dysgenesis with high incidence of gonadal cell tumors: clinical and genetic studies. J Med Genet 1983; 20:264.

111. Bricarelli FD, Fraccaro M, Lindstein J, et al. Sex-reversed XY females with campomelic dysplasia are H-Y negative. Hum Genet 1981; 57:15.

112. Bronson PC, Lewandowski RC, Toguri AG, et al. A new familial syndrome of 46,XY gonadal dysgenesis with anomalies of ectodermal and mesodermal structures. J Pediatr 1980; 97:586.

113. Elias S, Martin AO, Simpson JL. Longitudinal stability of sex chromosome mosaicism. J Pediatr 1980; 136:509.

114. Conte FA, Grumbach MM, Kaplan SL. A diphasic pattern of gonadotropin secretion in patients with the syndrome of gonadal dysgenesis. J Clin Endocrinol Metab 1975; 40:670.

115. Rebar RW, Yen SSC. Endocrine rhythms in gonadotropins and ovarian steroids with reference to reproductive processes. In: Krieger DT, ed. Endocrine rhythms. New York: Raven Press, 1979:259.

116. Rosenfeld RG, Hintz RL, Johanson AJ, et al. Methionyl human growth hormone and oxandrolone in Turner syndrome: preliminary results of a prospective randomized trial. J Pediatr 1986; 109:936.

117. Rosenfeld RG, Frane J, Attie KM, et al. Six-year results of a randomized prospective trial of human growth hormone and oxandrolone in Turner syndrome. J Pediatr 1992; 121:49.

118. Ross JL, Long LM, Skerda M, et al. Effect of low doses of estradiol on 6-month growth rates and predicted height in patients with Turner syndrome. J Pediatr 1986; 109:950.

119. Lucky AW, Marynick SP, Rebar RW, et al. Replacement oral ethinylestradiol therapy for gonadal dysgenesis: growth and adrenal androgen studies. Acta Endocrinol (Copenh) 1979; 91:519.

119a. Elshaikh M, Bird R, Casadei B, et al. The effect of hormone replacement therapy on cardiovascular hemodynamics in women with Turner's syndrome. J Clin Endocrinol Metab 2000; 85:614.

120. Rebar RW, Cedars MI. Hypergonadotropic amenorrhea. In: Filicori M, Flamigni C, eds. Ovulation induction. Basic science and clinical advances. Amsterdam: Elsevier Science, 1994.

121. Jacobs PA, Baikie AG, Court-Brown WM, et al. Evidence for the existence of the human "superfemale." Lancet 1959; 2:423.

122. Johnston AW, Ferguson-Smith MA, Handmaker SD, et al. The triple X syndrome: clinical, pathological and chromosomal studies in three mentally retarded cases. BMJ 1961; 2:1046.

123. Day RW, Larson W, Wright SW. Clinical and cytogenetic studies on a group of females with XXX sex chromosome complements. J Pediatr 1964; 64:24.

124. Villanueva AL, Rebar RW. Triple-X syndrome and premature ovarian failure. Obstet Gynecol 1983; 62:705.

125. Sills JA, Brown JK, Grace S, et al. XXX syndrome associated with immunoglobulin deficiency and epilepsy. J Pediatr 1978; 93:469.

126. Smith TF, Engel E. Marfan's syndrome with 47,XXX genotype and possible immunologic abnormality. South Med J 1981; 74:630.

127. Purtillo DT, DeFlorio D Jr, Hutt LH, et al. Variable phenotypic expression of an X-linked recessive lymphoproliferative syndrome. N Engl J Med 1977; 279:1077.

128. Noonan J. Hypertelorism with Turner phenotype: a new syndrome with associated congenital heart disease. Am J Dis Child 1968; 116:373.

129. Char F, Rodriguez-Fernandez HL, Scott CI Jr. The Noonan syndrome—a clinical study of forty-five cases. Birth Defects 1973; 8(5):110.

130. Miller M, Cotulsky AC. Noonan syndrome in an adult family presenting with chronic lymphedema. Am J Med 1978; 65:379.

131. Wilroy RS Jr, Summitt RL, Tipton RE. Phenotypic heterogeneity in the Noonan syndrome. Birth Defects 1979; 15(5B):305.

132. Hamerton JL, Canning N, Ray M, et al. A cytogenetic survey of 14,069 newborn infants. I. Incidence of chromosome abnormalities. Clin Genet 1975; 8:223.

133. Klinefelter HF Jr, Reifenstein EC Jr, Albright F. Syndrome characterized by gynecomastia, aspermatogenesis without A-Leydigism and increased excretion of follicle-stimulating hormone. J Clin Endocrinol 1942; 2:615.

134. Scheike O, Vaisfeld J, Peterson B. Male breast cancer III: breast carcinoma in association with Klinefelter syndrome. Acta Pathol Microbiol Scand 1973; 81:352.

135. Paulsen CA, Gordon DL, Carpenter RW, et al. Klinefelter's syndrome and its variants: a hormonal and chromosomal study. Recent Prog Horm Res 1968; 24:321.

136. De la Chapelle A. Analytical review: nature and origin of males with XX sex chromosomes. Am J Hum Genet 1972; 24:71.

137. De la Chapelle A. The etiology of maleness in XX men. Hum Genet 1981; 58:105.

138. Fechner PY, Marcantonio SM, Jaswaney V, et al. The role of the sex-determining region Y gene in the etiology of 46,XX maleness. J Clin Endocrinol Metab 1993; 76:690.

139. Del Castillo EB, Trabucco A, De La Balze FA. Syndrome produced by absence of the germinal epithelium without impairment of the Sertoli or Leydig cells. J Clin Endocrinol 1947; 7:493.

139a. Yaman O, Orzdiler E, Seckiner I, Gogus O. Significance of serum FSH levels and testicular morphology in infertile males. Int Urol Nephrol 1999; 31:519.

140. Hall JG, Morgan A, Blizzard RM. Familial congenital anorchia. Birth Defects 1975; 11(2):115.

141. Simpson JL, Horwith M, Morillo-Cucci G, et al. Bilateral anorchia: discordance in monozygotic twins. Birth Defects 1971; 7(6):196.

142. Bergada C, Cleveland WW, Jones HW, et al. Variants of embryonic testicular dysgenesis: bilateral anorchia and the syndrome of rudimentary testes. Acta Endocrinol (Copenh) 1962; 40:521.

143. Acien P. Reproductive performance of women with uterine malformations. Hum Reprod 1993; 8:122.

144. Buttram VC Jr, Gibbons WE. Müllerian anomalies: a proposed classification (an analysis of 144 cases). Fertil Steril 1979; 32:40.

145. Smith FR. The significance of incomplete fusion of the Müllerian ducts in pregnancy and parturition with a report on 35 cases. Am J Obstet Gynecol 1931; 22:714.

146. Barnes AB, Colton J, Gundersen J. Fertility and outcome of pregnancy in women exposed in utero to diethylstilbestrol. N Engl J Med 1980; 302:609.

147. Herbst AL, Hubby MM, Azizi F. Reproductive and gynecological surgical experience in diethylstilbestrol-exposed daughters. Am J Obstet Gynecol 1981; 141:1019.

148. Woolf RB, Allen WM. Concomitant malformations: the frequent simultaneous occurrence of congenital malformations of the reproductive and urinary tracts. Obstet Gynecol 1953; 2:236.

149. Buttram VC Jr, Reiter RC. Surgical treatment of the infertile female. Baltimore: Williams & Wilkins, 1985:89.

150. Pinsky L. A community of human malformation syndromes involving the Müllerian ducts, distal extremities, urinary tract and ears. Teratology 1974; 9:65.

151. McKusick VA, Weilbaecher RG, Gregg CW. Recessive inheritance of a congenital malformation syndrome. JAMA 1968; 204:113.

152. Stone DL, Agarwala R, Schaffer AA, et al. Genetic and physical mapping of the McKusick-Kaufman syndrome. Hum Mol Genet 1998; 7:475.

153. Chitayat D, Hahm SY, Marion RW, et al. Further delineation of the McKusick-Kaufman hydrometrocolpos-polydactyly syndrome. Am J Dis Child 1987; 141:1133.

154. Lurie IW, Wulfsberg EA. The McKusick-Kaufman syndrome: phenotypic variation observed in familial cases as a clue for the evaluation of sporadic cases. Genet Couns 1994; 5:275.

155. Edwards JA, Gale RP. Camptobrachydactyly: a new autosomal dominant trait with two probable homozygotes. Am J Hum Genet 1972; 24:464.

156. Winter JSD, Kohn G, Mellman WJ, et al. A familial syndrome of renal, genital and middle ear anomalies. J Pediatr 1968; 71:88.

157. King LA, Sanchez-Ramos L, Tallado OE, et al. Syndrome of genital, renal, and middle ear anomalies: a third family and report of pregnancy. Obstet Gynecol 1987; 69:491.

158. Fraser GR. Our genetical "load": a review of some aspects of genetic malformations. Ann Hum Genet 1962; 25:387.

159. Greenberg F, Keenan B, De Yanis V, et al. Gonadal dysgenesis and gonadoblastoma in situ in a female with Fraser (cryptophthalmos) syndrome. J Pediatr 1986; 108:952.

160. Geary WL, Weed JC. Congenital atresia of the uterine cervix. Obstet Gynecol 1973; 42:213.

161. Nivier DH, Barrett G, Jewelewicz R. Congenital atresia of the uterine cervix and vagina: three cases. Fertil Steril 1980; 33:25.

162. Page EW, Owsley JQ Jr. Surgical correction of vaginal agenesis. Am J Obstet Gynecol 1969; 105:774.

163. Wabrek AJ, Millard PR, Wilson WB Jr, et al. Creation of a neovagina by the Frank nonoperative method. Obstet Gynecol 1971; 37:408.

164. Shokeir MHK. Aplasia of the müllerian system: evidence for probable sex-limited autosomal dominant inheritance. Birth Defects 1978; 14(6c):147.

165. Carson SA, Simpson JL, Malinak LR, et al. Heritable aspects of uterine anomalies II: genetic analysis of Müllerian aplasia. Fertil Steril 1983; 40:86.

166. Petrozza JC, Gray MR, Davis AJ, et al. Congenital absence of the uterus and vagina is not commonly transmitted as a dominant genetic trait: outcomes of surrogate pregnancies. Fertil Steril 1997; 67:387.

167. O'Leary JL, O'Leary JA. Rudimentary horn pregnancy. Obstet Gynecol 1983; 22:371.

168. Heinonen PK, Saarikoshi S, Pystynen P. Reproductive performance of women with uterine anomalies. Acta Obstet Gynecol Scand 1982; 61:157.

169. Pellerito JS, McCarthy SM, Doyle MB, et al. Diagnosis of uterine anomalies: relative accuracy of MR imaging, endovaginal sonography, and hysterosalpingography. Genitourin Radiol 1992; 183:795.

170. Strassman EO. Fertility and unification of a double uterus. Fertil Steril 1966; 17:165.

171. Mercer CA, Long WN, Thompson JE. Uterine unification: indications and technique. Clin Obstet Gynecol 1981; 24:1199.

172. Buttram VC Jr. What sets the stage for intrauterine adhesions? Contemp Obstet Gynecol 1978; 11:1.

173. Valle RF, Sciarra JJ. Current status of hysteroscopy in gynecologic practice. Fertil Steril 1979; 32:619.

174. Chervenak FA, Neuwirth RS. Hysteroscopic resection of the uterine septum. Am J Obstet Gynecol 1981; 141:351.

175. Daly DC, Walters CA, Riddick DH. Hysteroscopic metroplasty and subsequent obstetric outcome. Fertil Steril 1983; 39(Suppl):416.

176. Elias S, Simpson JL, Carson SA, et al. Genetic studies in incomplete müllerian fusion. Obstet Gynecol 1984; 63:276.

177. Verp MS, Simpson JL, Elias S, et al. Heritable aspects of uterine anomalies I. Three familial aggregates with müllerian fusion anomalies. Fertil Steril 1983; 34:80.

178. Longmuir GA, Conley N, Nicholson DL, et al. The hand-foot-uterus syndrome: a case study. J Manipulative Physiol Ther 1986; 9:213.

179. Stern AM, Gall JC Jr, Perry BL, et al. The hand-foot-uterus syndrome: a new hereditary disorder characterized by hand and foot dysplasia, dermatoglyphic abnormalities, and partial duplication of the female genital tract. J Pediatr 1970; 77:109.

180. Mortlock DP, Post LC, Innis J. The molecular basis of hypodactyly (Hd): a deletion in Hoxa 13 leads to arrest of digital arch formation. Nat Genet 1996; 13:284.

181. Mortlock DP, Innis J. Mutation of HOXA13 in hand-foot-genital syndrome. Nat Genet 1997; 15:179.

182. Del Campo M, Jones MC, Veraksa AN. Monodactylous limbs and abnormal genitalia are associated with hemizygosity for the human 2q 31 region that includes the HOXD cluster. Am J Hum Genet 1999; 65:104.

183. Stillman RJ. In utero exposure to diethylstilbestrol: adverse affects on the reproductive tract and reproductive performance in male and female offspring. Am J Obstet Gynecol 1982; 42:905.

184. Herbst AL, Hubby MM, Blough RR. A comparison of pregnancy experience in DES-exposed and DES-unexposed daughters. J Reprod Med 1980; 24:62.

185. Kaufman RH, Adam E, Binder GL. Upper genital tract changes and pregnancy outcome in offspring exposed in utero to diethylstilbestrol. Am J Obstet Gynecol 1980; 137:299.

186. DeBraekeleer M, Férce C. Mutations in the cystic fibrosis gene in men with congenital bilateral absence of the vas deferens. Hum Mol Reprod 1976; 2:669.

187. Chillon M, Casals T, Mercier B, et al. Mutations in the cystic fibrosis gene in patients with congenital absence of the vas deferens. N Engl J Med 1995; 332:1475.

188. Schellen TM, van Straaten A. Autosomal recessive hereditary congenital aplasia of the vasa deferentia in four siblings. Fertil Steril 1980; 34:401.

189. Budde WJ, Verjaal M, Hamerlynck JV, et al. Familial occurrence of azoospermia and extreme oligozoospermia. Clin Genet 1984; 26:555.

190. Czeizel A. Congenital aplasia of the vasa deferentia of autosomal recessive inheritance in two unrelated sib-pairs. Hum Genet 1985; 70:288.

191. Imbeaud S, Carre-Eusebe D, Boussin L. Molecular biology of normal and pathologic anti-müllerian hormone. Ann Endocrinol 1991; 52:415.

192. Imbeaud S, Belville C, Messika-Zeitoun L, et al. A 27 base-pair deletion of the anti-müllerian type II receptor gene is the most common cause of the persistent müllerian duct syndrome. Hum Mol Genet 1996; 5:1269.

193. Imbeaud S, Carre-Eusebe D, Rey R, et al. Molecular genetics of the persistent müllerian duct syndrome: a study of 19 families. Hum Mol Genet 1994; 3:125.

194. Imbeaud S, Faure E, Lamarre I, et al. Insensitivity of anti-müllerian hormone due to a mutation in the human anti-müllerian hormone receptor. Nat Genet 1995; 11:382.

195. Meyers-Wallen V, Lee M, Manganaro T, Kuroda T. Müllerian inhibiting substance is present in embryonic testes of dogs with persistent müllerian duct syndrome. Biol Reprod 1993; 48:1410.

196. Simpson ER, Michael MD, Agarwal VR, et al. Cytochromes P450 11: expression of the CYP19 (aromatase) gene: an unusual case of alternative promoter usage. FASEB 1997; 11:29.

197. Ito Y, Fisher CR, Conte FA, et al. Molecular basis of aromatase deficiency in an adult female with sexual infantilism and polycystic ovaries. Proc Natl Acad Sci U S A 1993; 90:11673.

198. Carson SA, Simpson JL. Virilization of female fetuses following maternal ingestion of progestational and androgenic steroids. In: Mahesh VB, Greenblatt RB, eds. Hirsutism and virilization. Littleton, MA: PSG Publishing, 1984:177.

199. Schardein JL. Congenital abnormalities and hormones during pregnancy: a clinical review. Teratology 1980; 22:251.

200. Castro-Magana M, Cheruvansky T, Collipp PJ, et al. Transient androgenogenital syndrome due to exposure to danazol in utero. Am J Dis Child 1981; 135:1032.

201. Duck SC, Katayama K. Danazol may cause female pseudohermaphroditism. Fertil Steril 1981; 35:230.

202. Suchowsky GK, Jungmann K. A study of the virilizing effect of progestogens on the female rat fetus. Endocrinology 1961; 68:341.

203. Andrews FD, Staples RE. Prenatal toxicity of medroxyprogesterone acetate in rabbits, rats and mice. Teratology 1977; 15:25.

204. Burstein R, Wasserman HC. The effect of Provera on the fetus. Obstet Gynecol 1964; 23:931.

205. Rawlings WJ. Progestogens and the foetus. BMJ 1962; 1:336.

206. Yovich JL, Turner SR, Draper R. Medroxyprogesterone acetate therapy in early pregnancy has no apparent fetal effects. Teratology 1988; 38:135.

207. Franklin RR. In: Chez RA. Proceedings of the symposium "progesterone, progestins, and fetal development." Fertil Steril 1978; 30:16.

208. Jones GES. In: Chez RA. Proceedings of the symposium "progesterone, progestins, and fetal development." Fertil Steril 1978; 30:16.

209. Check JH, Rankin A, Teichman M. The risk of fetal anomalies as a result of progesterone therapy during pregnancy. Fertil Steril 1986; 45:575.

210. Resseguie LT, Hick JF, Bruen JA, et al. Congenital malformations among offspring exposed in utero to progestins, Olmsted County, Minnesota 1936–1974. Fertil Steril 1985; 43:514.

211. Sarto GE, Opitz JM. The XY gonadal agenesis syndrome. J Med Genet 1973; 10:288.

212. Ellis NA. The human Y chromosome. Semin Dev Biol 1991; 2:231.

213. Josso N, Briard MI. Embryonic testicular regression syndrome: variable phenotypic expression in siblings. J Pediatr 1985; 97:200.

214. Schulte MJ. Positive H-Y antigen testing in a case of XY gonadal absence syndrome. Clin Genet 1979; 16:438.

215. Duck SC, Sekkan GS, Wilbois R, et al. Pseudo-hermaphroditism with testes and 46,XX karyotypes. J Pediatr 1975; 87:58.

216. Berthezene F, Forest MG, Grimaud JA, et al. Leydig cell agenesis: a cause of male pseudohermaphroditism. N Engl J Med 1976; 295:969.

217. Brown DM, Markland C, Dehner LP. Leydig cell hypoplasia: a case of male pseudohermaphroditism. J Clin Endocrinol Metab 1978; 36:1.

218. Pérez-Palacios G, Scaglia HE, Kofman-Afaro S, et al. Inherited male pseudohermaphroditism due to gonadotrophin unresponsiveness. Acta Endocrinol (Copenh) 1982; 98:148.

219. Schwartz M, Imperato-McGinley J, Peterson RE, et al. Male pseudohermaphroditism secondary to an abnormality in Leydig cell differentiation. J Clin Endocrinol Metab 1981; 53:123.

220. Lee PA, Rock JA, Brown TR, et al. Leydig cell hypofunction resulting in male pseudohermaphroditism. Fertil Steril 1982; 37:675.

221. Saldanha PH, Arnhold IJP, Mendonca BB, et al. A clinico-genetic investigation of Leydig cell hypoplasia. Am J Med Genet 1987; 26:337.

222. Martens JW, Verhoef-Post M, Abelin N, et al. A homozygous mutation in the luteinizing hormone receptor gene causes partial Leydig cell hypoplasia: correlation between receptor activity and phenotype. Mol Endocrinol 1998; 12:775.

223. Themmen AP, Martens JW, Brunner HG. Activating and inactivating mutations in LH receptors. Mol Cell Endocrinol 1998; 145:137.

224. Salameh W, Shoukair M, Keswani A, et al. Evidence for a deletion in the LH receptor gene in a case of Leydig cell aplasia. Paper presented at: 77th Annual Meeting of the Endocrine Society; June 14–17, 1995; Washington, DC. Abstract P2-150:328.

225. Kirkland R, Kirkland JL, Johnson CM, et al. Congenital lipoid adrenal hyperplasia in an 8-year-old phenotypic female. J Clin Endocrinol Metab 1973; 36:488.

226. Degenhart HJ. Prader's syndrome (congenital lipoid adrenal hyperplasia). In: Laron Z, ed. Adrenal disease in childhood: pediatric adolescence endocrinology. Basel: S Karger, 1984:125.

227. Frydman M, Kauschansky A, Zamir R, et al. Familial lipoid adrenal hyperplasia: genetic marker data and an approach to prenatal diagnosis. Am J Med Genet 1986; 25:319.

228. Chung BC, Matteson KJ, Voutilainen R, et al. Human cholesterol side-chain cleavage enzyme P450scc: cDNA cloning assignment of the gene to chromosome 15 and expression in the placenta. Proc Natl Acad Sci U S A 1986; 83:892.

229. Lin D, Gitelman SE, Saenger P, et al. Normal genes for the cholesterol side chain cleavage enzyme. P450scc, in congenital lipoid adrenal hyperplasia. J Clin Invest 1991; 88:1955.

230. Bose HS, Sugawara T, Strauss JF III, Miller WL. The pathophysiology and genetics of congenital lipoid adrenal hyperplasia. N Engl J Med 1996; 335:1870.

231. Perrone L, Criscuolo T, Sinisi AA, et al. Male pseudohermaphroditism due to 3β-hydroxysteroid dehydrogenase-isomerase deficiency associated with atrial septal defect. Acta Endocrinol (Copenh) 1985; 110:532.

232. Bongiovanni AM. Further studies of congenital adrenal hyperplasia due to 3β-hydroxysteroid dehydrogenase deficiency. In: Vallet HL, Porter IH, eds. Genetic mechanisms of sexual development. New York: Academic Press, 1979:189.

233. Cravioto, MD, Ulloa-Aguirre A, Bermudez JA, et al. A new inherited variant of the 3 beta-hydroxysteroid dehydrogenase-isomerase deficiency syndrome: evidence for existence of two isoenzymes. J Clin Endocrinol Metab 1986; 63:360.

234. Chang YT, Kappy MS, Iwamoto K, et al. Mutations in the type II 3β-hydroxysteroid dehydrogenase gene in a patient with classic salt-wasting 3β-hydroxysteroid dehydrogenase deficiency congenital adrenal hyperplasia. Pediatr Res 1993; 34:698.

235. Rhéaume E, Simard J, Morel Y, et al. Congenital adrenal hyperplasia due to point mutations in the type II 3β-hydroxysteroid dehydrogenase gene. Nat Genet 1992; 1:239.

236. Simard J, Rhéaume E, Sanchez R, et al. Molecular basis of congenital adrenal hyperplasia due to 3 beta-hydroxysteroid dehydrogenase deficiency. Mol Endocrinol 1993; 7:716.

237. Heremans GFP, Moolenaar AJ, Van Geldren HM. Female phenotype in a male child due to 17α-hydroxylase deficiency. Arch Dis Child 1976; 51:721.

238. Yanase T, Simpson ER, Waterman MR. 17α-hydroxylase/17,20-lyase deficiency: from clinical investigation to molecular definition. Endocr Rev 1991; 12:91.

239. Zachmann M, Vollmin JA, Hamilton W, et al. Steroid 17,20-desmolase deficiency: a new cause of male pseudohermaphroditism. Clin Endocrinol (Oxf) 1972; 1:369.

240. Nebert DW, Nelson DR, Adesnik M, et al. The P-450 superfamily: updated listing of all genes and recommended nomenclature for the chromosomal loci. DNA 1989; 8:1.

241. Biason A, Mantero F, Scaroni C, et al. Deletion within the CYP17 gene together with insertion of foreign DNA is the cause of combined complete 17 alpha-hydroxylase/17,20-lyase deficiency in an Italian patient. Mol Endocrinol 1991; 5:2037.

242. Geller DH, Auchus RJ, Mendonca BB, et al. The genetic and functional basis of isolated 17,20-lyase deficiency. Nat Genet 1997; 17:201.

243. Scaroni C, Biason A, Carpene G, et al. 17-alpha-hydroxylase deficiency in three siblings: short- and long-term studies. J Endocrinol Invest 1991; 14:99.

244. Yanase T, Sasano H, Yubisui T, et al. Immunohistochemical study of cytochrome b5 in human adrenal gland and in adrenocortical adenomas from patients with Cushing's syndrome. Endocr J 1998; 5:89.

245. Yanase T, Sanders D, Shibata A, et al. Combined 17α-hydroxylase/17,20-lyase deficiency due to a 7-basepair duplication in the N-terminal region of the cytochrome P450 17alpha(CYP17) gene. J Clin Endocrinol Metab 1990; 70:1325.

246. Kagimoto K, Waterman MR, Kagimoto M, et al. Identification of a common molecular basis for combined 17α-hydroxylase/17,20-lyase deficiency in two Mennonite families. Hum Genet 1989; 82:285.

247. Rumsby G, Skinner C, Lee HA, et al. Combined 17α-hydroxylase/17,20-lyase deficiency caused by heterozygous stop codons in the cytochrome P450 17α-hydroxylase gene. Clin Endocrinol (Oxf) 1993; 39:483.

248. Balducci R, Toscano V, Wright F, et al. Familial male pseudohermaphroditism with gynecomastia due to 17β-hydroxysteroid dehydrogenase deficiency: a report of three cases. Clin Endocrinol (Oxf) 1985; 23:439.

249. Imperato-McGinley J, Peterson RE, Stoller R, et al. Male pseudohermaphroditism secondary to 17α-hydroxysteroid dehydrogenase deficiency: gender role with puberty. J Clin Endocrinol Metab 1979; 49:391.

250. Pang S, Softness B, Sweeney WJ III, New MI. Hirsutism, polycystic ovarian disease, and ovarian 17-ketosteroid reductase deficiency. N Engl J Med 1987; 316:1295.

251. Toscano V, Balducci R, Bianchi P, et al. Ovarian 17-ketosteroid reductase deficiency as a possible cause of polycystic ovarian disease. J Clin Endocrinol Metab 1990; 71:288.

252a. Luu-The V, Labrie C, Simard J, et al. Structure of two in tandem human 17β-hydroxysteroid dehydrogenase genes. Med Endocrinol 1990; 4:268.

253. Peterson RE, Imperato-McGinley J, Gautier T, et al. Male pseudohermaphroditism due to multiple defects in steroid-biosynthetic microsomal mixed-function oxidases: a new variant of congenital adrenal hyperplasia. N Engl J Med 1985; 313:1182.

254. Roger M, Merceron RE, Girard F. Dexamethasone-suppressible hypercortisteroidism in two 46,XX subjects with ambiguous genitalia and ovarian cysts: partial defect of 17α-hydroxylase or 17,20-desmolase. Horm Res 1982; 16:23.

255. Morris JM. The syndrome of testicular feminization in male pseudohermaphrodites. Am J Obstet Gynecol 1953; 65:1192.

256. Shull BL, Taylor PT. Testicular feminization syndrome: a case study of four generations. South Med J 1989; 82:251.

257. Brown CJ, Goss SJ, Lubahn DB, et al. Androgen receptor locus on the human X chromosome: regional localization to Xq11–12 and description of a DNA polymorphism. Am J Hum Genet 1989; 44:264.

258. Imperato-McGinley J, Ip NY, Gautier T, et al. DNA linkage analysis and studies of the androgen receptor gene in a large kindred with complete androgen insensitivity. Am J Med Genet 1990; 36:104.

258a. Choi C, Kim KC, Kim HO. Androgen receptor gene mutation identified by PCR–SSCP and sequencing in 4 patients with complete androgen insensitivity syndrome. Arch Gynecol Obstet 2000; 263:201.

259. Prior L, Bordet S, Trifèro MA, et al. Replacement of arginine 773 by cysteine or histidine in the human androgen receptor causes complete androgen insensitivity with different receptor phenotypes. Am J Hum Genet 1992; 51:143.

260. Griffin JE. Androgen resistance—the clinical and molecular spectrum. N Engl J Med 1992; 326:611.

261. Quigley CA, Friedman KJ, Johnson A, et al. Complete deletion of the androgen receptor gene: definition of the null phenotype of the androgen insensitivity syndrome and determination of carrier status. J Clin Endocrinol Metab 1992; 74:927.

262. Marcelli M, Zoppi S, Grino PB, et al. A mutation in the DNA-binding domain of the androgen receptor gene causes complete testicular feminization in a patient with receptor-positive androgen resistance. J Clin Invest 1991; 87:1123.

263. Sultan C, Lumbroso S, Poujol N, et al. Mutations of androgen receptor gene in androgen insensitivity syndromes. J Steroid Biochem Mol Biol 1993; 46:519.

264. Ulloa-Aquirre A, Mendez JP, Angeles A, et al. The presence of müllerian remnants in the complete androgen insensitivity syndrome: a steroid hormone-mediated defect? Fertil Steril 1987; 45:302.

265. Morris JM, Mahesh VB. Further observations on the syndrome "testicular feminization." Am J Obstet Gynecol 1963; 87:731.

266. Pinsky L, Kaufman M, Levitzsky LL. Partial androgen resistance due to a distinctive qualitative defect of the androgen receptor. Am J Med Genet 1987; 27:459.

267. Zoppi S, Marcelli M, Deslypere J-P, et al. Amino acid substitutions in the DNA-binding domain of the human androgen receptor are a frequent cause of receptor-binding positive androgen resistance. Mol Endocrinol 1992; 6:409.

268. McPhaul MJ, Marcelli M, Zoppi S, et al. Genetic basis of endocrine disease. 4. The spectrum of mutations in the androgen receptor gene that causes androgen resistance. J Clin Endocrinol Metab 1993; 76:17.

269. Sultan C. Androgen receptors and partial androgen insensitivity in male pseudohermaphroditism. Ann Genet 1986; 79:5.

270. Wilson JD, Harrod MJ, Goldstein JL, et al. Familial incomplete male pseudohermaphroditism, type 1. N Engl J Med 1974; 290:1097.

271. Wilson JD, Carlson BR, Weaver DD, et al. Endocrine and genetic characterization of cousins with male pseudohermaphroditism: evidence that the Lubs phenotype can result from a mutation that alters the structure of the androgen receptor. Clin Genet 1984; 26:363.

271a. Ahmed SF, Cheng A, Doves L, et al. Phenotypic features, androgen receptor binding, and mutational analysis in 278 clinical cases reported as androgen insensitivity syndrome. Clin Endocrinol Metab 2000; 85:658.

272. Bowen P, Lee CSN, Migeon CJ, et al. Hereditary male pseudohermaphroditism with hypogonadism, hypospadias, and gynecomastia (Reifenstein's syndrome). Ann Intern Med 1965; 62:252.

273. Amrhein JA, Klingensmith GJ, Walsh PC, et al. Partial androgen insensitivity: the Reifenstein syndrome revisited. N Engl J Med 1977; 297:350.

274. Smith EP, Boyd J, Frank GR, et al. Estrogen resistance caused by a mutation in the estrogen-receptor gene in a man. N Engl J Med 1994 331(16):1056.

275. Korach KS, Couse JF, Curtis SW, et al. Estrogen receptor gene disruption: molecular characterization and experimental and clinical phenotypes. Recent Prog Horm Res 1996; 51:159.

276. Simpson JL, New M, Peterson RE, et al. Pseudovaginal perineoscrotal hypospadias (PPSH) in sibs. Birth Defects 1971; 7(6):140.

277. Opitz JM, Simpson JL, Sarto GE, et al. Pseudovaginal perineoscrotal hypospadias. Clin Genet 1972; 3:1.

278. Imperato-McGinley J, Guerrero L, Gauiter T, et al. Steroid 5α-reductase deficiency: an inherited form of male pseudohermaphroditism. Science 1974; 186:1213.

279. Walsh PC, Madden JD, Harrod MJ, et al. Familial incomplete male pseudohermaphroditism, type 2. N Engl J Med 1974; 291:944.

280. Peterson RE, Imperato-McGinley J, Gautier T, et al. Male pseudohermaphroditism due to steroid 5α-reductase deficiency. Am J Med 1977; 62:170.

281. Fisher LK, Kogut MD, Moore RJ, et al. Clinical, endocrinological, and enzymatic characterization of two patients with 5α-reductase deficiency: evidence that a single enzyme is responsible for the 5α-reduction of cortisol and testosterone. J Clin Endocrinol Metab 1978; 47:653.

282. Akgun S, Ertel NH, Imperato-McGinley J, et al. Familial male pseudohermaphroditism in Turkish village due to 5α-reductase deficiency. Am J Med 1986; 81:267.

283. Labrie F, Sugimoto Y, Luu-The V, et al. Structure of human type II 5α-reductase gene. Endocrinology 1992; 131:1571.

284. Andersson S, Berman DM, Jenkins EP, Russell DW. Deletion of steroid 5α-reductase 2 gene in male pseudohermaphroditism. Nature 1991; 354:159.

285. Thigpen AE, Davis DL, Milatovich A, et al. Molecular genetics of steroid 5α-reductase 2 deficiency. Clin Invest 1992; 90:799.

286. Leshin M, Griffin JE, Wilson JD. Hereditary male pseudohermaphroditism associated with unstable form of 5α-reductase. J Clin Invest 1978; 62:685.

287. Greene S, Zachmann M, Manella B, et al. Comparison of two tests to recognize or exclude 5 alpha-reductase deficiency in prepubertal children. Acta Endocrinol (Copenh) 1987; 114:113.

288. Imperato-McGinley J, Gautier T, Pichardo M, et al. The diagnosis of 5 alpha-reductase deficiency in infancy. J Clin Endocrinol Metab 1986; 63:1313.

289. Cai L-Q, Fratianni CM, Gautier T, Imperato-McGinley J. Dihydrotestosterone regulation of semen in male pseudohermaphrodites with 5α-reductase-2 deficiency. J Clin Endocrinol Metab 1994; 79:409.

290. Pinsky L, Kaufman M. Genetics of steroid receptors and their disorders. Adv Hum Genet 1987; 16:299.

291. Mowszowicz I, Wright F, Vincens M, et al. Androgen metabolism in hirsute patients treated with cyproterone acetate. J Steroid Biochem 1984; 20:757.

292. Corvol P, Michaud A, Menard J, et al. Antiandrogenic effect of spironolactone: mechanism of action. Endocrinology 1975; 97:51.

293. Menard RH, Guenthner TM, Kon H, Gillette JR. Studies on the destruction of adrenal and testicular cytochrome P-450 by spironolactone. Requirement for the 7α-thio group and evidence for the loss of the heme and apoproteins of cytochrome P-450. J Biol Chem 1979; 254:1726.

294. Rittmaster RS. Finasteride. N Engl J Med 1994; 330:120.

295. Simard J, Luthy I, Guay J, et al. Characteristics of interaction of the antiandrogen flutamide and the androgen receptor in various target tissues. Mol Cell Endocrinol 1986; 44:261.

296. Brochu M, Belanger A, Dupont A, et al. Effects of flutamide and aminoglutethimide on plasma 5α-reduced steroid glucuronide concentrations in castrated patients with cancer of the prostate. J Steroid Biochem 1987; 28:619.

297. Sweet RA, Schrott HG, Kurland R, et al. Study of the incidence of hypospadias in Rochester, Minnesota, 1940–1970, and a case control comparison of possible etiologic factors. Mayo Clin Proc 1974; 49:52.

298. Curry CJR, Carey JC, Holland JS, et al. Smith-Lemi-Opitz syndrome: type II: multiple congenital anomalies with male pseudohermaphroditism and frequent early lethality. Am J Med Genet 1987; 26:45.

299. Lee MM, Donahoe PK. Ambiguous genitalia. In: Bardin CW, ed. Current therapy in endocrinology and metabolism, 5th ed. St. Louis: Mosby–Year Book, 1994:242.

300. Burstein S, Grumbach MM, Kaplan SL. Early determination of androgen responsiveness is important to the management of microphallus. Lancet 1979; 2:983.

301. Hricak H, Chang YCF, Thurnher S. Vagina evaluation with MR imaging. Part I: normal anatomy and congenital anomalies. Radiology 1991; 179:593.

# CHAPTER 91

# PHYSIOLOGY OF PUBERTY

PETER A. LEE

## DEFINITION OF PUBERTY

Puberty is the period of life from the first signs of sexual maturation until the final attainment of physical, mental, and emotional maturity. Numerous physical changes accompany the changes in the hypothalamic–pituitary–gonadal (HPG) axis and occur in an orderly sequence over a definite time during normal puberty.

Puberty represents the final step in the process of maturation of the HPG axis (Table 91-1); this process begins in fetal life, with control centered in the central nervous system (CNS). Gonadotropin release is episodic in response to the periodic release of gonadotropin-releasing hormone (GnRH) from cells within the hypothalamus.

GnRH is the releasing factor that controls the gonadotropin subunit gene expression of the pituitary and ultimately luteinizing hormone (LH) and follicle-stimulating hormone (FSH) release. GnRH is synthesized in only ~1000 neurons in the hypothalamus. The mechanisms regulating the control of the synthesis and secretion of GnRH in these neurons via the intricate interconnections of the neuroendocrine system are not well understood, partly because of the paucity of neurons scattered throughout the hypothalamus. The transcriptional and translational events that regulate GnRH biosynthesis are unknown.

The control of GnRH is believed to reside within a *GnRH oscillator* or *pulse generator*, a center involving intercommunications of GnRH-producing cells. Which neuronal structures and chemical interactions result in pulsatile GnRH release are unknown. The pulse generator appears to involve norepinephrine (NE) and NE transporter (the protein for presynaptic reuptake of NE). Numerous signals, both stimulatory and inhibitory, influence the pulse generator. Stimulatory signals for GnRH neuronal activities include NE and neuropeptide Y, and a subtype of glutamate receptor that selectively binds *N*-methyl-D-aspartate (NMDA). Inhibitory signals include β-endorphin, interleukin-1, and γ-aminobutyric acid (GABA). GABA inhibits GnRH secretion by NMDA receptors.

Pubertal maturation begins with a significant upsurge of the gonadotropin secretion that develops during fetal life, persists into infancy, and then enters a period of relative quiescence during childhood years. Enhanced intermittent release of LH and FSH, which marks the onset of puberty, is a result of, and reflective of, episodic release of GnRH from the hypothalamus in greater quantities and in more frequent pulses under CNS control.

Because damage to the CNS may result in early puberty, the facilitatory mechanisms appear to be operational during childhood, although during normal childhood the inhibitory or restraining mechanisms are superimposed.[1-4]

## HYPOTHALAMIC–PITUITARY–GONADAL DEVELOPMENT

### FETAL PERIOD

GnRH is present in the hypothalamus and LH and FSH are present in the pituitary, and responsive to GnRH, by 10 weeks of gestation.[1] Hypothalamic GnRH and pituitary and plasma LH and FSH levels increase until midgestation, progressively stimulating gonadal maturation and hormone production. After midgestation, hypothalamic GnRH content, pituitary LH and FSH content, and serum FSH levels are greater for several weeks in the female fetus than in the male fetus; this establishes a relative sex difference early and is related to the negative feedback of the testosterone synthesized by the fetal testes. Although fetal testosterone production is necessary for male genital differentiation, whether it causes gender-specific differentiation of the male hypothalamus and pituitary is unclear. For example, adults of both genders are capable of positive feedback gonadotropin release in response to estrogens; therefore, positive feedback in the ovulating female may arise from the hormonal milieu rather than from hypothalamic differentiation. Unlike in male development, ovarian steroidogenesis, although present during fetal life, is unnecessary for female

**TABLE 91-1.**
**Status of Hypothalamic–Pituitary–Gonadal Axis During Human Development**

| | Fetal | Infancy | Childhood | Onset of Puberty | Puberty | Adulthood |
|---|---|---|---|---|---|---|
| LH response to GnRH | | Present | ++ | ++ → +++ | +++ → ++++ | ++++ |
| FSH response to GnRH | | | +++ | +++ | +++, ++++ | ++++ |
| Circulating gonadotropins | | | | | | |
|   Mean | 0 → ++ | +++ | + | + → ++ | ++ → ++++ | ++++ |
|   Episodic | | | + | + → ++ | ++ → ++++ | ++++ |
|   Nocturnal | | | + | + | + | |
| Gonadal response to gonadotropins | 0 → +++ | +++ | + (↑ with priming) | + → ++ | ++ → ++++ | ++++ |
| Circulating gonadal steroids | 0 → ++++ | +++ → + | + | + → ++ | ++ → ++++ | ++++ |
| Circulating adrenal androgens | 0 → ++++ | ++++ → + | + → ++ | ++ → +++ | +++ → ++++ | ++++ |
| Feedback sensitivity to sex steroids | 0 → ++, + | + → +++ | ++++ | +++ | ++ → + | + |
| Positive feedback to estrogen | | | | | | |
|   Males | | | | | | + |
|   Females | | | | | − → + | + |

*LH*, luteinizing hormone; *GnRH*, gonadotropin-releasing hormone; *FSH*, follicle-stimulating hormone.

genital differentiation. Nevertheless, gonadotropin stimulation may be required for normal ovarian development with oocyte and primordial follicle production. Whether estrogen is required for sex-specific differentiation of the female hypothalamus and pituitary is unclear. Observations in humans and animal experiments suggest that gonadal steroids do affect differentiation of the CNS–hypothalamus–pituitary in the fetus and the timing of puberty.[5]

## NEONATAL AND CHILDHOOD PERIOD

Hormonal dynamics during the neonatal period reveal considerable HPG maturation.[1] At birth, gonadotropin and sex steroid levels are high, but these levels decline during the first few days. Gonadotropin levels begin to rise again before 1 week of life, suggesting a negative feedback response to the decline in circulating levels of sex steroids originating from the placenta. During the next several weeks, plasma levels of LH and FSH are higher than during the rest of childhood in both sexes (female levels, particularly of FSH, are greater than male levels). Levels of testosterone in males and, less dramatically, levels of estradiol in females are also higher for children at this age than for older children, a finding that suggests pituitary gonadotropin stimulation of gonadal steroidogenesis. These data indicate that gonadotropin secretion, gonadal response with steroid production, and negative feedback mechanisms are all functional at this age. Circulating levels of gonadotropins and sex steroids peak at 2 to 3 months, after which they begin to drop to the low levels that persist for several years.

*Inhibin B*, the biologically active inhibin among males that appears to be produced primarily by Sertoli cells, also rises to peak levels at ~3 months. Concentrations gradually fall over the next year or more; thus, the profile is more extended than for LH, FSH, or testosterone. Inhibin B may play a crucial role in seminiferous tubule development at this age.[6,7]

The fall in these hormone levels cannot be explained simply by an adjustment of the negative feedback mechanism, because a similar pattern with a drop in gonadotropin levels occurs among agonadal children. This phenomenon suggests that gonadotropin secretion is controlled by CNS differentiation and that sex steroid feedback is not an obligatory element in the decreased secretion during childhood. Although gonadotropin levels are lowest during midchildhood, levels usually are not only measurable and not completely suppressed but also indicate episodic release and diurnal (sleep-enhanced) variation.[2] Furthermore, gender differences persist, with female FSH levels being greater than male levels. Sex steroids, including estradiol,[8] and also inhibin may be detectable at very low levels in some children.

## PUBERTY

### GONADOTROPIN-RELEASING HORMONE AND GONADOTROPINS

As noted, the HPG axis is active beginning early in fetal life. Potentially, the gonad is capable of adult hormonal and germinal function throughout childhood and will respond if stimulated with pubertal or adult levels of gonadotropins. The pituitary in the prepubertal child can also secrete gonadotropin whenever stimulated with GnRH. The pituitary is capable of adult function; thus, the restraint of pubertal maturation lies at the level of GnRH secretion or higher CNS loci. Because the pituitary and gonad are ready to respond, the controlling level is expressed by the magnitude and frequency of GnRH stimulation.

The increasing mean levels of gonadotropins that precede the onset and continue during the progression of puberty result from increased secretion of gonadotropins in an episodic fashion, reflective of episodic GnRH secretion. This change in GnRH stimulation initiates the increased secretion of gonadotropins of puberty. Prepubertal children already have an episodic pattern of gonadotropin release, with infrequent pulses of low amplitude and greater secretion occurring during sleep. As pubertal maturation approaches, the episodic pattern becomes more regular and pulses attain a greater amplitude. This enhanced episodic pattern of puberty initially becomes apparent during sleep, already the time of increased activity during childhood.[1,2,9–13] Just before the clinical onset of puberty and during early puberty, episodic pulses and mean levels are distinctly higher during sleep than during wakefulness. These changes are more dramatic for LH than FSH, with the relative rise of LH being much greater than that of FSH during puberty. In the mature individual the LH episodic release occurs approximately every 90 minutes, with peak levels persisting for <20 minutes. The increases in FSH above the mean basal levels are less apparent, although episodic release occurs and values are greater during sleep than during waking hours.

The maturation of CNS-stimulating influences affecting the GnRH pulse generator or oscillator produces these episodic phenomena without the need for gonadal feedback, because a similarly enhanced episodic pattern occurs at the same age among agonadal individuals. The episodic release of gonadotropins causes mean gonadotropin levels to rise progressively throughout puberty in males and in females until the onset of menstrual cycling. This episodic release gradually becomes characteristic of the full 24-hour day, not only of sleep hours. Regular daytime pulses are first seen in females at the time of the onset of breast development.

Pubertal change of the hypothalamus and pituitary, therefore, involves the accentuation rather than the onset of the episodic secretion of GnRH, LH, and FSH. The intermittent bolus secretion of GnRH (12–18 per 24 hours) is regulated by a *neural "oscillator"* localized to the region of the arcuate nucleus of the medial basal hypothalamus. At the onset of puberty, the GnRH stimulus exerts a priming effect on the pituitary and causes a progressively greater release of gonadotropins. This increased responsiveness accompanies an increase in pituitary GnRH receptors. Both immunoreactive and bioactive LH increase during pubertal maturation, with a relatively greater rise of bioactive LH in both girls and boys.[14,15] The rise of immunoreactive FSH is more modest than that of LH in both sexes, with bioactive elevations significant in girls but not in boys. The difference in bioeffects may relate to changes in isoforms of gonadotropins during puberty.[16] Adult levels of LH and FSH are regulated by gonadal hormone secretions through a negative feedback effect and, in the presence of abrupt changes of estrogen and progesterone levels, as during the middle of the menstrual cycle, through a positive feedback. Inhibin concentrations, which rise throughout male and female puberty, also play a role in negative feedback of FSH secretion.[7,17–20] Müllerian inhibiting hormone levels progressively fall during puberty in males and appear to be inversely related to levels of gonadotropins and androgens.[21,22]

## SEX STEROIDS

The initial rise of circulating levels of gonadotropins and of the sex steroids of gonadal and adrenal cortical origin occurs before the clinical onset of puberty. The increase of adrenal androgen production, *adrenarche*, may be responsible for the onset of pubic hair growth, *pubarche*. The increase in gonadal sex steroid production in response to gonadotropin stimulation is known as *gonadarche*.

**Adrenarche.** Adrenarche is usually the first recognizable hormonal change of puberty. Elevated plasma levels of adrenal androgens, initially dehydroepiandrosterone sulfate[23] followed by dehydroepiandrosterone and androstenedione, are evident before any other hormonal evidence of pubertal maturation and precede the clinical evidence of adrenarche. The appearance of pubic and axillary hair, body odor, and mild acne may result from adrenal androgen secretion, because these findings may occur without gonadal steroidogenesis and before other clinical evidence of pubertal development.

The cause of adrenarche is uncertain. However, it does not occur because of increased gonadotropin stimulation. Although adrenocorticotropic hormone (ACTH) secretion does not increase at the age of adrenarche, the pattern of steroid response to ACTH stimulation changes. Proportionally greater adrenal androgen is produced in relation to other adrenal steroids, a phenomenon that parallels the development of the zona reticularis of the adrenal cortex. The developmental pattern of adrenal androgen production resembles that of HPG activity. After fetal development of this adrenal cortex zone, and the resultant fetal-neonatal adrenal androgen production, a regression of the zone occurs and androgen production decreases until puberty. Adrenarche generally precedes gonadarche; therefore, adrenal androgens possibly play a nonobligatory stimulatory role in the maturation of the HPG axis.

**Gonadarche.** Gonadarche is marked by the elevation of the mean circulating levels of testosterone in the male and of estrogen in the female. This change follows an increase in gonadotropin secretion, with testosterone levels peaking at night and estradiol levels peaking in the daytime.[24] FSH stimulates follicular growth and maturation in the female and seminiferous tubular growth and maturation in the male. Because the seminiferous tubules make up the bulk of the testis, testicular enlargement is the first sign of pubertal development among males.

## INFLUENCE OF OTHER FACTORS

*Leptin*, an adipocyte-derived hormone, appears to play a role in the regulation of body composition. Because leptin levels increase

### TABLE 91-2.
#### Sequence of First Occurrence of Events of Puberty Among Females

|  | Mean Age* (Years) | Age Range† (Years) |
|---|---|---|
| Stage 2 onset of breast development (breast budding and elevated contour, broadened areolar diameter) | 10.0–10.5 | 7.0–13.5 |
| Stage 2 onset of pubic hair growth (pigmented, primarily labial) | 10.3–10.8 | 7.5–13.5 |
| Maximum growth rate | 11.2–11.7 | 9.7–13.5 |
| Maximum rate of weight gain | 11.7–12.2 | 9.9–14.4 |
| Stage 3 breast development (enlargement of breast and areolae) | 11.3–11.8 | 9.0–14.0 |
| Stage 3 pubic hair (over mons pubis) | 11.4–11.9 | 9.2–14.0 |
| Onset of axillary hair | 12.3–12.8 | 10.0–14.5 |
| Onset of acne | 12.5–13.0 | 12.0–14.3 |
| Menarche | 12.6–13.1 | 10.0–16.0 |
| Stage 4 breast development (often secondary mound of areola) | 12.5–13.0 | 10.5–14.5 |
| Stage 4 pubic hair (adult density but not distribution) | 12.5–13.0 | 10.5–15.0 |
| Regular menstrual cycles | 13.7–14.2 | 12.0–17.0+ |
| Stage 5 pubic hair (adult) | 14.0–14.5 | 12.5–16.0 |
| Stage 5 breast development (adult) | 14.0–14.5 | 11.5–16.0 |

*Mean age is expressed as a half-year interval.
†Racial differences exist.

among both males and females before pubertal hormones increase, the hypothesis has been put forward that this molecule may trigger the onset of puberty. This is of interest in light of the long-held hypothesis that body mass and composition are related to the onset of puberty. Although most data do not support this hypothesis, clearly body fat distribution is related to hormone levels during early puberty. Nevertheless, no clear data exist to indicate that leptin is a factor related to the initiation of puberty. Leptin levels are always lower in boys than in girls, perhaps reflecting differences in body fat content. In fact, no gender differences are seen in leptin, independent of adiposity.[25,26] Leptin levels decline in boys when levels of testosterone, whether endogenous or exogenous, increase.[25,27]

A nonsteroidal peptide, *activin*,[19] appears to play an important role in regulation of follicular secretion and atresia. Another peptide, *follistatin*,[19] is activin bound and may contribute to reproductive physiology by regulating the bioactivity of activin. Circulating levels of follistatin do not change during puberty but are higher in adulthood than during childhood and puberty.[28]

Excessive exercise, inadequate protein-calorie nutrition (either because of unavailability, CNS-related anorexia, or chronic illness), psychiatric illness such as anorexia nervosa before or after nutritional insufficiency, and other forms of emotional or physical stress are associated with hypogonadotropic status, whether at the age of pubertal development or later (see Chap 128).

The clinical observation has also been made that exposure of prepubertal children to sex steroids may hasten the onset of pubertal hormone secretion. This may impact the GnRH pulse generator.[29]

# FEMALE PUBERTY

## PATTERN OF ONSET

The mean developmental pattern of female puberty is outlined in Table 91-2 and Figure 91-1*A*, with the mean ages and age ranges given for each event.[30–32] Pubertal events have occurred progressively earlier over this century, partly paralleling the generally better socioeconomic conditions, especially nutri-

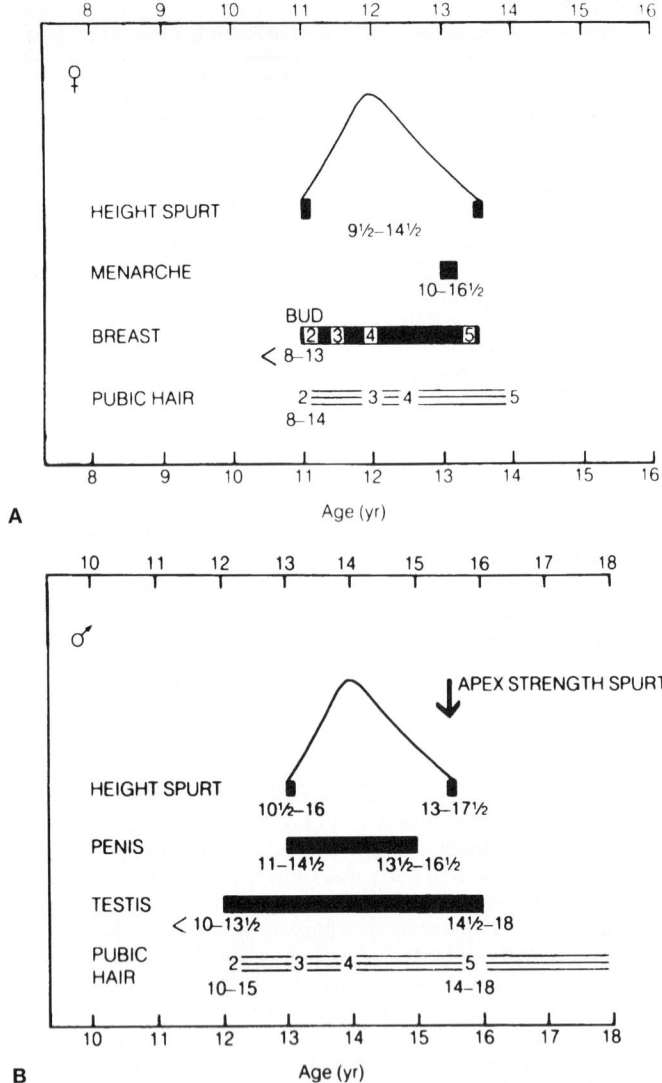

**A**

**B**

**FIGURE 91-1.** Typical sequence of events at adolescence in girls (**A**) and boys (**B**) in relation to average age. The range of age at which the changes occur is also given. The numbers within the pubic hair and breast developmental sequences refer to stages of puberty (see Fig. 91-2). The age ranges differ somewhat in different population groups. (Adapted from Marshall WA, Tanner JM. Variation in pattern of pubertal changes in boys. Arch Dis Child 1970; 45:13; Clin Endocrinol Metab 1986; 15:433.)

tional status. Racial differences exist in the onset and progression of puberty,[32] although no clearly representative longitudinal or cross-sectional data exist concerning the onset and progression of puberty. The initial physical signs of puberty, both breast and pubic hair development, begin among the earliest maturers at younger ages than previously thought.[32] This may occur because the ovaries are not completely quiescent during childhood and because FSH secretion is substantial during childhood, at least when compared with LH secretion. The transition from childhood to puberty appears to be subtle and gradual. Although physical changes of puberty may begin at younger ages than previously realized, significant progression may initially be slower, because the mean age and age range of menarche have not changed (see Table 91-2).

Pubertal development generally has been classified into *five stages*[33] (Fig. 91-2), with stage 1 being the prepubertal state and stage 5 adulthood. Mean plasma hormone levels correlated with the five stages of development for females are listed in Table 91-3.[2,20,24,34,35]

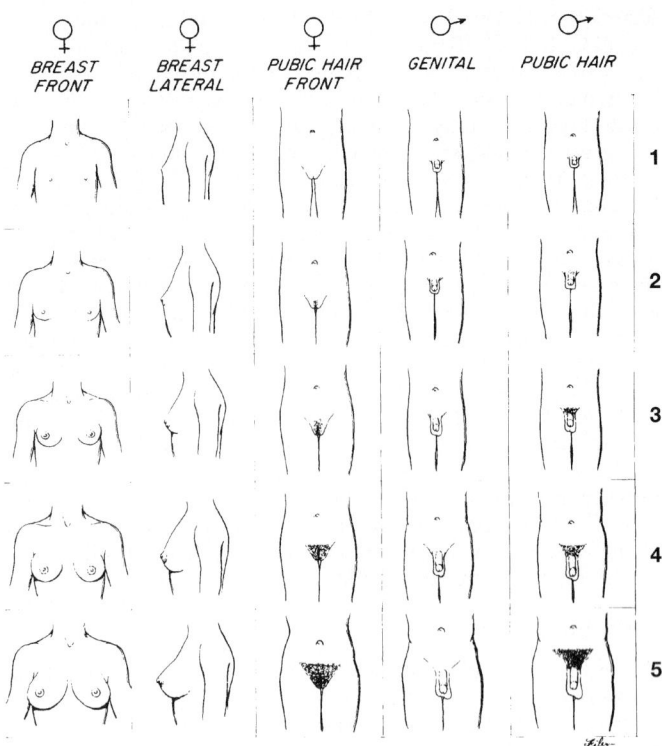

**FIGURE 91-2.** Five stages of puberty for females and males with two staging criteria for each sex. Stage 1 is prepuberty and stage 5 is adulthood.

The average age for the physical onset of puberty in girls is ~10 years, with the appearance of breast budding (*thelarche*). This occurs after a rise of mean circulating gonadotropin and estradiol levels and is marked by an increase of areolar diameter, a small elevation of the nipple and surrounding breast tissue, and the appearance of palpable tissue centered beneath the areolae (stage 2 of breast development). Breast budding may initially occur unilaterally; and in some instances, breast growth proceeds asymmetrically. Differences in size may persist past the pubertal years.

The next noticeable change in female puberty is usually the onset of pubic hair growth. The long pigmented pubic hair is considerably more coarse than the body hair of childhood, which may be more apparent in the genital region. Female pubic hair usually occurs first along the labia majora. This constitutes stage 2 of pubic hair development. Usually, pubic hair appears ~6 months after breast budding, although occasionally it precedes breast budding and constitutes the first evidence of pubertal development. Because breast development reflects the progressive increase of estrogen stimulation, whereas sexual hair reflects increased androgens, the five stages of breast development usually do not coincide exactly with the five stages of pubic hair development, although they generally overlap. Because of this nonparallelism, breast and pubic hair staging should be done separately.

## BREAST STAGING

The criteria for breast staging are illustrated in Figure 91-2. In stage 1, the prepubertal state, no breast tissue is palpable, and areolae are generally <2 cm in diameter. The nipples are only a few millimeters in diameter and may be relatively flat, inverted, or raised, although the papillae may be slightly raised from the chest contour. Stage 2 is first recognizable by the appearance of a visible and palpable mound of breast and papillae with increased areolar diameter. The skin of the areola becomes thinner. The nipple may be developed to various degrees. Stage 3 is expressed by further growth and elevation of the entire breast. Stage 4 includes further

**TABLE 91-3.**
**Mean and Range\* of Plasma Hormone Levels During Female Pubertal Development (Composite Breast–Pubic Hair Staging)**

| | Prepubertal Stage 1 | Stage 2 | Stage 3 | Stage 4 | Stage 5 *Phase* | |
|---|---|---|---|---|---|---|
| LH (mIU/mL) | 2.7 (<1.0–5.5) | 4.2 (<1.0–9.0) | 6.7 (<1.0–14.6) | 7.7 (2.8–15.0) | Follicular | 7.6 (3–18) |
| | | | | | Luteal | 6.6 (3–18) |
| (U/L)† | <0.1 (<0.1–0.2) | 0.7 (<0.1–2.8) | 2.1 (<0.1–6.8) | 3.6 (0.9–8.1) | Follicular | 3.8 (1.6–8.1) |
| | | | | | Luteal | 3.5 (1.5–8.0) |
| FSH (mIU/mL) | 4.0 (<1–5) | 4.6 (<1.0–7.2) | 6.8 (3.3–10.5) | 7.4 (3.3–10.5) | Follicular | 10.3 (6–15) |
| | | | | | Luteal | 6.0 (3.4–8.6) |
| (U/L)† | 2.1 (<0.5–5.4) | 3.5 (<0.5–6.6) | 4.9 (0.7–9.0) | 6.2 (1.1–11.3) | Follicular | 6.6 (1.9–10.8) |
| | | | | | Luteal | 5.4 (1.8–10.5) |
| Estradiol (pg/mL) | 9 (<9–20) | 15 (<9–30) | 27 (<9–60) | 55 (16–85) | Follicular | 50 (30–100) |
| | | | | | Luteal | 130 (70–300) |
| Estrone (pg/mL) | 13 (<9–23) | 18 (10–37) | 26 (17–58) | 36 (23–69) | Follicular | 44 (30–89) |
| | | | | | Luteal | 75 (39–160) |
| Progesterone (ng/dL) | 22 (<10–32) | 30 (10–51) | 36 (10–75) | 175 (<10–2500) | Follicular | 35 (13–75) |
| | | | | | Luteal | (200–2500) |
| 17-OH-progesterone (ng/dL) | 33 (<10–84) | 52 (10–98) | 75 (10–185) | 97 (17–235) | Follicular | 48 (12–90) |
| | | | | | Luteal | 178 (35–290) |
| DHEAS (μg/dL) | 49 (20–95) 106‡ (40–200) | 129 (60–240) | 155 (85–290) | 195 (106–320) | | 220 (118–320) |
| DHEA (ng/dL) | 35 (<10–70) 127‡ (72–180) | 297 (150–540) | 328 (190–620) | 394 (240–768) | | 538 (215–855) |
| Androstenedione (ng/dL) | 26 (<10–50) | 77 (40–112) | 126 (55–190) | 147 (70–245) | | 172 (74–284) |
| Testosterone (ng/dL) | 10 (<10–22) | 18 (<10–29) | 26 (<10–40) | 38 (24–62) | | 40 (27–70) |

*LH*, luteinizing hormone; *FSH*, follicle-stimulating hormone; *DHEAS*, dehydroepiandrosterone sulfate; *DHEA*, dehydroepiandrosterone.
\*Range is in parentheses.
†Sensitive third-generation assays.
‡Adrenarche, or increased adrenal androgen secretion, occurs as a separate event that may precede the increased gonadal secretion by 1 to 2 years. Therefore, the data are expressed as preadrenarche and postadrenarche.

but incomplete growth, which often includes a secondary mound formed by a projection of the areola and papilla above the general breast contour; however, the secondary mound may never appear. Stage 5 represents the adult breast, showing mature contour and proportions and considerable variation in size.

The duration of the developmental stages varies because it is related to the consistency of the pattern and the extent of estrogen secretion. Girls with early, but not rapid, progression of initial pubertal changes may take longer than average to complete puberty. Those with robust hormone secretion appear to complete puberty in a shorter than average duration, regardless of the age of onset.

## PUBIC HAIR STAGING

Pubic hair staging is based on quantity and distribution (see Fig. 91-2). Stage 1 is characterized by nonsexual general body hair, which may be more concentrated in the pubic area and may be present throughout childhood. No long, coarse, or heavily pigmented hair is present. Stage 2 is characterized by pigmented, straight or slightly curled hair, which is noticeably longer than the fine prepubertal hair and usually appears first along the labia majora. In stage 3, a greater concentration of dark, coarse, curly hair is seen that extends onto the mons pubis. Stage 4 hair is adult in texture and thickness but is not yet distributed in the full typical adult manner. Adult pubic hair, stage 5, is mature in quantity and type. Distribution is, at a minimum, an inverse triangle. Its extension laterally is variable, but it does not usually extend toward the umbilicus.

## GROWTH, SKELETAL MATURATION, AND BONE DENSITY

The growth spurt occurs relatively early in puberty among girls and occasionally precedes thelarche. Generally, the peak growth velocity is during the time when breast development is at stage 2 or 3. It arises from estrogen stimulation. Estrogen is a potent stimulator of somatic growth and is apparently the stimulator of skeletal maturation in both males and females.[36]

The evidence for this role of estrogen is the lack of skeletal maturity in a reported female with *aromatase deficiency*,[37] whereas males without estrogen effect show a lack of skeletal maturity and continue growth into adult life, eventually developing excessive height. (Examples of lack of estrogen effect in males include cases with an estrogen-receptor defect[38] and aromatase deficiency.[39])

The growth spurt occurs earlier among females in relation to overall pubertal development than among males, in whom the growth spurt occurs during midpuberty. When measured by an ultrasensitive assay, estradiol concentrations are found to be similar among males and females at the time of the pubertal growth spurt.[40] The difference between the genders is even more pronounced, in that female puberty begins at a younger age and the growth spurt progresses more rapidly. Females have a lesser relative height increase during puberty than do males. The peak height velocity ranges from 6.5 to 10.5 cm per year (mean, 8.5 cm per year) and occurs, on the average, at age 11 years.

*Bone mineral density (BMD)* progressively increases during puberty; peak bone mass (PBM) is attained in late puberty.[41,42] Estrogen plays a crucial role in accumulation of bone mass. Peak bone density follows *peak height velocity (PHV)* in both girls and boys. The interval between PHV and PBM in girls is ~1.5 years; the interval in boys is somewhat shorter. PHV and PBM occur ~2 years earlier in girls than in boys. The increase in BMD is greater in black girls than in white girls.[43]

Weight gain—with mature fat accumulation and distribution, particularly around the hips, thighs, and buttocks—is generally concurrent but peaks somewhat later. The mean maximum 6-month rate is 8 to 9 kg per year. The peak weight gain velocity may range from 5.5 to 10.5 kg per year for this 6-month interval. The increased pubertal velocity may begin as early as age 8 years or as late as age 12 years. If pubertal development is late or delayed, increased weight gain is also delayed.

Sex steroids obviously play a critical role in the acceleration of growth that occurs with pubertal development. That this effect is not entirely a direct one is also apparent, because growth hormone and insulin-like growth factor-I are necessary.[44] Evidence also suggests that estrogen in girls, and the aromatization of testosterone to estrogen in boys, is a likely stimulus, which amplifies the secretory activity of the growth hormone (GH) axis in puberty.[45]

## MENARCHE

The mean interval between the onset of stage 2 breast development and menarche is ~2 years. However, this time may vary considerably; the earlier thelarche, the longer the interval until menarche.[46] Generally, the interval correlates inversely with hormone levels in early puberty, with higher levels leading to earlier menarche.[47] Menarche most commonly occurs during late stage 3–early stage 4 breast development. Endometrial sloughing often occurs initially because of a wane in estrogen stimulation or after long-term unopposed estrogen stimulation, but it may follow ovulation and a normal luteal phase. Because menarche may not signal the institution of ovulation and menstrual cycling, and because biologic variation exists in the maturation of the menstrual cycle, the time of the initial period varies in relation to other aspects of pubertal development, including somatic growth. After menarche, growth may range from 1 to 10 cm, and the often-quoted rule of 5 cm (2 inches) of growth after menarche is only an average. Menarcheal age is a significant variable contributing to adult height.[48] Generally, the older a girl at menarche, the greater the adult height. Although ovulation, and hence potential fertility, may be present before menarche, in many females, regular ovulatory cycling does not occur for several months or years. At this age, irregular or long intervals between menses may occur and are often temporally related to emotional stress or environmental changes. (Also see ref. 48a and 48b.)

## VARIATIONS

The variation in the duration of female pubertal development reflects biologic diversification in the rate of maturation and attainment of full female adult reproductive function. Full breast development can occur within 3 years but may take longer. Pubic hair development progresses steadily from stage 2 to stage 5; adult female development is usually attained in 3 to 4 years. Further progression of hair development beyond stage 5 may occur because of the variations in adult female patterns. Severe acne and increased amounts of facial, periareolar, and abdominal hair may be normal, but such findings require assessment for possible hyperandrogenic states.

## PREMATURE PUBARCHE OR THELARCHE

Either pubarche or thelarche may occur considerably earlier than other signs of puberty. The prepubertal development of sexual hair as an isolated event (*premature pubarche*) or isolated premature breast development (*premature thelarche*) may actually represent the first evidence of precocious puberty. However, minimal breast development is usually a normal variation of late childhood. The diagnosis of premature pubarche or premature thelarche should be made only after precocious puberty has been ruled out. If no underlying pathology is present, both entities are benign. If premature pubarche is secondary to premature adrenarche, plasma dehydroepiandrosterone sulfate levels are above the range of prepubertal levels; dehydroepiandrosterone, testosterone, and androstenedione levels may not be elevated enough to detect levels above the prepubertal

range. Patients with premature pubarche may have increased oiliness of the skin and mild acne, with minimal or no increase in the growth rate, skeletal maturation, or clitoral size. The diagnosis is based on a finding of appropriate hormone levels for the stage of pubic hair without evidence of excessive androgen secretion or other pubertal development. No treatment is required. However, early development of pubic hair, if due to more than adrenarche, may be caused by abnormalities such as partial enzyme defects in adrenal steroidogenesis that may require treatment. (See also ref. 48.)

Premature thelarche, which is also considered a variant of the normal state, requires no specific treatment but must be differentiated from precocious puberty or abnormal estrogen stimulation. It may occur at any age but is seen most commonly before 2 years of age. It is secondary to the ovarian activity characteristic of childhood, especially of infancy. This activity may be characterized by minimal, intermittent, or sporadic estrogen secretion by the ovary related to the early stages of follicular maturation that occur throughout childhood, particularly during the first 2 years of life. Subsequently, the breast tissue may either regress or remain; regression is more common. Rarely, it progresses gradually. Generally, these cases should be considered to be a variation of prepubertal hypothalamic–pituitary–ovarian activity, with minimal gonadotropin secretion adequate to stimulate enough follicular maturity to result in estrogen secretion. Both low gonadotropin secretion and limited follicular maturity are part of normal infant-child physiology; however, in early thelarche estrogen secretion occurs to a degree sufficient to stimulate some breast growth. Growth acceleration, increased skeletal maturation, and vaginal bleeding usually do not occur in premature thelarche; when they do occur, it is only for a short duration. When an episode of vaginal bleeding or excessive growth does occur, it is likely secondary to an estrogen-secreting ovarian cyst; most of these cysts regress spontaneously. The presence and the regression of ovarian cysts can be documented by pelvic ultrasonography. Ovarian cysts may also occur in precocious puberty, but the regression of these cysts is not accompanied by regression of the signs of puberty. Ovarian cysts can be considered a variation of normal prepubertal or early pubertal follicular development and should be excised only if they are persistent or thought to be an impending surgical emergency. In the patient with premature thelarche, when the cyst regresses, growth rates normalize for age, and vaginal bleeding does not recur. Only rarely does a second cyst develop with a return of the clinical signs. Patients considered to have premature thelarche who have had an episode of progression of breast tissue, vaginal bleeding, and accelerated growth should be observed carefully, because full precocious puberty may become apparent.

Ovarian activity and FSH secretion are not quiescent among girls during childhood, and the line between prepuberty and puberty can be difficult to ascertain. Premature thelarche, at least in some instances, may represent cases in which activity is considerably higher than average. Although most such cases cannot be considered as precocious puberty, a greater than expected portion of these patients experience menarche at or before age 12.[49] However, patients with premature thelarche have normal adult height.[49]

## MALE PUBERTY

### PATTERN OF ONSET AND PROGRESSION

The initial physical evidence of puberty among boys is testicular growth (see Fig. 91-1B). Because seminiferous tubules make up the bulk of the testes, this change of testicular size is attributable primarily to seminiferous tubular growth. It follows an increase in circulating FSH levels with concomitant early elevation of testosterone levels. The long axis of the testis gradually

TABLE 91-4.
**Age of First Occurrence of Events of Puberty Among Males**

| | Mean Age* (Years) | Age Range (Years) |
|---|---|---|
| Stage 2 genital development (early testicular, penile, and scrotal growth) | 11.4–11.9 | 9.5–14.3 |
| Stage 2 pubic hair (pigmented at base of penis or on scrotum) | 12.0–12.5 | 10.7–14.0 |
| Onset of gynecomastia, palpable or visible | 13.0–13.5 | 11.7–14.8 |
| Stage 3 genital development (increased penile and testicular size) | 13.0–13.5 | 11.8–15.0 |
| Spermarche | 13.2–13.7 | 11.7–15.3 |
| Break in voice pitch | 13.3–13.7 | 11.6–15.7 |
| Maximum growth rate (height) | 13.6–14.1 | 11.7–16.0 |
| Maximum weight gain | 13.7–14.2 | 12.2–15.7 |
| Stage 3 pubic hair (adult in density around genitalia) | 13.7–14.2 | 12.2–15.8 |
| Onset of axillary hair | 13.7–14.2 | 11.8–16.2 |
| Change of voice pitch | 13.8–14.3 | 12.3–15.8 |
| Onset of acne | 14.0–14.5 | 11.7–15.7 |
| Stage 4 genital development (greater penile length and breadth) | 14.3–14.7 | 12.8–16.0 |
| Stage 4 pubic hair (full but less than adult distribution) | 14.5–15.0 | 13.0–16.5 |
| Onset of facial hair growth | 14.6–15.1 | 12.7–17.0 |
| Stage 5 genital development (adult) | 15.0–15.5 | 13.0–17.5 |
| Stage 5 pubic hair (adult; extending toward umbilicus, thighs, and anus) | 15.1–15.6 | 13.9–17.0 |

*Mean age is expressed as a half-year interval.

lengthens from ages 10 to 18. On average, the testis is 2.0 cm in its long axis in the boy approaching pubertal age; a testis longer than 2.5 to 3.0 cm is considered to have begun pubertal development and is present just before the 12th birthday in the average boy.[50] Testicular length gradually increases to a mean adult length of 5.0 cm, which is attained between 16 and 18 years of age. Testicular volume increases from ~2 mL at age 10 to a mean of 20 to 25 mL. Generally, testicular growth is bilaterally symmetric, although one testis may be disproportionally large. In most instances of unilateral hypertrophy, the contralateral testis is small for the stage of development and the patient has a history consistent with possible injury, such as herniorrhaphy or orchiopexy. Symmetric, fully developed testes rarely exceed 6 cm in length. In instances of true unilateral hypertrophy, the long axis of the testis may be as great as 8 cm (also see Chaps. 7 and 93).

## STAGING OF GENITAL SIZE AND PUBIC HAIR DEVELOPMENT

The staging of male pubertal sexual maturation is based on genital size and pubic hair development[33] (Table 91-4). The average and range of circulating levels of various hormones during the stages of male development are listed in Table 91-5.[2,9,18,20,35,51] Stage 2 of genital growth begins when testicular enlargement is recognizable. The criteria are a visible increase in the size of the penis, scrotum, and testes. The length of the longitudinal axis of the testes during stage 2 ranges from 2.5 to 3.2 cm. Stage 3 occurs subsequent to further growth, when the penis has increased in diameter as well as length, the scrotum is further developed, and the testes have increased in length to 3.3 to 4.0 cm. Stage 4 involves further growth of the genitalia. The penis becomes broader. The long axis of the testes reaches 4.0 to 4.5 cm. At this stage, the prostate is palpable by rectal examination. Stage 5 genitalia are within the adult range in size.

*Pubic hair staging* is as follows: stage 1—fine, prepubertal hair around the genitalia; stage 2—pigmented pubic hair around the base of the penis; stage 3—thicker hair, which is pigmented and curly and extends above the penis; stage 4—extension of hair over the genital area in less than adult distribution; and stage 5—spread of hair laterally onto the medial thighs. Adult male pubic hair varies considerably, as does general body hair. Hair may or may not extend from the pubic area toward the umbilicus and anus. The hair that extends toward the umbilicus may be as coarse and pigmented as pubic hair or less so.

Almost always, genital growth is the first sign of male puberty, particularly if testicular size is assessed. Although pigmented sexual hair is often the first recognized sign, this usually occurs ~6 months after genital growth is apparent on careful examination. Premature pubarche occurs much less

TABLE 91-5.
**Mean and Range* of Plasma Hormone Levels during Male Pubertal Development (Composite Genital–Pubic Hair Staging)**

| | Stage 1 | Stage 2 | Stage 3 | Stage 4 | Stage 5 |
|---|---|---|---|---|---|
| LH (mIU/mL) | 3.0 (<1.0–7.4) | 4.3 (<1.0–8.0) | 5.0 (1.7–11.5) | 6.1 (2.4–12.5) | 7.7 (3.0–18.9) |
| (U/L)† | 0.1 (<0.1–0.3) | 1.7 (0.2–4.1) | 2.0 (0.2–4.8) | 2.5 (0.7–6.0) | 2.9 (0.8–7.3) |
| FSH (mIU/mL) | 3.9 (<1.0–7.3) | 5.3 (1.6–10.7) | 6.1 (1.8–10.7) | 7.3 (2.0–11.4) | 7.5 (2.3–13.6) |
| (U/L)† | 1.0 (<0.5–2.9) | 2.3 (0.9–3.7) | 2.7 (1.0–5.0) | 3.7 (1.4–6.9) | 4.5 (1.8–8.2) |
| Testosterone (ng/dL) | <5 (<5–22) | 54 (20–250) | 190 (95–385) | 360 (180–650) | 611 (285–980) |
| Inhibin B (pg/mL) | 80 (35–182) | 175 (62–338) | 166 (78–323) | 171 (67–304) | 189 (95–349) |
| Estradiol (pg/mL) | <5 (<5–9) | 5.5 (<5–12) | 9.5 (<5–23) | 15.5 (10–28) | 19 (12–32) |
| Estrone (pg/mL) | 10 (<9–20) | 15 (<9–31) | 21 (15–38) | 30 (20–48) | 38 (20–51) |
| Progesterone (ng/dL) | 22 (<10–32) | 23 (<10–32) | 27 (<10–36) | 26 (<10–47) | 28 (<10–50) |
| 17-OH-progesterone (ng/dL) | 36 (<10–85) | 48 (<10–108) | 54 (<10–130) | 75 (<10–170) | 104 (<10–182) |
| Androstenedione (ng/dL) | 20 (<10–50) | 47 (18–89) | 76 (42–150) | 110 (60–198) | 142 (79–245) |
| DHEA (ng/dL) | 40 (<10–100) 175‡ (35–395) | 300 (128–550) | 392 (148–625) | 475 (175–694) | 555 (195–915) |
| DHEAS (µg/dL) | 49 (20–95) 73‡ (20–100) | 104 (60–190) | 112 (90–275) | 260 (140–360) | 278 (180–450) |
| DHT (ng/dL) | 3 (<2–4) | 8 (3–18) | 15 (9–26) | 36 (20–52) | 50 (30–85) |

*LH*, luteinizing hormone; *FSH*, follicle-stimulating hormone; *DHEA*, dehydroepiandrosterone; *DHEAS*, dehydroepiandrosterone sulfate; *DHT*, dihydrotestosterone.
*Range is in parentheses.
†Sensitive third-generation assays.
‡Adrenarche, or increased adrenal androgen secretion, occurs as a separate event that may precede the increased gonadal secretion by 1 to 2 years. Therefore, the data are expressed as preadrenarche and postadrenarche.

commonly than among females. After the development of the approximately simultaneous stage 2 events of puberty, the attainment of stage 3 genitalia is usually accompanied by the detectable presence of gynecomastia and the presence of sperm on urinalysis. The mean age of stage 3 genital development coincides with the mean age at onset of pubertal gynecomastia, which occurs in at least two-thirds of males and persists for an average of 12 to 18 months. At approximately this same phase of development, for the first time, mature sperm can be identified with microscopic urinalysis.[52] This coincides with the mean age of the first ejaculation, as self-reported retrospectively by adult men. The capacity for orgasm precedes pubertal development and may be experienced before the capability of ejaculation. The age of first orgasm and ejaculation varies considerably among males, correlating with psychosexual development as well as physical development. Masturbation yielding orgasm and ejaculation occurs in two-thirds of males by age 14 and in >90% by age 16. Although a marked increase is noted in the occurrence and frequency of masturbation at this age, normal males with subsequent normal reproductive functions and sexual behavior may not experience recognizable seminal discharge until late puberty. Evidence suggests that factors other than hormones play an important role in development of sexual behavior and response, with increased concentrations of sex hormones being one factor.[53]

Penile size and growth are frequent concerns, especially during puberty. A small-appearing penis during early pubertal years usually results from disproportionality in the size of genitalia compared with overall body size, particularly in a large or obese prepubertal or early pubertal boy. Penile growth lags behind general somatic growth from early infancy until puberty. To obtain a reproducible measurement of penile size, one should stretch the penis and measure along the dorsum. The mean penile length in centimeters before puberty (7 to 11 years) is $6.3 \pm 1.0$ (SD). Growth continues throughout puberty until an adult length of $15.7 \pm 1.9$ cm is attained (see also Chap. 93).[54]

## PUBERTAL GYNECOMASTIA

Gynecomastia is a normal phenomenon of male puberty. It is not related to the absolute concentration of estrogens but occurs when the ratio of estrogens to testosterone is greater than the usual male ratio. Breast tissue development occurs in two-thirds to three-fourths of all males. It may range in extent from a palpable disc of subareolar hyperplasia and protruding areola to varying amounts of raised breast tissue. Although it is usually first recognized 1 to 1.5 years after the onset of puberty, it may be an initial pubertal finding or, less commonly, may occur in later puberty. It may persist for various periods of time but usually eventually regresses until breast tissue is no longer palpable. The long-term presence of considerable breast tissue is seldom followed by complete regression, however. Rarely, breast development is so extensive that it requires surgical resection.

## OTHER PUBERTAL EVENTS

Other male midpubertal events include the attainment of stage 3 pubic hair, the presence of axillary hair, occurrence of the interval of maximum growth rate and weight gain, the onset of acne, and a change of voice pitch. The peak growth velocity occurs over a period of <12 months, whereas the entire period of accelerated growth may extend over several years. The maximal 6-month growth may be as great as 11 to 12 cm per year. For the average male, the peak rate is 9.5 cm per year for the 6-month maximal interval. The peak rate usually occurs from 13.6 to 14.1 years of age. The age of maximum height velocity ranges from 12 to 16 years; the growth spurt may begin as early as age 10 in some or last until age 17 in others. The accelerated

growth may not begin until age 15, concomitant with a later onset of other signs of puberty (also see Chap. 7).

Weight velocity patterns in males generally follow those of height velocity. The period of maximum gain also extends over approximately a 6-month period. The peak gain during this interval may be at a rate of as much as 12 to 13 kg per year (mean, 9 kg per year). The overall patterns differ for height and weight changes. The minimum rate for height occurs just before the onset of puberty, whereas weight gain velocity is minimal from between ages 3 and 5 years and gradually increases, with a considerable acceleration beginning at ~12 years. The period of increased pubertal weight gain may begin at 10 years and peak between 12 and 12.5 years or begin as late as 14 years and peak at 16 years. Full pubertal weight is attained by ~18 years in the average male.

The onset of acne is usually apparent at midpuberty and is related to a significant increase in circulating androgen levels. The progression of acne varies considerably. It may become more severe even during stage 4 or 5 of genital development (also see Chap. 101).

The onset of facial hair growth varies considerably. The appearance of a moustache and sideburns begins nearly concomitantly with pubic hair stage 4 and usually after the voice change and onset of acne. Further development and growth of the beard and chest hair vary and may progress over the next decade or longer.

## REFERENCES

1. Lee PA. Pubertal neuroendocrine maturation: early differentiation and stages of development. Adolesc Pediatr Gynecol 1988; 1:3.
2. Wu FCW, Butler GE, Kelnar CJH, et al. Patterns of pulsatile luteinizing hormone and follicle-stimulating hormone secretion in prepubertal (mid childhood) boys and girls and patients with idiopathic hypogonadotropic hypogonadism (Kallmann's syndrome): a study using an ultrasensitive time-resolved immunofluorometric assay. J Clin Endocrinol Metab 1991; 72:1229.
3. Bourguignon J-P, Jaeken J, Gerard A, de Zegher F. Amino acid neurotransmission and initiation of puberty: evidence from nonketotic hyperglycinemia in a female infant and gonadotropin-releasing hormone secretion by rat hypothalamic explants. J Clin Endocrinol Metab 1997; 82:1899.
4. Pau KY, Spies HG. Neuroendocrine signals in the regulation of gonadotropin-releasing hormone secretion. (Review). Chin J Physiol 1997; 40:181.
5. Kosut SS, Wood RI, Herbosa-Encarnación C, Foster DL. Prenatal androgens time neuroendocrine puberty in the sheep: effect of testosterone dose. Endocrinology 1997; 138:1072.
6. Andersson A-M, Toppari J, Haavisto A-M, et al. Longitudinal reproductive hormone profiles in infants: peak of inhibin B levels in infant boys exceeds levels in adult men. J Clin Endocrinol Metab 1998; 83:675.
7. Byrd W, Bennett MJ, Carr BR, et al. Regulation of biologically active dimeric inhibin A and B from infancy to adulthood in the male. J Clin Endocrinol Metab 1998; 83:2849.
8. Klein KO, Baron J, Colli MJ, et al. Estrogen levels in childhood determined by an ultra-sensitive recombinant cell bioassay. J Clin Invest 1994; 94:2475.
9. Dunkel L, Alfthan H, Ulf-Hoakan S, et al. Pulsatile secretion of LH and FSH in prepubertal and early pubertal boys revealed by ultrasensitive time-resolved immunofluorometric assays. Pediatr Res 1990; 27:215.
10. Goji K, Tanikaze S. Spontaneous gonadotropin and testosterone concentration profiles in prepubertal and pubertal boys: temporal relationship between luteinizing hormone and testosterone. Pediatr Res 1993; 34:229.
11. Wu FCW, Butler GE, Kelnar CJH, et al. Ontogeny of pulsatile gonadotropin releasing hormone secretion from midchildhood, through puberty, to adulthood in the human male: a study using deconvolution analysis and an ultrasensitive immunofluorometric assay. J Clin Endocrinol Metab 1996; 81:1798.
12. Apter D, Bützow GA, Laughlin GA, Yen SSC. Gonadotropin-releasing hormone pulse generator activity during pubertal transition in girls: pulsatile and diurnal patterns of circulating gonadotropins. J Clin Endocrinol Metab 1993; 76:940.
13. Demir A, Voutilainen R, Juul A, et al. Increase in first morning voided urinary luteinizing hormone levels precedes the physical onset of puberty. J Clin Endocrinol Metab 1996; 81:2963.
14. Kasa-Vubu JZ, Padmanabhan V, Kletter GB, et al. Serum bioactive luteinizing and follicle-stimulating hormone concentrations in girls increase during puberty. Pediatr Res 1993; 23:829.
15. Kletter GB, Padmanabhan V, Brown MB, et al. Serum bioactive gonadotropins during male puberty: a longitudinal study. J Clin Endocrinol Metab 1993; 76:432.
16. Phillips DJ, Albertsson-Wikland K, Eriksson K, Wide L. Changes in the isoforms of luteinizing hormone and follicle-stimulating hormone during puberty in normal children. J Clin Endocrinol Metab 1997; 82:3103.

17. Crofton PM, Illingworth PJ, Groome NP, et al. Changes in dimeric inhibin A and B during normal early puberty in boys and girls. Clin Endocrinol 1997; 46:109.

18. Andersson A-M, Juul AN, Petersen JH, et al. Serum inhibin B in healthy pubertal and adolescent boys: relation to age, stage of puberty, and follicle-stimulating hormone, luteinizing hormone, testosterone, and estradiol levels. J Clin Endocrinol Metab 1997; 82:3976.

19. Halvorson LM, DeCherney AH. Inhibin, activin, and follistatin in reproductive medicine. Fertil Steril 1996; 65:459.

20. Burger HG, McLachlan RI, Bangah M, et al. Serum inhibin concentrations rise throughout normal male and female puberty. J Clin Endocrinol Metab 1988; 67:689.

21. Baker ML, Hutson JM. Serum levels of Müllerian inhibiting substance in boys throughout puberty and in the first two years of life. J Clin Endocrinol Metab 1993; 76:245.

22. Lee MM, Donahoe PK, Hasegawa T, et al. Mullerian inhibiting substance in humans: normal levels from infancy to adulthood. J Clin Endocrinol Metab 1996; 81:571.

23. Šulcová J, Hill M, Hampl R, Stárka Š. Age and sex related differences in serum levels of unconjugated dehydroepiandrosterone and its sulphate in normal subjects. J Endocrinol 1997; 154:57.

24. Goji K. Twenty-four hour concentration profiles of gonadotropin and estradiol ($E_2$) in prepubertal and early pubertal girls: the diurnal rise of $E_2$ is opposite the nocturnal rise of gonadotropin. J Clin Endocrinol Metab 1993; 77:1629.

25. Garcia-Mayor RV, Andrade MA, Rios M, et al. Serum leptin levels in normal children: relationship to age, gender, body mass index, pituitary-gonadal hormones, and pubertal stage. J Clin Endocrinol Metab 1997; 82:2849.

26. Arslanian S, Suprasongsin C, Kalhan SC, et al. Plasma leptin in children: relationship to puberty, gender, body composition, insulin sensitivity, and energy expenditure. Metabolism 1998; 47:309.

27. Arslanian S, Suprasongsin C. Testosterone treatment in adolescents with delayed puberty: changes in body composition, protein, fat, and glucose metabolism. J Clin Endocrinol Metab 1997; 82:3213.

28. Kettel LM, DePaolo LV, Morales AJ, et al. Circulating levels of follistatin from puberty to menopause. Fertil Steril 1996; 65:472.

29. Belgorosky A, Rivarola MA. Irreversible increase of serum IGF-1 and IGFBP-3 levels in GnRH-dependent precocious puberty of different etiologies: implications for the onset of puberty. Horm Res 1998; 49:226.

30. Lee PA. Normal ages of pubertal events among American males and females. J Adolesc Health Care 1980; 1:26.

31. Harlan WR, Harlan EA, Grillo CP. Secondary sex characteristics of girls 12 to 17 years of age: the U.S. Health Examination Survey. J Pediatr 1980; 96:1074.

32. Herman-Giddens ME, Slora EJ, Wassermen RC, et al. Secondary sexual characteristics and menses in young girls seen in office practice: a study from the pediatric research in office settings network. Pediatrics 1997; 99:505.

33. Tanner JM. Issues and advances in adolescent growth and development. J Adolesc Health Care 1987; 8:470.

34. Hung W, August GP, Glasgow AM. Ovary. In: Pediatric endocrinology. New Hyde Park, NY: Medical Examination Publishing, 1983:324.

35. Neely EK, Hintz RL, Wilson DM. Normal ranges for immunochemiluminometric gonadotropin assays. J Pediatr 1995; 127:40.

36. Lee PA, Witchel SF. The influence of estrogen on growth. Curr Opin Pediatr 1997; 9:431.

37. Conte FA, Grumbach MM, Ito Y, et al. A syndrome of female pseudohermaphrodism, hypergonadotropic hypogonadism, and multicystic ovaries associated with missense mutations in the gene encoding aromatase (P450arom). J Clin Endocrinol Metab 1994; 78:1287.

38. Smith EP, Boyd J, Frank GR. Estrogen resistance caused by a mutation in the estrogen-receptor gene in men. N Engl J Med 1994; 331:1056.

39. Morishima A, Grumbach MM, Simpson ER. Aromatase deficiency in male and female siblings caused by a novel mutation and the physiological role of estrogens. J Clin Endocrinol Metab 1995; 80:3689.

40. Klein KO, Martha PM Jr, Blizzard RM. A longitudinal assessment of hormonal and physical alterations during normal puberty in boys. II. Estrogen levels as determined by an ultrasensitive bioassay. J Clin Endocrinol Metab 1996; 81:3203.

41. Martin AD, Bailey DA, McKay HA, et al. Bone mineral and calcium accretion during puberty. Am J Clin Nutr 1997; 66:611.

42. Takahashi Y, Minamitani K, Kobayashi Y, et al. Spinal and femoral bone mass accumulation during normal adolescence: comparison with female patients with sexual precocity and with hypogonadism. J Clin Endocrinol Metab 1996; 81:1248.

43. Gilsanz V, Roe TF, Mora S, et al. Changes in vertebral bone density in black girls and white girls during childhood and puberty. N Engl J Med 1991; 325:1597.

44. Juul A, Beng P, Hertel NT, et al. Serum insulin-like growth factor I in 1030 healthy adolescents and adults; relation to age, sex, stage of puberty, testicular size, and body mass index. J Clin Endocrinol Metab 1994; 78:744.

45. Veldhuis JD, Metzger DL, Martha PM Jr, et al. Estrogen and testosterone, but not a nonaromatizable androgen, direct network integration of the hypothalamus-somatotrope (growth hormone)-insulin-like growth factor I axis in the human: evidence from pubertal pathophysiology and sex-steroid hormone replacement. J Clin Endocrinol Metab 1997; 82:3414.

46. Marti-Henneberg C, Vizmanos B. The duration of puberty in girls is related to the timing of its onset. J Pediatr 1997; 131:618.

47. de Ridder CM, Thijssen JHH, Bruning PF, et al. Body fat mass, body fat distribution, and pubertal development: a longitudinal study of physical and hormonal sexual maturation of girls. J Clin Endocrinol Metab 1992; 75:442.

48. Shangold MM, Kelly M, Berkeley AS, et al. Relationship between menarcheal age and adult height. South Med J 1989; 82:443.

48a. van Hoof MH, Voorhost FJ, Kaptein MB, et al. Insulin, androgen, and gonadotropin concentrations, body mass index, and waist to hip ratio in the first years after menarche in girls with regular menstrual cycles, irregular menstrual cycles, or oligomenorrhea. Clin Endocrinol Metab 2000; 85:1394.

48b. Legro RS, Lin HM, Demers LM, Lloyd T. Rapid maturation of the reproductive axis during perimenarche independent of body composition. J Clin Endocrinol Metab 2000; 85:1021.

48c. Ibantz L, Potau N, De Zegher F. Endocrinology and metabolism after premature pubarche in girls. Acta Paediatr Suppl 1999; 88:73.

49. Salardi S, Cacciari E, Mainetti B, et al. Outcome of premature thelarche: relation of puberty and final height. Arch Dis Child 1998; 79:173.

50. Biro FM, Lucky AW, Huster GA, Morrison JA. Pubertal staging in boys. J Pediatr 1995; 172:100.

51. Raivio T, Perheentupa A, McNeilly AS, et al. Biphasic increase in serum inhibin B during puberty: a longitudinal study of healthy Finnish boys. Pediatr Res 1998; 44:552.

52. Kulin HE, Frontera MA, Demers LM, et al. The onset of sperm production in pubertal boys. Am J Dis Child 1989; 143:190.

53. Finkelstein JW, Susman EJ, Chinchilli VM, et al. Effects of estrogen or testosterone on self-reported sexual responses and behaviors in hypogonadal adolescents. J Clin Endocrinol Metab 1998; 83:2281.

54. Gebhard PH, Johnson AB. The Kinsey data: marginal tabulations of the 1938–1963 interviews conducted by the Institute of Sex Research. Philadelphia: WB Saunders, 1979.

## CHAPTER 92

# PRECOCIOUS AND DELAYED PUBERTY

EMILY C. WALVOORD, STEVEN G. WAGUESPACK, AND ORA HIRSCH PESCOVITZ

The human reproductive system begins to mature in fetal life and is remarkably active during the first months after birth. During childhood, the reproductive system becomes quiescent until subsequent reactivation begins pubertal development. Puberty is heralded by an increase in pulsatile secretion of gonadotropin-releasing hormone (GnRH) from the hypothalamus followed by an augmented pituitary response to GnRH and escalating secretion of luteinizing hormone (LH) and follicle-stimulating hormone (FSH). This sequence, which results in gonadal maturation (see Chap. 91) and increasing levels of sex steroids, leads to development of the secondary sexual characteristics, acceleration of growth, and ultimate fertility (see Chaps. 16 and 91). Although the mechanism of this reactivation has been largely elucidated, factors that determine the timing of pubertal onset remain elusive.

## PRECOCIOUS PUBERTY

The diagnosis of precocious puberty (PP) depends on a precise definition of the timing of normal puberty. It was previously accepted that normal puberty does not begin before age 8 years in girls and not before age 9 years in boys. A multicenter study of 17,077 girls revealed that the prevalence of breast development and/or pubic hair before age 8 years was 27% in black girls and 7% in white girls. By age 9 years, 48% of black girls and 15% of white girls showed some sign of pubertal development.[1] Interestingly, the mean age of menarche, 12.2 years in black girls and 12.9 years in white girls, did not differ significantly from previous reports. Therefore, new guidelines have been recommended redefining PP in girls as the onset of breast and/or pubic hair development before 7 years in white and 6 years in black girls.[2] Nonetheless, girls younger than 8 years old with rapid progression of puberty, poor adult height predictions, or psychosocial factors may still deserve evaluation and therapeutic intervention.

Long-term outcomes and therapeutic interventions differ depending on the etiology of premature pubertal development. Classic distinctions have been made between *gonadotropin-dependent* (i.e., central PP), *gonadotropin-independent* (i.e., peripheral PP), *premature thelarche*, and *premature pubarche*.

## PREMATURE THELARCHE

Premature thelarche is isolated premature breast development without other signs of estrogenization, such as growth acceleration or bone age advancement. It is not uncommon in the first 1 to 4 years of life,[3] with the peak prevalence in the first 2 years.[4,5] Premature thelarche is distinct from *neonatal breast hyperplasia*, which is common in the first few months of life, results from high levels of gestational hormones and spontaneously resolves over a few months.

Breast enlargement in premature thelarche may be unilateral or bilateral and often has a waxing and waning course. Complete regression is usually seen only if the onset is before age 2 years.[4,5] The etiology is unknown, but postulated mechanisms include abnormal sensitivity of breast tissue to small physiologic amounts of estrogen,[6] small autonomously functioning estrogen-producing ovarian cysts,[7] exogenous exposure to estrogens,[8] delayed inactivation of the hypothalamic–pituitary–gonadal axis after infancy,[4] or partial activation of GnRH neurons.[9] Traditionally, premature thelarche has been considered self-limited and a variant of normal. However, long-term follow-up of large cohorts of girls with premature thelarche reveals a 14% to 18% incidence of progression to gonadotropin-dependent PP,[5] which could not be predicted from clinical or laboratory features.

Girls with premature thelarche have elevated spontaneous and stimulated FSH levels, as compared to girls with central PP,[4] and a prepubertal pattern of LH secretion in response to GnRH stimulation.[4,9] However, patients with early central PP may also exhibit an FSH-predominant pattern before progressing to the LH-predominant response characteristic of gonadotropin-dependent central PP.[9] Thus, premature thelarche may be one point on the continuum between normal prepubertal development and gonadotropin-dependent PP.

## PREMATURE PUBARCHE

Premature pubarche is the development of pubic hair before the age of 7 years in girls and 9 years in boys. It occurs more commonly in children with obesity, a history of head trauma, or a central nervous system (CNS) lesion and is characterized by a rise in dehydroepiandrosterone (DHEA), DHEAS (the more stable sulfated form of DHEA), and $\Delta^5$-steroids. A minimally advanced bone age with mild growth acceleration, body odor, and acne may also be observed. The most frequent cause of premature pubarche is premature adrenarche, probably due to early maturation of the adrenal zona reticularis or an increase in peripheral sensitivity to androgens.[10]

Late-onset, nonclassical congenital adrenal hyperplasia (CAH), secondary to 21-hydroxylase, 3β-hydroxysteroid dehydrogenase, or rarely 11β-hydroxylase deficiencies, may be the etiology of premature pubarche in 12% to 40% of children, depending on the ethnic background of the population[11,12] (see Chap. 77). Other pathologic causes of premature pubarche include androgen-producing gonadal or adrenal tumors.

Premature adrenarche has also been long considered a benign variant of normal without long-term implications. However, although the subsequent timing of the entrance into puberty and final height are normal,[13] girls with a history of premature adrenarche have a 45% incidence of functional ovarian hyperandrogenism later in life.[14] The exaggerated adrenal hormone response to adrenocorticotropic hormone (ACTH) stimulation and the exaggerated ovarian androgen synthesis

**TABLE 92-1.**
**Differential Diagnosis of Gonadotropin-Dependent Precocious Puberty**

**IDIOPATHIC**
  Sporadic
  Familial
  Adoption from developing country
**CENTRAL NERVOUS SYSTEM DISORDER**
  *Hypothalamic Hamartoma*
  *Congenital Anomalies*
    Hydrocephalus
    Myelomeningocele
    Septo-optic dysplasia
  *Cysts*
    Arachnoid
    Glial
    Pineal
  *Neoplasms*
    Astrocytoma
    Craniopharyngioma
    Ependymoma
    Glioma
    Neuroblastoma
    Pinealoma
  *Head Trauma or Other Global Central Nervous System Injury*
  *Cranial Irradiation*
  *Infection*
    Abscess
    Encephalitis
    Meningitis
**SYNDROMES**
  Neurofibromatosis type 1
  Russell-Silver syndrome*
  Williams syndrome†
  Tuberous sclerosis

*Limb asymmetry, intrauterine growth retardation, small adult stature, downturned mouth, triangular shaped facial appearance, 5th finger clinodactyly.
†Hypercalcemia, supravalvular aortic stenosis, elfin facies, mental retardation, poor linear growth.

after GnRH stimulation, which is seen in some patients with premature adrenarche, suggest a dysregulation of cytochrome $P450_{c17}\alpha$ activity as the etiology. Abnormal enzymatic activity may involve the adrenals initially, but on maturation of the hypothalamic–pituitary–gonadal axis, may also occur during gonadal steroidogenesis.[14,15] There is also an increased incidence of hyperinsulinism in these individuals, even during childhood.[16]

## GONADOTROPIN-DEPENDENT/CENTRAL PRECOCIOUS PUBERTY

Gonadotropin-dependent PP (Table 92-1) results from premature activation of the hypothalamic–pituitary–gonadal axis. Girls may present with breast development alone or in combination with other secondary sexual development and menstrual bleeding. Since activation of the gonads, or *gonadarche*, is independent of adrenarche, pubic and axillary hair development may be less advanced than other secondary characteristics. Boys present first with testicular enlargement followed by phallic enlargement, pubic and axillary hair, body odor, and acne. Characteristic of this form of puberty, both girls and boys demonstrate accelerated growth velocities for age and advanced bone ages.

The etiology of gonadotropin-dependent PP is *idiopathic* in the vast majority of girls but in less than one-third of boys.[17,18] The reason for this is unclear. It has been postulated to be due to the relative ease with which reactivation of the hypothalamic–pituitary–gonadal axis occurs in girls as compared to boys.

Idiopathic PP has also been reported with increasing frequency in girls adopted from developing countries.[19] A correlation between the onset of early puberty and the rate of catch-up growth after adoption has been found, but the trigger of PP remains unknown. Final height may be compromised, worsening preexisting psychosocial adjustment problems.

*Hypothalamic hamartomas* are the most common identifiable causes of gonadotropin-dependent PP, being found in 10% to 44% of patients.[18] Hypothalamic hamartomas are congenital malformations made up of heterotopic, nonneoplastic CNS tissue found attached to the hypothalamus between the tuber cinereum and the mammillary bodies, just posterior to the optic chiasm. Magnetic resonance imaging (MRI) scanning can identify hamartomas initially missed on computed tomographic (CT) scanning alone. Hypothalamic hamartomas are comprised mostly of ectopic GnRH neurons that may act as autonomous GnRH-pulse generators. These neurons are not regulated by the normal CNS mechanisms that inhibit hypothalamic GnRH neuron activity during the prepubertal years. As a result, synchronous pulsatile firing often begins before the normal age of puberty, usually before 4 years.[18,20] Hypothalamic hamartomas can also be associated with gelastic (laughing) seizures, secondary generalized epilepsy, behavior problems, and variable cognitive degeneration.[20] Hypothalamic hamartomas usually do not enlarge with time and rarely cause mass effects. Because GnRH-analog therapy is extremely effective,[20,21] surgical resection is not recommended. Furthermore, long-term follow-up studies reveal that even if the hamartoma is completely resected, reversal of puberty is not always complete and pubertal advancement can resume prematurely.[21]

Many other CNS abnormalities can result in gonadotropin-dependent PP, most likely via disruption of tonic inhibitory input to the hypothalamus. Optic pathway gliomas are found frequently in association with neurofibromatosis type 1, but PP occurs only if the optic chiasm is involved[22] (Figs. 92-1 and 92-2). Conversely, patients with the syndrome of septo-optic dysplasia, myelomeningocele, or isolated hydrocephalus also have an increased incidence of PP.

High-dose *cranial irradiation* for childhood cancers can also cause PP in up to 25% of patients.[23] Even doses as low as 18 to 24 Gy, commonly used for CNS prophylaxis in patients with leukemia, can predispose children to gonadotropin-dependent PP. A direct correlation has been found between the age at radiation and the age at the onset of puberty. Concomitant growth hormone (GH) deficiency can mask the signs of a pubertal growth spurt. Thus, any sign of premature sexual development, even without growth acceleration, should prompt immediate evaluation, as final height may be severely compromised (see also Chap. 226).

## DIAGNOSIS

The evaluation of a girl presenting with early breast development should include a thorough physical examination to evaluate for other signs of secondary sexual development, such as pubarche or estrogenization of the vaginal mucosa, and careful plotting of height, as measured by a stadiometer, on a growth chart to determine if acceleration in linear growth velocity has occurred. If no abnormalities are found, no further testing is indicated. However, if any other feature of pubertal advancement is present, bone age radiography to assess skeletal maturation becomes the single most valuable test. A normal bone age is consistent with a diagnosis of *premature thelarche* and sup-

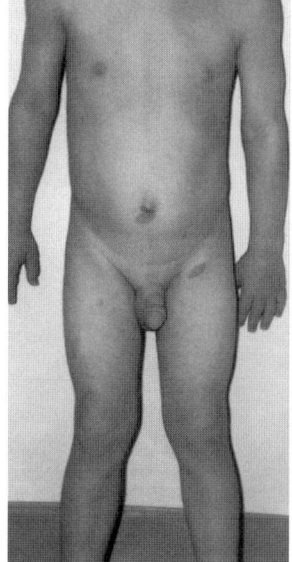
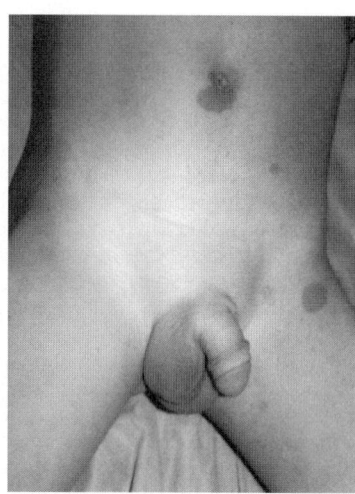

**FIGURE 92-1.** Four-year-old boy with neurofibromatosis type 1 and a history of testicular enlargement and growth acceleration. Note the multiple café au lait spots with smooth borders (coast of California). Gonadotropin-releasing hormone stimulation testing revealed a pubertal luteinizing hormone response.

ports careful observation only. If there is evidence of bone age advancement, a pelvic ultrasound may help in distinguishing between early central PP and premature thelarche. In girls with premature thelarche, the normal maximum uterine volume is 1.8 mL and the maximum ovarian volume is 1.2 mL.[24] Significant bone age advancement, growth acceleration, or progressive signs of pubertal advancement should prompt a more thorough evaluation.

Initial evaluation of *premature pubarche* should include a thorough physical examination, bone age radiography, DHEAS,

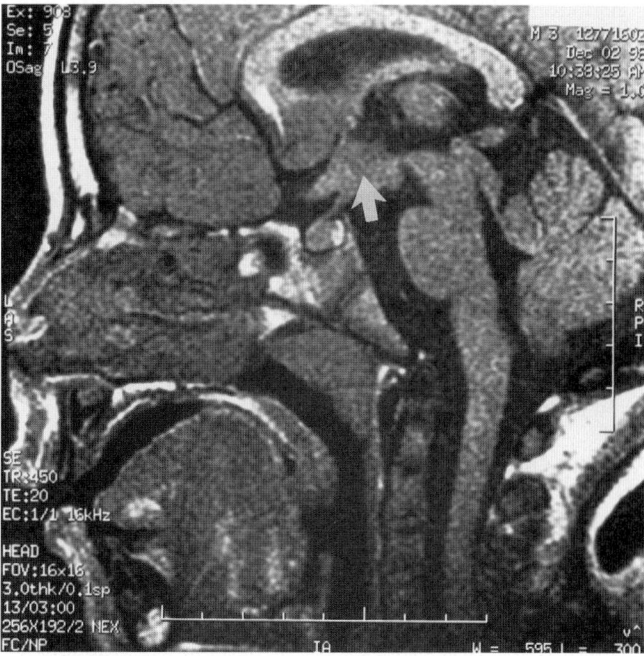

**FIGURE 92-2.** Head magnetic resonance imaging scan from the boy in Figure 92-1. Note the presence of a large glioma involving the optic chiasm (*arrow*).

testosterone, and 17α-hydroxyprogesterone (17-OHP) levels. DHEAS levels are typically elevated in accordance with the degree of pubarchal development. DHEAS levels above the early pubertal range or elevated testosterone levels should increase suspicions of a tumor and prompt radiologic evaluation of the adrenals and gonads. The presence of clitoromegaly also suggests pathology. Forty-six percent of patients with premature pubarche and clitoromegaly have defects in steroidogenesis.[12] ACTH-stimulation tests are recommended in children with clitoromegaly, abnormal baseline 17-OHP levels, or a bone age greater than two standard deviations (SD) above the mean for chronologic age.

Further evaluation is indicated in boys with testicular enlargement and in girls with breast development who are determined not to have isolated premature thelarche. The physical examination should also include a complete neurologic assessment including a visual field assessment and fundoscopic examination, an abdominal examination palpating for masses, precise Tanner staging, and an accurate height measurement. The diagnosis of *gonadotropin-dependent PP* is based on clinical findings in combination with laboratory and radiologic evaluations. Bone age radiography usually reveals advanced skeletal maturation. Pelvic ultrasound may be useful if it demonstrates a uterine length greater than the 97th percentile or a midline endometrial echo. However, one-third of patients with central PP have normal ultrasound findings.[25] The gold standard for confirming the onset of gonadotropin-dependent puberty is a traditional GnRH (Factrel)-stimulation test, with LH and FSH sampling every 15 or 20 minutes for at least 1 hour after an initial bolus of 100 μg GnRH. An LH predominant peak at any of the time points constitutes a positive test. A revised, simplified, GnRH-stimulation test, evaluating one sample for gonadotropin levels collected 40 minutes after a subcutaneous injection of 100 μg GnRH, was shown to have 88% of the sensitivity and 100% of the specificity of standard testing.[26,27] A third type of stimulation test, using the GnRH analog leuprolide (20 μg/kg or 500 μg) administered subcutaneously, results in peak LH levels 3 hours after the injection. Gonadotropin levels are equal to, or greater than, the response seen in traditional GnRH-stimulation testing, with a peak LH response >8 IU/L identifying those girls with progressive gonadotropin-dependent PP.[28] This test also has the advantage of inducing pubertal levels of estradiol 24 hours after injection in girls with gonadotropin-dependent PP, even in those who have not yet developed pubertal LH responses to conventional stimulation.[29]

Although still being tested in clinical practice, ultrasensitive hormone assays may increase the utility of random gonadotropin and estrogen levels. LH immunochemiluminometric assays (ICMA) are able to discriminate prepubertal from pubertal children when a single daytime specimen is analyzed.[30] Although currently used primarily only as a screening tool, random LH ICMA levels >0.1 IU/L are highly predictive of pubertal stimulated LH values. Estradiol levels as low as 0.02 pg/mL are now detectable by using an ultrasensitive recombinant yeast cell bioassay that is 100-fold more sensitive than conventional assays.[31] Unfortunately, this assay is not yet widely available.

After the diagnosis of gonadotropin-dependent PP is made, an MRI of the brain is necessary to rule out a tumor or other brain malformation.

## MANAGEMENT

Not all children with gonadotropin-dependent PP require pharmacologic therapy. Treatment is not necessary for girls, even with pubertal LH peaks, if their predicted adult height (based on the Bayley-Pinneau method) at the time of assessment is within one SD of their target height or of the population mean.[32] These girls often progress more slowly through the stages of puberty. However, careful follow-up is needed, and significant loss of predicted adult height should prompt initiation of therapy.

Therapy for gonadotropin-dependent PP is with long-acting GnRH analogs and is based on the paradoxical response of the pituitary gonadotrope to continuous GnRH stimulation. Modifications at the sixth and tenth positions of the GnRH decapeptide result in increased hormonal potency and duration of action. An initial surge in FSH and LH release in response to GnRH analog administration often results in a brief (4–6 weeks) stimulation of gonadal steroidogenesis. However, continuous receptor stimulation results in subsequent down-regulation of GnRH receptors on the gonadotropes and ultimately decreased gonadal sex steroid release. This results in variable regression of secondary sexual characteristics and slowing of growth velocity and bone age advancement. The most widely used GnRH analog in the United States is depot leuprolide acetate (Lupron) given at a dose of 0.2 to 0.3 mg/kg intramuscularly (im) every 28 days. Subcutaneous and intranasal formulations of various GnRH analogs are also available and more widely used in Europe. Side effects of therapy include erythema and local tenderness at the injection site and rare reports of anaphylaxis, sterile abscess formation, and cellulitis.[33]

The adequacy of therapy should be evaluated both clinically and biochemically. The simplified GnRH test or GnRH analog test can be performed after 6 months of treatment,[27] and should result in suppressed gonadotropin levels. Random estrogen levels usually are not helpful unless an ultrasensitive assay is used.[34] After 3 months of appropriate therapy, ovarian and uterine volumes return to age-appropriate sizes; thus, pelvic ultrasounds may provide an alternative to follow-up stimulation testing in patients with enlarged ovaries and uteri at the time of diagnosis. Long-term follow-up of children treated with GnRH analogs reveals significant improvements in adult height as compared to predicted adult height at the start of therapy and to untreated historic controls.[35-37] Final height remains the most relevant outcome measurement, as predicted adult height at the end of therapy invariably overestimates final height, in part because of the rapid progression through puberty that occurs once suppressive therapy is halted.[38] However, even with optimal therapy, some children do not attain their genetically predicted target height[36,37,39,40] (Fig. 92-3).

Disruptions of sex steroid influences on the growth axis are thought to result in marked growth deceleration in some children while on GnRH analog therapy. Thus, some investigators have treated poorly growing children with central PP with GH

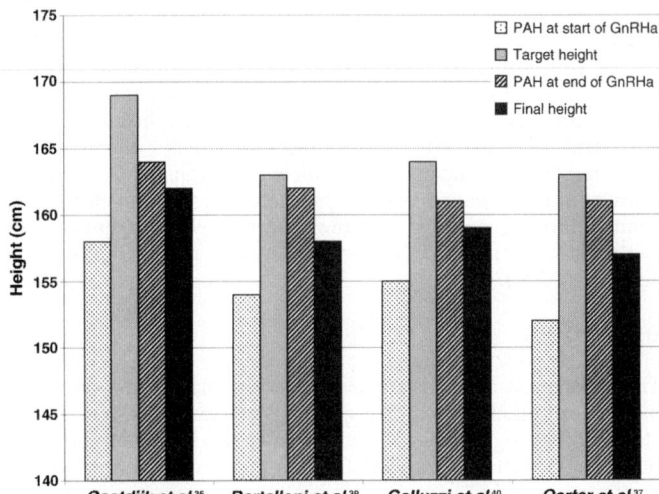

**FIGURE 92-3.** Graphic representation of the effect of gonadotropin-releasing hormone analog (*GnRHa*) therapy on gonadotropin-dependent precocious puberty. Note the poor initial predicted adult height with a marked improvement in final height. However, final height remained significantly lower than target height in all studies. (*PAH*, predicted adult height.)

in addition to GnRH analog therapy. Modest improvements in predicted adult heights are seen with this combination, but whether the effect on final height is sufficient to warrant the cost and complexity of therapy is still being debated.[41]

Concerns about the effect of GnRH analog therapy on bone mineral density (BMD) in growing children have arisen due to the marked osteopenia that is seen in adults treated with GnRH analogs. Although still controversial, most reports indicate that BMD remains normal for chronologic age and/or bone age[42] while the patient is on GnRH analog therapy. More important, GnRH analogs have not been shown to affect peak bone mass when treated girls reach their final heights.[39]

The decision to discontinue therapy must be individualized, based on adequacy of gain in predicted adult height and the appropriate timing of puberty. The authors recommend discontinuing therapy when the chronologic age and the bone age are equivalent, or the current height is acceptable to the family. After the discontinuation of therapy, most girls experience menarche and develop age-appropriate ovulatory cycles within 1 to 2 years.[43] Some investigators report an increased risk for the development of polycystic ovary syndrome in girls with a history of idiopathic central PP,[44] but this area is still under investigation.

# GONADOTROPIN-INDEPENDENT PRECOCIOUS PUBERTY

PP may also be caused by sex steroid hormone production independent of gonadotropin stimulation (Table 92-2).

*McCune-Albright syndrome* is characterized by the triad of polyostotic fibrous dysplasia, café au lait spots ("coast of Maine" configurations), and endocrinopathies, in particular PP (Fig. 92-4). This disorder results from a dominant, early embryonic, somatic activating mutation of the $\alpha$ subunit of the stimulatory guanine nucleotide-binding protein, Gs. The mutation results in decreased guanosine triphosphatase (GTPase) activity leading to constitutive cyclic adenosine monophosphate (cAMP) production, increased gene transcription, and subsequent endocrine hyperfunction.[45] Estrogen produced by autonomously functioning ovarian follicles leads to cyclical breast enlargement and uterine bleeding, occurring as early as infancy. Prolonged estrogen exposure also leads to growth acceleration, advanced bone age, and eventually secondary activation of the hypothalamic–pituitary–gonadal axis and central PP. Other endocrinologic problems include hyperthyroidism, GH excess, hyperprolactinemia, and nodular adrenal hyperplasia resulting in Cushing syndrome. Hypophosphatemic rickets, hepatobiliary disease, cardiac disease, and sudden death have also been reported.[46] The stage during embryonic development when the somatic mutation occurs determines the mosaic tissue distribution of the mutation and, thus, the clinical manifestations. In fact, a $G_s\alpha$ mutation restricted to the ovaries, diagnosed from ovarian cyst fluid analysis, has been reported in a young girl with recurrent ovarian cysts and sexual precocity without bony lesions or café au lait spots (see Chap. 66).[47]

McCune-Albright syndrome should be considered in any very young girl with signs of estrogenization. Skin hyperpigmentation may not be visible in early childhood. Bone scanning often reveals the pathognomonic lesions. In the presence of significantly elevated estrogen levels, LH levels are suppressed even below the prepubertal range.[48] Gonadotropin-independent PP also occurs in boys with McCune-Albright syndrome, but less commonly than in girls.

Current treatment of McCune-Albright syndrome results in somewhat disappointing long-term outcomes. Cyproterone acetate, a progestational agent used in Europe but not approved in the United States, is of minimal benefit.[49] Testolactone, a first-generation aromatase inhibitor, has been shown to be of some benefit in reducing estrogen levels, curtailing the frequency of menstrual bleeding, and increasing predicted adult height.[50]

**TABLE 92-2.**
**Differential Diagnosis of Gonadotropin-Independent Precocious Puberty**

**AUTONOMOUS GONADAL HYPERSECRETION**
  *McCune-Albright syndrome*
  *Familial male precocious puberty*
  *Ovarian cysts*
**GONADAL TUMORS**
  *Ovarian*
    Granulosa cell
    Theca cell
    Combination
  *Testicular*
    Leydig cell
    Sertoli cell
**EXOGENOUS STEROID INGESTION**
**HUMAN CHORIONIC GONADOTROPIN–SECRETING TUMORS**
  *Hepatoblastoma*
  *Pinealoma*
  *Germinoma*
    Thymic
    Testicular
  *Choriocarcinoma*
**ADRENAL DISORDERS**
  *Congenital adrenal hyperplasia*
  *Adenoma*
  *Carcinoma*
**SEVERE PRIMARY HYPOTHYROIDISM**

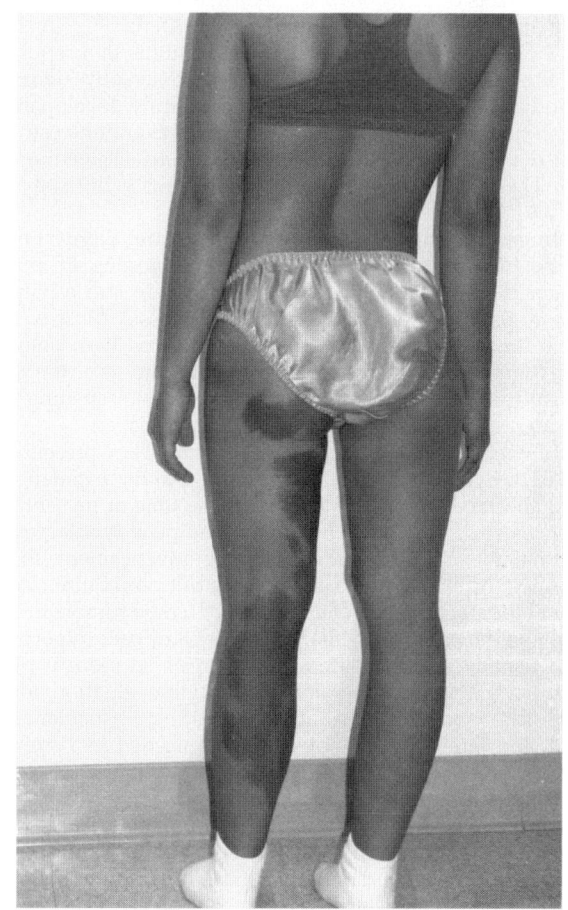

**FIGURE 92-4.** Fourteen-year-old girl with McCune-Albright syndrome. Note the rough borders to the café au lait spot (coast of Maine) and the significant scoliosis, due to extensive bony lesions causing a leg length discrepancy.

However, the therapeutic regimen is cumbersome and the response is usually unsustained.[51] More potent aromatase inhibitors, such as anastrozole (Arimidex), may prove more effective. Additionally, the estrogen-receptor antagonist tamoxifen has been reported to be useful in at least one patient.[52] GnRH agonists are beneficial only after secondary central puberty has been triggered by prolonged exposure to estrogens.[48,53]

*Familial male PP*, also known as *testotoxicosis*, results from a dominantly inherited mutation of the LH receptor, causing the receptor to remain constitutively active even in the absence of ligand binding.[54] Sixteen mutations have been identified to date. These point mutations allow continuous G-protein activation and high cAMP production leading to testosterone hypersecretion. Boys present in the first few years of life with pubic and axillary hair, modest testicular enlargement, penile growth, accelerated linear growth, bone age advancement, and spermatogenesis. The only adverse consequence appears to be severely compromised final height. Diagnosis is based on a positive family history, absence of other lesions, and an elevated testosterone level in the face of suppressed gonadotropin levels. Therapy for familial male PP is usually moderately effective.[55] Spironolactone, which blocks androgen action at the androgen receptor, and, thus, virilization, often results in gynecomastia because of the decreased androgen/estrogen ratio. The addition of testolactone, which causes competitive inhibition of aromatase, prevents androgen conversion to estrogen and decreases the risk of gynecomastia and rapid skeletal maturation, since estrogens, not androgens, cause acceleration of skeletal maturation.[56] Ketoconazole, which inhibits steroidogenesis including cortisol production, can be used as a single agent. Due to reports of significant hepatotoxicity, pneumonitis, and renal failure, frequent monitoring of patients on ketoconazole therapy is essential.[57] Adequacy of treatment is based primarily on clinical criteria.

Although small *ovarian cysts* are common in prepubertal girls, they rarely result in PP.[58] These cysts usually are unilateral and are larger than the cysts that frequently develop in central PP.[59] If an ovarian follicular cyst produces enough estrogen, breast development and occasionally menstrual bleeding may occur. These cysts often resolve spontaneously, but they may recur and require limited surgical resection.

Estrogen-producing *ovarian tumors* are rare. Eighty percent of these tumors present with rapidly progressing PP in girls younger than 4 years of age. Abdominal pain and a palpable mass are often present at the time of diagnosis. Most of these tumors are of granulosa cell origin, with less than one-third being composed of thecal cells, or a combination of the two.[60] Surgical removal alone is usually curative, with ensuing complete regression of secondary sexual characteristics.

*Leydig cell tumors* are also rare neoplasms. They present most often in boys between 5 and 9 years of age and are usually unilateral and large enough to palpate at the time of presentation. Gynecomastia frequently accompanies penile enlargement, pubic hair development, and bone age advancement. In children, most of these tumors are benign, but do require surgical removal for amelioration of symptoms.[61] These tumors must be differentiated from testicular adrenal rest cell hyperplasia, which usually occurs bilaterally, and may be seen in poorly controlled CAH (see Chap. 77). A thorough evaluation, including GnRH- and ACTH-stimulation testing, testicular ultrasound, and rarely even a biopsy may be needed to distinguish between the two. *Sertoli cell tumors* may present similarly and are primarily seen in association with Peutz-Jeghers syndrome.

*Exogenous ingestion* of steroid hormones may cause precocious sexual development. Use of oral contraceptive pills, topical estrogens, estrogen-contaminated foods, or hair care products or cosmetics that contain estrogens have all been shown to cause gonadotropin-independent PP.[8] Secondary sexual development often regresses after discontinued use of the product.

*Human chorionic gonadotropin (hCG)–secreting tumors* can cause PP because of the cross-reaction of hCG with LH, due to identical α subunits and markedly similar β subunits. In boys, hCG stimulates the production of testosterone and secondary sexual development. Rarely do hCG-producing tumors in girls result in PP, because LH and FSH are both needed to stimulate ovarian follicular development. However, a germ-cell tumor that secreted hCG, as well as possessing aromatase activity, has caused PP in a girl.[62] An hCG-secreting tumor should be suspected as the cause of PP when minimal testicular enlargement is present, as FSH stimulation of the seminiferous tubules is lacking, despite significant virilization. Hepatoblastomas are the most frequent etiology of hCG-secreting tumors. Other causes include tumors of the pineal gland, intracranial germinomas or choriocarcinomas, and thymic or testicular germ-cell tumors.[63] The discovery of an extragonadal germ-cell tumor in a boy necessitates that a karyotype be performed, since the incidence of germ-cell tumors is up to 50 times more common in boys with Klinefelter syndrome than in the general population.[64] Patients with even low-level mosaicism for Klinefelter syndrome have an increased tumor risk.[63]

*Adrenal disorders* may cause precocious sexual development in boys. Previously unrecognized CAH or adrenal tumors can cause virilization in the absence of gonadotropin stimulation (see Chap. 77). Tumors may be differentiated from CAH, as they do not respond to ACTH stimulation or to dexamethasone suppression. Adrenal adenomas produce predominantly DHEAS, whereas androstenedione and testosterone are the primary products of carcinomas. However, biopsy remains the most reliable means of definitive diagnosis. Girls may rarely present with feminizing, rather than virilizing, adrenal tumors.[65] Surgical removal alone is often curative. However, chemotherapy may be indicated if there is evidence of tumor extension or if there is a recurrence.

PP may rarely be seen in *severe hypothyroidism*, also known as the Van Wyk-Grumbach syndrome (see Chap. 45). Hypothyroidism is one of the few causes of PP in which children may have delayed or normal linear growth and skeletal retardation. Girls can have breast development, galactorrhea, ovarian cysts, and uterine bleeding.[66,67] Boys may develop macro-orchidism with minimal signs of virilization. Thyroid hormone replacement results in regression of secondary sexual characteristics, except macro-orchidism. The mechanism of PP in these children remains incompletely understood. Possible explanations include high levels of thyroid-stimulating hormone (TSH) acting at the FSH receptors in the gonads or thyrotropin-releasing hormone (TRH)–stimulating pulsatile bioactive FSH and α-subunit secretion from the pituitary.[68] Central activation of the hypothalamic–pituitary–gonadal axis can also occur.

## GONADOTROPIN-INDEPENDENT LEADING TO GONADOTROPIN-DEPENDENT PRECOCIOUS PUBERTY

Prolonged exposure to estrogens or androgens from a peripheral source may lead to early initiation of gonadotropin-dependent PP. Patients with virilizing adrenal tumors, uncontrolled or undiagnosed CAH, McCune-Albright syndrome, familial male PP, and ovarian tumors have been reported to progress to gonadotropin-dependent PP.[48,57,69,70] The mechanism seems to be secondary to inappropriate maturation of the hypothalamic–pituitary–gonadal axis after prolonged sex steroid exposure. The degree of bone age advancement has also been thought to correlate with the timing of the development of central puberty, as most reported cases have had bone ages of at least 10.5 years at the time of activation of the hypothalamic–pituitary–gonadal axis. However, a 5-year-old girl with a history of an ovarian tumor at the age of 7 months developed gonadotropin-dependent PP at a bone age of only 5.5 years.[71] Central activation of the hypothalamic–pituitary–gonadal axis usually occurs after the primary problem has been brought under control and sex steroid levels are lowered, relieving the hypothalamic–pituitary axis of negative feedback. Normal gonadotropin secretion then overrides the autonomous hormone production seen in McCune-Albright syndrome and familial male PP.[48,57]

## CONTRASEXUAL PRECOCIOUS PUBERTY

Contrasexual precocious puberty includes excessive virilization in girls and feminization in boys. Virilization in girls is primarily due to adrenal abnormalities and has already been discussed. Production of testosterone has also been reported in girls with ovarian juvenile granulosa cell tumors resulting in the development of pubic hair and clitoromegaly in the presence or absence of breast development and menstrual bleeding.[72] Feminization in boys presents primarily as gynecomastia. Some breast tissue develops in 50% to 100% of normal boys during early puberty, with a peak occurrence at age 13 years.[73] The tissue is firm and glandular in texture and may be quite tender. Gynecomastia develops as the result of an imbalance between estrogen and androgen levels. Spontaneous resolution is usually seen within 1 year, but breast tissue may persist into adulthood. Gynecomastia before the onset of puberty is always pathologic. Sertoli cell tumors associated with Peutz-Jeghers syndrome may cause gynecomastia due to increased tumor aromatase expression.[74] Additionally, any gonadal or adrenal tumor may produce estrogens or have significant aromatase expression that results in varying degrees of feminization. Other causes of gynecomastia in boys include marijuana or anabolic steroid use, hypogonadism, hCG-secreting tumors,[73] and the genetic aromatase excess syndrome.[75]

## DELAYED PUBERTY

The absence of breast development in a girl by the age of 13 years or a testicular volume <4 mL in a boy by the age of 14 is considered pubertal delay. Other definitions of delayed puberty include the absence of menarche by 16 years of age or a prolonged tempo of pubertal progression, >5 years from pubertal onset to completion. These conventional definitions are limited for several reasons. First, any definition of pubertal delay based on a gaussian distribution unavoidably includes a small percentage of normal children. Furthermore, although studies have attempted to define PP, no single study has clearly established the upper ranges of normal puberty. Finally, the definition of delayed puberty does not account for ethnic or other sociologic differences. For these reasons and given that some population studies have suggested an earlier onset of puberty,[1] the accepted definition of delayed puberty may eventually warrant reconsideration.

## DIFFERENTIAL DIAGNOSIS

Although not absolute, the simplest way to approach the diverse differential diagnosis of pubertal delay is to recognize it as occurring in two distinct groups. The first encompasses those children with primary pituitary or hypothalamic dysfunction and subsequently low or inappropriately normal gonadotropin levels (hypogonadotropic hypogonadism). The second group includes those with primary gonadal failure and consequent elevation of LH and FSH due to a lack of sex steroid inhibition at the level of the pituitary and hypothalamus (hypergonadotropic hypogonadism).

## HYPOGONADOTROPIC HYPOGONADISM

The term *hypogonadotropic hypogonadism* (Table 92-3) applies to a variety of diagnoses, all united by the feature of ineffective

**TABLE 92-3.**
**Differential Diagnosis of Hypogonadotropic Hypogonadism**

CONSTITUTIONAL DELAY OF GROWTH AND DEVELOPMENT

PRIMARY HYPOTHALAMIC/PITUITARY INSUFFICIENCY

Isolated gonadotropin-releasing hormone (GnRH) or gonadotropin deficiency
  Kallmann syndrome
  Idiopathic hypogonadotropic hypogonadism
  Partial gonadotropin deficiency/fertile eunuch syndrome
  Luteinizing hormone and follicle-stimulating hormone β-subunit mutations
  Adrenal hypoplasia congenita (DAX-1 mutation)
  GnRH-receptor gene mutation
Hypopituitarism of any cause
  Trauma, irradiation, infection, hypophysitis
  PROP-1 mutations
Central nervous system (CNS) abnormalities
  Empty sella
  Septo-optic dysplasia (de Morsier syndrome)
  Holoprosencephaly
Congenital syndromes (may also have primary hypogonadism)
  Prader-Willi syndrome
  Laurence-Moon syndrome
  Bardet-Biedl syndrome

SECONDARY HYPOTHALAMIC/PITUITARY INSUFFICIENCY

Chronic disease
Strenuous exercise
Malnutrition/weight loss
Eating disorders
Severe obesity
Space-occupying lesions
  Vascular lesions, craniopharyngioma, germinoma, pituitary adenoma, granulomatous disease, Langerhans cell histiocytosis, other CNS lesions
Endocrinopathies
  Hypothyroidism
  Hyperprolactinemia
  Cushing disease
  Isolated growth hormone deficiency
  Poorly controlled diabetes mellitus

gonadotropin production. It can result either from a true deficiency of gonadotropins due to primary disease in the hypothalamus or pituitary (primary hypothalamic/pituitary insufficiency) or as a consequence of a reversible gonadotropin deficiency that is due to another illness or condition (secondary hypothalamic/pituitary insufficiency).

## CONSTITUTIONAL DELAY

The majority of children with pubertal delay will have constitutional delay of puberty (CDP) (Table 92-4), a transient functional delay in sexual development that is a variant of normal. Although these adolescents ultimately progress through puberty normally, pubertal onset is sufficiently late to trigger concern and evaluation. CDP can occur either as an isolated finding, or, more commonly, it may be associated with concomitant short stature (constitutional delay of growth and puberty, or CDGP). In fact, many of these children initially come to medical attention because of height concerns, not pubertal delay. In either case, there often is a positive family history of similar developmental patterns, and physical examination and laboratory testing show the child to be without underlying disease.

**TABLE 92-4.**
**Constitutional Delay of Growth and Development**

Variant of normal
Boys present more frequently than girls
Delayed bone age
Short stature typical, but normal growth velocity
Positive family history
No underlying medical disease
Adrenarche and gonadarche are equally delayed
Puberty ultimately progresses normally
Normal final adult height, but short for midparental height

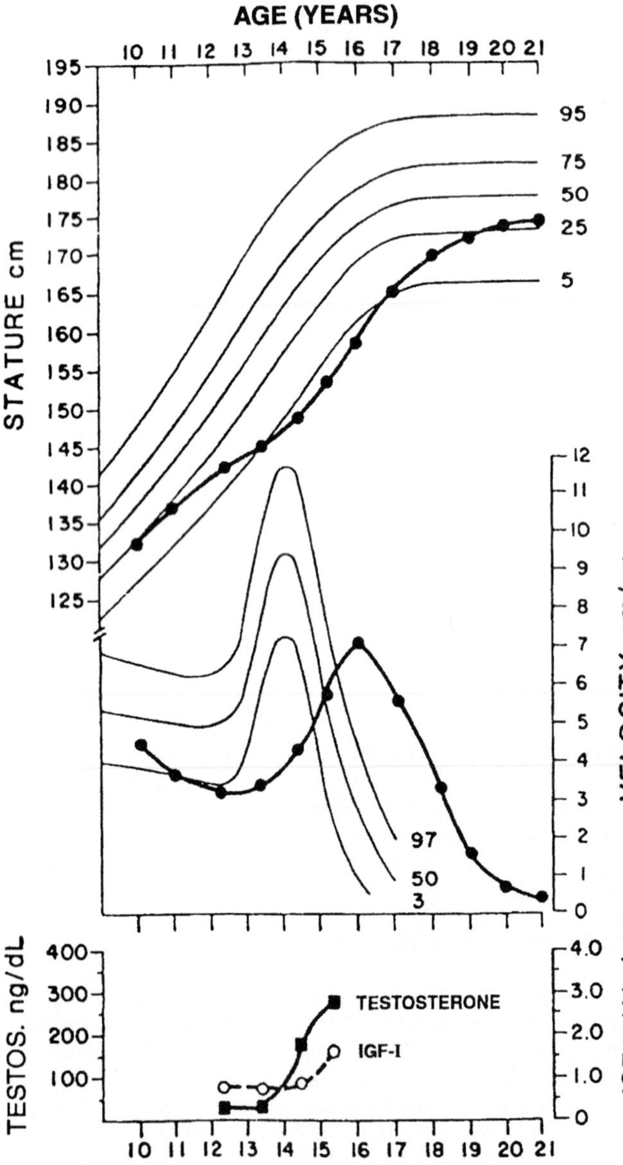

Children with constitutional delay have a temporary delay in the maturation of the hypothalamic–pituitary–gonadal axis and a protracted phase of prepubertal growth deceleration (Fig. 92-5). The exact etiology is not clear. Transient GH deficiency, relative to the chronologic age, is well described in children with constitutional delay. Whether low insulin-like growth factor-I (IGF-I) levels impair the gonadal response to gonadotropins[76] or whether GH deficiency is instead a consequence of the low sex steroid levels[77] is unknown. However, since GH secretion normalizes after the onset of puberty in most cases,[78] the latter seems more likely. Deficiency of the transcription factor, Otx1, has been implicated in transient hypogonadotropic hypogonadism and GH deficiency in mice[79]; this insight may someday lead to the identification of the genetic basis for constitutional delay in humans.

The prototypic adolescent with CDP is a boy, possibly short all of his life, who now seeks help for a delay in the onset of secondary sexual characteristics. Bone age is invariably delayed. In most cases, the growth velocity is within two SD of normal, especially for the bone age, and the height is also appropriate for bone age. Eventually, normal puberty will ensue before the bone age is 13 years. Children with CDGP should achieve a normal adult height, but there is controversy regarding whether these children achieve their genetic potential. Some studies demonstrate that final height is not significantly different from midparental height,[80] whereas others suggest that the target height is not achieved.[81]

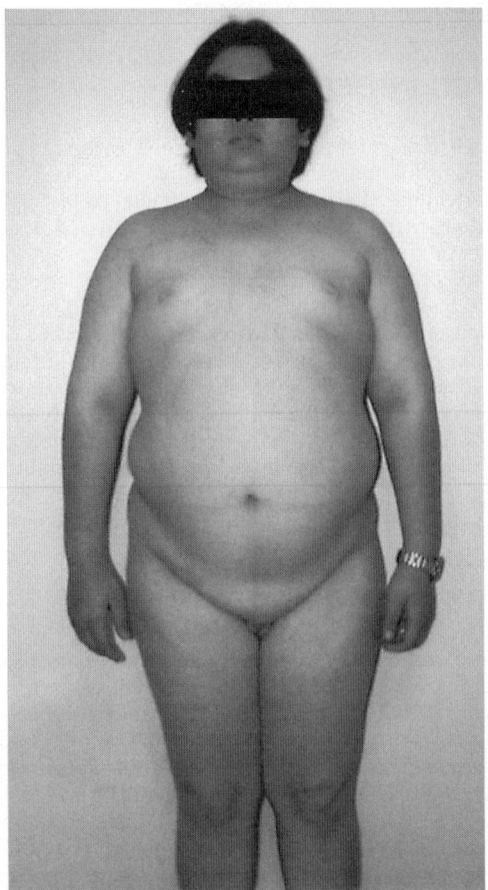

**FIGURE 92-5.** Growth pattern and hormonal changes in a boy with constitutional delay of growth and puberty. He ultimately entered puberty and achieved normal adult height, despite a delayed growth spurt. Testosterone and insulin-like growth factor-I (*IGF-I*) belatedly rose to normal levels. (Modified from Rosenfield RL. Clinical review 6: diagnosis and management of delayed puberty. J Clin Endocrinol Metab 1990; 70:559.)

**FIGURE 92-6.** Nineteen-year-old man with hypogonadotropic hypogonadism secondary to hypopituitarism. Height was 148 cm and bone age was 14 years. Central hypothyroidism and growth hormone deficiency were present; there was no adrenal insufficiency. Luteinizing hormone was 0.3 mIU/mL, follicle-stimulating hormone was 1.0 mIU/mL, and total testosterone was 6 ng/dL. Magnetic resonance imaging was normal except for the presence of a small pituitary gland.

Many more boys than girls are evaluated for delayed puberty. This may reflect the natural genetic and physiologic differences between boys and girls or, more likely, a societal bias regarding growth and development. Boys, particularly those with concomitant short stature, are more prone to teasing and stigmatization from a delay in pubertal development. The social repercussions and resultant psychological effects of constitutional delay can be quite severe; therefore, it is important that these issues always be thoughtfully addressed in these children.

## PRIMARY HYPOTHALAMIC/PITUITARY INSUFFICIENCY

Gonadotropin deficiency may occur either as an isolated event or as a component of multiple pituitary hormone deficiencies or hypothalamic dysfunction (Fig. 92-6). Essentially, any event or condition that results in hypopituitarism can cause hypogonadotropic hypogonadism. Predisposing factors include *head trauma, infection, CNS irradiation,* and intrinsic developmental or anatomic defects such as *septo-optic dysplasia* (de Morsier syndrome) or primary *empty sella* (Fig. 92-7). Most of these aforementioned problems are diagnosed before adolescence, since these children usually present earlier with associated endocrine deficiencies or growth failure. On the other hand, isolated gonadotropin deficiency may not be diagnosed until adolescence when pubertal delay is the primary complaint.

### ISOLATED GONADOTROPIN DEFICIENCY

*Kallmann syndrome* is isolated gonadotropin deficiency associated with anosmia or hyposmia. It is more common in boys and may be indistinguishable from CDGP, except that children with Kallmann syndrome often have normal stature in comparison to the short stature commonly seen in constitutional delay (see Chap. 115). A clinically heterogeneous disorder, Kallmann syndrome may occur sporadically or result from autosomal dominant, autosomal recessive, or X-linked modes of inheritance. X-linked Kallmann syndrome is secondary to mutations of the KAL gene, located at Xp22.3.[82,82a] The primary defect is the disordered migration, during embryogenesis, of GnRH-producing neurons to their normal location in the hypothalamus. An abnormal sense of smell is due to the simultaneous defective development of the olfactory bulbs and tracts. Often, the history and physical examination are entirely normal except for pubertal delay, eunuchoid body proportions (upper/lower segment ratio <0.9; arm span >5 cm greater than height), and an altered sense of smell that may not be identified unless formal testing is undertaken. Other midline defects and neurologic abnormalities, including cerebellar ataxia and synkinesis (mirror movements), may also be present. Furthermore, many boys with X-linked Kallmann syndrome have unilateral renal agenesis.

Kallmann syndrome is but one variant in a spectrum of disorders resulting from GnRH and gonadotropin deficiency. Other related conditions include isolated gonadotropin deficiency without an associated defect in olfaction (*idiopathic hypogonadotropic hypogonadism*) and incomplete GnRH deficiency, such as is thought to occur in the *fertile eunuch syndrome.* Men with the fertile eunuch syndrome have eunuchoid body proportions, varying degrees of virilization, and near normal-sized testes that have the capacity for spermatogenesis. It is believed that endogenous GnRH secretion is partially impaired but otherwise sufficient to stimulate Leydig cell secretion of testosterone. Although systemic levels of testosterone are inadequate for complete virilization, the local concentrations are sufficient for spermatogenesis and testicular growth.[82]

*Adrenal hypoplasia congenita* (AHC) is a rare genetic disorder that is inherited either in an X-linked or autosomal recessive fashion. In the X-linked type, boys typically present with primary adrenal insufficiency in infancy. In adolescence, these children fail to begin puberty as expected because of hypogonadotropic hypogonadism, which may be a result of defects both at the level

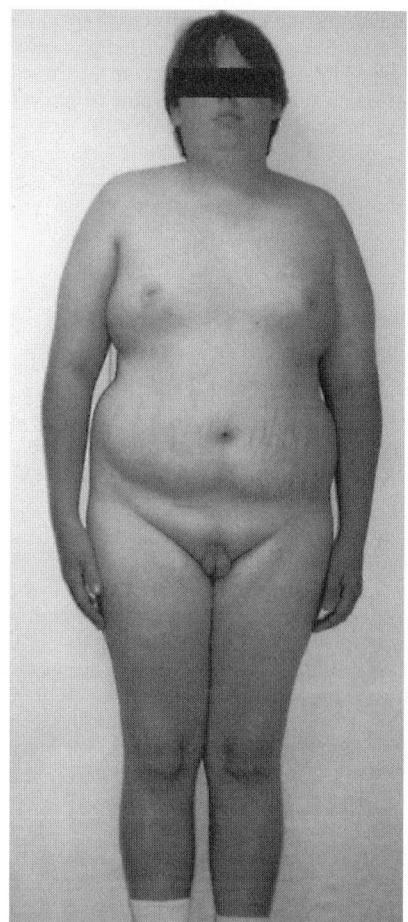

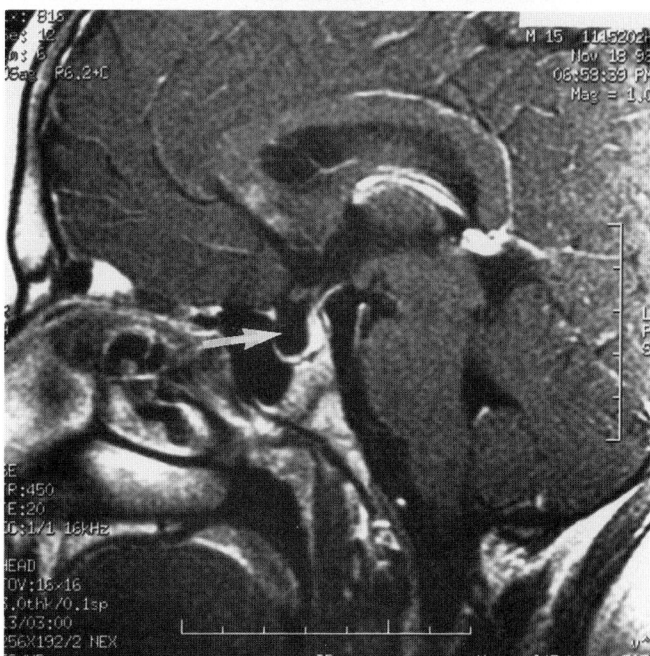

**FIGURE 92-7. A,** Fifteen-year-old boy with hypogonadotropic hypogonadism and a history of bilateral cryptorchidism. Sense of smell was normal. Height was 173 cm and eunuchoid body proportions were noted (upper/lower segment ratio of 0.86). Baseline luteinizing hormone was <0.7 mIU/mL, follicle-stimulating hormone was 0.6 mIU/mL, and testosterone was 9 ng/dL; there was no response to gonadotropin-releasing hormone stimulation. **B,** Magnetic resonance imaging revealed the presence of an empty sella (*arrow*). Note the normal posterior pituitary bright spot.

of the hypothalamus and of the pituitary.[83] This disorder occurs secondary to mutations in the DAX-1 gene, located on chromosome Xp21. The pubertal hypogonadism in these patients may actually represent a postnatal regression of hypothalamic–pituitary–gonadal function, as evidenced by the demonstration of a normal minipuberty of infancy in a child with AHC.[84]

Although specific genetic mutations account for some cases of hypogonadotropic hypogonadism,[84a] the exact molecular basis for most individuals remains unknown. Mutations in the GnRH gene have not yet been identified, but mutations in the gene encoding for the GnRH receptor have been discovered.[85] Defects in the genes encoding for the β subunits of LH and FSH have also been described.[86] Moreover, the discovery of transcription factors responsible for the ordered embryologic development of the anterior pituitary has provided further insight into the potential etiology for some cases of hypogonadotropic hypogonadism. Mutations in the PROP-1 gene, for example, have been implicated in combined pituitary hormone deficiencies, including gonadotropin deficiency.[87]

### CONGENITAL SYNDROMES

*Prader-Willi syndrome (PWS)*, the first congenital syndrome in which genomic imprinting was recognized, results from a defect of the paternally derived genes on chromosome 15 at the 15q11–q13 locus.[87a] Normally, the maternally derived genes at the 15q11–q13 locus are silent whereas those that are paternally inherited are expressed. In PWS, the paternally derived genes are absent. In 70% of cases, this absence is secondary to an interstitial deletion. Most of the remaining cases result from maternal uniparental disomy, in which both chromosomes 15 are inherited from the mother.[88] The syndrome is characterized by infantile hypotonia, onset of obesity in early childhood, insatiable hunger, behavioral problems, short stature, mental deficiency, small hands and feet, and characteristic facies (Fig. 92-8). Furthermore, hypoplastic external genitalia and delayed puberty occur in the majority of cases. In girls, menarche is typically delayed or absent altogether, and ovulation frequently does not occur. It is widely believed that the hypogonadism is secondary to hypothalamic dysfunction. However, GH deficiency is prevalent in children with PWS,[89] and this may be a contributing factor. Furthermore, boys with PWS occasionally have elevated gonadotropins that may result from primary testicular failure due to uncorrected cryptorchidism.

The *Laurence-Moon* and *Bardet-Biedl syndromes* are also characterized by hypogonadism and hypogenitalism, particularly in boys. Retinitis pigmentosa (see Chap. 215), varying degrees of mental deficiency, and autosomal recessive inheritance are additional features of both. In the Laurence-Moon syndrome, spastic paraparesis predominates, whereas obesity, dystrophic extremities (polydactyly, syndactyly), and renal abnormalities are found in children with the Bardet-Biedl syndrome. Historically believed to have hypogonadotropic hypogonadism, these children may also have concomitant primary gonadal failure.

## SECONDARY HYPOTHALAMIC/PITUITARY INSUFFICIENCY

Any chronic systemic disease can adversely affect normal gonadotropin secretion. This includes *renal disease* (e.g., renal failure or renal tubular acidosis), *chronic lung disease* (including cystic fibrosis and severe asthma), *gastrointestinal disease* (i.e., inflammatory bowel disease and celiac disease), and *hemoglobinopathies* (e.g., sickle cell disease and β-thalassemia major[84a,89a]). The exact pathophysiology is often multifactorial and, in many cases of chronic disease, unknown. Confounding factors often include inadequate nutrition or exposure to certain medications, such as glucocorticoids, that have profound effects on growth and development. Adequate treatment of the underlying disease and optimization of nutrition often reverse the hypogonadotropic hypogonadism seen in these disorders.

*Malnutrition* and *excessive weight loss* are clearly linked to delayed pubertal development[90] (see Chaps. 127 and 128). Similarly, children with *eating disorders* or those who engage in *vigorous exercise* may have disrupted hypothalamic-pituitary function. As exemplified by female athletes, menarche is frequently delayed and hypothalamic amenorrhea is a common problem, particularly in those girls who begin their training before the onset of menarche.[91]

Hypogonadotropic hypogonadism can also be caused by an underlying endocrinopathy. Normal gonadotropin secretion is disrupted in *hypothyroidism* and *hyperprolactinemia* (see Chaps. 13 and 45). Hyperprolactinemia results either from a pituitary adenoma or as a medication side effect, as seen with the neuroleptic agents. It is, however, an infrequent etiology for pubertal delay and is more commonly associated with galactorrhea and/or secondary amenorrhea. Although rare, *Cushing disease* has presented as isolated pubertal arrest and growth failure.[92] Pubertal development is often delayed in accordance with the degree of skeletal maturation delay in untreated children with *isolated GH deficiency* (see Chap. 12). Treatment with exogenous GH usually brings about normal pubertal development. However, it is unclear whether GH may actually accelerate the tempo of pubertal progression in these children.[93] *Poorly controlled type 1 diabetes mellitus*, as seen in the Mauriac syndrome, can also be associated with delayed puberty.

Finally, any lesion in the area of the hypothalamus or pituitary gland can cause pubertal delay. Clinical signs that may lead one to suspect this type of process include late onset of growth failure or a combination of anterior and posterior pituitary hormone deficiencies. The most common lesion is a *craniopharyngioma*, a congenital tumor originating from Rathke pouch. *Germinomas, pituitary adenomas, granulomatous disease* (sarcoidosis, tuberculosis), and *Langerhans cell histiocytosis* are other rare entities to consider.

## HYPERGONADOTROPIC HYPOGONADISM (TABLE 92-5)

### CONGENITAL DISORDERS

*Turner syndrome* (Ullrich-Turner syndrome; gonadal dysgenesis) is a relatively common disorder with a frequency in the range of 1 in 1500 to 1 in 2500 female births.[94] It is caused by an incomplete complement of X chromosomes, most commonly

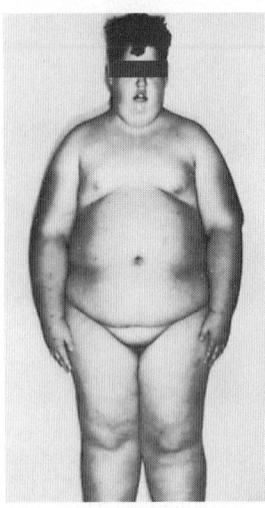
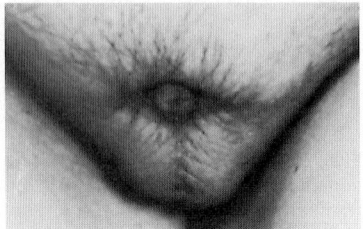

**A,B**

**FIGURE 92-8.** Prader-Willi syndrome. **A,** Characteristic physical features include obesity, relative short stature, and typical facies: fat face with prominent forehead, bitemporal narrowing, strabismus, open mouth, triangular upper lip, and submental adiposity. **B,** Puberty is typically delayed and external genitalia are often hypoplastic.

**TABLE 92-5.**
**Differential Diagnosis of Hypergonadotropic Hypogonadism**

**CONGENITAL DISORDERS**

Turner syndrome (45,XO) and its variants

Klinefelter syndrome (47,XXY) and its variants

46,XX Gonadal dysgenesis and its variants

Disorders of sexual differentiation

   5α-reductase deficiency

   Biosynthetic defects

     StAR deficiency (congenital lipoid adrenal hyperplasia)

     CYP-17 deficiency

       17α-hydroxylase deficiency (girls have pubertal delay)

       17,20-lyase deficiency

     3β-hydroxysteroid dehydrogenase deficiency

     17β-hydroxysteroid dehydrogenase deficiency

   Androgen insensitivity syndromes

     Complete androgen resistance (testicular feminization)

     Partial androgen resistance (Reifenstein syndrome)

   XY gonadal dysgenesis (Swyer syndrome)

   Testicular regression syndrome

   Leydig cell agenesis/luteinizing hormone (LH) receptor defect

Anorchia ("vanishing testes syndrome")

Resistant ovary syndrome/LH and follicle-stimulating hormone receptor gene mutations

Aromatase (CYP-19) deficiency

Metabolic disorders

   Galactosemia

   Carbohydrate-deficient glycoprotein syndrome type 1

   Nephropathic cystinosis

Other congenital syndromes

   Myotonic dystrophy

   Noonan syndrome

   Trisomy 21

   Ataxia-telangiectasia syndrome

   LEOPARD syndrome*

**ACQUIRED DISORDERS**

Irradiation

Cytotoxic therapy (e.g., alkylating agents)

Infection (mumps, Coxsackie, tuberculosis)

Gonadal injury/cryptorchidism

Autoimmune disorders

*\*Lentigines, electrocardiographic abnormalities, ocular hypertelorism, pulmonary stenosis, abnormal genitalia, retardation of growth, deafness.*

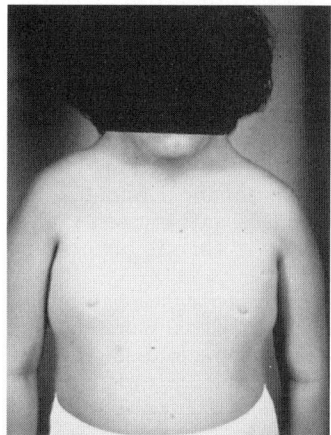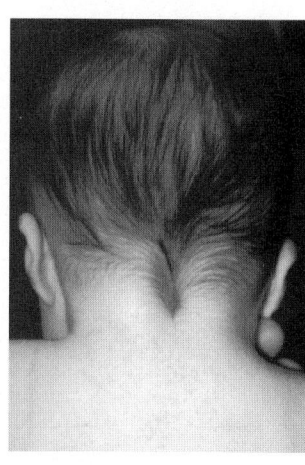

A,B

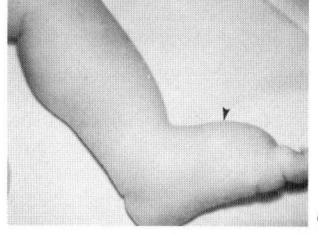

C

**FIGURE 92-9.** Turner syndrome. **A,** Webbed, short neck and broad, shield-like chest with the appearance of widely spaced nipples in a 10-year-old girl with Turner syndrome. Some features of Turner syndrome are obvious at birth and may include **(B)** low posterior hairline with tripartite appearance and **(C)** lymphedema of the extremities (*arrowhead*).

secondary to the complete absence of one of the X chromosomes (45,XO). Partial deletions of the X chromosome or mosaicism with multiple cell lines, at least one of which is 45,XO, are less frequent etiologies. Occasionally, there may be smaller deletions of the long arm of the X chromosome that result in primary gonadal failure without other phenotypic features of the syndrome[95]; these deletions may not be seen on a routine karyotype. Girls with Turner syndrome have short stature that may be due to haploinsufficiency of the SHOX (short-stature homeobox-containing) gene, located in the pseudoautosomal region of the sex chromosomes.[96] Other phenotypic features are variable in expression and include webbed neck, low posterior hairline, rotated ears, high arched palate, broad chest with the appearance of widely spaced nipples, increased carrying angle (cubitus valgus), short metacarpals, congenital lymphedema of the hands and feet, and dysplastic hyperconvex nails (Fig. 92-9). Congenital heart disease occurs in ~25% of cases, with bicuspid aortic valve and aortic coarctation being most frequent. Renal anomalies and autoimmune thyroid disease are also frequent findings, occurring in more than one-third of girls.[97]

As implied by its alternative name, gonadal dysgenesis, Turner syndrome is accompanied by primary gonadal failure in the majority of cases. This is due to a presumed acceleration of oocyte loss with a concomitant increase of stromal fibrosis, resulting in streak gonads.[97] These processes are not inevitable, however, and some women with Turner syndrome, particularly those girls with mosaicism or partial X deletions, may have normal pubertal development and even achieve fertility. As demonstrated in one study, up to 16% of girls may have spontaneous puberty, including menarche.[98] Gonadotropin levels are markedly elevated in a diphasic pattern (infancy to early childhood and after the age of 10 years) in girls with Turner syndrome.[99] Levels of LH and FSH measured at these ages, therefore, may serve as helpful markers of impaired gonadal function, if elevated (see Chap. 90). Furthermore, pelvic ultrasonography to assess ovarian size and appearance has been advocated by some as a prognostic indicator of future pubertal development.[100]

*Noonan syndrome*, often aberrantly referred to as male Turner syndrome, encompasses multiple congenital anomalies that resemble the phenotypic features of Turner syndrome. It is a genetic abnormality, linked to chromosome 12, which can be inherited in an autosomal dominant fashion.[101] It occurs in both boys and girls. Characteristic features include short stature, hypertelorism, low-set ears, webbed neck, chest deformity (pectus excavatum), and cardiac anomalies (chiefly pulmonic stenosis). Delayed puberty is common in both sexes. Fertility is preserved in females, but males have a high incidence of cryptorchidism, which appears to be the main factor in the high infertility rate seen in men with Noonan syndrome (see Chaps. 90 and 115).

Another chromosomal disorder that results in primary gonadal failure is *Klinefelter syndrome*. Affecting 1 in 500 to 1 in 1000 boys, it is the most frequent etiology of male hypogonadism.[102] The most common genotype is 47,XXY, although there are multiple variations (e.g., 48,XXXY; 48,XXYY; and mosaic genotypes) that may result in diverse phenotypes. Individuals who have Klinefelter syndrome tend to be tall with eunuchoid body proportions. There is an increased frequency of behavioral and learning problems. Primary gonadal failure results from hyalinization and fibrosis of the seminiferous tubules, a process that begins before puberty. As a result, the testes are typically small and firm in consistency. Due to variable Leydig cell function, testosterone production may be adequate to induce virilization. Thus, these boys often enter puberty normally but do not complete pubertal development as expected (see Chap. 115). Up to 60% of affected individuals have gynecomastia secondary to an abnormal estradiol/testosterone ratio.[102] In addition, there is an increased risk of malignancy, particularly mediastinal germ-cell tumors and breast carcinoma.

Genetic males with *disorders of sexual differentiation* (i.e., male pseudohermaphroditism) may occasionally present with delayed puberty, although they often come to medical attention sooner because of ambiguous genitalia. A variety of rare conditions responsible for this include the *androgen insensitivity syndromes*,[103] *5α-reductase deficiency*, *defects in androgen biosynthesis*, and *XY gonadal dysgenesis*. For example, pubertal delay and/or primary amenorrhea may be the presenting complaint in 46,XY individuals who are phenotypic females, as seen in pure XY gonadal dysgenesis and the complete androgen insensitivity syndrome.

In the *vanishing testes syndrome*, there is a presumed in utero insult to the testes late in gestation after sexual differentiation is complete. The child is born with a normal phallus, but the gonads are absent. This may differ from the *testicular regression syndrome*, a form of disordered sexual differentiation in which genetic XY males have testicular loss at an earlier, critical stage of development. Resulting in a lack of gonadal tissue and varying degrees of genital ambiguity, it may be part of the spectrum of pure XY gonadal dysgenesis.[104]

The *resistant ovary syndrome* is a poorly understood disorder in which otherwise normal girls present with delayed puberty and amenorrhea. On evaluation, they are found to have elevated gonadotropin levels and small ovaries with primordial follicles.[105] The primary defect is thought to lie at the gonadotropin-receptor level. In fact, inactivating mutations in both the FSH- and LH-receptor genes have now been described.[85]

Mutations in the aromatase gene (CYP-19) have been identified in both males and females,[106] and estrogen resistance due to a disruptive mutation of the estrogen receptor gene has also been found in a single male patient.[56] Girls with *aromatase deficiency* have no breast development or menses, whereas boys have normal sexual maturation. Both sexes lack pubertal growth spurts, however, and they have delayed bone ages, unfused epiphyses, and continued growth into adulthood.[106] BMD is invariably decreased in these cases despite high levels of androgens, and improved bone mass has been shown after estrogen therapy in a boy with aromatase deficiency.[107] These findings further support the notion that it is primarily estrogen that is responsible for pubertal growth, bone mineral accretion, and epiphyseal fusion.

## ACQUIRED GONADAL FAILURE

Acquired bilateral gonadal failure is an uncommon etiology of delayed puberty, and when it occurs, there is a marked elevation of the gonadotropins. Any insult to the gonads may result in testicular or ovarian failure (see Chap. 115). *Trauma*, *cryptorchidism*, and *testicular torsion* are possible etiologies, as is *infection* with the mumps or Coxsackie viruses. *Chemotherapy*, *surgery*, and *irradiation* for childhood malignancy are risk factors as well. *Autoimmune disease* is another cause of gonadal failure. It may be isolated, as seen in some cases of premature ovarian failure, or associated with other autoimmune endocrinopathies, namely adrenal insufficiency, as found in the polyglandular syndromes. Hypergonadotropic hypogonadism is also present in certain metabolic diseases, including nephropathic cystinosis in boys and galactosemia and carbohydrate-deficient glycoprotein syndrome type 1 in girls.

## PRIMARY AMENORRHEA

There is a unique subset of females who present with primary amenorrhea despite normal pubertal development. Separate consideration of these individuals is warranted, as the approach to diagnosis in these cases is often quite distinct from the typical assessment of delayed puberty. Common etiologies for this clinical scenario include *pregnancy*, *premature ovarian failure*, or *acquired hypothalamic/pituitary disease* after puberty has begun.[108] Developmental abnormalities of the genital tract, such as *vaginal septae* or *müllerian agenesis* (Rokitansky-Kuster-Hauser syndrome), may also be present in these girls. Additionally, an *imperforate hymen* or other outflow tract obstruction should be considered, particularly in those females with a history of cyclic abdominal pain. A complete physical examination to confirm normal vaginal anatomy and the presence of a cervix is clearly warranted in all cases of primary amenorrhea.

Females with the syndrome of *complete androgen insensitivity (testicular feminization)*[103] usually present with inguinal hernias in childhood or primary amenorrhea during adolescence (see Chap. 90). They have normal breast development and typically have normal external female genitalia. On closer examination, however, these children have absent or scant axillary and pubic hair. The vagina ends as a blind pouch, and the uterus and ovaries are absent. Karyotype will reveal that the patient is a genetic male with 46,XY chromosomes, and testes will be located anywhere from the abdominal cavity to the labia. Gonadotropins are elevated and testosterone levels will also be increased. These children are considered female, and there are usually no sexual identity problems, although psychological counseling is often required. Therapy should include estrogen replacement, vaginal dilatation to allow for intercourse, and gonadectomy, as the testes have a higher risk of malignant transformation.

## DIAGNOSIS

With a systematic approach, the clinician will often find an etiology for delayed puberty. The initial history and physical examination form the foundation of the investigation, and particular emphasis is given to the medical history, previous growth charts, and growth velocity over the previous 4 to 6 months. A thorough review of systems must be undertaken; questioning for symptoms of chronic disease and asking about the sense of smell are important. A review of the family history is vital and may support a diagnosis of constitutional delay if positive for similar pubertal delay. In addition, parental heights and the calculated target height are important components of the investigation. The physical examination must incorporate accurate anthropometric measurements (weight, height obtained with a stadiometer, upper/lower segment ratio, arm span) and Tanner staging. The presence of pubic hair does not reassure the clinician that puberty has been attained, since adrenarche alone could explain this milestone. Finally, one should search for stigmata of the various congenital syndromes associated with delayed puberty as well as for subtle evidence of chronic disease.

As most children with delayed puberty will represent variants of normal (i.e., constitutional delay), an involved costly investigation is not initially warranted. Instead, continued observation with accurate growth velocity assessment and well-documented physical examinations may be sufficient. However, if there are features of the presenting history or examination that indicate an underlying pathologic diagnosis, if growth velocity is much less than expected for bone age, or if further growth and development do not occur as anticipated, it is necessary to pursue a more complete evaluation.

Reasonable screening tests include a complete blood cell count and sedimentation rate, basic chemistry profile, urinaly-

**TABLE 92-6.**
**Hormonal Treatment in Delayed Puberty**

**MALE**

| Treatment | Induction of Puberty | Maintenance Dose |
|---|---|---|
| Testosterone enanthate or testosterone cypionate | 50–100 mg im q mo | 150–200 mg im q 2–3 wks |
| Testosterone undecanoate | 40 mg po qd | Up to 240 mg/d |
| Transdermal testosterone | Unknown | 4–6 mg/d |
| Androderm (2.5 mg; 5 mg) | | 5 mg qhs (back, upper arms, abdomen, or thighs) |
| Testoderm (4 mg; 6 mg) | | 4 mg or 6 mg qhs (scrotal skin) |
| Testoderm TTS (5 mg) | | 5 mg qhs (back, arms, or upper buttocks) |

**FEMALES**

| Treatment | Induction of Puberty | Maintenance Dose |
|---|---|---|
| Conjugated or esterified estrogens | 0.3 mg po qd | 0.6–1.25 mg po qd |
| Ethinyl estradiol | 2–5 μg po qd | 20–35 μg po qd |
| Transdermal 17β-estradiol | Unknown | 0.05–0.1 mg/d |
| Alora (0.05, 0.075, 0.1 mg/d) | | Applied 2×/wk |
| Estraderm (0.05, 0.1 mg/d) | | Applied 2×/wk |
| FemPatch (0.025 mg/d) | | Applied q wk |
| Vivelle (0.0375, 0.05, 0.075, 0.1 mg/d) | | Applied 2×/wk |
| Transdermal 17β-estradiol/norethindrone | Not used | 0.05 mg/d |
| CombiPatch (0.05/0.14 mg; 0.05/0.25 mg/d) | | Applied 2×/wk in women with an intact uterus |

sis, and thyroid function tests. IGF-I and insulin-like growth factor–binding protein-3 (IGFBP-3) levels should be considered if there is short stature or subnormal growth velocity, keeping in mind that these values are often low for chronologic age (although appropriate for bone age) in children with constitutional delay.[109] A bone age provides invaluable information, specifically in regard to the potential for continued growth. A karyotype should be considered in all girls (even in those without obvious stigmata of Turner syndrome) and in those boys with elevated gonadotropins or phenotypic features suggestive of a chromosomal disorder. MRI of the brain and sella turcica should be obtained in those individuals suspected of having permanent hypogonadotropic hypogonadism as well as those patients with visual field cuts or symptoms suggestive of an intracranial mass. Children with late onset of subnormal growth velocity or posterior pituitary insufficiency would also warrant CNS imaging.

Gonadotropin levels are helpful when elevated, for they suggest primary gonadal failure or end-organ resistance. When they are normal or low, however, the diagnostic challenge remains the differentiation of adolescents with constitutional delay from those with true gonadotropin deficiency, as both groups usually have prepubertal levels of LH and FSH. Certainly, the presence of physical signs such as anosmia, micropenis, or the stigmata of a particular syndrome may lead one to suspect permanent hypogonadotropic hypogonadism. However, despite the progress in endocrine testing, there has been no one test that has indisputably delineated these disorders,[110] although the advent of ultrasensitive assays for LH[30,111] may someday allow for more valid and reliable assessment.

Previous tests attempting to differentiate constitutional delay and isolated gonadotropin deficiency have included the measurement of adrenal androgens, testosterone levels after hCG stimulation, and the prolactin response to stimulation by TRH, metoclopramide, domperidone, and chlorpromazine.[112] However, each of these tests, as well as the use of random and GnRH-stimulated gonadotropin levels, has limitations that preclude definitive diagnosis. Some investigations have demonstrated a more promising distinction between the two groups by using frequent nocturnal sampling of LH,[113] gonadotropin levels after priming or stimulation with GnRH[114] or GnRH analogs,[113,115]

random early-morning testosterone levels,[116] and urinary excretion of gonadotropins.[117] Many of these tests are either too costly or have yet to be validated for routine clinical use.

Finally, although exogenous sex steroids should not increase testicular size, most boys with CDP have evidence of testicular growth a few months after a standard course of testosterone therapy.[118] It is believed that exogenous testosterone primes the hypothalamic–pituitary–gonadal axis. Thus, many clinicians use a course of testosterone not only as treatment, but also as a diagnostic tool in distinguishing CDP from true gonadotropin deficiency.

## MANAGEMENT

The management (Table 92-6) of delayed puberty depends on the underlying etiology, if one can be determined. In those cases in which there is an obvious correctable cause, simply treating the underlying problem should result in the attainment or the completion of puberty. In most other cases, the use of exogenous sex steroids will result in the induction and maintenance of the secondary sexual characteristics.

### CONSTITUTIONAL DELAY

Children with constitutional delay of growth and puberty do not require specific medical therapy. Emotional support for the child, counseling as indicated, and reassurance are often all that are needed. Pointing out early signs of puberty, often overlooked by the child, is also helpful. However, since most of these children are presumed by others to be younger than their chronologic age and are often ridiculed by their classmates, they may experience profound psychological effects, including poor self-esteem, social isolation, and prolonged parental dependence. Furthermore, pubertal delay has adverse effects on bone accretion, with decreased peak bone mass and consequent osteopenia in adulthood.[119] For these reasons, as well as for the diagnostic benefit previously discussed, it is appropriate to consider a brief course of sex steroids in children with CDGP to promote short-term growth and pubertal development. Studies have clearly shown the benefit of treatment on physical development and emotional well-being, and previous concerns about significant advancement of the bone age with resultant negative effects on final adult height are unfounded.[120]

The mainstay of therapy for boys with delayed puberty is testosterone, typically given as one of the long-acting esters, testosterone cypionate or testosterone enanthate. It is quite safe and has few side effects, except for the normal signs of puberty, including mood changes, gynecomastia, and increased erections. An oral testosterone ester, testosterone undecanoate, is available for use, but its efficacy may be limited by its variable oral absorption.[121] Testosterone patches are also widely available, but exact dosing for pubertal induction has not been established.

A typical course of testosterone enanthate for the boy with constitutional delay is 50 to 100 mg im every month for a period of 4 to 6 months. Six to 8 weeks after the last injection, the patient is reassessed with accurate documentation of the physical examination, growth velocity, and bone age. Most boys will have testicular enlargement, indicating endogenous pubertal progression. If testicular enlargement does not occur, further evaluation and an additional course of therapy may be indicated.

Fewer girls receive treatment for constitutional delay. However, similar to testosterone treatment in boys, a short course of estrogen therapy will result in the achievement of secondary sexual characteristics and accelerated growth without adverse effects on bone age or final adult height. Although potential side effects of thrombosis and hepatotoxicity can be seen with higher doses of estrogens as found in oral contraceptive pills, there are few data suggesting similar adverse effects at the low doses used for induction of puberty.[122]

Another approach to the treatment of constitutional delay is the use of the 17α-alkylated androgens, which include fluoxymesterone, methyltestosterone, and oxandrolone. These oral derivatives of testosterone do carry the risk of hepatotoxicity, however, which makes them less appealing. Oxandrolone is the best-studied and most frequently used anabolic steroid. It has weak androgenic action but is generally insufficient in inducing virilization. For this reason, its utility in constitutional delay has been more in its ability to accelerate growth, and it is considered a safe alternative (in both boys and girls) that does not advance bone age or compromise final adult height.[123,124]

hCG can also be used in the treatment of delayed puberty in boys, but it is inconvenient and must be given intramuscularly two to three times a week to maintain adequate testosterone levels. Finally, GH therapy is not indicated in the adolescent with isolated constitutional delay because available data suggest that there is no benefit on final height.[78]

## PERMANENT HYPOGONADISM

Children with permanent hypogonadism require therapy with sex steroids to induce and maintain the secondary sexual characteristics as well as to preserve bone mineral density. If the diagnosis is previously established, treatment should begin at the approximate age when puberty is expected to occur and when appropriate for the psychosocial milieu. However, those children receiving concomitant therapy with GH (e.g., girls with Turner syndrome) warrant separate consideration. In this setting, the benefit of sex steroids on bone accretion and feminization or masculinization must be weighed against its possible adverse effects on epiphyseal fusion and final adult height.

Testosterone or estrogen is initially administered in a fashion that attempts to mimic the natural rise of these hormone levels. Boys should begin testosterone at a dose of 50 mg im every month for 6 months. Typically, this is increased by 25 mg every 3 months until an adult replacement dose of 150 to 200 mg every 2 to 3 weeks is reached. At this point, testosterone patches are a good alternative for maintenance therapy. Girls are treated with esterified or conjugated estrogens at a dose of 0.3 mg per day for 3 to 6 months, followed by gradual increases up to 1.25

mg per day, based on the degree of breast maturation. Alternatively, escalating doses of unconjugated ethinyl estradiol (up to 20–35 µg per day) may be used, but the relative difficulty in obtaining ethinyl estradiol tablets makes this a less feasible option. Once breakthrough bleeding occurs, or by the second year of therapy, progesterone (e.g., medroxyprogesterone, 5–10 mg per day) should be added for 10 to 12 days per month, following which withdrawal bleeding can be expected to occur. Progesterone protects against endometrial hyperplasia and its attendant risk of adenocarcinoma. Other options are to start low-dose oral contraceptive pills at the time when a progestational agent is required or to utilize an estrogen patch, which has the advantage of no first-pass metabolism through the liver. Although transdermal therapy with 17β-estradiol has been used to induce puberty in girls with Turner syndrome,[125] its use may be most valuable in maintenance therapy.

Replacement therapy alone does not treat the infertility encountered in these patients, and the clinician must address this issue separately. Although many individuals with permanent hypogonadism will be unable to reproduce, the use of exogenous pulsatile GnRH via a pump is a valid choice for those patients with hypogonadotropic hypogonadism. In addition, fertility may also be achieved through the use of the gonadotropins, hCG and hMG (human menopausal gonadotropin).[126]

## REFERENCES

1. Herman-Giddens ME, Slora EJ, Wasserman RC, et al. Secondary sexual characteristics and menses in young girls seen in office practice: a study from the Pediatric Research in Office Settings network. Pediatrics 1997; 99:505.
2. Kaplowitz P, Oberfield SE. Reexamination of the age limit for defining when puberty is precocious in girls in the United States: implications for evaluation and treatment. Drug and Therapeutics and Executive Committees of the Lawson Wilkins Pediatric Endocrine Society. Pediatrics 1999; 104:936.
3. Volta C, Bernasconi S, Cisternino M, et al. Isolated premature thelarche and thelarche variant: clinical and auxological follow-up of 119 girls. J Endocrinol Invest 1998; 21:180.
4. Ilicki A, Prager Lewin R, Kauli R, et al. Premature thelarche—natural history and sex hormone secretion in 68 girls. Acta Paediatr Scand 1984; 73:756.
5. Pasquino AM, Pucarelli I, Passeri F, et al. Progression of premature thelarche to central precocious puberty. J Pediatr 1995; 126:11.
6. Jenner MR, Kelch RP, Kaplan SL, Grumbach MM. Hormonal changes in puberty. IV. Plasma estradiol, LH, and FSH in prepubertal children, pubertal females, and in precocious puberty, premature thelarche, hypogonadism, and in a child with a feminizing ovarian tumor. J Clin Endocrinol Metab 1972; 34:521.
7. Lyon AJ, De Bruyn R, Grant DB. Transient sexual precocity and ovarian cysts. Arch Dis Child 1985; 60:819.
8. Saenz de Rodriguez CA, Bongiovanni AM, Conde de Borrego L. An epidemic of precocious development in Puerto Rican children. J Pediatr 1985; 107:393.
9. Pescovitz OH, Hench KD, Barnes KM, et al. Premature thelarche and central precocious puberty: the relationship between clinical presentation and the gonadotropin response to luteinizing hormone-releasing hormone. J Clin Endocrinol Metab 1988; 67:474.
10. Rosenfield RL. Normal and almost normal precocious variations in pubertal development, premature pubarche, and premature thelarche revisited. Horm Res 1994; 41:7.
11. Temeck JW, Pang SY, Nelson C, New MI. Genetic defects of steroidogenesis in premature pubarche. J Clin Endocrinol Metab 1987; 64:609.
12. Siegel SF, Finegold DN, Urban MD, et al. Premature pubarche: etiological heterogeneity. J Clin Endocrinol Metab 1992; 74:239.
13. Ibanez L, Virdis R, Potau N, et al. Natural history of premature pubarche: an auxological study. J Clin Endocrinol Metab 1992; 74:254.
14. Ibanez L, Potau N, Virdis R, et al. Postpubertal outcome in girls diagnosed of premature pubarche during childhood: increased frequency of functional ovarian hyperandrogenism. J Clin Endocrinol Metab 1993; 76:1599.
15. Rosenfield RL, Barnes RB, Cara JF, Lucky AW. Dysregulation of cytochrome P450c 17 alpha as the cause of polycystic ovarian syndrome. Fertil Steril 1990; 53:785.
16. Ibanez L, Potau N, Francois I, de Zegher F. Precocious pubarche, hyperinsulinism, and ovarian hyperandrogenism in girls: relation to reduced fetal growth. J Clin Endocrinol Metab 1998; 83:3558.
17. Pescovitz OH, Comite F, Hench K, et al. The NIH experience with precocious puberty: diagnostic subgroups and response to short-term luteinizing hormone releasing hormone analogue therapy. J Pediatr 1986; 108:47.
18. Robben SG, Oostdijk W, Drop SL, et al. Idiopathic isosexual central precocious puberty: magnetic resonance findings in 30 patients. Br J Radiol 1995; 68:34.
19. Virdis R, Street ME, Zampolli M, et al. Precocious puberty in girls adopted from developing countries. Arch Dis Child 1998; 78:152.

20. Mahachoklertwattana P, Kaplan SL, Grumbach MM. The luteinizing hormone-releasing hormone-secreting hypothalamic hamartoma is a congenital malformation: natural history. J Clin Endocrinol Metab 1993; 77:118.
21. Stewart L, Steinbok P, Daaboul J. Role of surgical resection in the treatment of hypothalamic hamartomas causing precocious puberty. Report of six cases. J Neurosurg 1998; 88:340.
22. Habiby R, Silverman B, Listernick R, Charrow J. Precocious puberty in children with neurofibromatosis type 1. J Pediatr 1995; 126:364.
23. Oberfield SE, Chin D, Uli N, et al. Endocrine late effects of childhood cancers. J Pediatr 1997; 131:S37.
24. Haber HP, Wollmann HA, Ranke MB. Pelvic ultrasonography: early differentiation between isolated premature thelarche and central precocious puberty. Eur J Pediatr 1995; 154:182.
25. Griffin IJ, Cole TJ, Duncan KA, et al. Pelvic ultrasound findings in different forms of sexual precocity. Acta Paediatr 1995; 84:544.
26. Eckert KL, Wilson DM, Bachrach LK, et al. A single-sample, subcutaneous gonadotropin-releasing hormone test for central precocious puberty. Pediatrics 1996; 97:517.
27. Cavallo A, Richards GE, Busey S, Michaels SE. A simplified gonadotrophin-releasing hormone test for precocious puberty. Clin Endocrinol (Oxf) 1995; 42:641.
28. Ibanez L, Potau N, Zampolli M, et al. Use of leuprolide acetate response patterns in the early diagnosis of pubertal disorders: comparison with the gonadotropin-releasing hormone test. J Clin Endocrinol Metab 1994; 78:30.
29. Garibaldi LR, Aceto T Jr, Weber C, Pang S. The relationship between luteinizing hormone and estradiol secretion in female precocious puberty: evaluation by sensitive gonadotropin assays and the leuprolide stimulation test. J Clin Endocrinol Metab 1993; 76:851.
30. Pandian MR, Odell WD, Carlton E, Fisher DA. Development of third-generation immunochemiluminometric assays of follitropin and lutropin and clinical application in determining pediatric reference ranges. Clin Chem 1993; 39:1815.
31. Klein KO, Baron J, Colli MJ, et al. Estrogen levels in childhood determined by an ultrasensitive recombinant cell bioassay. J Clin Invest 1994; 94:2475.
32. Brauner R, Adan L, Malandry F, Zantleifer D. Adult height in girls with idiopathic true precocious puberty. J Clin Endocrinol Metab 1994; 79:415.
33. Neely EK, Hintz RL, Parker B, et al. Two-year results of treatment with depot leuprolide acetate for central precocious puberty. J Pediatr 1992; 121:634.
34. Klein KO, Baron J, Barnes KM, et al. Use of an ultrasensitive recombinant cell bioassay to determine estrogen levels in girls with precocious puberty treated with a luteinizing hormone-releasing hormone agonist. J Clin Endocrinol Metab 1998; 83:2387.
35. Oerter KE, Manasco PK, Barnes KM, et al. Effects of luteinizing hormone-releasing hormone agonists on final height in luteinizing hormone-releasing hormone-dependent precocious puberty. Acta Paediatr 1993; 388(Suppl):62; (Discussion):69.
36. Oostdijk W, Rikken B, Schreuder S, et al. Final height in central precocious puberty after long term treatment with a slow release GnRH agonist. Arch Dis Child 1996; 75:292.
37. Oerter KE, Manasco P, Barnes KM, et al. Adult height in precocious puberty after long-term treatment with deslorelin. J Clin Endocrinol Metab 1991; 73:1235.
38. Bar A, Linder B, Sobel EH, et al. Bayley-Pinneau method of height prediction in girls with central precocious puberty: correlation with adult height. J Pediatr 1995; 126:955.
39. Bertelloni S, Baroncelli GI, Sorrentino MC, et al. Effect of central precocious puberty and gonadotropin-releasing hormone analogue treatment on peak bone mass and final height in females. Eur J Pediatr 1998; 157:363.
40. Galluzzi F, Salti R, Bindi G, et al. Adult height comparison between boys and girls with precocious puberty after long-term gonadotrophin-releasing hormone analogue therapy. Acta Paediatr 1998; 87:521.
41. Walvoord EC, Pescovitz OH. Precocious puberty: combined use of GH and GnRH analogues: theoretical and practical considerations. Pediatrics 1999; 104:1010.
42. Neely EK, Bachrach LK, Hintz RL, et al. Bone mineral density during treatment of central precocious puberty. J Pediatr 1995; 127:819.
43. Jay N, Mansfield MJ, Blizzard RM, et al. Ovulation and menstrual function of adolescent girls with central precocious puberty after therapy with gonadotropin-releasing hormone agonists. J Clin Endocrinol Metab 1992; 75:890.
44. Lazar L, Kauli R, Bruchis C, et al. Early polycystic ovary-like syndrome in girls with central precocious puberty and exaggerated adrenal response. Eur J Endocrinol 1995; 133:403.
45. Weinstein LS, Shenker A, Gejman PV, et al. Activating mutations of the stimulatory G protein in the McCune-Albright syndrome. N Engl J Med 1991; 325:1688.
46. Shenker A, Weinstein LS, Moran A, et al. Severe endocrine and nonendocrine manifestations of the McCune-Albright syndrome associated with activating mutations of stimulatory G protein GS. J Pediatr 1993; 123:509.
47. Pienkowski C, Lumbroso S, Bieth E, et al. Recurrent ovarian cyst and mutation of the Gs alpha gene in ovarian cyst fluid cells: what is the link with McCune-Albright syndrome? Acta Paediatr 1997; 86:1019.
48. Foster CM, Comite F, Pescovitz OH, et al. Variable response to a long-acting agonist of luteinizing hormone-releasing hormone in girls with McCune-Albright syndrome. J Clin Endocrinol Metab 1984; 59:801.
49. Sorgo W, Kiraly E, Homoki J, et al. The effects of cyproterone acetate on statural growth in children with precocious puberty. Acta Endocrinol (Copenh) 1987; 115:44.
50. Feuillan PP, Foster CM, Pescovitz OH, et al. Treatment of precocious puberty in the McCune-Albright syndrome with the aromatase inhibitor testolactone. N Engl J Med 1986; 315:1115.
51. Feuillan PP, Jones J, Cutler GB Jr. Long-term testolactone therapy for precocious puberty in girls with the McCune-Albright syndrome. J Clin Endocrinol Metab 1993; 77:647.
52. Eugster EA, Shankar R, Feezle L, Pescovitz OH. Tamoxifen treatment of progressive precocious puberty in a patient with McCune-Albright syndrome. J Pediatr Endocrinol Metab 1999; 12:681.
53. Schmidt H, Kiess W. Secondary central precocious puberty in a girl with McCune-Albright syndrome responds to treatment with GnRH analogue. J Pediatr Endocrinol Metab 1998; 11:77.
54. Shenker A, Laue L, Kosugi S, et al. A constitutively activating mutation of the luteinizing hormone receptor in familial male precocious puberty. Nature 1993; 365:652.
55. Laue L, Kenigsberg D, Pescovitz OH, et al. Treatment of familial male precocious puberty with spironolactone and testolactone. N Engl J Med 1989; 320:496.
56. Smith EP, Boyd J, Frank GR, et al. Estrogen resistance caused by a mutation in the estrogen-receptor gene in a man. [Published erratum appears in N Engl J Med 1995 Jan 12; 12;332(2):131]. N Engl J Med 1994; 331:1056.
57. Holland FJ, Kirsch SE, Selby R. Gonadotropin-independent precocious puberty ("testotoxicosis"): influence of maturational status on response to ketoconazole. J Clin Endocrinol Metab 1987; 64:328.
58. Cohen HL, Eisenberg P, Mandel F, Haller JO. Ovarian cysts are common in premenarchal girls: a sonographic study of 101 children 2–12 years old. AJR Am J Roentgenal 1992; 159:89.
59. King LR, Siegel MJ, Solomon AL. Usefulness of ovarian volume and cysts in female isosexual precocious puberty. J Ultrasound Med 1993; 12:577.
60. Cronje HS, Niemand I, Bam RH, Woodruff JD. Granulosa and theca cell tumors in children: a report of 17 cases and literature review. Obstet Gynecol Surv 1998; 53:240.
61. Kim I, Young RH, Scully RE. Leydig cell tumors of the testis. A clinicopathological analysis of 40 cases and review of the literature. Am J Surg Pathol 1985; 9:177.
62. O'Marcaigh AS, Ledger GA, Roche PC, et al. Aromatase expression in human germinomas with possible biological effects. J Clin Endocrinol Metab 1995; 80:3763.
63. Leschek EW, Doppman JL, Pass HI, Cutler GB Jr. Localization by venous sampling of occult chorionic gonadotropin-secreting tumor in a boy with mosaic Klinefelter's syndrome and precocious puberty. J Clin Endocrinol Metab 1996; 81:3825.
64. Hasle H, Jacobsen BB, Asschenfeldt P, Andersen K. Mediastinal germ cell tumour associated with Klinefelter syndrome. A report of a case and review of the literature. Eur J Pediatr 1992; 151:735.
65. Comite F, Schiebinger RJ, Albertson BD, et al. Isosexual precocious pseudopuberty secondary to a feminizing adrenal tumor. J Clin Endocrinol Metab 1984; 58:435.
66. Van Wyk JJ, Grumbach MM. Syndrome of precocious menstruation and galactorrhea in juvenile hypothyroidism: an example of hormonal overlap in pituitary feedback. J Pediatr 1960; 57:416.
67. Lindsay AN, Voorhess ML, MacGillivray MH. Multicystic ovaries detected by sonography. Am J Dis Child 1980; 134:588.
68. Bruder JM, Samuels MH, Bremner WJ, et al. Hypothyroidism-induced macroorchidism: use of a gonadotropin-releasing hormone agonist to understand its mechanism and augment adult stature. J Clin Endocrinol Metab 1995; 80:11.
69. Pescovitz OH, Comite F, Cassorla F, et al. True precocious puberty complicating congenital adrenal hyperplasia: treatment with a luteinizing hormone-releasing hormone analog. J Clin Endocrinol Metab 1984; 58:857.
70. Soliman AT, AlLamki M, AlSalmi I, Asfour M. Congenital adrenal hyperplasia complicated by central precocious puberty: linear growth during infancy and treatment with gonadotropin-releasing hormone analog. Metabolism 1997; 46:513.
71. Kukuvitis A, Matte C, Polychronakos C. Central precocious puberty following feminizing right ovarian granulosa cell tumor. Horm Res 1995; 44:268.
72. Cameron FJ, Scheimberg I, Stanhope R. Precocious pseudopuberty due to a granulosa cell tumour in a seven-month-old female. Acta Paediatr 1997; 86:1016.
73. Glass AR. Gynecomastia. Endocrinol Metab Clin North Am 1994; 23:825.
74. Young S, Gooneratne S, Straus FH 2nd, et al. Feminizing Sertoli cell tumors in boys with Peutz-Jeghers syndrome. Am J Surg Pathol 1995; 19:50.
75. Stratakis CA, Vottero A, Brodie A, et al. The aromatase excess syndrome is associated with feminization of both sexes and autosomal dominant transmission of aberrant P450 aromatase gene transcription. J Clin Endocrinol Metab 1998; 83:1348.
76. Cara JF, Rosenfield RL. Insulin-like growth factor I and insulin potentiate luteinizing hormone-induced androgen synthesis by rat ovarian thecal-interstitial cells. Endocrinology 1988; 123:733.
77. Adan L, Souberbielle JC, Brauner R. Management of the short stature due to pubertal delay in boys. J Clin Endocrinol Metab 1994; 78:478.
78. Ferrandez Longas A, Mayayo E, Valle A, et al. Constitutional delay in growth and puberty: a comparison of final height achieved between treated and untreated children. J Pediatr Endocrinol Metab 1996; 9(Suppl 3):345.
79. Acampora D, Mazan S, Tuorto F, et al. Transient dwarfism and hypogonadism in mice lacking Otx1 reveal prepubescent stage-specific control of pituitary levels of GH, FSH and LH. Development 1998; 125:1229.
80. Arrigo T, Cisternino M, Luca De F, et al. Final height outcome in both

untreated and testosterone-treated boys with constitutional delay of growth and puberty. J Pediatr Endocrinol Metab 1996; 9:511.

81. LaFranchi S, Hanna CE, Mandel SH. Constitutional delay of growth: expected versus final adult height. Pediatrics 1991; 87:82.

82. Seminara SB, Hayes FJ, Crowley WF Jr. Gonadotropin-releasing hormone deficiency in the human (idiopathic hypogonadotropic hypogonadism and Kallmann's syndrome): pathophysiological and genetic considerations. Endocr Rev 1998; 19:521.

82a. Layman LC. Genetics of human hypogonadotropic hypogonadism. Am J Hem Genet 1999; 89:240.

83. Habiby RL, Boepple P, Nachtigall L, et al. Adrenal hypoplasia congenita with hypogonadotropic hypogonadism: evidence that DAX-1 mutations lead to combined hypothalamic and pituitary defects in gonadotropin production. J Clin Invest 1996; 98:1055.

84. Kaiserman KB, Nakamoto JM, Geffner ME, McCabe ER. Minipuberty of infancy and adolescent pubertal function in adrenal hypoplasia congenita. J Pediatr 1998; 133:300.

84a. Achermann JC, Gu WX, Kotlar TJ, et al. Mutational analysis of DAX1 in patients with hypogonadotropic hypogonadism or pubertal delay. J Clin Endocrinol Metab 1999; 84:4497.

85. Adashi EY, Hennebold JD. Single-gene mutations resulting in reproductive dysfunction in women. N Engl J Med 1999; 340:709.

86. Jameson JL. Inherited disorders of the gonadotropin hormones. Mol Cell Endocrinol 1996; 125:143.

87. Wu W, Cogan JD, Pfaffle RW, et al. Mutations in PROP1 cause familial combined pituitary hormone deficiency. Nature Genet 1998; 18:147.

87a. Saitoh S, Wada T. Parent-of-origin specific histone acetylation and reactivation of a key imprinted gene locus in Prader-Willi syndrome. Am J Hum Genet 2000; 66:1958.

88. Cassidy SB, Schwartz S. Prader-Willi and Angelman syndromes. Disorders of genomic imprinting. Medicine (Baltimore) 1998; 77:140.

89. Thacker MJ, Hainline B, St. Dennis-Feezle L, et al. Growth failure in Prader-Willi syndrome is secondary to growth hormone deficiency. Horm Res 1998; 49:216.

89a. Soliman AT, el Zalabany MM, Ragab M, et al. Spontaneous and GnRH-provoked gonadotropin secretion and testosterone response to human chorionic gonadotropin in adolescent boys with thalassaemia major and delayed puberty. J Trop Pediatr 2000; 46:79.

90. Pugliese MT, Lifshitz F, Grad G, et al. Fear of obesity. A cause of short stature and delayed puberty. N Engl J Med 1983; 309:513.

91. Henley K, Vaitukaitis JL. Exercise-induced menstrual dysfunction. Annu Rev Med 1988; 39:443.

92. Zadik Z, Cooper M, Chen M, Stern N. Cushing's disease presenting as pubertal arrest. J Pediatr Endocrinol 1993; 6:201.

93. Darendeliler F, Hindmarsh PC, Preece MA, et al. Growth hormone increases rate of pubertal maturation. Acta Endocrinol (Copenh) 1990; 122:414.

94. Saenger P. Turner's syndrome. N Engl J Med 1996; 335:1749.

95. Ponzio G, Chiodo F, Messina M, et al. Non-mosaic isodicentric X-chromosome in a patient with secondary amenorrhea. Clin Genet 1987; 32:20.

96. Rao E, Weiss B, Fukami M, et al. Pseudoautosomal deletions encompassing a novel homeobox gene cause growth failure in idiopathic short stature and Turner syndrome. Nature Genet 1997; 16:54.

97. Lippe B. Turner syndrome. Endocrinol Metab Clin North Am 1991; 20:121.

98. Pasquino AM, Passeri F, Pucarelli I, et al. Spontaneous pubertal development in Turner's syndrome. Italian Study Group for Turner's Syndrome. J Clin Endocrinol Metab 1997; 82:1810.

99. Conte FA, Grumbach MM, Kaplan SL. A diphasic pattern of gonadotropin secretion in patients with the syndrome of gonadal dysgenesis. J Clin Endocrinol Metab 1975; 40:670.

100. Matarazzo P, Lala R, Artesani L, et al. Sonographic appearance of ovaries and gonadotropin secretions as prognostic tools of spontaneous puberty in girls with Turner's syndrome. J Pediatr Endocrinol Metab 1995; 8:267.

101. Jamieson CR, van der Burgt I, Brady AF, et al. Mapping a gene for Noonan syndrome to the long arm of chromosome 12. Nature Genet 1994; 8:357.

102. Schwartz ID, Root AW. The Klinefelter syndrome of testicular dysgenesis. Endocrinol Metab Clin North Am 1991; 20:153.

103. Quigley CA, De Bellis A, Marschke KB, et al. Androgen receptor defects: historical, clinical, and molecular perspectives. [Published erratum appears in Endocr Rev 1995 Aug; 16(4):546.] Endocr Rev 1995; 16:271.

104. Marcantonio SM, Fechner PY, Migeon CJ, et al. Embryonic testicular regression sequence: a part of the clinical spectrum of 46,XY gonadal dysgenesis. Am J Med Genet 1994; 49:1.

105. Conway GS. Clinical manifestations of genetic defects affecting gonadotrophins and their receptors. Clin Endocrinol (Oxf) 1996; 45:657.

106. MacGillivray MH, Morishima A, Conte F, et al. Pediatric endocrinology update: an overview. The essential roles of estrogens in pubertal growth, epiphyseal fusion and bone turnover: lessons from mutations in the genes for aromatase and the estrogen receptor. Horm Res 1998; 49:2.

107. Bilezikian JP, Morishima A, Bell J, Grumbach MM. Increased bone mass as a result of estrogen therapy in a man with aromatase deficiency. N Engl J Med 1998; 339:599.

108. Braverman PK, Sondheimer SJ. Menstrual disorders. Pediatr Rev 1997; 18:17; quiz: 26.

109. Rosenfield RL. Clinical review 6: diagnosis and management of delayed puberty. J Clin Endocrinol Metab 1990; 70:559.

110. Styne DM. New aspects in the diagnosis and treatment of pubertal disorders. Pediatr Clin North Am 1997; 44:505.

111. Haavisto AM, Dunkel L, Pettersson K, Huhtaniemi I. LH measurements by in vitro bioassay and a highly sensitive immunofluorometric assay improve the distinction between boys with constitutional delay of puberty and hypogonadotropic hypogonadism. Pediatr Res 1990; 27:211.

112. Shalet SM. Treatment of constitutional delay in growth and puberty (CDGP). Clin Endocrinol (Oxf) 1989; 31:81.

113. Ehrmann DA, Rosenfield RL, Cuttler L, et al. A new test of combined pituitary-testicular function using the gonadotropin-releasing hormone agonist nafarelin in the differentiation of gonadotropin deficiency from delayed puberty: pilot studies. J Clin Endocrinol Metab 1989; 69:963.

114. Smals AG, Hermus AR, Boers GH, et al. Predictive value of luteinizing hormone releasing hormone (LHRH) bolus testing before and after 36-hour pulsatile LHRH administration in the differential diagnosis of constitutional delay of puberty and male hypogonadotropic hypogonadism. J Clin Endocrinol Metab 1994; 78:602.

115. Zamboni G, Antoniazzi F, Tato L. Use of the gonadotropin-releasing hormone agonist triptorelin in the diagnosis of delayed puberty in boys. J Pediatr 1995; 126:756.

116. Wu FC, Brown DC, Butler GE, et al. Early morning plasma testosterone is an accurate predictor of imminent pubertal development in prepubertal boys. J Clin Endocrinol Metab 1993; 76:26.

117. Kulin H, Demers L, Chinchilli V, et al. Usefulness of sequential urinary follicle-stimulating hormone and luteinizing hormone measurements in the diagnosis of adolescent hypogonadotropism in males. J Clin Endocrinol Metab 1994; 78:1208.

118. Kaplowitz PB. Diagnostic value of testosterone therapy in boys with delayed puberty. Am J Dis Child 1989; 143:116.

119. Finkelstein JS, Neer RM, Biller BM, et al. Osteopenia in men with a history of delayed puberty. N Engl J Med 1992; 326:600.

120. Richman RA, Kirsch LR. Testosterone treatment in adolescent boys with constitutional delay in growth and development. N Engl J Med 1988; 319:1563.

121. Zachmann M. Therapeutic indications for delayed puberty and hypogonadism in adolescent boys. Horm Res 1991; 36:141.

122. Heinrichs C, Bourguignon JP. Treatment of delayed puberty and hypogonadism in girls. Horm Res 1991; 36:147.

123. Stanhope R, Buchanan CR, Fenn GC, Preece MA. Double blind placebo controlled trial of low dose oxandrolone in the treatment of boys with constitutional delay of growth and puberty. Arch Dis Child 1988; 63:501.

124. Joss EE, Schmidt HA, Zuppinger KA. Oxandrolone in constitutionally delayed growth, a longitudinal study up to final height. J Clin Endocrinol Metab 1989; 69:1109.

125. Illig R, DeCampo C, Lang-Muritano MR, et al. A physiological mode of puberty induction in hypogonadal girls by low dose transdermal 17 beta-oestradiol. Eur J Pediatr 1990; 150:86.

126. Hayes F, Welt C, Martin K, Crowley W. Gonadotropin-releasing hormone deficiency: differential diagnosis and treatment. The Endocrinologist 1999; 9:36.

---

# C H A P T E R  9 3

# MICROPENIS, HYPOSPADIAS, AND CRYPTORCHIDISM IN INFANCY AND CHILDHOOD

WELLINGTON HUNG

## MICROPENIS

### DEFINITION AND EMBRYOLOGY

*Micropenis* is a normally formed penis, the stretched length of which is >2.5 standard deviations below the mean. It is a rare but important condition; not uncommonly, it is associated with abnormalities of testicular descent and growth.

Penile length measurements should be taken with the penis fully stretched rather than flaccid, because flaccid penile length varies excessively and thus is not reliable.[1-3] A firm rule or caliper should be pushed against the pubic ramis, depressing the suprapubic fat pad as completely as possible. The penis is stretched and the measurement is made along the dorsum to the top of the glans penis; the foreskin is not included. Stretched penis length measurements from birth through adulthood for normal males are given in Table 93-1.

**TABLE 93-1.**
**Penile and Testicular Size in Normal Males**

**Penis (Stretched Length in cm)***

| Age | Mean ± SD | Mean - 2.5 SD | Ref. |
|---|---|---|---|
| **Newborn** | | | |
| 30 weeks | 2.5 ± 0.4 | 1.5 | 1 |
| 34 weeks | 3.0 ± 0.4 | 2.0 | 1 |
| Full term | 3.5 ± 0.4 | 2.5 | 2 |
| 0–5 months | 3.9 ± 0.8 | 1.9 | 3 |
| 6–12 months | 4.3 ± 0.8 | 2.3 | 3 |
| 1–2 years | 4.7 ± 0.8 | 2.6 | 3 |
| 2–3 years | 5.1 ± 0.9 | 2.9 | 3 |
| 3–4 years | 5.5 ± 0.9 | 3.3 | 3 |
| 4–5 years | 5.7 ± 0.9 | 3.5 | 3 |
| 5–6 years | 6.0 ± 0.9 | 3.8 | 3 |
| 6–7 years | 6.1 ± 0.9 | 3.9 | 3 |
| 7–8 years | 6.2 ± 1.0 | 3.7 | 3 |
| 8–9 years | 6.3 ± 1.0 | 3.8 | 3 |
| 9–10 years | 6.3 ± 1.0 | 3.8 | 3 |
| 10–11 years | 6.4 ± 1.1 | 3.7 | 3 |
| 10.1–12.0 years | 5.2 ± 1.3 | 3.3 | 44 |
| 12.1–14.0 years | 6.2 ± 2.0 | 1.2 | 44 |
| 14.1–16.0 years | 8.6 ± 2.4 | 2.6 | 44 |
| 16.1–18.0 years | 9.9 ± 1.9 | 5.7 | 44 |
| 18.1–20.0 years | 11.0 ± 1.1 | 8.3 | 44 |
| Adult | 13.3 ± 1.6 | 9.3 | 44 |

**Testis (Volume in mL)†**

| Age | Left (Mean ± SE) | Right (Mean ± SE) | Ref. |
|---|---|---|---|
| **Birth** | 1.10 ± 0.14 | 1.10 ± 0.10 | 45 |
| 1 month | 1.80 ± 0.11 | 1.60 ± 0.10 | 45 |
| 2 months | 2.00 ± 0.12 | 2.05 ± 0.09 | 45 |
| 3 months | 2.05 ± 0.15 | 1.95 ± 0.11 | 45 |
| 4 months | 1.85 ± 0.13 | 1.80 ± 0.13 | 45 |
| 5 months | 1.75 ± 0.11 | 1.70 ± 0.11 | 45 |
| 6 months | 1.55 ± 0.13 | 1.50 ± 0.07 | 45 |
| **Tanner stage of sexual maturation** | | | |
| 1 | 4.76 ± 2.76 | 5.20 ± 3.86 | 46 |
| 2 | 6.40 ± 3.16 | 7.08 ± 3.89 | 46 |
| 3 | 14.58 ± 6.54 | 14.77 ± 6.1 | 46 |
| 4 | 19.8 ± 6.17 | 20.45 ± 6.79 | 46 |
| 5 | 28.31 ± 8.52 | 30.25 ± 9.64 | 46 |

*Data compiled from references 1–3 and 44.
†Data compiled from references 45 and 46. See Chapter 7 for testicular lengths.

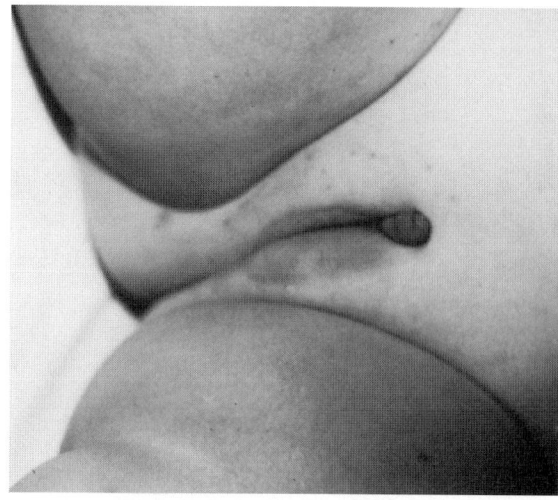

**FIGURE 93-1.** Infant with micropenis and septo-optic dysplasia (de Morsier syndrome; see Chap. 19).

## ETIOLOGY AND ASSOCIATIONS

The causes of micropenis include hypogonadotropic hypogonadism (pituitary or hypothalamic abnormality), hypergonadotropic hypogonadism (primary testicular disorder), partial androgen insensitivity, or idiopathic causes.[4a] Micropenis may be associated with any of the following: (a) specific syndromes such as Kallmann syndrome (hypogonadotropic hypogonadism and anosmia), Prader-Willi syndrome (short stature, obesity, mental retardation, hypotonia, hyperphagia, gonadotropin deficiency), Down syndrome (trisomy 21, mental retardation, flat occiput, simian creases), Ullrich-Noonan syndrome (male Turner syndrome), septo-optic dysplasia (hypopituitarism, absent septum pellucidum, hypoplastic optic discs, abnormal third ventricle) and Laurence-Moon-Biedl syndrome (short stature, retinal pigmentation, polydactyly, obesity, mental retardation); (b) syndromes associated with primary hypogonadism, such as Klinefelter syndrome, other X polysomies, or Robinow syndrome (fetal facies, brachymesomelic dwarfism); and (c) various other, poorly defined, congenital syndromes. Gonadotropin-releasing hormone (GnRH) and human chorionic gonadotropin (hCG) stimulation studies as well as studies of androgen receptor binding have been performed to determine if a defect in androgen biosynthesis or action could be responsible for isolated micropenis not associated with any of the previously mentioned syndromes.[4] No evidence of gonadotropin deficiency, defect in tes-

Accurate examination and measurement is essential in determining if micropenis is present. Micropenis (Fig. 93-1) must be differentiated from a *concealed penis* (Fig. 93-2), which is one buried in excessive suprapubic fat, and from a penis held in marked *chordee,* which is a downward bowing as a result of a congenital anomaly. Very rarely, the entire penis may be absent (aphallia).[4] Palpation and measurement of the length of the corporal bodies is the key to this differentiation; the length of the corpus in a concealed penis and one held in chordee is within the normal range.

Initially, the morphogenesis of the penis is independent of fetal pituitary gonadotropins. Starting at 8 weeks of gestation, placental chorionic gonadotropins stimulate the production of testosterone from the fetal Leydig cells. Under the influence of dihydrotestosterone, the penis differentiates; this process is complete by 12 weeks of gestation. During the second and third trimester, growth of the morphologically normal penis requires androgens, which are produced under stimulation by the fetal pituitary gonadotropins.

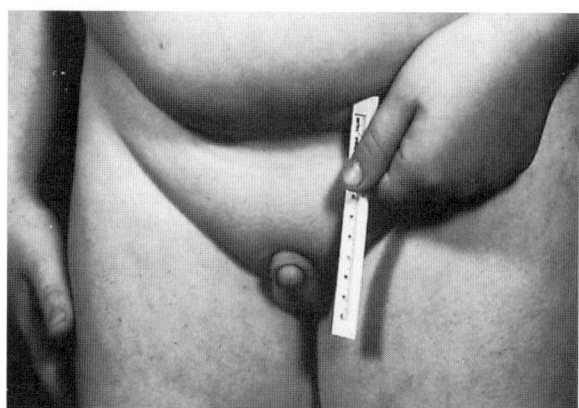

**FIGURE 93-2.** Ten-year-old boy with concealed penis secondary to obesity.

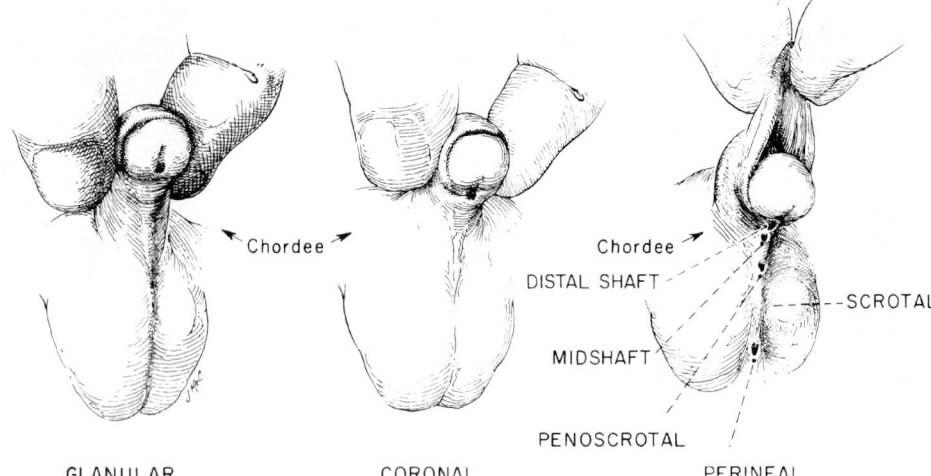

**FIGURE 93-3.** Classification of hypospadias. (From Kelalis PP, et al. Clinical pediatric urology. Philadelphia: WB Saunders, 1985:752.)

tosterone biosynthesis, or quantitative or qualitative defects in androgen binding have been found.

## DIAGNOSTIC EVALUATION AND TREATMENT

The management of micropenis in the neonate should be directed toward early diagnosis and therapy. The important question is whether the child will have sufficient penile growth to allow sexual function as an adult. Early neonatal evaluation is mandatory so that gender change can be an option. The workup includes karyotyping to rule out Klinefelter syndrome or variant forms of gonadal dysgenesis with a Y chromosome cell line. Conditions associated with fetal hypothalamic or pituitary disorders, such as growth hormone deficiency, with or without adrenocorticotropic hormone (ACTH) or thyroid-stimulating hormone (TSH) deficiencies, should be ruled out or treated before hypoglycemia or adrenocortical insufficiency or further harmful effects of hypothyroidism occur.[5] Plasma follicle-stimulating hormone, luteinizing hormone (LH), and testosterone levels, as well as the testosterone response to hCG stimulation, differentiate primary from secondary testicular deficiency.

An assessment should be made of the ability of the penis to respond to testosterone; testosterone enanthate in oil, 25 mg intramuscularly, may be given every 3 to 4 weeks for 3 months.[6] Androgen therapy is considered to be a failure if the penis does not increase in length. Generally, newborn males with the shortest penile length and those with no palpable corpora are least likely to respond. The side effects of this short course of testosterone therapy are minimal and include transient increase in growth velocity and bone age.

If testosterone administration does not produce significant penile growth, serious consideration should be given to sex reassignment and appropriate surgery. If sex reassignment is considered, the parents should be provided with diagnostic and prognostic information, and informed of the advantages and disadvantages of gender change. During this time, assuring the availability of psychological counseling for the parents is extremely important.

The role of long-term hormonal therapy for treatment of micropenis in young boys is controversial. Some have reported that early exposure of boys with micropenis to androgens might accelerate the loss of androgen receptors and prevent a subsequent pubertal response to endogenous hormone stimulation, thereby preventing maximum penile growth at that time.[7] These same investigators concluded that improved phallic growth occurs with delayed hormone therapy, that is, therapy given after age 11 compared to early treatment initiated before age 7.[8] Hormonal therapy consisted of the application of testosterone cream to the penis for >6 months or combined gonadotropin and testosterone therapy for >3 months.

## HYPOSPADIAS

### DEFINITION AND EMBRYOLOGY

*Hypospadias* is the term used to describe the abnormal anatomic location of the urethral meatus on the ventral aspect of the penis. Rarely, the urethral meatus is formed on the dorsal surface of the penis (*epispadias*). The incidence of hypospadias is approximately 8.2 in every 1000 male births.

The embryologic origin of the penis is a midline mesodermal mass called the *genital tubercle*, which appears at approximately the fifth week of fetal life. Elongation of the genital tubercle into the phallus is under the influence of androgens secreted by the fetal testes. Parallel urogenital folds form on the undersurface of the developing penis, with the urethral groove lying between them. By the 14th week of gestation, the urethral folds unite over the urethral groove, completing formation of the penile urethra. Development of the external genitalia is completed by the 12th week of gestation (see Chap. 90).

The formation of the ventral foreskin of the penis is related to normal urethral development; failure of the urethra to reach the tip of the glans penis is accompanied by absence of the ventral foreskin. The absence of this portion of the foreskin causes an abnormal ventral curvature of the penis known as chordee. Hypospadias is frequently accompanied by chordee.

If normal development of the urethra is arrested and the urethral folds fail to fuse, the meatus may be found anywhere along the course of the penis from the perineum to the glans. Hypospadias is best classified according to the anatomic site of the meatus, such as glanular; coronal; distal, mid, and proximal shaft; penoscrotal; scrotal; and perineal (Figs. 93-3 and 93-4).

### ETIOLOGY AND ASSOCIATIONS

Several nonendocrine and endocrine factors are considered to be involved in the development of hypospadias. Undoubtedly a genetic factor exists, most likely based on a multifactorial mode of inheritance. Delayed onset of androgen secretion or inadequate androgen synthesis by the fetal testes can lead to hypospadias. In most males with hypospadias who are otherwise normal, Leydig cell function can be either normal or abnormal, based on the determination of serum testosterone levels before and after hCG administration.[9,10] Whether any difference exists in pituitary Leydig cell function that is related to the various degrees of severity of hypospadias is unknown. Defects in the peripheral action of androgens on the target cells in the genital area may lead to hypospadias. The administration of extremely high doses of some progestins during early pregnancy may cause hypospadias.[11] However, in most boys with hypospadias, the cause is unknown.

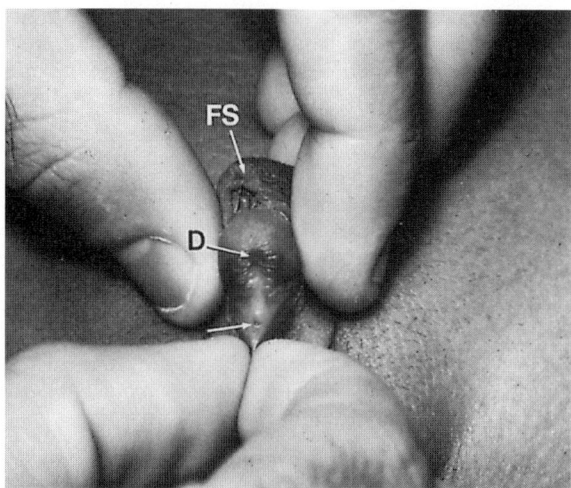

**FIGURE 93-4.** Glanular hypospadias demonstrated by pulling ventral penile tissue outward; hypospadiac meatus becomes more apparent. *Arrow* points to the hypospadias. (*FS,* foreskin; *D,* depression where urethra normally would be situated.) (From Kelalis PP, et al. Clinical pediatric urology. Philadelphia: WB Saunders, 1985:752.)

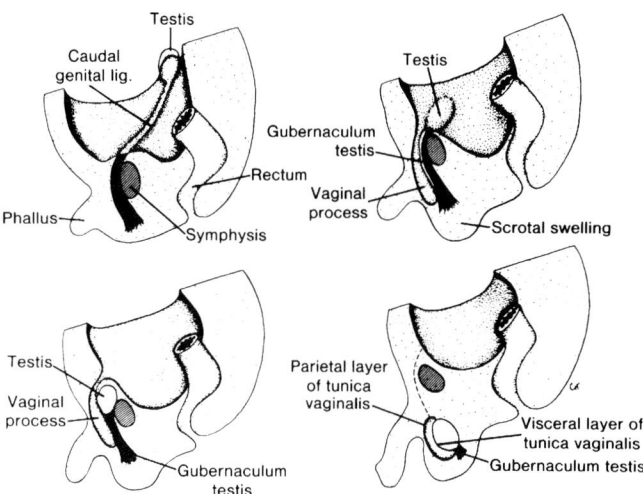

**FIGURE 93-5.** Descent of testis (see text for explanation). (*Lig.,* ligament.) (From Langman J. Medical embryology. Baltimore: Williams & Wilkins, 1981:263.)

An association is found between hypospadias and cryptorchidism; the incidence of cryptorchidism in boys with hypospadias is ~10%. Severe hypospadias, especially when associated with cryptorchidism, may occur in a patient with an intersex problem, and appropriate laboratory investigation is essential. Thus, one should look for other urogenital anomalies when one examines a patient with hypospadias. Also, this condition may be associated with chromosomal anomalies or may be part of many complex genetic syndromes, such as the cerebrohepatorenal syndrome (high forehead, flat facies, hepatomegaly, hypotonia, and hydroureter) and Smith-Lemli-Opitz syndrome (ptosis of the eyelids, anteverted nostrils, or both; syndactyly of the second and third toes; and cryptorchidism).[12] Rare reports are found of a slightly increased incidence of significant urinary anomalies in boys with hypospadias. Routine intravenous urography does not appear to be justified, however, although ultrasonographic studies of the urinary tract may be considered. Hypospadias repair is most commonly performed between 6 months and 1 year of age.[13]

### TREATMENT

If chordee is associated with hypospadias, surgical correction is necessary. Definitive urethroplasty should be performed before the boy enters school, so that he will be able to stand when urinating. Boys with hypospadias should *not* be circumcised, because the foreskin is used in the urethroplasty.

## CRYPTORCHIDISM

### DEFINITION AND EMBRYOLOGY

*Cryptorchidism,* a term derived from the Greek *cryptos* (hidden) and *orchis* (testis), is defined as a developmental defect characterized by the failure of the testis to descend completely into the scrotum. The development of the gonads and genital duct system begins at approximately the fifth week of gestation. The gonadal primordia develop as a thickening on the medial aspect of the mesonephros, forming a bulge in the dorsal wall of the coelomic cavity. At this early stage, the sex of the gonad is indifferent, and the organization of the primitive gonad into a testis is dependent on testis-determining factor (TDF). Differentiation of the primitive gonad into a testis begins at ~6 weeks of gestation (see Chaps. 90 and 113).

At ~3 months of gestation, the testis and mesonephros are attached to the posterior abdominal wall by the urogenital mesentery. Shortly thereafter, the mesonephros degenerates, and the mesentery becomes ligamentous and is known as the caudal genital ligament (Fig. 93-5). In the inguinal area, the caudal genital ligament becomes attached to the genital or scrotal swelling and becomes the gubernaculum. With later development, an extension of the peritoneum forms at the medial end of the inguinal ligament, and this traverses the inguinal canal and extends into the scrotum as the processus vaginalis. The distal end of the process normally reaches the scrotum at ~7 months. Usually, between the sixth and the eighth months of gestation, the testis descends behind the posterior wall of the processus vaginalis, passes through the inguinal canal, and descends into the scrotum; this process is accompanied shortly before birth by a shortening of the gubernaculum. The canal by which the processus vaginalis communicates with the peritoneal cavity usually becomes obliterated shortly after birth. Abdominal pressure is required to push the testis through the inguinal canal. Other essential anatomic factors include absence of any obstruction in the path of descent, an adequately long vas deferens and spermatic vessels, and a normal gubernaculum and epididymis.

Present evidence indicates that the process of descent is mediated by the fetal hypothalamic–pituitary–testicular axis.[14] Evidence exists that cryptorchidism is often associated with an abnormality of hormonal production. Infants with undescended testes have a deficient plasma LH response to LH-releasing hormone (LHRH, GnRH), and the usual response to the testosterone surge is blunted significantly. Possible causes of cryptorchidism include absence of the gubernaculum or abnormal gubernaculum attachment, abnormal epididymis, lack of abdominal pressure, mechanical obstruction, deficiency of LHRH, pituitary antigonadotropin-cell autoimmunity (deficient pituitary response to LHRH),[15] or failure of the testis to respond to LH. Immunogenetic investigations have demonstrated that the frequency of HLA-A11 and -A23 is significantly higher in cryptorchid boys than in control subjects.[16] The implications of this finding in the etiology of cryptorchidism are not known.

### CLASSIFICATION

A useful clinical classification of undescended testes is based on whether the testis is *palpable* or *nonpalpable.* Palpable undescended testes are either *retractile, ectopic,* or *undescended* within the inguinal canal. Nonpalpable testes may be truly *undescended* (intraabdominal) or *absent* (anorchia).

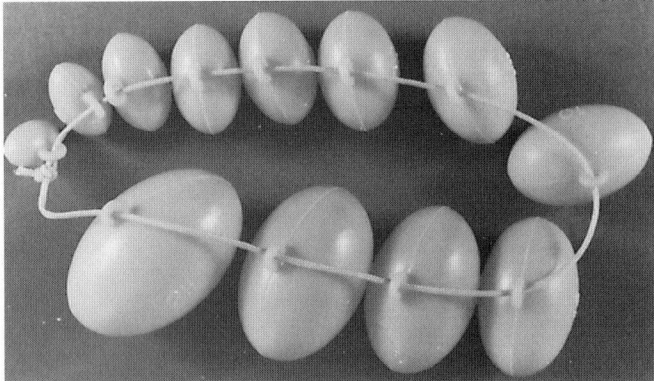

**FIGURE 93-6.** Orchidometer. To obtain true measurements, testicular volume should be estimated without inclusion of scrotal skin thickness. (Available from Resimed S.A., PO Box 775, CH 1211, Geneva 1, Switzerland.)

Retractile testes may be anywhere along the normal line of descent, although they are most commonly palpated in the inguinal area. The physician can manipulate the retractile testis into the scrotum with a stroking movement; the testis is retractile because of a very active cremasteric reflex, which causes the gonad to be withdrawn from the scrotum to a higher location. Retractile testes are frequently found in children but are never seen in the neonatal period. Retractile testes usually descend into the scrotum spontaneously when the child sleeps or when he relaxes, as in a warm bath; usually, they are bilateral, in contrast to true undescended testes. This condition does not require any treatment and, by puberty, the testes descend into the scrotum.

The assumption has always been that a descended testis remains descended permanently. However, well-documented instances exist in which previously fully descended testes have been found subsequently to "ascend" permanently out of the scrotum.[17] The mechanism of this ascent is unknown. An ascended testis is subject to the same degenerative processes as other cryptorchid testes undergo. The clinician must remember that the finding of a scrotal testes does not rule out the remote possibility of its ascending out of the scrotum.

An ectopic testis is one that has progressed normally through the inguinal canal and emerged from the external ring but has been directed from the scrotum into the suprapubic area, the thigh, or the perineum. In this case, the diagnosis is simple and the therapy is surgical.

Nonpalpable testes, particularly bilateral ones, present a difficulty in diagnosis. In boys with bilateral nonpalpable testes, various intersex anomalies must be ruled out. In addition to intersex problems, the possibility of anorchia must be considered. Monorchidism occurs more commonly than does bilateral anorchidism. Nonpalpable testes are less likely to descend spontaneously and are usually smaller than normal testes and testes whose descent is arrested closer to the scrotum. Testicular volume (see Table 93-1) may be obtained by comparing the testicular size determined by palpation with an orchidometer, which consists of testicular models of known volumes[18] (Fig. 93-6). From ages 7 to 12 years, very little increase in testicular volume occurs. After 12 years of age, size increases markedly until approximately 18 to 19 years of age, when the adult volume is achieved.

## INCIDENCE, LOCATION, AND ASSOCIATED ANOMALIES

Two percent to 3% of full-term and 15% to 30% of premature male neonates have a testis that has not completely descended to the scrotum. In ~25% of patients, the condition is bilateral. Many undescended testes descend by 1 year of age; the incidence of the anomaly is ~0.7% at 1 year of age. Most of the testes that descend during the first year of life do so within the first 3 months after birth. After 1 year of age, the incidence of cryptorchidism remains between 0.7% and 1.0%,[19,20] suggesting that spontaneous descent is unusual after 1 year of age.

In a series of 223 patients, the frequency and position of undescended testes were documented.[19] The most common abnormal location was the *high scrotal* position, which occurred in 44% of patients. In 26% of cases, the testis was in the *superficial inguinal pouch;* in 20%, it was within the *inguinal canal;* and in 10%, it was in the *abdomen.*

Certain well-established syndromes, particularly the more severe chromosomal anomalies, are characterized by cryptorchidism. It is present in half of all male infants with trisomy 13/15 (Patau syndrome, characterized by holoprosencephaly, mental retardation, and cleft lip and palate) and less frequently in those with trisomy 21 (Down syndrome) and trisomy 18 (Edward syndrome, characterized by neonatal hepatitis, mental retardation, skull abnormalities, micrognathia, low-set ears, corneal opacities, deafness, webbed neck, ventricular septal defects, short digits, Meckel diverticulum). Cryptorchidism also occurs in the Prader-Willi syndrome, Klinefelter syndrome, Laurence-Moon-Biedl syndrome, and Lowe syndrome (vitamin D–refractory rickets, hydrophthalmia, congenital glaucoma and cataracts, mental retardation, hypophosphatemia, acidosis, and aminoaciduria). Undescended testes may be associated with inguinal hernia, renal anomalies, Wilms tumor, and vasal and epididymal anomalies.[21]

## DIAGNOSIS

### HISTORY

The most important question to ask the parents is whether the testis that is undescended has been seen in the scrotum. If it has, the testis most likely is retractile, and the parents can be reassured that therapy is unnecessary. However, the patient should be examined frequently until it is confirmed that the testis is indeed retractile.

### PHYSICAL EXAMINATION

The examination should begin with inspection of the scrotum. Rugal folds or a fairly well developed scrotum suggest the prior presence of an intrascrotal testis and thus a retractile testis (Fig. 93-7). The genitalia should be examined for any anomaly that suggests an intersex disorder.

The diagnosis of cryptorchidism rests on the inability to palpate a testis or to manipulate a palpable testis into the scrotum. Repeat examinations in both the supine and standing positions

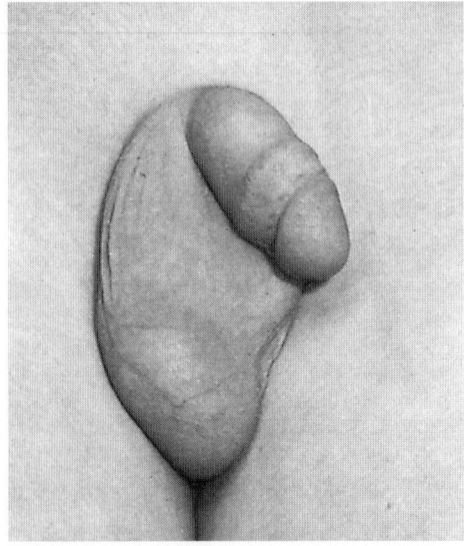

**FIGURE 93-7.** Note empty scrotum and scrotal atrophy on side of undescended testis. (From Schulze KA, Pfister RR. Evaluating the undescended testis. Am Fam Physician 1985; 31:135.)

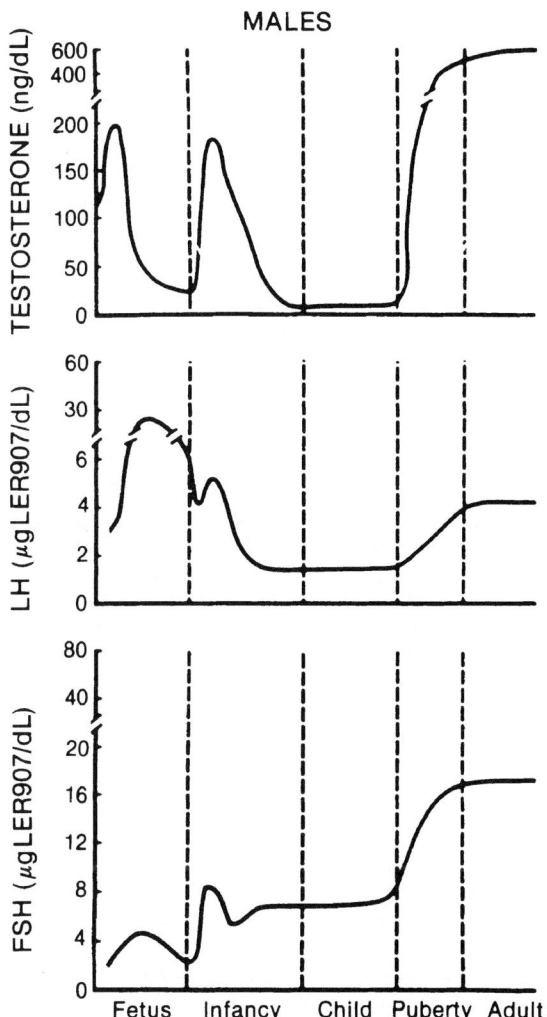

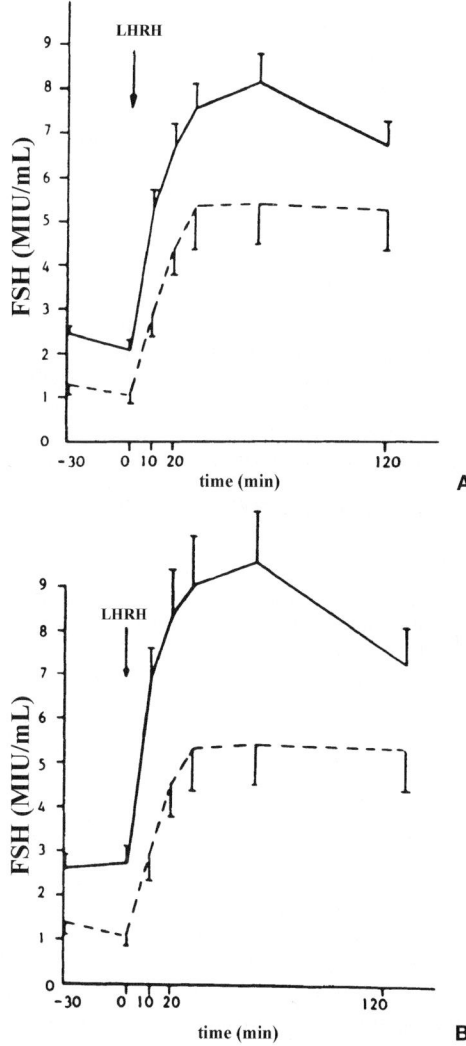

**FIGURE 93-8.** Mean concentrations of plasma testosterone, luteinizing hormone (*LH*), and follicle-stimulating hormone (*FSH*) in males during prenatal and postnatal development. Elevation of plasma FSH, LH, and testosterone concentrations is normal in male neonates and provides a simple in vivo assay for evaluation of the hypothalamic–pituitary–testicular axis. By 4 months of age, plasma FSH, LH, and testosterone levels decrease to the prepubertal range; this decline evidences increasingly sensitive negative feedback in the hypothalamic–pituitary–testicular axis in the male infant. (From Winter JS, Hughes IA, Reyes FI, Faiman C. Pituitary-gonadal relations in infancy: 2. Patterns of serum gonadal steroid concentrations in man from birth to two years of age. J Clin Endocrinol Metab 1976; 42:679.)

**FIGURE 93-9.** Plasma follicle-stimulating hormone (*FSH*) levels (mean + standard error of the mean) before and after administration of luteinizing hormone–releasing hormone (*LHRH*, or gonadotropin-releasing hormone) in boys with cryptorchidism (*solid lines*) compared with control subjects (*dotted lines*). **A,** Unilateral cryptorchidism. **B,** Bilateral cryptorchidism. Basal FSH levels and FSH response to LHRH were significantly higher in both groups of cryptorchid boys than in control groups ($p < .01$), but no difference was seen between the two categories of cryptorchid patients. (From Van Vliet G, Ceufriez A, Robyn C, et al. Plasma gonadotropin values in prepubertal cryptorchid boys: similar increase of FSH secretion in uni- and bilateral cases. J Pediatr 1980; 97:253.)

may be necessary to confirm the presence of a nonpalpable testis. Obesity may make the examination difficult.

In examining for undescended testes, ensuring that the examiner has warm hands, and that the examining room is warm, is extremely important to reduce cremasteric activity. Performing a gentle milking action from the superior iliac crest toward the scrotum may cause a nonpalpable testis to become palpable. The testis should then be brought down as far as possible into the scrotum by traction. If the testis can be brought into the scrotum and remains there, the diagnosis is retractile testis. An aid in palpating an undescended testis is to place the boy in the frog-leg or cross-legged position leaning slightly forward; this relaxes the cremasteric muscle, and the testis may become more easily palpable.

### LABORATORY EVALUATION

Generally, an uncomplicated, unilateral cryptorchid testis without accompanying symptoms or anomalies requires no further evaluation. The collected results of various endocrine studies in boys

with unilateral and bilateral cryptorchidism are contradictory.[22,23] Plasma LH and the postnatal rise in testosterone level are significantly lower in infants with either unilateral or bilateral cryptorchidism than in normal males (Fig. 93-8). A plasma follicle-stimulating hormone hyperresponse to LHRH (i.e., GnRH) has been found in prepubertal boys with both unilateral and bilateral cryptorchidism; no difference was found between the two cryptorchid groups[24] (Fig. 93-9). Abdominal ultrasonography and computed tomography may help in identifying intraabdominal testes. Gonadal arteriography and venography have been used to attempt to localize nonpalpable undescended testes, but these techniques have potential risks. Laparoscopy has been used more frequently to locate a nonpalpable cryptorchid testis.[25]

A boy with bilateral nonpalpable testes must be tested to determine whether he has bilateral anorchia or bilateral intraabdominal testes. Surgery has been used to make the diagnosis. However, the surgeon should perform extensive exploration before concluding that bilateral anorchia is present.

Classically, bilateral anorchia is characterized by elevated basal plasma gonadotropin levels and a lack of a plasma testosterone increase in response to adequate hCG stimulation.[26] After a course of hCG, boys with nonpalpable bilateral undescended testes respond with a significant increase in plasma testosterone concentration, whereas the testosterone level does not increase in boys with bilateral anorchia. Although endocrine tests appear to be able to predict bilateral anorchia reliably, making surgical exploration unnecessary,[27] this claim has been disputed by some investigators, who have suggested that unresponsiveness to hCG may be evidence of nonexistent or dysfunctional Leydig cells rather than of complete absence of testicular tissue.[28] These latter clinicians suggest that boys with bilateral nonpalpable testes who fail to show an increase in plasma testosterone levels after hCG stimulation should undergo laparoscopy. If testicular structures are seen, surgical exploration is indicated. Basal levels of serum inhibin B have been reported to be undetectable in boys with anorchia, in contrast to measureable levels in those with cryptorchidism.[28a]

## COMPLICATIONS OF CRYPTORCHIDISM

### TESTICULAR ATROPHY

Initially, the testicular volume in patients with cryptorchidism is relatively normal. However, long-term follow-up shows that testicular atrophy eventually results if the condition remains untreated. Also, contralateral testicular enlargement has been found in prepubertal and pubertal boys with unilateral cryptorchidism.[29] Testicular insufficiency in adulthood may occur despite such compensatory hypertrophy.

### EFFECTS ON FERTILITY

The failure of normal testicular descent from the abdomen into the scrotum, if uncorrected, may cause severe retardation of the maturation of the testis. The intrascrotal temperature is between 1.5 and 2.5°C lower than that of the abdomen; the higher temperature to which an intraabdominal testis is exposed may severely retard normal germinal maturation.

Most unilateral cryptorchid testes have normal morphology and spermatogonia content during the first 2 years of life.[30] However, by the beginning of the third year, cryptorchid testes have a statistically significant decrease in tubular growth and number of spermatogonia. Similarly, no ultrastructural differences in the seminiferous tubules were observed between scrotal and cryptorchid testes up to 1 year of age, but subsequently, significant differences were noted.[31] Thus, the most important complication of cryptorchidism is the failure of the seminiferous tubules to mature normally, with a resultant inability to produce normal mature sperm. Studies evaluating seminiferous tubule and Sertoli cell function in cryptorchid boys 1 to 4 years of age have been published.[32] The investigators measured serum inhibin levels before and after 6 weeks of hCG and human menopausal gonadotropins (hMG) injections before orchiopexy and testicular biopsy. Seminiferous tubular areas were measured and the numbers of spermatogonia were counted in the biopsies. After gonadotropin administration, serum inhibin levels were lower than in control boys. The number of spermatogonia were lower than in control biopsy specimens. The peak of inhibin concentration was positively correlated with the number of spermatogonia. The authors suggest that serum inhibin levels measured before and after gonadotropin stimulation are related to Sertoli cell function and provide a marker of testicular damage in cryptorchidism.

Some indirect evidence exists that unilateral cryptorchidism affects the contralateral descended testis at an early age. Studies have suggested that autoantibodies to the cryptorchid testis may be produced that can cause degenerative changes in the descended testis.[33]

### MALIGNANT POTENTIAL

An increased risk of malignancy in the undescended testis unquestionably exists[33a] (see Chap. 122); the probability of cancer is 20 to 48 times greater in an undescended testis than in a normally descended testis.[34,35] The location of the testis is also a factor in the development of malignancy; an intraabdominal testis is five times more likely to develop a malignancy than is an inguinal one.

Most tumors in cryptorchid testes are germinal in origin; seminoma is the most common and teratocarcinoma is the next most frequent. Among patients with bilateral undescended testes who have one germinal cell tumor, a second tumor develops in 25%. Interestingly, in patients with a unilateral cryptorchidism, the incidence of neoplasia in the descended testis is also increased.

The suggestion has been made that early orchiopexy offers some protection against the later development of malignancy.[34] Possibly, the risk of malignancy is related to the length of time the testis is retained in an abnormal location.

## TREATMENT

A testis that has not descended spontaneously or that cannot be manipulated into a low scrotal position by 1 year of age should be considered cryptorchid and requires therapy. However, disagreement exists regarding optimal treatment. The primary object is to bring the undescended testis into a scrotal position early enough to allow maximal development. In view of the data on early degenerative changes,[31] therapy should be instituted before 2 years of age. Another goal is to make the undescended testis easily accessible for examination to facilitate the early detection of malignancy. The treatment consists of either hormone administration or surgery.

### HORMONAL THERAPY

Exogenous hCG or GnRH has been used in cryptorchidism because of the role of the hypothalamic–pituitary–testicular axis in promoting normal testicular descent. Maximum stimulation may be obtained by as little as 100 U/kg of hCG administered intramuscularly every 5 days for 3 to 4 weeks.[36] The suggestion has been made that hCG should be the first choice of treatment for prepubertal boys older than 1 year of age.[37] If the testis has not descended after completion of this course of therapy, surgery is indicated, because excessive doses of hCG may be associated with sexual precocity and accelerated epiphyseal maturation. Also, hCG therapy is contraindicated in boys with associated inguinal hernias, in those with scar fixation after previous surgery, and in those with ectopic testes, because in these cases the gonads are mechanically prevented from entering the scrotum.

Intranasal GnRH has been used in the therapy for cryptorchidism; because of its simple and painless administration and the absence of adverse effects, this is a useful form of hormone therapy.[38] The contraindications to the use of GnRH are the same as those for hCG. Preliminary studies had suggested a success rate for GnRH approaching 80%. However, a placebo-controlled, double-blind study indicated that this agent may be no more effective than a placebo.

Most clinicians believe that hormonal therapy causes descent of those testes that ultimately would have descended without surgery. Some investigators have concluded that treatment of nonpalpable testes with hormones has a high risk of failure, and that surgery should be considered as an alternative primary treatment.[39]

### SURGERY

Orchiopexy is indicated when hormone therapy fails. The decision about the optimum time for orchiopexy depends on three factors: psychological, technical, and the risk of not operating early. Psychologically, the optimal time to operate on a child is between birth and 6 months of age. From 6 to 12 months of age, the infant becomes aware of separation from his mother. This awareness increases between 1 and 3 years of age, so that if surgery is performed during this period, the mother should stay with the patient in the hospital. From 3 to 6 years of age, separation from the mother and preparation for surgery can be more easily accomplished. After 6 years of age, the boy begins to feel anxiety about surgery on the genitalia.

Technically, successful orchiopexy can be performed at an early age by experienced surgeons with good pediatric anesthesia assistance.[39] Cryptorchidism may arise from an intrauterine endocrine disorder, and histologic abnormalities can be demonstrated as early as the second year of life. Also, data concerning malignancy in cryptorchidism indicate that subsequent tumor formation may be minimized, although not eliminated, by early surgery. Consideration of these issues, and the fact that spontaneous descent may take place during the first year of life, suggest that the optimum age for corrective surgery is during the second year.[40]

Studies of testicular endocrine function after orchiopexy have produced contradictory results; these uncertainties may be attributable to the small number of patients, the absence of control patients, the grouping of patients with unilateral and bilateral cryptorchidism, the grouping of patients who underwent surgery with those who did not, and the grouping of prepubertal with pubertal patients. Therefore, the effects of orchiopexy on endocrine testicular function are unknown. Fertility as a measure of success of orchiopexy is generally accepted but presents problems of its own. Other factors concerning the patient's partner are distinctly separate from the cryptorchidism itself, and these can be subject to reporting bias. One study compared paternity among men who underwent bilateral orchiopexy with paternity among a group of men who had unilateral orchiopexy and a control group.[41] In the group who had surgically corrected bilateral cryptorchidism, infertility was approximately 3.5 times as frequent as in the group with corrected unilateral cryptorchidism and >6 times as frequent as in the control group. (See also ref. 42.) Patients who have undergone orchiopexy should be informed about the increased risk of malignancy and the need for frequent self-examination.

Generally, for postpubertal patients with unilateral cryptorchidism, orchiopexy has been recommended. Studies suggest that orchiectomy is the treatment of choice for the majority of postpubertal males presenting with unilateral cryptorchidism.[43] The investigators cite the following reasons for recommending orchiectomy instead of orchiopexy: (a) the majority of cryptorchid testes have absent to very low numbers of spermatogonia, (b) a significant potential for malignancy exists, and (c) the chance of torsion of the undescended testicle is increased.

When anorchia is present, or after orchiectomy, a testicular prosthesis should be placed in the scrotum to minimize the psychological impact of an empty scrotum.

## REFERENCES

1. Feldman KW, Smith DW. Fetal phallic growth and penile standards for newborn male infants. J Pediatr 1975; 86:395.
2. Flatau E, Josefsberg Z, Reisner SH, et al. Penile size in the newborn infant. J Pediatr 1875; 87:663.
3. Schonfeld WA, Beebe GW. Normal growth and variation in the male genitalia from birth to maturity. J Urol 1942; 48:759.
4. Evans BAJ, Williams DM, Hughes IA. Normal postnatal androgen production and action in isolated micropenis and isolated hypospadias. Arch Dis Child 1991; 66:1033.
4a. Ludwig G. Micropenis and apparent micropenis—a diagnostic and therapeutic challenge. Andrologia 1999; 31(Suppl 1):27.
5. Lovinger RD, Kaplan SL, Grumbach MM. Congenital hypopituitarism associated with neonatal hypoglycemia and micropenis: four cases secondary to hypothalamic hormone deficiencies. J Pediatr 1975; 87:1171.
6. Burstein S, Kaplan SI, Grumbach MM. Early determination of androgen-responsiveness is important in the management of microphallus. Lancet 1979; 2:983.
7. Husmann DA, Cain MF. Microphallus: eventual phallic size is dependent on the timing of androgen administration. J Urol 1994; 152:734.
8. Ritchey ML, Bloom D. Summary of the urology section. Pediatrics 1995; 96:138.
9. Shima H, Yabumoto H, Okamoto E, et al. Testicular function in patients with hypospadias associated with enlarged prostatic utricle. Br J Urol 1992; 69:192.
10. Nonomura K, Fujieda K, Sakakibara N, et al. Pituitary and gonadal function in prepubertal boys with hypospadias. J Urol 1984; 132:595.
11. Aarskog D. Maternal progestins as a possible cause of hypospadias. N Engl J Med 1979; 300:76.
12. Barakat AY, Seikaly MG, Der Kaloustan VM. Urogenital abnormalities in genital disease. J Urol 1986; 136:778.
13. Zaontz MR, Packer MG. Abnormalities of the external genitalia. Pediatr Clin North Am 1997; 44:1267.
14. Hutson JM, Hasthorpe S, Heyms CF. Anatomical and functional aspects of testicular descent and cryptorchidism. Endocr Rev 1997; 18:259.
15. Pouplard MD, Job JC, Luxembourger I, et al. Antigonadotropic cell and antibodies in the serum of cryptorchid children and infants and of their mothers. J Pediatr 1985; 107:26.
16. Martinetti M, Maghnie, M, Salvaneschi L, et al. Immunogenetic and hormonal study of cryptorchidism. J Clin Endocrinol Metab 1992; 74:39.
17. Mayr J, Rune GM, Holas A, et al. Ascent of the testis in children. Eur J Pediatr 1995; 154:893.
18. Prader A. Testicular size: assessment and clinical importance. Triangle 1966; 7:240.
19. Scorer CG, Farrington GH. Congenital deformities of the testis and epididymis. New York: Appleton-Century-Crofts, 1972.
20. Berkowitz GS, Lapinski RH, Dolgin SE, et al. Prevalence and natural history of cryptorchidism. Pediatrics 1993; 92:44.
21. Rezvani I. Cryptorchidism: a pediatrician's view. Pediatr Clin North Am 1987; 34:735.
22. Sizonenko PC, Schindler A-M, Cuendet A. Clinical evaluation and management of testicular disorders before puberty. In: Burger H, de Kretser D, eds. The testes. New York: Raven Press, 1981:303.
23. De Muinck SMPF, Hazebroek FWJ, Drop SLS, et al. Hormonal evaluation of boys born with undescended testes during the first year of life. J Clin Endocrinol Metab 1988; 66:159.
24. Van Vliet G, Ceufriez A, Robyn C, et al. Plasma gonadotropin values in prepubertal cryptorchid boys: similar increase of FSH secretion in uni- and bilateral cases. J Pediatr 1980; 97: 253.
25. Atlas I, Stone N. Laparoscopy for evaluation of cryptorchid testis. Urology 1992; 40:256.
26. Rivarola MA, Bergada C, Cullen M. HCG stimulation test in prepubertal boys with cryptorchidism, bilateral anorchia and in male pseudohermaphroditism. J Clin Endocrinol Metab 1970; 31: 526.
27. Levitt SB, Kogan SJ, Schneider KM, et al. Endocrine tests in phenotypic children with bilateral impalpable testes can reliably predict "congenital" anorchism. Urology 1978; 11:11.
28. Bartone FF, Huseman CA, Maizels M, et al. Pitfalls in using human chorionic gonadotropin stimulation test to diagnose anorchia. J Urol 1984; 132:563.
28a. Kubini K, Zachman M, Albers N. Basal inhibin B and the testosterone response to human chorionic gonadotropin correlate in prepubertal boys. J Clin Endocrinal Metab 2000; 85:134.
29. Laron Z, Dickerman Z, Ritterman I, et al. Follow-up of boys with unilateral compensatory testicular hypertrophy. Fertil Steril 1980; 33:303.
30. Mengel W, Wronecki K, Schroeder J, et al. Histopathology of the cryptorchid testis. Urol Clin North Am 1982; 9:331.
31. Hadziselimovic F, Herzog B, Seguchi H. Surgical correction of cryptorchidism at 2 years: electron microscopic and morphometric investigations. J Pediatr Surg 1975; 10:19.
32. Longui CA, Arnhold IJP, Mendonca BB, et al. Serum inhibin levels before and after gonadotropin stimulation in cryptorchid boys under age 4 years. J Pediatr Endocrinol Metab 1998; 11:687.
33. Mengel W, Zimmerman FA. Immunologic aspects of cryptorchidism. In: Fonkalsaud EW, Mengel W, eds. The undescended testis. Chicago: Year Book Medical Publishers, 1981:57.
33a. Tekin A, Aygun YC, Aki FT, Ozen H. Bilateral germ cell cancer of the testis: a report of 11 patients with a long-term follow-up. BJU Int 2000; 85:864.
34. Martin DC. Malignancy in the cryptorchid testis. Urol Clin North Am 1982; 9:37.
35. Benson RC, Beard CM, Kelalis PP, Kurland LT. Malignant potential of the cryptorchid testis. Mayo Clin Proc 1991; 66:372.
36. Forest MG, David M, Lecoq A, et al. Kinetics of the HCG-induced steroidogenic response of the human testis. III: Studies in children of the plasma levels of testosterone and HCG: rationale for testicular stimulation test. Pediatr Res 1980; 14:819.
37. Christiansen P, Muller J, Buhl S, et al. Hormonal treatment of cryptorchidism—hCG or GnRH—a multicentre study. Acta Pediatr 1992; 81:605.
38. Gill B, Kogan S. Cryptorchidism: current concepts. Pediatr Clin North Am 1997; 44:1211.
39. Pyorala S, Huttunen NP, Uhari M. A review and meta-analysis of hormonal treatment of cryptorchidism. J Clin Endocrinol Metab 1995; 80:2795.
40. Rozanski TA, Bloom DA. The undescended testis. Urol Clin North Am 1995; 22:107.
41. Lee PA, O'Leary LA, Songer NJ, et al. Paternity after bilateral cryptorchism: a controlled study. Arch Pediatr Adolesc Med 1997; 151:260.
42. Gracia J, Sanchez Zalabardo J, Sanchez Garcia J, et al. Clinical, physical, sperm and hormonal data in 251 adults operated on for cryptorchidism in childhood. BJU Int 2000; 85:1100.
43. Rogers E, Teahan S, Gallagher H, et al. The role of orchiectomy in the management of postpubertal cryptorchidism. J Urol 1998; 159:851.
44. Winter JSD, Faiman C. Pituitary-gonadal relations in male children and adolescents. Pediatr Res 1972; 6:126.
45. Cassorla FG, Golden SM, Johnsonbaugh RE, et al. Testicular volume during early infancy. J Pediatr 1981; 99:742.
46. Daniel WA, Feinstein RA, Howard-Peebles R, et al. Testicular volumes of adolescents. J Pediatr 1982; 101:1010.

# PART VII

# ENDOCRINOLOGY OF THE FEMALE

ROBERT W. REBAR, EDITOR

# CHAPTER 94

# MORPHOLOGY AND PHYSIOLOGY OF THE OVARY

GREGORY F. ERICKSON AND JAMES R. SCHREIBER

Under normal conditions, women produce a *single dominant follicle* that participates in a single ovulation each menstrual cycle. The process begins when a cohort of *primordial follicles* is recruited to initiate growth. Successive recruitments give rise to a pool of growing follicles (i.e., primary, secondary, tertiary, graafian) in the ovaries. The ability to become dominant is not a characteristic shared by all follicles, and those that lack the property die by atresia. In the human female, only ~400 of the original 7 million follicles survive atresia. Recognition that only a few follicles survive and ovulate their eggs demonstrates the principle that folliculogenesis in mammals is a highly selective process.

After the dominant follicle ovulates its ovum, the follicle wall develops into a corpus luteum by a process called *luteinization*. If implantation does not occur, the corpus luteum is destroyed by luteolysis. This chapter reviews the structure of the various histologic units in the ovary, and analyzes the mechanisms that cause them to change during the menstrual cycle.

## MORPHOLOGY OF THE OVARY

The human ovary is organized into two principal parts: a central zone called the *medulla* and a predominant peripheral zone called the *cortex* (Fig. 94-1). The characteristic feature of the cortex is the presence of follicles, containing the female gamete or *oocyte*, and the corpus luteum. The number and size of the follicles change as a function of the age and reproductive stage of the female. Another feature of the cortex is the presence of clusters of differentiated steroidogenic cells called *secondary interstitial cells*. They arise from the *theca interna* of atretic follicles and remain as androgen-producing cells. Characteristically, the medulla contains blood tissue, nerves, and groups of hilus or ovarian Leydig cells (see Fig. 94-1).

## FOLLICLES

All follicles are located in the cortex, medial to the *tunica albuginea*, or ovarian capsule. There are two principal classes of follicles: nongrowing and growing. The nongrowing or *primordial* follicles comprise 90% to 95% of the ovarian follicles throughout the life of the woman. When a primordial follicle is recruited into the pool of growing follicles, its size and position in the cortex change (Fig. 94-2). Typically, the growing follicles are divided into four classes: *primary, secondary, tertiary, and graafian* (Fig. 94-3; see Fig. 94-2). Intrinsic signals are required for, and are important to, the development of preantral follicles (primary, secondary, early tertiary). Hence, the preantral stages of folliculogenesis are gonadotropin-independent. By contrast, the graafian stages (small, medium, large) are gonadotropin-dependent. The growing follicles that do not participate in ovulation undergo *apoptosis* (programmed cell death) and become atretic follicles.

### PRIMORDIAL FOLLICLE

The ability of a woman to have a menstrual cycle totally depends on having a pool of primordial follicles. Consequently, primordial follicles represent the fundamental reproductive units of the ovary. Histologically, primordial follicles possess a simple organization: a small oocyte arrested in diplotene of the first meiotic prophase, a surrounding layer of follicle cells (i.e., future granulosa cells), and a basal lamina (see Fig. 94-3). Primordial follicles do not have a theca and therefore do not have an independent blood supply.[1]

All primordial follicles are formed in the fetal ovaries[2] at between 6 and 9 months of gestation (Fig. 94-4). Because each germ cell has entered meiosis, there are no gametes capable of dividing mitotically. All oocytes capable of participating in reproduction during a woman's life are formed before birth. In human females, *recruitment* (i.e., the initiation of primordial follicle growth) begins in the fetus and continues until menopause.[2] As a result of recruitment, the size of the pool of primordial follicles becomes progressively smaller with age; between birth and menarche, the number of primordial follicles decreases from several million to several hundred thousand (see Fig. 94-4). The number of primordial follicles continues to decline until they are relatively rare at menopause.[3]

### PRIMARY FOLLICLE

A primary follicle contains a growing oocyte surrounded by one layer of granulosa cells (see Figs. 94-2 and 94-3). The pro-

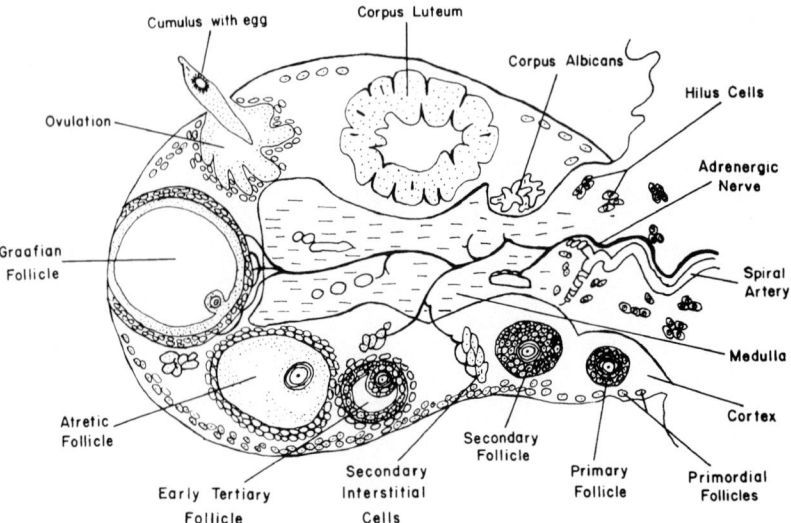

**FIGURE 94-1.** Morphology of the human ovary. The follicles, corpora lutea, and secondary interstitial cells are embedded in the outer cortex; hilus cells, autonomic nerves, and spiral arteries are found in the medulla. (From Erickson GF, Magoffin D, Dyer CA, et al. The ovarian androgen producing cells; a review of structure/function relationships. Endocr Rev 1985; 6:371.)

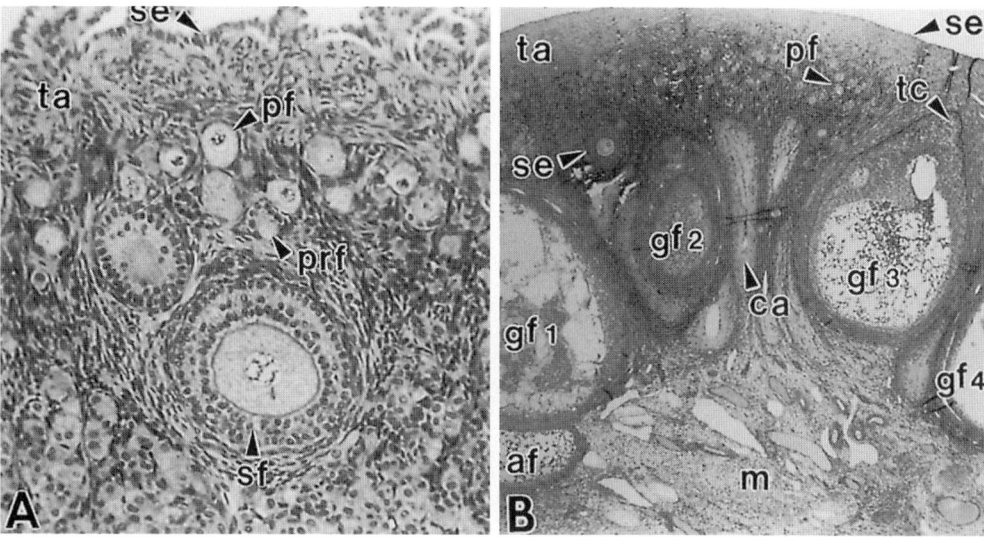

**FIGURE 94-2.** Photomicrographs of the adult ovary. **A,** High magnification of cortex shows nongrowing primordial follicles and their recruitment into the growing pool of preantral follicles. Notice the dramatic increase in oocyte size and the progressive migration of growing follicles toward the medulla. (*se,* surface epithelium; *ta,* tunica albuginea; *pf,* primordial follicle; *prf,* primary follicle; *sf,* secondary follicle.) **B,** Low magnification, showing diversity of follicles. Notice the follicle migration into the medulla, presumably by morphogenetic activities in the theca cone (*tc*). (*gf,* graafian follicles 1, 2, 3, 4; *ca,* corpus albicans; *af,* atretic follicle; *m,* medulla.)

cess of primary follicle formation begins when the squamous granulosa cells round up and appear cuboidal.[4] After this occurs, the meiotic chromosomes enter the lampbrush state, and the oocyte begins to increase in size by virtue of increased RNA and protein synthesis.[2,5] Small patches of oocyte-derived material appear between granulosa cells. Eventually, this extracellular matrix (i.e., *zona pellucida [ZP]*) covers the entire oocyte. By the late primary stage, the oocyte, encapsulated by the ZP, is almost full-grown (~100 μm in diameter). The human ZP is composed of three glycoproteins termed ZP-1, -2, and -3.[6] The ZP-3 glycoprotein functions as the primary sperm receptor and induces the *acrosome reaction*.[7] Anti–ZP-3 antibodies can block

fertilization, and attempts are under way to utilize ZP-3 as an immunogen to develop a human contraceptive vaccine.[8,9]

The development of primary follicles leads to an increase in the number and size of gap junctions between the granulosa cells (Fig. 94-5) as well as between the granulosa and the oocyte.[10] Gap junctions consist of a family of proteins called *connexins (Cx).*[10,11] In the case of animal follicles, Cx43 is the major gap junction protein between granulosa cells,[10] while Cx37 is the major gap junction protein between the oocyte and granulosa cells.[12] Cx37 is an oocyte-derived protein; results from studies of Cx37-deficient mice have shown that Cx37 is obligatory for folliculogenesis and fertility.[12] The role of Cx37

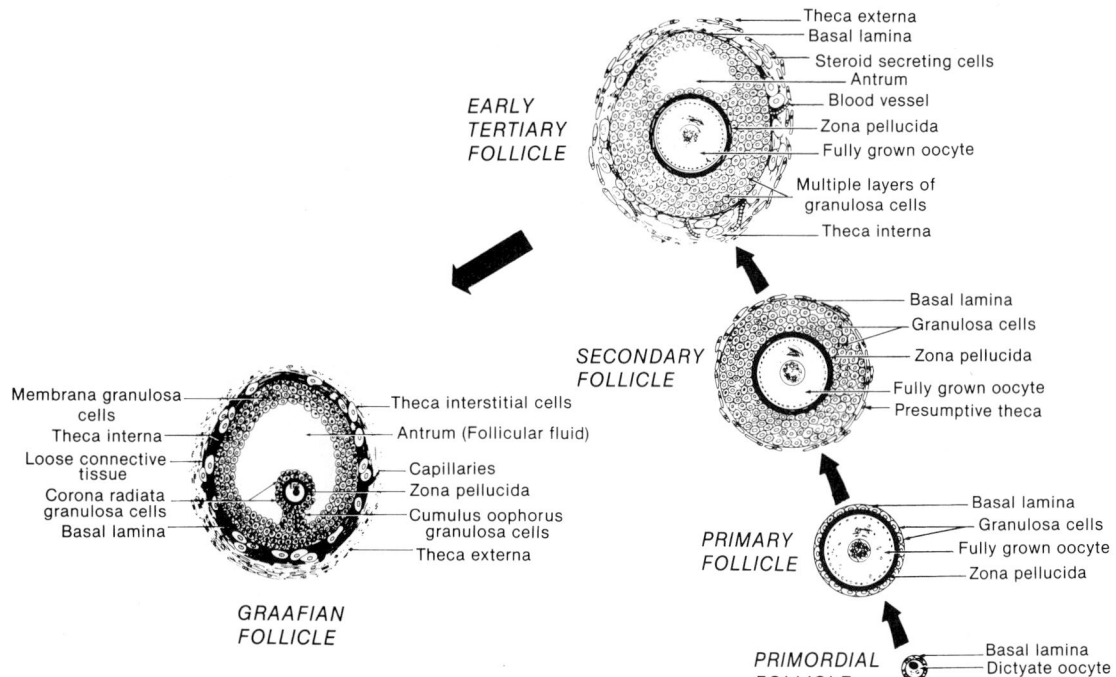

**FIGURE 94-3.** Architecture and classification of ovarian follicles during development: preantral (gonadotropin-independent) stages: primary, secondary, early tertiary; antral or graafian (gonadotropin-dependent). Recruitment occurs within the pool of primordial follicles, and selection of the dominant preovulatory follicle occurs at the graafian stage, when the follicle is ~5 mm in diameter. (From Erickson GF, Magoffin D, Dyer CA, et al. The ovarian androgen producing cells; a review of structure/function relationships. Endocr Rev 1985; 6:371.)

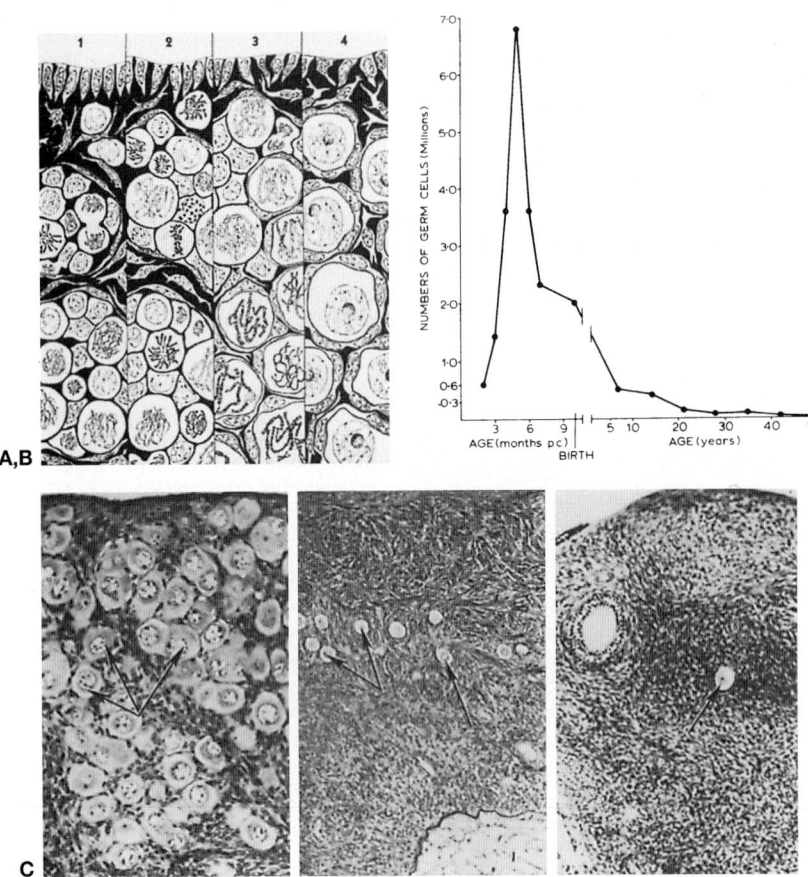

**FIGURE 94-4.** Changes in the pool of oocytes in human ovaries during aging. **A,** Stages of meiosis in human fetal ovaries leading to formation of primordial follicles: (1) At 3 months, oogonia are engaged in mitosis, and a few germ cells deep within the cortical cords enter meiosis; (2) at 4 months, more oocytes enter meiosis; (3) at 7 months, the cords are no longer distinct, and all germ cells are in meiotic prophase; (4) at 9 months, the cortex is packed with individual primordial follicles. (From Ohno S, Klinger HP, Atkin NB, et al. Human oogenenic. Cytogenetics 1962; 1:42.) **B,** Changes in the total number of germ cells in human ovaries during aging. (From Baker TG, Sum OW. Development of the ovary and oogenesis. Clin Obstet Gynecol 1967; 3:3.) **C,** The photomicrographs show a progressive decrease in the number of primordial follicles at different periods in a woman's life.

in human ovary physiology and pathophysiology remains to be determined.

## SECONDARY FOLLICLE

A secondary follicle contains two to eight layers of granulosa cells with no antrum. During secondary follicle development, the granulosa cells proliferate slowly,[4] and the oocyte completes its final growth.[13] By the end of the secondary stage, the follicle is a multilayered structure that is strikingly symmetric; in the center is a full-grown oocyte (~120 μm in diameter), eight layers of stratified low columnar granulosa cells, and a basal lamina (Fig. 94-6). When the follicle has two to three layers of granulosa cells, a signal (yet to be identified) is generated that causes a stream of mesenchymal cells to migrate toward the basal lamina.[14] They become organized into a layer of fibroblast-like cells (see Fig. 94-6) that ultimately develops into the *theca interna* and the *theca externa*. At about this time, the secondary follicle acquires a set of capillaries. The vessels form two sets of interconnected capillaries, an inner wreath located in the theca interna, which is supplied by branches from an outer wreath located in the theca externa.[1] *Call-Exner bodies* develop among the granulosa cells in the secondary follicle (see Fig. 94-6). Histologically, these bodies appear to be made of extracellular matrix. The physiologic function of Call-Exner bodies is unknown; however, given the importance of the extracellular matrix in proliferation and cytodifferentiation,[15] they may play a role in generating subtypes of granulosa cells by providing novel substrate-to-cell interactions.

## TERTIARY FOLLICLE

A characteristic feature of a tertiary follicle is the *antrum*.[16] When a follicle reaches ~400 μm in diameter, follicular fluid accumulates between some granulosa cells. This results in the formation of a small cavity or antrum at one pole of the oocyte (see Fig. 94-3). The initiation of antrum formation is controlled

by the follicle itself, but the nature of the regulatory factors remains unknown. As a consequence of beginning antrum formation, the follicle assumes a symmetry that remains throughout folliculogenesis (see Figs. 94-2 and 94-3). Simultaneously,

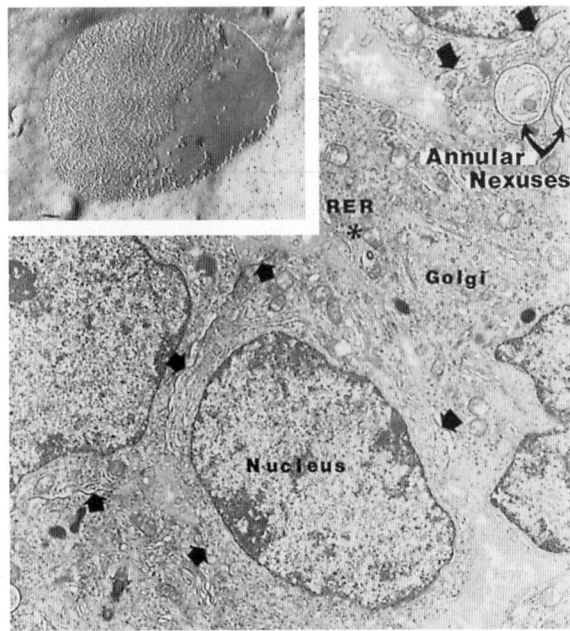

**FIGURE 94-5.** Electron micrograph shows the structure of gap junctions *(arrows)* between granulosa cells of a healthy graafian follicle. *Inset,* Replica of granulosa cell fracture shows the hexagonally ordered connexin proteins of the gap junction. (*RER,* rough endoplasmic reticulum.) (Courtesy of Dr. David Albertini, Tufts University, Boston, MA.)

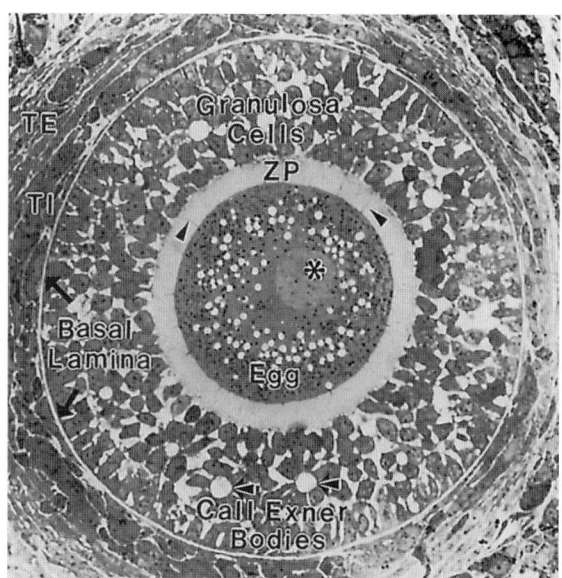

**FIGURE 94-6.** Photomicrograph of a fully grown secondary follicle with six to eight layers of granulosa cells. (*TE*, theca externa; *TI*, theca interna; *ZP*, zona pellucida; *, germinal vesicle or egg nucleus; *arrowheads*, cytoplasmic process of corona radiata granulosa cells traversing the ZP.) (Adapted from Anderson E. The ovary: basic principles and concepts. In: Felig P, Baxter JD, Broadus AE, Frohman LA, eds. Endocrinology and metabolism, 3rd ed. New York: McGraw-Hill, 1994.)

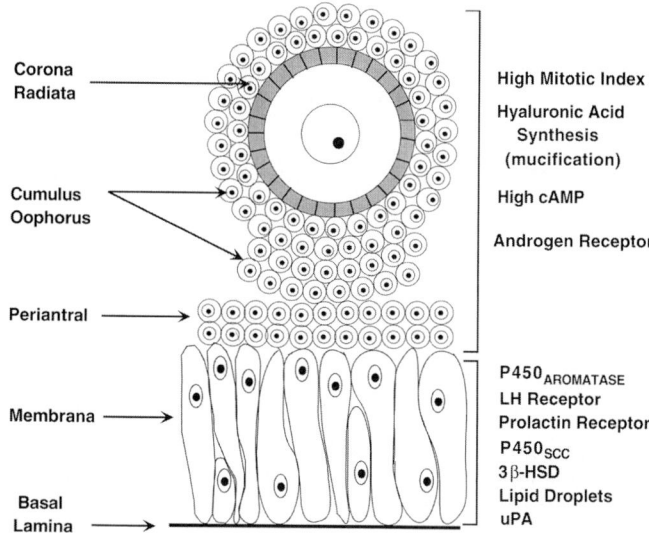

**FIGURE 94-7.** Diagram of the heterogeneity of the granulosa cells in a healthy graafian follicle. By virtue of their position or location in the follicle wall, the granulosa cells express different patterns of proliferation and cytodifferentiation in response to follicle-stimulating hormone stimulation. (*cAMP*, cyclic adenosine monophosphate; *LH*, luteinizing hormone; *HSD*, hydroxysteroid dehydrogenase.) (From Erickson GF. The graafian follicle: a functional definition. In: Adashi EY, ed. Ovulation: evolving scientific and clinical concepts. New York: Springer-Verlag, [in press 1999].)

histologic changes are initiated in the theca interna.[14] Subpopulations of fibroblasts transform into large epithelial-like cells called *theca-interstitial cells* (see Fig. 94-3), which produce a variety of ligands, most notably androgens in response primarily to luteinizing hormone (LH) and insulin stimulation. [17]

### GRAAFIAN FOLLICLE

The morphology of the early tertiary and graafian follicle is similar except that the graafian follicle is larger. In women, a graafian follicle can increase as much as 75-fold in diameter, from 0.4 mm to 30 mm.[18] The tremendous growth is caused by follicular fluid accumulation and proliferation of the granulosa and theca cells.[16,18] Follicular fluid is an exudate of plasma plus various regulatory factors produced by the follicle cells themselves.[19] The follicular fluid is the medium in which the granulosa cells are found and through which regulatory molecules must pass on their way to and from the microenvironment.

By virtue of the structure of the follicle, the granulosa cells become different from one another with respect to their position in the system (see Fig. 94-3). There are four granulosa cell domains[16]: Granulosa cells forming the corona radiata make contact with the oocyte and ZP, those comprising the cumulus make contact with the corona and membrana granulosa cells, and those forming the membrana granulosa make contact with the basal lamina and Call-Exner bodies (Fig. 94-7). It has been shown that the position of the granulosa cells determines the direction in which they differentiate in response to follicle-stimulating hormone (FSH).[16] For example, the membrana, but not cumulus, granulosa cells express the P450 enzyme aromatase ($P450_{AROM}$) and LH receptor in response to FSH stimulation (see Fig. 94-7). The significance of granulosa heterogeneity is unknown. Nonetheless, it is becoming clear that oocyte-derived regulatory proteins determine the way in which the granulosa cells differentiate.[20]

During the small (1–5 mm), medium (6–11 mm), and large (>12 mm) stages of graafian follicle development, the number of theca-interstitial cells increases progressively until there are five to eight layers in the dominant preovulatory follicle.[4,18] The increase results from mitosis, presumably within a population of undifferentiated stem cells. The theca externa (see Figs. 94-1 and 94-3) is composed of smooth muscle cells, and these contractile cells are innervated by the autonomic nervous system.[16,21]

### ATRETIC FOLLICLE

After a primordial follicle is recruited, it develops to the preovulatory stage or dies by atresia. Atresia results in the death and removal of the granulosa and the oocyte by a programmed cell death mechanism[22–24] called *apoptosis*. The discovery that atresia involves the activation of physiologic cell suicide mechanisms has opened up new ways to investigate the regulation and mechanisms underlying follicle death. Although the field is still in its infancy, it is clear that FSH is a major suppressor of apoptosis in granulosa cells.[22,23] The challenge is to understand the nature of the physiologic ligands that activate apoptosis in follicles during the menstrual cycle and in so doing understand the basis for selection of the dominant follicle. It is noteworthy that the theca cells appear to survive atresia, becoming islands of *secondary interstitial cells*.[14] Atresia is evident at all stages of graafian follicle growth, and at all stages of the cycle; however, atresia is rare or absent in the nongrowing primordial follicles and difficult to detect in the pool of preantral follicles.[4]

Morphologic data suggest that the sequence of atresia may be different for preantral and antral follicles.[14] Atresia of preantral follicles is most readily identified by precocious antrum formation (Fig. 94-8A); however, premature meiotic maturation and fragmentation of the oocyte are also seen in preantral atresia.[25] In the graafian follicles, the earliest morphologic sign of atresia involves a major shape change in the granulosa cells, which are attached to the basal lamina and the ZP.[26] In healthy graafian follicles,[16] the membrana granulosa cells consist of a uniform layer of pseudostratified epithelial cells, all of which are attached to the basal lamina. At or about the time atresia is initiated, these cells contract and become a simple stratified cuboidal epithelium (see Fig 94-8B).

The cause of this coordinated cell-contraction mechanism is unknown. A similar phenomenon occurs in the corona radiata cells. Another morphologic sign of early atresia in graafian follicles is that some of the periantral granulosa cells (those at the border of the antrum) lose contact with one another and are

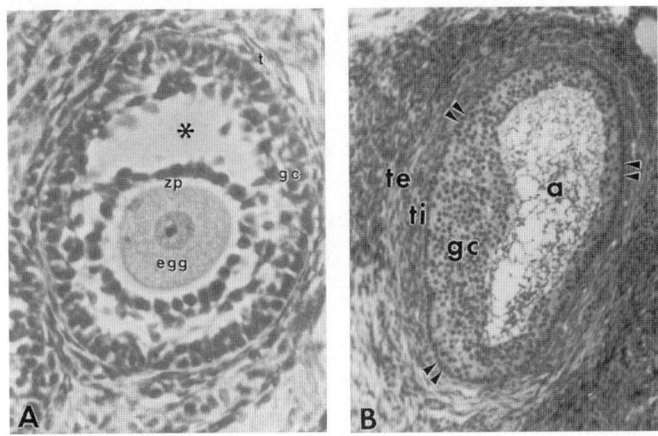

**FIGURE 94-8.** Photomicrographs showing the early histologic changes of atresia in preantral and graafian follicles. **A,** Preantral follicle (secondary stage), with three layers of granulosa cells (sc). A cavity (*) is already present, a phenomenon called *precocious antrum formation.* (*ZP,* zona pellucida; *t,* theca.) **B,** Graafian follicle. The membrana granulosa (outer layer) has contracted into a cuboidal epithelium that appears as a distinct bead of cells (*arrowheads*) around the periphery of the follicle. (*ti,* theca interna; *te,* theca externa; *a,* antrum.)

released into the follicular fluid, where they become apoptotic. As atresia progresses, the number of apoptotic cells increases to the point that no healthy granulosa cells are visible. Oocyte death occurs relatively late in the process of graafian follicle atresia by apoptotic mechanisms.[23]

## INTERSTITIAL CELLS

### THECA-INTERSTITIAL CELLS

Theca-interstitial cells are located in the theca interna of all graafian follicles. Morphologically, they have the ultrastructure that is typical of active steroidogenic cells.[14] In the human ovary, they are the primary site of androstenedione biosynthesis.[18,27]

Shortly after presumptive theca cells reach the secondary follicle, some begin a theca-interstitial cytodifferentiation.[14,28] Most notably, this developmental process involves the acquisition of the *steroid acute regulatory protein (StAR),* a protein that transfers cholesterol from the outer to the inner mitochondrial membrane; cholesterol side-chain cleavage enzyme (P450$_{c22}$); 3β-hydroxysteroid dehydrogenase-$\Delta^{4,5}$ isomerase enzyme (3β-HSD); and the LH receptor.[14,28] The initial differentiation of these cells is regulated by local autocrine/paracrine mechanisms operating within the secondary follicle.

In response to LH delivered by the theca capillaries, the interstitial cells transform from elongated mesenchymal cells into large epithelial-like cells that produce progesterone.[14,28] As the preantral follicle grows to the graafian stage, the interstitial cells express the 17α-hydroxylase C$_{17-20}$ lyase enzyme (P450$_{c17}$) and transform from progesterone-producing cells to cells that produce androstenedione (Fig. 94-9). As discussed later, there is a causal relationship between this switch into an androgen-producing cell and the ability of the developing follicle to produce aromatase substrate and, thus, estradiol.

It should be noted that an interesting role for insulin and lipoproteins in stimulating human theca progesterone and androstenedione production has been demonstrated by in vitro studies.[29] Thus, a much more complex endocrine regulation of theca-interstitial cells is emerging (Fig. 94-10).

### SECONDARY INTERSTITIAL CELLS

The secondary interstitial cells arise as a consequence of atresia.[14] Secondary interstitial cells maintain their specialized ultrastructure and can respond to LH with increased androstenedione production.[14,18]

One difference between the theca and the secondary interstitial cells is that the latter are the only endocrine cells in the ovary that are innervated[14] (see Fig. 94-1). Animal studies suggest that there is a point-to-point communication between neurons in the hypothalamus and the ovarian steroidogenic cells.[14,30] Moreover, in vitro studies indicate that catecholamines directly stimulate androgen synthesis in secondary interstitial cells.[14] There is strong evidence for neural and neurotrophic control of androgen production by ovarian secondary interstitial cells.[14,31] Evidence supports the proposition that the nervous system may play an important role in the physiology and pathophysiology of ovarian androgen production.

### CORPUS LUTEUM

After ovulation (see Fig. 94-1), the follicle wall transforms into the corpus luteum (Fig. 94-11). Cells that make up the corpus luteum are contributed by the membrana granulosa, theca interna, theca externa, and invading blood tissue. The white blood cells produce potent regulatory ligands, such as the cytokines, that can regulate ovulation and corpus luteum function.[32] Understanding how white blood cells influence these critical processes is a major goal of ovary research. Morphologically, there is a fibrin clot where the antrum and liquor folliculi were located, into which loose connective tissue and blood cells have invaded (see Fig. 94-11).

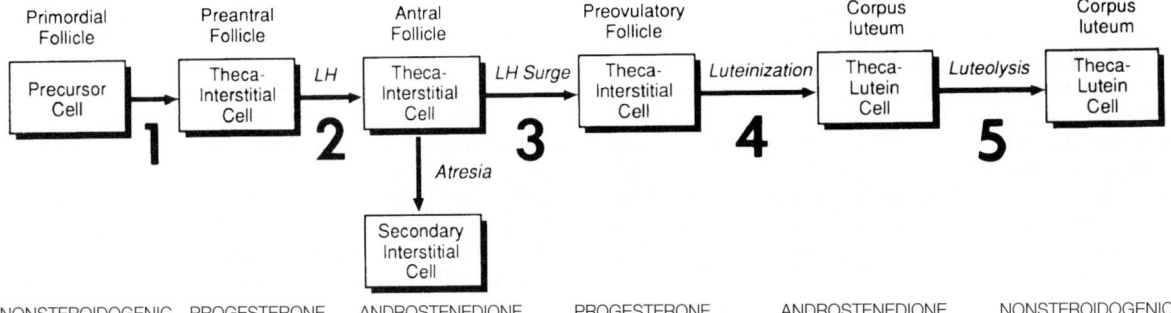

**FIGURE 94-9.** Flow pathway diagram of steroidogenesis of human interstitial cells during folliculogenesis. The first step is the conversion of prothecoblasts into theca-interstitial cells, which produce progesterone, which occurs in secondary follicles. The second step consists of luteinizing hormone (*LH*) induction of P450$_{c17}$, which results in the production of androstenedione. It begins in early tertiary follicles and continues through graafian follicle development (healthy and atretic). The third step is a switch back to a progesterone-producing cell, which occurs at ovulation. The fourth step is the reinduction of P450$_{c17}$ in theca-lutein cells during luteinization, which results in androstenedione production. (Adapted from Erickson GF. Normal regulation of ovarian androgen production. Semin Reprod Endocrinol 1993; 11:307.)

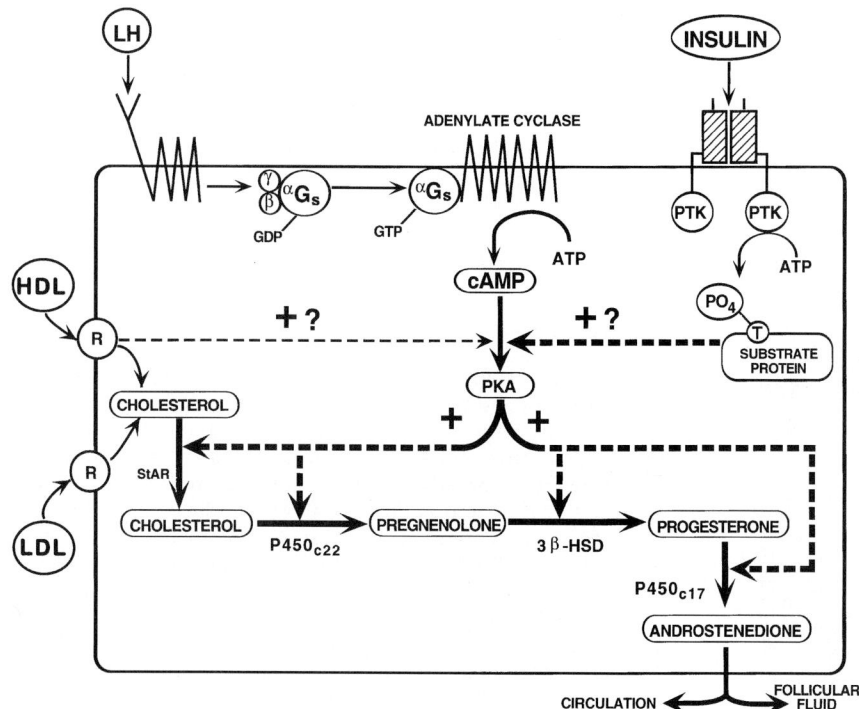

**FIGURE 94-10.** Diagram of the luteinizing hormone (*LH*) signal transduction pathway in differentiated theca-interstitial cells leading to androstenedione biosynthesis. Other regulatory molecules including insulin and low- and high-density lipoproteins (*LDL, HDL*) can interact with the LH signaling pathway to increase steroidogenesis further. (*GDP*, guanosine diphosphate; *GTP*, guanosine triphosphate; *PTK*, protein tyrosine kinase; *ATP*, adenosine triphosphate; *cAMP*, cyclic adenosine monophosphate; *R*, receptor; *StAR*, steroid acute regulatory protein; *HSD*, hydroxysteroid dehydrogenase.) (Redrawn from Erickson GF. Normal regulation of ovarian androgen production. Semin Reprod Endocrinol 1993; 11:307.)

During luteinization, the membrana and periantral granulosa cells attain a large size, ~35 μm in diameter.[33] These cells, now called *granulosa lutein cells,* have an ultrastructure typical of differentiated steroidogenic cells; they contain abundant smooth endoplasmic reticulum, tubular cristae in the mitochondria, and large clusters of lipid droplets containing cholesterol esters in the cytoplasm (Fig. 94-12).

The theca-interstitial cells also are incorporated into the corpus luteum, becoming the *theca-lutein cells* (see Fig. 94-12). They can be distinguished from granulosa lutein cells because they are smaller (~15 μm in diameter) and stain more darkly.[33] Theca-lutein cells also exhibit the ultrastructure of active steroid-secreting cells.[33] During the ovulatory phase, the theca cells lose the P450$_{c17}$ and become active in progesterone production (see Fig. 94-9). These cells reacquire the P450$_{c17}$ after luteinization and once again produce androstenedione (see Fig. 94-9). By virtue of the expression of androstenedione and P450$_{AROM}$ in the theca and granulosa lutein cells, respectively,[34] the corpus luteum also synthesizes and secretes estradiol.

If implantation does not occur, the corpus luteum degenerates. This process, called *luteolysis,* becomes apparent histologically at 8 days after ovulation. The first histologic indication of luteolysis is shrinkage of the granulosa lutein cells. The theca-lutein cells appear selectively hyperstimulated during early luteolysis, analogous to the theca-interstitial cell hypertrophy

associated with atresia. After day 23 of the cycle, apoptosis is activated,[35] and the corpus luteum dies. Histologically, all that remains is a nodule of dense connective tissue called the *corpus albicans* (see Figs. 94-1 and 94-2). The mechanism of luteolysis in women is poorly understood, but it has been proposed that prostaglandin F$_2$α might be involved.[36,37]

## PHYSIOLOGY OF THE OVARY

In women, the cyclic changes that occur in the menstrual cycle reflect structural and functional changes that occur within the follicle and corpus luteum. The dominant follicle begins as a primordial follicle and is slowly prepared for ovulation and luteinization by the action of the pituitary gonadotropins and ovarian growth factors. To understand the relationship of the dominant follicle to the events occurring in the menstrual cycle, the underlying physiologic mechanisms of folliculogenesis—recruitment, selection, atresia, ovulation, and luteogenesis (i.e., luteinization, luteolysis)—must be considered.

### NORMAL FOLLICULOGENESIS

Follicular growth and development in women is a very long process.[4] In each menstrual cycle, the ovulating follicle origi-

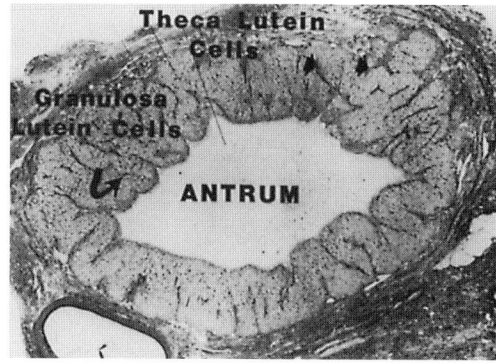
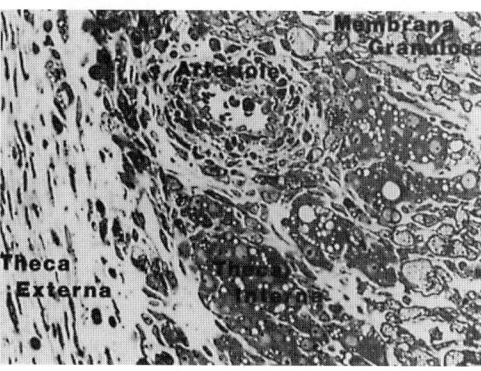

**FIGURE 94-11.** Photomicrographs of a section of human corpus luteum. **A,** Fibrin clot has formed in antrum, and collapsed follicle wall is composed of granulosa and theca-lutein cells. **B,** Theca externa, theca interna, and granulosa lutein tissues are readily distinguishable. (Courtesy of Dr. T. Crisp, USEPA, Washington, DC.)

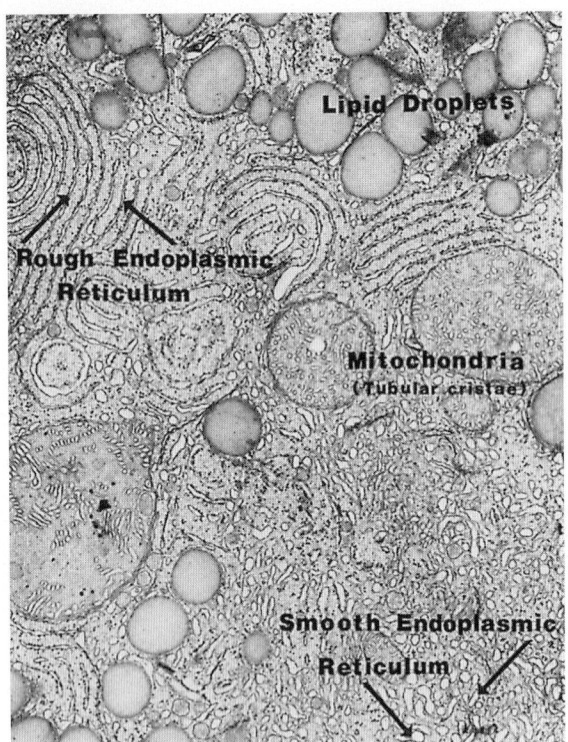

**FIGURE 94-12.** Electron micrograph of a section through a human granulosa lutein cell shows abundant rough and smooth endoplasmic reticulum, which synthesize proteins and steroids, respectively, and numerous lipid droplets composed of stored cholesterol esters. Notice the tubular cristae, the site of cholesterol side-chain cleavage enzyme (P450$_{c22}$) in mitochondria. (Courtesy of Dr. T. Crisp, USEPA, Washington, DC.)

nates from a primordial follicle that was recruited to grow ~1 year earlier (Fig. 94-13). At first, the recruited primordial follicle develops very slowly, requiring ~270 days to complete the preantral period and grow to the early tertiary stage (~0.4 mm). The basis of this slow growth is the very long doubling time (~250 hours) of the granulosa cells.[38]

When FSH enters the microenvironment of the early tertiary follicle, follicular fluid production by the granulosa cells is increased, and the graafian follicle begins to expand.[18] During the antral period, a graafian follicle may pass through the small, medium, and large stages (see Fig. 94-13). The follicles that survive to ovulate require ~85 days to complete the antral period (see Fig. 94-13).

Selection of the dominant follicle is one of the last steps in this long process. The dominant follicle is selected from a cohort of rapidly growing small graafian follicles in the late luteal phase of the menstrual cycle.[4,38,39] It requires ~15 to 19 days for the dominant follicle to complete its growth to the ovulatory stage (see Fig. 94-13). The 99.9% of all growing follicles that are not selected die by atresia (see Fig. 94-13).

### RECRUITMENT

In women, recruitment is a continuous process throughout life, and the mean age for total follicular exhaustion is ~51 years of age.[3,40,40a] The first indication that a primordial follicle has been recruited to grow is that the granulosa cells transform from a squamous to a cuboidal shape.[41] As the granulosa cells round up, they acquire the ability for DNA synthesis and division, albeit at a very slow rate.[41] When more than 90% of the granulosa cells are cuboidal, there occurs a dramatic increase in RNA synthesis in the arrested oocytes.[25] The increased transcription and translation lead to the marked growth of the oocyte that occurs during preantral follicle development (see Fig. 94-3). The fact that changes in the oocyte begin later than those in the granulosa suggests that the granulosa cells might produce or respond to a ligand that initiates the recruitment of the primordial follicle into the growing pool of follicles.

What is known about the mechanisms of recruitment? The evidence that recruitment continues in the absence of pituitary gonadotropins argues that the process is regulated by intrinsic ovarian factors.[3] Based on experiments in animals, it appears that the number of recruited primordial follicles varies with age—the highest level of recruitment occurs early in life, after which it decreases progressively with advancing age. This implies that the rate of recruitment is somehow determined by the actual number of primordial follicles and that the rate of recruitment can be suppressed by testosterone, thymectomy, starvation, and opioid peptides.[3] Although inconclusive, these results suggest that recruitment is an active process that can be modulated (i.e., inhibited) by ligands. What evokes or triggers a particular follicle to grow is totally obscure.

It is noteworthy that a *monotropic rise in FSH* (perhaps due to reduced plasma inhibin levels) occurs in women during aging, and this increase in FSH coincides with an accelerated loss in

**FIGURE 94-13.** Chronology of folliculogenesis in the human ovary. Follicle development is typically divided into two major periods. During the preantral period, the recruited primordial follicle develops to the early antral (tertiary) stage (class 2). Antrum formation occurs at this point, and the graafian follicle enters the antral period. Small antral (0.5–5.0 mm, class 4, 5), midantral (6–10 mm, class 6), large antral (10–15 mm, class 7), preovulatory (16–20 mm, class 8). The total time required for completion of preantral and antral periods is 355 days. The number of granulosa cells (GC), the follicle diameter in millimeters, and the percentage of atretic follicles in each class are indicated. (From Gougeon A. Dynamics of follicular growth in the human: a model from preliminary results. Hum Reprod 1986; 2:81.)

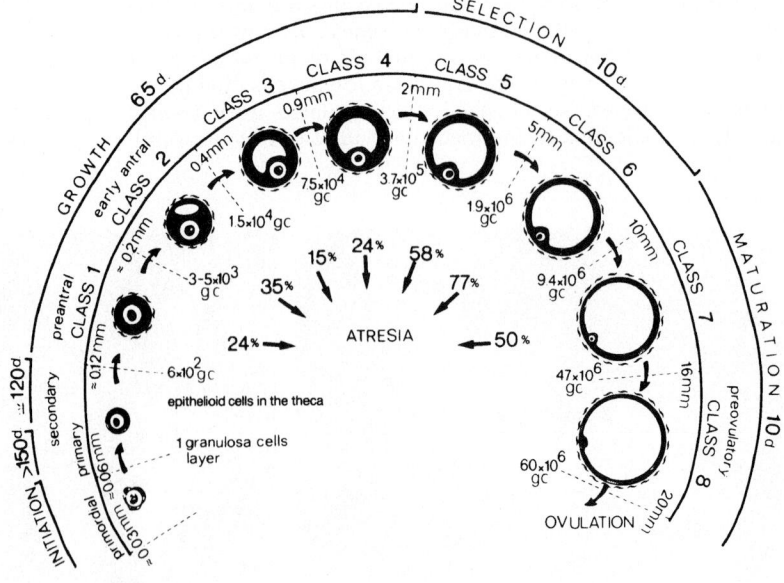

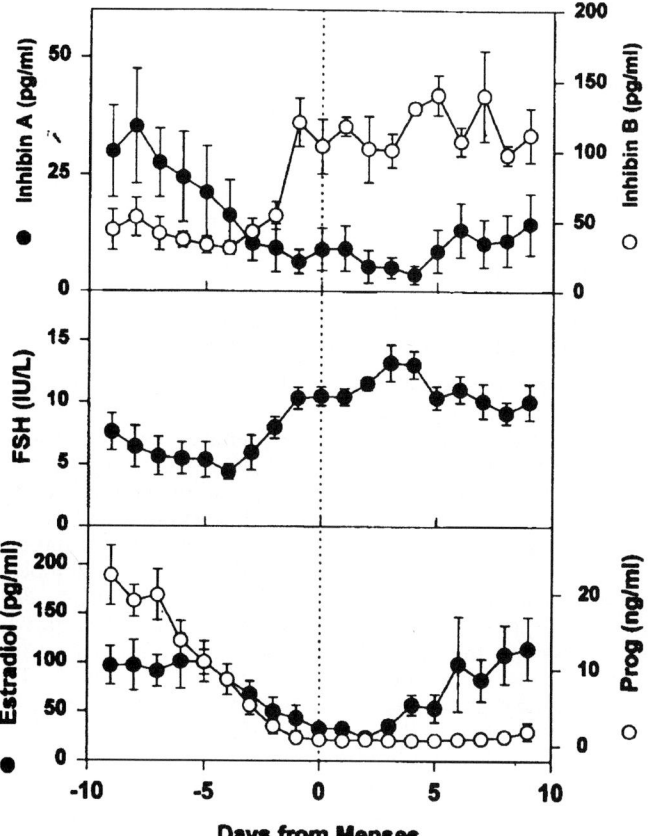

**FIGURE 94-14.** The secondary follicle-stimulating hormone (*FSH*) rise during the luteal-follicular transition. Data are mean (±SEM) of daily FSH, estradiol, progesterone, and inhibin A and B of normal cycling women (n = 5). Data are centered to the day of menses in the cycle. (From Welt CK, Martin KA, Taylor AE, et al. Frequency modulation of follicle stimulating hormone [FSH] during the luteal-follicular transition: evidence for FSH control of inhibin B in normal women. J Clin Endocrinol Metab 1997; 82:2645.)

primordial follicles or *ovary reserve (OR)*.[3] In this regard, studies of aging rats indicate that the monotropic rise in plasma FSH may be involved in the accelerated loss of OR in old rats.[3] This phenomenon could have clinical implications, because reduced OR leads to reduced fecundity in older women. Precisely how FSH might accelerate primordial follicle (OR) loss during aging is unknown, but it may involve the premature expression and/or activation of FSH receptors in granulosa cells of primordial follicles in aging ovaries.

## SELECTION

Morphometric studies of normal human ovaries indicate that the dominant follicle that will ovulate its egg the next cycle is selected from a cohort of small graafian follicles (4.7 ± 0.7 mm in diameter) at the end of the luteal phase of the menstrual cycle.[4,38,39] After the midluteal phase, there is an approximate doubling of the rate of mitosis in the granulosa cells of all cohort follicles. This suggests that the demise of the corpus luteum is followed by a dramatic stimulation of mitosis and granulosa cell division in the cohort follicles.

The first visible sign that one of the follicles has been selected is that the granulosa cells of the chosen follicle maintain a high rate of mitosis, but the mitotic rate falls significantly in the other follicles of the cohort.[4,38,39] This change becomes evident in the late luteal phase. The newly selected dominant follicle continues to grow and expand during the follicular phase and at a relatively rapid rate: 6.9 ± 0.5 mm at days 1 to 5;

13.7 ± 1.2 mm at days 6 to 10; and 18.8 ± 0.5 mm at days 11 to 14. The growth is caused by a progressive increase in follicular fluid and granulosa cell number.[18] As the dominant follicle undergoes its growth and development, the cohort of nondominant follicles becomes increasingly more atretic, and rarely does an atretic follicle reach ≥9 mm in diameter over the cycle.[39]

What do we know about the mechanisms underlying the selection process? There is compelling evidence that the *secondary rise in FSH* plays a central role in the selection process in rats.[42] In women, the secondary rise in plasma FSH begins at or about the time plasma progesterone levels fall to basal levels at the end of the luteal phase, and it continues through the first week of the follicular phase[43] (see Fig. 94-14). Evidence that suppression of the secondary rise in FSH prevents ovulation in monkeys supports the proposition that the secondary increase in FSH is critical for the continued growth and development of the dominant follicle in the primate.[44] It seems likely that the secondary rise in FSH is also critical for selection in women, but further proof is needed.

During this period, the concentration of FSH increases steadily in the microenvironment of the chosen follicle, and FSH levels become low or absent in the nondominant follicles.[45] In the dominant follicle, the FSH stimulates a sharp increase in the number of granulosa cells and apoptosis is suppressed. By contrast, the growth development of nondominant follicles is suppressed in the absence of adequate levels of FSH, and apoptosis is activated in the granulosa cells. In this way, the selected follicle achieves dominance. How is dominance established? In studies in the monkey, estradiol has been found to be a causative agent by virtue of negative feedback on the pituitary gonadotrope.[42,44] In this concept, the high intrafollicular levels of FSH lead to increased estradiol production, which, in turn, suppresses FSH secretion by the pituitary. When FSH becomes rate-limiting in the nondominant cohort follicles, they undergo atresia.[38] Human menopausal gonadotropins can stimulate granulosa cells to divide mitotically in nondominant follicles during the early follicular phase.[38] If FSH levels within the microenvironment are increased, it appears that the nondominant follicle can be rescued from atresia.[38] This *rescue phenomenon* could be involved in the generation of multiple large follicles in women undergoing ovulation induction with exogenous FSH.

The FSH rise that begins before the onset of menses also occurs with concomitant decreases in inhibin A produced by the corpus luteum.[43] The inverse relationship between inhibin A and FSH suggests an endocrine role for inhibin A in the regulation of the secondary FSH rise (see Fig. 94-14). In contrast to inhibin A, inhibin B increases before menses, coincident with the FSH rise (see Fig. 94-14). Although estradiol secretion by the follicle is primarily responsible for the negative-feedback regulation of FSH during the follicular phase of the cycle, it is possible that inhibin B produced by graafian follicles might play a role as well. However, the role of inhibin B in reproduction remains unknown. It should be mentioned that there is considerable interest in follistatin because it can specifically bind to activin and inhibin and modulate their activity.[46] Follistatin might, therefore, be a physiologically relevant protein in the control of folliculogenesis in the ovary. However, further work is needed to establish this concept.

## TWO-CELL, TWO-GONADOTROPIN CONCEPT

Because the estradiol produced by the selected follicle plays an important role in establishing follicle dominance,[42] an understanding of the mechanisms of follicular estradiol production is important. The process requires two cell types (i.e., theca and granulosa) and two gonadotropins (i.e., LH and FSH); it is called the *two-cell, two-gonadotropin concept for follicle estrogen synthesis* (Fig. 94-15).

When FSH and LH interact with transmembrane receptors in the granulosa and theca-interstitial cells, respectively, the bind-

## Theca Interstitial Cell

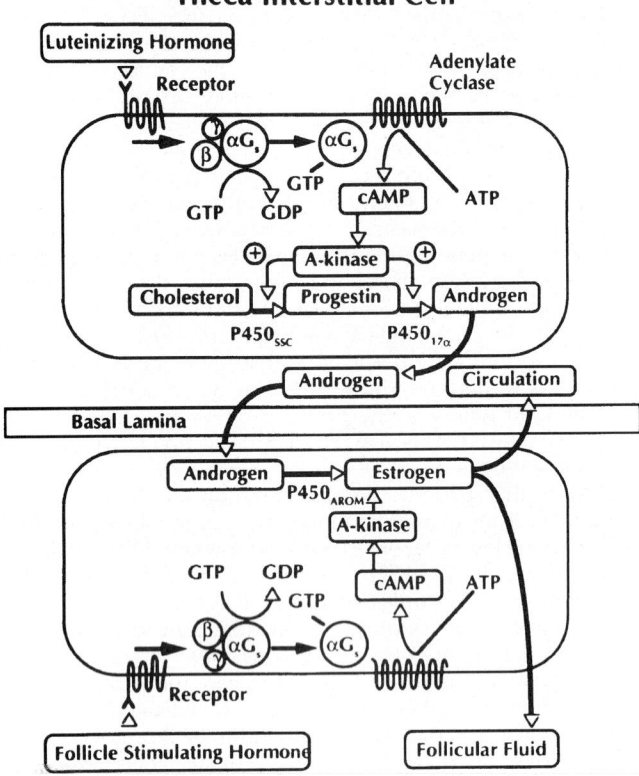

## Granulosa Cell

**FIGURE 94-15.** Diagram of the two-gonadotropin, two-cell concept of follicle estrogen biosynthesis. G proteins include αG-stimulatory (*αG_s*), β, γ, A kinase, cyclic adenosine monophosphate (*cAMP*)–dependent protein kinase A. (*GTP*, Guanine nucleotide triphosphate; *GDP*, Guanine nucleotide diphosphate; *ATP*, adenosine triphosphate.) (From Kettel LM, Erickson GF. Basic and clinical concepts of ovulation induction. In: Rock J, Alvarez-Murphy A, eds. Advances in obstetrics and gynecology. Chicago: Mosby, 1994.)

ing events are transduced into intracellular signals by means of the heterotrimeric G proteins. The LH-bound receptor is coupled to the αG-stimulatory (αG_s), cyclic AMP (cAMP), protein kinase A (PKA) pathway. The stimulation of this signal transduction pathway in the theca-interstitial cells leads to increased transcription of those genes involved in de novo androstenedione biosynthesis[28] (see Fig. 94-15). The FSH-bound receptor activates the αG_s/cAMP/PKA pathway in membrana granulosa cells (see Fig. 94-15), and the signal promotes the stimulation of the genes encoding P450_AROM and 17β–hydroxysteroid dehydrogenase (17β-HSD) type 1 enzyme,[47,48] which then results in the aromatization of androstenedione to estradiol. Because the dominant follicle contains large numbers of granulosa cells and relatively high levels of FSH, it is capable of producing large quantities of estradiol. Although nondominant follicles produce a high level of androstenedione, they have a paucity of granulosa cells and microenvironment FSH and, thus, produce very little estradiol.

The LH or human chorionic gonadotropin receptor (LH/hCG receptor) has been cloned, and its structure is similar to that of other G protein–coupled receptors.[49] The N terminus, which is the extracellular domain of the receptor, is glycosylated and binds circulating LH or hCG. As with other G protein–coupled receptors, this LH/hCG receptor contains seven membrane-spanning domains. The C-terminal domain is located intracellularly and is responsible for signal generation that begins with the activation of G proteins. The FSH receptor is structurally similar.[50] The extracellular domain binds FSH, there are seven membrane-spanning domains, and a short C-terminal cytoplasmic domain activates the heterotrimeric G

protein. The mechanism by which an increase in cAMP leads to increased gene expression is now understood in many instances. cAMP activates the catalytic subunit of protein kinase A. The kinase A phosphorylates *cAMP-response element–binding protein or other related DNA-binding proteins.*[51] When such proteins are phosphorylated, they bind to upstream DNA regulatory elements called *cAMP response elements.* The binding has been shown to increase gene transcription and the production of the LH/FSH-responsive proteins. The interaction among these various regulatory proteins is exceedingly complex but is described clearly in a review.[51]

### FOLLICLE-STIMULATING HORMONE REGULATION OF MITOSIS AND THE LUTEINIZING HORMONE RECEPTOR

Several other physiologically important effects of FSH occur in the dominant follicle, most notably the stimulation of mitosis and expression of LH receptor in the granulosa cells (Fig. 94-16). Based on in vivo[4,38] and in vitro[52,53] work, it appears that the rate of human granulosa cell division is stimulated directly by FSH in the human. Precisely how this occurs is unclear, but studies with growth factors indicate that human granulosa cells cultured in vitro respond to potent mitogens, such as fibroblast growth factor and epidermal growth factor, resulting in dramatic increases in mitosis.[54] The question of whether growth factors mediate the FSH-induced proliferation of human granulosa cells in vivo is an interesting, but unresolved, question. The ability of the dominant follicle to respond to the LH surge with ovulation depends on the expression of high levels of LH receptor in the membrana granulosa cells (see Figs. 94-7 and 94-16). Direct evidence that FSH induces LH receptors in the primate has been provided by in vitro experiments with monkey granulosa cells.[55] There is some evidence favoring this concept in women.[56] In examining the level of granulosa LH receptor during the follicular phase, the researcher finds that the number is low in small and medium graafian follicles but increases sharply to very high levels at the preovulatory stage.[57,58] Unlike the early effects of FSH on P450_AROM enzyme and mitosis, the FSH control of LH receptor appears to be restricted to the late

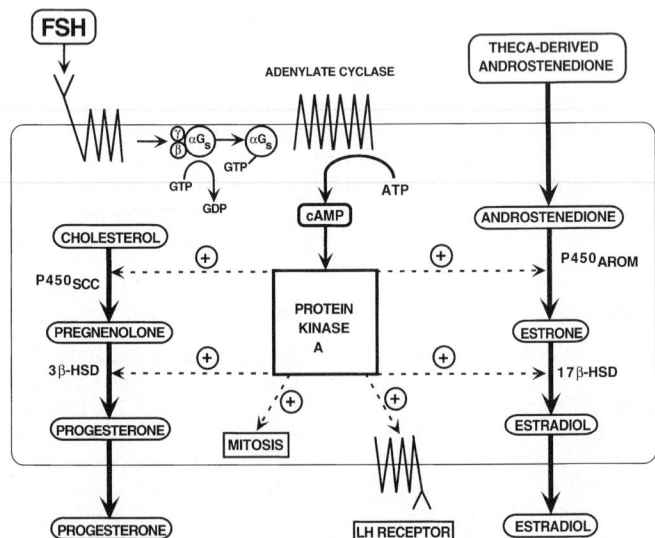

**FIGURE 94-16.** Diagram of the follicle-stimulating hormone (*FSH*) signaling pathway in granulosa cells of a dominant follicle that result in proliferation, steroid biosynthesis, and luteinizing hormone (*LH*)/human chorionic gonadotropin receptor expression. (*GTP*, guanosine triphosphate; *GDP*, guanosine diphosphate; *cAMP*, cyclic adenosine monophosphate; *HSD*, hydroxysteroid deoxygenase.) (From Erickson GF. Polycystic ovary syndrome: normal and abnormal steroidogenesis. In: Schats R, Schoemaker J, eds. Ovarian endocrinopathies. Proceedings of the 8th Reinier deGraaf Symposium. UK: Parthenon Publishing, 1994.)

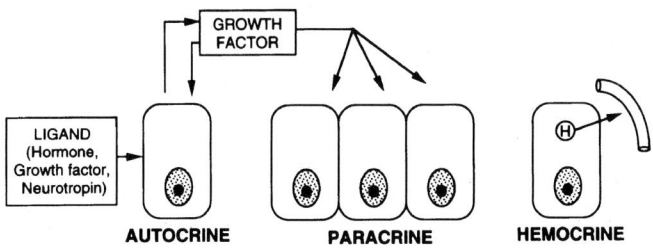

**FIGURE 94-17.** Growth factor or autocrine/paracrine concept. (From Erickson GF. Ovarian control of follicle development. Am J Obstet Gynecol 1995; 172:736.)

stages of folliculogenesis. How the stage-specific effects of FSH are achieved is unknown.

It is clear that the ability of the ovary to generate a dominant follicle depends on having sufficient amounts of FSH within the microenvironment and that the FSH functions in stimulating granulosa cell division and differentiation. A fundamental concept of ovarian physiology is that FSH is obligatory for dominant follicle formation and that no other ligand by itself can serve in this regulatory capacity.

### GROWTH FACTOR CONCEPT

One exciting and important concept to emerge in ovarian physiology is the awareness that folliculogenesis and luteogenesis are modulated by proteins that are produced by the ovaries themselves.[59,60,60a] The evidence has led to the novel idea that the actions of hormones (FSH, LH, progesterone, androgen, and estrogen) can be modulated, either amplified or attenuated, by ovary growth factors that act in autocrine/paracrine manners to control proliferation, differentiation, and apoptosis (Fig. 94-17).

Growth factors are regulatory proteins that control a wide variety of proliferative and developmental functions (see Chap. 173). All of them are ligands that interact with specific receptors in target cells, and the binding events generate signal transduction pathways that modulate cellular responses. All of the growth factors share the property of being modulators; they increase or decrease the responsiveness of target cells to ligands (e.g., hormones, growth factors, neurotransmitters). The results of a large number of studies have demonstrated that all five families of growth factors are expressed in the rat follicle, and there is increasing evidence for growth factors in the human ovary.[59,60] The potential importance of this rapidly emerging

field is illustrated by the gene knock-out studies in mice, which have demonstrated that specific growth factors are essential for FSH-dependent folliculogenesis and female fertility. For example, loss of function of insulin-like growth factor-I (IGF-I)[61] and *oocyte-derived growth differentiation factor-9 (GDF-9)*[62] results in the cessation of folliculogenesis at the preantral stage, and the females are infertile. Thus, it is becoming increasingly clear that ovary growth factors are fundamental players in female reproduction. The current challenges are to understand how specific growth factors affect ovarian function and how these actions are integrated into the overall effects of FSH and LH. The presence within the ovary of potent positive and negative regulatory proteins that function to modulate cell function could have far-reaching implications for physiology and pathophysiology in women; however, definitive evidence for an obligatory role of a growth factor in human fertility is still lacking.

## OVULATION

The expulsion of a mature oocyte from the ovary is tightly coupled to the generation of proteolytic activity.[63] This process occurs in a highly localized area called the *stigma* (Fig. 94-18). Morphologic and biochemical studies have shown that, during the ovulatory period, the surface epithelial cells in the presumptive stigma become filled with lysosome-like inclusions.[64] With increasing time, the inclusions fuse with the plasma membrane and release their contents toward the tunica albuginea. This process is accompanied by the progressive destruction of the basement membrane and the theca layers. In this way, the steps leading to the formation of the stigma are initiated in a specialized population of surface epithelial cells and involve the release of hydrolytic enzymes. How does this event occur?

The most important stimulating force in ovulation is the preovulatory surge of LH.[63] Although the basic mechanisms involved in LH-induced ovulation are still under investigation in women, some insights have been generated from studies carried out in rats. First, the LH surge starts the preovulatory follicle on the path of progesterone production. An important concept is that increased progesterone is obligatory for ovulation and that the progesterone response is mediated by the progesterone receptor induced in the follicle by the preovulatory surge of LH.[65,66] Thus, progesterone plays an essential physiologic role in the mechanism of ovulation, in part by acting as a mediator of LH action. Second, prostaglandins (i.e., PGE and PGF) are required for ovulation. After the ovulatory surge of LH and the stimulation of progesterone production,

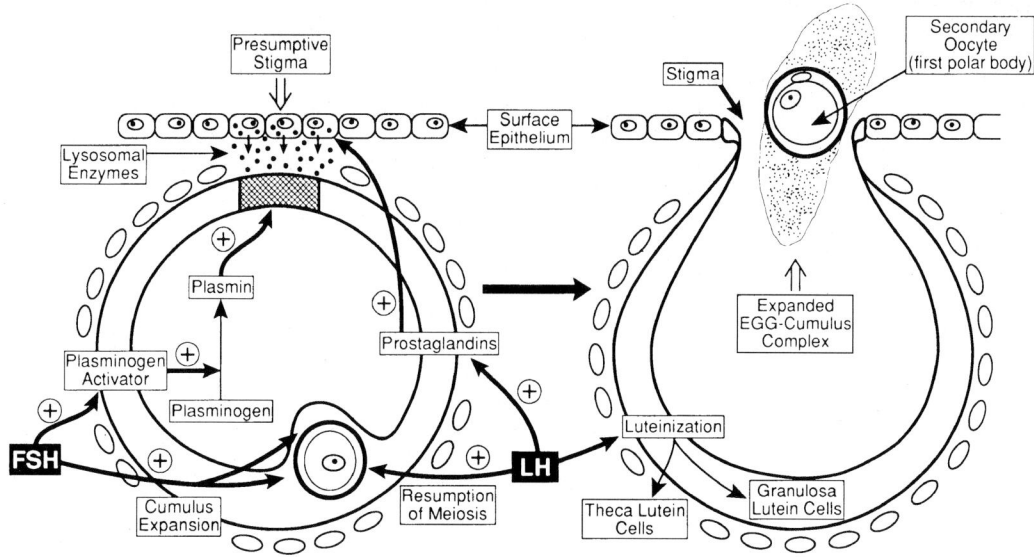

**FIGURE 94-18.** Progressive hormone-induced changes in the dominant follicle during ovulation. The preovulatory surge of follicle-stimulating hormone (*FSH*) causes cumulus expansion and participates in ovulation by virtue of stimulating plasminogen activator production. The preovulatory luteinizing hormone (*LH*) surge induces meiotic maturation, luteinization, and stigma formation; the latter depends on intrinsic progesterone and prostaglandin production. (From Erickson GF. The ovary: basic principles and concepts. In: Felig P, Baxter JD, Broadus AE, Frohman LA, eds. Endocrinology and metabolism, 3rd ed. New York: McGraw-Hill, 1994.)

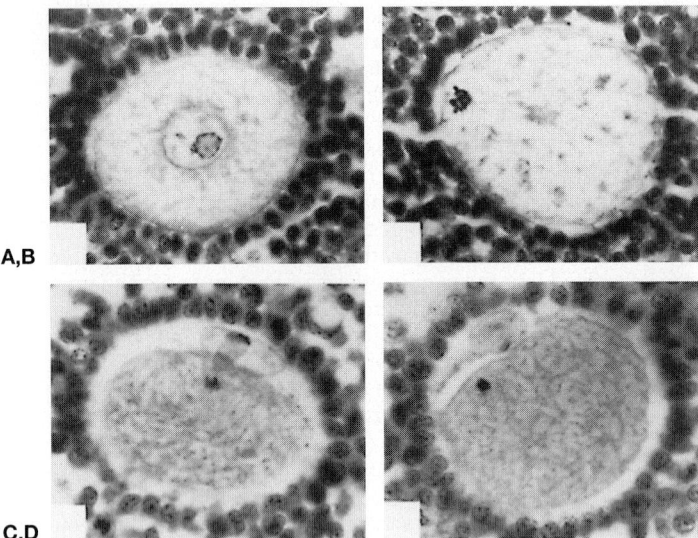

A,B

C,D

**FIGURE 94-19.** Process of meiotic maturation or resumption of meiosis. **A,** Germinal vesicle stage. **B,** Germinal vesicle breakdown followed by condensation of chromosomes into bivalents. **C** and **D,** Release of first polar body and arrest of meiotic process at metaphase II. (Courtesy of Dr. C. Banka.)

the synthesis of PGE and PGF is increased in the preovulatory follicle. If the follicle is injected with indomethacin or PG antibodies, ovulation is completely blocked. Furthermore, knocking out the key rate-limiting enzyme in PG synthesis, PG synthetase,[67] blocks ovulation, making the female mice infertile.[68,69] Morphologic studies of indomethacin-treated ovaries suggest that the prostaglandins are involved in stigma formation. Collectively, the data support the proposition that the elevated level of progesterone induced by LH serves to activate PG production, which, in turn, promotes the release of hydrolytic enzymes by a subpopulation of surface epithelial cells, which then causes stigma formation (see Fig. 94-18).

Another active protease relevant to ovulation is *plasmin*.[70] The follicular fluid of preovulatory follicles contains the plasmin precursor, *plasminogen*. The granulosa cells are stimulated specifically by FSH to release plasminogen activator, which converts plasminogen to the active protease, plasmin (see Fig. 94-18). After the process is initiated, holes are formed in the basal lamina, and there is a general weakening of the follicular wall, presumably caused by the proteolytic action of plasmin. More work is needed to elucidate the physiologic importance of plasminogen activator in ovulation in women.

High levels of LH at midcycle stimulate meiotic maturation, and the oocyte reaches the second meiotic metaphase or first polar body stage (Fig. 94-19). During this process, the cumulus granulosa cells undergo a series of structural and functional changes called *mucification* or *expansion*. The preovulatory surge of gonadotropins induces the granulosa cells in the cumulus to secrete a hyaluronidase-sensitive mucous substance.[71] This results in the dispersal of the cumulus cells and causes the oocyte-cumulus complex to expand tremendously. The specific stimulus for mucification is thought to be FSH, and the functional significance of mucification is thought to be critical for the pickup and transport of the oocyte-cumulus complex in the fallopian tube.

Therefore, a cascade of FSH- and LH-dependent progesterone and PG responses are involved in mediating the ovulation of a fertilizable oocyte at midcycle.

## DIFFERENTIATION OF THE OOCYTE

Oocyte differentiation involves two interrelated processes: *growth* and *meiotic maturation*.[71] Oocyte growth is associated with the accumulation and storage of nutritional and informa-

tional molecules. During growth, the oocyte increases in diameter from 20 μm to 120 μm (see Figs. 94-2 and 94-3). Oocyte growth depends on the transcription of selected genes in chromosomes that are in the so-called lampbrush stage.[2,4] Initially, oocyte and follicle growth are positively and linearly correlated until the follicle reaches the early tertiary stage; then, oocyte growth ceases while follicle growth continues.[23] The oocyte therefore completes its growth very early in follicle development, for example, when the early tertiary follicle reaches ~400 μm in diameter (see Figs. 94-2 and 94-6).

Granulosa cells are an absolute requirement for oocyte growth.[72,73] As growth progresses, the oocyte is surrounded closely by the corona radiata granulosa cells, which are metabolically coupled with the oocyte by means of gap junctions composed of Cx37. There is evidence that 85% of the metabolites in follicle-enclosed oocytes originally are taken up by the granulosa cells and then transferred into the oocyte through gap junctions.[72,73]

As discussed earlier, the oocyte-derived *ZP* (see Fig. 94-6) plays an important role in a number of vital biologic functions. It contains species-specific receptors for capacitated sperm, it participates in the block of polyspermy, and it is critical in allowing the embryo to move freely through the fallopian tube into the uterus.

There is increasing evidence that oocytes express growth factor ligands that control granulosa cytodifferentiation.[19] Indeed, a functional link between one such oocyte growth factor, GDF-9, and folliculogenesis and fertility has been established.[62] Hence, the emerging concept is that the oocyte may be at or near the apex in the mechanisms that control folliculogenesis in rats and, perhaps, humans.[74]

## MEIOTIC MATURATION

The capacity of the oocyte to resume meiosis is acquired at a specific stage in its growth, and the ability to complete meiotic maturation is acquired subsequently.[23] Meiotic maturation or resumption of meiosis (see Fig. 94-19) is a process characterized by the dissolution of the nuclear or germinal vesicle membrane, the condensation of dictyotene chromosomes into discrete bivalents, the separation of homologous chromosomes, the release of a first polar body, and the arrest of the meiotic process at metaphase II. After meiotic maturation, the completion of meiosis and release of the second polar body are triggered by fertilization.

In laboratory animals, the oocyte first acquires the capacity to resume meiosis at about the time of cavitation or early antrum formation, when the oocyte has completed its growth and is surrounded by the ZP and four or five layers of granulosa cells[23] (see Fig. 94-6). The acquisition of the capacity for meiotic maturation seems to be a two-step process. First, the oocyte acquires the capacity to undergo germinal vesicle breakdown and to progress to metaphase I. Subsequently, it acquires the capacity to complete the first reductional division and release the first polar body.[23] The mechanisms responsible for the acquisition of meiotic potential are unknown.

Although the oocyte is capable of resuming meiosis early in follicle development, it is kept from doing so by an inhibitory influence. Under physiologic conditions, meiotic maturation is a highly selective process; it occurs only in those oocytes that are in dominant preovulatory follicles, responding to the preovulatory surge of LH.[23] Fully grown oocytes from any tertiary or graafian follicle undergo meiotic maturation spontaneously if the oocyte is placed in tissue culture. Apparently, there is an inhibiting substance in follicular fluid that blocks meiotic maturation and that may be overridden by high levels of LH. The nature of the putative *oocyte meiotic inhibitor* remains to be elucidated.

## DIFFERENTIATION OF THE CORPUS LUTEUM

The life of the corpus luteum typically is divided into two periods: *luteinization* and *luteolysis*. Luteinization begins in

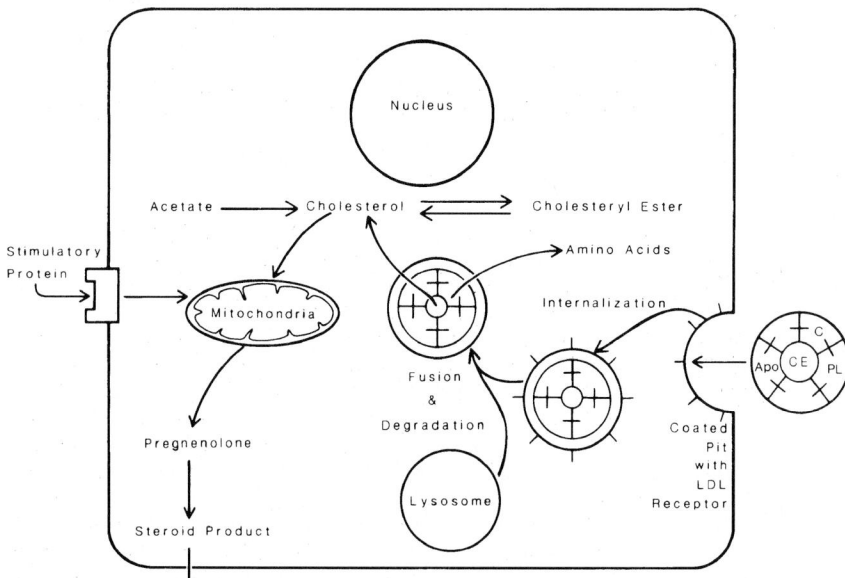

**FIGURE 94-20.** Lipoprotein-cell interaction is shown in this model for low-density lipoprotein (*LDL*) uptake by an ovary steroidogenic cell by means of the LDL receptor. (*C*, cholesterol; *CE*, cholesteryl ester; *PL*, phospholipid; *Apo*, apolipoprotein B.) (From Schreiber JR, Weinstein D. Receptors in stereogenic cells. In: Scanu A, Spector A, eds. Lipoproteins, receptors, and cell function. New York: Marcel Dekker Inc, 1986.)

response to the preovulatory surge of gonadotropins. Maximal differentiation is reached at the end of 1 week (i.e., day 21 or 22 of the cycle).[37] Subsequently, the corpus luteum normally undergoes apoptosis,[35] a process called *luteolysis*. The basis of luteal differentiation is reflected in the biphasic secretion of progesterone, 17α-hydroxyprogesterone, androstenedione, and 17β-estradiol. This biphasic steroid production is causally connected to biphasic changes of activities of key steroidogenic enzymes.

LH is the inducer of luteinization, and low levels of LH are critical for maintaining active luteal tissue during the early and midluteal phase. The hCG produced by the blastocyst can prevent luteolysis and promote further differentiation of the corpus luteum. The mechanism is totally obscure.

Because LH/hCG action is mediated by receptors, luteinization becomes intimately connected with how LH receptors are controlled by luteal cells.[36] LH receptors in the corpus luteum undergo a predictable pattern of activity. As ovulation approaches, a striking decrease in LH receptors occurs, and during the early luteal phase, LH receptors increase sharply, reaching near-maximum levels in the midluteal phase, and remain elevated until the end of the cycle.[75] It seems that LH receptors first are down-regulated and then are reinduced during luteinization.

Because reinduction of LH receptors is what renders the corpus luteum sensitive to hCG secreted by the implanting blastocyst, an important question is how LH receptors are reinduced in luteal cells. In the rat, FSH and prolactin are important in the induction and reinduction of LH receptors, respectively, in the granulosa cells.[76] Functional FSH and prolactin receptors are present in the highest concentration in the early human corpus luteum, when LH receptors are being replenished.[77] To what extent are FSH and prolactin involved in reinducing LH receptors during luteinization? Although the answer is unknown, it is important clinically, because foremost among luteal-phase defects in women is the inability of the corpus luteum to respond to LH/hCG. Could this defect be caused by inappropriate formation of new LH/hCG receptors?

At luteolysis, a program is initiated that leads to apoptosis ~5 to 7 days later.[35] After luteolysis is initiated, there occurs a striking decrease in progesterone production. Despite its physiologic importance, the mechanism regulating luteolysis in women is unknown. In laboratory animals, $PGF_2\alpha$ is a physiologic luteolysin[37]; however, the precise role of $PGF_2\alpha$ in human luteolysis remains equivocal.[36,37]

## OVARIAN STEROIDOGENESIS

### LIPOPROTEINS AS CHOLESTEROL SOURCE

Lipoproteins are complex particles containing a lipid core surrounded by amphiphilic proteins and phospholipids (see Chap. 162). Low-density lipoprotein (LDL; density = 1.019–1.063 g/mL) is the predominant cholesterol and cholesteryl ester carrier in human plasma and provides cholesterol to cells for membrane synthesis and as substrate for steroidogenesis in steroidogenic organs such as the ovary.[78] High-density lipoprotein (HDL; density = 1.063–1.21 g/mL) also carries cholesterol and cholesteryl ester. In humans, HDL cannot provide cholesterol for steroidogenesis.[79,80] In rats, a model often used in the study of the ovary, HDL and LDL can provide cholesterol for steroid hormone production.[81]

All cells can obtain cholesterol from two sources. Cholesterol can be synthesized de novo from acetate by the cell, or the cell can obtain the cholesterol from an external source such as lipoprotein.[79] The mechanism by which steroidogenic cells in the human ovary obtain LDL-cholesterol essentially is the pathway described by Brown and Goldstein[82] in their studies of the human fibroblast. LDL binds to ovarian steroidogenic cell-membrane receptors with high affinity and specificity. These receptors recognize apolipoprotein B, the predominant LDL apoprotein.[78] In studies of human ovarian corpora lutea membranes, the number of LDL receptors is highest in the midluteal phase, suggesting that LDL-receptor number and the rate of steroidogenesis are positively correlated.[83]

After the LDL particle binds to the receptor on the plasma membrane, particle and receptor are internalized by the cell inside coated vesicles, which fuse to form lysosomes. The lysosomes hydrolyze the components of the LDL particle; cholesteryl ester is hydrolyzed to free cholesterol, and apoproteins are hydrolyzed to amino acids. The free cholesterol can be stored in the cell as cholesteryl ester or can be converted to steroid hormone products. The increase in the cell concentration of free cholesterol or a metabolic product such as an oxygenated sterol acts as a major control point in cell cholesterol metabolism by decreasing the number of LDL receptors, decreasing de novo cholesterol synthesis from acetate and increasing esterification of cholesterol to cholesteryl ester.[84,85] In this way, the cell prevents the overaccumulation of cholesterol (Fig. 94-20).

The factor that down-regulates de novo synthesis of cholesterol and LDL receptors appears to be an oxysterol rather than cholesterol itself. A prime candidate for this regulatory role is 26-hydroxycholesterol. Luteinized human granulosa cells contain 26-hydroxylase messenger RNA (mRNA), and this enzyme is localized to mitochondria. Data suggest that, when steroidogenesis is active, the 26-hydroxylase enzyme is inhibited by the products of the side-chain cleavage enzyme, allowing de novo cholesterol synthesis and increased LDL-cholesterol uptake.[86] When steroidogenic activity is decreased in the ovary (i.e., follicle or corpus luteum), 26-hydroxylase activity remains, allowing the formation of 26-hydroxycholesterol and the resultant reduction in cholesterol synthesis and LDL-receptor gene expression. This finely tuned series of regulatory steps ensures enough cholesterol for cell function (e.g., membrane synthesis and specialized activities, such as steroid hormone production), but it prevents the overaccumulation of cholesterol in the cell.

Although there are receptors for HDL in the human ovary, HDL is unable to provide cholesterol for steroid hormone production. At high concentrations, HDL seems to inhibit steroidogenesis by cultured human ovarian cells.[80] This differential effect of HDL and LDL on steroid hormone synthesis by human ovarian cells could be of physiologic importance because of compartmentalization within the ovary. Granulosa cells in the preovulatory graafian follicle are bathed in follicular fluid but are separated from the ovarian vasculature by the basal lamina of the follicle. Human follicular fluid contains little or no LDL, but contains levels of HDL close to those in the plasma. The lack of available LDL probably limits progesterone synthesis before ovulation. After ovulation, the follicle becomes the vascularized corpus luteum, exposing these granulosa cells to plasma levels of LDL. The rapid rise in ovarian progesterone production after ovulation can be explained, at least in part, by the sudden availability of LDL-cholesterol as substrate by means of the LDL receptor.[87] Before ovulation, the theca is well vascularized, and LDL would be available to provide cholesterol for thecal androgen production. Androgen can cross through the basal lamina to provide substrate for estrogen production by follicle granulosa cells. The theca of the dominant follicle has the richest blood supply of all follicles, ensuring adequate substrate for estrogen synthesis.[88]

Rat ovarian steroidogenic cells also can use LDL-cholesterol by the pathway described for human cells. However, HDL also can provide cholesterol for rat ovarian steroidogenesis by a mechanism that is quite different from that described for LDL. For example, the HDL particle can provide cholesterol to the cell in the absence of degradation of the apolipoprotein surface coat.[81] The HDL (scavenger, type 1)-receptor mRNA is localized to theca cells of the rat ovary. Gonadotropic stimulation with hCG causes a marked increase in HDL receptor mRNA in theca interstitial cells and luteinized granulosa cells, consistent with a functional role for this receptor in rodent cholesterol transport and ovarian steroidogenesis.[89]

## MECHANISMS OF GONADOTROPIN EFFECTS

The $\alpha$ and the $\beta$ subunits of FSH and LH are required for binding to the specific membrane receptors. Theca cells have specific LH receptors, but granulosa cells contain FSH receptors. FSH stimulates production of granulosa cell LH receptors. Gonadotropin binding to its receptor stimulates the cAMP–A kinase regulatory system.[90] By this mechanism, gonadotropins increase available free cholesterol by increasing lipoprotein receptor number and by increasing hydrolysis of stored cholesteryl ester. In the absence of available lipoprotein (e.g., under serum-free in vitro conditions, perhaps within the follicle in the human ovary before ovulation), gonadotropins stimulate cholesterol synthesis de novo from acetate in the cell. The free cholesterol is transferred to mitochondria, which is the location of the rate-limiting enzyme in steroidogenesis, P450 side-chain cleavage enzyme (P450$_{scc}$), which converts cholesterol to pregnenolone.[81] There is evidence that cholesterol is carried to the

mitochondria by a carrier protein called *sterol carrier protein-2 (SCP-2)*. Gonadotropins then facilitate the transport of cholesterol from the outer to the inner mitochondrial membrane and continued transport to the P450$_{scc}$ enzyme on the inner mitochondrial membrane.[91] A protein named *steroidogenic acute regulatory protein (StAR)* has been implicated as the regulator of cholesterol translocation from the outer to inner mitochondrial membrane.[92] StAR mRNA transcripts are localized in the human ovary to the theca of preovulatory follicles, and luteinized granulosa and theca cells in the corpus luteum.[93] Mutations of the StAR gene result in *congenital lipoid adrenal hyperplasia*, in which synthesis of all gonadal and adrenal steroids is severely impaired.[94] This finding establishes the critical role of StAR protein in steroidogenesis. StAR gene expression is stimulated by cAMP.[93] Gonadotropins can stimulate acutely the transport of cholesterol to the P450$_{scc}$ enzyme and chronically increase the amount and activity of this enzyme. After conversion of cholesterol to pregnenolone in the mitochondria, the pregnenolone moves back out of the mitochondria and into the cell cytoplasm for conversion to progesterone in corpus luteum cells and androgen in theca cells. The enzymes for these conversions are located on the microsomes. A summary of cholesterol transport and metabolism within ovarian cells is shown in Figure 94-21.

## STEROID HORMONES PRODUCED BY THE OVARY

### ANDROGENS

Androgens, primarily androstenedione and testosterone, are secreted by interstitial and thecal cells. The secretion rate of androstenedione is ~3 mg per day, with one-half coming from the ovaries and the other half coming from the adrenal glands or from the peripheral conversion of circulating dehydroepiandrosterone.[95] The plasma androstenedione concentration is 40 to 240 ng/dL, with a small peak at ovulation and higher levels in the luteal than in the follicular phase. The secretion rate of testosterone is significantly less than that of androstenedione: ~0.25 mg per day, with a plasma concentration of ~19 to 70 ng/dL. Testosterone is bound tightly to testosterone-estradiol–binding globulin (TeBG; also known as sex hormone–binding globulin [SHBG]), and only ~1% of circulating testosterone is the biologically active free component (see Chap. 114).

The principal function of ovarian androgen production is to provide substrate to the granulosa cell aromatase enzyme for the synthesis of estrogen.[14] When ovarian androgen production is excessive (e.g., ovarian androgen-producing tumor, hyperthecosis) or when the conversion of androgen to estrogen in the ovary is inefficient (i.e., polycystic ovary syndrome), the excess androgen causes hirsutism or, at a higher concentration, virilism (see Chaps. 96, 101, and 102).

### ESTROGEN

Estrogen is produced predominantly in the ovarian follicle by the granulosa cell aromatization of thecal androgens.[90] The amount of estrogen production depends on the time of the menstrual cycle. During the early follicular phase, the secretion rates of estradiol and estrone are about equal at 60 to 170 µg per day. As the dominant follicle is selected in the second half of the follicular phase, the secretion rate of estradiol rises to 400 to 800 µg per day, with the estradiol coming almost exclusively from the dominant follicle.[96] The corpus luteum in the human ovary also produces significant quantities of estradiol, ~250 µg per day. In the late follicular and luteal phases, estrone secretion is one-fourth that of estradiol. Plasma concentrations of estradiol range from 50 to 60 pg/mL in the early follicular phase and rise to 250 to 400 pg/mL in the late follicular phase, but levels of estrone increase to only 150 to 200 pg/mL.

The dominant follicle and corpus luteum produce ~95% of circulating estradiol, and estrone has little clinical significance

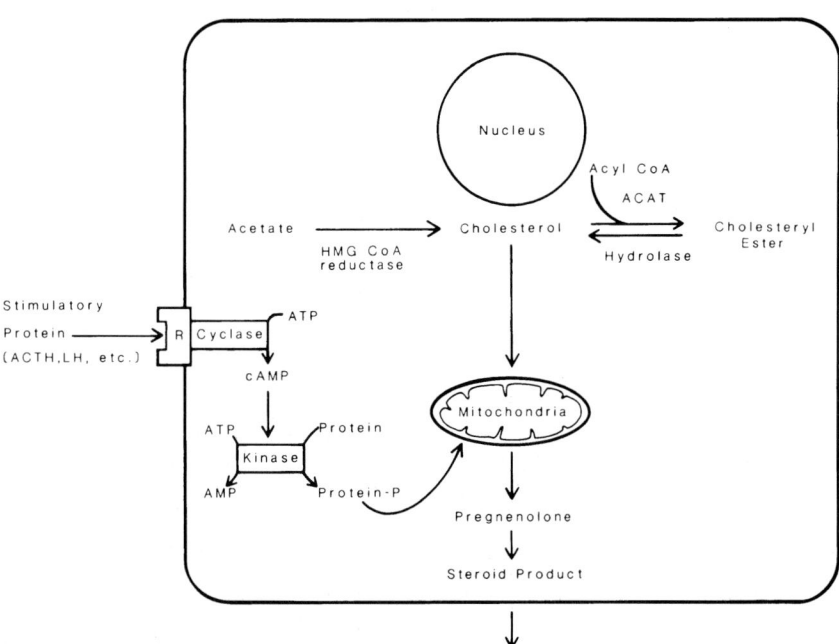

**FIGURE 94-21.** Cholesterol metabolism in a steroidogenic cell. (*ACTH*, adrenocorticotropic hormone; *LH*, luteinizing hormone; *R*, membrane receptor; cyclase, adenylate cyclase; *ATP*, adenosine triphosphate; *AMP*, adenosine monophosphate; *P*, phosphate; *kinase*, cyclic AMP–dependent protein kinase; *hydrolase*, cholesteryl ester hydrolase; *HMG*, human menopausal gonadotropin; *ACAT*, acyl CoA: cholesteryl acyltransferase.) Another source of cholesterol is low-density lipoprotein, as described in Figure 94-20. (From Schreiber JR, Weinstein D. Receptors in stereogenic cells. In: Scanu A, Spector A, eds. Lipoproteins, receptors, and cell function. New York: Marcel Dekker Inc, 1986.)

in cycling women. However, in the menopausal years, estrone becomes the predominant estrogen. Estrone comes from peripheral conversion (mostly in adipose tissue) of adrenal androgens, particularly of androstenedione[97] (see Chap. 100).

Estradiol and estrone are converted into at least 40 metabolic products. Most are conjugated to glucuronic acid for excretion in the urine, but sulfates and mixed conjugates also are found. The principal metabolites of estradiol and estrone are estriol (by 16-hydroxylation, plus reduction of the 17-keto group for estrone) and catechol estrogens (by hydroxylation at the 2 or 4 position; Fig. 94-22).

### PROGESTERONE

Progesterone production remains low until ovulation and corpus luteum formation. Just before ovulation, there is a slight rise in progesterone concentration; after ovulation, with the luteinization of granulosa cells and the influx of blood vessels carrying plasma levels of LDL, the production rate of progesterone rises to 10 to 40 mg each day.[95] Plasma concentrations rise to 5 to 25 ng/mL in the midluteal phase. The normal life span of the corpus luteum, in the absence of pregnancy, is ~14 days. The cause of the demise of the corpus luteum has been postulated to be the effects of intraovarian estrogen, prostaglandins,

and/or cytokines, but the mechanism remains unknown.[98] However, LH stimulation is required for corpus luteum progesterone production during the luteal phase.[99] Progesterone is cleared rapidly from plasma and is excreted mainly in the urine as pregnanediol.

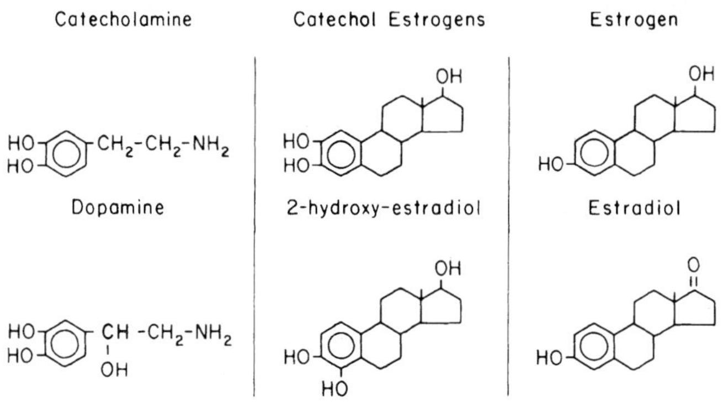

## EFFECTS OF OVARIAN STEROIDS

### ESTROGEN

Estrogen binds to specific estrogen receptors in target tissues and stimulates the production of particular mRNAs that direct the production of proteins that mediate the effects of estrogen.[100] Estrogen has various effects throughout the body (Table 94-1). In the rat ovary, estrogen stimulates granulosa cell division and subsequent follicle growth, increases the number of FSH receptors per follicle, and increases the follicle uptake of FSH. Estrogen has a positive effect on its own production within the ovary.[101] Estrogen sensitizes the human pituitary to

**FIGURE 94-22.** Structure of estrogens, catechol estrogens, and catecholamines. Notice the similarity of the left portion of these catechol estrogens to catecholamines.

**TABLE 94-1.**
**Functions of Estrogens and Progestins in Nonpregnant Women**

| Steroid | Organ | Function |
|---|---|---|
| **ESTROGENS** | Uterus | Stimulate endometrial gland proliferation |
| | | Increase endometrial cell progesterone receptor number |
| | Cervix | Stimulate production of large amounts of thin watery mucus |
| | Breast | Stimulate mammary gland duct growths |
| | Hypothalamus-pituitary | Sensitize gonadotropes to gonadotropin-releasing hormone |
| **PROGESTINS** | Uterus | Stop endometrial gland proliferation and stimulate gland secretion |
| | Cervix | Decrease mucus production and make mucus thick |
| | Breast | Along with prolactin and estrogen, stimulate development of lobuloalveolar system |
| | Hypothalamus-pituitary | May synergize with midcycle estrogen to assure luteinizing hormone surge |

the effects of gonadotropin-releasing hormone (GnRH or LHRH), increasing the secretion of LH in response to a given amount of GnRH. Estrogen stimulates the secondary sexual characteristics associated with female puberty, including breast development. It also stimulates uterine endometrial gland proliferation and induces the appearance of endometrial cell progesterone receptors. The hormone stimulates vaginal epithelial growth and secretions and cervical mucus production. It also has multiple effects on the liver, including the stimulation of hepatic synthesis of proteins such as renin substrate, TeBG, and others. In the postmenopausal woman, estrogen replacement can prevent hot flushes and bone loss (i.e., osteoporosis)[102] (see Chap. 100).

## PROGESTERONE

Progesterone also binds to specific receptors in target tissues. The hormone converts proliferative into secretory endometrium in estrogen-primed uteri (see Table 94-1). High levels of progesterone act as a smooth muscle relaxant and, in pregnancy, allow the uterus to expand. Progesterone counteracts the effect of estrogen on cervical mucus, making the estrogen-induced thin mucus thicker; it also has a mild thermogenic effect and is responsible for the increase in basal body temperature associated with ovulation.[102] The progesterone secreted by the ovary just before ovulation may synergize with estradiol to ensure the LH surge responsible for ovulation.[101]

## ANTIESTROGENS

Compounds that compete with estrogens for binding to the estrogen receptor and have little or no estrogenic effect themselves are antiestrogens. There are two groups: steroidal and nonsteroidal. Estrogen metabolites such as estriol bind weakly to the estrogen receptor and have little estrogenic activity themselves, but they can limit access of active estrogens to the receptor and behave as antiestrogens. Nonsteroidal antiestrogens have important therapeutic value. Clomiphene citrate, which structurally is related to diethylstilbestrol (DES), has found wide use as a fertility agent. Other nonsteroidal antiestrogens, such as tamoxifen and raloxifene, are members of a new class of drugs known as *selective estrogen receptor modulators (SERMs)*. These drugs work as estrogen in some tissues, but not in others, and offer new ways to treat osteoporosis and breast cancer.[103,104]

## CATECHOL ESTROGENS

Other metabolic products of estrogen include the catechol estrogens, which result from hydroxylation of estradiol or estrone at the 2 or 4 position (see Fig. 94-22). They have the potential for interacting with receptors for estrogen and catecholamines and with enzymes that degrade these two latter groups of compounds. Catechol estrogens are found in at least 10-fold higher concentrations in the hypothalamus and pituitary than are estradiol or estrone.[105] Although the functions of catechol estrogens remain unknown, it has been postulated that they may influence GnRH or LH release by acting as antiestrogens through the blockade of the binding of active estrogens to the estrogen receptor and by increasing the activity of endogenous catecholamines by competing for available catecholamine-degrading enzyme, catechol-O-methyltransferase.[106] Synergism of catechol estrogens and catecholamine and gonadotropin effect on progesterone production have also been reported.[107]

## INTRAOVARIAN STEROID EFFECTS

### ESTROGEN RECEPTOR

A novel estrogen receptor (ER), named *ER beta*, has been cloned from human tissue.[108] A comparison of the amino-acid sequence of ER beta with the classic ER *(ER alpha)* shows a high degree of conservation in the DNA-binding and ligand-binding domains. The rest of the protein is not conserved.[108] ER beta is expressed in human thymus, spleen, ovary, and testis. Estradiol-17 binds and activates both ER alpha and ER beta.

ER alpha has been identified in the ovarian surface epithelium cells. ER beta is most abundant in human fetal ovaries, suggesting that it perhaps plays a role in ovarian development.[109] Analysis of whole human ovaries shows equal amounts of ER alpha and ER beta mRNA.[108] Granulosa cells obtained at oocyte aspiration contain high levels of ER beta mRNA[109] and functional ERs.[110] These data are consistent with a direct role of estrogen on follicular granulosa cells. This is, however, an evolving and complex field.

## PROGESTERONE RECEPTOR

The progesterone receptor (PR) exists in two isoforms in the human, $PR_A$ and $PR_B$. $PR_A$ is an amino-terminal truncated variant of $PR_B$. PR has been identified in the epithelial and stromal cells in the ovaries of multiple species, including human.[111] The periovulatory expression of the PR gene in granulosa cells has been detected in all species examined thus far.[11] However, there are distinct species differences in the expression of PR in the corpus luteum (CL). PR has not been detected in the rat CL,[112] but is present in the CL of primates. PR mRNA is lowest in the primate CL cells in the early luteal phase, and increases threefold by the mid to late luteal phase.[113] hCG stimulates luteinized granulosa cell PR mRNA and PR expression, which is modulated by progesterone or a progesterone metabolite.[114] Interestingly, ovarian PR is not under estrogen control, as it is in most tissues.[111] These data suggest a role for intraovarian progesterone in primate ovarian function. The significance of the PR in the rodent ovary has been examined in the PR knock-out mouse. In the absence of PR, the ovary contains normal-appearing granulosa cells, but no corpora lutea, and no ovulation occurs in response to exogenous gonadotropin. These data suggest that PR plays a critical role in rodent ovulation and corpus luteum formation.[66]

## ANDROGEN RECEPTOR

Androgen receptor (AR) localization and abundance have been studied in primate ovary. In the ovary of the rhesus monkey, in situ hybridization demonstrates AR mRNA to be most abundant in granulosa cells of healthy preantral and antral follicles.[115] Theca interna and stromal cells also express AR mRNA, but to a lesser extent than granulosa cells. Granulosa cell AR mRNA abundance is positively correlated with granulosa cell proliferation and is negatively correlated with granulosa cell apoptosis, suggesting that intraovarian androgen stimulates early follicular development in the primate ovary.[115] Similar results were found in studies of the marmoset ovary, using immunohistochemistry. Granulosa cells of immature follicles had a 4.2-fold higher level of immunoreactive AR, as compared to preovulatory follicles. These and other data suggest that the paracrine action of androgen on granulosa cells converts from stimulation to inhibition as the follicle matures. It has been hypothesized that androgens stimulate early follicular development, and a development-related reduction in AR could then protect the follicle against a late inhibitory action of androgen, thus promoting preovulatory follicle dominance in the primate ovarian cycle.[116]

## RELAXIN

Relaxin is a 6-kilodalton (kDa) peptide hormone. The amino-acid sequence of relaxin from several species, including pig, rat, and shark, has been determined, and although the structure is conserved poorly across species lines, all the relaxins consist of two dissimilar peptide chains linked by disulfide bridges (Fig. 94-23). There is significant structural homology to insulin; as is

**B-chains**

Human Relaxin—1:   KWKDDVIKLCGRELVRAQIAICGMSTWSKRSL

Human Relaxin—2:   DSWMEEVIKLCGRELVRAQIAICGMSTWSKRSL

Porcine Relaxin:     QSTNDFIKACGRELVRLWVEICGSVSWGRTAL

**A-chains**

Human Relaxin—1:   RPYVALFEKCCLIGCTKRSLAKYC

Human Relaxin—2:   QLYSALANKCCHVGCTKRSLARFC

Porcine Relaxin:     RMTLSEKCCQVGCIRKDIARLC

**FIGURE 94-23.** Structure of relaxin. The amino- and carboxyl-terminal sequences of the A and B chains are based on probable sites of proteolytic cleavage. These sites have been confirmed for porcine relaxin (Schwabe C, McDonald JK, et al. Primary structure of the B-chain of porcine relaxin. Biochem Biophys Res Commun 1977; 75:503). Human relaxin-2 is a form of the hormone found in human ovaries during pregnancy. Cystine bridges for the A and B chains of relaxin are in the same relative amino-acid positions as in human insulin. (Sequence information obtained from Hudson P, John M, Crawford R, et al. Relaxin gene expression in human ovaries and the predicted structure of a human preprorelaxin by analysis of cDNA clones. EMBO J 1984; 3:2333.) Single-letter abbreviations for amino acids: A, alanine; B, asparagine or aspartic acid; C, cysteine; D, aspartic acid; E, glutamic acid; F, phenylalanine; G, glycine, H, histidine; I, isoleucine; K, lysine; L, leucine; M, methionine; N, asparagine, P, proline; Q, glutamine; R, arginine; S, serine; T, threonine; V, valine; W, tryptophan; Y, tyrosine; Z, glutamine or glutamic acid.

the case with insulin, relaxin is derived from a larger precursor in which the two chains are connected by a C peptide.[117]

Relaxin serves various functions and has different tissue sources in the species studied; therefore, extrapolation across species lines is unwise. Relaxin has been found in the peripheral blood of pregnant animals in all species studied (including women), and the principal tissue source is the corpus luteum, except in the pregnant mare, in which relaxin comes from the placenta. Relaxin has an obligatory role in cervical ripening, softening, and dilatation in pigs and rats, but no such role has been identified in women. Relaxin occasionally can be detected in the serum of nonpregnant women during the luteal phase and is found in the corpus luteum of nonpregnant women, but the concentration is only one-hundredth that in the corpus luteum of pregnant women.

In the rat, relaxin biologic activity is detected on day 14 of pregnancy and is maximal on day 20 (i.e., the last day of pregnancy in the rat). Relaxin is undetectable on day 1 of lactation. By immunocytochemical techniques, relaxin is localized exclusively in the rat ovary to the corpora lutea cells.[118] In the human, relaxin mRNA is localized to the corpus luteum of the cycling ovary, and is found in even much higher levels in the corpus luteum of pregnancy.[119] Relaxin is detectable in serum by postconception day 14. Relaxin concentrations in sera and corpora lutea are maximal in the first trimester and then fall by 20% at the end of the first trimester and remain stable through the end of pregnancy. Three days after delivery, relaxin falls to undetectable levels. Studies in the primate demonstrate that chorionic gonadotropin stimulates corpus luteum relaxin secretion.[120]

The effects of relaxin on the reproductive tract include actions that lead to changes that allow pregnancy to progress and that facilitate delivery. There are important species differences, and many questions remain. Relaxin facilitates delivery in rodents by causing a breakdown in the interpubic ligament that binds the pubic symphysis together.

Inhibition of uterine activity has been observed in guinea pigs, sheep, and hamsters. In the human, progesterone and relaxin synergistically decrease the amplitude of spontaneous myometrial contractions in vitro. Relaxin causes cervical softening in several species, including the rat and pig, but it does not seem to have this effect in primates.[117] Relaxin is also present in the male reproductive tract, and in seminal fluid, it may play a role in sperm motility.

## CONCLUSION

Knowledge of ovarian physiology leans heavily on findings in rodent species. The methods have been adapted by researchers working on the human ovary. Unfortunately, although many molecular processes found in the rat are also found in the human, many are not. The difficulty in this situation is the tendency to generalize the findings to all animals. The conclusion is that it is dangerous to attempt to generalize between the rodent and the human. Much more needs to be learned before the menstrual cycle can be fully understood. An understanding of folliculogenesis can lead to an understanding of fertility and the ability to alleviate the afflictions of infertility.

## REFERENCES

1. Reynolds SRM. The vasculature of the ovary and ovarian function. Recent Prog Horm Res 1950; 5:65.
2. Baker TG, Sum W. Development of the ovary and oogenesis. Clin Obstet Gynaecol 1976; 3:3.
3. Erickson GF. Basic biology: ovarian anatomy and physiology. In: Lobo R, Marcus R, Kelsey J, eds. Menopause. San Diego: Academic Press (in press 1999).
4. Gougeon A. Regulation of ovarian follicular development in primates: facts and hypotheses. Endocr Rev 1996; 17:121.
5. Bachvarova R. Gene expression during oogenesis and oocyte development in mammals. In: Browder L, ed. Developmental biology: a comprehensive synthesis. New York: Plenum Publishing, 1985.
6. Moos J, Faundes D, Kopf GS, Schultz RM. Composition of the human zona pellucida and modifications following fertilization. Hum Reprod 1995; 10:2467.
7. Wassarman PM. Zona pellucida glycoproteins. Annu Rev Biochem 1988; 57:415.
8. Skinner SM, Prasad SV, Ndolo TM, Dunbar BS. Zona pellucida antigens: targets for contraceptive vaccines. Am J Reprod Immunol 1996; 35:163.
9. Bagavant H, Fusi FM, Baisch J, et al. Immunogenicity and contraceptive potential of a human zona pellucida 3 peptide vaccine. Biol Reprod 1997; 56:764.
10. Grazul-Bilska AT, Reynolds LP, Redmer DA. Gap junctions in the ovaries. Biol Reprod 1997; 57:947.
11. Kumar NM, Gilula NB. The gap junction communication channel. Cell 1996; 84:381.
12. Simon AM, Goodenough DA, Li F, Paul DL. Female infertility in mice lacking connexin 37. Nature 1997; 385:525.
13. Green SH, Zuckerman S. Quantitative aspects of the growth of the human ovum and follicle. J Anat 1951; 85:373.
14. Erickson GF, Magoffin DA, Dyer C, Hofeditz C. The ovarian androgen producing cells: a review of structure/function relationships. Endocr Rev 1985;6:371.
15. Meredith JE Jr, Winitz S, Lewis JM, et al. The regulation of growth and intracellular signaling by integrins. Endocr Rev 1996; 17:207.
16. Erickson GF. The graafian follicle: a functional definition. In: Adashi EY, ed. Ovulation: evolving scientific and clinical concepts. New York: Springer-Verlag (in press 1999).
17. Erickson GF. Ovarian androgen biosynthesis: endocrine regulation. In: Azziz R, Nestler JE, Dewailly D, eds. Androgen excess disorders in women. New York: Lippincott–Raven Publishers, 1997.
18. McNatty KP, Moore-Smith D, Osathanondh R, Ryan KJ. The human antral follicle: functional correlates of growth and atresia. Ann Biol Anim Biochim Biophys 1979; 19:1547.
19. Edwards RG. Follicular fluid. J Reprod Fertil 1974; 37:189.
20. Eppig JJ, Chesnel F, Hirao Y, et al. Oocyte control of granulosa cell development: how and why. Hum Reprod 1997; 12:127.
21. Erickson GF. The ovary: basic principles and concepts. In: Felig P, Baxter JD, Frohman LA, eds. Endocrinology and metabolism, 3rd ed. New York: McGraw-Hill, 1995.
22. Hsueh AJ, Billig H, Tsafriri A. Ovarian follicle atresia: a hormonally controlled apoptotic process. Endocr Rev 1994; 15:707.
23. Tilly JL. Apoptosis and ovarian function. Rev Reprod 1996; 1:162.
24. Erickson GF. Defining apoptosis: players and systems. J Soc Gynecol Invest 1997; 4:219.
25. Erickson GF. Analysis of follicle development and ovum maturation. Semin Reprod Endocrinol 1986; 4:233.

26. Hirshfield AN, Midgley AR. Morphometric analysis of follicular development in the rat. Biol Reprod 1978; 19:597.

27. Erickson GF, Yen SSC. New data on follicle cells in polycystic ovaries: a proposed mechanism for the genesis of cystic follicles. Semin Reprod Endocrinol 1984; 2:231.

28. Magoffin DA, Erickson GF. Control systems of theca-interstitial cells. In: Findlay JK, ed. Molecular biology of the female reproductive system. New York: Academic Press, 1994.

29. Erickson GF, Magoffin DA, Jones KL. Theca function in polycystic ovaries of a patient with virilizing congenital adrenal hyperplasia. Fertil Steril 1989; 51:173.

30. Kawakami M, Kubo K, Uemura T, et al. Involvement of ovarian innervation in steroid secretion. Endocrinology 1981; 109:136.

31. Dissen GA, Dees WL, Ojeda SR. Neural and neurotrophic control of ovarian development. In: Adashi EY, Leung PCK, eds. The ovary. New York: Raven Press, 1993.

32. Brännström M, Norman RJ. Involvement of leukocytes and cytokines in the ovulatory process and corpus luteum function. Hum Reprod 1993; 8:1762.

33. Crisp TM, Dessouky DA, Denys FR. The fine structure of the human corpus luteum of early pregnancy and during the progestational phase of the menstrual cycle. Am J Anat 1970; 127:37.

34. Suzuki T, Sasano H, Tamura M, et al. Temporal and spatial localization of steroidogenic enzymes in premenopausal human ovaries: in situ hybridization and immunohistochemical study. Mol Cell Endocrinol 1993; 97:135.

35. Shikone T, Yamoto M, Kokawa K, et al. Apoptosis of human corpora lutea during cyclic luteal regression and early pregnancy. J Clin Endocrinol Metab 1996; 81:2376.

36. Michael AE, Abayasekara DR, Webley GE. Cellular mechanisms of luteolysis. Mol Cell Endocrinol 1994; 99:R1.

37. Auletta FJ, Flint AP. Mechanisms controlling corpus luteum function in sheep, cows, nonhuman primates, and women especially in relation to the time of luteolysis. Endocr Rev 1988; 9:88.

38. Gougeon A. Dynamics of follicular growth in the human: a model from preliminary results. Hum Reprod 1986; 1:81.

39. Gougeon A, Lefèvre B. Evolution of the diameters of the largest healthy and atretic follicles during the human menstrual cycle. J Reprod Fertil 1983; 69:497.

40. Gougeon A, Ecochard R, Thalabard JC. Age-related changes of the population of human ovarian follicles: increase in the disappearance rate of non-growing and early-growing follicles in aging women. Biol Reprod 1994; 50:653.

40a. McGee EA, Hsueb AJW. Initial and cyclic recruitment of ovarian regulatory system in health and disease. Endocr Rev 1999; 13:1018.

41. Gougeon A, Chainy GBN. Morphometric studies of small follicles in ovaries of women at different ages. J Reprod Fertil 1987; 81:433.

42. Zeleznik AJ. Dynamics of primate follicular growth: a physiologic perspective. In: Adashi EY, Leung PCK, eds. The ovary. New York: Raven Press, 1993.

43. Welt CK, Martin KA, Taylor AE, et al. Frequency modulation of follicle-stimulating hormone (FSH) during the luteal-follicular transition: evidence for FSH control of inhibin B in normal women. J Clin Endocrinol Metab 1997; 82:2645.

44. Zeleznik AJ. Premature elevation of systemic estradiol reduces serum levels of follicle-stimulating hormone and lengthens the follicular phase of the menstrual cycle in rhesus monkeys. Endocrinology 1981; 109:352.

45. McNatty KP, Hunter WM, McNeilly AS, Sawers RS. Changes in the concentration of pituitary and steroid hormones in the follicular fluid of human graafian follicles throughout the menstrual cycle. J Endocrinol 1975; 64:555.

46. Phillips DJ, deKretser DM. Follistatin: a multifunctional regulatory protein. Front Neuroendocrinol 1998; 19:287.

47. Sawetawan C, Milewich L, Word RA, et al. Compartmentalization of type I 17 beta-hydroxysteroid oxidoreductase in the human ovary. Mol Cell Endocrinol 1994; 99:161.

48. Zhang Y, Word RA, Fesmire S, et al. Human ovarian expression of 17 beta-hydroxysteroid dehydrogenase types 1, 2, and 3. J Clin Endocrinol Metab 1996; 8 1:3594.

49. Segaloff DL, Ascoli M. The lutropin/choriogonadotropin receptor...4 years later. Endocr Rev 1993; 14:324.

50. Simoni M, Gromoll J, Nieschlag E. The follicle-stimulating hormone receptor: biochemistry, molecular biology, physiology, and pathophysiology. Endocr Rev 1997; 18:739.

51. Meyer TE, Habener JF. Cyclic adenosine 3',5'-monophosphate response element binding protein (CREB) and related transcription-activating deoxyribonucleic acid–binding proteins. Endocr Rev 1993; 14:269.

52. McNatty KP, Sawers RS. Relationship between the endocrine environment within the graafian follicle and the subsequent rate of progesterone secretion by human granulosa cells in vitro. J Endocrinol 1975; 66:391.

53. Yong EL, Baird DT, Hillier SG. Mediation of gonadotrophin-stimulated growth and differentiation of human granulosa cells by adenosine-3',5'-monophosphate: one molecule, two messages. Clin Endocrinol (Oxf) 1992; 37:51.

54. Gospodarowicz D, Bialecki H. Fibroblast and epidermal growth factors are mitogenic agents for cultured granulosa cells of rodent, porcine, and human origin. Endocrinology 1979; 104:757.

55. Shaw HJ, Hillier SG, Hodges JK. Developmental changes in luteinizing hormone/human chorionic gonadotropin steroidogenic responsiveness in marmoset granulosa cells: effects of follicle-stimulating hormone and androgens. Endocrinology 1989; 124:1669.

56. Bar-Ami S, Haciski RC, Channing CP. Increasing 125I-human chorionic gonadotrophin specific binding in human granulosa cells by follicle-stimulating hormone and follicular fluid. Hum Reprod 1989; 4:876.

57. Channing CP. Steroidogenesis and morphology of human ovarian cell types in tissue culture. J Endocrinol 1969; 45:297.

58. Yamoto M, Shima K, Nakano R. Gonadotropin receptors in human ovarian follicles and corpora lutea throughout the menstrual cycle. Horm Res 1992; 37(Suppl 1):5.

59. Adashi F, Leung PCK, eds. The ovary: comprehensive endocrinology. New York: Raven Press, 1993.

60. Erickson GF, Danforth DR. Ovarian control of follicle development. Am J Obstet Gynecol 1995; 172:736.

60a. Abulafia O, Sherer DM. Angiogenesis of the ovary. Am J Obstet Gynecol 2000; 182:240.

61. Poretsky L, Catakio NA, Roseriwaks Z, et al. The insulin-related ovarian regulatory system in health and disease. Endocr Rev 1999; 20:535.

62. Elvin JA, Yan C, Wang P, et al. Molecular characterization of the follicle defects in the growth differentiation factor 9-deficient ovary. Mol Endocrinol 1999; 13:1018.

63. Tsafriri A, Chun SY, Reich R. Follicular rupture and ovulation. In: Adashi EY, Leung PCK, eds. The ovary: comprehensive endocrinology. New York: Raven Press, 1993.

64. Okamura H, Takenaka A, Yajima Y, Nishimura T. Ovulatory changes in the wall at the apex of the human graafian follicle. J Reprod Fertil 1980; 58:153.

65. Graham JD, Clarke CL. Physiological action of progesterone in target tissues. Endocr Rev 1997; 18:502.

66. Lydon JP, DeMayo FJ, Funk CR, et al. Mice lacking progesterone receptor exhibit pleiotropic reproductive abnormalities. Genes Dev 1995; 9:2266.

67. Herschman HR. Prostaglandin synthase 2. Biochim Biophys Acta 1996; 1299:125.

68. Dinchuk JE, Car BD, Focht RJ, et al. Renal abnormalities and an altered inflammatory response in mice lacking cyclooxygenase II. Nature 1995; 378:406.

69. Lim H, Paria BC, Das SK, et al. Multiple female reproductive failures in cyclooxygenase 2-deficient mice. Cell 1997; 91:197.

70. Beers WH. Follicular plasminogen and plasminogen activator and the effect of plasmin on ovarian follicle wall. Cell 1975; 6:379.

71. Eppig JJ. Regulation of mammalian oocyte maturation. In: Adashi EY, Leung PCK, eds. The ovary: comprehensive endocrinology. New York: Raven Press, 1993.

72. Helter DT, Cahill DM, Schultz RM. Biochemical studies of mammalian oogenesis: metabolic cooperativity between granulosa cells and growing mouse oocytes. Dev Biol 1981; 84:455.

73. Brower PT, Schultz RM. Intercellular communication between granulosa cells and mouse oocytes: existence and possible nutritional role during oocyte growth. Dev Biol 1982; 90:144.

74. McGrath SA, Esquela AF, Lee S-J. Oocyte-specific expression of growth/differentiation factor-9. Mol Endocrinol 1995; 9:131.

75. Nishimori K, Dunkel L, Hsueh AJ, et al. Expression of luteinizing hormone and chorionic gonadotropin receptor messenger ribonucleic acid in human corpora lutea during menstrual cycle and pregnancy. J Clin Endocrinol Metab 1995; 80:1444.

76. Richards JS. Hormonal control of gene expression in the ovary. Endocr Rev 1994; 15:725.

77. McNeilly AS, Kerin J, Swanston IA, et al. Changes in the binding of human chorionic gonadotrophin/luteinizing hormone, follicle-stimulating hormone and prolactin to human corpora lutea during the menstrual cycle and pregnancy. J Endocrinol 1980; 87:315.

78. Gwynne JT, Strauss JF 3rd. The role of lipoproteins in steroidogenesis and cholesterol metabolism in steroidogenic glands. Endocr Rev 1982; 3:299.

79. Miller GJ. High density lipoproteins and atherosclerosis. Ann Rev Med 1980; 31:97.

80. Tureck RW, Strauss JF 3rd. Progesterone synthesis by luteinized human granulosa cells in culture: the role of de novo sterol synthesis and lipoprotein-carried sterol. J Clin Endocrinol Metab 1982; 54:367.

81. Schreiber JR, Weinstein DB. Lipoprotein receptors in steroidogenesis. In: Scanu AM, Spector A, eds. Lipoproteins, receptors, and cell function. New York: Marcel Dekker Inc, 1985.

82. Brown MS, Goldstein JL. Receptor-mediated control of cholesterol metabolism. Science 1976; 191:150.

83. Ohashi M, Carr BR, Simpson ER. Lipoprotein-binding sites in human corpus luteum membrane fractions. Endocrinology 1982; 110:1477.

84. Kandutsch AA, Chen HW, Heiniger HJ. Biological activity of some oxygenated sterols. Science 1978; 201:498.

85. Brown MS, Goldstein JL. Receptor-mediated endocytosis: insights from the lipoprotein receptor system. Proc Natl Acad Sci U S A 1979; 76:3330.

86. Rennert H, Fischer RT, Alvarez JG, et al. Generation of regulatory oxysterols: 26-hydroxylation of cholesterol by ovarian mitochondria. Endocrinology 1990; 127:738.

87. Carr BR, MacDonald PC, Simpson ER. The role of lipoproteins in the regulation of progesterone secretion by the human corpus luteum. Fertil Steril 1982; 38:303.

88. diZerega GS, Hodgen GD. Fluorescence localization of luteinizing hormone/human chorionic gonadotropin uptake in the primate ovary. II. Changing distribution during selection of the dominant follicle. J Clin Endocrinol Metab 1980; 51:903.

89. Li X, Peegel H, Menon KM. In situ hybridization of high density lipoprotein (scavenger, type 1) receptor messenger ribonucleic acid (mRNA) dur-

ing folliculogenesis and luteinization: evidence for mRNA expression and induction by human chorionic gonadotropin specifically in cell types that use cholesterol for steroidogenesis. Endocrinology 1998; 139:3043.

90. Richards JS, Hedin L. Molecular aspects of hormone action in ovarian follicular development, ovulation, and luteinization. Annu Rev Physiol 1988; 50:441.
91. Privalle CT, Crivello JF, Jefcoate CR. Regulation of intramitochondrial cholesterol transfer to side-chain cleavage cytochrome P-450 in rat adrenal gland. Proc Natl Acad Sci U S A 1983; 80:702.
92. Clark BJ, Wells J, King SR, Stocco DM. The purification, cloning, and expression of a novel luteinizing hormone-induced mitochondrial protein in MA-10 mouse Leydig tumor cells. J Biol Chem 1994; 269:28314.
93. Kiriakidou M, McAllister JM, Sugawara T, Strauss JF 3rd. Expression of steroidogenic acute regulatory protein StAR in the human ovary. J Clin Endocrinol Metab 1996; 81:4122.
94. Lin D, Sugawara T, Strauss JF 3rd, et al. Role of steroidogenic acute regulatory protein in adrenal and gonadal steroidogenesis. Science 1995; 267:1828.
95. Lipsett M. Steroid hormones. In: Yen SSC, Jaffe RB, eds. Reproductive endocrinology. Philadelphia: WB Saunders, 1978.
96. Hodgen GD. The dominant ovarian follicle. Fertil Steril 1982; 38:281.
97. Grodin JM, Siiteri PK, MacDonald PC. Source of estrogen production in postmenopausal women. J Clin Endocrinol Metab 1973; 36:207.
98. Wuttke W, Theiling K, Hinney B, Pitzel L. Regulation of steroid production and its function within the corpus luteum. Steroids 1998; 63:299.
99. Hutchison JS, Zeleznik AJ. The rhesus monkey corpus luteum is dependent on pituitary gonadotropin secretion throughout the luteal phase of the menstrual cycle. Endocrinology 1984; 115:1780.
100. King WJ, Greene GL. Monoclonal antibodies localize oestrogen receptor in the nuclei of target cells. Nature 1984; 307:745.
101. Schreiber J. Current concepts of human follicular growth and development. Contemp Obstet Gynecol 1983; 26:125.
102. Henzl M. Natural and synthetic female sex hormones. In: Yen SSC, Jaffe RB, eds. Reproductive endocrinology. Philadelphia: WB Saunders, 1978.
103. Baker VL, Jaffe RB. Clinical uses of antiestrogens. Obstet Gynecol Surv 1996; 51:45.
104. Baynes KC, Compston JE. Selective oestrogen receptor modulators: a new paradigm for HRT. Curr Opin Obstet Gynecol 1998; 10:189.
105. Paul SM, Axelrod J. Catechol estrogens: presence in brain and endocrine tissues. Science 1977; 197:657.
106. Ball P, Knuppen R, Haupt M, Breuer H. Interactions between estrogens and catechol amines. 3. Studies on the methylation of catechol estrogens, catechol amines and other catechols by the catechol-O-methyltransferases of human liver. J Clin Endocrinol Metab 1972; 34:736.
107. Spicer LJ, Hammond JM. Mechanism of action of 2-hydroxyestradiol on steroidogenesis in ovarian granulosa cells: interactions with catecholamines and gonadotropins involve cyclic adenosine monophosphate. Biol Reprod 1989; 40:87.
108. Mosselman S, Polman J, Dijkema R. ER beta: identification and characterization of a novel human estrogen receptor. FEBS Lett 1996; 392:49.
109. Brandenberger AW, Tee MK, Jaffe RB. Estrogen receptor alpha (ER-alpha) and beta (ER-beta) mRNAs in normal ovary, ovarian serous cystadenocarcinoma and ovarian cancer cell lines: down-regulation of ER-beta in neoplastic tissues. J Clin Endocrinol Metab 1998; 83:1025.
110. Hurst BS, Zilberstein M, Chou JY, et al. Estrogen receptors are present in human granulosa cells. J Clin Endocrinol Metab 1995; 80:229.
111. Pinter JH, Deep C, Park-Sarge OK. Progesterone receptors: expression and regulation in the mammalian ovary. Clin Obstet Gynecol 1996; 39:424.
112. Park-Sarge OK, Parmer TG, Gu Y, Gibori G. Does the rat corpus luteum express the progesterone receptor gene? Endocrinology 1995; 136:1537.
113. Duffy DM, Stouffer RL. Progesterone receptor messenger ribonucleic acid in the primate corpus luteum during the menstrual cycle: possible regulation by progesterone. Endocrinology 1995; 136:1869.
114. Duffy DM, Molskness TA, Stouffer RL. Progesterone receptor messenger ribonucleic acid and protein in luteinized granulosa cells of rhesus monkeys are regulated in vitro by gonadotropins and steroids. Biol Reprod 1996; 54:888.
115. Weil SJ, Vendola K, Zhou J, et al. Androgen receptor gene expression in the primate ovary: cellular localization, regulation, and functional correlations. J Clin Endocrinol Metab 1998; 83:2479.
116. Hillier SG, Tetsuka M, Fraser HM. Location and developmental regulation of androgen receptor in primate ovary. Hum Reprod 1997; 12:107.
117. Weiss G. Relaxin. Annu Rev Physiol 1984; 46:43.
118. Golos TG, Weyhenmeyer JA, Sherwood OD. Immunocytochemical localization of relaxin in the ovaries of pregnant rats. Biol Reprod 1984; 30:257.
119. Bogic LV, Mandel M, Bryant-Greenwood GD. Relaxin gene expression in human reproductive tissues by in situ hybridization. J Clin Endocrinol Metab 1995; 80:130.
120. Duffy DM, Hutchison JS, Stewart DR, Stouffer RL. Stimulation of primate luteal function by recombinant human chorionic gonadotropin and modulation of steroid, but not relaxin, production by an inhibitor of 3 beta-hydroxysteroid dehydrogenase during simulated early pregnancy. J Clin Endocrinol Metab 1996; 81:2307.

# CHAPTER 95

# THE NORMAL MENSTRUAL CYCLE AND THE CONTROL OF OVULATION

ROBERT W. REBAR, GARY D. HODGEN, AND MICHAEL ZINGER

Perhaps the single feature that most clearly distinguishes the reproductive endocrinology of the female from that of the male is the dependence of female reproductive function on an entirely different set of endocrine rhythms. In considering abnormal female reproductive function, it is imperative to remember what is normal for that moment in the life of that individual.

An overview of the patterns of circulating concentrations of luteinizing hormone (LH), follicle-stimulating hormone (FSH), and estradiol ($E_2$) throughout the life of the normal woman is depicted in Figure 95-1. Rhythmic changes occur in the hormones secreted by all levels of the reproductive system. Moreover, hormonal secretion is modified through several phases of the life cycle.[1] Gonadotropin secretion is low in the prepubertal years, increases before and during pubertal development, assumes the characteristic monthly cyclicity of the reproductive years, and finally increases to high levels after the menopause (i.e., the final menstrual period). These changes are both temporally and causally related to simultaneous rhythms in the secretion of ovarian (especially $E_2$) and hypothalamic (particularly gonadotropin-releasing hormone [GnRH]) hormones. Superimposed on these long-term changes are the shorter-term rhythms that are so important to female reproduction.

Several distinctive rhythms become prominent as a female child progresses to sexual maturity. Female puberty is characterized by the resetting of the classic negative ovarian steroid feedback loop, the establishment of new circadian (24-hour) and ultradian (60- to 90-minute) gonadotropin rhythms, and

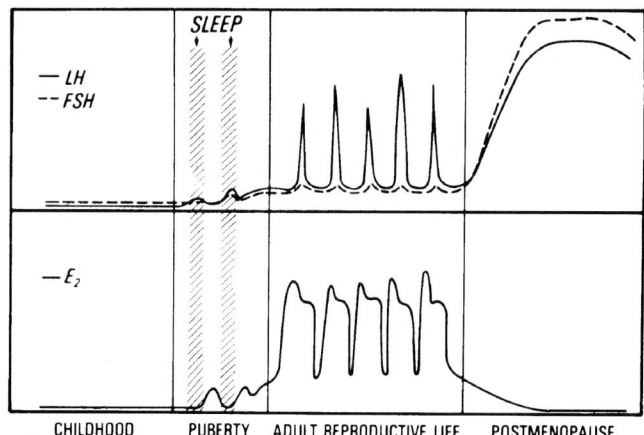

**FIGURE 95-1.** Changing patterns of luteinizing hormone (*LH*), follicle-stimulating hormone (*FSH*), and estradiol ($E_2$) concentrations in peripheral blood throughout the life of a typical woman. The pubertal period has been expanded to depict the sleep-induced increases in LH and FSH followed by morning increases in $E_2$ that are observed during puberty. Such sleep-associated increases also occur during the early follicular phase of the menstrual cycle. (From Rebar RW. Normal physiology of the reproductive system. In: Endocrine metabolism continuing education and quality control program. American Association of Clinical Chemistry, 1982.)

the development of a positive estrogen feedback loop control-ling the infradian (monthly) rhythm as an interdependent cyclic expression of the gonadotropins and the ovarian ster-oids.[2] Sleep-related increases in gonadotropins and gonadal steroids become evident during puberty and appear to play an important role in pubertal maturation (see Chap. 91).

Although changes in reproductive hormones during the menstrual cycle in adult women are common knowledge, it is not widely recognized that basal concentrations of several other hormones, including growth hormone (GH),[3,4] prolactin,[5,6] cor-ticotropin and cortisol, and parathyroid hormone and calcito-nin,[7] also are influenced by the stage of the menstrual cycle. Although the physiologic significance of these changes is unclear, they suggest that the menstrual cycle affects systems and functions throughout the body.

What is most remarkable about these separate and yet inter-dependent rhythms is that in most women, they are coordi-nated in an as yet incompletely defined manner to ensure ovulation and pregnancy. Because available data indicate the existence of finely controlled rhythms at all levels of the repro-ductive system, an abnormality at any level may lead to an abnormal state with altered rhythms.

## GENERAL CHARACTERISTICS OF THE NORMAL MENSTRUAL CYCLE

A series of cyclic and closely related events involving the repro-ductive organs occur in normal, nonpregnant adult women at about monthly intervals between *menarche*, at approximately age 12 years, and *menopause*, at approximately age 51 years. These events constitute the menstrual cycle. During each normal men-strual cycle, an ovum matures, is ovulated, and enters the uterine lumen through the fallopian tubes. Steroids secreted by the ova-ries effect endometrial changes, allowing implantation if the ovum is fertilized. In the absence of fertilization, ovarian secre-tion of progesterone and $E_2$ declines, the endometrium sloughs, and menstruation begins. The menstrual cycle requires the coor-dinated, functional interaction of the hypothalamus, the pitu-itary gland, and the ovaries (the hypothalamic–pituitary–ovarian axis) to produce associated changes in the target tissues of the reproductive tract (endometrium, cervix, and vagina), which then permit pregnancy and perpetuation of the species.[8] Although the individual units of the hypothalamic–pituitary–ovarian axis are innervated, the mediators of the communication also include autocrine, paracrine, and hemocrine mechanisms.

By definition, a menstrual cycle begins with the first day of genital bleeding and ends just before the next menstrual period begins. Although the median menstrual cycle length is 28 days, normal menstrual cycles may vary from ~21 to 40 days in length. Menstrual cycle length varies most in the years immedi-ately after menarche and in those immediately preceding meno-pause.[9] The average duration of menstrual flow is 5 ± 2 days, with typical blood loss ranging from 30 to 80 mL.[10–13] Tampons and pads each absorb an estimated 20 to 30 mL or more.

The normal menstrual cycle can be divided into the *follicular* and *luteal* phases. Sometimes an ovulatory phase is delineated as well.

The *follicular phase*, also known as the proliferative or preovu-latory phase, begins with the onset of menstruation and ends with ovulation (Fig. 95-2). It is variable in duration and accounts for the range in menstrual cycle length found in ovulatory women. The *luteal phase*, sometimes termed the postovulatory or secretory phase, begins with ovulation and ends with the onset of menses. It is the more constant half of the menstrual cycle and averages 14 days in length. The *ovulatory phase* extends from 1 day before the LH surge to the time of ovulation, ~32 to 34 hours after the onset of the preovulatory LH surge.

Some women experience dull, unilateral pelvic pain of a few minutes' to a few hours' duration near the time of ovulation.

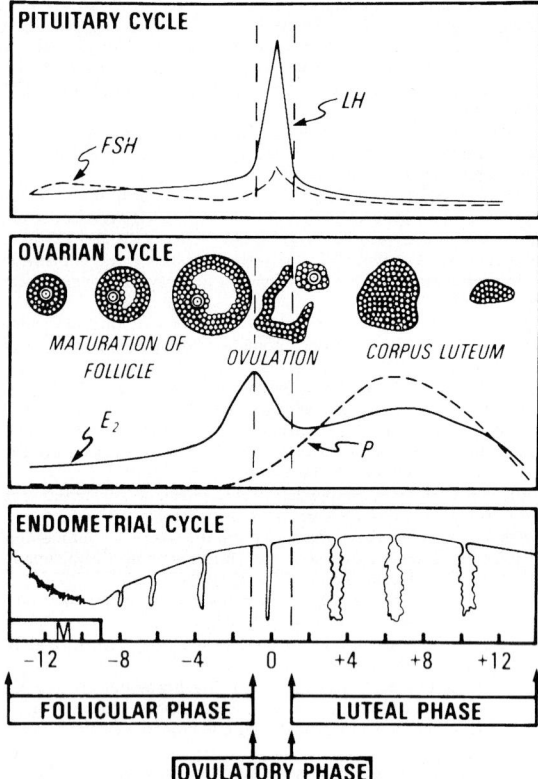

**FIGURE 95-2.** Idealized cyclic changes observed in pituitary secretion of gonadotropins, ovarian secretion of estradiol ($E_2$) and progesterone (*P*), and the uterine endometrium during the reproductive life of the woman. The data have been centered around the day of the luteinizing hormone (*LH*) surge (day 0). (*M*, days of menstrual bleeding; *FSH*, follicle-stimulating hormone.) (From Rebar RW. Normal physiology of the reproductive system. In: Endocrine and metabolism continuing educa-tion and quality control program. American Association of Clinical Chemistry, 1982.)

Such pain has been termed *mittelschmerz*. The pain may occur before, during, or after actual ovulation. Although the pain occurs on the side containing the ovary that releases the oocyte, it is not clear that the pain actually is caused by the physical act of ovulation itself.

## HORMONAL CHANGES DURING THE NORMAL MENSTRUAL CYCLE

Circulating concentrations of FSH begin to increase in the late luteal phase of the previous menstrual cycle[14–16] (see Fig. 95-2). The increase in FSH levels continues into the early follicular phase and is responsible for initiating the growth and develop-ment of a group of follicles. The oocyte that will be ovulated is selected from this cohort undergoing development, but the manner of selection is not understood. FSH levels then fall after the early follicular phase increase. Except for a brief peak at midcycle, FSH levels continue to fall until they reach their low-est levels in the midluteal phase, just before they begin to increase again before menses.

Circulating LH concentrations also begin to increase in the late luteal phase of the previous menstrual period.[14–16] How-ever, in contrast to FSH levels, LH concentrations continue to increase gradually throughout the follicular phase. At midcy-cle, there is a significant increase in circulating LH levels that lasts 1 to 3 days and triggers ovulation. Currently available urinary LH-testing kits detect the LH surge with reasonable accuracy. LH levels gradually decrease in the luteal phase to

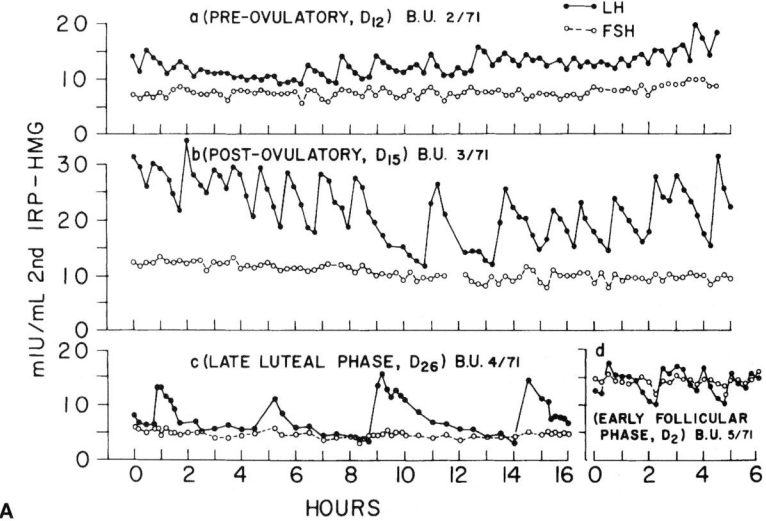

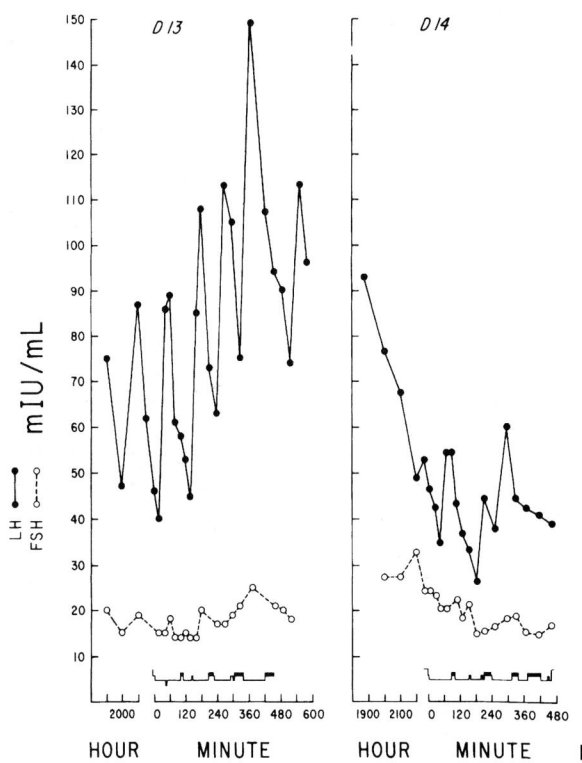

**FIGURE 95-3.** **A,** Variation in the frequency and magnitude of the pulsatile patterns of circulating luteinizing hormone (*LH*) and follicle-stimulating hormone (*FSH*) during different phases of the menstrual cycle. Results are presented in terms of the Second International Reference Preparation for Human Menopausal Gonadotropin (*2nd IRP-HMG*). **B,** LH and FSH concentrations by stages of sleep on cycle days 13 and 14. (From Yen SSC, Rebar RW, Vandenberg G, et al. Pituitary gonadotropin responsiveness to synthetic LRF in subjects with normal and abnormal hypothalamic-pituitary-gonadal axis. J Reprod Fertil 1973; 20[Suppl]:137.)

reach their lowest levels just before beginning to increase again before menses.

As is true for virtually all hormones, the gonadotropins (especially LH) are secreted in a pulsatile manner, with intervals of 1 to 4 hours between pulses, depending on the phase of the menstrual cycle.[17–19] (Fig. 95-3). LH pulse frequency is lowest during the luteal phase of the menstrual cycle, apparently because of the effects of progesterone.[20] The pulsatile secretion of the gonadotropins is dependent on the pulsatile secretion of GnRH by the hypothalamus.[21]

The ovary secretes numerous steroidal and nonsteroidal hormones. Several of the steroids secreted by the ovary also are secreted by the adrenal gland, and some are formed by peripheral conversion from other steroid precursors (Fig. 95-4). Consequently, circulating concentrations do not reflect ovarian production rates. Several steroids secreted by the ovary do vary throughout the menstrual cycle (Fig. 95-5, see Chap. 94).

$E_2$ may be the most important steroid secreted by the ovary because of its biologic potency and its many effects on peripheral target tissues. Circulating levels of $E_2$ are low during the first half of the follicular phase, begin to increase ~7 to 8 days before the preovulatory LH surge, and generally peak at levels of 250 to 350 pg/mL the day before or the day of the LH surge.[22–25] As peak LH levels are reached during the ovulatory phase, $E_2$ levels fall rapidly, only to increase again to a secondary peak 6 to 8 days after the LH surge during the midluteal phase[26] (Fig. 95-6). Parallel, but smaller, changes occur in circulating *estrone* levels. The dominant follicle and corpus luteum synthesize ~95% of circulating $E_2$. In contrast, a significant portion of the circulating estrone is converted from $E_2$ and from the peripheral conversion of androstenedione.

*Androstenedione* and *testosterone,* secreted by the interstitial and theca cells, are the primary ovarian androgens. Androstenedione, the major ovarian androgen, also can be converted to testosterone and estrogens in peripheral tissues. Both androstenedione and testosterone also are secreted in significant amounts by the adrenal gland, and both peak at the time of the midcycle LH surge, no doubt because of increased ovarian secretion.[23,24,27] In contrast, dehydroepiandrosterone and its sul-

fate, which are secreted almost entirely by the adrenal gland, do not vary with the menstrual cycle.

Circulating levels of *progesterone* and progesterone secretion remain low throughout the follicular phase and begin to increase just before the onset of the LH surge[26,28,29] (see Fig. 95-6). During the luteal phase, progesterone secretion increases to peak 6 to 8 days after the LH surge. Progesterone levels decrease toward menses unless the ovum is fertilized. Serum progesterone levels of 10 ng/mL or greater 1 week before menses generally indicate normal *ovulation.* Moreover, because progestins increase morning basal body temperature, an "upward shift" of more than 0.3°C orally after a midcycle nadir is a presumptive sign of ovulation and progesterone secretion. Unfortunately, daily measurement of basal temperature is tedious and not very reliable. *17α-Hydroxyprogesterone* concentrations actually begin to increase at midcycle, before progesterone and parallel changes in progesterone levels in the luteal phase.

*Insulin-like growth factor-I* (IGF-I) appears to play an important role in stimulating follicular growth and maturation as well as in augmenting steroid production. Although the majority of IGF-I production is peripheral,[30] IGF-I production by the ovary also occurs.[31] IGF-I levels in peripheral serum are lowest during menses and highest during the periovulatory period and the luteal phase.[32–34] Serum levels of IGF-I decline with age.[35] The main antagonist of IGF-I action is IGF-binding protein-3 (IGFBP-3), which decreases the amount of bioactive IGF-I through binding of the hormone.

Serum concentrations of *GH* have been correlated with those of $E_2$, peaking during the periovulatory period.[33,36] GH can potentiate the stimulatory effects of gonadotropins on ovarian follicles. It also stimulates the corpus luteum to increase progesterone production. These effects can be mediated by IGF-I.

*Inhibin* and *activin* are composed of a family of polypeptide subunits, α, β-A, and β-B, which are produced by follicular granulosa cells as well as the corpus luteum. Because earlier assays for inhibin were specific for the α subunit, they did not distinguish between *inhibin A,* which is composed of an α subunit and a β-A subunit, and *inhibin B,* which is composed of an α subunit and a β-B subunit. Therefore, care must be taken in

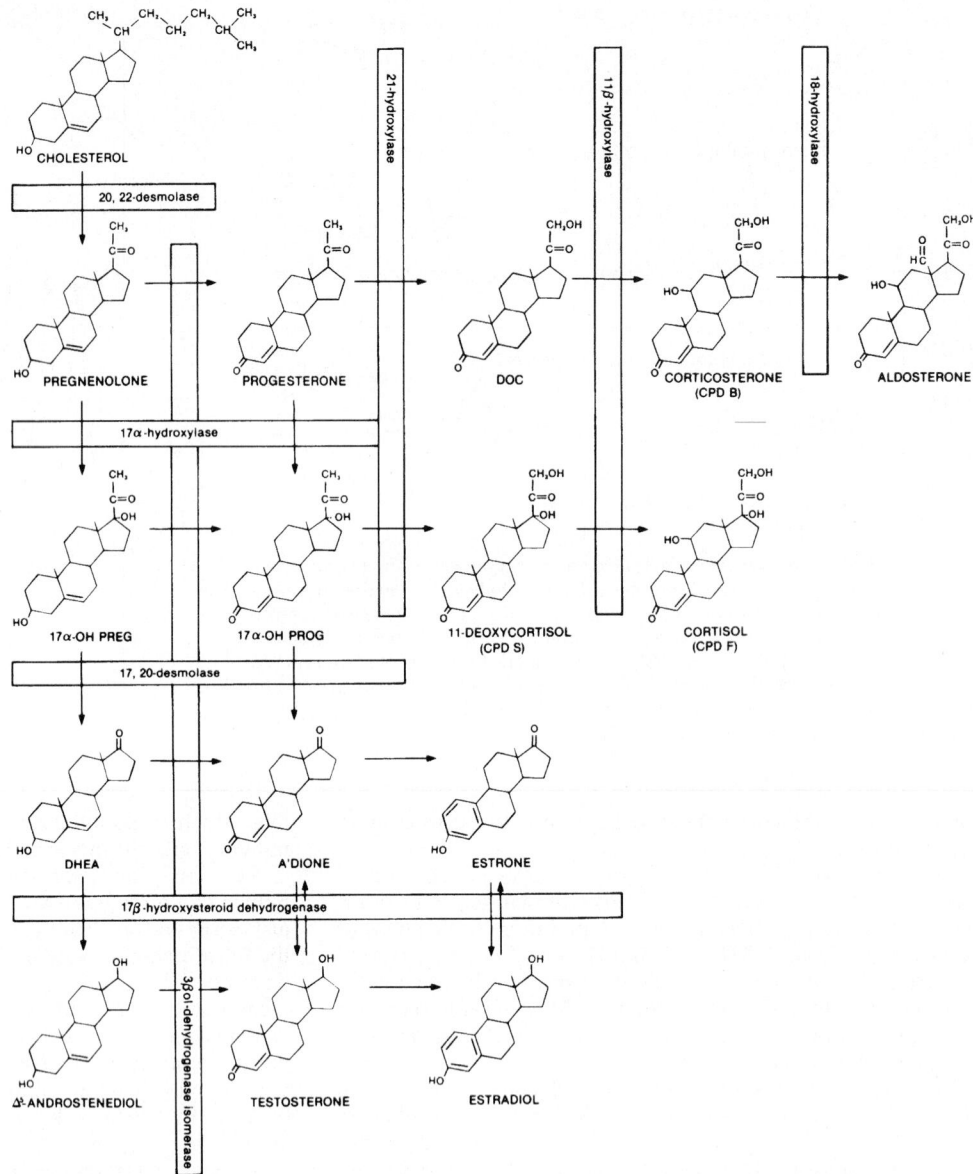

**FIGURE 95-4.** Pathways of steroidogenesis. The necessary enzymes are depicted as well as the steroids.

interpreting older studies that used this assay. Thus, although it was previously recognized that inhibin is often a negative regulator of FSH, current assays, which distinguish between inhibin A and B, provide a clearer delineation of their individual roles. Inhibin A begins to increase as the follicle grows and reaches its peak during the luteal phase. However, estradiol, not inhibin A, seems to be the predominant suppressor of FSH release during the luteal phase.[37] Serum inhibin B peaks during the follicular phase, apparently in response to increasing FSH.[38] Inhibin B is then critical for suppressing FSH release and inducing a plateau in FSH serum levels in the midfollicular phase; however, estradiol is instrumental in further reducing FSH levels.[37] The subsequent rise in LH and fall in FSH in the late follicular phase also are believed to be due in part to the fact that $E_2$ is more inhibitory of FSH than of LH secretion.[19]

Unlike inhibin, *activin*, a dimer composed of two β subunits in any combination, does not vary during the menstrual cycle.[39] The primary function of *follistatin*, which is concentrated 100-fold within follicular fluid, appears to be regulation of activin action by binding the hormone. FSH and prostaglandin $E_2$ promote follistatin production in granulosa cells.[40] However, reports of menstrual cycle variation of follicular fluid levels of follistatin have been inconsistent.

Circulating levels of several other hormones that do not seem to be directly related to ovulation (i.e., prolactin, cortisol, parathyroid hormone, calcitonin, estrogen-sensitive neurophysin, and catechol estrogens) appear to peak at midcycle.[20,41–44] Although the physiologic significance of such changes is unclear, the cyclic fluctuation of these hormones suggests that endogenous estrogen may modulate the secretion of other hormones.

## CYCLIC CHANGES IN THE TARGET ORGANS OF THE REPRODUCTIVE TRACT

### ENDOMETRIUM

During the menstrual cycle, the endometrium undergoes a series of histologic and cytologic changes that culminate in menstruation if pregnancy does not result[45–47] (see Fig. 95-2). The *basal layer* of the endometrium, nearest the myometrium, undergoes little change during the menstrual cycle and is not shed during menses. The basal layer regenerates an *intermediate spongiosa layer* and a *superficial compact epithelial cell layer*, both of which are sloughed at each menstruation. Under the influence of estrogen, with IGF-I likely acting as a paracrine mediator, the endometrial

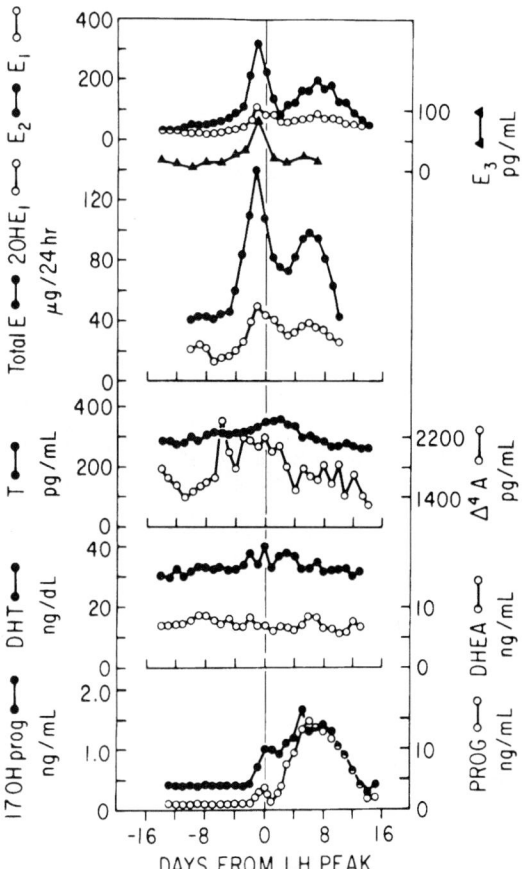

**FIGURE 95-5.** Steroid patterns during the menstrual cycle. All changes are those observed in circulating concentrations except for total estrogens (*Total E*) and 2-hydroxyestrone (*20HE₁*), for which changes in 24-hour urinary excretion are shown. (*E*, estrone; $E_2$, estradiol; $E_3$, estriol; *T*, testosterone; $\Delta^4 A$, $\Delta^4$-androstenedione; *DHT*, dihydrotestosterone; *DHEA*, dehydroepiandrosterone; *17OH prog*, 17-hydroxyprogesterone; *PROG*, progesterone; *LH*, luteinizing hormone.) (From Rebar RW, Yen SSC. Endocrine rhythms in gonadotropins and ovarian steroids with reference to reproductive processes. In: Krieger DT, ed. Endocrine rhythms. New York: Raven Press, 1979:259.)

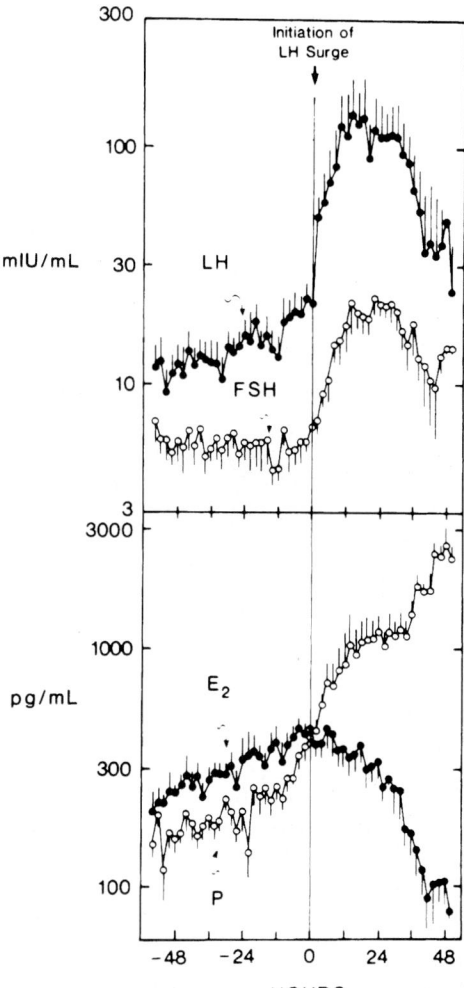

**FIGURE 95-6.** Mean (± SE) luteinizing hormone (*LH*), follicle-stimulating hormone (*FSH*), estradiol (*E₂*), and progesterone (*P*) concentrations in five women, measured at 2-hour intervals for 5 days at midcycle. The initiation of the LH surge has been used as the reference point (at time 0) from which data have been tabulated. The hormone concentrations are plotted on a logarithmic scale. (From Hoff JD, Quigley MD, Yen SSC. Hormonal dynamics at midcycle: a reevaluation. J Clin Endocrinol Metab 1983; 57:792.)

glands in these two functional layers proliferate during the follicular phase, leading to thickening of the mucosa. During the luteal phase, the glands become coiled and secretory under the influence of progesterone, with IGF-II being the suspected paracrine mediator.[48] The endometrium becomes much more edematous and vascular, largely because spiral arteries develop in the functional layers. With the decline of both $E_2$ and progesterone in the late luteal phase, endometrial and blood vessel necrosis occurs, and menstrual bleeding begins. The local secretion of prostaglandins appears to initiate vasospasm and consequent ischemic necrosis of the endometrium, as well as the uterine contractions that frequently occur with menstruation.[49] Thus, prostaglandin synthetase inhibitors can relieve dysmenorrhea (i.e., menstrual cramping).[50] Fibrinolytic activity in the endometrium also peaks during menstruation, thus explaining the noncoagulability of menstrual blood.[51] Because of the characteristic histologic changes that occur during the menstrual cycle, endometrial biopsies can be used to date the stage of the menstrual cycle and to assess the tissue response to gonadal steroids.[46,47] Transvaginal ultrasound is a less invasive modality that has a 76% accuracy in assessing endometrial stage as compared to biopsy.[52]

## CERVIX AND CERVICAL MUCUS

Under the influence of estrogen, cyclic changes occur in the diameter of the external cervical os, the dimensions of the exter-

nal cervical canal, the vascularity of the cervical tissues, and the amount and biophysical properties of cervical mucus[53,54] (Fig. 95-7). Normally, sex steroids are present in cervical mucus.[52a] During the follicular phase, there is a progressive increase in cervical vascularity, congestion, and edema, as well as in the secretion of cervical mucus. The external cervical os opens to a diameter of 3 mm at ovulation and then decreases to 1 mm. Under the influence of increasing levels of estrogen, several changes in cervical mucus occur. There is a 10- to 30-fold increase in the amount of cervical mucus. The elasticity of the mucus, also known as *spinnbarkeit*, increases. Just before ovulation, "palm leaf" arborization or ferning becomes prominent when cervical mucus is allowed to dry on a glass slide and is examined microscopically (Fig. 95-8). This ferning is a result of the increased sodium chloride concentration in the cervical mucus induced by rising levels of estrogen. The pH of the mucus increases to ~8.0 at midcycle as well. Under the influence of progesterone, during the luteal phase, cervical mucus thickens, becomes less watery, and loses its elasticity and ability to fern. These characteristics of cervical mucus can be used clinically to help evaluate the stage of the menstrual cycle, as in the Billings method,[55] to help a woman time her ovulation (although with poor precision).

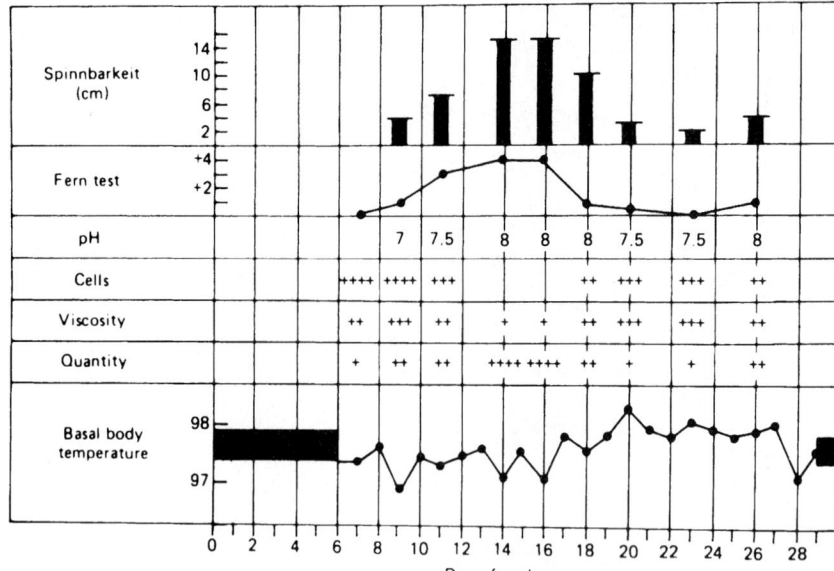

**FIGURE 95-7.** Changes in the composition and properties of cervical mucus during the menstrual cycle. (From Goldfien A, Monroe S. The ovaries. In: Greenspan FS, Forsham PH, eds. Basic and clinical endocrinology, 2nd ed. Los Altos, CA: Lange Medical Publications, 1986:400.)

## VAGINAL MUCOSA

Both proliferation and maturation of the vaginal epithelium are influenced by estrogens and progesterone.[56,57] Three types of vaginal cells are exfoliated: (a) mature *superficial cells,* which are squamous epithelial cells with pyknotic nuclei; (b) *intermediate cells,* which are relatively mature squamous epithelial cells with vesicular, nonpyknotic nuclei; and (c) *parabasal cells,* which are thick, small, round immature cells with large vesicular nuclei. Parabasal cells predominate before puberty, after menopause, and in women with estrogen-deficient forms of amenorrhea. When ovarian estrogen secretion is low in the early follicular phase, the vaginal epithelium is thin and pale. As $E_2$ levels increase in the follicular phase, there is an increase in the number of cells, the thickness of the epithelium, and the number of cornified superficial cells. Under the influence of progesterone during the luteal phase, the percentage of cornified cells decreases while the number of precornified intermediate cells increases, and there are increased numbers of polymorphonuclear leukocytes and increased cellular debris and clumping of shed (desquamated) cells. Thus, the ratio among the various desquamated vaginal cells, obtained by fixing a scraping from the upper third of the lateral vaginal wall on a microscope slide, can be used to evaluate estrogen effect. This ratio has been termed the *maturation index.*

Cytologic changes similar to those observed in vaginal cells also are seen in the lower urinary tract, particularly the urethra. This fact has been used clinically to examine the cells in the urinary sediment from children suspected of having prematurely increased estrogen levels.[58]

## CENTRAL AND GONADAL FEEDBACK MECHANISMS IN THE CONTROL OF OVULATION

### HYPOTHALAMIC-PITUITARY SIGNALS

For normal reproduction, the principal hormone that allows gonadotropin secretion from the pituitary gland is the decapeptide GnRH (also known as luteinizing hormone–releasing hormone).[21,59] Although GnRH is present in several hypothalamic regions, its greatest concentration is localized to the arcuate nucleus. The physiologic importance of this association is apparent from numerous observations that specific anatomic lesions within the arcuate nucleus result in hypogonadotropic hypogonadism secondary to either the absence of or deficiencies in gonadotropin secretion (see Chaps. 8, 16, and 96).

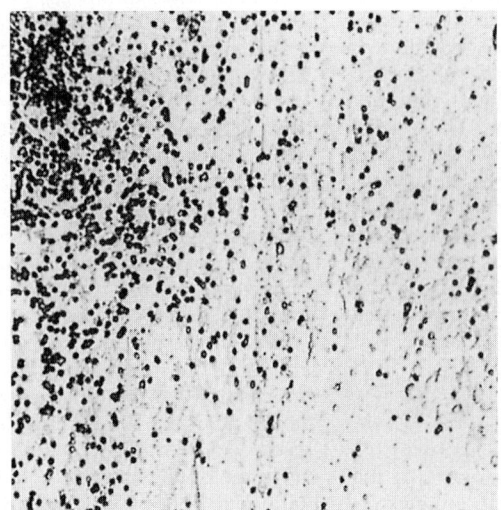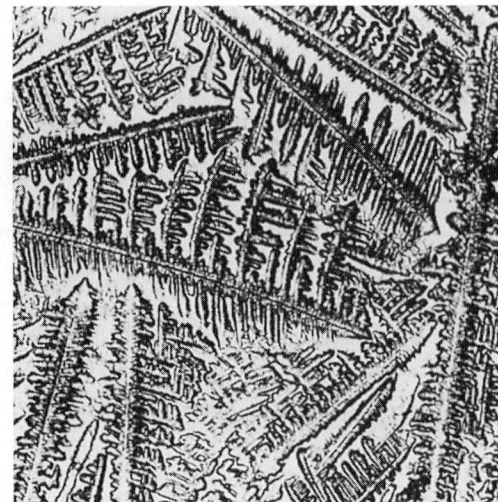

**FIGURE 95-8.** **A,** Absence of arborization (i.e., ferning) in a smear of cervical mucus obtained during the immediate postmenstrual period (day 5) from a normally menstruating woman (×88). **B,** Ferning in a smear obtained from the same woman just before ovulation (×88). The mucus was allowed to dry thickly on a microscope slide and then photographed through a microscope without staining or fixing. (From Rebar RW. Practical evaluation of hormonal status. In: Yen SSC, Jaffe RB, eds. Reproductive endocrinology: physiology, pathology and clinical management, 3rd ed. Philadelphia: WB Saunders, 1991:830.)

**A,B**

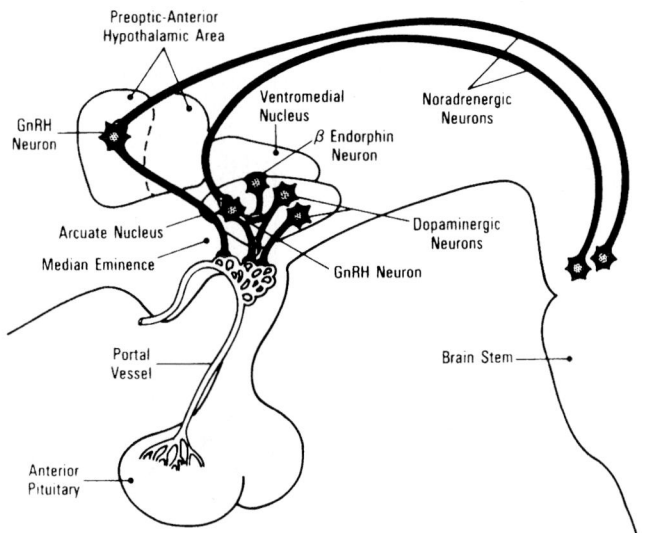

**FIGURE 95-9.** Neuroanatomic relationships among various neurons within the preoptic–anterior hypothalamic and arcuate nucleus–median eminence regions of the brain that affect gonadotropin secretion. (*GnRH*, gonadotropin-releasing hormone.) (Modified from Yen SSC. Neuroendocrine regulation of the menstrual cycle. Hosp Pract 1979; 14:83.)

GnRH from the arcuate nucleus is transported to the base of the hypothalamus, and more specifically to the median eminence, where it is released into the pituitary portal vascular bed (Fig. 95-9). This relatively closed vascular system directly links the hypothalamus to the pituitary and allows high concentrations of GnRH to affect pituitary gonadotropes directly without systemic passage. Thus, peripheral blood levels of GnRH and the other releasing hormones do not accurately reflect hypothalamic-pituitary interaction. Extremely high levels of GnRH may be present in the portal circulation when peripheral levels are undetectable.[60]

GnRH-secreting neurons in culture secrete GnRH in a pulsatile manner.[61] Furthermore, it is apparent that GnRH must be provided to the pituitary gland in such a pulsatile manner to stimulate normal adult ovarian function and ovulation.[62] The requirement for pulsatile GnRH presentation to the pituitary was proved when monkeys with endogenous GnRH secretion eliminated by selective placement of lesions in the hypothalamic arcuate nucleus were given replacement therapy with exogenous GnRH. GnRH given for 6 minutes every 60 minutes effectively induced ovulation and resulted in normal corpus luteum function.[21] Continuously administered GnRH was ineffective in inducing ovulation.

From the classic experimental model,[21] it is clear that the frequency and amplitude of infused GnRH pulses alter the quantitative secretion of LH and FSH. Continuous GnRH infusion results in less gonadotropin secretion (so-called down-regulation), either because of occupation of all receptors so that stimulation is impossible or because of internalization of receptors such that there is overt refractoriness to stimulation.

Information about responsiveness to exogenous GnRH is being used clinically. With commercially available portable pump technology, exogenous GnRH can be administered at regular intervals (60–120 minutes) either intravenously or subcutaneously over a dose range of 1 to 20 µg per pulse to induce ovulation[63,64] (see Chap. 97). Following an initial stimulation of gonadotropin secretion, long-acting GnRH agonists will, within 3 weeks of treatment, down-regulate gonadotropin release, creating a state termed *reversible menopause*.[65–67] The use of GnRH antagonists has been limited by incidental activation of mast-cell receptors, causing histamine release. Newer-generation

GnRH antagonists, however, show great promise, in producing much less mast-cell activation. Down-regulation with GnRH analogs can be used to treat steroid-dependent pathologic processes, including, among others, leiomyomas, endometriosis, hirsutism, precocious puberty, and dysfunctional uterine bleeding. Future applications of similar technologies may provide new strategies for female and male contraception (see Chaps. 104 and 123).

It appears that classic neurotransmitters (e.g., norepinephrine, dopamine, serotonin) as well as neuromodulators (e.g., endogenous opiates, prostaglandins) influence the secretion of GnRH by the hypothalamus.[62,68–75] In addition, estrogens and androgens can bind to receptors in cells in the hypothalamus and anterior pituitary,[76] and progestins[77] can bind to cells in the hypothalamus, to influence hypothalamic-pituitary regulation of ovarian function. Nonsteroidal ovarian factors, as noted previously, also play a role in the central control of ovulation.

In humans and other primates, the reproductive axis is seemingly dormant until puberty. It has become clear that this so-called immaturity of the reproductive axis is at the neural level of the brain, above the median eminence.[78] When exogenous GnRH is administered in appropriate fashion to juvenile primates, ovulation can be induced despite the chronologic and developmental age.[21]

This postnatal and prepubertal "off" stage of GnRH secretion in the juvenile has been likened to an electronic control system and termed a *gonadostat*.[78] The nature of this neuronal "clamp" is unclear, but such disparate stimuli as increased intracranial pressure or premature exposure to sex steroids (such as occurs in congenital adrenal hyperplasia) can prematurely lift the normal inhibition of GnRH secretion, leading to precocious puberty. With the onset of normal puberty, GnRH secretion first begins at night (see Chap. 91).

## STEROIDAL FEEDBACK

Gonadal steroids can exert both negative and positive feedback effects on gonadotropin secretion. Among ovarian steroids, $E_2$ is the most potent inhibitor of gonadotropin secretion. Thus, ovariectomy leads to a rapid increase in gonadotropins,[79] and the infusion of 17β-estradiol into women with hypoestrogenemia leads to almost immediate decreases in both LH and FSH[80] (Fig. 95-10). Although low concentrations of estrogen inhibit the secretion of gonadotropins by the pituitary, they also stimulate synthesis and storage of gonadotropins.

For women to ovulate, $E_2$ must have the ability to elicit a positive as well as a negative effect on gonadotropin secretion.[81–83] Although the ability of ovarian estrogen to exert both negative and positive feedback effects may seem paradoxical, the development of positive feedback is known to require an estrogenic stimulus of increasing strength and duration.[84] High concentrations of estrogen stimulate synthesis and storage of gonadotropin but also augment the effect of GnRH in eliciting release of gonadotropin.[85,86] In the normal menstrual cycle, the positive feedback action of $E_2$ leading to the LH surge is preceded by a period when lower $E_2$ levels are present, with their negative feedback effects (Fig. 95-11).

## PRESUMED MECHANISM FOR THE LUTEINIZING HORMONE SURGE

The basic activity of the pituitary gonadotropes is determined by the direct input of GnRH but is modulated by the feedback effects of $E_2$. Data now suggest the existence of two functionally separate pools of gonadotropin: one that is acutely releasable (and has been termed *sensitivity*) and a second that is released only with sustained stimulation (termed *reserve*).[86] Together, these pools define pituitary capacity. During the early follicular

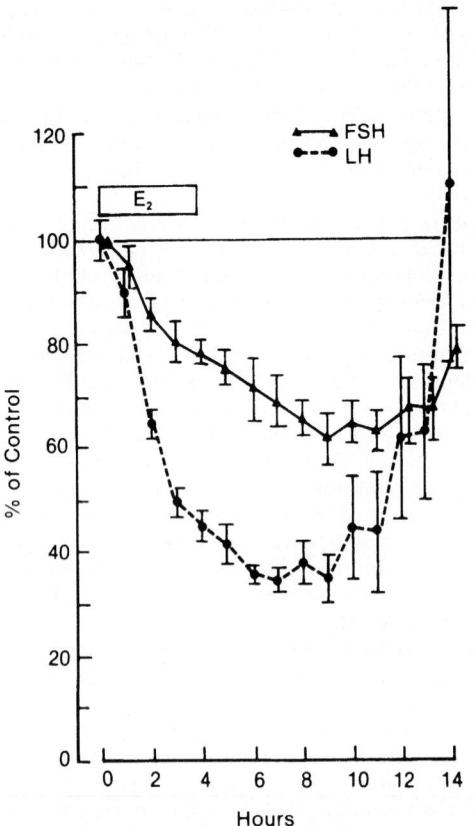

**FIGURE 95-10.** The inhibitory effect (i.e., negative feedback) of 17β-estradiol ($E_2$) on the release of luteinizing hormone (*LH*) and follicle-stimulating hormone (*FSH*) in agonadal women. The fall in circulating gonadotropin concentrations during and after a 4-hour infusion of $E_2$ (50 μg per hour) is expressed as percent of basal (i.e., control) concentrations. (From Yen SSC, Tsai CC, Vandenberg G, Rebar RW. Gonadotropin dynamics in patients with gonadal dysgenesis: a model for the study of gonadotropin regulation. J Clin Endocrinol Metab 1972; 35:897.)

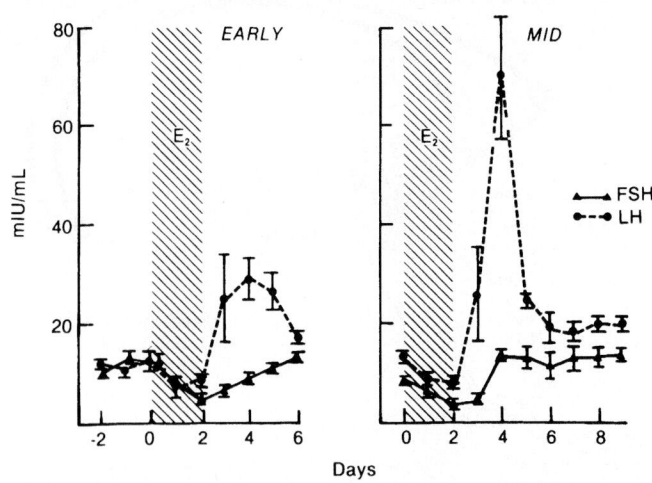

**FIGURE 95-11.** Differences in the feedback effects of exogenous estradiol ($E_2$) administered to normal women during the early (low endogenous estrogen) and midfollicular (moderately high endogenous estrogen) phases of the menstrual cycle. $E_2$ was administered at a dosage of 200 μg per day for 3 days on both occasions. Although these data are generally presented as depicting the stimulatory effects (i.e., positive feedback) of $E_2$ on gonadotropin secretion, the effects are really biphasic. (*FSH*, follicle-stimulating hormone; *LH*, luteinizing hormone.) (From Yen SSC, Vandenberg G, Tsai CC, Parker DC. Causal relationship between the hormonal variables in the menstrual cycle. In: Ferin M, Halberg F, Richart RM, Van de Wiele RL, eds. Biorhythms and human reproduction. New York: John Wiley and Sons, 1974:219.)

It is believed that the rising levels of progesterone at midcycle bring the LH surge to its end by inhibiting GnRH secretion in the hypothalamus and diminishing the sensitivity of the gonadotropes to GnRH in the pituitary.[91,92]

phase, when $E_2$ levels are low, both gonadotropin sensitivity and reserve are at a minimum. As $E_2$ levels increase during the midfollicular phase, a preferential increase in reserve occurs first. As $E_2$ increases further toward midcycle, both sensitivity and reserve become maximal until the sensitivity becomes such that the midcycle release of LH occurs. The surge also is partly a result of what is an estrogen-dependent self-priming effect of GnRH: A second pulse of GnRH elicits greater release of gonadotropin than does the first pulse in the estrogen-primed state[87] (Fig. 95-12).

Whether the pulsatile release of GnRH is increased at midcycle in women has not been determined. Studies with exogenous GnRH in both nonhuman primates and humans have demonstrated conclusively that the midcycle surge can occur without any increase in GnRH release.[21,63,64] However, a surge in GnRH has been shown to accompany the $E_2$-induced gonadotropin surge in monkeys.[88] On the other hand, the onset of the midcycle surge may merely reflect a rapid estrogen-stimulated increase in the number of GnRH receptors on the gonadotropes and the attainment of maximal capacity by the gonadotropes.[89]

Estrogen alone, when administered in a manner designed to mimic the physiologic blood levels that normally occur in the late luteal phase, induces an LH surge in women and monkeys. This surge, however, is not identical to that observed in ovulatory women.[26] The characteristics of the artificially induced surge are much more similar to those of the physiologic midcycle surge if progesterone is administered as well as $E_2$.[90]

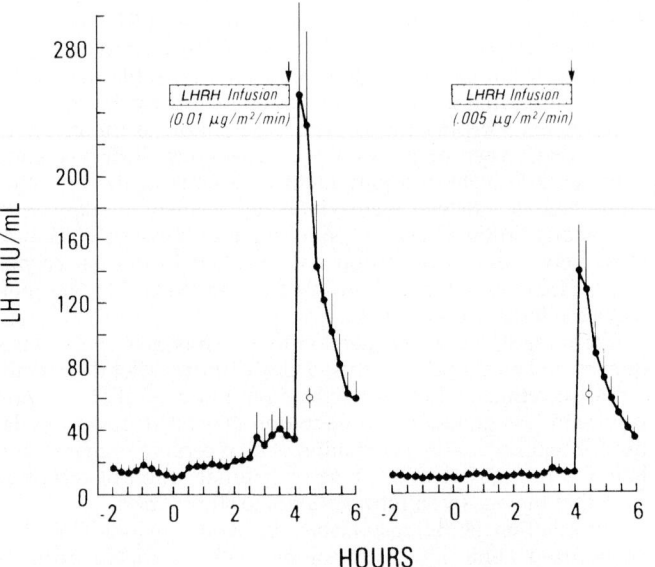

**FIGURE 95-12.** The self-priming effect of gonadotropin-releasing hormone (*GnRH*; i.e., luteinizing hormone–releasing hormone [*LHRH*]) appears to be separate from the ability of GnRH to release LH. Minute doses of GnRH, infused continuously for 4 hours, did not increase circulating levels of LH but did increase the response to a bolus of GnRH (10 μg intravenously administered at the *arrows*) compared to control responses to the bolus alone (*open circles*). (From Hoff JD, Lasley BL, Yen SSC. The functional relationship between priming and releasing actions of LRF [LHRH]. J Clin Endocrinol Metab 1979; 49:8.)

# EFFECT OF THE OVARY ON GONADOTROPIN SECRETION

According to Knobil,[21] the ovary is the "zeitgeber" for the timing of ovulation, with the hypothalamus stimulating pulsatile release of the gonadotropes. In turn, the follicular complex and corpus luteum of the ovary develop in response to gonadotropin stimulation as detailed in Chapter 94.

For appropriate ovarian regulation of reproductive function in women, at least five biologic characteristics appear necessary:

1. Appropriate negative and positive feedback actions of gonadal steroids on gonadotropin secretion
2. Differential feedback effects of ovarian secretions on the release of LH and FSH
3. Local intraovarian controls on follicular growth and maturation, separate from but interrelated to the effects of gonadotropins on the ovary
4. Appropriate development of oocytes so that ovulation may occur
5. Appropriate development of the endometrium so that implantation may occur if fertilization results

# RECRUITMENT AND SELECTION OF THE DOMINANT FOLLICLE IN OVULATORY MENSTRUAL CYCLES

In the absence of pharmacologic intervention, multiple ovulation is extremely atypical in women. The primordial follicle must slowly develop and grow for many months before it becomes a 5- to 8-mm antral follicle at the beginning of the cycle during which it will potentially ovulate.[93] Normally, many follicles reach this stage at the first half of each follicular phase (see Chap. 94). The process that follows has been termed *recruitment*[94,94a] (Fig. 95-13). Several morphologically identical follicles may be observed within the ovary before cycle days 5 to 7. The destruction of any

## TABLE 95-1.
### Granulosa Cell Survival Factors

| Substances Shown to Suppress Apoptosis | Partial Descriptions of Roles in Ovarian Function |
|---|---|
| Follicle-stimulating hormone | Its receptor uses cyclic adenosine monophosphate as second messenger; stimulates production of insulin-like growth factor-I (IGF-I) receptor |
| Insulin-like growth factor-I | Promotes FSH-stimulated production of steroids, luteinizing hormone (LH) receptors, and inhibin; no significant ovarian production; has been delineated in humans, but is present in follicular fluid |
| Insulin-like growth factor-II | Promotes cell replication and steroidogenesis; produced by both granulosa and theca cells; much more abundant in ovarian tissue than IGF-I |
| Epidermal growth factor | Likely acts through tyrosine kinase; stimulates proliferation of granulosa cells |
| Basic fibroblast growth factor | Likely acts through tyrosine kinase; stimulates proliferation of granulosa cells; inhibits production of estrogen and of LH receptors |
| Activin | Suppresses production of insulin-like growth factor–binding protein-4 and -5 |
| Interleukin-1β (IL-1β) | Effects mediated through nitric oxide production; inhibits production of estrogen; it is not clear whether IL-1β is produced by granulosa cells or by nearby white blood cells |
| Growth hormone | Ovarian effects likely mediated through stimulation of hepatic IGF-I production |

one of these follicles does not delay ovulation. In contrast, after about cycle day 7, the multipotentiality of these follicles is lost. Henceforth, only one follicle is capable of progressing to ovulation in the current cycle. This one follicle, destined to ovulate and form the corpus luteum, is known as the *dominant follicle*. Destruction of the dominant follicle, such as by selective cautery, delays ovulation by approximately the number of days that have passed from cycle onset to follicle destruction.[95] The point in time in the cycle at which all of the recruited follicles become qualitatively unequal in potential is the time of *selection*. That the process of selection is predetermined by some intrinsic aspect of a particular follicle seems unlikely. However, once acquired, dominance cannot be transferred. On selection of the single dominant follicle, all other follicles become destined for atresia.

Atresia of the nondominant follicles occurs through *apoptosis* or regulated cell death, most notably observed in granulosa cells. In the rodent model, a number of agents have a role in regulating apoptosis and in rescuing the dominant follicle from this fate (Tables 95-1 and 95-2). These actions are thought to be similar in

## TABLE 95-2.
### Granulosa Cell Apoptotic Factors

| Substances Shown to Promote Apoptosis | Partial Summaries of Roles in Ovarian Function |
|---|---|
| Tumor necrosis factor-α | Produced in the oocyte and in the granulosa cells; effects mediated through ceramide |
| Insulin-like growth factor–binding protein-1 | Prominent only in luteinized follicles |
| Insulin-like growth factor–binding protein-2, -4, -5 | Prominent only in granulosa cells of atretic follicles |
| Insulin-like growth factor–binding protein-3 | Produced in theca cells of all follicles and in granulosa cells of dominant follicles |
| Insulin-like growth factor–binding protein-6 | Not produced in any ovarian tissue, but is present in follicular fluid |
| Interleukin-6 | Found to be concentrated in follicular fluid; it is unclear whether produced by granulosa cells or by nearby white blood cells |
| Follistatin | Binds activin, thus reducing its bioavailability |

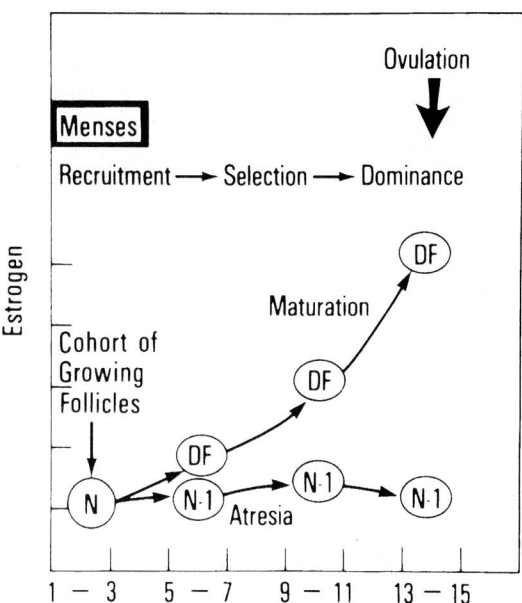

**FIGURE 95-13.** Time course for recruitment, selection, and ovulation of the dominant ovarian follicle (*DF*), with onset of atresia among other follicles of the cohort (*N-1*) in the natural ovarian/menstrual cycle. (From Hodgen GD. Fertil Steril 1982; 38:218.)

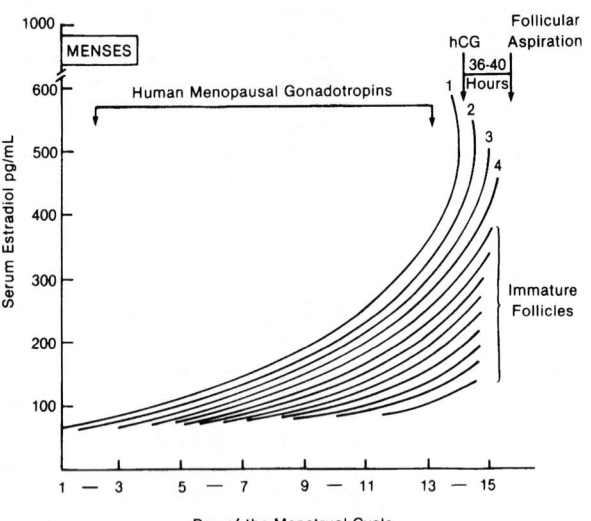

INDUCED FOLLICULAR MATURATION
hMG/hCG

**FIGURE 95-14.** Pattern of follicle growth during sustained elevations of follicle-stimulating hormone and luteinizing hormone (*LH*, with human menopausal gonadotropin [*hMG*]). Only a few follicles can develop quasisynchronously. Accordingly, if human chorionic gonadotropin (*hCG*) is given too late in the attempt to mimic the endogenous LH surge, follicles 1 and 2 may be postmature; if hCG is given too soon, other follicles will be immature. (From Hodgen GD. Physiology of follicular maturation. In: Jones HW Jr, Jones GF, Hodgen GD, Rosenwaks Z, eds. In vitro fertilization—Norfolk. Baltimore: Williams & Wilkins, 1986:8.)

humans. Activin, while it serves to help rescue the dominant follicle, counteracts the vital rescuing effects of FSH in preantral follicles. This seems to be part of the mechanism by which secondary follicles block the stimulation of primary follicles.[96]

The growth of the follicle, followed by the decrease in follicular diameter (which signals ovulation), and formation of the corpus luteum can be observed most accurately by transvaginal ultrasound.[97] Data from ultrasonographic studies in normal women indicate that the site of ovulation occurs randomly in consecutive cycles and does not alternate between the two ovaries.[98] With removal of one ovary, ovulation occurs in the single remaining ovary each month. At present, there is no good evidence that removal of one ovary (and even a small portion of the second) decreases the number of ovulatory menstrual cycles that the average woman has during her reproductive years.

The process of selection of the dominant follicle is overridden in the presence of supraphysiologic gonadotropin stimulation of the ovary. Typically, exogenous gonadotropin therapy allows several recruited follicles to avert atresia. Although the development of several stimulated follicles often is not perfectly synchronous, a few are likely to be mature enough for ovulation, fertilization, and implantation (Fig. 95-14). The ability of supraphysiologic stimulation to recruit several follicles is used effectively in ovulation induction and in in vitro fertilization (see Chap. 97).

Of interest is the observation that in women undergoing supraphysiologic stimulation with exogenous gonadotropins, the high levels of endogenous estrogens, with or without progesterone, frequently fail to promote a timely or full LH surge. This effect is likely due to a nonsteroidal substance, different from inhibin, that has been termed *gonadotropin surge-inhibiting or attenuating factor* (GnSI/AF) and can be isolated from follicular fluid by charcoal extraction. GnSI/AF has the ability to suppress GnRH-induced LH secretion in humans without affecting basal FSH production. Whether the putative factor is the C-terminal fragment of human serum albumin has not yet been confirmed.[99]

## ROLE OF ESTRADIOL IN FOLLICULAR DEVELOPMENT

It is clear that the secretion of $E_2$ by granulosa cells is critical for the occurrence of normal menstrual cycles. $E_2$ plays an essential role in feedback to the central nervous system and in preparing the endometrium for implantation of the developing blastocyst. It had been believed that $E_2$ also played a central role within the ovary in the developing dominant ovarian follicle. This concept, derived from experiments involving rodent models, has been questioned based on findings in women.

It has been observed that normal follicular growth and development, and successful fertilization in vitro, could be achieved using exogenous gonadotropins in a person with 17α-hydroxylase deficiency who, therefore, had no ability to synthesize androgens or estrogens.[100] Thus, in contrast to the rodent paradigm, estrogens are not essential for follicular development in humans. However, the finding that estradiol receptors are present in human granulosa cells has opened the possibility that estrogen may play a facilitory role in follicle development.

A number of already mentioned peptides appear to play more critical roles in intraovarian regulation. The physiologic roles of these peptides remain to be defined precisely, but data documenting their modulatory actions are accumulating.[101] It appears that FSH initially stimulates activin and inhibin synthesis by granulosa cells. In immature granulosa cells, activin augments FSH action, especially FSH-receptor expression and aromatase activity.[102] Inhibin appears to enhance LH stimulation of androgen synthesis in theca cells to serve as substrate for aromatization to estrogen in granulosa cells. Inhibin also inhibits FSH secretion centrally at the level of the gonadotrope. In the luteinizing granulosa cells of the dominant follicle just before ovulation, inhibin synthesis appears to come under control of LH. In the granulosa cells of growing follicles, IGF-I and IGF-II stimulate aromatase activity and cell proliferation.[103] These effects are modulated by several IGFBPs.

## MECHANISMS OF OVULATION

In normal ovulatory cycles, the mean interval from the late follicular phase peak estrogen level to the peak LH level is ~24 hours. Ovulation follows ~9 hours later, for a total interval of ~33 hours.[104] In in vitro fertilization protocols with human menopausal gonadotropin-induced ovarian stimulation and human chorionic gonadotropin (hCG) supplementation, follicular rupture seldom occurs until 36 hours after hCG administration (mimicking the endogenous LH surge). Similarly, initial ovulation seldom occurs until 34 or more hours after treatment with clomiphene citrate and hCG.

The actual events that lead to expulsion of the oocyte and that occur after either the natural or the induced LH surge are incompletely understood. It is not surprising that many of the biochemical and biophysical processes surrounding ovulation can be mimicked in vitro by cyclic adenosine monophosphate, in view of the fact that gonadotropins act by binding to receptors that are linked to cyclic adenosine monophosphate (see Chap. 94).

Several possible factors may play roles in extrusion of the oocyte and the granulosa cells immediately surrounding it (i.e., the *oocyte-cumulus complex*):

1. Granulosa cells produce large amounts of plasminogen activator, apparently stimulated by gonadotropins.[105] Because plasminogen is present in follicular fluid and plasmin can weaken follicle wall strips in vitro, LH-mediated enzymatic digestion of the follicle wall may be important in ovulation. Both interleukin-1β (IL-β) and tumor necrosis factor (TNF), which are in follicular fluid,

are known to suppress the plasminogen activator system, thereby likely helping to prevent premature follicular rupture.[106] However, they also stimulate prostaglandins, which are involved in promoting ovulation.

2. Maturation of the oocyte-cumulus complex involves the dispersal and expansion of the corona radiata (see Chap. 94). Before actual follicular rupture and oocyte extrusion, the oocyte-cumulus complex detaches itself from the granulosa cells of the follicle wall (i.e., the membrana granulosa). In mice, FSH-dependent deposition of a glycosaminoglycan is closely associated with cumulus expansion[107] and may be necessary for ovulation.

3. Because the outer structure of the follicle wall contains smooth muscle, muscular contractions may be important in oocyte extrusion. In this regard, LH and IL-1β can stimulate prostaglandin synthesis, and prostaglandin $F_{2\alpha}$ ($PGF_{2\alpha}$) stimulates ovarian smooth muscle activity.[108,109]

4. Follicular fluid has been found to contain an angiogenic factor.[110] It seems likely that this substance plays a role in the delivery of gonadotropins to the developing dominant follicle. Whether this substance also might promote follicular rupture remains to be explored.

It is possible that abnormalities in the process of oocyte extrusion account for the infrequent occurrence of "luteinized unruptured follicles" (see Chap. 96).

## LUTEAL FUNCTION AS THE SEQUEL TO FOLLICULOGENESIS

In most respects, the events of the luteal phase are consequences of preceding follicular phase activities. Indeed, the process of luteinization begins even before the time of ovulation (see Chap. 94). The granulosa and theca cells that, together with the oocyte, form the dominant follicle and secrete large amounts of estrogens and regulatory peptides are transformed into the corpus luteum after ovulation. In the luteal phase, these same cells produce progesterone as their primary secretory product, but estrogens still are produced in large amounts as well. The synergism of high estrogen levels and FSH in the late follicular phase induces LH receptors on granulosa cells and leads to progesterone secretion even before the LH surge. This change in granulosa cell function is known as *luteinization*.[111] It would seem, therefore, that the greater the proliferation of FSH-stimulated granulosa cells in the follicular phase, the greater will be the transformed luteinized cell mass for progesterone production and early pregnancy support.

Luteinization of granulosa and theca cells occurs only within the dominant follicle; nearby granulosa cells remain unaffected. Thus, intraovarian regulators have been suggested as important in causing this localized phenomenon as well. A *luteinizing inhibitor* is a convenient concept for explaining why other nearby ovarian cells do not undergo luteinization, especially because all granulosa cells removed from the ovary and cultured in vitro appear to luteinize spontaneously. Such a substance remains to be isolated and characterized.

The corpus luteum is not an autonomously functioning unit that is independent of gonadotropin stimulation. Primate models have provided evidence that LH is essential for the maintenance of the corpus luteum. If a GnRH antagonist that blocks LH secretion is administered during the midluteal phase, that menstrual cycle is significantly shortened and menses begins prematurely.[112] The neutralization of LH by antibody administration also causes premature demise of the corpus luteum.[113]

As is true for most other hormones, progesterone is secreted by the corpus luteum in a pulsatile fashion.[114,115] These pulses are most frequent in the early and midluteal phases, when progesterone secretion is greatest. The pulses appear to correlate with pulses of LH as well. Still, as noted previously, pulse frequency for LH is lowest during the luteal phase, so that progesterone pulses typically occur at 4- to 8-hour intervals. Progesterone production is also enhanced by IGF-I and IGF-II, likely through increasing levels of prostaglandin $E_2$ ($PGE_2$).[116]

The mechanisms responsible for regression of the corpus luteum (i.e., *luteolysis*) in women are unknown and are considered in more detail in Chapter 94.[117,118] The life span of the corpus luteum may depend in part on prostaglandins and prolactin, as well as on progestin. If fertilization does occur, hCG, which is biologically similar to LH, is secreted by the developing blastocyst and helps to support the corpus luteum until the fetoplacental unit can support itself (see Chap. 108). However, in the absence of a viable fetus, hCG supports the corpus luteum for only a short time in humans.

Despite the limits of current knowledge, an understanding of the corpus luteum and luteolysis is essential if rational therapies are to be provided to women with luteal phase defects (see Chap. 96).

## REFERENCES

1. Rebar RW, Yen SSC. Endocrine rhythms in gonadotropins and ovarian steroids with reference to reproductive processes. In: Krieger DT, ed. Endocrine rhythms. New York: Raven Press, 1979:259.
2. Rebar RW. Normal physiology of the reproductive system. In: Endocrine and metabolism continuing education and quality control program. American Association of Clinical Chemistry, 1982.
3. Genazzani AR, Lemarchand-Beraud T, Aubert ML, et al. Patterns of plasma ACTH, hGH and cortisol during the menstrual cycle. J Clin Endocrinol Metab 1975; 41:431.
4. Yen SSC, Vela P, Rankin J, et al. Hormonal relationships during the menstrual cycle. JAMA 1970; 211:1513.
5. Ehara Y, Suer T, VandenBerg G, et al. Circulating prolactin levels during the menstrual cycle: episodic release and diurnal variation. Am J Obstet Gynecol 1973; 117:962.
6. Vekemans M, Delvoye P, L'Hermite M, et al. Serum prolactin levels during the menstrual cycle. J Clin Endocrinol Metab 1977; 44:989.
7. Pitkin RM, Reynolds WA, Williams GA, et al. Calcium metabolism during the human menstrual cycle. Gynecol Obstet Invest 1977; 8:60.
8. Hodgen GD. Neuroendocrinology of the normal menstrual cycle. J Reprod Med 1989; 34(Suppl 1):68.
9. Treloar AE, Boynton RE, Benn BG, Brown BW. Variation of human menstrual cycle through reproductive life. Int J Fertil 1967; 12:77.
10. Baldwin RM, Whalley PJ, Pritchard JA. Measurements of menstrual blood loss. Am J Obstet Gynecol 1961; 81:739.
11. Hytten FE, Cheyne GA, Klopper AI. Iron loss at menstruation. J Obstet Gynaecol Br Commonw 1964; 71:255.
12. Hallberg L, Hogdahl A, Nilsson L, Rybo G. Menstrual blood loss—a population study. Acta Obstet Gynecol Scand 1966; 45:320.
13. Rybo G. Menstrual blood loss in relation to parity and menstrual pattern. Acta Obstet Gynecol Scand 1966; 7:119.
14. Midgley AR Jr, Jaffe RB. Regulation of gonadotropins. IV. Correlations of serum concentrations of follicle-stimulating and luteinizing hormones during the menstrual cycle. J Clin Endocrinol Metab 1968; 28:1699.
15. Ross GT, Cargille CM, Lipsett MB, et al. Pituitary and gonadal hormones in women during spontaneous and induced ovulatory cycles. Recent Prog Horm Res 1970; 26:1.
16. Vande Wiele RL, Bogumil RJ, Dyrenfurth I, et al. Mechanisms regulating the menstrual cycle in women. Recent Prog Horm Res 1970; 26:63.
17. Midgley AR Jr, Jaffe RB. Regulation of human gonadotropins. X. Episodic fluctuation of LH during the menstrual cycle. J Clin Endocrinol Metab 1971; 33:962.
18. Yen SSC, Tsai CC, Naftolin F, et al. Pulsatile patterns of gonadotropin release in subjects with and without ovarian function. J Clin Endocrinol Metab 1972; 34:671.
19. Yen SSC, VandenBerg G, Tsai CC, Parker DC. Ultradian fluctuations of gonadotropins. In: Ferin M, Halberg F, Richart RM, Vande Wiele RL, eds. Biorhythms and human reproduction. New York: John Wiley and Sons, 1974:203.
20. Soules MR, Steiner RA, Clifton DK, et al. Progesterone modulation of pulsatile luteinizing hormone secretion in normal women. J Clin Endocrinol Metab 1984; 58:378.
21. Knobil E. The neuroendocrine control of the menstrual cycle. Recent Prog Horm Res 1980; 36:53.
22. Mikhail G. Hormone secretion by the human ovaries. Gynecol Invest 1970; 1:5.
23. Lloyd CW, Lobotsky J, Baird DT, et al. Concentration of unconjugated estrogens, androgens and gestagens in ovarian and peripheral venous

plasma of women: the normal menstrual cycle. J Clin Endocrinol Metab 1971; 32:155.

24. Tagatz GE, Gurpide E. Hormone secretion by the normal human ovary. In: Greep PO, Astwood E, eds. Handbook of physiology, section 7. Endocrinology, vol II. Female reproductive system, part I. Washington, DC: American Physiological Society, 1973:603.

25. Baird DT, Fraser IS. Blood production and ovarian secretion rates of estradiol-17β and estrone in women throughout the menstrual cycle. J Clin Endocrinol Metab 1974; 38:1009.

26. Hoff JD, Quigley MD, Yen SSC. Hormonal dynamics at midcycle: a reevaluation. J Clin Endocrinol Metab 1983; 57:792.

27. Judd HL, Yen SSC. Serum androstenedione and testosterone levels during the menstrual cycle. J Clin Endocrinol Metab 1973; 36:475.

28. Yen SSC, Vela P, Rankin J, Littell AS. Hormonal relationships during the menstrual cycle. JAMA 1970; 211:1513.

29. Aido A-R, Landgren B-M, Cekan Z, Diczfalulsy E. Studies on the pattern of circulating steroids in the normal menstrual cycle. 2. Levels of 20α-dihydroprogesterone, 17-hydroxyprogesterone and 17-hydroxypregnenolone and the assessment of their value for ovulation prediction. Acta Endocrinol (Copenh) 1976;82:600.

30. Pellegrini S, Fuzzi B, Pratesi S, et al. In-vivo studies on ovarian insulin-like growth factor I concentrations in human preovulatory follicles and human ovarian circulation. Hum Reprod 1995; 10:1341.

31. Devoto L, Kohen P, Castro O, et al. Multihormone regulation of progesterone synthesis in cultured human midluteal cells. J Clin Endocrinol Metab 1995; 80:1566.

32. Helle SI, Anker GB, Meadows KA, et al. Alterations in the insulin-like growth factor system during the menstrual cycle in normal women. Maturitas 1998;28:259.

33. Ovesen P, Vahl N, Fisker S, et al. Increased pulsatile, but not basal, growth hormone secretion rates and plasma in insulin-like growth factor I levels during the periovulatory interval in normal women. J Clin Endocrinol Metab 1998; 83:1662.

34. Juul A, Scheike T, Pedersen AT, et al. Changes in serum concentrations of growth hormone, insulin, insulin-like growth factor and insulin-like growth factor–binding proteins 1 and 3 and urinary growth hormone excretion during the menstrual cycle. Hum Reprod 1997; 12:2123.

35. Klein NA, Battaglia DE, Miller PB, et al. Ovarian follicular development and the follicular fluid hormones and growth factors in normal women of advanced reproductive age. J Clin Endocrinol Metab 1996; 81:1946.

36. Amato G, Izzo A, Tucker A, Bellastella A. Insulin-like growth factor binding protein-3 reduction in follicular fluid in spontaneous and stimulated cycles. Fertil Steril 1998; 70:141.

37. Lahlou N, Chabbert-Buffet N, Christin-Maitre S, et al. Main inhibitor of follicle stimulating hormone in the luteal-follicular transition: inhibin A, oestradiol, or inhibin B? Hum Reprod 1999; 14:1190.

38. Fraser HM, Groome NP, McNeilly AS. Follicle-stimulating hormone–inhibin B interactions during the follicular phase of the primate menstrual cycle revealed by gonadotropin-releasing hormone antagonist and antiestrogen treatment. J Clin Endocrinol Metab 1999; 84:1365.

39. Demura R, Suzuki T, Tajima S, et al. Human plasma free activin and inhibin levels during the menstrual cycle. J Clin Endocrinol Metab 1993; 76:1080.

40. Tuuri T, Ritovs O. Regulation of the activin-binding protein follistatin in cultured human luteinizing granulosa cells: characterization of the effects of follicle stimulating hormone, prostaglandin E2, and different growth factors. Biol Reprod 1995; 53:1508.

41. Ebara Y, Siler T, VandenBerg G, et al. Circulating prolactin levels during the menstrual cycle: episodic release and diurnal variation. Am J Obstet Gynecol 1973; 117:962.

42. Genazzini AR, Lemarchand-Beraud TH, Aubert ML, Felber JP. Patterns of plasma ACTH, hGH and cortisol during the menstrual cycle. J Clin Endocrinol Metab 1975; 41:431.

43. Legros JJ, Franchimont P, Burger H. Variations of neurohypophyseal function in normally cycling women. J Clin Endocrinol Metab 1975; 41:54.

44. Vekemans M, Delvoye P, L'Hermite M, Robyn C. Serum prolactin levels during the menstrual cycle. J Clin Endocrinol Metab 1977; 44:989.

45. Noyes RW, Hertig AT, Rock J. Dating the endometrial biopsy. Fertil Steril 1950; 1:3.

46. Tredway DR, Mishell DR Jr, Moyer DL. Correlation of endometrial dating with luteinizing hormone peak. Am J Obstet Gynecol 1973; 117:1030.

47. Bulleti C, Gallassi A, Parmeggiani R, Polli V. Dating the endometrial biopsy by flow cytometry. Fertil Steril 1994; 62:96.

48. Guidice LC, Mark SP, Irwin JC. Paracrine actions of insulin-like growth factors and IGF binding protein-1 in non-pregnant human endometrium and at the decidual-trophoblast interface. J Reprod Immunol 1998; 39:133.

49. Henzl MR, Smith RE, Boost G, Tyler ET. Lysosomal concept of menstrual bleeding in humans. J Clin Endocrinol Metab 1972; 34:860.

50. Ylikorkala O, Dawood MY. New concepts in dysmenorrhea. Am J Obstet Gynecol 1978; 130:833.

51. Todd AS. Localization of fibrinolytic activity in tissues. Br Med Bull 1964; 20:210.

52. Forrest TS, Elyaderani MK, Muilenburg MI, et al. Cyclic endometrial changes: US assessment with histologic correlation. Radiology 1988; 167:233.

52a. Adamopoulos DA, Kapolla N, Abrahamian A, et al. Sex steroids in cervical mucus of spontaneous or induced ovulatory cycles. Steroids 2000; 65:1.

53. Moghissi KS, Syner FN, Evans TN. A composite picture of the menstrual cycle. Am J Obstet Gynecol 1972; 114:405.

54. Moghissi KS. Composition and function of cervical secretion. In: Greep RO, ed. Handbook of physiology. Endocrinology, vol II, part 2. Washington, DC: American Physiological Society, 1973:25.

55. Billings EL, Billings JJ, Brown JB, Burger HG. Symptoms and hormonal changes accompanying ovulation. Lancet 1972; 1:282.

56. Rakoff AE. Hormonal cytology in gynecology. Clin Obstet Gynecol 1961; 4:1045.

57. Frost JK. Gynecologic and obstetrics cytopathology. In: Novak ER, Woodruff JD, eds. Novak's gynecologic and obstetrics pathology, 7th ed. Philadelphia: WB Saunders, 1974:634.

58. Collett-Solberg PR, Grumbach MM. A simplified procedure for evaluating estrogenic effects and the sex chromatin patterns in exfoliated cells in urine: studies in premature thelarche and gynecomastia of adolescence. J Pediatr 1965; 66:883.

59. Halasz B. Hypothalamic mechanisms controlling pituitary function. Prog Brain Res 1972; 38:122.

60. Cannel PD, Araki S, Ferin M. Prolonged stalk portal blood collection in rhesus monkeys: pulsatile release of gonadotropin-releasing hormone (GnRH). Endocrinology 1976; 99:243.

61. Wetsel WC, Valenca MM, Merchenthaler I, et al. Intrinsic pulsatile secretory activity of immortalized luteinizing hormone-releasing hormone-secreting neurons. Proc Natl Acad Sci U S A 1992; 89:4149.

62. Pohl CR, Knobil E. The role of the central nervous system in the control of ovarian function in higher primates. Annu Rev Physiol 1982; 44:583.

63. Crowley WF, McArthur JW. Stimulation of the normal menstrual cycle in Kallmann's syndrome by pulsatile administration of luteinizing hormone-releasing hormone (LHRH). J Clin Endocrinol Metab 1980; 51:173.

64. Miller DS, Reid RR, Cetel NS, et al. Pulsatile administration of low-dose gonadotropin-releasing hormone: ovulation and pregnancy in women with hypothalamic amenorrhea. JAMA 1983; 250:2937.

65. Meldrum DR, Chang RJ, Lu J, et al. "Medical oophorectomy" using a long-acting GnRH agonist: a possible new approach to the treatment of endometriosis. J Clin Endocrinol Metab 1982; 54:1081.

66. Yen SSC. Clinical applications of gonadotropin-releasing hormone analogs. Fertil Steril 1983; 39:257.

67. Reissmann T, Felberbaum R, Diedrich K, et al. Development and application of luteinizing hormone-releasing hormone antagonists in the treatment of infertility: an overview. Hum Reprod 1995; 10:1974.

68. Fink G. Neuroendocrine control of gonadotropin secretion. Br Med Bull 1979; 35:155.

69. Gallo RV. Neuroendocrine control of pulsatile luteinizing hormone release in the rat. Neuroendocrinology 1980; 30:122.

70. Barraclough CA, Wise PM. The role of catecholamines in the regulation of pituitary luteinizing hormone and follicle-stimulating hormone secretion. Endocr Rev 1982; 3:91.

71. Yen SSC. Studies of the role of dopamine in the control of prolactin and gonadotropin secretion in humans. In: Fuxe K, Hökfelt T, Luff R, eds. Central regulation of the endocrine system. New York: Plenum Publishing, 1979:387.

72. Ropert JF, Quigley ME, Yen SSC. The dopaminergic inhibition of LH secretion during the menstrual cycle. Life Sci 1984; 34:2067.

73. Eskay RL, Warbert J, Mical RS, Porter JC. Prostaglandin E2-induced release of LHRH into hypophyseal portal blood. Endocrinology 1975; 97:816.

74. Quigley ME, Yen SSC. The role of endogenous opiates on LH secretion during the menstrual cycle. J Clin Endocrinol Metab 1980; 51:179.

75. Ropert JF, Quigley ME, Yen SSC. Endogenous opiates modulate pulsatile luteinizing hormone release in humans. J Clin Endocrinol Metab 1981; 52:583.

76. Stumpf WE, Sar M, Keeper DA. Anatomical distribution of estrogen in the CNS of mouse, rat, tree shrew and squirrel monkey. In: Raspe G, Bernhard A, eds. Central actions of estrogenic hormones. Oxford: Pergamon Press, 1975:77.

77. Sar M, Stumpf WE. Neurons of the hypothalamus concentrate ($^3$H) progesterone or its metabolites. Science 1973; 182(Suppl):1266.

78. Reiter EO, Grumbach MM. Neuroendocrine control mechanisms and the onset of puberty. Annu Rev Physiol 1982; 44:595.

79. Yen SSC, Tsai CC. The effect of ovariectomy on gonadotropin release. Clin Invest 1971; 50:1149.

80. Yen SSC, Tsai CC, VandenBerg G, Rebar RW. Gonadotropin dynamics in patients with gonadal dysgenesis: a model for the study of gonadotropin regulation. J Clin Endocrinol Metab 1972; 35:897.

81. Yen SSC, VandenBerg G, Tsai CC, Siler T. Causal relationship between the hormonal variables in the menstrual cycle. In: Fern M, Halberg F, Richart RM, Vande Wiele RL, eds. Biorhythms and human reproduction. New York: John Wiley and Sons, 1974:219.

82. Tsai CC, Yen SSC. Acute effects of intravenous infusion of 17β-estradiol on gonadotropin release in pre- and post-menopausal women. J Clin Endocrinol Metab 1971; 32:766.

83. Tsai CC, Yen SSC. The effect of ethinyl estradiol administration during early follicular phase of the cycle on the gonadotropin levels and ovarian function. J Clin Endocrinol Metab 1971; 33:917.

84. Lasley BL, Wang CF, Yen SSC. The effects of estrogen and progesterone on the functional capacity of the gonadotrophs. J Clin Endocrinol Metab 1975; 41:820.

85. Yen SSC, Lein A. The apparent paradox of the negative and positive feedback control system on gonadotropin secretion. Am J Obstet Gynecol 1976; 126:942.

86. Hoff JD, Lasley BL, Wang CF, Yen SSC. The two pools of pituitary gonadotropin: regulation during the menstrual cycle. J Clin Endocrinol Metab 1977; 44:302.

87. Hoff JD, Lasley BL, Yen SSC. The functional relationship between priming and releasing actions of LRF. J Clin Endocrinol Metab 1979; 49:8.

88. Xia L, Van Vugt D, Alston EJ, et al. A surge of gonadotropin-releasing hormone accompanies the estradiol-induced gonadotropin surge in the rhesus monkey. Endocrinology 1992; 131:2812.

89. Urban RJ, Veldhuis JD, Dufau ML. Estrogen regulates the gonadotropin-releasing hormone–stimulated secretion of biologically active luteinizing hormone. Clin Endocrinol Metab 1991; 72:660.

90. Liu JH, Yen SSC. Induction of midcycle gonadotropin surge by ovarian steroids in women: a critical evaluation. J Clin Endocrinol Metab 1983; 57:797.

91. Kasa-Vuvu JZ, Dahl GE, Evans NP, et al. Progesterone blocks the estradiol-induced gonadotropin discharge in the ewe by inhibiting the surge of gonadotropin-releasing hormone. Endocrinology 1992; 131:208.

92. Araki S, Chikazawa K, Motoyama M, et al. Reduction in pituitary desensitization and prolongation of gonadotropin release by estrogen during continuous administration of gonadotropin-releasing hormone in women: its antagonism by progesterone. J Clin Endocrinol Metab 1985; 60:590.

93. Gougeon A. Regulation of ovarian follicular development in primates: facts and hypothesis. Endocr Rev 1996; 17:121.

94. di Zerega GA, Hodgen GD. Folliculogenesis in the primate ovarian cycle. Endocr Rev 1981; 2:27.

94a. Yap C. Ontogeny: the evolution of an oocyte. Obstet Gynecol Surv 2000; 55:449.

95. Goodman AL, Hodgen GD. Between ovary interaction in the regulation of follicle growth, corpus luteum function, and gonadotropin secretion in the primate ovarian cycle. I. Effects of follicle cautery and hemiovariectomy during the follicular phase in cynomolgus monkeys. Endocrinology 1979; 104:1304.

96. Mizunuma H, Liu X, Andoh K, et al. Activin from secondary follicles causes small preantral follicles to remain dormant at the resting stage. Endocrinology 1999; 140:37.

97. Belaisch-Allart J, Dufetre C, Allan JP, De Mouzon J. Comparison of transvaginal and transabdominal ultrasound for monitoring follicular development in an in-vitro fertilization program. Hum Reprod 1991; 6:688.

98. Baird DT. A model for follicular selection and ovulation: lessons from superovulation. J Steroid Biochem 1987; 27:15.

99. Pappa A, Seferiadis K, Fotsis T, et al. Purification of a candidate gonadotropin surge attenuating factor from human follicular fluid. Hum Reprod 1999; 14:1449.

100. Rabinovici J, Blankstein J, Goldman B, et al. In vitro fertilization and primary embryonic cleavage are possible in 17α-hydroxylase deficiency despite extremely low intrafollicular 17β-estradiol. J Clin Endocrinol Metab 1989; 68:693.

101. Hillier SG. Paracrine control of follicular estrogen synthesis. Semin Reprod Endocrinol 1991; 9:332.

102. Miro F, Hillier SG. Relative effects of activin and inhibin on steroid hormone synthesis in primate granulosa cells. J Clin Endocrinol Metab 1992; 75:1556.

103. Yoshimura Y. Insulin-like growth factors and ovarian physiology. J Obstet Gynaecol Res 1998; 24:305.

104. Pauerstein CJ, Eddy CA, Croxatto HD, et al. Temporal relationships of estrogen, progesterone, and luteinizing hormone levels to ovulation in women and infrahuman primates. Am J Obstet Gynecol 1978; 130:876.

105. Strickland S, Beers WH. Studies on the role of plasminogen activator in ovulation: in vitro response of granulosa cells to gonadotropins, cyclic nucleotides, and prostaglandins. J Biol Chem 1976; 251:5694.

106. Terranova PF, Rice VM. Review: cytokine involvement in ovarian process. Am J Reprod Immunol 1997; 37:50.

107. Eppig JJ. Regulation of cumulus oophorus expansion by gonadotropins in vivo and in vitro. Biol Reprod 1980; 23:545.

108. Wallach EE, Wright KH, Hamada Y. Investigation of mammalian ovulation with an in vitro perfused rabbit ovary preparation. Am J Obstet Gynecol 1978; 132:728.

109. Adashi EY. The potential role of interleukin-1 in the ovulatory process: an evolving hypothesis. Mol Cell Endocrinol 1998; 140:77.

110. Frederick J, Shimanuki T, di Zerega GS. Initiation of angiogenesis by human follicular fluid. Science 1984; 224:389.

111. Hsueh AJW, Adashi EY, Jones PBC, Welsh TH Jr. Hormonal regulation of the differentiation of cultured ovarian granulosa cells. Endocr Rev 1984; 5:76.

112. Collins RL, Sopelak VM, Williams RF, Hodgen GD. Pulsatile GnRH treatment in mid-luteal phase: timely luteolysis despite enhanced steroidogenesis. In: Toft DO, Ryan RJ, eds. Proceedings of the fifth ovarian workshop. Champaign, IL: Ovarian Workshops, 1985:59.

113. Groff TR, Raj HGM, Talbert LM, Willis DL. Effects of neutralization of luteinizing hormone on corpus luteum function and cyclicity in Macaca fascicularis. J Clin Endocrinol Metab 1984; 59:1054.

114. Healy DL, Schenken RS, Lynch A, et al. Pulsatile progesterone secretion: its relevance to clinical evaluation of corpus luteum function. Fertil Steril 1984; 41:114.

115. Filicori M, Butler JT, Crowley WF. Neuroendocrine regulation of the corpus luteum in the human: evidence for pulsatile progesterone secretion. J Clin Invest 1984; 73:1638.

116. Apa R, Miceli F, Pierro E, et al. Paracrine regulation of insulin-like growth factor I (IGF-I) and IGF-II on prostaglandins F2α and E2 synthesis by human corpus luteum in vitro: a possible balance of luteotropic and luteolytic effects. J Clin Endocrinol Metab 1999; 84:2507.

117. Michael AE, Abayasekara DR, Webley GE. Cellular mechanisms of luteolysis. Mol Cell Endocrinol 1994; 99:R1.

118. Devoto L, Vega M, Kohen P, et al. Endocrine and paracrine-autocrine regulation of the human corpus luteum during the mid-luteal phase. J Reprod Fertil Suppl 2000; 55:13.

# CHAPTER 96

# DISORDERS OF MENSTRUATION, OVULATION, AND SEXUAL RESPONSE

ROBERT W. REBAR

Disorders of menstruation and ovulation are relatively common in women of reproductive age. Possible disorders range from minor to potentially life threatening. To diagnose and treat such menstrual disorders appropriately, an understanding of normal puberty and of the normal menstrual cycle is required (see Chaps. 91 and 95).

Although disorders of sexual response also occur with some frequency, they are often overlooked by physicians. Women seeking assistance may have other complaints, and only a sensitive clinician is able to discern the true reason for the visit. However, disorders of sexual response, although not life threatening, may significantly affect the life of the patient and her sexual partner. A knowledge of normal sexual responses and the willingness to discuss such issues openly with patients contribute to successful resolution of the problems.

## AMENORRHEA

### DEFINITION

Amenorrhea is generally defined as the absence of menstruation for 3 or more months in women with past menses or a failure to menstruate by girls 16 years of age who have never menstruated. Amenorrhea is merely a sign; it may suggest several disorders involving any of several organ systems. If the genital outflow tract is intact, amenorrhea indicates failure of the hypothalamic-pituitary-gonadal axis to interact to induce the cyclic changes in the endometrium that normally cause menses. Amenorrhea may be the result of an abnormality at any level of the reproductive tract.

Traditionally, amenorrhea is regarded as *primary* in women who have never menstruated and as *secondary* in women who have menstruated previously. Because such categorization may lead to diagnostic omission, whether the amenorrhea is primary or secondary should not be a major factor in the evaluation of an amenorrheic woman. Similarly, use of the term "postpill" amenorrhea to refer to women who fail to resume menses within 3 months of discontinuing oral contraceptives conveys nothing about the cause. Women who have fewer than 9 menstrual periods per calendar year should be evaluated identically to those with amenorrhea.

### CLINICAL EVALUATION

Most important to the clinical evaluation are the history and physical examination, with special attention to the possible effects of alterations in hormonal secretion on pubertal development. In general, the clinician should view the patient as a bioassay subject in whom gonadal steroids lead normally to the development of secondary sex characteristics. Breast development indicates exposure to estrogens. The presence of pubic and axillary hair indicates exposure to androgens. Any abnormality of the outflow tract should be eliminated by physical examination.

Patients should be questioned regarding the timing of pubertal milestones, and any abnormalities of growth and development should be pursued (see Chaps. 91 and 92).

Patients also should be asked about dietary and exercise habits; other aspects of lifestyle, environmental, and psychological stresses; and any family history of amenorrhea or genetic anomalies. It is also important to search for any signs of increased levels of androgen, including acne, hirsutism (i.e., increased sexually stimulated terminal hair; see Chap. 101), and even virilization, such as increased masculine and decreased feminine secondary sexual characteristics, including hirsutism, temporal balding, deepening of the voice, increased muscle mass, clitoromegaly, decreased breast size, and vaginal atrophy. Any history of *galactorrhea* (i.e., nonpuerperal secretion of milk) should be elicited.

Body dimensions and habitus, the distribution and extent of body hair, breast development and secretions, and the external and internal genitalia should be carefully evaluated. Because disorders of sexual development and reproduction frequently are manifested by changes in habitus, it is important to consider the patient's overall appearance. In normal adults, the arm span is similar to the height; in hypogonadal individuals, the arm span typically exceeds the height by 5 cm or more. In congenital hypothyroidism, the extremities are significantly shorter than in normal individuals.

The distribution and quantity of body hair should be evaluated, especially with reference to the family history. Hypertrichosis, or the excessive growth of terminal hair on the back and extremities, is almost invariably familial and must be differentiated from true hirsutism. Hypertrichosis is common in women of Mediterranean ancestry, but any facial hair growth in Asian and American Indian women demands evaluation. Although several semiquantitative methods of scoring hirsutism have been developed, it is perhaps most practical to grade facial hirsutism only (because this usually is of most concern to the patient) from 0 to 4+, assigning one point each for excess chin, upper lip, or sideburn hair, and 4+ for a complete beard.[1] For documentation, there is no substitute for photographs.

Breast development should be staged according to the method of Tanner[2] (see Chap. 91). The breasts should be examined for any secretion by applying pressure to all sections of the breast, beginning lateral to the nipple and working toward the nipple while the patient is seated. Secretions should be examined microscopically as a wet mount for the presence of thick-walled, perfectly round fat globules of various sizes, establishing that the discharge is milk (Fig. 96-1).

The female genitalia are the most sensitive indicators of hormonal status. The Tanner stage of pubic hair development should be recorded.[2] The extent of any virilization present indicates the stage in development when exposure to androgens occurred; in general, the sensitivity of the genitalia to androgens decreases with time from the early stages of fetal development to adulthood. The most significant changes, including fusion of the labia and enlargement of the clitoris with or without formation of a penile urethra, are found in women exposed to excess androgens during the first few months of fetal development, as in congenital adrenal hyperplasia (see Chap. 77). The development of significant clitoromegaly in an adult requires marked androgenic stimulation and strongly suggests the presence of an androgen-secreting neoplasm (see Chap. 102). The glans clitoris is definitely enlarged if it is 1 cm or more in diameter. A *clitoral index*, defined as the product of the sagittal and transverse diameters of the glans at the base, greater than 35 mm$^2$ falls outside the 95% confidence interval.[3] Under the influence of estrogen, the labia minora develop at puberty.

Examination of the internal genitalia should reveal any overt anomalies of müllerian duct derivatives, including imperforate hymen, vaginal and uterine aplasia, and vaginal septum (see Chap. 90). Obstruction to the escape of menstrual blood can cause *hematocolpos* (i.e., collection of blood in the vagina) and *hematometra* (i.e., distention of the uterus with blood). Although a bulging perineum and a pelvic mass are typically found on examination, differentiating vaginal agenesis from a vaginal septum or an imperforate hymen may be difficult. In all of these cases, the normal development of the external genitalia and of other secondary sex characteristics indicates normal ovarian function. The occurrence of intermittent abdominal pain suggests intra-abdominal bleeding. Müllerian dysgenesis (i.e., Rokitansky-Küster-Hauser syndrome) may be accompanied by bony abnormalities of the lumbar spine (e.g., spina bifida occulta), renal anomalies, and disorders of the eighth cranial nerve.[4]

If there is asynchronous pubertal development with significant breast development in the absence of much pubic and axillary hair, androgen insensitivity (i.e., 46,XY male pseudohermaphroditism) must be excluded. These disorders, including complete testicular feminization, are generally inherited as X-linked recessive or sex-linked autosomal-dominant traits. Complete virilization does not occur despite the presence of testes located inguinally or intraabdominally. Patients have a typical female habitus with normal female external genitalia, but breasts develop only to Tanner stage 3, and the vagina is absent or ends blindly (see Chap. 90).

Outflow tract obstruction associated with a normal uterus should be treated surgically to prevent tubal damage from intraabdominal menstruation. Individuals with testicular feminization should be reared as females and treated with an estrogen and a progestin after surgical removal of the testes. The testes should be removed because of the risk of malignancy. Girls lacking a vagina may undergo vaginoplasty (i.e., McIndoe procedure) when regular sexual activity is anticipated.[5] In motivated individuals, a vagina can also be created gradually by the daily use of dilators of increasing size (i.e., Frank nonoperative method).[6]

For individuals with a normal genital tract, visual inspection of the quality of the vaginal mucosa and of the cervical mucus is important because the two are sensitive to estrogen. In response to this hormone, the vaginal mucosa is transformed at puberty from a tissue with a shiny, smooth, bright red appearance to a dull, gray-pink, rugated surface. The cervical mucus increases in quantity and elasticity (i.e., *spinnbarkeit*) when estrogen is present. Pelvic examination may also reveal pelvic pathologic processes, including neoplasms.

The history and physical examination can differentiate several causes of amenorrhea in women of reproductive age, including *disorders of sexual differentiation* (e.g., distal genital tract obstruction such as müllerian agenesis and dysgenesis, gonadal dysgenesis, ambiguity of external genitalia as in male and female pseudohermaphroditism); *other peripheral causes* (e.g., pregnancy, gestational trophoblastic disease, amenorrhea traumatica as in Asherman syndrome); and *chronic anovulation* or *ovarian failure* (e.g., hypothalamic-pituitary dysfunction,

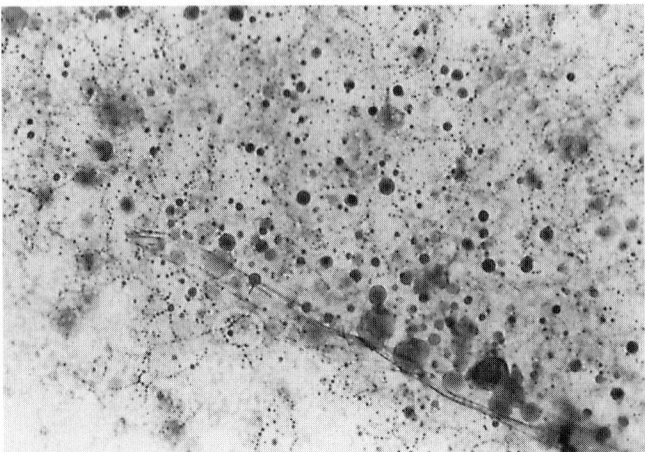

**FIGURE 96-1.** Perfectly round, thick-walled fat globules of various sizes are characteristic of galactorrhea when the breast secretion is viewed as a wet preparation under the microscope (original magnification, × 88). For photography, the oil red O stain was added to the specimen, accounting for the dark character of the fat droplets.

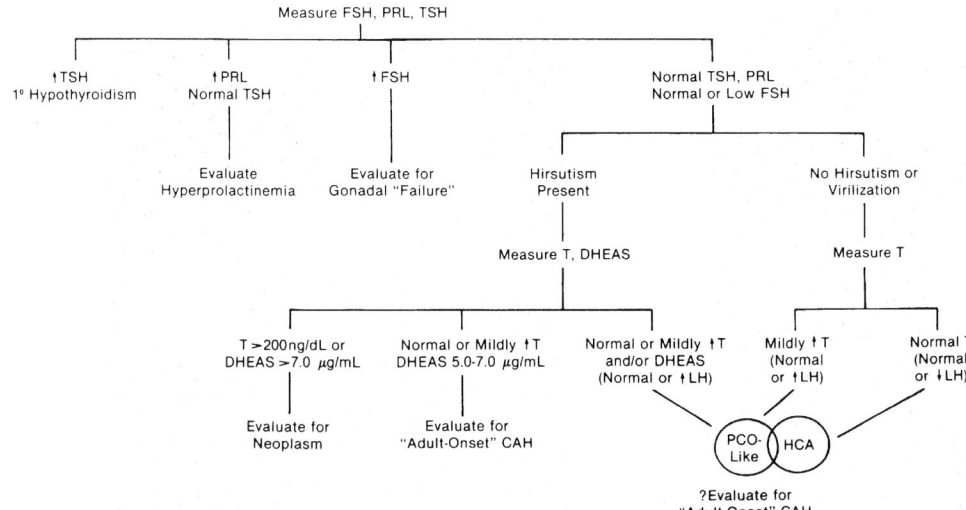

**FIGURE 96-2.** Flow diagram for the laboratory evaluation of amenorrhea. Such a scheme must be considered as an adjunct to the clinical evaluation of the patient. (*CAH*, congenital adrenal hyperplasia; *DHEAS*, dehydroepiandrosterone sulfate; *FSH*, follicle-stimulating hormone; *HCA*, hypothalamic chronic anovulation; *PCO*, polycystic ovarian syndrome; *PRL*, prolactin; *T*, thyroxine; *TSH*, thyroid-stimulating hormone.) (Reprinted from Rebar RW. The ovaries. In: Smith LH Jr, ed. Cecil textbook of medicine, 18th ed. Philadelphia: WB Saunders, 1992:1367.)

inappropriate feedback because of polycystic ovarian syndrome, adrenal or thyroid dysfunction, abnormal prolactin secretion, premature ovarian failure).

Any sexual ambiguity indicates the need for chromosomal karyotyping and the measurement of serum 17-hydroxyprogesterone to rule out 21-hydroxylase deficiency (e.g., congenital adrenal hyperplasia; see Chap. 77). Pregnancy and gestational trophoblastic disease may be confirmed by determining if circulating levels of human chorionic gonadotropin (hCG) are elevated. The existence of intrauterine synechiae or adhesions (i.e., *Asherman syndrome*) must be suspected in women who develop oligomenorrhea or amenorrhea after curettage or endometritis; tuberculous endometritis may also lead to this disorder.[7] The diagnosis can be made by performing hysterosalpingography or hysteroscopy. Hysteroscopic lysis of adhesions is effective in treating Asherman syndrome in more than 80% of affected individuals.

Unless serum follicle-stimulating hormone (FSH) levels are measured, it is frequently impossible to differentiate individuals with chronic anovulation, in whom hypothalamic–pituitary–ovarian function is disrupted, from those patients with ovarian failure in whom the ovaries are generally devoid of oocytes. However, it should be possible to form strong clinical impressions about the cause of the amenorrhea.

To determine with certainty whether the outflow tract is intact and to evaluate the levels of endogenous estrogen, exogenous progestin, in the form of progesterone in oil (100–200 mg given intramuscularly) or medroxyprogesterone acetate (5–10 mg taken orally each day for 5 to 10 days), can be administered. Any genital bleeding within 10 days of the completion of progestin administration makes the diagnosis of Asherman syndrome unlikely (although still possible) and suggests the presence of chronic anovulation rather than hypothalamic-pituitary or ovarian failure. If the patient does not bleed in response to the progestin, an estrogen and a progestin together (e.g., 2.5 mg of oral conjugated estrogen daily for 25 days with 5 to 10 mg of oral medroxyprogesterone acetate or 200 mg of micronized progesterone also given for the last 10 days) should produce bleeding if the endometrium is normal. Withdrawal bleeding in response to progestin does not exclude the diagnosis of hypergonadotropic amenorrhea, associated with ovarian failure.

## LABORATORY EVALUATION

After appropriate clinical evaluation, measurements of basal serum levels of FSH, prolactin, and thyroid-stimulating hormone (TSH) are indicated in all amenorrheic women to confirm the clinical impression (Fig. 96-2). Whenever the basal prolactin level is elevated (generally >20 ng/mL) on initial testing, the measurement should be repeated, because prolactin levels are increased by a number of nonspecific stimuli, including stress, sleep, and food ingestion. If thyroid function is normal and prolactin levels are elevated, further evaluation is warranted to rule out a pituitary tumor and other causes (see Chap. 13). Basal prolactin concentrations should be determined in all amenorrheic women, not just in those with galactorrhea, because prolactin levels are elevated in more than one-third of all amenorrheic women.[8]

Increased serum TSH levels (generally >5 μU/mL utilizing sensitive assays) with or without increased levels of prolactin indicate primary hypothyroidism (see Chaps. 15 and 45). The increased secretion of thyrotropin-releasing hormone (TRH) in this disorder stimulates increased secretion of prolactin and TSH in some affected women.

High serum FSH levels (>30 mIU/mL in most laboratories) imply ovarian failure. Chromosomal evaluation is indicated in all women with increased serum FSH levels who are younger than 30 years of age when the amenorrhea begins, because a number of karyotypic abnormalities have been identified in such women. Gonadectomy is indicated in any such individual who has a portion of a Y chromosome because of the malignant potential of the gonads.[9]

If prolactin, TSH, and FSH levels are normal or low, further evaluation is based on the clinical presentation. Circulating thyroid hormone levels should be determined if there is any suggestion of thyroid dysfunction. Serum total testosterone levels should be determined whether or not the patient is hirsute; not all hyperandrogenic women are hirsute because of relative insensitivity of the hair follicles to androgens in some women. Although slightly increased levels of serum testosterone and perhaps of dehydroepiandrosterone sulfate (DHEAS) suggest polycystic ovarian syndrome (PCO), androgen levels occasionally are not elevated in PCO, because of alterations in the metabolic clearance rates of androgens and in sex-hormone-binding-globulin (SHBG) concentrations.[10] Circulating levels of luteinizing hormone (LH) may also aid in differentiating PCO from hypothalamic-pituitary dysfunction or failure. LH levels often are increased in PCO such that the ratio of LH to FSH is increased, but this too is not always so.[11] However, LH and FSH levels are normal or slightly reduced in women with hypothalamic-pituitary dysfunction.[12]

There is some overlap between women with PCO-like disorders and those with hypothalamic-pituitary dysfunction. In an effort not to miss a serious cause of amenorrhea, some radiographic assessment of the region of the sella turcica is indicated in all amenorrheic women in whom LH and FSH levels are low (generally <10 mIU/mL) to exclude a pituitary or hypothalamic

**TABLE 96-1.**
**Proposed Classification of Gonadal Failure Arising before Birth**

| Disorder | Previous Nomenclature | Karyotype | Müllerian Duct | Wolffian Duct | External Genitalia | Days after Fertilization |
|---|---|---|---|---|---|---|
| DEFECTIVE GERM CELL MIGRATION | Pure gonadal dysgenesis<br>Swyer syndrome<br>Familial 46,XX dysgenesis<br>46,XX dysgenesis<br>46,XY dysgenesis | 46,XX or 46,XY | Present | Absent | Female | Before 43 |
| TESTICULAR REGRESSION | True agonadism<br>Testicular dysgenesis<br>Embryonic testicular regression<br>Testicular regression syndrome | 46,XY | Present to absent | Absent to present | Female to ambiguous male | 43–120 |
| TESTICULAR DYSGENESIS | Dysgenetic gonads<br>Mixed gonadal dysgenesis | 45,X or mosaic (commonly 45,X/46,XY) | Present to absent | Absent to present | Female to ambiguous | 43–84 |
| OVARIAN DYSGENESIS | Gonadal agenesis<br>Gonadal dysgenesis<br>Turner syndrome<br>Ovarian agenesis<br>Ovarian dysgenesis<br>Streak gonad | 45,X or mosaic (commonly 45,X/46,XX); submicroscopic changes in the X chromosome | Present | Absent | Female | After 80 |

(Modified from Coulam CB. Classification and treatment of premature gonadal failure. Semin Reprod Endocrinol 1983; 1:177; Rebar RW, Erickson GF, Coulam CB. Premature ovarian failure. In: Gondos B, Riddick D, eds. Pathology of infertility. New York: Thieme Medical Publishers, 1987:123.)

neoplasm. In addition to testosterone, serum DHEAS levels should be measured in women with evidence of hirsutism or virilization. Serum total testosterone levels of 200 ng/mL or greater should prompt an investigation for an androgen-producing neoplasm, most likely of ovarian origin. Serum DHEAS levels above 7.0 µg/dL should prompt an investigation for an adrenal neoplasm. Adult-onset or cryptic congenital adrenal hyperplasia (see Chap. 77) should be considered in women with severe hirsutism since puberty, a strong family history of hirsutism, stature shorter than expected compared with other family members, or serum DHEAS levels of 5.0 µg/mL or greater.

## HYPERGONADOTROPIC AMENORRHEA (PRIMARY HYPOGONADISM)

It is frequently impossible to diagnose hypergonadotropic amenorrhea, also called presumptive ovarian failure, without the measurement of basal serum gonadotropin levels. This is especially true because ovarian failure may occur at any time from embryonic development onward. The ovaries normally fail at the time of menopause, when virtually no viable oocytes remain. The premature loss of oocytes before age 40 results in premature ovarian failure. From what is known about follicular development and atresia, it appears that premature ovarian failure arises from abnormalities in the recruitment and selection of oocytes[13] (see Chap. 94). The follicles may undergo atresia at an accelerated rate or a smaller than normal pool may undergo atresia at the normal rate to yield early oocyte depletion. FSH must be involved, because it is the principal hormonal regulator of folliculogenesis. Circulating gonadotropin levels increase whenever ovarian failure occurs because of decreased negative estrogen feedback to the hypothalamic-pituitary unit. Gonadotropin levels sometimes increase even in the presence of viable oocytes, but the explanation for such increases is unclear. In principle, young women with hypergonadotropic amenorrhea must be considered potentially, if only rarely, fertile.

It is possible to identify disorders causing gonadal failure before birth that arise from gonadal abnormalities (Table 96-1; see Chap. 90). This classification emphasizes the need to consider genetic abnormalities in all young women with hypergo-

nadotropic amenorrhea. In ovarian dysgenesis, the normal complement of oocytes is present at 20 weeks of fetal age, but atresia accelerates until birth, and some affected girls may undergo sexual development, ovulate, and even conceive if some oocytes remain.[14,15] The classification in Table 96-1 is not ideal but should be viewed as an artificial categorization of a continuum. Excluding these disorders of gonadal development, premature ovarian failure still consists of several distinct disorders (Table 96-2).

## TYPES OF PREMATURE OVARIAN FAILURE

Inherited characteristics are important in the development of premature ovarian failure. Premature loss of oocytes could result from a reduced germ cell endowment in utero, accelerated atresia, or failure of all germ cells to migrate to the genital ridges in early development (see Chap. 90). There may be marked differences in oocyte endowment and rates of follicular atresia among women.[16,17] The cause of the ovarian failure that may accompany myotonia dystrophica is unknown but may involve decreased germ cell number or accelerated atresia.[18] An excess of X chromosomes may also be associated with decreased germ cell numbers or accelerated atresia.[19] The familial occurrence of premature ovarian failure with vertical transmission has been described, suggesting autosomal-dominant, sex-linked inheritance in some cases.[20] This observation has significant implications for the reproductive counseling of affected women who had children before developing ovarian failure.

At least two separate inherited enzymatic defects may also be associated with premature ovarian failure. Girls with 17α-hydroxylase deficiency who survive to their teens present with sexual infantilism; primary amenorrhea; increased circulating levels of LH, FSH, deoxycorticosterone, and progesterone; and hypertension with hypokalemic alkalosis[21–23] (see Chap. 77). Ovarian biopsy has revealed no evidence of orderly follicular maturation but instead has demonstrated numerous large cysts and primordial follicles. Presumably, the enzyme deficiency does not permit normal follicular development. The startling observation that normal follicular growth and development with successful fertilization in vitro can be achieved with exogenous gonadotropins in individuals with 17α-hydroxylase defi-

## TABLE 96-2.
### Tentative Classification of Premature Ovarian Failure

**GENETIC ALTERATIONS OR TENDENCIES**
  Structural alterations in or absence of an X chromosome
  Trisomy X with or without mosaicism
  Reduced germ cell number
  Accelerated atresia of germ cells (?)
  In association with myotonia dystrophica
  Enzymatic defects
  17β-Hydroxylase deficiency galactosemia

**DEFECTS IN GONADOTROPIN SECRETION OR ACTION**
  Secretion of biologically inactive gonadotropin
  α- or β-Subunit defects
  FSH receptor (FSHR) mutations
  Postreceptor defects (e.g., resistant ovary or Savage syndrome)

**IMMUNE DYSFUNCTION***
  Associated with other autoimmune disorders
  Isolated
  Congenital thymic aplasia

**PHYSICAL INSULTS**
  Chemotherapeutic (especially alkylating) agents
  Ionizing radiation
  Viral agents
  Cigarette smoking
  Surgical extirpation

**GONADOTROPIN-SECRETING PITUITARY TUMORS
  (EXTREMELY RARE)**

**IDIOPATHIC**

*Other conditions found in various combinations in association with premature ovarian failure include alopecia, anemia (acquired hemolytic and pernicious), Crohn disease, chronic active hepatitis, diabetes mellitus, hypoadrenalism (Addison disease), hypoparathyroidism, hypophysitis, idiopathic thrombocytopenic purpura, juvenile rheumatoid arthritis, keratoconjunctivitis and Sjögren syndrome, malabsorption syndrome, myasthenia gravis, primary biliary cirrhosis, quantitative immunoglobulin abnormalities, systemic lupus erythematous, thyroid disorders such as Graves disease and thyroiditis, and vitiligo.

(Modified from Rebar RW, Erickson GF, Coulam CB. Premature ovarian failure. In: Gondos B, Riddick D, eds. Pathology of infertility. New York: Thieme Medical Publishers, 1987:123.)

ciency raises significant questions about why there is no follicular development in affected girls[24] (see Chap. 95). Girls with galactosemia, a disorder in which galactose-1-phosphate uridyltransferase activity is decreased and that is characterized by mental retardation, cataracts, hepatosplenomegaly, and renal tubular dysfunction, may also develop premature ovarian failure with hypergonadotropinism even when a galactose-restricted diet is introduced early in infancy.[25]

At least one form of premature ovarian failure is caused by mutations of the FSH receptor (FSHR). (Because some clinicians regard this disorder as another form of XX gonadal dysgenesis, this disorder is also discussed in Chap. 90.) Because affected individuals present with primary or secondary amenorrhea and elevated levels of FSH and ovarian follicles may be detected during transvaginal ultrasound examination, it may be argued that the disorder is more appropriately included here.

One specific mutation on chromosome 2p (C566T:alanine to valine) in exon 7 of the FSHR has been identified in several Finnish families,[26,27] but the mutation must be very rare outside of Finland because it has not been detected in some other populations.[28,29]

The "resistant ovary" syndrome may be the result of a gonadotropin postreceptor defect. As originally described, the Savage syndrome (named after the first patient described) consisted of young amenorrheic women with elevated peripheral gonadotropin concentrations, normal but immature follicles in the ovaries on biopsy, 46,XX karyotype with no evidence of mosaicism, complete sexual development, and hyposensitivity

(i.e., "resistance") to exogenous gonadotropin stimulation.[30] Although the pathogenesis of this disorder remains obscure, it may be reasonable to consider affected individuals distinct from those with autoimmune disorders.

Premature ovarian failure may be associated with a number of autoimmune disorders.[13] The most common association may be with thyroiditis. Ovarian failure occurs commonly in women with polyglandular failure, including hypoparathyroidism, hypoadrenalism, and mucocutaneous candidiasis[31] (see Chap. 197). The heterogeneous nature of this disorder is suggested by the many different endocrinopathies that may be associated with premature ovarian failure. Autoimmune ovarian failure may occur independently of any other autoimmune disorder.[30a] Although the cause of autoimmune ovarian failure is unknown, circulating antibodies to ovarian tissue have been detected in many affected women, and FSH receptor antibodies have been detected in two women with myasthenia gravis and hypergonadotropic amenorrhea.[32] Immunoglobulins that block the trophic actions of FSH but not LH have also been reported.[33]

The thymus gland influences reproductive function[34] (see Chap. 193). Congenitally athymic girls have ovaries devoid of oocytes.[35]

Irradiation and an increasing number of chemotherapeutic (especially alkylating) agents used to treat various malignancies are causes of premature ovarian failure[36–38] (see Chap. 226). Inexplicably, both of these modalities have been associated with "reversible" ovarian failure. Ovulation and cyclic menses return in some individuals after prolonged intervals of hypergonadotropic amenorrhea associated with signs and symptoms of profound hypoestrogenism. Preliminary studies suggest that gonadotropin-releasing hormone analogs (but not oral contraceptive agents) may provide some protection from ovarian damage.[39] Rarely, the mumps virus can affect the ovaries and cause ovarian failure.[40]

Based on epidemiologic studies, there now appears to be an inverse dose-response relationship between the number of cigarettes smoked per day and the age at menopause. At any given age between 44 and 53 years, a woman who smokes one pack per day is more likely to have undergone menopause than a woman who smokes one-half pack per day or less[41] (see Chap. 234). However, because cigarette smoking is so prevalent and premature ovarian failure so uncommon, it is difficult to believe that smoking plays any significant role in inducing early ovarian failure. Moreover, because relatively few cases of premature ovarian failure appear to be the result of environmental factors, a cause distinct from an environmental cause should be sought in any affected woman without a history of systemic disease, radiation therapy, or chemotherapy.

### DIAGNOSIS AND THERAPY OF PREMATURE OVARIAN FAILURE

Individuals with premature ovarian failure warrant thorough evaluation to eliminate potentially treatable causes and to identify associated disorders that may require therapy. Chromosomal studies should be performed in affected women younger than 30 years of age to identify those with gonadal dysgenesis who have no signs of Turner syndrome. Surgical removal of the gonads is indicated in any individual in whom a Y chromosome is identified. A few simple laboratory studies can rule out endocrine disorders, such as thyroid disease, hypoparathyroidism, hypoadrenalism, and diabetes mellitus. Screening tests to eliminate autoimmune dysfunction are indicated as well. Measurement of circulating LH, FSH, and estradiol concentrations on more than one occasion may help to determine if any functional oocytes remain in the ovary. If the estradiol concentration is >50 pg/mL or if the LH level is significantly greater than the FSH level (in terms of mIU/mL) in any sample, the probability of viable oocytes is considerable. Irregular uterine bleeding, as an indication of estrogen stimulation, also provides good evidence of remaining functional ovarian follicles. It is not uncommon to

CHRONIC ANOVULATION OF CENTRAL ORIGIN
  HYPOTHALAMIC CHRONIC ANOVULATION (FUNCTIONAL)
    Anorexia nervosa and bulimia
    Amenorrhea associated with simple weight loss, diet, malnutrition
    Exercise-associated amenorrhea
    Psychogenic hypothalamic amenorrhea
    Pseudocyesis
    Due to systemic illness
  FORMS OF ISOLATED GONADOTROPIN DEFICIENCY (INCLUDING KALLMANN SYNDROME)
  HYPOPITUITARISM
    Idiopathic
    After hypothalamic-pituitary damage
    Neoplasms
    "Empty sella" syndrome
    After surgery
    After irradiation
    After trauma
    After infection
    After infarction
  HYPERPROLACTINEMIC CHRONIC ANOVULATION (GALACTOR-RHEA-AMENORRHEA) OF MULTIPLE CAUSES
CHRONIC ANOVULATION CAUSED BY INAPPROPRIATE FEED-BACK (i.e., POLYCYSTIC OVARY SYNDROME)
  EXCESSIVE EXTRAGLANDULAR ESTROGEN PRODUCTION (i.e., OBESITY)
  ABNORMAL BUFFERING INVOLVING SEX HORMONE–BINDING GLOBULIN (INCLUDING LIVER DISEASE)
  FUNCTIONAL ANDROGEN EXCESS OF ADRENAL OR OVARIAN ORIGIN
  NEOPLASMS PRODUCING ANDROGENS OR ESTROGENS
  NEOPLASMS PRODUCING CHORIONIC GONADOTROPIN
CHRONIC ANOVULATION CAUSED BY OTHER ENDOCRINE AND METABOLIC DISORDERS
  ADRENAL HYPERFUNCTION
    Cushing syndrome
    Congenital adrenal hyperplasia (female pseudohermaphroditism)
  THYROID DYSFUNCTION
    Hyperthyroidism
    Hypothyroidism

(Modified from Rebar RW. Chronic anovulation. In Serra GB, ed. The ovary. New York: Raven Press, 1983:217.)

identify women with intermittent menstruation, hypoestrogenism, and hypergonadotropinism. Because a number of pregnancies have occurred after biopsy of ovaries devoid of oocytes, ovarian biopsy cannot be recommended for affected women.

Even in women with intermittent ovarian failure, estrogen replacement is appropriate to prevent the accelerated bone loss that occurs in affected women.[42] The estrogen should always be given sequentially with a progestin to prevent endometrial hyperplasia (see Chap. 100). Because women with ovarian failure may conceive while on estrogen therapy (including combined oral contraceptive agents), affected women should be counseled appropriately and cautioned to have a pregnancy test if withdrawal bleeding does not occur or if signs and symptoms develop that are suggestive of pregnancy. Despite these considerations, probably no other contraceptive agent is required for those women who do not wish pregnancy but who are sexually active, because pregnancy occurs in far less than 10%.[13] Although rare pregnancies in women with premature ovarian failure have occurred after ovulation induction with human menopausal and chorionic gonadotropins, the low likelihood should lead the physician to discourage patients from selecting such therapy. Hormone replacement treatment to mimic the normal menstrual cycle, with oocyte donation for embryo transfer, may provide the greatest possibility for pregnancy in women desiring pregnancy.[43,44]

## CHRONIC ANOVULATION

Chronic anovulation may be viewed as a steady state in which the monthly rhythms associated with ovulation are not functional. Although amenorrhea is common, irregular menses and oligomenorrhea may occur as well. Chronic anovulation further implies that viable oocytes remain in the ovary and that ovulation can be induced with appropriate therapy.

Chronic anovulation is the most common endocrine cause of oligomenorrhea or amenorrhea in women of reproductive age (Table 96-3). Appropriate management requires determination of the cause of the anovulation. However, anovulation can be interrupted transiently by nonspecific induction of ovulation in most affected women.

### CHRONIC ANOVULATION OF CENTRAL ORIGIN

**Hypothalamic Chronic Anovulation.** Hypothalamic chronic anovulation may be defined as anovulation in which dysfunction of hypothalamic signals to the pituitary gland causes failure to ovulate. It remains unclear whether the primary abnormality is always present within the hypothalamus or sometimes occurs as a result of altered inputs to the hypothalamus. The term is used to refer to women who may be affected with suprahypothalamic or hypothalamic chronic anovulation. Although isolated gonadotropin deficiency frequently is caused by hypothalamic dysfunction, it is preferable to consider such individuals separately. However, it may be virtually impossible to differentiate partial forms of isolated gonadotropin deficiency from hypothalamic chronic anovulation.

Some reports have documented an increased incidence of amenorrhea in women who exercise strenuously, diet excessively, or are exposed to severe emotional or physical stresses of any kind[45-47] (see Chap. 128). Such amenorrheic persons fall into this group of women considered as having hypothalamic chronic anovulation, which is sometimes called *functional amenorrhea*. The diagnosis of hypothalamic chronic anovulation is suggested by the abrupt cessation of menses in women younger than 30 years of age who have no clinically evident anatomic abnormalities of the hypothalamic–pituitary–ovarian axis or any other endocrine abnormalities. The term *hypothalamic amenorrhea* was first proposed by Klinefelter and colleagues in 1943 for anovulation in which hypothalamic dysfunction is thought to interfere with the pituitary secretion of gonadotropin.[48]

Although hypothalamic chronic anovulation is a common cause of oligomenorrhea and amenorrhea, relatively little is known about its pathophysiologic basis. The diversity of women with hypothalamic chronic anovulation indicates that this is a heterogeneous group of disorders with similar manifestations. Compared with a matched control population, young women with secondary amenorrhea are more likely to be unmarried, to engage in intellectual occupations, to have had stressful life events, to use sedative and hypnotic drugs, to be underweight, and to have a history of previous menstrual irregularities.[45] Although it has been suggested that the percentage of body fat controls the maintenance of normal menstrual cycles, it is more likely that diet, exercise, stress, body composition, and other unrecognized nutritional and environmental factors contribute in various proportions to amenorrhea (Fig. 96-3).

Hormonally, basal circulating concentrations of pituitary (i.e., LH, FSH, TSH, prolactin, growth hormone), ovarian (i.e., estrogens, androgens), and adrenal hormones (i.e., dehydroepiandrosterone, DHEAS, cortisol) typically are within the normal range for women of reproductive age.[49] However, mean serum gonadotropin, gonadal steroid, and DHEAS levels often are

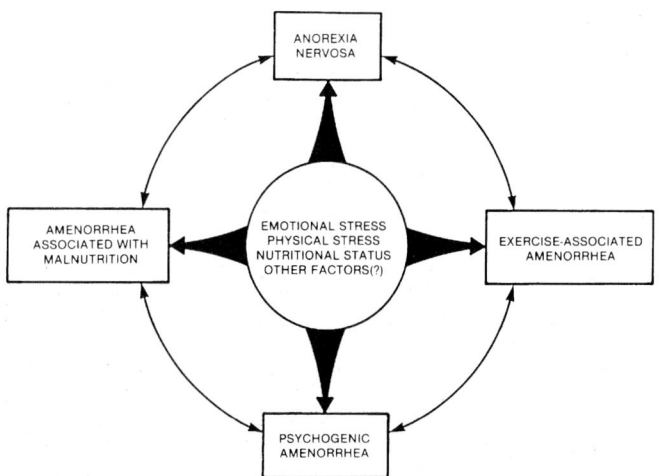

**FIGURE 96-3.** Schematic representation of postulated associations among various forms of hypothalamic chronic anovulation and common linked factors. These disorders appear to be closely interrelated. (Reprinted from Rebar RW. The reproductive age: chronic anovulation. In: Serra BG, ed. The ovary. New York: Raven, 1983:217.)

Peripheral gonadotropin and gonadal steroid levels generally are lower than in the early follicular phase of the menstrual cycle.[55] As patients undergo therapy, gain weight, and improve psychologically, sequential studies of the ultradian gonadotropin rhythms show progressive gonadotropin changes paralleling those normally seen during puberty. Initially, there is a nocturnal rise in gonadotropins, followed by an increase in mean basal gonadotropin levels throughout the 24-hour period.[56–58] The responses of severely ill anorectics to GnRH are also similar to those observed in prepubertal children and become adult-like with recovery or with treatment with pulsatile GnRH.[59,60] Because the metabolism of estradiol and testosterone is also abnormal, normalizing with weight gain, some of the gonadotropin changes may be secondary to peripheral alterations in steroids.[61]

Several abnormalities indicate hypothalamic dysfunction, including mild diabetes insipidus and abnormal thermoregulatory responses to heat and cold.[54] Affected individuals have altered body images as well.[62]

Still other central and peripheral abnormalities exist. There is evidence of chemical hypothyroidism, with affected patients having decreased body temperature, bradycardia, low serum triiodothyronine ($T_3$) levels, and increased reverse $T_3$ concentrations.[63–65] Circulating cortisol levels also are elevated, but the circadian cortisol rhythm is normal.[66] The increased cortisol seems to be caused by the reduced metabolic clearance of cortisol as a result of the reduced affinity constant for corticosteroid binding globulin (CBG) present in such patients.[67] Moreover, like women with endogenous depression, anorectics suppress significantly less after dexamethasone administration than do normal subjects.[68] Anorectics also have reduced ACTH responses to exogenous corticotropin-releasing hormone (CRH), suggesting normal negative pituitary feedback by the increased circulating cortisol.[69]

Although rigorous studies have not been performed of women with bulimia, presumably such individuals have endocrine disturbances similar to those of women with anorexia nervosa.

SIMPLE WEIGHT LOSS AND AMENORRHEA.    Societal attitudes encourage dieting and pursuit of thinness, particularly in young women. Several reproductive problems, including hypothalamic chronic anovulation, have been associated with simple weight loss. Affected women are distinctly different from anorectics in that they do not fulfill the psychiatric criteria for

slightly decreased, and circulating and urinary cortisol levels are generally increased compared with those in normal women in the early follicular phase of the menstrual cycle.[47,50] Despite low levels of circulating estrogen, affected women rarely have symptoms related to estrogen deficiency. Typically, the pulsatile secretion of gonadotropin is diminished, but these individuals respond normally to exogenous gonadotropin-releasing hormone (GnRH; Fig. 96-4).

ANOREXIA NERVOSA.    Anorexia nervosa may represent the severest form of functional hypothalamic chronic anovulation, or it may have one or more distinct pathophysiologic bases. The constellation of amenorrhea often preceding the weight loss, a distorted and bizarre attitude toward eating, food, or weight, extreme inanition, and a disordered body image makes the diagnosis of anorexia nervosa obvious in almost all cases[51–54] (see Chap. 128). Demographically, 90% to 95% of anorectic women are white and come from middle- and upper-income families.

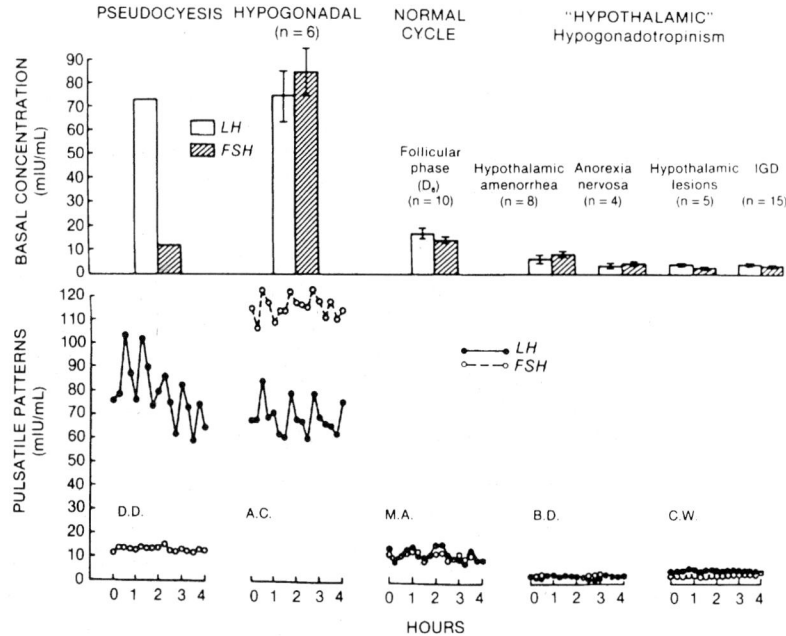

**FIGURE 96-4.** Basal concentrations of luteinizing hormone (*LH*) and follicle-stimulating hormone (*FSH*) and their pulsatile patterns during the early follicular phase of the normal menstrual cycle are compared with exaggerated patterns in subjects without ovarian feedback (hypogonadal), in patients with pseudocyesis, and in the absence of pulsatile fluctuations observed in various forms of hypothalamic hypogonadotropism. (*IGD*, isolated gonadotropin deficiency.) (Reprinted from Yen SSC, Lakely BL, Wang CF. The operating characteristics of the hypothalamic-pituitary system during the menstrual cycle and observations of biological action of somatostatin. Recent Prog Horm Res 1975; 31:321.)

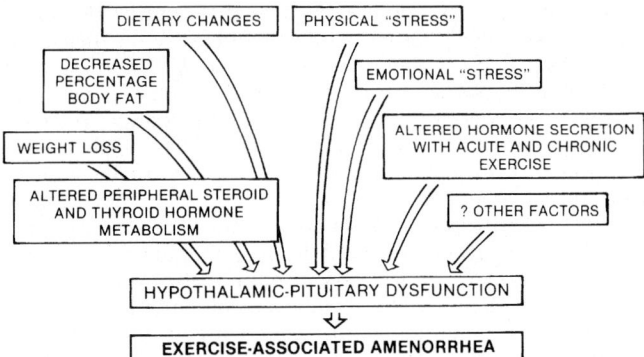

**FIGURE 96-5.** Some factors apparently involved in the pathophysiology of exercise-associated amenorrhea. (Reprinted from Rebar RW. Effect of exercise on reproductive function in females. In: Givens JR, ed. The hypothalamus in health and disease. Chicago: Year Book Medical Publishers, 1984:245.)

anorexia.[52] The cessation of menses does not occur before significant weight loss in such women, although this sequence is common in anorectics. The few studies that have been conducted in amenorrheic women with simple weight loss suggest that the abnormalities are similar to those observed in anorectics, but are more minor and more easily reversible with weight gain.[70] Although it has been suggested that the amenorrhea in these women is secondary to metabolic defects resulting from undernutrition, the possibility of separate central defects has not been excluded.[70] The importance of normal body weight to normal reproductive function is evident in studies of a tribe of desert-dwelling hunter-gatherers in Botswana.[71] The weights of the women vary markedly with the season, being greatest in the summer, and the peak incidence of parturition follows exactly 9 months after the attainment of maximal weight.

EXERCISE-ASSOCIATED AMENORRHEA.   Regular endurance training in women is associated with at least three distinct disorders of reproductive function: delayed menarche, luteal dysfunction, and amenorrhea.[72,73] The American College of Sports Medicine has coined the term the "female athletic triad" to describe the three disorders recognized as sometimes occurring together in female athletes: disordered eating, amenorrhea, and osteoporosis.[74,74a] Activities associated with an increased frequency of reproductive dysfunction include those favoring a slimmer, lower-body-weight physique such as middle and long distance running, ballet dancing, and gymnastics. Swimmers and bicyclists appear to have lower rates of amenorrhea despite comparable training intensities. The cause of these disorders remains to be established and may involve many factors. Dietary changes, the hormonal effects of acute and chronic exercise, alterations in hormone metabolism because of the increased lean to fat ratio, and the psychological and physical "stress" of exercise itself may all contribute and may vary in importance in different individuals (Fig. 96-5; see Chaps. 128 and 132).

Menstrual dysfunction was induced in untrained women who underwent a program of strenuous aerobic exercise (running 4–10 miles per day) combined with caloric restriction.[75] The spectrum of abnormalities in these women included luteal phase dysfunction, loss of the midcycle LH surge, prolonged menstrual cycles, altered patterns of gonadotropin secretion, and amenorrhea. Subsequent studies have indicated that luteal phase defects can occur soon after endurance training is begun in the majority of untrained women.[76] However, in contrast to these findings, others observed that a progressive exercise program of moderate intensity did not affect the reproductive system of gynecologically mature (mean age, 31.4 years), untrained, eumenorrheic women.[77] It was suggested that relatively young gynecologic age or an earlier age of training onset in particular adversely affects menstrual cyclicity.

Many amenorrheic athletes welcome the onset of amenorrhea. However, significant osteopenia, usually affecting trabecular bone, has been reported in these women.[78–80] It appears that the loss in bone density secondary to hypoestrogenism nullifies the beneficial effects of weight-bearing exercise in strengthening and remodeling bone.[79,81] Such women are at risk for stress fractures, particularly in the weight-bearing lower extremities, and bone density may remain below those of eumenorrheic athletes even after resumption of menses.[82]

Stress is generally acknowledged to play a role in the cause of this form of amenorrhea, even though it remains difficult to define the term *stress*. Amenorrheic runners subjectively associate greater stress with running than do runners with regular menses.[83] However, no increase in amenorrhea was observed in a competitive group of young classical musicians, who presumably were experiencing similar stress, compared with a group of young ballet dancers, in whom the incidence of amenorrhea was quite high.[84] Basal levels of circulating cortisol and urinary free cortisol excretion, which are indicative of increased stress, are increased in eumenorrheic and amenorrheic runners.[85] Because levels of CBG, the disappearance rate of cortisol from the circulation, and the response of cortisol to adrenocorticotropin (ACTH) were not altered in the women runners compared with sedentary control subjects, secretion of ACTH and possibly of CRH must be increased in women who run. Abnormalities of the hypothalamic–pituitary–adrenal axis also are indicated by the observations that serum ACTH and cortisol responses to exogenous CRH are blunted, as are the responses to meals.[86]

The observation that amenorrheic runners also have subtle abnormalities in hypothalamic–pituitary–adrenal function provides support for the concept that exercise-associated amenorrhea is similar to other forms of hypothalamic amenorrhea.[87]

PSYCHOGENIC HYPOTHALAMIC AMENORRHEA.   Amenorrhea may occur in women with a definite history of psychological and socioenvironmental trauma.[45,78–80] The incidence of amenorrhea is quite high among depressed women, and it is difficult to differentiate the effects of lifestyle and nutritional status from variables such as stress. Studies of individuals in whom a definite psychological traumatic event preceded the onset of amenorrhea have revealed low to normal basal levels of serum gonadotropins with normal responses to GnRH, prolonged suppression of gonadotropins in response to estradiol, and failure of a positive feedback response to estradiol.[78–97] Increased basal levels of cortisol and decreased levels of DHEAS also have been noticed in women with psychogenic amenorrhea compared with eumenorrheic women.[46] The mean levels of circulating cortisol are increased in such women largely because of an increase in the amplitude of the pulses of cortisol.[98] Moreover, studies of depressed women have revealed abnormal circadian rhythms of cortisol and early "escape" from dexamethasone suppression.[99–101]

The mechanism by which emotional states or stressful experiences cause psychogenic amenorrhea is not yet established. Evidence suggests, however, that a cascade of neuroendocrine events that may begin with limbic system responses to psychic stimuli impairs hypothalamic-pituitary activity.[102] It has been suggested that increased amounts of hypothalamic β-endorphin is important in inhibiting gonadotropin secretion.[102]

Psychological studies have found several social and psychological correlates of psychogenic amenorrhea: a history of previous pregnancy losses, including spontaneous abortion[103–105]; stressful life events within the 6-month period preceding the amenorrhea[106–108]; and poor social support or separation from significant family members during childhood and adolescence.[101,108,109] Many women with psychogenic amenorrhea report stressful events associated with psychosexual problems and socioenvironmental stresses during the teenage years.[89] Women with psychogenic amenorrhea also tend to have negative attitudes toward sexually related body parts, more partner-related sexual problems, and greater fear of or aversion to menstruation than do eumenorrheic women.[107] Distortions of body image and confusion about basic bodily functions, especially sexuality and reproduction, are common.[104]

DIMINISHED GONADOTROPIN-RELEASING HORMONE AND LUTEINIZING HORMONE SECRETION IN ALL FORMS. The various forms of hypothalamic chronic anovulation associated with altered lifestyles have several features in common. Altered GnRH and LH secretion seems to be the common result from altered hypothalamic input. It remains unclear if these disorders form a single disorder or several closely related disorders. Moreover, similar forms of amenorrhea are sometimes seen in women with severe systemic illnesses or with hypothalamic damage from tumors, infection, irradiation, trauma, or other causes.

TREATMENT. The treatment of patients with hypothalamic chronic anovulation is controversial. Psychological therapy and support or a change in lifestyle may cause cyclic ovulation and menses to resume. However, ovulation does not always resume, even after the lifestyle is altered. The treatment of affected women in whom menses do not resume and who do not desire pregnancy is difficult. Most physicians now advocate the use of exogenous sex steroids to prevent osteoporosis. Therapy consisting of oral conjugated estrogens (0.625–1.250 mg), ethinyl estradiol (20 μg), micronized estradiol-17β (1–2 mg), or estrone sulfate (0.625–2.500 mg) or of transdermal estradiol-17β (0.05–0.10 mg) continuously with oral medroxyprogesterone acetate (5–10 mg) or oral micronized progesterone (200 mg) added for 12 to 14 days each month is appropriate. Sexually active women can be treated with oral contraceptive agents. These women appear to be particularly sensitive to the undesired side effects of sex steroid therapy, and close contact with the physician may be required until the appropriate dosage is established. If sex steroid therapy is provided, patients must be informed that the amenorrhea may still be present after therapy is discontinued.

Some physicians believe that only periodic observation of affected women is indicated, with barrier methods of contraception recommended for fertility control. Contraception is necessary for sexually active women with hypothalamic chronic anovulation because spontaneous ovulation may resume at any time (before menstrual bleeding) in these mildly affected individuals. Women who refuse sex steroid therapy should be encouraged to have spinal bone density evaluated at intervals to document that bone loss is not accelerated. Adequate calcium ingestion should be encouraged in all affected women.

For women who desire pregnancy but who do not ovulate spontaneously, clomiphene citrate (50–100 mg per day for 5 days beginning on the third to fifth day of withdrawal bleeding) can be used. Treatment with human menopausal and chorionic gonadotropins (hMG-hCG) or with pulsatile GnRH may be effective in women who do not ovulate in response to clomiphene. Because the underlying defect in hypothalamic amenorrhea is decreased endogenous GnRH secretion, administration of pulsatile GnRH to induce ovulation can be viewed as physiologic; it offers the additional advantages of decreased need for ultrasonographic and serum estradiol monitoring, a decreased risk of multiple pregnancies, and a virtual absence of ovarian hyperstimulation. A starting intravenous dose of GnRH of 5 μg every 90 minutes is effective.[110] After ovulation is detected by urinary LH testing or ultrasound, the corpus luteum can be supported by continuation of pulsatile GnRH or by hCG (1500 IU every 3 days for four doses). Ovulation rates of 90% and conception rates of 30% per ovulatory cycle can be expected.[111]

**Isolated Gonadotropin Deficiency.** As originally described in 1944, Kallmann syndrome consisted of the triad of anosmia, hypogonadism, and color blindness in men.[112] Women may be affected as well, and other midline defects may be associated.[113–116] Because autopsy studies have shown partial or complete agenesis of the olfactory bulb, the term *olfactogenital dysplasia* has also been used to describe the syndrome.[117]

Because isolated gonadotropin deficiency may also occur in the absence of anosmia, the syndrome is considered to be quite heterogeneous.

Data indicate that the defect is a failure of GnRH neurons to form completely in the medial olfactory placode of the developing nose or the failure of GnRH neurons to migrate from the olfactory bulb to the medial basal hypothalamus during embryogenesis.[118] In some patients, structural defects of the olfactory bulbs can be seen on magnetic resonance imaging.[119] It appears likely that this disorder forms a structural continuum with other midline defects, with septo-optic dysplasia representing the severest disorder.

Clinically, affected individuals typically present with sexual infantilism and an eunuchoidal habitus, but moderate breast development may also occur. Primary amenorrhea is the rule. The ovaries usually are small and appear immature, with follicles rarely developed beyond the primordial stage.[120] These immature follicles respond readily to exogenous gonadotropin with ovulation and pregnancy, and exogenous pulsatile GnRH can also be used to induce ovulation.[121,122] Replacement therapy with estrogen and progestin should be given to affected women who do not desire pregnancy.

Circulating LH and FSH levels generally are quite low. The response to exogenous GnRH is variable, sometimes being diminished and sometimes normal in magnitude, but rarely may be absent.[123,124] Although the primary defect in most individuals appears to be hypothalamic, with reduced GnRH synthesis or secretion, a primary pituitary defect may occasionally be present. In addition, partial gonadotropin deficiency may be more frequent than has been appreciated (see Chap. 115).

**Hyperprolactinemic Chronic Anovulation.** Approximately 15% of amenorrheic women have increased circulating concentrations of prolactin, but prolactin levels are increased in more than 75% of patients with galactorrhea and amenorrhea.[8] Radiologic evidence of a pituitary tumor is present in ~50% of hyperprolactinemic women, and primary hypothyroidism must always be considered. Individuals with galactorrhea-amenorrhea (i.e., hyperprolactinemic chronic anovulation) frequently complain of symptoms of estrogen deficiency, including hot flushes and dyspareunia. However, estrogen secretion may be essentially normal.[125] It is not clear if it is the hyperprolactinemia or the "hypoestrogenism" that causes the accelerated bone loss seen in such individuals.[126] Signs of androgen excess are observed in some women with hyperprolactinemia; androgen excess may rarely result in PCO. In hyperprolactinemic women, serum gonadotropin and estradiol levels are low or normal.

Most hyperprolactinemic women have disordered reproductive function, and it appears that the effects on gonadotropin secretion are primarily hypothalamic. The mechanism by which hypothalamic GnRH secretion is disrupted is unknown but may involve an inhibitory effect of tuberoinfundibular dopaminergic neurons.[125,127] It has been proposed that increased hypothalamic dopamine is present in hyperprolactinemic women with pituitary tumors but is ineffective in reducing prolactin secretion by adenomatous lactotropes. The dopamine can, however, reduce pulsatile LH secretion and produce acyclic gonadotropin secretion through a direct effect on hypothalamic GnRH secretion (see Chap. 13).

It has been suggested that mild nocturnal hyperprolactinemia may be present in some women with regular menses and unexplained infertility.[128] Galactorrhea in women with unexplained infertility may reflect increased bioavailable prolactin and may be treated appropriately with bromocriptine.[129] Bromocriptine or cabergoline therapy may also be indicated in normoprolactinemic women with amenorrhea and increased prolactin responses to provocative stimuli.[130]

**Hypopituitarism.** Hypopituitarism may be obvious on cursory inspection or it may be quite subtle (see Chaps. 12 to 18). The clinical presentation depends on the age at onset, the

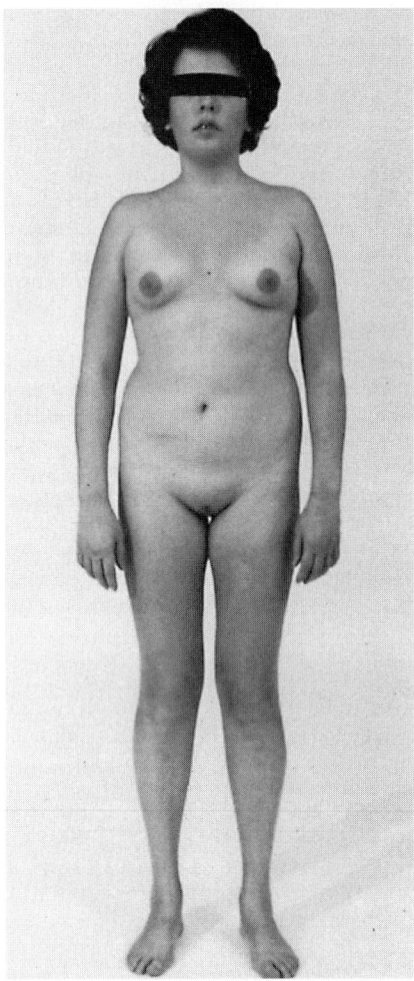

**FIGURE 96-6.** Hypopituitarism in a 28-year-old woman with a craniopharyngioma diagnosed at age 16 years. She had received total replacement therapy since the time of diagnosis. Breast development has not advanced beyond Tanner stage 3, little pubic hair is present, and the body habitus is not that of a mature adult. The deep pigmentation of the areolae occurred during therapy several years earlier with fluoxymesterone in an attempt to induce pubic and axillary hair growth.

cause, and the woman's nutritional status (Fig. 96-6). Loss of axillary and pubic hair and atrophy of the external genitalia should lead the physician to suspect hypopituitarism in a previously menstruating young woman who develops amenorrhea. In such cases, a history of past obstetric hemorrhage suggesting postpartum pituitary necrosis (i.e., Sheehan syndrome) should be sought.[131] Failure to develop secondary sexual characteristics or to progress in development once puberty begins must always prompt a workup for hypopituitarism (see Chap. 18).

Individuals with pituitary insufficiency often complain of weakness, easy fatigability, lack of libido, and cold intolerance. Short stature may occur in individuals developing hypopituitarism during childhood. Symptoms of diabetes insipidus may be observed if the posterior pituitary gland is involved. On physical examination, the skin is generally thin, smooth, cool, and pale (i.e., "alabaster skin") with fine wrinkling about the eyes; the pulse is slow and thready; and the blood pressure is low.

An evaluation of thyroid and adrenal function is of paramount importance in these individuals. Thyroid replacement therapy must be instituted and the patient must be euthyroid before adrenal testing is initiated (see Chaps. 14, 15, 18, and 74). Serum gonadotropin and gonadal steroid levels typically are low in hypopituitarism. Responses to exogenously adminis-

tered hypothalamic hormones have failed to localize the cause to the hypothalamus or the pituitary gland in affected patients.

Radiographic evaluation of the sella turcica is indicated in any individual with suspected hypopituitarism. The ovaries appear immature and unstimulated, but because oocytes still are present, ovulation can be induced with exogenous gonadotropins when pregnancy is desired. Exogenous pulsatile GnRH may also be used to induce ovulation if the disorder is hypothalamic. Moreover, oocytes may undergo some development, and even ovarian cysts may appear in the absence of significant gonadotropic stimulation (see Chap. 94). When pregnancy is not desired, maintenance therapy with cyclic estrogen and progestin is indicated to prevent signs and symptoms of estrogen deficiency (see Chap. 100).

### CHRONIC ANOVULATION RESULTING FROM INAPPROPRIATE FEEDBACK IN POLYCYSTIC OVARY SYNDROME

**Heterogeneous Disorder.** In 1935, Stein and Leventhal focused attention on a common disorder in which amenorrhea, hirsutism, and obesity were frequently associated.[132] With the development of radioimmunoassays for measuring reproductive hormones, it became clear that women with what is called PCO shared several distinctive biochemical features. Compared with eumenorrheic women in the early follicular phase of the menstrual cycle, affected women typically have elevated serum LH levels and low to normal FSH levels[11] (Fig. 96-7). Virtually all serum androgens are moderately increased, and estrone levels are generally greater than estradiol levels[133] (Fig. 96-8). Ovarian inhibin physiology is normal.[134]

Many women with the biochemical features of PCO have small or even morphologically normal ovaries and are not overweight or hirsute. Not all women with PCO have the characteristic features. Moreover, excess androgen from any source or increased conversion of androgens to estrogens can lead to the constellation of findings observed in PCO.[10] Included are such disorders as Cushing syndrome, congenital adrenal hyperplasia, virilizing tumors of ovarian or adrenal origin, hyperthyroidism and hypothyroidism, obesity, and type 2 diabetes.[134a] In all of these disorders, the ovaries may be morphologically polycystic.

Although no clinical and biochemical criteria describe the syndrome strictly, a conference convened by the National Institutes of Health[135] developed diagnostic criteria for PCO:

1. Clinical evidence of hyperandrogenism (e.g., hirsutism, acne, androgenetic alopecia) and/or hyperandrogemia (e.g., elevated total or free testosterone).
2. Oligoovulation (i.e., cycle duration >35 days or <8 cycles per year).
3. Exclusion of related disorders (e.g., hyperprolactinemia, thyroid dysfunction, androgen-secreting tumors, 21-hydroxylase-deficient nonclassical congenital adrenal hyperplasia).

PCO may be viewed as *a state of chronic anovulation associated with LH-dependent ovarian overproduction of androgens.* Clinically, the perimenarcheal onset of symptoms is a common feature. It has been estimated that PCO affects ~5% of women of reproductive age.[136,137] Although the cause of this disorder remains unknown, there is some evidence of autosomal-dominant transmission in some affected individuals.[138,139] Disorders presenting similarly but with different underlying causes can be considered as having chronic anovulation with inappropriate feedback.

**Polycystic Ovary.** Grossly, the ovaries of most women with PCO are bilaterally enlarged and globular (Fig. 96-9). They are often described as having an "oyster shell" appearance because they have smooth, glistening capsules and are the appropriate color. The tunica albuginea is often thickened diffusely, and many cysts 3 to 7 mm in diameter are present on cut section. Because ovulation rarely occurs, corpora lutea are rarely present. Histologically, the follicular cysts are usually

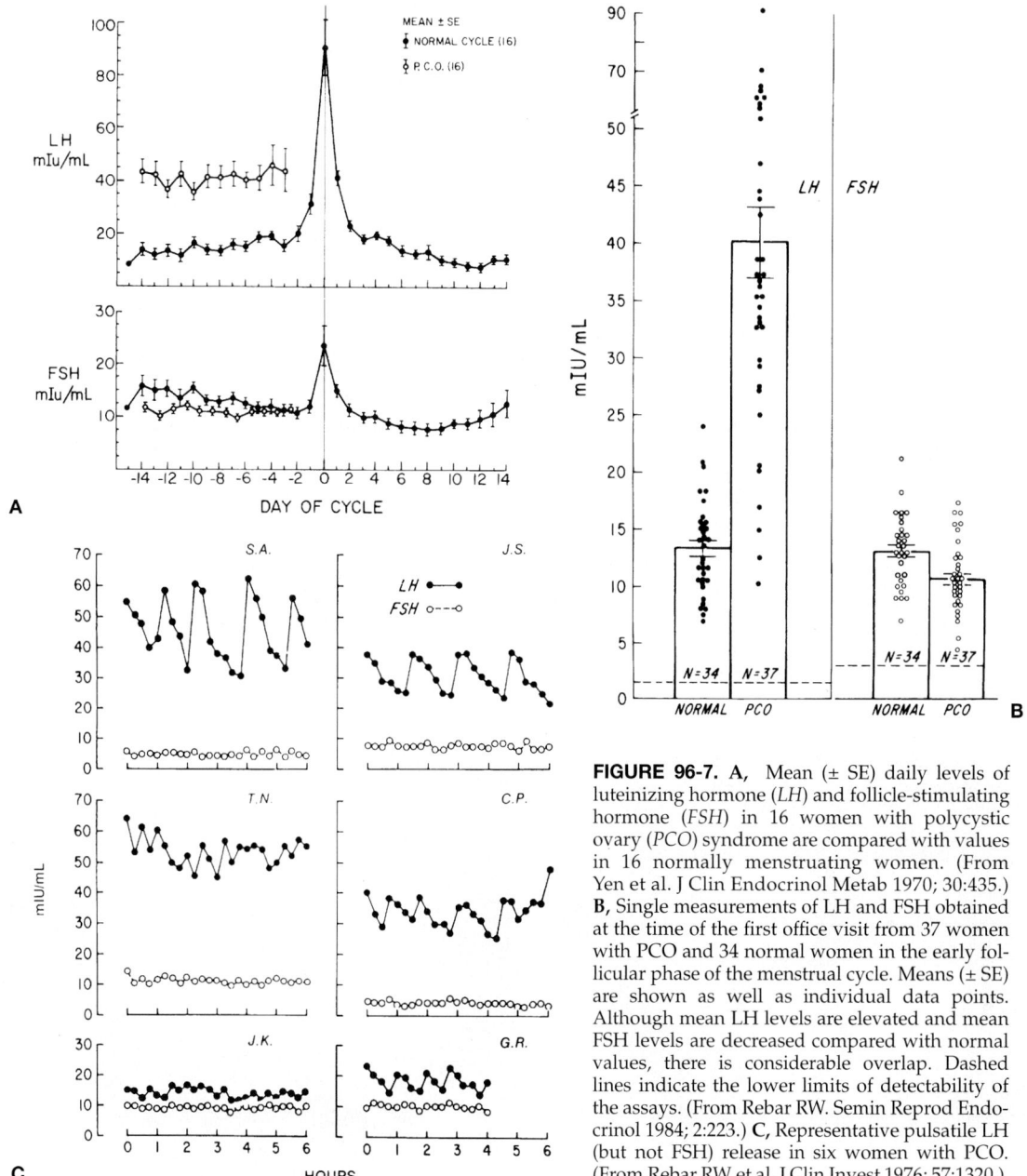

**FIGURE 96-7. A,** Mean (± SE) daily levels of luteinizing hormone (*LH*) and follicle-stimulating hormone (*FSH*) in 16 women with polycystic ovary (*PCO*) syndrome are compared with values in 16 normally menstruating women. (From Yen et al. J Clin Endocrinol Metab 1970; 30:435.) **B,** Single measurements of LH and FSH obtained at the time of the first office visit from 37 women with PCO and 34 normal women in the early follicular phase of the menstrual cycle. Means (± SE) are shown as well as individual data points. Although mean LH levels are elevated and mean FSH levels are decreased compared with normal values, there is considerable overlap. Dashed lines indicate the lower limits of detectability of the assays. (From Rebar RW. Semin Reprod Endocrinol 1984; 2:223.) **C,** Representative pulsatile LH (but not FSH) release in six women with PCO. (From Rebar RW et al. J Clin Invest 1976; 57:1320.)

lined by granulosa cells and surrounded by a thickened and luteinized theca interna and are in various stages of maturation and atresia. When islands of luteinized thecal cells are found scattered throughout the ovarian stroma, not just around the follicles, the term *hyperthecosis* is sometimes used. The clinical syndrome accompanying this pathologic finding is typically characterized by massive obesity, severe hirsutism reflecting particularly excessive ovarian overproduction of androgens, acanthosis nigricans, glucose intolerance with insulin resistance, and hyperuricemia (Fig. 96-10). Insulin action at the target cell appears defective in these patients, with some individuals having antibodies to insulin receptors and others apparently having a postreceptor defect.[140,141] PCO and hyperthecosis appear to represent facets of the same disease process rather than two distinct entities. Some authorities, however, maintain that the two represent different disorders.

The follicles in the ovaries of women with PCO do not mature completely. However, in vitro studies have failed to detect any primary defect in the steroidogenic capacity of polycystic ovaries.[142] Although there seems to be a relative deficiency in aro-

matase activity in the granulosa cells of polycystic ovaries, this deficiency can be corrected by FSH in vitro and in vivo.

**Other Clinical and Biochemical Features.**    Although all women with PCO produce androgens at increased rates compared with eumenorrheic women, only some have hirsutism, largely because of varying sensitivity at the level of the hair follicle (see Chap. 101). The hyperandrogenism is rarely sufficient to produce overt virilization. Signs of markedly elevated androgen levels, including clitoromegaly, temporal balding, and deepening of the voice, may suggest an androgen-producing tumor, especially if these features developed rapidly. Women with PCO invariably are well estrogenized, with normal breast development and abundant cervical mucus on examination. Because obesity is found in only ~50% of women with PCO, it is doubtful that obesity is central to its cause.

Approximately 50% of women with PCO have amenorrhea, ~30% have irregular bleeding, and ~12% have "cyclic menses."[143] No particular pattern of menstrual bleeding is characteristic of women with PCO, although a history of oligomenorrhea is probably most common. Because only ~75%

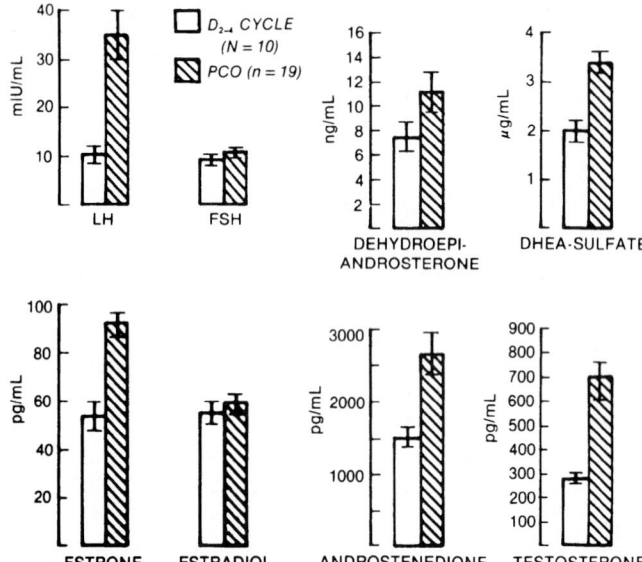

**FIGURE 96-8.** Mean (± SE) circulating levels of peptide and steroid hormone levels in women with polycystic ovary (*PCO*) syndrome compared with women in the early follicular phase of the menstrual cycle (days 2–4). (*FSH,* follicle-stimulating hormone; *LH,* luteinizing hormone.) (Reprinted from DeVane GW, Czekala NM, Judd HL, Yen SSC. Circulating gonadotropins, estrogens, and androgens in polycystic ovarian disease. Am J Obstet Gynecol 1975; 121:496.)

of women with PCO are infertile, women with PCO do ovulate occasionally.

Two other biochemical features warrant discussion. First, obese and normal-weight women with PCO generally release increased quantities of insulin in response to a standard glucose challenge compared with weight-matched eumenorrheic individuals.[144,145] Thus, regardless of body weight, 30% to 80% of women with PCO experience insulin resistance and compensatory hyperinsulinemia.[146,147] Based on studies in a very well-characterized subset of obese women with the disorder, the insulin resistance present in PCO appears to represent a postreceptor signaling aberration and differs from the insulin resistance observed in noninsulin-dependent (type 2) diabetes mellitus and simple obesity.[147] The compensatory hyperinsulinemia that results causes exaggerated effects in other tissues as well. These effects include increased ovarian androgen secretion; excessive growth of the basal cells of the skin leading to acanthosis nigricans in some women; increased vascular and endothelial reactivity, which may lead to hypertension and vascular disease; and abnormal hepatic and peripheral lipid metabolism, which may cause dyslipidemia. Thus, it is now recognized that women with PCO are at increased risk of cardiovascular disease and type 2 diabetes mellitus in addition to endometrial carcinoma because of anovulation. Because treatment with a GnRH analog reduces ovarian androgen secretion but does not correct the insulin resistance in women with PCO, the defect in insulin action presumably is not caused by abnormal sex steroid levels.[148] The possibility that a defect in the secretion or action of insulin or some related growth factor is

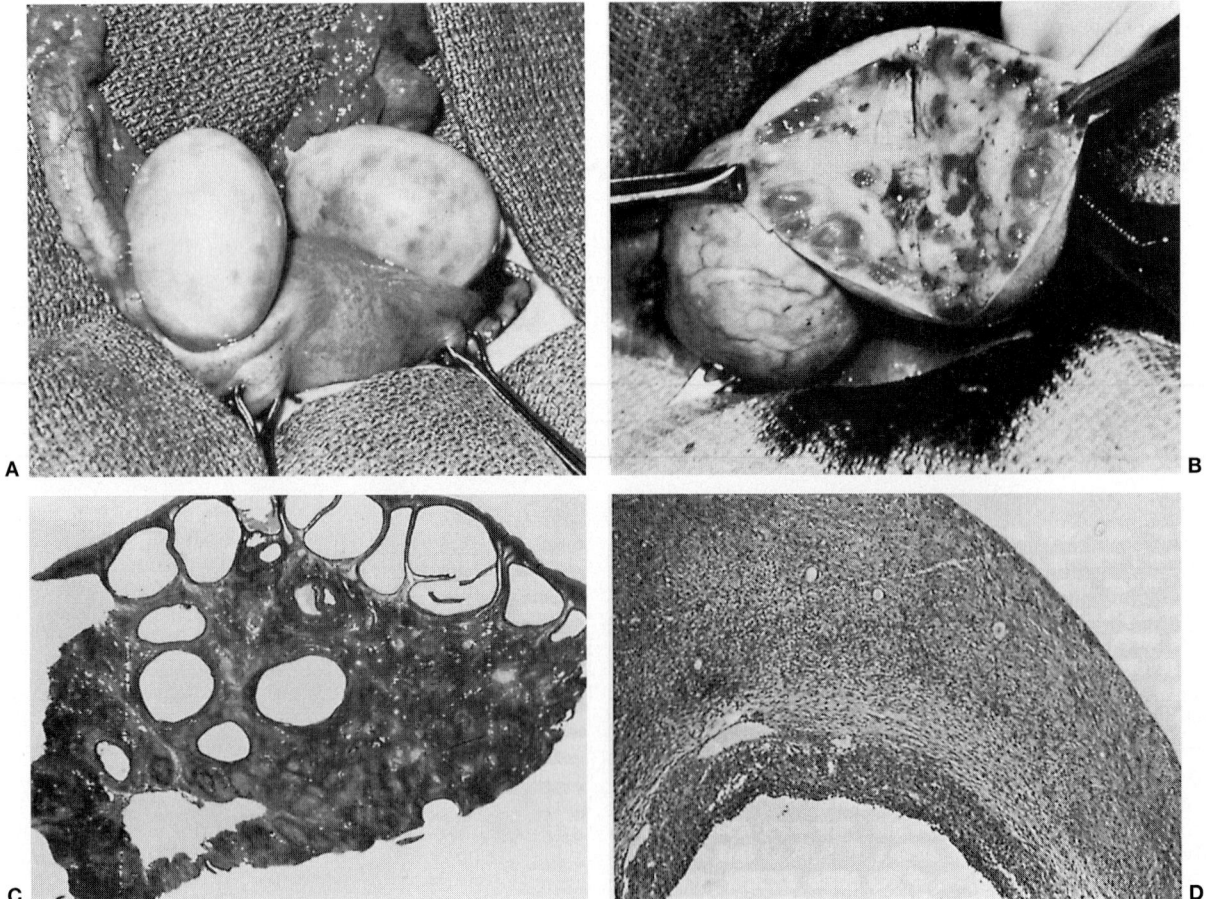

**FIGURE 96-9.** Polycystic ovaries. **A,** Grossly, the ovaries are enlarged and have a smooth, thickened capsule. **B,** Multiple follicular cysts are apparent throughout the cortex, and stroma is abundant on cut section. **C,** Microscopic appearance under low power (original magnification, × 10). **D,** Hyperplasia of the theca surrounding the granulosa cells is a characteristic feature under high magnification. (Courtesy of Dr. R. Jeffrey Chang, University of California, Davis.)

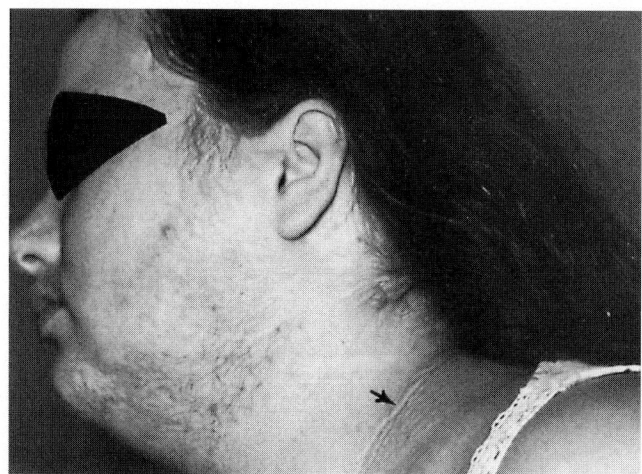

**FIGURE 96-10.** A 23-year-old woman had polycystic ovary syndrome, characterized by massive obesity, severe hirsutism, acanthosis nigricans (*arrow*), glucose intolerance with insulin resistance, hyperandrogenism, and hyperuricemia.

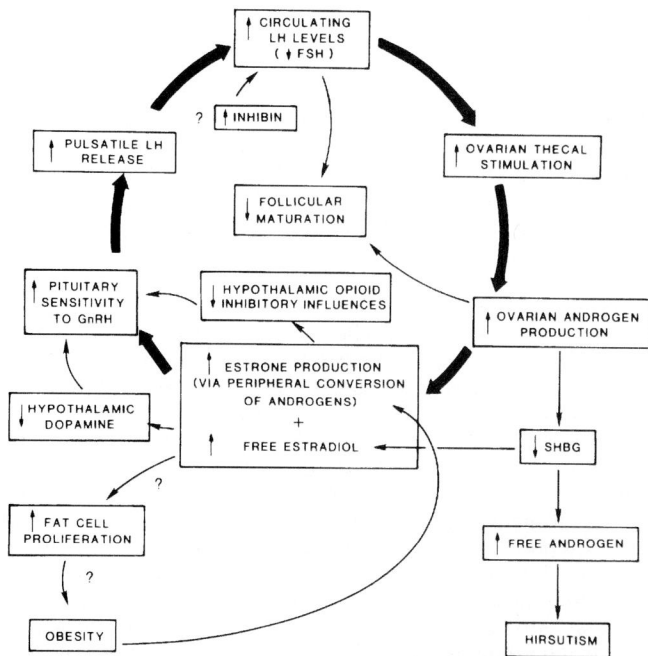

**FIGURE 96-11.** Proposed mechanism for persistent anovulation in polycystic ovary syndrome. (*FSH,* follicle-stimulating hormone; *LH,* luteinizing hormone; *SHBG,* sex hormone binding globulin.) (Reprinted from Rebar RW. The reproductive age: chronic anovulation. In: Serra GB, ed. The ovary. New York: Raven, 1983:217.)

central to the cause of PCO cannot be entirely excluded and is gaining increasing support as the cause of hyperandrogenemia in women with PCO.[149] The pivotal role of insulin resistance in PCO is strongly suggested by the beneficial effects of insulin-sensitizing agents (e.g., metformin and D-chiroinositol) on metabolic and reproductive function, regardless of the patient's weight.[150–153]

In addition, perhaps 10% to 15% of women with PCO have mild hyperprolactinemia in the absence of radiographic evidence of a pituitary tumor, possibly because of chronic acyclic estrogen secretion.[154] Although hyperprolactinemia is associated with increased adrenal production of DHEAS, the increased adrenal androgen production seen in women with PCO usually does not correlate with the hyperprolactinemia.

**Pathophysiology of the Chronic Anovulation.** A growing body of evidence indicates that disordered insulin action precedes the increase in androgens in PCO. The administration of insulin to women with PCO increases circulating androgen levels.[149,155] The administration of glucose to hyperandrogenic women increases circulating levels of insulin and androgen.[156] Weight loss decreases levels of insulin and androgens.[157] The suppression of circulating insulin levels experimentally by diazoxide reduces androgen levels.[158] The suppression of androgen secretion to normal levels with GnRH agonists does not lead to normal insulin responses to glucose tolerance testing in obese women with PCO.[148,159,160]

The hyperinsulinemia may cause hyperandrogenemia by binding to IGF-I receptors in the ovary.[161] Activation of ovarian IGF-I receptors by insulin can lead to increased androgen production by thecal cells.[162] Moreover, independent of any effect on ovarian steroid production, increased insulin inhibits the hepatic synthesis of SHBG.[163] Insulin directly inhibits insulin-like growth factor binding protein-1 in the liver, permitting greater local activity of IGF-I in the ovary.[164]

Regardless of the cause of PCO, it is possible to construct a rational pathophysiologic mechanism to explain the disorder. Regardless of the source or cause of androgen excess, a vicious cycle of events causing persistent anovulation commences (Fig. 96-11). The androgen is converted to estrogen, primarily estrone, in the periphery. The estrogen feeds back on the central nervous system–hypothalamic-pituitary unit to induce inappropriate gonadotropin secretion with an increased ratio of LH to FSH. The estrogen stimulates GnRH synthesis and secretion in the hypothalamus, causing preferential LH release by the pituitary gland. The estrogen may also increase GnRH by decreasing hypothalamic dopamine. Selective inhibition of FSH

secretion by increased ovarian inhibin may also occur in PCO. Possible inhibition of FSH secretion by increased androgen secretion has not been considered. The increased LH secretion stimulates thecal cells in the ovary to produce excess androgen. The androgen also inhibits production of SHBG, resulting in increased free androgen and predisposing affected women to hirsutism. The morphologic ovarian changes undoubtedly are secondary to hormonal changes. The absence of follicular maturation and the reduced estradiol production by the ovaries apparently result from a combination of inadequate FSH stimulation and inhibition by the increased concentrations of intra-ovarian androgen. The low levels of SHBG probably facilitate tissue uptake of free androgen, leading to increased peripheral formation of estrogen and perpetuating the acyclic chronic anovulation. The androgenic basis for the inappropriate estrogen feedback is partly shifted from the site of origin to the ovaries. The increased estrogens (and perhaps androgens) may also stimulate fat cell proliferation, leading to obesity. The current data suggest that there is no defect in the hypothalamic-pituitary axis in PCO but rather that peripheral alterations result in abnormal gonadotropin secretion.

**Therapy.** Appropriate therapy demands that potential causes such as neoplasms be eliminated. In addition to facilitating fertility, the aims of treatment in women with PCO are threefold: to control hirsutism, to prevent endometrial hyperplasia from unopposed acyclic estrogen secretion, and to prevent the long-term consequences of insulin resistance. The treatment must be individualized according to the needs and desires of each patient.

For an anovulatory woman with PCO who is not hirsute and who does not desire pregnancy, therapy with an intermittent progestin (e.g., medroxyprogesterone acetate, 5 to 10 mg orally, or micronized progesterone, 200 mg orally, for 10 to 14 days each month) or oral contraceptives if she is younger than 35 years of age, does not smoke, and has no other significant risk factor (see Chaps. 104 and 105) should be provided to reduce the increased risk of endometrial hyperplasia and carcinoma present in such a woman because of the unopposed estrogen secretion. A woman taking progestins intermittently should be informed of the need for effective barrier contraception if she is sexually active, because these agents as administered do not inhibit ovulation, and ovulation occasionally occurs in PCO. There is no evidence that the use of low-dose combined oral contraceptive agents increases the risks associated with insulin resistance in women with PCO, and the benefits in preventing endometrial hyperplasia are clearly established.

Therapy for a woman with PCO who is hirsute is described in Chapter 101. In general, oral contraceptives provide initial therapy for affected women with mild hirsutism and provide protection from endometrial hyperplasia.

For women with PCO who are overweight, it is reasonable to encourage lifestyle changes. Weight loss alone (of even <10%) may result in decreased insulin resistance and resumption of ovulation.[165–167] However, patients sometimes find it difficult to adopt lifestyle changes. The use of insulin-sensitizing agents such as metformin and other insulin sensitizers is more controversial and is not approved by the U.S. Food and Drug Administration. Whether the use of such agents will decrease the likelihood of the consequences of the metabolic alterations associated with insulin resistance is unclear. Presently, no data regarding the long-term safety and efficacy of these agents exist. What is clear is that only short-term trials of perhaps 3 months duration are needed to determine if insulin-sensitizing agents will be useful: responsive individuals will resume cyclic menstruation and ovulation in this short time frame, and insulin levels will fall substantially.[150,151,168,169,169a]

Predicting which individuals with PCO will respond is not possible presently. However, many clinicians believe that the therapy is low in risk, and the agents are relatively inexpensive. The use of these agents probably should be contemplated only in women with well-documented insulin resistance and PCO. Metformin should be administered only if the patient's creatinine level is normal and should be discontinued during illnesses to prevent the occurrence of lactic acidosis. Individuals should be cautioned that they may anticipate nausea or diarrhea on beginning metformin. Consequently, the drug should be increased slowly to the maximal dose of 2.5 g per day orally. Troglitazone has been taken off the market; whether other insulin sensitizers in this class would be effective is unknown.

The approach to a woman with PCO who wants to conceive is described in Chapter 97. Clomiphene citrate is used initially because of its high success rate and relative simplicity and inexpensiveness (Fig. 96-12). Other possible therapeutic approaches to ovulation induction include the use of hMG-hCG (perhaps preceded by a GnRH analog), purified FSH, pulsatile GnRH, and wedge resection of the ovaries at laparotomy. Wedge resection or any other surgical manipulation of the ovaries should be performed only after all other methods of ovulation induction fail, an ovarian tumor is possible because of ovarian size or circulating androgen levels, or fertility is unimportant, because pelvic adhesions frequently result from surgery and may contribute to infertility. Laparoscopic ovarian follicular cautery or laser vaporization can also be used successfully to induce ovulation.[170,171] However, these procedures also cause adhesion formation in a significant percentage of women. In addition, the success of medical therapy does not justify routine use of these procedures.

Preliminary data indicate that insulin-sensitizing agents, alone or in combination with clomiphene citrate, may improve both ovulatory function and fertility in some women with PCO.[150,151,168] A trial may be warranted in women who do not respond to clomiphene before the use of more expensive agents to induce ovulation is considered.

#### CHRONIC ANOVULATION CAUSED BY OTHER ENDOCRINE AND METABOLIC DISORDERS

**Cushing Syndrome.**    Along with the well-known physical manifestations in Cushing syndrome—central obesity, moon

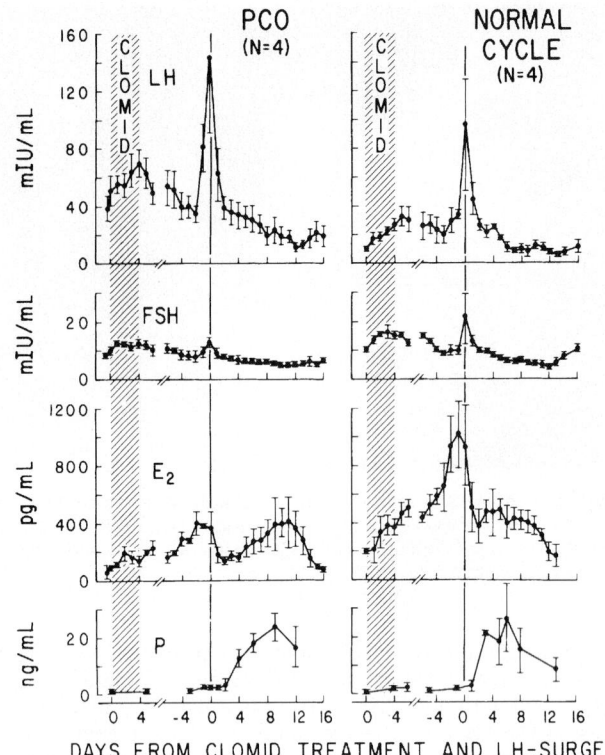

**FIGURE 96-12.** Effects of clomiphene citrate (Clomid, 100 mg per day for 5 days) on the release of gonadotropins and ovarian steroids in four women with polycystic ovary (*PCO*) syndrome and in four normal women receiving the same treatment during the early follicular phase of their menstrual cycles. Data are given in means ± SE. The high levels of estradiol ($E_2$) in the normal women suggest multiple follicular development. (*P*, progesterone.) (Reprinted from Rebar RW, Judd HL, Yen SSC. Characterization of the inappropriate gonadotropin secretion in polycystic ovary syndrome. J Clin Invest 1976; 57:1320.)

facies, and pigmented striae—are the less visible endocrinologic changes of amenorrhea, hirsutism, and infertility. The mechanisms responsible for the chronic anovulation are unclear, but several possibilities exist. The various degrees of adrenal androgen excess in Cushing syndrome of all causes together with obesity may cause excessive extraglandular conversion of androgens to estrogens in fat cells and inappropriate acyclic feedback to the hypothalamic-pituitary unit.[172] The increased levels of CRH and ACTH in Cushing disease may affect the hypothalamic-pituitary secretion of GnRH and LH, as suggested for hypothalamic chronic anovulation.

**Thyroid Dysfunction.**    As a result of significant changes in the metabolism and interconversion of androgens and estrogens, hyperthyroidism and hypothyroidism are associated with menstrual disorders ranging from excessive and prolonged uterine bleeding to amenorrhea. The altered sex steroid metabolism leads to inappropriate feedback and chronic anovulation. The changes are corrected by appropriate treatment of the underlying thyroid disease.

### DISORDERS OF THE LUTEAL PHASE

Subtle abnormalities of follicular development may result in disorders of the luteal phase: luteal-phase dysfunction and "luteinized unruptured follicle" syndrome. Other defects may be recognized in the future.

Luteal-phase defects are characterized by decreased secretion of progesterone after ovulation.[173] Progesterone secretion may be reduced in duration (i.e., *luteal-phase insufficiency*) or in amount (i.e., *luteal-phase inadequacy*). In an extremely rare but related disorder, the endometrium is unable to respond to secreted progesterone because of the absence of progesterone receptors. Any defect in follicular development or corpus luteum function could cause luteal-phase dysfunction. Such defects include but are not limited to inadequate or inappropriate FSH secretion in the follicular phase, inadequate or inappropriate estradiol secretion by granulosa cells, an inadequate LH surge, inadequate tonic LH secretion in the luteal phase, or defective progesterone secretion by luteal cells.[174] Evidence suggests that abnormalities in the frequency of gonadotropin pulses in the follicular phase account for most instances of luteal phase dysfunction.[175]

Clinical entities associated with luteal dysfunction include hyperprolactinemia (of any cause), strenuous physical exercise, inadequately treated 21-hydroxylase deficiency, and (presumably) recurrent abortion.[8,73,176,177] Luteal dysfunction is more common at the extremes of reproductive life and in the first menstrual cycles after delivery, abortion, and discontinuation of oral contraceptives. It can occur during ovulation induction with clomiphene citrate or hMG.[178,179]

Luteal-phase defects can be diagnosed by endometrial biopsy or from serial circulating progesterone or urinary pregnanediol determinations. Although fluctuations in basal body temperature have been used to diagnose luteal dysfunction, the technique is inaccurate. Endometrial biopsy specimens of the anterior uterine fundus in the late luteal phases (day 26) of two different cycles must be more than 2 days out of phase from the expected day of the menstrual cycle, as judged from the next menstrual period, for the diagnosis to be made. There is increasing evidence that more accurate dating can be achieved by counting forward from the LH surge.[180,181] Unfortunately, histologic dating of the endometrium is imprecise and inaccurate.[182–184] The absolute concentration that serum progesterone must achieve in the luteal phase to exclude luteal dysfunction is unclear, but a single value of 15 ng/mL or more precludes luteal dysfunction in most women. Endometrial biopsies and serum progesterone determinations together are probably complementary in establishing the diagnosis. In view of the inescapable conclusion that luteal phase dysfunction can occur in any single menstrual cycle by chance alone, it is important to reemphasize the need to document an abnormality in at least two cycles.

The treatment of luteal phase defects remains controversial. Any underlying defect, such as hyperprolactinemia, should be diagnosed and treated. Because subsequent luteal function depends on prior follicular development, modification of follicular development with clomiphene citrate (25 to 100 mg per day orally for 5 days, beginning on cycle day 3 to 5) is reasonable. Human chorionic gonadotropin (2500–5000 IU, given intramuscularly at 2- to 3-day intervals) or progesterone (12.5 mg, given intramuscularly in oil, or 25 mg twice daily as rectal or vaginal suppositories) beginning with the shift in basal body temperature also has been used. In general, synthetic progestational agents should not be used to treat luteal dysfunction, because these agents produce an abnormal endometrium. The potential teratogenicity of synthetic progestins also is undetermined. There is no good evidence that any treatment of luteal dysfunction increases the pregnancy rate. The treatment of early pregnancy with 17α-hydroxyprogesterone caproate (125 mg, given intramuscularly twice weekly) to prevent premature labor is also controversial.[185]

The *luteinized unruptured follicle syndrome* denotes the development of a follicle without subsequent disruption and ovum release.[186] The abnormality presumably can be diagnosed with ultrasound or from the absence of evidence of ovulation when the ovary is viewed at laparoscopy. Unfortunately, there is no direct evidence of a "trapped oocyte" within the follicle after diagnosis. Menstrual cycles in which no ovum is released should be characterized by biphasic basal body temperatures,

a normal LH surge, normal progesterone production in the luteal phase, and normal endometrial development. Because neither a corpus luteum nor signs of recent ovulation are always observed at laparoscopy, the existence of this disorder is presumptive even in the setting of considerable circumstantial evidence.[187] Ultrasound evidence suggests that luteinization of the unruptured follicle occurs uncommonly.[188] Should the disorder occur in repeated menstrual cycles, appropriate treatment may involve ovulation induction with exogenous gonadotropins.

## ABNORMAL GENITAL BLEEDING

Bleeding of presumed genital tract origin could also originate in the urinary or gastrointestinal tracts, and the source of the bleeding must be determined. Abnormal genital bleeding from organic causes occurs in ~25% of women. A functional abnormality of the hypothalamic–pituitary–ovarian axis, called *dysfunctional uterine bleeding*, exists in most women with abnormal genital bleeding. Dysfunctional uterine bleeding is anovulatory bleeding. No organic genital or extragenital cause can be demonstrated. However, the frequency of the various causes of abnormal genital bleeding varies with age. Dysfunctional uterine bleeding is more common early and late in the reproductive years. The frequency of organic causes, especially tumors, increases with advancing age.

Abnormal menstrual bleeding is generally described as excessive in duration or amount (i.e., *hypermenorrhea, menorrhagia*) or too frequent (i.e., *polymenorrhea*). Such bleeding may also occur intermenstrually (i.e., *metrorrhagia*). Postmenopausal uterine bleeding refers to any bleeding occurring 6 months or more after the last normal menstrual period at the menopause.

### PREPUBERTAL YEARS

Newborn girls sometimes spot for a few days after birth because of placental estrogenic stimulation of the endometrium in utero. Any other bleeding before puberty demands evaluation. Accidental trauma to the vulva or vagina is the most common cause of bleeding during childhood. Sexual abuse also must be considered. Vaginitis with spotting, most often because of irritation from a foreign body, may also occur. Prolapse of the urethral meatus and tumors of the genital tract must also be considered in the differential diagnosis of genital bleeding before puberty. For example, bleeding and vaginal discharge are the initial symptoms of most girls who have benign vaginal adenosis or clear cell adenocarcinoma of the vagina or cervix. These disorders have been linked to maternal ingestion of diethylstilbestrol during pregnancy and are diagnosed by Papanicolaou smear and colposcopically directed biopsy of suspicious areas.[189] Precocious puberty is a rare but real cause of bleeding in childhood and is generally recognized by the development of secondary sexual characteristics. If the bleeding is caused by ingestion of estrogen-containing drugs, there is rarely significant pubertal development.[190]

### REPRODUCTIVE YEARS

#### CAUSES OF BLEEDING

There are several causes of abnormal bleeding during the reproductive years:

Complications related to the use of hormonal contraceptive preparations
Complications related to pregnancy (i.e., threatened, incomplete, or missed abortion or ectopic pregnancy)
Coagulation disorders

Organic lesions of the genital tract, including intrauterine polyps, leiomyomas, and malignant tumors

Trauma (i.e., coital or other)

Foreign bodies

Systemic illnesses, including several endocrinopathies (i.e., diabetes mellitus, thyroid and adrenal disorders), leukemias, and renal and liver diseases.

Anovulatory or dysfunctional uterine bleeding is not infrequent in adolescents and in women in their fifth decade of life. Although perhaps one-half of menstrual cycles are anovulatory when menses begin, the incidence of dysfunctional bleeding in adolescents is low. Typically, anovulatory bleeding occurs at intervals longer than normal menstrual cycles, and bleeding from organic causes tends to occur more frequently than menstrual periods. In most cases, anovulatory bleeding resolves spontaneously. However, in a small number of adolescent girls and older women, anovulatory bleeding persists. For teenagers with continued bleeding, the eventual morbidity in terms of blood transfusions, operative procedures, and decreased reproductive potential is significant.[191] Older women frequently undergo hysterectomy if the bleeding cannot be controlled.

## EVALUATION OF ABNORMAL BLEEDING

All cases of abnormal genital bleeding demand evaluation, but treatment is not always necessary. A thorough history with emphasis on the pattern and quantity of bleeding is important, but most women are poor at estimating blood loss. All patients should be asked to keep a prospective menstrual calendar in which they record days and severity of bleeding. The normal volume of blood lost at each menses is ~30 mL; loss of more than 80 mL is abnormal.[192,193] Menses typically last 4 to 6 days, but normal menstrual flow may be as brief as 2 days or as long as 8 days. However, menses that commonly last 7 or more days warrant investigation. A pelvic examination is needed to rule out obvious organic causes.

Indicated laboratory tests include a complete blood cell count to assess hematologic status, a platelet count and other coagulation studies to rule out an underlying coagulation disorder, and thyroid function tests to rule out thyroid dysfunction. Dysfunctional uterine bleeding, although common, is a diagnosis of exclusion. An endometrial biopsy is indicated in any woman older than 35 years of age with abnormal uterine bleeding, a prolonged history of irregular bleeding, or severe bleeding.

## MANAGEMENT OF DYSFUNCTIONAL UTERINE BLEEDING

The management of dysfunctional bleeding depends on the severity of the problem, the age of the patient, and her desires regarding future fertility. Young affected women are treated much differently from those nearing the end of their reproductive years.

In young women in whom irregular bleeding is not a problem, reassurance and prospective charting of bleeding are indicated. In time, most adolescents begin or resume regular ovulatory menstrual cycles. In more severe cases, in which the bleeding has been more prolonged and erratic and there is some element of anemia but the hemoglobin is 10 g/dL or greater, therapy must be individualized. If the young woman is sexually active (but not pregnant), a progestin-dominant low-dose combined oral contraceptive agent can control the bleeding and provide contraception. Oral contraceptives can be used even if the patient is not sexually active. Alternatively, oral medroxyprogesterone acetate (5–10 mg daily) or micronized progesterone (200 mg daily) may be given for 12 to 14 days

every 30 to 60 days to induce intermittent "chemical curettage" and prevent chronic unopposed stimulation of the endometrium. Unfortunately, several months often are required before intermittent progestogens can control irregular uterine bleeding. Oral iron therapy is indicated for these women. Hormonal therapy may be discontinued in 6 months to 1 year. Most women have regular menses after therapy is stopped, but a thorough evaluation is warranted if irregular bleeding recurs.

In acute, severe menorrhagia (i.e., signs of acute blood loss and a hemoglobin level of <10 g/dL), blood transfusions may be necessary to restore hemodynamic homeostasis, but hormonal therapy is almost always effective in controlling the bleeding. The therapy of choice is a progestin-dominant low-dose combined oral contraceptive preparation at a dosage of one tablet every 6 hours. After bleeding stops, generally within 48 hours, the dosage may be tapered by reducing by one pill every other day. Withdrawal bleeding should be permitted after the dosage has been reduced to one tablet each day. The patient should then be maintained on oral contraceptives given in the usual fashion for 4 to 6 months. Oral contraceptives reduce menstrual bleeding by more than one-half in normal uteri.[194] Alternatively, high doses of conjugated estrogens (25 mg) can be given intravenously every 4 hours for a maximum of six doses.[195] Additional progestational therapy may be indicated initially to aid in stabilizing the endometrium. Norethindrone (5 mg orally four times each day) or medroxyprogesterone acetate (5–10 mg orally daily) should be given for 7 days with the onset of estrogen therapy. Withdrawal bleeding is then permitted, and oral contraceptives are administered in the standard manner for 4 to 6 months.

Neither high-dose estrogen nor progestin alone works effectively. The two hormones complement each other by promoting healing of and adding structural stability to the endometrium. If hormonal therapy cannot control the bleeding, the diagnosis of dysfunctional uterine bleeding is doubtful, and curettage is indicated.

Treatment of a woman older than 35 years of age with abnormal bleeding is more problematic. Organic causes of uterine bleeding are more common and mandate sampling of the endometrium. The risks of using oral contraceptives or estrogen to control the bleeding are increased because of the patient's age. Hormonal therapy with norethindrone or medroxyprogesterone acetate is a reasonable alternative. Curettage and hysterectomy are more common, particularly if the patient no longer desires childbearing. Endometrial ablation is also being carried out with increasing frequency, despite the absence of studies documenting long-term efficacy. In the future, GnRH analogs may be used to treat dysfunctional bleeding in all age groups.

Abundant data now document the efficacy of several medical therapies in the management of menorrhagia. Prostaglandin synthetase inhibitors decrease menstrual bleeding in a significant number of women and should be regarded as the first medications to use in those women who have no uterine abnormalities and are ovulatory but bleed heavily.[196,197] Side effects (e.g., nausea) are minimal because therapy is limited in duration, usually beginning with the onset of menses and continuing for 3 to 4 days. Such therapy also relieves other symptoms associated with menses. Danazol and inhibitors of fibrinolysis may also be effective but are not recommended or generally used because of significant side effects.[198] In comparative studies, the use of an intrauterine device that delivers progesterone or levonorgestrel to the endometrium in a local fashion is even more effective than prostaglandin synthetase inhibitors and antifibrinolytic agents.[198,199]

There is no role for the use of depot medroxyprogesterone acetate in the management of abnormal uterine bleeding. This is particularly true for the treatment of acute bleeding and for individuals in whom the cause of the bleeding has not been established. Although this agent may be effective in some women, the drug is also known to cause irregular bleeding and may compound the problem, especially because there is no effective therapy for drug-induced irregular bleeding. Other, more easily reversible forms of medical therapy are equally or more effective and should be used.

For reproductive-age women with irregular menses who desire childbearing, the use of clomiphene citrate to induce ovulation may be a reasonable alternative (see Chap. 97). An endometrial biopsy before therapy is indicated to eliminate the possibility of endometrial hyperplasia in women with a prolonged history of anovulation. Other causes of infertility should be considered as well (see Chap. 103). Simple and complex hyperplasia are reversible with adequate medical therapy. Progestins given continuously for 3 to 6 months or at intervals are appropriate, depending on the pathologic state of the endometrium. Therapy should be instituted only by individuals experienced in the treatment of these disorders.

More than one-half of functional ovarian cysts, most commonly follicular and corpus luteum cysts, incite some form of menstrual irregularity, ranging from amenorrhea to menorrhagia. In young women, it is common for cystic adnexal masses to disappear spontaneously. The administration of oral contraceptive agents for 1 to 2 months to suppress ovarian function has been advocated, but no data document that this approach effects resolution of the cyst.[200,201] Such ovarian suppression, however, should prevent development of other ovarian cysts. Adnexal masses more than 5 cm in diameter that persist for more than 1 to 2 months require surgical exploration to exclude a neoplasm. Although any ovarian tumor may cause abnormal uterine bleeding, bleeding is common only in endocrinologically active neoplasms. Transvaginal ultrasound is of value in distinguishing simple ovarian cysts from more complex masses; complex adnexal masses are much more apt to represent ovarian neoplasms.

Abnormal bleeding is also a common complaint of women using hormonal and other forms of contraception (see Chaps. 104 and 105). It is debated whether the incidence of menstrual irregularity is increased after tubal ligation (see Chap. 104). Thyroid dysfunction may cause any disorder of bleeding, ranging from amenorrhea to menorrhagia.

### POSTMENOPAUSAL YEARS

Any woman with genital bleeding in the postmenopausal years must be evaluated for a malignancy. Most causes of such bleeding are benign and include atrophic vaginitis, an atrophic endometrium, endometrial polyps, and endometrial hyperplasia. The finding of hyperplasia should lead to a search for a source of estrogen, from exogenous therapy or from an endogenous (commonly ovarian) neoplasm. Most cases of endometrial hyperplasia respond to progestational therapy, but hysterectomy may be preferred to exclude any possibility of recurrence.

Ovarian cysts occasionally occur even in postmenopausal women. Cysts that are less than 5 cm in diameter and do not contain any septations or solid components on ultrasound examination appear to have a very low potential for malignancy and may be observed serially by ultrasound scanning. Any increase in size necessitates surgical intervention. Such cysts are not commonly associated with bleeding, but data on this subject remain scanty.

## DYSMENORRHEA

Dysmenorrhea is the most common of all gynecologic disorders, affecting perhaps 50% of postpubescent women.[202] Dysmenorrhea is classified as primary or secondary. In primary dysmenorrhea, no pathologic cause for the pain can be identified. It occurs only in ovulatory menstrual cycles and may be more prevalent in women with the premenstrual syndrome (see Chap. 99). The pathogenesis of the dysmenorrhea is related to the prostaglandins that are released from the endometrium just before and during menstruation. The prostaglandins appar-

ently cause dysmenorrhea by inducing painful, exaggerated uterine contractions with myometrial ischemia. Associated systemic symptoms may include nausea, diarrhea, headache, and emotional changes.

Secondary dysmenorrhea has a pathologic cause for the discomfort. In severe cases, endometriosis is the most common cause. Other causes include pelvic inflammatory disease, congenital anomalies such as genital atresia and cystic duplication of the paramesonephric ducts, and cervical stenosis.

Treatment for dysmenorrhea begins with the use of prostaglandin synthetase inhibitors such as ibuprofen, mefenamic acid, indomethacin, and naproxen.[203] If the dysmenorrhea is incapacitating despite such therapy, an oral contraceptive agent should be added to inhibit ovulation and prostaglandin release. If intractable pain continues, additional evaluation is indicated. If thorough evaluation of the gastrointestinal and urinary tracts, including radiologic studies, fails to reveal a definitive cause, examination with the patient under anesthesia and diagnostic laparoscopy may be warranted.

Further treatment varies according to the diagnosis established. If endometriosis is diagnosed at laparoscopy, the treatment depends on the severity of the disease and the fertility goals of the patient (see Chap. 98). It may be possible to fulgurate implants or lyse adhesions through a laparoscope. In general, endometriosis should be treated medically, with any additional surgery deferred until fertility (if desired) becomes a problem. However, earlier surgery may be required for unrelenting pain, severe endometriosis, or ovarian cysts containing endometriosis (i.e., endometriomas).

Psychiatric evaluation is warranted if the dysmenorrhea continues despite adequate therapy or if psychologic overlay is apparent.[204] All medical causes of dysmenorrhea, however, should be identified and treated before the pain is viewed as psychologic only.

## IDIOPATHIC OR CYCLIC EDEMA

Idiopathic or cyclical edema, also called *periodic edema* or "swelling," occurs almost exclusively in adult women. It is characterized by excessive diurnal weight gain with development of peripheral edema when the patient is in the upright position.[205,206] It is more common in obese women and occurs in the absence of demonstrable cardiac, hepatic, or renal disease or abnormalities in serum protein levels. Idiopathic edema is often associated with headache, increased irritability, and depression and appears to occur more frequently just before menses. Because idiopathic edema is a diagnosis that was made much more commonly previously, it is possible that this disorder is a part of the syndrome comprising premenstrual tension (see Chap. 99). This possibility is made more likely by the observation that patients with significant periodic edema often have severe psychologic disturbances.

The essential pathophysiologic defect appears to be an abnormally great leakage of plasma from the intravascular compartment on standing. The hematocrit increases rapidly. The fall in plasma volume is compensated for by appropriate renal conservation of sodium as a result of increased reabsorption in the proximal tubules. Reduced urine output has been attributed to increased secretion of antidiuretic hormone.

The treatment of idiopathic edema frequently is unsatisfactory but should include a full explanation, weight reduction, moderate sodium restriction, psychiatric assessment, no smoking, and avoidance of prolonged standing. A mild diuretic may be added during episodes of fluid retention if these other measures are ineffective. However, the symptoms of idiopathic edema are frequently accentuated by the hypokalemia, hypomagnesemia, and postural hypotension that may accompany excessive use of diuretics.[207,208] The disorder usually is self-limited. It may persist for a few months or for as long as 25 years.[209]

## SEXUAL FUNCTION AND DYSFUNCTION

In women, complete sexual responses begin after puberty and can continue for the remainder of life. Sexual responses can be divided into four stages: excitement, plateau, orgasm, and resolution.[210,211] Visual, tactile, auditory, and olfactory stimuli lead to physical and emotional excitement and genital vasodilation in the responsive individual. Vasodilation of the blood vessels in the labia and tissues surrounding the vagina occurs with localized perivaginal edema and subsequent vaginal lubrication, followed by ballooning and expansion of the vagina and elevation of the uterus. A high state of sexual arousal is maintained during the plateau phase, which may be short or long. A brief series of involuntary, 0.9-second clonic contractions of the ischiocavernosus and pubococcygeal muscles occurs with orgasm or "climax." Although some women may resolve toward sleep after orgasm, many remain responsive to sexual stimulation and may undergo orgasm again with continued arousal.

Extragenital changes occur during sexual arousal as well, and responses may vary over time. Changes may occur in the breasts, with flushing and erection of the nipples. In some women, orgasm may be explosive and occur together with vocalization, and a few women may never experience orgasm. In many women, orgasm is intermittently absent. The intensity or even the presence of orgasm may be irrelevant to the satisfaction of the individual.

Sexual dysfunction may cause a woman to seek professional assistance or may be elicited or suspected when a patient has a complaint for which no abnormality is apparent.[212–215] A sexual dysfunction may be lifelong or may be acquired after a period of normal sexual function. It may affect both partners or only one, and it may be psychologic or physical.

In most cases in which a woman complains of sexual dysfunction, the problem is the result of interpersonal difficulties with her partner. For example, many instances of sexual incompatibility are based on insufficient foreplay. Psychic problems affecting sexual function may stem from past traumatic events in the life of a woman, including rape. Abnormalities of the reproductive organs may be viewed as a threat to normal reproductive functioning by some women. Avoidance of sex and unpleasant sexual experiences are seen frequently in women with debilitating or painful psychologic or somatic illnesses. Almost any chronic illness may affect sexual functioning adversely, directly by affecting neural and vascular pathways important in sexual arousal or indirectly by inhibiting the desire or the ability to respond to sexual stimuli. Any of various pelvic disorders, including vaginitis, cystitis, ovarian cysts, endometriosis, pelvic inflammatory disease, and uterine prolapse, may lead to dyspareunia and avoidance of sex. Mastectomy and hysterectomy may cause psychologic difficulties that interfere with sexual arousal. A variety of diseases affecting neurologic function, including diabetes mellitus and multiple sclerosis, also may prevent sexual arousal.

Women may vary in their sexual responsiveness through the menstrual cycle. Women appear to be more responsive at midcycle, and some women have an increased desire for sex just before the onset of menstruation. Pregnancy usually has no physical effect on sexual desire but may impair sexual relations because of resulting psychologic fears. Aging may affect sexual responsiveness as well. Menopause should not lead to any physiologic change in interest in sex, but some women may notice increased interest because they are no longer fearful of pregnancy. Alternatively, estrogen deficiency may lead to vaginal atrophy and dyspareunia and consequent sexual avoidance (see Chap. 100).

Several types of sexual dysfunction exist.[216] Commonly, the loss of desire is psychologic. Dyspareunia may be caused by inadequate vaginal lubrication because of sexual avoidance or inadequate arousal. Vaginismus involves involuntary contractions of the muscles surrounding the introitus and leads to dys-

pareunia or avoidance of penetration. Vaginismus is often a response conditioned by a previous imagined or real traumatic sexual experience. Failure to become excited has been discussed already. Failure to achieve orgasm should be viewed as a dysfunction if, as a result, the woman is frustrated or dissatisfied.

Management of patients with sexual dysfunction is best accomplished by eliminating organic causes and providing the patient, frequently together with her partner, with appropriate counseling. Behavior modification aimed at eliminating the emotional problems inhibiting appropriate sexual responses is often used.[213,214] A physician must show a nonjudgmental attitude in dealing with problems of sexual function. Treatment of sexual dysfunction is most often successful if patients and physicians establish definitive treatment objectives.

It is important to discuss sexual functioning with those who are physically disabled. A wide range of oral and manual sexual expressions are alternatives if they are not viewed as abnormal or unacceptable by the participants. There need be no handicap that precludes sexual satisfaction, and appropriate alternatives should be outlined for the handicapped.

## REFERENCES

1. Bardin CW, Lipsett MB. Testosterone and androstenedione blood production rates in normal women and women with idiopathic hirsutism or polycystic ovaries. J Clin Invest 1967; 46:891.
2. Marshall WA, Tanner JM. Variations in patterns of pubertal changes in girls. Arch Dis Child 1969; 44:291.
3. Tagatz GE, Kopher RA, Nagel TC, Okagaki T. The clitoral index: a bioassay of androgenic stimulation. Obstet Gynecol 1979; 54:562.
4. Pinsky L. A community of human malformation syndromes involving the müllerian ducts, distal extremities, urinary tract and ears. Teratology 1974; 9:65.
5. Page EW, Owsley JQ Jr. Surgical correction of vaginal agenesis. Am J Obstet Gynecol 1969; 105:774.
6. Wabrek AJ, Millard PR, Wilson WB Jr, Pion RJ. Creation of a neovagina by the Frank nonoperative method. Obstet Gynecol 1971; 37:408.
7. Asherman JG. Amenorrhea traumatica (atretica). J Obstet Gynaecol Br Emp 1948; 55:23.
8. Molitch ME, Reichlin S. Hyperprolactinemic disorders. Dis Mon 1982; 28:1.
9. Manuel M, Katayama KP, Jones HW Jr. The age of occurrence of gonadal tumors in intersex patients with a Y chromosome. Am J Obstet Gynecol 1976; 124:293.
10. Yen SSC. The polycystic ovary. Clin Endocrinol (Oxf) 1980; 12:177.
11. Rebar RW, Judd HL, Yen SSC, et al. Characterization of the inappropriate gonadotropin secretion in polycystic ovary syndrome. J Clin Invest 1976; 57:1320.
12. Rebar RW. Practical evaluation of hormonal status. In: Yen SSC, Jaffe RB, eds. Reproductive endocrinology, physiology, pathophysiology, and clinical management, 2nd ed. Philadelphia: WB Saunders, 1986:683.
13. Rebar RW, Erickson GF, Coulam CB. Premature ovarian failure. In: Gondos B, Riddick D, eds. Pathology of infertility. New York: Thieme Medical Publishers, 1987:123.
14. Singh RP, Carr DH. The anatomy and histology of XO human embryos and fetuses. Anat Rec 1966; 155:369.
15. Reyes FI, Koh KS, Faiman C. Fertility in women with gonadal dysgenesis. Am J Obstet Gynecol 1976; 126:668.
16. Block E. Quantitative morphological investigations of the follicular system in women: variations at different ages. Acta Anat 1952; 14:108.
17. Block E. A quantitative morphological investigation of the follicular system in newborn female infants. Acta Anat 1953; 17:201.
18. Harper PS, Dyken PR. Early onset dystrophica myotonia. Lancet 1972; 2:53.
19. Villanueva AL, Rebar RW. The triple X syndrome and premature ovarian failure. Obstet Gynecol 1983; 62:70S.
20. Mattison DR, Evans MI, Schwimmer WB, et al. Familial premature ovarian failure. Am J Hum Genet 1984; 36:1341.
21. Biglieri EG, Herron MA, Brust N. 17-Hydroxylation deficiency in man. J Clin Invest 1966; 45:1946.
22. Goldsmith O, Solomon DH, Horton R. Hypogonadism and mineralocorticoid excess: the 17-hydroxylase deficiency syndrome. N Engl J Med 1967; 277:673.
23. Mallin SR. Congenital adrenal hyperplasia secondary to 17-hydroxylase deficiency: two sisters with amenorrhea, hypokalemia, hypertension, and cystic ovaries. Ann Intern Med 1969; 70:69.
24. Rabinovici J, Blankstein J, Goldman B, et al. In vitro fertilization and primary embryonic cleavage are possible in 17α-hydroxylase deficiency despite extremely low intrafollicular 17β-estradiol. J Clin Endocrinol Metab 1989; 68:693.
25. Kaufman FR, Kogut MD, Donnel GN, et al. Hypergonadotropic hypogonadism in female patients with galactosemia. N Engl J Med 1981; 304:994.
26. Aittomaki K, Dieguez Luccena JL, Pakarinen P, et al. Mutation in the follicle-stimulating hormone receptor gene causes hereditary hypergonadotropic ovarian failure. Cell 1995; 82:959.

27. Aittomaki K, Herva R, Stenman UH, et al. Clinical features of primary ovarian failure caused by a point mutation in the follicle-stimulating hormone receptor gene. J Clin Endocrinol Metab 1996; 81:3722.
28. Layman LC, Amede S, Cohen DP, et al. The Finnish follicle-stimulating hormone receptor gene mutation is rare in North American women with 46,XX ovarian failure. Fertil Steril 1998; 69:300.
29. Liu JY, Gromoll J, Cedars MI. Identification of allelic variants in the follicle-stimulating hormone receptor genes of females with or without hypergonadotropic amenorrhea. Fertil Steril 1998; 70:326.
30. Jones GS, de Moraes-Ruehsen M. A new syndrome of amenorrhea in association with hypergonadotropism and apparently normal ovarian follicular apparatus. Am J Obstet Gynecol 1969; 104:597.
30a. van Kasteren YM, von Blomberg M, Hoek A, et al. Incipient ovarian failure and premature ovarian failure show the same immunological profile. Am J Reprod Immunol 2000; 43:359.
31. Drury MI, Keelán DM, Timoney FJ, Irvine WJ. Juvenile familial endocrinopathy. Clin Exp Immunol 1970; 7:125.
32. Chiauzzi V, Cigorraga S, Escobar ME, et al. Inhibition of follicle-stimulating hormone receptor binding by circulating immunoglobulins. J Clin Endocrinol Metab 1982; 54:1221.
33. van Weissenbruch MM, Hoek A, van Vliet-Bleeker I, et al. Evidence for existence of immunoglobulins that block ovarian granulosa cell growth in vitro. A putative role in resistant ovary syndrome. J Clin Endocrinol Metab 1991; 73:360.
34. Rebar RW. The thymus gland and reproduction: do thymic peptides influence reproductive lifespan in females? J Am Geriatr Soc 1982; 30:603.
35. Miller ME, Chatten J. Ovarian changes in ataxia telangiectasia. Acta Paediatr Scand 1967; 56:559.
36. Jacox HW. Recovery following human ovarian irradiation. Radiology 1939; 32:538.
37. Siris ES, Leventhal BG, Vaitukaitis JL. Effects of childhood leukemia and chemotherapy on puberty and reproductive function in girls. N Engl J Med 1976; 294:1143.
38. Koyama H, Wada J, Nishizawa Y, et al. Cyclophosphamide-induced failure and its therapeutic significance in patients with breast cancer. Cancer 1977; 39:1403.
39. Ataya KM, McKenna JA, Weintraub AM, et al. Treatment with LHRH agonist prevents chemotherapy induced follicular loss in rats. In: Abstracts of the 32nd annual meeting of the Society for Gynecologic Investigation, Arizona, 1985; 260.
40. Morrison JC, Givens JR, Wiser WL, Fish SA. Mumps oophoritis: a cause of premature menopause. Fertil Steril 1975; 26:655.
41. Jick H, Porter J, Morrison AS. Relation between smoking and age of natural menopause. Lancet 1977; 1:1354.
42. Cann CE, Martin MC, Genant HK, Jaffe RB. Decreased spinal mineral content in amenorrheic women. JAMA 1984; 251:626.
43. Lutjen P, Trounson A, Leeton J, et al. The establishment and maintenance of pregnancy using in vitro fertilization and embryo donation in a patient with primary ovarian failure. Nature 1984; 307:174.
44. Rebar RW, Cedars MI. Hypergonadotropic amenorrhea. In: Filicori M, Flamigni C, eds. Ovulation induction. Basic science and clinical advances. Amsterdam: Elsevier Science, 1994:115.
45. Fries HS, Nillius SJ, Petterson F. Epidemiology of secondary amenorrhea: II. A retrospective evaluation of etiology with special regard to psychogenic factors and weight loss. Am J Obstet Gynecol 1974; 118:473.
46. Warren MP. The effects of altered nutritional states, stress, and systemic illness on reproduction in women. In: Vaitukaitis J, ed. Clinical reproductive neuroendocrinology. New York: Elsevier Biomedical, 1981:177.
47. Rebar RW. The reproductive age: chronic anovulation. In: Serra GB, ed. The ovary. New York: Raven Press, 1983:217.
48. Klinefelter HF, Albright F Jr, Griswold GC. Experience with a quantitative test for normal or decreased amounts of follicle-stimulating hormone in the urine in endocrinological diagnosis. J Clin Endocrinol Metab 1943; 3:529.
49. Berga S, Mortola J, Gierton L, et al. Neuroendocrine aberrations in women with functional hypothalamic amenorrhea. J Clin Endocrinol Metab 1989; 68:301.
50. Suh BY, Liu JH, Berga SL, et al. Hypercortisolism in patients with functional hypothalamic-amenorrhea. J Clin Endocrinol Metab 1988; 66:733.
51. Bruch H. Perceptual and conceptual disturbances of anorexia nervosa. Psychosom Med 1962; 24:187.
52. Feighner JP, Robins E, Guze SB, et al. Diagnostic criteria for use in psychiatric research. Arch Gen Psychiatry 1972; 26:57.
53. Spitzer R, ed. Diagnostic and statistical manual of mental disorders, 4th ed.: American Psychiatric Association, 1994:53.
54. Vigersky RA, Loriaux DL, Andersen MB. Anorexia nervosa: behavioral and hypothalamic aspects. Clin Endocrinol (Oxf) 1976; 5:517.
55. Vigersky RA, Loriaux DL, Andersen AE, et al. Delayed pituitary hormone response to LRF and TRF in patients with anorexia nervosa and with secondary amenorrhea associated with simple weight loss. J Clin Endocrinol Metab 1976; 43:893.
56. Boyar R, Rosenfeld R, Kapen S, et al. Simultaneous augmented secretion of luteinizing hormone and testosterone during sleep. J Clin Invest 1974; 54:609.
57. Sherman BM, Halmi KA, Zamudio R. LH and FSH response to gonadotropin-releasing hormone in anorexia nervosa: effect of nutritional rehabilitation. J Clin Endocrinol Metab 1975; 41:135.
58. Katz JL, Boyar R, Roffwarg H, et al. Weight and circadian luteinizing hormone secretory pattern in anorexia nervosa. Psychosom Med 1978; 40:549.
59. Warren MP, Jewelewicz R, Dyrenfurth I, et al. The significance of weight loss in the evaluation of pituitary response to hypothalamic releasing hormones in patients with anorexia nervosa. J Clin Endocrinol Metab 1975; 40:601.
60. Marshall JC, Kelch RP. Low dose pulsatile gonadotropin-releasing hormone in anorexia nervosa: a model of human pubertal development. J Clin Endocrinol Metab 1979; 49:712.
61. Fishman J, Boyar RM, Hellman L. Influence of body weight on estradiol metabolism in young women. J Clin Endocrinol Metab 1975; 41:989.
62. Fries H. Studies on secondary amenorrhea, anorectic behavior, and body-image perception: importance for the early recognition of anorexia nervosa. In: Vigersky RA, ed. Anorexia nervosa. New York: Raven Press, 1977:163.
63. Mecklenberg RS, Loriaux DL, Thompson RH, et al. Hypothalamic dysfunction in patients with anorexia nervosa. Medicine (Baltimore) 1974; 53:147.
64. Warren MP, VandeWiele RL. Clinical and metabolic features of anorexia nervosa. Am J Obstet Gynecol 1973; 117:435.
65. Burman KD, Vigersky RA, Loriaux DL, et al. Investigations concerning thyroxine deiodinative pathways in patients with anorexia nervosa. In: Vigersky RA, ed. Anorexia nervosa. New York: Raven Press, 1977:255.
66. Boyar RM, Hellman LD, Roffwarg H, et al. Cortisol secretion and metabolism in anorexia nervosa. N Engl J Med 1977; 296:190.
67. Casper RC, Chatterton RT Jr, Davis JM. Alterations in serum cortisol and its binding characteristics in anorexia nervosa. J Clin Endocrinol Metab 1979; 49:406.
68. Takahara J, Hosogi H, Yunoki S, et al. Hypothalamic pituitary adrenal function in patients with anorexia nervosa. Endocrinol Jpn 1976; 23:451.
69. Gold PW, Gwirtsman H, Avgerinos PC, et al. Abnormal hypothalamic-pituitary-adrenal function in anorexia nervosa: pathophysiologic mechanisms in underweight and weight-corrected patients. N Engl J Med 1986; 314:1335.
70. Vigersky RA, Andersen AE, Thompson RH, Loriaux DL. Hypothalamic dysfunction in secondary amenorrhea associated with simple weight loss. N Engl J Med 1977; 297:1141.
71. Van der Walt LA, Wilmsen EN, Jenkins T. Unusual sex hormone patterns among desert-dwelling hunter-gatherers. J Clin Endocrinol Metab 1978; 46:658.
72. Rebar RW, Cumming DC. Reproductive function in women athletes. JAMA 1981; 246:1590.
73. Cumming DC, Rebar RW. Exercise and reproductive function in women: a review. Am J Ind Med 1983; 4:113.
74. American College of Sports Medicine. The female athlete triad: disordered eating, amenorrhea, and osteoporosis. Call to action. Sports Med Bull 1992; 27:4.
74a. Hobart JA, Smucker DR. The female athlete triad. Am Fam Physician 2000; 61:3357, 3367.
75. Bullen BA, Skrinar GS, Beitins IZ, et al. Induction of menstrual disorders by strenuous exercise in untrained women. N Engl J Med 1985; 312:1349.
76. Beitins IZ, McArthur JW, Turnbull BA, et al. Exercise induces two types of human luteal dysfunction: confirmation by urinary free progesterone. J Clin Endocrinol Metab 1991; 72:1350.
77. Rogol AD, Weltman A, Weltman JY, et al. Durability of the reproductive axis in eumenorrheic women during 1 year of endurance training. J Appl Physiol 1992; 72:1571.
78. Drinkwater BL, Nilson K, Chestnut CH III, et al. Bone mineral content of amenorrheic and eumenorrheic athletes. N Engl J Med 1984; 311:277.
79. Marcus R, Cann C, Madvig P, et al. Menstrual function and bone mass in elite women distance runners. Ann Intern Med 1985; 102:158.
80. Snead DB, Weltman A, Weltman JY, et al. Reproductive hormones and bone mineral density in women runners. J Appl Physiol 1992; 72:2149.
81. Myerson M, Gutin B, Warren MP, et al. Total body bone density in amenorrheic runners. Obstet Gynecol 1992; 79:973.
82. Jonnavithula S, Warren MP, Fox RP, Lazaro MI. Bone density is compromised in amenorrheic women despite return of menses. A 2-year study. Obstet Gynecol 1993; 81:669.
83. Schwartz B, Cumming DC, Riordan E, et al. Exercise-associated amenorrhea: a distinct entity? Am J Obstet Gynecol 1981; 141:662.
84. Warren MP. The effects of exercise on pubertal progression and reproductive function in girls. J Clin Endocrinol Metab 1980; 51:1150.
85. Villanueva AL, Schlosser C, Hopper B, et al. Increased cortisol production in women runners. J Clin Endocrinol Metab 1986; 63:126.
86. Loucks AB, Mortola JF, Girton L, Yen SSC. Alterations in the hypothalamic–pituitary–ovarian and the hypothalamic pituitary-adrenal axes in athletic women. J Clin Endocrinol Metab 1989; 68:402.
87. Loucks AB, Laughlin GA, Mortola JF, et al. Hypothalamic-pituitary-thyroidal function in eumenorrheic and amenorrheic athletes. J Clin Endocrinol Metab 1992; 75:514.
88. Yen SSC, Rebar R, VandenBerg G, Judd H. Hypothalamic amenorrhea and hypogonadotropinism: responses to synthetic LRF. J Clin Endocrinol Metab 1973; 36:811.
89. Lachelin GCL, Yen SSC. Hypothalamic chronic anovulation. Am J Obstet Gynecol 1978; 130:825.
90. Matsumoto S, Tamada T, Konuma S. Endocrinological analysis of environmental menstrual disorders. Int J Fertil 1979; 24:233.
91. Nillius SJ, Wide L. The LH-releasing hormone test in 31 women with secondary amenorrhea. Br J Obstet Gynaecol 1972; 79:874.
92. Vaitukaitis J, Becker R, Hansen J, Mecklenburg R. Altered LRF responsiveness in amenorrheic women. J Clin Endocrinol Metab 1974; 39:1005.
93. Keller E, Dahlén HG, Friedrich E, et al. Human pituitary gonadotropin index. I. Standardized LRH test criteria for evaluation of functional amenorrhea. J Clin Endocrinol Metab 1975; 40:959.

94. Santen RJ, Friend JN, Trojanoweki D, et al. Prolonged negative feedback suppression after estradiol administration: proposed mechanism of eugonadal secondary amenorrhea. J Clin Endocrinol Metab 1978; 47:1220.

95. Shaw RW, Butt WR, London DR. Pathological mechanisms to explain some cases of amenorrhea without organic disease. Br J Obstet Gynaecol 1975; 82:337.

96. Sherman BM, West JH, Zamudio R. Serum estradiol response to gonadotropin-releasing hormone: studies in normal women and in women with secondary amenorrhea. Fertil Steril 1976; 27:250.

97. Rakoff JS, Rigg LA, Yen SSC. The impairment of progesterone-induced pituitary release of prolactin and gonadotropin in patients with hypothalamic chronic anovulation. Am J Obstet Gynecol 1978; 130:807.

98. Suh BY, Liu JH, Berga SL, et al. College amenorrhea: aberrations of circadian and pulsatile secretory patterns of cortisol and luteinizing hormone. J Clin Endocrinol Metab 1988; 66:733.

99. Sachar EJ, Hellman L, Roffwarg H, et al. Disrupted 24 hour patterns of cortisol secretion in psychotic depression. Arch Gen Psychiatry 1973; 28:19.

100. Carroll BJ, Mendels J. Neuroendocrine regulation in affective disorders. In: Sachar EJ, ed. Hormones, behavior, and psychopathology. New York: Raven Press, 1976.

101. Amsterdam JD, Winokur A, Abelman E, et al. Cosyntropin (ACTH $\alpha_{1-24}$) stimulation test in depressed patients and healthy subjects. Am J Psychiatry 1983; 140:907.

102. Quigley ME, Sheenah KL, Casper RF, Yen SSC. Evidence for increased dopaminergic and opioid activity in patients with hypothalamic hypogonadotropic amenorrhea. J Clin Endocrinol Metab 1908; 50:949.

103. Ballenger JC, Post RM, Jimerson DC, et al. Biochemical correlates of personality traits in normals: an exploratory study. Personality Individ Differ 1983; 4:615.

104. Brown E, Bain J, Lerner P, Shaul D. Psychological, hormonal, and weight disturbances in functional amenorrhea. Am J Psychiatry 1983; 28:624.

105. Astor J, Pawson M. The value of psychometric testing in the investigation of infertility. J Psychosom Obstet Gynecol 1985; 5:107.

106. Osofsky HS, Fisher S. Psychological correlates of the development of amenorrhea in a stress situation. Psychosom Med 1967; 29:15.

107. Schreiber C, Florin I, Rost W. Psychological correlates of functional secondary amenorrhea. Psychother Psychosom 1983; 39:106.

108. Fava GA, Trombini G, Grandi S, et al. Depression and anxiety associated with secondary amenorrhea. Psychosomatics 1984; 25:905.

109. Drew FL, Seifel EN. Secondary amenorrhea among young women entering religious life. Obstet Gynecol 1968; 32:47.

110. Liu JH, Yen SSC. The use of gonadotropin-releasing hormone for the induction of ovulation. Clin Obstet Gynecol 1984; 27:975.

111. Martin K, Santoro N, Hall J, et al. Management of ovulatory disorders with pulsatile gonadotropin-releasing hormone. J Clin Endocrinol Metab 1990; 71:1081A.

112. Kallmann FJ, Schoenfeld WA, Barrera SE. The genetic aspects of primary eunuchoidism. Am J Ment Defic 1944; 48:203.

113. Odell WD. Isolated deficiencies of anterior pituitary hormones: symptoms and diagnosis. JAMA 1966; 197:1006.

114. Rosen SW. The syndrome of hypogonadism, anosmia and mid-line cranial anomalies. In: Abstracts of the 47th annual meeting of The Endocrine Society, 1965.

115. Spitz IM, Diamant Y, Rosen E, et al. Isolated gonadotropin deficiency: a heterogeneous syndrome. N Engl J Med 1974; 290:10.

116. Tagatz G, Fialkow PJ, Smith D, Spadoni L. Hypogonadotropic hypogonadism associated with anosmia in the female. N Engl J Med 1970; 283:1326.

117. De Morsier G. Etudes sur les dysraphies crânio-encéphaliques. 1. Agénésie des lobes olfactifs (télencéphaloschizis latéral) et des commissures calleuses et antérieures (télencéphaloschizis médian) la dysplasie olfacto-génitale. Schweiz Arch Neurol Psychiatr 1954; 74:309.

118. Schwanzel-Fukuda M, Pfaff DU. Origin of luteinizing hormone-releasing hormone neurons. Nature 1989; 338:161.

119. Klingmuller D, Dewes W, Krahe T, et al. Magnetic resonance imaging of the brain in patients with anosmia and hypothalamic hypogonadism (Kallmann's syndrome). J Clin Endocrinol Metab 1987; 65:581.

120. Goldenberg RL, Powell RD, Rosen SW, et al. Ovarian morphology in women with anosmia and hypogonadotropic hypogonadism. Am J Obstet Gynecol 1976; 126:91.

121. Crowley WF Jr, McArthur JW. Simulation of the normal menstrual cycle in Kallmann's syndrome by pulsatile administration of luteinizing hormone-releasing hormone (LHRH). J Clin Endocrinol Metab 1980; 51:173.

122. Leyendecker G, Struve T, Plotz EJ. Induction of ovulation with chronic intermittent administration of LHRH in women with hypothalamic and hyperprolactinemic amenorrhea. In: Abstracts of the 61st annual meeting of The Endocrine Society, 1979.

123. Yen SSC, Rebar RW, VandenBerg G, et al. Pituitary gonadotropin responsiveness to synthetic LRF in subjects with normal and abnormal hypothalamic-pituitary-gonadal axis. J Reprod Fertil 1973; 20:137.

124. Yeh J, Rebar RW, Liu JH, Yen SSC. Pituitary function in isolated gonadotropin deficiency. Clin Endocrinol 1989; 31:375.

125. Lachelin GCL, Abu-Fadil S, Yen SSC. Functional delineation of hyperprolactinemic-amenorrhea. J Clin Endocrinol Metab 1977; 44:1163.

126. Klibanski A, Neer RM, Beitins IZ, et al. Decreased bone density in hyperprolactinemic women. N Engl J Med 1980; 303:1511.

127. Leblanc H, Lachelin GC, Abu-Fadil S, Yen SSC. Effects of dopamine infusion on pituitary hormone secretion in humans. J Clin Endocrinol Metab 1976; 43:668.

128. Board JA, Storlazzi E, Schneider V. Nocturnal prolactin levels in infertility. Fertil Steril 1983; 36:720.

129. DeVane GW, Gusick DS. Bromocriptine therapy in normoprolactinemic women with unexplained infertility and galactorrhea. Fertil Steril 1986; 46:1026.

130. Suginami H, Hamada K, Yano K, et al. Ovulation induction with bromocriptine in normoprolactinemic anovulatory women. J Clin Endocrinol Metab 1986; 62:899.

131. Sheehan HL, Davis JC. Pituitary necrosis. Br Med Bull 1968; 24:59.

132. Stein IF, Leventhal ML. Amenorrhea associated with bilateral polycystic ovaries. Am J Obstet Gynecol 1935; 29:181.

133. DeVane GW, Czekala NM, Judd HL, Yen SSC. Circulating gonadotropins, estrogens, and androgens in polycystic ovarian disease. Am J Obstet Gynecol 1975; 121:496.

134. Buckler HM, McLachlan RI, MacLachlan VB, et al. Serum inhibin levels in polycystic ovary syndrome: basal levels and response to luteinizing hormone-releasing hormone agonist and exogenous gonadotropin administration. J Clin Endocrinol Metab 1988; 66:798.

134a. Conn JJ, Jacobs HS, Conway GS. The prevalence of polycystic ovaries in women with type 2 diabetes mellitus. Clin Endocrinol 2000; 52:81.

135. Zawadzki JK, Dunaif. Diagnostic criteria for polycystic ovary syndrome: towards a rational approach. In: Dunaif A, Givens JR, Haseltine F, Merriam GR, eds. Polycystic ovary syndrome. Boston: Blackwell Scientific, 1992:377.

136. Hull MGR. Epidemiology of infertility and polycystic ovarian disease: endocrinological and demographic studies. Gynecol Endocrinol 1987; 1:235.

137. Knochenhauer ES, Key TJ, Kahsar-Miller M, et al. Prevalence of the polycystic ovarian syndrome in unselected black and white women of the southeastern United States: a prospective study. J Clin Endocrinol Metab 1998; 83:3078.

138. Franks S, Gharani N, Waterworth D. The genetic basis of polycystic ovary syndrome. Hum Reprod 1997; 12:2641.

139. Legro RS, Driscoll D, Strauss JF III, et al. Evidence for a genetic basis for hyperandrogenemia in polycystic ovary syndrome. Proc Natl Acad Sci U S A 1998; 95:14956.

140. Taylor SI, Dons RF, Hernandez E, et al. Insulin resistance associated with androgen excess in women with autoantibodies to the insulin receptor. Ann Intern Med 1982; 97:851.

141. Bar RS, Muggeo M, Roth J, et al. Insulin resistance, acanthosis nigricans, and normal insulin receptors in a young woman: evidence for a postreceptor defect. J Clin Endocrinol Metab 1978; 47:620.

142. Erickson GF, Hsueh AJW, Quigley ME, et al. Functional studies of aromatase activity in human granulosa cells from normal and polycystic ovaries. J Clin Endocrinol Metab 1979; 49:514.

143. Goldzieher JW, Axelrod LR. Clinical and biochemical features of polycystic ovarian disease. Fertil Steril 1963; 14:631.

144. Burghen GA, Givens JR, Kitabchi AE. Correlation of hyperandrogenism with hyperinsulinism in polycystic ovarian disease. J Clin Endocrinol Metab 1980; 50:113.

145. Chang RJ, Nakamura RM, Judd HL, Kaplan SA. Insulin resistance in non-obese patients with polycystic ovarian disease. J Clin Endocrinol Metab 1983; 57:356.

146. Carmina E, Koyama T, Chang L, et al. Does ethnicity influence the prevalence of adrenal hyperandrogenism and insulin resistance in polycystic ovary syndrome? Am J Obstet Gynecol 1992; 167:1807.

147. Dunaif A. Insulin resistance and the polycystic ovary syndrome: mechanism and implications for pathogenesis. Endocr Rev 1997; 18:774.

148. Geffner ME, Kaplan SA, Bersch N, et al. Persistence of insulin resistance in polycystic ovarian disease after inhibition of ovarian sex steroid secretion. Fertil Steril 1986; 45:327.

149. Dunaif A, Graf M. Insulin administration alters gonadal steroid metabolism independent of changes in gonadotropin secretion in insulin-resistant women with polycystic ovary syndrome. J Clin Invest 1989; 83:23.

150. Velazquez EM, Acosta A, Mendoza SG. Menstrual cyclicity after metformin therapy in polycystic ovary syndrome. Obstet Gynecol 1997; 90:392.

151. Dunaif A, Scott D, Finegood D, et al. The insulin-sensitizing agent troglitazone improves metabolic and reproductive abnormalities in the polycystic ovary syndrome. J Clin Endocrinol Metab 1996; 81:3299.

152. Ehrmann DA, Schneider DJ, Sobel BE, et al. Troglitazone improves defects in insulin action, insulin secretion, ovarian steroidogenesis, and fibrinolysis in women with polycystic ovary syndrome. J Clin Endocrinol Metab 1997; 82:2108.

153. Nestler JE, Jakubowicz DJ, Reamer P, et al. Ovulatory and metabolic effects of D-chiro-inositol in the polycystic ovary syndrome. N Engl J Med 1999; 340:1314.

154. Luciano AA, Chapler FK, Sherman BM. Hyperprolactinemia in polycystic ovary syndrome. Fertil Steril 1984; 41:719.

155. Elkind-Hirsch KE, Valdes CT, McConnell TG, Malinak LR. Androgen responses to acutely increased endogenous insulin levels in hyperandrogenic and normal cycling women. Fertil Steril 1991; 55:486.

156. Smith S, Ravnikar V, Barbieri RL. Androgen and insulin response to an oral glucose challenge in hyperandrogenic women. Fertil Steril 1987; 48:72.

157. Kiddy DS, Hamilton-Fairley D, Seppala M, et al. Diet-induced changes in sex hormone binding globulin and free testosterone in women with normal or polycystic ovaries: correlation with serum insulin and insulin-like growth factor-I. Clin Endocrinol 1989; 31:757.

158. Nestler JC, Barlascini CO, Matt DW, et al. Suppression of serum insulin by diazoxide reduces serum testosterone levels in obese women with polycystic ovary syndrome. J Clin Endocrinol Metab 1989; 68:1027.

159. Dunaif A, Green G, Futterweit W, Dobrjansky A. Suppression of hyperandrogenism does not improve peripheral or hepatic insulin resistance in the polycystic ovary syndrome. J Clin Endocrinol Metab 1990; 70:699.

160. Dale PO, Tanbo T, Djoseland O, et al. Persistence of hyperinsulinemia in polycystic ovary syndrome after ovarian suppression by gonadotropin-releasing hormone agonist. Acta Endocrinol 1992; 126:132.

161. Poretsky L, Kalin MF. The gonadotropic function of insulin. Endocr Rev 1987; 8:132.

162. Bergh C, Carlsson B, Olsson J-H, et al. Regulation of androgen production in cultured human thecal cells by insulin-like growth factor I and insulin. Fertil Steril 1993; 59:323.

163. Nestler JE, Powers LP, Matt DW, et al. A direct effect of hyperinsulinemia on serum sex hormone-binding globulin levels in obese women with the polycystic ovary syndrome. J Clin Endocrinol Metab 1991; 72:83.

164. Conover CA, Lee PDK, Kanaley JA, et al. Insulin regulation of insulin-like growth factor binding protein-1 in obese and nonobese humans. J Clin Endocrinol Metab 1992; 74:1355.

165. Guzick DS, Wing R, Smith D. Endocrine consequences of weight loss in obese, hyperandrogenic anovulatory women. Fertil Steril 1994; 61:598.

166. Anderson P, Selifeflot I, Abdelnoor M, et al. Increased insulin sensitivity and fibrinolytic capacity after dietary intervention in obese women with polycystic ovary syndrome. Metabolism 1995; 44:611.

167. Jakubowicz DJ, Nestler JE. 17α-Hydroxyprogesterone responses to leuprolide and serum androgens in obese women with and without polycystic ovary syndrome after dietary weight loss. J Clin Endocrinol Metab 1997; 82:556.

168. Diamanti-Kandarakis E, Kouli C, Tsianateli T, et al. Therapeutic effects of metformin on insulin resistance and hyperandrogenism in polycystic ovary syndrome. Eur J Endocrinol 1998; 138:269.

169. Inzucchi SE, Maggs DG, Spollett GR, et al. Efficacy and metabolic effects of metformin and troglitazone in type 2 diabetes mellitus. N Engl J Med 1998; 338:867.

169a. Marca AL, Egbe TO, Morgante G, et al. Metformin treatment reduces ovarian cytochrome P-450c17α response to human chorionic gonadotrophin in women with insulin resistance–related polycystic ovary syndrome. Human Reproduction 2000; 15:21.

170. Greenblatt E, Casper RF. Endocrine changes after laparoscopic ovarian cautery in polycystic ovary syndrome. Am J Obstet Gynecol 1987; 156:279.

171. Daniell JF, Miller W. Polycystic ovaries treated by laparoscopic laser vaporization. Fertil Steril 1989; 51:232.

172. Smals AGH, Kloppenborg PWC, Benraad TJ. Plasma testosterone profiles in Cushing's syndrome. J Clin Endocrinol Metab 1977; 45:240.

173. Wentz AC. Physiologic and clinical considerations in luteal phase defects. Clin Obstet Gynecol 1979; 22:169.

174. Soules MR, McLachlan RI, Ek M, et al. Luteal phase deficiency: characterization of reproductive hormones over the menstrual cycle. J Clin Endocrinol Metab 1989; 69:804.

175. Soules MR, Clifton DK, Steiner RA, et al. The corpus luteum: determinants of progesterone secretion in the normal menstrual cycle. Obstet Gynecol 1988; 71:659.

176. Villanueva AL, Rebar RW. Congenital adrenal hyperplasia and luteal dysfunction. Int J Gynaecol Obstet 1985; 23:449.

177. Murthy YS, Arronet GH, Parekh MC. Luteal phase inadequacy. Obstet Gynecol 1970; 36:758.

178. Jones GS, Maffessoli RD, Strott CA, et al. The pathophysiology of reproductive failure after clomiphene-induced ovulation. Am J Obstet Gynecol 1970; 108:847.

179. Olson JL, Rebar RW, Schreiber JR, Vaitukaitis JL. Shortened luteal phase after ovulation induction with human menopausal gonadotropin and human chorionic gonadotropin. Fertil Steril 1983; 39:284.

180. Shoupe D, Mishell DR Jr, Lacarra M, et al. Correlation of endometrial maturation with four methods of estimating day of ovulation. Obstet Gynecol 1989; 73:88.

181. Batista MC, Cartledge TP, Merino MJ, et al. Midluteal phase endometrial biopsy does not accurately predict luteal function. Fertil Steril 1993; 59:294.

182. Noyes RW, Hertig AT, Rock J. Dating the endometrial biopsy. Fertil Steril 1950; 1:3.

183. Tredway DR, Mishell DR Jr, Moyer DL. Correlation of endometrial dating with luteinizing hormone peak. Am J Obstet Gynecol 1973; 117:1030.

184. Li T-C, Dockery P, Rogers AW, Cooke ID. How precise is histologic dating of endometrium using the standard dating criteria? Fertil Steril 1989; 51:759.

185. Johnson JWC, Austin KL, Jones GS, et al. Efficacy of 17α-hydroxyprogesterone caproate in the prevention of premature labor. N Engl J Med 1975; 293:675.

186. Jewelewicz R. Management of infertility resulting from anovulation. Am J Obstet Gynecol 1975; 122:909.

187. Koninckx PR, Heyns WJ, Corveloyn PA, Brosens IA. Delayed onset of luteinization as a cause of infertility. Fertil Steril 1978; 29:266.

188. Kerin JF, Kirby C, Morris D, et al. Incidence of the luteinized unruptured follicle phenomenon in cycling women. Fertil Steril 1983; 40:620.

189. Herbst AL, Ulfelder H, Poskanzer DC. Adenocarcinoma of the vagina: association of maternal stilbestrol therapy with tumor appearance in young women. N Engl J Med 1971; 284:878.

190. Hertz R. Accidental ingestion of estrogens by children. Pediatrics 1958; 221:203.

191. Southam AL, Richart RM. The prognosis for adolescents with menstrual abnormalities. Am J Obstet Gynecol 1966; 94:637.

192. Halberg L, Hogdahl A, Nilsson L, Rybo G. Menstrual blood loss: a population study. Acta Obstet Gynecol Scand 1966; 45:320.

193. Rybo G. Menstrual blood loss in relation to parity and menstrual pattern. Acta Obstet Gynecol Scand 1966; 7:119.

194. Nelson L, Rybo G. Treatment of menorrhagia. Am J Obstet Gynecol 1971; 110:713.

195. DeVore GR, Owens O, Kase N. Use of intravenous Premarin in the treatment of dysfunctional uterine bleeding: a double-blind randomized control study. Obstet Gynecol 1982; 59:285.

196. Vargyas JM, Campeau JO, Mishell DA. Treatment of menorrhagia with meclofenamate sodium. Am J Obstet Gynecol 1987; 157:944.

197. van Eijkeren MA, Christaens GCML, Geuze JH, et al. Effects of mefenamic acid on menstrual hemostasis in essential menorrhagia. Am J Obstet Gynecol 1992; 166:1419.

198. van Eijkeren M, Christaens GC, Sixma JJ, Haspels AA. Menorrhagia: a review. Obstet Gynecol Surv 1989; 44:421.

199. Milsom I, Andersson K, Andersch B, Rybo G. A comparison of flurbiprofen, tranexamic acid, and a levonorgestrel-releasing intrauterine contraceptive device in the treatment of idiopathic menorrhagia. Am J Obstet Gynecol 1991; 164:879.

200. Spanos WJ. Preoperative hormonal therapy of cystic adnexal masses. Am J Obstet Gynecol 1973; 116:551.

201. Goldstein SR, Subramanyam B, Snyder JR, et al. The postmenopausal cystic adnexal mass: the potential role of ultrasound in conservative management. Obstet Gynecol 1989; 7:8.

202. Ylikorkala O, Dawood MY. New concepts in dysmenorrhea. Am J Obstet Gynecol 1978; 130:833.

203. Smith RP. The dynamics of nonsteroidal anti-inflammatory therapy for primary dysmenorrhea. Obstet Gynecol 1987; 70:785.

204. Amodei N, Nelson RO, Jarrett RB, Sigmon S. Psychological treatments of dysmenorrhea: differential effectiveness for spasmodics and congestives. J Behav Ther Exp Psychiatry 1987; 18:95.

205. Thorn GW. Approach to the patient with "idiopathic edema" or "periodic swelling." JAMA 1968; 206:333.

206. Bailey RR. Water-logged women: idiopathic oedema. N Z Med J 1977; 85:129.

207. Thorn GW. Cyclical edema. Am J Med 1957; 23:507.

208. MacGregor GA, Markandu ND, Roulston JE, et al. Is "idiopathic" oedema idiopathic? Lancet 1979; 1:397.

209. Eisenstadt HB. Idiopathic edema. Tex State J Med 1966; 62:60.

210. Masters W, Johnson V. Human sexual response. Boston: Little, Brown & Co, 1966.

211. Green R. Human sexuality. In: Green R, ed. A health practitioner's guide, 2nd ed. Baltimore: Williams & Wilkins, 1979.

212. Masters W, Johnson V. Human sexual inadequacy. Boston, Little, Brown & Co, 1970.

213. Kolodny RC, Masters WH, Johnson VE. Textbook of sexual medicine. Boston, Little, Brown & Co, 1979.

214. Kaplan HS. The evaluation of sexual disorders: psychological and medical aspects. New York: Brunner-Mazel, 1983.

215. Nusbaum MR, Gamble G, Skinner B, Heiman J. The high prevalence of sexual concerns among women seeking routine gynecological care. J Fam Pract 2000; 49:229.

216. Basson R, Berman J, Burnett A, et al. Report of the international consensus development conference on female sexual dysfunction: definitions and classifications. J Urol 2000; 163:888.

# CHAPTER 97

# OVULATION INDUCTION

MICHAEL A. THOMAS

Ovulation induction is the primary method of ovarian stimulation in the 20% of infertile women who have an *ovulatory defect*. The World Health Organization (WHO) classifies those women with an inability to ovulate into three categories (Table 97-1).[1] Women for whom hypothalamic amenorrhea (HA) is the cause of their dysfunction comprise *WHO type I*. Such individuals, who generally have low to low-normal gonadotropin secretion with estradiol concentrations in the postmenopausal range, do not have withdrawal bleeding when administered exogenous progestin and have normal prolactin levels. Disorders in this category include Kallmann syndrome, isolated gonadotropin dysfunction, and some secondary causes of amenorrhea (anorexia nervosa, psychogenic or exercise-induced amenorrhea). Conception can be achieved most easily with pulsatile administration of gonadotropin-releasing hormone (GnRH) or administration of exogenous gonadotropins.

Individuals with *WHO type II* ovarian dysfunction are euestrogenic with an abnormal ratio of luteinizing hormone (LH) to follicle-stimulating hormone (FSH), although the gonadotropin levels are usually in the normal range. Most of these patients

**TABLE 97-1.**
**World Health Organization Classification of Ovarian Dysfunction**

**Type I: Hypothalamic Hypogonadism**
  Hypothalamic amenorrhea (idiopathic, anorexia nervosa, exercise-induced amenorrhea)
  Kallmann syndrome
  Isolated gonadotropin deficiency
**Type II: Euestrogenic Chronic Anovulation**
  Polycystic ovarian syndrome
  Hyperthecosis
**Type III: Hyperthalamic Hypogonadism**
  Premature ovarian failure
  Turner syndrome

have polycystic ovary syndrome (PCOS) with accompanying symptoms of obesity, hirsutism, and anovulation (see Chaps. 95 and 96). The most commonly used agents for ovulation induction in this group are clomiphene citrate and exogenous gonadotropins (see Chaps. 96 and 101). Investigators have used insulin receptor–sensitizing agents like metformin and troglitazone (no longer available) to increase the possibility of monofollicular development. This approach must be viewed as experimental.

Elevated levels of gonadotropins with hypoestrogenism occur in women of reproductive age who have WHO type III ovarian dysfunction. Premature ovarian failure and gonadal dysgenesis exemplify conditions found in this group. Ovulation induction is not indicated in this group of individuals because of the decreased possibility of ovarian response. Although the elevated gonadotropin levels in these patients can be reduced with administration of high-dose estrogens or GnRH agonists followed by exogenous gonadotropins, the ovarian response is inconsistent, and this treatment does not increase the pregnancy rate.[2]

## DETECTION OF OVULATION

Ovulation can be detected by *basal body temperature (BBT)* charting, measurement of *progesterone levels*, or *endometrial biopsy*. Although BBT charting is not considered a sensitive test for ovulatory defects, it shows a biphasic pattern with a rise in temperature that lasts for 11 to 16 days in most ovulatory women.[3] This rise in temperature is a progesterone-induced event. Basal body temperature charts are monophasic in 12% to 20% of patients who are ovulatory by serum testing; however, women who conceive typically have a biphasic pattern.[4,5]

Progesterone concentrations are elevated after ovulation. Although serum levels of >3 ng/mL are consistent with the development of secretory endometrium,[6] midluteal values of >8.8 ng/mL are typically observed in conception cycles.[7] These levels may be higher in ovulation induction cycles if development of multiple corpora lutea is demonstrated.

The routine use of endometrial biopsy to detect ovulatory response by noting secretory endometrium should be limited. Although endometrial biopsy is the gold standard in the histologic assessment of the ovarian stimulation of the endometrium, its use should probably be reserved for the detection of luteal-phase defects. Whether late luteal biopsies should ever be used is debatable, because women with proven fertility have the same incidence of abnormal biopsies as those with infertility problems.[8]

## CLOMIPHENE CITRATE

Clomiphene citrate, which was introduced in 1956, was first observed to achieve conception in humans in 1961.[9] It is used primarily in women with chronic anovulation secondary to PCOS or

with a luteal-phase defect, or to induce superovulation in eumenorrheic women with infertility. Clomiphene citrate is produced as a racemic mixture of two isomers: *trans* (62%) and *cis* (38%). The *cis* form is probably the one responsible for ovulation induction. Although it is available in a lower dose as a separate ovulation induction agent, no comparisons have been made between *cis*-clomiphene citrate and the commonly used racemic version.

Clomiphene has prolonged estrogen-receptor binding, with a plasma half-life of 5 to 7 days; indeed, it has been recovered in feces up to 6 weeks after discontinuation of treatment.[10] This binding to the estrogen receptor produces both antagonistic and agonistic effects. The first effect noted after the administration of clomiphene is an elevation in gonadotropin secretion that has been attributed to an antagonistic effect of this drug on the estrogen receptors in the hypothalamus. Clomiphene may also have a direct effect on the pituitary and ovary, both to enhance gonadotropin secretion and to induce aromatase activity synergistically with FSH. No stimulation of the cortisol, androgen, or progesterone receptor is noted.

## INDICATIONS FOR TREATMENT

The primary indication for clomiphene treatment is for induction of ovulation in the estrogenized, anovulatory woman, who usually has a history of reproductive dysfunction since puberty. Most of these women have PCOS, which includes symptoms of oligomenorrhea and hirsutism. In this group, FSH levels will increase to stimulate follicular development and ovulation in 70% of patients 5 to 10 days after taking the last dose.

Clomiphene is administered after a spontaneous menses or a progestin-induced withdrawal bleed. It is usually prescribed for 5 days starting between cycle days 2 and 5. The drug should be started early in the follicular phase to assure adequate follicular recruitment.

The starting dose of clomiphene for the majority of patients is 50 mg, but a dose of 25 mg may be considered for patients of lower body weight or a dose of 75 to 100 mg for obese patients. If no ovulatory response is noted, the dose should be increased by 25 to 50 mg during the next cycle, to a maximum dose of 250 mg. These doses are higher than those either approved or recommended by the FDA, but are consistent with clinical usage and experience. The lowest dose that causes ovulation should be used, because higher doses may have an antiestrogenic effect on the endometrial lining (preventing thickening) that may impede implantation. Follicular development may be monitored with the use of transabdominal or transvaginal ultrasonography. When the *leading follicle* (i.e., the largest) reaches a diameter of 17 to 20 mm, it is considered to be mature and close to ovulating. Although an increase in pregnancy rates has been noted when ultrasonography was used in cycle monitoring, its routine use is probably not cost effective.[11] *Human chorionic gonadotropin (hCG)* (10,000–20,000 IU intramuscularly) can be given to women with a mature follicle on ultrasonography, because it allows better cycle control and more precise timing of intercourse or the performance of inseminations. If ultrasonography is not used, intercourse should be initiated every other day starting 3 days after the last clomiphene dose, or it can be timed with a urinary LH surge detection kit. Some kits may give false-positive readings, however, even during clomiphene ingestion, because of the increase in gonadotropin secretion that clomiphene may cause.

The thickness of the entire lining of the endometrium ("endometrial stripe") is considered adequate for implantation on transvaginal ultrasonography if it is at least 6 mm in diameter. Clomophene has been shown to have an effect on the endometrium.[11a]

## RESULTS

In general, up to 80% of patients who use clomiphene will ovulate, and 40% of those women will achieve conception. If causes of infertility other than an ovulatory defect are excluded, the conception rate probably is higher. In more highly selected groups of infertile couples, the pregnancy rate has been as high as 90%. Other factors that also may influence the rate of conception are side effects from the clomiphene, including thickening of the cervical mucus and the induction of a luteal-phase defect.

When clomiphene is used in patients with an ovulatory dysfunction, the conception rate per ovulatory cycle is the same as that for couples achieving pregnancy spontaneously. After three cycles, the pregnancy rate with clomiphene in one study was 55.7%, which is comparable to that in the general population. A monthly fecundity rate of 15.7% has been noted if the drug is given for up to 10 cycles and 9% if it is given for up to 16 months. Because 95% of women who conceive will do so within the first six ovulatory cycles, treating for >6 months is not necessary.

Patients who do not ovulate after progressive increases in the dose of clomiphene should be reevaluated. If the patient is hyperandrogenic, adrenal androgens should be measured; if the serum level of dehydroepiandrosterone sulfate is found to be >2800 ng/mL, dexamethasone can be administered at a dose of 0.5 mg at bedtime, and clomiphene can be resumed at 50 mg with increases until ovulation is obtained. If the patient still does not ovulate, exogenous gonadotropins can be given. Because patients with PCOS can be very sensitive to human menopausal gonadotropins (hMG) or recombinant FSH, a starting dose of one ampule per day is often appropriate. Administration of the insulin-sensitizing agents metformin and troglitazone (no longer available) have produced an ovulatory response in some patients with PCOS.[12,13]

Tamoxifen, another nonsteroidal antiestrogen, has also been used for ovulation induction. The effective dosage of tamoxifen is 20 mg daily for 5 days, and the dosage can be increased to 80 mg per day. Higher rates of ovulation and lower adverse effects on cervical mucus have been noted in women taking tamoxifen than in those who used clomiphene.[14] This agent, however, is not approved for ovulation induction in the Unites States.

## ADVERSE EFFECTS

### HOT FLASHES

Hot flashes are one of the most common side effects of clomiphene use. Up to 11% of women experience hot flashes, which are usually mild and reversible on discontinuation of the medication.[15] The hot flashes associated with clomiphene are probably secondary to its antiestrogenic effect on the hypothalamus and are noted to increase in frequency with increasing doses.

### VISION SYMPTOMS

Less than 2% of women on clomiphene experience vision symptoms (e.g., night blindness, blurring, or scotomata).[16] These symptoms are usually seen with higher dosages of clomiphene and are reversible with discontinuation; however, rare instances of optic nerve injury have been reported in both men and women.[17,18] This type of injury is thought to be secondary to ischemia caused by vascular sludging.

### MULTIPLE BIRTHS

Clomiphene can cause a pronounced increase in the pulse frequency of gonadotropins, thereby increasing the number of follicles produced. Thus, the risk of multiple births is increased and ranges from 6.25% to 12.3%. Most of the multiple gestations are twins. Of the multiple births noted, 93% are twins.

### TERATOGENIC EFFECTS

Teratogenic effects have *not* been associated with clomiphene, although two studies suggest that it may increase the frequency of chromosomal anomalies in spontaneous abortions and recurrent molar pregnancies.[19,20]

### OTHER SIDE EFFECTS

Other side effects of clomiphene include thickening of the cervical mucus secondary to its antiestrogenic effect on the cervix and a delay in endometrial maturation that can lead to a luteal-phase defect. Clomiphene may lead to a higher incidence of *luteinized, unruptured follicle syndrome (LUFS).*[21]

## PULSATILE GONADOTROPIN-RELEASING HORMONE

Native GnRH is a decapeptide that is produced in the mediobasal and anterior hypothalamus and is transported via the portal vessels to the anterior pituitary to activate the secretion of the gonadotropins FSH and LH. When exogenous GnRH is administered in a pulsatile fashion, gonadotropin levels increase, causing ovarian stimulation.[22] If GnRH is given in a continuous manner, an initial stimulatory response is noted; later, FSH and LH secretion are suppressed, resulting in hypoestrogenism because of receptor down-regulation and desensitization.

Patients with HA (WHO type I), who are hypoestrogenic secondary to diminished GnRH release, respond to intravenous (IV) or subcutaneous (SC) GnRH administered in a pulsatile fashion via a pump.[23] The pumps used for ovulation induction generally are modified insulin pumps that allow a pulse frequency of 60 to 120 minutes with GnRH doses of 1 to 200 μg per pulse. The optimal IV dose is from 1 to 5 μg per pulse, whereas the equivalent dose given SC is 10 to 25 μg per pulse. When the proper dosage is achieved, 80% to 100% of HA patients ovulate, with a conception rate of 25% per treatment cycle. Although monofollicular development is most common with the use of the GnRH pump, when the amount of GnRH is increased, multiple follicles can be produced.[24]

Before the pump administration of exogenous GnRH, HA patients may be given exogenous estrogen for 2 months in an effort to increase GnRH receptors. The pharmacokinetics of IV GnRH is more physiologic than that obtained with SC administration, but IV use is associated with more patient discomfort and increased morbidity, including thrombophlebitis. Consequently, the IV site needs to be examined on a regular basis.

Patients using pulsatile GnRH can be monitored with transvaginal ultrasonography to detect follicular development. Once follicular growth is noted, an LH surge can be allowed to occur spontaneously, with the time of the surge identified by use of daily urinary tests to detect increased LH excretion. Luteal-phase support to maintain corpus luteal function and increased endogenous progesterone secretion can be provided by continued GnRH pump use or administration of low doses of hCG (1000–2000 IU) every 3 to 4 days. Without adequate luteal support, patients treated with pulsatile GnRH for ovulation induction have a spontaneous abortion rate of 24% to 32%.[25]

Women with HA are more likely to ovulate and conceive with pulsatile GnRH therapy than women with PCOS. In one study, women with HA had an ovulation rate of 89% and a pregnancy rate of 27%, whereas patients with PCOS had an ovulation rate of 43% and a pregnancy rate of 12%.[26] Possibly, patients with PCOS who use pulsatile GnRH may have more success if they are pretreated with a GnRH agonist[27] or GnRH antagonist[28] to decrease chronic androgen production, which can hamper ovarian follicular development.

## EXOGENOUS GONADOTROPINS

Initially, injectable gonadotropin used for ovarian stimulation was produced from animal pituitary extracts, but patients rapidly developed antibodies that eventually neutralized their clinical efficacy. Investigators then turned their attention to the use of postmortem *human pituitary gonadotropin (hPG)*, but lack of adequate amounts of pituitaries and the identification of Creutzfeldt-Jakob disease caused hPG to be banned from clinical use.[29,30] Gonadotropins (in a 1:1 ratio of LH to FSH) can be produced from the urine of menopausal women. Although one pituitary gland contains as much FSH as 2 to 5 liters of menopausal urine, the urinary extraction technique has been perfected. In 1962, three pregnancies were reported in women taking hMG after 16 cycles of use.[31] Since 1987, urinary-derived gonadotropins have been purified to significantly increase the percentage of FSH (uFSH). As the purification process has improved, the removal of other antigenic contaminants has allowed SC administration.

The advent of the availability of recombinant FSH (rFSH) products allows FSH receptor stimulation in the absence of LH. Production of rFSH takes place by the transfection of an ovarian cell line from the Chinese hamster with the genomic clone containing the complete human FSH-β coding sequence together with the α subunit minigene. Carbohydrate moieties, which are added after translation, make the product different from endogenous FSH. No differences have been noted between uFSH and rFSH in terms of rates of ovulation and pregnancy achieved.[31a]

In the early follicular phase of the menstrual cycle, exogenous gonadotropins directly stimulate the ovaries in an attempt to "rescue" from degeneration some of the 20 to 40 follicles with sufficient granulosa-cell FSH receptors. Because of this direct stimulation, follicular development is more pronounced, and estradiol levels are higher; therefore, the risk of multiple births and *ovarian hyperstimulation syndrome (OHSS)* is increased. When ultrasonographic monitoring demonstrates a lead follicle measuring 16 mm, hCG is given at a dose of 5000 to 20,000 units to mimic the LH surge and produce final follicular maturation and oocyte release. The suggestion has been made that FSH is needed only early in the follicular phase to "rescue" follicles and that a combination of LH and FSH (or LH alone) can be added subsequently to control follicular development more precisely.[32]

## INDICATIONS FOR TREATMENT

If patients with hypothalamic hypogonadism (WHO type I) do not respond to or refuse the use of pulsatile gonadotropin, exogenous gonadotropins can be used to induce ovulation. Because these patients have inadequate LH production, a combination of LH and FSH should be administered. The LH in this preparation allows the production of the androgen precursors needed for adequate estradiol production. When FSH alone is given to these individuals, follicular growth takes place, but inadequate estradiol production probably correlates with poor oocyte and endometrial development.[33,34] Ovulation is noted in up to 90% of these patients who use hMG, and the pregnancy rate is 25% to 30% per cycle, with a cumulative pregnancy rate of 70%.[35,36] Spontaneous abortions are noted to be as high as 25%, however, perhaps due to poor corpus luteal development. The use of luteal-phase progesterone or hCG administration 1 week after ovulation may be useful in decreasing pregnancy loss.

Anovulatory patients with PCOS (WHO type II) who do not ovulate with the use of clomiphene can be treated with exogenous gonadotropins. These women are very sensitive to gonadotropins, however, and *step-up protocols* (progressive increase in the number of ampules administered) should be used, with a starting dose of one ampule of hMG or FSH (75 IU). The dose of gonadotropins should be increased until a dominant follicle is seen to emerge from the multiple antral follicles associated with this disease state. A *step-down protocol* can also be used in which initial dosing with two ampules of gonadotropins is given, and the dose is then reduced to one ampule when two to three follicles begin to progress in development. The IV administration of gonadotropins at a dosage of 6 to 9 IU every 90 minutes has been used, but no advantages in ovarian stimulation have been

observed compared with intramuscular delivery.[37,38] The use of urinary and rFSH would theoretically be ideal for patients with hyperandrogenic anovulation because of the absence of the androgen stimulation, but clinical studies have not shown FSH to be more beneficial than hMG in this group of patients.

Protocols using both clomiphene and gonadotropins have been used in estrogenized anovulatory patients who have failed to respond adequately to clomiphene alone. Usually, clomiphene is started on cycle day 2 or 3 at a dose of 100 mg; then one or two ampules of exogenous gonadotropins are started 2 days later. Ovulation rates are noted to be higher on this regimen, but pregnancy rates are the same as those without the addition of clomiphene.[39]

Couples with unexplained infertility have had success in cycles in which they received empiric administration of hMG. Among 97 couples awaiting in vitro fertilization (IVF) who were treated for up to 4 cycles, the clinical pregnancy rate was 12.4% and the delivery rate was 8.2%.[40] This increased pregnancy rate in couples with unexplained infertility was also observed in a larger cohort of patients.[41] In another study, however, no difference in pregnancy rates was observed in gonadotropin-treated patients and in those who underwent expectant management.[42]

Because growth factors such as insulin-like growth factor-I (IGF-I) can regulate granulosa cell function in an autocrine fashion, growth hormone (GH) administration was thought to be able to enhance follicular growth. In a randomized, double-blind study, use of hMG stimulation plus GH (24 IU every other day) was compared to use of hMG plus placebo.[43] GH administration was associated with a decrease in the number of ampules of hMG used and the number of days of treatment. Other studies have not confirmed the clinical benefits of GH administration.[44,45]

## ADVERSE EFFECTS

### MULTIPLE BIRTHS

With increasing media and lay interest in multiple births, a national focus is now on this complication, which commonly occurs in response to ovulation induction with exogenous gonadotropins (Fig. 97-1). These pregnancies are of higher risk for both the mother and offspring, and account for a higher percentage of obstetrical interventions (breech extraction, vacuum and forceps use, and operative delivery) as well as increased neonatal intensive care admissions. Although the overall rate of multiple pregnancy is ~26% with these injectable medications, this incidence can be reduced with careful ultrasonography and estradiol monitoring. To prevent high-order multiples, hCG should not be administered when more than mature follicles (mean diameter ≥16 mm) are noted. Early ultrasonographic monitoring has shown evidence that some implantations may disappear naturally on future observation, indicating spontaneous resorption. The incidence of this "vanishing twin" phenomenon is unclear. Patients may also be given the option of transabdominal or transvaginal ultrasonography-guided selective reduction as a way to medically decrease the number of implantations to one or two.[46,47] This procedure has a rate of spontaneous abortion of <5% and is only offered in selected centers around the country. Because some patients may have a moral objection to this procedure, it should be discussed before the start of the ovulation induction process. (see ref. 47a for a review of pelvic ultrasound in women.)

### OVARIAN HYPERSTIMULATION SYNDROME

OHSS is one of the most serious complications associated with ovulation induction, especially when gonadotropins are used. This syndrome occurs after ovulation, particularly when induced with hCG, and is generally associated with varying degrees of ovarian cystic enlargement, which can cause abdominal fullness, weight gain, and pelvic pain.[48] The syndrome is

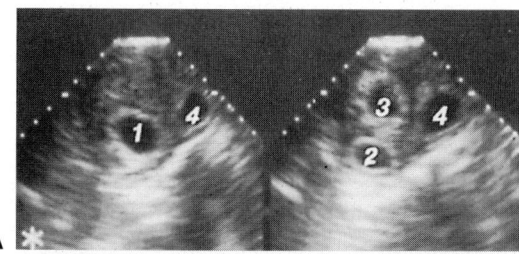

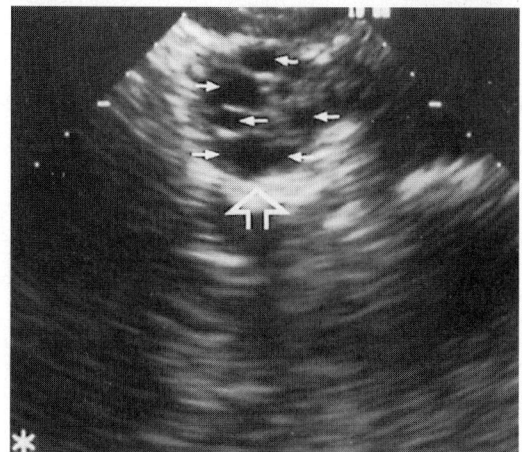

**FIGURE 97-1. A,** Pelvic ultrasonographic scans demonstrating a multiple (quadruplet) intrauterine pregnancy achieved with human menopausal gonadotropin (*hMG*)/human chorionic gonadotropin stimulation. Gestational sacs are numbered 1 through 4. **B,** Transvaginal pelvic ultrasonographic scan showing multiple ovarian follicles (*small solid arrows*) within the substance of the ovary (*large open arrow*) during hMG stimulation.

commonly self-limited, lasting 2 weeks or less. If the patient becomes pregnant, the OHSS symptoms may persist for many weeks longer.

In its mildest form (ovarian enlargement of <5 cm without ascites or pain), OHSS is self-limited and requires observation for possible fluid and electrolyte imbalances. Moderate OHSS is associated with ovaries of <10 cm with some degree of ascites as well as nausea and vomiting. In more severe forms of OHSS (ovarian enlargement of >10 cm), fluid shifts can lead to more hemoconcentration and accumulation of fluid in the third space, which can cause more pronounced ascites resulting in pleural and pericardial effusions. If poorly managed, severe OHSS can lead to renal failure, hypovolemic shock, thromboembolic phenomena, adult respiratory distress, and possibly death.[49]

When OHSS is suspected, a baseline complete blood cell count, coagulation parameters, electrolyte profile, and serum osmolarity should be determined. If hypokalemia is suspected or confirmed, an electrocardiogram should be taken. Daily hematocrit, weight, and fluid intake/output should be monitored. Patients who become dehydrated with a urine output of <30 mL per hour or show respiratory distress should be hospitalized. Because of severe friability of the ovaries, serial pelvic examinations should be avoided to decrease the possibility of ovarian torsion or intraperitoneal bleeding from a ruptured ovarian cyst. Administration of diuretics alone worsens the vasoconstriction. A decrease in ascites has been noted in patients given volume expanders followed by diuretics, but this method of treatment should be used sparingly. The prophylactic use of heparin to prevent venous thrombosis has not given consistent results. Paracentesis should be performed only in patients in respiratory distress.

### RISK OF CANCER

Questions have arisen about the safety of fertility drugs since a report of case-control findings in 1992.[50] In this study, a history of fertility drug use (no specific drug was mentioned) conferred a higher risk of ovarian cancer than was found in nonusers. Infertility patients who used drugs had an odds ratio of 2.8 compared with 0.91 in similar women who did not use drugs. A link between breast cancer and drugs that promote ovarian hyperstimulation has been proposed.[51] However, these studies did not adjust for age at first birth, family history, prior use of oral contraceptives, type of infertility, and dosage and duration of specific fertility drug use.

Other studies have demonstrated no increased risk of ovarian and breast cancers in users of clomiphene or exogenous gonadotropins compared with the general population.[52,53] However, larger multicenter clinical trials are needed to completely answer this question.

## DOPAMINE AGONISTS

Hyperprolactinemia causes a decrease in GnRH pulsatility through the direct effect of prolactin on the hypothalamus. Hyperprolactinemia occurs more often in women (1.2%) than in men (0.12%) and is found in 14% to 20% of women with secondary amenorrhea. Eumenorrheic women with hyperprolactinemia usually have infertility problems secondary to corpus luteal dysfunction.

Although surgical and radiologic interventions have been used in patients with prolactin-producing adenomas, medical therapy is more commonly used. Bromocriptine, the most commonly used dopamine agonist, interacts with the dopamine receptors in the brain and anterior pituitary (see Chaps. 13 and 21).[54] It is rapidly absorbed orally, with peak serum levels occurring in 2 to 3 hours. If bromocriptine causes nausea and vomiting, vaginal administration, which is equally efficacious and has a longer duration of action, can be used.[55] Other side effects include nasal congestion, headache, and fatigue. At least 68% of patients using bromocriptine have one of these side effects.

Bromocriptine is usually started at a dose of 1.25 mg given at dinner for the first 7 to 14 days to decrease possible side effects. The dose is then increased by 1.25 mg increments every 2 to 3 weeks until a euprolactinemic state is observed. Among hyperprolactinemic women treated with bromocriptine, 66% conceived, 80% of amenorrheic patients became eumenorrheic, and 76% had a decrease in galactorrhea.[56]

When pregnancy is noted during bromocriptine use, the dopamine agonist should be discontinued. In patients who unknowingly continued bromocriptine during a pregnancy, 50% discontinued use <4 weeks from the time of conception and 77% discontinued within 6 weeks.[57] No increase in spontaneous abortion, ectopic pregnancy, or multiple births was observed.

Other dopamine agonists include pergolide (daily use) or cabergoline (twice weekly use). Two studies have documented the occurrence of normal pregnancies in women who used cabergoline for hyperprolactinemia. Cabergoline was used in 455 male and female patients.[58] Of the 353 women in the study, 27 conceived, with 25 subsequent deliveries. How many of these women were actively attempting conception is unclear. In another study, cabergoline use restored menses in 7 of 10 patients with macroadenomas and all 22 individuals with microadenomas.[59] Of these, 5 of 6 infertile women became pregnant and had uneventful pregnancies.

## REFERENCES

1. Steinkampf MP, Hammond KR, Blackwell RE. Ovulation induction. In: Carr BR, Blackwell RE, eds. Textbook of reproductive medicine. Stamford, CT: Appleton & Lange, 1998:565.
2. Surrey ES, Cedars MI. The effect of gonadotropin suppression on induction of ovulation in premature ovarian failure. Fertil Steril 1989; 52:36.
3. Downs KA, Gibson M. Basal body temperature graph and the luteal phase defect. Fertil Steril 1983; 40:466.
4. Johanssen EDB, Larsson-Cohn U, Gemzell CA. Monophasic basal body temperature in ovulatory menstrual cycles. Am J Obstet Gynecol 1972; 113:933.

5. Moghissi KS. Accuracy of BBT for ovulation detection. Fertil Steril 1976; 27:1415.
6. Israel R, Mishell DR, Stone, et al. Single luteal phase serum progesterone assay as an indicator of ovulation. Am J Obstet Gynecol 1972; 112:1043.
7. Hull MGR, Savage PE, Bromham DR, et al. The value of a single serum progesterone measurement in the midluteal phase as a criterion of a potentially fertile cycle ("ovulation") derived from treated and untreated conception cycles. Fertil Steril 1982; 37:355.
8. Davis OK, Berkeley AS, Naus GF, et al. The incidence of luteal phase defect in normal, fertile women, determined by endometrial biopsies. Fertil Steril 1989; 51:582.
9. Greenblatt RB, Barfield WE, Jungck EC, Ray AW. Induction of ovulation with MMRI/41. JAMA 1961; 178:101.
10. Drug information for the health care provider. Easton, PA: Mack Publishing, 1986:541.
11. March CM. Improved pregnancy rates with monitoring of gonadotropin therapy by three modalities. Am J Obstet Gynecol 1987; 156:1473.
11a. Sereepapong W, Suwajanakorn S, Triratanachat S, et al. Effects of clomiphene citrate on the endometrium of regularly cycling women. Fertil Steril 2000; 73:287.
12. Glueck CJ, Wang P, Fontaine R, et al. Metformin-induced resumption of normal menses in 39 of 43 (91%) previously amenorrheic women with the polycystic ovary syndrome. Metabolism 1999; 48:511.
13. Dunaif A, Scott D, Finegood D, et al. The insulin-sensitizing agent troglitazone improves metabolic and reproductive abnormalities in the polycystic ovary syndrome. J Clin Endocrinol Metab 1996; 81:3299.
14. Bournstein R, Shoham Z, Vermini M, et al. Tamoxifen treatment in women with failure of clomiphene citrate therapy. Aust N Z J Obstet Gynaecol 1989; 29:173.
15. Jones GS, de Moraes-Ruehsen M. Induction of ovulation with human menopausal gonadotropins and with clomiphene. Fertil Steril 1965; 16:461.
16. Asch RH, Greenblatt RR. Update on the safety and efficacy of clomiphene citrate as a therapeutic agent. J Reprod Med 1976; 17:175.
17. Lawton AW. Optic neuropathy associated with clomiphene citrate. Fertil Steril 1994; 61:390.
18. Rock T, Dinar Y, Romen M. Retinal phlebitis after hormonal treatment. Ann Ophthalmol 1989; 21:75.
19. Boue JG, Boue A. Increased frequency of chromosomal anomalies in abortions after induced ovulation. Lancet 1973; 1:679.
20. Mor-Joseph S, Anteby SO, Granat M, et al. Recurrent molar pregnancies associated with clomiphene citrate and human menopausal gonadotropins. Am J Obstet Gynecol 1985; 151:1095.
21. Katz E. The luteinized unruptured follicle and other ovulatory dysfunctions. Fertil Steril 1988; 50:839.
22. Knobil E. The neuroendocrine control of the menstrual cycle. Recent Prog Horm Res 1980; 36:53.
23. Reid RL, Fretts R, Van Vugt DA. The theory and practice of ovulation induction with gonadotropin-releasing hormone. Am J Obstet Gynecol 1988; 158:176.
24. Liu JH, Durfee R, Muse K, et al. Induction of multiple ovulation by pulsatile administration of gonadotropin releasing hormone. Fertil Steril 1983; 40:18.
25. Santoro N. Efficacy and safety of intravenous pulsatile gonadotropin-releasing hormone: Lutrepulse for injection. Am J Obstet Gynecol 1990; 163:1959.
26. Filicori M, Flamigni C, Meriggiola MC, et al. Ovulation induction with pulsatile gonadotropin-releasing hormone: technical modalities and clinical perspectives. Fertil Steril 1991; 56:1.
27. Filicori M, Campaniello E, Michelacci L, et al. Gonadotropin-releasing hormone (GnRH) analog suppression renders polycystic ovarian disease patients more susceptible to ovulation induction with pulsatile GnRH. J Clin Endocrinol Metab 1988; 66:327.
28. Leroy I, d'Acremont MF, Brailly-Tabard S, et al. A single injection of a gonadotropin antagonist (Cetrolix) postpones the luteinizing hormone (LH) surge: further evidence for the role of GnRH during the LH surge. Fertil Steril 1994; 62:461.
29. Cochius JI, Mack K, Burns RJ. Creutzfeldt-Jakob disease in a recipient human pituitary derived gonadotropin. Aust N Z J Med 1990; 20:592.
30. Dumble LD, Klein RD. Creutzfeldt-Jakob disease legacy for Australian women treated with human menopausal gonadotropins. Lancet 1992; 340:848.
31. Hammond MG, Talbert LM. Therapeutic insemination. In: Seibel MM, ed. Infertility: a comprehensive text. Norwalk, CT: Appleton & Lange, 1997:309.
31a. Lenton E, Soltan A, Hewitt J, et al. Induction of ovulation in women undergoing assisted reproductive techniques: recombinant human FSH (follitropin alpha) versus highly purified urinary FSH. Hum Reprod 2000; 15:1021.
32. Sullivan MW, Stewart-Akers A, Krasnow JS, et al. Ovarian responses in women to recombinant follicle-stimulating hormone and luteinizing hormone (LH): a role for LH in the final stages of follicular maturation. J Clin Endocrinol Metab 1999; 84:228.
33. Sloham Z, Mannaerts B, Insler V, Coelingh-Bennink H. Induction of follicular growth using recombinant human follicle-stimulating hormone in two volunteer women with hypothalamic hypogonadism. Fertil Steril 1993; 59:738.
34. Fox R, Ekeroma A, Wardle P. Ovarian response to purified FSH in infertile women with long-standing hypogonadotrophic hypogonadism. Aust N Z Obstet Gynecol 1997; 37:92.
35. Dor J, Itzkowic DJ, Mashiach S, et al. Cumulative conception rates following gonadotropin therapy. Am J Obstet Gynecol 1980; 136:102.
36. Lam SL, Baker G, Pepperell R, et al. Treatment-independent pregnancies after cessation of gonadotropin ovulation induction in women with oligomenorrhea and anovulatory menses. Fertil Steril 1988; 50:26.
37. Nakamura Y, Yoshimure Y, Yamada H, et al. Clinical experience in the induction of ovulation and pregnancy with pulsatile subcutaneous administration of human menopausal gonadotropins: a low incidence of multiple pregnancy. Fertil Steril 1989; 51:423.
38. Nakamura Y, Yoshimura Y, Oda T, et al. Comparative study of hormonal dynamics during pregnant and nonpregnant cycles during pulsatile subcutaneous administration of human menopausal gonadotropin in anovulatory infertile women. Fertil Steril 1993; 60:254.
39. Jarrell J, McInnes R, Cooke R, Arronet G. Observations on the combination of clomiphene citrate-human menopausal gonadotropin-human chorionic gonadotropin in the management of anovulation. Fertil Steril 1981; 35:634.
40. Welner S, DeCherney AH, Polan ML. Human menopausal gonadotropin: a justifiable therapy in ovulatory women with long-standing idiopathic infertility. Am J Obstet Gynecol 1988; 158:111.
41. Aboulghar MA, Mansour RT, Serour GI, et al. Ovarian superstimulation and intrauterine insemination for the treatment of unexplained infertility. Fertil Steril 1993; 60:303.
42. Daly DC. Treatment validation of ultrasound-defined abnormal follicular dynamics as a cause of infertility. Fertil Steril 1989; 51:51.
43. Homburg R, Eshel A, Addulla HI, Jacobs HS. Growth hormone facilitates ovulation induction by gonadotropins. Clin Endocrinol 1988; 29:113.
44. Bergh C, Hillensjo T, Wikland M, et al. Adjuvant growth hormone treatment during in vitro fertilization: a randomized, placebo-controlled study. Fertil Steril 1994; 62:113.
45. Suikarra AM, MacLachlan V, Koistinen R, et al. Double-blind placebo-controlled study: human biosynthetic growth hormone for assisted reproductive technology. Fertil Steril 1996; 65:800.
46. Evans MI, Dommergues M, Wapner RJ, et al. Efficacy of transabdominal multifetal pregnancy reduction: collaborative experience of the world's largest centers. Obstet Gynecol 1993; 82:61.
47. Timor-Tritsch IE, Peisner DB, Monteagudo A, et al. Multifetal pregnancy reduction by transvaginal puncture: evaluation of the technique used in 134 cases. Am J Obstet Gynecol 1993; 168:799.
47a. Sivyer P. Pelvic ultrasound in women. World J Surg 2000; 24:188.
48. Rabau E, David A, Serr DM, et al. Human menopausal gonadotropins for anovulation and sterility. Am J Obstet Gynecol 1967; 98:92.
49. Golan A, Ron-El R, Herman A, et al. Ovarian hyperstimulation syndrome: an update review. Obstet Gynecol Surv 1989; 44:430.
50. Whittmore AS, Harris R, Itnyhre J. The collaborative ovarian cancer group. Characteristics related to ovarian cancer risk: collaborative analysis of twelve US case-control studies. II: Invasive epithelial cancer in white women. Am J Epidemiol 1992; 136:1184.
51. Brezezinski A, Peretz T, Mor-Yosef S, Schenker JG. Ovarian stimulation and breast cancer. Is there a link? Gynecol Oncol 1994; 52:292.
52. Potashnik G, Lerner-Geva L, Genkin L, et al. Fertility drugs and the risk of breast and ovarian cancers: results of a long-term follow-up study. Fertil Steril 1999; 71:853.
53. Venn A, Watson L, Bruinsma F, et al. Risk of cancer after use of fertility drugs with in-vitro fertilisation. Lancet 1999; 354:1586.
54. Hausler A, Rohr HP, Marbach P, et al. Changes in prolactin secretion in lactating rates assessed by correlative morphometric and biochemical methods. J Ultrastruct Res 1978; 64:74.
55. Katz E, Weiss BE, Hassell A, et al. Increased circulating levels of bromocriptine after vaginal compared to oral administration. Fertil Steril 1991; 55:882.
56. Cuellar FG. Bromocriptine mesylate (Parlodel) in the management of amenorrhea/galactorrhea associated with hyperprolactinemia. Obstet Gynecol 1980; 55:278.
57. Turkalj I, Baun P, Krupp P. Surveillance of bromocriptine in pregnancy. JAMA 1982; 247:1589.
58. Verheist J, Abs R, Maiter D, et al. Cabergoline in the treatment of hyperprolactinemia: a study in 455 patients. J Clin Endocrinol Metab 1999; 84:2518.
59. Cabergoline: a first-choice treatment in patients with previously untreated prolactin-secreting pituitary adenoma. J Endocrinol Invest 1999; 22:354.

# CHAPTER 98

# ENDOMETRIOSIS

ROBERT L. BARBIERI

Endometriosis is the *presence of endometrial glands and/or stroma outside the uterus*. The most common sites of endometriosis lesions are the pelvic peritoneum, ovary, uterosacral ligaments, bladder, bowel, and appendix.[1] Endometriosis is present in ~5% of women of reproductive age. Although it is a common disorder, it is an enigmatic disease that can be difficult to diagnose. There is a mean interval of 4 years from initial presentation to a physician with a symptom of endometriosis until the definitive diagnosis of the disease.

**TABLE 98-1.**

**Response of the Endometrium and Endometriosis Lesions to Steroids***

| Steroid | Response of Endometrium | Response of Endometriosis Lesions |
|---------|------------------------|-----------------------------------|
| Estrogen | Growth | Growth |
| Androgen | Atrophy | Atrophy |
| Progesterone | Differentiation and secretory changes | Many endometriosis lesions do not undergo secretory changes in response to physiologic concentrations of progesterone. There is evidence for resistance to progesterone |
| Synthetic progestins | Decidualization—a terminal differentiation pathway | Decidualization |

*Endometriosis lesions contain estrogen, progesterone and androgen receptors. Estrogen stimulates growth of the endometrium and endometriosis lesions. Androgens cause atrophy in the endometrium and endometriosis lesions.

Most women with endometriosis have pelvic pain, infertility, and/or an *endometrioma* (an ovarian endometriosis cyst). Pelvic pain caused by endometriosis lesions is best treated by suppression of ovarian estrogen production; infertility caused by endometriosis lesions is best treated by surgical resection of the endometriosis lesions, empirical stimulation of multifollicular development with clomiphene, administration of exogenous gonadotropins to increase fecundability, or in vitro fertilization (IVF). Nonfunctional cysts of the ovary, such as an endometrioma, are best treated by surgical removal. Surgical removal of nonfunctional ovarian cysts is both diagnostic and therapeutic. The likelihood of recurrence of an endometrioma is <10%.[2]

## ENDOMETRIOSIS LESIONS ARE STEROID RESPONSIVE

Mechanical (retrograde menstruation) and endocrine factors (estradiol, progesterone) contribute to the development of endometriosis lesions. In most women, the majority of menstrual effluent leaves the uterus through the cervical os, thereby entering the vagina.[3] In women with a reduced cervical os diameter, significant amounts of menstrual effluent exit the uterus through the fallopian tubes, thereby entering the peritoneal cavity.[4] The process of "retrograde" menstruation results in the transportation of small fragments of viable endometrium into the peritoneal cavity, where they can become implanted and grow. Women with endometriosis appear to have an eutopic endometrium, which has greater potential for implantation at distant sites than does that from women without endometriosis.[5]

Hemocrine, paracrine, and autocrine factors play major roles in regulating the growth of endometriosis lesions. The major endocrine regulators of endometriosis lesions are the steroid hormones, estrogen, androgens, and progestins.[6] Estrogens stimulate the growth of endometriosis lesions, whereas androgens inhibit lesion growth. The major paracrine and autocrine factors that regulate endometriosis lesions are cytokines[7,7a] and growth factors.[8] Endometriosis lesions are associated with the excessive secretion of chemotactic factors[9–11] and can grow in response to cytokines and growth factors secreted by activated immune cells.[12,13]

Endometriosis lesions contain estrogen, progesterone, and androgen receptors.[14,15] Usually, estrogen stimulates and androgens inhibit their growth.[16] Progestins have complex, dose-dependent effects on endometriosis lesions. At serum progesterone levels normally observed in the luteal phase of the menstrual cycle, progesterone may stimulate the differentiation of lesions. At very high serum concentrations, however, progestins can cause decidualization of endometriosis lesions and may inhibit their growth (Table 98-1). Multiple lines of evidence support the concept that endometriosis lesions are partially resistant to the action of progesterone.[17]

The steroid responsiveness of endometriosis lesions is the basis for most hormonal treatments. Available hormonal treatments include (a) suppression of estrogen production, (b) androgens, (c) synthetic progestins at high doses, and (d) combination estrogen-progestin contraceptives in a pseudopregnancy manner.

## TREATMENT OF ENDOMETRIOSIS BY SUPPRESSING ESTROGEN PRODUCTION AND ACTION

Suppression of ovarian estrogen production is the most reliable method for causing the regression of endometriosis lesions. For many years, surgical oophorectomy has been the main option for permanently reducing ovarian estrogen production. Long-term improvement in pelvic pain caused by endometriosis occurs in ~90% of women who have a bilateral oophorectomy.[18] In the United States, endometriosis is the second most common indication for hysterectomy and oophorectomy. For young women who have not completed their families, bilateral oophorectomy is not a good option. The gonadotropin-releasing hormone (GnRH) analogs—which can reversibly suppress ovarian estrogen production—have become the mainstay for the treatment of pelvic pain caused by endometriosis.

GnRH agonists are analogs of the native decapeptide, GnRH, with chemical changes in amino acids 6 and 10. The introduction of D-amino acids at position 6 of native GnRH can result in GnRH agonist analogs that are resistant to degradation by endopeptidases (and thus have long half-lives), have high affinity for the GnRH receptor, and have long receptor occupancy.[19] Paradoxically, initial treatment with a GnRH analog stimulates LH and FSH secretion, but prolonged treatment suppresses it (greater for LH than for FSH). The suppression of secretion results in suppression of ovarian follicle growth and a 95% decrease in estrogen production; the circulating estradiol concentration is in the range of that observed in menopausal women (15 pg/mL) (Table 98-2). Studies of surgical staging of endometriosis lesions before and after treatment with a GnRH

**TABLE 98-2.**

**Effects of Gonadotropin-Releasing Hormone (GnRH) Agonists on Serum Estradiol Concentrations in Women with Endometriosis***

| GnRH Agonist | Dose | Number of Subjects | Estradiol Concentration (pg/mL) | Variability of Patient Response to Treatment | Reference |
|--------------|------|--------------------|--------------------------------|---------------------------------------------|-----------|
| Nafarelin | 400 µg nasal spray | 77 | 28 | High | 20 |
| Nafarelin | 800 µg nasal spray | 79 | 15 | Moderate | 20 |
| Leuprolide acetate | 3.75 mg depot every 4 weeks | 52 | 15 | Low | 21 |
| Goserelin | 3.6 mg implant for 6 months | 40 | 13 | Low | 22 |

*The women were treated with the GnRH agonist for 20 to 24 weeks before measurement of the serum estradiol concentration.

analog demonstrated that serum estradiol levels in the range of 15 pg/mL reliably cause them to atrophy. In these studies, GnRH analogs produce significant decrease in pelvic pain in 85% of treated women and reduce the number and size of endometriosis implants.[20–23]

The hypoestrogenism induced by GnRH analogs is associated with vasomotor symptoms and decreased bone density. An important question in the endocrine management of endometriosis is: "To effectively treat endometriosis lesions, must the estradiol concentration be suppressed to the menopausal range (15 pg/mL)?" Suppression of serum estradiol to this concentration probably provides the most reliable and rapid suppression of endometriosis lesions, but suppression to 30 pg/mL can also be effective[24]; importantly, vasomotor symptoms and bone loss are less severe at a concentration of 30 pg/mL.

Thus, among women with endometriosis and pelvic pain who were randomized to receive either a GnRH agonist alone or a GnRH agonist plus low-dose estradiol (transdermal estradiol, 25 μg per day) plus low-dose progestin (oral medroxyprogesterone acetate, 2.5 mg per day), both groups had equivalent reductions in pain symptoms and in endometriosis lesions as determined by pretreatment and posttreatment laparoscopy.[25] The women who received GnRH agonist alone had more vasomotor symptoms and more bone loss than the women who received the GnRH agonist plus transdermal estradiol plus progestin. (Also see ref. 25a.)

Similar results have been obtained using other steroid "add-back" regimens.[26] Women with endometriosis and pelvic pain were randomized to four different hormone treatment groups: GnRH agonist alone, GnRH agonist plus progestin (norethindrone, 5 mg per day), GnRH agonist plus low-dose estrogen plus progestin (conjugated equine estrogen, 0.625 mg per day, and norethindrone acetate, 5 mg per day), or GnRH agonist plus high-dose estrogen plus progestin (conjugated equine estrogen, 1.25 mg per day, plus norethindrone acetate, 5 mg per day). Treatment was planned to continue for 1 year. The group receiving GnRH agonist plus high-dose estrogen had a higher rate of treatment discontinuation because of continuing pain than did any of the other treatment groups. The high-dose estrogen probably stimulated the continued functioning of the endometriosis implants. Consequently, GnRH agonist plus high-dose estrogen treatment is not recommended for most women with endometriosis and pelvic pain. The women in the other three groups had a similar decrease in their pelvic pain. Bone density decreased significantly in the women who received the GnRH agonist alone. Bone density was preserved in the groups that received a GnRH agonist plus the steroid add-back. Vasomotor symptoms were markedly reduced in the groups that received the steroid add-back. These studies and others[27] have demonstrated that the optimal treatment of pelvic pain caused by endometriosis may involve the use of GnRH agonists to suppress ovarian estrogen production followed by the "add-back" of *low doses* of estrogen-progestins or progestins alone (Table 98-3).

Novel strategies are being developed to treat the adverse effects of the hypoestrogenic state induced by the GnRH agonists. For example, the administration of a synthetic fragment of parathyroid hormone prevents the bone loss caused by the hypoestrogenism of GnRH agonist therapy.[28]

Estradiol is critical to the growth and functioning of endometriosis lesions, and the most common methods of reducing estrogen production are surgical bilateral oophorectomy or treatment with a GnRH agonist. A novel approach to reducing estrogen production in women with endometriosis is the use of *aromatase inhibitors*. In one study, the aromatase inhibitor anastrozole (1 mg per day) was administered to postmenopausal women with recurrent endometriosis after a bilateral oophorectomy. The aromatase inhibitor reduced circulating estradiol by 50%, and was associated with a decrease in pelvic pain.[29]

**TABLE 98-3.**
**Effective Low-Dose Steroid Hormone Plus Gonadotropin-Releasing Hormone (GnRH) Agonist Regimens**

| Low-Dose Steroid Hormone Regimen | Comments | Reference |
|---|---|---|
| Transdermal estradiol patch 25 μg/day, plus medroxyprogesterone acetate 2.5 mg daily | This regimen does not completely prevent bone loss. The estradiol concentration achieved is in the range of 30 pg/mL. | 25 |
| Norethindrone acetate 5 mg/day | This is a very high dose of progestin; it is associated with a decrease in HDL-cholesterol. | 41 |
| Conjugated equine estrogen 0.625 mg/day, norethindrone acetate 5 mg/day | This regimen prevents bone loss and markedly reduces the vasomotor symptoms reported. Pain relief was excellent. | 41 |

Note: GnRH agonist treatment combined with low-dose steroid "add-back" causes atrophy in endometriosis lesions, improves pelvic pain, and minimizes vasomotor symptoms and bone loss. These are the low-dose steroid hormone regimens that have been documented to be effective in randomized clinical trials when used in combination with a GnRH agonist.

Another approach to the treatment of endometriosis might be the use of *antiestrogens*. The original estrogen antagonists such as tamoxifen are weak estrogen agonists in the endometrium and have been demonstrated to lack efficacy in the treatment of endometriosis. In fact, there are numerous case reports of the onset of endometriosis in women receiving chronic tamoxifen therapy for breast cancer treatment or prevention.[30] The benzothiophene class of estrogen antagonists (raloxifene) are not estrogen agonists in the endometrium; therefore, these agents may have a role in the treatment of endometriosis.

## TREATMENT OF ENDOMETRIOSIS: ANDROGEN THERAPY

The first hormonal treatment of endometriosis was the intramuscular administration of testosterone. High-dose parenteral testosterone therapy was demonstrated to cause regression in endometriosis lesions. Unfortunately, many women became virilized. Androgen treatment was resurrected after the development of synthetic oral androgens, such as danazol, which have attenuated androgen properties.[31]

Danazol is a derivative of ethinyl testosterone and has moderate affinity for the androgen receptor, with a dissociation constant of $\sim 10^{-9}$ mol/L[32]; it also has weak affinity for the progesterone receptor, but no physiologically significant binding to estrogen or glucocorticoid receptors. At high doses, danazol directly suppresses cellular activity in endometriosis lesions, probably by acting through androgen and/or progestin receptors. In addition, the drug can modestly suppress pituitary secretion of LH and FSH, which in turn suppresses ovarian follicular growth, blocks ovulation (at doses >200 mg per day), and decreases the estradiol concentration to early follicular phase levels (30 pg/mL). The combination of an increase in androgen action and a decrease in estrogen action causes atrophy of the endometriosis lesions.

Randomized clinical trials that have directly compared the effects of danazol and the GnRH agonists demonstrated that both treatments improve pelvic pain in ~85% of treated women.[20] The side effects of these two treatments are very different. The main side effects of the GnRH agonists are those associated with hypoestrogenism, including vasomotor symptoms, diminished libido, dry vagina, and decreased bone density. The main side effects of danazol are weight gain (~4 kg at doses of 800 mg per day), muscle cramps, decrease in breast size, oily skin, and hirsutism.[33] Many of the side effects of danazol are dose-dependent; at doses of 50 mg, 100 mg, and 200 mg daily, it can be effective in relieving pelvic pain caused by endometriosis and is associated with less severe side effects than doses of 400 or 800 mg per day.[34] Doses of danazol of <400 mg per day do not reliably suppress ovulation. Danazol crosses the placenta and is a known teratogen. The clinician and patient must be sure that a pregnancy does not occur.

## TREATMENT OF ENDOMETRIOSIS BY INCREASING PROGESTIN ACTION

Many synthetic progestins are effective in the treatment of pelvic pain caused by endometriosis. High-dose progestin treatment produces an acyclic, hypoestrogenic environment by suppressing gonadotropin secretion. In addition, synthetic progestins have direct antiestrogenic effects on endometriosis lesions by binding to intracellular progesterone and androgen receptors. Synthetic progestins can be divided into two broad classes, the *C-21 progestins,* such as medroxyprogesterone acetate (MPA), and the *C-19 progestins,* such as gestrinone. In general, *the C-19 progestins have more androgenic activity* than the C-21 progestins.

Each of a group of women with endometriosis and pelvic pain who were treated with oral MPA (50 mg per day for 4 months) had pretreatment and posttreatment surgical staging of endometriosis.[35] Treatment resulted in an average serum estradiol concentration of 46 pg/mL and reduced serum estradiol levels to <20 pg/mL in some women. Eighty percent of the patients had improvement in their pelvic pain, and 70% had a decrease in their endometriosis lesions. The major side effect of treatment was irregular uterine bleeding, which occurred in 20%. Biopsy of the lesions before and after treatment demonstrated that MPA therapy induced atrophic and decidual changes. This study, although lacking a control group, suggests that MPA is effective in the treatment of endometriosis.

C-19 progestins, such as gestrinone, are also effective.[36] In one study, women with stage II and stage III endometriosis were randomized to receive gestrinone (1.25 mg once weekly or 2.5 mg once weekly). Most had improvement of their pelvic pain, and there was a better than 50% reduction in endometriosis lesions in both groups as determined by pretreatment and posttreatment laparoscopic examination. The major side effects were weight gain, headache, hirsutism, and irregular uterine bleeding.

## TREATMENT OF ENDOMETRIOSIS BY INCREASING ESTROGEN AND PROGESTIN ACTION

The combination estrogen-progestin birth control pill, when used in a continuous (pseudopregnancy) fashion, was found to be effective in the treatment of pelvic pain caused by endometriosis.[37] Subsequently, many clinicians noted that some women with endometriosis have some improvement in their dysmenorrhea and pelvic pain when treated with combination estrogen-progestin pills. However, few randomized clinical trials with oral contraceptives have been performed. One randomized clinical trial compared the effects of continuous (pseudopregnancy) combination estrogen-progestin oral contraceptive versus danazol therapy.[38] Symptomatic improvement occurred in 30% of the women given oral contraceptive; however, danazol treatment resulted in symptomatic improvement in 86%. Improvement in physical examination findings occurred in 84% of the women treated with danazol and in 18% of the women treated with continuous oral contraceptive.

In another randomized trial, an oral contraceptive was compared with a GnRH agonist in the treatment of pelvic pain caused by endometriosis. In this trial, the oral contraceptives and the GnRH agonist were equally effective for dysmenorrhea. However, the GnRH agonist was superior in the treatment of dyspareunia. A weakness of this study is that laparoscopic examination was not performed to assess the response of the endometriosis lesions.[39]

In a clinical trial, women with endometriosis were treated with a GnRH agonist (3.75 mg leuprolide acetate depot) or a GnRH agonist plus a low-dose oral estrogen-progestin contraceptive (20 µg ethinylestradiol and 0.15 mg desogestrel orally for 21 days every 4 weeks). The addition of the low-dose contraceptive reduced the efficacy of the GnRH agonist in the treatment of endometriosis[40]: pretreatment and posttherapy surgical staging of the endometriosis lesions demonstrated that treatment with the GnRH agonist plus oral contraceptive resulted in a 32% decrease (improvement) in the surgical staging score. In contrast, the GnRH agonist alone produced a superior, 76% decrease in the surgical staging score. Both treatment regimens produced a similar improvement in dysmenorrhea. However, the GnRH agonist produced better relief of dyspareunia.

Oral contraceptives probably are not as effective as GnRH agonists or danazol in the treatment of pelvic pain caused by endometriosis. However, given their safety and low cost, most clinicians treat women with pelvic pain with up to 3 months of these drugs, either in a cyclic or pseudopregnancy manner. If the patient has significant improvement in pain, treatment is continued for 6 to 12 months. If there is minimal improvement in pain, laparoscopy usually is offered to definitively diagnose the cause of the pain. At the time of the laparoscopy, an attempt is made to surgically excise the endometriosis lesions. GnRH agonists are often prescribed postoperatively to maximize the likelihood that the symptoms do not recur.[41] If pain recurs after the initial course of surgical-hormonal treatment, retreatment with a GnRH agonist is usually effective.

## INFERTILITY AND ENDOMETRIOSIS

The most common medical problem caused by endometriosis is pelvic pain. The second most common problem caused by endometriosis is a decrease in fecundability. *Fecundability is the chance of a couple conceiving during a single menstrual cycle.* The fecundability of a normal, young (25 years of age) couple is ~0.25. In couples with infertility and a female partner with early-stage endometriosis (stage I and II), the fecundability without treatment is ~0.03 per cycle, a marked reduction from normal.[42] In women with advanced endometriosis (stage III and IV), the fecundability is between 0.00 and 0.02. Surgical resection of endometriosis lesions in women with early-stage endometriosis has been demonstrated to increase fecundability from ~0.02 to 0.04 per cycle.[43] However, this requires general anesthesia and a major surgical procedure. An alternative to the surgical treatment of infertility associated with early-stage endometriosis is to empirically stimulate multifollicular development with clomiphene or gonadotropin therapy. When 40 women with infertility and stage I or II endometriosis were randomized to three treatment cycles of gonadotropin stimulation plus intrauterine insemination versus no treatment,[44] the cycle fecundability was 0.15 in the gonadotropin treatment group and 0.04 in the group that received no treatment. The relative effectiveness of gonadotropin versus clomiphene stimulation of multifollicular development was studied in women who were randomized to receive (a) no treatment, (b) clomiphene stimulation, or (c) clomiphene plus gonadotropin stimulation.[45] The cycle fecundability was 0.03 in the no treatment group, 0.07 in the clomiphene group, and 0.114 in the group receiving clomiphene plus gonadotropin. Both of these studies demonstrate the effectiveness of empirical stimulation of multifollicular development in the treatment of infertility caused by endometriosis.

In women with infertility and advanced endometriosis (stage III and IV), surgical resection of scar tissue[46] and endometriosis lesions or in vitro fertilization increases fecundability when compared with expectant management. After a primary surgical procedure, repeat surgery for infertility caused by endometriosis is unlikely to be effective. In women who have not become pregnant after a primary surgical procedure, IVF treatment is often effective.

For women with infertility and early-stage (stage I and II) or advanced endometriosis (stage III and IV), IVF may be highly effective. For women with infertility and endometriosis, IVF treatment results in ~0.30 deliveries per IVF cycle.[47] Although this therapy is resource intensive, the high pregnancy rate is likely to make it the primary treatment for infertility associated with endometriosis in the near future. Based on data from 1993, the cost of IVF per live birth is in the range of $22,000 to $43,000, depending on the clinical characteristics of the infertile couples.[48] These costs are within the range of current costs of adoption. Furthermore, since 1993, IVF success rates have increased and costs per cycle have decreased.

Endometriosis is a common gynecologic disorder that can be treated with surgical or hormonal interventions. It is likely that a complete elucidation of the pathophysiology of endometriosis will result in the development of novel and effective hormonal and medical treatments of endometriosis. As our hormonal armamentarium expands, the medical treatment of endometriosis will replace surgical treatment.

# REFERENCES

1. Hornstein MH, Barbieri RL. Endometriosis. In Ryan KJ, Berkowitz RS, Barbieri RL, eds. Kistner's gynecology: principles and practice, 6th ed. St. Louis: CV Mosby, 1995:187.
2. Ahmed MS, Barbieri RL. Re-operation rates for recurrent endometriomas after surgical excision. Gynecol Obstet Invest 1996; 43:53.
3. Barbieri RL, Callery M, Perez SE. Directionality of menstrual flow: cervical os diameter as a determinant of retrograde menstruation. Fertil Steril 1992; 57:727.
4. Barbieri RL. Stenosis of the external cervical os: an association with endometriosis in women with chronic pelvic pain. Fertil Steril 1998; 70:571.
5. Sugawara J, Fukaya T, Murakami T, et al. Increased secretion of hepatocyte growth factor by eutopic endometrial stromal cells in women with endometriosis. Fertil Steril 1997; 68:468.
6. Barbieri RL, Ryan KJ. Medical therapy for endometriosis: endocrine pharmacology. Semin Reprod Endocrinol 1985; 3:339.
7. Gazvani MR, Christmas S, Quenby S, et al. Peritoneal fluid concentrations of interleukin-8 in women with endometriosis: relationship to stage of disease. Hum Reprod 1998; 13:1957.
7a. Witz CA. Interleukin-6: another piece of the endometriosis-cytokine puzzle. Fertil Steril 2000; 73:212.
8. Shifren JL, Tseng JF, Zaloudek CJ, et al. Ovarian steroid regulation of vascular endothelial growth factor in the human endometrium: implications for angiogenesis during the menstrual cycle and in the pathogenesis of endometriosis. J Clin Endocrinol Metab 1996; 81:3112.
9. Murphy AA, Santanam N, Morales AJ, Parthasarathy S. Lysophosphatidyl choline, a chemotactic factor for monocytes/T-lymphocytes is elevated in endometriosis. J Clin Endocrinol Metab 1998; 83:2110.
10. Pellicer A, Albert C, Mercader A, et al. The follicular and endocrine environment in women with endometriosis: local and systemic cytokine production. Fertil Steril 1998; 70:425.
11. McLaren J, Prentic A, Charnock-Jones DS, et al. Vascular endothelial growth factor is produced by peritoneal fluid macrophages in endometriosis and is regulated by ovarian steroids. J Clin Invest 1996; 98:482.
12. Zhang RJ, Wild RA, Medders D, Gunupudi SR. Effects of peritoneal macrophages from patients with endometriosis on the proliferation of endometrial carcinoma cell line ECC-1. Am J Obstet Gynecol 1991; 165:1842.
13. Surrey ES, Halme J. Effect of platelet derived growth factor on endometrial stromal cell proliferation in vitro: a model for endometriosis. Fertil Steril 1991; 56:672.
14. Tamaya T, Motoyama T, Ohono Y. Steroid receptor levels and histology of endometriosis and adenomyosis. Fertil Steril 1979; 31:396.
15. Janne O, Kauppila A, Kokko E. Estrogen and progestin receptors in endometriotic lesions: comparison with endometrial tissue. Am J Obstet Gynecol 1981; 141:562.
16. DiZerga GS, Barber DL, Hodgen GD. Endometriosis: role of ovarian steroids in initiation, maintenance and suppression. Fertil Steril 1980; 33:649.
17. Metzger DA, Olive DL, Haney AF. Limited hormonal responsiveness of ectopic endometrium: histologic correlation with intrauterine endometrium. Hum Pathol 1988; 19:1417.
18. Ranney B. Endometriosis III. Complete operations. Am J Obstet Gynecol 1971; 109:1137.
19. Conn PM, Crowley WF Jr. Gonadotropin releasing hormone and its analogues. N Engl J Med 1991; 324:93.
20. Henzl MR, Corson SL, Moghissi K, et al. Administration of nasal nafarelin as compared with oral danazol for endometriosis. N Engl J Med 1988; 318:485.
21. Dlugi AM, Miller JS, Knittle J. Lupron Study Group. Lupron depot in the treatment of endometriosis: a randomized, placebo controlled double blind study. Fertil Steril 1990; 54:419.
22. Shaw RW. Goserelin depot preparation of LHRH analogue used in the treatment of endometriosis. In: Chadha DR, Buttram VC, eds, Current concepts in endometriosis. New York, Alan R. Liss, 1990; (323):383.
23. Bergqvist A, Bergh T, Hogstrom L, et al. Effects of triptorelin versus placebo on the symptoms of endometriosis. Fertil Steril 1998; 69:702.
24. Barbieri RL. Endometriosis and the estrogen threshold theory: relation to surgical and medical treatment. J Reprod Med 1998; 43:287.
25. Howell R, Edmonds D, Dowsett M, et al. Gonadotropin releasing hormone analogue plus hormone replacement therapy for the treatment of endometriosis: a randomized clinical trial. Fertil Steril 1995; 64:474.
25a. Parazzini F, Di Cintio E, Chatenad L, et al. Estroprogestin vs. gonadotrophin agonists plus estroprogestin in the treatment of endometriosis-related pelvic pain: a randomized trial. Europ J Obstet Gynecol Reprod Biol 2000; 88:11.
26. Hornstein MD, Surrey ES, Weinberg GW, et al. Leuprolide acetate depot and hormonal add-back in endometriosis: a 12-month study. Lupron Add-Back Study Group. Obstet Gynecol 1998; 91:16.
27. Moghissi KS, Scholar WD, Olive DL, et al. Goserelin acetate (Zoladex) with or without hormone replacement therapy for the treatment of endometriosis. Fertil Steril 1998; 69:1056.
28. Finkelstein JS, Klibanski A, Arnold AL, et al. Prevention of estrogen deficiency-related bone loss with human parathyroid hormone-(1-34): a randomized controlled trial. JAMA 1998; 280:1067.
29. Takayama K, Zeitoun K, Gunby RT, et al. Treatment of severe postmenopausal endometriosis with an aromatase inhibitor. Fertil Steril 1998; 69:709.
30. Ford MR, Turner MJ, Wood C, Soutter WP. Endometriosis developing during tamoxifen therapy. Am J Obstet Gynecol 1988; 158:1119.
31. Barbieri RL, Ryan KJ. Danazol: endocrine pharmacology and therapeutic applications. Am J Obstet Gynecol 1981; 141:453.
32. Barbieri RL, Lee H, Ryan KJ. Danazol binding to rat androgen, progestin, glucocorticoid and estrogen receptors. Correlation with biologic activity. Fertil Steril 1979; 31:182.
33. Barbieri RL, Evans S, Kistner RW. Danazol in the treatment of endometriosis: analysis of 100 cases with a 4-year follow-up. Fertil Steril 1982; 37:737.
34. Biberglou KO, Behrman SJ. Dosage aspects of danazol therapy in endometriosis: short-term and long-term effectiveness. Am J Obstet Gynecol 1981; 139:645.
35. Luciano AA, Turksoy RN, Carleo J. Evaluation of oral medroxyprogesterone acetate in the treatment of endometriosis. Obstet Gynecol 1988; 72:323.
36. Hornstein MD, Gleason RE, Barbieri RL. A randomized double blind prospective trial of two doses of gestrinone in the treatment of endometriosis. Fertil Steril 1990; 53:237.
37. Kistner RW. The treatment of endometriosis by inducing pseudopregnancy with ovarian hormones: a report of 58 cases. Fertil Steril 1959; 10:539.
38. Noble AD, Letchworth AT. Medical treatment of endometriosis: a comparative trial. Postgrad Med J 1979; 55(Suppl 5):37.
39. Vercellini P, Trespidi L, Colombo A, et al. A gonadotropin releasing hormone agonist versus a low dose oral contraceptive for pelvic pain associated with endometriosis. Fertil Steril 1993; 60:75.
40. Freundl G, Godtke K, Gnoth C, et al. Steroidal 'add-back' therapy in patients treated with GnRH agonists. Gynecol Obstet Invest 1998; 45 (Suppl 1):22.
41. Hornstein MD, Hemmings R, Yuzpe AA, Heinrichs WL. Use of nafarelin versus placebo after reductive laparoscopy surgery for endometriosis. Fertil Steril 1997; 68:860.
42. Berube S, Marcoux S, Langevin M, et al. Fecundity of infertile women with minimal or mild endometriosis and women with unexplained infertility. The Canadian Collaborative Group on Endometriosis. Fertil Steril 1998; 69:1034.
43. Marcoux S, Maheux R, Berube S, The Canadian Collaborative Group on Endometriosis. Laparoscopic surgery in infertile women with minimal or mild endometriosis. N Engl J Med 1997; 337:217.
44. Fedele L, Bianchi S, Marchini M, et al. Superovulation with human menopausal gonadotropins in the treatment of infertility associated with minimal or mild endometriosis. Fertil Steril 1992; 58:28.
45. Kemmann E, Chazi D, Corsan G, et al. Does ovulation stimulation improve fertility in women with minimal/mild endometriosis after laser laparoscopy. Int J Fertil 1993; 38:16.
46. Olive DL, Lee KL. Analysis of sequential treatment protocols for endometriosis associated infertility. Am J Obstet Gynecol 1986; 154:613.
47. Olivennes F, Feldberg D, Liu HC, et al. Endometriosis: a stage by stage analysis: role of in vitro fertilization. Fertil Steril 1995; 64:392.
48. Trad FS, Hornstein MD, Barbieri RL. In vitro fertilization: a cost-effective alternative for infertile couples? J Assist Reprod Genet 1995; 12:418.

# CHAPTER 99

# PREMENSTRUAL SYNDROME

ROBERT L. REID AND RUTH C. FRETTS

Most minor physical and psychological changes that mark the endocrine cyclicity of women of reproductive age (called *premenstrual molimina*) are normal phenomena that add to the uniqueness of the female personality. However, for a small percentage of women of reproductive age, cyclic variations in physical and behavioral symptoms may be pronounced.[1] The fact that such variations are often difficult to separate from physiologic changes makes an all-or-none accounting impossible; only the recognition of persistent premenstrual difficulties with quantifiable measures of functional or social impairment makes possible the designation of *premenstrual syndrome (PMS)* (formerly called *premenstrual tension*). The overlap of PMS symptoms with those of other disorders demands careful attention to the timing and cyclicity of symptoms.

## DEFINITION

Premenstrual syndrome is the cyclic recurrence in the luteal phase of the menstrual cycle of a combination of distressing physical, psychological, and/or behavioral changes of sufficient severity to result in deterioration of interpersonal relationships and/or interference with normal activities. The American Psychiatric Association has included as an appendix to the fourth revised edition of its *Diagnostic and Statistical Manual* diagnostic criteria for those persons in whom irritability, tension, dysphoria, or lability of mood are major components of premenstrual symptomatology, calling this condition *premenstrual dysphoric disorder (PMDD).*[2]

The classic manifestations of PMS may occur in the absence of menstrual bleeding if ovarian function and cyclicity have been preserved (e.g., after hysterectomy) and also in some anovulatory patients experiencing intermittent development and atresia of ovarian follicles.

Approximately 30% of women are sufficiently distressed by premenstrual symptoms to try over-the-counter remedies or to seek professional help; 3% to 8% report that their symptoms, although temporary, are severe or disabling.[3,4] Although PMS may span the complete age range from puberty until the menopause, many affected women report worsening of symptoms in the later reproductive years.

## CLINICAL MANIFESTATIONS

The symptoms of PMS fall into one of four temporal patterns (Fig. 99-1).[5] The most severely affected women report having only one symptom-free week per month; some may experience such a disruption of lifestyle in the affected weeks that a return to normal relationships and activities in the postmenstrual week is virtually impossible.

Often, the first noticeable changes include breast swelling and tenderness, together with lower abdominal bloating and constipation; some women change to looser clothing as the time of the menses approaches. A dramatic increase in appetite and cravings for chocolate or salty foods are also common.

Women troubled by the emotional changes may sleep longer, relinquish parental responsibility to the spouse, and cancel social commitments. Deterioration of interpersonal relationships and perceived inefficiency at work often precipitate feelings of personal inadequacy, hopelessness, and guilt. Some affected women

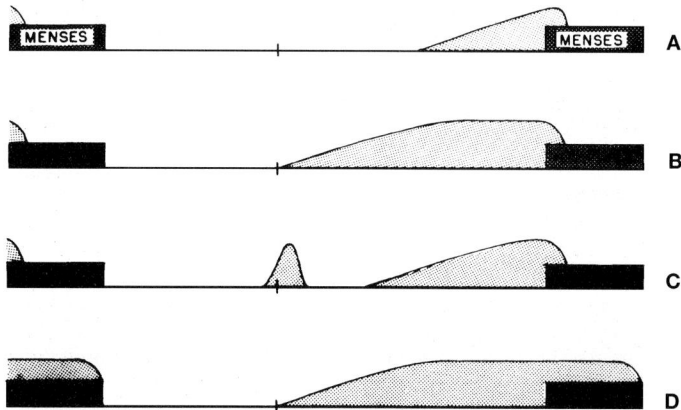

**FIGURE 99-1.** Schematic diagram showing variability in the onset and duration of premenstrual symptoms. Most patients experience patterns *A* or *B*. (From Reid RL, Yen SSC. Premenstrual syndrome. Clin Obstet Gynecol 1983; 26:710.)

experience an aversion to sexual relations in the midluteal phase with a rebound of sexual drive at or immediately before the onset of menstruation. Recurrent suicidal thoughts may occur.

In the final days of the cycle, particularly if the cycle is prolonged, inward tension, restlessness, and insomnia may become extreme. Some women have a burst of energy at this time and complete all of their previously neglected work; others describe associated confusion, inability to concentrate, and forgetfulness. Some avoid driving an automobile; others, believing their judgment to be impaired, may postpone important decisions until the days after menstruation. Depression or diminished impulse control in some women may result in alcohol or other substance abuse. There may be menopausal-like sweats and chills,[6] cardiac palpitations, sensitivity to noise, headaches, and a change from constipation to diarrhea in the final days of the cycle.

Some describe falling asleep at 10 p.m. and waking at 1 or 2 a.m. with their "engines revving." Unable to sleep, they may read or work for the remainder of the night, only to feel exhausted in the morning. Persistence of this pattern—for as long as a week before menstruation in some women—may result in prolonged periods of catch-up sleep after the menses begin.

Although some report the dramatic "lifting" of the inward tension and irritability several hours before the onset of menstrual flow, most experience relief only after the second or third day. Menorrhagia and dysmenorrhea are not features of PMS but, if present, may prolong or intensify the period of distress.

The predictable monthly recurrence of distressing premenstrual symptoms becomes an uncontrollable and unwanted intrusion into the personal and professional lives of afflicted women and may have important medical and legal implications.[5]

## PATHOPHYSIOLOGY

The pathophysiology of PMS is unknown. There appear to be two primary determinants. The first is cyclic function of the hypothalamic–pituitary–ovarian axis, because, without ongoing ovarian activity, the cyclic disruption in mood and behavior does not occur. The second factor is the intensity of coexisting life stresses. Together, they determine the timing and severity of PMS.

The linkage between the diverse manifestations of PMS and the cyclic changes in ovarian steroid production is unknown; some symptoms are probably a direct effect of circulating sex steroids, whereas others are mediated through changes in brain and hypothalamic neurotransmitters. Breast tenderness and enlargement are likely the result of direct sex steroid effects, leading to localized proliferation of ductal tissue and intralobular edema, whereas constipation and bloating reflect progestational effects on bowel function. The regulation of behavior, appetite, sleep, and temperature is more complex and probably involves a variety of neurotransmitter systems.

Numerous theories of pathophysiology have been advanced, some of which are invalid and none of which are entirely satisfactory.[7] Several are described in the following section.

## ABNORMALITIES OF ESTROGEN, PROGESTERONE, OR TESTOSTERONE

Studies purporting to show abnormal levels of estrogen, progesterone, and testosterone in PMS suffered from significant methodologic flaws. Subsequent investigations have confirmed normal circulating levels of gonadal steroids.[8,9] The demonstration of normal pulsatile luteinizing hormone secretion in the luteal phase challenged the long-held supposition that disordered neuroregulation of corpus luteal function could be implicated in PMS.[10] Treatment with progesterone vaginal suppositories was popularized as a means to correct the postulated progesterone deficiency; however, numerous randomized double-blind trials have since failed to demonstrate the efficacy of this therapy.[11,12]

Contrary to the widespread view that estrogen excess in the circulation triggers PMS, some evidence supports the concept that central (hypothalamic) estrogen deficiency may be the inciting factor.[13] Many women with PMS experience a brief period of intense symptoms coinciding with the drop in circulating estrogen that accompanies ovulation at midcycle (Fig. 99-1, pattern C). Women with PMS have a high incidence of hot flushes at the time they are symptomatic, in contrast to age-matched controls, who infrequently show this manifestation.[6] Whether central estrogen deficiency could occur in the face of normal circulating estradiol levels caused by progesterone-induced depletion of hypothalamic estrogen receptors is speculative; however, this might provide the "missing link" to connect ovarian cyclicity with changes in central neurotransmitters.[14]

## FLUID RETENTION

The popular notion that fluid retention explains symptoms of PMS is incorrect. Some women with PMS do experience minor peripheral edema premenstrually, but enlargement or tenderness of the breasts and abdominal bloating are more likely to result from fluid shifts within the body and not directly from a generalized overhydration. Most patients experience random fluctuations in weight over the course of the menstrual cycle; weight gain (as an indicator of fluid retention) does not correlate with the severity of other premenstrual manifestations. There is no convincing documentation of abnormal secretion of any fluid-retaining hormone in PMS.[7] Diuretic therapy, which transiently may help self-esteem by allowing the woman to fit into her tight clothing, may provoke further fluid retention by activating the renin-angiotensin-aldosterone system.

## HYPOGLYCEMIC-LIKE SYMPTOMS

Similarities between the symptoms of hypoglycemia and certain manifestations of PMS (fatigue, hunger, nervousness, sweating, and gastrointestinal complaints) led investigators to study hypoglycemia as a possible causative factor in PMS as early as the 1950s. A number of studies of glucose, insulin, and glucagon levels in response to either oral or intravenous glucose-tolerance tests at different phases of the menstrual cycle, in both PMS patients and controls, have failed to show significant differences,[15] thus casting doubt on this theory. However, more recent studies using sensitive analytic methods have shown declining insulin sensitivity in the luteal phase of the menstrual cycle.[16] In addition, the euglycemic insulin clamp technique has demonstrated premenstrual abnormalities of cellular glucose uptake in women with PMS, but not in normal controls.[17] Whether these changes can account for some of the varied clinical manifesta-

tions of PMS is uncertain. The role of "hypoglycemic" diets in the treatment of PMS is likewise unresolved.

## PROSTAGLANDIN E$_1$ DEFICIENCY

A defect in the conversion of essential free fatty acids to prostaglandin E$_1$ has been postulated to result from a competitive enzyme block at the conversion of γ-linoleic acid to dihomo-γ-linoleic acid, a precursor of prostaglandin E$_1$. Treatment with 9% γ-linoleic acid in the form of evening primrose oil has been suggested as therapy. Despite widespread promotion of this treatment for PMS in the lay literature, there has been no convincing documentation of its efficacy. Studies widely cited by proponents of this approach either fail to show superiority of evening primrose oil to placebo or contain serious methodologic flaws that cast doubt on the conclusions. Double-blind placebo-controlled trials have failed to establish the superiority of γ-linoleic acid supplements to placebo in the treatment of PMS.[18,19]

## SEROTONIN DEFICIENCY

The current consensus suggests that normal circulating levels of gonadal steroids can evoke manifestations of PMS in susceptible women through a psychoneuroendocrine mechanism. Of all the neurotransmitters studied to date, serotonin appears to be one of the most promising candidates as the "hypothalamic transducer."[20] The concept of a hypothalamic estrogen-serotonin connection has been reinforced by recent evidence that menopausal hot flashes resistant to estrogen can be alleviated in some women by selective serotonin reuptake inhibitors (SSRIs). Gamma-aminobutyric acid/benzodiazepine receptor complex abnormalities also may play a role.[20a]

## OTHER THEORIES

The continuation of PMS in women who have undergone a hysterectomy with preservation of ovarian function strongly argues against the concept that culturally derived negative beliefs about menstruation could lead to the development of severe recurrent premenstrual symptoms. The perpetuation of such a psychogenic theory for PMS has delayed the rational investigation and development of effective therapeutic interventions.

Prolactin levels are normal in PMS, and there is no evidence of pyridoxine (vitamin B$_6$) deficiency, although this substance is a coenzyme in the biosynthesis of certain neurotransmitters involved in the regulation of mood.

There are alleged cases of allergy to endogenous hormones, the most striking being those involving the appearance of rashes secondary to antibodies to 17-hydroxyprogesterone throughout the luteal phase of the cycle.[21] Nevertheless, there is no evidence that allergy provokes the manifestations of PMS or that allergies are more common in this condition.

Hypothyroidism is not a tenable hypothesis given the numerous studies reporting normal thyroid function.[22] Also, a report that calcium supplementation will relieve PMS should be viewed with skepticism until confirmed independently because the biologic plausibility of this approach is questionable.[23]

## DIAGNOSIS

### HISTORY AND PHYSICAL EXAMINATION

The investigation of PMS begins with a complete history and physical examination. A history detailing past reproductive events and current menstrual cyclicity sets the stage for a more informed discussion about menstrual cycle–related symptoms. Typically, women with PMS report feeling extremely well during past pregnancies. The nature, severity, and chronologic appearance of symptoms in the course of a menstrual cycle should be determined. Premenstrual manifestations should be distinguished from those involving menstruation, such as dysmenorrhea or menorrhagia, which may be addressed separately. It is extremely important to document the true sense of well-being in the postmenstrual week that most PMS sufferers describe to differentiate this condition from other chronic mood and behavioral disorders that surface under the guise of PMS merely because they show premenstrual exacerbation.

Information should be obtained about the stresses related to the woman's occupation and family life, because these may significantly affect premenstrual symptoms. Finally, past medical or psychiatric diagnoses and interventions for these should be reviewed. It is important to identify psychiatric illness unrelated to the menses. On the other hand, it is not uncommon for women with PMS to be inappropriately diagnosed as having neurotic depression or manic depressive disorders when the relationship of symptoms to menstruation has been overlooked.

Organic causes of PMS-like symptoms must be ruled out. Marked fatigue may result from anemia, leukemia, hypothyroidism, or diuretic-induced potassium deficiency; headaches may be caused by intracranial lesions. Pelvic examination may reveal tumors of the uterus or ovaries, endometriosis, or pelvic inflammatory disease. Typical menopausal-like hot flashes seen in the premenstrual week in PMS sufferers should not lead to an erroneous diagnosis of menopause.[23a]

### CHARTING

Retrospective recall by a patient correlates poorly with prospective records of symptoms. Daily records should be maintained for at least 2 months. A detailed record, the PRISM calendar (Prospective Record of the Impact and Severity of Menstrual Symptoms), is used in the authors' clinic (Fig. 99-2).[5] Patients begin charting on the first day of menstruation and indicate the number of days of bleeding or spotting. Each night they record the severity of any symptoms experienced on a scale of 1 to 3 and mark with an "X" the impact that these symptoms have had on their functioning on a given day. Additional information concerning external life events and use of medications is recorded. By reviewing 2 months of PRISM calendars, the woman and her physician can determine the duration and regularity of bleeding, the pattern and severity of premenstrual and menstrual symptomatology, and the degree of lifestyle disruption precipitated by these symptoms. The record of daily weight change is helpful to demonstrate to the bloated woman that weight change (hence fluid balance) usually fluctuates randomly in this disorder.

A concise 36-point self-rating scale has been developed that incorporates items with discriminating value in the diagnosis of PMS and its impact on lifestyle (Table 99-1).[24] When applied twice during the cycle (once before and once after menstruation), this rating scale allows easy identification of women with the on/off symptom profile typical of PMS. However, the self-rating scale does not replace the prospective record, because it lacks information on the duration or chronology of symptoms.

### SEEKING CONSULTATION

Gynecologic assessment is part of the initial evaluation of a woman with PMS because of the potential overlap of premenstrual complaints with symptoms of other pelvic disorders such as endometriosis and tubo-ovarian disease. Premenstrual pelvic pain, dysmenorrhea, dyspareunia, and menorrhagia are not usual features of PMS and warrant appropriate gynecologic evaluation.

Severe emotional symptoms lacking the on/off criteria of PMS, concern about suicidal intent or possible violence directed toward children or others, or psychotic behavior usually warrants psychiatric consultation. Additional consultation may be appropriate for unusual premenstrual complaints such as asthma, epilepsy, migraine, arthritis, and tinnitus or vertigo.[25]

## THERAPY

Education and counseling about the nature of premenstrual mood and behavioral changes is sufficient to allow many patients to cope with PMS. Most patients are embarrassed and frustrated by the skepticism with which their concerns are met by many within the medical profession. When their concerns are not taken seriously and they are simply advised to put "mind over matter," the recurrent monthly intrusion into their lives becomes a source of both fear and guilt. It is common for afflicted women to have fears that they are "going crazy" and to experience a loss of self-worth in their careers and their family roles. Validation of the woman's experience and letting her know that she is not alone is perhaps the most important first step in overcoming PMS. Women with PMS need to hear that although medicine has yet to unravel the complex interplay between reproductive hormones and mood, there are now effective interventions that will provide relief for this disorder.

Charting by itself may demonstrate to the patient the cyclicity of her symptoms, which is consistent with a hormonal cause (or, on the other hand, may indicate that she does not have PMS). Reassurance that other women experience similar problems is afforded by the fact that many of her symptoms are already listed on the PRISM calendar.

When an individual is suffering to a degree that requires more than simple counseling and assurance, measures aimed at lifestyle modification should be explored first. The woman and her family must develop strategies for coping and stress reduction. It is vital that she learn to anticipate times when she may be more vulnerable to emotional upset or confrontation with others by looking back at the previous month's calendar. Extra precautions at this time may reduce confrontations. For example, if a woman finds that drinking alcohol precedes temper flares or that drinking coffee induces anxiety, she should avoid these premenstrually. Ongoing charting is vital to this process of self-education.

A regular program of exercise should be encouraged as a useful outlet for tension and anxiety. All too often, the woman's best intentions are insufficient to keep her on track with an exercise program when the fatigue or depression of PMS sets in. Encouraging her to exercise with a friend who can provide continuing motivation at these times is helpful.

Group counseling in a program supervised by a clinical psychologist can be invaluable; however, participation in a "support group" of heterogeneous, self-diagnosed PMS sufferers is useless to women seeking reliable information and direction. The lay literature contains much misinformation.

Reduction of intake of salt and refined carbohydrates may help prevent edema and swelling in some women. There is anecdotal evidence that small, more frequent meals may alleviate some symptoms, perhaps by facilitating cellular glucose uptake.

Attention should be directed to the treatment of other menstrual cycle symptoms for which established treatments exist. For example, prostaglandin synthetase inhibitors afford effective relief from dysmenorrhea for most women. These agents may also attenuate other premenstrual symptoms when used on a regular basis in the 7 to 10 days before menstruation.[26] Caution must be exercised with the prescription of any drug in the luteal phase of the cycle if the possibility of pregnancy exists.

If the woman has contraceptive needs or experiences dysmenorrhea or menorrhagia, an oral contraceptive may be a good first choice, because it reduces the overall sum of premenstrual and menstrual symptoms. Nevertheless, it is important to remember that exposure to progestin begins 3 weeks before menstruation in oral contraceptive users, and some individuals will actually experience PMS symptoms occurring shortly after beginning their pill cycle until the onset of menstruation.[27] Women on the oral contraceptive who have distressing PMS should be counseled to consider an alternate means of contraception—at least on a trial basis—until the effect of the oral con-

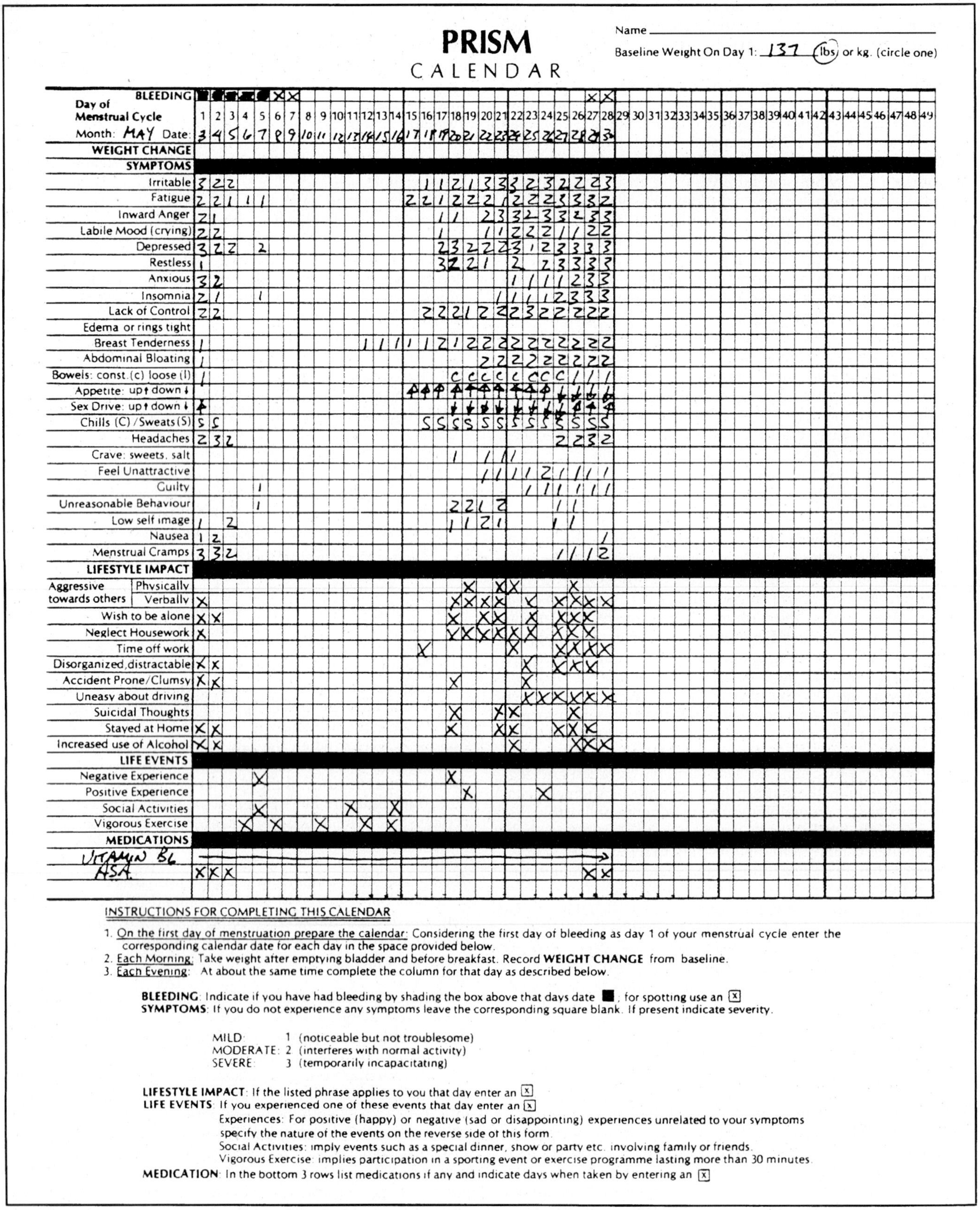

# PRISM CALENDAR

Name ____________

Baseline Weight On Day 1: 137 (lbs) or kg. (circle one)

BLEEDING

Day of Menstrual Cycle: 1 2 3 4 5 6 7 8 9 10 11 12 13 14 15 16 17 18 19 20 21 22 23 24 25 26 27 28 29 30 31 32 33 34 35 36 37 38 39 40 41 42 43 44 45 46 47 48 49

Month: MAY Date:

WEIGHT CHANGE

**SYMPTOMS**

- Irritable
- Fatigue
- Inward Anger
- Labile Mood (crying)
- Depressed
- Restless
- Anxious
- Insomnia
- Lack of Control
- Edema or rings tight
- Breast Tenderness
- Abdominal Bloating
- Bowels: const. (c) loose (l)
- Appetite: up ↑ down ↓
- Sex Drive: up ↑ down ↓
- Chills (C) / Sweats (S)
- Headaches
- Crave: sweets, salt
- Feel Unattractive
- Guilty
- Unreasonable Behaviour
- Low self image
- Nausea
- Menstrual Cramps

**LIFESTYLE IMPACT**

- Aggressive towards others: Physically / Verbally
- Wish to be alone
- Neglect Housework
- Time off work
- Disorganized, distractable
- Accident Prone/Clumsy
- Uneasy about driving
- Suicidal Thoughts
- Stayed at Home
- Increased use of Alcohol

**LIFE EVENTS**

- Negative Experience
- Positive Experience
- Social Activities
- Vigorous Exercise

**MEDICATIONS**

- VITAMIN B6
- ASA

INSTRUCTIONS FOR COMPLETING THIS CALENDAR

1. On the first day of menstruation prepare the calendar: Considering the first day of bleeding as day 1 of your menstrual cycle enter the corresponding calendar date for each day in the space provided below.
2. Each Morning: Take weight after emptying bladder and before breakfast. Record **WEIGHT CHANGE** from baseline.
3. Each Evening: At about the same time complete the column for that day as described below.

**BLEEDING**: Indicate if you have had bleeding by shading the box above that days date ■; for spotting use an ☒

**SYMPTOMS**: If you do not experience any symptoms leave the corresponding square blank. If present indicate severity.

MILD: 1 (noticeable but not troublesome)
MODERATE: 2 (interferes with normal activity)
SEVERE: 3 (temporarily incapacitating)

**LIFESTYLE IMPACT**: If the listed phrase applies to you that day enter an ☒

**LIFE EVENTS**: If you experienced one of these events that day enter an ☒

Experiences: For positive (happy) or negative (sad or disappointing) experiences unrelated to your symptoms specify the nature of the events on the reverse side of this form.
Social Activities: imply events such as a special dinner, show or party etc. involving family or friends.
Vigorous Exercise: implies participation in a sporting event or exercise programme lasting more than 30 minutes.

**MEDICATION**: In the bottom 3 rows list medications if any and indicate days when taken by entering an ☒

**FIGURE 99-2.** Prospective record of the impact and severity of menstrual symptomatology (PRISM calendar), developed by R. L. Reid and S. Maddocks. The calendar was completed by a patient for one complete menstrual cycle. Note the symptom-free interval after menstruation and the return of symptoms in the luteal phase.

**TABLE 99-1.**
**Self-Rating for Premenstrual Syndrome**

| Name: | | Date: | |
|---|---|---|---|
| Instructions: The following questions are concerned with the way you feel or act today. | | | |
| Please answer *all* questions by circling YES or NO as indicated. | | | |
| 1. Do you find yourself avoiding some of your social commitments? | | YES | NO |
| 2. Have you gained 5 or more pounds during the past week? | | YES | NO |
| 3. Is your coordination so poor that you are unable to use kitchen utensils, garden tools, or unable to drive? | | YES | NO |
| 4. Do you feel more angry than usual? | | YES | NO |
| 5. Do you avoid family activities and prefer to be left alone? | | YES | NO |
| 6. Do you doubt your judgment or feel that you are prone to hasty decisions? | | YES | NO |
| 7. Do you feel more irritable than usual? | | YES | NO |
| 8. Is your efficiency diminished? | | YES | NO |
| 9. Do you feel tense and restless? | | YES | NO |
| 10. Do you feel a marked change in your sexual drive or desire during the last week? | | YES | NO |
|    If YES, is it *increased* or *decreased*? | | ↑ | ↓ |
| 11. Are your present physical symptoms causing so much pain and discomfort that you are unable to function? | | YES | NO |
| 12. Have you recently cancelled previously scheduled social activities? | | YES | NO |
| 13. Do you feel as if you are unable to relax at all? | | YES | NO |
| 14. Do you feel confused? | | YES | NO |
| 15. Do you experience painful or tender breasts? | | YES | NO |
| 16. Do you have an increased desire for specific kinds of food (e.g., cravings for candy, chocolate, etc.)? | | YES | NO |
| 17. Do you scream/yell at family members (friends, colleagues) more than usual? Are you "short-fused"? | | YES | NO |
| 18. Do you feel sad, gloomy, and hopeless most of the time? | | YES | NO |
| 19. Do you feel like crying? | | YES | NO |
| 20. Do you have difficulty completing your daily household/job routine? | | YES | NO |
| 21. Was there a marked change in your sexual drive with definite change in your sexual behavior during the last week? | | YES | NO |
|    If YES, is it *increased* or *decreased*? | | ↑ | ↓ |
| 22. Do you find yourself being more forgetful than usual or unable to concentrate? | | YES | NO |
| 23. Do you happen to have more "accidents" with your daily housework/job (cut fingers, break dishes, etc.)? | | YES | NO |
| 24. Have you noticed significant swelling of your breasts and/or ankles and/or bloating of your abdomen? | | YES | NO |
| 25. Does your mood change suddenly without obvious reason? | | YES | NO |
| 26. Are you easily distracted? | | YES | NO |
| 27. Do you think that your restless behavior is noticeable by others? | | YES | NO |
| 28. Are you clumsier than usual? | | YES | NO |
| 29. Are you obviously negative and hostile toward other people? | | YES | NO |
| 30. Are you so fatigued that it interferes with your usual level of functioning? | | YES | NO |
| 31. Do you tend to eat more than usual or at odd irregular hours (sweets, snacks, etc.)? | | YES | NO |
| 32. Do you become more easily fatigued than usual? | | YES | NO |
| 33. Is your handwriting different (less neat than usual)? | | YES | NO |
| 34. Do you feel jittery or upset? | | YES | NO |
| 35. Do you feel sad or blue? | | YES | NO |
| 36. Have you stopped calling or visiting some of your best friends? | | YES | NO |

(From Steiner M, Haskett RF, Carroll BJ. Premenstrual tension syndrome: the development of research diagnostic criteria and new rating scales. Acta Psychiatr Scand 1980; 62:177.)

traceptive can be determined. Alternatively, an SSRI could be used in combination with the oral contraceptive.

For a woman in whom symptoms of anxiety, irritability, tension, or insomnia predominate, the use of short-acting anxiolytics or hypnotics such as alpazolam (0.25 mg orally twice or three times a day) or triazolam (0.25 mg orally each night), respectively, may provide substantial relief.[28]

Vitamin B$_6$ is of doubtful benefit and may cause peripheral neuropathy if dosing is excessive.[29] Herbal remedies are of unproven efficacy and some are unsafe.[29a] Disabling periovulatory or menstrual migraine headaches can be controlled with percutaneous or sublingual estradiol.[30] Bromocriptine, 2.5 mg twice a day, may relieve premenstrual mastodynia but does not relieve PMS in general.[31]

A range of newer antidepressant medications that augment central serotonin activity alleviate severe premenstrual syndrome. Because these agents will also relieve endogenous depression, a pretreatment diagnosis, achieved by prospective charting, is very important.

For patients in whom PMS symptoms are severe and menstrual cycle suppression is not a desired option, antidepressant therapy may provide excellent results. SSRIs such as fluoxetine, sertaline, paroxetine, fluvoxamine, and venlafaxine (a serotonin and norepinephrine reuptake inhibitor) have all been successfully used.[32,33]

Symptom profiles may help in selecting the most appropriate agent (e.g., fluoxetine in patients in whom fatigue and depression predominate; sertraline if insomnia, irritability, and anxiety are paramount). Preliminary data indicate that SSRIs may alleviate the menopausal-like hot flashes.[33a] SSRIs have been associated with loss of libido and anorgasmia, so appropriate pretreatment counseling is essential.

Tricyclic antidepressants (TCAs) have not generally been effective, with the exception of clomipramine, a TCA with strong serotoninergic activity. Intolerance to the side effects of TCAs is common.

Most PMS sufferers would prefer to medicate themselves only during the symptomatic phase of the menstrual cycle.

Recent studies suggest that luteal phase therapy may be as effective as continuous use of antidepressants.

For severely affected individuals and those with severe menstrual cycle–related conditions such as asthma, anaphylaxis, migraine, functional bowel disease, or sensorineural hearing loss, medical ovarian suppression with danazol, 200 mg twice daily,[34] on a continuous basis or a monthly injection of a gonadotropin-releasing hormone agonist (leuprolide [Depo Lupron], 3.75 mg, or goserelin [Zoladex], 3.6 mg) accompanied by low-dose estrogen-replacement therapy (Premarin, 1.25 mg or equivalent to obviate menopausal symptoms) will afford dramatic relief.[25]

If a woman who has completed her family suffers major lifestyle disruption and SSRIs are ineffective or poorly tolerated, a surgical option should be considered.[35,36] Obviously oophorectomy is only suited to women in whom long-lasting benefit from pharmacologic ovarian suppression has been documented but for whom continuing medical therapy is not a reasonable option because of inconvenience, side effects, or expense. Hysterectomy alone, with preservation of the ovaries, will not cure PMS, and cyclic symptoms in the luteal phase of the cycle will continue.[37] If the ovaries are to be removed, the uterus should also be removed to avoid the need for progestin treatment during subsequent hormone-replacement therapy. In the authors' experience, low-dose estrogen-replacement therapy is well tolerated without the return of PMS symptoms[38]; however, the addition of a progestin is often accompanied by recurrence of premenstrual symptoms.

## REFERENCES

1. Reid RL. Premenstrual syndrome. N Engl J Med 1991; 324:1208.
2. American Psychiatric Association. Diagnostic and statistical manual of mental disorders, 4th ed (DSM-IV). Washington, DC: APA, 1994.
3. Johnson SR, McChesney C, Bean JA. Epidemiology of premenstrual symptoms in a nonclinical sample. I. Prevalence, natural history, and help-seeking behavior. J Repro Med 1988; 33:340.
4. Rivera-Tovar AD, Frank E. Late luteal phase dysphoric disorder in young women. Am J Psychiatry 1990; 146:1634.
5. Reid RL. Premenstrual syndrome. Curr Probl Obstet Gynecol Fertil 1985; 8(2):1.
6. Hahn PM, Wong J, Reid RL. Menopausal-like hot flushes reported in women of reproductive age. Fertil Steril 1998; 70(5):913.
7. Reid RL, Yen SSC. The premenstrual syndrome. Am J Obstet Gynecol 1981; 139:85.
8. Rubinow DR, Hoban MC, Grovera GN, et al. Changes in plasma hormones across the menstrual cycle in patients with menstrually related mood disorder and in control subjects. Am J Obstet Gynecol 158(1):5; 1998.
9. Bloch M, Schmidt PH, Su TP, et al. Pituitary-adrenal hormones and testosterone across the menstrual cycle in women with premenstrual syndrome and controls. Biol Psychiat 1998; 43(12):897.
10. Reame NE, Marshall JC, Kelch RP. Pulsatile LH secretion in women with premenstrual syndrome (PMS): evidence for normal neuroregulation of the menstrual cycle. Psychoneuroendocrinology 1992; 17:205.
11. Maddocks SE, Hahn P, Moller F, Reid RL. A double-blind, placebo-controlled trial of progesterone vaginal suppositories in the treatment of premenstrual syndrome. Am J Obstet Gynecol 1986; 154:573.
12. Freeman E, Rickels K, Sondherimer SJ, Polansky M. Ineffectiveness of progesterone suppository treatment for premenstrual syndrome. JAMA 1990; 264(3):349.
13. Reid RL. Premenstrual syndrome. Am Assoc Clin Chem 1987; 5:1.
14. Schmidt PJ, Neiman LK, Danaceau MA, et al. Differential behavioral effects of gonadal steroids in women with and in those without premenstrual syndrome. N Engl J Med 1998; 338(4):209.
15. Reid RL, Greenaway-Coates A, Hahn P. Oral glucose tolerance (OGT) during the menstrual cycle in normal women (NW) and women with alleged premenstrual "hypoglycemic" attacks (PMHA): effects of naloxone. J Clin Endocrinol Metab 1986; 26:1167.
16. Valdes CT, Elkind-Hirsch KE. Intravenous glucose tolerance test–derived insulin sensitivity changes during the menstrual cycle. J Clin Endocrinol Metab 1991; 72:642.
17. Diamond M, Simonson DC, DeFronzo RA. Menstrual cyclicity has a profound effect on glucose homeostasis. Fertil Steril 1989; 52:204.
18. Collins A, Cerin A, Coleman G, Landgren BM. Essential fatty acids in the treatment of premenstrual syndrome. Obstet Gynecol 1993; 81:93.
19. Khoo SK, Munro C, Battistutta D. Evening primrose oil and treatment of premenstrual syndrome. Med J Aust 1990; 153:189.
20. Steiner M, Lepage P, Dunn EJ. Serotonin and gender-specific psychiatric disorders. Int J Psychiatry Clin Prac 1997; 1:3.
20a. Le Melledo JM, Van Driel M, Coupland NJ, et al. Response to flumazenil in women with premenstrual dysphoric disorder. Am J Psychiatry 2000; 157:821.
21. Cheesman KL, Gaynor LV, Chatterton RT, Radvany RM. Identification of a 17-OH progesterone-binding immunoglobulin in the serum of a woman with periodic rashes. J Clin Endocrinol Metab 1982; 55:597.
22. Schmidt PJ, Grover GN, Roy-Byrne PP, Rubinow DR. Thyroid function in women with premenstrual syndrome. J Clin Endocrinol Metab 1993; 76(3):671.
23. Thys-Jacobs S, Starkey P, Bernstein D, Tian J, and the PMS Study Group. Calcium carbonate and the premenstrual syndrome: effects on premenstrual and menstrual symptoms. Am J Obstet Gynecol 1998; 179(2):444.
23a. Hahn PM, Wong J, Reid RL. Menopausal-like hot flashes reported in women of reproductive age. Fertil Steril 1998; 70(5):913.
24. Haskett RF, Abplanalp JM. Premenstrual tension syndrome: diagnostic criteria and selection of research subjects. Psychiat Res 1983; 9:125.
25. Case AM, Reid RL. Effects of the menstrual cycle on medical disorders. Arch Intern Med 1998; 158:1405.
26. Mira M, McNeil D, Fraser IS, et al. Mefenamic acid in the treatment of premenstrual syndrome. Obstet Gynecol 1986; 68:395.
27. Forrest ARW. Cyclical variations in mood in normal women taking oral contraceptives. BMJ 1979; 1:1403.
28. Harrison WM, Endicott J, Nee J. Treatment of premenstrual dysphoria with alprazolam. A controlled study. Arch Gen Psychiat 1990; 47:270.
29. Schaumburg H, Kaplain J, Windebank A, et al. Sensory neuropathy from pyridoxine abuse. N Engl J Med 1983; 309:445.
29a. Bendich A. The potential for dietary supplements to reduce premenstrual syndrome (PMS) symptoms. J Am Coll Nutr 2000; 19:3.
30. de Lignieres B, Vincens M, Mas JL, et al. Prevention of menstrual migraine by percutaneous estradiol treatment. BMJ 1986; 293:1540.
31. Andersch B. Bromocriptine and premenstrual symptoms: a survey of double-blind trials. Obstet Gynecol Surv 1983; 38:643.
32. Steiner M, Steinberg S, Stewart D, et al, for the Canadian Fluoxetine/Premenstrual Dysphiria Collaborative Study Group. Fluoxetine in the treatment of premenstrual dysphoria. N Engl J Med 1995; 332(23):1529.
33. Freeman EW, Rickels K, Sondheimer SJ, Polansky M. Differential response to antidepressants in women with premenstrual syndrome/premenstrual dysphoric disorder: a randomized controlled trial. Arch Gen Psychiat 1999; 56:932.
33a. Loprinzi CL, Pisonsky TM, Fonseca R, et al. Pilot evaluation of venlafaxine hydrochloride for the therapy of hot flashes in cancer survivors. J Clin Oncol 1998; 16:2377.
34. Hahn PM, Van Vugt DA, Reid RL. A randomized placebo-controlled trial of danazol for the treatment of PMS. Psychoneuroendocrinology 1994; 60:297.
35. Reid RL. Use of GnRH agonists for menstrual cycle related disorders. J Soc Obstet Gynecol Canada 1992; 14(8):59.
36. Casson P, Hahn PM, Van Vugt DA, Reid RL. Lasting response to ovariectomy in severe intractable premenstrual syndrome. Am J Obstet Gynecol 1990; 162:99.
37. Casper RH, Hearn MT. The effect of hysterectomy and bilateral oophorectomy in women with severe premenstrual syndrome. Am J Obstet Gynecol 1991; 162:105.
38. Backstrom CT, Boyle H, Baird DT. Persistence of symptoms of premenstrual tension in hysterectomized women. Br J Obstet Gynaecol 1981; 88:530.

# CHAPTER 100

# MENOPAUSE

BRIAN WALSH AND ISAAC SCHIFF

## DEFINITION AND INCIDENCE

*Menopause* designates the permanent cessation of menses, which women experience at the average age of 51 years. This is but one aspect of the *climacteric*, the end of a woman's reproductive potential, when she experiences endocrinologic, somatic, and psychological changes. The changes that occur at menopause are related both to aging and to decreased estrogen levels, and it is difficult to quantify the respective effects of each.

It is incorrect to think that the ovary ages suddenly and dramatically at the time of menopause. Rather, the ovary begins to age from the start of life; it actually does so before birth. Throughout life there is a steady decline in the number of oocytes (see Chap. 95).

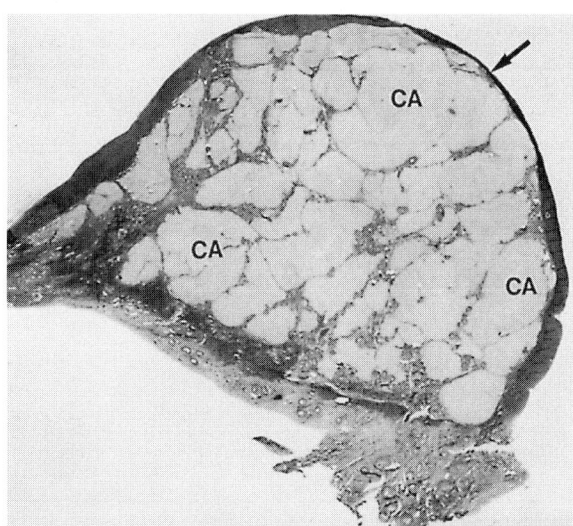

**FIGURE 100-1.** Normal transected postmenopausal ovary, showing a thin rim of cortex (*arrow*) with the center of the ovary filled with corpora albicantia (*CA*). (Hematoxylin and eosin stain; ×5) (Courtesy of Dr. Robert Scully, Massachusetts General Hospital.)

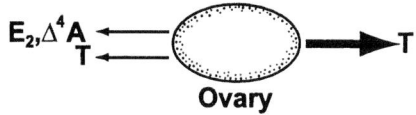

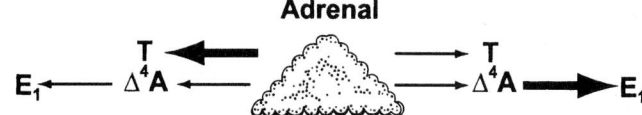

**FIGURE 100-2.** Changes in hormone secretion at menopause. Note loss of estradiol ($E^2$) and $\Delta^4$ androstenedione ($\Delta^4 A$) production by the ovary and a relative increase in ovarian secretion of testosterone ($T$). Adrenal secretion of testosterone is decreased, and there is continuing adrenal secretion of $\Delta^4$ androstenedione and an increased peripheral conversion of the latter steroid to estrone ($E_1$). (From Haas S, Schiff I. Physiology of estrogen deficiency. In: Riddick DH, ed. Reproductive physiology in clinical practice. New York: Thieme Medical Publishers, 1987:266.)

At the beginning of the twenty-first century, a woman who reaches the menopause can be expected to live until age 85 years. In contrast, in the first decade of the twentieth century, a woman's life expectancy was ~48 years. Thus, a woman can anticipate living about one-third of her life without ovarian hormones; this fact alone makes the well-being of postmenopausal women a major medical concern. Moreover, with the rise of the mean age in industrialized Western countries, the concern will become even greater. For example, in the United States, the proportion of the entire population older than age 65 years rose from ~9.2% in 1960, to ~9.8% in 1970, and to ~11.3% in 1980.[1] In 1990 there were 30 million persons in the United States aged 65 years and older.[2] This demographic group will more than double to reach 80 million between the years 2000 and 2050.[2]

## ENDOCRINE AND OTHER CHANGES OF THE MENOPAUSE

With follicular depletion, steroid production by ovarian follicles falls. The predominant estrogen produced by ovarian follicles is *estradiol*. When estradiol production ceases, the symptoms of menopause ensue. However, estrogen production in postmenopausal women does not stop completely; instead, production at low levels continues throughout life (Figs. 100-1 and 100-2). The estrogens produced after the menopause derive from androgens, specifically *androstenedione*, coming from the adrenal gland and, in part, from the stroma of the ovary. The androgens are converted into *estrone* by tissues such as the liver, the kidneys, and peripheral fat.[3] Estrone is a weaker estrogen than estradiol. The ratio of estrogens changes from the premenopausal situation, in which estradiol predominates over estrone, to the postmenopausal one, in which estrone predominates. Because androgens are converted to estrogens in peripheral fat, overweight women convert more of their adrenal androgens to estrogens than women of normal weight.[4] Thus, overweight women are less at risk for diseases associated with estrogen deficiency, such as osteoporosis, but are more at risk for diseases associated with estrogen excess, such as endometrial cancer.[5] Sex hormone–binding globulin is also relatively decreased in obese women, thereby increasing the proportion of bioactive (free) estradiol. As for androgens, the androstenedione concentration is little changed postmenopausally, but its peripheral conversion to estrone rises from 1.3% to 2.7%. Serum levels of testosterone are

slightly lower than in the premenopausal state. Nevertheless, there is relative androgen excess in the postmenopausal compared with the premenopausal situation (Table 100-1).

Menopause cannot be diagnosed by measuring plasma estrogens alone, because an overlap exists between the ranges of low normal estrogen levels in premenopausal women at the time of menses and the levels in postmenopausal women. To make the diagnosis of menopause, plasma follicle-stimulating hormone (FSH) concentrations can be measured; if they are >50 mIU/mL, then the diagnosis of menopause is likely.

The *perimenopause* begins with the onset of symptoms of hypoestrogenism and ends with the final menses. During this time, it is not uncommon for menstrual cycles to become more variable, lasting anywhere from 20 to 60 days. After age 40 years, it is more common for the follicular phase to be shortened. Anovulatory cycles may be interspersed with ovulatory cycles, and anovulatory bleeding may occur, indicated by variation and unpredictability in the amount of flow and in the duration and timing of the bleeding. Luteal phase defects also become more common as menopause is approached. Periods of amenorrhea with elevated plasma FSH levels suggesting menopause can occur, only to be followed a few months later by an ovulatory cycle. The decline in estrogen production by the perimenopausal ovarian follicle lessens the negative feedback on the hypothalamus and pituitary, causing FSH levels to rise. Moreover, the follicles themselves are less sensitive to FSH stimulation.

## PREMATURE MENOPAUSE

*Premature ovarian failure* is the onset of menopause before age 35 years, and is diagnosed by finding elevated plasma FSH levels. The reported incidence of this condition among women with amenorrhea varies from 4% to 10%. Women who pass through menopause at a younger age have the typical symptoms of estrogen deficiency, including vasomotor flushes and genital atrophy. However, it may not be permanent, and some women may ovulate again.[6,6a]

The causes of premature ovarian failure are many (see Chaps. 96 and 102). *Genetic abnormalities,* usually associated with deletions of the long arm of the X chromosome or mosaicism, may lead to depletion of oogonia.[7,8] *Autoimmune disorders,* either alone or in association with other autoimmune endocrine disorders such as Addison disease, may lead to ovarian failure. *Radiation or*

**TABLE 100-1.**
Representative Reproductive Hormone Levels in Women*

| Hormone | Premenopausal | | Postmenopausal | | % Tightly Bound |
|---|---|---|---|---|---|
| | *Plasma Level* | *Production Rate* | *Plasma Level* | *Production Rate* | |
| ANDROSTENEDIONE | 150 ng/dL | 2.7 mg/d | 90 ng/dL | 16 mg/d | 0 |
| TESTOSTERONE | 35 ng/dL | 200 μg/d | 25 ng/dL | 150 μg/d | >90 |
| DEHYDROEPIANDROSTERONE | 4–5 ng/mL | | 1.8 ng/mL | | 0 |
| DEHYDROEPIANDROSTERONE SULFATE | 1500 ng/mL | | 300 ng/mL | | 0 |
| ESTRONE | 40–200 pg/mL | 80–4000 μg/d | 35 pg/mL | 55 μg/d | 0 |
| ESTRADIOL | 40–350 pg/mL | 50–500 μg/d | 13 pg/mL | 12 μg/d | 50 |
| LUTEINIZING HORMONE | 10–40 mIU/mL | | 70 mIU/mL | | |
| FOLLICLE-STIMULATING HORMONE | 10–40 mIU/mL | | 80 mIU/mL | | |
| PROLACTIN | 10 ng/mL | | 8 ng/mL | | |

*Also see Chapter 237.
(From Korenman SG. Menopausal endocrinology and management. Arch Intern Med 1982; 142:1131. Copyright 1982, American Medical Association, reproduced by permission of the American Medical Association.)

*chemotherapy* can cause ovarian failure. There is evidence that chemotherapy administered before puberty and in the absence of radiation therapy does not affect the ovaries.[9] In a condition known as *Savage syndrome,* the ovarian follicles are resistant to the gonadotropins. The plasma gonadotropin levels are elevated. This disorder could be caused by a gonadotropin receptor or postreceptor defect within the ovary. *Galactosemia* is associated with primary ovarian failure; in this case, it is thought that an abnormal metabolite interferes with postreceptor activity. Another form of premature ovarian failure is *surgical menopause.*

In all of these cases, hormone-replacement therapy should be considered. Women with premature ovarian failure are vulnerable at an early age to develop genital atrophy, osteoporosis, vasomotor symptoms, and probably heart disease.

## GENITAL ATROPHY

### VULVA

The postmenopausal vulva has little subcutaneous fat and elastic tissue, resulting in a narrower opening, and sparser and coarser pubic hair than the premenopausal vulva. The labia majora shrink more than the labia minora, so that the relative proportions of the prepubertal organ are restored. The Bartholin glands secrete less fluids for lubrication, and vaginal dryness is often a problem. Moreover, the vulva may become more pruritic.

### VAGINA

The postmenopausal vaginal mucosa loses its papillae, the rugae flatten, and the vaginal walls become smoother and thinner. These changes often cause dyspareunia, burning, and occasional bleeding through breaks in the vaginal wall. For women who have ceased having intercourse, the vagina may become stenotic.[10]

With decreasing estrogen production, the vaginal glycogen content diminishes and the pH is increased, leading to inhibition of lactobacilli, which in turn permits other organisms to grow, including streptococci, staphylococci, diphtheroids, and coliforms. These bacteria are often responsible for vaginal discharge and vaginal infections after menopause. In such cases, antibiotics and other preparations provide temporary relief but are not curative. Estrogen treatment is more effective in providing long-term resolution of vaginal dryness and dyspareunia.

Some women passing through the menopause experience decreased intensity and duration of sexual response. However, many, if not most, postmenopausal women continue to be sexually active. If dryness is a problem, estrogens may be very helpful.[11] Nonhormonal vaginal lubricants (such as Replens, Columbia Pharmaceuticals) may also be useful.

### URETHRA

The urethra has the same biologic origin as the vagina (the urogenital sinus) and also undergoes postmenopausal atrophy. Some women experience problems with dysuria and frequency in the absence of infection; estrogen treatment is effective in providing relief.

### UTERUS

With estrogen depletion, the postmenopausal uterus becomes smaller and firmer. Vascularity is reduced, and uterine leiomyomas decrease in size. Inner migration of the squamocolumnar junction of the cervix occurs; thus, it may become more difficult to diagnose cervical cancer. The fallopian tubes show deciliation and decreased secretion.

### CARDIOVASCULAR DISEASE

Cardiovascular disease (CVD) is the leading cause of death among women in industrialized countries: >50% of postmenopausal women will die of CVD. Estrogens have been hypothesized to protect against atherosclerosis, because the incidence of CVD is quite low before the menopause. Premenopausal women have approximately one-fifth the CVD mortality of men, but after the menopause their mortality exponentially rises to approach that of men.[12] One explanation is that the estrogen of a premenopausal woman confers protection, which is lost at menopause; this is supported by the observation that women who undergo a premature surgical menopause (i.e., bilateral oophorectomy) and who do not use postmenopausal estrogens have twice as much CVD as age-matched premenopausal controls. If they use postmenopausal estrogens, however, their incidence of CVD is the same as that of premenopausal women of the same age.[13] Premature *natural* menopause, in contrast, has not been found to increase the risk of CVD when subjects are controlled for age, smoking, and estrogen use.[13]

Most epidemiologic studies have found that postmenopausal estrogen users have a lower incidence of CVD compared with nonusers. The Nurses' Health Study,[14] the largest cohort study, which followed 121,000 women for as long as 18 years, identified 425 cases of fatal myocardial infarction (MI). The adjusted relative risk of death from coronary heart disease was significantly reduced to 0.47 (95% CI, 0.32–0.69) for current hormone use but unchanged at 0.99 (95% CI, 0.75–1.30) for past use. The greatest decrease was seen in women who had at least one risk factor for heart disease (current tobacco use, hypercholesterolemia, hypertension, diabetes, parenteral history of premature MI, obesity). Substantially less benefit was seen in women with no risk factors. Concomitant progestin use did not appear to detract from this benefit.

Additional evidence for the benefit of estrogens was provided by a prospective study of more than 8000 postmenopausal women living in a moderately affluent retirement community in southern California.[15] After 7 years of observation, >1400 of these women had died. The investigators found that the women who had ever taken postmenopausal estrogens had 20% less all-cause mortality compared with women who did not (relative risk [RR] of death, 0.80; 95% CI, 0.70–0.87). The greatest reductions in mortality were seen with current use and with long durations of use: current use for more than 15 years was associated with a 40% reduction in mortality rates. This reduction in mortality rates was *not* dependent on the dosage of estrogen used: both high (i.e., ≥1.25 mg daily) and low (i.e., ≤0.625 mg daily) doses of oral conjugated equine estrogens (the most common estrogen used) were associated with nearly equal reductions in mortality. Few women took progestins or parenteral estrogens; therefore, the effect of those hormones on mortality cannot be determined from this study.

Most of the reduced mortality in estrogen users seen in this study[15] was the result of fewer deaths from occlusive arteriosclerotic vascular disease. Estrogen users were also found to have 20% less cancer mortality, which was observed for many malignancies, including breast cancer (RR, 0.81). One possible explanation is that estrogen users may have had greater health awareness and/or increased medical surveillance and consequently had less extensive disease at the time of diagnosis. As expected, estrogen users had excess mortality from endometrial cancer (RR, 3.0).

Women who underwent menopause before age 45 years showed the greatest benefit from estrogen use.[15] For the group of women whose menopause occurred after age 54 years, estrogen treatment did not reduce mortality rates. Estrogen use also appeared to reduce mortality for women who smoked, who had hypertension, or who had a history of angina or myocardial infarction, approaching that of healthy women who did not use estrogen. This appears to be a very important finding: at one time, hypertension, tobacco use, and coronary disease were thought to be relative contraindications to estrogen replacement. This was based on the increased incidence of stroke and heart attack seen with high-dose oral contraceptives, as well as with high-dose conjugated estrogens prescribed to men as secondary prevention of myocardial infarction.[16]

Conceivably, the results of this study[15] may argue for offering estrogen replacement to nearly all postmenopausal women, particularly those who underwent a relatively early menopause or who have risk factors for CVD. Perhaps the results may further argue for continuous, long-term treatment, because increasing durations of treatment were associated with further reductions in mortality. It should be remembered, however, that this study is an *epidemiologic observation* of estrogen users and nonusers and is *not a clinical trial*. Although the investigators controlled for many potential confounding factors, the possibility nevertheless exists that healthier women are more likely to seek and to be prescribed estrogens. Only randomized, placebo-controlled clinical trials are free of this bias (see later in this chapter).

Women with preexisting atherosclerosis may benefit from estrogen replacement.[17] In one study, estrogen users undergoing coronary catheterization were less likely to have demonstrable disease compared with nonusers (RR, 0.44; 95% CI, 0.29–0.67).[18] The investigators performed a retrospective analysis of the all-cause mortality of women who have undergone catheterization during the preceding 10 years. Relatively few women in this study were estrogen users, which was defined as estrogen use at the time of catheterization (5% subjects) or beginning some time thereafter (another 5% subjects). The adjusted 10-year survival of women with severe coronary stenosis who used estrogens was 97%, but it was only 60% for nonusers. For mild to moderate coronary stenosis, 10-year survival was 95% for users and 85% for nonusers. For women with normal coronary arteries, the 10-year survival was 98% for users and 91% for nonusers, a difference that was not statistically significant. These findings suggest that women with severe coronary atherosclerosis may

substantially benefit from estrogen use. However, this retrospective study may be biased by the fact that the decreased mortality seen in estrogen users may have been, in part, a self-fulfilling prophecy: estrogen nonusers who lived the longest after catheterization had the greatest opportunity to begin estrogen treatment and therefore became "estrogen users."

Initially, the only attempts to reduce CVD by estrogen treatment had all been performed in men. Early trials in which men were enrolled after a myocardial infarction showed estrogen treatment to reduce serum cholesterol but *not* the incidence of a second event.[19] The Coronary Drug Project, consisting of 1101 survivors of myocardial infarction, was terminated when excess thrombotic events (particularly pulmonary emboli) were seen in the group treated with estrogen; the incidence of CVD was not reduced.[16] This experience is similar to that seen in men with prostatic cancer treated with an estrogen, diethylstilbestrol, which appeared to increase CVD, possibly by causing excessive fluid accumulation leading to congestive heart failure or by increasing thromboembolism.[20] This adverse action of estrogen in men may have been the consequence of the high estrogenic potency of the doses used and may not reflect the physiologic action of estrogens.

Because men and women have an equal incidence of CVD when matched for lipoprotein concentrations,[21] the sex difference in CVD may be a consequence of the characteristic sex differences in serum lipoprotein concentrations. Thus, premenopausal women appear to be protected against CVD by their typically lower low-density lipoprotein (LDL) levels and higher high-density lipoprotein (HDL) levels compared with men of the same age. However, coincident with the loss of estrogen, female LDL levels rise at the time of the menopause and eventually exceed those of men.[22] It has been suggested that the loss of estrogen at the menopause causes this increase in LDL, because postmenopausal estrogen replacement has been found to lower LDL levels by 15% to 19% by increasing the clearance of LDL from the circulation.[23] In contrast, HDL levels in women decline by only 5% at menopause.[22] Thus, the HDL-raising effect of oral estrogens (typically 16% to 18%)[23] appears to be a pharmacologic action of the high portal estrogen concentrations presented to the liver after intestinal absorption, which stimulates the production of HDL particles.[24] Therefore, if endogenous estrogens protect against CVD, an effect on LDL levels that is greater than that on HDL levels is the likely mechanism. In contrast, the lower incidence of CVD among postmenopausal estrogen users may be the result of both increases in HDL levels and decreases in LDL levels. The magnitude of these lipid changes induced by oral estrogen treatment would be expected to lower the incidence of CVD by as much as 40%, using the regression coefficients determined by clinical trials in which cholesterol levels were improved by drug treatment. Reductions of this magnitude have been observed among estrogen users.[14,15] In addition, postmenopausal estrogen treatment has also been found to reduce plasma levels of lipoprotein(a), a highly atherogenic particle.[25]

Estrogens may also protect against CVD independent of their beneficial actions on lipoprotein levels. Estrogens may retard the oxidation of LDL, thereby decreasing its atherogenicity. This was demonstrated in healthy postmenopausal women who were infused with estradiol intravenously; LDL oxidation was significantly delayed.[26] Estrogens may also suppress the uptake of LDL by blood vessel walls, thereby impairing the development of endothelial atheroma.[27] There is also evidence that estrogens act directly to promote vasodilatation, as demonstrated in estrogen-treated castrated female monkeys.[28] This may be mediated indirectly by estrogen-induced alterations in prostacyclin metabolism, increasing the levels of prostacyclin, a vasodilator, and decreasing the levels of thromboxane, a vasoconstrictor.[29] The vasodilatory effect of estrogen may be more direct, because estrogen receptors are present throughout the vascular system.[30] The binding of estrogen to endothelial estrogen receptors could stimulate the release of nitric oxide, a potent endogenous vasodilator. This was suggested by work in female rabbits, in which endogenous estrogens were found to promote the rates of basal release of nitric oxide.[31]

Evidence from epidemiologic studies appears to suggest that estrogen use prevents the development of heart disease. However, the results of the first long-term randomized clinical trial of postmenopausal estrogen replacement *did not* prove this beneficial effect of estrogen.[32] The HERS study (Heart and Estrogen/Progestin Replacement Study) enrolled 2763 post-menopausal women with preexisting coronary disease and randomly assigned them to daily treatment with either a placebo or 0.625 mg conjugated equine estrogens and 2.5 mg medroxy-progesterone acetate. They noted a statistically significant 52% *increase* in myocardial infarction or cardiac death during the first year of treatment. By the third year, the women assigned hormone treatment began to have a *decrease* in the incidence of CVD. Overall, the incidence of CVD was nearly identical between the two groups when the entire 4.1-year study was considered. The explanation for these unexpected findings is unknown. One possibility is that estrogen treatment has a pro-thrombotic tendency, which increases the risk of a cardiac event in these high-risk women. Conceivably, after 2 years, the beneficial changes in the lipid profile induced by hormone-replacement therapy (HRT) may predominate over this prothrombotic effect, ultimately lowering the incidence of CVD. An alternative explanation is that the concomitant daily administration of the progestin, medroxyprogesterone acetate, detracts from the cardioprotective action of estrogen by adversely altering lipid levels or vasomotor function. The results of the Women's Health Initiative, which are not expected until 2008, will identify the effects of treatment with estrogen alone (and with progestin) in women not at high risk for CVD.

## OSTEOPOROSIS

Osteoporosis, the reduction in the mass of structural bone per unit volume, is a major affliction of older women. Osteoporosis can cause loss of height and an increased anterior-posterior diameter of the chest. Women may also develop a typical "dowager hump." It is estimated that 20% of women will experience a hip fracture by the time they reach age 90 years, nearly always because of osteoporosis. Moreover, up to 15% of women die within 3 months because of complications arising from the fracture, including pulmonary edema, myocardial infarction, and pulmonary embolism.[33] Spinal compression fractures are also associated with morbidity; this may affect up to 25% of women by the age of 60 years. The number of fractures of the radius also increases in older women, but the consequences are less serious. In all, it is estimated that in the United States, osteoporosis and its complications cost ~$14 billion annually.[34]

Osteoporosis occurs when the rate of bone resorption (by osteoclasts) exceeds the rate of bone formation (by osteoblasts). Thus, any successful therapy for the condition must either reduce bone resorption or promote bone production.

What is the evidence that osteoporosis is essentially a disease of the menopause? There is a dramatic increase in fractures among women after age 40 to 50 years,[35] a time when most women are passing through the menopause. Moreover, the bone mass of women tends to fall rapidly after age 50. When a woman's bone density falls below a "fracture threshold," minor trauma may cause a fracture. The critical event causing this accelerated bone loss is the depletion of estrogens. Indeed, it is now known that postmenopausal women lose less height if they take exogenous estrogens.

A double-blind prospective study conducted over a 5-year period demonstrated that mestranol decreased the rate of bone loss compared with a placebo; there was no appreciable increase in bone density. A 5-year follow-up to the same study found that women who stopped taking estrogens began to lose bone mass very rapidly, whereas women who remained on the drug maintained their bone density.[36]

Most important, however, is not whether estrogens prevent osteoporosis but whether estrogens indeed decrease the risk of fractures. Some studies have clearly shown this beneficial effect. For example, conjugated equine estrogens (0.625 mg) or ethinyl estradiol (20 μg), clearly reduced the risk of fracture in retrospective case-control studies. These studies indicate that to reduce bone fracture incidence by at least 50%, the estrogens must be started within 3 years of the menopause and must be continued for more than 6 years. It is not known how long estrogens must be continued for lasting benefits.[37–39]

Because progestins have antiestrogenic properties, it was believed formerly that addition of a progestin to an estrogen in postmenopausal women might negate the beneficial effects of estrogen on bone. However, it appears that combined estrogen and progestin therapy is at least as effective as estrogen alone in reducing bone loss and the risk of fracture in postmenopausal women.[40] Both estrogen and progestin receptors and messenger RNA transcripts have been found in human bone cells.[41–43] Estrogen has also been found to stimulate the proliferation and differentiation of cultured osteoblast-like cells derived from an osteogenic sarcoma in rats.[44] Thus, estrogens and progestins appear to have both direct and indirect actions on bone metabolism.

Osteoporosis may be prevented by therapies other than estrogen replacement. It appears that women who ingest more calcium than others are less at risk for the development of osteoporosis-related fractures. In addition, clinical trials of calcium supplementation combined with vitamin D have found a reduction in the incidence of hip fractures.[45] Premenopausal as well as postmenopausal women taking exogenous estrogen require ~1000 mg per day of calcium, whereas postmenopausal and castrate women not on estrogen require 1500 mg per day to be in calcium balance.[33] Most women do not reach this quota. Thus, dietary intake may be supplemented by calcium carbonate tablets, 500 mg of elemental calcium twice daily. Importantly, women who exercise moderately are found to have increased bone density.

Alendronate is a bisphosphonate that reduces osteoclastic activity, thereby reducing bone resorption. Ten milligrams given daily for 3 years increased the density of the spine by 8.8% and the femoral neck by 5.9%.[46] Vertebral fracture rates were reduced by 47%; there were similar decreases in hip and wrist fractures.[47] Because alendronate can cause esophagitis,[48] the patient should take it with a glass of water and remain upright for 30 minutes. The bisphosphonates may offer promise as (a) an alternative to estrogen in the prevention of osteoporosis; (b) an adjunctive treatment for women who nevertheless demonstrate bone loss while taking estrogen; and (c) treatment for established osteoporosis.

Although it might seem reasonable to give all women who pass through menopause some form of estrogen, *this must be balanced with the risks of estrogen therapy*. It may be prudent to target therapy to women at risk for osteoporosis. In addition to the risk factors listed in Chapter 64, women also at increased risk include those with premature menopause or early surgical castration, individuals with a strong family history of osteoporosis, and those taking corticosteroids. Sedentary women are also at increased risk, as are women who smoke[49] or have high caffeine intake.[50]

Measurement of bone density by bone biopsy is not practical. Of the different radiologic modalities available, quantitative digital radiography is the preferred technique. It is at least as accurate as other radiographic methods, is less costly, and can be performed rapidly with little radiation exposure.

Measurement of serum and urine markers for osteoporosis is usually not helpful.[51] For example, serum calcium levels are similar in osteoporotic and nonosteoporotic women. The 24-hour urinary excretion of hydroxyproline, which is a breakdown product of bone, is elevated in persons with osteoporosis and tends to decline when treatment is begun. The ratio of urinary calcium to creatinine also tends to decrease with estrogen administration. However, in individual patients, these values vary and are not specific.

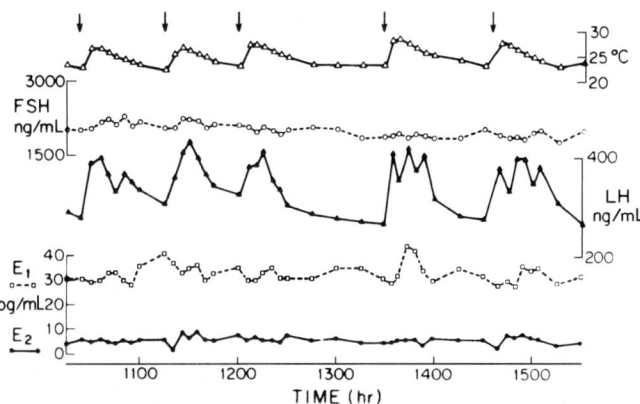

**FIGURE 100-3.** Serial measurements of finger temperature and serum follicle-stimulating hormone (*FSH*), luteinizing hormone (*LH*), estrone (*E$_1$*), and estradiol (*E$_2$*) levels in postmenopausal women during hot flushes. *Arrows* mark the hot flush episodes recorded by increases in finger temperature. (From Meldrum DR, et al. Gonadotropins, estrogens, and adrenal steroids during the menopausal hot flash. J Clin Endocrinol Metab 1980; 50:685.)

## VASOMOTOR FLUSHES

Vasomotor flushes are a common menopausal symptom[52] experienced by 75% of postmenopausal women. In ~20%, the flushes will be so severe that the woman will seek medical care. When they occur at night, they may awaken the patient. This may lead to chronic fatigue, poor concentration, emotional lability, and irritability.

Many women experience a premonition that they are about to have a flush. This is followed by a reddening of the face and upper body. The apparent vasodilation results in a rise in peripheral temperature and a subjective sensation of warmth; in fact, the temperature at the finger may increase by as much as 2° to 3°C and remain elevated for up to 20 minutes[53] and be associated with endocrine-metabolic alterations.[54] Because of the heat loss resulting from peripheral vasodilation, core temperature then falls and the woman will feel cold. These sensations of warmth followed by cold can be very disturbing.

The pathophysiology of vasomotor flushes is poorly understood. It is known, however, that the source of flushes is the thermoregulatory center in the hypothalamus (Fig. 100-3). Central catecholamines (norepinephrine and dopamine) may alter release of gonadotropin-releasing hormone (GnRH) and, because the GnRH neurons are in close proximity to the temperature control center, a vasomotor flush ensues (Fig. 100-4).[55] Thus, it is postulated that a change in neurotransmitters resulting from estrogen withdrawal stimulates GnRH release and alters the temperature control center to produce a flush. However, GnRH itself is not the primary source, because women with a deficiency of this hormone nevertheless can be symptomatic.[56] Based on studies with animal models, it has also been suggested that a decrease in gonadal steroids may cause a fall in endogenous opioid activity within the hypothalamus, thus inducing the symptoms of menopause that are similar to those of opiate withdrawal.[57]

Estrogen is effective therapy for vasomotor flushes; indeed, it is the standard to which all other therapies must be compared. Many double-blind, prospective, crossover, randomized studies have conclusively found that estrogens are more effective than placebo. Interestingly, the flushes return with increased frequency and severity on crossover from estrogens to placebo.[58] This suggests that the probable cause of the flushes is estrogen withdrawal rather than simply estrogen insufficiency; it further suggests that when estrogens are discontinued, they should be discontinued slowly over time. Importantly, when no therapy is used, the vasomotor flushes eventually disappear in most women.

Other forms of therapy with some reported effectiveness include medroxyprogesterone acetate at a dose of 10 to 20 mg per day, α-adrenergic agonists such as clonidine (0.1 mg, twice daily), and Bellergal (SANDOZ) (a nonspecific therapy containing ergotamine and belladonna, which are specific inhibitors of the sympathetic and parasympathetic nervous systems, respectively, reinforced by the synergistic action of phenobarbital in dampening cortical brain centers).[59] Currently the latter drug is seldom used.

## INSOMNIA

The possible relationship between hormone deprivation and sleep disturbance prompted a number of studies that examined estrogen's effect on insomnia. In one double-blind parallel study using estrone sulfate and placebo, an increase in rapid eye movement (REM) sleep was found but total sleep time was not affected.[60] In a second study with a double-blind crossover arrangement using conjugated estrogens (0.625 mg), women taking estrogens experienced fewer hot flushes, a shorter sleep latency period, and more REM sleep than women taking a placebo. The sleep latency decreased most in the patients ranked highest in psychological well-adjustment by the attending physician and nurse.[61] These results suggest that women experiencing the greatest number of hot flushes respond to estrogens by a decrease in flushing, with a resulting improvement in their insomnia. Women experiencing

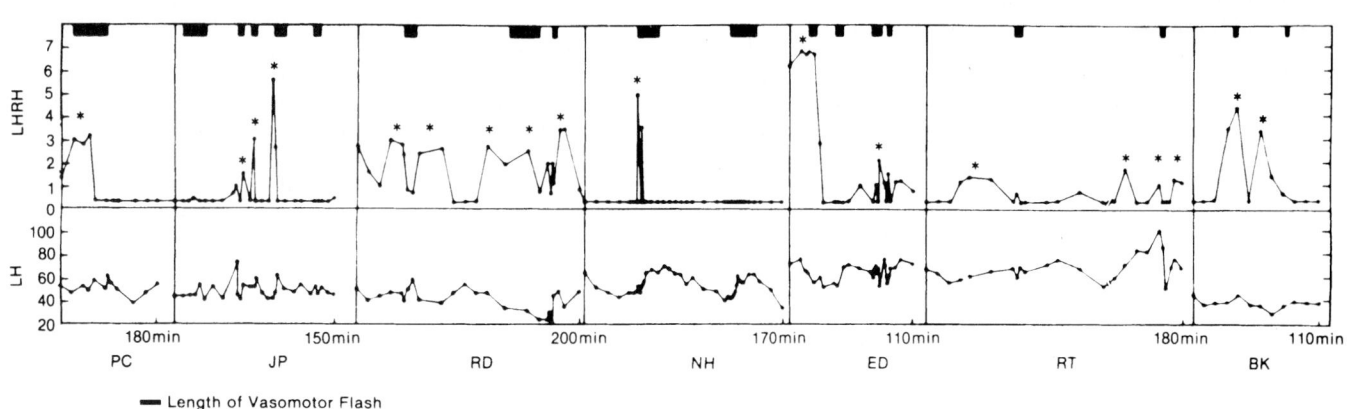

■— Length of Vasomotor Flash
• LHRH Pulse

**FIGURE 100-4.** Peripheral levels of luteinizing hormone–releasing hormone (*LHRH*) and luteinizing hormone (*LH*) during 3 hours of monitoring in seven women with vasomotor flushes. (From Ravnikar V, Elkind-Hirsch K, Schiff I, et al. Vasomotor flushes and the release of peripheral immunoreactive luteinizing hormone–releasing hormone in postmenopausal women. Fertil Steril 1984; 41:881.)

insomnia together with severe vasomotor flushes seem to respond best to estrogens. This has been confirmed in a study that found that women are indeed awakened by hot flushes.[62]

The concept of an association between vasomotor flushes and emotional state is not new. For example, one study that used a graphic scale to measure a subject's emotional state demonstrated that after beginning estrogen therapy, postmenopausal women who had experienced severe vasomotor flushes showed improvement in urinary frequency, vaginal dryness, insomnia, headaches, irritability, and other emotional variables such as decreased memory, anxiety, and worry; alternatively, among women who had not experienced flushes, estrogen therapy was followed by improvement only in memory, anxiety, and worry.[63] Thus, the amelioration noted in some psychological complaints may result from a domino-like effect initiated by the reduction in vasomotor flushes. Estrogens may also affect the emotional state by a biochemical effect on the brain. For example, estrogens may inhibit monoamine oxidase, an enzyme found in increased levels in some depressed women.[64] The alleged validity of a beneficial effect of estrogen replacement therapy on Alzheimer disease lacks adequate confirmation.[64a]

# ESTROGEN-REPLACEMENT THERAPY

## COMPLICATIONS

Hormone-replacement therapy may produce a number of undesirable side effects and complications. For example, it raises the risk of developing thromboembolic disease nearly three-fold, and increases the risk of gallbladder disease by 38%.[32] Complications such as coronary artery disease[18] and myocardial infarction have not been shown to occur with increased frequency in postmenopausal women as they have in younger women taking oral contraceptives, probably because the estrogen dose used for postmenopausal women is much lower than the one used in the standard oral contraceptive. However, *the major concern of exogenous estrogen use is the possible added risk of developing cancer* (see Chaps. 222 and 223).

### ENDOMETRIAL CANCER

In 1975, two published case-control studies showed an increased occurrence of endometrial cancer in postmenopausal women taking estrogens[65,66] (see Chap. 223). The occurrence of endometrial cancer appeared to be not only dose related but also duration related. It was possible to identify the estrogen-endometrial cancer relationship because the latency period between initial estrogen ingestion and the onset of the endometrial cancer was as short as 2 years. Some studies have suggested that after the estrogens are discontinued, the added risk disappears within 6 months. Estrogens seem to be associated with low-grade endometrial cancers; that is, although cancer is a frightening disease, perhaps prescribing estrogens does not increase the endometrial cancer mortality rate in women. Successful treatment, however, may require hysterectomy and possibly radiation therapy.[67]

It remained a paradox for a long time why older women given low-dose estrogens should develop endometrial cancer while younger women who are producing greater endogenous estrogen during pregnancy or taking high-estrogen birth control pills do not develop the disease. The explanation appears to be that the estrogens initially were given to postmenopausal women in an unopposed fashion, that is, without progesterone. This speculation led investigators to add a progestin to the prescribed estrogens given to older women, which lowered the incidence of endometrial cancer and of endometrial hyperplasia (considered a precursor of endometrial cancer). The progestins, used for at least 10 days a month within the estrogen regimen, may act by decreasing the estrogen receptors as well as by converting estradiol to estrone, which is a less potent estrogen.[68]

## BREAST CANCER

Breast cancer, which affects >10% of women in the United States, is a much more serious disease than endometrial cancer. Besides being common, breast cancer has a high mortality rate. This disease is frequently disfiguring and emotionally very disturbing. Whether estrogens actually cause breast cancer is presently unknown. Although some studies have found no increased risk of breast cancer.[69] Other large studies found excess risk among long-term users.[70] This observation was confirmed by the Nurses' Health Study, which analyzed 1935 cases of breast cancer prospectively seen during 725,000 person-years of observation.[71] They found that the risk of death due to breast cancer in women who had taken estrogen for five or more years was increased 45%. Other studies are in agreement.[71a] This conclusion is consistent with available animal data suggesting that breast cancer can be induced with high-dose estrogens (see Chap. 222). Also, estrogens can maintain breast tumor growth in tissue culture. They also found that the addition of a progestin to estrogen treatment did *not* influence the increased risk of breast cancer seen with long-term estrogen use.[71] Interestingly, hormone replacement therapy reduces the sensitivity of mammography.[71b]

## THERAPEUTIC ASPECTS

Theoretically, the ideal estrogen to administer should be the one the woman's own ovaries produced in the premenopausal years, namely, estradiol. Estradiol taken orally is converted to estrone in the gut and liver. However, estradiol given vaginally, by injection, or transdermally is absorbed rapidly; because it bypasses the liver, it appears in the plasma predominantly as estradiol. Estradiol remains biologically potent because it can suppress gonadotropins when given by any of the above routes.[72] The transdermal approach has the advantage of delivering constant physiologic levels of estradiol.[73] Because the liver is bypassed, it may be considered for women at risk for phlebitis or hypertension.

The most common form of estrogen-replacement therapy uses conjugated equine estrogens prescribed orally. The dose that is effective for osteoporosis and flushes is 0.3 to 0.625 mg daily. Estropipate (piperazine estrone sulfate) (1.25 mg per day) or micronized estradiol (Estrace) (0.5 mg) may also be used. Oral or injectable estrogens with prolonged half-lives generally should not be used. Transdermal estradiol is applied to the skin twice weekly. It is designed to deliver 0.05 to 0.10 mg per day of estradiol, which achieves a blood level in the range of the normal early follicular phase of the menstrual cycle. The drug avoids the first-pass hepatic metabolism of oral preparations; there is no stimulation of renin substrate, and no increase in sex hormone–binding globulin, corticosteroid-binding globulin, or thyroxine-binding globulin.[74] Oral estrogens do increase the levels of these globulins by their effect on the liver, but any long-term adverse reactions of these increases are unknown. On the other hand, with oral estrogen administration the liver produces more HDL-cholesterol[24] and clears more LDL-cholesterol[23] from the circulation, which is presumably a benefit.

The standard regimen adds a progestin[75] such as medroxyprogesterone acetate, 5 mg daily, from the 1st to the 13th days of the month to reduce the risk of endometrial cancer. A woman with a uterus will have a 90% chance of experiencing withdrawal bleeding. It has been shown that with continuous use of estrogens and progestins, this annoying side effect can be minimized.[76] However, irregular and unpredictable bleeding can occur in the first several months of continuous combined therapy and results in high dropout rates. The long-term safety of this regimen needs to be established. There are reports of endometrial cancer developing years later in women treated in this fashion.[77]

Endometrial biopsies need not be performed before estrogen therapy is begun unless irregular bleeding has occurred. Biopsies need only be performed during hormone treatment if withdrawal bleeding occurs before day 10 or after day 20 of monthly cyclic progestin therapy[78] or after 6 months of continuous progestin therapy. Vaginal probe ultrasonography may reduce the number of biopsies required; endometrial cancer is highly unlikely if endometrial thickness is <5 mm.[79]

In addition to uterine bleeding, there are a number of side effects to estrogen/progestin replacement therapy. Some weight gain (up to 2 kg) may occur at the outset. Breast tenderness may be relieved by reducing the dosage of estrogen. Alternatively, continued symptoms of estrogen deficiency indicate the need to increase the dose of estrogen. Progestins frequently cause bloating and depression, so that women may complain of typical premenstrual signs and symptoms just before withdrawal bleeding. Depression can be alleviated by reducing the frequency of medroxyprogesterone acetate administration to once every 2 or even 3 months. The patient must be informed, however, that decreasing the frequency of progestin administration may increase the risk of endometrial hyperplasia.[80] More careful surveillance with endometrial biopsies would be warranted. Depression may also be alleviated by using a different progestin, such as norethindrone at a dose of 1.25 to 2.5 mg daily. A major side effect of this 19-norsteroid, however, may be acne. Alternatively, megestrol acetate (Megace), 20 to 40 mg daily, or micronized progesterone, 100 to 200 mg daily, may be substituted.

## MONITORING

Women treated with estrogens should be seen regularly by their physicians, at which time an interim history should be taken and a complete physical examination (including height, weight, and blood pressure) performed. Additionally, the woman should be informed about the significant warning signs of the treatment, such as irregular bleeding. An endometrial biopsy should be performed when bleeding is irregular to rule out endometrial hyperplasia, and a mammogram should be obtained at regular intervals even in women not taking replacement hormones. Also, it is prudent to obtain a mammogram before estrogen treatment is begun because estrogens stimulate glandular breast tissue and may make the diagnosis of breast cancer more difficult. This also may prevent prescribing estrogen to a woman with a preexisting breast cancer. A lipid profile should be determined. Bone densitometry measurements may be clinically helpful.

## INDICATIONS AND CONTRAINDICATIONS

With the present state of knowledge, it is difficult to list indications for estrogen therapy of a postmenopausal woman. Treatment for each patient must be individualized. Benefits must be weighed against hazards.

Although several of the benefits of female sex hormones have been described, it must also be emphasized that *these hormones must be used selectively and with supervision*. Along with some of the unanswered questions concerning long-term effects, certain *contraindications* exist, including (a) breast cancer; (b) endometrial cancer, particularly within 2 years of diagnosis or if the tumor was not confined to the uterus; (c) pulmonary emboli; (d) phlebitis; and (e) active liver disease. A strong family history for breast cancer also merits consideration. There may be certain exceptions to these contraindications when the physician and patient both agree that the benefits of estrogen treatment substantially outweigh the risks.

# SELECTIVE ESTROGEN RECEPTOR MODULATORS

Postmenopausal estrogen use may protect against osteoporosis and heart disease, but may increase the risks of breast and endometrial cancers. Many women discontinue hormone treatment because of lingering concerns they have about these long-term hazards, or because of unacceptable side effects such as vaginal bleeding and breast tenderness.

Because estrogen is not an ideal treatment, drugs have been sought that have an estrogenic effect in some tissues, such as bone and the cardiovascular system, but not in others, such as the breast and endometrium. Drugs that have these tissue-specific effects have been termed *selective estrogen receptor modulators (SERMs)*.[81,81a] Potentially, the benefits of estrogen could be derived without the accompanying risks. This tissue selectivity is biologically possible, because the conformation of a drug-estradiol receptor complex determines the particular DNA response elements to which it can bind. Raloxifene, a benzothiophene that binds to the estrogen receptor,[81] is a SERM. The raloxifene-estrogen receptor complex does not bind to the estrogen-response element. Instead, it binds to a unique area of DNA, the raloxifene response element. The drug has an estrogen-antagonist effect on breast and endometrium and an estrogen-agonist effect on bone and cholesterol.

Raloxifene was first evaluated as a possible treatment for metastatic breast cancer. Large-scale clinical trials have been initiated to assess its efficacy in the prevention and treatment of osteoporosis in otherwise healthy postmenopausal women. To date, more than 14,000 women have been enrolled in raloxifene studies, of whom 8000 women were assigned treatment with raloxifene. Although most of these studies are ongoing, interim and short-term results indicate the following.

### EFFECT ON BONE

Raloxifene preserves bone density in postmenopausal women. Treatment with 60 mg daily for 2 years increases bone density (compared with a calcium-supplemented placebo) of the lumbar spine by 2.4%, the total hip by 2.4%, the femoral neck by 2.5%, and the total body by 2.0%. The 30-mg and 150-mg doses of raloxifene were equipotent with the 60-mg dose.[82] (Another study found that treatment with equine estrogen, 0.625 mg daily for 2 years, increased bone density of the total hip by 3%, compared with a placebo, greater than the 1.5% increase with 60 mg raloxifene daily.)[83] More recently, raloxifene also has been found to reduce the incidence of vertebral fractures by 47%. Based on these data, raloxifene, 60 mg daily, is approved in the United States for the *prevention* of osteoporosis.

### EFFECTS ON CARDIOVASCULAR RISK MARKERS

Lipids and coagulation factors were measured in 390 postmenopausal women after daily treatment for 6 months with either raloxifene, 60 mg or 120 mg, HRT (0.625 mg equine estrogen and 2.5 mg medroxyprogesterone), or a placebo.[84] Compared with the placebo, raloxifene lowered LDL-cholesterol by 12% (similar to the 14% reduction with HRT) and lipoprotein(a) by 7% (less than the 19% decrease with HRT). Because a 30% reduction in LDL by a lipid-lowering agent lowered cardiovascular events by 46% in women,[85] this 12% reduction in LDL might lower the incidence of heart disease by as much as 18%. The 7% reduction in lipoprotein(a) levels could further decrease this risk.

Raloxifene increased $HDL_2$-cholesterol levels by 15%, less than the 33% elevation with HRT. Raloxifene did not change HDL-cholesterol, triglycerides, and plasminogen activator inhibitor-1 (PAI-1) concentrations; whereas HRT increased HDL-cholesterol levels by 10% and triglycerides by 20%, and decreased PAI-1 by 19%. Raloxifene lowered fibrinogen levels by 10% to 12%, whereas HRT had no effect. This decline in fibrinogen may be cardioprotective. Fibrinogen levels are an independent risk factor for heart disease, with a reduction of 0.5% for every 0.01 g/L decrease in fibrinogen levels.[86] The 0.42 g/L reduction in fibrinogen induced by raloxifene could reduce cardiovascular events by 21%. For all these effects, there were no differences between the two raloxifene doses.

The effect of raloxifene on cardiovascular risk markers resembles that of tamoxifen more than it does HRT.[81,87,88] This similarity is noteworthy, because the changes induced by tamoxifen on cardiovascular risk markers could be responsible for its apparent cardioprotective effect. In randomized, controlled clinical trials, tamoxifen treatment reduced the incidence of fatal myocardial infarction (odds ratio, 0.37; 95% CI, 0.18–0.77)[89] and hospital admissions for cardiac disease (relative risk, 0.68; 95% CI, 0.48–0.97).[90] Proof that raloxifene reduces the risk of heart disease would require a clinical trial with a cardiovascular event end point. Such a study is currently under way.

### EFFECT ON VENOUS THROMBOEMBOLIC DISEASE

There have been 51 episodes of venous thromboembolic disease (VTE) in raloxifene studies: 19 pulmonary emboli and 32 deep vein thromboses.[91] The relative risk of VTE with raloxifene treatment is 3.4 (95% CI, 1.5–8.0) similar to that of 2.9 for postmenopausal estrogens[92] and 1.9 for tamoxifen. The greatest risk for VTE appeared during the first 4 months of treatment, usually in women with a prior history of thrombophlebitis. Thus, a past history of VTE is one of the few contraindications to raloxifene treatment (the others are hepatic dysfunction and premenopausal use). Patients should discontinue raloxifene at least 72 hours before immobilization (e.g., elective surgery) and resume taking it when ambulatory.

### EFFECT ON UTERUS

Raloxifene does not stimulate the endometrium. Endometrial biopsy specimens from 206 women given raloxifene for 1 year showed atrophy, whereas in 100 women given estrogen, 23 showed hyperplasia and 39 showed proliferation.[91] Endometrial thickness, assessed by transvaginal ultrasound over 2 years in 831 women, was unchanged by both raloxifene and the placebo.[82] The incidence of vaginal bleeding is 6% for both 60 mg raloxifene and for the placebo, considerably lower than the 64% incidence with hormone treatment.[84] Thus, vaginal bleeding that occurs with raloxifene warrants evaluation. There have been 12 new cases of endometrial cancer in women enrolled in raloxifene studies. However, the relative risk of endometrial cancer for raloxifene users was not increased at 0.84 (95% CI, 0.25–2.87).

### EFFECT ON BREAST

Raloxifene does not cause breast tenderness: the incidence was 4% for 60 mg raloxifene and 6% for the placebo, lower than the 38% incidence with hormone treatment.[84] There have been 45 new cases of breast cancer in women enrolled in raloxifene studies. Nevertheless, the relative risk of breast cancer for raloxifene users was significantly reduced at 0.33 (95% CI, 0.19–0.52). Of those 45 women, 25 were diagnosed after taking the study drug for more than 18 months. For this subgroup, the relative risk of breast cancer among raloxifene users was even lower at 0.23 (95% CI, 0.10–0.49). The protective effect of raloxifene was limited to estrogen receptor–positive tumors.[93]

### EFFECT ON CENTRAL NERVOUS SYSTEM

Raloxifene increases the incidence of hot flashes and is not a treatment for women who seek relief from menopausal symptoms. The difference in the incidence of hot flashes between raloxifene- and placebo-treated groups is 5% to 6%.[82,84] The effect of raloxifene on cognitive functioning and on the incidence of Alzheimer's disease is unknown.

## CONCLUSION

Each patient has to be informed about the possible benefits and risks of the currently available therapies, including alternatives. Only in this way can she share in making the decision about the treatment she is prescribed.

## REFERENCES

1. Statistical abstract of the United States: 1981, 102nd ed. Washington, DC: US Bureau of the Census, 1981.
2. U.S. Department of Commerce, Special Studies. 65+ in the United States. P23-190; 1996:2.
3. Grodin JN, Siiteri PK, MacDonald PC. Source of estrogen production in postmenopausal women. J Clin Endocrinol Metab 1973; 36:207.
4. Longcope C, Jaffee W, Griffing G. Production rates of androgens and estrogens in postmenopausal women. Maturitas 1981; 3:215.
5. MacDonald PC, Edman CD, Hemsell DL, et al. Effect of obesity on conversion of plasma androstenedione to estrone in postmenopausal women with and without endometrial cancer. Am J Obstet Gynecol 1978; 130:448.
6. Rebar RW, Erickson GF, Yen SSC. Idiopathic premature ovarian failure: clinical and endocrine characteristics. Fertil Steril 1982; 37:35.
6a. Kalantaridou SN, Nelson LM. Premature ovarian failure is not premature menopause. Ann NY Acad Sci 2000; 900:393.
7. Coulam CB. Premature gonadal failure. Fertil Steril 1982; 38:645.
8. Krauss CM, Turksoy RN, Atkins L, et al. Familial premature ovarian failure due to an interstitial deletion of the long arm of the X chromosome. N Engl J Med 1987; 317:125.
9. Stillman RJ, Schinfeld JS, Schiff I, et al. Ovarian failure in long-term survivors of childhood malignancy. Am J Obstet Gynecol 1981; 139:62.
10. Schiff I, Wilson E. Clinical aspects of aging of the female reproductive system. In: Schneider E, ed. Aging of the reproductive system. New York: Raven Press, 1978:9.
11. Morrell MJ, Dixen JM, Carter CS, Davidson JM. The influence of age and cycling status on sexual arousability in women. Am J Obstet Gynecol 1984; 148:66.
12. Lerner DJ, Kannel WB. Patterns of coronary disease morbidity and mortality: a 26-year follow-up of the Framingham population. Am Heart J 1986; 111(2):383.
13. Colditz GA, Willett WC, Stampfer MJ, et al. Menopause and the risk of coronary heart disease in women. N Engl J Med 1987; 316:1105.
14. Grodstein F, Stampfer MJ, Colditz GA, et al. Postmenopausal hormone therapy and mortality. N Engl J Med 1997; 336:1769.
15. Henderson BE, Paganini-Hill A, Ross RK. Decreased mortality in users of estrogen replacement therapy. Arch Intern Med 1991; 151:75.
16. The Coronary Drug Project Research Group. Findings leading to discontinuation of the 2.5 mg/day estrogen group. JAMA 1973; 226:652.
17. Sullivan JM, Vander Zwagg R, Hughes FP, et al. Estrogen replacement and coronary artery disease. Arch Intern Med 1990; 150:2557.
18. Sullivan JM, Vander Zwagg R, Lemp GF, et al. Postmenopausal estrogen use and coronary atherosclerosis. Ann Intern Med 1988; 108:358.
19. Stamler J, Katz LN, Pick R, et al. Effects of long-term estrogen therapy on serum cholesterol-lipid-lipoprotein levels and mortality in middle aged men with previous myocardial infarction. Circulation 1980; 22:658.
20. DeVogt HJ, Smith PH, Davone-Macaluso M, et al. Cardiovascular side effects of diethylstilbestrol, cyproterone acetate, and medroxyprogesterone acetate used for treatment of prostatic cancer. J Urol 1986; 135:303.
21. Gordon T, Castelli WP, Hjortland MC, et al. High density lipoprotein as a protective factor against coronary heart disease. Am J Med 1977; 62:707.
22. Matthews KA, Meilahn E, Kuller LH, et al. Menopause and risk factors for coronary heart disease. N Engl J Med 1989; 321:641.
23. Walsh BW, Schiff I, Rosner B, et al. Effects of postmenopausal estrogen replacement on the concentrations and metabolism of plasma lipoproteins. N Engl J Med 1991; 325:1196.
24. Walsh BW, Li H, Sacks FM. Effects of postmenopausal hormone replacement with oral and transdermal estrogen on high-density lipoprotein metabolism. J Lipid Res 1994; 35:2083.
25. Sacks FM, McPherson R, Walsh BW. Effect of postmenopausal estrogen replacement on plasma lipoprotein (a) concentrations. Arch Intern Med 1994; 154:1106.
26. Sack MN, Rader DJ, Cannon RO. Oestrogen and inhibition of oxidation of low-density lipoproteins in postmenopausal women. Lancet 1994; 343:269.
27. Wagner JD, Clarkson TB, St. Clair RW, et al. Estrogen and progesterone replacement therapy reduces low density lipoprotein accumulation in the coronary arteries of surgically postmenopausal cynomolgus monkeys. J Clin Invest 1991; 88:1995.
28. Williams JK, Adams MR, Herrington DM, Clarkson TB. Short-term administration of estrogen and vascular responses of atherosclerotic coronary arteries. J Am Coll Cardiol 1992; 20:452.
29. Steinleitner A, Stanzyk FZ, Levin JH, et al. Decreased in vitro production of 6-keto prostaglandin by uterine arteries from postmenopausal women. Am J Obstet Gynecol 1989; 161:1677.
30. McGill HC. Sex steroid hormone receptors in the cardiovascular system. Postgrad Med 1989; (April):64.
31. Hyashi T, Fukuto JM, Ignarro LJ, Chaudhuri G. Basal release of nitric oxide from aortic rings is greater in female rabbits than in male rabbits: implications for atherosclerosis. Proc Natl Acad Sci U S A 1992; 89:11259.
32. Hulley S, Grady D, Bush T, et al. Randomized trial of estrogen plus progestin for secondary prevention of coronary heart disease in postmenopausal women. JAMA 1998; 280:605.
33. Heaney RP. Estrogens in postmenopausal osteoporosis. Clin Obstet Gynecol 1976; 19:791.
34. World Health Organization. Research on menopause in the 1990's. Geneva, Switzerland, WHO, Series 1996; 866:40.
35. Gallagher JC, Nordin BEC. Calcium metabolism in the menopause. In:

Curry AS, Hewitt JV, eds. Biochemistry of women: current concepts. Cleveland: CRC Press, 1974:145.

36. Lindsay R, Herrington BS. Estrogens in osteoporosis. Semin Reprod Endocrinol 1983; 1:55.
37. Weiss NS, Ure CL, Ballard JH, et al. Decreased risk of fractures of the hip and lower forearm with postmenopausal use of estrogen. N Engl J Med 1980; 303:1195.
38. Paganini-Hill A, Ross RK, Gerkins VR, et al. Menopausal estrogen therapy and hip fractures. Ann Intern Med 1981; 95:28.
39. Felson DT, Zhang Y, Hannan MT, et al. The effect of postmenopausal estrogen therapy on bone density in elderly women. N Engl J Med 1993; 329:1141.
40. Gallagher JC, Kable WT, Goldgar D. Effect of progestin therapy on cortical and trabecular bone: comparison with estrogen. Am J Med 1991; 90:171.
41. Eriksen EF, Colvard DS, Berg NJ, et al. Evidence of estrogen receptors in normal human osteoblast-like cells. Science 1988; 241:84.
42. Komm BS, Teipening CM, Benz DJ, et al. Estrogen binding, receptor mRNA, and biologic response in osteoblast-like osteosarcoma cells. Science 1988; 241:81.
43. Kaplan FS, Fallon MD, Boden SD, et al. Estrogen receptors in bone in a patient with polyostotic fibrous dysplasia (McCune-Albright syndrome). N Engl J Med 1988; 319:421.
44. Gray TK, Flynn TC, Gray KM, Nabell LM. 17β-Estradiol acts directly on the clonal osteoblastic cell line UMR106. Proc Natl Acad Sci U S A 1987; 84:6267.
45. Chapuy MC, et al. Vitamin D, and calcium to prevent hip fractures in elderly women. N Engl J Med 1992; 327:1637.
46. Liberman UA, Weiss SR, Broll J, et al. Effect of oral alendronate on bone mineral density and the incidence of fractures in postmenopausal osteoporosis. N Engl J Med 1995; 333:1437.
47. Black DM, Cummings SR, Karpf DB, et al. Randomised trial of effect of alendronate on risk of fracure in women with existing vertebral fractures: Fracture Intervention Trial Research Group. Lancet 1996; 348:1535.
48. deGroen PC, Lubbe DF, Hirsh LJ, et al. Esophagitis associated with the use of alendronate. N Engl J Med 1996; 335:1016.
49. Hopper JL, Seeman E. The bone density of female twins discordant for tobacco use. N Engl J Med 1994; 330:387.
50. Barrett-Connor E, Chang JC, Edelstein SL. Coffee-associated osteoporosis offset by daily milk consumption. JAMA 1994; 271:280.
51. Christiansen C, Riis BJ, Rodbro P. Prediction of rapid bone loss in postmenopausal women. Lancet 1987; 1(8542):1105.
52. Tulandi T, Lal S. Menopausal hot flash. Obstet Gynecol Surv 1985; 40:553.
53. Tataryn IV, Lomax P, Meldrum DR, et al. Objective techniques for the assessment of postmenopausal hot flashes. Obstet Gynecol 1981; 57:340.
54. Cignarelli M, Cicinelli E, Corso M, et al. Biophysical and endocrine-metabolic changes during menopausal hot flashes: increase in plasma free fatty acid and norepinephrine levels. Gynecol Obstet Invest 1989; 27:34.
55. Ravnikar V, Elkind-Hirsch K, Schiff I, et al. Vasomotor flushes and the release of peripheral immunoreactive luteinizing hormone-releasing hormone in postmenopausal women. Fertil Steril 1984; 41:881.
56. Meldrum DR, Erlik Y, Lu JK, Judd HL. Objectively recorded hot flushes in patients with pituitary insufficiency. J Clin Endocrinol Metab 1981; 52:684.
57. Simpkins JW, Katovich MJ, Song IC. Similarities between morphine withdrawal in the rat and the menopausal hot flush. Life Sci 1983; 32:1957.
58. Coope J. Double-blind crossover study of estrogen replacement therapy. In: Campbell S, ed. The management of the menopause and postmenopausal years. Baltimore: University Park Press, 1976:159.
59. Schiff I, Tulchinsky D, Cramer D, Ryan KJ. Oral medroxyprogesterone treatment of postmenopausal symptoms. JAMA 1980; 244:1443.
60. Thompson J, Oswald I. Effect of estrogen on the sleep, mood, and anxiety of menopausal women. BMJ 1977; 2:1317.
61. Schiff I, Regestein Q, Tulchinsky D, Ryan KJ. Effects of estrogens on sleep and psychological state of hypogonadal women. JAMA 1979; 242:2405.
62. Erlik Y, Tartaryn I, Meldrum D, et al. Association of waking episodes with menopausal hot flushes. JAMA 1981; 245:1741.
63. Campbell S. Double-blind psychometric studies on the effects of natural estrogens on postmenopausal women. In: Campbell S, ed. The management of the menopausal and postmenopausal years. Baltimore: University Park Press, 1976:149.
64. Klaiber EI, Broverman DM, Vogel W, et al. Effects of estrogen therapy on plasma MAO activity and EEG during responses of depressed women. Am J Psychiatry 1972; 128:1492.
64a. Mulnard RA, Cotman CW, Kawas C, et al. Estrogen replacement therapy for treatment of mild to moderate Alzheimer disease: a randomized controlled trial. JAMA 2000; 283:10007.
65. Smith DC, Prentice R, Thompson DJ, Herrmann WL. Association of exogenous estrogens and endometrial cancer. N Engl J Med 1975; 293:1164.
66. Ziel HK, Finkle WD. Increased risk of endometrial carcinoma among users of conjugated estrogens. N Engl J Med 1975; 293:1167.
67. Chu J, Schweid AI, Weiss NS. Survival among women with endometrial cancer: a comparison of estrogen users and nonusers. Am J Obstet Gynecol 1982; 143:569.
68. Gambrell RD Jr. Clinical use of progestins in the menopausal patient. J Reprod Med 1982; 27(Suppl):531.
69. Sourander L, Rajala T, Raiha I, et al. Cardiovascular and cancer morbidity and mortality and sudden cardiac death in postmenopausal women on oestrogen replacement therapy (ERT). Lancet 1998; 352:1965.
70. Brinton LA, Hoover R, Fraumeni JF. Menopausal oestrogens and breast cancer risk: an expanded case-control study. Br J Cancer 1986; 54:825.
71. Colditz GA, Hankinson SE, Hunter DJ, et al. The use of estrogens and progestins and the risk of breast cancer in postmenopausal women. N Engl J Med 1995; 332:1589.
71a. Willet WC, Colditz G, Stampfer M. Postmenopausal estrogens—opposed, unopposed, or none of the above. JAMA 2000; 283:534.
71b. Kavanaugh AM, Mitchell AM, Giles GG. Hormone replacement therapy and accuracy of mammographic screening. Lancet 2000; 355:270.
72. Schiff I, Tulchinsky D, Ryan KJ. Vaginal absorption of estrone and estradiol-17β. Fertil Steril 1977; 28:1063.
73. Padwick ML, Endacott J, Whitehead MB. Efficacy, acceptability, and metabolic effects of transdermal estradiol in the management of postmenopausal women. Am J Obstet Gynecol 1985; 152:1085.
74. Haas S, Walsh B, Evans S, et al. The effect of transdermal estradiol on hormone and metabolic dynamics over a six-week period. Obstet Gynecol 1988; 71:671.
75. Whitehead MI, Siddle N, Lane G. The pharmacology of progestogens. In: Mishell DR, ed. Menopause, physiology and pharmacology. Chicago: Year Book Medical Publishers, 1987:326.
76. Archer DF, Pickar JH, Bottiglioni F. Bleeding patterns in postmenopausal women taking continuous combined or sequential regimens of conjugated estrogens with medroxyprogesterone acetate. Obstet Gynecol 1994; 83:686.
77. Leather AT, Savvas M, Studd JWW. Endometrial histology and bleeding patterns after 8 years of continuous combined estrogen and progestin therapy in postmenopausal women. Obstet Gynecol 1991; 78:1008.
78. Padwick ML, Pryse-Davies J, Whitehead MI. A simple method for determining the optimal dosage of progestin in postmenopausal women receiving estrogens. N Engl J Med 1986; 315:930.
79. Smith-Bindman R, Kerlikowske K, Feldstein V, et al. Endovaginal ultrasound to exclude endometrial cancer and other endometrial abnormalities. JAMA 1998; 280:1510.
80. Ettinger B, Selby J, Citron JT, et al. Cyclic hormone replacement therapy using quarterly progestin. Obstet Gynecol 1994; 83:693.
81. Grey AB, Stapleton JP, Evans MC, Reid IR. The effect of the anti-estrogen tamoxifen on cardiovascular risk factors in normal postmenopausal women. J Clin Endocrinol Metab 1995; 80:3191.
81a. Guzzo JA. Selective estrogen receptor modulators—a new age of estrogens in cardiovascular disease? Clin Cardiol 2000; 23:15.
82. Delmas PD, Bjarnason NH, Mitlak BH, et al. The effects of raloxifene on bone mineral density, serum cholesterol, and uterine endometrium. N Engl J Med 1997; 337:1641.
83. Eli Lilly and Company. Evista® (raloxifene hydrochloride) tablets prescribing information. Indianapolis, IN; 1997, Dec 10.
84. Walsh BW, Kuller LH, Wild RA, et al. Effects of raloxifene on serum lipids and coagulation factors in healthy postmenopausal women. JAMA 1998; 279:1445.
85. Sacks FM, Pfeffer MA, Moye LA, et al. The effect of pravistatin on coronary events after myocardial infarction in patients with average cholesterol levels. Cholesterol and Recurrent Events Trial investigators. N Engl J Med 1996; 335(14):1001.
86. Kannel WB, Wolf PA, Castelli WP, d'Augustino RB. Fibrinogen and risk of cardiovascular disease. JAMA 1987; 258:1183.
87. Mannucci PM, Bettega D, Chantarangkul V, et al. Effect of tamoxifen on measurements of hemostasis in healthy postmenopausal women. Arch Intern Med 1996; 156:1806.
88. Shewmon DA, Stock JL, Rosen CJ, et al. Tamoxifen and estrogen lower circulating lipoprotein(a) concentrations in healthy postmenopausal women. Arterioscler Thromb 1994; 14:1586.
89. McDonald CC, Stewart HJ, for the Scottish Breast Cancer Committee. Fatal myocardial infarction in the Scottish adjuvant tamoxifen trial. BMJ 1991; 303:435.
90. Rutqvist LE, Mattsson A, for the Stockholm Breast Cancer Study Group. Cardiac and thomboembolic morbidity among postmenopausal women with early stage breast cancer in a randomized trial of adjuvant tamoxifen. J Natl Cancer Inst 1993; 85:1398.
91. Data on file, Lilly Research Laboratories, Indianapolis, IN.
92. Hulley S, Grady D, Bush T, et al. Randomized trial of estrogen plus progestin for secondary prevention of coronary heart disease in postmenopausal women. JAMA 1998; 280:605.
93. Cummings SR, Eckert S, Krueger KA, et al. The effect of raloxifene on risk of breast cancer in postmenopausal women. JAMA 1999; 281:2189.

# CHAPTER 101

# HIRSUTISM, ALOPECIA, AND ACNE

ENRICO CARMINA AND ROGERIO A. LOBO

The effects of androgen on female skin include *acne, hirsutism,* and *alopecia.* Although derangements of androgen production and metabolism do not explain all such cases of dermatopathology, they often are of central importance in

OVARIES ADRENALS

Testosterone
(T)
. . . . . . . . . . . . . . . . . . .

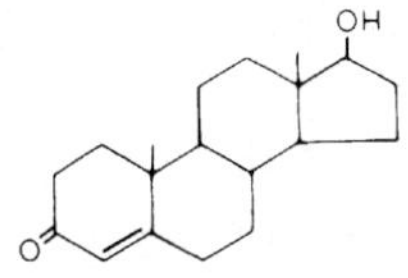

$\Delta^4$- Androstenedione
(Adione)

$\Delta^4$-Androstenedione

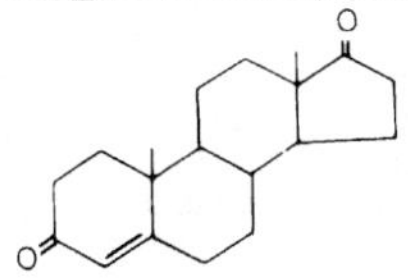

Dehydroepiandrosterone
(DHEA)

Dehydroepiandrosterone

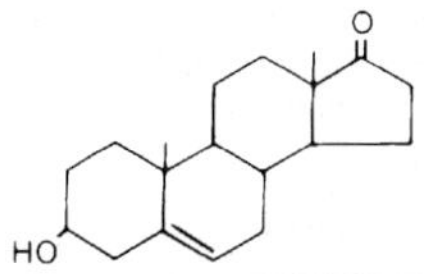

. . . . . . . . . . . . . . . . . . . . .

Dehydroepiandrosterone
**Sulfate** (DHEAS)

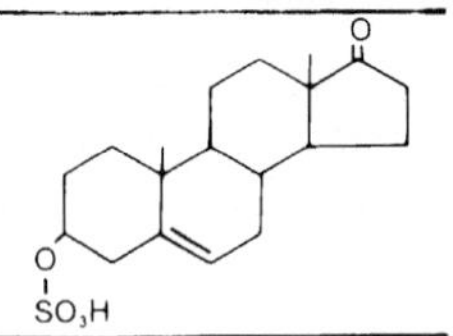

$\Delta^5$- Androstenediol
($\Delta^5$-diol)

$\Delta^5$-Androstenediol

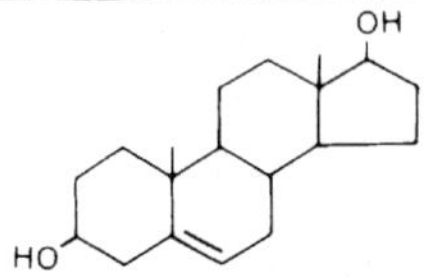

**FIGURE 101-1.** Androgens secreted by the normal ovaries and adrenals.

Commonly used abbreviations are in parentheses.

producing these abnormalities. To fully understand this interaction, the clinician must be familiar with androgen production in women and with the factors that modulate androgen action.

## ANDROGEN PRODUCTION IN WOMEN

Androgen production in women can be discussed in terms of three separate sources of production: the *ovaries* and the *adrenal glands,* which are glandular sources, and the *peripheral compartment,* which comprises all extrasplanchnic and nonglandular areas of androgen production. The peripheral compartment includes many tissues, the largest of which is the skin. The peripheral compartment modulates androgens produced by the ovaries and the adrenals.

The ovary directly secretes testosterone, $\Delta^4$-androstenedione (Adione), and, to a lesser degree, dehydroepiandrosterone (DHEA) (Fig. 101-1). The adrenal gland normally does not secrete testosterone but does secrete Adione in amounts equal to that produced by the ovary in the follicular phase.[1] The adrenal gland almost exclusively secretes dehydroepiandrosterone sulfate (DHEAS). DHEAS is secreted systemically in larger quantities than is any other androgen, and its serum concentration correlates significantly with urinary 17-ketosteroid excretion, but it appears to be a more specific marker of adrenal androgen production.[2] Another specific marker of adrenal androgen secretion is 11$\beta$-hydroxyandrostenedione. Under normal circumstances, the adrenal, but not the ovary, has the ability to 11-hydroxylate. The sensitivity of 11$\beta$-hydroxyandrostenedione as an adrenal marker is similar to that of DHEAS, but these two steroids are not correlated and probably reflect different aspects of adrenal androgen production.[3] DHEA and Adione are also secreted in greater quantities by the adrenal than by the ovary.[4]

## DIFFERENTIATION OF OVARIAN FROM ADRENAL ANDROGEN SECRETION

Investigators have used various stimulation and suppression protocols to determine the source of androgen production in normal and hyperandrogenic women. Selective catheterization of adrenal and ovarian veins also has been attempted. However, none of these techniques adequately shows the contribution of these glands to the total androgen pool. Selective venous catheterization data have confirmed that almost all exogenously administered agents (e.g., dexamethasone, human chorionic gonadotropin [hCG], adrenocorticotropin [ACTH]) affect the ovary and the adrenal.[5] Although these catheterization techniques may be useful in the detection of androgen-producing neoplasms, they have no place in the evaluation of other hyperandrogenic conditions.

The only probe that has the potential to differentiate ovarian from adrenal androgen secretion is the gonadotropin-releasing hormone (GnRH) agonist (see Chap. 16).[6,7] By down-regulating the gonadotrope and the ovary, ovarian androgens (i.e., testosterone and Adione) can be differentiated from adrenal androgens (i.e., DHEA, DHEAS) in normal women and those with polycystic ovary syndrome (PCOS) (Fig. 101-2). Because Adione can be secreted equally by the ovary and adrenal, serum testosterone is the better ovarian marker. Although only one-third of testosterone production (0.25–0.35 mg per day) is secreted directly by the ovary, the remaining two-thirds is derived in near-equal proportions from ovarian and adrenal precursors. Normally, two-thirds of circulating testosterone may originate from the ovary. These concepts, supported by data using a GnRH agonist, allow the conclusion that *serum testosterone is the primary marker of ovarian androgen production, and DHEAS and 11$\beta$-hydroxyandrostenedione are the best serum markers of adrenal androgen production.* However, DHEAS testing is more readily available, and the levels are not subject to diurnal variation.

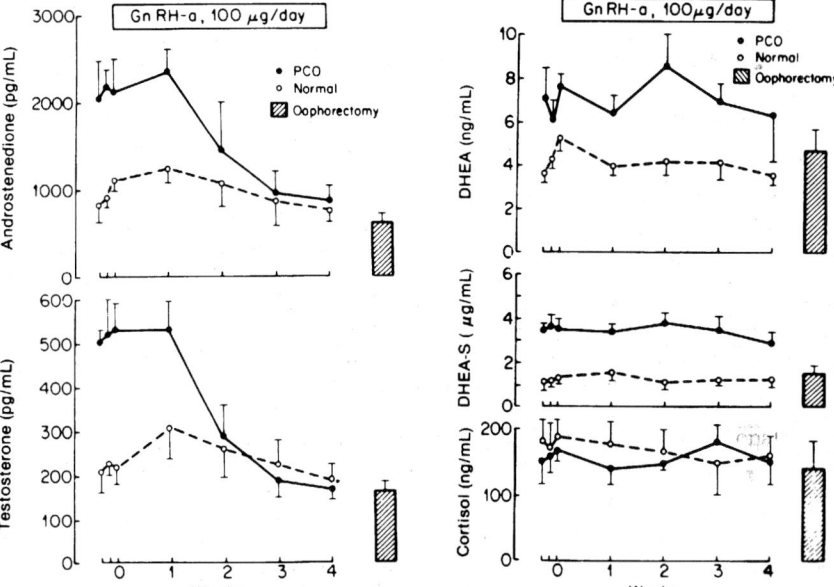

**FIGURE 101-2.** Mean (± standard error) androgen and cortisol levels with gonadotropin-releasing hormone agonist (*GnRH-a*) treatment (100 μg per day) in women with polycystic ovary (*PCO*) syndrome and normal ovulatory women compared with oophorectomized women (*shaded bars*). (*DHEA,* dehydroepiandrosterone; *DHEAS,* dehydroepiandrosterone sulfate.) (From Chang RJ. Ovarian steroid secretion in polycystic ovarian disease. Semin Reprod Endocrinol 1984; 2:244.)

Unlike in normal ovulatory women, in women with hyperandrogenic disorders such as PCOS, the ovary may contribute to the circulating pool of DHEAS and 11β-hydroxyandrostenedione.[8,9] Research using a GnRH agonist has shown that the ovary may be responsible for ~20% of circulating DHEAS.[10] The effort to differentiate ovarian from adrenal androgen secretion is also confounded by the fact that, in most hyperandrogenic conditions, both adrenal and ovarian androgen secretion are increased. In PCOS, 50% to 70% of patients present with adrenal hyperandrogenism,[9] whereas in nonclassic 21-hydroxylase deficiency, 50% to 80% present with evidence of ovarian hyperandrogenism.[11]

## SERUM MARKERS FOR ANDROGENICITY IN WOMEN

Testosterone exerts significant androgenic activity, whereas DHEAS is relatively inert as an androgen; however, 20 mg per day of DHEAS is produced, compared with only 3 mg per day of Adione and 8 mg per day of DHEA. These weak adrenal androgens exert their effects largely after conversion to more potent androgens. Testosterone, $\Delta^5$-androstenediol, dihydrotestosterone (DHT), and 3α-androstanediol (3α-diol) are classified as 17β-hydroxyandrogens and are the most potent circulating androgens; they are formed largely from other precursor androgens (Fig. 101-3).

To exert effects in the periphery, including skin and genitalia, even the more potent androgens such as testosterone must be converted to DHT. Androgen action in peripheral tissues requires receptor occupancy by DHT, which necessitates significant 5α-reductase activity (5α-RA) within the cell.[12] A more distal metabolite of DHT, 3α-diol, is also produced exclusively in peripheral tissues and is one of the 17β-hydroxyandrogens known to exert some biologic effect. Most of its activity, however, is linked to DHT production. In the peripheral compartment, other enzymatic activities, such as 17-ketoreductase and aromatase activities, are largely responsible for producing less potent androgens (e.g., Adione from testosterone) and estrogens. A balance appears to exist between the "step up" of androgen action when DHT is formed and the "step down" when less potent androgens and estrogens are formed. An understanding of the relative control of these enzymatic processes is key to an appreciation of the effects of androgen on skin (Fig. 101-4).

Two isoenzymes for 5α-reductase have been identified (types 1 and 2), and the genes are encoded on chromosomes 5 and 2, respectively.[13,14] Although some overlap between the localization of these enzymes within the body is probable, type 1 is found predominantly in the liver and nonsexual skin, and type 2 is the predominant 5α-reductase in the genitalia and prostate in men.

Logically, DHT should serve as the primary marker of peripheral androgen production; however, because of rapid cellular turnover of DHT and its great affinity for sex hormone–binding globulin (SHBG), serum DHT does not reflect the step-up phenomenon in peripheral tissues in terms of androgenicity.

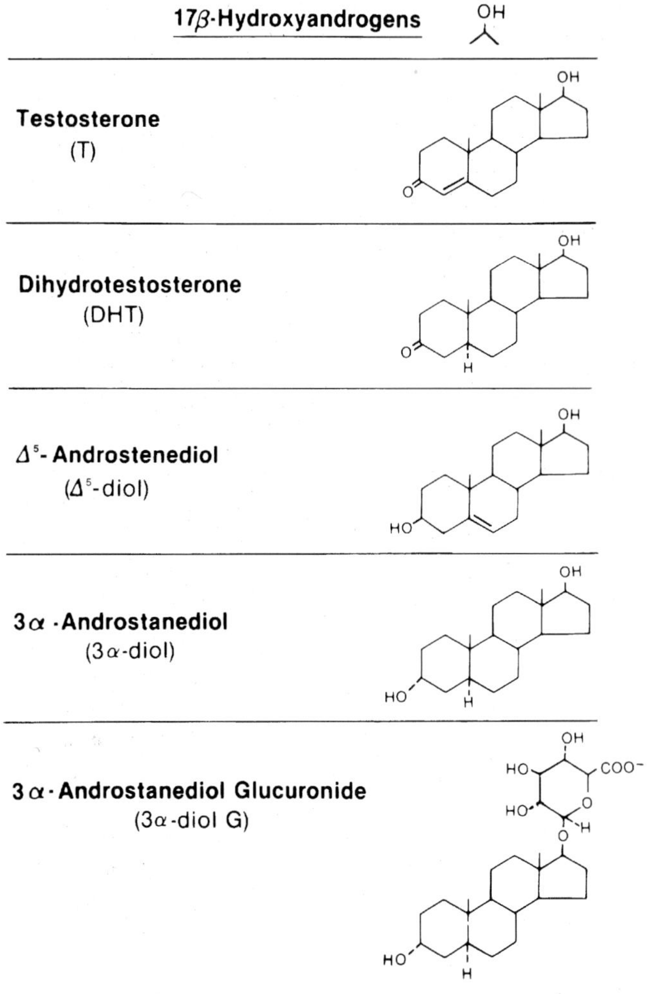

### 17β-Hydroxyandrogens

**Testosterone**
(T)

**Dihydrotestosterone**
(DHT)

**$\Delta^5$-Androstenediol**
($\Delta^5$-diol)

**3α-Androstanediol**
(3α-diol)

**3α-Androstanediol Glucuronide**
(3α-diol G)

**FIGURE 101-3.** Serum markers for androgenicity in women.

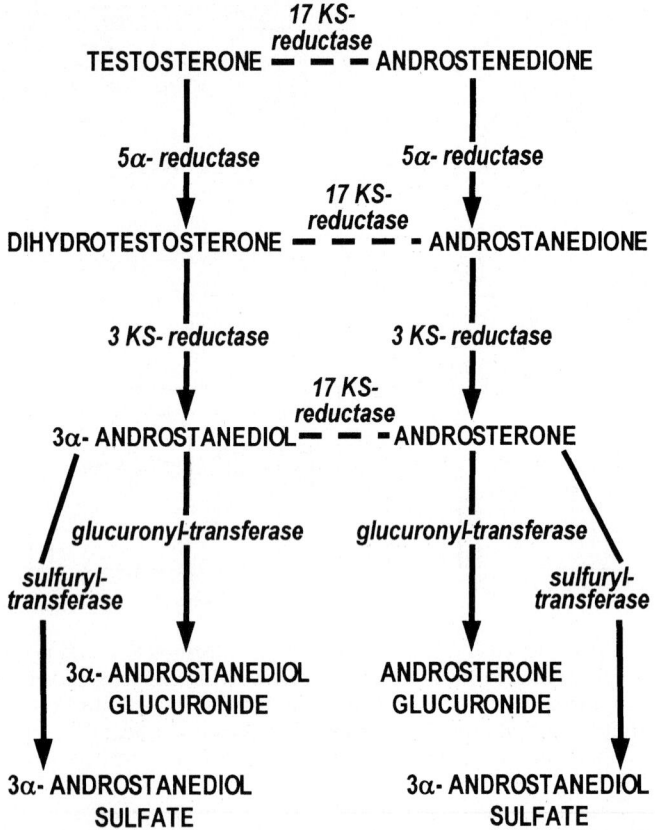

**FIGURE 101-4.** Peripheral metabolism of testosterone and androstenedione. (*KS*, ketosteroid.)

Investigators have focused on more distal metabolites of DHT. The most studied are 3α-diol and its glucuronide, 3α-androstanediol glucuronide (3α-diol G)[15] (see Fig. 101-4). Although 3α-diol and 3α-diol G are exclusively produced in peripheral tissues, 3α-diol G serves as a better marker of androgen action

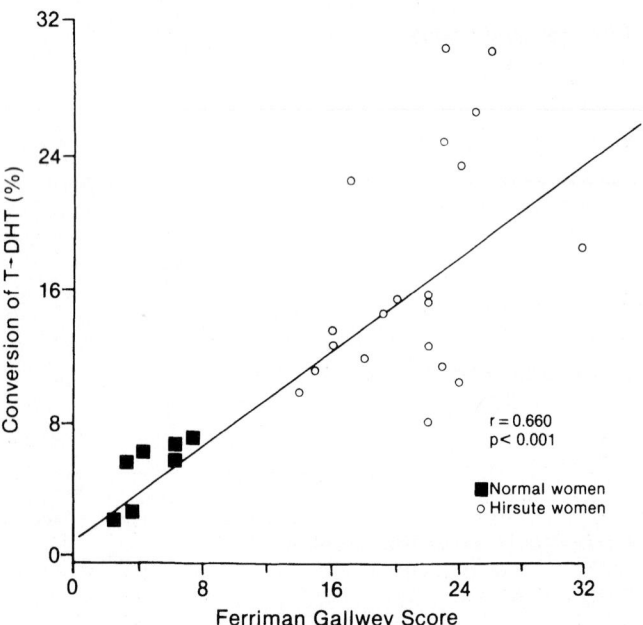

**FIGURE 101-5.** In vivo percentage conversion of testosterone (*T*) to dihydrotestosterone (*DHT*) by 5α-reductase in a genital skin preparation and relation to the clinical evaluation of hirsutism (Ferriman-Gallwey score). (From Serafini P, Lobo RA. Increased 5α-reductase activity in idiopathic hirsutism. Fertil Steril 1985; 43:74.)

because, once formed, no reconversion to DHT takes place. An excellent correlation is found between serum 3α-diol G level and the manifestation of androgenicity.[12,16] A good correlation is also seen between androgenicity and the level of skin 5α-RA[16] (Fig. 101-5). Although some investigators have argued that serum 3α-diol G may not exclusively reflect peripheral or skin activity and that it is largely derived from adrenal androgens,[17] data confirm the earlier observations. DHT produces much higher serum levels of 3α-diol G when it is applied to the skin than when it is delivered intravenously.[18] Serum 3α-diol G also shows excellent concordance with the improvement in hirsutism scores, which occurs with GnRH agonist treatment.[19]

Serum concentrations of androgen metabolites are also strongly influenced by the circulating levels of androgens.[20] In hirsute women, 3α-diol G levels depend both on levels of more potent androgens (e.g., testosterone and androstenedione) and on peripheral 5α-RA.[18,20]

Although serum 3α-diol G levels best reflect the presence and the severity of hirsutism, measurement of other androgen metabolites may be useful clinically. Assay of one of these metabolites, androsterone glucuronide, may be particularly helpful in patients with acne.[21]

## MODULATORS OF ANDROGEN ACTION

No correlation is found between androgen levels and the degree or severity of hirsutism. However, the modulation of androgen status by 5α-RA and the androgen receptor content in tissues are pivotal. Androgen receptor content appears to be less important than 5α-RA levels. Receptor concentrations alone do not explain differences in clinical androgenicity,[22] although some studies have suggested that polymorphisms of the androgen receptor may be implicated in the pathogenesis of some forms of alopecia and hirsutism[23] and may influence the peripheral expression of hyperandrogenism.[24]

The most important modulator of peripheral androgen action is 5α-reductase, (type 1 and 2)[13,14] (Table 101-1). The skin expression of 5α-reductase is highly influenced by racial and ethnic factors, as well as inheritance. Moreover, skin production of 5α-reductase is also regulated by local factors (e.g., transforming growth factor-β [TGF-β] and insulin-like growth factor-I [IGF-I] and its binding proteins) and circulating factors (e.g., circulating IGF-I and androgens).[25–27]

In blood, the primary modulator of the androgen signal is the transport protein SHBG, also known as testosterone-estradiol–binding protein (see Chap. 114). All conditions that decrease SHBG binding increase unbound concentrations of the active 17β-hydroxyandrogens, augmenting their effect. The percentage of unbound estradiol (normally 35% is SHBG bound) also increases. Although several factors regulate the liver production of SHBG, probably the most important factor is insulin, which reduces SHBG blood concentrations and, thus, increases unbound testosterone.[28] This effect may be important in some conditions in which insulin levels are increased (e.g., obesity and PCOS) and explains why weight reduction may be important to the treatment of hirsutism.

**TABLE 101-1.**
**Characteristics of Two 5α-Reductase Isoenzymes**

|  | 5α-Reductase Type 1 | 5α-Reductase Type 2 |
|---|---|---|
| **Structure** | 292 amino acids | 254 amino acids |
| **Molecular weight** | 29,000 | 29,000 |
| **pH** | Basic | Acid |
| **Gene** | Short arm of chromosome 8 | Short arm of chromosome 2 |
| **Localization** | Adult female genital skin, adult skin | Prostate, liver, male genital skin |
| **Sensitivity to finasteride** | + | + + |

Terminal Hair                                                    Vellus Hair

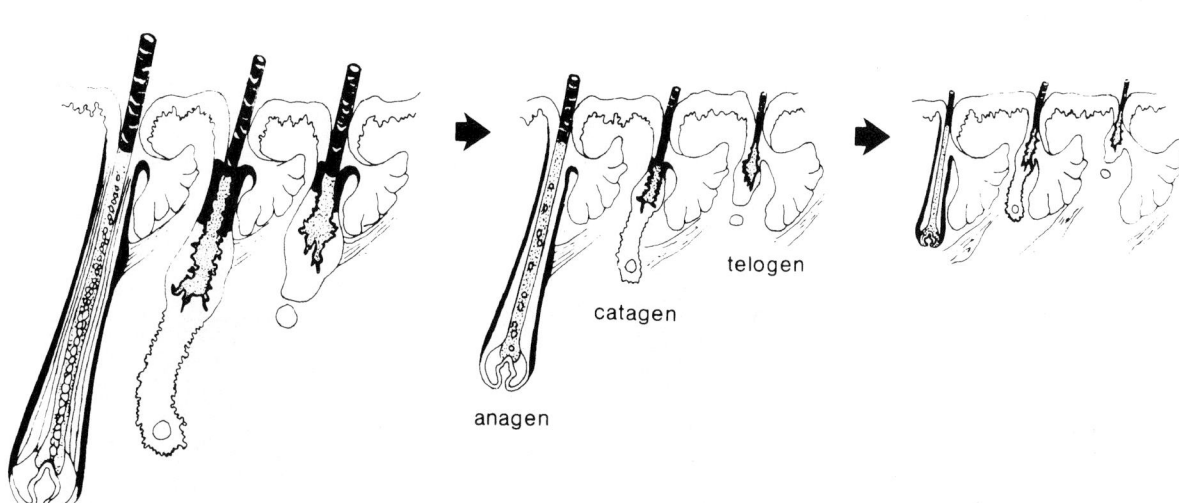

telogen

catagen

anagen

**FIGURE 101-6.** Changes occurring after several generations of hair cycles that result in the transition from terminal to vellus hair. During puberty, under the influence of androgens, some of the hair changes from vellus to terminal, especially in the axillary and pubic regions. However, after puberty, for uncertain reasons, an increase in the normally low level of 5α-reductase activity in the scalp may induce a transition from terminal to vellus hair, leading eventually to alopecia. (Modified from Montagna W, Parakkal PF. The structure and function of skin, 3rd ed. New York: Academic Press, 1974:250.)

The measurement of non–SHBG-bound or "free" testosterone has been advocated in the routine evaluation of androgen excess to more accurately detect subtle forms of hyperandrogenism.[29] However, the correlation of total and non–SHBG-bound testosterone is excellent and frequently can be predicted.[30] The assay of unbound testosterone generally is *not* necessary and should be used only in patients who have signs of androgen excess (i.e., hirsutism, acne, or alopecia) in the presence of normal levels of total testosterone and DHEAS. In an evaluation of 588 hirsute women, an increase of non-SHBG testosterone was found, with normal levels of total testosterone and DHEAS, in only 12 patients (1%).[31]

The normal serum levels for these sex steroids in women are as follows: *testosterone,* 20 to 70 ng/dL (some laboratories report values up to 100 ng/dL); *dialyzable free testosterone,* 1 to 8 pg/mL (free, by dialysis); *non–SHBG-bound testosterone,* 1 to 10 ng/dL (dialyzable free plus loosely bound); *androstenedione,* 20 to 250 ng/dL; *DHEA,* 130 to 980 ng/dL; *DHEAS,* 0.5 to 2.8 μg/mL (some laboratories report values to 3.3 μg/mL); *11β-hydroxyandrostenedione,* 15 to 200 ng/dL; *Δ5-androstenediol,* 20 to 80 ng/dL; *DHT,* 5 to 30 ng/dL; *3α-diol,* 0.5 to 6.5 ng/dL; and *3α-diol G,* 60 to 300 ng/dL (range has been extended with refinement in assay).

## PILOSEBACEOUS UNIT

An understanding of the clinical conditions associated with hyperandrogenism requires some background information about the pilosebaceous unit (PSU), the common structure in skin that gives rise to hair and sebaceous glands. PSUs and hair are distributed over virtually the entire body except the palms and soles. If the sebaceous component of the PSU is prominent, the hair is merely vellus—soft, fine, and unpigmented hair that may remain unrecognized (Fig. 101-6). If the pilary component is prominent, the terminal hair is differentiated from vellus hair by its darker color, greater length, and coarseness.

Before puberty, the predominant body hair is vellus. During puberty, some of the vellus hair normally is transformed into terminal hair, particularly in the pubic and axillary regions. After puberty, terminal hair undergoes normal cyclic changes, the control of which is only partly understood.

The characteristics and distribution of body hair differ greatly among women and are strongly influenced by ethnic and racial factors (i.e., Native Americans, Asians, fair-skinned whites, and some blacks have less hair). Body hair is also influenced by immediate genetic factors; family members frequently have similar hair characteristics. Elderly women often have increased facial hair, which may be associated with a diminution in pubic and axillary hair. Body hair is more noticeable in women with dark hair.

The attitude toward body hair varies among different societies and individuals. In some societies, a relatively large amount of body hair in women is admired; in others, it is considered unattractive. Similarly, the psychology and immediate environment of a woman may alter markedly her attitude toward a degree of body hair that most women would not consider excessive, but which she finds alarming or intolerable.

## GROWTH PHASES OF HAIR

*Anagen* is the growth phase of hair; the length of each phase of growth varies according to body site. This process is somewhat influenced by the hormonal environment. A primary feature of anagen hair is its pigmentation and medullary component (Fig. 101-7). After the growth phase, the transitional *catagen* phase ensues, in which the club-shaped bulb moves distally, eventually releasing the dermal papilla and becoming inactive. A resting stage, *telogen,* follows until the hair is shed and active follicular growth begins again.

## HORMONAL CONTROL

### ANDROGENS

Although the usual factors that control the transition between phases of hair growth remain elusive, androgens are probably the most important factors in determining the type and distribution of hair over the human body. Androgens may convert hair follicles into terminal hair and concomitantly prolong the anagen phase of hair growth.[32] Therefore, not only do androgens alter the type of hair, but they also increase its length and oiliness (because of their effects on sebaceous glands). As previously noted, most of this effect is determined by DHT, which is formed by the peripheral conversion of testosterone, via the action of 5α-

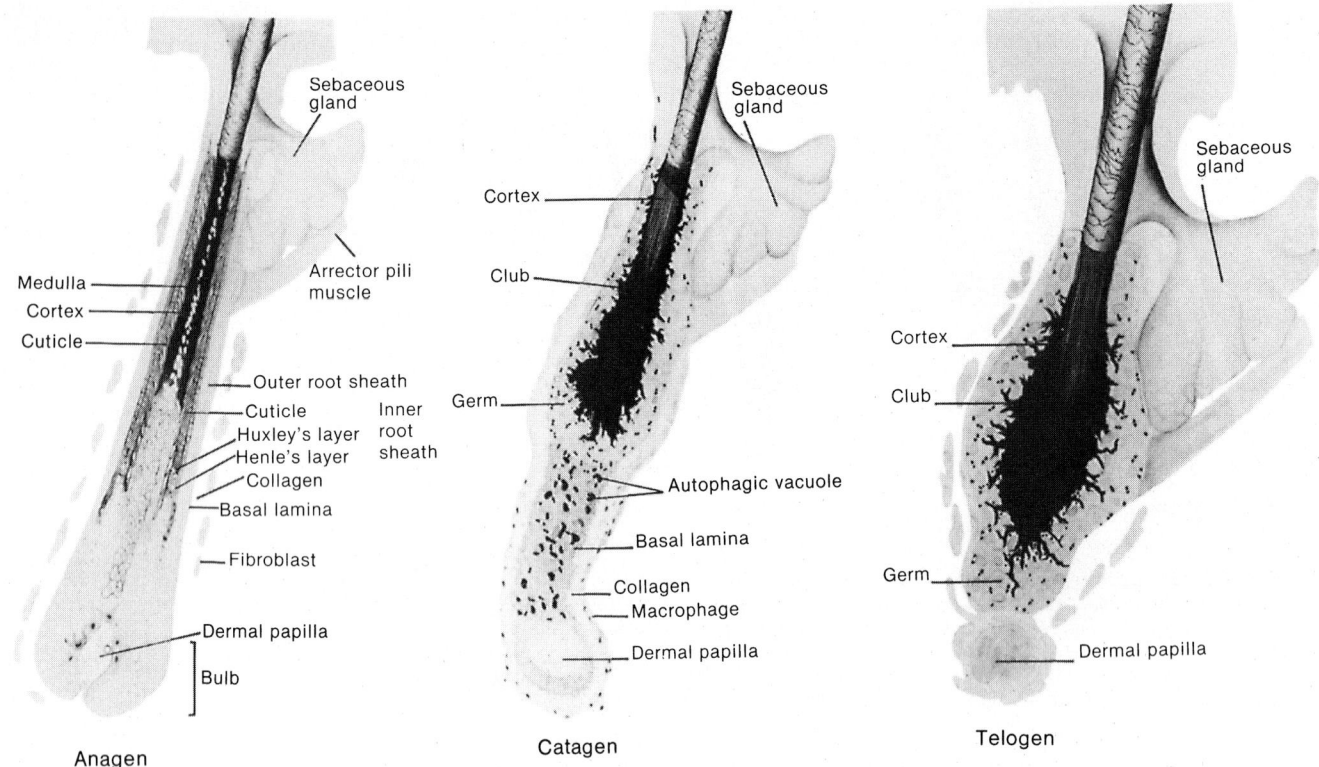

**FIGURE 101-7.** Changes in the hair follicle during growth (anagen), regression (catagen), and rest (telogen). (Adapted from Montagna W, Parakkal PF. The structure and function of skin, 3rd ed. New York: Academic Press, 1974:187.)

*reductase.* The two isoenzymes have different locations within the PSU; *type 1* is localized mostly in the distal portions of the sebaceous gland, in the dermal papilla and in the outer root sheaths, whereas *type 2* is found mostly in the dermal papilla.[33]

Other enzymes, mostly 17β-hydroxysteroid dehydrogenase type 2 (17β-HSD2), 17β-hydroxysteroid dehydrogenase type 1 (17β-HSD1), and 3β-hydroxysteroid dehydrogenase (3β-HSD) are also highly expressed within the PSU and are localized in the outer root sheath and sebaceous gland but not in the dermal papilla.[34] Thus, these two compartments may have the capacity to convert relatively weak androgens, such as DHEA, into testosterone. Finally, data are conflicting with respect to the presence of cytochrome P450 aromatase, which converts androgens to estrogens and may be viewed as providing a protective mechanism against the effects of androgens.[33,34]

One should keep in mind that different body areas may express different concentrations of these enzymes. Patients with adrenal androgen excess have lower 5α-RA in pubic skin than do patients with testosterone excess.[35] However, in the scalp, circulating DHEAS levels rather than testosterone levels correlate positively with the proliferation index of hair bulb cells.[36]

### OTHER FACTORS

Other factors that influence the PSU include growth hormone, insulin-like growth factors, adrenal steroids, and α-melanocyte–stimulating hormone.[37,38] Adrenal steroids alone appear to be sufficient for the normal production of hair in the axilla and pubis. Hair in these areas appears even in the absence of 5α-RA, but it is unlikely to be present in cases of androgen receptor deficiency (i.e., testicular feminization; see Chap. 90). This suggests that low levels of androgens are sufficient to stimulate some hair growth in pubic and axillary regions. However, some mechanism for androgen action is required, possibly one that does not need DHT or requires only a low level of DHT for receptor activation. The scalp does not require androgen for hair growth. Paradoxically, an increase in the normally low level of 5α-RA in the scalp may cause a transition from terminal to vellus hair (see Fig. 101-6) and the development of alopecia.

Various growth factors and cytokines may affect hair growth.[38–40] These factors generally act on cells of the dermal papilla as well as on follicular stem cells. They include fibroblast growth factor (FGF) and platelet-derived growth factor (PDGF) that potentiate the growth of dermal papilla cells, mostly by increasing the production of *stromolysin*, a metalloprotease that accelerates the growth of the PSU.[39] Other local factors such as TGF-β, IGF-I, interleukin-1, and epidermal growth factor (EGF) inhibit or attenuate the growth of the PSU.[40]

## ACNE

### HORMONAL CONTROL OF SEBUM

PSUs, which are primarily sebaceous, are influenced by many factors, and once they are stimulated, their actions may lead to oily skin and acne lesions. The density of PSUs is greatest on the face and scalp (400–800 glands/cm²) and lowest on the extremities (50 glands/cm²).[41] Androgen is unequivocally linked to stimulation of sebum *production.*[42] Androgen stimulates sebaceous gland cell division and intracellular lipid *synthesis.*[42] In animal studies that have examined the effects of testosterone and antiandrogens, estradiol has been shown to be an extremely potent inhibitor of sebum production. However, estradiol appears to have little or no effect on cell division. Corticosteroids have a stimulatory effect on sebaceous glands, and those progestins that have androgenic properties act at physiologic levels to stimulate sebaceous activity.

### PREVALENCE AND SCORING

Acne is present to some degree in almost all individuals but occurs most commonly during puberty, when it is found in as

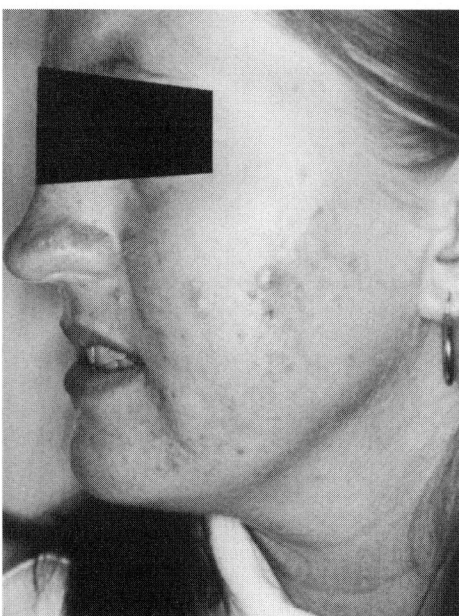

**FIGURE 101-8.** Cystic acne in a 20-year-old woman. (Courtesy of Dr. Maria L. Turner.)

many as 50% of adolescent girls and 85% of boys. After adolescence, acne disappears in most subjects but persists in some individuals. In other subjects, acne appears during adult life. Patients with persistent acne during adulthood (and patients with severe adolescent acne) can benefit from a systemic treatment (Fig. 101-8).

Acne may be graded according to several methods. An easy method is to score acne on a scale of 0 to 3.[43] In the modified method, the absence of lesions is scored as 0. Grade 1 (mild) lesions are characterized by comedones, with either no or only a few inflammatory papules or pustules. Grade 2 (moderate) lesions are characterized by numerous inflammatory lesions but with rare cystic activity. Grade 3 (severe) lesions are the worst lesions and are characterized by the presence of innumerable inflammatory papules or pustules as well as cysts. For research purposes, use of the method that scores the severity of lesions from 0 to 9 is preferable.[44]

## PATHOGENESIS

Acne is a multifactorial disease in which androgens have a central role. Four processes determine the appearance of the acneic skin lesions[45]: (a) excessive keratinization of the infra-infundibulum and cohesion of horny cell masses that lead to retention of hyperkeratosis; (b) increased sebum production; (c) bacterial colonization; and (d) inflammation (Fig. 101-9).

In this process, androgens appear to be key in the process of hyperkeratosis and the increased sebum production. Bacteria (e.g., *Propionibacterium acnes*) are implicated in the inflammatory process.[46] Obstruction to sebum excretion is a characteristic feature of comedone formation. Bacteria, specifically anaerobes such as *Corynebacterium* species in the deeper tissues and aerobes such as *Staphylococcus epidermidis* at the surface, are responsible for the breakdown of sebum by lipases, resulting in the liberation of irritant fatty acids.

In acne, the colonization correlates with sebum excretion, and sebaceous lipids are believed to be essential etiologic factors in *P. acnes* colonization of human skin.[46] Rupture of the cyst wall and expulsion of the irritant fatty acids into the dermis causes inflammatory and cystic lesions. Excessive bacterial counts in skin and surface irritants on the skin, such as cosmetic oils, also contribute to this process; diet is probably less important. A genetic predisposition is seen to the development of acne.

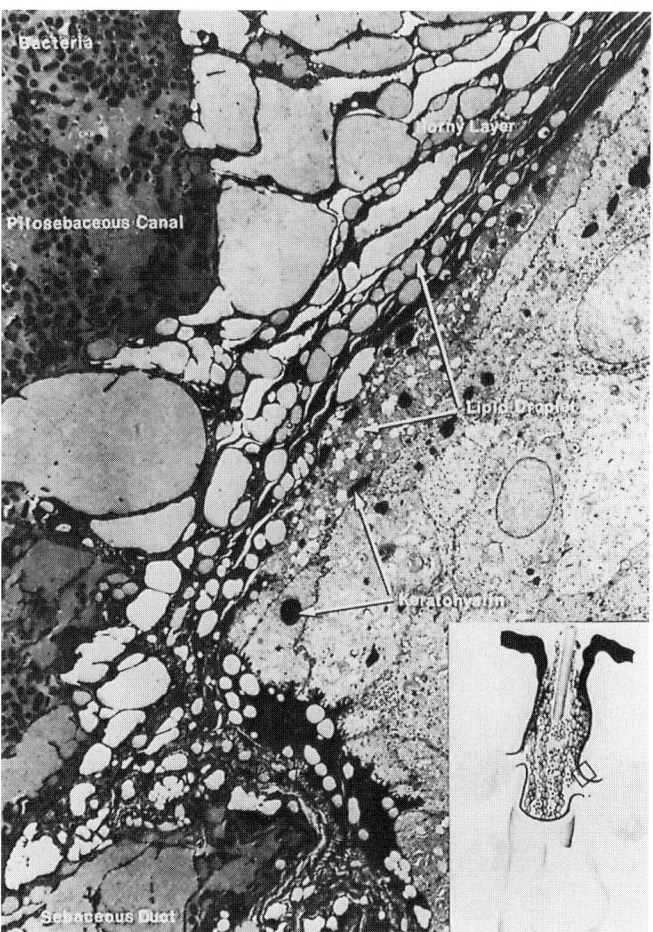

**FIGURE 101-9.** Electron photomicrograph of comedo formation beginning in infra-infundibulum. Large numbers of *Propionibacterium acnes* are present in the pilosebaceous canal. Keratohyalin is prominent. Cells of horny layer remain intact and begin to adhere to each other. Many cells contain lipid droplets not seen in normal infundibulum. (From Knutson DD. Comedo formation: ultrastructure. In: Frank SB, ed. Acne: update for the practitioner. New York: Yorke Medical Books, 1979:81.)

Whether this results from familial hyperandrogenemia during puberty, end organ (i.e., PSU) sensitivity, or both is uncertain.

## HYPERANDROGENISM AND ACNE

Several investigators have demonstrated a link between hyperandrogenism and acne; some studies have shown that most patients with acne have elevated serum androgens, reflecting increased ovarian and/or adrenal production.[47,48] Although some studies have reported specific correlations of acne with levels of serum free testosterone[49] or serum DHEAS,[50] the authors and others[21,51,52] have not observed any particular androgen profile in hyperandrogenic patients with acne. Also, no correlation exists between the degree of hyperandrogenism and the severity of acne. This suggests that peripheral factors are important in determining the appearance of acneic lesions in hyperandrogenic patients. These factors may include changes in peripheral androgen metabolism, alterations of some local factors, or both. Consistent with the first hypothesis, a particular profile of androgen metabolites has been shown to be present in hyperandrogenic acne patients characterized by relatively higher levels of androsterone glucuronide.[21] Indeed, although all studied androgen metabolites (including 3α-diol G) are increased in hyperandrogenic acne patients (because of the increase of androgen substrate), only androsterone glucuronide is higher in hyperandrogenic patients with acne as compared to hyperandrogenic

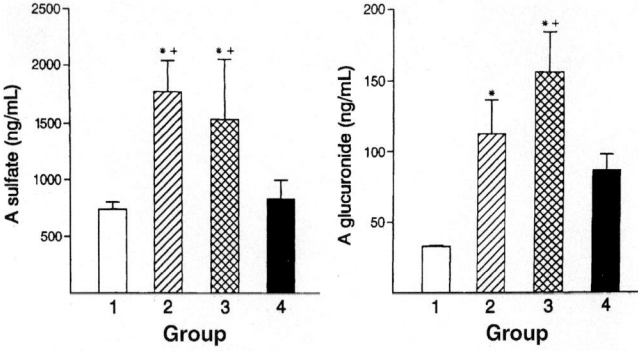

**FIGURE 101-10.** Mean serum levels of androsterone sulfate (A sulfate) and androsterone glucuronide (A glucuronide) in normal controls (group 1), hirsute hyperandrogenic patients with acne but no hirsutism (group 2), hirsute hyperandrogenic patients with acne (group 3), and hirsute hyperandrogenic women without acne (group 4). ($^{*+}$, $p$ <.01 vs. controls; $^*$, $p$ <.05 vs. controls; *bars*, standard errors.) (From Carmina E, Stanczyk FZ, Matteri RK, Lobo RA. Serum androsterone conjugates differentiate between acne and hirsutism in hyperandrogenic women. Fertil Steril 1991; 55:871.)

patients with hirsutism (Fig. 101-10). As expected, hyperandrogenic acne patients have high 5α-RA caused almost exclusively by an increase of the type 1 isoenzyme.[53]

Many patients with permanent or adult acne have normal androgen levels. In these patients, an increased sensitivity of the PSU (mostly the sebaceous component) to androgens has been hypothesized. As many as 60% of these patients respond to antiandrogen therapy.[54] In a study of the androgen metabolism of acne in patients who have normal androgen levels, an increased level of several androgen metabolites was demonstrated in 60%.[55] The most altered metabolite was serum androsterone glucuronide, a finding that suggests a link between altered androsterone metabolism and the development of acneic lesions[55] (Fig. 101-11).

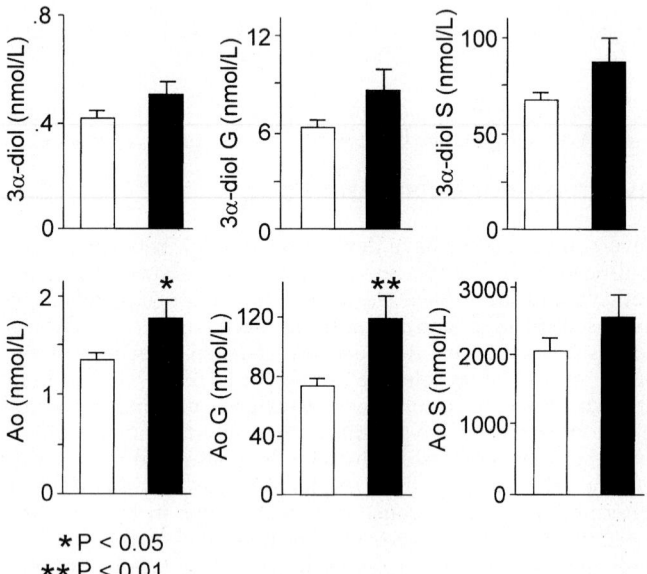

$\star$ P < 0.05
$\star\star$ P < 0.01

**FIGURE 101-11.** Mean levels of serum androgen metabolites in control subjects (*white bars*) and patients with normoandrogenic acne (*black bars*). Bars, standard errors. (*3α-diol*, 3α-androstanediol; *3α-diol G*, 3α-androstanediol glucuronide; *3α-diol S*, 3α-androstanediol sulfate; *Ao*, androsterone; *Ao G*, androsterone glucuronide; *Ao S*, androsterone sulfate.) (From Carmina E, Lobo RA. Evidence for increased androsterone metabolism in some normoandrogenic women with acne. J Clin Endocrinol Metab 1993; 76:1111.)

## THERAPY

Acne is usually treated with desquamative drugs such as benzoyl peroxide and antibacterial agents such as tetracycline or clindamycin. However, antiandrogen treatment is extremely successful. The most successful regimens have included the antiandrogens cyproterone acetate or spironolactone, used either locally or orally. Oral contraceptives are also effective. Cyproterone acetate is a progestin derivative that is used at a 2-mg dose in oral contraceptives and that has been marketed as Diane in Europe and Canada. In all oral contraceptives, the estrogen (e.g., ethinyl estradiol) is also important in inhibiting sebum production. The use of progestin ethynodiol diacetate in Demulen is most popular in the United States. However, even though Demulen lacks significant inhibitory effects on 5α-RA and the androgen receptor, it decreases ovarian and adrenal androgen secretion. Newer oral contraceptives marketed in the United States contain progestins with lower androgenicity. These progestins, norgestimate and desogestrel, are available in the formulations called Ortho-Cyclen, Ortho-Cept, and Desogen. All of these products offer a slight theoretical advantage for treatment of acne because they have inherently low androgenic activity. Ortho-Cyclen and Ortho Tri-Cyclen have received specific Food and Drug Administration approval for the treatment of acne. Other formulations are also likely to receive approval in the future. In Europe, the use of cyproterone acetate has yielded response rates of 90% or greater within a year.[56]

A standard treatment for resistant cystic acne is 13-*cis* retinoic acid (Accutane). This oral therapy, given in dosages of 0.5 to 2.0 mg/kg per day in two divided doses daily for 15 to 20 weeks, has proved to be extremely successful. However, marked adverse effects may occur. Also, because of a high risk of birth defects, pregnancy should be ruled out before therapy, and the patient should avoid pregnancy during therapy and for 1 month after treatment, by abstaining from sexual intercourse or by using two reliable forms of birth control at the same time. Data indicate that 5α-RA is substantially inhibited by this treatment.[57,58] These findings reinforce the notion that sebaceous 5α-RA is intricately involved in the pathophysiology of acne.

## HIRSUTISM

### DEFINITION

Hirsutism is the development of excessive androgen-stimulated terminal hair in a female in areas where terminal hair is not normally found. Various descriptive and quantitative scales have been used to document the process, but none is ideal. The modified Ferriman-Gallwey system is the most reliable (Fig. 101-12). However, this scale is subjective and requires grading of hair from specific body sites that may not include some important areas.

Hirsutism is characterized by increased numbers of terminal hairs in certain regions of the body. The chin, upper lip, and side-burn area often are involved, as are the neck, chest, shoulders, upper back, upper abdomen, and medial portions of the thighs. A diffuse increase in hair on the arms and legs may be noted. Hair on the knuckles and ears of women is unusual and may indicate the presence of virilization. Hirsutism can be a mild cosmetic problem that requires only reassurance and cosmetic therapy, or it can have considerable psychological impact necessitating other treatments. Hirsutism can also be an indication of an underlying illness.

### DIFFERENTIATION FROM VIRILIZATION

Although hirsutism often affects virilized individuals, the terms should not be used interchangeably. Virilization includes defeminizing signs (e.g., loss of female body contour, flattening of the breasts), increased libido, and frank masculinization (e.g., muscle mass increase, temporal balding, deepening of the

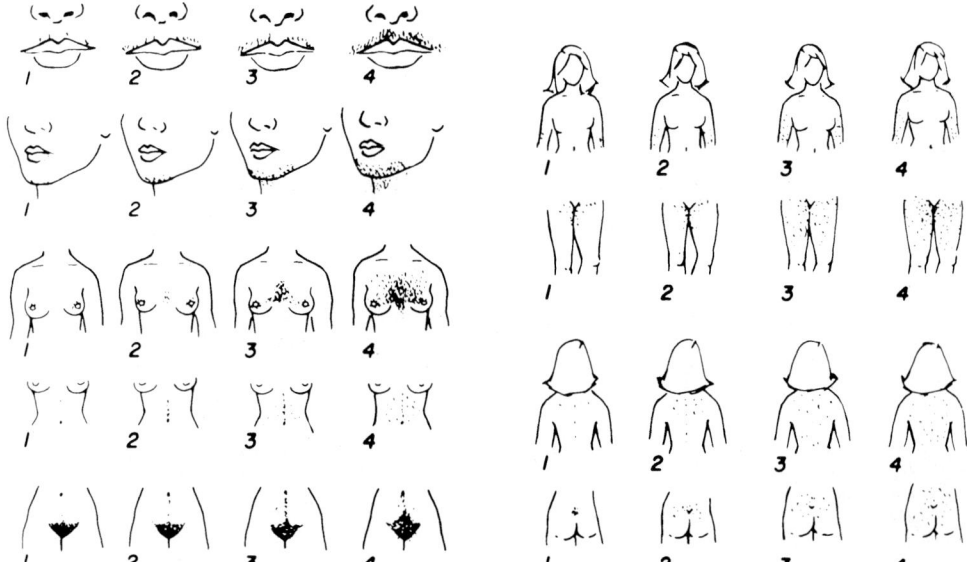

**FIGURE 101-12.** Semiquantitative system for the clinical assessment of the presence and severity of hirsutism in the premenopausal woman. Each of nine body areas is graded separately from no hirsutism (grade 0) to minimal hirsutism (grade 1) to marked hirsutism (grade 4). Then the grades of all areas are summed. In one study, 5% of premenopausal women had a score of 8 or more. (From Hatch R, Rosenfield RL, Kim MH, et al. Hirsutism: implications, etiology, and management. Am J Obstet Gynecol 1981; 140:815; as modified from Ferriman D, Gallwey JD. Familial study of hirsutism. J Clin Endocrinol Metab 1961; 21:1440, and Lorenzo E. Clinical assessment of body hair growth in women. J Clin Endocrinol Metab 1970; 31:556.)

voice, laryngeal hypertrophy, clitoromegaly). This extreme form of androgen excess is the product of time and hyperandrogenemia. Women rarely exhibit virilization unless serum testosterone levels are above 200 ng/dL. Interestingly, serum specific antigen (PSA) is statistically increased in hirsutism, and appears to be a marker of androgenation.[58a]

## CRYPTIC HYPERANDROGENISM

Cryptic hyperandrogenemia, characterized by absence of hirsutism or acne, can be encountered in anovulatory women and in women with the cryptic form of congenital adrenal hyperplasia (see Chap. 77).[59,60] The cause of this paradox is important to an understanding of the manifestations of androgen excess. In the expression of hyperandrogenism, the "signal" (in the form of secreted androgens) and the level of sensitivity of the PSU in the affected areas are important. This sensitivity, which includes 5α-RA, also involves genetic and other factors that can modulate the growth or regression of the PSU. In the case of cryptic hyperandrogenism, an elevated circulating androgen level (i.e., the signal) is not sufficient to cause hirsutism.

## HIRSUTISM AND HYPERANDROGENISM

Three major concepts link androgen with hirsutism:

1. Androgen is necessary to recruit terminal hair development.
2. Androgen prolongs the time spent in the anagen phase of hair growth.
3. 5α-RA within the PSU modulates the androgenic signal.

On the scalp, a generally androgen-unresponsive area, anagen lasts 3 years; on the face, it lasts ~4 months if not abnormally stimulated by androgen. Telogen phases average 3 months for scalp and facial hair. The prolonged anagen of scalp hair explains the greater length of hair in this area. Anagen on the thighs of men averages 54 days but is only 22 days in women. Moreover, axillary hair growth is 10% faster in men than in women.[61] With stimulation by androgen in androgen-responsive areas, the length of anagen is longer, terminal rather than vellus hairs appear, and the hair is thicker.

The latter findings, which explain hair density in hirsutism, have been inferred from antiandrogen therapy with cyproterone acetate and spironolactone. A major effect of antiandrogen therapy is to convert terminal hairs to vellus hairs. Figure 101-13 shows the dose-response change in thickness of anagen hair with spironolactone treatment.

Differences are seen in the expression of 5α-RA in men and in women. Male genital skin expresses both isoenzymes of 5α-reductase, but with a marked preponderance of isoenzyme type 2.[62] On the other hand, female genital skin expresses almost exclusively 5α-reductase type 1, and levels of 5α-reductase type 2 are very low.[62] Hirsute hyperandrogenic women exhibit a pattern of 5α-reductase isoenzymes that is similar to that of normal women, but in hirsutism a much higher concentration of 5α-reductase type 1 is found.[62,63] Therefore, both in acne and in hirsutism, an increase of the type 1 isoenzyme is found that probably occurs as a consequence of androgen excess.

## DIFFERENTIAL DIAGNOSIS OF ANDROGEN EXCESS

Patients with hirsutism must be evaluated for hyperandrogenemia. If hyperandrogenism is found, a differential diagnosis of androgen excess should be considered.

### DRUG EFFECTS AND SYSTEMIC CONDITIONS

Careful history-taking and a careful physical examination can eliminate the possibility of drug-induced androgen excess, the

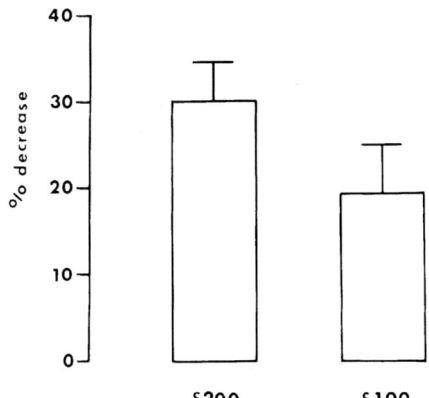

**ANAGEN HAIR SHAFT DIAMETERS**

**FIGURE 101-13.** Percentage decrease in anagen hair shaft diameters after therapy with 200 mg (*S200*) and 100 mg (*S100*) of spironolactone. *Bars,* standard errors. (From Lobo RA, Shoupe D, Serafini P, et al. The effects of two doses of spironolactone on serum androgens and anagen hair in hirsute women. Fertil Steril 1985; 43:200.)

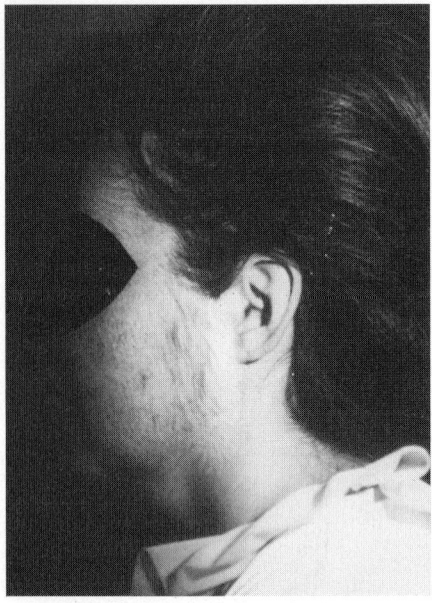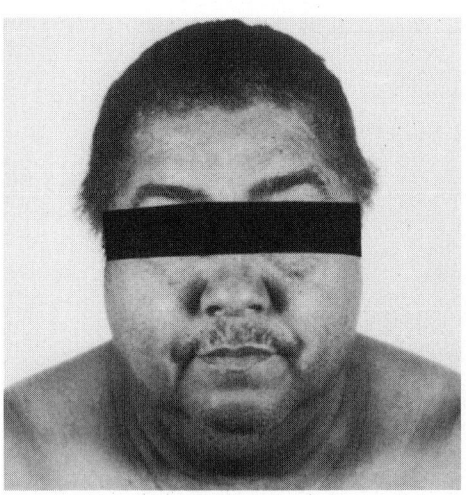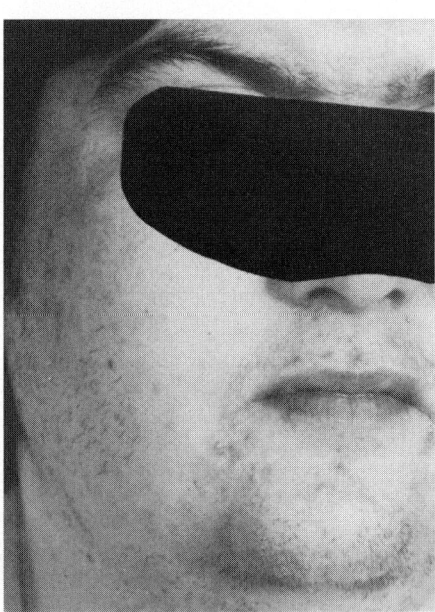

A–C

**FIGURE 101-14.** **A,** Long, thin, silk-like facial hair on a woman with Cushing disease. **B,** Hirsutism and virilization in a woman with an androgenizing ovarian tumor. Notice the male-pattern baldness. **C,** Coarse facial hair on a woman with polycystic ovary syndrome.

androgen insensitivity of genetic males, and several systemic conditions. Many preparations may contain androgen. Drugs such as diphenylhydantoin, some oral contraceptives, danazol, minoxidil, and diazoxide are known to cause hirsutism. Corticosteroid therapy can cause hirsutism; female athletes or women with conditions such as aplastic anemia who are taking anabolic agents may have hirsutism (see Chap. 119).

Not uncommonly, body hair increases in pregnant women, particularly during the first trimester; usually this condition resolves after delivery.

Some women with acromegaly are hirsute, as are some women with prolactinomas. Hypothyroidism, particularly in the young, may be associated with an increased growth of whorls of lanugo-like hair on the back. Women with anorexia nervosa (see Chap. 128) also may have large amounts of fine lanugo-like hair on the face, back, and shoulders.[63a] Porphyrin due to congenital erythropoietic porphyria, porphyria cutanea tarda, or toxic porphyria (see Chap. 235) is commonly associated with hypertrichosis. Certain extremely rare 46,XY individuals with ambiguous genitalia have been reared as females because of androgen-resistance syndromes (see Chap. 90); these persons may present in the peripubertal period as hirsute females. In congenital lipoatrophic diabetes (Berardinelli-Seip syndrome), the lipodystrophy may be accompanied by hirsutism and occasionally by hyperhidrosis. In many of these conditions, the primary suspected diagnosis can be established from the history and physical examination findings.

During history-taking, the patient may volunteer that she has been exposed to diethylstilbestrol (DES). Epidemiologically, DES exposure has been shown to be associated with hirsutism, although no direct cause has been established.

### CUSHING SYNDROME

Rarely, persons with Cushing syndrome present with hirsutism; other signs and symptoms usually predominate. Nevertheless, hirsutism is commonly present. In addition to increased terminal hairs, long, silky hair may be present on the face and extremities (Fig. 101-14). If this diagnosis is considered, an overnight dexamethasone-suppression test or urinary free cortisol assay are useful screening measures (see Chap. 75).

### NEOPLASIA AND HYPERANDROGENISM

An important reason for evaluating patients with androgen excess is to rule out neoplasms of the ovary or, less commonly, the adrenal gland. Measurement of blood levels of androgens and careful history-taking are of great importance. A history of sudden onset and rapid progression of the signs and symptoms in a previously asymptomatic woman is ominous. With rapidly increasing concentrations of androgens, defeminization usually occurs first: a decrease in breast size, a change in body contour, and menstrual disturbances precede acne and progressive hirsutism. Virilization is encountered because virtually all tumors secrete sufficient androgen to cause this finding. In the workup of a patient with hirsutism, a pelvic examination always should be performed.

**Ovarian Tumors.** Any ovarian neoplasm can produce androgen (see Chap. 102). Benign serous cysts and other nonfunctional tumors can cause excessive androgen production by stimulating the adjacent thecal-stromal tissue. The most frequently encountered functional tumors are the Sertoli-Leydig cell type (i.e., arrhenoblastoma), lipoid cell tumors, and hilus cell tumors (see Fig. 101-14). In premenopausal women, most tumors (e.g., arrhenoblastomas) become unilaterally palpable on pelvic bimanual examination. Functional ovarian tumors typically are unilateral masses.

In postmenopausal women, ovarian tumors often are small and not palpable. Any palpable ovary in this age group is of great concern. When the history is suggestive, attention is focused on the levels of serum testosterone. Most ovarian neoplasms are associated with serum testosterone levels above 200 ng/dL. However, because of episodic variation, some neoplasms are associated with serum testosterone levels between 150 and 200 ng/dL.[64] When androgen levels are in this range, tumor is a far less frequent diagnosis than in some other functional states, but the patient still requires thorough evaluation. Suppression and stimulation tests are unreliable for the diagnosis of an ovarian neoplasm.

Even the use of a GnRH agonist, which causes down-regulation of gonadotropins and ovarian suppression, has been shown to suppress androgen secretion in ovarian tumors.[65]

Nonsteroidal markers of ovarian tumors can also be evaluated but generally are of limited utility. Some Sertoli-Leydig–

cell tumors produce α-fetoprotein, and these tumors are often malignant. In these patients, measurements of α-fetoprotein may be useful in detecting recurrence and metastases.[66] Some granulosa-cell tumors produce androgens; in these tumors, circulating levels of inhibin are elevated and may be measured in postoperative follow-up.[67] Because pelvic examination may be difficult, especially in obese women (50% of patients with ovarian masses are obese), vaginal ultrasonography may be helpful to differentiate a unilateral mass.[68] Bilaterally enlarged ovaries are reassuring and suggest polycystic ovaries. With vaginal ultrasonography, the color flow Doppler technique has been helpful in diagnosing small ovarian tumors by measuring increased blood flow through the mass. If no ovarian mass is found and serum testosterone levels are >150 ng/dL, computed tomography (CT) or magnetic resonance imaging (MRI) of the adrenal should be performed. Rarely, a testosterone-secreting adrenal adenoma may be encountered. CT has limited value in the diagnosis of ovarian tumors,[69] but MRI may be useful for identifying small, solid ovarian tumors.[69] Iodomethylnorcholesterol scanning may also be useful and has been able to identify some small ovarian tumors.[70] Finally, if the results of these techniques are negative, selective venous catheterization studies should be considered but are dependent on the experience of the angiographer.

Further assessment of any virilized postmenopausal woman is mandatory, regardless of the serum androgen levels. Occasionally, a postmenopausal woman with an androgen-producing ovarian tumor complains only of postmenopausal bleeding, and virilization may not be obvious.[71]

**Adrenal Tumors.**    Adrenal adenomas and carcinomas may produce any or all of the steroids normally produced by the adrenal; attention should be directed to symptomatic signs of glucocorticoid and mineralocorticoid excess (see Chap. 75). Except for the testosterone-producing adenoma, an adrenal neoplasm virtually never is encountered with DHEAS levels <8 μg/mL. If serum DHEAS levels are >8 μg/mL, the differential diagnosis usually is between neoplasm and one of the enzymatic deficiencies causing congenital adrenal hyperplasia[72] (see Chap. 77).

The patient's history is important. Adrenal carcinomas often are debilitating and rapidly progressive. The history of the adult forms of congenital adrenal hyperplasia begins with peripubertal menstrual disturbances and hirsutism that is not rapidly progressive. Even the testosterone-producing adenomas lead to elevated serum levels of DHEAS, although these levels usually are between 3 and 5 μg/mL. In the presence of androgen excess, CT of the adrenal gland is the most sensitive diagnostic test for a neoplasm. Small lesions (1–2 cm) may be demonstrated. Lesions as small as 5 mm may be detected.[73] However, if the index of suspicion for congenital adrenal hyperplasia is high, initial screening tests for congenital adrenal hyperplasia may be performed first.

### IDIOPATHIC HIRSUTISM

Idiopathic hirsutism is perhaps the most common diagnosis in patients presenting with excessive hair. Other causes of hirsutism should be excluded. Idiopathic hirsutism includes conditions that have been called familial. Among whites, it is more common in women of Mediterranean ancestry. The diagnosis is most often made in women who have no menstrual complaints yet have hirsutism that cannot be explained on the basis of their normal serum levels of testosterone and DHEAS. Serum free or non–SHBG-bound testosterone levels should be normal.[31]

In spite of its name, nothing is idiopathic about this disorder in most patients. A subtle or even obvious source of increased androgen production may be documented.[74,75] Even if no signal-related disturbances are seen, skin sensitivity or a disorder of the peripheral compartment more than adequately explains the

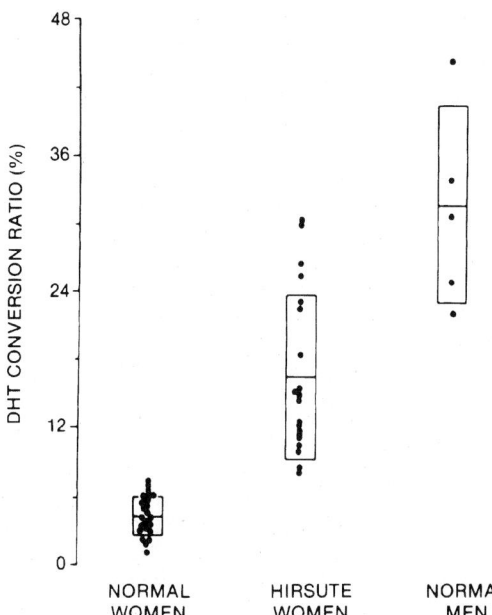

**FIGURE 101-15.** Percentage conversion of testosterone to dihydrotestosterone (*DHT*) in normal women, hirsute women, and normal men. Individual values are depicted together with the mean (± 1 standard deviation) in the three groups. (From Serafini P, Ablan F, Lobo RA. 5α-Reductase activity in the genital skin of hirsute women. J Clin Endocrinol Metab 1985; 60:349.)

hirsutism[12,76] (Fig. 101-15). High levels of serum 3α-diol G and genital skin 5α-RA are common in patients with idiopathic hirsutism[12,76] (Fig. 101-16). Moreover, peripheral androgen production (e.g., serum 3α-diol G) correlates well with the Ferriman-Gallwey score.

Idiopathic hirsutism may not be the result of disordered biochemistry. Examination of 5α-RA and other enzymes in individual anagen hair follicles has produced mixed results.[77]

Although idiopathic hirsutism is a misnomer for most patients because signal or tissue abnormalities in androgen pro-

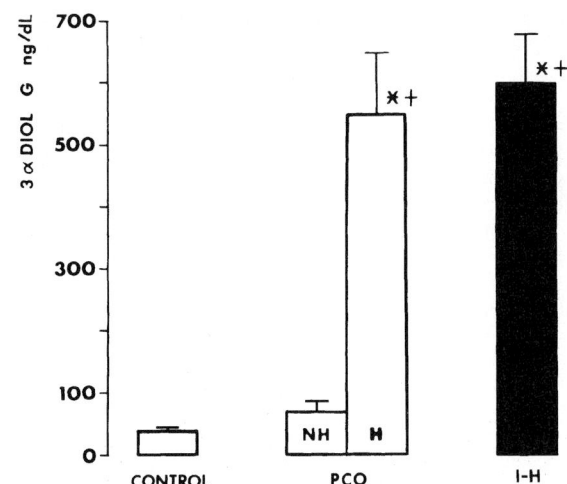

**FIGURE 101-16.** Serum levels of 3α-androstanediol glucuronide (*3α-diol G*) levels in control subjects, in nonhirsute (*NH*) and hirsute (*H*) women with polycystic ovary syndrome (*PCO*), and in women with idiopathic hirsutism (*I-H*). With assay modifications, absolute values for 3α-diol are reported to be higher than these data. (*, *p* <.01 vs. controls; +, *p* <.05 vs. nonhirsute group; *bars*, standard errors.)

TABLE 101-2.
Clinical Presentation of Polycystic Ovary Syndrome in 240 Women

| Symptom | Prevalence (%) |
|---|---|
| AMENORRHEA | 16 |
| OLIGOMENORRHEA | 64 |
| POLYMENORRHEA | 4 |
| NORMAL MENSES | 16 |
| HIRSUTISM | 70 |
| ACNE | 11 |
| OBESITY | 44 |
| ACANTHOSIS NIGRICANS | 2 |

(From Lobo RA, Carmina E. Polycystic ovary syndrome. In: Lobo RA, Mishell DH Jr, Paulson R, Shoupe D, eds. Mishell's textbook of infertility, contraception and reproductive endocrinology. Oxford: Blackwell, 1997:363.)

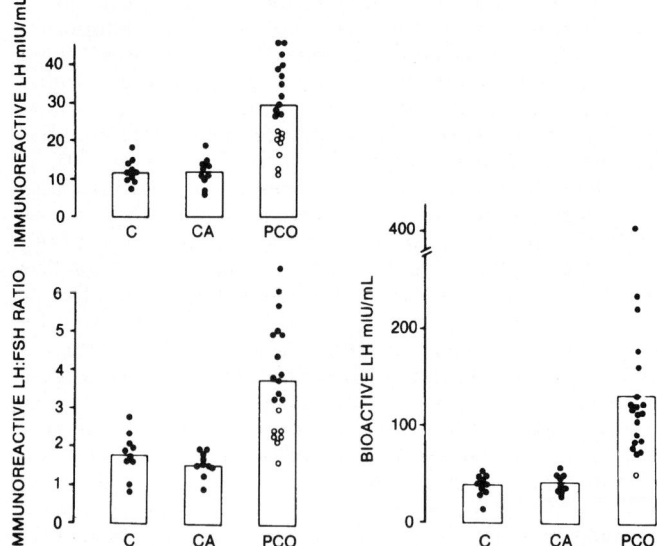

**FIGURE 101-17.** Serum levels of immunoreactive luteinizing hormone (*LH*), ratio of LH to follicle-stimulating hormone (*FSH*), and biologically active LH in control subjects (*C*), women with chronic anovulation (*CA*), and women with polycystic ovary syndrome (*PCO*). *Closed circles* for women with PCO indicate values exceeding 3 standard deviations of mean control levels. (From Lobo RA, Kletzky OA, Campeau JD, diZerega GS. Elevated bioactive luteinizing hormone in women with the polycystic ovary syndrome [PCO]. Fertil Steril 1983; 39:674.)

duction can be demonstrated, the disorder is truly idiopathic in a few persons. Patients with true idiopathic hirsutism have normal androgen production and normal skin 5α-RA. In these patients, the control of the hair cycle, which remains poorly understood, may be abnormal.

The treatment of idiopathic hirsutism is discussed in a subsequent section of this chapter.

## POLYCYSTIC OVARY SYNDROME

PCOS is the most common clinical disorder encountered in patients with hirsutism. PCOS, formerly called *Stein-Leventhal syndrome*, was historically diagnosed on the basis of ovarian morphologic abnormalities and has often been referred to as an ovarian disease. Although abnormal ovaries are common in this heterogeneous syndrome, to include or exclude this diagnosis on the basis of ovarian findings is no longer tenable. The syndrome is characterized by diversity, but the key features are hyperandrogenism and anovulation[78,78a] (Table 101-2).

**Ovarian Pathology.**   The ovary is characteristically enlarged, with multiple cysts occurring beneath a thickened capsule. However, similar morphologic abnormalities also may be encountered in children, in patients with Cushing syndrome, in patients with hypogonadotropic hypogonadism, in patients with congenital adrenal hyperplasia, and in 16% to 25% of normal women.[78–80] Patients with otherwise classic findings of PCOS may have ovaries of normal size. The ultrasonographic demonstration of polycystic ovaries may be helpful but is not necessary for the diagnosis. Ultrasonographic alterations of the ovary may be lacking, and the ovaries in PCOS show a spectrum of sonographic appearances.

In normal ovulatory women with polycystic ovaries, subtle endocrine and metabolic abnormalities may be encountered, although these women have normal fertility status.[81,82] Classically, the ovaries are defined as polycystic when the sonogram shows 10 or more small (2–8 mm) peripherally oriented cysts in one ultrasonographic plane, arranged around a dense stroma, which occupies at least one quarter of the ovarian volume.[83] Although stromal hyperplasia is considered the most specific sonographic criterion, in one study an increase of ovarian stroma could not be demonstrated in 26% of patients with PCOS.[84]

**Clinical Laboratory Findings.**   PCOS is an extremely heterogeneous clinical disorder that overlaps in many respects with other syndromes.[78] However, several primary features assist the clinician in making the diagnosis. The symptoms and signs begin perimenarchially and feature chronic anovulation (i.e., oligomenorrhea or amenorrhea) and hyperandrogenemia. The latter may occur without hirsutism in as many as 30% of patients. Many patients with PCOS are obese and have a body mass index of >27. If this is the classic clinical presentation of PCOS, many patients exhibit different clinical features. In fact,

PCOS may be diagnosed in many hyperandrogenic women with normal menses because of chronic anovulation or because of the presence of sonographic and hormonal features typical of the syndrome. The authors have calculated that ~20% of eumenorrheic hyperandrogenic women have chronic anovulation despite reporting "normal" menses, and another 50% have other features of PCOS.[85] Many women with PCOS also have normal body weight, and in the authors' experience obesity is present in only 44% of patients with classic PCOS (hyperandrogenism and chronic anovulation).[78]

The characteristic biochemical disturbance is inappropriate gonadotropin secretion with high serum luteinizing hormone (LH) levels, an exaggerated response of LH to GnRH, and normal or slightly low follicle-stimulating hormone (FSH) levels.[86] This usually yields elevated serum LH/FSH ratios. Abnormally high LH/FSH ratios may occur in only 75% of patients, but serum bioactive LH is elevated in most patients[87] (Fig. 101-17). Mild elevations in serum prolactin levels (between 22 and 40 ng/mL) may be found in a few patients (12% in the authors' experience).[88] The elevations in serum prolactin, coupled with GnRH and LH secretory abnormalities, have suggested a relative dopamine deficiency in this syndrome, but only suggestive data for some patients support this hypothesis. These abnormalities more probably are linked to increases in serum estrone and serum unbound estradiol.[89] PCOS is a disorder characterized by a chronic hyperestrogenic state, and it may contribute to the inappropriate gonadotropin secretion.[86]

Ovarian hyperandrogenism is a cardinal feature of PCOS. The ovaries produce increased amounts of testosterone, androstenedione, and DHEA, but elevations of serum testosterone are the most frequently encountered findings. The androgen excess in PCOS is milder than that observed in tumors or in ovarian hyperthecosis, and circulating levels of testosterone generally do not exceed 150 ng/dL. This may be demonstrated using a GnRH-agonist test. Interestingly, the most consistent alteration is the increase of serum 17-hydroxyprogesterone (17-OHP) that may help to distinguish women with PCOS from women with other forms of hyperandrogenism.[90]

That this syndrome has been considered to be ovarian does not exclude the presence of adrenal androgen secretory disturbances. In this regard, as many as 50% of patients with documented PCOS have increased adrenal androgen production.[9,91] In a prospective study in several countries, the prevalence of adrenal androgen excess in PCOS was 50% to 60%.[92] Several researchers have suggested that adrenal hyperandrogenism may be central to the pathogenesis of this syndrome. The best evidence, however, suggests that in most patients with PCOS, adrenal hyperandrogenism is secondary to the hormonal status of the syndrome.[93] Insulin resistance and ovarian steroid production (coupled with elevations in unbound estradiol) seem to be the main contributors to the development of adrenal hyperandrogenism in PCOS.[94]

Mild hyperinsulinemia and insulin resistance are characteristic features of PCOS that are worsened by obesity but also are present in ~50% of normal-weight women with the syndrome.[95] Excess circulating insulin influences the clinical presentation of PCOS in several major ways[78]: (a) direct stimulation of ovarian androgen secretion; (b) reduction of insulin-like growth factor–binding protein-1 production and, as a consequence, increase in bioavailable IGF-I activity; (c) influence on gonadotropin and adrenal androgen secretion; and (d) contribution to abnormalities in lipids and lipoproteins and to alterations in glucose tolerance.

The molecular mechanisms of insulin resistance in PCOS appear to be different from those found in other syndromes of insulin resistance. In many patients the mechanism consists of an abnormality of insulin receptor signaling and phosphorylation,[96] which is probably genetically transmitted.[95] This suggests that insulin resistance may play a central role in the pathogenesis of the syndrome.

**Pathogenesis of Hirsutism and Acne in Polycystic Ovary Syndrome.** Hirsutism and acne are common in PCOS but cannot be explained solely on the basis of elevated blood androgen levels. Serum androgen levels are similar in all patients with PCOS, whether or not hirsutism is present.[12] The response of the peripheral compartment appears to determine the manifestation of hirsutism. In one study, serum 3α-diol G levels were normal in nonhirsute patients with PCOS but were increased in the group with hirsutism (see Fig. 101-16). Genital skin 5α-RA is elevated to a similar degree in patients with PCOS and idiopathic hirsutism who have similar Ferriman-Gallwey scores. This further reinforces the concept that the immediate tissue environment of the PSU rather than the androgen substrate delivered to it is more pivotal in the expression of androgenicity. Some patients have responded to weight reduction by a resumption of ovulation and decreased androgen secretion.

The treatment of PCOS is discussed more extensively in Chapter 96. Central to the pathophysiology of PCOS is insulin resistance, which occurs in most women with PCOS and may or may not be associated with the finding of acanthosis nigricans. Although excessive body weight probably accentuates this abnormality, it may be found in women of normal weight. In studies in the United States, Italy, and Japan, insulin resistance was equally prevalent (~70%), even in the leaner Japanese women.[92]

As discussed, hyperinsulinemia has many ramifications in the pathophysiology of PCOS, which are beyond the scope of this review. However, an important association is found between hyperinsulinemia and ovarian hyperandrogenism. Insulin and IGF-I stimulate ovarian androgen production and decrease SHBG, leading to elevated levels of free testosterone. Moreover, evidence suggests that IGF-I may play a role in the control of skin 5α-RA. Evidence also suggests that insulin contributes to the hyperandrogenism by augmenting ovarian androgen production.

## STROMAL HYPERTHECOSIS

Hyperthecosis is an ovarian disorder that overlaps with true PCOS and ovarian tumors. The history is more compatible with that of PCOS, but onset is not sudden. Serum testosterone levels often exceed 150 to 200 ng/dL, however, and DHEAS and gonadotropin levels are usually normal. The disease is explained by luteinized thecal cells in the ovarian stroma that produce the excessive serum testosterone levels. The process is bilateral and usually diagnosed histologically only after oophorectomy. The ovaries are fleshy and do not resemble those seen in classic PCOS.[97] Patients with stromal hyperthecosis often respond poorly to suppression therapy, except for the use of a GnRH agonist, which is highly effective if therapy is prolonged. As these patients become older, and particularly for those who experience progression from hirsutism to frank virilization, bilateral oophorectomy often becomes the treatment of choice.

## NONCLASSIC 21-HYDROXYLASE DEFICIENCY

Nonclassic 21-hydroxylase deficiency (NC-21-OH) represents an attenuated form of classic congenital adrenal 21-hydroxylase deficiency and, as in the classic form, has an autosomal recessive mode of transmission.[98–100] The prevalence of NC-21-OH varies greatly according to ethnicity[100] and is very low in patients of Northern European ancestry, although it is relatively common in Southern Europe (~3% prevalence among hyperandrogenic women in Southern Italy[98]) and in some populations such as Ashkenazi Jews. In most cases, the clinical presentation is identical to that seen in PCOS,[98,101] and patients present with signs of hyperandrogenism during puberty or at menarche. Because of this later presentation, the disorder is also referred to as *late-onset 21-hydroxylase deficiency*. Most patients (70%) have menstrual irregularities and chronic anovulation; the androgen pattern is one of increased levels of androstenedione, testosterone, and unbound testosterone. DHEAS levels are often normal, because the adrenal gland produces mainly Δ4-androgens.[101] Up to 100% of patients with CAH have sonographic evidence of polycystic ovaries.

The diagnosis of NC-21-OH requires an elevation of *early morning* (8 a.m.) serum 17-OHP. Because serum 17-OHP rises during the luteal phase of the cycle, the blood sample should be obtained during the *follicular phase* in women with a menstrual factor. Basal levels of >10 ng/mL make the diagnosis clear, whereas in patients with 17-OHP levels from 3 to 10 ng/mL, the confirmation of the diagnosis requires an ACTH stimulation test. Importantly, very few patients with *normal* 17-OHP levels have an *exaggerated* response to ACTH. In some patients, a molecular study of the *CYP21* gene helps to establish the diagnosis.[102]

In the absence of clinical and androgen data characteristic of this disorder, a 17-OHP assay should be performed in all hyperandrogenic women. Most NC-21-OH patients must be considered to be affected by a mixed form of hyperandrogenism (both adrenal and ovarian).[101,103] This is probably a consequence of the effect of increased levels of estrogen (specifically unbound estradiol) on gonadotropin secretion.[104] Because of the increase of ovarian androgen secretion, glucocorticoid therapy may be relatively ineffective in many patients with NC-21-OH, and appropriate treatment of hirsutism may necessitate the administration of antiandrogens or GnRH-agonists.[103,105]

## OTHER LATE-ONSET ADRENAL ENZYMATIC DEFICIENCIES

Two other late-onset enzymatic deficiencies, 11-hydroxylase (11-OH) deficiency and 3β-ol-dehydrogenase-isomerase (3β-ol) deficiency, result in hyperandrogenism during adult life. However, *late-onset 11-OH deficiency* is very uncommon and few patients have been described.[106] In contrast, *late-onset 3β-ol deficiency* is relatively common (~1–2% of all hyperandrogenic women), and these patients present with high levels of DHEAS but with normal or even low levels of testosterone.[107] The diagnosis requires an ACTH stimulation test with comparison of the rises in $\Delta^4$ and $\Delta^5$ steroid precursors. In many patients, the defect may be sufficiently mild that the diagnosis is considered to be PCOS. Unlike for late-onset 21-OH deficiency, molecular studies have not shown any alteration of the type I or type II 3β-ol gene in patients with late-onset 3β-ol deficiency.[108,109] This has reinforced the notion that this disorder may be functional and represents an example of functional adrenal hyperandrogenism.

## TREATMENT OF HIRSUTISM

The evaluation of androgen excess should focus on establishing the cause and source of the hyperandrogenism. For treatment of hirsutism, the levels of serum testosterone and DHEAS must be known. Levels of these two hormones can serve as guides for suppression of ovarian or adrenal androgen production. This approach does not require a specific diagnosis for the more functional states, such as idiopathic hirsutism and PCOS, but instead focuses on the sources of production. A specific diagnosis such as congenital adrenal hyperplasia or a tumor warrants more specific treatment (i.e., corticosteroids or surgery, respectively).

Although measurements of serum 3α-diol G levels can confirm a peripheral source of hyperandrogenism, this evaluation is not essential. Normal testosterone and DHEAS levels imply a peripheral abnormality.

### ORAL CONTRACEPTIVES

If testosterone is elevated, ovarian hyperandrogenism is best suppressed with oral contraceptives. The combination of progestin and synthetic estrogen decreases LH-dependent ovarian androgen production. The estrogen also increases the production of SHBG, so that the lowered androgen (e.g., testosterone) is more avidly bound, yielding much lower serum non–SHBG-bound testosterone levels. Progestins alone are less effective than combination oral contraceptives. Certain oral contraceptives decrease adrenal androgen production by at least 30% and are helpful in cases of mild adrenal hyperfunction (DHEAS levels <5 μg/mL). Oral contraceptives may also have inhibitory effects on 5α-RA and on androgen receptor action. However, these latter effects are relatively mild.

With regard to the choice of an oral contraceptive, 35 μg of ethinyl estradiol is sufficient to significantly increase SHBG, and higher-dose estrogen pills should not be used routinely. However, much more latitude exists with the progestin component. The most androgenic 19-norgestogen is 1-norgestrel. Formulations such as Ovral and Lo/Ovral are best avoided. Ethynodiol diacetate (Demulen 1/35) is least androgenic and is somewhat estrogenic. Norethindrone and its acetate are only mildly androgenic, and Ortho-Novum 1-35, Modicon, and Brevicon have also been recommended. The oral contraceptives containing the newer, more potent, yet less androgenic progestins are considered by some to be more beneficial. These pills—Ortho-Cyclen, Ortho-Cept, and Desogen—may be considered the first choice for treatment of hirsutism if oral contraceptives are used. No data exist, however, that document a clinical advantage to any of the low-dose combination oral contraceptive preparations.

### CYPROTERONE ACETATE

Cyproterone acetate is a progestin with antiandrogen activity; it is taken up and released slowly by fat. To control menstrual disturbances, the drug has been administered as a "reverse sequential oral contraceptive." The original regimen included 50 to 100 mg per day of cyproterone acetate on days 5 to 15 and 50 μg of ethinyl estradiol on days 5 to 25.[110] Several different regimens may be used, and an equally effective regimen contains 50 mg of cyproterone acetate and 20 μg of ethinyl estradiol.[111] Patients with mild hirsutism or acne have benefited from treatment with Diane (2 mg of cyproterone acetate, 35 μg of ethinyl estradiol [not approved in the United States]). Patients with a major complaint of hirsutism usually require larger doses of cyproterone acetate (50–100 mg).

In the German experience, which is the most extensive, ~70% of patients demonstrated distinct improvement within 9 months of beginning treatment with cyproterone acetate. Acne and seborrhea improved in 96% and 89% of cases, respectively.[110] The mechanism of action is similar to that of oral contraceptives, but significant antiandrogenic effects also occur: receptor antagonism and inhibition of 5α-RA. Used in moderation, the drug does not appear to have significant side effects. A concern is that serum high-density lipoprotein and its subfractions decrease with use.[111,112] Cyproterone acetate is not approved for marketing in the United States because of the concern that the drug has the propensity to cause breast cancer in beagle dogs and teratogenicity in rodents when it is administered in extremely high doses during pregnancy.

### SPIRONOLACTONE

Spironolactone, which competitively inhibits aldosterone (see Chap. 80), has been used effectively for hirsutism.[113,114] As an antiandrogen, it has the same properties as cyproterone acetate, but it appears to cause greater antagonism of the androgen receptor. Moreover, inhibition of cytochrome P450–related steroidogenesis results in decreased ovarian testosterone and Adione production from adrenal and ovary. The clearance of serum testosterone is increased with spironolactone therapy.

Dosages of 50 to 200 mg per day have been used. However, the effect is dose related, and more than one-half of hirsute patients require 200 mg per day to benefit. The side effects are minimal, other than a transient initial diuresis. Hyperkalemia is extremely rare in healthy patients. The overall response rate is similar to that reported for cyproterone acetate, with 60% to 70% of patients responding as assessed by the Ferriman-Gallwey score (Fig. 101-18) or by the analysis of anagen hair diameters (see Fig. 101-13).[113,114] Not uncommonly, patients with idiopathic hirsutism who have regular menstrual cycles experience irregular bleeding with spironolactone; this is controlled by the addition of an oral contraceptive.[115] Because the effects of this

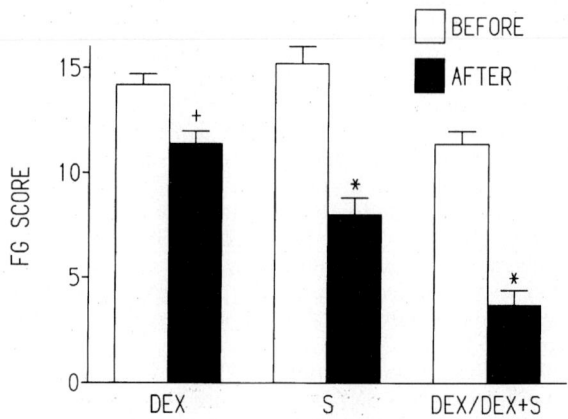

**FIGURE 101-18.** Mean and standard error of Ferriman-Gallwey (*FG*) scores for the severity of hirsutism before and after treatment for 1 year with dexamethasone (*DEX*) or spironolactone (*S*). The patients treated with DEX were then treated for an additional year with DEX plus S (*DEX/DEX + S*). (*, p <.01 compared to baseline; +, p <.05 compared to baseline.) (From Carmina E, Lobo RA. Peripheral androgen blockade versus glandular androgen suppression in the treatment of hirsutism. Obstet Gynecol 1991; 78:845.)

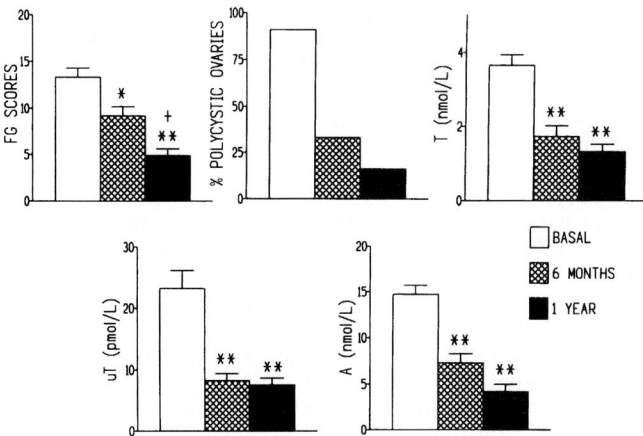

**FIGURE 101-19.** Results of treatment with a gonadotropin-releasing hormone agonist (Decapeptyl; Ipsen, France), with hormonal replacement using conjugated equine estrogens (0.625 mg on days 1–21 of each month) and medroxyprogesterone acetate (days 12–21 of each month) for 1 year in 12 patients with ovarian hyperandrogenism. Hirsutism was assessed by a modified Ferriman-Gallwey (FG) scale, and only those with scores of 8 or more were included in the study. Initially, 11 of the 12 patients had ultrasonographic findings consistent with polycystic ovaries (% polycystic ovaries). (**, p <.01 compared to baseline; *, p <.05 compared to baseline; +, p <.05 compared to 6-month value; T, total testosterone; uT, unbound testosterone; A, androstenedione; bars, standard errors.) (From Carmina E, Janni A, Lobo RA. Physiological estrogen replacement may enhance the effectiveness of the gonadotropin-releasing hormone agonist in the treatment of hirsutism. J Clin Endocrinol Metab 1994; 78:126.)

and other potent antiandrogens on the developing fetus have not been examined, spironolactone and also cyproterone acetate (which is not approved in the United States) should be used only in conjunction with effective contraception. Creams containing spironolactone or its active metabolite, canrenone, and cyproterone acetate have been used successfully for patients with more localized forms of hirsutism.

### GONADOTROPIN-RELEASING HORMONE AGONISTS

GnRH agonists are highly effective for treatment of severe hirsutism related to ovarian hyperandrogenism.[116,117] Estrogen and androgen levels are suppressed to the levels in oophorectomized women, and prolonged estrogen-replacement therapy is needed to avoid the adverse effects of prolonged hypoestrogenemia. Estrogen supplementation may be provided by low dosages (0.625 mg per day) of conjugated estrogens for 21 days[116] or by oral contraceptives[118] (Fig. 101-19). Because of the high costs of GnRH agonist therapy, its use should be reserved for patients who respond poorly to other therapies.

### CORTICOSTEROIDS

In the past, corticosteroid therapy was frequently used for the treatment of hirsutism. The improvement of hirsutism is only modest, however, and better results are obtained with the use of antiandrogens[119] (see Fig. 101-18). On the other hand, sensitivity to dexamethasone does not depend on the DHEAS levels.[120] When a mixed (adrenal and ovarian) hyperandrogenism is present, the normalization of adrenal androgens is not sufficient to produce an improvement in hirsutism. Because of this, many clinicians use corticosteroids only in the few hirsute patients who have a "pure" adrenal hyperandrogenism. In these patients and in those whose androgen levels are sensitive to corticosteroids, dexamethasone administration may provide an important advantage. Prolonged treatment (from 1 to 2 years of therapy) with low dosages of dexamethasone (0.375 mg per day) may result in a lasting remission of hyperandrogenism and hirsutism (up to 3 to 4 years).[121] This effect probably depends on the characteristics of adrenal function

and control. To permit better results in terms of the control of hirsutism, in these selected patients, dexamethasone may be combined with an antiandrogen (i.e., spironolactone, 100 mg per day).

### FLUTAMIDE

Flutamide is a nonsteroidal antiandrogen that inhibits nuclear binding of androgens and has been shown to be effective; it may decrease hirsutism to a greater extent than does spironolactone.[122–124] A dosage of between 250 and 750 mg per day has been used, but because significant hepatic toxicity may occur, lower dosages (250 or 375 mg per day) are currently preferred. At these dosages, the drug is generally safe and effective, although some patients may experience increases of transaminase enzymes. Flutamide does not inhibit gonadotropin and androgen secretion. It is currently used as an alternative to spironolactone.

### 5α-REDUCTASE INHIBITORS

Finasteride is the first product of a new class of drugs, 5α-reductase inhibitors. It is a 4-azasteroid that inhibits 5α-reductase type 2, with very little activity, at least in vitro, against the type 1 isoenzyme. In spite of this (as previously observed, hirsutism is primarily due to an increase of the type 1 isoenzyme), finasteride therapy improves hirsutism, and its effect is similar to that of spironolactone.[125,126] Most studies have used a dosage of 5 mg per day. At this dosage, finasteride suppresses DHT and 3α-diol G, whereas testosterone is increased. It has been shown that a dosage of 1 mg per day (similar to that used for treatment of alopecia) is equally effective in reducing chest hair growth in men.[127] Finasteride is not always effective; therefore, the authors use this product mostly in patients with idiopathic hirsutism, as a second choice to antiandrogens. Currently under study are new products (such as dutasteride) that have a mixed activity, inhibiting both type 1 and type 2 isoenzymes; these may offer advantages. (See also ref. 127a.)

### RESPONSE TO THERAPY AND SUBSEQUENT COURSE

Three to 4 months are required for a diminution of hair growth to be noticeable with any medical form of therapy. The goal is to diminish the rate of formation of new terminal hairs and the thickness and texture of the hair. The terminal hair of PSUs converts to the vellus type, but the hair shaft may not shed and the follicle remains intact.

Physiologic methods of controlling hirsutism should be encouraged, alone or as a supplement to drug therapy. Dark hair can be bleached to make it less obtrusive. Prominent hairs can be plucked, although this may stimulate adjacent hair growth. More extensive involvement can be treated by shaving. Chemical depilatories should be used with care, because they can irritate the skin. Wax depilation can be extremely useful. Electrolysis, if correctly performed, can give excellent results.

Hirsutism often is a lifelong problem and may be related to many still unidentified exogenous life influences in addition to factors that control the PSU and hair cycle. The condition may cause great psychological stress to some patients, and stress may have an adverse effect on the process. Emphasizing to the patient from the outset that treatment takes time and that existing hair may persist for a long time is extremely important. Therapy is inappropriate for women whose body hair is well within the normal range. In such women, reassurance concerning their normality is important. Any treatment needs to be reevaluated on an annual basis and according to the needs of the patient. To evaluate the response to therapy, a comparison with previous photographs of the affected areas is useful.

A few patients require treatment only for a short period, but most need continued attention. However, the long-term effects of many of the drugs mentioned previously have not been thoroughly evaluated.

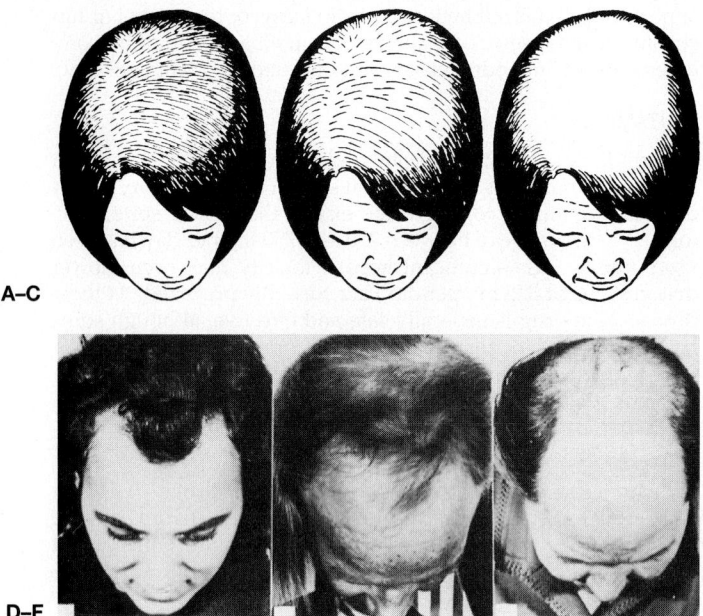

A–C

D–F

**FIGURE 101-20. A–C,** Three common stages of alopecia androgenica associated with near-normal androgen levels. Note sparing of the frontal fringes. **D–F,** Women with deep frontotemporal recession (**D**), severe alopecia androgenica (**E**), and "Hippocratic" baldness (**F**), all associated with other signs of hyperandrogenism and hyperandrogenemia. (From Ludwig E. Classification of the types of androgenetic alopecia [common baldness] occurring in the female sex. Br J Dermatol 1977; 97:247.)

## ALOPECIA

Whereas acne and hirsutism represent the results of stimulation of the PSU, *alopecia*, or the loss of hair, may represent the reverse process. Paradoxically, alopecia may also be related to hyperandrogenism.[128,129]

Alopecia usually occurs with various other disease states. Among these are systemic diseases such as systemic lupus erythematosus, dermatomyositis, and lymphomas. Endogenous or exogenous hypercortisolism, hyperthyroidism and hypothyroidism may be accompanied by alopecia. Near-complete alopecia may develop in early infancy in patients with severe hereditary resistance to 1,25-dihydroxyvitamin D. Severe febrile episodes may cause hair loss within 3 months, and alopecia may result from chemotherapy and radiation therapy. Infections of the hair follicles and scalp may also cause hair loss.

### ALOPECIA AREATA

Alopecia areata causes single or multiple round, bald patches on the scalp, which may be self-limiting and may respond to local corticosteroid treatment. This form of alopecia is thought to be autoimmune, with >40% of patients having antimicrosomal antibodies. Thyroid disease may coexist in this group; no androgen abnormality appears to be present.

### ALOPECIA ANDROGENICA

The most common form of alopecia is male-pattern baldness, called "alopecia androgenica." This process, which may be extremely gradual, occurs to some extent in virtually all men and many women, but in different patterns. In women, the frontal fringe remains intact[130] (Fig. 101-20). The characteristic abnormality is a gradual transition from terminal to vellus hair (see Fig. 101-6). However, frankly male-pattern baldness may also occur in women. This pattern is associated with significant elevations in circulating androgens, such as are observed when ovarian tumors are present. Two different types of androgen-related

hair loss are found in women. The first and most common type is not usually associated with an increase in androgen production. The second is associated with increased androgen production and may coexist with other virilizing features (see Fig. 101-20).

Although alopecia androgenica is thought to be related to functional hyperandrogenism, signal abnormalities or increases in glandular androgen production are not encountered in the more usual type of hair loss. This form of alopecia, which may have a genetic basis, appears to result from alterations in enzymatic activity of the PSU. Although hair growth on the scalp is not usually androgen dependent, some data suggest that the more potent androgens may be detrimental to the hair root. In the scalp, 5α-RA is generally low. However, the type 1 isoenzyme has been found to be increased in alopecia androgenica,[33] and its end product, DHT, may inhibit hair follicular adenylate cyclase activity.[131] This may cause the transition from terminal to vellus hair, the phenomenon observed in alopecia. In men with 5α-reductase deficiency, alopecia of the usual type does not occur, suggesting further that enhanced 5α-RA may be detrimental to scalp hair. Research has documented that the reverse transformation of terminal to vellus hair of the scalp is related to increased 5α-RA.[131a]

In the less common type of hair loss, in which alopecia results from high androgen production, the androgens may increase 5α-RA. Moreover, the detrimental effects of increased DHT production may be merely a consequence of the increased production of DHT precursor steroids such as androstenedione and testosterone. A common observation in men and women with androgenic alopecia is altered peripheral metabolism. Whether or not 5α-RA is increased, a tendency is seen for greater conversion of DHT to 3α-androstanediol sulfate rather than the glucuronide.[132] This observed decrease in glucuronide formation may be the cause of enhanced androgen action, leading to atresia of the hair root, or it may be the result of the atretic process.

A form of alopecia occurs in a relatively large number of postmenopausal women. At menopause, ovarian estrogen production decreases but androgen production changes very little. Administration of estrogen to postmenopausal women who are affected may also be of some benefit.

Women with androgenic alopecia may respond to antiandrogen therapy. In most patients the results are disappointing, however, and cannot be compared to those obtained in cases of acne and hirsutism.[110] This suggests that factors other than androgens may be operative. Flutamide appears to give the best results and may be preferred to cyproterone acetate or spironolactone. Generally, the effect obtained is a reduction of hair loss; the percentage of hair follicles that move to the anagen phase of growth is small. Interest has increased in the use of finasteride (1 mg per day) in the treatment (or prevention) of male alopecia.[133] However, no significant results have been reported in the treatment of female alopecia androgenica. Local application of minoxidil, a potent vasodilator, has been used in combination with antiandrogens to treat women with alopecia androgenica with some encouraging results.[134]

## REFERENCES

1. Bardin CW, Lipsett MB. Testosterone and androstenedione blood production rates in normal women and women with idiopathic hirsutism or polycystic ovaries. J Clin Invest 1967; 46:891.
2. Lobo RA, Paul WL, Goebelsmann U. Dehydroepiandrosterone sulfate as an indicator of adrenal androgen function. Obstet Gynecol 1981; 57:69.
3. Stanczyk FZ, Chang L, Carmina E, et al. Is 11β-hydroxyandrostenedione a better marker of adrenal androgen excess than dehydroepiandrosterone sulfate? Am J Obstet Gynecol 1991; 165:1837.
4. Bird CE, Morrow L, Fukumoto Y, et al. Δ5-Androstanediol: kinetics of metabolism and binding to plasma proteins in normal men and women. J Clin Endocrinol Metab 1976; 43:1317.
5. Moltz L, Schwartz UD. Gonadal and adrenal androgen secretion in hirsute females. In: Horton R, Lobo RA, eds. Androgen metabolism in normal and hirsute females. Clinics in Endocrinology and Metabolism 1986; 15:229.
6. Chang RJ, Laufer LR, Meldrum DR, et al. Steroid secretion in polycystic ovarian disease after ovarian suppression by a long-acting gonadotropin-releasing hormone agonist. J Clin Endocrinol Metab 1983; 56:897.

7. Barnes RB, Rosenfeld RL, Burstein S, Ehrmann DA. Pituitary-ovarian responses to nafarelin testing in the polycystic ovary syndrome. N Engl J Med 1989; 320:559.

8. Moltz L, Schwartz U, Sorensen R, et al. Ovarian and adrenal vein steroids in patients with nonneoplastic hyperandrogenism: selective catheterization findings. Fertil Steril 1984; 42:69.

9. Carmina E. Prevalence of adrenal androgen excess in PCOS. In: Azziz R, Nestler JE, Dewailly D, eds. Androgen excess disorders in women. Philadelphia: Lippincott–Raven Publishers, 1997:385.

10. Carmina E, Gonzalez F, Chang L, Lobo RA. Reassessment of adrenal androgen secretion in women with polycystic ovary syndrome. Obstet Gynecol 1995; 85:971.

11. Carmina E. Pathogenesis and treatment of hirsutism in late-onset congenital adrenal hyperplasia. Reprod Med Rev 1995; 4:179.

12. Lobo RA, Gobelsmann U, Horton R. Evidence for the importance of peripheral tissue events in the development of hirsutism in polycystic ovary syndrome. J Clin Endocrinol Metab 1983; 57:393.

13. Thigpen AE, Silver RI, Guilleyard JM, et al. Tissue distribution and ontogeny of steroid 5-reductase isoenzyme expression. J Clin Invest 1983; 92:903.

14. Russell DW, Wilson JD. Steroid 5α-reductase: two genes/two enzymes. Annu Rev Biochem 1994; 63:25.

15. Morimoto I, Edmiston A, Hawks D, Horton R. Studies on the origin of androstanediol and androstanediol glucuronide in young and elderly men. J Endocrinol Metab 1981; 52:772.

16. Serafini P, Lobo RA. Increased 5α-reductase activity in idiopathic hirsutism. Fertil Steril 1985; 43:74.

17. Rittmaster RS. Androgen conjugates: physiology and clinical significance. Endocr Rev 1993; 14:121.

18. Duffy DM, Legro RS, Chang L, et al. Metabolism of dihydrotestosterone to 5α-androstane-3α-17β diol glucuronide is greater in the peripheral compartment than in the plasmic compartment. Fertil Steril 1995; 64:736.

19. Carmina E, Stanczyk FZ, Gentzschein E, Lobo RA. Time-dependent changes in serum 3α-androstanediol glucuronide correlate with hirsutism scores after ovarian suppression. Gynecol Endocrinol 1995; 9:215.

20. Carmina E, Gentzschein E, Stanczyk FZ, Lobo RA. Substrate dependency of C19 conjugates in hirsute hyperandrogenic women and the influence of adrenal androgen. Hum Reprod 1995; 10:299.

21. Carmina E, Stanczyk FZ, Matteri RK, Lobo RA. Serum androsterone conjugates differentiate between acne and hirsutism in hyperandrogenic women. Fertil Steril 1991; 55:871.

22. Mowszowicz I, Melanitou E, Doukani A, et al. Androgen binding capacity and 5-reductase activity in pubic skin fibroblasts from hirsute patients. J Clin Endocrinol Metab 1983; 56:1209.

23. Sawaya ME, Shalita AR. Androgen receptor polymorphisms (CAG repeat lengths) in androgenetic alopecia, hirsutism and acne. J Cutan Med Surg 1998; 3:9.

24. Legro RS, Shalibahranir S, Lobo RA, Kovacs BW. Size polymorphisms of the androgen receptor among female Hispanics and correlations with androgenic characteristics. Obstet Gynecol 1994; 83:701.

25. Mauvais-Jarvis P. Regulation of androgen receptor and 5-reductase in the skin of normal and hirsute women. Clin Endocrinol Metab 1986; 15:307.

26. Cassidenti DL, Stanczyk FZ, Lobo RA. The relationship between insulin resistance, IGF-1 levels, adrenal androgens and peripheral androgen metabolism in polycystic ovary syndrome. Paper presented at 38th Annual Meeting of the Society for Gynecological Investigation; 1991; San Antonio, TX. Abstract 174.

27. Antonipillai I, Wake M, Yamamoto J, Horton R. Activin and inhibin have opposite effects on 5 alpha-reductase activity in genital skin fibroblasts. Mol Cell Endocrinal 1995; 107:99.

28. Plymate SR. Physiologic role of sex hormone binding globulin in androgen metabolism. In: Azziz R, Nestler JE, Dewailly D, eds. Androgen excess disorders in women. Philadelphia: Lippincott–Raven Publishers, 1997:47.

29. Cumming DC, Wall SR. Non-sex hormone binding globulin-bound testosterone as a marker for hyperandrogenism. J Clin Endocrinol Metab 1985; 61:18.

30. Schwartz U, Moltz L, Brotherton J, Hammerstein J. The diagnostic of plasma free testosterone in nontumorous and tumorous hyperandrogenism. Fertil Steril 1983; 40:66.

31. Carmina E. Prevalence of idiopathic hirsutism. Eur J Endocrinol 1998; 139:424.

32. Randall VA. Androgens and human hair growth. Clin Endocrinol (Oxf) 1994; 40:439.

33. Sawaya ME, Price VH. Different levels of 5α-reductase type 1 and 2, aromatase and androgen receptor in hair follicles of women and men with androgenetic alopecia. J Invest Dermatol 1997; 109:296.

34. Courchay G, Bpoyera N, Bernard BA, Mahe Y. Messenger RNA expression of steroidogenesis enzyme subtypes in the human pilosebaceous unit. Skin Pharmacol 1996; 9:169.

35. Kuttenn F, Mowszowicz I, Schaison G, Mauvais-Jarvis P. Androgen production and skin metabolism in hirsutism. J Endocrinol 1977; 75:83.

36. Kiesewetter F, Schell H. Cell kinetics of anagen scalp hairs under physiological and pathological conditions. Skin Pharmacol 1994; 7:55.

37. Ebling FJ, Rook A. Hair. In: Rook A, Wilkinson DS, Ebling FJG, eds. Textbook of dermatology. 3rd ed. Oxford: Blackwell Science, 1979:1733.

38. Akiyama M, Smith LT, Holbrook KA. Growth factor and growth factor receptor localization in the hair follicle bulge and associated tissue in human fetus. J Invest Dermatol 1996; 106:391.

39. Goodman LV, Ledbetter SR. Secretion of stromelysin by cultured dermal papilla cells: differential regulation by growth factors and functional role in mitogen induced cell proliferation. J Cell Physiol 1992; 151:41.

40. Slobodan M, Jankovi S, Jankovi V. The control of hair growth. Dermatol Online J 1998; 4:1.

41. Gzabo G. The regional anatomy of the human integument with special reference to the distribution of hair follicles, sweat gland and melanocytes. Physiol Trans R Soc Lond (Biol) 1967; 252:667.

42. Király C, Alen M, Korvola J, Horsmanheimo M. The effect of testosterone and anabolic steroids on the skin surface lipids and the population of propionic bacteria acnes in young postpubertal men. Acta Dermatol Venereol (Stockh) 1988; 68:21.

43. Lookingbill DP, Egan N, Santen RJ, Demers LM. Correlation of serum 3α-androstanediol glucuronide with acne and chest hair density in men. J Clin Endocrinol Metab 1988; 67:986.

44. Cook CH, Centner RL, Michaels SE. An acne grading method using photographic standards. Arch Dermatol 1979; 115:571.

45. Luderschmidt C. Pathogenesis of acne vulgaris. In: Hammerstein J, Lachnit-Fixson U, Neumann F, Plewig G, eds. Androgenization in women. Amsterdam: Excerpta Medica, 1980:75.

46. Holland KT, Aldana O, Bojar RA, et al. Propionibacterium acnes and acne. In: Sebaceous glands, acne and related disorders. Berlin, 1997. Abstract 46.

47. Lemay A, Dewailly SD, Grenier R, Huard J. Attenuation of mild hyperandrogenic activity in postpubertal acne by a triphasic oral contraceptive containing low doses of ethinylestradiol and d-l. norgestrel. J Clin Endocrinol Metab 1990; 71:8.

48. Slayden SM, Azziz R. The role of androgen excess in acne. In: Azziz R, Nestler JE, Dewailly D, eds. Androgen excess disorders in women. Philadelphia: Lippincott–Raven Publishers, 1997:131.

49. Lawrence D, Shaw M, Katz M. Elevated free testosterone concentrations in men and women with acne vulgaris. Clin Exp Dermatol 1986; 11:263.

50. Marynick SP, Chakmmakjian ZH, McCaffree DL, Herndo JH. Androgen excess in cystic acne. N Engl J Med 1983; 308:981.

51. Lucky AW, McGuire J, Rosenfield RL, et al. Plasma androgens in women with acne vulgaris. J Invest Dermatol 1983; 81:70.

52. Vexiau P, Husson C, Chivot M, Brerault JL. Androgen excess in women with acne alone compared with women with acne and/or hirsutism. J Invest Dermatol 1990; 94:279.

53. Thiboutot D, Harris G, Iles V, et al. Activity of the type 1 5-reductase exhibits regional differences isolated sebaceous glands and whole skin. J Invest Dermatol 1995; 105:209.

54. Hammerstein J, Moltz L, Schwartz U. Antiandrogens in the treatment of acne and hirsutism. J Steroid Biochem 1983; 19:591.

55. Carmina E, Lobo RA. Evidence for increased androsterone metabolism in some normoandrogenic women with acne. J Clin Endocrinol Metab 1993; 76:1111.

56. Colver GB, Mortimer PS, Dawber RPF. Cyproterone acetate and two doses of estrogen in female acne, a double-blind comparison. Br J Dermatol 1988; 118:95.

57. Hatch IE, Carmina E, Vijod MA, et al. Inhibition of the IGF axis and 5-alpha reductase activity by 13-cis retinoic acid in normal women. Paper presented at: 41st Annual Meeting of the Society for Gynecological Investigation; March 22–26, 1994; Chicago.

58. Boudou P, Chivot M, Vexiau P, et al. Evidence for decreased androgen 5α-reduction in skin and liver of men with severe acne after 13-cis-retinoic acid treatment. J Clin Endocrinol Metab 1994; 78:1064.

58a. Negri C, Tosi F, Dorizzi R, et al. Antiandrogen drugs lower prostate-specific antigen (PSA) levels in hirsute subjects: evidence that serum PSA is a marker of androgen action in women. J Clin Endocrinal Metab 2000; 85:81.

59. McKenna TJ, Moore A, Magee F, Cunningham S. Amenorrhea with cryptic hyperandrogenemia. J Clin Endocrinol Metab 1983; 56:893.

60. Levine LS, Dupont B, Lorenzen F, et al. Genetic and hormonal characterization of cryptic 21-hydroxylase deficiency. J Clin Endocrinol Metab 1981; 53:1193.

61. Pecoraro V, Astore I, Barman JM. Growth rate and hair density of the human axilla: a comparative study in normal males and females and pregnant and postpartum females. J Invest Dermatol 1971; 56:362.

62. Wang CY, Stanczyk FZ, Lobo RA. Quantitative measurements of mRNA encoding type 1 and type 2 5α-reductase genes in hirsute and nonhirsute women. Paper presented at 43rd Annual Meeting of the Society of Gynecological Investigation; 1996; Philadelphia. Abstract 51.

63. Carmina E. Role of 5α-reductase isoenzymes in the pathogenesis of acne and hirsutism. In: Dastidar SG, Chowdury NNR, eds. Proceedings of International Conference on Advances in Reproductive Medicine. Calcutta, 1997:154.

63a. Hediger C, Rost B, Itin P. Cutaneous manifestations in anorexia nervosa. Schweiz Med Wochenschr 2000; 130:565.

64. Friedman CI, Schmidt GE, Kim MH, Powell J. Serum testosterone concentrations in the evaluation of androgen-producing tumors. Am J Obstet Gynecol 1985; 153:44.

65. Miras-Mirakian P, Pugeat M, et al. Androgen suppressive effect of GnRH agonist in ovarian hyperthecosis and virilizing tumors. Clin Endocrinol 1994; 41:571.

66. Hammad A, Jasnosz KM, Olson PR. Expression of alpha-fetoprotein by ovarian Sertoli-Leydig cells tumors. Case report and review of the literature. Arch Pathol Lab Med 1995; 119:1075.

67. Healy DL, Burger HG, Mamers P, et al. Elevated serum inhibin concentrations in postmenopausal women with ovarian tumors. N Engl J Med 1993; 329:1539.

68. Cannistra SA. Cancer of the ovary. N Engl J Med 1993; 329:1550.

69. Occhipinti KA, Frankel SD, Hricak H. The ovary: computed tomography and magnetic resonance imaging. Radiol Clin North Am 1993; 31:1115.

70. Taylor L, Ayers KJW, Gross MD, et al. Diagnostic considerations in virilization: iodomethyl-norcholesterol scanning in the localization of androgen secreting tumors. Fertil Steril 1986; 46:1005.

71. Surrey ES, de Ziegler D, Gambone JC, Judd HL. Preoperative localization

of androgen-secreting tumors: clinical, endocrinologic, and radiologic evaluation of ten patients. Am J Obstet Gynecol 1988; 158:1313.

72. Derksen J, Nagesser SK, Meinders AE, et al. Identification of virilizing adrenal tumors in hirsute women. N Engl J Med 1994; 331:968.

73. Falke THM, Shaff MI, Seters AP, Sandler MP. Diagnostic imaging of adrenal disease. In: Scott HW, ed. Surgery of the adrenal gland. Philadelphia: Lippincott, 1990:85.

74. Paulson JD, Keller DW, Wiest WG, Warren JC. Free testosterone concentration in serum: elevation is the hallmark of hirsutism. Am J Obstet Gynecol 1977; 128:851.

75. Bouallouche A, Breault J-L, Fiet J, et al. Evidence for adrenal and/or ovarian dysfunction as a possible etiology of idiopathic hirsutism. Am J Obstet Gynecol 1983; 147:57.

76. Serafini P, Ablan F, Lobo RA. 5α-Reductase activity in the genital skin of hirsute women. J Clin Endocrinol Metab 1985; 60:349.

77. Glickman SP, Rosenfield RL. Androgen metabolism by isolated hairs from women with idiopathic hirsutism is usually normal. J Invest Dermatol 1984; 82:62.

78. Lobo RA, Carmina E. Polycystic ovary syndrome. In: Lobo RA, Mishell DR Jr, Paulson R, Shoupe D, eds. Mishell's textbook of infertility, contraception and reproductive endocrinology. Oxford: Blackwell, 1997:363.

78a. Lobo RA, Carmine E. The importance of diagnosing the polycystic ovary syndrome. Ann Intern Med 2000; 132:989.

79. Polson DW, Wodsworth J, Adams J, Franks S. Polycystic ovaries: a common finding in normal women. Lancet 1988; 1:870.

80. Farquhar CM, Birdsall M, Manning P, et al. The presence of polycystic ovaries on ultrasound scanning in a population of randomly selected women. Aust N Z J Obstet Gynecol 1994; 34:67.

81. Carmina E, Wong L, Chang L, et al. Endocrine abnormalities in ovulatory women with polycystic ovaries on ultrasound. Hum Reprod 1997; 12:905.

82. Wong LI, Morris RS, Legro R, et al. Isolated polycystic morphology in ovum donors predicts response to controlled hyperstimulation. Hum Reprod 1995; 10:524.

83. Adams J, Polson DW, Franks S. Prevalence of polycystic ovaries in women with anovulation and idiopathic hirsutism. BMJ 1986; 293:355.

84. Robert Y, Dubrulle F, Gaillandre L, et al. Ultrasound assessment of ovarian stroma hypertrophy in hyperandrogenism and ovulation disorders: visual analysis versus computerized quantification. Fertil Steril 1995; 64:307.

85. Carmina E, Lobo RA. Do hyperandrogenic women with normal menses have PCOS? Fertil Steril 1999; 71:319.

86. Rebar RW, Judd HL, Yen SSC, et al. Characterization of the inappropriate gonadotropin secretion in polycystic ovary syndrome. J Clin Invest 1976; 57:1320.

87. Lobo RA, Kletzky OA, Campeau JD, diZerega GS. Elevated bioactive luteinizing hormone in women with the polycystic ovary syndrome (PCO). Fertil Steril 1983; 39:674.

88. Carmina E. The role of extra-adrenal factors in adrenal androgen excess: in vivo studies. In: Azziz R, Nestler JE, Dewailly D, eds. Androgen excess disorders in women. Philadelphia: Lippincott–Raven Publishers, 1997:425.

89. Lobo RA, Granger L, Goebelsmann U, Mishell DR Jr. Elevations in unbound serum estradiol as a possible mechanism for inappropriate gonadotropin secretion in women with PCO. J Clin Endocrinol Metab 1981; 52:156.

90. Barnes RB, Rosenfield RL, Burstein S, Ehrmann DA. Pituitary-ovarian responses to nafarelin testing in the polycystic ovary syndrome. N Engl J Med 1989; 320:559.

91. Lobo RA. The role of the adrenal in polycystic ovary syndrome in polycystic ovary disease. Semin Reprod Med 1984; 2:251.

92. Carmina E, Koyama T, Chang L, et al. Does ethnicity influence the prevalence of adrenal hyperandrogenism and insulin resistance in polycystic ovary syndrome? Am J Obstet Gynecol 1992; 167:1807.

93. Carmina E, Lobo RA. Adrenal hyperandrogenism in the pathophysiology of polycystic ovary syndrome. J Endocrinol Invest 1998; 21:580.

94. Carmina E, Gonzalez F, Vidali A, et al. The contribution of estrogen and growth factors to increased adrenal androgen secretion in polycystic ovary syndrome. Hum Reprod 1999; 14:307.

95. Dunaif A. Insulin resistance and the polycystic ovary syndrome; mechanism and implications for the pathogenesis. Endocr Rev 1997; 774:800.

96. Dunaif A, Xia J, Book C, et al. Excessive insulin receptor serine phosphorylation in cultured fibroblasts and in skeletal muscle: a potential mechanism for insulin resistance in the polycystic ovary syndrome. J Clin Invest 1995; 96:801.

97. Judd HL, Scully RE, Herbst AL, et al. Familial hyperthecosis: comparison of endocrinologic and histologic findings with polycystic ovarian disease. Am J Obstet Gynecol 1973; 117:976.

98. Carmina E, Gagliano AM, Rosato F, et al. The endocrine pattern of late onset adrenal hyperplasia (21-hydroxylase deficiency). J Endocrinol Invest 1984; 7:89.

99. Speiser PW, New MI. Genotype and hormonal phenotype in nonclassical 21-hydroxylase deficiency. J Clin Endocrinol Metab 1987; 64:86.

100. Speiser PW, Dupont B, Rubinstein P, et al. High frequency of nonclassical steroid 21-hydroxylase deficiency. Am J Hum Genet 1986; 37:650.

101. Carmina E. Pathogenesis and treatment of hirsutism in late onset congenital adrenal hyperplasia. Reprod J Med Rev 1995; 4:179.

102. Azziz R, Owerbach D. Molecular abnormalities of the 21-hydroxylase gene in hyperandrogenic women with an exaggerated 17-hydroxyprogesterone response to acute adrenal stimulation. Am J Obstet Gynecol 1995; 172:914.

103. Carmina E, Lobo RA. Ovarian suppression reduces clinical and endocrine expression of late onset congenital adrenal hyperplasia due to 21-hydroxylase deficiency. Fertil Steril 1994; 62:738.

104. Levin JH, Carmina E, Lobo RA. Is the inappropriate gonadotropin secre-

tion of patients with polycystic ovary syndrome similar to that of patients with adult onset congenital adrenal hyperplasia? Fertil Steril 1991; 56:635.

105. Spitzer P, Billaud L, Thalabard JC, et al. Cyproterone acetate versus hydrocortisone treatment in late onset adrenal hyperplasia. J Clin Endocrinol Metab 1990; 70:642.

106. Carmina E, Malizia G, Pagano M, Janni A. Prevalence of late onset 11β-hydroxylase deficiency in hirsute patients. J Endocrinol Invest 1987; 11:595.

107. Lobo RA, Goebelsmann U. Evidence for reduced 3β-ol-hydroxysteroid dehydrogenase activity in some hirsute women thought to have polycystic ovary syndrome. J Clin Endocrinol Metab 1981; 53:394.

108. Chang YT, Zhang L, Alkaddour HS, et al. Absence of molecular defect in the type II 3β-hydroxysteroid dehydrogenase (3β-HSD) gene in premature pubarche children and hirsute female patients with moderately decreased adrenal 3β-HSD activity. Pediatr Res 1995; 37:820.

109. Zerah M, Rheaume E, Mani P, et al. No evidence of mutations in the genes for type I and type II 3β-hydroxysteroid dehydrogenase (3β-HSD) in nonclassical 3β-HSD deficiency. J Clin Endocrinol Metab 1994; 79:1811.

110. Hammerstein J. Possibilities and limits of endocrine therapy. In: Hammerstein J, Lachnit-Fixson U, Neumann F, Plewig G, eds. Androgenization in women. Amsterdam: Excerpta Medica, 1980:221.

111. Carmina E, Lobo RA. Effect of the estrogen dose in the treatment of hirsutism using cyproterone acetate. Paper presented at 46th Annual Meeting of the Society for Gynecological Investigation; 1999; Atlanta. Abstract 50.

112. Vexian P, Boudou P, Fiet J, et al. 17β-estradiol: oral or parenteral administration in hyperandrogenic women? Metabolic tolerance in association with cyproterone acetate. Fertil Steril 1995; 63:508.

113. Cumming DC, Yang JC, Rebar RW, Yen SSC. Treatment of hirsutism with spironolactone. JAMA 1982; 247:1295.

114. Lobo RA, Shoupe D, Serafini P, et al. The effects of two doses of spironolactone on serum androgens and anagen hair in hirsute women. Fertil Steril 1985; 43:200.

115. Helfer EL, Miller JL, Rose LI. Side-effects of spironolactone therapy in the hirsute woman. J Clin Endocrinol Metab 1988; 66:208.

116. Carmina E, Janni A, Lobo RA. Physiological estrogen replacement may enhance the effectiveness of the gonadotropin-releasing hormone agonist in the treatment of hirsutism. J Clin Endocrinol Metab 1994; 78:126.

117. Carmina E, Lobo RA. Gonadotropin releasing hormone agonist therapy for hirsutism is as effective as high dose cyproterone acetate but results in a longer remission. Hum Reprod 1997; 12:663.

118. Elkind-Hirsch KE, Anania C, Mack M, Malina KR. Combination gonadotropin releasing hormone agonist and oral contraceptive therapy improves treatment of hirsute women with ovarian hyperandrogenism. Fertil Steril 1995; 63:970.

119. Carmina E, Lobo RA. Peripheral androgen blockade versus glandular androgen suppression in the treatment of hirsutism. Obstet Gynecol 1991; 78:845.

120. Carmina E, Levin JH, Malizia G, Lobo RA. Ovine corticotropin releasing factor and dexamethasone responses in hyperandrogenic women. Fertil Steril 1990; 54:245.

121. Carmina E, Lobo RA. The addition of dexamethasone to antiandrogen therapy for hirsutism prolongs the duration of remission. Fertil Steril 1998; 69:1075.

122. Cusan L, Dupont A, Gomez J-L, et al. Comparison of flutamide and spironolactone in the treatment of hirsutism: a randomized controlled trial. Fertil Steril 1994; 61:281.

123. Ciotta L, Cianci A, Marletta E, et al. Treatment of hirsutism with flutamide and low-dosage oral contraceptive in polycystic ovarian disease patients. Fertil Steril 1994; 62:112.

124. Moghetti P, Castello R, Negri C, et al. Flutamide in the treatment of hirsutism: long term clinical effects, endocrine changes and androgen receptor behavior. Fertil Steril 1995; 64:51.

125. Wong IL, Morris RS, Chang L, et al. A prospective randomized trial comparing finasteride to spironolactone in the treatment of hirsute women. J Clin Endocrinol Metab 1995; 80:23.

126. Fruzzetti F, DeLorenzo D, Parrini D, Ricci C. Effects of finasteride, a 5-reductase inhibitor, on circulating androgens and gonadotropin secretion in hirsute women. J Clin Endocrinol Metab 1994; 79:83.

127. Rittmaster RS. Personal communication.

127a. Moghetti P, Tosi F, Tosti A, et al. Comparison of spironolactone, flutamide, and finasteride efficacy in the treatment of hirsutism: a randomized, double blind, placebo-controlled trial. J Clin Endocrinal Metab 2000; 85:89.

128. Futterweit W, Teh HC, Kingsley P. The prevalence of hyperandrogenism in 109 consecutive women presenting with diffuse alopecia. J Am Acad Dermatol 1988; 19:83.

129. Ludwig E. Classification of the types of androgenic alopecia (common baldness) occurring in the female sex. Br J Dermatol 1977; 97:247.

130. Adachi K, Takayasu S, Takashima I, et al. Human hair follicles: metabolism and control mechanisms. Soc Cosmet Chem 1970; 21:901.

131. Schweikert HU, Wilson JD. Regulation of human hair growth by steroid hormones. I. Testosterone metabolism in isolated hairs. J Clin Endocrinol Metab 1974; 38:811.

131a. Juricskay S, Telegdy E. Urinary steroids in women with androgenic alopecia. Clin Biochem 2000; 33:97.

132. Legro RS, Carmina E, Stanczyk FZ, et al. Alterations in androgen conjugate levels in women and men with androgenic alopecia. Fertil Steril 1994; 62:744.

133. Kaufman KD. Clinical studies on the effects of oral finasteride, a type II 5α-reductase inhibitor, on scalp hair in men with male pattern baldness. In: Van Neste D, Randall VA, eds. Hair research for the next millennium. Amsterdam: Elsevier Publications, 1996.

134. Sawaya ME. Alopecia: the search for novel agents continue. Exp Opin Therap Pat 1997; 7:859.

# CHAPTER 102

# FUNCTIONING TUMORS AND TUMOR-LIKE CONDITIONS OF THE OVARY

I-TIEN YEH, CHARLES ZALOUDEK, AND ROBERT J. KURMAN

## CLASSIFICATION OF OVARIAN NEOPLASMS

The World Health Organization histologic classification divides neoplasms of the ovary into 14 main categories (Table 102-1).[1] Of the listed classes, functioning tumors are most often surface epithelial–stromal, sex cord stromal, germ cell, secondary (metastatic) tumors, or a tumor-like condition. The clinical staging of ovarian cancer is based on the guidelines of the International Federation of Gynecologists and Obstetricians (Table 102-2).[2]

*Almost any tumor of the ovary may produce an endocrine effect,* either through functional activity of the tumor cells themselves or through activity of reactive nonneoplastic stromal cells.[3–5] Biochemical evidence of functional activity is extremely common, although only 5% to 6% of ovarian tumors show functional activity to a clinically significant level. The majority of the clinically functioning neoplasms are of the sex cord stromal type.

## DIAGNOSTIC EVALUATION

Most patients with *nonfunctional* ovarian tumors are asymptomatic early in the tumors' evolution; therefore, >70% of these lesions are diagnosed at an advanced stage. Patients with *functional* tumors commonly present with altered secondary sexual characteristics (e.g., hirsutism or virilization) or reproductive dysfunction; these lesions thus tend to be diagnosed at an earlier stage (Fig. 102-1).

### HISTORY AND PHYSICAL EXAMINATION

The clinical history in children should include growth rate and the time of onset and progression of puberty. In adults, the menstrual pattern, change in libido, body habitus, growth of hair, and pitch of the voice should be recorded. With tumor growth, abdominal distention occurs, and pressure on the bladder or rectum may cause a sensation of pelvic fullness and discomfort. Abdominal and pelvic pain is associated with torsion, hemorrhage, or rupture of a tumor.

A family history of ovarian cancer is the factor most strongly associated with ovarian cancer risk. Studies of inherited ovarian cancer have identified at least three syndromes: the *site-specific ovarian cancer syndrome*, the *breast/ovarian cancer syndrome*, and the *hereditary nonpolyposis colon cancer/ovarian cancer syndrome*.[6] Phenotypically, familial ovarian carcinomas are more frequently papillary serous tumors, and evidence exists that women with a genetic predisposition to ovarian cancer may be differentially affected by hormonal levels and metabolism. The occurrence of functioning ovarian tumors is not known to have any particular association with inherited ovarian risk.

The general physical examination should include measurement of height and weight, examination of the skin for excess

**TABLE 102-1.**
**World Health Organization Histologic Classification of Ovarian Tumors**

1. **SURFACE EPITHELIAL–STROMAL TUMORS**
   1.1 Serous
   1.2 Mucinous
   1.3 Endometrioid
   1.4 Clear cell
   1.5 Transitional cell
   1.6 Squamous cell
   1.7 Mixed epithelial
   1.8 Undifferentiated carcinoma
2. **SEX CORD STROMAL TUMORS**
   2.1 Granulosa stromal cell
   2.2 Sertoli-Leydig cell, androblastoma
   2.3 Sex cord tumor with annular tubules
   2.4 Gynandroblastomas
   2.5 Unclassified
   2.6 Steroid (lipid) cell
3. **GERM-CELL TUMORS**
   3.1 Dysgerminoma
   3.2 Yolk sac (endodermal sinus)
   3.3 Embryonal
   3.4 Polyembryoma
   3.5 Choriocarcinoma
   3.6 Teratoma
   3.7 Mixed germ cells
4. **GONADOBLASTOMA**
5. **GERM-CELL–SEX CORD STROMAL TUMOR OF NONGONADOBLASTOMA TYPE**
6. **TUMORS OF RETE OVARII**
7. **MESOTHELIAL TUMORS**
8. **TUMORS OF UNCERTAIN ORIGIN**
9. **GESTATIONAL TROPHOBLASTIC DISEASES**
10. **SOFT TISSUE TUMORS NOT SPECIFIC TO OVARY**
11. **MALIGNANT LYMPHOMAS, LEUKEMIAS, AND PLASMACYTOMA**
12. **UNCLASSIFIED TUMORS**
13. **SECONDARY (METASTATIC) TUMORS**
14. **TUMOR-LIKE LESIONS**
    14.1 Solitary follicular cyst
    14.2 Multiple follicular cysts
    14.3 Large solitary luteinized follicular cyst of pregnancy and puerperium
    14.4 Hyperreactio luteinalis
    14.5 Corpus luteum cyst
    14.6 Pregnancy luteoma
    14.7 Ectopic pregnancy
    14.8 Stromal hyperplasia
    14.9 Stromal hyperthecosis
    14.10 Massive edema
    14.11 Fibromatosis
    14.12 Endometriosis
    14.13 Cyst, unclassified
    14.14 Inflammatory lesions

production of sebum, assessment of distribution and quantity of hair, assessment of breast development, inspection of the external genitalia, and palpation of the gonads. Small tumors are difficult to detect on pelvic examination and, therefore, rectovaginal examination may be helpful. Evaluation of the breasts, gastrointestinal tract, and uterus is an important aspect of the examination, because ~10% of ovarian tumors are metastases from tumors in these sites. Ascites is typically associated with intraabdominal metastases.

**TABLE 102-2.**
**International Federation of Gynecologists and Obstetricians Staging of Carcinoma of the Ovary**

| | |
|---|---|
| STAGE I | Growth limited to the ovaries. |
| IA | Growth limited to one ovary; no ascites. No tumor on the external surface; capsule intact. |
| IB | Growth limited to both ovaries; no ascites. No tumor on the external surfaces; capsules intact. |
| IC | Tumor either stage IA or IB but with tumor on surface of one or both ovaries; or with capsule ruptured; or with ascites containing malignant cells or with positive peritoneal washings. |
| STAGE II | Growth involving one or both ovaries with pelvic extension. |
| IIA | Extension and/or metastasis to the uterus and/or tubes. |
| IIB | Extension to other pelvic tissues. |
| IIC | Tumor either stage IIA or IIB, but with tumor on surface of one or both ovaries; or with capsule(s) ruptured; or with ascites containing malignant cells or with positive peritoneal washings. |
| STAGE III | Tumor involving one or both ovaries with peritoneal implants outside the pelvis and/or positive retroperitoneal or inguinal nodes. Superficial liver metastasis equals stage III. |
| IIIA | Tumor grossly limited to the true pelvis with negative nodes but with histologically confirmed microscopic seeding of abdominal peritoneal surfaces. |
| IIIB | Tumor of one or both ovaries with histologically confirmed implants on abdominal peritoneal surfaces, none exceeding 2 cm in diameter. Nodes negative. |
| IIIC | Abdominal implants >2 cm in diameter and/or positive retroperitoneal nodes. |
| STAGE IV | Growth involving one or both ovaries with distant metastases. If pleural effusion is present, cytology must be positive to allot a case to stage IV. Parenchymal liver metastasis equals stage IV. |

(From International Federation of Gynecologists and Obstetricians Cancer Committee. Staging announcement. Gynecol Oncol 1986; 25:383.)

## LABORATORY EXAMINATION

Laboratory examination may include the measurement of serum levels of ovarian cancer–associated antigens such as CA125. CA125 measurement has also been used as a screening test for ovarian carcinoma, not only for women at high risk but also for the general population of women older than age 50 years. Although the serum levels of CA125 and carcinoembryonic antigen may be useful in monitoring the course of disease, their lack of specificity limits their diagnostic utility.[7] Alpha-fetoprotein, human chorionic gonadotropin (hCG), and human placental lactogen are present in germ-cell tumors, and measurement of their serum levels is valuable in monitoring tumor activity and directing treatment.[8,9] The measurement of steroid hormones and their metabolites peripherally, as well as locally (by retrograde catheterization), is particularly valuable in the differential diagnosis of virilizing ovarian versus adrenal neoplasms.[10] High serum levels of testosterone and low urine levels of 17-ketosteroids often are associated with ovarian tumors. Adrenal tumors usually produce high levels of dehydroepiandrosterone and its sulfate and low levels of testosterone. Consequently, urinary 17-ketosteroid concentrations are elevated, whereas serum testosterone levels may be only slightly elevated or normal.

Vaginal smear cytology, cervical mucus examination, and endometrial biopsy may demonstrate target organ effects, particularly those related to estrogen. Long-standing unopposed elevated estrogen levels cause an abnormal maturation of the vagina, which shows an increased proportion of superficial cells on cytologic examination. Stimulation of the endometrium may lead to various degrees of hyperplasia evident in endometrial biopsy specimens. Pelvic and abdominal study by ultrasonography, intravenous urography, computed tomography

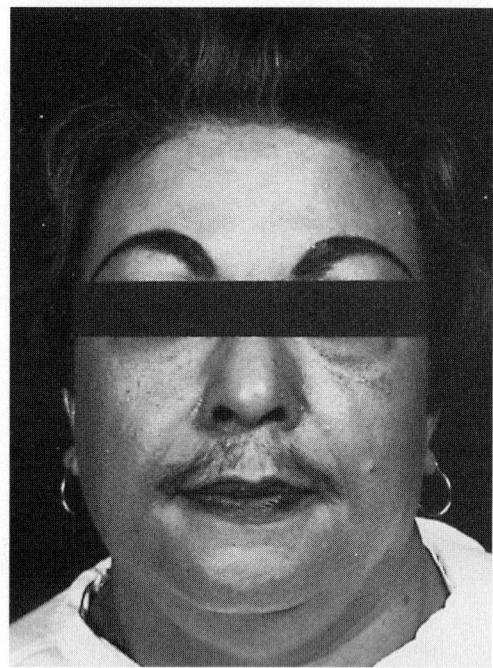

**FIGURE 102-1.** A 55-year-old woman with a 30-year history of amenorrhea, hirsutism, and clitoromegaly associated with a benign cystic teratoma. Note coarsening of the facial skin, seborrhea, temporal hair recession, and mustache.

(Fig. 102-2), or magnetic resonance imaging may aid in localizing disease to the ovaries or to the adrenals. Laparotomy is necessary for the diagnosis and appropriate clinical staging and treatment of ovarian neoplasms.

## THERAPY

Although therapy is dependent in part on the type of tumor and its stage, the primary treatment of ovarian neoplasms is surgical, ranging from unilateral salpingo-oophorectomy to hysterectomy and bilateral salpingo-oophorectomy in conjunction with cytoreductive surgery. Postoperative adjuvant chemotherapy or radiation is often used.[11]

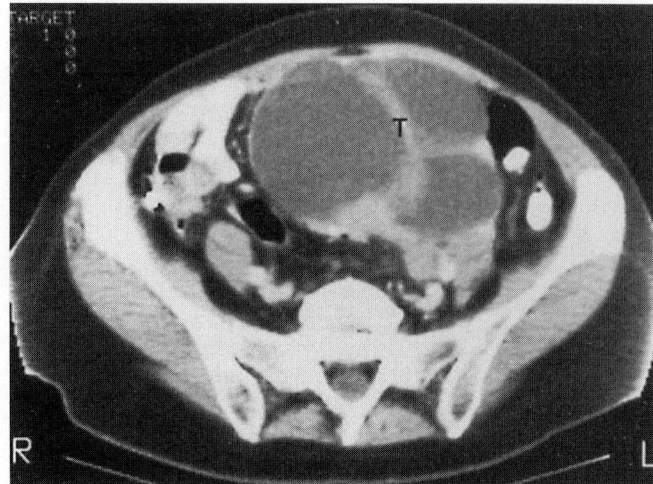

**FIGURE 102-2.** Ovarian carcinoma demonstrated in computed tomogram of pelvis. Large multiloculated tumor (*T*) with focal solid areas displaces other pelvic structures.

# COMMON EPITHELIAL TUMORS

Epithelial neoplasms account for >60% of all tumors arising in the ovary. These tumors are classified according to the predominant pattern of differentiation as *serous* (resembling fallopian tube epithelium), *mucinous* (resembling intestinal or endocervical glands), *endometrioid* (resembling endometrial glands), *clear cell*, or *Brenner* (urothelial). They are subdivided into *benign, low malignant potential,* and *malignant* types. Tumors of low malignant potential are distinguished from their benign counterparts by the presence of epithelial stratification, papillary tuft formation, nuclear atypia, and increased mitotic activity, and from the malignant tumors by the absence of stromal invasion. Tumors of low malignant potential have an excellent prognosis (as do stage IA or IB, well-differentiated tumors) with a >90% five-year survival rate; in contrast, advanced (stage III and IV) carcinomas have only a 20% five-year survival rate, even with current chemotherapeutic regimens.

Most epithelial tumors are nonfunctional and present as a pelvic mass with vague constitutional symptoms. Endocrinologically active stroma that produces steroid hormones, usually androgens, may be found in approximately one-third of epithelial neoplasms; however, only a few of the patients have symptoms. The surface epithelial tumors most often associated with functional stroma are mucinous or endometrioid in differentiation. Typically, the stroma surrounding the neoplasm is luteinized, with the stromal cells tending to be uniform, small, and polygonal with abundant eosinophilic cytoplasm and round nuclei with prominent nucleoli. These cells have the typical light-microscopic and ultrastructural features of steroid hormone–secreting cells. Functioning stroma is more frequent in pregnancy and in postmenopausal women.[12] (See also refs. 12a and 12b.)

# SEX CORD STROMAL TUMORS

Tumors given this designation are thought to be derived from the specialized ovarian stroma. They are the most common type of hormonally active neoplasm. The components include granulosa, theca, Sertoli, Leydig, and gonadal stromal cells.[13,14] (See also ref. 14a.)

## GRANULOSA TUMORS

The granulosa tumor is the most common malignant functioning tumor of the ovary. When functional, granulosa tumors almost always are estrinizing, although rare tumors are virilizing. These tumors occur in all age groups but are most frequent in women between 30 and 50 years of age. Approximately 5% of granulosa tumors occur in young girls. The symptoms differ with the age of the patient. Most young girls present with isosexual precocious pseudopuberty, whereas women in their reproductive years usually experience disturbances of the menstrual cycle that range from amenorrhea to menometrorrhagia. Occasionally, breast enlargement occurs. Postmenopausal women typically present with vaginal bleeding secondary to endometrial hyperplasia. The frequency of endometrial hyperplasia and carcinoma ranges from 10% to 20%, depending on the criteria used for the diagnosis of these lesions. Androgenic granulosa cell tumors are associated with recent onset of hirsutism.

Granulosa tumors are bilateral in 5% of patients and range in size from microscopic to >30 cm in diameter (median, 9 cm). Small neoplasms are solid, encapsulated by a thin fibrous layer, and located in the ovarian cortex, whereas larger tumors may replace the ovary and become focally cystic. Virilizing tumors tend to be thin-walled, cystic tumors. Blood is often present within the cysts and explains the presentation of hemoperitoneum secondary to rupture that occurs in 10% of cases.

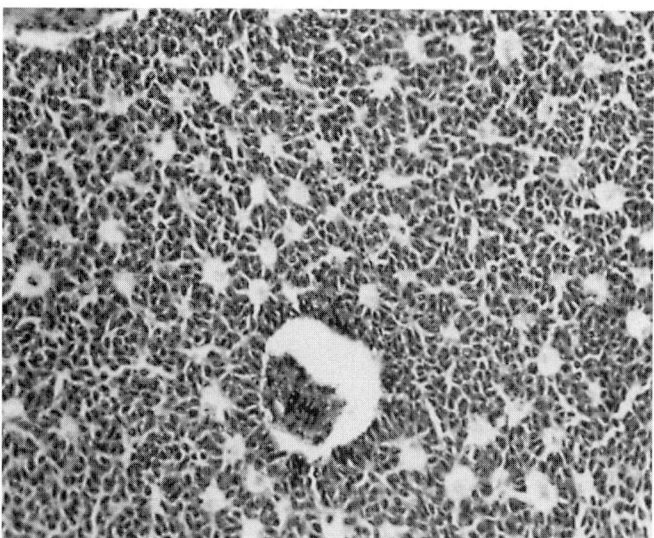

**FIGURE 102-3.** Granulosa tumor, microfollicular pattern. ×200

Granulosa tumors display many histologic patterns, including microfollicular (the most characteristic, showing many Call-Exner bodies; Fig. 102-3), macrofollicular, trabecular, insular, solid or diffuse, and juvenile. The pathologist must be aware of these patterns so that poorly differentiated carcinomas are not misdiagnosed as diffuse granulosa tumors. This relatively common error accounts for many of the examples of poor-prognosis granulosa tumors reported in the literature. Alpha-inhibin is expressed in granulosa cell tumors and other sex cord stromal tumors, but not in most carcinomas.[15] Immunohistochemical staining for this peptide may aid in the differential diagnosis. The histologic appearance of granulosa cell tumors does not correlate with the prognosis in most studies. The neoplastic cells resemble normal granulosa cells, being small, round to ovoid, and uniform. The nuclei have a characteristic longitudinal groove (a "coffee bean" appearance), and the cytoplasm is pale with poorly defined borders. Occasional cells are luteinized. Reactive thecal cells occur in ~25% of granulosa tumors. Anti-mullerian hormont (AMH) is a useful serum marker for these tumors.[15a]

The juvenile granulosa tumor, which accounts for 85% of granulosa cell tumors occurring before puberty, has distinctive features: the cells are larger, more pleomorphic, and often luteinized. Nuclear grooves are rare, and mitoses may be numerous.[16] Despite these ominous-appearing features, the prognosis is excellent.

Ultrastructural, immunocytochemical, and in vitro incubation studies have confirmed that the granulosa cells within these neoplasms can produce progesterone and testosterone in addition to estrogens, and receptors for these hormones may be detected as well.[17,18] These findings are in accord with the occasional virilizing and progestational activity displayed by these tumors.

Granulosa tumors are regarded as having low malignant potential, with a 5-year survival rate of >90%. However, these tumors recur in 10% to 33% of patients, and late recurrences (as much as 25 years after primary tumor resection) are characteristic. The prognosis is worse in patients with tumors >5 cm in diameter, bilateral tumors, rupture, and spread beyond the ovary.[19] Unilateral salpingo-oophorectomy is adequate treatment for premenopausal women with stage IA neoplasms, whereas postmenopausal women are treated by total abdominal hysterectomy and bilateral salpingo-oophorectomy.

## THECOMAS

Thecomas comprise 2% to 3% of all ovarian neoplasms and are found primarily in perimenopausal and postmenopausal women.

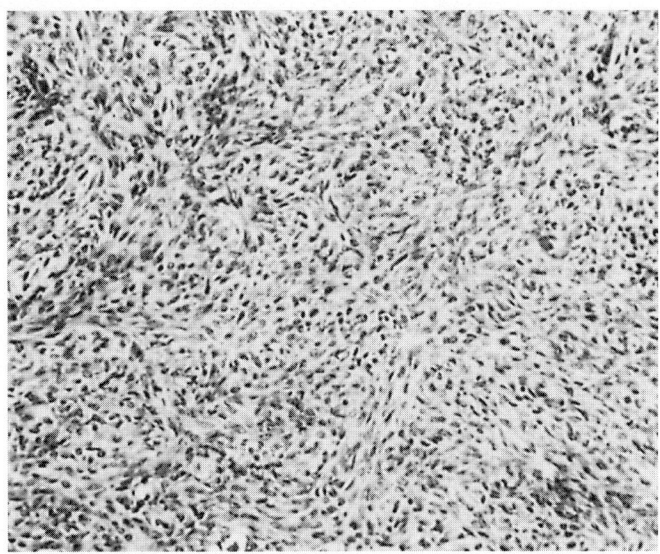

**FIGURE 102-4.** Thecoma. Spindle cells are in interlacing fascicles. Clear cytoplasm contains lipid. ×200

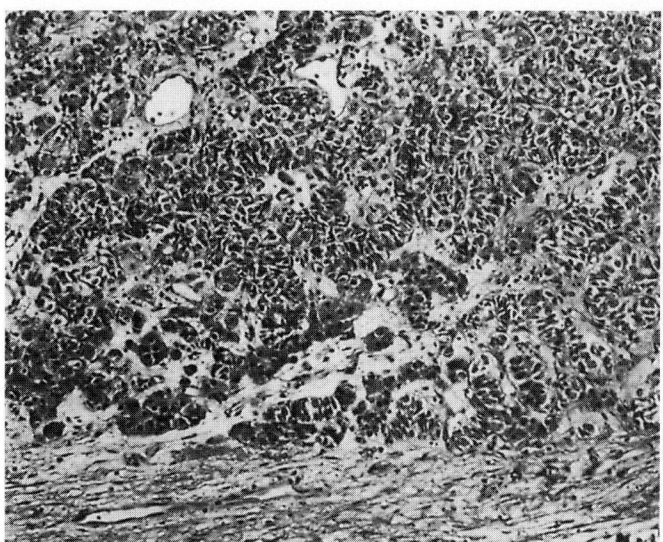

**FIGURE 102-5.** Sertoli-Leydig tumor. Cords of Sertoli cells are intermixed with plump, eosinophilic Leydig cells. ×200

Patients generally present with abnormal uterine bleeding and an abdominal mass. Most functional thecomas are estrinizing, but a few are virilizing.[20] Endometrial hyperplasia and carcinoma occur in association with these tumors but not as often as with granulosa tumors.

Grossly, these are solid, smooth, white to yellow tumors with occasional cysts and calcified areas. The tumors are bilateral in 5% of patients. Microscopically, thecomas have interlacing whorls of spindle cells, many containing abundant lipid (Fig. 102-4). Fibrocollagenous tissue makes up various proportions of these tumors, and if significant numbers of fibroblasts are present, the tumor may be designated a fibrothecoma.

These tumors are regarded as benign, and excision results in cure. A few cases of "malignant thecomas" have been said to show both clinical and pathologic features of malignancy, namely, invasion or metastases, atypical nuclei, and an increased mitotic rate.

## SERTOLI-LEYDIG TUMORS

Sertoli-Leydig cell tumors, also known as *androblastomas*, usually occur in women in the third or fourth decade of life. Less than 50% of the tumors are associated with androgenizing signs, including hirsutism and virilization (temporal balding, deepening of the voice, development of male body configuration, and clitoral enlargement) secondary to secretion of testosterone.[20,21] A few patients have estrinizing signs attributable to peripheral aromatization of androgens. The usual presentation is oligomenorrhea or amenorrhea. *Defeminization*, defined as regression of female secondary sex characteristics (amenorrhea, atrophy of endometrium and vaginal mucosa, decreased breast size), occurs initially and is followed by masculinization. The serum testosterone level is elevated, but because these tumors produce little or no androstenedione and dehydroepiandrosterone, urinary 17-ketosteroids are in the normal range. Masculinizing adrenal tumors produce high levels of androstenedione and dehydroepiandrosterone and small amounts of testosterone. Consequently, the urinary 17-ketosteroids are elevated in patients with masculinizing adrenal tumors.

Sertoli-Leydig cell tumors are unilateral in >95% of patients. The cut surface is homogeneous and gray-pink to yellow-orange, with occasional cysts, areas of hemorrhage, or necrosis. Well-differentiated tumors are usually <5 cm, whereas intermediate and poorly differentiated neoplasms are larger (10–15 cm). Microscopically, Sertoli tubules are lined by columnar epithelium and thus resemble immature seminiferous tubules.

Retiform tubules also may be present. Large polygonal eosinophilic or lipid-laden Leydig cells, some of which contain eosinophilic rod-like crystals (crystals of Reinke), are intermixed (Fig. 102-5). Pure Sertoli or Leydig tumors are composed of only one of the elements. Intermediate and poorly differentiated Sertoli-Leydig tumors have primitive gonadal stromal cells and contain heterologous elements, such as mucinous epithelium, cartilage, or striated muscle in nearly a fourth of cases. Immunocytochemical studies demonstrate testosterone, estradiol, and progesterone in all major cell components, although testosterone is most prominent in Leydig cells.[22]

The *sex cord tumor with annular tubules* (SCTAT) is considered a variant of the pure Sertoli tumor.[23] These tumors differ from the usual Sertoli tumor in their small size, bilaterality, ring arrangement of tubules, and frequent presence of calcification. One-third of patients with SCTAT have the Peutz-Jeghers syndrome (mucocutaneous pigmentation and intestinal polyposis). Unlike the usual Sertoli-Leydig tumor, the SCTAT typically secretes estrogens.

Sertoli-Leydig tumors rarely metastasize. Therefore, conservative surgical treatment—namely, excision of the involved ovary—is curative in most cases. Unfavorable prognostic features are extraovarian spread, poor or heterologous mesenchymal differentiation, and a high mitotic rate. Recurrences are usually detected within 5 years. In patients with the Peutz-Jeghers syndrome, SCTAT is an incidental finding and no therapy is necessary.

Rarely, Sertoli-Leydig and granulosa differentiation coexist in one tumor known as a *gynandroblastoma*. Patients may have either masculinizing or estrinizing clinical features. Histologically, well-differentiated granulosa and Sertoli-Leydig elements are present with minimal cellular atypia.

## STEROID (LIPID) CELL TUMORS

Lipid (lipoid) tumors are stromal lesions with abundant clear or granular cytoplasm.[13,24] When cytoplasmic Reinke crystals are identified, the neoplasm is termed a *Leydig cell tumor*.[24] Lipid cell tumors are rare, comprising <0.1% of all ovarian tumors, and are generally found in women in their fifth decade. Virilization occurs in 75% of the patients; the remainder show estrinizing effects. Features of Cushing syndrome are observed in ~10%. Urinary 17-ketosteroid levels are normal to slightly elevated, and the serum testosterone level is elevated. Microscopically, lipid cell tumors are composed of large, round cells

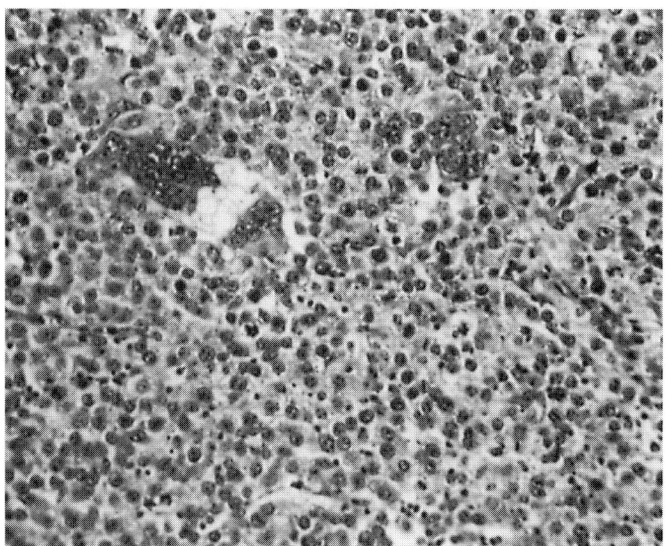

**FIGURE 102-6.** Dysgerminoma with syncytiotrophoblastic giant cells. ×200

resembling Leydig cells or adrenal cortical cells; a mixture of the two is common. The cytoplasm is clear or foamy and stains strongly positive for fat. Leydig cell tumors are rarely malignant, whereas lipid cell tumors in which Reinke crystals are not identified behave in a malignant fashion in a significant percentage of cases. The presence of Reinke crystals, therefore, is an important feature.

Unilateral salpingo-oophorectomy is sufficient treatment in a premenopausal patient whose tumor is confined to the ovary. Postmenopausal women and those with advanced disease are treated by total hysterectomy, bilateral salpingo-oophorectomy, and resection of any extraovarian tumor.

## GERM-CELL TUMORS

Any of the germ-cell tumors may produce steroid hormone effects, although some types do so with much greater frequency. Endocrine function depends on whether trophoblastic elements are present, because these secrete hCG, which, in turn, stimulates the opposite ovary to produce estrogen. Trophoblast may be present either in the form of isolated syncytiotrophoblastic giant cells (STGC) or as choriocarcinoma. The pathologist must distinguish these types, because the presence of STGC probably does not influence the prognosis of the tumor, whereas a significant amount of choriocarcinoma worsens the prognosis. The tumors that may contain isolated STGC are *embryonal carcinoma*,[25] *dysgerminoma*,[26] and, rarely, *teratoma*. STGC are present in ~5% of dysgerminomas (Fig. 102-6). Precocious puberty may be associated with any of these tumors when STGC are present because of gonadotropin production by these cells.[25] Patients with embryonal carcinoma usually have elevated serum levels of α-fetoprotein as well as hCG, and the measurement of both of these tumor markers is used to monitor treatment. *Primary ovarian choriocarcinoma* is very rare; it may arise because of an ectopic gestation (gestational trophoblastic disease) or from neoplastic germ cells.

The *gonadoblastoma* is a rare benign tumor composed of germ cells and gonadal stromal cells that arises in dysgenetic gonads (an indeterminate or streak gonad or cryptorchid dysgenetic testis).[27,28] This tumor is classified as a separate entity by the World Health Organization (see Table 102-1). Mild virilization is common secondary to hormone production by the gonadal stromal cells. More than 90% of patients with gonadoblastoma are chromatin-body negative and have a Y chromosome, although most patients are phenotypic females who present with amenorrhea (testicular feminization; see Chap. 90). Foci of calcification almost invariably are visible within the tumor by microscopy and in ~12% by radiography. The diagnosis of gonadoblastoma should be strongly considered in a female patient who presents with primary amenorrhea and an inappropriate karyotype. Calcification in the region of the gonads on abdominal radiographs is another useful clue. Treatment consists of total abdominal hysterectomy with bilateral salpingo-oophorectomy, because the tumor is bilateral in one-third of cases, the gonadal tissue is functionally abnormal, and the gonadoblastoma is overgrown by a malignant germ-cell tumor, usually a dysgerminoma, in nearly half the cases.

Other tumors composed of a mixture of germ cells and sex cord stromal cells have been associated with hormonal activity. These rare tumors may occasionally metastasize.[29]

The most common germ-cell tumor is the *benign cystic teratoma* (dermoid) (Fig. 102-7). Seven percent of these tumors contain thyroid tissue, and a fourth of these may be classified as *struma ovarii* (i.e., >50% of the neoplasm consists of thyroid tissue) (Fig. 102-8). A small proportion of patients with struma ovarii have thyroid enlargement and thyrotoxicosis.[30]

*Primary ovarian carcinoids* are extremely rare tumors that arise in conjunction with a teratoma.[31] One-third of the patients with carcinoids that display an insular pattern have the carcinoid syndrome (cutaneous flushing, telangiectasia, diarrhea, cardiac valvular lesions, and bronchoconstriction) (see Chap. 221). This syndrome

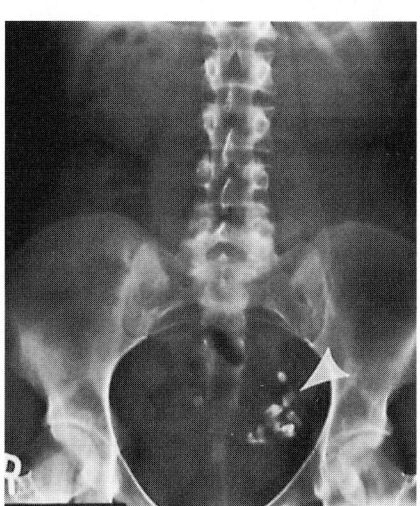
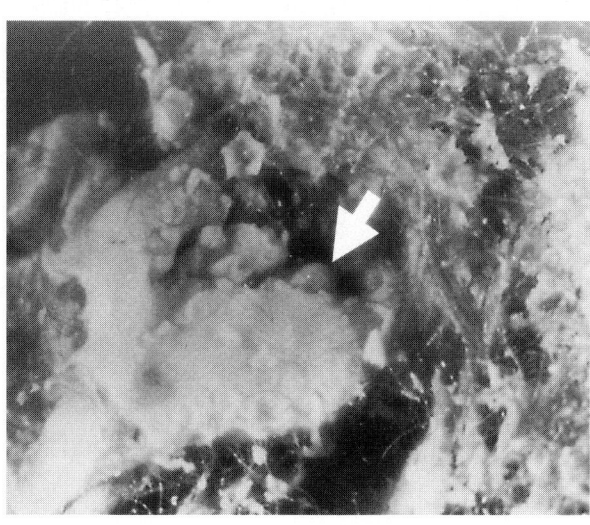

**A,B**

**FIGURE 102-7.** Benign cystic teratoma of ovary. **A,** Abdominal radiograph; note teeth (*arrowhead*). **B,** Gross photograph; hairs, keratin debris, and tooth (*arrow*) are seen.

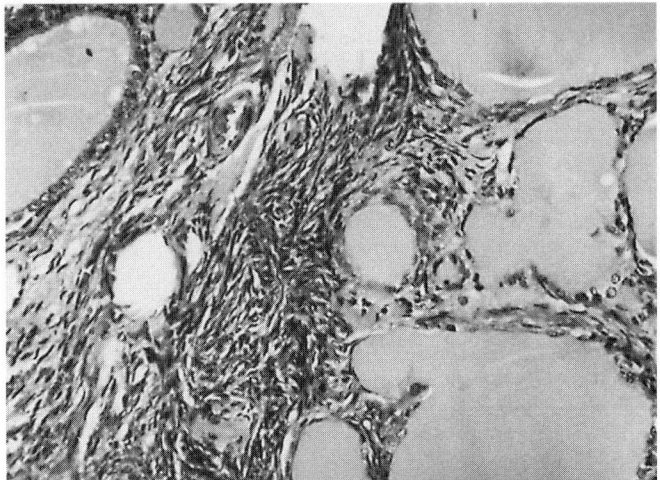

**FIGURE 102-8.** Struma ovarii. Normal thyroid follicles with ovarian stroma in background. ×400

occurs even in the absence of metastasis because the venous effluent from the ovarian tumor bypasses the portal system. Trabecular and strumal carcinoids (i.e., tumors with the combined features of struma ovarii and carcinoid) usually do not cause the carcinoid syndrome. In contrast to primary ovarian carcinoids, metastatic carcinoids, usually from the bowel, are bilateral, and patients frequently have the carcinoid syndrome. Serotonin has been identified immunohistochemically in both primary and metastatic tumors. Laboratory detection of increased amounts of 5-hydroxy-indoleacetic acid in the urine is useful in establishing the diagnosis and in monitoring the disease postoperatively.

## SECONDARY (METASTATIC) TUMORS

Carcinomas metastatic to the ovary can induce functional stroma (Fig. 102-9), possibly by means of tumor-produced gonadotropin. Functional stroma is most frequent in metastatic adenocarcinoma, generally from the colon or stomach, although sometimes from the breast. Patients may present with virilization. Most tumors metastatic to the ovary are bilateral, whereas functional primary tumors are generally unilateral. The pres-

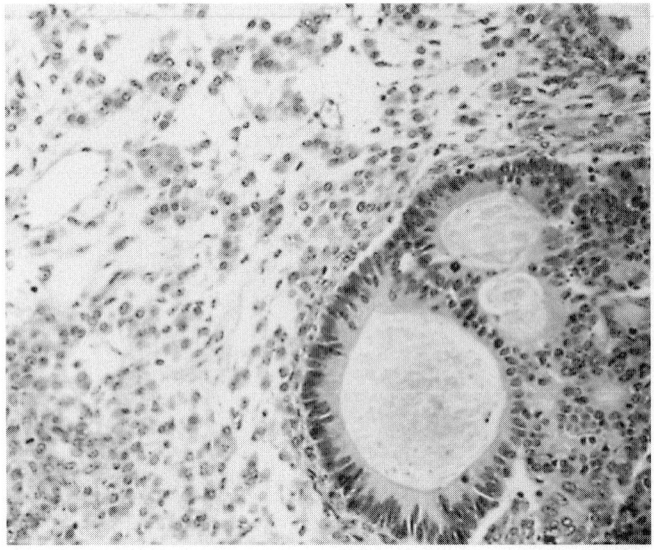

**FIGURE 102-9.** Metastatic colon carcinoma to ovary with functional activity; ovarian stromal cells are luteinized. ×200

ence of bilateral tumors in a patient with evidence of excess steroid hormone should alert the surgeon to look for a primary gastrointestinal neoplasm.[31a]

## TUMOR-LIKE CONDITIONS

*Follicular* and *luteal cysts* are the most frequent cause of an ovarian mass in women of reproductive age.[32] Follicular cysts are lined by granulosa cells that secrete estrogen. Luteal cysts contain luteinized granulosa cells that produce progesterone. A minority secrete sufficient estrogen and progesterone to cause symptoms. Typically, patients of reproductive age become anovulatory and present with menometrorrhagia. An endometrial biopsy or curettage performed for abnormal bleeding reveals endometrial stromal breakdown resulting from fluctuating levels of estrogen. In infants and prepubertal girls, precocious pseudopuberty may result from a functioning follicular cyst. These cysts often resolve spontaneously; consequently, conservative management is indicated. Patients with cysts that do not disappear after observation for 3 months require further studies, possibly surgical or laparoscopic exploration, to rule out neoplasm.

*Multiple luteinized thecal cysts* (hyperreactio luteinalis) cause bilateral ovarian enlargement and occur primarily in women with elevated levels of hCG in association with gestational trophoblastic disease. Hyperreactio luteinalis is also occasionally seen in normal pregnancies, multiple pregnancies, or ovulation induction therapy. Rarely, virilization occurs. Surgical removal is unwarranted because the cysts resolve once hCG levels normalize.

*Polycystic ovary syndrome (Stein-Leventhal syndrome)*[33,34] typically is characterized by enlarged cystic ovaries in women with amenorrhea, hirsutism, and obesity (see Chaps. 96 and 101). The ovarian cortex is thickened, and multiple follicular cysts are present. Corpora lutea may be found in 25% of patients. Laboratory findings may include increased serum levels of luteinizing hormone, decreased or normal levels of follicle-stimulating hormone, increased estrogen, and increased androgens. However, no single clinical, pathologic, or laboratory finding occurs in all affected women. Endometrial hyperplasia and, rarely, low-grade endometrial carcinoma may be found.

*Stromal hyperplasia* is an increase in the cellularity of the ovarian stromal cells. It occurs in approximately one-third of postmenopausal women and may be accompanied by estrinizing or androgenizing effects.

*Hyperthecosis* is a diffuse hyperplasia of the ovarian stroma within which clusters of lutein cells are found.[35] Most cases occur in women of reproductive age who present with marked virilization. Androgens, especially testosterone, are increased, but to a lesser degree than is usually seen with an androgen-producing tumor. As in other disorders associated with increased production of steroids, the frequency of endometrial hyperplasia and carcinoma is increased.

*Luteoma of pregnancy* is characterized by a hyperplasia of thecal cells that causes the formation of single or multiple nodules in one or both ovaries.[36] Approximately 80% of affected patients are black and multiparous. Androgenic signs are present in one-fourth of the women, and mild virilization of female infants can occur, with or without maternal functional signs. These nodules resolve spontaneously after delivery.

*Massive edema* can cause enlargement of the ovary to tumor-like proportions. Stromal luteinization occurs in association with this condition and can cause virilizing signs.[37]

## OTHER TYPES OF ENDOCRINE EFFECTS

Various peptides that induce endocrine or endocrine-like effects may be produced by a few ovarian tumors. The effects include hypercalcemia, hyperthyroidism, hypoglycemia, Cushing syndrome, and polycythemia (see Chap. 219).[38] Hypercalcemia has been described with clear cell carcinoma, serous carcinoma, dysgerminoma, and small cell undifferentiated carcinoma.[39] The latter is a rare, highly malignant tumor of young women. Thyroid-stimulating hormone may be produced by neoplastic cells, usually trophoblastic cells (see Chap. 112). Nontrophoblastic ovarian tumors can produce prolactin and hCG-like substances. Rarely, Cushing syndrome results from adrenocorticotropic hormone production by ovarian carcinoma or a malignant Sertoli cell tumor. Mild polycythemia may be associated with virilizing tumor.

## REFERENCES

1. Scully RE. Histological typing of ovarian tumors. In: Histological typing of female genital tract tumors. New York: Springer-Verlag, 1999; in press.
2. International Federation of Gynecologists and Obstetricians Cancer Committee. Staging announcement. Gynecol Oncol 1986; 25:383.
3. Hayes MC, Scully RE. Ovarian steroid cell tumors (not otherwise specified): a clinicopathologic analysis of 63 cases. Am J Surg Pathol 1987; 11:835.
4. Hayes MC, Scully RE. Stromal luteoma of the ovary: a clinicopathological analysis of 25 cases. Int J Gynecol Pathol 1987; 6:313.
5. Sasano H, Kaga K, Sato S, et al. Adrenal 4-binding protein in common epithelial and metastatic tumors of the ovary. Hum Pathol 1996; 27:595.
6. Claus EB, Schwartz. Familial ovarian cancer. Cancer 1995; 76:1998.
7. Schwartz P. The role of tumor markers in the preoperative diagnosis of ovarian cysts. Clin Obstet Gynecol 1993; 36:384.
8. Talerman A. Germ cell tumors of the ovary. In: Kurman RJ, ed. Blaustein's pathology of the female genital tract, 4th ed. New York: Springer-Verlag, 1994;849.
9. Matias-Guiu X, Prat J. Ovarian tumors with functioning stroma. Cancer 1990; 65:2001.
10. Freeman DA. Steroid hormone-producing tumors of the adrenal, ovary, and testes. Endocrinol Metab Clin North Am 1991; 20:751.
11. Cannistra SA. Medical progress: cancer of the ovary. N Engl J Med 1993; 329:1550.
12. Rome RM, Fortune DW, Quinn MA, et al. Functioning ovarian tumors in postmenopausal women. Obstet Gynecol 1981; 57:705.
12a. Markman M. The genetics, screening, and treatment of epithelial ovarian cancer: an update. Cleve Clin J Med 2000; 67:294.
12b. Maggino T, Gadducci A. Serum markers as prognostic factors in epithelial ovarian cancer: an overview. Eur J Gynaecol Oncol 2000; 21:64.
13. Fox H. Sex cord-stromal tumors of the ovary. J Pathol 1985; 145:127.
14. Young RH, Scully RE. Sex cord-stromal, steroid cell and other ovarian tumors with endocrine, paraendocrine and paraneoplastic manifestations. In: Kurman RJ, ed. Blaustein's pathology of the female genital tract, 4th ed. New York: Springer-Verlag, 1994:783.
14a. Choi YL, Kim HS, Ahn G. Immunoexpression of inhibin alpha subunit, inhibin/activin beta A subunit and CD99 in ovarian tumors. Arch Pathol Lab Med 2000; 124:563.
15. Zheng W, Luo MP, Welt C, et al. Imbalanced expression of inhibin and activin subunits in primary epithelial ovarian cancer. Gynecol Oncol 1998; 69:23.
15a. Long W-Q, Ranchin V, Pautier P, et al. Detection of minimal levels of serum anti-mullerian hormone during follow-up of patients with ovarian granulosa cell tumor by means of a highly sensitive enzyme-linked immunosorbent assay. J Clin Endocrinal Metab 2000; 85:540.
16. Young RH, Dickersin GR, Scully RE. Juvenile granulosa cell tumor of the ovary. Am J Surg Pathol 1984; 8:575.
17. Kurman RJ, Goebelsmann U, Taylor CR. Steroid localization in granulosa-theca tumors of the ovary. Cancer 1979; 43:2377.
18. Chadha S, Rao BR, Slotman BJ, et al. An immunohistochemical evaluation of androgen and progesterone receptors in ovarian tumors. Hum Pathol 1993; 24:90.
19. Bjorkholm E, Silfversward C. Prognostic factors in granulosa-cell tumors. Gynecol Oncol 1981; 11:261.
20. Zhang J, Young RH, Arseneau J, et al. Ovarian stromal tumors containing lutein or Leydig cells (luteinized thecomas and stromal Leydig cell tumors): a clinicopathologic study of 34 cases. Cancer 1981; 48:187.
21. Young RH, Scully RE. Ovarian Sertoli-Leydig cell tumors: a clinicopathological analysis of 207 cases. Am J Surg Pathol 1985; 9:543.
22. Kurman RJ, Andrade D, Goebelsmann U, et al. An immunohistological study of steroid localization in Sertoli-Leydig tumors of the ovary and testis. Cancer 1978; 42:1772.
23. Young RH, Welch WR, Dickersin GR, et al. Ovarian sex cord tumor with annular tubules. Cancer 1982; 50:1384.
24. Hayes MC, Scully RE. Ovarian steroid cell tumors (not otherwise specified). Am J Surg Pathol 1987; 11:835.
25. Kurman RJ, Norris HJ. Malignant germ cell tumors of the ovary. Hum Pathol 1977; 8:551.
26. Zaloudek CJ, Tavassoli FA, Norris HJ. Dysgerminoma with syncytiotrophoblastic giant cells: a histologically and clinically distinctive subtype of dysgerminoma. Am J Surg Pathol 1981; 5:361.
27. Scully RE. Gonadoblastoma: a review of 74 cases. Cancer 1970; 25:1340.
28. Roth LM, Eglen DE. Gonadoblastoma: immunohistochemical and ultrastructural observations. Int J Gynecol Pathol 1989; 8:72.
29. Lacson AG, Gillis DA, Shawwa A. Malignant mixed germ cell–sex cord–stromal tumors of the ovary associated with isosexual precocious puberty. Cancer 1988; 61:2122.
30. Hasleton PS, Kelehan P, Whittaker JD, et al. Benign and malignant struma ovarii. Arch Pathol Lab Med 1978; 102:180.
31. Robboy SJ, Norris HJ, Scully RE. Insular carcinoid primary in the ovary: a clinicopathologic analysis of 48 cases. Cancer 1975; 36:404.
31a. Sandmeier D, Lobrinus JA, Vial Y, et al. Bilateral Krukenberg tumor of the ovary during pregnancy. Eur J Gynaecol Oncol 2000; 21:58.
32. Eriksson L, Kjellgren O, von Schoultz B. Functional cyst or ovarian cancer: histopathological findings during 1 year of surgery. Gynecol Obstet Invest 1985; 19:155.
33. Goldzieher JW, Young RL. Selected aspects of polycystic ovarian disease. Endocrinol Metab Clin North Am 1992; 21:141.
34. McKenna JT. Pathogenesis and treatment of polycystic ovary syndrome. N Engl J Med 1988; 318:558.
35. Sasano H, Fukunaga M, Rojas M, et al. Hyperthecosis of the ovary: clinicopathologic study of 19 cases with immunohistochemical analysis of steroidogenic enzymes. Int J Gynecol Pathol 1989; 8:311.
36. Clement PB. Tumor-like lesions of the ovary associated with pregnancy. Int J Gynecol Pathol 1993; 12:108.
37. Young RH, Scully RE. Fibromatosis and massive edema of the ovary, possibly related entities: a report of 14 cases of fibromatosis and 11 cases of massive edema. Int J Gynecol Pathol 1984; 3:153.
38. Scully RE, Young RH, Clement PB. Paraendocrine, paraneoplastic, and other syndromes associated with ovarian tumors. In: Tumors of the ovary, maldeveloped gonads, fallopian tube and broad ligament. Atlas of tumor pathology, Series 3, fasc 23. Washington: Armed Forces Institute of Pathology, 1996.
39. Scully RE. Small cell carcinoma of hypercalcemic type. Int J Gynecol Pathol 1993; 12:148.

# C H A P T E R   1 0 3

# THE DIFFERENTIAL DIAGNOSIS OF FEMALE INFERTILITY

STEVEN J. ORY AND MARCELO J. BARRIONUEVO

## DEFINITION OF INFERTILITY

*Infertility* is the involuntary inability to conceive. *Sterility* is the permanent inability to reproduce. Infertility is a relative term, but sterility is not.

*Primary infertility* exists if a woman has never been pregnant after attempts at conception for 12 months without success. *Secondary infertility* connotes that a previous pregnancy has occurred, regardless of the outcome. The National Center for Health Statistics in 1988 estimated that 8.4% of women 15 to 44 years of age in the United States, or 4.9 million women, were infertile.[1] Approximately 45% experienced primary infertility,[1] and 25% experienced infertility at some time during their reproductive lives.[2] Approximately 10% to 15%, or 1 in 12 American couples, experience infertility. Half of these will require conventional therapy and the other 50% will require more advanced assisted reproductive techniques (ARTs). The rate of infertility has remained stable over the past 30 years.[2]

## NORMAL REPRODUCTIVE PERFORMANCE

*Fecundability* is the probability of achieving pregnancy within one menstrual cycle (20% to 25% per cycle). *Fecundity* is the ability to achieve pregnancy resulting in a live birth within one menstrual cycle (4% per cycle).

For *nulliparous* women (i.e., women who have never borne children), the average time during which the women and their partners engage in instances of unprotected intercourse from initiation to conception is 5.3 months. For *parous* women (i.e., those who have borne children), the duration is 2.7 months. Even after correction of the cause for infertility, achieving pregnancy may require several months.

Many couples presenting for assistance with fertility would conceive without any medical intervention: ~50% of women with infertility of 1 year's duration will conceive within 5 years without assistance, or a rate of ~3% per month. Any treatment may appear to increase fertility in the absence of comparison with an untreated control population. Most infertility studies lack such controls, and the statistical significance of the results often is not documented.

Four general factors influence the reproductive performance of couples: *the length of time the couple has been attempting to conceive; the age of the female partner; the age of the male partner; and the frequency of intercourse.*

The peak biologic fertility in women is in the late teens and early 20s. Among women in their mid-20s, the half-time to pregnancy averages 6 months. Thereafter, the mean time to conception is longer. A similar decline occurs in male reproductive performance after 25 years of age, but the decline is less marked. Conception occurs in <6 months in 75% of couples if the male partner is younger than 25 years of age, in 38% of couples if the man is 30 to 34, and in 23% if the man is 40 years of age or older.

Studies examining the effect of the age of the woman or man usually have not corrected for the age of the partner. Because older men tend to be married to older women, such data reflect the compound effects of age. Moreover, such data have not been corrected for the frequency of coitus. The frequency of intercourse affects the conception rate; 17% of couples having coitus less than once each week are likely to conceive in <6 months, but 51% of those having coitus three times per week will conceive.[3]

## REPRODUCTIVE PROCESSES IMPORTANT TO FERTILITY

Several requirements must be met for pregnancy. The male partner must produce adequate numbers of normal, motile spermatozoa; the man must be capable of ejaculating the sperm (i.e., patent ductal system); and the sperm must be able to traverse the female reproductive tract (i.e., no obstruction of the female tract). The female partner must ovulate and release an ovum; the sperm must be able to fertilize the ovum; the fertilized ovum must be transported from the distal fallopian tube, the site of fertilization, to the endometrial cavity in a timely manner; and the fertilized ovum must be capable of developing into an embryo and implanting.

Normally, several million to several hundred million spermatozoa are deposited in the posterior vagina during coitus. There, the ejaculate forms a gel that undergoes liquefaction within 20 to 30 minutes of its formation. Even before liquefaction, sperm gain entry to the upper female reproductive tract through the cervical mucus. Most of the sperm in the ejaculate that remains in the vagina are immobilized rapidly and killed in the acidic milieu. Fewer than 200 sperm per ejaculate ever reach the distal oviduct.

Cervical mucus is a relatively impermeable barrier to sperm throughout the menstrual cycle except during the periovulatory period, when access to the upper reproductive tract is permitted. During this interval, estrogen induces several clinically recognized changes, including an increase in the amount of cervical mucus; a decrease in its viscosity, manifested as increased *spinnbarkeit* (i.e., elasticity); a decrease in cellularity; and a prominent *ferning pattern* when dried on a slide. The ultrastructure of cervical mucus alters; the fibrous strands become oriented into channels through which the sperm travel into the endocervix and endocervical crypts. After ovulation, the mucus undergoes a progesterone-mediated change that renders it impenetrable again.

The sperm migrating into the cervix reside for various periods of time in the endocervical crypts before ascending into the uterus. The process of *capacitation,* which consists of three stages—(a) *acrosomal reaction,* (b) *zona pellucida binding of the sperm,* and (c) *hypermobility of the sperm*—is time dependent. This process originally was described in the rat and rabbit cervix, and its occurrence in the human is unconfirmed, although the *acrosome reaction* (i.e., orderly vesiculation process confined to the anterior acrosome) is thought to be essential to fertilization and may be an analogous phenomenon.[4] The acrosome reaction affects the sperm plasma membrane and the outer acrosomal membrane. After release, the acrosomal enzymes disperse the matrix of the cumulus oophorus before hydrolyzing the glycoprotein shell of the zona pellucida.[5] This prefertilization process does not require residence in the female reproductive tract, as proved by the success of in vitro fertilization.

After the surviving sperm leave the cervix, their migration through the endometrial cavity may be facilitated by uterine contractions. Sperm then enter the tubal ostia and later encounter the oocyte in the ampullary portion of the oviduct. Sperm have been recovered from the distal fallopian tube within 5 minutes of vaginal insemination.[6]

Egg retrieval by the oviduct in primates is not well understood. The tubal fimbria apparently come into approximation with the ovary at the time of ovulation, and the oocyte is extruded from the ovulatory follicle with its cumulus mass of follicular cells intact. The egg initially adheres to cilia on the fimbrial surface. Muscular movements of the tube and ciliary motion propel the oocyte and subsequent embryo toward the uterus.

The egg may be fertilized from 12 to 24 hours after ovulation; sperm probably retain fertilization potential for 48 hours and motility for 72 hours after ejaculation. The zona pellucida surrounding the egg regulates species specificity by restricting the access of sperm lacking binding sites for its surface receptors and prevents polyploidy by forming an impermeable barrier to additional sperm after fertilization. At fertilization, the newly formed embryo achieves a diploid number of chromosomes with the addition of the sperm's complement. Soon thereafter, the second polar body is extruded.

The embryo stays in the oviduct for almost 3 days, remaining at the ampullary isthmic junction for 30 hours. Transportation is accomplished primarily by ciliary action and is relatively rapid through the isthmic portion of the tube. Implantation occurs ~5 to 7 days after fertilization when the embryo reaches the blastocyst stage. Generally, estrogen delays embryo transport, and passage is facilitated by progesterone. Conception and implantation are discussed in detail in Chapter 107.

## CAUSES OF INFERTILITY

Conception and sustenance of early pregnancy require the integration of all of the steps described earlier. Clinical infertility management is directed toward elucidating abnormalities in reproduction, but many perturbations cannot be assessed directly or corrected, and their relevance to fertility potential is not well established. Nevertheless, several areas of clinical concern can be addressed. Possible causes of infertility are listed in Table 103-1. In general, they include 40% due to the *male factor*, 40% due to the *female factor*, 10% due to a *combined male/female factor*, and 10% due to unexplained causes.

### COITAL CAUSES OF INFERTILITY

Optimal fertility occurs with consistent midcycle coital exposure. Although this feature often is taken for granted in an infertility evaluation, establishing that coital technique and frequency are adequate is critical. The optimal frequency of intercourse is every other day during the periovulatory period; more frequent intercourse may lower the sperm count in some men.

Some couples may impair fertility by using lubricants with spermicidal properties. K-Y jelly and Surgilube immobilize sperm in vitro. Rarely, anatomic problems such as uterine descensus or hypospadias in the male contribute to infertility by impeding interactions between sperm and the cervical mucus.

**TABLE 103-1.**
**Causes of Infertility**

**INADEQUATE COITUS**
Frequency
Inadvertent use of spermicides (as lubricants)
Anatomic problems
  Male: hypospadias
  Female: uterine descensus
**MALE CAUSES** (see Chap. 118)
Pretesticular
Testicular
Posttesticular
**VAGINAL CAUSES**
Excessive acidity
**CERVICAL CAUSES**
Hormonal
  Inadequate estrogen
Infectious
  *Chlamydia trachomatis*
  *Ureaplasma urealyticum*
Anatomic
  Destruction by cone biopsy or cauterization
Immunologic
**UTERINE CAUSES**
Leiomyomas
Polyps
Intrauterine synechiae (Asherman syndrome)
Chronic endometritis
  *Ureaplasma urealyticum*
  *Tuberculosis*
**TUBAL CAUSES**
Infectious
  *Chlamydia trachomatis*
  *Neisseria gonorrhoeae*
  *Mycobacterium tuberculosis*
  *Streptococcus*
  Anaerobes
Inflammatory salpingitis isthmica nodosa
**CONGENITAL ABNORMALITIES**
Diethylstilbestrol exposure
Idiopathic
**ENDOMETRIOSIS**
Mild
Moderate
Severe
**OVULATORY DISORDERS**
Luteal phase deficiency
  Hypoprogesteronemia
  Hyperprolactinemia
Anovulation/oligoanovulation
  Chronic anovulation (polycystic ovary syndrome)
  Hypothalamic amenorrhea-anovulation
Pituitary disease (including hyperprolactinemia)
Adrenal disease
Thyroid disease
Luteinized unruptured follicle syndrome
Ovarian failure
Gonadal dysgenesis
**PELVIC ADHESIONS**
After intrauterine device use
Associated with pelvic inflammatory disease
Associated with appendicitis
Associated with other bowel disease
Idiopathic
**OTHER CAUSES**
Age related
Psychogenic

## MALE FACTOR IN INFERTILITY

The causes of male infertility are discussed in Chapter 118. Problems of the male partner are estimated to affect 30% to 40% of infertile couples.

## VAGINAL AND CERVICAL CAUSES OF INFERTILITY

Putative vaginal causes of infertility that have been proposed include excessive acidity. The normal vaginal milieu is lethal to sperm, and the small fraction of the ejaculate that enters the cervical mucus immediately after ejaculation is the only portion that normally survives. Nevertheless, a deleterious effect of low vaginal pH on fertility and the alleged benefit of alkalinization with sodium bicarbonate have not been documented. Common vaginal pathogens such as *Candida*, *Trichomonas*, and *Gardnerella vaginalis* are not thought to contribute to infertility.

"Cervical factor" infertility remains a controversial entity that encompasses potential infectious, hormonal, anatomic, and immunologic causes. *Chlamydia trachomatis* and *Ureaplasma urealyticum* infections may involve the cervix and have been implicated in infertility. Patients with deficient estrogen levels may not achieve optimal cervical mucus production, and sperm migration may be impeded. Ovulation induction with an estrogen antagonist such as clomiphene citrate also may adversely affect cervical mucus and, consequently, sperm migration. Some patients have had surgical excision or ablation of the endocervix or endocervical glands after cone biopsy or cryocauterization of the cervix, with resultant absent or diminished cervical mucus production. The presence of agglutinating and immobilizing sperm antibodies in cervical mucus has been postulated to cause infertility.[7,8] Some clinicians use the postcoital test to evaluate the interaction between cervical mucus and spermatozoa, but this test is more of historical interest than of true practical applicability as part of the infertility workup.

## UTERINE CAUSES OF INFERTILITY

Uterine abnormalities are implicated infrequently in infertility. Leiomyomas are common but rarely contribute to infertility. Intramural and submucosal myomas may distort the uterine cavity or obstruct the tubal lumen when located in the uterine cornu, or the endocervical canal when present in the lower segment. Abnormal vascular patterns have been associated with myomas.[9] Infertility and pregnancy loss have been postulated to result from faulty placentation and compromised placental perfusion. Premature labor and pregnancy wastage may occur when uterine compliance is reduced. Degenerating fibroids may produce irritable foci, leading to premature labor or abruptio placentae (i.e., premature detachment of a normally situated placenta).

Uterine scarring, also called *Asherman syndrome*, may produce infertility and pregnancy loss through mechanisms similar to leiomyomas; the patient usually has a history of endometritis after a delivery or an abortion. Many of these patients have amenorrhea or decreased menstrual flow, but some have clinically significant intrauterine synechiae without menstrual abnormalities.

Chronic endometritis has been implicated in infertility. *Ureaplasma urealyticum* has been isolated in chronic endometritis, but its relevance to infertility in the absence of scarring within the uterus or oviducts is unknown. Two conditions that are rare in the United States, *tuberculous* endometritis and salpingitis, have a devastating effect on fertility.

## TUBAL CAUSES OF INFERTILITY

The oviduct has several functions critical to reproduction. With extensive destruction of the fallopian tube, such as is seen with hydrosalpinx formation after gonococcal salpingitis, no obvious means exists for the sperm and egg to unite. However, more subtle abnormalities often cause infertility. Extrinsic adhesions may compromise tubal motility and prevent ovum pickup. Intraluminal adhesions may separate the sperm and egg or trap the embryo, leading to pregnancy wastage or ectopic pregnancy. Damage to or loss of the tubal cilia may have the same result. The diagnosis often is made in patients with a history of pelvic inflammatory disease, intrauterine device use, appendicitis with rupture, ectopic pregnancy, and septic abortion, although many patients with extensive tubal disease have no relevant history. Tubal disease may affect 20% to 40% of infertile couples.

Various infections can produce tubal disease.[10] Salpingitis isthmica nodosa consists of small diverticula in the proximal oviduct, usually in association with inflammation, which may lead to obstruction. The affected segment may form a palpable nodule. Its etiology is unknown. Müllerian anomalies and other congenital abnormalities may follow exposure to diethylstilbestrol in utero and can cause absent, hypoplastic, or occluded oviducts. Tubal adhesions may also follow pelvic surgery.

## OVULATORY FACTORS IN INFERTILITY

Various disorders of ovulation, ranging from luteal phase deficiency to anovulation, are estimated to account for 10% to 15% of all infertility problems (see Chaps. 96 and 97).

## ENDOMETRIOSIS AND INFERTILITY

Although the prevalence of endometriosis is unknown, 30% to 50% of women with the condition are thought to be infertile (see Chap. 98). Women with extensive inflammation and scar formation have obvious causes for infertility, but infertility in those with mild and moderate endometriosis is more puzzling. Proposed mechanisms to explain more subtle causes of infertility include interaction with macrophages, interleukins, integrins, and other inflammatory molecules as discussed in Chapter 96.[11,11a] However, previously advocated medical regimens may not be effective in treating infertility associated with endometriosis, even when the disease is eradicated. This is in contrast to the beneficial effect of laparoscopic resection or ablation of minimal and mild endometriosis, which enhances the fecundity in infertile women.[12,12a] Empiric approaches to treatment of infertility with ART appear to be effective treatments for endometriosis, even when the disease persists.

## OTHER CAUSES OF INFERTILITY

In women, an age-related decline in fertility precedes the hormonal changes characteristic of the climacteric and occurs while they are still ovulatory. This decline may result from a relative deficiency of fertilizable ova, an alteration of gonadotropin release or function, a change in uterine steroid receptors, impaired tubal function, or other, clinically unrecognized mechanisms. In older women (40 years of age or older) who are ovulatory, fertility is not improved by agents that induce ovulation. The observation that older women receiving embryos produced from oocytes that were donated from younger women have near-normal fertility potential suggests that age-related changes in the remaining oocytes is the principal mechanism for infertility.

Infertility is sometimes attributed to psychogenic causes.[13] Anxiety and apprehension can interfere with coital frequency and may be a factor in some instances of hypothalamic amenorrhea. Spasm at the tubal cornu, perhaps associated with anxiety, often is observed during hysterosalpingography but has not been directly implicated as a cause of infertility.

# EVALUATION OF THE INFERTILE COUPLE

## GENERAL CONSIDERATIONS

Treating the couple as a unit is important. Although infertility is not lethal, the desire to reproduce is a basic human instinct, and deprivation of fertility may lead to guilt and depression.

Because infertility is not a disease and the couple generally are otherwise healthy, they should be encouraged to be active in their evaluation and in determining their course of therapy after 1 year of unprotected intercourse, unless the female partner's age is 35 years of age or older, she has anovulatory cycles, or she has a history of pelvic pain, pelvic infection, or pelvic surgery. Evaluation of the male partner should be performed early on and he should definitely be evaluated if he has a history of testicular atrophy, testicular injury, undescended testicles, or sexual dysfunction. Most couples are anxious to learn the reason for their infertility even if it cannot be corrected.

Approximately 10% to 40% of couples have more than one cause for their infertility. In the United States, couples seeking evaluation and treatment have limited time as well as limited emotional and financial resources to invest. For these reasons, a comprehensive infertility evaluation should be completed as expeditiously as possible. The couple should be counseled regarding the diagnosis and prognosis, and the treatment alternatives should be presented in an objective, circumspect manner as soon as the tests are completed. When treatment is undertaken, end points should be determined, and periodic reassessment should be anticipated. The decision to terminate therapeutic efforts should be left to the patient; however, after a trial of reasonable duration, continuation of a therapeutic regimen should be discouraged.

The psychological aspects of the diagnosis of infertility and its treatment should be addressed early in the therapeutic alliance, and additional support should be offered to those needing it. The clinical condition of infertility must be presented to the couple as a problem shared by the partners without blaming one individual.

## ASSESSMENT OF OVULATION

Ovulatory function spans a spectrum from normal ovulation with optimal reproductive potential to frank anovulation. In between, various degrees of ovulatory dysfunction exist, encompassing entities such as *luteal phase deficiency, short luteal phase,* and *luteinized unruptured follicle syndrome.* The first two conditions result from insufficient progesterone production to permit normal endometrial maturational changes and implantation of the embryo, or normal levels of progesterone production that are not sustained long enough to allow complete endometrial maturation.[14] Luteinized unruptured follicle syndrome occurs when there is luteinization of the preovulatory follicle and progesterone production, but the ovum is not released from the preovulatory follicle.

The incidence, underlying pathophysiology, diagnostic evaluation, and treatment are controversial for all of these entities. Ovulation most commonly is evaluated by *basal body temperature* (BBT) charts, which rely on the thermogenic shift induced by pregnanediol, the principal metabolite of progesterone, to indicate the onset and duration of the luteal phase. Such charts lack sensitivity. One large study that measured serum levels of luteinizing hormone, follicle-stimulating hormone (FSH), estradiol, and progesterone noted that the time of ovulation was correctly identified by BBT in only 22% of cycles and that 22% of the charts were incorrectly interpreted as showing anovulation.[15]

Serum progesterone measurement and endometrial biopsy are more reliable methods of assessing ovulatory function. Most laboratories cite a serum progesterone value of 4 to 5 ng/mL as indicative of ovulation and a midluteal value of 10 ng/mL as consistent with normal luteal function. However, progesterone is secreted in a pulsate fashion, and a single value may not reflect luteal function adequately. A midluteal progesterone determination does not depict early or late luteal function, and a single determination may not be sensitive enough to detect subtle luteal dysfunction. Some physicians have proposed using three plasma luteal determinations, with a total value of 15 ng/mL or greater considered consistent with normal luteal function.[16]

Endometrial biopsy using a dating technique, such as urinary luteinizing hormone predictor kits, has been the tradi-

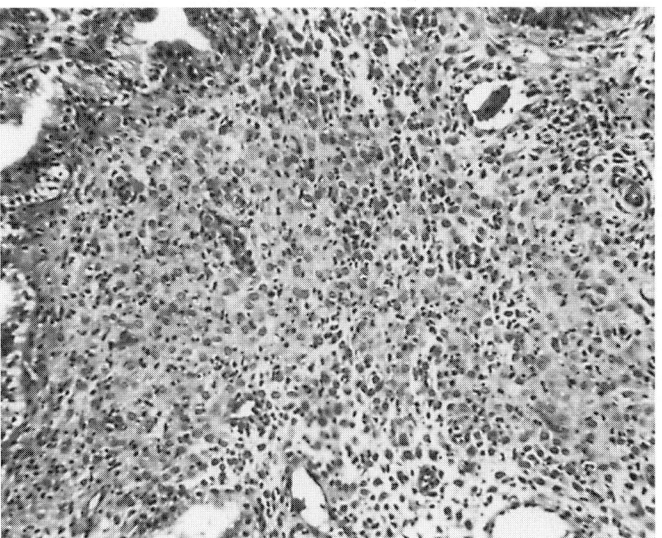

**FIGURE 103-1.** Endometrial biopsy is representative of day 27 of the menstrual cycle, with coalescent decidua and infiltration of leukocytes consistent with normal late luteal function. (Hematoxylin and eosin; ×100)

tional method of evaluating luteal function[17] (Figs. 103-1 and 103-2). Although some subjectivity exists in the interpretation, the test is less expensive than multiple progesterone determinations. However, it is invasive and may require repetition. Moreover, as documented in the original publication, an error in interpretation occurs in 20% to 25% of specimens. The specificity of endometrial biopsy and effectiveness of available treatment remain controversial.

Additional techniques for evaluating luteal function have been described. Prolactin production in endometrial explant culture is depressed in patients with luteal deficiency. Tissue obtained by endometrial biopsy in patients with luteal deficiency produces less prolactin, which is directly correlated with the amount of decidualization.[18] Luteal function has been

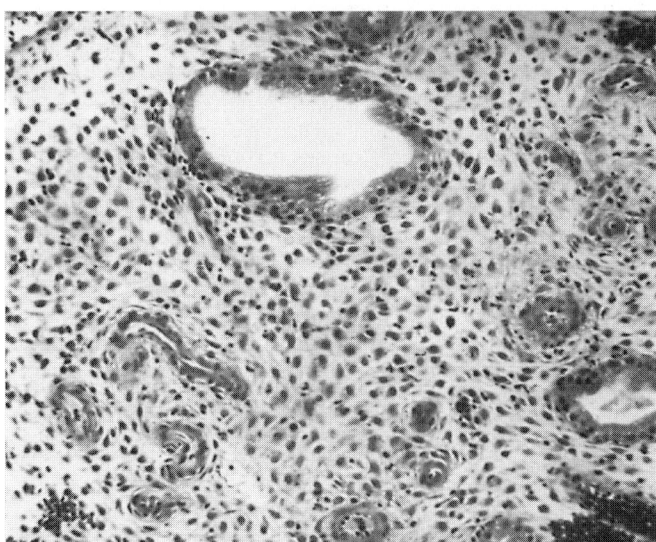

**FIGURE 103-2.** Endometrial biopsy, representative of day 24 of the menstrual cycle, shows periarteriolar and subcapsular pseudodecidual changes with stromal edema. If this specimen had been obtained the day before menstruation, it would be consistent with luteal-phase deficiency. However, to establish the diagnosis of luteal deficiency, the biopsy findings must be confirmed in two sequential cycles. (Hematoxylin and eosin; ×100)

assessed by daily pregnanediol radioimmunoassays of early morning urine specimens during the luteal phase. This technique is noninvasive and offers the opportunity to follow luteal function with daily measurements.[19]

Nineteen percent of fertile women have occasional cycles that display luteal deficiency; only those who have recurrent abnormalities should be treated.[20] Recurrent dysfunction is confirmed by repeating the studies in a subsequent cycle. Women who have two cycles with luteal deficiency satisfy the criteria for diagnosis and should receive therapy.

Hyperprolactinemia and hypothyroidism also have been associated with an inadequate luteal phase, and patients with luteal phase deficiency should be screened for these endocrinopathies.[21]

Sustained FSH levels of >40 mIU/mL are consistent with ovarian failure. A serum FSH determination obtained on the second or third day of the menstrual cycle reflects ovarian reserve. Patients with an abnormal serum FSH level, >15 mIU/mL, on cycle day 2 or 3 have a poor prognosis for success with in vitro fertilization and probably with other treatment modalities as well.[22]

## ASSESSMENT OF UTERINE CAVITY AND FALLOPIAN TUBES

Hysterosalpingography is the accepted standard for evaluating the uterine cavity and tubal lumen (Fig. 103-3). Water-soluble or oil-soluble radiopaque contrast material is injected through an endocervical cannula; the flow of contrast is followed with fluoroscopy; and radiographs are taken as a permanent record. Some researchers claim a therapeutic effect, with enhanced fertility 6 to 12 months after hysterosalpingography, but this benefit has not been documented in a controlled clinical trial.[23] Although the procedure is generally safe, the possible complications include uterine perforation, postexamination hemorrhage, hypersensitivity reactions to the iodine in the contrast material, exacerbation of pelvic inflammatory disease, granuloma formation, venous and lymphatic intravasation, and pain.

The uterine cavity also may be evaluated with hysteroscopy and ultrasonography using saline or Albunex (albumin microspheres) as a contrast medium. These techniques may be used when hysterosalpingography is contraindicated or for further study of a suspected abnormality.

## ASSESSMENT OF THE MALE FACTOR

Semen analysis remains the most accurate and widely used test to study male fertility. A small population of subfertile men with normal semen analyses has been identified, and new tests are being developed to assess the most critical element of sperm function: the ability to fertilize an ovum. Assessment of sperm morphology using the strict criteria of Kruger is more predictive of unsuspected male factor infertility; abnormalities are more often associated with failed in vitro fertilization and intrauterine insemination.[24,25] The presence of antisperm antibodies as well as tests of the 24-hour survival of the sperm are important predictors of male fertility potential. Sperm binding to the zona pellucida can be evaluated with hemizona assay; failure to bind is predictive of poor success with in vitro fertilization and intrauterine inseminations.[2,26]

## EVALUATION OF THE CERVICAL FACTOR

Assessment of the cervical factor in infertility remains one of the most controversial areas of investigation. The *postcoital test (Sims-Huhner test)* traditionally is used. This test has undergone modification since its original description, and considerable variation is seen in its performance and interpretation. It usually is performed at midcycle, as close to the time of ovulation as possible, within 8 hours of intercourse. A sample of cervical mucus is removed from the endocervix, with care taken to avoid vaginal contamination; the sample is placed on a slide for

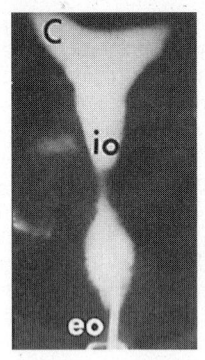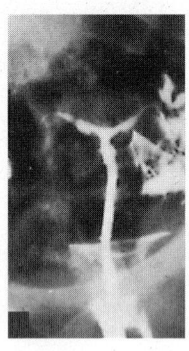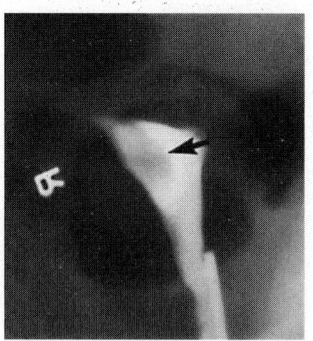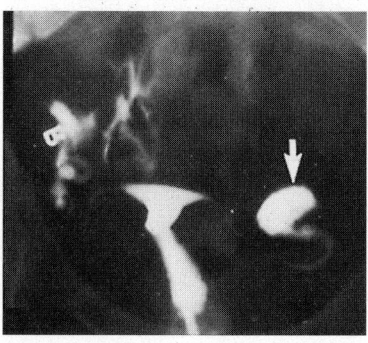

**FIGURE 103-3.** Hysterosalpingograms. **A,** Normal hysterosalpingogram. (*C*, uterine cornu; *io*, internal os of cervix; *eo*, external os of cervix.) **B,** T-shaped cavity characteristic of intrauterine diethylstilbestrol exposure. **C,** Endometrial polyp in the right cornu (*arrow*). **D,** Nonpatent hydrosalpinx, left oviduct (*arrow*).

evaluation of its estrogen effect (gauged by the volume, cellularity, spinnbarkeit, and ferning pattern of the mucus) to confirm the appropriateness of the timing of the test and is examined for the presence of motile sperm. Some women exhibit mucus receptiveness toward the sperm for only 1 day, with the mucus being relatively impermeable to the sperm at other times. A poor test result most often is due to performance of the test at a suboptimal time in the cycle.

After the mucus has been evaluated, sperm are identified. Considerable debate continues over the criteria for the minimum number of motile sperm present in a normal postcoital test: estimates range from 1 to >20 per high-power field. One review cited little difference in fertility rates when 1 to 5 motile sperm were seen per high-power field compared with 11 to 20.[27] Most sperm should demonstrate good forward motility; immobile sperm and rotary motion are abnormal.[28] Tests with the latter results should be repeated; often the sperm are found to be normal on reexamination. Less frequently, these patterns are present in patients with sperm immobilizing or sperm agglutinating antibodies.

Postcoital tests often are misleading. One study of fertile couples found abnormal postcoital tests (less than one sperm per high-power field) in 20%.[29] In another study, six of eight women with abnormal postcoital tests (i.e., persistently showing no sperm) had motile and presumably normal sperm recovered from the peritoneal cavity at laparoscopy.[30] In another study involving 355 infertile couples without severe defects in ovulation or seminal or tubal function, no correlation was found between the results of the postcoital test and subsequent pregnancy, with a minimum follow-up of 18 months.[31] The overall poor positive and negative predictive value of the postcoital test severely limits its clinical utility.

Although abnormal postcoital test results should be viewed with some skepticism, a normal study is helpful. It confirms that coital technique is appropriate and is associated with a more favorable prognosis.

Sperm antibody testing may be indicated when the sperm are nonmotile or demonstrate shaking movement without forward progression and when significant sperm agglutination has been observed in multiple semen specimens after infection has been excluded. Sperm agglutinating and immobilizing antibodies have been identified, and a diverse literature exists regarding their role in infertility. An association appears to exist between the presence of serum agglutinating antibodies and infertility in men, but a similar association does not appear to exist in women.[32] Sperm immobilizing antibodies in the serum and cervical mucus of infertile women also may be a reliable marker, because they are rarely detected in fertile controls.[33,34] An immunobead-binding assay may provide a semiquantitative means of assessing and localizing antibodies on the sperm.[35,36] The value and current role of sperm antibody testing remain controversial, because no specific antigen associated with immunologic infertility has been identified. Antibody-mediated infertility probably occurs in <1% of the infertile population.[37]

## EVALUATION OF THE PERITONEAL FACTOR

Laparoscopy is performed to assess possible peritoneal causes of infertility in patients in whom no cause of infertility is established by an otherwise comprehensive evaluation and to determine the feasibility of tubal reconstructive surgery or in vitro fertilization in patients in whom tubal disease is suspected by history, physical examination, or hysterosalpingogram. In one study, unanticipated pelvic pathology was encountered in 79% of patients undergoing laparoscopy for infertility evaluation; most reports describe abnormalities in at least 30% of cases.[38] Conversely, 37% of patients in whom tubal disease was suggested by hysterosalpingogram were found to have normal fallopian tubes at laparoscopy.[39] The diagnostic and therapeutic benefits of laparoscopy are well documented, and it has replaced culdoscopy and laparotomy in the direct assessment and treatment of the pelvic cavity.

## TREATMENT OF THE INFERTILE COUPLE

### TREATMENT OF OVULATORY DYSFUNCTION

After ovulatory dysfunction is established, treatment should begin. Some specialists recommend the use of simple means of inducing ovulation (e.g., clomiphene citrate) for 3 to 4 months before the completion of the infertility evaluation in an effort to save the couple effort and expense. However, because of the high incidence of multiple causes for infertility and the paradoxical potential of clomiphene to induce other causes of infertility (e.g., hostile cervical mucus, endometrial abnormalities, detrimental effects on oocyte maturation), the rationality of such an approach is unclear[40] (see Chap. 97).

Patients who ovulate with therapy but do not conceive should be reevaluated periodically to determine whether any other cause for the infertility exists. Individuals who become anovulatory after an initially favorable response also should be evaluated to exclude incipient thyroid disease and ovarian failure.

### SURGICAL TREATMENT

Significant uterine and tubal abnormalities usually necessitate surgical intervention. Many patients with uterine abnormalities such as fibroids and müllerian anomalies do not require surgery, and such surgery more often is considered for patients who have multiple pregnancy losses. The decision to proceed with tubal surgery is predicated on information obtained from a comprehensive infertility evaluation. Success rates for tubal patency range from 0% to 70%, depending on the location and the extent of disease and the presence of other infertility factors. For the

**TABLE 103-2.**
**Assisted Reproductive Technologies**

FERTILITY DRUGS
  Clomiphene citrate
  Gonadotropins
ARTIFICIAL INSEMINATION
  Intrauterine insemination
  Therapeutic donor insemination
ASSISTED REPRODUCTIVE TECHNIQUES
  In vitro fertilization–embryo transfer (IVF-ET)
  Gamete intrafallopian transfer (GIFT)
  Zygote intrafallopian transfer (ZIFT)
  Intracytoplasmic sperm injection (ICSI)
  Frozen embryo transfer (FET)

most common form of tubal factor infertility, distal tubal damage, the chance of successful pregnancy after surgery is 20% to 30%. For this reason, many patients now elect to proceed with in vitro fertilization, which yields a higher pregnancy rate (30% to 50%), rather than undergo tubal surgery. Significant predictive information usually can be obtained at diagnostic laparoscopy, and after this procedure, a more accurate appraisal of the prognosis and risks can be presented to the patient.

Significant improvements in atraumatic surgical technique, including the use of magnification, nonreactive suture material, and adhesion-inhibiting substances, have enhanced fertility potential compared with the macrosurgical methods used before 1970. However, many patients with extensive tubal destruction cannot be helped by reparative pelvic surgery. The advent of in vitro fertilization has been beneficial to these individuals.

## ASSISTED REPRODUCTIVE TECHNOLOGIES

ART includes techniques in which the ovaries are stimulated with fertility drugs and at the time of ovulation the sperm is introduced into the uterine cavity through a small catheter. This technique is called *superovulation with intrauterine insemination (IUI)* or *therapeutic donor insemination (TDI)* when donor sperm is used. More advanced reproductive techniques include those in which the oocytes are surgically aspirated from the ovary through a needle directed by transvaginal ultrasonography or at laparoscopy. These techniques include *in vitro fertilization (IVF), gamete intrafallopian transfer (GIFT),* and *zygote intrafallopian transfer (ZIFT)* (Table 103-2). The techniques have not been compared in a prospective, randomized fashion. Success rates with the different techniques vary widely among institutions.[41] IVF and *embryo transfer (ET)* technology has spawned several innovative approaches to the treatment of infertility. IVF and ET are the most successful ARTs, with pregnancy rates around 50% to 60% per cycle, and are most appropriate for patients with irreparable tubal damage, infertility attributed to the male factor, endometriosis, refractory ovulatory dysfunction, and idiopathic infertility.

The technique consists of inducing multiple follicles to develop by administering gonadotropins with or without gonadotropin-releasing hormone agonist therapy to prevent premature luteinizing hormone surge. Thirty-six hours after human chorionic gonadotropin administration, the ova are harvested by transvaginal ultrasonography-guided needle aspiration. Sperm from a fresh ejaculate, electroejaculation, or direct testicular aspiration are added to the oocytes, and they are incubated for fertilization to occur. In cases of male factor infertility, the fertilization of the ova can be performed with the direct injection of a single sperm into the cytoplasm. This technique is known as *intracytoplasmic sperm injection (ICSI).*[41a] Embryo transfer is usually accomplished 48 or 72 hours after oocyte retrieval and fertilization. Embryos not transferred at this time can be safely frozen and used in a later attempt.

In vivo embryos have usually developed to the morula or blastocyst stage when they appear in the uterus after spontaneous conception.[42] This knowledge and the use of special culture systems that allow the embryos to grow to a blastocyst stage over 5 or 6 days has enabled come investigators to achieve higher implantation and pregnancy rates and lower multiple gestation rates by transferring fewer embryos back to the uterus at this later stage.

GIFT is similar to IVF and ET in that ovulation-inducing agents are used to induce multiple follicles to develop, and the ova are then aspirated through the laparoscope, at laparotomy, or vaginally under ultrasonography guidance.[44] However, GIFT differs from IVF and ET in that normal oviducts are obligatory. The harvested oocytes and sperm are injected into the distal tubal ampulla through a small cannula, and fertilization occurs spontaneously within the fallopian tube. The resulting embryos are transferred to the uterus by the oviduct. This technique overcomes a potential failure of ovarian capture by the fallopian tube and may accomplish pregnancy rates on the order of 25% to 30% in patients with long-term idiopathic infertility or mild endometriosis, and perhaps in some couples with male factor infertility. These patients must have intact fallopian tubes, but the opportunity to confirm that fertilization has occurred is lost.

Other investigators have transferred embryos obtained from a donor's uterus before implantation to the uterus of another woman.[45] Fertilization in these situations is accomplished by artificial insemination using semen from the infertile woman's partner. This technique has been used successfully in women with ovarian failure who underwent treatment with estrogen and progesterone to prepare the endometrium before embryo transfer.[46] Several additional permutations of these techniques have been performed using semen donors and surrogate mothers for unique situations.

The empiric use of gonadotropin therapy and intrauterine insemination for idiopathic infertility has yielded success rates similar to those reported for GIFT. This approach has the advantages of being less expensive and less invasive than GIFT or IVF.

In November 1996, the Society of Assisted Reproductive Technology (SART) reported the 1994 registry data from the 249 centers offering ART in the United States, showing an overall live delivery rate per retrieval of 20.7% for IVF (33,700 retrievals), 28.4% for GIFT (4214 retrievals); and 29.1% for ZIFT (926 retrievals). Individual centers with superb in vitro fertilization laboratories are currently reporting pregnancy rates on the order of 66% for IVF/ET in specific patient populations in contrast to the 35% pregnancy rate for procedures such as GIFT or ZIFT.

## TREATMENT OF ENDOMETRIOSIS

The management of endometriosis has undergone significant change (see Chap. 98). Many infertile women with endometriosis conceive spontaneously within 1 year of diagnosis made by laparoscopy.[47] The use of laparoscopic resection or ablation of minimal to mild endometriosis enhances the fecundity of infertile women.[12] Hormonal suppressive therapy, including the use of gonadotropin-releasing hormone analogs and danazol, is not effective therapy for infertility, although it is effective treatment for pelvic pain associated with endometriosis. Patients with persistent infertility associated with endometriosis have the best chance of conceiving through the use of one of the ARTs or through superovulation therapy after the ablation or surgical removal of the endometriosis implants.

## TREATMENT OF CERVICAL ABNORMALITIES

Treatment of cervical factor infertility generally has proved unsatisfactory, except for eradication of cervicitis with antibiotics and, in selected cases, intrauterine inseminations. Therapy for immunologic infertility has included condom use for 6 months, followed by unprotected intercourse at midcycle. Other approaches are high-dose glucocorticoid suppression (i.e., 96 mg of methylprednisolone daily for 7 days) and intrauterine inseminations using washed semen in the hope of separating antibodies from the sperm and bypassing potential antibodies in the endocervix.[48] None of these regimens, except for intrauterine inseminations,[49] is documented to be effective.

## REFERENCES

1. Mosher WD, Pratt WF. Fecundity and infertility in the United States 1965–1988. Advance data from vital and health statistics, no. 192. Hyattsville, MD: Public Health Services, 1990. DHHS publication no. (PHS)91-1250.
2. Jones HW, Toner JP. The infertile couple. N Engl J Med 1993; 329:1710.
3. MacLeod J, Gold RZ. The male factor in fertility and infertility VI: semen quality and certain other factors in relation to ease of conception. Fertil Steril 1953; 4:10.
4. Chang MC. Fertilizing capacity of spermatozoa deposited into the fallopian tubes. Nature 1951; 168:697.
5. Stambaugh R, Buckley J. Zona pellucida dissolution enzymes of the rabbit sperm head. Science 1968; 161:585.
6. Settlage DSF, Motoshima M, Tredway DR. Sperm transport from the external cervical os to the fallopian tubes in women: a time and quantitation study. Fertil Steril 1973; 24:655.
7. Beer AE, Neaves WB. Antigenic status of semen from the viewpoint of the female and male. Fertil Steril 1978; 29:3.
8. Mathus S, Baker ER, Williamson HO, et al. Clinical significance of sperm antibodies in fertility. Fertil Steril 1981; 36:486.
9. Farner-Brown G, Beilby JO, Tarbit MH. Venous changes in the endometrium of myomatous uteri. Obstet Gynecol 1971; 38:743.
10. Henry-Suchet J, Utzman C, De Brux J, et al. Microbiologic study of chronic inflammation associated with tubal factor infertility: role of *Chlamydia trachomatis*. Fertil Steril 1987; 47:274.
11. Surrey ES, Halme J. Endometriosis as a cause of infertility. Obstet Gynecol Clin North Am 1989; 16:79.
11a. Abu JI, Konje JC. Leukotrienes in gynaecology: the hypothetical value of anti-leukotriene therapy in dysmenorrhea and endometriosis. Hum Reprod Update 2000; 6:200.
12. Maraacoux S, Maheux R, Berube S, and the Canadian Collaborative Group on Endometriosis. Laparoscopic surgery in the infertile woman with minimal or mild endometriosis. N Engl J Med 1997; 337:217.
12a. Maruyama M, Osuga Y, Momoeda M, et al. Pregnancy rates after laparoscopic treatment. Differences related to tubal status and presence of endometriosis. J Reprod Med 2000; 45:89
13. Rommer JJ. Sterility: its cause and its treatment. Springfield, IL: Charles C Thomas, 1952:271.
14. Dawood MY. Corpus luteal insufficiency. Curr Opin Obstet Gynecol 1994; 6:21.
15. Bauman JE. Basal body temperature: unreliable method of ovulation detection. Fertil Steril 1981; 36:729.
16. Abraham GE, Maroulis GB, Marshall JR. Evaluation of ovulation and corpus luteum function using measurement of plasma progesterone. Obstet Gynecol 1974; 44:522.
17. Noyes RW, Hertig A, Rock J. Dating the endometrial biopsy. Fertil Steril 1950; 1:30.
18. Daly DC, Maslar IA, Rosenberg SM, et al. Prolactin production by luteal phase defect endometrium. Am J Obstet Gynecol 1981; 140:587.
19. Chatterton RT Jr, Haan JN, Jenco JM, et al. Radioimmunoassay of pregnanediol concentration in early morning urine specimens for assessment of luteal function in women. Fertil Steril 1982; 37:361.
20. Israel SL. Diagnosis and treatment of menstrual disorders and sterility, 5th ed. New York: Hoeber Medical Division, Harper & Row, 1967:492.
21. Jones EE. Hyperprolactinemia and female infertility. J Reprod Med 1989; 34:117.
22. Scott RT, Toner JP, Muasher SJ, et al. Follicle-stimulating hormone levels on cycle day 3 are predictive of in vitro fertilization outcome. Fertil Steril 1989; 51:651.
23. Soules MR, Spadoni LR. Oil versus aqueous media for hysterosalpingography: a continuing debate based on many opinions and few facts. Fertil Steril 1982; 38:1.
24. Kruger TF, Menkveld R, Stander FSH, et al. Sperm morphologic features as a prognostic factor in in vitro fertilization. Fertil Steril 1986; 46:1118.
25. Oehninger S, Toner J, Muausher SJ, et al. Prediction of fertilization in vitro with human gametes: is there a litmus test? Am J Obstet Gynecol 1992; 167:1760.
26. Oehninger S, Acosta AA, Veeck LL, et al. Recurrent failure of in vitro fertilization: role of the hemizona assay in the sequential diagnosis of specific sperm-oocyte defects. Am J Obstet Gynecol 1991; 164:1210.
27. Jette NT, Glass RH. Prognostic value of the post-coital test. Fertil Steril 1972; 23:29.
28. Keel BA, Webster BW. Correlation of human sperm mobility characteristics with an in vitro cervical mucus penetration test. Fertil Steril 1988; 49:138.
29. Kovacs GT, Newman GB, Hanson GL. The post-coital test: what is normal? BMJ 1978; 1:818.
30. Asch RH. Laparoscopic recovery of sperm from peritoneal fluid in patients with negative or poor Sims-Huhner test. Fertil Steril 1976; 27:1111.
31. Collins JA, So Y, Wilson EH, et al. The postcoital test as a predictor of pregnancy among 355 infertile couples. Fertil Steril 1984; 41:703.
32. Rumke P, Van Amstel N, Messer EN, et al. Prognosis of fertility of men with sperm agglutinins in the serum. Fertil Steril 1974; 25:393.
33. Isojima S, Li T, Ashitaka Y. Immunologic analysis of sperm immobilizing factor found in sera of women with unexplained sterility. Am J Obstet Gynecol 1968; 101:677.
34. Witkin SS, David SS. Effect of sperm antibodies on pregnancy outcome in a subfertile population. Am J Obstet Gynecol 1988; 158:59.
35. Bronson RA, Cooper GW, Rosenfeld DL. Autoimmunity to spermatozoa: effect on sperm penetration of cervical mucus as reflected by postcoital testing. Fertil Steril 1984; 41:609.
36. Mandelbaum SL, Diamond MP, DeCherney AH. The impact of anti-sperm antibodies on human infertility. J Urol 1987; 138:1.
37. Haas GG Jr. Female immunologic factor. In: Garcia C-R, Mastroianni L Jr, Amelar RD, et al., eds. Current therapy of infertility, 1982–1983. Trenton, NJ: BC Decker, 1982:179.
38. Drake TS, Grunert GM. The unsuspected pelvic factor in the infertility investigation. Fertil Steril 1980; 34:27.
39. Musich JR, Behrmann SJ. Infertility laparoscopy in perspective: review of five hundred cases. Am J Obstet Gynecol 1982; 143:292.
40. Seibel MM, Smith DM. The effect of clomiphene citrate on human preovulatory oocyte maturation in vivo. J In Vitro Fertil Embryo Transfer 1989; 6:1.
41. Bouckert A, Psalti I, Loumaye E, et al. The probability of a successful treatment of infertility by in vitro fertilization. Hum Reprod 1994; 9:448.
41a. Bukulmez O, Yerali H, Yucel A, et al. Intracytoplasmic sperm injection versus in vitro fertilization for patients with a tubal factor as their sole cause of infertility: a prospective, randomized trial. Fertil Steril 1999; 73:38.
42. Croxatto HB, Fuentealba B, Diaz S, et al. A simple nonsurgical technique to obtain unimplanted eggs from human uteri. Am J Obstet Gynecol 1972; 112:662.
43. Jones GM, Trounson AL, Gardner DK, et al. Evolution of a culture protocol for successful blastocyst development and pregnancy. Hum Reprod 1998; 13:169.
44. Asch RH, Balmaceda JP, Ellsworth LR, et al. Gamete intra-fallopian transfer (GIFT): a new treatment for infertility. Int J Fertil 1985; 30:41.
45. Bustillo M, Busler JE, Freeman AG, et al. Nonsurgical ovum transfer as a treatment for intractable infertility: what effectiveness can we realistically expect? Am J Obstet Gynecol 1984; 149:371.
46. Lutjen P, Trounson A, Leeton J, et al. The establishment and maintenance of a pregnancy using in vitro fertilization and embryo donation in a patient with primary ovarian failure. Nature 1985; 307:174.
47. Schenken RS, Malinak LR. Conservative surgery versus expectant management for the infertile patient with mild endometriosis. Fertil Steril 1982; 37:183.
48. Shulman S, Harlin B, Davis P, et al. Immune infertility and new approaches to treatment. Fertil Steril 1978; 29:309.
49. Brasch JG, Rawlins R, Tarchalas S, Radwanska E. The relationship between total motile sperm count and success of intrauterine insemination. Fertil Steril 1994; 62:150.

# CHAPTER 104

# FEMALE CONTRACEPTION

ALISA B. GOLDBERG AND PHILIP DARNEY

## USE OF CONTRACEPTIVE METHODS

A worldwide revolution occurred in the early 1960s with the introduction of oral and intrauterine contraception. Use of these methods accounts for up to one-third of the subsequent decline in birth rate.

Fertility rates are a measure of timing and numbers of births as well as the population's preference for family size and acceptance of contraception. The U.S. fertility rate was at its peak (127 per 1000) in 1910, descended during the economic depression (89 per 1000 women), and then began an upward trend after World War II. By 1960, the rate was almost as high as it had been 50 years earlier (118 per 1000 women). The 1960s witnessed not only the introduction of modern contraceptive technologies but also a marked expansion in women's economic and social opportunities, resulting in preferences for childbearing at older ages and for smaller families. These societal changes, along with scientific advances, made possible the development of new methods of birth control.

As of 1995, ~39 million U.S. women 15 to 44 years of age (64%) were using some method of contraception. This total is

**TABLE 104-1.**
**Contraceptive Choices Among 39 Million U.S. Women Aged 15 to 44 Using Contraception**

| Method | Distribution (%) |
|---|---|
| Sterilization | |
| Female | 28 |
| Male | 11 |
| Oral contraception | 27 |
| Condoms | 20 |
| Injectable contraceptives (Depo-Provera) | 3 |
| Diaphragm | 1.9 |
| Implantable contraceptives (Norplant) | 1.4 |
| Intrauterine device | 0.8 |

(From Piccinino LJ, Mosher WD. Trends in contraceptive use in the United States: 1982–1995. Fam Plann Perspect 1998; 30:4–10,46.)

**TABLE 104-2.**
**Effectiveness of Various Contraceptive Methods During the First Year of Use**

| Method | Women Experiencing Unintended Pregnancy (%) | | Women Continuing Use at One Year (%) |
|---|---|---|---|
| | Typical Use | Perfect Use | |
| No method | 85 | 85 | |
| Oral contraception | 5 | | |
| Combined pills | | 0.1 | |
| Progestin-only pills | | 0.5 | |
| Depo-Provera | 0.3 | 0.3 | 70 |
| Norplant | 0.05 | 0.05 | 88 |
| Sterilization | | | |
| Female | 0.5 | 0.5 | 100 |
| Male | 0.15 | 0.10 | 100 |
| Intrauterine device | | | |
| Copper T380A | 0.8 | 0.6 | 78 |
| Progesterone T | 2.0 | 1.5 | 81 |
| Condoms (no spermicide) | | | |
| Male | 14 | 3 | 61 |
| Female | 21 | 5 | 56 |
| Diaphragm (with spermicide) | 20 | 6 | 56 |
| Cap (with spermicide) | | | |
| Parous | 40 | 26 | 42 |
| Nulliparous | 20 | 9 | 56 |
| Spermicides | 26 | 6 | 40 |
| Withdrawal | 19 | 4 | |
| Periodic abstinence | 25 | | 63 |
| Calendar | | 9 | |
| Ovulation method | | 3 | |
| Symptothermal | | 2 | |
| Postovulation | | 1 | |

(From Trussell J, Kowal D. The essentials of contraception. In: Hatcher RA, et al. Contraceptive technology, 17th ed. New York: Ardent Media, 1998:216.)

up from ~30 million users (56%) in 1982. Of the 36% not using contraception, 5% were at risk of unintended pregnancy (the remainder were either pregnant, trying to get pregnant, sterile for noncontraceptive reasons, or not sexually active).[1]

In the United States, *female sterilization* is currently the most common form of contraception, providing birth control to ~11 million women (28%).[1,1a] *Male sterilization* provides contraception for an additional 4 million couples (11%).[1] The *oral contraceptive pill* is the second most popular method with 10.4 million users (27%).[1] *Condom* use accounts for 20% of contraception, increasing significantly from 12% in 1982.[1] As of 1995, ~1.1 million women used *injectable contraception*, and 0.5 million women used *implants*.[1] Approximately 2 million women were using an *intrauterine device* (IUD) in 1982, but by 1995 IUD use had declined to <1 million[1] (Table 104-1). (Outside of the United States, the IUD continues to be very popular, with an estimated 90 million users worldwide.)

## CONTRACEPTIVE SELECTION

No contraceptive method is fully effective in preventing pregnancy, free of side effects, and acceptable to all couples. Every method has advantages and disadvantages. The best contraceptive choice is usually the method that can be used consistently.

*Contraceptive effectiveness* is measured by life tables that determine the probability of pregnancy in a given interval with the use of that method. *Failure rates* also have been expressed by a mathematical formula (Pearl index) that describes the number of pregnancies per 100 woman-years of use. *Theoretical effectiveness* is measured as failure rates in highly motivated study populations and represents failures in clinical trials with perfect use. *Use effectiveness* reflects failure rates with typical use and is always lower (i.e., more failures) than theoretical effectiveness.

Table 104-2 shows perfect and typical use effectiveness of the most common contraceptive methods during the first year of use. The percentages given are estimates from the means of many studies.[2] With long-term use, failure rates usually decline. A couple's motivation to avoid an unintended pregnancy also determines efficacy. For example, women who want no more children are better contraceptors than women who are delaying pregnancy.

## CONTRACEPTIVE COUNSELING

Couples differ socially, culturally, educationally, and economically as well as in their ages, lifestyles, and desires concerning family size. These individual differences make it imperative for clinicians to be informed about all methods of fertility control

so that they can help women reach the best decision by offering accurate and unbiased information.

When a woman presents for contraceptive counseling, the clinician should first ascertain whether she has completed her childbearing. If not, the clinician should determine whether she plans to try to conceive in the near or distant future. For women who desire future fertility, sterilization is not an option. For women hoping to conceive within a year or two, long-acting methods of contraception like depot medroxyprogesterone acetate (DMPA) may not be ideal. Next, the woman's risk for acquiring sexually transmitted infections (STIs) should be assessed; if her sexual practices place her at risk, she would not be a good candidate for an IUD and should be counseled to use condoms for disease prevention. Previously used methods should be discussed to determine which side effects were acceptable and which were intolerable. When helping the woman to choose a method, the clinician should address common side effects in advance and discuss the temporary and reversible nature of most common, minor side effects. For example, the nausea that is sometimes associated with combined oral contraceptive use often resolves after a few months, and the irregular bleeding associated with DMPA use is not harmful and is reversible.

Once a woman has made an informed decision and chosen a particular contraceptive method, she should receive clear, concise instructions on how to use that method. Any potential barriers to her continued successful use of the method should be eliminated. Her questions should be addressed, a follow-up evaluation should be scheduled, and she should receive the name and telephone number of a person she can contact if further questions or problems arise.

## HORMONAL CONTRACEPTION

### COMBINATION ORAL CONTRACEPTIVES

Combined oral contraceptive pills (COCs) contain various doses of synthetic estrogen (ethinyl estradiol or mestranol) and a synthetic progestin. All the synthetic estrogens and progestins used in oral contraceptives have an *ethinyl group on the 17 position* that enhances their oral activity by slowing hydroxylation and conjugation in the liver[3,4] (Fig. 104-1).

Table 104-3 lists all oral contraceptives (except some generic forms) currently marketed in the United States, ranked according to the dose of estrogen. *Low-dose COCs* contain <50 μg of estrogen and are the primary choice for oral contraception. COCs containing ≥50 μg of estrogen should *no longer* be routinely used for contraception. *Variable-dose* products are either biphasic or triphasic, depending on the number of dose regimens in a cycle, and are all low dose.

The introduction of the new progestins—desogestrel, norgestimate, dienogest, and gestodene (the latter two are not sold in the United States)—has created a new classification system for COCs. Pills containing ≥50 μg of estrogen are called "first-generation" COCs; COCs containing <50 μg of estrogen and any of the older progestins are termed "second generation"; and low-dose COCs containing the new progestins—desogestrel, dienogest, gestodene, and norgestimate—are called "third-generation" COCs. Classifying low-dose COCs by the androgenic effects of their progestins is clinically more useful than the "generational" approach[5]; the newest progestins (desogestrel, dienogest, gestodene, and norgestimate) are less androgenic than other progestins. (For an explanation, see later section on the noncontraceptive benefits of COCs.)

### MECHANISM OF ACTION

The progestin component is primarily responsible for the contraceptive effect of COCs. Synthetic progestins inhibit the midcycle luteinizing hormone (LH) surge, thereby suppressing ovulation. Progestins also cause changes in cervical mucus that retard sperm penetration and inhibit conception. Progestins alter the motility of the uterus and the fallopian tubes, hindering conception by altering the transport of sperm and ova. Progestins also affect glycogen production by the endometrium and ovarian steroidogenesis; whether this mechanism of action contributes to the contraceptive effect of progestins is unknown.

The estrogen component of COCs inhibits follicle-stimulating hormone (FSH), preventing the selection of a dominant follicle. It also potentiates the effects of the progestin, probably on an intracellular level, allowing use of a lower dose of progestin. Finally, the estrogen component of COCs provides stability to the endometrial lining and prevents the irregular bleeding that progestins provoke when used alone.

### USE OF COMBINED ORAL CONTRACEPTIVES

Table 104-4 lists for COCs the absolute and relative contraindications that have evolved over 30 years of experience with the pill. These contraindications are related primarily to the estrogen component of COCs. Much of the epidemiologic and physiologic evidence supporting these contraindications was obtained from the evaluation of COCs containing ≥50 μg of estrogen. Consequently, with the use of smaller doses of estrogen (and of progestin), several contraindications considered absolute for high-dose COCs are only relative contraindications with the lower-dose products.

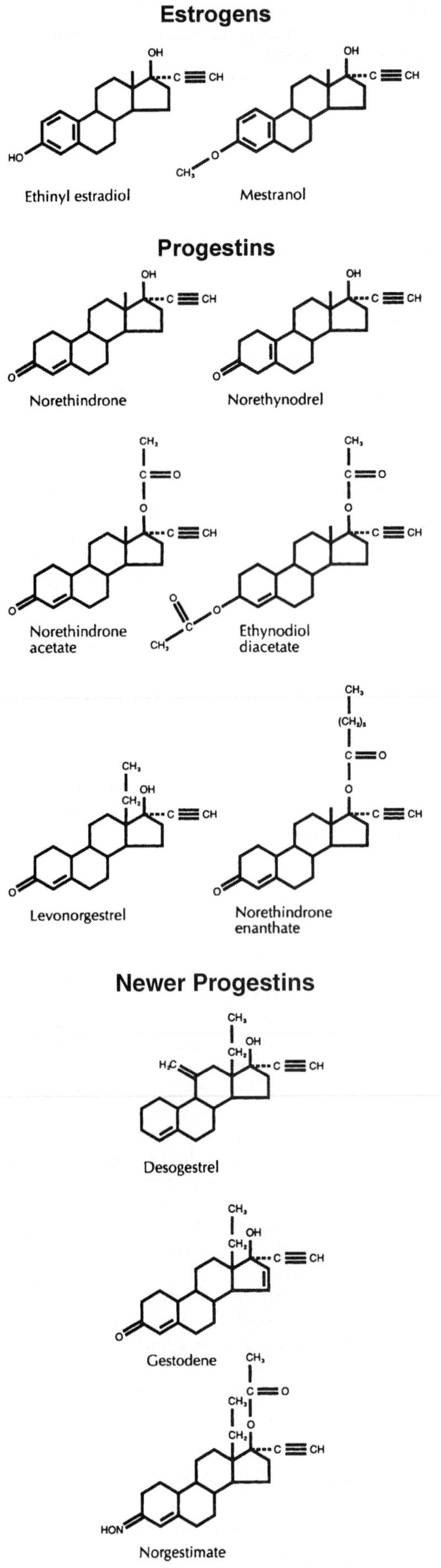

**FIGURE 104-1.** The biochemical structures of synthetic estrogens and progestins.

**TABLE 104-3.**
**Oral Contraceptives Available in the United States**

| Brand Name | Manufacturer | Estrogen | Dose (μg) | Progestin | Dose (mg) |
|---|---|---|---|---|---|
| **MONOPHASIC PILLS** | | | | | |
| *Containing 20 μg estrogen* | | | | | |
| Loestrin 1/20 | Parke-Davis | EE | 20 | NETA | 1.0 |
| Alesse | Wyeth-Ayerst | EE | 20 | LNG | 0.1 |
| Levlite | Berlex | EE | 20 | LNG | 0.1 |
| *Containing 30 μg estrogen* | | | | | |
| Loestrin 1/30 | Parke-Davis | EE | 30 | NETA | 1.5 |
| Nordette-21 | Wyeth-Ayerst | EE | 30 | LNG | 0.15 |
| Lo/Ovral | Wyeth-Ayerst | EE | 30 | NG | 0.3 |
| Ortho-Cept | Ortho | EE | 30 | DESO | 0.15 |
| Levlen | Berlex | EE | 30 | LNG | 0.15 |
| Desogen | Organon | EE | 30 | DESO | 0.15 |
| *Containing 35 μg estrogen* | | | | | |
| Ovcon 35 | Mead Johnson | EE | 35 | NET | 0.4 |
| Modicon | Ortho | EE | 35 | NET | 0.5 |
| Ortho-Novum 1/35 | Ortho | EE | 35 | NET | 1.0 |
| Ortho-Cyclen | Ortho | EE | 35 | NORG | 0.25 |
| Demulen | Searle | EE | 35 | EDDA | 1.0 |
| Norethin | Searle | EE | 35 | NET | 1.0 |
| Brevicon | Watson | EE | 35 | NET | 0.5 |
| Norinyl | Watson | EE | 35 | NET | 1.0 |
| *Containing 50 μg estrogen* | | | | | |
| Ovral | Wyeth-Ayerst | EE | 50 | NG | 0.5 |
| Ortho-Novum 1/50 | Ortho | ME | 50 | NET | 1.0 |
| Demulen 1/50 | Searle | EE | 50 | EDDA | 1.0 |
| Ovcon 50 | Mead Johnson | EE | 50 | NET | 1.0 |
| Norethin | Searle | EE | 50 | NET | 1.0 |
| Norinyl 1/50 | Watson | ME | 50 | NET | 1.0 |
| **PHASIC PILLS** | | | | | |
| Ortho-Novum 10/11 | Ortho | EE | 35 | NET | 0.5, 1.0 |
| Jenest | Organon | EE | 35 | NET | 0.5, 1.0 |
| Ortho-Novum 7/7/7 | Ortho | EE | 35 | NET | 0.5, 0.75, 1.0 |
| Ortho Tri-Cyclen | Ortho | EE | 35 | NORG | 0.18, 0.215, 0.25 |
| Tri-Norinyl | Searle | EE | 35 | NET | 0.5, 1.0, 0.5 |
| Mircette | Organon | EE | 20, 10* | DESO | 0.15 |
| Estrostep | Parke-Davis | EE | 20, 30, 35 | NETA | 0.10 |
| Triphasil | Wyeth-Ayerst | EE | 30, 40, 30 | LNG | 0.05, 0.075, 0.125 |
| Tri-Levlen | Berlex | EE | 30, 40, 30 | LNG | 0.05, 0.075, 0.125 |
| **PROGESTIN-ONLY PILLS** | | | | | |
| Micronor | Ortho | | | NET | 0.35 |
| Ovrette | Wyeth-Ayerst | | | NG | 0.075 |
| Nor-Q.D. | Watson | | | NET | 0.35 |

*EE*, ethinyl estradiol; *ME*, mestranol; *NETA*, norethindrone acetate; *LNG*, levonorgestrel; *NG*, norgestrel; *DESO*, desogestrel; *NET*, norethindrone; *NORG*, norgestimate; *EDDA*, ethynodiol diacetate.
*The 10-μg pills in Mircette are taken days 25–28.

The clinician should prescribe the lowest dose of estrogen and progestin consistent with high efficacy and few side effects. Only low-dose COCs (<50 μg of estrogen) should be prescribed routinely for contraception. When starting a woman on low-dose COCs, the clinician should consider whether she would benefit from low androgenic activity in the progestin component. Pills containing desogestrel or norgestimate are a good first choice for a woman who may be hyperandrogenic.[5] Other women may benefit from a COC with the lowest possible dose of estrogen. A woman who has successfully used a particular low-dose pill in the past should resume its use unless her health has changed.

Products containing 50 μg of estrogen are generally reserved for women who are taking a medication known to increase the metabolism, and, therefore, to decrease the efficacy of estrogen (i.e., barbiturates, phenytoin, carbamazepine, rifampin). The 50-μg pills are also used for emergency contraception (see later) and for the acute treatment of menorrhagia. Women taking pills containing 50 μg of estrogen for routine contraception should be switched to a low-dose pill; pills containing >50 μg of estrogen cause more side effects and are no more effective than lower dose pills. Moreover, most pharmaceutical companies have stopped selling high-dose pills for routine contraception.

## PILL TAKING AND MISSED PILLS

Combination oral contraceptives are taken for 21 days of the cycle, starting on day 1 of the menses or the first Sunday after the onset of menses. The 21 days of hormonally active pills are followed by 1 week without medication during which withdrawal bleeding occurs. Many preparations contain 21 active pills and 7 placebos for an easy-to-remember 28-day cycle.

**TABLE 104-4.**
**Contraindications to Combined Oral Contraceptive Use**

**ABSOLUTE**

*Presence or history of:*

Thromboembolic disease

Vascular disease

Thrombophlebitis

Cerebrovascular accident

Coronary artery disease

Breast cancer

Hepatic adenoma

Abnormal genital bleeding of unknown cause

Uncontrolled hypertension

Migraine headaches with associated neurologic symptoms

*Presence of:*

Pregnancy

Active liver disease

Active gallbladder disease

Hyperlipidemia

Smoking and age 35 or older

**RELATIVE**

*Presence of:*

Seizure disorder

Sickle cell disease

Infectious mononucleosis

Retinal vascular lesions

Initiation of breast-feeding

Smoking

*History of:*

Migraine headaches without neurologic symptoms

Pancreatitis

Family history of idiopathic thromboembolic disease

---

Some preparations (Loestrin Fe 1/20 and 1.5/30) contain 75 mg of iron per day for 7 days in place of the placebos. One preparation (Mircette) replaces the last 5 placebo days with 10 µg of estrogen per day.

The pills should be started no later than day 5 of the menstrual cycle, because pills missed early in the cycle increase the risk of breakthrough ovulation and contraceptive failure. If one pill is omitted at any time during the cycle, it should be taken as soon as remembered. Some vaginal bleeding may occur, but no backup method is necessary. If two pills are missed within the first two weeks of the cycle, then once the omission is remembered, two pills per day should be taken for 2 days. An additional method of contraception, such as a barrier method, should be used for 7 days and the rest of the pill cycle should be completed. If two pills are missed within the third week of the cycle by a woman who started her COCs on day 1 of her menses, she should start a new pack as soon as possible and use backup contraception for 7 days. If 2 pills are missed in the third week of the cycle by a woman who was a Sunday starter, she should continue taking the current pills until the next Sunday and then start a new package; she should also use backup contraception for 7 days. If three or more pills are missed at any time, a backup method should be started immediately and continued for 7 days. If the woman prefers not to have menses on weekends, she should continue the current pack until the next Sunday and then start the new pack. If the timing of menses is not a concern, or coordinating a Sunday start is too confusing, she should simply start a new package of pills immediately.

After women answer questions about possible contraindications to COCs and are given a baseline blood pressure check and screening physical examination, they may be prescribed pills. Within 3 months of beginning pill use, women should have their blood pressure and weight measured. Patients using oral contraceptives should be seen by a clinician once or twice a year, and at this visit a routine physical examination including abdominal, breast, and pelvic examinations should be performed.

No reason exists for patients to take a break from COC use, except when pregnancy is desired or a serious complication develops. The ability to conceive after discontinuing oral contraceptive use is not impaired.[6] In *nonsmoking* women, COC use can be continued until menopause.

## MINOR SIDE EFFECTS

The incidence of minor side effects varies significantly from one report to another. Nausea or vomiting is related to the dose of estrogen, is much reduced when products containing <50 µg of estrogen are used, and usually abates after 3 months of use. Management includes reassuring the patient, instructing the patient to take the pill at bedtime and to eat just before swallowing the pill, or, finally, changing to the lowest estrogen dose COC available (20 µg).

The most common pill-related side effect is breakthrough bleeding; it usually results from the inability of the hormones to maintain the endometrium for the full 21-day course of therapy and improves after 2 or 3 months. Bleeding can also occur because of failure to take the pill at the same time each day or omission of the pill for 1 or 2 days. Switching to another low-dose product containing a different progestin or from a phased to a steady dose COC often improves breakthrough bleeding. Should these measures not prove effective, possible pathologic causes of the bleeding should be investigated.

Some women using COCs experience amenorrhea. Once pregnancy has been ruled out, the patient can be reassured that the occurrence of amenorrhea while on COCs is not harmful. If the patient desires monthly withdrawal bleeding, changing to a low-dose pill with a higher estrogen dose or one containing a less androgenic progestin is recommended.

Weight gain is an often-cited side effect of pill use and is often a reason for discontinuation. Despite claims that COCs cause weight gain, studies have been unable to document a significant increase in mean weight in COC users.[7] Some perceived weight gain may represent bloating or fluid retention rather than an anabolic effect. Also, women tend to gain weight with increasing age, and age-related weight gain may be blamed on COC use. Nonetheless, some women do experience weight gain attributable to COCs. If the weight gain cannot be controlled with diet and exercise and is unacceptable, an alternative form of contraception may be necessary.

Mood changes, including depression, lethargy, loss of libido, irritability, sleep disturbances, and changes in appetite, occur in ~5% of oral contraceptive users. The severity of these symptoms, and the acceptability of contraceptive alternatives, should help women and their clinicians decide whether discontinuation is necessary.

## SERIOUS SIDE EFFECTS

Adverse effects reported with the use of COCs include thromboembolic disorders, cerebrovascular disorders, myocardial infarction, optic neuritis, hepatic adenoma, cervical dysplasia and carcinoma, exacerbation of biliary colic and cholecystitis, decreased carbohydrate tolerance, hypertension, migraine or vascular headache, psychic depression, and chloasma. These potentially serious side effects are estrogen related and are rare. Complications of steroidal contraception are discussed in further detail in Chapter 105.

Many of these adverse effects were initially observed among women taking COCs containing ≥50 µg of estrogen and markedly higher doses of progestins than are used today. Studies of COCs containing ≥50 µg of estrogen showed an increased risk of venous thromboembolism, stroke, myocardial infarction, and hypertension.[8,9]

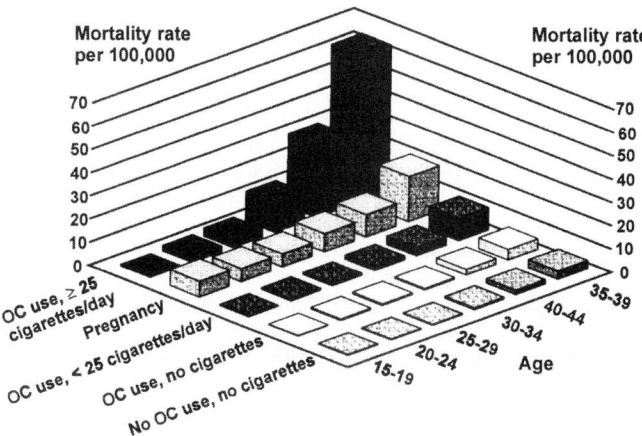

**FIGURE 104-2.** Estimated annual cardiovascular disease mortality rates per 100,000 women associated with oral contraceptive (*OC*) use, smoking, and pregnancy. (From Schwingl PJ, Ory HW, Visness CM. Estimates of the risk of cardiovascular death attributable to low-dose oral contraceptives in the United States. Am J Obstet Gynecol 1999; 180:241.)

Among healthy nonsmoking women, studies of low-dose COCs have shown an *increased risk of venous thromboembolic disease*, but no significantly increased risk of stroke, myocardial infarction, or hypertension.[8–12] In the long term, current and past COC users do not have an increased risk of mortality compared with those who never used COCs.[13]

*Smokers*, women with *genetic risk factors* (e.g., the factor V Leiden mutation), and those with medical problems that predispose them to *vasculopathies* are at higher risk than other subgroups.[14,15] Smoking appears to have a synergistic effect with COCs in increasing the risk of myocardial infarction, stroke, and venous thromboembolic disease.[16] This synergism has less impact on women aged younger than 35 years, whose overall risk for cardiovascular disease is extremely low. However, for women aged 35 years or older, the risk of dying from cardiovascular disease is 3.0 per 100,000 nonsmoking COC users; 10.0 per 100,000 smokers not using COCs; and 29.4 per 100,000 smokers using COCs[16] (Fig. 104-2). This level of risk is unacceptable; therefore, *COC use is contraindicated in smokers older than 35 years of age*. Among other high-risk populations, the use of COCs involves a fine balancing of benefit versus risk.[17]

### NONCONTRACEPTIVE BENEFITS OF ORAL CONTRACEPTIVE USE

Table 104-5 lists benefits to women using oral contraceptives. Some of these are well defined and may be of considerable significance to women's health.[18–30] Ovulation suppression by COCs causes regular menses, a decrease in menstrual flow, and a consequent protection against iron-deficiency anemia.[18] The use of COCs also has been shown to relieve premenstrual tension syndrome and improve dysmenorrhea.[18] Benign breast disease and ovarian and endometrial carcinoma are all less common in COC users.[21–23,25] COCs are the only known way to prevent ovarian cancer, aside from repeated pregnancy (see Chaps. 105 and 223).

Use of combined oral contraceptives has been shown to improve acne and hirsutism. The Food and Drug Administration (FDA) has approved the use of a triphasic pill containing norgestimate for the treatment of acne.[28] In particular, the new progestins have been shown to have a greater antiandrogenic effect than older progestins.

Given their biochemical similarity to testosterone, all progestins have both androgenic and antiandrogenic properties. Like testosterone, progestins decrease serum sex hormone–binding globulin (SHBG). A decrease in SHBG leads to more free testosterone and an androgenic effect. However, the estrogen component of COCs raises SHBG to a greater degree than

the progestin component lowers it. The overall effect of COCs is to raise SHBG. The new progestins (desogestrel, dienogest, gestodene, and norgestimate) counteract the estrogen-induced rise in SHBG less than older progestins and result in even higher levels of SHBG. Higher levels of SHBG are associated with lower levels of free testosterone and a decreased androgen effect. Progestins also compete with testosterone for the androgen receptor and for binding sites on SHBG. These latter biochemical actions are responsible for a proandrogenic effect, but usually are not large enough to overcome the estrogen-induced antiandrogenic effects of increasing SHBG.[32–34] In vivo, all COCs are predominantly antiandrogenic; however, expression of the androgenic/antiandrogenic biochemical properties of COCs varies among individuals.

### COMBINATION INJECTABLE CONTRACEPTIVES

Two combination estrogen-progestin monthly injectable contraceptives are in use around the world. Mesigna (norethisterone enanthate 50 mg and estradiol valerate 5 mg) and Lunelle or Cyclofem, formerly called Cyclo-Provera (medroxyprogesterone acetate 25 mg and estradiol cypionate 5 mg), are monthly combined injectable contraceptives. These injectable contraceptives have high contraceptive efficacy (0–0.4% failure rate in the first year of use) and are well tolerated.[35] They have similar

**TABLE 104-5.**
**Noncontraceptive Benefits of Oral Contraceptive Use**

| | Relative Risk or Odds Ratio (95% Confidence Interval) |
|---|---|
| **MENSTRUAL** | |
| Menstrual regulation | |
| Decreased dysmenorrhea[18] | |
| Relief of premenstrual tension syndrome | |
| Decreased menstrual flow[18] | |
| Decreased iron-deficiency anemia | |
| **PELVIC INFECTION** | |
| Decreased incidence of symptomatic pelvic inflammatory disease requiring hospitalization[19*†] | RR = 0.22 (0.08–0.64) |
| Decreased incidence of trichomonas vaginitis[20] | RR = 0.56 (0.39–0.81) |
| **BREAST** | |
| Decreased incidence of fibrocystic disease[21‡] | RR = 0.66 (0.4–0.9) |
| Decreased incidence of benign fibroadenomas[21‡] | RR = 0.35 (0.2–0.7) |
| **UTERUS** | |
| Decreased incidence of endometrial cancer[22,23§¶] | RR = 0.4 (0.3–0.6) |
| Decreased incidence of endometrial hyperplasia | |
| May decrease growth of uterine leiomyomas | |
| Decreased incidence of ectopic pregnancy[24] | RR = 0.19 (0.15–0.24) |
| **OVARY** | |
| Decreased incidence of ovarian cancer[25] | RR = 0.64 (0.6–0.7) |
| Decreased risk of death from ovarian cancer[13] | RR = 0.2 (0.1–0.8) |
| Decreased incidence of benign follicular cysts with high-dose COCs[26#] | RR = 0.24 (0.01–1.34) |
| **SKIN** | |
| Effective treatment for acne vulgaris[31] | RR = 0.44 (0.2–0.7) |
| Decreases hirsutism | |
| **MUSCULOSKELETAL** | |
| Decreased incidence of low bone mineral density in later life[29] | OR = 0.35 (0.2–0.5) |

*RR*, relative risk; *OR*, odds ratio; *COC*, combined oral contraceptive.
*May not be protective against subclinical endometritis.[30]
†Decreased incidence of tubal infertility not consistently found with COC use.[31]
‡Data from high-dose pills.[21]
§RR = 0.44 after 4 years, 0.33 after 8 years, and 0.28 after 12 years of use.[22]
¶Presented RR is for endometriod-type endometrial cancer.[23]
#Benefit does not appear to apply to low-dose COCs (RR = 1.3, 95% confidence interval = 0.5–3.6).[27]

contraindications and side effects as COCs but are associated with more irregular bleeding. Thus, most discontinuations in the first year of use have been due to irregular bleeding.[35]

## PROGESTIN-ONLY CONTRACEPTIVES

### PROGESTIN-ONLY ORAL CONTRACEPTIVES

Contraceptive pills that contain only a progestin are termed *minipills*. Worldwide, minipills are available containing norethindrone, norgestrel, levonorgestrel, lynestrenol, and ethynodiol diacetate. In the United States, only minipills containing norethindrone and levonorgestrel are available.

**Mechanism of Action.** Progestin-only minipills can inhibit ovulation, but not consistently. These agents primarily prevent conception by causing the formation of a thick, viscid cervical mucus that is impenetrable to sperm. They probably also increase the tubal transport time of gametes, allowing less opportunity for fertilization. The lack of consistent ovulation suppression leads to a higher failure rate with progestin-only oral contraceptives than with COCs. Progestins also cause atrophic-like changes of the endometrial lining that often result in irregular uterine bleeding.

**Use of Progestin-Only Pills.** Minipills are taken daily and continuously. The progestin-only minipill is less effective than combination oral contraceptives, and its efficacy is more reliant on regular pill taking. Minipills should be started on the first day of menses, and a backup method of contraception should be used for the first 7 days of use, as ovulation can occur. The minipill must be taken at the same time each day. A delay in pill-taking of >3 hours requires the use of a backup method for 2 days while continuing pill-taking.

The efficacy of minipills is excellent among women older than age 40 and lactating women. In women older than 40 years, decreased fecundity contributes to the efficacy of the minipill, whereas in lactating women, the prolactin-induced suppression of ovulation contributes to its efficacy. Another reason that the minipill is an excellent method of birth control in lactating women is that it does not decrease milk volume and has no negative impact on infant growth or development.[36–38]

**Side Effects.** The most common side effect associated with the minipill is irregular uterine bleeding. Women using the minipill may have irregular bleeding, spotting, or amenorrhea. Other side effects include acne and the development of functional ovarian follicular cysts.

### PROGESTIN-ONLY IMPLANTABLE CONTRACEPTIVES

Norplant, a progestin-only implantable contraceptive, was first introduced in Chile in 1972 and in the United States in 1990. The Norplant system is comprised of six silastic rods, each 34-mm long, filled with levonorgestrel. The semipermeable silastic rods allow for a slow release of levonorgestrel at an initial rate of 80 μg per day (equivalent to the amount in a progestin-only pill). After ~9 to 12 months of use, the rods release levonorgestrel at ~30 μg per day. They maintain excellent contraceptive efficacy (99.7% per year) and are FDA approved for 5 years of continuous use. In the near future, Implanon, a one-rod/3-year implant system containing 3-keto-desogestrel, and Norplant II, a two-rod/3-year implant system containing levonorgestrel, will be released.

**Mechanism of Action.** The principal mechanism by which progestin-only implants exert their contraceptive efficacy is by altering the cervical mucus and making it impenetrable to sperm. The continuous low levels of progestin also serve to suppress LH and prevent ovulation. Compared to cervical mucus changes, the prevention of ovulation is less reliable, and, as progestin levels decline over time, more ovulatory cycles are noted. With Norplant, in the first 2 years of use only 10% to 20% of cycles appear to be ovulatory, whereas in the fifth year of use, ~45% of cycles appear to be ovulatory. However, even

cycles that appear to be ovulatory are often not completely normal cycles. Women who have regular menstrual cycles on Norplant have been shown to have subnormal levels of LH, FSH, and progesterone.[39,40]

Progestin-only implants also induce changes in the endometrial lining. These changes are likely responsible for the irregular uterine bleeding associated with implant use. With Norplant, the endometrial lining has been found to be hypotrophic with an increased microvascular density of capillaries that appear to be particularly fragile.[41] The exact mechanism of these changes is unclear. Study has shown that postfertilization prevention of implantation on an unfavorable endometrial lining is not a mechanism for the contraceptive action of Norplant.[42]

**Use of Implants.** Contraceptive implants are inserted subdermally, in the upper inner arm, under local anesthesia using the provided trocar. Insertion is a simple procedure that usually takes 5 to 10 minutes. Special care must be taken to place the implants in the correct plane. Placement of all six implants in the same subdermal plane allows easy removal. Because the silastic rods are not biodegradable, after 5 years of use, or at the woman's request, the implants must be removed. Under local anesthesia, a small incision is made, and the implants can be removed either with finger pressure or with a pair of small hemostatic clamps. Removal of the implants can take from 5 to 60 minutes. The major advantage of one- and two-rod implant systems is faster and easier insertion and removal. Implant systems using biodegradable capsules are in development.

Absolute contraindications to progestin-only implants include undiagnosed vaginal bleeding, suspected or confirmed pregnancy, active liver disease or tumors, active thromboembolic disorders, and known or suspected breast cancer. Relative contraindications include severe acne, depression, vascular migraine headaches, and the concomitant use of medications that increase the hepatic metabolism of progestins—and, hence, decrease the efficacy of implants—such as phenytoin, carbamazepine, phenobarbital, and rifampin.

Progestin-only implants may be very well suited for women with hypertension, diabetes, a history of cardiovascular disease (such as stroke, myocardial infarction, or prior deep venous thrombosis), gallbladder disease, hypercholesterolemia, or hypertriglyceridemia. Implants are also appropriate contraception for heavy smokers, including women older than age 35 years.

**Side Effects.** The most common side effect of progestin-only implants, and the most commonly cited reason for removal of Norplant, is irregular menstrual bleeding. In the first year of use, 68% of women using Norplant report menstrual problems.[43] Of the women with these problems, 23% report increased bleeding, 16% report decreased bleeding or amenorrhea, and 29% report irregular bleeding or spotting.[43] Over time, bleeding patterns tend to improve, and many women report regular menstrual cycles. The Norplant 5-year cumulative removal rate for bleeding problems is 17.5%.[43] The cause of the irregular menstrual bleeding is not entirely clear. Under the influence of progestin-only contraception, the endometrial lining becomes hypotrophic, with an increased microvascular density of fragile capillaries.[41] These fragile capillaries may be especially prone to bleeding. Varying levels of estrogen, produced by partially stimulated follicles, may also contribute to the irregular bleeding associated with progestin-only implants.[39]

Other side effects occurring in 10% to 16% of Norplant users in the first year of use include headache, acne, weight gain, leukorrhea, pelvic pain, vaginal fungal infections, genital pruritus, and reaction at the implantation site.[43] The incidence of these side effects, with the exception of genital pruritus, decreases in later years. Of these side effects, only weight gain, mood changes, and headache lead to removal rates of >1%.[43] After 5 years of use, 59% of U.S. women with implants gained weight. The mean 5-year weight gain for these women was 5.2 kg.[43]

Another complication of implant use is difficulty in removing the rods. In a large U.S. study, 8% of Norplant removals were classified as difficult, and 3% were associated with adverse effects (including multiple incisions and a reaction to the local anesthetic).[43] The amount of difficulty encountered and the time required for removal are related to the provider's skill and experience. New systems with fewer implant rods should minimize difficulty with insertion and removal.

No adverse effects on fertility are seen after removal of the rods. Within 24 hours after removal, fertility returns to baseline.[40] No consistent effects on blood pressure, lipoproteins, or coagulation have been noted. Also, because hypoestrogenemia does not occur, bone density is not affected.

### PROGESTIN-ONLY INJECTABLE CONTRACEPTIVES

DMPA (Depo-Provera) is an injectable progestin-only contraceptive. It was first introduced in the mid-1960s and, since then, has been used extensively around the world. In 1992 it was approved by the FDA for use in the United States. It is an easy-to-use, private, and very effective (99.7%) method of birth control.

DMPA is given as an intramuscular injection every 3 months. Peak serum hormone levels occur shortly after injection and then progressively fall, yet remain in the effective contraceptive range, over the next 3 months.

**Mechanism of Action.** As do other progestin-only contraceptives, DMPA exerts its contraceptive effects by thickening the cervical mucus, making it impenetrable to sperm. However, compared with Norplant, which provides continuous low levels of levonorgestrel, DMPA provides much higher levels of progestin. These high levels of progestin are effective at inhibiting the LH surge, and as a result DMPA is effective at inhibiting ovulation. Despite the fact that DMPA is more effective at inhibiting ovulation than Norplant, both have similar contraceptive efficacy.

Although DMPA effectively inhibits the LH surge, it does not completely suppress FSH and, thus, stimulated follicles continue to make estrogen. Estrogen levels in DMPA users have been found to be approximately at the level found in the early follicular phase in a normal menstrual cycle.[44]

**Use of Depot Medroxyprogesterone Acetate.** DMPA is an aqueous solution of suspended crystals, given in a dose of 150 mg intramuscularly, either in the deltoid or gluteus maximus muscle. The first injection should be given within 5 days of the menstrual period to ensure the patient is not pregnant at that time. The next injection should be given 12 to 13 weeks after the first injection. If these guidelines are followed, ovulation is inhibited from the onset of use.

If the patient is not within 5 days of the onset of her menstrual period, or is beyond 13 weeks after her last injection, a pregnancy test is indicated. If a sensitive pregnancy test is negative and no episodes of unprotected intercourse have occurred in the prior 2 weeks, the injection can be given. If any doubt exists as to whether unprotected intercourse has occurred within the 2 weeks before the negative pregnancy test, a backup method of birth control should be used, and a second pregnancy test given 2 weeks later. If the sensitive pregnancy test is still negative, the injection may be given. In these situations, a backup method of birth control should be used for the first 2 weeks of DMPA use, as ovulation may not be inhibited during this time.

DMPA is contraindicated in women who are pregnant and those who have undiagnosed vaginal bleeding. Relative contraindications include active liver disease, breast cancer, severe depression, severe cardiovascular disease, and a desire to conceive within 1 year.

SIDE EFFECTS. The most common side effect associated with DMPA use is irregular menstrual bleeding.[44-46] Within the first year of use, ~70% of women using DMPA have irregular bleeding.[44] With continued use, a majority of women become amenorrheic. After 5 years of use, ~80% of women are amenorrheic.[47]

The irregular bleeding associated with DMPA use is usually not excessive in quantity, but can be of increased frequency or duration. Although average hemoglobin levels rise in women

**TABLE 104-6.**
**Known and Potential Noncontraceptive Benefits of Depot Medroxyprogesterone Acetate**

**KNOWN**
 Decreased incidence of sickling events in women with sickle cell disease
 Rise in seizure threshold and improvement in seizure control in women with seizure disorders
 Decreased incidence of endometrial cancer
 Decreased menstrual volume and anemia
 Increased volume of breast milk in lactating women
**POTENTIAL**
 Decreased incidence of pelvic inflammatory disease
 Decrease in symptoms associated with endometriosis
 Decreased incidence of ectopic pregnancy
 Halt in growth of uterine leiomyomas

using DMPA, frequent and prolonged bleeding are the most common reasons for discontinuation of DMPA.[47] As many as 25% of new DMPA users discontinue this contraceptive in the first year of use due to frequent or prolonged bleeding.[48]

Other side effects reported with DMPA use include weight gain, depression, decreased libido, headaches, dizziness, abdominal pain, anxiety, and delayed return to fertility. Systemic levels of the drug may persist for 9 months after injection, and long infertile periods of up to 18 months may occur.[49]

The increased risk of breast cancer found in beagle dogs treated with DMPA has not been observed in humans using DMPA. A multinational study of breast cancer risk in women using DMPA has shown no increased risk[50] (see Chap. 105).

In cross-sectional studies, DMPA use has been associated with decreased bone mineral density.[51-53] This loss in bone mineral density has been shown to be reversible with discontinuation of DMPA.[54] The long-term effect of a temporary loss of bone mineral density on osteoporosis and fractures later in life is unknown (see Chap. 105).

NONCONTRACEPTIVE BENEFITS OF DEPOT MEDROXYPROGESTERONE ACETATE. DMPA has been shown to have many noncontraceptive benefits (Table 104-6). Although DMPA is FDA approved only for use as a contraceptive and in the treatment of metastatic endometrial cancer, it has been shown to raise the seizure threshold and to improve seizure control in some women with seizure disorders, to decrease the incidence of sickling events in women with sickle cell disease, and to decrease the incidence of endometrial cancer. DMPA is also safe for use in lactating women. In contrast to COCs, DMPA causes an increased volume of breast milk in lactating women.

### POSTCOITAL "EMERGENCY" CONTRACEPTIVES

Postcoital contraception is an "emergency" aid that can be provided for women who have experienced a single *unprotected or inadequately protected act of intercourse within the previous 72 hours*. The mechanism of action of postcoital contraception is unclear. Studies have shown that emergency contraceptive pills (ECs) both alter the endometrium and delay ovulation.[55-58] Postcoital contraception also may prevent fertilization.

Various regimens containing either an estrogen-progestin combination (combined ECs) or a progestin alone (progestin ECs) have been used with considerable success (Table 104-7). The first dose of a combined EC regimen should be given within 72 hours of unprotected intercourse, and the second dose should be given 12 hours later. The reported failure (pregnancy) rate is ~2%. Women having unprotected intercourse during the second or third week of their menstrual cycle have an 8% chance of conceiving that cycle. Thus, postcoital contraception may decrease the risk of conception from 8% to 2%, a 75% decrease in risk.[59,60]

The principal side effects of combined ECs are nausea and vomiting. The prophylactic use of an antiemetic 1 hour before each dose

**TABLE 104-7.**
**Oral Contraceptives Used for Emergency Contraception\***

| Brand Name | Preparation | Tablets Per Dose and Color | Number of Doses |
|---|---|---|---|
| Ovral | EE 50 µg + NG 0.50 mg | 2 white | 2 |
| Preven | EE 50 µg + LNG 0.25 mg | 2 light blue | 2 |
| Lo/Ovral | EE 30 µg + NG 0.30 mg | 4 white | 2 |
| Levlen | EE 30 µg + LNG 0.15 mg | 4 light orange | 2 |
| Nordette | EE 30 µg + LNG 0.15 mg | 4 light orange | 2 |
| Tri-Levlen | EE 30 µg + LNG 0.05, 0.075, 0.125 mg | 4 yellow | 2 |
| Triphasil | EE 30 µg + LNG 0.05, 0.075, 0.125 mg | 4 yellow | 2 |
| Alesse | EE 20 µg + LNG 0.10 mg | 5 pink | 2 |
| Ovrette | NG 0.075 mg | 20 yellow | 2 |

*EE*, ethinyl estradiol; *NG*, norgestrel; *LNG* levonorgestrel.
\*Combined pills: begin within 72 hours of unprotected intercourse; doses 12 hours apart. Progestin-only pills: begin within 48 hours of unprotected intercourse; doses 12 hours apart.

can significantly reduce these symptoms.[60] Progestin ECs cause less nausea and vomiting. The only absolute contraindication to the use of postcoital contraception is confirmed or suspected ongoing pregnancy. Postcoital contraception with combined or progestin ECs does *not* terminate an ongoing pregnancy.

No data are available on the safety of combined ECs in women with contraindications to estrogen. The short duration of use make significant complications unlikely; however, the progestin-only regimen has similar efficacy and should be considered for these women.

In a woman planning to use an IUD for contraception, a copper IUD inserted within 5 days of unprotected intercourse is also a very effective method of emergency contraception (failure rates of <0.1%).[61]

Mifepristone (RU-486) is also effective for postcoital contraception. Mifepristone is an antiprogesterone steroid that acts at the receptor level.[62,62a] It interrupts the menstrual cycle and causes shedding of the endometrial lining whether fertilization and implantation have occurred or not. Compared with combined ECs, mifepristone has been shown to have similar contraceptive efficacy, cause less nausea and vomiting, and cause more frequent delay in the next menstrual period.[63]

In an effort to simplify use of emergency contraception, a new emergency contraception kit, Preven, has been FDA approved and marketed. The prescription-only kit contains a pregnancy test, 4 tablets (each containing 50 µg of ethinyl estradiol and 0.50 mg of norgestrel) and easy-to-follow instructions.

The advantage of postcoital hormonal contraception is obvious: a means of avoiding unwanted pregnancy and an opportunity for counseling regarding regular contraceptive use. (See refs. 63a and 63b.) However, in the event of contraceptive failure, high doses of hormones, plus perhaps an antiemetic, have been used at a critical stage of embryogenesis. Although no studies have looked specifically at teratogenesis after exposure to emergency contraception, epidemiologic studies of COCs containing as much as 150 µg of estrogen have not demonstrated a teratogenic effect with early embryonic exposure to these steroids.[64]

# NONHORMONAL CONTRACEPTION

## INTRAUTERINE DEVICE

The IUD is a highly effective method of contraception, with failure rates similar to those with female sterilization. Approximately 80% of women choosing an IUD for contraception

continue to use this method through the first year and ~60% continue through the second year. The incidence of complications differs with the device used, but overall morbidity is low. In the United States, the Cu-T380A and Progestasert are the only IUDs available.

### USE OF THE INTRAUTERINE DEVICE

The IUD is a safe, effective method of contraception for appropriate candidates. Women who are at low risk for STIs and who are without menstrual dysfunction or anatomic distortion of the uterine cavity are ideally suited to IUD use. Because the IUD provides no protection against STIs, and may increase the severity of existing infections, a thorough screening of women for STI risk factors is mandatory before IUD insertion.

Absolute contraindications to IUD insertion include a history of current, recent, or recurrent pelvic inflammatory disease, acute cervicitis, acute vaginitis, intrauterine pregnancy, allergy to copper (with copper IUDs), and immunosuppression. The relative contraindications to IUD use include multiple sexual partners, nulligravid condition, menometrorrhagia, hypermenorrhea, severe dysmenorrhea, uterine abnormalities distorting the cavity, anticoagulation therapy or a bleeding disorder, and valvular heart disease. Diabetes mellitus is not a contraindication to IUD use. Women with type 1 or type 2 diabetes mellitus (with no other contraindications to IUD use) may safely use this method of contraception.[65,66]

The IUD should be inserted during the last days of menstrual flow to ensure that the woman is not pregnant, and because the cervix is partially open at that time, allowing for easier insertion. An IUD may also be placed immediately after a first-trimester abortion without increased rates of expulsion or infection.[67,68] In the postpartum period, or after a second-trimester abortion, IUD insertion should be delayed 4 to 8 weeks because of the higher risk of IUD expulsion if performed sooner. Aside from an increased risk of expulsion, IUD insertion immediately postdelivery is not associated with an increased risk of complications.[69]

### COMPLICATIONS AND SIDE EFFECTS OF INTRAUTERINE DEVICE USE

Adverse effects of IUD use include expulsion, uterine or cervical perforation, syncope during insertion, severe uterine cramping, menometrorrhagia, chronic cervicitis or leukorrhea, and actinomycotic genital infection. During the first year of use, ~20% of patients request removal of the IUD because of heavy bleeding and cramping, and 5% to 10% spontaneously expel the IUD.

Among appropriately screened IUD users, pelvic infection is rare.[70,71] The risk of infection is highest immediately after insertion, at which time vaginal or cervical pathogenic organisms can be introduced into the uterus. If symptoms of upper genital tract infection develop, the IUD should be removed and sent for culture; cervical cultures should be taken, and antibiotic treatment should be instituted.

Given the high efficacy of the copper IUD in preventing pregnancy, women using a copper IUD have a markedly decreased risk of ectopic pregnancy compared with women not using contraception. A prior history of an ectopic pregnancy is not a contraindication to IUD use. In the rare event that a pregnancy does occur with an IUD in place, it is more likely to be an ectopic rather than an intrauterine pregnancy.[67] If an intrauterine pregnancy occurs with an IUD in place, the chance of spontaneous abortion is ~40% to 50%. If the IUD strings are visible, the IUD should be removed as soon as the pregnancy is diagnosed.

Studies indicate that fertility rates among monogamous women choosing to become pregnant after copper IUD removal are similar to those among women discontinuing the use of other contraceptives.[72,73]

# BARRIERS AND SPERMICIDAL AGENTS

The placement of various substances in the vagina either to act as a barrier to sperm transport or to exert spermicidal effects has been practiced for >2000 years. In addition to providing contraception, most barrier methods offer some protection against STIs.

## CONDOM

The use of a male or female condom, if made of latex, protects against the transmission of bacteria and viruses, including human immunodeficiency virus (HIV).[74] Between 1982 and 1995, condom use rose from 12% to 20% in the United States.[1] This rise likely reflects efforts to prevent STIs, specifically HIV. Many couples use a condom both for contraception and to prevent STIs. Others use condoms for disease prevention in addition to another, more effective contraception method.

## DIAPHRAGM

The diaphragm is a round latex barrier that is placed in the vagina before intercourse. The spring-like edges of the diaphragm allow it to collapse to enable placement in the vagina. Once it is properly positioned in front of the cervix, the spring opens and keeps the diaphragm in place. The three basic types of diaphragms are the *arcing spring*, the *coil spring*, and the *flat spring*. Diaphragms come in sizes between 50 and 105 mm in diameter and must be individually fitted for each woman. They must be refitted after childbirth.

Various clinical studies indicate typical use effectiveness rates ranging from 2 to 25 pregnancies per 100 woman-years. This broad range of contraceptive effectiveness is attributable to differences in the degree of motivation of the woman and to experience with the method.

The principal contraindications to diaphragm use are anatomic factors causing poor fit and allergies to latex or spermicide. The use of a diaphragm plus spermicide provides prophylaxis against many STIs and has been associated with a decrease in cervical dysplasia (likely due to decreased spread of human papilloma virus).

The principal complication of diaphragm use is recurrent cystitis, probably due to partial urethral blockage. If, despite adequate antibiotic treatment, the frequency of cystitis increases, another method of contraception should be considered.

A serious cause of concern among diaphragm users is the reporting of several nonfatal cases of toxic shock syndrome. In all of these cases, however, the patients had left the diaphragm in place for long periods of time. Women should be carefully instructed never to leave the diaphragm in the vagina longer than 24 hours.

## SPERMICIDAL PREPARATIONS

A great variety of spermicidal preparations are available as foams, creams, jellies, films, or suppositories. All spermicides contain a surfactant, which is responsible for the contraceptive effect. Surfactants have long-chain alkyl groups that easily penetrate the lipoprotein membrane of spermatozoa, increasing the permeability of the cell and leading to irreversible loss of motility.

The vagina absorbs some of the spermicidal chemicals. No human studies have reported deleterious effects resulting from the absorption of surfactants. A double-blind, placebo-controlled trial has colposcopically evaluated the local effects of the spermicide nonoxynol-9 on the vagina and cervix and found no increase in epithelial disruption.[75] Two studies have suggested a greater risk of congenital birth defects in the offspring of women using vaginal spermicides,[76,77] but other studies have not shown any association between spermicide exposure and congenital malformations.

Not only do spermicidal preparations provide a contraceptive benefit, but the incidence of cervical gonorrhea, vaginal candidiasis, trichomoniasis, and genital infection with herpes

**TABLE 104-8.**
**Failure Rates of Different Techniques of Tubal Sterilization**

| Type of Procedure | Number of Failures Per 100 Women |
|---|---|
| **Laparotomy (modified Pomeroy technique)** | |
| Postpartum | 0.75 |
| Interval | 2.0 |
| **Laparoscopy** | |
| Unipolar electrocautery | 0.75 |
| Silastic bands | 1.8 |
| Bipolar electrocautery | 2.5 |
| Hulka clips | 3.7 |

(From Petersen HB, Xia Z, Hughes JM, et al. The risk of pregnancy after tubal sterilization: findings from the U.S. Collaborative Review of Sterilization. Am J Obstet Gynecol 1996; 174:1161.)

simplex virus are all decreased by these chemical agents. Clinical trials to assess the efficacy of nonoxynol-9 in preventing HIV transmission are in progress.[75]

## FEMALE STERILIZATION

Sterilization has become the most common method of fertility regulation in the United States. It is an elective procedure that offers women permanent, nonreversible contraception. Female sterilization is performed by ligating, excising, cauterizing, banding, or clipping portions of both fallopian tubes. The majority of these procedures are performed either laparoscopically or via laparotomy. Failure rates for the most commonly used techniques of tubal sterilization are listed in Table 104-8.[78] The larger the amount of tube destroyed, the poorer the potential for a surgical reversal, should the woman desire to have this latter procedure later.

Although pregnancy after tubal sterilization is not common, when pregnancies do occur after sterilization, they are almost as likely to be ectopic as intrauterine pregnancies. The U.S. Collaborative Review of Sterilization found a 10-year cumulative probability of pregnancy of 18.5 per 1000 procedures (for all types of sterilization procedures combined). They found a 10-year cumulative probability of ectopic pregnancy of 7.3 per 1000 procedures. Women at highest risk for ectopic pregnancy after tubal sterilization are those sterilized under age 30 using the bipolar electrocautery technique.[79]

In the United States, deaths attributable to female sterilization are rare, with a case fatality rate of ~1.5 per 100,000 procedures.[80] This is markedly lower than the maternal mortality rate associated with childbearing, which is ~10 per 100,000 live births. Deaths associated with female sterilization have resulted from complications of general anesthesia as well as from infection and hemorrhage. Although major complications are infrequent, one study found that 1.7% of laparoscopic sterilizations are complicated by penetrating injuries, injuries to major abdominal and pelvic vessels, and bowel burns.[81] Complication rates are probably lower among clinicians with more laparoscopy experience.

# REFERENCES

1. Piccinino LJ, Mosher WD. Trends in contraceptive use in the United States: 1982–1995. Fam Plann Perspect 1998; 30:4.
1a. Westhoff C, Davis A. Tubal sterilization: focus on the U.S. experience. Fertil Steril 2000; 73:913.
2. Trussell J, Kowal D. The essentials of contraception. In: Hatcher RA, et al. Contraceptive technology, 17th ed. New York: Ardent Media, 1998:216.
3. Collins DC. Sex hormone receptor binding, progestin selectivity, and the new oral contraceptives. Am J Obstet Gynecol 1994; 170:1508.
4. Goldzieher JW. Selected aspects of the pharmacokinetics and metabolism of ethinyl estrogens and their clinical implications. Am J Obstet Gynecol 1990; 163:318.

5. Mishell DR, Darney PD, Burkman RT, Sulak PJ. Practice guidelines for OC selection: update. Dialogues Contracept 1997; 5(4):7.

6. Bagwell MA, Coker AL, Thompson SJ, et al. Primary infertility and oral contraceptive steroid use. Fertil Steril 1995; 63:1161.

7. Carpenter S, Neinstein LS. Weight gain in adolescent and young adult oral contraceptive users. J Adolesc Health Care 1986; 7:342.

8. Gerstman BB, Piper JM, Tomita DK, et al. Oral contraceptive estrogen dose and the risk of deep venous thromboembolic disease. Am J Epidemiol 1991; 133:32.

9. World Health Organization Collaborative Study of Cardiovascular Disease and Steroid Hormone Contraception. Ischaemic stroke and combined oral contraceptives: results of an international, multicentre, case-control study. Lancet 1996; 348:498.

10. World Health Organization Collaborative Study of Cardiovascular Disease and Steroid Hormone Contraception. Venous thromboembolic disease and combined oral contraceptives: results of international multicentre case-control study. Lancet 1995; 346:1575.

11. Pettiti DB, Sidney S, Bernstein A, et al. Stroke in users of low-dose oral contraceptives. N Engl J Med 1996; 335:8.

12. Sidney S, Pettiti DM, Quesenberry CP Jr, et al. Myocardial infarction in users of low-dose oral contraceptives. Obstet Gynecol 1996; 88:939.

13. Beral V, Hermon C, Kay C, et al. Mortality associated with oral contraceptive use: 25 year follow up of cohort of 46,000 women from Royal College of General Practitioners' oral contraception study. BMJ 1999; 318:96.

14. Croft P, Hannaford PC. Risk factors for acute myocardial infarction in women: evidence from the Royal College of General Practitioners' oral contraception study. BMJ 1989; 298:165.

15. Vandenbroucke JP, Koster T, Briet E, et al. Increased risk of venous thrombosis in oral-contraceptive users who are carriers of factor V Leiden mutation. Lancet 1994; 344:1453.

16. Schwingl PJ, Ory HW, Visness CM. Estimates of the risk of cardiovascular death attributable to low-dose oral contraceptives in the United States. Am J Obstet Gynecol 1999; 180:241.

17. Burkman RT Jr. Benefits and risks of oral contraceptives: a reassessment. J Reprod Med 1991; 36(Suppl):217.

18. Larsson G, Milsom I, Lindstedt G, Rybo G. The influence of a low-dose combined oral contraceptive on menstrual blood loss and iron status. Contraception 1992; 46:327.

19. Wolner-Hanssen P, Eschenbach DA, Paavonen J, Kiviat N, et al. Decreased risk of symptomatic chlamydial pelvic inflammatory disease associated with oral contraceptive use. JAMA 1990; 263:54.

20. Barbone F, Austin H, Louv WC, Alexander WJ. A follow-up study of methods of contraception, sexual activity, and rates of trichomoniasis, candidiasis, and bacterial vaginosis. Am J Obstet Gynecol 1990; 163:510.

21. Brinton LA, Vessey MP, Flavel R, et al. Risk factors for benign breast disease. Am J Epidemiol 1981; 113:203.

22. Schlesselman JJ. Risk of endometrial cancer in relation to use of combined oral contraceptives. A practitioner's guide to meta-analysis. Hum Reprod 1997; 12:1851.

23. Sherman ME, Sturgeon S, Brinton LA, et al. Risk factors and hormone levels in patients with serous and endometriod uterine carcinomas. Mod Pathol 1997; 10:963.

24. Mol BW, Ankum WM, Bossuyt PM, Van der Veen F. Contraception and the risk of ectopic pregnancy: a meta-analysis. Contraception 1995; 52:337.

25. Hankinson SE, Colditz GA, Hunter DJ, et al. A quantitative assessment of oral contraceptive use and ovarian cancer. Obstet Gynecol 1992; 80:708.

26. Lanes SF, Birmann B, Walker AM, Singer S. Oral contraceptive type and functional ovarian cysts. Am J Obstet Gynecol 1992; 166:956.

27. Grimes DA, Godwin AJ, Rubin A, et al. Ovulation and follicular development associated with three low-dose oral contraceptives: a randomized controlled trial. Obstet Gynecol 1994; 83:29.

28. Redmond GP, Olson WH, Lippman JS, et al. Norgestimate and ethinyl estradiol in the treatment of acne vulgaris: a randomized, placebo-controlled trial. Obstet Gynecol 1997; 89:615.

29. Kleerekoper M, Brienza RS, Schultz LR, Johnson CC. Oral contraceptive use may protect against low bone mass. Arch Intern Med 1991; 151:1971.

30. Ness RB, Keder LM, Soper DE, et al. Oral contraception and the recognition of endometritis. Am J Obstet Gynecol 1997; 176:580.

31. Cramer DW, Goldman M, Schiff I, et al. The relationship of tubal infertility to barrier method and oral contraceptive use. JAMA 1987; 257:2446.

32. Speroff L, Glass RH, Kase NG. Clinical gynecologic endocrinology and infertility, 5th ed. Baltimore: Williams & Wilkins, 1994:60.

33. Speroff L, Darney PD. Oral contraception. In: A clinical guide for contraception, 2nd ed. Baltimore: Williams & Wilkins, 1996.

34. Darney PD. The androgenicity of progestins. Am J Med 1995; 98(Suppl 1A):104.

35. World Health Organization Committee on Contraceptive Research for Human Reproduction. A multicentered phase III comparative clinical trial of Mesigna, Cyclofem and Injectable No. 1 given monthly by intramuscular injection to Chinese women. Contraception 1995; 51:167.

36. World Health Organization, Special Programme of Research, Development, and Research Training in Human Reproduction, Task Force on Oral Contraceptives. Effects of hormonal contraceptives on milk volume and infant growth. Contraception 1984; 30:505.

37. World Health Organization, Special Programme of Research, Development, and Research Training in Human Reproduction, Task Force for Epidemiological Research on Reproductive Health. Progestogen-only contraceptives during lactation. I. Infant growth. Contraception 1994; 50:35.

38. World Health Organization, Special Programme of Research, Development, and Research Training in Human Reproduction, Task Force for Epidemiological Research on Reproductive Health. Progestogen-only contraceptives during lactation. II. Infant development. Contraception 1994; 50:55.

39. Faundes A, Brache V, Tejada AS, et al. Ovulatory dysfunction during continuous administration of low-dose levonorgestrel by subdermal implants. Fertil Steril 1991; 56:27.

40. Walker DM, Darney PD. Implantable contraception. In: Sciarra JJ, ed. Gynecology and obstetrics. Philadelphia: Lippincott–Raven Publishers, 1998.

41. Fraser IS, Hickey M, Song J. A comparison of mechanisms underlying disturbances of bleeding caused by spontaneous dysfunctional uterine bleeding or hormonal contraception. Hum Reprod 1996; 11(Suppl 2):165.

42. Segal SJ, Alvarez-Sanchez F, Brache V, et al. Norplant implants: the mechanism of contraceptive action. Fertil Steril 1991; 56:273.

43. Sivin I, Mishell DR, Darney PD, et al. Levonorgestrel capsule implants in the United States: a 5-year study. Obstet Gynecol 1998; 92:337.

44. Speroff L, Darney PD. Injectable contraception. In: A clinical guide for contraception, 2nd ed. Baltimore: Williams & Wilkins, 1996.

45. Darney PD, Klaisle CM. Contraception-associated menstrual problems: etiology and management. Dialogues Contracept 1998; 5(5):1.

46. Grimes DA, Wallach M. Injectable contraception. In: Modern contraception: updates from the contraception report. Totowa, NJ: Emron, 1997.

47. Gardener JM, Mishell DR Jr. Analysis of bleeding patterns and resumption of fertility following discontinuation of a long-acting injectable contraceptive. Fertil Steril 1970; 21:286.

48. World Health Organization. Clinical evaluation of the therapeutic effectiveness of ethinyl oestradiol and oestrone sulphate on prolonged bleeding in women using depot medroxyprogesterone acetate for contraception. Hum Reprod 1996; 11(Suppl 2):1.

49. Kaunitz AM. Injectable depot medroxyprogesterone acetate contraception: an update for clinicians. Int J Fertil 1998; 43(2):73.

50. World Health Organization Collaborative Study of Neoplasia and Steroid Contraceptives. Breast cancer and depot–medroxyprogesterone acetate: a multinational study. Lancet 1991; 338:833.

51. Cundy T, Evans M, Roberts H, et al. Bone density in women receiving depot medroxyprogesterone acetate for contraception. BMJ 1991; 303:13.

52. Cromer BA, Blair JM, Mahan JD, et al. A prospective comparison of bone density in adolescent girls receiving depot medroxyprogesterone acetate (Depo-Provera), levonorgestrel (Norplant) or oral contraceptives. J Pediatr 1996; 129:671.

53. Scholes D, Lacroix AZ, Ott SM, et al. Bone mineral density in women using depot–medroxyprogesterone acetate for contraception. Obstet Gynecol 1999; 93:233.

54. Cundy T, Cornish J, Evans MC, et al. Recovery of bone density in women who stop using medroxyprogesterone acetate. BMJ 1994; 308:247.

55. Swahn ML, Westlund P, Johannisson E, Bygdeman M. Effect of post-coital contraceptive methods on the endometrium and the menstrual cycle. Acta Obstet Gynecol Scand 1996; 75:738.

56. Ling WY, Robichaud A, Zayid I, et al. Mode of action of DL-norgestrel and ethinyl estradiol combination in postcoital contraception. Fertil Steril 1979; 32:297.

57. Rowlands S, Kubba AA, Guillebaud J, Bounds W. A possible mechanism of action of danazol and an ethinyl estradiol/norgestrel combination used as postcoital contraceptive agents. Contraception 1986; 33:539.

58. Ling WY, Wrixon W, Acorn T, et al. Mode of action of dl-norgestrel and ethinyl estradiol combination in postcoital contraception. III. Effect of pre-ovulatory administration following the luteinizing hormone surge on ovarian steroidogenesis. Fertil Steril 1983; 40:631.

59. Trussell J, Ellertson C, Stewart F. The effectiveness of the Yuzpe regimen of postcoital contraception. Fam Plann Perspect 1996; 28(2):58.

60. American College of Obstetricians and Gynecologists. Practice patterns. Emergency oral contraception. Washington: American College of Obstetricians and Gynecologists, December 1996 (no. 3).

61. Trussell J, Ellertson C. Efficacy of emergency contraception. Fertil Control Rev 1995; 4(2):8.

62. Lockwood CJ, Krikin G, Papp C, et al. Biological mechanisms underlying RU486 clinical effects: inhibition. J Clin Endocrinol Metab 1994; 79:786.

62a. Baird DT. Clinical uses of antiprogestagens. J Soc Gynecol Investig 2000; 7(1 Suppl):S49.

63. Glasier A, Thong KJ, Dewar M, et al. Mifepristone (RU486) compared with high-dose estrogen and progestogen for emergency postcoital contraception. N Engl J Med 1992; 237:1041.

63a. Harvey SM, Beckman LJ, Sherman C, Petitti D. Women's experience and satisfaction with emergency contraception. Fam Plann Perspective 1999; 31:237.

63b. Hewitt G, Cromer B. Update on adolescent contraception. Obstet Gynecol Clin North Am 2000; 27:143.

64. Braken MB. Oral contraceptives and congenital malformations in offspring; a review and meta-analysis of the prospective studies. Obstet Gynecol 1990; 76:552.

65. Kjos SL, Ballagh SA, La Cour M, et al. The copper T380A intrauterine device in women with type II diabetes mellitus. Obstet Gynecol 1994; 84:1006.

66. Kimmerle R, Weiss R, Berger M, Kurz K. Effectiveness, safety and acceptability of a copper intrauterine device (Cu Safe 300) in type I diabetic women. Diabetes Care 1993; 16:1227.

67. Speroff L, Darney PD. Intrauterine contraception. In: A clinical guide for contraception, 2nd ed. Baltimore: Williams & Wilkins, 1996.

68. Querido L, Ketting E, Haspels AA. IUD insertion following induced abortion. Contraception 1985; 31:603.

69. Chi I-C, Farr G. Postpartum IUD contraception—a review of an international experience. Adv Contracept 1989; 5:127.

70. Lee NC. The intrauterine device and pelvic inflammatory disease revisited: new results from the Women's Health Study. Obstet Gynecol 1988; 72:1.

71. Kessel E. Pelvic inflammatory disease with intrauterine device use: a reassessment. Fertil Steril 1989; 51:1.

72. Cramer DW. Tubal infertility and intrauterine device. N Engl J Med 1985; 312:941.

73. Daling JR. Primary tubal infertility in relation to use of intrauterine device. N Engl J Med 1985; 312:937.

74. Laga M, Alary M, Nzila N, et al. Condom promotion, sexually transmitted disease treatment, and declining incidence of HIV-1 infection in female Zairian sex workers. Lancet 1994; 1:246.

75. Jick H. Vaginal spermicides and congenital disorders. JAMA 1981; 1245:1329.

76. Cordero JF, Layde PM. Vaginal spermicides, chromosomal abnormalities and limb reduction defects. Fam Plann Perspect 1983; 15:16.

77. Van Damme L, Niruthisard S, Atisook R, et al. Safety evaluation of nonoxynol-9 gel in women at low risk of HIV infection. AIDS 1998; 12:433.

78. Petersen HB, Xia Z, Hughes JM, et al. The risk of pregnancy after tubal sterilization: findings from the U.S. Collaborative Review of Sterilization. Am J Obstet Gynecol 1996; 174:1161.

79. Petersen HB, Xia Z, Hughes JM, et al. The risk of ectopic pregnancy after tubal sterilization. N Engl J Med 1997; 336:762.

80. Escobedo LG, Petersen HB, Grubb GS, Franks AL. Case-fatality rates for tubal sterilization in U.S. hospitals, 1979 to 1980. Am J Obstet Gynecol 1989; 160:147.

81. DeStefano F. Complications of interval laparoscopic tubal sterilization. Obstet Gynecol 1983; 61:163.

# CHAPTER 105

# COMPLICATIONS AND SIDE EFFECTS OF STEROIDAL CONTRACEPTION

ALISA B. GOLDBERG AND PHILIP DARNEY

All steroidal contraceptives are composed either of a progestin alone or a combination of an estrogen and a progestin. The side effects or complications observed with the use of hormonal contraception can be attributed either to the estrogen or progestin component. Understanding which effects are estrogen related and which are progestin related can help clinicians individualize hormonal contraceptive use for their patients.

## PHARMACOLOGY

Hormonal contraceptives are formulated from synthetic steroid 19-nortestosterone derivatives, which include *norethindrone, norethindrone acetate, norethynodrel, ethynodiol diacetate, norgestrel, levonorgestrel (LN), desogestrel, gestodene, norgestimate,* and *dienogest.* Exceptions are the injectable contraceptives *(Depo-Provera, Lunelle),* which use the progesterone derivative, *depot medroxyprogesterone acetate (MPA).* One of these progestins is combined with various dosages of an *estrogen,* either *ethinyl estradiol* or *ethinyl estradiol-3-methyl ether* (mestranol) in oral tablets and in some long-acting methods (injectables, vaginal rings, patches). The presence of a $C_{17}$ ethinyl group on all synthetic estrogens and progestins enhances the oral activities of these agents by slowing their rapid hydroxylation and conjugation in the hepatic portal system.[1,2]

Ethinyl estradiol and mestranol are fairly well absorbed; ~60% of the oral dose is recovered in the urine. In the liver, mestranol is demethylated to ethinyl estradiol. After oral administration, concentrations of both estrogens peak at 1 to 2 hours, with the areas under the plasma concentration time curves being equal. The metabolic degradation path of the two estrogens is identical, with the principal urinary metabolite being ethinyl estradiol glucuronide.

The progestins used in hormonal contraceptives are absorbed rapidly, with peak concentrations reached in ~1 hour after a pill is taken. The acetate compounds attain peak concentrations somewhat later because they must be deacetylated in the gastrointestinal tract before the progestin can be absorbed. All progestins are hydroxylated and conjugated in the liver before excretion primarily in the urine. Drugs that accelerate hepatic metabolism of steroids (rifampin, barbiturates, phenytoin, carbamazepine, fluconazole) can decrease the serum concentrations of low-dose hormonal contraceptives, such as the minipills or Norplant, and decrease efficacy.

## BIOLOGIC POTENCIES OF CONTRACEPTIVE STEROIDS

Various animal tissue responses (e.g., rat ventral prostate) have been used to assess the biopotency of contraceptive steroids. Much scientific criticism has been directed at these test systems, particularly at the extrapolation of dog and rodent data to humans. Specific steroid-receptor binding assays are now used. These allow in vitro comparisons of the androgenic, progestogenic, and estrogenic properties of sex steroids. In vivo, however, these effects are modulated by endogenous sex steroids and their binding globulins, notably sex hormone–binding globulin (SHBG).

Progestins differ in their bioactivities. This variation in bioactivity among different progestins is in large part due to modifications in the steroid structure that result in different receptor-binding affinities and different rates of metabolism. These factors require that different doses of each different progestin be used to achieve contraceptive efficacy. The administration of estrogen together with a progestin in combined contraceptives allows for use of a lower dose of progestin. The dose of progestin required for contraceptive efficacy in combined contraceptives is affected by the amount of estrogen administered. Because differences among progestin potencies are compensated for by dose adjustment, scales that attempt to correlate steroid dose with clinical effect are not useful.[3]

## METABOLIC EFFECTS

Pharmacologic doses of contraceptive hormones have widespread metabolic effects, but many of these are merely alterations in laboratory values without clinical significance. Nevertheless, some laboratory test alterations may reflect clinically significant metabolic changes. For example, changes in coagulation factors may predispose certain women to intravascular clotting, and changes in renin and angiotensin may affect blood pressure in a few users. Many of the metabolic alterations associated with steroid contraceptive use are attributable to the estrogenic component of the combination pill. These effects would not be expected with the use of progestin-only contraception. In contrast, the metabolic alterations caused by progestins, which would be expected in progestin-only contraceptive users, may be altered by the concomitant use of estrogen.[4] For example, the estrogen in *combined oral contraceptives (COCs)* raises triglycerides and high-density lipoprotein (HDL), whereas most progestins have the opposite effects.

### CARBOHYDRATE METABOLISM

**Combined Oral Contraception.** Early studies with high-dose COCs showed impairment of glucose tolerance and increased insulin resistance. However, multiple studies of low-dose COCs have not shown a clinically significant impact of COCs on carbohydrate metabolism.[5,6] Even women with a history of gestational diabetes have not been found to be at additional risk of developing diabetes due to COC use.[7,8] The small increase in insulin resistance seen with low-dose COC use may alter glucose metabolism in some women with overt diabetes mellitus; however, this effect has not been consistent among individual patients. Also, the use of COCs has not been found to increase the risk of development of nephropathy or retinopathy in patients with type 1 diabetes mellitus.[9] Current consensus opinion is that healthy diabetic women with no end-organ complications of diabetes mellitus may safely use low-dose COC.

The changes observed in carbohydrate metabolism with oral contraceptive use (increased insulin resistance and decreased glucose tolerance) are believed to be attributable almost entirely to the progestin component of combination pills, and are dose related. Ethinyl estradiol administered alone, even in high doses, does not cause glucose tolerance deterioration or abnormal insulin responses.

**Progestin-Only Contraceptives.** Progestin-only oral contraceptives, minipills or "POPs," may decrease carbohydrate tolerance in healthy women, but this effect is generally not clinically significant.[10] Because they do not adversely affect breast milk volume or quality, POPs are often used by lactating women. Those containing norethindrone have been found to increase the risk of developing diabetes among high-risk breast-feeding women (obese Latinas with a history of gestational diabetes; relative risk [RR] = 2.87, 95% confidence interval [CI] = 1.57–5.27).[8] The same study found no increase in the rate of development of diabetes on the basis of breast-feeding alone.[8] The predominantly progestogenic state of lactation combined with POPs may be enough to cause significant glucose intolerance in women at high risk. It remains unknown whether POPs will have a similar diabetogenic effect on high-risk, nonlactating women. One study of non–breast-feeding, type 1 diabetic women using POPs containing lynestrenol found no change in insulin requirements.[11]

LN implant contraceptives (e.g., Norplant, Jadelle) have been shown to have no clinically significant effect on carbohydrate metabolism in healthy women. In one study, 100 healthy women had a glucose-loading test before Norplant insertion, and then annually over 5 years of its use. The investigators found no significant changes in mean fasting serum glucose levels or in 2-hour postprandial serum glucose levels. The 1-hour postprandial glucose levels were elevated from baseline in years 1 and 2 of Norplant use, but not in years 3 through 5. These elevations were not above the normal range.[12] There is no evidence that LN implants increase the risk of developing diabetes among lactating or nonlactating women at high risk, as POPs containing norethindrone may.

Since depot MPA acetate injection (DMPA, Depo-Provera) results in higher serum concentrations of progestin at the beginning of each 3-month injection cycle, its effects on carbohydrate metabolism might differ from those of lower-dose POPs or continuous-release progestin implant systems. Studies have shown no deterioration in glucose tolerance in nondiabetic women using DMPA for contraception for short durations; however, after 4 to 5 years of continuous use, some studies show an increase in glucose intolerance.[13] Whether this is due to DMPA itself, or to associated weight gain, is unclear. DMPA is not contraindicated in diabetic women, and often is an excellent method of contraception for women with vascular disease; however, changes in glucose metabolism may occur.

### LIPID METABOLISM

**Combined Oral Contraceptives.** All estrogen-containing contraceptive pills increase serum triglyceride levels by an average of ~50%. The progestin-only pill has not been associated with such changes. The increased triglyceride levels are attributable mainly to an increase in very low-density lipoproteins (LDLs; see Chap. 162). Most low-dose COCs do not cause significant increases in mean serum cholesterol levels; however, high-dose estrogen-progestin formulations can decrease HDL while increasing LDL.[10] Although estrogens increase HDL levels and progestins decrease HDL levels, COCs may have various effects because of endogenous factors that modulate these effects.

COCs containing the less androgenic progestins (desogestrel, dienogest, gestodene, and norgestimate) moderately elevate triglycerides (as does the estrogen component of all COCs), as well as total cholesterol, but the increase in total cholesterol is all in the HDL fraction. LDL levels fall, so that except for women with very high triglycerides (>450 mg/dL), less androgenic COCs can improve the lipoprotein profile.[14–16] Whether this effect has consequences for cardiovascular health is undetermined. High-dose COCs can decrease HDL and increase LDL; however, they have not been associated with arteriosclerotic disease. In fact, the estrogen component of high-dose COCs protects against plaque deposition despite the adverse lipid effects of high doses of progestins.

**Progestin-Only Contraceptives.** Low-dose, sustained-release contraceptives (e.g., Norplant) do not perturb lipoprotein metabolism. A study of more than 20 LN implant users followed for 5 years showed that modest changes in the cholesterol/HDL ratio were accounted for by weight gain and aging. The low serum concentrations of LN (0.3–0.5 ng/mL) had no persistent effect on lipoprotein metabolism (Population Council, data on file). Other smaller, shorter-term studies also failed to show significant lipoprotein effects of LN implants.[12,17] With LN implant use, triglyceride levels fall slightly because no estrogen is administered, and endogenous estradiol production is modestly suppressed.

The effect of DMPA on lipid metabolism is not clear. Some studies have suggested that DMPA has a negative impact on lipids, because it has been associated with decreased HDL cholesterol and increased total and LDL cholesterol levels.[18] Other studies have not found DMPA to be associated with these negative changes in lipids.[19,20] Epidemiologic studies have not associated DMPA with cardiovascular disease.[21]

## CARDIOVASCULAR EFFECTS

### THROMBOEMBOLIC DISEASE

**Combined Oral Contraceptives.** Early epidemiologic studies[22–24] indicated a four-fold to eight-fold increase in the risk of venous thromboembolism (VTE) among oral contraceptive users. As the estrogen content of COCs declined, reported risks of VTE fell to approximately three-fold, but the increased risk of VTE remains the greatest health threat that COCs pose.[25,26, 26a]

A large World Health Organization (WHO) international multicenter hospital-based case-control study found an increased risk of VTE with low-dose COC use (Europe: odds ratio [OR] = 4.24, 95% CI 3.07–5.87; developing countries: OR = 3.02, 95% CI 2.28–4.00).[27] Further analysis of the data from this study,[28] as well as others,[26] has suggested an additional two-fold increase in VTE risk among users of COCs containing desogestrel and gestodene, compared to users of COCs containing LN. The additional risk of VTE observed with the use of desogestrel- or gestodene-containing COCs is best explained by selection and prescribing bias.[26] Women at highest risk of VTE, new starters, and women who have had complications on COCs in the past are most likely to have received COCs containing desogestrel or gestodene. In contrast, women who had been using COCs without complication for years comprise a population at low risk of complications, and were more likely to remain on older formulations. Whether selection and prescribing bias completely account for this observed effect is unknown.

Genetic predisposition also plays a role in modifying the risk of VTE associated with oral contraceptive use. The factor V Leiden mutation is a point mutation that results in resistance to the anticoagulant effects of activated protein C. The factor V

Leiden mutation is estimated to affect 4.4% of Europeans and 0.6% of Asians, and is extremely rare (or nonexistent) in populations from Africa and Southeast Asia.[29] Women with the factor V Leiden mutation have an eight-fold increased risk of VTE (RR = 7.9, 95% CI 3.2–19.4), compared to women without the mutation.[30] When a woman with the factor V Leiden mutation uses COCs, her baseline risk of VTE increases four-fold, and her overall risk of VTE is 35 times greater (RR = 34.7, 95% CI 7.8–154) than for women without the mutation who are not using COCs.[30] Screening the general population for the factor V Leiden mutation is currently not recommended; however, women who are known to have the mutation or a strong family history of thromboembolic disease should avoid COCs. Other thrombophilic disorders, such as protein C or S deficiency, also increase the risk of VTE with COC use.

The increased risk of VTE with COCs is largely due to the estrogen component. Progestin-only contraceptives do not appear to confer an increased risk of VTE.[21] Therefore, POPs, implants, and injectables are often reasonable contraceptive choices for women at high risk of VTE.

## MYOCARDIAL INFARCTION

**Combined Oral Contraceptives.** Several early epidemiologic studies of COCs containing 50 µg estrogen showed an increased risk of myocardial infarction (MI).[31] Much of the observed increased risk of MI among COC users was actually due to the increased incidence of smoking and hypertension among COC users in the past. More recent studies of low-dose COCs have not revealed an increased risk of MI among nonhypertensive COC users who do not smoke.[32,33] Similarly, current or past use of COCs has not been associated with an increased risk of mortality from MI.[34] Among women who smoke and use COCs, the RR of MI has been reported to range from 3.5 (1.3–9.5) for those who smoke <15 cigarettes per day to 20.8 (5.2–83.1) for those who smoke ≥15 cigarettes per day.[32] This risk is modified by age. For women younger than age 35 years, the overall risk of dying from all cardiovascular diseases due to COC use and smoking is exceedingly small (3.3 per 100,000 for smokers vs. 0.65 per 100,000 for nonsmokers).[35] Therefore, younger women who smoke can use COCs with little risk of cardiovascular complications. For women older than age 35 years using COCs, the risk of cardiovascular death among smokers is 29.4 per 100,000 compared to 6.21 per 100,000 for nonsmokers. This level of risk is unacceptably high, and COC use is contraindicated in women older than age 35 years who smoke.[35]

**Progestin-Only Contraceptives.** There does not appear to be any increased risk of MI with the use of progestin-only methods compared to nonhormonal methods (pills: RR = 0.98 [0.16–5.97]; injectables: RR = 0.66 [0.07–6.00]).[21]

## CEREBROVASCULAR ACCIDENTS

**Combined Oral Contraceptives.** The occurrence of stroke in young women is rare, with an estimated incidence of 11.3 cases per 100,000 woman-years of observation.[36] In the absence of smoking and hypertension, low-dose COC users do not have an increased risk of either hemorrhagic or thrombotic stroke.[36–39] Both smoking and hypertension appear to have a synergistic effect when combined with COC use to increase the risk of stroke.[36,38,39] In WHO studies,[38,39] smoking COC users had a seven-fold increased risk for ischemic stroke (RR = 7.2, 95% CI 3.23–16.1) and a three-fold increased risk for hemorrhagic stroke (RR = 3.1, 95% CI 1.65–5.83) when compared to nonsmoking, non-COC users. In the same studies, hypertensive women using COCs had a ten-fold increased risk for ischemic stroke (RR = 10.7, 95% CI 2.04–56.6) and for hemorrhagic stroke (RR = 10.3, 95% CI 3.27–32.3) as compared to nonhypertensive, non-COC users. In these studies, the risk of stroke among COC users with a history of hypertension was double the risk for hypertensive women not using COCs; however, approximately half the participants were using high-dose COCs.[38,39]

**Progestin-Only Contraception.** There is no increased risk of stroke among nonsmoking, nonhypertensive women using progestin-only contraception.[21] Smokers have a baseline increased risk of stroke, but this risk is not altered with progestin-only contraceptive use.[21] It is unclear whether progestin-only contraception increases the risk of stroke among hypertensive women; limited data suggest that this might be the case.[21]

## HYPERTENSION

**Combined Oral Contraceptives.** High-dose COCs have been found to induce hypertension in ~5% of users.[40] Low-dose COCs also can induce hypertension, although the risk is much lower. One study estimated that low-dose COCs induce hypertension in 0.42% of users (41.5 cases per 10,000 person-years).[40] The effect of COCs on blood pressure appears to be short-lived and reverses within 3 months after discontinuation of pills. The pathophysiologic mechanism for the oral contraceptive–induced hypertensive effect involves the renin-angiotensin system. In most women, the COC-induced increase in angiotensinogen is physiologically compensated for by a decrease in renin secretion, and normal blood pressure is maintained. Some women, however, do not make the necessary physiologic adjustments, and hypertension results. There are no good predictors of which patients will develop hypertension on COCs; therefore, all patients should have their blood pressure checked annually while on COCs. A history of pregnancy-induced hypertension is not associated with an increased risk of COC-induced hypertension.[41] It is likely that both the estrogen and progestin components of COCs can alter blood pressure.

**Progestin-Only Contraceptives.** Although past studies of high-dose COCs suggested that the progestin component was primarily responsible for the observed elevations in blood pressure, multiple studies of currently used POPs, implants, and injectables have not revealed an increased incidence of hypertension with these methods of contraception. Hypertensive women may use progestin-only contraception,[42] although their blood pressure should be closely followed, and if uncontrollable elevations result the method should be discontinued and nonhormonal methods considered.

## EFFECTS ON THE BREASTS

### BENIGN BREAST CHANGES

**Combined Oral Contraceptives.** The estrogen component of COCs can cause breast fullness and tenderness. Although the fullness often remains as long as COCs are taken, the tenderness usually resolves after a few months of use. If the tenderness persists, one should consider switching the patient to a COC containing a lower dose of estrogen.

The incidence of benign breast disease (fibrocystic changes and fibroadenomas) is decreased among women who have used high-dose COCs for more than 2 years.[43] Women using high-dose COCs for more than 6 years have an approximately 50% reduction in benign breast disease. Low-dose COCs may have an attenuated benefit.

The quantity and quality of milk produced during lactation have been found to be decreased with COC use.[44] Similarly, women using COCs have been found to breast-feed for shorter lengths of time postpartum. Both estrogens and progestins are secreted in the milk, and although these steroids decrease the levels of both proteins and fats in human milk, no adverse effects on the growth or development of infants have been identified.[45] Although COC use during lactation is not harmful to infants, it is not recommended because it makes breast-feeding more difficult.

**Progestin-Only Contraception.** LN implants (Norplant) have been associated with breast tenderness in 11% of users in a large U.S. study.[46] The tenderness may be due to temporarily elevated follicular estradiol levels in women with lower LN serum concentrations and usually resolves over time. After excluding pregnancy as a possible cause of the mastalgia, reassurance is usually all that is necessary. POPs and DMPA are rarely associated with breast complaints.

## BREAST CANCER

**Combined Oral Contraceptives.**    For many years a great deal of controversy surrounded the issue of breast cancer risk in COC users. Some epidemiologic studies have shown no increased risk of breast cancer with COC use,[47–49] whereas others have shown an increased risk of breast cancer in women using COCs before the age of 25 years.[50–53]

In 1996, a metaanalysis was performed using the data from 54 epidemiologic studies conducted in 25 countries.[54] This study analyzed data for >53,000 women with breast cancer and >100,000 controls. They found that women who are currently using COCs have a small increase (RR = 1.24, CI 1.15–1.33) in the risk of breast cancer as compared to nonusers. This risk remains slightly elevated within the first 10 years after discontinuation of use (1–4 years after stopping: RR = 1.16, CI 1.08–1.23; 5–9 years after stopping: RR = 1.07, CI 1.02–1.13). Beyond 10 years after discontinuation of use, there is no increased risk of breast cancer (10 or more years after stopping: RR = 1.01, CI 0.96–1.05). They found no significant effect of duration of use, age at first use, or the type of hormone contained in the COC on breast cancer risk.

In this study, although women currently using COCs were at increased risk of a new diagnosis of breast cancer, their tumors were significantly more likely to be confined to the breast at diagnosis than were those of nonusers (RR = 0.89 for spread to lymph nodes at diagnosis; RR = 0.70 for distant spread at diagnosis). Whether these effects are due to earlier diagnosis in current or recent COC users or due to a pathophysiologic effect of COCs on breast cancer remains unclear. The risk of breast cancer may be greater for younger than for older women.[54a] (See also Chaps. 222 and 223.)

**Progestin-Only Contraceptives.**    DMPA was initially found to cause malignant mammary tumors in beagle dogs. This finding created great fear as to whether DMPA would have the same effect in humans. Two large case-controlled studies, and one pooled analysis of these studies, have addressed this concern and have found no increased risk of breast cancer in ever-users of DMPA as compared to never-users.[55–57] The pooled analysis did show a slightly increased risk of breast cancer in DMPA users within the first 5 years of use (pooled analysis: RR = 2.0, CI 1.5–2.8).[57] Whether this is due to increased surveillance in DMPA users or stimulation of preexisting tumors is unclear. Two of the studies showed no increase in breast cancer risk with increasing duration of use.[55,57] The third study showed an increase in breast cancer risk with >6 years of DMPA use only in those women who began using DMPA before age 25 years (RR = 4.2, CI 1.1–16.2).[56]

Based on a few studies, POPs do not appear to increase breast cancer risk.[50,58] To date, there are no epidemiologic studies evaluating the effect of LN implants on breast cancer risk.

## EFFECTS ON THE REPRODUCTIVE TRACT

### OVARIAN EFFECTS

#### OVARIAN CYSTS

**Combined Oral Contraceptives.**    High-dose COCs have been shown to decrease the incidence of functional ovarian cysts.[59] Low-dose COCs have not demonstrated a similar effect, although an attenuated effect may exist.[60]

**Progestin-Only Contraceptives.**    An increased incidence of follicular cysts has been noted with LN implant (Norplant) use. The continuous low level of LN allows follicles to develop, and follicular cysts often result.[60a] These cysts only need to be evaluated sonographically or laparoscopically if they become large and painful. Similar to LN implants, the low dose of progestin in POPs allows follicles to develop and follicular cysts to form. However, one large cohort study evaluating ovarian cysts in COC users also looked at progestin-only pill users, and found no cases of follicular cysts in 219 person-months of observation.[59] In contrast to POPs and implants, DMPA effectively suppresses follicular development and ovulation; thus, follicular cysts are rare among DMPA users.

### OVARIAN CANCER

**Combined Oral Contraceptives.**    Women using COCs have a markedly reduced risk of ovarian cancer, with increasing duration of use increasing the protective effect.[61–63] A 10% decrease in risk is noted after 1 year of COC use, and a ~50% decrease in risk is achieved after 5 years of use.[62] This protective effect has been found to extend to women at highest risk of ovarian cancer, including women with BRCA-1 and BRCA-2 mutations[64] (see also Chap. 223).

**Progestin-Only Contraception.**    DMPA is probably associated with a slightly decreased risk of epithelial ovarian cancer, given that it effectively inhibits ovulation; however, studies have been unable to detect a difference in ovarian cancer risk largely because of the high parity of DMPA users.[65] There are no epidemiologic data evaluating the effects of POPs or implants on ovarian cancer risk.

## ENDOMETRIAL EFFECTS

### MENSTRUAL CHANGES

In the majority of COC users, menses are regular, and become shorter in duration, lighter in flow, and associated with less dysmenorrhea. Progestin-only contraceptives are usually associated with disruption of the menstrual cycle, but no overall increase in menstrual blood loss. Menstrual irregularity is one of the leading causes of dissatisfaction with progestin-only methods. (See Chap. 104 for a complete discussion of menstrual changes with hormonal contraceptives.)

### ENDOMETRIAL CANCER

**Combined Oral Contraceptives.**    Multiple studies indicate that the risk of endometrial cancer is reduced among users of COCs.[66,67] Longer duration of use is associated with increased protection against endometrial cancer. A metaanalysis found that women using COCs for 4 years had a 56% decreased risk of endometrial cancer; after 8 years of use, a woman's risk was reduced by 67%, and after 12 years of use, risk was reduced by 72%.[68] Although the greatest risk reduction is observed for women who are currently using COCs, even 20 years after discontinuation, the risk of endometrial cancer is ~50% lower in ever-users than never-users (see also Chap. 223).

**Progestin-Only Contraceptives.**    DMPA use has been associated with a decreased risk of endometrial cancer.[69] Although epidemiologic studies have not yet shown a decreased risk of endometrial cancer with POPs or LN implant use, given the protective effect of progestin on the endometrium, these agents may decrease endometrial cancer risk as well.

## CERVICAL EFFECTS

### CERVICAL CANCER

**Combined Oral Contraceptives.**    The relation of oral contraceptive use to cervical dysplasia, carcinoma in situ, and invasive squamous cell cervical cancer is unclear, since some studies show positive relations between cervical dysplasia and continuing oral contraceptive use, whereas other studies report no relation.[70,71] Cervical dysplasia, carcinoma in situ, and squamous cell carcinoma are thought to be at least partly of viral origin (human papilloma virus). Consequently, the confounding factors of coitus at early age, multiple sexual partners, sexually transmittable diseases, and oral contraceptive use are difficult to decipher. Similarly, women using COCs are subject to increased surveillance as compared to nonusers. Increased surveillance results in increased detection of cervical squamous cell disease, and although the association between COC use and cervical squamous cell disease may be real, it may reflect screening bias or confounding (see Chap. 223). Nonetheless, annual Papanicolaou (Pap) smear screening should be recommended for all women taking COCs, and women at highest risk because of multiple sexual partners or a history of sexually transmitted diseases should be screened twice a year.

There is convincing evidence suggesting a relationship between COC use and adenocarcinoma of the cervix.[72] Data from the Surveillance, Epidemiology and End Results (SEER) tumor registry for Los Angeles found ever-users of COCs to have an RR of 2.1 of adenocarcinoma of the cervix, compared to never-users (CI 1.1–3.8). With COC use of >12 years' duration, this rose to a RR of 4.4 for ever-users (CI 1.8–10.8). This association may be mediated directly via estrogen or progestin receptors on endocervical cells, or may be explained by the increased incidence of ectropion in oral contraceptive users. Ectropion results in exposure of endocervical cells to the vagina, which may result in increased exposure to carcinogens.

**Progestin-Only Contraceptives.** DMPA does not appear to have an independent effect on cervical cancer or dysplasia. One study found an increased risk of dysplasia among DMPA users; however, this increased risk was attributable to known risk factors for cervical dysplasia among DMPA users.[73] A WHO case-control study found a slightly higher risk of carcinoma in situ in DMPA users.[74] Although this may be a real finding, it may reflect confounding or screening biases. No epidemiologic data yet exist evaluating the effects of POPs and implants on cervical cancer risk. When these data become available, it is likely that similar issues of confounding and screening bias will make interpretation difficult.

## EFFECTS ON THE GASTROINTESTINAL TRACT

### LIVER AND BILIARY TREE EFFECTS

**Combined Oral Contraception.** COCs have a variety of effects on the liver. Estrogen influences the hepatic synthesis of DNA, RNA, enzymes, plasma proteins, lipids, and lipoproteins. It also influences the hepatic metabolism of carbohydrates and intracellular enzyme activity. Progestins have less, if any, effect on the liver. Although the liver is affected in a variety of ways by COCs, many of these changes have proved to be of no clinical significance, and others remain incompletely understood. Virtually all phase II and phase III studies of COCs have evaluated the effects of COCs on liver function tests, and have shown no effect.[75] Some studies have shown an increased incidence of gallbladder disease and gallstones among current COC users.[76] Other studies[77] and a metaanalysis[78] of the effect of COCs on biliary disease showed that COCs initially did increase the risk of biliary disease (RR = 1.36, 95% CI 1.15–1.62),[78] but over time the risk returns to baseline. This suggests that, under the influence of COCs, susceptible (or asymptomatic) women become symptomatic from biliary disease shortly after starting the pill, whereas nonsusceptible women do not develop biliary disease over time with continued use.

The mechanism by which estrogen has its cholestatic effects[79] is incompletely understood. Under the influence of estrogen, bile becomes increasingly saturated with cholesterol.[80] This effect is probably secondary to elevated cholesterol concentrations in the bowel caused by altered cholesterol and lipid metabolism dependent on estrogen dose. Given these effects, women with active hepatitis, jaundice, or cholestasis should avoid COCs. Women with a past history of hepatitis can safely be given COCs.

**Progestin-Only Contraceptives.** POPs, implants, and injectables do not alter liver function tests.[81,82] Women with a past history of liver disease may safely use these methods. Whether women with active hepatitis or cirrhosis should use progestin-only methods is controversial, and the decision should be strongly influenced by the likelihood of pregnancy with other methods. Clearly, nonhormonal methods are safest for these women; however, progestin-only methods are less likely to have an adverse effect on their liver disease than either COCs or pregnancy.[83] It is unlikely that progestin-only methods increase the risk of gallbladder disease.[83]

## LIVER TUMORS

**Combined Oral Contraceptives.** The use of COCs has been associated with an increased risk of hepatocellular adenoma, and risk may increase with longer duration of use.[84,85] Although hepatocellular adenomas are benign tumors, they may rupture, causing hemorrhage and death.

Several case-control studies have shown an increased incidence of hepatocellular carcinoma among COC users,[86] whereas other similar studies have not demonstrated the same effect.[85] A large population-based study evaluated trends in the incidence of primary liver cancer and concomitant oral contraceptive use in three countries, and found no association of oral contraceptive use with primary liver cancer.[87]

**Progestin-Only Contraceptives.** The WHO found no association between DMPA use and liver cancer.[69] There are no data linking POPs or implants to benign or malignant liver tumors.

## EFFECTS ON BONE MINERAL DENSITY

**Combined Oral Contraceptives.** Estrogen-replacement therapy has been proven to prevent bone loss and fractures in postmenopausal women. Similarly, women with a history of COC use are less likely to have low bone mineral density later in life (RR = 0.35, 95% CI 0.2–0.5).[88] The effect of COCs on increasing bone mineral density appears to be related to duration of use.[88] As the first large population of COC users pass into menopause, future epidemiologic studies will determine whether women with a history of COC use have fewer fractures than women who never used COCs. It also remains to be seen if a past history of COC use is protective against osteoporosis in the presence and absence of postmenopausal estrogen-replacement therapy.

**Progestin-Only Contraceptives.** In cross-sectional studies, DMPA use has been associated with a decrease in bone mineral density.[89–91a] This effect appears to be greater with a longer duration of use and among young women (ages 18–21).[91] This decrease in bone mineral density is likely the result of decreased endogenous estrogen secretion due to the suppression of follicular development by DMPA. With discontinuation of DMPA, bone mineral density recovers[92]; however, the long-term effects of a temporary loss in bone mineral density remain unknown.

Since POPs and implants do not completely suppress follicular development, endogenous estrogen secretion remains within the normal premenopausal range[93]; it is unlikely that progestin-only pills or implants adversely affect bone mineral density.

Different progestins also might directly affect bone mineral density differently. In vitro, osteoblasts have been found to have both estrogen and progesterone receptors.[94] In other cell lines, the nortestosterone derivatives (i.e., norethindrone, norgestrel) have been shown to stimulate the growth of estrogen-receptor–positive cells, whereas MPA did not.[95] Perhaps the nortestosterone group of progestins has an estrogenic effect on bone that MPA does not.

## COMMON MINOR SIDE EFFECTS

Other common side effects of hormonal contraception include weight gain,[96] nausea, headaches, skin changes, and changes in mood and libido. Although these side effects are usually not dangerous, they often limit the acceptability of a contraceptive method. These side effects are discussed in Chapter 104.

## REFERENCES

1. Goldzieher JW. Selected aspects of the pharmacokinetics and metabolism of ethinyl estrogens and their clinical implications. Am J Obstet Gynecol 1990; 163:318.
2. Collins DC. Sex hormone receptor binding, progestin selectivity, and the new oral contraceptives. Am J Obstet Gynecol 1994; 170:1508.
3. Upmalis D, Phillip A. Receptor binding and in vivo activities of the new progestins. J Soc Obstet Gynecol Can 1991; 13(Suppl):35.
4. Krauss RM, Burkman RT Jr. The metabolic impact of oral contraceptives. Am J Obstet Gynecol 1992; 167:1177.
5. Rimm EB, Manson JE, Stampfer MJ, et al. Oral contraceptive use and the risk of type 2 (non-insulin dependent) diabetes mellitus in a large prospective study of women. Diabetologia 1992; 35:967.
6. Duffy TJ, Ray R. Oral contraceptive use: prospective follow-up of women with suspected glucose intolerance. Contraception 1984; 30:197.
7. Kjos SL, Shoupe D, Douyan S, et al. Effect of low-dose oral contraceptives on carbohydrate and lipid metabolism in women with recent gestational diabetes: results of a controlled, randomized, prospective study. Am J Obstet Gynecol 1990; 163:1822.
8. Kjos SL, Peters RK, Xiang A, et al. Contraception and the risk of type 2 diabetes mellitus in Latina women with prior gestational diabetes mellitus. JAMA 1998; 280:533.
9. Garg SK, Chase HP, Marshall G, et al. Oral contraceptives and renal and retinal complications in young women with insulin-dependent diabetes mellitus. JAMA 1994; 271:1099.
10. Godsland IF, Crook D, Simpson R, et al. The effects of different formulations of oral contraceptive agents on lipid and carbohydrate metabolism. N Engl J Med 1990; 323:1375.
11. Radberg T, Gustafson A, Skryten A, Karlsson K. Oral contraception in diabetic women: a cross-over study on serum and high density lipoprotein (HDL) lipids and diabetes control during progestogen and combined estrogen/progestogen contraception. Horm Metab Res 1982; 14:61.
12. Singh K, Viegas OAC, Loke D, Ratnam SS. Effect of Norplant implants on liver, lipid and carbohydrate metabolism. Contraception 1992; 45:141.
13. Liew DF, Ng CS, Yong YM, Ratnam SS. Long-term effects of Depo-Provera on carbohydrate and lipid metabolism. Contraception 1985; 31:51.
14. Speroff L, De Cherney A. Evaluation of a new generation of oral contraceptives. Obstet Gynecol 1993; 81:1034.
15. Kloosterboer HJ, Vonk-Noordegraaf CA, Turpijn EW. Selectivity in progesterone and androgen receptor binding of progestins in oral contraceptives. Contraception 1988; 38:325.
16. Petersen KR, Skouby SO, Pedersen RG. Desogestrel and gestadene in oral contraceptives: 12 months assessment of carbohydrate and lipoprotein metabolism. Obstet Gynecol 1991; 78:666.
17. Viegas OAC, Singh K, Liew D, et al. The effects of Norplant on clinical chemistry in Singaporean acceptors after 1 year of use: metabolic changes. Contraception 1988; 38:79.
18. World Health Organization. A multicentre comparative study of serum lipids and apolipoproteins in long-term users of DMPA and a control group of IUD users. Contraception 1993; 47:177.
19. Mainwaring R, Hales HA, Stevenson K, et al. Metabolic parameter, bleeding and weight changes in U.S. women using progestin only contraceptives. Contraception 1995; 51:149.
20. Garza-Flores J, De la Cruz DL, Valles de Bourges V, et al. Long-term effects of depot medroxyprogesterone acetate on lipoprotein metabolism. Contraception 1991; 44:61.
21. World Health Organization Collaborative Study of Cardiovascular Disease and Steroid Hormone Contraception. Cardiovascular disease and use of oral and injectable progestogen-only contraceptives and combined injectable contraceptives. Contraception 1998; 57:315.
22. Royal College of General Practitioners. Oral contraceptives and health: interim report. New York: Pitman, 1974.
23. Collaborative Group for the Study of Stroke in Young Women. Oral contraception and increased risk of cerebral ischemia or thrombosis. N Engl J Med 1973; 288:871.
24. Collaborative Group for the Study of Stroke in Young Women. Oral contraceptives and stroke in young women: associated risk factors. JAMA 1975; 231:718.
25. Gerstman BB, Piper JM, Tomita DK, et al. Oral contraceptive estrogen dose and the risk of deep venous thromboembolic disease. Am J Epidemiol 1991; 133:32.
26. Lewis MA, Heinemann LAJ, MacRae KD, et al. The increased risk of venous thromboembolism and the use of third generation progestagens: role of bias in observational research. Contraception 1996; 54:5.
26a. Editorial. Oral contraceptives and cardiovascular risk. Drug Ther Bull 2000; 38:1.
27. World Health Organization Collaborative Study of Cardiovascular Disease and Steroid Hormone Contraception. Venous thromboembolic disease and combined oral contraceptives: results of international multicentre case-control study. Lancet 1995; 346:1575.
28. World Health Organization Collaborative Study of Cardiovascular Disease and Steroid Hormone Contraception. Effect of different progestagens in low oestrogen oral contraceptives on venous thromboembolic disease. Lancet 1995; 346:1582.
29. Rees DC, Cox M, Clegg JB. World distribution of factor V Leiden. Lancet 1995; 346:1133.
30. Vandenbrouke JP, Koster T, Briet E, et al. Increased risk of venous thrombosis in oral-contraceptive users who are carriers of factor V Leiden mutation. Lancet 1994; 344:1453.
31. Pettiti DB, Sidney S, Quesenberry CP. Oral contraceptive use and myocardial infarction. Contraception 1998; 57:143.
32. Croft P, Hannaford PC. Risk factors for acute myocardial infarction in women: evidence from the Royal College of General Practitioners' oral contraception study. Br Med J 1989; 298:165.
33. Sidney S, Pettiti DB, Quesenberry CP, et al. Myocardial infarction in users of low-dose oral contraceptives. Obstet Gynecol 1996; 88:939.
34. Beral V, Hermon C, Kay C, et al. Mortality associated with oral contraceptive use: 25 year follow up of cohort of 46,000 women from Royal College of General Practitioners' oral contraception study. Br Med J 1999; 318:96.
35. Schwingl PJ, Ory HW, Visness CM. Estimates of the risk of cardiovascular death attributable to low-dose oral contraceptives in the United States. Am J Obstet Gynecol 1999; 180:241.
36. Pettiti DB, Sidney S, Bernstein A, et al. Stroke in users of low-dose oral contraceptives. N Engl J Med 1996; 335:8.
37. Stampfer MJ, Willett WC, Colditz GA. A prospective study of past use of oral contraceptive agents and risk of cardiovascular diseases. N Engl J Med 1988; 319:1313.
38. World Health Organization Collaborative Study of Cardiovascular Disease and Steroid Hormone Contraception. Ischaemic stroke and combined oral contraceptives: results of an international, multicentre, case-control study. Lancet 1996; 348:498.
39. World Health Organization Collaborative Study of Cardiovascular Disease and Steroid Hormone Contraception. Haemorrhagic stroke, overall stroke risk, and combined oral contraceptives: results of an international, multicentre, case-control study. Lancet 1996; 348:505.
40. Chasan-Taber L, Willett WC, Manson JE, et al. Prospective study of oral contraceptives and hypertension among women in the United States. Circulation 1996; 94:483.
41. Pritchard JA, Pritchard SA. Blood pressure response to estrogen-progestin oral contraception after pregnancy-induced hypertension. Am J Obstet Gynecol 1977; 733.
42. Speroff L, Darney PD. Implant contraception: Norplant. In: A clinical guide for contraception, 2nd ed. Baltimore: Williams & Wilkins, 1996.
43. Brinton LA, Vessey MP, Flavel R, Yeates D. Risk factors for benign breast disease. Am J Epidemiol 1981; 113:203.
44. World Health Organization Task Force on Oral Contraceptives. Effects of hormonal contraceptives on milk volume and infant growth. Contraception 1984; 30:505.
45. Nillson S, Mellbin T, Hofvander Y, et al. Long-term follow-up of children breast-fed by mothers using oral contraceptives. Contraception 1986; 34:443.
46. Sivin I, Mishell DR, Darney P, et al. Levonorgestrel capsule implants in the United States: a 5-year study. Obstet Gynecol 1998; 92:337.
47. Centers for Disease Control Cancer and Steroid Hormone Study. Long-term oral contraceptive use and risk of breast cancer. JAMA 1983; 249:1591.
48. World Health Organization Collaborative Study of Neoplasia and Steroid Contraceptives. Breast cancer and combined oral contraceptives: results from a multinational study. Br J Cancer 1990; 61:110.
49. Huggins GR, Zucker PK. Oral contraceptives and neoplasia: 1987 update. Fertil Steril 1987; 47:733.
50. United Kingdom National Case-Control Study Group. Oral contraceptive use and breast cancer risk in young women. Lancet 1989; 1:1973.
51. Stadel BV, Schlesselman JJ, Murray PA. Oral contraceptives and breast cancer. Lancet 1989; 1:1257.
52. Vessey MP, McPherson K, Villard-Mackintosh L. Oral contraceptives and breast cancer: latest findings in a large cohort study. Br J Cancer 1989; 59:613.
53. White E, Malone KE, Weiss NS, Daling JR. Breast cancer among U.S. women in relation to oral contraceptive use. J NCI 1994; 86:505.
54. Collaborative Group on Hormonal Factors in Breast Cancer. Breast cancer and hormonal contraceptives: collaborative reanalysis of individual data on 53,297 women with breast cancer and 100,239 women without breast cancer from 54 epidemiological studies. Lancet 1996; 347:1713.
54a. Pathak DR, Osuch JR, He J. Breast carcinoma etiology: current knowledge and new insights into the effects of reproductive and hormonal risk factors in black and white populations. Cancer 2000; 88(5 Suppl):1230.
55. World Health Organization Collaborative Study of Neoplasia and Steroid Contraceptives. Breast cancer and depot-medroxyprogesterone acetate: a multinational study. Lancet 1991; 338:833.
56. Paul C, Skegg DCG, Spears GFC. Depot medroxyprogesterone (Depo-Provera) and risk of breast cancer. Br Med J 1989; 299:759.

57. Skegg DCG, Noonan EA, Paul C, et al. Depot medroxyprogesterone acetate and breast cancer. JAMA 1995; 273:799.
58. The Cancer and Steroid Hormone Study of the Centers for Disease Control and the National Institute of Child Health and Human Development. Oral contraceptive use and the risk of breast cancer. N Engl J Med 1986; 315:405.
59. Lanes SF, Birmann B, Walker AM, Singer S. Oral contraceptive type and functional ovarian cysts. Am J Obstet Gynecol 1992; 166:956.
60. Grimes DA, Godwin AJ, Rubin A, et al. Ovulation and follicular development associated with three low-dose oral contraceptives: a randomized controlled trial. Obstet Gynecol 1994; 83:29.
60a. Alvarez-Sanchez F, Brache V, Montes de Oca V, et al. Prevalence of enlarged ovarian follicles among users of levonorgestrel subdermal contraceptive implants (Norplant). Am J Obstet Gynecol 2000; 182:535.
61. Centers for Disease Control Cancer and Steroid Hormone Study. Oral contraceptive use and risk of ovarian cancer. JAMA 1983; 249:1596.
62. Hankinson SE, Colditz GA, Hunter DJ. A quantitative assessment of oral contraceptive use and risk of ovarian cancer. Obstet Gynecol 1992; 80:708.
63. Cancer and Steroid Hormone Study of the Centers for Disease Control and the National Institutes of Child Health and Human Development. The reduction in risk of ovarian cancer associated with oral contraceptive use. N Engl J Med 1987; 316:650.
64. Narod SA, Risch H, Moslehi R, et al. Oral contraceptives and the risk of hereditary ovarian cancer. N Engl J Med 1998; 339:424.
65. World Health Organization Collaborative Study of Neoplasia and Steroid Contraceptives. Depot-medroxyprogesterone acetate (DMPA) and risk of epithelial ovarian cancer. Int J Cancer 1991; 49:191.
66. Centers for Disease Control Cancer and Steroid Hormone Study. Oral contraceptive use and risk of endometrial cancer. JAMA 1983; 249:1600.
67. Cancer and Steroid Hormone Study of the Centers for Disease Control and the National Institutes of Child Health and Human Development. Combination oral contraceptive use and the risk of endometrial cancer. JAMA 1987; 257:796.
68. Schlesselman JJ. Risk of endometrial cancer in relation to use of combined oral contraceptives. A practitioner's guide to meta-analysis. Hum Reprod 1997; 12:1851.
69. World Health Organization Collaborative Study of Neoplasia and Steroid Contraceptives. Depot-medroxyprogesterone acetate (DMPA) and risk of endometrial cancer. Int J Cancer 1991; 49:186.
70. Brinton LA. Oral contraceptives and cervical neoplasia. Contraception 1991; 43:581.
71. World Health Organization Collaborative Study of Neoplasia and Steroid Contraceptives. Combined oral contraceptives and risk of cervical carcinoma in situ. Int J Epidemiol 1995; 24:19.
72. Ursin G, Peters RK, Henderson BE, et al. Oral contraceptive use and adenocarcinoma of the cervix. Lancet 1994; 344:1390.
73. The New Zealand Contraception and Health Study Group. History of long-term use of depot-medroxyprogesterone acetate in patients with cervical dysplasia; case-control analysis nested in a cohort study. Contraception 1994; 50:443.
74. Thomas DB, Ye Z, Ray RM, and the World Health Organization Collaborative Study of Neoplasia and Steroid Contraception. Cervical carcinoma in situ and use of depot-medroxyprogesterone acetate (DMPA). Contraception 1995; 51:25.
75. Goldzieher JW. Effects on other tissues. In: Fraser IS, ed. Estrogens and progestogens in clinical practice. London: Churchill Livingstone, 1998.
76. Grodstein F, Colditz GA, Hunter DJ, et al. A prospective study of symptomatic gallstones in women: relation with oral contraceptives and other risk factors. Obstet Gynecol 1994; 84:207.
77. Royal College of General Practitioners' Oral Contraception Study. Oral contraceptives and gallbladder disease. Lancet 1982; 2:957.
78. Thijs C, Knipschild P. Oral contraceptives and the risk of gallbladder disease: a meta-analysis. Am J Pub Health 1993; 83:113.
79. Sillem MH, Teichmann AT. The liver. In: Goldheizer J, Fotherby K (eds). Pharmacology of the contraceptive steroids. New York: Raven Press, 1994:247.
80. Bennion LJ, Ginsberg RL, Garnick MB, Bennett PH. Effects of oral contraceptives on the gallbladder bile of normal women. N Engl J Med 1976; 294:189.
81. Korba VD, Paulson SR. Five years of fertility control with microdose norgestrel: an updated clinical review. J Reprod Med 1974; 13:71.
82. Population Council. Norplant levonorgestrel implants: a summary of scientific data. New York: The Population Council, 1990.
83. McCann MF, Potter LS. Progestin-only oral contraception: a comprehensive review. Contraception 1994; 50(Suppl 1):S96.
84. Palmer JR, Rosenberg L, Kaufman DW, et al. Oral contraceptive use and liver cancer. Am J Epidemiol 1989; 130:878.
85. World Health Organization Collaborative Study of Neoplasia and Steroid Contraceptives. Combined oral contraceptives and liver cancer. Int J Cancer 1989; 43:254.
86. Prentice RL. Epidemiologic data on exogenous hormones and hepatocellular carcinoma and selected other cancers. Prev Med 1991; 20:38.
87. Waetjen LE, Grimes DA. Oral contraceptives and primary liver cancer: temporal trends in three countries. Obstet Gynecol 1996; 88:945.
88. Kleerekoper M, Brienza RS, Schultz LR, Johnson CC. Oral contraceptive use may protect against low bone mass. Arch Intern Med 1991; 151:1971.
89. Cundy T, Evans M, Roberts H, et al. Bone density in women receiving depot medroxyprogesterone acetate for contraception. Br Med J 1991; 303:13.
90. Cromer BA, Blair JM, Mahan JD, et al. A prospective comparison of bone density in adolescent girls receiving depot medroxyprogesterone acetate (Depo-Provera), levonorgestrel (Norplant®) or oral contraceptives. J Pediatr 1996; 129:671.
91. Scholes D, Lacroix AZ, Ott SM, et al. Bone mineral density in women using depot-medroxyprogesterone acetate for contraception. Obstet Gynecol 1999; 93:233.
91a. Petiti DB, Piaggio G, Mehta S, et al. for the WHO Study of Hormonal Contraception and Bone Health. Steroid hormone contraception and bone mineral density: a cross-sectional study in an international population. Obstet Gynecol 2000; 95:736.
92. Cundy T, Cornish J, Evans MC, et al. Recovery of bone density in women who stop using medroxyprogesterone acetate. BMJ 1994; 308:247.
93. Faundes A, Brache V, Tejada AS, et al. Ovulatory dysfunction during continuous administration of low-dose levonorgestrel by subdermal implants. Fertil Steril 1991; 56:273.
94. Eriksen EF, Colvard DS, Berg NJ, et al. Evidence of estrogen receptors in normal human osteoblast-like cells. Science 1988; 241:84.
95. Jordan VC, Jeng MH, Catherino WH, Parker CJ. The estrogenic activity of synthetic progestins used in oral contraceptives. Cancer 1993; 71(Suppl):1501.
96. Gluntz S, Gluntz JC, Campbell-Heider N, Schaff E. Norplant use among urban minority women in the United States. Contraception 2000; 61:83.

# CHAPTER 106

# MORPHOLOGY OF THE NORMAL BREAST, ITS HORMONAL CONTROL, AND PATHOPHYSIOLOGY

RICHARD E. BLACKWELL

## MORPHOLOGY AND HORMONAL CONTROL

### COMPARATIVE ANATOMY OF LACTATION

The constituents of milk products differ widely among species, undoubtedly reflecting differences in the nutritional requirements of the neonate and the environmental restrictions on the mother. The mammary gland is unique in the animal kingdom in that only 4200 species of mammals possess this organ. Most of these mammals (95%) belong to the subclass Eutheria; the remainder belong either to the subclass Monotremata, which contains the primitive egg-laying mammals such as the duck-bill platypus, or to the Metatheria, which contains the single-order Marsupilia (i.e., kangaroos).[1]

### HISTORY OF THE HORMONAL CONTROL OF THE BREAST

Haller, in 1765, was the first to conclude that milk was derived from blood. The relation of blood and milk production was investigated by Sir Astley Cooper, who first described the early physiologic occurrence of milk letdown and lactogenesis. In the 1930s, it was shown by means of pressure monitors that milk secretion and ejection are separate events.[2] In 1928, prolactin was extracted and demonstrated to be different from other known pituitary hormones.[3] In the 1940s, it was proposed that during pregnancy, estrogen and progesterone promote full mammary growth while progesterone inhibits estrogen stimulation of prolactin secretion, and that at parturition, an increase in circulating prolactin and cortisol accompanied by a fall in estrogen and progesterone trigger lactation.[4] Although incorrect in some aspects, this hypothesis endured for more than 20 years. It began to be challenged with the discovery that mammary growth occurs in the absence of steroid hormones in adrenalectomized and gonadectomized rats that are recipients of pituitary mammotrophic tumor xenografts secreting prolactin, growth hormone, and adrenocorticotropic

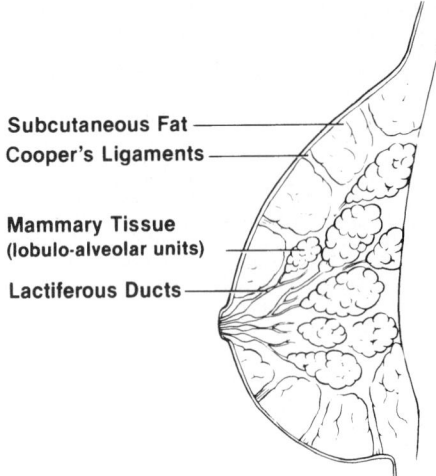

Subcutaneous Fat
Cooper's Ligaments

Mammary Tissue
(lobulo-alveolar units)

Lactiferous Ducts

**FIGURE 106-1.** Anatomy of the breast (sagittal view).

hormone.[5] Subsequent studies showed that estrogen stimulates the secretion of prolactin.[6] Partially inhibiting the response, progesterone suppresses prolactin secretion below baseline. It has been proposed that elevated progesterone levels during pregnancy prevent the secretion of milk and that the withdrawal of this hormone after parturition is in part responsible for lactogenesis.[7]

## ANATOMY OF THE MAMMARY GLAND

The mammary gland lies on the pectoralis fascia and musculature of the chest wall over the upper anterior rib cage (Fig. 106-1). It is surrounded by a layer of fat and encased in skin. The tissue extends into the axilla, forming the tail of Spence. The mammary gland consists of 12 to 20 glandular lobes or lobules that are connected by a ductal system. The ducts are surrounded by connective and periductal tissues, which are under hormonal control. The lactiferous ducts enlarge as they approach the nipple, which is pigmented and surrounded by the areola. The ductal tissue is lined by epithelial cells. The individual functional unit of the breast is the alveolar cell, which is surrounded by the hormonally responsive myoepithelial cells. Milk is produced at the surface of the alveolar cells and is ejected by the contraction of the myoepithelial cells under the influence of oxytocin. Fibrous septa run from the lobules into the superficial fascia. The suspensory ligaments of Cooper permit mobility of the breast.

The principal blood supply of the breast comes from the lateral thoracic and internal thoracic arteries, although components have been identified from the anterior intercostal vessels. The breast is innervated chiefly by the intercostal nerves carrying both sensory and autonomic fibers. The nipple and areola are innervated by the interior ramus of the fourth intercostal nerve. Seventy-five percent of the lymphatic drainage involves axillary pathways through the pectoral and apical axillary nodes. Drainage also occurs through parasternal routes.

## EMBRYOLOGY AND HISTOLOGY OF THE MAMMARY GLAND

The mammary gland can be identified 6 weeks after fertilization; it is derived from ectoderm. At 20 weeks' gestation, the 16 to 24 primitive lactiferous ducts invade the mesoderm. These ectodermal projections continue to branch and grow deeper into the tissue. Canalization occurs near term. Importantly, although the central lactiferous duct is present at birth, the gland does not differentiate until it receives the appropriate hormonal signals.

By the time an embryo is 7 mm in length, the mammary tissue has thickened to form a ridge (known as the *mammary crest* or *milk line*) extending along the ventrolateral body wall from the axillary to the inguinal region on each side. The caudal epithelium regresses, and the crest in the thoracic region thickens further to form a primordial mammary bud by the time the embryo is 10 to 12 mm in length. These embryologic origins account for the occasional development of supernumerary nipples and accessory breast tissue.

Although mammary tissue remains relatively unresponsive until pregnancy, it is responsive to systemic hormone administration during fetal life. In the third trimester, when fetal prolactin levels increase, terminal differentiation of ductal cells occurs. This hormonal milieu accounts for the *witch's milk* expressible from the nipples of some normal newborn girls. After birth, these cells revert slowly to a more primitive state.[8] The glands remain quiescent until the establishment of ovulatory menstrual cycles, at which time breast development proceeds in the manner described by Marshall and Tanner[9] (see Chap. 91). Although the hormonal regulation of mammogenesis is unclear, estrogen in vivo appears to bring about ductal proliferation, although it has little ability to stimulate lobuloalveolar development.[10] In vitro, however, estrogens do not promote mammary growth. It has been suggested that various epidermal growth factors participate in this process.[11] When progesterone is administered in vivo, lobuloalveolar development occurs.[12] However, the administration of estrogen and progesterone to hypophysectomized animals fails to promote mammogenesis.[13] These data strongly suggest that hormones other than estrogens and progestogens play a role in mammogenesis. For instance, if the pituitary and adrenal glands are removed from oophorectomized rats, the addition of estrogen plus corticoids and growth hormone restores duct growth similar to that seen in puberty.[14]

## NONPREGNANT (INACTIVE) MAMMARY GLAND

Before pregnancy, breast lobules consist of ducts lined with epithelium and embedded in connective tissue. The preponderance of the tissues in the gland are of the connective and adipose types. There is a scant contribution from glandular parenchyma, and a few bud-like sacculations arise from the ducts. The entire gland consists predominantly of the lactiferous ducts. The breast does undergo cyclic changes associated with normal ovulation, and the premenstrual breast engorgement noted by most women is probably secondary to tissue edema and hyperemia. Epithelial proliferation is also detectable during the menstrual cycle.[15]

## MAMMARY DEVELOPMENT IN PREGNANCY

After conception, the mammary gland undergoes remarkable development. Lobuloalveolar elements differentiate during the first trimester. Both in vitro and in vivo, it is possible to induce mammary development with either placental lactogen or prolactin in the absence of steroid hormones.[16] Although both placental lactogen and prolactin increase throughout pregnancy, data suggest that either of these hormones can stimulate complete mammogenesis. The role of estrogen in mammogenesis appears to be secondary, since lactation has been reported in pregnancies of women with placental sulfatase deficiency.[17] Progesterone, although stimulating lobuloalveolar development, also appears to antagonize the terminal effects induced by prolactin, at least in vitro. Cortisol, which potentiates the action of prolactin on mammary differentiation, apparently is unnecessary for either ductal or alveolar proliferation.[18]

Insulin and other growth factors also stimulate mammogenesis.[19] For example, insulin is required for the survival of postnatal mammary tissue in vitro. It is also possible that insulin-like molecules such as the insulin growth factors participate in this

**TABLE 106-1.**
**Hormone Regulation of the Breast**

**GROWTH**
*Ducts*
  Growth hormone
  Estrogen
  Cortisol
*Alveoli*
  Estrogen
  Progesterone
  Cortisol
  Prolactin
  Growth hormone
**LACTOGENESIS**
  Prolactin
  Insulin
  Insulin-like growth factor-I
  Cortisol

**TABLE 106-2.**
**Some Bioactive Substances in Milk of Humans and Other Mammals**

**PITUITARY HORMONES**
  Prolactin
  Growth hormone
  Thyroid-stimulating hormone
  Follicle-stimulating hormone
  Adrenocorticotropic hormone
  Oxytocin
**HYPOTHALAMIC HORMONES**
  Thyroid-releasing hormone
  Somatostatin
  Gonadotropin-releasing hormone
**GROWTH FACTORS**
  Insulin-like growth factors
  Insulin-like growth factor–binding proteins
  Nerve growth factor
  Epidermal growth factor
  Transforming growth factor-α
  Transforming growth factor-β
  Growth inhibitors macrophage-derived and macrophage-activating factor
  Relaxin
  Platelet-derived growth factor
**THYROID AND PARATHYROID HORMONES**
  Thyroxine
  Triiodothyronine
  Reverse triiodothyronine
  Calcitonin
  Parathyroid hormone
  Parathyroid hormone–related protein
**STEROID HORMONES**
  Estradiol
  Estriol
  Progesterone
  Testosterone
  Corticosterone
  Vitamin D
**GASTROINTESTINAL PEPTIDES**
  Vasoactive intestinal peptide
  Bombesin
  Cholecystokinin
  Gastrin
  Gastric inhibitory peptide
  Pancreatic peptide YY
  Substance P
  Neurotensin
**OTHERS**
  Prostaglandin E
  Prostaglandin $F_{2\alpha}$
  Cyclic adenosine monophosphate
  Cyclic guanosine monophosphate
  Delta sleep–inducing peptide
  Transferrin
  Lactoferrin
  Casomorphin
  Erythropoietin

(Modified from Grosvenor CE, Picciano MF, Baumrucker CR. Hormones and growth factors in milk. Endocr Rev 1993; 14:710.)

process. However, studies suggest that epidermal growth factor is involved in mammogenesis and, together with glucocorticoids, facilitates the accumulation of type IV collagen, a component of the basal lamina, on which epithelial cells are supported (Table 106-1).

## CONTROL OF LACTATION

Although milk letdown occurs fairly abruptly between the second and fourth postpartum days in the human, the transition from *colostrum* production to *mature milk* secretion is gradual. This process may take up to a month and seems to coincide with a fall in plasma progesterone and a rise in prolactin levels.

Twelve weeks before parturition, changes in milk composition begin[20]: increased production of lactose, proteins, and immunoglobulins and decreased sodium and chloride content. There is an increase in blood flow and in oxygen and glucose uptake in the breasts. There is also a marked increase in the amount of citrate at about the time of parturition. The composition of milk remains fairly stable until term, which is best exemplified by the stable production of α-lactalbumin, a milk-specific protein. At parturition, there is a marked fall in placental lactogen production, and progesterone levels reach nonpregnant levels within several days.[21] Plasma estrogen falls to basal levels in 5 days, whereas prolactin decreases over 14 days.[22] A fall in the progesterone level seems to be the most important event in the establishment of lactogenesis. Exogenous progesterone prevents lactose and lipid synthesis after ovariectomy in pregnant rats and in ewes.[23] Furthermore, progesterone administration inhibits casein and α-lactalbumin synthesis in vitro.[24]

The major proteins of human milk are α-lactalbumin (30% of the total protein content), lactoferrin (10–20%), casein (40%), and immunoglobulin A (IgA; 10%). Milk also contains many substances that are potentially capable of exerting biologic effects. Their physiologic role is, as yet, largely unexplored[25] (Table 106-2).

## MAINTENANCE OF LACTATION

In the human, lactation is maintained by the interaction of numerous hormones. After removal of either the pituitary or the adrenal glands from a number of animal species, milk production is terminated rapidly.[26] The species dictates the type of replacement therapy required to reinstitute milk production. For instance, in rabbits and sheep, prolactin is effective alone, whereas in ruminants, milk secretion is restored by the addition of corticosteroids, thyroxine, growth hormone, and prolactin. In humans, prolactin appears to be a key hormone in the maintenance of lactation, since the administration of bromocriptine

blocks lactogenesis.[27] The role of thyroid hormones in lactation is unclear. Thyroidectomy inhibits lactation, and replacement therapy with thyroxine increases milk yield. It has been suggested that growth hormone and thyroxine synergize to alter milk yield, and triiodothyronine acts directly on mouse mammary tissue in vitro to increase its sensitivity to prolactin.[28]

Despite species differences, in humans, prolactin levels reach a peak before delivery and subsequently rebound after the initiation of lactation. This phenomenon can be inhibited by progesterone. Despite the importance of declining progesterone levels in initiating this event, lactation fails to occur with inadequate prolactin production. Prolactin production becomes attenuated over time, with the most dynamic period being 8 to 41 days postpartum. By the 63rd day, the prolactin response will be attenuated by a factor of 5, and this is maintained to ~194 days postpartum.[29–32]

### SUCKLING AND MILK EJECTION

The integrated baseline level of prolactin is elevated in lactating women.[33] Suckling or manipulation of the breasts leads to elevation in prolactin within 40 minutes.[34] In rats, this response can be mimicked by electrical stimulation of the mammary nerves. Both growth hormone and cortisol are also increased. The response appears to be greatest in the immediate postpartum period and is attenuated over 6 months. If lidocaine is applied to the nipple, thus blocking nerve conduction, the rise in prolactin levels is abolished.[35] If two infants suckle simultaneously, the rise in prolactin is amplified. Along with prolactin release, suckling increases the secretion of oxytocin. After the application of a stimulus, there is an 8- to 12-hour delay before milk secretion is fully stimulated. This response seems to be correlated with the frequency and duration of vigorous suckling. There is no correlation between the amount of prolactin released and the milk yield.

Suckling of the breasts increases intramammary pressure bilaterally, secondary to contraction of the myoepithelial cells in response to the octapeptide oxytocin. This contraction follows the application of stimulation to the nipple, which activates sensory receptors transmitting impulses to the spinal cord and hypothalamus. Oxytocin-producing neurons are located both in the paraventricular and supraoptic nuclei (see Chap. 25). It is estimated that ~2 ng oxytocin is released per 2- to 4-second pulse interval.[36] The synthesis and release of oxytocin are rapid, because 90 minutes after injection of a radioactive amino acid into cerebrospinal fluid, radiolabeled oxytocin is released by exocytosis, and electrical pulse activity has been measured in oxytocic neurons 5 to 15 seconds before milk ejection. The response may be conditioned, since the cry of an infant or various other perceptions associated with nursing can trigger activity in the central pathways.

Thus, both oxytocin and prolactin are released in response to suckling, but the patterns of release clearly are different.[37] When nursing women are allowed to hold their infants but not to breast-feed, serum prolactin concentrations do not increase, despite the occurrence of the milk letdown reflex; prolactin levels rise only with nursing. The increase in prolactin with nursing is apparently sufficient to maintain lactogenesis and an adequate milk supply for the next feeding. This accounts for the ability of "wet nurses" to continue to breast-feed infants for years—even after the menopause—once lactation is established.

### RESOLUTION OF LACTATION

Postpartum lactation can be maintained over an extended period of time by discontinuing suckling. Nevertheless, prolactin levels decrease progressively over a number of weeks despite breast-feeding. The physiologic hyperprolactinemia is achieved by altering the endogenous secretory rate of each prolactin pulse. No alteration occurs in the number of bursts of prolactin or its half-life. A large group of Australian women breast-feeding for extended periods of time demonstrated a mean of 322 days of anovulation and 289 days of amenorrhea. Fewer than 20% of the women ovulated or had menstruated by 6 months postpartum. Ovulation was delayed to a maximum of 750 days and menstruation to 698 days.[38]

During pregnancy, luteinizing hormone (LH) and follicle-stimulating hormone (FSH) secretion are inhibited through hypothalamic mechanisms. The exogenous opioid tone is increased during the postpartum period, and the administration of exogenous gonadotropin-releasing hormone (GnRH) pulses restores gonadotropin secretion. All of this suggests a central blockade of folliculogenesis secondary to hyperprolactinemia.[39]

## BREAST FUNCTION AND AGING

In the reproductive-aged woman, glandular tissue makes up ~20% of the breast volume. The remainder of the breast is composed of connective and adipose tissue. Breast volume changes throughout the menstrual cycle by ~20% secondarily to vascular and lymphatic congestion. Adding to the increased volume of the breast is increased mitotic activity in nonglandular tissue. Breast engorgement and change in volume result in some element of mastalgia in most women, and this combined with an increase in tactile sensitivity of the breast results in the premenstrual tenderness found in most women.[40,41]

With the advent of menopause and a decrease in secretion of the gonadotropins estrogen and progesterone, involution of both glandular and ductal components of the breast occurs. Without replacement estrogen therapy there is a decrease in the number and size of glandular elements and both ducts and lobules become atrophic. Over time, the volume of the breast is primarily replaced with both adipose and stromal tissues, and as with most tissues there is a loss of both contour and structure, which makes the aging breast more amenable to surveillance with mammography.[42,43]

## PATHOPHYSIOLOGY

Any disorder of the breast is viewed by the patient with alarm. Although, with the exception of carcinoma, disorders of the breast are not life threatening, any deviation from normal size and appearance must be thoroughly evaluated. Because the development of the breasts is hormone dependent and breast disorders either may have a hormonal etiology or may be misconstrued as having a hormonal cause, the endocrinologist should be familiar with the pathophysiology of these organs.

### DEVELOPMENTAL ANOMALIES

It was not until 1969 that a system for classifying breast development was established by Marshall and Tanner[9] (see Chap. 91). In addition to its obvious use in evaluating the adequacy of breast development, this classification can be used to determine the presence of pathology.

#### CONGENITAL ANOMALIES

Congenital anomalies of the breast itself are uncommon; however, one frequently sees anomalies of development. Even so, *amastia*, congenital absence of the breast; *athelia*, congenital absence of the nipple; *polymastia*, multiple breasts; *polythelia*, multiple nipples; or some combination, occur in 1% to 2% of the population and may have a familial tendency.[44] If treatment is deemed necessary, surgical augmentation or excision is recommended (Fig. 106-2).

Young patients may present with the problem of *premature thelarche* (see Chap. 92). Many would define this condition as breast development beginning before age 8. Affected individuals may have either bilateral or unilateral development. The disorder may be differentiated from precocious puberty by the finding of prepubertal serum levels of gonadotropin and estrogen. Precocious thelarche is self-limited and demands no therapy other than assurance, once complete or incomplete isosexual precocity has been ruled out.

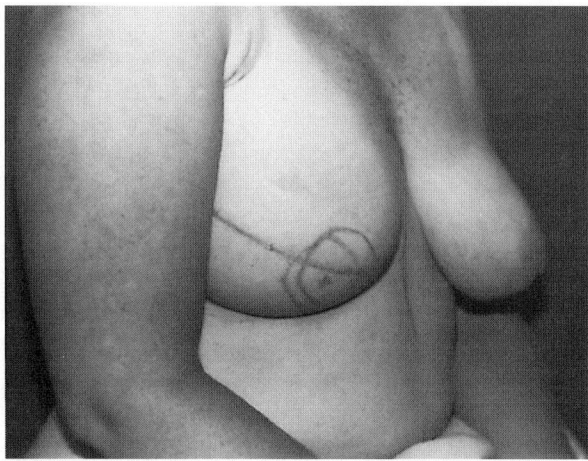

**FIGURE 106-2.** Patient with Poland syndrome (aplasia of the pectoralis muscles, rib deformities, webbed fingers, and radial nerve aplasia, often associated with unilateral amastia) after partial reconstruction. The areola and nipple remain to be reconstructed.

## BREAST ASYMMETRY

Breast asymmetry is fairly common (Fig. 106-3) and presumably is secondary to a difference in end-organ sensitivity to estrogen and progesterone. Occasionally, full symmetry is obtained in adolescents by the administration of an oral contraceptive agent, although either augmentation or reduction mammoplasty may be required if severe asymmetry does not resolve. Most patients with breast asymmetry do not require therapy other than reassurance that this is simply a variation of normal.

## HYPOPLASIA OF THE BREASTS

Perhaps one of the most common disorders of the breast involves hypoplasia. These individuals may simply have small

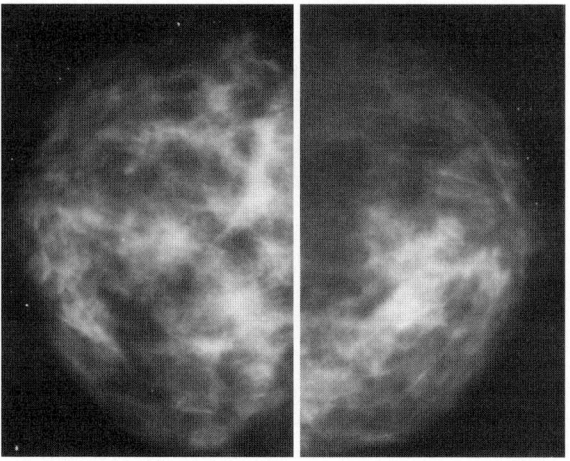

**FIGURE 106-3.** Normal mammogram showing breast asymmetry. Contemporary mammography uses a low kilovoltage–high milliamperage technique; the dose generally ranges from 20 to 30 kVp. Limitation of breast motion with a compression device allows decreased milliamperage and increased magnification to produce a more uniform image density. The breast image varies with the age of the patient. Virginal breasts are small and have near-consistent fibroglandular tissue. Breasts of a reproductive-aged individual, as shown in this figure, vary between well-developed fibroglandular and adipose tissues. Ducts and fibrous tissue are difficult to differentiate and are often found together. A wide variation is noted in the postmenopausal period, but there generally is increased fat content, making trabeculae, subareolar ducts, and veins easily visible. The atrophic breast shows a ground-glass homogeneity with prominent residual trabeculae.

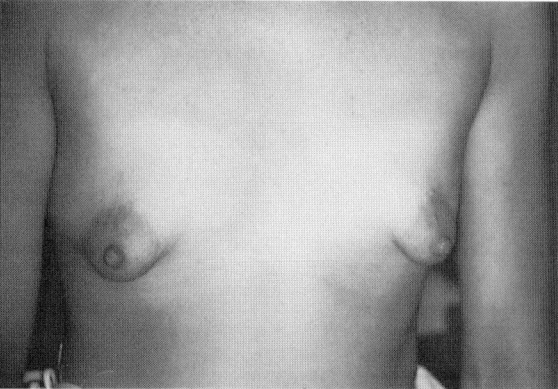

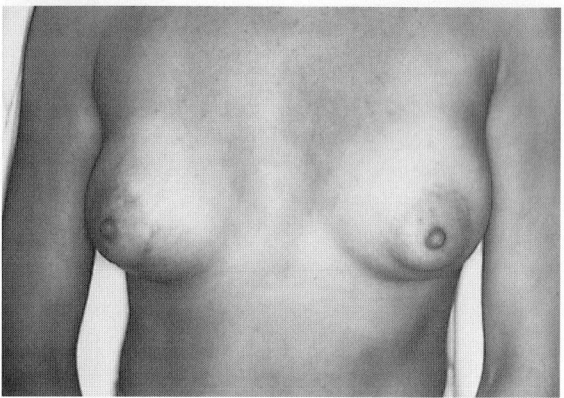

**FIGURE 106-4.** Breast hypoplasia (*top*) and same patient after augmentation mammoplasty (*bottom*).

breasts secondary to a transient delay in puberty or may have a genetic tendency toward hypoplasia, with other siblings having similar problems. Such breasts show a physiologic response to pregnancy, and lactation can follow. Not uncommonly, because of social pressure to have "normal-sized" breasts, augmentation is often sought by affected individuals (Fig. 106-4). Such augmentation will not interfere with lactation or breast-feeding but does increase the difficulty of self-examination and surveillance for breast malignancies. Breast hypoplasia is sometimes found in patients with severe anorexia nervosa and other variants of psychogenic amenorrhea associated with decreased body weight or extremes of exercise (see Chap. 128); such individuals have an altered fat/lean mass body ratio, which generally renders them hypogonadotropic and hypoestrogenic. The removal of estrogen-progesterone stimulation leads to breast atrophy. Reconstructive therapy is contraindicated in this group; correction of nutritional requirements is the therapy of choice, although this must often be accompanied by psychotherapy in patients with emotionally related weight loss.

Breast hypoplasia also occurs in the female pseudohermaphroditism of congenital adrenal hyperplasia (see Chap. 77) and in Turner syndrome (see Chap. 90). The early institution of corticosteroid therapy will greatly benefit the former patient; the latter should be treated at the appropriate time with cyclical estrogen and progesterone.

## BREAST HYPERTROPHY

Breast hypertrophy or *macromastia* is encountered commonly in both adolescents and adults. The breasts may be either symmetric or asymmetric. The patient frequently presents seeking advice on reduction mammoplasty (Fig. 106-5), perhaps because of chest wall pain secondary to the weight of the breasts, difficulty in finding clothes that fit the upper body, and difficulty with her self-image. Frequently, young women are under intense sexual pressure and are often embarrassed by

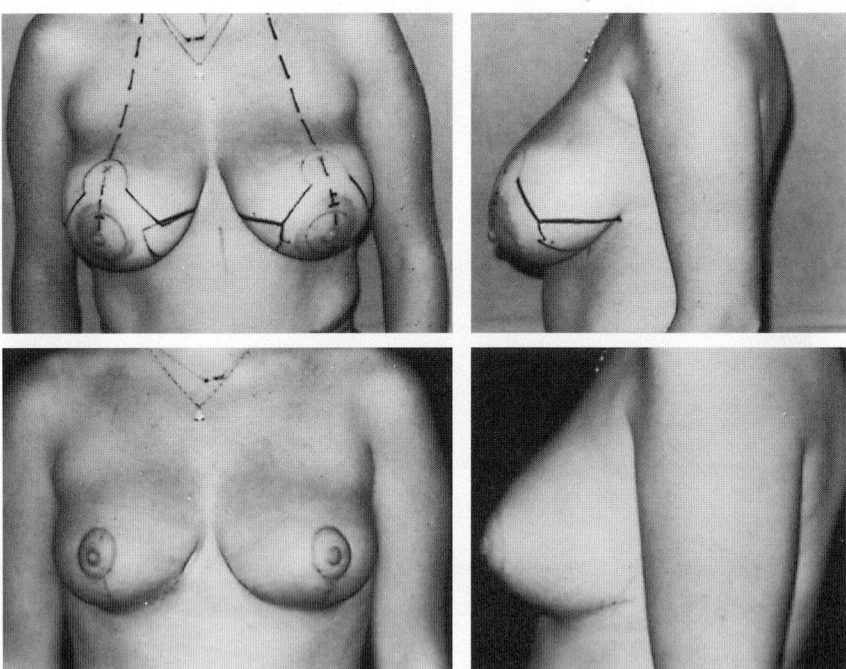

**FIGURE 106-5.** Patient before (*top left and right*) and after (*bottom left and right*) reduction mammoplasty.

peers during gymnasium classes or when wearing swimming suits. As an alternative to surgical correction, danazol has been tried.[45] Unfortunately, this drug has many side effects and definitely is not acceptable for long-term therapy.

### NIPPLE INVERSION

Nipple inversion is common but rarely presents as a complaint to the clinician. Cosmetic repair can be performed, but breast-feeding is difficult after such procedures.

### GALACTORRHEA

Galactorrhea, the inappropriate production and secretion of milk, may be intermittent or continuous, bilateral or unilateral, free flowing or expressible. By definition, *fat droplets* must be present on microscopic examination for a breast secretion to be considered milk and as evidence of galactorrhea. Galactorrhea is frequently associated with hyperprolactinemia (see Chap. 13),[46] which should be sought by repeatedly measuring serum prolactin levels, remembering that prolactin is a stress-related hormone whose secretion may be increased by breast examination and stimulation, acute exercise, food intake (particularly protein), and sleep.[47] Although the differential diagnosis of hyperprolactinemia is extensive, the common causes of this condition are prolactinoma, primary hypothyroidism, and drug intake. Galactorrhea should be evaluated by the measurement of multiple serum prolactin levels, thyroxine, and thyroid-stimulating hormone and by radiographic or magnetic resonance imaging studies of the pituitary. The prolactin level at which radiographic surveillance is begun is debated; however, computed tomography or magnetic resonance imaging should be done if basal prolactin levels exceed 100 ng/mL. Galactorrhea and its treatment are considered in more detail in Chapters 13, 21, 22, and 23.

### MASTODYNIA

Mastodynia, painful engorgement of the breasts, is usually cyclic, becoming worse before menstruation.[48] Although most women describe mastodynia at some times, they require no therapy. However, some patients require cyclic analgesics or nonsteroidal antiinflammatory drugs. Occasionally mastodynia is a complaint of women experiencing the premenstrual syndrome; some affected patients will sporadically obtain some

relief with nonspecific therapy, as discussed in Chapter 99. Mastodynia may also be treated effectively with danazol, but the side effects of the drug mandate its use only in severe cases.

In addition, a second generation of drugs, the GnRH analogs, have been used to induce hypogonadotropism and hypoestrogenism, thus treating disorders such as endometriosis, fibroids, hirsutism, and premenstrual syndrome. Treatment with these agents, either on a daily or monthly basis, will result in profound hypogonadism, breast atrophy, and relief of mastodynia. These drugs are not approved by the Food and Drug Administration for this purpose, and therapy beyond 6 months results in reversible bone demineralization. To compensate for this loss in other disorders, estrogen "add-back" therapy, cotreatment with progestogens, and the use of variable-dose estrogen-progestogen overlapping protocols have been used to counter this and other side effects.

### BREAST INFECTIONS

Breast infections are often confused with galactorrhea but require therapy with appropriate systemic antibiotics. Patients present with unilateral or bilateral breast drainage, which, when examined by microscopy, fails to show fat globules. Gram stain frequently will reveal *Staphylococcus*, *Streptococcus*, or *Escherichia coli*. If the discharge has a greenish tint, *Pseudomonas* should be suspected. If the discharge is accompanied by abscess formation, drainage as well as antibiotics should be used.

The *galactocele*, or retention cyst, which usually occurs after cessation of lactation, is caused by duct obstruction and can masquerade as mastitis. These lesions usually lie below the areola and are often tender to palpation. Such cysts occasionally can be emptied by properly placed pressure; however, drainage frequently must be carried out. Untreated galactoceles may be sites of future sepsis and can calcify and become confused with malignant lesions radiologically. The drainage from a galactocele may range from milky to clear to yellow-green purulent-appearing material; however, these lesions are usually sterile.

### MAMMARY DYSPLASIAS

Mammary dysplasia is perhaps the most common lesion of the female breast (Fig. 106-6). Historically, mammary dysplasias have carried the label fibrocystic disease, chronic lobular hyper-

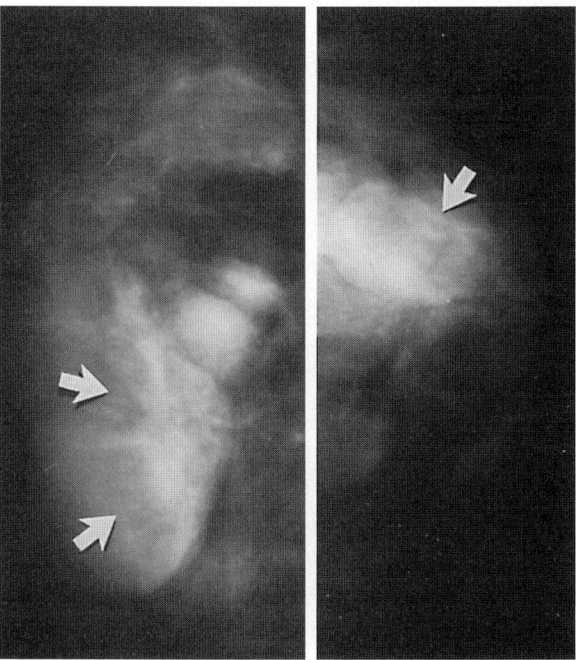

**FIGURE 106-6.** Composite mammogram showing bilateral fibrocystic disease. Note multiple large cysts in body of breast (*arrows*).

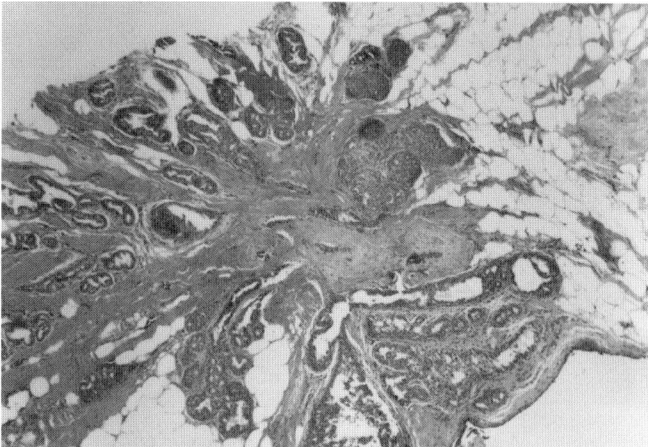

**FIGURE 106-7.** Light mammograph of tissue sample showing sclerosing adenosis.

plasia, cystic hyperplasia, or chronic cystic mastitis.[49] The term *cystic mastitis* should be discarded, since inflammation is not present in this disorder.

Mammary dysplasia may be unilateral or bilateral and most frequently occurs in the upper outer quadrants. The disorder tends to be exacerbated in the premenstrual period. Patients usually complain of pain or lumps in the breasts. The breasts may be tender in many locations; axillary adenopathy is generally not found. Palpable breast lumps are usually cystic and tense; they shrink after menstruation. The natural history of the disease varies; however, it tends to resolve at menopause. Mammary dysplasia may be accompanied by a nipple discharge, which may be clear or bloody, in up to 15% of patients. The disorder may be confused with carcinoma, and a Papanicolaou smear of the discharge, mammography, and perhaps needle aspiration may be necessary to rule out a malignancy. At the time of aspiration, one may evacuate a cyst filled with a dirty gray-green fluid. The management of this problem includes frequent breast examination, periodic mammography, use of a brassiere with good support, perhaps avoiding methylxanthines and chocolate, and, in extreme cases, the use of danazol therapy in daily doses of 100 to 800 mg in two divided doses. Although bromocriptine suppresses prolactin secretion, it has not been effective in the management of fibrocystic disease. It does decrease cyclic mastodynia, however. Likewise, GnRH analogs can be used in extreme cases. The dose of leuprolide acetate used to induce hypogonadism is 3.75 mg given intramuscularly every month.

## TUMORS OFTEN CONFUSED WITH BREAST CARCINOMA

A few lesions, such as fat necrosis, adenosis (especially the sclerosing type), intraductal papilloma (including juvenile papillomatosis), and fibroadenoma (including cystosarcoma phylloides), are often confused with carcinoma of the breast.[50]

### FAT NECROSIS

Fat necrosis may present as a hard lump that may be tender; it rarely enlarges. Skin retraction may be seen, along with irregularity of the edges; fine, stippled calcifications may be present on mammography. Approximately half the patients have a history of trauma. Excisional biopsy is the treatment of choice. At biopsy, one may note hemorrhage into the fatty tissue.

### SCLEROSING ADENOSIS

Breast adenosis may be confused with carcinoma, particularly if sclerosing adenosis is present. This latter condition is characterized by the proliferation of ductal tissue, producing a palpable lesion. These lesions are common in younger women, especially in the third and fourth decades of life; they are rarely seen postmenopausally. Grossly, breast carcinoma is often firm and gritty to palpation, whereas adenosis is usually rubbery. Microscopically, one sees a nodule or whorl pattern. In sclerosing adenomatous adenosis, one also sees circumscription of the lesion, central attenuation of ductal caliber, an organoid arrangement of the ducts, mild epithelial tissue surrounding the ducts, and absence of intraductal epithelial bridging (Fig. 106-7).

### INTRADUCTAL PAPILLOMA

Intraductal papilloma is a benign lesion of the lactiferous duct walls that occurs centrally beneath the areola in 75% of cases.[51] Such lesions present as pain or bloody discharge. They are soft, small masses that are difficult to palpate. Indeed, if the patient presents with a small palpable mass associated with a bloody nipple discharge, there is a 75% chance that an intraductal papilloma will be found. If no mass can be palpated, Paget disease of the nipple or a carcinoma must be considered. Intraductal papilloma is not premalignant and is best managed by excision of the duct by wedge resection. Although intraductal papillomas generally occur in women in the late childbearing years, they may present in the adolescent. In these younger patients, such lesions are generally found at the periphery of the breast; multiple ducts may be involved, and cystic dilation is noted. These lesions have been called "Swiss cheese disease" or *juvenile papillomatosis*. The treatment of juvenile papillomatosis involves excisional biopsy (Fig. 106-8).

### FIBROADENOMA

One of the most common benign neoplasms of the adolescent and adult breast is the *fibroadenoma*[52,53] (Fig. 106-9). These tumors may be small, firm nodules or large, rapidly growing masses that are multiple 20% of the time. They are more common in black than in white women. They may be painful. The fibroadenoma may be hormonally responsive; rapid growth occurs during pregnancy and lactation. These tumors are best treated by excisional biopsy. Rare variants of the fibroadenoma (cystosarcoma phylloides, also known as the giant fibroade-

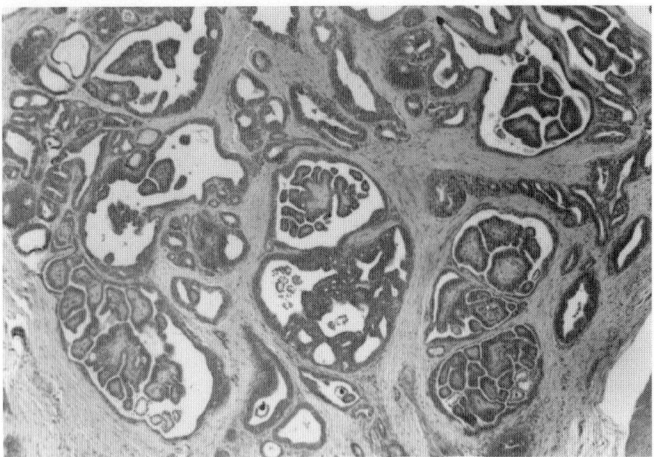

**FIGURE 106-8.** Light micrograph of tissue sample showing intraductal papilloma.

noma) have been described. Although these tumors are generally benign, a few have true sarcomatous potential.

## ASSESSMENT OF BREAST DISEASE

### SELF-EXAMINATION

Breast self-examination is still one of the most important methods for the diagnosis of diseases of the breast, either benign or malignant. A poll conducted for the American Cancer Society found that the physician plays a pivotal role in encouraging patients to practice breast self-examination.[53] It was noted that when patients received personal instruction from their physicians, 92% continued to practice breast self-examination regularly. Once taught self-examination, many patients can detect nodules in their own breasts before they are palpable by a skilled physician. Care must be taken to convince each patient that her breasts are not homogeneous but rather contain various structures and different degrees of nodularity, thickening, and small lumps. The texture of the breast changes throughout a woman's life and during the menstrual cycle (Table 106-3).

It is suggested that breast self-examination be practiced each month, preferably just after the menstrual period.[54] The examination should consist of inspection of the size, shape, and skin color and for puckering, dimpling, retraction of any of the surface, and any nipple discharge. The patient should look at her breasts by placing her hands on her hips and flexing the shoulders forward, then raising the hands behind her head. Breasts may be asymmetric in size, but asymmetry in movement is an indication of pathology. Next, palpation of the breast should be carried out in both the sitting and supine positions. Each quadrant should be palpated systematically, including the nipple and areolar area. Special attention should be paid to the upper

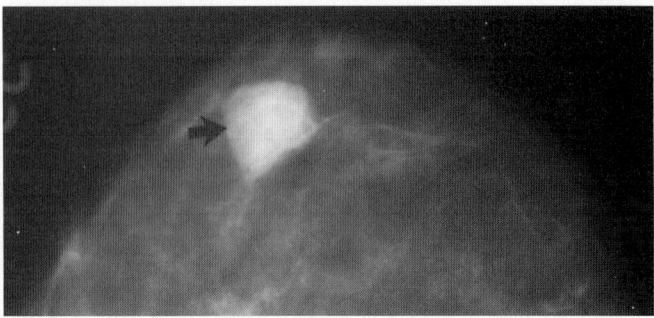

**FIGURE 106-9.** Mammogram showing fibroadenoma (*arrow*).

### TABLE 106-3.
### Breast Self-Examination

1. Begin at 20 years
2. Carry out exams at least once per month
3. Assess the following:
   a. Symmetry
   b. Size
   c. Lumps
   d. Skin discoloration, dimpling, puckering
   e. Nipple discharge
   f. Pain
   g. Nipple inversion

outer quadrant and the axilla, because this is the most frequent site of breast carcinoma. Examination can be carried out with the fingertips or with a rotary motion as suggested by the American Cancer Society. An annual physical examination also should be performed by a physician skilled in the diagnosis of breast disease. There are different variations and techniques of breast examination, but a consistent systematic examination is central to all.

### MAMMOGRAPHY

Breast imaging dates back to 1913. Mammography has been refined subsequently such that improved image, clarity, and contrast have increased its accuracy to well more than 90%.[55–59]

Despite widespread publicity urging the use of mammography and mass screening, breast cancer still strikes many women and is a common cause of death.[60] Although most recommendations relating to breast screening are aimed at women aged 35 or older, the incidence of breast cancer in women younger than 35 is not zero. An interdisciplinary task force in the United States has made the following recommendations[61]: First, mammography should be a part of clinical examination for breast disease and does not substitute for any part. Second, the mainstay of detection of breast disease remains self-examination and physician consultation. Third, women are candidates for mammography at any age if they have masses or nipple discharge, masses felt by the patient but not confirmed by a physician,[62] previous surgical alteration of the breast by augmentation procedures or implants, contralateral disease, previous breast cancer, history of breast cancer in a mother or sister, first pregnancy after age 30, and abnormal patterns in baseline mammography suggestive of increased risk[63] (Table 106-4). Women older than age 50 should receive regular breast examinations, including mammography, as determined by the physician. Baseline mammography should be performed on all women at some time between the ages of 35 and 50.

### BREAST IMAGING WITHOUT RADIATION

Because of concerns about the hazards of multiple radiation exposures for mammography, several other modes have been introduced in the field of breast imaging.

### TABLE 106-4.
### Principal Breast Cancer Risk Factors

**REPRODUCTIVE EXPERIENCE**
   Risk increases with increased age at which a woman bears her first full-term child
**OVARIAN ACTIVITY**
   70% risk reduction in women who undergo oophorectomy before age 35
**BENIGN BREAST DISEASE**
   Four-fold increase in risk in women with history of mammary dysplasia
**FAMILIAL TENDENCY**
   Two-fold to three-fold increased risk if female relative has breast cancer

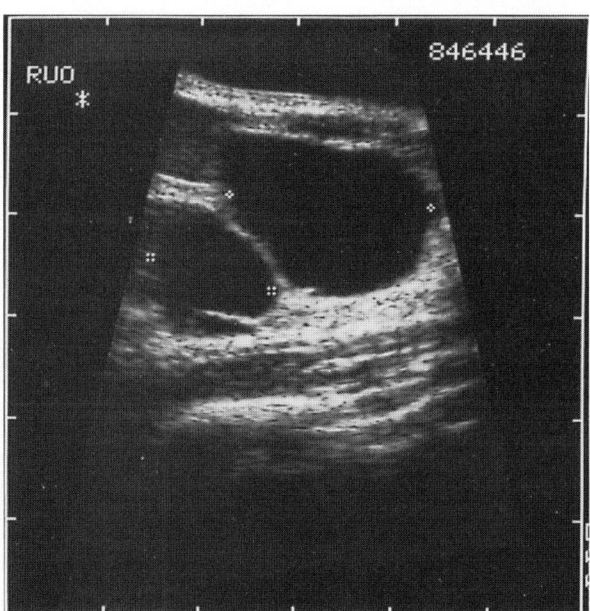

**FIGURE 106-10.** Breast sonogram showing fibrocystic disease. Multiple cysts are outlined by the *small white dots.*

**Thermography.** Thermography maps focal variations in skin temperature by various techniques.[64] Invasive breast cancers produce higher skin temperature, and thermography is accurate for detecting advanced disease. However, it is ineffective in the diagnosis of nonpalpable cancers, detecting only approximately one-half the cases that can be discovered by mammography. Thus it is not an acceptable modality for population screening.

**Ultrasound Mammography.** Breast ultrasound mammography can produce images in conjunction with immersion of the glands in a water bath[65] (Fig. 106-10). However, it has poor resolution; it will not image structures smaller than 1 mm or identify microcalcification. Ultrasonography seems to be most successfully applied to the diagnosis of breast disease in younger patients and is thought to be complementary to mammography.

## IMPORTANCE OF EARLY DIAGNOSIS OF BREAST ANOMALIES AND DISEASES

The endocrinologist should encourage early diagnosis of congenital and acquired breast disorders. Fear of breast disease and subsequent surgical mutilation often causes the patient to defer evaluation, often worsening the outcome. In particular, the mortality from breast cancer remains high, in part because of such delays.[66] It thus should be emphasized that both benign and malignant diseases of the breast are diagnosable at the most treatable stage by self-examination, early physician consultation, radiographic study, and, sometimes, other methods, and that the treatment of developmental anomalies and of benign and malignant breast disease may be hormonal as well as surgical (see Chap. 224). Moreover, even when surgery is mandated, early diagnosis plus available plastic surgery procedures can produce both cure and aesthetically satisfactory results.

## COMPLICATIONS OF BREAST AUGMENTATION

Major developments in breast augmentation such as silicone implants, mucocutaneous flaps, and autogenous tissue transfers have occurred within the past 20 years. When silicone implants were first introduced in 1964,[67] they were thought to be biocompatible products. However, it has been postulated that biomaterials such as silicone might behave like other immunogenic substances. Antibodies to silicone were described in sera of two patients who had severe chronic inflammatory reactions around implanted Silastic ventriculoperitoneal shunt tubing.[68] A study evaluating the sera of 79 women with breast implants who experienced a wide variety of problems found that half had antibody levels >2 standard deviations above the control group without implants.[69] Subsequent studies have been contradictory. Access to silicone implants has been restricted, and the Food and Drug Administration approved a protocol to evaluate silicone implants in women whose saline-filled implants are considered medically unsatisfactory.[70]

Augmentation mammoplasty creates a second problem, that is, the effect of capsular contracture on the quality of mammography. Moderate contracture has been predicted to result in a 50% reduction in the quality of visualization.[71,72] These factors need to be considered in advising patients about augmentation mammoplasty.

## BREAST CANCER

### ETIOPATHOLOGY

Despite the investments that have been made in the diagnosis and treatment of breast cancer over the last two decades, only modest headway has been made in managing this disease. Currently, women in the United States have a 1 in 8 risk, which is twice that found in 1940. In one study, at age 25, a woman had a 1 in 19,608 risk of developing breast cancer; by age 40 this had increased to 1 in 217; by age 70, 1 in 14; and by age 85, 1 in 9.[73]

Family history seems to play a major role in the development of breast cancer, with a two- to three-fold increased risk in the incidence of the disease being found in women who have female relatives with the disease. For instance, the patient with an affected mother or sister has a 2.3 relative risk and an affected aunt 1.5 relative risk, and a 14% incidence when both mother and sister are affected. Hereditary forms of breast cancer make up ~8% of the disease population, and those women who have a strong family history tend to develop the disease at a younger age.[74]

In this respect, perhaps the most exciting event to have occurred in breast cancer research is the identification of genes predisposing to breast cancer. BRCA-1 and BRCA-2 together account for approximately two-thirds of familial breast cancer or roughly 5% of all cases.[75–78] It also appears that BRCA-1 is associated with the predisposition of ovarian cancer. BRCA-1 is located on a locus on chromosome 17Q, and an analysis of 200 families has shown that BRCA-1 is responsible for multiple cases of breast cancer in ~33% of families but more than 80% of families in which there is both breast cancer and epithelial ovarian cancer. Women who inherit the BRCA genes have a 60% risk of acquiring breast cancer by age 50, and a 90% overall lifetime risk. BRCA-2 lies within a 6-centimorgan interval on chromosome 13Q12.13 centered on D13S260. The loss of this gene may also result in elimination of suppressor function. The discovery of these genes presents the possibility for genetic testing, which remains controversial at present.

Cigarettes, coffee, alcohol, and diet may play a role in the development of breast cancer. Tobacco-related cancers appear in the lung, esophagus, oral cavity, pancreas, kidney, bladder, and breast. Therefore, smoking remains the chief preventable cause of death and illness in the United States. It is responsible for ~70% of all deaths; however, although smoking decreased from 40% in 1965 to 29% in 1987, more than 5 million Americans continue to smoke. The incidence of smoking in women has risen at an alarming rate, and this parallels the increase in lung cancer found in women. Further, there has been an abrupt increase in smoking in girls aged 11 through 17.[79]

Methylxanthine-containing compounds have been implicated as a causative factor in the development of fibrocystic disease of the breast and cancer. The Boston Collaborative Drug Surveillance Program showed an increased risk in women who drank between one and three cups of coffee or tea per day.[80]

Several studies have evaluated the role of alcohol and its association with an increased risk of breast cancer. Women who consume more than three drinks per day have been reported to have a 40% increase in the risk of breast cancer.[81,82]

Dietary fat intake has been thought to be linked to breast cancer, but this relationship is controversial.[82a] It was noted that postmenopausal women in the United States are at a much higher risk for breast cancer than are Asian women. This does not appear to be a geographic phenomenon as movement of Asian women to either the Hawaiian Islands or Pacific Coast seems to eradicate the difference in incidence. The suppression, however, usually requires one to two generations to demonstrate significance. Other populations with high fat intake but relatively low risk of cancer such as seen in Greece or Spain use monounsaturated fats composed primarily of oleic acid. Likewise, fish oil which is rich in omega-3 fatty acids has been associated with a lower incidence of breast cancer in countries ranging from Greenland to Japan.[83]

Steroid hormones are thought to affect the expression of breast cancer. For instance, a woman who has a child at the age of 18 has approximately one-third the risk of a woman who delivers after age 35. However, pregnancy must occur before age 30 to be protective, but, in fact, a woman who gives birth after age 35 appears to be at greater risk than a woman who has never been pregnant. There is also a 70% reduction of risk in the incidence of breast cancer in women who undergo oophorectomy before the age of 35. There also appears to be a small increased risk in patients who experience early menarche as well as late menopause. It has been suggested that the endocrine milieu influences the susceptibility of the breast to environmental carcinogens.[84] This is the so-called *estrogen window hypothesis*, which suggests that an unopposed estrogen stimulation at certain periods of life favors tumor induction. The longer the unopposed estrogen stimulation acts on the breast, the greater is the risk factor. Perhaps pregnancy, a high progesterone state, closes the window, because progesterone is known to down-regulate the estrogen receptors in the endometrium and is protective against the development of endometrial cancer. Although the data appear to be inconclusive at present, one might speculate that a similar mechanism may be achieved at the level of the breast.

Various chemical agents have been implicated in a decrease or increase in breast cancer. Estrogens of all types and their analogs may stimulate tumorigenesis. Progestogens, while regulating estrogen expression, can induce significant mitosis of both epithelial and stromal components.[85] Historically, birth control pills have been evaluated using a variety of different study designs, and many, but not all reports have shown no increased risk of breast cancer.[86–88] GnRH analogs decrease estrogen production and therefore are thought to be protective against breast cancer. Tamoxifen is a weak estrogen agonist that antagonizes the biologic effect of 17β-estradiol. It is now used for the treatment of breast cancer in both menopausal and perimenopausal women, and current data suggest that this drug may in fact retard the expression of breast cancer. Raloxifene, a selective estrogen receptor modulator (SERM), used in hormonal replacement therapy, has also been shown to reduce the incidence of breast cancer and is given as a hormonal replacement therapy in menopause.[88a]

## POSTOPERATIVE REHABILITATION OF THE PATIENT WITH BREAST CANCER

Chapter 224 discusses the current therapy of breast cancer. Thirty years ago, radical mastectomy was considered by many surgeons to be the treatment of choice for resectable breast cancer. Reconstructive options were few, and required 3 to 4 stage procedures to create an adequate breast replacement. Usually, women were required to wear external breast prostheses. This resulted in surgical patients feeling disfigured, having a poor body image, lower self-esteem, and diminished feelings of sexual attractiveness and of femininity. Now, reconstructive techniques can be carried out immediately, or can be delayed. There has been a trend toward immediate reconstruction, as this tends to reduce the degree of psychological morbidity experienced by the patient, and the reconstructed breast is integrated into the body image. Further, the integrity of the soft tissue that envelops the breast is intact at the time of surgery; there is no fibrosis or contraction of the tissue, and a plastic surgeon can be involved in the surgery and the reconstruction to give the best cosmetic result, whether implant or autologous tissue is used.[89–92]

Following reconstruction, breast cancer patients are usually examined every 3 months for the first 5 years, at every 6 months for the next 5 years, and yearly thereafter. A metastatic survey including a complete blood cell count, blood chemistry, chest x-ray, and mammogram should be performed routinely in patients with stage I or II disease.

## REFERENCES

1. Mepham T. Physiological aspects of lactation. In: McPhan T, ed. Biochemistry of lactation. New York: Elsevier, 1983:3.
2. Peterson LV. Lactation. Physiol Rev 1944; 24:340.
3. Riddle O, Bates R, Dykshorn S. The preparation, identification and assay of prolactin-A hormone of the anterior pituitary. Am J Physiol 1933; 105:191.
4. Meites J, Turner C. Studies concerning the mechanism controlling the initiation of lactation at parturition: II. Why lactation is not initiated during pregnancy. Endocrinology 1942; 30:719.
5. Clifton K, Furth J. Ducto-alveolar growth in mammary glands of adrenogonadectomized male rats bearing mammotropic pituitary tumors. Endocrinology 1960; 66:893.
6. Chen C, Meites J. Effects of estrogen and progesterone on serum and pituitary levels in ovariectomized rats. Endocrinology 1970; 86:503.
7. Kuhn N. Progesterone withdrawal as the lactogenic trigger in the rat. J Endocrinol 1969; 44:39.
8. McKiernan J, Coyne J, Canglone S. Histology of breast development in early life. Arch Dis Child 1988; 63:136.
9. Marshall W, Tanner J. Variations in pattern of pubertal changes in girls. Arch Dis Child 1969; 44:291.
10. Cowie AT. Backward glances. In: Yokoyama A, Mizuno H, Nagasawa II, eds. Physiology of mammary glands. Baltimore: University Park Press, 1978:43.
11. Tonelli G, Sorof S. Epidermal growth factor: requirement for development of cultured mammary glands. Nature 1980; 285:250.
12. Ichinose R, Nandi S. Influence of hormones on lobulo-alveolar differentiation of mouse mammary glands in vitro. J Endocrinol 1966; 35:331.
13. Cowie A, Tindal J, Yokoyama A. The induction of mammary growth in the hypophysectomized goat. J Endocrinol 1966; 34:184.
14. Lyons WR. Hormonal synergism in mammary growth. Proc R Soc Biol 1958; 149:303.
15. Going JJ, Anderson TJ, Battersby S, et al. Proliferative and secretory activity in human breast during natural and artificial menstrual cycles. Am J Pathol 1988; 130:193.
16. Talwalker P, Meites T. Mammary lobulo-alveolar growth induced by anterior pituitary hormones in adreno-ovariectomized-hypophysectomized rats. Proc Soc Exp Biol Med 1961; 107:880.
17. France J, Seddon R, Liggins G. A study of a pregnancy with low estrogen production due to placental sulfatase deficiency. J Clin Endocrinol Metab 1973; 36:19.
18. Topper Y, Freeman C. Multiple hormone interactions in the developmental biology of the mammary gland. Physiol Rev 1980; 60:1049.
19. Elias J. Effect of insulin and cortisol on organ cultures of adult mouse mammary gland. Proc Soc Exp Biol Med 1959; 101:500.
20. Fleet I, Goode J, Hamon M, et al. Secretory activity of goat mammary glands during pregnancy and the onset of lactation. J Physiol 1975; 251:763.
21. Weiss G, Facog E, O'Byrne E, et al. Secretion of progesterone and relaxin by the human corpeus luteum at midpregnancy and at term. Obstet Gynecol 1977; 50:679.
22. Martin R, Glass M, Wilson G, Woods K. Human α-lactalbumin and hormonal factors in pregnancy and lactation. Clin Endocrinol (Oxf) 1980; 13:223.
23. Hartmann P, Trevethan P, Shelton J. Progesterone and oestrogen and the initiation of lactation in ewes. J Endocrinol 1973; 59:249.
24. Bruce J, Ramirez V. Site of action of the inhibitory effect of estrogen upon lactation. Neuroendocrinology 1978; 6:19.
25. Grosvenor CE, Picciano MF, Baumrucker CR. Hormones and growth factors in milk. Endocr Rev 1993; 14:710.
26. Hearn J. Pituitary inhibition of pregnancy. Nature 1973; 241:207.
27. Brun del Re R, del Pozo E, deGrandi P, et al. Prolactin inhibition and suppression of puerperal lactation by a Br-ergocriptine (CB 154): a comparison with estrogen. Obstet Gynecol 1973; 41:884.
28. Vonderhaar BK. Studies on the mechanism by which thyroid hormones enhance α-lactalbumin activity in explants from mouse mammary glands. Endocrinology 1977; 150:1423.

29. Riggs LA, Yen SSC. Multiphasic prolactin secretion during parturition in human subjects. Am J Obstet Gynecol 1977; 128:215.
30. Kuhn NJ. Lactogenesis. The search for trigger mechanisms in different species. Symp Zool Soc Lond 1977; 41:165.
31. Noel GL, Suh HK, Frantz AG. Prolactin release during nursing and breast stimulation in postpartum and non-postpartum subjects. J Clin Encocrinol Metab 1974; 38:413.
32. Nunley WL, Urban RT, Kitchin JD, et al. Dynamics of pulsatile prolactin release during the postpartum lactational period. J Clin Endocrinol Metab 1991; 72:287.
33. Gross B, Eastman C, Bowen C, McEldruff A. Integrated concentration of prolactin in breast-feeding mothers. Aust NZ J Obstet Gynaecol 1979; 19:150.
34. Howie P, McNeilly A, McArdle T, et al. The relationship between suckling-induced prolactin response and lactogenesis. J Clin Endocrinol Metab 1980; 50:670.
35. Tyson J. Nursing and prolactin secretion: principal determinants in the mediation of puerperal infertility. In: Crosignani P, Robyn C, eds. Prolactin and human reproduction. New York: Academic Press, 1977:97.
36. Lincoln O, Wakerley J. Electrophysiological evidence for the activation of supraoptic neuronics during the release of oxytocin. J Physiol (Lond) 1974; 242:533.
37. Brandts C, Rozenberg S, Meuris S. Advances in physiology of human lactation. In: Angeli A, Bradlow H, Dogliotti L, eds. Endocrinology of the breast. Ann NY Acad Sci 1986; 464:66.
38. Lewis PR, Brown JB, Renfree MB, et al. The resumption of ovulation and menstruation in a well-nourished population of women breast feeding for an extended period of time. Fertil Steril 1991; 55:529.
39. Matsuzaki T, Azuma K, Irabara M, et al. Mechanism of anovulation in hyperprolactinemic amenorrhea determined by pulsatile gonadotropin-releasing hormone injection combined with human chorionic gonadotropin. Fertil Steril 1994; 62:2254.
40. Milligan D, Drife JO, Short RV. Changes in breast volume during normal menstrual cycle and after oral contraceptives. Br Med J 1975; 4:494.
41. Robinson JE, Short RV. Changes in breast sensitivity at puberty, during the menstrual cycle, and at parturition. Br Med J 1977; 1:1188.
42. Cowie AT, Forsyth JA, Hart JC. Hormonal control of lactation. Berlin: Springer-Verlag, 1980.
43. Andolina V, Lille S, Wilson KM, eds. Mammographic imaging: a practical guide. Philadelphia: Lippincott, 1992.
44. Pellegrini J, Wagner R. Polythelia and associated conditions. Am Fam Physician 1983; 28:192.
45. Aksu MF, Tzingounis VA, Greenblatt RB. Treatment of benign breast disease with danazol: a follow-up report. J Reprod Med 1978; 31:181.
46. Blackwell RE. Diagnosis and treatment of hyperprolactinemic syndromes. In: Wynn RM, ed. Obstetrics and gynecology annual 1985. Norwalk, CT: Appleton-Century-Crofts, 1985:305.
47. Blackwell RE. Diagnosis and management of prolactinomas. Fertil Steril 1985; 43:5.
48. Pilnik S. Clinical diagnosis of benign breast disease. J Reprod Med 1979; 22:277.
49. Love S, Gelman R, Silen W. Fibrocystic "disease" of the breast: a nondisease? N Engl J Med 1982; 307:1010.
50. Oberman HA. Benign breast lesions confused with carcinoma. In: McDiuitt RW, Oberman HA, Ozzello L, Kaufman N, eds. International Academy of Pathology monograph: the breast. Baltimore: Williams & Wilkins, 1984:1.
51. Haagensen C, Stout A, Phillips J. Neoplasms of the breast: I. Benign intraductal papilloma. Am J Surg 1951; 133:18.
52. Hertel B, Zaloudek C, Kempson R. Breast adenomas. Cancer 1976; 37:2891.
53. Egan R. Breast imaging, 3rd ed. Baltimore: University Park Press, 1984:5.
54. Wilson RW. The breast. In: Sabiston D, ed. Davis-Christopher textbook of surgery, 10th ed. Philadelphia: WB Saunders, 1972:573.
55. Colman M, Mattheiem W. Imaging techniques in breast cancer: workshop report. Eur J Cancer Clin Oncol 1988; 24:69.
56. Maisey MN. Imaging techniques in breast cancer: what is new? What is useful? A review. Eur J Cancer Clin Oncol 1988; 24:61.
57. Bassett LW, Gold RH. The evolution of mammography. AJR Am J Roentgenol 1988; 150:493.
58. Salomon A. Beitrage zur Pathologie und Klinik des Mammarkarzinome. Arch Klin Chir 1913; 101:573.
59. Egan R. Mammography. Springfield, IL: Charles C Thomas Publisher, 1964:1.
60. Pietsch J. Breast disorders. In: Lavery J, Sanfilippo J, eds. Pediatric and adolescent obstetrics and gynecology. New York: Springer-Verlag, 1985:103.
61. Executive Board of the American Academy of Obstetrics and Gynecology. ACOG statement of policy mammography statement. Chicago: American College of Obstetrics and Gynecology, 1979:1.
62. Edeiken S. Mammography and palpable cancer of the breast. Cancer 1988; 61:263.
63. Solin LJ, Legoretta A, Schultz DJ, et al. The importance of mammographic screening relative to the treatment of women with carcinoma of the breast. Arch Intern Med 1994; 154:745.
64. Gauterie M, Gross C. Breast thermography and cancer risk prediction. Cancer 1980; 45:51.
65. Wild J. Review of the ultrasonic examination of the breast. In: Jellins J, Kobayashi T, eds. Ultrasonic examination of the breast. New York: John Wiley and Sons, 1983:21.
66. Carlson RW, Stockdale FE. The clinical biology of breast cancer. Annu Rev Med 1988; 39:453.
67. Cronin TD, Gerow F. Augmentation mammoplasty: a new "natural feel" prosthesis. In: Transactions of the Third International Congress of Plastic Surgeons. Amsterdam: Excerpta Medica, 1964.
68. Goldblum RM, Pelley RP, O'Donell AA, et al. Antibodies to silicone elastomers and reactions to ventriculoperitoneal shunts. Lancet 1992; 340:510.
69. Heggers JP, Goldblum RM, Pyron MT, et al. Immunologic responses to silicone implants: fact or fiction? Plast Surg Forum 1990; 8:13.
70. Randall T. First clinical study of breast implants launched. JAMA 1992; 268:1822.
71. Douglas KP, Bluth EI, Sauter ER, et al. Roentgenographic evaluation of the augmented breast. South Med J 1991; 64:49.
72. Handel N, Silverstein MJ, Gamagami P. Factors affecting mammographic visualization of the breast after augmentation mammaplasty. JAMA 1992; 268:1913.
73. Davis DL, Dinse GE, Hoel DG. Decreasing cardiovascular disease and increasing cancer among whites in the United States from 1973 through 1978. JAMA 1994;271:431.
74. Colton T, Greenberg ER, Noller K, et al. Breast cancer in mothers prescribed diethylstilbestrol in pregnancy. JAMA 1993; 269:2096.
75. Futreal PA, Liu Q, Shattuck-Eldens D, et al. BRCA1 mutations in primary breast and ovarian carcinomas. Science 1994; 266:120.
76. Miki Y, Swensen J, Shattuck-Eldens D, et al. A strong candidate for the breast and ovarian cancer susceptibility gene BRCA1. Science 1994; 266:66.
77. Nowak R. Breast cancer gene offers surprises. Science 1994; 265:1796.
78. Wooster R, Neuhausen SL, Mangion J, et al. Localization of a breast cancer susceptibility gene, BRCA2 to chromosome 13q12–13. Science 1996; 265:2088.
79. Rosenhert L, Schwingi PA. Breast cancer and cigarette smoking. N Engl J Med 1984; 310:92.
80. Welsch CW. Caffeine and the development of a normal and neoplastic mammary gland. Proc Soc Exp Biol 1994; 207:1.
81. Schotzkin A, Jones DY, Hoover RN, et al. Alcohol consumption and breast cancer in the epidemiologic followup study of the first national health and nutrition examination survey. N Engl J Med 1987; 316:1169.
82. Willett WC, Colditz G, Stampler MJ, et al. A prospective study of alcohol intake and risk of breast cancer. Am J Epidemiol 1986; 124:540.
82a. Velie E, Kulldorff M, Schaiver C, et al. Dietary fat, fat sib types, and breast cancer in postmenopausal women: a prospective cohort sudy. J Natl Cancer Inst 2000; 92:833.
83. Bland KI. Risk factors as an indicator for breast cancer screening in asymptomatic patients. Maturitas 1987; 9:135.
84. Korenmann SC. Estrogen window hypothesis of the etiology of breast cancer. Lancet 1980; 1:700.
85. Li JJ, Li SA. Estrogen carcinogenesis in hamster tissues: a critical review. Endocrinol Rev Monograph 1. Endocrine Aspects of Cancer 1993; 1:86.
86. Ramcharan S, Pellegrin FA, Ray RM, Hau J-P. The Walnut Creek Contraceptive Drug Study: a prospective study of the side-effects of oral contraceptives. J Reprod Med 1980; 25:366.
87. Royal College of General Practitioners Oral Contraceptive Study. Further analysis of mortality in oral contraceptive users. Lancet 1981; 1:541.
88a. Minton SE. Chemoprevention of breast cancer in the older patient. Hematol Oncol Clin North Am 2000; 14:113.
88. Kay CR, Hannaford PC. Breast cancer and the pill—a further report from the Royal College of General Practitioners Oral Contraceptive Study. Br J Cancer 1988; 58:675.
89. Lewis FM, Bloom JR. Psychosocial adjustment to breast cancer: a review of selected literature. Int J Psychiatry Med 1978; 9:1.
90. Stevens LA, McGrath MH, Druss RG, et al. The psychological impact of immediate breast reconstruction for women with early breast cancer. Plast Reconstr Surg 1984; 73:619.
91. Rowland JH, Holland JC, Chaglassian T, et al. Psychological response to breast reconstruction. Psychosomatics 1993; 34:241.
92. Moran SL, Herceg S, Kurtelawicz K, Serletti JM. TRAM flap breast reconstruction with expanders and implants. AORN J 2000; 71:354.

# CHAPTER 107

# CONCEPTION, IMPLANTATION, AND EARLY DEVELOPMENT

PHILIP M. IANNACCONE, DAVID O. WALTERHOUSE, AND KRISTINA C. PFENDLER

The hormonal milieu plays an essential role in the production of parental germ cells, the biology of the reproductive process, and the subsequent creation, development, and survival of the offspring. To understand fully the impact of hormones on the adult, the child, the newborn, and the as-yet-unborn, the endocrinologist must be aware of the processes of conception, implantation, and early fetal development.

Human loss through fetal wastage is significant. There are ~600,000 clinically apparent spontaneous abortions per year in the United States, and the 3 million live births probably represent 10 million conceptions.[1] Fetal loss can occur at any of the major steps in development. The probability of pregnancy in any given menstrual cycle under optimal conditions is ~30%.[2–4] The probability of successful fertilization may be as high as 85%, but 25% to 35% of conceptuses do not implant, and as many as 30% fail shortly after implantation. Undoubtedly, this loss represents a reproductive strategy. The rate-limiting feature of reproduction in mammals is the childbearing period. Therefore, if there is a possibility of loss of the individual during or immediately after the pregnancy, it is in the best interests of the species to eliminate the pregnancy as soon as possible and to make the mother available for another pregnancy. Thus, several critical steps of increasing sophistication of cellular coordination are required for the conceptus to enter midgestation and the organogenesis phase of development.

## OOCYTE MATURATION

Oocyte maturation in mammals proceeds from the development of a differentiated *gonadal ridge* in the fetus. For example, at approximately day 11 in the female mouse, *primordial germ cells* have located within the genital ridge, and ovarian development ensues.[5] In humans, primordial germ cells arise in the yolk sac in the fourth week of fetal life and begin migration caudally toward the genital ridge during the fifth week. The *first meiotic division* occurs in the fetal ovary, and the oocyte becomes arrested at the diplotene stage. A germinal vesicle (nucleus) then forms. The first meiotic division is completed in the adult ovary, and the onset of this process is heralded by germinal vesicle breakdown. After telophase I, the first polar body of the oocyte is formed.

The *second meiotic division* begins before ovulation, and the mature oocyte is fertilizable at the anaphase II stage. Fertilization occurs during anaphase II, and the completion of telophase II finds the zygote with two polar bodies and two pronuclei (Fig. 107-1). The oocyte and follicular maturation are discussed in Chapter 94.

Maturation of the oocyte and ovulation are regulated by hormone levels, notably those of follicle-stimulating hormone (FSH). The extruded oocyte and its closely adherent *cumulus adherens* (follicular cells; corona radiata) are collected by the fimbriated end of the oviduct. The adherent cells communicate with one another through a complex network of intercellular bridges that extends from the innermost cells through the zona pellucida to the perivitelline space and into the oocyte[6] (Fig. 107-2). These cells may have important nutritional functions for the oocyte and may control events in maturation or fertilization.[7] The cumulus cells can bind tightly to the epithelial cells of the tube and may help initiate tubal transport. Transport of the egg to fertilization sites at the distal end of the oviduct and transport of the fertilized ovum to the uterus appear to be the concerted effort of the ciliary movement of the epithelium and muscular contractions of the myosalpinx. These contractions are not peristaltic. The sperm at this time are moving in the opposite direction and, although the cilia beat in the direction of the uterus, the muscular contractions of the oviduct do not give direction to moving particles within it. Particles can be propelled in either direction in the fallopian tubes of most species.[8] The role of tubal secretions in the development of the early embryo has not been elucidated. These secretions do not have a demonstrable effect on the sperm because capacitation, which permits the acrosome reaction, can occur in chemically defined media.[9]

Because human oocytes can undergo spontaneous maturation in vitro, there appears to be an active inhibition of oocyte

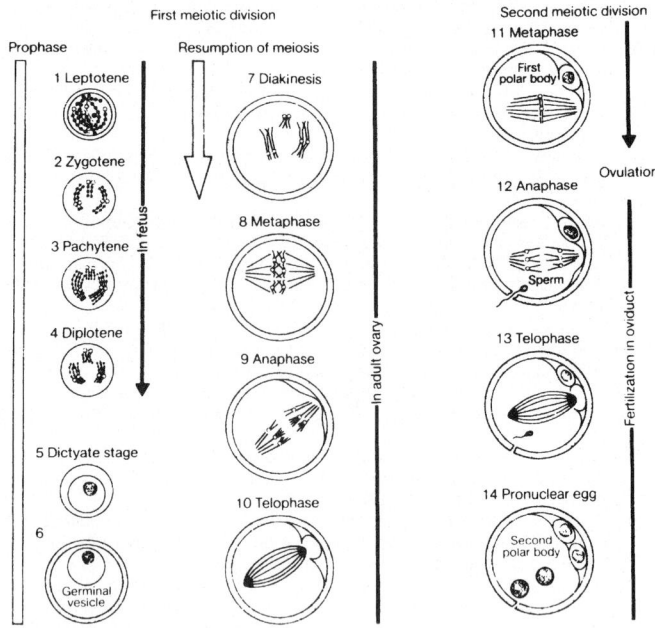

**FIGURE 107-1.** Diagram of oocyte maturation. Completion of the prophase of first meiotic division occurs in the fetal ovary of most animals. At zygotene (stage 2), homologous maternal and paternal chromosomes commence pairing; at pachytene (stage 3), pairing has occurred throughout their lengths, and they form bivalents. Each homologue separates longitudinally to create two sister chromatids; thus, each bivalent forms a tetrad. It is during this stage that crossing over occurs, causing an interchange of genetic material between the paternal and maternal chromatids. At the diplotene stage (stage 4), the chromosomes commence their separation; they remain connected at their points of interchange (chiasmata). The germinal vesicle appears after the first meiotic arrest after the diplotene stage. The dictyate stage is a quiescent period, which may last for many years. In the adult ovary, the first meiotic division is completed. Ovulation occurs after extrusion of the first polar body (stage 11), and the second meiotic division (stages 12–14) is completed after sperm penetration. The zona pellucida is shown as a stippled ring (see Chap. 87). (From Tsafiri A. Oocyte maturation in mammals. In: Jones RE, ed. The vertebrate ovary. New York: Plenum Publishing, 1978:410.)

maturation within the follicle. Meiosis is prevented by a maturation inhibitor produced by the granulosa cells of the follicle.[10] Meiosis is resumed within the follicle after a surge of luteinizing hormone. If oocytes are removed from cumulus cells, maturation inhibitors are ineffective. Moreover, receptors for luteinizing hormone have been demonstrated on cumulus cells but not on denuded oocytes. Therefore, the cumulus cells are important mediators of both maturation inhibition and resumption of meiosis, directed by the preovulatory luteinizing hormone surge.

Interestingly, in humans, oocyte maturation in vitro, as judged by germinal vesicle breakdown, is not necessary for sperm penetration, because penetration can be demonstrated at the first meiotic division. After sperm penetration of the mature oocyte, the sperm head swells and a pronucleus forms, with the sperm midpiece remaining visible. In immature oocytes, the sperm penetrates and swells but no pronucleus is formed. Thus, fertilization competence in humans is achieved only in fully mature oocytes at the time of the second meiotic division.

## SPERM CAPACITATION AND FERTILIZATION

The relatively thick and rigid structure that invests the mammalian egg, called the *zona pellucida*, has necessitated some

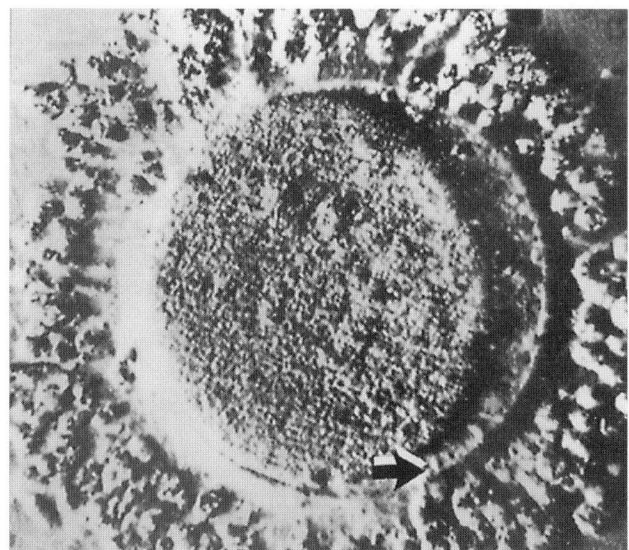

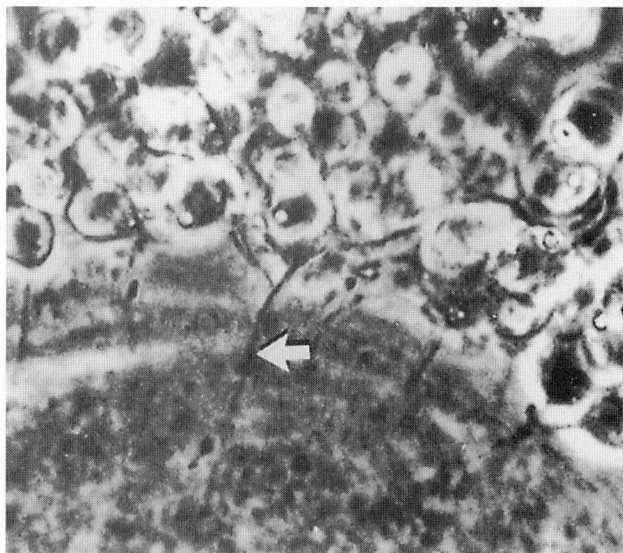

**FIGURE 107-2. A,** Photomicrograph of unfertilized, mature ovum with associated corona radiata cells. Coronal cells close to the ovum send processes through the zona pellucida. These processes (e.g., *arrow*) are evident as granules in the perivitelline space. **B,** Higher magnification in phase contrast shows these connecting processes of the corona radiata cells more clearly (*arrow*). (From Shettles LB. Ovum humanum. Munich: Urban und Schwarzenberg, 1960; 42:52.)

changes in the physiology of fertilization, particularly with respect to the sperm.

Mammalian sperm require the occurrence of two events before they can fertilize an oocyte. The first, known as *capacitation*, is the process by which sperm become competent for fertilization, an act they are not able to accomplish before an appropriate, species-dependent incubation time within the female reproductive tract milieu or similar in vitro medium.[11-13] During this time, the sperm not only mature but also attain a state of hyperactivated motility that is necessary for them to move through the length of the female reproductive tract and to generate the force necessary to pierce through the cumulus oophorus and the zona pellucida of the oocyte. In addition, certain incompletely defined factors known as *decapacitation factors* must be removed from the sperm before they become competent for fertilization. Presumably, these factors are macromolecules that are blocking certain receptor sites necessary for this functional change to occur, and there is evidence that removal of these factors increases the response of the sperm to extracellular $Ca^{2+}$.[11]

Once the sperm are capacitated, the acrosome reaction can begin, and it is through this process that the sperm can ultimately fuse with the oocyte. The morphology of the sperm head is such that an inner acrosomal membrane is immediately adjacent to the nuclear membrane of the cell, whereas an outer acrosomal membrane and the plasma membrane act as the limiting membrane of the acrosome.[14] The acrosome itself contains proteases, such as acrosin, and other enzymes necessary for the sperm to navigate the interstices of the corona radiata. The outer acrosomal membrane possesses specific molecules for attachment to the zona before penetration of the egg, including a receptor that binds to a glycoprotein named *ZP3* of the zona pellucida of the oocyte and a galactosyltransferase that recognizes *N*-acetylglucosamine residues.[15-18] This morphology necessitates some interesting adaptations during the fusion of the sperm to the oocyte. Because the surface molecules necessary for attachment to the zona must be retained, the outer membrane must remain intact after the release of enzymes. The spermatozoon joins with the egg by membrane fusion of a midportion membrane, the equatorial region of the sperm head. The acrosome reaction, then, seems designed to create the structural alterations required for these various constraints to be overcome. First, the sperm-limiting membrane changes to allow influx of calcium, presumably along an electrochemical gradient. Immediately thereafter, the acrosomal membrane becomes fenestrated, appearing to allow the acrosomal contents to be released while leaving the acrosomal membrane, with its putative zona attachment elements, largely intact. The equatorial portion of the membrane is left intact for fusion with the oolemma, the limiting membrane of the unfertilized egg. Once fusion has occurred, the sperm head swells rapidly and forms the male pronucleus, leaving the sperm midpiece visible within the fertilized egg.[19-22]

Numerous cations play distinctive roles in these processes of capacitation and acrosomal exocytosis.[22a] Moreover, it is thought that the female reproductive tract is instrumental in regulating these processes by forming gradients of the cations at different positions along its length, as well as allowing their concentrations to change during certain times of the menstrual cycle.[10] $Ca^{2+}$, one of the most studied of these cations, is necessary for achieving the hyperactivated motility and the fertilizing ability associated with capacitation, in addition to being required for the acrosome reaction. It has been postulated that the binding of sperm to ZP3 of the zona pellucida triggers a G-protein pathway that ultimately leads to the release of bound $Ca^{2+}$,[15] and that this $Ca^{2+}$ stimulates adenylate cyclase to produce cyclic adenosine monophosphate, which in turn activates cyclic adenosine monophosphate–dependent protein kinases that alter the sperm function during these prefertilization events.[11] $Na^+$ also has been shown to be critical for capacitation and the acrosome reaction, although much higher concentrations of $Na^+$ are required for the latter process. Finally, $K^+$ plays a crucial role in these events, albeit in a more regulatory capacity. High levels of $K^+$ do not inhibit capacitation, but they do suppress the fertilizing potential of the sperm. Before ovulation, $Ca^{2+}$ and $Na^+$ concentrations in the female reproductive tract are sufficient for capacitation, but the $K^+$ concentration is too high to permit either the acrosome reaction to proceed or fertilization to occur. Follicular fluids released during ovulation, however, are thought to cause a substantial decrease in $K^+$ concentration, as well as an added increase in $Na^+$ concentration, which result in the fulfillment of fertilizing potential. In addition to the increased potential for fertilization during ovulation that is regulated by the concentrations of these ions, concentrations also seem to vary along the length of the female reproductive tract to help ensure that sperm proceed through capacitation and the acrosome reaction at the proper time and place to optimize fertilization.[10,11]

Immediately after fertilization, the maternal genome is activated and forms the female pronucleus. The sperm nucleus reforms and is evident morphologically as the male pronucleus. As the cells enter mitosis, the nuclear membranes of the pronuclei break down, and the chromosomes comigrate to the poles of the cell, where they are packaged as a unit in the nuclei of the progeny blastomeres. Thus, at the first cleavage, there is a symmetric division of the fertilized egg, and the two blastomeres have fused nuclei containing the maternal and the paternal genomes.

It is clear that genetic information from both the mother and the father is an absolute requirement for normal development. When the maternal or paternal pronucleus is removed from fertilized mouse eggs and the egg is manipulated such that it contains either two maternal or two paternal pronuclei, development cannot proceed past midgestation. Bipaternal conceptions form only placenta, while bimaternal conceptions form disorganized embryonal tissue.[23,24] As a result of these types of experiments, it has become evident that the same gene derived from the mother may be functionally different when derived from the father, leading to the concept of *imprinting*.[25] Imprinting refers to a situation in which a gene is "marked" or "imprinted" during either female or male gametogenesis so that it is not expressed and, consequently, either the remaining paternal or maternal allele is exclusively expressed.[26]

The mechanism of imprinting remains uncertain, and it is not clear if each imprinted gene is imprinted using the same mechanism. Whatever the mechanism, the imprint must be maintained in somatic tissues during specific periods of development but must be reversible in the germline. Most imprinted genes are methylated in a parental-specific manner in the germline, and DNA methylation appears to be the most likely mechanism of imprinting.[27,28] In fact, mice deficient for DNA methyltransferase, an enzyme that helps maintain methylation stability, lose monoallelic expression of several imprinted genes and die in the early postimplantation period, probably because of instability of primary imprints.[29] Methylation may alter chromatin structure and modulate binding of transcriptional regulatory proteins to imprinted genes. The list of imprinted genes is expanding and includes *Wilms tumor 1 (WT1), insulin, insulin-like growth factor-II (IGF-II), insulin-like growth factor-II receptor (IGF-IIR), H19, X-inactive specific transcript (Xist),* and others.[28] The extent of monoallelic expression varies for different imprinted genes during development.

These discoveries are of great importance to medicine because aberrant imprinting has been demonstrated in the setting of human syndromes and cancer. *Biallelic expression* of an imprinted gene results in overexpression of the gene product compared with *monoallelic expression* as seen with imprinting. Expression from two alleles may occur by loss of the imprint or by deletion of the imprinted allele, with reduplication of the expressed allele resulting in uniparental disomy. Paternal uniparental disomy for the IGF-II locus has been described in Beckwith-Wiedemann syndrome (BWS).[30] BWS is an overgrowth disorder characterized by gigantism, macroglossia, and visceromegaly. Because IGF-II is maternally imprinted, reduplication of the paternal allele results in a double dose of IGF-II expression. Since IGF-II functions as a fetal growth factor, this may be in part responsible for the overgrowth phenotype. Loss of the maternal IGF-II imprint or paternal uniparental disomy, again resulting in a double dose of IGF-II expression, has also been described in Wilms tumor cells.[31] Here the excess growth factor may contribute to tumorigenesis. Finally, inheritance of a paternal deletion of chromosome region 15q11–13 is associated with Prader-Willi syndrome, characterized by obesity, hypogonadism, and mental retardation, whereas inheritance of this same deletion on the maternal chromosome is associated with Angelman syndrome, characterized by ataxic movements, inappropriate laughter, mental retardation, and hyperactivity.[32] In both cases, the allele located in this region on the one normal chromosome 15 is not capable of sustaining normal development, suggesting that imprinting occurs on a chromosome of particular parental descent. Clearly, imprinting plays a crucial

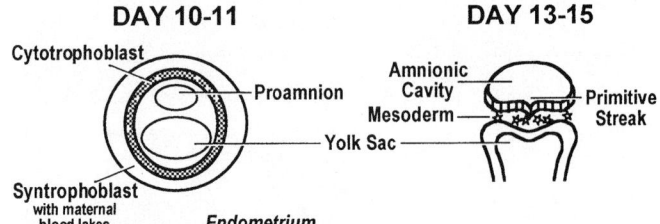

**FIGURE 107-3.** Early stages of mammalian development. The preimplantation stages shown are blastocysts with and without their zonae pellucidae. The embryonic end of the embryo contains the inner cell mass, which will form the fetus. Trophectodermal cells are fated to form the extraembryonic tissues, including the placenta. The primitive endoderm forms at the time of implantation and eventually will produce yolk sac structures. The primitive ectoderm will form the definitive ectoderm, endoderm, and mesoderm following the stages shown in the lower half of the diagram (postimplantation). The proamnion forms within the substance of the primitive ectoderm, and the trophoblast begins to differentiate into definitive placental structures (cytotrophoblast and syntrophoblast). By day 13, the primitive ectoderm has formed a single layer of columnar cells, and the craniocaudal groove (primitive streak) begins to form. Mesoderm differentiates from the primitive ectoderm at the point of the primitive streak in most primates.

role in determining nonequivalence of the maternal and paternal genomes and is necessary for normal development.

## PREIMPLANTATION DEVELOPMENT

The preimplantation period of development in mammals, the time from conception to nidation (implantation), has variable lengths in the various species. In humans, the preimplantation period lasts for ~7 days; in the mouse, it is 4 days, whereas in the rat, it is 5 days. The fertilized egg (Figs. 107-3 and 107-4) is morphologically similar to the mature unfertilized egg. The embryo at this stage is 100 μm in diameter, is associated with two polar bodies remaining from meiotic division, and is surrounded by the amorphous zona pellucida. The zona pellucida, which is composed primarily of three complex glycoproteins known as *ZP1, ZP2,* and *ZP3*, is important to early development for several, largely mechanical, reasons. First, there is evidence suggesting that certain glycoproteins of the zona pellucida may play a role in the recognition of the egg by the sperm. Competitive inhibition assays have shown that by incubating mouse sperm with ZP3 before fertilization, binding of the sperm to the zona pellucida is inhibited, thus suggesting that this glycoprotein is responsible for the recognition and binding of the sperm to the zona pellucida.[15] Second, the zona responds nearly instantaneously to sperm penetration and renders the egg impervious to additional penetration. Third, the zona provides a constraint to cleavage and ensures that as the

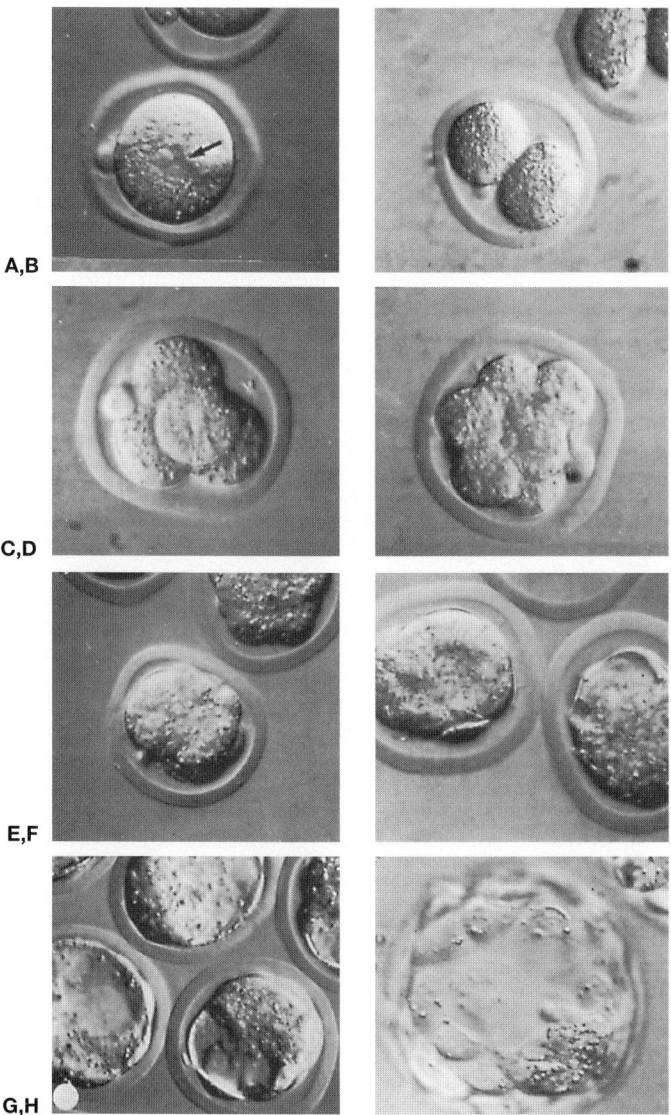

**FIGURE 107-4.** Photomicrographs (Hoffmann modulation contrast) of living preimplantation mouse embryos. **A,** One-cell pronuclear-stage egg ~12 hours after fertilization. A prominent pronucleus (*arrow*) and a polar body are evident. **B,** Two-cell cleavage stage. One of the two polar bodies is evident. **C,** Four-cell cleavage stage. One of the two polar bodies is evident. **D,** Eight-cell cleavage stage. **E,** Compacted 16-cell cleavage stage. **F,** Early blastocyst stage. A nascent blastocoele is evident. **G,** Mid-blastocyst stage. A well-formed blastocoele is evident in each embryo. Individual trophectodermal cells can be distinguished. The inner cell mass is apparent as an amorphous mass of cells. **H,** Expanded late blastocyst stage embryo. Inner cell mass is evident at lower right pole of the embryo. Individual trophectodermal cells are also evident. The embryos are surrounded by zonae pellucidae. The outside diameter of the embryos remains ~100 μm until the expanded blastocyst stage.

blastomeres divide, they remain together and in the proper orientation. Finally, the zona prevents the naturally sticky cleavage-stage embryo from adhering to the wall of the oviduct as it progresses to the uterus.

The mammalian oviduct also plays an important role in these early stages of preimplantation development. Not only does it provide a route through which the embryo is transported from the ovary to its site of implantation in the uterus, but it also provides a crucial timing mechanism for a process known as *cleavage division*.[33–35] At this stage of development, the embryo divides symmetrically and reductively such that a geometric increase in the number of cells (blastomeres) occurs without an actual increase in the overall size of the embryo.

These divisions occur entirely in the oviduct while the embryo is being propelled through its length as a result of ciliary action and muscular contractions in the oviduct wall. The primary function of development at this stage is to provide additional cells and membrane.

Beginning after the first division in the mouse embryo and after the second division in the human embryo, a critical transition occurs in the genetic control of development.[36] Before this time, the embryo contains a host of maternally derived mRNAs, ribosomes, and macromolecules that are sufficient to drive transcription and translation through the first (or second, as in the human embryo) cleavage division.[37] Further development, however, is dependent on the activation of embryonic control of transcription and the subsequent degradation of maternal mRNAs and proteins.[37] In the mouse, one population of polypeptides exhibits at least a two-fold decrease in abundance during the two-cell stage, whereas another population of polypeptides exhibits a similar increase in abundance.[38] Although this change most likely reflects the degradation of maternal mRNA and the appearance of new embryonic mRNA, it is possible that this transition is not complete and that some maternal products still may persist for a time after this transition.[37]

Once the embryonic genome has been activated, two important morphogenetic events occur in the embryo during the preimplantation period. The first, known as *compaction*, occurs late in the eight-cell stage when individual blastomeres condense and their boundaries become less prominent, thus forming a cellular mass known as a *morula* (see Fig. 107-4E). This process results in several profound changes in the embryo (Fig. 107-5). During this time, several new gene products are expressed that contribute to many of the morphologic manifestations of compaction. Included in this group are E-cadherin, gap junction proteins, tight junction proteins, growth factors, and components of the cytoskeleton.[39] E-cadherin (which originally was referred to as uvomorulin in the morula-stage mouse and later was identified as E-cadherin) acts as a $Ca^{2+}$-dependent cell adhesion molecule that binds adjacent blastomeres together and appears to facilitate the formation of junctional complexes, which include both gap junctions and tight junctions. Gap junctions form between all cells of the compaction-stage embryo and are constructed from a family of proteins known as the *connexins*, the structure of which creates channels between cells that allow for communication between blastomeres. During compaction, these gap junctions migrate from central regions of intercellular contact to peripheral locations of contact where tight junctions also form, thus creating junctional complexes between lateral surfaces of the outer blastomeres.[37,39,40] The tight junctions within these complexes serve a dual purpose. First, tight junctions play a critical role in the second preimplantation morphogenetic process known as *cavitation*. Second, they contribute to the polarization of the outer blastomeres by separating an apical region, where microvilli will form, from a basolateral region, to which the nuclei will migrate. By the 16-cell stage, these outer polar blastomeres form the trophectoderm, a cell lineage leading to the formation of extraembryonic tissues such as the placenta, whereas the inner apolar blastomeres form the inner cell mass, which ultimately will develop into the embryo proper.[41,42] This is the first stage of commitment of cells to a particular fate. Before this time, each blastomere in the two-cell, four-cell, and early eight-cell embryo is totipotent and, therefore, has the potential to develop into a complete organism when it is isolated from the remaining embryo. Once the 16-cell stage of development has been reached, however, the embryo has sufficient cells to form an inside and an outside, and thus establishes the conditions necessary for the first step of embryonic commitment. It is at this point that some of the embryo's cells lose their totipotency.

Although the details of the mechanism by which the morphologic change in cellular contact associated with compaction

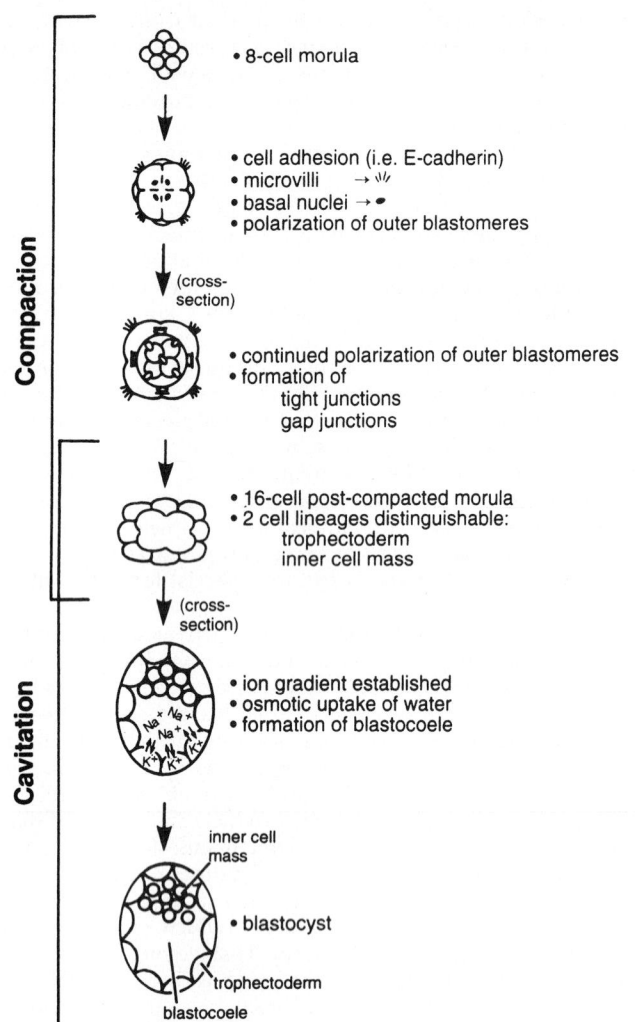

- 8-cell morula

- cell adhesion (i.e. E-cadherin)
- microvilli → ⋎⋎
- basal nuclei → •
- polarization of outer blastomeres

(cross-section)

- continued polarization of outer blastomeres
- formation of
    tight junctions
    gap junctions

- 16-cell post-compacted morula
- 2 cell lineages distinguishable:
    trophectoderm
    inner cell mass

(cross-section)

- ion gradient established
- osmotic uptake of water
- formation of blastocoele

inner cell mass

- blastocyst

trophectoderm

blastocoele

**Compaction**

**Cavitation**

**FIGURE 107-5.** Compaction and cavitation of the preimplantation mouse embryo. During the late eight-cell stage, embryos begin a morphogenetic process known as *compaction*, which ultimately results in the polarization of the outer blastomeres and the establishment of two cell lineages. During this process, individual blastomeres become less evident as the cell adhesion molecule E-cadherin functions to bind adjacent cells to one another. Simultaneously, microvilli form on the apical surfaces of the outer blastomeres, the nuclei migrate basolaterally, gap junctions form between all adjacent blastomeres, and tight junctions form between outer blastomeres, thus separating apical and basolateral regions. These changes result in the formation of two cell lineages by the 16-cell stage; the outer polar cells will form the trophectoderm, whereas the inner apolar cells will form the inner cell mass. The second morphogenetic event, cavitation, begins as soon as the two cell lineages are established and results in the formation of a blastocoelic cavity. The basolateral location of E-cadherin aids in restricting the distribution of Na$^+$/K$^+$–adenosine triphosphatases to this region, thus causing a Na$^+$ gradient to form within the embryo. Water flows into the embryo osmotically, and the presence of the tight junctions in the outer blastomeres prevents this fluid from leaking out. Thus, a blastocoelic cavity forms, and the embryo is now known as a *blastocyst*.

can induce all of these varied events are incompletely deciphered, evidence suggests that protein kinase C and subsequent phosphorylation of proteins may be involved.[43–45] Early activation of protein kinase C not only can trigger premature compaction through its effect on E-cadherin, but also can induce the migration of blastomere nuclei to a basolateral position.[43,44] If protein kinase C functions in the signal pathway leading to events of compaction much as it does in other signal pathways, it is possible that some type of surface signal is

detected by the blastomeres that causes a G protein to activate phospholipase C, which in turn cleaves phosphatidylinositol 4,5-bisphosphate. This results in the formation of two products: Ins (1,4,5)P$_3$, which causes an increase in intracellular calcium, and 1,2-diacylglycerol, which activates protein kinase C. The activated protein kinase C is then available to phosphorylate proteins involved in nuclear migration and cell adhesion.[43] It remains to be seen, however, what triggers this pathway, if indeed the phosphatidylinositol cycle functions to activate protein kinase C during compaction.

The second major morphogenetic event to occur in preimplantation development is known as cavitation. This process begins several days after conception (3 days in the mouse, 4 in the rat, and 6 in the human) and culminates in the formation of the blastocyst (see Fig. 107-4F through H). At least two factors are known to be critical to the proper execution of this event. First, the tight junctions that form between plasma membranes of the outer blastomeres not only provide an apical/basolateral polarization of the cells, but also prevent paracellular leakage of fluid from the nascent blastocoele. Second, the cell adhesion properties of E-cadherin, which is located in the basolateral regions of the plasma membrane, are crucial in restricting the distribution of Na$^+$/K$^+$–adenosine triphosphatases to this region as well. With these two factors in place, the polar distribution of Na$^+$/K$^+$–adenosine triphosphatases to this basolateral location causes a Na$^+$ gradient to be established within the interior of the embryo, and subsequently osmotic uptake of water occurs such that it accumulates in the extracellular space of the nascent blastocoele. Because the tight junctions prevent this fluid from leaking out, it accumulates until the blastocoelic cavity is fully expanded.[37,39] At this stage, the two cell types are easily distinguishable: The inner cell mass cells are located internally at the embryonic pole of the embryo, whereas the trophectodermal cells, which are extremely large, owing to acytokinetic cell division, surround both the inner cell mass cells and the blastocoele.

## OVIDUCT TRANSPORT

The role of oviduct transport in the maturation of the mammalian embryo is poorly understood. It is reasonable to assume that oviduct fluids have a central role in the nourishment of the embryo and in gas exchange; however, the fluids also may contain substances that control or somehow enhance the development of the cleavage-stage embryo. The mammalian embryo can survive and progress in various artificial media.

The embryo completes its passage through the oviduct at the early blastocyst stage and is propelled into the uterus. In the mouse, this occurs at day 3 of gestation, and in humans, at day 5 to 6. The blastocyst continues to develop in the uterus for another 24 to 48 hours, during which time it greatly expands its blastocoelic cavity until the inner cell mass is little more than a plaque of cells on the embryonic pole. Then, the embryo loses its zona pellucida. Despite attempts to isolate the factors involved in this process, little is known about the loss of the zona. In vitro, the zona can be removed by enzymatic digestion, mechanical disruption,[16,17] or an acid milieu.[46] In rabbits in vivo, the egg vestments are removed enzymatically at the implantation site and not while the blastocyst is free in the uterus.

## X CHROMOSOME INACTIVATION

In eutherian females (placental mammals, i.e., other than monotremes and marsupials), one of the two X chromosomes is inactivated early in embryonic development, thus providing a mechanism for genetic dosage compensation.[47] In eutherians, this inactivation begins in the trophectoderm in the early blastocyst stage and is characterized by a preferential paternal X chromosome inactivation. This also is true of X chromosome inactivation that subsequently occurs in the primitive endoderm during the midblastocyst stage. During the late blastocyst stage, however, X chromosome inactivation occurs randomly in the inner cell mass, with no paternal or maternal preference, thus resulting in mosaic females composed of a mixture of cells that have either a maternally or paternally active X chromosome. In somatic cells, this inactivation becomes fixed such that all descendants from a particular cell maintain the same inactivated X chromosome. In the germline, however, this inactivation must be reversed at the time of meiosis so that each X chromosome has an equal chance of contributing to the gametes.[48]

In marsupials, this pattern of X chromosome inactivation is different in that it is always the paternal X chromosome that is inactivated. This may not necessarily be a functional difference, however, because the marsupial blastocyst has no inner cell mass. The coincidence of the timing of X chromosome inactivation and cell commitment to either trophectoderm or inner cell mass lineages in eutherians strongly suggests that these two processes are linked in some meaningful way. Perhaps the preferential X chromosome inactivation may be part of a system that is necessary to prevent rejection of the conceptus. Alternatively, it also has been suggested that preferential X chromosome inactivation may prevent the accumulation of genes necessary to the proper development of extraembryonic membranes on the paternal X chromosome. This would adversely affect the development of boys because they do not possess a paternally derived X chromosome.[48,49]

X chromosome inactivation was first proposed as a mechanism of gene dosage control by Lyon.[50,51] The best evidence of it exists in women heterozygous at the glucose-6-phosphate dehydrogenase (G6PD) locus of the X chromosome. G6PD is a dimeric dimorphic enzyme; that is, there are two distinguishable allelic forms of the enzyme (isoenzymes) and the enzyme is composed of two subunits that must combine to form a holoenzyme. In heterozygous women, the two isoenzymes can combine to form heteropolymeric forms, which are distinguishable from the other two subunits. When X chromosome inactivation occurs in women heterozygous at the G6PD locus, two populations of cells are created: one with the paternal allele active and the other with the maternal allele active. The two isoenzymes can be distinguished by electrophoresis. No heteropolymeric form is present, however, indicating that the two alleles were not active simultaneously in the same cells at the time of sampling.[52]

Insights have been made into the multistep mechanism controlling X inactivation in mammals. First, the number of X chromosomes is counted by an as yet unknown process, tallying up the number of *X inactivation centers (Xic)*. Second, a single X chromosome is chosen to remain active, and inactivation of any additional X chromosomes is initiated by expression of the *Xist* from the *Xic*. Finally, this inactivation spreads over the length of each inactive chromosome.

*Xist* is only expressed on the inactive X in somatic cells of females, in male germ cells during spermatogenesis, and on the imprinted paternal X chromosome of the trophectoderm and primitive endoderm of the blastocyst. It does not encode a protein but instead remains as an RNA moiety that stays bound to the X chromosome undergoing inactivation. Furthermore, the expression of *Xist* coincides with the imprinted X inactivation that occurs in the trophectoderm and primitive endoderm of the blastocyst, which is then turned off before X inactivation in the embryonic lineage. DNA methylation of *Xist* correlates with its activity; it is unmethylated where it is expressed on an inactive X chromosome and methylated as an inactive allele on an active X chromosome.

*Xist* can operate from multiple promoters, resulting in production of either stable or unstable RNA, suggesting one mechanism whereby *Xist* can be developmentally regulated. Stable *Xist* forms as a result of activation of one promoter on the imprinted paternal X chromosome of the trophectoderm. Alternatively, unstable *Xist* RNA results from activation of a different promoter when the imprint is erased before random X inactivation of the somatic cells.[53,54]

Questions that remain to be answered about X inactivation are how *Xic*s are counted and how an inactivation signal can propagate throughout the entire length of the X chromosome and yet let certain genes escape this signal.

## IMPLANTATION

The embryo now undergoes implantation, which begins with attachment of the late blastocyst to the uterine tissue at a nidation site. The selection of this site is tightly regulated, because it usually occurs in a predictable manner, but little else is known. Implantation can be classified on the basis of the usual position of the site in the uterus and, hence, may be noninvasive and central, noninvasive and eccentric, or interstitial as in humans (Fig. 107-6). In humans, the embryo attaches to the lining of the uterine fundus, with the embryonic pole usually attaching to the antimesometrial lining. The endometrial cells of the uterus have microvilli on their luminal surfaces that begin to interdigitate with the microvilli of the trophectodermal cells. Pinocytosis (the cellular process of active engulfing of liquid) in the endometrial epithelial cells increases at this time and is thought to enhance or at least stabilize attachment, perhaps by removing uterine fluids from the attachment site. This pinocytosis is stimulated by progestins and inhibited by estrogens.[21] Actual cell fusion between the embryonic trophectoderm and the uterine epithelium does not occur in most species. The presence of the blastocyst in the uterus undoubtedly provides some signal to the uterus and to the ovary to maintain the pregnancy.[55] The blastocyst is capable of producing human chorionic gonadotropin, which supports the corpus luteum, and the luteal phase of human conception cycles maintains higher progesterone levels from day 3 through day 8 than in nonconception cycles.[56–58]

Implantation may be enhanced by proteases. These proteolytic enzymes are thought to have two functions: to cause the removal of the zona pellucida, which must precede the attachment of the embryo to the uterine lining, and to aid the embryo's invasion of the endometrial lining. The cells of the human trophoblast frankly invade uterine tissue as implantation proceeds. Early theories of the role of such enzymes suggested that they were necessary to digest maternal tissues; however, their actual role, if any, beyond the removal of the zona may be far more subtle. For example, such enzymes may act on the invasion process through limited proteolysis (e.g., blastolemmase) by beginning a cascade of activation of other enzymes.[34]

Implantation has at least three phases. The first is *attachment*, in which specific receptor sites may be responsible for binding of either the embryonic pole or the abembryonic pole, depending on the species, to the endometrial epithelium. The second phase is *invasion*. In humans, the trophectodermal cells invade through the basement membrane of the uterine epithelium to establish a nidation site in the stroma of the endometrium (see Fig. 107-6). The ability of the human embryo to invade tissue may explain the high frequency of ectopic pregnancies in women relative to other mammalian species. The third phase is the *endometrial response* to the implanted embryo. In a few eutherian species (including humans, other primates, and murine rodents), the uterine stromal cells undergo a specific reaction called *decidualization*. The name derives from the fact that these cells occasionally are shed at term. The stromal cells in the immediate area of the embryo become large, eosinophilic, and transcriptionally active. The cells of the decidual swelling may be important in the support of the pregnancy (e.g., by the production of luteotropin, which supports the corpus luteum); in

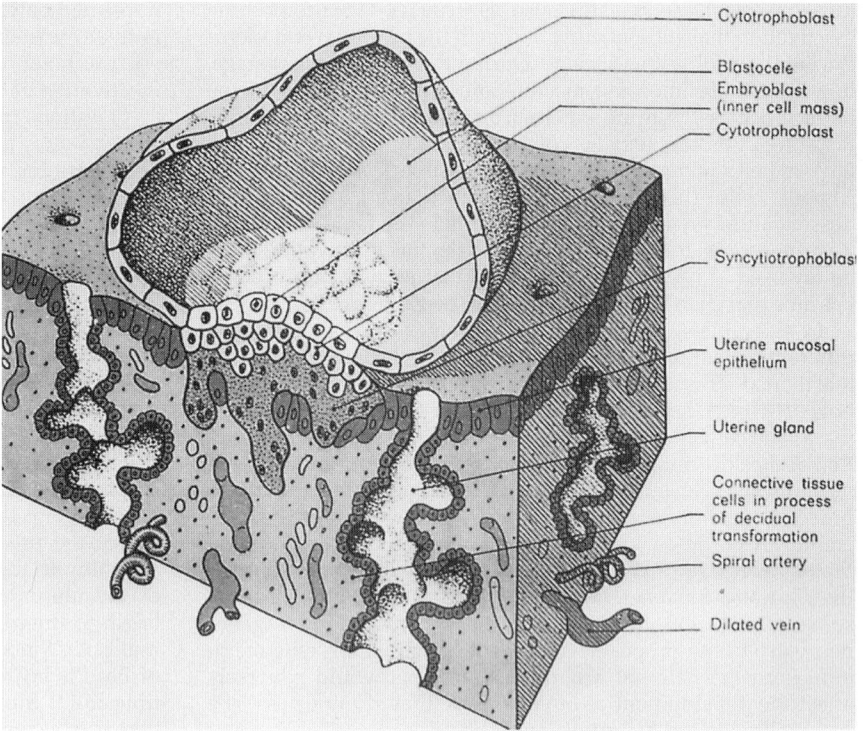

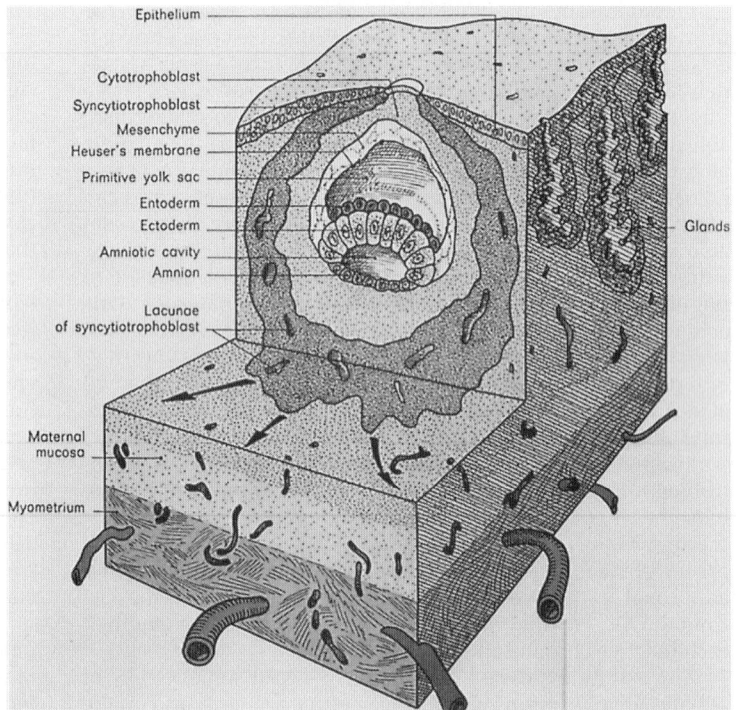

**FIGURE 107-6.** Diagram of human implantation site. **A,** Tropho-blast invasion of uterine epithelium at the time of attachment. **B,** Nidation site is completed with the embryo in its interstitial position. There is a single layer of abembryonic trophectoder-mal cells in contact with the uterine lumen. Primitive entoderm and primitive ectoderm are distinguishable. (From Tuchmann-Duplessis H, David G, Haegel P. Illustrated human embryology, vol I: embryogenesis. New York: Springer-Verlag, 1972.)

the prevention of immune rejection of the implanted embryo; or in some other, unknown capacity.[59]

Among mammals, there is a great variation in the specific details of development at this stage. Although many attempts at generalizations across species have been made, by and large, they are either not helpful or are actually incorrect. For example, much of what is known concerning reproductive endocrinology is derived from experiments in mouse and rat. These animals, like other *diapause* mammals (i.e., those that can delay implantation while keeping the embryo alive), express an estrogen surge, which seems to be necessary for the progesterone-primed uterus to accept the initiation of implantation. This is not true of humans. In the rabbit, the zona pellucida is removed

at the site of implantation, and the blastocyst is invested with additional coverings that must be removed enzymatically. In the mouse, the blastocyst can exist free in the uterine cavity without its zona pellucida. Virtually nothing is known about the removal of the zona in humans. One important reason for these variations is that there are several successful solutions to problems of early development in viviparous animals, and many of the specific details of reproductive strategy do not allow for clear winners or clear losers.

While the molecular control of implantation is not fully understood, many factors are necessary for proper implanta-tion of the embryo. Most of the factors identified to date are produced or released by the uterus (many in response to estrogen or progesterone), but it is becoming evident that embryonic factors are important as well. COX-1, leukemia inhibitory factor (LIF), HB-EGF, and amphiregulin are expressed by the uterine epithelium at the time of implantation, while adhesion molecules such as lectins, carbohydrate moieties, and heparin sulfate proteoglycan interact between the surfaces of the blastocyst and endometrium. Interleukin (IL)-1α and IL-1β are released by the blastocyst and adhere to the endometrial epithelial β$_3$-integrin subunit, while trophoblast giant cells produce proteinases such as gelatinases A and B and urokinase-type plasminogen activator (uPA) that mediate the invasion of the decidua.[60–64]

In diapause mammals such as the mouse or rat, there are uterine inhibitory factors that can prevent implantation. The blastocyst-stage embryo can overcome the inhibition by a process of activation, which occurs in response to the prenidation estrogen surge in these animals. This process does not occur in humans.

## POSTIMPLANTATION DEVELOPMENT

Development after implantation is rapid and complex. The embryo must establish both its placental compartment and its definitive fetal structures in a short time. The polar or embryonic trophectoderm (that overlying the inner cell mass) develops into an ectoplacental cone in the mouse, whereas in most primates, the trophoblast differentiates into *syncytiotrophoblast* and *cytotrophoblast*, the latter having a high mitotic rate. Rapid division produces a syncytial trophoblast surrounding the primate embryo, although the mural trophectoderm (that facing the uterine cavity) remains a single layer of cells. Lacunar spaces form within the syntrophoblast, which eventually becomes contiguous with the maternal capillary circulation, into which the chorionic villi will grow. The ectoplacental cone of the mouse and rat undergoes similar development, and the resulting placental structure is hemochorial, as in humans. The major placental classification among mammalian orders is derived from the number of tissue layers that separate the fetal and maternal circulations. There are six such potential barriers to exchange. Humans, like many other primates and murine species, have a *hemochorial* placenta in which three fetal tissues (endothelium, connective tissue, and chorionic epithelium) are bathed in maternal blood.[65]

As the process of placentation proceeds, definitive embryonic structures are developing. Immediately after implantation, a layer of cells appears at the blastocoele margin on the side of the inner cell mass. This layer is called the *endoderm*. The remaining cells of the inner cell mass are now called the *epiblast* or the primitive *ectoderm*. The endoderm proliferates rapidly and eventually surrounds the blastocoele. The epiblast cells (embryonic ectoderm) are now arranged in a columnar manner. Cells contiguous with the epiblast, called *amnioblasts*, appear; spaces between the amnioblasts develop (the proamnion) and eventually form the *amnionic cavity*. Although it is a matter of some debate, it seems possible that the amnioblast cells are the source of the amniotic fluid, which cushions and thereby protects the developing embryo. Apoptosis also plays a critical role in cavitation of the early embryo (not to be confused with cavitation of the blastocyst). A signal from the primitive endoderm acts over a short distance to induce apoptosis of the inner ectoderm cells, while survival of the outer ectodermal cells is mediated by interaction with the adjacent basement membrane that separates the ectoderm from the endoderm.[66]

By approximately 7 days in the mouse and 13 days in humans, all three germ layers are present. The primitive ectoderm (epiblast) gives rise to definitive ectoderm, definitive endoderm, and mesoderm, which appears between the primitive endoderm and the primitive ectoderm. The primitive endoderm gives rise to several extraembryonic tissues (see Fig. 107-3). The first indication of craniocaudal axis and bilateral symmetry

in the embryo appears as a longitudinal depression in the columnar embryonic ectoderm. This depression is called the *primitive streak* and, in most primates, it seems to be the site of origin of *mesodermal* cells (see Fig. 107-4). Most of the available information concerning cell lineage in the early embryo is derived from experiments performed in the mouse, and it is not clear whether these principal features of the fates of early cells are applicable to human development. It may be some time before this can be determined because, at present, the only way this information can be obtained is by experimental manipulation and disruption of the embryo. A case in point is a series of experiments that defined the ultimate fates of areas of the egg cylinder–stage embryo of the mouse (day 7). This work required microsurgical removal of some structures from the embryo with development in culture, or transplantation of radioactively labeled structures to unlabeled embryos, after the development of the combined structure.

Early postimplantation stages are responsible for establishing the structures that ultimately allow organogenesis to proceed.[33,35] An understanding of the molecular biology of the control of differentiation of the definitive structures will have far-reaching implications for many gestational diseases and certainly for human cancer.[67] Correct fetal development requires the coordinated expression of thousands of genes. The correct temporal and spatial expression of these genes could not occur without the intervention of some relatively small set of supervisor genes that can orchestrate the process. Such genes are being found based on information from diverse animal studies.[68]

## SPONTANEOUS ABORTION

The most common manifestation of the failure of embryonic and fetal development is *spontaneous abortion*: the failure of conception to produce a live birth. Spontaneous abortion, then, is either the disruption of pregnancy once it can be recognized or the expulsion of a nonviable fetus. Precise clinical definitions are much more difficult. Most often, these definitions must invoke low birth weight, because below certain weights, the fetus is unlikely to survive. Other definitions include loss of pregnancy before 20 or 28 weeks of gestation. Accurate estimates of the incidence of spontaneous abortion, therefore, are difficult to obtain. The frequency of clinically evident spontaneous abortion is ~15% of pregnancies. Undoubtedly, the risk is much higher in women with a previous spontaneous abortion, with the risk as high as 46% after three consecutive abortions. However, if the abortus is karyotypically abnormal, the risk of consecutive abortion is substantially lower.[69,70] The association of prior spontaneous abortion with subsequent poor pregnancy outcome has been well documented, even when all other risk factors have been controlled. The effects of specific risk factors seem to be much stronger than the history.

Early pregnancy losses are occult. Early abortion has many causes and must not be considered a single disease entity. One of the principal observations in human embryos that fail to cleave normally is the presence of structural abnormalities of chromosomes. In a large series of fetal deaths, the karyotypes of the offspring were compared with the morphology of the conception products.[71] More than half of the small or unformed fetuses had chromosomal abnormalities, whereas only 6% of fetuses of normal size with or without malformations had chromosomal aberrations (see Chap. 90). Intrauterine death may occur in association with chromosomal abnormalities that also can be seen in live births. These deaths result from the failure of embryonic development, not the gross anomalies frequently associated in live offspring with the deviant karyotype. There may exist a continuum of anomalies in the offspring into which spontaneous abortion fits, from failure of fetal development through to birth with malformations. Nonchromosomal causes of pregnancy loss include maternal metabolic disturbances such as endometrial growth factor disturbances or hyperglycemia.[72,73]

One potential source of disruption of pregnancy is exposure of the woman to toxic substances. Of particular concern are exposures in the early periods of pregnancy. Few data are available, however, in some measure because of the traditional view that preimplantation development is refractory to toxic insult. However, the general presumption that early-stage embryos are either killed or left unaffected to implant and develop normally is an oversimplification. For example, the blastocyst is sensitive to cyclophosphamide, heavy metals, and trypan blue. Such exposures decrease cell numbers in the early embryo and can lead to vascular anomalies in midgestation when exposure occurs at the blastocyst stage.

Exposure to toxic substances can be environmental, such as in the workplace, or self-inflicted, such as maternal smoking.[73a] Maternal smoking is important because of the numerous persons involved, and has been implicated by association in a wide array of pregnancy complications involving both the mother and the offspring. These complications include low birth weight, spontaneous abortion, sudden infant death syndrome, placenta previa, excessive maternal bleeding, and perinatal mortality.[74–76] Many laboratories have been investigating possible reasons for the adverse role of maternal smoking in pregnancy outcome (see Chap. 234), and several conclusions have emerged. First, the embryo can be affected directly by chemical exposure; there need not be any intervening maternal role. Nevertheless, injury to maternal pregnancy support systems, such as the corpus luteum, may occur, or maternal tissues may activate deleterious compounds in tobacco smoke. Second, the embryo is at risk for adverse effects much sooner than was previously suspected. The blastocyst-stage embryo is sensitive to compounds such as those in cigarette smoke with respect to implantation, decidual response, gross dysmorphogenesis, live birth rate, and perinatal mortality. These events can be manifested long after the exposure to the chemicals.[77–81] Because mothers are unaware of early pregnancy, these data may require a reevaluation of the advice given to women who are considering pregnancy: It is becoming clear that one should not wait for evidence of the pregnancy to refine the potential environment of the developing embryo.[82]

## PERSPECTIVES

The study of the progression of embryonic tissue is the study of evolution, organization, differentiation, and molecular control. It has attracted the attention of endocrinologists, biologists, clinicians, and amateur naturalists for centuries. There can be no doubt that detailed investigation of the issues surrounding reproductive strategies of species both related and unrelated to humans will yield abundant insight that will help alleviate human ailments as diverse as birth defects and cancer.

## REFERENCES

1. Fabro S. Reproductive toxicology: state of the art. Am J Ind Med 1983; 4:391.
2. Roberts CJ, Lowe CR. Where have all the conceptions gone? Lancet 1975; 1:498.
3. Hertig AT. The overall problem in man. In: Benirschke K, ed. Comparative aspects of reproductive failure. Berlin: Springer-Verlag, 1967:11.
4. King CR, Pernoll ML, Prescott G. Reproductive wastage. Obstet Gynecol Annu 1982; 11:59.
5. Newbold RR, Carter DB, Harris SE, et al. Molecular differentiation of the mouse genital tract: altered protein synthesis following prenatal exposure to diethylstilbestrol. Biol Reprod 1984; 30:459.
6. Shettles LB. Ovum humanum. Munich: Urban und Schwarzenberg, 1960:79.
7. Racowsky C, Satterlie RA. Metabolic, fluorescent dye and electrical coupling between hamster oocytes and cumulus cells during meiotic maturation *in vivo* and *in vitro*. Dev Biol 1985; 108:191.

8. Jansen RP. Endocrine response in the fallopian tube. Endocr Rev 1984; 5:525.
9. Chang MC. The meaning of sperm capacitation: a historical perspective. J Androl 1984; 5:45.
10. O'Neill C, Quinn P. Inhibitory influence of uterine secretions on mouse blastocysts decreases at the time of blastocyst activation. J Reprod Fertil 1983; 68:269.
11. Fraser LR, Umar G, Sayed S. Na+-requiring mechanisms modulate capacitation and acrosomal exocytosis in mouse spermatozoa. J Reprod Fertil 1993; 97:539.
12. Fraser LR. Requirements for successful mammalian sperm capacitation and fertilization. Arch Pathol Lab Med 1992; 116:345.
13. Spungin B, Levinshal T, Rubinstein S, Breitbart H. A cell free system reveals that capacitation is a prerequisite for membrane fusion during the acrosome reaction. FEBS Lett 1992; 311:155.
14. Oura C, Toshimori K. Ultrastructural studies on the fertilization of mammalian gametes. Int Rev Cytol 1990; 122:105.
15. Gilbert SF. Developmental biology, 3rd ed. Sunderland, MA: Sinauer Associates Inc, 1991:33.
16. Bleil JD, Wassarman PM. Identification of a ZP3-binding protein on acrosome-intact mouse sperm by photoaffinity crosslinking. Proc Natl Acad Sci U S A 1990; 87:5563.
17. Shur BD, Hall NG. A role for mouse sperm surface galactosyltransferase in sperm binding to the egg zona pellucida. J Cell Biol 1982; 95:574.
18. Shur BD, Neely CA. Plasma membrane association purification and partial characterization of mouse sperm β 1,4-galactosyltransferase. J Biol Chem 1988; 268:17706.
19. Bedford JM. Significance of the need for sperm capacitation before fertilization in eutherian mammals. Biol Reprod 1983; 28:108.
20. Hinrichsen-Kohane AC, Hinrichsen MJ, Schill WB. Molecular events leading to fertilization—a review. Andrologia 1984; 16:321.
21. Hendrickx AG. Disorders of fertilization, transport, and implantation. Prog Clin Biol Res 1984; 160:211.
22. Farooqui AA. Biochemistry of sperm capacitation. Int J Biochem 1983; 15:463.
22a. Espinosaal F, Lopez-Gonzaleza T, Munoz-Garaya C, et al. Dual regulation of the T-Type Ca (2+) current by serum albumin and beta-estradiol in mammalian spermatogenic cells. FEBS Lett 2000; 475:251.
23. Barton SC, Surani MAH, Norris ML. Role of paternal and maternal genomes in mouse development. Nature 1994; 311:374.
24. Spindle A, Sturm KS, Flannery M, et al. Defective chorioallantoic fusion in mid-gestation lethality of parthenogenone-tetraploid chimeras. Dev Dyn 1996; 173:447.
25. Sapienza C, Peterson AC, Rossant J, et al. Degree of methylation of transgenes is dependent on gamete of origin. Nature 1987; 328:251.
26. Pedersen RA, Sturm KS, Rappolee DA, Werb Z. Effects of imprinting on early development of mouse embryos. In: Bauister BD, ed. Preimplantation embryo development. New York: Springer-Verlag, 1993:212.
27. Surani MA. Imprinting and the initiation of gene silencing in the germ line. Cell 1998; 93:309.
28. Barlow DP. Gametic imprinting in mammals. Science 1995; 270:1610.
29. Li E, Beard C, Jaenisch R. Role for DNA methylation in genomic imprinting. Nature 1993; 366:362.
30. Junien C. Beckwith-Wiedemann syndrome, tumorigenesis and imprinting. Curr Opin Genet Dev 1992; 2:431.
31. Okawa O, Eccles MR, Szeto J, et al. Relaxation of insulin-like growth factor II gene imprinting implicated in Wilms' tumour. Nature 1993; 362:749.
32. Cassiday SB, Schwartz S. Prader-Willi and Angelman syndromes: disorders of genomic imprinting. Medicine 1998; 77:140.
33. McLaren A. Early mammalian development. Prog Clin Biol Res 1985; 163A:29.
34. Denker HW. Basic aspects of ovoimplantation. Obstet Gynecol Annu 1983; 12:15.
35. Swartz WJ. Early mammalian embryonic development. Am J Ind Med 1983; 4:51.
36. Telford NA, Watson AJ, Schultz GA. Transition from maternal to embryonic control in early mammalian development: a comparison of several species. Mol Reprod Dev 1990; 26:90.
37. Watson AJ, Kidder GM, Schultz GA. How to make a blastocyst. Biochem Cell Biol 1992; 70:849.
38. Latham KE, Garrels JI, Chang C, Solter D. Quantitative analysis of protein synthesis in mouse embryos I. Extensive reprogramming at the one- and two-cell stages. Development 1991; 112:921.
39. Watson AJ. The cell biology of blastocyst development. Mol Reprod Dev 1992; 33:492.
40. Becker DL, Leclerc-David C, Warner A. The relationship of gap junctions and compaction in the preimplantation mouse embryo. In: Stern C, Ingham P, eds. Gastrulation (Dev Suppl). Cambridge: The Company of Biologists Limited, 1992:113.
41. Rossant J, Papaioannou VE. The biology of embryogenesis. In: Sherman MI, ed. Concepts in mammalian embryogenesis. Cambridge, MA: MIT Press, 1977:36.
42. Sutherland AE, Calarco-Gillam PG. Analysis of compaction in the preimplantation mouse embryo. Dev Biol 1983; 100:328.
43. Winkel GK, Ferguson JE, Takeichi M, Nuccitelli R. Activation of protein kinase C triggers premature compaction in the four-cell stage mouse embryo. Dev Biol 1990; 138:1.
44. Ohsugi M, Ohsawa T, Yamamura H. Involvement of protein kinase C in nuclear migration during compaction and the mechanism of the migration: analyses in two-cell mouse embryos. Dev Biol 1993; 156:146.

45. Bloom T, McConnell J. Changes in protein phosphorylation associated with compaction of the mouse preimplantation embryo. Mol Reprod Dev 1990; 26:199.

46. Nicolson GL, Yanagimachi R, Yanagimachi H. Ultrastructural localization of lectin binding site on the zonae pellucidae and plasma membranes of mammalian eggs. J Cell Biol 1975; 66:263.

47. Migeon BR. X-chromosome inactivation: molecular mechanisms and genetic consequences. Trends Genet 1994; 10:230.

48. Gartler SM, Dyer KA, Goldman MA. Mammalian X-chromosome inactivation. Mol Genet Med 1992; 2:121.

49. Solter D. Differential imprinting and expression of maternal and paternal genomes. Annu Rev Genet 1988; 88:127.

50. Lyon MF. Mechanisms and evolutionary origins of variable X-chromosome activity in mammals. Proc R Soc Lond [Biol] 1974; 187:243.

51. Chapman VM, Shows TB. Somatic cell genetic evidence for X-chromosome linkage of three enzymes in the mouse. Nature 1976; 259:665.

52. Migeon BR. Glucose-6-phosphate dehydrogenase as a probe for the study of X-chromosome inactivation in human females. Curr Top Biol Med Res 1983; 9:189.

53. Goto T, Monk M. Regulation of X-chromosome inactivation in development in mice and humans. Microbiol Mol Biol Rev 1998; 62:362.

54. Johnston CM, Nesterova TB, Formstone EJ, et al. Developmentally regulated Xist promoter switch mediates initiation of X inactivation. Cell 1998; 94:809.

55. Kennedy TG. Embryonic signals and the initiation of blastocyst implantation. Aust J Biol Sci 1983; 36:531.

56. Casper RF, Wilson E, Collins JA, et al. Enhancement of human implantation by exogenous chorionic gonadotropin. (Letter). Lancet 1983; 2:1191.

57. Kusuda M, Nakamura G, Matsukuma K, et al. Corpus luteum insufficiency as a cause of nidatory failure. Acta Obstet Gynecol Scand 1983; 62:199.

58. Buster JE. Gestational changes in steroid hormone biosynthesis, secretion, metabolism, and action. Clin Perinatol 1983; 10:527.

59. Bazer FW, Roberts RM. Biochemical aspects of conceptus-endometrial interactions. J Exp Zool 1983; 228:373.

60. Rinkenberger JL, Cross JC, Werb Z. Molecular genetics of implantation in the mouse. Dev Genet 1997; 21:6.

61. Smith SE, French MM, Julian J, et al. Expression of heparan sulfate proteoglycan (Perlecan) in the mouse blastocyst is regulated during normal and delayed implantation. Dev Biol 1997; 184:38.

62. Cullinan EB, Abbondanzo SJ, Anderson PS, et al. Leukemia inhibitory factor (LIF) and LIF receptor expression in human endometrium suggests a potential autocrine/paracrine function in regulating embryo implantation. Proc Natl Acad Sci U S A 1996; 93:3115.

63. Das SK, Wang X-N, Paria BC, et al. Heparin-binding EGF-like growth factor gene is induced in the mouse uterus temporally by the blastocyst solely at the site of its apposition: a possible ligand for interaction with blastocyst EGF-receptor in implantation. Development 1994; 120:1071.

64. Schultz GA, Edwards DR. Biology and genetics of implantation. Dev Genet 1997; 21:1.

65. Benirschke K. Placentation. J Exp Zool 1983; 228:385.

66. Coucouvanis E, Martin GR. Signals for death and survival: a two-step mechanism for cavitation in the vertebrate embryo. Cell 1995; 83:279

67. Sanford JP, Chapman VM, Rossant J. DNA methylation in extraembryonic lineages of mammals. Trends Genet 1985; 1:89.

68. Utset MF, Awqulewitsch A, Ruddle FH, McGinnis W. Region-specific expression of two mouse homeo box genes. Science 1987; 235:1379.

69. Huisjes HJ. Spontaneous abortion. New York: Churchill Livingstone, 1984:205.

70. Wilcox AJ. Surveillance of pregnancy loss in human populations. Am J Ind Med 1983; 4:285.

71. Byrne J, Warburton D, Kline J, et al. Morphology of early fetal deaths and their chromosomal characteristics. Teratology 1985; 32:297.

72. Freinkel N, Lewis NJ, Akazawa S, et al. The honeybee syndrome: implications of the teratogenicity of mannose in rat-embryo culture. N Engl J Med 1984; 310:223.

73. Giudice LC. Growth factors and growth modulators in human uterine endometrium: their potential relevance to reproductive medicine. Fertil Steril 1994; 61:1.

73a. Zenzes MT. Smoking and reproduction: gene damage to human gametes and embryos. Hum Reprod Update 2000; 6:122.

74. Tovares R, Ramos P, Palminha J, et al. Transplacental exposure to genotoxins. Evaluation in hemoglobin of hydroxyethylvaline adduct levels in smoking and non-smoking mothers and their newborns. Carcinogenesis 1994; 15:1271.

75. Jacobson JL, Jacoboson SW, Sokol RJ, et al. Effects of alcohol use, smoking, and illicit drug use on fetal growth in black infants. J Pediatr 1994; 124:757.

76. Naeye RL. Common environmental influences on the fetus. Monogr Pathol 1981; 22:52.

77. Iannaccone PM, Tsao TY, Stols L. Effects on mouse blastocysts of *in vitro* exposure to methylnitrosourea and 3-methylcholanthrene. Cancer Res 1982; 42:864.

78. Iannaccone PM. Long-term effects of exposure to methylnitrosourea on blastocysts following transfer to surrogate female mice. Cancer Res 1984; 44:2785.

79. Iannaccone PM, Fahl WE, Stols L. Reproductive toxicity associated with endometrial cell mediated metabolism of benzo[a]pyrene: a combined *in vitro, in vivo* approach. Carcinogenesis 1984; 5:1437.

80. Bossert NL, Iannaccone PM. Midgestational abnormalities associated with in vitro preimplantation N-methyl-N-nitrosourea exposure with subsequent transfer to surrogate mothers. Proc Natl Acad Sci U S A 1985; 82:8757.

81. Dwivedi RS, Iannaccone PM. Effects of environmental chemicals on early development. In: Korach K, ed. Reproductive and developmental toxicology. New York: Marcel Dekker Inc, 1998:11.

82. Iannaccone PM, Bossert NL, Connelly CS. Disruption of embryonic and fetal development due to preimplantation chemical insults: a critical review. Am J Obstet Gynecol 1987; 157:476.

# CHAPTER 108

# THE MATERNAL-FETAL-PLACENTAL UNIT

BRUCE R. CARR

The hormonal changes and maternal adaptations of human pregnancy are among the most remarkable phenomena in nature. During pregnancy, the placenta, which is supplied with precursor hormones from the maternal-fetal unit, synthesizes large quantities of steroid hormones as well as various protein and peptide hormones and secretes these products into the fetal and maternal circulations. Near the end of pregnancy, a woman is exposed daily to ~100 mg estrogen, 250 mg progesterone, and large quantities of mineralocorticoids and glucocorticosteroids. The mother, and to a lesser extent the fetus, are also exposed to large quantities of human placental lactogen (hPL), human chorionic gonadotropin (hCG), prolactin, relaxin, and prostaglandins and to smaller amounts of proopiomelanocortin (POMC)-derived peptides such as adrenocorticotropic hormone (ACTH) and endorphin, gonadotropin-releasing hormone (GnRH), thyroid-stimulating hormone (TSH), corticotropin-releasing hormone (CRH), somatostatin, and other hormones.

Implantation, the maintenance of pregnancy, parturition, and finally lactation are dependent on a complex interaction of hormones in the maternal-fetal-placental unit. Moreover, there exists a complex regulation for the secretion of steroid hormones by means of protein and peptide hormones also produced within the placenta. In this chapter the discussion is focused on the hormones secreted by the placenta, the endocrinology of the fetus and the mother, the effect of various endocrine diseases on the maternal-fetal unit, and the use of endocrine tests to assess fetal well-being.

## PLACENTAL COMPARTMENT

In mammals, especially humans, the placenta has evolved into a complex structure that delivers nutrients to the fetus, produces numerous steroid and protein hormones, and removes metabolites from the fetus to the maternal compartment. The structure of the placenta is discussed in Chapter 111.

### PROGESTERONE

The principal source of progesterone during pregnancy is the placenta, although the corpus luteum is the major source during the first 6 to 8 weeks of gestation,[1] when progesterone is essential for the development of a secretory endometrium to receive and implant a blastocyst. Apparently, the developing trophoblast takes over as the principal source of progesterone by 8 weeks, since removal of the corpus luteum before this time, but not after, leads to abortion.[2] After 8 weeks, the corpus luteum contributes only a fraction of the progesterone secreted.

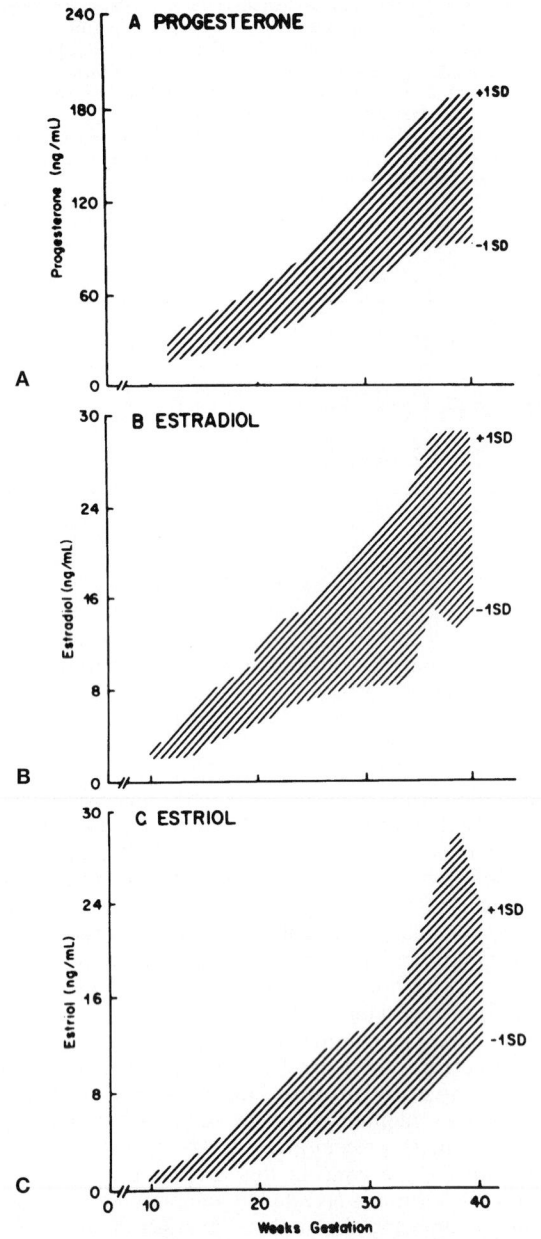

**FIGURE 108-1.** Range (mean ± 1 standard deviation) of progesterone (**A**), estradiol-17β (**B**), and estriol (**C**) in plasma of normal pregnant women as a function of a week of gestation. (Courtesy of Dr. C. Richard Parker, Jr.)

The placenta of a term pregnancy produces ~250 mg progesterone each day. Maternal progesterone plasma levels rise from 25 ng/mL during the late luteal phase to 40 ng/mL near the end of the first trimester to 150 ng/mL at term (Fig. 108-1A). Most progesterone (90%) secreted by the placenta enters the maternal compartment.

Although the placenta produces large amounts of progesterone, it normally has very limited capacity to synthesize precursor cholesterol from acetate. Radiolabeled acetate is only slowly incorporated into cholesterol in placental trophoblasts, and the activity of the rate-limiting enzyme of cholesterol biosynthesis—HMG-CoA reductase—in placental microsomes is low. Therefore, maternal cholesterol, in the form of low-density lipoprotein (LDL) cholesterol, is the principal substrate for the biosynthesis of progesterone.[3,4] LDL cholesterol attaches to its receptor on the trophoblast and is taken up and degraded to free cholesterol, which then is converted to progesterone and secreted. These findings not only have provided new insights into the biochemical basis for placental progesterone formation, but they have also provided clues to other aspects of maternal-placental physiology. For example, the rate of progesterone secretion may depend on the number of LDL receptors on the trophoblast and may be independent of placental blood flow: (a) Cholesterol side-chain cleavage by the placental mitochondria is in a highly activated state, perhaps meaning that the placenta is under constant trophic stimulation and that hCG and GnRH produced by the placenta are the trophic substances; (b) cholesterol synthesis from acetate is limited, as discussed earlier; (c) the fetus does not contribute precursors for placental biosynthesis; and (d) the levels of maternal LDL are not rate-limiting for the placental products of cholesterol or progesterone.[5]

A functioning fetal circulation is unimportant for the regulation of progesterone levels in the maternal unit. In fact, fetal death, ligation of the umbilical cord, or anencephaly—which all are associated with a decrease in estrogen production—have no significant effect on progesterone levels in the maternal compartment.[6,7]

The physiologic role of the large quantity of progesterone includes binding to receptors in uterine smooth muscle, thereby inhibiting contractility and leading to myometrial quiescence. Progesterone also inhibits prostaglandin formation, which is critical in human parturition[8] (see Chap. 109). Progesterone is essential for the maintenance of pregnancy in all mammals, possibly because of its ability to inhibit the T-lymphocyte cell-mediated responses involved in graft rejection. The high local levels of progesterone can block cellular immune response to foreign antigens such as a fetus, creating immunologic privilege for the pregnant uterus.[9]

## ESTROGEN

During human pregnancy, the rate of estrogen production and the levels of estrogen in plasma increase markedly (Fig. 108-1B and C), and the levels of urinary estriol increase 1000-fold.[10] In fact, it has been estimated that during a pregnancy, a woman produces more estrogen than a normal ovulatory woman could produce in 150 years![5] The corpus luteum of pregnancy is the principal source of estrogen during the first few weeks; subsequently, nearly all of the estrogen is formed by the trophoblast of the placenta.

The mechanism by which estrogen is synthesized by the placenta is unique (Fig. 108-2). The placenta cannot convert progesterone to estrogens because of a deficiency of 17α-hydroxylase (CYP17). Thus, it must rely on androgens produced in the maternal and fetal adrenal glands. Estradiol-17β and estrone are synthesized by the placenta by conversion of dehydroepiandrosterone sulfate (DHEAS) that reaches it from both the maternal and the fetal blood. Near term, 40% of the estradiol-17β and estrone is formed from maternal DHEAS and 60% of the estradiol-17β and estrone arises from fetal DHEAS precursor.[11] The placenta metabolizes DHEAS to estrogens through placental sulfatase, Δ4,5-isomerase and 3β-hydroxysteroid dehydrogenase, and aromatase enzyme complex. Estriol is synthesized by the placenta from 16α-hydroxydehydroepiandrosterone sulfate (16α-OHDS) formed in the fetal liver from circulating DHEAS. At least 90% of urinary estriol ultimately is derived from the fetal adrenal gland,[11] which secretes steroid hormones at a high rate, sometimes up to 100 mg per day, mostly as DHEAS. The principal precursor for this DHEAS is LDL cholesterol circulating in fetal blood. A minor source is formation from pregnenolone secreted by the placenta. Only 20% of fetal cholesterol is derived from the maternal compartment, and because amniotic fluid cholesterol levels are negligible, the principal source of cholesterol appears to be the fetus itself. The fetal liver synthesizes cholesterol at a high rate and may supply sufficient cholesterol to the adrenals to maintain steroidogenesis.[12]

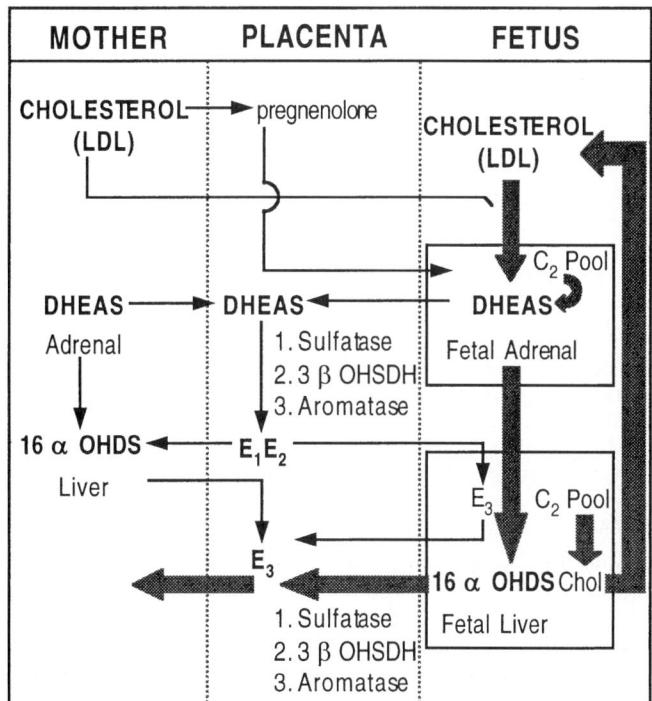

**FIGURE 108-2.** Sources of estrogen biosynthesis in the maternal-fetal-placental unit. (*LDL*, low-density lipoprotein; *chol*, cholesterol; *OHDS*, hydroxydehydroepiandrosterone sulfate; *OHSDH*, hydroxysteroid dehydrogenase; *C₂ pool*, carbon-carbon unit; *DHEAS*, dehydroepiandrosterone sulfate; $E_1$, estrone; $E_2$, estradiol-17β7; $E_3$, estriol.) (From Carr BR, Gant NE. The endocrinology of pregnancy-induced hypertension. Clin Perinatol 1983; 10:737.)

Estetrol is a unique estrogen, the 15α-hydroxy derivative of estriol, which is derived exclusively from fetal precursors and fetal metabolism. Although the measurement of estetrol in pregnant women had been proposed as an aid in monitoring a fetus at risk for intrauterine death, it is not superior to the measurement of urinary estriol.[13]

Several disorders lead to low urinary excretion of estriol by the mother. A particularly interesting one is *placental sulfatase deficiency*,[14] also known as the *steroid sulfatase deficiency syndrome*, an X-linked metabolic disorder characterized during fetal life by decreased maternal estriol production secondary to this deficient enzymatic activity (see Fig. 108-2), which renders the placenta unable to cleave the sulfate moiety from DHEAS. Placental sulfatase deficiency is associated with prolonged gestation and difficulty in cervical dilatation at term, often necessitating cesarean section. Steroid sulfatase deficiency is thought to occur in 1 of every 2000 to 6000 neonates. The male offspring are, of course, *sulfatase deficient*, manifest clinically by ichthyosis during the first few months of life. The genetic locus for steroid sulfatase deficiency is on the distal short arm of the X chromosome.[15]

Most of the estrogen secreted by the placenta is destined for the maternal compartment, as is true for progesterone: 90% of the estradiol-17β and estriol enters the maternal compartment. Interestingly, estrone is the estrogen preferentially secreted into the fetal compartment.[16] The physiologic role of the large quantity of estrogen produced by the placenta is not completely understood. It may regulate or fine-tune the events leading to parturition, because pregnancies are often prolonged when estrogen levels in maternal blood and urine are low, as in placental sulfatase deficiency or when the fetus is anencephalic. Estrogen stimulates phospholipid synthesis and turnover, increases incorporation of arachidonic acid into phospholipids, stimulates prostaglandin synthesis, and increases the number of lysosomes in the uterine endometrium.[8] Estrogens increase

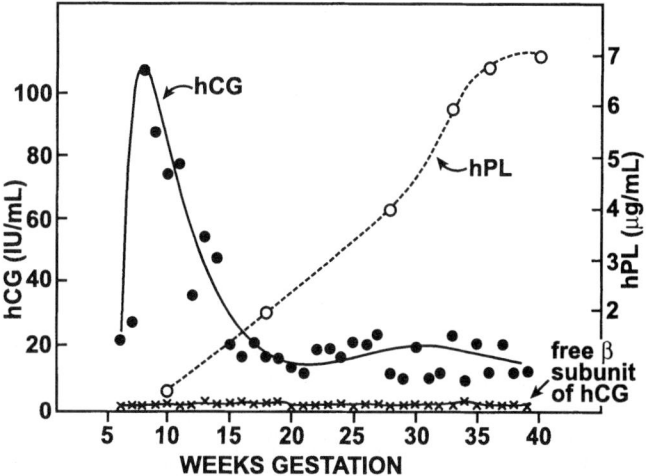

**FIGURE 108-3.** Mean concentration of chorionic gonadotropin (*hCG*) and placental lactogen (*hPL*) in sera of women throughout normal pregnancy. (From Pritchard JA, MacDonald PC, Gant NF. Williams obstetrics, 17th ed. Norwalk, CT: Appleton-Century-Crofts, 1985:121.)

uterine blood flow and may also play a role in fetal organ maturation and development.[17]

## HUMAN CHORIONIC GONADOTROPIN

The hCG secreted by the syncytiotrophoblast of the placenta is released into both the fetal and maternal circulation. This hormone is a glycoprotein with a molecular mass of ~38,000 daltons that consists of two noncovalently linked subunits: α and β.[18] It has been used extensively as a pregnancy test and can be detected in the serum as early as 6 to 8 days after ovulation. Plasma levels rise rapidly during normal pregnancy, with a doubling in concentration every 2 to 3 days,[19] reaching a peak between 60 and 90 days of gestation (Fig. 108-3). Thereafter, the maternal concentration declines and plateaus from ~120 days until delivery.[20] The levels of hCG are higher in multiple pregnancies, in pregnancies associated with Rh isoimmunization, and in diabetic women. Levels also are higher in pregnancies associated with hydatidiform moles or in women with choriocarcinoma (see Chap. 112).

There is some evidence that the rate of secretion of hCG is regulated by a paracrine mechanism involving the release of GnRH by the cytotrophoblast.[21] Fetal concentrations of hCG reach a peak at 11 to 14 weeks' gestation, thereafter falling progressively until delivery.

The most accepted theory regarding the role of hCG in pregnancy is the maintenance of the early corpus luteum to ensure continued progesterone and, possibly, relaxin secretion by the ovary until this function is taken over by the growing trophoblast. Likewise, some investigators have demonstrated that hCG promotes steroidogenesis (progesterone) by the trophoblast.[21] Others have suggested a role for hCG in promoting early growth and androgen secretion by the developing fetal zone of the human adrenal gland.[22] It is more likely that a primary role for hCG is to regulate the development as well as the secretion of testosterone by the fetal testes. Male sexual differentiation occurs at an early but critical time when hCG is present in fetal serum. At this time, fetal hCG levels are higher—before the vascularization of the fetal pituitary, when fetal plasma luteinizing hormone (LH) levels are low.[23] Another role may be to create immunologic privilege to the developing trophoblast.[24] Finally, the excess thyrotropic activity during the clinical development of hyperthyroidism observed in some women with neoplastic trophoblastic disease is secondary to excessive hCG secretion. hCG and TSH have similar structures, and purified hCG inhibits binding to thyroid membranes and stimulates adenylate cyclase in thyroid tissues[25] (see Chaps. 15 and 112).

## HUMAN PLACENTAL LACTOGEN

Placental lactogen is a single-chain polypeptide of 191 amino-acid residues with a molecular mass of ~22,000 daltons.[26] The hormone has both lactogenic and growth hormone (GH)–like activity and is also referred to as chorionic growth hormone or chorionic somatomammotropin. However, hPL exhibits principally lactogenic activity, having only 3% or less of the growth-stimulating activity of human GH. The amino-acid sequences of hPL and GH are similar,[27] and their genes are close together on chromosome 17: It has been proposed that the two hormones evolved from a similar ancestral polypeptide (see Chaps. 12 and 13). The nucleotide sequence for hPL has been reported, and the gene has been cloned.[28]

hPL is secreted by the syncytiotrophoblast and can be detected in serum by radioimmunoassay as early as the third week after ovulation.[26] The serum level of the hormone continues to rise with advancing gestational age and appears to plateau at term (see Fig. 108-3), the concentration closely following and being correlated with increasing placental weight.[29] The serum half-life of hPL is short. For example, although the serum level of hPL before delivery is the highest of all the protein hormones secreted by the placenta, hPL cannot be detected after the first postpartum day. The time sequence and peak of hPL secretion are significantly different from those of hCG (see Fig. 108-3), which suggests a different regulation for each hormone. This is interesting, because both are secreted by the syncytiotrophoblast rather than by the cytotrophoblast. Moreover, hPL secretion is not limited to the trophoblast, since immunoreactive hPL has been detected in patients with various malignant tumors including lymphomas, hepatomas, and bronchogenic carcinomas.

Interestingly, hPL appears to be secreted primarily into the maternal circulation; only low levels are found in cord blood of neonates. Thus, most of the physiologic roles proposed for hPL have centered on its sites of action in maternal tissues. It has been suggested that hPL has a significant effect on maternal glucose, thereby providing adequate and continued nourishment for the developing fetus.[27] It has been proposed that hPL exerts metabolic effects in pregnancy similar to those of GH, including stimulation of lipolysis, thus increasing the circulating free fatty acids available for maternal and fetal nutrition; inhibition of glucose uptake in the mother, yielding increased maternal insulin levels; development of maternal insulin resistance; and inhibition of gluconeogenesis, which favors transportation of glucose and protein to the fetus.[30] A few cases of deficient hPL in maternal serum have been described in otherwise normal pregnancies, however, raising issue with this proposed role of hPL.[31]

## HUMAN GROWTH HORMONE VARIANT

A "true" placental GH has been shown to be produced by the syncytiotrophoblast of the placenta and secreted in parallel with hPL.[32–35] This GH variant is now recognized to be the product of the hGH-V gene[34] and differs from the major 22-kDa GH in 13 amino-acid residues.[36] A glycosylated variant of this GH form has also been described in an in vitro system,[37] but it is not known if this form circulates. Because concentrations of the placental GH variant in maternal plasma correlate with plasma levels of insulin-like growth factor-I (IGF-I), it has been suggested that placental GH is involved in the control of serum IGF-I levels in normal pregnant women.[38]

## OTHER PLACENTAL PEPTIDE HORMONES

In addition to hCG and hPL, several other placental hormones that are similar or closely related to hypothalamic, pituitary, or other hormones in their biologic and immunologic activity have been described (e.g., POMC, human chorionic follicle-stimulating hormone [FSH], human chorionic gonadotropin–releasing hormone [hCGnRH], human chorionic thyrotropin [hCT]–releasing hormone, human chorionic corticotropin–releasing hormone, relaxin, somatostatin, gastrin, and vasoactive intestinal peptide). Information regarding these hormones is limited.[21] The regulation of their secretion is poorly understood, although it appears that classic negative feedback inhibition does not exist. Furthermore, their function and significance are speculative. Most of these hormones do not cross the placenta and are believed to enter primarily the maternal compartment.

### HUMAN CHORIONIC PROOPIOMELANOCORTIN PEPTIDES

Considerable evidence exists for a chorionic corticotropin or ACTH produced and secreted by placental tissue. Along with ACTH, other products that are processed from a similar 31-kDa POMC peptide are found in placental tissue, including β-endorphin, β-lipotropin, and α-melanocyte–stimulating hormone.[21,39,40]

### HUMAN CHORIONIC THYROTROPIN

A substance with TSH-like activity has been identified presumptively in placental tissue. However, the structure of this "hCT" is not identical to that of human pituitary TSH,[41] and its physiologic role is unclear. The increased thyroid activity observed in some women with gestational trophoblastic disease is believed to be secondary to the action of excessive hCG secretion and not to hCT.

### HUMAN CHORIONIC GONADOTROPIN–RELEASING HORMONE AND OTHER HORMONES

A substance with bioimmunoreactivity similar to that of hypothalamic GnRH has been localized to and shown to be synthesized by the cytotrophoblast layer of the placenta. It has been proposed that hCG secretion by the syncytiotrophoblast is regulated in part by hCGnRH.[21] Similarly, substances similar to thyrotropin-releasing hormone (TRH), somatostatin, and CRH are also synthesized by the trophoblast. CRH mRNA has been localized in the placenta, principally in the cytotrophoblast.[42] CRH levels increase in maternal plasma and amniotic fluid throughout pregnancy, but the role for this increase is unclear.[43] The FSH-suppressing hormone follistatin has been found in human placenta. Inhibin and activin are secreted by the placenta, and maternal levels increase near term.[44] (See Chap. 112 for a discussion of these and other placental hormones.)

## FETAL MEMBRANES AND DECIDUA

Fetal membranes consisting of amnion and chorion were originally thought to be inactive endocrinologically. The amnion is a thin structure (0.02–0.5 mm) and contains no blood vessels or nerves. However, the fetal membranes play important roles during pregnancy in the transport and metabolism of hormones and in the events that lead eventually to parturition.[45] Thus, although fetal membranes apparently do not synthesize hormones de novo, they have extensive enzymatic capabilities for regulating steroid hormone metabolism. Some of these enzymes are 5α-reductase, 3β-hydroxysteroid dehydrogenase, Δ4,5-isomerase, 20α-hydroxysteroid oxidoreductase, 17β-hydroxysteroid dehydrogenase, aromatase, and sulfatase. Also, fetal membranes contain large quantities of arachidonic acid, the obligate precursor of prostaglandins. Furthermore, they contain phospholipase $A_2$ and other enzymes that stimulate the release of arachidonic acid from glycerophospholipids in the amnion or chorion.[8]

The decidua is a complex structure of specialized endometrial stromal cells that proliferate in response to progesterone secreted during the luteal phase of the menstrual cycle and later in response to hormones secreted by the developing trophoblast. Evidence suggests that the decidua is also a rich source of enzymatic activity and secretion of hormones. The decidua may be important in fetal homeostasis and in the maintenance of pregnancy, since the decidua appears to communicate directly with the fetus via transport through the fetal membranes and into the amniotic fluid as well as directly into the myometrium by simple diffusion.

The hormones and enzymatic activities localized to the decidua include prolactin, relaxin, prostaglandins, and 1α-hydroxylase. The concentration of prolactin in amniotic fluid is extremely high compared with that in fetal or maternal plasma; it arises from the decidua.[46] Prolactin is secreted by decidual cells in culture but not by trophoblast or placental membranes. The prolactin secreted by the decidua is immunologically, structurally, and biologically similar to that from pituitary sources.[47] However, the regulation of decidual prolactin formation and secretion is more complex. Bromocriptine treatment of pregnant women reduces maternal and fetal plasma levels but not amniotic fluid levels of prolactin. Prolactin secretion by decidual cells or tissues is not affected by treatment with dopamine, dopaminergic agonists, or TRH. The function of decidual prolactin remains speculative. Because most of the prolactin synthesized and secreted by the decidua reaches amniotic fluid, a regulatory role in amniotic fluid osmolality and homeostasis has been proposed.[48]

Relaxin is a peptide consisting of two chains (A and B) of 22 and 31 amino acids covalently linked.[49] Relaxin is secreted by the corpus luteum, decidua, and basal plate and septa of the placenta.[50] The greatest source appears to be the corpus luteum of pregnancy, and it is thought to be regulated by hCG. That the decidua and placenta can synthesize relaxin is intriguing because of the proximity of the pregnant uterus. This is relevant because relaxin is believed to play a role along with progesterone in reducing uterine activity as well as in the softening of pelvic tissues and cervix before parturition (see Chap. 94).[50]

## FETAL COMPARTMENT

The understanding and elucidation of the human fetal endocrine system have required the development of assays for minute quantities of hormone. The regulation of the fetal endocrine system, like that of the placenta, is not completely independent, since synthesis relies to some extent on precursor hormones secreted directly by the placenta or obtained from the maternal unit. As the fetus develops, its endocrine system becomes more independent in preparation for extrauterine existence.

### HYPOTHALAMIC-PITUITARY AXIS

The fetal hypothalamus begins differentiation from the forebrain during the first few weeks of fetal life, and by 12 weeks, hypothalamic development is well advanced. Most of the hypothalamic-releasing hormones, including GnRH, TRH, dopamine, norepinephrine, and somatostatin, and their respective hypothalamic nuclei have been identified as early as 6 to 8 weeks of fetal life.[23] The neurohypophysis is detected first at 5 weeks, and by 14 weeks, the supraoptic and paraventricular nuclei are fully developed.[23,51]

Rathke pouch appears in the human fetus at 4 weeks. The premature anterior pituitary cells that develop from the cells lining Rathke pouch can secrete GH, prolactin, FSH, LH, and ACTH in vitro as early as 7 weeks of fetal life.[52] Evidence suggests that the intermediate lobe of the pituitary is a significant source of POMC hormones.[53,54]

The hypothalamic-pituitary portal system is the functional link between the hypothalamus and the anterior pituitary. Vascularization of the anterior pituitary begins by 13 weeks of fetal life, but a functioning intact portal system is absent until 18 to

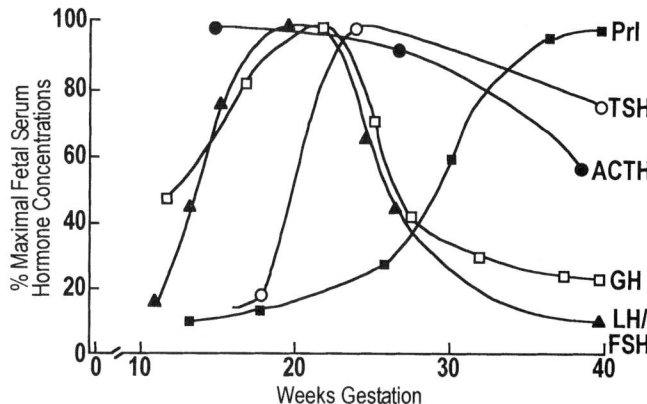

**FIGURE 108-4.** Ontogeny of pituitary hormones in human fetal serum. (*Prl*, prolactin; *TSH*, thyroid-stimulating hormone; *ACTH*, adrenocorticotropic hormone; *GH*, growth hormone; *LH*, luteinizing hormone; *FSH*, follicle-stimulating hormone.) (From Parker CR Jr. The endocrinology of pregnancy. In: Carr BR, Blackwell RE, eds. Textbook of reproductive medicine. Norwalk, CT: Appleton & Lange, 1993:17.)

20 weeks.[55] However, there is indirect evidence that hypothalamic secretion of releasing hormones influences anterior pituitary function before this time by simple diffusion, given their proximity in early fetal development. There is also evidence that fetal adrenal feedback is operative at the hypothalamic-pituitary axis as early as week 14 of fetal life. Elevated levels of fetal androgens are detected at this time in amniotic fluid in fetuses affected with congenital adrenal hyperplasia secondary to 21-hydroxylase deficiency.[56]

## GROWTH HORMONE, PROLACTIN, VASOPRESSIN, AND OXYTOCIN

GH is detected in the fetal pituitary as early as 12 weeks' gestation, and fetal pituitary GH concentrations increase until 25 to 30 weeks' gestation, thereafter remaining constant until term. Fetal plasma GH levels peak at 20 weeks and then fall rapidly until birth[57] (Fig. 108-4). However, fetal plasma concentrations of GH always exceed maternal concentrations, which are suppressed, possibly by the high circulating levels of hPL.

The regulation of GH release in the fetus appears to be more complex than in the adult. To explain the high levels of plasma GH at midgestation and a fall thereafter, unrestrained release of growth hormone–releasing hormone (GHRH) leading to excessive release of GH at midgestation has been postulated.[23] Thereafter, as the hypothalamus matures, somatostatin may increase and GHRH levels decline, reducing GH release. The role of GH in the fetus is also unclear. There is considerable evidence that GH is not essential to somatic growth in primates.[58] For example, in neonates with pituitary agenesis, congenital hypothalamic hypopituitarism, or familial GH deficiency, birth size and length are usually normal. However, the somatomedins, in particular IGF-I and IGF-II, increase in fetal plasma, and IGF-I and IGF-II levels correlate better than do GH levels with fetal growth.[59] Although GH is an important trophic hormone for somatomedin production in the fetus, somatomedin regulation may be independent of GH, depending instead on other factors. Prolactin, hPL, and insulin also stimulate somatomedin production.[23]

Prolactin is present in lactotropes by 19 weeks of life. The prolactin content of the fetal pituitary increases throughout gestation,[60] whereas plasma levels increase slowly until 30 weeks' gestation, when the levels rise sharply until term and remain elevated until the third month of postnatal life (see Fig. 108-4). In humans, TRH and dopamine as well as estrogens appear to affect fetal prolactin secretion. Bromocriptine both lowers maternal prolactin levels and crosses the placenta to inhibit fetal prolactin release and lower prolactin levels in fetal blood.[61] It has been suggested that prolactin in the fetus influences adrenal growth, lung maturation, and amniotic fluid volume.

Arginine vasopressin (AVP) and oxytocin are found in hypothalamic nuclei and in the neurohypophysis during early fetal development.[52] However, there are relatively few studies on the regulation and secretion of these hormones. The levels of AVP are high in fetal plasma and cord blood at delivery. The principal stimulus to AVP release appears to be fetal hypoxia, although acidosis, hypercarbia, and hypotension also play a role.[62] The elevated AVP levels in fetal blood may lead to increased blood pressure, vasoconstriction, and the passage of meconium by the fetus. Oxytocin levels in the fetus are not affected by hypoxia but appear to increase during labor and delivery (see Chap. 109).

## THYROID GLAND

The placenta apparently is relatively impermeable to TSH and thyroid hormone, so that the fetal hypothalamic–pituitary–thyroid axis develops and functions independently of the maternal system. Although thyroxine ($T_4$) may cross the placenta to a slight degree, human thyroid-stimulating immunoglobulins (TSI) as well as iodine and antithyroid drugs given to women with hyperthyroidism pass through the placenta and may affect fetal thyroid function.[63]

TRH is detectable in hypothalamic nuclei, and TSH is found in pituitary tissues by 10 to 12 weeks of fetal life.[64] High concentrations of TRH are detected in fetal blood, and the source is thought to be the fetal pancreas. However, this source of TRH appears to have little effect on the pituitary release of TSH, and the function of pancreatic TRH is unknown.[65]

The fetal thyroid has developed sufficiently by the end of the first trimester that it can concentrate iodine and synthesize iodothyronines. The levels of TSH and thyroid hormone are relatively low in fetal blood until midgestation. At 24 to 28 weeks' gestation, serum TSH concentrations rise abruptly to a peak but decrease slightly thereafter until delivery.[66] In response to the surge of TSH, $T_4$ levels rise progressively after midgestation until term (Fig. 108-5). During this time, both thyroid responsiveness to TRH and pituitary TRH content increase. At birth, there is an abrupt release of TSH, $T_4$, and triiodothyronine ($T_3$), and the levels of these hormones fall during the first few weeks after birth.[66] The relative hyperthyroid state of the fetus is believed to be necessary to prepare it for the thermoregulatory adjustments of extrauterine life. The abrupt changes of TSH and $T_4$ that occur at birth are believed to be stimulated by the cooling associated with delivery.[67] Finally, 3,3',5'-triiodo-L-thyronine (reverse $T_3$) levels are high during early fetal life, begin to fall at midgestation, and continue to fall after birth (see Chap. 47). The difference between the formation of $T_3$ and reverse $T_3$ is thought to be related to maturation of peripheral iodothyronine metabolism (see Chap. 30).

## GONADS

Bioactive and immunoreactive GnRH has been detected in the fetal hypothalamus by 9 to 12 weeks of life. The amount increases with fetal age, with the maximum noted between 22 and 25 weeks in females and between 34 to 38 weeks in males.[23] The dominant gonadotropin fraction in the fetal pituitary is the α subunit. However, the fetal pituitary in vitro is capable of secreting intact LH by 5 to 7 weeks.[53] The pituitary content of LH increases from 10 weeks to 24 weeks and then falls slowly near term. The content of LH is higher in females than in males, a difference thought to be secondary to a greater negative feedback in response to higher concentrations of plasma testosterone in fetal male plasma.[68] The FSH content of the fetal pituitary increases until midgestation, then falls until term. The FSH content is higher in female than in male fetuses because of greater negative feedback in the latter. The plasma concentra-

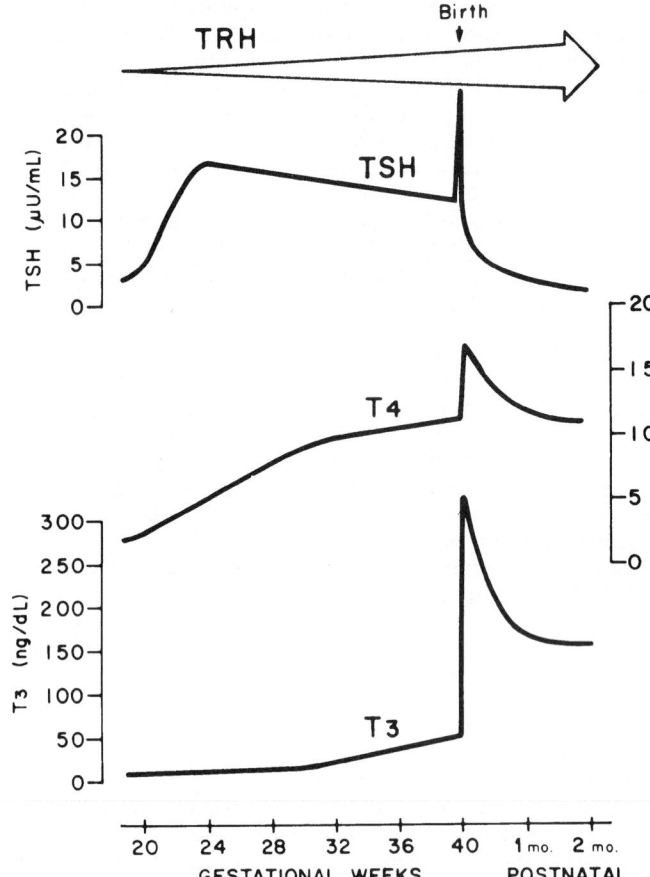

**FIGURE 108-5.** Maturation of serum thyroid-stimulating hormone (*TSH*), thyroxine (*T₄*), and triiodothyronine (*T₃*) during the last half of gestation and early neonatal life. The increase in thyrotropin-releasing hormone (*TRH*) effect or content is also illustrated. (From Fisher DA. Maternal-fetal neurohypophyseal system. Clin Perinatol 1983; 10:615.)

tion of FSH rises slowly to a peak near week 25 and then falls to low levels by term (see Fig. 108-4). The FSH levels parallel the pituitary content of FSH with respect to sexual dimorphism, being higher in females than in males. The pattern of LH levels in fetal plasma parallels that of FSH. The fall in gonadotropin pituitary content and plasma concentration after midgestation is thought to be attributable to the maturation of the hypothalamus.[23] The hypothalamus also becomes more sensitive to sex steroids circulating in fetal blood that originate in the placenta.

The differentiation of the bipotential fetal gonad into a testis or an ovary is discussed in Chapter 94. In the male, testosterone secretion begins soon after differentiation of the gonad into a testis and the formation of Leydig cells at 7 weeks of fetal life. Maximal levels are observed at ~15 weeks and decrease thereafter.[69] This early secretion of testosterone is important in regulating sexual differentiation. It is believed that hCG is the primary stimulus to the early development and growth of Leydig cells and the subsequent peak of testosterone. The pattern of hCG, the concentration of testicular hCG receptors, and the pattern of plasma testosterone are related closely.[70] Thus, it appears that sexual differentiation of the male does not rely solely on fetal pituitary gonadotropins. However, fetal LH and FSH are still required for complete differentiation of the fetal ovary and testis. For example, anencephalic fetuses with low levels of circulating LH and FSH have appropriate secretion of testosterone at 15 to 20 weeks secondary to adequate levels of hCG, but they have a decreased number of Leydig cells, exhibit hypoplastic external genitalia, and often have undescended testes.[71] Likewise, male fetuses with congenital hypopituitarism often have an associated micropenis. These observations suggest that beginning about midgestation fetal pituitary gonadotropins affect testosterone secretion from the testes. The regulation of testosterone secretion also appears to depend on fetal cholesterol, principally LDL cholesterol, to maintain maximal rates of testosterone secretion. Fetal testicular LDL receptors and rates of de novo synthesis of cholesterol also parallel the secretion of hCG and testosterone.[72]

The fetal ovary is involved primarily with the formation of follicles and germ cells. Although follicular development appears to be relatively independent of gonadotropins, the anencephalic female fetus has small ovaries and a decreased number of ovarian follicles. However, the fetal ovaries do not contain hCG receptors, at least by 20 weeks of gestation. The ovaries appear to be relatively inactive with respect to steroidogenesis during fetal life, but they can aromatize androgens to estrogens in vitro as early as 8 weeks of life.[73]

## ADRENAL GLAND

The human fetal adrenal glands secrete large quantities of steroid hormones (up to 200 mg per day near term).[74] This rate of steroidogenesis may be five times that observed in the adrenal glands of adults at rest. The principal steroids are C-19 steroids (mainly DHEAS), which serve as substrate for estrogen biosynthesis in the placenta.

It was recognized early that the human fetal adrenal gland contains a unique *fetal zone* that accounts for the rapid growth of the gland and that this zone disappears during the first few weeks after birth.[12] The fetal zone differs histologically and biochemically from the *neocortex* (also known as the definitive or *adult zone*). The uniqueness of a transient fetal zone has been reported in certain higher primates and some other species, but only humans possess the extremely large fetal zone that involutes after birth.

The cells of the adrenal cortex arise from coelomic epithelium. Those cells comprising the fetal zone can be identified in the 8- to 10-mm embryo and before the appearance of the cells of the neocortex (14-mm embryo).[75] Growth is most rapid during the last 6 weeks of fetal life. By 28 weeks' gestation, the adrenal gland may be as large as the fetal kidney and may be equal to the size of the adult adrenal by term (Fig. 108-6). The fetal zone accounts for the largest percentage of growth; after birth, the gland shrinks secondary to involution and necrosis of fetal zone cells.

Histologically, the central portion of the adrenal contains the fetal zone cells, which are eosinophilic cells with pale-staining nuclei that at term make up 80% to 85% of the volume of the gland. The neocortex is the outer rim of cells containing a small quantity of cytoplasm and dark-staining nuclei. The neocortex

is thought to originate the zona glomerulosa, zona fasciculata, and zona reticularis after birth.[12]

In vitro studies utilizing fetal adrenal tissues or cells, in vivo perfusion studies of previable fetuses, and cord blood measurements of steroid hormones demonstrate that the fetal zone can secrete the full complement of steroid hormones secreted by the adult adrenal cortex. However, the fetal zone has a reduced capacity to secrete C-21 steroids because of the low activity of 3β-hydroxysteroid dehydrogenase and $\Delta^{4,5}$-isomerase complex,[76] probably secondary to estrogen or other factors produced by the placenta that may inhibit enzyme action. Thus, the principal steroids secreted by the fetal zone cells are $\Delta^5$-sulfoconjugates, namely, DHEAS and pregnenolone sulfate.[77,78] In contrast, the principal secretory product of the neocortex is cortisol. Electron microscopic investigations suggest fetal zone activity as early as the seventh week and indicate that it is the most steroidogenic zone throughout gestation. The neocortex cells exhibit little steroidogenic activity until the third trimester.[79]

During gestation, DHEAS levels in fetal plasma rise, peaking between 34 and 40 weeks.[80] This pattern coincides with the marked increase in fetal adrenal growth. After birth, DHEAS levels decline, paralleling the regression of the fetal zone. Cortisol plasma levels also increase during fetal life, but there is little evidence after 25 weeks' gestation of a sharp rise like that of DHEAS. Moreover, a significant portion of the circulating cortisol in fetal plasma arises from placental transfer from the maternal compartment.[81]

### REGULATION OF FETAL ADRENAL GROWTH

ACTH stimulates steroidogenesis in vitro,[12] and there is clinical evidence that ACTH is the principal trophic hormone of the fetal adrenal gland in vivo. For example, in anencephalic fetuses, the plasma levels of ACTH are very low, and the fetal zone is markedly atrophic. Maternal glucocorticosteroid therapy suppresses fetal adrenal steroidogenesis by suppressing fetal ACTH secretion.[82] Further evidence that ACTH regulates steroidogenesis early in fetal life is provided by the observation of elevated levels of 17α-hydroxyprogesterone in the amniotic fluid of fetuses with congenital adrenal hyperplasia secondary to the absence of 21-hydroxylase. Despite these observations, other ACTH-related peptides (e.g., fetal pituitary or placental POMC derivatives) have been proposed as trophic hormones for the fetal zone, but the evidence is weak.[12] Other hormones or growth factors, including prolactin, hCG, GH, hPL, and epidermal and fibroblast growth factor, have no consistent significant effect on steroidogenesis or adenylate cyclase activity in cultures of fetal zone organs or monolayer cells or of membrane preparations. However, a role of these or other hormones in promoting growth of adrenal cells is possible.[83,84]

After birth, the adrenal gland shrinks by more than 50% secondary to regression of fetal zone cells. This suggests that a trophic substance other than ACTH is withdrawn from the maternal or placental compartment or that the secretion rates of some other trophic hormone are altered to initiate regression of this fetal zone.

### FETAL ADRENAL STEROIDOGENESIS

The availability of precursor substrates may assist ACTH in regulating the rate of steroid hormone production by the fetal zone. Circulating pregnenolone and progesterone have long been suggested as the principal precursors of fetal adrenal steroidogenesis, but a number of factors make this unlikely. For example, in view of the fetal adrenal blood flow and the levels of unconjugated pregnenolone in fetal plasma, <1% of the DHEAS produced by the fetal adrenal could be derived from pregnenolone.[12] Furthermore, estriol levels as well as fetal adrenal steroid secretion rates are reduced in pregnant women treated with glucocorticosteroids. Also, one would not expect pregnenolone or progesterone to be significant as a precursor hormone in adrenal steroidogenesis

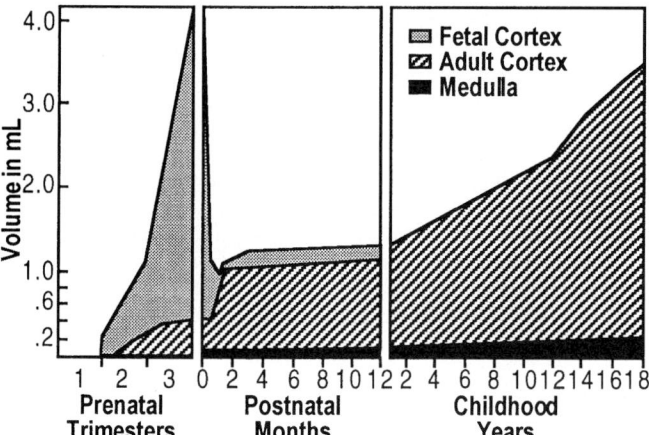

**FIGURE 108-6.** Size of adrenal gland and its component parts during fetal life, infancy, and childhood. (From Carr BR, Simpson ER. Lipoprotein utilization and cholesterol synthesis by the human fetal adrenal gland. Endocr Rev 1981; 2:306.)

if infants who have adrenal enzyme defects develop sexual ambiguity secondary to congenital adrenal hyperplasia.

Cholesterol is a major precursor for fetal adrenal steroidogenesis,[85] arising either from de novo synthesis from 2-carbon units (acetate) or from lipoprotein circulating in fetal plasma. Of the steroids secreted by the fetal adrenal, 50% to 75% are derived from cholesterol obtained from LDL.[86]

The fetal adrenal, particularly the fetal zone cells, contain the highest number of specific binding sites for LDL of any tissue studied.[87] ACTH binds to cell-surface receptors in the human fetal adrenal gland and stimulates adenylate cyclase activity. This leads to activation of protein hormones, which in turn increases phosphorylation of key enzymes in adrenal cholesterol metabolism. ACTH also increases the number of LDL receptors.[88] LDL binds to specific receptors on the cell surface (coated pits) and is internalized by *absorptive endocytosis.* The internalized coated vesicles fuse with lysosomes, and the cholesterol esters of LDL are liberated to yield free cholesterol, which is then available for the biosynthesis of steroid hormones and other cellular processes. ACTH also stimulates de novo synthesis of cholesterol; thus, cholesterol supplies are adequate for the high rate of steroid synthesis characteristic of the human fetal adrenal gland.[89] The plasma pool of LDL is turned over two to four times per day to meet steroidogenic requirements, five-fold to ten-fold greater than the turnover of the LDL pool in the adult.[12]

Measurement of the levels of LDL and DHEAS in cord blood in normal and anencephalic pregnancies has provided convincing evidence that cholesterol levels in fetal plasma are regulated partly by the degree of fetal adrenal activity: There is an inverse relation between cord blood levels of DHEAS and LDL.[90] That is, in normal pregnancies with normal fetuses, cord blood levels of DHEAS are high and LDL levels are low; in pregnancies with anencephalic fetuses who have atrophic adrenals, DHEAS levels are low and LDL levels are high. Furthermore, anencephalic adrenals have reduced numbers of LDL receptors and are unable to utilize LDL as a precursor for steroidogenesis in vitro.[91,92] Thus, normally, when the human fetal adrenal gland is utilizing LDL cholesterol maximally, factors regulating the formation of cholesterol in the fetal liver would be important, albeit indirectly, in determining the rate of DHEAS secretion by the fetal adrenal and the rate of estrogen formation by the placenta. Because glucocorticoids and estrogens formed by the maternal-fetal-placental unit also stimulate cholesterol synthesis by the fetal liver, these observations demonstrate the close interrelations of the regulation of the fetus and the rate of estrogen biosynthesis in the placenta[93] (see Fig. 108-2).

### FETAL ADRENAL MEDULLA

The medulla is formed by 10 weeks of gestation. Unlike the fetal adrenal cortex, the medulla is relatively immature at term.[94] The secretion of cortisol by the adrenal cortex, which surrounds the medulla, stimulates the formation of epinephrine from norepinephrine. However, most chromaffin tissue in the human fetus is formed in paraaortic paraganglia rather than in adrenal medullary tissue. Both epinephrine and norepinephrine can be detected in the human fetal medulla by 10 to 15 weeks' gestation.[95] Except for the effect of cortisol, the regulation of catecholamine secretion in the human fetus has not been completely elucidated. In other species, hypoxia and trauma, as well as advancing gestation and maturation, are related to the release of catecholamines by the adrenal medulla.

### PARATHYROID GLAND AND CALCIUM HOMEOSTASIS

The calcium levels in the fetus are regulated largely by transfer from the maternal compartment across the placenta. The maternal compartment undergoes a number of adjustments that ultimately permit a net transfer of sufficient calcium to sustain fetal bone growth. These changes include increases in maternal

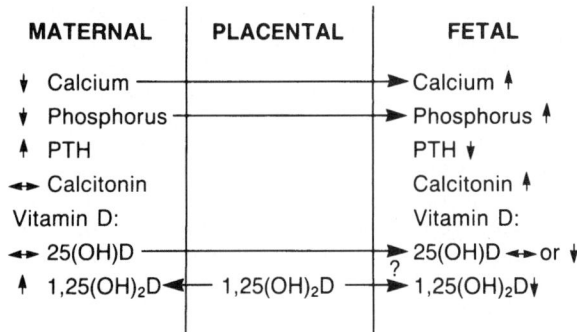

**FIGURE 108-7.** Regulation of calcium homeostasis in maternal-fetal-placental unit. *Arrows* designate major pathways and changes during pregnancy: ↑, increase; ↓, decrease; ←→, no change. (*PTH,* parathyroid hormone.) (Adapted in part from Schedewie HK, Fisher DA. In: Tulchinsky D, Ryan KJ, eds. Maternal-fetal endocrinology. Philadelphia: WB Saunders, 1980:365.)

dietary intake, in circulating maternal vitamin D [1,25(OH)₂D], and in circulating parathyroid hormone (PTH). Serum calcitonin levels increase (see Chap. 53). The levels of total calcium and phosphate decline, but ionized calcium levels remain unchanged.[96] The "placental calcium pump" creates a positive gradient of calcium and phosphorus to the fetus (Fig. 108-7). Circulating fetal calcium and phosphate levels increase steadily throughout gestation, and fetal levels of total and ionized calcium as well as of phosphate exceed maternal levels at term. The active transport of calcium to the fetus increases from 50 mg per day at 20 weeks to 350 mg per day by 35 weeks, and the total accumulation of calcium in the fetus is about 30 g.[97]

The fetal parathyroid gland contains PTH, and the gland can secrete hormone by 10 to 12 weeks' gestation.[98] The fetal plasma levels of PTH are low and increase after delivery. Likewise, the fetal thyroid contains calcitonin, and serum calcitonin levels in the fetus are elevated.[96,99] Because there is no transfer of PTH or calcitonin across the placenta, the consequences of the changes in these hormones on fetal calcium are consistent with an adaptation to conserve and stimulate bone growth within the fetus. Parathyroid hormone–related protein (PTHrP) is localized in the fetal parathyroid gland and plays a major role in fetal bone development and calcium homeostasis.[100] PTHrP knock-out mice die at birth with a number of skeletal anomalies.[101]

The levels of the various forms of vitamin D are lower in the fetus than in the maternal compartment. The placenta and decidua are capable of 1α-hydroxylation and of formation of the active metabolite 1,25(OH)₂D. However, the role, if any, of this hormone in the fetus is unknown, since its principal effect is on intestinal absorption of calcium.[102]

Serum calcium and phosphate levels fall in the neonate. Serum PTH levels begin to rise 48 hours after birth, and calcium and phosphate levels increase gradually over the following several days and are dependent on dietary intake of milk. Neonatal hypocalcemia, defined as a serum calcium concentration below 7 mg/dL, is a common complication of premature delivery, maternal diabetes, and birth asphyxia. The rare neonatal hypercalcemia may be caused by excessive maternal intake of calcium or vitamin D. Also, inadequate treatment of maternal hypoparathyroidism with resultant hypocalcemia may cause fetal hyperparathyroidism and elevated calcium levels early in neonatal life.

### PANCREAS

The human pancreas appears during the fourth week of fetal life. A cells, containing glucagon, and D cells, containing somatostatin, develop before B-cell differentiation, although insulin can be recognized in the developing pancreas before apparent

B-cell differentiation[103] (see Chaps. 133 and 134). The total pancreatic content of insulin and glucagon increases with fetal age and is higher than in the adult human pancreas.

Contrary to the pancreatic content of insulin, fetal insulin secretion is low and relatively unresponsive to acute changes in glucose in both in vitro studies of pancreatic cells and cord blood at delivery or blood obtained from the scalp of the fetus at term.[29,104] However, in vitro, fetal insulin secretion is responsive to amino acids and glucagon as early as 14 weeks of gestation.

Although the acute response to glucose is impaired in the fetal pancreas, when B cells are exposed chronically to elevated glucose levels (e.g., as in maternal diabetes mellitus), or in hypertrophy, the rate of secretion of insulin is increased (see Chap. 156).

Glucagon has been detected in human fetal plasma as early as 15 weeks' gestation. Although the secretion of glucagon is stimulated in late pregnancy by amino acids and catecholamines, acute changes in glucose appear to have little effect on fetal pancreatic glucagon secretion.[105]

## ROLE OF HORMONES IN LUNG MATURATION

The fetal lung undergoes dramatic changes near the end of gestation, owing to the significant anatomic and structural as well as biochemical maturation needed by the neonate to adapt to the extrauterine environment. Failure of normal maturation or, more often, premature delivery, may lead to significant morbidity and mortality secondary to the respiratory distress syndrome (RDS). It is widely accepted that failure of the fetal lung to produce sufficient surfactant, which reduces alveolar surface tension, is the principal defect in RDS[105] (see Chap. 202).

The human lung develops as a ventral diverticulum from the laryngotracheal groove of the foregut during the fifth week of gestation. This is followed by further differentiation into two lung buds and further branching. Between 20 and 24 weeks' gestation, differentiated type II pneumonocytes appear. The lamellar bodies, the intracellular structures in which surfactant are stored, are first visible at this time in these cells.[105,106]

The biochemical development of surfactant is crucial to fetal lung maturation. Surfactant is a lipoprotein consisting of glycerophospholipid (80%), neutral lipid (10%), and protein (10%). The phosphatidylcholines (lecithin) account for nearly 80% of the glycerophospholipid, and phosphatidylglycerol accounts for another 10%. There appears to be one major apoprotein that is critical in surfactant action and function. The formation of disaturated phosphatidylcholine, the principal lipoprotein of surfactant, involves a complex set of enzymatic actions in which the enzyme, phosphatidate phosphohydrolase (PAPase), appears to be critical[106] (Fig. 108-8). Surfactant concentrations that can sustain lung stability and extrauterine existence of the fetus are attained between 33 and 36 weeks of gestation.

The first sign that hormones might participate in fetal lung maturation was made by noting that premature fetal lambs treated with glucocorticosteroids had greater lung development than did controls.[107] Since then, evidence has accumulated that the production of surfactant in the human fetus involves the action of several hormones. Most investigations both in vivo and in vitro suggest a primary role for cortisol. The administration of glucocorticosteroids to the pregnant woman between weeks 29 and 33 of gestation and 24 to 48 hours before delivery significantly reduces the incidence of RDS in premature infants.[108] However, in vitro studies suggest that other hormones are required for lung maturation and surfactant expression. Among the agents suggested to act in concert with cortisol are prolactin, insulin, estrogen, thyroid hormone, and prostaglandins[106] (see Chap. 202). It has been suggested that estrogen stimulates fetal prolactin release to promote surfactant formation.[109] Although fetal prolactin levels parallel an increase in lecithin/sphingomyelin ratios, prolactin probably plays only a minor role in lung maturation. Women treated with bromocriptine have suppressed fetal prolactin levels, but the neonates do

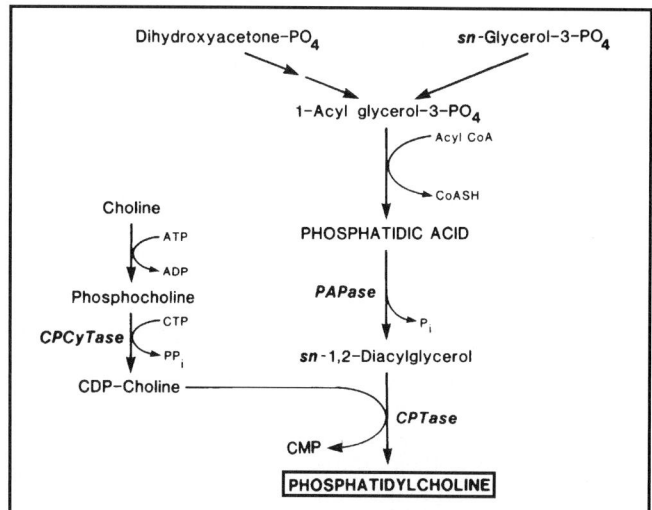

**FIGURE 108-8.** Biosynthetic pathway for phosphatidylcholine (lecithin) synthesis in type II pneumonocytes. (*ATP*, adenosine triphosphate; *ADP*, adenosine diphosphate; *PAPase*, phosphatidate phosphohydrolase; *CPTase*, choline phosphotransferase; *CPCyTase*, choline phosphate cytidylyltransferase; *CDP*, choline diphosphate; *CMP*, cytidine monophosphate.) (From Pritchard JA, MacDonald PC, Gant NF. Williams obstetrics, 17th ed. Norwalk, CT: Appleton-Century-Crofts, 1985:155.)

not develop RDS, whereas anencephalic fetuses, which are exposed to less estrogen and fetal androgen, have normal prolactin levels but appear to have delayed lung maturation.

A role for $T_4$ in the development of surfactant has been investigated.[110] Some investigators have observed that $T_4$ administration to subprimates accelerates fetal lung maturation; others have been unable to demonstrate increased surfactant formation. Because $T_4$ has only a limited ability to cross the placenta, intraamniotic administration of thyroid hormones would be required. At present, limited investigations with $T_4$ have suggested a stimulation of fetal lung maturation, but the role of thyroid hormones in the normal maturation of fetal surfactant remains unclear. TRH can cross the placenta; therefore, TRH administration may be an alternative to induce lung maturation.

The precise role of other hormones in fetal lung maturation and surfactant synthesis remains unclear. Evidence in vitro suggests that rather than acting independently, these hormones probably act in concert to promote lung maturation.[106]

## MATERNAL COMPARTMENT—ENDOCRINE ALTERATIONS AND ENDOCRINE DISEASES ASSOCIATED WITH PREGNANCY

Various maternal adaptations involving the endocrine system occur during pregnancy. Also, many of the diseases of the female endocrine system, if untreated, are associated with infertility and reduced conception rates. If conception does occur, the more serious the disorder (such as diabetes mellitus), the more likely it will affect the fetus adversely (see Chap. 156). Hormones or drugs used to treat the endocrine disorders may be transported across the placenta and alter the environment and development of the fetus.

### HYPOTHALAMUS AND PITUITARY GLAND

Little is known of the endocrine alterations of the maternal hypothalamus during pregnancy. Often, tumors of the hypothalamus or functional disorders of the hypothalamus cause infertility secondary to amenorrhea and chronic anovulation. The anterior pituitary undergoes a two-fold to three-fold enlargement due primarily to hyperplasia and hypertrophy of the lactotropes (prolactin-secreting cells) thought to result from estrogen stimulation (see Chap. 13). Thus, plasma prolactin levels parallel the increase in pituitary size, with a progressive increase throughout gestation. Maternal prolactin levels in plasma are 10- to 20-fold higher at term than in nonpregnant women.[111]

Contrary to lactotropes, the number of somatotrope cells in the pituitary decreases during pregnancy. Maternal levels of GH are low and do not change during pregnancy. The GH responses to insulin infusion appear blunted, suggesting that GH levels are suppressed.[112] Maternal levels of LH and FSH are also low during pregnancy. The response of gonadotropins to an infusion of GnRH is blunted severely. The loss of responsiveness to GnRH is thought to be secondary to a negative feedback inhibition from the elevated levels of estrogen and progesterone.[113] The levels of TSH are within the normal nonpregnant adult range. Furthermore, the response of TSH to a dose of TRH is similar to that in nonpregnant women.[63]

Numerous studies have examined the levels of ACTH- and POMC-related peptides in maternal blood throughout pregnancy. The maternal plasma levels of β-endorphin remain relatively low.[114] These levels increase with advancing labor, but levels of this hormone in cord blood are similar both in infants delivered vaginally and in those delivered by elective cesarean section from women not in labor. However, fetal hypoxia is associated with significant increases in β-endorphin levels in cord blood.[115] The plasma levels of maternal ACTH increase from early to late gestation.[116] The slight increases in ACTH levels that appear to occur during gestation might be explained by the increased secretion of placental ACTH that is not subject to feedback control or related to the increased levels of CRH of placental origin. Maternal ACTH rises to very high levels during labor and delivery. The levels of ACTH in umbilical cord plasma parallel those of β-endorphin and, because neither cross the placenta, offer further evidence that in the fetus these two peptides are processed from a common precursor, as is true in the adult.

Maternal plasma AVP levels remain low throughout gestation and are not believed to play a role in human parturition.[51] Maternal oxytocin levels are low and do not vary throughout pregnancy but increase during the later stages of labor (see Chaps. 25 and 109).

Women with idiopathic hypopituitarism who lack one or more pituitary hormones will continue to require replacement therapy (thyroid hormones and glucocorticoids) throughout pregnancy. Because the size of the pituitary as well as its vascularization increases, vascular accidents are more likely than in nonpregnant women. *Spontaneous pituitary necrosis*, which is rare, occurs most commonly in diabetic women. The principal clinical feature is a persistent midline headache. The diagnosis is often difficult but can be confirmed by pituitary testing with TRH or CRH. Once the diagnosis is confirmed, adequate replacement will usually not be associated with further fetal or maternal morbidity. In some women, hypopituitarism develops after a postpartum hemorrhage, in which an acute ischemic necrosis of the pituitary may occur and cause hormone insufficiency (*Sheehan syndrome*; see Chaps. 11 and 17). Finally, diabetes insipidus is a rare complication of pregnancy. Pregnant women who are treated with vasopressin replacement regimens appear to have no complications, and most treated women undergo spontaneous labor and delivery. Lactation occurs in some.[117,118]

The most common pituitary problem associated with pregnancy is growth of pituitary tumors, most commonly prolactinomas. Occasionally, women with small prolactinomas will become pregnant without treatment, but most will experience amenorrhea, galactorrhea, or infertility. Treatment with bromocriptine will increase the pregnancy rate in women with microprolactinomas or macroprolactinomas (see Chaps. 13 and 21). After conception, most women with these disorders exhibit no problems during the remainder of pregnancy.[119,120] The principal complications are headaches or visual disturbances secondary to tumor expansion, which usually respond rapidly to bromocriptine. The use of bromocriptine to induce ovulation or reinstitution of the drug during pregnancy does not appear to affect the fetus adversely.[121]

Other pituitary tumors associated with pregnancy include GH-secreting and ACTH-secreting tumors. Acromegaly secondary to excessive GH secretion is a very rare complication. In a few patients, a significant worsening of the disease has been reported.[122] Treatment includes medical therapy, irradiation, or surgical removal. Excessive ACTH secretion from a pituitary tumor is rarely associated with pregnancy. However, women with Nelson syndrome from previous bilateral adrenalectomy occasionally exhibit a marked increase in pituitary size and elevated ACTH levels. If hypophysectomy is required for tumor, it is usually not associated with adverse effects on the course of pregnancy or on the fetus, but the increased vascularization during pregnancy may increase perioperative blood loss.

## THYROID GLAND

The thyroid gland enlarges slightly during pregnancy secondary to increased vascularity and mild hyperplasia, but there is no true goiter. There is a modest (25%) increase in oxygen consumption (basal metabolic rate) caused by fetal requirements.

During pregnancy, the mother is in a euthyroid state. Serum total $T_4$ and $T_3$ increase markedly but do not indicate a hyperthyroid state, since a parallel increase in thyroxine-binding globulin (TBG) is also observed. The elevated TBG results from estrogen exposure. A similar change is observed in women on oral contraceptives. A lowered resin uptake of $T_3$ is also observed both in pregnancy and in women on oral contraceptives. However, the serum levels of free $T_3$ or $T_4$ are not increased in these circumstances[123] (see Chap. 30).

There is little, if any, transfer of $T_4$, $T_3$, or TSH across the placenta.[124] TRH can cross the placenta, but under normal conditions, there is little TRH circulating in the peripheral maternal plasma.

Hyperthyroidism occurs in ~2 of every 1000 pregnancies. Untreated thyrotoxicosis is associated with increased fetal loss.[125] The causes of hyperthyroidism in pregnancy include acute thyroiditis, Graves disease, toxic goiter, and gestational trophoblastic disease. The diagnosis is confirmed by finding increased total and free $T_3$ and $T_4$ levels as well as normal or increased $T_3$ resin uptake and elevated calculated free $T_4$ index. The therapy for hyperthyroidism during pregnancy includes antithyroid drugs alone or followed by surgery (see Chaps. 21 and 110). Radioactive iodine is contraindicated because iodine crosses the placenta and could affect fetal thyroid function. Antithyroid drugs also cross the placenta and can induce fetal hypothyroidism and goiter.[126] To prevent this complication, drug dosages are carefully titrated by following clinical symptoms and thyroid levels in maternal blood. Propranolol has also been used in pregnant women with hyperthyroidism, but adverse effects may occur in fetuses.[127] Long-acting thyroid stimulator and TSI can cross the placenta and cause transient neonatal thyrotoxicosis[123] (see Chap. 47).

Hypothyroidism is rarer in pregnancy than is hyperthyroidism, since infertility and early spontaneous abortion are common in hypothyroid women. The diagnosis is confirmed by clinical symptoms and lowered serum $T_3$ and $T_4$ levels as well as by elevated serum TSH levels.[128] Replacement with thyroid hormones is usually associated with a normal pregnancy.

## ADRENAL GLAND

Unlike the fetal adrenal, the maternal adrenal gland does not change morphologically during pregnancy. However, plasma adrenal steroid hormone concentrations increase with advancing gestation (Fig. 108-9).

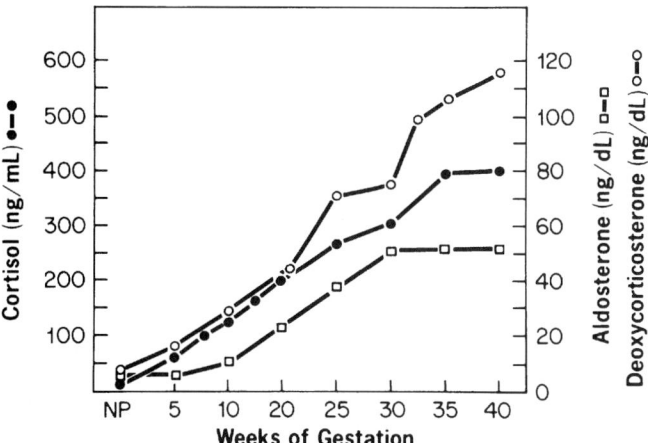

FIGURE 108-9. Mean concentrations of cortisol, aldosterone, and deoxy-corticosterone in sera of women throughout normal pregnancy. (*NP*, nonpregnant value.) (Adapted in part from data in Carr BR, Parker CR Jr, Madden JD, et al. Maternal plasma adrenocorticotropin [ACTH] and cortical relationships throughout human pregnancy. Am J Obstet Gynecol 1981; 139:416; Parker CR Jr, Everett RB, Whalley PJ, et al. Hormone production during pregnancy in the primigravid patient: II. Plasma levels of deoxycorticosterone throughout pregnancy of normal women and women who develop pregnancy-induced hypertension. Am J Obstet Gynecol 1980; 138:626; and Peterson RE. Corticosteroids and corticotropins. In: Fuchs F, Klopper A, eds. Endocrinology of pregnancy. Philadelphia: Harper & Row, 1983:112.)

The increase in total plasma cortisol is attributable principally to a concomitant increase in cortisol-binding globulin (CBG), also known as *transcortin*.[129] There is a slight increase in free plasma cortisol and urinary free cortisol, but pregnant women do not exhibit overt signs of hypercortisolism.[130] There continues to be a diurnal rhythm of cortisol secretion throughout pregnancy with a trend toward a greater morning to evening difference as pregnancy progresses.[116] The lower levels of serum ACTH in pregnancy probably reflect the higher levels of free cortisol. The changes in cortisol and CBG as well as in ACTH resemble those in women taking oral contraceptives.

Aldosterone levels increase with advancing gestation, reflecting an increased secretion rate by the zona glomerulosa. The levels of renin and angiotensinogen are increased, leading to elevated angiotensin II levels and consequently to markedly elevated levels of aldosterone.[131]

Finally, there is a marked increase in plasma levels of deoxy-corticosterone (DOC) during gestation.[132] The administration of dexamethasone or an infusion of ACTH has no effect on DOC levels in pregnant women. Increased maternal levels of DOC appear to arise from extraglandular 21-hydroxylation of circulating progesterone.[133] The activity of extraglandular 21-hydroxylase appears to be dependent on estrogen.

As with other endocrine disorders of women, abnormalities of adrenal function are usually associated with infertility. Thirty to 40 cases of Cushing syndrome have been reported during pregnancy,[134] approximately half of which were associated with adenomas or carcinomas of the adrenal gland and half with Cushing disease. The clinical diagnosis is difficult, because normal pregnant women have abdominal striae, weight gain, and fluid retention and may also have glucose intolerance and hypertension. Laboratory evaluations include measurement of free cortisol in a 24-hour urine collection, plasma ACTH assay, computed tomography or magnetic resonance imaging of the sella, and adrenal magnetic resonance imaging or ultrasonography. Adrenal computed tomography is contraindicated in pregnancy because of the relatively high radiation exposure to the pregnant uterus. The clinical symptoms and signs may become exacerbated by pregnancy but more often remit. There is a relatively high rate of fetal loss and premature birth in reported cases. If possible, treatment for Cushing syndrome is delayed until delivery; otherwise, the treatment is similar to that for nonpregnant subjects (see Chaps. 75 and 110).

Addison disease, or adrenal insufficiency, has been associated more frequently with pregnancy than has Cushing syndrome.[135] In those patients whose condition is diagnosed before pregnancy, adequate replacement therapy is sufficient, and there is often a slight amelioration of symptoms and decreased requirement for corticosteroid replacement during pregnancy. When the disease first appears during pregnancy, the diagnosis is often delayed because of the transfer of adrenal steroids from the fetus. Symptoms associated with pregnancy, such as nausea, vomiting, and lethargy, also increase the difficulty in establishing the diagnosis of Addison disease. The diagnosis and treatment are similar to that for nonpregnant women (see Chaps. 76 and 110). The woman with Addison disease should receive supplemental glucocorticoids at the onset of labor or before cesarean section.

Women given cortisol replacement since infancy for congenital adrenal hyperplasia have pregnancy rates near 60%. Continued close observation during pregnancy is important, because uncontrolled increased androgen production may virilize a female fetus in utero.

Pheochromocytomas rarely occur in pregnancy; fetal mortality in these cases is high. Maternal mortality is also high if a pheochromocytoma remains undiagnosed before the onset of labor. However, treatment is successful when the diagnosis is made before labor and pharmacologic treatment precedes resection of the tumor.[136]

## PARATHYROID GLAND

The reported incidence of hyperparathyroidism is low in pregnant women.[137] Usually, parathyroid adenoma is the cause. The incidence of complications, including hyperemesis, convulsions, and renal calculi, increases during pregnancy. Pregnancy loss is increased, and, occasionally, transient neonatal hypocalcemic tetany occurs secondary to oversuppression of fetal PTH by the increased transfer of calcium to the fetal compartment. The treatment is similar to that in nonpregnant women (see Chaps. 58 and 110).

Hypoparathyroidism associated with pregnancy is also rare and most often results from the previous removal of the parathyroids during thyroid surgery. There appears to be little effect of this disorder on the mother during pregnancy, but both primary hypoparathyroidism and pseudohypoparathyroidism may cause hypercalcemia and bone demineralization in the fetus. The treatment is similar to that in nonpregnant subjects (see Chaps. 60 and 110).

## OVARIAN ANDROGEN-SECRETING TUMORS

Maternal plasma levels of androstenedione and testosterone are increased during pregnancy, probably partly because of increased ovarian and adrenal secretion. Increased levels of sex hormone–binding globulin (SHBG) and active aromatization in the placenta prevent maternal and fetal masculinization. The most common causes of masculinization or virilization during pregnancy are benign luteomas or hyperreactio luteinalis, which may develop because of hCG secretion by the placenta. The primary risk, although rare, appears to be virilization of the fetus in utero. The diagnosis can be confirmed by ultrasonography (see Chap. 102).

## EVALUATION OF THE FETAL-PLACENTAL UNIT BY ENDOCRINE TESTING

Because of the enormous increases in hormone levels in pregnant women, it was originally hoped that fetal stress in utero could be detected by documenting changes in hormones secreted by the fetal-placental unit. The initial goal was to be

**TABLE 108-1.**

**Number of Days Required to Normalize β-Human Chorionic Gonadotropin Levels**

| Pregnancy Type | Days |
| --- | --- |
| Term delivery | 16 |
| Therapeutic abortion (first trimester) | 27 |
| Ectopic pregnancy (surgery) | 24 |
| Ectopic pregnancy (methotrexate) | 70 |
| Molar pregnancy (dilatation and curettage) | 115 |

(Adapted from Falcone T, Little AB. Placental polypeptides. In: Tulchinsky D, Little B, eds. Maternal-fetal endocrinology, 2nd ed. Philadelphia: WB Saunders, 1994:16.)

able to measure a single or group of hormone changes that would guide the physician in the management of high-risk pregnancies: If an abnormal level of a hormone or hormones were detected, the physician would interrupt the pregnancy to prevent death or significant morbidity to the fetus.

## EARLY PREGNANCY

To evaluate the newly implanted and growing embryo, quantitative serum β-hCG or serum progesterone has been used. These tests have been used most often to evaluate women with uterine bleeding in early pregnancy, ectopic pregnancy, luteal phase dysfunction, or a history of habitual abortion. Although serum levels of progesterone may decline before a spontaneous abortion, the clinical usefulness of this test is uncertain.[138] Because most spontaneous abortions are not the result of progesterone deficiency, declining progesterone levels often signify dying trophoblasts and a nonviable pregnancy.

With the development of accurate and rapid quantitative measurements of β-hCG in serum, these tests have been used extensively to confirm a normal developing embryo and trophoblast in women treated for various forms of infertility (see Chap. 112). A doubling of the β-hCG levels at ~48-hour intervals usually signifies a normal viable intrauterine pregnancy,[139] whereas low or falling levels are usually associated with an inevitable abortion or an ectopic pregnancy.[140] The number of days required for β-hCG levels to normalize following pregnancy and pregnancy complications is seen in Table 108-1.

## LATE PREGNANCY

As in early pregnancy, progesterone levels determined at or near maturity are not helpful in evaluating fetal status. The major emphasis of hormone testing during late pregnancy has been estrogen determinations. Estriol has been the primary estrogen studied, since estriol is formed predominantly by the placenta from fetal androgen precursors. Most centers have measured total plasma estriol, although plasma unconjugated estriol, urinary estriol, or the urinary estriol/creatinine ratio has also been widely used.[141,142] In clinical practice, however, single or multiple measurements of estriol are not totally reliable, and many factors besides fetal "stress" may cause decreased or low estriol. Thus, even in the absence of other causes, a low estrogen level may not mean fetal demise, and a normal level does not guarantee fetal well-being. The number of centers using estriol determination during pregnancy has declined. To be clinically useful, these tests need to be interpreted in light of other biophysical tests, including fetal size, age, activity, amount of amniotic fluid, response to oxytocin, ultrasonography, and clinical status of the mother.[138]

The DHEAS loading test was developed to assess the expected rise in estrogen levels.[143] The test is useful in confirming an anticipated diagnosis of placental sulfatase deficiency but is only a research tool for study of uteroplacental function.

hPL levels originally were thought to be predictive of fetal well-being in high-risk pregnancy. However, many conflicting reports of their usefulness caused a decline in popularity in most centers.[138,144]

## REFERENCES

1. Tulchinsky D, Hobel CJ. Plasma human chorionic gonadotropin, estrone, estradiol, estriol, progesterone and 17α-hydroxyprogesterone in human pregnancy III: early normal pregnancy. Am J Obstet Gynecol 1973; 117:884.
2. Csapo AL Pulkkinen MO, Wiest WG. Effects of luteectomy and progesterone replacement in early pregnant patients. Am J Obstet Gynecol 1973; 115:759.
3. Simpson ER, MacDonald PC. Endocrine physiology of the placenta. Annu Rev Physiol 1981; 43:163.
4. Winkel CA, Snyder JM, MacDonald PC, Simpson ER. Regulation of cholesterol and progesterone synthesis in human placental cells in culture by serum lipoproteins. Endocrinology 1980; 106:1054.
5. Pritchard JA, MacDonald PC, Gant NF. Williams obstetrics. Norwalk, CT: Appleton-Century-Crofts, 1985:119.
6. Bloch K. Biological conversion of cholesterol to pregnanediol. J Biol Chem 1945; 157:661.
7. Hellig H, Gattereau D, Lefebvre Y, Bolté E. Steroid metabolism from plasma cholesterol: I. Conversion of plasma cholesterol to placental progesterone in humans. J Clin Endocrinol Metab 1970; 30:624.
8. Casey ML, Winkel CA, Porter JC, MacDonald PC. Endocrine regulation of the initiation and maintenance of parturition. Clin Perinatol 1983; 10:709.
9. Siiteri PK, Febres F, Clemens LE. Progesterone and maintenance of pregnancy: is progesterone nature's immunosuppressant? Ann NY Acad Sci 1977; 186:384.
10. Brown JB. Urinary excretion of oestrogen during pregnancy, lactation and the re-establishment of menstruation. Lancet 1956; 1:704.
11. Siiteri PK, MacDonald PC. The utilization of circulating dehydroisoandrosterone sulfate for estrogen synthesis during human pregnancy. Steroids 1963; 2:713.
12. Carr BR, Simpson ER. Lipoprotein utilization and cholesterol synthesis by the human fetal adrenal gland. Endocr Rev 1981; 2:306.
13. Tulchinsky D, Frigoletto F, Ryan KJ, Fishman J. Plasma estetrol as an index of fetal well-being. J Clin Endocrinol Metab 1975; 40:560.
14. France JT, Liggins GC. Placental sulfatase deficiency. J Clin Endocrinol Metab 1969; 29:138.
15. Bradshaw KD, Carr BR. Placental sulfatase deficiency: maternal and fetal expression of steroid sulfatase deficiency and X-linked ichthyosis. Obstet Gynecol Surv 1986; 68:505.
16. Walsh SW, McCarthy MS. Selective placental secretion of estrogens into fetal and maternal circulations. Endocrinology 1981; 109:2152.
17. Rosenfeld CR. Consideration of the uteroplacental circulation in intrauterine growth. Semin Perinatol 1984; 8:42.
18. Ren SG, Braunstein G-D. Human chorionic gonadotropin. Semin Reprod Endocrinol 1992; 10:95.
19. Marshall JR, Hammond CB, Ross GT. Plasma and urinary chorionic gonadotropin during early human pregnancy. Obstet Gynecol 1968; 32:760.
20. Saxen BB, Landesman R. Diagnosis and management of pregnancy by the radioimmunoassay of hCG. Am J Obstet Gynecol 1978; 131:97.
21. Merz WE, Erlewein C, Licht P, Harbarth P. The secretion of human chorionic gonadotropin as well as the α- and β-messenger ribonucleic acids are stimulated by exogenous gonadoliberin pulses applied to first trimester placenta in a superfusion culture system. J Clin Endocrinol Metab 1991; 73:84.
22. Serón-Ferré M, Lawrence CC, Jaffe RN. Role of hCG in regulation of the fetal zone of the human fetal adrenal gland. J Clin Endocrinol Metab 1978; 46:834.
23. Grumbach MM, Gluckman PD. The human fetal hypothalamus and pituitary gland. In: Tulchinsky D, Little B, eds. Maternal-fetal endocrinology, 2nd ed. Philadelphia: WB Saunders, 1994:193.
24. Adcock EW III, Teasdale F, August CS, et al. Human chorionic gonadotropin: its possible role in maternal lymphocyte suppression. Science 1973; 181:845.
25. Kenimer JG, Hershman JM, Higgins P. The thyrotropin in hydatidiform moles is human chorionic gonadotropin. J Clin Endocrinol Metab 1975; 40:482.
26. Josimovich JB. Placental lactogen and pituitary prolactin. In: Fuchs F, Klopper A, eds. Endocrinology of pregnancy. Philadelphia: Harper & Row, 1983:144.
27. MacLeod JN, Worsley I, Ray J, et al. Human growth hormone-variant is a biologically active somatogen and lactogen. Endocrinology 1991; 128:1298.
28. Strauss JF III, Gafvels M, King BF. Placental hormones. In: DeGroot LJ, Besser M, Burger HG, et al, eds. Endocrinology, 3rd ed. Philadelphia: WB Saunders, 1995:2171.
29. Spellacy WN, Carlson KL, Birk SA. Human placental lactogen levels as a variable of placental weight and infant weight. Am J Obstet Gynecol 1966; 95:118.
30. Grumbach MM, Kaplan SL, Abramo CL. Plasma free fatty acid response to the administration of chorionic "growth hormone–prolactin." J Clin Endocrinol Metab 1966; 26:478.

31. Chard T. Placental lactogen: biology and clinical applications. In: Grudzinskas JG, Teisner B, Süppüla M, eds. Pregnancy proteins: biology, chemistry, and clinical application. New York: Academic Press, 1981:101.
32. Hennen G, Frankenne F, Pirens G, et al. New chorionic GH-like antigen revealed by monoclonal antibody radioimmunoassay. Lancet 1985; 1:399.
33. Frankenne F, Closset J, Gomez F, et al. The physiology of growth hormones (GHs) in pregnant women and partial characterization of the placental GH variant. J Clin Endocrinol Metab 1988; 66:1171.
34. Liebhaber SA, Urbanek M, Ray J, et al. Characterization and histologic localization of human growth hormone-variant gene expression in the placenta. J Clin Invest 1989; 83:1985.
35. Scippo ML, Frankenne F, Hooghe-Peters EL, et al. Syncytiotrophoblastic localization of the human growth hormone variant mRNA in the placenta. Mol Cell Endocrinol 1993; 92:R7.
36. Seeburg PH. The human growth hormone gene family: nucleotide sequences show recent divergence and predict a new polypeptide hormone. DNA 1982; 1:239.
37. Ray J, Jones BK, Liebhaber SA, Cooke NE. Glycosylated human growth hormone variant. Endocrinology 1989; 125:566.
38. Caufriez A, Frankenne F, Englert Y, et al. Placental growth hormone as a potential regulator of maternal IGF-I during human pregnancy. Am J Physiol 1990; 258(Endocrinol Metab 21):E1014.
39. Rees LH, Burke CW, Chard T, et al. Possible placental origin of ACTH in normal human pregnancy. Nature 1975; 254:620.
40. Liotta A, Osathanondtt T, Ryan KJ, Krieger DT. Presence of corticotropin in human placenta: demonstration of in vitro synthesis. Endocrinology 1977; 101:1552.
41. Hennen G, Pierce JG, Freychet P. Human chorionic thyrotropin: further characterization and study of its secretion during pregnancy. J Clin Endocrinol Metab 1969; 29:581.
42. Prager D, Webber MM, Herman-Bonert V. Placental growth factors and releasing/inhibiting peptides. Semin Reprod Endocrinol 1992; 10:83.
43. Emanuel RL, Robinson BG, Seely EW, et al. Corticotropin releasing hormone levels in human plasma and amniotic fluid during gestation. Clin Endocrinol 1994; 40:257.
44. Petroglio F, Gullinelli A, Grande A, et al. Local production and action of follistatin in human placenta. J Clin Endocrinol Metab 1994; 78:205.
45. MacDonald PC, Schultz FM, Duenhoelter JH, et al. Initiation of human parturition: I. Mechanisms of action of arachidonic acid. Obstet Gynecol 1974; 44:629.
46. Riddick DH, Kusmik WF. Decidua: a possible source of amniotic fluid prolactin. Am J Obstet Gynecol 1977; 127:187.
47. Riddick DH, Luciano AA, Kusmik WF, Maslar IA. De novo synthesis of prolactin by human decidua. Life Sci 1978; 23:1913.
48. Josimovich JB, Merisko K, Boccella L. Amniotic prolactin control over amniotic and fetal extracellular fluid water and electrolytes in the rhesus monkey. Endocrinology 1977; 100:564.
49. Schwabe C, Steinetz B, Weiss G, et al. Relaxin. Recent Prog Horm Res 1978; 34:123.
50. Bryant-Greenwood GD. Relaxin as a new hormone. Endocr Rev 1982; 3:62.
51. Fisher DA. Maternal-fetal neurohypophyseal system. Clin Perinatol 1983; 10:695.
52. Mulchahey JJ, Diblasio AM, Martin MC, et al. Hormone production and peptide regulation of the human fetal pituitary gland. Endocr Rev 1987; 8:406.
53. Siler-Khodr TM, Morgenstern LL, Greenwood FC. Hormone synthesis and release from human fetal adenohypophysis in vitro. J Clin Endocrinol Metab 1974; 39:891.
54. Silman RE, Chand T, Lowry PJ, et al. Human fetal corticotropin and related pituitary peptides. J Steroid Biochem 1977; 8:553.
55. Rinne UK. Neurosecretory material passing into the hypophyseal portal system in the human infundibulum and its foetal development. Acta Neuroreg 1962; 25:310.
56. Pang S, Levine LS, Decerquist LL, et al. Amnionic fluid concentrations of $\Delta^4\Delta^5$ steroids in fetuses with congenital adrenal hyperplasia due to 21-hydroxylase deficiency and in anencephalic fetuses. J Clin Endocrinol Metab 1980; 51:223.
57. Kaplan SL, Grumbach MM, Shepard TH. The ontogenesis of human fetal hormones: I. Growth hormone and insulin. J Clin Invest 1972; 51:3080.
58. Ducharme JT, Grumbach MM. Studies on the effects of human growth hormone in premature infants. J Clin Invest 1961; 40:243.
59. D'Ercole AJ. The insulin-like growth factors and fetal growth. In: Spencer EM, ed. Modern concepts of insulin-like growth. New York: McGraw-Hill, 1991:9.
60. Aubert ML, Grumbach MM, Kaplan SL. The ontogenesis of human fetal hormones: III. Prolactin. J Clin Invest 1975; 56:155.
61. Del Pozo E, Bigazzi M, Calaf J. Induced human gestational hypoprolactinemia: lack of action on fetal adrenal androgen synthesis. J Clin Endocrinol Metab 1980; 51:936.
62. DeVane GW, Porter JC. An apparent stress-induced release of arginine vasopressin by human neonates. J Clin Endocrinol Metab 1980; 51:1412.
63. Fisher DA. Maternal-fetal thyroid function in pregnancy. Clin Perinatol 1983; 10:615.
64. Fisher DA, Dussault JH, Sack J, Chopra IJ. Ontogenesis of hypothalamic-pituitary-thyroid function and metabolism in man, sheep and rat. Recent Prog Horm Res 1977; 33:59.
65. Engler P, Scanlon MF, Jackson IMD. Thyrotropin releasing hormone in the systemic circulation of the neonatal rat is derived from the pancreas and other extraneural tissues. J Clin Invest 1981; 67:800.
66. Fisher DA, Klein AH. Thyroid development and disorders of thyroid function in the newborn. N Engl J Med 1981; 304:702.
67. Fisher DA, Odell WD. Acute release of thyrotropin in the newborn. J Clin Invest 1969; 48:1670.
68. Kaplan SL, Grumbach MM. The ontogenesis of human foetal hormones II: luteinizing hormone (LH) and follicle stimulating hormone (FSH). Acta Endocrinol (Copenh) 1976; 81:808.
69. Rabinovici J, Jaffe RB. Development and regulation of growth and differentiation in human and subhuman primate fetal gonads. Endocr Rev 1990; 11:532.
70. Molsberry RL, Carr BR, Mendelson CR, Simpson ER. Human chorionic gonadotropin binding to human fetal testes as a function of gestational age. J Clin Endocrinol Metab 1982; 55:791.
71. Bearn JG. Anencephaly and the development of the male genital tract. Acta Paediatr Acad Sci Hung 1968; 9:159.
72. Carr BR, Parker CR Jr, Ohashi M, et al. Regulation of human fetal testicular secretion of testosterone: low density lipoprotein-cholesterol synthesized de novo as steroid precursor. Am J Obstet Gynecol 1983; 146:241.
73. George FW, Wilson JD. Conversion of androgen to estrogen by the human fetal ovary. J Clin Endocrinol Metab 1978; 47:550.
74. Simmer HH, Easterling WE, Pion RJ, Dignani WJ. Neutral C-19-steroids and steroid sulphates in human pregnancy. Steroids 1964; 4:125.
75. Uotila UU. The early embryological development of the fetal and permanent adrenal cortex in man. Anat Rec 1940; 76:183.
76. Doody KM, Carr BR, Rainey WE, et al. Endocrinology 1990; 126:2487.
77. Carr BR, Parker CR Jr, Milewich L, et al. Steroid secretion by ACTH-stimulated human fetal adrenal tissue during the first week in organ culture. Steroids 1980; 36:563.
78. Branchaud CT, Goodyer CG, Hall CStG, et al. Steroidogenic activity of hACTH and related peptides on the human neocortex and fetal adrenal cortex in organ culture. Steroids 1978; 31:557.
79. Johannisson E. The foetal adrenal cortex in the human. Acta Endocrinol (Copenh) 1968; 130(Suppl):7.
80. Parker CR Jr, Leveno KJ, Carr BR, et al. Umbilical cord plasma levels of dehydroepiandrosterone sulfate during human gestation. J Clin Endocrinol Metab 1982; 54:1216.
81. Beitins IZ, Bayard F, Ances IG, et al. The metabolic clearance rate, blood production, interconversion and transplacental passage of cortisol and cortisone in pregnancy near term. Pediatr Res 1973; 7:509.
82. Ballard PL, Ballard RA, Granberg JP, et al. Fetal sex and prenatal beta-methasone therapy. J Pediatr 1980; 97:451.
83. Pepe GJ, Albrecht E. Regulation of the primate fetal adrenal cortex. Endocr Rev 1990; 11:124.
84. Mesiano S, Jaffe R. Interaction of insulin-like growth factor-II and estradiol directs steroidogenesis in the human fetal adrenal toward dehydroepiandrosterone sulfate production. J Clin Endocrinol Metab 1993; 77:754.
85. Carr BR, Parker CR Jr, Milewich L, et al. The role of low-density, high-density and very low-density lipoproteins in steroidogenesis by the human fetal adrenal gland. Endocrinology 1980; 106:1854.
86. Carr BR, Simpson ER. De novo synthesis of cholesterol by the human fetal adrenal gland. Endocrinology 1981; 108:2154.
87. Brown MS, Kovanen PT, Goldstein JL. Receptor-mediated uptake of lipoprotein-cholesterol and its utilization for steroid synthesis in the adrenal cortex. Recent Prog Horm Res 1979; 35:215.
88. Ohashi M, Carr BR, Simpson ER. Effects of adrenocorticotropic hormone on low density lipoprotein receptors of human fetal adrenal tissue. Endocrinology 1981; 108:1237.
89. Carr BR, MacDonald PC, Simpson ER. The regulation of de novo synthesis of cholesterol in the human fetal adrenal gland by low density lipoprotein and adrenocorticotropin. Endocrinology 1980; 107:1000.
90. Parker CR Jr, Simpson ER, Bilheimer DW. Inverse relationship between LDL-cholesterol and dehydroisoandrosterone sulfate in human fetal plasma. Science 1980; 208:512.
91. Carr BR, Parker CR Jr, Porter JC, et al. Regulation of steroid secretion by adrenal tissue of a human anencephalic fetus. J Clin Endocrinol Metab 1980; 50:870.
92. Carr BR, Ohashi M, MacDonald PC, Simpson ER. Human anencephalic adrenal tissue: low-density lipoprotein metabolism and cholesterol synthesis. J Clin Endocrinol Metab 1981; 53:406.
93. Carr BR, Simpson ER. Cholesterol synthesis by human fetal hepatocytes: effect of hormones. J Clin Endocrinol Metab 1984; 58:1111.
94. Fisher DA. Fetal endocrinology: endocrine disease and pregnancy. In: DeGroot J, ed. Endocrinology, vol 3. New York: Grune & Stratton, 1979:1649.
95. Serón-Ferré M, Jaffe RB. The fetal adrenal gland. Annu Rev Physiol 1981; 43:141.
96. Pitkin RM, Reynolds WA, Williams GA, Hargia GK. Calcium metabolism in pregnancy: a longitudinal study. Am J Obstet Gynecol 1979; 133:781.
97. Forbes GB. Calcium accumulation by the human fetus. Pediatrics 1976; 57:976.
98. Leroyer-Alizon E, David L, Anast CS, Dubois PM. Immunocytological evidence for parathyroid hormone in human parathyroid glands. J Clin Endocrinol Metab 1981; 52:513.
99. Root A, Gruskin A, Reber RM, et al. Serum concentrations of parathyroid hormone in infants, children and adolescents. J Pediatr 1974; 85:329.

100. MacIsaac RJ, Caple IW, Danks JA, et al. Ontogeny of parathyroidectomy, parathyroid hormone and PTHrP on kidneys of ovine fetuses. Am J Physiol 1993; 264:E37.

101. MacIsaac RJ, Heath JA, Rodda CP, et al. Role of the fetal parathyroid glands and parathyroid hormone related protein in the regulation of placental transport of calcium, magnesium, and inorganic phosphate. Reprod Fertil Dev 1991; 3:337.

102. Pitkin RM. Endocrine regulation of calcium homeostasis during pregnancy. Clin Perinatol 1983; 10:575.

103. Sperling MA. Carbohydrate metabolism, glucagon, and insulin. In: Tulchinsky D, Little B, eds. Maternal and fetal endocrinology, 2nd ed. Philadelphia: WB Saunders, 1994:379.

104. Espinosa MMA, Driscoll SG, Steinke J. Insulin release from isolated human fetal pancreatic islets. Science 1970; 168:1111.

105. Farrell PM, Avery ME. Hyaline membrane disease. Am Rev Respir Dis 1975; 111:657.

106. Nelson GH. Lung biology in health and disease, vol 27, pulmonary development. New York: Marcel Dekker Inc, 1985:1.

107. Liggins GC. Premature delivery of foetal lambs infused with glucocorticoids. J Endocrinol 1969; 45:515.

108. Liggins GC, Howie MB. A controlled trial of antepartum glucocorticoid treatment and prevention of the respiratory distress syndrome in premature infants. Pediatrics 1972; 50:515.

109. Hauth JC, Parker CR Jr, MacDonald PC, et al. Role of fetal prolactin in lung maturation. Obstet Gynecol 1978; 51:81.

110. Smith BT, Post M. The influence of hormones in fetal lung development. In: Tulchinsky D, Little B, eds. Maternal-fetal endocrinology. Philadelphia: WB Saunders, 1994:365.

111. Rigg LA, Lein A, Yen SSC. The pattern of increase in circulating prolactin levels during human gestation. Am J Obstet Gynecol 1977; 129:454.

112. Spellacy WN, Buhi WC, Birk SA. Human growth hormone and placental lactogen levels in mid pregnancy and late post partum. Obstet Gynecol 1970; 36:238.

113. Reyes Fl, Winter JSD, Faiman C. Pituitary gonadotropin function during human pregnancy: serum FSH and LH levels before and after LHRH administration. J Clin Endocrinol Metab 1976; 42:590.

114. Goland RS, Wardlaw SL, Stark RI, Frantz AG. Human plasma β-endorphin during pregnancy, labor, and delivery. J Clin Endocrinol Metab 1981; 52:74.

115. Wardlaw SL, Stark RI, Baxi L, Frantz AG. Plasma β-endorphin and β-lipotropin in the human fetus at delivery: correlation with arterial pH and pO$_2$. J Clin Endocrinol Metab 1979; 79:888.

116. Carr BR, Parker CR Jr, Madden JD, et al. Maternal plasma adrenocorticotropin (ACTH) and cortisol relationships throughout human pregnancy. Am J Obstet Gynecol 1981; 139:416.

117. Chau SS, Fitzpatrick RJ, Jamison B. Diabetes insipidus and parturition. Br J Obstet Gynaecol 1969; 76:444.

118. Dürr JA. Diabetes insipidus in pregnancy. Am J Kidney Dis 1987; 9:226.

119. Jewelewicz R, VandeWeile RL. Clinical causes and outcome of pregnancy in twenty-five patients with pituitary microadenomas. Am J Obstet Gynecol 1980; 136:339.

120. Moltich ME, Elton RL, Blackwell RLEL, et al. Bromocriptine as primary therapy for prolactin-secreting macroadenomas: results of a prospective multi-center study. J Clin Endocrinol Metab 1985; 60:698.

121. Ruiz-Velasco V, Tolis G. Pregnancy in hyperprolactinemic women. Fertil Steril 1984; 41:793.

122. Abelove WA, Rubb JJ, Paschkis KE. Acromegaly and pregnancy. J Clin Endocrinol Metab 1954; 14:32.

123. Furth ED. Thyroid and parathyroid hormone function in pregnancy. In: Fuchs F, Klopper A, eds. Endocrinology of pregnancy. Philadelphia: Harper & Row, 1983:176.

124. Fisher DA, Lehman H, Lackey C. Placental transport of thyroxine. J Clin Endocrinol Metab 1964; 24:339.

125. Burrow GN. Hyperthyroidism during pregnancy. N Engl J Med 1978; 298:150.

126. Cheron RG, Kaplan MM, Larsen PR, et al. Neonatal thyroid function after propylthiouracil therapy for maternal Graves' disease. N Engl J Med 1981; 304:525.

127. Gladstone GR, Horclof A, Gersony WM. Propranolol administration during pregnancy: effects on the fetus. J Pediatr 1975; 86:962.

128. Davis LE, Leveno KL, Cunningham FG. Hypothyroidism complicating pregnancy. Obstet Gynecol 1988; 72:108.

129. Doe RP, Fernandez R, Seal US. Measurement of corticosteroid-binding globulin in man. J Clin Endocrinol Metab 1964; 24:1029.

130. O'Connell M, Welsh GW. Unbound plasma cortisol in pregnancy and Enovid-E treated women as determined by ultrafiltration. J Clin Endocrinol Metab 1969; 29:563.

131. Carr BR, Gant NF. The endocrinology of pregnancy-induced hypertension. Clin Perinatol 1983; 10:737.

132. Parker CR Jr, Everett RB, Whalley PJ, et al. Hormone production during pregnancy in the primigravid patient: II. Plasma levels of deoxycorticosterone throughout pregnancy of normal women and women who develop pregnancy-induced hypertension. Am J Obstet Gynecol 1980; 138:626.

133. Casey ML, MacDonald PC. Extraadrenal formation of a mineralocorticosteroid: deoxycorticosterone and deoxycorticosterone sulfate biosynthesis and metabolism. Endocr Rev 1982; 3:396.

134. Peterson RE. Corticosteroids and corticotropins. In: Fuchs F, Klopper A, eds. Endocrinology of pregnancy. Philadelphia: Harper & Row, 1983:112.

135. Osler M. Addison's disease and pregnancy. Acta Endocrinol (Copenh) 1962; 41:67.

136. Schenker JG, Granat M. Pheochromocytoma and pregnancy: an updated appraisal. Aust NZ J Obstet Gynaecol 1982; 22:1.

137. Lowe DK, Orwoll ES, McClung MR, et al. Hyperparathyroidism and pregnancy. Am J Surg 1983; 145:611.

138. Tulchinsky D. Endocrine assessments of fetal-placental well-being. Clin Perinatol 1983; 10:763.

139. Ackerman R, Deutch S, Krunholz B. Levels of human chorionic gonadotropin in unruptured and ruptured ectopic pregnancy. Obstet Gynecol 1982; 60:13.

140. Hussa RO. Clinical utility of human chorionic gonadotropin and β-subunit measurements. Obstet Gynecol 1982; 60:1.

141. Tulchinsky D. Endocrine evaluation in the diagnosis in intrauterine growth retardation. Clin Obstet Gynecol 1977; 20:969.

142. Seibel MM, Levesque LA, Seidenberg EJ, Ransil BJ. Serial first morning estriol determinations in evaluating the high risk obstetric patient. Obstet Gynecol 1982; 59:27.

143. Tulchinsky D, Osathanondh R, Finn A. Dehydroepiandrosterone sulfate loading test in the diagnosis of complicated pregnancies. N Engl J Med 1976; 294:517.

144. Neilson JP, Cloherty LJ. Hormonal placental function tests for fetal assessment in high risk pregnancies. Cochrane Database Syst Rev 2000; 2:CD000108.

# CHAPTER 109

# ENDOCRINOLOGY OF PARTURITION

JOHN R. G. CHALLIS

The duration of human pregnancy, counting from the first day of the last menstrual period, is ~280 days, or 40 weeks. The expected date of delivery can be estimated by counting back 3 months from the first day of the last menstrual period and adding 7 days (Nägele's rule). Approximately 40% of women begin labor within 5 days of the *estimated date of confinement (EDC)* and nearly two-thirds do so within 10 days.

In most species, including the human, the uterus remains relatively quiescent for most of the pregnancy. The contractions that occur are poorly synchronized and of low amplitude and develop only small increases in uterine pressure. This pattern contrasts with the high-frequency, high-amplitude contractions of the myometrium that occur at the time of labor. Thus, the uterine changes can be divided into distinct phases. For most of pregnancy, the myometrium is relatively quiescent, corresponding to phase 0 of parturition. In late gestation, the myometrium undergoes a transition from a state of quiescence to one of activation, which physiologically corresponds to phase 1 of parturition. Clinically, the first stage of labor begins with the first uterine contraction and ends with complete dilatation of the cervix. The second stage begins with complete dilatation of the cervix and ends with the birth of the baby. During this phase, the activated uterus responds to stimulation by a variety of uterotonins. Involution of the uterus postpartum is termed phase 3. This stage begins with delivery of the baby and ends with the expulsion of the placenta. The mean duration of labor in primigravid women is ~14 hours; the duration of labor in multiparous women is ~6 hours shorter. In this sequence, the term "initiation of parturition" most closely corresponds to the transition from phase 0 to phase 1.

During the first stage of labor the cervix undergoes progressive effacement in which the cervical canal shortens from a structure ~2 cm in length to one in which the edges of the orifice are paper thin, and dilatation in which the orifice to the uterus (internal cervical os) enlarges from a few millimeters in diameter to an aperture large enough to permit passage of the baby (10 cm or complete dilatation). At labor, the uterus gradually differentiates into an upper, actively contracting portion, which thickens as labor advances, and a lower portion composed of the lower uterine segment and cervix, which thins remarkably. Spontaneous rupture of the membranes usually occurs during labor, generally manifested by a sudden gush of clear or slightly turbid fluid. The uterus changes in shape during each contraction and as labor progresses towards the final expulsion of the infant.

Profound changes occur in the cervix during pregnancy, and these include softening and cyanosis, which may be detected as early as 1 month after conception. The hydroxyproline content of the cervix decreases as pregnancy advances. A marked decrease in the compactness and cohesiveness of the collagen fibers also occurs immediately after vaginal delivery. The mechanisms for these changes are poorly understood, as are the mechanisms underlying parturition, which occurs either at term or preterm.

*Preterm birth*, defined as birth before 37 weeks of completed pregnancy, occurs in 5% to 10% of all pregnancies in North America. It is associated with 70% of all neonatal deaths and up to 75% of neonatal morbidity. Babies born preterm have an increased incidence of neurologic, metabolic, and respiratory disorders. The cost of caring for preterm babies has been estimated in the United States at $5 billion to $6 billion annually. The incidence of preterm birth has remained relatively unchanged over the past 20 to 30 years. At present, ~30% of preterm births are believed to be associated with an underlying infective process. Of the remainder, 20% to 30% may be elective, and ~50% are idiopathic, of unknown cause. Clearly, preterm birth is more correctly described as a syndrome, representing a myriad of causes. The factors contributing to preterm birth may differ at different times of gestation, and understanding these factors is key to the diagnosis of preterm birth, to the recognition of those patients in true preterm labor, and to the development of effective methods of treatment.

## PREGNANCY—PHASE 0 OF PARTURITION

Myometrial activity is inhibited during pregnancy by a variety of substances, including progesterone, prostacyclin (PGI2), relaxin, parathyroid hormone–related protein (PTHrP), and nitric oxide. These substances act in different ways, although in general they increase the intracellular levels of cyclic nucleotides, which in turn inhibit release of calcium ($Ca^{2+}$) from intracellular stores or reduce the activity of the enzyme *myosin light-chain kinase (MLCK)*. Myometrial contractions depend on conformational changes in the actin and myosin filaments that allow these to slide over each other, a process that requires adenosine triphosphate. This, in turn, is generated by myosin after phosphorylation of the myosin light chains by MLCK. MLCK is activated by interaction with the calcium-binding protein calmodulin, which in turn requires four $Ca^{2+}$ ions for its own activation. Thus, agents that inhibit release of calcium from intracellular stores or reduce the levels of MLCK result in reductions of uterine contractility.

Progesterone inhibits spontaneous myometrial contractility and reduces stimulated activity during pregnancy. In species in which the ovary continues as a major source of progesterone throughout pregnancy, ovariectomy results in increased myometrial contractility—an effect that can be reversed by administration of exogenous progesterone. In primates, however, including the human, little evidence is seen for systemic progesterone withdrawal prepartum, and local, intrauterine changes in progesterone production or action have been postulated to occur at the time of labor. In women, ovarian progesterone production predominates during the first 5 to 6 weeks of pregnancy, and ovariectomy or administration of a progesterone receptor antagonist, such as mifepristone (RU-486), during this time results in increased myometrial contractility. The placenta becomes the major site of progesterone production after the sixth week of gestation. A key enzyme is 3β-hydroxysteroid dehydrogenase (3β-HSD) type 2, expressed in syncytiotropho-

blast and responsible for the conversion of pregnenolone to progesterone. Pregnenolone is derived from low-density lipoprotein from the maternal circulation, and the syncytiotrophoblast layer of the placental villi contains low-density lipoprotein receptors allowing uptake from the intervillous pool of blood. The chorion, one of the membranes surrounding the fetus inside the uterus, also produces progesterone from pregnenolone within trophoblast cells, and this may provide a local source of progesterone to regulate production of uterotonins within the fetal membranes.

PTHrP is produced in intrauterine tissues, particularly in the myometrium, during gestation. Expression of PTHrP is up-regulated by estrogen and by stretch. The suggestion has been made that PTHrP acts locally through specific myometrial receptors to generate increased intracellular cyclic adenosine monophosphate (cAMP) and to inhibit myometrial contractility. Nitric oxide, synthesized from L-arginine by one or more of the various isoforms of nitric oxide synthase, is generated in amnion, chorion, decidua, and myometrium. Nitric oxide acts through cyclic guanosine monophosphate to alter the level of intracellular calcium. Thus, it can function in a paracrine fashion, potentially in conjunction with progesterone, to suppress myometrial contractility. In several species, a decrease in nitric oxide synthase expression and/or activity by uterine tissue has been reported prepartum. In the rat, decreased myometrial nitric oxide synthase activity in late gestation is accompanied by an increase in nitric oxide synthase activity in the cervical inflammatory cells. This observation suggests that nitric oxide might be involved in promoting cervical effacement and dilatation at the time of birth, an activity that increases as the inhibitory influence of nitric oxide on the myometrium is diminished.

Relaxin has long been regarded as an inhibitor of uterine contractility, although its precise role has remained something of an enigma. Relaxin acts by elevating myometrial cAMP and by inhibiting oxytocin-induced turnover of phosphoinositide by the action of cAMP-dependent protein kinase. Relaxin is expressed in fetal membranes, placenta, and decidua, and is up-regulated in these sites in patients with premature rupture of the membranes. Relaxin increases levels of the matrix metalloproteinase enzymes, which are normally involved in remodeling cervical connective tissue, suggesting a further mechanism by which hyperrelaxinemia can be associated with prematurity.

Clearly, withdrawal of one or more of these compounds may occur in relation to labor at term. Furthermore, premature withdrawal of one of these compounds may predispose to premature delivery. Although the concept of withdrawal of the progesterone block to the myometrium is well established in animals, and is demonstrable in early human pregnancy, considerable debate remains as to whether the process of labor in women results from withdrawal of the influence of progesterone on the myometrium, or from the active imposition of factors that stimulate myometrial contractility. Parturition may result from a combination of these processes.

## ACTIVATION OF THE MYOMETRIUM— PHASE 1 OF PARTURITION

Activation of the myometrium (phase 1 of parturition) can be considered as an active process involving the fetal genome. This influence may be exerted through a growth pathway that predisposes to uterine stretch and activation, or through an endocrine pathway (involving the fetal hypothalamic–pituitary–adrenal, or HPA, axis and increased output of cortisol), or through a combination of these processes. Phase 1 activation is manifested through up-regulation in the myometrium of a cassette of contraction-associated proteins (CAPs), including connexin-43 (CX-43; the major protein of gap junctions), and receptors for oxytocin and stimulatory prostaglandins. Expression of increased gap junction protein allows formation of gap junctions, which permit cell-to-cell coupling, whereas expression of proteins that are constituents of ion channels determine the resting membrane potential and, hence, the excitability of the uterine myocytes.

## EFFECTS OF STRETCH ON UTERINE ACTIVATION

The effects of uterine stretch on CAP gene activation has been demonstrated in animal studies and is partly dependent on the prevailing endocrine environment. The normal prepartum increase in myometrial expression of CX-43, oxytocin receptor, and prostaglandin F receptor (FP) mRNA can be inhibited by administration of progesterone or induced by administration of the progesterone receptor antagonist mifepristone or by ovariectomy at earlier times in gestation. When a small (3-mm) inert tube was placed within one uterine horn of nonpregnant ovariectomized rats, a significant increase in CX-43 mRNA was seen compared with the contralateral horn, and this effect was blocked by progesterone. In rats made unilaterally pregnant, insertion of the inert tube into the nonpregnant horn increased expression of CX-43 and oxytocin receptor mRNA levels at the time of labor but was ineffective at earlier times of gestation when the endogenous, prevailing progesterone concentration was elevated.

Estrogen is also regarded as a uterotropin that promotes activation of myometrial function. In human pregnancy, estrogen production in the placenta depends on the provision of C-19 precursor steroids, predominantly from the fetal adrenal gland. The fetal zone of the fetal adrenal gland, which occupies ~85% of the fetal adrenal cortex, is deficient in the enzyme 3β-HSD; therefore, it produces predominantly $\Delta^5$ steroids such as dehydroepiandrosterone (DHEA) that is secreted as its sulfoconjugate (DHEAS). Fetal DHEAS can be converted to estrone and estradiol in the placenta, and ~50% of circulating maternal estrone and estradiol is derived from the placental aromatization of fetal DHEAS; the remainder is formed from maternal adrenal C-19 steroids. Activation of the pituitary-adrenal axis of the fetus occurs in late gestation. In subhuman primate species, the concentration of DHEAS in the fetal circulation shows a progressive increase at this time. This mirrors an increase in the maternal plasma estriol concentration (maternal estriol is formed in the placenta from the precursor 16α-hydroxy DHEAS, which is 90% of fetal origin and is formed in the fetal liver from adrenal DHEAS). The pattern of fetal adrenal activation reflected in DHEAS output resembles that seen in ruminant species, such as the sheep, in which a progressive increase in cortisol output occurs from the late-gestation fetal adrenal gland. In primates, the fetal adrenal is divided into the outer adult zone that produces predominantly aldosterone, the inner fetal zone that produces DHEAS, and a transitional zone, which is interposed between the adult and fetal cortex and is thought to produce cortisol. Adrenocorticotropic hormone (ACTH) stimulates steroidogenesis in the transitional and fetal zones. During pregnancy, fetal ACTH output may be relatively suppressed by the negative feedback of cortisol derived from the maternal circulation after transplacental transfer. In late gestation, increased activity of 11β-HSD (the type-2 isoform) in the placenta leads to increased conversion of maternal cortisol to cortisone, which is bioinactive. Therefore, less maternal cortisol enters the fetal compartment, and less negative feedback occurs, allowing fetal ACTH concentrations to rise.

## FETAL INPUT TO THE PROCESS OF PARTURITION—ACTIVATION OF FETAL HYPOTHALAMIC–PITUITARY–ADRENAL FUNCTION

The changes in uterotropin (estrogen) and uterine inhibitor (progesterone) described earlier depend in large part on endocrine activities within the fetus. Early studies of the sheep and goat clearly demonstrated that the fetus triggered the onset of parturition through activation of the fetal HPA axis, with increased output of cortisol from the fetal adrenal gland. Lesions in the basal region of the fetal hypothalamus, fetal hypophysectomy, or adrenalectomy in utero lead to prolonged pregnancy, whereas infusion of ACTH or glucocorticoids into the fetal lamb results in premature parturition. Fetal cortisol acts on the placenta to initiate a sequence of events that decreases the placental output of progesterone and increases the output of estrogen. Concomitantly with this change in steroid milieu, the output of stimulatory prostaglandins (PGs) from the uterus increases, noted initially as an increase in the concentration of $PGF_{2\alpha}$ into the utero-ovarian venous blood.

Activation of fetal HPA function is associated with increased levels of mRNA encoding corticotropin-releasing hormone (CRH) (in the parvocellular neurons of the paraventricular nucleus of the fetal hypothalamus) and of proopiomelanocortin (POMC), the precursor to ACTH (in the corticotropes of the fetal pars distalis). ACTH is the major trophic factor for the fetal adrenal gland. It increases expression of its own receptor in fetal adrenal cortical cells and up-regulates key enzymes in the steroidogenic pathway. These include P450 C17, P450 C21, and P450 C11. Activation of the fetal HPA axis can also take place in response to an adverse intrauterine environment, for example hypoxemia. Short-term hypoxemia results in increases in plasma ACTH and cortisol concentrations in the fetal circulation, in association with increased levels of CRH mRNA and POMC mRNA in the fetal hypothalamus and pituitary, respectively. After prolonged hypoxemia, further increases occur in pituitary POMC mRNA levels, and fetal plasma cortisol concentrations rise, reflecting up-regulation of key enzymes for cortisol biosynthesis in the fetal adrenal gland.

The primate fetus may play a similar role in the initiation of parturition. During late gestation, levels of POMC mRNA in the fetal pituitary are increased, and this increase probably is evoked by increased input or action from hypothalamic CRH. In the monkey, the length of "placental pregnancy" is prolonged considerably after removal of the fetus. Levels of C-19 estrogen precursor steroids increase in the circulation of the intact fetal monkey during late pregnancy, in parallel with cortisol, mimicking the changes that occur in fetal sheep. Infusion of androstenedione to pregnant monkeys at approximately three-quarters through gestation results in premature birth, which is inhibited by concurrent infusion of an aromatase inhibitor. This suggests that the effect of androstenedione is dependent on conversion to estrogen. However, systemic estrogen infusion fails to induce premature delivery in late pregnant rhesus monkeys; for estrogen to be active, it must be formed and act in a local paracrine or autocrine fashion at, or near, the site of production. Thus, in both primates and sheep evidence is found linking the fetal HPA axis and the placenta through the provision of C-19 steroids and synthesis of estrogen, in mechanisms leading to parturition. In primates, cortisol of fetal origin acts in additional ways to promote delivery. For example, glucocorticoids stimulate prostaglandin output in trophoblast-derived tissues (i.e., fetal membranes) in late human gestation by up-regulating prostaglandin synthesis and by decreasing rates of prostaglandin metabolism. In addition, glucocorticoids up-regulate expression of CRH in the human placenta, and, in turn, CRH serves as a stimulus to prostaglandin production by intrauterine structures (see later).

In both primate and sheep pregnancy a functional fetal adrenal-placental unit is found. A critical difference is that in the primate, the fetal adrenal gland secretes C-19 precursors for placental aromatization to estrogen, whereas in the sheep, the fetal adrenal secretes predominantly cortisol, which leads to up-regulation of P450 C17 in the placenta, and it is then the placenta which becomes capable of converting C-21 steroids to C-19 estrogen precursors that can be converted to estrogen.

# STIMULATION OF THE MYOMETRIUM—PHASE 2 OF PARTURITION

## PROSTAGLANDINS

Prostaglandins play a role in the labor process at term and preterm in animal species and in primates. Mice lacking the ability to generate prostaglandins (PGHS-1 knock-outs) have protracted labors. The capacity for prostaglandin production by intrauterine tissues increases before the onset of labor. Furthermore, inhibitors of prostaglandin synthesis, such as indomethacin, effectively block uterine contractility and prolong gestation. Prostaglandins, including $PGE_2$ and $PGF_{2\alpha}$, are formed from the obligate precursor arachidonic acid, which is liberated from membrane phospholipids through the activities of one or more isoforms of phospholipase C or phospholipase $A_2$. Arachidonic acid is converted to prostaglandins through prostaglandin $H_2$ synthase (PGHS) activity. There are two forms of PGHS: PGHS-1, which is described as constitutive, and PGHS-2, which is inducible by growth factors, cytokines, and glucocorticoids in human fetal membrane cells. Arachidonic acid can also be metabolized to compounds such as leukotrienes. Current evidence suggests that conversion of arachidonic acid to leukotrienes predominates in fetal membranes for much of gestation but decreases at term, at the time of increased PGHS activity, resulting in an increased output of primary prostaglandins.

In turn, the primary prostaglandins are metabolized through a nicotinamide adenine dinucleotide (NAD)–dependent 15-hydroxyprostaglandin dehydrogenase (PGDH) enzyme to inactive metabolites. PGDH activity is especially high in human chorion trophoblast, and this may provide an important metabolic barrier that prevents the passage of unmetabolized prostaglandins—generated during pregnancy in amnion and chorion—from reaching the underlying decidua and myometrial tissue.

Prostaglandin action is effected through specific receptors, including the four main subtypes of receptors for $PGE_2$—EP-1, EP-2, EP-3, and EP-4—and the FP receptors for $PGF_{2\alpha}$. EP-3 receptors exist in several isoforms produced by alternative splicing of a single gene product. EP-1 and EP-3 receptors mediate contractions of smooth muscle in several tissues through mechanisms that lead to increased calcium mobilization and to inhibition of intracellular cAMP. Activation of EP-2 and EP-4 receptors increases cAMP formation and relaxes smooth muscle. These different receptor subtypes are expressed in human myometrium throughout gestation. Thus, it is evident why a single ligand, $PGE_2$, may have different effects in different areas of the uterus, producing contractions (through EP-1 and EP-3) or relaxation (through EP-2 or EP-4), wherever a predominance of a particular receptor subtype occurs.

In human pregnancy, prostaglandin production is discretely compartmentalized between layers of the fetal membranes. PGHS activity predominates in amnion, $PGE_2$ is the major prostaglandin formed, and levels of mRNA and activity of the PGHS-2 isoform increase at the time of labor, both term and preterm. Chorion expresses both PGHS and PGDH enzyme activity. At term parturition, output of prostaglandins from chorion increases as PGHS-2 activity rises and PGDH declines. At preterm labor, activities of both PGHS-1 and PGHS-2 increase in chorion. Both PGHS enzymes are produced in decidua, although little change occurs in the levels of mRNA encoding these enzymes in this tissue at the time of labor. Studies have shown that human myometrium also expresses PGHS enzymes. Whether those prostaglandins that stimulate myometrial contractility are generated in myometrium, decidua, or the amniochorion layers is unclear.

Regulation of prostaglandin production from human fetal membranes is multifactorial. Remarkably, output of $PGE_2$ and increased levels of PGHS mRNA in amnion and chorion are stimulated by glucocorticoids. No glucocorticoid-responsive element (GRE) sequence is recognized in the PGHS-2 promoter, suggesting that this activity of glucocorticoids may be mediated through a locally produced neuropeptide (for example, CRH) or through specific generation of other transcription factors. Cytokines, such as interleukin-1, exert a similar activity and increase levels of PGHS-2 mRNA and immunoreactive PGHS-2 within the fibroblast and epithelial cell layers of amnion primary cultures. Prostaglandin production is increased in in vitro studies through agents that increase availability of calcium (e.g., calcium ionophores such as A23187). Epidermal growth factor (EGF) increases rates of PGHS synthesis and potentiates arachidonic acid–stimulated $PGE_2$ output. Importantly, amnion cells and decidual tissue also express $\beta_2$ receptors and respond to catecholamines with increases in cAMP production. The promoter region of PGHS-2 contains a cAMP response element. Thus, it is not surprising that agents that stimulate production of cAMP, dibutyryl cAMP, or the phosphodiesterase inhibitor methylxanthine all increase outputs of prostaglandins by amnion and decidual cells maintained in culture. This may explain, at least in part, the limited efficacy of β-sympathomimetic drugs in sustaining inhibition of uterine activity in women in preterm labor. The likelihood is that these compounds in fact stimulate production of prostaglandins, the very uterotonins that their infusion is designed to inhibit.

## PROSTAGLANDINS AND INFECTION

Many studies have suggested that infection may be associated with 30% to 40% of preterm labor, although others have suggested that infection-driven prostaglandin release is a result rather than a cause. In patients presenting in preterm labor with infection, concentrations of various cytokines in amniotic fluid are generally increased. In animal models of infection-associated premature delivery, administration of cytokines induces preterm birth, and output of prostaglandins by fetal membranes collected from patients with preterm labor and underlying infection is increased. A currently accepted model is that, in the presence of an ascending bacterial infection, organisms passing between the fetal membranes may later reach the amniotic cavity. Bacteria themselves produce phospholipases that provoke arachidonic acid release and stimulate the pathway leading to prostaglandin production. Bacterial organisms may also produce endotoxins such as lipopolysaccharide (LPS), which act on macrophages to stimulate prostaglandin or cytokine release; macrophage-stimulated cytokines stimulate further prostaglandin release from amnion stromal cells and/or decidual tissue.

## PROSTAGLANDIN METABOLISM

The chorion trophoblast expresses abundant PGDH mRNA and protein, and the presence of this enzyme may serve as a metabolic barrier preventing prostaglandins generated within amnion or chorion from reaching the underlying decidua and myometrium. Hence, absence of PGDH in chorion trophoblasts may predispose to premature delivery. Approximately 10% to 15% of patients presenting in idiopathic preterm labor have diminished levels of PGDH, and many patients presenting in preterm labor with underlying infection have virtual or complete absence of PGDH, associated with loss of chorionic trophoblast cells. Diminished activity of PGDH in chorion trophoblast at term or preterm suggests that the enzyme may be regulated. Progestogens sustain PGDH activity, whereas glucocorticoids (e.g., cortisol or betamethasone) and cytokines (e.g., tumor necrosis factor-α or interleukin-1β) down-regulate PGDH activity. In circumstances in which PGDH in chorion trophoblast is reduced, this would facilitate transfer of prostaglandins across the membranes, resulting in premature stimulation of myometrial contractility. The ability of progesterone to maintain PGDH activity can be reversed in the presence of mifepristone (a progesterone receptor antagonist) or inhibitors of progesterone synthesis within trophoblast cells. An attractive possibility is that progesterone helps maintain PGDH activity during pregnancy. Progesterone action on PGDH at term and in some circumstances of preterm labor may result from local inhibition of its production or action. For example, progesterone action in endometrial tissues may be inhibited by antiprogestins such as transforming growth factor-β (TGF-β). The possibility that up-regulation of TGF-β expression antagonizes progesterone action on PGDH at term is an attractive one. Alternatively, the effect of progesterone on PGDH (and other genes) may be effected through binding to the glucocorticoid receptor (GR), and this activity is antagonized as cortisol levels rise in later gestation. Also, a selective decrease in PGDH expression occurs in chorion trophoblasts overlying the internal os of the cervix in patients at the time of active labor. This raises the possibility that reduced PGDH activity in fetal membranes in this region of the uterus may allow prostaglandins generated in the amnion or chorion to reach the underlying cervix and help promote cervical effacement and dilatation.

## UTERINE PEPTIDES AND PARTURITION

A variety of peptides are produced within intrauterine tissues and placenta, and these may exert local paracrine, autocrine, or intracrine actions as well as systemic effects on events associated with increased myometrial contractility at term. Among such peptides, CRH has been studied extensively, particularly in view of its potential role as a marker in the patient presenting in preterm labor.

CRH mRNA and peptide levels increase exponentially in placental tissue during late gestation. These changes give rise to the progressive increase in maternal peripheral plasma CRH concentrations. In maternal plasma, CRH bioactivity is diminished by binding to a high-affinity circulating binding protein, CRH-binding protein (CRH-BP). Toward term, as plasma CRH concentrations increase, CRH-BP concentrations decrease; this decrease presumably increases the concentrations of free CRH in the maternal circulation.

Regulation of placental CRH output is multifactorial. Progesterone and nitric oxide decrease placental CRH output by placental cells in culture, whereas neuropeptides and cytokines up-regulate CRH expression. Importantly, glucocorticoids also increase CRH mRNA levels in placental cells and increase output of CRH from placental cells in vitro, and increase maternal plasma CRH concentrations in vivo. This relationship likely is important in relation to mechanisms at term and preterm birth. For example, circumstances of maternal stress that may predispose to elevations of maternal plasma cortisol may give rise to early increases in maternal CRH concentrations. Similarly, the fetus exposed to acute or chronic hypoxemia responds with up-regulation of fetal HPA function and increased glucocorticoid output from the fetal adrenal gland, in addition to increased DHEAS output. Perhaps cortisol acts on the placenta and fetal membranes to stimulate CRH synthesis and release. In turn, CRH stimulates prostaglandin production from fetal membranes in vitro, raising the possibility that elevations of CRH may predispose to stimulated production of uterotonins and premature myometrial contractility. Measurements of CRH have been used to discriminate patients presenting in preterm labor who are in true labor from those who are not. Maternal CRH is elevated in patients who deliver prematurely within 24 to 48 hours, whereas levels are not different from those of controls in patients who continue through pregnancy to deliver at term, despite the earlier diagnosis of threatened premature labor. Thus, maternal plasma CRH concentrations might be used to discriminate precisely those patients who are indeed in premature labor and would, therefore, be appropriate candidates for receiving antenatal glucocorticoid therapy for fetal pulmonary maturation.

## INVOLUTION OF THE UTERUS—PHASE 3 OF PARTURITION

The third stage of labor is defined as the time from delivery of the baby to delivery of the placenta. For practical purposes one should also include the hour after delivery of the placenta as a component of the third stage, because during this time the patient is at greatest risk for postpartum hemorrhage.

Placental separation generally occurs by cleavage along the plane of the decidua basalis and is usually complete within the space of relatively few contractions. Uterine contraction is essential to prevent bleeding from large venous sinuses that are exposed after delivery of the placenta, and the average blood loss at the time of a normal vaginal delivery may be around 500 mL. Phase 3 of labor is associated with the release and action of maternal oxytocin. Uterine atony is generally managed with administration of intravenous oxytocin or $PGF_{2\alpha}$.[10,11]

The modest changes in maternal plasma oxytocin concentrations in late gestation are offset by a substantial increase in expression of the oxytocin receptor in endometrium and in myometrium and by a dramatic increase in uterine sensitivity to oxytocin stimulation. These changes can be induced experimentally by uterine stretch, by progesterone withdrawal, and by estrogen stimulation. The choriodecidual tissue itself produces oxytocin, and levels of oxytocin mRNA and peptide increase three- to fivefold at the time of parturition. The stimulus to increased uterine oxytocin expression appears to be increased activity of estrogen, either from the systemic circulation, or generated locally within choriodecidual tissue from sulphoconjugated precursors derived from maternal plasma, or from the amniotic fluid. Oxytocin promotes myometrial contractility by increasing the concentration of free calcium in myocytes, secondary to increases in phosphoinositide turnover and generation of inositol triphosphate. These actions can be inhibited by activators of protein kinase A, indicating the close relationship between the protein kinase A (PKA) and protein kinase C (PLC) pathways.

## CONCLUSION

The process of labor is clearly complex. Extrapolation of mechanisms of normal labor to an understanding of premature parturition is simplistic. The clinical condition of preterm labor may arise from one or more of several underlying causes. Recognition of the specific underlying cause of preterm labor in individual patients is essential to development of appropriate therapy and management for that patient. The current failure to achieve effective *tocolysis* (inhibition of uterine contractions) in many circumstances results from an inability to understand the underlying cause of preterm labor in a particular patient, and the use of a singular, often inappropriate treatment modality for all patients. Further advances through basic and clinical research should allow the development of tocolytic strategies that are appropriate, on a patient by patient basis, and hopefully provide and allow effective tocolysis for those patients who truly are in preterm labor at the beginning of treatment.

## SUGGESTED READINGS

1. Challis JRG, Lye SJ, Gibb W. Prostaglandins and parturition. Ann N Y Acad Sci 1997; 828:254.
2. Chwalisz K, Garfield RE. Regulation of the uterus and cervix during pregnancy and labor. Role of progesterone and nitric oxide. In: Bulleti C, de Ziegler D, Guller S, Levitz M, eds. The uterus: endometrium and myometrium. Ann N Y Acad Sci 1997; 828:238.
3. Karalis K, Majzoub JA. Regulation of placental corticotrophin-releasing hormone by steroids—possible implication in labor initiation. Ann N Y Acad Sci 1995; 551.
4. MacDonald PC, Casey ML. The accumulation of prostaglandins (PG) in amniotic fluid is an after effect of labor and not indicative of a role for PGE2 or $PGF_{2\alpha}$ in the initiation of human parturition. J Clin Endocrinol Metab 1993; 77:805.

5. Patel FA, Clifton VL, Chwalisz K, Challis JRG. Steroidal regulation of prostaglandin dehydrogenase activity and expression in human term placenta and choriodecidua in relation to labor. J Clin Endocrinol Metab 1999; 84:291.
6. Riley SC, Walton JC, Herlick JM, Challis JRG. The localization and distribution of corticotrophin-releasing hormone in the human placental and fetal membranes throughout gestation. J Clin Endocrinol Metab 1991; 72:1001.
7. Romero R, Avila C, Brekus CA, Morotti R. The role of systemic and intrauterine infection in preterm parturition. Ann N Y Acad Sci 1991; 622:355.
8. Sangha RK, Walton JC, Ensor CM, et al. Immunohistochemical localization, mRNA abundance and activity of 15-hydroxyprostaglandin dehydrogenase in placenta and fetal membranes during term and preterm labor. J Clin Endocrinol Metab 1994; 78:982.
9. Van Meir CA, Sangha RK, Walton JC, et al. Immunoreactive 15-hydroxyprostaglandin-dehydrogenase (PGDH) is reduced in fetal membranes from patients at preterm delivery in the presence of infection. Placenta 1996; 17:291.
10. Main DM, Main EK, Moore DH 2nd. The relationship between maternal dye and uterine dysfunction: a continuous effect throughout reproductive life. Am J Obstet Gynecol 2000; 182:1312.
11. Ngai SW, Chan YM, Lam SW, Lao TT. Labour characteristics and uterine activity: misprostol compared with oxytocin in women at term with prelabour rupture of the membranes. Br J Obstet Gynecol 2000; 107:222.

# CHAPTER 110

# ENDOCRINE DISEASE IN PREGNANCY

MARK E. MOLITCH

## POSTERIOR PITUITARY GLAND AND PREGNANCY

### ALTERATIONS IN WATER BALANCE IN PREGNANCY

Pregnancy is associated with a lowering of the osmostat, the setpoint for plasma osmolality at which arginine vasopressin (AVP) is secreted, by ~10 mOsm/kg. Thus, pregnant women experience thirst and release AVP at lower levels of plasma osmolality than do nonpregnant women.[1] The physiologic basis for this reset osmostat is not clear, but some studies suggest that it is related to high levels of human chorionic gonadotropin (hCG).[1] In a patient with polyuria and polydipsia, therefore, the finding of lower than expected serum sodium levels should not exclude the diagnosis of diabetes insipidus (DI).[2] Testing of urinary concentrating ability (see Chaps. 25 and 26) in a pregnant woman should be performed with the patient in the sitting position, because the lateral recumbent position results in an inhibition of maximal urinary concentrating ability.[1,2]

The placenta produces vasopressinase, an enzyme that inactivates AVP rapidly. Vasopressinase levels increase 1000-fold between the 4th and 38th weeks of gestation.[3] This increased metabolic clearance of AVP interferes with the determination of plasma AVP levels during pregnancy and may explain the blunted rise in these levels seen during hypertonic saline infusion in the last trimester.[1] Therefore, nomograms that indicate "normal" relationships between plasma osmolality and AVP for nonpregnant patients cannot be used for pregnant patients.

### DIABETES INSIPIDUS

DI usually worsens during pregnancy,[2] probably because of the increased clearance of AVP resulting from the increased levels of vasopressinase. Thus, patients with mild disease who are treated with either increased fluid intake or chlorpropamide are likely to deteriorate considerably. In addition, because chlorpropamide readily crosses the placenta and can cause hypoglycemia in the fetus, this agent should be discontinued whenever

pregnancy is contemplated or discovered. Rarely, patients with asymptomatic DI begin to experience symptoms during pregnancy.[4] The AVP analog desmopressin (DDAVP) is resistant to vasopressinase. Many women have been treated satisfactorily with this medication,[2] although a higher dosage may be required. Transient AVP-resistant forms of DI that occurred sporadically during one pregnancy but did not recur during another have also been reported.[5] Some of these patients responded to DDAVP and others did not, but symptoms always resolved by several weeks after delivery.[2,5] Regardless of the cause of the DI, vasopressinase may play a substantial role in these cases; thus, the prompt use of DDAVP is indicated. No adverse effects on the fetus have been described in pregnancies in which the mother took DDAVP throughout the pregnancy.[6] Minimal transference of DDAVP into breast milk occurs, and its use is not a contraindication to breast-feeding.[2]

In patients with idiopathic DI, oxytocin levels are normal and labor begins spontaneously and proceeds normally.[7] In patients with DI resulting from tumor, trauma, or infiltrative disease, the oxytocinergic pathways may be affected, resulting in poor progression of labor and uterine atony.

An important finding in women with transient DI of pregnancy is the simultaneous occurrence of acute fatty liver of pregnancy in some patients. Six such patients presented at 35 to 39 weeks of gestation with nausea, vomiting, and polyuria; preeclampsia was diagnosed in four.[8] In four cases, polyuria developed before delivery, and in two, it developed postpartum. All six had complete resolution of their DI and liver abnormalities by the fourth week postpartum. The hypothesis is that the acute liver dysfunction in these patients reduces the degradation of vasopressinase, thereby increasing vasopressinase levels even more than usual with yet greater clearance of vasopressin.[8] Thus, women presenting with DI very late in gestation should also be screened for liver function abnormalities.

DI that develops initially postpartum is usually the result of Sheehan syndrome, especially if the patient has a history of obstetric hemorrhage (see later). However, two cases of transient DI have been reported that occurred within the first 2 weeks postpartum and lasted for only days to weeks. The mechanisms in these instances are not clear.[9]

Congenital nephrogenic DI is a rare disorder that predominantly affects males. However, female carriers of this disease have had significant polyuria during pregnancy. As in the nonpregnant state, treatment is with thiazide diuretics,[2] although these should be used carefully in pregnant women.

## ANTERIOR PITUITARY GLAND AND PREGNANCY

The normal pituitary gland enlarges during pregnancy, predominantly because of the estrogen-stimulated hyperplasia and hypertrophy of the prolactin (PRL)-producing lactotropes.[10] PRL levels rise gradually throughout gestation.[11] This stimulatory effect of pregnancy on the pituitary has important implications for the patient with a preexisting prolactinoma who desires pregnancy.

In the second half of pregnancy, pituitary growth hormone (GH) secretion falls, and levels of a GH variant made by the syncytiotrophoblastic epithelium of the placenta increase in the circulation to as high as 10 to 20 ng/mL.[12,13] The decreased production of normal pituitary GH presumably results from negative feedback effects of the placentally produced variant.[12,13] In patients with acromegaly who have autonomous GH secretion and become pregnant, both forms of GH persist in the blood throughout pregnancy.[14]

### PROLACTINOMA

Hyperprolactinemia is responsible for approximately one-third of all cases of female infertility.[15,16] Hyperprolactinemia impairs

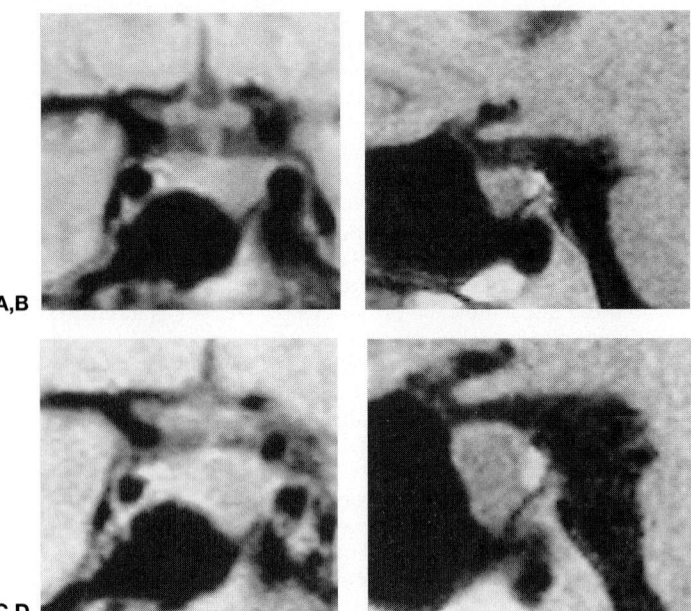

**A,B**

**C,D**

**FIGURE 110-1.** Magnetic resonance imaging scans with coronal (**A, C**) and sagittal (**B, D**) views demonstrating a prolactin-secreting macroadenoma before pregnancy (**A, B**) that progressively enlarged during pregnancy. Scan taken during the third trimester is shown here (**C, D**). The patient had been complaining of increasing headaches.

the hypothalamic–pituitary–ovarian axis at several levels, the primary site of inhibition being at the hypothalamus.[16] The differential diagnosis of hyperprolactinemia is extensive (see Chap. 13).

For patients with prolactinomas, the choice of therapy may have important consequences for decisions regarding pregnancy. Transsphenoidal surgery is curative in 50% to 60% of cases and rarely causes hypopituitarism when it is performed on women with microadenomas. However, it cures a much smaller number with a considerably greater risk of causing hypopituitarism when it is performed for macroadenomas, and may affect fertility.[16]

Bromocriptine therapy restores ovulatory menses in 80% to 90% of women (see Chaps. 13 and 21). Once this has been accomplished, and if pregnancy is desired, mechanical contraception is used until the first two or three cycles have occurred, so that an intermenstrual interval can be established. In this way, a woman will know when she has missed a menstrual period, a pregnancy test can be performed quickly, and the precise gestational age of the fetus will be known. Moreover, bromocriptine will have been given for only 3 to 4 weeks of the gestation. In addition to its efficacy in lowering PRL levels, bromocriptine reduces the size of PRL-secreting macroadenomas by at least 50% in more than half of all patients.[16]

Cabergoline is a dopamine agonist that is given just once or twice weekly. Cabergoline is as effective as, if not more effective than, bromocriptine in lowering PRL levels and is clearly better tolerated.[17] In addition, cabergoline has similar efficacy to bromocriptine in reducing tumor size.[18,19]

### EFFECTS OF PREGNANCY ON PROLACTINOMA GROWTH

In women with prolactinomas, the stimulatory effect of the hormonal milieu of pregnancy may result in significant tumor enlargement during gestation (Fig. 110-1). In a survey of 19 reported series,[20] symptomatic tumor enlargement (producing headaches, visual field disturbance) occurred during pregnancy in 5 of 376 women with PRL-secreting microadenomas treated only with bromocriptine (Table 110-1). The reviewed series included 86 pregnant women with macroadenomas; 20 (23.3%) had symptomatic tumor enlargement. Of 71 women with macroadenomas treated with irradiation or surgery before conception, only 2 (2.8%) had symptomatic tumor enlargement, and none had asymptomatic tumor enlargement during gestation. Twenty-five percent to 50% of patients with symptomatic tumor enlargement require intervention. Bromocriptine therapy usually is successful in reducing the size of the tumor, but transsphenoidal surgery may be necessary.[19]

### EFFECTS OF HYPERPROLACTINEMIA AND ITS TREATMENT ON PREGNANCY

Bromocriptine taken for only the first few weeks of gestation has not been associated with any increase in spontaneous abortions, ectopic pregnancies, trophoblastic disease, multiple pregnancies, or congenital malformations[20,21] (Table 110-2). The experience with bromocriptine given throughout pregnancy is limited, however. One malformation (talipes) has been reported in 114 such pregnancies,[21] which is not an unexpected frequency. However, because bromocriptine crosses the placenta,[22] it should not be used any longer than necessary during pregnancy. The effects of cabergoline usage on fetal outcome has been documented in just over 200 cases; it appears to be safe.[23] Because of this relatively limited experience, however, bromocriptine would appear to be the preferred dopamine agonist when fertility is the primary concern of therapy. The effects of transsphenoidal surgery during gestation are not known specifically but would not be expected to be significantly different from the effects of other types of surgery (unless hypopituitarism should ensue).

### MANAGEMENT OF PROLACTINOMA

The risks of surgery versus medical therapy for prolactinoma should be explained in detail to each patient. For patients with microadenomas or intrasellar macroadenomas, bromocriptine therapy is generally preferred to surgery because it is safe for the fetus when discontinued early in gestation and poses only a small risk of tumor enlargement for the mother. Such patients should be seen each trimester and assessed for symptoms such

**TABLE 110-1.**
**Effect of Pregnancy on Prolactinomas**

| Tumor Type | Prior Therapy* | Number | Symptomatic Enlargement† |
|---|---|---|---|
| MICROADENOMAS | None | 376 | 5 |
| MACROADENOMAS | None | 86 | 20 |
| MACROADENOMAS | Yes | 71 | 2 |

*Surgery or irradiation.
†Requiring intervention—surgery or bromocriptine therapy.
(Adapted from Molitch ME. Management of prolactinomas during pregnancy. J Reprod Med 1999; 44:1121.)

**TABLE 110-2.**
**Effects of Bromocriptine Therapy on Pregnancy**

|  | Bromocriptine Therapy | | Normal Population |
|---|---|---|---|
|  | Number | Percent | Percent |
| PREGNANCIES | 6239 | 100.0 | 100.0 |
| Spontaneous abortion | 620 | 9.9 | 10.0–15.0 |
| Termination | 75 | 1.25 | — |
| Ectopic pregnancy | 31 | 0.5 | 0.5–1.0 |
| Hydatidiform mole | 11 | 0.2 | 0.05–0.7 |
| DELIVERIES (KNOWN DURATION) | 4139 | 100.0 | 100.0 |
| At term (>38 weeks) | 3620 | 87.5 | 85.0 |
| Before term (<38 weeks) | 519 | 12.5 | 15.0 |
| DELIVERIES (KNOWN OUTCOME) | 5120 | 100.0 | 100.0 |
| Single births | 5031 | 98.3 | 98.7 |
| Multiple births | 89 | 1.7 | 1.3 |
| BABIES (KNOWN DETAILS) | 5213 | 100.0 | 100.0 |
| Normal | 5030 | 96.5 | 95.0 |
| With malformations | 93 | 1.8 | 3.0–4.0 |
| With perinatal disorders | 90 | 1.7 | >2.0 |

(Adapted from Krupp P, Monka C, Richter K. In: Program of the Second World Congress of Gynecology and Obstetrics, Rio de Janeiro, 1988:9.)

as headaches or vision problems; visual field testing need be done only when clinically indicated. When the tumor is large or extends to the optic chiasm or into the cavernous sinus, the following approaches should be considered: (a) surgical debulking, (b) intensive monitoring without bromocriptine therapy, or (c) continuous bromocriptine therapy. The safety of the last approach has not been established, but based on the small number of cases cited earlier, it probably is not harmful. Patients with macroadenomas should be seen monthly for such assessments, and visual fields should be tested each trimester. PRL levels, which normally increase in pregnancy, may not rise in women with prolactinomas. Furthermore, PRL levels may not always rise with pregnancy-induced tumor enlargement[24]; therefore, periodic measurements of PRL levels are of little benefit.

When evidence of tumor enlargement is seen during pregnancy, bromocriptine therapy should be reinstituted immediately and the dosage increased as rapidly as tolerated. Such therapy must be monitored closely, and transsphenoidal surgery or delivery (if the pregnancy is far enough advanced) should be considered if the patient does not respond to bromocriptine therapy.[20]

Although suckling stimulates PRL secretion in normal women for the first few weeks to months postpartum,[16] no data have been reported to suggest that breast-feeding can cause tumor growth. Thus, no reason exists to discourage nursing in women with prolactinomas.

### CONTRACEPTION

Withholding bromocriptine and allowing a woman to remain anovulatory may be the most efficacious mode of contraception. However, such women have hypoestrogenemia and are predisposed to the development of osteoporosis,[16] so this form of contraception is not recommended. The estrogens in oral contraceptives can increase PRL levels modestly in normal women, and estrogens clearly can stimulate normal lactotropes (see earlier). However, oral contraceptive administration, with and without concomitant bromocriptine therapy, does not usually lead to the growth of preexisting microadenomas or their initial development in women with idiopathic hyperprolactinemia.[25] Thus, oral contraceptives and estrogen/progestin

replacement therapy can be used safely when fertility is not desired. Nevertheless, women on this regimen should be followed carefully with periodic monitoring of PRL levels to detect the rare tumor that may be unusually estrogen sensitive.

### ACROMEGALY

Reports of pregnancy in patients with acromegaly are uncommon,[14,22,26,27] perhaps because ~40% of such patients have hyperprolactinemia.[28] Correction of hyperprolactinemia with bromocriptine therapy may be necessary to permit ovulation and conception in these patients.[23]

Conventional radioimmunoassays for GH cannot distinguish between normal pituitary GH and the placental GH variant.[12] Special radioimmunoassays using antibodies that recognize specific epitopes on the two hormones[12] must be used. When such specific assays are not available, testing may need to be delayed until after delivery to assess pituitary GH secretion accurately, because the placental variant falls to undetectable levels within 24 hours.[12] However, two differences exist between the secretion of the placental GH variant and the secretion of pituitary GH during acromegaly that may allow a distinction to be made during pregnancy. First, pituitary GH secretion in acromegaly is highly pulsatile, with 13 to 19 pulses per 24 hours,[29] whereas secretion of the pregnancy GH variant is nonpulsatile.[13] Second, in acromegaly, ~70% of patients have a GH response to thyrotropin-releasing hormone,[28] whereas the placental GH variant does not respond to this hormone.[14]

Only two patients with tumors secreting GH have been reported to have enlargement of their tumors, with a resultant visual field defect in one, during pregnancy.[26,30] Therefore, patients with acromegaly should be monitored for symptomatic tumor enlargement as are patients with PRL-secreting macroadenomas.

Certain complications of acromegaly are potentially harmful to both the mother and the fetus. Carbohydrate intolerance is present in as many as 50% of patients with acromegaly, and overt diabetes is seen in 10% to 20%.[28] Insulin resistance secondary to the increased levels of GH may increase the risk of gestational diabetes. Salt retention is increased, and hypertension occurs in 25% to 35% of patients. In addition, cardiac disease is present in approximately one-third of patients. A specific cardiomyopathy associated with acromegaly may be present, and coronary artery disease may be increased.[28]

The considerations regarding the use of bromocriptine in women with prolactinomas also apply to those with acromegaly. Data on the use of octreotide during pregnancy are limited. Only three pregnant patients treated with octreotide have been reported; no malformations were found in their children.[31–33] Because of the limited data, octreotide use should be discontinued if pregnancy is considered, and contraception should be used when octreotide is administered.

### OTHER PITUITARY TUMORS

Adrenocorticotropic hormone (ACTH)–secreting pituitary tumors are discussed later (see Adrenal Cortex and Pregnancy). Little information is available concerning pregnancies occurring in patients with nonsecreting tumors or those with tumors that secrete thyroid-stimulating hormone (TSH), gonadotropin, or the glycoprotein subunit. In these patients, pregnancy is unlikely to have any influence on tumor size, although a patient with a nonsecreting tumor that enlarged during pregnancy has been reported.[26] Only one case of pregnancy occurring in a women with a TSH-secreting tumor has been reported, and in this patient, octreotide therapy, which had been stopped, had to be reinstituted to control tumor size.[33] The specific problems regarding potential hypopituitarism and hyperthyroidism are discussed later.

**TABLE 110-3.**
**Symptoms and Signs of Sheehan Syndrome**

| Acute Form | Chronic Form |
| --- | --- |
| Hypotension | Light-headedness |
| Tachycardia | Fatigue |
| Failure to lactate | Failure to lactate |
| Hypoglycemia | Persistent amenorrhea |
| Failure to regrow shaved pubic hair | Decreased body hair |
| Extreme fatigue | Dry skin |
| Nausea and vomiting | Loss of libido |
| | Nausea and vomiting |
| | Cold intolerance |

(From Molitch ME. Pituitary, thyroid, adrenal and parathyroid disorders. In: Barron WM, Lindheimer MD, eds. Medical disorders during pregnancy. Chicago: Mosby–Year Book, 1991.)

## HYPOPITUITARISM

### CHRONIC HYPOPITUITARISM

Hypopituitarism can result from many causes, including tumors, trauma, and infiltrative and vascular diseases (see Chaps. 3, 11, and 12). The hormone deficits can be partial or complete, with loss of gonadotropin secretion being common. Ovulation often is difficult to induce and usually is best accomplished by an experienced reproductive endocrinologist, so that a planned pregnancy results. In adult women, the only hormones that may need to be replaced are thyroid and adrenal hormones; these are described in the sections on hypothyroidism and adrenal insufficiency. Those patients with hypothalamic disease should also be monitored for the development of symptomatic DI (see earlier).

### SHEEHAN SYNDROME

The term *Sheehan syndrome* refers to the development of pituitary necrosis due to ischemia within a few hours of delivery.[34] Usually, antecedent hypotension and shock are present, resulting most commonly from obstetric hemorrhage and occasionally from retained placenta.[34] Sheehan believed that the ischemia is caused by occlusive spasm of the arteries that supply the anterior lobe and the hypothalamic-pituitary stalk.[34] Estrogen- and pregnancy-induced pituitary enlargement has also been implicated in the pathogenesis.[34] The degree of ischemia and necrosis dictates the subsequent course of the patient. Both acute and chronic forms exist (Table 110-3).

**Acute Form of Sheehan Syndrome.** In the acute form of Sheehan syndrome, patients may have persistent hypotension, tachycardia, failure to lactate, and hypoglycemia.[34,35] The diagnosis should be considered and treatment started in patients with obstetric hemorrhage and a prolonged course of hypotension that is not responsive to appropriate blood product replacement. Blood should be obtained for determination of ACTH, cortisol, thyroxine ($T_4$), and PRL levels in the basal state. An ACTH stimulation test is of no value because the adrenal glands are not yet atrophied. $T_4$ levels may not be decreased because of the 7-day half-life of this hormone. PRL levels, which normally are five- to ten-fold elevated in the puerperium, are low in patients with Sheehan syndrome.

Treatment should be initiated with stress doses of intravenous glucocorticoids and saline after blood has been drawn, without waiting for the test results. Once the patient has recovered, additional testing can be done to assess the need for other hormone replacement, as in patients who have the more usual, chronic form of Sheehan syndrome. In the acute form, usually <10% of normal pituitary tissue remains,[34] and CT scans show either a partially or completely empty sella turcica.[36]

**Chronic Form of Sheehan Syndrome.** Patients with the chronic form of Sheehan syndrome have lesser degrees of pituitary infarction[35] and come to medical attention weeks to years after delivery (see Table 110-3). Amenorrhea and loss of libido are common, but many women menstruate and ovulate normally. Spontaneous pregnancies have been reported.[35] Patients frequently have a history of failure to lactate postpartum and some breast atrophy. Fatigue, loss of axillary and pubic hair, nausea, vomiting, abdominal pain, and diarrhea may suggest a secondary adrenal insufficiency. A full pituitary evaluation is indicated in such patients.

DI also may be caused by vascular occlusion with resultant atrophy and scarring of the neurohypophysis[37] and lesions in the supraventricular and paraventricular nuclei.[38] Many patients recall transient polydipsia and polyuria in the postpartum period with subsequent recurrence of these symptoms. Although most have no symptoms when they are seen in later years, many demonstrate impaired urinary concentrating ability and deficient vasopressin secretion when tested with dehydration or hypertonic saline.[39]

## LYMPHOCYTIC HYPOPHYSITIS

Lymphocytic hypophysitis is characterized by a massive infiltration of the pituitary by lymphocytes and plasma cells, with destruction of the normal parenchyma. The disorder is thought to have an autoimmune basis. Most cases occur in association with pregnancy, and women are seen during or after pregnancy with symptoms of varying degrees of hypopituitarism, or with symptoms related to the mass lesion, such as headaches or visual field defects. Mild hyperprolactinemia and DI also may be found. On CT or magnetic resonance imaging (MRI) scanning, a sellar mass is present that may extend in an extrasellar fashion and may cause visual field defects. The condition usually is confused with that of a pituitary tumor and cannot be distinguished from a tumor except by biopsy.[40,41]

The diagnosis of lymphocytic hypophysitis should be entertained in women who develop symptoms of hypopituitarism and/or mass lesions of the sella during or after pregnancy, especially in the absence of a history of obstetric hemorrhage or previous infertility or menstrual disorder. An evaluation of pituitary function is warranted, as well as a CT or MRI scan. In the presence of a large mass, if PRL levels are only modestly elevated (<150 ng/mL), the diagnosis is unlikely to be an enlarging prolactinoma and more likely to be lymphocytic hypophysitis or a nonsecreting tumor. Hormone-replacement therapy should be instituted promptly when hypopituitarism is determined to be present. Unless visual field defects, uncontrollable headaches, or radiologic evidence of progressive enlargement of the sellar mass are present, rapid surgical intervention is not warranted, because some women may undergo a spontaneous regression of the mass and have a return of pituitary function.[40,41]

## THYROID GLAND AND PREGNANCY

Numerous changes occur in the thyroid gland and in the levels of thyroid hormones during pregnancy.[42] When iodine intake is marginal, increased renal clearance results in iodine deficiency, and minimal enlargement of the thyroid may ensue.[43] The iodine in iodized salt and in prenatal vitamins usually prevents this deficiency and the resultant thyroid enlargement. These small amounts of iodine (6–40 mg daily) cause only a transient, mild fall in fetal free $T_4$ levels, and the fetus soon escapes this inhibition, as does the mother.[44] Excessive iodine ingestion should be avoided, however, because iodine crosses the placenta and may cause neonatal goiter (see later).

The belief is widespread that a goiter commonly develops during pregnancy. This belief is based on uncontrolled observations in the early literature made in iodine-deficient areas.[45] In iodine-replete regions, no increase is seen in the frequency of goiters during pregnancy.[45,46] Of 309 pregnant adolescents in one study, 19 had goiters,[46] 2 had Graves disease and hyperthyroidism, 3 had Hashimoto thyroiditis (1 with hyperthyroidism), 4 had subacute thyroiditis (1 with hyperthyroidism), and 9 had simple nontoxic goiters. Thus, the presence of a palpable goiter in iodine-replete areas indicates significant disease in ~50% of patients and always requires evaluation.

The fetal thyroid and the fetal hypothalamic–pituitary–thyroid axis develop independently of the maternal thyroid status. The components of this axis are functioning after 10 weeks of gestation. By 11 to 12 weeks of gestation, the fetal thyroid begins to concentrate iodine, and $T_4$ and TSH are present in the fetal circulation.[47] The placenta is permeable to iodine and to medications used to treat hyperthyroidism, such as propylthiouracil (PTU), methimazole, and propranolol. Triiodothyronine ($T_3$) and TSH cross the placenta only minimally.[42,48] When fetal thyroid disease is suspected, the assessment for a goiter can be performed using ultrasonography[48]; percutaneous cord blood sampling can be carried out to evaluate fetal thyroid hormone status,[47] and therapy can be initiated to forestall problems. $T_4$ crosses the placenta in somewhat larger amounts than $T_3$, and its administration to mothers late in gestation leads to amelioration of the effects of hypothyroidism in infants with congenital hypothyroidism resulting from enzyme defects or agenesis of the thyroid.[49]

Thyroid-stimulating activity as measured by serum bioassay is increased in the first trimester because of the intrinsic thyroid-stimulating activity of hCG.[42,43,50] The hCG may cause increased $T_4$ and $T_3$ levels, as well as a transient hyperthyroidism associated with hyperemesis gravidarum (see later). Markedly elevated levels of hCG secreted by trophoblastic neoplasms also may cause hyperthyroidism.[50] In addition, a human chorionic thyrotropin may be made by the placenta, but it has little thyroid-stimulating activity and probably plays no physiologic role.[51]

The increased estrogens produced by the fetal-placental unit raise thyroid hormone–binding globulin levels in the mother by stimulating its hepatic production, as well as by decreasing its degradation through altered glycosylation.[42,51] The increased thyroid hormone–binding globulin levels result in higher levels of bound $T_4$, beginning by 4 to 6 weeks of gestation[51] (Fig. 110-2).

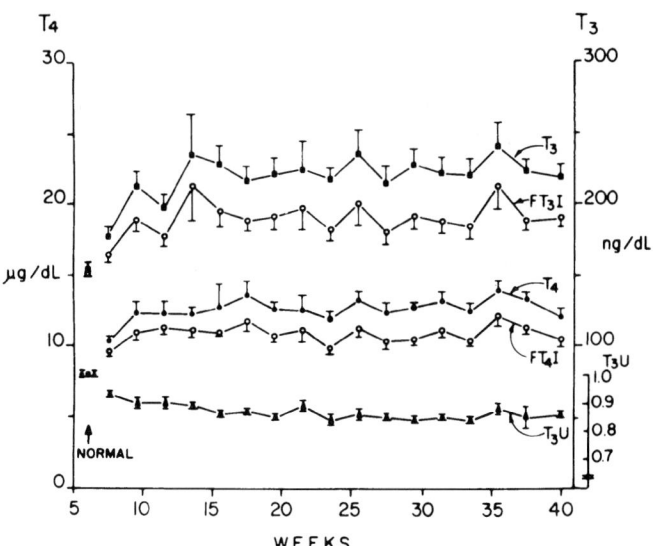

**FIGURE 110-2.** Mean levels (± standard error) of serum thyroxine ($T_4$), serum triiodothyronine ($T_3$), $T_3$ uptake ($T_3U$), free $T_4$ index ($FT_4I$), and free $T_3$ index ($FT_3I$) at various weeks of pregnancy. Nonpregnant control values are shown on the left. Serum $T_4$, $T_3$, $FT_4I$, and $FT_3I$ were significantly elevated and $T_3U$ was reduced throughout pregnancy. (From Harada A, Hershman JM, Reed AW, et al. Comparison of thyroid stimulators and thyroid hormone concentrations in the sera of pregnant women. J Clin Endocrinol Metab 1979; 48:793.)

Free $T_4$ levels have been reported to be unchanged, increased, or decreased during pregnancy, although they remain within the normal range in most patients.[42,43,51] These differences may relate to relative iodine deficiencies in the populations studied[43] and to the stage of pregnancy being assessed. The slightly elevated free $T_4$ levels seen in some persons may result from the stimulating activity of the high levels of hCG.[43,50,51] $T_3$ is bound to thyroid hormone–binding globulin with somewhat less affinity than $T_4$, but increases in total $T_3$ levels similar to those of $T_4$ are observed during pregnancy.[51] TSH levels are decreased minimally during pregnancy, possibly because of the increased free $T_4$ levels.[51]

## HYPERTHYROIDISM

Hyperthyroidism occurs in ~2 of every 1000 pregnancies.[42,52] Approximately 95% of these cases are caused by Graves disease (see Chap. 42). Preexisting Graves disease often ameliorates during pregnancy, as do other autoimmune disorders, perhaps due to the gestationally mediated alterations in immune mechanisms.[42,52] Clinical improvement is most likely to occur in the second half of pregnancy, paralleling the fall in circulating levels of the stimulatory immunoglobulins.[52] However, Graves disease also may present initially or may relapse during pregnancy.[42,52] Hyperthyroidism may be exacerbated postpartum, possibly because the pregnancy had an ameliorating effect on the disease that was lost with delivery.

Untreated hyperthyroidism clearly has an adverse consequence on fetal outcome. Among 57 patients with uncontrolled hyperthyroidism, 25 had low-birth-weight infants (a nine-fold increase in relative risk), 19 had premature deliveries (a 16.5-fold increase in relative risk), and 8 developed preeclampsia (a 4.74-fold increase in relative risk); however, no perinatal deaths occurred.[53] In patients who were hyperthyroid but whose condition was brought under control during the pregnancy, these numbers were considerably improved but still not normal. Patients whose hyperthyroidism was under control throughout the pregnancy had no increased risk of these complications.[53]

### DIAGNOSIS OF HYPERTHYROIDISM DURING PREGNANCY

The hyperdynamic state of pregnancy may make the clinical diagnosis of hyperthyroidism more difficult; tachycardia, warm skin, systolic flow murmurs, and heat intolerance are common to both. Even the presence of a goiter may not be specific. However, weight loss, marked tachycardia, eye signs, and a bruit over the thyroid are more suggestive of hyperthyroidism.[42,52]

The diagnosis is confirmed by documenting completely suppressed TSH levels and elevated free $T_4$ and $T_3$ indices in the blood. If, in the face of strong clinical suspicion, the calculated free $T_4$ and $T_3$ indices are not elevated, then free $T_4$ and free $T_3$ levels should be measured by equilibrium dialysis. Scanning or uptake with radioactive tracers such as iodine-131 ($^{131}$I) or technetium-99 ($^{99}$Tc) should be avoided to prevent exposure to the developing fetus. However, the small tracer doses used in these studies are not sufficient to cause demonstrable harm to the fetus in the event of inadvertent administration to someone not known to be pregnant.[42,52]

### TREATMENT OF HYPERTHYROIDISM DURING PREGNANCY

**Medical Therapy.** Medical therapy is generally considered the treatment of choice for hyperthyroidism during pregnancy. The thionamide derivatives PTU and methimazole are equally efficacious. The suggestion that infants exposed to methimazole have an increased chance of developing a scalp anomaly known as aplasia cutis have not been confirmed by analyses of large numbers of offspring.[54,55] Methimazole crosses the placenta at a four-fold greater rate than PTU,[56] so that it has potentially greater effects on the fetus. Primarily for this reason, as well as because of anecdotal case reports of aplasia cutis with methimazole, PTU has become the preferred thionamide for use in pregnancy. Studies in which pregnancy outcomes have been compared, however, demonstrate no essential clinical differences in the safety or efficacy of the two drugs.[55,57,58]

After initial attainment of the euthyroid state, the lowest dosage of PTU or methimazole that maintains thyroid hormone levels in the upper normal to minimally elevated range should be used to minimize fetal hypothyroidism.[42,58] An earlier practice of using higher dosages of antithyroid drugs plus supplementation with thyroid hormone has been abandoned because thyroid hormones are now known to cross the placenta only in small amounts. Such combined therapy yields a euthyroid mother at the expense of a hypothyroid infant. A small neonatal goiter sometimes may be apparent at delivery, but this is not clearly related to the dosage of PTU or methimazole. Such goiters usually reflect fetal hypothyroidism due to the thionamide,[42,52] and hormone levels in these infants should be determined immediately. Long-term follow-up of children exposed in utero to PTU has shown no ill effects with respect to physical or intellectual development.[59]

The β-adrenergic receptor–blocking drugs may be useful in patients with severe hyperthyroidism and in those with marked tachycardia (>120 beats per minute) or tachyarrhythmias. The β-blockers also cross the placenta. Although some early reports suggested an association with neonatal bradycardia and hypoglycemia, these concerns have not been borne out.[60] Unlike the thionamides, β-blockers do not reduce the increased basal metabolic rate and the protein catabolism that occur during hyperthyroidism, and patients have gone into thyroid storm during labor when their sole therapy has been β-blockade (see later).[61]

Iodides cross the placenta readily and can cause fetal hypothyroidism and large goiters.[62] They should be used only for a short time to aid in the preparation of patients for surgery or for rare cases of thyroid storm. In pregnancies in which iodide has been used, the size of potential fetal goiters should be assessed by ultrasonography.[48]

Lithium carbonate is teratogenic when given in the first trimester and may cause neonatal lithium intoxication and goiters when given near term.[63] In general, this drug should not be used in pregnancy, even during thyroid storm, unless toxic reactions to the many other antithyroid drugs preclude their use.

**Surgery.** Although a retrospective review of the literature suggested that the results of treatment with antithyroid drugs were equivalent to those of surgery performed in the second trimester,[64] in the United States, medical therapy is generally used for hyperthyroidism during pregnancy because surgery may pose an increased risk to the fetus.[42,52,65] Surgery is reserved for those patients who do not respond well to or develop an intolerance for medication (e.g., rash, allergy, agranulocytosis). As in the nonpregnant state, patients should be prepared medically with thionamides, β-blockers, and iodide before surgery to prevent thyroid storm.

**Radioactive Iodine Therapy.** Radioactive iodine can cross the placenta and permanently ablate the gland of the fetus as well as that of the mother. Therapeutic doses of radioactive iodine, therefore, are contraindicated during pregnancy. A pregnancy test should be performed before the administration of radioactive iodine to all women at risk for being pregnant.

## THYROID STORM DURING PREGNANCY

Thyroid storm is a medical emergency that is still associated with an appreciable mortality for both the mother and the fetus. Most commonly, it is precipitated by stress, such as infection, labor, or cesarean section or other surgery, in a previously undiagnosed patient. The diagnosis and treatment of this condition are discussed in Chapter 42, and no specific problems unique to pregnancy are seen. However, the clinician should not hesitate to use inorganic iodide because of theoretic risks to the fetus; the benefits of acute reduction of thyroid hormone release and

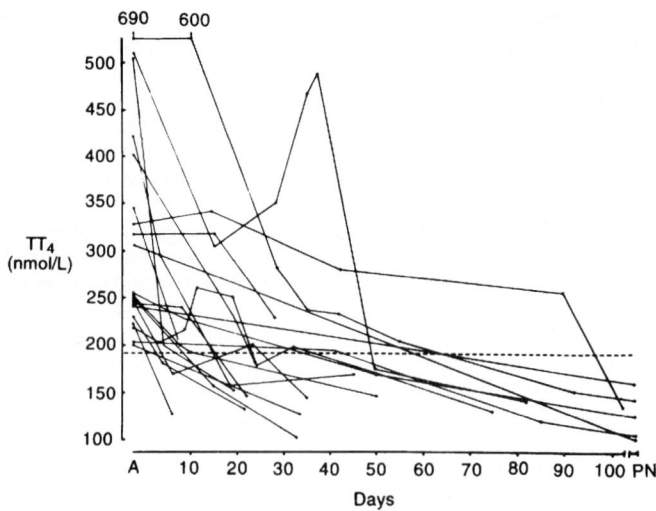

**FIGURE 110-3.** Changes in plasma total thyroxine ($TT_4$) concentration in 20 subjects with hyperemesis on admission to the hospital (*A*) and during the course of their pregnancy. The interrupted line represents the value of the mean + 1 standard deviation seen in normal pregnancy. (*PN*, postnatal.) (From Swaminathan R, Chin RK, Lao TH, et al. Thyroid function in hyperemesis gravidarum. Acta Endocrinol [Copenh], 1989; 120:155.)

amelioration of the overall condition greatly outweigh possible occurrence of goiter. In women who receive a large iodide load, the fetus should be monitored for the presence of a large goiter by ultrasonography.

## HYPERTHYROIDISM AND HYPEREMESIS GRAVIDARUM

Nausea and vomiting occasionally may be the predominant presenting symptoms in patients with hyperthyroidism. In pregnancy, the severe nausea and vomiting that sometimes begins in the first trimester, known as *hyperemesis gravidarum*, may be associated with biochemical hyperthyroidism.[50] In one series of 39 patients with hyperemesis gravidarum, 2 were found to be clinically thyrotoxic.[66] However, elevated free $T_4$ levels associated with suppressed TSH levels, without clinical evidence of hyperthyroidism, may be found transiently in 30% to 60% of subjects with severe hyperemesis gravidarum, and these levels return to normal by 18 weeks of gestation[66,67] (Fig. 110-3). Patients with hyperemesis have much higher levels of hCG than do matched control subjects. The degree of biochemical hyperthyroidism and severity of vomiting correlate with the level of hCG, and hCG may play a causative role in both the hyperemesis and the hyperthyroidism.[68] Careful evaluation of clinical features and thyroid function as well as close follow-up are indicated in these patients to distinguish true hyperthyroidism, which may appear initially in pregnancy and requires treatment, from the much more common biochemical hyperthyroidism, which is associated with hyperemesis gravidarum and does not require therapy.

A very rare cause of recurrent gestational hyperthyroidism occurring in families is a missense mutation in the extracellular domain of the TSH receptor that is more sensitive than the wild-type receptor to hCG and occurs with normal rather than elevated levels of hCG.[69]

## GRAVES DISEASE AND THYROID FUNCTION IN THE NEONATE

Fetal and neonatal hypothyroidism and goiters may result from the passage of thionamides across the placenta. Cord blood should be obtained for the measurement of $T_4$ and TSH levels. These measurements should be repeated 3 days later because transient hypothyroidism resulting from thionamide passage across the placenta usually has resolved by that time.[58]

Approximately 10% of infants may develop transient hyperthyroidism resulting from the passage of thyroid-stimulating immunoglobulins and, possibly, thyrotropin-binding inhibitor immunoglobulins across the placenta.[42] Although the finding of a high titer of such immunoglobulins in the blood of an infant is highly predictive of the development of hyperthyroidism, the absence of such titers does not mean that hyperthyroidism will not develop. The hyperthyroidism also may manifest in utero as an increased fetal heart rate. In a few cases, intrauterine fetal hyperthyroidism has been treated by increasing the maternal thionamide dosage, titrating it to the fetal heart rate[70] (see Chap. 47).

## HYPERTHYROIDISM AND BREAST-FEEDING

Radioiodine treatment is contraindicated during breast-feeding because of passage of the isotope into the breast milk. Scanning should not be performed, even though the doses used are small and the amount found in the breast milk is minimal. In a description of an infant who breast-fed 4 hours after the mother had received $^{99m}$Tc, the exposure to the thyroid was 300 mRad, to the upper large intestine was 180 mRad, and to other organs was considerably less.[71] The total dose received by the infant was 82.5 µCi. However, a feeding 30 minutes after the isotope was given was estimated to result in the ingestion of 728 µCi. These authors suggest that at least 48 hours be allowed to elapse after scanning before breast-feeding is resumed, and that formula be substituted in the interim.

Both methimazole and PTU appear in breast milk. However, the amounts are small and should not affect neonatal thyroid function. Nevertheless, monitoring of thyroid function in breast-feeding infants is recommended.[71] Theoretically, infants could also have idiosyncratic reactions to these drugs, which may not be dose-dependent. However, jaundice, rash, and agranulocytosis have not been reported in such infants.[72]

## HYPOTHYROIDISM

Some series have found that women with hypothyroidism have a higher incidence of spontaneous abortion, preeclampsia, abruptio placentae, stillbirth, premature birth, postpartum hemorrhage, pregnancy-induced hypertension, and congenital anomalies.[73,74] In general, patients with mild to moderate hypothyroidism tolerate well stresses such as labor and delivery, and other surgery.[75] Nevertheless, sedatives and analgesics must be administered cautiously because of their slow metabolism. These patients may require intubation and ventilator support for extended periods because of their depressed hypoxic and ventilatory drives. They also may have a decreased ability to clear free water, leading to hyponatremia, and postoperative ileus may be prolonged.

### TREATMENT OF HYPOTHYROIDISM DURING PREGNANCY

Because virtually all women of childbearing age with hypothyroidism have normal coronary arteries, therapy can be started on L-thyroxine at 0.1 mg per day and increased by 0.025- to 0.05-mg increments at 2-week intervals. The dosage is increased gradually until the TSH level and the free $T_4$ index are normal. Because of the 60% to 80% absorption of oral L-thyroxine,[76] patients who are unable to take oral medication should be given approximately two-thirds of the usual dosage by the intravenous route.

$T_4$ turnover is increased during gestation.[42] In pregnant patients who are receiving $T_4$ replacement, serum TSH levels should be checked each trimester to determine whether the dosage needs to be increased.[77] In one study, the $T_4$ dosage had to be increased in 75% of patients during pregnancy.[77] Some of this increased $T_4$ requirement may be due to intestinal complexing of $T_4$ with ferrous sulfate[78] or with calcium,[78a] which are frequent components of prenatal vitamins. The importance of careful testing and thyroid hormone replacement is demonstrated by the finding that even mild maternal hypothyroidism is associated with lowered childhood intelligence quotients.[78b]

## MYXEDEMA COMA

Myxedema coma is extremely rare in pregnancy because it primarily affects older patients, and when it is present in younger patients, the severity of the hypothyroidism usually results in anovulation and infertility. When myxedema coma occurs, however, it is a true medical emergency, with a 20% mortality even when treated properly. Therapy is the same as in nonpregnant individuals (see Chap. 45).

## POSTPARTUM THYROIDITIS

Postpartum, subacute lymphocytic thyroiditis occurs in ~5% of women[79–81]; this figure increases to 25% in women with type 1 diabetes mellitus.[82] Characteristically, the syndrome consists of hyperthyroidism associated with a low radioactive iodine uptake that occurs 6 to 12 weeks postpartum and lasts for 1 to 2 months, followed by transient hypothyroidism associated with a goiter that generally resolves spontaneously by 6 to 9 months postpartum.[81] The hyperthyroid phase is observed in approximately two-thirds of patients and may not cause symptoms, although many patients complain of fatigue, shoulder stiffness, increased appetite, sweating, and nervousness.[79–81]

Approximately two-thirds of all patients with postpartum thyroiditis have hypothyroidism. In one-third of these, the hypothyroidism occurs without preceding hyperthyroidism. The hypothyroidism resolves spontaneously in ~80% of cases but persists in 20%.[81] The titer of antimicrosomal antibodies appears to be predictive, with higher titers tending to be associated with persistent hypothyroidism.[79] The hypothyroid phase may cause no symptoms, or it may cause fatigue, lack of initiative, weight gain, and depression.[81] Many women with "postpartum depression" actually may have thyroiditis, and thyroid function tests always should be performed.

The laboratory evaluation for postpartum thyroiditis includes the measurement of serum $T_4$, $T_3$, and TSH levels. Because of the changing course of the condition, these measurements should be repeated at intervals of 4 to 8 weeks. Treatment should be reserved for symptomatic cases, because most resolve spontaneously. Women with significant hyperthyroid symptoms should undergo radioactive iodine uptake testing to differentiate the condition from Graves disease, which also may develop during the postpartum period. Thionamide antithyroid drugs are not effective in treating postpartum thyroiditis; β-blockers are indicated for symptomatic relief. Postpartum hypothyroidism that causes symptoms should be treated with L-thyroxine. Because this disorder usually is transient, however, therapy should be decreased or discontinued after 6 months and repeat thyroid function testing should be performed 6 weeks later. If hypothyroidism persists at that point, therapy should be restarted, then decreased or discontinued after 6 more months and followed again in 6 weeks by thyroid function testing.[80,81] Often, women who have a complete return to normal function continue to maintain positive antimicrosomal antibody levels in their blood and manifest organification defects.[83] If they are exposed to excess iodide (e.g., radiocontrast media), they may develop hypothyroidism, as do patients with more typical Hashimoto thyroiditis.[83] Thus, iodine should not be used in such patients, and they should be considered to be at risk for the development of more permanent hypothyroidism in the future. Recurrent hypothyroidism has been noted in 23% of patients with histories of postpartum thyroiditis 2 to 4 years previously[84] (see Chap. 46).

## THYROID NODULES AND THYROID CANCER DURING PREGNANCY

The risk of malignancy in a solitary thyroid nodule is ~10%. A history of previous head and neck irradiation greatly increases this risk[85] (see Chap. 39). Of cancers found in the childbearing

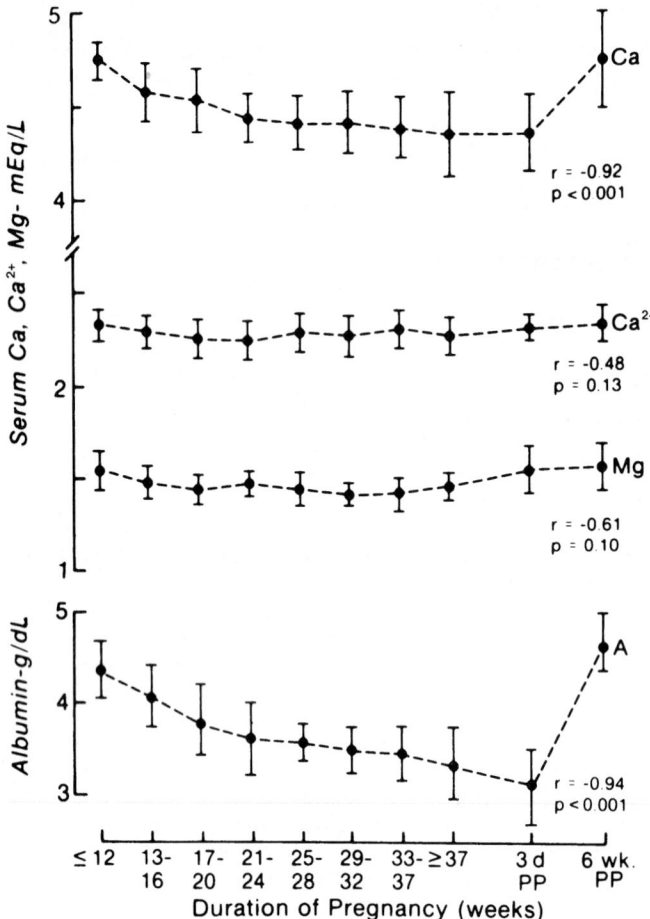

**FIGURE 110-4.** Mean levels (± standard deviation) of Ca, $Ca^{2+}$, Mg, and albumin (A) during pregnancy and the puerperium (PP). (From Pitkin RM, Reynolds WA, Williams GA, et al. Calcium metabolism in normal pregnancy: a longitudinal study. Am J Obstet Gynecol 1979; 133:781.)

age group, ~65% are papillary, 30% are follicular, 3% are medullary, 1% are anaplastic, and 1% are other types, such as metastatic disease to the thyroid or lymphoma.[85]

Because radioisotopic scanning is contraindicated during pregnancy, fine-needle aspiration should be performed; it has excellent sensitivity and specificity. Surgery should be undertaken immediately if the aspirate reveals medullary or anaplastic carcinoma or lymphoma (see Chap. 44). However, waiting until after delivery to perform surgery does not alter the prognosis for differentiated carcinoma[85,86]; all such patients should have their thyroid glands suppressed with exogenous L-thyroxine until surgery. Pregnancy itself appears to have no effect on the prognosis of thyroid cancer.[86,87]

## CALCIUM BALANCE DURING PREGNANCY

Twenty-five to 30 g of calcium is transferred from the mother to the fetus during gestation; ~300 mg per day is transferred in the third trimester.[88] A net loss of calcium into the urine also occurs because of the increased glomerular filtration that is associated with pregnancy.[89] Serum total calcium levels decrease modestly from 2.4 mmol/L to 2.2 mmol/L, in parallel with a fall in serum albumin levels from 4.7 to 3.2 g/dL. Ionized calcium levels remain unchanged[88–90] (Fig. 110-4).

The primary adaptational event to counter this negative calcium balance is an increase in circulating 1,25-dihydroxyvitamin D levels; this results in increased intestinal absorption

of calcium.[91,92] Although this augmented formation of 1,25-dihydroxyvitamin D has been thought to result from increases in parathyroid hormone, serum levels have been reported to be low, normal, and high,[88–92] probably because of differences in the detection of parathyroid hormone cleavage products.[91,92] Women who have poor calcium intake during gestation probably develop significant negative calcium balance despite these adaptive changes; thus, an intake of at least 1200 to 1600 mg per day has been recommended.[93]

Serum calcium levels in the fetus are greater than those in the mother, suggesting active transport of calcium across the placenta.[88,89] The fetal hypercalcemia suppresses the fetal parathyroids, so that the neonate is relatively hypoparathyroid at birth.[88,89] The elevated calcium levels present in cord blood fall to a nadir at 24 to 48 hours of age. In the absence of confounding factors such as maternal diabetes mellitus, preterm birth, or birth hypoxia, the parathyroid glands in the neonate generally recover quickly[88,89] (see Chap. 49).

## HYPERCALCEMIA

Most pregnant patients with hypercalcemia do not have symptoms, and the condition is discovered on routine screening. The occurrence of renal calculi, peptic ulcer disease, bone disease, or mental dysfunction in these patients is uncommon. Rarely, the diagnosis in the mother is made only after an evaluation is performed because of hypocalcemia in the neonate.[94]

Many conditions are associated with hypercalcemia, and increased calcium levels are common, being present in 0.1% to 0.6% of the general nonpregnant population. Although a careful investigation is always warranted, most women in this age group are found to have hyperparathyroidism. (For a discussion of the evaluation of patients with hypercalcemia, see Chaps. 58 and 59.)

Although fewer than 100 cases of hyperparathyroidism occurring in pregnant women have been reported in the literature, this is likely to be the result of considerable bias, because the condition often either is not detected or is not reported because patients have no symptoms. Hypercalcemia can affect both the mother and the fetus. Rarely, women may have severe hypercalcemia ("hypercalcemic crisis"), with rapidly progressive anorexia, nausea, vomiting, weakness, fatigue, dehydration, and stupor. This condition may be fatal and demands emergency treatment. Another, less common, but severe, complication of hypercalcemia is acute pancreatitis.[89,94–96] Clinical findings include hypertension, nausea, and vomiting; the last of these may be mistaken for hyperemesis gravidarum.[89,94–96] Patients with persistent vomiting must be hydrated rapidly to prevent worsening of the hypercalcemia from dehydration. In general, pregnancy has an ameliorating effect on hypercalcemia because of the shunting of calcium from the mother to the fetus. This may lead to dramatic worsening and even hypercalcemic crisis after delivery when such shunting is lost.[94–96]

Infants of mothers with hypercalcemia have a 15% to 25% risk of severe hypocalcemia with or without tetany, as well as a risk of spontaneous abortion (8%), premature birth (10%), stillbirth (2%), and neonatal death (2%).[89,94–96] The neonatal hypocalcemia results from the placental transfer of elevated calcium levels with resulting suppression of the fetal parathyroid glands. At delivery, the calcium transfer stops, but the involuted parathyroid glands cannot maintain adequate calcium levels. The hypocalcemia generally is transient, lasting as long as 3 to 5 months; it can be managed with calcium and vitamin D supplementation.[89,94–96]

Because of the potential hazards to both mother and child, all patients with known primary hyperparathyroidism should undergo surgery before conceiving. Major difficulties arise when hyperparathyroidism is diagnosed during gestation. The literature[96] was reviewed to compare the outcome of surgery with that of expectant therapy for this condition. Among 12 patients operated on between 1975 and 1987, one fetal death occurred (in a mother who had severe hypercalcemic crisis with pancreatitis [calcium level 19 mg/dL] and who underwent emergency neck exploration) but no other instances of fetal complications were seen. Mothers and fetuses usually tolerate parathyroidectomy well. Among 15 patients treated either expectantly or with oral phosphates over this period, no fetal deaths occurred but six instances of neonatal hypocalcemia were seen. Treatment with oral phosphate (Fleet Phospho-Soda, 15–50 mL per day in divided doses) has been used to control hypercalcemia when it is discovered late in gestation.[89,94–96] A reasonable course is to reserve surgery for patients who do not achieve stable calcium levels with oral phosphate.[89,94–96] Close follow-up is necessary for such patients, with calcium level determinations every 2 to 4 weeks. If hypocalcemia develops in the neonate, it generally can be treated easily.

In patients with severe hypercalcemia (calcium level >14 mg/dL or obtundation), initial therapy consists of adequate rehydration with saline. Furosemide may be added to increase calcium excretion further. Glucocorticoids and oral phosphate may be given during pregnancy, but the safety of other agents (e.g., pamidronate, gallium, plicamycin) has not been established.

## HYPOCALCEMIA

The most common cause of hypocalcemia is hypoparathyroidism secondary to surgery performed for hyperparathyroidism or thyroid disease. Idiopathic, autoimmune, and infiltrative causes are rare. Vitamin D deficiency and other causes also are extremely uncommon.

Maternal hypocalcemia results in inadequate transfer of calcium to the fetus, with consequent fetal hypocalcemia. This fetal hypocalcemia stimulates the fetal parathyroids and may cause generalized skeletal demineralization, subperiosteal resorption, and even osteitis fibrosa cystica.[97]

Because of the continued drain of calcium from the mother by the fetus, increased dosages of calcium and vitamin D may be necessary to maintain normal maternal calcium levels. The dosage of 1,25-dihydroxyvitamin D may need to be increased as much as four- to six-fold over the course of gestation.[98] Dosage adjustments should be made to keep the serum calcium level in the normal range. The fetus can tolerate large changes in 1,25-dihydroxyvitamin D dosage. In one reported case of a woman receiving 1,25-dihydroxyvitamin D at a dosage of 17 to 36 μg per day because of hereditary insensitivity to 1,25-dihydroxyvitamin D, considerable transplacental passage of this compound occurred, resulting in 20-fold elevation in cord blood levels. Despite such levels, the neonate had only minimal and transient hypercalcemia and showed no other abnormalities.[99] As in the treatment of hypoparathyroidism in nonpregnant individuals, use of 1,25-dihydroxyvitamin D is preferable to use of vitamin $D_3$ itself because of the rapidity of its onset and offset of action, which allows more precise modulation of serum calcium levels (see Chap. 60).

## ADRENAL CORTEX AND PREGNANCY

Cortisol levels rise progressively over the course of gestation, resulting in a two- to three-fold increase by term[100] (Fig. 110-5). Most of the elevation of cortisol levels is due to the estrogen-induced increase in cortisol-binding globulin levels,[101] but the bioactive "free" fraction also is elevated three-fold and the cortisol production rate is increased.[100,101] This is reflected in two- to three-fold elevations in urinary free cortisol levels.[100,101]

ACTH levels have been variously reported as being normal, suppressed, or elevated early in gestation.[100,102] During pregnancy, a progressive rise is seen, followed by a final surge of ACTH and cortisol levels during labor.[100] ACTH does not cross

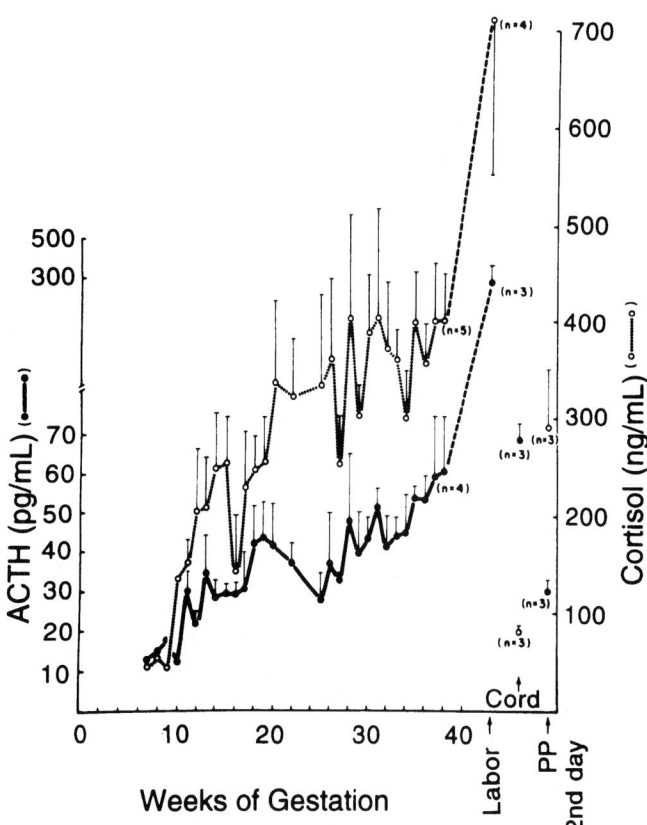

**FIGURE 110-5.** Mean plasma concentrations (± standard error) of adrenocorticotropic hormone (*ACTH*) and cortisol during normal pregnancy. Blood samples were obtained from five normal pregnant women weekly at 8:00 to 9:00 a.m. and from three women during labor and on the second postpartum (*PP*) day. In addition, umbilical cord plasma was obtained from the newborn infants of three of these subjects. The mean plasma concentrations for ACTH are denoted by the solid circles; plasma cortisol levels are denoted by open circles. (From Carr BR, Parker CT Jr, Madden JD, et al. Maternal plasma adrenocorticotropin and cortisol relationships throughout human pregnancy. Am J Obstet Gynecol 1981; 139:416.)

the placenta but is manufactured by the placenta.[102] The amounts of ACTH in serum that are of placental as compared to pituitary origin at various stages of gestation are not known. Corticotropin-releasing hormone (CRH) is also produced by the placenta and is released into maternal plasma.[103] The CRH is bioactive and may release ACTH both from the placenta, in a paracrine fashion, and from the maternal pituitary[103] (although the latter source is not absolutely proven).

## CUSHING SYNDROME DURING PREGNANCY

Just under 100 cases of Cushing syndrome in pregnancy have been reported.[104–110] The distribution of causes in pregnant women differs from that in the nonpregnant population. Less than 50% of the patients described had pituitary adenomas, a similar number had adrenal adenomas, and 10% had adrenal carcinomas.[104–110] Only one report described a pregnancy associated with the ectopic ACTH syndrome.[106] In many cases, the hypercortisolism first became apparent during pregnancy, with improvement after parturition; this leads to the speculation that unregulated placental CRH was instrumental in causing this pregnancy-induced exacerbation.[105,106]

Diagnosing Cushing syndrome during pregnancy may be difficult. Both conditions may be associated with weight gain in a central distribution, fatigue, edema, emotional upset, glucose intolerance, and hypertension. The striae associated with the weight gain and increased abdominal girth are usually white in normal pregnancy and red or purple in Cushing syndrome. Hirsutism and acne may point to excessive androgen production.

The laboratory evaluation of Cushing syndrome during pregnancy is not straightforward. Elevated total and free serum cortisol and ACTH levels, and urinary free cortisol excretion are compatible with that of normal pregnancy. The overnight dexamethasone test usually demonstrates inadequate suppression during normal pregnancy.[107] At least in the latter part of the third trimester, the elevated cortisol levels are not suppressed during the low-dose dexamethasone test but are suppressed during the high-dose test, as in patients with Cushing disease.[105] ACTH levels are normal to elevated in pregnant patients with all forms of Cushing syndrome.[104–110] These "normal" rather than suppressed levels of ACTH in patients with adrenal adenomas may result from the production of ACTH by the placenta or from the nonsuppressible stimulation of pituitary ACTH by placental CRH.

A persistent circadian variation in the elevated levels of total and free serum cortisol during normal pregnancy may be most helpful in distinguishing Cushing syndrome from the hypercortisolism of pregnancy, because this finding is characteristically absent in all forms of Cushing syndrome.[101] In many cases, radiologic imaging is necessary. An adrenal mass often is visible with ultrasonography; however, CT or MRI scanning of the pituitary or adrenal may be required. Most adrenal lesions are unilateral, so that localization is important. Little experience has been reported with newer techniques such as CRH stimulation testing or petrosal venous sinus sampling during pregnancy (see Chap. 75). However, in a case study, a woman with Cushing disease who had the typical exaggerated ACTH response to CRH experienced no ill effects from such testing.[108] CRH testing during petrosal sinus sampling was performed without ill effects in a woman at 14 weeks' gestation, but catheterization was performed via the direct internal jugular vein approach rather than the femoral vein approach to minimize fetal irradiation.[111]

Cushing syndrome is associated with a fetal mortality of 25% due to spontaneous abortion, stillbirth, and early neonatal death because of extreme prematurity.[104–110] Premature labor occurs in >50% of cases, regardless of etiology.[104–110] The passage of cortisol across the placenta occasionally results in suppression of the fetal adrenals.[112] This appears to be uncommon, but the neonate should be tested for this potential problem and given exogenous corticosteroids until the results of the evaluation are known.

Maternal complications also may occur. Hypertension develops in most patients. Diabetes and myopathy are frequent. Postoperative wound infection and dehiscence are common after cesarean section. The pregnancy appears to induce an amelioration of Cushing syndrome in some patients, but an exacerbation in others.[104–110]

In data from the literature summarized in two reviews,[104,107] fetal loss rates of 9% and 24%, and premature labor rates of 20% and 47% were found in the 11 and 17 women, respectively, who were treated during pregnancy; in comparison, fetal loss rates were 30% and 38%, and premature labor rates were 48% and 72% in the 26 and 43 women, respectively, in whom treatment was delayed. Therefore, treatment during pregnancy has been advocated.

Medical therapy for Cushing syndrome during pregnancy is not effective.[106,107,110] A few case reports have documented the efficacy of metyrapone therapy. No experience exists with other agents, such as ketoconazole or aminoglutethimide.

Surgical removal of an adrenal adenoma through a flank incision can be performed safely even early in the third trimester.[104,106,107,110] Because of the high incidence of adrenal carcinomas among adrenal masses, and their poor prognosis, early surgery may offer additional benefit to the mother. Transsphenoidal resection of a pituitary ACTH-secreting adenoma has

been carried out successfully at 22 weeks of gestation.[105] Transsphenoidal surgery has been performed for an expanding prolactinoma many times during pregnancy with no untoward consequences. Although any surgery poses risks for the mother and fetus, with Cushing syndrome, the risks of not operating appear to be considerably higher than the risks of proceeding with surgery (see Chaps. 23, 75, and 89).

## ADRENAL INSUFFICIENCY DURING PREGNANCY

Primary adrenal insufficiency uncommonly presents during pregnancy.[113] Secondary adrenal insufficiency may be seen in patients with pituitary lesions or those in whom the hypothalamic–pituitary–adrenal axis has been suppressed by exogenous glucocorticoids.

During the first trimester, the features commonly associated with adrenal insufficiency, including fatigue, nausea, and vomiting, may be difficult to distinguish. However, the persistence of these symptoms in association with weight loss should at least prompt a screening diagnostic evaluation. Increased pigmentation similar to that seen with increased ACTH and lipotropin levels also may occur during normal pregnancy. Mild cases of adrenal insufficiency may go undetected during pregnancy, only to progress to adrenal crisis with the stress of labor or other illness, such as urinary tract infection.[113] In some cases, severe adrenal insufficiency may not develop until the postpartum period, possibly due to maintenance of maternal cortisol levels by fetal adrenal production.[114] Maternal adrenal insufficiency has been associated with fetal growth retardation.[114]

If the signs, symptoms, and laboratory data suggest adrenal insufficiency, diagnostic and therapeutic procedures should be carried out quickly and simultaneously. A blood sample should be obtained for serum cortisol and ACTH measurements, and an ACTH (cosyntropin) stimulation test should be performed. The cortisol level should be inappropriately low for the stage of pregnancy. ACTH levels are elevated if the disease is primary, but may not be low in acquired hypopituitarism, because of placental production. However, placental production of ACTH is not sufficient to maintain normal adrenal function in these circumstances, and patients may die of secondary adrenal insufficiency, especially in the setting of lymphocytic hypophysitis.

Patients with previously diagnosed adrenal insufficiency will have been stabilized on glucocorticoid therapy before conceiving. Because of the known increased cortisol production rate during pregnancy, the dosage theoretically should be increased. However, this does not seem to be necessary in most patients. Additional glucocorticoids are needed in times of stress, such as during labor and delivery. Patients who have what appears to be acute adrenal crisis are treated in essentially the same way as patients who are not pregnant (i.e., with high doses of intravenous hydrocortisone and fluids).

Patients who have received greater than physiologic replacement doses of glucocorticoids as antiinflammatory therapy for >1 month should be considered to have insufficient adrenal function for as long as 1 year after such treatment is discontinued.[115] With steroid treatment of <1 month, >90% recover their adrenal responsiveness within 2 weeks.[115a] These patients should be given high doses of corticosteroids during labor and delivery. They also are subject to the postoperative difficulties experienced by patients with endogenous Cushing syndrome, including the development of transient adrenal insufficiency in the neonate (see earlier). Although there is some suggestion of an increased risk of cleft palate in infants born of mothers who have received pharmacologic doses of corticosteroids before the 14th week of gestation, this risk is <1%, and whether a cause-and-effect relationship truly exists is difficult to know. A review of the literature suggests that corticosteroid use during pregnancy is safe; prednisone, but not prednisolone, appears to cross the placenta readily.[116] Suppression of neonatal adrenal function in offspring of women taking prednisone during pregnancy is uncommon.[117] Glucocorticoids also may pass to the neonate in breast milk, but in amounts (0.14% of maternal blood levels) that are not sufficient to alter neonatal adrenal function, even with large maternal doses of prednisone[118] (see Chap. 76).

## CONGENITAL ADRENAL HYPERPLASIA DURING PREGNANCY

Ninety percent to 95% of patients with congenital adrenal hyperplasia have 21-hydroxylase deficiency[119,120] (see Chap. 77). Menarche is often delayed.[121,122] In one series of such women desiring pregnancy, the fertility rate was 64%.[121] Of the 15 pregnancies reported in this group, there were 8 full-term deliveries, 2 premature deliveries (one normal infant and another with multiple skeletal anomalies and a meningomyelocele who died of sepsis at 2 weeks of age), 2 elective terminations, and 3 spontaneous abortions. A trial of labor is warranted. However, in all the full-term pregnancies, cesarean section was required because of cephalopelvic disproportion. Glucocorticoid replacement dosages were not altered during these pregnancies except for an increase during labor and delivery. In patients with non-classic (late-onset) 21-hydroxylase deficiency who have hirsutism, sterility, or irregular menses, successful pregnancy is often possible without glucocorticoid treatment. However, fertility may improve with glucocorticoid treatment, with a tendency toward a decrease in spontaneous abortions.[123]

Adequate suppression of adrenal androgens in a fetus with classic, virilizing 21-hydroxylase deficiency is important. Virilization of the fetus does not appear to occur with the nonclassic variety of the disorder.[124] In fetuses with classic 21-hydroxylase deficiency, successful suppression of fetal androgen production in the first trimester requires the administration of dexamethasone to the mother, 1.5 mg per day in two or three divided doses, beginning at approximately the fifth week of gestation.[125] Maternal cortisol and estriol levels are measured to monitor compliance. Only 25% of female fetuses are affected in any family with congenital adrenal hyperplasia, so therapy should be discontinued as soon as possible to avoid suppressing the adrenal glands of unaffected females and males. This requires making the diagnosis in utero. When it is available, chorionic villus sampling for karyotyping, determination of sex, and direct molecular analysis of the 21-hydroxylase locus should be performed at 8 to 10 weeks of gestation to determine whether the fetus is an affected female.[119,120,125] When this test is not available, dexamethasone should be withheld for 5 days and 17-OH progesterone and androstenedione levels should be measured in amniotic fluid that has been obtained by amniocentesis at 16 to 18 weeks of gestation.[125] Side effects of dexamethasone therapy are significant, consisting of excessive weight gain, severe striae resulting in permanent scarring, gestational diabetes, hypertension, gastrointestinal intolerance, and severe irritability.[126] Lowering the dosage of dexamethasone to 0.75 to 1.0 mg per day in the second half of pregnancy has been advocated to decrease maternal side effects while still maintaining activity against virilization in the fetus.[126]

## PRIMARY HYPERALDOSTERONISM DURING PREGNANCY

Primary hyperaldosteronism has been reported in only 20 pregnant women.[127–130] Although the elevated aldosterone levels found in pregnant patients with these tumors are similar to those found in normal pregnant women, plasma renin activity is suppressed rather than elevated.[127–130]

During pregnancy, the normally increased basal aldosterone levels are appropriately suppressed by salt loading,[112] so these maneuvers have diagnostic utility.[127–130] If the results of base-

line serum renin and aldosterone determinations or of suppression tests are equivocal, or if CT or MRI scanning does not suggest unilateral disease, the recommendation has been to treat these patients medically until delivery, when more definitive isotope scanning can be done, and when aldosterone and renin levels should fall.[129] In the nonpregnant individual, the usual medical therapy is with spironolactone, an aldosterone antagonist. However, spironolactone can cross the placenta; it is a potent antiandrogen and may cause abnormal development of the genitalia.[130] Therefore, spironolactone use is contraindicated during pregnancy. If the hypertension responds to other agents that are safe to use during pregnancy, surgery for an adenoma may be deferred to the postpartum period. In any event, gestation sometimes ameliorates the potassium-losing aspect of the disease, perhaps because of the high levels of progesterone that are present in the circulation during pregnancy.[131] If the hypertension cannot be controlled, surgery may be necessary (see Chap. 80).

# PHEOCHROMOCYTOMA AND PREGNANCY

Some patients with pheochromocytoma have such infrequent episodes that suspicion of the condition first arises with an increase in blood pressure during the induction of anesthesia, during labor, or during surgery. Failure to recognize this possibility may result in the death of the patient. Some pregnant patients with pheochromocytoma have sudden shock that appears spontaneously or is induced by anesthesia or by labor and delivery.[132–135] Extraadrenal tumors, which constitute ~10% of cases, may provoke paroxysmal symptoms after particular activities. A frequent site is the organ of Zuckerkandl, located at the bifurcation of the aorta. The enlarging uterus may cause pressure on a tumor at this site, with hypertensive episodes occurring with changes in position, uterine contractions, fetal movement, and execution of Valsalva maneuvers.[136]

The rate of maternal mortality from undiagnosed pheochromocytoma is ~50%; the rate falls to 11% if the condition is diagnosed before delivery.[133–135] The rate of fetal loss is similar, even if the diagnosis is made during pregnancy.[133–135] Catecholamines cross the placenta only minimally,[133] and the fetus appears to be unaffected by the high maternal levels. However, some element of hypoxia, caused by vasoconstriction of the uterine vascular bed, may be present.[135]

## DIAGNOSIS OF PHEOCHROMOCYTOMA DURING PREGNANCY

The diagnosis of pheochromocytoma is established primarily by biochemical means and is presented in detail in Chapter 86. A key consideration in a pheochromocytoma occurring during pregnancy is differentiating it from preeclampsia. The onset of hypertension in the first two trimesters is not characteristic of preeclampsia. Careful evaluation will reveal the absence of proteinuria, edema, or hyperuricemia. Urinary and plasma epinephrine and norepinephrine levels are normal in uncomplicated pregnancy,[137–139] as well as in preeclampsia.[137] However, urinary and plasma catecholamine levels may be elevated two- to four-fold for >24 hours after a seizure in eclampsia.[140] Therefore, to make a diagnosis in a pregnant woman who does not have eclampsia, a 24-hour urine collection can be analyzed for vanillylmandelic acid and fractionated metanephrines and catecholamines, as in a nonpregnant patient. Because stimulation tests have been associated with fetal demise, their use has been discouraged.[133–135]

Once the diagnosis has been established by biochemical means, efforts should be made to localize the tumor. Both CT and MRI scanning are excellent in detecting the presence of tumors. Isotopic scanning with [131]I-metaiodobenzylguanidine (I-MIBG) generally is contraindicated during pregnancy. However, if the clinical and biochemical indications are strong, and the tumor cannot be localized by other techniques, this scan may be necessary because of the significant risks to the mother and fetus associated with delaying operation.

## TREATMENT OF PHEOCHROMOCYTOMA DURING PREGNANCY

Once the diagnosis of pheochromocytoma has been made, long-term α-adrenergic blockade should be initiated with phenoxybenzamine, as for nonpregnant patients. No reports have been published of teratogenesis with α-blockers, and the fetus appears to tolerate these medications well.[133,141] If treatment with phenoxybenzamine does not lower the blood pressure satisfactorily, metyrosine, a substance that interferes with catecholamine synthesis, may prove helpful and has been used in one pregnant patient with a pheochromocytoma with no apparent ill effects on the fetus.[141] However, because this drug interrupts normal catecholamine synthesis, it cannot be considered free of adverse effects on the fetus on the basis of one case. Nevertheless, because of the potentially lethal nature of an uncontrolled pheochromocytoma, the use of metyrosine in this circumstance is justified. If arrhythmias or severe tachycardia is a problem, propranolol can be added in dosages of 10 to 40 mg four times a day after the establishment of α-blockade. If hypertensive emergencies occur, they can be treated with intravenous administration of phentolamine or nitroprusside. The prolonged use of nitroprusside should be avoided because fetal cyanide toxicity may ensue.

When the patient is medically stabilized, surgery to remove the tumor should be considered. No definitive data exist to guide the timing of surgery for pheochromocytoma. Surgery before 24 weeks of gestation has been recommended.[133,142] Because surgery could result in premature labor, after 24 weeks prolonged medical therapy has been advised until the fetus is viable, at which time combined cesarean section and exploration for the pheochromocytoma could be done.[133–135,142] A commonsense approach might be to locate the tumor and determine how well the patient responds to medical therapy. A tumor at the organ of Zuckerkandl might be expected to become progressively more difficult to manage as the uterus continues to enlarge. A patient who is monitored closely and responds well to medical therapy might be maintained until fetal viability is achieved. Any patient in whom the condition is difficult to control should undergo surgery more quickly. The intraoperative and postoperative care of the patient with pheochromocytoma is discussed in Chapter 89.

## OBESITY AND PREGNANCY

Obese individuals are at increased risk for hypertension, diabetes mellitus, hypertriglyceridemia, and coronary artery disease, all of which may affect the health of a pregnant woman (see Chap. 126). Operative wound infections and dehiscence, and postoperative thromboembolic disease also are more common among these patients.

In patients with morbid obesity (>100 lb overweight or >200% of ideal body weight), respiratory impairment, which may be a major source of morbidity, takes three forms. The first is directly related to increased chest wall and abdominal fat, and consists of a reduction in lung and chest wall compliance. In an ambulatory setting, these patients do not retain carbon dioxide, but they may be slightly hypoxic, especially when supine.[143] After abdominal surgery, such as a cesarean section, massively obese patients have a further reduction in arterial partial pressure of oxygen ($PaO_2$), with the nadir appearing on the second postoperative day.[143] A much smaller group of massively obese patients have hypoventilation, hypercapnia,

hypoxia, somnolence, and markedly reduced lung compliance—a constellation of findings that has been referred to as the *pickwickian syndrome*. Finally, some patients with obesity develop upper airway obstruction when asleep (or sedated) and have hypoxia and even apnea.

These concerns have important implications for obese women who become pregnant. Several series reporting data in such women have been published. In women in the top fifth percentile for weight (>90 kg at term), the incidence of hypertension and gestational diabetes was increased two- to eightfold.[144–146] Slight increases also were noted in the rates of other complications, including thrombophlebitis, preeclampsia, urinary tract infection, and infection of an episiotomy or other wound.[144–146] Although an increased rate of respiratory complications related to the influence of the expanding uterine contents on an already impaired respiratory apparatus would be expected, this was not found in these series.[144–146] The rate of cesarean section was increased in these women in one series,[146] but not in the other two.[144,145] Thus, obese women should be screened periodically for gestational diabetes and monitored carefully for the development of hypertension, urinary tract infection, and preeclampsia. For obese women with complicated deliveries who may remain at bed rest for extended periods, prophylactic subcutaneous heparin may be indicated. In massively obese women, care also must be taken to prevent respiratory compromise.

Fetal complication rates also are increased by maternal obesity. Birth weights are higher, and this is not due to the associated gestational diabetes.[144–146] Follow-up shows that, at 12 months, the infants of obese mothers are significantly more obese than the infants of nonobese mothers.[145] Increased shoulder dystocia, meconium, and late deceleration during labor also are noted.[146] Although one series found an increase in perinatal mortality due to obesity,[146] this was not found in the other two series.[144,145]

Estimates are that 40,000 to 80,000 additional calories are required during pregnancy.[147] The normal, nonobese woman usually gains little during the first trimester, 0.36 kg per week between weeks 13 and 18, 0.45 kg per week between weeks 18 and 28, and 0.36 kg per week between week 28 and term.[147] Of the recommended 9- to 13.5-kg weight gain during pregnancy, ~3.6 kg is actually maternal fat.[147] Many obese women resist diets that cause them to gain the recommended amount of weight during pregnancy, and 10% to 40% gain <5.4 kg.[147] This may not be harmful, however, because the birth weights of term infants of obese mothers who actually lose weight are greater than the birth weights of term infants of normal-weight mothers who gain the recommended amount of weight.[147] Thus, obese mothers may be able to mobilize nutrient stores and transmit nutrients to the fetus better than normal-weight women, who generally would have infants with fetal growth restriction if their weight gain was inadequate. Because of these findings, a weight gain of 4.5 to 9.0 kg has been recommended for obese women, although careful attention to fetal growth through serial ultrasonographic measurements is necessary.[147] Strenuous efforts may be required to prevent excessive weight gain, because it only exacerbates the risks of gestational diabetes and hypertension, and results in more permanent weight gain.

## LIPID DISORDERS AND PREGNANCY

Total serum cholesterol and low-density lipoprotein (LDL) cholesterol levels begin to rise at the end of the first trimester and eventually reach levels ~150% above prepregnancy levels[148] (see Chaps. 162 through 166). High-density lipoprotein (HDL) cholesterol levels increase by 25% to 45% within the first trimester and then decline nearly to prepregnancy levels by term.[148] Triglyceride levels begin to rise toward the end of the first trimester and continue to increase, reaching levels three-fold greater than prepregnancy levels by term.[148] In patients with preexisting elevations of LDL cholesterol, the increases during pregnancy are exaggerated.[148] Although an initial fall in LDL cholesterol and triglycerides occurs within the first few days postpartum, levels may not return completely to their prepregnancy status for several weeks to months.[148]

The changes in the hormonal milieu that occur with pregnancy appear to be responsible for the elevated lipid fractions, with the increase in triglycerides correlating with estriol levels, the increase in HDL cholesterol correlating with levels of estradiol and progesterone, and the level of LDL cholesterol correlating negatively with progesterone level.[148] The rate of lipolysis of the elevated triglycerides increases, and the resultant increase in free fatty acids results in their increased transport across the placenta to serve as nutrient substrate for the fetus.[148]

In patients with gestational, non–insulin-dependent and insulin-dependent diabetes, the increases in triglycerides are exaggerated, and HDL cholesterol levels are reduced even further.[148]

Most patients with preexisting dyslipidemias who are being treated with medications have their therapy discontinued for the duration of pregnancy and rely on dietary modification alone. Inhibitors of 3-hydroxy-3-methyl glutaryl-coenzyme A (HMG-CoA) reductase are contraindicated during pregnancy because of the potential for impairing fetal neural lipid synthesis. The safety of nicotinic acid therapy during pregnancy is not established, and because of its potential to cause hepatic toxicity and insulin resistance, it should not be used. The safety of gemfibrozil also has not been established. Although no toxicity has been seen when it is given to pregnant rats, it has been shown to be tumorigenic in rats and, therefore, should not be used unless absolutely necessary. Because bile acid–binding resins are not absorbed, they may be given, although care must be taken to avoid vitamin K deficiency.

Rarely, severe hypertriglyceridemia (2000–10,000 mg/dL) may occur during gestation due to a combination of lipoprotein lipase deficiency and the increased triglyceride production of pregnancy.[149] The hypertriglyceridemia may lead to pancreatitis, which carries a 20% rate of maternal mortality.[149] In such situations, drastic dietary fat restriction occasionally is successful, but patients sometimes must be treated with total parenteral nutrition, plasma exchange, or lipoprotein apheresis.[149,150]

## REFERENCES

1. Lindheimer MD, Davison JM. Osmoregulation, the secretion of arginine vasopressin and its metabolism during pregnancy. Eur J Endocrinol 1995; 132:133.
2. Durr JA. Diabetes insipidus in pregnancy. Am J Kidney Dis 1987; 9:276.
3. Davison JM, Shiells EA, Barron WM, et al. Changes in the metabolic clearance of vasopressin and of plasma vasopressinase throughout human pregnancy. J Clin Invest 1989; 83:1313.
4. Soule SG, Monson JP, Jacobs HS. Transient diabetes insipidus in pregnancy—a consequence of enhanced placental clearance of arginine vasopressin. Hum Reprod 1995; 10:3322.
5. Barron WM, Cohen LH, Ulland LA, et al. Transient vasopressin-resistant diabetes insipidus of pregnancy. N Engl J Med 1984; 310:442.
6. Källén BAJ, Carlsson SS, Bengtsson BKA. Diabetes insipidus and use of desmopressin (Minirin) during pregnancy. Eur J Endocrinol 1995; 132:144.
7. Hawker RW, North WG, Colbert IC, Lang LP. Oxytocin blood levels in two cases of diabetes insipidus. Br J Obstet Gynaecol 1987; 74:430.
8. Kennedy S, Hall PM, Seymour AE, Hague WM. Transient diabetes insipidus and acute fatty liver of pregnancy. Br J Obstet Gynaecol 1994; 101:387.
9. Raziel A, Rosenberg T, Schreyer P, et al. Transient postpartum diabetes insipidus. Am J Obstet Gynecol 1991; 164:616.
10. Goluboff LG, Ezrin C. Effect of pregnancy on the somatotroph and the prolactin cell of the human adenohypophysis. J Clin Endocrinol Metab 1969; 29:1533.
11. Rigg LA, Lein A, Yen SSC. Pattern of increase in circulating prolactin levels during human gestation. Am J Obstet Gynecol 1977; 129:454.
12. Frankenne F, Closset J, Gomez F, et al. The physiology of growth hormones (GHs) in pregnant women and partial characterization of the placental GH variant. J Clin Endocrinol Metab 1988; 66:1171.
13. Eriksson L, Frankenne F, Eden S, et al. Growth hormone 24-h serum profiles during pregnancy—lack of pulsatility for the secretion of the placental variant. Br J Obstet Gynaecol 1989; 106:949.
14. Beckers A, Stevenaert A, Foidart J-M, et al. Placental and pituitary growth hormone secretion during pregnancy in acromegalic women. J Clin Endocrinol Metab 1990; 71:725.
15. Kredentser JV, Hoskins CF, Scott JZ. Hyperprolactinemia: a significant factor in female infertility. Am J Obstet Gynecol 1981; 139:264.
16. Molitch ME. Diagnosis and treatment of prolactinomas. Adv Intern Med 1999; 44:117.
17. Webster J, Piscitelli G, Polli A, et al. A comparison of cabergoline and bromocriptine in the treatment of hyperprolactinemic amenorrhea. N Engl J Med 1994; 331:904.
18. Biller BMK, Molitch ME, Vance ML, et al. Treatment of prolactin-secreting macroadenomas with the once-weekly dopamine agonist cabergoline. J Clin Endocrinol Metab 1996; 81:2338.
19. Verhelst J, Abs R, Maiter D, et al. Cabergoline in the treatment of hyperprolactinemia. J Clin Endocrinol Metab 1999; 84:2518.
20. Molitch ME. Management of prolactinomas during pregnancy. J Reprod Med 1999; 44:1121.
21. Krupp P, Monka C, Richter K. The safety aspects of infertility treatments. In: Program of the Second World Congress of Gynecology and Obstetrics, Rio de Janeiro, Brazil, 1988:9.
22. Bigazzi M, Ronga R, Lancranjan I, et al. A pregnancy in an acromegalic woman during bromocriptine treatment: effects on growth hormone and prolactin in the maternal, fetal, and amniotic compartments. J Clin Endocrinol Metab 1979; 48:9.
23. Robert E, Musatti L, Piscitelli G, Ferrari CI. Pregnancy outcome after treatment with the ergot derivative, cabergoline. Reprod Toxicol 1996; 10:333.
24. Divers WA, Yen SSC. Prolactin-producing microadenomas in pregnancy. Obstet Gynecol 1983; 62:425.
25. Corenblum B, Donovan L. The safety of physiological estrogen plus progestin replacement therapy and with oral contraceptive therapy in women with pathological hyperprolactinemia. Fertil Steril 1993; 59:671.
26. Kupersmith MJ, Rosenberg C, Kleinberg D. Visual loss in pregnant women with pituitary adenomas. Ann Intern Med 1994; 121:473.
27. Herman-Bonert V, Seliverstow M, Melmed S. Pregnancy in acromegaly: successful therapeutic outcome. J Clin Endocrinol Metab 1998; 83:727.
28. Molitch ME. Clinical manifestations of acromegaly. Endocrinol Metab Clin North Am 1992; 21:597.
29. Barkan AL, Stred SE, Reno K, et al. Increased growth hormone pulse frequency in acromegaly. J Clin Endocrinol Metab 1989; 69:1225.
30. Okada Y, Morimoto I, Ejima K, et al. A case of active acromegalic woman with a marked increase in serum insulin-like growth factor-1 levels after delivery. Endocr J 1997; 44:117.
31. Landolt AM, Schmid J, Wimpfheimer C, et al. Successful pregnancy in a previously infertile woman treated with SMS 201-995 for acromegaly. N Engl J Med 1989; 320:671.
32. Montini M, Pagani G, Gianola D, et al. Acromegaly and primary amenorrhea: ovulation and pregnancy induced by SMS 201-995 and bromocriptine. J Endocrinol Invest 1990; 13:193.
33. Caron P, Gerbeau C, Pradayrol L, et al. Successful pregnancy in an infertile woman with a thyrotropin-secreting macroadenoma treated with somatostatin analog (octreotide). J Clin Endocrinol Metab 1996; 81:1164.
34. Sheehan HL, Davis JC. Pituitary necrosis. Br Med Bull 1968; 24:59.
35. Ozbey N, Inanc S, Aral F, et al. Clinical and laboratory evaluation of 40 patients with Sheehan's syndrome. Isr J Med Sci 1994; 30:826.
36. Bakiri F, Bendib S-E, Maoui R, et al. The sella turcica in Sheehan's syndrome: computerized tomographic study in 54 patients. J Endocrinol Invest 1991; 14:193.
37. Sheehan HL. The neurohypophysis in post-partum hypopituitarism. J Pathol Bacteriol 1963; 85:145.
38. Whitehead R. The hypothalamus in post-partum hypopituitarism. J Pathol Bacteriol 1963; 86:55.
39. Iwasaki Y, Oiso Y, Yamauchi K, et al. Neurohypophyseal function in post-partum hypopituitarism: impaired plasma vasopressin response to osmotic stimuli. J Clin Endocrinol Metab 1989; 68:560.
40. Pressman EK, Zeidman SM, Reddy UM, et al. Differentiating lymphocytic adenohypophysitis from pituitary adenoma in the peripartum patient. J Reprod Med 1995; 40:251.
41. Thodou E, Asa SL, Kontogeorgos G, et al. Lymphocytic hypophysitis: clinicopathological findings. J Clin Endocrinol Metab 1995; 80:2302.
42. Burrow GN. Thyroid function and hyperfunction during gestation. Endocr Rev 1993; 14:194.
43. Glinoer D, De Nayer P, Bourdoux P, et al. Regulation of maternal thyroid during pregnancy. J Clin Endocrinol Metab 1990; 71:276.
44. Momotani N, Hisaoka T, Noh J, et al. Effects of iodine on thyroid status of fetus versus mother in treatment of Graves disease complicated by pregnancy. J Clin Endocrinol Metab 1992; 75:738.
45. Levy RP, Newman DM, Rejai LS, et al. The myth of goiter in pregnancy. Am J Obstet Gynecol 1980; 137:701.
46. Long TJ, Felice ME, Hollingsworth DR. Goiter in pregnant teenagers. Am J Obstet Gynecol 1985; 152:670.

47. Thorpe-Beeston JF, Nicoladies KH, Felton CV, et al. Maturation of the secretion of thyroid hormone and thyroid-stimulating hormone in the fetus. N Engl J Med 1991; 324:532.
48. Utiger RD. Recognition of thyroid disease in the fetus. N Engl J Med 1991; 324:550.
49. Nicolini U, Venegoni E, Acaia B, et al. Prenatal treatment of hypothyroidism: is there more than one option? Prenat Diagn 1996; 16:443.
50. Goodwin TM, Hershman JM. Hyperthyroidism due to inappropriate production of human chorionic gonadotropin. Clin Obstet Gynecol 1997; 40:32.
51. Harada K, Hershman JM, Reed AW, et al. Comparison of thyroid stimulators and thyroid hormone concentrations in the sera of pregnant women. J Clin Endocrinol Metab 1979; 48:793.
52. Mestman JH. Hyperthyroidism in pregnancy. Clin Obstet Gynecol 1997; 40:45.
53. Millar LK, Wing DA, Leung AS, et al. Low birth weight and preeclampsia in pregnancies complicated by hyperthyroidism. Obstet Gynecol 1994; 84:946.
54. Van Dijke CP, Heydendael RJ, De Kleine MJ. Methimazole, carbimazole, and congenital skin defects. Ann Intern Med 1987; 106:60.
55. Mitsuda N, Tamaki H, Amino N, et al. Risk factors for developmental disorders in infants born to women with Graves disease. Obstet Gynecol 1992; 80:359.
56. Marchant B, Brownlie BEW, Hart DM, et al. The placental transfer of propylthiouracil, methimazole and carbimazole. J Clin Endocrinol Metab 1977; 45:1187.
57. Wing DA, Millar LK, Koonings PP, et al. A comparison of propylthiouracil versus methimazole in the treatment of hyperthyroidism in pregnancy. Am J Obstet Gynecol 1994; 170:90.
58. Momotani N, Noh JY, Ishikawa N, Ito K. Effects of propylthiouracil and methimazole on fetal thyroid status in mothers with Graves' hyperthyroidism. J Clin Endocrinol Metab 1997; 82:3633.
59. Messer MP, Hauffa BP, Olbricht T, et al. Antithyroid drug and Graves' disease in pregnancy. Long term effects on somatic growth, intellectual development and thyroid function of the offspring. Acta Endocrinol 1990; 123:311.
60. Magee LA, Ornstein MP, Von Dadel P. Management of hypertension in pregnancy. BMJ 1999; 318:1332.
61. Eriksson M, Rubenfeld S, Garber AJ, et al. Propranolol does not prevent thyroid storm. N Engl J Med 1977; 296:263.
62. Senior B, Chernoff HL. Iodide goiter in the newborn. Pediatrics 1971; 47:510.
63. Linden S, Rich CL. The use of lithium during pregnancy and lactation. J Clin Psychiatry 1983; 44:358.
64. Pekonen F, Lamberg B-A. Thyrotoxicosis during pregnancy. Ann Chir Gynaecol 1978; 67:165.
65. Brodsky JB, Cohen EN, Brown BW, et al. Surgery during pregnancy and fetal outcome. Am J Obstet Gynecol 1980; 138:1165.
66. Swaminathan R, Chin RK, Lao TTH, et al. Thyroid function in hyperemesis gravidarum. Acta Endocrinol (Copenh) 1989; 120:155.
67. Goodwin TM, Montoro M, Mestman J. Transient hyperthyroidism and hyperemesis gravidarum: clinical aspects. Am J Obstet Gynecol 1992; 167:648.
68. Goodwin TM, Montoro M, Mestman JH, et al. The role of chorionic gonadotropin in transient hyperthyroidism of hyperemesis gravidarum. J Clin Endocrinol Metab 1992; 75:1333.
69. Rodien P, Brémont C, Sanson M-LR, et al. Familial gestational hyperthyroidism caused by a mutant thyrotropin receptor hypersensitive to human chorionic gonadotropin. N Engl J Med 1998; 339:1823.
70. Hatjis CG. Diagnosis and successful treatment of fetal goitrous hyperthyroidism caused by maternal Graves disease. Obstet Gynecol 1993; 81:837.
71. Rumble WF, Aamodt RL, Jones AE, et al. Case reports. Accidental ingestion of Tc-99m in breast milk by a 10-week-old child. J Nucl Med 1978; 19:913.
72. Cooper DS. Antithyroid drugs. To breast-feed or not to breast-feed. Am J Obstet Gynecol 1987; 157:234.
73. Leung AS, Millar LK, Koonings PP, et al. Perinatal outcome in hypothyroid pregnancies. Obstet Gynecol 1993; 81:349.
74. Wasserstrum N, Anania CA. Perinatal consequences of maternal hypothyroidism in early pregnancy and inadequate replacement. Clin Endocrinol 1995; 42:353.
75. Ladenson PW, Levin AN, Ridgway EC, et al. Complications of surgery in hypothyroid patients. Am J Med 1984; 77:261.
76. Wenzel KW, Kirschsieper HE. Aspects of the absorption of oral L-thyroxine in normal man. Metabolism 1977; 26:1.
77. Mandel SJ, Larsen PR, Seely EW, Brent GA. Increased need for thyroxine during pregnancy in women with primary hypothyroidism. N Engl J Med 1990; 323:91.
78. Campbell NRC, Hasinoff BB, Stalts H, et al. Ferrous sulfate reduces thyroxine efficacy in patients with hypothyroidism. Ann Intern Med 1992; 117:1010.
78a. Singh N, Singh PN, Hershman JM. Effect of calcium carbonate on the absorption of levothyroxine. JAMA 2000; 283:2822.
78b. Haddow JE, Palomak GE, Allan WC, et al. Maternal thyroid deficiency during pregnancy and subsequent neuropsychological development of the child. N Engl J Med 1999; 341:549.
79. Nikolai TF, Turney SL, Roberts RC. Postpartum lymphocytic thyroiditis. Prevalence, clinical course, and long-term follow-up. Arch Intern Med 1987; 147:221.
80. Lazarus JH, Hall R, Rothman S, et al. The clinical spectrum of postpartum thyroid disease. Q J Med 1996; 89:429.
81. Terry AJ, Hague WM. Postpartum thyroiditis. Semin Perinatol 1998; 22:497.
82. Gerstein HC. Incidence of postpartum thyroid dysfunction in patients with type I diabetes mellitus. Ann Intern Med 1993; 118:419.
83. Roti E, Minelli R, Gardini E, et al. Impaired intrathyroidal iodine organification and iodine-induced hypothyroidism in euthyroid women with a previous episode of postpartum thyroiditis. J Clin Endocrinol Metab 1991; 73:958.
84. Othman S, Phillips DIW, Parkes AB, et al. A long-term follow-up of postpartum thyroiditis. Clin Endocrinol (Oxf) 1990; 32:559.
85. Molitch ME, Beck JR, Dreisman M, et al. The cold thyroid nodule. An analysis of diagnostic and therapeutic options. Endocr Rev 1984; 5:185.
86. Herzon FS, Morris DM, Segal MN, et al. Coexistent thyroid cancer and pregnancy. Arch Otolaryngol Head Neck Surg 1994; 120:1191.
87. Hill CS Jr, Clark RL, Wolf M. The effect of subsequent pregnancy on patients with thyroid carcinoma. Surg Gynecol Obstet 1966; 122:1219.
88. Pitkin RM. Calcium metabolism in pregnancy and the perinatal period. A review. Am J Obstet Gynecol 1985; 151:99.
89. Mestman JH. Parathyroid disorders of pregnancy. Semin Perinatol 1998; 22:485.
90. Rasmussen N, Rolich A, Hornnes PJ, Hegedus L. Serum ionized calcium and intact parathyroid hormone levels during pregnancy and postpartum. Br J Obstet Gynaecol 1990; 97:857.
91. Wilson SG, Retallack RW, Kent JC, et al. Serum free 1,25-dihydroxyvitamin D and the free 1,25-dihydroxyvitamin D index during a longitudinal study of human pregnancy and lactation. Clin Endocrinol (Oxf) 1990; 32:613.
92. Seely EW, Brown EM, DeMaggio DM, et al. A prospective study of calciotropic hormones in pregnancy and postpartum: reciprocal changes in serum intact parathyroid hormone and 1,25-dihydroxyvitamin D. Am J Obstet Gynecol 1997; 176:214.
93. Rush D, Johnstone FD, King JC. Nutrition and pregnancy. In: Burrow GN, Ferris TF, eds. Medical complications during pregnancy, 3rd ed. Philadelphia: WB Saunders, 1988:117.
94. Salem R, Taylor S. Hyperparathyroidism in pregnancy. Br J Surg 1979; 66:648.
95. Shangold MM, Dor N, Welt SL, et al. Hyperparathyroidism and pregnancy. A review. Obstet Gynecol Surv 1982; 37:217.
96. Mansberger JA, Mansberger AR Jr. Hyperparathyroidism and pregnancy. Case report and therapy update. J Med Assoc Ga 1988; 77:309.
97. Aceto T Jr, Batt RE, Bruck E, et al. Intrauterine hyperparathyroidism: a complication of untreated maternal hypoparathyroidism. J Clin Endocrinol Metab 1966; 26:487.
98. Sadeghi-Nejad A, Wolfsdorf JI, Senior B. Hypoparathyroidism and pregnancy treatment with calcitriol. JAMA 1980; 243:254.
99. Marx SJ, Swart EG Jr, Hamstra AJ, et al. Normal intrauterine development of the fetus of a woman receiving extraordinarily high doses of 1,25-dihydroxyvitamin D. J Clin Endocrinol Metab 1980; 51:1138.
100. Carr BR, Parker CR Jr, Madden JD, et al. Maternal plasma adrenocorticotropin and cortisol relationships throughout human pregnancy. Am J Obstet Gynecol 1981; 139:416.
101. Nolten WE, Lindheimer MD, Rueckert PA, et al. Diurnal patterns and regulation of cortisol secretion in pregnancy. J Clin Endocrinol Metab 1980; 51:466.
102. Rees LH, Burke CW, Chard T, et al. Possible placental origin of ACTH in normal human pregnancy. Nature 1975; 254:620.
103. Sasaki A, Shinkawa O, Yoshinaga K. Placental corticotropin-releasing hormone may be a stimulator of maternal pituitary adrenocorticotropic hormone secretion in humans. J Clin Invest 1989; 84:1997.
104. Bevan JS, Gough MH, Gillmer MDG, et al. Cushings syndrome in pregnancy. The timing of definitive treatment. Clin Endocrinol (Oxf) 1987; 27:225.
105. Casson IF, Davis JC, Jeffreys RV, et al. Successful management of Cushings disease during pregnancy by transsphenoidal adenectomy. Clin Endocrinol (Oxf) 1987; 27:423.
106. Aron DC, Schnall AM, Sheeler LR. Cushings syndrome and pregnancy. Am J Obstet Gynecol 1990; 162:244.
107. Buescher MA, McClamrock HD, Adashi EY. Cushings syndrome in pregnancy. Obstet Gynecol 1992; 79:130.
108. Ross RJ, Chew SL, Perry L, et al. Diagnosis and selective cure of Cushing's disease during pregnancy by transsphenoidal surgery. Eur J Endocrinol 1995; 132:722.
109. Chico A, Manzanares JM, Halperin I, et al. Cushing's disease and pregnancy. Eur J Obstet Gynecol Reprod Biol 1996; 64:143.
110. Guilhaume B, Sanson ML, Billaud L, et al. Cushing's syndrome and pregnancy: aetiologies and prognosis in twenty-two patients. Eur J Med 1992; 1:83.
111. Pinette MG, Pan YQ, Oppenheim D, et al. Bilateral inferior petrosal sinus corticotropin sampling with corticotropin-releasing hormone stimulation in a pregnant patient with Cushing's syndrome. Am J Obstet Gynecol 1994; 171:563.
112. Kreines K, DeVaux WD. Neonatal adrenal insufficiency associated with maternal Cushings syndrome. Pediatrics 1971; 47:516.
113. Albert E, Dalaker K, Jorde R, Berge LN. Addison's disease and pregnancy. Acta Obstet Gynecol Scand 1989; 68:185.
114. Drucker D, Shumak S, Angel A. Schmidt's syndrome presenting with intrauterine growth retardation and postpartum Addisonian crisis. Am J Obstet Gynecol 1984; 149:229.
115. Schlaghecke R, Kornely E, Santen RT, Ridderskamp P. The effect of long-term glucocorticoid therapy on pituitary-adrenal responses to exogenous corticotropin-releasing hormone. N Engl J Med 1992; 326:226.

115a. Henzen C, Suter A, Lerch E, et al. Suppression and recovery of adrenal response after short-term high dose glucocorticoid treatment. Lancet 2000; 355:542.

116. Turner ES, Greenberger PA, Patterson R. Management of the pregnant asthmatic patient. Ann Intern Med 1980; 93:905.

117. Kenny FM, Preeyasombat C, Spaulding JS, et al. Cortisol production rate. IV. Infants born of steroid-treated mothers and of diabetic mothers. Infants with trisomy syndrome and with anencephaly. Pediatrics 1966; 37:960.

118. McKenzie SA, Selley JA, Agnew JE. Secretion of prednisolone into breast milk. Arch Dis Child 1975; 50:894.

119. Speiser PW, New MI. Prenatal diagnosis and management of congenital adrenal hyperplasia. Clin Perinatol 1994; 21:631.

120. Garner PR. Congenital adrenal hyperplasia in pregnancy. Semin Perinatol 1998; 22:446.

121. Klingensmith GJ, Garcia SC, Jones HW Jr, et al. Glucocorticoid treatment of girls with congenital adrenal hyperplasia. Effects on height, sexual maturation, and fertility. J Pediatr 1977; 90:996.

122. Premawardhana LD, Hughes IA, Read GF, Scanlon MF. Longer term outcome in females with congenital adrenal hyperplasia (CAH): the Cardiff experience. Clin Endocrinol 1997; 46:327.

123. Feldman S, Billaud L, Thalabard J-C, et al. Fertility in women with late-onset adrenal hyperplasia due to 21-hydroxylase deficiency. J Clin Endocrinol Metab 1992; 74:635.

124. Azziz R, DeWailly D, Owerbach D. Nonclassic adrenal hyperplasia: current concepts. J Clin Endocrinol Metab 1994; 78:810.

125. Pang A, Pollack MS, Marshall RN, Immken LD. Prenatal treatment of congenital adrenal hyperplasia due to 21-hydroxylase deficiency. N Engl J Med 1990; 322:111.

126. Pang S, Clark AT, Freeman LC, et al. Maternal side effects of prenatal dexamethasone therapy for fetal congenital adrenal hyperplasia. J Clin Endocrinol Metab 1992; 75:249.

127. Baron F, Sprauve ME, Huddleston JF, Fisher AJ. Diagnosis and surgical treatment of primary aldosteronism in pregnancy: a case report. Obstet Gynecol 1995; 86:644.

128. Solomon CG, Thiet M-P, Moore F Jr, Seely EW. Primary hyperaldosteronism in pregnancy. A case report. J Reprod Med 1996; 41:255.

129. Webb JC, Bayliss P. Pregnancy complicated by primary hyperaldosteronism. Southern Med J 1997; 90:243.

130. Robar CA, Poremba JA, Pelton JJ, et al. Current diagnosis and management of aldosterone-producing adenomas during pregnancy. Endocrinologist 1998; 8:403.

131. Ehrlich EN, Lindheimer MD. Effects of administered mineralocorticoids on ACTH in pregnant women. Attenuation of kaliuretic influence of mineralocorticoids during pregnancy. J Clin Invest 1972; 51:1301.

132. Tremblay RR. Treatment of hirsutism with spironolactone. Clinics in Endocrinol Metab 1986; 15:363.

133. Schenker JG, Granat M. Phaeochromocytoma and pregnancy—an updated appraisal. Aust N Z J Obstet Gynaecol 1982; 22:1.

134. Oishi S, Sato T. Pheochromocytoma in pregnancy: a review of the Japanese literature. Endocr J 1994; 41:219.

135. Lau P, Permezel M, Dawson P, et al. Phaeochromocytoma in pregnancy. Aust N Z J Obstet Gynaecol 1996; 36:472.

136. Levin N, McTighe A, Abdel-Aziz MIE. Extra-adrenal pheochromocytoma in pregnancy. Maryland State Med J 1983; 32:377.

137. Castren O. Urinary excretion of noradrenaline and adrenaline in late normal and toxemic pregnancy. Acta Pharmacol Toxicol 1963; 20(Suppl 2):1.

138. Zuspan FP. Urinary excretion of epinephrine and norepinephrine during pregnancy. J Clin Endocrinol 1970; 30:357.

139. Tunbridge RDG, Donnai P. Plasma noradrenaline in normal pregnancy and in hypertension of late pregnancy. Br J Obstet Gynaecol 1981; 88:105.

140. Moodley J, McFadyen ML, Dilraj A, Rangiah S. Plasma noradrenaline and adrenaline levels in eclampsia. S Afr Med J 1991; 80:191.

141. Devoe LD, O'Dell BE, Castillo RA, et al. Metastatic pheochromocytoma in pregnancy and fetal biophysical assessment after maternal administration of alpha-adrenergic, beta-adrenergic, and dopamine antagonists. Obstet Gynecol 1986; 68:155.

142. Fudge TL, McKinnon WMP, Geary WL. Current surgical management of pheochromocytoma during pregnancy. Arch Surg 1980; 115:1224.

143. Vaughan RW, Engelhardt RC, Wise L. Postoperative hypoxemia in obese patients. Ann Surg 1976; 180:877.

144. Calandra C, Abell DA, Beischer NA. Maternal obesity in pregnancy. Obstet Gynecol 1981; 57:8.

145. Edwards LE, Dickes WF, Alton IR, et al. Pregnancy in the massively obese. Course, outcome, and obesity prognosis of the infant. Am J Obstet Gynecol 1978; 131:479.

146. Galtier-Dereure F, Boegner C, Bringer J. Obesity and pregnancy: complications and cost. Am J Clin Nutr 2000; 71(5 suppl):1242S.

147. Kliegman RM, Gross T. Perinatal problems of the obese mother and her infant. Obstet Gynecol 1985; 66:299.

148. Knopp RH, Warth MR, Charles D, et al. Lipoprotein metabolism in pregnancy, fat transport to the fetus and the effects of diabetes. Biol Neonate 1986; 50:297.

149. Roberts IM. Hyperlipidemic gestational pancreatitis. Gastroenterology 1993; 104:1560.

150. Saravanan P, Blumenthal S, Anderson C, et al. Plasma exchange for dramatic gestational hyperlipidemic pancreatitis. J Clin Gastroenterol 1996; 22:295.

# CHAPTER 111

# TROPHOBLASTIC TISSUE AND ITS ABNORMALITIES

CYNTHIA G. KAPLAN

## PLACENTAL AND TROPHOBLASTIC DEVELOPMENT

Trophoblasts, the principal component of the placenta, are the earliest cells to differentiate in the cleaving, fertilized egg. Four to 5 days after fertilization, they become differentiated from the external cells of the morula as it becomes a blastocyst. Thereafter, trophoblastic cells proliferate rapidly and surround the inner cell mass. Attachment to the surface and implantation occur at 5 to 6 days. In human implantation, the blastocyst sinks and becomes surrounded by endometrium in an interstitial location (Fig. 111-1). The endometrial stroma throughout the uterus soon undergoes decidual change. Several regions are defined: the decidua between the blastocyst and myometrium is the *decidua basalis,* that covering the surface defect is the *decidua capsularis,* and that lining the rest of the uterus is the *decidua parietalis.*[1-3]

The trophoblast soon differentiates into three forms—*cytotrophoblast, syncytiotrophoblast,* and *intermediate trophoblast.* The first two are often called *villous trophoblast,* whereas the latter is designated *extravillous.* Although not wholly accurate, this categorization does denote their predominant sites. The cytotrophoblastic cells are uninucleate with clear cytoplasm, occupying a central location in the villi. Although they retain the capacity for mitosis throughout gestation, little functional differentiation occurs. The peripheral syncytiotrophoblast is nonmitotic and grows through incorporation of cytotrophoblastic nuclei. The cells are irregular and multinucleate with abundant dense cytoplasm. The nuclei are usually small and dark, although, soon after

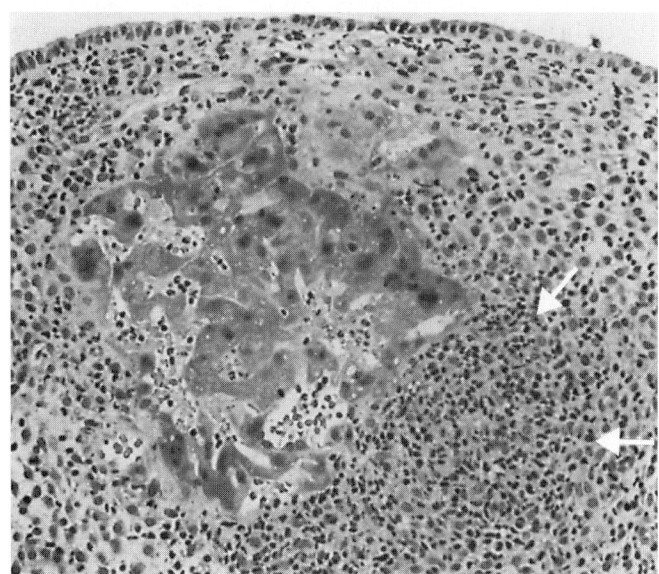

**FIGURE 111-1.** Edge of early implantation site found in an endometrial biopsy and estimated to be 9 days postovulatory. Surface defects are covered completely, and the early-differentiated syncytiotrophoblast forms rudimentary vascular spaces. A chronic inflammatory infiltrate is present (*arrows*), typical of implantation site. (Hematoxylin and eosin; ×160)

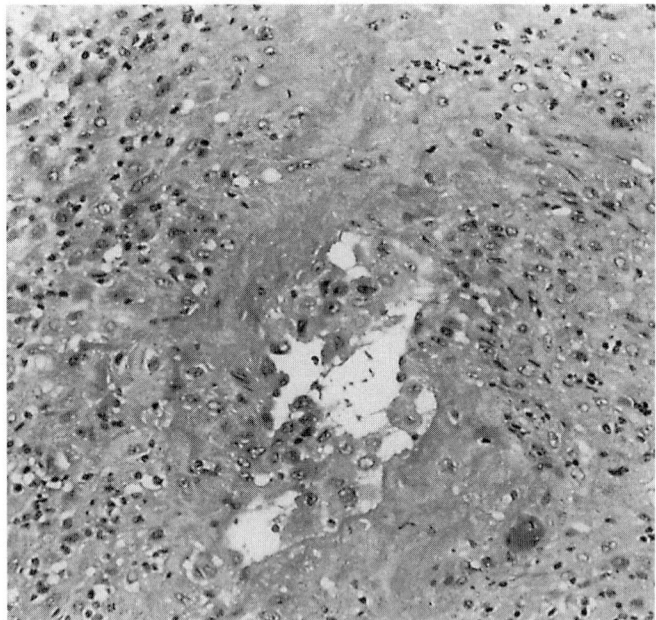

**FIGURE 111-2.** Section of implantation site from a first-trimester spontaneous abortion reveals abundant intermediate trophoblast with relatively clear cytoplasm. The wall of a spiral arteriole is largely replaced by these cells. (Hematoxylin and eosin; ×100)

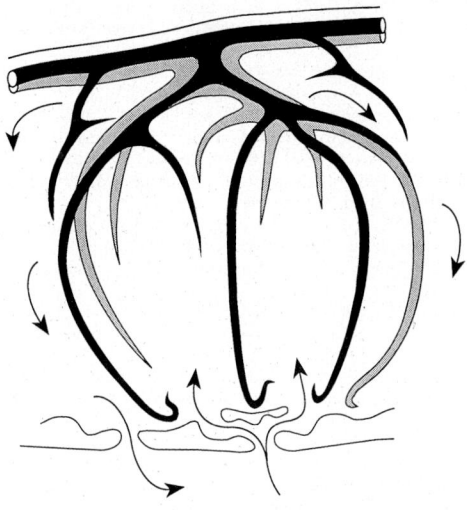

**FIGURE 111-3.** In this schematic of a placental lobule, maternal blood is shown being injected into the intervillous space centrally. The blood flows toward the fetal surface and drains back passively to decidual veins. The midzone of the placenta is the best perfused, with poorer flow at the base, under the fetal surface, and at the margins. The fetal arteries (*solid*) run over fetal veins (*shaded*), and both branch to capillaries at the villus level. (Courtesy of Cynthia G. Kaplan, M.D. From Color atlas of gross placental pathology. New York: Igaku-Shoin Medical Publishers, 1994.)

implantation, they may have inclusion-like nucleoli. The syncytiotrophoblast is functionally active, making large amounts of human chorionic gonadotropin (hCG). The intermediate trophoblast is found predominantly in the implantation site, often admixed with fibrin. The cells are polygonal and uninucleate or multinucleate with abundant amphophilic cytoplasm. Intermediate trophoblast synthesizes predominantly human placental lactogen. All types of trophoblast are epithelial in origin and show such markers (e.g., keratins).[3–5]

The *fetomaternal circulation* is initiated through the formation of lacunae in the syncytiotrophoblast and invasion of intermediate trophoblast into maternal vessels. This leads to loss of muscle and elastic, creating the typical physiologic change (Fig. 111-2). The *primary villi* are cords of cytotrophoblast covered by syncytiotrophoblast. With the invasion of avascular extraembryonic mesenchyme from the embryonic body stalk into the columns, the villi become *secondary villi* and, finally, with the establishment of the capillary network, *tertiary villi,* which are present by the third developmental week. Capillaries form within the villi, probably from mesenchyme, coalesce, and connect to the fetus by means of the vessels differentiating from the inner chorion and from the embryonic body stalk. With growth, branching of villi occurs. Primary stem villi break up below the chorionic plate to form secondary and tertiary stem villi. Each primary stem forms a fetal lobule and is supplied by a branch of a fetal surface vessel. On the surface, arteries always cross over veins. No cross-fetal circulation occurs between villus districts. In situ, most villi float free in the intervillus space, supplied by blood injected from maternal spiral arterioles, generally into the center of the lobules (Fig. 111-3). The villi at the base of the placenta, called *anchoring villi,* retain large cords of cytotrophoblast capped by syncytiotrophoblast. The peripheral syncytiotrophoblast degenerates and is replaced by fibrin (Nitabuch layer).[2–3]

Most commonly, implantation occurs in the upper portion of the uterus. The developing conception, mostly placenta, enlarges rapidly and protrudes into the endometrial cavity. At first, the entire sac is covered by chorion frondosum. As growth continues, the surface thins, forming the placental membranes composed of decidua capsularis and atrophied flat chorion of the sac. These eventually appose the decidua parietalis of the

opposite side of the uterus, obliterating the endometrial cavity. The definitive placenta is left at the base. Until 12 weeks of gestation, the amnion is a smaller sac within the chorionic sac. With growth, these two layers eventually lie adjacent but do not fuse[2,3] (Fig. 111-4).

The umbilical cord forms in the region of the body stalk where the embryo is attached to the chorion. This area contains the allantoic duct, evolving umbilical arteries and veins, omphalomesenteric duct, and vitelline vessels. The expanding amnion surrounds these and covers the umbilical cord. Eventually, most of the embryonic structures, as well as the right umbilical vein, disappear. The mature umbilical cord is an amnion-covered mesenchymal structure containing two arteries and one vein and usually inserts into a location central to the placental disc.[2,3]

The gross morphology of the placenta is established before the end of the first trimester, and further change is limited

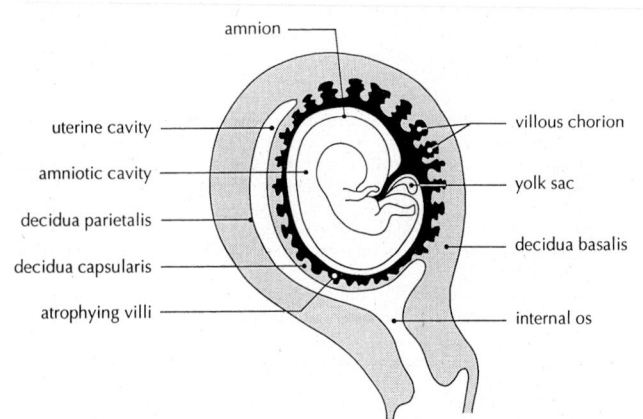

**FIGURE 111-4.** The embryo lies within the chorionic and amniotic sacs. Note the yolk sac between them. The capsular chorionic villi associated with the eventual peripheral membranes are undergoing atrophy, creating a discoid placenta at the base into which the umbilical cord inserts. (Courtesy of Cynthia G. Kaplan, M.D. From Color atlas of gross placental pathology. New York: Igaku-Shoin Medical Publishers, 1994.)

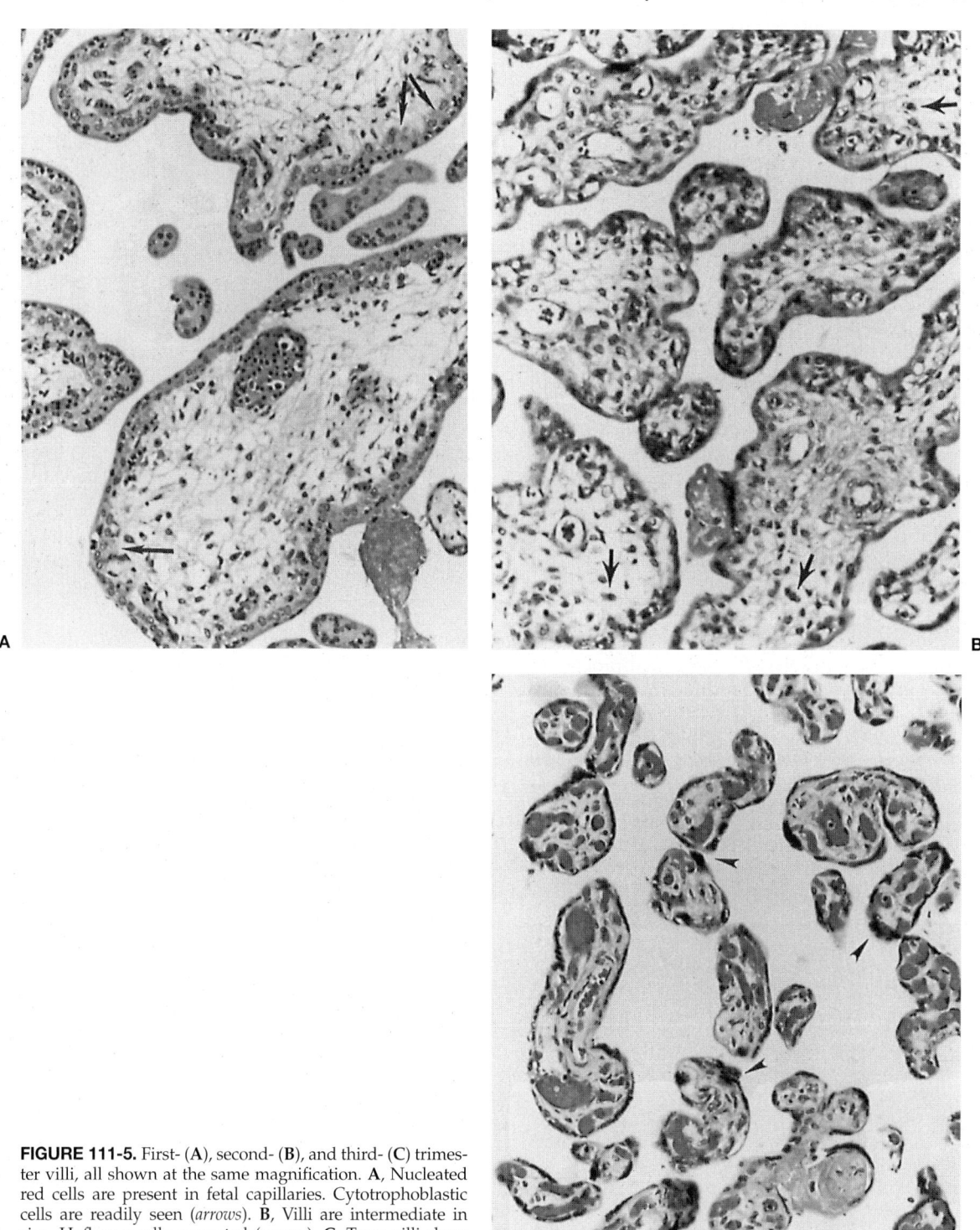

**FIGURE 111-5.** First- (**A**), second- (**B**), and third- (**C**) trimester villi, all shown at the same magnification. **A**, Nucleated red cells are present in fetal capillaries. Cytotrophoblastic cells are readily seen (*arrows*). **B**, Villi are intermediate in size. Hofbauer cells are noted (*arrows*). **C**, Term villi show typical knots (*arrowheads*). Capillaries are close to surface. (Hematoxylin and eosin; ×160)

largely to overall growth and histologic maturation of villi. The placenta becomes a discoid organ that weighs 400 to 600 g at term and is ~19 cm diameter by 2 cm thick. The maternal surface divides into 15 to 20 lobes by decidual septa from the basal plate, but these are of no functional significance; the circulatory unit is the lobule already described. Studies indicate that the weight and DNA content of the placenta continue to grow throughout pregnancy.[3]

The chorionic villi undergo a series of histologic changes during the course of gestation. In the first trimester, the villi are relatively large, with well-defined cytotrophoblast covered by syncytiotrophoblast. Abundant central mesenchyme is present

containing small blood vessels. Subsequently, reduction occurs in villus size and in the volume of mesenchyme. Cytotrophoblasts become less apparent by light microscopy. The syncytiotrophoblastic nuclei aggregate into groups known as *knots*, which may be found free in the circulation. Electron microscopy has shown that cytotrophoblast is present at term and does not truly disappear. The number of villus capillaries increases, and these come to appose thinned regions of trophoblast close to the villus surface, called *vasculosyncytial membranes*. Hofbauer cells, or tissue macrophages, are found in the villus stroma throughout gestation. The distinction among first-, second-, and third-trimester placentas is readily apparent (Fig. 111-5). Villus

**TABLE 111-1.**
**World Health Organization Classification of Gestational Trophoblastic Disease**

Hydatidiform mole
   Complete
   Partial
**Invasive hydatidiform mole**
**Choriocarcinoma**
**Placental site trophoblastic tumor**
**Trophoblastic lesions, miscellaneous**
   Exaggerated placental site
   Placental site nodule or plaque
**Unclassified trophoblastic lesion**

(From Silverberg SG, Kurman RJ. Tumors of the uterine corpus and gestational trophoblastic disease. Washington: Armed Forces Institute of Pathology, 1992.)

appearance is different in different regions of the placenta. In the center of the lobule, the villi tend to be larger and less well differentiated, whereas at the periphery, they appear more mature. Maturation often is altered in disease states.[2,3]

## GESTATIONAL TROPHOBLASTIC DISEASE

Gestational trophoblastic disease is an abnormal proliferation of trophoblastic tissue, reflecting its inherent capacity for invasiveness. Some lesions contain villus structures, whereas others are avillus. Historically, gestational trophoblastic disease was classified into three well-defined types: hydatidiform mole, invasive mole, and choriocarcinoma. Today, additional categories are recognized, some of which show overlap with spontaneous abortions and implantation site reactions. The World Health Organization classification of trophoblastic disease is presented in Table 111-1.[4]

### HYDATIDIFORM MOLE

The classic *complete hydatidiform mole* is readily recognized. It is composed of free vesicles ("bunches of grapes") without recognizable placenta or fetus (Fig. 111-6). All villi are dilated to

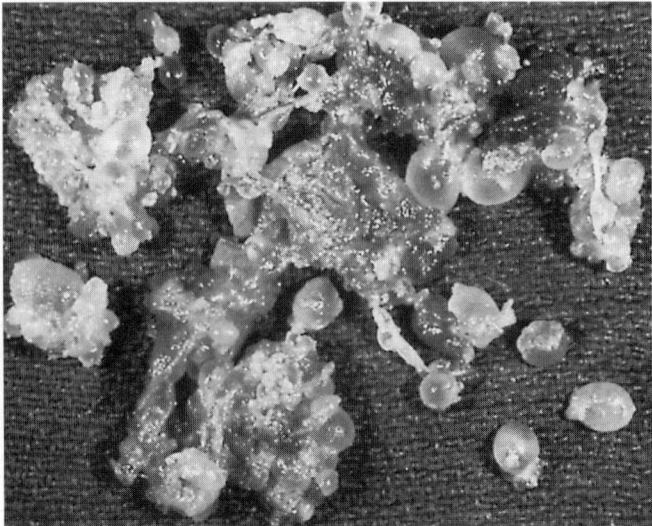

**FIGURE 111-6.** Gross appearance of complete hydatidiform mole. Villi are dilated as individual free, grape-like vesicles.

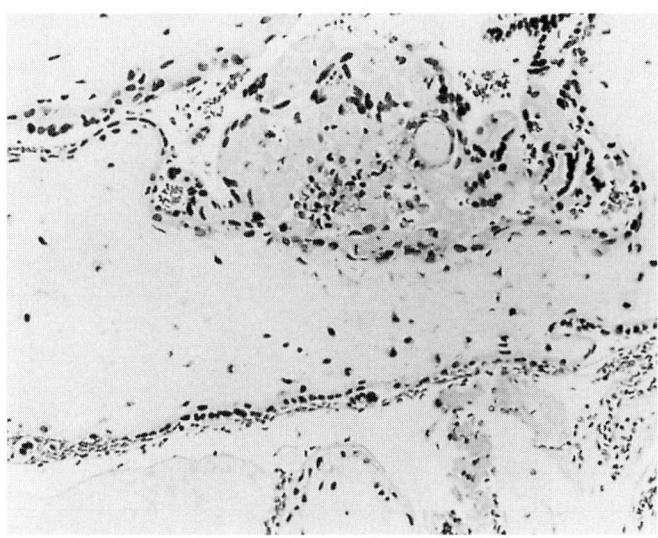

**FIGURE 111-7.** Section of hydropic villus from a partial hydatidiform mole. Macerated embryo was present, and tissue culture showed the karyotype to be 69,XXY. Villus outline is irregular, and mildly proliferated syncytiotrophoblast is present on the surface. Adjacent small villi were present. (Hematoxylin and eosin; ×400)

varying degrees, ranging from a few millimeters to several centimeters. Histologically, the villi are largely avascular, and larger ones show central cisternae. No blood is present in the occasional vessel. Proliferation of cytotrophoblast and syncytiotrophoblast is present on the surface of the villi. This shows a haphazard arrangement without the typical cap of syncytiotrophoblast on cytotrophoblast noted on the young avascular villi of an early pregnancy. Free aggregates of trophoblast are also noted in the intervillus space. An exaggerated placental site reaction with numerous giant cells in the myometrium is often present.[4–7]

A syndrome of *partial hydatidiform mole* has been distinguished from complete mole. In these, the villus tissue is organized into a placenta, and a fetus or embryo is often found. The villi display a variable pattern. Some show hydatidiform change, whereas others are small. Capillaries are frequently present and may contain blood. The surface trophoblast, predominantly syncytiotrophoblast, is somewhat hyperplastic. The outlines of the villi tend to be irregular and map-like, leading to the frequent presence of stromal trophoblastic inclusions on section (Fig. 111-7).

Cytogenetic studies reveal that partial moles are usually triploid (69,XXX,XXY,XYY), and most originate through fertilization by two sperm. The typical complete hydatidiform mole is diploid and totally of paternal origin (androgenetic). Usually, an empty egg is fertilized by a haploid spermatozoa that duplicates its DNA, resulting in a 46,XX karyotype. Thus, both types of moles show a predominance of paternal genes, which is implicated in causing the placental hyperplasia. Flow cytometry on molar pregnancies can also be used to determine the ploidy of an individual case.[3,6,7] Triploidy is common, occurring in ~20% of all chromosomally abnormal spontaneous abortions.[8] Not all triploids are partial moles, largely due to the maternal origin of the extra chromosome set.[6]

The clinical presentation of mole is frequently vaginal bleeding. Complete mole may be associated with increased uterine size for date, toxemia, thyrotoxicosis, theca lutein cysts, and hyperemesis. The incidence of complete molar pregnancy varies throughout the world. In the United States, it is 1 in 4500 deliveries, whereas in Mexico, it is 1 in 200 deliveries. Treatment of all moles is by uterine evacuation.[8] A pla-

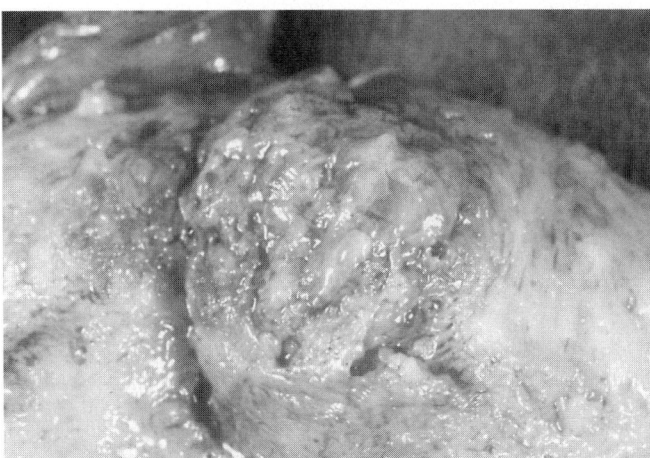

**FIGURE 111-8.** Uterine tissue from hysterectomy performed because of persistently elevated levels of human chorionic gonadotropin after a complete hydatidiform mole. Villous structures can be seen extending into the myometrium in this invasive mole.

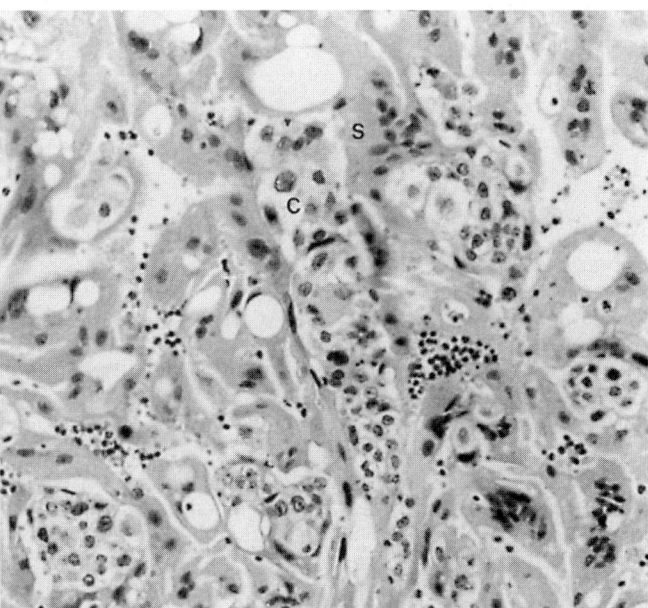

**FIGURE 111-9.** Choriocarcinoma is characterized by irregularly interlacing aggregates of syncytiotrophoblast (*S*) and cytotrophoblast (*C*). Villus structures are not found. (Hematoxylin and eosin; ×400)

teau or rise in β-subunit human chorionic gonadotropin (hCG) levels indicates persistent disease requiring chemotherapy.[4,6,7] The incidence of such disease is 10% to 20% after a complete mole but 5% or less after a partial mole. Choriocarcinoma is extremely rare after a partial mole. Most patients with complete and partial moles later have normal pregnancies.[6]

## INVASIVE MOLE

The invasive mole is the most common form of persistent trophoblastic disease. It is usually diagnosed through persistent hCG elevation. This lesion is rarely seen as a pathologic specimen unless complications necessitate hysterectomy (Fig. 111-8). In such cases, histology shows villi, typical of a classic mole, extending into the uterine wall. The diagnosis cannot usually be made on evacuated material. Most invasive moles are adequately treated by chemotherapy.[3,4,6]

## CHORIOCARCINOMA

Choriocarcinoma is a true malignant neoplasm of trophoblastic cells. Approximately half of cases follow molar pregnancies. The remainder occur after spontaneous abortions and ectopic or normal pregnancies. Grossly, choriocarcinoma is an extremely hemorrhagic lesion in both primary and metastatic sites. Microscopically, it is a haphazard mixture of cytotrophoblast and syncytiotrophoblast (Fig. 111-9). The syncytiotrophoblast may be extensively vacuolated. In general, anaplasia is not striking, although it may be present. No molar villi are seen, and their presence precludes the diagnosis. Such patients usually present with bleeding after a molar or other pregnancy. Treatment with multiagent chemotherapy is usually curative, and later normal pregnancy is possible.[3,4,6]

## PLACENTAL SITE TROPHOBLASTIC TUMOR

Placental site trophoblastic tumor is an avillous lesion composed of uninucleate intermediate trophoblastic cells that invade myometrium and blood vessels. The cells secrete predominantly human placental lactogen and a small amount of hCG. This tumor tends to present with amenorrhea and a uterine mass. It may perforate the uterus. Ten percent to 15% of cases behave in a malignant fashion. Treatment is surgical because response to chemotherapy is poor.[3,4,8]

## PLACENTAL SITE LESIONS

As described previously, the placental site is largely composed of intermediate trophoblastic cells. These cells are involved in several benign placental site processes. The exaggerated placental site reaction (syncytial endometritis) contains multinucleate as well as uninucleate intermediate cells. Although large masses of cells may be present, the underlying architecture is retained. Placental site nodules and plaques show hyalinized material surrounding the intermediate cells. These are remnants of former gestations and may be found years later.[3,10]

## REFERENCES

1. Jirasek JE. Atlas of human prenatal morphogenesis. Boston: Martinus Nijhoff, 1983:23.
2. Popek EJ. Normal anatomy and histology of the placenta. In: Lewis SH, Perrin E, eds. Pathology of the placenta, 2nd ed. Philadelphia: Churchill Livingstone, 1999.
3. Benirschke K, Kaufmann P. Pathology of the human placenta, 3rd ed. New York: Springer-Verlag, 1990.
4. Silverberg SG, Kurman RJ. Tumors of the uterine corpus and gestational trophoblastic disease. Washington: Armed Forces Institute of Pathology, 1992.
5. Wells M, Bulmer JN. The human placental bed: histology, immunohistology, and pathology. Histopathology 1988; 13:483.
6. Szulman AE. Trophoblastic diseases: complete and partial hydatidiform mole. In: Lewis SH, Perrin E, eds. Pathology of the placenta, 2nd ed. Philadelphia: Churchill Livingstone, 1999.
7. Lage JM, Wolf NF. Gestational trophoblastic disease: new approaches to diagnosis. Clin Lab Med 1995;15:631.
8. Gillespie AM, Kumar S, Hancock BW. Treatment of persistent trophoblastic disease later than 6 months after diagnosis of molar pregnancy. Br J Cancer 2000; 82:1393.
9. Carr DH. Cytogenetics of human reproductive wastage. In: Kalter H, ed. Issues and reviews in teratology. New York: Plenum, 1983.
10. Baergen RN. Trophoblastic lesions of the placental site. Gen Diagn Pathol 1997; 143:143.

# CHAPTER 112

# ENDOCRINOLOGY OF TROPHOBLASTIC TISSUE

Z. M. LEI AND CH. V. RAO

The placenta develops from trophectoderm of the blastocyst through the processes of cell proliferation and differentiation. It consists of an outer layer of trophoblasts and an inner connective tissue core with macrophages (Hofbauer cells), fibroblasts, and blood vessels branched out from the umbilical vessels. The trophoblast layer and connective tissue core communicate with each other through the molecules made by each of them. The trophoblast cell layer contains *outer syncytiotrophoblasts* and *inner mononuclear cytotrophoblasts* and *extravillous mononuclear trophoblasts* that invade the uterus to establish a vascular connection with the maternal circulation.[1] Signals of invasion may come from syncytiotrophoblasts through human chorionic gonadotropin (hCG).[2–5] Villus and extravillus cytotrophoblasts can proliferate and are relatively inactive in the synthesis of many placental hormones. Upon appropriate stimulation, villus cytotrophoblasts can undergo aggregation and fusion of their plasma membranes to become syncytiotrophoblasts, which are terminally differentiated and serve as the primary source of many placental hormones and other regulatory agents. The placenta deters the noxious agents and yet allows nutrients to enter the fetal circulation and fetal metabolic waste to empty into the maternal circulation, while preventing maternal immune system cells from attacking the fetus. Structural features, and the ability to produce a wide array of regulatory molecules, allow the placenta to grow, to differentiate, and to perform numerous diverse functions, including possible communications with the brain.[6–9]

## TROPHOBLAST HORMONES

The placenta produces a wide variety of regulatory hormones. In fact, it is difficult to find anything not made by placenta that is produced elsewhere in the body. Many regulatory molecules produced by human trophoblastic tissue are summarized in Table 112-1.[7,8,10–16] These hormones have diverse functions in the fetoplacental unit and in maternal and fetal tissues. Interestingly, some have similar functions, suggesting there might be a hierarchy. Having more than one regulatory hormone may allow for more control points in the regulation. Control of cytotrophoblastic differentiation is one example of multiple regulatory agents having a similar function with one playing a central role. Like hCG, epidermal growth factor (EGF), transforming growth factor-α (TGF-α), and leukemia inhibitory factor (LIF) promote differentiation and also increase the synthesis of hCG.[17–21] Inhibiting hCG-receptor synthesis by treatment with 21 mer phosphorothioate antisense oligodeoxynucleotide prevents not only hCG action, but also the actions of EGF, TGF-α, and LIF in promoting differentiation of cytotrophoblasts.[22,23]

## HUMAN CHORIONIC GONADOTROPIN

*hCG is the signature hormone of the placenta.* It is produced in *large amounts*, has *pervasive actions*, and has a profile of an *early rise followed by a decrease to low steady-state levels.* Although trophoblast is the major source, a wide variety of normal tissues, including anterior pituitary, can make hCG. Nontrophoblastic hCG is not glycosylated and its levels are very low in the circu-

**TABLE 112-1.**
**Regulatory Molecules Produced by Human Trophoblast Tissue**

| | |
|---|---|
| Steroid hormones | Estrogens, progesterone |
| Protein hormones | Human chorionic gonadotropin (hCG), human placental lactogen (HPL), prolactin (PRL), growth hormone (GH), corticotropin, thyrotropin (TSH), parathyroid hormone (PTH), calcitonin (CT), relaxin, leptin, renin, inhibins, follistatin, activins, leptin |
| Neuropeptides | Gonadotropin-releasing hormone (GnRH), thyrotropin-releasing hormone (TRH), growth hormone–releasing hormone (GHRH), somatostatin, corticotropin-releasing hormone (CRH), CRH-binding protein, oxytocin, neuropeptide Y, opioids |
| Growth factors/ cytokines | Epidermal growth factor (EGF), fibroblast growth factor (FGF), transforming growth factor (TGF)-α and -β, platelet-derived growth factor (PDGF), placental growth factor, vascular endothelial growth factor (VEGF), insulin, insulin-like growth factor (IGF)-I and -II, IGF-binding proteins (IGFBPs), macrophage colony-stimulating factor (MCSF), erythropoietin, stem cell factor Interleukins (IL-1, IL-2, IL-6, IL-8, IL-10, IL-13), leukemia inhibitory factor (LIF), tumor necrosis factor (TNF)-α, interferon-α, -β, and -γ |
| Eicosanoids | Prostaglandins, thromboxane A₂, leukotrienes, and 5-, 12-, and 15-hydroxyeicosatetraenoic acids |

lation due to rapid clearance. Some nontrophoblastic tissues may not even release hCG, so that it will serve as a local ligand for hCG/luteinizing hormone (LH) receptors.[24,25] This chapter focuses on trophoblastic hCG and some of its newly discovered actions in the fetoplacental unit and elsewhere in the body that are necessary for completion of a successful full-term pregnancy.

## STRUCTURE AND REGULATION OF HUMAN CHORIONIC GONADOTROPIN SYNTHESIS

hCG is a heterodimeric glycoprotein hormone consisting of noncovalently bound α and β subunits.[26] The α subunit is identical to that of others in the glycoprotein hormone family, which consists of LH, follicle-stimulating hormone (FSH), and thyroid-stimulating hormone (TSH) (see Chaps. 15 and 16). The β subunit, on the other hand, is hormone specific and, while similar, is not identical to the β subunit of LH.[26] The primary difference is that the hCG-β subunit contains 30 additional amino acids at the carboxyterminus with four O-linked oligosaccharide chains, enabling intact hCG to survive in the circulation longer than does LH and also establishing a basis for developing highly specific immunoassays. The β-hCG assay measures not only the β subunit but also intact hCG. The circulatory half-life of intact hCG, 24 to 36 hours, is much longer than that for LH (2–3 hours), for free hCG-α (10–15 minutes), and for free hCG-β (35–45 minutes). Thus, not only the amount of carbohydrate on the protein backbone but also the conformation of the native hormone plays an important role in the clearance from the circulation.[11,26,27]

The α subunit of hCG contains 92 amino acids with 10 half-cystine residues, forming five intrachain disulfide linkages. The β subunit of hCG contains 145 amino acids with 12 half-cystines that form six conserved disulfide bridges.[27] The folding pattern of the α and β subunits, with three disulfide bonds, forms a distinct seatbelt-like motif that is found in a family of cystine-knot growth factors, which include nerve growth factor, TGF-β, and platelet-derived growth factor-β.[28]

A single gene on chromosome 6q21.1–23 encodes the α subunit of hCG.[29] It contains five introns, four exons, and a consensus TATA box located 30 base pairs (bp) upstream from a single transcription initiation site. The β subunit of hCG is encoded by a cluster of six genes spanning more than 52 kbp on chromo-

**TABLE 112-2.**
*Trans*-Acting Factors and *Cis*-Acting Elements in the Transcription of Human Chorionic Gonadotropin Subunit Genes

| *Trans*-Acting | *Cis*-Acting | Subunit | Interaction |
|---|---|---|---|
| **ACTIVATION** | | | |
| Ap-2 | URE | α & β | Direct binding |
| CREB | CRE(s) | α & β | Direct binding |
| CAT-binding proteins | CAT box | α | Direct binding |
| JREB | JRE | α | Direct binding |
| GATAB | GATA | α | Direct binding |
| TSEB(s) | TSE | α | Direct binding |
| SF-1 | GSE | α | Direct binding |
| LH-2 | PGBE | α | Direct binding |
| **INHIBITION** | | | |
| c-Jun | CRE(s) | α & β | Direct binding |
| Oct-3/4 | Octamer | α & β | Direct binding to the β promoter |
| *Indirect action on the α promoter* | | | |
| Glucocorticoid receptor | GRE | α | Indirect action |
| T₃ receptor | TRE | α | Indirect action |

*AP-2*, activator protein-2; *URE*, upstream regulatory element; *CREB*, cyclic adenosine monophosphate (*cAMP*) response element-binding protein; *CRE(s)*, cAMP response elements; *JREB*, junctional regulatory element-binding protein; *JRE*, junctional regulatory element; *GATAB*, GATA-binding protein; *TSEB(s)*, trophoblast-specific element-binding proteins; *TSE*, trophoblast-specific element; *SF-1*, steroidogenic factor-1; *GSE*, gonadotrope-specific element; *PGBE*, pituitary glycoprotein hormone basal element; *GRE*, glucocorticoid response element; *TRE*, thyroid hormone response element.

**TABLE 112-3.**
Regulators of Human Chorionic Gonadotropin Biosynthesis

| Regulator | Effect |
|---|---|
| β-Adrenergic agonists | Stimulation |
| cAMP | Stimulation |
| DHEA | Stimulation |
| EGF & TGF-α | Stimulation |
| Glucocorticoids | Stimulation |
| GnRH | Stimulation |
| IL-1 & -6 | Stimulation |
| Insulin | Stimulation |
| LIF | Stimulation |
| MCSF | Stimulation |
| Retinoic acid | Stimulation |
| Thyroid hormone | Stimulation |
| Activin | Potentiation of GnRH effect |
| hCG | Biphasic effect |
| Phorbol ester | Synergistic effect with cAMP |
| Dopamine | Inhibition |
| GnRH antagonists | Inhibition |
| Inhibin | Inhibition |
| Prolactin | Inhibition |
| Progesterone | Inhibition |
| Mifepristone | Inhibition |
| TGF-β | Inhibition |
| TSH | Inhibition |

*DHEA*, dehydroepiandrosterone. See Table 112-1 for explanations of the peptide abbreviations.

some 19q13.3.[30,31] The genes are a closely spaced array of tandem inverted copies. The hCG-β subunit genes 5, 3, and 8 contain a natural promoter and have high transcriptional activity. The 5'-flanking region of other hCG-β subunit genes contains several gaps and deletions that make them transcriptionally less active; sensitive methods are required to detect their expression.[32]

Analysis of sequence divergence in the coding and noncoding regions of hCG-β subunit genes suggests that multiple copies are probably derived from duplication of the ancestral LH-β subunit gene.[33] During this duplication, deletion of a single base resulted in read-through of the translation stop codon. Thus, a part of the 3'-untranslated region became the coding sequence for the additional 30 amino acids in the carboxyterminus of the hCG-β subunit.[34] Unlike the gonadotropin-α subunit gene, which contains a single promoter site, the evolution of the hCG-β subunit gene introduced a new promoter and a number of *cis*-acting elements that confer cell-specific transcription.[35] The α subunit gene is transcriptionally more active than are the hCG-β subunit genes. However, the hCG-β subunit is rate limiting in the synthesis of intact hCG.[27,36] The *trans*-acting factors and *cis*-acting elements that are involved in transcriptional activation or inhibition of the α and β subunit genes of hCG are summarized in Table 112-2.[35–38] These confer the specificity of regulation by agents that modulate the hCG synthesis. The regulation of hCG synthesis also involves posttranscriptional mechanisms such as the stability of the hCG-subunit mRNA and protein and posttranslational modifications.[30–41]

The placenta primarily secretes intact hCG and, to a small extent, the free α subunit, nicked hCG, and the β-core fragment.[26,27] The control mechanisms for their release are probably different and are not well understood. Intact hCG is bioactive by virtue of its ability to bind to hCG/LH receptors. The free subunits, on the other hand, are bioinactive because they cannot bind to hCG/LH receptors. It is difficult to reconcile the few reports[42–44] claiming that free subunits are also bioactive because no separate receptors for subunits have been identi-

fied. The functional relevance of nicked hCG and β-core fragment is unknown.

A number of agents produced by the placenta can regulate the synthesis of hCG. Some of them inhibit, whereas others stimulate; depending on the concentration, hCG can do both. Many of the regulatory agents that control hCG synthesis are listed in Table 112-3.[2,8,15,36,41]

hCG synthesis can be controlled at two different levels: (a) by increasing the number of syncytiotrophoblasts that produce large amounts of hCG[45] (these are formed from cytotrophoblasts, which produce very little hCG) and (b) by regulating the expression of hCG-subunit genes in syncytiotrophoblasts. The self-regulation of hCG synthesis is a new concept, which has developed from the discovery that cyto- and syncytiotrophoblasts contain hCG/LH receptors and that exogenous, as well as endogenous, hCG can promote the differentiation of cytotrophoblasts and the expression of hCG-subunit genes by both transcriptional and posttranscriptional mechanisms. The effects of hCG are concentration dependent. Lower concentrations stimulate and higher concentrations inhibit the differentiation of cytotrophoblasts as well as the expression of hCG-subunit genes.[17,40] Although hCG/LH receptors are present in the first-trimester placenta, they are not functional in self-regulation of hCG biosynthesis.

Self-regulation can potentially explain the pregnancy profile of hCG. Its rapid increase to peak levels is probably due to lack of feedback inhibition by hCG during the first trimester. Once peak levels are reached, feedback inhibition results in a drop in hCG levels. When they decrease, they can never fall to zero because low levels stimulate synthesis. When they begin to rise, they can never return to previous high levels because high concentrations inhibit synthesis. Thus, low steady-state levels are maintained throughout the second and third trimester of pregnancy.[2] This profile is quite different from that of other placental hormones (i.e., human placental lactogen and the steroid hormones; see Chaps. 108 and 109), which *progressively increase* throughout pregnancy.

**TABLE 112-4.**
**Human Chorionic Gonadotropin/Luteinizing Hormone Receptor Distribution**

Ovary
Placenta
Fetal membranes
Decidua
T cells, monocytes, and macrophages
Umbilical cord
Uterus
Oviduct
Urinary bladder
Skin
Adrenal cortex–zona reticularis
Brain
Neural retina
Breast

**TABLE 112-5.**
**Actions of Human Chorionic Gonadotropin during Pregnancy**

Support luteal synthesis of progesterone through 6–9 weeks
Inhibit cyclic release of luteinizing hormone
Induce behavioral changes, i.e., nausea and vomiting, craving, drowsiness, and decreased physical activity, etc.
Promote early embryonic growth and development
Promote implantation
Maintain myometrial quiescence
Increase uterine blood flow
Regulate placental steroid and eicosanoid biosynthesis
Increase invasion of extravillous trophoblasts
Prevent maternal T-cell activation through up-regulation of 2,3-indoleamine dioxygenase in syncytiotrophoblasts
Regulate the differentiation of cytotrophoblasts
Regulate the expression of human chorionic gonadotropin subunit genes
Facilitate nutrient and metabolite exchange between maternal and fetal circulation through its actions on umbilical vessels
Promote weakening of fetal membranes and softening of cervix toward the end of pregnancy through increased prostaglandin production

The self-regulation of hCG biosynthesis is probably not an all-or-none phenomenon. Its onset may be gradual, potentially explaining the decrease in doubling times as hCG levels rapidly increase during the first trimester. The presence or absence and the strength of self-regulation may explain individual variations in hCG levels, variations in the same woman during different pregnancies, and the high hCG levels in preeclampsia and Down syndrome as compared to those found in normal pregnancy.[7,9,46]

## SHIFT IN THE CURRENT PARADIGM FOR HUMAN CHORIONIC GONADOTROPIN ACTIONS

For a long time, it was believed that the only function of hCG was to rescue and maintain the corpus luteum from regression in a fertile cycle until the placenta could start producing adequate amounts of progesterone. Once this luteoplacental shift was completed, hCG was considered a vestigial hormone. The persistence of hCG throughout pregnancy should have aroused suspicions that it might have other functions. However, this possibility was not considered since it was not known that hCG has pervasive actions throughout the body,[9,46,47] as evidenced by the low levels of functional hCG/LH receptors found in several nongonadal tissues[9,46–49] (Table 112-4).

The receptors in nongonadal tissues, as in gonadal tissues, have been demonstrated by mRNA, protein, and hormone-binding studies.[9,46–49] The existence of these receptors indicates that hCG can regulate nongonadal tissue functions. Indeed, studies have substantiated this possibility. The actions of hCG from early embryonic growth and development to the end of pregnancy are summarized in Table 112-5.[9,46,47,49]

The absence of cyclic LH release during pregnancy could be due to hCG reaching gonadotropin-releasing hormone (GnRH) neurons in hypothalamus to inhibit its synthesis.[6,50,51] Many pregnancy-associated behaviors can be induced in the rat model by injecting hCG into the peripheral circulation or into brain ventricles.[52,53] This implies that peripheral hCG is transported into cerebrospinal fluid by receptors in choroid plexus to act on brain areas that are associated with behavioral regulation.[6,52,53] Locally made, peripherally and/or blastocyst-derived hCG/LH may promote early embryonic growth, development, and implantation.[54,55] hCG derived from placenta may maintain myometrial quiescence,[56,57] increase the uterine blood flow,[58,59] and induce numerous other changes in the fetoplacental unit.[60,61]

hCG levels are very low in the fetal circulation, suggesting that hCG secretion is directed into the maternal circulation and is prevented from entering into the fetus. The reason for this could be that the hCG surge may interfere with growth and developmental programs in the fetus. The low fetal hCG levels

are derived primarily from the fetal kidney and liver.[62] Fetal hCG is structurally and functionally similar to, but not identical to, the maternal hormone. Fetal hCG may control fetal adrenal androgen synthesis, gonadal steroid production,[62,63] and brain growth and differentiation,[64–66] and may relax the umbilical vessels, keeping the umbilical cords from becoming too rigid.[60]

hCG reportedly has antiviral properties, which may protect the fetus from certain viral infections.[67] Although this may depend on the stage of pregnancy, the viral load, and the type of virus, studies on a human immunodeficiency virus (HIV) transgenic mouse model may support these observations.[68] In this model, heterozygous mothers bear homozygous and heterozygous litters that cannot be differentiated until ~3 days after birth. Then, homozygous pups begin to show severe signs of wasting syndrome and 100% of them die in a few weeks. If these pups have been treated with hCG, the disease progression slows and the animals survive. Thus, transgenic HIV mice fetuses are protected in utero, and this protection can be extended by hCG administration after birth. Although the mechanisms have not been worked out, a number of different ones could be involved in this protective action of hCG.[68,69]

The influence of hCG on myometrium should diminish toward the end of pregnancy, so that active labor can begin. In fact, the myometrial hCG/LH receptors appear to decrease as labor approaches.[70] hCG acts on the fetal membranes to increase the synthesis of prostaglandins, possibly weakening them by collagen breakdown.[61] Since fetal membranes lie in the cervical canal during active labor, any prostaglandins produced by the fetal membranes will have an opportunity to cause cervical softening through collagenolysis. Thus, the waning influence of hCG on the myometrium and its increasing influence on the fetal membranes and the cervix are probably meant for smooth progression of labor and delivery. These opposing influences of hCG on different tissues at the same time may occur through interactions with other agents present within the fetomaternal environment.

Table 112-5 does not include some of the predictable changes during pregnancy. For example, the presence of hCG/LH receptors predicts pregnancy-associated skin changes.[71] The presence of receptors in the urinary bladder and the possible smooth muscle-relaxing activity of hCG suggest that frequent urination during early pregnancy could be caused by hCG.[72] Changes in visual processing during pregnancy may occur through the actions of hCG/LH receptors contained in the neural retina.[73] The synthesis of maternal and fetal adrenal androgens may, in part, be controlled by hCG.[62] Since fetal adrenal androgens are precursors of estriol synthesis in the placenta, and urinary estriol reflects fetal well-being, ultimate fetal and placental well-being could be determined by actions of hCG.

## PRODUCTION AND ACTION OF HUMAN CHORIONIC GONADOTROPIN IN TUMOR TISSUES

hCG belongs to a family of embryonically related marker proteins that include carcinoembryonic antigen and α-fetoprotein.[74] Thus, a wide variety of cancers and cancer cells contain intact hCG and/or one of its subunits; to date, >70 different cancer cell lines have been shown to contain them.[25,75–78,78a] The presence of hCG and/or one of its subunits in cancer cells is probably due to synthesis rather than sequestration. The regulatory mechanisms involved in the expression of hCG-subunit genes in cancer cells is not known.

Ectopic production of hCG is considered a recapitulation of the embryonic state, as is cancer. The expression of hCG and/or one of its subunits increases in advanced cancers, suggesting that they might be involved in the progression of the disease. In fact, contraceptive hCG vaccine is now being tested, especially against cancers of the colon and pancreas.[79–81]

Like other hormones, hCG acts via binding to its receptors. A demonstration of hCG/LH receptors in cancers of nongonadal tissues has reinforced a belief that hCG may indeed play a role. In fact, studies suggest that hCG may have dual roles in cancers. It promotes some cancers (endometrial cancer,[82–86] choriocarcinomas[4,5] [see Chap. 111], and lung cancer[87,88]), whereas it inhibits others (prostate cancer[89–92] and breast cancer[93–96]). Some controversies on whether hCG prevents or promotes cancers could be due to whether they produce intact hCG or just its β subunit, which may have a stimulatory effect, probably due to the formation of homodimers.[97–99]

When intact hCG or LH promotes cancer, its presence in cancer tissues can be expected to be associated with a poor prognosis. When these hormones protect against cancer, their presence indicates a good prognosis. In the latter case, injection of the hormone into the lesion may slow the cancer progression.

Gestational trophoblastic neoplasms (GTNs) contain high hCG/LH receptor levels, which further increase in more malignant phenotypes such as choriocarcinomas.[100] These high receptor levels are due to a loss of self-regulation of hCG biosynthesis. This may explain how GTNs can produce much higher levels of hCG than do normal trophoblasts.[101] The high hCG levels produced by choriocarcinomas may promote their growth, development, and metastasis in the host body.[5]

hCG-producing tumors (see Chaps. 120 and 219) in young boys can cause precocious puberty by virtue of constant stimulation of the testis to produce testosterone[102] (see Chap. 92). Such tumors in young girls usually do not have obvious adverse effects unless they are associated with the ovaries. The reason for this gender difference is that both LH and FSH are required for ovarian estradiol synthesis, whereas LH alone is capable of stimulating testicular synthesis of testosterone. This gender difference is also seen when there is an activating LH receptor mutation.[103] hCG-producing tumors in some men can cause gynecomastia, possibly due to direct actions of hCG on the breast. hCG-producing tumors in women cause disruption of the menstrual cycle and dysfunctional uterine bleeding.

## POTENTIAL THERAPEUTIC USES OF HUMAN CHORIONIC GONADOTROPIN

There are several potential therapeutic uses of hCG. Since hCG has pervasive actions during pregnancy, some unexplained pregnancy losses could be due to aberrant or inadequate

actions of hCG; this may be corrected by the administration of hCG. hCG levels progressively decrease during threatened abortion, but whether this is a cause or consequence is not known. Administration of hCG also may help in some of these cases. hCG treatment may work by increasing the placental endocrine activity, by preventing immunologic mechanisms that promote fetal rejection, by increasing uterine blood flow, by decreasing uterine activity, and so forth.[49] This treatment may not work if infection, anatomic defects, fetal anomalies, and so forth, are responsible for these conditions.

The ability of hCG to maintain myometrial quiescence suggests it may be used in the treatment of preterm labor and delivery, unless it is caused by infection, premature rupture of membranes, and so forth. In fact, administration of hCG has a tocolytic effect in a mouse preterm-labor model.[104] If it is proved that hCG works in women, it would be the most natural means of preventing preterm labor. The rationale for giving hCG when women already have it in their circulation is that perhaps their levels are not adequate, and increasing levels by giving exogenous hormone might delay events that lead to preterm labor and delivery.

Epidemiologic data, the rat breast cancer model studies, and the anticancer effects of hCG in human breast cancer cells suggest that the decreased incidence of breast cancer in women who complete a full-term pregnancy before 20 years of age could be due to hCG.[105–108] This hormone may act on breasts to promote nonreversible differentiation of proliferation-competent epithelial cells into secretory cells in terminal end buds. Coincidentally, this differentiation, which is a physiologic phenomenon to prepare the breast for lactation, also makes the cells less susceptible to carcinogenic transformation.[109] Additional mechanisms, such as inhibition of cell growth and invasion,[94,95,110] increase of apoptosis,[111,112] and the cell's ability to repair DNA damage, also may play roles in the protective actions of hCG in the breast.[113,114] Increased inhibin and insulin-like growth factor (IGF)–binding proteins and/or decreased IGF-I and its receptors may mediate hCG actions in breast cancer cells.[109,115,116]

These findings do not necessarily mean that every woman who completes a full-term pregnancy at a young age will never get breast cancer. Several other factors, such as family history, radiation, environment, and so forth, contribute to the development of this disease; therefore, pregnancy may not be able to overcome some or all of these factors.

Potential uses of hCG in the treatment of HIV infections and Kaposi sarcomas are controversial.[117,118] Nonetheless, these treatment strategies may have some merit because of the reported antiviral properties of hCG as well as its ability to act on cells of the immune system and numerous other target tissues throughout the body.[46,49,67,119–121]

## SUMMARY AND PERSPECTIVES

Trophoblastic tissue is a transient and unique endocrine organ that is capable of producing a vast array of bioactive substances. Among them, hCG is the best known and perhaps most important. hCG is not just a gonadal-regulating hormone as once was believed. It is a pluripotent regulatory molecule with the actions of a classic hormone, a growth factor, and a cytokine. It plays a pivotal role in the regulation of the functions of the fetoplacental unit and of a number of other tissues during pregnancy. Although the evolutionary significance of the broad spectrum of hCG actions is unknown, it could have evolved to orchestrate numerous functions during pregnancy in women. LH may fulfill some of the roles of hCG in other species. These far-ranging actions are not unique to hCG, as prolactin is another example of a hormone having multiple targets in the body. hCG research has helped to explain many unknown, and to rationalize several known, effects of hCG.

# REFERENCES

1. Bernischke K, Kaufmann P. Pathology of the human placenta, 3rd ed. New York: Springer-Verlag. 1995.
2. Rodway MR, Rao ChV. A novel perspective on the role of human chorionic gonadotropin during pregnancy and in gestational trophoblastic disease. Early Pregnancy Biol Med 1995; 1(3):176.
3. El-Hendy KA, Subramanian MG, Diamond MP, Yelian FD. hCG modulates MMP-9 activity in first trimester trophoblast cells. J Soc Gynecol Invest 1998; 5:118A.
4. Zygmunt M, Hahn D, Munstedt K, et al. Invasion of cytotrophoblastic JEG-3 cells is stimulated by hCG in vitro. Placenta 1998; 19(8):587.
5. Lei ZM, Taylor DD, Gercel-Taylor C, Rao ChV. Human chorionic gonadotropin promotes tumorigenesis of choriocarcinoma JAR cells. Trophoblast Res 1999; 13:147.
6. Lei ZM, Rao ChV, Kornyei JL, et al. Novel expression of human chorionic gonadotropin/luteinizing hormone receptor gene in brain. Endocrinology 1993; 132(5):2262.
7. Kliman HJ. Placental hormones. Endocrinol Pregnancy 1994; 5(4):591.
8. Petraglia F, Florio P, Nappi C, Genazzani AR. Peptide signaling in human placenta and membranes: autocrine, paracrine, and endocrine mechanisms. Endocr Rev 1996; 17(2):156.
9. Rao ChV. Potential novel roles of luteinizing hormone and human chorionic gonadotropin during early pregnancy in women. Early Pregnancy Biol Med 1997; 3(1):1.
10. Walsh SW. Prostaglandins in pregnancy. In: Sciarra JJ, ed. Gynecology and obstetrics. Philadelphia: JB Lippincott Co, 1992.
11. Reyes FI. Protein hormones of the placenta. In: Sciarra JJ, ed. Gynecology and obstetrics. Philadelphia: JB Lippincott Co, 1992.
12. Guilbert L, Robertson SA, Wegmann TG. The trophoblast as an integral component of a macrophage-cytokine network. Immunol Cell Biol 1993; 71(Pt 1):49.
13. Senaris R, Garcia-Caballero T, Casabiell X, et al. Synthesis of leptin in human placenta. Endocrinology 1997; 138(10):4501.
14. Conrad KP, Benyo DF. Placental cytokines and the pathogenesis of pre-eclampsia. Am J Reprod Immunol 1997; 37(3):240.
15. Petraglia F, Santuz M, Florio P, et al. Paracrine regulation of human placenta: control of hormonogenesis. J Reprod Immunol 1998; 39(1–2):221.
16. He Y, Smith SK, Day KA, et al. Alternative splicing of vascular endothelial growth factor (VEGF)-R1 (FLT-1) pre-mRNA is important for the regulation of VEGF activity. Mol Endocrinol 1999; 13(4):537.
17. Shi QJ, Lei ZM, Rao ChV, Lin J. Novel role of human chorionic gonadotropin in differentiation of human cytotrophoblasts. Endocrinology 1993; 132(3):1387.
18. Sawai K, Azuma C, Koyama M, et al. Leukemia inhibitory factor (LIF) enhances trophoblast differentiation mediated by human chorionic gonadotropin (hCG). Biochem Biophys Res Commun 1995; 211(1):137.
19. Sawai K, Matsuzaki N, Kameda T, et al. Leukemia inhibitory factor produced at the fetomaternal interface stimulates chorionic gonadotropin production: its possible implication during pregnancy, including implantation period. J Clin Endocrinol Metab 1995; 80(4):1449.
20. Mochizuki M, Maruo T, Matsuo H, et al. Biology of human trophoblast. Int J Gynaecol Obstet 1998; 60(Suppl 1):S21.
21. Morrish DW, Dakour J, Li H. Functional regulation of human trophoblast differentiation. J Reprod Immunol 1998; 39(1–2):179.
22. Yang M, Lei ZM, Rao ChV. Mechanism of leukemia inhibitory factor induced differentiation of human cytotrophoblasts into syncytiotrophoblasts. In: The Endocrine Society Annual Meeting, San Diego, CA; 1999. Abstract P1–6.
23. Yang M, Lei ZM, Rao ChV. How does epidermal growth factor promote the differentiation of human cytotrophoblasts into syncytiotrophoblasts. J Soc Gynecol Invest 1999; 6(Suppl 1):Abstract 31.
24. Lei ZM, Toth P, Rao ChV, Pridham D. Novel coexpression of human chorionic gonadotropin (hCG)/human luteinizing hormone receptors and their ligand hCG in human fallopian tubes. J Clin Endocrinol Metab 1993; 77:863.
25. Acevedo HF, Hartsock RJ, Maroon JC. Detection of membrane-associated human chorionic gonadotropin and its subunits on human cultured cancer cells of the nervous system. Cancer Detect Prev 1997; 21(4):295.
26. Pierce JG, Parsons TF. Glycoprotein hormones: structure and function. Annu Rev Biochem 1981; 50:465.
27. Iles RK, Chard T. Molecular insights into the structure and function of human chorionic gonadotrophin. J Mol Endocrinol 1993; 10(3):217.
28. Lapthorn AJ, Harris DC, Littlejohn A, et al. Crystal structure of human chorionic gonadotropin. Nature 1994; 369(6480):455.
29. Fiddes JC, Goodman HM. The gene encoding the common alpha subunit of the four human glycoprotein hormones. J Mol Appl Genet 1981; 1(1):3.
30. Boorstein WR, Vamvakopoulos NC, Fiddes JC. Human chorionic gonadotropin beta-subunit is encoded by at least eight genes arranged in tandem and inverted pairs. Nature 1982; 300(5891):419.
31. Policastro P, Ovitt CE, Hoshina M, et al. The beta subunit of human chorionic gonadotropin is encoded by multiple genes. J Biol Chem 1983; 258(19):11492.
32. Bo M, Boime I. Identification of the transcriptionally active genes of the chorionic gonadotropin beta gene cluster in vivo. J Biol Chem 1992; 267(5):3179.
33. Talmadge K, Vamvakopoulos NC, Fiddes JC. Evolution of the genes for the beta subunits of human chorionic gonadotropin and luteinizing hormone. Nature 1984; 307(5946):37.
34. Fiddes JC, Goodman HM. The cDNA for the beta-subunit of human chorionic gonadotropin suggests evolution of a gene by readthrough into the 3'-untranslated region. Nature 1980; 286(5774):684.
35. Albanese C, Colin IM, Crowley WF, et al. The gonadotropin genes: evolution of distinct mechanisms for hormonal control. Recent Prog Horm Res 1996; 51:23.
36. Jameson JL, Hollenberg AN. Regulation of chorionic gonadotropin gene expression. Endocr Rev 1993; 14(2):203.
37. Liu L, Roberts RM. Silencing of the gene for the beta subunit of human chorionic gonadotropin by the embryonic transcription factor Oct-3/4. J Biol Chem 1996; 271(28):16683.
38. Liu L, Leaman D, Villalta M, Roberts RM. Silencing of the gene for the alpha-subunit of human chorionic gonadotropin by the embryonic transcription factor Oct-3/4. Mol Endocrinol 1997; 11(11):1651.
39. Fuh VL, Burrin JM, Jameson JL. Cyclic AMP (cAMP) effects on chorionic gonadotropin gene transcription and mRNA stability: labile proteins mediate basal expression whereas stable proteins mediate cAMP stimulation. Mol Endocrinol 1989; 3(7):1148.
40. Licht P, Cao H, Lei ZM, et al. Novel self-regulation of human chorionic gonadotropin biosynthesis in term pregnancy human placenta. Endocrinology 1993; 133(6):3014.
41. Merz WE. Biosynthesis of human chorionic gonadotropin: a review. Eur J Endocrinol 1996; 135(3):269.
42. Blithe DL, Richards RG, Skarulis MC. Free alpha molecules from pregnancy stimulate secretion of prolactin from human decidual cells: a novel function for free alpha in pregnancy. Endocrinology 1991; 129(4):2257.
43. Moy E, Kimzey LM, Nelson LM, Blithe DL. Glycoprotein hormone alpha-subunit functions synergistically with progesterone to stimulate differentiation of cultured human endometrial stromal cells to decidualized cells: a novel role for free alpha-subunit in reproduction. Endocrinology 1996; 137(4):1332.
44. Wolkersdorfer GW, Bornstein SR, Hilbers U, et al. The presence of chorionic gonadotrophin beta subunit in normal cyclic human endometrium. Mol Hum Reprod 1998; 4(2):179.
45. Ringler GE, Strauss JF. In vitro systems for the study of human placental endocrine function. Endocr Rev 1990; 11(1):105.
46. Rao ChV. The beginning of a new era in reproductive biology and medicine: expression of low levels of functional luteinizing hormone/human chorionic gonadotropin receptors in nongonadal tissues. J Physiol Pharmacol 1996; 47(Suppl 2):41.
47. Rao ChV. Novel concepts in neuroendocrine regulation of reproductive tract functions. In: Bazer FW, ed. The endocrinology of pregnancy. Totowa, NJ: Humana Press, 1998:125.
48. Ziecik AJ, Derecka-Reszka K, Rzucidlo SJ. Extragonadal gonadotropin receptors, their distribution and function. J Physiol Pharmacol 1992; 43(4 Suppl 1):33.
49. Rao ChV. A paradigm shift on the targets of luteinizing hormone/human chorionic gonadotropin actions in the body. J Bellevue Obstet Gynecol Soc 1999; 15:26.
50. Lei ZM, Rao ChV. Signaling and transacting factors in the transcriptional inhibition of gonadotropin releasing hormone gene by human chorionic gonadotropin in immortalized hypothalamic GT1-7 neurons. Mol Cell Endocrinol 1995; 109(2):151.
51. Lei ZM, Rao ChV. Cis-acting elements and trans-acting proteins in the transcriptional inhibition of gonadotropin-releasing hormone gene by human chorionic gonadotropin in immortalized hypothalamic GT1-7 neurons. J Biol Chem 1997; 272(22):14365.
52. Toth P, Lukacs H, Hiatt ES, et al. Administration of human chorionic gonadotropin affects sleep-wake phases and other associated behaviors in cycling female rats. Brain Res 1994; 654(2):181.
53. Lukacs H, Hiatt ES, Lei ZM, Rao ChV. Peripheral and intracerebroventricular administration of human chorionic gonadotropin alters some hippocampus-associated behaviors in cycling female rats. Horm Behav 1995; 29(1):42.
54. Han SW, Lei ZM, Rao ChV. Up-regulation of cyclooxygenase-2 gene expression by chorionic gonadotropin during the differentiation of human endometrial stromal cells into decidua. Endocrinology 1996; 137(5):1791.
55. Han SW, Lei ZM, Rao ChV. Treatment of human endometrial stromal cells with chorionic gonadotropin promotes their morphological and functional differentiation into decidua [In Process Citation]. Mol Cell Endocrinol 1999; 147(1–2):7.
56. Ambrus G, Rao ChV. Novel regulation of pregnant human myometrial smooth muscle cell gap junctions by human chorionic gonadotropin. Endocrinology 1994; 135(6):2772.
57. Eta E, Ambrus G, Rao ChV. Direct regulation of human myometrial contractions by human chorionic gonadotropin. J Clin Endocrinol Metab 1994; 79(6):1582.
58. Toth P, Li X, Rao ChV, et al. Expression of functional human chorionic gonadotropin/human luteinizing hormone receptor gene in human uterine arteries. J Clin Endocrinol Metab 1994; 79(1):307.

59. Toth P, Gimes G, Rao ChV. hCG treatment in early gestation: its impact on uterine blood flow and pregnancy outcome. In: 16th World Congress on Fertility and Sterility and 54th Annual Meeting of the American Society for Reproductive Medicine; 1998, San Francisco, CA; Abstract S46.

60. Rao ChV, Li X, Toth P, et al. Novel expression of functional human chorionic gonadotropin/luteinizing hormone receptor gene in human umbilical cords. J Clin Endocrinol Metab 1993; 77(6):1706.

61. Toth P, Li X, Lei ZM, Rao ChV. Expression of human chorionic gonadotropin (hCG)/luteinizing hormone receptors and regulation of the cyclooxygenase-1 gene by exogenous hCG in human fetal membranes. J Clin Endocrinol Metab 1996; 81(3):1283.

62. McGregor WG, Kuhn RW, Jaffe RB. Biologically active chorionic gonadotropin: synthesis by the human fetus. Science 1983; 220(4594):306.

63. Dobozy O, Brindak O, Csaba G. Influence of pituitary hormones (hCG, TSH, Pr, GH) on testosterone level and on the functional activity of the Leydig cell in rat fetuses. Acta Physiol Hung 1988; 72(2):159.

64. Al-Hader AA, Lei ZM, Rao ChV. Novel expression of functional luteinizing hormone/chorionic gonadotropin receptors in cultured glial cells from neonatal rat brains. Biol Reprod 1997; 56(2):501.

65. Al-Hader AA, Lei ZM, Rao ChV. Neurons from fetal rat brains contain functional luteinizing hormone/chorionic gonadotropin receptors. Biol Reprod 1997; 56(5):1071.

66. Al-Hader AA, Tao YX, Lei ZM, Rao ChV. Fetal rat brains contain luteinizing hormone/human chorionic gonadotropin receptors. Early Pregnancy Biol Med 1997; 3(4):323.

67. Harris PJ. Human chorionic gonadotropin hormone is antiviral. Med Hypotheses 1996; 47(2):71.

68. De SK, Wohlenberg CR, Marinos NJ, et al. Human chorionic gonadotropin hormone prevents wasting syndrome and death in HIV-1 transgenic mice. J Clin Invest 1997; 99(7):1484.

69. Shapira A, Bao S, Lei ZM, et al. Treatment of homozygous HIV-1 transgenic mouse pups with human chorionic gonadotropin (hCG) upregulates the skin hCG/luteinizing hormone receptor levels. In the program of The Endocrine Society Annual Meeting, 1998, Abstract P2–149.

70. Zuo J, Lei ZM, Rao ChV. Human myometrial chorionic gonadotropin/luteinizing hormone receptors in preterm and term deliveries. J Clin Endocrinol Metab 1994; 79(3):907.

71. Bird J, Li X, Lei ZM, et al. Luteinizing hormone and human chorionic gonadotropin decrease type 2 5 alpha-reductase and androgen receptor protein levels in women's skin. J Clin Endocrinol Metab 1998; 83(5):1776.

72. Tao YX, Heit M, Lei ZM, Rao ChV. The urinary bladder of a woman is a novel site of luteinizing hormone–human chorionic gonadotropin receptor gene expression. Am J Obstet Gynecol 1998; 179(4):1026.

73. Thompson DA, Othman MI, Lei ZM, et al. Localization of receptors for luteinizing hormone/chorionic gonadotropin in neural retina. Life Sci 1998; 63(12):1057.

74. Jacobs EL, Haskell CM. Clinical use of tumor markers in oncology. Curr Probl Cancer 1991; 15(6):299.

75. Acevedo HF, Krichevsky A, Campbell-Acevedo EA, et al. Expression of membrane-associated human chorionic gonadotropin, its subunits, and fragments by cultured human cancer cells. Cancer 1992; 69 (7):1829.

76. Acevedo HF, Krichevsky A, Campbell-Acevedo EA, et al. Flow cytometry method for the analysis of membrane-associated human chorionic gonadotropin, its subunits, and fragments on human cancer cells. Cancer 1992; 69(7):1818.

77. Acevedo HF, Tong JY, Hartsock RJ. Human chorionic gonadotropin-beta subunit gene expression in cultured human fetal and cancer cells of different types and origins [see comments]. Cancer 1995; 76(8):1467.

78. Lazar V, Diez SG, Laurent A, et al. Expression of human chorionic gonadotropin beta subunit genes in superficial and invasive bladder carcinomas. Cancer Res 1995; 55(17):3735.

78a. Fujikawa K, Matsui Y, Oka H, et al. Prognosis of primary testicular seminoma: a report of 57 new cases. Cancer Res 2000; 60:2152.

79. Triozzi PL, Martin EW, Gochnour D, Aldrich W. Phase Ib trial of a synthetic beta human chorionic gonadotropin vaccine in patients with metastatic cancer. Ann N Y Acad Sci 1993; 690:358.

80. Triozzi PL, Stevens VC, Aldrich W, et al. Effects of a beta-human chorionic gonadotropin subunit immunogen administered in aqueous solution with a novel nonionic block copolymer adjuvant in patients with advanced cancer. Clin Cancer Res 1997; 3(12 Pt 1):2355.

81. Triozzi PL, Stevens VC. Human chorionic gonadotropin as a target for cancer vaccines. Oncol Rep 1999; 6(1):7.

82. Lin J, Lei ZM, Lojun S, et al. Increased expression of luteinizing hormone/human chorionic gonadotropin receptor gene in human endometrial carcinomas. J Clin Endocrinol Metab 1994; 79(5):1483.

83. Bax CR, Chatzaki E, Davies S, Gallagher CJ. Elucidating the role of gonadotropins in endometrial cancer cell growth. Biochem Soc Trans 1996; 24:443S.

84. Konishi I, Koshiyama M, Mandai M, et al. Increased expression of LH/hCG receptors in endometrial hyperplasia and carcinoma in anovulatory women. Gynecol Oncol 1997; 65(2):273.

85. Nagamani M, Cao HA. Specific binding and proliferative effects of luteinizing hormone in human endometrial cancer cell lines. J Soc Gynecol Invest 1997; 4:132A.

86. Han SW, Zhou XL, Lei ZM, Rao ChV. Role of luteinizing hormone in human endometrial carcinoma. In: The Endocrine Society Annual Meeting; 1999, Abstract P1–593.

87. Rivera RT, Pasion SG, Wong DT, et al. Loss of tumorigenic potential by human lung tumor cells in the presence of antisense RNA specific to the ectopically synthesized alpha subunit of human chorionic gonadotropin. J Cell Biol 1989; 108(6):2423.

88. Kumar S, Talwar GP, Biswas DK. Necrosis and inhibition of growth of human lung tumor by anti-alpha human chorionic gonadotropin antibody. J Natl Cancer Inst 1992; 84(1):42.

89. Tao YX, Bao S, Ackermann DM, et al. Expression of luteinizing hormone/human chorionic gonadotropin receptor gene in benign prostatic hyperplasia and in prostate carcinoma in humans. Biol Reprod 1997; 56(1):67.

90. Bao S, Lei ZM, Rao ChV. The presence of functional luteinizing hormone/chorionic gonadotropin receptors in human prostate cell lines. In: The Endocrine Society Annual Meeting; 1997, Abstract P3–403.

91. Dirnhofer S, Berger C, Hermann M, et al. Coexpression of gonadotropic hormones and their corresponding FSH- and LH/CG-receptors in the human prostate. Prostate 1998; 35(3):212.

92. Lei ZM, Rao ChV. Direct luteinizing hormone regulation of male reproductive tract In: Coutinho EMSP, ed. Reproductive medicine: a millennium review. The proceedings of the 10th World Congress on Human Reproduction; 2000. London: Parthenon Publishing. 2000, In press.

93. Russo IH, Russo J. Chorionic gonadotropin: a tumoristatic and preventive agent in breast cancer. In: Teicher BA, ed. Drug resistance in oncology. New York: Marcel Dekker Inc, 1993:537.

94. Lojun S, Bao S, Lei ZM, Rao ChV. Presence of functional luteinizing hormone/chorionic gonadotropin (hCG) receptors in human breast cell lines: implications supporting the premise that hCG protects women against breast cancer. Biol Reprod 1997; 57(5):1202.

95. Li X, Lei ZM, Rao ChV. The actions of human chorionic gonadotropin in MCF-7 cells support the premise that it may protect woman against breast cancer. In: The Endocrine Society Annual Meeting, 1999. Abstract P3.

96. Lei ZM, Rao ChV. Protective role of human chorionic gonadotropin and luteinizing hormone against breast cancer. In: Barnea ER, Jaunaiux JE, Schwartz PE, Schofield PN, eds. Cancer and pregnancy. London: Springer-Verlag, 2000.

97. Gillott DJ, Iles RK, Chard T. The effects of beta-human chorionic gonadotrophin on the in vitro growth of bladder cancer cell lines. Br J Cancer 1996; 73(3):323.

98. Bieche I, Lazar V, Nogues C, et al. Prognostic value of chorionic gonadotropin beta gene transcripts in human breast carcinoma. Clin Cancer Res 1998; 4(3):671.

99. Butler SA, Laidler P, Porter JR, et al. The beta-subunit of human chorionic gonadotrophin exists as a homodimer [In Process Citation]. J Mol Endocrinol 1999; 22(2):185.

100. Lei ZM, Rao ChV, Ackerman DM, Day TG. The expression of human chorionic gonadotropin/human luteinizing hormone receptors in human gestational trophoblastic neoplasms. J Clin Endocrinol Metab 1992; 74(6):1236.

101. Licht P, Cao H, Zuo J, et al. Lack of self-regulation of human chorionic gonadotropin biosynthesis in human choriocarcinoma cells. J Clin Endocrinol Metab 1994; 78(5):1188.

102. Perilongo G, Rigon F, Murgia A. Oncologic causes of precocious puberty. Pediatr Hematol Oncol 1989; 6(4):331.

103. Themmen AP, Martens JW, Brunner HG. Activating and inactivating mutations in LH receptors. Mol Cell Endocrinol 1998; 145(1–2):137.

104. Kurtzman JT, Spinnato JA, Zimmerman MJ, et al. Human chorionic gonadotropin exhibits potent inhibition of preterm delivery in a small animal model. Am J Obstet Gynecol 1999; 181:853.

105. Hildreth NG, Shore RE, Dvoretsky PM. The risk of breast cancer after irradiation of the thymus in infancy. N Engl J Med 1989; 321(19):1281.

106. Tokunaga M, Land CE, Tokuoka S. Follow-up studies of breast cancer incidence among atomic bomb survivors. J Radiat Res (Tokyo) 1991; 32 (Suppl):201.

107. MacMahon B, Cole P, Lin TM, et al. Age at first birth and breast cancer risk. Bull WHO 1970; 43(2):209.

108. Trapido EJ. Age at first birth, parity, and breast cancer risk. Cancer 1983; 51(5):946.

109. Russo J, Russo IH. Hormonally induced differentiation: a novel approach to breast cancer prevention. J Cell Biochem Suppl 1995;22:58.

110. Alvarado MV, Alvarado NE, Russo J, Russo IH. Human chorionic gonadotropin inhibits proliferation and induces expression of inhibin in human breast epithelial cells in vitro. In Vitro Cell Dev Biol Anim 1994; 30A(1):4.

111. Srivastava P, Russo J, Russo IH. Chorionic gonadotropin inhibits rat mammary carcinogenesis through activation of programmed cell death. Carcinogenesis 1997; 18(9):1799.

112. Srivastava P, Russo J, Mgbonyebi OP, Russo IH. Growth inhibition and activation of apoptotic gene expression by human chorionic gonadotropin in human breast epithelial cells. Anticancer Res 1998; 18(6A):4003.

113. Huang Y, Bove B, Wu Y, et al. Microsatellite instability during the immortalization and transformation of human breast epithelial cells in vitro. Mol Carcinog 1999; 24(2):118.

114. Russo J, Yang X, Hu YF, et al. Biological and molecular basis of human breast cancer. Front Biosci 1998; 3:D944.

115. Alvarado MV, Russo J, Russo IH. Immunolocalization of inhibin in the mammary gland of rats treated with hCG. J Histochem Cytochem 1993; 41(1):29.

116. Huynh H. In vivo regulation of the insulin-like growth factor system of mitogens by human chorionic gonadotropin. Int J Oncol 1998; 13(3):571.

117. Bourinbaiar AS, Nagorny R. Inhibitory effect of human chorionic gonadotropin (hCG) on HIV-1 transmission from lymphocytes to trophoblasts. FEBS Lett 1992; 309(1):82.

118. Darzynkiewicz Z. The butler did it: search for killer(s) of Kaposi's sarcoma cells in preparations of human chorionic gonadotropin. J Natl Cancer Inst 1999; 91(2):104.

119. Lin J, Lojun S, Lei ZM, et al. Lymphocytes from pregnant women express human chorionic gonadotropin/luteinizing hormone receptor gene. Mol Cell Endocrinol 1995; 111:R13.

120. Zhang YM, Lei ZM, Rao ChV. Human macrophages contain luteinizing hormone and chorionic gonadotropin receptors. J Soc Gynecol Invest 1998; 5(Suppl 1):Abstract 212.

121. Zhang YM, Lei ZM, Rao ChV. Functional importance of human monocyte luteinizing hormone and chorionic gonadotropin receptors. J Soc Gynecol Invest 1999;6(Suppl 1):Abstract 46.

# PART VIII

# ENDOCRINOLOGY OF THE MALE

WILLIAM J. BREMNER, EDITOR

# CHAPTER 113

# MORPHOLOGY AND PHYSIOLOGY OF THE TESTIS

DAVID M. DE KRETSER

## STRUCTURAL ORGANIZATION OF THE TESTIS

In most mammalian species, the testis is located within the scrotum, having descended from an intraabdominal position during fetal development[1] (see Chap. 93). The intrascrotal position allows the testis to function at a lower temperature than is found within the abdomen. This is a requirement for normal spermatogenesis in many mammals including humans, although in some, such as the elephant, the testes do not descend and spermatogenesis is unaffected by the higher temperature within the abdomen. Because of testicular descent, the vascular supply originates relatively proximally, from the aorta near the origin of the renal arteries. The venous drainage, commencing as an anastomotic plexus of veins (the pampiniform plexus that surrounds the testicular artery), terminates in the renal vein on the left and in the inferior vena cava on the right.

This arrangement of vessels acts as a countercurrent mechanism to maintain lower testicular temperature; the cooler venous blood surrounds the testicular artery, decreasing its temperature as it approaches the testis.

The remnant of the peritoneal sac, the *processus vaginalis*, surrounds the testis on its anterior and lateral sides as the *tunica vaginalis*. The outer dense connective tissue covering, the *tunica albuginea*, sends septa, which run posteriorly toward the mediastinum of the testis and divide the testis into a series of *lobules*. Within these lobules lie the *seminiferous tubules*, which are coiled, extending as loops from the region of the mediastinum of the testis, from which they drain by straight tubules into an anastomotic network of ducts, the *rete testis*[2] (Fig. 113-1). The products of the tubules drain from the rete testis by a series of 15 to 20 ducts, the *ductuli efferentes*, which in humans constitute part of the *head of the epididymis*. In turn, the ductuli drain into the *duct of the epididymis*, whose coils form the remainder of the *head, body, and tail of the epididymis*.

The connective tissue surrounding the seminiferous tubules contains vascular and lymphatic vessels and the *Leydig cells*, which are responsible for the androgenic output of the testis.

## SPERMATOGENESIS

The sequence of cytologic changes that produce spermatozoa from spermatogonia is called *spermatogenesis*. It can be subdi-

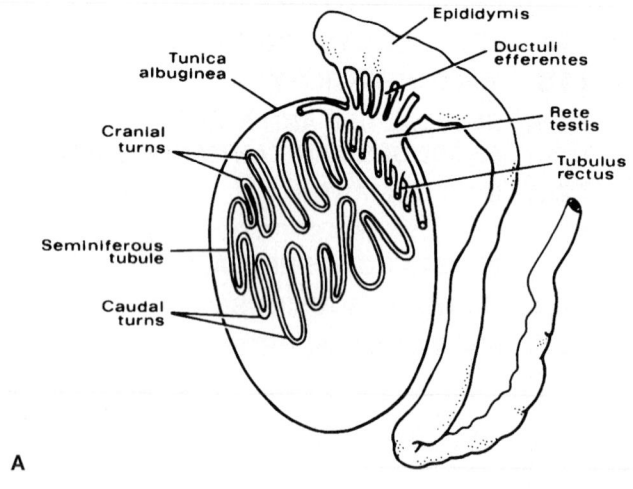

**A**

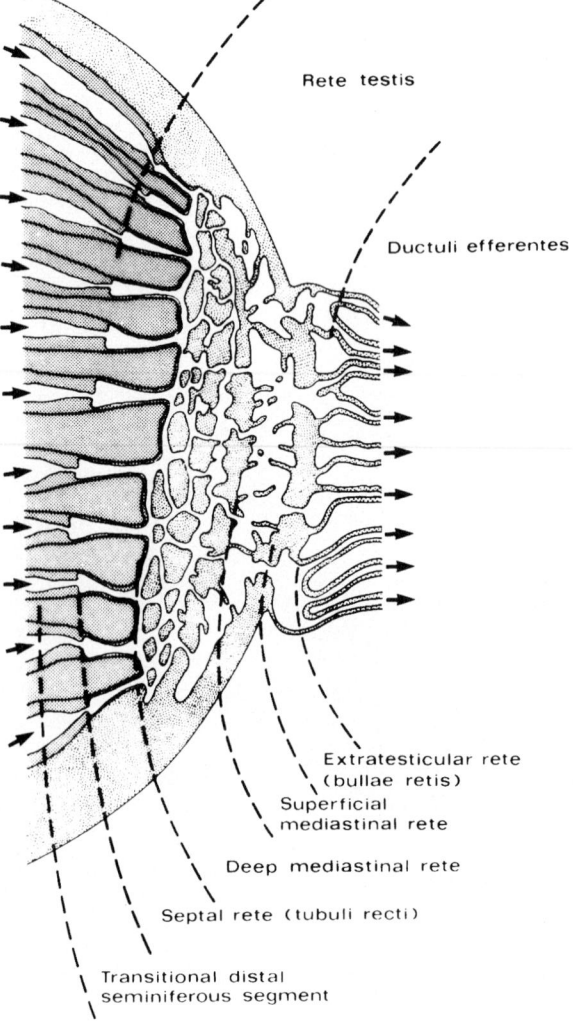

Rete testis

Ductuli efferentes

Extratesticular rete (bullae retis)
Superficial mediastinal rete
Deep mediastinal rete
Septal rete (tubuli recti)
Transitional distal seminiferous segment

**B**

**FIGURE 113-1. A,** The arrangement of the seminiferous tubules, rete testis, efferent ducts, and epididymis is illustrated. **B,** The structure of the rete testis is detailed. (From de Kretser DM, Temple-Smith PD, Kerr JB, et al. Anatomical and functional aspects of the male reproductive organs. In: Bandhauer K, Frick J, eds. Handbuch der Urologie, vol XVI. Berlin: Springer-Verlag, 1982:1.)

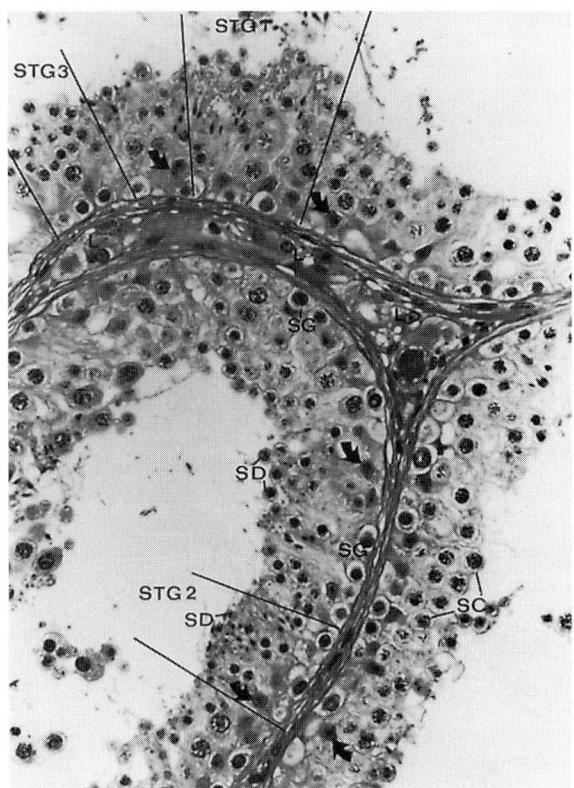

**FIGURE 113-2.** Light micrograph of a section from a normal human testis illustrates spermatogonia (*SG*), primary spermatocytes (*SC*), spermatids (*SD*), Sertoli cell nuclei (*arrows*), and Leydig cells (*L*). Stages of the human seminiferous cycle are denoted where identifiable (*STG*). ×950

vided into three major phases: the *replication of stem cells, meiosis,* and *spermiogenesis.*

## REPLICATION OF STEM CELLS

The replication of stem cells commences in fetal life with the migration of the *primordial germ cells* into the mesenchyme of the *gonadal ridge.* There is evidence that this migration is controlled by stem cell factor and its receptor *c-kit.*[3] After a period of prenatal mitotic division, the gonocytes, which populate the seminiferous cords at birth, remain quiescent until immediately before puberty, when they divide by mitosis to form the spermatogonial population.[4] The types of *spermatogonia* (Fig. 113-2) that can be characterized cytologically vary with each species. However, a feature common to all is the division of the stem cell population to provide two pools of cells, one that moves through the subsequent steps of spermatogenesis and the other

that retains its stem cell function.[5,6] In the human male, three types of spermatogonia are recognized classically: the A dark, thought to represent the most primitive; the A pale; and the B spermatogonia. They lie adjacent to the basement membrane of the tubule, interspersed with the basal aspects of the *Sertoli cells.* During cell division, the spermatogonia do not complete cytokinesis and remain linked by intercellular bridges.[7] Populations of spermatogonia that are injected into tubules devoid of germ cells will partially restore spermatogenesis.[8] These studies will provide the experimental basis for further evaluation of the nature and control of the stem cells in the testis.

## MEIOSIS

Responding to unknown signals, groups of type B spermatogonia begin meiosis, which involves two cell divisions. The spermatogonia lose their contact with the basement membrane of the tubule and are then called *primary spermatocytes.*[9] During the prophase of the first division (see Chap. 90), the primary spermatocytes, which have already replicated their DNA and contain twice the diploid content, undergo a series of characteristic nuclear changes consistent with the appearance and pairing of homologous chromosomes (Fig. 113-3). During the *leptotene* stage, the chromosomes appear as single, randomly coiled threads, which thicken and commence pairing during *zygotene.* During *pachytene,* the chromosomes appear as condensed, closely paired structures, which begin to repel each other during *diplotene. Diakinesis* is associated with further repulsion of the pairs of chromosomes, which each consist of a pair of daughter chromatids. During the metaphase of this *first division,* each member of the pair of homologous chromosomes moves to each daughter cell, reducing the number of chromosomes to the diploid number; however, because each chromosome is composed of two chromatids, the DNA content of a diploid cell is retained. Incomplete cytokinesis causes the formation of a pair of joined *secondary spermatocytes* from each primary spermatocyte.

During the *second division,* the 23 chromosomes, each comprising a pair of *chromatids,* attach to the spindle, and the chromatids separate. This yields a cell, a *spermatid,* containing the haploid DNA and chromosomal complement.

## SPERMIOGENESIS

Cell division stops after the formation of the spermatids. However, a dramatic metamorphosis, *spermiogenesis,* transforms a conventional cell into a highly specialized cell with the capability of flagellar-derived motility (Figs. 113-4 and 113-5). Little is known of the mechanisms by which these dramatic cytologic changes are controlled. The developmental phases are termed the $Sa_1$, $Sb_1$, $Sb_2$, $Sc_2$, $Sd_1$, and $Sd_2$ stages according to Clermont, but many of the details can be determined only by electron microscopy.[9–11] With the increasing use of spermatids extracted directly from the testis by biopsy, the specific features that characterize each of the above stages become crucial in identifying

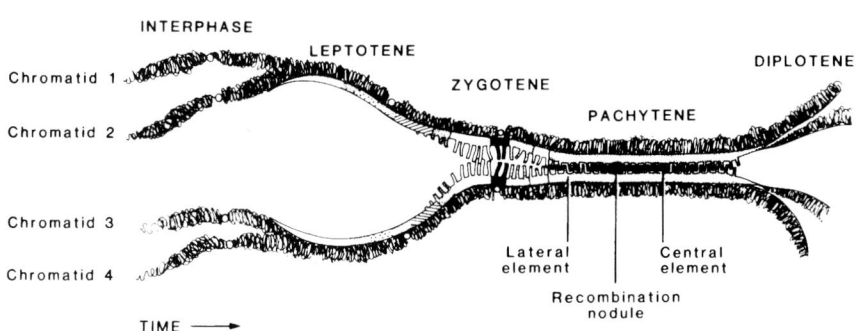

**FIGURE 113-3.** This diagram illustrates the process by which homologous chromosomes pair in the first meiotic division involving the primary spermatocytes. In the *leptotene* phase, the chromosomes are represented by unpaired fine "threads." These pair during *zygotene* and thicken during *pachytene,* eventually repelling each other during *diplotene.* The pairing process involves the formation of a tripartite structure, *synaptinemal complex,* which can be identified under the electron microscope. During the pairing, exchange of genetic material occurs between the maternal and paternal chromosomes in a process called *crossing over.* (From de Kretser DM, Kerr JB. The cytology of the testes. In: Knobil E, Neill JD, eds. The physiology of reproduction, 2nd ed. New York: Raven Press, 1994.)

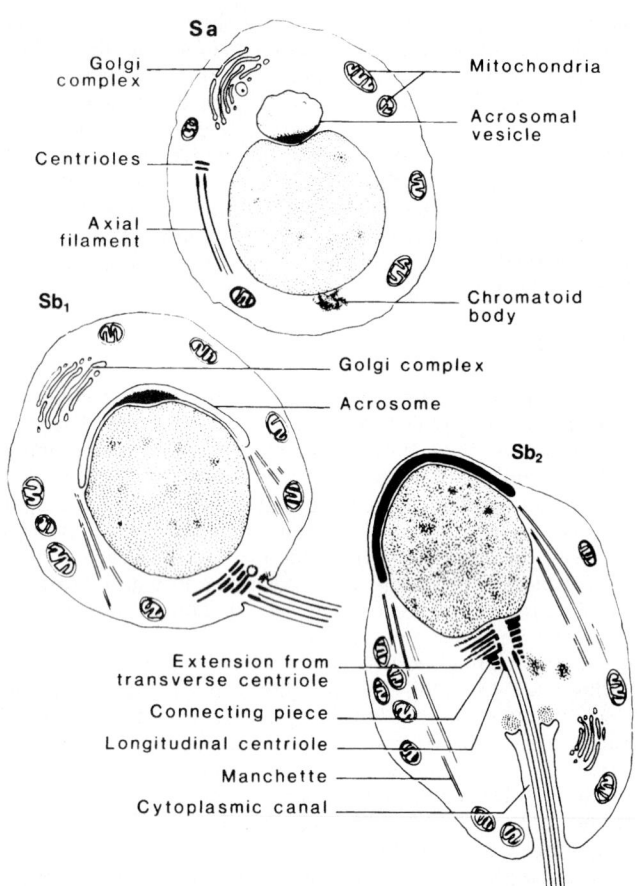

**FIGURE 113-4.** Initial cytologic changes during spermiogenesis are shown. See Figure 113-7 for explanation of Sa, Sb$_1$, and Sb$_2$. (From de Kretser DM. The light and electron microscope anatomy of the normal human testis. In: Santen RJ, Swerdloff RS, eds. Male sexual dysfunction: diagnosis and management of hypogonadism, infertility and impotence. New York: Marcel Dekker Inc, 1986:3.)

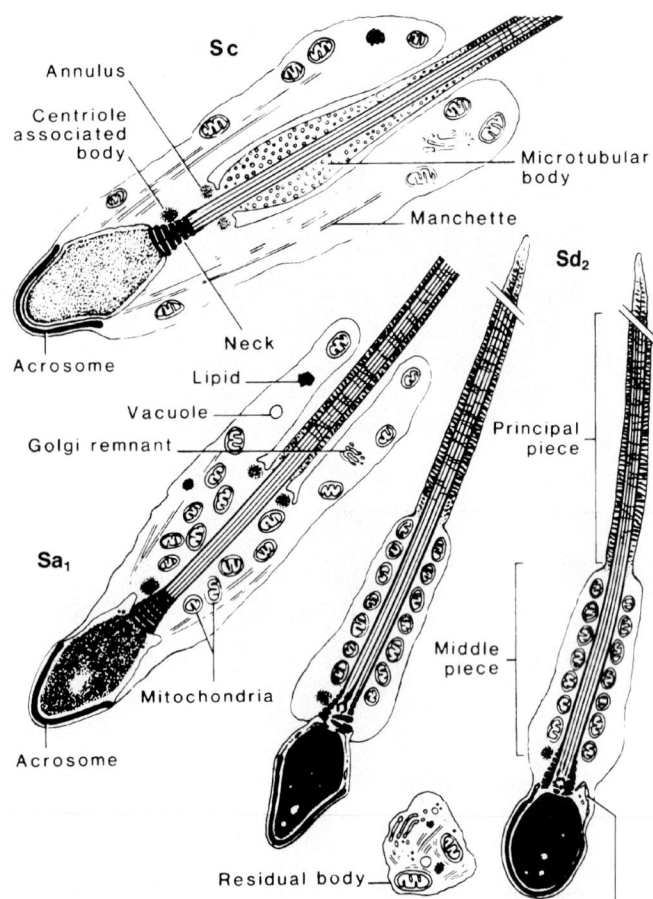

**FIGURE 113-5.** Subsequent cytologic changes during spermiogenesis. (See also Fig. 113-7.) (From de Kretser DM. The light and electron microscope anatomy of the normal human testis. In: Santen RJ, Swerdloff RS, eds. Male sexual dysfunction: diagnosis and management of hypogonadism, infertility and impotence. New York: Marcel Dekker Inc, 1986:3.)

the nature of the cell type injected into the cytoplasm of the oocyte to achieve fertilization. The changes can be subdivided into *nuclear, acrosome formation, flagellar development, redistribution of cytoplasm*, and *spermiation*.

### NUCLEAR CHANGES

During the Sa$_1$ and Sb$_1$ stages, the nucleus, which ultimately forms the *head of the sperm*, remains centrally placed, but it is subsequently displaced peripherally, coming into apposition with the cell membrane, separated only by the *acrosomal cap*. There is also a progressive decrease in nuclear volume associated with chromatin condensation, causing the development of resistance by the DNA to degradation by the enzyme DNAase.

### ACROSOME FORMATION

During the Sa$_1$ and Sb$_1$ stages, the Golgi complex of the spermatid produces several large vacuoles, which are applied to one pole of the nucleus. These vacuoles form a cap-like structure, the *acrosome*, which contains substances for penetration of the ovum during fertilization.[11a] Sperm that do not contain an acrosome cannot fertilize the ovum; because of the globular shape of the sperm head, the condition is known as *globozoospermia*. The Golgi complex subsequently migrates to the abacrosomal pole of the spermatid and is lost in the residual cytoplasm.

### FLAGELLAR DEVELOPMENT

The initial development of the *tail* occurs from the pair of centrioles located near the Golgi complex of the Sa$_1$ spermatid. The

microtubular structure, comprising nine peripheral doublets surrounding a pair of single microtubules, grows out from the distal centriole and forms the *axoneme* or core of the tail. The developing axoneme lodges in a facet at the abacrosomal pole of the nucleus by a complex articulation called the *neck* of the spermatid. Initially, the axoneme distal to the neck is surrounded by the cell membrane, but several specializations develop. Immediately adjacent to the outer nine doublets, a set of nine electron-dense fibers develop, which are connected cranially to the neck but distally taper to disappear eventually. A pair of these dense fibers, which lie diametrically opposite to each other, persist distally and become surrounded by a collection of microtubules. These microtubules form the precursors for solid electron-dense fibers, or ribs, which run transversely around the axoneme, joining the pair of longitudinal, dense fibers. The region of the tail surrounded by these ribs is the *principal piece*. The region between the principal piece and the neck is the last segment to become organized. Some of the genes, which encode the proteins comprising the outer dense fibers and the fibrous sheath, have been identified; these will provide the basis for future studies on the formation and function of the components.[12-15] Relatively late in spermiogenesis, between the Sd$_1$ and Sd$_2$ stages, the mitochondria that lie in the peripheral regions of the cell coalesce to form several helical arrays around the axoneme, forming the *midpiece* of the sperm.

The axoneme is identical to the core structure of cilia throughout the plant and animal kingdoms. The two centrally placed, single microtubules appear to be connected to the nine

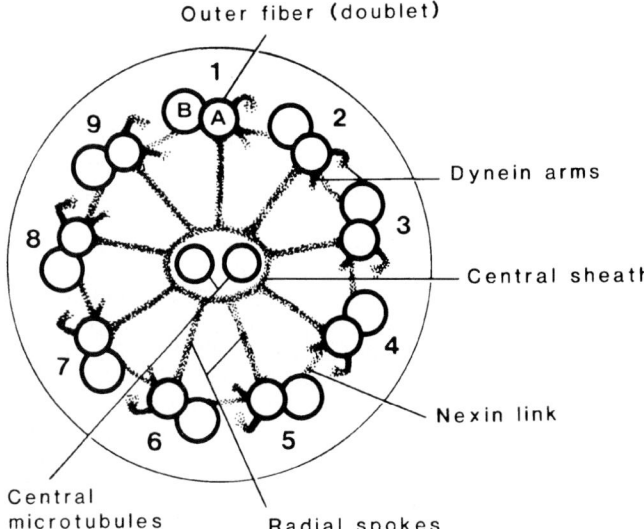

**FIGURE 113-6.** The structure of a typical axoneme of a sperm tail.

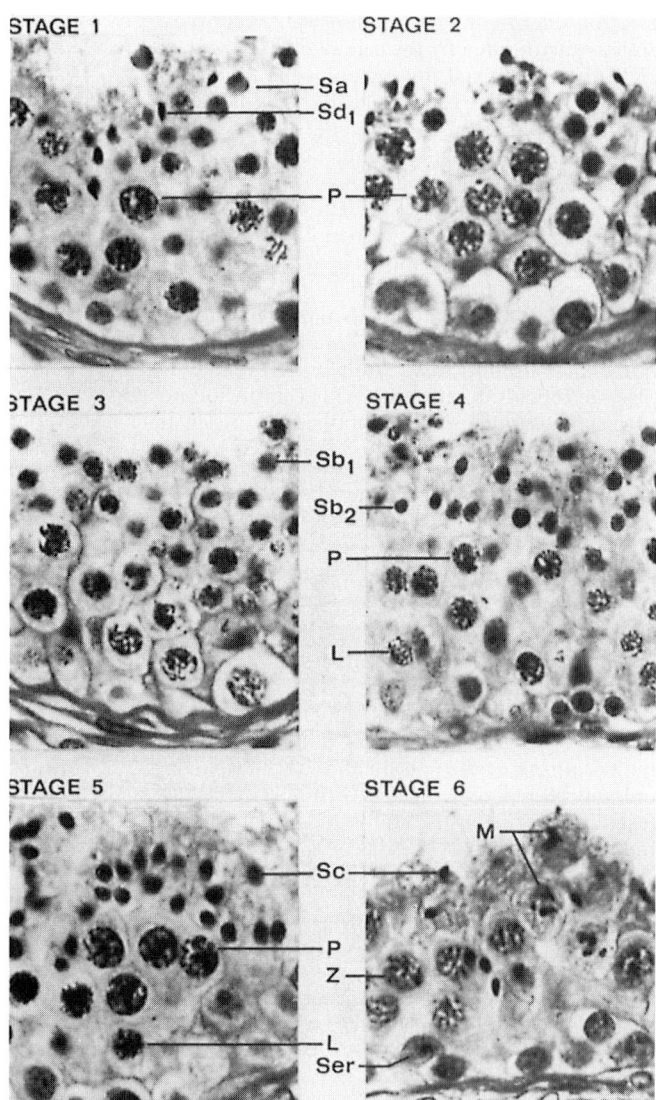

**FIGURE 113-7.** The light microscopic features of the stages of the human seminiferous cycle are illustrated. (*L*, leptotene primary spermatocyte; *M*, spermatocytes in meiosis; *P*, pachytene primary spermatocyte; *Z*, zygotene primary spermatocyte; $Sa_1$, $Sb_1$, $Sb_2$, $Sc$, $Sd_1$, spermatids at different steps of spermiogenesis; *Ser*, Sertoli cell nucleus.) (From de Kretser DM, Temple-Smith PD, Kerr JB, et al. Anatomical and functional aspects of the male reproductive organs. In: Bandhauer K, Frick J, eds. Handbuch der Urologie, vol XVI. Berlin: Springer-Verlag, 1982:1.)

peripheral doublets by a series of radial spokes (Fig. 113-6). One of each pair of doublets, termed *subfiber A*, is smaller and more electron dense; it sends a pair of hook-like extensions, or dynein arms, toward the adjacent doublet. They represent condensations of the protein, dynein, which has adenosine triphosphatase activity and is vital to the generation of flagellar motility; the absence of dynein arms is associated with immobility of sperm and cilia.[16,17]

### REDISTRIBUTION OF CYTOPLASM

Associated with the eccentric placement of the nucleus is a significant repositioning of the cytoplasm and organelles. This probably is caused by a palisade of microtubules, the *manchette*, which extends as a cylindrical collection from the head, in the region where the acrosome ends, to the caudal pole of the spermatid. Ultimately, most of this cytoplasm is shed by the spermatid and effectively appears to be pulled off by processes of Sertoli cell cytoplasm, which invaginate into pouches developing in the spermatid cytoplasm.[10] This cytoplasmic remnant, the *residual body*, is phagocytosed and degraded by the adjacent Sertoli cells.

### SPERMIATION

The release of spermatids at the $Sd_2$ stage occurs in association with the loss of the residual cytoplasm.

### SPERMATOGENIC CYCLE

Careful and extensive cytologic studies have demonstrated a characteristic sequence of cell associations through which the seminiferous epithelium passes and that constitute the cycle of the seminiferous epithelium.[6] In the rat, this consists of 14 cell associations, each of which may extend over several millimeters of tubule. However, in the human, six cell associations or stages have been identified, and each may occupy only 25% to 33% of a cross section of a seminiferous tubule[9] (Fig. 113-7). Studies in which dividing cells are labeled by tritiated thymidine have shown that the time taken for the daughter cells of spermatogonial divisions to mature to $Sd_2$ spermatids released from the seminiferous tubule is 64 ± 6 days or 4.5 cycles of the human seminiferous cycle.[18] The time for spermatogenesis is unique for each species and represents a biologic constant. The germ cells either pass through these stages at a specified speed or degenerate.

It is uncertain whether these time constraints are an innate function of each cell or whether they are imposed by other con-

trolling factors. Coordination of the spermatogenic process may be achieved by the unusual organization of the seminiferous epithelium, wherein the germ cells remain joined by intercellular bridges.[7] Additionally, coordination may be achieved by the Sertoli cells, whose arborizing branches maintain contact with many germ cell stages around the radial axis of the seminiferous tubules.

### SERTOLI CELLS

**Sertoli Cell Cytology.**    The general features of the Sertoli cell are similar in most mammalian species.[19,20] The cells extend from the basement membrane of the tubule to the luminal surface of the epithelium, and, although the base of the cell is clearly identifiable, the central portions cannot be distinguished by light microscopy. This results from the formation of many thin cytoplasmic prolongations that extend in an arborizing network around the germ cells undergoing spermatogenesis.

Electron microscopy has demonstrated that these processes are always surrounded by the cell membrane of the Sertoli cell.

In the Sertoli cell, the cytoplasmic organelles exhibit some degree of polarity. The basal aspects, which abut the basement membrane of the tubule, interspersed between spermatogonia, often show collections of mitochondria. The nucleus is pleomorphic, is aligned perpendicular to the basal lamina, and contains a prominent nucleolus. The nucleolus is a feature of the postpubertal Sertoli cell, probably related to the follicle-stimulating hormone (FSH)–induced maturation of the protein synthetic capacity of the mature Sertoli cell.[21,22]

In the perinuclear region, small collections of rough endoplasmic cisternae and Golgi membranes can be seen. Significant numbers of lipid inclusions, often surrounded by smooth endoplasmic reticulum, are found adjacent to the nucleus; in some species, these inclusions exhibit significant changes in number with the stages of the seminiferous cycle. Lysosomes, lipofuscin pigment, and residual bodies, which are the phagocytosed cytoplasmic remnants of the spermatids, may be seen deep within the Sertoli cell cytoplasm. The shape of the Sertoli cell is probably maintained by the cytoskeleton, consisting of a perinuclear array of fine filaments and microtubules that often extend into the smaller processes of cytoplasm surrounding the germ cells.

**Inter–Sertoli Cell Junctions.** One of the characteristic features of the Sertoli cell is the specialized inter–Sertoli cell junction, which occurs where adjacent Sertoli cells abut. These usually commence at a level in the epithelium just luminal to the basal row of the spermatogonia and extend centrally. This unique cell junction consists of small occluding junctions, representing points of fusion of the cell membranes that obliterate the intercellular space. Adjacent to these points of occlusion, smooth-membraned cisternae run parallel to the cell membrane and demarcate a narrow band of cytoplasm containing bundles of fine filaments.[23] The effect of these complexes is to prevent transport by way of the intercellular space to the centrally placed germ cells.[23] The inter–Sertoli cell junctions divide the seminiferous epithelium into two compartments: a basal one containing the spermatogonia and preleptotene primary spermatocytes and an adluminal one containing the subsequent stages of germ cell maturation. The cell junctions represent the site of the blood–testis barrier; by preventing intercellular transport, they create a highly selective permeability barrier based on transport systems within the Sertoli cell.[24] These cell junctions and the blood–testis barrier are absent in the immature testis but develop during pubertal maturation.[21,25] The resultant development of the cell junctions and barrier coincides with the onset of meiosis and seminiferous fluid secretion.[22,26] These cell junctions are not permanent structures since they must disassemble and re-form basally as preleptotene spermatocytes lose their attachment to the basement membrane and move centrally.

**Sertoli Cell Function.** There has been a great expansion in the knowledge of Sertoli cell function.[27] Because of the intimate relationship of the Sertoli cells to germ cells, the function of these cells is probably crucial for the successful completion of spermatogenesis. The concept that the number of Sertoli cells determines the spermatogenic output of the testis has gained considerable support, and clearly, the Sertoli cell is critically important for the transport of substances into the seminiferous tubule. Numerous examples indicate that the Sertoli cells are essential for the metabolic activities of the germ cells: For example, the germ cells, which are unable to metabolize glucose, are provided with lactate by the Sertoli cells.[28] Key roles of the Sertoli cells are discussed later.

**Sertoli Cell Replication.** Studies in the rat demonstrate that the Sertoli cell population divides by mitosis in fetal and postnatal life until day 15 but remains stable thereafter.[29] Neonatal hypothyroidism in the rat can extend the period of Sertoli cell replication, and in adult life the increased numbers of Ser-

toli cells lead to a marked increase in sperm output.[30] These data strongly suggest that the number of Sertoli cells in the testis is a major factor in controlling the spermatogenic potential of the testis. Use of this model has also shown that the functional maturation of the Sertoli cells is delayed during hypothyroidism[31] and that there is a marked delay in the process of spermatogenesis.[32] The control of Sertoli cell proliferation involves FSH, thyroid hormones, and growth factors such as activin A.[33]

**Seminiferous Tubule Fluid Production.** The Sertoli cells secrete a fluid, with characteristics distinct from plasma, into the lumen of the seminiferous tubule.[34] This secretion commences during sexual maturation, after the formation of the blood–testis barrier; it is dependent on FSH for its production.[35,36] In animals, the production of seminiferous tubule fluid can be measured by unilateral efferent duct ligation; the increasing difference in weight, with time, between the ligated and unligated sides provides this index.[35] Under such conditions, fluid production is maintained for 24 hours, after which a pressure atrophy of the seminiferous epithelium occurs and fluid production decreases, eventually ceasing altogether.[35,36]

**Androgen-Binding Protein.** The discovery that the Sertoli cell produces an androgen-binding protein (ABP) that is capable of binding dihydrotestosterone and testosterone with high affinity has provided a biochemical marker of Sertoli cell function.[27,37] Purification and characterization have revealed that, in the rat, ABP is a protein with a molecular mass of 85,000 daltons, for which a radioimmunoassay has been developed.[38] The amount of ABP secreted by the Sertoli cells varies among species; it is absent in some, and in others, such as humans, it is uncertain whether it is produced in the testis, because there is contamination of testis tissue with blood, which contains an ABP formed in the liver. ABP and the sex steroid–binding globulin (SSBG) found in some species are very similar, and represent the same protein produced in the liver and testis under different regulatory mechanisms.[39,40] ABP/SSBG acts as a hormone or growth factor, as evidenced by several studies that have identified high-affinity binding sites.[41,42] Furthermore, there are multiple alternate RNA transcripts of ABP in different tissues, and one of these encodes a nuclear targeting signal.[43,44] The secretion of ABP occurs principally into the lumen of the seminiferous tubules (Fig. 113-8), but it also passes across the basal aspect of the Sertoli cells into interstitial fluid and blood.[38] ABP may provide a mechanism for ensuring a large store of testosterone within the tubule, stabilizing fluctuations in testosterone secretion by the Leydig cells. It may also provide a mechanism for ensuring a high concentration of testosterone for the caput epididymis, because ABP and its bound testosterone are transported into the epididymis, where they are absorbed by the principal cells.

**Secretion of Other Plasma Proteins.** The Sertoli cell may produce a number of other proteins found in plasma, perhaps circumventing the presence of the blood–testis barrier and ensuring adequate local concentrations. Albumin, transferrin, and plasminogen activator are such proteins secreted by the Sertoli cell.[45–47] Their specific functions are unclear. Plasminogen activator has been proposed as a mechanism for enabling the discrete disruption of the inter–Sertoli cell junctions to allow germ cells to pass through from the basal to the adluminal compartments. Transferrin production by the Sertoli cells facilitates the transport of iron across the blood–testis barrier and enables the provision of adequate amounts of iron for the metabolism of germ cells.[47]

**Inhibins.** The Sertoli cell secretes inhibin (see Fig. 113-8), which increases in the testis after efferent duct ligation.[48–50] Inhibin, originally isolated from follicular fluid, is a disulfide-linked dimer of two dissimilar subunits termed $\alpha$ and $\beta$.[51] Two forms exist that share a common $\alpha$ subunit but distinct $\beta$ subunits: These forms are *inhibin A* ($\alpha\beta_A$) and *inhibin B* ($\alpha\beta_B$).[51] Both forms suppress FSH, whereas dimers of the $\beta$ subunits—

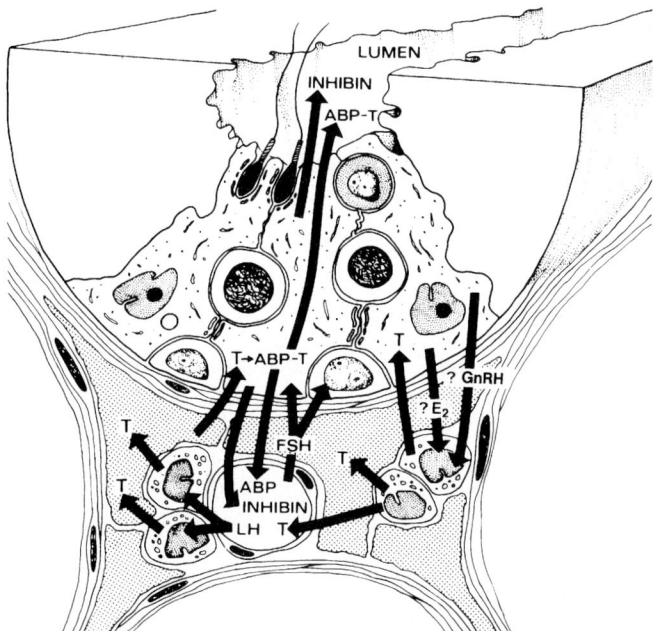

**FIGURE 113-8.** A diagram of the testis shows the relationship of Sertoli cells to germ cells. Factors controlling the testicular compartments are outlined. Evidence for the secretion of estradiol (*E₂*) and gonadotropin-releasing hormone (*GnRH*) by the adult Sertoli cell is tentative, but the hormones have been suggested as local modulators of Leydig cell function. (*T*, testosterone; *ABP*, androgen binding protein; *FSH*, follicle-stimulating hormone; *LH*, luteinizing hormone.)

termed *activins* (activin A [$\beta_A\beta_A$], activin AB [$\beta_A\beta_B$], activin B [$\beta_B\beta_B$])—all stimulate FSH. The genes coding the subunits produce larger precursor molecules that dimerize and are proteolytically cleaved to form the mature substances.[52,53] The subunits of inhibin show significant homology to transforming growth factor-β, antimüllerian hormone (AMH), and numerous other proteins, such as the protein coded for by the decapentaplegic gene complex of *Drosophila*.[52–54]

The Sertoli cells secrete inhibin B as the principal protein feedback on FSH secretion, and there is a good correlation between sperm output and inhibin B levels in the circulation.[55,56] Inhibin B levels are inversely correlated to FSH concentrations; therefore, there have been suggestions that inhibin B is a useful marker for *Sertoli cell function*.[57] Experiments using recombinant inhibin A indicate that, although both testosterone and inhibin modulate FSH, inhibin can normalize FSH levels in castrated rams in the absence of testosterone.[58,59]

**Antimüllerian Hormone.** Antimüllerian hormone is produced by the Sertoli cell during fetal and early postnatal life.[60,60a] It has been purified and shown to be a glycoprotein. In fetal life it directs the regression of the müllerian ducts during male sexual differentiation (see Chap. 90).

**Steroidogenic Function.** The presence of smooth endoplasmic reticulum, lipid droplets, and mitochondria with tubular cristae in the cytoplasm of the Sertoli cells led to the proposal that the Sertoli cells could be the site of steroid biosynthesis.[61] By separating seminiferous tubules from interstitial tissue, it was demonstrated that the tubules do not have the capacity to metabolize cholesterol to products more distant in the steroidogenic pathway. However, if provided with substrates such as progesterone, the seminiferous tubules have the capacity to metabolize these materials to androgens.[62] Unique metabolites of C-19 steroids have been identified in Sertoli cells, and the pattern of metabolism can be altered by FSH treatment. Despite the uncertainty about the steroidogenic capacity of the seminiferous tubules and Sertoli cells, cultures of immature rat Sertoli cells have the ability to metabolize androgens, with the enzyme aro-

matase, to estradiol.[63] However, in the rat, this activity decreases rapidly with age and is not detectable 20 days after birth. Evidence suggests that estradiol production by the testis after this time occurs within the Leydig cells.[64] In the immature rat, the activity of aromatase is FSH inducible, and this reaction has been used as a basis for an in vitro bioassay for FSH.[65]

**Age-Dependent Changes in Sertoli Cell Function.** Before 20 days, the Sertoli cells can respond dramatically to FSH by an increase in cyclic adenosine monophosphate (AMP) and in protein synthesis, together with the stimulation of the enzyme aromatase. Additionally, the immature Sertoli cells produce AMH in fetal life and for a short period after birth. These functions disappear ~20 days after birth in the rat and are replaced by increases in ABP secretion, the onset of fluid production, and an increase in inhibin secretion.[66] The mechanisms causing these changes in Sertoli cell function are unknown, but some may be related to the onset of pubertal secretion of FSH by the pituitary.

**Stage-Dependent Changes in Sertoli Cell Function.** The seminiferous tubule undergoes a sequence of cytologic changes, causing the formation of specific cell associations, which have been identified as the seminiferous cycle. In association with these changes in the germ cell complement of the seminiferous tubule, there are distinct cytologic changes that have been identified within the Sertoli cell, particularly in the rat, in which there is a very well-defined seminiferous cycle. In this species, a number of biochemical parameters vary according to the stage of the seminiferous cycle.[67] Thus, FSH-receptor levels, ABP production, and cyclic AMP production change according to the stage of the seminiferous cycle in response to FSH stimulation.[9] The nature of the products from germ cells that modulate Sertoli cell function is still unknown. The concept that these may arise from late spermatids, possibly through the phagocytosis of residual bodies, has been reviewed.[68]

## CONTROL OF THE SEMINIFEROUS TUBULE

**Hormonal Control.** The function of the testis depends on the secretion of the gonadotropic hormones, FSH and luteinizing hormone (LH), by a functional hypothalamic-pituitary unit (see Chap. 16). Moreover, the action of LH on spermatogenesis is mediated through the secretion of testosterone by the Leydig cells. However, there is considerable controversy concerning the relative roles of FSH and testosterone in the control of seminiferous tubule function.

**Initiation of Spermatogenesis.** The role of testosterone in this process is not questioned, and current data indicate that constitutive-activating mutations in the LH receptor cause precocious puberty, while inactivating mutations result in familial testosterone resistance and male pseudohermaphroditism.[69,70] The earlier view that, in humans and other mammalian species, both FSH and LH are required for the initiation of spermatogenesis during pubertal maturation[71–73] has been challenged by three studies in mice. First, testosterone alone has been shown to induce spermatogenesis in the *hpg* mouse, which lacks the capacity to secrete gonadotropin-releasing hormone and, thus, cannot produce both FSH and LH.[74] Secondly, inactivation of the gene encoding the β subunit of FSH did not prevent the onset of full spermatogenesis during pubertal maturation in these mice.[75] The third study of several males with inactivating mutations of the FSH receptor found that the males were able to complete spermatogenesis, but in most, the testicular volumes and sperm counts were very significantly impaired.[76]

In all these studies it was noted that the testes were smaller and that the sperm output was lower than normal. The possibility that this results from an impairment of Sertoli cell multiplication (normally stimulated by FSH) is being explored.

The view that both FSH and LH were required originated from studies of patients with hypogonadotropic hypogonadism during the induction of spermatogenic activity using FSH and LH. Some patients respond to LH or human chorionic gonadotropin (hCG) alone, but most require the action of both gonadotropic hormones.[77] There are conflicting data for the rat, suggesting that LH, through the action of testosterone, may play a more dominant role during pubertal maturation; however, the rat is a very poor model for studies of sexual maturation because it does not have a prepubertal period. The spermatogenic process in the rat occupies 48 to 50 days, and mature spermatozoa can be seen in the rat 45 to 50 days after birth. Consequently, changes closely related to the time of birth in the rat may be involved in the initiation of spermatogenesis.

**Maintenance of Spermatogenesis.**    Given the results of the studies in the *hpg* mouse and those in genetically modified mice in which the β subunit of FSH is not produced, the controversy regarding the role of FSH in the maintenance of spermatogenesis after its establishment at puberty is still unresolved. In the rat, the observations that testosterone alone, given immediately after hypophysectomy, could maintain spermatogenesis without FSH have received some support from experiments in humans using an alternative design. In these studies, the suppression of FSH and LH secretion by the administration of contraceptive doses of testosterone caused azoospermia or severe oligospermia. These changes could be reversed by the administration of hCG or LH, which presumably act by stimulating Leydig cells to increase the intratesticular levels of testosterone.[77,78] However, when researchers used the same design to suppress spermatogenesis, highly purified FSH was also able to restore the sperm count, presumably without altering intratesticular levels of testosterone.[79] Several studies have shown that the levels of testosterone normally found within the testis are not required to maintain spermatogenesis, which can proceed successfully at concentrations ~10% of normal.[80,81] Nonetheless, these levels still represent twice the normal circulating concentrations, in turn raising questions as to why the testicular androgen receptor requires significantly greater stimulation than other androgen-dependent tissues, for example, prostate.

Both in rats and in humans, if regression of the spermatogenic epithelium has occurred after hypophysectomy, testosterone alone is insufficient to restore spermatogenesis.[80–82] However, this view has been challenged by studies in stalk-sectioned monkeys in whom testosterone treatment alone reversed the testicular regression that had occurred, although testicular volumes returned to only 60% of presurgical levels.[83]

The claim that no biochemical action of FSH was found in the adult rat testis[84] has now been shown to be erroneous since the sensitivity to FSH stimulation varies with the stage of the seminiferous cycle within the seminiferous tubule.[67] These studies demonstrate that an FSH-induced effect can be obtained in the adult testis provided an FSH-sensitive phase of the seminiferous cycle is selected. Positive evidence for the role of FSH in the spermatogenic process includes the fact that receptors for FSH have been identified on the Sertoli cell and on spermatogonia.[85] The action of FSH is mediated by the cyclic AMP–protein kinase system and stimulates protein synthesis by the Sertoli cell. A number of proteins, such as ABP, aromatase, plasminogen activator, RNA polymerase, inhibin, and proteoglycan, are responsive to FSH or cyclic AMP.[49,66,84] Studies in primates and in normal men have shown that FSH is important in maintaining the transition of type A to type B spermatogonia.[86,87]

Testosterone is clearly important in maintaining the seminiferous epithelium. This action of testosterone is mediated through androgen receptors found within the Sertoli cell and on peritubular and Leydig cells.[88–90] Further evidence for the role of androgens in the stimulation of Sertoli cell function was obtained from Sertoli cells in culture, in which RNA polymerase and ABP production could be stimulated independently of any action of FSH.[91,92] After hypophysectomy, testosterone alone can maintain fluid production and the secretion of inhibin by the rat testis.[36,93] Unfortunately, the rat proves

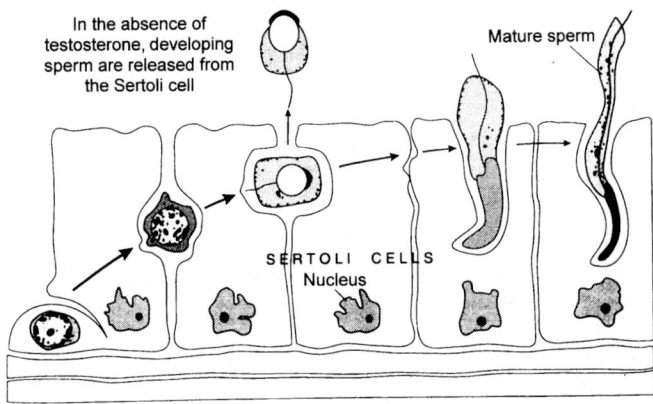

**FIGURE 113-9.** The relationship between germ cells and Sertoli cells in the rat is shown. In the presence of low intratesticular testosterone levels, spermatids at stages VII to VIII of the cycle are shed from the epithelium. (From McLachlan RI, Wreford NG, Robertson DM, et al. Hormonal control of spermatogenesis. Trends Endocrinol Metab 1995; 6:95.)

to be a difficult model in which to explore the effect of high doses of testosterone, since these stimulate FSH secretion.[94]

Morphometric studies have shown that spermiogenesis is exquisitely sensitive to testosterone,[81,94] and further data suggest that withdrawal of testosterone disrupts the conversion of step 7 to 8 because of premature sloughing of round spermatids into the epididymis.[95,96] It is likely that this cell loss is due to disruption of the ectoplasmic specializations between spermatids and Sertoli cells (Fig. 113-9). Further, the studies in the *hpg* model indicate that testosterone is important in facilitating the survival of primary spermatocytes.[74]

The relative role of testosterone and dihydrotestosterone in spermatogenesis has been perplexing, given that the concentrations of intratesticular testosterone are significantly greater. However, studies with 5α-reductase inhibitors have shown that dihydrotestosterone is a significant stimulator of spermatogenesis when intratesticular testosterone concentrations decline.[96]

It is recognized that the testis secretes estradiol, arising from the conversion of androgens by the enzyme aromatase. Evidence for an effect of estradiol on spermatogenesis has emerged from gene-targeted disruption of the P450 aromatase gene, which demonstrated that the initially fertile mice progressively became infertile as a result of decreases in spermatid numbers, increased apoptosis, and abnormal acrosome development.[97–99] More direct evidence of the actions of estradiol was obtained from gene knock-out of the estradiol α receptor: These mice were infertile due to the actions of estradiol on fluid reabsorption in the epithelium of the efferent ductules.[100] The resultant back pressure resulted in loss of germ cells from the seminiferous epithelium. However, estradiol can still act on the seminiferous epithelium in these mice, since a functional estradiol β receptor remains in the testis.[101] Initial reports of the knock-out of this gene indicate that the mice are fertile at 6 weeks of age.[102]

In summary, while recent studies shed some doubt as to the critical importance of FSH in enabling spermatogenesis to proceed to completion, others have defined specific points at which FSH appears to be very important in maintaining a normal throughput of germ cells. These points appear to be in its action on Sertoli cell mitosis and in facilitating the formation and survival of type B spermatogonia.

**Nonhormonal Control.**    There are numerous steps that must be successfully completed before the testis can successfully produce a normal sperm output. These involve molecular mechanisms that require key regulators that are not hormones. As these molecular controllers are identified, usually through experiments that involve the exploration of the function of a protein through gene-targeted disruption, additional regulators of spermatogenesis emerge. It is not possible to consider these proteins exhaustively in this chapter, but a few examples are given that illustrate these developments.

For successful sperm production, the development and differentiation of the testis must proceed normally. Any mutation or rearrangement in genes, which is crucial for normal testis development, will impair sperm output or testicular development. Mutations in key domains of the androgen receptor can disrupt hormone binding and result in testicular feminization, but data indicate that there are mutations that occur in other regions of the gene encoding the receptor that do not interfere with sexual differentiation but can impair spermatogenesis. These include expansions of the CAG repeat sequence in the amino-terminal region of the protein.[103]

The deletion of genes on the long arm of the Y chromosome has demonstrated the presence of testis-specific genes that are essential to enable normal sperm production. One of these, DAZ (deleted in azoospermia), encodes an apparent RNA-binding protein and exhibits homology to the boule gene in *Drosophila*, mutations that cause sterility in flies. Mutations or deletions of the DAZ genes, for which there are multiple copies in humans, result in severe disruption of spermatogenesis, without any effect on sexual differentiation.[104,105]

Numerous studies in mice have shown that mutations in the gene encoding stem cell factor or its receptor c-*kit* result in testes devoid of germ cells because of disruption of the migration of the primordial germ cells and their transformation into spermatogonia.[3,106]

Later stages of spermatogenesis can show disruption by interference in molecular mechanisms. For instance, targeted disruption of the gene encoding heat shock protein 70-2, a molecular chaperone, results in the arrest of spermatogenesis at the primary spermatocyte stage since this protein appears to be crucial to enabling the completion of meiosis.[107]

There are numerous studies to indicate that apoptotic mechanisms are important regulatory pathways in the testis, especially following hormonal modulation.[108] Evidence supporting this view has emerged from studies of targeted disruption of the gene encoding bcl-w, a cell survival molecule; the first wave of spermatogenesis in mice almost progressed to completion but collapsed, resulting in infertility and ultimately in a Sertoli cell–only phenotype.[109] Whether there are hormonal mechanisms that regulate this and other proteins, which control cell survival, remains to be established.

## INTERTUBULAR TISSUE

The seminiferous tubules are supported by a loose connective tissue, which is supplied by a rich vascular network. It is bounded by the basement membrane of the seminiferous tubule, which is surrounded by a varying number of layers of contractile *myoid cells* interspersed with collagen fibers and a basement membrane–type material that is applied to some of the layers of the myoid cells. The myoid cells are modified smooth muscle cells that cause the contraction of the seminiferous tubules. The general organization of the intertubular tissue varies among species, based on the number of Leydig cells, which are responsible for androgen secretion, the arrangement of the lymphatics, and the extent of the connective tissue.[110] The intertubular tissue contains varying numbers of Leydig cells, fibroblasts, macrophages, mast cells, and small unmyelinated nerve fibers.

## LEYDIG CELLS

The Leydig cells are derived from the mesenchyme of the gonadal ridge; two generations of Leydig cells are developed. In fetal life, the differentiation of mesenchyme into Leydig cells induces the secretion of androgens that generate the sexual differentiation of the external genitalia. These *fetal Leydig cells* degenerate shortly after birth, and the prepubertal period is characterized by the absence of Leydig cells from the intertubu-

lar tissue. Associated with the pubertal secretion of gonadotropins, *adult Leydig cells* redifferentiate from connective tissue precursors[111] within the intertubular tissue. In other species, such as the rat, in which the interval from birth to sexual maturation is short, some overlap occurs between the fetal and adult generations. The testosterone is secreted into the intertubular tissue, where it is absorbed by blood vessels, lymphatics, and the seminiferous tubules.

**Leydig Cell Cytology.**    Leydig cells form small collections around blood vessels and have a variable appearance by light microscopy, usually attributed to the lipid inclusions, which cause a variable vacuolation (see Fig. 113-2). The Leydig cells are characterized by an ovoid nucleus exhibiting a conspicuous nucleolus. The cytoplasm contains a large amount of smooth endoplasmic reticulum in the form of interconnected tubules. Mitochondria contain both lamellar and tubular cristae, the latter being typical of steroid-secreting cells. The content of lipid, lysosomes, and lipofuscin pigment is variable. The human Leydig cells are characterized by the presence of crystalloid inclusions, the *crystals of Reinke*, the functional significance of which is unknown. The amount of smooth endoplasmic reticulum and mitochondria declines after hypophysectomy and increases after LH or hCG stimulation.[112]

**Leydig Cell Function.**    The Leydig cells secrete testosterone and are able to synthesize cholesterol from acetate, with the cholesterol acting as a substrate for steroidogenesis. The amount of cholesterol obtained by lipoprotein uptake relative to synthesis from acetate varies among species. The enzymatic steps involved in the synthesis of testosterone from cholesterol are outlined in Figure 113-10. Besides the secretion of testosterone, the Leydig cells secrete estradiol, contributing 20% to 30% of the total circulating estradiol; the remainder is derived from the peripheral aromatization of androgenic substrates. There is a subcellular localization of the enzymes involved in steroidogenesis, with the conversion of cholesterol to pregnenolone localized in mitochondria; the remaining steps of steroid biosynthesis in the testis depend on enzymes located within the smooth endoplasmic reticulum of the Leydig cell.

Several studies have expanded the understanding of the mechanisms underlying cholesterol transport into the mitochondria, a step that is critical in enabling cleavage of the side chain of pregnenolone. The isolation and characterization of *steroidogenic acute regulatory protein (StAR)*[113] and the cloning of the gene encoding this protein demonstrated that it had a crucial role in the transport of cholesterol into mitochondria. Mutations in this gene or its targeted disruption profoundly interfered with steroid hormone biosynthesis in all steroid-secreting endocrine tissues; in humans, mutations were shown to be responsible for the condition of lipoid congenital adrenal hyperplasia.[114,115]

**Influence of Luteinizing Hormone.**    The Leydig cell contains receptors for LH on its cell membrane; this hormone controls testosterone secretion by means of cyclic AMP.[116] The principal enzyme controlled by LH is the side-chain cleavage enzyme involved in the conversion of cholesterol to pregnenolone. Besides the immediate events initiated through the phosphorylation of proteins that induce testosterone secretion, LH is trophic to the Leydig cell and stimulates the incorporation of labeled amino acids into specific proteins. This trophic activity causes a hypertrophy of the Leydig cells and probably increases the number of Leydig cells.

The stimulation of Leydig cells with large doses of LH or hCG rapidly reduces the number of their receptors, a phenomenon termed *down-regulation*.[116,117] Although these changes decrease testosterone secretion 24 to 48 hours after an injection, repeated stimulation does not yield the same results. Additionally, a single injection of hCG is followed by a prolonged steroidogenic response characterized by two phases of testosterone secretion, one initially occurring over the first 6 to 18 hours and the second occurring 48 to 72 hours later.[117] The

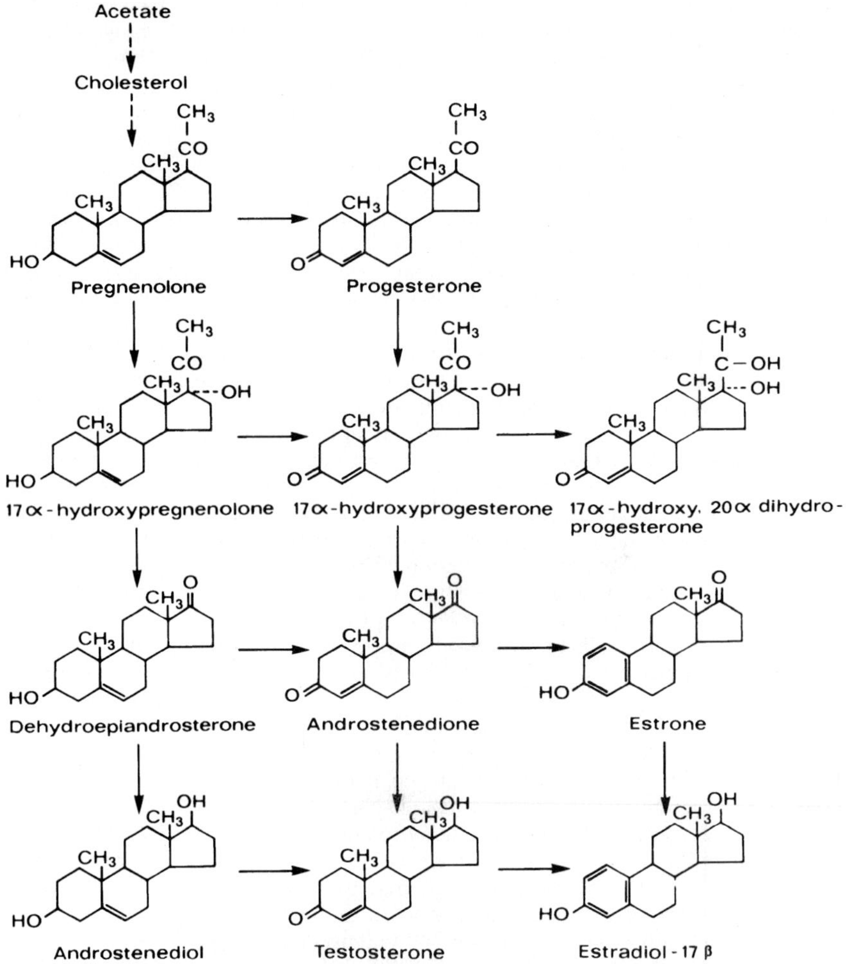

**FIGURE 113-10.** These are the biochemical pathways in the synthesis of testosterone.

results indicate that hCG can be administered at 6- to 7-day intervals due to the prolonged steroidogenic response. The nadir between the two phases of testosterone secretion is due to the block in testosterone production induced by the large injection of hCG, and recovery from the inhibition allows restimulation of testosterone secretion by the existing plasma hCG, because of the long half-life of hCG.

INFLUENCE OF OTHER FACTORS. There is increasing evidence, principally from rat studies, that other factors may be involved in the stimulation of testosterone secretion by Leydig cells. This concept originated from observations that damage to the seminiferous tubules by a number of experimental agents caused changes within the Leydig cells,[118] which included Leydig cell hypertrophy, partial loss of LH receptors, and a hyperresponsiveness of the Leydig cells to hCG stimulation in vitro. If unilateral damage to the testis was induced, such as after unilateral cryptorchidism, the Leydig cell changes were present exclusively in the damaged testis, thereby ruling out circulating humoral factors, such as LH, participating in these changes. The resultant hypothesis suggested that the seminiferous tubules somehow modulate the Leydig cells (see Fig. 113-8).

Reasoning that any factor passing from the seminiferous tubules to the Leydig cells must pass across the lymphatic sinusoidal system in the rat, investigators have demonstrated a proteinaceous factor that was not LH and that stimulated steroidogenesis.[119] This substance stimulates testosterone more than the maximum levels generated by LH or hCG. Also, a number of studies have suggested that the macrophages present in both the testis and ovary may secrete substances capable of stimulating steroidogenesis, thereby increasing the potential for local control of Leydig cells.[118] This view has been substantiated by the impaired development and function of Leydig cells in mice wherein the gene encoding CSF-1 has been disrupted.[120] The relative importance of these local factors and of LH in the physiology of testosterone secretion requires clarification. The possibility that these changes may be explained by modulation of StAR or the peripheral benzodiazepine receptor[121] requires further work.

## INTERCOMPARTMENTAL MODULATION IN THE TESTIS

Throughout this chapter, the seminiferous tubules and intertubular tissue have been considered as independent entities. However, there is increasing evidence that this approach is unwarranted. It is well documented that testosterone is required for the process of spermatogenesis, indicating that the Leydig cells at a local level are able to influence the seminiferous tubules.[122] Additionally, the seminiferous tubules are involved in the modulation of Leydig cell function. There is also evidence that the Leydig cells exhibit changes in size according to the stage of the seminiferous cycle in the tubules immediately adjacent to them.[123] Furthermore, the Sertoli cells show marked changes in function in association with spermatogenic damage and the stage of the seminiferous cycle.[124] All of the agents used to induce experimental damage to spermatogenesis decrease the parameters of Sertoli cell function, such as seminiferous tubule fluid production, ABP production, and inhibin production. These changes occur despite a relatively well-maintained morphology of the Sertoli cell; they indicate the importance of obtaining sensitive biochemical indices of Sertoli cell function.

The testis should be considered as a functional unit and not as individual compartments with few functional interrelationships. Consideration of these factors may soon provide explanations about why spermatogenesis in certain infertile men does not proceed to completion despite a well-maintained stem cell population within the seminiferous epithelium.

## IMMUNOLOGIC CONTROL IN THE TESTIS

There is increasing interest in the concept that the testis is an immunologically privileged site; this is based on observations that grafts in the testis survive for prolonged periods.[125,126] The maintenance of this environment may be crucial in preventing the formation of autoantibodies to sperm components. Attention has been drawn to the large population of macrophages in the intertubular tissue of the testis that have an impaired capacity to respond to an inflammatory stimulus by the secretion of proinflammatory cytokines. The reason for this observation is still unclear but may involve the production of unidentified substances by the Leydig and Sertoli cells. These cells have the capacity to produce cytokines such as interleukin (IL)-1 and IL-6 in response to inflammatory stimuli.[127]

## REFERENCES

1. Wartenberg H. Differentiation and development of the testes. In: Burger HG, de Kretser DM, eds. The testis. New York: Raven Press, 1981:39.
2. de Kretser DM, Temple-Smith PD, Kerr JB. Anatomical and functional aspects of the male reproductive organs. In: Bandhauer K, Frick J, eds. Handbuch der Urologie, vol XVI. Berlin: Springer-Verlag, 1982:1.
3. Marziali G, Lazzaro D, Sorrentino V. Binding of germ cells to mutant SI^d Sertoli cells is defective and is rescued by expression of the transmembrane form of the c-*kit* ligand. Dev Biol 1993; 157:182.
4. Muller J, Skakkebaek NE. Quantification of germ cells and seminiferous tubules by stereological examination of testicles from 50 boys who suffered from sudden death. Int J Androl 1983; 6:143.
5. Huckins C. The spermatogonial stem cell population in adult rats: I. Their morphology, proliferation and maturation. Anat Rec 1971; 169:533.
6. Clermont Y. Kinetics of spermatogenesis in mammals: seminiferous epithelium cycle and spermatogonial renewal. Physiol Rev 1972; 52:198.
7. Dym M, Fawcett DW. Further observations on the numbers of spermatogonia, spermatocytes and spermatids connected by bridges in the mammalian testis. Biol Reprod 1971; 4:195.
8. Brinster RL, Zimmerman JW. Spermatogenesis following male germ-cell transplantation. Proc Natl Acad Sci U S A 1994; 11298.
9. Clermont Y. The cycle of the seminiferous epithelium in man. Am J Anat 1963; 112:35.
10. de Kretser DM. Ultrastructural features of human spermiogenesis. Z Zellforsch 1969; 98:477.
11. Holstein AF, Roosen-Runge EC. Atlas of human spermatogenesis. Berlin: Grosse Verlag, 1981.
11a. Abou-Haila A, Tulsiani DR. Mammalian sperm acrosome: formation, contents, and function. Arch Biochem Biophys 2000; 379:173.
12 Fulcher KD, Mori C, Welch JE, et al. Characterization of *FSC-1* complementary deoxyribonucleic acid for a mouse sperm fibrous sheath component. Biol Reprod 1995; 52: 41.
13. Schalles U, Shao X, van der Hoorn FA, Oko R. Developmental expression of the 84 kDa ODF sperm protein: localization to both the cortex and medulla of outer dense fibers and to the connecting piece. Develop Biol 1998; 199:250.
14. Burfeind P, Hoyer-Fender S. Sequence and developmental expression of a mRNA encoding a putative protein of rat sperm outer dense fibers. Develop Biol 1991; 148:195.
15. O'Bryan MK, Loveland KL, Herzfield D, et al. Identification of a rat testis specific gene encoding a potential rat outer dense fibre protein. Mol Reprod Develop 1998; 50:313.
16. Gibbons IRL. Mechanisms of flagellar motility. In: Afzelius BA, ed. The functional anatomy of the spermatozoon. Oxford: Pergamon Press, 1975:127.
17. Afzelius BA, Eliasson R, Johnsen O, Lindholmer C. Lack of dynein arms in immotile human spermatozoa. J Cell Biol 1975; 66:225.
18. Heller CG, Clermont Y. Kinetics of the germinal epithelium in man. Recent Prog Horm Res 1964; 20:545.
19. Fawcett DW. Ultrastructure and function of the Sertoli cell. In: Hamilton DW, Greep RO, eds. Handbook of physiology, section 7, vol 5. Baltimore: Williams & Wilkins, 1975:21.
20. de Kretser DM, Kerr JB. The cytology of the testis. In: Knobil E, Neill JD, eds. Physiology of reproduction. New York: Raven Press, 1994:1177.
21. de Kretser DM, Burger HG. Ultrastructural studies of the human Sertoli cell in normal men and males with hypogonadotropic hypogonadism before and after gonadotropic treatment. In: Saxena BB, Beling CG, Gandy HM, eds. Gonadotropins. New York: Wiley Interscience, 1972:640.
22. Means AR, Fakunding JL, Huckins C, et al. Follicle stimulating hormone, the Sertoli cell and spermatogenesis. Recent Prog Horm Res 1976; 32:477.
23. Dym M, Fawcett DW. The blood–testis barrier in the rat and the physiological compartmentation of the seminiferous epithelium. Biol Reprod 1970; 3:308.
24. Setchell BP, Waites GMH. The blood–testis barrier. In: Hamilton DW, Greep RO, eds. Handbook of physiology, section 7, vol 5. Baltimore: Williams & Wilkins, 1975:143.
25. Flickinger CJ. The postnatal development of the Sertoli cells of the mouse. Z Zellforsch 1967; 78:92.
26. Gilula NB, Fawcett DW, Aoki A. The Sertoli cell occluding junctions and gap junctions in mature and developing mammalian testis. Dev Biol 1976; 50:142.
27. Russell LD. Form, dimensions and cytology of mammalian Sertoli cell. In: Russell LD, Griswold MD, eds. The Sertoli cell. Vienna, IL: Cache River Press, 1993:1.
28. Jutte NHPM, Jansen R, Grootegoed AJ, et al. Regulation of survival of rat pachytene spermatocytes by lactate supply from Sertoli cells. J Reprod Fertil 1982; 65:431.
29. Orth JM, Gunsalus GL, Lamperti AA. Evidence from Sertoli cell–depleted rats indicates that spermatid number in adults depends on numbers of Sertoli cells. Endocrinology 1988; 122:787.
30. Cooke PS, Hess RA, Porcelli J, Meisami E. Increased sperm production in adult rats after transient neonatal hypothyroidism. Endocrinology 1991; 129:244.
31. Bunick KD, Kirby J, Hess RA, Cooke PS. Developmental expression of testis messenger ribonucleic acids in the rat following propylthiouracil–induced neonatal hypothyroydism. Biol Reprod 1994; 51:706.
32. Simorangkir DR, Wreford NG, de Kretser DM. Impaired germ cell development in the testis of immature rats with neonatal hypothyroidism. J Androl 1997; 18:186.
33. Boitani C, Stefanini M, Fragale A, Morena AR. Activin stimulates Sertoli cell proliferation in a defined period of rat testis development. Endocrinology 1995; 136:5438.
34. Setchell BP. Do Sertoli cells secrete fluid into the seminiferous tubules? J Reprod Fertil 1969; 19:391.
35. Jégou B, Le Gac F, de Kretser DM. Seminiferous tubule fluid and interstitial fluid production: I. Effects of age and hormonal regulators in immature rats. Biol Reprod 1982; 27:590.
36. Jégou B, Le Gac F, Irby D, de Kretser DM. Studies on seminiferous tubule fluid production in the adult rat: effect of hypophysectomy and treatment with FSH, LH, and testosterone. Int J Androl 1983; 6:249.
37. French FS, Ritzen EM. A high-affinity androgen binding protein (ABP) in rat testis: evidence for secretion into efferent duct fluid and absorption by epididymis. Endocrinology 1973; 93:88.
38. Gunsalus GL, Musto NA, Bardin CW. Immunoassay of androgen binding protein in blood: a new approach for study of the seminiferous tubule. Science 1978; 200:65.
39. Hansson V, Ritzen EM, French FS, et al. Testicular androgen-binding protein (ABP): comparison of ABP in rabbit testis and epididymis with a similar androgen-binding protein (TeBG) in rabbit serum. Mol Cell Endocrinol 1975; 3:1.
40. Joseph DR, Hall SH, French FS. Rat androgen binding protein: evidence for identical subunits and amino acid sequence homology with human sex hormone binding globulin. Proc Natl Acad Sci U S A 1987; 84:337.
41. Hryb DJ, Khan MS, Romus NA, Rosner W. The solubilization and partial characterization of the sex hormone–binding globulin receptor from human prostate. J Biol Chem 1989; 264:5378.
42. Porto CS, Abreu LC, Gunsalus GL, Bardin CW. Binding of sex hormone–binding globulin (SHBG) to testicular membranes and solubilized receptors. Mol Cell Endocrinol 1992; 89:33.
43. Joseph BR, Becchis M, Fenstermacher DA, Petrusz P. The alternate N-terminal sequence of rat androgen binding protein/sex hormone binding globulin contains a nuclear targetting signal. Endocrinology 1996; 137:1138.
44. Joseph DR, Wang YM, Sullivan PS. Characterization and sex hormone regulation of multiple alternate androgen–binding protein/sex hormone-binding globulin RNA transcript in rat brain. Endocr J 1994; 2:749.
45. Wright WW, Musto NA, Mather JP, Bardin CW. Sertoli cells secrete both testis-specific and serum proteins. Proc Natl Acad Sci U S A 1981; 78:7565.
46. Lacroix M, Smith FE, Fritz IB. Secretion of plasminogen activator by Sertoli cell enriched cultures. Mol Cell Endocrinol 1977; 9:227.
47. Huggenvik J, Sylvester SR, Griswold MD. Control of transferrin in RNA synthesis in Sertoli cells. Ann NY Acad Sci 1984; 438:1.
48. Steinberger A, Steinberger E. Secretion of an FSH-inhibiting factor by cultured Sertoli cells. Endocrinology 1976; 99:918.
49. Le Gac F, de Kretser DM. Inhibin production by Sertoli cells. Mol Cell Endocrinol 1982; 28:487.
50. Au CL, Robertson DM, de Kretser DM. An in vivo method for estimating inhibin production by adult rat testes. J Reprod Fertil 1985; 71:259.
51. Robertson DM, Foulds LM, Leversha L, et al. Isolation of inhibin from bovine follicular fluid. Biochem Biophys Res Commun 1985; 126:220.
52. Mason AJ, Hayflick JS, Ling N, et al. Complementary DNA sequences of ovarian follicular fluid inhibin show precursor structure and homology with transforming growth factor. Nature 1985; 318:659.
53. Forage RG, Ring JM, Brown RW, et al. Cloning and sequence analysis of cDNA species coding for the two subunits of inhibin from bovine follicular fluid. Proc Natl Acad Sci U S A 1986; 83:3091.

54. Massague J. The TGF-β family of growth and differentiation factors. Cell 1987; 49:437.

55. Jensen TK, Andersson AM, Hjollund NHI, et al. Inhibin B as a serum marker of spermatogenesis: correlation to differences in sperm concentration and follicle stimulating hormone levels. A study of 349 Danish men. J Clin Endocrinol Metab 1997; 82:4059.

56. Anderson RA, Wallace EM, Groome NP, et al. Physiological relationships between inhibin B, follicle stimulating hormone secretion and spermatogenesis in normal men and response to gonadotrophin suppression by exogenous testosterone. Hum Reprod 1997; 12:746.

57. Anawalt BD, Bebb RA, Matsumoto AM, et al. Serum inhibin B levels reflect Sertoli cell function in normal men and men with testicular dysfunction. J Clin Endocrinol Metab 1996; 81:3341.

58. Tilbrook AJ, de Kretser DM, Clarke IJ. Human recombinant inhibin A suppresses plasma follicle stimulating hormone to intact levels but has no effect on luteinizing hormone in castrated rams. Biol Reprod 1993; 49:779.

59. Tilbrook AJ, de Kretser DM, Clarke IJ. Human recombinant A and testosterone act directly at the pituitary to suppress plasma concentrations of FSH in castrated rams. J Endocr 1993; 138:181.

60. Josso N, Picard J, Tran D. The antimullerian hormone. Recent Prog Horm Res 1977; 33:117.

60a. de Santa Barbara P, Moniot B, Poulat K, Berta P. Expression and subcellular localization of SF-1, Sox 9, WT1, and AMH proteins during early human testicular development. Dev Dyn 2000; 217:293.

61. Brokelmann J. Fine structure of germ cells and Sertoli cells during the cycle of the seminiferous epithelium in the rat. Z Zellforsch 1963; 59:820.

62. Christensen AK, Mason NR. Comparative ability of seminiferous tubules and interstitial tissue of rat testes to synthesize androgen from progesterone-4-$^{15}$C in vitro. Endocrinology 1965; 76:646.

63. Dorrington JH, Armstrong DT. Follicle stimulating hormone stimulates estradiol-17β synthesis in cultured Sertoli cells. Proc Natl Acad Sci U S A 1975; 72:2677.

64. Tsai-Morris CH, Aquilano DR, Dufau ML. Cellular localization of rat testicular aromatase activity during development. Endocrinology 1985; 116:38.

65. Van Damme MP, Robertson DM, Marana R, et al. A sensitive and specific in vitro bioassay method for the measurement of follicle stimulating hormone activity. Acta Endocrinol (Copenh) 1979; 91:224.

66. Hodgson Y, Robertson DM, de Kretser DM. The regulation of testicular function. In: Greep RO, ed. International review of physiology, vol 27, reproductive physiology IV. Baltimore: University Park Press, 1983:275.

67. Parvinen M. Regulation of the seminiferous epithelium. Endocr Rev 1982; 3:404.

68. Jégou B, Syed V, Sourdaine P, et al. The dialogue between late spermatids and Sertoli cells in vertebrates: a century of research. In: Nieschlag E, Habernicht UF, eds. Spermatogenesis, fertilization, contraception. Berlin: Springer-Verlag, 1992:57.

69. Toledo SP. Leydig cell hypoplasia leading to two different phenotypes: male pseudohermaphroditism and primary hypogonadism not associated with this. Clin Endocrinol 1992; 36:521.

70. Latronico AC, Anasti J, Arnhold IJ, et al. Brief report: testicular and ovarian resistance to luteinizing hormone caused by inactivating mutations of the luteinizing hormone–receptor gene. N Engl J Med 1996; 334:507.

71. Steinberger E, Root A, Ficher M, Smith KD. The role of androgens in the initiation of spermatogenesis in man. J Clin Endocrinol Metab 1973; 37:746.

72. Burger HG, Baker HWG. Therapeutic considerations and results of gonadotropin treatment in male hypogonadotropic hypogonadism. Ann N Y Acad Sci 1984; 438:447.

73. Paulsen CA. The effect of human menopausal gonadotropin on spermatogenesis in hypogonadotropic hypogonadism. In: Gual C, ed. Proceedings of the sixth Pan-American Congress in Endocrinology: International Congress Series 112. Amsterdam: Excerpta Medica, 1966:398.

74. Singh J, O'Neill C, Handlesman DJ. Induction of spermatogenesis by androgens in gonadotropin deficient (hpg) mice. Endocrinology 1995; 136:5311.

75. Kumar TR, Wang Y, Lu N, Matzuk M. Follicle stimulating hormone is required for ovarian follicle maturation but not male fertility. Nature Genet 1997; 15:201.

76. Tapanainen JS, Aittomaki K, Min J, et al. Men homozygous for an inactivating mutation of the follicle stimulating hormone (FSH) receptor gene present variable suppression of spermatogenesis and fertility. Nature Genet 1997; 15:205.

77. Bremner WJ, Matsumoto AM, Paulsen CA. Gonadotropin control of spermatogenesis in man: studies of gonadotropin administration in spontaneous and experimentally induced hypogonadotropic states. Ann N Y Acad Sci 1984; 438:465.

78. Matsumoto AM, Paulsen CA, Bremner WJ. Stimulation of sperm production by human luteinizing hormone in gonadotrophin-suppressed normal men. J Clin Endocrinol Metab 1984; 55:882.

79. Matsumoto AM, Karpas AE, Bremner WJ. Chronic human chorionic gonadotropin administration in normal men: evidence that follicle stimulating hormone is necessary for the maintenance of quantitatively normal spermatogenesis in man. J Clin Endocrinol Metab 1986; 62:1184.

80. Cunningham GR, Huckins C. Persistence of complete spermatogenesis in the presence of low intra-testicular concentration of testosterone. Endocrinology 1979; 105:177.

81. Sun YT, Wreford NG, Robertson DM, de Kretser DM. Quantitative cytological studies of spermatogenesis in intact and hypophysectomised rats: identification of androgen-dependent stages. Endocrinology 1990; 127:1215.

82. Macleod J, Pazianos A, Ray B. The restoration of human spermatogenesis and of the reproductive tract with urinary gonadotropins following hypophysectomy. Fertil Steril 1966; 17:7.

83. Marshall GR, Wickings EJ, Lüdecke DK, Nieschlag E. Stimulation of spermatogenesis in stalk-sectioned rhesus monkeys by testosterone alone. J Clin Endocrinol Metab 1983; 57:152.

84. Means AR, Dedman JR, Tash JS, et al. Regulation of the testis Sertoli cell by follicle stimulating hormone. Annu Rev Physiol 1980; 42:59.

85. Orth J, Christensen AK. Autoradiographic localization of specifically bound $^{125}$I-labelled follicle stimulating hormone on spermatogonia of the rat testis. Endocrinology 1978; 103:1944.

86. Zhengwei Y, Wreford NG, Royce P, et al. Stereological evaluation of human spermatogenesis following suppression by testosterone treatment: heterogeneous pattern of spermatogenic impairment. J Clin Endocrinol Metab 1998; 83:1284.

87. Zhengwei Y, Wreford NG, Schlatt S, et al. GnRH antagonist-induced gonadotropin withdrawal acutely and specifically impairs spermatogonial development in the adult macaque (Macaca fascicularis). J Reprod Fertil 1998; 112:139.

88. Grootegoed JA, Peters MJ, Mulder E, et al. Absence of nuclear androgen receptor in isolated germinal cells of rat testes. Mol Cell Endocrinol 1977; 9:159.

89. Sanborn BM, Steinberger A, Tcholakian RK, Steinberger E. Direct measurement of androgen receptors in cultured Sertoli cells. Steroids 1977; 29:493.

90. Bremner WJ, Millar MR, Sharpe RM. Immunohistochemical localization of androgen receptors in the rat testis: evidence of a stage-dependent expression and regulation by androgens. Endocrinology 1994; 135:1227.

91. Lamb DJ, Tsai YH, Steinberger A, Sanborn BM. Sertoli cell nuclear transcriptional activity: stimulation by follicle stimulating hormone and testosterone in vivo. Endocrinology 1981; 108:1020.

92. Louis BG, Fritz IB. FSH and testosterone independently increase the production of ABP by Sertoli cells in culture. Endocrinology 1979; 104:454.

93. Au CL, Irby DC, Robertson DM, de Kretser DM. Effects of testosterone on testicular inhibin and fluid production in intact and hypophysectomized adult rats. J Reprod Fertil 1986; 76:257.

94. Sun YT, Irby DC, Robertson DM, de Kretser DM. The effects of exogenously administered testosterone on spermatogenesis in intact and hypophysectomised rats. Endocrinology 1989; 125:1000.

95. O'Donnell L, McLachlan RI, Wreford NG, et al. Testosterone withdrawal promotes stage-specific detachment of round spermatids from the rat seminiferous epithelium. Biol Reprod 1996; 55:895.

96. O'Donnell L, Stanton PG, Wreford NG, et al. Inhibition of 5α reductase activity impairs T-dependent restoration of spermiogenesis in rats. Endocrinology 1996; 137:2703.

97. Janulis L, Bahr JM, Hess RA, et al. Rat testicular germ cells and epididymal sperm contain active P450 aromatase. J Androl 1998; 19:65.

98. Carreau S, Bilinska B, Levallet J. Male germ cells: a new source of estrogens in the mammalian testis. Ann Endocrinol (Paris) 1998; 59:79.

99. Robertson DM, O'Donnell L, Jones ME, et al. Impairment of spermatogenesis in mice lacking a functional aromatase (cyp 19) gene. Proc Natl Acad Sci U S A 1999; 96:7986.

100. Hess RA, Bunick D, Lee KH, et al. A role for oestrogens in the male reproductive tract. Nature 1997; 390:509.

101. Saunders PTK, Maguire SM, Gaughan J, Millar MR. Expression of oestrogen receptor beta (ER beta) in multiple cell types including some germ cells, in the rat testis. J Endocrinol 1997; 156:R13.

102. Krege JG, Hodgin JB, Couse JF, et al. Generation and reproductive phenotypes of mice lacking estrogen receptor beta. Proc Natl Acad Sci U S A 1998; 95:15677.

103. Yong EL, Wang Q, Tut TG, et al. Male infertility and the androgen receptor: molecular, clinical and therapeutic aspects. Reprod Med Rev 1997; 6:113.

104. Reijo R, Lee TY, Salo P, et al. Diverse spermatogenic defects in humans caused by Y chromosome deletions encompassing a novel RNA-binding protein gene. Nature Genet 1995; 10:383.

105. Eberhart CG, Maines JZ, Wasserman SA. Meiotic cell cycle requirement for a fly homologue of human deleted in azoospermia. Nature 1996; 381:783.

106. Loveland KL, Schlatt S. Stem cell factor and c-kit in the mammalian testis: lessons originating from mother nature's gene knockouts. J Endocr 1997; 153:337.

107. Dix DJ, Allen JW, Collins BW, et al. Targetted disruption of Hsp 70-2 results in failed meiosis, germ cell apoptosis and male infertility. Proc Natl Acad Sci U S A 1996; 93:3264.

108. Sinha Hikim AP, Swerdloff RS. Hormonal and genetic control of germ cell apoptosis in the testis. Rev Reprod 1999; 4:38.

109. Print CG, Loveland K, Gibson L, et al. Apoptosis regulator Bcl-w is essential for spermatogenesis but is otherwise dispensable. Proc Natl Acad Sci U S A 1998; 95:12424.

110. Fawcett DW, Neaves WB, Flores MN. Comparative observations on intertubular tissue of the mammalian testis. Biol Reprod 1973; 9:500.

111. Lording DW, de Kretser DM. Comparative ultrastructural and histochemical studies of the interstitial cells of the rat testis during fetal and postnatal development. J Reprod Fertil 1972; 29:261.

112. Ewing LL, Zirkin B. Leydig cell structure and steroidogenic activity. Recent Prog Horm Res 1983; 39:599.

113. Clark BJ, Wells J, King SR, Stocco DM. The purification, cloning, and expression of a novel LH-induced mitochondrial protein in MA-10 mouse Leydig tumor cells: characterization of the steroidogenic acute regulatory protein (StAR). J Biol Chem 1994; 269:28314.

114. Bose HS, Pescovitz OH, Miller WL. Spontaneous feminization in a 46XX

female patient with congenital lipoid adrenal hyperplasia due to a homozygous frameshift mutation in the acute steroid regulatory protein. J Clin Endocrinol Metab 1997; 82:1511.

115. Fujieda K, Tajima T, Nakae J, et al. Spontaneous puberty in 46XX subjects with congenital lipoid adrenal hyperplasia. J Clin Invest 1997; 99:1265.

116. Catt KJ, Harwood JP, Aguilera G, Dufau ML. Hormonal regulation of peptide receptors and target cell responses. Nature 1979; 280:109.

117. Padron RS, Wischusen J, Hudson B, et al. Prolonged biphasic response of plasma testosterone to single intramuscular injections of human chorionic gonadotropin. J Clin Endocrinol Metab 1980; 50:1100.

118. de Kretser DM. Sertoli cell-Leydig cell interaction in the regulation of testicular function. Int J Androl 1982; 5(Suppl):11.

119. Sharpe RM, Cooper I. Intratesticular secretion of a factor(s) with major stimulating effects on Leydig cell testosterone secretion in vitro. Mol Cell Endocrinol 1984; 37:159.

120. Cohen PE, Hardy MP, Pollard JW. Colony-stimulating factor-1 plays a major role in the development of reproductive function in male mice. Mol Endocrinol 1997; 11:1636.

121. Papadopoulos V. Peripheral-type benzodiazepine/diazepam binding inhibitor receptor: biological role in steroidogenic cell function. Endocrinol Rev 1993;14:222.

122. McLachlan RI, Wreford NG, de Kretser DM, Robertson DM. The effects of testosterone on spermatogenic cell populations in the adult rat. Biol Reprod 1994;51:945.

123. Bergh A. Local differences in Leydig cell morphology in the adult rat testis: evidence for a local control of Leydig cells by adjacent seminiferous tubules. Int J Androl 1982; 5:325.

124. Rich KA, de Kretser DM. Spermatogenesis and the Sertoli cell. In: de Kretser DM, Burger HG, Hudson B, eds. The pituitary and testis: clinical and experimental studies. Berlin: Springer-Verlag, 1983:85.

125. Head JR, Billingham RE. Immune privilege in the testis. II: evaluation of potential local factors. Transplantation 1985; 40:269.

126. Hedger MP. Testicular leucocytes: what are they doing? Rev Reprod 1997; 2:38.

127. Cucicini C, Kercret H, Touzlain AM, et al. Vectorial production of interleukin 1 and interleukin 6 by rat Sertoli cells cultured in a dual culture compartment system. Endocrinology 1997; 138:2863.

# CHAPTER 114

# EVALUATION OF TESTICULAR FUNCTION

STEPHEN J. WINTERS

Male hypogonadism signifies impaired production of testosterone by Leydig cells, or deficient spermatogenesis, but in most clinical disorders both compartments of the testis are abnormal. This is not surprising because extensive biochemical communication occurs between the Leydig cells and the seminiferous tubules (see Chap. 113). Hypogonadism due to pathology intrinsic to the testis (primary testicular failure) or to deficient gonadotropin drive to the testis (hypogonadotropic hypogonadism) may produce similar clinical features, and the tests used to diagnose most forms of hypogonadism overlap. Therefore, a general clinical and laboratory approach to evaluating testicular function will be presented.

## CLINICAL EVALUATION

Patients with impaired testicular function present variably, depending on the *age at onset* of their disease. Hypogonadism in the *fetus* results in *genital ambiguity* (see Chap. 90). When the disturbance begins in childhood, puberty is delayed or does not occur (see Chap. 92). Adult men with hypogonadism often present with a decrease in libido and energy, or with infertility, among other symptoms (Table 114-1), and although these symptoms are sensitive indicators of androgen deficiency, they are nonspecific. For example, a reduced libido in men is also a characteristic of depression as well as of performance anxiety.

**TABLE 114-1.**
**Symptoms and Signs of Hypogonadism in Adult Men**

| Symptoms | Signs |
|---|---|
| Decreased libido | Soft smooth skin |
| Asthenia | Decreased beard, axillary, and pubic hair |
| Erectile dysfunction | Decreased muscle mass and strength |
| Infertility | Small testes |
| Osteopenia/fractures | Gynecomastia |
| | Small prostate |

A complete physical examination is needed to evaluate hypogonadal males. Prepubertal Leydig cell insufficiency causes eunuchoidism, including a juvenile voice; childlike facies; scant facial, pubic, and body hair; smooth skin; poorly developed skeletal musculature; fat accumulation in the hips, buttocks, and lower abdomen; a small prostate; and failure of epiphyseal closure of the long bones, resulting in an arm span that exceeds the height by >6 cm and disproportionately long legs. The testis size is readily measured by approximating its length and width with a ruler or with a commercially available series of ovoids (see Chap. 93). The testes generally reach adult size by 18 years of age. The median testis length among normal men is 5 cm, equivalent to 25 mL in volume.[1] The left testis is often slightly smaller than the right. Although testes that are 4 cm long may be normal, many men with hypospermatogenesis will have testes of this size. There are genetic differences in testis size, with smaller testes found among Asian men. Testis size declines with aging.[2] *Varicocele* (see Chap. 118), a distention of the pampiniform plexus within the scrotum due to dysfunctional valves within the spermatic vein, is a common finding in infertile men, and is associated with a reduction in testis size beginning in adolescence, particularly on the left.[3,4] Usually, the venous distention is visible or palpable in the upright posture, increases if the patient performs a Valsalva maneuver, and disappears as soon as the patient is recumbent. Color Doppler ultrasonography can be used to confirm the presence of a varicocele.[5]

The skin of hypogonadal men may be soft and smooth. Muscle mass may decline, and fat mass may increase. Gynecomastia is a frequent finding in hypogonadal teenagers and in adults. Examination of the male breast can be difficult, however, because the distinction between fat and breast tissue is often inexact. Galactorrhea, on the other hand, is a rare finding in males (see Chap. 13). Physical changes regress slowly in sexually mature men who acquire Leydig cell dysfunction. If some of the physical changes of eunuchoidism in previously normal men are present, androgen deficiency is both severe and long standing. Therefore, testosterone deficiency is often present in men with limited physical findings. Reduced visual acuity or a visual field disturbance suggests a mass lesion in the hypothalamus-pituitary (see Chap. 19). The digital rectal examination is useful in assessing sphincter tone in men with erectile dysfunction, and for estimating prostate size.

## LABORATORY EVALUATION

### TESTOSTERONE

**Physiologic Aspects of Testosterone Testing.**    Testosterone is both a paracrine regulator of spermatogenesis (see Chap. 113) and a hemocrine hormone. The testicular content of testosterone is ~50 μg (1 μg/g testis), whereas the blood production rate is ~5000 μg per day, indicating that only a small portion of the testosterone produced each day is stored in the testes. The testosterone precursor steroids, including pregnenolone, 17-OH pregnenolone, dehydroepiandrosterone (DHEA), progesterone, 17α-hydroxyprogesterone, and

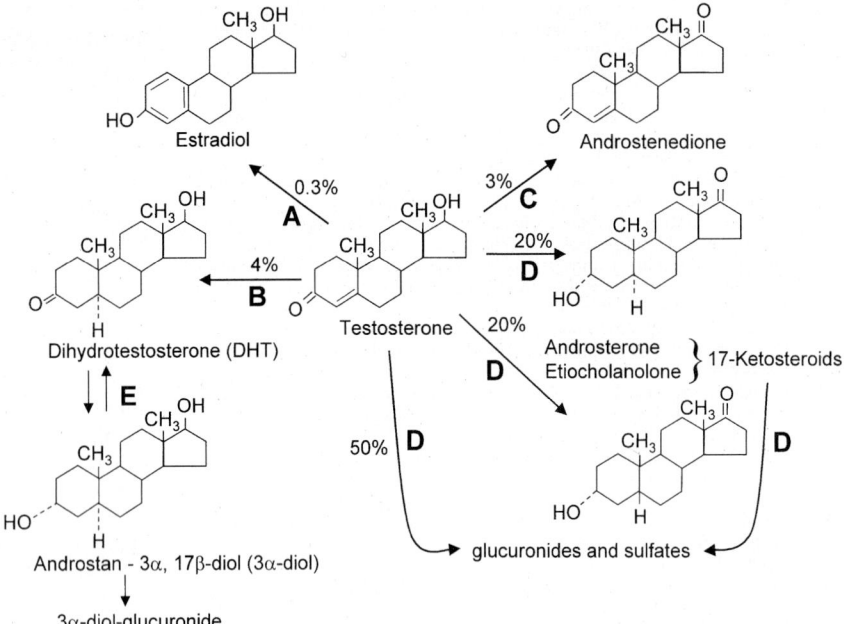

**FIGURE 114-1.** Metabolic pathways for testosterone. Enzymes are (A) aromatase, (B) 5α-reductase, (C) 17β-hydroxysteroid dehydrogenase, (D) various hydroxylases and transferases, and (E) 3α-hydroxysteroid dehydrogenase. The percentages represent the average percent bioconversion in normal men to these active and inactive metabolities.

androstenedione, are also secreted by the testis, and the relative concentrations of these steroids in spermatic vein blood are proportional to their testicular concentrations.[6] The release of precursor steroids into the circulation may indicate that they are unnecessary by-products in the orderly biotransformation of pregnenolone to testosterone, because none is known to have a physiologic action in the male. Androstenedione is of special interest because it is used as a performance-enhancing drug. Androstenedione is bioconverted to testosterone and to estrone, but there is little published information on the endocrine profile following androstenedione administration.

A single sample of blood, generally drawn in the morning, can be used to measure testosterone. The usual normal range in morning samples is 3 to 10 ng/mL (10–40 nmol/L). There is a diurnal variation in testosterone in adult men, with *highest levels in the early morning,* followed by a progressive fall throughout the day, reaching the lowest levels in the evening and during the first few hours of sleep. Peak and nadir values differ by ~15%, although more pronounced differences are sometimes observed.[7] The diurnal rhythm is blunted with aging[8] and in men with testicular failure.[9] The metabolic clearance of testosterone is not thought to vary throughout the day, so that the diurnal testosterone rhythm is presumed to result from a day-night difference in testosterone production. Because there are no parallel changes in serum LH levels, however, the origin as well as physiologic significance of the diurnal testosterone rhythm remains uncertain. *It is important to measure testosterone in the morning,* because reference ranges are based on morning values. Frequent sampling of spermatic venous blood reveals testosterone secretory pulses at a frequency of ~1 pulse per hour,[6] but because of this rapid frequency and relatively low pulse amplitude only small fluctuations occur in peripheral plasma. Testosterone secretory bursts are more readily defined in the peripheral blood when pulse frequency is low.[7] There is a good correlation between the plasma testosterone level at first sampling and the mean of multiple samples taken over 1 year, so that one morning sample is reasonably representative,[10] although abnormal and borderline values should be confirmed.

There is a prominent sleep-related increase in serum testosterone in pubertal boys, with abrupt rises from female to adult male levels.[11] This difference can be used clinically to evaluate boys with delayed puberty (see Chap. 92), because the rise to a higher testosterone value in the morning may precede pubertal testis growth and indicates that puberty has begun.[12]

Men with hypogonadism and hyperprolactinemia have an exaggerated diurnal testosterone rhythm, leading to very low levels in the afternoon and evening, which can explain clinical hypogonadism despite a normal morning total testosterone level,[9] as sometimes occurs in men with a prolactinoma. The testosterone level tends to rise during intense exercise because of hemoconcentration[13] and to decline 12 to 24 hours later because gonadotropin-releasing hormone (GnRH) secretion is reduced.[14] *Testosterone levels are also reduced in acute and chronic illness*[15] and *with fasting* for at least 48 hours. These factors can confound an evaluation of testicular function.

**Testosterone Metabolism.**    The metabolism of testosterone is shown in Figure 114-1. Testosterone is metabolized into two biologically important products, dihydrotestosterone (DHT) and estradiol, by the enzymes 5α-reductase and aromatase, respectively. Most of the metabolism of testosterone occurs in the liver, however, via 3α- and 3β-hydroxysteroid dehydrogenase, 5α- and 5β-steroid reductase, and oxidation of the D-ring to the 17-ketosteroids androsterone (3α-hydroxy-5α-androstane-17-one) and etiocholanolone (3α-hydroxy-5β-androstane-17-one), which are then excreted in the urine. Most of the 10 to 25 mg per day of ketosteroids in the urine of men is of adrenal origin, however, so that the urinary 17-ketosteroid excretion is not a test of testicular function. Testosterone metabolites are also conjugated to sulfuric and glucuronic acids at the 3- or 17-position and excreted in the urine and bile. A small fraction (2%) of the circulating testosterone is excreted unchanged in the urine.

## SEX HORMONE–BINDING GLOBULIN

Of the circulating testosterone in normal men, <4% is free (not protein bound), 1% to 2% is bound to cortisol-binding globulin, ~50% is loosely bound to albumin, and ~45% is bound with high affinity to *sex hormone–binding globulin (SHBG),* a β-globulin produced by the liver[16] (Fig. 114-2). (SHBG is also referred to as testosterone-binding globulin [TeBG] or sex steroid–binding protein [SBP]). The level of SHBG in plasma is a strong predictor of the total testosterone level in normal men (Fig. 114-3), accounting for 50% of the variance in total testosterone. SHBG is present in plasma as a 100-kDa heterodimer of variably glycosylated subunits.[17,18] *Androgen-binding protein* is a nearly identical protein that is produced by Sertoli cells of the testis.[19] Androgen-binding protein and SHBG differ in carbohydrate content. Although SHBG binds testosterone and other steroids and prolongs their metabolic clearance, its function remains

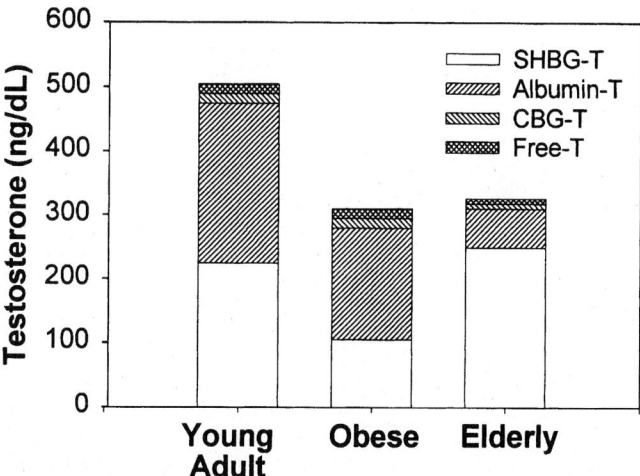

**FIGURE 114-2.** Distribution of testosterone in blood plasma. The free fraction represents 1% to 4% of the total testosterone (*T*). The albumin-bound testosterone represents a loosely bound complex of albumin and testosterone that dissociates readily. Together the free and albumin-bound testosterone have been termed *bioavailable testosterone*. Sex hormone–binding globulin (*SHBG*) has a high affinity for testosterone and dihydrotestosterone, and its role in androgen action remains controversial. When the level of SHBG is reduced, as in obesity, the total testosterone is low, but the bioavailable and free testosterone levels are generally normal. In older men, the mean total testosterone level declines, but because SHBG increases with aging, the decrease in total testosterone is less than the decrease in free and bioavailable testosterone. (*CBG*, cortisol-binding globulin.)

controversial. The finding of membrane-binding sites for androgen-binding protein in the epididymis and for SHBG in testis, prostate, and other tissues *and the activation of the cyclic adenosine monophosphate (cAMP)/protein kinase A (PKA) pathway, which is a coactivator of androgen receptors (ARs), suggest* that these binding proteins could play a direct role in androgen action. However, according to the free hormone hypothesis, which states that only free steroid enters target cells, SHBG functions solely as a reservoir for testosterone.

## FREE OR BIOAVAILABLE TESTOSTERONE

For most clinical applications the measurement of the total testosterone level is entirely satisfactory. However, when circulat-

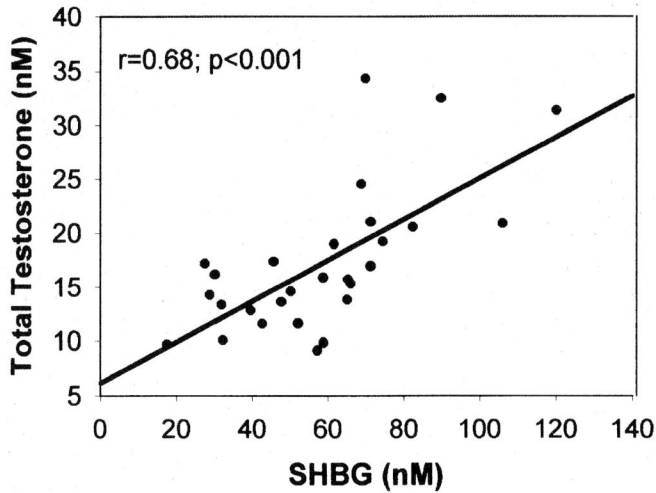

**FIGURE 114-3.** Relationship between the level of sex hormone–binding globulin (*SHBG*) and total testosterone in plasma from normal-weight and obese men. (Plasma samples were kindly provided by Drs. Bret Goodpaster and David Kelley of the University of Pittsburgh; republished with the permission of *Clinical Chemistry.*)

**TABLE 114-2.**
**Conditions with Abnormal Sex Hormone–Binding Globulin Concentrations**

| Increased | Decreased |
|---|---|
| Aging | Hyperinsulinemia |
| Androgen deficiency | Obesity |
| Estrogen treatment | Androgen treatment |
| Thyrotoxicosis | Hypothyroidism |
| Alcoholic cirrhosis | Hypercortisolism |
| Hepatitis | Nephrotic syndrome |
| Growth hormone deficiency | Acromegaly |
| | Familial |

ing SHBG levels are altered (Table 114-2), this change may be reflected as an increase or a decrease in the measured serum total testosterone concentration. For example, a low testosterone level in an obese man may be misinterpreted to suggest androgen deficiency (see Fig. 114-2). Because there is considerable evidence that the non–SHBG-bound portion of circulating testosterone represents the biologically active fraction, *many methods* for determining non–SHBG-bound or free testosterone have been developed.[20]

### METHODOLOGY

**Total Testosterone.** Total testosterone can be measured *directly in serum* by immunoassay, *or after extraction* with organic solvents with or without further chromatographic separation. Commercial kits for the direct assay of testosterone in unextracted serum or plasma using an iodine-125 ($^{125}$I)-labeled tracer are technically easy to use, precise, and sufficiently accurate for most purposes. *When SHBG levels are low,* however (see later), *the result for testosterone may be overestimated,* whereas *high SHBG levels may lead to underestimation* of the actual testosterone value. This artifact appears to result from differences between the SHBG levels in the assay standards and samples, with nonlabeled testosterone binding to both SHBG and to the testosterone antiserum, whereas the $^{125}$I-testosterone tracer binds primarily to the antiserum.[21] Direct assays also tend to *overestimate the true values of testosterone at low concentrations.*

To discriminate among low levels more accurately, or to control for the effects of abnormal SHBG concentrations, immunoassays using organic solvent extraction and chromatographic separation may be needed, *but are more costly and difficult to perform.*

Fully automated immunoassay analyzers have been introduced into clinical laboratories for competitive and two-site assays.[22] These electrochemiluminescence immunoassays (ECLIAs) use nonradiolabeled detection methods, and have very short incubation times. Thus, they are attractive for clinical laboratories. The precision and accuracy are quite acceptable for samples from adult men, with results similar to those of radioimmunoassays (RIAs). At low levels, however, ECLIAs may produce values that are 50% to 100% *higher* than those of RIAs. *Lipemia* may also produce inaccurate high values.

**Equilibrium Dialysis Assay.** The *equilibrium dialysis assay* is used to calculate the percent free testosterone. The diffusion across a semipermeable membrane of tracer amounts of $^3$H-testosterone added to the sample is measured. *The free testosterone concentration is then calculated from the product of the total testosterone level and the percentage of tracer crossing the dialysis membrane (percent free testosterone).* The latter is usually 1% to 4%, with a free testosterone level commonly ranging from 4 to 20 ng/dL. This assay is complex, with potential errors due to temperature, sample dilution, and tracer impurities. (Testosterone can also be measured by RIA in the dialysate, avoiding the use of $^3$H-testosterone, but a very sensitive immunoassay is needed.) *Centrifugal ultrafiltration* is a variation of equilibrium

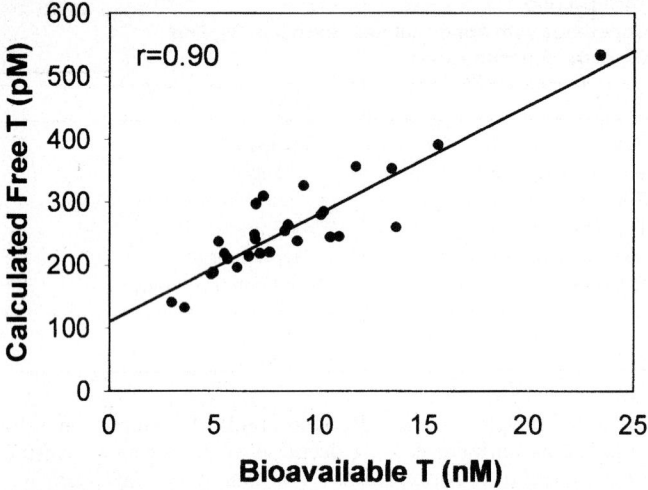

**FIGURE 114-4.** Relation between the free testosterone (*T*) level calculated from the plasma levels of total testosterone and sex hormone–binding globulin (*SHBG*) and the non-SHBG testosterone among normal thin and overweight men, determined by ammonium sulfate precipitation.

dialysis in which high-speed centrifugation is used to separate bound from free hormone across a dialysis membrane.

**Calculated Free Testosterone.** Another approach for correcting the total testosterone value for variations in SHBG concentrations is to *calculate the free testosterone level from the levels of total testosterone and SHBG*, using binding constants for SHBG and albumin.[23] This value appears to correlate quite well with the value obtained by equilibrium dialysis.

**Free Testosterone Index.** The *"free testosterone index"* has been calculated as the ratio: total testosterone/SHBG using units of nmol/L. *Although the calculation is easy to perform and is believed to be valid in women, it appears to be less useful in men,* because most of the SHBG in men is bound to testosterone.[24]

**Analog Kits.** The free testosterone level has been determined directly using *solid-phase free testosterone RIA analog kits*, which use an [125]I-labeled testosterone analog as the tracer. This assay is based on the selective binding of the analog tracer to the testosterone antiserum, but not to SHBG, and is a popular, high-precision, single-step, nonextraction method. Although there is a strong positive correlation between free testosterone levels measured by these analog kits and by equilibrium dialysis assay, the kits produce substantially (75%) *lower values.*[24a] Moreover, the level of SHBG is a positive predictor of the free testosterone level as measured by analog methods. The percentage of free testosterone (determined by the analog method) does not decrease as SHBG increases, and this free testosterone level is almost perfectly positively correlated with the total testosterone. Thus, both the total testosterone and the free testosterone (determined by the analog method) appear to provide essentially the same clinical information.[25]

**Non–Sex Hormone–Binding Globulin Assay (Bioavailable Testosterone).** The concept of the *non–SHBG–testosterone assay* (sometimes referred to as *bioavailable testosterone*) is that the testosterone bound to albumin, because of its low-affinity binding, is as readily available to target tissues as is free testosterone.[26] The most widely used technique to measure non–SHBG-bound testosterone involves the precipitation of tracer amounts of [3]H-testosterone bound to SHBG using ammonium sulfate. *The non-SHBG testosterone is calculated by multiplying the total testosterone level times the percent of [3]H-testosterone remaining in the supernatant after precipitation.* Figure 114-2 shows that the decline in bioavailable testosterone as men grow older is substantially *greater* than the fall in total testosterone, whereas the bioavailable testosterone level is *normal in obesity* although SHBG is reduced. On the other hand, SHBG increases as men grow older.[27] Figure 114-4 illustrates the excellent correlation

between the non-SHBG testosterone (i.e., bioavailable testosterone) and the free testosterone calculated from the level of SHBG and total testosterone in normal men, suggesting that the measures provide equally useful information.

**Salivary Testosterone.** Testosterone concentrations have also been measured in saliva in which the testosterone level is 2% to 3% of the concentration in serum. This approach is useful in field studies. Because the salivary gland basement membrane excludes proteins, salivary testosterone correlates with free testosterone. Differences between salivary and free testosterone levels have been explained by enzymes in salivary glands or saliva that convert androstenedione to testosterone, or that metabolize testosterone further, and by meal-related changes in saliva production.

**Sex Hormone–Binding Globulin.** Several two-site immunoradiometric assays (IRMAs) for SHBG, which use rabbit and mouse polyclonal antibodies, are available.[28] The normal range for men is 10 to 50 nmol/L, children 45 to 90 nmol/L, and women 30 to 90 nmol/L. SHBG can also be measured indirectly using radioligand binding assays based on the specific binding of [3]H-testosterone or [3]H-DHT by serum.[29] The range of normal values for men approximates 0.3 to 1.2 µg bound DHT/dL, indicating that most of the circulating SHBG in plasma in men is complexed to androgens. Aging and various medical disorders alter plasma levels of SHBG (see Table 114-2). Measurement of SHBG in plasma is useful in interpreting testosterone concentrations, and as a marker for insulin resistance and cardiovascular risk.[30]

## LUTEINIZING HORMONE AND FOLLICLE-STIMULATING HORMONE

The pituitary gonadotropins, luteinizing hormone (LH) and follicle-stimulating hormone (FSH)—like thyroid-stimulating hormone (TSH) and human chorionic gonadotropin (hCG)—are heterodimeric glycoproteins composed of a common α subunit and a hormone-specific β subunit.[31] LH activates Leydig cells, whereas FSH stimulates Sertoli cells. Gonadotropin synthesis is up-regulated by GnRH, and suppressed by gonadal steroids. FSH-β mRNA and thereby FSH secretion are also regulated at the pituitary level by testicular inhibin, and perhaps by pituitary activin and follistatin.[32] LH is secreted into the circulation in normal adult men in discrete pulses approximately once every 1 to 2 hours throughout the day and night.[33] This mode of secretion results from the pulsatile release of GnRH into the portal blood by the anterior hypothalamus (see Chap. 19). To estimate mean serum LH levels for a given patient, three blood samples can be drawn at 20-minute intervals. These can be assayed individually, or equal aliquots of each sample can be pooled, and the pool assayed. FSH levels are more constant in peripheral blood,[34] presumably because the FSH response to GnRH is of lesser magnitude, and because the clearance of FSH from blood is slow, as compared to LH.

Highly sensitive and specific two-site immunoassays for LH and FSH are now widely available. Specificity results from the use of two distinct antibodies, which bind to separate sites on the protein. Often, one antibody is to the α subunit, and the other antibody is to the β subunit. One antibody, which is present in excess, is immobilized to facilitate separation of bound from free label; it is known as the *capture antibody.* The other antibody, which is coupled to a detectable label, is the *detection antibody.* The signal increases in proportion to the level of hormone, rather than decreasing in proportion to the level of hormone, as in RIAs. The detection antibody is radiolabeled with [125]I in IRMAs, whereas ion-chelated antibodies are used in immunofluorometric assays (IFMAs). Delayed addition of an enhancement solution dissociates the metal from the antibody. The metal then binds to other constituents of the enhancement solution, forming a highly fluorescent chelate. Because the low molecular weight metal chelates to an antibody without altering its binding affinity, IFMAs tend to be more sensitive than are IRMAs. In addition, with IFMAs there are no radioactive materials to dispose of, and the shelf life of the reagents is longer. However, reagents for IFMAs tend to be more expensive, and the interassay variation tends to be greater than for IRMAs. Enzyme-linked immunosorbent assays (ELISAs) for gonadotropins are also available. These assays are also nonisotopic, but are generally less sensitive than are IRMAs or IFMAs because of the coupling of the macromolecular enzyme to the antibody, and they have a higher nonspecific binding. Two-site assays using monoclonal antibodies may be too specific. For example, an LH-β sequence variant, which appears to represent a polymorphism, was identified when a specific monoclonal antiserum to the LH-α/β dimer was unable to recognize LH in the sera and urine of healthy Finnish men and women.[35]

LH levels as measured by two-site immunoassays are detectable in all adult male serum samples and in most samples from normal prepubertal boys, especially nighttime samples, whereas LH levels are often below the normal range in gonadotropin-deficient patients.[36] Nevertheless, the diagnosis of gonadotropin deficiency should not be made based on the serum LH level alone. Instead, the serum testosterone level should also be low. In contrast to their barely detectable LH levels, serum FSH levels in patients with GnRH deficiency are readily measurable,[37] consistent with paracrine stimulation of FSH-β mRNA and FSH secretion by activin, as occurs in cultured rat pituitary cells.

The finding of elevated LH and FSH concentrations in serum indicates primary testicular failure. Serum LH levels rise when testosterone production falls because the negative feedback effects of testosterone on GnRH secretion are reduced. Elevated serum FSH concentrations, which generally indicate a disturbance of seminiferous tubule function, are now known to result from deficient secretion of *testicular inhibin B* as well as sex steroids.[38] LH levels are rarely increased in men without a concomitant increase in FSH concentrations because seminiferous tubules are more readily damaged than are Leydig cells, but elevated FSH and normal LH levels are often found in severely oligospermic men.[39] Pituitary tumors may produce FSH,[40] and rarely dimeric LH.[41]

## DIHYDROTESTOSTERONE

The concentration of DHT in the circulation of adult men is ~10% that of testosterone. Of the circulating DHT, ~25% is secreted by the testis, and the remainder arises from the bioconversion of testosterone in liver, kidney, muscle, prostate, and skin.[42] The DHT concentration in prostate is 5- to 10-fold greater than that in the peripheral blood.[43] There are two isoenzymes that convert testosterone to DHT, *5α-reductase types 1 and 2*. The type 1 enzyme is found in the liver and skin, and perhaps in other tissues. The type 2 enzyme predominates in genital and male accessory gland tissues in which 5α-reduction is a prerequisite for normal androgen-mediated function.[44] Unlike testosterone, DHT levels in plasma do not decrease as men grow older.[45] Because serum DHT levels are usually normal in men with testicular dysfunction, the measurement of DHT is not recommended for routine clinical purposes. Moreover, antisera to DHT may cross-react with testosterone, making the complete separation of these two steroids difficult.

Only a small fraction of the DHT produced in target tissues reenters plasma; rather it is metabolized by 3α reduction to 5α-androstane 3β-17β-diol (3α-diol), which reenters plasma and is further metabolized by glucuronide conjugation and by other pathways.[46] 3α-Diol-G is present in significantly reduced concentrations in plasma from hypogonadal and elderly men, and in patients with androgen resistance and 5α-reductase deficiency. Plasma 3α-diol-G levels are increased in men with severe acne or dense chest hair,[47] and in hirsute women. Plasma 3α-diol-G is derived from ketosteroids secreted by the adrenals as well as from DHT, however, so that interpretation

of plasma 3α-diol-G levels is complex. Therefore, its measurement remains a research tool.

## PROLACTIN

The measurement of prolactin in serum is of great importance in the evaluation of men with sexual dysfunction, impaired libido, or delayed adolescence, because these symptoms are common in men with prolactin-producing pituitary tumors[48] (see Chap. 13). Slight elevations of prolactin, which become more pronounced after stimulation with dopamine antagonists or thyrotropin-releasing hormone (TRH), may be found in men with primary testicular failure,[49] perhaps because of androgen deficiency and unchanged or increased estrogen production, because prolactin (PRL) gene expression is stimulated by estradiol. On the other hand, men with complete GnRH deficiency, with very low circulating levels of testosterone and estradiol, have low prolactin levels that normalize after treatment with hCG or testosterone.[50] Prolactin levels are rarely increased in otherwise healthy men with infertility.[51]

## ESTROGENS

Most of the estrogens in the circulation in normal adult men are derived from the bioconversion of testosterone to estradiol, and androstenedione to estrone, by the aromatase enzyme complex in fat, muscle, kidney, and liver. Thus, plasma estrogen concentrations in men are determined by both testicular and adrenal substrate production, and by the aromatase enzyme activity in several tissues. The normal range is generally <50 pg/mL for total estradiol and <60 pg/mL for estrone. Serum estradiol levels are relatively constant throughout the day and night, and unlike testosterone, plasma estrogens are unchanged with aging.[45] Estrogens in plasma are found bound mainly to albumin. Estradiol also binds to SHBG but with only 10% the affinity of testosterone, and at an order of magnitude lower affinity than are circulating estradiol levels. Therefore, changes in circulating SHBG levels would be predicted to have little influence on measured estrogen levels or on estrogen bioactivity. Nevertheless, adding serum to culture media reduced the uptake of estradiol by MCF-7 breast cancer cells,[52] and bioavailable estrogen levels are more positively correlated with bone mineral density than is total plasma estrogen.[53] Therefore, measuring bioavailable estradiol levels may be useful in research studies in men that seek to relate estradiol levels to clinical outcomes.

**Clinical Applicability in Men.** The measurement of serum estradiol and estrone levels may be useful in the clinical evaluation of men with hypogonadism and gynecomastia. Table 114-3 lists

**TABLE 114-3.**

**Conditions Associated with Increased Serum Estradiol or Estrone Levels in Adult Men**

**NEOPLASMS**
　Testicular Leydig cell and Sertoli cell tumors
　Adrenal adenomas and carcinomas
　Choriocarcinomas
　Hepatomas
**PRIMARY TESTICULAR FAILURE**
**ALCOHOLIC LIVER DISEASE**
**HYPERTHYROIDISM**
**OBESITY**
**ANDROGEN-INSENSITIVITY SYNDROME**
**FAMILIAL AROMATASE EXCESS**
**MEDICATIONS**
　Antiandrogens
　Antiestrogens

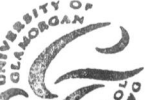

clinical conditions commonly associated with increasing circulating estrogen levels. Obesity is the most common cause of mildly increased circulating estradiol and estrone levels in men, and correction occurs with weight loss.[54] To monitor ovulation induction in women, commercial kits for the direct assay of estradiol in serum have been developed. They are optimized for high values and for rapidity of performance. However, *at the low values characteristic of male plasma*, these assays *may be imprecise and inaccurate*; they may *overestimate* the true values,[55] and between-laboratory variation may be substantial. The determination of the low levels of estradiol and estrone in male plasma may require preliminary extraction with organic solvents, and sometimes chromatographic separation of interfering steroids, before immunoassay.

## GONADOTROPIN SUBUNITS

The α subunit of the glycoprotein hormones is found in the serum of normal men and women. Serum α-subunit levels are elevated in postmenopausal women and in men and women with gonadal failure, and increase following administration of GnRH. α-Subunit levels are also low in children and increase at puberty in parallel with LH. α Subunit is secreted into peripheral blood in normal men in pulses that parallel LH pulses. Together, these data suggest that the gonadotrope is an important source of uncombined α subunit.[56] The presence of α subunit in serum from men with complete hypogonadotropic hypogonadism, who produce little or no LH, suggests that factors in addition to GnRH regulate α-subunit secretion, however.[57,58] A portion of the plasma α-subunit levels is from thyrotropes; α-subunit levels are increased in hypothyroid patients, and are increased further by TRH.[59] No physiologic role for secreted α subunit has so far been described. Pituitary tumors often produce α subunit alone, or together with GH, FSH, and/or TSH,[40] and various malignancies may produce α subunit ectopically. Serum α-subunit concentrations are markedly increased in patients with chronic renal failure,[60] presumably because renal clearance mechanisms are reduced. Uncombined β subunits, LH-β, FSH-β, and hCG-β are also present in sera from men with pituitary tumors, especially after TRH stimulation,[61] and in patients with germ-cell neoplasms.[62,63]

## INHIBIN

Inhibin is a glycoprotein hormone produced by the testes and ovaries that functions in the feedback control of FSH secretion and presumably as an intragonadal regulator.[64,65,65a] After many years of controversy surrounding its existence, inhibin was purified from porcine and bovine follicular fluids, and found to be a 32-kDa heterodimer composed of an α and one of two β subunits, $\beta_A$ or $\beta_B$. Inhibin B ($\alpha$-$\beta_B$) is the form produced by the Sertoli cells of the human testis.[66] Inhibin production by Leydig cells and germ cells has been suggested, but remains controversial. A larger (55–60 kDa) molecular mass form of inhibin B and various molecular weight forms of the inhibin α subunit are also present in human male plasma,[67] but probably are not bioactive. Inhibin is part of a family of proteins that includes transforming growth factor-β (TGF-β), activin, and anti-müllerian hormone (AMH). Inhibin suppresses FSH secretion by decreasing FSH-β mRNA levels, possibly by blocking stimulation by pituitary activin.

Specific two-site ELISAs to measure plasma inhibin B[66] as well as inhibin α subunit–related proteins[68] have been developed. Circulating inhibin-B levels are low in prepubertal boys[69] and in gonadotropin-deficient men.[70] Inhibin-B levels decline within a few months after cancer chemotherapy[71] and testicular irradiation,[72] each of which disrupts spermatogenesis. Although there is overlap among patient groups, inhibin-B levels are reduced in oligospermic and azoospermic men (Fig. 114-5), and inhibin-B levels correlate positively with testicular volume among infertile men, and with germ-cell score in testicular biopsy specimens.[73] Thus, inhibin B appears to be a marker for

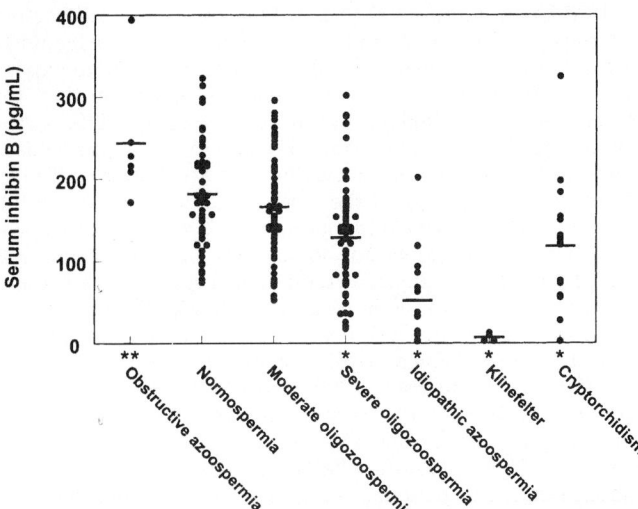

**FIGURE 114-5.** Serum levels of inhibin B in men with various causes of infertility. Inhibin-B levels in men with obstructive azoospermia (in whom spermatogenesis may be normal), a surrogate group for normal men, were significantly higher than those in all other groups. Mean levels in men with severe oligospermia, idiopathic azoospermia, and cryptorchidism as well as Klinefelter syndrome were lower than those in infertile men with normospermia. Substantial overlap between patient groups is evident, however. (From Pierik FH, Vreeburg JTM, Stijnen T, et al. Serum inhibin B as a marker of spermatogenesis. J Clin Endocrinol Metab 1998; 83:3110.)

Sertoli cell number and function, and is a useful research tool, but its usefulness for clinical purposes is not well defined. Although inhibin α subunit is sometimes produced by ovarian tumors, inhibin levels in men with testicular cancer have not been increased,[74] although some testicular neoplasms stain positively for inhibin α subunit.

## MÜLLERIAN INHIBITORY HORMONE

Testicular müllerian inhibitory hormone, a member of the TGF-β family of proteins, causes regression of müllerian structures during fetal development in males.[74a] This hormone is readily detectable in the serum of boys in concentrations of 10 to 70 ng/mL but declines to levels of 2 to 5 ng/mL with maturation to adolescence and adulthood, and is nearly undetectable in girls. Müllerian inhibitory hormone is also absent from the plasma of most boys with congenital anorchia, but is generally detectable in boys with bilateral cryptorchidism. Thus, its measurement in plasma is useful in deciding whether testes are present, and whether surgical exploration for cryptorchidism is indicated.[75]

## GONADOTROPIN RADIORECEPTOR ASSAYS AND IN VITRO BIOASSAYS

Isoforms of the glycoprotein hormones, which differ in size and charge, are present in the pituitary and plasma.[31,76] The variation is in the carbohydrate chains with differences in terminal sialic acid and sulfate groups. Different isoforms may have different biologic properties, such as half-life and receptor-binding activity, and the synthesis and secretion of isoforms may be physiologically regulated and altered by pathologic mechanisms. Gonadotropin function can be estimated in vitro using radioreceptor assays and bioassays, or these assays can be used to analyze gonadotropins, which have been fractionated by electrophoresis or by other methods. The production of testosterone by dispersed mouse or rat Leydig cells is used as a bioassay for LH,[77] and the production of estradiol by Sertoli cells or granulosa cells serves as a bioassay for FSH.[78] Bioassays based on primary cell cultures are expensive and sometimes inaccurate because of serum effects, and are subject to substantial between-assay variation. In fact, many statements about the bioactivity of plasma gonadotropins—including effects of aging, sex steroids, GnRH, and GnRH analogs—may have been inaccurate.[79] Newer bioassays, in which recombinant LH or FSH receptors are co-transfected in Chinese hamster ovary cells together with cAMP reporter systems, have now been developed.[80] Receptor assays and bioassays can also be used to test for substances that block receptor binding or hormone action and to measure gonadotropins in species in which no immunoassays are available.

## ANDROGEN RECEPTORS

ARs, which are expressed ubiquitously in genital and nongenital tissues, mediate the actions of testosterone and DHT. The AR protein has a molecular mass of ~110 kDa and binds DHT with higher affinity than T. Like other members of the steroid hormone receptor superfamily, the AR contains a transcription-regulating amino-terminal domain, a DNA-binding domain, and a steroid-binding domain near its carboxyl terminus.[81] Unliganded receptors are maintained in an inactive state by binding other intracellular proteins. Subsequent to androgen binding, the receptor dimerizes and shuttles to the nucleus. It binds to DNA-target sequences and initiates transcription of androgen-responsive genes, or represses transcription (e.g., feedback inhibition of α-subunit gene expression). The AR is encoded by a gene located on the X chromosome; therefore, there are carrier females of mutant genes and hemizygous affected males with androgen-insensitivity syndromes (see Chap. 90).

Cultured genital skin fibroblasts can be used to study AR function. Radiolabeled androgens, in increasing concentrations, are incubated with whole cells or with broken cell preparations until equilibrium. When receptor-bound and unbound ligand is separated, the affinity and receptor-binding capacity can be calculated. AR mRNA can be detected by Northern analysis, and AR structure can be studied by polymerase chain reaction (PCR) amplification of individual exons. AR function can be examined by cotransfection of a plasmid expressing a normal or mutant receptor together with a second plasmid expressing an androgen-responsive DNA sequence upstream of a reporter gene, such as luciferase or CAT.[82] Numerous AR mutations, in both the steroid-binding and DNA-binding domains, disrupt AR function totally or partially, causing androgen-insensitivity syndromes.[83]

Testosterone is important for the initiation and maintenance of spermatogenesis, and decreased AR binding has been detected in skin fibroblast cultures from phenotypically normal men with azoospermia,[84] but few AR mutations in men with defective spermatogenesis have so far been identified.[85] The AR gene contains a stretch of CAG repeats in exon 1 that code for glutamine. Men with *spinal and bulbar muscular atrophy (Kennedy disease)* have an expansion of this stretch (to 40–60 triplet codons) as compared to an average of 21 in normal men. Men with this condition develop gynecomastia, clinical signs of androgen deficiency, and small testes with hypospermatogenesis later in life with increased serum LH and testosterone levels, indicating androgen insensitivity. The mutations appear to impair transactivation of androgen-responsive genes.[86] Increased CAG repeats in exon 1 of the AR may also predispose to male infertility in the absence of neurologic disease.[87] On the other hand, fewer CAG repeats in exon 1 of the AR are associated with increased transcriptional activity and have been associated with increased risk for aggressive prostate cancer.[88]

## FUNCTIONAL TESTS

**Response to Human Chorionic Gonadotropin.**   Stimulation of testosterone secretion by hCG is a useful diagnostic test for examining Leydig cell function in prepubertal boys who secrete little or no endogenous gonadotropin. A variety of clinical protocols have been used. In one study, serum testosterone levels rose to >300 ng/dL in prepubertal boys given seven intramuscular injections of hCG, 1500 IU, every other day.[89] Testosterone levels usually fail to increase in plasma in boys with congenital bilateral anorchia, but increase somewhat in boys with bilateral intraabdominal testes.[90] Based on the results of this test, as well as the level of müllerian inhibitory substance, the latter patients will undergo laparoscopy followed by orchidopexy or orchiectomy[91] (see Chap. 93). The change in the circulating level of testosterone and its precursor steroids after hCG stimulation has been used to distinguish between boys with primary hypogonadism, defects in testosterone biosynthesis, and boys with androgen-insensitivity syndromes.[92]

Adult men with primary testicular failure have elevated serum LH concentrations. The administration of hCG to these men predictably increases serum testosterone levels less than in normal men.[93] In gonadotropin-deficient men, the short-term administration of hCG will also produce a blunted testosterone response because Leydig cells have been exposed to subnormal LH stimulation. Overall, little clinically useful information is gained from hCG testing in either group of adult men.

**Response to Antiestrogens.**   The estrogen antagonists, clomiphene and tamoxifen, have been used to assess the integrity of the hypothalamic–pituitary–testicular unit in adult men with borderline low testosterone levels and possible hypogonadotropic hypogonadism. This clinical situation often is encountered in obese[94] and in elderly men.[95] Endogenous estrogens suppress gonadotropin secretion in normal men, and blocking this suppression increases gonadotropin concentrations. Dosages of 100 to 200 mg per day of clomiphene for 7 days produce a mean two-fold increase in serum LH, FSH, and testosterone levels in normal men.[96] A normal response implies the functional integrity of GnRH-LH pathways, but responses among subjects are variable, and the test is probably not useful clinically.

**Gonadotropin-Releasing Hormone Test.**   GnRH is used as a research tool to examine the ability of the gonadotrope cells to release LH and FSH in response to their hypophysiotropic stimulus (see Chap. 16). The GnRH test was introduced as a method for diagnosing hypogonadism and for discriminating hypothalamic from pituitary disorders. In normal adult men given 100 μg GnRH intravenously, serum LH levels increase three- to- sixfold, and serum FSH levels rise by 50%. Generally, the total and incremental release of LH and FSH after GnRH administration is proportional to the basal hormone level,[97] although exceptions occur. In adult men with either hypothalamic or pituitary disease, the release of gonadotropins after GnRH stimulation usually is reduced, but may be normal. Overall, in evaluating gonadotropin-deficient men, the GnRH test provides little information beyond that of the basal testosterone, LH, and FSH levels; therefore, it is not recommended. Furthermore, the presence of a hypothalamic or pituitary mass is most directly demonstrated by magnetic resonance imaging. Treatment with GnRH will increase LH and FSH secretion in GnRH-deficient men, but is less effective in men with hypogonadotropic hypogonadism due to GnRH-receptor mutations.

Peak serum gonadotropin levels after GnRH stimulation are increased in patients with primary testicular failure. Subtle testicular dysfunction may produce an exaggerated response even with normal basal LH and FSH levels.[98] The LH response to a subcutaneous dose of a potent GnRH agonist in boys with delayed puberty may exceed that of patients with congenital hypogonadotropic hypogonadism, and may be useful in distinguishing between these two patient groups,[99] although not all studies are in agreement.

## SEMEN ANALYSIS

The semen analysis is a simple, inexpensive, and useful test to evaluate testicular function. Complete details of the laboratory

**TABLE 114-4.**
**World Health Organization Criteria of Normality for a Semen Sample (1992)**

| Criterion | Value |
|---|---|
| Volume | $\geq 2.0$ mL |
| pH | 7.2–7.8 |
| Sperm concentration | $\geq 20 \times 10^6$ spermatozoa/mL |
| Total sperm count | $\geq 40 \times 10^6$ spermatozoa/ejaculate |
| Motility | $\geq 50\%$ sperm with forward progression, or 25% with rapid linear progression within 60 min after collection |
| Morphology | $\geq 30\%$ with normal morphology |
| Viability | $\geq 75\%$ living (i.e., excluding dye) |
| White blood cells | $< 1 \times 10^6$/mL |
| Immunobead test | $< 20\%$ of sperm with adherent particles |

methods for semen analysis are available in a comprehensive manual published by the World Health Organization[100] (Table 114-4). There is an effect of duration of abstinence on semen volume and sperm output. Accordingly, a fixed abstinence interval of 2 to 3 days is suggested to standardize results. There is also day-to-day variability in sperm output. Therefore, if the initial sample is not entirely normal, three samples may be obtained during one sperm cycle (72 days). Since acute and chronic illness and surgery suppress gonadal function, semen samples should be evaluated at a time when the patient has been in good health.

The patient should be given precise written instructions for the collection and transport of the sample. The ejaculate should be obtained by masturbation, and collected in a wide-mouth laboratory glass jar. Semen collected by interrupted coitus is less desirable, because the sperm-rich early fraction may be lost during collection. Samples should not be collected in condoms because recovery will be incomplete, and most condoms contain spermicidal compounds. The sample jar should be kept warm adjacent to the body, and transported to the laboratory within 1 to 2 hours, because in vitro motility declines thereafter. The ejaculate coagulates immediately, and will liquefy within 10 to 30 minutes; failure to do so is consistent with prostatitis.

Semen is first examined for motility. At least 100 sperm are viewed in a drop of undiluted semen on several different microscopic slides. The percentage of sperm that are moving forward is determined, and is usually at least 40%. Decreased motility is termed *asthenozoospermia*. Motility can be graded semiquantitatively using a scale of 0 to 3. Sperm of grade 3 have active forward progression, grade 2 have moderate forward progression, grade 1 have only tail movement without progression, and grade 0 are immotile.

Sperm density is determined with a hemocytometer after appropriate dilution. Both sperm density and total sperm output should be reported. Sperm density partly depends on semen volume, which may vary from 2 to 6 mL in normal men. Small volumes suggest incomplete collection, retrograde ejaculation, or androgen deficiency, or may be idiopathic. The definition of what constitutes "normal" sperm output is arguable. Based on the results of populations of men requesting vasectomy, normal has been defined as >20 million sperm per milliliter, or a total sperm output of 40 million.[101] Some men with consistently fewer sperm are fertile, however. An epidemiologic study found that the likelihood of conception increased with increasing sperm concentration up to 40 million/mL.[102]

Sperm morphology is determined in smears that are air dried, fixed in formalin, and stained with Harris hematoxylin, or by the Papanicolaou staining method, which is decidedly more complex. The sperm can be divided into two major parts: head and tail. The head consists of the acrosome and the nucleus. The tail can be divided into the neck, middle piece,

principal piece, and end piece. Normal human sperm are ~50 μm long, of which 10 μm represents a symmetric oval head. The assessment of sperm morphology is highly subjective, and normal values vary considerably. All ejaculates appear to contain a mixture of "normal" and "abnormal" sperm. Abnormal forms include those with large oval heads, small oval heads, tapered heads, double heads, amorphous heads, and double tails. The distinction between spermatids (immature sperm without tails that often appear in the ejaculate of infertile men) and leukocytes is difficult, requiring special staining techniques. More detailed morphologic study has been accomplished with computer digitization, scanning, and transmission electron microscopy.

Automated equipment for the determination of sperm morphology, motility, and density is commercially available. *Computer-aided semen analysis* eliminates examiner error and provides an array of semen parameters for objective analysis, but the results so far are of no greater clinical benefit than is the traditional semen analysis.

Because the diagnosis of male-factor infertility is often difficult, due to overlap in semen parameters among fertile and infertile men, various tests of sperm function have been developed with the hope that a test would reliably predict a successful or unsuccessful pregnancy outcome.[103,103a] Among these tests are the motility of sperm in cervical mucus, the ability of sperm to penetrate zona pellucida–free hamster eggs, the binding of sperm to human zona pellucida (*hemizona assay*), and the *hypoosmotic swelling test*, which provides information concerning the integrity of sperm membranes. Although abnormal test results tend to predict poor fertilization, there are no absolute diagnostic criteria. Therefore, in spite of the results, many couples choose in vitro fertilization or intracytoplasmic sperm injection with the hope that it will be successful.

### SPERM ANTIBODIES

Sperm antibodies in the male or female are proposed to cause infertility.[104] Antibodies bound to sperm antigens are found in 1% to 10% of infertile men and are thought to impair sperm motility and zona pellucida binding, thereby disrupting fertilization. Sperm antibodies are generally detected using the immunobead test, in which beads coated with anti–immunoglobulin G (IgG) or anti–immunoglobulin A (IgA) are mixed with washed sperm. The mixture is then placed on a slide and examined by phase-contrast microscopy. Values among fertile men are usually <10% of sperm bound to one or more beads. High-titer sperm antibodies have been reported to reduce the fertilization rate with conventional in vitro fertilization, whereas intracytoplasmic sperm injection was equally effective in couples with and without sperm antibodies,[105] so that the latter treatment approach may be preferred when sperm antibodies are present.

### GENITAL TRACT INFECTION

Genital tract infection remains a controversial cause of male infertility. Leukocytospermia has been defined as the presence of >1 million white blood cells (WBCs)/mL semen, and finding >6 WBCs per high-power microscopic field in expressed prostatic secretions suggests infection. Seminal plasma pH may be elevated. Cytokines produced by WBCs in response to infection could damage sperm cell membrane integrity and impair fertilization. Infection with *Chlamydia trachomatis* is now the most common sexually transmitted disease, and is known to cause symptomatic pelvic inflammatory disease in women. Chlamydia urethritis in men has been proposed to produce chronic prostatitis and seminal vesicle infection. Detection of chlamydia in a first-void urine sample or in semen can be accomplished by specific PCR or ligase chain reaction assays. *C. trachomatis* seems to be rare in the semen and urine of asymptomatic infertile men, however.[106]

## BIOCHEMICAL ANALYSIS OF SEMEN

There is a tremendous array of seminal plasma constituents, each of which presumably plays a role in maintaining the proper milieu for fertilization.[107] After ejaculation, human semen coagulates because of the formation of a dense fibrous network. Proteolytic enzymes of prostatic origin lyse the fibers in 10 to 30 minutes. Sperm can then be separated from seminal plasma by gentle centrifugation. Because of cell breakage, however, intracellular constituents invariably are present in seminal plasma, and specific seminal plasma constituents may be reduced or absent because they bind to the sperm surface and are removed.

The protein content of seminal plasma ranges from 3.5 to 5.0 g/dL. Some of these proteins are identical to that of blood plasma, including transferrin, insulin-like growth factor (IGF)-I and -II, and inhibin; others are specific for semen such as *sperm adherins*, which are glycoproteins that are thought to play a role in sperm binding to the zona pellucida. The prostate contributes protective redox enzymes such as superoxide dismutase as well as a number of peptidases such as prostate-specific antigen, which, although a marker for prostate cancer, plays a physiologic role in semen liquefaction. Carbohydrates are present in semen, both free and associated with proteins. Fructose is the principal sugar of seminal plasma. Bilateral agenesis or complete obstruction of the seminal vesicles results in ejaculates that are nearly free of fructose. Androgen deficiency impairs the function of the accessory organs, with a reduction in the concentrations of many substances normally present in semen. Among the steroid hormones, testosterone, several of its precursor steroids, DHT, and 17β-estradiol are present in semen.[108] Seminal plasma contains many trace elements, with calcium and zinc being the most abundant.[109] Carnitine, acetyl-carnitine, glycerylphosphorylcholine, and citric acid are among the products of the human prostate. Carnitine is also present in sperm, and treatment with oral carnitine has been proposed to improve sperm motility.

High levels of the cytokine interleukin-6 (IL-6) in semen have been proposed as a marker for infection of the male accessory glands, although no relationship has been shown between seminal plasma IL-6 levels and sperm parameters.[110] Prostaglandins of both the E and F series are produced by the testis and throughout the excurrent duct system, and presumably regulate ejaculatory function. There is substantial concern that environmental pollutants damage the male reproductive system. An estimation of internal dosing can be made by measuring chemicals in serum or semen. Blood lead levels have been a better indicator of seminiferous tubule dysfunction than is the level of lead in semen,[111] whereas the concentration of aluminum in spermatozoa may be a more reliable biomarker of aluminum toxicity.[112]

## STUDY OF TESTICULAR TISSUE

Over the past 30 years, physical examination of the testes and measurement of plasma testosterone, LH, and FSH levels have replaced testicular biopsy for distinguishing gonadotropin deficiency from primary testicular failure. The use of routine testicular biopsy in men with unexplained infertility has also declined because the finding of damaged seminiferous tubular epithelium with incomplete spermatogenesis has provided little insight into the pathogenesis of male infertility, and the ultimate therapeutic impact of the biopsy results has been limited. However, testicular biopsy is performed in azoospermic men with normal plasma FSH levels in an effort to identify genital tract obstruction, which can be successfully treated by microsurgery. In many centers, fine-needle aspiration biopsy of the testis has replaced open biopsy.[113] In addition, transrectal ultrasonography and transurethral vasography can be used to localize the site of an obstruction.[114] In men with marked hypospermatogenesis, testicular sperm aspiration (TESA) and epididymal sperm aspiration (PESA) are used to obtain sperm for intracytoplasmic sperm injection (ICSI) when few or no sperm are present in the ejaculate.[115]

## GENETIC STUDIES

Cytogenetic studies are helpful in clarifying the cause of primary testicular failure, and for genetic counseling in men planning ICSI because mutations can be passed on to the progeny. Standard chromosomal analyses were abnormal in 13.7% of azoospermic men and 4.6% of oligospermic men.[116] Klinefelter syndrome (47,XXY) and its variants (e.g., 46,XY/47,XXY) are the most common cause of azoospermia and are detected by peripheral blood leukocyte karyotyping with banding procedures, and no longer by the examination of buccal mucosal cells for condensed chromatin (Barr body).

Genes on the long arm of the Y chromosome are required for spermatogenesis. This region of the Y is known as the *AZF region* because it contains genes related to azoospermia. Using the PCR to analyze DNA from peripheral blood leukocytes, small deletions of AZF genes, which escape detection under the microscope, can be identified in 15% to 30% of men with azoospermia.[117] The absence of these deletions in the fathers of infertile men indicates that they represent de novo mutations, and provides good evidence that they relate to male infertility. Because, with ICSI, Y microdeletions will be passed on to sons, screening tests for Y microdeletions have been recommended.

Congenital bilateral absence of the vas deferens accounts for 3.5% to 8.0% of cases of azoospermia, and represents a mild form of cystic fibrosis in ~70% of cases.[118] This autosomal recessive disorder results from mutations involving the cystic fibrosis transmembrane conductase regulator gene, which codes for a membrane protein that functions as an ion channel, and appears to play a role in the development of the epididymis, seminal vesicles, and vas deferens. Testing for this mutation should be performed in men with obstructive azoospermia. Computed tomographic (CT) scans of the paranasal sinuses, chest radiography, and pulmonary function tests should also be obtained, and affected men should be cautioned not to smoke cigarettes.

## REFERENCES

1. Takihara H, Sakatoku J, Fujii M, et al. Significance of testicular size measurement. In: Andrology. I. A new orchiometer and its clinical application. Fertil Steril 1983; 39:836.
2. Stearns EL, MacDonnell JA, Kaufman BJ, et al. Decline of testicular function with age: hormonal and clinical correlates. Am J Med 1974; 57:761.
3. Sawczun IS, Hensle TW, Burbie KA, Nagler HM. Varicoceles: effect on testicular volume in prepubertal and pubertal males. Urology 1993; 41:466.
4. Haans LCF, Laven JSE, Mali WPThM, et al. Testis volumes, semen quality, and hormonal patterns in adolescents with and without a varicocele. Fertil Steril 1991; 56:731.
5. Chiou RK, Anderson JC, Wobig RK, et al. Color Doppler ultrasound criteria to diagnose varicoceles: correlation of a new scoring system with physical examination. Urology 1997; 50:953.
6. Winters SJ, Takahashi J, Troen P. Secretion of testosterone and its delta-4 precursor steroids into spermatic vein blood in men with varicocele-associated infertility. J Clin Endocrinol Metab 1999; 84:997.
7. Spratt DI, O'Dea L St L, Schoenfeld D, et al. Neuroendocrine-gonadal axis in men: frequent sampling of LH, FSH and testosterone. Am J Physiol 1988; 254:E658.
8. Tenover JS, Matsumoto AM, Clifton DK, Bremner WJ. Age-related alterations in the circadian rhythms of pulsatile luteinizing hormone and testosterone secretion in healthy men. J Gerontol 1988; 43:M163.
9. Winters SJ. Diurnal rhythm of testosterone and luteinizing hormone in hypogonadal men. J Androl 1991; 12:185.
10. Vermeulen A, Verdonck G. Representativeness of a single point plasma testosterone level for the long term hormonal milieu in men. J Clin Endocrinol Metab 1992; 74:939.
11. Boyar RN, Rosenfeld RS, Kapen S, et al. Human puberty: simultaneous augmented secretion of luteinizing hormone and testosterone during sleep. J Clin Invest 1974; 54:609.

12. Wu F, Brown DC, Butler GE, et al. Early morning plasma testosterone is an accurate predictor of imminent pubertal development in prepubertal boys. J Clin Endocrinol Metab 1993; 76:26.

13. Zmuda JM, Thompson PD, Winters SJ. Exercise increases serum testosterone and sex hormone-binding globulin levels in older men. Metabolism 1996; 45:935.

14. Kujala H, Alem M, Huhtaniemi IT. Gonadotrophin-releasing hormone and human chorionic gonadotropin tests reveal that both hypothalamic and testicular endocrine functions are suppressed during acute prolonged exercise. Clin Endocrinol 1990; 33:219.

15. Turner HE, Wass JAH. Gonadal function in men with chronic illness. Clin Endocrinol 1997; 47:379.

16. Dunn JF, Nisula BC, Rodbard D. Transport of steroid hormones: binding of 21 endogenous steroids to both testosterone-binding globulin and corticosteroid-binding globulin in human plasma. J Clin Endocrinol Metab 1981; 53:58.

17. Petra PH. The plasma sex steroid binding protein (SBP or SHBG). A critical review of recent developments on the structure, molecular biology and function. J Steroid Biochem Molec Biol 1991; 40:735.

18. Terasaki T, Nowlin DM, Pardridge WM. Differential binding of testosterone and estradiol to isoforms of sex hormone-binding globulin: selective alteration of estradiol binding in cirrhosis. J Clin Endocrinol Metab 1988; 67:639.

19. Joseph DR. Structure, function, and regulation of androgen-binding protein/sex hormone-binding globulin. Vitam Horm 1994; 49:197.

20. Wheeler MJ. The determination of bioavailable testosterone. Ann Clin Biochem 1995; 32:345.

21. Masters AM, Hahnel R. Investigation of sex-hormone binding globulin interference in direct radioimmunoassays for testosterone and estradiol. Clin Chem 1989; 35:979.

22. Wheeler MJ, D'Souza A, Matadeen J, et al. Ciba Corning ACS:180 testosterone assay evaluated. Clin Chem 1996; 42:1445.

23. Sodergard R, Backstrom T, Shanbhag V, Carstensen H. Calculation of free and bound fractions of testosterone and estradiol 17-β to human plasma proteins at body temperature. J Steroid Biochem 1982; 16:810.

24. Kapoor P, Luttrell BM, Williams D. The free androgen index is not valid for adult males. J Steroid Biochem 1993; 45:325.

24a. Rosner W. Errors in the measurement of plasma free testosterone. J Clin Endcrinol Metab 1997; 82:2014.

25. Winters SJ, Kelley DE, Goodpaster B. The analog free testosterone assay: are the results in men clinically useful? Clin Chem 1998; 44:2178.

26. Manni A, Pardridge WM, Cefalu W, et al. Bioavailability of albumin-bound testosterone. J Clin Endocrinol Metab 1985; 61:705.

27. Vermeulen A, Kaufman JM, Giagulli. Influence of some biological indexes on sex hormone-binding globulin and androgen levels in aging or obese males. J Clin Endocrinol Metab 1996; 81:1821.

28. Cox C, Caulier C, Havelange G, et al. Two-sites immunoradiometric assay using monoclonal antibodies for the determination of serum human sex hormone binding globulin. J Immunoassay 1992; 13:355.

29. Nisula BC, Loriaux DL, Wilson YA. Solid phase method for measurement of the binding capacity of testosterone-estradiol binding globulin in human serum. Steroids 1979; 31:681.

30. Pugeat M, Crave JC, Tournaire J, Forest MG. Clinical utility of sex hormone-binding globulin measurement. Horm Res 1996; 45:148.

31. Chin WW, Boime I, eds. Glycoprotein hormones. Norwell, MA: Serono Symposia, 1990.

32. Shupnik MA. Gonadotropin gene modulation by steroids and gonadotropin-releasing hormone. Biol Reprod 1996; 54:279.

33. Nankin HR, Troen P. Repetitive luteinizing hormone elevations in serum in normal men. J Clin Endocrinol Metab 1971; 33:558.

34. Veldhuis JD, King JC, Urban RJ, et al. Operating characteristics of the male hypothalamo-pituitary-gonadal axis: pulsatile release of testosterone and follicle-stimulating hormone and their temporal coupling with luteinizing hormone. J Clin Endocrinol Metab 1987; 65:929.

35. Haavisto A-M, Pettersson K, Bergendahl M, et al. Occurrence and biological properties of a common genetic variant of luteinizing hormone. J Clin Endocrinol Metab 1995; 80:1257.

36. Wu FCW, Butler GE, Kelnar CJH, et al. Patterns of pulsatile luteinizing hormone and follicle-stimulating hormone secretion in prepubertal (midchildhood) boys and girls and patients with idiopathic hypogonadotropic hypogonadism (Kallmann's syndrome): a study using an ultrasensitive time-resolved immunofluorometric assay. J Clin Endocrinol Metab 1991; 72:1229.

37. Odink RJ, Schoemaker J, Schoute E, et al. Predictive value of serum follicle-stimulating hormone levels in the differentiation between hypogonadotropic hypogonadism and constitutional delay of puberty. Horm Res 1998; 49:279.

38. Anawalt BD, Bebb RA, Matsumoto AM, et al. Serum inhibin B levels reflect Sertoli cell function in normal men and men with testicular dysfunction. J Clin Endocrinol Metab 1996; 81:3341.

39. Rosen SW, Weintraub BD. Monotropic increase of serum FSH correlated with low sperm count in young men with idiopathic oligospermia and aspermia. J Clin Endocrinol Metab 1972; 32:410.

40. Snyder PJ. Gonadotroph cell adenomas of the pituitary. Endocr Rev 1985; 6:552.

41. Vos P, Croughs RJM, Thijssen JHH, et al. Response of luteinizing hormone secreting pituitary adenoma to a long-acting somatostatin analog. Acta Endocrinol 1988; 118:587.

42. Ito T, Horton R. The source of plasma dihydrotestosterone in man. J Clin Invest 1971; 50:1621.

43. McConnell JD, Wilson JD, George FW, et al. Finasteride, an inhibitor of 5α-reductase, suppresses prostatic dihydrotestosterone in men with benign prostatic hyperplasia. J Clin Endocrinol Metab 1992; 74:505.

44. Thigpen AE, Silver RI, Guileyardo JM, et al. Tissue distribution and ontogeny of steroid 5α-reductase isozyme expression. J Clin Invest 1993; 92:903.

45. Belanger A, Candas B, Dupont A, et al. Changes in serum concentrations of conjugated and unconjugated steroids in 40- to 80-year old men. J Clin Endocrinol Metab 1994; 79:1086.

46. Horton R. Dihydrotestosterone is a peripheral paracrine hormone. J Androl 1992; 13:23.

47. Lookingbill DP, Egan N, Santen RJ, Demers LM. Correlation of serum 3α-androstenediol glucuronide with acne and chest hair density in men. J Clin Endocrinol Metab 1988; 67:986.

48. Perryman RL, Thorner MO. The effects of hyperprolactinemia on sexual and reproductive function in men. J Androl 1981; 2:233.

49. Spitz IM, LeRoith D, Livshin J, et al. Exaggerated prolactin response to TRH and metoclopramide in primary testicular failure. Fertil Steril 1980; 34:573.

50. Winters SJ, Johnsonbaugh RE, Sherins RJ. The response of prolactin to chlorpromazine stimulation in men with hypogonadotropic hypogonadism and early pubertal boys: relationship to sex steroid exposure. Clin Endocrinol (Oxf) 1982; 10:321.

51. Sigman M, Jarow JP. Endocrine evaluation of infertile men. Urology 1997; 50:659.

52. Nagel SC, vom Saal FS, Welshons WV. The effective free fraction of estradiol and xenoestrogens in human serum measured by whole cell uptake assays: physiology of delivery modifies estrogenic activity. Proc Soc Exp Biol Med 1998; 217:300.

53. Khosla S, Melton LJ, Atkinson EJ, et al. Relation of serum sex steroid levels and bone turnover markers with bone mineral density in men and women: a key role for bioavailable estrogens. J Clin Endocrinol Metab 1998; 83:2266.

54. Stanik S, Dornfeld LP, Maxwell MH, et al. The effect of weight loss on reproductive hormones in obese men. J Clin Endocrinol Metab 1981; 53:828.

55. Schioler V, Thode J. Six direct radioimmunoassays of estradiol evaluated. Clin Chem 1988; 34:949.

56. Winters SJ, Troen P. Pulsatile secretion of immunoreactive α-subunit in man. J Clin Endocrinol Metab 1985; 60:344.

57. Winters SJ, Troen P. α-Subunit secretion in men with idiopathic hypogonadotropic hypogonadism. J Clin Endocrinol Metab 1988; 66:338.

58. Pralong FP, Pavlou SN, Waldstreicher J, et al. Defective regulation of glycoprotein free α-subunit in males with isolated gonadotropin-releasing hormone deficiency—a clinical research center study. J Clin Endocrinol Metab 1995; 80:3682.

59. Kourides IA, Weintraub BD, Ridgway EC, Maloof F. Pituitary secretion of free alpha and beta subunit of human thyrotropin in patients with thyroid disorders. J Clin Endocrinol Metab 1975; 40:872.

60. Blackman MR, Weintraub BD, Kourides IA, et al. Discordant elevation of the common α-subunit of the glycoprotein hormones compared to β-subunits in serum of uremic patients. J Clin Endocrinol Metab 1981; 53:39.

61. Somjen D, Tordjman K, Kohen F, et al. Combined beta FSH and beta LH response to TRH in patients with clinically non-functioning pituitary adenomas. Clin Endocrinol 1997; 46:555.

62. Fein HG, Rosen SW, Weintraub BD. Increased glycosylation of serum human chorionic gonadotropin and subunits from eutopic and ectopic sources: comparison with placental and urinary forms. J Clin Endocrinol Metab 1980; 50:1111.

63. Saller B, Clara R, Spottl G, et al. Testicular cancer secretes intact human choriogonadotropin (hCG) and its free β-subunit: evidence that hCG (+hCG-β) assays are the most reliable in diagnosis and follow-up. Clin Chem 1990; 36:234.

64. Burger HG. Inhibin in the male: progress at last. Endocrinology 1997; 138:1361.

65. Hayes FJ, Hall JE, Boepple PA, Crowley WF Jr. Differential control of gonadotropin secretion in the human: endocrine role of inhibin. J Clin Endocrinol Metab 1998; 83:1835.

65a. Anderson RA, Sharpe RM. Regulation of inhibin production in the human male and its clinical applications. Int J Androl 2000; 23:136.

66. Illingworth PJ, Groome NP, Byrd W, et al. Inhibin-B: a likely candidate for the physiologically important form of inhibin in men. J Clin Endocrinol Metab 1996; 81:1321.

67. Robertson DM, Cahir N, Findlay JK, et al. The biological and immunological characterization of inhibin A and B forms in human follicular fluid and plasma. J Clin Endocrinol Metab 1997; 82:889.

68. Groome NP, Illingworth PJ, O'Brien M, et al. Quantification of inhibin pro-αC-containing forms in human serum by a new ultrasensitive two-site enzyme-linked immunosorbent assay. J Clin Endocrinol Metab 1995; 80:2926.

69. Andersson AM, Toppari J, Haavisto AM, et al. Longitudinal reproductive hormone profiles in infants: peak of inhibin B levels in infant boys exceeds levels in adult men. J Clin Endocrinol Metab 1998; 83:675.

70. Nachtigall LB, Boepple PA, Seminara SB, et al. Inhibin B secretion in males with gonadotropin releasing hormone (GnRH) deficiency before and during long-term GnRH replacement: relationship to spontaneous puberty, testicular volume, and prior treatment—a clinical research center study. J Clin Endocrinol Metab 1996; 81:3520.

71. Wallace EM, Groome NP, Riley SC, et al. Effects of chemotherapy-induced testicular damage on inhibin, gonadotropin and testosterone secretion: a prospective longitudinal study. J Clin Endocrinol Metab 1997; 82:3111.

72. Petersen P, Andersson A-M, Rorth M, et al. Undetectable inhibin B serum levels in men after testicular irradiation. J Clin Endocrinol Metab 1999; 84:213.

73. Pierik FH, Vreeburg JTM, Stijnen T, et al. Serum inhibin B as a marker of spermatogenesis. J Clin Endocrinol Metab 1998; 83:3110.

74. Petersen PM, Skakkebaek NE, Vistisen K, et al. Semen quality and reproductive hormones before orchiectomy in men with testicular cancer. J Clin Oncol 1999; 17:941.

74a. Hiort O, Holterhus PM. The molecular basis of male sexual differentiation. Eur J Endocrinol 2000; 142:101.

75. Lee MM, Donahoe PK, Silverman BL, et al. Measurements of serum müllerian inhibiting substance in the evaluation of children with nonpalpable gonads. N Engl J Med 1997; 336:1480.

76. Pierce JG, Parsons TF. Glycoprotein hormones: structure and function. Annu Rev Biochem 1982; 50:465.

77. van Damme M-P, Robertson DM, Diczfalusy E. An improved in vitro bioassay method for measuring luteinizing hormone (LH) activity using mouse Leydig cell preparations. Acta Endocrinol 1974; 77:655.

78. Dahl KD, Stone MP. FSH isoforms, radioimmunoassays, bioassays, and their significance. J Androl 1992; 13:11.

79. Jaakkola T, Ding Y-Q, Kellokumpu-Lehtinen P, et al. The ratios of serum bioactive/immunoreactive luteinizing hormone and follicle-stimulating hormone in various clinical conditions with increased and decreased gonadotropin secretion: reevaluation by a highly sensitive immunometric assay. J Clin Endocrinol Metab 1990; 70:1496.

80. Christin-Maitre S, Bouchard P. Bioassays of gonadotropins based on cloned receptors. Mol Cell Endocrinol 1996; 125:151.

81. Beato M, Truss M, Chavez S. Control of transcription by steroid hormones. Ann NY Acad Sci 1996; 784:93.

82. Deslypere JP, Young M, Wilson JD, McPhaul MJ. Testosterone and 5 alpha-dihydrotestosterone interact differently with the androgen receptor to enhance transcription of the MMTV-CAT reporter gene. Mol Cell Endocrinol 1992; 88:15.

83. Quigley CA, de Bellis A, Marschke E, et al. Androgen receptor defects: historical, clinical and molecular perspectives. Endocr Rev 1995; 16:27.

84. Aiman J, Griffin JE. The frequency of androgen receptor deficiency in infertile men. J Clin Endocrinol Metab 1982; 54:725.

85. Wang Q, Ghadessy FJ, Yong EL. Analysis of the transactivation domain of the androgen receptor in patients with male infertility. Clin Genet 1998; 54:185.

86. MacLean HE, Warne GL, Zajac JD. Spinal and bulbar muscular atrophy: androgen receptor dysfunction caused by a trinucleotide repeat expansion. J Neurol Sci 1996; 135:149.

87. Tut TG, Ghadessy FJ, Trifiro MA, et al. Long polyglutamine tracts in the androgen receptor are associated with reduced trans-activation, impaired sperm production, and male infertility. J Clin Endocrinol Metab 1997; 82:3777.

88. Kantoff P, Giovannucci E, Brown M. The androgen receptor CAG repeat polymorphism and its relationship to prostate cancer. Biochim Biophys Acta 1998; 1378:C1.

89. Forest MG. Pattern of the response of testosterone and its precursors to human chorionic gonadotropin stimulation in relation to age in infants and children. J Clin Endocrinol Metab 1979; 49:132.

90. Aynsley-Green A, Zachmann M, Illig R, et al. Congenital bilateral anorchia in childhood: a clinical, endocrine and therapeutic evaluation of twenty-one cases. Clin Endocrinol (Oxf) 1976; 5:381.

91. Cisek LJ, Peters CA, Atala A, et al. Current findings in diagnostic laparoscopic evaluation of the nonpalpable testis. J Urol 1998; 160:1145.

92. Lee PA, Danish RK, Mazur T, Migeon CJ. Micropenis III. Primary hypogonadism, partial androgen insensitivity syndrome, and idiopathic disorders. Johns Hopkins Med J 1980; 147:175.

93. de Kretser DM, Burger HG, Hudson B, Keogh EJ. The hCG stimulation test in men with testicular disorders. Clin Endocrinol (Oxf) 1975; 4:591.

94. Vermeulen A. Decreased androgen levels and obesity in men. Ann Med 1996; 28:135.

95. Korenman SG, Morley JE, Mooradian AD, et al. Secondary hypogonadism in older men: its relation to impotence. J Clin Endocrinol Metab 1990; 71:963.

96. Tenover JS, Matsumoto AM, Plymate SR, Bremner WJ. The effects of aging in normal men on bioavailable testosterone and luteinizing hormone secretion: response to clomiphene citrate. J Clin Endocrinol Metab 1987; 65:1118.

97. Harman SM, Tsitouras PD, Costa PT, et al. Evaluation of pituitary gonadotropic function in men: value of luteinizing hormone-releasing hormone response versus basal luteinizing hormone level for discrimination of diagnosis. J Clin Endocrinol Metab 1982; 54:196.

98. Hudson RW. The endocrinology of varicoceles. Fertil Steril 1988; 49:199.

99. Ghai K, Cara JF, Rosenfield RL. Gonadotropin releasing hormone agonist (nafarelin) test to differentiate gonadotropin deficiency from constitutionally delayed puberty in teen-age boys—a clinical research center study. J Clin Endocrinol Metab 1995; 80:2980.

100. World Health Organization. WHO laboratory manual for the examination of human semen and sperm-cervical-mucus interaction, 3rd ed. Cambridge, England: Cambridge University Press, 1992.

101. Zuckerman Z, Rodriguez-Rigau L, Smith KD, Steinberger E. Frequency distribution of sperm counts in fertile and infertile males. Fertil Steril 1977; 28:1310.

102. Bonde JPE, Ernst E, Jensen EK, et al. Relation between semen quality and fertility: a population-based study of 430 first-pregnancy planners. Lancet 1998; 352:1172.

103. Critser JK, Noiles EE. Bioassays of sperm function. Semin Reprod Endocrinol 1993; 11:1.

103a. Carrell DT. Semen analysis at the turn of the century: an evaluation of potential uses of new sperm function assays. Arch Androl 2000; 44:65.

104. Adeghe JH. Male subfertility due to sperm antibodies: a clinical overview. Obstet Gynecol Surv 1993; 48:1.

105. Clarke GN, Bourne J, Baker HWG. Intracytoplasmic sperm injections for treating infertility associated with sperm immunity. Fertil Steril 1997; 68:112.

106. Fujisawa M, Nakano Y, Matsui T, et al. *Chlamydia trachomatis* detected by ligase chain reaction in the semen of asymptomatic patients without pyospermia or pyuria. Arch Androl 1999; 42:41.

107. Mann T, Lutwak-Mann C. Male reproductive function and semen. New York: Springer-Verlag, 1981.

108. Garcia Diez LC, Gonzalez Buitrago IM, Corrales IJ, et al. Hormone levels in serum and seminal plasma of men with different types of azoospermia. J Reprod Fertil 1983; 67:208.

109. Abou-Shakra FR, Ward NI, Everard DM. The role of trace elements in male infertility. Fertil Steril 1989; 52:307.

110. Matalliotakis I, Kirakou D, Fragouli I, et al. Interleukin-6 in seminal plasma of fertile and infertile men. Arch Androl 1998; 41:43.

111. Alexander BH, Checkoway H, Faustman EM, et al. Contrasting associations of blood and semen lead concentrations with semen quality among lead smelter workers. Am J Industr Med 1998; 34:464.

112. Hovatta O, Venalainen ER, Kuusimaki L, et al. Aluminum, lead, and cadmium concentrations in seminal plasma and spermatozoa, and semen quality in Finnish men. Hum Reprod 1998; 13:115.

113. Dajani YF, Kilani Z. Role of testicular fine needle aspiration in the diagnosis of azoospermia. Int J Androl 1998; 21:295.

114. Kuligowska E, Baker CE, Oates RD. Male infertility: role of transrectal US in diagnosis and management. Radiology 1992; 185:353.

115. Belker AM, Sherins RJ, Dennison-Lagos L, et al. Percutaneous testicular sperm aspiration: a convenient and effective office procedure to retrieve sperm for in vitro fertilization with intracytoplasmic sperm injection. J Urol 1998; 160:2058.

116. Van Assche E, Bonduelle M, Tournaye H, et al. Cytogenetics of infertile men. Hum Reprod 1996; 11(Suppl 4):1.

117. Roberts KP. Y-chromosome deletions and male infertility. State of the art and clinical implications. J Androl 1998; 19:255.

118. Durieu I, Bey-Omar F, Rollet J, et al. Diagnostic criteria for cystic fibrosis in men with congenital absence of the vas deferens. Medicine 1995; 74:42.

# CHAPTER 115

# MALE HYPOGONADISM

STEPHEN R. PLYMATE

Male hypogonadism may be defined as a failure of the testes to produce testosterone, spermatozoa, or both (Table 115-1). This may be caused by a failure of the testes or of the anterior pituitary. Hypogonadism may also occur if a testicular product is unable to exert an effect, as in the androgen-resistance syndromes (Table 115-2).

## CLINICAL CHARACTERISTICS OF HYPOGONADISM

The clinical presentation of hypogonadism depends on whether the onset was in utero, prepubertal, or postpubertal. If hypogonadism is present because of a defect that occurred in utero, the individual will have ambiguous genitalia (see Chaps. 77 and 90). The clinical pictures of testicular androgen failure of prepubertal and postpubertal onset are presented in Table 115-2.

Although the findings on physical examination may be normal, a problem with seminiferous tubule function may manifest

**TABLE 115-1.**
**Classification of Male Hypogonadism**

**PRIMARY HYPOGONADISM**
> Klinefelter syndrome
> XX males
> XY/XO mixed gonadal dysgenesis
> XYY syndrome
> Ullrich-Noonan syndrome
> Myotonic dystrophy (myotonia dystrophica)
> Sertoli-cell-only syndrome
> Functional prepubertal castrate syndrome
> Enzymatic defects involving testosterone biosynthesis
> 5α-reductase deficiency
> Luteinizing hormone/gonadotropin–resistant testis
> Persistent müllerian duct syndrome
> Male pseudohermaphroditism involving androgen receptor defects
> Testicular feminization
> Reifenstein syndrome
> Infertility due to a receptor defect
> After orchitis
> Cryptorchidism
> Leprosy
> Testicular trauma
> After testicular irradiation
> Autoimmune testicular failure
> After chemotherapy

**SECONDARY HYPOGONADISM**
> Hypogonadotropic hypogonadism
> Isolated luteinizing hormone or follicle-stimulating hormone deficiency
> Acquired gonadotropin deficiencies
> Prolactin-secreting pituitary tumors
> Severe systemic illness
> Uremia
> Hemochromatosis

**COMBINED PRIMARY AND SECONDARY CAUSES**
> Aging
> Hepatic cirrhosis
> Sickle cell disease

**TABLE 115-2.**
**Manifestations of Testicular Androgen Failure**

**PREPUBERTAL TESTICULAR FAILURE**
> Testes, <2.5 cm long; volume <5 mL
> Penis, <3–5 cm long
> Lack of scrotal pigmentation and rugae
> Prepubertal subcutaneous fat distribution over hips, face, and chest
> Eunuchoidal skeletal proportions: crown to pubis/pubis to floor ratio is decreased; arm span is considerably greater than height (normally black men have a decreased ratio and relatively longer arm span than whites)
> Female escutcheon
> No terminal facial hair; decreased body hair
> No temporal hair recession
> High-pitched voice
> Decreased muscle mass
> Delayed bone age
> Small prostate
> Cross-hatching over skin lateral to the orbits
> Decreased libido
> Osteoporosis later in life

**POSTPUBERTAL TESTICULAR FAILURE**
> Normal skeletal proportions and penile length
> Loss of libido
> Decrease in strength and muscle mass
> Decrease in rate of growth of facial hair
> Normal distribution of pubic hair
> Testes are soft; volume <15 mL
> Prostate is adult size, although may be smaller than average
> No change in voice
> Diminished aggressivity
> Decreased amount of axillary and pubic hair
> Osteoporosis later in life

as infertility. With the development of sensitive assays for testosterone, an increasing number of circumstances have been described in which serum testosterone levels are lower than normal without any obvious end-organ deficiencies. Examples of this phenomenon are seen in aging or stressed men who have low levels of serum testosterone without definitive evidence of end-organ deficiency. In the case of stress, end-organ deficiency may not be seen, because the period of hypogonadism is transient. Deciding whether these men really are androgen deficient or whether they simply are displaying a physiologic response to stress or age may be difficult. These situations pose further difficulties for clinicians who must decide whether androgen replacement is needed. The classic states of androgen deficiency are discussed in this chapter; androgen replacement therapy, described in Chapter 119, is mentioned. In those situations in which obvious deficiency states are not present, however, the indication for replacement therapy may not be clear-cut. In some of these patients, the finding of an exaggerated gonadotropin response to luteinizing hormone–releasing hormone (LHRH) may help to define the presence of testicular failure.

Functionally, the hypogonadal states may be classified according to the level at which the hypothalamic–pituitary–testicular axis is defective. Briefly, the control of testicular function begins with the release, in a pulsatile fashion, of LHRH from the hypothalamus (see Chap. 16). LHRH, transported by the hypothalamic-pituitary portal system, then causes the release of luteinizing hormone (LH) and follicle-stimulating hormone (FSH) from the anterior pituitary. An optimal rate of pulsation (3.8 pulses every 6 hours) appears to be necessary for adequate secretion of both LH and FSH for normal gonadal function. When the rate is slower than optimal, FSH may be preferentially released in greater amounts than normal and LH in lesser amounts. When the pulse frequency of LHRH is more rapid than normal, serum FSH levels may be suppressed and LH release preferentially stimulated. LH subsequently binds to the Leydig cell to initiate testosterone synthesis and secretion. FSH binds to the Sertoli cell and stimulates the production of several factors that, with testosterone from the Leydig cell, induce and maintain normal spermatogenesis (see Chap. 113). LH and FSH release also are regulated by a negative feedback system (i.e., serum testosterone and estradiol). Inhibin, an FSH-stimulated Sertoli cell peptide, can partially block FSH release from the pituitary without influencing LH release. Serum testosterone and inhibin also may affect the release of LHRH from the hypothalamus. However, the precise role of inhibin in the feedback process in men is not completely defined.

In addition to the direct effects of testosterone on sexual tissues, the secretion of androgens is related to other endocrine systems that may affect body habitus during both puberty and adulthood. This is especially true for the somatotropin axis, in which androgens are necessary for normal growth hormone and insulin-like growth factor-I secretion. Furthermore, in normal men, components of the gonadal axis are regulated by other endocrine systems (e.g., insulin pulsation closely determines the blood levels of sex hormone–binding globulin [SHBG]). Therefore, hypogonadism may result from abnormalities in multiple systems, and its manifestations are evident in most physiologic systems.[1–3]

Based on this understanding of the hypothalamic–pituitary–gonadal axis, male hypogonadal disorders may be classified into two broad categories. The first is *primary hypogonadism*, in which

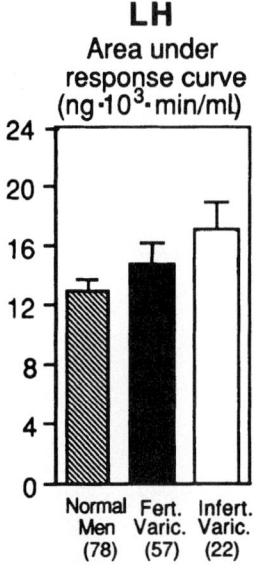
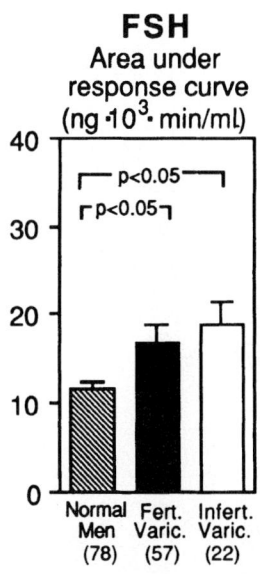

**LH**
Area under
response curve
(ng·10³·min/mL)

**FSH**
Area under
response curve
(ng·10³·min/mL)

**FIGURE 115-1.** Exaggerated luteinizing hormone (*LH*) and follicle-stimulating hormone (*FSH*) response to gonadotropin-releasing hormone in fertile and infertile men with a varicocele is compared with that of normal men. Results suggest impairment of both seminiferous tubule and Leydig cell function. Bars indicate standard error of the mean. (*Fert. Varic.*, fertile men with varicocele; *Infert. Varic.*, infertile men with varicocele.) (From Nagao RR, Plymate SR, Berger RE, et al. Comparison of gonadal function between fertile and infertile men with varicoceles. Fertil Steril 1986; 46:930.)

the dysfunction is in the testis. Primary hypogonadism is manifested by a deficiency in the main testicular products, testosterone or sperm. The basis for the primary hypogonadism is a testicular defect. In states of primary hypogonadism, negative feedback by testicular products such as testosterone or inhibin on the hypothalamus and pituitary is lost, so that serum LH and FSH levels are elevated in the basal state or, despite normal basal gonadotropin levels, an exaggerated gonadotropin response to LHRH occurs.

The presence of testosterone alone is not enough to achieve normal male development. A portion of the Y chromosome also is needed for normal testicular development and regression. In humans, this testis-determining factor has been mapped to a 35-kilobase (kb) segment on the short arm of the Y chromosome close to the pseudoautosomal region. The gene isolated from this locus that equates with the testis-determining factor has been called sex-determining region Y (*SRY*).[4,5]

*Secondary hypogonadism* (i.e., decreased gonadotropin stimulation of potentially normal testes) presents with low serum testosterone levels or decreased sperm production and low serum gonadotropin levels (or values inappropriately low for the level of serum testosterone, sperm production, or both). Since the discovery of LHRH, some authors have divided secondary hypogonadism into pituitary failure and hypothalamic failure ("tertiary hypogonadism"). In this chapter, the division into primary and secondary hypogonadism is used, with the latter including both pituitary and hypothalamic disorders. Table 115-1 lists the categories of diseases discussed.

# PRIMARY HYPOGONADISM

Including infertile men, primary testicular failure affects 5% to 10% of the male population.[4] Although male infertility is commonly considered a problem that involves exclusively seminiferous tubular function and spermatogenesis, evidence from men with varicoceles has demonstrated the presence of an exaggerated response of both serum LH and FSH to LHRH.[6] Although total serum testosterone levels are normal in these

patients, the augmented gonadotropin response to LHRH indicates a failure in both Leydig cell and seminiferous tubular function (Fig. 115-1). Some compensation for the impaired Leydig cells must occur that is sufficient to return testosterone levels to normal under the influence of increased LH stimulation. These findings confirm that infertile men often possess primary gonadal failure of a subtle nature. Because the incidence of male infertility is fairly high, primary testicular dysfunction in the male population is an important issue.

## KLINEFELTER SYNDROME

The chromosomal constitution of 47,XXY epitomizes the classic form of male primary testicular failure. This abnormality is present in ~1 in 400 men. Klinefelter syndrome was first described in 1942 in nine male patients who, at puberty, experienced the onset of bilateral gynecomastia, small testes with Leydig cell dysfunction and azoospermia, and increased urinary gonadotropin excretion.[7] Later, Leydig cell failure was shown to be variable in its magnitude. In 1956, the X chromatin body (Barr body) was found in these individuals, and in 1959, the XXY chromosome constitution was first described, demonstrating that the disease was the result of an extra X chromosome (see Chap. 90).[8,9]

### PHENOTYPIC MANIFESTATIONS

The phenotypic manifestations of Klinefelter syndrome are characteristic for the classic form of the disease in which all cells carry the XXY karyotype. Many men with Klinefelter syndrome have a *mosaic* form, in which some cell lines are XXY and others are XY. In these mosaic individuals, all cell lines are from a single zygote, and the XXY cell lines arise from mitotic nondisjunction after fertilization. Manifestation of the disease may not be typical or consistent. Before puberty, the only physical findings are the small testes; in the classic form of Klinefelter syndrome, a gonadal volume of <1.5 mL after the age of 6 years is usual.[10,11] Regardless of the patient's age, a decreased testicular size is the most diagnostic clinical feature of classic Klinefelter syndrome. A suggested cause for the small prepubertal testicular size is a loss of germ cells before puberty; thus, the prepubertal testis is small. In secondary forms of hypogonadism, the number of germ cells is normal, and the prepubertal testicular size is indistinguishable from that of normal boys.

Microcephaly also has been described in some cases of Klinefelter syndrome. After puberty, the more characteristic features of the syndrome appear (Figs. 115-2 and 115-3). These include varying degrees of gynecomastia. The gynecomastia is of interest because it is due primarily to an increase in periductal tissue rather than ductal tissue; increased ductal tissue often is found in gynecomastia of acute onset, whatever the cause. If the gynecomastia were due only to the increased estrogen production in Klinefelter syndrome, an increase in ductal tissue might be expected. Nonetheless, the histopathologic appearance of the breast tissue is not consistently separable from that of other patients with long-standing gynecomastia.

After puberty, an abnormality in skeletal proportions becomes manifest. The lower extremities show exaggerated growth, resulting in a decreased crown-to-pubis/pubis-to-floor ratio, such as that seen in eunuchoid men (see Chap. 18). However, unlike in the true eunuchoid state, in which the arm span often is at least 6 cm more than the height, in Klinefelter syndrome, the arm span/height ratio usually is not abnormal. The reason for the abnormal growth in the lower extremities is unknown. The phenotypic manifestations, such as the gynecomastia, pattern of hair distribution, muscle mass, and subcutaneous fat distribution, vary even among patients with classic Klinefelter syndrome.

### LABORATORY FINDINGS

In patients with Klinefelter syndrome, serum testosterone levels range from low to well into the normal range[12,13] (Fig. 115-4). The

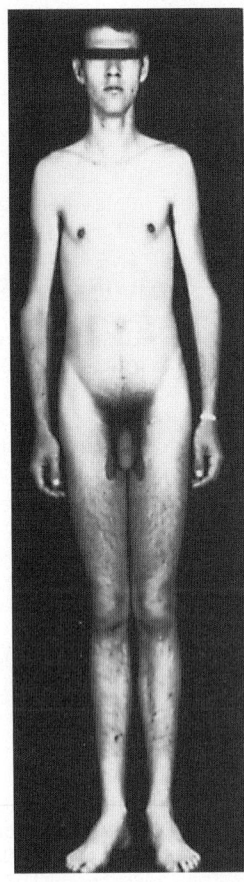 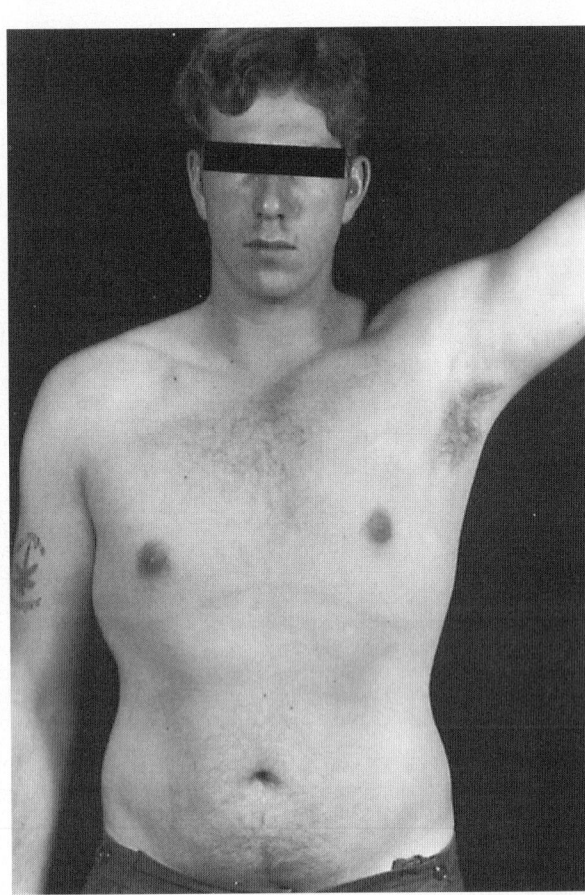

**FIGURE 115-2.** Two patients with Klinefelter syndrome. The man on the left has the phenotypic features of a markedly increased lower body segment. He has XXY/XY mosaicism in all tissues, including the testes. On semen analysis, his sperm count was 300,000/mL. The patient on the right has moderate gynecomastia, but a relatively normal masculine appearance. He has an XXY karyotype.

relatively decreased serum testosterone is the result of deficient testosterone production (3.27 ± 1.35 mg per 24 hours vs. 7.04 ± 2.47 mg per 24 hours in normal persons).[14] An increase in SHBG also occurs in Klinefelter syndrome; thus, the bioavailable, or free, testosterone is further suppressed.[12,15] As men with Klinefelter syndrome age, a further decline in testicular function often occurs.[16]

Patients with Klinefelter syndrome may have serum estradiol levels higher than those of normal men. The increase in estradiol has been shown to come from an augmented peripheral conversion of testosterone to estradiol.[12,14] After puberty, serum gonadotropin levels are elevated, even when serum testosterone levels are normal.[13] Before puberty, serum gonadotropin levels are

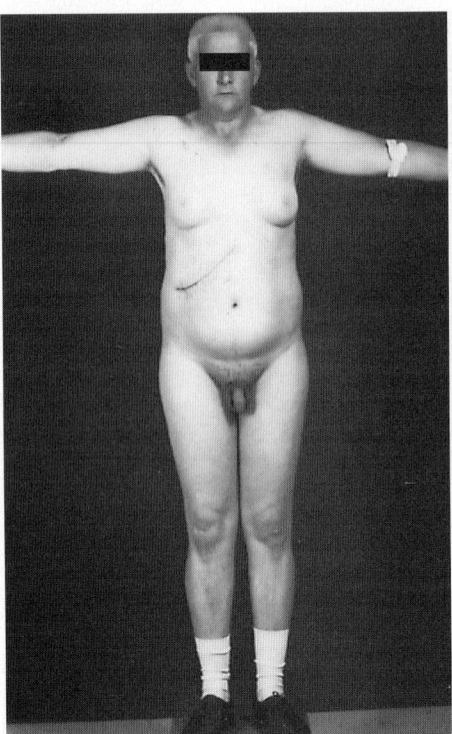 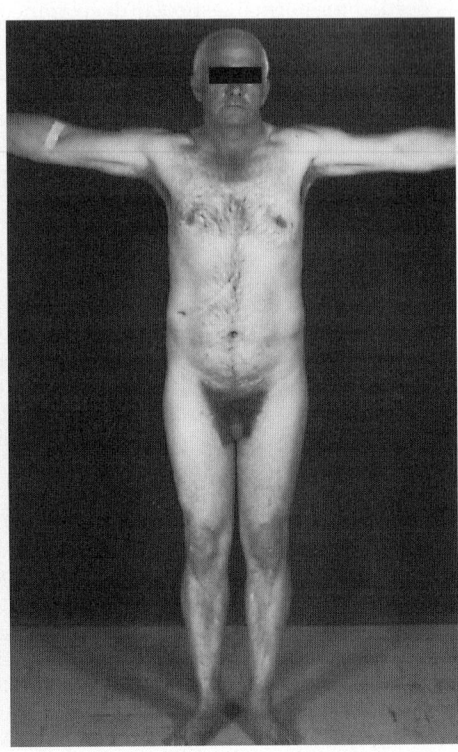

**FIGURE 115-3.** Patient with Klinefelter syndrome before and after treatment with testosterone. He had a sparsity of body hair and marked gynecomastia. Note the diminution of subcutaneous fat, the increased body hair, and the increased muscle mass after therapy. In addition, the patient had breast tissue removed. (From Becker KL. Clinical and therapeutic experiences with Klinefelter syndrome. Fertil Steril 1972; 23:568.)

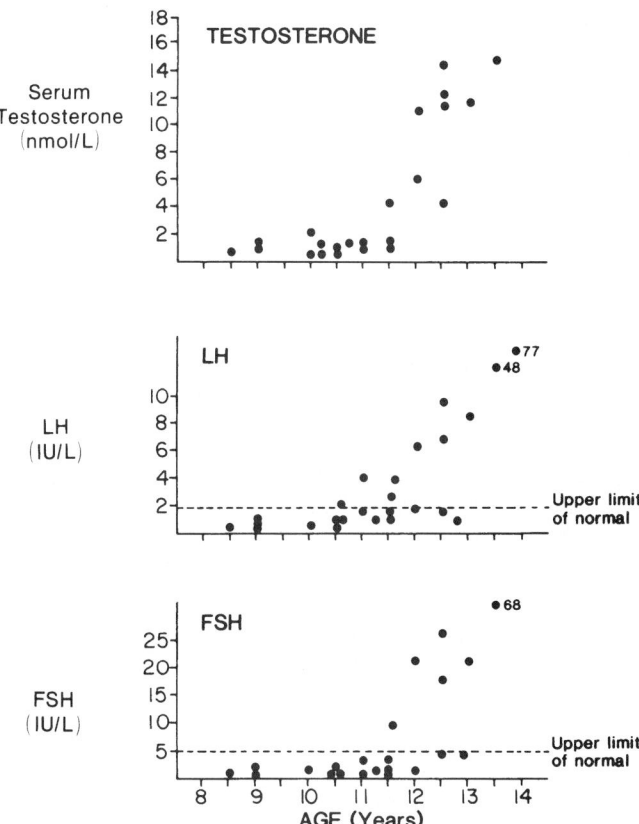

FIGURE 115-4. Changes in serum gonadotropin and testosterone levels in boys with Klinefelter syndrome as they are followed up through puberty. Note the lack of differentiation from normal values until after puberty has supervened. (*LH,* luteinizing hormone; *FSH,* follicle-stimulating hormone.) The numbers represent actual values for three patients whose values (77, 48, and 68) exceeded the scale of the graph. (From Ratcliffe SG. Klinefelter's syndrome in children: a longitudinal study of 47 XXY boys identified by population screening in Klinefelter's syndrome. In: Bandmann HJ, Breit R, Perwein E, eds. Klinefelter's syndrome. New York: Springer-Verlag, 1984:38.)

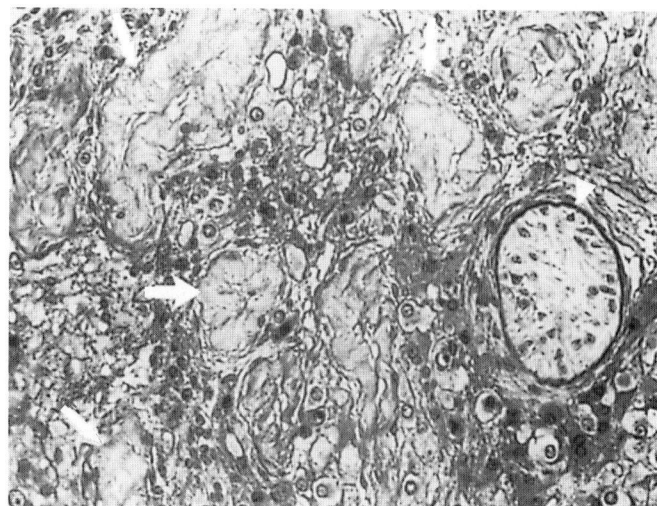

FIGURE 115-5. Testis biopsy specimen from a patient with XXY Klinefelter syndrome demonstrating hyalinized tubules (*arrows*) with focal areas of immature seminiferous tubules (*arrowhead*).

normal[17] (see Fig. 115-4). Interestingly, in spite of the relatively normal masculine appearance of some young men with Klinefelter syndrome, their physical strength often is significantly less than that of their peers because of the deficient androgen action on muscle. Men with Klinefelter syndrome usually do not have the ability to grow a full beard or a mustache; however, like muscle strength, androgen-dependent hair growth is variable.

The abnormal serum testosterone levels and the diminished response of serum testosterone to human chorionic gonadotropin (hCG) is a reflection of the disturbance of Leydig and Sertoli cell function. Of the two compartments in the testes, the seminiferous tubules are the most affected by the presence of the extra X chromosome.[18–20] Clinically, this is manifested by azoospermia, which occurs in virtually all patients with classic Klinefelter syndrome. Testicular biopsy specimens consistently demonstrate seminiferous tubule hyalinization and fibrosis (Fig. 115-5). Because the seminiferous tubule basement membrane is so crucial to spermatogenesis, the defect in basement membrane formation may explain why the initial testicular damage is to the seminiferous epithelium.

In some patients with Klinefelter syndrome, usually the mosaic forms, testicular biopsy specimens have demonstrated focal areas of spermatogenesis. On occasion, sperm have been noted in the ejaculate, and these patients may be fertile. However, most of the reported impregnations have been single events occurring early in the individual's reproductive life, with azoospermia developing in later years.[21] Is it the lack of normal androgen environment in the testes or the chromosomal abnormality that impairs spermatogenesis? In part, the answer to this question has come from studies of XXY and XX sex-reversed mice in which sperm can develop but are always diploid, with an XX or XY content.[22] In these animals, during spermatogonial mitosis, the XY and XX daughter cells are not viable, but an occasional nondisjunctional event takes place and the extra chromosome is lost. Thus, in subsections of the germinal epithelium, a normal haploid germ cell develops and full spermatogenesis may take place. The testicular biopsy specimens of these animals, as well as of patients with Klinefelter syndrome, show focal areas of spermatogenesis. Interestingly, the XXY fetal testis may be unaffected.[23] Meiotic segregation of sperm nuclei has been evaluated in sperm obtained from a patient with Klinefelter syndrome; by fluorescence in situ hybridization analysis, 958 cells contained the X chromosome and 1077 cells contained the Y chromosome. This ratio is significantly different from the 1:1 ratio that was expected (chi$^2$ test, $p < .01$). The frequency of 24,XX, 24,XY, and diploid cells was significantly increased. These results suggest that the 47,XXY cells are able to complete meiosis and produce mature sperm nuclei.[24]

## PSYCHOPATHOLOGY

Decreased intellectual development and antisocial behavior occur with a high frequency in Klinefelter syndrome.[25–27] In this regard, the incidence of Klinefelter syndrome in subsets of the population with mental retardation ranges from ~0.5% to 2.5%. Studies from Denmark, in which the records of all men taller than 184 cm were surveyed, show that the incidence of criminal offense was 9.3% in men with an XY chromosome pattern, 18.8% in men with an XXY chromosome pattern, and 41.7% in men with an XYY chromosome pattern.[28] Furthermore, the incidence of criminal behavior was inversely related to the subjects' full intelligence quotient (IQ). Studies of boys with Klinefelter syndrome have found that a significant reduction in verbal IQ is present at the age of 7 years.[29] Interestingly, as the number of X chromosomes increases in the poly-X disorders, the degree of mental retardation also increases. The mechanism by which the extra X chromosome impairs central nervous system (CNS) function has not been delineated, although an inverse relationship exists between the ability to cope and antisocial behavior. Furthermore, although androgen production by the Leydig cells is decreased, low androgen production does not appear to be responsible for all the characteristic clinical manifestations of the syndrome (other states of androgen deficiency are not necessarily associated with increased criminal behavior and mental retardation). The extra X chromosome may affect neuronal function directly, which then leads to behavioral abnormalities related to decreased IQ and other, nondefined factors.

Other areas of psychiatric dysfunction, such as personality traits of timidity, introspective behavior, and social drive, are more clearly related to the androgen deficiency and often improve after androgen replacement.[30] The lack of self-restraint and aggressiveness shown by some subjects appears to be related to the effects of the extra X chromosome on CNS function.

### ETIOLOGY

The development of the XXY chromosome constitution may occur by several mechanisms. The most common of these is *nondisjunction during the first and second meiotic division* in parental oogenesis or spermatogenesis (see Chap. 90). A second possibility for the development of the classic syndrome is *nondisjunction during the first postzygotic mitosis*. Nondisjunction in mitosis after this time results in mosaic forms of Klinefelter syndrome. A third, and rare, mechanism is *anaphase lag during mitosis or meiosis*, with the lagging chromatid included in the daughter nucleus. Reports have been published of six men with an XXY chromosome pattern (including one set of brothers) whose mothers had XX/XXX chromosomes.[9] These family data suggest a *nondisjunctional event during maternal zygotic development*, and this may have been present in a grandparent. Because Klinefelter syndrome usually is not recognized until after puberty, most mothers of affected men have not had chromosome analyses performed.

The reason for the nondisjunction is not known, although maternal age has been shown to be a factor. The incidence of Klinefelter syndrome increases from 0.6% when the maternal age is 35 years or less to 5.4% when the maternal age is >45 years.[31,32] Sixty-five percent of patients with Klinefelter syndrome have a maternal origin for their extra X chromosomes. Maternal age is thought to be a factor because of the longer diplotene stage of the ova in older women (see Chap. 94). The existence of mothers with an XX/XXX chromosome pattern (see earlier) and an increased incidence of twins with Klinefelter syndrome, as well as the finding of an increased frequency of Klinefelter syndrome in patients with Down syndrome, suggest that some families may have a factor predisposing to chromosomal nondisjunction.

### DISEASE ASSOCIATIONS AND MEDICAL COMPLICATIONS

Numerous disease associations have been made with Klinefelter syndrome; especially prominent are malignancies and autoimmune diseases. Malignancies include breast carcinoma (with an incidence 20 times greater than that of men with an XY chromosome pattern and 20% that of women), nonlymphocytic leukemia, lymphomas, marrow dysplastic syndromes, and extragonadal germ cell neoplasms.[33–37] Autoimmune diseases, especially chronic lymphocytic thyroiditis and rare syndromes such as Takayasu arteritis, have been reported in Klinefelter syndrome.[38–42] Whether this results from an effect of decreased androgens on the OKT4/OKT8 lymphocyte ratios or from the combined effect of decreased immune surveillance and increased X chromosome material is unknown.[43,44]

Taurodontism (enlargement of the molar teeth by an extension of the pulp) is present in 40% of men with Klinefelter syndrome, compared with ~1% of men with an XY chromosome pattern.[45] Varicose veins, with or without hypostatic ulceration, are seen in 40%; this, along with the 55% incidence of mitral valve prolapse, suggests a connective tissue defect.[46,47] Abnormal glucose tolerance due to a postreceptor defect in insulin action is seen in 10% of patients with Klinefelter syndrome.[48] The incidence of asthma and chronic bronchitis is also increased. Although osteoporosis is increased, the frequency is no greater than in other male hypogonadal states.[49–52]

As with most hypogonadal syndromes, sexual activity or sexual orientation is of concern to these patients and their family members or spouses. The patients with marked hypogo-

nadism tend to associate less in adolescence with male peer groups because of their physical inability to compete. However, patients with Klinefelter syndrome do not have any greater homosexual tendencies than do men with an XY chromosome pattern. Usually, heterosexual activity is less frequent among patients with Klinefelter syndrome; many do not attain orgasm during sexual activity.[53]

### VARIANT FORMS

In certain patients, the sex chromosome configuration may show two or more stem cell lines (*mosaicism*). For example, in a testicular biopsy prepared for chromosome analysis, the predominant cell line may be XXY but another line of normal XY cells also may be present. Thus, on metaphase analysis, an XXY/XY cell pattern is found. This lack of a pure XXY cell line may result in a modification of the phenotypic characteristics of the patient such that the only clinical manifestation of classic Klinefelter syndrome is infertility (Table 115-3). On the other hand, if most cells are XXY, the patient may appear to have the classic Klinefelter syndrome, yet because of a normal XY cell line in some testicular germ cells, spermatogenesis and fertility may occur[54] (see Fig. 115-5). Approximately 10% of patients with Klinefelter syndrome have a mosaic chromosomal constitution.

The existence of mosaic forms may be suspected in men who are infertile with small testes or who have primary hypogonadism and normal buccal smears. In these patients, if more than one tissue specimen is examined for the presence of an XXY chromosome constitution (e.g., leukocytes and testicular tissues), and an extra X chromosome is found in one cell line but not the other, evidence for mosaicism exists.

Importantly, the examination for chromatin in tissues often is poorly performed and may lead to erroneous conclusions. For example, many laboratories allow "normal" men to have an occasional X-chromatin body in a buccal smear. These are not true X-chromatin bodies but folds in cells (or bacteria). Therefore, when Klinefelter syndrome, especially the mosaic form, is suspected, confirmation should be made by a formal karyotyping (Fig. 115-6).

Several additional variant forms of Klinefelter syndrome have been reported (see Table 115-3). These usually arise from consecutive nondisjunctional events in oogenesis or spermatogenesis. Individuals with the poly-X chromosomal syndromes (e.g., XXXY, XXXXY) display more severe abnormalities than do those with the classic Klinefelter syndrome[55] (Fig. 115-7). A clue to these disorders is the presence of more than one chromatin body on buccal smear preparations. Often, marked mental retardation is present. The seminiferous tubules may have undergone hyalinization before puberty, and the testes commonly are undescended. Skeletal abnormalities, including proximal radioulnar synostosis and overgrowth of the radioulnar head, are characteristic of these disorders. As evidence of more severe androgen deficiency, the development of the genitalia may be retarded and a bifid scrotum or hypoplastic penis may be present.

The XXYY syndromes can combine the gonadal and associated features of Klinefelter syndrome with the skeletal height and social aggressiveness of the XYY syndrome.[56] All patients in these categories may have social problems, which usually are related to the decreased IQ. Indeed, when these patients have normal IQs, they may be socially sensitive and model citizens. The specific skeletal feature is their mean height of 190 cm, which is 6 cm taller than the mean height of 184 cm of those with XXY Klinefelter syndrome. Both these mean heights are significantly greater than the mean height of normal men. This probably is due to the excessive growth of the lower extremities.

### THERAPY

The treatment of patients with Klinefelter syndrome must address three major facets of the disease: hypogonadism,

**TABLE 115-3.**
**Karyotype and Clinical Features of Classic and Variant Forms of Klinefelter Syndrome**

| XXY Group* | XX Group | XX Group (XXYY, XXXYY, XX$_i$[Y$_p$]Y/XY/X$_i$[X$_{pi}$]Y) |
|---|---|---|
| Prepubertal: No definite decrease in germinal cells, although most testes in these subjects are smaller than those of age-matched controls. | Very uncommon. Patients possess the same features of the syndrome, except they may be somewhat shorter. | Not common. Clinical and laboratory features similar to those seen in classic form except for the following: |
| Incidence of cryptorchidism not increased. | The key laboratory findings to explain the male phenotype and testes is the presence of the transposed testis-determining portion of a Y chromosome onto one of the X chromosomes. | More severe mental retardation. |
| Subnormal intelligence of varying degrees, but deficit usually mild. | | Tendency to be tall, >183 cm (6 ft). |
| Bone abnormalities (not consistent). | | Increased incidence of "antisocial" behavior and varicose veins. |
| Buccal smear: one sex chromatin body. | | |

*The XXY karyotype is the classic form; all other groups are variants.

| | Poly X + Y Chromosomal Group | |
|---|---|---|
| *Mosaicism* | *Mosaicism* | *Poly X + Y Disorder* |
| XXY/XX | XXXY/XY | XXXY |
| XXY/XY | XXXY/XXY | XXXYY |
| XXY/XYY | XXXY/XXY/XY | XXXXY |
| XXY/XXYY | XXXXY/XXXY | XXX$_i$(X$_p$)Y |
| XX$_i$(X$_p$)Y/XY/Y$_i$(X$_p$)Y | XXXXY/XXXXY/XXY | X$_i$(X$_q$)Y |
| 46XX/47,XX,+Y(q12-7qter) | | XX,invY(p+q-) |
| | | XXq-Y |

Clinical and pathologic features vary. In patients with sex chromosomal mosaicism, spermatogenesis may be active and sperm present in the ejaculate. Testes may be virtually normal in size. This is particularly true when the normal stem cell line (XY) is present in the testes. Patients with other forms of mosaicism usually demonstrate testicular damage that extends to that observed in the classic form.

Prepubertal: definite decrease in immature germinal cells, with hypoplastic tubules and increased connective tissue stroma.
Incidence of cryptorchidism increased.
Subnormal intelligence, usually severely so.
Bone abnormalities are common. Radioulnar synostosis and other abnormalities of the elbow.
Buccal smear: two sex chromatin bodies in XXY and XXXYY; three sex chromatin bodies in XXXXY.

gynecomastia, and psychosocial problems. Androgen therapy is the most important aspect of treatment. Androgens are necessary to prevent the physical consequences of androgen deficiency, such as diminished libido and physical endurance, decreased muscle strength, and osteoporosis.[57-61] Maintaining or increasing muscle strength and improving libido usually result in an enhanced self-image and an improved ability to cope with life (see Fig. 115-3). Treatment with testosterone should begin at puberty or as soon after puberty as the diagnosis is made. Androgen therapy should not be used in cases of severe mental retardation in which management of a more aggressive individual could be a problem. The presence of breast cancer or prostatic carcinoma demands special consider-

ation before androgen therapy is maintained or initiated. Patients and their sexual partners should be counseled before treatment with androgens is begun, because a sudden increase in libido may present the couple with adjustment problems.

Because the infertility does not appear to be related directly to the decreased intratesticular androgen levels, androgen therapy does not improve infertility, and because of the suppression of gonadotropins, this therapy could further diminish any spermatogenesis that is taking place. Specific information on androgen replacement therapy is found in Chapter 119.

The gynecomastia of Klinefelter syndrome may be disfiguring and can cause significant social problems. Treatment with testosterone does not significantly diminish or worsen the con-

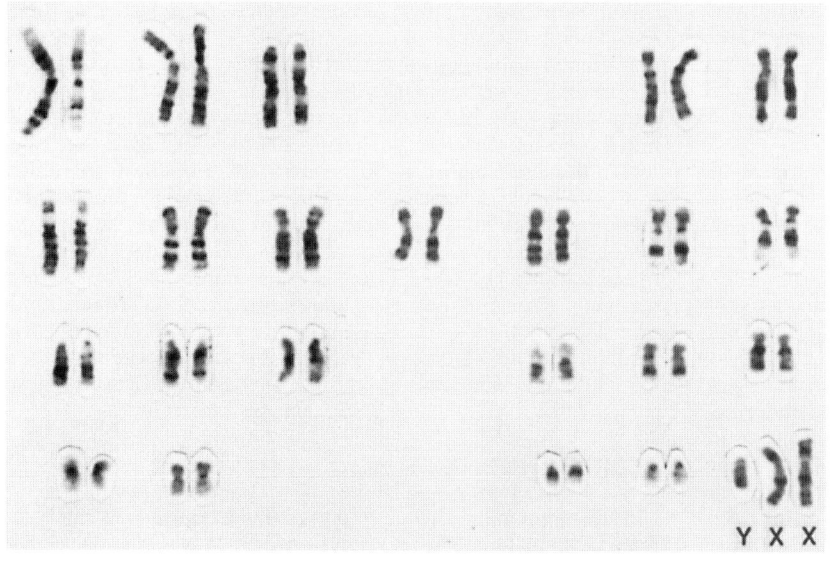

**FIGURE 115-6.** Karyotype with Giemsa banding from a peripheral lymphocyte of a patient with Klinefelter syndrome. Note the similar banding patterns of the duplicated X chromosome. (Courtesy of C. M. Disteche, Department of Pathology, University of Washington, Seattle, WA.)

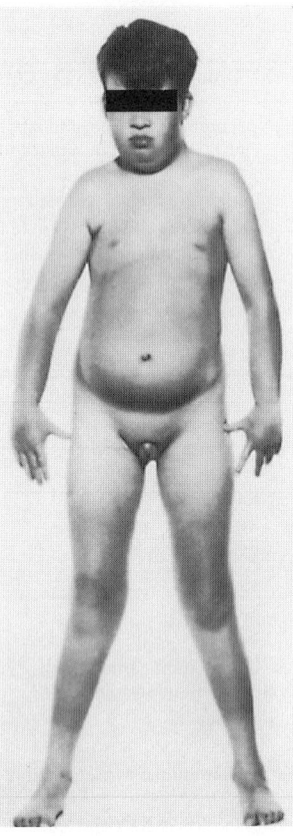

**FIGURE 115-7.** Youth with the XXXXY syndrome. Epicanthal folds, a hypoplastic midface, and prognathism are seen. The neck is short, the penis is small, and the scrotum is hypoplastic. (From Goodman RM, Gorlin RJ. The face in genetic disorders. St. Louis: CV Mosby, 1977:722.)

dition, and no medical therapy is available. Therefore, if the breast enlargement concerns the patient, cosmetic surgery is required. Correction of the gynecomastia should help improve the patient's self-image.

No long-term prospective studies are available regarding therapy for the learning disabilities and psychological problems associated with Klinefelter syndrome.[62,63] With the increased use of amniocentesis, more cases with this disease are being identified, and the development of prepubertal support programs should be possible. Screening for earlier diagnosis may be considered in certain groups of young boys, such as those with learning disabilities who have testes smaller than 1.5 mL. Most patients have only mild problems in their verbal IQ, and early educational support may help prevent frustration and isolation.

## XX MALES

Patients with XX chromosomal configurations may appear as normal females, females with gonadal dysgenesis, true hermaphrodites, or males with gonadal dysgenesis. Only those manifesting as phenotypic males are discussed here. These men proceed through puberty and subsequently present with small testes, infertility, and gynecomastia. As in patients with Klinefelter syndrome, serum testosterone levels may be low to normal, but serum gonadotropin levels are invariably elevated.[63,64] These patients tend to be shorter than normal men. A high incidence of hypospadias is found, but no mental retardation. The abnormal skeletal proportions and many of the other associated features of Klinefelter syndrome are absent. The incidence of the syndrome ranges from 1 in 9000 to 1 in 20,000 live births.

In approximately two-thirds of cases, XX males result from the translocation of the SRY gene to the X chromosome. In the remaining cases, no SRY has been detected. In the latter individuals, a mutation is thought to have occurred in an autosome that triggered the same series of events as SRY, leading to testicular development. Evidence for this is found in the fact that SRY-negative men with the XX chromosome pattern often have other congenital abnormalities, especially cardiac problems. These abnormalities suggest autosomal mutations close to an SRY-like region of an autosome, although this region has not been identified.[65] The treatment of XX males includes surgery for gynecomastia, androgen replacement therapy, and psychological support, as described for Klinefelter syndrome.

## XY/XO MIXED GONADAL DYSGENESIS

Patients with XY/XO mixed gonadal dysgenesis who have the 45,XO/46,XY genotype may appear as phenotypic males, although most patients with this chromosomal constitution are phenotypic females.[66] They have been considered to be H-Y antigen positive. Before the report of the translocation in XX males, the suggestion was made that, because such men were H-Y antigen positive but had gonadal dysgenesis, they must have lost the Y chromosome from the cell in the zygote. This issue is now somewhat clouded, and these patients need further study.

Usually, the gonads are located within the abdomen. Both testes may be defective, or one may be a streak gonad. Depending on the gestational timing of the arrested gonadal development of the ipsilateral gonad, a paramesonephric duct may be present. In addition, a rudimentary uterus may be present. At birth, the external genitalia may range from female appearing, with clitoral enlargement, to male appearing, with some degree of hypospadias. These patients usually have been raised during their prepubertal years as females; they are discovered at the time of puberty, when primary amenorrhea is noted, or when, because of the increased pubertal stimulation of the defective testis and subsequent androgen production, marked virilization occurs.

Treatment consists of supporting the sex of rearing with appropriate hormone replacement and castration. Castration is done to prevent the development of a malignancy in the defective gonad (20% incidence) and, if the individual has been raised as a female, to prevent the virilization that may occur after puberty. Fertility is extremely rare and should not be considered in the decision to remove an intraabdominal testis. The tumors that develop may be either dysgerminomas, gonadoblastomas, or embryonal cell carcinomas (see Chap. 122).

## XYY SYNDROME

Individuals with the XYY syndrome have erroneously been called "supermales"; this is a misnomer, because testicular function may be normal or associated with varying degrees of impaired spermatogenesis.[67–69] These individuals, with a mean height of 189 cm, are markedly taller than normal men and are more prone to antisocial behavior. Serum testosterone levels may be normal or elevated. Serum LH and FSH levels are normal unless spermatogenesis is markedly impaired, in which case FSH levels are elevated. Findings in testicular biopsy specimens have ranged from normal to markedly impaired spermatogenesis with seminiferous tubules that have undergone hyalinization. The sex chromosomal abnormalities arise from meiotic nondisjunction in the male or from zygotic nondisjunction. The impaired spermatogenesis alone, therefore, may be the result of diploid YY or XY spermatogonia, as has been described for Klinefelter syndrome. No specific therapy exists for these patients unless they have decreased testosterone levels.

## ULLRICH-NOONAN SYNDROME

Ullrich-Noonan syndrome (Noonan syndrome) often has been referred to as "male Turner syndrome."[70] This is because of the

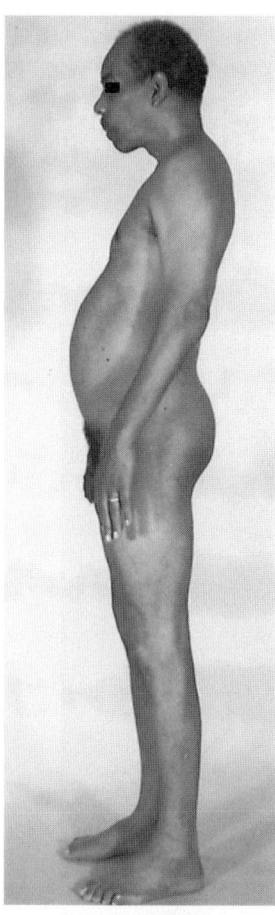
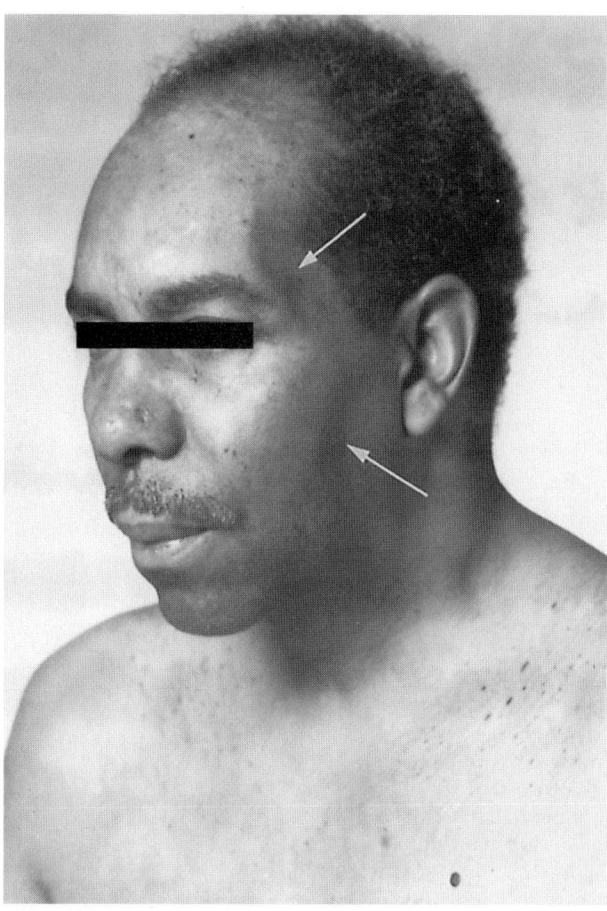

**FIGURE 115-8.** Patient with myotonic dystrophy (myotonia dystrophica, Steinert disease). Weakness of the muscles, wasting of the limbs, and slumped posture are present. Note the expressionless facies, the frontal balding, and the marked atrophy of the temporal and masseter musculature (*arrows*).

phenotypic characteristics commonly shared with women who have Turner syndrome: webbed neck, low hairline, short stature, shield chest, and cubitus valgus (see Chap. 90).[71] However, these men have a normal chromosome pattern. In Noonan syndrome, commonly encountered cardiac abnormalities include pulmonary artery stenosis and atrial septal defects. Although testicular function may be normal, primary gonadal failure usually is present. Infertility, if present, generally is associated with cryptorchidism. Serum levels of testosterone, LH, and FSH may be normal or consistent with primary testicular failure (i.e., decreased serum testosterone and increased LH and FSH). Mental retardation, ptosis, hypertelorism, and low-set ears also are prominent in this disorder. Rarely, autosomal dominant transmission may occur. Treatment is directed toward any cardiac abnormalities; if androgen deficiency exists, testosterone replacement therapy should be instituted.

## MYOTONIC DYSTROPHY

Myotonic dystrophy is an autosomal dominant disorder characterized by an inability to relax the striated muscles after contraction (myotonia). The disorder results in muscle atrophy and eventual death. In addition to the myotonia, frontal balding, lenticular opacities, and primary testicular failure are commonly associated abnormalities[72] (Fig. 115-8). Because the disease usually is not manifest until after puberty, most commonly in the late 30s and mid-40s, these men do not have an eunuchoid body habitus. The most prominent physical manifestation of their gonadal failure is the small testes and sometimes the other signs of postpubertal gonadal failure. Many cases demonstrate low serum levels of testosterone and azoospermia. In such patients, testicular biopsy specimens reveal complete hyalinization of the seminiferous tubules. Although serum testosterone levels usually are decreased, LH is increased in only 50% of the patients.[73] Occasionally, only seminiferous tubule

failure is present, which is characterized by a monotropic increase in serum FSH with normal testosterone levels.

The pathogenesis of the testicular failure is unknown; however, the (CTG)n amplification in the myodystrophy (*MD*) and *MT-PK* gene mutations varies from 70 to 1520. The length of the repeat correlated significantly ($p < .001$) with the LH and FSH levels, suggesting that the severity of hypogonadism in myotonic dystrophy is related to the *MT-PK* gene mutation.[74] No therapy is available for the seminiferous tubule failure. Studies indicate that testosterone replacement may result in some improvement in muscle mass and strength. However, the duration of this effect and the resultant functional changes are unknown. Therefore, this therapy should be considered experimental.[75]

## SERTOLI-CELL-ONLY SYNDROME

Sertoli-cell-only syndrome (del Castillo syndrome) is a histologic diagnosis that is made only when a testicular biopsy is performed in an infertile man. The characteristic features are complete, or almost complete, absence of germ cells in all seminiferous tubules[76] (Fig. 115-9). Occasionally, a focal area of spermatogenesis may be identified. The basement membrane may be slightly thickened and, under electron microscopy, the Sertoli cells are vacuolated.[77] Because Leydig cell function is only mildly impaired, these men present clinically with infertility; the testes are slightly smaller than normal but are of normal consistency. The patients have azoospermia and elevated serum levels of FSH. Mean serum testosterone levels are within the normal range, but lower than the mean for fertile individuals. Furthermore, the response of serum testosterone to hCG is diminished and, although serum LH levels are normal, the values tend to cluster in the upper range for normal men. This finding indicates that a relationship exists between normal seminiferous tubule function and normal Leydig cell function, and that in this syndrome, in which sem-

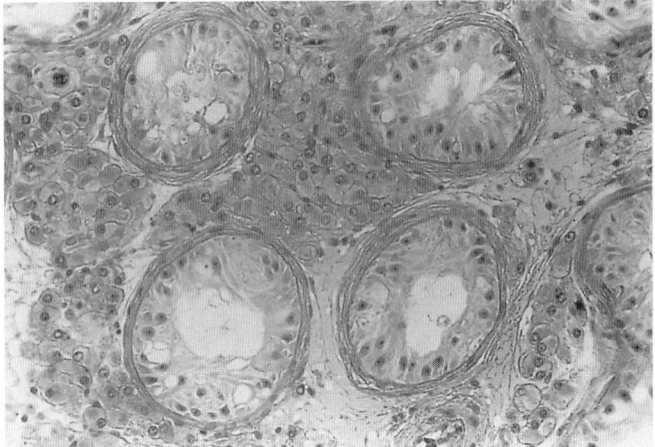

**FIGURE 115-9.** Testicular biopsy specimen from a patient with Sertoli-cell-only syndrome. Note the complete lack of germ cells, with tubular support maintained by Sertoli cells. (From Paulsen CA. The testis. In: Williams RH, ed. Textbook of endocrinology. Philadelphia: WB Saunders, 1974:315.)

iniferous tubule function is impaired, some compromise of testosterone production is seen.

The cause of Sertoli-cell-only syndrome has not been defined, and it may be the end result of one of several inducing factors. However, the prevailing theory is that most of these cases are caused by congenital absence or early neonatal loss of the germ cells. This may result from abnormal Sertoli cell function that is unable to support the germ cells. The elevated serum LH levels and the abnormal responses to hCG stem from the fact that normal Leydig cell function also requires normal paracrine activity between the Sertoli and Leydig cells. This form of infertility cannot be reversed.

## FUNCTIONAL PREPUBERTAL CASTRATE SYNDROME

The functional prepubertal castrate syndrome (vanishing testes syndrome) is a relatively rare condition that manifests as prepubertal testicular failure. On physical examination, any discernible testicular tissue is completely lacking.[78] Usually, serum testosterone levels are low, similar to those of castrated men. No response is seen to hCG administration. Castrate levels of serum LH and FSH, normal male wolffian derivatives, an absence of müllerian structures, a eunuchoid body habitus, and a normal XY karyotype also are present[79] (Fig. 115-10). Infrequently, when a slight testosterone response to hCG occurs, a testicular remnant may be found in the abdomen or inguinal canal. Because no müllerian structures are present, testes must have been present in utero to produce antimüllerian hormone and to allow normal wolffian structures to develop. This has led to the hypothesis that events such as torsion of the testes in utero, trauma, infection, or an early manifestation of the polyglandular autoimmune deficiency syndrome may be responsible for the disorder.

Regardless of the cause, recognition of this condition is important for two reasons. First, if hCG administration increases serum testosterone levels, a search should be undertaken for the presence of abdominal testes. Usually, testicular remnants can be found in the scrotum. A computed tomographic (CT) scan shows this and may alleviate the need for abdominal surgery to determine the source of testosterone production. However, abdominal testes should be removed because of the potential for malignant degeneration. Second, androgen replacement should be undertaken at the normal time for puberty (see Chap. 119 and Fig. 115-10). Because this syndrome can be recognized before puberty, these boys should not be made to suffer hypogonadism

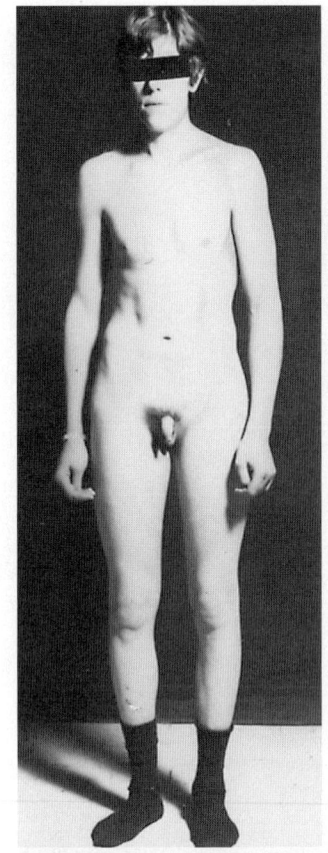
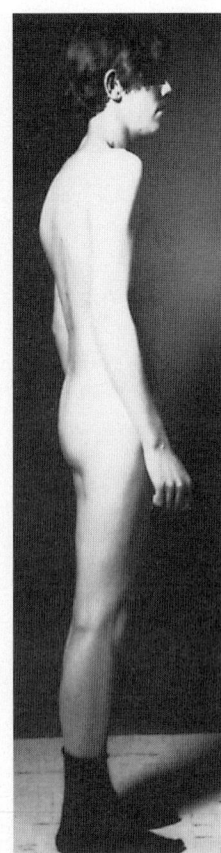
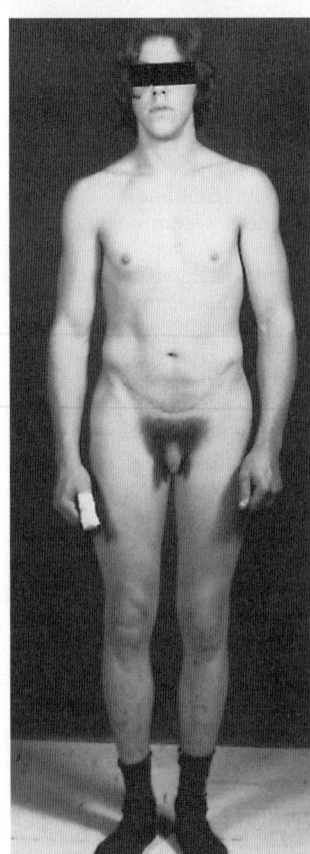
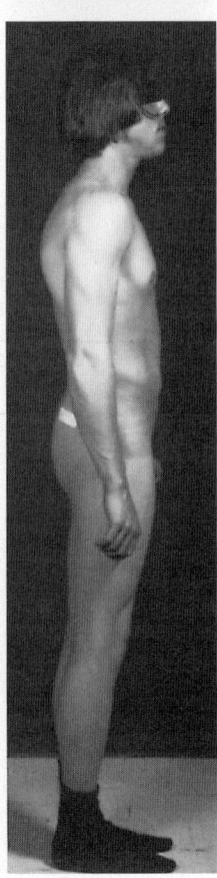

**FIGURE 115-10.** *Above,* In a 24-year-old man with the vanishing testes syndrome, serum testosterone levels were nearly undetectable, and no testes were found on exploration. The karyotype was XY. *Below,* After 1 year of testosterone therapy, note the great increase in body musculature, the darkening of the skin, and widening of the jaw.

**TABLE 115-4.**
**Mode of Inheritance and Characteristics of Enzyme Defects of Testosterone Production**

| Defect | Inheritance | Genitalia | Pubertal Development | Hormone Status |
|---|---|---|---|---|
| 20,22-Desmolase | AR | Ambiguous | None | ↑ LH, FSH<br>↓ Cortisol<br>↓ Mineralocorticoids<br>↓ Androgens |
| 3β-Hydroxydehydrogenase | AR | Male hypospadias | None or poor | ↑ Or normal LH, FSH<br>↓ Cortisol (severe at birth)<br>↓ Androgens<br>↓ Mineralocorticoids (variable) |
| 17α-Hydroxylase | AR | Ambiguous | None or poor | ↓ LH, ↑ FSH<br>↓ Androgens<br>↓ Cortisol<br>↑ Mineralocorticoids (patients are hypertensive) |
| 17,20-Desmolase | AR | Male | Genitalia are prepubertal | ↓ T<br>↑ LH, FSH<br>↑ 17-Hydroxyprogesterone<br>Normal cortisol |
| 17-Ketosteroid reductase | AR | Female or ambiguous | Partial puberty | ↓ T<br>↑ LH, FSH<br>Normal cortisol |

*AR,* autosomal recessive; ↓, decreased; ↑, increased; *LH,* luteinizing hormone; *FSH,* follicle-stimulating hormone; *T,* testosterone.

at the chronologic time of adolescence; artificial testes can be placed in the scrotum to facilitate normal scrotal expansion. The infertility is irreversible.

## ENZYMATIC DEFECTS INVOLVING TESTOSTERONE BIOSYNTHESIS

Defects of testosterone biosynthesis (see Chap. 90) are reviewed only briefly. These defects can be divided into two categories: those that involve steroidogenesis in the production of both testosterone and cortisol, and those that involve testosterone biosynthesis alone.[80] Suspicion of one of these enzyme deficiencies should be raised in cases of male pseudohermaphroditism. The sex chromosomal analysis reveals an XY karyotype. In the case of disorders involving both testosterone and cortisol production (20,22-desmolase deficiency, 3β-dehydrogenase deficiency, 17α-hydroxylase deficiency) (Table 115-4 and Fig. 115-11), the serum cortisol deficiency may be severe, and these infants appear with adrenal crisis soon after birth. The disorders that primarily affect testicular testosterone production include 17,20-desmolase and 17-ketosteroid reductase deficiency (see Table 115-4). These patients also manifest as male pseudohermaphrodites and may have relatively normal-appearing female external genitalia. Because such patients can produce cortisol normally, the condition may not be detected until they are adults, when they present with primary amenorrhea. The 17,20-desmolase deficiency has been shown to involve either the Δ⁴ or the Δ⁵ pathway.

The 17β-hydroxysteroid dehydrogenase enzyme is responsible for the conversion of androstenedione to testosterone.[81–83] The enzyme is present in the testes and in peripheral tissues. Whether the enzyme in the testes is controlled by the same gene as that in the adrenal gland is unknown. Patients with 17β-hydroxysteroid dehydrogenase deficiency present clinically with ambiguous genitalia and usually are raised as females before puberty. However, at puberty, marked virilization occurs. This probably is due to the marked increase in secretion of androstenedione from the testes and its subsequent peripheral conversion to testosterone. Often, the diagnosis is first made at this time. However, because the patient already has been raised as a female and fertility is not attainable, the best course is to remove the testes to decrease the androgen effect

and to eliminate the risk of testicular carcinoma if the testes are located within the abdomen. If the specific diagnosis is made before puberty (i.e., by noting an increase in serum androstenedione after hCG administration), castration before puberty is preferable if the child has been raised as a female. Alternatively, if the child has been raised as a male and the testes are in the scrotum, testosterone treatment should be undertaken at puberty to achieve appropriate virilization and to reduce breast enlargement, which is thought to be caused by the conversion of the weak androgen, androstenedione, to estrone.[84]

Any of these enzymatic defects should be considered in a male pseudohermaphrodite if no uterus can be demonstrated. The diagnosis can be made before puberty by stimulating the testes with hCG and measuring the precursor steroid for the enzyme that is deficient. For example, in 17-ketosteroid reductase deficiency, the level of Δ⁴ androstenedione is elevated because it cannot be further reduced to testosterone. These enzyme deficiencies may not be complete and the disorders may present in a more heterogeneous fashion. Although the disorder is commonly thought of as causing pseudohermaphroditism, a late-onset form of 17-ketosteroid reductase deficiency does not manifest until after puberty. These men present with hypogonadism rather than pseudohermaphroditism. Because the concentrations of estrone and androstenedione are elevated in their sera, these men have low LH and FSH levels, suggestive of hypogonadotropic hypogonadism.[84]

If both testosterone and cortisol pathways are defective, treatment includes cortisol replacement. Testosterone should be given if the genitalia are primarily male or are ambiguous in an individual who has a male gender identity. If the patient is older when the problem is first recognized (as often may be the case if the only defect is in testosterone synthesis), and if the individual has been raised as a female, castration should be considered; subsequently, estrogen replacement can be started. Surgical correction of the external genitalia should be performed to maintain the female identification. Defects in testosterone production also exist in these patients (unlike the situation in congenital adrenal hyperplasia [see Chaps. 77 and 83], in which only cortisol synthesis is involved). Consequently, corticosteroid replacement therapy does not permit fertility to occur because of the inability to reproduce the high intratesticular levels of testosterone.

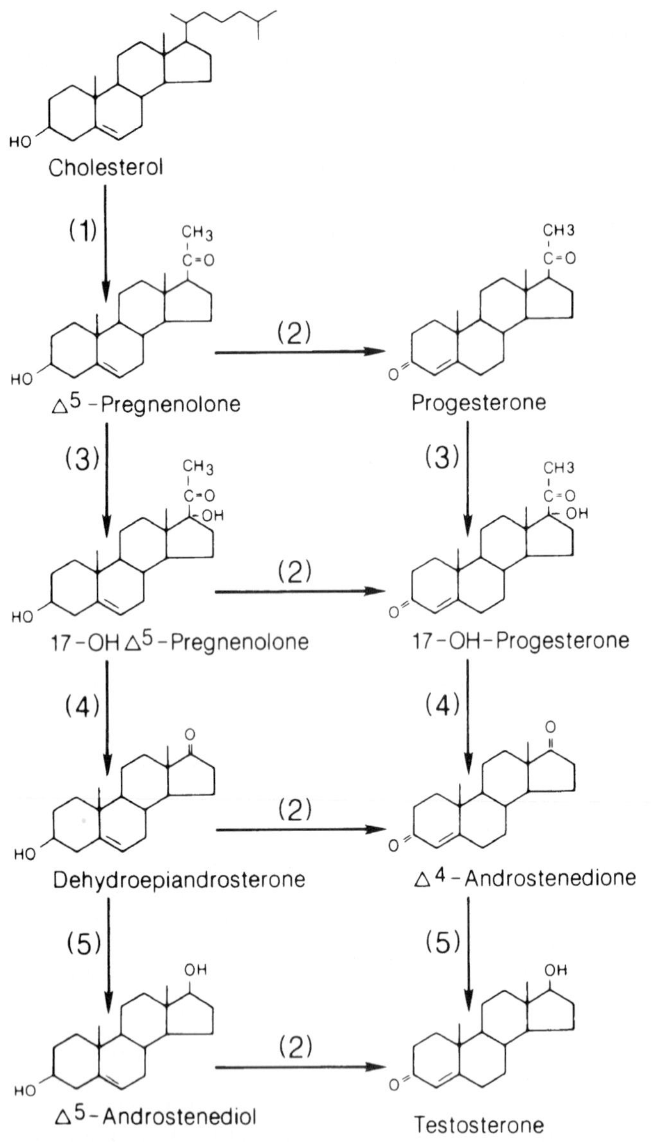

**FIGURE 115-11.** Testicular enzymatic defects in synthesis of testosterone. (1), 20,22-desmolase system; (2), 3βol-dehydrogenase; (3), 17α-hydroxylase; (4), 17,20-desmolase; (5), 17βol-oxidoreductase (17-ketosteroid reductase).

## 5α-REDUCTASE DEFICIENCY

The 5α-reductase deficiency syndrome (pseudovaginal perineoscrotal hypospadias, penis at 12 syndrome, type II incomplete androgen resistance) originally was described in 1961 as a defect in the conversion of testosterone to dihydrotestosterone resulting from the absence or lability of the 5α-reductase enzyme.[85] This disorder is most prevalent in certain rural villages in the Dominican Republic. However, it has been described sporadically in other countries throughout the world.[86] This is an autosomal recessive disorder that occurs in individuals with an XY chromosome pattern. The testes function normally insofar as androgen production and antimüllerian hormone are concerned; consequently, normal wolffian structures are formed and complete regression of the müllerian structures occurs. Because of the deficiency of dihydrotestosterone, however, the scrotum is usually bifid and the phallus displays severe hypospadias and may even appear as a moderately enlarged clitoris (see Chap. 90). Furthermore, a blind, vagina-like pouch (the bifid scrotum) may be present that opens just behind the urogenital sinus. The testes may be located anywhere from within the abdomen in the inguinal canal to within the bifid scrotum. At birth, these individuals appear to be girls who have moderately ambiguous genitalia (Fig. 115-12). At puberty, however, testosterone production by the testes is normal. Because no receptor problem exists, the full testosterone effect occurs, and masculinization, manifest by a deepening of the voice, marked phallic enlargement, loss of subcutaneous fat, and an increase in muscle mass, takes place. However, the sexual tissues that respond primarily to dihydrotestosterone, such as the scrotum, prostate, and testes, remain prepubertal. In adults with this syndrome, serum levels of testosterone are normal or mildly elevated, but dihydrotestosterone concentrations are low. Postpubertal serum gonadotropin levels are slightly increased.

The definitive diagnosis is made by the demonstration of an abnormal basal serum testosterone/dihydrotestosterone ratio.[87] After puberty, this ratio is <20 in normal men, but >35 in men with 5α-reductase deficiency. When the diagnosis is suspected before puberty, it can be confirmed by measuring the testosterone/dihydrotestosterone ratio after hCG stimulation. In such circumstances, normal boys maintain a ratio of <20, but boys with this enzyme deficiency develop a ratio of >50.

The 5α-reductase deficiency syndrome has been of particular interest because of the endocrine abnormalities and because several large kindreds have been found in two isolated agricultural villages in the Dominican Republic, where male and female gender roles are well defined.[88] This setting has provided a unique opportunity to determine the contribution of androgens to male gender identity. These psychosocial studies have demonstrated that, in the absence of sociocultural factors that could interrupt the change from female to male sexual orientation, the presence of male levels of testosterone overrides the effects of having been raised as a female. At puberty, these men take on traditional male roles.

Unfortunately, because the testes are usually undescended, and because dihydrotestosterone levels are low, sperm production is absent or proceeds to completion in only a few focal areas of the gonad. If the diagnosis has been made before puberty and if the children appear to have the female gender identity, they should be raised as females. The testes should be removed and estrogens should be administered at an appropriate pubertal age (see Chap. 91). If these patients have proceeded through puberty, they usually should be permitted to continue with their current gender identity, assuming that their phenotype is sufficiently male or female and their chosen gender is appropriate for their social situation. Because an undescended testis is at risk for the development of malignancy, and because these individuals are infertile, consideration should be given to removal of the testes and initiation of replacement therapy with sex steroids appropriate to the identified gender.

The defects in 5α-reductase described thus far have dealt with the most severe form, in which serum testosterone is unable to bind to the enzyme. The defect is genetically heterogeneous, however, and two additional abnormalities in expression of the 5α-reductase enzyme have been described.[89,90] These include an unstable 5α-reductase with a decreased affinity for testosterone, and an unstable 5α-reductase with a decreased affinity for the cofactor NADPH (nicotinamide-adenine dinucleotide phosphate, reduced form). These two defects result in milder clinical forms of the disease. Patients have more male-appearing genitalia at birth, allowing for an earlier diagnosis.

## LUTEINIZING HORMONE/GONADOTROPIN–RESISTANT TESTIS

The LH/gonadotropin–resistant testis is a rare defect characterized by a lack of receptors or receptor response to LH and hCG.[91] In general, these patients have genitalia that appear female. Occasionally, they may have more ambiguous structures, including microphallus, severe hypospadias, a bifid scro-

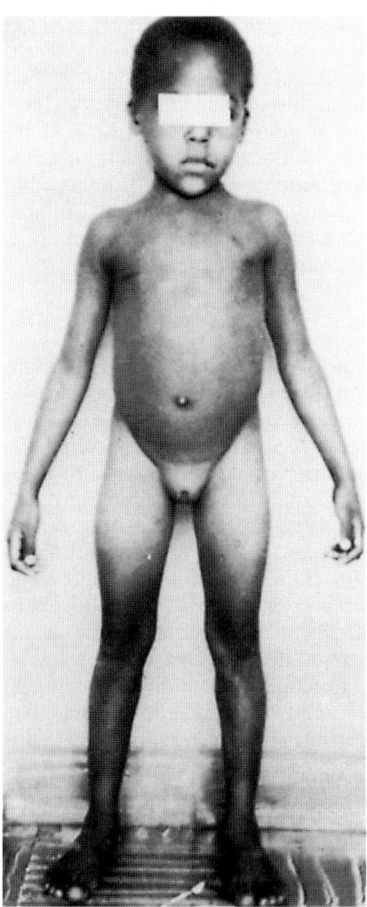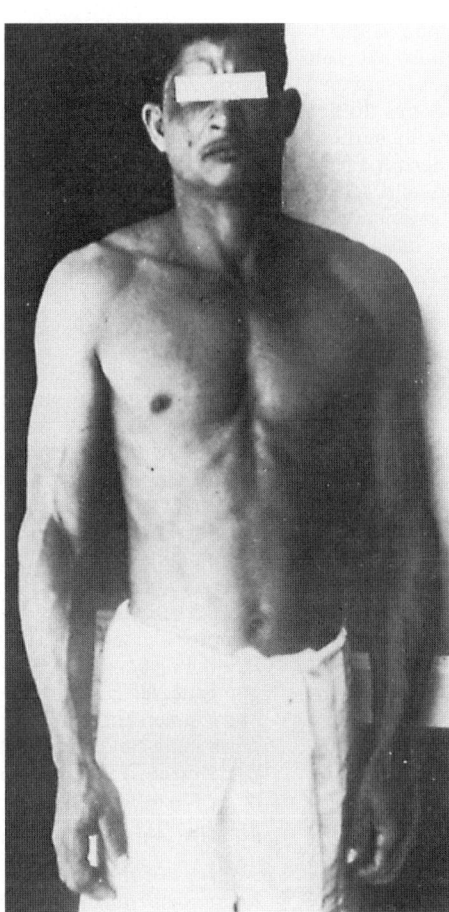

A,B

**FIGURE 115-12.** Two patients with 5α-reductase deficiencies. **A,** Before puberty, the patient has a female phenotype. **B,** After puberty, a normal male body habitus develops. Note the muscular development and masculine appearance in response to endogenous testosterone. See Chapter 90 for appearance of genitalia of such patients. (From Peterson RE. Male pseudohermaphroditism due to 5α-reductase deficiency. Am J Med 1977; 61:251.)

tum, and a urogenital sinus. If a vagina is present, it ends in a blind pouch, because complete regression of the müllerian structures has occurred due to the normal presence of anti-müllerian hormone from the testes. Because no testosterone production occurs in utero, the wolffian structures do not develop. Normally, the fetal testes respond to maternal hCG, and the wolffian structures develop. This is evident especially in patients with hypogonadotropic hypogonadism or Kallmann syndrome, in which, in utero, the fetus does not produce LH but the fetal testes respond to maternal hCG. Because androgens are necessary for the completion of spermatogenesis, histologic examination of the testes reveals spermatogenic arrest.

These patients have elevated serum gonadotropin levels and no increase in either serum testosterone or 17-hydroxyprogesterone levels after the administration of hCG. They can respond to exogenous androgens if these are indicated. For example, if a patient has been raised as male, he should be treated with testosterone. Alternatively, if the patient has been reared as a female, estrogen therapy should be considered. Because exogenous testosterone cannot achieve the intratesticular levels of testosterone that are necessary to support spermatogenesis, these patients are infertile.

## PERSISTENT MÜLLERIAN DUCT SYNDROME

Persistent paramesonephric structures often are part of the syndromes associated with defective gonads.[92] Sometimes, normal-appearing males are found at the time of herniorrhaphy or laparotomy to have a cervix, uterus, fallopian tubes, or enlarged prostatic utricle. Occasionally, they may have fathered children, although they often have a history of an undescended testis and infertility. The persistence of the paramesonephric system with otherwise normal testicular development suggests an abnormality of Sertoli cell maturation and deficient production of anti-müllerian hormone. Although the reported cases are few, in some

families, the data suggest autosomal recessive inheritance. These men also are at increased risk for testicular tumors and, when identified, should have gonadal examinations at regular intervals.

## MALE PSEUDOHERMAPHRODITISM INVOLVING ANDROGEN-RECEPTOR DEFECTS

Androgens enter the target cells and bind to the intracellular receptor, which subsequently attaches to the appropriate site on the gene to initiate translation (see Chaps. 4 and 114). If an absence of or defect in this receptor is present, androgenization cannot occur in spite of a normal or supranormal level of testosterone. The complete absence or lack of dihydrotestosterone binding by the receptor results in the complete female phenotype, which is seen in the testicular feminization syndrome. Variants of this syndrome depend on the degree of receptor defect.

### TESTICULAR FEMINIZATION

Classically, patients with the testicular feminization syndrome appear to be well-developed females who are identified only after they have gone through a normal puberty and are seen for evaluation of amenorrhea (see Chap. 90). These patients are chromosomally normal males who have a complete absence of androgen receptors.[93,94] At puberty, they have normal breast development because of the unopposed estrogen effects.[95,96] On physical examination, the clitoris is of normal size, but pelvic examination reveals a blind vaginal pouch. The testes may present as masses in the labia or may be located within the abdomen. At times, the testes are in the canal of Nuck, and patients have what appear to be bilateral inguinal hernias. Because the testes are not in their normal scrotal position, the potential for malignancy exists, and these gonads should be removed.[97] In general, these individuals have been raised as females; they do not respond to exogenous androgens, and the female gender identity should be continued. Treatment consists of castration and estrogen replacement. Because they have an XY karyotype with testes, antimüllerian hormone is present and müllerian structures are absent. The wolffian structures do not develop. Because the Leydig cells can function normally in these men, testosterone levels are normal or elevated. Serum LH is increased because of the lack of androgen feedback and serum FSH is increased because of seminiferous tubular dysfunction.

The classic form of this disease results in a complete lack of binding of androgens to the receptor. However, multiple defects in the androgen-receptor gene have been described. These defects may be in either the hormone-binding domain or the DNA-binding domain of the receptor; the latter defect accounts for those forms of testicular feminization in which hormone binding is intact.[98] These defects in the androgen receptor have been reviewed.[99] The inheritance of testicular feminization is X-linked recessive. Although these patients have a more severe biochemical syndrome, they usually have less difficulty with social adjustment than do patients with other types of pseudohermaphroditism because their phenotypic sex is less ambiguous.

## REIFENSTEIN SYNDROME

Individuals with Reifenstein syndrome have partial androgen resistance and are detected at birth with variable degrees of pseudohermaphroditism, ranging from hypospadias and undescended testes to a urogenital sinus with perineal opening of the urethra and complete lack of fusion of the scrotum.[100,101] The karyotype is XY. At puberty, when the testes are physiologically stimulated by endogenous gonadotropins to produce testosterone, an incomplete androgen effect may be noted. Subsequently, the penis remains small, the testes usually remain undescended, and the scrotum is poorly developed. Androgen-sensitive hair growth is decreased, and muscle mass and strength are diminished in these patients. The estrogen receptors function normally. Therefore, the increased testosterone production at puberty provides an increased sex steroid substrate for the peripheral production of estrogen in either the liver or fat, and marked gynecomastia usually develops. Most commonly, the testes remain within the abdomen. Light-microscopic examination shows an absence of normal spermatogenesis and hyalinization of most seminiferous tubules. The Leydig cells appear normal. Serum levels of testosterone and dihydrotestosterone are normal or elevated. Because functional androgen receptors in the pituitary are also decreased, serum LH and FSH levels are elevated. This experiment of nature further demonstrates that serum testosterone, as well as estradiol, contributes to normal gonadotropin regulation.

Men with Reifenstein syndrome present a difficult problem in gender selection. Unlike their more severely affected counterparts with testicular feminization, these men are usually raised as males. Studies have shown that, although some response may occur to exogenous testosterone therapy, very high dosages (e.g., 400 mg of testosterone enanthate intramuscularly each week) are required to achieve an androgenizing effect. Unfortunately, these dosages have not been proven to be safe for long-term treatment; in addition, they provide sex steroid substrate for estrogen production. Even high dosages of testosterone usually result in only a partial androgenization. Thus, the long-term treatment of these individuals requires adequate psychological support. Consideration should be given to removing testes if they are located within the abdomen, because they are prone to malignant transformation.

If patients with Reifenstein syndrome have been reared as females, castration and estrogen replacement result in a relatively normal phenotypic female and a more satisfactory outcome than does conversion to a male. Castration prevents partial virilization, which may occur at puberty (especially in cases of 17-ketosteroid reductase deficiency).

Reifenstein syndrome has been shown to have a heterogeneous etiology, with some patients demonstrating a decreased number of normal receptors and others having receptors that are defective, as evidenced by their decreased affinity for dihydrotestosterone, their heat lability, and their failure to be stabilized by molybdate.[102–105,105a] This variability of receptor number or activity may be due to the varied genetic defects that are found in Reifenstein syndrome.[106,107] An X-linked inheritance is predominant, but in some cases, distinction between X-linked and autosomal recessive inheritance is not clear.

## KENNEDY SYNDROME

Kennedy syndrome is a disorder of primary hypogonadism and progressive motor neuron disease caused by a polynucleotide repeat, (CAG)n, expansion in the androgen-receptor gene.[108] Although the androgen-receptor sequence is normal, the expanded polyglutamine (polyGln) region suppresses androgen-receptor transreactivity.[109] Interestingly, although the androgen-receptor normally contains a polyGln tract, when the repeat number is reduced to 0, further transactivation by the androgen-receptor occurs. This suggests that within the whole male human population, variable transactivation by the androgen-receptor occurs. The potential effect of a decrease in CAG repeat length has been associated with an increase in incidence of prostate cancer.[110,111] The repeat length correlates with the incidence of prostate cancer in younger men, with the increased incidence of prostate cancer in the African-American population, and with the decreased incidence of prostate cancer in Asian populations.

## INFERTILITY DUE TO AN ANDROGEN-RECEPTOR DEFECT

A group of men with severe oligospermia have been reported to possess unstable androgen receptors.[112] These men were described as phenotypically normal, and the condition was found only when they underwent evaluation for infertility with androgen-receptor measurements. Usually, they were noted to have serum testosterone levels in the upper normal range and LH values that were high normal or mildly elevated. The incidence of this syndrome among infertile men has not been determined because screening for abnormal androgen receptors is not usually required in the workup of male infertility. Since the original description of this defect, subsequent investigators have not been able to confirm the results of the original study. Unfortunately, no treatment is available for this problem.

The syndromes associated with androgen-receptor defects have been described as separate entities; however, their mode of inheritance (i.e., autosomal recessive) is similar. Whether these syndromes are distinctly different or simply represent varying degrees of the same disease process awaits identification of the specific causative gene defect.

## POSTPUBERTAL ORCHITIS (EPIDEMIC PAROTITIS)

Although prepubertal mumps is almost never associated with orchitis, men who acquire mumps during or after puberty have approximately a 25% chance of developing orchitis.[113] The orchitis is usually clinically apparent; nevertheless, some men being evaluated for infertility give a history of postpubertal mumps without a recollection of orchitis. Orchitis is commonly unilateral. However, testicular biopsy (Fig. 115-13) at the time of the orchitis demonstrates bilateral involvement. Furthermore, both testes are damaged if the patient has abnormal spermatogenesis and infertility. Of those men who have postpubertal mumps orchitis, as many as 60% will be infertile. During the acute infection, these patients demonstrate sloughing of the germinal seminiferous epithelium. On physical examination, they have atrophic testes. At that time, the biopsy shows tubular sclerosis and hyalinization, which may be focal or diffuse. Although the usual testicular consequence of mumps orchitis is seminiferous

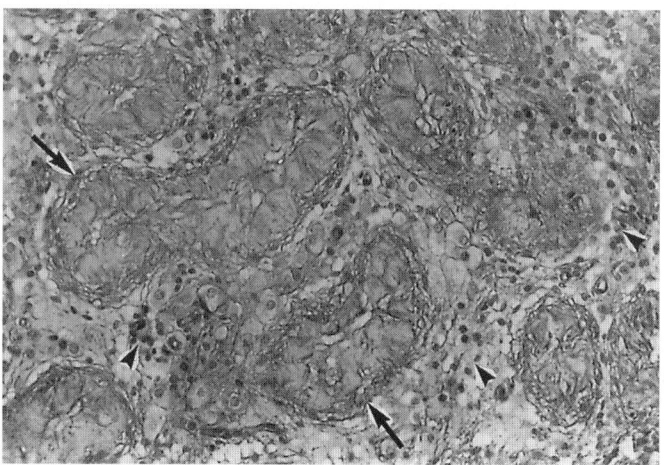

**FIGURE 115-13.** Testicular biopsy specimen from a patient after mumps orchitis. Notice the completely hyalinized seminiferous tubules (*arrows*) and the "mulberry" appearance to the clumped Leydig cells (*arrowheads*) similar to that seen in Klinefelter syndrome.

tubule failure, some of these men also have Leydig cell failure and androgen deficiency. In view of the evidence that local paracrine factors from the Sertoli cells are necessary for adequate Leydig cell function, the finding of decreased testosterone production in these patients is not surprising. These patients usually show a monotropic increase in serum FSH levels but may have elevated LH levels, depending on the degree of androgen deficiency. Stimulation tests with LHRH may be necessary to reveal the exaggerated rise in gonadotropins if the testicular damage is mild and the basal FSH levels are normal.

Since the development of a mumps vaccine, the incidence of mumps orchitis has decreased significantly. This means that many individuals who do have mumps are adults who did not receive the vaccine as children and are more prone to orchitis. Treatment with androgens or estrogens during the acute phase of the infection to suppress and protect the germinal seminiferous tubular epithelium has been suggested. This approach is of dubious benefit, however, and no definitive studies have been performed.[114] Corticosteroid treatment has been shown to decrease the inflammation and severity of the acute orchitis; whether long-term follow-up treatment would diminish the damage to the seminiferous tubules is unknown.[115] If spermatogenesis has been severely impaired, no successful therapy for the infertility is available. If androgen levels are deficient, testosterone substitution therapy should be instituted. Other viral infections may cause similar problems (see Chap. 213).

## CRYPTORCHIDISM

At birth, as many as 10% of male infants have an undescended testis. By 1 year of age, 70% to 90% of these testes descend into the scrotum, and after puberty, only 0.3% to 0.4% of men continue to have one or both testes undescended (see Chap. 93).[116] Undescended testes have been associated with numerous gonadal disorders, including hypogonadotropic hypogonadism, Ullrich-Noonan syndrome, Klinefelter syndrome, and Reifenstein syndrome.[117] Nevertheless, most patients with cryptorchidism have no readily discernible endocrine disease. The association of the true cryptorchid testis and the high incidence of infertility with these syndromes indicates that, in most patients, the problem does not lie within the anatomic structures associated with testicular descent but arises from an endocrine-related developmental abnormality. This is particularly true for unilateral cryptorchidism.

In animals made cryptorchid, infertility develops, further confirming the damage caused by an abdominal testicle. Human cryptorchidism is associated with infertility in ~70% of

cases.[118] The cryptorchid testicle is treated by bringing it into the scrotum surgically as soon as the abnormality is detected. This decreases the 8% risk of carcinoma of the testis that is associated with this disorder (see Chap. 122) and places the testis in a location where it can more easily be observed. Another reason to bring the testis into the scrotum is to increase the possibility of fertility. Unfortunately, even when the once-cryptorchid testis is placed in the scrotum, infertility is common.

Various nonsurgical maneuvers (e.g., hCG or LHRH administration) have been tried to stimulate the testis to migrate permanently into the scrotum. These maneuvers have not been proven successful.[119]

## LEPROSY

Although leprosy occurs infrequently in the United States, it remains a common problem in many countries and affects many men, who require years of therapy for the disease. The *Mycobacterium leprae* organism has been shown to invade the testis directly and cause primary testicular failure. This occurs in as many as 75% of men with the disease.[120] Although leprosy most often affects both testicular compartments and causes infertility and decreased testosterone production with elevated serum gonadotropin levels, the disease may result in selective destruction of either compartment, causing isolated increases in serum LH or FSH levels.[121] Most other infectious processes of the testes affect primarily the seminiferous epithelium. In addition, even when serum LH levels are elevated selectively, affected men still have decreased sperm counts. In leprosy, the greatest damage is to the interstitial compartment. Serum testosterone responses to hCG are blunted to a degree that is proportional to the elevation of serum estradiol.

The severity of testicular damage appears to be related somewhat to the type of leprosy, with lepromatous and borderline leprosy causing the greatest degree of Leydig cell failure and tuberculoid leprosy causing the least. The recognition of androgen deficiency is important in a chronic catabolic disease such as this, because androgen replacement may hasten the overall rate of recovery (see Chap. 213).

## TESTICULAR TRAUMA

The traumatic loss of both testes results in hypogonadism (posttraumatic testicular dysfunction) that requires androgen replacement. However, injury to one testicle that disrupts the continuity of the blood–testis barrier also appears to result in damage to the unaffected, contralateral testis. Sometimes, this damage manifests as infertility. The mechanism for the infertility is unknown, but it may be similar to the cause of infertility in the case of a single undescended testis. Clinically, the appearance of the individual depends on the degree of androgen deficiency and whether the injury occurred before or after puberty.

One of the most common reasons for the loss of a testicle before puberty is testicular torsion. This problem, which tends to be recurrent and often is bilateral, results from a developmental defect. The torsion may be reversed and the testis fixed in place. If the testis is not viable, it should be removed. After correction of the torsion, the viability of the testis depends on the length of time the blood supply has been interrupted. Unfortunately, as may occur with an undescended testis, fertility of the unaffected testis may be compromised.

## TESTICULAR IRRADIATION EFFECTS

Irradiation of the testes usually is associated with a treatment program for an associated disease, such as Hodgkin disease or prostatic carcinoma. Most of the current data regarding the effects of irradiation on seminiferous tubule dysfunction are derived from two investigations in which otherwise normal

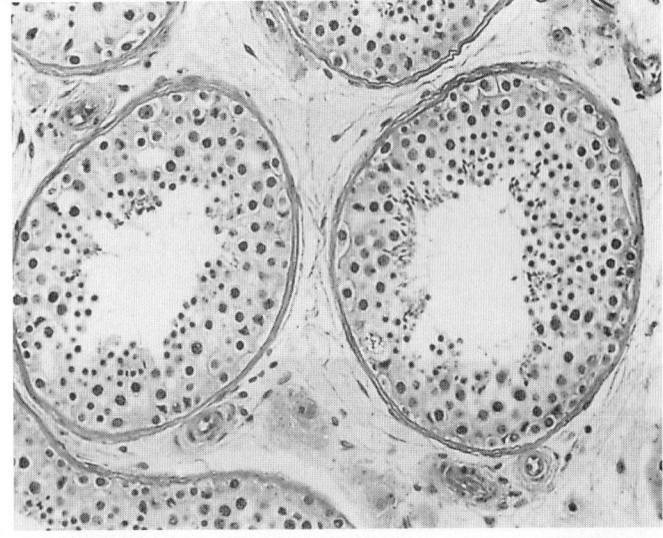

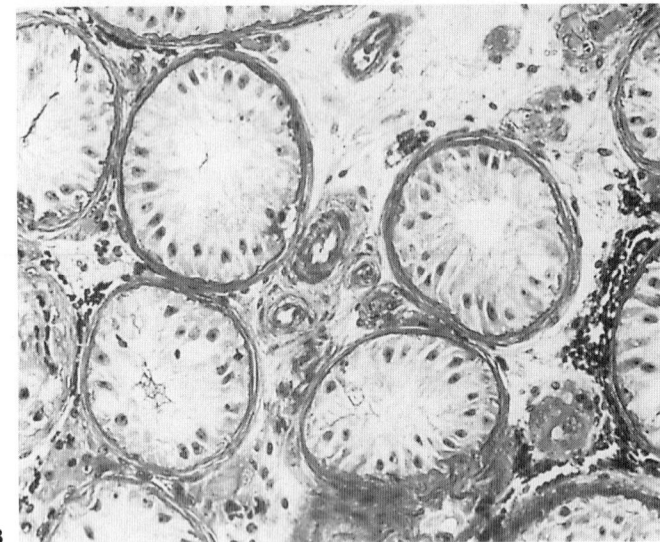

**FIGURE 115-14.** Testicular biopsy before (**A**) and 228 days after exposure to 100 rad of x-ray irradiation (**B**). Note the loss of germ cells except for a few type A spermatogonia.

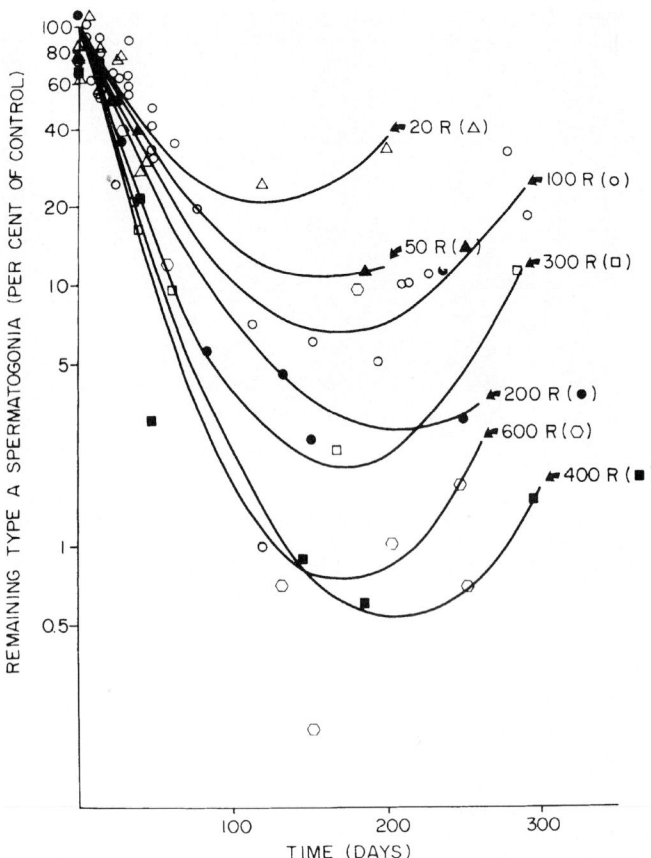

**FIGURE 115-15.** The effects of various doses of testicular x-ray irradiation on type A spermatogonia over time. Lines represent least squares regression over data points for each dose group. The return of spermatogenesis depends on the degree of loss of spermatogonia. (*R*, rads.) (Modified from Clifton DK, Bremner WJ. The effect of testicular x-irradiation on spermatogenesis in man. J Androl 1983; 4:387.)

men who were undergoing vasectomies had semen analyses, testicular biopsies, and serum hormone measurements made before, during, and while recovering from graded doses of x-ray irradiation[122,123] (Fig. 115-14). These studies demonstrated that doses as small as 15 rad may cause a marked fall in the sperm count, and that doses of 50 rad may cause azoospermia. After doses as high as 400 rad, sperm counts and testicular biopsy results returned to normal.[124] The time required for normalization correlated directly with the radiation dose and depended on the number of type A spermatogonia remaining after irradiation. A failure to recover was noted at doses of 600 rad or more, and the biopsy specimens from these men demonstrated a complete loss of type A spermatogonia. Disappearance of spermatocytes did not occur consistently until doses were in the range of 200 rad (Fig. 115-15). Serum measurements of FSH began to show significant increases at doses >30 rad, and the return of serum FSH levels to normal paralleled the return to normal spermatogenesis. No significant change in the levels of serum LH or testosterone occurred at any of these doses.

If a patient is scheduled to receive therapeutic irradiation, suppression of spermatogenesis with testosterone or testosterone and an LHRH agonist or antagonist has been suggested to protect against infertility, because dividing cells are more sensitive to the effects of irradiation. This preventive treatment has not been tested. The only acceptable methods of preventing the damage are testicular shielding during irradiation or sperm banking before treatment. Consideration must be given to the increased numbers of chromosomal breaks that will occur during the irradiation, which may lead to an increase in fetal anomalies.

Leydig cell dysfunction is not seen until doses of >800 rad are administered. However, these are common doses of therapeutic irradiation.[124] In studies performed on men who had received therapeutic irradiation for prostate cancer without testicular shielding (the usual procedure), a significant decrease in basal serum testosterone levels, compared with age-matched men, was noted. A single, large dose was more deleterious than were fractional doses of similar total magnitude. Serum LH and FSH levels were found to be significantly increased, which indicates primary testicular damage. Treatment of the testosterone deficiency should be considered, because this should improve the anabolic state and enable patients to tolerate chemotherapy. However, in the case of prostate carcinoma, an androgen-responsive tumor, replacement therapy should not be given.

Radioiodine therapy for thyroid cancer also has been associated with testicular dysfunction, primarily a loss of spermatogenesis.[125] Because comprehensive studies have not been done, however, the frequency of significant damage is unknown (see Chap. 226).

## AUTOIMMUNE TESTICULAR FAILURE

Two types of autoimmune testicular failure have been described. The most common of these is infertility resulting from the production of antibodies to sperm.[126] This situation has been described most convincingly after vasovasostomy in men who have had a vasectomy. The antibody reaction may be responsible for the persistence of infertility in spite of normal sperm counts after vasovasostomy.

The presence of antisperm antibodies of the immunoglobulin A (IgA) class in semen and of the immunoglobulin G (IgG) class in the peripheral blood may be a cause of idiopathic infertility. The mechanism for the appearance of these antibodies in infertile men without histories of testicular damage or genital infections is unknown. Because of the high incidence of antisperm antibodies in the normal fertile population, however, this hypothesis may not be valid (see Chap. 118). Treatment of this form of infertility with high-dose glucocorticoids has been attempted.

The second, and less common, form of autoimmune testicular failure is that which occurs with steroid cell antibodies and subsequent loss of testosterone production.[127] This type of steroid cell antibody has been recognized most commonly in women with ovarian failure but is found in men in rare cases. Usually, this condition is seen with other endocrine gland autoimmune diseases, especially Addison disease. The antibody is directed against the microsomal portion of the cell and not against the steroid hormone. Thyroid disease (e.g., Graves disease, hypothyroidism, or Hashimoto thyroiditis); hypoparathyroidism; pernicious anemia; diabetes mellitus; and alopecia totalis also have been associated with Leydig cell failure due to steroid cell antibodies (see Chap. 197). This form of autoimmune disease has been linked with the HLA-B8 major histocompatibility locus on chromosome 6. Because of the small number of men described with autoimmune Leydig cell failure, specific types of HLA associations are unknown. Androgen replacement treatment is required for these patients.

## CHEMOTHERAPY EFFECTS

Similar to radiation exposure, chemotherapy also may damage the testes (see Chap. 226). Alkylating agents, such as nitrogen mustards, cyclophosphamide, and chlorambucil, consistently harm spermatogenesis in a dose-related fashion.[128,129] Other agents, such as procarbazine and various combinations of drugs, also affect spermatogenesis in most individuals.[130] The appearance of gynecomastia provides a clue that Leydig cell function may be affected.[131,132]

The same recommendations for prevention of damage described in the section on irradiation also apply to the use of chemotherapeutic agents. Sperm banking may be considered in young men who undergo curative chemotherapy for malignancies such as Hodgkin disease or germ cell carcinoma. In some of these tumors, especially Hodgkin disease, testicular function may be affected by the disease itself. The effects of chemotherapy on Leydig cell function have not been well described; however, the association of gynecomastia with chemotherapy suggests a defect in testosterone production.

## SECONDARY HYPOGONADISM

### HYPOGONADOTROPIC HYPOGONADISM

Hypogonadotropic hypogonadism may be caused by acquired or congenital defects. The presentation of the acquired forms of the disorder varies depending on whether the individual has gone through puberty and whether other anterior or posterior pituitary hormone deficiencies are involved. If the individual acquires the disorder before the onset of puberty, the presentation is that of a prepubertal male, as noted in Table 115-2. If puberty has occurred before the onset of the disorder, the presentation is with signs and symptoms of postpubertal testicular failure. The acquired forms of the disorder and some congenital forms have additional anterior pituitary deficiencies. If growth

hormone is deficient, it is of clinical significance only if the individual is prepubertal and has not reached his adult height. After puberty, when the epiphyses of the long bones have fused and linear growth has ceased, growth hormone deficiency will no longer be apparent.

## CLASSIC HYPOGONADOTROPIC EUNUCHOIDISM

Just as Klinefelter syndrome has become the prime example of hypergonadotropic hypogonadism, congenital hypogonadotropic eunuchoidism is the classic example of hypogonadotropic hypogonadism. As originally described by Kallmann and colleagues, this syndrome (Kallmann syndrome) is characterized by isolated gonadotropin deficiency and anosmia or hyposmia due to defective development of the olfactory bulbs.[132,133] Other findings occasionally described with this disorder include midline cleft palate and lip, congenital deafness, cerebellar seizures, a short fourth metacarpal, and cardiac abnormalities.[134,135]

Kallmann syndrome is most commonly associated with autosomal dominant inheritance.[134] The associated defects, especially anosmia, have enabled tracing of father-to-son transmission.[136] However, kindreds have been reported that suggest an autosomal recessive or X-linked form of inheritance.[137] The X-linked form of Kallmann syndrome is due to point mutations and exon deletions of the *KAL* gene located on the X chromosome at location Xp22.3.[138–140] The gene consists of 14 exons and produces a 680-amino-acid, 76-kDa protein (anosmin-1) that can be glycosylated to form an 85-kDa protein product. The protein contains four fibronectin type III repeats associated with cellular adhesion functions, and a four-disulfide core motif that is commonly associated with antiprotease activity. The question of other forms of inheritance will be further defined as more men and women with the syndrome become fertile as a result of newer modes of therapy, and their progeny are studied.

The incidence of this syndrome is ~1 in 10,000 male births.[134] These men present as prepubertal eunuchs. They usually have no evidence of pubertal physical findings and their skeletal proportions are eunuchoid, with the ratio of upper body segment (pubis to vertex) to lower body segment (pubis to floor) decreased; the arm span is at least 6 cm greater than the height. These body proportions result from a failure of epiphyseal fusion and continued long bone growth. Beard and pubic hair growth are absent or minimal. Most patients retain their prepubertal subcutaneous body fat (Fig. 115-16). Hyposmia is present in most cases but may be missed unless specifically tested using appropriate olfactory sensation materials[141] (Fig. 115-17). Muscle mass and strength remain at prepubertal levels. Although some CNS problems have been described,[142] mental retardation is not one of them. A small phallus and temporal facial wrinkling caused by hypogonadism are common in this disorder. Gynecomastia may occur; peripheral aromatization of adrenal androgens may be contributory. Testicular development remains at prepubertal levels, with a few patients showing some testicular enlargement at puberty.[143] However, unlike in Klinefelter syndrome, the testes are of normal prepubertal size because no tubular scarring or loss of germ cells is present. The Leydig cells are immature (as would be seen without LH stimulation), although normal numbers of interstitial cells are present, and the development into mature testosterone-producing Leydig cells occurs with gonadotropin stimulation (Fig. 115-18).

Basal serum gonadotropin levels are low normal or undetectable in these men. When multiple samples are taken over a 24-hour period, however, some subjects demonstrate occasional small pulses of LH.[144] When a single bolus dose of gonadotropin-releasing hormone is administered, the response of the pituitary gonadotropins usually is minimal. However, if repeated pulses of gonadotropin-releasing hormone are given, a normal rise in serum LH and FSH levels eventually occurs.[143,145,146]

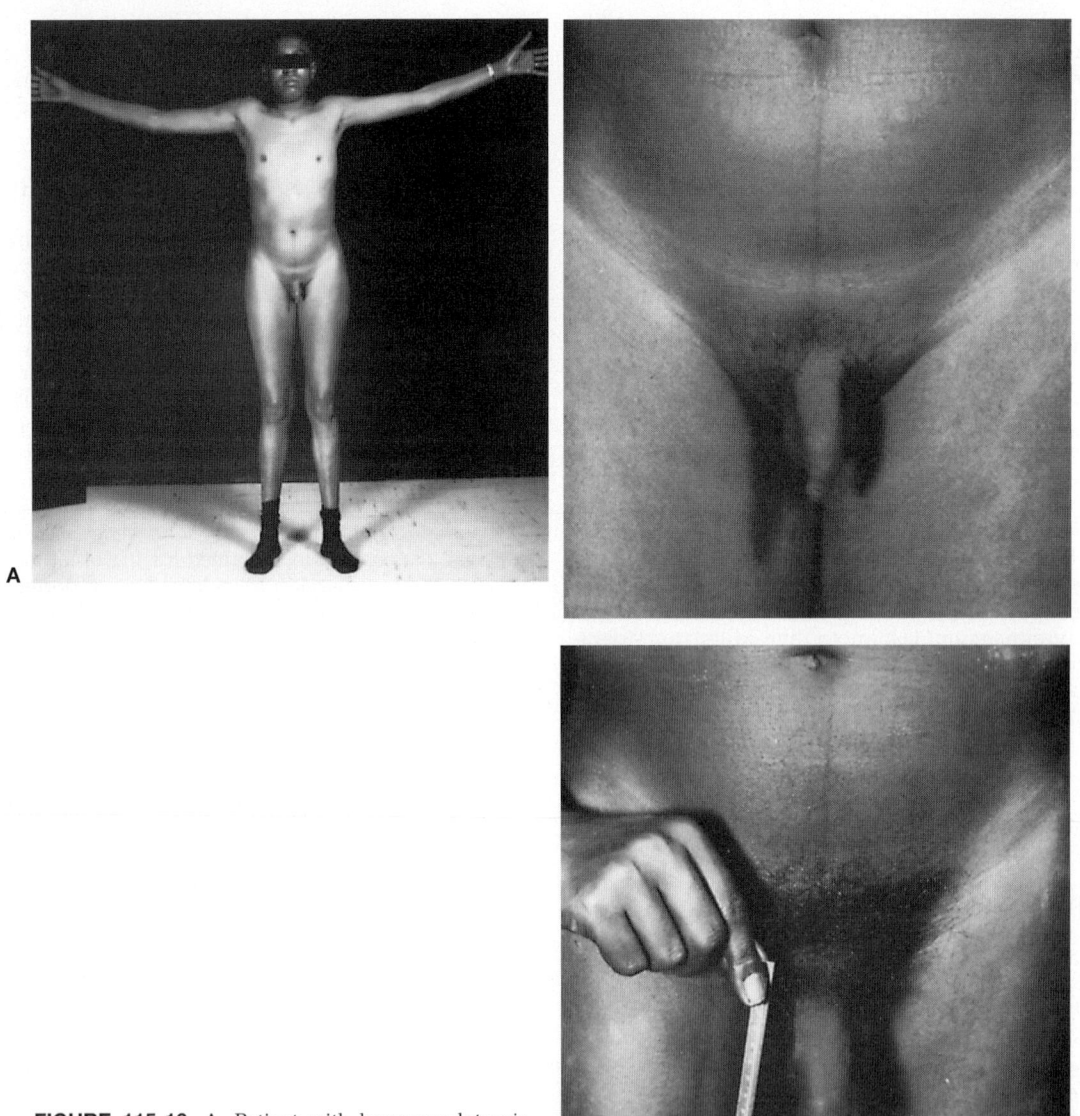

**FIGURE 115-16. A,** Patient with hypogonadotropic hypogonadism (Kallmann syndrome). Note the long legs and the increased arm span. Body hair is sparse, and the penis is small (**B**). **C,** Note the increase in penile size and pubic hair after 6 months of therapy with testosterone.

These studies indicate that the most likely defect is a deficiency in LHRH secretion by the hypothalamus. Furthermore, autopsy studies have demonstrated anatomically normal pituitary glands.[147] Serum testosterone levels remain in the middle of the female range in most patients with this condition before treatment, although they may have shown partial progression through puberty. No other pituitary hormonal defect has been documented in these patients.

Approximately 10% of men with idiopathic hypogonadotropic hypogonadism provide a history of some pubertal development with subsequent regression. This diagnosis should be suspected in any man who has passed the normal pubertal age and remains prepubertal.[144] Serum gonadotropin levels are low, testosterone levels are low, and prolactin levels are normal.[148,149] If one of the associated abnormalities, such as anosmia, cleft palate, and cleft lip, is present, the diagnosis can be made with some assurance. If these findings are absent, however, differentiating between delayed puberty and idiopathic hypogonadotropic eunuchoidism can be extremely difficult, because puberty does not occur until 18 or 19 years of age in some normal men. Several maneuvers have been described that purport to differ-

entiate this condition from delayed puberty.[147,150,151] These include a subnormal serum prolactin response to thyrotropin-releasing hormone or to a phenothiazine, a decreased serum testosterone response to exogenous hCG, and a normal LH response to pulsatile stimulation by LHRH. None of these tests has been consistently reliable. If the differentiation cannot be made and the circumstances warrant, treatment with testosterone or hCG for 3 or 6 months may be indicated. After this, therapy can be discontinued and the patient observed to see whether spontaneous puberty progresses.

The treatment of idiopathic hypogonadotropic eunuchoidism has two goals: to provide adequate androgen replacement and to achieve fertility.[151a] Androgen replacement may be accomplished as indicated in Chapter 119. Androgen replacement therapy does not impair subsequent therapeutic stimulation of spermatogenesis. In contrast to most of the causes of primary testicular failure in which improvement of fertility is not possible, in secondary hypogonadism fertility may be initiated. Several methods are available. One method of restoring spermatogenesis involves the use of hCG and then FSH in the form of human menopausal gonadotropins (hMGs).[152–155] Ini-

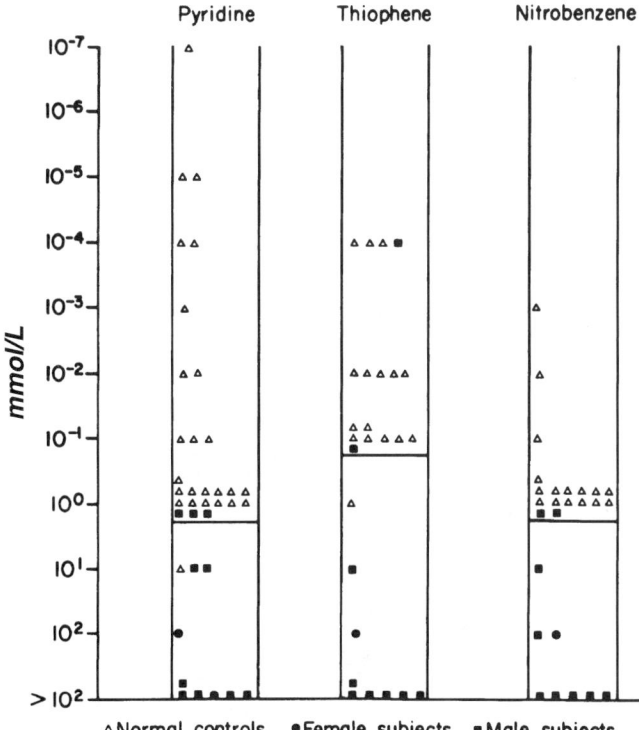

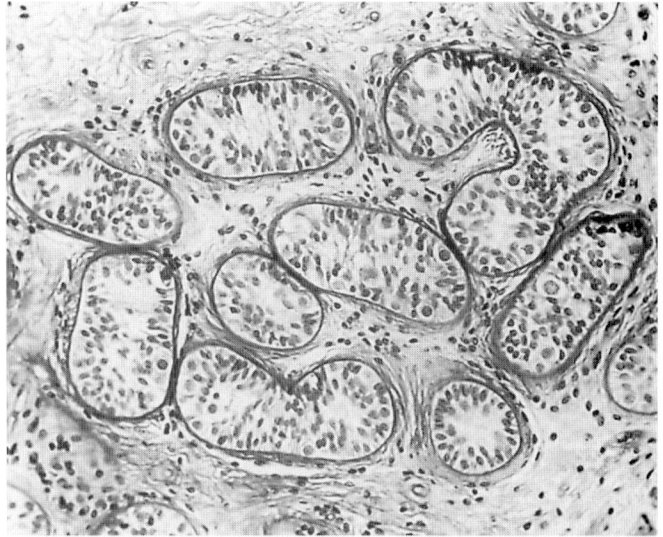

A

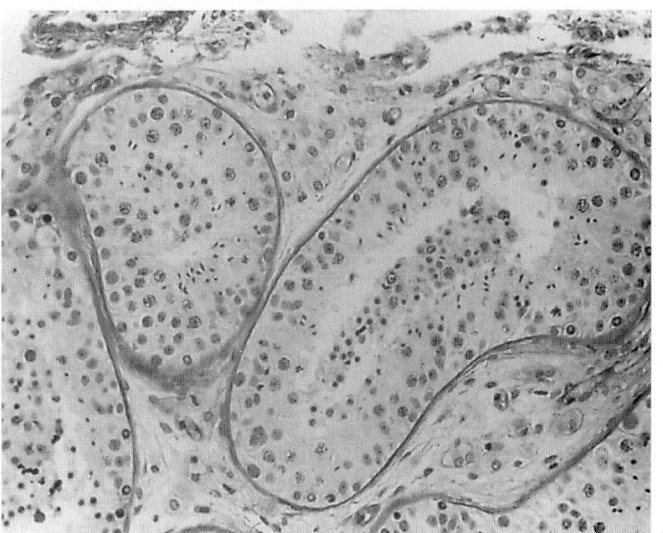

B

**FIGURE 115-17.** Olfactory thresholds for various molar concentrations of aromatic solutions in patients with hypogonadotropic hypogonadism (Kallmann syndrome). Transverse lines indicate the olfactory thresholds for normal adults. This test is performed by making separate molar solutions of the three substances indicated. The subjects are blinded to the contents of the containers and, after they are presented in random order, are asked to indicate whether a solution has an identifiable odor. Solutions should be made fresh weekly and the consistency of the investigator's threshold should be noted to determine loss of aroma of the test solutions. The molar concentration at which the test subject can no longer consistently detect an aroma is noted. This threshold then is compared with that of a group of normal controls and to the threshold of the normal investigator. Patients with anosmia consistently fall below the normal threshold, but not all patients with hypogonadotropic hypogonadism have anosmia. (From Santen RJ, Paulsen CA. Hypogonadotropic eunuchoidism. I. Clinical study of the mode of inheritance. J Clin Endocrinol Metab 1973; 36:47.)

**FIGURE 115-18.** Initiation of spermatogenesis with administration of human chorionic gonadotropin (*hCG*) and human menopausal gonadotropin (*hMG*) in a patient with hypogonadotropic hypogonadism as demonstrated by serial testicular biopsy specimens. **A,** Initial state. **B,** After 6 months of therapy with hCG plus hMG. (From Paulsen CA. The testis. In: Williams RH, ed. Textbook of endocrinology. Philadelphia: WB Saunders, 1981:333.)

tially, hCG is administered at a dosage of 1000 to 2000 IU intramuscularly three times a week to stimulate Leydig cell function; this increases intratesticular testosterone levels. After the dosage of hCG that achieves normal serum testosterone levels has been determined and the patient has been treated for 8 to 12 weeks, hMG may be added (see Fig. 115-18). The initial regimen is 75 IU intramuscularly three times a week while continuing hCG therapy. Once spermatogenesis is initiated, the dosage of hMGs can be decreased to 12 to 25 IU three times weekly. In some men, especially those with an initial testicular volume >5 mL, spermatogenesis can be maintained without continuing hMG. A history of undescended testes or of multiple pituitary hormone defects in syndromes other than hypogonadotropic eunuchoidism may result in treatment failure.

A second method, which takes advantage of the knowledge of the pulsatile release of LH and FSH in these patients, has been used to stimulate spermatogenesis and Leydig cell function.[144,156,157] By administration of a subcutaneous pulse of LHRH every 90 to 120 minutes through an infusion pump worn by the patient, a normal pattern of gonadotropin pulsation can be induced and spermatogenesis subsequently occurs.[144,145] The dose of LHRH given with each pulse depends on the number of pulses administered each day. Usually, a pulse is given every 90 minutes. Thus, the average dose per pulse is between 1.5 and 10 ng/kg, assuming an average of 16 pulses each day. The dosage

generally is determined by what is needed to produce a normal serum testosterone level. Spermatogenesis can be expected to occur after 2 to 3 months. The administration of LHRH at intervals faster or slower than 90 to 120 minutes produces inappropriate secretion of LH and FSH. The cost of pulsatile LHRH administration and hCG/hMG therapy is similar. A clear reason for one therapy or the other is not apparent.

In addition to inducing fertility in these men, androgen replacement therapy is needed to develop muscle mass, prevent osteoporosis, provide psychological support, and produce full pubertal development. Any of the methods for inducing spermatogenesis also replace androgens by stimulating the Leydig cells. However, once fertility has been achieved, exogenous androgen therapy probably is the most satisfactory and economic choice for the patient. Then, if another pregnancy is desired, the patient can be switched back to gonadotropin or LHRH therapy.

Idiopathic hypogonadotropic eunuchoidism may occur in women. The condition may be isolated or inherited as an autosomal dominant or autosomal recessive trait. It presents simi-

**TABLE 115-5.**
**Syndromes Associated with Congenital Gonadotropin Deficiency**

| Syndrome | Typical Features |
|---|---|
| Laurence-Moon-Biedl | Retinitis pigmentosa polydactyly, mental retardation, hypogonadotropic hypogonadism, and Sertoli-cell-only syndrome.[204–206] |
| Lowe | Fanconi syndrome, cataracts, glaucoma, buphthalmos, hypotonia, mental retardation, and hypogonadotropic hypogonadism.[207] |
| Multiple lentigines (leopard syndrome) | Generalized lentigines, sensorineural hearing loss, hypertelorism, short stature, pulmonic stenosis, and hypogonadotropic hypogonadism.[208] |
| Prader-Willi | Hypomentia, hypotonia, obesity, short stature, small hands and feet, hypogonadotropic hypogonadism, and primary testicular deficiency.[209] |
| RUD* | Hyposmia, congenital ichthyosis, mental retardation, epilepsy, and hypogonadotropic hypogonadism.[210] |
| CHARGE† | Coloboma, heart disease, atresia of the choanae, retarded growth and development, and hypogonadotropic hypogonadism.[211] |
| Steroid sulfatase deficiency | Hypogonadism associated with steroid sulfatase and arylsulfatase C deficiency, congenital ichthyosis, nystagmus, strabismus, decreased visual acuity, hypopigmentation of the iris, unilateral renal hypoplasia or agenesis, and hypogonadotropic hypogonadism.[212] |
| Martsolf | Short stature, severe mental retardation, and hypogonadotropic hypogonadism; patients mainly of Jewish ancestry; X-linked or autosomal recessive inheritance.[213] |
| Rothmund-Thomson | Hypodontia, soft-tissue contractures, short stature, anemia, osteogenic sarcoma, and hypogonadotropic hypogonadism.[214] |
| Börjeson-Forssman-Lehmann | Prominent supraorbital ridges, ptosis, large ears, hypotonia, severe mental retardation, and hypogonadotropic hypogonadism.[215] |

*Retardation, underdeveloped gonads, dermatoses.
†Coloboma, heart disease, atresia of choanae, retarded growth and development, genital hyperplasia, ear anomalies.

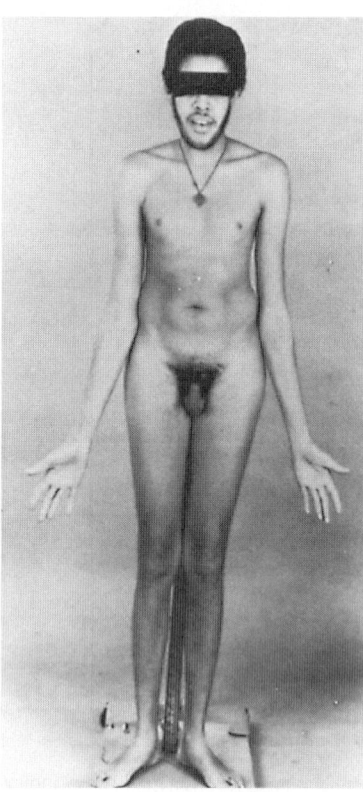

**FIGURE 115-19.** Patient with isolated deficiency of luteinizing hormone ("fertile eunuch"). Note the eunuchoidal body proportions but pubertal development and partial masculinization. Serum testosterone levels ranged from 1 to 2 ng/mL, which are well above the normal female range and those seen in hypogonadotropic hypogonadism, but below those of a normal man. (From Killinger DW. The testis. In: Ezrin C, Godden JO, Volpé R, eds. Systematic endocrinology, 2nd ed. Hagerstown, MD: Harper & Row, 1979:232.)

larly in women and men, with a failure to proceed through puberty. These patients usually appear as normal prepubertal females and only rarely have had any signs of pubertal development. In addition, they may have other characteristic somatic features, including anosmia, short fourth metacarpals, and midline defects.

Other syndromes manifest as isolated gonadotropin deficiency. Most of these are associated with severe neurologic damage and mental retardation (Table 115-5).

## ISOLATED DEFICIENCY OF LUTEINIZING HORMONE OR FOLLICLE-STIMULATING HORMONE

The original reports of isolated LH deficiency occurred in eunuchoid men with testicular volumes, suggesting some development greater than that seen in patients with idiopathic hypogonadotropic hypogonadism.[158,159] The term *fertile eunuch* was applied to these men, although most are infertile because the low intratesticular concentrations of testosterone do not support complete spermatogenesis.[160] In these patients, testicular biopsy specimens reveal some progression of spermatogenesis. The serum testosterone levels are also low, accounting for the eunuchoid body habitus (Fig. 115-19). Therapy with hCG restores normal serum testosterone levels and completes spermatogenesis.[161] Because data have shown that some men with classic idiopathic hypogonadotropic hypogonadism and low levels of both serum LH and FSH may have testicular volumes >5 mL and may demonstrate complete spermatogenesis with hCG alone, these syndromes most likely are a part of the spectrum of the same disease. A group of older men who manifest impotence, low serum testosterone levels, low LH levels, and normal FSH levels has been described (see Chap. 114).

These men have gone through normal puberty and fathered children, and whether their LH deficiency is acquired or is a late expression of a congenital disorder has not been determined.

Isolated deficiency of FSH also has been reported.[162,163] Men with this disorder are seen for infertility and are normally androgenized. They are not eunuchoid in appearance, have normal serum testosterone levels, and have sperm counts ranging from azoospermia to oligospermia.

In addition to syndromes of isolated FSH deficiency, male hypogonadism has been reported to be due to mutations in the β subunit of FSH that result in an inactive protein.[164]

## ACQUIRED FORMS OF GONADOTROPIN DEFICIENCY

Gonadotropin deficiency may result from numerous acquired disorders, as noted in Table 115-6. These lesions had been thought to be caused by the loss of gonadotropin secretion by compression and necrosis of pituitary tissue. This especially appears to be true in the case of tumors or granulomatous disease. However, some pituitary lesions can cause hypogonadism without anatomically affecting the pituitary tissue. For instance, tumors that produce corticotropin-releasing hormone, cortisol, or prolactin may directly inhibit gonadotropin secretion. Clinically, the appearance of these patients depends on whether or not they have gone through puberty (see Table 115-2).

Patients who have space-occupying lesions of the sella may lose secretion of other pituitary hormones and have symptoms of multiple hormone deficiencies (i.e., hypothyroidism due to thyroid-stimulating hormone deficiency, hypoadrenalism due to adrenocorticotropic hormone deficiency). Before puberty,

## TABLE 115-6.
### Causes of Acquired Gonadotropin Deficiency

**CONDITIONS THAT OFTEN OCCUR BEFORE PUBERTY**
  Craniopharyngioma
  Eosinophilic granuloma
**CONDITIONS THAT USUALLY OCCUR AFTER PUBERTY**
  Functioning pituitary tumors
    Prolactinoma
    Growth hormone–secreting tumor
    Adrenocorticotropic hormone–secreting tumor
  Nonfunctioning pituitary tumors
    Chromophobe adenoma
    Sarcoma
  Irradiation
  Granulomatous disease: eosinophilic granuloma, sarcoidosis, tuberculosis
  Tumors metastasized to the pituitary
  Pituitary abscess
  Pituitary apoplexy, often with the degeneration of pituitary tumor or cyst
  Postpartum pituitary hemorrhage: Sheehan syndrome
  Arteriovenous malformations
  Hemochromatosis
  Autoimmune pituitary hypophysitis

manifestations of growth hormone deficiency may be present. However, clinical growth hormone deficiency is not seen after puberty because maximum growth has already occurred. Some of the causes of acquired gonadotropin deficiency are listed in Table 115-5.

## PROLACTIN-SECRETING PITUITARY TUMORS

Prolactin-producing tumors of the pituitary have been divided into microadenomas (<10 mm in diameter) and macroadenomas (>10 mm in diameter) (see Chap. 13). In women, >80% of the tumors are microadenomas; in men, 80% are macroadenomas.[165,166] This difference may result from earlier detection in women (due to the occurrence of galactorrhea or of irregular menstrual cycles) or from a difference between the two sexes in the character of tumor growth. Because galactorrhea occurs so rarely in men, even in men with high serum prolactin levels, early clinical signs of the tumor are not available. Therefore, the tumor may not be manifest until symptoms caused by the mass of the lesion are present.[167] In some men, temporal lobe epilepsy has been associated with hyperprolactinemia.[168]

The mechanism by which prolactin-producing pituitary adenomas cause hypogonadism has not been well defined. Prolactin had been thought to lower basal serum LH and FSH levels, but this has been an inconsistent finding. A change in LH pulse amplitude or frequency has occurred in some men.[169] Another possibility is that a single neurotransmitter, such as dopamine (see Chap. 16) or γ-aminobutyrate, may be involved. The latter may both stimulate serum prolactin and suppress serum LH, in which case the prolactin itself may have little direct effect on gonadal function.[170]

The diagnosis of a prolactinoma requires the finding of an elevated serum prolactin level. Most men with demonstrable prolactinomas have serum prolactin levels of >50 ng/mL. Computerized tomography of the sella is the current standard for demonstrating the tumor mass and should be performed in men with elevated serum prolactin levels. Although magnetic resonance imaging (MRI) of the sella may be useful, instruments of <1.5 tesla usually cannot achieve the resolution necessary to define a tumor <10 mm in diameter. The exclusion of other causes of hyperprolactinemia (e.g., hypothyroidism, medication, renal failure) is obligatory. As with any large pituitary tumor, the testing of visual fields and of other pituitary functions should be considered (see Chaps. 17 and 19).

The treatment of prolactinoma is discussed in Chapters 13, 21, 22, and 23. Changes in Leydig cell function usually correlate well with reductions in serum prolactin levels, and normal levels of testosterone and potency are associated with a decrease in serum prolactin levels to normal. The resumption of spermatogenesis and subsequent fertility have been less consistent, however; the rate of restored fertility after the treatment of prolactinomas in men is 50% or less.[171] As is the case in many forms of male infertility, the reasons are not entirely clear. Although isolated case reports suggest that a clinical trial of therapy with gonadotropins may be justified, such a study has not yet been accomplished.

A report of a prolactinoma enlarging during testosterone replacement therapy suggests that tumor size should be reassessed periodically if androgen replacement is necessary in a man with a prolactinoma.[171]

## INFECTIONS OF THE HYPOTHALAMUS AND PITUITARY

Although it is uncommon, systemic infections such as tuberculosis and leptospirosis may destroy either the hypothalamus or pituitary and result in the loss of gonadotropin secretion.

## SEVERE SYSTEMIC ILLNESS

Severe systemic illness has a profound effect on gonadal function (see Chap. 116). Only a few specific entities are examined in this section.

A marked decrease in testosterone is seen early in the course of thermal injury.[172] This decrease in serum testosterone is associated with a modest decrease in serum immunoassayable LH and a marked decrease in serum bioactive LH. This difference may be related to the high levels of serum estradiol that are present. Estradiol can cause increased secretion of a form of LH that is not bioactive.[173,174] In addition, the high level of cortisol seen with stress may inhibit the output of LHRH. The suppression of testosterone in these men is proportional to the surface area of the burn and, therefore, correlates inversely with survival. Of further interest are the markedly decreased levels of SHBG immediately after the burn; however, the levels of biologically available testosterone also are low because of the extremely low levels of total testosterone. As the patient recovers from the burn and total testosterone rises, SHBG rises, so that bioavailable testosterone does not increase for a prolonged period after the burn. In these men, the serum LH and FSH responses to exogenous LHRH are normal.[175] Autopsy studies of men who have died of burns but did not have scrotal injury reveal disordered spermatogenesis.

The illness may result from physical injury or a systemic medical disorder. In some circumstances, the defects in testicular function are a result of treatment (e.g., head irradiation for CNS tumors). In most of these situations, the hypogonadism is reversible with resolution of the illness.[176,177]

Although obesity is not considered an acute illness, free and total testosterone levels are decreased in men with a body mass index of 30 or greater. This is accompanied by an attenuated LH pulse amplitude, suggesting that these men may be truly hypogonadal because of their weight.[178]

Similar mechanisms for decreased serum levels of gonadal steroids are encountered in normal individuals who are subjected to severe physical stress.[173]

No studies have shown benefit from testosterone treatment of critically ill men. Although administration of androgen therapy to reverse their catabolic state may be tempting, until controlled studies demonstrate benefit, even short-term therapy should not be tried because it may be harmful (as is the case for thyroid hormone replacement therapy in the critically ill).

## UREMIA

Hypogonadism is a common finding in men undergoing dialysis.[179–181] Uremia often is associated with marked hyperpro-

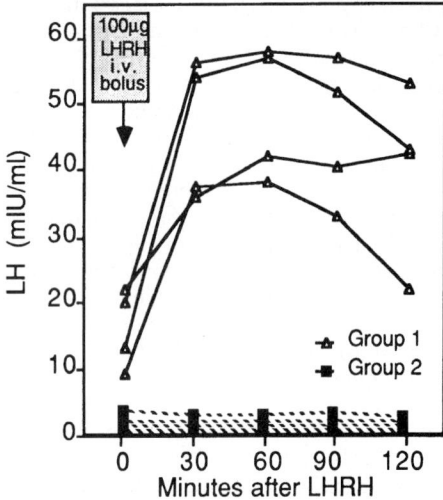

**FIGURE 115-20.** Luteinizing hormone (*LH*) response to luteinizing hormone–releasing hormone (*LHRH*) in two groups of men with hemochromatosis. Patients in group 1 (*solid lines* and *triangles*) had lower serum ferritin levels than patients in group 2 (*dotted lines* and *squares*) and, presumably, a lesser degree of pituitary failure.

lactinemia, and originally this was thought to be the reason for the hypogonadism. However, if the prolactin level is decreased with bromocriptine, the serum testosterone level remains low, although the libido is improved.[181] Two other factors in uremia may contribute to the hypogonadism. One is zinc deficiency, although zinc replacement has not corrected the hypogonadism completely.[182] An accumulation of a toxic product also occurs in uremia that impairs testicular function (see Chap. 209).[183] Use of androgen replacement therapy in patients with uremia who are receiving dialysis has been a standard practice, primarily as a means of increasing erythrocyte production.

## LYMPHOCYTIC HYPOPHYSITIS

Lymphocytic hypophysitis has been described as a cause for secondary hypogonadism with no defined infectious agent. On CT or MRI scan, the disease may mimic a pituitary adenoma. Surgical removal does not restore function, and treatment is replacement therapy.[184]

## HEMOCHROMATOSIS

In hemochromatosis, excessive tissue iron stores are present (see Chap. 131). Usually, hemochromatosis is clinically manifest by the presence of liver disease, and the hypogonadism that occurs in as many as 60% of these men originally was thought to be secondary to the hepatic abnormalities. More recent investigations have shown that the causative lesion resides in the pituitary and is related to the severity of iron overload.[185] Serum testosterone, LH, and FSH levels are low. The response of serum gonadotropins to LHRH stimulation decreases as the severity of the systemic disease increases, and is totally absent in severe cases of hemochromatosis. However, the testes respond normally to hCG. Thus, the primary defect appears to be pituitary failure (Fig. 115-20).

Treatment of the hemochromatosis with phlebotomy in young men results in a partial normalization of hypothalamic–pituitary–gonadal function. This improvement occurs in a minority of men, however, and is only partial. The younger the man, the greater is the likelihood of improvement; amelioration of established disease in men older than 40 years is rare.[186]

## COMBINED PRIMARY AND SECONDARY HYPOGONADISM

### AGING

Women undergo a marked change in gonadal function with age, as evidenced by menopause, but the situation in men is less clear. Early studies demonstrated a well-defined change in total serum testosterone levels with age.[187] However, because many of these studies involved men with systemic illnesses, and because these illnesses by themselves may significantly affect gonadal function, the results probably were not representative of the normal aging process without superimposed disease (see Chap. 199). Studies involving normal, older, healthy men have demonstrated few differences compared to younger men.[188] Nevertheless, a small difference persists, especially when diurnal variations in total testosterone are examined.[189] When the bioavailable (non–SHBG-bound) testosterone was measured, a more marked difference between young and elderly populations was discovered.[190] Part of the reason for the greater difference in non–SHBG-bound testosterone than in total testosterone is the slight fall in total serum testosterone that occurs with age and the increase in SHBG, which further decreases the available testosterone.[191] The reason for the increase in SHBG is not well understood. Explanations include stimulation by the increased serum estrogen that occurs with age, possible alteration in response to decreased thyroid hormones, or a change in glycosylation of the SHBG that might prolong the circulating half-life of this protein.

One aspect of male gonadal function that changes significantly with age is potency. Some investigators have interpreted this change in potency as indicating a change in gonadal function.[192] When these men have been examined critically, however, their serum testosterone levels and other aspects of gonadal function have been found to be only minimally different from those of potent age-matched men, suggesting that hypogonadism alone is an uncommon cause of impotence in elderly men.[193] The most common finding in this group is a high incidence of chronic systemic disease, which may involve the neurologic or vascular systems necessary for potency, or may necessitate the use of medications such as antihypertensive agents, which affect potency. In addition to an effect on Leydig cell function, age also appears to cause a decline in spermatogenesis.

The reason for the decline in gonadal function in healthy older men is not clear. The rat demonstrates a decline with age in LH output from the pituitary and a decreased response of the testes to hCG.[194] In older men, basal serum LH levels usually are increased, and the output of gonadotropins in response to LHRH is greater than occurs in younger men.[195] The decreased response of the testes to hCG stimulation in older men suggests a primary testicular cause for the age-related decline in testosterone. Thus, two factors appear to contribute to hypogonadism in aging men: a decrease in testosterone production and an increase in binding of circulating testosterone. The consequences of these decreased testosterone levels on the aging process have not been defined. Although serum testosterone levels may be somewhat below the normal range in normal, potent, older men, such a finding in impotent men does not mean that other factors, such as neurologic or vascular disease, should be excluded.

The efficacy or safety of routine testosterone therapy for otherwise healthy older men with low serum testosterone levels and normal gonadotropin levels has not been supported by long-term studies. Preliminary studies in older men with low testosterone levels suggest that some improvement in bone and muscle status may occur; however, no clinical improvement in frailty has been demonstrated.[196,197] Several long-term studies are being conducted to resolve this issue. Until these studies are completed, testosterone therapy for older men who have only modest decreases in testosterone is not indicated.

The routine treatment of otherwise normal elderly men with testosterone is not indicated. This is particularly important because subclinical carcinoma of the prostate could be aggravated and cardiovascular risk factors are exacerbated by such therapy.

## HEPATIC CIRRHOSIS

Both cirrhosis and significant ethanol ingestion have major effects on testicular function (see Chaps. 205 and 233). Acute ethanol ingestion lowers serum testosterone levels and raises LH levels, findings that suggest a primary effect on the testes.[198,199] One way in which ethanol may acutely inhibit spermatogenesis is by interfering with alcohol dehydrogenase. This enzyme is necessary for the metabolism of retinol, an important substrate for normal spermatogenesis; ethanol has an affinity for this enzyme that is 50 times greater than the affinity for retinol. Therefore, ethanol ingestion alone without any secondary damage to the liver may inhibit testicular function. Normal men who ingest significant amounts of ethanol and achieve blood alcohol levels >0.10 mg/dL have a temporary decrease in serum testosterone and a rise in LH.

If the long-term ingestion of ethanol results in cirrhotic changes of the liver, permanent alterations in gonadal function occur. These include suppression of gonadotropin release and decreased testosterone production.[200] In addition, a rise in SHBG may lead to a further decrease in bioavailable testosterone. The SHBG in these individuals may be abnormal; inhibition of transport of testosterone is retarded, as would be expected by a rise in SHBG, but no inhibition of estradiol transport occurs.[201] Estradiol production is increased and provides an additional explanation for the gynecomastia. Furthermore, although serum testosterone levels are decreased, the increased availability of estradiol also may provide a mechanism for the suppression of gonadotropin output.

## SICKLE CELL DISEASE

Men with sickle cell disease display characteristics of prepubertal hypogonadism.[202,203] They have eunuchoid skeletal proportions, small testes, decreased muscle mass, and decreased hair growth. Because most patients with sickle cell disease are black, however, their eunuchoid skeletal proportions may not be abnormal. Normal black men may have skeletal proportions that tend to fit the definition of eunuchoid measurements in whites. In some patients with sickle cell disease, serum testosterone levels are low, but LH and FSH levels may be inappropriately normal. LHRH tests have yielded equivocal results.

These findings suggest that several possible causes probably exist for the hypogonadism, including hypogonadotropic hypogonadism of chronic stress and specific destruction of testicular tissue because of interruption of the blood supply by the sickling process. Hypogonadism also may be caused by malnutrition and, possibly, zinc deficiency. Treatment with androgens has not been studied systematically in these patients.

## REFERENCES

1. Hobbs C, Plymate S, Rosen C, Adler R. Testosterone administration increases insulin-like growth factor I levels in normal men. J Clin Endocrinol Metab 1993; 77:776.
2. Peiris A, Stagner J, Plymate S, Vogel R. Relationship between secretory pulses to sex hormone binding globulin in normal men. J Clin Endocrinol Metab 1993; 76:279.
3. Weissberger A, Ho K. Activation of the somatotropic axis by testosterone in adult males: evidence for the role of aromatization. J Clin Endocrinol Metab 1993; 76:1407.
4. Mosher WD. Infertility trends among U.S. couples: 1965–1976. Family 1982; 14:22.
5. Goodfellow P, Lovell-Badge R. SRY and sex determination in mammals. Annu Rev Genet 1993; 27:71.
6. Nagao RR, Plymate SR, Berger RE, et al. Comparison of gonadal function between fertile and infertile men with varicoceles. Fertil Steril 1986; 46:930.
7. Klinefelter HG Jr, Reifenstein EC Jr, Albright F. Syndrome characterized by gynecomastia, aspermatogenesis without a-Leydigism and increased excretion of follicle-stimulating hormone. J Clin Endocrinol Metab 1942; 2:615.
8. Plunkett ER, Barr ML. Cytologic tests of sex in congenital testicular hypoplasia. J Clin Endocrinol Metab 1956; 16:829.
9. Lodi A, Monti D, Gaspari G, et al. Klinefelter's syndrome in nontwin brothers and maternal XX/XXX mosaicism. J Endocrinol Invest 1979; 2:419.
10. Laron Z, Hochman H. Small testes in prepubertal boys with Klinefelter's syndrome. J Clin Endocrinol Metab 1971; 32:671.
11. Ratcliffe SG. The sexual development of boys with the chromosome constitution of 47 XXY (Klinefelter's syndrome). In: Bancroft J, ed. Clinics in endocrinology and metabolism, vol 11. Philadelphia: WB Saunders, 1982:703.
12. Plymate SR, Leonard JM, Paulsen CA, et al. Sex hormone-binding globulin changes with androgen replacement. J Clin Endocrinol Metab 1983; 57:645.
13. Plymate SR, Paulsen CA. Klinefelter's syndrome. In: King R, Motulsky A, eds. The genetic basis of common disease. New York: Oxford University Press, 1989: 127.
14. Wang C, Baker HW, Burger HG, et al. Hormonal studies in Klinefelter's syndrome. Clin Endocrinol (Oxf) 1975; 4:399.
15. Wieland RG, Zorn EM, Johnson MW. Elevated testosterone-binding globulin in Klinefelter's syndrome. J Clin Endocrinol Metab 1980; 51:1199.
16. Gabrilove JL, Freiberg EK, Thornton JC, Nicholis GL. Effect of age on testicular function in Klinefelter's syndrome. Clin Endocrinol (Oxf) 1979; 11:343.
17. Ratcliffe SG, Bancroft J, Axworthy D, McCloren W. Klinefelter's syndrome in adolescence. Arch Dis Child 1982; 57:6.
18. Nistal M, Santamaria L, Paniagua R. Quantitative and ultrastructural study of Leydig cells in Klinefelter's syndrome. J Pathol 1985; 146:323.
19. Nistal M, Paniagua R, Abaurrea MA, Santamaria L. Hyperplasia and the immature appearance of Sertoli cells in primary testicular disorders. Hum Pathol 1982; 13:3.
20. Sasagawa I, Katayama T. Ultrastructural study of Leydig cells in cases with Klinefelter's syndrome. J Clin Electron Microsc 1985; 18:163.
21. Schill WB, Strasser R, Krassnigg F, et al. Spermatological investigation in men with Klinefelter's syndrome. In: Bandmann HJ, Breit R, Perwein E, eds. Klinefelter's syndrome. New York: Springer-Verlag, 1984:147.
22. Ohno S. Control of meiotic processes. In: Troen P, Nankin H, eds. The testis in normal and infertile men. New York: Raven Press, 1976:1.
23. Jequirer AM, Bullimore NJ. Testicular and epididymal histology in a fetus with Klinefelter's syndrome at 22 weeks' gestation. Br J Urol 1989; 11:214.
24. Guttenbach M, Michekmann H, Hinney B, et al. Segregation of sex chromosomes into sperm nuclei in a man with 47,XXY Klinefelter's karyotype: a FISH analysis. Hum Genet 1997; 4:474.
25. Swanson DW, Stipes AN. Psychiatric aspects of Klinefelter's syndrome. Am J Psychiatry 1969; 126:814.
26. Ferguson-Smith MA. The prepubertal testicular lesion in chromatin-positive Klinefelter's syndrome (primary micro-orchidism) as seen in mentally handicapped children. Lancet 1959; 1:219.
27. de la Chapelle A. Sex chromosome abnormalities among the mentally defective in Finland. J Ment Defic Res 1963; 7:129.
28. Witkin HA, Mednick SA, Schulsinger F, et al. Criminality in XYY and XXY men. Science 1976; 193:547.
29. Ratcliffe SG. Klinefelter's syndrome in children: a longitudinal study of 47,XXY boys identified by population screening in Klinefelter's syndrome. In: Bandmann HJ, Breit R, Perwein E, eds. Klinefelter's syndrome. New York: Springer-Verlag, 1984:38.
30. Becker KL. Clinical and therapeutic experiences with Klinefelter's syndrome. Fertil Steril 1972; 23:568.
31. Ferguson-Smith MA, Yates JRW. Maternal age specific rates for chromosome aberrations and factors influencing them. Prenat Diagn 1984; 4:5.
32. Carothers AD, Collyer S, de Mey R, Frackiewicz A. Parental age and birth order in the aetiology of some sex chromosome aneuploidics. Ann Hum Genet 1979; 41:227.
33. van Geel AN, van Slooten EA, Mavrunac M, Hart AA. A retrospective study of male breast cancer in Holland. Br J Surg 1985; 72:724.
34. Meister P. Klinefelter's syndrome and testicular tumors. In: Bandmann HJ, Briet R, Perwein E, eds. Klinefelter's syndrome. New York: Springer-Verlag, 1984:115.
35. Becher R. Klinefelter syndrome and malignant lymphoma. Cancer Genet Cytogenet 1986; 21:271.
36. Abidi SM, Griffiths M, Oscier DG, et al. Primary myelodysplastic syndrome with complex chromosomal rearrangements in a patient with Klinefelter's syndrome. J Med Genet 1986; 23:183.
37. Arens R, Marcus D, Engelberg S, et al. Cerebral germinomas and Klinefelter's syndrome. Cancer 1988; 61:1228.
38. Price WH, Clayton JF, Wilson J, et al. Causes of death in X chromatin positive males (Klinefelter's syndrome). J Epidemiol Community Health 1985; 39:330.
39. Schelberger T, Kekow J, Gross WL. Impaired T-cell-independent B-cell maturation in systemic lupus erythematosus. Coculture experiments in monozy-

gotic twins concordant for Klinefelter's syndrome but discordant for systemic lupus erythematosus. Clin Immunol Immunopathol 1986; 40:365.

40. Alarcon-Segovia D, Sauza J. Systemic lupus erythematosus and Klinefelter's syndrome. In: Bandmann HJ, Breit R, Perwein E, eds. Klinefelter's syndrome. New York: Springer-Verlag, 1984:109.

41. Berginer VM, Paran E, Hirsch M, Abelliovich D. Klinefelter's and Takayasu's syndromes in one patient—a pure coincidence? Angiology 1983; 34:170.

42. Armstrong RD, Macfarlane DG, Panayi GS. Ankylosing spondylitis and Klinefelter's syndrome: does the X chromosome modify disease expression? Br J Rheumatol 1985; 24:277.

43. Bizzaro A, Valentini G, DiMartino G, et al. Influences of testosterone therapy on clinical and immunological features of autoimmune disease associated with Klinefelter's syndrome. J Clin Endocrinol Metab 1987; 64:32.

44. Grossman CJ. Regulation of the immune system by sex steroids. Endocr Rev 1984; 5:435.

45. Jorgenson RJ. The conditions manifesting taurodontism. Am J Med Genet 1982; 11:435.

46. Verp MS, Simpson JL, Martin AO. Hypostatic ulcers in 47,XXY Klinefelter's syndrome. J Med Genet 1983; 20:100.

47. Fricke GR, Mattern HJ, Schweikert HU, Schwanitz G. Klinefelter's syndrome and mitral valve prolapse, an echocardiographic study in twenty-two patients. Biomed Pharmacother 1984; 38:88.

48. Geffner ME, Kaplan SA, Bersch N, et al. Insulin resistance in Klinefelter's syndrome. Clin Res 1985; 33:128A.

49. Rohde RA. Klinefelter's syndrome with pulmonary disease and other disorders. Lancet 1964; 2:149.

50. Bomers-Marres AJML. Klinefelter's syndrome with asthma. Lancet 1964; 2:364.

51. Delmas P, Meunier PJ. Osteoporosis in Klinefelter's syndrome. Quantitative bone histological data in 5 cases and relationship with hormonal deficiency. Nouv Presse Med 1981; 10:687.

52. Foresta C, Zanatta GP, Busnardo B, et al. Testosterone and calcitonin plasma levels in hypogonadal osteoporotic young men. J Endocrinol Invest 1985; 8:377.

53. Vogt HJ. Sexual behavior in Klinefelter's syndrome. In: Bandmann HJ, Breit R, Perwein E, eds. Klinefelter's syndrome. New York: Springer-Verlag, 1984:163.

54. Paulsen CA, Gordon DL, Carpenter RW, et al. Klinefelter's syndrome and its variants: a hormonal and chromosomal study. Recent Prog Horm Res 1968; 24:321.

55. Sarkar R, Marimathu KM. Association between the degree of mosaicism and the severity of syndrome in Turner's mosaics and Klinefelter's mosaics. Clin Genet 1983; 24:420.

56. Morishima A, Grumbach MM. The interrelationship of sex chromosome constitution and phenotype in the syndrome of gonadal dysgenesis and its variants. Ann N Y Acad Sci 1968; 155:695.

57. Forbes G, Porta C, Herr B, Griggs R. Sequence of changes in body composition induced by testosterone and reversal of changes after drug is stopped. JAMA 1992; 267:397.

58. Burris A, Banks S, Carter C, et al. A long-term prospective study of the physiologic and behavioral effects of hormone replacement in untreated hypogonadal men. J Androl 1992; 13:297.

59. Carani C, Bancroft J, Granata A, et al. Testosterone and erectile function, nocturnal penile tumescence and rigidity, and erectile response to visual erotic stimuli in hypogonadal and eugonadal men. Psychoneuroendocrinology 1992; 17:647.

60. Scane A, Francis R. Risk factors for osteoporosis in men. Clin Endocrinol (Oxf) 1993; 38:15.

61. Isaia G, Mussetta M, Pecchio F, et al. Effect of testosterone on bone in hypogonadal males. Maturitas 1992; 15:47.

62. Frey C. Klinefelter syndrome: is early diagnosis by screening study necessary? Monatsschr Kinderheilkd 1986; 134:78.

63. Borelli JB, Bender BG, Puck MH, et al. The meaning of early knowledge of a child's infertility in families with 47,XXY and 45,X children. Child Psychiatry Hum Dev 1984; 14:215.

64. Perez-Palacios G, Medina M, Ullao-Aguirre A, et al. Gonadotropin dynamics in XX males. J Clin Endocrinol Metab 1981; 53:254.

65. Fechner P, Marcantonio S, Jaswaney V, et al. The role of the sex-determining region Y gene in the etiology of 46, XX maleness. J Clin Endocrinol Metabol 1993; 76:690.

66. Davidoff F, Federman DD. Mixed gonadal dysgenesis. Pediatrics 1973; 52:725.

67. Philip J, Lundsteen C, Owen D. The frequency of chromosome aberrations in tall men with special reference to 47,XYY and 47,XXY. Am J Hum Genet 1976; 28:404.

68. Santen RJ, de Kretser DM, Paulsen CA, Vorhees J. Gonadotrophins and testosterone in the XYY syndrome. Lancet 1970; 2:371.

69. Skakkebaek NE, Hulten M, Jacobsen P, Mikkelsen M. Quantification of human seminiferous epithelium. II. Histological studies in eight 47,XYY men. J Reprod Fertil 1973; 32:391.

70. Noonan JA. Hypertelorism with Turner phenotype. Am J Dis Child 1968; 116:373.

71. Mendez HM, Opitz JM. Noonan syndrome: a review. Am J Med Genet 1985; 21:493.

72. Takeda R, Ueda M. Pituitary-gonadal function in male patients with myotonic dystrophy—serum luteinizing hormone, follicle-stimulating hor-

mone and testosterone levels, and histological damage of the testis. Acta Endocrinol (Copenh) 1977; 84:382.

73. Sagel J, Distiller LA, Morley JE, Isaacs H. Myotonia dystrophica: studies on gonadal function using luteinizing hormone-releasing hormone (LHRH). J Clin Endocrinol Metab 1975; 40:1110.

74. Mastrogiacomo I, Pagani E, Novelli G, et al. Male hypogonadism in myotonic dystrophy is related to (CTG)n triplet mutation. J Endocrinol Invest 1994; 17:381.

75. Wells S, Josefowicz R, Forbes G, Griggs R. Effect of testosterone on metabolic rate and body composition in normal men and men with muscular dystrophy. J Clin Endocrinol Metab 1992; 74:332.

76. de Kretser DM, Burger HG, Fortune D, et al. Hormonal, histological and chromosomal studies in adult males with testicular disorder. J Clin Endocrinol Metab 1972; 35:392.

77. de Kretser DM, Kerr JB, Paulsen CA. The peritubular tissue in the normal and pathological human testis: an ultrastructural study. Biol Reprod 1975; 12:317.

78. Green AA, Dynsley-Green A, Zachman M, et al. Congenital bilateral anorchia in childhood: a clinical, endocrine, and therapeutic evaluation of 21 cases. Clin Endocrinol (Oxf) 1976; 5:381.

79. Bergada C, Cleveland WW, Jones HW, Wilkins L. Variants of embryonic testicular dysgenesis: bilateral anorchia and the syndrome of rudimentary testes. Acta Endocrinol (Copenh) 1962; 40:521.

80. Forest MG. Inborn errors of testosterone biosynthesis in the intersex child. In: Josso N, ed. Pediatric and adolescent endocrinology, vol 8. Basel: Karger, 1981:133.

81. Goebelsmann U, Horton R, Mestman JH, et al. Male pseudohermaphroditism due to testicular 17β-hydroxysteroid dehydrogenase deficiency. J Clin Endocrinol Metab 1973; 36:867.

82. Saez JM, Morera AM, de Peretti E, Bertrand J. Further in vivo studies in male pseudohermaphroditism with gynecomastia due to a testicular 17-ketosteroid defect (compared to a case of testicular feminization). J Clin Endocrinol Metab 1972; 34:598.

83. Saez JM, de Peretti E, Morera AM, et al. Familial male pseudohermaphroditism with gynecomastia due to a testicular 17-ketosteroid reductase defect. I. In vivo studies. J Clin Endocrinol Metab 1971; 32:604.

84. Castro-Magana M, Angulo M, Uy J. Male hypogonadism with gynecomastia caused by late-onset deficiency of 17-ketosteroid reductase. N Engl J Med 1993; 328:1297.

85. Imperato-McGinley JL, Guerrero L, Gautier T, Peterson RE. Steroid 5α-reductase deficiency in man: an inherited form of male pseudohermaphroditism. Science 1974; 186:1213.

86. Walsh PC, Madden JD, Harrod MJ, et al. Familial incomplete male pseudohermaphroditism, type 2. Decreased dihydrotestosterone formation in pseudovaginal perineoscrotal hypospadias. N Engl J Med 1974; 291:944.

87. Peterson RE, Imperato-McGinley J, Gauiter T, Sturla E. Male pseudohermaphroditism due to steroid 5α-reductase deficiency. Am J Med 1977; 62:170.

88. Imperato-McGinley JL, Peterson RE. Male pseudohermaphroditism: the complexities of male phenotypic development. Am J Med 1976; 61:251.

89. Leshin M, Griffin JE, Wilson JD. Hereditary male pseudohermaphroditism associated with an unstable form of 5α-reductase. J Clin Invest 1978; 62:685.

90. Fisher KL, Kogut MD, Moore RJ, et al. Clinical, endocrinological, and enzymatic characterization of two patients with 5α-reductase deficiency: evidence that a single enzyme is responsible for the 5α-reduction of cortisol and testosterone. J Clin Endocrinol Metab 1978; 47:653.

91. David R, Yoon DJ, Landin L, et al. A syndrome of gonadotropin resistance possibly due to a luteinizing hormone receptor defect. J Clin Endocrinol Metab 1984; 59:156.

92. Josso N, Fetcke C, Cachin O, et al. Persistence of müllerian ducts in male pseudohermaphroditism and its relationship to cryptorchidism. Clin Endocrinol (Oxf) 1983; 19:247.

93. Kovacs WJ, Griffin JE, Weaver DD, et al. A mutation that causes lability of the androgen receptor under conditions that normally promote transformation to the DNA-binding state. J Clin Invest 1984; 73:1095.

94. Griffin JE, Wilson JD. The syndromes of androgen resistance. N Engl J Med 1980; 302:198.

95. Boyar RM, Moore RJ, Rosner W, et al. Studies on gonadotropin-gonadal dynamics in patients with androgen insensitivity. J Clin Endocrinol Metab 1978; 47:1116.

96. MacDonald PC, Madden JD, Brenner PF, et al. Origin of estrogen in normal men and in women with testicular feminization. J Clin Endocrinol Metab 1979; 49:905.

97. O'Leary JA. Comparative studies of the gonad in testicular feminization and cryptorchidism. Fertil Steril 1965; 16:813.

98. Kaufman M, Pinsky L, Baird PH, McGillivray BC. Complete androgen insensitivity with a normal amount of 5α-dihydrotestosterone-binding activity in labium majus skin fibroblasts. Am J Med Genet 1983; 4:401.

99. McPhaul MJ, Marcelli M, Zoppi S, et al. Genetic basis of endocrine disease: the spectrum of mutations in the androgen gene that causes androgen resistance. J Clin Endocrinol Metabol 1993; 76:17.

100. Reifenstein EC Jr. Hereditary familial hypogonadism. Clin Res 1947; 3:86.

101. Amrhein JA, Klingensmith GJ, Walsh PC, et al. Partial androgen insensitivity: Reifenstein syndrome revisited. N Engl J Med 1977; 297:350.

102. Wilson JD, Harrod MJ, Goldstein JL, Griffin JE. Familial incomplete male pseudohermaphroditism, type I. N Engl J Med 1974; 290:1097.

103. Griffin JE, Punyashthiti K, Wilson JD. Dihydrotestosterone binding by cultured human fibroblasts: comparison of cells from control subjects and from patients with hereditary male pseudohermaphroditism due to androgen resistance. J Clin Invest 1976; 57:1342.

104. Gyorki S, Warne GL, Khalid BAK, Funder JW. Defective nuclear accumulation of androgen receptors in disorders of sexual differentiation. J Clin Invest 1983; 72:819.

105. Eil C. Familial incomplete male pseudohermaphroditism associated with impaired nuclear androgen retention. J Clin Invest 1982; 71:850.

105a. Ahmed SF, Cheng A, Dovey L, et al. Phenotypic features, androgen receptor binding, and mutational analysis in 278 clinical cases reported as androgen insensitivity syndrome. J Clin Endocrinol Metab 2000; 815:658.

106. Bremner WJ, Ott J, Moore DJ, Paulsen CA. Reifenstein's syndrome: investigation of linkage to X-chromosomal loci. Clin Genet 1974; 6:216.

107. Wooster R, Mangion J, Eeles R, et al. A germline mutation in the androgen receptor gene in two brothers with breast cancer and Reifenstein syndrome. Nat Genet 1992; 2:132.

108. Fischbeck K. Kennedy disease. J Inherit Metab Dis 1997; 20(2):152.

109. Kazemi-Esfarjani P, Trifiro MA, Pinsky L. Evidence for a repressive function of long polyglutamine tract in the human androgen receptor: possible pathogenetic relevance for the (CAG)n-expanded neuronopathies. Hum Mol Genet 1995; 4:523.

110. Schoenberg MP, Hakimi JM, Wang S, et al. Microsatellite mutation (CAG 24-18) in the androgen receptor gene in human prostate cancer. Biochem Biophys Res Commun 1994; 198(1):74.

111. Hardy DO, Scher HI, Bogenreider T, et al. Androgen receptor CAG repeat lengths in prostate cancer: correlation with age of onset. J Clin Endocrinol Metab 1996; 81:4400.

112. Aiman J, Griffin JE, Gazak JM, et al. Androgen insensitivity as a cause of infertility in otherwise normal men. N Engl J Med 1979; 300:223.

113. Ballew JW, Masters WH. Mumps, a cause of infertility. I. Present consideration. Fertil Steril 1954; 5:536.

114. Savran J. Diethylstilbestrol in prevention of orchitis following mumps. Rhode Island Med J 1946; 29:662.

115. Mongon ES. The treatment of mumps orchitis with prednisone. Am J Med Sci 1959; 237:749.

116. Charney CW. The spermatogenic potential for the undescended testis before and after treatment. J Urol 1960; 83:697.

117. Rajfer J, Walsh PC. Testicular descent: normal and abnormal. Urol Clin North Am 1978; 5:223.

118. Albescu JZ, Bergada C, Cullen M. Male fertility in patients treated for cryptorchidism before puberty. Fertil Steril 1971; 22:829.

119. Rajfer J, Handelsman DJ, Swerdloff RS, et al. Hormonal therapy of cryptorchidism. A randomized double-blind study comparing human chorionic gonadotropin and gonadotropin releasing hormone. N Engl J Med 1986; 314:466.

120. Shilo S, Livshin Y, Sheskin J, Spitz IM. Gonadal function in lepromatous leprosy. Lepr Rev 1981; 52:127.

121. Kannan V, Vijaya G. Endocrine testicular functions in leprosy. Horm Metab Res 1984; 16:146.

122. Rowley MJ, Leach DR, Warner GA, Heller CG. Effect of graded doses of ionizing radiation in the human testis. Radiat Res 1974; 59:665.

123. Paulsen CA. The study of irradiation effects on the human testis, including histologic, chromosomal and hormonal aspects. Final progress report of AEC contract AT(45-1)-2225, Task Agreement 6. Atomic Energy Commission, 1973. RLO-2225-2.

124. Clifton DK, Bremner WJ. The effect of testicular x-irradiation on spermatogenesis in man. J Androl 1983; 4:387.

125. Handelsman DJ, Turtle JR. Testicular damage after radioactive iodine ($^{131}$I) therapy for thyroid cancer. Clin Endocrinol (Oxf) 1983; 18:465.

126. Haas GGJ, Cines DB, Schreiber AD. Immunologic infertility: identification of patients with antisperm antibody. N Engl J Med 1980; 303:722.

127. Elder M, Maclaren N, Riley W. Gonadal autoantibodies in patients with hypogonadism and/or Addison's disease. J Clin Endocrinol Metab 1981; 52:1137.

128. Schilsky RL, Lewis BJ, Sherins RJ, Young RC. Gonadal dysfunction in patients receiving chemotherapy for cancer. Ann Intern Med 1980; 93:109.

129. Shalet SM. Disorders of the endocrine system due to radiation and cytotoxic chemotherapy. Clin Endocrinol (Oxf) 1983; 18:637.

130. Chapman RM, Sutcliffe SB, Rees LH, et al. Cyclical combination chemotherapy and gonadal function. Lancet 1979; 1:285.

131. Friedman NM, Plymate SR. Leydig cell dysfunction and gynaecomastia in adult males treated with alkylating agents. Clin Endocrinol (Oxf) 1980; 12:553.

132. Kallmann FJ, Schoenfeld WA, Barrera SE. The genetic aspects of primary eunuchoidism. Am J Ment Defic 1944; 48:203.

133. Takeda T, Takasu N, Yamauchi K, et al. Magnetic resonance imaging of the hypoplasia of the rhinencephalon in a patient with Kallmann's syndrome. Intern Med 1992; 31:394.

134. Santen RJ, Paulsen CA. Hypogonadotropic eunuchoidism, I. Clinical study of the mode of inheritance. J Clin Endocrinol Metab 1973; 36:47.

135. Herzog AG, Seibel MM, Schomer DL, et al. Reproductive endocrine disorders in men with partial seizures of temporal lobe origin. Arch Neurol 1986; 43:347.

136. Merriam GR, Beitins IZ, Bode HH. Father-to-son transmission of hypogonadism with anosmia: Kallmann's syndrome. Am J Dis Child 1977; 131:1216.

137. Hermanussen M, Sippell WG. Heterogeneity of Kallmann's syndrome. Clin Genet 1985; 28:106.

138. Legouis R, Cohen-Salmon M, Del Castillo I, et al. Isolation and characterization of the gene responsible for the X chromosome-linked Kallmann syndrome. Biomed Pharmacother 1994; 48:241.

139. de Zoysa P, Helliwell R, Duke VM, et al. Contrasting expression of KAL in cell-free systems: 5′ UTR and coding region structural effects on translation. Protein Expr Purif 1998; 13:235.

140. Maya-Nunez G, Zenteno J, Ulloa-Aguirre A, et al. A recurrent missense mutation in the KAL gene in patients with x-linked Kallmann's syndrome. J Clin Endocrinol Metab 1998; 83:1650.

141. Henkin RF, Barter FC. Olfactory thresholds in normal men and in patients with adrenocortical insufficiency. J Clin Invest 1966; 45:1631.

142. Schwankhaus JD, Currie J, Jaffe MJ, et al. Neurological findings in men with isolated hypogonadotropic hypogonadism. Neurology 1989; 39:223.

143. Yoshimoto Y, Moridera K, Imura H. Restoration of normal pituitary gonadotropin reserve by administration of luteinizing-hormone-releasing hormone in patients with hypogonadotropic hypogonadism. N Engl J Med 1975; 292:242.

144. Spratt DI, Finkelstein JS, O'Dea LS, et al. Long-term administration of gonadotropin-releasing hormone in men with idiopathic hypogonadotropic hypogonadism. A model for studies of the hormone's physiologic effects. Ann Intern Med 1986; 105:848.

145. Hoffman AR, Crowley WF Jr. Induction of puberty in men by long-term pulsatile administration of low-dose gonadotropin-releasing hormone. N Engl J Med 1982; 307:1237.

146. Bremner WJ, Fernando NN, Paulsen CA. The effect of luteinizing hormone-releasing hormone in hypogonadotrophic eunuchoidism. Acta Endocrinol (Copenh) 1977; 85:1.

147. Gauthier G. Olfacto-genital dysplasia (agenesis of the olfactory lobes) with absence of gonadal development at puberty. Acta Neurochurg 1960; 21:345.

148. Bardin CW, Ross GT, Rifkind AB, et al. Studies of the pituitary-Leydig cell axis in young men with hypogonadotrophic hypogonadism and hyposmia: comparison with normal men, prepubertal boys, and hypopituitary patients. J Clin Invest 1969; 48:2046.

149. Boyar RM, Finkelstein JW, Witkin M, et al. Studies of endocrine function in isolated gonadotropin deficiency. J Clin Endocrinol Metab 1973; 36:64.

150. Dunkel L. Metoclopramide test in the diagnosis of isolated hypogonadotrophic hypogonadism. Acta Endocrinol (Copenh) 1986; 111:241.

151. Winters SJ. How to diagnose delayed puberty? Int J Androl 1984; 7:177.

151a. Zitzman M, Nieschlag E. Hormone substitution in male hypogonadism. Mol Cell Endocrinal 2000; 161:73.

151b. Yesilova Z, Ozata M, Kocar IH, et al. The effects of gonadotropin treatment on the immunological features of male patients with idiopathic hypogonadotropic hypogonadism. J Clin Endocrinol Metab 2000; 85:66.

152. Paulsen CA. The effect of human menopausal gonadotrophin on spermatogenesis in hypogonadotrophic hypogonadism. In: Proceedings of the Sixth Pan-American Congress of Endocrinology. Amsterdam: Excerpta Medica, 1966.

153. Paulsen CA, Espeland DH, Michals EL. Effect of HCG, HMG, HLH and HGH administration on testicular function. In: Rosenberg E, Paulsen CA, eds. The human testis. New York: Plenum Press, 1970:547.

154. Sherins RJ. Clinical aspects of treatment of male infertility with gonadotropins: testicular response of some men given HCG with and without pergonal. In: Mancini RE, Mortini L, eds. Male infertility and sterility. New York: Academic Press, 1974:545.

155. Ley SB, Leonard JM. Male hypogonadotropic hypogonadism: factors influencing response to human chorionic gonadotropin and human menopausal gonadotropin, including prior exogenous androgens. J Clin Endocrinol Metab 1985; 61:746.

156. Hazard J, Rozenberg I, Perlemuter L, et al. Gonadotropin responses to low-dose pulsatile administration of GnRH in a case of anosmia with hypogonadotropic hypogonadism associated with gonadal dysgenesis 47 XXY. Acta Endocrinol (Copenh) 1986; 113:593.

157. Santoro N, Filicori M, Crowley WF Jr. Hypogonadotropic disorders in men and women: diagnosis and therapy with pulsatile gonadotropin-releasing hormone. Endocr Rev 1986; 7:11.

158. Pasqualini RW, Bur GE. Hypoandrogenic syndrome with spermatogenesis. Fertil Steril 1955; 6:144.

159. Faiman C, Hoffman RJ, Ryan RJ, Albert A. The "fertile eunuch" syndrome: demonstration of isolated luteinizing hormone deficiency by radioimmunoassay technique. Mayo Clin Proc 1968; 43:661.

160. McCullagh EP, Beck JC, Jones HW. A syndrome of eunuchoidism with spermatogenesis, normal urinary FSH and low or normal ICSH (fertile "eunuchs"). J Clin Endocrinol Metab 1953; 13:489.

161. Al-Ansari AA, Khalil TH, Kelani Y, Mortimer CH. Isolated follicle-stimulating hormone deficiency in men: successful long-term gonadotropin therapy. Fertil Steril 1984; 42:618.

162. Mozaffarian GA, Higley M, Paulsen CA. Clinical studies in an adult male patient with "isolated follicle stimulating hormone (FSH) deficiency." J Androl 1983; 4:393.

163. Maroulis G, Parlow AF, Marshall JR. Isolated follicle-stimulating hormone deficiency in man. Fertil Steril 1977; 28:818.

164. Phillip M, Arbelle JE, Segev Y, Parvari R. Male hypogonadism due to a mutation in the gene for the beta-subunit of follicle-stimulating hormone. N Engl J Med 1998; 338:1729.

165. Rodman EF, Goodman R. Prolactinomas in males. In: Olefsky JM, Robbins RJ, eds. Prolactinomas—contemporary issues in endocrinology and metabolism, vol 2. New York: Churchill Livingstone, 1986:115.

166. Carter JN, Tyson JE, Tolis G, et al. Prolactin-secreting tumors and hypogonadism in 22 men. N Engl J Med 1978; 299:847.
167. Greenspan SL, Neer RM, Ridgway EC, Klibanski A. Osteoporosis in men with hyperprolactinemic hypogonadism. Ann Intern Med 1986; 104:777.
168. Spark RF, Wills CA, Royal H. Hypogonadism, hyperprolactinaemia, and temporal lobe epilepsy in hyposexual men. Lancet 1984; 1:413.
169. Winters SJ, Troen P. Altered pulsatile secretion of luteinizing hormone in hypogonadal men with hyperprolactinemia. Clin Endocrinol (Oxf) 1984; 21:257.
170. Fuchs E, Mansky T, Stock KW, et al. Involvement of catecholamines and glutamate in GABAergic mechanisms regulatory to luteinizing hormone and prolactin. Neuroendocrinology 1984; 38:484.
171. Murray FT, Cameron DF, Ketchum C. Return of gonadal function in men with prolactin-secreting pituitary tumors. J Clin Endocrinol Metab 1984; 59:79.
172. Plymate SR, Vaughan GM, Mason AD Jr, Pruitt BA Jr. Central hypogonadism in burned men. Horm Res 1987; 27:152.
173. Friedl KE, Plymate SR, Bernhard WN, Mohr LC. Elevation of plasma estradiol in healthy men during a mountaineering expedition. Horm Metab Res 1988; 20:239.
174. Veldhuis JD, Sowers JR, Rogol AD, et al. Pathophysiology of male hypogonadism associated with endogenous hyperestrogenism. Evidence for dual defects in the gonadal axis. N Engl J Med 1985; 312:1371.
175. Dolecek R, Dvoracek C, Jezek M, et al. Very low serum testosterone levels and severe impairment of spermatogenesis in burned male patients. Correlations with basal levels and levels of FSH, LH and PRL after LHRH + TRH. Endocrinol Experimentalis 1983; 17:33.
176. Constine L, Woolf P, Cann D, et al. Hypothalamic-pituitary dysfunction after irradiation for brain tumors. N Engl J Med 1993; 328:87.
177. Spratt D, Bigos S, Beitens I, et al. Both hyper- and hypogonadotropic hypogonadism occur transiently in acute illness: bio- and immunoreactive gonadotropins. J Clin Endocrinol Metab 1992; 75:1562.
178. Vermeulen A, Kaufman J, Deslypere J, Thomas G. Attenuated luteinizing hormone (LH) pulse amplitude but normal LH pulse frequency, and its relation to plasma androgens in hypogonadism of obese men. J Clin Endocrinol Metab 1993; 76:1140.
179. Lim VS, Fang VS. Gonadal dysfunction in uremic men. A study of the hypothalamo-pituitary testicular axis before and after renal transplantation. Am J Med 1975; 58:655.
180. Sawin CT, Longcope C, Schmitt GW, Ryan RJ. Blood levels of gonadotropins and gonadal hormones in gynecomastia associated with chronic hemodialysis. J Clin Endocrinol Metab 1973; 36:988.
181. Handelsman DJ. Hypothalamic-pituitary gonadal dysfunction in renal failure, dialysis and renal transplantation. Endocr Rev 1985; 6:151.
182. Mahajan SK, Abbasi AA, Prasad AS, et al. Effect of oral zinc therapy on gonadal function in hemodialysis patients. A double-blind study. Ann Intern Med 1982; 97:357.
183. Massry SC, Goldstein DA, Procci WR, Keltzky OA. Impotence in patients with uremia: a possible role for parathyroid hormone. Nephron 1977; 19:305.
184. Farah JO, Rossi M, Foy PM, MacFarlane IA. Cystic lymphocytic hypophysitis, visual field defects and hypopituitarism. Int J Clin Pract 1999; 53:643.
185. Sparacia G, Iaia A, Banco A, et al. Transfusional hemochromatosis: quantitative relation of HIR imaging pituitary signal intensity reduction to hypogonadotropic hypogonadism. Radiology 2000; 215:818;
186. Cundy T, Butler J, Bomford A, Williams R. Reversibility of hypogonadotrophic hypogonadism associated with genetic haemochromatosis. Clin Endocrinol (Oxf) 1993; 38:617.
187. Vermeulen A. Androgen secretion after age 50 in both sexes. Horm Res 1983; 18:37.
188. Harman SM, Tsitouras PD. Reproductive hormones in aging men. I. Measurement of sex steroids, basal luteinizing hormone, and Leydig cell response to human chorionic gonadotropin. J Clin Endocrinol Metab 1980; 51:35.
189. Bremner WJ, Vitiello MV, Prinz PN. Loss of circadian rhythmicity in blood testosterone levels with aging in normal men. J Clin Endocrinol Metab 1983; 56:1278.
190. Tenover JS, Matsumoto AM, Plymate SR, Bremner WJ. The effects of aging in normal men on bioavailable testosterone and luteinizing hormone secretion: response to clomiphene citrate. J Clin Endocrinol Metab 1987; 65:1118.
191. Nankin HR, Calkins JH. Decreased bioavailable testosterone in aging normal and impotent men. J Clin Endocrinol Metab 1986; 63:1418.
192. Davidson JM, Chen JJ, Crapo L, et al. Hormonal changes and sexual function in aging men. J Clin Endocrinol Metab 1983; 57:71.
193. Knussman R, Christiansen K. Relations between sex hormone levels and sexual behaviour in men. Arch Sex Behav 1986; 15:429.
194. Karpas AE, Bremner WJ, Clifton DK, et al. Diminished LH pulse frequency and amplitude with aging in the male rat. Endocrinology 1983; 112:788.
195. Nieschlag E, Lammers U, Freischem CW, et al. Reproductive functions in young fathers and grandfathers. J Clin Endocrinol Metab 1982; 55:676.
196. Tenover J. Effects of testosterone supplementation in the aging male. J Clin Endocrinol Metab 1992; 75:1092.
197. Morley J, Perry H, Kaiser F, et al. Effects of testosterone replacement therapy in old hypogonadal males. J Am Geriatr Soc 1993; 41:149.
198. Galvao-Teles A, Monteiro E, Gavaler JS, Van Thiel DH. Gonadal consequences of alcohol abuse: lessons from the liver. Hepatology 1986; 6:135.
199. Ida Y, Tsujimaru S, Nakamaura K, et al. Effects of acute and repeated alcohol ingestion on hypothalamic-pituitary-gonadal and hypothalamic-pituitary-adrenal functioning in normal males. Drug Alcohol Depend 1992; 31:57.
200. Bannister P, Handley T, Chapman C, Losowsky MS. Hypogonadism in chronic liver disease: impaired release of luteinising hormone. BMJ 1986; 293:1191.
201. Sakiyama R, Pardridge WM, Judd HL. Effects of human cirrhotic serum or estradiol and testosterone transport into rat brain. J Clin Endocrinol Metab 1982; 54:1140.
202. Landefeld CS, Schambelan M, Kaplan SL, Embury SH. Clomiphene-responsive hypogonadism in sickle cell anemia. Ann Intern Med 1983; 99:480.
203. el-Hazami M, Bahakim H, al-Fawaz I. Endocrine functions in sickle-cell anemia patients. J Trop Pediatr 1991; 38:307.
204. Perez-Palacios G, Uribe M, Scaglia H, et al. Pituitary and gonadal function in patients with the Laurence-Moon-Biedl syndrome. Acta Endocrinol (Copenh) 1977; 84:191.
205. Riise R. Laurence-Moon-Bardet-Biedl syndrome. Clinical, electrophysiological and genetic aspects. Acta Ophthalmol Scand Suppl 1998; 226:1.
206. Rimoin DL, Schimke RN. The gonads. In: Rimoin DL, Schimke RN, eds. Genetic disorders of the endocrine glands. St. Louis: CV Mosby, 1971:241.
207. Gorlin RJ, Anderson RL, Blaw M. Multiple lentigines syndrome. Am J Dis Child 1969; 117:652.
208. Bray GH, Dahms WJ, Swerdloff RS, et al. The Prader-Willi syndrome: a study of 40 patients and a review of the literature. Medicine (Baltimore) 1983; 62:59.
209. Marxmiller J, Trenkle I, Ashwal S. RUD syndrome revisited: ichthyosis, mental retardation, epilepsy and hypogonadism. Dev Med Child Neurol 1985; 27:335.
210. Davenport SC, Hefner MA, Mitchell JA. The spectrum of clinical features in the Charge syndrome. Clin Genet 1986; 4:298.
211. Sunohara N, Sakuragawa N, Satoyoshi E, et al. A new syndrome of anosmia, ichthyosis, hypogonadism and various neurological manifestations with deficiency of steroid sulfatase and arylsulfatase C. Ann Neurol 1986; 19:174.
212. Sanchez JM, Barreiro C, Freilij H. Two brothers with Martsolf's syndrome. J Med Genet 1985; 22:308.
213. Starr DG, McClure JP, Connor JM. Non-dermatological complications and genetic aspects of the Rothmund-Thompson syndrome. Clin Genet 1985; 27:102.
214. Ardinger HH, Hanson JW, Zellweger HV. Borjeson-Forssman-Lehmann syndrome: further delineation in five cases. Am J Med Genet 1984; 19:653.
215. Killinger DW. The testis. In: Ezrin C, Godden JO, Volpé R, eds. Systematic endocrinology, 2nd ed. Hagerstown, MD: Harper & Row, 1979:232.

# CHAPTER 116

# TESTICULAR DYSFUNCTION IN SYSTEMIC DISEASE

H. W. GORDON BAKER

Deficient testicular function is classically associated with certain severe chronic disorders, such as hepatic cirrhosis, but many acute and chronic illnesses alter testicular function in a nonspecific manner. The mechanisms probably are multifactorial, including accelerated aging, increased sensitivity to toxins, adaptation to reduced energy supply, nutritional deficiencies, stress responses, overproduction of cytokines, and autoimmune or vascular changes.[1] Many drugs and toxins also affect testicular function,[1,2] and these may contribute to the hypogonadism that accompanies systemic disease (see Chaps. 205, 233, 235, and 239).

## PATHOPHYSIOLOGY OF TESTICULAR DYSFUNCTION

Control of the pituitary-testicular axis is discussed in detail in Chapters 16, 113, and 114. Figure 116-1 is a schematic outline to aid understanding of the changes that occur with hypogonadism. The pituitary-testicular axis displays a limited range of responses to stress. Generally, *acute stresses* are associated with gonadotropin suppression and secondary testicular failure, and *chronic stresses* are associated with primary testicular failure and elevated gonadotropin levels. Both patterns of abnormal testicular function appear to be reversible. Studies performed in

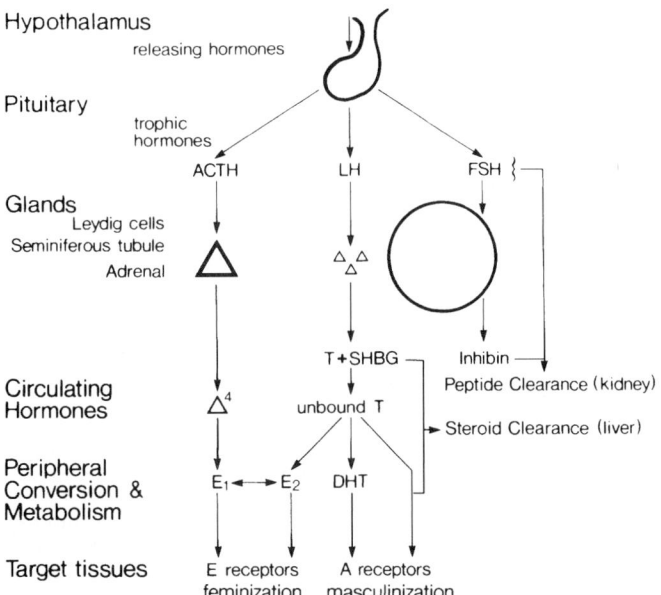

**FIGURE 116-1.** Schematic outline of the pituitary-testicular axis showing the relation between the trophic hormones: adrenocorticotropic hormone (*ACTH*), luteinizing hormone (*LH*), and follicle-stimulating hormone (*FSH*); the target gland hormones: androstenedione ($\Delta^4$), testosterone (*T*), and inhibin B; and estrone ($E_1$), estradiol ($E_2$), and dihydrotestosterone (*DHT*), produced mainly by peripheral conversions. (*SHBG*, sex hormone–binding globulin.)

patients after kidney or liver transplantation show that recovery of testicular function is possible.[3–7]

Most studies of testicular function in various systemic diseases have been small and cross-sectional, and it sometimes is difficult to know whether the hormone patterns are stable or evolving. For example, low testosterone and high luteinizing hormone (LH) levels may indicate either primary Leydig cell dysfunction or a recovery phase after gonadotropin suppression.

## CLINICAL FEATURES
## OF TESTICULAR FAILURE

Testicular failure with an onset before the end of childhood prevents the full development of masculine features; the genitalia remain infantile in appearance, and secondary sex characteristics, such as deepening of the voice and pubic, beard, and body hair, do not develop. Epiphyseal fusion is delayed, and long bone growth is proportionately greater than that of the axial skeleton, causing eunuchoidal proportions (see Chap. 115). Deterioration of testicular function after normal puberty decreases sperm and testosterone production, manifesting clinically as the loss of libido, impotence, infertility, reduced hair growth, atrophy of the prostate and other accessory sex organs, and a reduced semen volume if ejaculation is possible (Fig. 116-2). There may be dryness of the skin from reduced sebum production and wrinkling of the skin on the face. Atrophy and depigmentation of the genital skin and hot flushes also may occur, but the latter are less marked symptoms of gonadal failure in men than they are in women. Other features possibly attributable to androgen deficiency include lethargy and weakness with loss of muscle bulk and increased subcutaneous fat on the trunk. Anemia and osteoporosis may result from prolonged androgen deficiency. Gynecomastia commonly accompanies hypogonadism of many causes (see Chap. 120). Spider nevi may be seen with testicular failure unassociated with liver disease or alcoholism, although rarely in large numbers[8] (see Fig. 116-2).

## DEVELOPMENT OF THE CLINICAL FEATURES
## OF TESTICULAR FAILURE

### SUPPRESSION OF GONADOTROPIN SECRETION

Severe, acute illnesses are associated with low gonadotropin levels.[1,9] Presumably, the output of gonadotropin-releasing hormone (GnRH) is reduced by a central mechanism[9] (see Fig. 116-1). It is suggested that there is a common underlying mechanism termed *ontogenic regression* similar to seasonal regression of reproductive function in animals, which acts to conserve the individual under adverse circumstances.[5] However, many mechanisms may contribute, including the effects of fever, drugs, cytokines, or stress hormones either directly on the testes or indirectly on the hypothalamus and pituitary.[1,5–17] Primary and secondary hypogonadism may alternate or may be superimposed. For example, a suppression of previously high gonadotropin levels occurs during the terminal stages of cirrhosis with the onset of hepatic coma.[8] Conversely, gonadotropin levels, which are suppressed during severe starvation, may be elevated with refeeding, causing a transient excess of estrogen production and *refeeding gynecomastia.* The mechanism of this

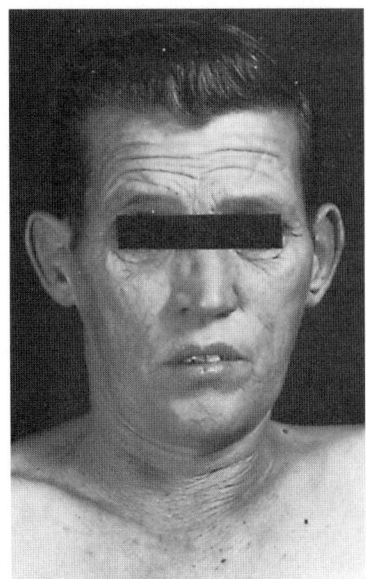

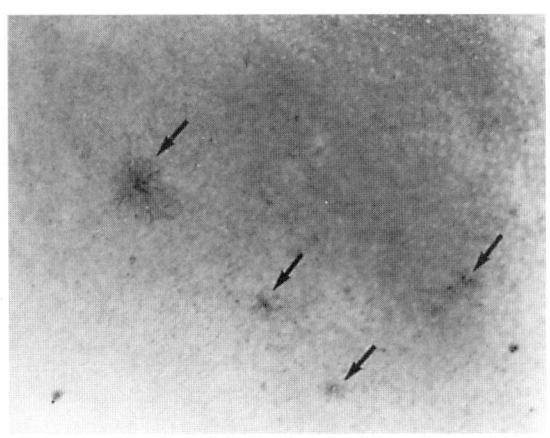

**FIGURE 116-2. A,** Hypogonadal facies of a 45-year-old man with alcoholic cirrhosis and severe hypogonadism. Note the wrinkled, parchment-like skin and the sparse facial hair. **B,** Close-up of spider angiomata (*arrows*) of this patient. These telangiectatic lesions blanch with pressure but immediately refill when the pressure is removed.

A,B

condition may be similar to that of the physiologic gynecomastia of puberty.[18,19]

## GONADOTROPINS IN PRIMARY HYPOGONADISM

The hypogonadism that accompanies most chronic systemic diseases is associated with high gonadotropin levels, indicating reduced feedback inhibition of the hypothalamus and pituitary by sex steroids and inhibin B from the damaged testis (see Fig. 116-1). There also may be some insufficiency of gonadotropin secretion, because the pattern of change in serum LH and follicle-stimulating hormone (FSH) levels are different and their relative responses to clomiphene or GnRH are less than expected.[5,8,11,19–21] This combination of subnormal LH and FSH secretion and primary testicular failure is described as a double defect.[20] However, the results of stimulation tests are difficult to interpret when baseline hormone levels and secretion kinetics are different, and it may be impossible to distinguish low from normal responses.

## BLOOD LEVELS AND CLEARANCE OF GONADOTROPIN-RELEASING HORMONE AND GONADOTROPINS

The patterns of LH pulses have been studied in hypogonadal disorders.[21–23] If the serum LH levels are low, pulses are difficult to detect. In certain conditions with high LH levels, the amplitude may be reduced, but the pulse frequency is similar to that of men with normal LH levels.[21,22] However, in testicular failure, LH pulse frequency and amplitude are both increased.[23] The metabolism and clearance of peptide hormones involve enzyme degradation and some urinary excretion. There is increased urinary output of LH and FSH during carbohydrate starvation, reflecting altered renal handling.[22] Urinary excretion is altered in chronic renal failure, and the clearance of LH, in particular, is reduced.[11] A delay in the peak and the slow falloff of LH levels after the administration of GnRH have been noticed in other hypergonadotropic patients. This may result from an abnormality of secretion rather than delayed clearance.[8,11,21] Gonadotropin levels measured by radioimmunoassay may not reflect their bioactivity. Bioassays of gonadotropins have produced conflicting results.[24] For example, it has been suggested that the bioactivity of LH in old age is reduced, but some studies show no change.[25,26]

## LEYDIG CELL AND SEMINIFEROUS TUBULE FUNCTION

Human chorionic gonadotropin (hCG) is used to test Leydig cell responsiveness to LH. In both primary and secondary testicular failure, the rise in testosterone levels after a maximally effective dose of hCG (1500 IU given intramuscularly) is usually less than the normal doubling of pretreatment levels. Defective Leydig cell function may result from altered paracrine signals from damaged seminiferous tubules.[14] Inhibin-B levels reflect Sertoli cell function and are inversely related to spermatogenesis and the change in FSH levels with age.[26–29] Semen analyses have been performed in a few studies of men with systemic disease, and they are severely abnormal if there are signs of hypogonadism.[4,6,7] Testis biopsies show nonspecific impairment of spermatogenesis, ranging from hypospermatogenesis to germ-cell aplasia and hyalinized tubules.

## SEX HORMONE–BINDING GLOBULIN

The plasma protein binding of steroid hormones affects their bioactivity and clearance rates to different degrees.[30,31] For example, serum androstenedione is bound only to albumin, and its metabolic clearance rate is high (about equal to hepatic blood flow). Serum estradiol is bound to albumin and sex hormone–binding globulin (SHBG), but the dissociation rate of the SHBG-estradiol complex is so rapid at 37°C that the metabolic clearance rate of estradiol is high and relatively uninfluenced by

SHBG.[32] In contrast, the binding of dihydrotestosterone (DHT) and testosterone to SHBG does affect the metabolic clearance rate of these hormones significantly. The consequence of these differential effects is that changes in SHBG levels modulate the effective estrogen/androgen ratio. This is accentuated by the fact that sex steroids control the production of SHBG by the liver; androgens suppress and estrogens stimulate production. An increase in estrogen increases serum SHBG levels, reducing the free testosterone and DHT with only a limited effect on the bioavailability of estrogens. This has been called the *estrogen amplification effect of SHBG* and may contribute to the signs of feminization in conditions such as cirrhosis, senescence, and thyrotoxicosis, in which serum SHBG levels are elevated[33] (see Chaps. 114 and 115). Other factors altering SHBG levels may influence the hormone changes seen with illness. Low androgens and increased thyroid hormone or insulin augment SHBG levels. High glucocorticoids or progestins, and low estrogens, thyroid hormone, insulin, or insulin sensitivity, reduce SHBG levels. SHBG is also high in liver disease and low in obesity. The regulation of SHBG is related to growth hormone, insulin-like growth factor (IGF), insulin, and leptin levels in metabolic disturbances such as diabetes, obesity, and weight loss.[31,34,35] There are racial variations, and low SHBG levels are seen in some men for unknown reasons.[36] Low SHBG levels are related to increased cardiovascular risk factors, adverse lipid profiles, visceral obesity, and risk of developing familial essential hypertension and type 2 diabetes.[31,36]

## STEROID HORMONE METABOLISM

Steroid hormone metabolism includes reversible conversions between serum androstenedione and testosterone and between estradiol and estrone, as well as irreversible conversions, such as androgens to estrogens and testosterone to DHT. Hydroxylations and conjugations of steroids increase their water solubility and facilitate their urinary excretion. The liver in particular is important in the degradative metabolism of steroids, and there is considerable biliary excretion and enterohepatic recirculation of steroid conjugates. With chronic renal failure, there is a massive accumulation of steroid conjugates in the bloodstream.[11] The activity of the 5α-reductase enzymes, which convert testosterone to DHT, is maintained in androgen target tissues with aging.[37] Virtually all circulating estradiol in men derives from the peripheral conversion of testosterone or estrone.[38] Estrone arises by peripheral conversion from androstenedione, which is secreted by both the adrenal cortex and Leydig cells (see Fig. 116-1). These steroids are not directly involved in the feedback control of the trophic hormones of the adrenal cortex and Leydig cell and therefore may reach excessive levels if the control systems are perturbed. The peripheral conversion of androgens to estrogens is increased in many forms of hypogonadism, including cirrhosis, chronic renal failure, thyrotoxicosis, old age, Klinefelter syndrome, and testicular atrophy after mumps orchitis.[8,38–40]

## MECHANISMS OF FEMINIZATION AND DECREASED VIRILIZATION

The features of feminization are believed to result from estrogen action, but circulating estrogen levels correlate poorly with the signs, such as gynecomastia.[8,11,39] This has led some to suggest that it is the ratio of estrogen to androgen that is important in the genesis of gynecomastia. However, it also is probable that there is a wide range of responsiveness of male breast tissue to estrogen, as shown by the great variability in the extent of gynecomastia in men given estrogens for metastatic prostatic cancer. Variability in tissue responsiveness to androgen also may account for the different degrees of virilization seen in men. Androgen-receptor defects have been reported in men with idiopathic seminiferous tubular failure, and an acquired androgen resistance or 5α-reductase deficiency has been described in celiac disease.[41–43]

**TABLE 116-1.**
Conditions Associated with Suppression of Pituitary-Testicular Function

| Acute | Chronic |
|---|---|
| Surgery/anesthesia[9,13] | Liver disease[4,5,7,8,20,38,51,53,55-64,142,143] |
| Intensive care patients[48,49,139] | Alcoholism[52,54,64-70] |
| Hepatic coma[8] | Hemochromatosis[8,71-76] |
| Head injury or stroke[9,146] | Chronic anemia[77-83,144] |
| Acute renal failure[11,86] | Chronic renal failure[11,36,84,85,87] |
| Respiratory failure[9,146,147] | Chronic lung disease[146-148,159-161] |
| Myocardial infarction[9] | Neoplasia[88-95,141] |
| Congestive cardiac failure[9] | Spinal cord injury[97-104] |
| Burns[10,47,149] | Thyrotoxicosis[38,107,108,110,111] |
| Alcohol intoxication[150] | Hypothyroidism[106,109] |
| Psychological stress[151-155] | Cushing syndrome[16,113-115] |
| Physical exhaustion[129,136,156] | Obesity[122-126] |
| Acute fever[1,44-46] | Starvation[18,19,22,127-136,145] |
| War trauma[157] | Systemic lupus erythematosus[162] |
| Glucoprivation[158] | Rheumatoid arthritis[163,164] |

**TABLE 116-2.**
Miscellaneous Associations with Testicular Disorders

**SUPPRESSION OF GONADOTROPINS**
  Congenital adrenal hyperplasia
  Estrogen-producing tumors
  Hyperprolactinemia
**DIRECT TESTICULAR INVOLVEMENT**
  Polyarteritis nodosa
  Leprosy
  Amyloidosis
  Leukemia
  Polyglandular autoimmune diseases
**NEUROLOGIC DISORDERS WITH HYPOGONADISM**
  Prader-Willi syndrome
  Myotonic dystrophy
  Demyelination, hypoadrenalism, and hypogonadism
  Cerebellar ataxia and hypogonadotropic hypogonadism
  Temporal lobe lesions and gynecomastia
**OTHER**
  Renal tumor (varicocele)
  Celiac disease (androgen resistance)
  Cystic fibrosis (agenesis of the vas deferens)
  Immotile cilia (zero sperm motility)
  Bronchiectasis (epididymal obstruction)

(From Baker HWG, Burger HG, de Kretser DM, Hudson B. Relative incidence of etiological disorders in male infertility. In: Santen RJ, Swerdloff RS, eds. Male reproductive dysfunction: diagnosis and management of hypogonadism, infertility and impotence. New York: Marcel Dekker Inc, 1986:341.)

# DISEASES THAT ALTER TESTICULAR FUNCTION

The major acute and chronic systemic diseases that alter testicular function are listed in Table 116-1. Several conditions associated with testicular disorders by means of pituitary suppression, direct testicular involvement, generalized structural abnormalities, or unknown mechanisms are listed in Table 116-2. Details of the interaction between the male reproductive system and disorders in other body systems are covered in other sections of the textbook (see Chaps. 13, 77, 115, and 118, and Parts XIV–XVII). A summary of the principal hormonal changes in several conditions affecting gonadal function is shown in Table 116-3.

## ACUTE CONDITIONS WITH PERTURBATION OF HORMONE SECRETION OR SPERMATOGENESIS

Fever or heating the testes can suppress spermatogenesis.[1,44-46] The suppression of serum gonadotropin or testosterone levels has been demonstrated during severe acute physical and psychological insults (see Table 116-1). The reduction in testosterone levels is related directly to the severity of the critical condition and inversely to the prognosis.[13,47-49] Recovery is usually associated with a transient rebound rise in serum LH before eventual normalization. Presumably, all result primarily from the temporary inhibition of GnRH secretion; however, altered hormone clearance and direct impairment of testicular function may contribute if circulatory changes, fever, activa-

tion of cytokine cascades, or other factors are influencing paracrine regulation.[44-50]

## CHRONIC DISORDERS ASSOCIATED WITH TESTICULAR FAILURE

### LIVER DISEASE

Hepatic cirrhosis, classically, is associated with hypogonadism and signs of feminization[4,5,7,8,20] (see Chaps. 205 and 233). Testicular atrophy, impotence, reduced secondary sex hair, gynecomastia, spider nevi, and palmar erythema are seen in 50% to 75% of men with alcoholic cirrhosis. These signs also are common in cirrhosis of other causes. Compared with healthy men of comparable ages, men with cirrhosis have reduced production and clearance rates of testosterone, low total and free serum testosterone levels, and high serum estrone, estradiol, LH, FSH, and SHBG levels. Also, there is increased peripheral conversion of testosterone to estradiol, androstenedione to testosterone, and androstenedione to estrone, which may be the main reason for the hyperestrogenism of cirrhosis. The produc-

**TABLE 116-3.**
Summary of Serum Hormone Changes in Patients with Cirrhosis, Alcoholism, and Other Illnesses

| Patient Group | Number of Patients | Follicle-Stimulating Hormone | Luteinizing Hormone | Estradiol | Testosterone | Sex Hormone–Binding Globulin |
|---|---|---|---|---|---|---|
| Cirrhosis, men | 117 | ↑ | ↑ | ↑ | ↓ | ↑ |
| Cirrhosis, postmenopausal women | 10 | ↓ | ↓ | ↑ | N | ↑ |
| Other liver disease | 10 | N | ↑ | ↑ | ↓ | ↑ |
| Alcoholism without liver disease | 19 | ↑ | ↑ | ↑ | ↓ | N |
| Miscellaneous chronic illness without alcoholism | 17 | ↑ | ↑ | ↑ | ↓ | N |
| Impotence with organic disease | 45 | ↑ | ↑ | ↑ | ↓ | — |
| Impotence without organic disease | 37 | N | N | ↑ | ↓ | — |

(From Baker HWG, Burger HG, de Kretser DM, et al. A study of the endocrine manifestations of hepatic cirrhosis. Q J Med 1976; 45:145.)

tion rate of estradiol is increased, but the clearance rate is not reduced.[8,38,51] The response of the Leydig cells of cirrhotics to administered hCG is reduced. The LH pulses and responses to GnRH and clomiphene are decreased.[8,20,52,53] Several other factors may contribute to the hormonal changes in cirrhosis, including hepatic overproduction of SHBG, changed SHBG isoforms with different steroid-binding affinities, elevated prolactin levels, direct suppression of Leydig cell function by estrogen, increased estrogen receptors in the liver, and cyclic variations in the severity of the liver illness producing the hormone changes of refeeding gynecomastia.[8,54–56]

In early studies of cirrhosis, serum FSH and LH levels were normal or elevated despite the high serum estrogen levels, except in severely ill patients.[8,20,52,57,58] Elevated levels of FSH and LH are noted less frequently than in the past.[5,59–63] Possibly there was a preponderance of patients with alcoholic cirrhosis in the original studies, and alcohol has a direct toxic effect on the testis. Impaired testicular histology may be more related to alcoholism than the severity of the liver disease.[64,65] However, in some studies there may be patients with suppressed gonadotropin levels because of advanced hepatic decompensation, transfusion siderosis, or treatment with drugs such as aldosterone blockers.[5,57,61,62] Testicular function can recover after liver transplantation, but the recovery may be less with alcoholic cirrhosis.[4,5,7,61,62] Other studies show that men with severe viral and autoimmune liver disease can display the same range of abnormalities of the pituitary testicular axis as those with alcoholic cirrhosis.[59,60,62,63] Also, noncirrhotic chronic liver disease is associated with the same clinical and hormonal changes, but these are less marked (see Table 116-3).

## CHRONIC ALCOHOLISM WITHOUT LIVER DISEASE

As a group, alcoholics have reduced serum testosterone, free testosterone levels and sperm production, and high serum LH, FSH, and estradiol levels[52,64–70] (see Table 116-3 and Chap. 233). When compared with men with other nonhepatic illnesses without alcoholism, alcoholics may have slightly higher estradiol levels. Infertile men with severe oligospermia and alcoholism may recover after stopping drinking, and their sexual performance also may improve.[66,67,70]

## HEMOCHROMATOSIS

Hereditary hemochromatosis is usually caused by mutations in the HFE gene. The HFE gene product modulates the uptake of transferrin by cells, and defects can cause excessive iron accumulation and toxicity.[71] Several mechanisms may operate to produce hypogonadism in hemochromatosis[8,71–76] (see Chaps. 131 and 205). A hypothalamic defect has been described early before there is severe iron overload.[75] Most commonly, serum LH and FSH levels are low and unresponsive to GnRH.[8,73,76] This secondary hypogonadism results from iron deposits in the gonadotropes, and gonadotropin secretion is selectively impaired. With this gonadotropin-deficient form, there usually is no estrogen overproduction or feminization and patients may present with impotence or infertility with low testosterone, azoospermia or low semen volume, and sperm motility with normal sperm concentration (*fertile eunuch syndrome*).[74,76] In these forms testicular function may recover with removal of the iron overload, but often does not.[73,75] Hypogonadism with high serum LH and FSH levels is also found with hemochromatosis; however, it is possible that the diagnosis may have been based on the amount of iron in liver biopsies alone in these cases.[72]

## CHRONIC ANEMIA

Several forms of chronic anemia, especially sickle cell disease and thalassemia major, are associated with hypogonadism, mainly manifesting as delayed puberty[77–83] (see Chap. 212).

Modern treatment with chelation therapy has reduced the frequency of hypogonadotropic hypogonadism from pituitary siderosis.[82] Semen quality is often poor in adults with sickle cell disease.[80] Possible mechanisms include the hypothalamic suppression from the severity of the illness, direct testicular or pituitary damage from ischemia, and pituitary siderosis from frequent blood transfusions.[77–82]

## CHRONIC RENAL DISEASE

Reduced libido and impotence occur in most men with chronic renal failure (see Chap. 209). Gynecomastia is common. These features usually persist or worsen during dialysis but often disappear after successful renal transplantation.[3,5,6,84–87] Semen quality, spermatogenesis, and fertility are impaired to a severe but somewhat variable degree. It is believed there is a double defect in chronic renal failure: primary testicular failure combined with inadequate LH secretion.[5,87] In acute renal failure, FSH and testosterone are low but recover after diuresis.[86] With chronic renal failure, testosterone levels and production rates are low, but the clearance rate is normal or high, and the response to hCG is only slightly reduced.[5] Serum LH levels are increased proportionately to the severity of the renal failure or the duration of dialysis. Serum FSH levels are normal or high. The clearance of the serum gonadotropins, particularly LH, is reduced, and this contributes to the higher serum levels and to the increased LH/FSH ratio. Analysis of LH pulses indicates reduced GnRH secretion.[87] The LH response to administered GnRH shows a delayed peak and a slower return to baseline values. The serum gonadotropin response to clomiphene is normal or reduced. Serum estrone and prolactin levels are increased in some subjects. Estradiol, SHBG, and androstenedione levels usually are normal. The reduction or cessation of renal clearance of hormones contributes to the elevated LH levels and also has a major impact on circulating conjugated steroids, which become very high.[5] Although testicular function often improves after successful renal allografts, the vasa may be damaged and become obstructed during the transplantation surgery.[3,5,6,84]

## NEOPLASIA

Untreated Hodgkin disease and other cancers may be associated with testicular atrophy, spermatogenic defects, abnormal semen analyses, low serum testosterone, and increased SHBG levels. Serum gonadotropin levels are variable.[88–94] Gonadotropin secretion is impaired.[88,92] The hypogonadism is more frequent and severe with Hodgkin disease and testicular cancer.[93,94] Otherwise it correlates poorly with the clinical severity and extent of the disease but tends to be greater in patients with general symptoms and weight loss.[90] The changes in testicular function may, in part, result from the effects of cytokines on the testis.[12,14,15] Semen cryopreservation before chemotherapy or radiotherapy was of limited value in the past because it was often too poor after thawing to produce pregnancies by artificial insemination. Intracytoplasmic sperm injection has improved the outlook for paternity.[95] Some therapeutic regimens in cancer treatment may eventuate in hypogonadism.[95a]

## PARAPLEGIA

Gynecomastia and testicular atrophy were common accompaniments of chronic spinal cord injury in the past and occasionally showed a refeeding pattern, but these now are rare because the nutritional state of the patients is better maintained.[96–103] Testosterone levels may be reduced in the acute phase of the injury.[96] Some men with chronic spinal cord injuries have hypogonadism.[97–99,103] In most, serum LH, FSH, estradiol, and testosterone levels and the response to hCG are usually in the normal range, but, occasionally, LH and FSH levels are elevated.[89,97,103] Those men with chronic spinal cord injuries who also have a spermatogenic disorder may have an obvious cause such as episodes of epididymoorchitis or other testicular damage. A spermatogenic disorder associated with a particular level of spinal cord lesion has been suggested.[99]

Attempts to obtain sperm for insemination from paraplegic patients by assisted emission or ejaculation have variable success rates.[97,98,100,102] Shortly after injury, semen is unable to be collected during the phase of spinal shock. Once bowel sounds return, electroejaculation may produce normal semen for several days, but semen quality deteriorates after the first 2 weeks.[101] It is possible that this deterioration is associated with testicular hyperthermia caused by defective thermoregulation in the testes.[97]

With chronic spinal cord injury of greater than 6 months' duration, semen can be collected by electroejaculation and occasionally by vibration ejaculation in those patients with lesions above T6.[101,102] However, the semen is characterized by very poor sperm motility and viability. The semen is usually heavily contaminated with white blood cells, and the reactive oxygen species production is very high.[104] Sperm motility may improve with repeated ejaculation. Patients with necrospermia of unknown cause also show an improvement in sperm motility with frequent ejaculation, suggesting that there is a defect of epididymal storage.[105]

## THYROID DISORDERS

Thyroid hormones have a direct stimulating effect on SHBG production by the liver.[31] Thyroid disorders may alter testicular function.[31,38,106–111] With thyrotoxicosis, serum SHBG, total testosterone, LH, and FSH levels are elevated, but free testosterone is usually normal once compensation is complete. Gynecomastia may occur with elevated estradiol levels, resulting from the increased conversion of androgens to estrogens.[38,107] Reduced libido, potency, and sperm concentration or sperm motility have been reported.[108,110] There may be a reduced testosterone response to hCG and an increased LH response to GnRH, indicating a degree of primary testicular failure[108] (see Chap. 42).

SHBG levels are low in hypothyroidism.[31] Reduced libido and hypogonadism related to concomitant hyperprolactinemia may occur[109] (see Chap. 45). However, semen quality may be normal in severe primary myxedema.[106]

## CUSHING SYNDROME

Oligospermia and symptoms of androgen deficiency can occur with Cushing disease or glucocorticoid administration.[16,17,112–115] Gynecomastia occasionally occurs with Cushing disease or adrenal tumors. Reduced gonadotropin levels, pulsatility, and GnRH responsiveness have been found.[16,114] Administration of prednisolone, 50 mg per day for 2 to 6 months, to healthy men with sperm autoimmunity produced a fall of ~25% in SHBG, testosterone, and estradiol levels.[17] The low hormone levels may contribute to muscle and bone atrophy (see Chap. 75).

## DIABETES MELLITUS

Autonomic neuropathies causing neurogenic impotence and retrograde ejaculation are important adverse effects of diabetes on the male reproductive system. Impotence may be the presenting symptom of diabetes. In many instances, this form of impotence recovers with control of the diabetes (see Chap. 148).

Although male reproductive function usually is normal in well-controlled diabetes, some abnormalities have been described. Testosterone levels are low with ketosis and increase with insulin treatment.[116] Some evidence of mild primary hypogonadism has been found in diabetic men younger than 50 years of age, particularly in those with poor glycemic control.[117] Similarly, low free testosterone levels and increased urinary excretion of LH have been reported in diabetic men with organic impotence of neurologic or vascular origin.[118] Impo-

tent men with features of hypogonadism have been treated with clomiphene.[119] Strong associations exist between insulin action and sensitivity, SHBG, bioavailable sex steroids, obesity, and the risk of developing type 2 diabetes and cardiovascular disease.[31,35,120,121]

## OBESITY

A number of effects of simple obesity on the hypothalamic–pituitary–testicular axis and direct impairment of scrotal thermoregulation are postulated (see Chap. 126). The main confirmed changes are in hormone metabolism with increased conversion of androgens to estrogens in peripheral tissues and low SHBG.[122–126] The reduction in both total testosterone and SHBG levels is related to severity of obesity.[125] Testosterone metabolic clearance rates are normal or high.[122] Gonadotropin levels are normal or low for age.[125] LH-pulse amplitude is reduced, but responses to pituitary and Leydig cell stimulation are normal.[122,125] The low total testosterone levels and high SHBG and estrogen levels are reversed by weight loss.[125,126] Insulin resistance may cause the low SHBG levels.[31] Whether leptin is involved in the gonadal hormone changes of obesity remains to be determined.[35]

## STARVATION

Starvation as a result of famine, catabolic states, excessive exercise, or psychological disturbances (as in anorexia nervosa) has a profound suppressive effect on gonadotropin secretion and testicular function[18,19,90,127–136] (see Chaps. 127 and 128). The mechanism of gonadotropin suppression involves inhibition of GnRH secretion.[132,134,135] Serum testosterone levels are low, with a poor response to hCG.[19] Experiments in fasted men show that testosterone secretion can be maintained by pulsatile GnRH therapy.[134] Renal clearance of gonadotropins is altered.[131] SHBG levels rise rapidly, at least in fasted obese men.[130]

The androgen deficiency–induced loss of sex drive may be a useful adaptation to starvation. Often spermatogenesis continues, but there is low semen volume and poor sperm motility, probably because of reduced accessory sex organ function. With recovery and weight gain, pulsatile secretion of gonadotropins increases in a manner reminiscent of the changes with puberty.

During an improvement in nutritional status, gynecomastia and, rarely, spider nevi may develop.[18] The breast development is called *refeeding gynecomastia*. It was seen in starved prisoners of World War II. Sometimes, there was fatty infiltration of the liver, and it has been suggested that there was an additional hepatic mechanism operating in the patients.[18]

Studies of protein and calorie malnutrition indicate changes similar to those occurring in chronic illnesses; for example, gonadotropin levels can be high from a rebound rise during refeeding.[19] Anorexia nervosa occurs rarely in men but appears to have the same hormone changes as expected from studies in women: low serum LH and FSH levels and a poor response to GnRH if starvation is severe and an excessive response during weight gain that normalizes with attainment of normal weight.[127,128] Endurance athletes may have similar changes if their energy balance is marginal[129,133] (see Chap. 132). Low free testosterone and low sperm motility have been reported in men with very heavy training programs.[133,136]

Deficiencies of specific nutrients, especially vitamins, amino acids, and metals, can be associated with disordered spermatogenesis and Leydig cell function[136a] (see Chaps. 130 and 131). Some of these disorders can be produced experimentally, for example, zinc deficiency.[137,138]

## MISCELLANEOUS ILLNESSES

Mild features of primary hypogonadism with a tendency to high serum estradiol, LH, and FSH and reduced testosterone levels are common accompaniments of illnesses. They are found in groups of hospitalized men with chronic respiratory and cardiac conditions, diabetes, hypertension, and peptic ulcer as well as in men with alcoholism and impotence not associated with obvious severe hypogonadism (see Table 116-3). Severe chronic illnesses in childhood, including multisystem diseases such as juvenile chronic arthritis (Still disease), malabsorption syndromes, chronic respiratory diseases, and the psychological trauma of emotional deprivation, are known to be associated with delayed puberty and retarded skeletal growth (see Chaps. 92 and 198). Additional information about the effect of systemic illnesses on testicular function is in Chapters 115 and 118, aging in Chapter 199, acquired immunodeficiency syndrome (AIDS) in Chapter 214, and critical illness in Part XVI; some extra references are cited in Table 116-1.

## CLINICAL PERSPECTIVE OF TESTICULAR DYSFUNCTION IN SYSTEMIC DISEASES

### ACUTE DISEASES

The disturbances in testicular function accompanying severe, acute systemic conditions are transient but may contribute to or regulate the catabolic state. Whether treatment with anabolic agents is useful is unresolved.[139] The possibility of an illness affecting gonadotropin and sex steroid levels or semen analysis is important to consider in the interpretation of results of tests.

### CLINICAL COURSE OF HYPOGONADISM WITH CHRONIC ILLNESS

Although impotence may be the presenting symptom of a chronic illness, such as hemochromatosis or diabetes, the symptoms of hypogonadism associated with most systemic diseases—loss of libido, impotence, and lethargy—frequently are unnoticed by the patient among the more serious symptoms of the underlying disease. Few patients are aware of testicular atrophy, gynecomastia, or loss of male pattern hair. It is likely that the hypogonadism often is a nonspecific response to the illness and that the features are more florid in certain conditions because of their severity and their duration.[8,11,140,141]

## TREATMENT OF TESTICULAR DYSFUNCTION IN SYSTEMIC DISEASE

The testicular suppression accompanying chronic systemic disorders may be reversible with recovery or correction by organ transplantation. Drugs used for managing the disorder may also contribute to the reduced testicular function.[1] In patients with stable underlying disorders, androgen therapy may be effective in improving virility (see Chap. 119). The possibility that androgen deficiency contributes to the overall disease state has been investigated. For example, controlled trials of androgen therapy have been conducted in men with cirrhosis. While gynecomastia was reduced, there was no effect on survival or sexual function.[142,143] Gynecomastia can be treated by plastic surgery if necessary.[143a] In hemochromatosis with gonadotropin deficiency, spermatogenesis usually can be reestablished with hCG, but occasionally additional FSH is needed (see Chap. 115). Patients with hyperprolactinemia may respond to dopaminergic agents (see Chap. 13). There are case reports showing that patients with gonadotropin suppression from dietary restriction and exercise or illness respond to long-term clomiphene treatment.[144,145] However, a controlled trial of clomiphene for secondary hypogonadism in men did not demonstrate an improvement

in sexual function although gondadotropin and testosterone levels were increased.[119]

## REFERENCES

1. Baker HWG. Reproductive effects of nontesticular illness. Endocrinol Metab Clin North Am 1998; 27:831.
2. Irvine DS. Declining sperm quality: a review of facts and hypotheses. Baillieres Clin Obstet Gynaecol 1997; 11:655.
3. Samojlik E, Kirschner MA, Ribot S, Szmal E. Changes in the hypothalamic-pituitary-gonadal axis in men after cadaver kidney transplantation and cyclosporine therapy. J Androl 1992; 13:332.
4. Madersbacher S, Grunberger T, Maier U. Andrological status before and after liver transplantation. J Urol 1994; 151:1251.
5. Handelsman DJ, Strasser S, McDonald JA, et al. Hypothalamic-pituitary-testicular function in end-stage non-alcoholic liver disease before and after liver transplantation. Clin Endocrinol 1995; 43:331.
6. Prem AR, Punekar SV, Kalpana M, et al. Male reproductive function in uraemia: efficacy of haemodialysis and renal transplantation. Br J Urol 1996; 78:635.
7. Madersbacher S, Ludvik G, Stulnig T, et al. The impact of liver transplantation on endocrine status in men. Clin Endocrinol 1996; 44:461.
8. Baker HWG, Burger HG, de Kretser DM, et al. A study of the endocrine manifestations of hepatic cirrhosis. Q J Med 1976; 45:145.
9. Woolf PD, Hamill RW, McDonald JV, et al. Transient hypogonadotrophic hypogonadism caused by critical illness. J Clin Endocrinol Metab 1985; 60:444.
10. Semple CG, Robertson WR, Mitchell R, et al. Mechanisms leading to hypogonadism in men with burn injuries. Br Med J 1987; 295:403.
11. Handelsman DJ, Dong Q. Hypothalamo-pituitary gonadal axis in chronic renal failure. Endocrinol Metab Clin North Am 1993; 22:145.
12. van de Poll T, Romijn JA, Endert E, Sauerwein HP. Effect of tumour necrosis factor on the hypothalamic-pituitary-testicular axis in healthy men. Metabolism 1993; 43:303.
13. Dong Q, Hawker F, McWilliam D, et al. Circulating immunoreactive inhibin and testosterone level in men with critical illness. Clin Endocrinol 1992; 36:399.
14. Leung PC, Steele GL. Intracellular signaling in the gonads. Endocr Rev 1992; 13:476.
15. Meikle AW, Cordoso de Sousa JC, Ward JH, et al. Reduction of testosterone synthesis after high dose interleukin-2 therapy of metastatic cancer. J Clin Endocrinol Metab 1991; 73:931.
16. Samuels MH, Luther M, Henry P, Ridgway EC. Effects of hydrocortisone on pulsatile pituitary glycoprotein secretion. J Clin Endocrinol Metab 1994; 78:211.
17. Pearce G, Tabensky DA, Delmas PD, et al. Corticosteroid-induced bone loss in men. J Clin Endocrinol Metab 1998; 83:801.
18. Zubiran S, Gomez-Mont F. Endocrine disturbances in chronic human malnutrition. Vitam Horm 1953; 11:97.
19. Smith SR, Chhetri MK, Johanson AJ, et al. The pituitary-gonadal axis in men with protein-caloric malnutrition. J Clin Endocrinol Metab 1975; 41:60.
20. Van Thiel DH, Lester R, Sherins RJ. Hypogonadism in alcoholic liver disease: evidence for a double defect. Gastroenterology 1974; 67:1188.
21. Winters SJ, Troen P. Episodic luteinizing hormone (LH) secretion and the response of LH and follicle-stimulating hormone to LH releasing hormone in aged men: evidence for coexistent primary testicular insufficiency, endocrine insufficiency and impairment of gonadotropin secretion. J Clin Endocrinol Metab 1982; 55:560.
22. Kyung NH, Barkan A, Klibanski A, et al. Effect of carbohydrate supplementation on reproductive hormones during fasting in men. J Clin Endocrinol Metab 1985; 60:827.
23. Matsumoto AM, Bremner WJ. Modulation of pulsatile gonadotropin secretion by testosterone in man. J Clin Endocrinol Metab 1984; 58:609.
24. Jockenhovel F, Kahn SA, Nieschlag E. Varying dose-response characteristics of different immunoassays and an in-vivo bioassay for FSH are responsible for changing ratios of biologically active immunologically active FSH. J Endocrinol 1990; 127:523.
25. Warner BA, Dufau ML, Santen RJ. Effects of aging and illness on the pituitary testicular axis in men: qualitative as well as quantitative changes in luteinizing hormone. J Clin Endocrinol Metab 1985; 60:263.
26. Mitchell R, Hollis S, Rothwell C, Robertson WR. Age related changes in the pituitary-testicular axis in normal men—lower serum testosterone results from decreased bioactive LH drive. Clin Endocrinol 1995; 42:501.
27. Jensen TK, Andersson AM, Hjollund NHI, et al. Inhibin B as a serum marker of spermatogenesis—correlation to differences in sperm concentration and follicle-stimulating hormone levels—a study of 349 Danish men. J Clin Endocrinol Metab 1997; 82:4059.
28. Byrd W, Bennett MJ, Carr BR, et al. Regulation of biologically active dimeric inhibin A and B from infancy to adulthood in the male. J Clin Endocrinol Metab 1998; 83:2849.
29. Pierik FH, Vreeburg JTM, Stijnen T, et al. Serum inhibin B as a marker of spermatogenesis. J Clin Endocrinol Metab 1998; 83:3110.
30. Porto CS, Lazari MFM, Abreu LC, et al. Receptors for androgen-binding proteins—internalization and intracellular signalling. J Steroid Biochem Molec Biol 1995; 53:561.
31. Pugeat M, Crave JC, Tourniaire J, Forest MG. Clinical utility of sex hormone-binding globulin measurement. Horm Res 1996; 45:148.

32. Heyns W, De Moor P. Kinetics of dissociation of 17 β-hydroxysteroids from the steroid binding globulin of human plasma. J Clin Endocrinol Metab 1971; 32:147.

33. Burke CW, Anderson DC. Sex-hormone-binding globulin is an oestrogen amplifier. Nature 1972; 240:38.

34. Behre HM, Simoni M, Nieschlag E. Strong association between serum levels of leptin and testosterone in men. Clin Endocrinol 1997; 47:237.

35. Van Gaal LF, Wauters MA, Mertens IL, et al. Clinical endocrinology of human leptin. Int J Obes 1999; 23:29

36. Wu AH, Whittemore AS, Kolonel LN, et al. Serum androgens and sex hormone-binding globulins in relation to lifestyle factors in older African-American, white, and Asian men in the United States and Canada. Cancer Epidemiol Biomarkers Prev 1995; 4:735.

37. Morimoto I, Eto S, Inoue S, et al. Dihydrotestosterone accumulation in genital skin fibroblasts derived from elderly men with prostatic hyperplasia. J Clin Endocrinol Metab 1992; 75:632.

38. Olivo J, Gordon GG, Raffi F, Southern AL. Estrogen metabolism in hyperthyroidism and in cirrhosis of the liver. Steroids 1975; 26:47.

39. Baker HW, Burger HG, de Kretser DM, et al. Changes in the pituitary-testicular system with age. Clin Endocrinol (Oxf) 1976; 5:349.

40. Wang C, Baker HWG, Burger HG, et al. Hormonal studies in Klinefelters syndrome. Clin Endocrinol 1975; 4:399.

41. Farthing MJG, Rees LH, Edwards CRW, Dawson AM. Male gonadal function in coeliac disease. 2: Sex hormones. Gut 1983; 24:127.

42. Sher KS, Jayanthi V, Probert CS, et al. Infertility, obstetric and gynaecological problems in coeliac sprue. Dig Dis 1994; 12:186.

43. Patterson MN, McPhaul MJ, Hughes IA. Androgen insensitivity syndrome. Baillieres Clin Endocrinol Metab 1994; 8:379.

44. Mieusset R, Bujan L. Testicular heating and its possible contribution to male infertility: a review. Int J Androl 1995; 18:169.

45. Brown-Woodman PDC, Post EJ, Goss GC, et al. The effect of a single sauna exposure on spermatogenesis. Arch Androl 1984; 12:9.

46. Mieusset R, Grandjean H, Mansat A, et al. Inhibiting effect of artificial cryptorchidism on spermatogenesis. Fertil Steril 1985; 43:589.

47. Plymate SR, Vaughan GM, Mason AD, et al. Central hypogonadism in burned men. Horm Res 1987; 27:152.

48. Luppa P, Munker R, Nagel D, et al. Serum androgens in intensive care patients: correlations with clinical findings. Clin Endocrinol 1991; 34:305.

49. Spratt D, Bigos S, Beitens I, et al. Both hyper- and hypogonadotropic hypogonadism occur transiently in acute illness: bio- and immunoreactive gonadotropins. J Clin Endocrinol Metab 1992; 75:1562.

50. Reed MJ, Cheng RW, Beranek PA, James VHT. The influence of stress-related factors on the distribution of sex steroids in plasma—implications for endocrine-dependent cancers. Endocrine-Related Cancer 1994; 1:43.

51. Longcope C, Pratt JH, Schneider S, Fineberg E. Estrogen and androgen dynamics in liver disease. J Endocrinol Invest 1984; 7:629.

52. Van Thiel DH, Lester R, Vaitukaitis J. Evidence for a defect in pituitary secretion of luteinizing hormone in chronic alcoholic men. J Clin Endocrinol Metab 1978; 47:499.

53. Bannister P, Handley T, Chapman C, Losowsky MS. Hypogonadism in chronic liver disease: impaired release of luteinising hormone. Br Med J (Clin Res) 1986; 293:1191.

54. Basile A, Proto G, Laperchia N, et al. Increased prolactin reserve in alcoholics. Drug Alcohol Depend 1981; 7:99.

55. Villa E, Baldini GM, Rossini GP, et al. Ethanol-induced increase in cytosolic estrogen receptors in human male liver: a possible explanation for biochemical feminization in chronic liver disease due to alcohol. Hepatology 1988; 8:1610.

56. Terasaki T, Nowlin DM, Pardridge WM. Differential binding of testosterone and estradiol to isoforms of sex hormone-binding globulin: selective alteration of estradiol binding in cirrhosis. J Clin Endocrinol Metab 1988; 67:639.

57. Van Thiel DH, Gavaler JS, Spero JA, et al. Patterns of hypothalamic-pituitary-gonadal dysfunction in men with liver disease due to differing etiologies. Hepatology 1981; 1:39.

58. Cornely CM, Schade RR, Van Thiel DH, Gavaler JS. Chronic advanced liver disease and impotence: cause and effect? Hepatology 1984; 4:1227.

59. Bannister P, Oakes J, Sheridan P, Losowsky MS. Sex hormone changes in chronic liver disease: a matched study of alcoholic versus non-alcoholic liver disease. Q J Med 1987; 63:305.

60. Wang YJ, Wu JC, Lee SD, et al. Gonadal dysfunction and changes in sex hormones in postnecrotic cirrhotic men: a matched study with alcoholic cirrhotic men. Hepatogastroenterology 1991; 38:531.

61. Van Thiel DH, Kumar S, Gavaler JS, Tarter RE. Effect of liver transplantation on the hypothalamic-pituitary-gonadal axis of chronic alcoholic men with advanced liver disease. Alcohol Clin Exp Res 1990; 14:478.

62. Guechot J, Chazouilleres O, Loria A, et al. Effect of liver transplantation on sex-hormone disorders in male patients with alcohol-induced or post-viral hepatitis advanced liver disease. J Hepatol 1994; 20:426.

63. Kaymakoglu S, Okten A, Cakaloglu Y, et al. Hypogonadism is not related to the etiology of liver cirrhosis. J Gastroenterol 1995; 30:745.

64. Kuller LH, May SJ, Perper JA. The relationship between alcohol, liver disease, and testicular pathology. Am J Epidemiol 1978; 108:192.

65. Lindholm J, Fabricius-Bjerre N, Bahnsen M, et al. Sex steroids and sex-hormone binding globulin in males with chronic alcoholism. Eur J Clin Invest 1978; 8:273.

66. Van Thiel DH, Gavaler JS, Sanghvia A. Recovery of sexual function in abstinent alcoholic men. Gastroenterology 1983; 84:677.

67. Brzek A. Alcohol and male fertility (preliminary report). Andrologia 1987; 19:32.

68. Pajarinen JT, Karhunen PJ. Spermatogenic arrest and "Sertoli cell-only" syndrome—common alcohol-induced disorders of the human testis. Int J Androl 1994; 17:292.

69. Martinezriera A, Santolariafernandez F, Reimers EG, et al. Alcoholic hypogonadism—hormonal response to clomiphene. Alcohol 1995; 12:581.

70. Iturriaga H, Valladares L, Hirsch S, et al. Effects of abstinence on sex hormone profile in alcoholic patients without liver failure. J Endocrinol Invest 1995; 18:638.

71. Cox TM, Kelly AL. Haemochromatosis: an inherited metal and toxicity syndrome. Curr Opin Genet Dev 1998; 8:274.

72. Simon M, Franchimont P, Murie N, et al. Study of somatotropic and gonadotropic pituitary function in idiopathic haemochromatosis (31 cases). Eur J Clin Invest 1972; 2:384.

73. Kelly TM, Edwards CQ, Meikle AW, Kushner JP. Hypogonadism in hemochromatosis: reversal with iron depletion. Ann Intern Med 1984; 101:629.

74. Stremmel W, Niederau C, Berger M, et al. Abnormalities in estrogen, androgen, and insulin metabolism in idiopathic hemochromatosis. Ann NY Acad Sci 1988; 526:209.

75. Piperno A, Rivolta MR, D'Alba R, et al. Preclinical hypogonadism in genetic hemochromatosis in the early stage of the disease: evidence of hypothalamic dysfunction. J Endocrinol Invest 1992; 15:423.

76. Duranteau L, Chanson P, Blumberg-Tick J, et al. Non-responsiveness of serum gonadotropins and testosterone to pulsatile GnRH in hemochromatosis suggesting a pituitary defect. Acta Endocrinol (Copenh) 1993; 128:351.

77. Soliman AT, elZalabany MM, Ragab M, et al. Spontaneous and GnRH-provoked gonadotropin secretion and testosterone response to human chorionic gonadotropin in adolescent boys with thalassaemia major and delayed puberty. J Trop Pediatr 2000; 46:79.

78. Osegbe DN, Akinyanju OO. Testicular dysfunction in men with sickle cell disease. Postgrad Med J 1987; 63:95.

79. Wang C, Tso SC, Todd D. Hypogonadotropic hypogonadism in severe β-thalassemia: effect of chelation and pulsatile gonadotropin-releasing hormone therapy. J Clin Endocrinol Metab 1989; 68:511.

80. Modebe O, Ezeh UO. Effect of age on testicular function in adult males with sickle cell anemia. Fertil Steril 1995; 63:907.

81. Valenti S, Giusti M, McGuinness D, et al. Delayed puberty in males with β-thalassemia major: pulsatile gonadotropin-releasing hormone administration induces changes in gonadotropin isoform profiles and an increase in sex steroids. Eur J Endocrinol 1995; 133:48.

82. Papadimas J, Mandala E, Pados G, et al. Pituitary-testicular axis in men with β-thalassemia major. Hum Reprod 1996; 11:1900.

83. Beris P, Samii K, Darbellay R, et al. Iron overload in patients with sideroblastic anaemia is not related to the presence of the haemochromatosis Cys282Tyr and His63Asp mutations. Br J Haematol 1999; 104:97.

84. Lim VS, Fang VS. Gonadal dysfunction in uremic men. A study of the hypothalamo-pituitary-testicular axis before and after renal transplantation. Am J Med 1975; 58:655.

85. Holdsworth S, Atkins RC, de Kretser DM. The pituitary-testicular axis in men with chronic renal failure. N Engl J Med 1977; 296:1245.

86. Levitan D, Moser SA, Goldstein DA, et al. Disturbances in the hypothalamic-pituitary-gonadal axis in male patients with acute renal failure. Am J Nephrol 1984; 4:99.

87. Veldhuis JD, Wilkowski MJ, Zwart AD, et al. Evidence for attenuation of hypothalamic gonadotropin-releasing hormone (GnRH) impulse strength with preservation of GnRH pulse frequency in men with chronic renal failure. J Clin Endocrinol Metab 1993; 76:648.

88. Vigersky RA, Chapman RM, Berenberg J, Glass AR. Testicular dysfunction in untreated Hodgkins disease. Am J Med 1982; 73:482.

89. Ragni G, Bestetti O, Armando S, et al. Evaluation of semen and pituitary gonadotropin function in men with untreated Hodgkins disease. Fertil Steril 1985; 43:927.

90. Handelsman DJ, Staraj S. Testicular size: the effects of aging, malnutrition and illness. J Androl 1985; 6:144.

91. Aasebo U, Bremnes RM, Dejong FH, et al. Pituitary-gonadal dysfunction in male patients with lung cancer—association with serum inhibin levels. Acta Oncologica 1994; 33:177.

92. Magnanti M, Malizia S, Garufi G, et al. Luteinizing hormone pulsatility and computer-assisted analysis of sperm features in patients with Hodgkin's disease. J Cancer Res Clin Oncol 1996; 122:416.

93. Padron OF, Sharma RK, Thomas AJ Jr, Agarwal A. Effects of cancer on spermatozoa quality after cryopreservation: a 12-year experience. Fertil Steril 1997; 67:326.

94. Petersen PM, Skakkebaek NE, Rorth M, Giwercman A. Semen quality and reproductive hormones before and after orchiectomy in men with testicular cancer. J Urol 1999; 161:822.

95. Apperley JF, Reddy N. Mechanism and management of treatment-related gonadal failure in recipients of high dose chemotherapy. Blood Reviews 1995; 9:93.

95a. Pfeilschifter J, Diel IJ. Osteoporosis due to cancer treatment: pathogenesis and management. J Clin Oncol 2000; 18:1570.

96. Claus-Walker J, Scurry M, Carter RE, Campos RJ. Steady state hormonal secretion in traumatic quadriplegia. J Clin Endocrinol Metab 1977; 44:530.

97. Linsenmeyer TA, Perkash I. Infertility in men with spinal cord injury. Arch Phys Med Rehabil 1991; 72:747.

98. Wang YH, Huang TS, Lien IN. Hormone changes in men with spinal cord injuries. Am J Phys Med Rehabil 1992; 71:328.

99. Chapelle PA, Roby-Brami A, Jondet M, et al. Trophic effects on testes in paraplegics. Paraplegia 1993; 31:576.
100. Lim TC, Mallidis C, Hill ST, et al. A simple technique to prevent retrograde ejaculation during assisted ejaculation. Paraplegia 1994; 32:142.
101. Mallidis C, Lim TC, Hill ST, et al. Collection of semen from men in acute phase of spinal cord injury. Lancet 1994; 343:1072.
102. Sonksen J, Ohl DA, Giwercman A, et al. Quality of semen obtained by penile vibratory stimulation in men with spinal cord injuries: observations and predictors. Urology 1996; 48:453.
103. Huang TS, Wang YH, Lee SH, Lai JS. Impaired hypothalamus-pituitary-adrenal axis in men with spinal cord injuries. Am J Phys Med Rehabil 1998; 77:108.
104. de Lamirande E, Leduc BE, Iwasaki A, et al. Increased reactive oxygen species formation in semen of patients with spinal cord injury. Fertil Steril 1995; 63:637.
105. Wilton LJ, Temple-Smith PD, Baker HWG, de Kretser DM. Human male infertility caused by degeneration and death of sperm in the epididymis. Fertil Steril 1988; 49:1052.
106. Griboff SI. Semen analysis in myxedema. Fertil Steril 1962; 13:436.
107. Southren AL, Olivo J, Gordon GG, et al. The conversion of androgens to estrogens in hyperthyroidism. J Clin Endocrinol Metab 1974; 38:207.
108. Kidd GS, Glass AR, Vigersky RA. The hypothalamic-pituitary-testicular axis in thyrotoxicosis. J Clin Endocrinol Metab 1979; 48:798.
109. Wortsman J, Rosner W, Dufau ML. Abnormal testicular function in men with primary hypothyroidism. Am J Med 1987; 82:207.
110. Hudson RW, Edwards AL. Testicular function in hyperthyroidism. J Androl 1992; 13:117.
111. Lovejoy JC, Smith SR, Bray GA, et al. Effects of experimentally induced mild hyperthyroidism on growth hormone and insulin secretion and sex steroid levels in healthy young men. Metabolism 1997; 46:1424.
112. Mancini RE, Lavieri JC, Muller F, et al. Effect of prednisolone upon normal and pathologic human spermatogenesis. Fertil Steril 1966; 17:500.
113. Smals AG, Kloppenborg PW, Benraad TJ. Plasma testosterone profiles in Cushing's syndrome. J Clin Endocrinol Metab 1977; 45:240.
114. Luton JP, Thieblot P, Valcke JC, et al. Reversible gonadotropin deficiency in male Cushing's disease. J Clin Endocrinol Metab 1977; 45:488.
115. Cuerda C, Estrada J, Marazuela M, et al. Anterior pituitary function in Cushing's syndrome: study of 36 patients. Endocrinol Jpn 1991; 38: 559.
116. Gluud C, Madsbad S, Krarup T, Bennett P. Plasma testosterone and androstenedione in insulin dependent patients at time of diagnosis and during the first year of insulin treatment. Acta Endocrinol (Copenh) 1982; 100:406.
117. Handelsman DJ, Conway AJ, Boylan LM, et al. Testicular function and glycemic control in diabetic men. A controlled study. Andrologia 1985; 17:488.
118. Murray FT, Wyss HU, Thomas RG, et al. Gonadal dysfunction in diabetic men with organic impotence. J Clin Endocrinol Metab 1987; 65:127.
119. Guay AT, Bansal S, Heatley GJ. Effect of raising endogenous testosterone levels in impotent men with secondary hypogonadism: double blind placebo-controlled trial with clomiphene citrate. J Clin Endocrinol Metab 1995; 80:3546.
120. Ebeling P, Stenman UH, Seppala M, Koivisto VA. Androgens and insulin resistance in type 1 diabetic men. Clin Endocrinol 1995; 43:601.
121. Haffner SM. Sex hormone-binding protein, hyperinsulinemia, insulin resistance and noninsulin-dependent diabetes. Horm Res 1996; 45:233.
122. Schneider G, Kirschner MA, Berkowitz R, Ertel HH. Increased estrogen production in obese men. J Clin Endocrinol Metab 1979; 46:633.
123. Zumoff B, Strain GW, Miller LK, et al. Plasma free and non-sex-hormone-binding-globulin-bound testosterone are decreased in obese men in proportion to their degree of obesity. J Clin Endocrinol Metab 1990; 71:929.
124. Gray A, Feldman HA, McKinlay JB, Longcope C. Age, disease, and changing sex hormone levels in middle-aged men: results of the Massachusetts male aging study. J Clin Endocrinol Metab 1991; 73:1016.
125. Vermeulen A. Decreased androgen levels and obesity in men. Ann Med 1996; 28:13.
126. Pasquali R, Vicennati V, Scopinaro N, et al. Achievement of near-normal body weight as the prerequisite to normalize sex hormone-binding globulin concentrations in massively obese men. Int J Obes 1997; 21:1.
127. Garfinkel PE, Brown GM, Stancer HC, Moldofsky H. Hypothalamic-pituitary function in anorexia nervosa. Arch Gen Psychiatry 1975; 32:739.
128. Wheeler MJ, Crisp AH, Hsu LK, Chen CN. Reproductive hormone changes during weight gain in male anorectics. Clin Endocrinol 1983; 18:423.
129. Ayers JW, Komesu Y, Romani T, Ansbacher R. Anthropomorphic, hormonal, and psychologic correlates of semen quality in endurance-trained male athletes. Fertil Steril 1985; 43:917.
130. Tegelman R, Lindeskog P, Carlstrom K, et al. Peripheral hormone levels in healthy subjects during controlled fasting. Acta Endocrinol (Copenh) 1986; 113:457.
131. Hoffer LJ, Beitins IZ, Kyung NH, Bistrian BR. Effects of severe dietary restriction on male reproductive hormones. J Clin Endocrinol Metab 1986; 62:288.
132. Cameron JL, Helmreich DL, Schreihofer DA. Modulation of reproductive hormone secretion by nutritional intake: stress signals versus metabolic signals. Hum Reprod 1993; 8(Suppl 2):162.
133. De Souza MJ, Arce JC, Pescatello LS, et al. Gonadal hormones and semen quality in male runners. A volume threshold effect of endurance training. Int J Sports Med 1994; 15:383.
134. Aloi JA, Bergendahl M, Iranmanesh A, Veldhuis JD. Pulsatile intravenous gonadotropin-releasing hormone administration averts fasting-induced hypogonadotropism and hypoandrogenemia in healthy, normal weight men. J Clin Endocrinol Metab 1997; 82:1543.
135. Bergendahl M, Aloi JA, Iranmanesh A, et al. Fasting suppresses pulsatile luteinizing hormone (LH) secretion and enhances orderliness of LH release in young but not older men. J Clin Endocrinol Metab 1998; 83:1967.
136. Elias AN, Wilson AF. Exercise and gonadal function. Hum Reprod 1993; 8:1747.
136a. Longcope C, Feldman HA, McKinlay JB, Araujo AB. Diet and sex hormone binding globulin. J Clin Endocrinol Metab 2000; 85:293.
137. Hunt CD, Johnson PE, Herbel J, Mullen LK. Effects of dietary zinc depletion on seminal volume and zinc loss, serum testosterone concentrations, and sperm morphology in young men. Am J Clin Nutr 1992; 56:148.
138. Martin GB, Markey CM, White CL. Roles of zinc and other nutrients in testicular development. In: Waites GMH, Frick J, Baker HWG, eds. Current advances in andrology. Bologna: Monduzzi Editorie, 1997:317.
139. Chang DW, DeSanti L, Demling RH. Anticatabolic and anabolic strategies in critical illness: a review of current treatment modalities. Shock 1998; 10:155.
140. Semple CG, Gray CE, Beastall GH. Male hypogonadism—a non-specific consequence of illness. Q J Med 1987; 64:601.
141. Blackman ML, Weintraub BO, Rosen SW, Harman SM. Comparison of the effects of lung cancer, benign lung disease, and normal aging on pituitary-gonadal function in men. J Clin Endocrinol Metab 1988; 66:88.
142. Copenhagen Study Group for Liver Diseases. Testosterone treatment of men with alcoholic cirrhosis: a double-blind study. Hepatology 1986; 6:807.
143. Gluud C, Wantzin P, Eriksen J. No effect of oral testosterone treatment on sexual dysfunction in alcoholic cirrhotic men. Gastroenterology 1988; 95:1582.
143a. Gasperoni C, Salgarello M, Gasperoni P. Technical refinements in the surgical treatment of gynecomastia. Ann Plast Surg 2000; 44:455.
144. Landefeld CS, Schambelan M, Kaplan SL, Embury SH. Clomiphene-responsive hypogonadism in sickle cell anemia. Ann Intern Med 1983; 99:480.
145. Burge MR, Lanzi RA, Skarda ST, Eaton RP. Idiopathic hypogonadotropic hypogonadism in a male runner is reversed by clomiphene citrate. Fertil Steril 1997; 67:783.
146. Jeppesen LL, Jorgensen HS, Nakayama H, et al. Decreased serum testosterone in men with acute ischemic stroke. Arterioscler Thromb Vasc Biol 1996; 16:749.
147. Aasebo U, Gyltnes A, Bremnes RM, et al. Reversal of sexual impotence in male patients with chronic obstructive pulmonary disease and hypoxemia with long term oxygen therapy. J Steroid Biochem Molec Biol 1993; 46:799.
148. Hjalmarsen A, Aasebo U, Aakvaag A, Jorde R. Sex hormone responses in healthy men and male patients with chronic obstructive pulmonary disease during an oral glucose load. Scand J Clin Lab Invest 1996; 56:635.
149. Vogel AV, Peake GT, Rada RT. Pituitary-testicular axis dysfunction in burned men. J Clin Endocrinol Metab 1985; 60:658.
150. Heikkonen E, Ylikahri R, Roine R, et al. The combined effect of alcohol and physical exercise on serum testosterone, luteinizing hormone, and cortisol in males. Alcohol Clin Exp Res 1996; 20:711.
151. Aakvaag A, Bentdal O, Quigstad K, et al. Testosterone and testosterone binding globulin (TeBG) in young men during prolonged stress. Int J Androl 1978; 1:22.
152. Nilsson PM, Moller L, Solstad K. Adverse effects of psychosocial stress on gonadal function and insulin levels in middle-aged males. J Intern Med 1995; 237:479.
153. Schulz P, Walker JP, Peyrin L, et al. Lower sex hormones in men during anticipatory stress. Neuroreport 1996; 7:3101.
154. Chatterton RT Jr, Vogelsong KM, Lu YC, Hudgens GA. Hormonal responses to psychological stress in men preparing for skydiving. J Clin Endocrinol Metab 1997; 82:2503.
155. Chatterton RT Jr, Dooley SL. Reversal of diurnal cortisol rhythm and suppression of plasma testosterone in obstetric residents on call. J Soc Gynecol Invest 1999; 6:50.
156. Kuoppasalmi K, Naveri H, Harkonen M, Adlercreutz H. Plasma cortisol, androstenedione, testosterone and luteinizing hormone in running exercise of different intensities. Scand J Clin Lab Invest 1980; 40:403.
157. Cernak I, Savic J, Lazarov A. Relations among plasma prolactin, testosterone, and injury severity in war casualties. World J Surg 1997; 21:240.
158. Elman I, Breier A. Effects of acute metabolic stress on plasma progesterone and testosterone in male subjects: relationship to pituitary-adrenocortical axis activation. Life Sci 1997; 61:1705.
159. Semple PD, Beastall GH, Watson WS, Hume R. Hypothalamic-pituitary dysfunction in respiratory hypoxia. Thorax 1981; 36:605.
160. Semple PD, Beastall GH, Brown TM, et al. Sex hormone suppression and sexual impotence in hypoxic pulmonary fibrosis. Thorax 1984; 39:46.
161. Handelsman DJ, Conway AJ, Boylan LM, van Nunen SA. Testicular function and fertility in men with homozygous α-1 antitrypsin deficiency. Andrologia 1986; 18:406.
162. Mackworth-Young CG, Parke AL, Morley KD, et al. Sex hormones in male patients with systemic lupus erythematosus: a comparison with other disease groups. Eur J Rheumatol Inflamm 1983; 6:228.
163. Gordon D, Beastall GH, Thomson JA, Sturrock RD. Androgenic status and sexual function in males with rheumatoid arthritis and ankylosing spondylitis. Q J Med 1986; 60:671.
164. Gordon D, Beastall GH, Thomson JA, Sturrock RD. Prolonged hypogonadism in male patients with rheumatoid arthritis during flares in disease activity. Br J Rheumatol 1988; 27:440.

# CHAPTER 117

# ERECTILE DYSFUNCTION

GLENN R. CUNNINGHAM AND MAX HIRSHKOWITZ

## DEFINITIONS OF ERECTILE DYSFUNCTION

The literal definition of *impotence* is loss of power. This term emphasizes the enormous psychological effect sexual problems can have on some men. Furthermore, impotence also concerns the sexual partner and can play a critical role in a relationship. Nevertheless, the word "impotence" carries a very negative connotation; therefore, the term *sexual dysfunction* is preferred.

Human sexual activity involves four processes: *desire, arousal* (both attaining and maintaining erections), *consummation*, and *fertilization*. Significant difficulty in any of these processes can produce sexual problems. In men, sexual dysfunction most often denotes *erectile dysfunction (ED)*. However, loss of sexual desire (libido), nonconsummation (ejaculatory or orgasmic problems), and even infertility are sometimes referred to as "impotence" in the medical and lay literature. Thus, to avoid ambiguity, *specific designations*, rather than the term "impotence," are used in this chapter.

*Libido* is sexual desire, calling for relief through sexual activity. *Erectile dysfunction* may be defined as difficulty obtaining or maintaining a penile erection sufficient to permit vaginal penetration and satisfactory conclusion of sexual intercourse. (In men, ED is the most common sexual problem.) *Orgasm* is the pleasurable sensation marking the climax of sexual activity. *Failure to ejaculate* (emit seminal fluid) raises concern primarily in situations in which fertility is desired (see Chap. 118).

In the not too distant past, ED was seldom addressed. Shame, guilt, ignorance, and lack of effective therapy perpetuated the patient's practice of concealing problems and the clinician's practice of overlooking them. However, treatment of ED has steadily progressed into mainstream medicine. Reasons for this include (a) the liberalization of society's attitude toward sex, (b) the increasing mean age of the population, (c) the greater emphasis on maximizing quality of life, (d) the recognition that most ED stems from organic conditions, (e) availability of more precise diagnostic methods, and (f) development of improved therapies.

## PREVALENCE OF ERECTILE DYSFUNCTION

The revolutionizing effect of improved therapeutics became readily apparent following the introduction of sildenafil (Viagra), the orally administered agent for treating ED. The widespread public media attention produced a flood of patients presenting with ED and seeking this treatment from primary care physicians. Commonly, the drug is administered as first-line empirical therapy with little regard for cause or diagnosis. If it provides relief, its use is continued. The availability of this drug altered (a) the population seeking treatment, (b) the persons who administer treatment, and (c) the overall treatment algorithms used in medical practice. Interestingly, availability of this compound has helped verify the high prevalence estimates of previous studies.

Early estimates of the prevalence of ED were relatively low. In 1948, Kinsey reported that 1.9% of 40-year-old men complained of ED; this number increased to 6.7% by age 50, 18.4% by age 60, and 27.4% by age 70. A household survey of men found that 35.3% of married men older than 60 years of age had ED.[1] Another large study confirmed the frequency of ED and reported a higher frequency among those with cardiovascular

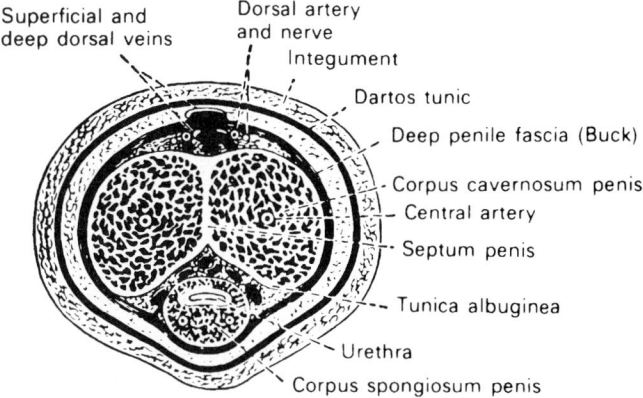

**FIGURE 117-1.** Transverse section of the penis. The two corpora cavernosa become engorged with blood, resulting in penile erection. They are surrounded by the relatively inelastic tunica albuginea, which helps to provide rigidity. (From Clemente CD, ed. Gray's anatomy, 30th ed. Philadelphia: Lea & Febiger, 1985:1564.)

risk factors and among smokers.[2] The age-adjusted probability of ED also increases as the level of high-density lipoprotein (HDL) cholesterol decreases; however, no association is found with the total cholesterol level. The risk for developing ED is ~2.6% per year for men 40 to 69 years of age.

## ANATOMY AND PHYSIOLOGY

### PENILE ANATOMY

Because of its anatomy, the penis has the potential for rapid engorgement with blood, an increase in size, and the development of rigidity. The two corpora cavernosa become engorged with blood during erection (Fig. 117-1). They contain lacunae lined by endothelium possessing contractile elements and have septa that are rich in smooth-muscle cells, elastin, nerves, and small blood vessels.[3] The two corpora have a vascular communication and, unlike the corpus spongiosum, are surrounded by a relatively inelastic tunica albuginea. This arrangement enables the generation of very high intracavernosal pressure and rigidity of the penis when venous outflow is reduced and the lacunae are engorged. The glans penis is an extension of the corpus spongiosum.

The arterial supply of the penis derives from the *internal pudendal arteries*, which are branches of the internal iliac vessels. Each pudendal artery provides a branch to the bulbourethra, a deep artery to one of the corpora cavernosa, and a dorsal artery. Venous blood eventually drains into the deep pelvic veins.

A complex array of autonomic and somatic nerves innervates the penis. *Sympathetic fibers* originate from thoracolumbar and sacral levels. They reach the pelvic plexus through hypogastric and pudendal nerves. *Parasympathetic innervation* derives from S2 to S4. The glans penis is rich in nerve endings that convey touch, pain, temperature, and vibration. Although *local neural centers* in the lumbosacral spinal cord can cause erection in response to stimulation of the penis, penile erections usually are stimulated by olfactory, auditory, visual, and other sensory inputs that are *perceived centrally* by the frontal, temporal, parietal, or occipital lobes. These areas may be stimulated by memory and fantasy. Signals are sent to the visceral brain, to the rhinencephalon, and subsequently to the centers in the spinal cord.

### PHYSIOLOGY OF THE ERECTILE PROCESS

#### VASCULAR ASPECTS

The normal erectile process requires an increase in blood flow to the corpora cavernosa. Studies have demonstrated that the direct injection of 20 to 50 mL of saline per minute into the corpus cavernosum of fresh cadavers can initiate an erection. Furthermore, the erection can be maintained by an infusion rate of 12 mL per minute, although infusion into the internal pudendal artery is ineffective.[4] Shunting of blood from the deep artery of the cavernosum into the vascular spaces, relaxation of the smooth muscles of the cavernous tissues, and impeded drainage are important factors in the erectile process.[5]

## NEUROMUSCULAR ASPECTS

Histochemical studies indicate that the corpora cavernosa are rich in adrenergic fibers. In vitro studies have demonstrated contractile responses to norepinephrine in the presence of phentolamine, implying *β-adrenergic as well as α-adrenergic stimulation*.[3] The adrenergic nerves are responsible for detumescence. In this respect, *endothelin-1*, which is present in erectile tissue,[6] can, like adrenergic stimulation, increase cytosolic $Ca^{2+}$ and cause smooth muscle contraction. In the corpora cavernosa, acetylcholinesterase-positive fibers are few, and the contraction of the smooth muscle in the presence of high concentrations of acetylcholine is minimal. Interestingly, *vasoactive intestinal peptide (VIP)*, a potent dilator of smooth muscle, is found in the corpora,[7] although neither adrenergic nor cholinergic nerves innervate the VIP-containing cells. Levels of VIP in the cavernous spaces of the corpora cavernosa increase during tumescence, and the direct injection of VIP into the corpora cavernosa induces an erection in some normal men and in some men with ED (see Chaps. 182 and 184). *Nitric oxide* is the primary endothelium-derived relaxing factor,[8] and it causes the smooth muscle in the corpora cavernosa to relax. Nitric oxide synthase has been identified in the neurons and endothelium in the corpora cavernosa.[9] Nitric oxide synthase and VIP immunoreactivity colocalize to perivascular and trabecular nerve fibers in the corpus cavernosa.[10] Importantly, positive staining for nitric oxide synthase is positively correlated with a clinical history of cavernous nerve integrity.[11]

## ENDOCRINE INFLUENCE

In humans, testosterone (T) and dihydrotestosterone (DHT) play critical roles during the embryogenesis of the testes, epididymis, vas deferens, seminal vesicles, prostate, and external genitalia. Furthermore, evidence implicates the sex steroids in imprinting *gender identification* on the central nervous system (see Chap. 176).[12] The development of the accessory sex glands, testes, and external genitalia depend on normal circulating levels of androgen and on the androgen responsiveness of the target tissues. This is also the case for the development of secondary sex characteristics at puberty. In addition, androgen mediates the development and maintenance of libido and erectile function.

Antiestrogens do not appear to inhibit libido or potency in man. Moreover, DHT alone is as effective as T in maintaining potency in agonadal men.[13] This differs from the situation in rodents, in which aromatization of androgens to estrogen is required for normal sexual function. Humans appear not to require this process to maintain sexuality. Indeed, sexual desire and erectile function remain intact in men with 5α-reductase deficiency type 2, who have extremely low DHT levels.

Early studies in mixed populations indicate several age-related changes. Serum total T levels fall, T-binding globulin (TeBG) binding capacity increases, free T levels fall, and estradiol levels increase or remain constant after the fifth decade of life. Similar hormonal changes have been observed in healthy monks living in a monastery, where environmental factors were minimal.[14] On the other hand, some reports have demonstrated normal levels of total and free serum T in extremely healthy aging men. Usually, serum T levels exhibit less circadian rhythm in older men than in younger men.[15] A large metaanal-

ysis found that, in healthy men, aging was accompanied by a fall in T levels when samples were drawn in the morning.[16] Thus, health status and age can affect total and free T levels as well as their diurnal variations. The changes are greatest in patients aged 70 years or older (see Chap. 199).

## RELATIONSHIP BETWEEN SLEEP-RELATED ERECTIONS AND SERUM TESTOSTERONE

Objective direct measurement of penile erections can be accomplished using strain gauges to monitor changes in circumference. Applying a force to the penile tip during an erection and assessing its resistance to buckling provides an index for rigidity, sometimes referred to as *erectile quality*. Thus, frequency, magnitude, duration, and quality of erections can be studied with continuous monitoring. Spontaneous erections occur in association with rapid-eye-movement (REM) sleep. These *sleep-related erections (SREs)* are used to study nonvolitional physiologic processes associated with sexuality; some of this research has addressed endocrine mechanisms.

The gonadotropin-releasing hormone (GnRH) agonist leuprolide initially stimulates and later decreases gonadotropin secretion; within three weeks of injection, serum T levels are suppressed. In one study, leuprolide injection was followed by varying dosages of replacement T (using microspheres) to achieve serum T levels in either the low-normal or the high-normal ranges.[17] No posttreatment differences were found in the number, magnitude, or duration of nocturnal erections. With respect to involuntary SREs, men with induced low-normal T levels did not differ from those with high-normal T levels. Another study in which either leuprolide or a placebo was administered examined whether induced T suppression altered SREs in normal men.[18] The percentage of REM sleep and sleep efficiency did not differ between groups, but a significant reduction in total tumescence was observed at 2 and 3 months in the group receiving leuprolide. Another study compared SRE changes in response to supplemental testosterone enanthate (TE) (150 mg given intramuscularly) and to placebo in normal men.[19] SREs were recorded when T levels were high or supernormal (2 days after injection). No significant differences were noted in frequency, magnitude, or duration of SREs; however, penile rigidity and duration of maximal rigidity were increased in those receiving TE. Antagonists to GnRH can also be used to suppress T levels. Healthy young adult men made hypogonadal in this manner complain of sexual dysfunction within a month.[20] T replacement with as little as 50 mg of TE per week prevents symptoms. This collection of studies suggests that a *T threshold exists for sexual behaviors and that this threshold is slightly below the normal range of serum T levels for young adult men*. Little or no change is found in erections at widely varying T levels within the normal range. This finding is consistent with data indicating that the threshold level for ED is ~200 ng/dL in men with diseases producing hypogonadism.[21]

The associations between SREs and T levels may be mediated directly by T, or indirectly by its metabolites (DHT and estradiol). (At least two 5α-reductase enzymes are found; therefore, to ascertain DHT's role in erection would require inhibiting both.) The central nervous system effects of 5α-reductase inhibitors or of aromatase inhibitors depend on the permeability of the blood–brain barrier. Many such inhibitors are steroids and should cross that barrier. Males with inherited 5α-reductase defect type 2 develop a normal libido and erections; however, their penile development is delayed (occurring at puberty). Furthermore, these men have only rudimentary prostates.[22] Because of the latter phenomenon, inhibitors of the activity of both 5α-reductase type 1 and 5α-reductase type 2 have been developed in hopes of treating prostatic hyperplasia and cancer. Reduced libido or erections are found in 3% to 4% of men treated with finasteride[23] (a type 2 inhibitor) or with GI198745 (unpublished data) (an inhibitor of both the type 1

## TABLE 117-1.
### Evaluation of Erectile Dysfunction (ED)

**HISTORY**
  Marital status
  Extramarital experiences
  Homosexual activity
  Erectile history
    Early morning erections
    Masturbation
    Nocturnal erections and emissions
    Pain or curvature of penis
    Previous priapism
    Prior trauma or surgery of genitalia, perineum, pelvis, or lower abdomen
    Ejaculatory disturbance
    Libido
    Estimate of penile size during erection
    Penile or genital sensation
    Onset of ED
      Gradual and progressive?
      Sudden?
      After major surgery?
    Prior history of urologic, vascular, or neurologic disorders
    History of diabetes, hypertension, increased low-density lipoprotein cho-lesterol, or pulmonary, liver, renal, or other systemic disease
    Drug use, excessive alcohol intake, smoking
    Psychological factors
      Was ED acute in onset?
      Is ED intermittent?
      Is ED selective for one sex partner?
      Sex partner's reaction to ED?
**PHYSICAL EXAMINATION**
  Body habitus
  Hair patterns
  Penile abnormalities
  Testicular size
  Testicular sensitivity
  Femoral pulses
  Somatic motor and sensory examination
  Supine and erect blood pressures and pulses

## TABLE 117-2.
### Drugs Associated with Erectile Dysfunction

| | |
|---|---|
| Antiandrogen | Cimetidine, cyproterone acetate, estrogens, finas-teride, ketoconazole, progestins, spironolactone |
| Anticholinergic | Atropine, butyrophenones, disopyramide, gangli-onic blocking agents |
| Antidepressants | Monamine oxidase inhibitors, tricyclic antidepres-sants, selective serotonin reuptake inhibitors |
| Antihypertensives | α-Methyldopa, reserpine, clonidine, propranolol, thiazides, prazosin, phenoxybenzamine, phen-tolamine |
| Antipsychotics | Phenothiazines, thioridazine |
| Central nervous sys-tem depressants | Barbiturates, benzodiazepines, carbamazepine, methadone, morphine, phenytoin, primidone |
| Substances of abuse | Amphetamines, cocaine, heroin, ethanol, tobacco |

and type 2 enzymes). In this regard, in a double-blind, placebo-controlled trial of sexually active men, no consistent changes were found in SRE frequency, magnitude, duration, or quality in response to finasteride, 5 mg daily, or placebo administered for 3 months.[24]

Animal models are also useful for studying erectile physiology. Androgen receptors are present in nerves that innervate the corpora cavernosa. Androgen can modulate nitric oxide (NO) synthase activity and NO production by these neurons.[25–28] Interestingly, DHT is required for normal penile erections in the rat.

# EVALUATION OF ERECTILE DYSFUNCTION

## OVERVIEW

The diagnostic testing and treatment options for ED are intimately related. Invasive therapy necessitates greater reliance on diagnostic testing than do benign therapeutic interventions. Consequently, practice conventions have changed radically now that a relatively safe, orally administered medication for treatment of ED is available.

For years, the evaluation and treatment of ED was the purview of specialists. The complexity of the erectile and ejaculatory processes often required evaluation by clinicians from several disciplines. With the introduction of sildenafil, however,

most men are seen initially by their primary care physicians. Commonly, empirical treatment ensues, and referral to a specialist is made only after treatment failure. This approach provides treatment to a large number of men at lowest cost, but it shifts efficacy and risk assessments to primary care providers.

Before any treatment is initiated, the assessment should begin with a careful history-taking and physical examination, recording of the sexual history, and a thorough review of the sexual problem. Use of questionnaires can be particularly helpful for the sexual history-taking and problem documentation. These procedures allow informed determination of (a) the need for treatment, (b) the nature of the dysfunction, (c) the severity of the condition, and (d) the potential contraindications for treatment. Sometimes problems are related to medication side effects, and at other times they may stem directly from relationship issues. If the physician has a high clinical suspicion of a specific pathologic condition (e.g., hypothyroidism), appropriate laboratory testing should be performed. Further diagnostic assessment usually is considered only after the initial treatment challenge fails. Additional diagnostic tests are indicated, as interventions become more invasive.

## HISTORY AND PHYSICAL EXAMINATION

The history-taking and physical examination seek to evaluate the severity of the patient's erectile problems and determine the cause. Whether the ED is due primarily to *organic* or *psychogenic factors* helps direct the therapeutic approach. Aspects of the history and physical examination are outlined in Table 117-1. Use of a short questionnaire may help identify specific sexual complaints. Many drugs that act on the central or autonomic nervous system have been associated with ED[29–31] (Table 117-2); however, most of these drugs have not been tested using objective measures of erectile function. For example, questionnaire studies addressing the effects of the use of selective serotonin reuptake inhibitors in 152 men and 192 women revealed greater delayed orgasm and ED with paroxetine than with fluvoxamine, fluoxetine, and sertraline. Overall, sexual dysfunction correlated with dosage. On the other hand, patients with premature ejaculation benefited from ejaculatory delay and had improved sexual satisfaction.[32] This latter result supports the laboratory-demonstrated therapeutic benefit realized by patients with premature ejaculation from the use of clomipramine[33,34] and fluoxetine.[35] Nonetheless, objective studies of drug-related iatrogenic ED are largely lacking.

The clinician should consider relevant comorbid factors (Table 117-3). Many endocrine disorders, genitourinary diseases, and neurologic dysfunctions are associated with ED. Importantly, aging per se does not cause ED; however, the incidence of many ED-causing diseases increases as a function of age. In the community-based Massachusetts Male Aging Study, hypertension, diabetes, cigarette smoking, and low levels of

**TABLE 117-3.**
**Diseases Associated with Organic Erectile Dysfunction**

| | |
|---|---|
| Endocrine | 17-Ketoreductase deficiency, Cushing syndrome, diabetes, feminizing testicular or adrenal tumor, hyperthyroidism, hyperprolactinemia, hypogonadism (primary or secondary), hypothyroidism, pituitary tumor |
| Genitourinary | Hypospadias, medical therapies for testicular cancer, micropenis, pelvic fracture, penectomy, penile trauma, perineal prostatectomy, Peyronie disease, phimosis, priapism, prostate irradiation, prostatitis, retroperitoneal lymphadenectomy, rectosigmoid surgery, systemic sclerosis, urethritis |
| Neurologic | Amyotrophic lateral sclerosis, arachnoiditis, autonomic neuropathy, Friedreich ataxia, general paresis, herniated disc, hypothalamic disease, multiple sclerosis, parkinsonism, pelvic or retroperitoneal lymphadenectomy, peripheral neuropathy, pernicious anemia, Shy-Drager syndrome, spina bifida, spinal cord transection, spinal cord tumor, spinal cord syrinx, sympathectomy, tabes dorsalis, temporal lobe disorders, transverse myelitis |
| Vascular | Aneurysm, aortoilial arteriosclerosis and atherosclerosis, arteritis, Leriche syndrome, aortoiliac surgery, hypertension |
| Organ system | Cardiac, hepatic, pulmonary, or renal failure |

HDL lipoprotein cholesterol increased the risk of ED.[2] Cigarette smoking increased the probability of total ED in men with heart disease and hypertension. Increased Lp(a) lipoprotein levels also have been correlated with ED of vascular origin.[36]

## QUESTIONNAIRES

Sexual function inventories and psychometric tests provide valuable clinical information even though they do not reliably differentiate the cause of ED as being organic, psychological, or behavioral. Most specialized clinics assess attitudes toward sex, knowledge about sexual matters, prior sexual experience, self-perception, relationship dynamics, and performance anxiety. Exploring, at least in general, certain psychiatric issues—especially mood, general anxiety, and personality—is also helpful. Several standardized sexual functioning questionnaires are available. Widely recognized sexual history and functioning instruments designed for men include the Florida Sexual History Questionnaire, the Sexual Arousability Inventory, the Sexual Anxiety Inventory, the Pittsburgh Sexual Functioning Inventory, and the Derogatis Sexual Functioning Inventory. Relationship issues can be investigated using the Dyadic Adjustment Scale or the more elaborate Family Adaptability and Cohesion Evaluation Scales III (FACES-III). Commonly used self-administered instruments for assessing mood, anxiety, and personality include the Beck and Zung depression inventories, the Spielberger State-Trait Anxiety Inventory, and the Minnesota Multiphasic Personality Inventory. Alternatively, a psychiatric interview can provide the skilled clinician with comparable information.

The use of information obtained from the questionnaires mentioned previously helps to optimize the treatment plan. However, a positive psychological test finding does not necessarily indicate a psychogenic basis for ED. Distress arising from an organically based intermittent erectile failure is understandable. Performance anxiety is likely to emerge, mood may suffer, and changes in relationship dynamics will follow. Denial, avoidance, projection, guilt, reaction formation, or depression may accompany organic ED. For many men, the development of ED, regardless of its cause, constitutes a crisis. Psychological or behavioral measures reflect this fact.

If ED is primarily psychogenic, evaluating the nature and scope of psychological, relationship, and behavioral disruption can identify problems and suggest appropriate ways to intervene. If the primary mechanism underlying ED is organic, psychometric instruments can identify factors compounding the condition. Moreover, psychological and relationship issues may

render physiologically targeted therapies ineffective unless the clinician addresses secondary behavioral factors. Therefore, because psychiatric, relationship, and behavioral influences can predispose to, precipitate, or perpetuate ED, these nonorganic factors must not be overlooked.

## LABORATORY AND ENDOCRINE TESTS

Usually, a complete blood count and screening serum chemistries will detect systemic diseases that can cause ED, and measurement of serum T level can detect androgen deficiency (Fig. 117-2). If the initial T level is <350 ng/dL, early morning serum T, luteinizing hormone, and prolactin levels should be obtained. Because T and prolactin values are higher in the early morning, blood specimens should be collected between 8:00 and 10:00 a.m. The age-related increase in TeBG or sex hormone–binding globulin produces a reduction in non–TeBG-bound T. This is the fraction that is bioactive; therefore, measurement or calculation of non–TeBG-bound T in men who are older than 60 years or have altered levels of TeBG may be useful. (However, commercially available free T assays are influenced by the level of TeBG and often are unreliable.) Thyroid and adrenal disease can cause ED and, if suspected, should be considered in the evaluation.

## SLEEP-RELATED ERECTION TESTING

SREs were first reported in adults in 1944.[37] The association between SREs and *REM sleep* was established 21 years later, and the term *nocturnal penile tumescence (NPT)* was coined. Although the function of REM sleep erections is unknown, they have proven useful for assessing erectile capability in men complaining of ED.[38] Erectile activity can be measured directly and objectively in terms of increases in penile length, circumference, and volume, duration of erection, and firmness of the penis during erection. Procedures used to measure activity during the initiation and maintenance phases of erection need to be as unobtrusive as possible to minimize alterations in erection produced by the apparatus. Measuring penile length or volume is both difficult and expensive; by contrast, expandable strain gauges provide easily transduced electronic signals that are linearly related to *circumference* change.[39] Other instruments measure penile circumference by measuring lengths of inelastic band encircling the penis.[40] Measuring circumference increase is the most common method for indexing the presence and duration of erections.

Compared to other techniques, SRE testing provides several advantages for assessing erectile function. Sleep erections occur naturally and are virtually independent of psychological influences.[41,42] Patients with anxiety disorders who experience intermittent erectile failure during the day have normal SRE patterns. By contrast, SRE patterns reveal erectile impairment in patients with a wide variety of *comorbid organic conditions*. These include diabetes, spinal cord injury, end-stage renal disease, Shy-Drager syndrome, alcoholism, peripheral autonomic deficits, subnormal T levels, supernormal prolactin levels, aqueductal stenosis, narcolepsy, hypertension, sleep apnea, periodic limb movement disorder, chronic obstructive pulmonary disease, cigarette smoking, and atherosclerosis.[43] The interpretation of sleep erection changes associated with major depression (formerly termed "organic depression") are controversial.[44] Some clinicians characterize depression-related decrements as evidence for a psychological effect. Others interpret these same data as support for the contention that major depression has an organic basis, noting that other REM sleep alterations are associated with major depressive disorder.

### LABORATORY SLEEP-RELATED ERECTION TESTING

The current *gold standard* for evaluating SREs combines penile circumference measurement with comprehensive *polysomnogra-*

## PART I: SPECIFIC TREATMENTS

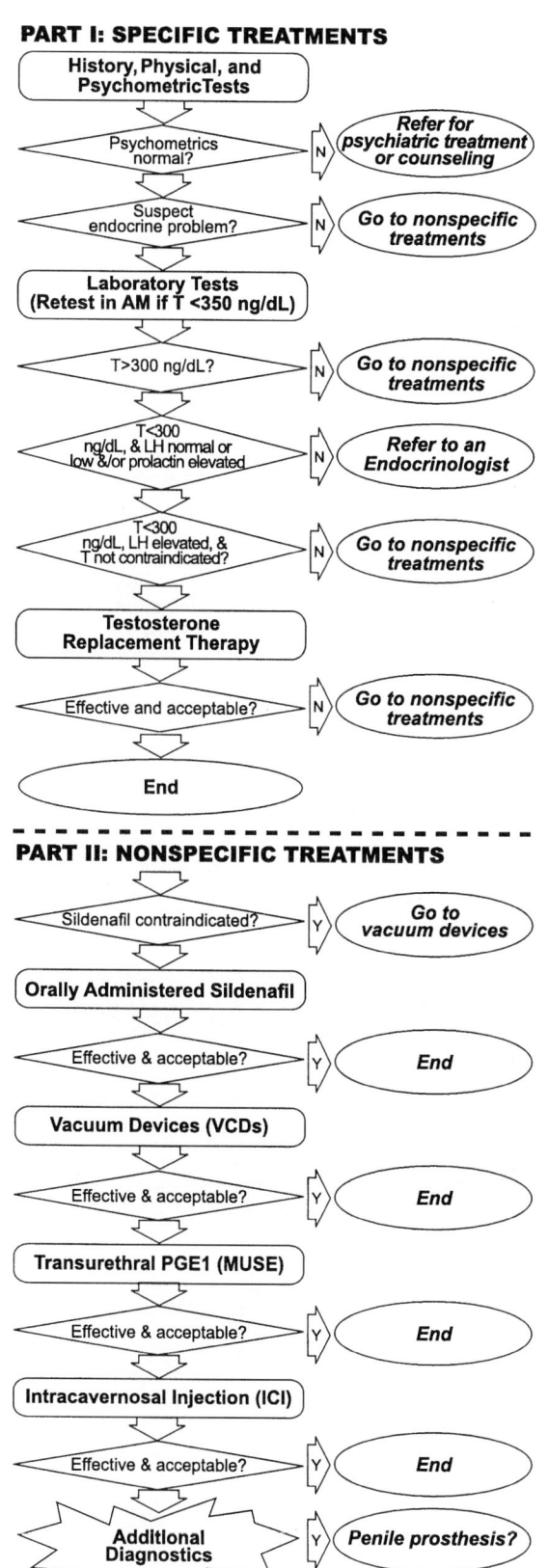

**FIGURE 117-2.** Proposed treatment algorithm for erectile dysfunction. Part I shows etiologically specific treatments and part II illustrates a hierarchical cascade of nonspecific treatments. Nonspecific treatments begin with noninvasive approaches and continue with minimally invasive (Medicated Urethral System for Erection, *MUSE*), moderately invasive (intracavernosal injection, *ICI*), and very invasive (prosthesis) therapeutics. (*T*, testosterone; *LH*, luteinizing hormone; *PGE₁*, prostaglandin E₁.)

*phy.*[45] To measure circumference, strain gauges are placed around the penile base and just behind the glans. To assess sleep, noninvasive measures of brain activity, eye movements, skeletal muscle tone, airflow, respiratory effort, leg movement, and heart rhythm are recorded. Polysomnography documents the sleep patterns, allowing reliable interpretation and recognition of sleep disorders that are common in men with ED (e.g., obstructive sleep apnea syndrome and periodic limb movement disorder).

*Penile rigidity* is the most important SRE measure. It is determined during the maximal circumference of one or more representative erections. A calibrated force is applied to the tip of the penis (parallel to the shaft), and the amount of force required to bend the penile shaft is noted (force stops at 1000 g). This penile resistance to buckling indexes rigidity. Most healthy, sexually functional men have values >1000 g. The average minimum force needed to achieve penetration, under optimal circumstances, is ~500 g.[46] Rigidity between 500 and 750 g usually indicates some organic involvement but enough residual function to achieve penetration in situations made maximally conducive for sexual activity.

Other critically important measures concern the *erectile pattern* in relation to REM. An erection should achieve full magnitude soon after the transition to REM sleep. In potent men, a maximum-increase plateau phase continues throughout most of the REM sleep episode. With REM sleep termination, detumescence occurs, and the penile circumference rapidly falls to baseline (Fig. 117-3). Detumescence during ongoing REM sleep can indicate organic problems. Complaints of an inability to maintain erections are verified when sleep erections do not persist for at least 5 to 10 minutes. Age-related normative values for SREs are available.[47] Overall, SREs persist across the life span in sexually potent men. Some decline may occur with age, but critical measures change little. Importantly, penile rigidity and duration of maximal erectile phase remain within the functional range in healthy, sexually active men, regardless of age.

### NONLABORATORY SLEEP-RELATED TESTING

Laboratory SRE testing is expensive and labor intensive. In an attempt to contain costs, alternative techniques have evolved to *detect or record erections in the home*. Devices that slide, snap, or break in response to penile expansion can detect erections. In theory, a sufficiently large or rigid erection will expand or break the device. In home studies, a patient inspects the device in the morning and reports the results. In practice, these devices are known to yield substantial false-positive and false-negative results.[48]

Another approach is to *continuously monitor penile circumference* and record the information. These devices do not depend on the patient to record test results. One such device (RigiScan) also measures *compressibility* (Fig. 117-4). The original technique used for indexing rigidity sufficient to achieve vaginal penetration was measurement of buckling resistance (Fig. 117-5).[46] The subsequent adoption of the same term, rigidity, to describe tissue compressibility has produced confusion, especially when earlier work is cited as rationale for the importance of this indicator. Both methods index rigidity, but the difference must be kept in mind when interpreting clinical test results.

Table 117-4 compares information obtained using laboratory procedures to that obtained using various portable devices. Two issues are critical: (a) determination of sleep state, and (b) susceptibility to tampering. The relationship between REM sleep and erection is critical, because REM sleep provides the prerequisite underlying nervous system activity needed for nocturnal erections. Thus, a normal pattern of erections registered on a continuous circumference recorder raises clinical suspicion of psychogenic ED. However, reduced or absent REM sleep leads to diminished sleep erections. Therefore, test results that show reduced penile activity are inconclusive unless ade-

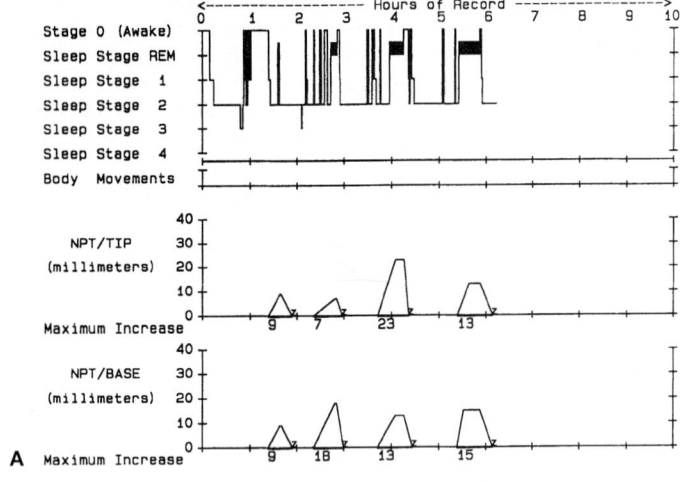

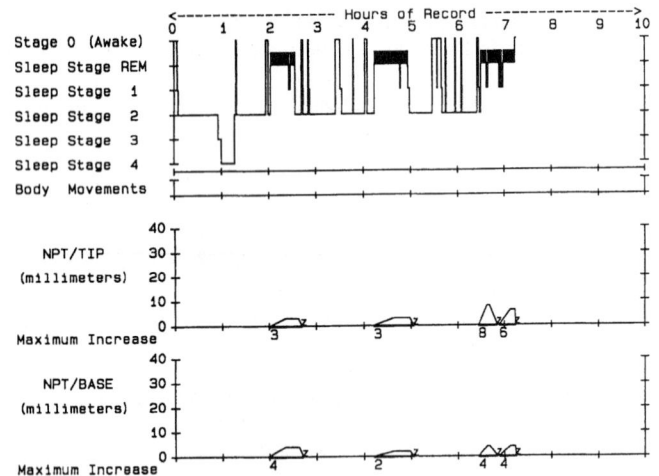

**FIGURE 117-3.** Normal and abnormal sleep-related erection (*SRE*) profiles. **A,** Sleep-stage patterns and penile circumference increase in a hypogonadal man with effective androgen replacement. **B,** Diminished SRE profile present 2 months after cessation of testosterone therapy in the same patient. (*REM,* rapid eye movement; *NPT,* nocturnal penile tumescence.)

quate REM sleep is documented. Importantly, middle-aged men, especially those with obesity and hypertension, are at significant risk (>15%) for sleep apnea,[49] a condition that can profoundly disrupt REM sleep. SRE testing is popular in cases involving litigation concerning personal injury or accusations of rape. Nonlaboratory test results are too easily manipulated for application in this arena. A man need only remain awake all night to suppress erections. Thus, laboratory studies with polysomnography provide the most optimal information, but at considerable expense. Although home monitoring may preserve some essential features of SRE testing, it falls short in other aspects. False-negative results can be avoided with laboratory sleep studies.[43]

## ADDITIONAL DIAGNOSTIC TESTS

### PENILE BLOOD PRESSURE

The early attempts to develop objective indices for documenting vasculogenic ED investigated pressure in the flaccid penis. Using a Doppler system, systolic blood pressure is measured in the left and right dorsal and cavernosal arteries. These pressures are expressed as a percentage of brachial pressure to produce a penile-brachial index (PBI).[50–52] Studies of PBI in patients with

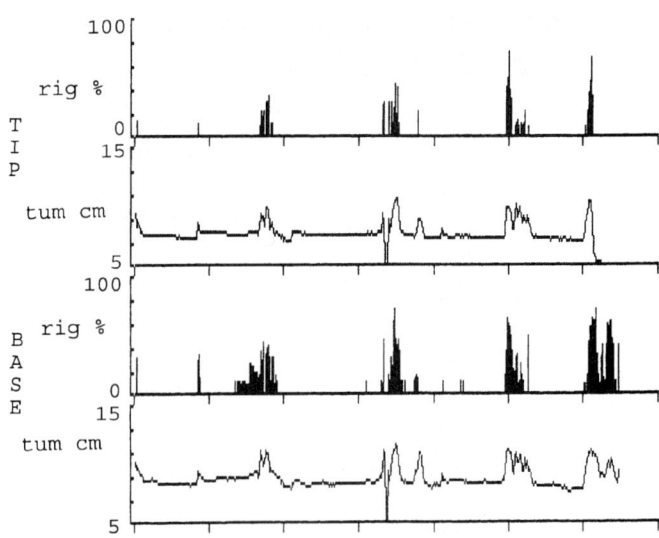

**FIGURE 117-4.** Normal RigiScan histogram. Penile circumference (*Tum*) in centimeters and compressibility (*Rig*) recorded from coronal sulcus (*Tip*) and penile base (*Base*) in a young adult, potent volunteer subject. A normal pattern of erections, presumably during rapid-eye-movement sleep, can be seen. The absence of such a normal pattern could derive from either organic erectile dysfunction or disturbed sleep and, therefore, would be diagnostically inconclusive.

different conditions associated with organic ED reveal statistically significant differences. The intersubject variance is large, however, so that the clinical usefulness of this test is limited. If practice demographics are weighted toward severe vasculogenic ED, this inexpensive test may be useful. In general, values <0.70 are abnormal, those between 0.70 and 0.75 are borderline, those between 0.76 and 0.80 are at the low end of the normal

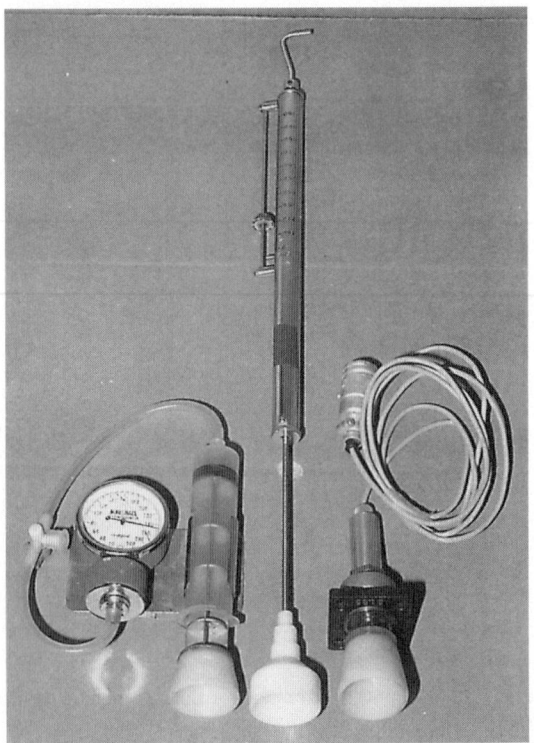

**FIGURE 117-5.** Rigidity meters. Three devices for measuring penile rigidity are shown. The instrument used in the authors' original studies assessed firmness by indexing pressure (*left*). This device was replaced with a spring-loaded mechanical force meter (*middle*). Electronic force gauges also are used to determine penile buckling resistance (*right*).

**TABLE 117-4.**
**Sleep-Related-Erection (SRE) Recording Protocols
and What They Measure**

| PARAMETER | Laboratory | Unattended, Overnight Erection Tests | |
|---|---|---|---|
| | SREs with Polysomnography | Continuous Monitors | Devices That Snap or Break |
| Erection occurred | Yes | Yes | Yes |
| Number of erections | Yes | Yes | No |
| Circumference increase | Yes | Yes | No |
| Duration of erections | Yes | Yes | No |
| Coordination with REM sleep | Yes | No | No |
| Penile compressibility | No | Yes | No |
| Penile buckling resistance | Yes | No | No |

REM, rapid eye movement.

range, and those >0.80 are normal. Note that certain conditions (e.g., cigarette smoking) can produce transient decreases in PBI.[53] Therefore, results need cautious interpretation.

## ERECTILE RESPONSE TO VASODILATOR INJECTION

When injected into the penis, agents that relax smooth muscle commonly produce erections (see Therapeutic Approaches). *Intracavernosal injection (ICI) of a vasodilator* is popular as a diagnostic challenge. Failure to attain full erection after injection of papaverine or prostaglandin $E_1$ ($PGE_1$) has been interpreted as suggesting vascular problems. By contrast, men with ED of neurogenic etiology often have a heightened response. However, some reports challenge the usefulness of this procedure.

Differential diagnosis of ED using ICI of papaverine or $PGE_1$ has been compared with classification based on SRE findings using a RigiScan device.[54] One hundred and fifty-nine men with ED were evaluated. Satisfactory sleep erections were observed in 58%; 15% definitely had impaired SREs. Of 92 men (58%) with satisfactory SREs, 40% had clearly impaired and 41% had satisfactory responses to ICI testing. Of the 51 men with normal ICI responses, 8% had clearly impaired SREs and 74.5% had satisfactory SREs. Thus, the high incidence of abnormal responses to ICI challenge in men with normal SREs limits the diagnostic value of ICI testing. In another study, men who had diabetes and ED were compared with an age-matched, nondiabetic group with ED.[55] RigiScan recordings classified 29% of the diabetic men who had complained of erectile failure as having satisfactory SREs, compared with 58% of the men without diabetes. Twenty-seven of 41 men in the diabetic group (66%) who underwent ICI challenge had satisfactory responses. By contrast, only 7 (23%) of the 31 nondiabetic men tested with ICI had a satisfactory response. Only in the diabetic group was impairment of SREs associated with a good ICI response. Of the 21 (33%) men with diabetes and impaired SREs, 16 (76%) had a satisfactory response to ICI testing. None of the 7 SRE-impaired nondiabetic men had satisfactory responses to ICI challenge. Of the 17 diabetic men with known vascular disease, 14 (82%) had a satisfactory ICI response. These observations supported the use of SRE results, rather than a positive ICI response, to identify men with psychogenic ED.

## DUPLEX DOPPLER IMAGING

The combination of color Doppler and duplex ultrasonography provides information about the vascular supply and drainage of the penis. Individual arteries can be analyzed for peak flow rates, changes in arterial diameter, and pulsations. These measurements are of limited value when collected only when the penis is in the flaccid state, but provide useful information when obtained during a pharmacologically induced erection. In normal men, the diameter of the superficial arteries increases by 20% and the diameter of the deep arteries increases by 70%.[56] The blood flow increases three-fold in the superficial penile arteries and four-fold in the deep cavernous arteries. Peak flow velocity doubles for the superficial arteries and triples for the deep arteries. This information can be used to calculate arterial resistance.

Clinicians often infer the diagnoses of arterial insufficiency and venous leakage from duplex Doppler imaging. Peak velocities of <25 cm/sec are associated with arterial disease, whereas values of >35 cm/sec indicate normal arterial supply.[57] In some cases, however, anxiety and failure of the cavernosal smooth muscles to relax completely result in reduced flow. A strong correlation is seen with findings on pudendal arteriography; anatomic variations make arteriography necessary before revascularization is undertaken.[58] In a study of men with ED, venous insufficiency was diagnosed by a persistent diastolic velocity of >7 cm/sec. Normal findings were observed in 30% of patients, arterial insufficiency was found in 39%, and venous insufficiency was seen in 24%.[59] Others reported similar results.[60] Because Peyronie disease usually is obvious during an erection, the fact that this procedure, which involves a pharmacologically induced erection, can be used to make the diagnosis is not surprising. Interestingly, in another study, 55 of 280 men with ED who were thus tested were found to have Peyronie disease; 58% of these latter patients also had arterial or venous abnormalities.[61] Infusion cavernosography or injection of a radiopaque contrast agent coupled with radiography can also be used to document venous leakage.

Duplex ultrasonographic measurements taken after pharmacologic stimulation must be viewed cautiously, especially in men who may have psychogenic ED.[62] In a study of 40 men with ED, 20 men had abnormal results on duplex ultrasonography, and 9 of these men had normal SREs. Of the 20 men with normal duplex ultrasonographic findings, 11 had abnormal SREs. None of 14 men with normal SREs and other evidence of psychogenic ED had an abnormal result on duplex ultrasonography. Only 2 of 11 men in whom both studies were abnormal had evidence of psychogenic ED.

## NEUROLOGIC TESTING

Measurement of the *bulbocavernosus reflex (BCR)* in response to penile coronal stimulation can be used to evaluate the autonomic afferent nerves if autonomic neuropathy is suspected.[63,64] BCR latency is thought to reflect pudendal nerve function; however, in a group of men with ED, no reliable relationship was found between BCR and pudendal evoked responses.[65] By contrast, tibial and peroneal motor conduction studies hold promise as useful techniques. Prolonged latency indicates compromise of the sacral-spinal reflex arc, and somatic feedback mechanisms are believed necessary to maintain erection during intercourse. However, dysfunction of this pathway is neither necessary nor sufficient to produce diminished sleep erections. Frequently, an abnormal BCR can be observed in men with normal SREs.[66] Recording of cortical brain potentials to the same stimulus may also provide information about the resulting innervation of somatic pathways.

Autonomic dysfunction also correlates with ED, especially in men with diabetes.[67] Cardiac responses to deep breathing and orthostatic changes in blood pressure can be used to examine parasympathetic and sympathetic innervation. Severely impaired autonomic regulation correlates with SRE impairment. Another autonomic marker, electrodermal response, shows high activity during slow-wave sleep but is virtually absent during REM sleep erections.[68] Dysregulation in this pattern (i.e., electrodermal activity intrusions into REM sleep) is found in some patients with ED.

### ERECTILE RESPONSE TO VISUAL SEXUAL STIMULATION

The presentation of erotic films or videotapes fairly reliably produces penile erections in men with normal sexual function.[69] When visual sexual stimulation fails to evoke a full erection, the question of cause remains. Organic ED is not the only reason that a patient may be unable to achieve a full, firm, adequately sustained erection in a laboratory or hospital setting. Sympathetic activation and anxiety are known to inhibit volitional erections, and men with marginal erectile problems may be more susceptible to such factors. Furthermore, a disparity between what is depicted in the videotape and the patient's sexual preferences, gender identity, religiosity, and sensibilities also can inhibit response. Nonetheless, if a man achieves a full, firm, and sustained erection with visual stimulation, organic cause is ruled out, with rare exceptions. In such cases, psychological, behavioral, or relationship issues become the therapeutic focus.

## ETIOLOGY OF ERECTILE DYSFUNCTION

### OVERVIEW

The literature contains several studies in which men with ED were evaluated with SRE testing to differentiate organic and psychogenic causes for their condition. Other tests were used to further classify the organic causes. Two hundred and fifty-six men with ED were examined by a psychiatrist and a urologist, and then studied in a sleep laboratory using measurements of SREs. Thirty-six percent had organic ED, 38% had psychogenic ED, and 26% had a mixed or uncertain diagnosis.[70] Androgen deficiency or hyperprolactinemia was noted in 17.5%. Another study evaluated 172 men with ED aged 19 to 60 years.[71] Patients taking drugs strongly suspected of causing ED were excluded from the sample. Abnormal SREs and abnormal penile rigidity were observed in 62% of the patients, low penile blood pressure was noted in 37%, low serum T or mildly to moderately elevated prolactin values were observed in 22%, and Peyronie disease was noted in 8%. The evaluation of 121 *older* men with ED (mean age 68 ± 5.3 years) revealed 21% with a vascular cause for the ED, 28% with a neurogenic cause, and 30% with combined vasculogenic and neurogenic causes.[72] Drug-induced ED accounted for 4%, hypogonadism for 2.9%, and Peyronie disease for 1.3%. Abnormal SREs without identifiable cause occurred in 3.9% of these patients. Thus, the frequency of specific causes varies. Differences likely depend on referral patterns and how the reported group is defined. In nearly all reports, however, organic causes predominate. Other disease associations are listed in Table 117-3. Because many patients have benign prostatic hypertrophy (BPH) and prostate cancer, noting reported incidents of ED with different treatments for these conditions is useful.

### BENIGN PROSTATE HYPERTROPHY AND PROSTATE CANCER

Treatment of BPH and prostate cancer frequently is associated with ED. In one study, patients were treated with one of several therapies.[73] ED was noted in 1 of 40 patients treated by open prostatectomy, in 3 of 89 men treated with transurethral prostatectomy after 6 months, in 1 of 33 men treated with doxazosin for 6 months, and in 12 of 36 men treated with finasteride for 6 months. (This incidence of ED with finasteride therapy is much higher than that noted in the large multicenter trials [<5%].) In the Veterans Affairs cooperative study that compared management with watchful waiting and transurethral prostatectomy (TURP), TURP was not associated with increased ED.[74]

Prostate cancer is the second most common nonskin cancer diagnosed in men. The widespread use of prostate-specific antigen (PSA) testing to screen for prostate cancer has resulted in increased diagnosis at an earlier age and, consequently, at a stage when the disease is localized to the prostate. *Radical prostatectomy* and *external beam radiotherapy* are the modalities with the potential for curing this disease. Although some differences are noted in the incidence of ED between patients undergoing radical bilateral nerve-sparing surgery and those undergoing either unilateral or non–nerve-sparing prostatectomy,[75,75a] and between those receiving conventional radiotherapy and those receiving conformational radiotherapy,[76] available data suggest that severe ED is common after *both* radical prostatectomy and radiotherapy. After surgery, ED is more likely to improve after several months. By contrast, ED tends to be less at 3 months than at 12 months after radiotherapy.[77] In a metaanalysis, the probability of maintaining erectile function after radiotherapy was found to be 0.69 and after surgery was 0.42.[78] In a study of Medicare beneficiaries, only 33% of men younger than 70 years of age who had radiotherapy and 11% of men who had surgery had erections sufficient for intercourse at follow-up, 3 or more years later.[79,79a] For men older than 70 years of age, only 27% of those who had radiotherapy and 12% of those who had surgery were potent. A randomized trial with sufficient sample size is sorely needed, however, to clarify the most curative and least detrimental therapies for different subsets of patients with prostate cancer. In addition to reflecting physician and patient biases that influence therapeutic choice, metaanalysis comparisons are limited to data available from studies that assessed pretreatment erectile function, stage of disease, age at treatment, and period of follow-up. Nonetheless, in men younger than 70 years of age, external beam radiation appears less likely to cause ED than surgery.[80] Patients who had partial ED preoperatively and those with preexistent diabetes or vascular disease are more likely to experience severe ED after surgery. Thus, ED is a likely side effect in men being treated for prostate cancer. Neurologic injury best explains surgically related ED in the majority of cases; vascular and neurologic injury represent probable causes after radiotherapy. Therefore, because the causes differ, the treatment response for ED also will likely differ for men undergoing different prostate cancer treatments.

### ANDROGEN DEFICIENCY

Androgen deficiency is widely recognized as a cause of sexual dysfunction (see Chaps. 115 and 116). Diminished libido, reduced ejaculate volume, and ED are common when androgen deficiency develops after puberty. If androgen deficiency occurs in the presence of gynecomastia, a late-onset deficiency of 17-ketosteroid reductase should be considered.[81] ED and symptoms of androgen deficiency are usually manifest when T levels are <300 ng/dL. One study including 68 hypogonadal men and 105 eugonadal men concluded that the threshold for normal SREs is ~200 ng/dL.[21] The estimated incidence of androgen deficiency in unselected men with ED ranges from 2.1% to 23%.[71,82-85] In a study of 1022 men presenting with ED, serum T was low (<300 ng/dL) in 107; however, *repeat testing* found normal values in 40% of these men.[86] Therefore, *confirmation* of androgen deficiency is important. Limiting T assessment to patients with low sexual desire or abnormal physical examination misses 40% of the men with low T levels. This includes 37% of the men whose symptoms improved with androgen replacement.

A significant number of bona fide hypogonadal patients presenting with ED and T deficiency have secondary or tertiary hypogonadism.[84] A major issue is whether or not imaging studies of the pituitary and hypothalamus are warranted. In a study of 164 men presenting with ED in whom the T level was <230 ng/dL, 11 had anatomical abnormalities.[87] Five patients had pituitary microadenomas, four had pituitary macroadenomas, and two had hypothalamic lesions. T levels were <104 ng/dL in all of the patients with macroadenomas as well as in those with hypothalamic lesions. (To minimize negative radiologic evaluations, one could limit imaging to patients having morning T levels of <150 to 200 ng/dL.)

## HYPERPROLACTINEMIA

ED is a common presenting symptom in men with pituitary tumors (see Chap. 13). Seventy-six percent of patients with a tumor in the region of the sella turcica reported decreased or absent libido or potency.[88] Usually, these patients have subnormal serum T levels. Prolactinomas, the most common pituitary tumors, are more rare in men than in women. Nonetheless, of men with ED referred to urologists or psychiatrists, ~16% had mild hyperprolactinemia (16–25 ng/mL) and 3% had modest hyperprolactinemia (25–50 ng/mL) in the absence of liver or renal disease or the use of drugs known to increase serum prolactin levels.[71,89] Prolactin levels are >50 ng/mL in most patients with prolactinomas; normalization of minimal hyperprolactinemia does not ameliorate ED. Therefore, prolactin levels of <50 ng/mL should alert the physician to evaluate thyroid, liver, and renal function. Studies performing routine measurement of serum prolactin find a low yield of prolactinomas (<1% of patients).[86,90] A reasonable course is to measure the morning prolactin level when a T level is <300 ng/dL and sexual desire is low, or when gynecomastia is found.

## DIABETES MELLITUS

ED is common among men with diabetes mellitus.[91] The prevalence in three large studies was ~50% at 50 years of age.[92] Among 365 men older than 21 years of age who had had a diagnosis of diabetes for a minimum of 10 years before age 30,[93] only 1.1% of those aged 21 to 30 years were afflicted with ED compared with 55% of those aged 50 years and 75% of those aged older than 60 years. Individuals with diabetes who are smokers are 1.4 times more likely to have ED than are nonsmokers; nevertheless, ED is also more common among nonsmokers, as well as the obese diabetics.[2] Furthermore, in diabetes, glycosylated hemoglobin is inversely related to ED. The age-adjusted probability of ED increases as HDL cholesterol decreases; however, there is no association with total cholesterol.

In men with diabetes, ED progresses gradually, and other symptoms and signs of autonomic neuropathy may be present (see Chap. 148). ED is more common in men with severe vascular or neurologic complications. In a study of diabetic and nondiabetic men with erectile complaints,[67] measurements were obtained for BCR latency, heart rate responses to deep breathing, postural blood pressure changes, penile and brachial blood pressures, and SREs with rigidity during overnight sleep studies. Of the 100 men with diabetes, 28 had penile rigidity of >500 g. Men with diabetes and rigidity of <500 g had diminished SREs compared to those with rigidity of >500 g, although no sleep architecture differences were found. Among all men with rigidity of <500 g, those with diabetes had less change in heart rate during deep breathing and lower penile blood pressure than did those without diabetes. Thus, organic ED with evidence of autonomic dysregulation is more common in men with diabetes than in those with other causes of ED. However, abnormal SRE findings associated with diabetes must be interpreted cautiously, because potent men with diabetes frequently have a subclinical decline in erectile function detectable with SRE testing.[94]

Thirty-four percent of diabetic men with ED had evidence of neuropathy on the basis of cystometrogram or BCR latency prolongation.[95] Other investigators found that 68% of men with ED and diabetes had vascular abnormalities noted on arteriography, whereas only 19% had neurologic pathology.[96] Thus, although organic ED is common among men with diabetes, its origin may be vascular, neuropathic, or both.

In addition to the vascular and neuropathic abnormalities, other changes may limit development of normal erections in diabetes. More glycation end products, which are associated with collagen in the tunica and the corpora cavernosa, are found in tissue from diabetic men than in tissue from nondiabetic men.[97] However, electron microscopic examination of corpora cavernosal tissue obtained from men with erectile failure with and without diabetes revealed no structural differences except for mitochondrial swelling in tissue taken from men with diabetes.[98] Specimens from both groups contained increased fibroblasts and thickened basement membranes in smooth muscle cells. Whether glycation of collagen in the cavernosum limits intracavernosal pressure during an erection is not known. In vitro studies of corporal smooth muscle indicate that isolated strips from men with diabetes and ED are less responsive to electrical stimulation but equally responsive to nitroprusside and papaverine compared to strips from nondiabetic men with ED.[99]

Diabetes-prone BB/WOR rats and streptozotocin-treated rats are used as models of type 1 diabetes, and insulin-resistant, BBZ/WOR rats are used to model type 2 diabetes mellitus. These diabetic rodents develop changes in sexual behavior that are thought to be analogous to sexual dysfunction in men.

Penile neuronal nitric oxide synthase activity is 47% lower in BB/WOR diabetic rats and 33% lower in BBZ/WOR rats than in controls.[100] This is partially explained by reduced serum T levels in both models. (In contrast, penile nitric oxide synthase activity is increased in streptozotocin-induced diabetic rats.[101]) Other studies reveal reduced hydrolysis of both cyclic guanosine monophosphate (cGMP) and cyclic adenosine monophosphate (cAMP) in penile and aortic tissue compared to that in controls.[102] The resulting elevation in penile cGMP and cAMP levels suggests that abnormal distal mechanisms affecting smooth muscle may play a role in nonrelaxation of corporal muscle. These changes typically produced reduced cavernosal tissue responsiveness.

In a study using a different approach, New Zealand white rabbits were made diabetic with alloxan.[103] A significant increase in endothelin-B receptor-binding sites was found in cavernosal tissue obtained from these diabetic animals. The suggestion was made that autocrine release of endothelin-1 coupled with the increase in receptor-binding sites could lead to increased smooth muscle contraction. Interestingly, peripheral plasma endothelin-1 levels were higher in diabetic men, both with and without ED, than in healthy control subjects.[104] When erections were induced with PGE$_1$, however, intracavernosal endothelin-1 levels were similar in men with and without diabetes who suffered from ED. Thus, whether or not increased endothelin-1 and its receptors contribute to ED in men is not known.

## HYPERTENSION

Men with hypertension frequently report difficulty in initiating or maintaining erections that are adequate for sexual intercourse. Clinicians widely believe this to be a side effect of antihypertensive medication. The reported incidence of erectile failure is 9% with hydrochlorothiazide, 20% with α-methyldopa, 46% with reserpine, 24% with guanethidine, 1% to 41% with clonidine, and 13.8% with propranolol.[105] However, *untreated hypertension* is also associated with an increased prevalence of ED in men.

A study of spontaneous sleep-related bulbocavernosus activity in potent men with untreated hypertension found reductions in activity during sleep erections compared with control subjects.[106] This change in erectile physiology preceded the clinical manifestation of ED. Interestingly, penile blood flow measured during sleep erections was reduced in potent men with untreated hypertension. The study also found a further reduction in blood flow in men with untreated hypertension and ED. The pathophysiologic mechanism is not known; however, the authors have hypothesized the involvement of neurologic and vascular mechanisms. Peripheral vasoconstriction, autonomic dysfunction, or vascular bed damage seems a likely candidate.

# TREATMENT FOR ERECTILE DYSFUNCTION

## OVERVIEW

Ideally, therapy should be selected based on the cause of ED. However, the techniques for identifying specific causes of ED are not fully refined, are not readily available to many physicians, and are expensive. Furthermore, many patients have multiple causes of ED. *These factors and the availability of noninvasive and minimally invasive therapies make it more practical to minimize initial evaluation before therapeutic challenge.* Until recently, few studies included placebo controls, and no studies have evaluated the outcome for patients randomly assigned to different treatments. A National Institutes of Health consensus conference presented guidelines for treating ED (prior to the introduction of sildenafil).[107,108] Nevertheless, the importance of conducting controlled studies and of informing patients of the therapeutic options was emphasized.

## AVAILABLE TREATMENTS

### PSYCHOLOGICAL, BEHAVIORAL, AND RELATIONSHIP THERAPY

Selection of appropriate psychological therapy for ED depends entirely on factors concerning the patient, the partner, and the relationship. Therapy can play either a primary role (as in the case of performance anxiety) or a secondary role. If anxiety or depression is prominent, psychiatric or psychological attention is needed. Major depressive disorders are associated with physiologic alterations of sleep as well as changes in erectile profiles.

In many instances, sex therapy is helpful, even when the ED has an organic origin. Optimizing sexual performance using different techniques or positions often is beneficial. Behavioral methods, most commonly systemic desensitization, may be required to treat sexual performance anxiety. Finally, because sex is still largely a taboo subject among many in society, misinformation, inaccurate expectations, and general ignorance abound. Correcting misconceptions and misinformation can help tremendously.

When relationship problems are prominent, treatment of the couple is essential. In some cases, adequate correction of organic erectile failure may not produce potency. Tremendous anger and contention may exist in the relationship, and the male partner's loss of sexual potency may symbolically initiate his loss of power in the relationship.

### ENDOCRINE APPROACHES

**Testosterone Replacement Therapy.** Sexual activity, as assessed by subjective measures, is increased by T therapy.[109] Treatment of six hypogonadal men with parenteral TE (400 mg every 4 weeks) increased their total erections, nocturnal erections, and coital attempts as compared with placebo treatment. Similarly, hypogonadal men given oral testosterone undecanoate experienced an increase in the number of sexual acts per week, number of ejaculations per week, frequency of sexual thought, and sexual excitement, compared with men receiving a placebo.[110]

T treatment of men with low total T levels can improve daytime erectile rigidity and SREs. One group of investigators reported that untreated hypogonadal men had erections while observing erotic films. They had circumference changes similar to those of controls, but diminished maximum rigidity. The penile rigidity of erections stimulated by visual erotic material improved significantly after T therapy.[111] In a group of six severely hypogonadal men (aged 25 to 40 years) who had not previously received

androgen replacement therapy, nocturnal erections were absent or severely impaired. SREs increased progressively into the normal range with androgen replacement therapy over 6 to 12 months.[112] The authors studied six hypogonadal men who received 200-mg injections of testosterone cypionate.[113] SRE studies were conducted during the week after an injection and again after 7 to 8 weeks without further replacement therapy. Androgen withdrawal was associated with a significant reduction in the number of erections, total tumescence time, penile circumference changes during erections, and penile rigidity. In 20 hypogonadal men, the duration and rigidity of nocturnal erections, as measured by RigiScan, were greater during transdermal T replacement therapy than at the end of 8 weeks of androgen withdrawal.[114]

The contraindications to and complications of androgen replacement therapy must be considered carefully before treatment is recommended. Men older than 50 years must be evaluated for benign prostatic hyperplasia and prostate cancer before and during androgen therapy. Sleep apnea or polycythemia may worsen with androgen therapy. Careful history-taking and periodic assessment of hematocrit, serum PSA, and the prostate are essential.

**Dopamine Agonists.** The normalization of hyperprolactinemia by the surgical removal of a prolactinoma or by administration of dopamine agonists may increase serum T levels and restore potency. Eight patients with prolactinomas were studied using nonpolysomnographic SRE monitoring before and after therapy.[115] Before treatment, circumference increases during tumescence episodes were smaller and total tumescence time was lower in the patients with prolactinomas than in age-matched control subjects. Treatment was associated with a greater penile circumference increase during SREs. One study reported a 17% incidence of mild hyperprolactinemia (16–22 ng/mL) in 47 men with ED.[89] The patients were randomly assigned to bromocriptine or placebo treatment groups. Clinical response did not differ between the two groups; thus, the normalization of mild hyperprolactinemia in the presence of normal T levels is unlikely to restore potency. Normalization of more marked hyperprolactinemia (>50 ng/mL), however, *even in the presence of normal T levels,* improves libido and potency.

Dopamine agonists may exert erectogenic effects by acting on D2 receptors and oxytocin neurons.[116] Apomorphine tablets (3 or 4 mg) caused erections in 8 of 12 men with ED. Seven of the 11 men who used apomorphine at home reported successful erections.[117] This agent currently is undergoing clinical trials. Melatonin II, a synthetic α-melanocyte-stimulating hormone analog, seems to work downstream from the dopamine receptor. This peptide, when administered subcutaneously, initiated erections in men with psychogenic ED.[118] Its role as a therapeutic agent is not defined.

### OTHER MEDICAL THERAPIES

**Orally Administered Therapies.** Orally administered agents to treat ED have long been sought. Sildenafil is a selective inhibitor of cGMP-specific phosphodiesterase type 5. Cyclic GMP phosphodiesterase type 5 is the predominant isozyme found in corporal smooth muscle involved in the breakdown of cGMP. Smooth muscle relaxation in cavernosal bodies is triggered by sexual stimuli. This leads to nitric oxide release from nonadrenergic noncholinergic nerves that, in turn, innervate the cavernosal smooth muscle. Sildenafil, therefore, appears to potentiate erections induced by physiologic mechanisms. Unlike PGE$_1$, it does *not independently* evoke penile erections. Furthermore, oral L-arginine, a substrate for NO synthase, is not an effective treatment for ED.[118a]

In a placebo-controlled, double-blind, randomized parallel group study, use of sildenafil improved vaginal penetration (93% versus 10%) and ability to maintain erections (140% versus 13%) compared to placebo.[119] The ability to achieve erections, maintain erections, or both during intercourse improved in groups with presumed organic, psychogenic, or mixed etiologies. A dose-escalation study revealed the following adverse events for sildenafil compared to placebo: headaches (18% vs. 4%), flushing (18% vs. 1%), dyspepsia (6% vs. 2%), rhinitis (5% vs. 1%), and visual disturbances (2% vs. 1%). No patient had priapism. Initially, several deaths occurred that were attributed to sildenafil among patients taking nitrates for angina pectoris, and the FDA issued an advisory warning. In a subsequent report of 123 deaths possibly related to sildenafil use,[120] details were available for 69 men, including 46 who experienced cardiovascular events, 2 who had strokes, and 21 for whom the cause of death was unknown. The mean age was 64 years (range, 29–87 years). At least 36% of these men began experiencing symptoms within 4 to 5 hours of ingestion of the drug, and 18 died during or soon after sexual intercourse. The vast majority of these men had one or more cardiovascular risk factors in addition to age and sex. Most deaths probably occurred in men with greater cardiovascular risk than those participating in the clinical trials, because the studies restricted enrollment of men using nitrates, those with comorbid systemic disease, and those who had had myocardial infarcts or strokes within the previous 6 months.

Animal studies provide insight into the mechanism of action of sildenafil. For example, in dogs N omega-nitro-L-arginine, a nitric oxide synthesis inhibitor, blocks the usual increased blood flow and intracavernosal pressure induced by pelvic nerve stimulation.[121] By contrast, sildenafil (1–100 µg/kg) increases these parameters. Thus, inhibition of cGMP-specific phosphodiesterase type 5 augments the neuronal mechanisms of erection in dogs. In a study of rabbits, corpus cavernosum strips were stimulated with phenylephrine. Sildenafil reduced spontaneous tone in unstimulated tissue; the drug sensitized tissue to sodium nitroprusside but had little effect in the absence of sodium nitroprusside.[122]

Other orally administered agents have been tested for treating ED. Oral PGE$_1$ (30 µg, three times a day) was administered to 25 men with mild ED while an herbal medicine (gosyajinkigan) was given to a second group.[134] Eleven men who received PGE$_1$ and 4 men taking the herbal preparation achieved penetration. SREs increased in the group taking PGE$_1$. However, patients apparently did not achieve full erections. When pentoxifylline (400 mg three times daily) was used to treat 18 men with ED, 9 had erections sufficient for vaginal intercourse, 3 experienced no change, and 6 did not attempt intercourse.[135] Yohimbine, an α-adrenergic inhibitor, is another substance that for many years has been regarded as a potentially useful oral agent. Conflicting reports concerning its use have been published, and the American Urological Association guidelines do not endorse its use. Nonetheless, metaanalysis of all randomized placebo-controlled trials of yohimbine did find support for its use.[136] In seven studies that were considered, yohimbine was found more effective than placebo for treating ED, and serious adverse reactions were infrequent and reversible. A double-blind controlled trial[137] involving 86 patients with ED found subjective and objective evidence (SRE measures) that yohimbine was more effective than placebo for treating ED (71% showed improvement with yohimbine vs. 45% with placebo). In contrast, another study[138] found yohimbine no better than placebo in a randomized controlled trial. Therefore, the use of yohimbine remains controversial, but it may have a place in treating psychogenic ED.

**Vacuum Constriction Devices.**  External vacuum constriction devices (VCDs) are cylinder-like chambers that use a pump to create a vacuum around the penis. This increases penile blood flow into the corpora cavernosa. The erection is maintained by restricting outflow by placing a constricting band at the base of the penis. The use of VCDs is successful in selected patients with ED.[123]

In two studies, 75% of patients achieved adequate erections with a VCD.[124] Subjects included men with organic and psy-

chogenic ED. The long-term satisfaction rates, however, dropped to 43% and 68% in the two studies. Complications included mild numbness in the penis, mild cyanosis, painless ecchymoses, petechiae, and blocked ejaculation. Some men and spouses complained of a cool penis. Although the penis is rigid during intercourse, this therapy may create a "hinge-like" effect at the base of the penis. Encouraging patients to use the device on loan before purchase helps to identify those likely to accept and use it. VCDs have been effective in as many as 69% of men with venous leakage[125] and 57% of men with both traumatic and nontraumatic neurologic disorders.[126]

Comparisons of the use of VCDs and ICIs in the same patients are limited. In one study involving 44 patients, the two treatments had similar efficacy.[127] However, subgroup analysis suggested a preference for ICI among younger men, men who had had ED for <12 months, and men who had undergone radical prostatectomy for prostate cancer. (See later for a discussion of ICI.)

**Topical Preparations.**  Topical treatment, if effective, would likely be more acceptable to patients than ICI or transurethral approaches. Therefore, formulations of nitroglycerin,[128] prostaglandin E$_2$,[129] PGE$_1$,[130] papaverine,[131] stearyl-VIP,[132] and minoxidil are being evaluated. They show promise, but these agents may have systemic effects when applied topically in quantities sufficient to effect erections.

Topical PGE$_1$ was evaluated in 9 men with ED secondary to spinal cord injury and in 1 man with mild arterial insufficiency.[130] The preparation was applied to the scrotum, perineum, and penis. Color flow Doppler ultrasonography was used for measurements. Mean cavernous artery diameter and peak systolic flow velocity increased. Clinical erections occurred in 2 men using PGE$_1$ and in none using a placebo. In another study, a non-blinded, placebo-controlled trial of a papaverine topical gel for treating ED was evaluated in men (some with spinal injury).[131] When the papaverine topical gel was applied to the scrotum, perineum, and penis, the cavernous artery diameter increased 36%, as determined by color Doppler ultrasonography. Peak systolic flow velocity increased 26%, and full erections occurred in 3 of 17 patients. The investigators found this result hopeful for the development of a topical therapy.

Transdermal nitroglycerin and ICI of papaverine were compared for the treatment of ED in men with spinal cord lesions.[133] ICI produced responses in 93% and transdermal nitroglycerin produced responses in 61% of patients. ICI complications occurred in 32% of patients. The main side effect with the nitroglycerin patch was headache, which occurred in 21% of the men.

**Transurethral Drug Administration.**  Transurethral PGE$_1$ was approved for treating ED after its efficacy and safety were demonstrated in a large-scale, double-blind, placebo-controlled clinical trial.[139] Transurethral administration of alprostadil using the Medicated Urethral System for Erection (MUSE) was tested in 1511 men with ED. Trial doses were administered in the clinic (125, 250, 500, 1000 µg), and responders were randomly assigned either to their effective dose or to a placebo. Study subjects used MUSE for 3 months at home. In the clinic, 65.9% of men attained intercourse-sufficient erections, and ~70% of home-trial MUSE administrations were followed by intercourse. Effectiveness was independent of the presence of comorbid factors. Approximately 11% of subjects experienced penile pain and 3.3% experienced hypotension (during the clinic test session). Thus, for those men who responded to MUSE in the clinic, it was reasonably effective as an ongoing therapy at home. Other studies reported similar results.[140]

MUSE response also has been compared with ICI of alprostadil.[141] A 43% response rate was attained with MUSE compared to 70% with ICI. Completely rigid erections occurred in 10% of patients using MUSE and 48% using ICI. Burning sensation side effects were more common with MUSE than with ICI (31.4% vs. 10.6%, respectively). Interestingly, some patients who rejected or failed to respond to ICI (alprostadil, papaverine, phentolamine, or a combination) responded to MUSE.[142] Of 95 such men with ED, 58% attained an erection sufficient for intercourse with transurethral alprostadil therapy in the clinic. Among ICI therapy patients who found ICI sometimes effective, 68% had adequate erections with MUSE. Thus, transurethral alprostadil therapy is effective in many men and may work even when ICI fails.

**Intracavernosal Injection.**    Patients with neurogenic, vasculogenic, and psychogenic ED usually obtain erections in response to ICI of vasodilators. Reports vary on the efficacy of administering intracavernosal VIP in men with ED.[143] However, administration of PGE$_1$, alone[144] or in combination with papaverine and phentolamine,[145] produced erections initially in 70% and long term in ~50% of men with ED.[146,147] Dose-response studies of PGE$_1$ (ranging from 2.5 to 20 μg), indicate that 20 μg is the maximum dose for monotherapy.[144] PGE$_1$ produces a slower onset of action and a longer duration of action than does papaverine.[148] PGE$_1$ and nitroprusside were compared in 100 men with ED (mean age, 55 years).[149] PGE$_1$ (20 μg) was administered, and after 1 to 7 days sodium nitroprusside (600 μg) was tried. Shorter latency to erection, longer duration of erection, and better self-rating of erection were found for PGE$_1$. Thus, ICI of sodium nitroprusside is *less effective* than ICI of PGE$_1$. In a single-blind study involving 129 men with ED, PGE$_1$ was found subjectively and objectively to be *more effective than papaverine*.[150] Of 249 patients, 72% responded to PGE$_1$, 31% responded to papaverine, and 29% responded to papaverine plus phentolamine.[147] Side effects (including plaque formation and priapism) appear less often with PGE$_1$. The injections are more expensive, however, and may be painful. Pain can be reduced by alkalinization of the solution before injection. The risk of priapism is higher in patients with psychogenic and neurogenic ED. Treatment success in older men (mean age, 70 years) was similar to that in a younger group (mean age, 47 years).[151] In most studies, only 50% of patients continue ICI for >1 year.[152] In itself, priapism is a rare condition; however, data indicate that its incidence has increased in recent years. This increase is attributed to the use of vasoactive drugs to treat ED. In a case series from Finland, 207 patients with priapism were reported from two 9-year surveys between 1973 and 1990.[153]

### SURGICAL THERAPY

Surgical therapy is most often offered to some men with vasculogenic ED and to men with neurogenic or psychogenic ED who do not respond to less invasive treatments. Attempts to surgically correct venous leaks improved erections in *only* 11% of patients.[154,155] Similarly, efforts to revascularize the penis have *limited* success *unless* there is obstruction to flow in the distal aorta, internal iliac, or pudendal arteries.

### PENILE PROSTHESES

Patients with neurologic causes, genital abnormalities, or vascular disease who cannot be treated medically may be candidates for penile prostheses[156–158] (Fig. 117-6). In addition, some patients thought to have psychogenic ED that is refractory to psychotherapy and behavior therapy have been treated successfully with penile prostheses. In experienced hands, satisfactory implantation of either a semirigid or an inflatable penile prosthesis is achieved in >95% of patients. Usually, a penoscrotal incision is used; many surgeons operate using local anesthesia. In one study, the semirigid Jonas penile prosthesis was implanted in 77 patients.[159] Of the 31 who responded to a questionnaire, 74% of the patients and 65% of the partners were satisfied. Complications, though rare, include infection and perforation of the prosthesis through the penile skin. Mechanical failure is more common with inflatable than with semirigid prostheses, and the total costs of an inflatable prosthesis are two to three times greater. However, inflatable prostheses are more acceptable to patients. The current rate of mechanical failure is <5%. No mechan-

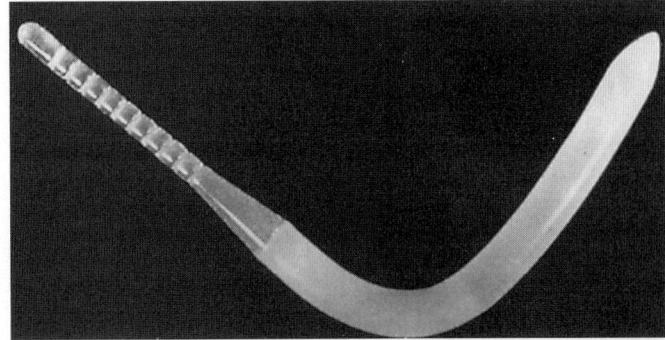

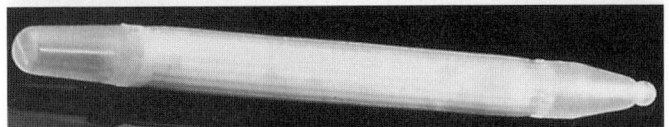

**FIGURE 117-6.** Penile prostheses. Two implantable devices used to treat erectile dysfunction. **A,** Finney semirigid rod. **B,** Dynaflex prosthesis (American Medical Systems), a more advanced inflatable device.

ical failures were reported after 1 year in 43 men implanted with Hydroflex prostheses,[160] and all patients reported successful intercourse. Complications were reported in only 5 of 150 consecutively treated patients who were evaluated at a mean of 19 months after implantation of a Mentor Alpha 1 penile prosthesis. Complications included infection (1%) and cylinder aneurysm (2%).[161] Evaluation of 80 men implanted with the Mark II inflatable penile prosthesis revealed no mechanical problems for up to 27 months; however, six required repositioning of the reservoir pump.[162] Questionnaires indicated that >80% of the patients and 70% of the partners were satisfied with the inflatable prostheses.[163] Multicomponent inflatable prostheses are reported to have fewer mechanical problems and produce higher patient satisfaction than self-contained prostheses.[164,164a]

*Long-term* follow-up reports for *all* treatment modalities have been sparse. Telephone interviews and chart reviews were conducted for 115 patients treated with ICI and 65 men treated with surgical prostheses.[165] The mean age of patients was 57 and 60 years, respectively. The average follow-up time was 5.4 years (range, 3.3–16 years) after treatment. Nineteen percent of men treated with ICI and 18% of those treated with prostheses were lost to follow-up. Six percent of the ICI group and 19% of the prosthetic group had died. Only 41% of men given ICI continued with that therapy, and 61% of those who discontinued ICI used other therapies to remain sexually active. Seventy percent of the prosthetic patients remained sexually active.

### TREATMENT ALGORITHM

A proposed treatment algorithm is depicted in Figure 117-2, parts I and II. Based on history-taking, physical examination, and psychometric testing, the clinician should form a clinical hypothesis about the underlying cause. If the patient has a mood disturbance, performance anxiety, an obvious relationship problem, or current alcohol or drug abuse, referral for psychiatric treatment or counseling is warranted. If androgen deficiency is suspected clinically, laboratory tests should be performed and referral should be made to an endocrinologist, as needed. Otherwise, unless the use of sildenafil is contraindicated, a pharmacologic challenge can be performed. If the drug is ineffective or is not tolerated, another noninvasive therapy may be tried (specifically, VCDs).[166] If this also fails, a minimally invasive treatment challenge follows with MUSE. Treatment failure with MUSE, or intolerable side effects, would lead to more invasive procedures. ICI with alprostadil is effective in 85% of men who fail initial treatment with sildenafil.[167] Comparisons of transurethral vs. intracavernous delivery of alprostadil indicate that the latter is more efficacious and better tolerated.[168]

Clearly, a very large population of patients complain of ED. The experience with sildenafil indicates that they will seek medical therapy if it can be given orally, is effective, and is safe. Although the availability of sildenafil represents a major breakthrough in the treatment of ED, it is not effective for many patients, and many others are taking nitrates or have complicating illnesses that are contraindications to its use. Therefore, at the present time, other treatment modalities may need to be used. One hopes that the large public response to the introduction of sildenafil and the knowledge that is achieved through further research will result in the development of more effective oral therapies in the future.

# REFERENCES

1. Diokno AC, Brown MB, Herzog AR. Sexual function in the elderly. Arch Intern Med 1990; 150:197.
2. Feldman HA, Goldstein I, Hatzichristou DG, et al. Impotence and its medical and psychosocial correlates: results from the Massachusetts Male Aging Study. J Urol 1994; 151:54.
2a. Johannes CB, Araujo AB, Feldman HA, et al. Incidence of erectile dysfunction in men 40 to 69 years old: longitudinal results from the Massachusetts male aging study. J Urol 2000; 163:460.
3. Benson GS, McConnell J, Lipshultz L. Neuromorphology and neuropharmacology of the human penis. J Clin Invest 1980; 65:506.
4. Newman HF, Northrup JD, Devlin J. Mechanism of human penile erection. Invest Urol 1964; 1:350.
5. Wagner G. Vascular mechanisms involved in erection and erectile disorders. Clin Endocrinol Metab 1983; 11:717.
6. Zhao W, Christ GJ. Endothelin-1 as a putative modulator of erectile dysfunction. II. Calcium mobilization in cultured human corporal smooth muscle cells. J Urol 1995; 154:1571.
7. Ottesen B, Wagner G, Virag R, Fahrenkrug J. Penile erection: possible role for vasoactive intestinal polypeptide as a neurotransmitter. BMJ 1984; 288:9.
8. Rajfer J, Aronson WJ, Bush PA, et al. Nitric oxide as a mediator of relaxation of the corpus cavernosum in response to nonadrenergic, noncholinergic neurotransmission. N Engl J Med 1992; 326:90.
9. Bloch W, Klotz T, Sedlaczek P, et al. Evidence for the involvement of endothelial nitric oxide synthase from smooth muscle cells in the erectile function of human corpus cavernosum. Urol Res 1998; 26:129.
10. Ehmke H, Junemann KP, Mayer B, Kummer W. Nitric oxide synthase and vasoactive intestinal polypeptide colocalization in neurons innervating the human penile circulation. Int J Impot Res 1995; 7(3):147.
11. Brock G, Nunes L, Padma-Nathan H, et al. Nitric oxide synthase: a new diagnostic tool for neurogenic impotence. Urology 1993; 42:412.
12. Ehrhardt AA, Meyer-Bhalung WSL. Prenatal sex hormones and the developing brain. Effects on psychosocial differentiation and cognitive function. Annu Rev Med 1979; 30:417.
13. Gooren LJG. Human male sexual functions do not require aromatization of testosterone: a study using tamoxifen, testolactone, and dihydrotestosterone. Arch Sex Behav 1985; 14:539.
14. Deslypere JP, Vermeulen A. Leydig cell function in normal men: effect of age, life-style, residence, diet, and activity. J Clin Endocrinol Metab 1984; 59:955.
15. Bremner WJ, Vitiello MV, Prinz PN. Loss of circadian rhythmicity in blood testosterone levels with aging in normal men. J Clin Endocrinol Metab 1983; 56:1278.
16. Gray A, Berlin JA, McKinlay JB, Longcope C. An examination of research design effects on the association of testosterone and male aging: results of a meta-analysis. J Clin Epidemiol 1991; 44:671.
17. Buena F, Swerdloff RS, Steiner BS, et al. Sexual function does not change when serum testosterone levels are pharmacologically varied within the normal male range. Fertil Steril 1993; 59(5):1118.
18. Hirshkowitz M, Moore CA, O'Connor S, et al. Androgen and sleep-related erections. J Psychosom Res 1997; 42(6):541.
19. Carani C, Scuteri A, Marrama P, Bancroft J. Brief report—the effects of testosterone administration and visual erotic stimuli on nocturnal penile tumescence in normal men. Horm Behav 1990; 24:435.
20. Bagatell CJ, Heiman JR, Rivier JE, Bremner WJ. Effects of endogenous testosterone and estradiol on sexual behavior in normal young men. J Clin Endocrinol Metab 1994; 7:711.
21. Granata AR, Rochira V, Lerchl A, et al. Relationship between sleep-related erections and testosterone levels in men. J Androl 1997; 18:522.
22. Imperato-McGinley J, Peterson RE, Gautier T, Sturla E. Androgens and the evolution of male-gender identity among male pseudohermaphrodites with 5 α-reductase deficiency. N Engl J Med 1979; 300:1233.
23. Gormley GJ, Stoner E, Bruskewitz RC, et al. The effect of finasteride in men with benign prostatic hyperplasia. N Engl J Med 1992; 327:1185.
24. Cunningham GR, Hirshkowitz M. Inhibition of steroid 5α-reductase with finasteride: sleep-related erections, potency, and libido in healthy men. J Clin Endocrinol Metab 1995; 80(6):1934.
25. Lugg JA, Rajfer J, Gonzalez-Cadavid NF. Dihydrotestosterone is the active androgen in the maintenance of nitric oxide-mediated penile erection in the rat. Endocrinol 1995; 36(4):1495.
26. Reilly CM, Zamorano P, Stopper VS, Mills TM. Androgenic regulation of NO availability in rat penile erection. J Androl 1997; 18(2):110.
27. Schirar A, Bonnefond C, Meusnier C, Devinoy E. Androgens modulate nitric oxide synthase messenger ribonucleic acid expression in neurons of the major pelvic ganglion in the rat. Endocrinology 1997; 138:3093.
28. Melvin JE, Hamill RW. The major pelvic ganglion: androgen control of postnatal development. J Neurosci 1987; 7:1607.
29. Mills LC. Drug-induced impotence. Clin Pharmacol 1975; 12:104.
30. Horowitz ID, Goble AJ. Drugs and impaired male sexual function. Drugs 1979; 18:206.
31. Brock G, Lue TF. Drug-induced male sexual dysfunction. An update. Drug Saf 1993; 8:414.
32. Montejo-Gonzalez AL, Llorca G, Izquerdo JA, et al. SSRI-induced sexual dysfunction: fluoxetine, paroxetine, sertraline, and fluvoxamine in a prospective, multicenter and descriptive clinical study of 344 patients. Sex Marital Ther 1997; 23:176.
33. Althof SE, Levine SB, Corty EB, et al. A double-blind crossover trial of clomipramine for rapid ejaculation in 15 couples. J Clin Psychiatry 1995; 56: 402.
34. Haensel SM, Rowland DL, Kallan KT. Clomipramine and sexual dysfunction in men with premature ejaculation and controls. Urology 1996; 156:1310.
35. Haensel SM, Klem TM, Hop WC, Slob AK. J Clin Psychopharmacol 1998; 18:72.
36. Atahan O, Kayigil O, Metin A. Modified four corner bladder neck suspension in anatomical stress incontinence with moderate cystocele. Int Urol Nephrol 1998; 30:439.
37. Ohlmeyer P, Brilmayer H, Hullstrung H. Periodisch vorgange im schlaf. Pflugers Arch 1944; 248:559.
38. Karacan I. Clinical value of nocturnal erection in the prognosis and diagnosis of impotence. Med Aspects Hum Sex 1970; 4:27.
39. Karacan I. Evaluation of nocturnal penile tumescence and impotence. In: Guilleminault C, ed. Sleep and waking disorders: indications and techniques. Menlo Park, CA: Addison-Wesley, 1982:343.
40. Bradley WE, Timm GW, Gallagher JM, Johnson BK. New method for continuous measurement of nocturnal penile tumescence and rigidity. Urology 1985; 26:4.
41. Karacan I, Williams RL, Salis PJ. The effect of sexual intercourse on sleep patterns and nocturnal penile erections. Psychophysiology 1970; 7:338.
42. Karacan I, Ware JC, Salis PJ, et al. Sexual arousal and activity: effect on subsequent nocturnal penile tumescence patterns. Sleep Res 1979; 8:61.
43. Hirshkowitz M, Ware JC. Studies of nocturnal penile tumescence and rigidity. In: Singer C, Weiner WJ, eds. Sexual dysfunction: a neuro-medical approach. Armonk, NY: Futura, 1994:77.
44. Thase ME, Reynolds CF III, Glanz LM, et al. Nocturnal penile tumescence in depressed men. Am J Psychiatry 1987; 144:89.
45. Ware JC, Hirshkowitz M. Recording nocturnal penile tumescence. In: Kryger M, Roth T, Dement WC, eds. Principles and practice of sleep medicine, 2nd ed. Philadelphia: WB Saunders, 1994:967.
46. Karacan I, Moore CA, Sahmay S. Measurement of pressure necessary for vaginal penetration. Sleep Res 1985; 14:269.
47. Ware JC, Hirshkowitz M. Characteristics of penile erections during sleep recorded from normal subjects. J Clin Neurophysiol 1992; 9:78.
48. Allen R, Brendler CB. Snap-gauge compared to a full nocturnal penile tumescence study for evaluation of patients with erectile impotence. J Urol 1990; 143:51.
49. Young T, Palta M, Dempsy J, et al. The occurrence of sleep-disordered breathing among middle-aged adults. N Engl J Med 1993; 328:1230.
50. Karacan I, Ware JC, Dervent B, et al. Impotence and blood pressure in the flaccid penis: relationship to nocturnal penile tumescence. Sleep 1978; 1:125.
51. Buvat J, Lemaire A, Buvat-Herbaut M, et al. Comparative investigations in 26 impotent and 26 nonimpotent diabetic patients. J Urol 1985; 133:34.
52. Virag R, Bouilly P, Frydman D. Is impotence an arterial disorder? Lancet 1985; 1:181.
53. Hirshkowitz M, Karacan I, Howell JW, et al. Nocturnal penile tumescence in cigarette smokers with erectile dysfunction. Urology 1992; 39:101.
54. Bancroft J, Malone N. The clinical assessment of erectile dysfunction: a comparison of nocturnal penile tumescence monitoring and intracavernosal injections. Int J Impot Res 1995; 7:123.
55. Bancroft J, Gutierrez P. Erectile dysfunction in men with and without diabetes mellitus: a comparative study. Diabet Med 1996; 13:84.
56. Lee B, Sikka SC, Randrup ER, et al. Standardization of penile blood flow parameters in normal men using intracavernous prostaglandin E1 and visual sexual stimulation. J Urol 1993; 149:49.
57. Benson CB, Aruny JE, Vickers MA Jr. Correlation of duplex sonography with arteriography in patients with erectile dysfunction. AJR Am J Roentgenol 1993; 160:71.
58. Jarow JP, Pugh UW, Routh WD, Dyer RB. Comparison of penile duplex ultrasonography to pudendal arteriography. Variant penile arterial anatomy affects interpretation of duplex ultrasonography. Invest Radiol 1993; 28:806.
59. Patel U, Amin Z, Friedman E, et al. Colour flow and spectral Doppler imaging after papaverine-induced penile erection in 220 impotent men: study of temporal patterns and the importance of repeated sampling, velocity asymmetry and vascular anomalies. Clin Radiol 1993; 48:18.

60. Shabsigh R, Fishman IJ, Quesada ET, et al. Evaluation of vasculogenic erectile impotence using penile duplex ultrasonography. J Urol 1989; 142:1469.

61. Amin Z, Patel U, Friedman EP, et al. Colour Doppler and duplex ultrasound assessment of Peyronie's disease in impotent men. Br J Radiol 1993; 66:398.

62. Allen RP, Engel RM, Smolev JK, Brendler CB. Comparison of duplex ultrasonography and nocturnal penile tumescence in evaluation of impotence. J Urol 1994; 151(6):1525.

63. Ertekin C, Reel F. Bulbocavernosus reflex in normal men and in patients with neurogenic bladder and/or impotence. J Neurol Sci 1976; 28:1.

64. Sarica Y, Karacan I. Bulbocavernosus reflex to somatic and visceral nerve stimulation in normal subjects and in diabetics with erectile impotence. J Urol 1987; 138:55.

65. Nogueira MC, Herbaut AG, Wespes E. Neurophysiological investigations of two hundred men with erectile dysfunction. Interest of bulbocavernosus reflex and pudendal evoked responses. Eur Urol 1990; 18:37.

66. Lavoisier P, Proulx J, Courtois F, DeCarufel F. Bulbocavernosus reflex: its validity as a diagnostic test of neurogenic impotence. J Urol 1989; 141:311.

67. Hirshkowitz M, Karacan I, Rando KC, et al. Diabetes, erectile dysfunction, and sleep-related erections. Sleep 1990; 13:53.

68. Ware JC, Karacan I, Salis PJ, et al. Sleep-related electrodermal activity patterns in impotent patients. Sleep 1984; 7:247.

69. Wincze JP, Bansal S, Malholtra C, et al. Comparison of nocturnal penile tumescence and penile response to erotic stimulation during waking states in comprehensively diagnosed groups of males experiencing erectile difficulties. Arch Sex Behav 1988; 17:333.

70. Nickel IC, Morales A, Condra M, Fenemore J. Endocrine dysfunction in impotence: incidence, significance and cost-effective screening. J Urol 1984; 132:40.

71. Cunningham GR, Karacan I, Ware JC, et al. The relationships between serum testosterone and prolactin levels and nocturnal penile tumescence (NPT) in impotent men. J Androl 1982; 3:241.

72. Mulligan T, Katz PG. Why aged men become impotent. Arch Intern Med 1989; 149:1365.

73. Uygur MC, Gur E, Arik AI, et al. Erectile dysfunction following treatments of benign prostatic hyperplasia: a prospective study. Andrologia 1998; 30:5.

74. Wasson JH, Reda DJ, Bruskewitz RC, et al. A comparison of transurethral surgery with watchful waiting for moderate symptoms of benign prostatic hyperplasia. The Veterans Affairs Cooperative Study Group on Transurethral Resection of the Prostate. N Engl J Med 1995; 332:75.

75. Talcott JA, Rieker P, Propert KJ, et al. Patient-reported impotence and incontinence after nerve-sparing radical prostatectomy. J Natl Cancer Inst 1997; 89:1117.

75a. Stanford JL, Feng Z, Hamilton AS, et al. Urinary and sexual function after radical prostatectomy for clinically localized prostate cancer: the Prostate Cancer Outcome Study. JAMA 2000; 283:354.

76. Nguyen LN, Pollack A, Zagars GK. Late effects after radiotherapy for prostate cancer in a randomized dose-response study: results of a self-assessment questionnaire. Urology 1998; 51:991.

77. Talcott JA, Rieker P, Clark JA, et al. Patient-reported symptoms after primary therapy for early prostate cancer: results of a prospective cohort study. J Clin Oncol 1998; 16:275.

78. Robinson JW, Dufour MS, Fung TS. Erectile functioning of men treated for prostate carcinoma. Cancer 1997; 79:538.

79. Fowler FJ Jr, Barry MJ, Lu-Yao G, et al. Outcomes of external-beam radiation therapy for prostate cancer: a study of Medicare beneficiaries in three surveillance, epidemiology, and end results areas. J Clin Oncol 1996; 14:2258.

79a. Benoit RM, Naslund MJ, Cohen JK. Complications after prostate brachytherapy in the Medicare population. Urology 2000; 55:91.

80. Mantz CA, Song P, Farhangi E, et al. Potency probability following conformal megavoltage radiotherapy using conventional doses for localized prostate cancer. Int J Radiat Oncol Biol Phys 1997; 37:551.

81. Castro-Magana M, Angulo M, Uy J. Male hypogonadism with gynecomastia caused by late-onset deficiency of testicular 17-ketosteroid reductase. N Engl J Med 1993; 328:1297.

82. Johnson AR, Jarrow JP. Is routine endocrine testing of impotent men necessary? J Urol 1992; 147:1542.

83. Carroll JL, Ellis DJ, Bagley DH. Age-related change in hormones in impotent men. Urology 1990; 36:42.

84. Korenman SG, Morley JE, Mooradian AD, et al. Secondary hypogonadism in older men: its relation to impotence. J Clin Endocrinol Metab 1990; 71:963.

85. Grovier FE, McClure RD, Kramer-Levien D. Endocrine screening for sexual dysfunction using free testosterone determinations. J Urol 1996; 156:405.

86. Buvat J, Lemaire A. Endocrine screening in 1,022 men with erectile dysfunction: clinical significance and cost-effective strategy. J Urol 1997; 158:1764.

87. Citron JT, Ettinger B, Rubinoff H, et al. Prevalence of hypothalamic-pituitary imaging abnormalities in impotent men with secondary hypogonadism. J Urol 1996; 155:529.

88. Lundberg PO, Wide L. Sexual function in males with pituitary tumors. Fertil Steril 1978; 29:175.

89. Ambrosi B, Banra R, Travaglini P, et al. Study of the effects of bromocriptine on sexual impotence. Clin Endocrinol (Oxf) 1977; 7:417.

90. Akpunonu BE, Mutgi AB, Federman DJ, et al. Routine prolactin measurement is not necessary in the initial evaluation of male impotence. J Gen Intern Med 1994; 9:336.

91. Carlin BW. Impotence and diabetes. Metabolism 1988; 37:19.

92. McCullough DK, Campbell IW, Wu FC. The prevalence of diabetic impotence. Diabetologia 1980; 18:279.

93. Klein R, Klein BEK, Lee KE, et al. Prevalence of self-reported erectile dysfunction in people with long-term IDDM. Diabetes Care 1996; 19(2):135.

94. Schiavi RC, Stimmel BB, Mandell J, Rayfield EJ. Diabetes mellitus and male sexual function: a controlled study. Diabetologia 1993; 36:745.

95. Levtich MJ, Edson M, Larman WD, Herrera HH. Vascular factor in erectile failure among diabetics. Urology 1982; 19:163.

96. Lehman TP, Jacobs IA. Etiology of diabetic impotence. J Urol 1983; 129:291.

97. Seftel AD, Vaziri ND, Ni Z, et al. Advanced glycation end products in human penis: elevation in diabetic tissue, site of deposition, and possible effect through iNOS or eNOS. Urology 1997; 50:1016.

98. Basar MM, Sargon MF, Basar H, et al. Comparative study between corpus cavernosum-electromyography findings and electron microscopy of cavernosal muscle biopsies in erectile dysfunction patients. Int J Urol 1998; 5:252.

99. Saenz de Tejada I, Goldstein I, Azadzoi K, et al. Impaired neurogenic and endothelium-mediated relaxation of penile smooth muscle from diabetic men with impotence. N Engl J Med 1989; 320(16):1025.

100. Vernet D, Cai L, Garban H, et al. Reduction of penile nitric oxide synthase in diabetic BB/WORdp (type I) and BBZ/WORdp (type II) rats with erectile dysfunction. Endocrinology 1995; 136(12):5709.

101. Elabbady AA, Gagnon C, Hassouna MM, et al. Diabetes mellitus increases nitric oxide synthase in penises but not in major pelvic ganglia of rats. Br J Urol 1995; 76:196.

102. Miller MAW, Morgan RJ, Thompson CS, et al. Hydrolysis of cyclic guanosine monophosphate and cyclic adenosine monophosphate by the penis and aorta of the diabetic rat. Br J Urol 1996; 78:252.

103. Sullivan ME, Dashwood MR, Thompson CS, et al. Alterations in endothelin B receptor sites in cavernosal tissue of diabetic rabbits: potential relevance to the pathogenesis of erectile dysfunction. J Urol 1997; 158:1966.

104. Francavilla S, Properzi G, Bellini C, et al. Endothelin-1 in diabetic and nondiabetic men with erectile dysfunction. J Urol 1997; 158:1770.

105. Segraves RT, Schoenberg HW, Segraves KAB. Evaluation of the etiology of erectile failure. In: Segraves RT, Schoenberg HW, eds. Diagnosis and treatment of erectile disturbances: a guide for clinicians. New York: Plenum Press, 1985:165.

106. Karacan I, Salis PJ, Hirshkowitz M, et al. Erectile dysfunction in hypertensive men: sleep-related erections, penile blood flow, and musculovascular events. J Urol 1989; 142:56.

107. National Institutes of Health Consensus Development Panel on Impotence. Impotence. JAMA 1993; 270:83.

108. Skolnick A, for Medical News & Perspectives. Guidelines for treating erectile dysfunction issued (American Urological Assn). JAMA 1997; 277:7.

109. Davidson JM, Camargo CA, Smith ER. Effects of androgen on sexual behavior in hypogonadal men. J Clin Endocrinol Metab 1979; 45:955.

110. Skakkebaek J, Bancroft J, Davidson DW, Warner P. Androgen replacement with oral testosterone undecanoate in hypogonadal men: a double-blind controlled study. Clin Endocrinol (Oxf) 1981; 14:49.

111. Carani C, Granata AR, Bancroft J, Marrama P. The effects of testosterone replacement on nocturnal penile tumescence and rigidity and erectile response to visual erotic stimuli in hypogonadal men. Psychoneuroendocrinology 1995; 20:743.

112. Burris AS, Banks SM, Carter CS, et al. A long-term, prospective study of the physiologic and behavioral effects of hormone replacement in untreated hypogonadal men. J Androl 1992; 13:297.

113. Cunningham GR, Hirshkowitz M, Korenman SG, Karacan I. Testosterone replacement therapy and sleep-related erections in hypogonadal men. J Clin Endocrinol Metab 1990; 70:792.

114. Arver S, Dobs AS, Meikle AW, et al. Improvement of sexual function in testosterone deficient men treated for 1 year with a permeation enhanced testosterone transdermal system. J Urol 1996; 155:1604.

115. Murray FT, Cameron DF, Ketchum C. Return of gonadal function in men with prolactin-secreting pituitary tumors. J Clin Endocrinol Metab 1984; 59:79.

116. Segraves RT, Bari M, Segraves K, Spirnak P. Effect of apomorphine on penile tumescence in men with psychogenic impotence. J Urol 1991; 145:1174.

117. Heaton JP, Morales A, Adams MA, et al. Recovery of erectile function by the oral administration of apomorphine. Urology 1995; 45:200.

118. Wessells H, Fuciarelli K, Hansen J, et al. Synthetic melanotropic peptide initiates erections in men with psychogenic erectile dysfunction: double-blind, placebo controlled crossover study. J Urol 1998; 160:389.

118a. Klotz T, Mathers MJ, Braun M, et al. Effectiveness of oral L-arginine in first-line treatment of erectile dysfunction in a controlled crossover study. Urol Int 1999; 63:220.

119. Goldstein I, Lue TF, Padma-Nathan H, et al. Oral sildenafil in the treatment of erectile dysfunction. N Engl J Med 1998; 338(20):1397.

120. Food and Drug Administration Web site. Available at: http://www.fda.gov/fdahomepage.html.

121. Carter S, Zvara P, Nunes L, et al. Regeneration of nitric oxide synthase-containing nerves after cavernous nerve neurotomy in the rat. J Urol 1998; 160:242.

122. Chuang AT, Strauss JD, Merphy RA, Steers WD. Sildenafil, a type-5 CGMP phosphodiesterase inhibitor, specifically amplifies endogenous cGMP-dependent relaxation in rabbit corpus cavernosum smooth muscle in vitro. J Urol 1998; 160:257.

123. Witherington R. Vacuum constriction device for management of erectile impotence. J Urol 1989; 141:320.

124. Segenreich E, Shmuely J, Israilov S, et al. Treatment of erectile dysfunction with vacuum constriction device. Harefuah 1993; 124:326.

125. Blackard CE, Barkon WD, Lima JS, Nelson J. Use of vacuum tumescence device for impotence secondary to venous leakage. Urology 1993; 41:225.

126. Aloni R, Heller L, Keren O, et al. Noninvasive treatment for erectile dysfunction in the neurogenically disabled population. J Sex Marital Ther 1992; 18:243.

127. Soderdahl DW, Thrasher JB, Hansberry KL. Intracavernosal drug-induced erection therapy versus external vacuum devices in the treatment of erectile dysfunction. Br J Urol 1997; 79:952.

128. Sonksen J, Biering-Sorensen F. Transcutaneous nitroglycerine in the treatment of erectile dysfunction in spinal cord injured. Paraplegia 1992; 30:554.

129. Wolfson B, Pickett S, Scott NE, et al. Intraurethral prostaglandin E-2 cream: a possible alternative treatment for erectile dysfunction. Urology 1993; 42:73.

130. Kim ED, McVary KT. Topical prostaglandin-E1 for the treatment of erectile dysfunction. J Urol 1995; 153:1828.

131. Kim ED, el-Rashidy R, McVary KT. Papaverine topical gel for treatment of erectile dysfunction. J Urol 1995; 153:361.

132. Gazes I, Fridkim M. A fatty neuropeptide. Potential drug for noninvasive impotence treatment in a rat model. J Clin Invest 1992; 90:810.

133. Renganathan R, Suranjan B, Kurien T. Comparison of transdermal nitroglycerin and intracavernous injection of papaverine in the treatment of erectile dysfunction in patients with spinal cord lesions. Spinal Cord 1997; 35:99.

134. Sato Y, Horita H, Adachi H, et al. Effect of oral administration of prostaglandin E1 on erectile dysfunction. Br J Urol 1997; 80:772.

135. Korenman SG, Viosca SP. Treatment of vasculogenic sexual dysfunction with pentoxifylline. J Am Geriatr Soc 1993; 41:363.

136. Ernst E, Pittler MH. Yohimbine for erectile dysfunction: a systematic review and meta-analysis of randomized clinical trials. J Urol 1998; 159:433.

137. Vogt HJ, Brandl P, Kockott G, et al. Double-blind, placebo-controlled safety and efficacy trial with yohimbine hydrochloride in the treatment of nonorganic erectile dysfunction. Int J Impot Res 1997; 9:155.

138. Kunelius P, Hakkinen J, Lukkarinen O. Is high-dose yohimbine hydrochloride effective in the treatment of mixed-type impotence? A prospective, randomized, controlled double-blind crossover study. Urology 1997; 49:441.

139. Padma-Nathan H, Hellstrom WJ, Kaiser FE, et al. Treatment of men with erectile dysfunction with transurethral alprostadil. Medicated Urethral System for Erection (MUSE) Study Group. N Engl J Med 1997; 336:1.

140. Williams G, Abbou CC, Amar ET, et al. Efficacy and safety of transurethral alprostadil therapy in men with erectile dysfunction. Br J Urol 1998; 81: 889.

141. Porst H. Transurethral alprostadil with MUSE (medicated urethral system for erection) vs intracavernous alprostadil—a comparative study in 103 patients with erectile dysfunction. Int J Impot Res 1997; 9:187.

142. Engel JD, McVary KT. Transurethral alprostadil as therapy for patients who withdrew from or failed prior intracavernous injection therapy. Urology 1998; 51:687.

143. Sundaram CP, Thomas W, Pryor LE, et al. Long-term follow-up of patients receiving injection therapy for erectile dysfunction. Urology 1997; 49:932.

144. von Heyden B, Donatucci CF, Marshall GA, et al. A prostaglandin E1 dose-response study in man. J Urol 1993; 150:1825.

145. Govier FE, McClure RD, Weissman RM, et al. Experience with triple-drug therapy in a pharmacological erection program. J Urol 1993; 150:1822.

146. Gerber GS, Levine LA. Pharmacological erection program using prostaglandin E1. J Urol 1992; 146:786.

147. Porst H. Prostaglandin E1 in erectile dysfunction. Urologe A 1989; 28:94.

148. Chen JK, Hwang TI, Yang CR. Comparison of effects following the intracorporeal injection of papaverine and prostaglandin E1. Br J Urol 1992; 69:404.

149. Martinez-Pineiro L, Cortes R, Cuervo E, et al. Prospective comparative study with intracavernous sodium nitroprusside and prostaglandin E1 in patients with erectile dysfunction. Eur Urol 1998; 34:350.

150. Earle CM, Keogh EJ, Wisniewski ZS, et al. Prostaglandin E1 therapy for impotence, comparison with papaverine. J Urol 1990; 143:57.

151. Kerfoot WW, Carson CC. Pharmacologically induced erections among geriatric men. J Urol 1991; 146:1022.

152. Casabe A, Bechara A, Cheliz G, et al. Drop-out reasons and complications in self-injection therapy with a triple vasoactive drug mixture in sexual erectile dysfunction. Int J Impot Res 1998; 10:5.

152a. Vardi Y, Sprecher E, Gruenwald I. Logistic regression and survival analysis of 450 impotent patients treated with injection therapy: long-term dropout parameters. J Urol 2000; 163:467.

153. Kulmala R. Treatment of priapism: primary results and complications in 207 patients. Ann Chir Gynaecol 1994; 83: 309.

154. Schultheiss D, Truss MC, Becker AJ, et al. Long-term results following dorsal penile vein ligation in 126 patients with veno-occlusive dysfunction. Int J Impot Res 1997; 9:205.

155. Freedman AL, Costa-Neto F, Mehringer CM, Rajfer J. Long-term results of penile vein ligation for impotence from venous leakage. J Urol 1993; 149:1301.

156. Scott FB, Byrd GJ, Karacan I, et al. Erectile impotence treated with an implantable, inflatable prosthesis. Five years of clinical experience. JAMA 1979; 241:2609.

157. Narayan P, Lange PH. Semirigid penile prostheses in erectile dysfunction. Urol Clin North Am 1981; 8:181.

158. Furlow WL. Use of the inflatable penile prosthesis in erectile dysfunction. Urol Clin North Am 1981; 8:181.

159. Tegelaar RJ, Kycklama-a-Nijeholt AA, Kropman RF. Experiences of patients with semi-rigid Jonas penile prosthesis. Ned Tijdschr Geneeskd 1991; 135:514.

160. Kabalin JN, Kessler R. Experience with the Hydroflex penile prosthesis. J Urol 1989; 141:58.

161. Garber BB. Inflatable penile prosthesis: results of 150 cases. Br J Urol 1996; 78:933.

162. Fein RL. The G.F.S. Mark II inflatable penile prosthesis. J Urol 1992; 147:66.

163. McLaren RH, Barrett DM. Patient and partner satisfaction with the AMS 700 penile prosthesis. J Urol 1992; 147:62.

164. Wilson SK, Cleves M, Delk JR 2nd. Long-term results with Hydroflex and Dynaflex penile prostheses: device survival comparisons to multicomponent inflatables. J Urol 1996; 155:162.

164a. Montorsi F, Rigatti P, Carmignani G, et al. AMS three-piece inflatable implants for erectile dysfunction: a long-term multi-institutional study in 2000 consecutive patients. Eur Urol 2000; 37:50.

165. Sexton WJ, Benedict JF, Jarow JP. Comparison of long-term outcomes of penile prostheses and intracavernosal injection therapy. J Urol 1998; 159:811.

166. Tan HL. Economic cost of male erectile dysfunction using a decision analytic model: for a hypothetical managed-care plan of 100,000 members. Pharmacoeconomics 2000; 17:77.

167. Shabsigh R, Padma-Nathan H, Gittleman M, et al. Intracavernous alprostadil alfadex (EDEX/VIRIDAL) is effective and safe in patients with erectile dysfunction after failing sildenafil (Viagra). Urology 2000; 55:477.

168. Shabsigh R, Padma-Nathan H, Gittleman M, et al. Intracavernous alprostadil alfadex is more efficacious, better tolerated, and preferred over intraurethral alprostadil plus optional actis: a comparative, randomized, crossover, multicenter study. Urology 2000; 55:109.

# CHAPTER 118

# MALE INFERTILITY

RICHARD V. CLARK

The evaluation and management of the infertile man have evolved considerably because of the development of new methodologies associated with procedures for in vitro fertilization (IVF), particularly *intracytoplasmic sperm injection* (ICSI), and an increase in our understanding of the genetics of sperm function.[1] Nevertheless, the physician is often confronted with a patient in whom the diagnosis of "unexplained infertility" is the most appropriate description of his condition. The treatment for this has remained mostly empirical and somewhat controversial because of the paucity of effective medical therapies and the expense of procedures such as IVF with ICSI.

The treatment regimen for an infertile man requires a secure diagnostic foundation to allow appropriate selection from potential therapies. In the past, there were few measures of sperm function in the laboratory.[2,3] Historically, semen analysis has been used to estimate fertility potential in men.[4] However, errors in interpreting the semen analysis occur frequently because such measures do not directly assess sperm function or define what constitutes the "minimally adequate ejaculate." Moreover, there is variability in semen quality among different specimens, and there are temporal changes in sperm output and semen quality. The consideration of the reproductive potential of the sexual partner is equally important, and the evaluation of a potentially infertile man necessitates a thorough gynecologic review of the sexual partner to recognize any coexisting reproductive dysfunction.

## DIAGNOSTIC APPROACH

### DEFINITION OF INFERTILITY

A *couple* is considered infertile if *no pregnancies have occurred during at least 1 year of unprotected intercourse.* However, studies on the probability of fertility over time suggest that this interval may be too short, because 15% of couples fail to achieve pregnancy in 1 year but only 6% fail by the end of 2 years.[5,6] Basic evaluation reasonably can begin after 1 year of infertility, as can relatively low-cost appropriate therapy, but the use of expensive and specialized procedures should probably be reserved until after 2 or more years of infertility.

At the initial evaluation, the man and his partner should be questioned about libido and erection (see Chap. 117), coital technique, frequency, and timing of intercourse. Although uncommon, people who lack understanding of simple reproductive physiology can reduce fertility by the practice of premature withdrawal, coitus associated with the time of menses rather than midcycle, or abstinence except for an erroneously perceived fertility period. Obviously, the timing of intercourse close to the time of ovulation is essential. For most couples, this optimal time is ~11 to 13 days after the onset of menses. Basal body temperature records can be useful, relying on the progesterone-induced temperature rise, but these records are often confusing for patients. Home kits are available to assist the timing of intercourse by monitoring for the appearance of luteinizing hormone (LH) in a woman's urine, indicating the preovulatory surge of LH.

A critical feature of the initial assessment is consideration of the female partner's reproductive potential. Although obvious menstrual irregularity can be ascertained by history, subtle dysfunction may require careful gynecologic evaluation. Female factors that frequently may be unrecognized include abnormal coital habits, cervical factors, tubal obstruction, anovulation, oligomenorrhea, short luteal phase, hyperprolactinemia, and age. The evaluation of both partners should proceed simultaneously. Frequently, correction of a female factor markedly improves fertility rates among couples in whom the problem initially had been assumed to be a male factor (see Chaps. 97 and 103).

## MALE HISTORY

The medical history of the infertile man should focus on identifying factors that are known to impair erectile or testicular function and excluding mild forms of systemic illness that can be associated with reduced sperm production[7,8] (see Chap. 116). Major risk factors include late or incomplete testicular descent, abnormal pubertal development, inadequate libido or potency, retrograde ejaculation, genital infections, drugs (including alcohol and marijuana), toxins (including pesticides and radiation), heat (including prolonged fever), cancer therapy, and systemic illness. Failure of complete testicular descent or late descent can cause permanent germ-cell injury (see Chap. 93). In utero exposure to diethylstilbestrol is associated with epididymal abnormalities that can cause obstructive azoospermia.[9] Late or incomplete puberty can indicate hypogonadism, especially when associated with partial or complete impotence (see Chaps. 92 and 115). Failure to ejaculate, despite a normal erection and the sensation of orgasm, indicates retrograde ejaculation.[10] Genital infections, especially chronic epididymitis and prostatitis, can markedly diminish sperm motility and fertility.[11] Mumps orchitis can cause progressive tubular sclerosis and irreversible damage to the seminiferous epithelium and to Leydig cells.[12] Personal habits can lead to testicular injury, especially heavy alcohol intake, bathing in hot water, and frequent marijuana use.[13,14] Occupational exposures to radiation, certain pesticides such as dibromochloropropane, and aromatic solvents are associated with reduced fertility[15–17,17a] (see Chap. 235). Treatment of cancer by radiation or chemotherapy can severely impair sperm production.[18] Pelvic trauma or pelvic surgery can injure the gonads, or the accessory organs and ducts, or damage pelvic nerves, causing erectile or ejaculatory dysfunction. The effects of systemic illnesses on testicular function are discussed in Chapter 116.

## PHYSICAL EXAMINATION

The infertile man usually has a normal physical examination; nevertheless, a thorough examination is important to detect any evidence of hypogonadism or potential causes of infertility.[7] The degree of virilization can be a useful index of hypogonadism. Usually, the normal male has full axillary and pubic hair with a male pattern escutcheon; terminal hair on the face, upper chest, upper abdomen, and frequently over the shoulders; male muscle pattern and mass; deep, "adult male" voice; and often temporal balding. The nipples and pectoral area should be palpated for any evidence of gynecomastia or galactorrhea (see Chap. 120).

**TABLE 118-1.**
**Classification of Testicular Size**

| Volume (mL) | Dimensions (cm) | Adult Condition |
|---|---|---|
| 2 | 2.0 × 1.2 | Severe hypogonadism, such as Klinefelter syndrome |
| 4 | 2.5 × 1.5 | |
| 6 | 2.9 × 1.8 | Moderate hypogonadism, such as gonadotropin deficiency or maturation arrest |
| 10 | 3.4 × 2.1 | |
| 15 | 4.1 × 2.5 | |
| 20 | 4.3 × 2.8 | Normal size, but may include obstruction or idiopathic oligospermia |
| 25 | 4.7 × 3.1 | |
| 30 | 5.2 × 3.3 | |

The genitals should be examined carefully for phallic size (normal, >6 cm flaccid), location of the urethral opening with any evidence of hypospadias, completeness of testicular descent, and normal thinning of scrotal skin with rugal folds.

Testicular size and consistency are important indices of germ-cell content. The testis grows from a neonatal size of 1 to 3 mL to an adult size of 20 to 30 mL[19] (see Chaps. 91 and 93). The normal adult seminiferous tubules are composed of several stages of development, with germ cells making up >95% of the testicular volume and Leydig cells contributing <1%. Adult testes that are soft in consistency or are <20 mL in volume suggest hypogonadism and warrant a complete endocrinologic evaluation. Testicular size is measured by volume with an orchidometer (see Chap. 93) or by linear dimensions (short and long axes) with a ruler. Corresponding volumes and linear dimensions are shown in Table 118-1. Most examiners find the orchidometer easier to use, and the measurements are more reproducible. The testis, epididymis, and vas deferens should be palpated bilaterally for continuity, masses, nodules, or tenderness. The presence of a varicocele can be assessed by palpation of the spermatic cord while the patient is standing and by performing the Valsalva maneuver to induce filling of a potential varicocele. The prostate should be palpated for size, consistency, tenderness, and evidence of masses or nodules. The examination should also exclude any evidence of systemic illness that may affect testicular function (see Chap. 116). Testicular ultrasound can provide useful imaging to evaluate nodules (irregular texture, possible hydrocele) and to confirm volume estimates.[20]

## INTERPRETATION OF LABORATORY DATA

The use of laboratory data to evaluate testicular function is discussed in Chapter 114. This section focuses on the interpretation of certain laboratory tests in evaluating the infertile man.

### SEMEN ANALYSIS

The semen analysis remains a critical part of the evaluation of an infertile man.[21] Although standard semen characteristics do not provide a strong prediction of fertility, more functional assays, such as hamster ova penetration and zona binding, are also indirect measures that have variably predictive values.[2,3] The methodology for semen analyses is well standardized using specialized chambers for determining sperm density and motility.[21] Automated semen analysis using video recording of semen samples with computer analysis has become widely used for more objective evaluation of sperm motility.[22,23] However, the interpretation of a single semen sample is difficult because of the marked variability in sperm count, motility, morphology, and semen volume among samples from a particular man.[24,25] This variability appears to be accentuated with poorer semen characteristics. The source of the variability is poorly understood and may reflect subtle endogenous factors. Length of abstinence can be a confounding factor, as abstinence of more than a few days can induce a false elevation of sperm count and depression of

**TABLE 118-2.**
**Semen Characteristics***

| Semen Characteristic | Category | | |
|---|---|---|---|
| | *Good* | *Equivocal* | *Poor* |
| Total sperm | $>60 \times 10^6$ | $40–59 \times 10^6$ | $<40 \times 10^6$ |
| Sperm density | $>20 \times 10^6/\text{mL}$ | $10–19 \times 10^6/\text{mL}$ | $<10 \times 10^6/\text{mL}$ |
| Volume | $>2.0$ mL | $1.0–1.9$ mL | $<1.0$ mL |
| Motility | $>60\%$ | $40–59\%$ | $<40\%$ |
| Motility grade | $>3.0$ | $2.5–2.9$ | $<2.5$ |
| Oval forms | $>60\%$ | $40–59\%$ | $<40\%$ |

*Based on multiple analyses of 119 men, 30 fertile and 89 infertile.
(From Sherins RJ, Brightwell D, Steruthal PM. Longitudinal analysis of semen of fertile and infertile men. In: Troen P, Nankin HR, eds. The testis in normal and infertile men. New York: Raven Press, 1977.)

sperm motility.[26,27] The author recommends the collection of at least three to six semen samples during 2 to 4 months to get a reasonable impression of a patient's semen characteristics. Samples should be collected after 24 to 48 hours of abstinence.

Semen characteristics can be grouped into broad categories, based on sperm count, motility, morphology, and semen volume, as having good, poor, or equivocal probability of fertility. Suggested limits based on multiple analyses of 119 men are presented in Table 118-2.[28] No single semen characteristic (except perhaps azoospermia) has an absolute correlation with fertility. This is shown in Table 118-3, which lists the percentage of men who had a particular semen characteristic that was presumed to be associated with either infertility or fertility. Only 75% of 89 infertile men had low sperm counts, and only 20% of 30 fertile men had a normal percentage of motile sperm.

The concept of a minimally adequate ejaculate for fertility has undergone progressive decrements in absolute numbers since it was first introduced in the 1920s. To highlight this point, pregnancies have been induced by men with counts of <1 million/mL (e.g., normal men who had spermatogenesis suppressed as part of a male contraceptive study or men treated for hypogonadotropic hypogonadism).[29,30] In practice, *a total sperm count of <20 million/mL, motility <40%, normal oval morphology <40% by World Health Organization (WHO) criteria or <10% by strict criteria, or semen volume <1 mL is associated with impaired fertility.*[6,28,31] Table 118-4 shows the probable causes of seminiferous tubule dysfunction based on semen analysis characteristics.

### HORMONAL DATA

The hormonal data provide another important assessment of testicular function. Four patterns are common in infertile men: patients with normal values for serum testosterone, LH, and

**TABLE 118-3.**
**Semen Characteristics of Infertile versus Fertile Men**

| Semen Characteristic | Infertile (Men in Poor Category) | | Fertile (Men in Good Category) | |
|---|---|---|---|---|
| | %* | *Limit* | % | *Limit* |
| Total sperm | 75 | $<40 \times 10^6$ | 80 | $>60 \times 10^6$ |
| Sperm density | 58 | $<10 \times 10^6/\text{mL}$ | 76 | $>20 \times 10^6/\text{mL}$ |
| Volume | 5 | $<1.0$ mL | 73 | $>2.0$ mL |
| Motility | 58 | $<40\%$ | 20 | $>60\%$ |
| Quality | 53 | $<2.5$ | 43 | $>3.0$ |
| Oval forms | 44 | $<40\%$ | 80 | $>60\%$ |

*Percentage of infertile men (89) and fertile men (30) whose mean semen characteristics fell into the expected category.
(From Sherins RJ, Brightwell D, Sternthal PM. Longitudinal analysis of semen of fertile and infertile men. In: Troen P, Nankin HR, eds. The testis in normal and infertile men. New York: Raven Press, 1977.)

**TABLE 118-4.**
**Causes of Male Infertility Based on Semen Analysis**

**AZOOSPERMIA**
  Seminiferous tubule sclerosis
  Germinal aplasia
  Maturation arrest
  Ductal obstruction
  Absent ejaculation
**NONMOTILE SPERM**
  Kartagener syndrome
  Metabolic defect
  Prolonged abstinence
  Idiopathic
**OLIGOSPERMIA**
  Drug/toxin
  Varicocele
  Cryptorchidism
  Genital infection
  Systemic illness
  Idiopathic
**NORMAL BUT INFERTILE**
  Female abnormality
  Inadequate coital habits
  Immunologic
  Idiopathic

follicle-stimulating hormone (FSH); patients with elevated serum gonadotropins and a low testosterone, suggesting severe primary testicular failure; patients with elevated serum FSH but normal LH and testosterone seen in milder forms of germ-cell depletion; and patients with low or normal serum gonadotropins and low testosterone, indicating gonadotropin deficiency (secondary testicular failure).[32] *Inhibin* has been shown to serve as a *marker* of *seminiferous epithelial function*, and inhibin levels are elevated in conditions of epithelial dysfunction.[33] Secondary hypogonadism can be induced by hyperprolactinemia, possibly by inhibiting the pulsatile release of gonadotropin-releasing hormone (GnRH), although direct effects on the Leydig cells and seminiferous tubules may also be a factor.[34] However, hyperprolactinemia typically presents as impotence rather than as infertility (see Chap. 13). Hormonal evaluation of infertile men with poor semen characteristics should include serum testosterone, LH, FSH, and possibly estradiol. Prolactin levels should be reserved for men with suspected gonadotropin deficiency or impotence. Because gonadotropins are secreted in pulses, and a single blood sample can represent a peak or a nadir, the author recommends drawing three samples during 45 to 60 minutes. Pooling the sera significantly reduces the cost of the hormone assays and gives a reasonable estimate of the mean for the three samples.

### TESTICULAR BIOPSY

A testicular biopsy can provide direct information about the degree of spermatogenesis in the area sampled. This can be extremely useful in demonstrating obstructive azoospermia, which shows normal spermatogenesis within the tubules.[35,36] However, there are few other conditions in which information from the biopsy directs a therapeutic decision that may improve sperm production or fertility. The response of the seminiferous epithelium to a variety of injuries can be similar, and the usual finding is one of maturation arrest or variable germ-cell depletion. However, a biopsy or testicular sperm aspiration can allow sperm retrieval for ICSI. Usually, the author reserves a diagnostic testicular biopsy for evaluation of azoospermia in a man with normal-sized testes and with normal LH, FSH, and testosterone.

# IDENTIFIABLE CAUSES OF MALE INFERTILITY

A variety of factors have been identified that can impair sperm production and cause infertility. Many of these are associated with reduced Leydig cell function and may present as hypogonadism rather than infertility (see Chap. 115). This section reviews the major causes of infertility based on pathophysiology.

## HORMONAL DISORDERS

Several hormonal disorders are associated with testicular dysfunction. The most common of these is gonadotropin deficiency, either congenital, as in idiopathic hypogonadotropic hypogonadism (IHH, Kallmann syndrome) in which there is a failure of GnRH secretion, adult-onset IHH, or acquired, as by a mass or infiltrative lesion interfering with pituitary or hypothalamic function and normal gonadotropin stimulation of the testes.[37,38] These patients may present with loss of libido and impotence and usually have small or soft testes and an inadequate or absent ejaculate. The hormone profile shows low serum gonadotropins and a low testosterone. A similar clinical picture is produced by hyperprolactinemia because excess prolactin depresses GnRH secretion.[34] Prolactin levels two to three times the upper limits of normal are usually associated with impaired testicular function and impotence, while the effects of slight elevations are unclear. So far, gonadotropin-receptor defects, as for FSH, have not been demonstrated to be a cause of hypogonadism.[39]

Patients with hypogonadotropic hypogonadism respond well to therapy, with many becoming fertile. Intramuscular gonadotropins (human chorionic gonadotropin [hCG], human menopausal gonadotropin [hMG], recombinant FSH [rFSH]) directly stimulate the testis to produce testosterone and sperm. These are usually administered as hCG alone, 1200 to 2000 IU given intramuscularly thrice weekly, or with hMG or rFSH, 37.5 to 75.0 IU given intramuscularly thrice weekly.[32] Normal testosterone production is achieved in >90% of cases, while sperm production depends on testicular size. Men with testicular volumes >4 mL produce sperm and are fertile in ~80% of cases, while those with initial gonadal volumes of <4 mL become fertile in fewer than half of cases and require combination therapy (hCG plus hMG or rFSH). Alternatively, pulsatile GnRH can be administered by a pump and can stimulate pituitary gonadotropin release, although response rates seem similar.[37]

Subtle forms of androgen resistance also may exist in which the presentation is infertility with azoospermia, although this was not duplicated in a separate study.[40,41] Subsequent studies of the androgen receptor trans-activation domain have shown that point mutation polymorphisms do not affect sperm production, but long polyglutamic tracts can.[42,43] Hyperthyroidism is associated with elevated sex hormone–binding globulin, altering the ratio of free testosterone to free estradiol.[44] In severe cases, this can cause gynecomastia and reduced sperm output. Hypothyroidism may be associated with a reversible hypogonadism.[44a] Hypercortisolism can be associated with depressed testicular function, probably by suppression of the hypothalamic-pituitary axis.[45]

## CHROMOSOMAL ABNORMALITIES

Certain specific chromosomal abnormalities are associated with impaired testicular function. Klinefelter syndrome (47,XXY) is the most common of these (see Chap. 115). The classic form—small firm testes, inadequate virilization, gynecomastia, and azoospermia—is relatively easy to recognize. However, patients can present with impaired sperm production and azoospermia but with adequate androgen levels inducing normal virilization, libido, and potency.[46,47] This is especially true

of mosaic forms (e.g., 46,XY/47,XXY). In mosaics, the testes are small, and serum gonadotropins usually are elevated, but the spectrum can extend to near normal values. A karyotype should be considered in men with reduced testicular size and azoospermia to rule out Klinefelter syndrome or a variant.

Another disorder of sex chromosome number is the XYY syndrome (47,XYY), in which there is an extra Y chromosome. Typically, these men have normal virilization and normal serum gonadotropins and testosterone but show variable tubular abnormalities (from maturation arrest to tubular sclerosis) and have severe oligospermia or azoospermia.[48,49] Autosomal chromosome abnormalities can be associated with testicular dysfunction, notably Down syndrome (trisomy 21) and balanced autosomal translocations.[50] Specific causes of nonmotile sperm (necrospermia) have been identified that are associated with infertility. One form of nonmotile sperm is caused by a lack of dynein arms in the microtubule filaments forming the sperm tail (Kartagener syndrome: includes sinusitis, bronchiectasis, and situs inversus).[51] Another form of necrospermia is caused by a deficiency of a specific metabolic enzyme, protein–carboxyl methylase, resulting in a metabolic basis for the loss of motility.[52]

Several groups have demonstrated the presence of microdeletions in the Y chromosome, some of which are associated with infertility.[53,54] These may account for 10% to 15% of cases of "idiopathic infertility." As these microdeletions can be transmitted by IVF-ICSI, consideration for genetic screening and counseling should be given to men who are candidates for these procedures.[55]

## CRYPTORCHIDISM

Cryptorchidism is associated with infertility and impaired testicular function (see Chap. 93), whether the disorder is bilateral or unilateral. This suggests that factors in addition to the effect of increased temperature on the undescended testis are responsible for the testicular injury. The location of the cryptorchid testis is important because testes at the external inguinal ring have a more advanced germ-cell component than do abdominal testes. The age of the patient at orchiopexy also appears to be important for later testicular development; those performed before the age of 3 years appear to result in better function than those done at puberty.[56,57] Other than orchiopexy or the use of exogenous GnRH to induce descent, no therapy is available. Typically, these men have normal levels of serum testosterone and LH, but an elevated FSH and inhibin consistent with primary testicular failure.

## VARICOCELE

Varicocele is clearly associated with infertility, and marked testicular atrophy can be found with large varicoceles[58] (Fig. 118-1). The incidence of varicocele appears to be ~10%, and roughly half of the men with varicoceles show reduced semen quality—either low sperm counts or reduced motility. Nevertheless, varicoceles are not uniformly associated with impaired fertility even in men with suboptimal semen characteristics.[59] Men with varicoceles have evidence of a primary testicular defect and either elevated basal serum FSH or an exaggerated response of FSH and LH to GnRH stimulation, whether they have normal or impaired semen characteristics or infertility.[60,61]

Varicoceles affect testicular function by increased testicular temperature, altered blood flow, and venous reflux of metabolic wastes from the kidneys or of organ-specific compounds, such as adrenal steroids or catecholamines. Varicoceles occur on the left side in ~90% of cases, probably related to the insertion of the left testicular vein into the left renal vein rather than the inferior vena cava, as on the right side. The semen characteristics of infertile men with varicocele are not specific, showing variable reductions in sperm count motility and an increased percentage of tapered sperm and immature or amorphous forms.[58,62]

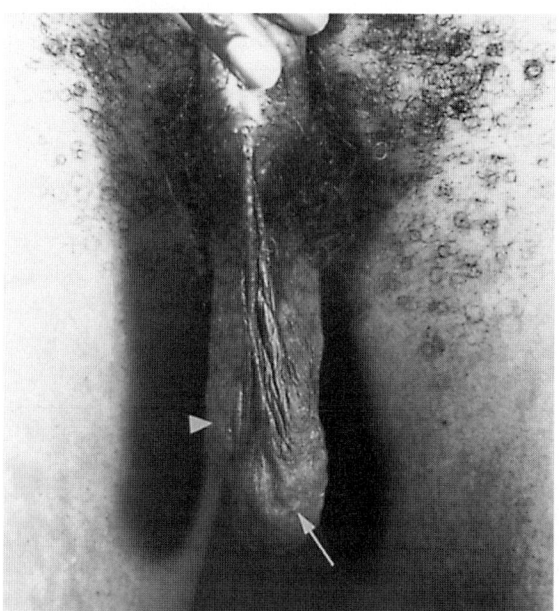

**FIGURE 118-1.** Left varicocele (*arrow*) in a patient with oligospermia. The *arrowhead* points to the right testis for comparison.

Compared with other therapies for oligospermia, surgical repair of a varicocele may offer promising results. However, responses to treatment are not consistent.[63] Published reports indicate an improvement of semen quality in 30% to 70% of patients and pregnancy in up to 25% of treated couples.[64,65] Unfortunately, reported series differ in patient selection, in the degree of evaluation before and after varicocelectomy, and in the exclusion of female factors. Although there is no well-controlled study demonstrating statistically significant improvement in fertility after varicocele repair, studies comparing men electing surgery or medical therapy suggest a positive response to surgery. Even more controversial is the issue of subclinical varicoceles identified only by special studies, and whether these subclinical changes represent physiologically significant alterations, which may be amenable to surgical correction.

## EJACULATORY DYSFUNCTION

Ejaculatory dysfunction can cause infertility by preventing the deposition of semen in the vagina. The failure of emission, or retrograde ejaculation, can be caused by interference with sympathetic innervation of the musculature of the bladder neck sphincter.[10] Retrograde ejaculation should be suspected if orgasm occurs with little or no ejaculate, and confirmed by demonstrating abundant sperm in a postejaculation urine specimen.

Ejaculation depends on three processes for completion: movement of semen into the posterior urethra, bladder neck closure, and propulsion of semen from the posterior urethra to the outside. This requires a combination of sympathetic autonomic and somatic innervation. As shown in Figure 118-2, fibers from the thoracolumbar sympathetic outflow induce smooth muscle contraction of the epididymis, vas deferens, seminal vesicles, and prostate, moving semen and sperm to the posterior urethra and causing closure of the bladder neck. Propulsion of the semen through the urethra is based on somatic

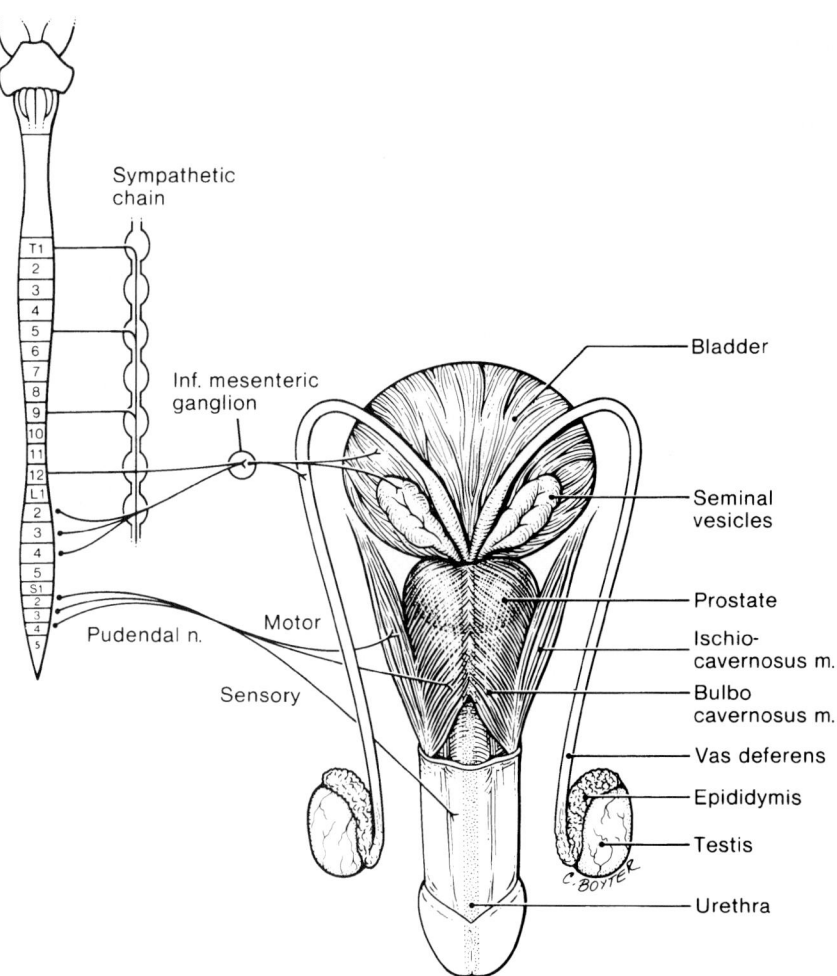

**FIGURE 118-2.** Schematic diagram of sympathetic and somatic innervation to urogenital organs necessary for ejaculation.

pudendal motor efferents to striated muscles forming the pelvic floor and the bulbocavernosus and ischiocavernosus muscles.

Retrograde ejaculation most commonly is associated with diabetic neuropathy or prostatic resection, but it can result from pelvic surgery, retroperitoneal lymph node dissection, and drug treatment (especially with adrenergic antagonists like phenoxybenzamine and guanethidine), or it may occur spontaneously. Sympathomimetic drugs and imipramine can be effective in treating postsurgical or diabetic retrograde ejaculation.[66] Alternatively, sperm can be recovered from the urine, concentrated, and used for intrauterine insemination.[67,68]

Ductal obstruction can cause azoospermia with normal or reduced ejaculatory volume. Ductal obstruction is frequently a postinfectious complication of epididymitis or urethritis with subclinical spread up the vas and can also be due to congenital strictures anywhere along the outflow tract.[11] This should be suspected in patients with azoospermia and can be documented by a vasogram and a testicular biopsy confirming adequate spermatogenesis. Young syndrome is a rare condition, characterized by chronic sinopulmonary infections and obstructive azoospermia, in which thickened mucous secretions lead to blockage of the bronchioles and epididymis.[69] Cystic fibrosis can be associated with congenital absence of the vas deferens and azoospermia or epididymal obstruction.[70] However, vasectomy is the most common cause of obstructive azoospermia.

## IMMUNOLOGIC FACTORS

Immunologic factors have been associated with infertility.[71,71a] Sperm antibodies have been reported in infertile men and their partners, although the incidence is low.[72] These also can be found in fertile couples, and the association with infertility has not been shown to be directly causative. However, sperm-specific antigens can be present in semen and may be related to sperm agglutination or poor sperm motility despite normal sperm counts. Therapy with glucocorticoids has been used with some success, although well-controlled studies are not available.[73] However, these drugs can cause significant side effects as glucose intolerance, hypertension, fluid retention, myopathy, and aseptic necrosis of the hip, and should be used with caution (see Chap. 78). ICSI seems to offer the best therapeutic approach in difficult cases.[74]

## INFECTIONS

Infections in the male reproductive tract can cause infertility (see Chap. 213).[74a] Clinically apparent infections of the testis, epididymis, or prostate can lead to reduced sperm count or motility. Epididymitis is considered secondary to urethritis or cystitis, and the ipsilateral testis usually is involved. Causative organisms typically are *Neisseria gonorrhoeae* and *Chlamydia trachomatis* in sexually active men younger than 35 years of age and coliform bacteria in men older than 35 years of age.[11] A variety of other organisms have been associated with epididymitis, including *Mycobacterium tuberculosis, Ureaplasma urealyticum*, herpes simplex virus, and mumps virus. Mumps orchitis virtually always occurs in postpubertal males in ~33% of cases of mumps parotitis.[12] Mumps orchitis can cause progressive, severe, irreversible tubular damage and presents with soft testes, oligospermia, and elevated gonadotropins. Prostatitis can take several forms: acute or chronic, bacterial or nonbacterial, symptomatic or asymptomatic. The presence of excess leukocytes in the semen suggests prostatitis (>1 leukocyte/100 sperm).[75] The physical examination often reveals a soft, tender, enlarged prostate gland. Culture is best obtained using a two- or four-glass urine collection with prostatic massage.[76] The most common infectious organism is *Escherichia coli*. Ureaplasm infections have been implicated in infertility, and treatment with doxycycline improves sperm function or fertility, although a controlled study did not show an effect.[77]

**TABLE 118-5.**
**Medications Associated with Impaired Testicular Function**

**ANTIANDROGENS**
  Spironolactone
  Cyproterone
  Cimetidine
  Flutamide
**ANDROGEN SYNTHESIS INHIBITORS**
  Ketoconazole
  Leuprolide
**ANTINEOPLASTIC DRUGS**
  Cyclophosphamide
  Cisplatin
  Melphalan
  Chlorambucil
  Nitrosoureas
  Busulfan
  Procarbazine
**ANTIHYPERTENSIVES/CARDIOVASCULAR AGENTS**
  α-Methyldopa
  Digoxin
  Calcium-channel blockers
  Reserpine
  Amiodarone
**PSYCHOACTIVE AGENTS**
  Tricyclic antidepressants
  Amphetamines
  Narcotics
  Major tranquilizers
  Minor tranquilizers
**OTHER DRUGS**
  Anabolic steroids
  Phenytoin
  Ethanol
  Penicillamine
  Isoniazid

## DRUGS, TOXINS, AND RADIATION

Several drugs, chemicals, and radiation can cause damage to the seminiferous epithelium (Table 118-5). Many of the anticancer drugs cause direct damage to the germ cells[17] (see Chap. 226). Particularly toxic are the alkylating agents, including cyclophosphamide, nitrosoureas, chlorambucil, melphalan, busulfan, and cisplatin, and other agents such as procarbazine, doxorubicin, and cytosine arabinoside. Antimetabolites, such as methotrexate, 5-fluorouracil, and 6-mercaptopurine, do not appear to affect testicular function significantly. Alcohol can suppress Leydig cells, germ cells, and gonadotropin release by the pituitary, leading to a spectrum of hypogonadism[13] (see Chaps. 205 and 233). Crude marijuana is a potential suppressant of testicular function, although available data are not definitive[14] (see Chap. 234). Radiation at doses as low as 15 rad can transiently decrease sperm output, and doses >200 rad can produce prolonged azoospermia.[15] Although only a few drugs, such as sulfa drugs and cimetidine, have been shown to cause testicular injury, the chronic use of any drug may be a factor in infertility.[78,79]

## MANAGEMENT OF MALE INFERTILITY

The primary management decision is whether there is an identifiable and treatable cause for the infertility. The causes of testicular dysfunction are listed in Table 118-6.

The failure to identify a known factor leads to the unsatisfying diagnosis of idiopathic infertility. This category probably

**TABLE 118-6.**
**Causes of Male Infertility**

**USUALLY IRREVERSIBLE**
  Chromosomal abnormality
  Absent vas deferens
  Young syndrome
  Nonmotile sperm
  Mumps orchitis
  Cryptorchidism
  Drugs/toxins
  Epididymal dysfunction
**POTENTIALLY REVERSIBLE**
  Vas or epididymal occlusion
  Retrograde ejaculation
  Prostatitis, epididymitis
  Gonadotropin deficiency
  Varicocele
  Drugs/toxins
  Heat or irradiation
  Sexual dysfunction
  Immunologic dysfunction
  Systemic illness

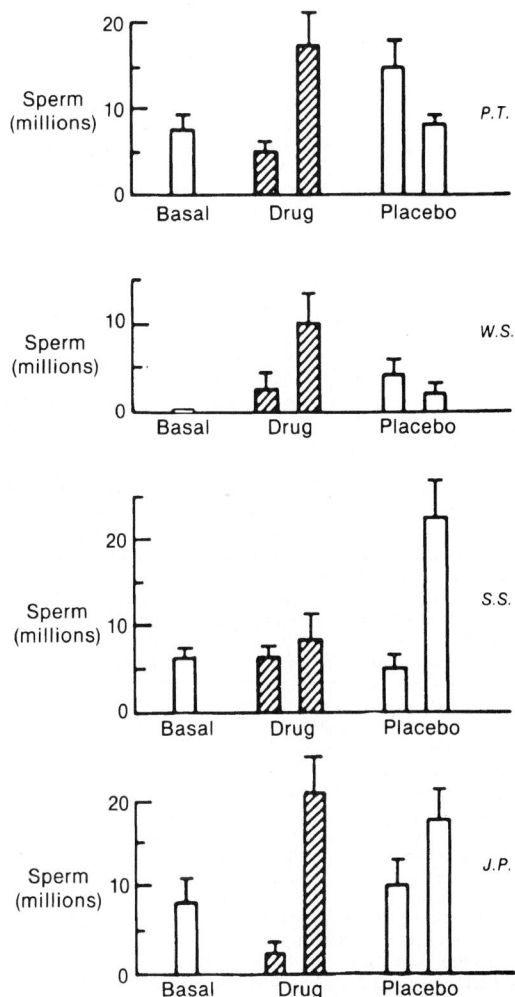

**FIGURE 118-3.** Changes in mean sperm output over time. Mean total sperm output is plotted for 4-month intervals in individual patients on therapeutic protocol for oligospermic infertility. Means are based on the minimum of four samples from each treatment period: basal, drug, or placebo. Note that marked increases in output occurred while the patient was on either drug or placebo therapy. (Based on data from Clark RV, Sherins RJ. Use of semen analysis in the evaluation of the infertile couple. In: Santen RJ, Swerdloff RS, eds. Male reproductive dysfunction. New York: Marcel Dekker Inc, 1986:253.)

includes various factors, not yet identified, that produce a similar clinical picture of low sperm count, poor sperm motility, and infertility.

Numerous agents have been proposed for the treatment of idiopathic infertility. An evaluation of their efficacy is difficult because of the scarcity of well-conducted therapeutic trials that exclude spousal factors and improper coital techniques and include adequate basal evaluation with three to six semen samples collected during the 4 to 6 months before therapy, plus an adequate number of semen samples during and after therapy to document any effect. The treatment period should be at least 3 months to span one germ-cell cycle. Moreover, a double-blind placebo control is necessary because spontaneous pregnancies may occur that are unrelated to treatment.[80] A review using metaanalyses of randomized controlled trials concluded that there is no demonstrable efficacy of medical treatments for idiopathic male infertility.[81]

Despite controversial efficacy, three hormonal approaches to therapy are often empirically employed: exogenous gonadotropins, antiestrogens, and aromatase inhibitors, which reduce conversion of androgens to estrogens.[82–87a] Gonadotropins have been used to provide an additional stimulus to the germinal epithelium and Leydig cells by increasing intratesticular testosterone with hCG or by stimulating germ-cell maturation with hMG or rFSH. Some studies indicate a positive response to exogenous gonadotropins, but this has not been confirmed in several carefully studied series.[82,83] Clomiphene is an antiestrogen that increases gonadotropin release. Controlled studies with clomiphene at a dosage between 25 and 50 mg per day for 3 to 6 months have reported both negative and positive responses, and the present data must be regarded as discouraging.[84,85] An aromatase inhibitor, testolactone, has been used, based on the possibility that excess estrogen may impair the germinal epithelium. An initial study without a control group reported success, but a subsequent study with placebo controls and patient crossover showed no effect on sperm count or fertility.[86,87] Random, sustained increases in sperm count occur during both placebo and drug therapy (Fig. 118-3), illustrating the importance of controls in therapeutic trials.

Therapies designed to isolate more functional sperm, such as sperm washing for intrauterine insemination or IVF, are proving to be more useful in treating male factor infertility.[88] Microinjection of sperm into ooplasm, ICSI, is performed at a

number of centers and appears to be effective without increased risk of fetal abnormalities or loss.[64,89,90,91] Such specialized reproductive techniques currently offer the greatest chance for success in treating idiopathic male infertility.

## REFERENCES

1. Forti G, Krausz C. Evaluation and treatment of the infertile couple. J Clin Endocrinol Metab 1998; 83:4177.
2. Franken DR, Acosta AA, Kruger TF, et al. The hemizona assay: its role in identifying male factor infertility in assisted reproduction. Fertil Steril 1993; 59:1075.
3. Barratt CLR, St. John JC. Diagnostic tools in male infertility. Hum Reprod 1998; 13(Suppl 1):51.
4. Clark RV, Sherins RJ. Use of semen analysis in the evaluation of the infertile couple. In: Santen RJ, Swerdloff RS, eds. Male reproductive dysfunction. New York: Marcel Dekker Inc, 1986:253.
5. Bostofte E, Bagger P, Michael A, Stakemann G. Fertility prognosis for infertile men: results of follow-up study of semen analysis in infertile men from two populations evaluated by the Cox regression model. Fertil Steril 1990; 54:1100.
6. Collins JA, Burrows EA, Willan AR. Prognosis for live birth among untreated infertile couples. Fertil Steril 1995; 64:22
7. Clark RV. Clinical andrology: history and physical examination. Endocrinol Metab Clin North Am 1994; 23:699.
8. Irvine DS. Epidemiology and aetiology of male infertility. Hum Reprod 1998; 13(Suppl 1):33.

9. Whitehead ED, Leiter E. Genital abnormalities and abnormal semen analyses in male patients exposed to diethylstilbestrol in utero. J Urol 1981; 125:47.

10. Thomas AJ Jr. Ejaculatory dysfunction. Fertil Steril 1983; 39:445.

11. Berger RE, Holmes KK. Infection and male infertility. In: Santen RJ, Swerdloff RS, eds. Male reproductive dysfunction. New York: Marcel Dekker Inc, 1986:407.

12. Beard CM, Benson RC, Kelalis PP, et al. The incidence of mumps orchitis in Rochester, Minnesota, 1935 to 1974. Mayo Clin Proc 1977; 52:3.

13. Van Thiel DH, Lester R, Sherins RJ. Hypogonadism in liver disease: evidence for a double defect. Gastroenterology 1974; 67:1188.

14. Hembree WC, Zeidenberg P, Nahas G. Marihuana effects on human gonadal function. In: Nahas G, Poton WDM, Idanpaan-Heittila J, eds. Marihuana: chemistry, biochemistry, and cellular effects. New York: Springer-Verlag, 1976:521.

15. Clifton DK, Bremner WJ. The effect of testicular X-irradiation on spermatogenesis in man. J Androl 1983; 4:387.

16. Tas S, Lauwerys R, Lison D. Occupational hazards for the male reproductive system. Crit Rev Toxicol 1996; 26:26.

17. Tielemans E, Burdorf A, te Velde ER, et al. Occupationally related exposures and reduced semen quality: a case control study. Fertil Steril 1999; 71:690.

17a. De Celis R, Feria-Kelasco A, González-Unzaga M, et al. Semen quality of workers occupationally exposed to hydrocarbons. Fertil Steril 2000; 73:221.

18. Sherins RJ. Adverse effects of treatment: gonadal dysfunction. In: DeVita VT Jr, Hellman S, Rosenberg SA, eds. Cancer: principles and practice of oncology, 4th ed. Philadelphia: JB Lippincott Co, 1993:2395.

19. Winters JSD, Faiman C. Pituitary-gonadal relations in male children and adolescents. Pediatr Res 1972; 6:126.

20. Lenz S, Giwercman A, Elsborg A, et al. Ultrasonic testicular texture and size in 444 men from the general population: correlated to semen quality. Eur Urol 1993; 24:231.

21. World Health Organization. WHO laboratory manual for the examination of human semen and sperm-cervical mucus interaction, 3rd ed. Cambridge, UK: Cambridge University Press, 1992.

22. Davis RO, Katz DF. Operational standards for computer-aided sperm analysis instruments. J Androl 1993; 14:385.

23. Vantman D, Zinaman M, Koukoulis G, et al. Computer-assisted semen analysis: evaluation of method and assessment of the influence of sperm concentration on linear velocity determination. Fertil Steril 1988; 49:510.

24. Baker HWG, Burger HC, de Kretser DM, et al. Factors affecting the variability of semen analysis results in infertile men. Int J Androl 1981; 4:609.

25. Tielemans E, Heederik D, Burdorf A. Intraindividual variability and redundancy of semen parameters. Epidemiology 1997; 8:99.

26. Tyler JPP, Crockett NG, Driscoll L. Studies of human seminal parameters with frequent ejaculation. I. Clinical characteristics. Clin Reprod Fertil 1982; 1:273.

27. Cooper TG, Keck C, Oberdieck U, Nieschlag E. Effects of multiple ejaculations after extended periods of sexual abstinence on total, motile, and normal sperm numbers from healthy normal and oligospermic men. Hum Reprod 1993; 8:1251.

28. Sherins RJ, Brightwell D, Steruthal PM. Longitudinal analysis of semen of fertile and infertile men. In: Troen P, Nankin HR, eds. The testis in normal and infertile men. New York: Raven Press, 1977:473.

29. Barfield A, Melo J, Coutinho E, et al. Pregnancies associated with sperm concentrations below 10 million/mL in clinical studies of a potential male contraceptive method, monthly depot medroxyprogesterone acetate and testosterone esters. Contraception 1979; 20:121.

30. Burris AS, Clark RV, Vantman DJ, et al. A low sperm concentration does not preclude fertility in men with isolated hypogonadotropic hypogonadism after gonadotropin therapy. Fertil Steril 1988; 50:343.

31. Ombelet W, Bosmans E, Janssen M, et al. Semen parameters in a fertile versus subfertile population: a need for change in the interpretation of semen testing. Hum Reprod 1997; 12:987.

32. Burris AS, Rodbard HW, Winters SJ, Sherins, RJ. Gonadotropin therapy in men with isolated hypogonadotropic hypogonadism: the response to human chorionic gonadotropin is predicted by initial testicular size. J Clin Endocrinol Metab 1988; 66:1144.

33. Anawalt BD, Bebb RA, Matsumoto AM, et al. Serum inhibin B levels reflect Sertoli cell function in normal men and men with testicular dysfunction. J Clin Endocrinol Metab 1996; 81:3341.

34. Bouchard P, Lagoguey M, Brailly S, Schaisan G. Gonadotropin-releasing hormone pulsatile administration restores luteinizing hormone pulsatility and normal testosterone levels in males with hyperprolactinemia. J Clin Endocrinol Metab 1985; 60:258.

35. Silber SJ, Rodriguez-Rigau LJ. Quantitative analysis of testicle biopsy: determination of partial obstruction and prediction of sperm count after surgery for obstruction. Fertil Steril 1981; 36:480.

36. Tournaye H, Liu J, Nagy PZ, et al. Correlation between testicular histology and outcome after intracytoplasmic sperm injection using testicular spermatozoa. Hum Reprod 1997; 11:127.

37. Whitcomb RW, Crowley WF. Diagnosis and treatment of isolated gonadotropin-releasing hormone deficiency in men. J Clin Endocrinol Metab 1990; 70:3.

38. Nachtigall LB, Boepple PA, Pralong FP, Crowley WF. Adult-onset idiopathic hypogonadotropic hypogonadism, a treatable form of male infertility. N Engl J Med 1997; 336:410.

39. Simoni M, Gromoll J, Hoppner W, et al. Mutational analysis of FSH receptor in normal and infertile men: identification and characterization of two discrete FSH receptor isoforms. J Clin Endocrinol Metab 1999; 84:751.

40. Aiman J, Griffin JE. The frequency of androgen receptor deficiency in infertile men. J Clin Endocrinol Metab 1982; 54:725.

41. Eil C, Gamblin GT, Hodge JW, et al. Whole cell and nuclear androgen uptake in skin fibroblasts from infertile men. J Androl 1985; 6:365.

42. Tut TG, Ghadessy FJ, Trifiro MA, et al. Long polyglutamine tracts in the androgen receptor are associated with reduced trans-activation, impaired sperm productions, and male infertility. J Clin Endocrinol Metab 1997; 82:3777.

43. Wang Q, Ghadessy FJ, Yong EL. Analysis of the trans-activation domain of the androgen receptor in patients with male infertility. Clin Genet 1998; 54:185.

44. Kidd GS, Glass AR, Vigersky RA. The hypothalamic-pituitary testicular axis in thyrotoxicosis. J Clin Endocrinol Metab 1979; 48:798.

44a. Donnelly P, White C. Testicular dysfunction in men with primary hypothyroidism; reversal of hypogonadotropic hypogonadism with replacement thyroxine. Clin Endocrinol 2000; 52:197.

45. Luton JP, Thieblot P, Valcke JC, et al. Reversible gonadotropin deficiency in male Cushings disease. J Clin Endocrinol Metab 1977; 45:488.

46. Paulsen CA, Gorden DL, Carpenter RW, et al. Klinefelters syndrome and its variants: a hormonal and chromosomal study. Recent Prog Horm Res 1968; 24:321.

47. Wang C, Baker HWG, Burger HW, et al. Hormonal studies in Klinefelters syndrome. Clin Endocrinol (Oxf) 1975; 4:399.

48. Santen RJ, de Kretser DM, Paulsen CA, Vorhees J. Gonadotropins and testosterone in the XYY syndrome. Lancet 1970; 2:371.

49. Skakkebaek NE, Zeuthen E, Nielsen J, Yde H. Abnormal spermatogenesis in XYY males: a report on four cases ascertained through a population study. Fertil Steril 1973; 24:390.

50. Hasen J, Boyar RM, Shapiro LR. Gonadal function in trisomy 21. Horm Res 1980; 12:345.

51. Afzelius BA. A human syndrome caused by immotile cilia. Science 1976; 193:317.

52. Gagnon C, Sherins RJ, Phillips DM, Bardin CW. Deficiency of protein carboxyl methylase in immotile spermatozoa in infertile men. N Engl J Med 1982; 306:821.

53. Najmabadi H, Huang V, Yen P, et al. Substantial prevalence of microdeletions of the Y-chromosome in infertile men with idiopathic azoospermia and oligozoospermia detected using a sequence-tagged site-based mapping strategy. J Clin Endocrinol Metab 1996; 81:1347.

54. Pryor JL, Kent-First M, Muallem A, et al. Microdeletions in the Y chromosome of infertile men. N Engl J Med 1997; 336:534.

55. Kim ED, Bischoff FZ, Lipshultz LI, Lamb DJ. Genetic concerns for the subfertile male in the era of ICSI. Prenat Diagn 1998; 18:1349.

56. Lipshultz LI, Caminos-Torres R, Greenspan C. Testicular function after unilateral orchiopexy. N Engl J Med 1976; 295:15.

57. Alpert PF, Klein RS. Spermatogenesis in the unilateral cryptorchid testis after orchiopexy. J Urol 1983; 129:301.

58. Gorelick JI, Goldstein M. Loss of fertility in men with varicocele. Fertil Steril 1993; 59:613.

59. Fariss BL, Fenner DK, Plymate SR, et al. Seminal characteristics in the presence of a varicocele as compared with those of expectant fathers and prevasectomy men. Fertil Steril 1981; 35:325.

60. Nagao RR, Plymate SR, Berger RE, et al. Comparison of gonadal function between fertile and infertile men with varicoceles. Fertil Steril 1986; 46:930.

61. Hudson RW. The endocrinology of varicoceles. Fertil Steril 1988; 49:199.

62. Rodriguez-Rigau LJ, Smith KD, Steinberger E. Varicocele and the morphology of spermatozoa. Fertil Steril 1981; 35:54.

63. Nieschlag E, Hertle L, Fischedick A, Behre HM. Treatment of varicocele: counselling as effective as occlusion of the vena spermatica. Hum Reprod 1995; 10:347.

64. Dubin L, Amelar RD. Varicocelectomy: 986 cases in a twelve-year study. Urology 1977; 10:446.

65. Madgar I, Weissenberg R, Lunenfield B, et al. Controlled trial of high spermatic vein ligation for varicocele in infertile men. Fertil Steril 1995; 63:120.

66. Proctor KG, Howards SS. The effect of sympathomimetic drugs on postlymphadenectomy aspermia. J Urol 1983; 129:837.

67. Urry RL, Middleton RG, McGavin S. A simple and effective technique for increasing pregnancy rates in couples with retrograde ejaculation. Fertil Steril 1986; 46:1124.

68. Scammell GE, Stedronska-Clark J, Edmonds DK, Hendry WF. Retrograde ejaculation: successful treatment with artificial insemination. Br J Obstet Gynaecol 1989; 63:198.

69. Handelsman DJ, Conway AJ, Boylan LM, Turtle JR. Young's syndrome: obstructive azoospermia and chronic sinopulmonary infections. N Engl J Med 1984; 310:3.

70. van der Ven K, Messer L, van der Ven H, et al. Cystic fibrosis mutation screening in healthy men with reduced sperm quality. Hum Reprod 1996; 11:513.

71. Marshburn PB, Kutteh WH. The role of antisperm antibodies in infertility. Fertil Steril 1994; 61:799.

71a. Dickman AB, Norton EJ, Westbrook VA, et al. Anti-sperm antibodies from infertile patients and their cognate sperm antigens: a review. Am J Reprod Immunol 2000; 43:134.

72. Clarke GN, Eliott PJ, Smaila C. Detection of sperm antibodies in semen using the immunobead test: a survey of 813 consecutive patients. Am J Reprod Immunol Microbiol 1985; 7:118.

73. Bals-Pratsch M, Doren M, Karbowski B, et al. Cyclic corticosteroid immunosuppression is unsuccessful in the treatment of sperm-antibody-related male infertility: a controlled study. Hum Reprod 1992; 7:99.

74. Clarke GN, Bourne H, Baker HW. Intracytoplasmic sperm injection for treating infertility associated with sperm autoimmunity. Fertil Steril 1997; 68:112.

74a. Diemer T, Ludwig M, Huwe P, et al. Influence of urogenital infection on sperm function. Curr Opin Urol 2000; 10:39.

75. Branigan EF, Muller CH. Efficacy of treatment and recurrence rate of leukocytospermia in infertile men with prostatitis. Fertil Steril 1994; 62:580.

76. Berger RE, Karp LE, Williamson RA, et al. The relationship of pyospermia and seminal fluid bacteriology to sperm function as reflected in the sperm penetration assay. Fertil Steril 1982; 37:557.

77. Toth A, Lesser ML, Brooks C, Labriola D. Subsequent pregnancies among 161 couples treated for T-mycoplasma genital tract infection. N Engl J Med 1983; 308:505.

78. Toth A. Reversible toxic effect of salicylazosulfapyridine on semen quality. Fertil Steril 1979; 31:538.

79. Van Thiel DH, Gavaler JS, Smith WJ. Hypothalamic-pituitary-gonadal dysfunction in men using cimetidine. N Engl J Med 1979; 300:1012.

80. Collins JA, Wrixon W, Janes LB, Wilson EH. Treatment-independent pregnancy among infertile couples. N Engl J Med 1983; 309:1201.

81. O'Donovan PA, Vandekerchove P, Lilford RJ, Hughes E. Treatment of male infertility: is it effective? Review and meta-analyses of published randomized controlled trials. Hum Reprod 1993; 8:1209.

82. Schill WB, Jungst D, Unterburger P, Braun S. Combined hMG/hCG treatment in subfertile men with idiopathic normagonadotropic oligospermia. Int J Androl 1982; 5:467.

83. Knuth UA, Hönigl W, Bals-Pratsch M, et al. Treatment of severe oligospermia with human chorionic gonadotropin/human menopausal gonadotropin: a placebo-controlled, double blind trial. J Clin Endocrinol Metab 1987; 65:1081.

84. Newton R, Schinfeld JS, Schiff I. Clomiphene treatment of infertile men: failure of response with idiopathic oligospermia. Fertil Steril 1980; 34:399.

85. Sokol RZ, Steiner B, Bastillo M, et al. Controlled comparison of the efficacy of clomiphene citrate in male infertility. Fertil Steril 1988; 49:865.

86. Vigersky RA, Glass AR. Effects of testolactone on the pituitary-testicular axis in oligospermic men. J Clin Endocrinol Metab 1981; 52:897.

87. Clark RV, Sherins RJ. Treatment of men with idiopathic oligospermic infertility using the aromatase inhibitor, testolactone: results of a double blinded, randomized placebo controlled trial with crossover. J Androl 1989; 10:240.

87a. Vandekerekhove P, Lilford R, Vail A, Hughes E. Clomiphene or tamoxifen for idiopathic oligolashenospermia. Cochrane Database Syst Rev 2000; 2:CD000151.

88. Schlegel PN, Girardi SK. In vitro fertilization for male factor infertility. J Clin Endocrinol Metab 1997; 82:709.

89. Palermo G, Joris H, Devroey P, Steirteghem AC. Pregnancies after intracytoplasmic injection of single spermatozoon into an oocyte. Lancet 1992; 340; 17.

90. Nagy Z, Liu J, Verheyen G, et al. The results of intracytoplasmic sperm injection are not related to any of the three basic sperm parameters. Hum Reprod 1995; 10:1123.

91. Givens CR. Intracytoplasmic sperm injection: what are the risks? Obstet Gynecol Surv 2000; 55;58.

92. Tarlatzis BC, Bili H. Intracytoplasmic sperm injection. Survey of world results. Ann N Y Acad Sci 2000; 900:336.

# CHAPTER 119

# CLINICAL USE AND ABUSE OF ANDROGENS AND ANTIANDROGENS

ALVIN M. MATSUMOTO

## ANDROGENS: PAST AND PRESENT

The popular belief that failure of testicular function was responsible for symptoms of old age in men stimulated early attempts to isolate an active testicular substance that would rejuvenate aging men. In 1889, Brown-Sequard reported that an extract he prepared from dog and guinea pig testes and administered to himself resulted in increased vigor, strength, intellectual capacity, and sexual potency.[1] Because of his stature in the scientific community, many people in the public and medical profession began using testicular extracts, but others castigated Brown-Sequard. Although his aqueous extract probably was devoid of steroid hormone and bioactivity, the controversy concerning his "elixir of life" stimulated further studies of internal secretions of glands, from which evolved the science of modern endocrinology.

Soon after the discovery of androgenic substances in the urine, urinary extracts were reported to increase the frequency of erections and improve well-being in hypogonadal men. Because of their limited availability and weak activity, however, urinary androgens were not widely used. In the mid-1930s, testosterone was isolated and identified as the major androgenic principle of the testes. Soon thereafter, the chemical structure of testosterone was elucidated, and the hormone was synthesized and came to be used clinically in the treatment of male hypogonadal states. Because of the short duration of action of testosterone, numerous analogs and derivatives of testosterone with greatly prolonged action were developed.

Today, the principal clinical use of androgens remains the treatment of androgen deficiency resulting from hypogonadism and delayed puberty.[2–4] Androgens are also used to stimulate erythropoiesis in hypoproliferative anemias related to renal or bone marrow failure; to treat micropenis and microphallus (see Chap. 93); to treat hereditary angioneurotic edema; as adjuvant hormonal therapy for female breast cancer (see Chap. 224); topically to treat vulvar lichen sclerosus; and to stimulate bone formation in the treatment of osteoporosis.[2–4]

Preliminary studies have suggested a number of potential uses of androgens for treatment of clinical syndromes associated with wasting syndromes (e.g., acquired immunodeficiency syndrome [AIDS] and cancer); chronic illnesses, such as renal failure and chronic obstructive pulmonary disease (COPD); long-term use of certain medications (e.g., glucocorticoid therapy); autoimmune rheumatologic diseases (e.g., rheumatoid arthritis); and aging. Evidence is also emerging that androgens may be useful in treating reduced libido and in increasing bone mass in postmenopausal women. Finally, interest is renewed in investigating the use of androgens to promote protein anabolism in catabolic states (e.g., after major trauma or surgery, burns, space travel, and spinal cord injury). Although the short- and long-term benefits and risks of androgen therapy in these conditions are not fully established, the potential for expanded clinical uses of androgens has stimulated interest in the development of new androgens and alternative androgen formulations, and has once again sparked both public and physician enthusiasm for the use of testosterone as an agent to prevent frailty in aging men.

Although androgens have been used to treat children with short stature, their value for this purpose is dubious, and such a use is inappropriate. Extremely high dosages of androgenic, anabolic steroids are increasingly consumed by athletes to improve performance and by adolescents to enhance appearance. Whether androgens improve athletic performance is uncertain, and the high dosages are often associated with severe side effects. Despite condemnation by the medical community and by athletic organizations, this form of androgen abuse remains widespread. The potential for androgen abuse has resulted in reclassification of androgen and androgenic anabolic steroid preparations as Schedule III controlled substances by the U.S. Food and Drug Administration (FDA). With the enactment of the Dietary Supplement Health and Education Act of 1994, however, preparations containing the androgens dehydroepiandrosterone (DHEA) and $\Delta^4$-androstenedione (androstenedione), both of which may be converted to testosterone in the body, became available over the counter as "dietary supplements" free of FDA regulation. Despite the lack of evidence for their benefits or risks, DHEA and androstenedione are being abused by athletes to enhance strength and performance, and by men and women in the hope of "preventing the aging process."

*Antiandrogens* are compounds that bind to the androgen receptor and competitively inhibit androgen binding, thereby antagonizing androgen action at target organs. Clinically, they are useful in the treatment of androgen-dependent malignancies (e.g., prostate and male breast cancer) and conditions such as hirsutism and acne (see Chaps. 101 and 225).

## PHARMACOLOGY OF ANDROGEN PREPARATIONS

Because of the short duration of testosterone action, pharmacologic strategies have been developed to achieve more sustained blood levels of testosterone and thereby prolong its androgenic action. The development of novel methods of testosterone administration and chemically modified analogs of the native testosterone molecule are the two major pharmacologic strategies used to prolong androgen action.[2] In general, the chemical modifications of testosterone involve esterification of the 17β-hydroxyl group or alkylation of the 17α-position of the D ring, with or without other modifications of the ring structure of native testosterone (Table 119-1). Mesterolone and dihydrotestosterone (DHT) are androgen preparations that have A-ring modifications without any alterations at the 17-position of the D ring (see Table 119-1).

## TESTOSTERONE

Orally administered testosterone is rapidly absorbed from the gastrointestinal tract into the portal blood and accumulated in the liver. Because it is efficiently degraded by the liver, very little testosterone reaches the systemic circulation, and sustained blood levels are very difficult to maintain. No oral forms of unmodified testosterone are available in the United States. A microparticulate form of testosterone has been administered to a small number of hypogonadal men in Europe and has been shown to achieve therapeutic blood levels of testosterone in some patients.[5] Absorption of this preparation is erratic, however, and very large dosages (200–400 mg per day) taken several times a day are required to maintain adequate serum testosterone levels. Furthermore, the long-term toxicity to the liver of this large burden of testosterone is unknown. Intramuscular injections of aqueous native testosterone are also rapidly absorbed from the injection site and promptly degraded by the liver. Therefore, unmodified testosterone administered either orally or parenterally is impractical for achieving sustained physiologic testosterone levels in blood and androgenic effects on target organs.

### TRANSDERMAL TESTOSTERONE DELIVERY

Currently, three transdermal testosterone patches are approved for use in androgen replacement therapy for hypogonadal men (see Table 119-1): a scrotal matrix patch (*Testoderm*), the first to be marketed; a nonscrotal, permeation-enhanced, reservoir patch (*Androderm* or Andropatch [United Kingdom]); and a nonscrotal reservoir patch that does not contain permeation enhancers (*Testoderm TTS*).[6] Because a normal adult man produces ~7 mg per day of testosterone (i.e., up to 100-fold the daily production of estradiol), testosterone patches are larger and require more frequent (daily) application than do estrogen patches.

The scrotal Testoderm patch consists of an ethylene-vinyl acetate copolymer containing testosterone within this matrix.[7,8] When applied to scrotal skin, the 40 cm$^2$ or 60 cm$^2$ patches deliver 4 or 6 mg of testosterone over 24 hours, respectively. The unusual superficial vascularity of scrotal skin permits 5- to 40-fold greater testosterone absorption from this site than from other skin sites. Because of initial problems with adhesion of these patches to scrotal skin, thin, lightly adhesive strips were incorporated onto the patch. Daily application in the morning on the scrotum of hypogonadal men produces physiologic levels of testosterone that mimic the normal circadian rhythm of testosterone in young men, with peak testosterone levels reached within 2 to 4 hours. Because these patches do not contain permeation enhancers, they are generally well tolerated, with only occasional itching (~7%) and moderate skin irritation (~5%). The use of this patch, however, does require an adequate-size scrotum that is clean, dry, and shaven for optimal adhesion and effectiveness; this limits its acceptability and clinical utility. Also, supraphysiologic concentrations of DHT are produced, as a result of the high 5α-reductase activity in scrotal skin. The physiologic significance of high circulating DHT levels on androgen-responsive target organs (e.g., prostate) is not

known, but careful monitoring for adverse androgenic effects is recommended.

The nonscrotal Androderm transdermal system consists of an adhesive patch with a central reservoir containing testosterone and permeation enhancers in an alcohol-based gel that are delivered to skin through a microporous polyethylene membrane.[9–11] Permeation enhancers facilitate testosterone absorption through nonscrotal sites (e.g., back, abdomen, thighs, or upper arm). In hypogonadal men, nightly application of a single 5 mg (44 cm$^2$) or two 2.5 mg (37 cm$^2$) patches on nonscrotal skin also maintains serum testosterone concentrations in the normal physiologic range with a circadian rhythm similar to that of young men. The Androderm patch causes more local skin irritation (~30% of users) than do scrotal Testoderm patches (~5%).[12] Unlike scrotal patches, they may cause allergic contact dermatitis (~12%) and, uncommonly, a burn-like blister reaction, which is usually associated with placement of the patch over bony prominences. The severity and incidence of skin irritation is reduced by coapplication of triamcinolone acetonide (0.1%) cream under the drug reservoir. However, skin irritation limits the acceptability and use of this nonscrotal patch. Unlike with the scrotal testosterone patch, serum DHT levels remain within the physiologic range during Androderm use.

Another nonscrotal transdermal testosterone delivery system, the Testoderm TTS patch, is available for androgen replacement therapy.[13–15] It is composed of a relatively large (72 cm$^2$) lightly adhesive patch with a reservoir (60 cm$^2$ contact area) containing testosterone in an alcohol-based gel that does not contain permeation enhancers. Nightly application of the Testoderm TTS patch on nonscrotal skin (arms, upper buttocks, or torso) in hypogonadal men results in physiologic serum testosterone and DHT levels with pharmacokinetics similar to that of the Androderm patch. Early clinical experience in hypogonadal men suggests that this patch is associated with less skin irritation but is also less adherent to skin than the permeation-enhanced Androderm patch.

Currently available testosterone patches are also being tested for treatment of other patient populations (e.g., adolescent boys with hypogonadism and men and women with muscle wasting associated with AIDS).[16–18] Because of problems with skin adherence and irritation associated with available transdermal testosterone patches, other matrix and reservoir patches are being developed and tested for androgen therapy (e.g., in hypogonadal men and postmenopausal women).[19,20]

A transdermal 1% hydroalcoholic gel preparation of tesosterone (AndroGel) has been approved and become available for androgen replacement therapy in hypogonadal men. In initial studies in hypogonadal men, the application of 50 to 100 mg per day of AndroGel divided over four different sites increased serum testosterone levels and maintained them in the physiologic range for 180 days.[21] Unlike testosterone creams or ointments, the testosterone gel dried rapidly, left no residue and, more importantly, did not cause skin irritation. A caution with testosterone gel is the transfer of androgens and induction of androgenic effects in female and childhood contacts. AndroGel also produces a disproportionate increase in serum DHT levels. Long-term studies have demonstrated continued efficacy (improved sexual function, mood, body composition, and bone mineral density) and safety without significant skin irritation.[21a,21b] AndroGel offers an easy, acceptable, rapidly reversible, and titratable method for delivering androgen therapy for a variety of disorders in men, and perhaps in women and children.

### TESTOSTERONE IMPLANTS

Subcutaneous surgical implantation of fused *pellets* or *capsules* of unmodified testosterone has been used to achieve a prolonged, sustained release of physiologic levels of testosterone for 4 to 6 months for androgen replacement therapy of hypogonadal men.[22–25] This form of testosterone administration is used rarely

**TABLE 119-1.**
**Common Androgen Preparations**

### TESTOSTERONE

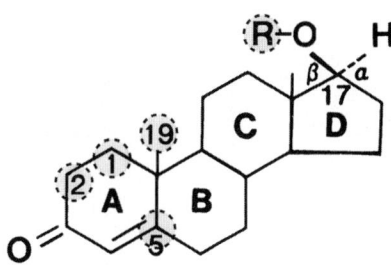

*I. Modalities currently available:*

| Treatment Modality | Trade Name | Route |
|---|---|---|
| Transdermal testosterone | Testoderm (Alza) | Scrotal patch |
|  | Androderm (Watson) | Nonscrotal patch |
|  | Testoderm TTS (Alza) | Nonscrotal patch |
|  | AndroGel (Unimed) | Hydroalcoholic gel |
| Testosterone pellets | Testosterone pellets (Organon)* | SC implant |
|  | Testopel pellets (Bartor) |  |
| *II. Modalities being developed (not currently available):* |  |  |
| Testosterone microspheres[†] (testosterone microencapsulated in biodegradable matrix [85:15, DL-lactide: glycolide copolymer]) | — (BioTek) | IM |
| Testosterone-cyclodextrin complex[†] (testosterone complexed with hydroxypropyl-β-cyclodextrin) | — (Bio-Technology) | SL |
| Transbuccal testosterone[†] | —(Watson; Columbia) | Buccal |

### TESTOSTERONE DERIVATIVES

*I. 17β-hydroxyl esterification (with or without other ring modifications)*

| Generic Name | Trade Name | Route | Modification |
|---|---|---|---|
| Testosterone propionate | (Generic) | IM | $R = COCH_2CH_3$ |
| Testosterone cypionate (cyclopentylpropionate) | Depo-Testosterone (Pharmacia Upjohn)[‡] (Generic) | IM | $R = COCH_2CH_2$ ⬠ |
| Testosterone enanthate (heptanoate) | Delatestryl (Bio-Technology) (Generic) | IM | $R = CO(CH_2)_5CH_3$ |
| Testosterone undecanoate*[¶] | Restandol, Andriol (Organon) | PO | $R = CO(CH_2)_5CH=CH_2$ |
| Nandrolone phenpropionate | Durabolin (Organon) Hybolin Improved (Hyrex) (Generic) | IM | $R = COCH_2CH_2$ ⬡ Position 19: removal of —$CH_3$ |
| Nandrolone decanoate | Deca-Durabolin (Organon) (Generic) Hybolin Decanoate (Hyrex) | IM | $R = CO(CH_2)_4CH_3$ Position 19: removal of—$CH_3$ |
| Testosterone buciclate*[†] (butylcyclohexylcarboxylate, 20 Aet-1) |  | IM | $R$ —CO—⬡—$(CH_2)_3CH_3$ |

(continued)

**TABLE 119-1. (continued)**

**TESTOSTERONE DERIVATIVES**

*II. 17α-alkylation (with or without other ring modifications)#*

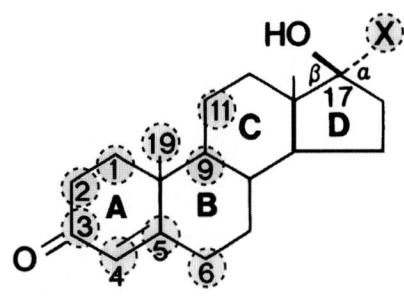

| Generic Name | Trade Name | Route | Modification |
|---|---|---|---|
| **Methyltestosterone** | Android (ICN) | PO | $X = CH_3$ |
| | Testred (ICN) | | |
| | Oreton Methyl (Schering) | | |
| | Virilon (Star) | | |
| | Oreton Methyl Buccal | Buccal | |
| **Fluoxymesterone** | Halotestin (Pharmacia Upjohn) | PO | $X = CH_3$ |
| | (Generic) | | Position 9: — —F |
| | | | Position 11: —OH |
| **Oxandrolone** | Oxandrin (Bio-Technology) | PO | $X = CH_3$ |
| | | | Position 2: occupied by oxygen |
| | | | Position 5: — —H |
| **Oxymetholone** | Anadrol-50 (Unimed) | PO | $X = CH_3$ |
| | | | Position 2: =CHOH |
| | | | Position 5: — —H |
| **Stanozolol** | Winstrol (Sanofi) | PO | $X = CH_3$ |
| | | | Position 5: — —H |
| | | | Position 2, 3: |
| **Danazol** | Danocrine (Sanofi) | PO | $X = CH=CH$ |
| | Danazol (Barr) | | |
| | | | Position 2, 3: |

**TESTOSTERONE DERIVATIVES**

*III. Ring Modification Without Position 17 Modifications*

| | | | |
|---|---|---|---|
| **Mesterolone\*** | Mestoranum (Schering) | PO | Position 1: — —CH$_3$ |
| | Pro-viron | | Position 5: — —H |
| **Dihydrotestosterone††** | Andractim (Besins-Iscovesco) | Percutaneous | Position 5: — —H |
| | Gelovit | | |

*SC*, subcutaneous; *SL*, sublingual; *IM*, intramuscular; — —, alpha substitution; —, beta substitution; ● (shaded circles), position of modifications.
\*Not available in the United States.
†Being developed; not currently available.
‡Other trade names for testosterone cypionate include: Dep Andro (Forest); Duratest (Hauck); Depotest (Hyrex); Testred Cypionate (ICN); Andro Cyp (Keene); T-Cypionate (Legere); Andronate (Pasadena); Virilon IM (Star).
§Other trade names for testosterone enanthate include: Testro LA (CO Truxton); Andro LA (Forest); Durathate (Hauck); Everone (Hyrex); Testrin (Pasadena); Andropository (Rugby).
¶Also being developed in oil for IM injections.
#Because of limited clinical usefulness, potential hepatotoxicity, and possibility for abuse, many oral 17α-alkylated androgens have been withdrawn from the market in the United States and in some countries in Europe. Some preparations such as methandrostenolone (Dianabol, Nerobol, Danabol, Metanabol), norethandrolone (Nilevar), methenolone (Primobolan), bolasterone (Tes-10), formebolone (Esiclene, Hubernol), and oxymesterone (Oranabol), ethylestrenol (Maxibolin), and methandriol (Stenediol) remain available in some foreign countries. These preparations are not listed in the table.
††Also being developed as a 0.7% hydroalcoholic gel formulation in the United States.

in the United States and is not acceptable to many hypogonadal men because of the large number and/or size of the implants, the need for a minor surgical procedure using a large trocar, extrusion of the pellets (8–9% of cases), and, although it is small, the risk of bleeding (2–3%) and infection (<1%). With the development of injectable, biodegradable matrices for drug administration, the potential exists for developing more practical and acceptable injectable preparations that would slowly release unmodified testosterone and sustain physiologic levels for prolonged periods.

## TESTOSTERONE FORMULATIONS UNDER DEVELOPMENT

Testosterone has been complexed with hydroxypropyl-β-cyclodextrin (see Table 119-1) to enhance its solubility and absorption. Sublingual administration of this formulation to hypogonadal men results in a prompt rise in serum testosterone concentrations that peak in ~20 min at supraphysiologic levels and then fall to baseline levels in 4 to 6 hours.[26,27] In short-term studies, sublingual *testosterone cyclodextrin*, 2.5 or 5.0

mg administered three times daily, improved sexual function and mood; increased lean body mass and leg strength; and decreased bone-resorption and increased bone-formation markers.[27,28] In a preliminary study, short-term administration of a *buccal testosterone* formulation in hypogonadal men resulted in a pharmacokinetic profile similar to that of sublingual testosterone cyclodextrin and improved sexual function.[29]

Despite the seemingly unfavorable pharmacokinetics, the clinical effects induced by sublingual and buccal testosterone administration support the concept that circulating testosterone concentrations may not reflect its biological actions on target tissues. This is similar to the case with oral hydrocortisone, which also has a short plasma half-life but a sufficiently sustained biological action to permit twice-daily administration for replacement therapy of patients with adrenal insufficiency. Both sublingual and buccal testosterone formulations have a bitter taste, which may limit their acceptability as preparations for long-term androgen replacement therapy. Because of the relative ease of administration, lower average daily testosterone concentrations, and rapid reversibility of their effects, these short-acting formulations may be most suitable for boys with delayed puberty, postmenopausal women with reduced libido, and elderly men with hypoandrogenism.

Customized topical formulations of testosterone in creams, ointments, or gels prepared by local pharmacies have been used by some clinicians to administer testosterone to patients with a variety of conditions, including men with hypogonadism, women with vulvar lichen sclerosus, postmenopausal women with reduced libido, and children with delayed puberty, micropenis, or microphallus. Anecdotally, these formulations seem to be effective, but no formal studies have been performed of the absorption, bioavailability, pharmacokinetics, pharmacodynamics, or clinical utility of these custom-formulated topical preparations. A *testosterone cream* or *ointment* has been used for the treatment of micropenis and microphallus in children and vulvar lichen sclerosus in women.[30-33] Although they are applied directly on the skin, testosterone from these topical formulations is absorbed into the circulation and probably acts systemically as well as locally.

The intramuscular injection of testosterone, microencapsulated in a biodegradable 85:15 molar lactide/glycolide copolymer (*testosterone microcapsules*) in hypogonadal men results in a rapid rise and maintenance of serum testosterone levels in the eugonadal range for 10 to 11 weeks.[34] Despite its long duration of action and zero-order kinetics, the pain and discomfort from the two large-volume (2.5-mL) deep intramuscular injections required to administer the microcapsules, as well as batch-to-batch variability, limit the appeal of this testosterone formulation for long-term androgen replacement.

## 17β-HYDROXYL ESTERIFICATION

Esterification at the 17β-hydroxyl group of testosterone (with or without other ring modifications) prolongs the duration of action compared with unmodified testosterone. By decreasing the polarity of the molecule, 17β-hydroxyl esterification increases its solubility in hydrophobic injection vehicles (sesame or cottonseed oil) and slows its release into the circulation. The 17β-hydroxyl esters of testosterone lack androgenic activity; they all require hydrolysis to native testosterone to permit bioaction. Thus, measurements of serum testosterone levels may be used to monitor the adequacy of therapy.

The three testosterone preparations most commonly used in clinical applications, and the only 17β-hydroxyl esters of testosterone available in the United States, are *testosterone propionate*, a relatively short-acting parenteral preparation, and *testosterone enanthate* and *testosterone cypionate*, both longer-acting parenteral preparations (see Table 119-1). Testosterone propionate is usually administered by intramuscular injection every other day. After injection, testosterone enanthate and testosterone cypi-

onate produce similar testosterone levels and durations of action, and are clinically equivalent. Typically, both of these esters are administered every 2 to 3 weeks in hypogonadal men to maintain testosterone levels within the normal range.[35]

Testosterone enanthate and testosterone cypionate are the mainstays of androgen replacement therapy because they are effective, safe, and inexpensive. However, the intramuscular injection of either preparation usually produces supraphysiologic testosterone levels for 1 to 2 days after administration that gradually fall to low-normal or subnormal levels before the next injection. These large variations in serum testosterone levels may produce noticeable fluctuations in energy level, mood, and sexual function. For these reasons, new short-acting androgen preparations that maintain physiologic testosterone concentrations and longer-acting forms with zero-order release kinetics and extended durations of action are being developed.

Preparations containing a combination of short- and long-acting 17β-hydroxyl testosterone esters are available in Europe (e.g., Testoviron Depot 50 and 100, which contain a combination of testosterone propionate and enanthate; and Sustanon 100 and 250, which contain combinations of testosterone propionate, phenylpropionate, isocaproate, and decanoate). These formulations produce much higher peak testosterone levels and larger fluctuations of levels without prolonging the duration of action, and are not recommended over testosterone enanthate or testosterone cypionate alone for androgen replacement therapy.

*Testosterone undecanoate* is an oral 17β-hydroxyl testosterone ester that has been used in dosages of 80 to 240 mg per day for androgen replacement therapy and 40 mg per day for delayed puberty in Europe, Canada, and Australia.[36-38] The long aliphatic side chain of the ester makes it very hydrophobic. The nonpolar nature of this ester, together with its oleic acid vehicle, favor its absorption from the gastrointestinal tract directly into the lymphatics on chylomicrons, and then into the systemic circulation, so that initial inactivation by the liver is bypassed. Although testosterone undecanoate is effective in the treatment of male hypogonadism and is not hepatotoxic, the large dosages administered several times daily, the highly variable blood levels of testosterone achieved, the need for refrigerated storage and the uncommon but often unacceptable gastrointestinal side effects (e.g., flatus, oily stools, diarrhea, and anorexia) limit its practical use in long-term androgen therapy. Testosterone undecanoate also gives rise to a disproportionate increase in serum DHT relative to testosterone levels, as a result of intestinal 5α-reductase activity.

Initial pharmacokinetic studies in hypogonadal men have demonstrated that intramuscular injection of testosterone undecanoate, 500 to 1000 mg in tea seed oil or castor oil, yields testosterone concentrations that are initially at or above the upper limits of normal and that are maintained within the normal range for 6 to 8 weeks.[39,40] As the preparation is formulated currently, the volume of intramuscular injection (4–8 mL) and the need for more than one injection site are factors that may limit the acceptability of this preparation for androgen replacement therapy or other applications, such as male contraception.

*Testosterone buciclate* (20 Aet-1; see Table 119-1) is another 17β-hydroxyl ester with a prolonged duration of action. It was developed by the World Health Organization. In preliminary studies, a single 600-mg intramuscular injection of testosterone buciclate in hypogonadal men maintains serum testosterone levels in the low normal range for ~12 weeks.[41] Whether the relatively low testosterone levels achieved with this preparation are adequate for androgen replacement therapy of hypogonadal men is unclear. The large volume of the injections (2.4 mL/600 mg) is also a limiting factor with this formulation.

*Nandrolone phenylpropionate* and *nandrolone decanoate* are 17β-hydroxyl esters of 19-nortestosterone (see Table 119-1). The 17β-hydroxyl esterification of 19-nortestosterone and the injection in an oil vehicle prolong the duration of action of these steroids.[42] Nandrolone decanoate (1 mL) injected into the gluteal muscle results in the greatest bioavailability and physiologic effect. Because of their reduced androgenic potency, these long-acting, parenteral, 19-nortestosterone esters are not used in the treatment of androgen deficiency, but rather as anabolic agents (e.g., in the treatment of osteoporosis, anemia of renal failure, and wasting states, such as AIDS).

## 17α-ALKYLATION

The alkylation of testosterone at the 17α-position (with or without other ring modifications) reduces hepatic inactivation, allowing sufficient levels of drug to reach the systemic circulation and permitting oral administration. *Methyltestosterone* is a 17α-alkylated derivative of testosterone that has been used for androgen replacement therapy (see Table 119-1). It can be administered orally or buccally. Most orally active androgen preparations have incorporated other modifications of the ring structure of testosterone (e.g., 5α-reduction; oxidation at positions 1 or 2; removal of the methyl group at position 19; substitutions at positions 2, 3, 4, 6, 9, or 11; and substitution of the A ring) to modify their androgenic potency and metabolic clearance (see Table 119-1). *Fluoxymesterone* is another orally active androgen preparation that has been used for the treatment of androgen deficiency. Because ring modifications in the other 17α-alkylated derivatives reduce their androgenic potency, these preparations are used as anabolic, rather than androgenic, agents or for the treatment of specific clinical conditions (e.g., *oxandrolone* for promoting weight gain, *stanozolol* for osteoporosis and *danazol* for hereditary angioneurotic edema, endometriosis, and fibrocystic breast disease).

In contrast to 17β-hydroxyl esters of testosterone, 17α-alkylated androgens are not dealkylated or 5α-reduced before their action at target organs or excretion. Because these preparations exhibit little cross-reactivity in testosterone radioimmunoassays, measurements of serum testosterone levels cannot be used to monitor therapy.

Oral androgens cannot be recommended for androgen replacement therapy in hypogonadal men.[2-4] All orally active androgen preparations available in the United States are 17α-alkylated derivatives of testosterone (e.g., *methyltestosterone* and *fluoxymesterone*) that have the potential for serious hepatotoxicity (cholestasis, peliosis hepatis, benign and malignant liver tumors). On the other hand, liver toxicity is not found with replacement dosages of parenteral 17β-hydroxyl esters of testosterone. Also, because oral preparations are usually less potent than parenteral preparations, achieving full androgenic effects using oral androgens is often difficult.[2-4] Finally, the cost of oral androgen replacement therapy is much greater than the cost of parenteral preparations. Because oral androgens entail greater risk for less therapeutic benefit and at a greater cost than parenteral preparations, *long-acting 17β-hydroxyl esters of testosterone (testosterone enanthate* and *testosterone cypionate) are the preparations of choice for androgen replacement therapy for hypogonadal men. Although it is more expensive than testosterone esters and requires daily application, AndroGel is a useful alternative to parenteral testosterone esters for androgen replacement therapy in hypogonadal men who prefer or do not tolerate injections.* Because they are more expensive, are less convenient, acceptable, and/or effective for some men, and may cause significant skin irritation, currently available transdermal testosterone patches should be considered a second choice to testosterone esters or testosterone gel for androgen replacement therapy in selected hypogonadal men.

## RING MODIFICATIONS WITHOUT MODIFICATIONS OF POSITION 17

*Mesterolone* is an orally effective androgen that contains only modifications of the A ring, without 17β-hydroxyl esterification or 17α-alkylation (see Table 119-1). It is a 1α-methyl derivative

of 5α-DHT, the active intracellular metabolite of testosterone in certain tissues (such as prostate, seminal vesicles, epididymides, and skin) (see Chap. 114). In some target organs (e.g., brain and the central nervous system [CNS]), a part of testosterone action may require intracellular aromatization of testosterone to estradiol. Like 17α-alkylated androgens (see earlier), DHT and mesterolone cannot be aromatized to estrogens. Because aromatization may be important in androgen action in some tissues (e.g., bone and brain), the clinical effects of these steroids in some tissues may be attenuated or absent. Mesterolone has been used in Europe to treat androgen deficiency in hypogonadal men, but it is a relatively weak androgen.[43]

In Belgium and France, *DHT* is available in a 2% hydroalcoholic gel formulation for androgen replacement therapy for hypogonadal men.[44] After the daily application of DHT gel on a large area of skin, DHT is rapidly absorbed and forms a depot in the dermis from which it is released into the circulation in sufficient quantities to maintain sexual function in hypogonadal men. DHT gel treatment is most useful in treating patients with 5α-reductase deficiency and microphallus.[45,46] Concerns with this formulation include transfer of DHT to contacts and induction of androgenic effects in female partners, as reported with earlier topical DHT formulations (e.g., creams); lack of aromatization to estrogens; suppression of endogenous estradiol concentrations; consequences of relative estrogen deficiency by DHT induction (e.g., on bone, lipids, and brain function); and effects of long-term elevations in circulating DHT levels (e.g., on the prostate). Interestingly, prostate volume is reported to decrease, and prostate-specific antigen (PSA) is unchanged, with long-term DHT gel treatment in older men; perhaps this is related to suppression of endogenous testosterone and estradiol with exogenous DHT administration.[47] A 0.7% hydroalcoholic DHT gel formulation is being developed for androgen therapy in older men.[48,49] In initial short-term studies in healthy elderly men, the daily application of DHT gel increases serum DHT and suppresses serum testosterone and estradiol levels in a dose-dependent fashion that is maintained over 14 days.

## SELECTIVE ANDROGENS AND NONSTEROIDAL ANDROGENS

"Designer" androgens that are aromatized to estrogens but are not 5α-reduced or selective androgen-receptor modulators (SARMs) analogous to selective estrogen-receptor modulators (SERMs), such as raloxifene, probably will be developed in the future. The therapeutic goal in developing these agents is to maintain the beneficial actions of androgens (e.g., on muscle, bone, brain, and sexual function) but to reduce or prevent adverse effects (e.g., on the prostate, lipids, and cardiovascular risk).

An androgen synthesized over 20 years ago, *7α-methyl-19-nortestosterone (MENT)*, is a modified androgen that can be aromatized to estrogen but is not 5α-reduced. In orchidectomized monkeys, MENT is ten times more potent than testosterone in stimulating body weight gain and suppressing gonadotropins, but only twice as potent in stimulating prostate growth.[50] The relative sparing of the prostate with MENT compared with testosterone suggests that MENT may be useful in androgen therapy and male contraceptive development. MENT is being formulated as a long-acting subcutaneous implant. Clinical trials in hypogonadal men are ongoing. In hypogonadal men, use of two MENT acetate implants maintained stable plasma MENT concentrations, sexual function, and mood for 6 weeks.[51]

Initial studies to identify novel human androgen receptor modulators have identified a series of derivatives of 2(1H)-pyrrolidino[3,2-g]quinolone that are potent nonsteroidal human androgen receptor agonists and antagonists.[52] These drug discovery strategies and programs may eventually yield clinically useful *nonsteroidal* androgens with tissue-selective actions (SARMs) for androgen therapy for a variety of conditions (see later).

# ANDROGEN TREATMENT OF MALE HYPOGONADISM AND DELAYED PUBERTY

The principal use of androgens is as replacement therapy for androgen-deficient hypogonadal men.[2,4] The therapeutic goal of androgen replacement therapy is to restore the normal physiologic effects of testosterone, which depend on the individual's stage of development.[53] In prepubertal androgen deficiency, which delays the onset of pubertal development, the aim of androgen therapy is to induce and maintain normal male secondary sexual characteristics, somatic development, and sexual behavior. Androgens stimulate the normal male pattern of hair growth (face, chest, abdominal, perianal area, and inner thighs); growth of the penis and scrotum; development of accessory sexual organs (prostate and seminal vesicles) with an increase in ejaculatory volume; enlargement of the larynx with consequent deepening of the voice; development of skeletal musculature and an increase in strength, especially in the shoulder and pectoral muscles; decrease and redistribution of body fat; growth of the long bones and eventual closure of epiphyses; erythropoiesis; and libido and potency. An important goal of androgen therapy in prepubertal children is to induce the pubertal growth spurt without compromising adult height by premature closure of the epiphyses. In adult male hypogonadism, the goal of androgen treatment is to restore and maintain secondary male sexual characteristics and sexual behavior.

Androgen treatment cannot correct ambiguous external genitalia resulting from androgen deficiency during fetal development, although testosterone has been used as adjunctive treatment to surgery in selected cases of microphallus and hypospadias.[54,55] Also, exogenous testosterone cannot be administered practically in sufficiently high dosages to achieve the high intratesticular levels required to stimulate and maintain spermatogenesis. Despite its inability to restore sperm production in hypogonadal men, androgen treatment does increase the volume of ejaculate by stimulating the development of accessory sexual organs (prostate and seminal vesicles).

# TREATMENT OF ADULT MALE HYPOGONADISM

## TESTOSTERONE FORMULATIONS

The long-acting 17β-hydroxyl esters of testosterone, testosterone enanthate and testosterone cypionate, are the most practical, effective, and safe, and least expensive preparations available for androgen replacement therapy for hypogonadal men. The intramuscular administration of 200 mg of testosterone enanthate induces peak serum testosterone levels at or just above the upper limits of the normal adult male range within 1 to 2 days of administration (Fig. 119-1).[35] Testosterone levels usually remain within the normal range for 2 weeks. By increasing the dose of testosterone enanthate to 300 mg, eugonadal levels of testosterone in blood are maintained for 3 weeks (see Fig. 119-1). However, the administration of 400 mg of testosterone enanthate does not maintain normal serum testosterone levels for >3 weeks (see Fig. 119-1). No formal evaluations of the optimal dosage of testosterone cypionate have been reported. Because the kinetics of serum testosterone levels after a single intramuscular injection of testosterone cypionate are similar to those after a single injection of testosterone enanthate, however, the two preparations are thought to be therapeutically equivalent in terms of duration of action and potency.

In adults, androgen replacement therapy is usually instituted with testosterone enanthate or testosterone cypionate at a dosage of 200 mg, intramuscularly, every 2 weeks. Patients can usually be taught to self-administer intramuscular injections, or a family

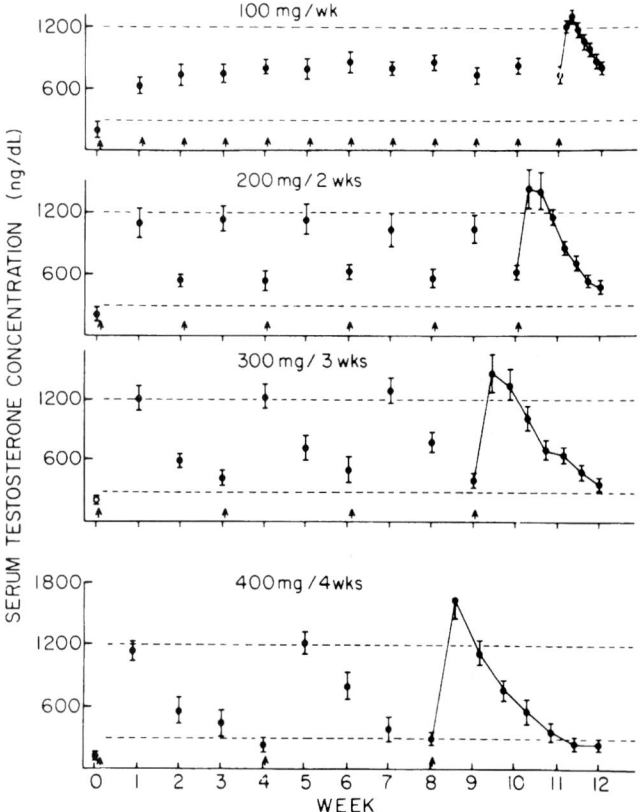

**FIGURE 119-1.** Serum testosterone concentrations (mean ± SEM) during testosterone replacement therapy in adult men with primary hypogonadism. Testosterone enanthate was administered by intramuscular injection (*arrows*) for 12 weeks in four dosage regimens: 100 mg weekly; 200 mg every 2 weeks; 300 mg every 3 weeks; and 400 mg every 4 weeks. Blood was sampled weekly until the last dose and more frequently thereafter. The dashed lines define the normal range of testosterone concentrations. Note that the regimen of 400 mg every 4 weeks does not maintain testosterone concentrations within the normal range for the entire period between injections as do the other regimens. (From Snyder PJ, Lawrence DA. Treatment of male hypogonadism with testosterone enanthate. J Clin Endocrinol Metab 1980; 51:1335.)

member or friend may be trained to give them. The assessment of therapeutic efficacy is accomplished by careful monitoring of the clinical response. Ideally, serum testosterone concentrations should be in the midnormal range 1 week after a testosterone ester injection and above the lower limit of the normal range immediately before the next injection. In some hypogonadal men, the large fluctuations in serum testosterone concentrations between intramuscular injections of testosterone enanthate or testosterone cypionate given every 2 to 3 weeks produce disturbing fluctuations in sexual function, energy, and mood.[56] Patients may complain of reduced libido, erectile dysfunction, and diminished energy a few days before their next testosterone injection. The documentation of low serum testosterone levels at that time may be useful to justify an adjustment of the dosage interval (e.g., from every 2 weeks to every 10 days).

In elderly hypogonadal patients with symptoms of bladder outlet obstruction or enlarged prostate glands, the prudent approach is to begin testosterone therapy gradually and at a reduced dosage (e.g., testosterone enanthate or cypionate 50–100 mg intramuscularly every 2–4 weeks). Alternatively, a short-acting testosterone ester may be used, such as testosterone propionate, 25 to 50 mg given intramuscularly three times weekly. The shorter duration of action permits rapid withdrawal if androgen-induced prostatic growth, urinary obstruction, or a prostatic nodule develops, but the need for frequent injections limit the practicality and acceptability of this approach.

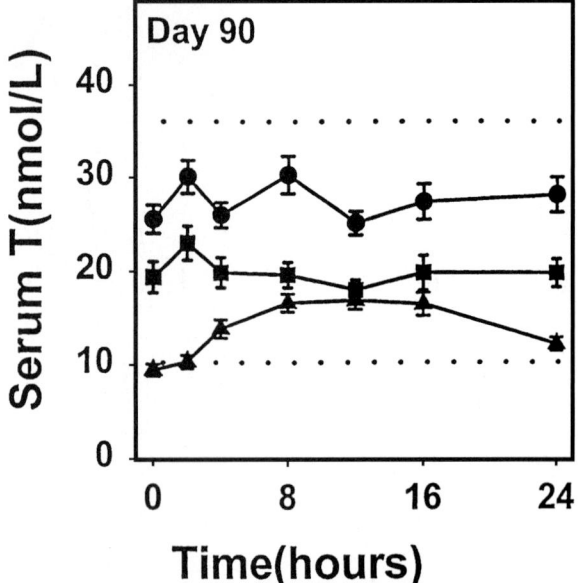

**FIGURE 119-2.** Serum total testosterone concentrations (mean ± SEM) over 24 hours after 90 days of daily application of testosterone in a 1% hydroalcoholic gel (AndroGel) 50 mg daily (n=67, n) or 100 mg daily (n=75, l), or a permeation-enhanced testosterone patch (Androderm) 5 mg daily (n=65, s) in 207 hypogonadal men. Time 0 hours is 8:00 a.m. Serum testosterone levels were relatively constant in the mid-normal range (19.2 ± 1.1 nmol/L) and mid- to upper-normal range (27.5 ± 1.1 nmol/L) in hypogonadal men treated with AndroGel 50 mg and 100 mg daily, respectively, and in the lower normal range (14.5 ± 0.7 nmol/L) in those treated with the Androderm patch daily. In the latter, serum testosterone levels exhibited a circadian variation from the low- to mid-normal range.

Transdermal testosterone gel or patches (see earlier) provide alternatives to testosterone ester injections for androgen replacement in adult hypogonadal men who refuse or cannot tolerate intramuscular injections every 2 to 3 weeks; cannot administer injections to themselves or logistically arrange for injections to be given; have a bleeding diathesis; or have a personal preference.

A transdermal testosterone gel formulation (AndroGel) is a useful alternative to testosterone ester injections for androgen replacement therapy in hypogonadal men. Daily application of 50, 75, or 100 mg of testosterone in a 1% hydroalcoholic gel for 180 days in men with androgen deficiency produced relatively constant serum testosterone levels in the middle to upper physiologic range throughout the entire day (Fig. 119-2). By comparison, nightly application of a permeation-enhanced nonscrotal patch (Androderm) produced testosterone levels that exhibited a normal circadian variation in the lower normal range. AndroGel treatment increased energy and a sense of well being; improved libido and sexual function; increased lean body mass, muscle mass and strength, bone turnover markers, bone mineral density, and hematocrit; and decreased fat mass in a dose-dependent fashion, generally to a greater extent than did the testosterone patch. Compared to Androderm, AndroGel caused relatively little skin irritation and was associated with better compliance. However, AndroGel caused a disproportionate elevation in serum DHT levels, probably because of the large surface area of skin (containing 5 α-reductase) on which it is applied.

Compared with testosterone esters, the patches provide comparable symptomatic relief of androgen deficiency; increase energy, libido, and sexual function; and improve bone mineral density.[6,14] In contrast to injections of testosterone enanthate or testosterone cypionate, daily application of a testosterone patch in hypogonadal men produces physiologic serum testosterone concentrations that mimic the normal circadian variation of levels found in young men (Fig. 119-2).[6,14] As a result, hypogonadal men using patches do not

experience the fluctuation in symptoms that some men on testosterone injections encounter and have fewer androgenic side effects (e.g., erythrocytosis).[6,10,11] Compared with testosterone ester injections, however, the currently available testosterone patches require more attention (daily application on clean, dry skin) and care (a shaven scrotum is preferable for the Testoderm patch); may be associated with relatively poor adherence to skin (greater with the Testoderm and Testoderm TTS patches) and/or significant skin irritation and contact allergy (greater with the Androderm patch); and are considerably more expensive.[6,14] Also, the scrotal (Testoderm) patch requires an adequate scrotal skin surface area and causes elevations in circulating DHT levels.

Because available oral preparations have greater risk of hepatotoxicity, greater cost, and reduced clinical efficacy, oral androgens should not be used in the treatment of male hypogonadism. Only rarely is a patient unwilling or unable to take parenteral or transdermal androgen treatment. In these unusual circumstances, methyltestosterone (25–50 mg given orally or 10–25 mg delivered buccally daily) or fluoxymesterone (10–20 mg per day given orally) may be used, with the realization that full androgen replacement will *not* be achieved and that *hepatotoxicity* is a significant risk.

## CLINICAL EFFECTS OF TESTOSTERONE REPLACEMENT

The beneficial effects of testosterone treatment are most remarkable in men with severe hypogonadism and androgen deficiency. The effects of androgen replacement therapy on sexual behavior in adult hypogonadal men show considerable variability. Libido (sexual interest and drive) is improved more consistently than is erectile dysfunction, because the latter is more commonly caused by vascular and/or neurologic disease, especially in older men. In the absence of other causes of reduced sexual function, however, most hypogonadal men experience a stimulation of libido and erectile function, and a resumption of normal sexual activity after adequate androgen replacement.[57–59] Androgen treatment improves energy level, overall feeling of well-being, and mood; increases physical and social drive, motivation, and initiative; improves spatial and verbal memory; improves sleep quality; and reduces central vasomotor instability, which may cause hot flushes (in men with acute and/or severe androgen deficiency).[59–63] In hypogonadal men, testosterone treatment has significant effects on body composition, increasing lean body mass, muscle mass and strength; decreasing total and visceral fat mass; and increasing bone mineral density.[27,64–67] Hypogonadism increases and testosterone treatment suppresses high-density lipoprotein (HDL) cholesterol, resulting in a more atherogenic lipid profile.[68,69] However, epidemiologic studies suggest that higher testosterone levels are associated with reduced coronary artery disease risk.[70,71] Finally, androgen replacement stimulates erythropoiesis and normalizes the hematocrit and hemoglobin concentration.[72–74] The stimulation of erythropoiesis by testosterone primarily is responsible for the normal difference between men and women in hematocrit and hemoglobin.[72]

The changes in sexual behavior and aggressiveness experienced by a hypogonadal man treated with testosterone may be distressing to the patient and his partner, both of whom may have grown accustomed to the patient's behavior before androgen replacement. Often, problems in sexual adjustment may be avoided if patients and their partners are counseled before and during testosterone replacement.

## TREATMENT OF DELAYED PUBERTY

In sexually immature, eunuchoidal patients, androgen therapy stimulates the development of normal male secondary sexual characteristics and somatic growth (see Chap. 115). These effects of androgens are less dramatic in older eunuchoidal patients and adult hypogonadal men. androgen replacement therapy for patients with delayed puberty who have not achieved full adult height is complex and should be undertaken with great care (see Chap. 92).[75] Overzealous androgen therapy, although it results in virilization and increased long bone growth, can lead to premature closure of the epiphyses of long bones, resulting in a compromise of the final, achievable adult height. Furthermore, it is difficult clinically to differentiate patients with constitutional delay of puberty, who require only temporary androgen replacement to induce pubertal changes, from those with permanent idiopathic hypogonadotropic hypogonadism, who require lifelong androgen treatment to stimulate puberty and to maintain sexual functioning.

Boys with constitutional delay of puberty present with short stature and delayed pubertal development relative to their peers, and demonstrate delayed height and bone age relative to their chronologic age. Although these boys eventually undergo puberty spontaneously without treatment, studies suggest that delay or omission of therapy may permanently affect acquisition of peak bone mass and have profound, long-lasting psychological effects, considerations that argue for early androgen treatment of constitutional delay of puberty.[76]

In boys with delayed pubertal development, androgen therapy is begun at reduced dosages and is usually intermittent.[76] If the patient's height is far below the expected adult height (by 10–15 cm), androgen therapy is usually begun with testosterone enanthate or testosterone cypionate, 50 to 100 mg intramuscularly every month, to stimulate bone growth and mild virilization in younger patients (e.g., in boys whose chronologic age is 14 years and bone age is 12 years). The dosage is raised to 50 to 100 mg intramuscularly every 2 weeks over the next year and then gradually increased to full adult androgen replacement dosages over the subsequent few years. Treatment goals should be individualized and should consider both growth and virilization, as well as the psychological state of the patient and family. The monthly administration of testosterone enanthate or testosterone cypionate may stimulate adequate growth, but sufficient virilization usually requires larger, more frequent doses. Neither approach has been demonstrated to compromise final adult height. With either approach, careful monitoring of growth, virilization, and psychological adjustment is necessary. The recommendation is that androgen therapy be withheld until the chronologic age is 14 years or the bone age is >10.5 years. The severe emotional stress and trauma of delayed sexual maturation to patients and families, however, often requires androgen treatment at an earlier age. In patients with delayed onset of puberty, androgen therapy is instituted for 3 to 6 months and then stopped for 3 to 6 months to determine whether the spontaneous onset and progression of puberty will occur. An increase of testis size is the most important clinical indicator of spontaneous pubertal development. If no increase occurs during the period the patient is off androgen treatment, another course of androgen therapy is initiated. For boys on monthly testosterone injections, testis growth may occur during treatment. Increases in serum testosterone and gonadotropin levels (initially at night) may also help in detecting spontaneous pubertal onset.

Prepubertal boys who have coexistent growth hormone (GH) deficiency exhibit reduced stimulation of secondary sexual characteristics and somatic growth in response to androgen therapy alone.[77] In these boys, normal pubertal growth and development are restored by simultaneous GH and androgen treatment. Testosterone that is aromatized to estradiol enhances pulsatile GH secretion and serum insulin-like growth factor-I (IGF-I) levels in prepubertal boys.[78,79] This may explain some of the growth-promoting effects of testosterone during puberty. In contrast, nonaromatizable oral 17α-alkylated androgens (e.g., methyltestosterone and oxandrolone) and DHT do not increase GH or IGF-I secretion, but stimulate growth to a similar degree as does testosterone treatment.[77,79] The consequences of relative estrogen deficiency induced by the use of nonaromatizable

androgens (e.g., on bone and brain function) are not known. This, together with the small but significant risk of hepatotoxicity, make use of these agents less desirable than testosterone therapy for treatment of delayed puberty.

## OTHER USES OF ANDROGENS

### ANEMIAS

The effect of androgens in enhancing erythropoiesis is mediated primarily by the indirect stimulation of erythropoietin secretion from renal and extrarenal sources (see Chap. 212).[72,73] Moreover, androgens act directly on the bone marrow to increase red blood cell production in response to erythropoietin. The demonstration that erythropoiesis was stimulated by replacement dosages of androgens in hypogonadal men prompted the use of androgens to treat a variety of other anemias. The anemia of chronic renal failure and hypoproliferative anemias due to bone marrow dysfunction (e.g., aplastic anemia, myelofibrosis, and anemia caused by hematologic malignancies) are the most common conditions in which androgen therapy has been used.

Androgens are beneficial in the treatment of anemia in patients with chronic renal failure who are on adequate maintenance hemodialysis and whose iron and folate stores are normal.[80–82] Parenterally administered androgen preparations (e.g., testosterone enanthate and nandrolone decanoate) are more effective than oral androgens (e.g., fluoxymesterone and oxymetholone). Anephric patients do not respond to androgen treatment.[81]

The androgen formulations that are used to treat anemia in hemodialysis patients are intramuscular testosterone enanthate (4 mg/kg per week) or nandrolone decanoate (1.5 mg/kg per week for women; 3 mg/kg per week for men). Typical dosages are testosterone enanthate 200 to 250 mg intramuscularly weekly and nandrolone decanoate 100 to 200 mg intramuscularly weekly. The typical response to these pharmacologic doses is a rise in hemoglobin of 1 to 2 g/dL.[80,81] Because nandrolone decanoate has reduced androgenic activity, it is the preferred preparation to treat women with renal failure. Long-term androgen therapy should be limited to patients who demonstrate symptomatic and hematologic responses after a 6-month trial of androgen treatment. Therapy should be stopped periodically in all patients to assess the continued need for treatment. In many instances, the anemia of chronic renal failure responds to androgen treatment because patients are relatively androgen deficient (i.e., men with hypogonadism commonly associated with uremia, or women).

Because it is more effective and does not cause virilization in women, in comparison with androgens, recombinant human erythropoietin is becoming the treatment of choice for the anemia of renal failure. Erythropoietin is expensive, however, and may be associated with significant side effects (e.g., severe hypertension and arteriovenous fistula thrombosis).[83] Because androgens stimulate erythropoiesis directly, they have been used to augment the action of exogenous erythropoietin, so that lower doses of erythropoietin are needed to achieve an adequate hematopoietic response.[84,85] Thus, androgens remain useful as a primary treatment (particularly in men) or adjunctive treatment for the anemia of end-stage kidney disease.

Androgen therapy has been useful in ameliorating some anemias resulting from bone marrow dysfunction, including aplastic anemia and primary refractory anemias; anemias secondary to hematologic malignancies, such as multiple myeloma and chronic lymphocytic leukemia; and myelophthisic anemias such as myelofibrosis.[72,73] In unselected patients, the response rate of these anemias to androgens has been ~50%.[86] Patients with mild or moderate hypocellular bone marrows or myelofibrosis respond more consistently than those with severely aplastic bone marrows, hypercellular marrows (e.g., secondary to malignancies), or marrows demonstrating ineffective erythropoiesis (e.g., in primary refractory anemias or agnogenic myeloid metaplasia). Because many of the acquired causes of hypoplastic or aplastic anemias resolve spontaneously, attributing the responses totally to androgen administration is difficult. In fact, two small, prospective, randomized trials of androgen therapy in patients with refractory or aplastic anemia did not demonstrate any benefit of androgen treatment.[87,88]

Androgens have been used as adjunctive therapy to stimulate erythropoiesis in patients with hemolysis due to sickle cell disease and paroxysmal nocturnal hemoglobinuria.[73,89] In these conditions, androgens do not affect the hemolytic process. However, danazol, a weak oral 17α-alkylated androgen (600–800 mg per day), has been used successfully to treat patients with autoimmune hemolytic anemia and idiopathic thrombocytopenic purpura by directly lowering autoantibody titers.[73,90] Maintenance therapy with low-dose danazol (50 mg per day) for the latter condition has been successful.[90]

## MICROPENIS AND MICROPHALLUS

A micropenis is a small but normal-appearing penis (see Chap. 93). A microphallus is a small, ambiguous-appearing penis, often seen in male pseudohermaphroditic children in association with hypospadias. Enlargement of a micropenis or microphallus has been achieved by parenteral administration of 25 to 50 mg of testosterone enanthate or testosterone cypionate intramuscularly every 3 to 4 weeks for 3 months.[54,91,92] Others have used topical application of 1.25% to 5.0% testosterone cream, 5% dihydrotestosterone cream, or 10% testosterone propionate cream applied twice daily for 3 months.[29,30,45,46,54,55] Although topical testosterone preparations may be easier to administer to children, their lack of availability, need for frequent administration, and variable absorption and bioavailability make them less practical than parenteral preparations. The enlargement of a microphallus with testosterone therapy is a useful adjunct to surgical repair of associated hypospadias.[55]

High-dose androgen therapy has improved virilization, masculine self-image, and sexual functioning in patients with male pseudohermaphroditism caused by 5α-reductase deficiency and certain androgen-receptor defects.[93] Because these patients are androgen resistant, very high dosages of testosterone (e.g., 500 mg testosterone enanthate or mixed esters weekly) are required to sustain androgen effects.

## HEREDITARY ANGIONEUROTIC EDEMA

Hereditary angioneurotic edema is an autosomal dominant disorder characterized by a nonfunctional or markedly reduced circulating level of the serum inhibitor of the first component of complement (C1-esterase inhibitor). Biochemically, patients with this disorder have unimpeded activation of the first (C1), fourth (C4), and second (C2) components of the complement cascade. Uninhibited activation of the complement system causes increased vascular permeability and a clinical syndrome characterized by episodic angioedema of the skin and mucous membranes, most commonly affecting the extremities, face, pharynx, and gastrointestinal tract.[94]

The 17α-alkylated androgens increase C1-esterase inhibitor activity in serum and normalize serum levels of the complement components that are depleted.[94] Androgens that are not 17α-alkylated, such as testosterone and 17β-hydroxyl esters of testosterone, do not increase serum C1-esterase inhibitor activity. Because the toxicity of 17α-alkylated androgens results in increased levels of several other plasma proteins synthesized by the liver (e.g., transferrin, haptoglobin, and plasminogen), the therapeutic benefit of these androgen preparations in stimulating C1-esterase inhibitor activity may be a manifestation of their liver toxicity.[95]

Because of its very weak androgenic action, the 17α-alkylated testosterone derivative danazol has been used to prevent attacks of hereditary angioneurotic edema.[96] Long-term prophylaxis against attacks is achieved with maintenance dosages of

danazol ranging from 200 mg every other day to 600 mg daily. The objective evidence of response is the presence of increased serum levels of C2. The short-term prevention of attacks of angioedema for patients not on long-term maintenance therapy is obtained by administering 600 mg daily for 10 days before surgical trauma or stress. Despite a high incidence of side effects (menstrual disturbances, weight gain, muscle cramps, and elevated liver function test results), danazol has proven to be a relatively safe and effective therapy for women with hereditary angioneurotic edema.[97] Danazol suppresses gonadotropin secretion and inhibits gonadal steroid synthesis, and is also used to treat a variety of other conditions, most notably endometriosis and cystic disease of the breast (see Chaps. 98 and 106).[96]

## BREAST CANCER

Androgens have been used in the treatment of premenopausal or early postmenopausal women with metastatic carcinoma of the breast whose tumors demonstrate estrogen receptors (see Chap. 224).[98] Usually, these women are treated initially with the estrogen antagonist tamoxifen. Approximately 40% of premenopausal women with estrogen-receptor–positive breast cancer respond to tamoxifen. These women have a high probability of responding to further hormonal therapy, such as oophorectomy, aminoglutethimide treatment, adrenalectomy or hypophysectomy, and androgen administration. The antitumor effects of the various androgen preparations correlate well with their androgenic effects; therefore, testosterone esters are the most effective preparations. Androgen therapy for metastatic breast carcinoma invariably has virilizing side effects. For this reason, and because of lower response rates compared with other forms of hormonal and chemotherapy, androgen treatment of breast cancer has been markedly curtailed.

## LICHEN SCLEROSUS

Lichen sclerosus is a chronic skin disorder that most commonly occurs on the vulva of postmenopausal white women. If left untreated, this condition causes chronic pruritus and progresses to atrophy and contracture of the introitus, causing dyspareunia. Topical androgen in the form of 2% testosterone propionate in petrolatum or 2% testosterone cream applied to the affected areas twice daily is an effective treatment for lichen sclerosus.[31,32] However, the use of high-potency corticosteroid creams (e.g., clobetasol dipropionate 0.05%) probably is more effective than topical testosterone or testosterone propionate in the treatment of severe vulvar lichen sclerosus.[31,32]

## OSTEOPOROSIS

In men, testosterone and its aromatization to estradiol play important roles in the attainment of peak bone mass and maintenance of bone density in adulthood.[99] Delayed puberty is associated with reduced peak cortical and trabecular bone mass, and testosterone therapy increases bone mineral density.[100,101] However, the increase in bone mass with testosterone treatment is greater in individuals with open epiphyses than in those with closed epiphyses, and the absolute bone mass achieved may be below that of normal men, a result that emphasizes the importance of the timing of testosterone exposure for normal bone development.

In hypogonadal men, androgen deficiency increases bone turnover, which may result in osteopenia or osteoporosis and in increased risk of vertebral and hip fractures. Testosterone treatment of androgen-deficient men improves levels of bone turnover markers and increases both trabecular and cortical bone mineral density.[64,66,99] Whether testosterone therapy reduces the risk of fractures in osteoporotic hypogonadal men, however, is not known. Nevertheless, because it may have other beneficial effects, testosterone is the initial treatment of choice in hypogonadal men with osteoporosis.

Uncontrolled preliminary studies suggest that testosterone treatment also increases lumbar spine bone mineral density in eugonadal men with idiopathic osteoporosis and in men receiving glucocorticoid therapy (who often have low serum testosterone levels).[102,103] Further longer-term, placebo-controlled studies involving larger numbers of men are needed, however, before testosterone therapy can be recommended for eugonadal men or men receiving glucocorticoids.

Androgens also have an important role in the maintenance of bone mass in women. In postmenopausal women, administration of pharmacologic doses of androgens increases both trabecular and cortical bone mineral density. Androgen preparations that have been shown to increase bone mass include implants containing testosterone and estradiol (50 mg each); combinations of oral conjugated equine estrogen (0.625 or 1.25 mg) and methyltestosterone (1.25 or 2.5 mg) (Estratest HS or Estratest); intramuscular nandrolone decanoate (50 mg every 2 to 3 weeks); oral tibolone (a steroid with androgenic, estrogenic, and progestogenic activity available in Europe); and oral stanozolol (a 17α-alkylated androgen, 2 to 6 mg per day).[104–112] The combined administration of estrogen and androgen increases levels of bone formation markers and bone mineral density to a greater extent than does estrogen replacement alone.[105–107,112] However, long-term studies demonstrating their efficacy in reducing fracture rate and defining the risks of androgen therapy have not been performed. Because of the potential for hepatotoxicity and suppression of HDL cholesterol with 17α-alkylated androgens and their virilizing side effects, the use of androgenic steroids should probably be reserved for women with progressive, severe, symptomatic osteoporosis that has not responded to other forms of treatment.

# POTENTIAL USES OF ANDROGENS

## REPLACEMENT THERAPY FOR POSTMENOPAUSAL WOMEN

Circulating concentrations of androgens decline gradually with aging before menopause and, unlike estrogen levels, do not decrease precipitously during the menopausal transition.[112] In contrast, androgen levels decline sharply by ~50% after surgical or medical oophorectomy (e.g., induced by administration of gonadotropin-releasing hormone [GnRH] analog). Estrogen replacement therapy also suppresses circulating free testosterone levels and probably contributes to postmenopausal symptoms of androgen deficiency (i.e., reduced libido and sexuality). Among surgically and spontaneously menopausal women with significant sexual dysfunction, androgen replacement therapy stimulates libido and improves the feeling of well-being and sexuality.[105,112–114] Androgen treatment may also increase bone formation and density (see earlier). The major identifiable risk of androgen treatment in women is the potential for masculinizing side effects (e.g., acne, hirsutism, hair loss, and deepening of the voice). The effects and consequences of androgen therapy on body adiposity, fat distribution, muscle mass and strength, and risk of coronary artery disease and breast cancer are unknown.

## REPLACEMENT THERAPY FOR AGING MEN

With increasing age, otherwise healthy men experience a gradual decline in testicular function, and in total and free testosterone concentrations, so that levels in a significant proportion of elderly men (~30%) fall below the normal range for young men.[115] Testosterone production is compromised further by conditions such as illness, administration of some medications (e.g., glucocorticoids, CNS-acting drugs), and malnutrition, which occurs commonly in aging men. In addition to the decrease in testosterone levels, aging is associated with a functional decline in a number of androgen-dependent tissues, which results in diminished libido and erectile function; increased adiposity; reduced muscle mass and strength; decreased bone mass; increased risk of fractures; mood changes; diminished vigor; and alterations in sleep quality.[115,116] Therefore, the age-related decrease in testosterone concentrations may contribute to these functional declines with aging. Short-term preliminary studies of the administration of testosterone enanthate to mildly androgen-deficient elderly men have revealed beneficial effects on lean body mass, muscle strength, bone turnover, libido, and mood, without significant adverse clinical effects, notably on either the prostate or serum lipid profiles, except polycythemia.[117–119b] Larger longer-term, randomized, placebo-controlled studies are needed, however, to determine the benefits and risks of androgen replacement therapy in elderly men (especially effects on the prostate and cardiovascular risk).

## WASTING AND CATABOLIC STATES

The demonstration that testosterone increases fat-free muscle mass and strength both in hypogonadal men receiving androgen replacement therapy and in eugonadal men who were using supraphysiologic dosages (matched for diet and exercise) has renewed interest in studying the anabolic effects of androgen administration in clinical states associated with muscle wasting (sarcopenia) and protein catabolism.[63,64,120,121] These states include AIDS, cancer, chronic illness (e.g., end-stage renal disease, COPD), conditions due to use of medications (e.g., glucocorticoids), normal aging, muscle disease, autoimmune disease (e.g., rheumatoid arthritis, systemic lupus erythematosus), major trauma and surgery, burns, immobilization, and zero-gravity conditions during space travel. Many patients with these conditions also have low serum testosterone concentrations, providing a further rationale for considering androgen treatment to increase muscle mass and strength, and most important, to improve muscle performance, physical function, and quality of life.

Preliminary studies have demonstrated that androgen therapy may have beneficial effects in some sarcopenic states. In most but not all studies, the administration of supraphysiologic dosages of testosterone, nandrolone decanoate, or oxandrolone in men and women with AIDS-related wasting increased lean body mass, sexual function, general well-being, mood, and quality of life.[17,18,122–127a] In other short-term studies, the administration of nandrolone decanoate to patients with end-stage renal disease on hemodialysis increased lean body mass and measures of physical performance; administration of nandrolone decanoate or stanozolol to patients with COPD increased fat-free mass, and use of the latter androgen in combination with nutritional support also improved respiratory muscle function; and administration of oxandrolone to patients with major burns who were given a high-protein diet increased the rate of weight gain during recovery.[128–131] As discussed earlier, in preliminary studies of elderly men with mild androgen deficiency, testosterone supplementation increased lean body mass and muscle strength.

The clinical conditions associated with wasting and protein catabolism described earlier are complex, and the pathophysiology of sarcopenia in these states involves a number of factors other than androgen deficiency. Important factors that contribute to the pathophysiology of wasting in these conditions are nutritional status, activity and exercise, the natural history of the underlying condition, comorbid illnesses, cytokine and immune responses, other anabolic factors (e.g., levels of GH and IGF-I), and medication use (e.g., glucocorticoids). In particular, the importance of adequate nutrition, activity, and exercise has been a focus in many of the studies that have investigated the anabolic effects of androgens in various clinical states.[120,121,125–127,129–132]

Although preliminary studies suggest potential short-term benefits of androgen therapy in promoting anabolism (increase in lean body and muscle mass), and in some instances strength, whether these changes produce long-lasting, clinically meaningful improvements in muscle performance, physical function, independent living, and quality of life without significant adverse effects is not known.

## MALE CONTRACEPTION

Androgens, mostly testosterone enanthate, either alone or in combination with progestogens or GnRH analogs, have been used to suppress endogenous gonadotropin and sperm production in male contraceptive development trials (see Chap. 123).[133] Androgen administration is an absolute requirement for hormonal male contraception, both to suppress gonadotropin secretion and to replace endogenous testosterone suppressed by other agents. Because it plays such a key role in male contraceptive strategies, more practical androgen preparations with zero-order kinetics and longer durations of action are being developed and evaluated.

## CORONARY ARTERY DISEASE

A number of uncontrolled reports in the 1940s suggested that testosterone administration may improve symptoms of angina pectoris.[134] In one placebo-controlled study, short-term intramuscular administration (4 to 8 weeks) of testosterone cypionate 200 mg weekly improved electrocardiographic ST segment depression after a modified two-step exercise test.[135] Subsequent epidemiologic studies have suggested an association between low testosterone levels and increased risk of atherosclerotic coronary and carotid artery disease.[69,70] These studies suggest a potential beneficial effect of testosterone on coronary artery disease. However, the administration of physiologic doses of testosterone to hypogonadal men decreases HDL cholesterol, producing a more atherogenic lipid profile.[68,69] Nevertheless, evidence in animals has indicated that testosterone induces endothelium-independent relaxation of isolated coronary arteries. Placebo-controlled studies of men with both normal and low serum testosterone levels found that the acute intravenous infusion of testosterone during a treadmill exercise test increased the time to develop significant ST segment depression and total exercise time.[136,137a] These early studies suggest that testosterone may have beneficial effects on exercise-induced myocardial ischemia in men with coronary artery disease.

# INAPPROPRIATE USES OF ANDROGENS

## IMPROVEMENT OF ATHLETIC PERFORMANCE

Androgens are commonly used in high-dosage combinations by competitive athletes who hope that these steroids will improve muscle strength, endurance, and athletic performance.[138,139] Their use has been prohibited by local, national, and international athletic organizations (e.g., the International Olympic Committee), but the covert use (i.e., abuse) of very high dosages of androgens has become widespread, despite a lack of objective evidence for the long-term risks and benefits of their use. In the late 1950s, androgens were used almost exclusively by weight lifters, bodybuilders, and heavy throwers. Today, their use has spread to football players, swimmers, and track and field participants at all levels of athletic competition. Surveys also reveal a relatively high prevalence of androgenic anabolic steroid abuse in peripubertal boys, not only to enhance athletic performance but also to improve their appearance.[140]

Whether androgen administration improves athletic performance is controversial. One review of 25 well-documented studies of the effects of anabolic steroids on athletic performance concluded that androgen use alone did not increase muscle strength or improve athletic performance.[141] Anabolic steroids did significantly increase strength in athletes who had intensive weight training before and during steroid treatment and who maintained a high-protein diet.[141] Many of these studies were not blinded or placebo-controlled, however, and most did not control for energy and protein intake or training.[121] A randomized, double-blind, placebo-controlled study demonstrated that short-term administration (10 weeks) of a supraphysiologic dosage of testosterone enanthate (600 mg weekly) with or without resistance exercise increased fat-free mass, muscle size, and muscle strength in normal men.[120] When high-dosage testosterone was combined with exercise, the increases in strength were greater than those found with either testosterone or exercise alone. This study clearly demonstrated the short-term anabolic effects of supraphysiologic testosterone administration in normal men in whom diet and exercise were carefully controlled. However, the longer-term effects on muscle strength and risks of high-dosage androgen use are not known. Moreover, the effects of androgens on muscle and athletic performance remain to be demonstrated in carefully controlled studies. Uncontrolled studies investigating the effect of androgens on strength and athletic performance may be confounded by the covert use of other androgenic steroids and/or anabolic agents, such as GH.

Athletes often take multiple androgenic anabolic agents in combination, including 17α-alkylated androgens, in extremely high dosages (10–100 times the therapeutic dosages) with little regard for potentially serious side effects. Abnormalities in liver function as well as more life-threatening hepatotoxicity (e.g., peliosis hepatis and hepatocellular carcinoma), impaired spermatogenesis causing infertility, gynecomastia, cardiomyopathy, thrombotic events, severe mood and behavioral disturbances, and, in women, hirsutism and virilization have been observed in athletes taking anabolic steroids, especially 17α-alkylated androgens.[138,139,142–144] Moreover, the long-term sequelae of huge dosages of the safer testosterone esters is unknown. For example, self-administration of high dosages of androgenic steroids by weight lifters and bodybuilders sharply reduces HDL cholesterol and elevates low-density lipoprotein cholesterol, producing an atherogenic lipoprotein profile, despite high-level exercise training.[145] Effects on lipoproteins occur to a greater extent with oral 17α-alkylated androgens than with parenteral 17β-hydroxyl testosterone esters, but supraphysiologic doses of the latter significantly suppress HDL cholesterol.[1,20,146,147] Whether the continued, long-term use of androgenic steroids will cause premature atherosclerotic cardiovascular disease is unknown.

The potential risks of high-dosage androgenic anabolic steroid abuse outweigh their potential benefits, and the use of these agents to improve athletic performance or appearance should be strongly discouraged.

## USE OF DEHYDROEPIANDROSTERONE AND ANDROSTENEDIONE

DHEA, DHEA sulfate (DHEAS), and androstenedione are weak androgens produced by the adrenal cortex. DHEA and DHEAS are produced in very large quantities and are the most abundant circulating steroid hormones in humans. Both DHEA and androstenedione can be converted within most peripheral tissues to testosterone, DHT, estrone, and estradiol. Therefore, they are precursors for more potent androgens and estrogens.[148,149] Furthermore, the actions of these androgens may depend on the capability of individual target tissues to convert them into more potent androgens and estrogens, independent of their circulating concentrations. DHEA administration also increases levels of serum IGF-I, which may act independently on certain target organs.

Preparations of these androgens are sold alone or in combination with other "natural" substances as "dietary supplements." Therefore, they are easily available over the counter and are *not regulated by the FDA*. In combination with other androgens and performance-enhancing substances, both DHEA and androstenedione are being increasingly abused by athletes in the hopes of improving strength and athletic performance. Thus, use of these androgens has been prohibited by most but not all local, national, and international athletic organizations.

Beginning at ~30 years of age, serum DHEA concentrations decrease progressively with increasing age in both men and women.[148,149] This decline is associated with age-related decreases in muscle mass and strength (sarcopenia); increases in osteoporosis; increases in adiposity, insulin resistance, and type 2 diabetes mellitus; declines in cognitive function; increases in atherosclerotic cardiovascular disease; increases in malignancy; and decreases in immune function. Studies that demonstrated beneficial effects of DHEA administration in preventing these age-related illnesses and declines in function have used *pharmacologic doses in rodents that produce very little DHEA.* Therefore, these studies have limited applicability to humans. Nevertheless, based primarily on these studies, dietary supplements containing DHEA are being popularized and used to prevent these age-related problems and to impede the aging process itself.

*No conclusive scientific evidence* exists to support the use of DHEA or androstenedione to increase muscle strength and athletic performance or to prevent age-associated functional decline and disease. The results of short-term preliminary studies using replacement dosages of DHEA (50–100 mg per day) in small numbers of subjects have been inconsistent. Some have demonstrated small improvements in general well-being, levels of bone turnover markers, muscle strength, and levels of immune markers, whereas others have not.[149–152] A placebo-controlled trial in older men and women aged 60 to 79 years found that DHEA (50 mg/day for 1 year) produced small increases in serum testosterone and estradiol levels; improved bone mineral density; decreased osteoclastic activity; and increased libido and skin status in women older than 70 years old.[152a] A double-blind study in women with adrenal insufficiency found that DHEA (50 mg/day for months) increased both serum androstenedione and testosterone concentrations; improved the sense of well-being; and increased the frequency of sexual thoughts, interest, and satisfaction with both mental and physical aspects of sexuality.[152b] A pharmacologic dosage of androstenedione (300 mg per day) given cyclically in young men undergoing resistance training did not increase muscle size or strength.[153]

Replacement and pharmacologic doses of DHEA and androstenedione increase serum estradiol levels in men and testosterone levels in women, and may result in estrogenic or androgenic side effects, respectively, in users.[150,153a] Because DHEA may be converted within target tissues to testosterone, DHT, or estradiol, concern exists regarding possible adverse effects of long-term use on benign and malignant prostate growth in men and adverse effects on the breast and masculinization in women. Both DHEA and androstenedione treatment may suppress HDL cholesterol and produce a more atherogenic profile.[149,153] The long-term effects of increased IGF-I levels with DHEA replacement (e.g., on tumor growth) is unknown. Finally, the *quantity* of DHEA and androstenedione in preparations, particularly those containing other dietary supplements, and their *quality* are *highly variable.* This raises concerns regarding excessive or inadequate dosing, and more importantly, the presence of *impurities or contaminants* that may pose health risks.

Because the long-term benefits and risks of DHEA and androstenedione are unknown, the use of these weak androgens should be *strongly discouraged.*

## TREATMENT OF SHORT AND TALL STATURE

The administration of androgen before epiphyseal closure accelerates long bone growth in children with short stature. However, no evidence exists that androgen therapy increases the eventual adult height. In fact, premature androgen treatment of short children may compromise adult height.[154] With the exception of children with pituitary insufficiency, androgens are not indicated for the treatment of children with short stature. In some European countries, supraphysiologic dosages of testosterone (e.g., testosterone ester 500 mg every 2 weeks for 1–4 years until epiphyseal closure) is used with variable success to treat constitutional tall stature in boys.[155] In contrast to short stature, however, tall stature in boys is not socially unacceptable and is sometimes desirable in the United States. Therefore,

high-dosage testosterone treatment of excessively tall boys is rarely indicated except in very unusual circumstances.

## CONTRAINDICATIONS TO ANDROGEN USE

Androgen therapy is absolutely contraindicated in men with prostatic carcinoma and breast carcinoma. These are androgen-sensitive cancers, and androgen administration can cause rapid tumor growth that may lead to acute urinary obstruction, bone pain, or spinal cord compression. Accordingly, a careful examination of the prostate gland and breast should be performed before and during androgen therapy. Androgen use is also contraindicated in pregnant women. Because androgenic steroids cross the placenta, the sexual differentiation of a female fetus may be affected by the administration of these drugs to the mother.

Full replacement dosages of androgens may be inappropriate for hypogonadal men with severe psychopathology or mental retardation and for elderly, androgen-deficient men with severe bladder outlet obstruction from benign prostatic hyperplasia who are not good surgical candidates. Lower dosages of androgens may be administered to preserve muscle mass and strength, and bone mineral mass. Androgens should be administered with great caution to women or children who use their voices professionally.

## SIDE EFFECTS OF ANDROGENS

Adverse effects of androgens may be caused by their androgenic actions or, if they are aromatizable, by their estrogenic effects.[156] Other side effects are related to the particular androgen formulation (e.g., hepatotoxicity with 17α-alkylated androgens).

### ANDROGENIC SIDE EFFECTS

Complaints of excessive stimulation of libido and erections induced by androgen replacement therapy are uncommon. This complication usually occurs in young boys and men with long-standing, severe androgen deficiency. In these patients, symptoms usually resolve spontaneously or with a reduction in the dosage of testosterone. Contrary to popular belief, androgen administration in physiologic or moderately supraphysiologic dosages does not cause excessive aggressiveness or anger. Social aggressiveness, motivation, initiative, energy, and well-being improve, and anger and irritability are *reduced* with androgen replacement therapy in hypogonadal men.[156,157] In normal men, short-term administration of moderately high dosages of testosterone (testosterone enanthate up to 600 mg per week) causes a slight increase in sexual arousal but no change in sexual activity and no increase in angry behavior.[156,158] However, the appearance of normal sexual and aggressive behavior in hypogonadal men as a result of testosterone replacement may cause distress in patients and their partners, who may require careful counseling.

Acne and increased oiliness of the skin often develop in patients receiving androgen therapy for the induction of puberty and is usually treated satisfactorily with local skin measures, retinoic acid cream, and antibiotics. Acne nearly always resolves spontaneously with continued androgen treatment. Frontal balding or androgenic alopecia may develop in genetically predisposed individuals during androgen therapy.

Testosterone and its intraglandular conversion to DHT by 5α-reductase are important determinants of normal prostate growth. In hypogonadal men, testosterone replacement therapy increases prostate volume and PSA levels to values comparable to those of age-matched eugonadal men.[159] Androgen therapy in elderly men has not been associated with a greater rate of benign prostatic hyperplasia (BPH), but exposure times have been relatively short (2 to 3 years).[119] Thus, the prudent course is to undertake androgen treatment in elderly men with great care, especially in those with enlarged prostate glands or symptoms of bladder outlet obstruction. Although acute urinary retention may occur because of androgen-induced prostatic growth in patients with BPH, it is extremely uncommon in the absence of prostatic carcinoma.[160] Because prostate cancer is the most common cancer in men and its growth is stimulated by androgens, older men (older than 45 years of age) treated with testosterone should have a digital rectal examination and serum PSA measurement at least yearly.

Androgen use may cause mild or moderate weight gain as a result of protein anabolic effects and sodium and water retention induced by these agents.[56] Patients with underlying edematous states (e.g., congestive heart failure, nephrotic syndrome, or hepatic cirrhosis) may have worsening edema during androgen treatment.

All of the available androgen preparations, including those with reduced androgenic potency (anabolic steroids), may cause unwanted virilizing side effects when administered to women or young children. None of the anabolic steroids is completely free of androgenic effects. Depending on the androgenic potency, dosage and duration of administration, and individual susceptibility, the virilizing side effects of androgen therapy may be mild (e.g., acne and mild hirsutism) or severe (e.g., severe acne and hirsutism, frontal balding, deepening of the voice, and clitoromegaly). In children, excessive androgen exposure may also cause premature closure of long bone epiphyses and shorten eventual adult height.

In hypogonadal men androgen replacement therapy normally stimulates erythropoiesis and increases the hemoglobin concentration and hematocrit into the normal adult male range.[72] Occasionally, excessive erythrocytosis or polycythemia occurs during testosterone replacement therapy that may require therapeutic phlebotomy and lowering of the testosterone dosage. Although such effects have not been documented, persistently elevated hematocrit, red blood cell volume, and blood viscosity may predispose some patients, particularly elderly men, to vascular thromboses. Some men who develop polycythemia have predisposing conditions, such as hypoxia due to COPD or obstructive sleep apnea, that independently increase erythropoietin production. In other men, no predisposing factors are apparent. Excessive erythrocytosis is less common with transdermal testosterone patches that produce physiologic serum testosterone levels than with injections of testosterone esters that produce slightly supraphysiologic testosterone concentrations initially after administration.

Replacement dosages of testosterone in hypogonadal men can induce or worsen obstructive sleep apnea.[161,162] On testosterone replacement, these men demonstrate erythrocytosis and have normal oxygen saturation, pulmonary function testing, and respiratory drives while awake. During sleep, however, they exhibit frequent apneic episodes associated with arousals, significant oxygen desaturation, and cardiac dysrhythmias. Apneic episodes decrease markedly after the discontinuation of testosterone therapy. The development of signs and symptoms of the obstructive sleep apnea syndrome during androgen therapy should prompt a formal sleep study. If sleep apnea is documented, treatment should be instituted (e.g., continuous positive airway pressure). If the patient is unresponsive or cannot tolerate treatment, androgens should be reduced in dosage or discontinued.

By suppressing endogenous gonadotropin secretion, exogenous testosterone or androgen administration suppresses spermatogenesis to various degrees, depending on the specific preparation, dosage, and duration of treatment.[163] The suppression of sperm production may impair fertility in patients on androgen therapy. Discontinuance of androgens restores normal spermatogenesis. This reversible suppression of sperm production by exogenous testosterone is the basis for clinical trials of androgens as male contraceptive agents (see Chap. 123). In patients with hypogonadotropic hypogonadism, long-term testosterone replacement therapy does not impair the subsequent induction of spermatogenesis with gonadotropin therapy (see Chap. 115).[56]

## ESTROGENIC SIDE EFFECTS

Because testosterone is aromatized to estradiol in many tissues, the administration of testosterone or testosterone esters increases blood levels of estradiol as well as of testosterone. The ratio of estradiol to testosterone levels usually remains normal during androgen therapy. Occasionally, gynecomastia develops in patients receiving testosterone therapy, especially in boys receiving androgens for the induction of puberty and in adult hypogonadal men who receive high dosages of testosterone or who have a predisposing condition, such as cirrhosis of the liver. With a careful examination of the breast, gynecomastia in hypogonadal men and small amounts of palpable breast tissue (2 to 3 cm in diameter) in eugonadal men are commonly detectable before the initiation of androgen therapy. Although the mechanism by which gynecomastia develops is poorly understood, the hormonal milieu in which it usually occurs is an abnormally high ratio of serum estradiol to testosterone levels (see Chap. 120).

## HEPATOTOXICITY

All 17α-alkylated androgens can cause hepatic cholestasis with elevations of serum alkaline phosphatase and conjugated bilirubin, occasionally resulting in clinical jaundice.[164] During treatment with oral androgens, disordered hepatic function is manifested by increases in various plasma proteins (e.g., haptoglobin, plasminogen, and C1-esterase inhibitor, sex hormone–binding globulin) and decreases in serum clotting factors (I, V, VII, and X) and thyroid-binding globulin, all of which normally are synthesized by the liver.[95] Although preexisting liver disease predisposes to the development of abnormal liver function during oral androgen therapy, these abnormalities may occur in the absence of previous hepatic dysfunction.

Although they are very rare, more serious and potentially life-threatening complications of oral androgen therapy may occur, including the development of peliosis hepatis (hemorrhagic cysts in the liver), hepatic adenoma, hepatoma, and hepatic angiosarcoma.[164] Most patients who develop liver tumors on oral androgen therapy have coexistent underlying illnesses (e.g., Fanconi anemia, aplastic anemia, or hematologic malignancies). Hepatic tumors also have been reported, however, in patients receiving androgens at relatively high dosages for hypogonadism and various other disorders. Peliosis hepatis and hepatic adenomas usually regress with discontinuation of oral androgens, but the course of hepatic malignancies may sometimes be rapidly fatal.

Hepatotoxicity does not occur with replacement dosages of parenteral 17β-hydroxyl esters of testosterone. Although rare cases of peliosis hepatis and hepatic angiosarcoma have been associated with testosterone ester therapy, high-dosage testosterone enanthate regimens usually were used in these patients, who had severe underlying hematologic illnesses.[164] If oral 17α-alkylated androgens are used, the liver should be examined frequently, and liver function tests should be monitored routinely.

## OTHER SIDE EFFECTS

As discussed earlier, transdermal testosterone patches may cause itching, skin irritation, and contact dermatitis. Skin reactions occur most commonly with the nonscrotal permeation-enhanced adhesive testosterone patch (Androderm), less commonly with the nonscrotal testosterone patch that does not contain permeation enhancers (Testoderm TTS) and scrotal testosterone patch (Testoderm) and least commonly with testosterone gel (AndroGel).[10–12,15,33]

Occasionally, local pain, hemorrhage, or irritation is experienced at the site of injection of testosterone esters. These local side effects usually occur in patients who self-administer testosterone and can be avoided with a proper instruction in intramuscular injection technique. Subcutaneous administration of testosterone esters can cause local irritation and pain.

Rarely, patients may experience an allergic reaction to the injection vehicles of testosterone enanthate (sesame oil) or testosterone cypionate (cottonseed oil). Certain preparations of methyltestosterone or fluoxymesterone contain tartrazine for coloring. This dye may cause allergic reactions, including bronchial asthma, in susceptible patients.

## DRUG INTERACTIONS

Caution is required when oral 17α-alkylated androgens are administered to patients receiving anticoagulation therapy. Oral androgens may prolong the prothrombin time in patients on warfarin, thereby increasing the risk of hemorrhage. With the addition or withdrawal of any androgenic steroid in a patient receiving warfarin, more frequent prothrombin time determinations should be made, and warfarin dosage should be changed appropriately. Oral 17α-alkylated androgens may also increase cyclosporine levels and predispose patients to cyclosporine toxicity (e.g., renal dysfunction and neurotoxicity).

## ANTIANDROGENS

Antiandrogens are drugs that antagonize the actions of androgens by binding to or interacting with androgen receptors and competitively or noncompetitively inhibiting the binding of endogenous androgens. These drugs were developed for use in hormonal treatment of androgen-dependent malignancies, such as prostatic carcinoma and breast carcinoma in men. Subsequently, antiandrogens have been used to treat a variety of nonmalignant androgen-dependent conditions, such as acne, hirsutism, hyperandrogenism in women, male pattern baldness, and hypersexuality in men. The thera-

peutic advantage of antiandrogens over gonadal androgen suppression (e.g., with a GnRH analog) in the treatment of androgen-dependent disorders is that they antagonize the actions of both gonadal and adrenal androgens. When they are administered alone to patients with intact hypothalamic–pituitary–gonadal axes, however, the activation of normal feedback mechanisms may lead to increased testosterone production, which counteracts the actions of antiandrogens. Fortunately, many antiandrogens also have suppressive effects on pituitary gonadotropin secretion that limit the normal feedback increase of gonadotropins.

## PROGESTERONE

Progesterone (Fig. 119-3) and other progestogens are weak antiandrogens. Their interactions with androgen target tissues are complex, however, because they also have inhibitory effects on androgen production, potent direct progestational actions of their own on these tissues, some antiestrogenic action, and suppressive effects on gonadotropin secretion (antigonadotropic action). Some derivatives of progesterone (e.g., megestrol acetate and cyproterone acetate) have potent antiandrogenic action.

## MEGESTROL ACETATE

The progestational antiandrogen megestrol acetate (see Fig. 119-3) significantly blocks androgen production and androgen-mediated action at doses of 120 to 160 mg per day.[165] When administered alone, megestrol acetate profoundly suppresses serum gonadotropin and testosterone levels. In patients with intact hypothalamic–pituitary–gonadal axes, however, partial escape from this suppressive effect occurs, with serum testosterone levels returning toward control levels after 5 months. The

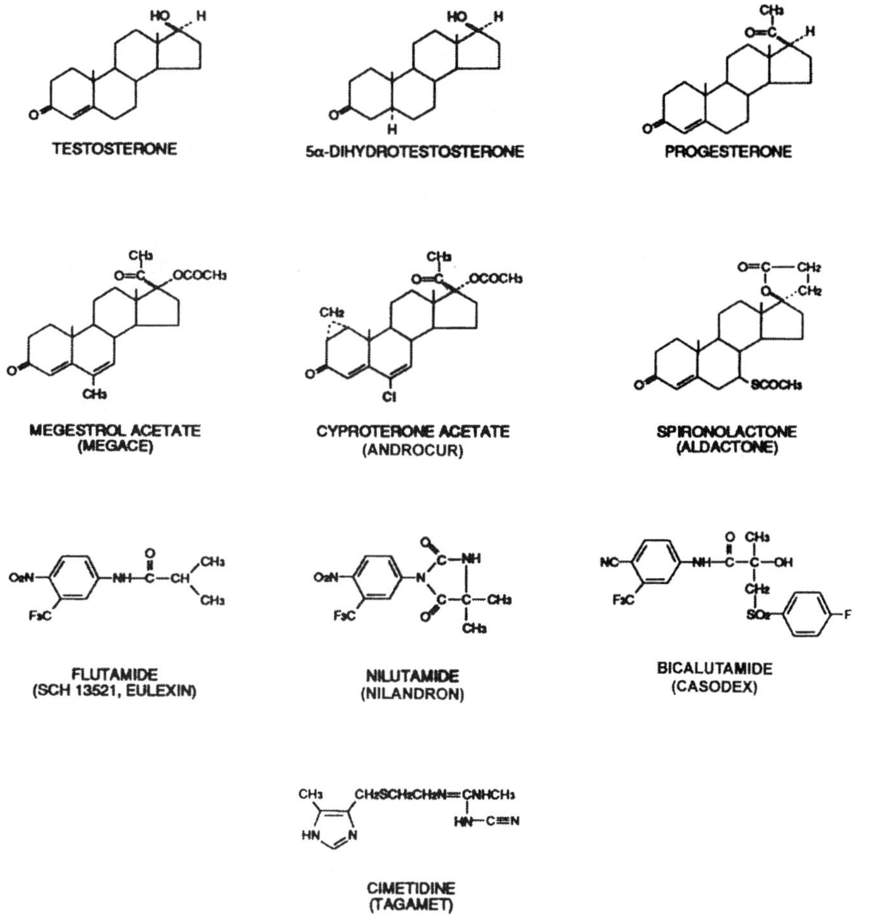

**FIGURE 119-3.** Structural formulas of common antiandrogens compared with those of testosterone and dihydrotestosterone.

addition of estradiol (0.5–1.5 mg per day) or diethylstilbestrol (0.1–0.2 mg per day) to the megestrol acetate (80–160 mg per day) maintains castrate levels of serum testosterone. These combinations have been used in the treatment of metastatic prostate cancer (see Chap. 225).[165] Megestrol acetate has also been used in the treatment of breast cancer and in management of the anorexia and cachexia associated with malignancy and AIDS, and for prevention of hot flashes.[98,166,167] One should note, however, that megestrol acetate may suppress endogenous gonadotropin and testosterone secretion in men, resulting in decreases in muscle mass and increases in fat mass.[168] Because it has glucocorticoid-like activity, high-dosage megestrol acetate may also cause clinical adrenal insufficiency and Cushing syndrome.[169,170]

## CYPROTERONE ACETATE

Cyproterone acetate (see Fig. 119-3) is a synthetic hydroxy-progesterone derivative that has potent antiandrogenic, progestational, and antigonadotropic actions.[171] It also suppresses gonadal testosterone biosynthesis by inhibiting 17,20-desmolase enzyme activity. It is commonly used in many countries but is not available in the United States. At doses of 200 to 300 mg per day, cyproterone acetate has been used to achieve short-term responses in the treatment of prostatic and male breast carcinoma and, in combination with GnRH analogs or orchidectomy, to achieve complete androgen blockade in patients with metastatic prostate cancer.[172,173] The potent progestational and antigonadotropic actions of cyproterone acetate inhibit feedback stimulation of gonadotropin secretion during its administration. A combination of low-dose cyproterone acetate (2 mg) and cyclical ethinyl estradiol (e.g., 35 µg [Dianette] and 50 µg [Diane]) has been used with variable success to treat acne, hirsutism, and hyperandrogenism in women (see Chap. 101).[171,174,175] No significant difference is found in the overall efficacy of high-dose (100 mg) compared with low-dose cyproterone acetate in the treatment of acne and hirsutism. More severe degrees of androgenization in women, however, may require higher dosage regimens (50–100 mg). Because of its potent progestational and antigonadotropic actions, cyproterone acetate causes menstrual abnormalities (e.g., oligomenorrhea, amenorrhea, and dysmenorrhea), as well as breast engorgement and gastrointestinal upset, which limit its use in nonmalignant conditions. In high doses, it may cause impairment of adrenocortical function. To reduce side effects, a topical cyproterone acetate lotion is being tested for the treatment of acne. The combination of cyproterone acetate and testosterone enanthate suppresses sperm production very effectively in normal men, suggesting that combinations of an androgen plus an antiandrogenic progestogen may hold promise for male contraceptive development.[176]

## PURE NONSTEROIDAL ANTIANDROGENS

Flutamide (Eulexin; see Fig. 119-3) is a nonsteroidal, substituted anilide. Despite the lack of structural homology of this compound with androgens, it behaves as a pure antiandrogen. Unlike steroid antiandrogens, it is devoid of androgenic, estrogenic, antiestrogenic, progestational, adrenocortical, and antigonadotropic activity. Thus, serum testosterone levels increase into the high normal adult male range in patients receiving flutamide. Although flutamide has been used as monotherapy, it generally is used in combination with GnRH analogs or orchidectomy to achieve complete androgen blockade in patients with metastatic prostatic carcinoma.[177,178] At present, the use of complete androgen blockade in patients with metastatic prostate cancer is controversial, with some studies, but not others, finding a clinically meaningful improvement in survival. Complete androgen blockade is also associated with more side effects and greater costs. At the dosages used for prostate cancer, the most troublesome side effects are gastrointestinal upset (diarrhea and nausea), dizziness,

gynecomastia, hot flushes, hepatic dysfunction, and occasional severe hepatotoxicity. The short-term coadministration of flutamide or other antiandrogens is used to prevent the acute stimulation of gonadotropins and testosterone induced by GnRH agonists that can cause an increase in tumor growth and symptoms. Flutamide (250 mg twice daily) was found to be more effective than spironolactone in treating hirsutism and acne, and lower dosages (125 to 250 mg daily) were also found to be effective.[179,180] Given the potential for more side effects and serious hepatotoxicity, however, flutamide should not be a first-line therapy for benign conditions such as hirsutism and acne.

Bicalutamide (Casodex; see Fig. 119-3) is a new nonsteroidal antiandrogen that has a long half-life (~1 week), permitting once-daily administration.[177,181] It is being used at a dosage of 50 mg per day in combination with GnRH agonists to achieve complete androgen blockade in patients with metastatic prostate cancer. In comparison with regimens of flutamide (250 mg three times daily) plus the GnRH agonist goserelin, the use of bicalutamide (50 mg per day) plus goserelin is better tolerated (less diarrhea) and is associated with a similar time to disease progression and survival in patients with stage D2 prostate cancer. Except for the occurrence of hot flushes, gynecomastia, breast tenderness, and diarrhea, it is tolerated well (see Chap. 225). It may also cause transient elevations in liver enzymes. The use of bicalutamide monotherapy at a dosage of 150 mg per day for patients with prostate cancer is being tested. Preliminary studies suggest that bicalutamide therapy may preserve sexual interest better than orchidectomy in patients with nonmetastatic disease.

Nilutamide (Nilandron; see Fig. 119-3) is a nonsteroidal antiandrogen that also has a long half-life (~40 hours), allowing once-daily oral administration (150–300 mg per day).[177,182] It is also being used primarily in combination with orchidectomy or a GnRH agonist for complete androgen blockade in men with metastatic prostate cancer. Although no comparative studies have been performed with other nonsteroidal antiandrogens, nilutamide appears to produce a higher frequency of side effects than bicalutamide and flutamide. Side effects of nilutamide include impaired ocular dark adaptation and color vision, mild nausea, alcohol intolerance, and occasional acute interstitial pneumonitis.

## SPIRONOLACTONE

Spironolactone (see Fig. 119-3), an aldosterone antagonist, is also an antiandrogen. It competitively blocks the interaction of androgen with its receptor, inhibits androgen biosynthesis by inhibiting 17α-hydroxylase and 17,20-desmolase activity, and interferes with the binding of testosterone to sex hormone–binding globulin.[183] Spironolactone has been used successfully in dosages of 100 to 200 mg daily for the treatment of idiopathic hirsutism and hirsutism associated with polycystic ovarian disease (see Chaps. 96 and 101).[184] Because it has very little antigonadotropic activity, the spironolactone-induced decrease in androgen negative feedback causes compensatory increases in gonadotropin secretion that may reduce its long-term clinical efficacy. Spironolactone, in combination with dexamethasone or oral contraceptives (both of which suppress gonadotropin secretion), has been used in the management of unresponsive hirsutism.[185] Spironolactone has also been used in combination with testolactone and the GnRH agonist deslorelin to treat patients with familial male-limited precocious puberty.[186]

## CIMETIDINE

Cimetidine (see Fig. 119-3), a histamine $H_2$ receptor antagonist used primarily for the treatment of peptic ulcer disease, also has weak antiandrogenic action. Despite initial reports of its effectiveness in treating hirsute women, controlled trials have failed to support any significant benefit of cimetidine in the treatment of hirsutism.[187]

## KETOCONAZOLE

Ketoconazole is a synthetic, orally active, imidazole dioxolone derivative that is used in doses of 200 to 400 mg per day for the treatment of superficial and deep fungal infections. Although ketoconazole does not interact with the androgen receptor and therefore is not an antiandrogen, in high doses (>800 mg per day) it is a potent inhibitor of gonadal and adrenal steroidogenesis, inhibiting both 17α-hydroxylase and 17,20-desmolase activity[188,189] (see Chaps. 21 and 75). In a dosage of 400 mg every 8 hours, ketoconazole has been used with some success as a second-line agent to treat metastatic prostate cancer (see Chap. 225).[190,191] After an initial suppression to castrate levels, testosterone levels rise moderately, concomitant with the activation of feedback mechanisms, resulting in increased luteinizing hormone secretion. Combining ketoconazole with an antigonadotropic agent, such as a GnRH analog, may help to prevent this secondary rise in serum testosterone levels. Because adrenal steroid synthesis is inhibited, glucocorticoid replacement is needed in conjunction with the high dosages of ketoconazole used for the treatment of prostate cancer. Ketoconazole has also been used in lower dosages to treat hirsutism and, combined with a GnRH agonist, to treat male-limited precocious puberty.[192,193] The potential idiosyncratic hepatotoxicity of ketoconazole, however, although uncommon, limits its use in benign conditions.

## REFERENCES

1. Wilson JD. Charles-Edouard Brown-Sequard and the centennial of endocrinology. J Clin Endocrinol Metab 1990; 71:1403.
2. Bagatell CJ, Bremner WJ. Androgens in men—uses and abuses. N Engl J Med 1996; 334:707.
3. Bhasin S, Bremner WJ. Emerging issues in androgen replacement therapy. J Clin Endocrinol Metab 1997; 82:3.
4. Matsumoto AM. Androgen treatment of male hypogonadism. In: Bagdade JD, ed. 1998 Yearbook of endocrinology. St. Louis: Mosby, 1998:xix.
5. Daggett PR, Wheeler MJ, Nabarro JDN. Oral testosterone, a reappraisal. Horm Res 1978; 9:121.
6. Amory JK, Matsumoto AM. The therapeutic potential of testosterone patches. Exp Opin Invest Drugs 1998; 7:1977.
7. Findlay JC, Place VA, Snyder PJ. Treatment of primary hypogonadism in men with the transdermal administration of testosterone. J Clin Endocrinol Metab 1989; 68:369.
8. Place VA, Atkinson L, Prather DA, et al. Transdermal testosterone replacement through genital skin. In: Nieschlag E, Behre HM, eds. Testosterone: action, deficiency, substitution. Berlin: Springer-Verlag, 1990:165.
9. Meikle AW, Mazer NA, Moellmer JF, et al. Enhanced transdermal delivery of testosterone across nonscrotal skin produces physiological concentrations of testosterone and its metabolites in hypogonadal men. J Clin Endocrinol Metab 1992; 74:623.
10. Arver S, Dobs AS, Meikle AW, et al. Long-term efficacy and safety of a permeation-enhanced testosterone transdermal system in hypogonadal men. Clin Endocrinol (Oxf) 1997; 47:727.
11. Parker S, Armitage M. Experience with transdermal testosterone replacement therapy for hypogonadal men. Clin Endocrinol (Oxf) 1999; 50:57.
12. Jordan WP Jr. Allergy and topical irritation associated with transdermal testosterone administration: a comparison of scrotal and nonscrotal transdermal systems. Am J Contact Derm 1997; 8:108.
13. Yu A, Gupta SK, Hwang SS, et al. Transdermal testosterone administration in hypogonadal men: comparison of pharmacokinetics at different sites of application and at the first and fifth days of application. J Clin Pharmacol 1997; 37:1129.
14. Yu A, Gupta SK, Hwang SS, et al. Testosterone pharmacokinetics after application of an investigational transdermal system in hypogonadal men. J Clin Pharmacol 1997; 37:1139.
15. Jordan Jr WP, Atkinson LE, Lai C. Comparison of the skin irritation potential of two testosterone transdermal systems: an investigational system and a marketed product. Clin Ther 1998; 20:80.
16. De Sanctis V, Vullo C, Urso L, et al. Clinical experience with Androderm® testosterone transdermal system in hypogonadal adolescents and young men with β-thalassemia major. J Pediatr Endocrinol Metab 1998; 11:891.
17. Miller K, Corcoran C, Armstrong C, et al. Transdermal testosterone administration in women with acquired immunodeficiency syndrome wasting: a pilot study. J Clin Endocrinol Metab 1998; 83:2717.
18. Bhasin S, Storer TW, Asbel-Sethi N, et al. Effects of testosterone replacement with a nongenital, transdermal system, Androderm, in human immunodeficiency virus-infected men with low testosterone levels. J Clin Endocrinol Metab 1998; 83:3155.
19. Rolf C, Gottschalk I, Behre HM, et al. Pharmacokinetics of new testosterone transdermal therapeutic systems in gonadotropin-releasing hormone antagonist-suppressed normal men. Exp Clin Endocrinol Diabetes 1999; 107:63.
20. Buckler HM, Robertson WR, Wu FCW. Which androgen replacement for women? J Clin Endocrinol Metab 1998; 83:3920.
21. Swerdloff RS, Wang C, Cunningham G, et al. Long-term pharmacokinetics of transdermal testosterone gel versus testosterone patch in hypogonadal men [abstract]. In: Proceedings of The Endocrine Society 82nd Annual Meeting, Toronto, Ontario, Canada, June 21–24, 2000; 2347.
21a. Wang C, Swerdloff RS, Iranmanesh A, et al. Transdermal testosterone gel improves sexual function, mood, muscle strength, and body composition parameters in hypogonadal men. J Clin Endocrinol Metab 2000; in press.
21b. Wang C, Swerdloff RS, Iranmanesh A, et al. Effects of transdermal testosterone gel on bone turnover markers and bone mineral density in hypogonadal men [abstract]. In: Proceedings of The Endocrine Society 82nd Annual Meeting, Toronto, Ontario, Canada, June 21–24, 2000; 2348.
22. Conway AJ, Boylan LM, Howe C, et al. Randomized clinical trial of testosterone replacement therapy in hypogonadal men. Int J Androl 1988; 11:247.
23. Handelsman DJ, Conway AJ, Boylan LM. Pharmacokinetics and pharmacodynamics of testosterone pellets in man. J Clin Endocrinol Metab 1990; 71:216.
24. Jockenhovel F, Vogel E, Kreutzer M, et al. Pharmacokinetics and pharmacodynamics of subcutaneous testosterone implants in hypogonadal men. Clin Endocrinol (Oxf) 1996; 45:61.
25. Handelsman DJ, Mackey M-A, Howe C, et al. An analysis of testosterone implants for androgen replacement therapy. Clin Endocrinol (Oxf) 1997; 47:311.
26. Stuenkel CA, Dudley RE, Yen SSC. Sublingual administration of testosterone-hydroxypropyl-β-cyclodextrin inclusion complex simulates episodic androgen release in hypogonadal men. J Clin Endocrinol Metab 1991; 72:1054.
27. Salehian B, Wang C, Alexander G, et al. Pharmacokinetics, bioefficacy, and safety of sublingual testosterone cyclodextrin in hypogonadal men: comparison to testosterone enanthate—a clinical research center study. J Clin Endocrinol Metab 1995; 80:3567.
28. Wang C, Eyre DR, Clark R, et al. Sublingual testosterone replacement improves muscle mass and strength, decreases bone resorption, and increases bone formation markers in hypogonadal men—a clinical research center study. J Clin Endocrinol Metab 1996; 81:3654.
29. Dobs AS, Hoover DR, Chen M-C, Allen R. Pharmacokinetic characteristics, efficacy, and safety of buccal testosterone in hypogonadal males: a pilot study. J Clin Endocrinol Metab 1998; 83:33.
30. Ben-Galim E, Hillman RE, Weldon VV. Topically applied testosterone and phallic growth. Am J Dis Child 1980; 134:296.
31. Klugo RC, Cerny JC. Response of micropenis to topical testosterone and gonadotropin. J Urol 1978; 119:667.
32. Bracco GL, Carli P, Sonni L, et al. Clinical and histologic effects of topical treatments of vulval lichen sclerosus. A critical evaluation. J Reprod Med 1993; 38:37.
33. Bornstein J, Heifetz S, Kellner Y, et al. Clobetasol dipropionate 0.05% versus testosterone propionate 2% topical application for severe vulvar lichen sclerosus. Am J Obstet Cynecol 1998; 178:80.
34. Bhasin S, Swerdloff RS, Steiner B, et al. A biodegradable testosterone microcapsule formulation provides uniform eugonadal levels of testosterone for 10-11 weeks in hypogonadal men. J Clin Endocrinol Metab 1992; 74:75.
35. Snyder PJ, Lawrence DA. Treatment of male hypogonadism with testosterone enanthate. J Clin Endocrinol Metab 1980; 51:1335.
36. Skakkebaek NE, Bancroft J, Davidson DW, Warner P. Androgen replacement with oral testosterone undecanoate in hypogonadal men: a double-blind controlled study. Clin Endocrinol (Oxf) 1981; 14:49.
37. Butler GE, Sellar RF, Walker RF, et al. Oral testosterone undecanoate in the management of delayed puberty in boys: pharmacokinetics and effects on sexual maturation and growth. J Clin Endocrinol Metab 1992; 75:37.
38. Gooren LJG. A ten year safety study of the oral androgen testosterone undecanoate. J Androl 1994; 15:212.
39. Zhang G-Y, Gu Y-Q, Wang X-H, et al. A pharmacokinetic study of injectable testosterone undecanoate in hypogonadal men. J Androl 1998; 19:761.
40. Behre HM, Abshagen K, Oettel M, et al. Intramuscular injection of testosterone undecanoate for the treatment of male hypogonadism: phase I studies. Eur J Endocrinol 1999; 140:414.
41. Behre HM, Nieschlag E. Testosterone buciclate (20 Aet-1) in hypogonadal men: pharmacokinetics and pharmacodynamics of the new long-acting androgen ester. J Clin Endocrinol Metab 1992; 75:1204.
42. Minto CF, Howe C, Wishart S, et al. Pharmacokinetics and pharmacodynamics of nandrolone esters in oil vehicle: effects of ester, injection site and injection volume. J Pharmacol Exp Ther 1997; 281:93.
43. Luisi M, Franchi F. Double blind group comparative study of testosterone undecanoate and mesterolone in hypogonadal male patients. J Endocrinol Invest 1980; 3:305.
44. Schaison G, Nahoul G, Couzinet B. Percutaneous dihydrotestosterone system. In: Nieschlag E, Behre HM, eds. Testosterone: action, deficiency and substitution. Berlin: Springer Verlag, 1990:155.
45. Mendonca BB, Inacio M, Costa EM, et al. Male pseudohermaphroditism due to steroid 5alpha-reductase 2 deficiency. Diagnosis, psychological evaluation, and management. Medicine 1996; 75:64.
46. Choi SK, Han SW, Kim DH, de Lignieres B. Transdermal dihydrotestosterone therapy and its effects on patients with microphallus. J Urol 1993; 150:657.
47. de Lignieres B. Transdermal dihydrotestosterone treatment of "andropause." Ann Med 1993; 25:235.
48. Wang C, Iranmanesh A, Berman N, et al. Comparative pharmacokinetics of three doses of percutaneous dihydrotestosterone gel in healthy elderly men—a clinical research center study. J Clin Endocrinol Metab 1998; 83:2749.

49. Swerdloff RS, Wang C. Dihydrotestosterone: a rationale for its use as a non-aromatizable androgen replacement therapeutic agent. Baillières Clin Endocrinol Metab 1998; 12:501.
50. Cummings DE, Kumar N, Bardin CW, et al. Prostate-sparing effects in primates of the potent androgen 7α-methyl-19-nortestosterone: a potential alternative to testosterone for androgen replacement and male contraception. J Clin Endocrinol Metab 1998; 83:4212.
51. Anderson RA, Martin CW, Kung AW, et al. 7α-methyl-19-nortestosterone maintains sexual behavior and mood in hypogonadal men. J Clin Endocrinol Metab 1999; 84:3356.
52. Edwards JP, West SJ, Pooley CLF, et al. New nonsteroidal androgen receptor modulators based on 4-(trifluoromethyl)-2(1H)-pyrrolidino[3,2-g]quinolone. Bioorg Med Chem Lett 1998; 8:745.
53. Matsumoto AM. The testis. In: Bennett JC, Plum F, eds. Cecil textbook of medicine, 20th ed. Philadelphia: WB Saunders, 1996:1325.
54. Burstein S, Grumbach MM, Kaplan SL. Early determination of androgen responsiveness is important in the management of microphallus. Lancet 1979; 2:983.
55. Tsur H, Shafir R, Shachar J, Eshkol A. Microphallic hypospadias: testosterone therapy prior to surgical repair. Br J Plast Surg 1983; 36:398.
56. Matsumoto AM. Hormonal therapy of male hypogonadism. Endocrinol Metab Clin North Am 1994; 23:857.
57. Davidson JM, Kwan M, Greenleaf W. Hormonal replacement and sexuality in men. Clin Endocrinol Metab 1982; 11:599.
58. Burris AS, Banks SM, Carter CS, et al. A long-term prospective study of the physiologic and behavioral effects of hormone replacement in untreated hypogonadal men. J Androl 1992; 13:297.
59. Bagatell CJ, Heiman JR, Rivier JE, Bremner WJ. Effects of endogenous testosterone and estradiol on sexual behavior in normal young men. J Clin Endocrinol Metab 1994; 78:711.
60. Wang C, Alexander G, Berman N, et al. Testosterone replacement therapy improves mood in hypogonadal men—a clinical research center study. J Clin Endocrinol Metab 1996; 81:3578.
61. Janowsky JL, Oviatt SK, Orwoll ES. Testosterone influences spatial cognition in older men. Behav Neurosci 1994; 108:325.
62. Alexander GM, Swerdloff RS, Wang C, et al. Androgen-behavior correlations in hypogonadal and eugonadal men. II. Cognitive abilities. Horm Behav 1998; 33:85.
63. Leibenluft E, Schmidt PJ, Turner EH, et al. Effects of leuprolide-induced hypogonadism and testosterone replacement on sleep, melatonin, and prolactin secretion in men. J Clin Endocrinol Metab 1997; 82:3203.
64. Katznelson L, Finkelstein JS, Schoenfeld DA, et al. Increase in bone density and lean body mass during testosterone administration in men with acquired hypogonadism. J Clin Endocrinol Metab 1996; 81:4358.
65. Bhasin S, Storer TW, Berman N, et al. Testosterone replacement increases fat-free mass and muscle size in hypogonadal men. J Clin Endocrinol Metab 1997; 82:407.
66. Behre HM, Kliesch S, Leifke E, et al. Long-term effect of testosterone therapy on bone mineral density in hypogonadal men. J Clin Endocrinol Metab 1997; 82:2386.
67. Marin P, Arver S. Androgens and abdominal obesity. Baillières Clin Endocrinol Metab 1998; 12:441.
68. Bagatell CJ, Knopp RH, Vale WW, et al. Physiologic testosterone levels in normal men suppress high-density lipoprotein cholesterol levels. Ann Intern Med 1992; 116:967.
69. Zgliczynski S, Ossowski M, Slowinska-Srzednicka J, et al. Effect of testosterone replacement therapy on lipids and lipoproteins in hypogonadal and elderly men. Atherosclerosis 1996; 121:35.
70. Bagatell CJ, Bremner WJ. Androgen and progestogen effects on plasma lipids. Prog Cardiovasc Dis 1995; 38:255.
71. English KM, Steeds R, Jones TH, Channer KS. Testosterone and coronary heart disease: is there a link? QJM 1997; 90:787.
72. Shahidi NT. Androgens and erythropoiesis. N Engl J Med 1973; 289:72.
73. Ammus SS. The role of androgens in the treatment of hematologic disorders. Adv Intern Med 1989; 34:191.
74. Jockenhovel F, Vogel E, Reinhardt W, Reinwein D. Effects of various modes of androgen substitution therapy on erythropoiesis. Eur J Med Res 1997; 2:293.
75. Kulin HE. Delayed puberty in boys. Curr Ther Endocrinol Metab 1997; 6:346.
76. Houchin LD, Rogol AD. Androgen replacement in children with constitutional delay of puberty: the case for aggressive therapy. Baillières Clin Endocrinol Metab 1998; 12:427.
77. Aynsley-Green A, Zachman M, Prader A. Interrelation of the therapeutic effects of growth hormone and testosterone on growth in hypopituitarism. J Pediatr 1976; 89:992.
78. Parker MW, Johanson AJ, Rogol AD, et al. Effect of testosterone on somatomedin C concentrations in prepubertal boys. J Clin Endocrinol Metab 1984; 58:87.
79. Veldhuis JD, Metzger DL, Martha PM Jr, et al. Estrogen and testosterone, but not non-aromatizable androgen, direct network integration of the hypothalamo-somatotrope (growth hormone)-insulin-like growth factor I axis in the human: evidence from pubertal pathophysiology and sex-steroid hormone replacement. J Clin Endocrinol Metab 1997; 82:3414.
80. Hendler ED, Goffinet JA, Ross S, et al. Controlled study of androgen therapy in anemia of patients on maintenance hemodialysis. N Engl J Med 1974; 291:1046.
81. Neff MS, Goldberg J, Slifkin RF, et al. A comparison of androgens for anemia in patients on hemodialysis. N Engl J Med 1981; 304:871.
82. Teruel JL, Aguilera A, Marcen R, et al. Androgen therapy for chronic renal failure. Indications in the erythropoietin era. Scand J Urol Nephrol 1996; 30:403.
83. Teruel JL, Marcen R, Navarro-Antolin J, et al. Androgen versus erythropoietin for the treatment of anemia in hemodialyzed patients: a prospective study. J Am Soc Nephrol 1996; 7:140.
84. Ballal SH, Domoto DT, Polack DC, et al. Androgens potentiate the effects of erythropoietin in the treatment of anemia of end-stage renal disease. Am J Kidney Dis 1991; 17:29.
85. Gaughan WJ, Liss KA, Dunn SR, et al. A 6-month study of low-dose recombinant human erythropoietin alone and in combination with androgens for the treatment of anemia in chronic hemodialysis patients. Am J Kidney Dis 1997; 30:495.
86. Van Hengstrum M, Steenbergen J, Haanen C. Clinical course in 28 unselected patients with aplastic anemia treated with anabolic steroids. Br J Haematol 1979; 41:323.
87. Branda RF, Amsden TW, Jacob HS. Randomized study of nandrolone therapy for anemias due to bone marrow failure. Arch Intern Med 1977; 137:65.
88. Camitta BM, Thomas ED, Nathan DG, et al. A prospective study of androgens and bone marrow transplantation for treatment of severe aplastic anemia. Blood 1979; 53:504.
89. Harrington WJ Sr, Kolodny L, Horstman LL, et al. Danazol therapy for paroxysmal nocturnal hemoglobinuria. Am J Hematol 1997; 54:149.
90. Ahn YS. Efficacy of danazol in hematologic disorders. Acta Hematol 1990; 84:122.
91. Guthrie RD, Smith DW, Graham CB. Testosterone treatment of micropenis during early childhood. J Pediatr 1973; 83:247.
92. Gearhart JP, Jeffs RD. The use of parenteral testosterone therapy in genital reconstructive surgery. J Urol 1987; 138:1077.
93. Price P, Wass JAH, Griffin JE, et al. High-dose androgen therapy in male pseudohermaphroditism due to 5 α-reductase deficiency and disorders of the androgen receptor. J Clin Invest 1984; 74:1496.
94. Frank MM, Gelfand JA, Atkinson JP. Hereditary angioedema: the clinical syndrome and its management. Ann Intern Med 1976; 84:580.
95. Barbosa J, Seal US, Doe RP. Effects of anabolic steroids on haptoglobin, orosomucoid, plasminogen, fibrinogen, ceruloplasmin α1 antitrypsin, β-glucuronidase, and total serum proteins. J Clin Endocrinol Metab 1971; 33:388.
96. Madanes AE, Farber M. Danazol. Ann Intern Med 1982; 96:625.
97. Zurlo JJ, Frank MM. The long-term safety of danazol in women with hereditary angioedema. Fertil Steril 1990; 54:64.
98. Allegra JC. Rationale approaches to the hormonal treatment of breast cancer. Semin Oncol 1983; 10(Suppl 4):25.
99. Katznelson L. Therapeutic role of androgens in the treatment of osteoporosis in men. Baillières Clin Endocrinol Metab 1998; 12:453.
100. Finkelstein JS, Klibanski A, Neer RM, et al. Increases in bone density during treatment of men with idiopathic hypogonadotropic hypogonadism. J Clin Endocrinol Metab 1989; 69:776.
101. Finkelstein JS, Neer RM, Biller BM, et al. Osteopenia in men with a history of delayed puberty. N Engl J Med 1992; 326:600.
102. Anderson FH, Francis RH, Faulkner K. Androgen supplementation in eugonadal men with osteoporosis—effects of six months' treatment on bone mineral density and cardiovascular risk factors. Bone 1996; 18:171.
103. Reid IR, Wattie DJ, Evans MC, Stapleton JP. Testosterone therapy in glucocorticoid-treated men. Arch Intern Med 1996; 156:1173.
104. Savvas M, Studd JW, Norman S, et al. Increase in bone mass after one year of percutaneous oestradiol and testosterone implants in post-menopausal women who have previously received long-term oral oestrogens. Br J Obstet Gynaecol 1992; 99:757.
105. Davis SR, McCloud P, Strauss BJ, Burger H. Testosterone enhances estradiol's effects on post-menopausal bone density and sexuality. Maturitas 1995; 21:227.
106. Watts NB, Notelovitz M, Timmons MC, et al. Comparison of oral estrogens and estrogens plus androgen on bone mineral density, menopausal symptoms, and lipid-liporotein profiles in surgical menopause. Obstet Gynecol 1995; 85:529.
107. Barrett-Connor E. Efficacy and safety of estrogen/androgen therapy. Menopausal symptoms, bone, and cardiovascular parameters. J Reprod Med 1998; 43(Suppl 8):746.
108. Need AG, Horowitz M, Bridges A, et al. Effects of nandrolone decanoate and antiresorptive therapy on vertebral density in osteoporotic post-menopausal women. Arch Intern Med 1989; 149:57.
109. Passeri M, Pedrazzoni M, Pioli G, et al. Effects of nandrolone decanoate on bone mass in established osteoporosis. Maturitas 1993; 17:211.
110. Studd J, Arnala I, Kicovic PM, et al. A randomized study of tibolone on bone mineral density in osteoporotic post-menopausal women with previous fractures. Obstet Gynecol 1998; 92:574.
111. Chesnut CH, Ivey JL, Gruber HE, et al. Stanozolol in post-menopausal osteoporosis: therapeutic efficacy and possible mechanisms of action. Metabolism 1983; 32:571.
112. Davis SR, Burger HG. The rationale for physiological testosterone replacement in women. Baillières Clin Endocrinol Metab 1998; 12:391.
113. Burger HG, Hailes J, Menelaus M, et al. The management of persistent menopausal symptoms with oestradiol-testosterone implants: clinical, lipid and hormonal results. Maturitas 1984; 6:351.
114. Sherwin BB, Gelfand MM, Brender W. Androgen enhances sexual motivation in females: a prospective, crossover study of sex steroid administration in the surgical menopause. Psychosom Med 1985; 47:339.
115. Tenover JS. Androgen administration to aging men. Endocrinol Metab Clin North Am 1994; 23:877.

116. Bhasin S, Bagatell CJ, Bremner WJ, et al. Issues in testosterone replacement in older men. J Clin Endocrinol Metab 1998; 83:3435.

117. Tenover JS. Effects of testosterone supplementation in the aging male. J Clin Endocrinol Metab 1992; 75:536.

118. Sih R, Morley JE, Kaiser FE, et al. Testosterone replacement in older hypogonadal men: a 12-month randomized controlled trial. J Clin Endocrinol Metab 1997; 82:1661.

119. Hajjar RR, Kaiser FE, Morley JE. Outcomes of long-term testosterone replacement in older hypogonadal males: a retrospective analysis. J Clin Endocrinol Metab 1997; 82:3793.

119a. Snyder PJ, Peachey H, Hannoush P, et al. Effect of testosterone treatment on bone mineral density in men over 65 years of age. J Clin Endocrinol Metab 1999; 84:1966.

119b. Snyder PJ, Peachey H, Hannoush P, et al. Effect of testosterone treatment on body composition and muscle strength in men over 65 years of age. J Clin Endocrinol Metab 1999; 84:2647.

120. Bhasin S, Storer TW, Berman N, et al. The effects of supraphysiologic doses of testosterone on muscle size and strength in normal men. N Engl J Med 1996; 335:1.

121. Bross R, Casaburi R, Storer TW, Bhasin S. Androgen effects on body composition and muscle function: implications for the use of androgens as anabolic agents in sarcopenic states. Baillières Clin Endocrinol Metab 1998; 12:365.

122. Coodley GO, Coodley MK. A trial of testosterone therapy for HIV-associated weight loss. AIDS 1997; 11:1347.

123. Grinspoon S, Corcoran C, Askari H, et al. Effects of androgens in men with AIDS wasting syndrome. A randomized, double-blind, placebo-controlled trial. Ann Intern Med 1998; 129:18.

124. Rabkin JG, Wagner GJ, Rabkin R. Testosterone therapy for human immunodeficiency virus-positive men with and without hypogonadism. J Clin Psychopharmacol 1999; 19:19.

125. Sattler FR, Jaque SV, Schroder ET, et al. Effects of pharmacological doses of nandrolone decanoate and progressive resistance training in immunodeficient patients infected with human immunodeficiency virus. J Clin Endocrinol Metab 1999; 84:1268.

126. Strawford A, Barbieri T, Van Loan M, et al. Resistance exercise and supraphysiological androgen therapy in eugonadal men with HIV-related weight loss. JAMA 1999; 281:1282.

127. Corcoran C, Grinspoon S. Treatments for wasting in patients with the acquired immunodeficiency syndrome. N Engl J Med 1999; 340:1740.

127a. Bhasin S, Storer TW, Javanbakht M, et al. Testosterone replacement and resistance exercise in HIV-infected men with weight loss and low testosterone levels. JAMA 2000; 283:763.

128. Johansen KL, Mulligan K, Schambelan M. Anabolic effects of nandrolone decanoate in patients receiving dialysis. A randomized controlled trial. JAMA 1999; 281:1275.

129. Schols AM, Soeters PB, Mostert R, et al. Physiological effects of nutritional support and anabolic steroids in patients with chronic obstruction pulmonary disease. A placebo-controlled randomized trial. Am J Respir Crit Care Med 1995; 152:1268.

130. Ferreira IM, Verreschil T, Nery LE, et al. The influence of 6 months of oral anabolic steroids on body mass and respiratory muscles in undernourished COPD patients. Chest 1998; 114:19.

131. Demling RH, DeSanti L. Oxandrolone, an anabolic steroid, significantly increases the rate of weight gain in the recovery phase after major burns. J Trauma 1997; 43:47.

132. Zachwieja JJ, Smith SR, Lovejoy JC, et al. Testosterone administration preserves protein balance but not muscle strength during 28 days of bed rest. J Clin Endocrinol Metab 1999; 84:207.

133. Amory JK, Bremner WJ. The use of testosterone as a male contraceptive. Baillières Clin Endocrinol Metab 1998; 12:471.

134. Lesser MA. Testosterone propionate therapy in one hundred cases of angina pectoris. J Clin Endocrinol 1946; 6:549.

135. Jaffe MD. Effect of testosterone cypionate on postexercise ST segment depression. Br Heart J 1977; 39:1217.

136. Rosano GMC, Leonardo F, Pagnotta P, et al. Acute anti-ischemic effect of testosterone in men with coronary artery disease. Circulation 1999; 99:1666.

137. Webb CM, Adamson DL, de Zeigler D, Collins P. Effect of acute testosterone on myocardial ischemia in men with coronary artery disease. Am J Cardiol 1999; 83:437.

137a. Webb CM, McNeill JG, Hayward CS, et al. Effects of testosterone on coronary vasomotor regulation in men with coronary artery disease. Circulation 1999; 100:1690.

138. Wilson JD. Androgen abuse by athletes. Endocr Rev 1988; 9:181.

139. Yesalis CE, Bahrke MS. Anabolic-androgenic steroids. Current issues. Sports Med 1995; 19:326.

140. American Academy of Pediatrics. Committee on Sports Medicine and Fitness. Adolescents and anabolic steroids: a subject review. Pediatrics 1997; 99:904.

141. Haupt HA, Rovere GD. Anabolic steroids: a review of the literature. Am J Sports Med 1984; 12:469.

142. Wu FC. Endocrine aspects of anabolic steroids. Clin Chem 1997; 43:1289.

143. Sullivan ML, Martinez CM, Gennis P, Gallagher EJ. The cardiac toxicity of anabolic steroids. Prog Cardiovasc Dis 1998; 41:1.

144. Porcerelli JH, Sandler BA. Anabolic-androgenic steroid abuse and psychopathology. Psychiatr Clin North Am 1998; 21:829.

145. Webb OL, Laskarzewski PM, Glueck CJ. Severe depression of high-density lipoprotein cholesterol levels in weight lifters and body builders by self-administered exogenous testosterone and anabolic-androgenic steroids. Metabolism 1984; 33:971.

146. Thompson PD, Cullinane EM, Sady SP, et al. Contrasting effects of testosterone and stanozolol on serum lipoprotein levels. JAMA 1989; 261:1165.

147. Glazer G. Atherogenic effects of anabolic steroids on serum lipid levels. Arch Intern Med 1991; 151:1925.

148. Labrie F, Belanger A, Luu-The V, et al. DHEA and the intracrine formation of androgens and estrogens in peripheral tissues: its role during aging. Steroids 1998; 63:322.

149. Nippoldt TB, Nair KS. Is there a case for DHEA replacement? Baillières Clin Endocrinol Metab 1998; 12:507.

150. Morales AJ, Haubrich RH, Hwang JY, et al. The effect of six months of treatment with a 100 mg daily dose of dehydroepiandrosterone (DHEA) on circulating sex steroids, body composition and muscle strength in age-advanced men and women. Clin Endocrinol (Oxf) 1998; 49:421.

151. Gordon CM, Grace E, Jean Emans S, et al. Changes in bone turnover markers and menstrual function after short-term oral DHEA in young women with anorexia nervosa. J Bone Miner Res 1999; 14:136.

152. Flynn MA, Weaver-Osterholtz D, Sharpe-Timms KL, et al. Dehydroepiandrosterone replacement in aging humans. J Clin Endocrinol Metab 1999; 84:1527.

152a. Baulieu EE, Thomas G, Legrain S, et al. Dehydroepiandrosterone (DHEA), DHEA sulfate, and aging: contribution of the DHEAge Study to a sociobiomedical issue. Proc Natl Acad Sci U S A 2000; 97:4279.

152b. Arlt W, Callies F, van Vlijmen JC, et al. Dehydroepiandrosterone replacement in women with adrenal insufficiency. N Engl J Med 1999; 341:1013.

153. King DS, Sharp RL, Vukovich MD, et al. Effect of oral androstenedione on serum testosterone and adaptations to resistance training in young men. A randomized controlled trial. JAMA 1999; 281:2020.

153a. Leder BZ, Longcope C, Catlin DH, et al. Oral androstenedione administration and serum testosterone concentrations in young men. JAMA 2000; 283:779.

154. Bettman HK, Goldman HS, Abramowicz M, Sobel EH. Oxandrolone treatment of short stature: effect on predicted mature height. J Pediatr 1971; 79:1018.

155. Binder D, Grauer ML, Wehner AV, et al. Outcome in tall stature. Final height and psychological aspects in 220 patients with and without treatment. Eur J Pediatr 1997; 156:905.

156. Rolf C, Nieschlag E. Potential adverse effects of long-term testosterone therapy. Baillières Clin Endocrinol Metab 1998; 12:521.

157. Wang C, Alexander G, Berman N, et al. Testosterone replacement therapy improves mood in hypogonadal men—a clinical research center study. J Clin Endocrinol Metab 1996; 81:3578.

158. Tricker R, Casaburi R, Storer TW, et al. The effects of supraphysiological doses of testosterone on angry behavior in healthy eugonadal men—a clinical research center study. J Clin Endocrinol Metab 1996; 81:3754.

159. Behre HM, Bohmeyer J, Nieschlag E. Prostate volume in testosterone-treated and untreated hypogonadal men in comparison to age-matched normal controls. Clin Endocrinol (Oxf) 1994; 40:341.

160. Jackson JA, Waxman J, Spiekerman AM. Prostatic complications of testosterone replacement therapy. Arch Intern Med 1989; 149:2365.

161. Matsumoto AM, Sandblom RE, Schoene RB, et al. Testosterone replacement in hypogonadal men: effects on obstructive sleep apnoea, respiratory drives, and sleep. Clin Endocrinol (Oxf) 1985; 22:713.

162. Schneider BK, Pickett CK, Zwillich CW, et al. Influence of testosterone on breathing during sleep. J Appl Physiol 1986; 61:618.

163. Matsumoto AM. Effects of chronic testosterone administration in normal men: safety and efficacy of high dosage testosterone and parallel dose-dependent suppression of luteinizing hormone, follicle-stimulating hormone, and sperm production. J Clin Endocrinol Metab 1990; 70:282.

164. Ishak KG, Zimmerman HJ. Hepatotoxic effects of anabolic/androgenic steroids. Semin Liver Dis 1987; 7:230.

165. Geller J. Megestrol acetate plus low-dose estrogen in the management of advanced prostatic carcinoma. Urol Clin North Am 1991; 18:83.

166. Ottery FD, Walsh D, Strawford A. Pharmacologic management of anorexia/cachexia. Semin Oncol 1998; 25(Suppl 6):35.

167. Loprinzi CL, Michalak JC, Quella SK, et al. Megestrol acetate for the prevention of hot flashes. N Engl J Med 1994; 331:347.

168. Grinspoon S, Corcoran C, Lee K, et al. Loss of lean body and muscle mass with androgen levels in hypogonadal men with acquired immunodeficiency syndrome and wasting. J Clin Endocrinol Metab 1996; 81:4051.

169. Subramanian S, Goker H, Kanji A, Sweeney H. Clinical adrenal insufficiency in patients receiving megestrol therapy. Arch Intern Med 1997; 157:1008.

170. Mann M, Koller E, Murgo A, et al. Glucocorticoidlike activity of megestrol. A summary of Food and Drug Administration experience and a review of the literature. Arch Intern Med 1997; 157:1651.

171. Neumann F. The antiandrogen cyproterone acetate: discovery, chemistry, basic pharmacology, clinical use and tool in basic research. Exp Clin Endocrinol (Oxf) 1994; 102:1.

172. Barradell LB, Faulds D. Cyproterone acetate. A review of its pharmacology and therapeutic efficacy in prostate cancer. Drugs Aging 1994; 5:59.

173. Lopez M. Cyproterone acetate in the treatment of metastatic cancer of the male breast. Cancer 1985; 55:2334.

174. Shaw JC. Antiandrogen and hormonal treatment of acne. Dermatol Clin 1996; 14:803.

175. Barth JH, Cherry CA, Wojnarowska F, et al. Cyproterone acetate for severe hirsutism: results of a double-blind dose-ranging study. Clin Endocrinol (Oxf) 1991; 35:5.

176. Meriggiola MC, Bremner WJ, Paulsen CA, et al. A combined regimen of cyproterone acetate and testosterone enanthate as a potentially highly effective male contraceptive. J Clin Endocrinol Metab 1996; 81:3018.

177. Goktas S, Crawford ED. Optimal hormonal therapy for advanced prostate carcinoma. Semin Oncol 1999; 26:162.

178. Eisenberger MA, Blumenstein BA, Crawford ED, et al. Bilateral orchidectomy with of without flutamide for metastatic prostate cancer. N Engl J Med 1998; 339:1036.

179. Cusan L, Dupont A, Gomez J-L, et al. Comparison of flutamide and spironolactone in the treatment of hirsutism: a randomized controlled trial. Fertil Steril 1994; 61:281.

180. Muderris II, Bayram F. Clinical efficacy of lower dose flutamide 125 mg/day in the treatment of hirsutism. J Endocrinol Invest 1999; 22:165.

181. Goa KL, Spencer CM. Bicalutamide in advanced prostate cancer. A review. Drugs Aging 1998; 12:401.

182. Dole EJ, Holdsworth MT. Nilutamide: an antiandrogen for the treatment of prostate cancer. Ann Pharmacother 1997; 31:65.

183. Givens J. Treatment of hirsutism with spironolactone. Fertil Steril 1985; 43:841.

184. Jeffcoate W. The treatment of women with hirsutism. Clin Endocrinol (Oxf) 1993; 39:143.

185. Pittaway DE, Maxson WS, Wentz AC. Spironolactone in combination drug therapy for unresponsive hirsutism. Fertil Steril 1985; 43:878.

186. Werber Leschek E, Jones J, Barnes KM, et al. Six-year results of spironolactone and testolactone treatment of familial male-limited precocious puberty with addition of deslorelin after central puberty onset. J Clin Endocrinol Metab 1999; 84:175.

187. Lissak A, Sorpkin Y, Calderon I, et al. Treatment of hirsutism with cimetidine: a prospective randomized controlled trial. Fertil Steril 1989; 51:247.

188. Pont A, Graybill JR, Craven PC, et al. High-dose ketoconazole therapy and adrenal and testicular function in humans. Arch Intern Med 1984; 144:2150.

189. Rajfer J, Sikka SC, Rivera F, Handelsman DJ. Mechanism of inhibition of human testicular steroidogenesis by oral ketoconazole. J Clin Endocrinol Metab 1986; 63:1193.

190. Small EJ, Vogelzong NJ. Second-line hormonal therapy for advanced prostate cancer: a shifting paradigm. J Clin Oncol 1997; 15:382.

191. Bok RA, Small EJ. The treatment of advanced prostate cancer with ketoconazole: safety issues. Drug Saf 1999; 20:451.

192. Venturoli S, Marescalchi O, Colombo FM, et al. A prospective randomized trial comparing low dose flutamide, finasteride, ketoconazole, and cyproterone acetate-estrogen regimens in the treatment of hirsutism. J Clin Endocrinol Metab 1999; 84:1304.

193. Holland FJ, Kirsch SE, Selby R. Gonadotropin-independent precocious puberty ("testotoxicosis"): influence of maturational status on response to ketoconazole. J Clin Endocrinol Metab 1987; 64:328.

# CHAPTER 120

# GYNECOMASTIA

ALLAN R. GLASS

## GENERAL CONSIDERATIONS

Gynecomastia (enlargement of the male breast secondary to an increase in glandular tissue and stroma) can be a vexing clinical problem.[1-3] Often, it is a benign finding, but sometimes it is an important clue to disease elsewhere[4] (Table 120-1). Thus, the condition cannot be dismissed as a simple cosmetic defect, although, in a substantial number of cases, no underlying cause is ever found.

On physical examination, it is necessary to distinguish between *pseudogynecomastia*, which is breast enlargement caused by increased adipose tissue, and *true gynecomastia* (Fig. 120-1). In the latter condition, there is enlargement of the mammae. The glandular tissue can be palpated as radially arranged cords, usually around the nipple, and may form a discrete button-like mass or merge gradually with the surrounding adipose tissue. The areolae may be enlarged and convex, and the small areolar glands (glands of Montgomery) often are prominent. Frequently, the mammary papilla or nipple is enlarged and protuberant (Fig. 120-2). Breast tenderness (mastodynia) may be present, particu-

**TABLE 120-1.**
**Causes of Gynecomastia**

**PHYSIOLOGIC**
  Neonatal
  Pubertal
  Senescent
**NEOPLASMS**
  Steroid-producing (adrenal, testis)
  Human chorionic gonadotropin–producing (especially testis and lung)
**DRUGS**
  (see Table 120-2)
**CONGENITAL DISORDERS**
  Klinefelter syndrome and variants
  Anorchia (vanishing testis syndrome)
  Cryptorchidism
  Defects in enzymes of testosterone biosynthesis
  Defects in androgen action
  True hermaphroditism
**ACQUIRED TESTICULAR DAMAGE**
  Surgery
  Trauma
  Irradiation
  Infection (mumps and other viruses, leprosy)
**ENVIRONMENTAL**
  Phytoestrogens
  Hepatotoxic agents
**SYSTEMIC DISORDERS**
  Renal failure
  Hepatitis
  Cirrhosis
  Thyrotoxicosis
**MISCELLANEOUS**
  Spinal cord injury
  Myotonic dystrophy
  Refeeding after starvation
  Increased aromatization of androgens
  Psychological stress
  Human immunodeficiency virus infection
  Chest wall trauma

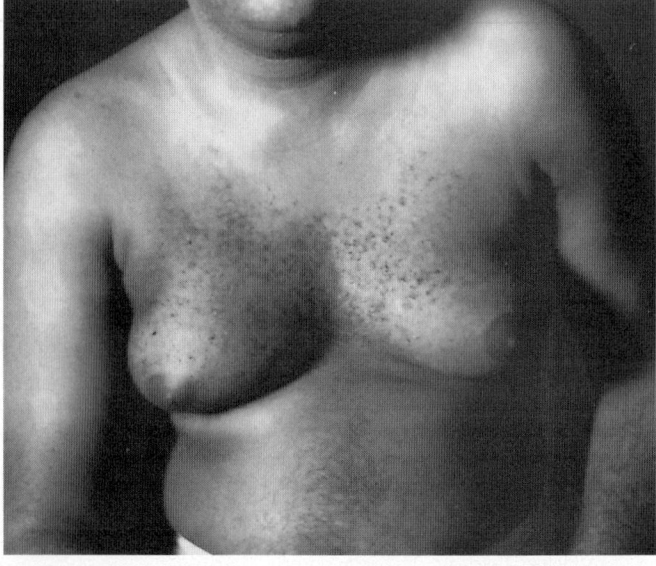

**FIGURE 120-1.** Gynecomastia in 30-year-old man who had unilateral testicular atrophy after postpubertal mumps orchitis.

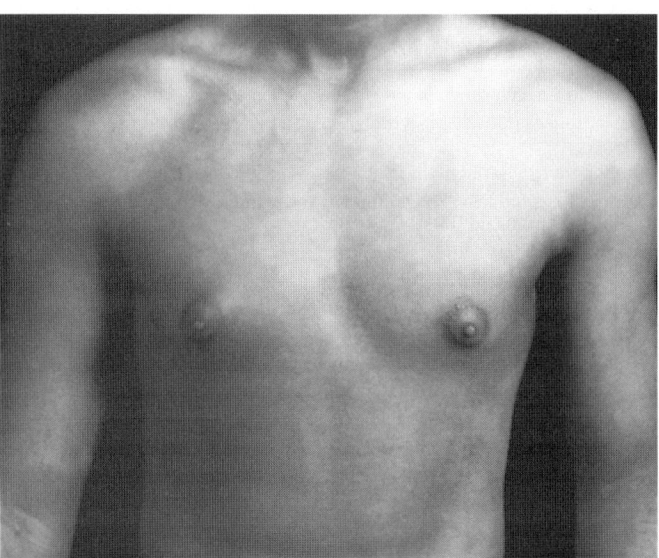

**FIGURE 120-2.** Gynecomastia in 36-year-old man with renal failure. Note enlarged and convex areolae and protuberant nipples.

larly if the onset is recent. Although commonly bilateral and symmetric, gynecomastia of any cause may be unilateral or markedly asymmetric, either initially or throughout its course (Fig. 120-3).

Histologically, there may be hyperplasia of the epithelial or stromal cells or an increase in fibrous tissue. The appearance tends to correlate with the duration of the condition (Fig. 120-4). Thus, gynecomastia of more recent onset tends to show cellular hyperplasia that, over time, progresses to increased fibrous tissue without increased cellularity, including new induction of type VI collagen.[5-7] This increase in fibrous tissue explains why long-standing gynecomastia is so difficult to treat by nonsurgical means.

Because so many conditions can cause gynecomastia, it is not unusual to encounter the condition clinically. In addition, several studies have reported a high prevalence of gynecomastia in the normal population (>40% of young, healthy men[8]) and in hospitalized patients.[1] Often, gynecomastia represents the quiescent residual enlargement attributable to a condition that is no longer present.

# HORMONAL CONTEXT OF GYNECOMASTIA

Given the long-recognized role of estrogens in stimulating mammary growth, it is not surprising that high circulating estrogen levels of exogenous or endogenous origin can be associated with gynecomastia. More recently, however, gynecomastia has been noted in disorders with deficient androgen production even when estrogen production is normal, leading to the concept that gynecomastia often may be related to increases in the circulating estrogen/androgen ratio rather than to absolute increases in estrogen per se. Finally, the occurrence of gynecomastia in conditions in which the androgen sensitivity of peripheral target tissues is reduced, even without significant changes in circulating androgens or estrogens, has refined this concept to suggest that gynecomastia is related to the resultant estrogen/androgen ratio effect at the breast. Although experimental evidence is inconclusive, this has proved to be a useful framework for evaluating gynecomastia.

In men, the principal circulating androgenic activity resides in testosterone, which originates almost exclusively from testicular secretion. By contrast, the major estrogenic effect in men is related to circulating estradiol and estrone, most of which originate from the conversion of circulating androgenic precursors to estrogens by peripheral tissues such as fat. Because a substantial fraction of these androgen precursors is of adrenal origin, an endocrine dysfunction limited to the testis can cause significant reductions in circulating androgens with less effect on circulating estrogens, and the resulting increase in the estrogen/androgen ratio can lead to gynecomastia. This general scheme is thought to apply in a variety of testicular disorders.

Primary increases in estrogen production also have secondary effects that can further elevate the estrogen/androgen ratio and enhance gynecomastia: stimulation of sex hormone–binding globulin (SHBG) levels or suppression of androgen production by direct inhibition of testicular biosynthetic enzymes or by inhibition of luteinizing hormone (LH). Increased activity of the enzyme aromatase, which converts androgens to estrogens, has been noted in tissues from some patients with gynecomastia,[9] suggesting that local production of estrogen within the breast may also play a contributory role.

In addition to the role of androgens and estrogens, the role of gonadotropins in relation to gynecomastia needs to be considered. LH and human chorionic gonadotropin (hCG) increase

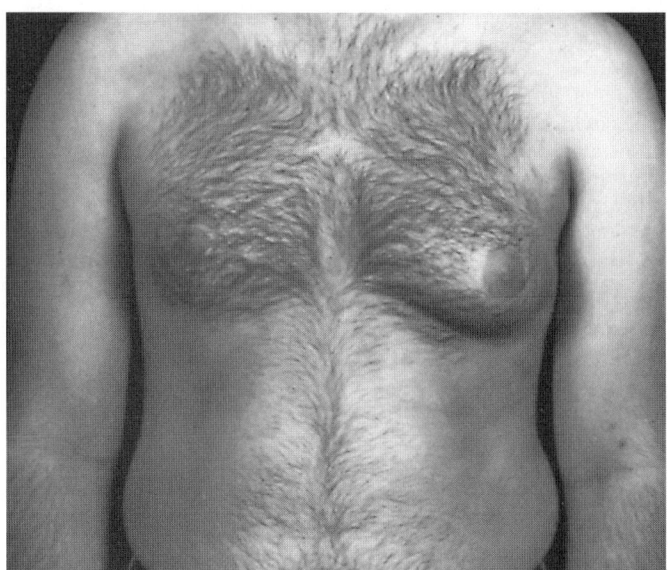

**FIGURE 120-3.** Unilateral gynecomastia secondary to spironolactone therapy in 38-year-old man.

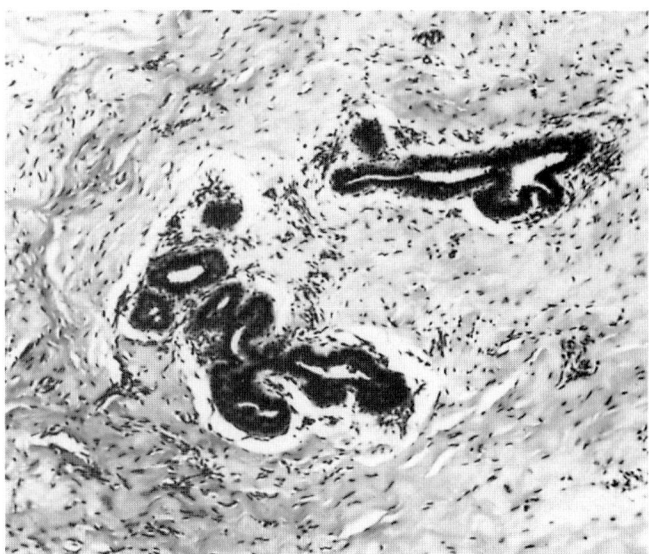

**FIGURE 120-4.** Histologic appearance of gynecomastia of relatively acute onset. There is epithelial proliferation of the ducts and loose periductal fibroblastic tissue. There also is a mild inflammatory infiltrate. (Courtesy of Dr. Nirmal Saini.)

the secretion of estradiol from Leydig cells in the testis; therefore, gynecomastia is particularly common in forms of testicular dysfunction in which circulating gonadotropin levels are elevated (primary testicular failure). Conversely, gynecomastia is less common when testicular dysfunction is accompanied by low circulating gonadotropin levels, as may occur in some pituitary disorders. Also, in the latter condition, coexistent impairment of adrenocorticotropic hormone (ACTH) release may decrease the adrenal output of the androgens that serve as precursors for circulating estrogens, thus decreasing further the estrogen/androgen ratio.

Hyperprolactinemia, which is implicated strongly in *galactorrhea* (milky breast discharge), rarely is a cause of gynecomastia. However, disorders causing increases in the circulating estrogen/androgen ratio may result in both hyperprolactinemia and gynecomastia as independent secondary effects. In addition, a patient with hyperprolactinemia may have gynecomastia from secondary hypogonadism consequent to the prolactin excess or from another cause totally unrelated to the hyperprolactinemia. Galactorrhea appears more likely to occur in a hyperprolactinemic man who happens to have concurrent gynecomastia.

## CAUSES OF GYNECOMASTIA

### PHYSIOLOGIC GYNECOMASTIA

Physiologic gynecomastia can be seen at the extremes of life. Neonatal gynecomastia usually is transient, reflecting the effect of the high level of estrogens in the maternal-fetal unit. The gynecomastia seen in senescence may be related to several factors. Older people may be more likely to develop (or to have developed) some of the various disorders associated with gynecomastia. Further, aging seems to be associated with a progressive primary testicular dysfunction, including low-normal or low serum testosterone levels, increases in serum LH and follicle-stimulating hormone (FSH), and normal or increased serum estrogen levels.[10,11] The resulting increase in the circulating estrogen/androgen ratio then could account for gynecomastia. Some controversy revolves around whether this progressive loss of testicular function is related solely to aging per se or also reflects underlying diseases to which older people become susceptible[12] (see Chap. 199). In addition, aging is associated with accumulation of adipose tissue, which is an important source of the aromatase enzyme that converts circulating androgen precursors to estrogens.

Physiologic gynecomastia is most common during sexual maturation; such pubertal gynecomastia can affect as many as two-thirds of normal adolescents. It usually lasts for only a few months to a few years but sometimes persists into adulthood. A wide variety of alterations in androgens, estrogens, or estrogen/androgen ratios have been described in subjects with pubertal gynecomastia,[13–16] but their etiology and causative relation to the breast enlargement remain largely speculative. Persistent pubertal gynecomastia also has been called *essential gynecomastia*. In some cases, the breasts become female-appearing in size and conformation, and these otherwise hormonally normal adults have been said to have *persistent pubertal macromastia*.

### TUMORS

Tumors of the steroid-producing organs (adrenal, testis) are an uncommon cause of gynecomastia but one that must be ruled out in a male with breast enlargement (see also Chap. 219). Feminizing adrenal tumors usually are malignant. Commonly, such tumors are large. Many are palpable, and they are easily seen by computed tomography or magnetic resonance imaging. Biochemically, they produce large amounts of various steroid precursors that can be detected as elevated plasma dehydroepiandrosterone sulfate (DHEAS) and serve as the substrate for peripheral conversion to estrogens. Serum estradiol levels are high.

**TABLE 120-2.**
**Drugs Associated with Gynecomastia***

Angiotensin-converting enzyme inhibitors (captopril, enalapril)

Antiandrogens (flutamide, cyproterone, zanoterone, finasteride, spironolactone)

Antihypertensives (methyldopa, reserpine)

Antiinfectives (minocycline, indinavir, ketoconazole, ethionamide, metronidazole, isoniazid [INH])

Arthritis drugs (auranofin, sulindac)

Calcium-channel blockers (verapamil, nifedipine, diltiazem, amlodipine)

Cancer chemotherapy drugs (alkylating agents, methotrexate)

Cardiac drugs (digitalis, amiodarone)

Central nervous system (CNS)-acting drugs (diazepam, phenytoin, phenothiazines, tricyclic antidepressants)

Diuretics (spironolactone)

Drugs of abuse (marijuana, heroin, methadone, amphetamines, anabolic steroids)

Gastric motility enhancers (metoclopramide, domperidone)

Miscellaneous (clomiphene, penicillamine, etretinate, theophylline)

Peptide hormones (gonadotropins, growth hormone)

Steroids (estrogens, aromatizable androgens, anabolic steroids)

Ulcer drugs (cimetidine, omeprazole [rare])

*Some of these drug associations are clearly evident and others are anecdotal.

In contrast to feminizing adrenal tumors, estrogen-producing tumors of the testis often are small and can be benign. If not palpable, they may be imaged by testicular ultrasound. Although estrogen-producing testicular tumors are usually of Leydig-cell origin, there is an association between gynecomastia, feminizing Sertoli cell tumors, and the Peutz-Jeghers syndrome.[17]

The gynecomastia associated with some tumors has been related to high levels of aromatase activity (which converts androgens to estrogens) within the tumor itself; this phenomenon has been noted in some testicular tumors[18,19] as well as in hepatocellular carcinoma.[20]

Clinically, one should suspect an estrogen-producing neoplasm if gynecomastia is of rapid onset, if serum estrogen levels are very high, or if a mass is found in the abdomen or testis. Often, the autonomous estrogen production has suppressed the pituitary, leading to low serum LH and FSH levels and, consequently, to secondary hypogonadism and testicular atrophy.

More commonly, tumors lead to gynecomastia through the paraneoplastic production of gonadotropin, particularly hCG. This hormone and LH in high levels tend to stimulate testicular estrogen production disproportionate to androgen production, leading to increases in the circulating estrogen/androgen ratio. Testicular tumors are the most common neoplasm with clinically evident hCG production (7% of all testicular tumors are associated with gynecomastia[21]), but many other tumors can produce this hormone[22] (see Chaps. 122 and 219). Serum estrogen levels tend to be high, and serum hCG-β virtually always is elevated. Occasionally, the source of the ectopic hCG production is not evident, in which case catheterization of veins draining various organs to determine the source of the hormone can be helpful. In such cases, one should pay particular attention to the possibility of an occult testicular tumor.[23]

### DRUGS

Medications commonly are implicated in gynecomastia[24] (Table 120-2). For some drugs, studies have revealed the mechanism by which the estrogen/androgen ratio effect at the breast is increased. For exogenous estrogens, as in the treatment of prostate cancer, the mechanism of gynecomastia is self-evident. Other exposures to exogenous estrogen are not so apparent, however, such as estrogen-containing creams used by a spouse or mother or designed to treat baldness, foods prepared from estrogen-treated animals, or occupational exposure during the manufacture of estrogen-containing medications.[24a] Crude marijuana extracts, but not the purified active ingredient tetrahydrocannabinol, interact with estrogen receptors, suggesting that marijuana-associated gynecomastia may reflect the presence of plant estrogens.[25] Digitalis preparations also may have estrogen-like effects.

Other drugs may produce gynecomastia by interfering with androgen production or action, thus increasing the estrogen/androgen ratio effect at the breast.[25a] The antifungal agent ketoconazole is a potent inhibitor of testosterone biosynthesis and can cause gynecomastia.[26] However, because of its pharmacokinetics, the incidence of gynecomastia is low when the drug is given in a once-a-day dosage because this regimen allows the serum testosterone levels to normalize before each succeeding dose. Traditional antiandrogens (cyproterone, flutamide), as well as the H$_2$-blocker cimetidine, appear to cause gynecomastia by blocking androgen receptors at the breast rather than by decreasing androgen production; they cause an increased effective estrogen/androgen ratio in the breast tissue. This side effect of cimetidine is most common when high doses are used to treat Zollinger-Ellison syndrome and is seen much less frequently with other antiulcer drugs, such as ranitidine or omeprazole. The blockade of androgen action at the breast by a commercial insecticide has been implicated in an epidemic of gynecomastia in Haitian immigrants.[27] The aldosterone antagonist spironolactone, frequently used as a diuretic, may block androgen receptors as well as interfere with androgen production, thereby leading to an increased effective estrogen/androgen ratio at the breast.[28] Here, too, the breast enlargement is seen most commonly at high dosages, as in the treatment of primary hyperaldosteronism. Finasteride, which is used in the treatment of prostate disorders and which inhibits 5-α reductase and reduces intracellular levels of active androgen (dihydrotestosterone) in target tissues, has also been associated with gynecomastia[29] (see Chap. 115).

A wide variety of neurotransmitter agonists, antagonists, or modulators that are used to treat hypertension or psychiatric disorders have been associated with gynecomastia, but the nature and mechanism of this connection are largely unexplored. Also, such agents commonly are associated with hyperprolactinemia, which may cause secondary hypogonadism.

An increasingly frequent cause of drug-related gynecomastia is cancer chemotherapeutic agents. Gynecomastia associated with such medications may be increasing in prevalence as their spectrum of use is extended to nonmalignant conditions (e.g., gynecomastia following methotrexate treatment of rheumatoid arthritis). It has been known for many years that such drugs, particularly alkylating agents, are highly toxic to the spermatogenic epithelium, causing primary testicular failure with azoospermia, small testicles, and high serum LH and FSH levels.[30] Serum testosterone levels, however, usually are normal or low normal, but in some cases of chemotherapy-related gynecomastia, serum estrogen levels have been elevated.[31] A reasonable, but unproved, theory is that chemotherapeutic agents produce compensated Leydig cell failure, with normal or low-normal serum testosterone levels maintained only with the stimulus of high serum LH. This increased serum LH then causes a relative increase in testicular estrogen output, leading to an increase in the circulating estrogen/androgen ratio and then to gynecomastia. Such chemotherapy-related gynecomastia can occur during or after cancer treatment, often resolves spontaneously, and has no prognostic significance with regard to the effectiveness of chemotherapy or recurrence of tumor. If the chemotherapy is given for a tumor that produces hCG, a chemotherapy-induced gynecomastia then must be differentiated from tumor recurrence by means of the measurement of serum hCG-β, which does not cross-react with LH.

## CONGENITAL DISORDERS

Any congenital or acquired defect of androgen production or of androgen action at target tissues can cause gynecomastia. The most common congenital disorder associated with gynecomastia

is Klinefelter syndrome, in which the abnormal karyotype (usually 47,XXY) is associated with primary testicular failure (see Chap. 115). Serum free testosterone levels are low normal or frankly low, whereas serum estradiol levels are normal or elevated.[32] The resulting increase in the circulating estrogen/androgen ratio leads to gynecomastia, which is seen in more than half of these patients. Moreover, the incidence of breast cancer is markedly increased in men with Klinefelter syndrome.[33]

Another congenital disorder leading to gynecomastia is anorchia (vanishing testis syndrome), in which no testes can be located. In this condition, the presence of the testis during fetal development may be inferred from the male phenotype of the external genitalia; the reasons for the subsequent testicular disappearance are unknown.

In two other genetic disorders associated with the development of hypogonadism, namely myotonic dystrophy and sickle cell anemia, gynecomastia is uncommon (<10%). In the former condition, this infrequency of breast enlargement may reflect low levels of adrenal androgens,[34] which otherwise may serve as precursors for peripheral conversion to estrogens.

A congenital defect in one of the enzymes of testosterone biosynthesis may lead to gynecomastia, but this is rare because most such enzyme defects, with the exception of 17-ketosteroid reductase deficiency, also lead to impaired estrogen production and thus do not cause large increases in the circulating estrogen/androgen ratio. Several cases have been reported in which such defects in enzymes of testosterone biosynthesis, although presumably congenital, do not present clinically until adulthood, with gynecomastia a prominent finding.[35,36] Conversely, a primary increase in peripheral tissue aromatase activity, with enhanced conversion of circulating androgen precursors to estrogens, appears to be a rare cause of gynecomastia.[37] The nature of this disorder is unknown. Isotopic determination of conversion rates of androgen to estrogen and exclusion of all other causes are necessary to make this diagnosis.

A somewhat more common group of congenital disorders associated with gynecomastia includes the defects in androgen action.[38] In these disorders, such as testicular feminization and Reifenstein syndromes, testosterone production is not decreased, but testosterone action on target tissues, including the breast, is impaired (see Chap. 90). Frequently, this impairment in androgen action is related to quantitative or qualitative abnormalities in the androgen receptors, and this lack of androgen effect on the breast may contribute directly to gynecomastia.[39] For example, the X-linked *Kennedy syndrome* of spinobulbar muscular atrophy is associated with gynecomastia and a genetic abnormality in the androgen receptor. Molecular studies of the androgen receptor in Kennedy syndrome have shown an expansion in the number of the CAG tandem repeats, a finding reminiscent of the genetic alterations in other congenital neuromuscular disorders. In these disorders of androgen action, the lack of the usual inhibitory androgen effect at the pituitary gland leads to increased gonadotropin output and consequently to increased testicular estrogen production, which may contribute to gynecomastia. Many subjects with such defects in androgen action also have some form of ambiguous genitalia because the defect is present in the fetus.

Individuals with true hermaphroditism or related conditions may develop gynecomastia related to estrogen production by their ovarian tissue.

## ACQUIRED DISORDERS

Acquired defects of testicular function or of testosterone production are common causes of gynecomastia. In damage related to trauma or radiation of the testis, the pathogenesis of testicular hypofunction is apparent. Moreover, postpubertal mumps infection frequently causes orchitis, which can lead to testicular atrophy, hypogonadism, and gynecomastia. Another infectious disease, lepromatous leprosy, frequently is associated with testicular failure and consequent gynecomastia. Studies of men with spinal cord injury, which may be associated with testicular dysfunction, reveal a modest incidence (<10%) of gynecomastia.[40]

A variety of systemic disorders are associated with gynecomastia, although the specific pathogenesis may differ. For example, the gynecomastia commonly seen in renal failure is associated with small testes, low serum testosterone, and elevated serum LH and FSH, suggesting that the breast enlargement is related to primary testicular failure.[41] Because serum estrogen levels are not elevated, the gynecomastia presumably is secondary to an increased estrogen/androgen ratio rather than to excessive estrogen production. The cause of the hypogonadism in uremia is controversial, with etiologic roles being suggested for hyperprolactinemia, secondary hyperparathyroidism, and zinc deficiency (see Chaps. 131 and 209). The manifestations of hypogonadism appear to be reversed by renal transplantation but not by dialysis.

Conversely, the gynecomastia commonly seen in cirrhosis of the liver is associated with increased estrogen production and high serum estrogen levels, particularly elevated serum estrone.[42] These high estrogen levels appear to be the result of increased peripheral conversion of adrenal androgen precursors to estrogens. Further, the tendency toward low serum free testosterone levels raises the circulating estrogen/androgen ratio. Despite these hormonal abnormalities, one study revealed that gynecomastia was no more frequent in patients with cirrhosis than in the population at large, an issue that remains unresolved.

Also associated with high serum estradiol levels is the gynecomastia commonly observed in men with thyrotoxicosis.[43,44,44a] Despite usually normal serum free testosterone levels, the circulating estrogen/androgen ratio often is very high, causing the breast enlargement. The increased estrogen levels may reflect a direct effect of thyroid hormone excess in increasing the conversion of androgens to estrogens in peripheral tissues because thyroid hormone enhances various enzyme activities. High serum LH levels in thyrotoxicosis also may facilitate estrogen production.

Gynecomastia has been associated with diabetes. In such cases, lymphocytic infiltration of the breast tissue raises the possibility of an autoimmune etiology.[45]

## MISCELLANEOUS CAUSES

Prisoners of war develop gynecomastia, particularly when their poor diet during captivity is corrected after liberation. Similarly, gynecomastia sometimes occurs in men who have become emaciated by coexisting disease and subsequently return to normal weight. The etiology of such "refeeding" gynecomastia is unknown but may be similar to that of pubertal gynecomastia.

Lung cancer may be accompanied by gynecomastia, sometimes secondary to hCG production by the tumor and, in other cases in which any known hormone overproduction is absent, in conjunction with hypertrophic pulmonary osteoarthropathy (see Chap. 219). Transient gynecomastia has also been reported in men with human immunodeficiency virus infection.[46] Chest wall trauma has rarely been associated with gynecomastia,[47] and psychological stress has been linked to transient increases in the estrogen/androgen ratio and gynecomastia.[48]

## EVALUATION OF THE PATIENT WITH GYNECOMASTIA

The evaluation should focus initially on identifying patients in whom the breast enlargement is a manifestation of a treatable underlying disease. In particular, special emphasis must be given to excluding a neoplasm whose sole external manifestation may be gynecomastia. In this regard, a history of a recent onset of gynecomastia is particularly pertinent. In taking the patient's history, one should pay particular attention to prescribed medications or illicit drugs known to be related to gynecomastia, pubertal development, symptoms of hypogonadism, fertility, and symptoms of a systemic disease (e.g., liver disease, thyrotoxicosis) that can be associated with gynecomastia. On physical examination, the patient should be carefully evaluated for secondary sexual characteristics, testicular size, presence of abdominal or testicular masses, and ambiguous genitalia, including hypospadias. One should verify gynecomastia (distinguish from fat) and its nature. Unilateral, very hard, nontender, irregular breast enlargement suggests the possibility of male breast cancer, which is extremely unusual before age 50. Sometimes, the history and physical examination alone suffice to establish rapidly the cause of gynecomastia (e.g., recent use of spironolactone, normal pubertal boy, long-standing cirrhosis with generalized feminization).

The initial laboratory evaluation should include measurements of serum LH, FSH, testosterone, estradiol, prolactin, and hCG-β; tests of liver, kidney, and thyroid function also are appropriate in many cases. Such screening identifies most disorders associated with gynecomastia. Thus, small testes, low serum testosterone, and high serum LH and FSH suggest that the gynecomastia is related to one of the causes of primary testicular failure. The finding of a high serum estradiol level, in conjunction with either high serum hCG-β or low serum LH and FSH (the latter suggesting suppression of gonadotropins by autonomous estrogen production), makes it essential to exclude a testicular or adrenal neoplasm. Abdominal computed tomographic scan and testicular ultrasound can be particularly useful in this regard. Evaluation of estrogen receptor status of the gynecomastia breast may prove useful.[49]

Fine-needle aspiration cytology of the breast may be quite helpful when breast neoplasia is suspected; the finding of aneuploidy or increases in argyrophilic nucleolar organizing regions[50] may suggest malignancy. Imaging procedures (mammography, ultrasound) may also be quite useful when breast cancer is suspected (see Chaps. 106 and 224). When malignancy is not a consideration, the role of aspiration cytology has not been clearly established, although some histologic findings may suggest a particular cause of gynecomastia (e.g., apocrine metaplasia in gynecomastia associated with anabolic steroid abuse[51]).

## TREATMENT

The treatment of gynecomastia depends on the underlying cause. Surgical removal of estrogen-producing or hCG-producing tumors usually is required and may be curative. Offending medications should be stopped. The treatment of any underlying systemic disorders (e.g., radioiodine for thyrotoxicosis, renal transplantation) may be helpful. Radiotherapy of the breast may prevent the development of gynecomastia in circumstances in which its occurrence can be predicted (e.g., treatment with estrogens or antiandrogens[52]). In severe cases of gynecomastia of any cause, particularly in boys and younger men, mammoplasty may be required (Figs. 120-5 and 120-6). Advances in surgery for gynecomastia have included new anatomic approaches (transaxillary), new instrumentation (cannulas, endoscopes), and new surgical techniques (liposuction, pedicle grafting, pull-through procedure). Because such surgery is not completely risk-free, it is important to choose a plastic surgeon who is experienced with the procedure. In less severe cases of gynecomastia, treatment may be withheld in anticipation of spontaneous resolution (pubertal, postchemotherapy) or when it may not be appropriate (end-stage cirrhosis).

The pharmacologic treatment of gynecomastia is an attempt to decrease the circulating estrogen/androgen ratio or to alter hormonal effects on target tissues. When androgen deficiency is

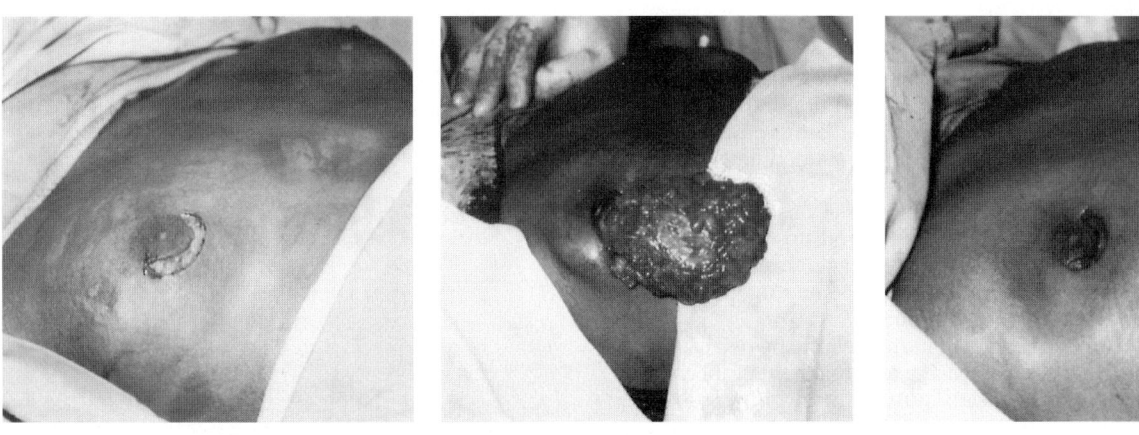

**A–C**

**FIGURE 120-5.** Operation for removal of gynecomastic breasts. **A,** Incision is made at the periphery of the areola. **B,** Breast tissue is removed through the periareolar incision. **C,** Appearance of chest after removal of both breasts and before incision closure.

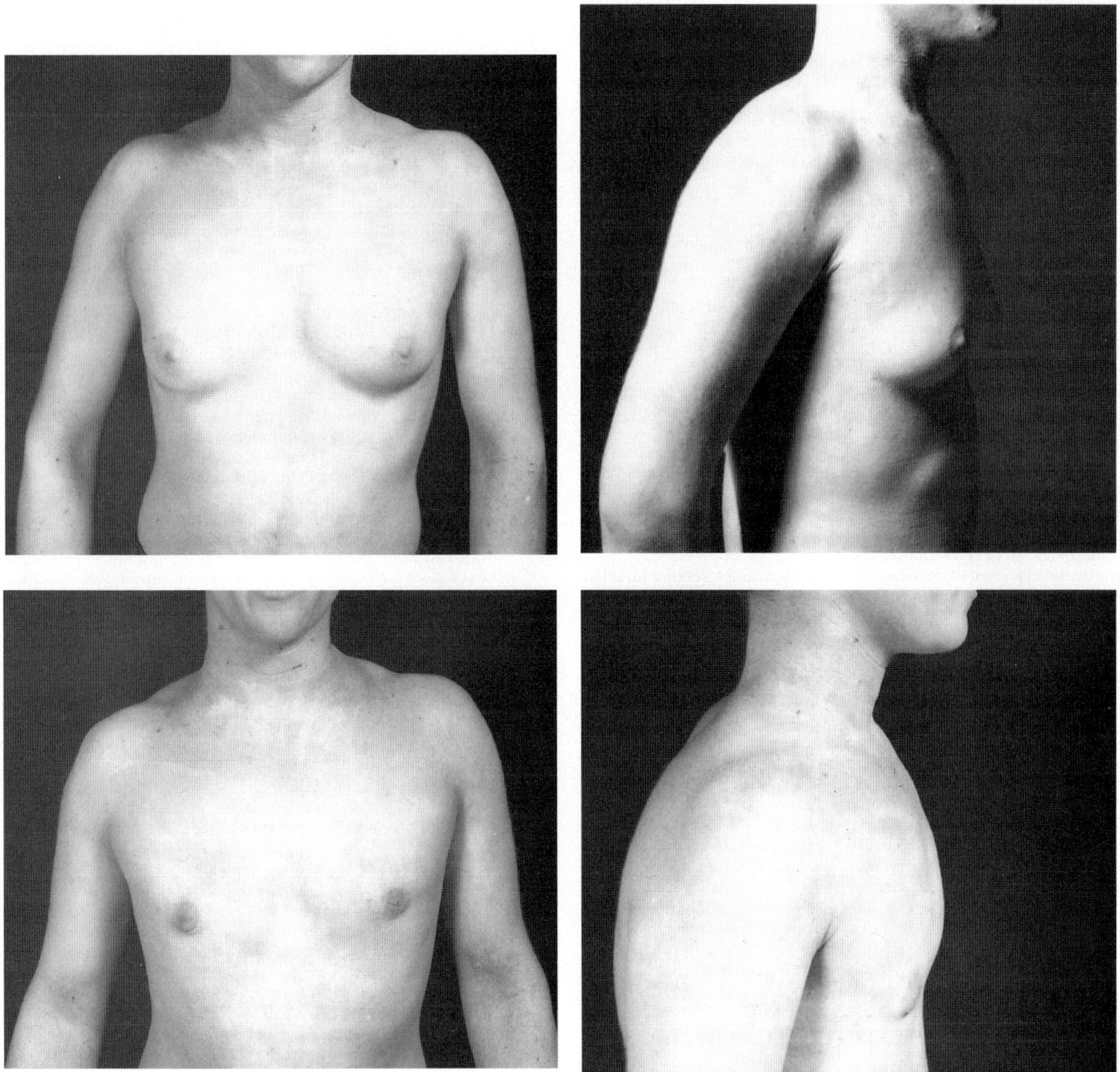

A

B

C

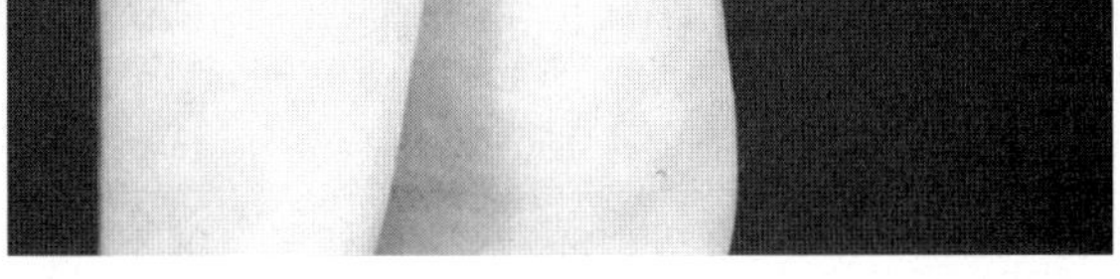

D

**FIGURE 120-6.** Eighteen-year-old youth with marked gynecomastia that occurred 4 months after a several-week period of bilateral testicular pain and a viral orchitis. **A and B,** Before surgery. **C and D,** Subsequent to surgery similar to that shown in Figure 120-5.

a prominent component, as in severe primary testicular failure, androgen treatment not only corrects the androgen deficiency but also may lead to resolution or diminution of the gynecomastia. In addition, one controlled study reported that testosterone treatment also decreased gynecomastia in cirrhosis.[53] Because the most readily available androgen, namely testosterone, can be converted to estrogen by peripheral tissues, its usefulness in gynecomastia of most other causes has not been established. One study suggested that dihydrotestosterone, an androgen that cannot be metabolized to estrogen, leads to the resolution of gynecomastia. Danazol, a modified androgen, also is useful in the treatment of gynecomastia.[54]

Attempts to decrease the estrogen/androgen ratio by decreasing estrogen rather than by increasing androgen have been tried as therapy for gynecomastia. Thus, both uncontrolled[55] and controlled studies[56,57] of the estrogen blocker tamoxifen have suggested effectiveness, as have uncontrolled studies of the antiestrogen clomiphene[58] and the aromatase inhibitor testolactone.[59] Such antiestrogens have a low side-effect profile, but their effectiveness has been variable (they seem to be most useful in decreasing pain rather than in reducing breast size), and they tend to be expensive.

# REFERENCES

1. Braunstein GD. Gynecomastia. N Engl J Med 1993; 328:490.
2. Williams MJ. Gynecomastia: its incidence, recognition and host characterization in 447 autopsy cases. Am J Med 1963; 34:100.
3. Hands LJ, Greenall MJ. Gynaecomastia. Br J Surg 1991; 78:907.
4. Cespedes RD, Caballero RL, Peretsman SJ, Thompson IM. Cryptic presentations of germ cell tumors. J Am Coll Surg 1994; 178:261.
5. Becker KL, Matthews MJ, Winnacker J, Higgins GA Jr. Sequential histological study of the regression of gynecomastia in a patient with alcoholic liver disease. Am J Med Sci 1967; 254:685.
6. Nicolis G, Modlinger R, Gabrilove J. A study of the histopathology of human gynecomastia. J Clin Endocrinol Metab 1971; 32:173.
7. Lanzafame S, Magro G, Colombatti A. Expression and distribution of type VI collagen in gynecomastia. Acta Histochem 1994; 96:219.
8. Georgiadis E, Papandreou L, Evangelopoulou C, et al. Incidence of gynaecomastia in 954 young males and its relationship to somatometric parameters. Ann Hum Biol 1994; 21:579.
9. Sasano H, Kimura M, Shizawa S, et al. Aromatase and steroid receptors in gynecomastia and male breast carcinoma: an immunohistochemical study. J Clin Endocrinol Metab 1996; 81:363
10. Pirke KM, Doerr P. Age related changes and interrelationships between plasma testosterone, oestradiol and testosterone-binding globulin in normal adult males. Acta Endocrinol (Copenh) 1973; 74:792.
11. Stearns EL, MacDonnell JA, Kaufman BJ, et al. Declining testicular function with age: hormonal and clinical correlates. Am J Med 1974; 57:761.
12. Harman SM, Tsitouras PD. Reproductive hormones in aging men. I. Measurement of sex steroids, basal luteinizing hormone, and Leydig cell response to human chorionic gonadotropin. J Clin Endocrinol Metab 1980; 51:35.
13. Large DM, Anderson DC. Twenty-four hour profiles of circulating androgens and estrogens in male puberty with and without gynaecomastia. Clin Endocrinol 1979; 11:505.
14. Moore DC, Schlaepfer LV, Paunier L, Sizonenko PC. Hormonal changes during puberty. V. Transient pubertal gynecomastia: abnormal androgen-estrogen ratios. J Clin Endocrinol Metab 1984; 58:492.
15. Biro F, Lucky A, Huster G, et al. Hormonal studies and physical maturation in adolescent gynecomastia. J Pediatr 1990; 116:450.
16. Villalpando S, Mondragon L, Barron C, et al. Role of testosterone and dihydrotestosterone in spontaneous gynecomastia of adolescents. Arch Androl 1992; 28:171.
17. Hertl MC, Wiebel J, Schafer H, et al. Feminizing Sertoli cell tumors associated with Peutz-Jeghers syndrome: an increasingly recognized cause of prepubertal gynecomastia. Plast Reconstr Surg 1998; 102:1151.
18. Coen P, Kulin H, Ballantine T, et al. An aromatase-producing sex-cord tumor resulting in prepubertal gynecomastia. N Engl J Med 1991; 324:317.
19. Kirschner M, Cohen F, Jesperson D. Estrogen production and its origin in men with gonadotropin-producing neoplasms. J Clin Endocrinol Metab 1974; 39:112.
20. Agarwal VR, Takayama K, VanWyk JJ, et al. Molecular basis of severe gynecomastia associated with aromatase expression in a fibrolamellar hepatocellular carcinoma. J Clin Endocrinol Metab 1998; 83:1797.
21. Hernes EH, Harstad K. Changing incidence and delay of testicular cancer in southern Norway (1981–1992). Eur Urol 1996; 30:349.
22. Braunstein GD, Vaitukaitis JL, Carbone PP, Ross GT. Ectopic production of human chronic gonadotropin by neoplasms. Ann Intern Med 1973; 78:39.
23. Rudnick P, Odell WD. In search of a cancer. N Engl J Med 1971; 284:405.
24. Thompson DF, Carter JR. Drug-induced gynecomastia. Pharmacotherapy 1993; 13:37.
24a. Felner EI, White PC. Prepubertal gynecomastia: indirect exposure to endocrine cream. Pediatrics 2000; 105:E55.
25. Saver MA, Rifka SM, Hawks RL, et al. Marijuana: interaction with the estrogen receptor. J Pharmacol Exp Ther 1983; 224:404.
25a. Zimmerman RL, Fogt F, Cronin D, Lynch R. Cytologic atypia in a 53-year-old man with finasteride-induced gynecomastia. Arch Pathol Lab Med 2000; 124:625.
26. Pont A, Williams PL, Azhar S, et al. Ketoconazole blocks testosterone synthesis. Arch Intern Med 1982; 142:2137.
27. Brody SA, Winterer J, Drum MA, et al. An epidemic of gynecomastia among Haitian refugees: possible exposure to an anti-androgen. Endocrinology 1983; 112(Suppl):261.
28. Loriaux DL, Menard R, Taylor A, et al. Spironolactone and endocrine dysfunction. Ann Intern Med 1976; 85:630.
29. Wilton L, Pearce G, Edet E, et al. The safety of finasteride used in benign prostatic hypertrophy: a non-interventional observational cohort study in 14,772 patients. Br J Urol 1996; 78:379.
30. Shalet SM. Disorders of the endocrine system due to radiation and cytotoxic chemotherapy. Clin Endocrinol 1983; 18:637.
31. Trump DL, Pary MD, Staal S. Gynecomastia in men following antineoplastic therapy. Arch Intern Med 1982; 142:511.
32. Wang C, Baker HWG, Burger HG, et al. Hormonal studies in Klinefelter's syndrome. Clin Endocrinol 1975; 4:399.
33. Jackson A, Muldal S, Ockley C, et al. Carcinoma of the male breast in association with the Klinefelter syndrome. Br Med J 1965; 1:223.
34. Carter JN, Steinbeck KS. Reduced adrenal androgens in patients with myotonic dystrophy. J Clin Endocrinol Metab 1985; 60:611.
35. Castro-Magan M, Angulo M, Uy J. Male hypogonadism with gynecomastia caused by late-onset deficiency of testicular 17-ketosteroid reductase. N Engl J Med 1993; 328:1297.
36. Cavanah S, Dons R. Partial 3-beta hydroxysteroid dehydrogenase deficiency presenting as new-onset gynecomastia in a eugonadal adult male. Metabolism 1993; 42:65.
37. Berkovitz G, Buerami A, Brown T, et al. Familial gynecomastia with increased aromatization of plasma carbon 19 steroids. J Clin Invest 1985; 75:1763.
38. Griffin JE, Wilson JD. The syndromes of androgen resistance. N Engl J Med 1980; 302:198.
39. Grino PB, Griffin JE, Cushard WG Jr, Wilson JD. A mutation of the androgen receptor associated with partial androgen resistance, familial gynecomastia, and fertility. J Clin Endocrinol Metab 1988; 66:754.
40. Heruti RJ, Dankner R, Berezin M, et al. Gynecomastia following spinal cord disorder. Arch Phys Med Rehabil 1997; 78:534.
41. Holdsworth S, Atkins RC, de Kretser DM. The pituitary-testicular axis in men with chronic renal failure. N Engl J Med 1977; 296:1245.
42. Valimaki M, Salaspuro M, Harkonen M, Ylikahri R. Liver damage and sex hormones in chronic male alcoholics. Clin Endocrinol 1982; 17:469.
43. Becker KL, Matthews MJ, Higgins G, Mohamadi M. Histologic evidence of gynecomastia in hyperthyroidism. Arch Pathol 1974; 98:257.
44. Kidd GS, Glass AR, Vigersky RA. The hypothalamic-pituitary-testicular axis in thyrotoxicosis. J Clin Endocrinol Metab 1979; 48:798.
44a. Abalovich M, Levalle O, Hermes R, et al. Hypothalamic-pituitary-testicular axis and seminal parameters in hyperthyroid males. Thyroid 1999; 9:857.
45. Hunfeld KP, Bassler R, Kronsbein H. Diabetic mastopathy in the male breast—a special type of gynecomastia. Pathol Res Pract 1997; 193:197.
46. Couderc LJ, Clauvel JP. HIV-infection-induced gynecomastia. Ann Intern Med 1987; 107:257.
47. Field J, Solis R, Dear W. Case report: unilateral gynecomastia associated with thoracotomy following resection of carcinoma of the lung. Am J Med Sci 1989; 298:402.
48. Gooren L, Daantje C. Psychological stress as a cause of intermittent gynecomastia. Horm Metab Res 1986; 18:424.
49. Adersen J, Orntoft TF, Andersen JA, Poulsen HS. Gynecomastia: immunohistochemical demonstration of estrogen receptors. Acta Pathol Microbiol Immunol Scand 1987; 95:263.
50. Wolman SR, Sanford J, Ratner S, Dawson PJ. Breast cancer in males: DNA content and sex chromosome constitution. Mod Pathol 1995; 8:239.
51. Fowler LJ, Smith SS, Snider T, Schultz MR. Apocrine metaplasia in gynecomastia by fine needle aspiration as a possible indicator of anabolic steroid use. A report of two cases. Acta Cytol 1996; 40:734.
52. Eriksson T, Eriksson M. Irradiation therapy prevents gynecomastia in sex offenders treated with antiandrogens. J Clin Psychiatry 1998; 59:432.
53. Copenhagen Study Group for Liver Diseases. Testosterone treatment of men with alcoholic cirrhosis: a double-blind study. Hepatology 1986; 6:807.
54. Jones D, Davison D, Holt S, et al. A comparison of danazol and placebo in the treatment of adult idiopathic gynaecomastia: results of a prospective study in 55 patients. Ann R Coll Surg Engl 1990; 72:296.
55. Staiman VR, Lowe FC. Tamoxifen for flutamide/finasteride-induced gynecomastia. Urology 1997; 50:929.
56. Parker LN, Gray DR, Lai MK, Levin ER. Treatment of gynecomastia with tamoxifen: a double-blind crossover study. Metabolism 1986; 35:705.
57. McDermott M, Hofeldt F, Kidd G. Tamoxifen therapy for painful idiopathic gynecomastia. South Med J 1990; 83:1283.
58. Plourde PV, Kulin HE, Santner SJ. Clomiphene in the treatment of adolescent gynecomastia: clinical and endocrine studies. Am J Dis Child 1983; 137:1080.
59. Zachmann M, Eiholzer U, Muritano M, et al. Treatment of pubertal gynecomastia with testolactone. Acta Endocrinol 1986; 279(Suppl):218.

# CHAPTER 121

# ENDOCRINE ASPECTS OF BENIGN PROSTATIC HYPERPLASIA

ELIZABETH A. MILLER AND WILLIAM J. ELLIS

Benign prostatic hyperplasia (BPH) is a common disorder of the aging male that is a benign enlargement of the prostate gland. Histologic evidence of BPH is rare under the age of 30, but by the eighth decade of life the disease can be found in nearly all men.[1,2] An abnormal proliferation of both stromal and glandular elements in an area of the prostate known as the transition zone is responsible for the disease. The etiology of this proliferation is unknown at the present time.[3] A genetic predisposition to the proliferation appears to exist, as a family history of BPH is a significant risk factor for the development of BPH. An endocrine basis for the disease also exists. Men who have been castrated do not develop BPH. Furthermore, as is discussed later, endocrine manipulation can cause involution of BPH.

BPH produces symptoms, which are classified as either obstructive or irritative. The obstructive symptoms include urinary hesitancy, a weak stream, double voiding, and an inability to empty the bladder. The irritative symptoms, which consist of frequency, urgency, and dysuria, are the most bothersome and are the reason most men seek treatment. A poor correlation is found between prostate size and the magnitude of voiding symptoms, although larger glands in general do produce more prostatic symptoms.

In men with mild to moderate voiding symptoms, observation is a reasonable option.[4,5] Results of a multicenter randomized trial show that most men do not develop serious complications such as retention or urinary tract infections if such an approach is followed.[6] Growth of the prostate is relatively slow, averaging 1.6% per year in a prospective population-based trial.[7] In larger prostates, the growth rate is higher.

Surgical resection or enucleation of the prostatic adenoma has been the mainstay of treatment for BPH until the past decade. Transurethral resection of the prostate (TURP) remains the gold standard of treatment for BPH, as it produces the greatest improvements in urinary flow rate and symptom improvement. TURP is an invasive procedure, however, requiring a 1- to 3-day hospital stay, and is associated with a 70% to 75% incidence of retrograde ejaculation, a 5% to 10% incidence of impotence, and a 2% to 4% risk of urinary incontinence.[8–11] In addition, the reoperation rate is estimated at 15% to 10%.[12] For smaller prostates, transurethral incision of the prostate is an effective procedure.[13]

The prevalence of this disease has produced tremendous interest in the development of alternative treatments. These include minimally invasive surgical procedures and medical treatments. Broadly, the medical treatments for BPH may be subdivided into treatments based on androgen deprivation and treatments based on blockade of the α1 receptors.

Alpha-adrenergic stimulation is responsible for maintaining the smooth muscle tone within the bladder neck and prostate.[14] Thus, the α-adrenergic pathway is an ideal target for modulating bladder outlet obstruction. Terazosin hydrochloride (Hytrin) and doxazosin mesylate (Cardura) are two selective $\alpha_1$-adrenergic antagonists that are used for the treatment of both hypertension and BPH.[15,16] These agents cause a relaxation in the prostatic smooth muscle, resulting in improvements in urinary flow rates and decreases in voiding symptoms. A newer agent, tamsulosin hydrochloride (Flomax), is an antagonist selective for the $\alpha_1$A receptor.[17] This receptor subtype is located primarily in the prostatic stroma. Blockade of this receptor improves urinary symptoms with a smaller decrease in blood pressure.

Herbal treatments of BPH are becoming increasingly popular. Little data on these treatments have been published in the mainstream literature. One of the most popular treatments is an extract from the saw palmetto plant (Serenoa repens). A review has suggested that use of the extract is, indeed, efficacious in the treatment of BPH.[18] Originally, this extract was thought to act as a 5α-reductase inhibitor; however, one study has indicated that saw palmetto extract has noncompetitive $\alpha_1$-adrenoreceptor antagonist activity.[19]

Minimally invasive surgical procedures have also been designed for the treatment of BPH. Most of these procedures involve the administration of thermotherapy to ablate the prostatic adenoma. Interstitial laser therapy administers energy in the form of light to the prostate.[20] Transurethral needle ablation of the prostate (TUNA) uses radiofrequency energy to heat the prostate.[21] Transurethral microwave therapy (TUMT) radiates energy into the prostate via a microwave antenna within a urethral catheter.[22] High-intensity focused ultrasound (HIFU) directs ultrasonic energy into the prostate via a transrectal ultrasonic probe.[23] An alternative approach to BPH management has been placement of prostatic stents to open the prostatic lumen.[24] All of these treatment modalities are efficacious to various degrees. The nuances of the various treatments are beyond the scope of the present chapter. The remainder of this chapter focuses on the current status of endocrine therapy for the treatment of symptomatic BPH.

## ANDROGEN DEPRIVATION THERAPY

Although the exact pathogenesis of BPH is not well defined, clearly aging and the presence of androgens are required for the development of this condition. Numerous laboratory and clinical studies have demonstrated that the prostate gland is an androgen-sensitive organ. If the androgenic stimulation to the prostate is eliminated, the prostatic adenoma decreases in size, outflow resistance through the prostatic urethra diminishes, and the ability to urinate improves.[25–27] The predominant histologic effect is involution of the glandular epithelium of the prostate. To produce a state of androgen deprivation, the hypothalamic–pituitary–gonadal axis must be interrupted.

Under normal physiologic conditions, testicular androgen production is under the control of the hypothalamus.[28] Neurons in the preoptic area of the hypothalamus secrete the decapeptide luteinizing hormone–releasing hormone (LHRH) (also called gonadotropin-releasing hormone [GnRH]) in a pulsatile fashion directly from their terminals into the hypophysioportal circulation. GnRH then interacts with its high-affinity receptor on the plasma membrane of the anterior pituitary cells to stimulate them to release the heterodimeric gonadotropins—follicle-stimulating hormone (FSH) and luteinizing hormone (LH). LH travels through the peripheral circulation to reach the testes, where it binds to its high-affinity receptor on the surface of the Leydig cells. These Leydig cells are stimulated to produce and secrete primarily testosterone (4-androsten-17β-ol-3-one), which travels in the bloodstream either in a free state or bound to sex hormone–binding globulin (SHBG) and albumin. At the target organ (the prostate gland), unbound testosterone binds to its high-affinity receptor within the prostatic cell, where the majority is converted to dihydrotestosterone (DHT) by the enzyme 5α-reductase.[29] Inside the prostatic cell, the remaining testosterone and DHT bind to the same high-affinity androgen-receptor protein, enter the nucleus, and interact with specific DNA-binding sites. Androgen-dependent genes undergo transcription, and the resulting mRNA is translated into specific proteins. Overall, protein biosynthesis increases, leading to cellular hypertrophy and hyperplasia. Each of the three agents

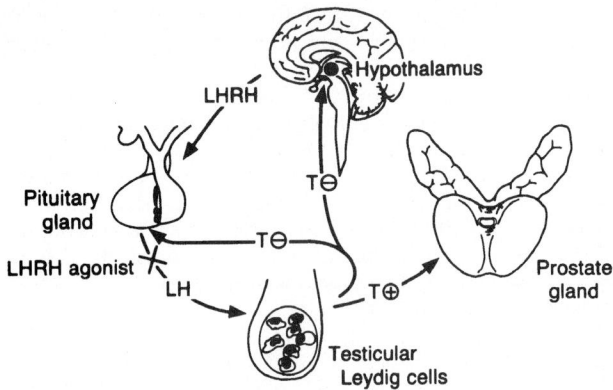

**FIGURE 121-1.** Hypothalamic–pituitary–gonadal axis. (*LHRH*, luteinizing hormone–releasing hormone; *LH*, luteinizing hormone; *T*, testosterone.) (From Oesterling JE. LHRH agonists. A nonsurgical treatment for benign prostatic hyperplasia. J Androl 1991; 12:381.)

most commonly used to inhibit testicular androgen production (GnRH agonists, antiandrogens, and 5α-reductase inhibitors) interferes with the hypothalamic–pituitary–gonadal axis (Figs. 121-1 and 121-2) to exert an effect on the enlarged prostate gland.

## GONADOTROPIN HORMONE–RELEASING HORMONE AGONISTS

GnRH agonists bind to the GnRH receptor of the gonadotropic cells of the anterior pituitary gland. Normally GnRH is released in a pulsatile fashion by the hypothalamus and stimulates the production of LH. Paradoxically, administration of a GnRH agonist in a continuous fashion results in internalization of the GnRH receptor complex in the cells of the anterior pituitary. As the number of receptors on the plasma membrane decreases, the stimulation of these cells and subsequent LH release decrease.[30,31] The administration of GnRH agonists is associated with an LH and testosterone flare, which rapidly reverses, and in several weeks castrate levels of serum testosterone and serum DHT are achieved.[32] Like surgical castration, this medical castration decreases the size of the prostatic adenoma.

A number of clinical trials of GnRH agonists have been carried out. Initially, the use of the GnRH agonist buserelin was described for patients with BPH.[33] Later nafarelin acetate was reported to be effective for patients treated for 6 months.[34] In a subsequent uncontrolled study evaluating 17 patients in a 6-

month trial of goserelin,[35] many patients elected to continue the treatment for a year. Prostate size reached its nadir at 9 months with a mean decrease of 63%; this size decrease was accompanied by a significant improvement in peak urinary flow rates. No significant change was seen in the postvoid residual volume. Urinary symptoms decreased within the first month, with a mean decrease of 33% at 6 months. Six of the 17 patients experienced no improvement in urinary symptoms during the treatment period, and 3 months after the treatment was withdrawn, prostate volumes returned to 95% of the pretreatment volumes. Symptoms and urinary flow rates also worsened, indicating that the improvements could not be maintained in the absence of continuous treatment.

In most men the side effects associated with GnRH agonist therapy outweigh the benefits. Impotence and loss of libido occur in nearly all treated men, and hot flashes and gynecomastia develop in ~50%. Other side effects include weight gain and a loss of energy. Treatment with GnRH agonists is also expensive (~$5000 per year). For these reasons, and because of the availability of other treatment modalities, GnRH agonists are rarely used in the treatment of BPH.

## ANTIANDROGENS

Androgen-receptor–blocking agents directly interfere with the ability of testosterone and DHT to bind to the androgen receptor within the prostate (see Fig. 121-2). The result is prostatic involution with normal serum testosterone levels.[36] Thus, many of the side effects associated with GnRH agonists can be avoided.

Three antiandrogens for which clinical trials have been conducted are flutamide (Eulexin), bicalutamide (Casodex), and zanoterone. All three compounds are orally administered, nonsteroidal compounds. Flutamide is metabolized in the liver to its active form, hydroxyflutamide. Both hydroxyflutamide and bicalutamide compete effectively with testosterone and DHT for the cytosolic androgen receptor.[37,38] In rat models, bicalutamide has an affinity for the androgen receptor that is four times greater than flutamide.[39] In addition, the serum half-life is one week, allowing for once-a-day dosing at a lower dosage than flutamide.[37] The antiandrogens have no androgenic, estrogenic, antiestrogenic, progestational, or antiprogestational action; therefore, the serum testosterone level is not decreased, and fewer hormonally related side effects occur.[40] Serum LH and testosterone levels may be elevated by flutamide because of the loss of central inhibition by the negative hypothalamic–pituitary–gonadal feedback loop. This effect is not seen with bicalutamide use because it is peripherally selective and has no effect on the hypothalamus. Both flutamide and bicalutamide have been approved by the Food and Drug Administration for use in the treatment of advanced prostate cancer.

In the first report on the use of flutamide in the treatment of symptomatic BPH,[41] improvements in both urinary symptoms and peak urinary flow rates were noted after 12 weeks of flutamide therapy (300 mg per day). In a subsequent study, subjects treated for 6 months with flutamide (750 mg per day) showed a 41% decrease in prostate volume and a 46% improvement in peak urinary flow rates.[42] Interestingly, no difference was seen between the treatment and placebo control groups in reported symptom score improvements.

The largest study to date was designed to assess the efficacy of flutamide in the treatment of BPH.[43] This randomized, placebo-controlled study of 367 men with BPH demonstrated a 9% improvement in urinary flow from baseline and a 27% reduction in prostate volume in patients taking 250 mg of the drug three times a day for 24 weeks. A corresponding improvement in total urinary symptom score was not shown, however, and 39% of study patients discontinued the drug because of adverse reactions. In addition, the improvement in urinary flow rates was not statistically significant beyond 6 weeks; this was attrib-

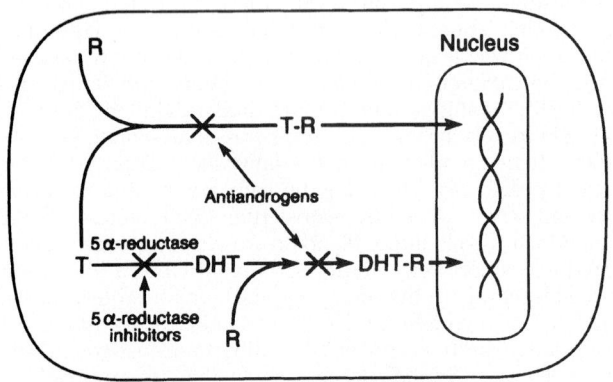

**FIGURE 121-2.** Diagram of prostate cell, showing the mechanism of testosterone (*T*) stimulation and its blockage by 5α-reductase inhibitors. (*R*, cytoplasmic receptor for androgens; *T-R*, testosterone receptor complex; *DHT*, dihydrotestosterone; *DHT-R*, dihydrotestosterone receptor complex.) (From Monda JM, Oesterling JE. Curr Probl Urol 1992; 2:100.)

uted to the high rate of study discontinuation after 6 weeks, primarily due to side effects.

Bicalutamide has also been evaluated as a treatment for BPH. In a 24-week trial at a dosage of 50 mg per day,[44] prostate volume decreased by 26% in patients taking the drug. Peak flow rates and pressure flow examinations were not significantly different in treatment and control groups. A significantly greater improvement in irritative symptom scores was noted in the treatment group than in the control group by week 24.

Another androgen-receptor antagonist, zanoterone, has been evaluated at multiple dosages ranging from 100 to 800 mg daily for 6 months.[45] Significant differences were not noted between the treatment and control groups with regard to decreased prostate volume or improved symptom scores. An improvement in peak urinary flow rates was noted for one treatment group (taking 200 mg per day) compared with the placebo group.

Prostate-specific antigen (PSA) levels can be decreased by antiandrogen therapy. In one study, the serum PSA level decreased by 65% in patients receiving flutamide, whereas no change occurred in the placebo cohort ($p < .001$).[46] No correlation was found between the decrease in serum PSA level and the improvement in peak urinary flow rate or the symptom score. In a similar study of 390 patients with prostate cancer, administration of bicalutamide (50 mg per day) for at least 12 weeks produced a 90% decrease in serum PSA.[47] Serum testosterone levels ranged from normal to 60% elevated.

Side effects are an important deterrent to antiandrogen therapy. The major side effects of flutamide therapy include gynecomastia and breast tenderness, which occur in ~50% of patients.[43] Gastrointestinal upset, manifested by nausea, diarrhea, and flatulence, also is seen frequently. Bicalutamide has a similar side-effect profile, except that gastrointestinal side effects occur less frequently.[47] Libido and potency are affected only rarely by antiandrogen treatment (in 8% and 7% of patients, respectively) because the serum testosterone level is not decreased.[46]

Antiandrogen therapy represents an improvement over GnRH-agonist therapy in that antiandrogens are oral medications and have no significant effect on sexual function. However, they are associated with breast and gastrointestinal side effects in many patients. Like GnRH agonists, they decrease prostatic size by ~20% to 25%, improve voiding function in 30% of patients, cause lowering of the serum PSA concentration, and are expensive to administer. The annual cost of flutamide therapy is ~$2500. Currently, their use in the treatment of BPH is limited, primarily because of the adverse reactions and cost.

## 5α-REDUCTASE INHIBITORS

Studies of male pseudohermaphroditism led to what is today considered the most promising endocrine treatment of BPH.[48,49] Boys with this autosomal recessive disorder present with ambiguous genitalia and normal but undescended testes. The disorder, most commonly found in the Dominican Republic, is linked to a deficiency in the enzyme 5α-reductase (see Chaps. 114 and 115). This enzyme is responsible for the conversion of testosterone to the more active androgen DHT. External genitalia are abnormal due to failure of the urogenital sinus structures to fully develop. Wolffian structures are able to develop normally. At puberty, a marked increase in testosterone levels allows for virilization. Interestingly, men with this deficiency do not develop clinical evidence of BPH or male-pattern baldness. Thus, the link between 5α-reductase activity and the development of BPH was established.

Two subtypes of 5α-reductase receptors are found[50]: 5α-reductase type 1 receptors are found primarily in the skin and hair follicles; 5α-reductase type 2 receptors are present primarily in the prostate. Thus, receptor selectivity may be useful in producing different therapeutic effects. Currently, the role of

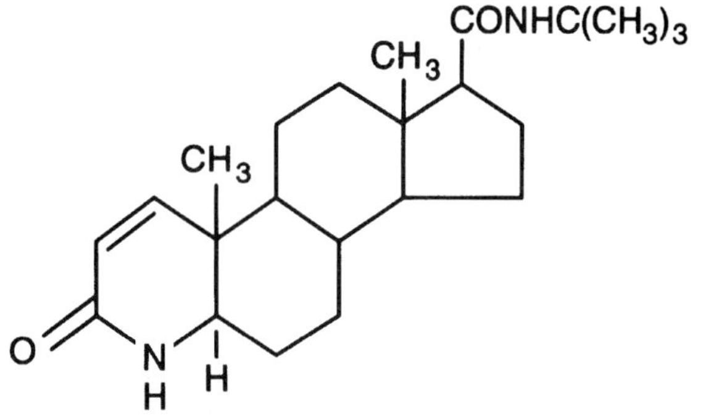

**FIGURE 121-3.** Structure of finasteride.

5α-reductase type 2 in the prostate is unknown. Studies are ongoing to determine if blockade of both isoenzymes of 5α-reductase is more effective than blockade of only the type 2 enzyme in patients with BPH.

Finasteride is a potent oral 5α-reductase type 2 inhibitor that has been studied extensively (Fig. 121-3). This synthetic 4-azasteroid compound does not interfere with the binding of testosterone or DHT to the androgen receptor and does not possess any androgenic, antiandrogenic, or other hormonally related properties.[51] The selective nature of the 5α-reductase inhibitors in decreasing DHT without causing other hormonal effects makes them potentially ideal medications for the treatment of BPH.

The efficacy of finasteride in the treatment of symptomatic BPH was first evaluated in a multicenter, double-blind trial in which 895 men were randomized to receive placebo or finasteride (5 mg per day).[52] A modified symptom score was used for evaluation. The finasteride-treated group had a decrease of 2.5 units in the symptom score, whereas the placebo group had a decrease of 1 unit ($p < .5$). Peak urinary flow rates increased by 1.6 mL per second in the treatment group but did not change in the placebo group. The mean decrease in prostatic volume for the finasteride-treated men was 19% after 12 months of therapy. Similar results have been observed in the Canadian PROSPECT study, the Scandinavian SCARP studies, and two larger international studies, those of the finasteride and PROWESS study groups.[53-56]

Interestingly, finasteride appears to reduce voiding pressures to a greater degree than it improves flow rates. In pressure-flow studies of 27 patients,[57] the mean detrusor pressures at maximum urine flow decreased by >60% after 4 years of finasteride treatment.

Nevertheless, the Veterans Affairs Cooperative Studies BPH study group found that finasteride was no more effective than placebo in the treatment of symptomatic BPH.[58] In a 52-week study, 1229 veterans were randomized to receive either terazosin (an $\alpha_1$-adrenergic antagonist), finasteride (5 mg per day), a combination of terazosin and finasteride, or placebo. The average change in symptom score (3.2 in the finasteride group vs. 2.6 in the placebo group) was not statistically significant. The average increase in urinary flow rate was 1.6 mL per second in the finasteride group and 1.4 mL per second in the placebo group. Consistent with other reports, however, the mean decrease in prostate volume in the finasteride group after 52 weeks of treatment was 6.1 mL (27%). The placebo group had an increase in prostate volume of 0.5 mL. The conclusion drawn was that finasteride, although effective in reducing the volume of the prostate gland, was not as effective in the treatment of BPH as had been previously reported. However, the average baseline prostate volume in this study was noted to be 50% less than that in previous studies.

The premise that the efficacy of finasteride depends on the baseline prostate volume has been tested in a metaanalysis of data from six different studies in which the efficacy of finasteride treatment of men with large prostates was evaluated.[59]

Improvements in urinary flow rates and symptom scores were found to be proportional to prostate volume. Patients with prostate glands of ≥40 mL experienced a statistically significant improvement in urinary flow and symptoms, whereas those with smaller glands did not. The conclusion was that finasteride treatment of BPH is more effective in those men with large prostates.

The finding that finasteride therapy is more effective in men with larger prostates is further supported by evaluation of the tissue composition of prostates treated with this medication. Analysis of serial prostate biopsy specimens from men treated with finasteride for 24 to 30 months revealed a progressive decrease in the epithelial component.[60] Furthermore, epithelium comprised a greater percentage of prostate volume in large prostates than it did in small prostates. Thus, that larger prostates with a greater epithelial component should respond best to finasteride therapy is logical.

Finally, finasteride treatment reduces the incidence of acute urinary retention and the requirement for surgical intervention in men with BPH. In a 4-year study, 2.8% of study patients taking finasteride experienced acute urinary retention compared with 6.6% in a placebo group ($p < .001$).[61] The largest BPH study completed to date has confirmed this finding.[62] In this multicenter randomized, placebo-controlled study, 3040 men with moderate to severe BPH symptoms and enlarged prostates were assigned to receive finasteride (5 mg per day) or placebo, and outcomes—including urinary retention and surgical intervention—were assessed. During the 4-year study, 4.6% of the finasteride patients underwent surgery for an enlarged prostate compared with 10.1% of the control group. Acute urinary retention developed in 2.8% of finasteride-treated men and in 6.7% of controls. Finasteride has also been shown to reduce hematuria in men with BPH. In a study of men with BPH and hematuria, hematuria recurred within 1 year in 63% of control patients vs. 14% of finasteride treated patients.[62a]

Two to 6 months of continuous therapy are required to achieve an improvement in BPH symptoms. In those patients who respond to treatment, a greater symptomatic improvement is observed with time. Studies of the long-term efficacy of finasteride treatment have shown that the benefits are maintained for 4 or 5 years.[63] If finasteride treatment is withdrawn, the prostate slowly enlarges and symptoms of bladder obstruction return.

Finasteride has an excellent side-effect profile. The reported rate of impotence is ~2% greater than in the placebo control group.[52] Some men report a decrease in libido. A demonstrable decrease occurs in ejaculatory volume.

Serum PSA has played a major role in prostate cancer screening. This analyte is produced by the prostatic epithelium. By reducing the prostatic epithelium, finasteride also reduces serum PSA. A multicenter trial indicated that the PSA level decreases by ~50% within 6 months.[64] Thus, the PSA level in men receiving finasteride therapy should be doubled to properly compare this level with reference ranges. Free PSA appears to be decreased proportionately to total PSA, so the ratio is not significantly changed.[65]

The favorable side-effect profile of finasteride has made this agent attractive for the treatment of BPH. For men with a larger prostate, finasteride may be an appropriate treatment option. Patients should be counseled not to expect improvement for 3 to 6 months. Therapy must be continued for life to maintain efficacy.

## AROMATASE INHIBITORS

Both the prevalence and magnitude of BPH increase with age; therefore, by the eighth decade, nearly all men have developed BPH.[2] Because of the hormonal sensitivity of the prostate, numerous studies have attempted to associate the hormonal changes of aging with BPH. Serum free (bioactive) testosterone concentrations begin a slow, continuous decline after the third

decade of life.[66,67] Conversely, the free estrone and 17-estradiol concentrations maintain a constant level.[68,69] Thus, the ratio of free estrogen to free testosterone increases at the same time that BPH is developing. In a group of men undergoing radical prostatectomy for low-volume prostate carcinoma, sera were assayed for 23 different hormones.[70] These hormone concentrations were correlated with the volume of BPH found within the prostate and corrected for age. The volume of BPH found in the specimens correlated with levels of serum free testosterone, 17β-estradiol, and estriol.

Aromatase inhibitors are compounds that selectively inhibit the enzyme aromatase, which converts testosterone to 17β-estradiol [1,3,5 (10)-estratrien-3, 17β-diol] and androstenedione to estrone [1,3,5 (10)-estratrien-3-ol-17-one].[71] The association between estrogens and BPH aromatase activities in the prostate has been investigated. Indeed, aromatase levels are higher in the prostates of men with BPH than in the prostates of men without BPH.[72,73]

Two aromatase inhibitors, testolactone and atamestane, have been investigated as therapeutic agents for BPH. In single-armed nonrandomized studies, these agents appeared to have some efficacy in treating BPH with no significant adverse side effects.[74–77] These preliminary findings led to a multicenter, double-blind trial involving 292 men with symptoms of BPH.[78] The men were randomized to treatment with either placebo or atamestane at 100 mg or 300 mg per day. Although reductions in serum estrone and estradiol levels were shown, no statistically significant difference was seen in symptom improvement or in urinary flow rate between the placebo group and either atamestane treatment group. Thus, although early studies suggested a possible role for aromatase and estrogens in the pathogenesis of prostatic hyperplasia, aromatase inhibitors do not appear to have a beneficial clinical effect in men with BPH. Additional studies to evaluate the efficacy of aromatase inhibitors in the treatment of men with BPH have not been performed.

## CONCLUSIONS

An endocrine component is at least partially responsible for the development of BPH. Medical therapy has become the first-line treatment for this disorder. The most effective endocrine treatment for BPH available at this time is 5α-reductase inhibition; finasteride is the only 5α-reductase inhibitor currently approved for this use. A major advantage of this medication is its excellent side-effect profile. There is compelling evidence that finasteride is most effective in those men with larger prostates. Improvement generally occurs within 3 to 6 months, and long-term efficacy has been demonstrated after 5 years.

The future of endocrine treatments is bright. Evaluation of other 5α-reductase inhibitors is in progress; these include agents that block the type 1 enzyme. Further investigation of the pathogenesis of BPH will provide better insights into promising directions for the development of future endocrine treatments of BPH.

## REFERENCES

1. Oesterling JE. Benign prostatic hyperplasia: its natural history, epidemiologic characteristics, and surgical treatment. Arch Fam Med 1992; 1:257.
2. Barry MJ. Epidemiology and natural history of benign prostatic hyperplasia. Urol Clin North Am 1990; 17:495.
3. Walsh PC. Human benign prostatic hyperplasia: etiological considerations. Prog Clin Biol Res 1984; 145:1.
4. Birkhoff JD, Wiederhorn AR, Hamilton ML, Zinsser HH. Natural history of benign prostatic hypertrophy and acute urinary retention. Urology 1976; 7:48.
5. Ball AJ, Feneley RCL, Abrams PH. The natural history of untreated prostatism. Br J Urol 1981; 53:613.
6. Wasson JH, Bruskewitz RC, Elinson J, et al. A comparison of transurethral surgery with watchful waiting for moderate symptoms of benign prostatic hyperplasia. The Veterans Affairs Cooperative Study Group on transurethral resection of the prostate. N Engl J Med 1995; 332:75.

7. Rhodes T, Girman CJ, Jacobsen SJ, et al. Longitudinal prostate growth rates during 5 years in randomly selected community men 40 to 79 years old. J Urol 1999; 161:1174.

8. Lepor H, Rigaud G. The efficacy of transurethral resection of the prostate in men with moderate symptoms of prostatism. J Urol 1990; 143:533.

9. Mebust WK, Holtgrewe HL, Cockett AT, and Writing Committee. Transurethral prostatectomy: immediate and postoperative complications. A cooperative study of 13 participating institutions evaluating 3,885 patients. J Urol 1989; 141:243.

10. Holtgrewe HL, Mebust WK, Dowd JB, et al. Transurethral prostatectomy: practice aspects of the dominant operation in American urology. J Urol 1989; 141:248.

11. Fowler FJ Jr, Wennberg JE, Timothy RP, et al. Symptom status and quality of life following prostatectomy. JAMA 1988; 259:3018.

12. Wennberg JE, Roos N, Sola L, et al. Use of claims data systems to evaluate health care outcomes: mortality and reoperation following prostatectomy. JAMA 1987; 257:933.

13. Sirls LT, Ganabathi K, Zimmern PE, et al. Transurethral incision of the prostate: an objective and subjective evaluation of long-term efficacy. J Urol 1993; 150:1615.

14. Caine M, Pfau A, Perlberg S. The use of alpha-adrenergic blockers in benign prostatic obstruction. Br J Urol 1976; 48:255.

15. Roehrborn CG, Oesterling JE, Auerbach S, et al. The Hytrin community assessment trial study: a one-year study of terazosin versus placebo in the treatment of patients with symptomatic benign prostatic hyperplasia (BPH). Urology 1996; 47:159.

16. Gillenwater JY, Conn RL, Chrysant SG, et al. Doxazosin for the treatment of benign prostatic hyperplasia in patients with mild to moderate essential hypertension: a double-blind placebo-controlled, dose-response multicenter study. J Urol 1995; 154:110.

17. Lepor H. Phase III multicenter, placebo-controlled study of tamsulosin in benign prostatic hyperplasia. Urology 1998; 51:892.

18. Wilt TJ, Ishani A, Stark G, et al. Saw palmetto extracts for the treatment of benign prostatic hyperplasia: a systemic review. JAMA 1998; 280:1604.

19. Goepel M, Hecker U, Krege S, et al. Saw palmetto extracts potently and noncompetitively inhibit human alpha adrenoreceptors in vitro. Prostate 1999; 38:208.

20. Muschter R, de la Rosette JJ, Whitfield H, et al. Initial human clinical experience with diode laser interstitial treatment of benign prostatic hyperplasia. Urology 1996; 48:223.

21. Bruckewitz R, Issa MM, Roerhborn CG, et al. A prospective, randomized 1-year clinical trial comparing transurethral needle ablation to transurethral resection of the prostate for the treatment of symptomatic benign prostatic hyperplasia. J Urol 1998; 159:1588.

22. Blute ML, Tomera KM, Hellerstein DK, et al. Transurethral microwave thermotherapy for management of benign prostatic hyperplasia: results of the United States Prostatron cooperative study. J Urol 1993; 150:1591.

23. Madersbacher S, Kratzik C, Susani M, Marberger M. Tissue ablation in benign prostatic hyperplasia with high intensity focused ultrasound. J Urol 1995; 152:1956.

24. Oesterling JE, Kaplan SA, Epstein HB, et al. The North American experience with the UroLume™ endoprosthesis as a treatment for benign prostatic hyperplasia: long-term results. Urology 1994; 44:353.

25. White JW. The results of double castration in hypertrophy of the prostate. Ann Surg 1995; 22:1.

26. Huggins C, Clark PJ. Quantitative studies of prostatic secretion: II. The effect of castration and of estrogen injection on the normal and on the hyperplastic prostate glands of dogs. J Exp Med 1940; 72:747.

27. Cabot AT. The question of castration for enlarged prostate. Ann Surg 1996; 24:265.

28. Huggins C, Stevens RA. The effect of castration on benign hypertrophy of the prostate in man. J Urol 1940; 43:705.

29. Griffin JE, Wilson JD. Disorders of the testes and male reproductive tract. In: Wilson JD, Foster DW, eds. Textbook of endocrinology, 7th ed. Philadelphia: WB Saunders, 1985:259.

30. Conn PM, Crowley WF Jr. Gonadotropin-releasing hormone and its analogues. N Engl J Med 1991; 324:93.

31. Blum JJ, Conn PM. Gonadotropin-releasing hormone stimulation of luteinizing hormone release: a ligand-receptor-effector model. Proc Natl Acad Sci U S A 1982; 79:7307.

32. Eri LM, Haug E, Tveter KJ. Effects on the endocrine system of long-term treatment with the luteinizing hormone–releasing hormone agonist leuprolide in patients with benign prostatic hyperplasia. Scand J Clin Lab Invest 1996; 56(4):319.

33. Schrüder FH, Westerhof M, Bosch RJLH, Kurth KH. Benign prostatic hyperplasia treated by castration or the LHRH analogue buserelin: a report on 6 cases. Eur Urol 1986; 12:318.

34. Peters CA, Walsh PC. The effect of nafarelin acetate, a luteinizing hormone–releasing hormone agonist, on benign prostatic hyperplasia. N Engl J Med 1987; 317:599.

35. Matzkin H, Chen J, Lewysohn O, Braf Z. Treatment of benign prostatic hypertrophy by a long-acting gonadotropin-releasing hormone analogue: one-year experience. J Urol 1991; 145:309.

36. McConnell JD. Androgen ablation and blockade in the treatment of benign prostatic hyperplasia. Urol Clin North Am 1990; 17:661.

37. Sufrin G, Coffey DS. Flutamide: mechanism of action of a new nonsteroidal antiandrogen. Invest Urol 1976; 13:429.

38. Blackledge GR, Cockshott ID, Furr BJ. Casodex (bicalutamide): overview of a new antiandrogen developed for the treatment of prostate cancer. Eur Urol 1997; 31(Suppl 2):30.

39. Furr BJ, Tucker H. The preclinical development of bicalutamide: pharmacodynamics and mechanism of action. Urology 1996; 47(Suppl 1A):13.

40. Neri R. Pharmacology and pharmacokinetics of flutamide. Urology 1989; 34(Suppl):19.

41. Caine M, Perlberg S, Gordon R. The treatment of benign prostatic hypertrophy with flutamide (SCH 13521): a placebo-controlled study. J Urol 1975; 114:564.

42. Stone N. Flutamide in treatment of benign prostatic hypertrophy. Urology 1989; 39(Suppl):64.

43. Narayan P, Trachtenberg J, Lepor H, et al. A dose-response study of the effect of flutamide on benign prostatic hyperplasia: results of a multicenter study. Urology 1996; 47(4):497.

44. Eri LM, Kjell JT. A prospective, placebo-controlled study of the antiandrogen Casodex as treatment for patients with benign prostatic hyperplasia. J Urol 1993; 150:90.

45. Berger BM, Naadimuthu A, Boddy A. The effect of zanoterone, a steroidal androgen receptor antagonist, in men with benign prostatic hyperplasia. J Urol 1995; 154:1060.

46. Stone NN, Clejan SJ. Response of prostate volume, prostate-specific antigen, and testosterone to flutamide in men with benign prostatic hyperplasia. J Androl 1991; 12:376.

47. Tyrrell CJ, Denis L, Newling D, et al. Casodex 10–200 mg daily, used as monotherapy for the treatment of patients with advanced prostate cancer. An overview of the efficacy, tolerability and pharmacokinetics from three phase II dose-ranging studies. Eur Urol 1998; 33(1):39.

48. Walsh PC, Madden JD, Harrod MJ, et al. Familial incomplete male pseudohermaphroditism, type 2. Decreased dihydrotestosterone formation in pseudovaginal perineoscrotal hypospadias. N Engl J Med 1974; 291:944.

49. Imperato-McGinley J, Guerrero L, Gautier T, Peterson RE. Steroid 5α-reductase deficiency in man: an inherited form of male pseudohermaphroditism. Science 1974; 186:1213.

50. Russell DW, Wilson JD. Steriod 5 alpha reductase: two genes/two enzymes. Annu Rev Biochem 1994; 63:25.

51. Bartsch G, Rittmaster RS, Klocker H. Dihydrotestosterone and the concept of 5alpha-reductase inhibition in human prostatic hyperplasia. Eur Urol 2000; 37:367.

52. Gormley GJK, Stoner E, Bruskewitz RC, et al. The effect of finasteride in men with benign prostatic hyperplasia. N Engl J Med 1992; 327:1185.

53. Nickel JC, Fradet Y, Boske RC, et al. Efficacy and safety of finasteride therapy for benign prostatic hyperplasia: result of a 2-year randomized controlled study. Can Med Assoc J 1996; 155:1251.

54. Andersen JT, Ekman P, Wolf H, et al. Can finasteride reverse the progress of benign prostatic hyperplasia? A two-year placebo-controlled study. The Scandinavian BPH Study Group. Urology 1995; 46:631.

55. The Finasteride Study Group. Finasteride (MK-906) in the treatment of benign prostatic hyperplasia. Prostate 1993; 22:291.

56. Marberger JM. Long-term effects of finasteride in patients with benign prostatic hyperplasia: a double-blind, placebo-controlled, multicenter study. Urology 1998; 51:677.

57. Tamella TLJ, Kontturi MJ. Long-term effects of finasteride on invasive urodynamics and symptoms in the treatment of patients with bladder outflow obstruction due to benign prostatic hyperplasia. J Urol 1995; 154:1466.

58. Lepor H, Williford WO, Barry MJ, et al. The efficacy of terazosin, finasteride, or both in benign prostatic hyperplasia. N Engl J Med 1996; 335(8):533.

59. Boyle P, Gould AL, Roerhrborn CG. Prostate volume predicts outcome of treatment of benign prostatic hyperplasia with finasteride: meta-analysis of randomized clinical trials. Urology 1996; 48:398.

60. Marks LS, Partin AW, Dorey FJ, et al. Long-term effects of finasteride on prostate tissue composition. Urology 1999; 53:574.

61. Roehrborn CG, Bruskewitz R, Nickel GC, et al. Urinary retention in patients with BPH treated with finasteride or placebo over 4 years. Characterization of patients and ultimate outcomes. The PLESS Study Group. Eur Urol 2000; 37:528.

62. McConnell JD, Bruskewitz R, Walsh P, et al. The effect of finasteride on the risk of acute urinary retention and the need for surgical treatment among men with benign prostatic hyperplasia. N Engl J Med 1998; 338:557.

62a. Foley SJ, Soloman LZ, Wedderburn AW, et al. A prospective study of the natural history of hematuria associated with benign prostatic hyperplasia and the effect of finasteride. J Urol 2000; 163:496.

63. Hudson PB, Boak R, Trachtenberg J, et al. Efficacy of finasteride is maintained in patients with benign prostatic hyperplasia treated for 5 years. Urology 1999; 53:690.59.

64. Guess HA, Gormley GJ, Stoner E, et al. The effect of finasteride on prostate specific antigen. J Urol 1996; 155:3

65. Pannek J, Marks LS, Pearson JD, et al. Influence of finasteride on free and total serum prostate specific antigen levels in men with benign prostatic hyperplasia. J Urol 1998; 159:449.

66. Vermeulen A, Rubens R, Verdonck L. Testosterone secretion and metabolism in male senescence. J Clin Endocrinol Metab 1972; 34:730.

67. Rubens R, Dhont M, Vermeulen A. Further studies on Leydig cell function in old age. J Clin Endocrinol Metab 1974; 39:40.

68. Harman SM, Tsitouras PD. Reproductive hormones in aging men. I. Measurement of sex steroids, basal luteinizing hormone, and Leydig cell response to human chorionic gonadotropin. J Clin Endocrinol Metab 1980; 51:35.

69. Deslypere JP, Vermeulen A. Leydig cell function in normal men: effect of age, lifestyle, residence, diet and activity. J Clin Endocrinol Metab 1984; 59:955.

70. Partin AW, Oesterling JE, Epstein JI, et al. Influence of age and endocrine factors on the volume of benign prostatic hyperplasia. J Urol 1991; 145:405.

71. Henderson D, Habenicht UF, Nishino Y, El Etreby MF. Estrogens and benign prostatic hyperplasia: the basis for aromatase inhibitor therapy. Steroids 1987; 50:219.

72. Stone NN, Fair WR, Fishman J. Estrogen formation in human prostatic tissue from patients with and without benign hyperplasia. Prostate 1986; 9:311.

73. Perel E, Killinger DW. The metabolism of androstenedione and testosterone to C19 metabolites in normal breast, breast carcinoma and benign prostatic hypertrophy tissue. J Steroid Biochem 1983; 19:1135.

74. Habenicht U-F, Tunn UW, Senge TH, et al. Management of benign prostatic hyperplasia with particular emphasis on aromatase inhibitors. J Steroid Biochem Mol Biol 1993; 44:557.

75. El Etreby MF. Atamestane: an aromatase inhibitor for the treatment of benign prostatic hyperplasia: a short review. J Steroid Biochem Mol Biol 1993; 44:565.

76. El Etreby MF, Habenicht UF, Henderson D, et al. Atamestane: a new aromatase inhibitor. Berlin: Diesbach Verlag, 1991:49.

77. Schweikert HU, Tunn UW. Effects of the aromatase inhibitor, testolactone on human benign prostatic hyperplasia. Steroids 1987; 50:191.

78. Radlmaier A, Eickenberg HU, Fletcher MS, et al. Estrogen reduction by aromatase inhibition for benign prostatic hyperplasia: results of a double-blind, placebo-controlled, randomized clinical trial using two doses of the aromatase-inhibitor atamestane. Prostate 1996; 29(4):199.

# CHAPTER 122

# TESTICULAR TUMORS

NIELS E. SKAKKEBAEK AND MIKAEL RØRTH

Although tumors of the testis may originate from several types of cells in the seminiferous tubules or the interstitial tissue, most testicular tumors are *germ-cell neoplasms*.[1] Approximately 25% to 30% of all germ-cell tumors produce human chorionic gonadotropin (hCG), α-fetoprotein (AFP), or both. Tumors originating from Leydig cells or Sertoli cells often produce sex steroids (testosterone or estrogen). Therefore, germ-cell tumors as well as Leydig- and Sertoli-cell neoplasms may be associated with clinical signs of abnormal hormone production (e.g., gynecomastia; Fig. 122-1). Moreover, testicular cancer is associated with an increased risk of infertility. Hence, these lesions are of considerable importance to the clinical endocrinologist.

# GERM-CELL TUMORS

## ETIOLOGY AND EPIDEMIOLOGY

The etiology of testicular germ-cell cancer is unclear, although genetic, hormonal, and environmental factors seem important.[1a] For example, the morbidity of testicular cancer in Finland, which has an ethnic background different from that of other Nordic countries, is far lower than in Denmark,[2] although the economic, social, and cultural conditions are rather similar. Likewise, the morbidity of testicular cancer is many times less among blacks in both the United States and Africa than in the white population in the United States.[2] Familial testicular cancer occurs rarely.[3,4]

It appears from several lines of evidence that endocrine factors play a role in the development of testicular cancer.[5–8] First, germ-cell cancer is extremely rare during childhood except for the first 1 to 2 years after birth. Similarly, blood levels of gonadotropins and sex steroids are extremely low during childhood except for the perinatal period through the first half-year. The increase in the production of follicle-stimulating hormone, luteinizing hormone, and testosterone during puberty is followed by an increase in the incidence of testicular cancer, which peaks 10 to 20 years later.[2] Second, germ-cell cancer is extremely rare in patients with hypogonadotropic hypogonadism, although this syndrome is associated with a high incidence of cryptorchidism, which generally increases the risk of germ-cell tumors (see later). Third, an association between gonadotropin or clomiphene administration and testicular cancer has been reported occasionally.[5–8] Fourth, hCG-producing tumors have a more aggressive course than do other nonseminomas. Fifth, it has been suggested that exogenous estrogens given during pregnancy can lead to testicular cancer of the offspring.[9] Nevertheless, the direct role of hormones in the pathogenesis of testicular cancer is unclear.

The average annual age-adjusted testicular cancer incidence rates, which among North American whites and most West Europeans are 3 to 9 per 100,000, have increased two-fold to four-fold during the last few decades.[2,10] This increase also has occurred in countries with stable populations; this and other evidence suggest that environmental factors play a role.[11]

## HISTOLOGY: CLASSIFICATION AND DIAGNOSIS

Traditionally, germ-cell tumors are classified as *seminomas* or *nonseminomas*[12] (Table 122-1; Figs. 122-2 through 122-5).

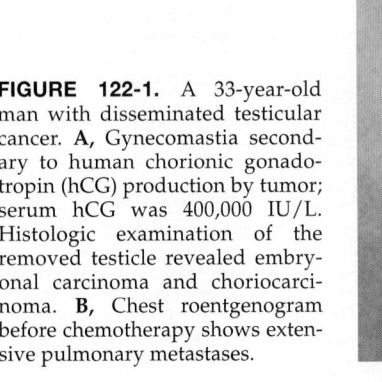

**FIGURE 122-1.** A 33-year-old man with disseminated testicular cancer. **A,** Gynecomastia secondary to human chorionic gonadotropin (hCG) production by tumor; serum hCG was 400,000 IU/L. Histologic examination of the removed testicle revealed embryonal carcinoma and choriocarcinoma. **B,** Chest roentgenogram before chemotherapy shows extensive pulmonary metastases.

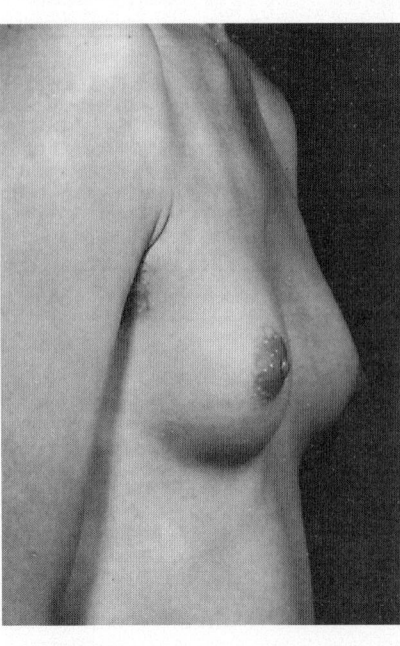

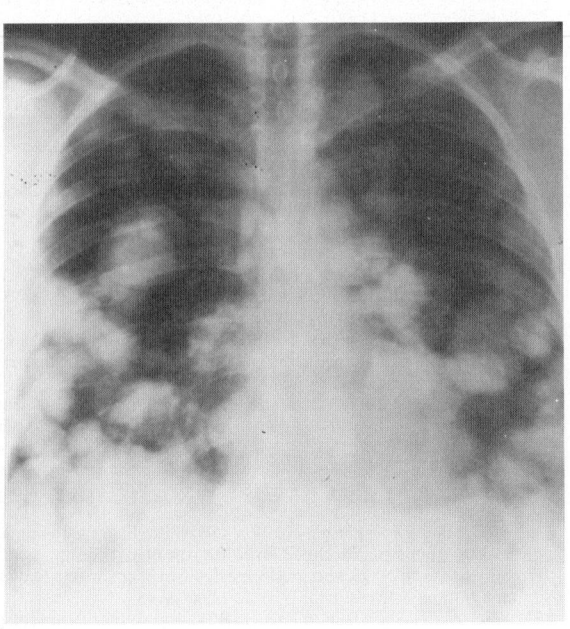

**A,B**

**TABLE 122-1.**
**Nomenclature of Testicular Germ-Cell Tumors**

**SEMINOMA**
　Classic
　Spermatocytic
**NONSEMINOMA**
　Teratoma
　　Mature
　　Immature
　Teratoma with malignant transformation
　Embryonal carcinoma
　Choriocarcinoma
　Yolk sac tumor
**COMBINED TUMOR**

(From World Health Organization. Histological typing of testis tumours. Geneva: WHO, 1977:1.)

Although one type of lesion has been called *spermatocytic seminoma*,[12] there is strong biologic evidence that it is different from seminoma,[13,14] so the term *spermatocytoma* should be used[16] (also see later).

The classic seminoma and the nonseminomatous germ-cell tumors seem to have the same biology. First, several studies have shown that morphologically identical precursor cells, *carcinoma in situ* (CIS) of the testis, originate both seminomas and nonseminomas[15–17] (see Figs. 122-2 and 122-5). Second, approximately one-third of germ-cell tumors contain mixed elements of seminomas and nonseminomas.[18] Third, the seminoma cells sometimes have functional properties similar to those of choriocarcinoma cells, including hCG production,[19–21] thus indicating that intermediate forms exist. Nevertheless, practically, especially in relation to treatment, it remains appropriate to maintain the distinction between seminomas and nonseminomas.

Several new histologic techniques are available for the diagnosis of different components in germ-cell tumors, including the immunocytochemical demonstration of cytoplasmic AFP, hCG, and placenta-like alkaline phosphatase.[20,22,23] The diagnosis of CIS requires special histologic techniques (see later).

## CARCINOMA IN SITU OF THE TESTIS

CIS of the testis is a characteristic abnormal histologic pattern of intratubular germ cells that may precede by many years the development of a palpable tumor.[16,24–27] The testicle harboring this lesion usually is one-half or one-third the size of the normal organ.[28] Sometimes, it is slightly tender, although no clinical signs or symptoms are present in most patients. CIS is not associated with tumor markers in serum, although the platelet-derived growth factor α-receptor has been suggested as a molecular marker.[29] Thus, a standard surgical biopsy procedure is the only way to detect CIS.

### DIAGNOSIS OF CARCINOMA IN SITU

The diagnosis of CIS requires appropriate fixatives (i.e., Stieve or Bouin fixative). Several staining methods can be used. For routine purposes, the iron hematoxylin stain is best. In specimens, which have been handled appropriately,[30] the CIS germ cells can be identified easily inside the seminiferous tubules.[25,31] In typical cases, they are located along the tubular membrane in one layer

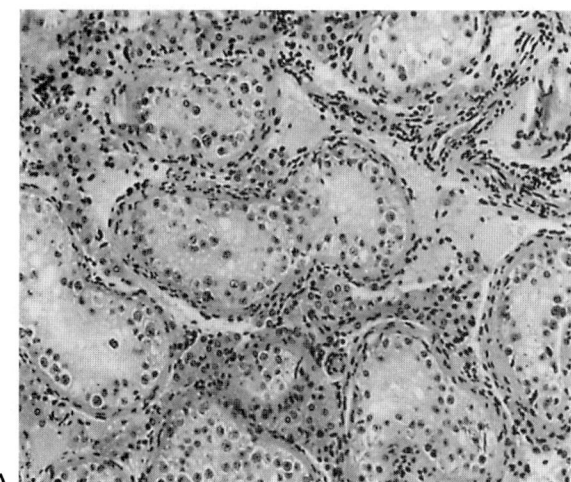
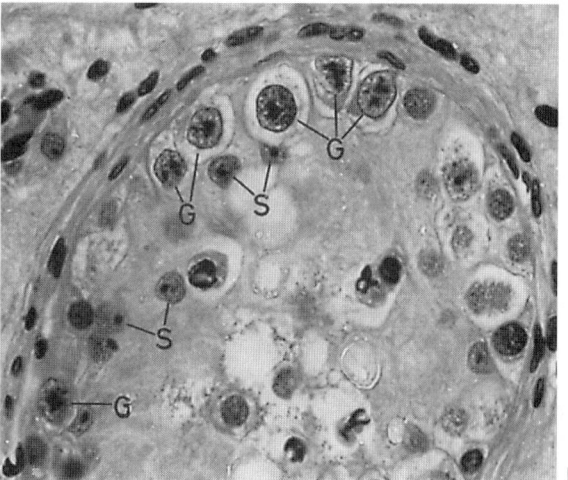
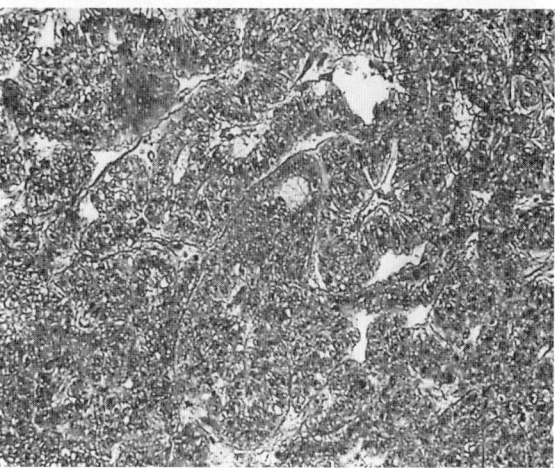

**FIGURE 122-2.** A 30-year-old oligozoospermic man. **A,** Testicular biopsy shows seminiferous tubules with carcinoma in situ. No invasion of interstitial tissue. ×180 **B,** Higher magnification of seminiferous tubules containing germ-cell carcinoma in situ (G) and Sertoli cells (S). **C,** Same testis excised 4 years later for palpable tumor shows mixed non-seminomatous germ-cell tumor containing embryonal carcinoma elements. (From Skakkebaek NE. Carcinoma-in-situ of the testis: frequency and relationship to invasive germ-cell tumours in infertile men. Histopathology 1978; 2:157.)

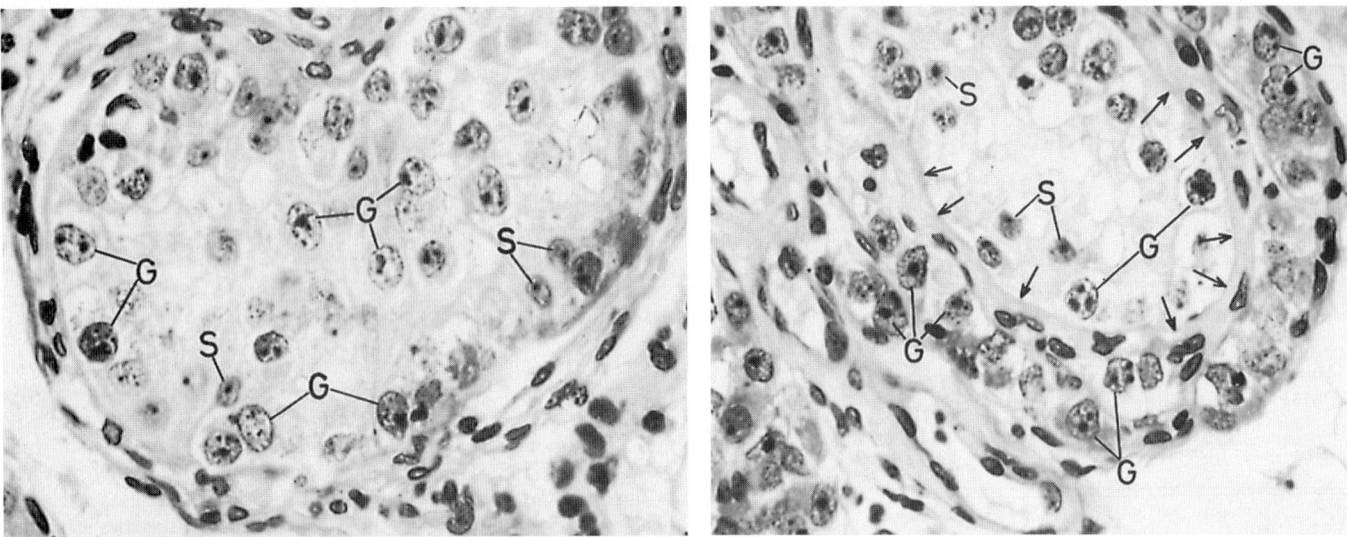

**FIGURE 122-3.** Excised testis of a 36-year-old oligozoospermic, infertile man. **A,** Seminiferous tubule from area with carcinoma in situ pattern. No invasive growth. Identical to testicular biopsy taken 4 years previously. (*G,* carcinoma in situ of germ cells; *S,* Sertoli cells.) ×700 **B,** Area with invasive growth of germ cells (*G*), which are located both inside the seminiferous tubule and in the interstitial tissue. (*S,* Sertoli cells.) *Arrows* indicate basal membrane of the tubule. ×700 (From Skakkebaek NE. Carcinoma-in-situ of the testis: frequency and relationship to invasive germ cell tumours in infertile men. Histopathology 1978; 2:157.)

of cells. The nucleus of each CIS cell is ~10 μm in diameter (normal spermatogonia have nuclei of 6 μm). The chromatin pattern is coarse, and one or two nucleoli usually are visible in each cell. The DNA content is aneuploid[32]; the isochromosome 12p, a marker chromosome in germ-cell tumors, has also been demonstrated in CIS, which overexpresses cyclin D2.[33] The cytoplasm of the CIS cell is rich in glycogen and placenta-like alkaline phosphatase.[22,34,35] The monoclonal antibodies (439F, M2A, TRA60, and c-*kit*) also can be used as immunohistochemical markers for CIS because these antigens are not expressed in normal germ cells.[36–39] The Sertoli cells, which in typical cases are the only other cells present, are found in a layer closer to the lumen (see

Figs. 122-2 and 122-3). Ultrastructural studies show that the CIS cells have characteristics of primordial germ cells.[15,40,41]

CIS of the testis is a dispersed process. In an extensive study of material from excised testicles with CIS, it was found that a conventional surgical biopsy specimen measuring ~3 mm in diameter usually is representative of the whole testicle.[42] In almost all cases, CIS was found at follow-up biopsy in patients who had CIS at the time of initial biopsy.[25] The incidence of CIS in the general population is unknown, although preliminary evidence suggests that it is much rarer than in the special at-risk groups (<0.2%). CIS cells of the seminiferous epithelium may be exfoliated into the seminal fluid.[43]

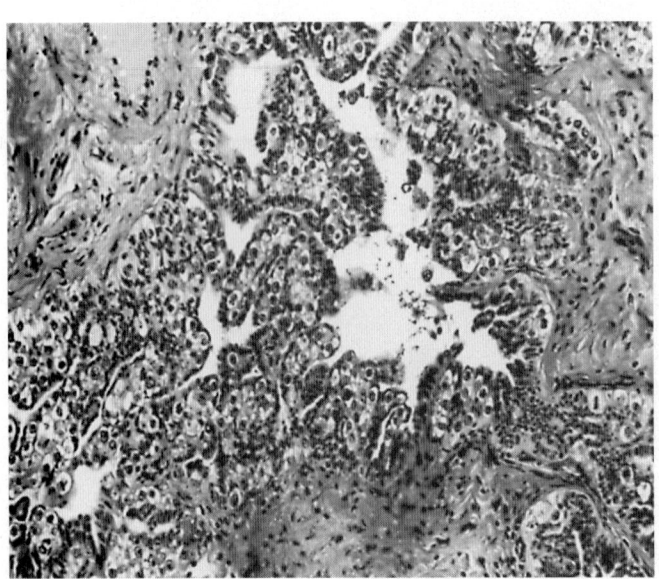
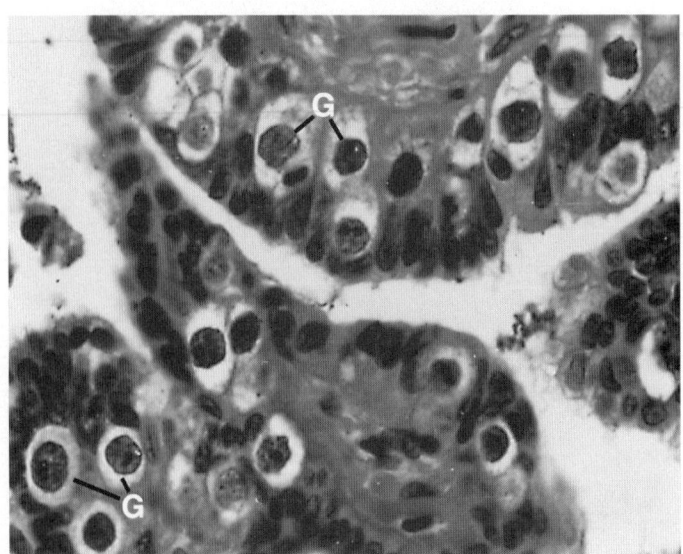

**FIGURE 122-4.** Excised testis of a 35-year-old oligozoospermic, infertile man. Germ cells had invaded the interstitial tissue in several parts of the testis. **A,** Section of rete testis showing invasive growth of germ cells. ×180 **B,** Higher magnification; note that germ cells are identical to carcinoma in situ cells underneath cylindrical epithelium of rete testis. (*G,* germ cells.) ×700 (From Skakkebaek NE. Carcinoma-in-situ of the testis: frequency and relationship to invasive germ cell tumours in infertile men. Histopathology 1978; 2:157.)

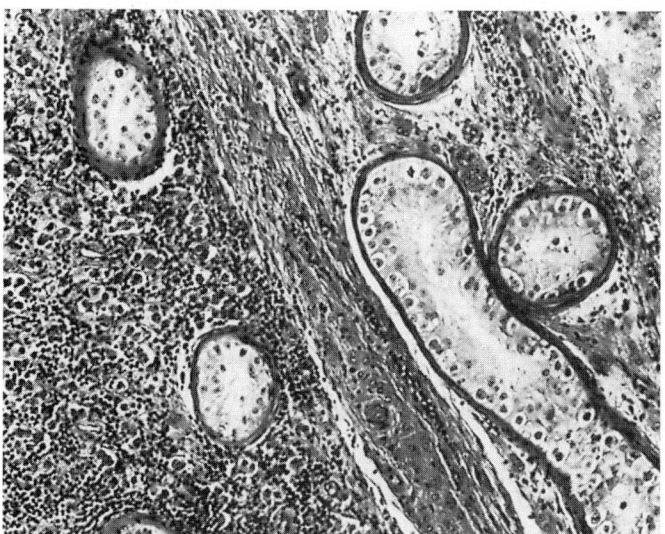

**FIGURE 122-5.** Seminoma in testis of an 18-year-old man with maldescended testis, showing the border between the seminoma (*left*) and adjacent testicular tissue. Note carcinoma in situ of germ cells inside seminiferous tubules. ×150 (From Krabbe S, Skakkebaek NE, Berthelsen JG, et al. High incidence of undetected neoplasia in maldescended testes. Lancet 1979; 1:999.)

### CARCINOMA IN SITU IN INFERTILE MEN

CIS first was diagnosed in infertile men as a chance finding in biopsy specimens removed as part of an infertility evaluation[24–27,44] (see Figs. 122-2 and 122-3). Among ~1300 infertile men selected for testicular biopsy because of oligozoospermia or azoospermia, CIS was found in 1%.[25,45] Similar studies in other countries also have revealed CIS as a chance finding in testicular biopsies of infertile men.[24,26,27] The incidence of CIS probably is highest in biopsy series comprising a relatively high number of infertile patients with very low sperm counts, because the CIS pattern usually is associated with severe oligozoospermia (sperm counts of <5 million/mL; on average, 1–2 million/mL).[28] However, the observed variation in the incidence of CIS as a chance finding in testicular biopsy specimens from infertile men (0.4–1.1%)[24,26,45] also may correspond to the variation in the incidence of testicular cancer in various countries.

It is important to diagnose CIS, because invasive cancer develops in 50% of the patients within 5 years.[45,46] If the CIS is unilateral, orchiectomy should be performed without further treatment except clinical follow-up. In bilateral CIS, irradiation of both testicles is recommended.

### CARCINOMA IN SITU IN THE CONTRALATERAL TESTIS OF PATIENTS WITH GERM-CELL CANCER

In men with unilateral germ-cell cancer of the testis, the risk of cancer developing in the contralateral gonad is significantly increased.[47,48] Therefore, patients with unilateral testicular cancer should have a biopsy specimen from the contralateral testis examined for CIS. In Danish and German studies, the incidence of CIS in the contralateral testis was 5%.[49–51] Intensive chemotherapy given because of dissemination of contralateral testicular cancer sometimes eradicates the CIS germ cells.[52–55] However, CIS in the contralateral testis of patients who receive irradiation of the regional lymph nodes or no postorchiectomy therapy for their initial testicular cancer persists and, in half of the cases, is followed by invasive cancer within 5 years.[50,51] Data show that irradiation of a testis with CIS using a dose of 16 to 20 Gy delivered as 8 to 10 fractions within 2 weeks eradicates the CIS germ cells.[51,56] Leydig cell function and, hence, testosterone production are affected little by this treatment, which, in men with one previous tumor, is standard therapy to avoid bilateral orchiectomy and subsequent androgen replacement.[55] The authors are evaluating the effects of lower doses (14 Gy) that may be sufficient to eradicate CIS cells without impairing Leydig cell function.[57]

### CARCINOMA IN SITU IN PATIENTS WITH MALDESCENDED TESTES

Men with current or corrected cryptorchidism have an increased risk of testicular cancer[58,59] (see Chap. 93). Previous reports, which were based on retrospective studies, overestimated this risk. More recent investigations, which also include one cohort study,[60] show that men with maldescended testes have a four-fold to nine-fold increased risk of germ-cell cancer development.[61,62] Several researchers have reported on CIS in cryptorchid testes.[28,44,61–63] However, the incidence of CIS in the population of men with maldescended testes remains to be established. Thus, the place of testicular biopsy in the follow-up of patients with maldescended testes is unclear.

Intraabdominal testes, which cannot be placed in the scrotum by hormonal or surgical therapy, pose a special problem. Several authors recommend orchiectomy in such cases, especially if the patient is younger than 40 years.[58] However, the finding, discussed earlier, that a moderate dose of irradiation can eradicate the germ cells, including the CIS cells, without significantly impairing Leydig cell function makes this treatment a possible alternative to orchiectomy, especially for patients with bilateral intraabdominal testes or intraabdominal monorchia.

### CARCINOMA IN SITU IN THE ANDROGEN-INSENSITIVITY SYNDROME AND 45,X/46,XY GONADAL DYSGENESIS

Patients with androgen insensitivity and those with 45,X/46,XY gonadal dysgenesis are at extremely high risk for the development of germ-cell cancer.[64] CIS germ cells also seem to be associated with the cancer in these syndromes.[65–70] It is common to recommend prophylactic orchiectomy in patients with these conditions, although in the case of the androgen-insensitivity syndrome, it is unsettled whether the orchiectomy should be carried out during childhood or after the pubertal development of the breasts has occurred.[64,68]

### CARCINOMA IN SITU IN PATIENTS WITH EXTRAGONADAL GERM-CELL TUMORS

CIS has been found in the testis of 42% of patients with primary retroperitoneal tumors as compared to patients with primary tumors in the mediastinum or central nervous system. These findings indicate that these tumors are not always truly extragonadal. Therefore, bilateral surgical biopsies of the testes are needed to exclude testicular malignancy in patients with assumed extragonadal primaries in the retroperitoneum.[71]

## SEMINOMATOUS AND NONSEMINOMATOUS GERM-CELL TUMORS

### SYMPTOMATOLOGY AND PHYSICAL FINDINGS

The usual presentation of testicular cancer is a painless mass, but pain occurs in 15% to 35% of the cases.[72] A scrotal mass can be caused by several nonmalignant conditions, such as epididymitis, orchitis, inguinal hernia, hydrocele, varicocele, and spermatocele, and a correct initial diagnosis of testicular cancer is made in only 55% to 60% of the cases.[73] The most frequent erroneous diagnosis is urogenital infection, especially epididymitis. Ultrasonography can improve the diagnostic differentiation between scrotal abnormalities. This procedure is particularly useful when the tumor is small and centrally located. If a tumor cannot be ruled out, surgical exploration through an inguinal incision should be done. A biopsy is insufficient.

In 5% to 10% of the cases, the presenting symptoms or physical signs of testicular cancer are secondary to metastatic disease.[74] Symptoms such as pain in the lumbar region and uncharacteristic discomfort can be caused by retroperitoneal metastases. Pulmonary symptoms attributable to metastases are rare and generally related to massive pulmonary infiltration.

Although effective therapy is available for testicular cancer, it is important to diagnose these tumors as early as possible. The presence of a scrotal mass always should raise the suspicion of a germ-cell tumor. Furthermore, signs and symptoms such as gynecomastia (see Fig. 122-1*A*), lumbar pain, or a retroperitoneal, mediastinal, pulmonary (see Fig. 122-1*B*), or left supraclavicular tumor in a young male always should lead to a thorough investigation for a germ-cell tumor. The evaluation includes careful examination of the testes, ultrasound, and measurements of serum tumor markers. Germ-cell tumors in the testis can be present without physical signs. Furthermore, germ-cell tumors may originate in extragonadal structures. Delays by patients and by physicians often amount to several months and adversely affect the prognosis.[73,75]

### BIOCHEMICAL MARKERS IN SERUM ("TUMOR MARKERS")

Sixty percent of nonseminomatous germ-cell tumors produce AFP, hCG, or both. Although some seminomas excrete small amounts of hCG, large amounts of hCG or AFP in the serum generally indicate the presence of a nonseminomatous germ-cell tumor. Smaller increases in serum AFP (<200 μg/L) are found in some patients with benign liver diseases. Higher levels can be seen in hepatomas (sometimes on the order of grams per liter). If the level in serum exceeds 200 to 300 μg/L, the AFP of germ-cell origin can be distinguished from that of hepatic origin by lectin-affinity immunoelectrophoresis.[76] Certain tumors of non–germ-cell origin (e.g., large cell carcinoma of the lung) can produce hCG, although usually in relatively small amounts.

The proportion of patients with tumors who have markers in the serum increases with advancing stage of disease. The half-life of tumor markers in the serum is ~1 day for hCG and 5 days for AFP. Therefore, if tumor markers do not disappear within days (hCG) or weeks (AFP) after the removal of the testicular lesion, residual tumor tissue must be present. Thus, the measurement of tumor markers during and after treatment is a valuable tool for the detection of residual or relapsing tumor. New markers, especially for seminomas and embryonal carcinomas, are needed. TRA-1-60 is of interest, although its value remains to be confirmed.[77]

### STAGING

Careful staging is always mandatory in testicular cancer, primarily because the treatment strategy and prognosis depend on the extent of disease.[78,79] Noninvasive procedures include roentgenography of the thorax, and computed tomography (CT), ultrasonography, or both, of the retroperitoneal area. The evaluation also should include the measurement of serum tumor markers.

When metastases are present, the retroperitoneal lymph nodes are involved in 85% of the cases. Therefore, study of these lymph nodes is essential, and CT scan or ultrasonography always should be done. Positron emission tomography scanning is being performed, especially for visualization of retroperitoneal metastases.[80] This procedure is likely to lead to better detection of small metastases.

Until recently, it was common practice to carry out a staging laparotomy in patients with nonseminomatous tumors. In many medical centers, this procedure has been replaced by a "wait and see" policy. By performing a thorough retroperitoneal lymph node dissection, ~20% of patients thought to be without extragonadal disease are found to have micrometastases in the lymph nodes.

Conventional chest films usually are sufficient to identify pulmonary metastases; however, metastatic involvement of mediastinal lymph nodes can be difficult to visualize. Therefore, a CT scan of the thorax should be a part of the staging procedure.

On the basis of the results of the staging procedure, the disease can be classified into stages: stage I (no metastases), stage IIA (retroperitoneal node metastases <2 cm), stage IIB (retroperitoneal node metastases ≤5 cm), stage IIC (retroperitoneal node metastases >5 cm), stage IIIA (supradiaphragmatic node metastases), or stage IIIB (extranodal metastases; e.g., lung).[78,79]

## TREATMENT AND PROGNOSIS

The primary treatment of testicular cancer is orchiectomy. In the rare cases in which systemic treatment is begun without orchiectomy, this operative procedure should be carried out subsequently.

Treatment after orchiectomy differs according to the type of testicular tumor (i.e., seminoma vs. nonseminoma) and the stage of disease. A few decades ago, surgery and radiotherapy were the only effective therapies for testicular cancer. The prognosis for patients with nonseminomatous testicular cancer was poor; most eventually died of their disease. With the advent of modern systemic treatment and with the optimal use of combined modalities, the outlook for patients with testicular cancer has improved dramatically: More than 90% can be cured by appropriate treatment.

Germ-cell tumors are among the most sensitive of the malignant diseases to cytotoxic drugs. Active single agents include cisplatin, vinblastine, bleomycin, etoposide, ifosfamide, dactinomycin, methotrexate, and mithramycin. However, cures seldom are achieved with single-agent chemotherapy; to obtain long-term survival, combination chemotherapy should be used. A combination of cisplatin, etoposide, and bleomycin is recommended as standard treatment,[81] but other cisplatin-based combinations also can be used.

### SEMINOMA

Seminomas are highly radiosensitive.[82] The standard treatment of patients with stage I disease includes irradiation of the retroperitoneal, ipsilateral pelvic, and inguinal lymph nodes. Usually, a dose of 25 to 35 Gy is sufficient. More recent studies indicate that 25 Gy is sufficient and that paraaortic irradiation is adequate.[83] The basis for this treatment is the assumption that micrometastases are present in many cases, although the actual incidence is unknown. The long-term survival rate with this treatment strategy is >98%.[84,85] A surveillance strategy is used for patients with stage I disease, based on the assumptions that more than 70% of these patients would be cured by orchiectomy and that "relapses" can be cured.[86] This strategy has yielded good results, but still should be considered experimental (i.e., restricted to clinical trials). In stage II seminomas, the radiotherapy is directed to the same area. In the final part of this treatment, a boost of 5 to 10 Gy is delivered to the retroperitoneal tumor area. However, ~30% of patients with a retroperitoneal tumor diameter exceeding 5 cm cannot be cured by radiotherapy alone, and many centers recommend chemotherapy as a primary treatment in these cases. Others still prefer to give radiotherapy initially.[87] With either strategy, long-term survival for patients with stage II seminoma exceeds 90%.[85]

All patients with stage III seminoma should be assumed to have disseminated disease and, therefore, should be given systemic treatment. The results of such treatment are similar to those of nonseminomatous testicular cancers in stage III, with a long-term survival rate of ~70%.[88,89]

### NONSEMINOMA

Whenever embryonal carcinoma, choriocarcinoma, teratoma, or endodermal sinus tumor is present, the disease should be characterized as a nonseminomatous testicular cancer and treated accordingly. This also holds true for patients with apparent seminoma who have significant amounts of serum AFP (i.e., >20 µg/L) or high amounts of serum hCG (i.e., >300–500 IU/L). Nonseminomas generally are less radiosensitive than are seminomas. Therefore, radiotherapy as the only treatment after orchiectomy has been less rewarding. In stage I, radiotherapy has been standard treatment in some countries (e.g., the United Kingdom and Denmark), whereas retroperitoneal lymph node dissection has been the treatment of choice in many other countries, including the United States. The progress in diagnosis and treatment of this disease has formed the basis for a "wait and see" treatment policy: Patients are observed closely after orchiectomy, and only those in whom signs of metastases develop receive further treatment (combination chemotherapy). The reported relapse frequency is 15% to 30%.[90–93] In most cases, chemotherapy has effectively eradicated the residual disease. The prognosis for patients with stage I nonseminomatous tumors is as good as that for patients with stage I seminomas. This implies a long-term survival rate of more than 98%. The choice of treatment should be based on the possibility of careful control. Thus, factors such as diagnostic facilities and patient compliance play a part in planning the strategy.[94–96]

The treatment strategy for patients with stage II disease is dependent on the tumor size. If the tumor is larger than 5 cm in diameter, treatment should be combination chemotherapy. Debulking surgery in such cases is ineffective.[97] The treatment strategy for patients with stage IIA and IIB disease varies. Most centers in the United States and many in Europe recommend retroperitoneal lymph node dissection with adjuvant chemotherapy. In other countries, such as Denmark, primary systemic treatment always is applied for stage II disease. Both strategies give excellent results, with projected long-term survival rates of >90%.[84] In 15% to 20% of the cases, residual tumor is found in the retroperitoneal area after the scheduled systemic treatment. These tumors should be removed. Usually, such tumors consist of benign elements such as fibrous tissue or teratoma.[98,99]

Patients with stage III disease should receive systemic treatment according to the principles outlined earlier. With cisplatin-based regimens, cure rates of 60% to 70% are obtained.[100–103] The outcome of the therapy depends on several prognostic factors, which should be used to determine the intensity of the treatment.[104,105] An international study, which included 10 countries, evaluated 5202 patients with nonseminomatous germ-cell tumors and 660 patients with seminomas. The following independent adverse factors were identified: mediastinal primary site; degree of elevation of AFP, hCG, and lactic acid dehydrogenase (LDH); and presence of nonpulmonary visceral metastases. Three prognostic groups have been identified using these factors: good, intermediate, and poor prognosis. The 5-year survival rates for these groups are 91%, 79%, and 48%, respectively.[106] By tailoring the therapy according to prognostic factors, the results can be improved.[107] Long-term disease-free survival can be obtained in more than 90% of patients with good or intermediate prognostic factors. In a randomized trial in which standard-dose cisplatin was compared to double-dose therapy in *high-risk* patients, no significant effect of increasing dose intensity could be shown.[107] Thus, intensive treatment of patients with a high risk of relapse is still at issue. Significant increases in the applied myelosuppressive drugs, such as etoposide, carboplatin, and ifosfamide, can be achieved by the use of peripheral blood stem cells and colony-stimulating factors. With this strategy, a significant number of patients with relapse can be salvaged.[108] The high-dose treatment is now being applied as primary treatment to patients with a high risk of relapse in several centers.[109] Paclitaxel (Taxol) has shown efficacy in refractory germ-cell tumors with and without cisplatin.[110–112]

Current treatment regimens have several important side effects, including nephrotoxicity (cisplatin), pulmonary toxicity (bleomycin), bone marrow suppression (vinblastine and etoposide), and neurotoxicity (cisplatin and vinblastine). Secondary leukemia has been reported after the use of high-dose etoposide.[113]

All patients treated for germ-cell tumors should be observed closely. Most regimens include follow-up every month for the first year and at longer intervals thereafter. The follow-up includes clinical examination, roentgenography of the thorax, CT scanning, and measurements of serum tumor markers.

## SPERMATOCYTOMA (SPERMATOCYTIC SEMINOMA)

Traditionally, the "spermatocytic" seminoma has been considered a subgroup of seminomas. As noted earlier, it is the authors' contention that this view is not justified. The tumor should be called *spermatocytoma* and should be considered a disease entity with specific clinical and biologic features. In contrast to the other germ-cell tumors, it occurs only in older men. Furthermore, it always presents in pure form, and it rarely metastasizes.

## EXTRAGONADAL TUMORS

Germ-cell tumors occasionally occur outside the gonads, most frequently in the retroperitoneum, mediastinum, and pineal body, although other sites can be involved. It has been suggested that the cells of origin are primordial germ cells displaced during embryogenesis.[114] Therapy for these patients should be designed according to the principles outlined earlier for systemic treatment of nonseminomatous germ-cell tumors. Many of these patients have a poor prognosis, primarily because they often have a considerable tumor burden at the time of diagnosis. Improvement of treatment results also has been noted in this group of patients.[115]

Although it is clear that extragonadal tumors exist as a disease entity, small invasive tumors or CIS sometimes are found in the testes of patients with presumed extragonadal primary tumors.[71] Such patients should be considered to have metastatic testicular cancer. Accordingly, all patients with germ-cell metastases should be evaluated for testicular cancer. This evaluation includes ultrasonography and biopsy of the testes.

## EMBRYOLOGY AND HISTOGENESIS OF TESTICULAR CANCER

All types of germ-cell tumors except the spermatocytoma seem to originate from CIS germ cells, which probably arise from primitive, fetal stem cells in the yolk sac.[11,13,15,16] Several findings support this theory. First, abnormal germ cells identical to adult CIS cells have been identified in infantile and neonatal testes of patients at risk for testicular cancer.[63,67,69] Second, both by light microscopy and ultrastructurally, CIS germ cells are morphologically similar to the germ cells that migrate from the yolk sac to the testis during fetal life.[17,40,41] Third, the enzyme placenta-like alkaline phosphatase and the protein product of the protooncogene c-*kit* and other markers of primordial germ cells are overexpressed in CIS cells, but not in normal spermatogonia[39,116] (Fig. 122-6).

## INFERTILITY AND TESTICULAR CANCER

Although it has been known for decades that patients with certain testicular problems are at greater risk for the development of testicular cancer, it only recently was shown that patients with testicular cancer generally have poor semen quality and impaired spermatogenesis.[55,117–122] The authors have studied semen, biopsy specimens, or both, of the contralateral testis before radiotherapy and chemotherapy in 73 consecutive

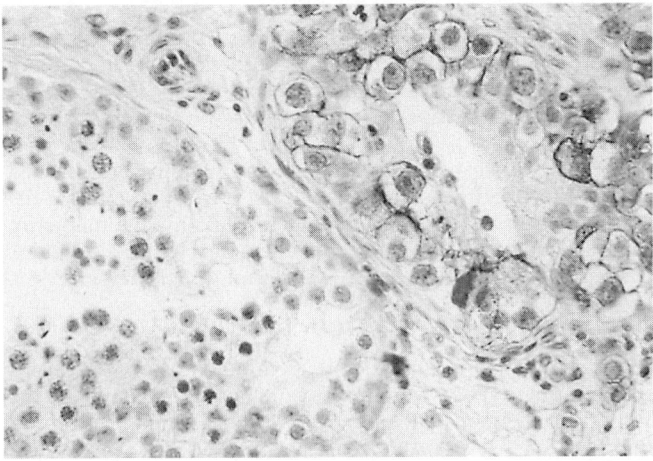

**FIGURE 122-6.** Expression of the protein product of the c-*kit* protoon-cogene in carcinoma in situ (cells with dark staining of membranes). For comparison, a neighboring seminiferous tubule with normal spermatogenesis also is shown. (From Rajpert-De Meyts E, Skakkebaek NE. Expression of the c-kit protein product in carcinoma in situ and invasive testicular germ cell tumours. Int J Androl 1994; 17:85.)

patients with testicular cancer. In general, the semen quality was poor. Biopsy of the contralateral testis in 200 consecutive patients showed that 24% had severe, and presumably permanent, changes in the testis (i.e., partial or complete Sertoli cell–only pattern, spermatogenic arrest, hyalinized tubules, or CIS).[123]

The reduced semen quality may be caused by one of the following factors: (a) premorbid defects in spermatogenesis or (b) high circulating levels of hCG, radiation, or chemotherapy. Evidence indicates that the semen quality is best before orchiectomy in patients with testicular cancer.[124,125] Currently, sperm banking is recommended to all testicular patients who want to have children. Sperm banking should preferably be carried out before orchiectomy.[124,125] At least 75% of all men who undergo therapy for testicular cancer have azoospermia at the end of treatment. In one study, a median of 540 days passed before spermatozoa were again found in semen samples, and a median of 1250 days passed before the sperm counts reached the pretreatment level.[50] Analysis of serum testosterone and luteinizing hormone showed that Leydig cell function was slightly impaired before treatment in some patients with testicular cancer. This endocrine dysfunction apparently can be aggravated temporarily by the treatment, although the contralateral testis usually is able to maintain normal or near normal serum testosterone levels both before and after radiotherapy and chemotherapy.[50] Patients with hCG-producing testicular tumors or metastases generally have normal serum testosterone levels, although higher than normal levels are encountered occasionally.[50,126]

Infertility also can result from damage of the sympathetic nerves during lymphadenectomy. Dry orgasms, probably attributable to retrograde ejaculation, have been reported in 40% to 90% of patients after operation, with some spontaneous later return of ejaculations. Possibly, a modified operative technique can prevent some ejaculatory failures.[121]

## NON–GERM-CELL TUMORS

### LEYDIG CELL TUMORS

Only 3% of testicular tumors originate from the Leydig cells; 90% of these are benign and usually produce steroid hormones.[127,128] Consequently, symptoms such as gynecomastia and precocious puberty can be seen. Treatment consists of surgical enucleation in children and orchiectomy in adults (in children, tumors are usually benign, but in adults 10% to 15% seem

to progress to malignancy). In cases of malignancy, the staging procedures outlined earlier should be applied. No large series of chemotherapy or radiotherapy have been published, and the few available reports indicate lack of efficacy of both these treatment modalities.

## SERTOLI CELL TUMORS

Another type of stromal tumor of the gonads is the Sertoli cell tumor. These lesions are extremely rare, accounting for ~1% of testicular tumors. In most cases, Sertoli cell tumors are found in association with multiple neoplasia syndromes, such as Peutz-Jeghers syndrome and Carney complex. Fifteen percent are malignant, with metastases reported to the retroperitoneum, lung, and liver. Estrogens, androgens, or both sometimes are produced by the tumor. Therapy consists of orchiectomy. The role of radiotherapy and chemotherapy in the treatment of patients with metastatic disease is unclear.[127,129]

## MALIGNANT LYMPHOMAS AND LEUKEMIA

Although malignant lymphoma of the testis is rare, it is the most common testicular tumor in men older than 60 years. Its presence in the testis should be considered an indication of disseminated lymphoma. A careful evaluation according to the principles of staging of lymphomas always should be carried out[130]; more than 90% of patients with primary lymphoma in the testis are found to have tumor deposits at other sites, and in the remaining fraction of patients, the tumor eventually turns out to be systemic. Thus, it remains controversial whether malignant lymphoma truly can be considered a local testicular disease or is always a local expression of a disseminated disease.

As in lymphoma, the testis can be a sanctuary for malignant leukemia cells.[131] As an initial sign of disease, an acute lymphoblastic leukemia may present as a testicular swelling. Testicular relapses in childhood leukemia are fairly frequent.

## OTHER TUMORS

Rarely, tumors originate from other structures in the testicular and adjacent tissues. These tumors include adenocarcinoma of the rete testis, malignant mesothelioma of the tunica vaginalis testis,[130,132,133] and rhabdomyosarcomas. Such lesions should be treated with orchiectomy. Postorchiectomy treatment depends on the nature and extent of disease.

## REFERENCES

1. Damjanov I. Male reproductive system. In: Damjanov I, Lindner J, eds. Anderson's pathology. St. Louis: Mosby, 1996:2166.
1a. Rupley EA, Crockford GP, Teare D, et al. Localization to Xq27 of a susceptibility gene for testicular germ-cell tumours. Nat Genet 2000; 24:197.
2. Clemmesen J. Testis cancer incidence: suggestion of a world pattern. Int J Androl 1981; 4(Suppl 4):111.
3. Han S, Peschel RE. Father-son testicular tumors: evidence for genetic anticipation? A case report and review of the literature. Cancer 2000; 88:2319.
4. Gedde-Dahl T, Hannisdal E, Klepp OH, et al. Testicular neoplasms occurring in four brothers. A search for a genetic predisposition. Cancer 1985; 55:2005.
5. Henderson BE, Ross PK, Pike MC, Casagrande JT. Endogenous hormones as a major factor in human cancer. Cancer Res 1982; 42:3232.
6. Skakkebaek NE, Berthelsen JG. Carcinoma in situ testis and development of different types of germ cell tumours. Fortschr Androl 1981; 7:89.
7. Reyes FI, Faiman C. Development of a testicular tumour during cisclomiphene therapy. Can Med Assoc J 1973; 109:502.
8. Rubin SO. Malignant teratoma of testis in a subfertile man treated with hCG and hMG. Scand J Urol Nephrol 1972; 7:81.
9. Depue RH, Pike MC, Henderson BE. Estrogen exposure during gestation and risk of testicular cancer. J Natl Cancer Inst 1983; 71:1151.
10. Adami H-O, Bergström R, Möhner M, et al. Testicular cancer in nine Northern European countries. Int J Cancer 1994; 59:33.
11. Skakkebaek NE, Rajpert-De Meyts E, Jørgensen N, et al. Germ cell cancer and disorders of spermatogenesis: an environmental connection? APMIS 1998; 106:3.

12. Mostofi FK, Sobin LH. Histological typing of testis tumours: International Histological Classification of Tumours No. 16. Geneva: WHO, 1977.

13. Skakkebaek NE, Berthelsen JG. Carcinoma-in-situ of the testis and invasive growth of different types of germ cell tumours: a revised germ cell theory. Int J Androl 1981; 4(Suppl 4):26.

14. Müller J, Skakkebaek NE, Parkinson MC. The spermatocytic seminoma: views on pathogenesis. Int J Androl 1987; 10:147.

15. Skakkebaek NE, Berthelsen JG, Müller J. Histopathology of human testicular tumours: carcinoma-in-situ germ cells and invasive growth of different types of germ cell tumours. INSERM 1984; 123:445.

16. Skakkebaek NE, Berthelsen JG, Giwercman A, Müller J. Carcinoma-in-situ of the testis: possible origin from gonocytes and precursor of all types of germ cell tumours except spermatocytoma. Int J Androl 1987; 10:19.

17. Nielsen H, Nielsen M, Skakkebaek NE. The fine structure of a possible carcinoma-in-situ in the seminiferous tubules in the testis of four infertile men. APMIS 1974; 82:235.

18. Jacobsen GK, Barlebo H, Olsen J, et al. Testicular germ cell tumours in Denmark 1976–1980: pathology of 1058 consecutive cases. Acta Radiol Oncol 1984; 23:239.

19. Skrabanek P, Kirrane J, Powell DA. Unifying concept of chorionic gonadotrophin production in malignancy. Invest Cell Pathol 1979; 2:75.

20. Grigor KM. Extraembryonic elements in testicular tumours. Int J Androl 1981; 4(Suppl 4):35.

21. Lange PH. Serum and tissue markers of testicular tumours. Int J Androl 1981; 4:191.

22. Paiva J, Damjanov I, Lange P, Harris H. Immunohistochemical localization of placental-like alkaline phosphatase in testis and germ-cell tumors using monoclonal antibodies. Am J Pathol 1983; 111:156.

23. Jacobsen GK, Jacobsen M. Alpha-fetoprotein (AFP) and human chorionic gonadotropin (HCG) in testicular germ cell tumours. APMIS 1983; 91:165.

24. Nüesch-Bachmann IH, Hedinger C. Atypische Spermatogonien als Präkanzerose. Schweiz Med Wochenschr 1977; 107:795.

25. Skakkebaek NE. Carcinoma in situ of the testis: frequency and relationship to invasive germ cell tumours in infertile men. Histopathology 1978; 2:157.

26. Pryor JP, Cameron KM, Chilton CP, et al. Carcinoma in situ in testicular biopsies from men presenting with infertility. Br J Urol 1983; 55:780.

27. West AB, Butler MR, Fitzpatrick J, O'Brien A. Testicular tumors in subfertile men: report of 4 cases with implications for management of patients presenting with infertility. J Urol 1985; 133:107.

28. Skakkebaek NE, Berthelsen JG, Müller J. Carcinoma-in-situ of the undescended testis. Urol Clin North Am 1982; 9:377.

29. Oosterhuis JW, Gillis AJM, Van Roozendaal CEP, et al. The platelet-derived growth factor α-receptor 1.5 kb transcript: target for molecular detection of testicular germ cell tumours of adolescents and adults. APMIS 1998; 106:207.

30. Rowley MJ, Heller CG. The testicular biopsy: surgical procedure, fixation, and staining technics. Fertil Steril 1966; 17:177.

31. Skakkebaek NE. Abnormal morphology of germ cells in two infertile men. APMIS 1972; 80:374.

32. Müller J, Skakkebaek NE. Microspectrophotometric DNA measurements of carcinoma-in-situ germ cells in the testis. Int J Androl 1981; 4(Suppl 4):211.

33. Chaganti RSK, Houldsworth J. The cytogenetic theory of the pathogenesis of human adult male germ cell tumors. APMIS 1998; 106:80.

34. Holstein AF, Körner F. Light and electron microscopical analysis of cell types in human seminoma. Virchows Arch [Pathol Anat] 1974; 363:97.

35. Müller J, Berthelsen JG, Skakkebaek NE. Carcinoma in situ and invasive growth of testicular cancer. In: Javadpour N, ed. Principles and management of testicular cancer. New York: Thieme Medical Publishers, 1986:120.

36. Giwercman A, Marks A, Bailey D, et al. A monoclonal antibody as a marker for carcinoma in situ germ cells of the human adult testis. APMIS 1988; 96:667.

37. Giwercman A, Andrews PW, Jørgensen N, et al. Immunohistochemical expression of embryonal marker TRA-1-60 in carcinoma in situ and germ cell tumors of the testis. Cancer 1993; 72:1308.

38. Giwercman A, Lindenberg S, Kimber SJ, et al. Monoclonal antibody 43-9F as a sensitive immunohistochemical marker of carcinoma in situ of human testis. Cancer 1990; 65:1135.

39. Rajpert-De Meyts E, Skakkebaek NE. Expression of the c-kit protein product in carcinoma-in-situ and invasive testicular germ cell tumours. Int J Androl 1994; 17:85.

40. Albrechtsen R, Nielsen MH, Skakkebaek NE, Wewer U. Carcinoma in situ of the testis. Some ultrastructural characteristics of germ cells. APMIS 1982; 90:301.

41. Gondos B, Berthelsen JG, Skakkebaek NE. Intratubular germ cell neoplasia (carcinoma in situ): a preinvasive lesion of the testis. Ann Clin Lab Sci 1983; 13:185.

42. Berthelsen JG, Skakkebaek NE. Distribution of carcinoma-in-situ in testes from infertile men. Int J Androl 1981; 4(Suppl 4):172.

43. Giwercman A, Marks A, Skakkebaek NE. Carcinoma-in-situ germ-cells exfoliated from seminiferous epithelium into seminal fluid. Lancet 1988; 1:530.

44. Skakkebaek NE. Possible carcinoma-in-situ of the testis. Lancet 1972; 2:516.

45. Skakkebaek NE, Berthelsen JG, Visfeldt J. Clinical aspects of testicular carcinoma-in-situ. Int J Androl 1981; 4(Suppl 4):153.

46. Skakkebaek NE, Berthelsen JG. Carcinoma-in-situ of testis and orchiectomy. Lancet 1978; 2:204.

47. Hamilton JB, Gilbert JB. Studies in malignant tumors of the testis. IV. Bilateral testicular cancer. Incidence, nature, and bearing upon management of the patient with a single testicular cancer. Cancer Res 1942; 2:125.

48. Østerlind A, Berthelsen JG, Abildgaard N, et al. Risk of bilateral testicular germ cell cancer in Denmark: 1960–1984. J Natl Cancer Inst 1991; 83:1391.

49. Doeckmann K, Loy V. The value of the biopsy of the contralateral testis in patients with testicular germ cell cancer: the recent German experience. APMIS 1998; 106:13.

50. Berthelsen JG. Thesis. Andrological aspects of testicular cancer. Int J Androl 1984; 7:451.

51. von der Maase H, Rørth M, Walbom-Jørgensen S, et al. Carcinoma in situ of contralateral testis in patients with testicular germ cell cancer: study of 27 cases in 500 patients. Br Med J 1986; 293:1398.

52. von der Maase H, Berthelsen JG, Jacobsen GK, et al. Carcinoma-in-situ of testis eradicated by chemotherapy. Lancet 1985; 1:98.

53. Christensen TB, Daugaard G, Geertsen PF, von der Maase H. Effect of chemotherapy on carcinoma in situ of the testis. Ann Oncol 1998; 9:657.

54. von der Maase H, Meinecke B, Skakkebaek NE. Residual carcinoma-in-situ of contralateral testis after chemotherapy. Lancet 1988; 1:477.

55. Giwercman A, von der Maase H, Skakkebaek NE. Epidemiological and clinical aspects of carcinoma in situ of the testis. Eur Urol 1993; 23:104.

56. Giwercman A, von der Maase H, Berthelsen JG, et al. Localized irradiation of testes with carcinoma in situ: effects on Leydig cell function and eradication of malignant germ cells in 20 patients. J Clin Endocrinol Metab 1991; 73:596.

57. Skakkebaek NE, Grigor KM, Giwercman A, Rørth M, eds. Management and biology of carcinoma in situ and cancer of the testis. In: Proceedings of the 3rd Copenhagen Workshop. Basel: Karger, 1993:129.

58. Farrer JH, Rajfer J. Cryptorchidism and testicular cancer. In: Javadpour N, ed. Principles and management of testicular cancer. New York: Thieme Medical Publishers, 1986:133.

59. United Kingdom Testicular Cancer Study Group. Aetiology of testicular cancer: association with congenital abnormalities, age at puberty, infertility, and exercise. Br Med J 1994; 308:1393.

60. Giwercman A, Grindsted J, Hansen B, et al. Testicular cancer risk in boys with maldescended testis: a cohort study. J Urol 1987; 138:1214.

61. Williams TR, Brendler H. Carcinoma in situ of the ectopic testis. J Urol 1977; 117:610.

62. Krabbe S, Skakkebaek NE, Berthelsen JG, et al. High incidence of undetected neoplasia in maldescended testes. Lancet 1979; 1:999.

63. Müller J, Skakkebaek NE, Nielsen OH, Graem N. Cryptorchidism and testis cancer: atypical infantile germ cells followed by carcinoma in situ and invasive carcinoma in adulthood. Cancer 1984; 54:629.

64. Scully RE. Neoplasia associated with anomalous sexual development and abnormal sex chromosomes. Pediatr Adolesc Endocrinol 1981; 8:203.

65. Skakkebaek NE. Carcinoma-in-situ of testis in testicular feminization syndrome. APMIS 1979; 87:87.

66. Nogales FF Jr, Toro M, Ortega I, Fulwood HR. Bilateral incipient germ cell tumours of the testis in the incomplete testicular feminization syndrome. Histopathology 1981; 5:511.

67. Müller J, Skakkebaek NE. Testicular carcinoma-in-situ in children with the androgen insensitivity (testicular feminization) syndrome. Br Med J 1984; 288:1419.

68. Müller J. Morphometry and histology of gonads from twelve children and adolescents with the androgen insensitivity (testicular feminization) syndrome. J Clin Endocrinol Metab 1984; 59:785.

69. Müller J, Skakkebaek NE, Ritzén EM, et al. Carcinoma in situ of the testis in children with 45,X/46,XY gonadal dysgenesis. J Pediatr 1985; 106:431.

70. Müller J, Visfeldt J, Philip J, Skakkebaek NE. Carcinoma in situ, gonadoblastoma, and early invasive neoplasia in a nine-year-old girl with 46,XY gonadal dysgenesis. APMIS 1992; 100:170.

71. Daugaard G, Rørth M, von der Maase H, Skakkebaek NE. Management of extragonadal germ-cell tumors and the significance of bilateral testicular biopsies. Ann Oncol 1992; 3:283.

72. Nilsson S, Anderström C, Hedelin H, Unsgaard B. Signs and symptoms of adult testicular tumours. Int J Androl 1981; 4(Suppl 4):146.

73. Fosså SD, Klepp O, Elgjo RF, et al. The effect of patients delay and doctors delay in patients with malignant germ cell tumours. Int J Androl 1981; 4(Suppl 4):134.

74. Dieckmann KP, Krain J, Gottschalk W, Buttner P. Atypical symptoms in patients with germinal testicular tumors. Urologe A 1994; 33:325.

75. Hernes EH, Harstad K, Fossa. Changing incidence and delay of testicular cancer in southern Norway (1981–1992). Eur Urol 1996; 30:349.

76. Toftager-Larsen K, Petersen PL, Nørgaard-Pedersen B. Carbohydrate microheterogeneity of human alpha-fetoprotein: oncodevelopmental aspects. Biol Biochem Clin Biochem 1981; 1:283.

77. Gels ME, Marrink J, Visser P, et al. Importance of a new tumor marker TRA-1-60 in the follow-up of patients with clinical stage I nonseminomatous testicular germ cell tumors. Ann Surg Oncol 1997; 4:321.

78. Schultz HP, Arends J, Barlebo H, et al. Testicular carcinoma in Denmark 1976–1980. Acta Radiol Oncol 1984; 23:249.

79. Roth BJ, Nichols CR. Testicular cancer. Semin Oncol 1992; 19:117.

80. Cremerius U, Effert PJ, Adam G, et al. FDG PET for detection and therapy control of metastatic germ cell tumor. J Nucl Med 1998; 39:815.

81. Peckham MJ, Barrett A, Liew KH, et al. The treatment of metastatic germ-cell testicular tumours with bleomycin, etoposide and cis-platin (BEP). Br J Cancer 1983; 47:613.

82. Horwich A, Bell J. Mortality and cancer incidence following radiotherapy for seminoma of the testis. Radiother Oncol 1994; 30:193.

83. Sultanem K, Souhami L, Benk V, et al. Para-aortic irradiation only appears to be adequate treatment for patients with stage I seminoma of the testis. Int J Radiat Oncol Biol Phys 1998; 40:455.

84. Schultz HP, von der Maase H, Rørth M, et al. Testicular seminoma in Denmark 1976–1980: results of treatment. Acta Radiol Oncol 1984; 23:263.

85. Bauman GS, Venkatesan VM, Ago CT, et al. Postoperative radiotherapy for stage I/II seminoma: results for 212 patients. Int J Radiat Oncol Biol Phys 1998; 42:313.

86. von der Maase H, Specht L, Jacobsen GK, et al. Surveillance following orchidectomy for stage I seminoma of the testis. Eur J Cancer 1993; 29A:1931.

87. Smalley SR, Evans RG, Richardson RL, et al. Radiotherapy as initial treatment for bulky stage II testicular seminomas. J Clin Oncol 1985; 3:1333.

88. van Oosterom AT, Williams SD, Funes HC, et al. Treatment of seminomas with chemotherapy. In: Kürth KH, ed. Progress and controversies in oncological urology. New York: Alan R Liss, 1984:103.

89. Friedman EL, Garnick MB, Stomper PC, et al. Therapeutic guidelines and results in advanced seminoma. J Clin Oncol 1985; 3:1325.

90. Peckham MJ, Husband JE, Barrett A, Hendry WF. Orchidectomy alone in tesicular stage I non-seminomatous germ-cell tumours. Lancet 1982; 2:678.

91. Rørth M. Therapeutic alternatives in clinical stage I non-seminomatous disease. Semin Oncol 1992; 19:190.

92. Rørth M, Krag Jacobsen G, von der Maase H, et al. Surveillance alone versus radiotherapy after orchiectomy for clinical stage I nonseminomatous testicular cancer. J Clin Oncol 1991; 9:1543.

93. Klepp O, Dahl O, Flodgren P, et al. Risk-adapted treatment of clinical stage I non-seminoma testis cancer. Eur J Cancer 1997; 7:1038.

94. Williams SD, Einhorn LH. Clinical stage I testis tumors: the medical oncologists view. Cancer Treat Rep 1982; 66:15.

95. Sharir S, Jewett MA, Sturgeon JF, et al. Progression in detection of stage I nonseminomatous testis cancer on surveillance: implications for followup protocol. J Urol 1999; 161:472.

96. Hao D, Seidel J, Brant R, et al. Compliance of clinical stage I nonseminomatous germ cell tumor patients with surveillance. J Urol 1998; 160:768.

97. Javadpour N, Ozols RF, Anderson T, et al. A randomized trial of cytoreductive surgery followed by chemotherapy versus chemotherapy alone in bulky stage III testicular cancer with poor prognostic features. Cancer 1982; 50:2004.

98. Einhorn LH, Williams SD, Mandelbaum I, Donohue JP. Surgical resection in disseminated testicular cancer. Cancer 1981; 48:904.

99. Rasmussen OV, Daugaard G, Christiansen S, et al. Secondary surgery in patients with malignant germ cell tumors. J Urol 1992; 147:393.

100. Einhorn LH, Donohue JP. Improved chemotherapy in disseminated testicular cancer. J Urol 1977; 117:65.

101. Stöter G, Vendrik CPJ, Struyvenberg A, et al. Combination therapy with cis-diamine-dichloro-platinum, vinblastine, and bleomycin in advanced testicular non-seminoma. Lancet 1979; 1:941.

102. Peckham MJ, Barrett A, McElwain TJ, Hendry WF. Combined management of malignant teratoma of the testis. Lancet 1979; 2:267.

103. Nichols CR. Testicular cancer. Curr Probl Cancer 1998; 22:187.

104. Daugaard G, Hansen HH, Rørth M. Treatment of malignant germ cell tumors. Ann Oncol 1990; 1:195.

105. Medical Research Council Working Party on Testicular Tumours: prognostic factors in advanced non-seminomatous germ-cell testicular tumours: results of a multicentre study. Lancet 1985; 1:8.

106. International Germ Cell Cancer Collaborative Group. International Germ Cell Consensus Classification: a prognostic factor-based staging system for metastatic germ cell cancers. J Clin Oncol 1997; 15:594.

107. Rørth M. Dose escalation of cisplatin in the chemotherapy of poor risk germ cell tumour patients. In: Horwich A, ed. Testicular cancer. London: Chapman & Hall, 1991:221.

108. Broun ER, Nichols CR, Gize G, et al. Tandem high dose chemotherapy with autologous bone marrow transplantation for initial relapse of testicular germ cell cancer. Cancer 1997; 79:1605.

109. Motzer RJ, Mazumdar M, Bajorin DF, et al. High-dose carboplatin, etoposide, and cyclophosphamide with autologous bone marrow transplantation in first-line therapy for patients with poor-risk germ cell tumors. J Clin Oncol 1997; 15:2546.

110. Sandler AB, Cristou A, Fox S, et al. A phase II trial of paclitaxel in refractory germ cell tumors. Cancer 1998; 82:1381.

111. Motzer RJ. Paclitaxel in salvage therapy for germ cell tumors. Semin Oncol 1997; 24:15.

112. Tjulandin SA, Titov DA, Breder VV, et al. Paclitaxel and cisplatin as salvage treatment in patients with non-seminomatous germ cell tumour who failed to achieve a complete remission on induction chemotherapy. Clin Oncol 1998; 10:297.

113. Pedersen-Bjerregaard J, Daugaard G, Werner Hansen S, et al. Increased risk of myelodysplasia and leukaemia following etoposide, cisplatin and bleomycin for germ cell tumours. Lancet 1991; 338:359.

114. Friedman NB. The comparative morphogenesis of extragenital and gonadal teratoid tumors. Cancer 1951; 4:265.

115. Daugaard G, Rørth M, Hansen HH. Therapy of extragonadal germ-cell tumors. J Cancer Clin Oncol 1983; 19:895.

116. Jacobsen GK, Nørgaard-Pedersen B. Placental alkaline phosphatase in testicular germ cell tumours and in carcinoma-in-situ of the testis. APMIS 1984; 92:323.

117. Skakkebaek NE, Berthelsen JG, Grigor KM, Visfeldt J. Early detection of testicular cancer. Copenhagen: Scriptor, 1981.

118. Fosså SD, Klepp O, Molne K, Aakvaag A. Testicular function after unilateral orchiectomy for cancer and before further treatment. Int J Androl 1982; 5:179.

119. Jewett MAS, Thachil JV, Harris JF. Exocrine function of testis with germinal testicular tumour. Br Med J 1983; 286:1849.

120. Berthelsen JG, Skakkebaek NE. Gonadal function in men with testis cancer. Fertil Steril 1983; 39:68.

121. Chiou R-K, Fraley EE, Lange PH. Newer ideas about fertility in patients with testicular cancer. World J Urol 1984; 2:26.

122. Petersen PM, Giwercman A, Skakkebaek NE, Rørth M. Gonadal function in men with testicular cancer. Semin Oncol 1998; 25:224.

123. Jørgensen N, Giwercman A, Müller J, Skakkebaek NE. Immunohistochemical markers of carcinoma in situ of the testis also expressed in normal infantile germ cells. Histopathology 1993; 22:373.

124. Petersen PM, Skakkebaek NE, Rørth M, Giwercman A. Semen quality and reproductive hormones before and after orchiectomy in men with testicular cancer. J Urol 1999; 161:822.

125. Lampe H, Horwich A, Norman A, et al. Fertility after chemotherapy for testicular germ cell cancer. J Clin Oncol 1997; 15(1):239.

126. Kirschner MA, Wider JA, Ross GT. Leydig cell function in men with gonadotrophin-producing testicular tumors. J Clin Endocrinol Metab 1970; 30:504.

127. Kim I, Young RH, Scully RE. Leydig cell tumors of the testis: a clinicopathological analysis of 40 cases and review of the literature. Am J Surg Pathol 1985; 9:177.

128. Cheville JC, Sebo TJ, Lager DJ, et al. Leydig cell tumor of the testis: a clinicopathologic, DNA content, and MIB-1 comparison of nonmetastasizing and metastasizing tumors. Am J Surg Pathol 1998; 22:1361.

129. Young RH, Koelliker DD, Scully RE. Sertoli cell tumors of the testis, not otherwise specified: a clinicopathologic analysis of 60 cases. Am J Surg Pathol 1998; 22:709.

130. Ferry JA, Harris NL, Young RH, et al. Malignant lymphoma of the testis, epididymis, and spermatic cord. A clinicopathologic study of 69 cases with immunophenotypic analysis. Am J Surg Pathol 1994; 18:376.

131. de Almeida MM, Chagas M, de Sousa JV, Mandoca ME. Fine-needle aspiration cytology as a tool for the early detection of testicular relapse of acute lymphoblastic leukemia in children. Diagn Cytopathol 1994; 10:44.

132. Chen KTK, Arhelger RB, Flam MS, Hanson JH. Malignant mesothelioma of tunica vaginalis testis. Urology 1982; 20:316.

133. Plas E, Riedl CR, Pfluger H. Malignant mesothelioma of the vaginalis testis: review of the literature and assessment of prognostic parameters. Cancer 1998; 83:2437.

# CHAPTER 123

# MALE CONTRACEPTION

JOHN K. AMORY AND WILLIAM J. BREMNER

Currently available nonendocrine options for male contraception are *vasectomy* and *condoms*. Vasectomy is a safe, simple outpatient surgery performed under local anesthesia in which a small scrotal incision is made, the ductus deferens severed, and the ends ligated. Vasectomies are extremely effective and safe, with a failure rate of <1% and a low incidence of complications. However, they are invasive and difficult to reverse, with 30% to 40% of men remaining infertile even after microsurgical reversal. Happily, earlier reports of associations with cardiovascular disease and prostate cancer have not been substantiated[1] (see Chap. 225).

Condoms have been used as a means of male fertility control for several hundred years. They are relatively inexpensive and free from adverse side effects. Unfortunately, condoms suffer from poor long-term compliance and efficacy, mainly because of improper or inconsistent usage. When made of latex, condoms offer some protection against sexually transmitted disease; however, many couples in stable relationships view condoms as only a temporary means of contraception.[2]

Because existing methods of male contraception have shortcomings, efforts have been made to develop a hormonally derived male contraceptive. A hormonally derived contraceptive analogous to estrogen/progesterone birth control pills for women should be safe, easy to use, and reversible. Ongoing research demonstrates that such methods are likely to become available.

# ENDOCRINE APPROACH TO MALE CONTRACEPTION

The administration of testosterone (T) to normal men functions as a contraceptive by suppressing secretion of the pituitary gonadotropins, luteinizing hormone (LH) and follicle-stimulating hormone (FSH) (see Chap. 119). Low levels of LH and FSH deprive developing sperm of the signals required for normal maturation, leading to reversible infertility in most, but not all, men. In the normal male, FSH acts on Sertoli cells in the seminiferous tubules of the testis to facilitate sperm maturation. The absence of FSH, or blockade of the FSH receptor, has a deleterious effect on sperm counts, but mature sperm capable of fertilization persist.[3] LH stimulates the production of T by Leydig cells in the testis. Blockade of LH production shuts down the testicular production of T and leads to the cessation of sperm production; however, the absence of T is harmful since T is necessary to maintain normal male health.

Therefore, attempts at the formulation of a hormonal contraceptive must (a) contain some androgen activity to prevent hypogonadism and (b) suppress LH and FSH levels low enough to block spermatogenesis. T alone accomplishes both goals, but, nevertheless, some men remain fertile on contraceptive regimens using only T. Compounds such as gonadotropin-releasing hormone (GnRH) analogs or progestins that synergistically suppress pituitary gonadotropin production or directly block sperm production have, therefore, been combined with T in attempts to optimize its contraceptive efficacy further.

## TESTOSTERONE CONTRACEPTIVE TRIALS: GENERAL CONSIDERATIONS

In assessing the efficacy of potential male contraceptives, it is important to determine what level of sperm inhibition is necessary to achieve infertility; however, this is not precisely known. Sperm counts in normal men vary from 20 to 200 million sperm per milliliter of ejaculate. The absence of spermatozoa in the ejaculate, a condition termed *azoospermia*, renders fertilization impossible and is, therefore, the ultimate goal of male contraception. Unfortunately, azoospermia has not been achieved reliably in all men in studies using existing hormonal techniques. Most studies have some subjects who sustain partial but incomplete reduction of their sperm counts, a condition called *oligozoospermia*. There is good evidence that sperm counts <3 million sperm per milliliter of ejaculate are associated with decreased rates of pregnancy.[4] This "severe oligozoospermia" decreases the chances of conception considerably, and is considered a reasonable short-term goal for male contraceptive research.

Additional factors important in the design of a hormonal contraceptive include time until onset of action and method of administration. Most hormonal contraceptives do not incapacitate existing sperm; they block sperm production. Since sperm take an average of 72 days to reach maturity, it is likely that any contraceptive based on manipulation of the hormonal axis will be associated with some delay in the onset of full contraceptive efficacy. In addition, it is important to consider ethnic differences in interpreting results of contraceptive trials. Study volunteers in Asia are more susceptible to T-induced suppression of spermatogenesis than are men studied in Europe, North America, and Australia.[4,5] While the reason for this difference remains to be elucidated, it is important in the interpretation of trial results and complicates extrapolation of data to different populations.

## THE CONTRACEPTIVE ANDROGEN

Administration of native T is impractical because when given orally or by injection it is promptly degraded by the liver. In addition, many orally active androgens (those with a 17-ethinyl group) can cause liver damage and are, therefore, not considered safe for long-term use in oral contraceptives.[6] Most current regimens use T esters such as T enanthate (TE), given by intramuscular (im) injection on a weekly to fortnightly basis.

Other methods of sustained delivery for T that are suitable for use in a contraceptive regimen are being examined. T buciclate, a synthetic ester given by depot injection, maintains physiologic androgen levels for up to 3 months in hypogonadal men.[7] T undecanoate (TU), an ester that is absorbed via lymphatics and therefore escapes first-pass hepatic metabolism,[8] can be given orally twice a day; it can also be used by injection where it maintains serum T levels for at least 6 weeks in hypogonadal men.[9] In addition, research into injectable steroid polymer microparticles or fused crystalline T implants reveals a similar ability to maintain T levels in hypogonadal men.[10–12]

Other esters such as 19-nortestosterone (19-NT) have been evaluated as potential substitutes for TE. In addition to its potent androgen effects, 19-NT has ten times the progestational activity of T and therefore inhibits FSH and LH production to a greater degree than TE.[13]

A derivative of 19-NT, 7α-methyl-19-nortestosterone (MENT), is also of interest. The 7-methylation of this compound prevents 5α-reduction, thus preventing its dihydrotestosterone (DHT)-like effects.[14] This is of particular importance in spermatogenesis, as it has been shown that men who remain oligospermic after TE administration have higher DHT levels.[15] To date, 5-MENT has not been used in contraceptive trials, but seems a likely candidate for future studies.

## CONTRACEPTIVE TRIALS: I. TESTOSTERONE ALONE

As early as 1939, T administration was shown to suppress sperm counts[16]; however, the first systematic studies of T alone as a contraceptive date from the 1960s and 1970s[17–19] and used TE given by intramuscular injection. In these trials of white men, more than half the subjects were rendered azoospermic, and most of the others became severely oligospermic. The onset of azoospermia was around 72 days, and recovery of normal sperm counts occurred 3 to 4 months after T was discontinued.

Based on these initial encouraging results, two large, multicenter trials of TE were conducted by the World Health Organization (WHO).[4,20] The first study enrolled 271 subjects who were given 200 mg TE intramuscularly weekly for a 6-month induction phase. Sixty-five percent of these men achieved azoospermia, and an additional 30% were rendered severely oligospermic. The fertility of the azoospermic men was then tested in a 12-month efficacy phase. Of the 119 couples who became azoospermic, continued the injections, and used no other form of birth control, only one pregnancy occurred. This pregnancy rate of 0.8 pregnancies per 100 person-years demonstrates that in men rendered azoospermic, TE is an effective contraceptive. Volunteers discontinued involvement with the study mainly because of regimen failure and dislike of the injection schedule.

The second WHO study examined the fertility of both the men who became azoospermic and those who achieved severe oligozoospermia on the TE regimen.[4] A total of 399 men were enrolled in this study. Of these, all but 8 (2%) became severely oligospermic or azoospermic. In terms of fertility, there were no pregnancies fathered by the men who became azoospermic; in men whose sperm counts were suppressed to <3 million/mL, fertility was reduced to 8.1 pregnancies per 100 person-years.

The combined fertility rate for oligospermic and azoospermic men was 1.4 per 100 person-years. Therefore, the overall failure rate (including men who failed to suppress to oligozoospermia) was 3.4%, for an overall contraceptive efficacy of 96.6%.

This research demonstrated that T is safe, fully reversible, and effective as a contraceptive in the majority of men. Drawbacks to T-alone methods, however, are apparent. While effective in those who achieve azoospermia, some men fail to suppress to <3 million sperm per milliliter, and, therefore, presumably remain fertile. In addition, the necessity of weekly intramuscular injections using TE is a deterrent. Twelve percent of patients in the second WHO study discontinued involvement for personal or medical reasons or because of dislike of the injection schedule. Lastly, high-dose T has been shown to decrease serum high-density lipoprotein (HDL) cholesterol, and this could contribute to accelerating atherosclerosis.[21,22] Current research using TU given by injection is ongoing in China. The long half-life of this compound allows injections to be given at 10- to 12-week intervals, reducing the need for frequent injections. In white men, the failure to achieve uniform azoospermia with T alone has led to the study of second agents, either a GnRH analog or a progestin, added to the contraceptive androgen to improve its contraceptive efficacy.

## CONTRACEPTIVE TRIALS: II. TESTOSTERONE AND GONADOTROPIN-RELEASING HORMONE ANALOGS

The decapeptide structure of GnRH was first discovered in 1971.[23] Since then, many analogs with both agonist and antagonist properties have been synthesized. Compounds with agonist properties cause an initial stimulation of gonadotropin secretion. After 2 to 3 weeks of use, the pituitary loses its ability to respond to GnRH, causing a marked fall in gonadotropin levels. At least 12 trials using three different GnRH agonists with T have been reported.[24] The results of these studies, however, were disappointing, with roughly 25% of men achieving azoospermia, a third achieving severe oligozoospermia, and the remainder suppressing only partially to levels of <30 million sperm per milliliter; this degree of suppression is inadequate for use as a reliable contraceptive. These results have led to the abandonment of trials using GnRH agonists as male contraceptives.

Some synthetic GnRH analogs have been shown to possess potent antagonist properties and suppress the production of FSH and LH.[24a] These GnRH antagonists can suppress FSH and LH production within hours of administration, and their inhibition of the gonadotropins is more complete than can be produced by agonists. Three human trials have been conducted using the GnRH antagonist "Nal-Glu" with T. The first two trials showed promise, with seven of eight subjects in one study achieving azoospermia by 6 to 10 weeks of treatment.[25,26] A third trial, however, demonstrated no difference in azoospermia when compared to TE alone.[27] The time required to reach azoospermia was roughly 7 to 10 weeks. Normal sperm counts returned in roughly the same amount of time, demonstrating the reversibility of this approach. GnRH antagonists may be useful in the initiation of spermatogenic arrest. It has been demonstrated that administration of Nal-Glu in conjunction with T for 12 weeks can be used to induce azoospermia, which can then be maintained by TE alone for a subsequent period of 20 weeks.[28]

GnRH antagonists have some drawbacks. Since they are peptides, they are expensive to make and must be injected subcutaneously to avoid degradation in the intestines; also, most have very short half-lives. Side effects noted by trial volunteers included mild burning sensations at the injection site and occasional, nontender, subcutaneous nodules at the injection site, which resolve within weeks. Because GnRH antagonists are very effective, however, additional work should be undertaken to develop less expensive analogs that are easier to administer.

An orally active (probably nonpeptide) analog would be an ideal compound for male contraceptive trials.

## CONTRACEPTIVE TRIALS: III. TESTOSTERONE AND PROGESTINS

The idea of using a progestin synergistically with T to block sperm production was first tested in the 1970s, mostly using depot medroxyprogesterone acetate (DMPA). More than 35 studies were carried out and showed that progestins possessed the ability to inhibit LH and FSH secretion in men.[29] Furthermore, it has been suggested that progestins may also have a direct suppressive effect on spermatogenesis.[30,31]

In five studies conducted by the Population Council, 100 volunteers were given monthly injections of DMPA in combination with 100 to 250 mg TE intramuscularly for 4 to 16 months.[32-36] These combinations were able to induce azoospermia in half of the subjects, and some degree of oligozoospermia in most others; however, the contraceptive efficacy of these combinations was poor, with nine couples conceiving while on therapy despite simultaneous use of other contraceptives.[37] Drawbacks to this class of 17-hydroxyl progestational agents were significant; patients experienced weight gain, transient decreases in HDL cholesterol, and gynecomastia.

Following these first studies, compounds with fewer side effects, such as the potent oral progestin, levonorgestrel (LNG), were tested as an adjuvant agent for male contraception. A randomized, controlled trial of LNG (500 μg orally per day) with TE (100 mg im per week), showed that the LNG-TE combination was superior to TE alone in terms of azoospermia (67% vs. 33%) by 6 months.[38] In addition, the total who achieved either severe oligozoospermia or azoospermia was 94% in the LNG-TE group compared to 61% of the TE-alone group. Drawbacks to the LNG-TE regimen included greater weight gain and decreases in HDL cholesterol when compared to the TE-alone group. Encouraged by this result, the same research group is evaluating lower doses of LNG, in the hopes that side effects can be minimized while contraceptive efficacy is maintained.

In early, small-scale studies of 19-NT, rates of azoospermia were in the 80% to 90% range when combined with the progestin DMPA.[39] A large multicenter trial was conducted by the WHO in Indonesia using weekly injections of either TE or 19-NT in combination with the progestin DMPA. Both groups had >95% azoospermia, showing 19-NT to be at least as effective as TE with no untoward side effects.[40]

Progestins with antiandrogenic effects such as cyproterone acetate (CPA) have also been tested as potential male contraceptives. CPA functions as an antiandrogen by blocking the binding of T and DHT to androgen receptors[41]; therefore, it may interfere with androgen-dependent spermatogenesis in the testis. In addition, CPA suppresses FSH and LH production at the pituitary by means of its progestational activity.[31] It was initially tried as a single agent for contraception,[42,43] but caused intolerable hypogonadism.

The combination of TE and CPA was tried in monkeys,[44] and a few humans,[45] in the mid-1980s. In a promising trial, two groups of men received CPA at either 50 or 100 mg orally per day, and 100 mg TE intramuscularly per week, while a third group received weekly TE alone.[46] All men who received CPA became azoospermic, whereas only three of five in the TE-alone group attained azoospermia. In addition, the time required to achieve azoospermia in the CPA groups was half that needed in the T-alone group (49 vs. 98 days). This result is encouraging, given the 72-day maturation time of sperm; it implies that this regimen both blocks the generation of new spermatids and prevents the maturation of already developing sperm. Happily, no major adverse side effects, such as changes in HDL cholesterol, liver function, libido, or sexual potency, were noted in this small sample of men. The sole drawbacks noted were slight decreases in body weight and serum hemoglobin level that were dependent on the dose of CPA.

The same group has reported on the first oral combination of CPA with TU.[47] In this study, CPA was combined with oral TU twice a day. Of eight subjects, one became azoospermic, five were suppressed <3 million sperm per milliliter, and the two remaining subjects were suppressed to 4 and 6 million sperm per milliliter. It is hoped that alterations in the regimen will lead to more complete and reliable spermatogenic suppression and the eventual availability of an oral male contraceptive.

Given the positive results from combinations of T and progestins, many researchers now feel that this combination is the most likely to result in a viable contraceptive method. Current research is focused on both improving the method of androgen administration and finding dose combinations that optimize sperm count suppression in all populations, while minimizing side effects.

## NEWER ANDROGENS

Newer androgens such as MENT, a derivative of 19-NT, show promising properties in animal studies. In one study in monkeys, MENT showed a ten-fold greater potency (vs. T) in terms of LH inhibition, but only two-fold greater potency at stimulating prostate growth.[48] This tissue selectivity could be advantageous in efforts to maximize the long-term safety of a hormonally derived male contraceptive.

Furthermore, tissue-selective, nonsteroidal androgenic compounds have been described.[49] Such compounds, analogous to the selective estrogen receptor modulators tamoxifen and raloxifene, have the potential to block spermatogenesis and prostatic enlargement while simultaneously providing for the beneficial effects of androgens on other tissues such as bone and muscle (see Chap. 225). These nonsteroidal androgens can be administered orally and could easily be incorporated into a contraceptive regimen. Further animal testing will be required before these compounds can be tested in humans; however, their potential role in male contraception is great.

## CONCLUSIONS

Research has demonstrated the feasibility of the hormonal approach to male contraception. Androgen-based sex steroid combinations are able to suppress human spermatogenesis reversibly without severe side effects in most men; however, a regimen with 100% effectiveness has remained elusive. GnRH antagonists improve the efficacy of T, but are presently impractical for widespread use. T combinations with progestins appear promising. Ongoing trials with T plus LNG and CPA may offer a usable option for men, but difficulties in T delivery continue to hinder commercial use. New steroidal and nonsteroidal androgens may help improve T delivery and aid in the generation of a more marketable contraceptive regimen.[50] Now that research has proved that the principle of hormonal male contraception is viable, the time has come for the pharmaceutical industry to take an active interest in male contraceptive development and bring the promise of a hormonal male contraceptive to the public.

## REFERENCES

1. Goldstein M, Girardi SK. Vasectomy and vasectomy reversal. Curr Ther Endocrinol Metab 1997; 6:371
2. Feldblum PJ, Fortney JA. Condoms, spermicides, and the transmission of human immunodeficiency virus: a review of the literature. Am J Public Health 1988; 78:52.
3. Matsumoto AM, Bremner WJ. Endocrine control of human spermatogenesis. J Steroid Biochem 1989; 33:789.
4. World Health Organization Task Force on Methods for the Regulation of Male Fertility. Contraceptive efficacy of T-induced azoospermia and oligozoospermia in normal men. Fertil Steril 1996; 65:821.
5. Handelsman DJ, Farley TM, Peregoudov A, et al. Factors in nonuniform induction of azoospermia by testosterone enanthate in normal men. Fertil Steril 1995; 63:125.
6. Bagatell CJ, Bremner WJ. Androgens in men—uses and abuses. N Engl J Med 1996; 334:707.
7. Behre HM, Nieschlag E. Testosterone buciclate (20 Aet-1) in hypogonadal men: pharmacokinetics and pharmacodynamics of the new long-acting androgen ester. J Clin Endocrinol Metab 1992; 75:1204.
8. Coert A, Geelen J, de Visser J, et al. The pharmacology and metabolism of testosterone undecanoate (TU), a new orally active androgen. Acta Endocrinol 1975; 79:789.
9. Zhang GY, Gu YQ, Wang XH, et al. A pharmacokinetic study of injectable testosterone undecanoate in hypogonadal men. J Androl 1998; 19:761.
10. Bhasin S, Swerdloff RS, Steiner B, et al. A biodegradable testosterone microcapsule formulation provides uniform eugonadal levels of testosterone for 10–11 weeks in hypogonadal men. J Clin Endocrinol Metab 1992; 74:75.
11. Handelsman DJ, Conway AJ, Boylan LM. Suppression of human spermatogenesis by testosterone implants. J Clin Endocrinol Metab 1992; 75:1326.
12. Handelsman DJ, Conway AJ, Howe CJ, et al. Establishing the minimum effective dose and additive effects of depot progestin in suppression of human spermatogenesis by a testosterone depot. J Clin Endocrinol Metab 1996; 81:4113.
13. Schurmeyer T, Knuth UA, Belkien L, et al. Reversible azoospermia induced by the anabolic steroid 19-nortestosterone. Lancet 1984; 417:875.
14. Sundaram K, Kumar N, Bardin CW. 7-α-methyl-19-nortestosterone: an ideal androgen for replacement therapy. Recent Prog Horm Res 1994; 49:373.
15. Anderson RA, Wallace AM, Wu FC. Comparison between testosterone enanthate-induced azoospermia and oligozoospermia in a male contraceptive study. III. Higher 5α-reductase activity in oligospermic men administered supraphysiological doses of testosterone. J Clin Endocrinol Metab 1996; 81:902.
16. Heckel NJ. Production of oligozoospermia in a man by the use of testosterone propionate. Proc Soc Exp Biol Med 1939; 40:658.
17. Steinberger E, Smith KD. Effect of chronic administration of testosterone enanthate on sperm production and plasma testosterone, FSH and LH levels: a preliminary evaluation of a possible male contraceptive. Fertil Steril 1977; 28:1320.
18. Steinberger E, Smith KD. Testosterone enanthate: a possible reversible male contraceptive. Contraception 1977; 16:261.
19. Swerdloff RS, Campfield LA, Palacios A, et al. Suppression of human spermatogenesis by depot androgen: potential for male contraception. J Steroid Biochem 1979; 11:663.
20. WHO. Contraceptive efficacy of testosterone-induced azoospermia in normal men. Lancet 1990; 336:995.
21. Bagatell CJ, Heiman JR, Matsumoto AM, et al. Metabolic and behavioral effects of high-dose, exogenous testosterone in healthy men. J Clin Endocrinol Metab 1994; 79:561.
22. Meriggiola MC, Marcovina S, Paulsen CA, Bremner WJ. Testosterone enanthate at the dose 200 mg/week decreases HDL-cholesterol levels in healthy men. Int J Androl 1995:18:237.
23. Matsuo H, Baba Y, Nair RM, et al. Structure of the porcine LH and FSH releasing hormone. Biochem Biophys Res Commun 1971; 43:1334.
24. Cummings DE, Bremner WJ. Prospects for new hormonal male contraceptives. Endocrinol Metab Clin North Am 1994; 23:893.
24a. Schally AV. LH-RH analogies: I. Their impact on reproductive medicine. Gynecol Endocrinol 1999; 13:401.
25. Pavlou SN, Brewer K, Farely MG, et al. Combined administration of a gonadotropin-releasing hormone antagonist and testosterone in men induces reversible azoospermia without loss of libido. J Clin Endocrinol Metab 1991; 73:1360.
26. Tom L, Bhasin S, Salameh W, et al. Induction of azoospermia in normal men with combined Nal-Glu gonadotropin-releasing hormone and testosterone enanthate. J Clin Endocrinol Metab 1992; 75:476.
27. Bagatell CJ, Matsumoto AM, Christensen RB, et al. Comparison of a gonadotropin-releasing hormone antagonist plus testosterone (T) versus T alone as potential male contraceptive regimens. J Clin Endocrinol Metab 1993; 77:427.
28. Swerdloff RS, Bagatell CJ, Wang C, et al. Suppression of spermatogenesis in man induced by Nal-Glu gonadotropin-releasing hormone antagonist and testosterone enanthate (TE) is maintained by TE alone. J Clin Endocrinol Metab 1998; 83:3527.
29. Schearer SB, Alvarez-Sanchez F, Anselmo J, et al. Hormonal contraception for men. Int J Androl 1978; 2:680.
30. Fotherby K, Davies JE, Richards DJ, Bodin M. Effect of low doses of synthetic progestagens on testicular function. Int J Fertil 1972; 17:113.
31. Meriggiola MC, Bremner WJ. Progestin-androgen combination regimens for male contraception. J Androl 1997; 18:240.
32. Alvarez-Sanchez F, Faundes A, Brache V, et al. Attainment and maintenance of azoospermia with combined monthly injections of depot medroxy-

progesterone acetate and testosterone enanthate. Contraception 1977; 15:635.

33. Brenner PF, Mishell DR, Bernstein GS, et al. Study of medroxyprogesterone acetate and testosterone enanthate as a male contraceptive. Contraception 1977; 15:679.

34. Frick J, Bartsch G, Weiske WH. The effects of monthly depot medroxyprogesterone acetate and testosterone on human spermatogenesis. I. Uniform dosage levels. Contraception 1977; 15:649.

35. Frick J, Bartsch G, Weiske WH. The effects of monthly depot medroxyprogesterone acetate and testosterone on human spermatogenesis. II. High initial dose. Contraception 1977; 15:669.

36. Melo JF, Coutinho EM. Inhibition of spermatogenesis in men with monthly injections of medroxyprogesterone acetate and testosterone enanthate. Contraception 1977; 15:627.

37. Barfield A, Melo J, Coutinho E, et al. Pregnancies associated with sperm concentrations below 10 million/mL in clinical studies of a potential male contraceptive method, monthly depot medroxyprogesterone acetate and testosterone esters. Contraception 1977; 20:121.

38. Bebb RA, Anawalt BD, Christensen RB, et al. Combined administration of levonorgestrel and testosterone induces more rapid and effective suppression of spermatogenesis than testosterone alone: a promising male contraceptive approach. J Clin Endocrinol Metab 1996; 81:757.

39. Knuth UA, Yeung C, Nieschlag E. Combination of 19-nortestosterone-hexoxyphenylpropionate (Anadur) and depot medroxyprogesterone-acetate (Clinovir) for male contraception. Fertil Steril 1989; 51:1011.

40. WHO. Comparison of two androgens plus depot-medroxyprogesterone acetate for suppression to azoospermia in Indonesian men. Fertil Steril 1993; 60:1062.

41. Neumann F, Topert M. Pharmacology of antiandrogens. J Steroid Biochem 1986; 25:885.

42. Moltz L, Rommler A, Post K, et al. Medium dose cyproterone acetate (CPA): effects on hormone secretion and on spermatogenesis in normal men. Contraception 1980; 21:393.

43. Wang C, Yeung KK. Use of low-dosage cyproterone acetate as a male contraceptive. Contraception 1980; 21:245.

44. Lohiya NK, Sharma OP, Sharma RC, Sharma RS. Reversible sterility by cyproterone acetate plus testosterone enanthate in monkey with maintenance of libido. Biomed Biochem Acta 1987; 46:259.

45. Roy S. Experience in the development of hormonal contraceptive for the male. In: Asch RH, ed. Recent advances in human reproduction. Rome: Fondazione per gli Studi sulla Riproduzione Umana, 1985:95.

46. Meriggiola MC, Bremner WJ, Paulsen CA, et al. A combined regimen of cyproterone acetate and testosterone enanthate as a potentially highly effective male contraceptive. J Clin Endocrinol Metab 1996; 81:3018.

47. Meriggiola MC, Bremner WJ, Constantino A, et al. An oral regimen of cyproterone acetate and testosterone for spermatogenic suppression in men. Fertil Steril 1997; 68:844.

48. Cummings DE, Kumar N, Bardin CW, et al. Prostate-sparing tissue specific effects of the potent androgen $7\alpha$-methyl-19-nortestosterone (MENT) in primates. J Clin Endocrinol Metab 1998; 83:4212.

49. Hamann LG, Higuchi RI, Zhi L, et al. Synthesis and biological activity of a novel series of nonsteroidal, peripherally selective androgen receptor antagonists derived from 1,2-dihydropyridonon[5,6-g] quinolines. J Med Chem 1998; 41:623.

50. Gambineri A, Pasquali R. Testosterone therapy in men: clinical and pharmacological perspectives. J Endocrinol Invest 2000; 23:196.

# DISORDERS OF FUEL METABOLISM

C. RONALD KAHN, EDITOR

# S E C T I O N   A

# FOOD AND ENERGY

## C H A P T E R   1 2 4

# PRINCIPLES OF NUTRITIONAL MANAGEMENT

ROBERTA P. DURSCHLAG AND ROBERT J. SMITH

## ESSENTIAL NUTRIENTS

The provision of essential nutrients to humans in correct amounts is necessary for both the maintenance of existing tissues and the generation of new tissues. Required nutrients include *nitrogen,* several *minerals,* and an appropriate and adequate *source of energy.* Because their biosynthetic pathways are lacking or inadequate, *essential amino acids,* two *fatty acids,* and *vitamins* must be included in the diet. Recommended dietary allowances (RDAs), published by the National Research Council, have defined requirements for energy, protein, vitamins, and minerals, as well as general recommendations for intake of carbohydrate, fiber, and lipids in healthy Americans.[1] The National Academy of Sciences has begun to report *dietary reference intakes* (DRIs) for nutrients, which eventually will replace the old RDAs.[2] DRIs encompass two standards that can be used to assess the intake of individuals (RDAs and adequate intakes [AIs]) and one that can be used to assess the intake of groups (estimated average requirements [EARs]). In addition to more traditional parameters of sufficient nutrient intake, DRIs take into consideration evidence concerning the role of nutrients in the prevention of disease and developmental disorders. Currently DRIs are available for calcium, phosphorus, magnesium, vitamin D, fluoride, thiamine, riboflavin, niacin, vitamin $B_6$, folate, vitamin $B_{12}$, pantothenic acid, biotin, choline, vitamin C, vitamin E, selenium, and carotenoids. These values establish for the first time upper limits for nutrient consumption. The upper limit is defined as the maximal level of nutrient intake that is unlikely to pose risks of adverse health effects in almost all individuals. In considering the established requirements for nutrients, it is important to appreciate that nutritional requirements can be altered by endocrinologic and metabolic disorders. Conversely, certain types of nutritional support, such as parenteral hyperalimentation, can cause endocrinologic or metabolic disease. For these reasons, optimal patient care requires a knowledge of normal nutritional requirements and of the relations between nutrition and disease.

## ENERGY BALANCE

### ENERGY INTAKE

The energy content of ingested food can be estimated from its *carbohydrate, fat,* and *protein* content; a correction for the efficiency of digestion and absorption; and an allowance for the loss of some of the energy of protein molecules in the urine, primarily as urea. When these factors are combined, values of 4, 9, and 4 kcal/g are obtained for carbohydrate, fat, and protein, respectively. Proteins can be catabolized as a source of energy and, thus, are included in calculations of energy intake, but dietary proteins have a much more important function in providing essential and nonessential amino acids as precursors for endogenous protein synthesis. Thus, the bulk of metabolic energy is derived from ingested carbohydrates and fats.

### CARBOHYDRATES

Nutritionally important carbohydrates in foods occur as *monosaccharides, disaccharides,* and *polysaccharides.* Quantitatively important monosaccharides are glucose and fructose; disaccharides include sucrose (glucose plus fructose) and lactose (galactose plus glucose). Dietary starches, which include amylose (unbranched glucose chains) and amylopectin (branched glucose chains), yield free glucose after digestion. The polysaccharide glycogen, also composed of branched glucose chains, is found exclusively in animal products at very low levels. Besides digestible saccharides, dietary carbohydrate also includes various forms of *undigestible fiber,* which has little nutritional value but may influence the digestion, absorption, or metabolism of ingested foods.

The substitution for sucrose, the principal form of sugar in the Western diet, with other sugars and sugar alcohols has been suggested to be of advantage when the reduction of dietary glucose (diabetes) or energy (obesity) is a goal. Although fructose produces a smaller rise in plasma glucose than isocaloric amounts of sucrose, its use in a diet for diabetes is limited because of its adverse effects on total and low-density-lipoprotein cholesterol levels.[3] The energy value of fructose is identical to that of sucrose (4 kcal/g), thereby providing *no* benefit as a means of reducing energy intake in obesity. The sugar alcohols sorbitol, mannitol, and xylitol also do *not* appear to offer any significant metabolic advantages in the treatment of diabetes.[3] Their energy values range from 1.6 to 2.6 kcal/g, but their utility in weight reduction diets is limited by a laxative effect when consumed in large quantities and their reduced sweetening ability when compared with sucrose.[4]

*Nonnutritive sugar substitutes* approved by the U.S. Food and Drug Administration in the United States include *aspartame, saccharin, acesulfame K,* and *sucralose.* Aspartame is a dipeptide of aspartic acid and the methyl ester of phenylalanine, which is ~200 times as sweet as sucrose.[4] If used alone as a sweetener, it would contribute negligible calories. However, because it is sold with a dextrose and corn syrup filler, it contributes approximately one-eighth as many kilocalories as does sucrose. Saccharin is truly a nonnutritive artificial sweetener, with no caloric value and no effects on plasma glucose.[4] Although a ban on saccharin use was proposed by the U.S. Food and Drug Administration in 1977 because of evidence of carcinogenicity, the U.S. Congress subsequently reversed the ban in response to public pressure.[4] Acesulfame K (5,6-dimethyl-1,2,3-oxathiazin-4[3H]-one, 2,2-dioxide) is 200 times sweeter than sugar and provides no calories. Sucralose, synthesized by substituting three chlorine atoms for three hydroxyl groups on sucrose, is 600 times sweeter than sucrose and also yields no calories. When sold as a tabletop sweetener, sucralose contains 2 kcal per teaspoon as a result of added fillers.

## FATS

Dietary lipid consists almost entirely (98% to 99%) of triglycerides, with the remainder being monoglycerides, diglycerides, free fatty acids, phospholipids, and cholesterol. Humans are capable of synthesizing all the fatty acids needed for endogenous triglyceride synthesis from carbohydrate and protein precursors, except for linoleic acid and linolenic acid.[5,6] As the parent compounds of the omega-6 and omega-3 families of fatty acids, respectively, these two *essential fatty acids* are converted to polyunsaturated 20-carbon eicosanoids, which are the precursors of prostaglandins, thromboxanes, and leukotrienes.[7] DRIs have not yet been formally established for linoleic acid and linolenic acid. However, clinical and biochemical symptoms of linoleic acid deficiency can be prevented by its inclusion in amounts approximating 1% to 2% of total kilocalories in the diets of adults. Based on similar criteria, the requirement for linolenic and other omega-3 fatty acids has been proposed to be 10% to 25% of the linoleic acid requirement.[1] Typical American diets meet these preliminary recommendations.

Food composition tables are available that specify not only the carbohydrate, protein, and lipid content of foods, but also the amounts of fiber, cholesterol, and individual amino acids and fatty acids.[8,9] The use of this information in dietary analysis has become more common as it has been compiled into computer databases. Currently available databases vary considerably in the number of food items included and the exact values used in computing nutrient intake, so care must be taken in choosing a software package.[10,11] Computer databases have made it possible to convert information rapidly from standardized dietary histories into reasonably accurate, comprehensive descriptions of total nutrient intake. With this type of analysis, it has been possible to document changes over

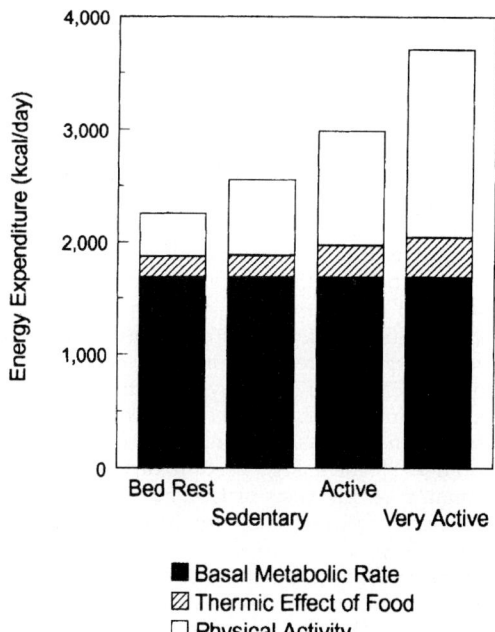

**FIGURE 124-1.** Total energy expenditure at various physical activity levels.

time in food consumption patterns in the United States. For example, the average daily percentage of kcal from carbohydrates has been shown to increase from 42.6% in 1977–1978 to 48.9% in 1989–1991. Over the same period, the average daily percentage of kcal from fat decreased from 40.5% to 34.8%, and the total intake decreased slightly from 1826 to 1774 kcal per day.[12]

## ENERGY EXPENDITURE

In addition to energy intake, a determination of energy expenditure is essential for the formulation of human energy needs. If body weight is constant, all the energy ingested in food must be expended (as heat and work) or lost in excreted substances. Total energy expenditure depends on three factors: *basal metabolic rate* (BMR), the *thermic effect of food* (TEF), and *physical activity*. The BMR, defined as the amount of energy needed to maintain body processes at rest after a 12-hour fast, correlates with lean body mass (higher in men than in women) and is influenced by thyroid hormone, growth hormone, and norepinephrine.[13] During prolonged starvation, the BMR may drop as much as 50%, and it increases 13% with each degree centigrade rise in body temperature.

The TEF refers to an increase in heat production during the absorptive phase after food ingestion, apparently resulting from the energy cost of digesting, absorbing, and metabolizing food substances. Typically, the TEF causes the loss of ~10% of the potential caloric value of a mixed diet. This represents the integrated energy expenditure related to the handling of ingested carbohydrate and lipid (5%), and of protein (25%).[13] The process of adaptive thermogenesis, or an increase in energy expenditure in response to overfeeding, appears to play little role in energy balance in humans.[14]

*Physical activity* accounts for a substantial but variable fraction of total energy expenditure, ranging from 10% of the total in a bedridden person to 50% in an extremely active person (Fig. 124-1). Besides the level of activity, body weight and efficiency of movement determine the caloric cost of physical activity.

## MEASUREMENT OF ENERGY EXPENDITURE

Energy expenditure can be measured by *direct calorimetry,* which requires placing a person in a sealed chamber where heat production, work done, and the energy of excreta can be determined. Alternatively, two methods of indirect calorimetry are available. One method relies on a determination of oxygen consumption; energy expenditure is then determined using the experimental observation that a person ingesting a mixed diet expends 4.82 kcal/L of $O_2$ consumed.[13] The second technique relies on water labeled with both deuterium and $^{18}O$ to measure $CO_2$ production.[15]

Without any direct determinations, it also is possible to calculate energy expenditure by estimating and combining the contributions of BMR, TEF, and physical activity. Energy expenditure resulting from BMR totaled over 24 hours, referred to as *basal energy expenditure,* is calculated based on body weight, height, and age.[1,16] The energy used in various physical activities is estimated on the basis of tabulated values; the sum of BMR and the cost of physical activity then are increased by 10% to include the TEF.[13]

Using measured and estimated rates of energy expenditure, the National Research Council has established ranges of recommended energy intake for persons based on sex, height, and weight.[1] Realizing that an imbalance in energy intake and expenditure with resulting obesity is an enormous public health problem, the formulation of these allowances for energy differs from that of other nutrients in that the energy allowances do not contain a safety factor but rather represent the minimum caloric intake thought to be appropriate for good health.

## REGULATION OF ENERGY BALANCE

Most healthy adults are able to balance energy intake and expenditure such that body weight is maintained at a stable level. The regulation is remarkably precise, considering that the average adult ingests ~1 million kcal/year. An excess of intake over expenditure of only 1% would yield a yearly weight gain of ~3 pounds.[17] The nature of the control mechanisms and the issue of whether regulation occurs at the level of intake or expenditure or both are subjects that have received much investigation.

There is no doubt that energy intake is regulated, as evidenced by fluctuating sensations of hunger and satiety. The original view that the hypothalamus has discrete feeding and satiety centers that sense the need for energy intake and regulate eating behavior has been modified to include contributions of other components of the nervous system, hormonal factors such as cholecystokinin and insulin,[18,19] and peripheral organs such as the stomach and liver.[20,21] The brain is thought to have an important role in the integration of internal and external stimuli to produce appropriate metabolic and behavioral responses through neural and hormonal signals.[20]

A number of neuroendocrine factors have been identified that appear to have important roles in the modulation of energy intake through their effects on the hypothalamic centers controlling satiety or hunger. Leptin, a peptide hormone secreted by adipose tissue, suppresses appetite and activates pathways that increase energy expenditure following its binding to hypothalamic receptors.[22,23] Loss of function mutations in leptin or leptin receptors results in obesity in murine models (*ob/ob*[22] and *db/db* mice,[24] respectively), and similar mutations have been identified as rare causes of human obesity.[25] In addition to modulating energy intake and expenditure, leptin has effects on growth hormone–releasing hormone and gonadotropin-releasing hormones that suggest roles in linking nutritional status to growth and reproductive capacity.[23] Another substance, the hypothalamic hormone neuropeptide Y, is a potent central appetite stimulator that may have even more important effects than leptin on energy intake.[26] Leptin may exert part of its actions by decreasing serum levels of neuropeptide Y,[27] which

**TABLE 124-1.**
**Nutritional Classification of Amino Acids**

| Essential | Nonessential |
|---|---|
| Arginine | Alanine |
| Histidine | Asparagine |
| Isoleucine | Aspartic acid |
| Leucine | Cysteine |
| Lysine | Cystine |
| Methionine | Glutamic acid |
| Phenylalanine | Glutamine* |
| Threonine | Glycine |
| Tryptophan | Proline |
| Valine | Serine |
| | Tyrosine |

*It has been suggested that glutamine be placed in a special category as a conditionally essential amino acid, because it commonly appears to become deficient during severe clinical illnesses (Smith RJ, Wilmore DW. Glutamine nutrition and requirements. JPEN 1990; 12:94S; Smith RJ. Glutamine-supplemented nutrition. JPEN 1997; 21:183).

appears to be regulated by factors other than leptin.[28] There are also a number of other hormones and receptors that have been found to have effects on the control of energy intake,[29] and it is likely that further work in this area will lead to substantial progress in the understanding of the integrated processes that control energy balance.

Although increased energy intake currently is thought to be the most important factor leading to human obesity, energy expenditure also appears to differ among individuals and to be regulated. When caloric intake is limited, decreases in both the BMR and physical activity result in diminished energy expenditure.[30] Unfortunately, analogous increases in BMR and activity are limited and not adequate to offset excess caloric intake. *Facultative thermogenesis,* the dissipation of some of the energy of ingested food as heat, has been the focus of considerable interest, but still has *not* been clearly established as a mechanism for expending excess energy in humans.[16,31] The uncoupling of oxidative phosphorylation from adenosine triphosphate generation through the action of inducible uncoupling proteins in brown fat appears to be an important mechanism of energy expenditure in nonhuman species. The discovery of an uncoupling protein isoform (UCP2) with significant expression in human skeletal muscle and white adipose tissue has led to an interest in the potential importance of uncoupled oxidative phosphorylation as a determinant of energy expenditure in humans. Further study is required, however, to determine the importance of this mechanism for overall energy balance.

In looking to the future, the development of pharmacologic strategies for weight reduction targeted to specific molecules that regulate energy intake and expenditure has become a major research goal, with considerable promise for defining new and more effective approaches to body weight control.

## DIETARY PROTEIN AND NITROGEN BALANCE

Protein is required in the diet to provide nitrogen for the synthesis of nonessential amino acids and other nitrogen-containing compounds, such as purines and pyrimidines, and to provide essential amino acids that cannot be synthesized endogenously in adequate amounts (Table 124-1). Moreover, amino acids derived from dietary protein may have important effects in addition to serving as precursors for protein synthesis. For example, glutamic acid acts as a central nervous system neurotransmitter.[32] Excessive glutamic acid ingestion, typically as a component of Asian cuisine, can produce a toxic response that is

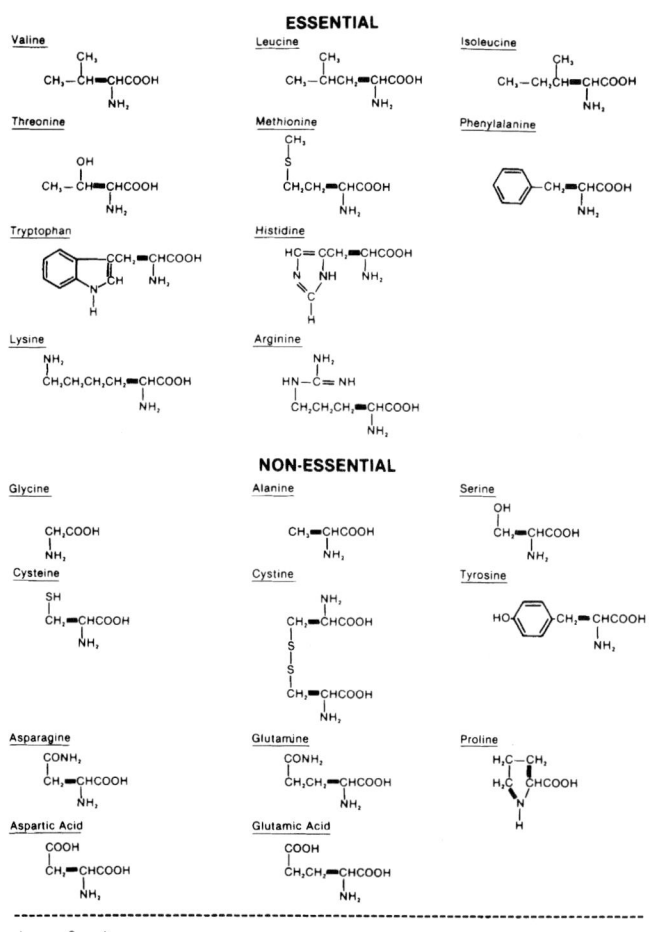

**ESSENTIAL**

Valine, Leucine, Isoleucine, Threonine, Methionine, Phenylalanine, Tryptophan, Histidine, Lysine, Arginine

**NON-ESSENTIAL**

Glycine, Alanine, Serine, Cysteine, Cystine, Tyrosine, Asparagine, Glutamine, Proline, Aspartic Acid, Glutamic Acid

*Note that the common denominator of each amino acid is the presence of the glycyl group (—CHCOOH), as indicated by the bold dash.

NH₂

**FIGURE 124-2.** Common amino acids in protein.

thought to be related to altered neurotransmission (designated the "Chinese restaurant syndrome").[33]

## ESSENTIAL AMINO ACIDS

Dietary proteins differ in their content of essential amino acids (Fig. 124-2). *"Complete" proteins* contain all of the essential amino acids in the right proportions necessary for protein synthesis. These proteins are found in animal products such as eggs, milk, meat, fish, and poultry. The *"incomplete" proteins* found in legumes, nuts, seeds, and grains provide insufficient amounts of some essential amino acids. Because the specific amino acids missing in commonly consumed plants differ, mixtures of plant proteins can be used to complement each other, which is an important consideration in the design of vegetarian diets. Common vegetarian diets include *lacto-ovo-vegetarian* (composed of milk, eggs, and plant products, and potentially deficient in iron and zinc), *lacto-vegetarian* (composed of milk and plant products, and also potentially deficient in iron and zinc), and *total vegetarian* or *vegan* (consisting of plant products, and potentially deficient in iron, zinc, calcium, vitamin B₁₂, riboflavin, and vitamin D). All of these vegetarian diets meet essential amino-acid requirements if a variety of plants—including grains, legumes, seeds, and nuts—are included.[34,35]

The minimum dietary protein requirement for adults currently recommended by the National Research Council is 0.8 g per kilogram of body weight per day.[1] At this level, protein

**TABLE 124-2.**
**Representative Food Choices for Low-, Medium-, and High-Fiber Diets**

| Low (~15 g/d) | Medium (~30 g/d) | High (~45 g/d) |
|---|---|---|
| 1½ cups cornflakes | 1 cup 40% bran flakes | ½ cup 100% bran |
| 2 slices white bread | 4 slices whole wheat bread | 6 slices whole wheat bread |
| 1 cup raw carrots | 1 cup raw carrots | 1 cup raw carrots |
| ½ cup canned corn | ½ cup canned corn | 1 cup broccoli |
| 2 apples | 2 apples | 1 cup canned corn |
| 1 orange | 2 oranges | 2 apples |
| | ½ cup canned kidney beans | 2 oranges |
| | | ½ cup canned kidney beans |

accounts for 8% to 9% of total caloric intake, a proportion well below the average amount consumed in the United States (17% in 1988–1991).[12] This estimated requirement is based on the observed loss of body protein that occurs on a protein-free diet (0.45 g per kilogram of body weight per day), plus an increase by 30% to correct for the efficiency with which dietary protein is used, and an additional 33% correction for the quality of protein in the average American diet.[1] Efficient utilization of dietary protein requires the inclusion of sufficient calories so that amino acids are not catabolized as a source of energy.

## ASSESSMENT OF PROTEIN STATUS

To assess the adequacy of dietary protein intake and body protein status, several procedures are available. Measurements of nitrogen balance, which is the difference between dietary intake and nitrogen loss, is the most direct method for determining whether intake is sufficient to cover losses. However, nitrogen balance gives information only about current intake and excretion, and may not reflect accurately the body protein status during states of physiologic change, such as recovery from illness. As an alternative, the determination of upper arm circumference and calculation of arm muscle area gives reliable insight into muscle protein status.[36] This measurement can be supplemented with determinations of circulating proteins, such as serum albumin, transferrin, prealbumin, or retinol-binding protein. Urinary creatine and the creatine-height index also can be used to assess muscle mass. Because nonnutritional factors can affect each of these end points, it is best to use several different parameters in estimating body protein status.[37]

## DIETARY FIBER

### TYPES OF FIBER

Dietary fiber is comprised of polysaccharides and lignins of plant origin that are not digested by the endogenous secretions of the human digestive tract.[38] This includes *water-soluble fibers* (pectins, gums, mucilages, algal polysaccharides, storage polysaccharides, and some hemicelluloses) and *insoluble fibers* (cellulose, lignins, and certain hemicelluloses). The term *crude fiber,* which appears in some nutritional literature, refers to a fraction of dietary fiber (15–25%) that is resistant to vigorous treatment with acid and alkali.[39] Recognition of this terminology is important for the correct interpretation of the reported fiber content of different foods. Important sources of dietary fiber include cereal grains, vegetables, and fruits, which differ considerably in their content of soluble and insoluble fiber. A summary of fiber sources in representative low-, medium-, and high-fiber diets is presented in Table 124-2. It has been difficult to establish quantitative recommendations for dietary fiber intake because of analytic problems in determining the many contributors to total dietary fiber, as well as uncertainty about the physiologic effects of each dietary fiber fraction. As a result, accurate dietary fiber levels have been established for only a few foods.[39,40] Daily dietary fiber intake of adults in the United States (age 20–59 years) was found to be 18.9 g for men and 13.1 g for women in 1980–1981.[12] The American Dietetic Association recommends a daily fiber intake of 20 to 35 g.[41]

## EFFECTS OF FIBER

Interest in the physiologic effects of dietary fiber stems from the observation that many diseases common in Western cultures are rare in African countries where fiber intake is high.[42] The principal effects of water-insoluble fiber appear to result from a decreased intestinal transit time and an increase in fecal bulk. This is associated with a modest decrease in blood cholesterol levels and in the plasma glucose response to oral glucose tolerance testing or meal ingestion.[43–45] Water-soluble fiber increases intestinal transit time and generally causes greater decreases in cholesterol levels and postprandial plasma glucose levels.[42–47] The lowered glucose levels have been postulated to result from delayed absorption of glucose and diminished secretion of glucagon and gastric inhibitory polypeptide in response to a meal.[43,45] Many reviews of the physiologic effects of fiber that include discussions of relationships between dietary fiber and various chronic diseases are available.[41,43,48,49]

# APPLICATION OF THE PRINCIPLES OF NUTRITIONAL MANAGEMENT TO SPECIFIC DISORDERS

Many endocrinologic and metabolic disorders alter nutritional needs. In disorders such as diabetes mellitus, obesity, or anorexia nervosa, appropriate nutritional management is a fundamental part of successful treatment (see Chaps. 126 and 127), whereas in disorders such as hyperthyroidism, optimal nutritional support complements the primary treatment of the disease, reducing morbidity and hastening complete recovery.

## HYPERTHYROIDISM

In patients with hyperthyroidism, excess heat production and increased motor activity elevate caloric requirements (see Chap. 42). The prominence of weight loss as a symptom of uncontrolled hyperthyroidism is indicative of the failure of most patients to fully compensate by increasing caloric intake, although appetite commonly is increased.[50] The elevations of metabolic rate and caloric requirements are highly variable, with the greatest increases typically occurring in young patients with Graves disease.

The primary treatment of hyperthyroidism is not nutritional. However, in patients who remain hyperthyroid for a period before definitive therapy takes effect or in patients who have experienced significant weight loss, it may be beneficial to increase caloric intake. Besides increasing the size of meals, the substitution of high-calorie for low-calorie foods and the consumption of concentrated calorie sources between meals (e.g., ice cream and nuts) can effectively increase intake by 500 to 2000 kcal per day. Based on the degree of hyperthyroidism and the estimated loss of body mass, caloric intake should be increased above normal by 15% to 75%.

## OBESITY

Obesity currently is defined as *a body mass index ≥30 kg/m²* (see Chap. 126).[51] The medical risks and social stigma associated with obesity have provided impetus for the design of myriad

dietary treatments that illustrate many of the consequences of extreme changes in caloric intake or dietary composition.[52]

## TOTAL STARVATION

The most dramatic nutritional intervention for obesity is prolonged total starvation. Because of metabolic adaptations that allow the brain to use ketone bodies rather than glucose for fuel and the conservation of body protein mass, obese persons can undergo total fasting for as long as 8 weeks, often without serious medical consequences.[53] Weight reduction is marked, averaging ~0.5 kg per day, but the costs are significant.[54] Patients must stay in either a hospital or a supervised facility. They need mineral supplements, multivitamins, medication to prevent gout, and frequent observation by medical personnel.[55] Besides the expense and the disruption of patients' normal lives, the principal problem with total fasting for weight reduction is that it does not provide a mechanism for the long-term maintenance of reduced body weight. In follow-up studies, most patients return to their original weight.[56]

## VERY-LOW-CALORIE DIETS

Very-low-calorie diets include a variety of regimens that commonly are structured as protein-sparing modified fasts containing 200 to 800 kcal per day, with high-protein foods or commercially available liquid protein formulas as the only source of nutrient intake. In the former, protein intake is derived from lean meat, fish, and fowl, providing 1.5 g of protein per kilogram of ideal body weight per day plus the small amount of fat contained in these foods.[57] Liquid protein diets are available in several formulations that generally contain greater than 50% of calories as protein and a total of less than 500 kcal per day. As with total starvation, vitamin and mineral supplements should be provided. The rationale for these diets is that the dietary protein replaces body protein that is being degraded as a source of glucose and energy, and thereby minimizes the wasting of lean body mass. Weight loss is extremely rapid (~0.25 kg per day).[58] However, the diets carry significant risks, as evidenced by the deaths of 58 people on these regimens in 1977 and 1978.[59] Although a definite link was not established between the high-protein diets and cardiac complications in the affected individuals, the most consistent pathologic finding was myocardial atrophy, a condition that also develops in protein-calorie malnutrition.[60] Subsequent experience has demonstrated an absence of these severe complications with diets containing higher-quality protein, but it still is advisable to use high-protein, very-low-calorie diets only in the morbidly obese and under close medical supervision.[58,61]

## HIGH-PROTEIN, LOW-CARBOHYDRATE DIETS

Less extreme high-protein, low-carbohydrate diets have been introduced under many names. They generally contain <50 g of carbohydrate, <1000 total kilocalories, and >120 g of protein per day. The combination of a reduction in total calories and carbohydrate leads to a state of mild ketosis, and it has been claimed that the loss of calories as ketones in the urine contributes to weight loss. In reality, however, a maximum of 50 kcal per day is excreted in the urine as ketone bodies.[62] Even with the high protein intake, muscle protein wasting may occur as amino acids are mobilized to provide gluconeogenic substrate. Other potential adverse effects of the diets include fatigue, nausea, postural hypotension, hyperuricemia, and complications related to high dietary fat intake.[62] Vitamin and mineral deficiencies also can occur, so supplements should be provided.[63] Fundamentally, high-protein, low-carbohydrate diets appear to depend on the same principle as do other diets, which is a reduction of caloric intake below expenditure. Food intake may decrease, because a low-carbohydrate diet is not very palatable, but for this reason, patients also may fail to adhere to the diets for long periods.

## SUCCESSFUL APPROACHES

Although these approaches to weight reduction are interesting metabolically, their success rates are disappointingly low.[64] Programs that provide multiple strategies for achieving and maintaining weight loss seem to meet with more success. These approaches take into consideration patients' readiness for behavior change, incorporate an exercise plan, provide problem-solving strategies when progress is threatened, and emphasize behavior modification and social support.[51,65,66] The meal plan should be reduced in caloric content, while assuring compatibility with good health and acceptability to patients. Specifically, a daily deficit of 500 to 1000 kcal combined with a modified fat diet should be implemented.[51] Finally, it must be emphasized that behavioral changes are necessary if weight reduction is to be permanent.

## DIABETES MELLITUS

Close adherence to a defined diet is essential for good metabolic control in type 1 diabetes, because it assures that a given insulin regimen is neither deficient nor excessive from one day to the next. Moreover, diets are intended to serve several other functions in patients with both type 1 and type 2 diabetes (see Chap. 141). Ideally, a diabetic diet minimizes postprandial plasma glucose excursions, lowers lipid levels, and either maintains body weight or reduces weight to normal levels.

Diabetic diets traditionally were limited in carbohydrate content, because it was thought that there would be a direct correlation between the amount of ingested carbohydrate and the degree of elevation of plasma glucose levels after a meal.[67] Between 1921 and 1986, the percent of kilocalories from carbohydrate recommended in the treatment of diabetes increased from 20% to 60%, based on findings demonstrating no deterioration in blood glucose control as the carbohydrate content of the diet increased, and progressive realization of the importance of reducing dietary lipid. The 1994 recommendations of the American Diabetes Association do not assign a specific percent distribution for carbohydrate and fat, but emphasize the principle of meeting metabolic, nutritional, and lifestyle goals that include near-normal blood glucose levels, optimal serum lipid levels, reasonable body weight, prevention of hypoglycemia, and improvement of overall health through optimal nutrition.[68]

### IS CARBOHYDRATE RESTRICTION JUSTIFIED?

The rationale for carbohydrate-restricted diets in patients with diabetes has been questioned for two major reasons. First, several studies have suggested that an increase in dietary carbohydrate actually might improve the control of plasma glucose. Second, raising the carbohydrate content of the diet makes it possible to lower the fat content. This, in turn, could decrease circulating lipids and lower the risk of coronary artery disease and peripheral vascular disease. Although many studies have been carried out with the goal of assessing the metabolic effects of high-carbohydrate diets in diabetes mellitus, the interpretation of the results of most of these investigations is confounded by coincident changes in body weight and dietary fiber, both of which probably have independent effects on metabolic control. The effects of increasing dietary carbohydrate exclusive of changes in other dietary constituents have been investigated with liquid formula diets.[69,70] This work showed that large increases in carbohydrate intake (up to 85% of calories) were not accompanied by increased insulin requirements, and fasting blood glucose levels actually were noted to decrease in one study.[70] Effects were noted in patients with both type 1 and type 2 diabetes. Although triglyceride levels increased two-fold

to four-fold initially, there was a downward trend with time. These studies with liquid formula diets demonstrate that patients with diabetes can tolerate extremely high levels of carbohydrate intake without a deterioration in metabolic control, and perhaps even with improved control. It is unclear from this work, however, whether more normal diets with more palatable carbohydrate levels would have similar effects.

Studies with diets composed of natural foods and more moderately increased carbohydrate content generally have yielded unimpressive or conflicting results. For example, in type 1 and type 2 diabetes patients, a comparison of diets containing 42% and 53% carbohydrate revealed no decrease in 2-hour postprandial or daily plasma glucose levels on the higher-carbohydrate diet.[71] In patients with type 2 diabetes, when two diets containing 35% and 60% carbohydrate were studied, mean basal blood glucose levels decreased, but 2-hour postprandial glucose levels increased with the 60% carbohydrate diet.[72] There were no changes in hemoglobin $A_{1c}$, mean plasma cholesterol, or fasting plasma triglyceride levels. Although this work does not demonstrate a metabolic advantage of diets high in carbohydrate, there is a consistent absence of deleterious effects. Thus, there appears to be no justification for restricting the carbohydrate content of diabetic diets.

### SIMPLE VERSUS COMPLEX CARBOHYDRATES

The recommendation that patients with diabetes should limit the consumption of simple sugars and should consume varied sources of complex carbohydrate also has been questioned. When standardized amounts of carbohydrate-containing foods are given, the plasma glucose response varies with different foods but is not predictable on the basis of the fiber or sugar content of the food.[73] In particular, some foods containing simple sugars cause glucose elevations no greater than those observed with complex carbohydrates. These findings are reflected in the 1994 recommendations of the American Diabetes Association, which emphasize attention to total amount rather than type of carbohydrate in the diet.[68]

### INCREASED FIBER CONTENT

The observation that diabetes mellitus is rare among rural African populations that consume large amounts of high-fiber foods has led to interest in increasing the fiber content of diabetic diets.[74] As was the case with the studies on dietary carbohydrate content, because foods containing generous amounts of fiber tend to be high in carbohydrate, much of the subsequent work has failed to separate these two variables. The problem is complicated even further by the potentially different effects of soluble and insoluble fiber. Both soluble fibers (such as guar) and insoluble fiber (bran) significantly lower postprandial blood glucose levels.[44] Although the mechanisms of action of the different forms of fiber are not clear, several subsequent studies with fiber-supplemented diets have confirmed these beneficial effects in the metabolic control of patients with diabetes.[75–80]

As with high-carbohydrate diets, high-fiber diets tend to be either difficult to prepare or unappealing in composition. For this reason, the 1994 guidelines of the American Dietetic Association acknowledge that the level of dietary fiber, particularly soluble fiber, necessary to blunt the glycemic response is impractical to consume from food sources and recommend the same dietary intake for patients with diabetes as for nondiabetic patients.[68] This reinforces the point that the demonstration of a beneficial effect of a specific dietary regimen on diabetic control does not necessarily translate into a practical therapeutic tool. The high-fiber diets that are most acceptable to patients have been evaluated in studies in which the carbohydrate and fiber content of the diet were altered simultaneously. Although this design makes it impossible to distinguish the effects of carbohydrate and fiber, such studies provide a valid analysis of diets that can be used in clinical practice. Controlled trials are few, but the results generally have been favorable.[80–83] With some variation, different measures of plasma glucose control such as fasting plasma glucose concentrations, postprandial glucose levels, and mean plasma glucose values have decreased modestly on high-carbohydrate, high-fiber diets. Finally, people with diabetes could benefit from the other suggested advantages of a diet rich in fiber: the prevention/improvement of gastrointestinal disorders and the reduction of serum lipids.[84] More work is needed, but it seems advisable to modify traditional diabetic diets by liberalizing carbohydrate-containing foods that are a good source of dietary fiber.

## ENTERAL AND PARENTERAL NUTRITION

The use of enteral feeding (through a nasogastric, gastrostomy, or jejunostomy tube) and parenteral feeding (through a central or peripheral vein) has increased steadily in hospitalized patients as complication rates have decreased and the importance of optimal nutritional support has been recognized.[85–88] Further, patients with chronic diseases often are maintained as outpatients with enteral or parenteral nutritional support. With the widespread use of these forms of nutrition and the consequent increase in the sophistication of the techniques, it is uncommon for deficiencies of vitamins or specific nutrients to develop. Nevertheless, it is important to be aware of the endocrinologic problems that could occur with "incomplete" nutritional support. For example, osteomalacia can develop in patients who do not receive adequate vitamin supplements, especially if they are being fed intravenously or have steatorrhea and malabsorption.[85]

The most common endocrinologic disorder in nutritionally supported patients is hyperglycemia. This can develop in patients being fed enterally,[89] but is especially common with parenteral hyperalimentation.[90] The combination of a high rate of glucose administration plus the insulin resistance that characterizes severe illnesses appears to overwhelm the pancreatic secretory reserve, causing a relative insulin deficiency. Because endogenous insulin is present, ketoacidosis is rare, but hyperglycemia can be marked. In the extreme, a hyperglycemic, hyperosmolar state with coma may develop.[91]

In general, the control of hyperglycemia resulting from nutritional support is not difficult. Patients receiving enteral nutrition can be given small doses of subcutaneous regular insulin (usually every 6 hours) or intermediate-acting insulin (every 12 hours). A similar approach can be used with patients receiving total parenteral hyperalimentation, but it generally is better to add regular insulin directly to each bottle of parenteral nutrition solution as needed (typically 6 to 8 U/L). With this approach, the potential hazard of hypoglycemia resulting from the continued absorption of subcutaneous insulin after the infusion of nutrients has been intentionally or accidentally interrupted is minimized, because interruption of the insulin infusion occurs simultaneously with cessation of nutrient administration. The incidence of hyperglycemia during parenteral hyperalimentation can be decreased by providing a portion of total calories as lipid. Infused lipids appear to have nitrogen-sparing ability similar to that of glucose; they diminish plasma glucose excursions and may have advantages in patients with compromised respiratory function by decreasing carbon dioxide production.[92] Hypoglycemia occasionally develops if the infusion of a concentrated glucose solution is discontinued suddenly, even in patients who are not receiving exogenous insulin.

Most patients in whom hyperglycemia develops during parenteral nutritional support are not diabetic and do not exhibit glucose intolerance after resuming a normal oral diet. Other patients, however, may have previously undetected diabetes or may remain glucose intolerant. Thus, it always is necessary to monitor plasma glucose levels carefully as patients recover. In patients who have a return to normal fasting and normal 2-hour postprandial plasma glucose levels, formal glucose tolerance testing generally is not indicated.

## REFERENCES

1. National Research Council. Recommended dietary allowances, 10th ed. Washington, DC: National Academy Press, 1989:21.
2. Food and Nutrition Board, Institute of Medicine. Dietary reference intakes. Washington, DC: National Academy Press, 1997, 1998, 2000.
3. American Dietetic Association. Nutrition recommendations and principles for people with diabetes mellitus. J Am Diet Assoc 1994; 94:504.
4. American Dietetic Association. Position paper: Use of nutritive and nonnutritive sweeteners. J Am Diet Assoc 1998; 98:580.
5. Conner WE, Conner SL. The dietary treatment of hyperlipidemia: rationale, techniques and efficacy. Med Clin North Am 1982; 66:485.
6. Holman RT, Johnson SB, Hatch TF. A case of human linolenic acid deficiency involving neurological abnormalities. Am J Clin Nutr 1982; 35:617.
7. Murray RK, Granner DK, Mayes PA, Rodwell VW. Harper's biochemistry, 24th ed. Norwalk, CT: Appleton & Lange, 1996.
8. Pennington JAT. Bowes' and Church's food values of portions commonly used. Philadelphia: JB Lippincott, 1994.
9. Adams CF. Nutritive value of American foods. Agriculture handbook number 456. Washington, DC: United States Department of Agriculture, 1975.
10. Rand WH. Food composition data: problems and plans. J Am Diet Assoc 1985; 85:1081.
11. Lee RD, Nieman DC, Rainwater M. Comparison of eight microcomputer dietary analysis programs with the USDA nutrient data base for standard reference. J Am Diet Assoc 1995; 95:858.
12. Federation of American Societies for Experimental Biology, Life Science Research Office. Third report on nutrition monitoring in the United States. Washington, DC: U.S. Government Printing Office, 1995.
13. Mahan LK, Escott-Stump S. Food, nutrition and diet therapy, 9th ed. Philadelphia: WB Saunders, 1996.
14. Stubbs RJ. Appetite, feeding behaviour and energy balance in human subjects. Proc Nutr Soc 1998, 57:341.
15. Schoeller DA. Measurement of energy expenditure in free-living humans by using doubly labeled water. J Nutr 1988; 118:1278.
16. Harris HA, Benedict FG. A biometric study of basal metabolism in man. Washington, DC: Carnegie Institute of Washington, 1919.
17. Bray GA, Campfield LA. Metabolic factors in the control of energy stores. Metabolism 1975; 24:99.
18. Stricker EM. Biological bases of hunger and satiety: therapeutic implications. Nutr Rev 1984; 42:333.
19. Smith GP, Gibbs J. Brain-gut peptides and the control of food intake. In: Martin JB, Reichlin S, Bick KL, eds. Neurosecretion and brain peptides. New York: Raven Press, 1981:389.
20. Hernandez L, Hoebel BG. Basic mechanisms of feeding and weight regulation. In: Stunkard AJ, ed. Obesity. Philadelphia: WB Saunders, 1980:25.
21. Widdowson EM. Nutritional individuality. Proc Nutr Soc 1962; 21:121.
22. Zhang Y, Proenca R, Maffei M, et al. Positional cloning of the mouse ob gene and its human homologue. Nature 1994; 372:425.
23. Flier JS. What's in a name? In search of leptin's physiologic role. J Clin Endocrinol Metab 1998; 83:1407.
24. Chen H, Charlat O, Tartaglia LA, et al. Evidence that the diabetes gene encodes the leptin receptor: identification of a mutation in the leptin receptor gene in *db/db* mice. Cell 1996;84:491.
25. Montague CT, Farooqi IS, Whitehead JP, et al. Congenital leptin deficiency is associated with severe early-onset obesity in humans. Nature 1997; 387:903.
26. Billington CJ, Briggs JE, Harker S, et al. Neuropeptide Y in hypothalamic paraventricular nucleus: a center coordinating energy metabolism. Am J Physiol 1994; 266:R1765.
27. Stephens TW, Basinski M, Bristow PK, et al. A role for neuropeptide Y in the antiobesity action of the obese gene product. Nature 1995; 377:530.
28. Zukowska-Grojec Z. Neuropeptide Y: a novel sympathetic stress hormone and more. Ann NY Acad Sci 1995; 77:219.
29. Rosenbaum M, Leibel RL, Hirsch J. Obesity: medical progress. N Engl J Med 1997; 337:396.
30. James WP. Energy requirements and obesity. Lancet 1983; 2:386.
31. Rothwell NJ, Stock MS. Luxuskonsumption, diet-induced thermogenesis and brown fat: the case in favor. Clin Sci 1983; 64:19.
32. Shank RP, Aprison MH. Biochemical aspects of the neurotransmitter function of glutamine. In: Filer LJ, Garrattini S, Kare MP, et al., eds. Glutamic acid: advances in biochemistry and physiology. New York: Raven Press, 1979:139.
33. Schaumburg HH, Byck R, Gerstl R, Mashman JH. Monosodium glutamate: its pharmacology and role in the Chinese restaurant syndrome. Science 1969; 163:826.
34. American Dietetic Association. Position paper: vegetarian diets. J Am Diet Assoc 1997; 1317.
35. Barnes LA, American Academy of Pediatrics Committee on Nutrition. Nutritional aspects of vegetarianism, health foods and fad diets. Nutr Rev 1977; 35:153.
36. Heymsfield SB, McManus C, Smith J, et al. Anthropometric measurement

of muscle mass: revised equations for calculating bone-free arm muscle area. Am J Clin Nutr 1982; 36:680.

37. Gibson RS. Principles of nutritional assessment. New York: Oxford University Press, 1990.
38. Vahouny GV. Conclusions and recommendations of the Symposium on Dietary Fibers in Health and Disease, Washington, DC, 1981. Am J Clin Nutr 1982; 35:152.
39. Anderson JW, Bridges SR. Dietary fiber content of selected foods. Am J Clin Nutr 1988; 47:440.
40. Marlett JA. Content and composition of dietary fiber in 117 frequently consumed foods. J Am Diet Assoc 1992; 92:175.
41. American Dietetic Association position paper: health implications of dietary fiber. J Am Diet Assoc 1997; 97:1157.
42. Burkitt DP, Walker ARP, Painter NS. Dietary fiber and disease. JAMA 1974; 229:1068.
43. Anderson JW, Chen W-J. Plant fiber: carbohydrate and lipid metabolism. Am J Clin Nutr 1979; 32:346.
44. Jenkins DJA, Wolever TMS, Leeds AR, et al. Dietary fibres, fibre analogues and glucose tolerance: importance of viscosity. BMJ 1978; 1:1392.
45. Munoz JM. Fiber and diabetes. Diabetes Care 1984; 7:297.
46. Jenkins DJ, Jenkins AL, Wolever TM, et al. Starchy foods and fiber: reduced rate of digestion and improved carbohydrate metabolism. Scand J Gastroenterol 1987; 129:132.
47. Madar Z, Thorne R. Dietary fiber. Prog Food Nutr Sci 1987; 11:153.
48. Kelsay JL. A review of research on effects of fiber intake on man. Am J Clin Nutr 1978; 31:142.
49. National Research Council. Diet and health: implications for reducing chronic disease risk. Washington, DC: National Academy Press, 1989.
50. Oddie TH, Boyd CM, Fisher DA, Hales IB. Incidence of signs and symptoms in thyroid disease. Med J Aust 1972; 2:981.
51. National Heart, Lung and Blood Institute, National Institute of Digestive, Diabetes and Kidney Diseases. Clinical guidelines on the identification, evaluation and treatment of overweight and obese adults. Obesity Res 1998; 6(Suppl 2):51S.
52. Van Itallie TJ. Obesity: adverse effects on health and longevity. Am J Clin Nutr 1979; 32:2723.
53. Aoki TT. Metabolic adaptations to starvation, semistarvation and carbohydrate restriction. In: Selvey N, White PL, eds. Nutrition in the 1980s: constraints on our knowledge. New York: Alan R Liss, 1981:161.
54. Drenick EJ, Swendseid MD, Blahd WH, Tuttle SG. Prolonged starvation as treatment for severe obesity. JAMA 1964; 187:100.
55. Drenick EJ, Smith R. Weight reduction by prolonged starvation. Postgrad Med 1964; 36:A-95.
56. Drenick EJ, Johnson D. Weight reduction by fasting and semistarvation in morbid obesity: long-term follow-up. Int J Obes 1978; 2:123.
57. Bistrian BR. Clinical uses of a protein-sparing modified fast. JAMA 1978; 240:2299.
58. Wadden TA, Stunkard AJ, Brownell KP. Very low calorie diets: their efficacy, safety and structure. Ann Intern Med 1983; 99:675.
59. Sours HE, Frattali VP, Brand CD, et al. Sudden death associated with very low calorie weight reduction regimes. Am J Clin Nutr 1981; 34:453.
60. Van Itallie TB, Yang M-U. Cardiac dysfunction in obese dieters: a potentially lethal complication of rapid, massive weight loss. Am J Clin Nutr 1984; 39:695.
61. National Task Force on the Prevention and Treatment of Obesity. Very low-calorie diets. JAMA 1993; 270:967.
62. American Medical Association Council on Food and Nutrition. A critique of low carbohydrate ketogenic weight reduction regimes: a review of "Dr. Atkins' Diet Revolution." JAMA 1973; 224:1415.
63. Fisher MC, Lachance PA. Nutrition evaluation of published weight reducing diets. J Am Diet Assoc 1985; 85:450.
64. American Medical Association, Council on Scientific Affairs. Treatment of obesity in adults. JAMA 1988; 260:2547.
65. Brownell KD, Wadden TA. Etiology and treatment of obesity: understanding a serious prevalent and refractory disorder. J Consult Clin Psychol 1992; 60:505.
66. Kayman S, Bruvold W, Stern JS. Maintenance and relapse after weight loss in women: behavioral aspects. Am J Clin Nutr 1990; 52:800.
67. Fajans SS. Current unsolved problems in diabetes management. Diabetes 1972; 21(Suppl 2):678.
68. American Dietetic Association. Nutrition recommendations and principles for people with diabetes mellitus. J Am Diet Assoc 1994; 94:504.
69. Bierman EL, Hamlin JT. The hyperlipemic effect of a low-fat, high-carbohydrate diet in diabetic subjects. Diabetes 1961; 10:432.
70. Brunzell JD, Lerner RL, Porte D, Bierman EL. Effect of a fat free, high carbohydrate diet on diabetic subjects with fasting hyperglycemia. Diabetes 1974; 23:138.
71. Riccardi G, Rivellesi A, Pacioni D, et al. Separate influence of dietary carbohydrate and fiber on the metabolic control in diabetes. Diabetologia 1984; 26:116.
72. Simpson HCR, Carter RD, Lousley S, Mann JI. Digestible carbohydrate: an independent effect on diabetic control in type 2 (non-insulin-dependent) diabetic patients? Diabetologia 1982; 23:235.
73. Jenkins DJA, Wolever TM, Taylor RH, et al. Glycemic index of foods: a physiological basis for carbohydrate exchange. Am J Clin Nutr 1981; 34:362.
74. Trowell HC. Dietary fiber hypothesis of the etiology of diabetes mellitus. Diabetes 1975; 24:762.

75. Jenkins DJA, Leeds AR, Wolever TMS, et al. Unabsorbable carbohydrates and diabetes: decreased post-prandial hyperglycemia. Lancet 1976; 2:172.
76. Jenkins DJA, Wolever TMS, Nineham R, et al. Guar crispbread in the diabetic diet. BMJ 1978; 2:1744.
77. Hall SEH, Bolton TM, Hetenyi G. The effect of bran on glucose kinetics and plasma insulin in non-insulin-dependent diabetes mellitus. Diabetes Care 1980; 3:520.
78. Villaume C, Beck B, Gariot P, et al. Long term evaluation of the effect of bran ingestion on meal-induced glucose and insulin responses in healthy man. Am J Clin Nutr 1984; 40:1023.
79. Kay RM, Grobin W, Track NS. Diets rich in natural fibre improve carbohydrate tolerance in maturity-onset non-insulin–dependent diabetics. Diabetologia 1981; 20:18.
80. Rivellese A, Giacco A, Genovese S, et al. Effect of dietary fibre on glucose control and serum lipoproteins in diabetic patients. Lancet 1980; 2:447.
81. Anderson JW, Ward K. High-carbohydrate, high-fiber diets for insulin-treated men with diabetes mellitus. Am J Clin Nutr 1979; 32:2312.
82. Simpson RW, Mann JI, Eaton J, et al. Improved glucose control in maturity-onset diabetes treated with high-carbohydrate-modified fat diet. BMJ 1979; 1:1753.
83. Simpson RW, Mann JI, Eaton J, et al. High carbohydrate diets and insulin-dependent diabetics. BMJ 1979; 2:523.
84. Franz MJ, Horton ES, Bantle JP. Nutrition principles for the management of diabetes and related complications. Diabetes Care 1995; 17:490.
85. Elia M. Home enteral nutrition: general aspects and a comparison between the United States and Britain. Nutrition 1994; 10:115.
86. Kalfarentzos F. Intraperitoneal nutrition. Nutrition 1994; 10:85.
87. Wolfson M. Use of intradialytic parenteral nutrition in hemodialysis patients. Am J Kidney Dis 1994; 23:856.
88. Wright J. Total parenteral nutrition and enteral nutrition in diabetes. Curr Opin Clin Nutr Metab Care 2000; 3:5.
89. Vanlandingham S, Simpson S, Daniel P, Newmark SR. Metabolic abnormalities in patients supported with enteral tube feeding. JPEN 1981; 5:322.
90. Ryan JA. Complications of total parenteral nutrition. In: Fischer JE, ed. Total parenteral nutrition. Boston: Little, Brown, 1976:55.
91. Michel L, Serrano A, Malt RA. Nutritional support of hospitalized patients. N Engl J Med 1981; 304:1147.
92. Greig PD, Baker JP, Jeejeebhoy KN. Metabolic effects of total parenteral nutrition. Annu Rev Nutr 1982; 2:179.

# CHAPTER 125

# APPETITE

ANGELICA LINDÉN HIRSCHBERG

*Appetite* is the sensation of hunger or desire for specific food. The behavioral response to this sensation is *food intake*, which eventually leads to *satiety*. Many factors are involved in the regulation of appetite, both on a meal-to-meal basis and longer term. The mechanisms consist of peripheral factors from the gastrointestinal tract that signal satiety when the stomach is full and hormones (secreted in proportion to body adipose tissue mass) that provide feedback information on body fat stores. These peripheral signals reach the brain and act on central effectors that either reduce food intake and promote weight loss or stimulate food intake and promote weight gain. The overall purpose of all appetite-regulating mechanisms is to adjust food intake so that caloric intake balances energy expenditure, with the result that body weight is maintained at a certain *setpoint*. The hypothalamus has a key function in the central mechanisms of appetite and body weight regulation.

## HYPOTHALAMIC CENTERS

In the early 1940s, it was demonstrated that bilateral lesions in the ventromedial hypothalamus (VMH) of animals caused hyperphagia and obesity (see Chaps. 8 and 9).[1] Some years later it was shown that lesions in the lateral hypothalamus (LH) resulted in aphagia and finally death.[2] These results led to the

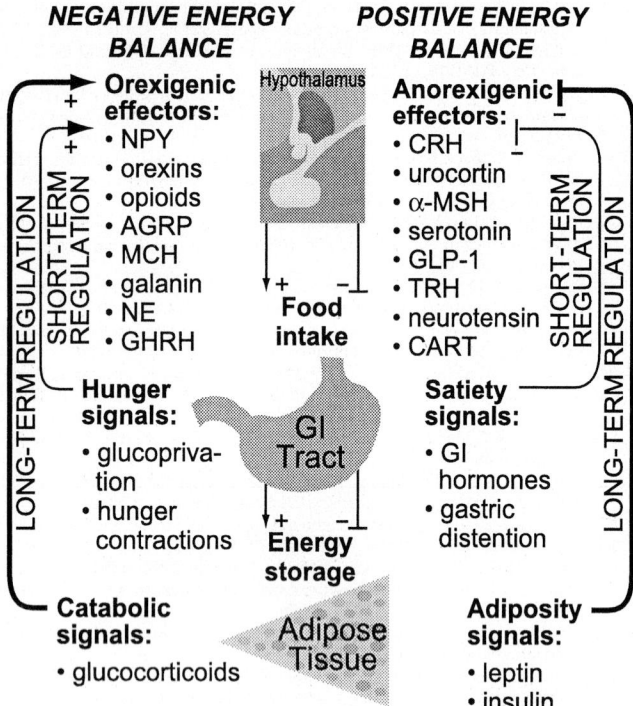

**FIGURE 125-1.** Schematic representation of the major mechanisms in the short-term and long-term regulation of appetite and energy homeostasis. *Short-term* mechanisms regulate appetite in connection with every meal. During conditions of *negative energy balance*, food intake is stimulated by glucoprivation and hunger contractions through promotion of orexigenic systems in the hypothalamus. In response to meal ingestion, satiety signals—including gastrointestinal hormones and gastric distention—are evoked. These signals are transmitted through vagal afferent fibers and through the blood to the brain, where they promote anorexigenic systems, leading to termination of a meal. *Long-term* mechanisms regulate food intake to achieve energy homeostasis. During conditions of *positive energy balance* and increased adipose mass, adiposity signals secreted in proportion to adipose tissue provide negative feedback to the brain and favor hypothalamic anorexigenic systems leading to decreased food intake and energy storage. On the other hand, in the presence of a low amount of body fat, increased secretion of glucocorticoids provides positive feedback to the brain, which favors central orexigenic systems, resulting in increased food intake and energy storage. ← indicates increased food intake and/or energy storage, whereas ⊥ indicates decreased food intake and/or energy storage. (*AGRP*, agouti-related peptide; *CART*, cocaine and amphetamine-regulated transcript; *CRH*, corticotropin-releasing hormone; *GHRH*, growth hormone–releasing hormone; *GI*, gastrointestinal; *GLP-1*, glucagon-like peptide-1; *MCH*, melanin-concentrating hormone; *α–MSH*, melanocyte-stimulating hormone; *NE*, norepinephrine; *NPY*, neuropeptide Y; *TRH*, thyrotropin-releasing hormone.)

simplified general concept of the LH as a "feeding center" and the VMH as a "satiety center."

During the 1990s, several new neurohumoral substances that regulate food intake were identified, and knowledge about how different transmitters, receptors, and cell systems in the hypothalamus interact has increased dramatically. The hypothalamus is the relay and integrator of afferent inputs, including somatic sensory signals (e.g., smell and taste), gastrointestinal signals (e.g., mechanical distention and gastrointestinal hormone release), circulating glucose and free fatty acids, and adiposity signals (e.g., hormones secreted in proportion to the amount of body fat) (Fig. 125-1). These signals influence hormones and neuropeptides within the hypothalamus that mediate appetite changes and moderate efferent pathways that control energy expenditure. It has become clear that many hypothalamic cell systems are involved in this process. In addition to VMH and LH, the arcuate nucleus (ARC), the paraventricular nucleus

(PVN), and the dorsomedial nucleus have been implicated in appetite and body-weight regulation.

## AFFERENT MECHANISMS IN THE CONTROL OF APPETITE

Different hypotheses have been advanced about the mechanisms involved and the signals that are sensed by the hypothalamus in the control of appetite. The *glucostatic hypothesis* proposes that a reduced availability of glucose in the hypothalamus stimulates food intake, whereas increased glucose utilization produces a sensation of satiety.[3] This hypothesis is supported by several studies that have established that the transient decline in blood glucose is a signal for meal initiation. The *lipostatic hypothesis* postulates that adipose tissue secretes a humoral signal—in proportion to the amount of body fat—that acts on the hypothalamus to decrease food intake and increase energy output.[4] The *thermostatic hypothesis* suggests that a fall in body temperature below a given setpoint stimulates appetite, and a rise above the setpoint inhibits appetite.[5] Food intake increases in cold weather and decreases in warm weather. There is, however, little evidence that body temperature is a major regulator of food intake. The *gut-peptide hypothesis* postulates that food in the gastrointestinal tract causes the release of satiety signals from the intestine that act on the hypothalamus to inhibit food intake.[6] Besides different physiologic factors, it is important to remember that food intake is a complex behavior. In humans, it is also influenced by cultural factors, environment, stress, mood, and past experiences related to the sight, smell, and taste of foods.

## SHORT-TERM REGULATION OF APPETITE

The mechanisms involved in the regulation of appetite during a meal (*short-term regulation*) differ from those acting over a longer period in the control of energy homeostasis (*long-term regulation*) (see Fig. 125-1). Short-term regulation of appetite serves to adjust food intake to the immediate need for nutrition. Hunger is elicited by the contractions of the empty stomach. A transient decline in blood glucose, as proposed by the glucostatic hypothesis, is also involved in short-term regulation of hunger and meal initiation. Satiety mechanisms involve gastrointestinal peptides that signal satiety and contribute to meal termination when released in response to food ingestion. These satiety factors support the gut peptide hypothesis. In addition, gastric distention produces satiety through activation of the vagal nerve.[7]

### SATIETY SIGNALS

Several gastrointestinal peptides (see Chap. 182) are considered as meal-related satiety signals (Table 125-1).

#### CHOLECYSTOKININ

Cholecystokinin (CCK) is the most studied gastrointestinal satiety factor. In the early 1970s, it was found that peripheral administration of the gut-brain peptide CCK caused a dose-dependent decrease in meal size in fasted rats.[8] Since then, several studies, including human studies, have confirmed the satiety effect of CCK, which may inhibit food intake via various mechanisms.[9]

In response to a meal, CCK is released from the intestine and reaches the stomach, where it activates vagal afferent fibers through CCK-A receptors. CCK may also influence food intake by the inhibition of gastric emptying. Activation of CCK-A receptors on the pylorus contracts the pyloric sphincter and produces gastric distention, which also activates vagal afferents. Meal-related information from the gut to the brain is

**TABLE 125-1.**
**Effects of Hormones and Neuropeptides on Appetite and Body Weight**

| Hormone | Appetite | Body Weight |
|---|---|---|
| **SATIETY SIGNALS** | | |
| CCK | ↓ Considered a physiologic satiety peptide in both animals and humans. | 0 Decreases meal size but increases the number of meals, thereby maintaining body weight. |
| Bombesin, gastrin-releasing peptide | ↓ Decrease food intake in both animals and humans by mechanisms involving vagal and splanchnic afferents. | ↓ |
| Somatostatin | ↓ Decreases food intake via a vagally dependent mechanism. | ↓ Decreased weight gain may be attributed to decreased food intake, reduced nutrient absorption, and increased metabolism. |
| Glucagon | ↓ Decreases food intake both in animals and humans. This mechanism seems to involve glucosensitive cells in the liver, as well as the vagal nerve. | ↓ Stimulates thermogenesis. |
| Amylin, calcitonin gene-related peptide | ↓ Decrease food intake by both peripheral and central mechanisms. | ↓ |
| Enterostatin | ↓ Decreases fat intake selectively. Uncertain role in humans. | ↓ Weight loss associated with increased corticosterone secretion and decreased insulin secretion. |
| **ADIPOSITY SIGNALS** | | |
| Leptin | ↓ Secreted from adipocytes in proportion to the amount of body fat and acts on the brain to decrease food intake. | ↓ Decreases adipose mass by increasing SNS activity. |
| Insulin | ↓ Decreases food intake in experimental animals when administered into the CNS at concentrations that do not produce hypoglycemia. | ↓ Decreases body weight to a greater extent than can be accounted for by decreased food intake; mechanism not yet elucidated. |
| **METABOLIC SIGNALS** | | |
| Glucocorticoids | ↑ Favor fat intake. | ↑ Increase the storage of abdominal fat by stimulating LPL activity in visceral adipose tissue. |
| Estrogen | ↓ Decreases food intake by central mechanisms involving increased activity of CRH and decreased activity of NPY. | ↓ Increases lipolysis. Promotes gluteofemoral fat distribution. |
| Progesterone | ↑ Increases food intake in the presence of estrogen. | ↑ Increases body weight in the presence of estrogen by a lipogenic action. |
| Testosterone | ↑ Increases food intake by mechanisms involving increased NPY activity. | ↑ Promotes weight gain by increasing lean body mass. |
| **OREXIGENIC EFFECTORS** | | |
| NPY | ↑ Favors carbohydrate intake. Interacts with β-endorphin and galanin. | ↑ Increases fat storage by reducing SNS activity and increasing white fat LPL activity. |
| Orexins A, B | ↑ Probably a physiologic role in stimulating appetite. | ? |
| Endogenous opioids, especially β-endorphin | ↑ Favor fat intake and highly palatable food. | ↓ Increase lipolysis. |
| Agouti-related peptide | ↑ Increases food intake by antagonist actions on melanocortin-4 receptors. | ↑ Obesity associated with hyperinsulinemia and hyperglycemia. |
| MCH | ↑ Uncertain physiologic role as appetite stimulator. | 0 |
| Galanin | ↑ Favors fat intake. The release of NE may mediate galanin-induced feeding. | 0 |
| NE | ↑ Increases carbohydrate intake specifically through α-2-receptors. | ↑ Reduces energy expenditure. |
| Growth hormone–releasing hormone | ↑ Favors protein intake. | ↑ |
| **ANOREXIGENIC EFFECTORS** | | |
| CRH, urocortin | ↓ CRH inhibits NPY-induced feeding. | ↓ CRH increases SNS activity. |
| α-MSH, α-melanocortin | ↓ Decreases food intake through melanocortin-4 receptors. Inhibits MCH-induced feeding. | ↓ Increases SNS activity. |
| Serotonin | ↓ Decreases carbohydrate intake selectively. Inhibits NPY release. | ↓ Decreased weight gain due to decreased food intake and metabolic effects. |
| Glucagon-like peptide-1 | ↓ Gut-brain peptide that reduces meal size only if given by intracerebral injection. Inhibits feeding induced by NPY and MCH. | ↓ Induces weight loss; mechanism not yet elucidated. |
| Thyrotropin-releasing hormone | ↓ | ↓ Increases energy expenditure. |
| Neurotensin | ↓ Inhibits feeding induced by NE and MCH. | |
| CART | ↓ May be one of the mediators of leptin action. Inhibits NPY-induced feeding. | ↓ Increases SNS activity. |

*CART*, cocaine and amphetamine-regulated transcript; *CCK*, cholecystokinin; *CNS*, central nervous system; *CRH*, corticotropin-releasing hormone; *LPL*, lipoprotein lipase; *MCH*, melanin-concentrating hormone; *α-MSH*, α-melanocyte-stimulating hormone; *NE*, norepinephrine; *NPY*, neuropeptide Y; *SNS*, sympathetic nervous system.

transmitted to the nucleus of the solitary tract in the brainstem, which is a primary sensory relay for taste and afferent signals from the gastrointestinal tract. Neuronal information then passes anteriorly to the parabrachial nucleus in the pons, which is connected with the hypothalamus. CCK peptides and receptors are found along the entire gut-brain pathway. There is evidence that peripheral CCK mechanisms via CCK-A receptors, as well as central CCK mechanisms via brain-type so-called CCK-B receptors, are involved in the regulation of food intake. The necessary neuronal circuitry for the satiety action of CCK is, however, contained within the lower brainstem, because CCK is also effective in reducing meal size in chronic decerebrate animals.[10]

There are substantial data to support CCK as an important endogenous meal-related appetite regulator, but CCK has limited or no influence on body weight. It has been shown that chronic administration of CCK consistently suppresses meal size in rats, but the animals compensate by increasing the number of meals, thereby maintaining body weight.[11]

## LONG-TERM REGULATION OF APPETITE AND ENERGY HOMEOSTASIS

Long-term regulation of appetite serves to compensate for temporary inadequacies in food intake and to control energy homeostasis (see Chap. 129) so that body weight is maintained at a certain setpoint. The mechanisms controlling energy homeostasis involve hormones secreted in proportion to the size of the body adipose tissue mass and the number of central nervous system (CNS) targets on which they act (see Fig. 125-1).

### ADIPOSITY SIGNALS

Leptin and insulin are both peripheral signals proportional to adiposity that act on the same brain mechanisms to decrease food intake and increase energy output. These adiposity signals provide support for the lipostatic hypothesis (see Table 125-1).

#### LEPTIN

The protein product of the obese (*ob*) gene has been cloned and a 167 amino-acid hormone produced in adipose tissue discovered.[12] This hormone, which acts on the hypothalamus to reduce food intake and increase energy expenditure, has been named *leptin*, from the Greek word for *thin*. Obese *ob/ob* mice have a mutation of the *ob* gene resulting in a lack of active leptin. Another type of obese and diabetic mice has a mutation of the diabetes (*db*) gene, which produces a defective leptin receptor.[13] This leads to a compensatory increase in *ob* gene expression and in plasma leptin levels. Consequently, leptin administration has no effect on *db/db* mice, whereas it reverses obesity in *ob/ob* mice. Weight loss is entirely due to loss of fat mass.

Leptin acts in the brain by binding to specific receptors, which have been found mainly in the ARC and the VMH—the region known as the satiety center.[14] Several central effectors of feeding are influenced by leptin. The highly potent appetite stimulator neuropeptide Y (NPY) is inhibited by leptin, whereas the anorectic agents corticotropin-releasing hormone (CRH), α-melanocyte-stimulating hormone, and cocaine and amphetamine-regulated transcript are stimulated by leptin (see Table 125-1).[14,15] Circulating leptin enters the brain via a saturable receptor-mediated transport process that is less efficient when plasma concentrations are elevated. In humans, leptin levels strongly correlate with the amount of body fat, and obese subjects have an approximately four-fold increase in leptin as compared with lean subjects.[16] These observations suggest resistance to endogenous leptin in obese humans by analogy with *db/db* mice. To date, however, no defects in the leptin receptor or in the coding region of the ob gene have been associated with

human obesity. It remains to be determined whether human obesity can be treated with leptin administration.

Insulin stimulates ob gene expression, and a simultaneous increase in leptin and insulin appears to be a common marker of obesity in humans. It has been suggested that endogenous insulin and leptin may be involved in a negative feedback circuit of energy homeostasis, acting as satiety signals on the CNS to reduce food intake and body weight during conditions of positive energy balance (see also Chap. 186).

### CATABOLIC SIGNALS

#### GLUCOCORTICOIDS

Glucocorticoids secreted by the adrenal cortex preferentially stimulate the intake of fat and increase the storage of abdominal fat (see Chaps. 72 and 73). Several mechanisms seem to be involved. Central effectors that stimulate food intake are potentiated by glucocorticoids, such as the activity of norepinephrine and NPY.[17] On the other hand, the activity of anorectic agents like insulin and leptin is inhibited.[18] Glucocorticoids also provide negative feedback on hypothalamic CRH secretion, as part of the hypothalamic–pituitary–adrenal (HPA) axis. Furthermore, the expression of the enzyme lipoprotein lipase (LPL) is increased by glucocorticoids, which promote storage of triglycerides in adipose tissue. The presence of glucocorticoid receptors has been demonstrated in visceral abdominal fat in humans, and through these receptors the expression of LPL increases.[19] Cortisol levels are inversely related to the amount of body fat in humans; thus, hypercortisolism is seen in anorectic patients and female athletes, whereas low cortisol levels are seen in obese people.[20,21] However, severely increased cortisol levels (as observed in Cushing disease) are associated with abdominal obesity and protein catabolism. Taken together, these findings suggest that endogenous glucocorticoids are involved in a feedback circuit of energy homeostasis that favors central anabolic pathways under conditions of negative energy balance. Sex steroids also play an important role in the regulation of appetite and energy metabolism, particularly during growth and reproduction (see Table 125-1).

## CENTRAL EFFECTORS IN THE CONTROL OF APPETITE AND ENERGY HOMEOSTASIS

The hypothalamus contains many hormones and neuropeptides that are targets for peripheral signals. Some of these central effectors stimulate appetite (orexigenic effectors), while others inhibit appetite (anorexigenic effectors). They are involved in a neural circuitry of orexigenic and anorexigenic networks that interact in a complex way in the control of appetite and energy homeostasis (see Table 125-1 and Fig. 125-1).

### OREXIGENIC EFFECTORS

#### NEUROPEPTIDE Y

The 33-amino-acid peptide NPY, which is the most potent stimulant of food intake known, is produced by cell bodies in the ARC with axons that project to the PVN (which is thought to be the main site of its action). Centrally administered NPY causes hyperphagia with a preference for carbohydrates and promotes increased fat storage and obesity by reducing the activity of the sympathetic nervous system and by increasing the expression of LPL in white adipose tissue.[22] Among several influences, there is evidence that the hypothalamic NPY system is negatively regulated by insulin, leptin, and CRH and positively regulated by glucocorticoids.[14,17,23,24] NPY activity is increased in conditions associated with energy deficiency, such as caloric restriction, lactation, and intense exer-

**TABLE 125-2.**
**Clinical Abnormalities of Appetite**

| DISEASE | APPETITE | BODY WEIGHT |
|---|---|---|
| Kleine-Levin syndrome | ↑ Hypersomnia, hyperphagia, hypersexuality; probably due to intermittent hypothalamic dysfunction. | ↑ |
| Prader-Willi syndrome | ↑ Autosomal dominant disorder characterized by hypotonia, hyperphagia, obesity, hypogonadism, mental retardation, and short stature. | ↑ Consequence of both an abnormal appetite and a tendency toward calorie conservation. |
| Malignancy-associated anorexia | ↓ Evidence for cytokine-induced satiety mechanisms. | ↓ The mechanism is multifactorial and may involve decreased appetite, increased basal metabolism, and malabsorption. |
| Anorexia nervosa | ↓ Associated with increased activity of satiety factors, such as CRH, serotonin, and CCK. | ↓ |
| Bulimia nervosa | ↑ Evidence for a role of serotonin and endogenous opioids. | 0 Patients are often of normal weight but may exhibit large weight fluctuations. |
| Obesity | ↑ A primary disturbance of the hypothalamic–pituitary–adrenal axis has been suggested. | ↑ The result of excess energy intake in relation to energy expenditure. Etiologies may be environmental, biologic, and genetic. |

*CCK*, cholecystokinin; *CRH*, corticotropin-releasing hormone.

cise. This response seems to be mediated by reduced negative feedback from insulin and leptin and positive feedback from glucocorticoids.

### OREXINS

A family of novel hypothalamic peptides called *orexins* have recently been discovered and characterized. The Greek word *orexis* means appetite, and intracerebroventricular administration of orexins is found to stimulate appetite in rats. The orexin genes are expressed in the LH, the region known as a feeding center.[25] The two peptides, orexin A (33 amino acids) and orexin B (28 amino acids) are derived from a common preproorexin precursor and bind to specific G-protein–coupled orexin receptors—termed OX-1R and OX-2R—within the CNS.[26] Like hypothalamic NPY mRNA, preproorexin mRNA levels increase with fasting. It is therefore possible that orexins play a physiologic role as mediators of central anabolic pathways in the regulation of energy balance.

### ANOREXIGENIC EFFECTORS

#### CORTICOTROPIN-RELEASING HORMONE AND UROCORTIN

CRH, a 41-amino-acid peptide produced in the PVN, is a potent anorectic substance when injected into the brain.[27] Furthermore, CRH augments energy expenditure by increasing sympathetic nervous system outflow. CRH production is positively regulated by CCK and leptin and negatively regulated by glucocorticoids.[14,28] Endogenous CRH is increased in response to starvation and exercise. Overproduction of CRH is also implicated in anorexia nervosa and in stress-related disorders.[29]

A new mammalian CRH-like peptide—urocortin—has been discovered. This 40-amino-acid peptide binds with high affinity to the CRH-2 receptor, which is abundant in hypothalamic areas that are of importance for appetite regulation. Central administration of urocortin produces appetite-suppressing effects that are even more potent than CRH.[30]

## CLINICAL ABNORMALITIES OF APPETITE

### KLEINE-LEVIN SYNDROME

The Kleine-Levin syndrome (see Chap. 128) is a rare disease comprising periodic hypersomnia, hyperphagia, and abnormal behavior frequently associated with sexual disinhibition (Table 125-2).[31] This syndrome classically occurs in an adolescent man in his early 20s and vanishes in his 30s. The etiology and pathogenesis of the disease are unknown, although intermittent hypothalamic dysfunction has been proposed. Endocrinologic analysis, which has been carried out on a few patients, has revealed abnormalities of the HPA axis, and growth hormone and prolactin secretion during the symptomatic phase that normalized in the asymptomatic phase.[32]

### PRADER-WILLI SYNDROME

The Prader-Willi syndrome is another rare syndrome characterized by congenital onset of hypotonia, childhood-onset hyperphagia and obesity, hypogonadism, mental retardation, and short stature (see Chap. 92) (see Table 125-2).[33] This syndrome, which is associated with a deletion of the paternal chromosome 15, may represent a defect in early hypothalamic development. The hyperphagia is characterized by continuous eating as long as food is available, suggesting deficient satiety mechanisms. However, postprandial secretion of CCK is not impaired in patients with Prader-Willi syndrome.[33] Furthermore, serum leptin levels and adipose tissue leptin mRNA have not been found to differ between children with Prader-Willi syndrome and obese nonsyndromal children.[34]

### MALIGNANCY-ASSOCIATED ANOREXIA

The etiology of malignancy-associated anorexia is multifactorial. It involves endocrine, metabolic, and immune changes induced by the tumor, and toxicity of the antitumor therapy. It is proposed that cytokines play a major role in this process (see Table 125-2). The mechanism seems to consist of cytokine-induced inhibition of hypothalamic NPY and stimulation of CRH.[35] Taste abnormalities may also be cytokine-mediated. However, weight loss in patients with cancer may result not only from anorexia, but also from malabsorption and increased basal metabolism. Progestogens such as megestrol acetate as well as glucocorticoids have been used to improve appetite and prevent weight loss in cachectic patients.

### EATING DISORDERS

Anorexia nervosa and bulimia nervosa are disorders of multiple etiologies (i.e., cultural, environmental, and biologic) (see Chap. 128). The disorders are associated with extensive abnormalities in hormones and neurotransmitters that usually resolve with normalization of body weight (see Table 125-2).[36] Consequently, while there is little support for the possibility that neuroendocrine abnormalities are of etiologic importance, they may serve to establish the disease.

The essential features of anorexia nervosa may be ascribed to hypothalamic dysfunction, including disturbances in appetite regulation, hypothyroidism, and amenorrhea. These patients also have activation of the HPA axis, as shown by increased concentrations of CRH in the cerebrospinal fluid and by basal hypercortisolism.[29] The anorectic agent CRH is released in response to food restriction and increased physical activity—two main features of anorexia nervosa. Furthermore, it is known that glucocorticoids have rewarding effects. Therefore, it has been suggested that self-starvation is rewarding and leads to a vicious cycle maintained by behavior and neurohumoral mechanisms. In addition, other satiety systems may be involved in the pathogenesis of anorexia nervosa. Low-weight patients have low levels of the serotonin metabolite 5-hydroxyindoleacetic acid in the cerebrospinal fluid, whereas long-term weight-recovered patients have greater than normal levels.[37]

It has been suggested that increased activity of the serotonin system might be a premorbid disturbance and a risk factor for the development of anorexia nervosa. There is evidence that bulimic patients also have abnormalities in serotonergic function, as supported by the effectiveness of serotonin reuptake blockers, such as fluoxetine, in reducing binge frequency.

Meal-related secretion of CCK is increased in anorectic patients, which is in agreement with increased satiety and delayed gastric emptying in these patients.[38] On the other hand, bulimic patients have an impaired meal-related secretion of CCK, which can be related to decreased satiety. The disturbed CCK secretion in eating disorders is normalized after recovery.

Some evidence also exists that the endogenous opioid system is involved in bulimia nervosa, because opioid antagonists have been shown to reduce experimentally induced binges in bulimic patients.[39] Leptin appears to have no specific role in eating disorders.

## OBESITY

There are several endocrine abnormalities found in obese patients (see Chap. 126).[40] Most altered endocrine functions—including hyperinsulinemia, increased levels of leptin,[41] and decreased secretion of growth hormone[42]—appear to be secondary to the obese state. However, abnormalities of the HPA axis have been suggested to be a primary cause of abdominal obesity (see Table 125-2). It has been demonstrated that a pathologic HPA axis—including decreased secretion of cortisol and flattening of the diurnal cortisol rhythm—is associated with abdominal obesity, hyperinsulinemia, hyperlipidemia, and hypertension (i.e., the metabolic syndrome [see Chap. 145]).[21] The development of this syndrome has been explained by a stress reaction that initially activates the HPA axis with increased cortisol secretion, which in turn promotes fat accumulation in visceral depots and increases intake and preference of fat. The activity of the HPA axis gradually deteriorates, leading to burnout of the feedback mechanisms. This deleterious response to stress seems to be genetically determined. From animal experiments, there is support for the concept that glucocorticoids may induce leptin resistance, thereby causing obesity.[18] Whether partial resistance to leptin in obese humans can be overcome by sufficient exogenous leptin therapy is not known. However, a weight-reducing drug will probably not solve the problem of obesity, because it has many causes and largely depends on environmental factors.

## REFERENCES

1. Brobeck JR, Tepperman J, Long CNH. Experimental hypothalamic hyperphagia in the albino rat. Yale J Biol Med 1943; 15:831.

2. Anand B, Brobeck J. Hypothalamic control of food intake in rats and cats. Yale J Biol Med 1951; 24:123.

3. Mayer J, Thomas D. Regulation of food intake and obesity. Science 1967; 156(773):328.

4. Kennedy G. The role of depot fat in the hypothalamic control of food intake in the rat. Proc R Soc Lond B Biol Sci 1953; 140:578.

5. Garland H. Altered temperature. In: Case RM, Waterhouse JM, eds. Human physiology: age, stress, and the environment, 2nd ed. Oxford: Oxford University Press, 1994.

6. Gibbs J, Smith GP. Satiety: the roles of peptides from the stomach and the intestine. Fed Proc 1986; 45:1391.

7. Robinson P, McHugh P, Moran T, Stephenson J. Gastric control of food intake. J Psychosom Res 1988; 32(6):593.

8. Gibbs J, Young R, Smith G. Cholecystokinin decreases food intake in rats. J Comp Physiol Psychol 1973; 84:488.

9. Lindén A. Role of cholecystokinin in feeding and lactation. Acta Physiol Scand 1989; 137(Suppl):585.

10. Seeley R, Grill H, Kaplan J. Neurological dissociation of gastrointestinal and metabolic contributions ot meal size control. Behav Neurosci 1994; 108(2):347.

11. West D, Fey D, Woods S. Cholecystokinin persistently suppresses meal size but not food intake in free-feeding rats. Am J Physiol 1984; 246: R776.

12. Zhang Y, Proenca R, Maffei M, et al. Positional cloning of the mouse obese gene and its human homologue. Nature 1994; 372:425.

13. Lee G, Proenca R, Montez J, et al. Abnormal splicing of the leptin receptor in diabetic mice. Nature 1996; 379:632.

14. Schwartz M, Seeley R, Campfield L, et al. Identification of targets of leptin action in rat hypothalamus. J Clin Invest 1996; 98:1101.

15. Cheung C, Clifton D, Steiner R. Proopiomelanocortin neurons are direct targets for leptin in the hypothalamus. Endocrinology 1997; 138(10):4489.

16. Considine R, Sinha M, Heiman M, et al. Serum immunoreactive-leptin concentrations in normal-weight and obese humans. N Engl J Med 1996; 334(5):292.

17. Larsen P, Jessop D, Chowdrey H, et al. Chronic administration of glucocorticoids directly upregulates prepro-neuropeptide Y and Y1-receptor mRNA levels in the arcuate nucleus of the rat. J Neuroendocrinol 1994; 6(2):153.

18. Zakrewska K, Cusin I, Sainsbury A, et al. Glucocorticoids as counterregulatory hormones of leptin: towards an understanding of leptin resistance. Diabetes 1997; 46:717.

19. Rebuffé-Scrive M, Brönnegård M, Nilsson A, et al. Steroid hormone receptors in human adipose tissues. J Clin Endocrinol Metab 1990; 71:1215.

20. Lindén Hirschberg A, Lindholm C, Carlström K, von Schoultz B. Reduced serum cholecystokinin response to food intake in female athletes. Metabolism 1994; 43:217.

21. Rosmond R, Dallman M, Björntorp P. Stress-related cortisol secretion in men: relationships with abdominal obesity and endocrine, metabolic and hemodynamic abnormalities. J Clin Endocrinol Metab 1998; 83:1853.

22. Stanley B, Kyrkouli S, Lampert S, Leibowitz S. Neuropeptide Y chronically injected into the hypothalamus: a powerful neurochemical inducer of hyperphagia and obesity. Peptides 1986; 7(6):1189.

23. Schwartz M, Figlewicz D, Baskin D, et al. Insulin in the brain: a hormonal regulator of energy balance. Endocr Rev 1992; 13(3):387.

24. Heinrichs S, Menzaghi F, Merlo Pich E, et al. Corticotrophin releasing factor in the paraventricular nucleus modulates feeding induced by neuropeptide Y. Brain Res 1993; 611:18.

25. De Lecea L, Kilduff T, Peyron C, et al. The hypocritins: hypothalamic-specific peptide with neuroexcitatory activity. Proc Natl Acad Sci U S A 1998; 95:322.

26. Sakurai T, Amemiya A, Ishii M, et al. Orexins and orexin receptors: a family of hypothalamic neuropeptides and G protein-coupled receptors that regulate feeding behavior. Cell 1998; 92:573.

27. Morley J, Levine J. Corticotrophin releasing factor, grooming and ingestive behavior. Life Sci 1982; 31(14):1459.

28. Kamilaris T, Johnson E, Calogero A, et al. Cholecystokinin-octapeptide stimulates hypothalamic-pituitary-adrenal function in rats: role of corticotrophin-releasing hormone. Endocrinology 1992; 130:1764.

29. Hotta M, Shibasaki T, Masuda A, et al. The response of plasma adrenocorticotropin and cortisol to corticotrophin-releasing hormone (CRH) and cerebrospinal fluid immunoreactive CRH in anorexia nervosa patients. J Clin Endocrinol Metab 1986; 62:319.

30. Spina M, Merlo-Pich E, Chan R, et al. Appetite-suppressing effects of urocortin, a CRF-related neuropeptide. Science 1996; 273:1561.

31. Critchley M. Periodic hypersomnia and megaphagia in adolescent males. Brain 1962; 85:628.

32. Fernandez J, Lara I, Gila L, et al. Disturbed hypothalamic-pituitary axis in idiopathic recurring hypersomnia. Acta Neurol Scand 1990; 82(6):361.

33. Holland A, Treasure J, Coskeran P, et al. Measurement of excessive appetite and metabolic changes in Prader-Willi syndrome. Int J Obes 1993; 17:527.

34. Lindgren A, Marcus C, Skwirut C, et al. Increased leptin messenger RNA and serum leptin levels in children with Prader-Willi syndrome and non-syndromal obesity. Pediatr Res 1997; 42(5):593.

35. Plata-Salamán C. Anorexia during acute and chronic disease. Nutrition 1996; 12:69.

36. Lindén Hirschberg A. Hormonal regulation of appetite and food intake. Ann Med 1998; 30:7.

37. Jimerson D, Lesem M, Kaye W, et al. Eating disorders and depression: is there a serotonin connection? Biol Psychiatry 1990; 28(5):443.

38. Geraioti T Jr, Kling M, Joseph-Vanderpool J, et al. Meal-related cholecystokinin secretion in eating and affective disorders. Psychopharmacol Bull 1989; 25(3):444.

39. Mitchell J, Laine D, Morley J, Levine A. Naloxone but not CCK-8 may attenuate binge-eating behavior in patients with the bulimia syndrome. Biol Psychiatry 1986; 21:1399.
40. Bioletto S, Golay A, Munger R, et al. Acute hyperinsulinemia and very-low-density and low-density lipoprotein subfractions in obese subjects. Am J Clin Nutr 2000; 71:443.
41. Ahima RS, Flier JS. Leptin. Annu Rev Physiol 2000; 62:413.
42. Kamel A, Norgren S, Elimam A, et al. Effects of growth hormone treatment in obese prepubertal boys. J Clin Endocrinol Metab 2000; 85:1412.

# CHAPTER 126

# OBESITY

JULES HIRSCH, LESTER B. SALANS, AND LOUIS J. ARONNE

Obesity continues to be a major clinical problem throughout the world. Treatment remains difficult and often unsuccessful; however, refinements in methods for measuring energy metabolism in humans and a rapid increase in the application of molecular genetics to human metabolism have combined to clarify a number of aspects of the pathogenesis of obesity. An exclusively psychosocial approach to the etiology of obesity is no longer tenable, as previous theories of pathogenesis have been enriched by new cellular and metabolic considerations.[1] The new findings hold promise for better methods of treatment and prevention. This chapter is a selective review of past and recent findings of particular relevance to endocrinology.

## PREVALENCE OF OBESITY

An expert panel assembled by the National Institutes of Health (NIH) stated, "An estimated 97 million adults in the United States are overweight or obese, a condition that substantially raises their risk of morbidity from hypertension, dyslipidemia, type 2 diabetes, coronary heart disease, stroke, gallbladder disease, osteoarthritis, sleep apnea and respiratory problems, and endometrial, breast, prostate, and colon cancers. Higher body weights are also associated with increases in all-cause mortality. Obese individuals may also experience social stigmatization and discrimination. As the second leading cause of preventable death in the United States today, overweight and obesity pose a major public health challenge."[2] This high prevalence of obesity was affirmed at an NIH-sponsored Technology Assessment Conference, at which conferees noted, "33% to 40% of adult women and 20% to 24% of men are currently trying to lose weight."[3]

## DEFINITION AND COMPLICATIONS OF OBESITY

### DETERMINATION OF OBESITY

Obesity is an excess of body fat (adipose tissue), and ideally the diagnosis should be based on the direct demonstration of an excess amount of fat. Many sophisticated laboratory procedures have been applied to the direct measurement of body fat content in humans and experimental animals. These include underwater weighing to determine body density; compartmental analysis by measurement of the in vivo dilution of isotopes, such as tritiated or deuterated water[4]; and the determination of cytoplasmic mass from the number of naturally occurring isotopes, such as potassium-40, as counted in a total body liquid-

scintillation apparatus.[5] These methods are based on assumptions and equations that are not always valid across the spectrum of body weight. Newer techniques such as dual x-ray absorptiometry (DEXA) and computed tomography (CT) or magnetic resonance imaging (MRI) scanning are more accurate. The DEXA method passes two very low energy x-ray beams through a supine subject. The beams are differentially attenuated by lean body mass, body fat, and bone mineral density. Measurement of regional body fat distribution is most reliably determined by imaging the abdomen with CT or MRI, which can distinguish subcutaneous from visceral fat. For maximum accuracy, serial scans can be performed, but often, a single cut in the L4–L5 region is used. *Total body electrical conductivity* (TOBEC) is a method of evaluating fat content through changes in electromagnetic fields. Like the other methods, it is expensive, but involves no radiation and, thus, may be useful for evaluating children. *Bioelectrical impedance* is a less expensive method for assessing body composition, but measures are a complex function of electrolyte and water content, and are not accurate without careful standardization. Simpler measures, such as the determination of skinfold thickness (see Chap. 7) are appealing but are highly dependent on technique and require a number of assumptions to estimate body fat.

No matter which method is used, body fat is a continuous variable, skewed to the more obese side of the distribution, with no clear bimodality that would enable the separation of a clearly obese group from the remaining normal population.

Body weight is the most widely used estimator of body fatness. Individuals can shrink or enlarge fat stores by a factor of 10 or more with starvation or with the development of obesity. During such changes, lean body mass changes as well, but to a much smaller degree. Thus, weight is to some degree a valid measure of fatness. However, estimates are made more accurate by a consideration of height.

A simple mathematical manipulation of ordinary height and weight data obtained without shoes and clothing is now generally used. The body mass index (BMI), (weight in kilograms)/(height in meters)$^2$, or (weight in pounds × 703)/(height in inches)$^2$ tends to be constant for individuals of a given degree of leanness or fatness within wide ranges of heights. Thus, a change in the weight/height$^2$ ratio is useful as a measure of fatness, independent of height. Since BMI, like weight, is a continuous variable skewed to the right, there is no a priori method for ascertaining where obesity begins. Hence, impact of the accumulation of excess fat on health must be reviewed to determine at what point its pathologic effects begin.

## HAZARDS OF OBESITY

Data accumulated over many years by the National Center for Health Statistics, referred to as the National Health and Nutrition Examination Survey (NHANES), have been used to estimate the risks of excess body fat. The second survey, NHANES II, conducted from 1976 to 1980, examined ~20,000 people in a carefully selected sample. NHANES II analyzed the evidence of adverse consequences to health of various degrees of overweight. A modest, even conservative, definition of obesity, roughly corresponding to weights 20% or more in excess of desirable, showed definite and sizable adverse consequences for health. Thus, those ≥20% overweight who were 20 to 44 years of age had a 5.6-fold greater likelihood of hypertension (blood pressure >160/95), a 2.1-fold greater likelihood of hypercholesterolemia (>250 mg/dL), and a 3.8-fold greater likelihood of diabetes than the non-overweight sample. Admittedly, it is an arbitrary judgment, but at this stage of understanding, the Expert Panel on the Identification, Evaluation and Treatment of Overweight and Obesity in Adults convened by the NIH, in concordance with the World Health Organization, defines *overweight* as a BMI between 25 and 29.9 and *obesity* as a BMI >30.[2] While return to a BMI in the normal range is probably optimal for an individual losing weight, evidence suggests that weight loss of a lesser degree, in some cases as little as 10% to 20% of total body weight, may suffice to lessen the morbidity associated with diabetes[6] and hypertension.[7] It has been suggested that this finding is due to a disproportionate loss of visceral fat with small amounts of weight loss. Thus, in any evaluation of the hazards of obesity, the *distribution of adipose tissue* can be an important consideration in addition to the BMI.

## DISTRIBUTION OF FAT

An abdominal or "potbelly" distribution in either sex must elicit more concern than fat in other distributions. *Central distribution of adipose tissue*, characterized by an increase in the ratio of the waist to hip (W/H) circumference, or in the abdominal sagittal diameter, has been associated with an increased risk of medical complications, including angina pectoris, stroke, and type 2 diabetes.[8–10] As a result, it has been suggested that waist circumference should be part of the evaluation of the overweight and obese individual. Between a BMI of 25 and 35, a waist circumference >102 cm (40 inches) in men and 88 cm (35 inches) in women represents a significant and probably independent risk to health (Table 126-1). The possible reasons for this unusual association of regional adiposity with diabetes, hypertension, and plasma lipoproteins are dealt with in the Obesity and Diabetes Mellitus section.

The list of health hazards of obesity unfortunately is not restricted to those risk factors already enumerated but also includes hiatal hernia, gastroesophageal reflux, pickwickian syndrome, and gout. The specific contribution of obesity to coronary artery disease and to reduction in longevity has been more difficult to demonstrate because it is mediated via its impact on other risk factors such as dyslipidemia, type 2 diabetes, and hypertension, but is now clear enough for the American Heart Association to have declared obesity a "major, modifiable risk factor" for coronary artery disease. Finally, the obvious adverse psychosocial consequences of obesity in society are by no means trivial.

## PATHOGENESIS

### THERMODYNAMIC CONSIDERATIONS

It has become customary to remind all who deal with obesity that it is a disease of energy storage and as such must obey the laws of thermodynamics. The first law mandates that the amount of energy in any system cannot vary unless the inflow or egress of energy from the system becomes unequal. In mathematical terms, $\Delta E = Q - W$. For our purposes this formula translates into the following: Any change in adipose tissue mass (E) cannot come about unless there is a change of Q (food intake) or W (caloric expenditure).

A brief perspective on the history of thermodynamics may be relevant.[11] Engineers, mechanics, and scientists before the nineteenth century earnestly labored to develop a perpetual motion machine. In fact, the history of science is strewn with the wrecks of plans and models for such machines. The second law of thermodynamics, enunciated in the nineteenth century, ordained that entropy rises with the operation of these machines, and, thus, the machines must stop unless more energy is supplied; however, this did not curtail efforts to create engines that might subdue entropy. The history of obesity research and the first law of thermodynamics are similar.[12] At the end of the eighteenth century, Lavoisier had shown that respiration and oxidation are not different from combustion. There is no vital heat production in living organisms, different from the production of heat by the burning of fuels in ovens or bonfires. Nevertheless, the search for ways to extract more energy from ingested food or burn away more energy than can be

**TABLE 126-1.**

**Classification of Overweight and Obesity by Body Mass Index, Waist Circumference, and Associated Disease Risk\***

| | BMI (kg/m²) | Obesity Class | Disease Risk* (Relative to Normal Weight and Waist Circumference) | |
|---|---|---|---|---|
| Men | | | ≤40 in. (≤102 cm) | >40 in. (>102 cm) |
| Women | | | ≤35 in. (≤88 cm) | >35 in. (>88 cm) |
| Under-weight | <18.5 | | | — |
| Normal† | 18.5–24.9 | | — | — |
| Over-weight | 25.0–29.9 | | Increased | High |
| Obesity | 30.0–34.9 | I | High | Very high |
| | 35.0–39.9 | II | Very high | Very high |
| Extreme obesity | ≥40 | III | Extremely high | Extremely high |

*BMI*, body mass index.
\*Disease risk for type 2 diabetes mellitus, hypertension, and cardiovascular disease.
†Increased waist circumference can also be a marker for increased risk, even in persons of normal weight.
(Adapted from World Health Organization. Preventing and managing the global epidemic of obesity. Report of the World Health Organization Consultation of Obesity. Geneva: WHO, June 1997.)

explained by simple chemical considerations remains active. Periodically, new diets allege to "burn away fat" or to enable one to "eat all you want without weight gain."

Consider for a moment the formula, $\Delta E = Q - W$. It should be evident that, over long periods of time, $\Delta E = 0$. This means that weight is generally stable whether one is obese or lean. With weight stability, however, passage of calories through the system is high; during an average lifetime one can expect that >50 million calories will come in as Q and disappear as W. Hence, very small alterations in the system can make for great obesity or remarkable leanness. The most interesting phenomenon from the standpoint of energy storage is the reason why Q and W are so often precisely equal. Most clinicians have chosen to focus on the possibility that some individuals eat a lot and remain thin whereas others eat very little yet become obese. These observations that appear to violate thermodynamic principles have carried the name *endogenous* obesity. Other observers have focused on the fact that obese individuals are driven by remarkable psychological or hedonic drives and supposedly do this in secret. This would be considered *exogenous* obesity.

Classic studies nearly 70 years ago demonstrated clearly that all individuals, obese or not, respond to diets in lawful ways.[13] One might have hoped that bizarre notions about diets and obesity would have vanished. However, perusals of studies of nutrition and obesity done in recent years still level accusing fingers at either the sedentary nature of our lives or our propensity to overeat as though in some way these two behaviors can become completely disarticulated from each other. To be sure, the presence of obesity means that at some point $\Delta E$ rose above 0. It is not often realized, however, that such changes in $\Delta E$ must have been quite small since the acquisition of obesity is measured in months or, more frequently, many years. *The extra bites of food eaten each day or the slight diminutions in physical activity that create obesity have been difficult to measure.* When precise measures of total 24-hour energy expenditure were made in obese and nonobese individuals in a hospital setting, utilizing various techniques for measuring energy expenditure, it was found that differences between the obese and nonobese, when expressed per kilogram fat-free mass, were small.[14] For example, the obese expended 51 ± 7 kcal/kg fat-free mass, as compared to 47 ± 7 kcal/kg fat-free mass in the nonobese. Since these studies were done in a circumstance in which weight was kept stable by giving a sufficient amount of food intake to maintain stability, clearly Q = W; therefore, the food intake of the obese is only very slightly larger than that of the nonobese and is matched by the slight increase in energy expenditure. This increased caloric exchange of the obese may well be the necessary additional energy required for carrying a larger fat mass or the need for more cardiopulmonary activity than in the lean.

The previous data do not speak to any deficiency of caloric expenditure in the obese. One theory, which has been prominent since early in this century, is that all individuals have "luxus konsumption," which permits them to overeat and burn more calories in response to overeating, as a control against becoming obese. The fault of obesity was believed by some to be found in an inability to exercise this special control mechanism with precision. Extrapolating from brown adipose tissue, which in some animals and in the premature human infant create nonshivering thermogenesis by excess caloric burning, it has been thought that the obese experience a dysfunction of brown adipose tissue or a deficiency in amount. Yet, the data clearly show no deficiency in energy production in the obese, but rather a slight increase.

Since the obese usually maintain obese weight at a constant level, energy outgo equals intake and, thus, the data do not implicate a sedentary nature of the obese as the cause of this unfortunate state. What may, however, be observed is a high intake of calories in the obese, when they have dieted and lost weight and are "breaking away" from the diet and regaining. Such hyperphagia can easily be misinterpreted as a natural state of hyperphagia in the obese. The more usual slight differences in food intake of the obese required to maintain the additional caloric needs of their obesity do not suggest that they have unusual hedonic or psychological needs that have to be met by large amounts of food intake.

With precise measures of energy homeostasis, the effect of artificial increases in body weight of 10% above "usual" or 10% below showed unanticipated changes in caloric expenditure.[14] The increase in caloric expenditure with weight increase is disproportionately high for the small accompanying changes in lean body mass. A reverse situation is the decline in caloric need per unit of lean body mass when weight is lowered 10%. The most likely explanation for these findings is that usual body weight is arrived at by a complex of forces, which detect body fatness and equalize the rate of energy expenditure and food intake. When alterations are made in weight by increasing or decreasing the level of fat storage, the same homeostatic mechanisms act to restore body fat to its previous state. When $\Delta E = 0$, however, there is a reduction in caloric expenditure (and intake) when weight is lowered and an increase in caloric expenditure (and intake) when weight is elevated.

The previous energy changes with weight change are largely in nonresting energy expenditure. There are smaller changes in the thermic effect of food and resting metabolic rate when weight declines. These changes in the efficiency of caloric expenditure as weight is changed may be due to alterations in metabolism, substituting oxidative for glycolytic metabolism, or as yet unknown mechanisms whereby muscle metabolism can vary in the efficiency of caloric disposal. Whatever the mechanism, it has become clear that there is a complex system maintaining constant body weight, which functions well in the obese but at a higher level of fat storage than in the nonobese. After obese or nonobese is changed from "usual" weight, Q and W must change coordinately if $\Delta E$ remains 0. This can be considered as a setpoint mechanism, which maintains the lean at their "set" and the obese at a higher set. Efforts to change body weight are resisted by the system.

Thus, *no laws of thermodynamics are contravened in human obesity*. However, the system involved in the maintenance of a constant level of energy (fat) storage in adults is complex. How the system adjusts during growth and development and how the

adult "set" may be altered by events in infancy, childhood, or even adolescence remain important topics for investigation.

## OPERATION OF THE SYSTEM MAINTAINING ENERGY STORAGE

The above description of energy metabolism in humans implicates the existence of a coordinated and complex mechanism controlling body fat. There is no reason to believe that a system of such great importance (i.e., the storage of energy for the prevention of starvation) would be any less complex than systems for the control of other physiologic variables such as body sodium, osmotic pressure, or blood pressure.[15] Short-term regulators involve cognitive functions as well as gastrointestinal signals. Endocrine signals, signals from adipose tissue, and possibly signals from the liver are involved in both short- and long-term controls of fat storage in adipose tissue. The hypothalamus is considered the central signal-processing center with afferents from the above and efferents, which utilize the endocrine and autonomic nervous systems for control of both energy intake and outgo.

An interesting aspect of this system is the relative ease with which it can be bypassed in the short run by the overeating of particularly attractive foods, by starvation imposed by illness, or by impeded access to food. It is generally observed that overriding of the system in the short term is readjusted over time to the original level of fat storage by operation of the central control center. It is also worth noting that the complexity of the system makes it likely that there are redundant loops so that the administration of a novel diet or a new drug for the treatment of obesity may affect one loop and be effective in the short run, but is often overridden in time by operation of other loops.

### HYPOTHALAMIC OBESITY

Damage to the ventromedial hypothalamus has been shown to produce obesity in experimental animals. Hypothalamic injury is a rare cause of human obesity, but it can occur, after surgical removal of craniopharyngiomas or other tumors impinging upon the hypothalamus. In this event there is a marked increase in appetite and the rapid accession of fat along with hyperinsulinemia, similar to what is found in the experimental production of ventromedial lesions in animals. More subtle hypothalamic injuries may also produce obesity. In experimental animals it has been shown that canine distemper virus can infect the central nervous system early in life and, with little residual evidence of neural damage, produce obesity at a later age. Whether viral infections can produce obesity in humans remains uncertain.

### HORMONAL OBESITY

Other chapters in this textbook describe the effects of growth hormone, thyroid hormone, and adrenal steroids on general metabolism and fat storage, and it must be remembered that these are rare causes of obesity. The central obesity of hyperadrenocorticism, with striae, hypertension, acne, and hirsutism, produces a recognizable syndrome of obesity. Subtle changes in the "set" for fat storage independent of specific endocrine abnormalities are more usual causes for obesity than any antecedent hormonal change.

### DRUGS

A number of drugs can produce a weight increase. Most notable are some antidepressants. Other drugs that may lead to weight gain include progestational agents, cyproheptadine, and valproate.

### GENETIC OBESITY

For many years it has been recognized that a number of Mendelian disorders are associated with marked obesity. The most commonly considered are the *Prader-Willi* and the *Bardet-Biedl syndromes*. The former is related to a deletion of 15q 11.2q-12 in the father of affected individuals or to uniparental disomy for maternal chromosome, and separate cases of the latter have been linked with markers on chromosomes 3, 11, and 15. There are many uncertainties as to precisely how these chromosomal aberrations lead to obesity. The small nuclear ribonucleoprotein-associated polypeptide N (SNRPN) gene has been implicated in the Prader-Willi syndrome. Clinical descriptions of other Mendelian disorders with obesity are numerous; one review listed no fewer than 24.[1]

It has become clear that "ordinary" human obesity occurring in the absence of known endocrine states or specific syndromes also shows a high degree of heritability. Furthermore, precise molecular lesions have been found in experimental rodent obesities that have been studied for many years by traditional physiologic and biochemical techniques.[16] Genes responsible for rodent genetic obesities and their protein products are:

**Yellow Obesity.** Yellow obesity occurs in the yellow mouse as the result of a dominant mutation in the agouti locus on mouse chromosome 2 that leads to widespread expression of a protein known as the *agouti signaling protein*. The relevant site in humans is 20q13, although examples of this obesity in humans have not been described.

**Ob.** The ob mouse has been studied for many years, but it was not until recently that the nature of a specific recessive mutation on mouse chromosome 6 was found. A peptide termed *leptin* cannot be elaborated or secreted from adipose tissue. It is believed that leptin is sensed in the central nervous system to modulate the complex mechanism for the control of body fat. The homologous site for this gene in humans is 7q31.3. Although a few families have been found with leptin deficiency, most obese humans have a large increase in plasma leptin levels (proportionate to body fat storage) rather than a deficiency of leptin (see Chap. 186).

**Db.** In this animal there are abnormalities of the central leptin receptor, leading to obesity. The genetic lesion is found on mouse chromosome 4. The locus for the production of leptin receptor in humans is 1p21–p31. Whether leptin receptor abnormalities are present in humans remains uncertain. Lesions downstream to the receptor may also be a factor in human obesity. Leptin detected by the leptin receptor affects the JAK/STAT system. Neuropeptide Y figures prominently in this pathway and is a current focus of research (see Chap. 125).

**Zucker Rat.** The Zucker obese rat has a leptin-receptor lesion on chromosome 5 similar to that of the db mouse.

**Tubby.** The tubby mouse obesity (tub) leads to maturity-onset obesity. It is due to a recessive mutation found on chromosome 7. The mechanism of action of the gene product remains uncertain.

**Fat.** This is due to a recessive mutation on mouse chromosome 8 with a related site on human 4q32. It is due to a mutation in the carboxypeptidase E gene. A similar abnormality of prohormone convertase in humans has been described. An inability to cleave large prohormones leads to hyperproinsulinemia, associated with obesity. The obesity may be related to the inability to cleave prohormones other than insulin.

Each of the above genetic abnormalities in mice has been important in enriching the study of the control mechanisms for fat storage. As of this time, it appears unlikely that single mutations, as found in mice, will be frequent causes for human obesity. However, genomic scans in families with obesity or in special subgroups of obese individuals are uncovering molecular lesions that may be related to obesity. A linkage of obesity to a peroxisome proliferator-activated receptor (PPARγ) gene has been uncovered[17]; likewise, the possibility that uncoupling proteins (UCPs) may be related to obesity is under active study.[18] It was originally thought that these proteins existed only in brown adipose tissue and were of importance only for thermoregulation during hibernation and infancy. Currently, UCPs found in white adipose tissue and muscle are being evaluated.

Thus, genetic studies have been more revealing for uncovering the details of the mechanisms controlling fat storage than in discovering major causes for human obesity. It is likely that human obesity comes about by virtue of early life adjustment of the "set" for fat storage, which involves many genes. Given the complex nature of the system responsible for the "set," there is abundant opportunity for early environmental influences to fashion lifelong changes in fat storage.

# ADIPOSE TISSUE GROWTH AND DEVELOPMENT

## EARLY GROWTH OF ADIPOSE TISSUE

Normal growth of human adipose tissue is achieved through an increase in adipocyte size and number. Histologic studies, as well as studies of adipocyte development in tissue culture, strongly suggest that the precursor cell, or adipoblast, is a cell that is indistinguishable from the fibroblast. The replication of preadipocytes and their differentiation into mature adipocytes have been shown to be affected by epidermal growth factor, insulin, glucocorticoids, and PPARγ.[19] This gene encodes two proteins, PPARγ1 and PPARγ2. The latter is found in adipose tissue and is believed to play a role in adipocyte differentiation. Adipose cells first appear at approximately the 15th week of human gestation, continue to appear in large numbers until approximately 23 weeks of gestation, and then appear more slowly throughout the remainder of gestation. During the first 2 years of life, adipose tissue mass grows by an increase in both cell size and number. Cell number rises slowly from 2 years of age until close to the onset of puberty, and during adolescence, there is another sharp elevation in cell number that accounts for a second spurt in the growth of the adipose tissue mass. Thereafter, the size of adipose tissue of nonobese adults maintaining constant body weight remains stable, as do adipose cell size and number. The size of adipose cells within nonobese individuals can differ considerably from one fat depot to another. In a large group of nonobese healthy subjects, cell size in six separate fat depots ranged from 0.14 to 0.68 μg of lipid per cell, with a mean size of 0.41 μg lipid per cell.[20] The average total cell number in this nonobese population was $30 \times 10^9$.

## ADIPOSE CELL NUMBER AND SIZE

Modest changes in fat cell size occur with small changes in body weight. Greater expansion of the adipose tissue can be achieved either by an alteration in adipose cell size (*hypertrophic, normal cell-number obesity*) or in both adipose cell number and size (*hyperplastic-hypertrophic obesity*). Hyperplastic obesity in humans usually has its onset in early life, often before the age of 20 years. Obesity of later onset usually is accompanied by adipose cellular enlargement and normal cell number, but there is evidence that adult rodents can, under some circumstances, markedly increase their cell number. When adult body weight exceeds 170% of ideal, a maximum cell size (1.0–1.2 μg lipid per cell) is reached, after which cell number and obesity are highly correlated.[21]

Both the age of onset and severity of obesity appear to contribute to adipose hyperplasia. Although hypercellularity most often is found in those with early-onset obesity, patients have been observed with increased cell number in whom obesity apparently developed during adult life. These individuals usually are massively obese.

Weight loss and reduction in the adipose tissue mass of all adult obese patients and of obese children, regardless of the age of onset or the degree and duration of obesity, are accompanied by a change in adipose cell size alone. Cell number remains constant, even in the face of dramatic weight loss. Thus, adipose hypercellularity appears to inflict a permanent, irreversible abnormality on the patient suffering from hyperplastic obesity.

It has been hypothesized for nearly 30 years that fat-cell size and number may play a role in the control of human energy metabolism. The study of substances secreted by adipocytes has led to the addition of a new chapter in this textbook on the endocrine adipocyte (see Chap. 186). The contributions of fat-cell size and number to the newly discussed endocrine functions of adipose tissue are yet to be elucidated.

# ENDOCRINE AND METABOLIC CONSEQUENCES OF OBESITY

Various alterations in endocrine and metabolic function can be observed in obese individuals, including disturbances of growth hormone, changes of thyroid function, adrenal hormone metabolism, and insulin secretion and insulin action and alterations in lipid metabolism that may lead to hyperlipidemia. These are thought to be secondary to, rather than a primary characteristic of, obesity.

## OBESITY AND GROWTH HORMONE

Growth hormone secretion in response to hypoglycemia or arginine is decreased in obese compared with lean patients, but weight reduction restores normal responses and plasma levels.

## OBESITY AND THYROID FUNCTION

Thyroid function is normal in most obese patients, but subtle changes in thyroid hormone metabolism may occur. Plasma triiodothyronine ($T_3$) levels are increased and reverse triiodothyronine levels ($rT_3$) are decreased in many obese patients, whereas plasma thyroxine ($T_4$) and thyroid-stimulating hormone levels are normal (see Chap. 33). The plasma $T_3$ and $rT_3$ changes are reversed by weight loss and $T_3$ may even become subnormal although thyroid-stimulating hormone (TSH) remains normal. Hypothyroidism is rarely a cause of obesity, but it should be considered in the differential diagnosis. The obesity caused by hypothyroidism usually is mild, and restoration of euthyroidism eliminates the problem.

## OBESITY AND ADRENAL FUNCTION

Cortisol secretion rates are increased in obesity, but normal plasma cortisol concentration, normal diurnal variation in secretion, and normal response to dexamethasone suppression distinguish obesity-associated alterations in adrenal function from Cushing syndrome (see Chap. 75). Total 24-hour urinary 17-hydroxycorticosteroids generally are increased in obese patients but are normal when expressed per kilogram of body weight. Twenty-four–hour urinary 17-ketosteroids may be normal or slightly increased in obesity. Weight reduction normalizes the cortisol secretion rate and 24-hour urinary 17-hydroxysteroid and 17-ketosteroid levels, indicating that these changes are secondary to obesity. However, hyperadrenocorticism (Cushing syndrome) can cause obesity; thus, it always should be considered and ruled out in an obese person (see Chap. 74). When Cushing syndrome is the cause of obesity, it tends to be mild and completely reversible after definitive treatment.

## OBESITY AND SEX HORMONES

The onset of menarche is earlier in obese than in nonobese girls, and obese women often suffer from a variety of menstrual cycle abnormalities, including hypermenorrhea, oligomenorrhea, amen-

orrhea, irregular or anovulatory cycles, infertility, and premature menopause. Obesity is often associated with polycystic ovarian disease, hyperandrogenism, and hirsutism (see Chaps. 96 and 101). Although the mechanism of these disorders in obese women is unknown, the disorders could be secondary to alterations in hypothalamic-pituitary function, to abnormalities in the synthesis or secretion of estrogens or androgens from the ovaries or adrenals, or to alterations in the metabolism of sex steroids by non–steroid-producing peripheral tissues. Elevation of plasma luteinizing hormone, reduction of plasma follicle-stimulating hormone, and increased luteinizing hormone/follicle-stimulating hormone ratios have been reported in some obese women. Elevated circulating levels of estrogens and androgens also have been reported in some obese women. These hormones may be of either ovarian or adrenal origin. Alterations in sex steroid metabolism, specifically increased conversion of androstenedione of adrenal origin to estrone and its metabolites by non–steroid-producing peripheral tissues, also may play a role in some of the menstrual cycle abnormalities and in the increase in prevalence of breast cancer in obese women.[22] Conversely, an increased conversion of estrogen to androgen, which has been postulated to occur, may be a factor in creating hirsutism or abnormal menstruation. Most of these changes are reversible by weight loss.

In men with severe obesity, both serum total and free testosterone levels may be mildly decreased. Increased conversion of androgens to estrogens may result in increased serum estrogen levels. Usually, libido and potency remain normal.

Amenorrhea of hypothalamic origin, such as is found in starvation, occurs frequently in obese women who lose a great deal of weight. This is often accompanied by low $T_3$ levels, leukopenia, and cold sensitivity. This may persist for long periods of time after weight loss and cannot be safely repaired by hormone therapy.

## OBESITY AND DIABETES MELLITUS

Obesity is a major risk factor for type 2 diabetes. On average, >70% of type 2 diabetics studied in various populations throughout the world are obese, with prevalence variation dependent upon the population studied.

The alarming increase in the worldwide prevalence of type 2 diabetes, especially in recently industrialized developing countries, in minority groups, and in children, appears, in large part, to be attributable to overnutrition and overweight. Other lifestyle factors—such as decreased physical activity and a general increase in longevity—all contribute to the emergence of type 2 diabetes as a serious worldwide medical and public health problem.

### INTERACTION OF GENES AND ENVIRONMENT

For obesity to induce overt type 2 diabetes in a given individual, a genetic susceptibility must exist. Multiple genes are likely to be involved including those inducing insulin resistance and defective pancreatic B-cell function. It is upon this genetic background that obesity produces its "diabetogenic" effect.

### ADIPOSE TISSUE AND INSULIN RESISTANCE

There is a close relationship between increased adipose-cell size, and insulin resistance or plasma insulin levels in both rodents and humans.[23] The relationship is stronger than that between total body fat mass and either insulin resistance or plasma insulin levels. With weight loss and reduction in fat-cell size, insulin sensitivity usually improves, and there is almost always a decline in plasma insulin levels. The mechanism by which an enlarged adipocyte causes insulin resistance, increases plasma insulin levels, and impairs glucose metabolism is not known. Several factors are postulated to contribute. For example, release of increased amounts of free fatty acids (FFA) from enlarged, insulin-resistant adipocytes results in increased plasma FFA levels, and flux of FFA to peripheral tissues, the liver, and pancreatic B cells. Increased oxidation of FFA decreases insulin-stimulated glucose uptake into skeletal muscle due to inhibition of glucose transport.[24] This adds to already existing insulin resistance in type 2 diabetes and can precipitate hyperglycemia. Decreased insulin action caused by increased FFA oxidation leads to an even greater rate of lipolysis in adipose tissue and further elevation of plasma FFA levels, creating a vicious cycle. In addition, increased flux of FFA to the liver increases hepatic gluconeogenesis and hepatic glucose output, adding to the already existing abnormalities in hepatic glucose metabolism in type 2 diabetes.[25] Elevated levels of FFA also stimulate insulin secretion, placing a further burden on genetically compromised and stressed B-cell function in individuals susceptible to type 2 diabetes. Furthermore, elevated FFAs have been reported to impair early insulin secretion, a characteristic B-cell abnormality in type 2 diabetes.[26]

Other factors associated with the enlarged adipose depot of the obese have been postulated to contribute to the link between obesity and diabetes. Release of increased amounts of the peptide leptin from the expanded adipose depot may play some role. Plasma leptin levels are elevated in most obese patients, and an inverse relationship between plasma leptin levels and insulin sensitivity has been reported.[27] Studies in laboratory animals and humans, however, report conflicting data.[28] In both db/db and ob/ob mice, roughly equivalent degrees of carbohydrate intolerance can develop in the presence of obesity, but in the former, plasma leptin levels are increased while in the latter they are reduced. In obese humans, plasma leptin levels are almost always elevated, whether diabetes is present or not; thus, a role for plasma leptin in the obesity-diabetes connection remains to be established. The enlarged adipose depot also produces increased amounts of tumor necrosis factor-α (TNF-α), which has been shown to impair insulin action and is postulated to play a role in the link between obesity and diabetes.[29]

### ROLE OF BODY-FAT DISTRIBUTION

The "diabetogenic" effects of obesity depend not only on an increased total body adipose tissue mass or fat-cell size, but also on the distribution of the excess fat. Excessive accumulation of abdominal fat (*central obesity, android* or *"apple shape"* body type) is associated with a much greater likelihood of diabetes and other metabolic derangements than equal amounts of fat in the gluteal-femoral region (*peripheral obesity, gynoid* or *"pear shape"* body type).[9] Increased values of the W/H ratios are associated with increased plasma insulin levels, decreased glucose disposal, increased hepatic glucose output, glucose intolerance, dyslipidemias, especially hypertriglyceridemia, increased small dense low-density lipoprotein (LDL) cholesterol particles, decreased high-density lipoprotein (HDL), atherosclerosis, hypertension, and type 2 diabetes.[8] It is postulated that the delivery to the liver of high levels of FFA from the enlarged, lipolytically active visceral adipose mass causes hepatic insulin resistance and hepatic triglyceride and very low-density lipoprotein (VLDL) overproduction; increased FFA delivery to the B cell causes hyperinsulinemia, secondarily leading to peripheral insulin resistance.

Insulin resistance, whether due to increased rates of FFA oxidation, hyperleptinemia, excess TNF-α, or other factors, provokes increased insulin secretion to overcome impaired insulin action and to maintain normal blood glucose levels. Chronic hyperinsulinemia leads to down-regulation of insulin receptors, further worsening insulin resistance. Chronic exposure to excess insulin levels is thought to be a major factor in the development of the metabolic syndrome described below.

### OVERNUTRITION, EXCESSIVE CALORIC INTAKE, AND DECREASED PHYSICAL ACTIVITY

Increased adiposity alone may not fully account for the "diabetogenic" effect of obesity. Chronic overeating—stimulating insulin secretion from defective pancreatic B cells in individuals who are genetically susceptible to type 2 diabetes—could produce hyperinsulinemia, which down-regulates insulin receptors, thereby contributing to insulin resistance. Chronic demand for increased insulin secretion from genetically defective B cells may lead to B-cell decompensation. Hyperinsulinemia triggers counterregulatory glucagon, catecholamine, and growth hormone responses known to be hyperglycemic. For these reasons, caloric restriction alone, independent of weight loss, significantly improves glycemic control. Decreased physical activity, characteristic of sedentary lifestyles in economically developed and "modernized" societies, is also thought to play an important role in the link between diabetes and obesity.

### OTHER POTENTIAL "DIABETOGENIC" EFFECTS OF OBESITY

Hypothalamic controls mediated by the activity of various neuropeptides, hormones, and the autonomic nervous system, acting in concert to maintain a given level of adipose tissue and normal blood glucose concentration, may be deranged and may contribute to the relationship of obesity to diabetes.[15] Adipose tissue *UCP*—reported to play an important role in regulating energy homeostasis and, therefore, in intermediary carbohydrate and lipid metabolism—has been implicated in the coexistence of obesity and diabetes.[18] It should be noted that activation of PPARγ by the thiazolidinedione class of drugs increases insulin sensitivity and decreases insulin resistance in type 2 diabetics. Finally, membrane glycoprotein PC-1 is expressed in tissues with insulin resistance, and PC-1 expression in skeletal muscle and adipose tissue has been reported to correlate inversely with insulin sensitivity.[30]

### METABOLIC SYNDROME

Abdominal obesity is associated not only with an increased risk of type 2 diabetes, but also with a number of other disorders with serious medical consequences, including atherosclerosis, dyslipidemia (most commonly hypertriglyceridemia, decreased HDL, increased small dense LDL, and increased FFA), increased plasminogen activator inhibitor and fibrinogen levels, hypertension, and vascular smooth muscle cell proliferation. This complex of disorders has been variously referred to as *syndrome X, Reaven syndrome, metabolic syndrome,* or the *New World syndrome*. This combination of disorders poses a major public health problem (see Chap. 145).

### CONTROL OF OVERNUTRITION AND OBESITY

It seems highly likely that avoidance of overnutrition, overweight, or obesity, or successful long-term weight reduction in obese individuals, will significantly reduce the incidence and prevalence of type 2 diabetes and associated disorders. Indeed, a diet and/or exercise intervention in a population with impaired glucose tolerance (IGT) has been found to decrease significantly the incidence of type 2 diabetes over a 6-year period.[31]

### OBESITY AND LIPIDS

Obesity is typically associated with hypertriglyceridemia, decreased HDL cholesterol, and, to a lesser extent, hypercholesterolemia, abnormalities considered to be important risk factors for coronary heart disease (see Chaps. 162 and 163). Elevation of plasma triglycerides very likely arises from increased influx of nutrient substrate (glucose, glycerol, FFA) into the liver of obese patients and the consequent production of triglyceride-rich VLDL at a rate greater than that of peripheral tissue utilization. Weight reduction often restores plasma triglycerides to normal or near-normal levels.

There is an inverse relationship between HDL cholesterol and BMI in obese patients, especially if they also are diabetic.

Low HDL, which constitutes a risk for atherosclerosis, is also negatively correlated with high W/H ratios. After weight loss, plasma HDL levels transiently decrease and then usually rise above pre–weight-reduction levels.

The relationship between obesity and hypercholesterolemia is less clear-cut than is the relationship between obesity and hypertriglyceridemia and HDL. Total body cholesterol synthesis and plasma cholesterol levels increase with increasing body weight, but in general, there is a poor correlation between weight loss and reduction in total or LDL plasma cholesterol.

# TREATMENT OF OBESITY

## WEIGHT-REDUCTION MEASURES

In most obese individuals, specific aberrations of the weight-control mechanism described under Pathogenesis cannot be identified and, thus, treatment must be nonspecific. Short-term weight loss often can be achieved, but obese patients tend to regain their lost weight: Only ~20% of obese patients maintain their weight loss over a 5- to 15-year period after initial treatment.[32] Greater success is likely to be achieved through programs that lead to permanent changes both in eating habits and in physical activity. Achievement of this goal requires new approaches that extend beyond the confines of traditional medical settings, involving not only the physician but also various nonphysician resources in the community.

It is important to remember that obesity is a medical as well as a cosmetic problem. Treatment should be considered for all with a BMI in excess of 27 or with lesser degrees of obesity in those with associated disorders, such as type 2 diabetes, hyperlipidemia, cardiovascular disease, hypertension, gout, pulmonary disease, and severe osteoarthritis.

Management of type 2 diabetes associated with obesity requires not only aggressive control of blood glucose with pharmacologic agents, but also healthy nutrition, weight reduction, and exercise. Weight loss in overweight, obese individuals with type 2 diabetes (even if only partially successful) is imperative in the treatment of type 2 diabetes. As little as 5% weight loss has been shown to improve blood glucose and lipid levels in overweight and obese type 2 diabetics.

### DIETARY THERAPY

The cornerstone of treatment is dietary therapy (see Chap. 124). Weight loss depends on caloric deficit, and caloric deficit depends on the total number, not the kind, of calories consumed relative to calories expended. Many different types of calorie-restricted diets have been advanced for the treatment of obesity, some of which are in the form of liquid formulas, and others that use bizarre combinations of foods or nutrients based on unfounded theories that may be hazardous. *None of these fad diets offers advantages over a calorie-restricted diet of normal foods that is balanced to provide the conventional distribution of carbohydrate (45–50% of total calories), fat (35% of calories), and protein (15% of calories).* Low-carbohydrate, high-fat, ketogenic diets and diets very high in protein cannot be recommended for long-term treatment of obesity. The more rapid initial weight loss induced by some fad diets during the first few weeks of treatment is secondary to a loss of sodium, water, and body protein rather than fat, and after the first 2 or 3 weeks, the rate of weight loss may be disappointing. Furthermore, these diets can be associated with serious health hazards.[33] Finally, *the ingestion of unbalanced diets does nothing to modify eating habits or to develop healthy long-term nutritional practices, which are essential for successful long-term management of obesity.*

The extent to which calories should be restricted in a given patient depends on the degree of obesity and the age, sex, physical activity, and general health of the patient. A loss of ~2 pounds per week is a reasonable goal in most patients and can usually be accomplished by a daily deficit of ~1000 kcal. If the obesity is associated with severe, debilitating, or life-threatening disease, such as the pickwickian syndrome, severe congestive heart failure, or severe hyperglycemia, a more drastic reduction in calorie intake may be indicated.

### EXERCISE

Daily exercise is an important adjunct to caloric restriction in achieving and maintaining reduced weight. However, exercise is not an effective means of inducing weight loss unless combined with the reduction of caloric intake. When combined with a hypocaloric diet, a daily exercise program, carefully planned and tailored to the patient's physical condition and ability, is important for long-term weight reduction. However, a sudden increase in physical activity in obese patients or a strenuous exercise program is hazardous and contraindicated. Exercise should begin gradually in the form of a low-level aerobic activity such as walking, swimming, or cycling. After normal or near-normal body weight is achieved, the degree of physical activity can be increased, depending on the patient's physical condition (see Chap. 132).

### LIFESTYLE CHANGES

Successful long-term outcome of the treatment of obesity requires that an individual change or modify attitudes, beliefs, and behavior with respect to eating and physical activity. Although unusual dietary excesses and sedentary behavior may or may not be "causes" for obesity (see Thermodynamic Considerations, above), there is no way to combat obesity other than by increasing physical activity and diminishing caloric intake. These efforts may be opposed by hormonal and neural mechanisms; yet, a lifelong effort to combat any adverse feelings that may be associated with weight loss is essential. Therefore, a program of formal behavioral modification may be helpful. A behavioral modification program individualized to the person's needs and abilities, combined with a program of diet and exercise, can be advantageous. A wide variety of groups, such as Weight Watchers, TOPS, and Overeaters Anonymous, are available throughout the United States. A useful manual for the evaluation of treatment programs, entitled "Weighing the Options," was published by the National Academy Press for the Institute of Medicine.[34] Even the best of these programs has not been uniformly successful in achieving the long-term goal of maintaining reduced weight. Thus, an NIH Technology Assessment Panel concluded that, "For most weight loss methods, there are few scientific studies evaluating their effectiveness and safety. The available studies indicate that persons lose weight while participating in such programs, but after completing the program, tend to regain the weight over time."[3]

### WEIGHT CYCLING

A number of investigators have examined the possibility that repeated bouts of weight loss and regain, termed *cycling*, may have deleterious consequences on energy metabolism and perhaps on the morbidity of obesity. In one study,[35] it was found that rats subjected to cycling regained their lost weight more easily than did controls. However, careful review of the animal literature on this subject and the few relevant human experiments do not support this contention.[36,37]

Although there is continued concern about the relationship of weight variability to mortality in some epidemiologic studies,[38] there is no reason to restrain a person's effort to lose weight, with its known attendant benefits, for alleged lesser, long-term hazards, for which there is no known pathogenesis and which have not been conclusively demonstrated.

### DRUG THERAPY

Drug therapy in the treatment of obesity is of limited utility. Drugs are ineffective as the sole approach to the treatment of obesity, and it is unclear whether the modest benefits of adding drugs to caloric restriction, exercise, and behavioral modification outweigh their cost and untoward effects.

Although some evidence suggests that medication can increase the weight loss achieved by caloric restriction, prolong weight maintenance, and decrease comorbidity in at least a portion of patients treated for years,[39] larger, long-term studies must be performed before medication can be recommended as a primary treatment.

After reviewing the available evidence, the Expert Panel on the Identification, Evaluation, and Treatment of Overweight and Obesity issued the following recommendation about the drug treatment of obesity in its report:

"Weight loss drugs approved by the FDA [Food and Drug Administration] may only be used as part of a comprehensive weight loss program, including dietary therapy and physical activity, for patients with a BMI of ≥30 with no concomitant obesity-related risk factors or diseases, and for patients with a BMI of ≥27 with concomitant obesity-related risk factors or diseases. Weight loss drugs should never be used without concomitant lifestyle modifications. Continual assessment of drug therapy for efficacy and safety is necessary. If the drug is efficacious in helping the patient lose and/or maintain weight loss and there are no serious adverse effects, it can be continued. If not, it should be discontinued."[2]

Two medications have been approved for long-term use by the FDA: sibutramine (Meridia), a norepinephrine and serotonin reuptake inhibitor that enhances satiety,[40] and orlistat (Xenical), an inhibitor of pancreatic lipase.[41]

Thyroid hormone, diuretics, and digitalis should be used in the treatment of obesity only when specific indications exist (e.g., hypothyroidism, edema, hypertension, or congestive heart failure), and never for the achievement of weight reduction. Diabetes and hypertension occurring in obesity should be treated aggressively. Human chorionic gonadotropin and growth hormone have no place in the treatment of obesity.

### SURGICAL TECHNIQUES

Surgical techniques, such as the vertical-banded gastroplasty and Roux en Y gastric bypass, have been used for the treatment of morbid obesity.[42] An NIH Consensus Conference on Gastrointestinal Surgery for Severe Obesity had evaluated the need for this treatment.[43] Surgery was only recommended for cooperative patients who have been at least twice their ideal body weight for at least 5 years, have failed all other treatment modalities, have no psychiatric, alcohol, or drug abuse problems, and have no medical contraindications to surgery. Substantial improvement in comorbid conditions has been reported; however, short- and long-term complications of surgery are common, and the risk/benefit ratio must be carefully examined for each patient. Referral of suitable patients to a medical center specializing in this type of procedure is recommended. Of note, laparoscopic techniques to accomplish stomach restriction are under investigation. However, their safety and efficacy await evaluation.

## CONCLUSION

The treatment of obesity is unsatisfactory and frequently unsuccessful. Nevertheless, the evidence is overwhelming that obesity is a significant risk factor for many illnesses. The physician and the obese patient must recognize that nothing short of a change in lifestyle (nutritional change, increase in physical activity, diminution of stressful life situations, etc.) is needed for treatment. No pill, formula, or unusual dietary manipulation is available to provide certain success. It may not be possible to correct all of the obesity; however, even *some* weight loss may ameliorate concurrent diabetes, hypertension, or other complicating diseases. The recent rapid growth of biomedical

science and increasing attention to the understanding of the basics of energy metabolism may eventually provide further insights and better therapies for this unfortunate situation.

## REFERENCES

1. Bray GA, Bouchard C, James WP. Handbook of obesity. New York: Marcel Dekker Inc, 1995.
2. Clinical guidelines on the identification, evaluation, and treatment of overweight and obesity in adults—the evidence report. Obes Res 1998; 6(Suppl 2):51S.
3. NIH Technology Assessment Conference Panel. Methods for voluntary weight loss and control. Ann Intern Med 1993; 119:764.
4. Brozek J, Henschel A, eds. Techniques for measuring body composition: proceedings of a conference, Quartermaster Research and Engineering Center, January 22–23, 1959. Washington, DC: National Academy of Sciences–National Research Council, 1961.
5. Anonymous. Proceedings of a panel on the clinical uses of whole-body counting, Vienna, June 28–July 2, 1965. Vienna: International Atomic Energy Agency, 1966.
6. Wing RR, Marcus MD, Epstein LH, et al. Long-term effects of modest weight loss in type II diabetic patients. Arch Intern Med 1987; 147:1749.
7. Eliahou HE, Iana A, Gaon T. Body weight reduction necessary to attain normotension in the overweight hypertensive patient. Int J Obese 1981; 5(Suppl 1):157.
8. Kalkhoff RK, Hartz AH, Rupley D, et al. Relationship of body fat distribution to blood pressure, carbohydrate tolerance and plasma lipids in healthy obese women. J Lab Clin Med 1983; 102:61.
9. Björntorp P. Regional obesity. In: Björntorp P, Brodoff B, eds. Obesity. Philadelphia: JB Lippincott Co, 1992; 579–586.
10. Pouliot MC, Despres JP, Lemieux S, et al. Waist circumference and abdominal sagittal diameter: best simple anthropometric indexes of abdominal visceral adipose tissue accumulation and related cardiovascular risk in men and women. Am J Cardiol 1994; 73(7):460.
11. Van Baeyer HC. Maxwell's dream. New York: Random House Inc, 1998.
12. Kleiber M. The fire of life: an introduction to animal energetics. New York: Robert E Krieger Publishing Co, 1975.
13. Newburgh LH, Johnston MW. Endogenous obesity—a misconception. Ann Intern Med 1993; 3:815.
14. Leibel RL, Rosenbaum M, Hirsch J. Changes in energy expenditure resulting from altered body weight. N Engl J Med 1995; 332:621.
15. Rosenbaum M, Leibel RL, Hirsch J. Obesity. Medical progress. N Engl J Med 1997; 337:396.
16. Hirsch J, Leibel RL. The genetics of obesity. Hosp Pract 1998; 33(3):55.
17. Ristow M, Muller-Wieland D, Pfeffer A, et al. Obesity associated with a mutation in a genetic regulator of adipocyte differentiation. N Engl J Med 1998; 339:953.
18. Ricquier D, Fleury C, LaRose M, et al. Contributions of studies on uncoupling proteins to research on metabolic disease. J Intern Med 1999; 245:637.
19. Freake HC. A genetic mutation in PPARγ is associated with enhanced fat cell differentiation: implications for human obesity. Nutr Rev 1999; 1:154.
20. Salans LB, Cushman SW, Weismann RE. Studies of human adipose tissue: adipose cell size and number in nonobese and obese patients. J Clin Invest 1973; 52:929.
21. Hirsch J, Batchelor BR. Adipose tissue cellularity in human obesity. Clin Endocrinol Metab 1976; 5(2):299.
22. Nimrod A, Ryan KJ. Aromatization of androgens by human abdominal and breast fat tissue. J Clin Endocrinol Metab 1975; 40:367.
23. Salans LB, Knittle JL, Hirsch J. Obesity, glucose intolerance and diabetes mellitus. In: Ellenberg M, Rifkin H, eds. Diabetes mellitus: theory and practice. New York: Medical Examination Publishing, 1983:469.
24. Boden G. Role of fatty acids in the pathogenesis of insulin resistance and NIDDM. Diabetes 1990; 39:226.
25. Rebrin K, Steil GM, Getty L, Bergman RN. Free fatty acids as a link in the regulation of hepatic glucose output by peripheral insulin. Diabetes 1995; 44:1038.
26. Paolissa G, Gambardeira A, Amato L, et al. Effect of long-term fatty acid infusion on insulin secretion in healthy subjects. Diabetologia 1995; 38:1295.
27. Segal KR, Landt M, Klein S. Relationship between insulin sensitivity and plasma leptin concentration in lean and obese man. Diabetes 1996; 45:988.
28. Auwerx J, Staels B. Leptin. Lancet 1998; 351:737.
29. Hotamisligil GS, Spiegelman BM. Tumor necrosis factor, as key component in the obesity–diabetes link. Diabetes 1994; 43:1271.
30. Frittitta L, Youngren JF, Sbraccia P, et al. Increased adipose tissue PC-1 protein content, but not tumor necrosis factor-gene expression, is associated with a reduction of both whole body insulin sensitivity and insulin receptor tyrosine–kinase activity. Diabetologia 1997; 40:282.
31. Pan XR, Li GW, Hu YH, et al. Effects of diet and exercise in preventing NIDDM in people with impaired glucose tolerance: the Da Qing IGT and Diabetes Study. Diabetes Care 1997; 20:537.
32. Drenick E. The prognosis of conventional treatment in severe obesity. In: Björntorp P, Cairella M, Howard A, eds. Recent advances in obesity research III. London: John Libbey, 1981:80.
33. National Task Force on the Prevention and Treatment of Obesity. Very low calorie diets. JAMA 1993; 270:967.

34. Thomas PR. Weighing the options—criteria for evaluating weight management programs. Washington, DC: National Academy Press, 1995.

35. Brownell KD, Greenwood MRC, Stellar E, Shrager EC. The effects of repeated cycles of weight loss and regain in rats. Physiol Behav 1986; 38:459.

36. Reed GW, Hill JO. Weight cycling: a critical review of the animal literature. Obes Res 1993; 1:392.

37. Wing RR. Weight cycling in humans: a critical review of the literature. Ann Behav Med 1992; 14:113.

38. Lissner L, Odell PA, D'Agostino RB, et al. Variability of body weight and health outcomes in the Framingham population. N Engl J Med 1991; 324:1839

39. Weintraub M. Long-term weight control: the National Heart, Lung, and Blood Institute funded multimodal intervention study. Clin Pharmacol Ther 1992; 51:581.

40. Fanghanel G, Cortinas L, Sanchez-Reyes L, Berber A. A Clinical trial of the use of sibotramine for the treatment of patients suffering essential obesity. Int J Obes Related Metab Disord 2000; 24:144.

41. Heymsfield SB, Segal KR, Hauptman J, et al. Effects of weight loss with orlistat on glucose tolerance and progression to type 2 diabetes in obese adults. Arch Intern Med 2000; 160:1321.

42. Balsiger BM, Murr MM, Poggio JL, Sarr MG. Bariatric surgery. Surgery for weight control in patients with morbid obesity. Med Clin North Am 2000; 84:477.

43. Gastrointestinal surgery for severe obesity: Proceedings of an NIH Consensus Development Conference, March 25–27, 1991. Am J Clin Nutr 1992; 55(Suppl 2):615S.

# CHAPTER 127

# STARVATION

RUTH S. MACDONALD AND ROBERT J. SMITH

Protein-energy malnutrition is a major public health problem in many parts of the world. Severe protein-energy malnutrition is characterized by cessation of growth in children, body wasting, mental apathy, and loss of pigmentation of the hair and skin.[1] When both dietary energy sources and protein are deficient, the syndrome called *marasmus* develops, characterized by generalized emaciation, an absence of subcutaneous fat, muscle wasting, and wrinkled and dry skin (Fig. 127-1, *left*). A severe deficiency of protein, with either low or adequate energy intake, causes the syndrome called *kwashiorkor*, characterized by emaciated limbs as evidence of a loss of lean body mass but a swollen abdomen sec-

ondary to edema and hepatomegaly[2] (see Fig. 127-1, *right*). Features of marasmus and kwashiorkor often occur simultaneously or at different times in one person. Both conditions are associated with reduced resistance to disease and infection, and with diminished capacity for recovery from concurrent illnesses.[1,3,4]

Periods of partial or total starvation and resulting malnutrition often occur during the course of catabolic illnesses or after injury. During starvation in otherwise normal persons, there is a coordinated adaptive response within different tissues such that nutrient stores (glycogen, triglycerides, and protein) are used efficiently. These metabolic changes occur in response to alterations in nutrient availability and in the levels of several hormones. In treating patients with both malnutrition and an additional illness, it is important to understand these normal nutrient and hormonal control mechanisms and the possible alterations in the normal adaptive responses.

## METABOLIC RESPONSE TO STARVATION

The metabolic adaptation to starvation can be divided into four temporal phases: the *postabsorptive period* (5–6 hours after a meal), *early starvation* (1–7 days), *intermediate starvation* (1–3 weeks), and *prolonged starvation* (more than 3 weeks). During the first three phases, a series of metabolic changes occurs progressively, until a more stable, near steady state is reached during prolonged starvation.[5]

Metabolic fuel use and production by liver, muscle, adipose tissue, kidney, and brain during the four phases of starvation are summarized in Table 127-1. During the postabsorptive period and early in starvation, glucose is readily available from hepatic stores of glycogen and is consumed as a principal fuel by the brain, muscle, kidney, and other tissues. As hepatic glycogen stores become depleted during the first 24 hours of fasting, plasma levels of glucose decrease modestly, gluconeogenesis becomes a progressively more important source of glucose, and alternative substrates begin to replace glucose as a metabolic

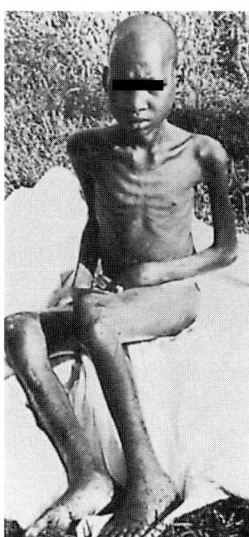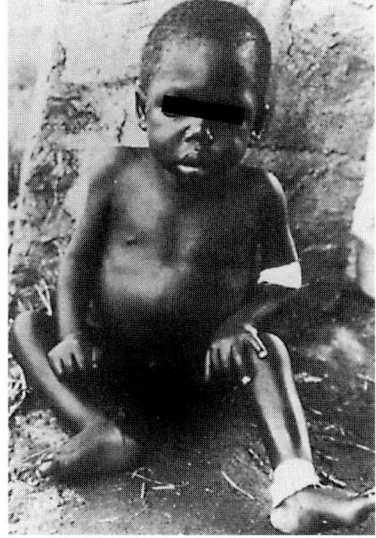

**FIGURE 127-1.** Typical appearance of children with advanced protein-energy malnutrition. *Left,* Marasmus. *Right,* Kwashiorkor. (Photograph from Kivu region, Republic of the Congo, by R. J. Smith.)

**TABLE 127-1.**
**Adaptations in Metabolic Fuel Use and Production during Progressive Starvation**

Postabsorptive, 5–6 hr
  Glucose is primary fuel in tissues such as skeletal muscle, kidney, and brain.
  Primary source of glucose is hepatic glycogenolysis.
Early starvation, 1–7 d
  Fatty acids assume increasing importance as fuels for muscle and kidney.
  Ketone bodies partially replace glucose as a fuel for the brain.
  Primary source of fatty acids is adipose tissue triglyceride.
  Ketone bodies are synthesized in the liver from fatty acid precursors.
  Hepatic glycogen stores become depleted and gluconeogenesis from amino acids and glycerol becomes the primary source of glucose.
Intermediate starvation, 1–3 wk
  Fatty acids and ketone bodies predominate as fuels for muscle and kidney.
  Ketone bodies become more important and glucose less important as fuels for brain.
  Adipose tissue lipolysis and hepatic ketogenesis increase.
  Glucose is derived from both hepatic and renal gluconeogenesis.
Prolonged starvation, >3 wk
  Fatty acids and ketone bodies remain the predominant fuels for muscle and kidney.
  Ketone body utilization further increases and glucose utilization decreases in brain.
  Adipose tissue triglyceride becomes the primary fuel source.
  Hepatic gluconeogenesis decreases as muscle proteolysis and the release of amino acids from muscle decreases.
  Renal gluconeogenesis from glutamine increases.

fuel.[6] It has been estimated that ≤90% of available glucose derives from gluconeogenesis after a 40-hour fast.[7] Free fatty acid release from adipose tissue triglyceride stores is augmented progressively during fasting, resulting in increased plasma fatty acid levels, consumption of fatty acids by skeletal muscle and kidney, and sparing of glucose. The synthesis of ketone bodies by the liver is activated by the increased availability of fatty acids and a rising glucagon/insulin ratio, elevating circulating levels of ketone bodies as starvation continues.[8] Skeletal muscle, kidney, and brain begin to metabolize ketone bodies in proportion to their plasma concentrations, further reducing the requirement for glucose.

The net breakdown of muscle protein during starvation reflects the requirements of the liver and kidney for substrates for gluconeogenesis and ammoniagenesis, respectively. Alanine and other amino acids released from muscle are converted into glucose in the liver,[9] whereas muscle-derived glutamine[10] is utilized primarily in renal ammoniagenesis or as a fuel and precursor of gluconeogenic amino acids in the gastrointestinal tract.[11] During early starvation, the increased urinary levels of metabolically generated anions in the form of ketone bodies require an accompanying excretion of sodium. This probably explains the natriuresis and diuresis, correlated with rapid weight loss, that occur during the first days of a fast.[12] As total body sodium becomes depleted and ketone body production increases, ammonium derived primarily from glutamine replaces sodium as the primary urinary cation.

As starvation progresses and the levels of ketone bodies and free fatty acids continue to rise, diminished requirements for endogenous glucose production enable an adaptive conservation of body protein.[13] Thus, during long-term fasting, amino-acid conversion to glucose is minimized, and the net breakdown of muscle protein is governed largely by the glutamine requirement for maintenance of acid-base balance through renal ammoniagenesis pathways.[14]

This series of metabolic adaptations during fasting assures adequate metabolic fuels for all tissues and the efficient utilization of nutrient stores. The net result is a remarkable capacity for survival in the absence of food intake. The maximal duration of fasting compatible with life in initially normal-weight persons is demonstrated by the unfortunate example of political protesters in Northern Ireland, who died after 45 to 76 days of essentially total fasting.[15] Obese patients, who may have as much as four times the normal caloric reserve, have been treated clinically with total fasting for more than 200 days without serious complications,[16] although the apparent risk of sudden death from cardiac failure makes fasting of this duration inadvisable.[17] Thus, the length of time a person can survive starvation differs with body composition. Generally, the loss of one-third to one-half of body nitrogen is incompatible with life in lean or obese patients, but the large fat stores in obesity allow longer-term sparing of body nitrogen. Patients with debilitating illnesses or malnourished, wasted persons may have a markedly decreased tolerance for nutrient deprivation.

## HORMONAL CONTROL AND ADAPTATION DURING STARVATION

The most important factor controlling the metabolic adaptation to starvation is insulin. Without a regulated decrease in the secretion and the circulating levels of insulin, endogenous glucose-generating pathways cannot be activated, and alternative fuel stores cannot be mobilized. Superimposed on these dominant actions of insulin are the effects of multiple other catabolic and anabolic hormones, including glucagon, growth hormone, growth factors, thyroid hormone, and glucocorticoids. Regulated change in the levels of each of these hormones is essential for effective metabolic adaptation during fasting.

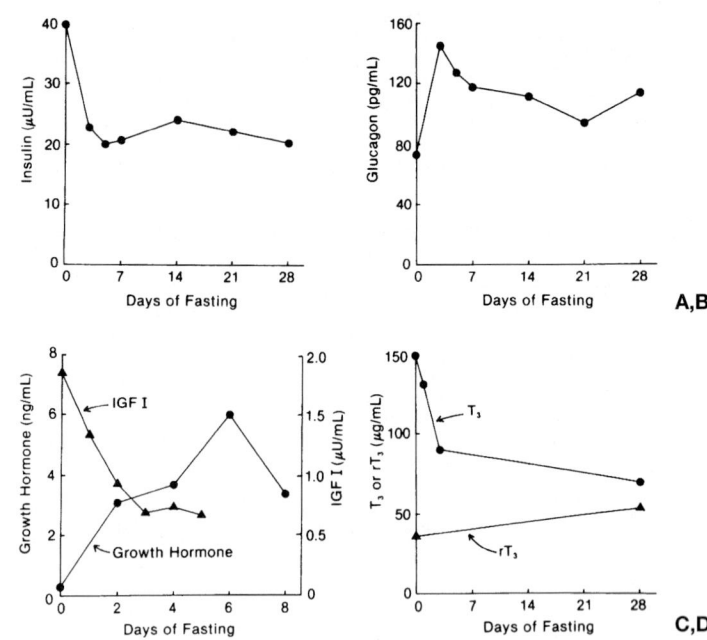

**FIGURE 127-2.** Changes in hormone levels during fasting. **A,** Insulin. **B,** Glucagon. (Data in **A** and **B** from Marliss EB, Aoki TT, Unger RH, et al. Glucagon levels and metabolic effects in fasting man. J Clin Invest 1970; 49:2256.) **C,** Growth hormone and insulin-like growth factor-I (*IGF-I*). (Data in **C** from Cahill GF Jr, Herrera MG, Morgan AP, et al. Hormone-fuel interrelationships during fasting. J Clin Invest 1966; 45:1751; and Isley WL, Underwood LE, Clemmons DR. Dietary components that regulate serum somatomedin-C concentrations in humans. J Clin Invest 1983; 71:175.) **D,** Triiodothyronine ($T_3$) and reverse triiodothyronine ($rT_3$). (Data in **D** from Merimee TJ, Fineberg ES. Starvation-induced alterations of circulating thyroid hormone concentrations in man. Metabolism 1976; 25:79; and Gardner DF, Kaplan MM, Stanley CA, Utiger RD. Effect of triiodothyronine replacement on the metabolic and pituitary responses to starvation. N Engl J Med 1979; 300:579.)

## INSULIN

The changes in circulating hormone levels during starvation are illustrated in Figure 127-2. Plasma insulin levels decrease to approximately half the normal postabsorptive levels during the first 3 days of food withdrawal and then stabilize at low but physiologically significant concentrations.[18] This adaptation in insulin secretion develops gradually during fasting and, in turn, normalizes only after several days of refeeding. Thus, when glucose or other food is ingested after a period of fasting, there is a subnormal insulin secretory response.[19] In some nondiabetic persons, glucose intolerance may be observed after periods of inadequate food ingestion; therefore, the results of glucose tolerance tests can be difficult to interpret unless patients have had adequate carbohydrate and total caloric intake for several days before testing.

## GLUCAGON

During starvation, the blood glucose concentration is maintained in part through the action of glucagon. Serum glucagon levels increase within the first 48 hours and continue to rise throughout the first several days of fasting in normal humans.[18] In obese persons undergoing prolonged fasting, plasma glucagon concentrations rise initially but return toward prefast levels after 3 to 4 weeks.[20] Probably, in early starvation, hyperglucagonemia is attributable to decreased clearance of the hormone rather than to increased secretion.[20] During prolonged starvation, glucagon levels return toward normal because of a decrease in secretion, with continued decreased clearance of the hormone. Pancreatic stores of glucagon do not appear to be diminished after short-term fasting, as evidenced by an exaggerated glucagon secretory response to arginine infusion.[21]

With low concentrations of insulin in the fasting state, glucagon contributes to the maintenance of glucose homeostasis by stimulating hepatic gluconeogenesis and glycogenolysis.[8,22] An increase in the plasma glucagon/insulin ratio during early starvation also promotes the generation of alternative fuels by increasing hepatic synthesis of ketone bodies and mobilizing free fatty acids from adipose tissue.[23] In prolonged starvation, circulating glucagon returns to postabsorptive levels concurrent with the reduced demand for glucose (see Chap. 134).

## GROWTH HORMONE AND INSULIN-LIKE GROWTH FACTOR-I

Serum growth hormone levels also become elevated early in starvation.[24] The role of growth hormone as a metabolic regulator during fasting is unclear, however, because individual values are variable and do not correlate closely with metabolic adaptations. Because patients with growth hormone deficiency can become hypoglycemic during fasting,[25] it seems reasonable to conclude that adequate levels of the hormone are important for the maintenance of blood glucose in the fasting state but that elevated concentrations have an otherwise minor role in the metabolic adaptation to fasting.

Possibly, elevated growth hormone secretion during fasting is a consequence, in part, of the normal feedback relation between insulin-like growth factor-I (IGF-I) and growth hormone.[26,26a] IGF-I (designated somatomedin C in earlier literature) is a peptide growth factor that functions as an important mediator of the anabolic actions of growth hormone[27] (see Chaps. 12 and 173). Growth hormone stimulates IGF-I synthesis in the liver and some peripheral tissues, and there is evidence that IGF-I in turn exerts negative feedback inhibition on growth hormone secretion.[28] Although growth hormone appears to be the principal regulator of IGF-I, other factors, such as thyroid hormone, insulin, estrogens, and nutritional status, also influence IGF-I levels.[29] As a consequence, circulating levels of IGF-I decrease during fasting in spite of elevated growth hormone levels (see Fig. 127-2),[30,31] and feedback inhibitory effects of IGF-I on growth hormone secretion do not occur. During fasting, growth hormone binding in the liver is reduced in parallel with decreased IGF-I mRNA synthesis, suggesting growth hormone resistance as a mechanism contributing to decreased circulating IGF-I.[32] Decreased IGF-I also occurs during protein restriction, however, even though liver growth hormone binding is not altered.[33] Thus, protein restriction appears to affect growth hormone regulation of circulating IGF-I through a postreceptor mechanism. In addition to these effects on the liver, fasting reduces IGF-I mRNA levels in peripheral tissues, including kidney, muscle, gut, and brain, while simultaneously increasing IGF-I–receptor mRNA.[34] The combination of low IGF-I and high growth hormone levels may have adaptive value by diminishing the energy expenditure necessary for growth-related processes and yet enabling growth hormone to promote the mobilization of alternative fuels through its lipolytic actions.[31] The availability of IGF-I to tissues is directly influenced by circulating IGF-binding proteins (IGFBPs). IGFBP-3 is thought to be the major carrier of IGFs in the circulation. Prolonged fasting or protein depletion is correlated with decreased concentrations of IGFBP-3.[35] IGFBP-2 and IGFBP-1 may mediate cellular transport of the IGFs. Both IGFBP-2 and IGFBP-1 tend to increase during prolonged fasting, likely as a consequence of decreased insulin concentrations.[35]

In malnourished patients given nutritional support, the direction of changes in serum IGF-I levels correlates closely with the direction of changes in nitrogen balance. Refeeding adequate energy but low protein only partially restores circulating IGF-I concentrations. When total parenteral nutrition is provided to nutritionally deprived patients, serum IGF-I levels rise at a rate corresponding to the improvement in nitrogen balance.[36] This does not appear to reflect simply increased synthesis of hepatic proteins secondary to improved nutrition, because the levels of other hepatic secretory proteins are not consistently raised during the time IGF-I increases. IGF-I may prove to be a sensitive indicator of the response to nutritional rehabilitation.[37]

## THYROID HORMONE

One of the energy-conserving adaptations during prolonged starvation is a decrease in the basal metabolic rate, which is mediated at least in part by altered levels of triiodothyronine ($T_3$). In normal humans undergoing a short-term fast, serum $T_3$ levels decrease, whereas levels of thyroxine ($T_4$), thyroid-stimulating hormone, and the response of thyroid-stimulating hormone to thyroid-releasing hormone are unchanged.[38–40] Experimentally, starvation causes an increased sensitivity of pituitary thyrotrope cells to $T_3$.[41] The decrease in serum $T_3$ coincides with an increase in less biologically potent reverse $T_3$ (see Fig. 127-2), suggesting that peripheral tissues convert a greater proportion of $T_4$ into reverse $T_3$ during fasting (see Chaps. 30 and 36). A similar hormonal pattern develops in adults with protein-energy malnutrition.[42] If $T_3$ levels are maintained by the administration of $T_3$ during fasting, an increase in the catabolism of nutrient stores occurs, as demonstrated by elevated levels of glucose, free fatty acids, and ketone bodies,[43] and by increased urinary urea excretion.[39] Therefore, it is thought that diminished levels of $T_3$ are an important determinant of the decreased oxygen consumption observed in prolonged starvation and may be protective in limiting muscle protein breakdown. Reduced thyroid receptor protein levels also occur in starvation,[43] and thus, by reducing tissue responsiveness to the catabolic effects of $T_3$, may also have a role in the adaptation to starvation.

## GLUCOCORTICOIDS

Although early work provided evidence for an absence of changes in the pituitary-adrenal axis in obese patients undergoing prolonged starvation,[45] more recent studies have demonstrated modest elevations in glucocorticoid levels during fasting.[46] In catabolic states associated with injury or systemic illness (see later), more marked glucocorticoid elevations are believed to contribute to tissue breakdown. It is possible that the effects of glucocorticoids in starvation as compared to systemic disease states may depend on the magnitude of change in circulating levels. Patients with glucocorticoid deficiency frequently have fasting hypoglycemia, because adequate glucocorticoid levels are necessary to maintain the activity of pyruvate carboxylase, a rate-limiting enzyme for gluconeogenesis,[47] and for the release of gluconeogenic amino acids from skeletal muscle.[48] Thus, it appears that normal or modestly elevated levels are necessary for the adaptive response to starvation.

## CATECHOLAMINES

Increased sympathetic nervous system activity may contribute to the elevation of plasma free fatty acids and glucagon concentrations, and to the maintenance of blood glucose levels during fasting, but several lines of evidence suggest that this is not an important factor.[49] For example, normal elevations in free fatty acid levels occur during fasting in patients who have undergone adrenalectomy, adrenergic blockade, or even complete disruption of the sympathetic efferent pathways at the level of the cervical cord.[50–52] Similarly, catecholamine deficiency has not been associated with the development of fasting hypoglycemia. Therefore, it appears that sympathetic activity neither initiates nor maintains the metabolic adaptations to starvation.

## LEPTIN

The obesity gene product, leptin, is released from adipose tissue, and circulating concentrations increase with increased body fat content. Leptin has been proposed as an afferent signal between adipose tissue and the central nervous system that regulates body composition. In accordance with this role, leptin levels decrease with loss of body weight and reduction in adipose tissue mass.[52a] In short-term fasting, however, leptin levels decrease more rapidly and are more rapidly restored with refeeding than is body fat.[53,54] In mice, repletion of leptin during fasting partially reverses changes in thyroid, adrenal, and gonadal hormones, suggesting a role for decreasing leptin as an activator of neuroendocrine adaptations to starvation.[55,56] The regulation of leptin may involve both glucose and insulin concentrations, as no decrease in leptin occurs during fasting when glucose or insulin concentrations are maintained.[54]

## IMPACT OF STARVATION ON ENDOCRINE AND NONENDOCRINE DISEASE

The adaptive metabolic responses to starvation make it possible for humans to survive long periods of inadequate nutrient intake.[57] Because the metabolic adaptation to fasting is largely the result of endocrinologic regulation, the normal response can be markedly altered by endocrine disorders. For example, lack of a single hormone, such as cortisol[58] or growth hormone,[59] can cause severe hypoglycemia within a few hours of food deprivation. Fortunately, these primary endocrinologic diseases are relatively uncommon and generally recognized early.

Much more commonly, patients with nonendocrine disease are nutritionally depleted but unable to generate a normal endocrine response to partial or total fasting. Consequently, malnutrition can have a significant effect on morbidity and mortality. For example, after traumatic injuries, major operative procedures, burns, systemic infections, or other serious illnesses, a well-characterized catabolic stress response develops.[60] An important adaptive function of this response appears to be the accelerated mobilization of body nutrient stores, which are used in tissue repair, by inflammatory cells, and for processes such as acute-phase protein synthesis. The metabolic alterations of stress depend in large part on changes in hormone levels, which, as illustrated in Figure 127-3,

are different from the endocrine response to fasting. Levels of sympathetic nervous system activity and circulating catecholamines rise early,[61] followed somewhat later by more sustained elevations of glucocorticoids,[62] glucagon,[63] and growth hormone.[64] Insulin levels may be decreased early but ultimately are normal or elevated.[65] In addition, wounds, sepsis, or inflammation induce a variety of hormonal mediators, or cytokines, such as tumor necrosis factor and the interleukins, which exacerbate skeletal muscle breakdown and debilitation.[66] Attenuation of the metabolic effects of these stress mediators through nutritional intervention is limited, although specific nutrient formulas in combination with trophic hormones potentially may provide beneficial effects.[67]

When decreased nutrient intake or total fasting coincides with severe injury or illness, the normal metabolic adaptation to fasting does not develop. Instead of decreased energy requirements and a lowered basal metabolic rate, energy requirements remain increased as a result of the demands for tissue repair processes, inflammatory cell formation and function, hyperdynamic circulation, and, sometimes, fever-associated shivering. Increased concentrations of stress hormones, in particular glucocorticoids, greater than the levels characteristic of fasting may lead to the net catabolism of tissue protein and may increase negative nitrogen balance.[68] Insulin levels remain normal or elevated in spite of fasting, reflecting a state of insulin resistance that prevents insulin from counteracting the catabolic effects of the stress hormones. In spite of this insulin resistance, there may be enough antilipolytic action of insulin in some patients to diminish free fatty acid mobilization and ketone body synthesis and, thus, an impaired transition to lipid fuel consumption during fasting. Consequently, in some patients with multiple traumatic injuries, levels of plasma ketone bodies remain low during fasting.[69] This is associated with increased urinary nitrogen excretion and, probably, less effective protein conservation.

As in starvation, adaptation to a catabolic stress ultimately is characterized by a reduction of muscle protein catabolism and increased use of free fatty acids and ketone bodies.[70] Depending on the demands for glucose consumption and overall energy use, and on the effectiveness of alternative fuel mobilization, however, the adaptation may be delayed for many weeks. Thus, even modest degrees of undernutrition or short periods of total fasting can lead to significant nutritional depletion, such that the provision of adequate nutritional support in the setting of catabolic diseases may be essential for optimal recovery or even survival.[71] For this reason, parenteral feeding should be considered early in the course of critically ill patients if oral food intake is inadequate.

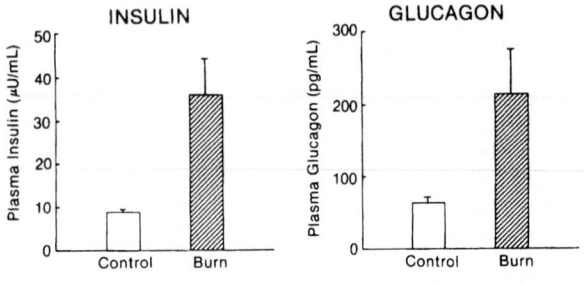

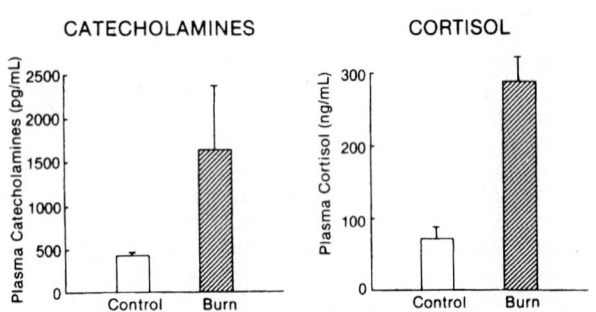

**FIGURE 127-3.** Effects of burn injury on basal hormone levels. Plasma hormone concentrations were determined after 8 hours of fasting in 15 subjects with 25% to 90% burns. (Redrawn from Wolfe RR, Durkot MJ, Allsop JR, Burke JF. Glucose metabolism in severely burned patients. Metabolism 1979; 28:1031.)

## REFERENCES

1. Olsen RE. Protein-calorie malnutrition. New York: Academic Press, 1975.
2. Winick M. Long term effects of kwashiorkor. J Pediatr Gastroenterol Nutr 1987; 6:833.
3. Wolstenholme GEW, O'Connor M. Nutrition and infection. Boston: Little, Brown, 1967.
4. Adhikari M, Gita-Ramjee, Berjak P. Aflatoxin, kwashiorkor, and morbidity. Nat Toxins 1994; 2:1.
5. Cahill GF, Owen OE, Morgan AP. The consumption of fuels during prolonged starvation. Adv Enzyme Regul 1968; 6:143.
6. Webber J, Macdonald IA. The cardiovascular, metabolic and hormonal changes accompanying acute starvation in men and women. Br J Nutr 1994; 71:437.
7. Katz J, Tayek JA. Gluconeogenesis and the Cori cycle in 12-, 20-, and 40-h-fasted humans. Am J Physiol 1998; 275:E537.
8. Gelfand RA, Sherwin RS. Glucagon and starvation. In: Lefebvre PJ, ed. Glucagon II. Handbook of experimental pharmacology, vol 66[II]. Berlin: Springer-Verlag, 1983:223.
9. Felig P, Marliss E, Owen OE, Cahill GF Jr. Blood glucose and gluconeogenesis in fasting man. Arch Intern Med 1969; 123:293.
10. Marliss EB, Aoki TT, Pozefsky T, et al. Muscle and splanchnic glutamine and glutamate metabolism in postabsorptive and starved man. J Clin Invest 1971; 50:814.
11. Windmueller HG. Glutamine utilization by the small intestine. Adv Enzymol Relat Areas Mol Biol 1982; 53:202.

12. Sigler MH. The mechanism of the natriuresis of fasting. J Clin Invest 1975; 55:377.
13. How ketones spare protein in starvation. (Editorial). Nutr Rev 1989; 3:80.
14. Aoki TT, Mueller WA, Brennan MF, Cahill GF Jr. Metabolic effects of glucose in brief and prolonged fasted man. Am J Clin Nutr 1975; 28:507.
15. Kerndt PR, Naughton JL, Driscoll CE, Loxterkamp DA. Fasting: the history, pathophysiology and complications. West J Med 1982; 137:379.
16. Thomson TJ, Runcie J, Miller V. Treatment of obesity by total fasting for up to 249 days. Lancet 1966; 2:992.
17. Garnett ES, Barnard DL, Ford J, et al. Gross fragmentation of cardiac myofibrils after therapeutic starvation for obesity. Lancet 1969; 1:914.
18. Marliss EB, Aoki TT, Unger RH, et al. Glucagon levels and metabolic effects in fasting man. J Clin Invest 1970; 49:2256.
19. Fink G, Gutman RA, Cresto JC, et al. Glucose-induced insulin release patterns: effect of starvation. Diabetologia 1974; 10:421.
20. Fisher M, Sherwin RS, Hendler R, Felig P. Kinetics of glucagon in man: effects of starvation. Proc Natl Acad Sci U S A 1976; 73:1735.
21. Aguilar-Parada E, Eisentraut AM, Unger RH. Effects of starvation on plasma pancreatic glucagon in normal man. Diabetes 1969; 18:717.
22. Ven de Werve G, Hue L, Hers HG. Hormonal and ionic control of the glycogenolytic cascade in rat liver. Biochem J 1977; 162:135.
23. McGarry JD, Foster DW. Regulation of hepatic fatty acid oxidation and ketone body production. Annu Rev Biochem 1980; 493:395.
24. Cahill GF Jr, Herrera MG, Morgan AP, et al. Hormone-fuel interrelationships during fasting. J Clin Invest 1966; 45:1751.
25. Merimee TJ, Felig P, Marliss E, et al. Glucose and lipid homeostasis in the absence of human growth hormone. J Clin Invest 1971; 50:574.
26. Abe H, Molitch ME, Van Wyk JJ, Underwood LE. Human growth hormone and somatomedin C suppress the spontaneous release of growth hormone in unanesthetized rats. Endocrinology 1983; 113:1319.
26a. Thissen JP, Underwood LE, Ketelslegers JM. Regulation of insulin-like growth factor-I in starvation and injury. Nutr Rev 1999; 57:167.
27. Chochinov RH, Daughaday WH. Current concepts of somatomedin and other biologically related growth factors. Diabetes 1976; 25:994.
28. Clemmons DR, Underwood LE. Somatomedin-C/insulin-like growth factor I in acromegaly. J Clin Endocrinol Metab 1986; 15:629.
29. Phillips LS, Goldstein S, Gavin JR III. Nutrition and somatomedin XVI: somatomedins and somatomedin inhibitors in fasted and refed rats. Metabolism 1988; 37:209.
30. Isley WL, Underwood LE, Clemmons DR. Dietary components that regulate serum somatomedin-C concentrations in humans. J Clin Invest 1983; 71:175.
31. Merimee TJ, Zapf J, Froesch ER. Insulin-like growth factors in the fed and fasted states. J Clin Endocrinol Metab 1982; 55:999.
32. Straus DS, Takemoto CD. Effect of fasting on insulin-like growth factor-I (IGF-I) and growth hormone receptor mRNA levels and IGF-I gene transcription in rat liver. Mol Endocrinol 1990; 4:91.
33. Maiter DM, Maes M, Underwood LE, et al. Early changes in serum concentrations of somatomedin-C induced by dietary protein deprivation: contributions of growth hormone receptor and post-receptor defects. J Endocrinol 1988; 118:113.
34. Lowe WJ, Adamo M, Werner H, et al. Regulation by fasting of insulin-like growth factor-I and its receptor: effects on gene expression and binding. J Clin Invest 1989; 84:619.
35. Clemmons DR, Underwood LE. Nutritional regulation of IGF-I and IGF binding proteins. Annu Rev Nutr 1991; 11:393.
36. Clemmons DR, Underwood LE, Dickerson RN, et al. Use of plasma somatomedin-C/insulin-like growth factor I measurements to monitor the response to nutritional repletion in malnourished patients. Am J Clin Nutr 1985; 41:191.
37. Unterman TG, Vazquez RM, Slas AJ, et al. Nutrition and somatomedin XIII: usefulness of somatomedin-C in nutritional assessment. Am J Med 1985; 78:228.
38. Merimee TJ, Fineberg ES. Starvation-induced alterations of circulating thyroid hormone concentrations in man. Metabolism 1976; 25:79.
39. Gardner DF, Kaplan MM, Stanley CA, Utiger RD. Effect of triiodothyronine replacement on the metabolic and pituitary responses to starvation. N Engl J Med 1979; 300:579.
40. Vagenakis AG. Thyroid hormone metabolism in prolonged experimental starvation in man. In: Vigersky RA, ed. Anorexia nervosa. New York: Raven Press, 1977:243.
41. Hugues JN, Enjalbert A, Burger AG, et al. Sensitivity of thyrotropin (TSH) secretion to 3,5,3'-triiodothyronine and TSH-releasing hormone in rats during starvation. Endocrinology 1986; 119:253.
42. Chopra IJ, Smith SR. Circulating thyroid hormones and thyrotropin in adult patients with protein-calorie malnutrition. J Clin Endocrinol Metab 1975; 40:221.
43. Carter WJ, Shakir KM, Hodges S, et al. Effect of thyroid hormone on metabolic adaptation to fasting. Metabolism 1975; 24:1177.
44. Tagami T, Nakamura H, Sasaki S, et al. Starvation-induced decrease in the maximal binding capacity for triiodothyronine of the thyroid hormone receptor is due to a decrease in the receptor protein. Metabolism 1996; 45:970.
45. Sabeh G, Alley RA, Robbins TJ, et al. Adrenocortical indices during fasting in obesity. J Clin Endocrinol Metab 1969; 29:373.
46. Bergendahl M, Vance ML, Iranmanesh A, et al. Fasting as a metabolic stress paradigm selectively amplifies cortisol secretory burst mass and delays the time of maximal nyctohemeral cortisol concentrations in men. J Clin Endocrinol Metab 1996; 81:692.
47. Baxter JD, Forsham PH. Tissue effects of glucocorticoids. Am J Med 1972; 53:573.
48. Bondy PK, Ingle DJ, Meeks RC. Influence of adrenal cortical hormones upon the level of plasma amino acids in eviscerate rats. Endocrinology 1954; 55:354.

49. Jung RT, Shetty PS, James WPT. Nutritional effects on thyroid and catecholamine metabolism. Clin Sci 1980; 58:183.
50. Levy AC, Ramey ER. Effect of autonomic blocking agents on depot fat mobilization in normal and adrenalectomized animals. Proc Soc Exp Biol Med 1958; 99:637.
51. Misbin RI, Edgar PJ, Lockwood DH. Adrenergic regulation of insulin secretion during fasting in normal subjects. Diabetes 1970; 19:688.
52. Brodows RG, Campbell RG, Al-Aziz AJ, Pi-Sunyer FX. Lack of central autonomic regulation of substrate during early fasting in man. Metabolism 1976; 25:803.
52a. Klein S, Horowitz JF, Landt M, et al. Leptin production during early starvation in lean and obese women. Am J Physiol Endoc Metab 2000; 278:E280.
53. Weigle DS, Duell PB, Connor WE, et al. Effect of fasting, refeeding, and dietary fat restriction on plasma leptin levels. J Clin Endocrinol Metab 1997; 82:561.
54. Boden G, Chen X, Moxxoli M, Ryan I. Effect of fasting on serum leptin in normal human subjects. J Clin Endocrinol Metab 1996; 81:3419.
55. Ahima RS, Prabakaran D, Mantzoros C, et al. Role of leptin in the neuroendocrine response to fasting. Nature 1996; 382:250.
56. Flier JS. What's in a name? In search of leptin's physiologic role. J Clin Endocrinol Metab 1998; 83:1407.
57. Joslin EP. Treatment of diabetes mellitus. Philadelphia: Lea & Febiger, 1916:243.
58. Bondy PK. Disorders of the adrenal cortex. In: Wilson JD, Foster DW, eds. Williams textbook of endocrinology, 7th ed. Philadelphia: WB Saunders, 1985:816.
59. Goodman HG, Grumbach MM, Kaplan SJ. Growth and growth hormone II: a comparison of isolated growth-hormone deficiency and multiple pituitary-hormone deficiencies in 35 patients with idiopathic hypopituitary dwarfism. N Engl J Med 1968; 278:57.
60. Wolfe RR, Durkot MJ, Allsop JR, Burke JF. Glucose metabolism in severely burned patients. Metabolism 1979; 28:1031.
61. Jaattela A, Alho A, Avikainen V, et al. Plasma catecholamines in severely injured patients: a prospective study on 45 patients with multiple injuries. Br J Surg 1975; 62:177.
62. Vaughan GM, Becker RA, Allen JP, et al. Cortisol and corticotrophin in burned patients. J Trauma 1982; 22:263.
63. Wilmore DW, Lindsey CA, Moylan JA, et al. Hyperglucagonaemia after burns. Lancet 1974; 1:73.
64. Ross H, Johnston IDA, Welborn TA, Wright AD. Effect of abdominal operation on glucose tolerance and serum levels of insulin, growth hormone, and hydrocortisone. Lancet 1966; 2:563.
65. Black PR, Brooks DC, Bessey PQ, et al. Mechanisms of insulin resistance following injury. Ann Surg 1982; 196:420.
66. Hardin TC. Cytokine mediators of malnutrition: clinical implications. Nutr Clin Pract 1993; 8:55.
67. Wilmore DW. Catabolic illness. N Engl J Med 1991; 325:695.
68. Tishler ME, Leng E, Al-Kanhal M. Metabolic response of muscle to trauma: altered control of protein turnover. In: Dietze G, Kleinberger W, eds. Clinical nutrition and metabolic research proceedings, 7th congress. Munich: ESPEN, 1985:40.
69. Smith R, Fuller DJ, Wedge JH, et al. Initial effect of injury on ketone bodies and other blood metabolites. Lancet 1975; 1:1.
70. Krause MV, Mahan LK. The metabolic stress response and methods for providing nutritional care to stressed patients. In: Food, nutrition, and diet therapy, 6th ed. Philadelphia: WB Saunders, 1979:694.
71. Ingenbleek Y, Bernstein LH. The nutrionally dependent adaptive dichotomy (NDAD) and stress hypermetabolism. J Clin Ligand Assay 1999; 22:259.

# CHAPTER 128

# ANOREXIA NERVOSA AND OTHER EATING DISORDERS

MICHELLE P. WARREN AND REBECCA J. LOCKE

Starvation engenders various adaptive metabolic and endocrine changes that decrease caloric demands and permit survival. The starvation associated with the syndrome of *anorexia nervosa* combines medical, endocrine, and psychological manifestations. The abnormality is partly hypothalamic in origin and represents an adaptation to the starvation state.[1,2] Although not associated with starvation, *bulimia* (abnormal means of purging calories or weight) similarly involves endocrine and behavioral symptoms.

# ANOREXIA NERVOSA

## CHARACTERISTICS

Anorexia nervosa usually occurs during adolescence and in women younger than 25 years. *Amenorrhea, weight loss,* and *behavioral changes* constitute the classic triad, any one of which may precede the others. The incidence differs greatly among population groups, and high-risk populations are found.[3] For example, 1 in 100 middle-class adolescent girls and 1 in 20 to 1 in 5 professional ballet dancers have anorexia.[4-6] The *Diagnostic and Statistical Manual of Mental Disorders, Revised Third Edition*, estimates that the rate of anorexia in girls between the ages of 12 and 18 years ranges from 1 in 800 to 1 in 100.[7] The high incidence of this disorder in dancers derives from the rigid standards for thinness as well as the many hours of exercise this profession entails.[5] (Increased levels of activity and restricted eating can induce self-starvation in rats, providing an interesting animal model.[8]) On the other hand, the condition is rare among blacks, including black ballet dancers, despite their exposure to the rigid standards of competition and weight restriction.[5,9] This difference may relate to different social or cultural influences or, perhaps, to more efficient metabolic mechanisms. The risk that a sister of a patient with anorexia nervosa will acquire the illness is 6%; this fact, along with studies of monozygous twins, suggests that inborn metabolic factors contribute to the syndrome.[10] The incidence of anorexia nervosa is increased in Turner syndrome, diabetes mellitus, and Cushing disease.[6,11] Family histories of depression, alcohol, and drug abuse or dependence may be risk factors for the disorder.[12] The female/male ratio is 9:1.[13] The condition has been reported in men who are training for competitive activity while restricting their weight.[14]

The age of onset shows a bimodal pattern, with a high incidence between 13 and 14 years, and again between 17 and 18 years. The dieting behavior is related to pubertal maturational development and may coincide with the rapid accumulation of fat that is normal at that time. Dieting in this age group also is related to negative feelings about body image independent of weight.[15,16]

## CLINICAL SYNDROME

Anorexia nervosa represents a prototype of "hypothalamic amenorrhea." The reproductive and physiologic adjustments appear to be an adaptive phenomenon appropriate for the semistarved state. Generally, recovery from the amenorrhea and the psychiatric disturbance parallels the weight gain.

The criteria for the diagnosis of anorexia nervosa appear in the *Diagnostic and Statistical Manual of Mental Disorders, Fourth Edition*.[17] This new definition contains bulimic subgroups. The diagnosis of anorexia nervosa depends on finding a symptom complex that includes severe weight loss (usually to less than 80% of ideal body weight; Fig. 128-1); behavioral changes such as hyperactivity and preoccupation with food; and perceptual changes, in particular, a distorted view of the body accompanied by an unreasonable concern about being "too fat." The amenorrhea may occur at any time, even preceding the syndrome, but often is related to the start of the food restriction, even if weight loss has been slight. If the weight is lost before menarche, patients may have primary amenorrhea.

The hyperactivity may begin in the guise of an athletic pursuit. Excessive exercise is often an integral aspect of the disorder in its acute phases. Moreover, the combination of strenuous physical activity and immoderate dieting has been found to lead to comorbidity.[18] Anorectic patients may demonstrate an intense interest in low-calorie foods, with a large intake of diet sodas and raw vegetables, and avoidance of fried foods or other products high in calories. Hypercarotenemia may give a yellow cast to the skin, especially on the palms and soles; the sclerae remain clear. The high serum carotene level is only partly attributable to

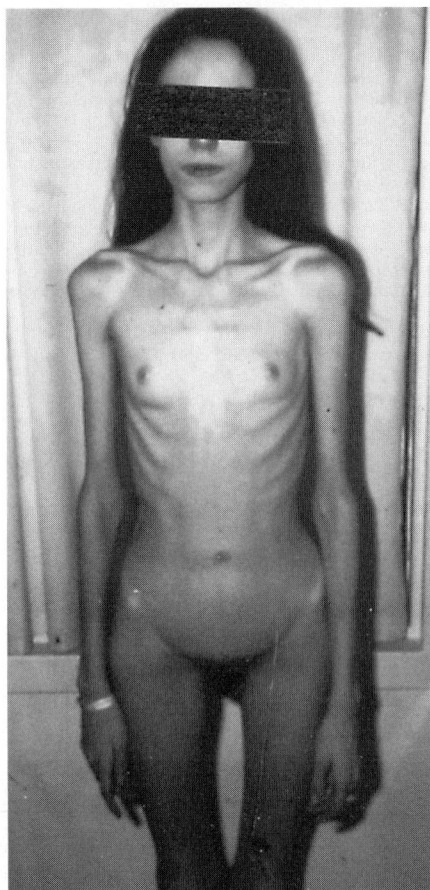

**FIGURE 128-1.** Young woman with severe anorexia nervosa.

an increased intake of raw vegetables; metabolism of carotene, a precursor of vitamin A, also is decreased.[6] The possible complaints and physical findings of the anorectic patient include abdominal pain, intolerance to cold, vomiting, hypotension, hypothermia, dry skin, lanugo-type hair, bradycardia, a systolic murmur, pedal edema, petechiae, and acrocyanosis.

Despite the frequent leukopenia, which may be marked, the risk of infection is not increased, and cell-mediated immunity is intact. Anemia, thrombocytopenia, and hypoplastic bone marrow may be present. Severe hypoalbuminemia is rare; nevertheless, pitting edema may occur, especially with refeeding. Dehydration may cause an elevated blood urea nitrogen level, which returns to normal after rehydration. Electrolyte abnormalities and hypophosphatemia may occur. Occasionally, hypoglycemia has been severe enough to cause coma.[11] Hematologic abnormalities, including decreased total leukocyte, monocyte, neutrophil, and platelet counts, appear to be correlated with total body fat–mass depletion.[19]

Numerous medical problems occur in anorexia nervosa, including salivary gland enlargement, pericardial effusion, pancreatitis, pancreatic insufficiency, delayed gastric emptying, poor intestinal motility, liver dysfunction with increased hepatic enzyme levels, pneumomediastinum, kidney stones, coagulopathies, bilateral peroneal nerve palsies, and deficiencies of thiamine and zinc. As a heat-conserving mechanism, marked vasoconstriction of the extremities may be present. If the weight loss occurs at or before the growth spurt, permanent growth deficiency may result. Duodenal ulcers may occur, and disregarding complaints of abdominal pain is unwise.[6] Electrocardiographic changes include low-voltage, inverted T waves and, sometimes, arrhythmias. Hypoglycemia has been associated with coma and with low or absent insulin and C peptide levels, suggesting that this problem results from malnutrition.[20]

Osteoporosis and fractures occur as a result of long-term poor nutritional intake and prolonged estrogen deficiency.[6,21–23] Computed tomographic scanning or magnetic resonance imaging of the brain occasionally demonstrates enlargement of the cortical sulci and subarachnoid spaces, as well as cerebral atrophy; surprisingly, in one patient, the atrophy was reversed with weight gain.[6] Changes in the brain due to anorexia nervosa may be irreversible. Weight recovery does not seem to reverse unilateral temporal lobe hypoperfusion, gray matter volume deficits, or various localized brain dysfunction.[24–26]

## ENDOCRINOPATHY

### HYPOTHALAMIC DYSFUNCTION

Low serum levels of luteinizing hormone (LH) and follicle-stimulating hormone (FSH) are associated with a profound estrogen deficiency.[3] Serum levels of triiodothyronine ($T_3$) and thyroxine ($T_4$) may be low. The serum cortisol concentration may be high, a finding that differentiates anorexia nervosa from pituitary insufficiency.

**Gonadotropin Abnormalities.** In anorexia nervosa, the normal episodic, pulsatile variation in the secretion of LH is absent, and a pattern typical of early puberty may be seen[27] (Fig. 128-2). These abnormalities normalize with weight gain. In addition, the pattern of gonadotropin secretion can be normalized by the pulsatile administration of luteinizing hormone–releasing hormone (LHRH)[28]; if this hormone is injected every 2 hours, menstrual bleeding and ovulation also can be induced. Interestingly, similar disturbances in LH secretion are noted in normal women who are exposed to a low-calorie diet.[29]

The amenorrhea probably is secondary to altered signals reaching the medial central hypothalamus from the arcuate nucleus or higher levels. (The arcuate nucleus probably is the center responsible for the episodic stimulation of LHRH.) In a subset of patients, pulsations of LH are restored by administration of naloxone, suggesting that increased opioid activity participates in the suppressed LHRH pulsations. Experiments with another opioid inhibitor, naltrexone, have shown variable effects on LH secretion, a finding which indicates that the suppression of LH is not consistently opioid linked.[30,31] The pattern of response to injected LHRH is immature, resembling that seen in prepubertal children—the FSH response is much greater than that of LH. The normalization of LH/FSH ratios with repeated injections of LHRH suggests that the pituitary gonadotropes have become sluggish because of the lack of endogenous stimulation, and that the episodic stimulation is important in determining the relative amounts of LH and FSH secreted. Moreover, patients who recover partially from anorexia nervosa tend to have exaggerated responses to injected LHRH.[32] These changes are seen in normal children during early puberty. Thus, all of these changes indicate that the hypothalamic signals of the central nervous system revert to a prepubertal or pubertal state.

**Hypometabolic Manifestations.** Despite their marked cachexia, patients with anorexia nervosa have clinical and metabolic signs suggestive of hypothyroidism: constipation, cold intolerance, bradycardia, hypotension, dry skin, prolonged ankle reflexes, low basal metabolic rate, and carotenemia.[3] In addition, the altered metabolism of certain sex steroids, such as testosterone, is analogous to that seen in hypothyroidism.[3] Some of these changes suggest a compensatory hypometabolism.

Studies of the circulatory system show that, during maximal exercise, the attainable oxygen uptake and heart rate are low in children with anorexia nervosa; the maximal aerobic power ($VO_{2max}$) appears to be decreased disproportionately to the circulatory and body dimensions.[3] An adaptation to caloric restriction, with metabolic rates reduced in proportion to the absolute reduction in body weight, has been documented in animals; this mechanism of energy conservation also may be operative in persons with anorexia. The hypometabolism that occurs in anorexia nervosa reverses with refeeding. Resting energy expenditure and thermic response to food are decreased.[33] This hypometabolism appears to be an appropriate mechanism to conserve energy.

The low serum $T_3$ levels in anorexia nervosa may be explained by an alteration in $T_4$ conversion (see Chaps. 30 and 36). In anorexia nervosa, as in starvation, the peripheral deiodination of $T_4$ is diverted from the formation of the active $T_3$ to the production of the inactive reverse $T_3$. Fasting decreases the hepatic uptake of $T_4$, with a proportionate decrease in $T_3$ production. (This "low $T_3$ syndrome" rarely may mask hyperthyroidism.) The low serum $T_4$ value in some patients with anorexia nervosa is somewhat more difficult to explain. Low $T_4$ euthyroidism has been seen in seriously ill patients in whom there is a dysfunctional state of deficient $T_4$ binding with a normal availability of peripheral tissue sites for free $T_4$. Presumably, a similar mechanism may be operative in anorexia nervosa. The secretion of thyroid-stimulating hormone (TSH) is normal, but an augmented serum TSH response to thyrotropin-releasing hormone (TRH) stimulation is seen, and the peak is delayed from 30 to between 60 and 120 minutes.[3] This change may reflect an altered setpoint for endogenous TRH regulation. One study shows a subnormal response of $T_4$ and $T_3$ to TRH, with a normal TSH response, suggesting chronic understimulation of the thyroid as a consequence of hypothalamic hypothyroidism.[34] In another study, the level of TRH in cerebrospinal fluid was found to be low.[35]

**Hypothalamic-Adrenal Interrelations.** Levels of serum cortisol often are elevated in anorexia nervosa; 24-hour studies demonstrate normal episodic and circadian rhythms of serum cortisol, but considerably higher levels[36] (Fig. 128-3). This change, which also can be seen in malnutrition, is secondary to prolongation of the half-life of cortisol because of reduced metabolic clearance. The urinary levels of corticosteroids, including

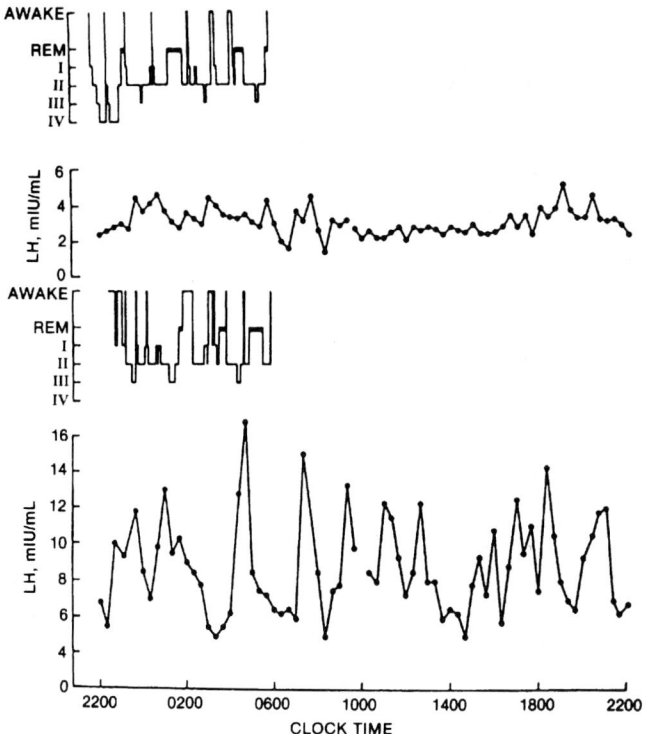

**FIGURE 128-2.** Plasma luteinizing hormone (*LH*) concentration measurements taken every 20 minutes for 24 hours during acute exacerbation of anorexia nervosa (*upper panel*) and after clinical remission with return of body weight to normal (*lower panel*). The latter represents a normal adult pattern. (*REM*, rapid eye movement.) (Boyar RN, Katz J, Finkelstein JW, et al. Anorexia nervosa: immaturity of the 24-hour luteinizing hormone secretory pattern. N Engl J Med 1974; 291:861.)

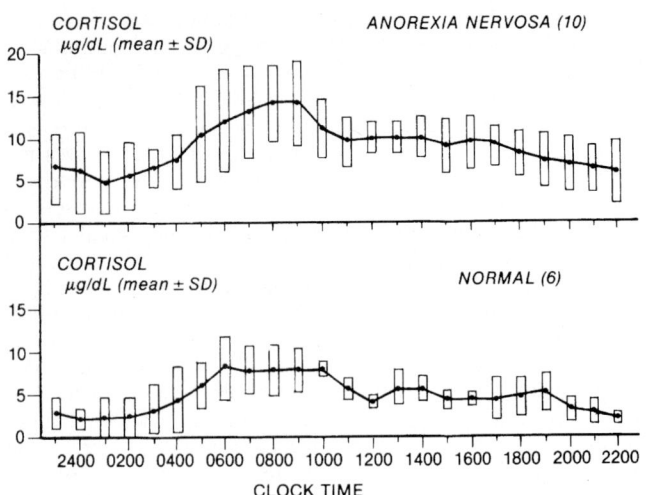

**FIGURE 128-3.** Hourly mean serum cortisol level derived from average of samples obtained 20 minutes before, on, and after the hour in 10 patients with anorexia nervosa, compared with 6 normal controls matched for age and sex. Circadian rhythm of cortisol remains intact in anorexia nervosa but the level is higher. (*SD*, standard deviation.) (From Boyar RM, Hellman LD, Roffwang H, et al. Cortisol secretion and metabolism in anorexia nervosa. N Engl J Med 1977; 296:190.)

17-hydroxysteroids and 17-ketosteroids, usually are low. The production rate of cortisol may be elevated; suppression with dexamethasone is inadequate, and the cortisol concentrations may exceed the binding capacity of cortisol-binding globulin.[2] In addition, affinity of serum cortisol-binding globulin for cortisol is decreased. Thus, unbound serum cortisol may be increased, so that it becomes available to the tissues. Higher levels of cortisol might be expected to suppress corticotropin secretion. However, the circadian rhythm that is maintained at the higher serum cortisol levels suggests that a new setpoint has been determined by the hypothalamic–pituitary–adrenal axis. Work on the hypothalamic–pituitary–adrenal pathways suggests activation of this axis. Cortisol level is elevated and responses to corticotropin-releasing hormone (CRH) are abnormal. CRH is increased in the cerebrospinal fluid of patients with anorexia.[37] CRH is known to suppress LH pulses in both humans and animals, and may augment dopaminergic and opiodergic inhibition of gonadotropin-releasing hormone.

Miscellaneous hypothalamic abnormalities in anorexia nervosa include a deficiency in the handling of a water load (probably as a result of a mild diabetes insipidus, characterized by an erratic serum vasopressin response to osmotic challenge); abnormal thermoregulatory responses with exposure to temperature extremes; and a lack of shivering.

**Leptin Levels.** An intriguing aspect of the disorder involves leptin, the hormone secreted by the adipocyte that seems to be a critical link between metabolic and reproductive pathways. Leptin appears to modulate food intake by affecting appetite, energy requirements, and eating behavior.[38] Low leptin levels, which have been reported in hypothalamic amenorrhea,[39,40] have been linked to low bone mass.[40,41] *Ob/ob* rodents lacking an active form of leptin tend to be not only overweight but also amenorrheic and infertile.[42,43] A critical leptin level exists below which menstruation stops.[44] Leptin levels are reduced in both cycling and amenorrheic athletes, and a diurnal pattern of 24-hour leptin levels is strikingly absent in amenorrheic athletes.[45]

Anorexia nervosa patients consistently exhibit hypoleptinemia.[46-49] A threshold effect for leptin occurs at low body weights. Leptin levels correlate linearly with body mass index in normal persons and recovering anorectic patients[49a] but uncouple in a nonlinear fashion in untreated anorectics.[46] A strong correlation is found between leptin levels and absolute body fat mass; however, fasting behavior, regardless of body fat, may also be correlated with low leptin levels.[50,51] A rapid, disproportional lowering of leptin levels often accompanies starvation.[50,52] Anorectic patients, thus, may have three factors leading to hypoleptinemia: low body fat, excessive exercise, and fasting behavior itself. However, leptin levels normalize and can even peak above normal levels with incomplete weight gain.[47,48] As leptin acts to reduce food intake, this premature restoration of leptin levels with only minor weight gain can be extremely detrimental to anorectic patients by actually perpetuating the disorder.

### OTHER PITUITARY HORMONE ABNORMALITIES

Serum growth hormone levels are elevated in starvation or any other restriction of food beyond the normal 12- to 15-hour overnight fast. Generally, basal serum growth hormone levels are higher than normal in anorexia nervosa but respond normally to provocative stimuli. These high levels are associated with a decreased level of somatomedin C (i.e., insulin-like growth factor-I), as is also found in starvation. Occasionally, low serum growth hormone levels are seen, with blunted responses to insulin-induced hypoglycemia.[6] Insulin-like growth factor is decreased, and both these abnormalities resolve with nutritional therapy. Nutritional deprivation may alter the growth hormone–insulin-like growth factor axis by down-regulation of growth hormone receptor or postreceptor.[53] A comparison of normal and anorectic subjects found that the elevation of growth hormone secretion in anorexia nervosa may be due to an increased frequency of secretory pulses superimposed on heightened tonic growth hormone secretion. Thus, the elevation may not simply result from a malnutrition-induced impairment of insulin-like growth factor-I production. Instead, it may reflect a complex hypothalamic dysregulation of growth hormone release.[54]

Sleep in anorexia nervosa has been the subject of ongoing investigation.[55] Growth hormone levels associated with delta-wave sleep are normal.[6] A paradoxic growth hormone secretory response to the infusion of TRH has been observed in underweight persons in both anorexia nervosa and starvation. The basal serum prolactin levels are normal, and TRH-stimulated prolactin levels also are normal, although the time of the peak prolactin level is delayed. With recovery (weight gain), all of these endocrine changes normalize. However, despite the normalization of serum gonadotropin secretory patterns, amenorrhea persists in 30% of patients.[6]

### ESTROGEN ABNORMALITIES

Sonographic imaging of the ovaries of patients with anorexia nervosa demonstrates cystic involvement resembling that seen at adolescence.[56,57] The low serum estradiol levels are partly attributable to the lack of ovarian stimulation. However, estrogen metabolism also is altered: the metabolism of estradiol, which normally proceeds with 16α-hydroxylation, is decreased in favor of 2-hydroxylation and the resulting formation of catechol estrogen (2-hydroxyestrone).[2] This latter compound has features of an antiestrogen because it has no intrinsic bioactivity. Thus, the extraordinarily low serum estrogen levels sometimes seen in anorexia nervosa are compounded by an endogenously produced antiestrogen. Furthermore, the lack of adipose tissue may deny to patients extraovarian sources of estrogen: normally, fat converts androstenedione to estrone.

## NEUROENDOCRINE AND PSYCHOLOGICAL CHARACTERISTICS AND INTERRELATIONS

The altered behavior patterns in anorexia nervosa are distinctive. Sometimes, periods of gorging alternate with food avoidance and starvation. Altered food intake combined with activity changes also may accompany hypothalamic tumors and other hypothalamic syndromes. Such changes also have been documented in rats with lesions of the ventromedial nucleus of the hypothalamus, a finding which led investigators to conclude that the ventromedial nucleus inhibits food intake and promotes activity—similar to the pattern seen in anorexia nervosa.[3]

Some of the changes of anorexia nervosa, including the lowered metabolic rate, a decrease in attainable oxygen uptake and $VO_{2max}$, an increase in serum cortisol (which stimulates gluconeogenesis and decreases peripheral glucose utilization), and the diminished serum gonadotropin levels (with a consequent loss of fertility), are appropriate adaptations to starvation.[3] Because of these neuroendocrine changes, the speculation had been that abnormalities of neurotransmission participate in the pathogenesis of the condition. In particular, excess dopamine and norepinephrine have known effects on behavior and appetite. In addition, β-endorphin affects feeding behavior; this hormone is thought to modulate the secretion of LHRH from the hypothalamus, and administration of its antagonist, naloxone, can restore LH pulsations in some persons with anorexia nervosa.

Patients with anorexia nervosa and those with secondary amenorrhea due to a hypothalamic cause commonly share a need for achievement and approval. On fear-of-failure scales, patients with anorexia score the highest.

Another early marker for anorexia nervosa is perceptual distortion. These patients consider themselves to be too fat despite their low weights. They consistently overestimate body size; this overestimation tends to disappear with weight gain. The perceptual distortion may reinforce dieting behavior, perpetuating the condition.

Anorexic behavior scales have been said to aid in differentiating persons with anorexia nervosa from those with secondary amenorrhea of other causes. Often, the scale consists of a psychological profile that is either self-administered or administered by a physician, nurse, or clinical psychologist. One study indicated that this scale is useful and accurate in distinguishing healthy persons from those with anorectic behavior.[58] Thus, it may prove useful in the early diagnosis of anorexia nervosa, particularly in patients with secondary amenorrhea only and little, if any, weight loss.

### OSTEOPOROSIS

A leading complication of amenorrhea seen with anorexia and weight loss is osteopenia. This is present in spinal, radial, and femoral sites, and is associated with fractures.[59–65] After 12 years, 67% of chronic anorectic patients suffered from medical comorbidity, most often involving osteoporosis and renal disease.[66] Longitudinal studies on bone density show little or no reversal with resolution of the amenorrhea.[60,63] These observations are important because hypoestrogenism in young adulthood may predispose to premature osteoporosis in later life. Increases in bone mass may occur in young persons before the return of normal menses, but bone mass remains below that of normal control subjects, possibly because of prolonged hypoestrogenism in adolescence, and, thus, may have permanent effects on peak bone mass.[64] Loss of bone mass also may occur. The effects of estrogen replacement on these changes need to be studied to determine whether the trend toward decreased bone mass can be reversed by therapy. Unfortunately, estrogen replacement does not restore bone mass in patients with anorexia nervosa.[67,68]

In general, 25-hydroxyvitamin D, 1,25 dihydroxyvitamin D, and osteocalcin levels are normal, although osteocalcin levels may be depressed because of lower bone turnover.[62] When reversal of osteoporosis occurs, it is seen more often with recovery from anorexia and is associated more tightly with weight gain than with return of menses. Some studies suggest, however, that bone mass does not appear to recover even with weight gain,[68a] calcium supplementation, and exercise. One study found that 14 out of 18 recovered anorexia nervosa patients exhibited osteope-

nia.[69] The increased cortisol levels seen in anorexia have been suggested as a mechanism for the osteopenia.[70]

## BULIMIA

### CHARACTERISTICS

Bulimia usually is a condition of young women, often related to previous anorectic behavior. These persons gorge themselves and use unusual means to lose weight, such as vomiting, enemas, and abuse of laxatives or diuretics. Gorging episodes may alternate with periods of severe food restriction. Most commonly, this syndrome occurs in high school and college students. Among males, bulimia is more common than is anorexia nervosa. According to the *Diagnostic and Statistical Manual of Mental Disorder, Revised Third Edition*, 4.5% of girls and women younger than 20 years of age have bulimia, whereas other sources estimate that at least 20% of this population exhibits bulimic behaviors.[71] This syndrome may occur in 3% to 15% of university students.[72,73] The weight may fluctuate, but usually not to dangerously low levels. The patient often has a history of other impulsive behavior, such as alcohol or drug use. Depression is common. Stealing and shoplifting, as well as unrestrained sexual promiscuity, may be part of the syndrome—unlike in anorexia nervosa, in which patients generally are sexually inactive. Depression and obsessive-compulsive behavior often coexist with eating disorders, particularly when bulimia is also present. Other comorbid problems include drug abuse and alcoholism.[74] Patients with bulimia tend to be slightly older than those with anorexia, usually between 17 and 25 years. A separate condition, known as *bulimia nervosa*, has been described, in which bulimic behavior has evolved from the prior, more restrictive anorexia nervosa–type pattern.

### CLINICAL MANIFESTATIONS

Persons with bulimia have a wide variety of superimposed medical problems, including vomiting-related tooth decay, parotid enlargement, stomach rupture, pancreatitis, metabolic alkalosis, and carpal-pedal spasm.

Occasionally, persons with bulimia have menstrual irregularities despite normal weight.[6] Some patients are anovulatory, yet have adequate estrogen secretion. Evidence exists for hormonal defects in CRH and cholecystokinin regulation.[75,76] Bulimic behavior often is secretive; many patients do not admit to these patterns even when questioned directly. The condition often is chronic, and increased anxiety, irritability, depression, and poor social functioning are common. The relapse rate for bulimia nervosa can be as high as 30%, although risk of relapse declines after approximately 4 years.[77] Eventually, protein and calorie malnutrition may supervene and contribute to the development of the reproductive disorder.

Several neurologic problems are associated with bulimia, including Huntington chorea and seizure disorders. Bulimia also may follow encephalitis and can be seen in association with the hypersomnia of Kleine-Levin syndrome (periodic attacks of hypersomnia and bulimia, often secondary to encephalitis, head injury, or hypothalamic tumor) and with parkinsonism; the latter patients improve in their eating patterns with treatment.[3]

## TREATMENT OF ANOREXIA NERVOSA AND BULIMIA

The treatment of anorexia nervosa and bulimia is controversial. All treatment modalities are directed toward the reestablishment of normal weight and eating habits. Treatment has included combinations of psychotherapy, including family therapy, psychoanalysis, and drug therapy. Tricyclic antidepressants, cyproheptadine, L-dopa, and metoclopramide have been used with variable success. Antidepressants may be the most successful, particularly for bulimia, in which drugs such as fluoxetine have a 30% success rate.[78] Behavior modification has been attempted, again with variable efficacy.

The early recognition of anorectic behavior is essential so that patients may be treated before the full-blown syndrome sets in. Because amenorrhea occurs early in the disease process, it often is the first symptom that causes patients to seek help. Thus, physicians should be particularly attentive to a history of dieting and weight loss in their young patients with amenorrhea. Patients who are 75% of ideal body weight or below need immediate and aggressive intervention. Dietary therapy is important because the response to psychotherapy is improved with nutritional rehabilitation. Usually, this is best accomplished in a hospital setting by a team consisting of a psychiatrist or a psychologist, an internist or a pediatrician, and, if possible, a nutritionist with special interest and expertise in anorexia nervosa and related eating disorders. Ninety percent of standard body weight may be a reasonable target weight for treatment, as it seems to be an average weight at which menses resume. Research shows that 86% of patients who reach this target resume menstruating within 6 months. Interestingly, the resumption does not depend on body fat, but rather on restoration of hypothalamic–pituitary–ovarian function.[79]

Considerable caution should be taken when treating severely malnourished patients. Rapid refeeding of patients who are <70% of ideal body weight may lead to hypophosphatemia, cardiac arrest, and delirium.[80] In addition, patients' exercise levels should be closely monitored, as refeeding restores muscle performance long before nutritional status normalizes. This improved muscle performance enables high levels of physical activity concomitant with sustained malnutrition.[81] Mortality from anorexia nervosa ranges from 8% to 18%, with lower rates in pediatric and adolescent groups. Morbidity persists with eating disorders concomitant with depression, obsessive-compulsive behavior, and poor sexual adjustment, although one study found that concomitant obsessive-compulsive disorder did not indicate a poorer prognosis for anorectic or bulimic patients.[82] Eating problems persist in more than half of all cases. Death results from starvation or its complications, including infection, renal or cardiac failure, arrhythmia, and complications of fluid imbalance.[83] Suicide also occurs, with an incidence of 5% to 7%. Laboratory findings obtained on initial diagnosis may predict a fatal or chronic prognosis. Low serum albumin levels and a low weight may prove lethal, whereas high serum creatinine and uric acid levels may predict a chronic course.[66]

Recovery from anorexia nervosa may take several years. Longitudinal studies highlight the extent to which treatment must be tailored to the individual symptoms and history of the patient.[84,85] More long-term follow-up studies should eventually help improve chances of recovery. In patients who do not have a return of menstrual function, fertility may be restored by the therapeutic induction of ovulation using clomiphene citrate or human menopausal gonadotropins. (Other causes of amenorrhea, such as pituitary tumors or premature ovarian failure, must be ruled out.) Cyclic menstrual function may be restored with LHRH administered intravenously or subcutaneously in a pulsatile manner through a pump. Despite a return to normal weight, some patients have permanent problems. A continuing preoccupation with food and persistent dieting behavior are common.[4]

For those patients who have recovered from anorexia nervosa but who never menstruate again, cyclic estrogen and progesterone replacement is indicated to prevent premature osteoporosis.[86] Such patients may refuse estrogen therapy, however, because of anxiety about gaining weight.

## REFERENCES

1. Warren MP. Anorexia nervosa and bulimia. In: Sciarra JJ, ed. Gynecology and obstetrics. Philadelphia: Harper & Row, 1988:1.
2. Morley JE, Blundell JE. The neurological basis of eating disorders: some formulations. Biol Psychiatry 1988; 23:53.
3. Warren MP. The effects of undernutrition on reproductive function in the human. Endocr Rev 1983; 4:363.
4. Garner DM, Garfinkel PE. Sociocultural factors in the development of anorexia nervosa. Psychol Med 1980; 10:647.
5. Hamilton LH, Brooks-Gunn J, Warren MP. Sociocultural influences on eating disorders in professional female ballet dancers. Int J Eat Disord 1985; 4(4):465.
6. Warren MP. Anorexia nervosa. In: DeGroot LJ, ed. Endocrinology, 3rd ed. Philadelphia: WB Saunders, 1995:2679.
7. American Psychiatric Association. Diagnostic and statistical manual of mental disorders, 3rd ed, rev. Washington: American Psychiatric Association, 1987.
8. Epling WF, Pierce WD, Stephen L. A theory of activity-based anorexia. Int J Eat Disord 1983; 3:27.
9. Aumariega AJ, Edwards P, Mitchell CB. Anorexia nervosa in black adolescents. J Am Acad Child Adolesc Psychiatry 1984; 1:111.
10. Askevold F, Heiberg A. Anorexia nervosa: two cases in discordant MZ twins. Psychother Psychosom 1979; 32:223.
11. Zelin AM, Lant AF. Anorexia nervosa presenting as reversible hypoglycemic coma. J R Soc Med 1984; 77:193.
12. Lyon M, Chatoor I, Atkins D, et al. Testing the hypothesis of the multidimensional model of anorexia nervosa in adolescents. Adolescence 1997; 32:101.
13. Warren MP, Vande Wiele RL. Clinical and metabolic features of anorexia nervosa. Am J Obstet Gynecol 1973; 117(3):435.
14. Smith NJ. Excessive weight loss and food aversion in athletes simulating anorexia nervosa. Pediatrics 1980; 66:139.
15. Halmi KA, Casper RC, Eckert ED, et al. Unique features associated with age of onset of anorexia nervosa. Psychiatry Res 1979; 1:209.
16. Brooks-Gunn J, Warren MP. Biological and social contributions to negative affect in young adolescent girls. Child Dev 1989; 60:40.
17. Wilson GT, Walsh BT. Eating disorders in the DSM-IV. J Abnorm Psychol 1991; 100(3):362.
18. Davis C, Katzman DK, Kaptein S, et al. The prevalence of high-level exercise in the eating disorders: etiological implications. Compr Psychiatry 1997; 38:321.
19. Lambert M, Hubert C, Depresseux G, et al. Hematological changes in anorexia nervosa are correlated with total body fat mass depletion. Int J Eat Disord 1997; 21:329.
20. Rich LM, Caine MR, Findling JW, Shaker JL. Hypoglycemic coma in anorexia nervosa. Case report and review of literature. Arch Intern Med 1990; 150:894.
21. McAnarney ER, Greydanus EE, Campanella VA, Hoekelman RA. Rib fractures and anorexia nervosa. J Adolesc Health 1983; 4:40.
22. Ayers JW, Gidwani GP, Schmidt IM, Gross M. Osteopenia in hypoestrogenic women with anorexia nervosa. Fertil Steril 1984; 41:224.
23. Rigotti NA, Nussbaum SR, Herzog DB, Neer RM. Osteoporosis in women with anorexia nervosa. N Engl J Med 1984; 311:1601.
24. Lambe EK, Katzman DK, Mikulis DJ, et al. Cerebral gray matter volume deficits after weight recovery from anorexia nervosa. Arch Gen Psychiatry 1997; 54:537.
25. Kato T, Shiiori T, Murashita J, Inubushi T. Phosphorus-31 magnetic resonance spectroscopic observations in 4 cases with anorexia nervosa. Prog Neuropsychopharmacol Biol Psychiatry 1997; 21:719.
26. Bradley SJ, Taylor MJ, Rovet JF, et al. Assessment of brain function in adolescent anorexia nervosa before and after weight gain. J Clin Exp Neuropsychol 1997; 19:20.
27. Boyar RM, Katz J, Finkelstein JW, et al. Anorexia nervosa: immaturity of the 24-hour luteinizing hormone secretory pattern. N Engl J Med 1974; 291:861.
28. Marshall JC, Kelch RP. Low dose pulsatile gonadotropin-releasing hormone in anorexia nervosa: a model of human pubertal development. J Clin Endocrinol Metab 1979; 49:712.
29. Pirke KM, Schweiger U, Strowitzki T, et al. Dieting causes menstrual irregularities in normal weight young women through impairment of episodic luteinizing hormone secretion. Fertil Steril 1989; 51:263.
30. Grossman A, Moulte PJA, McIntyre H, et al. Opiate mediation of amenorrhea in hyperprolactinemia and in weight loss-related amenorrhea. Clin Endocrinol (Oxf) 1982; 17:379.
31. Giusti M, Cavagnaro P, Torre R, et al. Endogenous opioid blockade and gonadotropin secretion: role of pulsatile luteinizing hormone-releasing hormone administration in anorexia nervosa and weight loss amenorrhea. Fertil Steril 1988; 49:797.
32. Warren MP, Jewelewicz R, Dyrenfurth I, et al. The significance of weight loss in the evaluation of pituitary response to LH-RH in women with secondary amenorrhea. J Clin Endocrinol Metab 1975; 40:601.
33. Vaisman N, Clark R, Rossi M, et al. Protein turnover and resting energy expenditure in patients with undernutrition and chronic lung disease. Am J Clin Nutr 1992; 55:63
34. Kiyohara K, Tamai H, Takaichi Y, et al. Decreased thyroidal triiodothyronine secretion in patients with anorexia nervosa: influence of weight recovery. Am J Clin Nutr 1989; 50:767.
35. Lesem MD, Kaye WH, Bissette G, et al. Cerebrospinal fluid TRH immunoreactivity in anorexia nervosa. Biol Psychiatry 1994; 35:48.

36. Boyar RM, Hellman LD, Roffwarg H, et al. Cortisol secretion and metabolism in anorexia nervosa. N Engl J Med 1977; 296:190.

37. Gold P, Gwirtsman H, Avgerinos P, et al. Abnormal hypothalamic-pituitary-adrenal function in anorexia nervosa. N Engl J Med 1986; 314:1335.

38. Flier JS. What's in a name? In search of leptin's physiologic role. J Clin Endocrinol Metab 1998; 83:1407.

39. Miller KK, Parulekar MS, Schoenfeld E, et al. Decreased leptin levels in normal weight women with hypothalamic amenorrhea: the effects of body composition and nutritional insults. J Clin Endocrinol Metab 1998; 83:2309.

40. Warren MP, Voussoughian F, Geer EB, et al. Functional hypothalamic amenorrhea: hypoleptinemia and disordered eating. J Clin Endocrinol Metab 1999; 84:873.

41. Warren MP, Voussoughian F, Geer EB, et al. Functional hypothalamic amenorrhea: hypoleptinemia and disordered eating. J Clin Endocrinol Metab 1999; 84(3):873.

42. Zamorano PL, Mahesh VB, DeSevilla LM, et al. Expression and localization of the leptin receptor in endocrine and neuroendocrine tissues of the rat. Neuroendocrinology 1997; 65:223.

43. Yu WH, Kimura M, Walczewska A, et al. Role of leptin in hypothalamic-pituitary function. Proc Natl Acad Sci U S A 1997; 94:1023.

44. Kopp W, Blum WF, von Prittwitz S, et al. Low leptin levels predict amenorrhea in underweight and eating disordered females. Mol Psychiatry 1997; 2:335.

45. Laughlin GA, Yen SSC. Hypoleptinemia in women athletes: absence of a diurnal rhythm with amenorrhea. J Clin Endocrinol Metab 1997; 82:318.

46. Eckert ED, Pomeroy C, Raymond N, et al. Leptin in anorexia nervosa. J Clin Endocrinol Metab 1998; 83:791.

47. Hebebrand J, Blum WF, Barth N, et al. Leptin levels in patients with anorexia nervosa are reduced in the acute stage and elevated upon short-term weight restoration. Mol Psychiatry 1997; 2:330.

48. Mantzoros C, Flier JS, Lesem MD, et al. Cerebrospinal fluid leptin in anorexia nervosa: correlation with nutritional status and potential role in resistance to weight gain. J Clin Endocrinol Metab 1997; 82:1845.

49. Casanueva FF, Dieguez C, Popovic V, et al. Serum immunoreactive leptin concentrations in patients with anorexia nervosa before and after partial weight recovery. Biochem Molec Med 1997; 60:116.

49a. Frey J, Hebebrand J, Muller B, et al. Reduced body fat in long-term followed-up female patients with anorexia nervosa. Journal of Psychiatric Research 2000; 34(1):83

50. Boden G, Chen X, Mozzoli M, Ryan I. Effect of fasting on serum leptin in normal human subjects. J Clin Endocrinol Metab 1996; 81:3419.

51. Rosenbaum M, Nicolson M, Hirsch J, et al. Effects of gender, body composition, and menopause on plasma concentrations of leptin. J Clin Endocrinol Metab 1996; 81:3424.

52. Geldszus R, Mayr B, Horn R, et al. Serum leptin and weight reduction in female obesity. Eur J Endocrinol 1996; 135:659.

53. Counts DR, Gwirtsman H, Carlsson LMS, et al. The effect of anorexia nervosa and refeeding on growth hormone-binding protein, the insulin-like growth factors (IGFs), and the IGF-binding proteins. J Clin Endocrinol Metab 1992; 75:762.

54. Scacchi M, Pincelli AI, Caumo A, et al. Spontaneous nocturnal growth hormone secretion in anorexia nervosa. J Clin Endocrinol Metab 1997; 82:3225.

55. Levy AB, Dixon KN, Schmidt H. Sleep architecture in anorexia nervosa and bulimia. Biol Psychiatry 1988; 23:99.

56. Adams J, Franks S, Polson DW, et al. Multifollicular ovaries: clinical and endocrine features and response to pulsatile gonadotropin releasing hormone. Lancet 1985; 2:1375.

57. Treasure JL, Gordon PAL, King EA, et al. Cystic ovaries: a phase of anorexia nervosa. Lancet 1985; 2:1379.

58. Fries H. Studies on secondary amenorrhea, anorectic behavior and body image perception: importance for the early recognition of anorexia nervosa. In: Vigersky R, ed. Anorexia nervosa. New York: Raven Press, 1977:163.

59. Bachrach LK, Guido D, Katzman D, et al. Decreased bone density in adolescent girls with anorexia nervosa. Pediatrics 1990; 86:440.

60. Rigotti NA, Neer RM, Skates SJ, et al. The clinical course of osteoporosis in anorexia nervosa: a longitudinal study of cortical bone mass. JAMA 1991; 265:1133.

61. Salisbury JJ, Mitchell JE. Bone mineral density and anorexia nervosa in women. Am J Psychiatry 1991; 148:768.

62. Davies KM, Pearson PH, Huseman CA, et al. Reduced bone mineral in patients with eating disorders. Bone 1990; 11:143.

63. Bachrach LK, Katzman DK, Litt IF, et al. Recovery from osteopenia in adolescent girls with anorexia nervosa. J Clin Endocrinol Metab 1991; 72:602.

64. Jonnavithula S, Warren MP, Fox RP, Lazaro MI. Bone density is compromised in amenorrheic women despite return of menses: a 2-year study. Obstet Gynecol 1993; 81:669.

65. Fonseca VA, D'Souza V, Houlder S, et al. Vitamin D deficiency and low osteocalcin concentrations in anorexia nervosa. J Clin Pathol 1988; 41:195.

66. Herzog W, Deter HC, Fiehn W, Petzold E. Medical findings and predictors of long-term physical outcome in anorexia nervosa: a prospective, 12-year follow-up study. Psychol Med 1997; 27:269.

67. Kreipe RE, Hicks DG, Rosier RN, Puzas JE. Preliminary findings on the effects of sex hormones on bone metabolism in anorexia nervosa. J Adolesc Health 1993; 14:319.

68. Klibanski A, Biller BMK, Schoenfeld DA, et al. The effects of estrogen administration on trabecular bone loss in young women with anorexia nervosa. J Clin Endocrinol Metab 1995; 80:898.

68a. Baker D, Roberts R, Towell T. Factors predictive of bone mineral density in eating-disordered women: a longitudinal study. International Journal of Eating Disorders 2000; 27(1):29.

69. Ward A, Brown N, Treasure J. Persistent osteopenia after recovery from anorexia nervosa. Int J Eat Disord 1997; 22:71.

70. Biller BMK, Saxe V, Herzog DB, et al. Mechanisms of osteoporosis in adult and adolescent women with anorexia nervosa. J Clin Endocrinol Metab 1989; 68:548.

71. Schwartz DM, Thompson MG, Johnson CL. Anorexia nervosa and bulimia: the sociocultural context. In: Emmett SW, ed. Theory and treatment of anorexia nervosa and bulimia. New York: Brunner/Mazel, 1985:95.

72. Stangler RS, Printz AM. DSM-III: psychiatric diagnosis in a university population. Am J Psychiatry 1980; 137:937.

73. Halmi KA, Falk JR, Schwartz E. Binge-eating and vomiting: a survey of a college population. Psychol Med 1981; 11:697.

74. Holderness CC, Brooks-Gunn J, Warren MP. The co-morbidity of eating disorders and substance abuse: a review of the literature. Int J Eat Disord 1994; 16:1.

75. Mortola JF, Rassmussen DD, Yen SSC. Alterations of the adrenocorticotropin-cortisol axis in normal weight bulimic women: evidence for a central mechanism. J Clin Endocrinol Metab 1989; 68:517.

76. Geracioti TDJ, Liddle RA. Impaired cholecystokinin secretion in bulimia nervosa. N Engl J Med 1988; 319:689.

77. Keel PK, Mitchell JE. Outcome in bulimia nervosa. Am J Psychiatry 1997; 154:313.

78. Walsh BT, Devlin MJ. The pharmacologic treatment of eating disorders. In: Shaffer D, ed. Pediatric psychopharmacology. Philadelphia: WB Saunders, 1992:149.

79. Golden NH, Jacobson MS, Schebendach J, et al. Resumption of menses in anorexia nervosa. Arch Pediatr Adolesc Med 1997; 151:16.

80. Kohn MR, Golden NH, Shenker IR. Cardiac arrest and delirium: presentations of the refeeding syndrome in severely malnourished adolescents with anorexia nervosa. J Adolesc Health 1998; 22:239.

81. Rigaud D, Moukaddem M, Cohen B, et al. Refeeding improves muscle performance without normalization of muscle mass and oxygen consumption in anorexia nervosa patients. Am J Clin Nutr 1997; 65:1845.

82. Thiel A, Zuger M, Jacoby GE, Schussler G. Thirty-month outcome in patients with anorexia or bulimia nervosa and concomitant obsessive-compulsive disorder. Am J Psychiatry 1998; 155:244.

83. Comerci GD. Medical complications of anorexia nervosa and bulimia nervosa. Med Clin North Am 1990; 74(5):1293.

84. Herzog W, Schellberg D, Deter HC. First recovery in anorexia nervosa patients in the long-term course: a discrete-time survival analysis. J Consult Clin Psychol 1997; 65:169.

85. Strober M, Freeman R, Morrell W. The long-term course of severe anorexia nervosa in adolescents: survival analysis of recovery, relapse, and outcome predictors over 10–15 years in a prospective study. Int J Eat Disord 1997; 22:339.

86. Locke RJ, Warren MP. How to prevent bone loss in women with hypothalamic amenorrhea. Women's Health in Primary Care 2000; 3(4):270.

# CHAPTER 129

# FUEL HOMEOSTASIS AND INTERMEDIARY METABOLISM OF CARBOHYDRATE, FAT, AND PROTEIN

NEIL B. RUDERMAN, KEITH TORNHEIM, AND MICHAEL N. GOODMAN

## FUEL HOMEOSTASIS

### ENERGY RESERVOIRS

A basic problem in human fuel homeostasis is that the body requires a constant expenditure of energy to maintain cellular metabolism, yet intake of food (energy) is intermittent. To deal with this, humans, like all mammals, ingest more calories during a meal than they require for their immediate metabolic needs and store the excess in readily mobilized reservoirs of carbohydrate, fat, and protein[1-3] (Table 129-1).

The principal storage form of carbohydrate in humans is glycogen. Approximately 80 g of carbohydrate is stored as glycogen in liver and 400 g is stored in muscle in the postabsorp-

**TABLE 129-1.**
**Fuel Reservoirs of Normal 70-kg Man after Overnight Fast**

| Fuel (Organ) | Mass (g) | Energy Content (kcal) |
|---|---|---|
| **TISSUE** | | |
| Fat (adipose tissue) | 12,000 | 110,000 |
| Protein (mainly muscle) | 6000 | 24,000 |
| Glycogen (muscle) | 400 | 1600 |
| Glycogen (liver) | 80 | 320 |
| **CIRCULATING** | | |
| Glucose* | 20 | 80 |
| Free fatty acids | 0.3 | 3 |
| Triglycerides | 3 | 30 |
| Ketone bodies | 0.2 | 0.8 |
| Amino acids | 6 | 24 |

*Circulating glucose, ketone bodies, and amino acids assume equal concentrations in plasma and interstitial fluid. During starvation, the amount of ketone bodies in the circulation may increase as much as 100-fold.

(Data from Cahill GF. Starvation in man. N Engl J Med 1970; 282:688; and from Cahill GF, Aoki T, Rossini AA. Metabolism in obesity and anorexia nervosa. In: Wurtman RJ, Wurtman JJ, eds. Nutrition and the brain, vol 3. New York: Raven Press, 1979:1.)

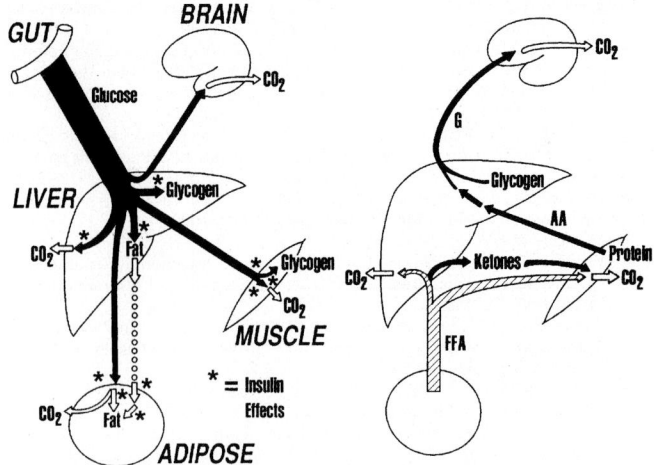

**FIGURE 129-1. A,** Fuel metabolism during a carbohydrate meal. Soon after the ingestion of a carbohydrate meal, insulin levels rise and stimulate the uptake of glucose by muscle and adipose tissue. Glucose is the major oxidative fuel of all major tissues at this time. Glucose that is present in excess of the oxidative needs of tissues is stored as glycogen or lipid. *Asterisks* indicate steps enhanced by insulin. **B,** Fuel metabolism after an overnight fast (postabsorptive). After ~12 hours of starvation, insulin concentrations have returned to basal levels, and glucose entering the circulation is derived from both hepatic glycogen and gluconeogenesis. Free fatty acids (*FFA*) produced from adipocyte lipolysis have become a principal fuel for skeletal muscle. (*G,* glucose; *AA,* amino acids.) (Reprinted from Joslin's Diabetes Mellitus, Thirteenth Edition, 1994. Copyright 1994 by Joslin Diabetes Center.)

tive state. Hepatic glycogen can be used to generate free glucose for release into the circulation. In contrast, muscle does not possess the enzymatic machinery needed to generate free glucose; instead, its glycogen serves principally as a fuel for muscle itself and as a source of lactate, pyruvate, and alanine for gluconeogenesis during early starvation and exercise.[4]

The 6 kg of protein in a 70-kg man hypothetically could provide an additional 24,000 kcal of fuel. However, unlike the glucose stored as glycogen and the lipid stored as triglyceride, the amino acids in body protein do not constitute a true reservoir of expendable energy. Rather, each protein molecule appears to have a function, whether it be an enzyme, a structural component of a tissue such as collagen, or an element of a contractile system such as actin and myosin in skeletal muscle. Nevertheless, some breakdown of body protein occurs during a fast, and many of the amino acids released are used by the liver for gluconeogenesis.

By far the largest energy reservoir in humans is fat. A nonobese 70-kg man has ~12 kg of adipose tissue triglyceride, the equivalent of roughly 110,000 kcal. In a totally starved person, this amount would be sufficient to supply fuel needs for ~60 days. As well as being more abundant, fat is a more efficient energy store than is either glycogen or protein: ~9.5 kcal is generated per gram of fat oxidized versus only 4 kcal/g for protein and glycogen. Furthermore, fat exists in a nearly anhydrous environment in the adipocyte, whereas each gram of protein and glycogen is associated with ~3 g of water. Thus, the caloric density of adipose tissue is ~8.5 kcal/g, whereas a gram of glycogen or protein provides only 1 kcal. If an equicaloric amount of glycogen were to be substituted for the fat in the man described in Table 129-1, his weight would increase from 70 to 196 kg. Clearly, fat has evolved as the principal fuel reservoir in all mobile terrestrial organisms that carry out sustained activity.[2,3]

## FUEL CONSUMPTION: BRAIN AND MUSCLE

Although all human tissues require energy, fuel homeostasis is understood most easily in terms of its principal function of serving the needs of brain and muscle, the major consumers of fuel. The brain uses glucose exclusively as its fuel except during prolonged starvation and other ketotic states, when it also uses the lipid-derived fuels, acetoacetate and β-hydroxybutyrate (ketone bodies).[1–3,5,6] In a 70-kg man, the brain oxidizes ~120 g of glucose per day, the equivalent of ~25% of the body's total caloric expenditure. As is discussed later, because of the brain's

dependence on glucose as a fuel, blood glucose levels must be carefully regulated to maintain central nervous system function under most conditions.

Muscle makes up 40% of the body's mass and accounts for 20% to 30% of its oxygen consumption at rest and for as much as 90% during exercise. Unlike brain, muscle can use fatty acids as well as glucose as a fuel and, like brain, it can use ketone bodies.[7–9] The relative use of these fuels depends on a person's nutritional and hormonal status and, if exercise is being performed, on the duration and intensity of that exercise. Generally, glucose is the principal fuel of resting muscle after a carbohydrate meal, and fatty acids and ketone bodies are the principal fuels during periods of caloric deprivation.[7–10] During exercise of mild to moderate intensity, fatty acids tend to be the predominant fuel of muscle, especially when the exercise is prolonged. In contrast, carbohydrate is used to a greater extent during the initial phases of exercise and when the exercise is intense.[7–10]

## REGULATORY CONTROLS

The regulation of fuel homeostasis in humans is complex. Hormonal and neural factors, plasma levels of specific fuels, and, in muscle, ongoing or prior contractions all play a role.[7,9,10] Numerous hormonal factors control the mobilization of fuels from their reservoirs (catabolism); however, only one of them, insulin, controls both their formation (anabolism) and mobilization.[11,12] Insulin stimulates glycogen synthesis and inhibits its breakdown in both muscle and liver, and it stimulates the synthesis and inhibits the degradation of triglycerides and proteins in many tissues. Thus, insulin is the principal anabolic and anticatabolic hormone. Concordantly, insulin levels invariably are increased in the absorptive state when exogenous substrates are used both for energy metabolism and the repletion of fuel reservoirs (Fig. 129-1A), and they are decreased in the postabsorptive state and during starvation, when fuel reservoirs are broken down to provide for the needs of vital organs (Fig. 129-1B).

Catabolic factors counter the effects of insulin and cause fuels to be mobilized from their reservoirs. They appear to differ from one tissue to another. Thus, hepatic glycogenolysis is stimulated by glucagon and epinephrine, hepatic protein degradation by glucagon, and muscle glycogenolysis by epinephrine and $Ca^{2+}$ released during contraction. In the fat cell, triglyceride lipolysis is enhanced by a wide variety of endogenous stimuli, one of the most important being norepinephrine released from sympathetic nerve endings.[7,13]

In general, gradual changes in the balance between insulin and counterinsulin hormones allow for a smooth transition of fuel metabolism when humans go from the fed to a starved state (see Fig. 129-1). As is discussed later, substantial imbalances between insulin and counterinsulin hormones can lead to major derangements of fuel homeostasis such as hypoglycemia and diabetic ketoacidosis.

# GLUCOSE HOMEOSTASIS IN NORMAL HUMANS

The concentration of glucose in the circulation is more closely regulated than that of any other fuel. In normal humans, it is generally maintained between 70 and 120 mg/dL (3.8–6.7 mmol/L), whereas variations in plasma free fatty acids (FFAs) and ketone bodies may be as great as 10- and 100-fold, respectively.[1,6] Plasma glucose must be maintained above a certain level because it is the sole fuel of the central nervous system under most physiologic conditions. This presents no problem at normal plasma glucose concentrations because the metabolism of glucose by brain rather than its transport across the blood–brain barrier is rate limiting. As the plasma glucose concentration falls, however, brain glucose transport diminishes and, at hypoglycemic levels (typically <3.6 mmol/L in a previously normoglycemic person), it becomes limiting for brain glucose utilization.[14,15] Even moderate degrees of hypoglycemia can cause substantial cerebral dysfunction in some individuals, and severe hypoglycemia can lead to seizures, coma, and even brain death. The precise glucose concentration at which central nervous system dysfunction occurs may differ considerably in different individuals; symptoms tend to occur at higher concentrations of glucose in patients with diabetes mellitus, and at lower concentrations in patients with chronic or recurrent hypoglycemia.[15] Studies of animals suggest that this difference may be secondary to adaptations in glucose transport at the blood–brain barrier.[16]

The upper level of plasma glucose also is closely regulated in normal humans. This is presumably because moderate elevations in blood glucose are disadvantageous for survival. In keeping with this notion, moderate degrees of hyperglycemia in pregnant women (i.e., gestational diabetes) are associated with an increased incidence of congenital malformations, morbidity, and mortality in the fetus. Furthermore, prevention of such hyperglycemia appears to prevent these complications[17] (see Chap. 156).

## ROLE OF LIVER

Maintenance of the plasma glucose concentration in the postabsorptive state is largely the responsibility of the liver. The liver can provide glucose for other tissues, either by breaking down its own glycogen stores or by synthesizing it from amino acids, lactate, pyruvate, and glycerol (*gluconeogenesis*). It occupies this unique role in metabolism because it contains the enzyme glucose-6-phosphatase, which catalyzes the conversion of glucose-6-phosphate to free glucose. Other tissues, including muscle, adipose tissue, and brain, also possess the enzymatic apparatus to degrade glycogen and to synthesize glucose-6-phosphate from amino acids and lactate; however, they either lack glucose-6-phosphatase, or they possess too little of it to release free glucose into the circulation in significant amounts.[7,13,18,19]

Increases in glucagon and epinephrine and a decrease in insulin appear to be the principal hormonal stimuli for glyco-

genolysis whenever blood glucose levels are falling. Insulin inhibits the stimulation of glycogen breakdown by both glucagon and epinephrine, and substantial evidence suggests that it is the relative balance between insulin and these counterinsulin hormones that determines the rate of glycogenolysis under most physiologic conditions. Acting within this hormonal framework, hepatic glycogen metabolism also is modulated by the concentration of glucose. High concentrations of glucose, such as occur after a meal, stimulate hepatic glycogen synthesis and inhibit its breakdown, whereas low glucose concentrations have the reverse effect.[18–20]

Gluconeogenesis, like glycogenolysis, is stimulated by glucagon and catecholamines and inhibited by insulin, and its rate is largely determined by the balance between these hormones.[18–20] Glucocorticoids are permissive; when they are lacking, as in an adrenalectomized rat, the ability of glucagon and catecholamines to stimulate hepatic gluconeogenesis is lost, and the release of amino acids and other gluconeogenic precursors from the periphery is diminished. The principal gluconeogenic precursors are amino acids released from muscle and other tissues, lactate, and glycerol, which is derived principally from the hydrolysis of adipose tissue triglyceride.[1,6,19,21] Lactate accounts for ~50% of gluconeogenic precursor in the postabsorptive state and an even higher percentage during exercise. It arises principally from red blood cells, platelets, and the renal medulla, which derive all of their energy from anaerobic glycolysis, and, more importantly, from tissues in which either glycolysis is accelerated beyond the capacity for pyruvate oxidation (e.g., exercising muscle) or pyruvate dehydrogenase is inhibited (e.g., muscle during starvation). Under all of these circumstances, much of the glucose taken up by a tissue is metabolized only as far as lactate and pyruvate, which are reconverted to glucose in the liver. This sequence of events is referred to as the *Cori cycle*.[6,7,13]

Studies in rats suggest that the amino acids used for gluconeogenesis are derived from protein breakdown in muscle, liver, and gut during early starvation, and almost exclusively from muscle during longer starvation.[22] This protein breakdown is decreased when plasma insulin levels are high, such as after a meal rich in carbohydrate and protein. Conversely, it is increased when plasma insulin levels are low, such as in early starvation and untreated type 1 diabetes, or when insulin is bioineffective, such as after trauma or when cytokines and other factors counter its action during sepsis. The role of other hormones in regulating protein metabolism is less clear. Glucagon can stimulate hepatic protein degradation directly, but it has no direct effect on muscle.[1] Glucocorticoids in large amounts inhibit protein synthesis and probably stimulate protein degradation in muscle and other tissues.[23] However, the role of physiologic alterations in plasma glucocorticoid levels in the regulation of protein catabolism is not clear.

Alanine is the principal amino acid used for gluconeogenesis in humans.[24] Alanine and glutamine account for 50% of the amino acids released from muscle even though they make up <15% of muscle protein.[1,24] The additional alanine arises from the amination of pyruvate generated principally by glycolysis; thus, alanine is a vehicle for the transfer of nitrogen from muscle to liver. Glutamine is formed primarily from the amidation of glutamate in muscle, a reaction catalyzed by glutamine synthetase.[1] Glutamine is used primarily by the gut and kidney, and under most circumstances, it is not a significant gluconeogenic substrate for the liver.[6,25,26]

## ROLE OF KIDNEY AND INTESTINE

Kidney, like liver, possesses the complete enzymatic apparatus for gluconeogenesis. During brief periods of starvation, it accounts for 10% to 25% of gluconeogenesis. During longer starvation and other states in which the kidney has to cope with a large acid load (e.g., metabolic acidosis), renal gluconeogene-

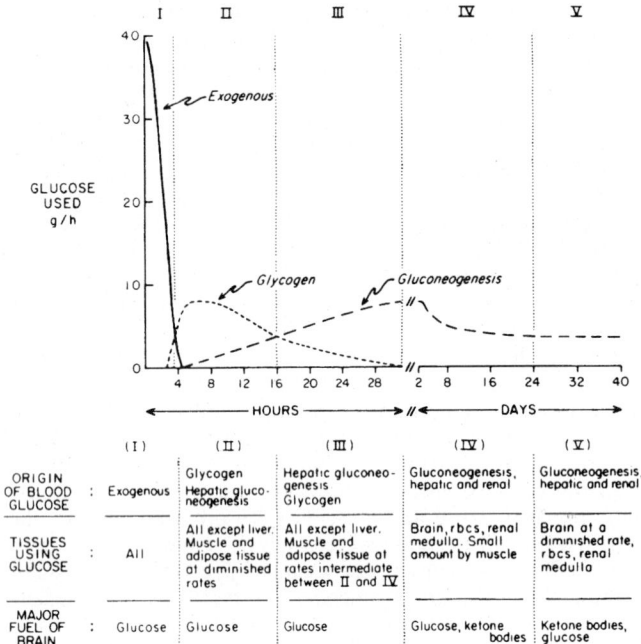

| | (I) | (II) | (III) | (IV) | (V) |
|---|---|---|---|---|---|
| ORIGIN OF BLOOD GLUCOSE : | Exogenous | Glycogen Hepatic gluconeogenesis | Hepatic gluconeogenesis Glycogen | Gluconeogenesis, hepatic and renal | Gluconeogenesis, hepatic and renal |
| TISSUES USING GLUCOSE : | All | All except liver. Muscle and adipose tissue at diminished rates | All except liver. Muscle and adipose tissue at rates intermediate between II and IV | Brain, rbcs, renal medulla. Small amount by muscle | Brain at a diminished rate, rbcs, renal medulla |
| MAJOR FUEL OF BRAIN : | Glucose | Glucose | Glucose | Glucose, ketone bodies | Ketone bodies, glucose |

**FIGURE 129-2.** Five phases of glucose homeostasis. (*rbcs*, red blood cells.) (From Ruderman NB, Aoki TT, Cahill GF. Gluconeogenesis and its disorders in man. In: Hanson R, Mehlman M, eds. Gluconeogenesis. New York: John Wiley and Sons, 1975:515.)

sis is accelerated. The principal gluconeogenic substrates for the kidney are glutamine, which also is its principal source of free ammonia; lactate; and glycerol.[25,26] During long-term starvation, when hepatic gluconeogenesis is diminished, the kidney may be responsible for as much as 50% of the glucose entering the circulation.[4]

It has been demonstrated that the small intestine has the capability of being a gluconeogenic organ[26a] and that it may contribute 20% to 25% of total endogenous glucose production in fasted and diabetic rats.[26b] Interestingly, glutamine appears to be its major gluconeogenic precursor. The importance of intestinal gluconeogenesis in humans remains to be established.

## FIVE PHASES OF GLUCOSE HOMEOSTASIS

The roles of hepatic glycogen metabolism and gluconeogenesis in the regulation of blood glucose are best illustrated by a description of glucose homeostasis in fed and fasted human beings. Glucose homeostasis can be divided into five phases on the basis of the origin of blood glucose, as depicted in Figure 129-2, in which glucose utilization is plotted against time in a theoretical person who ingests 100 g of glucose and then fasts for 40 days.[1,6]

### ABSORPTIVE PHASE

For 3 to 4 hours after glucose ingestion (*phase I*, the absorptive period), blood glucose is derived principally from exogenous carbohydrate. The concentrations of insulin and glucose are increased, whereas that of glucagon is depressed. Glucose in excess of the fuel needs of the liver and peripheral tissues is stored as glycogen, predominantly in liver and muscle, or is converted to lipid. This is the only phase in which the liver is a net user of glucose.

### POSTABSORPTIVE PHASE AND EARLY STARVATION

By the end of the absorptive period, insulin, glucose, and glucagon return to basal (12 hours postabsorptive) levels (*phase II*) and the liver produces glucose, which is derived principally from stored glycogen. The major user of glucose now is the brain. Tissues that derive all or most of their energy from anaer-

obic glycolysis, such as red and white blood cells and the renal medulla, also use glucose. Muscle and adipose tissue use glucose at a decreased rate. Further, the oxidation of glucose is inhibited in these tissues at the pyruvate dehydrogenase step, which causes increased release of lactate, pyruvate, and alanine, all of which can be used for gluconeogenesis. This decrease in glucose oxidation is the first of the body's adaptations to conserve protein while maintaining the brain's glucose supply during starvation.

After an overnight fast, a substantial part of the glucose released by liver is still derived from glycogen.[27] The approximately 80 g of glycogen in the liver are adequate to meet the fuel needs of peripheral tissues (~180 g per day, of which 120 g is used by brain) for only 12 hours; therefore, gluconeogenesis must rapidly replace glycogen as the major provider of glucose. Concordantly, the ability of the liver cell to carry out gluconeogenesis is enhanced after 12 to 48 hours of starvation (*phase III* and early *phase IV*), apparently secondary to both a further decrease in insulin and an increase in glucagon. Likewise, the release of gluconeogenic precursors from peripheral tissues and of FFA from fat (for which oxidation enhances hepatic gluconeogenesis) is increased because of lack of insulin. At this point, liver glycogen is depleted, the brain is not yet using significant amounts of ketone bodies, and the demand for gluconeogenesis is at its peak. Thus, this also is the time of greatest susceptibility to hypoglycemia because of impaired gluconeogenesis. Children[28] and pregnant women[17] are particularly susceptible to hypoglycemia during this period—the child because of the disproportionate size of the brain relative to tissues that provide gluconeogenic substrate (e.g., muscle) and the mother because she has to supply glucose to the fetus as well as to herself.

### PROLONGED STARVATION

During the latter part of phase IV and in phase V, the rate of hepatic gluconeogenesis diminishes, ketone bodies partially replace glucose as a fuel for the brain,[1–3,5] and body protein is conserved. The mechanism by which protein is conserved is unclear; however, animal studies indicate that the presence of lipid stores is required and that protein catabolism is accelerated once plasma FFA and ketone bodies begin to fall.[29]

### EXERCISE

The ability of normal humans to maintain glucose homeostasis is most severely tested during exercise. During intense exercise, the glucose demand by muscle can increase ten-fold or more, yet plasma glucose levels must be maintained for the central nervous system. This increased demand for glucose is met by the liver.[8] Liver provides glucose initially by breaking down its glycogen stores and later by rapid gluconeogenesis. In many respects, the response of the liver during exercise is a telescoped version of its response during starvation, with many of the same hormonal alterations, including diminished insulin levels and increased glucagon levels in plasma.[30,31] Significant differences exist, however, including a more important role for catecholamines in glucose homeostasis during exercise.[30–32] Interestingly, exercise may increase the sensitivity of skeletal muscle to insulin for many hours postexercise,[33] an effect that may contribute to its beneficial effects on glucose tolerance in some patients with type 2 diabetes (see later).

## GLUCOSE HOMEOSTASIS IN DIABETES MELLITUS

### TYPE 1 DIABETES

The most common cause of glucose dysregulation in humans is diabetes mellitus. Patients with type 1 diabetes, because of an absolute deficiency of insulin, have both an accelerated rate of hepatic glucose production and a decreased rate of glucose utilization by peripheral tissues. Insulin therapy corrects the hyperglycemia; however, glycemic control equivalent to that of persons without diabetes rarely is achieved. An added therapeutic problem in patients with type 1 diabetes is that the counterregulatory response to insulin-induced hypoglycemia may be abnormal.[15] Thus, in certain patients, glucagon secretion in response to a decreasing plasma glucose level is deficient. Epinephrine serves as a backup to glucagon in this circumstance; however, in some patients with type 1 diabetes, such as those with autonomic neuropathy, its secretion also may be abnormal. These patients are poor candidates for intensive insulin therapy.

Patients with type 1 diabetes also may become hypoglycemic during and after exercise. Hypoglycemia occurs during exercise when plasma insulin levels are high as a result of previous injections of insulin, and because of this hepatic glucose production is suppressed in the face of increased glucose utilization by muscle.[30,34] A similar mechanism probably accounts for the hypoglycemia that sometimes occurs in patients with type 1 diabetes many hours after exercise.[30,35] To prevent this hypoglycemia, patients with type 1 diabetes often must ingest supplemental carbohydrate or diminish their insulin dose on days they exercise.[35]

## TYPE 2 DIABETES

The basis for impaired glucose homeostasis is more complex in patients with type 2 diabetes than in those with type 1 diabetes. Abnormalities in insulin secretion and peripheral resistance to the action of insulin may both be present in patients with type 2 diabetes. Insulin resistance is particularly important in patients with obesity and mild type 2 diabetes (see section on Insulin-Resistance Syndrome; see Chaps. 137 through 139, and 146); such patients are more likely to benefit from diet and exercise.[36] In contrast, diminished insulin secretion is more prominent in nonobese patients and patients with severe hyperglycemia. Both factors are present in many patients, and their relative importance may vary not only with obesity, but with duration and severity of disease. Many studies suggest that, in patients with type 2 diabetes, fasting hyperglycemia is principally the result of increased hepatic glucose production and that postprandial hyperglycemia is due to diminished peripheral glucose utilization.[37]

## INSULIN-RESISTANCE SYNDROME (SYNDROME X)

Type 2 diabetes in many persons is preceded by a period in which skeletal muscle and possibly other peripheral tissues are resistant to the action of insulin.[38,39] Thus, many first-degree relatives of patients with type 2 diabetes[40] and persons followed up longitudinally who later become diabetic[41] have been shown to be hyperinsulinemic and insulin resistant, as have persons at risk for essential hypertension, certain dyslipidemias, and premature coronary heart disease.[38,41] This insulin-resistance syndrome is sometimes referred to as syndrome X (see Chap. 145).[41] It is often, although not invariably, associated with obesity, particularly obesity in which intraabdominal fat is disproportionately increased,[42,43] although many affected individuals are normal weight.[44] The metabolic defects causing this insulin resistance are still unclear; however, higher plasma FFA levels, alterations in cellular lipids (see later) and an impaired ability of insulin to activate glycogen synthase in muscle may be early events.[39-44] An important and unresolved question is whether this insulin resistance is reversible with diet and exercise or pharmacologic therapy, and, if so, whether this will prevent the development of diabetes and the other disorders associated with this syndrome.[44,45] In this regard, two studies showing diminished progression from impaired glucose toler-

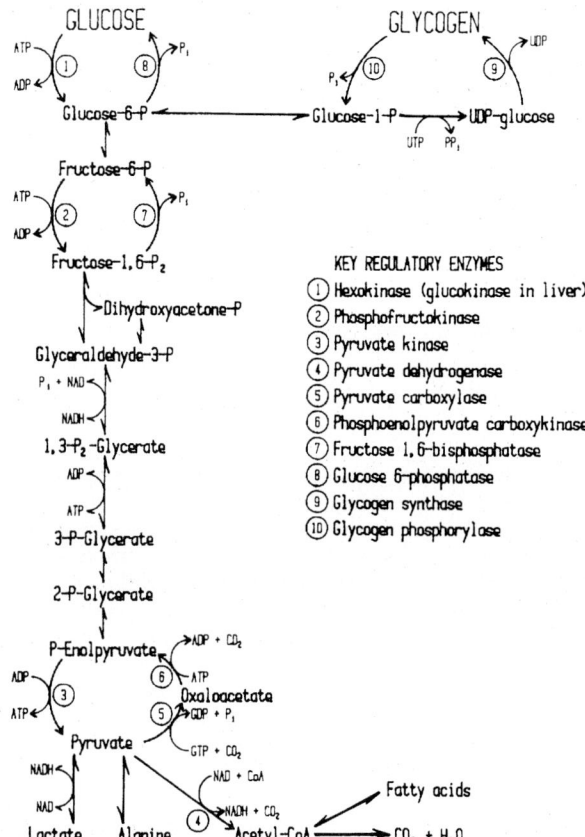

**FIGURE 129-3.** General scheme of glucose and glycogen metabolism. Amounts of various enzymes and their regulatory properties can differ considerably depending on the tissue (see text). In particular, glucose-6-phosphatase is absent in muscle and most other tissues except liver and kidney. (*ATP*, adenosine triphosphate; *ADP*, adenosine diphosphate; *P$_i$*, inorganic phosphate; *P*, phosphate; *UDP*, uridine diphosphate; *UTP*, uridine triphosphate; *PP$_i$*, pyrophosphate; *NAD*, nicotinamide adenine dinucleotide, oxidized form; *NADH*, nicotinamide adenine dinucleotide, reduced form; *GDP*, guanosine diphosphate; *GTP*, guanosine triphosphate; *CoA*, coenzyme A.)

ance to type 2 diabetes in subjects placed on diet and/or exercise regimens for 6 years are noteworthy.[46,47]

## INTERMEDIARY METABOLISM OF GLUCOSE AND GLYCOGEN

### GENERAL REMARKS

The major pathways of glucose and glycogen metabolism are connected at glucose-6-phosphate (Fig. 129-3). Thus, glucose-6-phosphate is both the precursor for glycogen synthesis and glycolysis, and the product of glycogen breakdown and gluconeogenesis. Moreover, it is the immediate substrate for the pentose phosphate pathway, which supplies the reduced form of nicotinamide-adenine dinucleotide phosphate (NADPH), needed for fatty acid biosynthesis and other processes, and ribose-5-phosphate, needed for nucleotide and nucleic acid biosynthesis. Glucose transport into the cell is important in the regulation of its metabolism in muscle and some other nonhepatic tissues.[7,13]

Although the pathways of glucose and glycogen metabolism are similar in muscle and liver (see Fig. 129-3), profound differences exist in their control and coordination in the two tissues. For instance, in muscle, when glycogenolysis occurs during exercise, it is accompanied by an increase in glycolysis, whereas hepatic glycogenolysis (e.g., in response to low blood glucose) usually occurs when glycolysis is inhibited and gluconeogenesis is enhanced. Likewise, insulin-mediated glucose transport may be rate limiting for both glycogen synthesis and glycolysis in muscle, whereas hepatic glucose transport is far more rapid and is not acutely dependent on insulin.

## MECHANISMS OF METABOLIC REGULATION

Nearly all biochemical reactions, including those of glucose metabolism, are catalyzed by specific enzymes. Enzyme regulation can occur in several ways.

### ALTERATION OF ENZYME CONCENTRATION

The abundance of an enzyme in a cell may be altered by changing its rate of synthesis or degradation. Such enzymes are called "adaptive" and are analogous to the "inducible" enzymes in bacteria. For example, a high-carbohydrate diet increases the concentrations of the glycolytic and fatty acid–synthesizing enzymes in the liver, whereas starvation or a low-carbohydrate diet increases the concentrations of the gluconeogenic enzymes. Such adaptive changes can be mediated by hormones and/or fuels; they occur slowly, taking hours to days; and they often are the result of increases or decreases of enzyme synthesis at the level of transcription. A more rapid change in enzyme concentration can be produced by proteolytic activation, such as occurs with digestive enzyme precursors (e.g., conversion of trypsinogen to trypsin) and blood-clotting factors.

### SUBSTRATE CONCENTRATION

Changing the concentration of the substrate for an enzyme also can change the rate of a reaction, provided the concentration of substrate is not already saturating (i.e., $[S] < K_M$ or $K_{0.5}$). This simple control is important in certain instances. For example, the sensitivity of both the liver[18,20,21] and pancreatic B cell[48] to changes in blood glucose concentration, such as occur after a meal, is partly attributable to the presence of the high-$K_M$ (10 mmol/L or 180 mg/dL) hexokinase, usually referred to as glucokinase. Other hexokinases are saturated at submillimolar concentrations of glucose and, therefore, are insensitive to changes within the physiologic range. Another example of substrate regulation is the negative effect of ethanol on gluconeogenesis, a matter of clinical importance in malnourished persons with alcoholism. Hypoglycemia in such individuals is attributed to a decrease in the hepatic concentration of the gluconeogenic substrate pyruvate, due to the shift of the lactate dehydrogenase equilibrium more strongly in favor of lactate during ethanol oxidation.[49]

### ALLOSTERIC REGULATION

Allosteric activators and inhibitors (effectors) are typically small intracellular molecules that affect the rate of a given enzymatic reaction. Many of these effectors bind to a site distinct from the catalytic site and alter the conformation of the enzyme. Highly regulated enzymes such as phosphorylase (adenosine monophosphate [AMP]), phosphofructokinase (adenosine triphosphate [ATP], AMP, fructose-2,6-bisphosphate, and citrate) and acetyl-coenzyme A (CoA) carboxylase (citrate, long-chain fatty acyl CoA) (see later) have activators and inhibitors of this type. In addition, simple product inhibition at the catalytic site is significant in the regulation of some enzymes. In general, the effects of allosteric effectors are lost during tissue processing; as a result, this type of regulation, in contrast to covalent modification, is not detected by standard enzyme assays.

### COVALENT MODIFICATION

Covalent modification of enzymes, such as by phosphorylation, acetylation, adenylation, or methylation, is a means of altering enzyme activity that lasts until the covalently attached group is removed. Phosphorylation and dephosphorylation of key enzymes is an important aspect of the regulation of carbohydrate, lipid, and protein metabolism and mediates the effects of many hormones (see later).[50] In most instances, phosphorylation involves serine and threonine residues; however, the importance of reactions involving tyrosine phosphorylation is now recognized. Thus, the receptors for insulin and many growth factors (e.g., insulin-like and platelet-derived growth factors) possess an intrinsic tyrosine kinase that is activated by ligand binding.[51] A variety of experiments indicate that these tyrosine kinases catalyze the phosphorylation of both the receptor of which they are a part (autophosphorylation) and specific substrates within the cell. In the case of insulin, among the principal intracellular substrates are proteins referred to as insulin receptor substrates, of which at least four have been identified.[51]

### PROTEIN-PROTEIN INTERACTIONS

Many events in signal transduction and metabolic regulation are now known to be mediated by protein-protein interactions. With respect to insulin, one example of this is the interaction of insulin with its receptor; another is the interaction of protein substrates of the insulin receptor such as insulin receptor substrate-1 (IRS-1) with other proteins in the cell. For instance, after it is tyrosine phosphorylated at two or more sites, IRS-1 is able to interact with proteins that contain specific amino-acid sequences referred to as SH-2 (src-homology 2) regions.[52] One of these proteins is the 85-kDa subunit of phosphatidylinositol 3-kinase, an enzyme that has been implicated in the regulation of nearly all of the metabolic actions of insulin.[52] Numerous protein-protein interactions occur in the insulin-signaling cascade, and they almost certainly play a key role in explaining much of the diversity of insulin action.[53]

### ISOENZYMES

The metabolic differences between tissues are partly attributable to differing amounts of specific enzymes or, in the extreme case, to their absence. For example, muscle cannot perform gluconeogenesis because of the near absence of glucose-6-phosphatase. A more subtle difference can be due to the presence of isoenzymes (i.e., enzymes that catalyze the same reaction but have different amino-acid sequences and, consequently, can have different kinetic or regulatory properties). Such isozymes can be derived from different genes (e.g., acetyl-CoA carboxylases that predominate in liver and muscle) or they can result from gene splicing. The presence in liver and the pancreatic B cell of glucokinase, the high-$K_M$ isoenzyme of hexokinase, already has been noted. Another example is pyruvate kinase. In liver, for gluconeogenesis to proceed, pyruvate kinase must be strongly inhibited, so that the phosphoenolpyruvate generated by the phosphoenolpyruvate carboxykinase reaction is not reconverted to pyruvate. This inhibition is made possible by the sensitivity of the liver isoenzyme to allosteric effectors and reversible phosphorylation. The muscle isoenzyme lacks these regulatory properties.

## REGULATION OF GLYCOGEN METABOLISM

### GLYCOGENOLYSIS

Hormonal stimulation of glycogenolysis (e.g., by glucagon in liver and by epinephrine in muscle) occurs by a cascade mechanism (Fig. 129-4).[18,54,55] Binding of the hormone to its receptor activates the membrane enzyme adenylate cyclase, which catalyzes the formation of cyclic adenosine monophosphate (cAMP) from ATP. The cAMP activates the cAMP-dependent protein kinase by binding to regulatory subunits and releasing active catalytic subunits. The active protein kinase then phos-

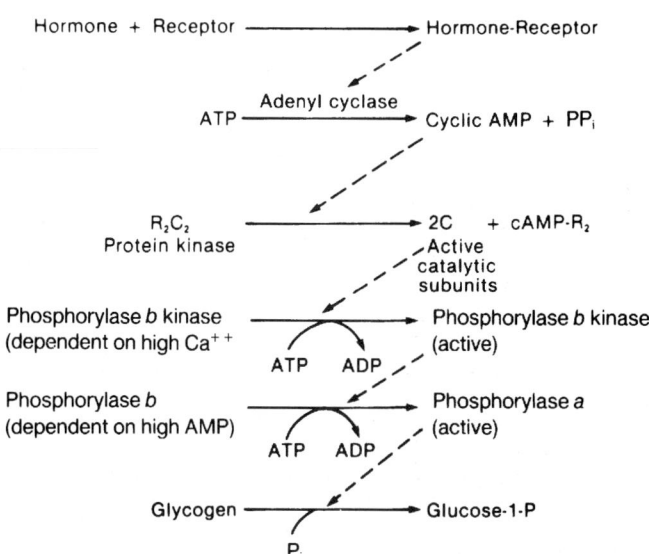

**FIGURE 129-4.** Cascade mechanism for hormonally induced glycogenolysis in muscle (by epinephrine) and liver (by glucagon). See text for discussion of the simultaneous effects of these hormones on glycogen synthase and other enzymes through phosphorylation by the cyclic adenosine monophosphate (cAMP)–dependent protein kinase, which has regulatory (R) and catalytic (C) subunits. (ATP, adenosine triphosphate; PP$_i$, pyrophosphate; ADP, adenosine diphosphate; P, phosphate; P$_i$, inorganic phosphate.)

phorylates, and thereby activates phosphorylase $b$ kinase, which in turn phosphorylates glycogen phosphorylase $b$ to yield the more active phosphorylase $a$, which then degrades glycogen. Such a cascade mechanism has the advantages of increased sensitivity to and amplification of the hormone signal, as well as coordinated regulation of opposing enzymes and related pathways.[56]

In reversing the cascade signal, the phosphorylated proteins are dephosphorylated by phosphoprotein phosphatases. In addition, cAMP is hydrolyzed to AMP by a cyclic nucleotide phosphodiesterase. The pharmacologic action of the methylxanthines—caffeine, theophylline, and theobromine, found in coffee, tea, and cocoa—is attributable partly to their inhibition of this phosphodiesterase. Insulin action may involve stimulation of phosphoprotein phosphatase, the phosphodiesterase, or both.[57]

A second means of triggering the phosphorylation, and hence the activation, of phosphorylase is by raising the intracellular $Ca^{2+}$ concentration. Calmodulin, a calcium-binding regulatory protein, also is a subunit of phosphorylase $b$ kinase. If the intracellular free calcium concentration is raised ten-fold or more to $10^{-6}$ mol/L, as occurs in exercising muscle, calcium binding to calmodulin is increased, and the nonphosphorylated phosphorylase $b$ kinase is activated. The phosphorylated form of phosphorylase $b$ kinase also is dependent on $Ca^{2+}$, but the low levels of free calcium ($10^{-8}$ to $10^{-7}$ mol/L) in resting muscle are sufficient to activate it. The phosphorylation of phosphorylase $b$ kinase increases its affinity for the activator $Ca^{2+}$. Under some conditions, calcium also may be an important modulator of glycogenolysis in the liver. Thus, in rat liver, epinephrine at physiologic concentrations binds to $\alpha$-adrenergic receptors and stimulates glycogenolysis by increasing $Ca^{2+}$ levels.[58] An increase in cAMP, such as occurs when epinephrine binds to $\beta$-adrenergic receptors, is observed only at supraphysiologic concentrations of the hormone.

The mechanism by which epinephrine raises cytoplasmic $Ca^{2+}$ levels involves activation of phospholipase C to cleave inositol-containing phospholipids in the plasma membrane, thereby generating inositol triphosphate, which releases $Ca^{2+}$

from intracellular stores[59] (see Chap. 4). Glycosylated inositol derivatives, similarly generated from glycosylated phosphoinositides, have been suggested as mediators of insulin action. Diacylglycerol, the residual moiety from the phospholipid cleavage, also can serve as a second messenger, most notably by activating protein kinase C.

In concert with control by phosphorylation and dephosphorylation, glycogen phosphorylase is modulated by allosteric regulators. Phosphorylase $b$ is inhibited by ATP and glucose-6-phosphate, and requires high concentrations of AMP or inosine monophosphate for activity. Phosphorylase $a$ also is dependent on AMP under inhibitory conditions, but much lower concentrations suffice.[60] Thus, phosphorylation increases the affinity of phosphorylase for this activator. Besides directly altering its activity, the allosteric regulators affect the phosphorylation and dephosphorylation of phosphorylase. Binding of AMP causes a change in conformation of phosphorylase $a$ such that the phosphate groups are "tucked in" and become resistant to removal by the phosphoprotein phosphatase.[61] Conversely, binding of glucose displaces AMP and exposes the phosphate groups to attack. Glucose-6-phosphate both activates the phosphatase reaction and inhibits the phosphorylase $b$ kinase reaction by binding to phosphorylase.

The relative importance of allosteric effectors versus the phosphorylation cascade in the regulation of glycogenolysis probably is greatest in exercising muscle. There, increases in phosphorylase $a$ levels are relatively small and transient in comparison with the large stimulation of glycogenolysis.[20,60] Likewise, I-strain mice, which lack muscle phosphorylase $b$ kinase and therefore must depend on allosteric activation of phosphorylase $b$ for glycogenolysis, are little affected by this defect during exercise. Their rate of glycogenolysis can exceed that of a normal mouse, and they exercise without difficulty; in fact, they have more endurance, presumably because of their larger reserves of glycogen.[62]

### GLYCOGEN SYNTHESIS

Glycogen synthase, the rate-limiting enzyme for glycogen synthesis, also is regulated by phosphorylation-dephosphorylation and by allosteric effectors.[20,54] The classic view held that glycogen synthase was phosphorylated by cAMP-dependent protein kinase, and thus converted from the active $a$ (or I, for independent of the activator glucose-6-phosphate) form to the inactive or less active $b$ (or D, for dependent) form of the enzyme. Therefore, hormonal stimulation of cAMP generation would both activate glycogen breakdown and inhibit glycogen synthesis. The situation is now known to be somewhat more complex. Whereas phosphorylase has a single phosphorylation site per subunit, glycogen synthase can be phosphorylated at more than ten sites, and at least nine protein kinases may be involved, including cAMP-dependent, calmodulin-dependent, phosphorylase $b$ kinase, casein kinases I and II, and glycogen synthase kinase 3.[20,54] Generally, a greater degree of phosphorylation decreases the affinity of glycogen synthase for the activator glucose-6-phosphate and for its substrate uridine diphosphoglucose. However, the precise effects of phosphorylation and dephosphorylation at specific sites remain unclear.

Insulin induces the dephosphorylation and activation of glycogen synthase at the same time it stimulates glucose disposal, especially in muscle. This could be due to its ability to activate Akt/PKB (protein kinase B), the enzyme that phosphorylates and inhibits glycogen synthase kinase 3 (GSK3).[20,54] In addition, insulin can activate phosphoprotein phosphatase 1, which dephosphorylates and, therefore, activates glycogen synthase. Derangements of one or both of these mechanisms could contribute to the impaired activation of glycogen synthase in patients who have type 2 diabetes or are at high risk for developing it. In this regard, insulin-resistant Pima Indians who have an extremely high prevalence of type 2 diabetes have been shown to have defects in phosphoprotein phosphatase 1 activity.[63]

## COORDINATE REGULATION OF GLYCOGEN SYNTHASE AND PHOSPHORYLASE

Coordinate control of glycogen synthase and phosphorylase involves phosphoprotein phosphatase as well as protein kinases. In liver, phosphorylase *a* appears to inhibit dephosphorylation (and hence activation) of glycogen synthase by binding preferentially to the phosphatase—even when its phosphate group is tucked in and cannot be hydrolyzed. Thus, only after a rise in glucose has exposed the phosphate group and most of the phosphorylase *a* has been converted to the *b* form is the phosphatase free to act on glycogen synthase.[20] This probably is a means of restricting operation of a futile cycle of simultaneous glycogen synthesis and breakdown. In this regard, the suggestion has been made that glucose could be a significant determinant of glycogen breakdown or synthesis in liver, with phosphorylase *a* functioning as an intracellular glucose receptor or sensor. Adding to this complexity is the finding that the regulation of the protein phosphatase(s) involves inhibitory proteins, which themselves are subject to phosphorylation and dephosphorylation.[57]

## REGULATION OF GLYCOLYSIS

### PHOSPHOFRUCTOKINASE

Control of glycolysis is discussed first in the context of a non-gluconeogenic tissue such as muscle.

Once glucose has been transported into the cell, the primary functional control point of glycolysis appears to be the phosphofructokinase reaction. This enzyme is affected by various metabolites that reflect the fuel and energy status of the cell.[64] ATP, a major product of glycolysis, serves as a classic feedback inhibitor of phosphofructokinase. (No confusion should exist over the second function of ATP, as a substrate: inhibition by ATP occurs when it binds to a regulatory site distinct from the catalytic site.) Conversely, AMP, adenosine diphosphate (ADP), and inorganic phosphate ($P_i$), which are products of ATP breakdown, all are activators of phosphofructokinase. They are present in lower concentrations than ATP and, during conditions of altered energy demand, the percentage changes in their concentrations are much greater. (AMP is generated from ADP in the myokinase reaction: 2 ADP = AMP + ATP.) ATP inhibition of phosphofructokinase is potentiated by low pH; this may be a "safety switch" to turn off glycolysis and thereby prevent an excessive drop in pH from the continued generation of lactic acid. Inhibition of phosphofructokinase by a decrease in pH probably occurs in vivo in ischemic tissue. A second end product of glycolysis is acetyl-CoA, which can be used for fatty acid synthesis or as a substrate for the citric acid cycle. Citrate derived from the condensation of acetyl-CoA and oxaloacetate serves as a feedback inhibitor of phosphofructokinase and probably mediates the inhibitory effects of fatty acids and ketone bodies on glycolysis in the heart and other tissues[65] as well as the autoregulation by glucose of its use as a fuel.[66] Other activators of phosphofructokinase include ammonia (from working muscle); fructose-1,6-bisphosphate (involved in the generation of glycolytic oscillations, which may be of advantage in the maintenance of a high-energy state and in the pulsatile release of insulin[67,68]); and fructose-2,6-bisphosphate (of uncertain importance in muscle[67,69] but of great importance in liver[69–73]). Most of these activators and inhibitors affect the affinity of the enzyme for its substrate fructose-6-phosphate. The concentration of the latter, therefore, is an important determinant of enzyme activity. Sometimes, a rise in hexose monophosphate secondary to rapid glycogenolysis may be an important stimulator of glycolysis.

## HEXOKINASE AND GLUCOSE TRANSPORT

Phosphofructokinase is the logical control point of glycolysis because it is the first nonequilibrium reaction ("committed step") after the branch point at glucose-6-phosphate. However, it is preceded by nonequilibrium steps at hexokinase and (although not in liver) glucose transport. Hexokinase is inhibited noncompetitively by glucose-6-phosphate at a regulatory locus distinct from the catalytic site. Consequently, a block at phosphofructokinase (or excessive glycogenolysis) could secondarily inhibit hexokinase through a rise in the hexose monophosphates, and, conversely, activation of phosphofructokinase could release such inhibition. Glucose transport in muscle and adipose tissue is activated by insulin, but the hormone appears to have no direct effect on muscle phosphofructokinase. Insulin may stimulate hexokinase activity by promoting binding of that enzyme to mitochondria for more efficient energy transfer.[59,74] Anoxia also stimulates glucose transport, but whether this is related to the concurrent increases in allosteric effectors of phosphofructokinase such as AMP and $P_i$ is unknown. Secondary regulation of the glycolytic pathway downstream from phosphofructokinase involves product inhibition of glyceraldehyde-3-phosphate dehydrogenase by 1,3-bisphosphoglycerate and the reduced form of nicotinamide adenine dinucleotide (NADH), and of pyruvate kinase by ATP.

## CONTROL OF GLUCONEOGENESIS AND GLYCOLYSIS IN LIVER

### SUBSTRATE CYCLES

The opposing glycolytic and gluconeogenic enzymes form ATP-consuming "substrate cycles" (see Fig. 129-3). These frequently were termed "futile cycles" when it was assumed such energy wastage would be prevented by tight regulation, so that only one opposing pathway would proceed at a given time. In cellular metabolism, however, a greater premium seems to be placed on responsiveness and flexibility of control than on minimizing energy costs—witness, for example, the synthesis of mRNA precursor forms that are much larger than the final product, even though the addition of each extra nucleotide residue effectively costs twice as much as one turn of a metabolic "futile cycle." Coordinate regulation of simultaneously operating glycolytic and gluconeogenic pathways could have advantages in sensitivity to metabolic needs, and significant rates of recycling have been demonstrated under some conditions by sophisticated radiolabel experiments.[7,18,75,76]

### REGULATORY PROPERTIES

The direction and magnitude of the flux between glucose and pyruvate are determined by the balance of regulatory effects on the key glycolytic and gluconeogenic enzymes.[55] These enzymes are adaptive in liver in response to alterations in the nutritional and hormonal state, and this is a key means by which they are regulated over the long term. Pertinent allosteric effects on gluconeogenic enzymes include the inhibition of fructose-1,6-bisphosphatase by AMP and fructose-2,6-bisphosphate, both of which activate the opposing glycolytic enzyme, phosphofructokinase; and the absolute dependence of the pyruvate carboxylase reaction on the activator acetyl-CoA. The latter property provides a regulatory link between gluconeogenesis and fatty acid oxidation.

Generally, the key glycolytic enzymes appear to be subject to more stringent control than are their gluconeogenic counterparts, and probably are the principal sites of regulation of net gluconeogenic as well as glycolytic flux. Glucokinase, by virtue of its high $K_M$, is sensitive to changes in glucose concentration in the physiologic range and has an adaptive response to insulin. In low-insulin states, such as starvation or diabetes, the amount of glucokinase is diminished greatly. Liver phosphofructokinase has the same wide range of allosteric effectors noted for muscle; nutritional and hormonal regulation of the enzyme in liver, in particular, involves fructose-2,6-bisphosphate. Liver pyruvate kinase has a requirement for the activator fructose-1,6-bisphosphate: only in the presence of this metabolite does it have as great an affinity for its substrate, phosphoenolpyruvate, as the muscle isoenzyme has with or without fructose-1,6-bisphosphate. Thus, a decrease in phosphofructokinase activity would decrease fructose-1,6-bisphosphate levels and, therefore, inhibit liver pyruvate kinase. Liver pyruvate kinase also is strongly inhibited by ATP (feedback inhibition) and by alanine, a major gluconeogenic precursor released by muscle and gut. In addition, liver pyruvate kinase is subject to phosphorylation by the cAMP-dependent protein kinase. Phosphorylation inhibits the enzyme by decreasing its affinity for phosphoenolpyruvate and for the required activator, fructose-1,6-bisphosphate.

## FRUCTOSE-2,6-BISPHOSPHATE AND GLUCAGON ACTION

A prime example of the reciprocal regulation of glycolytic and gluconeogenic enzymes is the action on the liver by glucagon, a hormone long known to stimulate gluconeogenesis. Activation of the cAMP-dependent protein kinase by glucagon inhibits the phosphofructokinase reaction by reducing the hepatic concentration of the potent activator fructose-2,6-bisphosphate.[69-73] Fructose-2,6-bisphosphate is synthesized from fructose-6-phosphate and ATP by 6-phosphofructo-2-kinase. The same protein also has the fructose-2,6-bisphosphatase activity (at a second site) that cleaves fructose-2,6-bisphosphate to fructose-6-phosphate and $P_i$. Phosphorylation of this multifunctional enzyme by the cAMP-dependent protein kinase decreases the kinase activity and enhances the phosphatase activity, and this causes a decrease in fructose-2,6-bisphosphate. Because fructose-2,6-bisphosphate is an activator of phosphofructokinase, as well as an inhibitor of fructose-1,6-bisphosphatase, a fall in its concentration decreases the conversion of fructose-6-phosphate to fructose-1,6-bisphosphate and increases the conversion of fructose-1,6-bisphosphate to fructose-6-phosphate, thus favoring net gluconeogenesis. Moreover, fructose-1,6-bisphosphatase can be phosphorylated by the cAMP-dependent protein kinase, and the phosphorylated enzyme is more active by virtue of a reduced affinity for the inhibitors AMP and fructose-2,6-bisphosphate.[77] Glucose opposes glucagon and raises fructose-2,6-bisphosphate levels partly by raising the concentration of fructose-6-phosphate, the substrate for 6-phosphofructo-2-kinase.

## COORDINATION WITH GLYCOGEN METABOLISM

The underlying mechanism for the multisite and coordinate control of glycogen and glucose metabolism in liver now can be seen: activation of cAMP-dependent protein kinase by glucagon leads to phosphorylation of phosphorylase kinase, phosphorylase, and glycogen synthase (thus promoting glycogenolysis), as well as pyruvate kinase, fructose-1,6-bisphosphatase, and 6-phosphofructo-2-kinase/fructose-2,6-bisphosphatase (thus decreasing fructose-2,6-bisphosphate and inhibiting glycolysis and promoting gluconeogenesis). Alternatively, glucose or insulin promotes the dephosphorylation of these enzymes and, hence, promotes glycogen synthesis and glycolysis. Thus, the balance between insulin and glucagon is perhaps the principal determinant of the setting of hepatic carbohydrate metabolism at a given time. Finally, some controversy exists over whether the immediate precursor for hepatic glycogen synthesis after carbohydrate administration is circulating glucose or gluconeogenic precursors, largely derived from the peripheral catabolism of the glucose.[20,78,79]

## PYRUVATE DEHYDROGENASE

Pyruvate dehydrogenase catalyzes the conversion of pyruvate to acetyl-CoA, which, in turn, is oxidized to carbon dioxide and water in the citric acid cycle or is used for lipogenesis. Conversion of pyruvate to acetyl-CoA by this multienzyme complex is under stringent control, because any carbon passing through this reaction no longer can be used for the resynthesis of glucose.[55,80,81] The enzyme is inhibited by its products, acetyl-CoA and NADH, and this inhibition is countered by CoA and nicotinamide adenine dinucleotide (NAD). Thus, the acetyl-CoA/CoA and NADH/NAD ratios are important determinants of its activity in situ. The enzyme is subject to inactivation and activation by phosphorylation and dephosphorylation reactions, respectively. The kinase that catalyzes the phosphorylation reaction is activated by high ratios of ATP/ADP, acetyl-CoA/CoA, and NADH/NAD. The corresponding phosphatase is stimulated by high concentrations of calcium and pyruvate. Thus, pyruvate dehydrogenase is sensitive to the relative need for acetyl-CoA for fatty acid synthesis, the generation of energy by the citric acid cycle, and the supply of pyruvate. Concordantly, pyruvate dehydrogenase activity is increased in liver, muscle, and heart in the fed state and decreased in starvation and diabetes when abundant lipid fuels (increased acetyl-CoA/CoA and NADH/NAD) are available. Pyruvate dehydrogenase activity also is markedly increased in muscle during exercise, presumably because of the activation of pyruvate dehydrogenase phosphatase by $Ca^{2+}$ and changes in intramitochondrial ATP, ADP, and redox state.[82]

## SORBITOL PATHWAY

Present in many tissues are aldose reductases, enzymes that convert glucose to the sugar alcohol sorbitol. Aldose reductases have a very low affinity for glucose ($K_M$ ~20 mmol/L); therefore, the reactions that they catalyze are of interest principally in patients with diabetes, in whom plasma and intracellular glucose concentrations are elevated. Increases in sorbitol have been linked to the pathogenesis of cataracts, neuropathy, and vascular disease in patients with diabetes.[83,84] This may involve associated decreases in myoinositol, or nitric oxide,[85] which in turn affect the plasma membrane sodium-potassium adenosine triphosphatase that is responsible for the ion gradients essential for nerve conduction and certain transport processes. Galactose also is converted to its corresponding sugar alcohol (galactitol) by aldose reductases, and pathologic changes similar to those produced by diabetes have been noted in galactose-fed animals. Therefore, aldose reductase inhibitors are being tested for their ability to prevent or reverse long-term complications of diabetes.[83]

## LIPID METABOLISM[7,13,86]

The largest caloric reservoir in humans is triglyceride stored in adipose tissue. Triglycerides are degraded to FFAs and glycerol in all persons, and their degradation is increased during starvation and in other situations (e.g., exercise) in which plasma insulin levels are low and glucose cannot meet all the fuel needs of the body (Fig. 129-5). When FFAs enter the circulation, they are complexed to albumin, which facilitates their interorgan transport and diminishes their potential toxicity. In liver, muscle, and most other organs, FFAs can be esterified to form triglycerides or oxidized to carbon dioxide and water to generate ATP. Liver can also metabolize FFA to form ketone bodies (acetoacetate and β-hydroxybutyrate) that can be used by the brain (which does not oxidize appreciable quantities of FFA) and muscle during starvation. During prolonged starvation, the brain uses ketone bodies in even greater quantity; indeed, they can replace glucose as its principal fuel (see later).

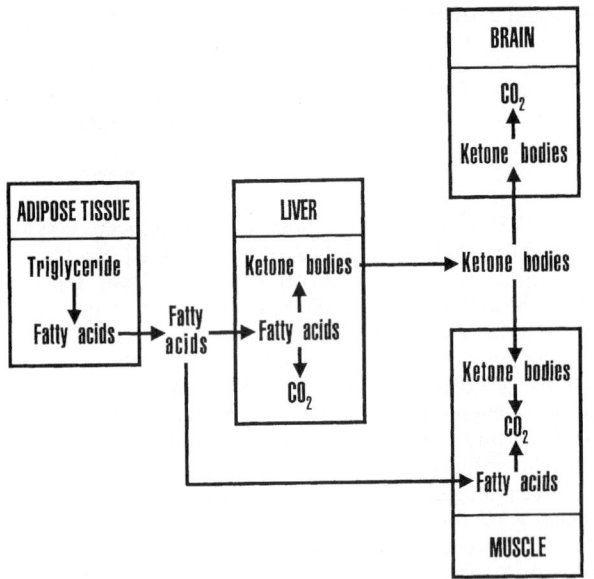

**FIGURE 129-5.** Overview of free fatty acid and ketone body metabolism during brief and prolonged starvation. In the fed state, the liver tends to esterify fatty acids to form triglycerides and phospholipids that it can export as constituents of very low density lipoproteins. During starvation it primarily oxidizes fatty acids, and the principal lipid-derived exports are the ketone bodies, acetoacetate and β-hydroxybutyrate. Ketone bodies are principally used as a fuel by muscle during early starvation (1–5 days) and during more prolonged starvation. (See text for details.)

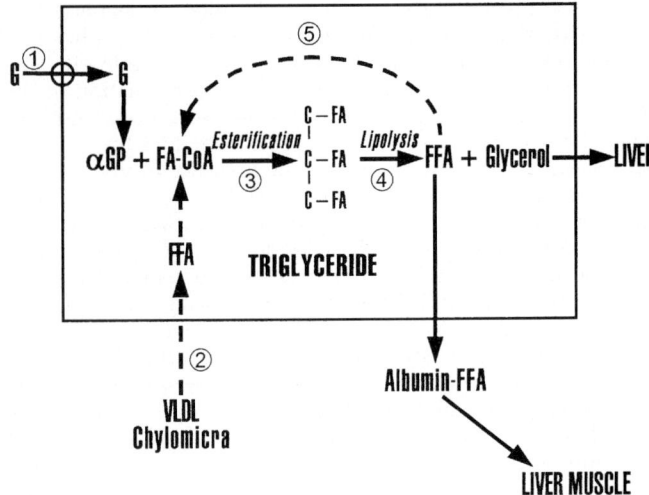

**FIGURE 129-6.** Triglyceride metabolism in adipose tissue. Insulin stimulates triglyceride accumulation by enhancing glucose ($G$) transport (1), activating lipoprotein lipase (2) and glycerol phosphate ($GP$) acyltransferase (3), and inhibiting hormone-sensitive lipase (4). By virtue of its effects on (1) and (3), insulin also stimulates the reesterification of free fatty acids ($FFAs$) (5) derived from the lipolysis of intracellular triglyceride. Counterinsulin hormones appear to inhibit the three processes (steps 1–3), stimulated by insulin. FFAs that are released from the adipocyte are complexed to albumin in the circulation. Principal sites at which FFAs are used include muscle and liver. The glycerol released during lipolysis is not metabolized in the adipocyte, which lacks glycerol kinase. Most of this glycerol appears to be used by the liver for gluconeogenesis. (*FA*, fatty acyl; *CoA*, coenzyme A; *VLDL*, very low density lipoprotein.)

## FREE FATTY ACID METABOLISM

### MOBILIZATION FROM ADIPOSE TISSUE AND TRANSPORT IN PLASMA

The fall of insulin levels in the plasma during starvation or diabetes orchestrates a series of events that leads to the breakdown of triglycerides stored in adipose tissue (i.e., lipolysis) and the elevation of plasma FFA levels. The breakdown of these triglyceride stores is regulated by a hormone-sensitive lipase within the adipocyte. Several lipases interact to degrade the triglyceride molecule completely to form three molecules of fatty acid plus one of glycerol. The initial cleavage of the triglyceride molecule by triglyceride lipase appears to be the rate-limiting step, because the breakdown of diglyceride to free glycerol is ~10 times faster than the breakdown of triglyceride to diglyceride. Thus, the release of the first fatty acid molecule from triglyceride is followed by rapid complete hydrolysis to FFAs and glycerol.

Insulin diminishes the release of FFA from the adipocyte both by inhibiting lipolysis and by enhancing fatty acid esterification (Fig. 129-6). The activity of triglyceride lipase in adipose tissue is regulated by the phosphorylation state of the enzyme and is subject to hormonal modulation in much the same manner as glycogen phosphorylase. Phosphorylation of the lipase is catalyzed by a cAMP-dependent protein kinase and is associated with activation of the enzyme. Catecholamines, glucagon, and several other hormones that increase cAMP by activating adenylate cyclase activate triglyceride lipase by this means.[87] Dephosphorylation, catalyzed by a phosphoprotein phosphatase, inactivates the enzyme. As with phosphorylase, insulin facilitates inactivation of the lipase either by decreasing intracellular cAMP or by increasing the activity of a phosphoprotein phosphatase.[88] It can diminish cAMP by increasing the activity of a cyclic guanosine monophosphate–dependent phosphodiesterase (PDE3$_b$) that converts cAMP to AMP,[88] or by a direct effect on the activity of adenylate cyclase. Alternatively, the antilipolytic effect of insulin can occur when no change in cAMP levels occurs within the adipocyte, suggesting that it can alter phosphatase activity by

other mechanisms.[89] Whatever the mechanism, the antilipolytic effect of insulin appears to require activation of phosphatidylinositol 3-kinase by insulin.[90] Interestingly, a limiting enzyme for triglyceride formation, α-glycerophosphate acyltransferase, becomes inactive when phosphorylated by a cAMP-dependent protein kinase and active when dephosphorylated by a phosphoprotein phosphatase. Thus, the control is opposite to that of triglyceride lipase, which permits a tight control of triglyceride formation and breakdown.

The principal long-chain fatty acids (at least 14 carbon atoms) found in human plasma are oleic (43%), palmitic (24%), stearic (13%), linoleic (10%), and palmitoleic (5%). At least 10 fatty acid molecules may be bound by each albumin molecule, although this capacity is never reached under physiologic (0.2–2 mmol/L) or even pathologic (2–3 mmol/L) conditions. Three of these 10 sites have a high affinity for fatty acids and, when they are fully occupied (at a fatty acid concentration of ~2 mmol/L), the concentration of fatty acids not bound to the albumin increases markedly.[91]

### FREE FATTY ACID TURNOVER AND OXIDATION

The concentration of FFAs in plasma is low (~10 mg/L) compared with that of glucose. The half-life of FFAs in the circulation is <2 minutes, however, and their concentration increases several-fold during starvation and other situations in which triglyceride hydrolysis is accelerated. Consequently, FFA turnover in a normal human approximates 250 g per day, a value comparable to that for glucose. Fatty acids are oxidized by most tissues.[92] Liver, kidney, heart, brown adipose tissue, and aerobic muscles (slow-twitch and fast-twitch oxidative fibers) have a high capacity for fatty acid oxidation, whereas fatty acid oxidation is low in brain, white adipose tissue, and fast-twitch white muscle (tissues with relatively few mitochondria). Controversy exists over whether transport of FFAs from

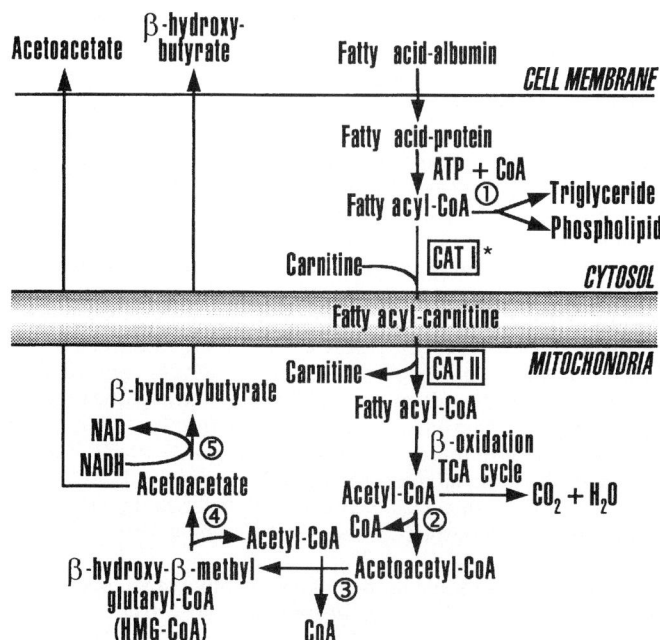

**FIGURE 129-7.** Free fatty acid metabolism to acetyl–coenzyme A (*CoA*) and its oxidation in the citric acid cycle. These processes are similar in liver and muscle, except that liver possesses the enzymes (steps 2–5) to synthesize acetoacetate and β-hydroxybutyrate in significant quantities. Malonyl-CoA, an inhibitor of carnitine acyltransferase I (*CAT I*; also referred to as carnitine palmitoyl transferase I), is a major determinant of whether fatty acyl–CoA enters the mitochondria, where it is oxidized, or remains in the cytosol, where it can be used for triglyceride and phospholipid synthesis. Enzymes: (*1*), α-glycerophosphate acyltransferase; (*2*), acetoacetyl-CoA acetyl transferase; (*3*), β-hydroxy-β-methylglutaryl-CoA (*HMG-CoA*) synthetase; (*4*), HMG-CoA lyase; (*5*), β-hydroxybutyrate dehydrogenase. (*ATP*, adenosine triphosphate; *NAD*, nicotinamide adenine dinucleotide, oxidized form; *NADH*, nicotinamide adenine dinucleotide, reduced form; *TCA*, tricarboxylic acid cycle.)

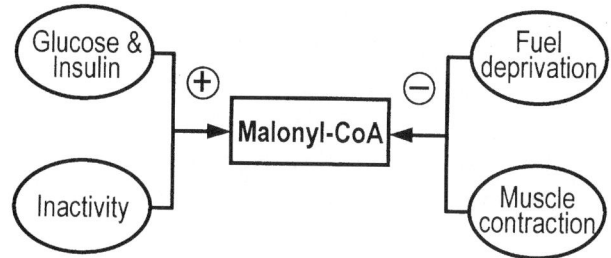

**FIGURE 129-8.** The malonyl-CoA fuel-sensing and signaling mechanism in skeletal muscle. According to this scheme, malonyl-CoA is a component of a fuel-sensing and signaling mechanism that responds to changes in glucose availability and energy expenditure. Thus, when the muscle is provided with a surplus of glucose and fuels other than fatty acids, or when it does not use available glucose because of inactivity, malonyl-CoA levels increase. Conversely, malonyl-CoA levels decrease when the muscle is glucose deprived or energy use is increased by contraction. In the proposed mechanism, acetyl-CoA carboxylase functions as the sensor and malonyl-CoA is the signal. (From Ruderman NB, Saha AK, Vavvas D, Witters LA. Malonyl CoA, fuel sensing, and insulin resistance. Am J Physiol 1999; 39:E1.)

the circulation into cells is a passive process, occurring by simple diffusion across the plasma membrane, or whether it involves specific transporters.[93] Whatever the mechanism, a rise in plasma FFAs during starvation increases their transport into cells such as muscle.

Before entering the mitochondria where they are oxidized (Fig. 129-7), long-chain fatty acids are activated to acyl-CoA derivatives by appropriate acyl-CoA synthetases (note that medium- and short-chain fatty acids can be activated within the mitochondria). Because the mitochondrial inner membrane is impermeable to CoA and its derivatives, a specific transport system is required to transfer long-chain fatty acyl–CoA across this membrane. This system is generally held to have three components[86,94]: (a) the enzyme carnitine palmitoyltransferase I (CPT1), located in the outer mitochondrial membrane, that transfers the activated acyl unit from fatty acyl–CoA to carnitine and perhaps is the principal determinant of whether fatty acids entering certain cell types, such as liver or muscle, are oxidized or esterified; (b) a translocase system for the exchange diffusion of fatty acyl–carnitine into the mitochondrial matrix in exchange for carnitine (not shown in figure); and (c) a second transferase, termed carnitine palmitoyltransferase II, located principally on the inner surface of the inner mitochondrial membrane, that catalyzes the transfer of the fatty acyl unit from fatty acyl–carnitine back to CoA before β-oxidation. The compartmentalization of carnitine acyltransferases I and II allows interaction of these enzymes with metabolites or regulatory factors in the extramitochondrial and intramitochondrial

compartments, respectively. The CPT1 step appears to be the rate-limiting intracellular event for fatty acid oxidation. A key factor controlling this enzyme is probably its allosteric inhibitor malonyl-CoA.

### METABOLISM IN MUSCLE

Muscle can either oxidize fatty acids or use them to synthesize triglycerides and other glycerolipids. Studies in the rat indicate that during starvation, fatty acid oxidation is favored due, at least in part, to a decrease in the intracellular concentration of malonyl-CoA. Malonyl-CoA is an allosteric inhibitor of CPT1, and changes in its concentration appear to parallel changes in the rate of fatty acid oxidation in rat muscle.[95–97] Malonyl-CoA levels in muscle can be acutely regulated by changes in its fuel supply or energy expenditure (Fig. 129-8). Thus, exposure to insulin or glucose, or inactivity caused by denervation leads to rapid increases in malonyl-CoA in rat muscle, whereas exercise (muscle contraction) and glucose deprivation have the opposite effect, in keeping with the rates of fatty acid oxidation in these situations.[66] Whether similar events occur in humans is less certain, although increases in malonyl-CoA and decreases in fatty acid oxidation have been observed in humans during a hyperinsulinemic euglycemic clamp.[98]

Malonyl-CoA levels in muscle appear to be governed by changes in the activity of the β isoform of acetyl-CoA carboxylase (ACCβ) (Fig. 129-9). Studies suggest that increases in malonyl-CoA induced in rat and human muscle by insulin and glucose may be due to increases in the cytosolic concentration of citrate, an allosteric activator of ACC. In contrast, exercise decreases malonyl-CoA levels by activating an AMP-activated protein kinase (see also section on Fuel-Sensing Mechanisms) that phosphorylates and inhibits ACC.[66,99] Interestingly, neither changes in ACC phosphorylation nor changes in cytosolic citrate appear to account for the alterations in malonyl-CoA caused by starvation or refeeding.[99]

### METABOLISM IN LIVER

The liver has a high capacity to remove fatty acids from the circulation and either oxidize or esterify them. Unlike most other tissues, it can either use the fatty acids for its own needs (e.g., oxidation, fuel storage) or export the products of fatty acid metabolism either as ketone bodies or as triglycerides and phospholipids in very low density lipoproteins (VLDLs). In general, esterification and VLDL production are favored in the fed state when insulin levels are high, and fatty acid oxidation and

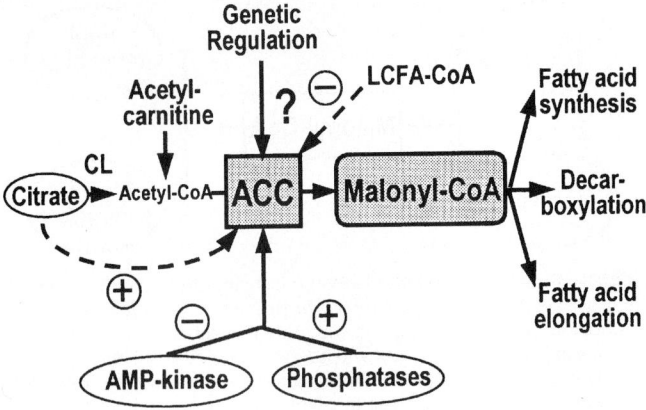

**FIGURE 129-9.** Control of acetyl–coenzyme A (*CoA*) carboxylase β isoform (*ACC<sub>β</sub>*) activity and malonyl–CoA concentration in skeletal muscle. $ACC_\beta$ is regulated by phosphorylation-dephosphorylation via adenosine monophosphate (*AMP*) activated kinase and phosphatases and by changes in the cytosolic concentration of citrate, an allosteric activator. Studies in rat muscle suggest that AMP kinase activation is responsible for the decrease in malonyl-CoA during exercise. The suggestion has been made that $ACC_\beta$ activity may also be governed by changes in the cytosolic concentration of long-chain fatty acyl–coenzyme A (*LCFA-CoA*), an allosteric inhibitor. Whether $ACC_\beta$ abundance is regulated at a genetic level is uncertain. (*CL*, citrate lyase.) (From Ruderman NB, Saha AK, Vavvas D, Witters LA. Malonyl CoA, fuel sensing, and insulin resistance. Am J Physiol 1999; 39:E1.)

ketone body formation are favored during starvation when insulin levels are low (see Fig. 129-5). As in muscle, regulation of CPT1 by malonyl-CoA appears to play a major role in determining whether fatty acids are esterified or oxidized,[94] although other factors are probably involved.[100] In contrast to muscle, the decreases in malonyl-CoA observed in liver during starvation are due to rapidly occurring (in hours) and slowly occurring (over days) decreases in the activity of $ACC_\alpha$, the acetyl-CoA carboxylase isoform that predominates in liver.[101] The slow changes are due to regulation at the level of transcription and the rapid changes to alterations in phosphorylation.[102]

## FUEL-SENSING MECHANISMS AND METABOLIC REGULATION

### ADENOSINE MONOPHOSPHATE–ACTIVATED PROTEIN KINASE

An increasing body of evidence indicates that the AMP-activated protein kinases (AMPKs) that phosphorylate and inhibit ACC may be components of a fuel-sensing mechanism by which a cell can respond to a change in its energy state. As reviewed elsewhere,[66,102] AMPKs could occupy this role, because changes in their activity are modulated by increases in the concentration of AMP and decreases in creatine phosphate, either or both of which occur in muscle during exercise and in other cells in response to various stresses. AMPK-like proteins have been shown in nearly all cell types including yeast, in which their activity is increased by glucose deprivation.[102] The targets for the AMPKs include ACC (which links them to the oxidation of fatty acids) and hydroxymethylglutaryl-CoA synthase (the rate-limiting enzyme in cholesterol synthesis), which they also phosphorylate and inhibit. Incubation or perfusion of muscle with aminoimidazole carboximide riboside (AICAR), which leads to activation of AMPK, increases glucose transport into muscle by a non–insulin-dependent mechanism. This has led to the interesting speculation that activation of an AMPK modulates the increase in glucose transport and possibly other metabolic changes observed in muscle during exercise. Studies to test this hypothesis and to examine how AMPK activation affects signaling and gene expression in muscle and other tissues will clearly be of interest.

## GLUCOSE-SENSING MECHANISMS: MALONYL-COENZYME A/ LONG-CHAIN FATTY ACYL–COENZYME A AND HEXOSAMINES

Changes in the concentration of malonyl-CoA provide another mechanism by which alterations in energy state (glucose supply) could modulate cellular signaling and function. Such a mechanism was first demonstrated in the pancreatic B cell, in which glucose-induced insulin secretion was linked to increases in malonyl-CoA[103]; however, it very likely occurs in skeletal muscle and other cells in which the use of glucose as a fuel is determined by its availability.[104] Increases in malonyl-CoA might act in these cells by inhibiting fatty acid oxidation and increasing the cytosolic concentration of long-chain fatty acyl–CoA (LCFA-CoA).[95] LCFA-CoA in turn could affect cellular signaling by exerting a direct action on specific enzymes or by increasing the formation of diacylglycerol, an activator of protein kinase C. The suggestion has been made that sustained increases in malonyl-CoA, particularly if associated with other factors that increase cytosolic LCFA-CoA, such as high plasma FFA or muscle triglyceride levels, could contribute to the pathogenesis of insulin resistance in skeletal muscle.[45,105]

Other glucose-sensing mechanisms have also been proposed. One of them involves the generation (by excess glucose) of increases in the content of hexosamines and secondarily uridine diphosphate acetylhexosamines.[106] The latter, like increases in malonyl-CoA and LCFA-CoA, have been implicated in the pathogenesis of insulin resistance induced by sustained hyperglycemia.

## KETONE BODY METABOLISM

Most peripheral tissues can use ketone bodies (acetoacetate and β-hydroxybutyrate) as well as FFA and glucose for their fuel needs[107]; indeed, ketone bodies are now widely recognized to play an extremely important role in caloric homeostasis.[108] Ketone bodies are important respiratory fuels for muscle and for brain during starvation, and they appear to be crucial in the adaptation leading to protein conservation during prolonged starvation. A near-total insulin lack, such as in untreated type 1 diabetes, can yield extremely high levels of ketone bodies in plasma secondary to an imbalance between hepatic production and peripheral utilization. This pathologic ketosis, in contrast to the physiologic ketosis arising during starvation, causes severe metabolic acidosis that can be fatal if not treated quickly (see Chap. 127).

### KETOGENESIS IN THE LIVER

Ketone bodies are formed by a specific biosynthetic pathway in the liver from incoming FFAs (see Fig. 129-7). FFAs enter liver mitochondria, where they are converted to acetyl-CoA and synthesized into ketone bodies by the hydroxymethylglutaryl-CoA pathway. In the fed state, when insulin levels are high and glucagon levels are low, the liver uses FFAs predominantly for triglyceride synthesis; during starvation and in diabetes, the hormonal pattern is reversed, and fatty acid oxidation and ketone body formation are favored. The differences between the fed and fasted states appear to reflect differences in the activity of the carnitine-mediated fatty acid transport system, at least in part caused by changes in the concentration of malonyl-CoA.[109] As already noted, malonyl-CoA levels are high in the fed state, thus favoring triglyceride synthesis, whereas in the starved or diabetic condition, malonyl-CoA levels are low and fatty acid oxidation and ketogenesis are favored. The possibility that alterations in CPT1 in liver occur in starvation or diabetes, which change its response to malonyl-CoA, has also been suggested.[100]

### PATHWAY OF KETONE BODY UTILIZATION

With the exception of the liver, which does not use acetoacetate or β-hydroxybutyrate as fuels, most tissues can oxidize ketone

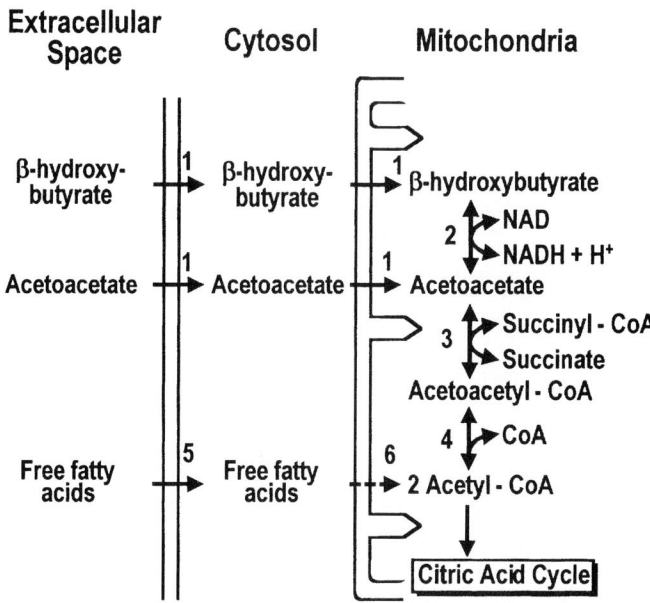

**FIGURE 129-10.** Utilization of ketone bodies and free fatty acids by muscle. *1*, Diffusion or transport of ketone bodies across the cell and mitochondrial membrane; *2*, β-hydroxybutyrate dehydrogenase; *3*, 3-oxoacid-coenzyme A (CoA) transferase; *4*, acetoacetyl-CoA thiolase; *5*, movement of free fatty acids across cell membrane and binding to cytosolic protein(s) for translocation; and *6*, carnitine-dependent transport of long-chain fatty aids into mitochondria. Note interaction of free fatty acid oxidation and pathway of ketone body utilization at the level of acetyl-CoA. (*NAD*, nicotinamide adenine dinucleotide, oxidized form; *NADH*, nicotinamide adenine dinucleotide, reduced form.)

bodies by the pathway shown in Figure 129-10. After entering the mitochondria, acetoacetate reacts with succinyl-CoA to form acetoacetyl-CoA by a reaction catalyzed by 3-oxoacid-CoA transferase. Acetoacetyl-CoA then is cleaved to form two molecules of acetyl-CoA by acetoacetyl-CoA thiolase. The CoA for this reaction is derived from the free CoA pool within the mitochondria; in this respect, acetoacetate is competing with pyruvate and fatty acyl–carnitine, which also must react with CoA to be metabolized. In muscle and brain, most acetyl-CoA formed from acetoacetate and β-hydroxybutyrate is oxidized to carbon dioxide and water in the citric acid cycle. In adipose tissue, a significant portion may be used for the synthesis of fatty acids. The metabolism of β-hydroxybutyrate is identical to that of acetoacetate, except that it first must be converted to acetoacetate by β-hydroxybutyrate dehydrogenase, an enzyme located on the inner mitochondrial membrane.

The utilization of ketone bodies by peripheral tissues usually appears to be dependent on their concentration in plasma and does not appear to be regulated by changes in the activities of the enzymes involved in their oxidation, at least in adult organisms. Carrier-mediated translocation of ketone bodies across the blood–brain barrier and the mitochondrial membrane of liver, heart, and brain could be important in regulating ketone body metabolism in these tissues.

#### KETONE BODY USAGE BY MUSCLE AND BRAIN IN STARVATION AND DIABETES

Ketone bodies are the principal fuels of muscle in both humans and animals during a brief fast, once their blood levels increase to 1 to 3 mmol/L. The utilization of ketone bodies by muscle is dependent on their concentration in plasma. That other factors play a role is suggested by observations made in obese humans undergoing therapeutic starvation.[110] The total ketone body concentration in the blood of these persons is ~3 mmol/L after fasting for 3 days; ketone bodies are the principal fuel of mus-

cle. By 24 days of starvation, ketone body levels increase to 7 mmol/L (vs. 4 mmol/L of glucose); however, their utilization by muscle is markedly decreased. Presumably, FFAs have replaced ketone bodies as the dominant fuel of muscle at this time (see Figs. 129-2 and 129-5). The biochemical basis for this switch in fuels is not known; however, it is clearly an important means of increasing plasma ketone bodies during prolonged starvation, so as to enhance their uptake by brain and thereby spare glucose. In keeping with this notion, the secondary decrease in muscle ketone body utilization occurs at the same time during prolonged starvation that muscle protein catabolism and hepatic gluconeogenesis are decreasing.

Another situation in which ketone bodies in plasma reach levels as high as 5 to 10 mmol/L is diabetic ketoacidosis (see Chap. 155), when ketone body usage by muscle is depressed; this condition can be corrected by insulin administration.[111] Studies in the rat suggest that FFAs are the principal fuel of muscle in diabetic ketoacidosis, because glucose oxidation is also depressed, but oxygen consumption is maintained or even increased.[111] This diminished utilization of ketone bodies by muscle, as well as their overproduction by liver, accounts for the sometimes profound hyperketonemia in this disorder.

## PROTEIN METABOLISM

Compared with the metabolism and biochemistry of carbohydrates and lipids, protein metabolism is not well understood, and details of the regulation of protein synthesis and degradation in tissues are only partially known. The regulation of protein synthesis involves the transport of amino acids into cells, their activation to form aminoacyl–transfer RNA complexes, and, finally, polymerization of activated amino acids into protein. The last process involves several ribosome-catalyzed reactions that are referred to collectively as peptide chain initiation, elongation, and termination. Each of these steps involves a variety of enzymes and protein factors (e.g., for initiation), as well as energy in the form of guanosine triphosphate and ATP.[112]

Proteolytic enzymes capable of degrading many different proteins are found both inside and outside lysosomes. The degradation of membrane proteins and endocytosed proteins occurs within the lysosome, and the size, density, and fragility of this organelle may change during states of altered protein breakdown. Important nonlysosomal proteases or proteolytic complexes that degrade protein in a wide variety of tissues, including skeletal muscle, include the calcium-activated proteases and the ubiquitin proteolytic complex. The ubiquitin-proteasome pathway is now thought to be responsible for the degradation of the majority of cellular proteins, including abnormal proteins, short-lived normal proteins, and long-lived normal proteins (i.e., contractile proteins in muscle). This pathway has been identified as being responsible for accelerated proteolysis in a number of catabolic conditions associated with the loss of lean tissue mass. Other factors that may regulate or signal the breakdown of a specific protein include its chemical and physical properties, as well as its molecular features such as specific amino-acid sequences.

#### FACTORS AFFECTING PROTEIN METABOLISM IN MUSCLE

The complexity of protein metabolism can be illustrated by focusing on muscle. Various factors, including both hormones and substrates, can either increase or decrease protein synthesis or degradation (Table 129-2).[23] In the fed state, dietary carbohydrate (i.e., glucose) and protein (i.e., amino acids) stimulate insulin secretion, and this largely is responsible for the increase in protein synthesis and the decrease in protein breakdown in muscle. The availability of amino acids, especially the

**TABLE 129-2.**
**Factors Affecting Protein Synthesis and Degradation in Muscle**

| Factor | Synthesis | Degradation |
|---|---|---|
| Insulin | ↑ | ↓ |
| Growth hormone | ↑ | — |
| Thyroid hormone | ↑ | ↑ |
| Glucocorticoids | ↓ | ↑ |
| Prostaglandin $PGF_{2\alpha}$ | ↑ | — |
| Prostaglandin $PGE_2$ | — | ↑ |
| β-Adrenergic transmitters | — | ↓ |
| Serotonin | — | ↓ |
| Glucose | — | ↓ |
| Amino acids | ↑ | ↓ |
| Ketone bodies | — | ↓ |
| Free fatty acids | ↑ | ↓ |
| Exercise | ↓ | ↑, ↓ |
| Starvation | ↓ | ↑ |
| Diabetes | ↓ | — |
| Fever | — | ↑ |
| Trauma | — | ↑ |

(Adapted from Mitch WE, Clark AS. Muscle protein turnover in uremia. Kidney Int 1983; 24:S2.)

branched-chain amino acids, of growth hormone, and of thyroid hormone, as well as generation of the prostaglandin $PGF_2$ within muscle, also may play a role. During brief starvation, insulin levels decrease, decreasing protein synthesis and increasing protein breakdown. This causes a greater efflux of amino acids from muscle, an important adaptation that provides precursor for gluconeogenesis in the liver. Such an increase in amino-acid efflux cannot go unabated, because a loss of more than one-third of the protein stores of muscle is incompatible with survival. To solve this problem, the brain and other peripheral tissues begin to use ketone bodies (see Fig. 129-2). After 1 to 2 weeks of starvation, the fuel mix of the brain consists of about equal amounts of glucose and ketone bodies. This adaptation effectively reduces the requirement of many brain cells for glucose and diminishes the need for hepatic gluconeogenesis. Concurrently, amino-acid efflux from muscle decreases, and protein is conserved. The biochemical mechanism by which protein is conserved in muscle during prolonged starvation is unknown but appears to be related to a decrease in protein degradation. Studies in the rat suggest that the use by muscle of ketone bodies early in starvation and of FFAs later plays a key role.[113]

# REFERENCES

1. Cahill G Jr, Herrera M, Morgan A, et al. Hormone-fuel interrelationships during fasting. J Clin Invest 1966; 45:1751.
2. Cahill G Jr. Starvation in man. N Engl J Med 1970; 282:668.
3. Cahill GF, Aoki T, Rossini AA. Metabolism in obesity and anorexia nervosa. In: Wurtman RJ, Wurtman JJ, ed. Nutrition and the brain. New York: Raven Press, 1979:1.
4. Ruderman N. Muscle amino acid metabolism and gluconeogenesis. Annu Rev Med 1975; 26:245.
5. Owen OE, Morgan AP, Kemp HG. Brain metabolism during fasting. J Clin Invest 1966; 48:574.
6. Ruderman NB, Aoki TT, Cahill GF. Gluconeogenesis and its disorders in man. In: Hanson R, Mehlman M, ed. Gluconeogenesis. New York: John Wiley and Sons, 1975:515.
7. Newsholme EA, Leech AR. Regulation of glucose and fatty acid oxidation in relation to energy demand in muscle. In: Biochemistry for the medical sciences. Chichester, England: John Wiley, 1983:300.
8. Felig P, Wahren J. Fuel homeostasis in exercise. N Engl J Med 1975; 293:1078.
9. Ruderman N, Goodman M, Conover C, Berger M. Substrate utilization in perfused skeletal muscle. Diabetes 1979; 28:13.
10. Holloszy JO, Kohrt WM, Hansen PA. The regulation of carbohydrate and fat metabolism during and after exercise. Front Biosci 1998; 3:D1011.
11. Chipkin SR, Kelly KL, Ruderman NB. Hormone-fuel interrelationships: fed state, starvation and diabetes. In: Kahn CR, Weir GC, Bussy RK, eds. Joslin's diabetes mellitus. Philadelphia: Lea & Febiger, 1993:97.
12. Felig P. Physiological action of insulin. In: Ellenberg M, Rifkin H, eds. Diabetes mellitus: theory and practice. New York: Medical Examination Publishing, 1983:77.
13. Frayn KN. Metabolic regulation: a human perspective. In: Frontier in metabolism. London: Portland Press, 1996.
14. Boyle PJ. Alteration in brain glucose metabolism induced by hypoglycaemia in man. Diabetologia 1997; 40:S69.
15. Cryer P, Gerich J. Glucose counterregulation, hypoglycemia, and intensive insulin therapy in diabetes mellitus. N Engl J Med 1985; 313:232.
16. McCall A, Fixman L, Fleming N, et al. Chronic hypoglycemia increases brain glucose transport. Am J Physiol 1986; 251:E442.
17. Freinkel N, Metzger BE, et al. The offspring of the mother with diabetes. In: Ogata E, Rifkin H, Porte D Jr, eds. Diabetes mellitus: theory and practice, 4th ed. New Hyde Park, NY: Medical Examination Publishing, 1990:651.
18. Hers H, Hue L. Gluconeogenesis and related aspects of glycolysis. Annu Rev Biochem 1983; 52:617.
19. Exton J. Hormonal control of gluconeogenesis. Adv Exp Med Biol 1979; 111:125.
20. Bollen, Keppens S, Stalmans W. Review: specific features of glycogen metabolism in liver. Biochem J 1998; 336:19.
21. Pilkis S, Granner D. Molecular physiology of the regulation of hepatic gluconeogenesis and glycolysis. Annu Rev Physiol 1992; 54:885.
22. Goodman M, Lowell B, Belur E, Ruderman N. Sites of protein conservation and loss during starvation: influence of adiposity. Am J Physiol 1984; 246:E383.
23. Tischler M. Hormonal regulation of protein degradation in skeletal and cardiac muscle. Life Sci 1981; 28:2569.
24. Felig P. Amino acid metabolism in man. Annu Rev Biochem 1975; 44:933.
25. Stumvoll M, Meyer C, Mitrakou A, et al. Renal glucose production and utilization: new aspects in humans. Diabetologia 1997; 40:749.
26. Stumvoll M, Meyer C, Perriello G, et al. Human kidney and liver gluconeogenesis: evidence for organ substrate selectivity. Am J Physiol 1998; 274:E817.
26a. Rajas F, Croset M, Zitoun C, et al. Induction of the phosphoenolpyruvate carboxykinase gene expression in insulinopenia states in rat small intestine. Diabetes 2000; 49:1165.
26b. Mithieux G, Croset M, Zitoun C, Hurot JM. Contribution of small intestine to endogenous glucose production in insulinopenia states in rats. Diabetologia 2000; 42(Suppl 1):165A.
27. Rothman D, Magnusson I, Katz L, et al. Quantitation of hepatic glycogenolysis and gluconeogenesis in fasting humans with $^{13}$C NMR. Science 1991; 254:573.
28. Pagliara A, Karl I, Haymond M, Kipnis D. Hypoglycemia in infancy and childhood. Part I. J Pediatr 1973; 82:365.
29. Goodman M, Lowell B, Ruderman N. Protein conservation during starvation: possible role of lipid fuels. Prog Clin Biol Res 1982; 102:317.
30. Richter E, Ruderman N, Schneider S. Diabetes and exercise. Am J Med 1981; 70:201.
31. Galbo H. Hormonal and metabolic adaptation to exercise. Stuttgart: Georg Thieme Verlag, 1983.
32. Christensen N, Galbo H. Sympathetic nervous activity during exercise. Annu Rev Physiol 1983; 45:139.
33. Richter EA, Garetto LP, Goodman MN, Ruderman NB. Muscle glucose metabolism following exercise in the rat: increased sensitivity to insulin. J Clin Invest 1982; 69:785.
34. Vranic M, Berger M. Exercise and diabetes mellitus. Diabetes 1979; 28:147.
35. Berger M. Adjustment of insulin therapy. In: Ruderman N, Devlin J, ed. Health professional's guide to diabetes and exercise. Alexandria, VA: American Diabetes Association, 1995:115.
36. American Diabetes Association. Position statement: diabetes mellitus and exercise. Diabetes Care 1999; 22:S49.
37. Olefsky JM. Pathogenesis of insulin resistance and hyperglycemia in non-insulin-dependent diabetes mellitus. Am J Med 1985; 79:1.
38. DeFronzo RA, Ferrannini E. Insulin resistance. A multifaceted syndrome responsible for NIDDM, obesity, hypertension, dyslipidemia, and atherosclerotic cardiovascular disease. Diabetes Care 1991; 14:173.
39. Beck-Nielsen H, Hother-Nielsen O, Vaag A, Alford F. Pathogenesis of type 2 (non-insulin-dependent) diabetes mellitus: the role of skeletal muscle glucose uptake and hepatic glucose production in the development of hyperglycaemia. A critical comment. Diabetologia 1994; 37:217.
40. Vaag A, Henriksen JE, Beck-Nielsen H. Decreased insulin activation of glycogen synthase in skeletal muscles in young non-obese Caucasian first-degree relatives of patients with non-insulin-dependent diabetes mellitus. J Clin Invest 1992; 89:782.
41. Reaven GM. Role of insulin resistance in human diabetes. Diabetes 1988; 37:1595.
42. Kissebah AH. Central obesity: measurement and metabolic effects. Diabetes Rev 1997; 5:8.
43. Bjorntorp P. Metabolic implications of body fat distribution. Diabetes Care 1991; 14:1132.
44. Ruderman N, Chisholm D, Pi-Sunyer X, Schneider S. The metabolically obese, normal-weight individual: revisited. Diabetes 1998; 47:699.

45. Ruderman N, Apelian AZ, Schneider SH. Exercise in therapy and prevention of type II diabetes. Implications for blacks. Diabetes Care 1990; 13:1163.
46. Pan DA, Lillioja S, Kriketos AD, et al. Skeletal muscle triglyceride levels are inversely related to insulin action. Diabetes 1997; 46:983.
47. Eriksson J, Saloranto C, Groop L. Non-esterified fatty acids do not contribute to insulin resistance in persons at increased risk of developing type 2 (non-insulin dependent) diabetes mellitus. Diabetologia 1991; 34:192.
48. Matschinsky F, Liang Y, Kesavan P, et al. Glucokinase as pancreatic beta cell glucose sensor and diabetes gene. J Clin Invest 1993; 92:2092.
49. Krebs HA. The effects of ethanol on the metabolic activities of the liver. Adv Enzyme Regul 1968; 6:467.
50. Krebs EG, Beavo JA. Phosphorylation-dephosphorylation of enzymes. Annu Rev Biochem 1979; 48:923.
51. White MF. The insulin signalling system and the IRS proteins. Diabetologia 1997; 40:S2.
52. Shepherd PR, Withers DJ, Siddle K. Phosphoinositide 3-kinase: the key switch mechanism in insulin signalling. Biochem J 1998; 333:471.
53. Coffer PJ, Jin J, Woodgett JR. Protein kinase B (c-Akt): a multifunctional mediator of phosphatidylinositol 3-kinase activation. Biochem J 1998; 335:1.
54. Lawrence JC Jr, Roach PJ. New insights into the role and mechanism of glycogen synthase activation by insulin. Diabetes 1997; 46:541.
55. Harris RA. Carbohydrate metabolism I: major metabolic pathways and their control. In: Devlin TM, ed. Textbook of biochemistry with clinical correlations, 4th ed. New York: Wiley-Liss, 1997:267.
56. Chock PB, Rhee SG, Stadtman ER. Interconvertible enzyme cascades in cellular regulation. Annu Rev Biochem 1980; 49:813.
57. Lawrence JC Jr. Signal transduction and protein phosphorylation in the regulation of cellular metabolism by insulin. Annu Rev Physiol 1992; 54:177.
58. Exton JH. Mechanisms involved in alpha-adrenergic phenomena: role of calcium ions in actions of catecholamines in liver and other tissues. Am J Physiol 1980; 238:E3.
59. Berridge MJ. Inositol trisphosphate and diacylglycerol: two interacting second messengers. Annu Rev Biochem 1987; 56:159.
60. Aragon JJ, Tornheim K, Lowenstein JM. On a possible role of IMP in the regulation of phosphorylase activity in skeletal muscle. FEBS Lett 1980; 117(Suppl):K56.
61. Madsen NB, Kasvinsky PJ, Fletterick RJ. Allosteric transitions of phosphorylase a and the regulation of glycogen metabolism. J Biol Chem 1978; 253:9097.
62. Rahim ZH, Perrett D, Lutaya G, Griffiths JR. Metabolic adaptation in phosphorylase kinase deficiency: changes in metabolite concentrations during tetanic stimulation of mouse leg muscles. Biochem J 1980; 186:331.
63. Nyomba BL, Brautigan DL, Schlender KK, et al. Deficiency in phosphorylase phosphatase activity despite elevated protein phosphatase type-1 catalytic subunit in skeletal muscle from insulin-resistant subjects. J Clin Invest 1991; 88:1540.
64. Uyeda K. Phosphofructokinase. Adv Enzymol 1979; 48:193.
65. Parmeggiani A, Bowman RH. Regulation of phosphofructokinase activity by citrate in normal and diabetic muscle. Biochem Biophys Res Commun 1963; 12:268.
66. Ruderman NB, Saha AK, Vavvas D, Witters LA. Malonyl CoA, fuel sensing, and insulin resistance. Am J Physiol 1999; 39:E1.
67. Tornheim K. Fructose 2,6-bisphosphate and glycolytic oscillations in skeletal muscle extracts. J Biol Chem 1988; 263:2619.
68. Tornheim K. Are metabolic oscillations responsible for normal oscillatory insulin secretion? Diabetes 1997; 46:1375.
69. Winder WW, Carling JM, Duan C, et al. Muscle fructose-2,6-bisphosphate and glucose-1,6-bisphosphate during insulin-induced hypoglycemia. J Appl Physiol 1994; 76:853.
70. Hers HG, Van Schaftingen E. Fructose 2,6-bisphosphate 2 years after its discovery. Biochem J 1982; 206:1.
71. Claus TH, El-Maghrabi MR, Regen DM, et al. The role of fructose 2,6-bisphosphate in the regulation of carbohydrate metabolism. Curr Top Cell Regul 1984; 23:57.
72. Hue L, Rider MH. Role of fructose 2,6-bisphosphate in the control of glycolysis in mammalian tissues. Biochem J 1987; 245:313.
73. Van Schaftingen E. Fructose 2,6-bisphosphate. Adv Enzymol Relat Areas Mol Biol 1987; 59:315.
74. Bessman SP, Geiger PJ. Compartmentation of hexokinase and creatine phosphokinase, cellular regulation, and insulin action. Curr Top Cell Regul 1980; 16:55.
75. Hue L. The role of futile cycles in the regulation of carbohydrate metabolism in the liver. Adv Enzymol Relat Areas Mol Biol 1981; 52:247.
76. Tejwani GA. Regulation of fructose-bisphosphatase activity. Adv Enzymol Relat Areas Mol Biol 1983; 54:121.
77. Ekdahl KN, Ekman P. Fructose-1,6-bisphosphatase from rat liver. A comparison of the kinetics of the unphosphorylated enzyme and the enzyme phosphorylated by cyclic AMP-dependent protein kinase. J Biol Chem 1985; 260:14173.
78. Katz J, McGarry JD. The glucose paradox: is glucose a substrate for liver metabolism? J Clin Invest 1984; 74:1901.
79. Scofield RF, Kosugi K, Schumann WC, et al. Quantitative estimation of the pathways followed in the conversion to glycogen of glucose administered to the fasted rat. J Biol Chem 1985; 260:8777.
80. Randle PJ. Phosphorylation-dephosphorylation cycles and the regulation of fuel selection in mammals. Curr Top Cell Regul 1981; 18:107.
81. Reed LJ. Regulation of mammalian pyruvate dehydrogenase complex by a phosphorylation-dephosphorylation cycle. Curr Top Cell Regul 1981; 18:95.
82. Hagg SA, Taylor SI, Ruderman NB. Glucose metabolism in perfused skeletal muscle. Pyruvate dehydrogenase activity in starvation, diabetes, and exercise. Biochem J 1976; 158:203.
83. Greene DA, Sima AA, Stevens MJ, et al. Aldose reductase inhibitors: an approach to the treatment of diabetic nerve damage. Diabetes Metab Rev 1993; 9:189.
84. Williamson JR, Chang K, Frangos M, et al. Hyperglycemic pseudohypoxia and diabetic complications. Diabetes 1993; 42:801.
85. Gupta S, Sussman I, McArthur CS, et al. Endothelium-dependent inhibition of $Na^+K^+$ ATPase activity in rabbit aorta by hyperglycemia. Possible role of endothelium-derived nitric oxide. J Clin Invest 1992; 90:727.
86. McGarry JD. Lipid metabolism I: utilization and storage of energy in lipid form. In: Devlin TM, ed. Textbook of biochemistry with clinical correlations, 4th ed. New York: Wiley-Liss, 1997:361.
87. Khoo JC, Steinberg D, Thompson B, Mayer SE. Hormonal regulation of adipocyte enzymes: the effects of epinephrine and insulin on the control of lipase, phosphorylase kinase, phosphorylase, and glycogen synthase. J Biol Chem 1973; 248:3823.
88. Manganiello VC, Degerman E, Taira M, et al. Type III cyclic nucleotide phosphodiesterases and insulin action. Curr Top Cell Regul 1996; 34:63.
89. Kather H, Bieger W, Michel G, et al. Human fat cell lipolysis is primarily regulated by inhibitory modulators acting through distinct mechanisms. J Clin Invest 1985; 76:1559.
90. Lam K, Carpenter CL, Ruderman NB, et al. The phosphatidylinositol 3-kinase serine kinase phosphorylates IRS-1. Stimulation by insulin and inhibition by Wortmannin. J Biol Chem 1994; 269:20648.
91. Spector AA, Fletcher JE. Transport of fatty acids in the circulation. In: Dietschy JM, Gotto AM, Ontko JA, ed. Disturbances in lipid and lipoprotein metabolism. Bethesda, MD: American Physiological Society, 1979:229.
92. Fredrickson DS, Gordon RS. Transport of fatty acids. Physiol Rev 1958; 38:585.
93. Hamilton JA. Fatty acid transport: difficult or easy? J Lipid Res 1998; 39:467.
94. McGarry J, Brown N. The mitochondrial carnitine palmitoyltransferase system. From concept to molecular analysis. Eur J Biochem 1997; 244:1.
95. Alam N, Saggerson ED. Malonyl-CoA and the regulation of fatty acid oxidation in soleus muscle. Biochem J 1998; 334:233.
96. Dean D, Chien D, Saha A, et al. Malonyl CoA acutely regulates fatty acid oxidation in rat muscle in vivo. Diabetes 2000; 49.
97. Merrill GF, Kurth EJ, Hardie DG, Winder WW. AICA riboside increases AMP-activated protein kinase, fatty acid oxidation, and glucose uptake in rat muscle. Am J Physiol 1997; 273:E1107.
98. Bavenholm P, Pigon G, Saha A, et al. Fatty acid oxidation in humans is regulated by malonyl-CoA in muscle. Diabetes 2000; 49:1078.
99. Winder WW, MacLean PS, Lucas JC, et al. Effect of fasting and refeeding on acetyl-CoA carboxylase in rat hindlimb muscle. J Appl Physiol 1995; 78:578.
100. Zammit V. Role of insulin in hepatic fatty acid partitioning: emerging concepts. Biochemistry 1996; 314:1.
101. Kim KH. Regulation of mammalian acetyl-coenzyme A carboxylase. Annu Rev Nutr 1997; 17:77.
102. Hardie DG, Carling D. The AMP-activated protein kinase. Fuel gauge of the mammalian cell. Eur J Biochem 1997; 246:259.
103. Prentki M, Corkey BE. Are the beta-cell signaling molecules malonyl-CoA and cystolic long-chain acyl-CoA implicated in multiple tissue defects of obesity and NIDDM? Diabetes 1996; 45:273.
104. Saha AK, Kurowski TG, Ruderman NB. A malonyl-CoA fuel-sensing mechanism in muscle: effects of insulin, glucose, and denervation. Am J Physiol 1995; 269:E283.
105. Ruderman NB, Saha AK, Vavvas D, et al. Lipid abnormalities in muscle of insulin-resistant rodents. The malonyl-CoA hypothesis. Ann N Y Acad Sci 1997; 827:221.
106. McClain DA, Crook ED. Hexosamines and insulin resistance. Diabetes 1996; 45:1003.
107. Keller U, Lustenberger M, Muller-Brand J, et al. Human ketone body production and utilization studied using tracer techniques: regulation by free fatty acids, insulin, catecholamines, and thyroid hormones. Diabetes Metab Rev 1989; 5:285.
108. Robinson AM, Williamson DH. Physiological roles of ketone bodies as substrates and signals in mammalian tissues. Physiol Rev 1980; 60:143.
109. McGarry JD, Foster DW. Regulation of hepatic fatty acid oxidation and ketone body production. Annu Rev Biochem 1980; 49:395.
110. Owen OE, Reichard GAJ. Human forearm metabolism during progressive starvation. J Clin Invest 1971; 50:1536.
111. Ruderman NB, Goodman MN. Inhibition of muscle acetoacetate utilization during diabetic ketoacidosis. Am J Physiol 1974; 226:136.
112. Moldave K. Eukaryotic protein synthesis. Annu Rev Biochem 1985; 54:1109.
113. Goodman MN, McElaney MA, Ruderman NB. Adaptation to prolonged starvation in the rat: curtailment of skeletal muscle proteolysis. Am J Physiol 1981; 241:E321.

# CHAPTER 130

# VITAMINS: HORMONAL AND METABOLIC INTERRELATIONSHIPS

ALAA ABOU-SAIF AND TIMOTHY O. LIPMAN

Vitamins are micronutrient chemical compounds that cannot be synthesized by an organism and that are essential for life processes.[1] They act as required intermediaries, cofactors, or coenzymes in many processes of normal metabolism or may have distal effects. In physiologic or pharmacologic amounts, vitamins may affect hormonal function. Conversely, much vitamin metabolism is hormone dependent.[2]

## WATER-SOLUBLE VITAMINS

### THIAMINE (VITAMIN B₁)[3–6]

The active coenzyme form of thiamine is thiamine pyrophosphate, which is required for the oxidative decarboxylation of α-ketoacids (including pyruvate and α-ketoglutarate) and ketoanalogs of branched-chain amino acids. Thiamine pyrophosphate is required for the action of transketolase in the pentose monophosphate shunt; it also functions as a coenzyme in other enzyme systems.

Thyroid hormones affect both the need for thiamine and its metabolism. Thyroxine (tetraiodothyronine, T₄) administered to rats increases the degradation of thiamine. Thiamine-deficient rats become anorectic and show growth retardation. If hypothyroidism is induced in such rats, the anorexia and decreased growth are mitigated, suggesting decreased thiamine requirements. Conversely, hyperthyroid thiamine-deficient rats have exaggerated growth retardation. T₄ appears to increase the depletion of liver thiamine but does not affect thiamine metabolism in muscle or erythrocytes (i.e., multiple pools of thiamine exist that are affected differently by thyroid hormone). Thus, the need for thiamine is decreased in hypothyroid states, whereas patients with hyperthyroidism may require thiamine supplementation. As an example, gestational thyrotoxicosis has presented as Wernicke encephalopathy, a state of acute thiamine deficiency.

Thiamine also may affect the metabolism of thyroid hormones. When calf thyroid slices are incubated in vitro with thiamine, formation of monoiodotyrosine and diiodotyrosine, and of organic iodide is decreased. In addition, pharmacologic doses of thiamine in rats reduce the uptake of radioiodine into the formation of organic iodine compounds.

Although beriberi is rare in Western society, refractory lactic acidosis has occurred in patients receiving thiamine-free total parenteral nutrition. Thiamine deficiency should be considered in the differential diagnosis of severe metabolic acidosis of obscure cause. (See Tables 130-1 and 130-2.)

### RIBOFLAVIN (VITAMIN B₂)[7–11]

Riboflavin functions primarily as a precursor for two important metabolically active coenzymes: flavin mononucleotide (FMN) and flavin adenine dinucleotide (FAD). The flavin coenzymes are necessary for mitochondrial integrity, fatty acid oxidation, and phospholipid composition. They are coenzymes in the conversion of pyridoxine to pyridoxal-5-phosphate (PLP) as well as in the activation of folic acid, niacin, and vitamin A.

Thyroid hormones appear to have major regulatory control of flavokinase, which regulates the conversion of riboflavin to

**TABLE 130-1.**

**Additional Interactions of Vitamins with Hormonal or Metabolic Systems**

| Vitamin | Effect |
|---|---|
| **WATER-SOLUBLE VITAMINS** | |
| Thiamine | Chronic pharmacologic administration anatomically alters the paraventricular and supraoptic hypothalamic nuclei in rats. |
| | Hypophysectomy in the rat prolongs the half-life of exogenous thiamine. |
| | A thiamine-binding protein has been demonstrated, which may be important for placental vitamin transport. |
| | Weak correlation of blood thiamine levels in diabetic rabbits and humans suggests possible decreased use in diabetes. |
| Riboflavin | Hypophysectomy in rats prolongs the half-life of exogenous riboflavin. |
| | a. Partial effect reproduced by adrenalectomy. |
| | b. Not reproduced by thyroidectomy. |
| | Specific flavin-binding protein has been demonstrated, which may be involved with placental riboflavin transport. |
| | Spontaneous riboflavin deficiency occurs in genetically diabetic mice, suggesting an increased requirement for riboflavin in diabetes. |
| | Absorption of pharmacologic doses of riboflavin is increased in hypothyroid children and decreased in hyperthyroid children. |
| Niacin | Hypophysectomy in the rat prolongs half-life of exogenous nicotinic acid. |
| | Nicotinamide restores the phosphaturic effect of parathyroid hormone and calcitonin in phosphate-depleted rats; the proposal has been made that nicotinamide-adenine dinucleotide formation inhibits tubular reabsorption of phosphate. |
| Pyridoxine | Pharmacologic amounts of pyridoxine have been reported to (a) decrease urinary calcium oxalate stones by decreasing oxalate excretion and (b) increase urinary calcium oxalate stones by increasing oxalate excretion. |
| | Pharmacologic doses of pyridoxine have been reported, without confirmation, to be effective in the treatment of premenstrual depression. |
| | Toxemic placentas have markedly decreased pyridoxine content. |
| Folic acid | Folate deficiency in pregnancy is associated with defective trophoblast, fetal abnormalities (neural tube defects), abruptio placentae, and spontaneous abortion. Women of childbearing age may need to take a folic acid supplement. |
| | Low serum cholesterol has been correlated with low serum folate. |
| Vitamin B₁₂ | Improvement of semen in infertile men reported with vitamin B₁₂ administration (increased total sperm count, increased motility, decreased immature forms). |
| | Bone metabolism is affected by vitamin B₁₂ deficiency. |
| Ascorbic acid | Vitamin C mobilizes bone calcium in young chicks. |
| | Pharmacologic doses of vitamin C reported to decrease fracture rates in osteogenesis imperfecta. |
| | Vitamin C with calcitonin reported to relieve the bone pain of Paget disease. |
| | Pathologic semen reported to contain decreased vitamin C. |
| | Low vitamin C intake reported to be an independent risk factor in cervical dysplasia. |
| **FAT-SOLUBLE VITAMINS** | |
| Vitamin A | Growth hormone may enhance uptake of vitamin A by peripheral tissues. |
| | Short-term pharmacologic doses of vitamin A to rats decrease adrenal ascorbate and cholesterol content. |
| | Menorrhagia can be associated with vitamin A deficiency and improved with vitamin A supplementation. |
| | Cervical dysplasia and neoplasia may be associated with carotenoid or vitamin A status. |
| | Retinoic acid activates osteocalcin gene expression in human osteoblasts. |
| Vitamin E | Pharmacologic doses of vitamin E are reported to ameliorate symptoms of premenstrual syndrome, but do not appear to act through alterations in sex hormones. |
| | Pharmacologic administration of vitamin E reported to lessen menorrhagia associated with intrauterine devices. |
| | Platelet vitamin E content reported to be both elevated and depressed in diabetics, perhaps affecting function. |
| | Pharmacologic doses of vitamin E may enhance insulin action in type 2 diabetes. |
| Vitamin K | Estrogens improve vitamin K absorption in rats and decrease the clotting abnormalities in vitamin K deficiency. |
| | In general, mild hypovitaminosis occurs in well-nourished persons. |

**TABLE 130-2.**
**Effects of Oral Contraceptives (OCs) on Vitamin Status**

| Vitamin | Effect |
|---|---|
| Thiamine | In general, mild hypovitaminosis occurs in well-nourished women. No clinical deficiencies are noticed. Populations at risk (e.g., alcoholics, those with impaired intake) may need supplementation. |
| Riboflavin | Mild laboratory evidence of deficiency found. No clinical deficiency documented. Pathogenesis may be hepatic sequestration of riboflavin and increased conversion to flavin coenzymes. |
| Pyridoxine | Abnormalities in tryptophan metabolism caused by the estrogen component of OCs and reversed with pyridoxine suggest functional deficiency. However, other methods for determining pyridoxine nutriture do not confirm deficiency. The pyridoxine-responsive tryptophan abnormalities have been implicated in OC-induced mental depression. Whether pyridoxine supplementation is necessary remains unclear. |
|  | No adverse effect on pyridoxine status seen with seven different low-dose OC preparations. |
| Folic acid | In the presence of insufficient folate intake or interference with its metabolism, OCs may exacerbate folate deficiency and induce a megaloblastic anemia. |
| Vitamin $B_{12}$ | Vitamin $B_{12}$ levels often tend toward lower limits of normal. |
| Ascorbic acid | OCs may decrease plasma, leukocyte, and platelet ascorbic acid, but this is controversial. Vitamin C supplementation does not seem necessary. |
| Vitamin A | Serum levels of vitamin A are increased, although this may be secondary to increased retinol-binding protein. The fate of human hepatic stores of vitamin A is unclear. The clinical consequence of increased serum vitamin A levels appears to be minimal. |
|  | Combined cigarette smoking and oral contraceptive use associated with low β-carotene levels. |
| Vitamin D | OCs appear to have little effect on vitamin D requirements. |
| Vitamin E | Vitamin E levels have been found inconsistently to be low. Supplementation is not needed. |
| Vitamin K | Requirement for vitamin K appears to be reduced. |
| Multivitamins | Supplementation not necessary for healthy young women taking oral contraceptives. |

(Data from Tonkin SY. In: Briggs MH, ed. Vitamins in human biology and medicine. Boca Raton, FL: CRC Press, 1981:30.)

FMN. $T_4$ augments rat flavokinase and increases the formation of FMN. In addition, thyroid hormones increase the conversion of FMN to FAD by augmenting the converting enzyme, FAD pyrophosphorylase. Conversely, in hypothyroid states decreased formation of the riboflavin coenzymes FMN and FAD occurs, which produces a hepatic coenzyme profile that mimics true riboflavin deficiency.

Because of the regulatory control of thyroid hormone on riboflavin metabolism, extra riboflavin may be needed in both hypothyroid and hyperthyroid states. This is true in hypothyroidism because of the decreased synthesis of FMN and FAD, and in hyperthyroidism because of the increased utilization of riboflavin and its conversion to active forms.

Erythrocyte glutathione reductase, an FAD-dependent enzyme, can be used to define riboflavin nutriture. In hypothyroid humans, erythrocyte glutathione reductase activity is reduced. $T_4$ therapy results in normal levels of this enzyme, demonstrating that thyroid hormone regulates the enzymatic conversion of riboflavin to its active coenzyme forms in the human adult.

Thyroid hormones also appear to control the formation of another class of flavins that is covalently bound to tissue protein. The rate of formation of these covalently bound flavins is increased in the brains of rats that are stimulated with triiodothyronine ($T_3$) and $T_4$. This is striking, in that brain tissue is thought to be resistant to the metabolic effects of thyroid hormones.

Riboflavin deficiency affects thyroid hormonal function and metabolism. Thyroid hormones control flavoprotein enzymes but are less effective as enzyme inducers in riboflavin deficiency

because the necessary FMN and FAD are not available for enzyme stabilization. Riboflavin deficiency retards the hepatic deiodination of $T_4$, which is a flavin coenzyme–dependent process.

Riboflavin metabolism also depends on pituitary and adrenal hormones. Administration of adrenocorticotropic hormone (ACTH) to rats increases the formation of FMN and FAD from riboflavin in the adrenal cortex, kidney, and liver. Aldosterone increases the renal incorporation of riboflavin into FAD; spironolactone blocks this effect. Structural analogs of riboflavin inhibit the formation of FMN and the action of aldosterone, suggesting that part of aldosterone function is flavin coenzyme dependent. (See Tables 130-1 and 130-2.)

## NIACIN[12–15]

Niacin is the generic description of nicotinic acid and its primary derivative, nicotinamide. The nutritional role of niacin was established when it was shown to cure "black tongue" in dogs and pellagra in humans.

Niacin acts as a precursor for two important coenzymes of many metabolic pathways: (a) Nicotinamide adenine dinucleotide is a coenzyme for dehydrogenases that are active in the metabolism of fat, carbohydrates, and amino acids. (b) Nicotinamide adenine dinucleotide phosphate is a coenzyme in dehydrogenation reactions, particularly the hexose monophosphate shunt of glucose metabolism.

Nicotinic acid (at a dose of 1.5–3.0 g per day), but not nicotinamide, decreases levels of very low density lipoprotein cholesterol, intermediate-density lipoprotein cholesterol, and low-density lipoprotein cholesterol, and increases levels of high-density lipoprotein cholesterol (see Chap. 164). The usefulness of nicotinic acid in pharmacologic doses has been impaired by the occurrence of severe flushing reactions. Long-term concerns include peptic ulcer disease, liver dysfunction, and alteration of glucose tolerance. The treatment of hyperlipidemia with nicotinic acid can result in the deterioration of glucose control in patients with diabetes.

Nicotinamide may interfere with nitrous oxide production and immune destruction of B cells, directly preserving B-cell function. Nicotinamide prevents chemically induced and spontaneous insulin-dependent diabetes in animal models. Small-scale studies have shown nicotinamide therapy to prevent or delay the development of type 1 diabetes mellitus in humans at high risk. Nicotinamide use has had no efficacy in early-onset type 1 diabetes, however. Large-scale randomized trials are needed to establish a potential role for this agent in the treatment of diabetes.

Nicotinic acid is a component of the "glucose tolerance factor." Synthetic glucose tolerance factor with bioactivity comparable to that of natural glucose tolerance factor can be produced from chromium and nicotinic acid. (See Table 130-1.)

## PYRIDOXINE (VITAMIN $B_6$)[16–21]

Pyridoxine is converted to its active coenzyme form, PLP. More than 60 PLP-dependent enzymes are known, including amino transferases and others that participate in important decarboxylation reactions.

PLP is the coenzyme in the decarboxylation of DOPA to dopamine and of 5-hydroxytryptophan to serotonin. Theoretically, providing excess PLP as a coenzyme may drive one or both systems. In fact, pharmacologic amounts of pyridoxine and PLP decrease serum prolactin, luteinizing hormone, and thyroid-stimulating hormone levels, and increase growth hormone release. These effects are blocked by the administration of a dopamine receptor–blocking agent. Furthermore, these responses to pyridoxine are absent or diminished in pathologic states such as pituitary adenomas and galactorrhea syndromes. Attempts have been made to use this response in clinical diagnosis or therapy, but they have generally been unsuccessful. Intravenous administration of pyridoxine has not been useful in the assessment of hypothalamic-pituitary status in children with short stature. Initial reports of improvement in the galactorrhea-amenorrhea syndrome in women after the administration of pharmacologic doses of pyridoxine have not been substantiated. Pyridoxine deficiency leads to defective transport of amino acids into cells, which may arise from the deficient growth hormone levels seen in this condition.

By various measures, pyridoxine nutriture is deficient in hyperthyroid conditions, suggesting the need for pyridoxine supplementation.

PLP may have a noncoenzymatic role in cellular physiology and corticosteroid hormone action. After entering cells, corticosteroids bind to specific binding proteins (or receptors) with high affinity, forming an activated steroid-receptor complex (see Chap. 4). This activated complex normally is transported to the cell nucleus and binds to either DNA or chromatin, or both. In the liver, PLP reacts with activated glucocorticoid steroid-receptor complex and inhibits its binding to the cell nucleus. In pyridoxine deficiency, more liver cytosolic glucocorticoid-receptor complex is available for binding to the cell nucleus.

Xanthurenic acid is a metabolic by-product of pyridoxine insufficiency and has been postulated to complex with insulin, producing glucose intolerance. Serum pyridoxine levels are lower in patients with diabetes than in normal control subjects. Attempts to treat gestational diabetes with pharmacologic doses of pyridoxine, however, have not been fruitful.

A randomized trial of pyridoxine, 50 mg daily, demonstrated benefit for psychologic symptoms (depression, irritability, fatigue) seen in the premenstrual syndrome but no benefit for any other premenstrual symptoms. (See Tables 130-1 and 130-2.)

## FOLATE[22-26]

Folate consists of a family of coenzymes whose function is to transfer one-carbon units in the metabolism of amino acids. Folic acid is the synthetic form used for food fortification and supplements. Folates are active in the metabolic interconversion of amino acids and in the biosynthesis of the purine and pyrimidine components of nucleic acids.

Thyroid status may affect folate metabolism. In the rat, excretion of formiminoglutamic acid is increased when low folate intake is accompanied by excess thyroid hormone administration. In addition, thyrotoxic rats have inefficient liver conversion of folate to its active forms, and changes are noted in the liver storage of folate coenzymes. Conversely, in thyroidectomized rats, changes occur in several hepatic folate-metabolizing enzymes.

In humans, clearance of intravenous folic acid is increased in patients with hyperthyroidism, with a return toward normal in the euthyroid state. The suggestion has been made that hyperthyroidism causes depletion of folate and can cause subclinical deficiency, presumably secondary to the hypermetabolic state.

Testosterone affects folate metabolism. Castrated rats show inhibition of the conversion of folic acid to active forms in the liver, prostate, and seminal vesicles. In these organs, the enzymatic activities that are involved with folate coenzyme synthesis are abnormal, and these abnormalities can be reversed with the administration of exogenous testosterone. (See Tables 130-1 and 130-2.)

Folate deficiency is thought to cause fetal neural tube defects, primarily spina bifida but also anencephalopathy. For this reason, since January 1, 1998, in the United States enriched cereal grains have been supplemented with folic acid at the level of 1.4 μg per gram of grain. Low folate intake results in elevated plasma total homocysteine levels, which have been associated with the development of occlusive vascular disease.

## VITAMIN B$_{12}$ (COBALAMIN)[27-30]

Vitamin B$_{12}$ is synthesized by bacteria and is required for normal hematopoiesis; it facilitates the cyclic metabolism of folic acid. Its methyl group transfer activity is essential for a normally functioning nervous system.

Abnormalities in vitamin B$_{12}$ metabolic enzymes are found after experimental thyroidectomy as well as in hyperthyroidism. Vitamin B$_{12}$ deficiency occurs frequently in patients with hyperthyroidism, reflecting an increased requirement for the vitamin; the level normalizes with the return to a euthyroid state. Pernicious anemia, the classic disease of vitamin B$_{12}$ deficiency, is known to be associated with both hyperthyroidism and hypothyroidism. In addition, vitamin B$_{12}$ may be malabsorbed in hypothyroidism in the absence of intrinsic factor abnormalities.

After administration of vitamin B$_{12}$ to mice, the weight of the thyroid gland increases, peroxidase activity of the thyroid increases, and iodination is stimulated. (See Tables 130-1 and 130-2.)

Vitamin B$_{12}$ deficiency induces elevated plasma total homocysteine levels as does folate deficiency. Five percent to 20% of the elderly population may have B$_{12}$ deficiency because of malabsorption of food-bound B$_{12}$ or intrinsic factor deficiency. Thus, because of the association between elevated total homocysteine and occlusive vascular disease, B$_{12}$ deficiency may be a cause of occlusive vascular disease in the elderly.

## ASCORBIC ACID (VITAMIN C)[31-37]

Ascorbic acid is an essential nutrient in humans, although it can be synthesized in several animals, including the rat. It is required for proline hydroxylation in collagen synthesis. It also is required in other enzymatic reactions that necessitate reducing equivalents (i.e., it acts as an electron donor). The normal daily requirements are debatable, because a recommended daily allowance of ~10 mg per day would prevent scurvy, whereas ~200 mg per day would saturate tissue stores.

The pituitary has a high vitamin C content. The vitamin C content of the rat pituitary varies little, however, decreasing only after intense hypertrophy. Generally, the stimulation or inhibition of pituitary hormone release causes no change in pituitary vitamin C levels. In the hypophysectomized rat, however, uptake of vitamin C is lower in many peripheral tissues.

Vitamin C deficiency in guinea pigs increases deiodination of both T$_3$ and T$_4$, decreases inorganic and organic iodine uptake, and decreases organification of iodine. In rats with normal or increased protein intake, the administration of low-dose vitamin C stimulates thyroid activity, whereas the administration of high-dose vitamin C inhibits thyroid activity. Thyroidectomized rats show decreased serum and tissue levels of vitamin C, increased excretion, and increased hepatic degrading enzyme activity, results which suggest that vitamin C needs may be increased in hypothyroid states.

The highest tissue concentration of vitamin C is in the adrenal glands. Although ascorbic acid alters various reactions of corticosteroid synthesis in vitro, its function in the adrenals remains unclear. Chronic ACTH stimulation causes a decrease in adrenal vitamin C; however, the acute administration of ACTH increases the adrenal uptake of vitamin C. Vitamin C deficiency does not cause any clinical adrenal abnormality. Because of the affinity of the adrenal gland for vitamin C, radiolabeled vitamin C has been suggested as an adrenal scintigraphic agent.

Rats given pharmacologic doses of vitamin C have no change in basal corticosterone levels; when they are stressed with ether, however, vitamin C inhibits the normal stress corticosteroid response. Therefore, vitamin C may have inhibitory actions in adrenal steroid synthetic pathways.

Adrenal mineralocorticoids (deoxycorticosterone, aldosterone) appear to influence vitamin C metabolism. Adrenalectomized rats display increased vitamin C catabolism and excretion, which can be reversed by supplementation with mineralocorticoids.

Ascorbic acid acts as a cofactor and functions as an electron donor for the enzyme dopamine β-hydroxylase, which converts dopamine to norepinephrine.

A close relationship may exist between the metabolism of glucose and vitamin C. Scorbutic guinea pigs have impaired glucose tolerance, and the suggestion has been made that similarities exist between the clinical lesions seen in scurvy and the capillary fragility seen in diabetic microangiopathy. Treatment of diabetic rats with ascorbic acid prevented the decreased activity of the collagen-associated enzyme prolyl hydroxylase. This enzyme may be involved in some of the changes seen in the collagen of patients with diabetes. The level of dehydroascorbic acid, the oxidized form of vitamin C, is elevated in the serum of patients with diabetes and prediabetes. This compound has a chemical structure moderately similar to that of alloxan and has caused diabetes when given to rats. Other studies have not found abnormalities in ascorbic acid or dehydroascorbic acid in patients with diabetes. When ascorbic acid supplements have been given to patients with abnormal ascorbic acid and dehydroascorbic acid levels, these values normalized, with no changes in glucose levels. Finally, decreased platelet levels of vitamin C occur in patients with diabetes. When ascorbic acid was added to these platelets in vitro, platelet aggregation was inhibited, suggesting that decreased platelet vitamin C may be a factor in the platelet hyperaggregation of these patients.

The relationship of vitamin C to lipid metabolism is controversial. Several animal models have shown increased serum and tissue lipids in vitamin C deficiency and mobilization of lipids with aggressive vitamin C repletion. Several human studies have correlated low levels of vitamin C with cholesterol or triglyceride metabolic abnormalities. Researchers have observed decreases in lipoproteins with vitamin C given in doses higher than those required to treat scurvy. Serum vitamin C levels have been found to be positively associated with high-density lipoprotein cholesterol levels in women, suggesting that vitamin C is a cofactor in cholesterol homeostasis. Not all studies have confirmed the putative benefits in human lipid metabolism.

Oxalic acid is an end product of normal ascorbic acid metabolism. Excessive intake of vitamin C may produce oxalate kidney stones, although this may occur only in persons predisposed to oxalate stone formation. (See Tables 130-1 and 130-2.)

## FAT-SOLUBLE VITAMINS

### VITAMIN A[38-46]

Vitamin A is a generic term for all retinoids that exhibit the bioactivity of all-*trans* retinol. Vitamin A is a visual pigment precursor, and it prevents xeromalacia. It also serves as a growth factor in somatic cells, is important for epithelial differentiation, and has roles in sexual function.

In severe hypothyroidism or myxedema, the serum is deep orange and patients have an orange hue to the skin; both characteristics are the result of increased concentrations of carotenoids. Although the carotenemia was originally thought to arise from impaired conversion of carotene to vitamin A in the absence of thyroid hormone, it is now attributed to changes in the metabolism of low-density lipoproteins, which act as carriers for carotene.

In hyperthyroidism, liver vitamin A storage is increased and plasma vitamin A is decreased as a result of lower plasma retinol-binding protein levels. Impaired dark adaptation has been associated with low vitamin A levels in patients with thyroid dysfunction.

Vitamin A excess depresses the metabolic rate and induces thyroid atrophy in normal rats treated with thiouracil and $T_4$. Multiple changes in thyroid hormone homeostasis occur in such animals, including alterations in the thyroid hormone–binding capacity of serum proteins, decreases in total circulating thyroid hormone concentrations, increases in iodine-125 uptake by the thyroid gland, and increases in the conversion of $T_4$ to $T_3$ in hepatic homogenates. Prolonged treatment with vitamin A improves experimental immune thyroiditis.

Vitamin A–deficient rats have increased serum $T_3$ and $T_4$ levels as well as elevated serum thyroid-stimulating hormone and thyroid-releasing hormone levels. Vitamin A deficiency has been postulated to induce disturbances in the hypothalamic–pituitary–thyroid axis. Further, the proposal has been made that vitamin A deficiency, because it causes disturbances in this axis, may be a causal factor in the genesis of goiter.

Vitamin A deficiency affects the osseous system by causing changes in bone matrix, including decreased calcium, increased sulfated glycosaminoglycan, and bony overgrowth.

Vitamin A excess can produce bone toxicity, including hypercalcemia, thinning and resorption of long bones, periosteal calcification, and spontaneous fractures (see Chap. 59). The clinical picture may mimic hyperparathyroidism. Vitamin A appears to have direct osteoclastic stimulating activity that is mediated through increased release of lysosomal enzymes as well as direct stimulation of parathyroid hormone secretion. High vitamin A intake is associated with decreased bone mineral density (osteoporosis) and increased risk of hip fractures in women. The metabolic bone disease seen in chronic renal failure has been attributed to vitamin A toxicity, although this is controversial.

Retinol deficiency in rats affects male reproduction by causing atrophy of accessory sex organs, small edematous testes, degeneration of germinal epithelium, decreased size of seminiferous tubules, and cessation of spermatogenesis; all are reversed by replacement with retinol but not by replacement with retinoic acid. Retinoic acid stimulates the testosterone output of Leydig cells. Serum follicle-stimulating hormone (FSH) levels increase in rats after prolonged vitamin A deficiency. These changes in FSH levels appear to be testosterone independent.

Hypervitaminosis A in rats induces hypogonadism, decreased to absent spermatogenesis, and seminiferous tubule degeneration. Morphologic examination of such testes shows focal lesions in the germinal epithelium, delayed spermatogenesis, and decreased nuclear volume of the Leydig cells. Excess vitamin A given to maternal rats induces abnormalities in spermatogenesis in the nursing weanlings.

Both vitamin A deficiency and vitamin A excess can induce endometrial metaplasia in rats. Rats deficient in retinol, but not in retinoic acid, have normal growth and life spans, but pregnancy is terminated with fetal resorption despite normal estrous cycles and mating. This is not corrected with estrogen or progesterone levels. The long-term treatment of female rats with high but nontoxic doses of vitamin A induces polycystic anovulatory ovaries. (See Tables 130-1 and 130-2.)

### VITAMIN D[47,48]

Thyroid hormone decreases the serum concentration of 1,25-dihydroxyvitamin D, although the changes in calcium metabolism seen with thyroid dysfunction may result from direct effects on bone. Administration of 1-α-hydroxyvitamin D together with methimazole may be a useful adjunct in the treatment of Graves disease.

Growth hormone appears to stimulate intestinal calcium absorption. This may occur by way of increased production of 1,25-dihydroxyvitamin D. The elevated serum calcitonin levels that occur in medullary thyroid carcinoma can be associated with alterations in vitamin D metabolites (increased 1,25-dihydroxyvitamin D and decreased 25-hydroxyvitamin D). Abnormal levels return to normal after surgical removal of the medullary carcinoma.

## VITAMIN E[49]

Vitamin E includes ~30 tocol and tocotrienol derivatives, including α-, β-, γ-, and δ-tocopherols. Vitamin E acts as an antioxidant to prevent the peroxidation of unsaturated fatty acids in cells through a free radical scavenger mechanism. Its antioxidant function may be important in platelet function and prostaglandin synthesis.

Vitamin E–deficient rats display decreased pituitary and serum FSH and luteinizing hormone levels, whereas vitamin E–supplemented rats show increased pituitary FSH and luteinizing hormone levels without changes in serum levels. Vitamin E supplementation in humans appears to increase responsiveness of plasma testosterone to human chorionic gonadotropin.

Serum vitamin E levels are low in hyperthyroidism and elevated in hypothyroidism. Thyroid hormone in rats appears to redistribute the vitamin E content of heart and skeletal muscle and of liver tissue.

The rat adrenal gland has a high vitamin E content. In isolated adrenal cell preparations, vitamin E abolishes the inhibitory effect of ascorbic acid on ACTH-stimulated steroidogenesis.

## VITAMIN K[50]

A low-molecular-weight protein, osteocalcin, has been isolated from bone; this protein binds calcium (see Chap. 56). Osteocalcin contains four residues of γ-carboxyglutamic acid, which is the calcium-binding moiety of prothrombin. Osteocalcin appears to be vitamin K dependent in the chick embryo. Neither vitamin K deficiency nor administration of vitamin K antagonists, however, appears to induce abnormal bone growth or abnormal bone mineralization. (See Tables 130-1 and 130-2.)

## FREE RADICALS AND ANTIOXIDANT VITAMINS[51–59]

A free radical is a chemical species possessing an unpaired electron. In animals, free radicals most commonly relate to oxygen metabolism and include superoxide ($O_2^-$), hydrogen peroxide ($H_2O_2$), and hydroxyl radical ($OH^-$).

Free radical generation is essential for the survival of organisms. For example, superoxide production by the white cell is necessary for microbial killing. Oxidation in excess or free radical formation can be toxic, however, resulting in lipid peroxidation, protein degradation, and DNA damage. Free radicals may be generated by normal metabolism of oxygen as well as by such "oxidative" stresses as inflammation, exercise, radiation, air pollution, smoking, and dietary intake. Phenomena attributed to free radical toxicity include autoimmune disease, inflammatory bowel disease, coronary artery disease, stroke, cataract, aging, and cancer.

Antioxidants are substances—endogenous enzymes, vitamins, minerals—that, when present, inhibit substrate oxidation and free radical damage. The antioxidant vitamins include vitamin E (tocopherol), vitamin C (ascorbic acid), and β-carotene.

Antioxidant status is particularly relevant to lipid metabolism. Lipid peroxidation creates a variety of products, including mutagenic lipid epoxides, lipid hydroperoxides, lipid alkoxyl and peroxyl radicals, and enols (α,β-unsaturated aldehydes). Oxidized low-density lipoprotein, resulting from lipid peroxidation, is implicated in the development of atherosclerosis. Antioxidant vitamins and minerals may limit the extent or rate of this lipid peroxidation, thus modulating the development of atherosclerosis.

Antioxidant nutrient status also may be relevant in diabetes mellitus. Oxidants, also termed "reactive oxygen species," have been implicated in the pathogenesis of diabetes (oxidative damage to pancreatic B cells) and diabetic complications, including increased lipid peroxidation in patients with angiopathy, poor glycemic control, cataract development, protein degradation (increased glycosylation), and alterations in glutathione metabolism. Not all studies, however, have confirmed increased free radical activity in diabetes, with or without complications.

Vitamin E may reduce protein glycosylation in patients with diabetes independent of changes in plasma glucose. Vitamin E also may inhibit platelet aggregation in these patients. Furthermore, it reduces vascular reactivity and improves endothelial function.[60–62] Vitamin C levels may be depressed in patients with diabetes who have complications, and a protective role for supplemental vitamin C has been postulated. Not all studies, however, have been able to correlate antioxidant vitamin status with diabetic complications.

Intake of β-carotene, vitamin C, and vitamin E has been associated with decreased risk of thyroid carcinoma in an observational study.

Although observational and epidemiologic data suggest a reduction in cardiovascular as well as other disease risks associated with antioxidant vitamins, randomized clinical trials remain inconclusive. Significantly more research with good-quality prospective, randomized, controlled clinical trials is needed before any therapeutic recommendations can be made with respect to lipid metabolism, diabetes, or cancer prevention. The best advice is to follow recommended dietary guidelines, with reduction in total fat, reduced emphasis on protein, and increased consumption of fruits and vegetables (at least five servings per day).

## MEGAVITAMIN THERAPY[63,64]

Although many effects of pharmacologic doses of vitamins (megavitamins) have been reported in this chapter, none (other than nicotinic acid for hyperlipidemia) have proven efficacy in humans. Reports often involve short-term use, animal experimentation, or extrapolation from retrospective, observational, or epidemiologic studies. Megavitamin therapy is potentially toxic. Use of pharmacologic doses of nutrients should await properly performed prospective, randomized, controlled clinical trials assessing safety and efficacy.

## REFERENCES

1. Ziegler E, Filer LJ Jr, eds. Present knowledge in nutrition, 7th ed. Washington: International Life Sciences Institute, 1996.
2. Kutsky RJ. Handbook of vitamins, minerals and hormones, 2nd ed. New York: Van Nostrand Reinhold, 1981.
3. Appledorf H, Newberne PM, Tannenbaum SR. Influence of altered thyroid status on the food intake and growth of rats fed a thiamine-deficient diet. J Nutr 1969; 97:271.
4. Appledorf H, Tannenbaum SR. Metabolism of thiamine in the hyperthyroid rat. J Nutr 1970; 100:193.
5. Velez RJ, Myers B, Guber MS. Severe acute metabolic acidosis (acute beriberi): an avoidable complication of total parenteral nutrition. J Parenter Enteral Nutr 1985; 9:216.
6. Otsuka F, Tada K. Gestational thyrotoxicosis manifesting as Wernicke encephalopathy: a case report. Endocr J 1997; 44(3):447.
7. Rivlin RS. Medical progress: riboflavin metabolism. N Engl J Med 1970; 283:463.
8. Rivlin RS. Hormones, drugs and riboflavin. Nutr Rev 1979; 37:241.
9. Cimino JA, Jhangiani S, Schwartz E, Cooperman JM. Riboflavin metabolism in the hypothyroid human adult. Proc Soc Exp Biol Med 1987; 184(2):151.
10. Rivlin RS, Fazekas AG, Huang YP, Chaudhuri R. Flavin metabolism and its control by thyroid hormones. In: Singer TP, ed. Flavins and flavoproteins: proceedings of the Fifth International Symposium on Flavins and Flavoproteins. New York: Elsevier, 1976:747.
11. Trachewsky D. Aldosterone stimulation of riboflavin incorporation into rat renal flavin coenzymes and the effect of inhibition by riboflavin analogues on sodium absorption. J Clin Invest 1978; 62:1325.
12. Wahlgvist ML. Effects on plasma cholesterol of nicotinic acid and its analogues. In: Briggs MH, ed. Vitamins in human biology and medicine. Boca Raton, FL: CRC Press, 1981:82.
13. Drood JM, Zimetbaum PJ, Frishman WH. Review: nicotinic acid for the treatment of hyperlipoproteinemia. J Clin Pharmacol 1991; 31:641.
14. Henderson LM. Niacin. Annu Rev Nutr 1983; 3:289.

15. Pociot F, Reimers JI, Anderson HU. Workshop report: nicotinamide—biological actions and therapeutic potential in diabetes prevention. Diabetologia 1993; 36:574.

16. Bigazzi M, Ferraro S, Ronga R, et al. Effect of vitamin $B_6$ on the serum concentration of pituitary hormones in normal humans and under pathologic conditions. J Endocrinol Invest 1979; 2:117.

17. Kidd GS, Dimond R, Kark JA, et al. The effects of pyridoxine on pituitary hormone secretion in amenorrhea-galactorrhea syndromes. J Clin Endocrinol Metab 1982; 54:872.

18. Anonymous. The role of growth hormone in the action of vitamin $B_6$ on cellular transfer of amino acids. Nutr Rev 1979; 37:300.

19. Anonymous. The function of a vitamin $B_6$ coenzyme in the activation and nuclear binding of steroid receptors. Nutr Rev 1980; 38:350.

20. Rao RH, Vigg BL, Rao KS. Failure of pyridoxine to improve glucose tolerance in diabetics. J Clin Endocrinol Metab 1980; 50:198.

21. Doll H, Brown S, Thurston A, Vessey M. Pyridoxine (vitamin B6) and the premenstrual syndrome: a randomized crossover trial. J R Coll Gen Pract [Occas Pap] 1989; 39:364.

22. Lindenbaum J, Klipstein FA. Folic acid clearances and basal serum folate levels in patients with thyroid disease. J Clin Pathol 1964; 17:666.

23. Pasquali P, Landi L, Bovina C, Marchetti M. Effects of thyroxine on the synthesis of folate coenzymes in rat liver. Biochem J 1970; 116:217.

24. Rovinetti C, Bovina C, Tolomelli B, Marchetti M. Effects of testosterone on the metabolism of folate coenzymes in the rat. Biochem J 1972; 126:291.

25. Anonymous. Folic acid fortification. Nutr Rev 1996; 54:94.

26. Pietrzik K, Bronstrup A. Folate in preventive medicine: a new role in cardiovascular disease, neural tube defects and cancer. Ann Nutr Metab 1997; 41(6):331.

27. Stokstad EL, Chan MM, Watson JE, Brody T. Nutritional interactions of vitamin $B_{12}$, folic acid, and thyroxine. Ann N Y Acad Sci 1980; 355:119.

28. Biggs JC, Witts LJ. Altered thyroid function in the rat. Effects on gastric secretion and vitamin $B_{12}$ metabolism. Gastroenterology 1967; 52:494.

29. Carmel R, Lau K-HW, Baylink DJ, et al. Cobalamin and osteoblast-specific proteins. N Engl J Med 1988; 319:70.

30. Stabler SP, Lindenbaum J, Allen RH. Vitamin B-12 deficiency in the elderly: current dilemmas. Am J Clin Nutr 1997; 66:741.

31. Englard S, Seifter S. The biochemical functions of ascorbic acid. Annu Rev Nutr 1986; 6:365.

32. Anonymous. An ascorbate shuttle drives catecholamine formation by adrenal chromaffin granules. Nutr Rev 1986; 44:248.

33. Nath N, Nath M, Muddeshwar MG. Ascorbic acid in thyroidectomized rats. I. Biosynthesis and catabolism. Acta Vitaminol Enzymol 1984; 6:83.

34. Mooradian AD, Morley JE. Micronutrient status in diabetes mellitus. Am J Clin Nutr 1987; 45:877.

35. McLennan S, Yue DK, Fisher E, et al. Deficiency of ascorbic acid in experimental diabetes. Diabetes 1988; 37:359.

36. Hemilü H. Vitamin C and plasma cholesterol. Crit Rev Food Sci Nutr 1992; 32:33.

37. Simon JA, Hudes ES. Relation of serum ascorbic acid to serum lipids and lipoproteins in US adults. J Am Coll Nutr 1998; 17:250.

38. Walton KW, Campbell DA, Tonks EL. The significance of alterations in serum lipids in thyroid dysfunction. I. The relation between serum lipoproteins, carotenoids, and vitamin A in hypothyroidism and thyrotoxicosis. Clin Sci 1965: 29:199.

39. Melhus H, Michaelsson K, Kindmark A, et al. Excessive dietary intake of vitamin A is associated with reduced bone mineral density and increased risk for hip fracture. Ann Intern Med 1998; 129:770.

40. Anonymous. Vitamin A and the thyroid. Nutr Rev 1979; 37:90.

41. Morley JE, Melmed S, Reed A, et al. Effect of vitamin A on the hypothalamo-pituitary-thyroid axis. Am J Physiol 1980; 238:E174.

42. Navia JM, Harris SS. Vitamin A influence on calcium metabolism and calcification. Ann N Y Acad Sci 1980; 355:1.

43. Anonymous. The function of retinol and retinoic acid in the testes. Nutr Rev 1982; 40:187.

44. Carvalho TLL, Lopes RA, Azoubel R, Ferreira AL. Morphometric study of testicle alterations in rats submitted to hypervitaminosis A. Int J Vitam Nutr Res 1978; 48:307.

45. Olson JA. Biological actions of carotenoids. J Nutr 1989; 119:94.

46. Evain-Brian D, Porquet D, Therand P, et al. Vitamin A deficiency and nocturnal growth hormone secretion in short children. Lancet 1994; 343:87.

47. Pahuja DN, De Luca HF. Thyroid hormone and vitamin D metabolism in the rat. Arch Biochem Biophys 1982; 213:293.

48. Kawakami-Tani T, Fukawa E, Tanaka H, Abe Y, Makino I. Effect of 1 alpha-hydroxyvitamin $D_3$ on serum levels of thyroid hormones in hyperthyroid patients with untreated Graves' disease. Metabolism 1997 46:1184.

49. Umeda F, Kato K, Muta K, Ibayashi H. Effect of vitamin E on function of pituitary-gonadal axis in male rats and human subjects. Endocrinol Jpn 1982; 29:287.

50. Hauscaka PV. Osteocalcin: the vitamin K-dependent $Ca^{2+}$-binding protein of bone matrix. Haemostasis 1986; 16:258.

51. Ames BN, Shigenaga MK, Hagen TM. Review: oxidants, antioxidants, and the degenerative diseases of aging. Proc Natl Acad Sci U S A 1993; 90:7915.

52. Abbey M, Nestel PJ, Baghurst PA. Antioxidant vitamins and low-density-lipoprotein oxidation. Am J Clin Nutr 1993; 58:525.

53. Packer L. Protective role of vitamin E in biological systems. Am J Clin Nutr 1991; 53:1050S.

54. Strain JJ. Disturbances of micronutrient and antioxidant status in diabetes. Proc Nutr Soc 1991; 50:591.

55. Sinclair AJ, Lunec J, Girling AJ, Barnett AH. Modulators of free radical activity in diabetes mellitus: role of ascorbic acid. In: Emerit I, Chance B, eds. Free radicals and aging. Basel: Birkhauser Verlag, 1992:342.

56. Alpha Tocopherol, Beta Carotene Cancer Prevention Study Group. The effect of vitamin E and beta carotene on the incidence of lung cancer and other cancers in male smokers. N Engl J Med 1994; 330:1029.

57. Jacob RA. The case for vitamin supplementation. (Editorial). J Am Coll Nutr 1994; 13:111.

58. Lonn EM, Yusuf S. Is there a role for antioxidant vitamins in prevention of cardiovascular disease? An update on epidemiological and clinical trials data. Can J Cardiol 1997; 13(10):957.

59. D'Avanzo B, Ron E, La Vacchia C, et al. Selected micronutrient intake and thyroid carcinoma risk. Cancer 1997; 79(11):2186.

60. Paolisso G, Tagliamonte MR, Barbieri M, et al. Chronic vitamin E administration improves brachial reactivity and increases intracellular magnesium concentration in type II diabetic patients. J Clin Endocrinol Metab 2000; 85:109.

61. Skyrme-Jones RAP, O'Brien RC, Luo M, Meredith IT. Endothelial vasodilator function is related to low-density to lipoprotein size and low-density lipoprotein vitamin E content in type 1 diabetes. J Am Coll Cardiol 2000; 35:292.

62. Neuntevfl T, Priglinger U, Heher S, et al. Effects of vitamin E on chronic and acute endothelial dysfunction in smokers. J Am Coll Cardiol 2000; 35:277.

63. Rudman D, Williams PJ. Megadose vitamins: use and misuse. N Engl J Med 1983; 309:488.

64. Weight LM, Myburgh KH, Noakes TD. Vitamin and mineral supplementation: effect on the running performance of trained athletes. Am J Clin Nutr 1988; 47:192.

# CHAPTER 131

# TRACE MINERALS: HORMONAL AND METABOLIC INTERRELATIONSHIPS

ROBERT D. LINDEMAN

## TRACE MINERALS IN HUMAN NUTRITION

For several decades, trace elements have been recognized as essential substances for animal nutrition. Recognition of their place in human nutrition, however, has been much slower. Our knowledge of the requirements for these substances remains incomplete, largely because of the shortcomings of the methods available for analysis and the difficulty in diagnosing deficiency states. The trace minerals identified as important in metabolic processes are iron, zinc, copper, manganese, chromium, selenium, vanadium, tin, nickel, molybdenum, cobalt, and silicon. The quantities of the four bulk cations (calcium, potassium, sodium, and magnesium) and 11 of 12 of the essential trace elements present in a typical 70-kg man are as follows: calcium, 1000 g; potassium, 140 g; sodium, 110 g; magnesium, 20 g; iron, 4200 mg; zinc, 2300 mg; copper, 72 mg; vanadium, 30 mg; tin, 17 mg; selenium, 13 mg; manganese, 12 mg; nickel, 10 mg; molybdenum, 9 mg; chromium, 1.7 mg; and cobalt 1.5 mg.[1]

Recommended daily allowances or requirements have been established for iron, zinc, copper, manganese, and chromium.[2,3] The most striking examples of clinical deficiency have been recognized in patients on long-term total parenteral nutrition (TPN), in which often no mineral supplements have been provided.

Most manifestations of mineral deficiencies, especially the endocrine and metabolic derangements, can be attributed to decreases in concentration (or activity) of specific enzymes. Many enzymes contain trace amounts of mineral that are required for their full activity. Removal of the metal from an enzyme often reduces its activity to zero; sometimes repletion of the mineral restores the activity, although occasionally an irreversible denaturation occurs. A high degree of specificity is seen in metal requirements; some enzymes, however, allow for substitutions of the naturally occurring metal, but with reduc-

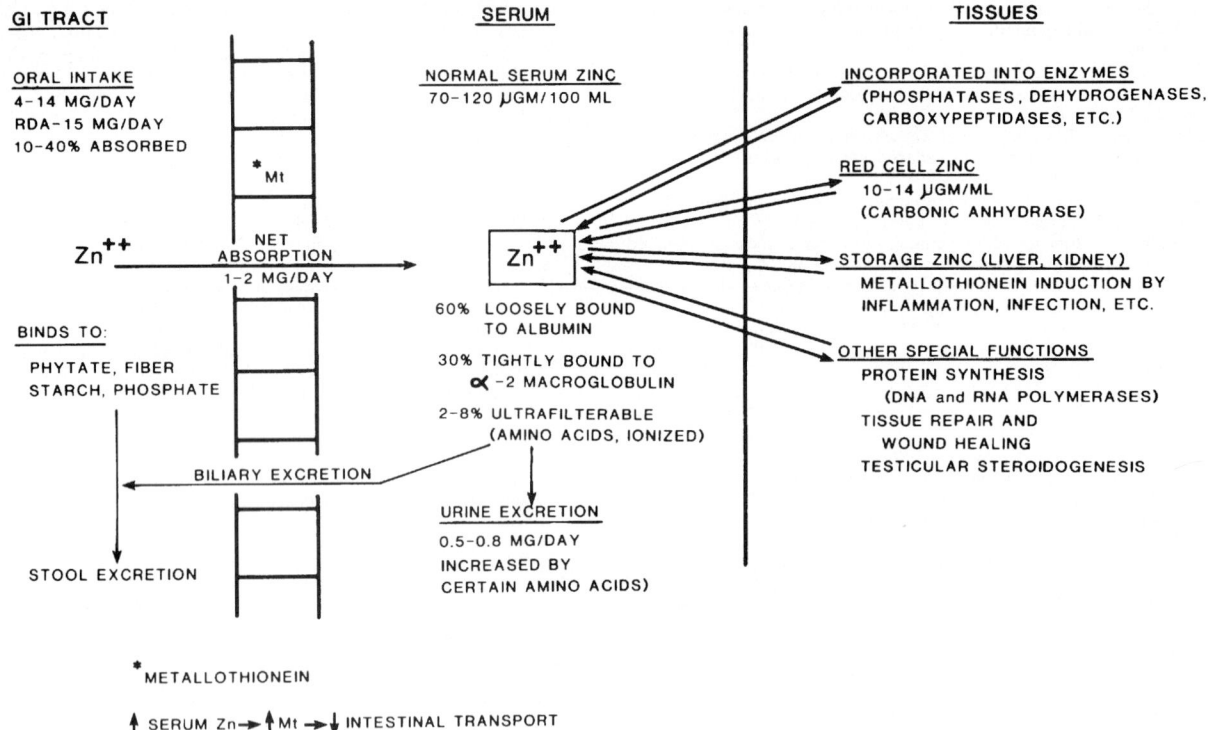

**FIGURE 131-1.** Zinc kinetics in a 70-kg male. All of the trace minerals have similar mechanisms for absorption, transport, metabolism, and excretion. (*GI*, gastrointestinal; *RDA*, recommended daily allowance.) (From Lindeman RD. Mineral metabolism, aging, and the aged. In: Young EA, ed. Nutrition, aging and health. New York: Alan R Liss, 1986:198.)

tion or loss of activity. Much investigative work remains to be done to define the importance of mineral deficiencies that occur in disease entities in which impaired absorption (e.g., malabsorption), increased excretion (e.g., salt-losing nephritis), or abnormal distribution occurs.

## ABSORPTION

The absorption of all trace minerals appears to be at the level of the intestinal mucosa of the small intestine (Fig. 131-1) and is regulated by the concentrations of low-molecular-weight binding proteins. Examples are gastroferrin (iron) and metallothionein (zinc, copper). As the mineral concentration increases in the circulation, the intestinal mucosal cells synthesize these proteins more rapidly. When the minerals attempt to move from the intestinal lumen into the circulation, they are trapped inside the cell and bound to the protein, and, thereby, absorption is inhibited. Dietary components also can bind minerals and prevent their absorption, as illustrated by the binding of zinc by phytates, fiber, starch, and phosphates.

## EXCRETION

For most minerals, excretion is predominantly through the enterohepatic circulation (biliary and pancreatic secretions). Although urinary excretion is not quantitatively important in most instances, notable exceptions occur under certain conditions and in certain disease states. For example, in TPN patients, urinary losses of zinc may become large because of the binding of zinc to amino acids and to other excreted organic complexes.

## PLASMA TRANSPORT

In plasma, all minerals are bound to carrier proteins, either specific proteins such as transferrin (iron) and ceruloplasmin (copper), or nonspecific proteins such as albumin. Only a small

percentage of the mineral remains ultrafiltrable. Most of this, if not all, exists bound to low-molecular-weight substances such as amino acids.

## ENDOCRINE AND METABOLIC DISORDERS ASSOCIATED WITH MINERAL DEFICIENCIES AND EXCESSES

The endocrine and metabolic disorders associated with mineral deficiencies are summarized in Table 131-1.

### IRON

The recommended dietary allowance of iron is 15 mg per day for menstruating females; 30 mg per day for pregnant females; and 10 mg per day for children, all men, and women older than 50 years.[3] Sixty percent to 70% of body iron is found in hemoglobin and myoglobin. Another 20% is stored in a labile form (ferritin, hemosiderin) in the liver, spleen, bone marrow, and other tissues, to be used for the regeneration of hemoglobin in case of blood loss. The remaining iron is firmly fixed in tissues, with small amounts incorporated in the heme-containing mitochondrial enzymes, the flavin-iron enzymes such as succinic dehydrogenase, and red-cell catalase.[4] A hypochromic, microcytic anemia, identified by decreased serum iron concentration and normal to increased iron-binding capacity, is the primary manifestation of iron deficiency. This entity needs to be distinguished from sideroblastic anemia, in which a defect in erythropoiesis but no lack of iron stores is found, and the anemias of malignancy, chronic renal failure, infections, and inflammatory disease, in which iron reutilization is defective and in which both serum iron concentrations and iron-binding capacities are decreased.

Hemochromatosis is a disorder of iron metabolism characterized by the gradual accumulation of excessive tissue iron

**TABLE 131-1.**
**Endocrine and Metabolic Aberrations Associated with Essential Trace Mineral Deficiencies**

| Deficiency | Endocrine | Metabolic |
|---|---|---|
| ZINC | *Growth*—Growth hormone fails to enhance growth rate unless zinc sufficient.<br>*Gonadal function*—Altered steroidogenesis occurs with decreases in serum testosterone and sperm count. Zinc content of testes is decreased. Serum thyroid-stimulating hormone and luteinizing hormone increased. High serum prolactin levels in dialysis patients lowered by zinc supplements.<br>*Somatomedin*—Activity appears to be zinc dependent.<br>*Thymopoietin*—Activity is decreased, affecting thymic-dependent lymphocytes adversely. | *Night blindness*—This may be related to vitamin A deficiency or depletion of retinene reductase, a zinc metalloenzyme.<br>*Impaired taste and smell*<br>*Carbohydrate metabolism*—Rate of insulin secretion in response to glucose administration is decreased. Total insulin-like activity and immunoreactive insulin decreased (? enhanced insulin degradation vs. impaired synthesis or release of insulin from pancreatic B cells). |
| COPPER | *Reproductive failure* | *Brain metabolism of catecholamines*—Low epinephrine levels may be explained by impaired activity of dopamine β-hydroxylase (copper-dependent enzyme).<br>*Abnormal bone formation*—Osteoporosis, probably caused by decreased activity of lysyl oxidase, a copper-dependent enzyme necessary for cross-linking of collagen.<br>*Hypopigmentation*—Results from decreased tyrosinase, the copper-dependent enzyme necessary for melanin synthesis.<br>Hypoproteinemia |
| SELENIUM | *Reproductive abnormalities*—Selenoproteins exist in sperm and testes. Rats fed low-selenium diets reproduce normally; their offspring show impaired sperm motility and morphology (separation of heads and tails).<br>*Thyroid abnormalities*—Decreased glutathione peroxidase in thyroid predisposes to cytotoxicity and thyroid atrophy in iodine-deficient states.[31] Decreased activity of iodothyronine 5'-deiodinase decreases thyroxine degradation. | *Biomembrane protection*—Selenium is the cofactor in glutathione peroxidase that protects biomembranes against oxidative destruction. |
| MANGANESE | Growth impaired<br>Reproductive abnormalities | *Hypocholesterolemia*—Observed in a volunteer made manganese deficient.<br>*Carbohydrate intolerance*—Pancreatic abnormalities and diabetic glucose tolerance.<br>*Lipotropic action*—Increased deposits of fat in abdomen and liver.<br>*Cartilage and bone formation*—Decreased synthesis of normal cartilage and bone matrix rich in mucopolysaccharides (glycosaminoglycans); related to depressed glycosyl transferase, manganese-requiring enzyme.<br>*Biomembrane protection*—Superoxide dismutase protects cells from the deleterious effects of superoxide radicals. |
| CHROMIUM | | *Abnormal glucose tolerance*—Insulin resistance results from deficiency of glucose tolerance factor, a dinicotinic acid–glutathione complex that increases the influx of glucose in response to insulin.<br>Hypercholesterolemia |
| NICKEL | *Perinatal mortality increased*<br>*Growth impaired* | *Skeletal calcium decreased*<br>Hepatic enzymes and concentration of hepatic metabolites decreased<br>Serum proteins and lipids (cholesterol) decreased<br>Iron metabolism impaired (anemia) |
| VANADIUM | | *Hypercholesterolemia, insulin-mimetic* |
| SILICON | | *Connective tissue and bone abnormalities*—Related to depressed collagen content and mucopolysaccharide formation; also, impaired cross-linking in collagen and elastin |

*Observed in humans; all others are documented only in animal studies.

stores associated with parenchymal damage and fibrosis. The principal organs involved are the liver, pancreas, heart, and gonads. Total body iron stores may increase from the normal level of 4 g to as much as 60 g. The excess iron accumulation is due to an undefined increase in iron absorption from the gut.

Family studies suggest that some cases of hemochromatosis are transmitted as an autosomal dominant trait with variable penetrance. Eighty percent of cases are males, and most cases manifest between the ages of 40 and 60 years. Manifestations include hepatosplenomegaly, diabetes mellitus, congestive heart failure, arrhythmia, skin pigmentation, lassitude and weakness, and impotence with testicular atrophy. The last not only is related to direct iron deposition in the testes, but also may be due to anterior pituitary insufficiency.

The diagnosis of hemochromatosis is made by a finding of elevation of the serum iron level (>220 mg/dL), saturation of iron-binding capacity (>90%), elevation of the serum ferritin

level, and demonstration of increased tissue stores on liver biopsy. Phlebotomy is the most satisfactory form of therapy. When hemochromatosis is secondary to a chronic refractory anemia, chelating agents (deferoxamine) can be used.

Aceruloplasminemia is a systemic degenerative disorder characterized by mutations in the ceruloplasmin gene, the absence of serum ceruloplasmin, and iron accumulation in the brain, liver, and other tissues. Patients develop late-onset diabetes as well as neurologic symptoms.[5] Basal lipid peroxide values are greatly elevated. Because iron is an important catalyst of oxyradical-mediated cellular and tissue injury, the speculation has been that B cells become susceptible to the cytotoxic effects of oxidative stress (lipid peroxidation).

In an epidemiologic study of Finnish men, a significant inverse association was found between body iron stores, as determined by serum ferritin concentration, and serum glucose ($p <.001$), insulin ($p <.001$), and fructosamine ($p <.01$).[6]

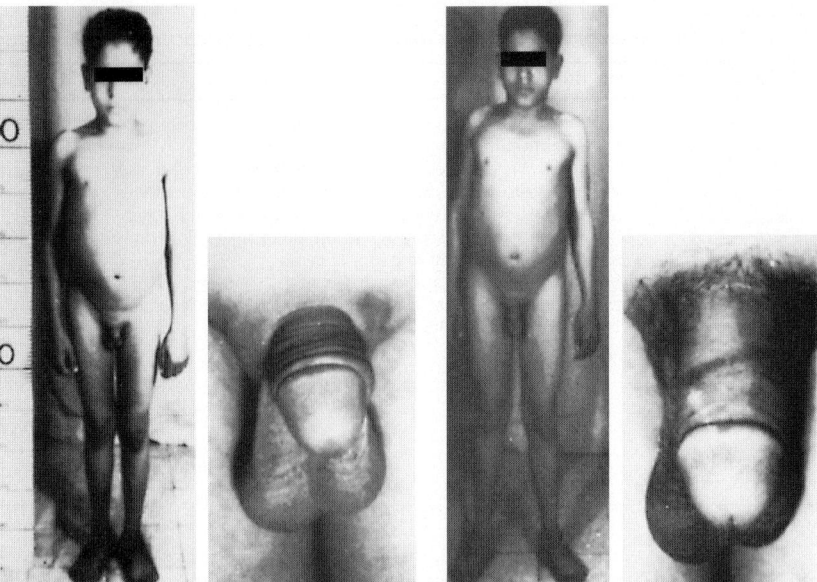

**FIGURE 131-2. A,** A 17-year-old zinc-deficient youth from Egypt with dwarfism was treated with supplemental zinc for 3 months. **B,** Note the striking growth spurt and change in gonadal development. (From Prasad AS. Metabolism of zinc and its deficiency in human subjects. In: Prasad AS, ed. Zinc metabolism. Springfield, IL: CC Thomas, 1966:264, 283.)

**A,B**

Endocrine function was described in nine hemodialysis patients with iron overload, as evidenced by high serum ferritin concentrations, high hepatic density on computerized tomography, and excessive iron stores in the bone marrow.[7] Initially, eight had gonadal failure, six had hypothalamopituitary (HTP) dysfunction, and four manifested thyroid abnormalities. Aggressive iron mobilization improved HTP and thyroid function in all but one patient, but gonadal failure persisted.

## ZINC

The recommended dietary allowance of zinc is 15 mg per day for males and 12 mg per day for females, with an increase for women who are pregnant or lactating.[3] Zinc is the intrinsic metal component or activating cofactor for >70 important enzyme systems, including carbonic anhydrase, the alkaline phosphatases, the dehydrogenases, and the carboxypeptidases. Zinc governs the rate of synthesis of the nucleoproteins (DNA and RNA polymerases are zinc-dependent enzymes) and other proteins, thereby influencing growth and the reparative processes. Zinc is also an important regulator of the activity of various inflammatory cells (macrophages, polymorphonuclear leukocytes) and plays a role in several endocrine functions (growth and sex hormones) and carbohydrate tolerance.[4] The last effect appears to be related to a decreased rate of insulin secretion in response to glucose administration, which could be due either to enhanced insulin degradation or to impaired synthesis or release of insulin from pancreatic B cells. Finally, zinc appears to be an important regulator of bone growth, bone repair, and ectopic bone formation through mechanisms that remain poorly understood.[8,8a]

Animals with restricted dietary zinc develop a moist eczematoid dermatitis, most pronounced in the nasolabial folds and around the orifices; alopecia; retarded growth; anorexia; emaciation; testicular atrophy; and ocular lesions. They fail to gain weight comparably to pair-fed controls. Along with decreased testicular size, a decreased number of spermatozoa is seen, with a late-stage spermatogenic arrest; Leydig cells, however, remain intact. In severe atrophy, the changes are irreversible. The principal defect is a decrease in the release of pituitary gonadotropins.[8] Zinc deficiency in pregnant rats causes fetal abnormalities, behavioral impairment in the offspring, and difficulty in parturition.

Zinc-deficient adolescent males in Iran and Egypt develop a syndrome of severe growth retardation (dwarfism), anemia, hypogonadism, rough skin, and apathy or general lethargy[9] (Fig. 131-2). In these patients, the zinc depletion results from both an inadequate zinc intake and the binding of ingested zinc to foods that contain fiber and phytates (e.g., unleavened bread) and to clay. The impaired growth and hypogonadism respond dramatically to zinc supplementation. Patients with thyroid disease develop aberrations in zinc homeostasis of unknown significance.[10]

Acrodermatitis enteropathica is an inherited (autosomal recessive) partial defect in intestinal zinc absorption that causes severe zinc depletion. Infants develop an erythematous and vesiculobullous dermatitis, alopecia, ophthalmic disorders, diarrhea with malabsorption, severe growth retardation with cachexia, delayed sexual maturation, neuropsychiatric manifestations (irritability, tremors, cerebellar ataxia), and frequent infections.[11] Oral zinc supplements are effective in treating this disorder.

Manifestations similar to those described in infants with acrodermatitis enteropathica are seen in patients with severe hypozincemia associated with TPN (Fig. 131-3), chronic infection, or penicillamine therapy. Clinical manifestations consistent with zinc deficiency are observed in a number of disease states in which it may be difficult to eliminate metabolic dysfunctions associated with the underlying primary disease.[12,13] For example, patients with cirrhosis, nephrotic syndrome, and chronic renal failure have low serum zinc concentrations and nonspecific symptomatology, such as anorexia, growth failure, apathy, and mental aberrations. They also have impaired dark adaptation (night blindness), taste and smell dysfunction, and testicular atrophy with low serum testosterone levels—findings that would appear to be more specific for zinc deficiency. Attempts to improve these manifestations by zinc supplementation have provided highly suggestive but inconclusive results.[14-16] Experimental zinc deficiency has been induced in normal volunteers by placing them on a zinc-restricted diet.[17] A decrease in serum androgens, increase in serum gonadotropins, and oligospermia were observed similar to that seen in patients with zinc deficiency, findings which confirm that these changes were related to the zinc deficiency rather than to the underlying disease.

One of the most studied thymic hormones is serum thymic factor (STF), which is responsible for the maturation and differentiation of the thymus-derived T-lymphocyte line. STF is biologically active only when bound to zinc ions, and in this form it is called *thymulin*. Type 1 diabetics with low plasma and tissue zinc concentrations have marked serum reductions in the active form of thymulin and corresponding increases in the inactive form. Total STF levels in diabetics are comparable to those in normal controls.[18] The low thymulin levels in diabetics and in other patients who have conditions characterized by low plasma zinc concentra-

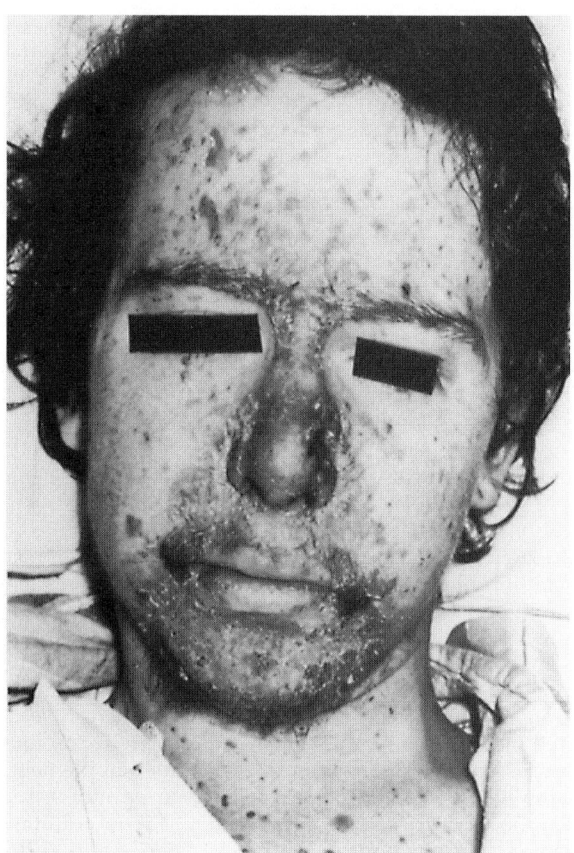

**FIGURE 131-3.** A 23-year-old man with Crohn disease (regional enteritis) was placed on total parenteral nutrition (*TPN*) without supplemental trace minerals. After 3 weeks, he developed lesions, first in the nasolabial folds on the chin and later on the face, perineum and scrotum, extensor aspects of the elbows, the back, and the fingers and toes. After 7 weeks, he had lost most of his hair. Serum zinc was 12 μg/100 mL (normal, 80–130 μg/mL) and serum copper was 62 μg/100 mL (normal, 80–140 μg/mL). Urinary zinc excretion was above normal. The lesions resolved with restoration of hair growth after proctocolectomy and trace mineral supplementation that normalized serum zinc and copper concentrations. (From Kay RG, Tasman-Jones C, Pybus I, et al. A syndrome of acute zinc deficiency during total parenteral alimentation in man. Ann Surg 1976; 183:331.)

tions are due not to a thymic failure in synthesizing and secreting STF, but to a peripheral defect in zinc saturation of the hormone.

An interplay has been demonstrated between serum zinc, prolactin, and thymulin concentrations. Patients with prolactinomas (high serum prolactin levels) have reduced serum zinc and thymulin concentrations with normal levels of STF.[19] Administration of zinc sulfate to patients with prolactinomas raises serum zinc and thymulin levels and produces a small but not significant decrease in serum prolactin levels. Bromocriptine, which suppresses prolactin levels, increases serum zinc and thymulin concentrations. Depletion of total zinc stores, as determined by leukocyte zinc content, has been highly inversely correlated with plasma prolactin levels in patients with chronic renal insufficiency and those on dialysis.[20,21] Zinc supplementation of hemodialysis patients also significantly decreases serum prolactin levels.[20] In one study,[20] the serum prolactin levels in zinc-supplemented dialysis patients were 11 ± 4 ng/mL, compared with 29 ± 7 ng/mL in unsupplemented dialysis patients (normal level is <20 ng/mL). The elevated levels, which persist despite adequate dialysis, often lead to galactorrhea and gynecomastia and may explain the gonadal dysfunction. In contrast, studies of normal and hyperprolactinemic women who were administered a single dose of 50 mg of zinc failed to show any suppression of plasma prolactin concentrations.[22]

In patients with zinc deficiency and normal thyroxine ($T_4$) but low free triiodothyronine ($T_3$) concentrations, free $T_3$ levels normalized after zinc supplementation, suggesting that zinc, like selenium, may contribute to the conversion of $T_4$ to $T_3$ in humans.[23] Furthermore, these patients also showed enhanced reactions of serum thyrotropin (TSH) after thyroid-releasing hormone (TRH) injections; these reactions also normalized after zinc supplementation. Serum selenium concentrations were not affected by the zinc supplementation.

Erythrocyte zinc concentrations are decreased in hyperthyroid patients.[24] They are not comparably increased in hypothyroidism, however. These results suggest that the erythrocyte zinc concentration in hyperthyroid patients reflects a patient's mean thyroid hormone level over the preceding several months, somewhat analogous to the way in which a glycosylated hemoglobin level reflects serum glucose in diabetic patients.

Zinc deficiency occurs frequently in patients with type 2 diabetes mellitus.[25,26] In animal studies zinc deficiency lowers insulin-like growth factor-I (IGF-I), which in turn could alter energy metabolism. Short-term zinc supplementation in postmenopausal women with type 2 diabetes mellitus increased IGF-I only when IGF-I concentrations were initially low (<165 mg/L), but not if they were above this level.[25] Because nutrient intake is the main regulator of IGF-I, another study examined the relationship between nutrient intake and IGF-I concentrations in postmenopausal women; this study found that, after adjusting for age, weight, and intake of protein and other nutrients, zinc intake remained the major determinant of the serum IGF-I concentration.[27]

Zinc plays an imortant role in appetite regulation. Zinc restriction decreases serum leptin levels, and zinc supplementation increases leptin concentrations.[27a] Zinc may influence serum leptin levels by increasing the production of interleukin-2 (IL-2) and tumor necrosis factor-α (TNF-α). On the other hand, it protects against the endothelial cell apoptosis induced by TNF-α.[27b]

## COPPER

Copper is the metal component of the respiratory enzyme cytochrome oxidase and various other enzymes important in human metabolism (e.g., superoxide dismutase, lysyl oxidase, and tyrosinase). It is involved in such diverse enzymatic and metabolic activities as hemoglobin synthesis, bone and elastic tissue development, and the normal function of the central nervous system.[28]

Animals with induced copper deficiency develop central nervous system abnormalities (ataxia, mental deficiency, hypogeusia), skeletal defects (osteoporosis with fractures), heart failure and aortic rupture, infertility, diarrhea, and skin and hair changes. Adrenal steroidogenesis is affected, with decreased conversion of cholesterol to progesterone, corticosterone, and cortisol.[28] Catecholamine synthesis is impaired owing to a deficiency of the copper-containing enzyme dopamine β-hydroxylase. Hypercholesterolemia (increased low-density and decreased high-density lipoproteins) also has been observed in copper-deficient animals.

Menkes kinky hair syndrome is a sex-linked, recessive genetic disorder in which copper absorption from the intestine is defective.[29] These infants develop progressive mental deterioration, hypothermia, defective keratinization of hair, metaphyseal lesions, hyperlipidemia, and degenerative changes in aortic elastin along with hypocupremia and decreased tissue (liver) concentration of copper.

A degenerative neurologic disease has been described in siblings in association with hypocupremia and hypobetalipoproteinemia. Serum copper levels failed to increase despite administration of copper sulfate both orally and intravenously, yet copper concentrations in fibroblasts cultured from these patients were higher than in those from controls.[30]

A hypochromic, microcytic (iron-deficiency) anemia and neutropenia are the principal manifestations of copper deficiency in humans. This syndrome has been observed most frequently in infants with chronic diarrhea or malabsorption or those who are almost exclusively on a cow's milk diet. Both iron and copper replacements are needed to adequately treat these infants. When challenged with bacterial infections, these infants have the capacity to increase polymorphonuclear leukocytes in the blood. Older patients given TPN and sickle cell patients taking zinc supplements to treat hypozincemia also develop anemia and neutropenia secondary to copper deficiency. Experimental copper deficiency induced in a healthy volunteer has produced hyperlipidemia.[31] Marginal deficiencies of this mineral have been implicated in the epidemiology of ischemic heart disease.

Wilson disease, or hepatolenticular degeneration, is a rare inborn error of copper metabolism inherited as an autosomal recessive trait; it is characterized by central nervous system degenerative changes, cirrhosis, and renal dysfunction owing to copper deposits in the affected organ systems. The neurologic abnormalities usually start with an intention tremor and progress to rigidity, choreoathetoid movements, and ataxia. The hepatic involvement may suggest a chronic active hepatitis, or only asymptomatic liver function abnormalities may be present. The renal manifestations are those of acquired Fanconi syndrome (aminoaciduria, glycosuria, renal tubular acidosis, phosphaturia, and uricosuria). The phosphaturia may produce an osteomalacia. A pathognomonic finding is the presence of greenish brown (Kayser-Fleischer) rings in the limbus of the cornea (Descemet membrane) owing to copper deposition.

The histopathologic abnormalities can be related directly to increased accumulations of copper in the brain, liver, kidney, and other organ systems, and they appear to be caused by an impairment in biliary excretion rather than by an increased absorption of copper. The primary defect is theorized to be an abnormality in hepatic lysosomal enzymes involved in the excretion of copper, although the suggestion has also been made that the ability to incorporate copper into protein may be impaired or the synthesis of ceruloplasmin may have failed.

The biochemical manifestations of Wilson disease are a deficiency in plasma ceruloplasmin, the principal copper-binding protein, and an increase in urinary copper excretion. The total serum copper concentration may be high, normal, or low, but the free (unbound) copper is markedly increased. The diagnosis is established by the demonstration of a reduced plasma ceruloplasmin concentration (<20 mg/100 mL) and an increase in hepatic copper concentration (>250 μg/g dry weight). Excess copper stores can be reduced by administering the copper-chelating agent D-penicillamine (1 g per day). Pyridoxine supplements may be necessary to avoid a deficiency of this vitamin.

Zinc supplementation also has been used as a lifelong treatment to prevent reaccumulation of copper, especially in patients unable to tolerate penicillamine. Zinc therapy works by stimulating synthesis of intestinal metallothionein, thereby blocking zinc absorption as well as copper absorption.[32] Although zinc therapy lowers serum high-density lipoprotein cholesterol concentrations in these patients, as in normal subjects, this therapy does not appear to be atherogenic.[33]

## SELENIUM

Selenium is concerned with growth, muscle function, the integrity of the liver, and fertility in ways that are poorly understood. It is closely associated with vitamin E, because the vitamin and the mineral appear synergistic in correcting deficiency states. This may be because they both function as antioxidants, protecting against oxidation injury. Selenium is the metal component of glutathione peroxidase, an enzyme important in preventing red-cell damage.

Retarded growth, infertility, liver necrosis, and myopathy occur in animals made selenium deficient. Weight loss, listlessness, and alopecia, along with myopathy and hepatic degeneration that ultimately leads to death, are observed when primates are made selenium deficient. Interestingly, selenoproteins ranging in size from 15,000 to 20,000 Da have been characterized in spermatozoa and testes. In this regard, rats fed a low-selenium diet reproduce normally, but their offspring on the same diet show impaired sperm motility and morphology.[34]

Several patients on long-term TPN developed muscle pain, tenderness, and weakness.[35,36] They had undetectable serum selenium concentrations, and their myopathy responded to replacement of selenium. Other patients on TPN developed a cardiomyopathy that responded to selenium replacement therapy.[37] This latter entity is common in the Keshan province of China, where the environment appears deficient in selenium. The cardiomyopathy is selenium responsive.

Children with phenylketonuria (PKU) are at risk of selenium deficiency because of their synthetic diets. A group of children with PKU were observed to have significantly lower plasma and erythrocyte selenium and glutathione peroxidase activities than matched controls. They also had significantly higher levels of lipid peroxidation products (plasma malondialdehyde concentrations).[38] Oral administration of sodium selenite to the children with PKU caused all these differences to disappear.

Iodothyronine 5'-deiodinase, which is mainly responsible for peripheral $T_3$ production, is a selenium-containing enzyme. Reduced peripheral conversion of $T_4$ to $T_3$ with a lower $T_3/T_4$ ratio and overt hypothyroidism is common in the elderly (see Chap. 199). A highly significant direct linear correlation has been observed between the $T_3/T_4$ ratio, and serum selenium and red blood cell glutathione peroxidase activity (an index of selenium status).[39] Furthermore, selenium supplementation with improved selenium status resulted in an increase in the $T_3/T_4$ ratio, primarily due to a lowering of $T_4$ concentrations.[40]

Low serum selenium concentrations and decreased thyroid function are often seen in chronic uremic patients. In one study, serum selenium correlated directly with free $T_3$ and inversely with TSH concentrations; moreover, selenium supplementation increased free $T_3$ and reduced TSH concentrations.[41] In another study of patients with acute renal failure, serum selenium, $T_4$, $T_3$ and free $T_3$ concentrations were all reduced, but free $T_4$ and TSH concentrations were normal, and no clinical manifestations of hypothyroidism were present.[42]

Interesting observations have been reported on the development of endemic myxedematous cretinism in a population in northern Zaire with combined selenium and iodine deficiencies. The postulation was that, by decreasing glutathione peroxidase activity, selenium deficiency might increase the hydrogen peroxide supply in the thyroid, leading to cytotoxicity and thyroid atrophy.[43] Selenium supplementation alone was further speculated to possibly aggravate hypothyroidism by increasing the activity of the selenoenzyme type I iodothyronine 5'-deiodinase and thereby increasing thyroxine degradation.[44] This hypothesis was tested by showing that selenium supplementation produced a dramatic decrease in the already impaired thyroid function of clinically hypothyroid subjects.[45]

## MANGANESE

Manganese is the metal component of two critically important enzymes: pyruvate carboxylase and superoxide dismutase. Pyruvate carboxylase regulates the first step of carbohydrate synthesis from pyruvate, and superoxide dismutase protects cells from the deleterious effects of free superoxide radicals. Although manganese can activate many metal-enzyme complexes, other metals (e.g., magnesium) may substitute for manganese.

Manganese-deficient animals exhibit defective growth, bone abnormalities, reproductive dysfunction, and central nervous system abnormalities (ataxia). The synthesis of normal cartilage or of bone matrix rich in mucopolysaccharides (glycosaminoglycans) is depressed in manganese deficiency, presumably because of the depressed activity of glycosyl transferase, a manganese-requiring enzyme.

In female rodents, decreased manganese intake is associated with inability to mate, sterility, and absent or irregular estrous cycles; in the male, it is accompanied by decreased or absent spermatozoa, seminal tubule degeneration, hypogonadism, sterility, and lack of libido. Manganese-deficient animals also develop pancreatic abnormalities and show a diabetic glucose tolerance curve and abnormal deposits of fat in the abdomen and liver (lipotropic effect).

Manganese deficiency was first noted in humans[46] when manganese was inadvertently omitted from a purified synthetic diet fed to a volunteer under study for vitamin K deficiency for 7 months. The person developed weight loss, reddening of his normally black hair and beard, slowed growth of hair and nails, and a transient dermatitis. Most striking was the marked decrease in serum cholesterol; other lipids (phospholipids and triglycerides) showed lesser decreases. These manifestations and lipid levels all normalized after repletion with manganese.

## CHROMIUM

Chromium is an integral and active part of the glucose tolerance factor (GTF), a dinicotinic acid glutathione complex, which increases the influx of glucose into cells in response to insulin. Because of the low levels of chromium normally present in tissue and blood and the difficulty in accurately quantifying these amounts, chromium deficiency is best documented by demonstrating a response to chromium supplementation.[47]

A deficiency of chromium or GTF in animals produces an abnormal glucose tolerance (insulin resistance). Chromium deficiency in humans occurs after prolonged TPN.[48] Cases are characterized by impaired glucose tolerance, insulin resistance not responsive to added exogenous insulin, decreased high-density lipoprotein cholesterol and increased low-density lipoprotein cholesterol, and peripheral neuropathy or encephalopathy. All signs and symptoms disappear when chromium intake is increased.

Interestingly, diabetics have an increased turnover of chromium; increased intestinal absorption and urinary losses have been documented. Diabetic children have lower hair and liver chromium concentrations than do matched controls. Age appears to be associated with a gradual depletion of body chromium stores, suggesting suboptimal intakes or absorption over long periods.[49] Males have significantly lower levels than females. Supplements of GTF contained in brewer's yeast or chromium chloride have been reported to improve glucose tolerance in some populations of elderly subjects.[50] In a more recent double-blind, randomized trial involving 180 patients with type 2 diabetes, supplementation with chromium, either as picolinate or chloride, had significant beneficial effects on glucose, insulin, glycosylated hemoglobin, and cholesterol variables after 4 months of treatment.[51] On the other hand, other studies involving elderly patients with type 2 diabetes have failed to show improvement in carbohydrate metabolism (plasma glucose and insulin, glycosylated hemoglobin, C peptide), or total cholesterol with chromium supplementation.[52–54] Two of these studies, however, did show that chromium supplementation lowered serum triglyceride concentrations significantly,[52,53] and one of these found an increase in high-density lipoprotein cholesterol.[52] Corticosteroid treatment increases urinary chromium losses; corticosteroid-induced diabetes can be reversed by chromium supplementation.[54a]

## MOLYBDENUM

Molybdenum is a cofactor of xanthine, sulfite, and aldehyde oxidases, and is a copper antagonist. Molybdenum deficiency in animals reduces the conversion of hypoxanthine and xanthine to uric acid (dependent on xanthine oxidase), causing the development of xanthine renal calculi. Thus, the effects of molybdenum deficiency resemble those of allopurinol. An increase in dental caries and defective growth have also been attributed to a deficiency of molybdenum.

One case of apparent molybdenum deficiency was reported in a patient on TPN.[55] The patient appeared intolerant of the sulfur amino acids and developed tachycardia, tachypnea, central scotomas, night blindness, irritability, and, finally, coma that cleared when the amino acids were discontinued. Serum uric acid levels were low. Urinary sulfite, thiosulfite, xanthine, and hypoxanthine excretions were increased, and urinary sulfate and uric acid excretions were low. Sulfite and thiosulfite are converted to sulfate by sulfite oxidase, and xanthine and hypoxanthine are converted to uric acid by xanthine oxidase, both molybdenum-dependent enzymes. Treatment with molybdenum improved the patient's clinical condition, reversed the sulfur-handling defect, and normalized uric acid production.

## COBALT

Cobalt is the metal cofactor in vitamin $B_{12}$. Some evidence also indicates that it may play a role in immunity. Because it is such a commonly available nutrient and such a small amount is needed to meet demands, no cobalt deficiency in animals or humans has been reported.

## VANADIUM

Vanadium deficiency appears to impair growth, affect bone development and reproduction adversely, and have an impact on lipid metabolism. As a deficiency is induced, a decrease in serum cholesterol is observed, but later a hypercholesterolemia develops. When pharmacologic quantities of vanadium are given to normal volunteers, a striking decrease in serum cholesterol concentrations is observed.[56] Insulin-mimetic, anti-diabetic, and antihypertensive effects have been demonstrated with pharmacologic doses of vanadium. Organic vanadium complexes are 2 to 3 times more potent than inorganic vanadium.[56a]

## NICKEL

Nickel deficiency in animals produces an impaired growth rate, hair changes, decreased skin pigmentation, shortening of the long bones, anemia, impaired reproduction, hypocholesterolemia, and ultrastructural changes in hepatocytes. Nickel may play a role in metabolism, or it may affect the structure of membranes, possibly by stabilizing the structure of nucleic acids. Nickel nutriture does not appear to be a problem in normal humans, but plasma nickel concentrations are decreased in patients with cirrhosis and chronic renal failure.[57] This could be due to either nickel deficiency or a decrease in plasma carrier protein concentrations.

## SILICON

Silicon is one of the elements most recently reported to be essential for animals. It is necessary for an early stage of bone calcification involving the cartilage matrix.[58] Silicon is a constituent of certain glycosaminoglycans and polysaccharide matrices, suggesting a role for silicon in mucopolysaccharide metabolism.

## TIN

Tin is essential for the growth of rats maintained on purified amino-acid diets in a trace element–controlled environment. Other trace elements (e.g., aluminum and titanium) ultimately may be shown to be essential minerals.

## FLUORIDE

Although not strictly a trace mineral, fluoride, like iodide (see Chap. 37), has an important role in preventing disease and promoting health, and yet, when given in excess, produces toxicity.

Interest in the biologic importance of fluoride has initially focused on the toxic effects in animals and humans (*chronic endemic fluorosis*). The beneficial effect of fluoride on the incidence of dental caries first was recognized with the observation that children with mottled enamel were relatively free from dental decay. Subsequently, a quantitative relation between caries incidence and fluoride in drinking water was shown, with optimal levels of fluoride in drinking water for dental health found to be 1 to 2 ppm. Mechanisms suggested to explain the cariostatic properties of fluoride include (a) alteration of tooth crown morphology, (b) formation of large, perfect crystals of apatite, (c) stimulation of processes at the enamel surface, (d) decreased solubility of enamel, and (e) decreased bacterial enzymatic activity in dental plaque.

As much as 95% of body fluoride is incorporated into skeletal and dental tissues. Chronic exposure to excessive fluoride leads to fibrosis of the bones, characterized by an increase in the radiologic density of the axial skeleton, starting with a coarsening of the trabecular pattern of the lumbar vertebrae and progressing to the marble-white appearance of osteosclerosis. New periosteal growth occurs, and osteophytes form. Nerve compression as well as kyphosis may ensue.

Fluoride may be a possible factor in the prevention and therapy of osteoporosis.[59] Osteoporosis appears to be less common in high-fluoride regions. Therapeutically, the predominant effect of fluoride on the skeleton is to stimulate osteoblastic activity. Osteoid is laid down, and unless calcium supplements are provided, osteomalacia develops. The osteogenic effect of fluoride contrasts with that of estrogen and calcium, which maintain bone mass by retarding resorption rather than by stimulating accretion. Fluoride stimulates positive calcium balance; it is incorporated into the crystalline structure of bone as fluoroapatite. Although fluoride treatment appears to result in a gain in axial trabecular bone, osteoporotic patients treated with fluoride show a loss of radial and metacarpal cortical bone.

Two controlled trials of fluoride treatment of osteoporosis have shown no reduction in fracture rates; in neither was calcium supplementation provided with the fluoride, and this might have influenced the results. In a subsequent study that used various combinations of calcium and fluoride, a considerable reduction in vertebral fracture rate was observed.[60] The results were even more striking when estrogen was added to this combination (see Chap. 64).

Finally, the incidence of urolithiasis is higher in areas in which the fluoride content of water is high. The ingestion of fluoride increases susceptibility to crystalluria and bladder stone formation in rats, further suggesting that fluoride intake may be a factor in urinary tract stone formation.[61]

## SOME OTHER EFFECTS OF EXCESS ESSENTIAL TRACE ELEMENTS

Each of the essential trace elements can produce acute or chronic signs and symptoms of toxicity when given in sufficient quantities. Most toxicity is related to specific organ damage (liver, kidney, brain), gastrointestinal irritation, and systemic manifestations. The endocrine and metabolic evidence of toxicity is primarily related to effects on testicular and reproductive functions. Iron, molybdenum, selenium, and nickel all have their adverse effects.[8] Trace mineral toxicity also can result from inherited metabolic diseases that cause an abnormal accumulation of the minerals in susceptible organs or sites. Examples are hemochromatosis and aceruloplasminemia (iron) and Wilson disease (copper), in which these minerals produce damage and fibrosis in such sites as the liver, kidney, brain, eyes, and heart.

## ENDOCRINE AND METABOLIC DISORDERS THAT AFFECT SERUM MINERAL CONCENTRATIONS

Endocrine and metabolic disturbances may affect trace mineral concentrations in serum, red cells, or other tissues. Specifically,

**TABLE 131-2.**

**Influence of Hormones and Metabolic Disorders on Serum Trace Mineral Concentrations**

| Hormone or Metabolite | Serum Trace Mineral Concentrations |
|---|---|
| **Growth hormone** (acromegaly) | Increases serum copper and decreases serum zinc concentrations[8] |
| **Thyroid hormone** (hyperthyroidism) | Increases serum copper and decreases serum selenium concentrations[62] |
| **Adrenocortical hormones** (Cushing syndrome) | Decreases serum zinc and copper concentrations[8,63] |
| **Estrogen, oral contraceptives** | Increases serum copper (and ceruloplasmin) and iron concentrations[8] (also iron-binding capacity) |
| **Progesterone** | Increases serum copper (and ceruloplasmin) and decreases serum zinc concentrations[8,63a] |
| **Carbohydrate metabolism** (diabetes mellitus type 2) | Decreases serum zinc concentrations[64-66] and increases serum copper concentrations[66] |

*Note*: Other pituitary hormones (luteinizing hormone, thyroid-stimulating hormone, follicle-stimulating hormone) do not appear to influence trace mineral concentrations.

the hormones can affect metal distribution, ligand binding, absorption, or excretion. Examples are listed in Table 131-2.

In some cases, the cause of the deviations from normal has been identified. For example, adrenal corticosteroids increase urinary zinc and copper excretions, accounting for at least some of the decrease in serum concentrations of these minerals.[63] Corticosteroids also induce metallothionein synthesis in hepatic and other cells, causing an intracellular shift of zinc. Although the increased serum iron and iron-binding capacity in women on oral contraceptives has been attributed to decreased menstrual blood loss, these also are seen in pregnancy, a finding which suggests that estrogen and progesterone increases alter serum iron concentrations in other ways. Finally, patients with type 2 diabetes have both increased urinary losses and impaired absorption of zinc, which may explain the decreased serum concentrations.[25,26,64] Patients with type 1 diabetes also have increased urinary zinc excretions that return to near normal with improved glycemic control.[64a]

## TOXIC TRACE MINERALS

Five nonessential trace elements (cadmium, lead, mercury, arsenic, and aluminum) can accumulate acutely or chronically to the point of producing toxicity.

### CADMIUM

Chronic cadmium poisoning (itai-itai disease) produces proximal renal tubular disease with tubular proteinuria, bone demineralization owing to phosphate wasting, glycosuria, aminoaciduria, and renal tubular acidosis owing to bicarbonate loss.[67] This entity gets its name from the tendency to develop bone fractures (translation of the Japanese is "ouch-ouch" disease). Animals given oral cadmium over the long term develop hypertension related to salt retention and hyperreninemia.[68] Investigators have speculated that excessive cadmium in the environment attaches preferentially to metallothionein located in the kidney and produces nephrotoxicity, which may be a significant cause of hypertension in humans. Single injections of cadmium produce severe testicular necrosis in most animals. Pretreatment with zinc or a number of other metals is protective.

### LEAD

Lead poisoning can cause gastrointestinal, neuromuscular, or encephalopathic symptomatology. Two distinct types of renal involvement are seen in humans. One is a Fanconi-type proximal tubular disorder characterized by glycosuria, phosphaturia, aminoaciduria, and renal tubular acidosis. The other is a progressive interstitial nephritis, with a high incidence of hyperuricemia and gout, and hypertension.

Excessive lead intake impairs thyroid function, affecting both the pituitary (TSH) and the thyroid gland. It also decreases the secretion of other pituitary hormones.[8] "Moonshine" whiskey drinkers with lead poisoning related to the preparation of whiskey in lead-coated stills have decreased metyrapone responsiveness (decreased pituitary reserve) and decreased immunoreactive serum adrenocorticotropic hormone.[8] Decreased serum levels of 17-hydroxycorticosteroids and aldosterone also occur in association with lead toxicity. The former generally return to normal after adrenocorticotropic hormone administration, suggesting that the defect is pituitary or hypothalamic in origin. Evidence also exists of gonadal dysfunction in individuals with high lead exposure; both men and women have decreased fertility, and the incidence of spontaneous abortion is increased (see Chap. 235). Men younger than 40 years of age and those exposed for <10 years to lead (moderate exposure) have high levels of luteinizing hormone and follicle-stimulating hormone and normal testosterone concentrations, whereas older men and those with longer exposure to greater amounts of lead tend to have normal levels of luteinizing hormone and follicle-stimulating hormone and low testosterone concentrations.[69]

## MERCURY

Mercury poisoning can be due to either inorganic or organic mercury compounds; the symptomatology varies according to the type of exposure, with considerable overlap. Neurotoxicity (memory loss, tremors, cerebral palsy–like picture, sensory deficit) and nephrotoxicity (proteinuria of glomerular and tubular origin) are the most common manifestations.

## ARSENIC

Acute arsenic poisoning is characterized by cramping abdominal pain, diarrhea, nausea and vomiting, dysphagia, cyanosis, headache, hematuria, and weakness, but hyperesthesia, muscle cramps, conjunctivitis, syncope, polydipsia, epistaxis, tinnitus, and periorbital swelling also may occur. A metallic taste and garlic odor to the breath may be present, but are not pathognomonic. Anemia, leukopenia, thrombocytopenia, and eosinophilia also may develop. Subsequent developments may include hepatic enzyme abnormalities with jaundice, electrocardiographic abnormalities from a cardiomyopathy or pericarditis, encephalopathy, kidney failure from acute tubular necrosis, and seizures. A symmetric polyneuropathy (stocking-glove distribution) characterized by a burning sensation and muscle weakness is common.

Chronic exposure to arsenic is associated with hyperpigmentation (arsenic melanosis) and hyperkeratoses located primarily on the palms and soles. Ultimately, the incidence of squamous cell and basal cell carcinoma is increased. Late manifestations to arsenic exposure include a variety of chronic liver lesions leading to portal hypertension, splenomegaly, and esophageal varices.

In Taiwan, high concentrations of arsenic in well water have been associated with peripheral vascular disease and various malignancies. A dose-response relationship also was found between cumulative arsenic exposure and the prevalence of type 2 diabetes.[70] Similarly, in Bangladesh, where individuals with keratosis, indicative of exposure to arsenic, were compared with unexposed individuals, the risk ratio for type 2 diabetes was 5.2 (95% confidence interval, 2.5–10.5) after adjustment for age, sex, and body mass index using multiple regression.[71] Furthermore, the significant trend in risk for diabetes was strongly dependent on dose and duration of arsenic exposure ($p < .001$).

## ALUMINUM

Although aluminum may or may not be toxic in the presence of normal renal function, no doubt exists about its importance in patients with chronic renal failure on treatment with hemodialysis (see Chap. 61). In this group of patients, the tissue accumulation of aluminum causes encephalopathy, osteomalacic osteodystrophy, and, possibly, other complications such as a normocytic, normochromic anemia and metastatic calcification.[72] Although most reports describe the development of aluminum toxicity in patients treated with aluminum-containing dialysates, oral aluminum, which is absorbed from antacids given as phosphate binders or through the use of aluminum-containing cooking utensils, substantially increases aluminum levels in patients with chronic renal failure. Exposure to acid increases ionized aluminum levels.[73] Suppressed parathyroid activity appears to be both a cause and a consequence of aluminum toxicity. Aluminum blocks parathyroid hormone release and causes failure to respond to hypocalcemic stress. Thus, parathyroidectomy accentuates the deposition of aluminum in bone and other tissues.

Dialysis encephalopathy is widely accepted to be caused by the excessive deposition of aluminum in the central nervous system.[72] The first manifestation is a speech defect, followed by dementia, convulsions, and myoclonus. This condition generally develops 3 to 7 years after the patient starts dialysis, but its occurrence has diminished with the recognition of the cause and the use of proper measures to reduce aluminum intake. Aluminum also has been thought to be a neurotoxin associated with Alzheimer disease.[74]

The bone disease in aluminum intoxication is that of a vitamin D–resistant osteomalacia with severe axial bone pain and spontaneous fractures with muscle weakness (see Chap. 61). It often develops or progresses, and serum calcium and magnesium concentrations are normal. The administration of aluminum-containing medications can induce phosphate deficiency, which accentuates the osteodystrophy. Histologically, two variants of bone involvement are noted: an osteomalacic form with widened osteoid seam and an aplastic form with a normal osteoid seam. Both are associated with high bone aluminum concentrations. Once established, aluminum intoxication can be treated with the chelating agent deferoxamine, thereby producing symptomatic relief of the encephalopathy and osteomalacia.

## REFERENCES

1. Schroeder HA, Nason AP. Trace element analysis in clinical chemistry. Clin Chem 1971; 17:461.
2. Guidelines for essential trace element preparations for parenteral use: a statement by the Nutritional Advisory Group. J Parenter Enteral Nutr 1979; 3:263.
3. Recommended dietary allowances, 10th ed. Washington: National Academy Press, 1989.
4. Prasad AS. Trace elements and iron in human metabolism. New York: Plenum Publishing, 1978.
5. Miyajima H, Takahashi Y, Shimizu H, et al. Late onset diabetes mellitus in patients with hereditary aceruloplasminemia. Intern Med 1996; 35:641.
6. Tumainen TP, Nyyssonen K, Salonen R, et al. Body iron stores are associated with serum insulin and blood glucose concentrations. Population study in 1,013 eastern Finnish men. Diabetes Care 1997; 20:426.
7. el-Reshaid K, Seshadri MS, Hourani H, et al. Endocrine abnormalities in hemodialysis patients with iron overload; reversal with iron depletion. Nutrition 1995; 11(Suppl 5):521.
8. Henkin RI. Trace metals in endocrinology. Med Clin North Am 1976; 60:779.
8a. Kirsch T, Harrison G, Worch KP, Golub EE. Regulatory roles of zinc in matrix vesicle-mediated mineralization of growth plate cartilage. Bone Mineral Rts 2000; 15:261.
9. Prasad AS, Miale A Jr, Farid A, et al. Zinc metabolism in patients with a syndrome of iron deficiency anemia, hypogonadism and dwarfism. J Lab Clin Med 1963; 61:537.
10. Dolev E, Deuster PA, Solomon B, et al. Alterations in magnesium and zinc metabolism in thyroid disease. Metabolism 1988; 37:61.
11. Neldner KH, Hambidge KM. Zinc therapy of acrodermatitis enteropathica. N Engl J Med 1975; 292:879.

12. Lindeman RD, Mills BJ. Zinc homeostasis in health and disease. Miner Electrolyte Metab 1980; 3:223.

13. Prasad AS. Clinical and biochemical spectrum of zinc deficiency in human subjects. In: Prasad AS, ed. Current topics in nutrition and disease, vol 6. Clinical, biochemical and nutritional aspects of trace elements. New York: Alan R Liss, 1982:3.

14. Morrison SA, Russell RM, Carney EH, Oakes EV. Zinc deficiency as a cause of abnormal dark adaptation in cirrhosis. Am J Clin Nutr 1978; 31:276.

15. Mahajan SK, Abbasi AA, Prasad AS, et al. Improvements of uremic hypogeusia by zinc: a double blind study. Am J Clin Nutr 1980; 33:1517.

16. Mahajan SK, Abbasi AA, Prasad AS, et al. Effect of oral zinc therapy on gonadal function in hemodialysis patients: a double blind study. Ann Intern Med 1982; 97:357.

17. Abbasi AA, Prasad AS, Rabbani P, Dumouchelle E. Experimental zinc deficiency in man: effect on testicular function. J Lab Clin Med 1980; 96:544.

18. Mocchegiani E, Boemi M, Fumelli P, Fabris N. Zinc-dependent low thymic hormone level in type 1 diabetes. Diabetes 1989; 38:932.

19. Travaglini P, Mocchegiani E, DeMin C, et al. Zinc and bromocriptine long-term administration in patients with prolactinomas: effects on prolactin and thymulin circulating levels. J Neurosci 1991; 59:119.

20. Mahajan SK, Hamburger RJ, Flamenbaum W, et al. Effect of zinc supplementation of hyperprolactinemia in uremic men. Lancet 1985; 2:750.

21. Caticha O, Norato DY, Tambascia MA, et al. Total body zinc depletion and its relationship to the development of hyperprolactinemia in chronic renal insufficiency. J Endocrinol Invest 1996; 19:441.

22. Koppelman MC, Greenwood V, Sohn J, Deuster P. Zinc does not acutely suppress prolactin in normal or hyperprolactinemic women. J Clin Endocrinol Metab 1989; 68:215.

23. Nishiyama S, Futagoishi-Suginohara Y, Matsukura M, et al. Zinc supplementation alters thyroid hormone metabolism in disabled patients with zinc deficiency. J Am Coll Nutr 1994; 13:62.

24. Yoshida K, Kiso Y, Watanabe TK, et al. Erythrocyte zinc in hyperthyroidism: reflection of integrated thyroid hormone levels over the previous few months. Metabolism 1990; 39:182.

25. Blostein Fujii A, Disilvestro RA, Frid D, et al. Short-term zinc supplementation in women with non-insulin-dependent diabetes mellitus: effects on plasma 5'-nucleotidase activities, insulin-like growth factor 1 concentrations, and lipoprotein oxidation rates in vitro. Am J Clin Nutr 1997; 66:639.

26. Sandstead HH, Egger NG. Is zinc nutriture a problem in persons with diabetes mellitus? Am J Clin Nutr 1997; 66:681.

27. Devine A, Rosen C, Mahan S, et al. Effects of zinc and other nutritional factors on insulin-like growth factor binding proteins in post-menopausal women. Am J Clin Nutr 1998; 68:200.

27a. Mantzoros CS, Prasad AS, Beck FW, et al. Zinc may regulate serum leptin concentrations in humans. J Am Coll Nutr 1998; 17:270.

27b. Meerarani P, Ramadass P, Toborele M, et al. Zinc protects against apoprosis of endothelial cells induced by linoleic acid and tumor necrosis factoral. Am J Clin Nutr 2000; 71:81

28. Mason KE. A conspectus of research on copper metabolism and requirements in man. J Nutr 1979; 109:1979.

29. Danks DM, Campbell PE, Stevens BJ, et al. Menkes kinky hair syndrome: an inherited defect in copper absorption with widespread effects. Pediatrics 1972; 50:188.

30. Iwakawa Y, Shimohira M, Kohyama J, Kodama H. Sibling cases of a degenerative neurological disease associated with hypocupremia and hypobetalipoproteinemia. Eur J Pediatr 1993; 152:368.

31. Klevay LM, Inman L, Johnson LK, et al. Increased cholesterol in plasma of a young man during experimental copper depletion. Metabolism 1984; 33:1112.

32. Yuzbasiyan-Gurkan V, Grider A, Nostrant T, et al. Treatment of Wilson's disease with zinc. X. Intestinal metallothionein induction. J Lab Clin Med 1992; 120:380.

33. Brewer GJ, Yuzbasiyan-Gurkan V, Johnson V. Treatment of Wilson's disease with zinc. IX. Response of serum lipids. J Lab Clin Med 1991; 118:466.

34. Levander OA. Selenium: biochemical actions, interactions and some human health implications. In: Prasad AS, ed. Current topics in nutrition and disease, vol 6. Clinical, biochemical, and nutritional aspects of trace elements. New York: Alan R Liss, 1982:345.

35. Thompson CD, Robinson MF. Selenium in human health and disease with emphasis on those aspects peculiar to New Zealand. Am J Clin Nutr 1980; 33:303.

36. King WW. Reversal of selenium deficiency with oral selenium. N Engl J Med 1981; 304:1305.

37. Johnson RH. An occidental case of cardiomyopathy and selenium deficiency. N Engl J Med 1981; 30:1210.

38. Wilke BC, Vidailhet M, Favier A, et al. Selenium, glutathione peroxidase and lipid peroxidation products before and after selenium supplementation. Clin Chim Acta 1992; 207:137.

39. Olivieri O, Girelli D, Stanzial AM, et al. Selenium, zinc, and thyroid hormones in healthy subjects: low $T_3/T_4$ ratio in the elderly is related to impaired selenium status. Biol Trace Element Res 1996; 51:31.

40. Olivieri O, Girelli D, Azzini M, et al. Low selenium status in the elderly influences thyroid hormones. Clin Sci 1995; 89:637.

41. Napolitano G, Bonomini M, Bomba G, et al. Thyroid function and plasma selenium in chronic uremic patients on hemodialysis treatment. Biol Trace Element Res 1996; 55:221.

42. Makropoulos W, Heintz B, Stefanidis I. Selenium deficiency and thyroid function in acute renal failure. Ren Fail 1997; 19:129.

43. Courvilain B, Contempre B, Longombe AO, et al. Selenium and the thyroid: how the relationship was established. Am J Clin Nutr 1993; 57:2445.

44. Vanderpas JB, Contempre B, Duale NL, et al. Selenium deficiency mitigates hypothyroxinemia in iodine deficient subjects. Am J Clin Nutr 1993; 57:2715.

45. Contempre B, Dumont JE, Ngo B, et al. Effect of selenium supplementation in hypothyroid subjects of an iodine and selenium deficient area: the possible danger of indiscriminate supplementation of iodine-deficient subjects with selenium. J Clin Endocrinol Metab 1991; 73:213.

46. Doisy FA Jr. Micronutrient control on biosynthesis of clotting, protein and cholesterol. In: Hemphill DD, ed. Trace substances in environmental health. Columbia: University of Missouri Press, 1973:193.

47. Anonymous. Is chromium essential for humans? Nutr Rev 1988; 46:17.

48. Jeejeebhoy KK, Chu RC, Marliss EB, et al. Chromium deficiency, glucose intolerance, and neuropathy reversed by chromium supplementation, in a patient receiving long-term total parenteral nutrition. Am J Clin Nutr 1977; 30:581.

49. Davies S, McLaren Howard J, Hunnisett A, Howard M. Age related decreases in chromium levels in 51,665 hair, sweat, and serum samples from 40,872 patients—implications for the prevention of cardiovascular disease and type II diabetes mellitus. Metabolism 1997; 46:469.

50. Offenbacher EG, Rinko CJ, Pi-Sunyer FX. The effects of inorganic chromium and brewers yeast on glucose tolerance, plasma lipids and plasma chromium in elderly subjects. Am J Clin Nutr 1985; 42:454.

51. Anderson RA, Ching N, Bryden NA, et al. Elevated intakes of supplemental chromium improve glucose and insulin variables in individuals with type 2 diabetes. Diabetes 1997; 46:1786.

52. Abraham AS, Brooks BA, Eylath V. The effects of chromium supplementation on serum glucose and lipids in patients, with and without non-insulin-dependent diabetes. Metabolism 1992; 41:768.

53. Uusitupa MI, Mykkanen L, Siitonen O, et al. Chromium supplementation in impaired glucose tolerance of elderly: effects on blood glucose, plasma insulin, C-peptide and lipid levels. Br J Nutr 1992; 68:209.

54. Lee NA, Reasner CA. Beneficial effect of chromium supplementation on serum triglyceride levels in NIDDM. Diabetes Care 1994; 17:1449.

54a. Ravina A, Siezak L, Mirsky N, et al. Reversal of corticosteroid-induced diabetes mellitus with supplemental chromium. Diabet Med 1999; 16:164.

55. Abrumrad NN, Schneider AJ, Steel D, Rogers LS. Amino acid intolerance during prolonged total parenteral nutrition reversed by molybdate therapy. Am J Clin Nutr 1981; 34:2551.

56. Curran GL, Azarnoff DL, Bolinger RE. Effect of cholesterol synthesis inhibition in normocholesterolemic young men. J Clin Invest 1959; 38:1251.

56a. Verma S, Cam MC, McNeill JH. Nutritional factors that can favorable influence the glucose/insulin system: vanadium. J Am Coll Nutr 1998; 17:11.

57. McNeely MD, Sunderman FW Jr, Nechay MW, Levine H. Abnormal concentrations of nickel in serum in cases of myocardial infarction, stroke, burns, hepatic cirrhosis and uremia. Clin Chem 1971; 17:1123.

58. Nielsen FH, Sandstead HH. Are nickel, vanadium, silicon, fluorine and tin essential for man? Am J Clin Nutr 1974; 27:515.

59. Fluoride and the treatment of osteoporosis. (Editorial). Lancet 1984; 1:547.

60. Riggs BL, Seeman E, Hodgson ST, et al. Effect of fluoride/calcium regimen on vertebral fracture occurrence in post-menopausal osteoporosis. N Engl J Med 1982; 306:446.

61. Role of fluoride and silicon in urinary calculi disease. (Editorial). Nutr Rev 1985; 43:140.

62. Aihara K, Nishi Y, Hatano S, et al. Zinc, copper, manganese and selenium metabolism in thyroid disease. Am J Clin Nutr 1984; 40:26.

63. Henkin RI, Foster DM, Aamodt RL, Berman M. Zinc metabolism in adrenal cortical insufficiency: effects of carbohydrate-active steroids. Metabolism 1984; 33:491.

63a. Berg G, Kohlmeier L, Brenner H. Effect of oral contraceptive progestins on serum copper concentration. Eur J Clin Nutr 1998; 52:711.

64. Kurlow WB, Levine AS, Morley JE, et al. Abnormal zinc metabolism in type II diabetes mellitus. Am J Med 1983; 75:273.

64a. Pedrosa LF, Ferreira SR, Cesarini PR, et al. Influence of glycemic control on zinc urinary excretion in patients with type 1 diabetes. Diabetes Care 1999; 22:362.

65. Sjögren A, Florén C-H, Nilsson A. Magnesium, potassium and zinc deficiency in subjects with type II diabetes mellitus. Acta Med Scand 1988; 224:461.

66. Walter RM Jr, Uriu-Hare JY, Olin KL, et al. Copper, zinc, manganese, and magnesium status and complications of diabetes mellitus. Diabetes Care 1991; 14:1050.

67. Perry HM Jr. Review of hypertension induced in animals by chronic ingestion of cadmium. In: Prasad AS, ed. Trace elements in human health and disease, vol 2. New York: Academic Press, 1976:417.

68. Friberg L, Piscator M, Hordberg GF, Kjellstrom T, eds. Cadmium in the environment, 2nd ed. Cleveland: CRC Press, 1974.

69. Ng TP, Goh HH, Ng YL, et al. Male endocrine functions in workers with moderate exposure to lead. Br J Industr Med 1991; 48:485.

70. Rahman M, Tondel M, Ahmad SA, Axelson O. Diabetes mellitus associated with arsenic exposure in Bangladesh. Am J Epidemiol 1998; 148:198.

71. Lai MS, Hsueh YM, Chen CJ, et al. Ingested inorganic arsenic and prevalence of diabetes mellitus. Am J Epidemiol 1994; 139:484.

72. Wills MR, Savory J. Aluminum poisoning: dialysis encephalopathy, osteomalacia and anemia. Lancet 1983; 2:29.

73. Kirschbaum BB, Schoolwerth AC. Acute aluminum toxicity associated with oral citrate and aluminum-containing antacids. Am J Med Sci 1989; 297:9.

74. Newman PE. Alzheimer's disease revisited. Cancer Treat Rev 2000; 54:774.

# CHAPTER 132

# EXERCISE: ENDOCRINE AND METABOLIC EFFECTS

JACQUES LEBLANC

## DEFINITIONS APPLICABLE TO EXERCISE

For various reasons, a growing portion of the population has acquired the habit of doing physical work in the form of exercise. When a person does maximal work, the *oxygen consumption* ($VO_2$) is increased many-fold over the *resting metabolic rate*. A relatively high percentage of this increase is explained by *aerobic energy expenditure,* which refers to metabolic processes that require oxygen for the adequate supply of adenosine triphosphate to contracting muscles (Fig. 132-1).[1] The production of adenosine triphosphate primarily depends on the utilization of glucose by various processes, in which the end products are pyruvic acids. These substances diffuse into the mitochondria and combine with coenzyme A (CoA) to form acetyl-CoA. When fatty acids are used as substrate, after being catabolized inside the mitochondria (β-oxidation), they also are converted into acetyl-CoA. Once the step of acetyl-CoA formation is reached in the transformation of glucose and fatty acids, a common oxidation takes place in the Krebs cycle. This form of

energy is available for work at up to 50% to 60% of $VO_2$ max (maximum oxygen consumption); therefore, many activities, such as light jogging, golf, or domestic work, can be classified as aerobic work. *Aerobic exercise* corresponds to activities at which the heart rate remains below 120 to 130 beats per minute—a level of exertion that satisfies most persons. Normative data have been generated for aerobic and anaerobic exercise.[2]

In 1967, Borg and Linderholm[3] defined a scale of exertion corresponding to the heart rate that is attained during work. They observed that when physical work is performed at a heart rate of 120 beats per minute or lower, the effort is perceived as being fairly light, whereas with a heart rate of 140 beats per minute and above, it is perceived as being strenuous. Only persons with considerable motivation voluntarily endure levels of exertion sufficient to increase heart rates above 130 beats per minute and the corresponding expending of energy at levels at which anaerobic processes come into play. This is the level of work (>130 beats per minute) at which evidence for adaptive processes is observed, as commonly demonstrated by an increase in $VO_2$ max and improved performance.

*Anaerobic energy expenditure,* which is less efficient than aerobic work, does not require oxygen. In this case, pyruvic acid that is derived from glucose utilization is transformed into lactic acid, which overflows into the circulation. At this point, it is either transported to aerobic muscles to be transformed into pyruvic acid and completely oxidized in the Krebs cycle or it is converted into glucose in the liver. This transformation of lactic acid, and also of amino acids, into glucose is termed *gluconeogenesis.* The increased blood lactate that occurs during exercise is proportional to the level of anaerobic work. Increased arterial

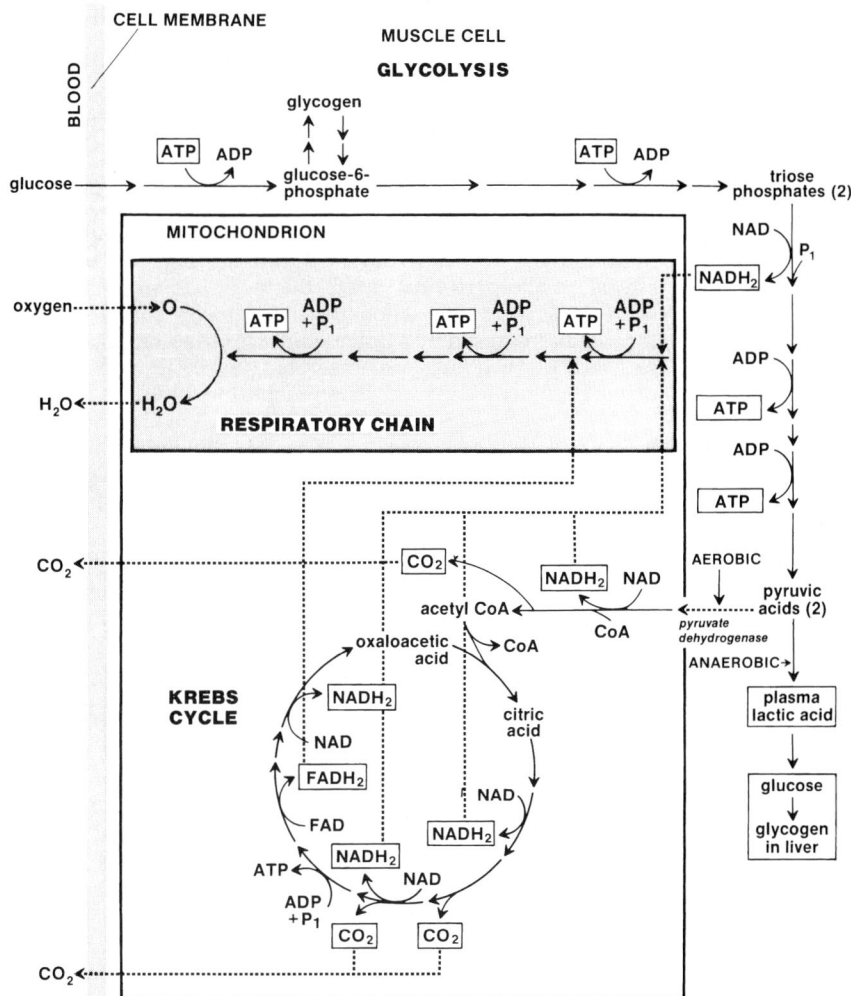

**FIGURE 132-1.** Metabolic pathways for glucose oxidation in the cell. (*ATP,* adenosine triphosphate; *ADP,* adenosine diphosphate; *NAD,* nicotinamide adenine dinucleotide; *NADH_2,* reduced nicotinamide adenine dinucleotide; $P_1$, phosphorus; *CoA,* coenzyme A; *FADH_2,* reduced flavin adenine dinucleotide; *FAD,* flavin adenine dinucleotide.) (From Strauss RH. Sports medicine and physiology. Philadelphia: WB Saunders, 1979.)

lactate concentrations are also found in submaximal effort, particularly when the energy expenditure is sustained by relatively small muscle groups.[4] This level of arterial lactate is an indicator of the extent of the oxygen debt. The *oxygen debt* refers to the excess oxygen intake after exercise; it is calculated as the oxygen consumed above resting requirements. The oxygen debt is proportional to both the intensity and the duration of anaerobic work that is performed. The point at which blood lactate production begins to increase is called the *anaerobic threshold.* Many studies have demonstrated that the percentage of $VO_2$ max at which this threshold is observed increases with training; this finding thus explains the enhanced capacity and the greater ease of performing a given exercise that one acquires after habitually practicing a sport (see Chaps. 129 and 141).[5]

## ADAPTATIONS TO EXERCISE

The adaptive regulatory changes that result from repeated exercise include enhanced blood flow to active muscles, increased blood volume, and more efficient sweating. Cardiac and skeletal muscle hypertrophy is also observed, along with increased density of mitochondria and myoglobin content of individual muscle fibers. The overall functioning of the cardiovascular system is improved, as evidenced by characteristic changes in heart rate, stroke volume, and cardiac output. The reported changes in breathing patterns, pulmonary blood flow, and respiratory minute volume are also indicative of improved pulmonary function because of training.[5,6]

### ENDOCRINE AND METABOLIC ADAPTATION

The regulatory and adaptive responses to exercise result from important changes in endocrine functions, especially those related to substrate metabolism (Fig. 132-2), and are of essential importance in the various processes of energy utilization.[7]

### CATECHOLAMINES

The sympathetic nervous system (see Chap. 85) plays an important role in supporting the energy requirements during physical activities by controlling various cardiovascular adjustments and allowing energy substrate mobilization.[8] The variations of plasma catecholamine concentrations, which are secondary to an overflow into the circulation caused by an increased activity of nerve endings, are acceptable indices of the level of sympathetic activity. The urinary and plasma elevations of norepinephrine are proportional to the intensity of work accomplished by a given muscle mass.[9–12] For example, an increase in oxygen consumption resulting from work done by one arm causes a larger elevation of plasma catecholamines than doing the same work with both legs.[13] Also, plasma catecholamine levels start to increase during running when the work intensity exceeds 50% of $VO_2$ max.[14] For various workloads, this elevation is smaller in trained than in nontrained subjects.[15–18] The capacity for enduring prolonged work at high intensity is primarily controlled by the availability of energy substrates, and in this regard the lipolytic and glycolytic actions of catecholamines are essential. They also exert selective influences on the type of energy sources that are used, such as glycogen. The amount of this substrate that can be stored by the liver and muscles is relatively small; consequently it becomes a limiting factor.[19] One of the ways in which training increases work capacity is through a reduction of glycogen utilization. This sparing effect that is observed in athletes is aided by an enhanced capacity to mobilize lipids in response to catecholamine levels.[20–22] Moreover, the time to exhaustion can be delayed when stored glycogen is increased.[4] Such an effect occurs when the glycogen is first depleted by

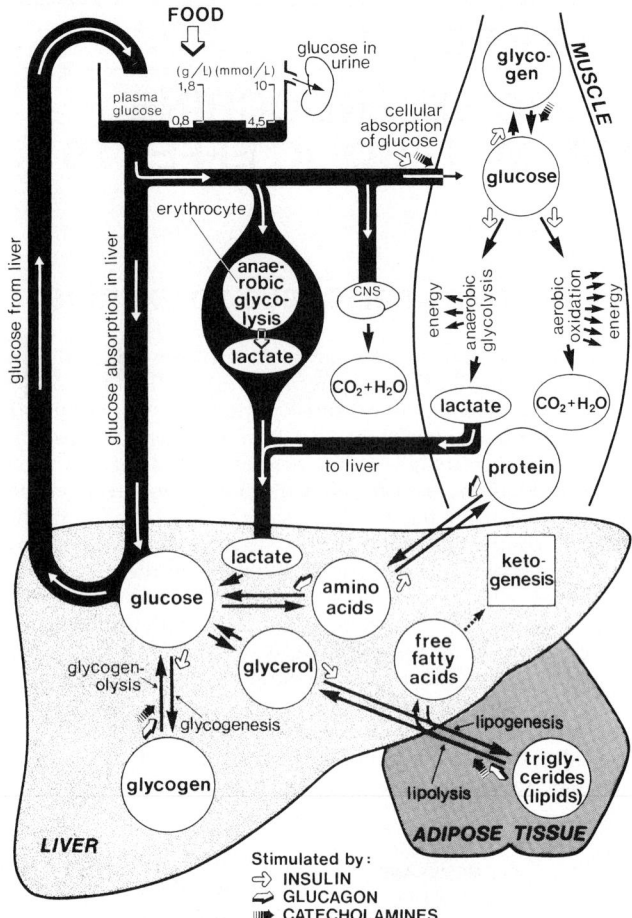

**FIGURE 132-2.** Various hormonal influences on glucose metabolism. (*CNS*, central nervous system.) (From Silbernagl S, Despopoulos A. Atlas de poche de physiologie. Paris: Flammarion, 1985. Copyright Georg Thieme Verlag, Stuttgart, 1989.)

exercise and then is allowed to be replenished by high-carbohydrate diets for a few days.[23,24] Caffeine also has beneficial effects on the performance of athletes.[25] The suggestion has been made that this action is related to an enhanced lipid mobilization caused by a larger epinephrine secretion.[26] At levels of activity above the anaerobic threshold, increases of plasma epinephrine and norepinephrine are observed. In trained subjects at comparable workloads these increases are less, whereas lipid mobilization by catecholamines is significantly enhanced.

### INSULIN

At levels of exercise that increase oxygen consumption to 50% or more of $VO_2$ max, a significant fall in plasma insulin and C peptide is observed.[27,28] Perhaps this decreased insulin secretion is due to sympathetic-receptor stimulation of the pancreas. Indeed, a significant activation of the sympathetic nervous system is found during exercise when oxygen consumption is 50% or more of the $VO_2$ max. Thus, insulin and the sympathetic nervous system respond in parallel and are mutually influenced. Interestingly, the insulin and C-peptide response to a meal or to injected glucose is significantly smaller in trained than in sedentary subjects despite a comparable plasma glucose increase (Fig. 132-3).[29] This finding suggests either an increased sensitivity to insulin in well-trained subjects or a reduced requirement for this hormone. Indeed, various studies have shown greater insulin binding in athletes. However, the hypoglycemic response to injected insulin does not seem to be greatly affected by the

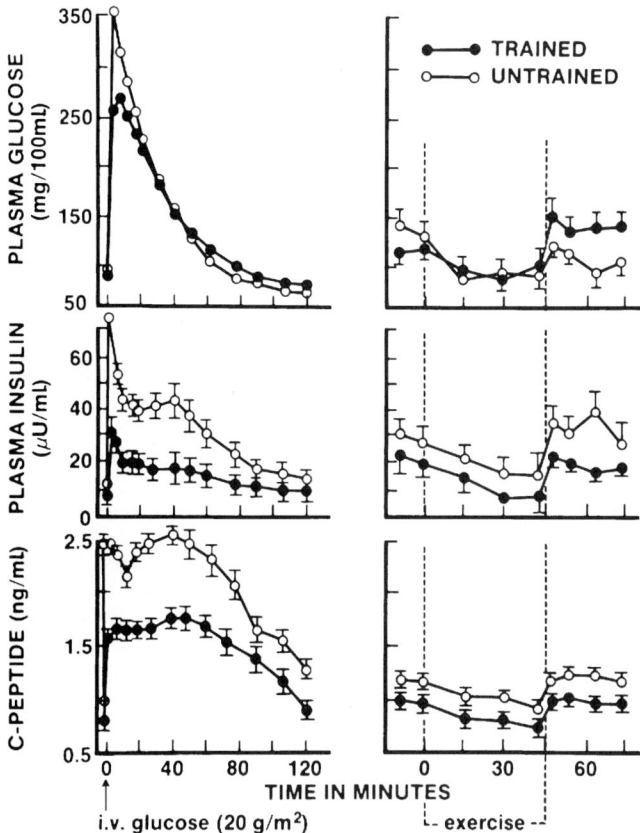

TRAINED
UNTRAINED

**FIGURE 132-3.** Acute effect of exercise and intravenous glucose (20 g/m² body surface) on plasma glucose, insulin, and C-peptide levels in trained and nontrained subjects. (*iv,* intravenous.) (From LeBlanc J, Jobin M, Côté J, et al. Enhanced metabolic response to caffeine in exercise-trained human subjects. J Appl Physiol 1985; 59:832; and from Wirth A, Diehm C, Mayer H, et al. Plasma C-peptide and insulin in trained and untrained subjects. J Appl Physiol 1981; 50:71.)

level of training.[30] Thus, the available evidence would seem to favor the possibility of reduced requirements.[30a] The reason for a reduced need for insulin is unknown. One explanation may be the greater transformation of glucose into glycogen, a process that requires less insulin than its incorporation into lipids. This is suggested by the fact that exercise training causes a "glucose storage space" supported by an enhanced glycogen synthetase activity.[31]

Studies made in vivo as well as with the isolated pancreas have shown a reduced insulin secretion in trained rats in response not only to glucose but also to tolbutamide or arginine, a finding which suggests that the reduced insulin secretion observed with training is possibly due to a direct blunting action on pancreatic B cells rather than to extrinsic autonomic influences (see Chap. 134).[32] Weight loss induced by diet plus exercise has positive effects on the lowering of insulin values obtained during fasting and on oral glucose-tolerance tests; these effects are greater than those achieved with diet alone.[33] Interestingly, there are gender differences in the glucoregulatory response to exercise.[33a,33b]

## THYROID HORMONES

The assessment of thyroid function in acute situations is always difficult because of the very large differences in turnover rates among thyroid-stimulating hormone (TSH), triiodothyronine ($T_3$), thyroxine ($T_4$), and other hormones. Possibly for this reason, the elevation of plasma TSH that is induced by a single bout of exercise is not paralleled by significant changes in plasma $T_4$ and $T_3$ concentrations.[34] If this acute effect of exercise on TSH secre-

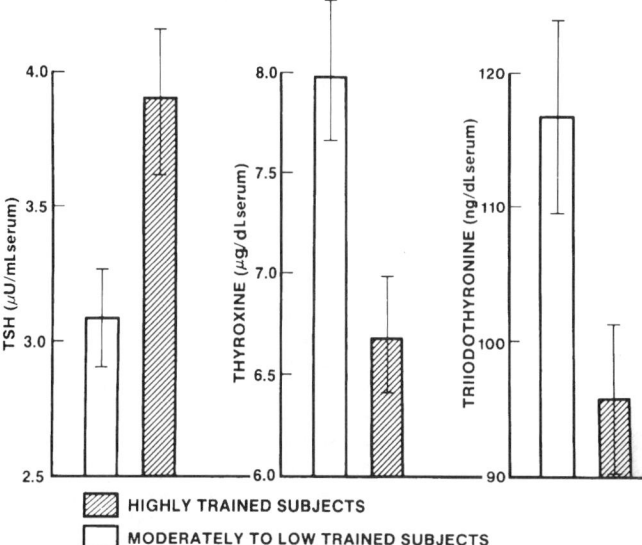

HIGHLY TRAINED SUBJECTS
MODERATELY TO LOW TRAINED SUBJECTS

**FIGURE 132-4.** Plasma levels of thyroid-stimulating hormone (*TSH*), thyroxine, and triiodothyronine in exercise-trained and sedentary subjects.

tion is repeated many times over days, however, a new equilibrium in thyroid hormone activity likely would be established, as shown by the significant lowering of both plasma $T_4$ and $T_3$ and the elevation of plasma TSH, which does indeed occur (Fig. 132-4). These findings are compatible with a feedback-controlled action.[35] Studies of racehorses and of athletes indicate that the lower plasma concentrations of thyroid hormones associated with exercise training are due to increased turnover rather than to enhanced clearance.[36,37] Although the elevated plasma TSH level might increase thyroid hormone secretion, possibly the enhanced sympathetic activity associated with high-intensity physical activity could also contribute to this action.[38] The purpose of an increase in thyroid hormone turnover in exercise training is unknown. One possibility involves the synthesis of protein. Both $T_3$ and $T_4$ restore the depressed degradation and synthesis of protein in muscles of thyroidectomized animals. Also, increased plasma $T_3$ levels cause an increase in anaerobic activity in the soleus muscle paralleled by changes in fiber types. In addition, several studies have revealed an increase in the activity of mitochondrial enzymes when thyroid activity is increased. Thyroid action would also be needed to permit fatty acid oxidation, which is increased by training.[39] These various actions of thyroid hormones are compatible with the greatly enhanced energy metabolism induced in muscles by repetitive physical training, and it might be expected that these actions would manifest themselves primarily in the tissues that are called on during exercise (i.e., muscle and heart) (see Chap. 30).

## GROWTH HORMONE

Marked elevations of plasma growth hormone occur in subjects exercising at levels corresponding to 50% and greater of their $VO_2$ max.[40] As in the case of TSH[41] and catecholamines,[14] this increase may be linked to anaerobic work production. The elevation of core temperature that is often observed with work of high intensity and the psychological stress that is also present in performing athletes are other possible factors responsible for the growth hormone elevation. The beneficial effect of growth hormone during exercise results from its anabolic and protein synthesis–promoting properties, as well as increased bone and collagen turnover.[41a] These actions would be especially useful in strengthening ligaments, tendons, and muscles in persons who are frequently engaged in physical activities.[6,34,42] Another effect of growth hormone is to activate glycolysis and increase plasma levels of free fatty acids. The increased secretion of growth hormone during exercise also diminishes with exercise training (see Chap. 12).[40,43]

## GLUCAGON

Glucagon, as well as the catecholamines, helps to furnish an adequate supply of glucose when its requirements are increased by exercise. Although adrenergic hormones contribute to ensuring an adequate source of glucose in cases of an acute increase of need, glucagon appears to exert this same action in situations when the need is experienced for more prolonged periods. Glucagon increases glycogenolysis through an effect on cyclic adenosine monophosphate and increases gluconeogenesis by stimulating the transformation of lactic acid, glycerol, and amino acids in the liver.[34,42] Thus, this hormone has the important function of transforming various substrates into glucose, which is a limiting energy source during exercise. Glucagon simultaneously activates the release of free fatty acids into the circulation. These actions are shared by catecholamines, which are themselves modulators of glucagon secretion. In exercise training, the needs for glucagon are significantly reduced, because exercising at 60% of VO$_2$ max (which in nontrained subjects causes a two-fold increase of this hormone in the plasma) has no effect in athletes.[40]

## PROLACTIN

Like growth hormone, plasma prolactin levels are increased during exercise, although to a lesser extent (see Chap. 13).[44] In some well-trained athletes, exercise fails to change plasma prolactin levels; therefore, the suggestion has been made that this may be related to an alteration in the release of β-endorphins, which antagonize the inhibitory action of dopamine on prolactin secretion.[45]

## GLUCOCORTICOIDS

The glucocorticoid response to exercise resembles that described for catecholamines. The plasma changes in these hormones reflect the various psychological and physical components associated with physical activity. Only intensive work increases secretion of glucocorticoids. Furthermore, daytime multiple exercise produces suppressed cortisol levels at night.[46] The potential usefulness of these hormones in these circumstances is suggested by their known actions on glycogen formation, hepatic gluconeogenesis, and lipolysis. Some studies have indicated that exercise training may attenuate the glucocorticoid response to exercise.

## SEX HORMONES

Thirty minutes of exercise at 74% of VO$_2$ max was found to cause a significant increase in both progesterone (37%) and estradiol (13.5%), whereas no change in plasma follicle-stimulating hormone and luteinizing hormone was observed in exercising women[47]; others have confirmed these findings.[48] Another exercise study found a simultaneous decrease of the metabolic clearance rate of estradiol,[49] suggesting that the elevation of plasma ovarian hormone levels during heavy exercise is due to their reduced plasma clearance rather than to an enhanced secretion caused by gonadotropins. Physical training may cause menstrual irregularities, and abbreviated anovulatory menstrual cycles have often been observed in elite athletes. Plasma testosterone levels are increased in competitive male athletes.[50] This action does not seem to be caused by an enhanced secretion from the interstitial cells, because gonadotropin levels do not rise, nor from the adrenal cortex, because the suppression of adrenocorticotropic hormone by drugs fails to reduce the testosterone level elevation. Possibly both the ovarian hormone and testosterone elevations after heavy exercise arise from a reduced plasma clearance.

## LIPIDS

In marathon runners, the triglycerides and very-low-density lipoprotein cholesterol levels were significantly reduced, whereas high-density lipoprotein cholesterol was increased[51,52]; no change was observed in total cholesterol level. A single session of exercise several hours before a high-fat meal reduced postprandial lipemia.[53] Low to moderate physical activity caused no such change in serum lipid levels unless it was associated with a negative energy balance leading to the loss of body fat (see also Chap. 162).[6] On the other hand, a study of adolescent females found that one month of exercise was a more important factor in improving the ratio of total cholesterol to high-density lipoprotein cholesterol than concomitant body fat reduction.[54]

## EFFECT OF EXERCISE ON BODY WEIGHT

A method often used in attempting to reduce body fat is to engage in a program of regular physical activity.[55] During the period of training, athletes with high VO$_2$ max consume up to 1000 more calories per day, and yet clearly their adiposity is significantly less than that of a comparable sedentary population. Exercise markedly influences energy balance in male animals, primarily by reducing energy intake, although exercise has no apparent effects on female animals. This anorectic effect of exercise is probably mediated by the release of corticotropin-releasing hormone, because it is prevented by the corticotropin-releasing hormone antagonist α-helical corticotropin-releasing factor.[56] With time, however, a new equilibrium is reached, a normalized energy balance is achieved, and body fat remains at a constant low level. Facilitation of lipid mobilization occurs through an enhanced lipolytic activity of various hormones, especially catecholamines. Concomitantly, the secretion of hormones such as catecholamines, growth hormone, prolactin, and TSH, which are normally increased by physical activity, is significantly reduced by prolonged exercise training. Interestingly, the daily insulin requirement for an individual on a normal mixed diet is reduced up to 40% in well-trained subjects.[57] These hormonal adaptations tend to disappear soon after physical training is discontinued. It is unclear, however, whether this is due to reduced physical activity or to the fact that detraining is often associated with an excess energy intake, which gradually contributes to restoration of a higher percentage of body fat (see Chap. 126).

## CONCLUSION

In prolonged exercise the initial source of energy is muscle glycogen,[58] and after some time glycogen from the liver is mobilized as well. This source of energy gradually becomes limiting, and plasma glucose levels fall slightly. Concomitantly, a larger proportion of the energy is supplied by adipose tissue, from which lipids are mobilized through the action of various hormones such as catecholamines, glucagon, growth hormone, and prolactin. One peculiarity of exercise is that muscles can extract glucose from the circulating blood without requiring insulin. Because of adaptation to exercise, the insulin requirements during the feeding period are greatly reduced. Similarly, training diminishes the secretion of catecholamines, glucagon, prolactin, and glucocorticoids, which are normally increased by exercise. This abatement of stimulation is a general adaptive response that is common to many hormonal secretions. Perhaps, because many endocrine responses to exercise are observed primarily during the anaerobic phase, exercise training reduces endocrine secretions by raising the anaerobic threshold. The fact that the various processes of energy mobilization continue to function adequately despite reduced hormonal secretions would seem to indicate a general enhanced hormonal sensitivity associated with exercise training.

# REFERENCES

1. Strauss RH. Sports medicine and physiology. Philadelphia: WB Saunders, 1979.
2. Washington RL, van Gundy JC, Cohen C, et al. Normal aerobic and anaerobic exercise data for North American school-age children. J Pediatr 1988; 112:223.
3. Borg G, Linderholm H. Perceived exertion and pulse rate during exercise in various age groups. Acta Med Scand 1967; 472(Suppl):194.
4. Shephard RJ, Allen C, Banade AJS, et al. Standardization of sub-maximal exercise tests. Bull World Health Organ 1968; 38:765.
5. Astrand PO, Rodahl K. Textbook of work physiology. New York: McGraw-Hill, 1977.
6. Shephard RJ. Physiology and biochemistry of exercise. New York: Praeger, 1985.
7. Silbernagl S, Despopoulos A. Atlas de poche de physiologie. Paris: Flammarion, 1985.
8. Sigal RJ, Purdon C, Bilinski D, et al. Glucoregulation during and after intense exercise: effects of β-blockade. J Clin Endocrinol Metab 1994; 78:359.
9. Von Euler US, Hellner S. Excretion of noradrenaline and adrenaline in muscular work. Acta Physiol Scand 1952; 26:183.
10. Banister EW, Jackson RC. The effect of speed and load charges on oxygen intake for equivalent power outputs during bicycle ergometry. Int Z Angew Physiol 1967; 24:284.
11. Péronnet F, Cousineau D, Nadeau R, et al. Adrenal medulla activity in exercising dogs. Med Sci Sports Exerc 1978; 10:40.
12. Greine JS, Hickner RC, Shah SD, et al. Norepinephrine response to exercise at the same relative intensity before and after endurance exercise training. J Appl Physiol 1999; 86:531.
13. Davies CTM, Few J, Foster KG, Sargeant AJ. Plasma catecholamine concentration during dynamic exercise involving different muscle groups. Eur J Appl Physiol 1974; 32:195.
14. Galbo H, Holst JJ, Christensen NJ. Glucagon plasma catecholamine responses to graded and prolonged exercise in man. J Appl Physiol 1975; 38:70.
15. Hartley LH, Mason JW, Hogan RP, et al. Multiple responses to graded exercise in relation to physical training. J Appl Physiol 1972; 33:602.
16. Péronnet F, Nadeau RA, de Champlain J, et al. Plasma norepinephrine response to exercise before and after training in humans. J Appl Physiol 1981; 51:812.
17. Kjaer M, Galbo H. Effect of physical training on the capacity to secrete epinephrine. J Appl Physiol 1988; 64:11.
18. McMurray RG, Forsythe WA, Mar MH, Hardy CJ. Exercise intensity–related responses of beta-endorphin and catecholamines. Med Sci Sports Exerc 1987; 19:57.
19. Hultman E. Muscle glycogen stores and prolonged exercise. In: Shephard RJ, ed. Frontiers of fitness. Springfield, IL: Charles C Thomas, 1971.
20. Shepherd RE, Noble EG, Klug GA, Collnick PD. Lipolysis and cyclic-AMP accumulation in adipocytes in response to training. J Appl Physiol 1981; 50:143.
21. Ashew EW, Hecker AL. Adipose tissue cell size and lipolysis in the rat: response to exercise intensity and food restriction. J Nutr 1976; 106:1351.
22. Bukowiecki L, Lupien J, Follea N, et al. Mechanism of enhanced lipolysis in adipose tissue of exercise-trained rats. Am J Physiol 1980; 239:E422.
23. Saltin B, Hermansen L. Glycogen stores and prolonged severe exercise. In: Blix G, ed. Nutrition and physical activity. Uppsala: Almqvist & Wiksell, 1967:32.
24. Bergström J, Hultman E. Muscle glycogen synthesis after exercise: an enhancing factor localized in the muscle cells in man. Nature 1966; 210:309.
25. Costill DL, Dalsky GP, Fink WJ. Effect of caffeine ingestion on metabolism and exercise performance. Med Sci Sports Exerc 1978; 10:155.
26. LeBlanc J, Jobin M, Côté J, et al. Enhanced metabolic response to caffeine in exercise-trained human subjects. J Appl Physiol 1985; 59:832.
27. Pruett EDR. Plasma insulin concentrations during prolonged work stress in men living on different diets. J Appl Physiol 1970; 28:199.
28. Wirth A, Diehm C, Mayer H, et al. Plasma C-peptide and insulin in trained and untrained subjects. J Appl Physiol 1981; 50:71.
29. LeBlanc J, Nadeau A, Boulay M, Rousseau-Migneron S. Effects of physical training and adiposity on glucose metabolism and $^{125}I$ insulin binding. J Appl Physiol 1979; 46:235.
30. LeBlanc J, Nadeau A, Richard D, Tremblay A. Variations in plasma glucose, insulin, growth hormone and catecholamines in response to insulin in trained and nontrained subjects. Metabolism 1982; 31:453.
30a. Ryan AS, Pratley RE, Elahi D, Goldberg AP. Changes in plasma leptin and insulin action with resistive training in postmenopausal women. Intl J Obesity 2000; 24:27.
31. Ivy CH, Holloszy JO. Persistent increase in glucose uptake by rat skeletal muscles following exercise. Am J Physiol 1981; 241:200.
32. Richard D, LeBlanc J. Pancreatic insulin response in relation to exercise training. Can J Physiol Pharmacol 1983; 61:1194.
33. Rice B, Jannsen I, Hudson R, Ross R. Effects of aerobic or resistance exercise and/or diet on glucose tolerance and plasma insulin levels in obese men. Diabetes Care 1999; 22:684.
33a. Marliss EB, Kreisman SH, Manzon A, et al. Gender differences in glucoregulatory responses to intense exercise. J Appl Physiol 2000; 88:457.
33b. Davis SN, Galassetti P, Wasserman PH, Tate D. Effects of gender on neuroendocrine and metabolic counterregulatory responses to exercise in normal man. J Clin Endocrinol Metab 2000; 85:224.
34. Terjung R. Endocrine response to exercise. Med Sci Sports Exerc 1979; 9:153.
35. LeBlanc J, Jobin M, Diamond P. Plasma thyroid hormones of sedentary and trained subjects in resting state and in response to norepinephrine. (Unpublished data.)
36. Irvine CHG. Thyroxine secretion in the horse in various physiological states. J Endocrinol 1967; 39:313.
37. Irvine CHG. Effect of exercise on thyroxine degradation in athletes and non-athletes. J Clin Endocrinol Metab 1968; 28:942.
38. Melander A, Rankley E, Sundler F, Westgren U. Beta₂-adrenergic stimulation of thyroid hormone secretion. Endocrinology 1975; 97:332.
39. Paul P. Uptake and oxidation of substrates in the intact animal during exercise. In: Pernow B, Saltin B, eds. Muscle metabolism during exercise. New York: Plenum Publishing, 1971.
40. Bloom SR, Johnson RH, Park DM, et al. Differences in the metabolic and hormonal response to exercise between racing cyclists and untrained individuals. J Physiol (Lond) 1976; 258:1.
41. Galbo H, Hummer L, Petersen IB, et al. Thyroid and testicular hormone responses to graded and prolonged exercise in man. Eur J Appl Physiol 1977; 36:101.
41a. Wallace JD, Cuneo RC, Lundberg PA, et al. Response of markers of bone and collagen turnover to exercise, growth hormone (GH) administration, and GH withdrawal in trained adult males. J Clin Endocrinol Metab 2000; 85:124.
42. Galbo H. Hormonal and metabolic adaptation to exercise. New York: Georg Thieme, 1983.
43. Sutton JR, Young JD, Lazarus L. The hormonal response to physical exercise. Aust Ann Med 1969; 18:85.
44. Brisson GR, Ledoux M, Péronnet F, et al. Prolactinemia in exercising male athletes. Horm Res 1981; 15:218.
45. Grossman A, Sutton JR. Endorphins: what are they? how are they measured? what is their role in exercise? Med Sci Sports Exerc 1985; 17:74.
46. Hockney AC, Viru A. Twenty-four-hour cortisol response to multiple daily exercise sessions of moderate and high intensity. Clin Physiol 1999; 19:178.
47. Bonen A, Ling WY, MacIntyre KP, et al. Effects of exercise on the serum concentrations of FSH, LH, progesterone and estradiol. Eur J Appl Physiol 1979; 43:15.
48. Jurkowski JE, Jones NL, Walker C, et al. Ovarian hormonal responses to exercise. J Appl Physiol 1978; 44:109.
49. Keizer HA, Poortman J, Bunnik GSJ. Influence of physical exercise on sex-hormone metabolism. J Appl Physiol 1980; 45:765.
50. Sutton JR, Coleman MT, Casey JH. Testosterone production rate during exercise. In: Landry F, Orban WAR, eds. Third International Symposium of Biochemistry of Exercise. Miami: Symposium Specialists, 1978:227.
51. Woods PDS, Haskell WL, Lewis S, et al. Concentration of plasma lipids and lipoproteins in male and female long-distance runners. In: Landry F, Orban WAR, eds. Third International Symposium on Biochemistry of Exercise. Miami: Symposium Specialists, 1978:301.
52. Lamon-Fava S, Fischer EC, Nelson ME, et al. Effect of exercise and menstrual cycle status on plasma lipids, low density lipoprotein particle size, and apolipoproteins. J Clin Endocrinol Metab 1989; 68:17.
53. Malkova D, Hardman AE, Bonness RJ, Macdonald IA. The reduction in postprandial lipemia after exercise is independent of the relative contributions of fat and carbohydrate to energy metabolism during exercise. Metabolism 1999; 48:245.
54. Hanoi T, Takado H, Magamisha M, et al. Effects of exercise for 1 month on serum lipids in adolescent females. Pediatr Int 1999; 41:253.
55. Brownell KD, Steen SN, Wilmore JH. Weight regulation practices in athletes: analysis of metabolic and health effects. Med Sci Sports Exerc 1987; 19:546.
56. Richard D, Rivest S. The role of exercise in thermogenesis and energy balance. Can J Physiol Pharmacol 1989; 67:402.
57. LeBlanc J, Nadeau A, Richard D. Daily variations of plasma glucose and insulin in physically trained and sedentary subjects. Metabolism 1983; 32:552.
58. Bonen A, Homanko DA. Effects of exercise and glycogen depletion on glyconeogenesis in muscle. J Appl Physiol 1994; 76:1753.

# SECTION B

# DIABETES MELLITUS

---

## CHAPTER 133

# MORPHOLOGY OF THE ENDOCRINE PANCREAS

SUSAN BONNER-WEIR

## PANCREATIC ISLETS

The endocrine pancreas consists of numerous clusters of cells called *islets of Langerhans,* which are scattered throughout the exocrine tissue in vertebrates phylogenetically higher than fish. The relative volume of the islet cell mass differs with age; it is much greater in fetuses and in the young, presumably because the growth of the islet and exocrine tissues is discordant. In newborn humans, islets constitute 20% of the pancreatic tissue; in children (1.5–11 years), 7.5%; and in adults, 1%[1]; similar data have been reported for cattle and rats. An adult human has roughly 1 g of islet tissue, or 500,000 to 1,000,000 islets. Islets range in size from clusters of only a few cells with a total diameter of <40 μm to oblate spheroids of perhaps >5000 cells totaling 400 μm in diameter. Whereas islets 300 μm or larger make up only 15% of the islet population, they account for 60% of the mass.

Each islet is a highly vascularized cluster of several cell types in a nonrandom organization. Four cell types are common to all species: B, or *insulin producing;* A, or *glucagon producing;* D, or *somatostatin producing;* and PP, or *pancreatic polypeptide producing* (Fig. 133-1). Specific islet staining techniques, used since early in this century, include aldehyde fuchsin for B cells, Grimelius silver for A cells, and modified Davenport silver for D cells. B cells in insulinomas and in nesidioblastosis also may stain with the Grimelius technique.[1] However, these staining methods have been largely supplanted by the more sensitive immunoperoxidase and immunofluorescent techniques, with which immunoreactivity for several other peptides (gastric inhibitory peptide, cholecystokinin [CCK], secretin, corticotropin, thyrotropin-releasing hormone, and glicentin) has been detected in islet cells. What role, if any, these peptides have in the islet is unclear. More importantly, use of these immunohistochemical techniques has demonstrated that islets are heterogeneous,[2] usually having either A or PP cells, and that the distribution of such islets is regional: those with A cells or that are glucagon rich are limited to the body and tail of the pancreas (dorsal pancreas), whereas those with PP cells are limited to the head or uncinate process (ventral pancreas).

The cells within a mammalian islet have a consistent pattern of organization, with the D, A, or PP (non-B) cells occurring as a discontinuous mantle one to three cells thick around a central core of B cells. In humans, the pattern is more complex but can be thought of as a composite of several subunits with the same pattern seen in other species. The nonrandomness of the organization of islet cells indicates a functional basis.

## PANCREATIC EMBRYOLOGY

The pancreas is derived from outpocketings of the *digestive endoderm* (primitive gut).[3] Two or three pancreatic anlagen or primordia are found: a dorsal outpocketing of the gut across from the budding liver and, after a short temporal lag, one or two ventral buds (which often fuse very early) from the base of the biliary floor of the gut. The dorsal anlage, which gives rise to the splenic portion (tail and body) of the pancreas, fuses to various degrees with the ventral anlage(n), which gives rise to

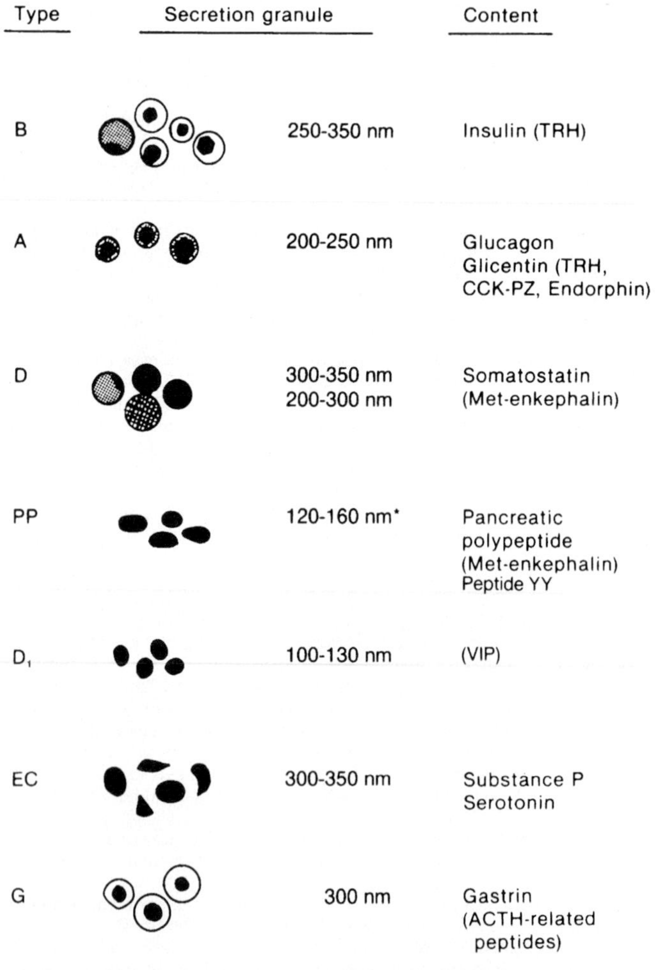

| Type | Secretion granule | | Content |
|---|---|---|---|
| B | | 250-350 nm | Insulin (TRH) |
| A | | 200-250 nm | Glucagon Glicentin (TRH, CCK-PZ, Endorphin) |
| D | | 300-350 nm 200-300 nm | Somatostatin (Met-enkephalin) |
| PP | | 120-160 nm* | Pancreatic polypeptide (Met-enkephalin) Peptide YY |
| D₁ | | 100-130 nm | (VIP) |
| EC | | 300-350 nm | Substance P Serotonin |
| G | | 300 nm | Gastrin (ACTH-related peptides) |

**FIGURE 133-1.** Cell types found in islets of Langerhans. B, A, D, and PP cells are found in all species. B cells usually constitute 60% to 80% of the islet cells and D cells are 5% to 10%. A cells and PP cells, usually mutually exclusive, make up 15% to 20% of the cell number. D₁, EC, and G cells are found only infrequently in most species. Hormones enclosed in parentheses are ones that have been identified immunocytochemically in at least some species. (*TRH,* thyrotropin-releasing hormone; *CCK-PZ,* cholecystokinin-pancreozymin; *VIP,* vasoactive intestinal peptide; *ACTH,* adrenocorticotropic hormone.) *Human PP granules are smaller and more dense than those seen in dog and other species, in which granules are 300 nm in diameter and more flocular in density.

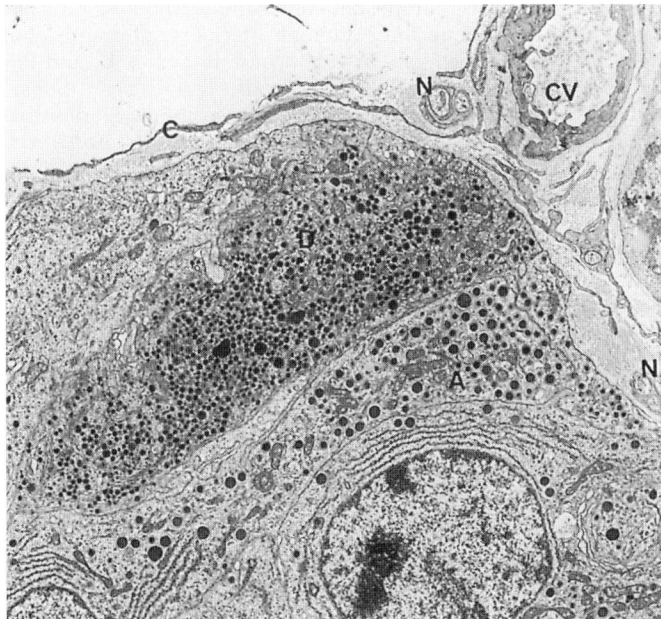

**FIGURE 133-2.** Electron micrograph of periphery of rat islet showing capsule (*C*), nerves (*N*), and collecting venule (*CV*) within islet capsule. D cell (*D*) full of variable, dense granules (120–160 nm in diameter) is between several A cells (*A*) with the typical glucagon granule (200–250 nm in diameter). ×6000

the head or duodenal portion of the pancreas. Islet cells are seen first as single cells among the exocrine cells of the terminal pancreatic tubules and then as clusters of cells within the exocrine basement membrane.[3] These clusters become separated from the exocrine tissue to form islets. At times, the only separation between exocrine and islet cells arises from their respective basement membranes. Usually, however, islets have at least a partial capsule of fibroblasts and collagen fibers (Fig. 133-2).

The A cells appear before the others, followed by the B cells and finally by the D cells. (PP cells have been reported several days before birth in rats.) Initially, endocrine cells may express more than one islet hormone, with a progressive restriction to just one hormone.[3,4] Exciting ongoing studies are defining the cascade of the transcription factors involved in the differentiation of pancreas from endoderm and subsequently to the varied pancreatic cell types (exocrine and endocrine).[4]

The origin of the pancreas as separate buds is thought to be the basis of the regional distribution of glucagon and pancreatic peptide cells. The dorsal pancreas, supplied with blood by the celiac trunk through the gastroduodenal and splenic arteries and drained by one main pancreatic duct, contains the glucagon-rich islets with few pancreatic peptide-rich cells. The opposite distribution is found in the ventral pancreas, which is supplied with blood from the superior mesenteric artery through the inferior pancreaticoduodenal artery and drained by a separate exocrine duct. The degree of fusion of the ducts differs among species.

## ISLET GROWTH AND DEVELOPMENT

Until late gestation, most B cells result from the differentiation of precursor cells in the ducts to islet cells, a process called *neogenesis*. From birth to adulthood, the volume of islet tissue with respect to that of the pancreas as a whole (relative volume) decreases, but the actual volume of islet tissue increases; the more slowly growing islet tissue is diluted by the exuberant postnatal growth of the exocrine tissue. The low replication rate seen in adult islets has led many to assume that the B-cell mass does not turn over significantly and that one is born with all the

B cells one will ever have. Such reasoning ignores the fact that the B-cell mass continues to grow well into adulthood. Thus, with a B-cell birthrate of just under 3% of new cells per day, the rodent B-cell mass would double in 1 month if cell death were negligible.[5] Likewise, if the rate of B-cell death approached the replication rate of 3%, then complete replacement of the B-cell population could occur. Because the B-cell mass does not continue to double on a monthly basis throughout life, the B cell, like most other cell types, must have a finite life span.[6]

In the adult, the B-cell mass can increase or decrease to maintain euglycemia. Although some of this compensation can be functional, with the amount of insulin each B cell secretes changing, the B-cell mass itself is the major factor in the amount of insulin that can be secreted. The mechanisms involved in this compensatory regulation of B-cell mass are (a) changes in replication rate, (b) changes in individual cell size (hypertrophy), (c) changes in cell death rate, and (d) changes in rates of neogenesis.[6] Neogenesis has been described in humans with type 1 (insulin-dependent) diabetes mellitus or severe liver disease,[7] and also in the adult rodent after experimental manipulations, such as partial pancreatectomy. The enlargement of individual cells with increased age or activity has been reported, but no estimate has been made of the contribution this growth could make to the islet mass.

The different islet cells do not have the same pattern of growth. The proportions of the different cell types vary with age; the functional significance of these changes is unclear. For example, D cells in the rat and human make up a considerably greater percentage of the islet cell number in the fetus and neonate than in the adult. In the adult mammal, the islet composition is 70% to 80% B cells, 15% to 20% A or PP cells (usually mutually exclusive), and 5% to 10% D cells.

Studies using isolated rat islets synchronized in culture by temporary exposure to hydroxyurea have found the cycle of the B cell to be 14.9 hours.[5] The length of the cell cycle does not change under glucose stimulation or when islets of different-aged animals are used. Instead, the growth rate is regulated by the number of B cells that can enter the division phase from the resting ($G_0$) phase. The size of this proliferative pool varies with age and stimulus; it is 10% in the fetus and neonate, and only 3% in the adult. The growth capacity of the B cell depends on the stimulus and the cell's ability to recognize that stimulus, as well as on the number of B cells that can enter the cell cycle and undergo mitosis.

Although numerous stimuli for B-cell growth may exist, glucose and members of the growth hormone family (prolactin, placental lactogen, growth hormone) are stimuli both in vivo and in vitro.[8] In vitro studies, however, have never achieved the B-cell growth seen in the in vivo models.

## NEURAL RELATIONS

The pancreas is innervated by sympathetic fibers from the celiac ganglion and by parasympathetic fibers from the vagus nerve. Nerve fibers terminate in perivascular, periacinar, and periinsular areas (see Fig. 133-2). Within the islet, nerves are unmyelinated and can be surrounded by Schwann cells. They may be closely apposed to islet cells, in the pericapillary space, or even under the capillary endothelial basement membrane. Because no specialized synapses are found, the suggestion has been made that neurotransmitters released into the interstitial space may affect several neighboring islet cells.[9]

The autonomic nervous system modulates islet hormone secretion. Cholinergic stimulation elicits increased insulin, glucagon, and pancreatic polypeptide secretion. Its effects on somatostatin are less clear but appear to be inhibitory. Similarly, β-adrenergic stimulation elicits increased secretion of insulin, glucagon, pancreatic polypeptide, and somatostatin; however, the effects of α-adrenergic stimulation are less evident. The effects of stimulation of peptidergic nerves have not been stud-

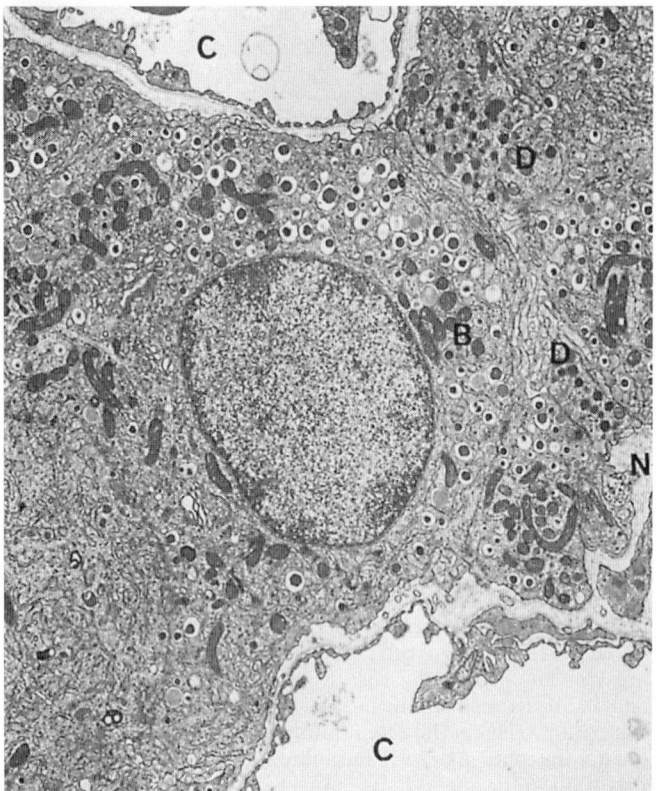

**FIGURE 133-3.** Electron micrograph of B cell (*B*) facing two fenestrated capillaries (*C*). Adrenergic nerve fibers (*N*) are closely apposed to B cell. D cell (*D*), showing the often dendritic nature, is sectioned incompletely between two B cells. ×10,000

ied as closely, but vasoactive intestinal peptide (VIP), CCK, and galanin can affect islet cell secretion.

The distribution and number of the different types of nerve fibers vary among species.[9] Cholinergic nerves are common in rat, cat, and rabbit islets. Adrenergic nerves are common in the hamster, dog, and cat. Peptidergic nerves containing substance P, enkephalin, VIP, or CCK are found in the human, rat, and dog. In the human and the rat, VIP neurons form a periinsular network. However, the relation of this network to the islet vasculature is uncertain; therefore, whether these nerves influence islet secretion through changes in the islet blood flow remains unknown.

## ISLET BLOOD SUPPLY

The islets of Langerhans have a glomerular-like capillary network with a direct arteriolar blood supply. With nonradioactive microspheres, the blood flow to the islets has been estimated as 10% to 15% of the total pancreatic blood flow, although islet tissue accounts for only 1% to 2% of the pancreatic mass.[5,10] Blood equal to the volume of an islet passes through the islet every 3 seconds. Factors regulating islet blood flow may affect islet hormone secretion, and one such factor may be a high concentration of glucose, which enhances pancreatic blood flow and preferentially increases islet blood flow.

Islet capillaries are fenestrated (Fig. 133-3), whereas capillaries in surrounding exocrine tissue have few or no fenestrations. Islet capillaries are highly permeable: horseradish peroxidase passes into the islet pericapillary space within 45 seconds, whereas it takes 5 minutes to pass into the cardiac pericapillary space. Islet capillaries also have a greater luminal diameter than do exocrine capillaries.

Research using a combination of a three-dimensional view of the islet microvasculature gained by scanning electron microscopic examination of methacrylate corrosion casts and

reconstructions of immunostained paraffin sections in rat islets has found that one to three afferent arterioles enter an islet at gaps in the discontinuous mantle of non-B (i.e., A, D, and PP) cells, thereby entering directly into the B-cell core.[11] Subsequently, the arterioles branch into numerous capillaries that traverse the B-cell core before passing through the non–B-cell mantle. In small islets (<160 μm in diameter), the efferent capillaries pass through exocrine tissue before coalescing into collecting venules. In intermediate or large islets, however, the collecting venules form a network under the islet capsule.

## ULTRASTRUCTURE OF THE ISLET

With electron microscopy, the islet cells are distinguishable from each other by the appearance and size of their secretion granules, although significant interspecies variation is seen. Besides the more frequently occurring B, A, D, and PP cells, many less common but distinct cells have been described (see Fig. 133-1).

### B CELLS

B cells are polyhedral and are arranged in tubes of eight to ten around a capillary. Each B cell has a second capillary face.[11] In well-granulated B cells, the rough endoplasmic reticulum (RER) is scanty and scattered among the numerous secretory granules, which are 250 to 350 nm in diameter (see Fig. 133-3). Two forms of granules are seen: the "mature," which have an electron-dense core, often of crystalline nature, within a loosely fitting granule-limiting membrane and have the appearance of a spacious empty halo; and the "immature," which have little or no halo and moderately electron-dense contents. In the mature granules, the form of the crystal differs across species; for example, it is stellate in the dog and chicken. In more degranulated B cells, the RER is more extensive, as are the Golgi complex and polysomes. The remaining granules are accumulated in a polar fashion distal to the nucleus. The two faces on the capillaries and this polarity of the B cell provide an anatomic basis for the intraislet compartmentalization that has been suggested by physiologic data.[11] Such compartmentalization allows a segregation of sensing and secretory functions.

### A CELLS

A cells are more columnar and smaller than B cells and have many granules, which are 200 to 250 nm in diameter (see Fig. 133-2). The granules are electron dense with a narrow halo of less dense material and a tightly fitting granule-limiting membrane; little species variation is seen. With immunogold techniques, glicentin has been found in the periphery of glucagon-containing granules.[2] A cells have abundant stacks of RER that often are in the perinuclear region. A cells form the islet mantle and are interspersed with D cells. A capsule of fibroblasts and collagen fibrils may separate these mantle cells from the exocrine cells. However, great expanses of islet A and D cells are separated from the exocrine tissue only by two basement membranes (one from the islet cell, the other exocrine) and by the islet efferent blood vessels.

### D CELLS

D cells usually are smaller than either of the previous types and often are dendritic and well granulated (see Fig. 133-2). The granules (200–250 nm in diameter) contain a homogeneous, moderately electron-dense material that fills the granule-limiting membrane. Within an individual D cell, the electron density of the granules is variable. The RER is not prominent in these cells.

### PP CELLS

The PP cells are variable, depending on the species. In the human, the granules are electron dense, elongate, and 120 to

160 nm in diameter. In the dog and cat, the granules are spherical, 300 nm in diameter, and variable in electron density.

## MORPHOLOGY OF THE ISLET IN DIABETES MELLITUS

In type 1 (insulin-dependent) diabetes mellitus, the islet size is severely reduced; most, if not all, of the B cells are destroyed, leaving A, PP, and D cells. Neogenesis is now known to occur, yielding islets that are predominantly B cells.[7,12] However, where these islets are found, often round-cell infiltrates or *insulitis* is present, suggesting a continuation of the B-cell destruction. Surprisingly, in a few cases of type 1 diabetes mellitus, the pancreas has as much as 20% of the normal B-cell mass.

In type 2 (non–insulin-dependent) diabetes mellitus, the B-cell mass is reduced to 40% to 60% of normal, but the mass of non-B cells seems to be unchanged. Interestingly, no B-cell or islet hyperplasia is present, as might be expected from chronic hyperglycemia, although obese persons without diabetes have a 40% increase in B-cell mass compared with lean persons without diabetes.[13] Obese persons with diabetes have double the B-cell mass of lean persons with diabetes, but still have only 70% of that seen in lean persons without diabetes. Rodent studies using mice with known genetic causes of insulin resistance also showed markedly increased B-cell mass compared to wild-type mice.[14] Previously, hydropic degeneration or vacuolization of the B cells from patients with diabetes often was reported; however, this is now recognized to be an artifact resulting from the extraction of large glycogen stores by the techniques used to process the tissue. Fibrosis along the intraislet capillaries often is increased. In at least 50% of persons with type 2 diabetes mellitus, deposits of amyloid (formerly called *hyaline*) are found along the capillaries. The amount of amyloid seems to be correlated with the severity and duration of disease and with patient age, but amyloid also is found in older patients without diabetes. The aggregation of the human islet amyloid polypeptide (IAPP, also called *amylin*) into fibrils has been shown to be toxic to B cells in vitro, suggesting that amyloid deposition in vivo may cause a loss of B cells.[15] (See also Chap. 53.)

## THE ISLET AS AN ORGAN

The interrelations of the islet cells and their relations with the microvasculature have functional implications. Although the secretory products of most of the islet cells are capable of influencing the other cells, certain restrictions are imposed by the complex nonrandom organization of the islet.[11] Because the blood flows directly into the B-cell core, that blood-borne insulin could affect the A, D, or PP cells downstream seems reasonable; however, the hormones from these peripheral cells are unlikely to have a vascularly mediated effect on the B cells. This is not to say, however, that these hormones could not exert paracrine effects on B cells. The dynamics and direction of flow of the interstitial fluid are unknown, but one could speculate that diffusion in the interstitial space allows somatostatin and glucagon to influence not only each other (adjacent cells), but also B cells that are within a certain distance. If this is the case, then peripheral B cells may be directly influenced by the non–B-cell hormones, whereas more centrally located B cells are protected. A further extrapolation is that in small islets, all B cells are essentially peripheral, whereas in larger islets, a substantial core of central B cells are protected. In addition, in vitro evidence is increasing that not all B cells are the same functionally: individual B cells have different thresholds for glucose-induced insulin response.[16]

Another level of paracrine interaction could be through gap junctions, the morphologic entity responsible for electrical coupling of cells and for the transfer of small ions and molecules

(up to 1200 Da), which have been found in clusters on islet cells between both homologous and heterologous cells. These junctions may have a role in the synchronizing or amplifying of a response, because the islet functions as an organ.[17,18]

Similarly, intrinsic intrapancreatic ganglia, which contain cholinergic, adrenergic, and peptidergic neurons, may be the pacemakers involved in the synchronization of islet secretion within the whole pancreas. Physiologic data showing intrinsic patterns of oscillation of hormone secretion have suggested such a pancreatic pacemaker.[11]

The hypothesis has been put forward that one reason the endocrine pancreas is dispersed as islets throughout the exocrine pancreas is that the islet hormones regulate exocrine function and growth locally through an insulo-acinar portal system. Physiologically, somatostatin, insulin, and pancreatic polypeptide can affect exocrine function and, in turn, can be influenced by CCK, gastric inhibitory peptide, and other gastrointestinal peptides. Histologic evidence of periinsular halos, or the enlarged exocrine cells adjacent to islets, has been cited as evidence of trophic effects of islet hormones. The early studies using microvascular corrosion casts described efferent vessels from islets passing through the exocrine tissue before coalescing into venules; these vessels were called the *insulo-acinar portal system*. More recent studies on rat islet microvasculature confirmed the presence of such vessels, but only from smaller islets (160 μm in diameter and smaller). These smaller islets usually are embedded in exocrine tissue and constitute 75% of the islet population, although they make up only 40% of the total islet volume. Even in the larger islets without these efferent capillaries, however, the postcapillary and collecting venules at the periphery are the type considered the "leakiest" or most permeable in other tissues, so that they possibly allow diffusion of the hormones into the surrounding tissue.

## REFERENCES

1. Witte DP, Greider MH, DeSchryver-Kecshemeti K, et al. The juvenile human endocrine pancreas: normal vs. idiopathic hypoinsulinemic hypoglycemia. Semin Diagn Pathol 1984; 1:30.
2. Orci L. Banting Lecture 1981: macro- and micro-domains in the endocrine pancreas. Diabetes 1982; 31:538.
3. Pictet R, Rutter WJ. Development of the embryonic pancreas. In: Steiner DF, Freinkel N, eds. Handbook of physiology, vol 1. The endocrine pancreas. Baltimore: Williams & Wilkins, 1972:25.
4. Edlund H. Transcribing pancreas. Diabetes 1998; 47:1817.
5. Hellerstrom C, Swenne I, Andersson A. Islet cell replication and diabetes. In: Lebvre PJ, Pipeleers DG, eds. The pathology of endocrine pancreas in diabetes. Heidelberg: Springer-Verlag, 1988:141.
6. Finegood DT, Scaglia L, Bonner-Weir S. Dynamics of β-cell mass in the growing rat pancreas: estimation with a simple mathematical model. Diabetes 1995; 44:249.
7. Gepts W, Lecompte PM. The pancreatic islets in diabetes. Am J Med 1981; 70:105.
8. Bonner-Weir S, Smith FE. Islet cell growth and the growth factors involved. Trends Endocrinol Metab 1994; 5:60.
9. Sundler F, Bottcher G. Islet innervation with special reference to neuropeptides. In: Samols E, ed. The endocrine pancreas. New York: Raven Press, 1991:29.
10. Lifson N, Lassa CV, Dixit PK. Relation between blood flow and morphology in islet organ of rat pancreas. Am J Physiol 1985; 249:E43.
11. Samols E, Bonner-Weir S, Weir GC. Intra-islet insulin-glucagon-somatostatin relationships. Clin Endocrinol Metab 1986; 15:33.
12. Pipeleers D, Ling Z. Pancreatic beta cells in insulin dependent diabetes. Diabetes Metab Rev 1992; 8:209.
13. Kloppel G, Lohr M, Habich K, et al. Islet pathology and pathogenesis of type 1 and type 2 diabetes mellitus revisited. Surv Synth Pathol Res 1985; 4:110.
14. Bruning JC, Winnay J, Bonner-Weir S, et al. Development of a novel polygenic model of noninsulin dependent diabetes mellitus in mice heterozygous for insulin receptor and IRS-1 null alleles. Cell 1997; 88:561.
15. Lorenzo A, Razzaboni B, Weir GC, Yankner BA. Pancreatic cell toxicity of amylin associated with type 2 diabetes mellitus. Nature 1994; 368:756.
16. Pipeleers DG. Heterogeneity in pancreatic β-cell population. Diabetes 1992; 41:777.
17. Salomon D, Meda P. Heterogeneity and contact dependent regulation of hormone secretion by individual β-cells. Exp Cell Res 1986; 162:507.
18. Dunne MJ. Ions, genes, and insulin release: from basic science to clinical disease. Diabet Med 2000; 17:91.

# CHAPTER 134

# ISLET CELL HORMONES: PRODUCTION AND DEGRADATION

GORDON C. WEIR AND PHILIPPE A. HALBAN

The concentration of a hormone in the circulation at a given time is a reflection of both its rate of production and its rate of destruction or clearance. Therefore, understanding the broad molecular principles and significant regulatory features of these two processes is important. The metabolic status of an individual is influenced profoundly by the extraordinary integration of the opposing effects of glucagon and insulin. Furthermore, the regulation of the release of glucagon and insulin from the pancreatic A and B cells is consistent with the diverse bioeffects of these hormones. The molecular and ultrastructural events involved in the synthesis, storage, and release of insulin and the ultimate degradation of this hormone by its target tissues have been studied in great detail and serve as a model system for the other islet cell types.

## INSULIN PRODUCTION BY THE B CELL

Insulin production is initiated by transcription of the gene in the nucleus of the B cell. Thereafter, a cascade of molecular[1-3] and subcellular events culminates in the secretion of insulin by exocytosis (extrusion of the secretory granule contents) (Fig. 134-1; see Chap. 3). The initial gene transcript, the mRNA precursor, is processed within the nucleus to remove the nontranslated introns (two introns are found in most insulin genes). Once processed, the mRNA is transferred to the cytosol, where it becomes associated with ribosomes in the rough endoplasmic reticulum (RER). Polyribosomal mRNA is the substrate for translation of the initial peptidic insulin precursor, *preproinsu-*

lin, which is characterized by a peptide (*signal,* or *leader, sequence*) that typically extends some 23 amino acids from the N terminus of the insulin B chain. The leader sequence becomes associated with the membrane of the RER, thereby facilitating penetration of the nascent preproinsulin molecule into the lumen of the RER. Preproinsulin has a very short half-life. The leader sequence is rapidly cleaved off to form *proinsulin.* This may occur before translation is complete (i.e., as soon as this portion of the molecule has served its purpose as a vector for transfer across the RER membrane). Proinsulin then is transported in small membrane-limited vesicles (transitional elements) from the RER to the Golgi complex. In secretory cells, the trans-Golgi network (TGN) channels secretory products to their correct destination.[4] For the B cell, the TGN complex is responsible for ensuring that proinsulin received from the RER is delivered to, and packaged in, nascent secretory granules.[5] This segregation procedure must be sufficiently selective to ensure that only proinsulin and other desirable granule constituents, but no other products being handled in parallel by the TGN (i.e., lysosomal enzymes, plasma membrane proteins), are directed toward granules.

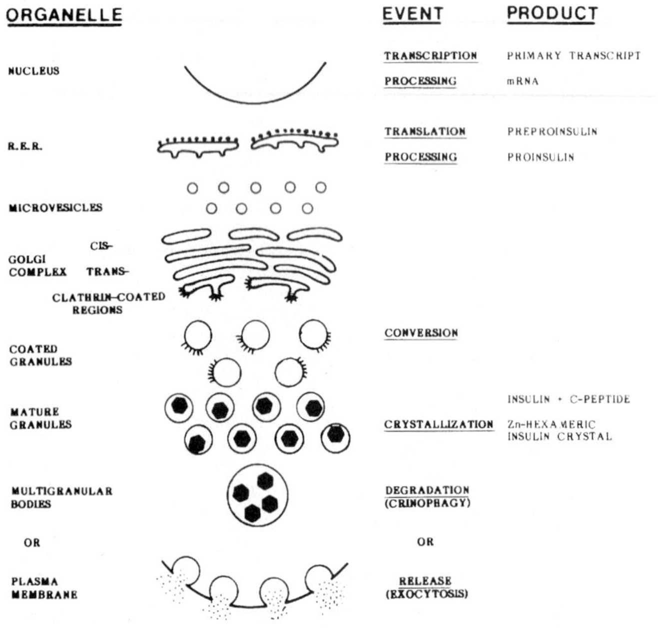

Secretory granules are formed by the budding of selective, *clathrin*-coated regions of the TGN. Clathrin, a complex aggregate of protein subunits, is found on the cytosolic face of the limiting membrane of many vesicles and is thought to facilitate intracellular shuttling. The clathrin of coated granules is shed rapidly to form mature granules.[2] By electron microscopy, secretory granules in B cells from most species appears with an electron-dense central core, well separated from the limiting membrane.[2] This core is thought to consist of the insulin crystal. Proinsulin, although it can be crystallized in vitro under certain stringent conditions, would not be expected to crystallize within secretory granules. Theoretically, the insulin crystal would be expected to allow for both orderly and compact packaging of insulin, permitting relatively large amounts of the hormone to be released, and stability of the insulin molecule in the face of proteases that may reside within the granule.

The insulin molecule consists of two peptide chains linked by two sulfhydryl bridges (Fig. 134-2). Proinsulin is synthesized as one peptide chain. Conversion of proinsulin to insulin involves the removal of the segment connecting the two insulin chains (*C peptide,* or connecting peptide).[1] Conversion arises within secretory granules and is thought not to occur to any significant extent outside the B cell. Theoretically, granules can be expected to contain proinsulin, proinsulin mixed with equimolar amounts of insulin and C peptide, or only C peptide and insulin (again in equimolar amounts) if conversion has gone to completion. The enzymes responsible for conversion have now been identified. The proinsulin-processing endopeptidase PC3 (also known as PC1) cleaves specifically at the Arg31, Arg32 site of proinsulin, whereas PC2 prefers the Lys64, Arg65 site. These enzymes are members of a family of subtilisin-like endoproteases homologous to the yeast Kex2 gene product.[6] The pairs of basic amino acids that are exposed by PC3 and PC2 are then removed by the exopeptidase carboxypeptidase H. Little convincing evidence is found of a biologic role for the C peptide; however, this molecule theoretically is released into the circulation in the same amount as insulin. Proinsulin also can be released from B cells, presumably reflecting exocytosis of granules in which conversion either has not occurred or has not gone to completion. Alternatively, proinsulin could be released through the constitutive pathway. This secretory pathway involves rapid transfer of products from the Golgi complex to the plasma membrane in small vesicles.[7] No storage compartment exists, and release is not regulated by secretagogues. Although proinsulin is released essentially only through the regulated (secretory granule) pathway in native B cells, it probably is released to a much greater extent through the constitutive pathway in insulinoma cells.[8]

| ORGANELLE | EVENT | PRODUCT |
|---|---|---|
| NUCLEUS | TRANSCRIPTION | PRIMARY TRANSCRIPT |
| | PROCESSING | mRNA |
| R.E.R. | TRANSLATION | PREPROINSULIN |
| | PROCESSING | PROINSULIN |
| MICROVESICLES | | |
| GOLGI COMPLEX CIS- TRANS- | | |
| CLATHRIN-COATED REGIONS | | |
| COATED GRANULES | CONVERSION | |
| MATURE GRANULES | CRYSTALLIZATION | INSULIN + C-PEPTIDE Zn-HEXAMERIC INSULIN CRYSTAL |
| MULTIGRANULAR BODIES | DEGRADATION (CRINOPHAGY) | |
| OR | OR | |
| PLASMA MEMBRANE | RELEASE (EXOCYTOSIS) | |

**FIGURE 134-1.** Key events in insulin production by the B cell. (*RER,* rough endoplasmic reticulum.)

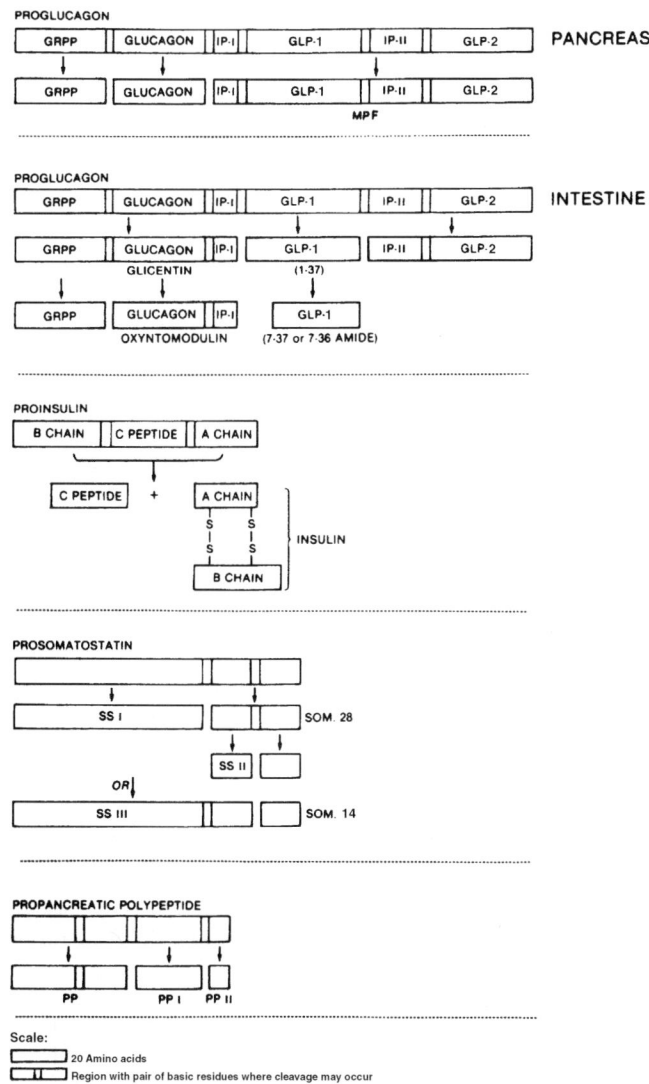

**FIGURE 134-2.** Processing of pancreatic prohormones. Processing of proglucagon is tissue specific. Proinsulin assumes a correct secondary structure, with disulfide bridge formation between the A and B chains, before conversion. Somatostatin-28 is an identifiable intermediate in humans. In the rat, an alternative pathway for direct cleavage of somatostatin-14 has been documented. Pancreatic polypeptide I (*PPI*) often is referred to as pancreatic eicosapeptide. Cleavage site between PPI and pancreatic polypeptide II (*PPII*) is, exceptionally, at a single arginine residue rather than a pair of basic residues. (*GRPP*, glicentin-related pancreatic peptide; *IP*, intervening peptide; *GLP*, glucagon-like peptide; *MPF*, major proglucagon fragment; *S*, sulfhydryl; *SS*, somatostatin; *Som*, somatostatin.)

Insulin release is achieved by *exocytosis* (or *emiocytosis*) of granule contents.[2] The granule membrane fuses with the plasma membrane, and its contents then are extruded from the cell. Exocytosis is succeeded by *endocytosis* (the reverse process), so that a relatively constant amount of membranous material is ensured at the plasma membrane and in the intracellular pool.[2] The mechanism by which granules are channeled to the plasma membrane and by which their release is enhanced in response to a stimulus remains unknown. Granules have been postulated to become associated with microtubules or microfilaments; certainly, this would provide one means of directional movement.[9] When insulin release is stimulated from the pancreas of a normal individual by glucose, release is biphasic: the first phase is short-lived and prompt (peaking by 5 minutes), whereas the second phase is of slower onset but is maintained for considerable periods under experimental conditions. An additional level of

complexity is provided by the functional heterogeneity noted among B cells in any single islet. Although such heterogeneity has been well documented in dispersed single cells, its physiologic significance remains to be defined.[10]

The degradation of insulin within B cells is a mechanism to diminish stored insulin when its release is inhibited.[2] Degradation is thought to proceed primarily by *crinophagy* (fusion of granules with lysosomes), a pathway common to many secretory cell types.[2] Once introduced into the lysosome, the insulin molecules become exposed to lysosomal proteases. The factors influencing the rate of crinophagy are unknown.

## THE INSULIN GENE: SPECIES VARIATIONS AND MUTANT HUMAN FORMS

The insulin molecule (and, to a lesser extent, proinsulin, which displays considerable species variation in the C peptide) has been remarkably conserved throughout evolution, a fact with important theoretic and practical (clinical) implications. Those regions of the primary sequence of the insulin A and B chains conserved in most species correspond to regions involved in (a) the folding of the molecule into its secondary structure (i.e., disulfide bridge formation), (b) the association of monomers and dimers to form the hexamer or of hexamers to pack into a crystal form, and (c) correct structure, conformation, and presentation of the regions thought to be involved in receptor binding and, thus, bioactivity. One result of such conservation of structure and function is the successful therapeutic use in the past of animal insulins (notably beef and pork) in humans. Pork insulin differs from its human counterpart by only one amino acid (at the C terminus of the B chain). Beef insulin, differing by three amino acids, appears to be intrinsically more immunogenic than pork insulin in humans. Human insulin, which is now in widespread clinical use, is manufactured by the introduction of the human insulin gene into the microorganisms *Escherichia coli* and yeast. Proinsulin is extracted from the microorganism, converted to insulin in vitro, and then purified.

Individuals (and, in some instances, families) displaying *abnormal proinsulin* or *insulin* as a result of a mutation in the insulin gene have been studied.[11,12] Such mutations have become evident through the analysis of circulating (and, in one case, pancreatic) forms of insulin in individuals displaying, typically, hyperinsulinemia or hyperproinsulinemia of obscure origin (i.e., no insulinoma and no insulin-receptor defects). Two major types of mutations have been characterized. The first causes an amino-acid substitution in the region of the insulin molecule critical for bioactivity. These include insulin Chicago (Phe-B25-Leu), insulin Los Angeles (Phe-B24-Ser), and insulin Wakayama (Val-A3-Leu). These mutations almost completely obliterate bioactivity. Only heterozygotes have been found, and some do not even have diabetes; this finding provides insight into the capacity of only one normal allele to provide sufficient insulin for decades. Other mutations lead to hyperproinsulinemia, which may also be associated with type 2 diabetes mellitus. Individuals with these mutations have insulin secretory characteristics virtually identical to those of subjects with type 2 diabetes. This can occur with an Arg-C65-His mutation that interferes with the normal processing of proinsulin to insulin, resulting in a circulating moiety consisting of proinsulin cleaved between the C peptide and the B chain, but with the A-chain–C-peptide link still intact.[13] Through another mechanism, a His-B10-Asp mutation leads to increased circulating levels of this mutated proinsulin-like molecule.[14] This mutant proinsulin appears to be diverted to the constitutive pathway of release in B cells, thus avoiding the processing to insulin and C peptide that occurs in regulated secretory granules. Mutations leading to functionally altered proinsulin or insulin are rare. Other mutations may arise more frequently but lead either to no change in the amino-acid sequence (silent mutations) or to changes that do not affect bioactivity and, therefore, do not produce an identifiable phenotype.

# REGULATION OF INSULIN PRODUCTION

## INSULIN BIOSYNTHESIS

Insulin biosynthesis can be regulated by glucose at the level of either transcription or translation.[1] Translation is more important for controlling the short-term changes in the rate of insulin biosynthesis—glucose can exert effects on translation within only 20 minutes. Glucose effects on transcription can take hours, but are certainly important for the long-term control of insulin production, such as that associated with changes in diet. Although a close correlation is found between the regulation of insulin biosynthesis and insulin release, some factors affect one pathway but not the other; for example, decreasing extracellular calcium inhibits release without affecting biosynthesis. The dose-response curve for glucose stimulation of insulin biosynthesis in rat islets has a threshold of ~2.5 mmol/L, whereas the threshold for glucose-induced secretion is ~4.5 mmol/L.

Much has been learned about the transcriptional control of insulin secretion.[15] In adult mammals, insulin is selectively expressed in pancreatic B cells. Although the insulin gene may be regulated far upstream from the transcription start site, a smaller highly conserved region of ~400 base pairs contains the major glucose control elements. The enhancer elements that seem particularly important include E1, A2-C1, A4-A3, and E2. Transcription factors that form complexes and bind to these elements include those that are ubiquitous and those that are cell specific. Transcription factors that are relatively cell specific are BETA2 and PDX-1, with the latter probably being especially important for control by glucose. Other notable transcription factors include C/EBPβ, which has an inhibitory effect, CREB, which is largely controlled by cyclic adenosine monophosphate (cAMP), and STAT5, which is influenced by growth hormone. The effects of glucose on translation are exerted at multiple steps, including the initiation phase, the elongation phase, and the transfer to the endoplasmic reticulum via the signal recognition particle (SRP).[1] The molecular signals that link glucose metabolism to changes in transcription and translation remain to be determined.

## INSULIN RELEASE

The regulation of insulin release has been studied extensively both in vivo (in humans and animals) and in vitro (using the perfused pancreas or isolated islets of Langerhans).[16] Regulatory factors can be classed into three major groups: (a) metabolic (i.e., glucose), (b) hormonal (i.e., glucagon), and (c) neural (i.e., acetylcholine). The effect of any of these agents on B-cell function is either to stimulate or to inhibit exocytosis (Table 134-1). The manner in which a given stimulus to the B cell is coupled with the change in the rate of insulin release (*stimulus-secretion coupling*) probably is different for the three major groups of factors listed earlier (Fig. 134-3). The regulation of insulin secretion by glucose is somehow controlled by glucose metabolism.[16] A high-capacity glucose transporter (GLUT) in B cells, GLUT2 in rats and possibly GLUT1 in humans, allows rapid equilibration of extracellular and cytosolic glucose concentrations. The rate of glucose metabolism, which is closely coupled with the rate of insulin secretion, is determined by glucokinase, the enzyme in the rate-limiting step of glycolysis.[17,18] Metabolism leads to several intracellular events that culminate in an increase in cytosolic calcium. A key step is known to be depolarization of the B cell evoked by blocking of the adenosine triphosphate (ATP)–sensitive potassium channel in the plasma membrane, which probably is controlled mainly by the

**TABLE 134-1.**

**Effects of Various Major Modulators of Pancreatic Hormone Secretion**

|  | Glucagon | Insulin | Somatostatin |
| --- | --- | --- | --- |
| **ISLET HORMONES** | | | |
| Glucagon | ↓ | ↑ | ↑ |
| Insulin | ↓ | ↓ | ↓ |
| Somatostatin | ↓ | ↓ | ↓ |
| **NUTRIENTS/METABOLITES** | | | |
| Glucose | ↓ | ↑ | ↑ |
| Amino acids | ↑ | ↑ | ↑ |
| Fatty acids | ↓ | ↑ | ↑ |
| **NEURAL MEDIATORS** | | | |
| α-Adrenergic | ↑ | ↓ | ↓ |
| β-Adrenergic | ↑ | ↑ | ↑ |
| Cholinergic | ↑ | ↑ | ↓ |
| **GUT HORMONES** | | | |
| Gastrin | ↑ | ↑ | ↑ |
| Cholecystokinin | ↑ | ↑ | ↑ |
| Gastric inhibitory peptide | ↑ | ↑ | ↑ |
| Secretin | ↓ | ↑ | ↑ |
| Gastrin-releasing peptide* | 0 | ↑ | ↑ |
| Vasoactive intestinal peptide | ↑ | ↑ | ↑ |

↑, stimulates release; ↓, inhibits release; 0, has no effect.
*The amphibian equivalent, bombesin, often is used experimentally.

ratio of ATP to adenosine diphosphate (ADP). This depolarization leads to the opening of voltage-dependent calcium channels that allows extracellular calcium, which has a relatively high concentration, to enter B cells. This increase in cytosolic calcium then triggers the complex process of distal release that culminates in exocytosis with extrusion of insulin. The produc-

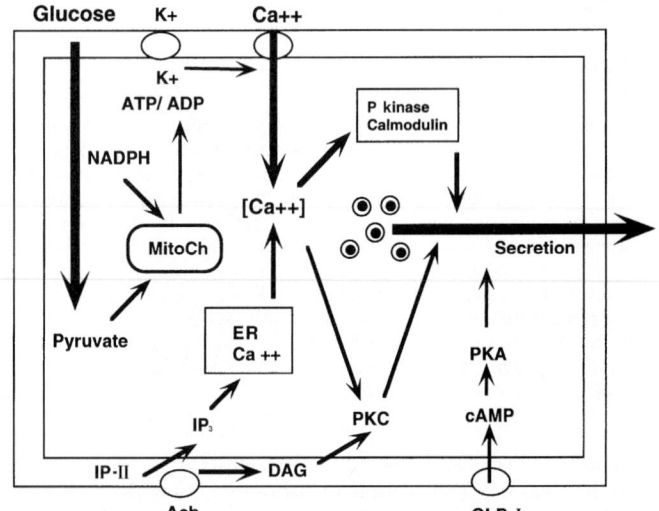

**FIGURE 134-3.** Mechanisms of insulin release. The metabolism of glucose increases the ratio of adenosine triphosphate (*ATP*) to adenosine diphosphate (*ADP*), closing the ATP-sensitive potassium channel. The subsequent depolarization opens the voltage-dependent calcium channel, allowing calcium to enter the B cell. Increased cytosolic calcium then triggers secretion by activating protein kinases. (*P kinase*, protein kinase; *NADPH*, reduced form of nicotinamide-adenine dinucleotide phosphate; *MitoCh*, mitochondria; *ER*, endoplasmic reticulum; *PKA*, protein kinase A; *IP₃*, inositol trisphosphate [note that the active form is inositol 1,4,5-trisphosphate]; *PKC*, protein kinase C; *cAMP*, cyclic adenosine monophosphate; *IP₂*, inositol diphosphate; *Ach*, acetylcholine; *DAG*, diacylglycerol; *GLP-I*, glucagon-like peptide-I.) (This scheme was modified from the original version provided by Dr. Claes Wollheim, University of Geneva, Switzerland.)

tion of ATP is not entirely from metabolism of pyruvate originating from glucose; a major contribution also comes from the generation of NADPH (reduced form of nicotinamide-adenine dinucleotide phosphate) by glycolysis, which can send reducing equivalents to the mitochondria via specialized shuttles that are uniquely active in B cells.[19–21] Moreover, the effects of glucose cannot be explained entirely by depolarization. The likelihood that glucose stimulates the production of as yet unidentified lipid mediators that could act on separate pathways has generated much interest.[22,23]

Another less well understood pathway for raising cytosolic calcium would be by the stimulation of calcium mobilization from intracellular storage in the endoplasmic reticulum.[16,24] Much attention has focused on the role of phospholipid, and in particular the inositol trisphosphates ($IP_3$) on stimulus-secretion coupling. $IP_3$ mobilizes calcium directly from the endoplasmic reticulum, and diacylglycerol, a second product of the action of phospholipase C on phosphatidylinositol bisphosphate, participates in stimulus-secretion coupling by stimulating protein kinase C (see Chap. 4). Finally, the cAMP-dependent protein kinase also can participate in stimulation of release.

The outlines of the distal steps of insulin secretion are now emerging.[25] Insulin-containing secretory granules are associated with microtubules and move to the cell surface via further interactions with the microfilaments of the cortical actin web. Increased cytosolic calcium plays a key role in several distal steps. Initially calcium binds to calmodulin (CaM), which can then bind CaM kinases. CaM kinase II has been localized to insulin secretory granules. These kinases can then phosphorylate proteins such as microtubule-associated protein-2 (MAP-2) and synapsin I that may be involved in the exocytosis of synaptic-like microvesicles (SLMV). They also may regulate the key proteins involved in the docking of granules, v-SNARES (*synaptobrevin* [VAMP] and *cellubrevin*) and t-SNARES (SNAP-25 and *syntaxin*). The docking complex binds to NSF (*N*-ethyl-maleimide-sensitive fusion protein) and α-SNAP (soluble NSF attachment protein). NSF has adenosine triphosphatase activity that probably allows the formation of fusion-competent granules that are primed for release as the first phase of insulin secretion.

Insulin is normally secreted in coordinated secretory bursts. In humans, pulses occur approximately every 10 to 13 min. Although the variations in peripheral circulating insulin levels are modest, marked variations can be found in the portal vein.[26] Metabolic oscillation of glycolysis, probably controlled by the enzyme phosphofructokinase, must play a key role, but some kind of neural network may also exist that can coordinate communication between islets in different parts of the pancreas.[27–29] Because the variations in the concentrations of insulin (and glucagon) in the portal veins are substantial,[26] the possibility that these fluctuations have an important influence on hepatic metabolism is attractive. The oscillations of insulin levels in arterial plasma are more modest, and further dampening must occur when insulin leaves the vasculature to reach muscle or fat cells. Thus, the influence of pulsatile insulin secretion on peripheral metabolism may be inconsequential.

## INTEGRATED REGULATION OF B-CELL FUNCTION

The plasma concentration of insulin in the fasting state usually is between 5 and 20 μU/mL. C peptide, which is secreted in equimolar amounts with insulin, has a higher molar concentration in plasma because its half-life is considerably longer than that of insulin (30 vs. 5 minutes). Generally, the amount of proinsulin secreted by B cells is small—<3% that of insulin—but because of its long half-life (~17 minutes), it can account for as much as 30% of the insulin immunoreactivity in plasma.[30] When B-cell secretion is stimulated by food intake, the concen-

trations of all three plasma components increase, but the proportions change because of the different half-lives and because the actual ratio of proinsulin to insulin released from the B cell may increase, reflecting faster turnover. Insulin is the most important secretory product of the B cell; C peptide has not been shown to have significant bioactivity, and the effects of proinsulin probably are negligible, because it has only 10% to 15% of the bioactivity of insulin.

Interestingly, patients with insulinomas (insulin-producing pancreatic islet cell tumors) usually have a disproportionate amount of circulating proinsulin-like material. Presumably, neoplasia somehow disrupts the precisely ordered mechanisms of normal processing and secretion, causing the release of abnormally large amounts of insulin precursor.

Insulin plays a critical role in the anabolic events that accompany nutrient intake because it is the principal promoter of the synthesis and storage of glycogen, fat, and protein. Nutrient storage is efficient, and the mechanisms responsible for this are both complex and elegant. The liver is the key organ for nutrient deposition; therefore, the fact that its major blood supply comes from the portal venous system, which drains the gastrointestinal tract, is particularly advantageous. Furthermore, because of the location of the pancreas, insulin and glucagon are released directly into the portal vein, so that the liver is exposed to particularly high concentrations of these hormones. Even the anticipation of food intake may trigger insulin secretion (*cephalic phase*) and allow some insulinization of the liver to take place at a very early stage. The contribution of the cephalic phase may be a modest one and is thought to be exerted by the vagus nerve. A more potent effect is exerted by various gut factors that are not fully elucidated but are assigned the general term *incretin*.[31] The most attractive candidates for this incretin role are gastric inhibitory peptide (see Chap. 182) and glucagon-like peptide 1. Once a meal is absorbed, the plasma concentrations of both glucose and amino acids increase, providing an additional stimulus for insulin secretion. The entire process can be extraordinarily efficient, as evidenced by the virtual absence of a rise in plasma glucose levels in some normal persons after the oral ingestion of a 100-g glucose load. Even in the absence of a rise in glucose concentrations, enough insulin presumably is secreted to stimulate hepatic and peripheral glucose uptake and also to inhibit hepatic glucose output—with these combined effects being sufficient to preserve euglycemia.

The autonomic nervous system exerts an important influence on islet hormone secretion, and the sympathetic branch appears to play a particularly prominent role during stress and exercise. Epinephrine secreted by the adrenal medulla and norepinephrine released from nerve terminals within the islet can inhibit insulin secretion through α-adrenergic receptors.[32] Beta-adrenergic stimulation actually can stimulate insulin secretion, but this effect is obscured by the dominant α activity. The peptide galanin, which has an inhibitory effect on the B cell, is also released by sympathetic nerve terminals. Because stress is part of the "fight or flight" process, it is often accompanied by muscular activity. Muscular exercise consumes glucose, and yet plasma glucose levels must be kept up to provide the brain with a continuous supply of this fuel. Fortunately, hepatic glucose output is increased, and this is accomplished partly through the inhibition of insulin secretion. Another important mechanism is the increase in glucagon secretion stimulated by the sympathetic nervous system, with the effect being exerted by both α and β receptors. If stress occurs in the absence of muscular activity, hyperglycemia can result. This condition is termed *stress hyperglycemia* and often is seen during such situations as trauma, major surgery, burns, and febrile illness. Many individuals do not become hyperglycemic during such events; those who do may have a tendency toward the development of diabetes, perhaps related to marginal B-cell reserve. Pheochromocytomas (see Chaps. 86 and 87) also can be associated with hyperglycemia, presumably because of the ability of catecholamines, both epinephrine and norepinephrine, to inhibit insulin secretion, stimulate glucagon release, and independently enhance hepatic glucose output. Parasympathetic nervous stimulation, mediated by vagal release of acetylcholine and probably vasoactive intestinal peptide (VIP), stimulate both insulin and glucagon secretion and may be important during nutrient intake.

## INSULIN SECRETION AND DIABETES

Insulin secretion in non–insulin-dependent diabetes mellitus (type 2 diabetes) has been studied in considerable detail, and various abnormalities have been identified.[33,34] In contrast, little information is available about B-cell function in insulin-dependent diabetes mellitus (type 1 diabetes) or pre–type 1 diabetes; however, the fact that some of the secretory characteristics resemble those found in type 2 diabetes is of interest.

Some investigators have found that fasting plasma insulin concentrations are elevated in persons with type 2 diabetes. In only moderately severe forms of this disease, the mean plasma insulin levels over a 24-hour period are essentially normal. Nonetheless, individuals with type 2 diabetes can be considered to be insulin deficient in a relative sense, because a pancreas with normal B-cell function and mass would secrete considerably larger amounts of insulin when confronted with a similar degree of hyperglycemia. This relative insulin deficiency is confounded by unusually high levels of proinsulin and of the conversion intermediate des 31.32 split proinsulin.[1] Both of these peptides are less biologically active than is fully processed insulin. The cause of this elevation of insulin precursors in type 2 diabetes remains to be established.[35] The fundamental role of the B cell in type 2 diabetes cannot be underestimated, because "normal" B-cell function usually can maintain euglycemia even in the face of a substantial amount of insulin resistance. Another defect found in type 2 diabetes is an inability of the B cell to respond to an acute glucose challenge, which is seen most prominently as a loss of first-phase release. Nonetheless, responses to various nonglucose secretagogues such as isoproterenol, arginine, and secretin are preserved, although the ability of glucose to potentiate these responses is partially lost. The mechanisms responsible for these secretory abnormalities are uncertain. An attractive hypothesis is that these defects result mainly from the adverse effects of chronic hyperglycemia, but the elevated free fatty acids of the diabetic state may also exert an inhibitory influence. The mechanisms responsible for the B-cell dysfunction found in the diabetic state are not completely understood, but B cells chronically exposed to the diabetic milieu undergo dedifferentiation, which appears to selectively damage the unique mechanisms required for glucose-induced insulin secretion.[36]

## INSULIN DEGRADATION

Insulin exerts its effects on target cells after binding to specific plasma membrane receptors. An important consequence of the insulin-receptor interaction is that this forms the first step in insulin degradation by most target tissues.[37] The insulin-receptor complex becomes internalized by the cell, and insulin subsequently is degraded. Although lysosomes generally are thought to be largely responsible for the degradation, nonlysosomal proteases displaying considerable activity against insulin may be critical for the early steps in the degradative pathway.[37] Under physiologic conditions, the liver is the single most important organ for insulin destruction: as much as 50% of the insulin entering the liver is estimated to be degraded in a single passage. This degradation occurs almost exclusively through the receptor-mediated pathway. An interesting consequence is the dramatically reduced rate of insulin clearance (and resulting hyperinsulinemia) in patients displaying severely diminished insulin-receptor binding capacity. The other important site of degradation is the kidney, in which insulin is cleared from the circulation by a combination of a saturable, receptor-mediated pathway and a nonsaturable pathway.[38] The latter pathway, in which receptors are not implicated, assumes greater importance under pathologic conditions of elevated plasma insulin levels. Both proinsulin and C peptide, in contrast to insulin, are degraded primarily in the kidneys through a nonsaturable pathway. Because C peptide is not taken up by the liver, its measurement in plasma can be used to calculate insulin secretory rates.[39]

To understand insulin degradation, as well as its bioactivity, one must recall the anatomic location of the pancreas with respect to the liver. Direct secretion of insulin into the portal vein causes as much as 50% of the newly produced insulin to be cleared immediately by the liver. Such is not the case when insulin is injected subcutaneously. The physiologic significance of portal insulin delivery is not well understood, but the inability to deliver exogenous insulin in a physiologic fashion surely is a compounding factor in the inadequate minute-to-minute control of type 1 diabetes. Finally, it should be noted that insulin is degraded to some extent before its delivery to the circulation, whether within the pancreatic B cell (under physiologic conditions) or in the subcutaneous depot (after insulin injection).

## GLUCAGON PRODUCTION

Proglucagon is synthesized in the pancreatic A cell and the gastrointestinal tract, and is processed in a tissue-specific manner (see Fig. 134-2). The full complexity of this processing has not been defined. The most prominent secretory product of the pancreatic and gastric A cells is glucagon. The intestinal L cells contain and secrete glicentin, oxyntomodulin, and glucagon-like peptide 1.[40] Glicentin and oxyntomodulin have no known biologic role. The naturally occurring truncated form of glucagon-like peptide 1 (7-36-amide), which is a potent insulin secretagogue,[41] is released by the intestine during food ingestion and may serve the important physiologic function of enhancing insulin secretion during meals—the *incretin* effect.[42]

Glucagon has a potent and important influence on hepatic glycogenolysis, gluconeogenesis, and ketogenesis. The critical experiments proving glucagon's fundamental role in carbohydrate metabolism used somatostatin as a tool. Somatostatin inhibits glucagon secretion efficiently, allowing the effects of glucagon deficiency to be studied (see Chap. 169). When somatostatin is infused into fasting humans, the release of both glucagon and insulin is inhibited, and the plasma glucose level falls. This indicates that the short-term influence of glucagon on the maintenance of basal glucose levels is more important than that of insulin, a finding that was surprising at the time it was made.[43] Over a longer period, however, the effects of insulin deficiency outweigh those of glucagon deficiency, because after somatostatin is infused for a few hours, hyperglycemia develops—a result predicted from the fact that surgical pancreatectomy causes diabetes.

That glucagon is required for survival still is not totally accepted, because identification of convincing cases of glucagon deficiency has been so difficult. Nevertheless, because the amino-acid sequence of this peptide is almost perfectly preserved in vertebrates, glucagon can be presumed to be an essential hormone. Glucagon may be of particular importance during food ingestion, particularly in carnivores, because, in the absence of glucagon, a large protein load could cause hypoglycemia through the unopposed stimulation of insulin secretion. Glucagon also has an important, perhaps critical, role in maintaining hepatic glucose output during prolonged exercise and fasting. Finally, glucagon may be important in preventing hypoglycemia in infants.

The fasting concentration of pancreatic glucagon in plasma is 25 to 50 pg/mL. This level is increased by a high-protein meal and usually is modestly decreased by a high-carbohydrate meal. As is the case with insulin, glucagon release probably is influenced by gut hormones; this may account for the observation that intravenous administration of glucose inhibits glucagon release more effectively than does oral glucose administration. In the normal state, little circulating proglucagon is present. However, glucagon-producing pancreatic tumors (glucagonomas; see Chap. 220) release a disproportionate amount of proglucagon-like material; their behavior is thus analogous to that of insulinomas, which also secrete a precursor form (see Chap. 158).

The inhibitory influence of glucose on glucagon secretion is well known, but the mechanisms involved are unclear. One critical issue is whether the glucose effect is exerted directly on the pancreatic A cell.[44] Several situations are seen in which B-cell function is either absent or impaired, and in these, the A cell appears to be blind to the suppressive effects of glucose. These situations include human and experimentally induced diabetes, experiments that take advantage of the loss of insulin secretion produced by streptozocin, and studies of gastric A cells that do not have adjacent B cells. These observations provided the basis for the hypothesis that glucose-induced glucagon suppression is exerted indirectly by intraislet secretion of insulin, which is carried from the B cell–containing islet core to the A cell–containing islet mantle by islet blood vessels.[45,46] This hypothesis has been strengthened considerably by the demonstration that infusion of insulin antiserum into the isolated perfused rat pancreas causes an abrupt increase in glucagon secretion. Some evidence exists, however, that isolated A cells can respond directly to glucose, and whether islet somatostatin exerts a significant paracrine effect is still unknown. A potential explanation for the hypoglycemia-induced increase of glucagon is the release of norepinephrine from intraislet adrenergic nerve terminals, which causes catecholamine-induced glucagon release.[32] Interestingly, this has been found in an isolated pancreas preparation, a finding which indicates that the central nervous system may not have to participate in the process.[47]

Many substances have been found to exert either a stimulatory or inhibitory effect on glucagon secretion[48] (see Table 134-1). Because the study of isolated A cells is so difficult, whether these agents are acting directly or indirectly is not known. However, most amino acids stimulate glucagon secretion. Moreover, most gut hormones have a stimulatory effect, although secretin, which is inhibitory in some species, is a notable exception. The effects of the other islet hormones are presumed to be important, and both insulin and somatostatin exert an inhibitory influence. With regard to the autonomic nervous system, parasympathetic activation stimulates glucagon secretion, but the effects of the sympathetic division of the system are more complex. The overall effect of sympathetic activation is to stimulate glucagon release, but disagreement exists about the relative roles of α- and β-adrenergic receptors, partly because results have been obtained in different species and preparations. Usually both α and β stimulation are found to elicit glucagon secretion. Free fatty acids have an inhibitory effect, but the physiologic importance of this is unclear. Relatively little is known about the cellular mechanisms responsible for glucagon secretion. The effects of various agents have been partially elucidated, and glucagon secretion is likely mediated in some circumstances by an increase in cytosolic calcium, an increase in cAMP, or both. Until proved otherwise, the mechanisms of A cell secretion should be assumed to resemble those of other secretory cells.

## GLUCAGON AND DIABETES

The contribution of glucagon to the metabolic derangements seen in diabetes mellitus has generated considerable interest. Clearly, glucagon secretion is inappropriately elevated in diabe-

tes, because hyperglycemia normally would be expected to suppress plasma glucagon levels. Why glucagon levels are increased in either an absolute or a relative sense is not completely understood, but intraislet or systemic insulin deficiency appears important. Another interesting possibility is that hyperglycemia somehow desensitizes the A cell, perhaps in a fashion similar to that in the B and D cells, thus making it nonresponsive to the effects of hyperglycemia. Although the mechanisms responsible for the hyperglucagonemia of diabetes are unclear, the contributions of glucagon to the hyperglycemia and hyperketonemia of diabetes are substantial. In type 1 diabetes, when insulin therapy is discontinued suddenly, plasma glucose and ketone levels increase rapidly; however, if glucagon secretion is inhibited with somatostatin, these increases are markedly attenuated.[49] Therefore, particularly in uncontrolled diabetes but even in relatively well-controlled diabetes, glucagon exerts an important stimulatory effect on hepatic glucose output through its influence on gluconeogenesis and glycogenolysis, an effect that clearly is enhanced by insulin deficiency. Alterations in both hormones also are critical in the generation of ketone bodies. Insulin deficiency is the primary factor responsible for the release of free fatty acids from adipose tissue, and this provides substrate for hepatic ketogenesis, which is stimulated primarily by glucagon.

Thus, the metabolic derangements of diabetes can be considered to be the result of a *bihormonal* disturbance. Even though the importance of glucagon in diabetes now is well accepted, the fundamental contribution of insulin deficiency remains paramount. Not only does insulin deficiency contribute either directly or indirectly to the hyperglucagonemia of diabetes, but also, even if plasma glucagon levels are either zero or extremely low (as may be found after a pancreatectomy), if insulin secretion is low enough, diabetes still will be present.

In humans without diabetes, insulin-induced hypoglycemia elicits a clear increase in the plasma glucagon concentration, but in those with diabetes, this rise often is missing. Although glucagon provides an important defense against hypoglycemia, its loss usually does not have serious consequences, because catecholamines provide a satisfactory backup mechanism.[50] Some patients, however, also have an inadequate catecholamine response, perhaps secondary to autonomic neuropathy, and they are especially vulnerable to hypoglycemia. The mechanisms responsible for this lost glucagon response in diabetes have not been elucidated.

## SOMATOSTATIN PRODUCTION

Shortly after somatostatin was discovered in the hypothalamus, it also was found in many other tissues, including the gastrointestinal tract and the D cells of pancreatic islets (see Chap. 169). The peptide that was described first consists of 14 amino acids and has been called *somatostatin-14*; an N-terminal–extended form also has been identified, which is called *somatostatin-28* (see Fig. 134-2). The somatostatin peptides have a remarkably diverse range of actions, including potent inhibitory effects on insulin and glucagon secretion. Although islets contain much more somatostatin-14 than somatostatin-28, the latter is far more potent in its inhibition of the other islet hormones. In contrast to islet D cells, those of the gastrointestinal tract contain a relatively greater proportion of somatostatin-28, a finding which indicates that the intracellular processing mechanisms differ in these two sites.

The importance of the islet somatostatins has not been established. Although suggestions have been made that circulating somatostatins exert some physiologic effects, the contribution of the islet somatostatins undoubtedly is inconsequential, because the amounts coming from islets are much less than those coming from the gastrointestinal tract.[51] The most likely role for the pancreatic somatostatins is an intraislet one. They may inhibit insulin and glucagon secretion through paracrine mechanisms, so that the locally secreted peptides reach B and A cells through the interstitial space.[46] However, the somatostatins secreted from D cells in the islet mantle might have difficulty penetrating very far into the central B-cell core; therefore, the influence of this hormone on insulin secretion probably is not significant. Glucagon or pancreatic polypeptide (PP) secretion seems more likely to be modulated by secretion from adjacent D cells, but proving that this occurs has been difficult. Interestingly, in vertebrates such as birds and fish, islets contain a larger proportion of D cells than is found in mammals. This finding has generated speculation that mammalian D cells in islets may be becoming vestigial. Because the structure of somatostatin is well preserved in most vertebrate species, the peptide should be assumed to have an essential function, but perhaps this is true only in tissues such as the nervous system and the gastrointestinal tract.

The secretory characteristics of the pancreatic D cell have been reasonably well characterized (see Table 134-1). With only a few exceptions, the direction of secretion—either increased or decreased—is the same in both D and B cells. As is the case with the other islet hormones, somatostatin secretion is influenced by nutrients such as glucose and amino acids, by gastrointestinal hormones, and by autonomic nervous system mediators. Moreover, glucagon is able to stimulate somatostatin secretion, and in some species, insulin appears to have an inhibitory influence. As with A cells, little is known about the cellular mechanisms of somatostatin secretion, because sufficient D cell tissue cannot be obtained to carry out biochemical studies. At present, no evidence exists that somatostatin plays any role in the pathogenesis of diabetes.

## PANCREATIC POLYPEPTIDE

In humans, PP consists of 36 amino acids and is found in PP cells, which are concentrated in the mantle of the islets of the ventral lobe of the pancreas. In common with the other islet hormones, this peptide is synthesized in precursor form. Processing of the precursor yields not only mature PP itself but also two other peptides, one of which often is called *pancreatic eicosapeptide* (see Fig. 134-2). PP has received relatively little attention because its biologic significance is undetermined. Perhaps it is involved in suppressing secretions from the exocrine pancreas. Studies using the radioimmunoassay for PP have led to some understanding of its secretory characteristics.[52] Various gastrointestinal hormones can stimulate PP secretion; vagal stimulation is a particularly potent stimulus for its release. Because of this marked sensitivity to vagal stimulation, diminished PP secretion in response to hypoglycemia has been suggested to predict the development of diabetic autonomic neuropathy.[53] This peptide has not been shown to be important in diabetes, although plasma levels are elevated in insulin-treated patients with type 1 and type 2 diabetes.

## ISLET AMYLOID–ASSOCIATED PEPTIDE

At autopsy, amyloid deposits have been found in the islets of most patients with type 2 diabetes.[54,55] The amyloid is formed by a 37-amino-acid peptide called *islet amyloid polypeptide* (IAPP), or amylin. An 89-amino-acid precursor form of IAPP is synthesized in B cells. The sequence between positions 20 and 29, with position 25 being particularly important, determines the ability of this peptide to form amyloid. Because of these structural requirements, amyloid deposits are found in primates and cats but not in many other species. Production of IAPP is restricted to B cells and its stored content is only ~1% of that of insulin, with this ratio being reflected in the amount secreted. IAPP has no known functional role, and although various pharmacologic effects have been demonstrated, no persuasive evidence exists that secreted IAPP has any physiologic effect on peripheral tissues, particularly because the circulating

levels are so low. The mechanisms responsible for the deposition of amyloid in type 2 diabetes are unknown, but this fibrillar material has been shown to have a toxic effect on B cells in vitro.[56] Moreover, questions have been raised about whether intracellular IAPP accumulation can exert a toxic effect in normal B cells.[55,57] Such processes occurring slowly over years could contribute to a gradual decline in B-cell mass.

## REFERENCES

1. Rhodes CJ. Processing of the insulin molecule. In: LeRoith D, Taylor SI, Olefsky JM, eds. Diabetes mellitus, 2nd ed. Philadelphia: Lippincott Williams & Wilkins, 2000:20.
2. Orci L. The insulin factory: a tour of the plant surroundings and a visit to the assembly line. Diabetologia 1985; 28:528.
3. Orci L, Vassali JD, Perrelet A. The insulin factory. Sci Am 1988; 259:85.
4. Mellman I, Simons K. The Golgi complex: in vitro veritas? Cell 1992; 68:829.
5. Guest PC, Bailyes EM, Rutherford NG, Hutton JC. Insulin secretory granule biogenesis. Biochem J 1991; 274:73.
6. Halban PA, Irminger J-C. Sorting and processing of secretory proteins. Biochem J 1994; 299:1.
7. Kelly RB. Pathways of protein secretion in eukaryotes. Science 1985; 230:25.
8. Rhodes CJ, Halban PA. Newly synthesized proinsulin/insulin and stored insulin are released from pancreatic B cell predominantly via a regulated, rather than a constitutive pathway. J Cell Biol 1987; 105:145.
9. Howell SL. The mechanism of insulin secretion. Diabetologia 1984; 26:319.
10. Pipeleers DG. Heterogeneity in pancreatic beta-cell population. Diabetes 1992; 41:777.
11. Tager H. Abnormal products of the human insulin gene. Diabetes 1984; 33:693.
12. Steiner DF, Tager HS, Chan SJ, et al. Lessons learned from molecular biology of insulin-gene mutations. Diabetes Care 1990; 13:600.
13. Oohashi H, Ohgawara H, Nanjo K, et al. Familial hyperproinsulinemia associated with NIDDM. Diabetes Care 1993; 16:1340.
14. Chan SJ, Seino S, Gruppuso PA, et al. A mutation in the B chain coding region is associated with impaired proinsulin conversion in a family with hyperproinsulinemia. Proc Natl Acad Sci U S A 1987; 84: 2194.
15. Sander M, German MS. The β-cell transcription factors and development of the pancreas. J Mol Med 1997; 75:327.
16. Henquin J-C. Cell biology of insulin secretion. In: Kahn CR, Weir GC, eds. Joslin's diabetes mellitus, 13th ed. Philadelphia: Lea & Febiger, 1994:56.
17. Matschinsky F, Liang Y, Kesavan P, et al. Glucokinase as pancreatic B cell glucose sensor and diabetes gene. J Clin Invest 1993; 92:2092.
18. Matschinsky FM, Glaser B, Magnuson MA. Pancreatic beta-cell glucokinase: closing the gap between theoretical concepts and experimental realities. Diabetes 1998; 47:307.
19. Eto K, Tsubamoto Y, Terauchi Y, et al. Role of NADH shuttle system in glucose-induced activation of mitochondrial metabolism and insulin secretion. Science 1999; 283:981.
20. MacDonald MJ. Elusive proximal signals of beta cells for insulin secretion. Diabetes 1990; 39:1461.
21. MacDonald MJ. Feasibility of a mitochondrial pyruvate malate shuttle in pancreatic islets. J Biol Chem 1995; 270:20051.
22. McGarry JD, Dobbins RL. Fatty acids, lipotoxicity and insulin secretion. Diabetologia 1999, 42:128.
23. Prentki M, Corkey BE. Are the β-cell signaling molecules malonyl-CoA and cytosolic long-chain acyl-CoA implicated in multiple tissue defects of obesity and NIDDM? Diabetes 1996, 45:273.
24. Wolf BA, Colca JR, Turk J, et al. Regulation of Ca$^{2+}$ homeostasis by islet endoplasmic reticulum and its role in insulin secretion. Am J Physiol 1988; 254:E121.
25. Easom RA. CaM Kinase II: a protein kinase with extraordinary talents germane to insulin exocytosis. Diabetes 1999; 48: 675.
26. Porksen N, Munn S, Steers J, Velhuis JD, Butler PC. Effects of glucose ingestion versus infusion on pulsatile insulin secretion. Diabetes 1996, 45:1317.
27. Tornheim K. Are metabolic oscillations responsible for normal oscillatory insulin secretion? Diabetes 1997; 46:1375.
28. Gilon P, Shepherd RM, Henquin JC. Oscillations of secretion driven by oscillations of cytoplasmic Ca$^{2+}$ as evidenced in single pancreatic islets. J Biol Chem 1993; 268:22265.
29. Stagner J, Samols E, Weir GC. Sustained oscillations of insulin, glucagon and somatostatin from the isolated canine pancreas during exposure to a constant glucose concentration. J Clin Invest 1980; 65:939.
30. Robbins DC, Tager HS, Rubenstein AH. Biologic and clinical importance of proinsulin. N Engl J Med 1984; 310:1165.
31. Creutzfeld W, Ebert R. New developments in the incretin concept. Diabetologia 1985; 28:565.
32. Taborsky GJ, Ahren B, Havel PJ. Autonomic mediation of glucagon secretion during hypoglycemia: implications for impaired alpha cell responses in type 1 diabetes. Diabetes 1998; 47:995.
33. Weir GC, Leahy JL. Pathogenesis of non-insulin-dependent diabetes mellitus. In: Kahn CR, Weir GC, eds. Joslin's diabetes mellitus, 13th ed. Philadelphia: Lea & Febiger, 1994:240.
34. Weir GC, Bonner-Weir S. Insulin secretion in non-insulin-dependent diabe-

tes mellitus. In: LeRoith D, Taylor SI, Olefsky JM, eds. Diabetes mellitus, 2nd ed. Philadelphia: Lippincott Williams & Wilkins, 2000:595.

35. Rhodes CJ, Alarcon C. What beta cell defect could lead to hyperproinsulinemia in NIDDM? Diabetes 1994; 43:511.
36. Jonas J-C, Sharma A, Hasenkamp W, et al. Chronic hyperglycemia triggers loss of pancreatic β cell differentiation in an animal model of diabetes. J Biol Chem 1999; 274:14112.
37. Duckworth WC, Kitabchi AE. Insulin metabolism and degradation. Endocr Rev 1981; 2:210.
38. Rabkin R, Ryan MP, Duckworth WC. The renal metabolism of insulin. Diabetologia 1984; 27:351.
39. Polonsky KS, Given BD, VanCauter E. Twenty-four hour profiles and pulsatile patterns of insulin section in normal and obese subjects. J Clin Invest 1988; 81:442.
40. Philippe J, Mojsov S, Drucker DJ, Habener JF. Proglucagon processing in a rat islet cell line resembles phenotype of intestine rather than pancreas. Endocrinology 1986; 119:2833.
41. Weir GC, Mojsov S, Hendrick GK, Habener JF. Glucagon-like peptide I (7-37) actions on endocrine pancreas. Diabetes 1989; 38:338.
42. Kreymann B, Williams G, Ghatei MA, Bloom SR. Glucagon-like peptide-I 7-36: a physiological incretin in man. Lancet 1987; 2:1300.
43. Liljenquist JE, Mueller GL, Cherrington AD, et al. Evidence for an important role of glucagon in the regulation of hepatic glucose production in normal man. J Clin Invest 1977; 59:369.
44. Samols E, Weir GC, Bonner-Weir S. Intraislet insulin-glucagon-somatostatin relationships. In: Lefebvre P, ed. Handbook of experimental pharmacology 66/II. Berlin: Springer-Verlag, 1983:133.
45. Stagner JI, Samols E, Bonner-Weir S. Beta, alpha, delta pancreatic islet cellular perfusion in dogs. Diabetes 1988; 37:1715.
46. Weir GC, Bonner-Weir S. Islets of Langerhans: the puzzle of intraislet interactions and their relevance to diabetes. J Clin Invest 1990; 85:983.
47. Hisatomi A, Maruyama H, Orci L, et al. Adrenergically mediated intrapancreatic control of the glucagon response to glucopenia in the isolated rat pancreas. J Clin Invest 1985; 75:420.
48. Dobbs RE. Control of glucagon secretion: nutrients, gastroenteropancreatic hormones, calcium, and prostaglandins. In: Unger RM, Orci L, eds. Glucagon. New York: Elsevier, 1981:115.
49. Gerich J, Lorenzi M, Bier D, et al. Prevention of human diabetic ketoacidosis by somatostatin: evidence for an essential role for glucagon. N Engl J Med 1975; 292:985.
50. Cryer PE. Hypoglycemia: the limiting factor in the management of IDDM. Diabetes 1994; 43:1378.
51. Weir GC, Bonner-Weir S. Pancreatic somatostatin. In: Patel YC, Tannenbaum GS, eds. Somatostatin. New York: Plenum Publishing, 1985:403.
52. Floyd JC Jr, Fajans SS, Pek S, Chance RE. A newly recognized pancreatic polypeptide: plasma levels in health and disease. Recent Prog Horm Res 1976; 33:519.
53. Kennedy FP, Go VLW, Cryer PE, et al. Subnormal pancreatic polypeptide and epinephrine response to insulin-induced hypoglycemia identify patients with insulin-dependent diabetes mellitus predisposed to develop overt autonomic neuropathy. Ann Intern Med 1988; 108:54.
54. Kahn SE, Andrikopoulos S, Verchere CB. Islet amyloid: a long-recognized but underappreciated pathological feature of type 2 diabetes. Diabetes 1999; 48:241.
55. Butler PC. Islet amyloid and its potential role in the pathogenesis of type II diabetes mellitus. In: LeRoith D, Taylor SI, Olefsky JM, eds. Diabetes mellitus, 2nd ed. Philadelphia: Lippincott Williams & Wilkins, 2000:141.
56. Lorenzo A, Razzaboni B, Weir GC, Yankner BA. Pancreatic islet cell toxicity associated with type-2 diabetes mellitus. Nature 1994; 368:756.
57. Hayden MR, Tyagi SC. Remodeling of the endocrine pancreas: The central role of amylin and insulin resistance. South Med J 2000; 93:24.

# CHAPTER 135

# GLUCOSE HOMEOSTASIS AND INSULIN ACTION

C. RONALD KAHN

## GLUCOSE HOMEOSTASIS

Glucose homeostasis depends on a balance between glucose production by the liver and glucose utilization by insulin-dependent tissues, such as fat and muscle, and insulin-independent tissues, such as brain and kidney.[1,2] In normal individuals, these are in a correct balance such that, despite periods of feeding and fasting,

blood glucose concentrations are kept in a relatively narrow range between 70 and 120 mg/dL (4 and 7 mmol/L; Fig. 135-1A). Prevention of hypoglycemia in the fasting state is important, because glucose serves as a critical fuel for the central nervous system, and impairment of central nervous system function can potentially occur if plasma glucose concentrations fall below 40 mg/dL. Likewise, prevention of hyperglycemia is important to avoid the loss of calories that would occur through glycosuria if glucose concentrations were to rise above the renal threshold (~180 mg/dL). This pattern of glucose utilization is highly regulated, particularly through hormones secreted by the pancreatic islet, insulin from the B cell, and glucagon from the A cell. Although the fine-tuning of glucose metabolism may be influenced by many hormones and metabolic intermediates, normal glucose disposal depends primarily on three factors: the ability of the body to secrete insulin both immediately and in a sustained fashion; the ability of insulin to inhibit hepatic glucose output and to promote glucose disposal (i.e., insulin sensitivity); and the ability of glucose to enter the cells in the absence of insulin, sometimes referred to as *glucose sensitivity* or *glucose effectiveness*.

During the period immediately after a carbohydrate meal, the glucose absorbed from the gastrointestinal tract provides for the metabolic needs of the brain, and any excess glucose is stored as energy in liver, muscle, or fat. After the ingestion of a pure glucose load (i.e., during a glucose-tolerance test), the absorbed glucose far exceeds the immediate needs of the brain; most is taken up by skeletal muscle.[3-6] Skeletal muscle makes up 40% of the body mass but has been estimated to account for between 80% and 95% of glucose disposal at high insulin concentrations or after an oral glucose load.[6,7] These data suggest an extremely important role for skeletal muscle in glucose disposal. Studies of genetically engineered mice with selective insulin resistance in muscle only, however, have challenged this concept.[8]

Alterations in glucose homeostasis are the sine qua non of diabetes mellitus and occur in both the type 1 and type 2 forms of the disease. In the mildest forms of diabetes, this alteration is detected only after challenge with a carbohydrate load, whereas in moderate to severe forms of the disease, hyperglycemia is present in both the fasting and postprandial states. In type 1 diabetes, a loss of insulin secretion occurs due to destruction of the pancreatic B cell (see Fig. 135-1B). In type 2 diabetes, at least two pathophysiologic defects are present: one is a decreased ability of insulin to act on peripheral tissues to stimulate glucose metabolism or inhibit hepatic glucose output, a phenomenon known as *insulin resistance*; the other is the inability of the endocrine pancreas to fully compensate for this insulin resistance (i.e., relative insulin deficiency; see Chap. 137 and Fig. 135-1C).

Insulin is the primary hormone responsible for regulating glucose metabolism and signaling the storage and use of many basic nutrients. Insulin acts as an anabolic hormone, activating transport systems and enzymes involved in intracellular utilization and storage of glucose, amino acids, and fatty acids. It also is a potent inhibitor of the catabolic processes evoked by counterregulatory hormones, such as breakdown of glycogen, fat, and protein. Although the physiologically important target tissues for insulin with respect to glucose homeostasis are liver, muscle, and fat, insulin has effects on cell growth and metabolism in many tissues. Insulin exerts its actions through insulin receptors and, to a lesser extent, insulin-like growth factor-I (IGF-I) receptors. Both of these receptor types are expressed in classic target tissues for insulin action, such as liver, fat, and skeletal muscle, as well as in nontarget tissues.

The insulin and IGF-I receptors are members of the class of receptors known as *protein tyrosine kinases*.[9] After stimulation by insulin or IGF-I binding, these receptors activate a complex network of events involving phosphorylation and dephosphorylation, as well as possible mediator generation to promote glucose uptake, to stimulate metabolism and conversion of glucose to glycogen by activating glycogen synthase, and to regulate a variety of intracellular enzymes involved in carbohydrate

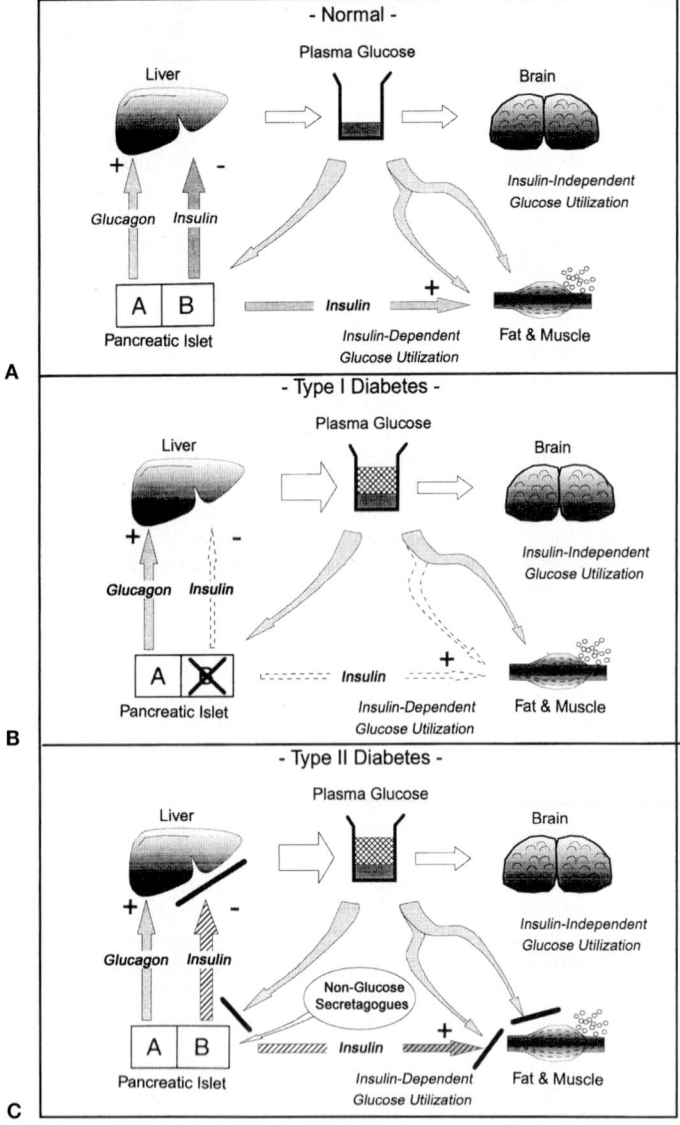

**FIGURE 135-1.** Regulation of glucose homeostasis. **A,** Glucose homeostasis in the normal person is a balance between glucose production by the liver and glucose utilization by insulin-independent tissues, such as the brain, and insulin-dependent tissues, such as muscle and fat. Both these processes are regulated by insulin secretion from the pancreatic B cell, and at the liver are counterbalanced by glucagon secretion by the A cell. **B,** Glucose homeostasis in a patient with type 1 diabetes. Pancreatic B cells are destroyed by the autoimmune process. Glucose production by the liver is not inhibited and glucose utilization is not stimulated. **C,** Glucose homeostasis in a patient with type 2 diabetes. Insulin resistance occurs in liver, muscle, and fat. The B cell initially responds by increasing insulin secretion, but then fails because of desensitization of the glucose stimulus. Nonglucose secretagogues, however, continue to stimulate insulin secretion.

metabolism.[9,10] In addition, insulin acts at the level of muscle to modify lipid and protein metabolism through effects on membrane transport, enzyme activity, and gene expression.[11,12] This chapter briefly reviews some of the newer concepts regarding the mechanism of insulin action and insulin degradation and their possible alterations in diabetes.

## CELLULAR ACTION OF INSULIN

The effects of insulin at the cellular level may be classified into three groups based on the time course of action. The *immediate effects* of insulin occur within seconds after the addition of the hormone and include the activation of glucose and ion transport systems and the covalent modification (i.e., phosphorylation and dephosphorylation) of preexisting enzymes. The *intermediate effects* involve the induction of genes and the expression of some proteins, such as the induction of ornithine decarboxylase and tyrosine aminotransferase activity; these can be detected within 5 to 60 minutes, but reach a maximum 3 to 6 hours after stimulation by insulin. The *long-term effects* of insulin require many hours to several days. This category includes insulin's effects to stimulate DNA synthesis, cell proliferation, and cell differentiation, as well as some gene expression events. The rapid, intermediate, and long-term actions of insulin are the results not of a simple linear pathway but of the multiple diverging and converging pathways mediated by the insulin and insulin-like growth factor receptors.

## THE INSULIN RECEPTOR AND ITS SIGNALING NETWORK

Like other peptide hormones, insulin initiates its action by binding to a cell-surface receptor. These receptors are expressed on the plasma membranes of virtually all mammalian cells, including the classic target tissues for insulin, such as liver, muscle, and fat, and nonclassic target tissues, such as circulating blood cells, brain cells, and gonadal cells. Structurally, the receptor is a glycoprotein composed of two α subunits (135,000 Da each) and two β subunits (95,000 Da each) linked by disulfide bonds to form a β-α-α-β heterotetramer[9,13,14] (Fig. 135-2). Both subunits are coded for by a single gene and are derived from a single-chain precursor molecule, or proreceptor, that contains the entire sequence of the α and β subunits separated by a processing site consisting of four basic amino acids. The insulin receptor gene is on the short arm of chromosome 19.[15]

The two subunits of the insulin receptor are specialized to perform the two functions of the receptor. The α subunits are entirely extracellular and contain the insulin-binding site. The β subunits are transmembrane proteins and possess tyrosine protein kinase activity on their intracellular domains. An important advance in the field of insulin action was the discovery that the insulin receptor, like several other growth factor receptors, was a hormone-activated protein tyrosine kinase.[14,16] Protein tyrosine kinases are enzymes that catalyze the transfer of phosphate groups from adenosine triphosphate (ATP) to tyrosine residues of proteins. Other growth factor receptors exhibiting tyrosine kinase activity include the receptors for epidermal growth factor, IGF-I, platelet-derived growth factor, colony-stimulating factor-I, and fibroblast growth factor.[17]

Transmission of an insulin signal after receptor kinase activation involves a complex network of pathways. Insulin binding stimulates autophosphorylation and activation of the receptor kinase, and the activated receptor phosphorylates several endogenous cellular substrate proteins (see Fig. 135-2). The best characterized of the endogenous substrates of the insulin receptor is a family of cytosolic proteins termed *IRS-1 (insulin-receptor substrate-1), IRS-2, IRS-3,* and *IRS-4.*[9,18–20] These proteins range in molecular mass from 60 to 185 kDa and have two structural features that are important for their action. First, at the amino-terminal end of the molecule are two domains (the *plextrin homology [PH]* and *phosphotyrosine-binding [PTB] domains*), causing these substrates to bind to the insulin receptor with high affinity. Second, dispersed through the molecule are many tyrosine residues that are readily phosphorylated after insulin stimulation.[1,18] These tyrosine residues have a special function in signal transduction, because after phosphorylation they serve as intracellular docking sites for other downstream molecules in the signal-transduction cascade.

Most of these downstream partners of the IRS proteins contain specific recognition sequences that promote protein-protein

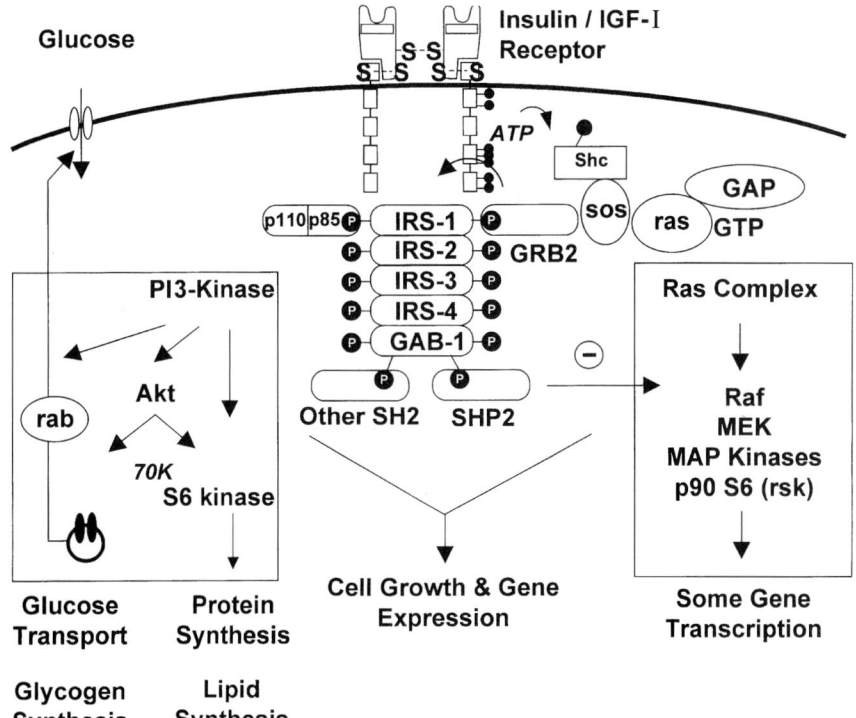

**FIGURE 135-2.** Model of insulin signaling pathways. Insulin binds to the α subunit of the insulin receptor and stimulates autophosphorylation of the β subunit. Once activated, the receptor kinase phosphorylates several intracellular substrates, including the insulin-receptor substrates IRS-1 to IRS-4, GAB1, and Shc. These substrates act as an intracellular docking protein for several enzymes and adapter proteins and eventually stimulate a cascade of phosphorylation and dephosphorylation reactions, centering around the enzymes phosphatidylinositol 3-kinase (*PI3-kinase*) and microtubule-associated protein (*MAP*) kinase. These mediate other endogenous cell-signaling mechanisms, causing a translocation of glucose transporters to the cell surface and increased glucose transport, as well as other cellular responses, such as stimulation of glycogen synthesis. PI3-kinase appears to be most closely linked to the metabolic actions of insulin. (*IGF-I*, insulin-like growth factor-I; *ATP*, adenosine triphosphate; *GTP*, guanosine triphosphate.)

interaction between the partner protein and the *sites of tyrosine phosphorylation*, called *SH2 domains* (*src homology 2 domains*).[20,21] The three best studied of the SH2 domain proteins involved in insulin signaling are a lipid-metabolizing enzyme, *phosphatidylinositol 3-kinase (PI3-kinase)*; a *phosphotyrosine phosphatase* called *SHP2*; and an *adapter molecule (GRB2)*, which links insulin signaling to a pathway involving Ras and a cascade of intracellular serine kinases centering around an enzyme called *microtubule-associated protein (MAP) kinase*.[1,20,21] Most current studies indicate that the PI3-kinase pathway is the critical pathway for most metabolic events, including stimulation of glucose transport, glycogen synthesis, lipid synthesis, and protein synthesis. The MAP kinase pathway, on the other hand, probably plays a major role in regulation of expression of some insulin-responsive genes and stimulation of cell growth.

## GLUCOSE TRANSPORT REGULATION

The effect of insulin to stimulate glucose uptake into muscle and adipose tissue forms a central point in its physiologic role. Now-classic studies demonstrated that one major component in the mechanism of insulin stimulation of glucose transport is a temperature- and energy-dependent translocation of intracellular vesicles containing glucose transporter proteins to the plasma membrane.[22–26] The effect is reversible, and once insulin is removed, the glucose transporters return to the intracellular pool. Seven distinct mammalian glucose transporters have been cloned and sequenced. Five of these are molecules believed to be involved in the sodium-independent facilitative transport of glucose into cells, and two are the sodium-glucose cotransporters involved in the absorption of glucose from the intestine and reabsorption of glucose from the kidney tubule. The first *facilitative transporter* to be cloned (*GLUT1*) was called the *erythroid cell–brain glucose transporter*. It is present in large amounts in erythrocytes, in the endothelial cells that form the blood–brain barrier, and in some hepatoma cells in culture. It is not expressed in normal liver and is at low levels in fat and muscle.[27] The second transporter, termed *GLUT2*, has a similar, but not identical, structure and is found mainly in liver plasma

membranes and pancreatic B cells, where it may participate in glucose-stimulated insulin secretion.[28–30] This transporter has a slightly higher Michaelis constant ($K_M$) for transport (5–7 mmol/L) than the other glucose transporters; this may account for the difference in B-cell stimulation compared with peripheral tissue uptake of glucose. From the point of view of insulin action, the most important transporter is the *GLUT4 glucose transporter*. This transporter is expressed predominantly in tissues where glucose transport is sensitive to insulin, including striated muscle, cardiac muscle, and adipose tissue.[31–33] Additional types of transporters are expressed in fetal muscle, small intestine, and many nonmuscle adult tissues.

All of the facilitative glucose transporter–related proteins are integral membrane glycoproteins with molecular masses of 45 to 55 kDa. They share a large degree of sequence identity (50–65%) and presumably also share structural homologies. Based on sequence analysis, each is thought to contain 12 membrane-spanning α-helical domains that presumably form a channel through which glucose passes (Fig. 135-3). Exactly how receptor kinase activation is coupled to transporter translocation is unknown and is one of the most important questions in insulin action. At least two intermediate steps appear to involve the enzyme *PI3-kinase* and one of its downstream partners, a *serine kinase* termed *Akt*.[34] Once inside the muscle, the glucose is rapidly phosphorylated by hexokinase to form glucose-6-phosphate. Although the rate-limiting step for glucose uptake is at the level of transport, evidence is increasing that the major control of carbohydrate metabolism is exerted after the glucose-6-phosphate step.[35] Depending on the hormonal milieu and metabolic state, the glucose-6-phosphate can enter either oxidative or nonoxidative pathways. The major nonoxidative pathway involves conversion of the glucose to glycogen. The rate-limiting enzyme of this reaction is glycogen synthase. The activity of glycogen synthase is regulated primarily by phosphorylation and dephosphorylation, and by the presence of the allosteric regulator glucose-6-phosphate. In catabolic states, glucose is metabolized through the glycolytic pathway to pyruvate, which in turn is either converted to lactate (under anaerobic conditions) or oxidized to carbon dioxide and acetyl–coenzyme A. The latter reaction is catalyzed by the multienzyme complex *pyruvate dehydrogenase (PDH)*. PDH activity also is regu-

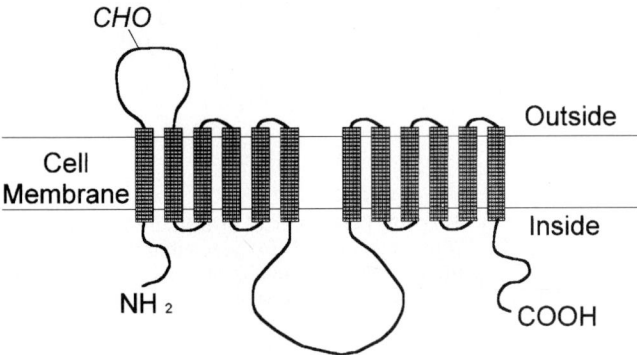

**FIGURE 135-3.** Schematic structure of glucose transporter. Glucose transporters are membrane-associated glycoproteins with 12 transmembrane α-helical domains (*rectangular boxes*), cytoplasmic $NH_2$ and COOH terminus, a large extracellular loop between helix 1 and 2 containing the site of glycosylation (*CHO*), and a long intracellular loop between helix 6 and 7.

lated by the level of the enzyme, phosphorylation and dephosphorylation, and several allosteric modifiers. Most of the enzymes and proteins involved in glucose metabolism have been identified and purified, and many have been cloned at a molecular level.

## DEGRADATION OF INSULIN

Like most peptide hormones, insulin circulates in blood as the free monomeric hormone. The volume of distribution approximates the volume of extracellular fluid, although the concentration of insulin in lymph and cerebrospinal fluid is lower than that in blood. Under basal conditions, the pancreas secretes 1 mg insulin per day, or 40 μg (1 U) per hour, into the portal vein; this provides a concentration of insulin in portal blood of 2 to 4 ng/mL (50 to 100 μU/mL). More than half of this insulin is cleared in the liver, so that the peripheral circulation concentration is ~0.5 ng/mL (12 μU/mL), or ~$10^{-10}$ mol/L. After ingestion of a meal, a rapid rise in portal insulin occurs, followed by a parallel, but smaller, rise in the peripheral insulin level.

The plasma half-life of insulin injected intravenously is 5 to 6 minutes in normal persons and about the same in patients with uncomplicated diabetes.[36] In those patients with diabetes in whom antiinsulin antibodies develop, the plasma half-life may be increased. Although the pancreatic content and the amount of secreted proinsulin is only 1% to 3% that of insulin, proinsulin has a longer half-life (~17 minutes) and, therefore, may account for 10% to 25% of the immunoreactive "insulin" in plasma.[37] In patients with insulinoma, the percentage of proinsulin in the circulation usually is increased and may be as much as 80%.[38] Because proinsulin has only 2% to 3% of the intrinsic bioactivity of insulin, the biologically effective concentration of insulin is somewhat lower than that estimated by immunoassay. C peptide, which is secreted in equimolar amounts with insulin, also has a higher molar concentration in plasma because of its considerably longer half-life (~30 minutes).[37] Although most studies have indicated that C peptide has no bioactivity, one study has suggested a potential role for C-peptide deficiency in the long-term vascular and neurologic complications of diabetes.[39] In any case, C peptide serves as a useful surrogate for endogenous insulin secretion in both diabetic and normal individuals, as well as in patients with insulin-secreting tumors, in whom C-peptide levels are high (see Chap. 158).

The primary sites for insulin degradation are the liver, kidney, and muscle, in that order.[40] At least 50% of the insulin that reaches the liver through the portal vein is taken up in a single passage, thus never reaching the general circulation. Insulin is filtered by the renal glomeruli and reabsorbed by the tubules, which also degrade it. Severe impairment of renal function appears to affect the rate of disappearance of circulating insulin to a greater extent than does hepatic disease. This is because the liver operates closer to its capacity to destroy the hormone and cannot compensate for such loss of renal catabolic function. Proteolytic degradation of insulin in the liver occurs both at the cell surface and after internalization of insulin with its receptor. The extent to which the internalized insulin is degraded by the cell varies considerably depending on the cell type. In hepatocytes, most of the internalized insulin is degraded, whereas in endothelial cells, most internalized insulin appears to be released intact. In the latter case, this intact release appears to be related to the role of these cells in transcytosis of the insulin molecule from the intravascular to extracellular space.[41] Several enzymes have been suggested to be involved in insulin degradation.[42,43]

## ALTERATIONS IN INSULIN ACTION IN DIABETES

Defects in insulin action in diabetes mellitus are a feature common to most forms of the disease and are central to the pathogenesis of type 2 diabetes and other insulin-resistant states. At the clinical research level, these defects in insulin action can be identified by decreased response to intravenous glucose injection during an insulin-tolerance test, by the euglycemic clamp technique, or by nuclear magnetic resonance spectroscopy. In addition, a limited number of studies have been performed on biopsies of tissues taken from normal and diabetic individuals. In type 2 diabetes, abnormalities have been described in insulin receptor binding, receptor kinase activation, glycogen synthase activation, and glucose transporter translocation[45–48] (see Chap. 137).

In patients taking insulin, insulin resistance may also occur due to the presence of antiinsulin antibodies or increased subcutaneous degradation of the hormone. With the introduction of highly purified recombinant human insulin, both of these problems have become relatively rare. Some of the patients in whom a presumed increase in subcutaneous destruction is associated with insulin resistance have even been treated with protease inhibitors, such as aprotinin, with an improvement in insulin sensitivity.[44] Many physicians debate whether this syndrome truly exists, however, because no direct evidence has been found of increased protease activity in subcutaneous extracts from these patients, and many have psychosocial disturbances that suggest poor compliance with the insulin regimen.

## REFERENCES

1. Kahn CR. Banting lecture. Insulin action, diabetogenes, and the cause of type II diabetes. Diabetes 1994; 43 (8):1066.
2. Bergman RN. Lilly lecture 1989. Toward physiological understanding of glucose tolerance. Minimal model approach. Diabetes 1989; 38:1512.
3. Klip A, Paquet MR. Glucose transport and glucose transporters in muscle and their metabolic regulation. Diabetes Care 1990; 13:228.
4. Caro JF, Dohm LG, Pories WJ, Sinha MK. Cellular alterations in liver, skeletal muscle, and adipose tissue responsible for insulin resistance in obesity and type II diabetes. Diabetes Metab Rev 1989; 5:665.
5. Bogardus C. Does insulin resistance primarily affect skeletal muscle? Diabetes Metab Rev 1989; 5:527.
6. Beck-Nielsen H. Insulin resistance in skeletal muscles of patients with diabetes mellitus. Diabetes Metab Rev 1989; 5:487.
7. Baron AD, Brechtel G, Wallace P, Edelman SV. Rates and tissue sites of non-insulin- and insulin-mediated glucose uptake in humans. Am J Physiol 1988; 255:E769.
8. Bruning JC, Michael MD, Winnay JN, et al. A muscle specific insulin receptor knockout challenges the current concepts of glucose disposal and NIDDM pathogenesis. Mol Cell 1998; 2(5):559.
9. Cheatham B, Kahn CR. Insulin action and the insulin signaling network. Endocr Rev 1995; 16(2):117.
10. Mandarino LJ, Wright KS, Verity LS, et al. Effects of insulin infusion on human skeletal muscle pyruvate dehydrogenase, phosphofructokinase, and glycogen synthase. Evidence for their role in oxidative and nonoxidative glucose metabolism. J Clin Invest 1987; 80:655.

11. Kimball SR, Jefferson LS. Cellular mechanisms involved in the action of insulin on protein synthesis. Diabetes Metab Rev 1988; 4:773.
12. Alexander MC, Lomanto M, Nasrin N, Ramaika C. Insulin stimulates glyceraldehyde-3-phosphate dehydrogenase gene expression through cis-acting DNA sequence. Proc Natl Acad Sci U S A 1988; 85:5092.
13. Czech MP. The nature and regulation of the insulin receptor: structure and function. Annu Rev Physiol 1985; 47:357.
14. White MF, Kahn CR. The insulin signaling system. J Biol Chem 1994; 269:1.
15. Seino S, Seino M, Nishi S, Bell GI. Structure of the human insulin receptor gene and characterization of its promoter. Proc Natl Acad Sci U S A 1985; 86:114.
16. Kasuga M, Karlsson FA, Kahn CR. Insulin stimulates the phosphorylation of the 95,000 dalton subunit of its own receptor. Science 1982; 215:185.
17. Yarden Y, Ullrich A. Growth factor receptor tyrosine kinases. Annu Rev Biochem 1988; 57:443.
18. Myers MG Jr, White MF. New frontiers in insulin receptor substrate signaling. Trends Endocrinol Metab 1995; 6(6):209.
19. Liu SC, Wang Q, Lienhard GE, Keller SR. Insulin receptor substrate 3 is not essential for growth or glucose homeostasis. J Biol Chem 1999; 274(25):18093.
20. Pawson T, Olivier P, Rozakis-Adcock M, et al. Proteins with SH2 and SH3 domains couple receptor tyrosine kinases to intracellular signalling pathways. Philos Trans R Soc Lond B Biol Sci 1993; 340(1293):279.
21. Koch CA, Anderson D, Moran MF, et al. SH2 and SH3 domains: elements that control interactions of cytoplasmic signaling proteins. Science 1991; 252:668.
22. Suzuki K, Kono T. Evidence that insulin causes translocation of glucose transport activity of the plasma membrane from an intracellular storage site. Proc Natl Acad Sci U S A 1980; 77:2542.
23. Karnieli E, Zarnowski MJ, Hissin PJ, et al. Insulin-stimulated translocation of glucose transport systems in the isolated rat adipose cell. Time course, reversal, insulin concentration dependency, and relationship to glucose transport activity. J Biol Chem 1981; 256:4772.
24. Holman GD, Cushman SW. Subcellular localization and trafficking of the GLUT4 glucose transporter isoform in insulin-responsive cells. Bioessays 1994; 16(10):753.
25. Olson AL, Pessin JE. Structure, function, and regulation of the mammalian facilitative glucose transporter gene family. Annu Rev Nutr 1996; 16:235.
26. Czech MP, Corvera S. Signaling mechanisms that regulate glucose transport. J Biol Chem 1999; 274(4):1865.
27. Mueckler M, Caruso C, Baldwin SA, et al. Sequence and structure of a human glucose transporter. Science 1985; 229:941.
28. Thorens B, Sarker HK, Kaback HR, Lodish HF. Cloning and functional expression in bacteria of a novel glucose transporter present in liver, intestine, kidney and β-pancreatic islet cells. Cell 1988; 55:281.
29. Burant CF, Sivitz WI, Fukumato H, et al. Mammalian glucose transporters: structure and molecular regulation. Recent Prog Horm Res 1991; 47:349.
30. Mueckler M. Facilitative glucose transporters. Eur J Biochem 1994; 219:713.
31. Charron MJ, Brosius FC III, Alper SL, Lodish HF. A glucose transport protein expressed predominantly in insulin-responsive tissues. Proc Natl Acad Sci U S A 1989; 86:2535.
32. Birnbaum MJ. Identification of a novel gene encoding an insulin-responsive glucose transporter protein. Cell 1989; 57:305.
33. Kahn BB. Lilly lecture 1995. Glucose transport: pivotal step in insulin action. Diabetes 1996; 45(11):1644.
34. Avruch J. Insulin signal transduction through protein kinase cascades. Mol Cell Biochem 1998; 182(1–2):31.
35. Mandarino LJ. Regulation of skeletal muscle pyruvate dehydrogenase and glycogen synthase in man. Diabetes Metab Rev 1989; 5:475.
36. Hachiya HL, Treves ST, Kahn CR, et al. Altered insulin distribution and metabolism of type I diabetics assessed by [123]I-insulin scanning. J Clin Endocrinol Metab 1987; 64:801.
37. Robbins DC, Tager HS, Rubenstein AH. Biologic and clinical importance of proinsulin. N Engl J Med 1984; 310:1165.
38. Gorden P, Skarulis MC, Roach P, et al. Plasma proinsulin-like component in insulinoma: a 25-year experience. J Clin Endocrinol Metab 1995; 80(10):2884.
39. Ido Y, Vindigni A, Chang K, et al. Prevention of vascular and neural dysfunction in diabetic rats by C-peptide. Science 1997; 277(5325):563.
40. Duckworth WC. Insulin degradation: mechanisms, products and significance. Endocr Rev 1988; 9:319.
41. King GL, Johnson SM. Receptor mediated transport of insulin across endothelial cells. Science 1985; 219:865.
42. Shii K, Yokono K, Baba S, Roth RA. Purification and characterization of insulin-degrading enzyme from the human erythrocytes. Diabetes 1986; 35:675.
43. Authier F, Posner BI, Bergeron JJ. Insulin-degrading enzyme. Clin Invest Med 1996; 19(3):149.
44. Schade DS, Duckworth WC. In search of the subcutaneous-insulin resistance syndrome. N Engl J Med 1986; 315:147.
45. Strack V, Hennige AM, Krutzfeldt J, et al. Serine residues 994 and 1023/25 are important for insulin receptor kinase inhibition by protein kinase C isoforme beta 2 and theta. Diabetologia 2000; 43:443.
46. Sozen I, Arici A. Hyperinsulinism and its interaction with hyperandrogenism in polysystic ovary syndrome. Obstet Gynecol Surv 2000; 55:321.
47. Auclair M, Vigouroux C, Desbois-Mouthan C, et al. Antiinsulin receptor autoantibodies induce insulin receptors to constitutively associate with insulin receptor substrate -1 and -2 and cause severe cell resistance to both insulin and insulin-like growth factor I. J Clin Endocrinol Metab 1999; 84:3197.
48. Tirosh A, Rudich A, Bashan N. Regulation of insulin transporters—implications for insulin resistance states. J Pediatr Endocrinol Metab 2000; 13:115.

# CHAPTER 136

# CLASSIFICATION, DIAGNOSTIC TESTS, AND PATHOGENESIS OF TYPE 1 DIABETES MELLITUS

GEORGE S. EISENBARTH

## CLASSIFICATION

Diabetes mellitus is a complex of syndromes characterized metabolically by hyperglycemia and altered glucose metabolism and associated pathologically with specific microvascular complications, macrovascular disease secondary to accelerated atherosclerosis, and various other complications, including neuropathy, complicated pregnancy, and an increased susceptibility to infection. Heterogeneity in the presentation of patients with diabetes has been recognized for more than 2000 years. In its classic form, two common forms of diabetes are recognized: type 1 (formerly termed insulin-dependent diabetes mellitus [IDDM] or juvenile-onset diabetes) and type 2 diabetes (formerly termed non–insulin-dependent diabetes mellitus [NIDDM] or maturity-onset diabetes). A committee of the American Diabetes Association has revised the classification to begin to encompass the expanding knowledge with respect to the etiology of diabetes (Table 136-1). Type 1 diabetes is divided into type 1A and type 1B diabetes, both of which are associated with a severe deficiency of insulin secretion that often leads to a tendency to ketosis and absolute dependence on insulin for survival and maintenance of health. Type 1A diabetes is considered immune-mediated diabetes and is characterized by the presence of antiislet autoantibodies. Type 1B is defined as "idiopathic" insulin-deficient diabetes. Type 2 diabetes is characterized by an association with obesity, a lesser likelihood of ketoacidosis, and the absence of an absolute dependence on insulin for survival. Both forms of the disease may exist in the same family, and persons with either type are subject to the same long-term complications, albeit with somewhat differing frequencies.

In addition, a large group of other specific types of diabetes are defined. These defined forms of diabetes include those due to mutations of identified genes, such as those causing several forms of maturity-onset diabetes of youth (MODY3–hepatic nuclear factor [HNF]–1α; MODY1-HNF-4α; MODY2-glucokinase), genetic defects in insulin action, endocrinopathies, and so on. A fourth major category is that of gestational diabetes mellitus.

**TABLE 136-1.**
**American Diabetes Association 1997 Classification of Diabetes Mellitus**

| ETIOLOGIC CLASSIFICATION | CHARACTERISTICS |
|---|---|
| I. Type 1A | Immune-mediated |
| Type 1B | Insulin deficient, not autoimmune |
| II. Type 2 | Insulin resistance ± insulin secretory deficiency |
| III. Other Specific Types | Mitochondrial, maturity-onset diabetes of youth, lipoatrophic, type A insulin resistant, endocrinopathies, drug induced, etc. |
| IV. Gestational Diabetes | Glucose intolerance with first recognition or onset during pregnancy |

Over the next decade the definition of the forms of diabetes likely will become more commonly based on genetic analysis (potentially sequencing of relevant genes) and immunologic tests. Which specific form of diabetes is present can have an important influence on the risk of diabetes in relatives, the form of therapy that may be necessary, and the prognosis. For example, MODY2, which is caused by mutations in the glucokinase gene, is inherited as an autosomal dominant trait. The diabetes is often relatively mild and nonprogressive and, thus, usually is not associated with microvascular complications. The distinction between type 1 and type 2 diabetes is often clinically apparent, but significant clinical overlap is seen, particularly at the onset of disease. For example, ~50% of black and Hispanic *children* presenting with diabetes have no antiislet autoantibodies, and the majority appear not to have type 1 diabetes. Between 5% and 10% of *adults* presenting with what appears to be type 2 diabetes express antiislet autoantibodies, and most of these individuals progress to insulin dependence.

This chapter considers the diagnostic tests for diabetes and current concepts regarding the origin of type 1 diabetes, states of impaired glucose tolerance, and other melliturias. Secondary forms of diabetes, such as those related to diseases of the pancreas, hormonal overactivity, or drug-induced conditions, are described in Chapter 139. Diabetes secondary to genetic or acquired alterations in insulin receptors and in insulin action is discussed in Chapter 146, and gestational diabetes is included in Chapter 156.

# DIAGNOSTIC PROCEDURES AND CRITERIA

## ORAL GLUCOSE-TOLERANCE TEST

The diagnosis of diabetes mellitus may be made on the basis of classic symptoms and an unequivocal elevation on more than one occasion of fasting or postprandial glucose levels.[1] In the absence of this picture, the most useful diagnostic test is the oral glucose-tolerance test (Table 136-2). Although the appropriate carbohydrate load has been debated, current recommendations by the National Diabetes Data Group are 75 g in adults or 1.75 g per kilogram of body weight (maximum 75 g) in children, given in water at a concentration of no greater than 25 g/dL and ingested in ~5 minutes. The test should be performed after an overnight fast and should be preceded for 3 days by consumption of a diet containing at least 150 g of carbohydrate per day. Only two blood samples need to be collected: the first at time zero and the second at 2 hours. The diagnostic criteria recommended by the American Diabetes Association Expert Committee (see Table 136-2) are similar to those recommended by the World Health Organization Expert Committee[2] and have supplanted most previous criteria.

Several caveats apply in the evaluation of the test results.[3] First, the values presented in Table 136-2 are for venous plasma. Capillary whole-blood values are lower in the basal state and are considered abnormal if they exceed 120 mg/dL. Second, the criteria for the diagnosis of gestational diabetes are somewhat lower (see Chap. 156). Third, as with any test, some persons have nondiagnostic results. This problem can be minimized by standardizing the conditions of the test as much as possible, because many factors can influence the outcome[1] (see footnote to Table 136-2).

## OTHER DIAGNOSTIC TESTS

### INTRAVENOUS GLUCOSE-TOLERANCE TEST

The intravenous glucose-tolerance test allows an assessment of the body's ability to dispose of a glucose load without worry about alterations in the rate of absorption, such as may occur in hypothyroidism, hyperthyroidism, or malabsorption syndromes,

**TABLE 136-2.**
**Criteria for Diagnosis of Diabetes**

**DIABETES IN NONPREGNANT INDIVIDUALS**

Classic symptoms of diabetes, such as polyuria, polydipsia, ketonuria, and rapid weight loss, together with gross and unequivocal elevation of plasma glucose (e.g., postprandial or random plasma glucose concentration >200 mg/dL)

OR

Fasting plasma glucose concentration of ≥126 mg/dL on more than one occasion

OR

Glucose concentration at 2 hours of ≥200 mg/dL during an oral glucose-tolerance test

One or more of these diagnostic criteria must be met on a subsequent day for diagnosis of diabetes.

**GESTATIONAL DIABETES**

Two or more of the following plasma glucose concentrations after fasting and a 100-g oral glucose dose:

Fasting ≥105 mg/dL

1 hour ≥190 mg/dL

2 hour ≥165 mg/dL

3 hour ≥145 mg/dL

**IMPAIRED GLUCOSE TOLERANCE**

Fasting ≥110 mg/dL and <126 mg/dL

2 hour ≥140 mg/dL and <200 mg/dL following oral glucose-tolerance test*

*The glucose-tolerance test should be standardized as follows: (a) consumption of diet containing at least 150 g of carbohydrate for at least 3 days before test; (b) discontinuance, if possible, of drugs that alter glucose tolerance (e.g., benzothiadiazines, salicylates, corticosteroids, nicotinic acid, oral contraceptive agents, as well as insulin and oral hypoglycemic agents); (c) treatment of any infections (both overt and occult infection may alter glucose tolerance); (d) assessment of physical activity (prolonged inactivity and bed rest decrease carbohydrate tolerance, a significant factor in the increased percentage of abnormal glucose-tolerance tests in the elderly); (e) testing at proper time of day (plasma glucose responses to oral glucose are substantially higher in the afternoon; all criteria are based on morning tests); and (f) identification of other diseases present. Even with standardization, the range of normal glucose tolerance is considerable.

(Adapted from National Diabetes Data Group. Classification and diagnosis of diabetes and other categories of glucose intolerance. Diabetes 1979; 28:1039.)

or after gastrectomy. Glucose (0.5g/kg of body weight) is injected intravenously as a 25% solution within 1 to 3 minutes, and blood is collected every 10 minutes for 1 hour. Under these conditions, the plasma glucose level decreases exponentially from its initial height, and the glucose disappearance rate can be calculated.[4] Normally, the rate (kilogram value) exceeds 1.2% per minute; values below 1% are indicative of diabetes, and values between 1.2% and 1.0% are considered borderline.

Although this test still has tremendous research value in the evaluation of both the insulin secretory response to glucose[5] and insulin insensitivity,[6,7] it generally is not used for diagnostic purposes because the oral test is considered more physiologic. In addition, the oral test usually is more sensitive than the intravenous test to changes in carbohydrate metabolism. Early-phase insulin release (at 1 and 3 minutes) after intravenous glucose administration has been used to predict the onset of overt type 1 diabetes (see later).

### CORTICOSTEROID-PRIMED ORAL GLUCOSE-TOLERANCE TEST

The glucocorticoid-primed oral test was introduced to identify persons who have a "tendency" to diabetes at a time when no evidence of glucose intolerance can be detected in the standard oral glucose-tolerance test.[8] However, subsequent follow-up of the tested individuals revealed that this test is not of great predictive value and is no more sensitive than the standard oral glucose-tolerance test.

### GLYCOSYLATED HEMOGLOBIN TEST

Glucose condenses with the N-terminal valine residue of the β chain of hemoglobin to form a stable ketamine in the form of glycosylated hemoglobin.[9] This reaction provides a valuable method for the evaluation of ambient plasma glucose concentrations over long periods because both the formation and the degradation of glycosylated hemoglobin are relatively slow, and because hemoglobin has the same half-life as the circulating erythrocytes. Thus, this test provides an index of the average plasma glucose level over ~2 months.

Although it is an extremely sensitive and useful measure of diabetic control, glycosylated hemoglobin testing has not proved more sensitive than the oral glucose-tolerance test in the diagnosis of diabetes.[10] In patients with a first episode of hyperglycemia, however, measurement of glycosylated hemoglobin can provide some insight into the minimum duration of the diabetic state.

### MEASUREMENT OF URINARY GLUCOSE AND KETONES

Before the advent of simple and reliable methods for the measurement of plasma glucose on small volumes of blood, the measurement of urinary glucose was an important adjunct to the diagnosis and follow-up of patients with diabetes. Currently, however, except when plasma glucose testing is impossible, urinary glucose measurements are not particularly helpful in the diagnosis of diabetes because, in most persons, significant amounts of glucose do not appear in the urine until the plasma concentration exceeds 180 mg/dL. Normal persons excrete small amounts of glucose (up to ~100 mg per 24 hours) in their urine, as well as numerous other sugars and reducing substances that are not detected by standard methods. The amount of sugar in the urine is increased in diabetes; in renal glycosuria; in states in which the renal threshold for glucose is decreased (e.g., pregnancy); and in the nondiabetic melliturias. Many drugs, especially antibiotics, also may alter urine testing for glucose if nonspecific methods (Benedict reagent or Clinitest) are used, and some interfere even with the more specific glucose oxidase methods. The measurement of urine ketones, however, is by far the most convenient method of detecting early ketosis (see Chap. 155). Devices that will enable continuous glucose monitoring are finally coming to the market.[11]

## IMPAIRED GLUCOSE TOLERANCE AND RELATED DISORDERS

Regardless of the criteria used for diagnosis or the nature of the testing performed, some persons do not meet the criteria for the diagnosis of diabetes mellitus, yet do not have (or did not have) totally normal glucose tolerance. Their disorders fall into several categories.[1,2]

### IMPAIRED GLUCOSE TOLERANCE

The term *impaired glucose tolerance* is used to describe the condition in which the fasting glucose level is ≥110 mg/dL and <126 mg/dL, and the 2-hour value during an oral glucose-tolerance test lies between the normal and diabetic values (≥140 mg/dL and <200 mg/dL; see Table 136-2). Previously, such persons were said to have "chemical diabetes" or "borderline diabetes." Many of them are elderly or have syndromes related to secondary diabetes such as drug-induced impaired glucose tolerance.

The intent of this intermediate classification was to identify persons who might be at higher risk for diabetes without forcing on them the diagnosis of diabetes. Although many of these persons do not appear to develop diabetes, even after 20 years of follow-up,[1,2] this group does have an increased frequency of progression to NIDDM similar to that observed in patients with gestational diabetes.[12]

### PREVIOUS ABNORMALITY OF GLUCOSE TOLERANCE

The designation *previous abnormality of glucose tolerance* is applied to persons who have normal glucose tolerance at the time of testing but who previously had hyperglycemia or impaired glucose tolerance. The abnormality may have occurred in response to an identifiable factor or may have resolved spontaneously without an apparent cause having been determined. Previously, this condition was termed *latent diabetes*; it is applied to persons who have had gestational diabetes, to obese "diabetic" individuals whose glucose tolerance normalizes with weight loss, and to persons with histories of abnormal glucose tolerance after stress such as surgery, trauma, or myocardial infarction.

### POTENTIAL ABNORMALITY OF GLUCOSE TOLERANCE

*Potential abnormality of glucose tolerance* is a diagnosis used for persons who have never had glucose intolerance but who are considered to be at greater risk for the development of diabetes or impaired glucose tolerance. This group includes monozygotic twins of patients with diabetes, the offspring of two diabetic parents, mothers of children with a high birth weight, and members of racial or ethnic groups with a high prevalence of diabetes, such as the Pima Indians.

## INSULIN-DEPENDENT (TYPE 1) DIABETES MELLITUS

Type 1 diabetes mellitus is characterized by an insulin deficiency secondary to B-cell destruction. In the absence of insulin therapy, the resulting metabolic abnormalities eventually lead to death. In the preinsulin era, patients were treated with the Allen starvation diet and sometimes lived without insulin therapy for 5 or more years after diagnosis. Despite this, these patients actually were insulin dependent because they ultimately were dependent on insulin for survival. Although the terms *insulin-dependent diabetes* and *type 1 diabetes* commonly were used synonymously in the past, the author prefers to use the term *type 1A* to signify the autoimmune disease associated with IDDM, because any process that destroys enough B cells will cause IDDM, including extensive pancreatectomy, the ingestion of toxins such as the rodenticide pyriminil (Vacor), and certain genetic disorders such as Wolfram syndrome.

The typical pancreatic lesion of type 1A diabetes is a selective loss of almost all B cells, whereas other islet cell types (A, D, and PP cells) are intact.[13] Such "end-stage" islets are characterized by an absence of the inflammatory infiltrate (insulitis) that is present in many islets in children who die shortly after the onset of type 1A diabetes. Significantly, islet inflammation and B-cell destruction are a spotty process, in many ways resembling the lesions of early vitiligo, in which melanocytes in seemingly random regions of the skin are destroyed, and normal and vitiliginous skin are interspersed. Insulitis is not seen in the islets of patients with type 2 diabetes, but B-cell mass appears to be ~50% lower than in the pancreases of weight-matched control subjects.[14]

Not all spontaneous type 1 diabetes is the result of autoimmune mechanisms.[15] In db/db mice, after a period of hyperinsulinemia, B-cell destruction occurs. Introduction of a gene for severe combined immunodeficiency into mice with the db/db mutation blocks the production of several autoantibodies but has no influence on the loss of B cells. Conversely, in nonobese diabetic (NOD) mice, an animal model of type 1 diabetes, the introduction of an immunodeficiency gene prevents diabetes, as would be expected for an autoimmune disease.[16] Selective B-cell destruction in humans also can occur in the absence of known immunologic pathogenesis. For example, persons with Wolfram syndrome inherit an autosomal recessive gene that

TABLE 136-3.
**Genetics of Type 1 Diabetes Mellitus in Humans and Rodent Models**

**NOD MOUSE**

Recessive MHC gene (chromosome 17)

Diabetes more frequent in females than in males

More than 12 other contributing loci

**BB RAT**

MHC gene

Recessive T lymphopenia gene on chromosome 4

At least one other gene

**HUMAN**

DR3- and DR4-associated MHC genes (DQA1*0501, DQB1*0201; DQA1*0301, DQB1*0302)

Other high risk DQ alleles: DQA1*0401, DQB1*0402 and DQA1*0102, DQB1*0502 and DQA1*0101 and DQB1*0501

Protective HLA alleles:

DQA1*0102, DQB1*0602

DRB1*1401

DRB1*0403, DQA1*0201, DQB1*0303

Insulin regulatory gene polymorphism

Gene outside MHC: >10 loci proposed including CTLA-I$_g$

*NOD*, nonobese diabetic; *MHC*, major histocompatibility complex; *BB*, biobreeding.

leads to extensive B-cell destruction as well as to numerous neurologic deficits.[17] This constellation is designated by the acronym *DIDMOAD syndrome* (*d*iabetes *i*nsipidus, *d*iabetes *m*ellitus, *o*ptic *a*trophy, and nerve *d*eafness). No HLA-DR3 or HLA-DR4 association with this syndrome is seen, and no autoantibodies can be detected. In addition, in animals, streptozotocin, alloxan, and several viruses selectively destroy B cells.[18] Clinically, Vacor poisoning often leads to transient insulin dependence, as well as to severe neuropathy.[19]

The number of pathologic processes whose result is selective B-cell destruction is remarkable. Whether this reflects the ability to detect B-cell destruction more easily than a loss of, for instance, A cells, or whether it reflects a unique metabolic sensitivity of B cells is unknown.

## ROLE OF THE MAJOR HISTOCOMPATIBILITY COMPLEX

### AUTOIMMUNITY IN PATHOGENESIS OF TYPE 1A DIABETES

A large body of information indicates that autoimmune mechanisms lead to B-cell destruction in most persons in whom insulin dependence develops. In humans with type 1A diabetes and in the two animal models of this disease (the NOD mouse and the BB [biobreeding] rat), this destruction is associated with a gene within the major histocompatibility complex[15,20] (MHC) (Table 136-3). The MHC is ~2 × 10$^6$ nucleotide base pairs long and presumably contains more than 100 different genes.[21,22] Included in this region of the human genome are three classes of genes that profoundly affect immune function.

Class I genes (HLA-A, HLA-B, and HLA-C) are the classic strong transplantation antigens. The class I genes code for single-chain glycoproteins. These molecules also are recognized by cytotoxic T lymphocytes when they destroy virus-infected cells.

In humans, at least three expressed class II molecules are found, termed *DP, DQ,* and *DR*.[23] These molecules are dimeric glycoproteins and also are termed *Ia* (immune-associated) or *Ir* (immune-response) molecules. Once thought to be restricted in their tissue distribution, these molecules now are known to be expressed on many cells at different stages of development or in response to various stimuli. In particular, nondividing human macrophages and B lymphocytes express Ia antigens, whereas T lymphocytes express Ia antigens only after activation. Fibroblasts, thyrocytes, and many epithelial cells express

Ia antigens if exposed to γ-interferon (a T-lymphocyte product). Erythroid precursor cells and some other bone marrow cells express DR early in their life cycles. Myoblasts within atheromas express Ia antigens. In type 1A human diabetes after extensive B-cell destruction, but not in early lesions of BB rats and NOD mice, a small proportion of the B cells may express Ia. This is a controversial area, because such cells may represent dead B cells ingested by macrophages.

The class III genes code for components of the complement cascade. This subject is discussed in Chapter 194.

In addition to class I, II, and III genes, other genes are found within the MHC, such as the gene coding for the enzyme 21-hydroxylase. A defect of this gene leads to congenital adrenal hyperplasia. Although the specific gene within the MHC associated with type 1A diabetes is unknown, it is most likely a class II or Ir gene. Ninety-five percent of white patients with IDDM express the HLA alleles DR3 or DR4. Although ~40% of normal persons express DR3 or DR4, this huge excess of DR3/DR4 heterozygotes in patients with IDDM indicates that >90% of persons with type 1A diabetes have a histocompatibility-related gene contributing to the disease.[24,25]

The different alleles of the histocompatibility genes also are nonrandomly associated with each other (i.e., in linkage disequilibrium).[21] Thus, many different histocompatibility genes are associated with diabetes. For example, because DR3 is associated with type 1 diabetes, and alleles A1 and B8 are associated with DR3, alleles A1 and B8 also are associated with type 1 diabetes.

Several alleles appear to be protective (e.g., DQB1*0602, DRB1*1401). Persons heterozygous for both DR3 and DR4 are at highest risk for the development of type 1A diabetes. The excess risk of DR3 and DR4 heterozygotes extends even to identical twins. Almost 70% of monozygotic twins expressing both DR3 and DR4 alleles are concordant for type 1A diabetes, compared with 30% to 40% of twins not expressing both DR3 and DR4. This synergistic effect suggests that more than one gene within the MHC contributes to the development of type 1 diabetes.

Persons who have inherited the same HLA haplotypes as a sibling with type 1A diabetes are at increased risk for the development of diabetes (Fig. 136-1). Thus, persons who are HLA-identical to a sibling with diabetes have approximately a 1:10 to 1:20 chance of developing diabetes, whereas siblings sharing neither HLA haplotype have less than a 1:100 chance of developing diabetes. The excess of persons who are HLA-identical to a diabetic sibling suggests that one diabetogenic gene in the MHC functions in a recessive manner. Not all diabetic siblings express identical HLA haplotypes, however. This may be explained by the relatively large number of parents (e.g., 20%) who are potentially homozygous for diabetogenic MHC genes. Such a high percentage of homozygous parents is suggested by the observations that 5% of parents of children with type 1A

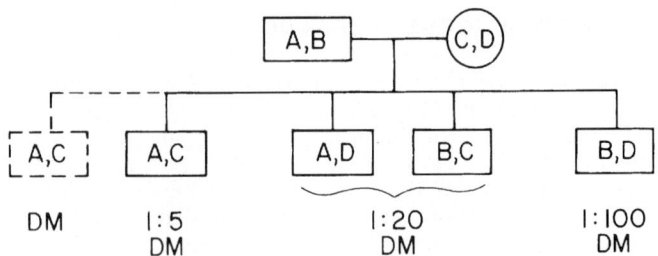

**FIGURE 136-1.** HLA haplotype sharing versus approximate concordance for type 1 diabetes mellitus (*DM*) in a family in which neither parent has type 1A diabetes. Letters refer to four major histocompatibility complex (*MHC*) haplotypes in the family, with each parent passing on one of the two sixth chromosomes to each child (MHC region marked by HLA typing). Siblings HLA-identical to the proband have the highest risk of type 1 diabetes (1:10 to 1:5) and siblings sharing neither HLA haplotype have the lowest risk (1:100). (From Eisenbarth GS. Autoimmune beta cell insufficiency. Triangle 1984; 24:111.)

diabetes develop overt type 1A diabetes, and that penetrance even in HLA-identical siblings is <1:4.

Although DR alleles are associated with risk for type 1A diabetes, DQ molecules appear to be more important in determining diabetes susceptibility,[24] DR and DQ molecules are closely linked, and both function to bind peptides for presentation to CD4-positive T lymphocytes. Each DQ molecule has two chains, α and β. For DQ molecules, both chains are polymorphic. Each different amino-acid sequence (polymorphism) of these chains is assigned a number. With DNA-based technology, small amounts of blood can be typed rapidly (within hours) for DQ alleles. One hypothesis related the presence of aspartic acid at position 57 on the DQ β chain to diabetes risk (DQ alleles lacking aspartic acid at position 57 are frequently associated with diabetes[26]). Too many exceptions exist to this rule, however, for it to be useful (e.g., DQB1*0402),[26] given the ease of typing for specific alleles with current technology.

Certain DQ molecules appear to provide almost complete protection from type 1A diabetes, such as DQA1*0102/ DQB1*0602.[27,28] This molecule is usually associated with DR2, but when DR2 is associated with other DQ molecules (e.g., DR2, DQB1*0502, which is found among patients with type 1 diabetes on the island of Sardinia), the haplotype is diabetogenic. Of >800 patients with type 1A diabetes, the author and his associates have typed five who have had DQB1*0602, and one 0602 patient had the polyendocrine autoimmune type I syndrome with its coexistent mucocutaneous candidiasis. The manner in which this DQ molecule protects against type 1A diabetes is unknown.

The highest-risk DQ alleles associated with type 1A diabetes are DQA1*0501/DQB1*0201 associated with DR3, and DQA1*0301/DQB1*0302 associated with DR4. Persons in the general population heterozygous for these two alleles have a risk of diabetes similar to that of an offspring of a parent with type 1 diabetes (~1:16). Such persons make up ~2% of the U.S. population, but account for 40% of patients with type 1A diabetes. A research program to identify these persons at birth is under way. Subsequent studies will define the timing and sequence of the appearance of autoantibodies, with the long-term goal of predicting type 1A diabetes in the general population.

The fact that the incidence of diabetes in HLA-identical siblings (16%) is less than that in identical twins (40–50%) strongly suggests that another gene outside the MHC contributes to diabetes susceptibility. This is similar to the genetics of diabetes susceptibility of BB rats and NOD mice. When either of these animals is crossed with normal-strain animals, only offspring inheriting a "diabetogenic" MHC gene and other autosomal genes develop diabetes. Multiple other genes influence the susceptibility of NOD mice, and a gene on chromosome 4 influences susceptibility associated with a T-cell immunodeficiency of BB rats (see Table 136-3).

Too many false-positive results occur with HLA typing (30–40% of the general population express DR3 or DR4) for this study to aid in clinical decision making. Moreover, HLA typing is relatively expensive and can never indicate a risk for diabetes greater than that of DR3/4 HLA-identical siblings (25–40%). (Within a family, nondiabetic siblings who are HLA-identical by serologic typing to a sibling with type 1A diabetes are usually [>99% of the time] identical at all HLA loci; nevertheless, their risk of developing diabetes is only ~17%.) The imprecision of HLA typing for predicting diabetes even within families probably results in part from the inability to identify another genetic linkage group for type 1A diabetes. Even when such a linkage group is discovered, genetic prediction of the risk of type 1A diabetes cannot exceed the concordance rate of identical twins (50%).

In addition to alleles within the MHC on chromosome 6, alleles of the insulin gene on chromosome 11 contribute to diabetes susceptibility.[29] Approximately 90% of persons with type

1A diabetes are homozygous for a common allele compared with 60% of the general population. Some controversy exists regarding whether this insulin-gene polymorphism shows "imprinting" (i.e., a differential influence on diabetes susceptibility depending on whether it is inherited from the father or the mother). These insulin alleles differ not in their coding sequence but in the 5' region of the gene. Thus, differential regulation of expression of insulin, particularly for expression in the thymus, may have an important influence on diabetes risk.

In addition to genes within the MHC and insulin alleles, other genes probably influence diabetes risk. With molecular and computational tools provided by the Genome Project, and shared national repositories of cell lines and DNA from families with multiple affected members, the search for these additional genes is under way and has identified multiple loci that may be associated with diabetes risk. Environmental factors may not be necessary for the triggering of type 1A diabetes. As in many cancers, somatic mutations may randomly trigger disease expression. Testing of this hypothesis will likely depend on the localization of major susceptibility genes.

## GENETIC AND ENVIRONMENTAL FACTORS

The lack of 100% concordance for type 1A diabetes in identical twins has been used to argue that environmental factors must contribute to the development of this disease.[30,31] One environmental factor known to increase the incidence of type 1A diabetes is congenital rubella. After prenatal infection with this virus, as many as 20% of children later develop diabetes. As in those who spontaneously develop type 1A diabetes, individuals with congenital rubella who later develop diabetes express HLA alleles DR3 and DR4.[32] These children often also have thyroiditis and other immunologic disorders (e.g., agammaglobulinemia) in association with an abnormal T-lymphocyte phenotype that differs from that in both normal persons and usual patients with type 1A diabetes.

No epidemiologically defined environmental factors other than congenital rubella have been clearly associated with type 1A diabetes. Viral infections, in particular those that occur close to the time of onset of overt diabetes, are known to precipitate hyperglycemia (secondary to insulin resistance associated with infection), but they are unlikely to play a primary pathogenic role. Although coxsackievirus B4 has been isolated from the pancreas of a child with recent-onset diabetes,[33] the pancreas had multiple pseudoatrophic islets (islets with no B cells but abundant A and D cells) with no inflammation, indicating chronic B-cell destruction preceding the viral infection. Any search for environmental factors that may trigger autoimmunity, such as drugs, unknown viruses, or dietary components (e.g., milk proteins), must focus on factors that act months to years before the onset of diabetes rather than on acutely diabetogenic factors.

## ISLET CELL ANTIBODIES AND OTHER IMMUNOLOGIC MARKERS

Approximately 5% of first-degree relatives of patients with type 1A diabetes also develop diabetes. Immunologic and endocrinologic assays capable of identifying those relatives most likely to develop diabetes and predicting approximately when overt diabetes will occur include the immunofluorescence assay for cytoplasmic islet cell antibody, the results of which are positive in 70% to 80% of patients with new-onset type 1A diabetes. Some assays for islet cell antibodies[34–36] and a few radioimmunoassays for antiinsulin autoantibodies[37,38] have the requisite specificity to identify persons at high risk. Examples are the complement-fixation tests for cytoplasmic islet cell antibodies, variants of the standard cytoplasmic islet cell antibody assays, fluid-phase antiinsulin autoantibody assays, and autoantibodies to a 64-kDa islet protein (predominantly antibodies to glutamic acid decarboxylase [GAD]) and antibodies to a molecule termed ICA512(IA-2).[38] Autoantibody assays using defined

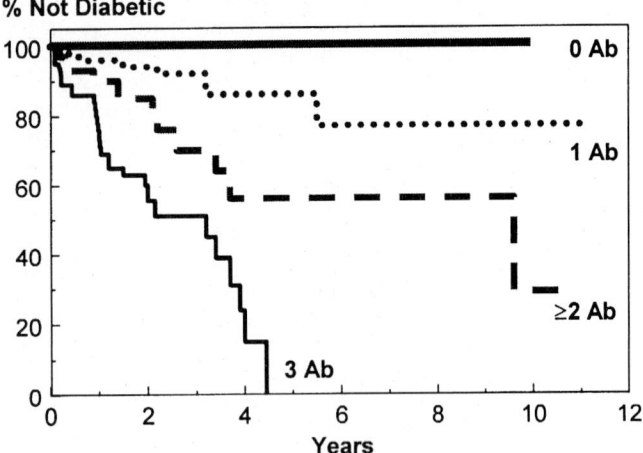

**% Not Diabetic**

**FIGURE 136-2.** Progression to type 1A diabetes of first-degree relatives of patients with diabetes based on the number of defined antiislet autoantibodies (*Ab*; of GAD65 [glutamic acid decarboxylase], ICA512, and insulin). One relative (of ~500) lacking autoantibodies progressed to diabetes. (From Verge CF, Gianani R, Kawasaki E, et al. Prediction of type 1 diabetes in first-degree relatives using a combination of insulin, GAD and ICA512bdc/IA-2 autoantibodies. Diabetes 1996; 45:926.)

islet autoantigens (GAD65, ICA512, or insulin) have improved so much (Fig. 136-2) that for most clinical settings the difficult-to-standardize cytoplasmic islet cell antibody assay should be abandoned.

The presence of antiislet cell antibodies can precede the development of overt diabetes by more than a decade[34,39] (Fig. 136-3). HLA typing of antibody-positive relatives and even antibody-positive "normal" persons indicates that they have the same HLA distribution as do patients with type 1A diabetes, and within 7 years, ~50% develop overt diabetes.

The appearance of autoantibodies to human insulin also can precede by years the development of type 1A diabetes.[40] Anti-insulin antibodies are present in both cytoplasmic antibody–positive and antibody–negative persons who develop diabetes; these antibodies provided the first radioimmunoassay aid for

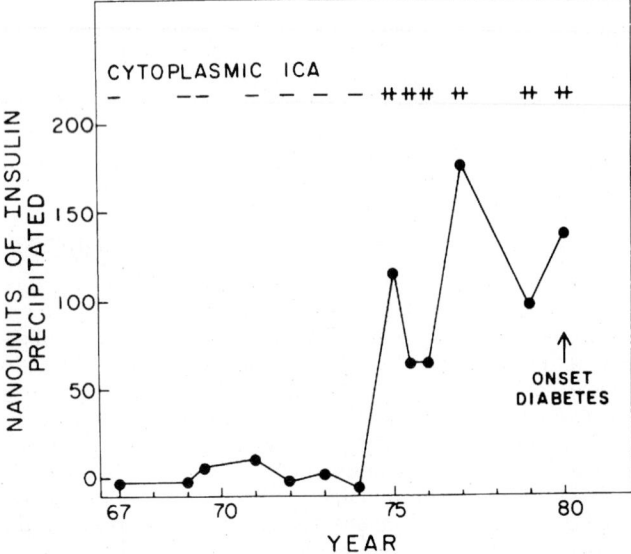

**FIGURE 136-3.** Development of insulin autoantibodies and cytoplasmic islet cell antibodies (*ICA*) in overt diabetes. (Adapted from Soeldner JS, Tuttleman M, Srikanta S, et al. Insulin dependent diabetes mellitus and initiation of autoimmunity: islet cell autoantibodies, insulin autoantibodies and beta cell failure. N Engl J Med 1985; 313:893.)

predicting type 1A diabetes. Antiinsulin autoantibodies are found in ~60% of persons who develop diabetes. When this test is combined with assays for cytoplasmic islet cell antibodies, 90% of patients with new-onset type 1A diabetes are found to have evidence of autoimmune disease.

In addition to the presence of cytoplasmic islet cell antibodies and insulin autoantibodies, many immunologic abnormalities are present in patients with type 1A diabetes and their relatives.[41] Many of these abnormalities (e.g., presence of anti-thyroglobulin and microsomal antibodies, antibodies to single-stranded DNA, antibodies to the surface of rat islet cells and a rat insulinoma cell line) are inherited independently of the HLA susceptibility to type 1A diabetes and are present in as many as 30% of first-degree relatives. Such abnormalities provide relatively little prognostic information but appear to be related to the autoimmune background of type 1A diabetes.

A major advance in the past several years has been the biochemical characterization of a series of islet autoantigens, including insulin, GAD (a major component of the 64-kDa autoantigen),[42] carboxypeptidase H,[43] a milk-related islet protein (ICA69),[44] ICA512,[45] and ganglioside GM2-1.[46] Biochemical assays are now available that use recombinant human proteins to measure antibodies to insulin, GAD, and ICA512. When just these three assays are used, >98% of patients with new-onset type 1A diabetes and prediabetes express at least one antibody, and >80% express two or more. Specificity and sensitivity are much higher with these biochemical assays than with cytoplasmic islet cell antibody testing. In contrast to cytoplasmic islet cell antibody testing, with its inherent problems of reproducibility, biochemical determination of autoantibodies is remarkably stable in the prediabetic phase. International workshops to standardize insulin and GAD radioassays are under way. Such assays should rapidly replace standard cytoplasmic islet cell antibody testing in both the diagnosis and prediction of type 1A diabetes.

## FIRST-PHASE INSULIN SECRETION AS AN INDEX OF EARLY TYPE 1 DIABETES MELLITUS

Approximately 3% of nondiabetic relatives of patients with type 1A diabetes have positive results on screening assays for islet cell autoantibodies. When such antibodies are detected, intravenous glucose-tolerance testing can be used to assess first-phase insulin release as a measure of subclinical B-cell dysfunction (Fig. 136-4). The loss of first-phase insulin secretion, as well as its rate of fall, aids in predicting the time of onset of overt diabetes.[47,48] At the time of initial detection of islet cell antibodies, one of four patients has first-phase insulin secretion below the first percentile of normal persons. Almost all persons who develop type 1A diabetes lose first-phase insulin secretion before they develop overt diabetes. For patients with initially normal insulin release, intravenous glucose-tolerance testing is performed again in 3 to 6 months and, depending on its stability, at subsequent 3- to 12-month intervals. Immunologically and endocrinologically, persons with abnormal results may be alerted to the risk of type 1A diabetes and advised concerning routine home monitoring for glucosuria or capillary blood glucose determination.

To aid in predicting the time of onset of type 1A diabetes among antibody-positive relatives of persons with type 1A diabetes, the following mathematic formula has been developed: years to diabetes = $-0.12 + 1.35 \times \log_e$ (insulin secretion) $-0.59 \log_e$ (insulin autoantibody concentration). This simple formula appears to account for ~50% of the variance in the time of diabetes onset.[48]

Immunologic assays also are being used to aid in the classification of patients with diabetes. Insulin dependence is a physiologic state that can evolve slowly, even in type 1A diabetes, from a stage in which hyperglycemia is controlled with diet or oral medication to a stage in which death occurs in the absence

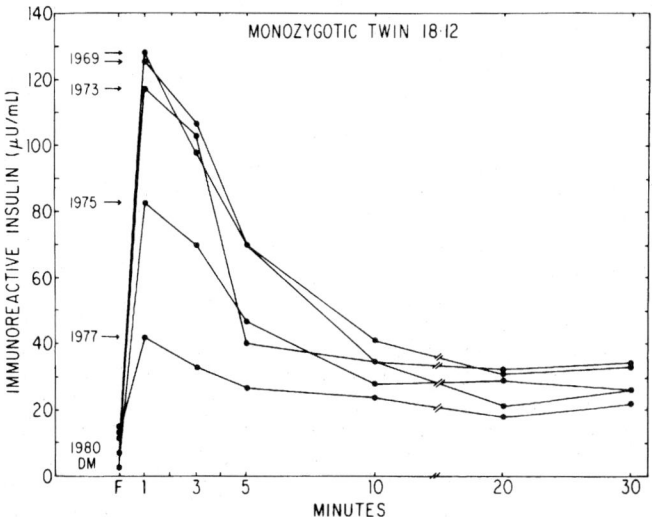

**FIGURE 136-4.** Loss of first-phase insulin secretion in a prediabetic twin with islet cell antibody. The y-axis gives insulin concentrations at the times indicated after the intravenous injection of glucose. Initial phase of insulin release (1 and 3 minutes) is progressively lost. (*DM*, diabetes mellitus; *F*, fasting.) (Adapted from Srikanta S, Ganda OP, Eisenbarth GS, Soeldner JS. Islet cell antibodies and beta cell function in monozygotic triplets and twins initially discordant for type I diabetes. N Engl J Med 1983; 308:322.)

of insulin therapy (Fig. 136-5). Antiislet antibodies are found in as many as 10% of patients with classic type 2 diabetes at the time of diagnosis, and over the ensuing 5 years, many of these patients become insulin dependent.[35]

Epidemiologic data from Japan, Pittsburgh, the Netherlands, and Poland indicate that 1 in 200 children die of ketoacidosis at the time of diagnosis of their diabetes. Such deaths probably could be prevented by early detection and treatment of diabetes.

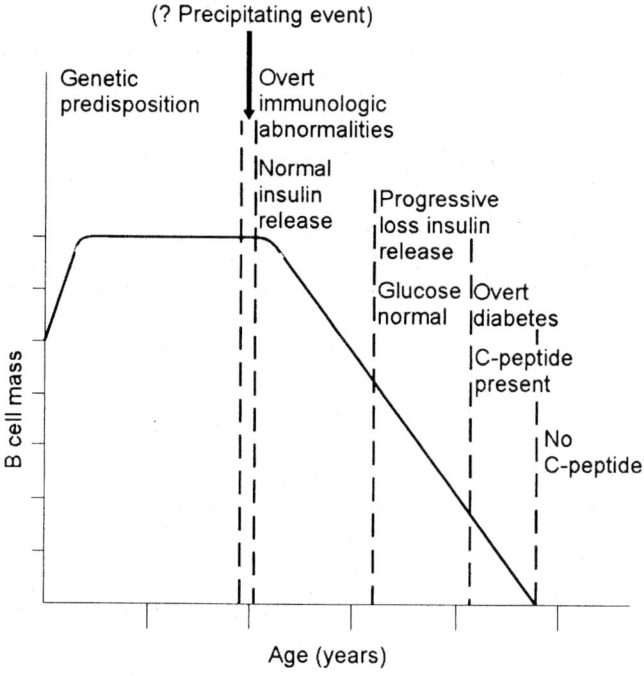

**FIGURE 136-5.** Stages in the development of type 1 diabetes, beginning with genetic predisposition and ending with insulin-dependent diabetes with essentially complete B-cell destruction. (Adapted from Eisenbarth GS. Type I diabetes mellitus: a chronic autoimmune disease. N Engl J Med 1986; 314:1360.)

## IMPLICATIONS FOR PREVENTIVE THERAPY

The newer immunologic knowledge concerning type 1A diabetes and the success of a wide variety of immunotherapies in preventing the diabetes of BB rats and NOD mice have led to trials of immunotherapy in patients with recent-onset type 1A diabetes, and to a few trials in persons at high risk for the development of type 1A diabetes. These trials indicate that limiting B-cell destruction is possible. Toxic side effects of the most powerful (and most effective) drugs are a serious problem, however. For example, cyclosporine A is nephrotoxic at the dosages that appear to be required to induce remissions of type 1A diabetes,[49,50] and azathioprine may be associated with epithelial malignancies. Prednisone given after the onset of type 1A diabetes is ineffective, and a series of other therapies, such as plasmapheresis and treatment with antithymocyte globulin or monoclonal antibody T12, produce no long-term benefit.

A series of new agents that are not significantly immunosuppressive yet are able to limit B-cell destruction in animal models of type 1A diabetes are being studied. All immunologic attempts to limit B-cell destruction are considered investigational and should be used only under the oversight of a human investigation committee.[51]

Trials investigating the prevention of type 1A diabetes and the amelioration of further B-cell loss after diabetes onset are concentrating on nonimmunosuppressive therapies. Such trials include administration of the vitamin nicotinamide,[52] which modestly delays diabetes onset in NOD mice; vaccination with bacille Calmette-Guérin[53]; administration of oral insulin[54]; and therapy with parenteral insulin.[55] Nicotinamide may have an effect by limiting free radical damage to B cells. In the NOD mouse model, a single injection of bacille Calmette-Guérin (BCG) prevents diabetes but not insulitis. Such therapy may limit B-cell destruction by altering cytokines produced by infiltrating T cells. A completed German trial of nicotinamide found no benefit, but a larger European trial is continuing. In randomized trials, BCG had no beneficial effect. Oral administration of insulin delays or prevents type 1 diabetes in NOD mice. Its effect is likely due to the generation of T cells (by peptides of insulin present in the intestinal mucosa) that suppress inflammation. The most dramatic prevention of diabetes in both the NOD mouse and the BB rat has been obtained with parenteral administration of insulin. Such therapy prevents not only diabetes, but also infiltration of islets by T cells and destruction of B cells. A small pilot trial[53] of intravenous insulin and low-dose subcutaneous insulin for the prevention of diabetes in high-risk relatives of patients with diabetes suggests that such therapy may delay the onset of type 1 diabetes, and a large U.S. prevention trial (DPT-1 [Diabetes Prevention Trial-1]) is under way.

## AUTOIMMUNE POLYGLANDULAR FAILURE

Approximately 20% of patients with type 1A diabetes develop other organ-specific autoimmune diseases (see Chap. 197), such as celiac disease, Graves disease, hypothyroidism, Addison disease, and pernicious anemia.[56,57] Some patients develop multiple disorders as a part of two inherited polyendocrine autoimmune syndromes (type I and type II). The type I syndrome usually has its onset in infancy, with hypoparathyroidism, mucocutaneous candidiasis, and, somewhat later, Addison disease and other organ-specific disorders. Fifteen percent of these children develop type 1A diabetes. This disorder is inherited in an autosomal recessive manner with no HLA association due to mutations of a gene (*AIRE*) located on chromosome 21. This mutated gene codes for a DNA-binding protein that is expressed in the thymus. The type II polyendocrine autoimmune syndrome (Addison disease, type 1 diabetes [50% of patients], Graves disease, hypothyroidism, myasthenia gravis, and other organ-specific diseases) is strongly HLA-associated and has an onset from late childhood to middle age. In these families, a high prevalence of undiagnosed organ-specific autoimmune disease is seen, and, at a minimum, thyroid function tests should be performed in the first-degree relatives of these patients. Biochemical evaluation for adrenal insufficiency and pernicious anemia should be performed if any suggestive symptom or sign is present (e.g., decreasing insulin requirements can herald the development of Addison disease in a patient with type 1 diabetes before electrolyte abnormalities or hyperpigmentation develop). Excellent autoantibody tests can facilitate the detection of Addison disease (21-hydroxylase autoantibodies) or celiac disease (transglutaminase autoantibodies) in patients with type 1A diabetes. As many as 1 in 200 patients with type 1A diabetes develop Addison disease, and 1 in 20 develop celiac disease.

# REFERENCES

1. Report of the Expert Committee on the Diagnosis and Classification of Diabetes Mellitus. Diabetes Care 1997; 20:1183.
2. World Health Organization Expert Committee on Diabetes Mellitus. Second report. Geneva: World Health Organization, 1980:646. Technical report series 1980.
3. Marble A, Ferguson BD. Diagnosis and classification of diabetes mellitus and the non-diabetic melliturias. In: Marble A, Krall LP, Bradley RF, et al., eds. Joslin's diabetes mellitus, 12th ed. Philadelphia: Lea & Febiger, 1985:332.
4. Polonsky KS, Stuns J, Bell GI. Non-insulin-dependent diabetes mellitus: a genetically programmed failure of the beta cell to compensate for insulin resistance. N Engl J Med 1996; 334:777.
5. Nelson RL. Oral glucose tolerance test: indications and limitations. Mayo Clin Proc 1988; 63:263.
6. Ganda OP, Srikanta S, Brink SJ, et al. Differential sensitivity to beta cell secretagogues in "early" type I diabetes. Diabetes 1984; 33:516.
7. Bergman RN, Finegood DJ, Ader M. Assessment of insulin sensitivity in vivo. Endocr Rev 1985; 6:45.
8. Fajans SS, Conn JW. An approach to the prediction of diabetes mellitus by modification of the glucose tolerance test with cortisone. Diabetes 1954; 3:296.
9. Koenig RJ, Cerami A. Hemoglobin A$_{1c}$ and diabetes mellitus. Annu Rev Med 1980; 31:29.
10. Starkman HS, Soeldner JS, Gleason RE. Oral glucose tolerance—relationship with hemoglobin A$_{1c}$. Diabetes Res Clin Pract 1987; 6:343.
11. Garg SK, Potts RO, Ackerman NR, et al. Correlation of fingerstick blood glucose measurements with Gluco Watch biographer glucose results in young subjects with type 1 diabetes. Diabetes Care 1999; 22:1708.
12. Agner E, Thorsteinssen B, Eriksen M. Impaired glucose tolerance and diabetes mellitus in elderly subjects. Diabetes Care 1982; 5:600.
13. Gepts W. The pathology of the pancreas in human diabetes. In: Adreani D, Federlin KF, DiMario U, Heding LG, eds. Immunology in diabetes. London: Kimpton Publishers, 1984:21.
14. Gepts W. Islet cell morphology in type I and type II diabetes. In: Irvine WJ, ed. Immunology in diabetes. Edinburgh: Teviot Scientific Publications, 1982:255.
15. Eisenbarth GS. Type I diabetes mellitus: a chronic autoimmune disease. N Engl J Med 1986; 314:1360.
16. Makino S, Harada M, Kishimoto Y, Hayashi Y. Absence of insulitis and overt diabetes in athymic nude mice with NOD genetic background. Jikken Dobitsu Exp Anim 1986; 35:495.
17. Inoue H, Tanizawa Y, Wasson J, et al. A gene encoding a transmembrane protein is mutated in patients with diabetes mellitus and optic atrophy (Wolfram syndrome). Nat Genet 1998; 20:143.
18. Mordes JP, Greiner DL, Rossini AA. Animal models of autoimmune diabetes mellitus. In: LeRoith D, Taylor SI, Olefsky JM, eds. Diabetes mellitus. Philadelphia: Lippincott–Raven Publishers, 1996:349.
19. Feingold KR, Lee TH, Chug MY, et al. Muscle capillary basement membrane width in patients with Vacor-induced diabetes mellitus. J Clin Invest 1986; 78:102.
20. Jackson RA, Buse JB, Rifai R, et al. Two genes required for diabetes in BB rats. J Exp Med 1984; 159:1629.
21. Nepom GT, Kwok H-W. Perspectives in diabetes: molecular basis for HLA-DQ associations with IDDM. Diabetes 1998; 47:1177.
22. Todd JA. From genome to aetiology in a multifactorial disease, type 1 diabetes. Bioessays 1999; 21:164.
23. Bellgrau D, Eisenbarth GS. Immunobiology of autoimmunity. In: Eisenbarth GS, ed. Molecular mechanisms of endocrine and organ specific autoimmunity. Austin: RG Landes Company, 1991:1.
24. Redondo MJ, Kawasaki E, Mulgrew CL, et al. DR and DQ associated protection from type 1 diabetes: comparison of DRB1*1401 and DQA1*0102-DQB1*0602. J Clin Endocrinol Metab 2000; in press.
25. Nepom GT. Immunogenetics and IDDM. Diabetes Rev 1993; 1:93.
26. Kawasaki E, Noble J, Erlich H, et al. Transmission of DQ haplotypes to patients with type 1 diabetes. Diabetes 1998; 47:1971.
27. Erlich HA, Griffith RL, Bugawan TL, et al. Implication of specific DQB1 alleles in genetic susceptibility and resistance by identification of IDDM siblings with novel HLA-DQB1 allele and unusual DR2 and DR1 haplotypes. Diabetes 1991; 40:478.
28. Greenbaum CJ, Cuthbertson D, Eisenbarth GS, et al. Islet cell antibody positive relatives with HLA-DQA1*0102, DQB1*0602: Identification by the Diabetes Prevention Trial-1. J Clin Endocrinol Metab 2000; 85:1255.
29. Bennett ST, Lucassen AM, Gough SCL, et al. Susceptibility to human type I diabetes at IDDM2 is determined by tandem repeat variation at the insulin gene minisatellite locus. Nat Genet 1995; 9:284.
30. Barnett AH, Eff C, Leslie RDG, Pyke DA. Diabetes in identical twins: a study of 200 pairs. Diabetologia 1981; 20:87.
31. Blom L, Dahlquist G, Nyström L, et al. The Swedish childhood diabetes study—social and perinatal determinants for diabetes in childhood. Diabetologia 1989; 32:7.
32. Menser MA, Forrest JM, Brensby RD. Rubella infection and diabetes mellitus. Lancet 1981; 1:57.
33. Yoon JW, London WT, Curfman BL, et al. Coxsackie virus B4 produces transient diabetes in non-human primates. Diabetes 1986; 35:712.
34. Bingley PJ, Gale EAM. Current status and future prospect for prediction of IDDM. In: Palmer JP, ed. Prediction, prevention, and genetic counseling in IDDM. Chichester, England: John Wiley, 1996:227.
35. Turner R, Stratton I, Horton V, et al. UKPDS 25: autoantibodies to islet-cell cytoplasm and glutamic acid decarboxylase for prediction of insulin requirement in type 2 diabetes. UK Prospective Diabetes Study Group. Lancet 1997; 30:1288.
36. Gorsuch AN, Spencer KM, Lister J, et al. Evidence for a long prediabetic period in type I (insulin-dependent) diabetes mellitus. Lancet 1981; 2:1363.
37. Palmer JP, Asplin CM, Clemons P, et al. Insulin antibodies in insulin-dependent diabetics before insulin treatment. Science 1983; 222:1337.
38. Vardi P, Tuttleman M, Grinbergs M, et al. Consistency of anti-islet autoimmunity in "pre-type I diabetics" and genetically susceptible subjects: evidence from an ultrasensitive competitive insulin autoantibody (CIAA) radioimmunoassay. Diabetes 1986; 35(Suppl 1):86A.
39. Gale EAM. Islet cell autoantibodies: a family story. Eur J Endocrinol 1996; 135:643.
40. Kuglin B, Bertrams J, Linke C, et al. Prevalence of cytoplasmic islet cell antibodies and insulin auto-antibodies is increased in subjects with genetically defined high risk for insulin-dependent diabetes mellitus. Klin Wochenschr 1989; 67:66.
41. Radetti G, Paganini C, Gentili L, et al. Frequency of Hashimoto's thyroiditis in children with type 1 diabetes mellitus. Acta Diabetol 1995; 32:121.
42. Baekkeskov S, Aanstoot H, Christgau S, et al. Identification of the 64K autoantigen in insulin dependent diabetes as the GABA-synthesizing enzyme glutamic acid decarboxylase. Nature 1990; 347:151.
43. Castano L, Russo E, Zhou L, et al. Identification and cloning of a granule autoantigen (carboxypeptidase H) associated with type I diabetes. J Clin Endocrinol Metab 1991; 73:1197.
44. Pietropaolo M, Castano L, Babu S, et al. Islet cell autoantigen 69 kDa (ICA69): molecular cloning and characterization of a novel diabetes associated autoantigen. J Clin Invest 1993; 92:359.
45. Verge CF, Stenger D, Bonifacio E, et al. Combined use of autoantibodies (IA-2ab, Gadab, IAA, ICA) in type 1 diabetes: combinatorial islet autoantibody workshop. Diabetes 1998; 47:1857.
46. Nayak RC, Omar MAK, Rabizadeh A, et al. "Cytoplasmic" islet cell antibodies: evidence that the target antigen is asialoglycoconjugate. Diabetes 1985; 34:617.
47. Srikanta S, Ganda OP, Soeldner JS, Eisenbarth GS. First-degree relatives of patients with type I diabetes: islet cell antibodies and abnormal insulin secretion. N Engl J Med 1985; 313:461.
48. Eisenbarth GS, Gianani R, Yu L, et al. Dual parameter model for prediction of type 1 diabetes mellitus. Proc Assoc Am Physicians 1998; 110:126.
49. Stiller CR, Dupré J, Gent M, et al. Effect of cyclosporine immunosuppression in insulin-dependent mellitus of recent onset. Science 1984; 223:1362.
50. Feutren G, Asson G, Karsenty G, et al. Cyclosporine increases the rate and length of remissions in insulin-dependent diabetes of recent onset: results of a multi-center trial. Lancet 1986; 2:119.
51. Gottlieb PA, Eisenbarth GS. Diagnosis and treatment of pre-insulin dependent diabetes (IDDM). Annu Rev Med 1998; 49:391.
52. Lampeter EF, Klinghammer A, Scherbaum WA, et al. The Deutsche Nicotinamide Intervention Study: an attempt to prevent type 1 diabetes. DENIS Group. Diabetes 1998; 47:980.
53. Sadelain MWJ, Qin H-Y, Lauzon J, Singh B. Prevention of type I diabetes in NOD mice by adjuvant immunotherapy. Diabetes 1990; 39:583.
54. Zhang JZ, Davidson L, Eisenbarth G, Weiner HL. Suppression of diabetes in nonobese diabetic mice by oral administration of porcine insulin. Proc Natl Acad Sci U S A 1991; 88:10252.
55. Keller RJ, Eisenbarth GS, Jackson RA. Insulin prophylaxis in individuals at high risk of type I diabetes. Lancet 1993; 341:927.
56. Nuefeld M, Maclaren N, Blizzard RM. Two types of autoimmune Addison's disease associated with different polyglandular autoimmune (PGA) syndromes. Medicine (Baltimore) 1981; 60:355.
57. Verge C, Eisenbarth GS. Autoimmune polyendocrine syndromes. In: Wilson JD, Foster DW, eds. Williams textbook of endocrinology, 9th ed. Philadelphia: WB Saunders, 1998:1651.

# CHAPTER 137

# ETIOLOGY AND PATHOGENESIS OF TYPE 2 DIABETES MELLITUS AND RELATED DISORDERS

C. RONALD KAHN

## NON–INSULIN-DEPENDENT (TYPE 2) DIABETES MELLITUS

Type 2 diabetes mellitus is by far the most prevalent endocrine disease. It is estimated to affect >15 million people in the United States, approximately one-third of whom are undiagnosed.[1,2] The prevalence increases with age, and >9% of those older than 65 years have the disease. The prevalence is higher in Mexican Americans, blacks, and Native Americans, reaching as high as 50% among adult Pima Indians. Development of type 2 diabetes is strongly influenced by genetic factors and environmental factors, including obesity, decreased physical activity, and a low level of physical fitness.[3]

### PATHOGENESIS

Although type 2 or non–insulin-dependent diabetes mellitus is the more common form of the disease, the exact nature of its pathogenesis remains controversial, and in contrast to type 1 diabetes, in which immunologic markers confirm the pathogenesis of the disease, no specific diagnostic tests are available for type 2 diabetes.

Type 2 diabetes has strong genetic influences and occurs in identical twins with almost total concordance[4,5]; however, defining the exact genes involved has posed a great challenge. In type 2 diabetes, B-cell mass is relatively well preserved, but insulin secretion in response to specific secretagogues such as glucose is reduced, and clear evidence exists for resistance to insulin action in the peripheral tissues.[6–9] The precise genetic defects have been identified in some of the minor forms of type 2 diabetes, including those in rare patients with genetic syndromes of insulin resistance (see Chap. 146) and in patients with *maturity-onset diabetes of youth (MODY)*.

For the common form of type 2 diabetes, controversy continues over whether the decreased insulin secretion or insulin resistance is the principal factor in the pathogenesis of the disease, and which occurs first in the longitudinal development of the syndrome. Uncertainty also exists about the extent of the heterogeneity and the identity of the primary lesion.

### INSULIN SYNTHESIS AND SECRETION

Even before the introduction of radioimmunoassays, morphologic studies suggested that the pancreas of a patient with type 2 diabetes has at least 50% (and sometimes up to 100%) of the normal B-cell mass, whereas that of a patient with type 1 diabetes of more than a few years' duration has virtually no B cells.[6] This finding is consistent with the data on extractable insulin as measured in bioassay and radioimmunoassay. Immunoassay of plasma insulin and of C peptide has confirmed the presence of functioning B cells in patients with this disease, but the extent of function varies considerably depending on the type of stimulus used, the body weight of the patient, and the stage of disease.[8–10] In long-standing disease, islets do produce amyloid deposits, which are partly comprised of a second hormone

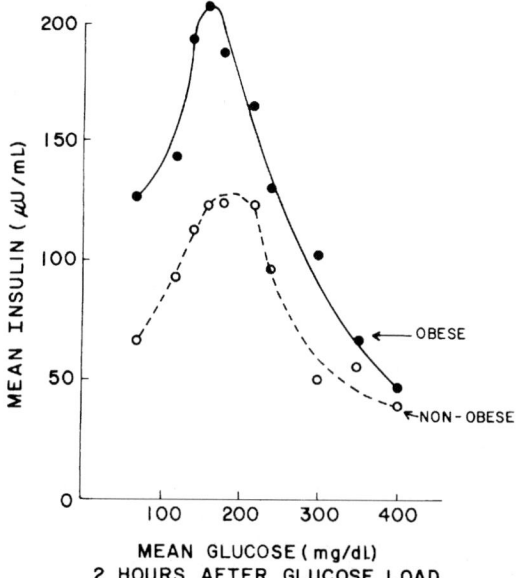

**FIGURE 137-1.** Relation between insulin secretion and glucose level 2 hours after a glucose load. Data were obtained for Pima Indians with various degrees of glucose intolerance. Similar results have been observed in whites. (Data from Savage PJ, Dippe SE, Bennett PH, et al. Hyperinsulinemia and hypoinsulinemia: insulin responses to oral carbohydrate over a wide spectrum of glucose tolerance. Diabetes 1975; 24:262.)

(termed *islet amyloid polypeptide* or *amylin*), which is secreted by B cells.[10] Although some studies have implicated this peptide in the abnormal B-cell function of type 2 diabetes, this hypothesis remains unproven, and it seems more likely that the amyloid deposits are a marker of chronic insulin hypersecretion.

In most individuals with type 2 diabetes, basal insulin levels are normal or elevated, and the degree of elevation correlates with the degree of obesity.[11] Elevated insulin levels also occur in thin individuals with type 2 diabetes. Although a few patients have been identified with a defect in the conversion of proinsulin to insulin or mutant insulin molecules, in most patients with type 2 diabetes, the proportion of proinsulin to insulin is normal or only slightly increased, and the insulin and proinsulin have normal receptor binding and bioactivity.

Although basal insulin levels usually are elevated in patients with type 2 diabetes, the insulin secretory responses to oral glucose differ considerably, depending on the extent of glucose intolerance. In patients with normal fasting glucose levels and 2-hour postprandial levels of <220 mg/dL, insulin secretion is increased in proportion to the degree of glycemia (Fig. 137-1). With more severe degrees of glucose intolerance, the secretion of insulin in response to an oral glucose load is reduced. This bell-shaped curve is reminiscent of the Starling curve for cardiac function. Insulin response to mixed meals often is preserved in patients with type 2 diabetes, even those with fasting glucose levels of >200 mg/dL.[7,8]

In contrast to the relative preservation of insulin response to meals and to oral glucose, a loss of acute-phase (first-phase) insulin release in response to intravenous glucose occurs in virtually all patients with significant fasting hyperglycemia.[9] Acute insulin release in response to β-adrenergic stimuli, amino acids, and other insulin secretagogues in these same individuals often is normal, suggesting a specific defect in glucorecognition rather than a general defect in B-cell function.[12,13] This pattern of response resembles that seen in patients in the early, preclinical phase of type 1 diabetes. In studies of perfused pancreases from animal models of type 2 diabetes, although first-phase secretion may be lost, glucose maintains its ability to potentiate arginine-induced insulin secretion.[14] The preservation of response to an oral glucose load probably is a reflection of the importance in this response of the potentiation of the glucose effect by gastrointestinal hormones. In humans with type 2 diabetes, however, the glucose potentiation is also blunted.[12] The lost first-phase response to glucose can be restored, at least partially, by α-adrenergic blockade, opiate-receptor blockade, inhibitors of prostaglandin synthesis, reduction of plasma glucose by dietary restriction, use of oral hypoglycemic agents, or even administration of insulin.[15] The fact that this lesion is functional and at least partially reversible makes it potentially amenable to therapeutic manipulation. A fragment of glucagon-like peptide-1 (GLP-1) may potentiate glucose-induced insulin secretion in persons with type 2 diabetes; this offers a possible new avenue for therapy that is currently being explored in clinical trials.[16]

## INSULIN RESISTANCE

Virtually all patients with type 2 diabetes have some degree of insulin resistance.[17] Conditions associated with the development of insulin resistance, especially obesity and advancing age, greatly increase the risk of type 2 diabetes. Insulin resistance correlates with certain patterns of obesity and is greater in individuals with central obesity than in those with more generalized obesity.[18] At any given body weight, a high waist-to-hip ratio correlates with insulin resistance and increased risk of type 2 diabetes. Insulin resistance and hyperinsulinemia are also associated with hypertension and hypertriglyceridemia, deceased high-density lipoprotein cholesterol, and increased risk of atherosclerosis and cardiovascular disease.[19,20] The association of insulin resistance with these features in the absence of clinical diabetes has been referred to as the *metabolic syndrome* or *syndrome X* (see Chap. 145).[19]

In cases of type 2 diabetes and syndrome X, insulin resistance is suggested by the elevated insulin levels and the fact that the patient develops glucose intolerance with circulating insulin levels well above those seen in the type 1 diabetic. The simplest test of insulin sensitivity is the measurement of the fall in plasma glucose in response to a given dose of exogenous insulin (i.e., an insulin-tolerance test). In normal individuals, glucose usually falls by >50% in response to a dose of 0.05 to 0.1 U per kilogram of body weight. In type 2 diabetics, this response may be markedly blunted, and as much as 0.3 U/kg may be required to produce a 50% fall in glucose.

Because the variability of endogenous insulin secretion and the counterregulatory hormones released during hypoglycemia may modify the response to the insulin test, more sophisticated measures of insulin resistance have been developed in which these factors are minimized. These tests include the measurement of steady-state glucose during simultaneous insulin and glucose infusion in which pancreatic insulin is suppressed with propranolol and epinephrine or somatostatin or the use of the euglycemic insulin clamp technique.[21] In the latter, dose-response curves for the effect of insulin on glucose disposal in normal humans can be constructed (Fig. 137-2). When this test is used, the nature of the insulin resistance can be dissected into changes in median effective dose (ED$_{50}$) on dose-response curves (i.e., changes in insulin sensitivity) and changes in maximal insulin effect (i.e., changes in insulin responsiveness).[21,22] In type 2 diabetes, decreased sensitivity in insulin action to decreased splanchnic glucose output (i.e., an effect primarily on the liver) and decreased sensitivity and decreased responsiveness of insulin action to increased glucose utilization (i.e., effects primarily on muscle and fat tissue) are seen.[21,23]

The resistance to insulin that occurs in the patient with type 2 diabetes mellitus could result from defects at several levels of insulin action (see Chap. 135). To produce a signal at the target cell, insulin must bind to its receptor, generate a transmembrane signal by activation of the insulin-receptor kinase, and initiate a complex network of intracellular signals that ulti-

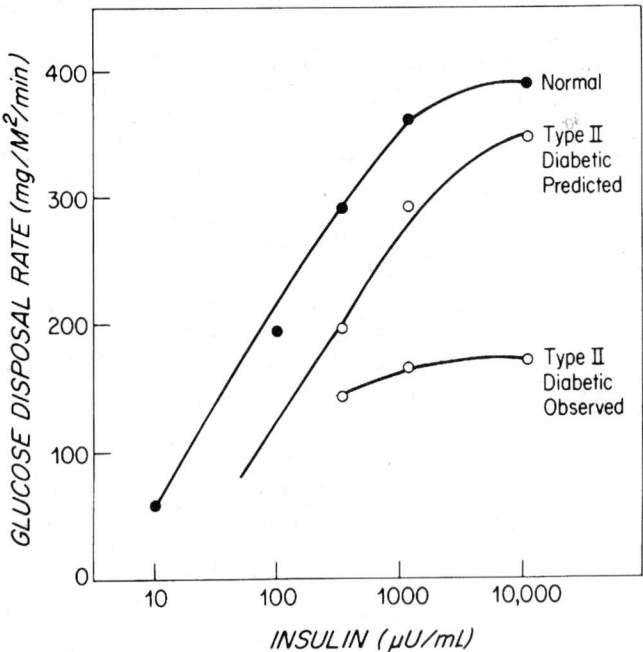

**FIGURE 137-2.** Glucose disposal during a euglycemic clamp in normal patients and in those with type 2 diabetes. Predicted level of insulin resistance, assuming the only defect to be that of insulin binding, was compared with the observed data. The observed data indicate more severe insulin resistance and thus suggest the presence of a postbinding defect as well. (Redrawn from data of Scarlett JA, Gray RS, Griffin J, et al. Insulin treatment reverses the insulin resistance of type II diabetes mellitus. Diabetes Care 1982; 5:353.)

mately culminate in the activation and inhibition of the different cellular processes responsible for the physiologic effects of insulin. Studies of tissues taken from animal models of type 2 diabetes, as well as biopsies of tissues from humans with the disease, have revealed multiple alterations, including defects at the insulin receptor (e.g., binding and kinase activation) and at several of the postreceptor steps involved in insulin action.

Decreased insulin-receptor binding has been described in obese and thin individuals with type 2 diabetes[23,24] (Fig. 137-3). This decrease in binding is attributable to a decrease in receptor

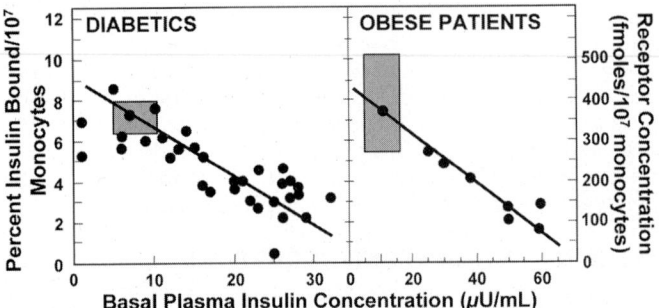

**FIGURE 137-3.** Defect in insulin-receptor binding in diabetes and obesity. The negative relation between receptor concentration and plasma insulin concentration is illustrated. Data are plotted as insulin binding versus plasma insulin concentration. *Shaded areas* indicate the normal range. Data on the left are from thin and obese patients with type 2 diabetes and data on the right are from obese individuals with and without diabetes. (Data for diabetic patients from Kahn CR. Insulin action, diabetogenes, and the cause of type II diabetes [Banting lecture]. Diabetes 1994; 43[8]:1066; and from Ferrannini E, Mari A. How to measure insulin sensitivity. J Hypertens 1998; 16[7]:895. Data for obese patients from Caro JF, Sinha MK, Raju SM, et al. Insulin receptor kinase in human skeletal muscle from obese subjects with and without non–insulin-dependent diabetes. J Clin Invest 1987; 79:1330.)

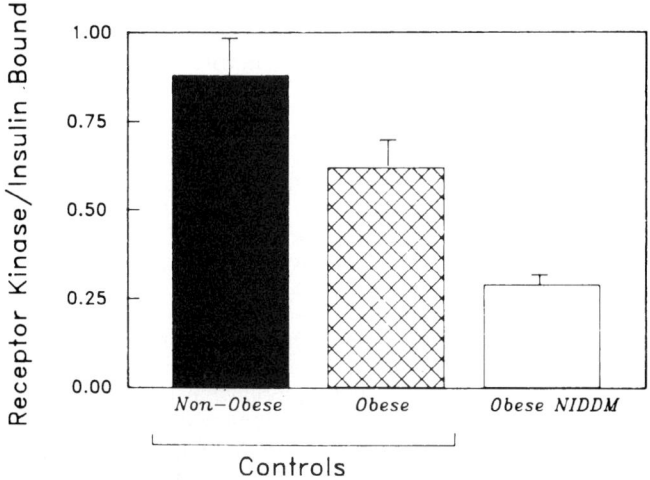

**FIGURE 137-4.** Defect in insulin-receptor kinase activity in type 2 diabetes, in which the activity of this enzyme in liver is decreased by ~50%, even when expressed per receptor. (*NIDDM*, non–insulin-dependent diabetes mellitus.) (Redrawn from Caro JF, Ittoop O, Pories WJ, et al. Studies in the mechanism of insulin resistance in the liver from humans with non–insulin-dependent diabetes. J Clin Invest 1986; 78:249.)

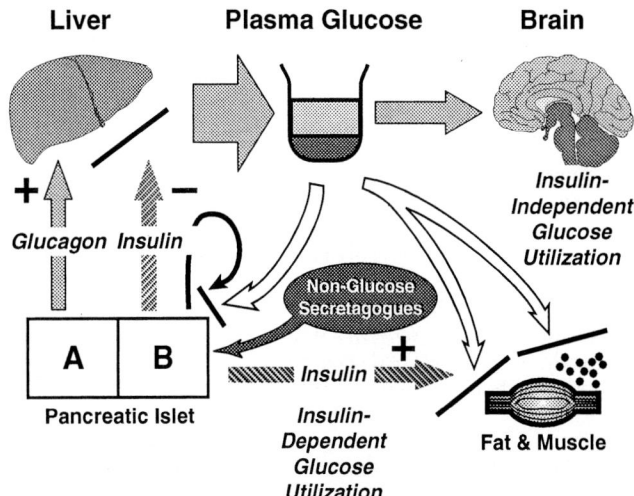

**FIGURE 137-5.** Schema for pathogenesis of type 2 diabetes, illustrating insulin resistance to glucose uptake at muscle and fat and failure of insulin to suppress hepatic glucose output, coupled with a defect in glucose sensing at the B cell.

number, with no changes in receptor affinity, and is thought to be secondary to *down-regulation* of the receptor by the elevated basal endogenous insulin level.[16,24] Similar decreases in insulin binding are observed in patients with impaired glucose tolerance and in some obese individuals with normal glucose tolerance. These findings indicate that the decrease in insulin receptors alone probably does not entirely account for the insulin resistance. Because "spare" receptors for insulin action are present in many tissues, a decrease in receptors would be expected to produce only a shift in the dose-response curve, with no changes in maximal response (i.e., decreased sensitivity).[22]

As noted previously, euglycemic clamp studies have indicated that both decreased sensitivity and decreased responsiveness to insulin are present, indicating postbinding defects in insulin action.[23] These include defects in activation of the insulin-receptor kinase and phosphorylation of intracellular substrates.[23,25–28] Sequence variations have been identified in several of the proteins involved in insulin signaling, and in the case of insulin-receptor substrate-1 (IRS-1), these occur with increased frequency in patients with type 2 diabetes.[29] Most studies have indicated that a defect in glucose transport is also present due to a defect in glucose transporter translocation[30,31] (Fig. 137-4). Finally, a defect also is present in glycogen synthesis, which forms the major component of nonoxidative glucose metabolism.[6,31] Which of these defects is primary and whether other defects are present in the intracellular steps of insulin action remain unknown; however, some of these alterations can be found in normoglycemic offspring of parents with type 2 diabetes.[31]

Studies in both animal models and cell culture have demonstrated that a number of defects in insulin signaling may be secondary to different metabolic abnormalities present in the type 2 diabetic patient. For example, prolonged exposure to high insulin levels produces postbinding desensitization and receptor down-regulation, suggesting a role for increased basal insulin levels in these defects.[32] The increased levels of tumor necrosis factor-α (TNF-α) and free fatty acids (FFAs), which are also found in obesity, produce insulin resistance by inhibiting the insulin-receptor kinase and by altering postreceptor metabolism, respectively.[33–35] Hyperglycemia, both directly and through the production of intermediates like glucosamine, can also contribute to increasing levels of insulin resistance.[36] Thus, like the defects in insulin secretion, the defects in insulin action are largely reversible when the diabetes is treated and the metabolic abnormalities are corrected. This is true whether the treat-

ment involves diet, oral hypoglycemic agents, or intensive insulin treatment.[36–38] A schematic diagram illustrating the various factors involved in the pathogenesis of type 2 diabetes is shown in Figure 137-5.

## EVENTS IN THE DEVELOPMENT OF TYPE 2 DIABETES

Like type 1 diabetes, type 2 diabetes is preceded by a long prediabetic phase in which glucose-tolerance tests are normal, but insulin resistance is present[17,39-40] (Fig. 137-6). Many patients also pass through a stage of impaired glucose tolerance in which basal and stimulated insulin levels are increased, findings which further suggest that insulin resistance precedes the functional insulin deficiency. At this stage, decreases in insulin-receptor binding and insulin action in muscle and fat can be detected. Fasting hyperglycemia suggests unsuppressed gluco-

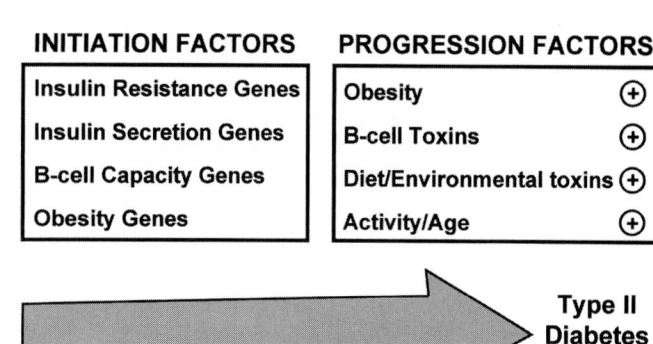

**FIGURE 137-6.** Model of the progressive pathogenesis of type 2 diabetes mellitus.

neogenesis and indicates further resistance to insulin action at the liver. These patients also have a significant functional defect in insulin secretion, especially in glucose recognition.[12,13]

## GENETICS OF TYPE 2 DIABETES

Although type 2 diabetes has a very strong genetic influence, the genes leading to development of this disease are poorly understood. In most patients, type 2 diabetes probably is polygenic in nature, and the polygenes involved may be different among different families or population groups. However, a small number of patients show a monogenic form of type 2 diabetes. These include patients with maturity-onset diabetes of youth (MODY; described below), a few families in whom genetic defects in the insulin molecule lead to generation of a mutant insulin or a failure to process proinsulin and hyperproinsulinemia,[41,42] patients with defects in mitochondrial DNA, and patients with genetic defects in the insulin receptor. In each of these cases, the resulting syndrome usually has clinical features that are distinct from typical type 2 diabetes.

Genetic defects in the insulin receptor have been described in at least 100 individuals, virtually all with different mutations in the gene. Most of these patients have syndromes of severe insulin resistance (e.g., leprechaunism, Rabson-Mendenhall syndrome, or the type A syndrome of insulin resistance and acanthosis nigricans).[43,44] These patients are discussed in Chapter 146.

A variant of type 2 diabetes associated with a point mutation in the gene encoding the transfer RNA for leucine has been described. This gene is present in *mitochondrial DNA rather than in nuclear DNA*. Because mitochondrial DNA is inherited almost exclusively from the mother, this form of diabetes is characterized by a maternal inheritance pattern.[45,46] This condition of diabetes is also associated with nerve deafness and some somatic defects, and may represent as much as 0.8% of type 2 diabetes in some populations.

## RELATED CONDITIONS

### IMPAIRED GLUCOSE TOLERANCE

*Impaired glucose tolerance (IGT)* is present in 7% to 11% of the population, depending on the diagnostic criteria used and the group studied. Recommendations by the American Diabetes Association Expert Committee on the Diagnosis and Classification of Diabetes Mellitus suggested that this diagnosis be based simply on a fasting glucose level of 110 to 125 mg/dL.[47] Many of the characteristics of this population, other than the level of hyperglycemia, are similar to those of patients with type 2 diabetes, suggesting that IGT may be an intermediate step in the development of overt type 2 diabetes.[47,48] IGT may also be a component of syndrome X. The presence of IGT significantly increases the risk of subsequent development of type 2 diabetes, although in many individuals, IGT is transient or does not progress. Researchers at the National Institutes of Health are about to undertake a major study to determine if the progression of IGT to type 2 diabetes can be prevented by changes in lifestyle or pharmacologic intervention.

### GESTATIONAL DIABETES MELLITUS

*Gestational diabetes mellitus* is defined as the development of diabetes during pregnancy in a woman with no previous history of disease (see Chap. 156).[49–52] Gestational diabetes may occur in 2% to 5% of all pregnancies. Although some of these cases represent the coincidence of detection of type 1 or type 2 diabetes with pregnancy, in most patients with true gestational diabetes, the hyperglycemia disappears after delivery. These women have an increased risk of developing type 2 diabetes, which is usually estimated at 2% to 3% per year of follow-up.[49,50] Pathophysiologically, women with gestational diabetes have insulin resistance, as measured in a euglycemic clamp, and decreased early

insulin response to intravenous glucose.[51] These changes are similar to those observed in type 2 diabetes and may reflect an unmasking of the diabetic state by the hormonal milieu of pregnancy, particularly the increased levels of placental lactogen.

### MATURITY-ONSET DIABETES OF YOUTH

From a genetic perspective, the best-characterized subset of patients with type 2 diabetes are those with MODY.[53–59] As implied by the name, this form is characterized by an early age of onset and a strong family history, with affected members in at least three generations, suggesting an autosomal dominant mode of inheritance. Although the typical patient in these kindreds is first found to be diabetic in the teens or 20s, some may be diagnosed as early as 5 years of age. As in other forms of type 2 diabetes, the level of hyperglycemia increases gradually, allowing treatment with diet or sulfonylureas, although in the latter stages of disease some patients require insulin for control of blood glucose. These patients develop the typical chronic complications of diabetes mellitus, including retinopathy, nephropathy, and neuropathy. Pathophysiologically, the disorder is heterogeneous, but in many families, the major defect appears to be relatively low insulin secretion.

Genetic studies have revealed at least five subtypes of MODY. These have been designated *MODY1* through *MODY5*, based on the order in which the genetic loci were identified. All five forms of MODY thus far identified are due to genetic defects impairing B cell function. The most common form of MODY in the United States and in most European countries is MODY3, which is present in 25% to 50% of families that meet the clinical criteria for MODY. This form is due to genetic defects in the nuclear transcription factor *hepatic nuclear factor-1α (HNF-1α)*, a gene that plays a major role in control of insulin synthesis and B-cell function.[53,54] From 10% to 40% of the kindreds have MODY2, in which the molecular abnormalities are genetic defects in the enzyme *glucokinase*.[55,56] Glucokinase is the major form of hexokinase, the enzyme responsible for phosphorylation of glucose to glucose-6-phosphate in the liver and in islets of Langerhans. In the latter site, the enzyme is one of the rate-limiting steps in glucose sensing by the B cell. In comparison with other forms of type 2 diabetes, MODY2 is usually characterized by relatively mild degrees of hyperglycemia and glucose intolerance. *MODY1, MODY4, and MODY5* are also due to defects in the transcription factors HNF-4α, PDX-1, and HNF-1β, respectively. Each of these affects only a few families. In all forms of MODY, the gene involved may have a wide variety of mutations, including point mutations, nonsense mutations leading to premature termination, and splicing defects. This makes screening for these defects more difficult in individual patients. Almost all patients are heterozygous for the mutation, with one normal allele and one mutant allele. The mechanism by which the mutant enzyme becomes dominant over the normal enzyme is poorly understood. The genetic defect in 15% to 30% of families has not yet been determined.[57–59]

## NONDIABETIC MELLITURIA

The presence of some form of sugar in the urine is not necessarily diagnostic of diabetes. At one time, the forms of nondiabetic mellituria were confused with diabetes, but this occurs rarely now that the diagnosis of diabetes is based primarily on blood glucose measurement. Moreover, urinary glucose is determined with more specific glucose oxidase detection systems (e.g., Tes-Tape, Clinistix, Diastix, Chemstrip uG). Nonetheless, sugar in the urine may be due to diseases other than diabetes.

### RENAL GLUCOSURIA

The most commonly recognized nondiabetic mellituria is renal glucosuria.[60] This disorder accounted for as many as 1 of 500 patients referred for evaluation of diabetes when the diagnosis depended primarily on urine glucose measurements. The diagnosis of renal glycosuria requires the detection of glucosuria with simultaneous normal plasma glucose on timed urine samples taken during an oral glucose-tolerance test. Renal glucosuria usually is not associated with other urinary tubular absorptive defects (e.g., aminoaciduria of the Fanconi syndrome should be excluded) and appears to be benign. Some patients with renal glucosuria have mistakenly been treated for decades with insulin. With increased reliance on measurements of serum and capillary glucose and on hemoglobin $A_{1C}$, such mistaken diagnoses should be extremely rare.

Normally, glucose is actively reabsorbed at the proximal renal tubule after filtration at a concentration equal to that in plasma. In normal individuals, the reabsorptive capacity of the proximal tubule exceeds the filtered load of glucose, and little glucosuria occurs with a plasma glucose concentration of <180 mg/dL. Renal glucosuria results predominantly from autosomal recessive abnormalities of glucose transport that decrease the maximum tubular reabsorptive capacity (type A) or decrease the threshold for glucosuria with a normal maximal reabsorptive capacity (type B). A subset of patients with type B renal glycosuria also have intestinal glucose-galactose malabsorption, which presents as watery diarrhea in infants fed diets containing lactose, sucrose, glucose, or galactose. Small bowel biopsies from such patients indicate loss of active transporters for glucose and galactose.

In addition to inherited abnormalities of renal carbohydrate transport, *renal glucosuria* can occur during pregnancy because of a reduced renal threshold for glucose. One cause of renal glycosuria is MODY, because HNF-1α is also important in the development of normal nephron mass; thus, patients with MODY3 diabetes may have a reduced renal threshold for glucose.

## NONGLUCOSE MELLITURIA

Nonglucose melliturias are rare disorders that include hereditary fructose intolerance, congenital galactosemia, essential fructosuria, and essential pentosuria. These disorders are now identified by specific tests but could also be identified by a positive reaction for reducing sugars using alkaline copper reagents in the *absence* of a concomitant positive reaction with glucose oxidase reagent strips. False-positive tests for these reducing sugars may occur when the copper reagents are used, however, because various drugs (e.g., cephalosporins, chloramphenicol, isoniazid, phenacetin, and salicylates) appear in the urine as reducing substances.

### HEREDITARY FRUCTOSE INTOLERANCE

Hereditary fructose intolerance is an autosomal recessive disorder characterized by the lack of fructose-1-phosphate aldolase.[61-63] The deficiency of this enzyme causes an accumulation of fructose-1-phosphate within tissues when foods containing fructose are ingested. Infants usually present with the disease after they have been weaned. The accumulated fructose metabolites are toxic to several tissues, and hepatic cirrhosis and renal proximal tubular damage can result from continued fructose or sorbitol ingestion. Children with fructose intolerance present with severe vomiting and diarrhea and failure to thrive, which resolve after fructose avoidance.

### GALACTOSEMIA

Galactosemia results from autosomal recessive disorders that produce a deficiency of galactose-1-phosphate uridyltransferase (i.e., classic galactosemia) or galactokinase.[64,65] The classic disease is associated with mental retardation and cirrhosis, and both diseases lead to cataract formation. In patients with galactosemia, the ingestion of milk, in which the major carbo-

hydrate is lactose (a disaccharide containing glucose and galactose), elevates serum galactose levels, with attendant vomiting, failure to thrive, jaundice, hepatomegaly, and cataracts. Diagnosis depends on specifically demonstrating galactosemia, galactosuria, and, for the classic disease, a deficiency of the enzyme galactose-1-phosphate uridyltransferase in red blood cells. Therapy consists of consumption of a galactose-free diet.

### ESSENTIAL FRUCTOSURIA

Essential fructosuria results from a deficiency of the enzyme fructokinase, which catalyzes the first step in the metabolism of fructose to fructose-1-phosphate.[66] The disease is transmitted as an autosomal recessive characteristic. After the ingestion of fructose, a large proportion of the saccharide remains in the blood and is cleared in the urine. Perhaps because the initial step in metabolism is blocked and cellular metabolites do not accumulate, essential fructosuria is a benign, asymptomatic condition requiring no therapy.

### ESSENTIAL PENTOSURIA

Essential pentosuria has been found in ~1 in 40,000 persons receiving insurance examinations and in ~1 of 2000 American Jews.[67] A benign condition inherited as an autosomal recessive trait, it results from a deficiency of the enzyme converting xylitol to xylulose; L-xylulose is excreted in the urine.[64]

## REFERENCES

1. U.S. Department of Health & Human Services, Centers for Disease Control and Prevention. Diabetes in the United States: a strategy for prevention. 1994.
2. Harris MI. Epidemiology of diabetes mellitus among the elderly in the United States. Clin Geriatr Med 1990; 6:703.
3. Pi-Sunyer FX. Medical hazards of obesity. Ann Intern Med 1993; 119:655.
4. Barnett AH, Eff C, Leslie RDG, Pyke DA. Diabetes in identical twins: a study of 200 pairs. Diabetologia 1981; 20:87.
5. Leslie RDG, Pyke DA. Genetics of diabetes. In: Alberti KGGM, Krall LP, eds. The diabetes annual III. New York: Elsevier, 1987:39.
6. Gepts W. The pathology of the pancreas in human diabetes. In: Andreani D, Federlin KF, DiMario U, Heding LG, eds. Immunology in diabetes. London: Kimpton Publishers, 1984:21.
7. DeFronzo RA. The triumvirate B-cell, muscle, liver: a collusion responsible for NIDDM. Diabetes 1988; 37:667.
8. Savage PJ, Dippe SE, Bennett PH, et al. Hyperinsulinemia and hypoinsulinemia: insulin responses to oral carbohydrate over a wide spectrum of glucose tolerance. Diabetes 1975; 24:262.
9. Porte D. Beta-cells in type II diabetes mellitus. Diabetes 1990; 40:166.
10. Clark A, Wells CA, Buley ID, et al. Islet amyloid, increased A-cells, reduced B-cells and exocrine fibrosis: quantitative changes in the pancreas in type 2 diabetes. Diabetes Res 1988; 9(4):151.
11. Sims EAH, Danforth E Jr, Horton ES, et al. Endocrine and metabolic effects of experimental obesity in man. Recent Prog Horm Res 1973; 29:457.
12. Porte D Jr. Banting lecture 1990. B-cells in type II diabetes mellitus. Diabetes 1991; 40(2):166.
13. Polonsky KS, Sturis J, Bell GI. Non-insulin dependent diabetes mellitus—a genetically programmed failure of the beta cell to compensate for insulin resistance. N Engl J Med 1996; 334(12):777.
14. Leahy JL, Bonner-Weir S, Weir GC. B-cell dysfunction induced by chronic hyperglycemia—current ideas on mechanisms of impaired glucose-induced insulin secretion. Diabetes Care 1992; 15:442.
15. Vague P, Moulin J. The defective glucose sensitivity of the β-cell in non-insulin dependent diabetes: improvement after 20 hrs. of normoglycemia. Metabolism 1982; 31:139.
16. Todd JF, Wilding JP, Edwards CM, et al. Glucagon-like peptide-1 (GLP-1): a trial of treatment in non-insulin-dependent diabetes mellitus. Eur J Clin Invest 1997 June; 27(6):533.
17. Kahn CR. Insulin action, diabetogenes, and the cause of type II diabetes (Banting lecture). Diabetes 1994; 43(8):1066.
18. Kissebah AH, Vydelingum N, Murray R. Relation of body fat distribution to metabolic complications of obesity. J Clin Invest 1982; 54:254.
19. Reaven GM. Role of insulin resistance in human disease. Diabetes 1988; 37:1595.
20. Karam JH. Type II diabetes and syndrome X. Pathogenesis and glycemic management. Endocrin Metab Clin North Am 1992; 21:329.
21. Ferrannini E, Mari A. How to measure insulin sensitivity. J Hypertens 1998; 16(7):895.
22. Kahn CR. Insulin resistance, insulin insensitivity and insulin unresponsiveness: a necessary distinction. Metabolism 1978; 27:1893.

23. Olefsky JM, Nolan JJ. Insulin resistance and non insulin-dependent diabetes mellitus: cellular and molecular mechanisms. Am J Clin Nutr 1995; 61(Suppl 4):980S.

24. Bar RS, Harrison LC, Muggeo M, et al. Regulation of insulin receptors in normal and abnormal physiology in humans. Adv Intern Med 1979; 24:23.

25. Caro JF, Sinha MK, Raju SM, et al. Insulin receptor kinase in human skeletal muscle from obese subjects with and without non-insulin-dependent diabetes. J Clin Invest 1987; 79:1330.

26. Mandarino LJ, Campbell PJ, Gottesman IS, et al. Abnormal coupling of insulin receptor binding in non-insulin dependent diabetes. Am J Physiol 1987; 247:E688.

27. Caro JF, Ittoop O, Pories WJ, et al. Studies in the mechanism of insulin resistance in the liver from humans with non-insulin-dependent diabetes. J Clin Invest 1986; 78:249.

28. Obermaier-Kusser B, White MF, Pongrantz DE, et al. A defective intramolecular autoactivation cascade may be the cause of reduced kinase activity in the skeletal muscle insulin receptor from patients with non-insulin dependent diabetes mellitus. J Biol Chem 1989; 264:9497.

29. Alnund KB, Orback C, Vestergaard H, et al. Amino acid polymorphisms of insulin receptor substrate-1 in non-insulin dependent diabetes mellitus. Lancet 1993; 342:828.

30. Rondinone CM, Carvalho E, Wesslau EC, et al. Impaired glucose transport and protein kinase B activation by insulin, but not okadaic acid, in adipocytes from subjects with Type II diabetes mellitus. Diabetologia 1999; 42:819.

31. Rothman DL, Magnusson I, Cline G, et al. Decreased muscle glucose transport/phosphorylation is an early defect in the pathogenesis of non-insulin-dependent diabetes mellitus. Proc Natl Acad Sci U S A 1995; 92:983.

32. Inoue G, Cheatham B, Kahn CR. Different pathways of post-receptor desensitization following chronic insulin treatment and in cells overexpressing constitutively active insulin receptors. J Biol Chem 1996; 271(45):28206.

33. Hotamisligil GS, Budavari A, Murray D, et al. Reduced tyrosine kinase activity of the insulin receptor in obesity-diabetes. Central role of tumor necrosis factor alpha. J Clin Invest 1994; 94(4):1543.

34. Groop LC, Saloranta C, Shank M, et al. The role of free fatty acid metabolism in the pathogenesis of insulin resistance in obesity and noninsulin-dependent diabetes mellitus. J Clin Endocrinol Metab 1991; 72(1):96.

35. Jucker BM, Rennings AJM, Cline GW, et al. $^{13}$C and $^{31}$P NMR studies on the effects of increased plasma free fatty acids on intramuscular glucose metabolism in the awake rat. J Biol Chem 1997; 272(16):10464.

36. Baron AD, Zhu JS, Zhu JH, et al. Glucosamine induces insulin resistance in vivo by affecting GLUT4 translocation in skeletal muscle: implications for glucose toxicity. J Clin Invest 1995; 96(6):2792.

37. Simonson DC, Ferranini E, Bevilacqua S, et al. Mechanism of improvement in glucose metabolism after chronic glyburide therapy. Diabetes 1984; 33:838.

38. Andrews WJ, Vasques B, Nagulesparan M, et al. Insulin therapy in obese, non-insulin dependent diabetes induces improvements in insulin action and secretion that are maintained for two weeks after insulin withdrawal. Diabetes 1984; 33:634.

39. Gavey WT, Olefsky JM, Griffin J, et al. The effect of insulin treatment on insulin secretion and insulin action in type II diabetes mellitus. Diabetes 1985; 34:222.

40. Knowler WC, Pettitt DJ, Saad MF, et al. Diabetes mellitus in the Pima Indians: incidence, risk factors and pathogenesis. Diabetes Metab Rev 1990; 6:1027.

41. Martin BC, Warram JH, Krolewski AS, et al. Role of glucose and insulin resistance in development of Type II diabetes mellitus: results of a 25-year follow-up study. Lancet 1992; 340:925.

42. Tager HS. Lilly lecture 1983: abnormal products of the human insulin gene. Diabetes 1984; 33:693.

43. Sanz N, Karam JH, Horita S, et al. Prevalence of insulin-gene mutations in non-insulin-dependent diabetes mellitus. (Letter). N Engl J Med 1986; 314:1322.

44. Flier JS. Lilly lecture: syndromes of insulin resistance from patient to gene and back again. Diabetes 1992; 41:1207.

45. Taylor SI. Lilly lecture: molecular mechanisms of insulin resistance—lessons from patients with mutations in the insulin receptor gene. Diabetes 1992; 41:1473.

46. Reardon W, Ross RJ, Sweeney MG, et al. Diabetes mellitus associated with a pathogenic point mutation in mitochondrial DNA. Lancet 1992; 340:1376.

47. Kadowaki T, Kadowaki H, Mori Y, et al. A subtype of diabetes mellitus associated with a mutation of mitochondrial DNA. N Engl J Med 1994; 330:962.

48. Report of the Expert Committee on the Diagnosis and Classification of Diabetes Mellitus. Diabetes Care 1997; 20:1183.

49. Harris MI. Impaired glucose tolerance in the United States population. Diabetes Care 1989; 12:464.

50. Kjos SL, Buchanan TA, Greenspoon JS, et al. Gestational diabetes mellitus: the prevalence of glucose intolerance and diabetes mellitus in the first two months postpartum. Am J Obstet Gynecol 1990; 163:93.

51. O'Sullivan JB. Diabetes mellitus after GDM. Diabetes 1993; 40:131.

52. Catalano PM, Tyzbir ED, Wolfe RR, et al. Carbohydrate metabolism during pregnancy in control subjects with gestational diabetes. Am J Physiol 1993; 264:E60.

53. Fajans SS, Bell GI, Bowden DW. MODY: a model for the study of the molecular genetics of NIDDM. J Lab Clin Med 1992; 119:206.

53a. Costa A, Bescos M, Velho G, et al. Genetic and clinical characterization of maturity-onset diabetes of the young in Spanish families. Eur J Endocrinol 2000; 142:380.

54. Yamagata K, Oda N, Kaisaki PJ, et al. Mutations in the hepatocyte nuclear factor-1alpha gene in maturity-onset diabetes of the young. Nature 1996; 384(6608):455.

55. Lehto M, Tuomi T, Mahtani MM, et al. Characterization of the MODY3 phenotype. Early-onset diabetes caused by an insulin secretion defect. J Clin Invest 1997; 99(4):582.

56. Froguel P, Zouali H, Vionnet N, et al. Familial hyperglycemia due to mutations in glucokinase. Definition of a subtype of diabetes mellitus. N Engl J Med 1993; 328:697.

57. Hattersley AT, Turner RC, Permutt MA, et al. Linkage of type 2 diabetes to the glucokinase gene. Lancet 1992; 339:1307.

58. Bell GI, Xiang KS, Newman MV, et al. Gene for non-insulin-dependent diabetes mellitus (maturity-onset diabetes of the young subtype) is linked to DNA polymorphism on human chromosome 20q. Proc Natl Acad Sci U S A 1991; 88:1484.

59. Doria A, Yang Y, Malecki M, et al. Phenotypic characteristics of early-onset autosomal-dominant type 2 diabetes unlinked to known maturity-onset diabetes of the young (MODY) genes. Diabetes Care 1999; 22(2): 253.

60. Brodehl J, Oemar BS, Hoyer PF. Renal glucosuria. Pediatr Nephrol 1987; 1(3):502.

61. Froesch ER. Essential fructosuria, hereditary fructose intolerance and fructose-1,6-diphosphatase deficiency. In: Stanbury JB, Wyngaarden JB, Frederickson DS, eds. The metabolic basis of inherited disease, 4th ed. New York: McGraw-Hill, 1978:121.

62. Chambers RA, Pratt RTC. Idiosyncrasy to fructose. Lancet 1956; 2:340.

63. Rellos P, Sygusch J, Corx TM. Expression, purification, and characterization of natural mutants of human aldolase B. Role of Quaternary structure in catalysis. J Biol Chem 2000; 275:1145.

64. Segal S. Disorders of galactose metabolism. In: Stanbury JB, Wyngaarden JB, Frederickson DS, eds. The metabolic basis of inherited disease, 4th ed. New York: McGraw-Hill, 1978:160.

65. Kolosha V, Anoia E, de Cespedes C, et al. Novel mutations in 13 probands with galactokinase deficiency. Hum Mutat 2000; 15:447.

66. Schapira F, Schapira G, Dreyfus JC. La lésion enzymatique de la fructosuria bénigne. Enzymol Biol Clin (Basel) 1970; 1:1961.

67. Hiatt HH. Pentosuria. In: Stanbury JB, Wyngaarden JB, Frederickson DS, eds. The metabolic basis of inherited disease, 4th ed. New York: McGraw-Hill, 1978:110.

# CHAPTER 138

# NATURAL HISTORY OF DIABETES MELLITUS

ANDRZEJ S. KROLEWSKI AND JAMES H. WARRAM

Knowledge of the natural history of diabetes and its complications is important both to the practicing endocrinologist and to the diabetes researcher. For example, advice to patients about the value of various preventive actions depends on an awareness of the probability that a patient will develop diabetes or its complications. Also, any valuable etiologic hypothesis must account for features of the natural history of diabetes and its complications in humans, not animals.

## MEASURES OF OCCURRENCE

Information on how diabetes occurrence differs in human populations according to age, sex, socioeconomic status, geography, or DNA polymorphisms may be useful in generating etiologic hypotheses as well as in testing hypotheses generated in clinical and laboratory settings.

The *incidence rate* measures the effect of a force of nature (force of morbidity) acting on a population to produce some number of transitions from health to disease.[1] Incidence rates of diabetes during the 1960s are shown in Table 138-1 for various age categories of the population of Rochester, Minnesota.[2,3] In the span of a year, between 6 and 25 of every 100,000 healthy individuals (depending on the age) developed diabetes and required treatment with insulin. Most of these patients can be considered to have insulin-dependent (IDDM) or type 1 diabetes. The incidence rate for non–insulin-dependent diabetes

**TABLE 138-1.**

**Age-Specific Incidence Rates of Diabetes Per 100,000 Per Year in Rochester, Minnesota, in 1960–1969 According to Type of Diabetes**

| Age (Years) | Type 1 Diabetes | Type 2 Diabetes |
|---|---|---|
| 0–9 | 6.5 | 0.0 |
| 10–19 | 12.5 | 7.5 |
| 20–29 | 9.6 | 9.6 |
| 30–39 | 6.9 | 66.8 |
| 40–49 | 17.2 | 155.2 |
| 50–59 | 25.8 | 322.2 |
| 60–69 | 26.9 | 612.8 |
| Cumulative incidence by age 70 per 1000* | **10.5** | **111.0** |

*Net cumulative incidence by the life-table method.[4] For a cumulative incidence of <10%, a good approximation can be obtained simply by summing the incidence rates over the age groups after multiplying them by 10 (the number of years in the age intervals).
(Data from Melton LJ, Palumbo PJ, Chu C. Incidence of diabetes mellitus by clinical type. Diabetes Care 1983; 6:75; and from Melton LJ, Palumbo PJ, Dwyer MS, Chu C. Impact of recent changes in diagnostic criteria on the apparent natural history of diabetes mellitus. Am J Epidemiol 1983; 117:559.)

(NIDDM, or type 2 diabetes) in the same community was similar for the population between the ages of 10 and 29, then rose rapidly to 613 per 100,000 by the seventh decade of life. Incidence rates for both type 1 and type 2 diabetes are slightly higher in men than in women.[4,5]

An informative technique for summarizing this set of age-specific incidence rates is the *cumulative incidence*.[6] For illustration, suppose 1000 individuals were followed from birth to age 70, and they were subject at each age to the age-specific rates shown in Table 138-1. Ten would have developed type 1 diabetes by age 70 and >10 times as many (i.e., 111) would have developed type 2 diabetes by this age.

In many situations, however, the time of onset of the diabetes cannot be determined. All one can do is count individuals with diabetes (preexisting as well as recent cases) in the population at a specific point in time and express this number as a proportion or *prevalence*. Figure 138-1 shows the prevalence of diabetes in a random sample of adults in the U.S. population from 1988 to 1994.[7] Whereas Table 138-1 shows the incidence rates of diagnosed diabetes, Figure 138-1 shows the prevalence of diagnosed and undiagnosed diabetes together, and the prev-

alence of impaired fasting glucose. The prevalence of each condition increased with age. Because type 1 diabetes is very rare in the population in comparison with type 2 diabetes, the prevalence data in Figure 138-1 reflect mainly type 2 diabetes. The prevalence of undiagnosed diabetes was ~50% of that of diagnosed diabetes. In addition, almost the same proportion of the U.S. population in each age category had impaired fasting glucose, a condition carrying a high risk of progression to type 2 diabetes. In the total adult U.S. population, 5.3% had diagnosed diabetes, 2.8% had undiagnosed diabetes, and an additional 6.9% had impaired fasting glucose.

## DISTRIBUTION OF TYPE 1 DIABETES

Type 1 diabetes results from the selective destruction of the B cells responsible for insulin secretion within the islets of Langerhans in the pancreas. The disease develops as a result of an autoimmune reaction directed against the B cells[8,9] (see Chap. 136). The destruction of B cells persists for years and possibly decades before the disease is manifested.[10–12] The autoantigen that triggers the initial activation of the immune system remains unknown.

The incidence rates of type 1 diabetes listed in Table 138-1 show two peaks: the first in the second decade of life (around puberty) and the second during the sixth and seventh decades. This pattern suggests that the factors responsible for destruction of B cells might be different in one or more ways in the young and in the elderly. Little is known about the occurrence of the disease in middle or old age because most studies have concentrated on its occurrence in the young.

The incidence rate of the illness in children and teenagers in the United States has increased several-fold during the past 30 years.[13,14] Similar secular trends have been reported in many European countries, particularly the United Kingdom, Denmark, Norway, Sweden, and Finland.[15,16] Despite these similar trends, the actual incidence rates vary considerably among countries (Fig. 138-2).[17,18] During the 1980s the incidence rate was 29 per 100,000 per year in Finland (i.e., northern Europe), 6

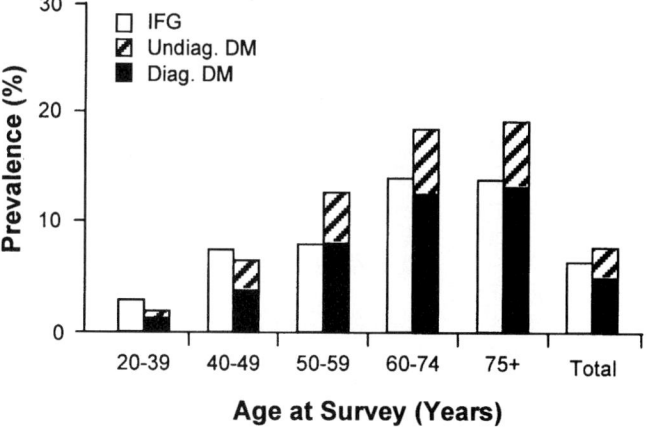

**FIGURE 138-1.** Prevalence of diagnosed diabetes (*Diag. DM*), undiagnosed diabetes (*Undiag. DM*), and impaired fasting glucose (*IFG*) in U.S. adults by age. (Adapted from data in Harris MI, Goldstein DE, Flegal KM, et al. Prevalence of diabetes, impaired fasting glucose, and impaired glucose tolerance in U.S. adults. The third National Health and Nutrition Examination Survey, 1988–1994. Diabetes Care 1998; 21:518.)

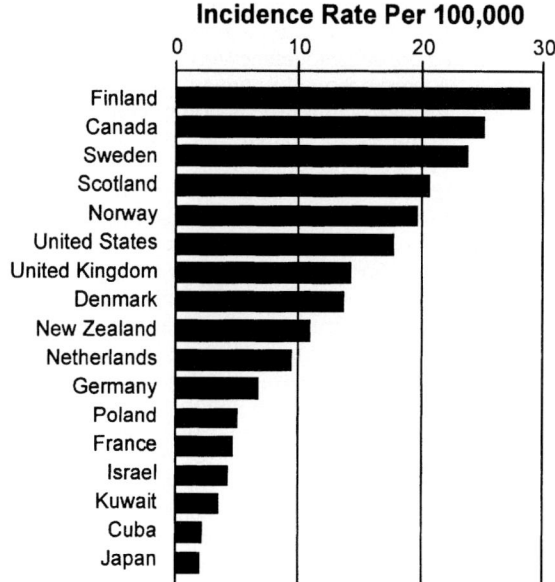

**FIGURE 138-2.** Incidence rate of type 1 diabetes in children younger than 15 years of age (per 100,000) in various populations. (Adapted from Patrick SL, Moy CS, LaPorte RE. The world of insulin-dependent diabetes mellitus: what international epidemiologic studies reveal about the etiology and natural history of IDDM. Diabetes Metab Rev 1989; 5:571.)

to 10 in central Europe, and around 3 in the south and in Israel. Sardinia was an exception to this gradient and had an incidence rate equal to that of Finland.[18] In the United States, the incidence rate of type 1 diabetes in Allegheny County, Pennsylvania, was 19 per 100,000 per year.[17]

## ENVIRONMENTAL FACTORS

The secular trend and geographic variation in the occurrence of type 1 diabetes in young populations resembles the gradual emergence of poliomyelitis as an important childhood disease early in this century. In the wake of improvements in sanitation, the first exposure to the poliovirus was delayed from infancy, when susceptibility to neurologic involvement is low, to an age when it is greater.[19] By analogy, delayed infection with some agent may be a cause of the rising incidence of type 1 diabetes. Although attempts to associate the occurrence of the disease with a specific infectious agent or other environmental exposure have been unsuccessful so far,[20–22] the hypothesis needs further evaluation. Following the analogy with poliomyelitis, these efforts assumed a short latent period, which is not the case for type 1 diabetes. The clinical manifestation of the illness is preceded by a very long preclinical period (years to decades) of autoimmune destruction of B cells.[23]

Breast-feeding is a factor that protects children from the development of type 1 diabetes.[24,25] The lack of it, however, accounts for only a small proportion of the disease cases. Interestingly, when the period of breast-feeding is short, children are exposed very early in life to cow's milk proteins. The latter have been implicated as factors that might increase the risk of the disease.[26,27] The evidence is still only circumstantial, and further studies are required.[22,28,29]

## GENETIC FACTORS

The development of type 1 diabetes is influenced by genetic factors. In a population-based study of twins, the risk of diabetes in the twins of probands with type 1 diabetes was 53% if the twins were monozygous and 11% if they were dizygous.[30] The latter figure is similar to the risk to nontwin siblings of probands with type 1 diabetes.[5] Examination of the risk to other categories of relatives of the probands led to the conclusion that the mode of inheritance of susceptibility to type 1 diabetes is complex and involves a major gene effect together with polygenes.[31]

As of now, 18 chromosomal regions have been linked with type 1 diabetes in studies that used genome-wide mapping and examine affected sib pairs.[32,33] Only the one on chromosome arm 6p, the HLA class II region, contains a major locus, which accounts for at least 40% of the familial clustering of the illness. The other regions, not all of which have been replicated, seem to have minor effects.[32,33]

The first evidence for the role of HLA was the association of type 1 diabetes with HLA-B8 and HLA-B15 and then with the HLA-DR3 and HLA-DR4 antigens.[34,35] Regardless of the overall risk of the illness in a population, almost 95% of patients with type 1 diabetes have HLA-DR3 or HLA-DR4 antigens.[5,34,35] Subsequent studies based on DNA genotypes showed that certain alleles of the DQB1 and DQA1 genes were even more strongly associated with type 1 diabetes.[36,37]

Studies have demonstrated that haplotypes formed by alleles at all three loci (i.e., DRB1, DQA1, and DQB1) influence type 1 diabetes susceptibility.[38] Haplotypes formed of the following alleles predispose to the illness: at DRB1*0301 & *0405, at DQA1*0301 & *0501, and at DQB1*0302 & *0201.[38] Haplotype analysis also showed that among different combinations of the DRB1-DQA1-DQB1 alleles a single dose of certain alleles (i.e., DRB1*0403 or DQB1*0301) is sufficient to confer protection against the illness.[38]

Some have hypothesized that the frequency of susceptible as well as protective haplotypes may account for a significant part of variability in the incidence of type 1 diabetes among coun-

tries (see Fig. 138-2). Results consistent with this hypothesis were obtained when prevalences of HLA risk alleles (not whole haplotypes) were investigated in countries with different risk of the disease.[39,40] In all populations, however, only a small proportion of carriers of HLA susceptibility alleles develop type 1 diabetes.[5,39,40] This implies that susceptibility alleles at other non-HLA loci (or unknown environmental factors) must interact (have an epistatic effect) with risk alleles at HLA loci to cause the development of the disease.

## DISTRIBUTION OF TYPE 2 DIABETES

Two processes underlie the development of type 2 diabetes: insulin resistance and failure in insulin secretion.[41,42] The rise in the incidence rate of the condition from 8 per 100,000 per year at age 15 to 613 per 100,000 per year at age 65 (see Table 138-1) dramatically illustrates the powerful effect of age on these processes. Research has shown lessening insulin secretory capacity with age, but the mechanisms are unknown.[43,44] Resistance to insulin action also increases with age,[45–47] but how much of this increase is attributable merely to diminished physical activity or the relative increase in fat that accompanies aging is not clear.

Variability is seen among populations in the occurrence of type 2 diabetes (Fig. 138-3).[5] A higher prevalence of the illness is seen in Native Americans, Mexican Americans, and blacks than in Americans of European origin. The prevalence of type 2 diabetes in this last group, however, is two to three times higher than in Europe. Part of this variability can be explained by differences among populations in the frequency of obesity, level of physical activity, and dietary habits—all factors that are associated with the level of affluence. Much of it remains unexplained, however, and must be attributed to unknown environmental or genetic factors.

### OBESITY

The major risk factor influencing the incidence of type 2 diabetes is the degree of obesity. Figure 138-4 shows that the risk of

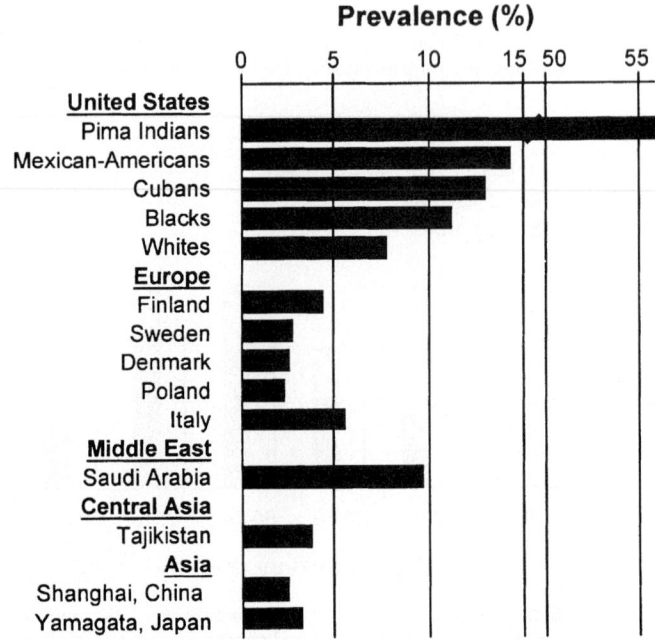

**FIGURE 138-3.** Prevalence of type 2 diabetes in men aged 45 to 54 years in various populations screened for undiagnosed diabetes. (Adapted from Warram JH, Rich SS, Krolewski AS. Epidemiology and genetics of diabetes mellitus. In: Kahn CR, Weir GC, eds. Joslin's diabetes mellitus, 13th ed. Philadelphia: Lea & Febiger, 1994:201.)

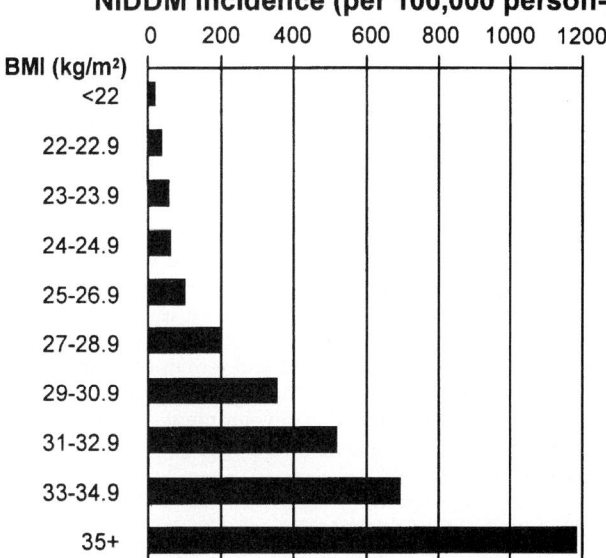

**NIDDM Incidence (per 100,000 person-yr)**

FIGURE 138-4. Incidence rate of type 2 diabetes according to body mass index (*BMI*) in a large cohort of U.S. women followed for 14 years. (*NIDDM*, non–insulin-dependent diabetes or type 2 diabetes.) (Adapted from data in Colditz GA, Willett WC, Rotnitzky A, Manson JE. Weight gain as a risk factor for clinical diabetes mellitus in women. Ann Intern Med 1995; 122:48.)

the illness rose exponentially with increasing body mass index (BMI) in a large cohort study of U.S. women followed for 14 years.[48] The incidence rate increased from 13 per 100,000 person-years for women with a BMI of <22, to 104 for those with a BMI of 25 to 26.9, and then to 1190 for those with a BMI of ≥35. Similar findings were reported in men.[49,50] In addition, a pattern of *centrally distributed body fat* (also called *visceral adiposity*) appears to increase the risk of type 2 diabetes more than does a similar degree of excess that is more uniformly distributed.[49,51] Potentially important issues, such as the duration of obesity, the role of obesity in diminished physical activity, and the source of excess calories, have not been fully explored (see also Chap. 126).

### GENETIC FACTORS

The distribution of type 2 diabetes is influenced by familial factors that are interpreted as genetic susceptibilities. A high prevalence of diabetes among relatives of affected individuals has been demonstrated in many studies.[52–55] Also, a history of diabetes in relatives is a significant risk factor for the condition in population studies.[48,56] Compared with the general population, the risk of type 2 diabetes is four times higher in the siblings of persons with diabetes and about eight times higher in the offspring of two parents with the condition.[5,57,58] The risk seems to be even higher in monozygotic twins of index cases.[59]

A series of genetic models have been evaluated, using these data, to estimate the number of genes involved in type 2 diabetes susceptibility.[31] The conclusion was that the pattern of risk to relatives of persons with the illness is compatible with inheritance based on only a few interacting loci plus polygenes (many genes having small additive effects) or shared family environment. This result suggests the possibility of identifying several single genes with moderate effects on type 2 diabetes susceptibility.

Over the last decade, an intensive effort has been under way to identify these genes. In studies using a *candidate genes* approach, mutations in several genes have been found to be responsible for segregation of diabetes in families with an auto-

somal dominant pattern of inheritance and young age of manifestation of diabetes. These are termed *MODY* (maturity-onset diabetes of youth) genes.[60,61] Mutations in these genes account for the development of diabetes in only a small proportion of patients with type 2 diabetes.

Genome-wide linkage in several family collections with onset of type 2 diabetes in middle age found some evidence for linkage but, unfortunately, linkage with different chromosomal regions. In Pima Indians, suggestive evidence for linkage was found on chromosome arm 11q.[62] In Mexican Americans, strong evidence for linkage was found on the long arm of chromosome 2.[63] In whites, in separate studies, evidence for linkage has been found on 1q, 12q, and 20q.[64–66] The region on chromosome arm 20q had been found previously to be linked with type 2 diabetes.[67–69] Overall, the linkage data are consistent with the hypothesis that several susceptibility genes that have moderate additive effects may exist for the illness.[31] So far, none of the described linkages has led to the identification of any of these genes.

## DISTRIBUTION OF LATE DIABETIC COMPLICATIONS

Diabetes is truly a chronic disease, one in which the complications of the kidney, eyes, and heart develop over many years, sometimes decades, after the onset of hyperglycemia. The patterns of the development of these complications according to duration of type 1 diabetes are shown in Figure 138-5. As can be seen, the pattern of occurrence of each of these complications is different, a finding which suggests that different etiologies must be involved. Although the level of glycemic control plays a role in the development of each of these complications,[70–72] other organ-specific genetic or environmental factors are also necessary.[73]

### NEPHROPATHY

Diabetic nephropathy can be recognized clinically as persistent proteinuria, which subsequently progresses (at a variable rate) to end-stage renal failure. The incidence rate of persistent proteinuria in patients with type 1 diabetes increases with the duration of diabetes during the first 15 years and then declines (see Fig. 138-5*A*).[74] Overall, only one of three individuals with the illness ever develops nephropathy, suggesting that the susceptibility to this complication is limited to a subset of diabetic patients that is depleted over time.[73] The accumulating evidence favors genetic factors as the underlying determinant of this susceptibility.[75,75a] Uncontrolled diabetes (hyperglycemia), however, is a necessary factor for the development of nephropathy,[70–72] although other environmental factors as well as the previously mentioned genetic factors may be required to complete a sufficient set of causes. The ability to identify individuals who are at high risk for diabetic nephropathy due to genetic predisposition or environmental damage would be very useful. With this knowledge, a target group can be identified, and special effort can be undertaken to control hyperglycemia or to treat patients with angiotensin-converting enzyme inhibitors (see also Chap. 150).

### RETINOPATHY

All patients with type 1 diabetes and many of those with type 2 diabetes develop some degree of background retinopathy within the first 5 to 15 years of diabetes.[76,77] Once patients reach this stage, they become susceptible to proliferative retinopathy. The incidence rate of proliferative retinopathy is almost nil during the first 10 years of diabetes[78] (see Fig. 138-5*B*), but thereafter it increases rapidly to 30 per 1000 per year and remains at this level during the subsequent 30 years. The absence of any decline in risk over that span of years suggests that all patients

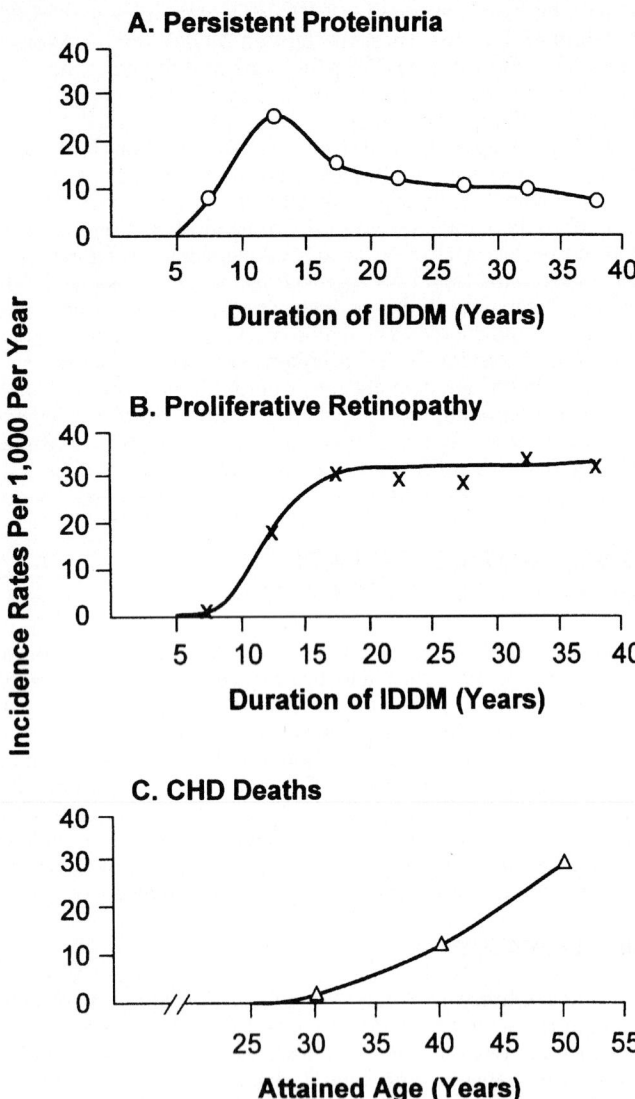

**FIGURE 138-5.** Incidence rates of late complications of type 1 diabetes according to years of duration based on data from a 40-year follow-up of 292 patients with a juvenile onset. **A,** Persistent proteinuria was defined as albuminuria >30 mg/dL in random specimens on three consecutive clinic visits. **B,** Proliferative retinopathy was diagnosed if any of the following lesions was observed: new vessels (regardless of the location in the retinal fundus), vitreous or preretinal hemorrhage, or fibrous proliferation. **C,** Coronary heart disease (*CHD*) death was defined as death with documented myocardial infarction (regardless of the immediate cause of death) or history of angina with subsequent sudden death or congestive heart failure. (*IDDM*, insulin-dependent or type 1 diabetes.) (Data from Krolewski AS, Warram JH, Christlieb AR, et al. The changing natural history of nephropathy in type I diabetes. Am J Med 1985; 78:785; Krolewski AS, Warram JH, Rand LI, et al. Risk of proliferative retinopathy in juvenile onset type I diabetes: 40 years follow-up study. Diabetes Care 1986; 9:443; and Krolewski AS, Kosinski E, Warram JH, et al. Magnitude and determinants of coronary artery disease in juvenile-onset, insulin-dependent diabetes mellitus. Am J Cardiol 1987; 59:750.)

are susceptible to this severe eye complication and will develop it if followed long enough. The actual rate of development of proliferative retinopathy is related to the level of glycemic control[78–80]; therefore, the incidence rates shown in Figure 138-5B reflect the distribution of glycemic control achieved by this particular study population. Thus, whereas 60% had proliferative retinopathy after 40 years of diabetes, that proportion would have been reached in a shorter time if more individuals with poor control had been included. Conversely, perhaps 50 or

60 years would have been required to reach this level if patients' control had been better (see Chap. 151).

## NEPHROPATHY–RETINOPATHY INTERRELATIONS

Comparison of the incidence rates of persistent proteinuria and severe eye complications (see Figs. 138-5A and B) reveals quite different patterns according to the duration of diabetes. However, a peculiar association is found between the two. In a study of 292 patients with type 1 diabetes at the Joslin Diabetes Center who were followed for 20 to 40 years, almost all patients who developed nephropathy also developed proliferative retinopathy either at the same time or within a few years. In the same cohort, however, a similar number of individuals developed only proliferative retinopathy and remained without any clinical evidence of nephropathy through many years of subsequent follow-up.[78] Whether the development of proliferative retinopathy in these two situations is attributable to the same causal factors is unknown.

## CORONARY HEART DISEASE

In many countries, most notably the United States, the ultimate complication for patients with diabetes is coronary heart disease (CHD).[81,82,82a] Morphologically, atherosclerosis in the coronary arteries has the same characteristics in diabetic patients as in nondiabetic individuals. However, the changes are more frequent and their distribution more diffuse, particularly in patients with type 1 diabetes.[83–86] Consequently, individuals with diabetes have a higher incidence rate of CHD and a lower chance of surviving a myocardial infarction than do nondiabetic persons. Regardless of the age at onset of diabetes (0 to 20 years in this study), symptoms or death from CHD are rare before age 35. Thereafter, the mortality rate increases rapidly with increasing age, so that, by age 55, one of three patients with diabetes may die of CHD (see Fig. 138-5C).[85] Males and females are affected equally.

This cumulative risk constitutes an enormous excess over the comparable figures for the Framingham population at that age (8% for men and 4% for women). High incidence rates of CHD and mortality rates attributable to CHD also occur in individuals with diabetes diagnosed after age 30.[81,87–89] In most studies, a moderate excess in the mortality rate from CHD in comparison with the nondiabetic population is evident soon after the diagnosis of diabetes. With longer duration of diabetes, the excess increases significantly.[81,87] Whereas the excess in CHD among men is independent of the type of treatment, diabetic women treated with insulin have significantly higher CHD risks than those treated with oral agents or diet.[81,87,88] At present, no explanation exists for this intriguing interaction.

Thus, CHD is the principal cause of premature death in persons with type 1 and type 2 diabetes (see Chap. 147). Investigations into mechanisms that might explain this have demonstrated excess frequencies of several risk factors for cardiovascular disease in patients at the time of diagnosis of diabetes.[90,91] Once diabetes is established, the levels of these factors increase, and their effect may be magnified in some way, perhaps by some influence (as yet unidentified) peculiar to diabetes. Given these insights into the pathogenesis of atherosclerosis in diabetes, reports that the risk of CHD is low among diabetic patients in Japan and among Pima Indians are particularly interesting.[92,93] Perhaps the putative diabetic factors that significantly accelerate the progression of atherosclerosis cannot initiate it.[85]

## PROGNOSIS OF DIABETES

Although the distributions of particularly late complications of diabetes are extremely important for understanding these outcomes, data on prognosis provide an integrated index of the

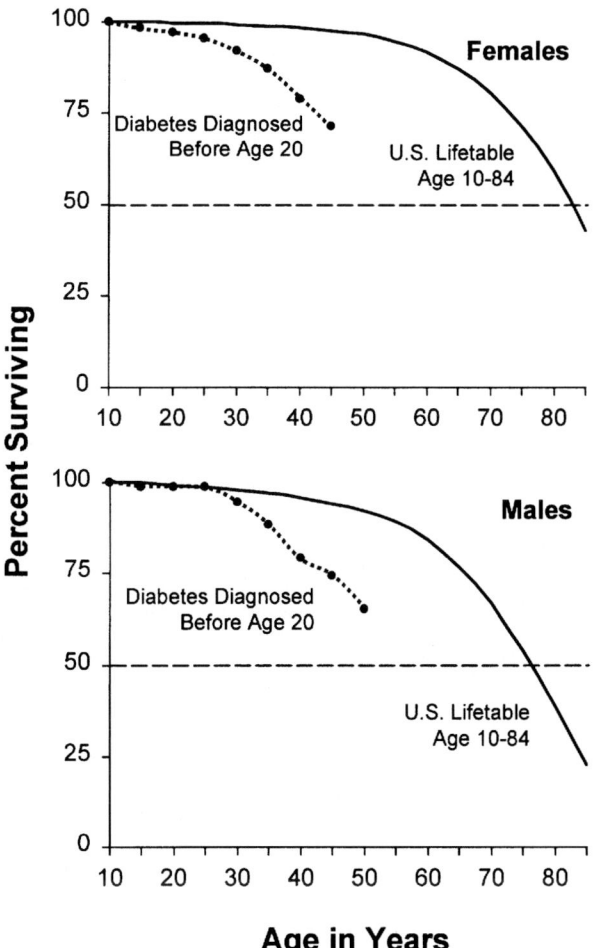

**FIGURE 138-6.** Prognosis of diabetes diagnosed before age 20. Cumulative survival rates according to gender and attained age in comparison with gender-specific survival rates from age 10 to 84 in the general population, based on the U.S. life table for 1989–1991 for whites. (Unpublished data from Krolewski M, Eggers PW, Warram JH. Magnitude of end-stage renal disease in IDDM: a 35 year follow-up study. Kidney Int 1996; 50:2041. Population data are from the National Center for Health Statistics, www.cdc.gov/nchswww/data/life89ri.pdf).

are still alive would be 70 years, which is 20 years older than the age at which an equal percentage of diabetic men are alive. As the age at diagnosis of the diabetes increases, the difference between the survival of a diabetic population and that of the general population becomes progressively smaller.[89] Individuals with diabetes diagnosed after age 70 have a life expectancy almost identical to that of the general population.

consequences of all these health problems for the population of diabetic patients. Pragmatically, the age at death is the primary outcome of interest. A standard technique for examining survival patterns in a population with a chronic disease is *life table analysis*, a procedure that allows the calculation of the proportion of the population with the disease that is surviving at each anniversary after the diagnosis.[6]

Survival rates for a cohort of patients who came to the Joslin Clinic in 1959 with newly diagnosed juvenile-onset type 1 diabetes and were followed until 1994 are plotted in Figure 138-6 according to age. Regardless of the age at onset of type 1 diabetes, few deaths occurred before age 30. However, thereafter, the proportion surviving declined rapidly, and by age 50 only 71% of the women and 65% of the men were still alive. The cause of death was about equally divided between renal disease and CHD, with only 12% due to other causes.

If the same method is applied to calculate survival rates for a hypothetical sample of children aged 10 and survival data for the general population are used, then 96% of the women and 92% of the men would be found to survive to age 50. The age at which 71% of the women in the general population are still alive would be 75 years, which is 25 years older than the age at which the same percentage of diabetic women are alive. Similarly, the age at which 65% of the men in the general population

## REFERENCES

1. Rothman KJ. Modern epidemiology. Boston: Little, Brown and Company, 1986.
2. Melton LJ, Palumbo PJ, Chu C. Incidence of diabetes mellitus by clinical type. Diabetes Care 1983; 6:75.
3. Melton LJ, Palumbo PJ, Dwyer MS, Chu C. Impact of recent changes in diagnostic criteria on the apparent natural history of diabetes mellitus. Am J Epidemiol 1983; 117:559.
4. Karvonen M, Tuomilehto J, Libman I, et al. A review of the recent epidemiological data on the worldwide incidence of type 1 (insulin-dependent) diabetes mellitus. Diabetologia 1993; 36:883.
5. Warram JH, Rich SS, Krolewski AS. Epidemiology and genetics of diabetes mellitus. In: Kahn CR, Weir GC, eds. Joslin's diabetes mellitus, 13th ed. Philadelphia: Lea & Febiger, 1994:201.
6. Merrell M, Shulman LE. Determination of prognosis in chronic disease, illustrated by systemic lupus erythematosus. J Chronic Dis 1955; 1:12.
7. Harris MI, Goldstein DE, Flegal KM, et al. Prevalence of diabetes, impaired fasting glucose, and impaired glucose tolerance in U.S. adults. The third National Health and Nutrition Examination Survey, 1988–1994. Diabetes Care 1998; 21:518.
8. Atkinson MA, Maclaren NK. The pathogenesis of insulin-dependent diabetes mellitus. N Engl J Med 1994; 331:1428.
9. Boitard C, Timsit J, Larger E, Dubois D. Immune mechanisms leading to Type 1 insulin-dependent diabetes mellitus. Horm Res 1997; 48(suppl.4):58.
10. Gorsuch AN, Spencer KM, Lister J. Evidence for a long prediabetic period in type I (insulin-dependent) diabetes mellitus. Lancet 1981; 2:1363.
11. Srikanta S, Ganda OP, Eisenbarth GS, Soeldner JS. Islet cell antibodies and beta-cell function in monozygotic triplets and twins initially discordant for type I diabetes mellitus. N Engl J Med 1983; 308:322.
12. Yamamoto AM, Deschamps I, Garchon HJ, et al. Young age and HLA markers enhance the risk of progression to Type 1 diabetes in antibody-positive siblings of diabetic children. J Autoimmun 1998; 11:643.
13. Krolewski AS, Warram JH, Rand LI, Kahn CR. Epidemiologic approach to the etiology of type I diabetes mellitus and its complications. N Engl J Med 1987; 317:1390.
14. Libman IM, Dorman JS, LaPorte RE, et al. Was there an epidemic of diabetes in nonwhite adolescents in Allegheny County, Pennsylvania? Diabetes Care 1998; 21:1278.
15. Bingley PJ, Gale EAM. Rising incidence of IDDM in Europe. Diabetes Care 1989; 12:289.
16. Tuomilehto J, Virtala E, Karvonen M, et al. Increase in incidence of insulin-dependent diabetes mellitus among children in Finland. Int J Epidemiol 1995; 24:984.
17. Patrick SL, Moy CS, LaPorte RE. The world of insulin-dependent diabetes mellitus: what international epidemiologic studies reveal about the etiology and natural history of IDDM. Diabetes Metab Rev 1989; 5:571.
18. Green A, Gale EAM, Patterson CC. Incidence of childhood-onset insulin-dependent diabetes mellitus: the EURODIAB ACE study. Lancet 1992; 339:905.
19. Hillis A. Does insulin-dependent diabetes mellitus (IDDM) follow the poliomyelitis pattern? Am J Epidemiol 1980; 112:452.
20. Gamble DR. The epidemiology of insulin dependent diabetes with particular reference to the relationship of virus infection to its etiology. Epidemiol Rev 1980; 2:49.
21. Yoon JW. Induction and prevention of IDDM by viruses. Diabetes Metab 1992; 18:378.
22. Akerblom HK, Knip M. Putative environmental factors in type 1 diabetes. Diabetes Metab Rev 1998; 14:31.
23. Graves PM, Norris JM, Pallansch MA, et al. The role of enteroviral infections in the development of IDDM. Limitations and current approaches. Diabetes 1997; 46:161.
24. Borch-Johnsen K, Joner G, Mandrup-Poulsen T, et al. Relation between breast-feeding and incidence rates of insulin-dependent diabetes mellitus: a hypothesis. Lancet 1984; 2(8411):1083.
25. Mayer EJ, Hamman RF, Gay EC, et al. Reduced risk of IDDM among breast-fed children: The Colorado IDDM registry. Diabetes 1988; 37:1625.
26. Kostraba JN, Cruickshanks KJ, Lawler-Heavner J, et al. Early exposure to cow's milk and solid foods in infancy, genetic predisposition, and risk of IDDM. Diabetes 1993; 42:288.
27. Virtanen SM, Rasanen L, Ylonen K, et al. Early introduction of dairy products associated with increased risk for insulin-dependent diabetes mellitus in Finnish children. Diabetes 1993; 42:1786.
28. Gerstein HC. Cow's milk exposure and type 1 diabetes mellitus: a critical overview of the clinical literature. Diabetes Care 1994; 17:13.

29. Norris JM, Scott FW. A meta-analysis of infant diet and insulin-dependent diabetes mellitus: do biases play a role? Epidemiology 1996; 7:87.

30. Kyvik KO, Green A, Beck-Nielsen H. Concordance rates of insulin dependent diabetes mellitus: a population based study of young Danish twins. BMJ 1995; 311:913.

31. Rich SS. Mapping genes in diabetes. Genetic epidemiological perspective. Diabetes 1990; 39:1315.

32. Schranz DB, Lernmark A. Immunology in diabetes: an update. Diabetes Metab Rev 1998; 14:3.

33. Concannon P, Gogolin-Ewens KJ, Hinds DA, et al. A second-generation screen of the human genome for susceptibility to insulin-dependent diabetes mellitus. Nat Genet 1998; 19:292.

34. Nerup J, Mandrup-Poulsen T, Molving J. The HLA-IDDM association: implications for etiology and pathogenesis of IDDM. Diabetes Metab Rev 1987; 3:779.

35. Svejgaard A, Ryder LP. HLA and insulin dependent diabetes: an overview. Genet Epidemiol 1989; 6:1.

36. Todd JA, Bell JI, McDevitt HO. HLA-DQ beta gene contributes to susceptibility and resistance to insulin-dependent diabetes mellitus. Nature 1987; 329:599.

37. Khalil I, d'Auriol L, Gobet M, et al. A combination of HLA-DQbeta Asp57-negative and HLA-DQ alpha Arg52 confers susceptibility to insulin-dependent diabetes mellitus. J Clin Invest 1990; 85:1315.

38. She JX. Susceptibility to type 1 diabetes: HLA-DQ and DR revisited. Immunol Today 1996; 17:323.

39. Dorman JS, LaPorte RE, Stone RA, Trucco M. Worldwide differences in the incidence of type 1 diabetes are associated with amino acid variation at position 57 of the HLA-DQ beta chain. Proc Natl Acad Sci U S A 1990; 87:7370.

40. Dorman JS, McCarty B, McCanlies E, et al. Molecular IDDM epidemiology: international studies. WHO DiaMond Molecular Epidemiology Sub-Project Group. Diabetes Res Clin Pract 1996; 34(Suppl.):S107.

41. Martin BC, Warram JH, Krolewski AS, et al. Role of glucose and insulin resistance in the development of type II diabetes: results of a 25-year follow-up study. Lancet 1992; 340:925.

42. Weir GC, Leahy JL. Pathogenesis of non–insulin-dependent (type II) diabetes mellitus. In: Kahn CR, Weir GC, eds. Joslin's diabetes mellitus, 13th ed. Philadelphia: Lea & Febiger, 1994:240.

43. Crockford PM, Harbeck RJ, Williams RH. Influence of age on intravenous glucose tolerance and serum immunoreactive insulin. Lancet 1966; 1:465.

44. Chen M, Bergman RN, Pacini G, Porte D Jr. Pathogenesis of age-related glucose intolerance in man: insulin resistance and decreased B-cell function. J Clin Endocrinol Metab 1985; 60:13.

45. Himsworth HP, Kerr RB. Age and insulin sensitivity. Clin Sci 1942; 4:153.

46. DeFronzo RA. Glucose intolerance and aging: evidence for tissue insensitivity to insulin. Diabetes 1979; 28:1095.

47. Fink RI, Kolterman OG, Griffin J, Olefsky JM. Mechanisms of insulin resistance in aging. J Clin Invest 1983; 71:1523.

48. Colditz GA, Willett WC, Rotnitzky A, Manson JE. Weight gain as a risk factor for clinical diabetes mellitus in women. Ann Intern Med 1995; 122:481.

49. Chan JM, Rimm EB, Colditz GA, et al. Obesity, fat distribution, and weight gains as risk factors for clinical diabetes in men. Diabetes Care 1994; 17:961.

50. Perry IJ, Wannamethee SG, Walker MK, et al. Prospective study of risk factors for development of non-insulin dependent diabetes in middle-aged British men. BMJ 1995; 3:560.

51. Hartz AJ, Rupley DC, Rimm AA. The association of girth measurements with disease in 32,856 women. Am J Epidemiol 1984; 119:71.

52. Pincus G, White P. On the inheritance of diabetes mellitus. I. An analysis of 675 family histories. Am J Med Sci 1933; 186:1.

53. Krolewski AS, Czyzyk A, Kopczynski J, et al. Prevalence of diabetes mellitus, coronary heart disease and hypertension in the families of insulin dependent and insulin independent diabetics. Diabetologia 1981; 21:520.

54. Thomas F, Balkau B, Vauzelle-Kervroedan F, et al. Maternal effect and familial aggregation in NIDDM. Diabetes 1994; 43:63.

55. Weijnen CF, Krolewski AS, Warram JH. Maternal and paternal diabetes confer similiar risk of type II diabetes to children. J Diabetologia 1997; 40 (Suppl 1):A201 (abstract).

56. Knowler WC, Pettitt DJ, Savage PJ, Bennett PH. Diabetes incidence in Pima Indians: contribution of obesity and parental diabetes. Am J Epidemiol 1981; 113:144.

57. Gottlieb MS. Diabetes in offspring and siblings of juvenile- and maturity-onset type diabetes. J Chronic Dis 1980; 33:331.

58. Warram JH, Martin BC, Soeldner JS, Krolewski AS. Study of glucose removal rate and first phase insulin secretion in the offspring of two parents with non–insulin-dependent diabetes. In: Camerini-Davalos RA, Cole HS, eds. Advances in experimental medicine and biology, vol 246. Prediabetes. New York: Plenum Publishing, 1988:175.

59. Pyke DA. Development of diabetes in identical twins. In: Camerini-Davalos RA, Cole HS, eds. Advances in experimental medicine and biology, vol 246. Prediabetes. New York: Plenum Publishing, 1988:255.

60. Hattersley AT. Maturity-onset diabetes of the young: clinical heterogeneity explained by genetic heterogeneity. Diabetes Med 1998; 15:15.

61. Doria A, Yang Y, Malecki M, et al. Phenotypic characteristics of early-onset autosomal-dominant type 2 diabetes unlinked to known maturity-onset diabetes of the young (MODY) genes. Diabetes Care 1999; 22:253.

62. Hansen RL, Ehm MG, Pettitt DJ, et al. An autosomal genomic scan for loci linked to type II diabetes mellitus and body-mass index in Pima Indians. Am J Hum Genet 1998; 63:1130.

63. Hanis CL, Boerwinkle E, Chakraborthy R, et al. A genome-wide search for human non-insulin-dependent (type 2) diabetes genes reveals a major susceptibility locus on chromosome 2. Nat Genet 1996; 13:161.

64. Mahtani MM, Widen E, Lehto M, et al. Mapping a gene for type 2 diabetes associated with an insulin secretion defect by a genome scan in Finnish families. Nat Genet 1996; 14:90.

65. Elbein SC, Hoffman MD, Teng K, et al. A genome-wide search for Type 2 diabetes susceptibility genes in Utah Caucasians. Diabetes 1999; 48(5):1175.

66. Ghosh S, Watanabe RM, Hauser ER, et al. Type 2 diabetes: evidence for linkage on chromosome 20 in 716 Finnish affected sib pairs. Proc Natl Acad Sci U S A 1999; 96:2198.

67. Li J, Malecki M, Warram JH, et al. New susceptibility locus for NIDDM is localized to human chromosome 20q. Diabetes 1997; 46:876.

68. Bowden DW, Sale M, Howard TD, et al. Linkage of genetic markers on human chromosome 20 and 12 to NIDDM Caucasian sib pairs with a history of diabetic nephropathy. Diabetes 1997; 46:882.

69. Zouali H, Hani EH, Philippi A, et al. A susceptibility locus for early-onset non-insulin dependent (type 2) diabetes mellitus maps to chromosome 20q, proximal to the phosphoenolpyruvate carboxykinase (PCK1) gene. Hum Mol Genet 1997; 6:1401.

70. The effect of intensive treatment of diabetes on the development and progression of long-term complications in insulin-dependent diabetes mellitus. The Diabetes Control and Complications Trial Research Group. N Engl J Med 1993; 329:977.

71. Krolewski AS, Laffel LMB, Krolewski M, et al. Glycated hemoglobin and risk of microalbuminuria in patients with insulin-dependent diabetes mellitus. N Engl J Med 1995; 332:1251.

72. United Kingdom Prospective Diabetes Study (UKPDS) Group. Intensive blood-glucose control with sulphonylureas or insulin compared with conventional treatment and risk of complications in patients with type 2 diabetes (UKPDS 33). Lancet 1998; 352:837.

73. Krolewski AS, Warram JH, Freire MB. Epidemiology of late diabetic complications. Endocrinol Metab Clin North Am 1996; 25:217.

74. Krolewski AS, Warram JH, Christlieb AR, et al. The changing natural history of nephropathy in type I diabetes. Am J Med 1985; 78:785.

75. Krolewski AS. Genetics of diabetic nephropathy: evidence for major and minor gene effects. Kidney Int 1999; 55(4):1582.

75a. Moczulski DK, Scott L, Antonellis A, et al. Aldose reductase gene polymorphisms and susceptibility to diabetic nephropathy in type 1 diabetes mellitus. Diabet Med 2000; 17:111.

76. Klein R, Klein BEK, Moss SE, et al. The Wisconsin epidemiologic study of diabetic retinopathy: II. Prevalence and risk of diabetic retinopathy when age at diagnosis is less than 30 years. Arch Ophthalmol 1984; 102:520.

77. Klein R, Klein BEK, Moss SE, et al. The Wisconsin epidemiologic study of diabetic retinopathy: III. Prevalence and risk of diabetic retinopathy when age at diagnosis is 30 or more years. Arch Ophthalmol 1984; 102:527.

78. Krolewski AS, Warram JH, Rand LI, et al. Risk of proliferative retinopathy in juvenile onset type I diabetes: 40 years follow-up study. Diabetes Care 1986; 9:443.

79. Klein R, Klein BEK, Moss SE, et al. Glycosylated hemoglobin predicts the incidence and progression of diabetic retinopathy. JAMA 1988; 260:2864.

80. Janka HU, Warram JH, Rand LI, Krolewski AS. Risk factors for progression of background retinopathy in long-standing IDDM. Diabetes 1989; 38:460.

81. Krolewski AS, Warram JH. Epidemiology of late complications of diabetes. In: Kahn CR, Weir GC, eds. Joslin's diabetes mellitus, 13th ed. Philadelphia: Lea & Febiger, 1994:605.

82. Stamler J, Vaccaro O, Neaton JD, et al. Diabetes, other risk factors, and 12-yr cardiovascular mortality for men screened in the multiple risk factor intervention trial. Diabetes Care 1993; 16:434.

82a. Gillum RF, Mussolino ME, Madans JH. Diabetes mellitus, coronary heart disease incidence, and death from all causes in African American and European American women: The NHAMES I epidemiologic follow-up study. J Clin Epidemiol 2000; 53:511.

83. Robertson WB, Strong JP. Atherosclerosis in persons with hypertension and diabetes mellitus. Lab Invest 1968; 18:538.

84. Crall FV, Roberts WC. The extramural and intramural coronary arteries in juvenile diabetes mellitus: analysis of nine necropsy patients aged 19 to 38 years with onset of diabetes before age 15 years. Am J Med 1978; 64:221.

85. Krolewski AS, Kosinski E, Warram JH, et al. Magnitude and determinants of coronary artery disease in juvenile-onset, insulin-dependent diabetes mellitus. Am J Cardiol 1987; 59:750.

86. Valsania P, Zarich SW, Kowalchuk GJ, et al. Severity of coronary artery disease in young patients with insulin-dependent diabetes mellitus. Am Heart J 1991; 122:695.

87. Warram JH, Kopczynski J, Janka HU, Krolewski AS. Epidemiology of non-insulin-dependent diabetes mellitus and its macrovascular complications. Endocrinol Metab Clin North Am 1997; 26:165.

88. Manson JE, Colditz GA, Stampfer MJ, et al. Prospective study of maturity-onset diabetes mellitus and risk of coronary heart disease and stroke in women. Arch Intern Med 1991; 151:1141.

89. Krolewski AS, Warram JH, Christlieb AR. Onset, course, complications, and prognosis of diabetes mellitus. In: Marble A, Krall LP, Bradley RF, et al., eds. Joslin's diabetes mellitus, 12th ed. Philadelphia: Lea & Febiger, 1985:251.

90. Wingard DL, Barrett-Connor E, Criqui H, Suarez L. Clustering of heart disease risk factors in diabetic compared to nondiabetic adults. Am J Epidemiol 1983; 117:19.

91. Pyorala K, Laakso M, Uusitupa M. Diabetes and atherosclerosis: an epidemiologic view. Diabetes Metab Rev 1987; 3:463.

92. Nelson RG, Sievers MI, Knowler WC, et al. Low incidence of fatal coronary heart disease in Pima Indians despite high prevalence of non–insulin-dependent diabetes. Circulation 1990; 81:987.

93. Matsumoto T, Ohashi Y, Yamada N, et al. Coronary heart disease mortality is actually low in diabetic Japanese by direct comparison with the Joslin cohort. Diabetes Care 1994; 17:1062.

# C H A P T E R  1 3 9

# SECONDARY FORMS OF DIABETES MELLITUS

VERONICA M. CATANESE AND C. RONALD KAHN

## DEFINITION

In addition to primary forms of diabetes mellitus (see Chaps. 136 through 138), glucose intolerance is associated with various other disorders and is commonly termed *secondary diabetes*. In many cases, the distinction between the simultaneous occurrence of a disease with primary diabetes or glucose intolerance and diabetes secondary to another disease cannot be made with certainty because no known independent genetic markers exist for primary diabetes mellitus. Epidemiologic data, as well as the reversal of the glucose intolerance in some patients with treatment of the primary disorder, indicate that secondary diabetes is a real phenomenon. This distinction between secondary diabetes and coincident primary diabetes is important, because the proper treatment of such patients may also influence their risk for diabetic complications.

## CAUSES

Secondary diabetes may occur in association with endocrine or nonendocrine disorders (Table 139-1). The most common endocrine diseases associated with glucose intolerance are those involving overproduction of counterregulatory hormones: growth hormone, glucagon, cortisol, and catecholamines. In these diseases, the secondary diabetes is usually reversible with successful treatment of the underlying disorder, and it is characterized by the absence of ketosis and the preservation of endogenous insulin secretion. Secondary diabetes resulting from insulin underproduction is far less common. This may occur in the setting of autoimmune polyendocrine disease or pheochromocytoma and can be accompanied by ketoacidosis.

Nonendocrine conditions associated with glucose intolerance fall into three general categories. Pancreatic diseases may be accompanied by variable amounts of insulin deficiency and the potential for occurrence of ketoacidosis, giving rise to the term "pancreoprivic diabetes." Pancreatitis, pancreatectomy, and hemochromatosis are the major causal factors within this group. A second, large category includes drug-induced diabetes and glucose intolerance. This may occur in the presence of "adequate" levels of insulin (i.e., corticosteroids) or because of impaired insulin secretion (i.e., B-cell toxins). Finally, several complex genetic syndromes, as well as diseases affecting hepatic or renal function, dietary composition, body weight (from obesity to malnutrition), serum electrolytes (particularly K⁺), or muscle function may cause impaired glucose tolerance (see Table 139-1).

## TABLE 139-1.
### Causes of Secondary Diabetes

**ENDOCRINE DISEASES**
  Acromegaly
  Cushing syndrome
  Glucagonoma
  Pheochromocytoma
  Hyperthyroidism
  Carcinoid syndrome
  Primary hyperaldosteronism
  Hyperprolactinemia
  Autoimmune polyendocrine syndromes

**PANCREATIC DISEASES**
  Pancreatectomy
  Pancreatitis—acute and chronic
  Tropical or J-type diabetes
  Hemochromatosis

**DRUG-INDUCED DIABETES**
  *Drugs That Impair Insulin Secretion*
    α-Adrenergic agents
    Diuretics (by K⁺ depletion)
    Phenytoin
  *Drugs That Impair Insulin Action*
    Glucocorticoids
    Oral contraceptive agents

**GENETIC SYNDROMES THAT MAY BE ASSOCIATED WITH IMPAIRED GLUCOSE TOLERANCE**
  Acute intermittent porphyria
  Alström syndrome (obesity, deafness, retinitis pigmentosa)
  Ataxia-telangiectasia
  Cockayne syndrome
  Cystic fibrosis
  Friedreich ataxia (spinocerebellar ataxia)
  Glycogen storage disease type I
  Herrmann syndrome (photomyoclonus, nerve deafness, nephropathy, cerebral dysfunction)[135]
  Huntington chorea
  Isolated growth hormone deficiency
  Klinefelter syndrome
  Laurence-Moon-Biedl syndrome
  Leprechaunism
  Lipoatrophic diabetes
  Machado disease (ataxia, nystagmus, dysarthria, depressed tendon reflexes, distal muscle atrophy)[136]
  Myotonic dystrophy
  Panhypopituitary dwarfism
  Prader-Willi syndrome
  Trisomy 21
  Turner syndrome
  Werner syndrome
  Wolfram syndrome (hereditary optic atrophy, visual loss, neurosensory deafness)

## DIABETES SECONDARY TO HORMONE OVERPRODUCTION

### ACROMEGALY

Excessive secretion of growth hormone (GH) causes gigantism in the prepubertal child and acromegaly in the adult (see Chaps. 12 and 18). Most commonly, GH overproduction results from autonomous secretion of the hormone by a pituitary adenoma; rarely, however, GH-releasing hormone (GHRH) may be produced "ectopically" by tumor cells, with resultant stimulation of GH production by the pituitary (see Chap. 219).

## METABOLIC EFFECTS OF GROWTH HORMONE

Growth hormone has multiple effects on both cell growth and intermediary metabolism. Although the importance of GH in childhood is well established, its physiologic role in adults is unknown. GH levels rise in response to fasting and during insulin-induced hypoglycemia.[1] When patients with isolated GH deficiency fast, plasma glucose and insulin levels decrease to a greater extent than do the same factors in fasting normal persons, whereas free fatty acid (FFA) and ketone levels increase to higher levels than in normal persons.[2] In adults, physiologic levels of GH enhance lipolysis and ketonemia,[3] but these actions are inapparent when physiologic levels of insulin are present. GH also plays a tonic role in the control of insulin and glucagon release; this is a rapid, direct effect of GH that does not appear to be mediated by insulin-like growth factor-I (IGF-I).[4]

At pathologic levels, GH has both acute and delayed effects on carbohydrate metabolism. During the first 4 hours after the intravenous administration of GH, insulin-like effects occur, including increased glucose uptake and utilization, with a concomitant fall in plasma glucose and FFA levels.[5,6] These effects are explained by direct, GH-stimulated insulin secretion, GH-mediated increase in hepatic IGF-I production, or GH-induced activation of some of the early steps in insulin-receptor signal transduction.[7] The delayed effects of high concentrations of GH are "counterinsulin" actions. Thus, several hours after rats are injected with GH, glucose uptake and utilization in adipocytes are impaired.[5] FFA levels rise in only fasted rats, supporting the notion that, even with pharmacologic doses of GH, significant lipolysis does not occur in the presence of adequate insulin. Insulin resistance is present at the tissue level, similar to that which occurs in patients with acromegaly or in normal persons given exogenous GH.[6,8,9]

The cellular mechanism for the insulin resistance occurring in patients with chronic GH excess appears to be complex. Rats treated with supraphysiologic doses of GH demonstrate a decrease in the number of hepatic insulin receptors, but this is almost completely compensated for by an increased affinity of these receptors for insulin.[10] Conversely, hypophysectomized rats show an increased receptor concentration and a decreased affinity that are only partially corrected by GH. Similar abnormalities have been noted in insulin receptors on monocytes from patients with acromegaly.[11] The receptor number varies inversely with the basal plasma insulin level, and the affinity of the unoccupied receptor is increased, whereas that of the filled receptor is unchanged. Usually, these reciprocal changes produce normal amounts of insulin binding at basal insulin concentrations but a decrease in the amount bound at "stimulated" insulin concentrations.

The cellular observations described earlier suggest an as yet undefined, pathophysiologic, postreceptor mechanism for the insulin resistance associated with sustained GH excess. Continuous administration of recombinant human GH to normal rats reduces insulin-mediated suppression of hepatic glucose output and produces significant decreases in the steady-state glucose infusion rate and the glucose disposal rate during hyperinsulinemic glucose clamping.[12] Similar results have been obtained in normal humans studied under conditions of continuous GH infusion.[13] In both rats and humans, fasting plasma glucose and insulin levels during GH treatment were not different from those in controls, providing an experimental correlate of those acromegalic patients with evidence of impaired insulin action in the postabsorptive state. Although the mechanisms responsible for this insulin resistance remain unclear, impairment of early events in insulin signaling in liver and skeletal muscle is a likely contributing factor. Both the tyrosine phosphorylation of insulin-receptor substrate-1 (IRS-1) and IRS-2, and association of these substrates with phosphatidylinositol 3-kinase (PI3-kinase) are reduced in the livers and muscles of rats

treated over the long term with GH.[14] Whether the thiazolidinedione drugs—which may ameliorate the GH-induced alterations in hepatic glucose output, glucose infusion rate, and glucose disposal rate[12]—affect the changes in IRS-1 and IRS-2 phosphorylation and PI3-kinase association observed in liver or muscle of GH-treated rats is unknown.

## CLINICAL FEATURES

Approximately 60% of acromegalic patients demonstrate glucose intolerance during an oral glucose-tolerance test.[9] The majority of acromegalic patients with abnormal oral glucose tolerance have normal fasting plasma glucose levels but an impaired response to a glucose load associated with elevated basal and/or stimulated insulin levels.[9a] In addition, 20% of acromegalic patients with normal glucose tolerance have elevated plasma insulin levels in the basal or in the stimulated state. Both acromegalic individuals with normal and those with abnormal glucose tolerance demonstrate impaired muscle glucose uptake and nonoxidative glucose metabolism in the postabsorptive state or after glucose challenge.[15] Thus, the oral glucose-tolerance test underestimates the prevalence of insulin resistance in patients with acromegaly. A small subgroup of acromegalic patients have low basal insulin levels and dramatically impaired insulin responses, and they demonstrate severe hyperglycemia and insulin dependency. Whether these patients have coincident type 1 diabetes mellitus or whether they represent a group of patients with B-cell desensitization to the prolonged hyperglycemic state is unclear.

The glucose intolerance and insulin resistance in most acromegalic patients is improved or completely ameliorated by the reversal of the acromegalic state. Longitudinal studies have shown that preradiotherapy and postradiotherapy plasma GH levels correlate directly with the fasting plasma glucose levels, as well as with the plasma glucose level after an oral glucose load, and indirectly with the maximal percentage fall in glucose during insulin-tolerance testing.[16] Approximately one-third of acromegalic patients display abnormally increased insulin secretion during an oral glucose-tolerance test up to 2 years after successful transsphenoidal surgery, despite having normal plasma glucose values and normal GH and IGF-I levels.[17] These findings suggest that, even after the normalization of GH secretion, secretagogue-induced hyperinsulinemia may persist in some patients with acromegaly. Whether this is secondary to an alteration in B-cell mass or response, to a mild persistent abnormality of GH secretion, or to decreased peripheral sensitivity to insulin is unknown. Furthermore, whether this is of any significance in predicting recurrence of disease or the subsequent development of type 2 diabetes mellitus is also unknown.

In contrast to transsphenoidal surgery and radiotherapy, another effective treatment option for acromegaly—the synthetic, long-acting somatostatin analog octreotide—has complex effects on multiple hormonal factors that affect carbohydrate metabolism. In addition to inhibiting GH and IGF-I hypersecretion, octreotide inhibits insulin and glucagon secretion, delays gastrointestinal glucose absorption, and increases production of the insulin antagonist, IGF-binding protein-1 (IGFBP-1).[18] Consequently, octreotide therapy may result in concomitant improvement in glucose tolerance with control of the GH hypersecretion; or, alternatively, it may worsen glucose tolerance, particularly if GH secretory profiles remain abnormal.[19]

## CUSHING SYNDROME

Cushing syndrome results from a chronic increase in plasma glucocorticoids (see Chap. 75). The source of the glucocorticoids may be exogenous or endogenous due to autonomous adrenal cortical hyperfunction, pituitary hypersecretion of adrenocorticotropic hormone (ACTH) (i.e., Cushing disease), or paraneoplastic production of ACTH by tumor cells (see Chap. 219).

## METABOLIC EFFECTS OF GLUCOCORTICOIDS

Generally, glucocorticoids are glucose sparing, that is, they promote release of amino acids from muscle and FFA from fat, as well as utilization of these as precursors for gluconeogenesis.[20] Several key enzymes controlling the production and utilization of metabolic fuels are directly regulated by glucocorticoids at the level of gene transcription. Phosphoenolpyruvate carboxykinase (PEPCK), a critical enzyme in gluconeogenesis, is positively regulated by glucocorticoids.[21] Transgenic mice overexpressing PEPCK, in fact, exhibit impaired glucose tolerance.[22] In addition, exposure of pregnant rats during late gestation to glucocorticoid excess permanently increases hepatic PEPCK and glucocorticoid-receptor expression, and causes glucose intolerance in adult offspring.[23] Under normal physiologic conditions, however, PEPCK is down-regulated even more potently and dominantly by insulin,[24] which promotes glucose uptake, inhibits hepatic gluconeogenesis, and blocks lipolysis and amino-acid release from muscle. When insulin is replete, therefore, enhanced gluconeogenesis as a result of glucocorticoid excess is prevented. In the presence of insulin deficiency or impaired insulin action, however, the stimulatory effects of glucocorticoids on glucose production become apparent. Because insulin resistance is almost invariably present in patients with Cushing syndrome,[25,26] the stage is set for glucocorticoid-enhanced carbohydrate intolerance, secondary to poorly restrained gluconeogenesis.

The mechanism of the decreased peripheral glucose utilization and insulin resistance observed during glucocorticoid excess is multifactorial. Glucocorticoids induce resistance to insulin-stimulated glucose uptake in rat adipocytes.[27] This effect may be brought about, at least in part, by direct glucocorticoid-mediated inhibition of insulin-induced protein kinase C translocation from cytosol to plasma membrane. Glucocorticoids also inhibit activation of glucose transport in rat skeletal muscle by insulin, IGF-I, and hypoxia.[28] In rat soleus muscle, this effect is associated with preservation of the total content of GLUT4 glucose transporters but reduced translocation of GLUT4 transporter units to the plasma membrane.[29] In addition to these effects on GLUT4 subcellular trafficking, glucocorticoids also affect early steps in insulin-receptor signaling in skeletal muscle, as well as in liver.[30] As a result, both basal and insulin-stimulated glucose uptake and utilization are subject to modulation by excess glucocorticoids.

Although insulin resistance has long been a recognized consequence of glucocorticoid excess, effects of glucocorticoids on insulin secretion have only recently been described. Transgenic mice that overexpress the glucocorticoid receptor under control of the insulin promoter have increased glucocorticoid sensitivity restricted to their pancreatic B cells.[31] These animals have normal fasting and postabsorptive blood glucose levels, but a dramatically reduced insulin response and impaired glucose tolerance during intravenous glucose testing. This in vivo evidence suggests a diabetogenic effect of glucocorticoids, mediated not solely through their effects on glucose production and peripheral insulin sensitivity, but also through an effect on insulin secretion. This hypothesis is supported by in vitro evidence for dexamethasone-induced, posttranslational degradation of B-cell GLUT2 glucose transporters,[32] and dexamethasone-induced inhibition of exocytotic insulin release from cultured rodent islet cells.[33] The diminished glucose utilization in Cushing syndrome, therefore, may be a composite result of both deficient insulin secretion and impaired insulin action. Although the relative contributions of impaired insulin secretion and action to the decreased glucose utilization in humans with Cushing syndrome have not been investigated, possibly a spectrum exists, similar to that in patients with type 2 diabetes, that

defines subgroups of patients with diabetes secondary to glucocorticoid excess.

## CLINICAL FEATURES

Although fasting hyperglycemia occurs in only 5% of patients with Cushing syndrome, glucose intolerance with varying degrees of basal or stimulated hyperinsulinemia occurs in up to 90% of patients.[34] This is not simply due to obesity. Patients with Cushing disease have disproportionately higher plasma insulin levels than do obese nondiabetic subjects of similar weight and height.[35] Attempts to define the group of patients who are most likely to develop corticosteroid diabetes have met with limited success. The development of "diabetes" in nondiabetic renal transplant patients correlates with age and body weight, corticosteroid dose, and a positive family history of diabetes.[36,37] Corticosteroid-induced insulin resistance may occur in patients receiving daily or alternate-day therapy (see Chap. 78). Regardless of whether endogenous or exogenous corticosteroids are responsible for the hypercortisolism, patients may present in a hyperosmolar, nonketotic state[38] (see Chap. 155). In addition, the mortality of patients with Cushing disease who have impaired glucose metabolism is higher than that of those with Cushing disease and normal glucose metabolism.[39]

## GLUCAGONOMA

Glucagon-secreting tumors of the pancreas (see Chap. 220) have been recognized with increasing frequency since their original description in 1966.[40] Unlike other islet cell tumors, these neoplasms are frequently malignant and are associated with a characteristic clinical syndrome that includes normochromic normocytic anemia, stomatitis, weight loss, glucose intolerance, and the pathognomonic rash, necrolytic migratory erythema[41,42] (see Chap. 220).

## METABOLIC EFFECTS OF GLUCAGON

The major target for glucagon action is the liver, where receptor-mediated cyclic adenosine monophosphate (cAMP)–dependent mechanisms increase glycogenolysis and gluconeogenesis.[43,44] Glucagon also has effects on muscle and adipose tissue, promoting the release of amino acids and FFAs that serve as gluconeogenic precursors.[45] Thus, glucagon helps maintain plasma glucose levels in the fasted state and after the ingestion of a protein-rich meal.[46,47] In the presence of insulin, however, these catabolic effects of glucagon on muscle and fat are limited. Therefore, an increased glucose-production rate alone is unlikely to cause glucose intolerance in the absence of an absolute or relative decrease in glucose-disposal rate.

In patients with glucagonoma, plasma glucagon levels are markedly elevated.[48,49] Infusions or injections of glucagon to produce similar blood levels cause prompt hyperglycemia. The elevated plasma glucagon levels also are directly responsible for the hypoaminoacidemia noted in the glucagonoma syndrome and can be reproduced by the infusion of glucagon into normal individuals.[50] The characteristic skin lesion associated with glucagonoma (see Chap. 218) may be secondary to amino-acid deficiency, because these lesions improve after the infusion of parenteral amino acids, despite continued hyperglucagonemia.[51]

In contrast to GH or cortisol excess, insulin resistance is not a major feature of the carbohydrate intolerance associated with glucagon excess. Rather, hyperglucagonemia is associated with enhanced glucose production caused by increased hepatic glycogenolysis and gluconeogenesis. Moreover, glucagon is a potent stimulus to epinephrine release from the adrenal medulla,[52] and the glucose production rate can be augmented further by adrenergic-receptor mechanisms. An increase in glucose production rate alone is unlikely to cause glucose intolerance unless the glucose disposal rate is absolutely or relatively diminished. Decreased insulin secretion and/or insulin resistance could result in diminished glucose utilization. Because insulin resistance has not been described in patients with glucagonoma, a relative decrease in insulin secretion, either by a direct paracrine effect of glucagon or by α-adrenergic receptor–mediated inhibition of insulin secretion, may be responsible for a mismatch between glucose production and disposal rates.[53] On the other hand, direct paracrine stimulatory effects of excess glucagon on B-cell insulin secretion also occur. B cells in the nontumoral endocrine pancreatic tissue of patients with glucagonoma have reduced immunoreactive insulin content, and ultrastructural features suggestive of accelerated insulin synthesis and secretion.[54] Therefore, the balance of multiple effects of hyperglucagonemia on insulin secretion may determine the degree of impairment in glucose disposal rate and, ultimately, the severity of the combined defects in glucose production and glucose utilization that result in glucose intolerance.

## CLINICAL FEATURES

The incidence of glucose intolerance in patients with glucagonoma approaches 100%. The metabolic defect varies in intensity from very mild to quite severe,[40,41] but, generally, it is not associated with the development of ketoacidosis.[47,48] This probably reflects the stimulatory effect of glucagon on insulin secretion and the importance of the relative concentrations of both insulin and glucagon to hepatic glucose production and ketogenesis. Plasma levels of glucagon are markedly elevated (900–7800 pg/mL), but the absolute value alone does not always distinguish those patients with A-cell tumors from patients with other causes of hyperglucagonemia (i.e., diabetic and alcoholic ketoacidosis, hyperosmolar syndrome, renal failure, acute pancreatitis).[48] Although the characteristic skin lesion or the persistence of a markedly elevated plasma glucagon value in a patient with poorly controlled diabetes should suggest the diagnosis of glucagonoma, further evidence for the disease may be obtained by biochemical analysis of the circulating glucagon. Total immunoreactive glucagon comprises several fractions, including native pancreatic glucagon (3500 Da) and other species with apparent molecular masses of ~40,000, 9000, and 2000 Da.[48] The 3500- and 40,000-Da forms are the predominant circulating species in normal humans and in subjects with "secondary hyperglucagonemia," whereas in studies of patients with glucagonoma, high levels of the 9000-Da component are found. The successful surgical resection of the tumor has been associated with cure of the insulin-requiring diabetes.[48,55] Malignant tumors may respond to therapy with streptozocin[56] or somatostatin infusion[57] (see Chap. 169) with a reduction of the proglucagon-like component in plasma and an improvement in glucose tolerance.

## PHEOCHROMOCYTOMA

Pheochromocytomas are associated with the continuous or intermittent overproduction of epinephrine and norepinephrine (see Chap. 86). Ninety percent are located in the adrenal medulla, with the remainder situated along the abdominal aorta, in the organ of Zuckerkandl, in the urinary bladder, or in the mediastinum.[58] Ninety-five percent are benign, and up to 10% of those in the adrenal medulla may be bilateral (see Chap. 188).

### METABOLIC EFFECTS OF CATECHOLAMINES

Many of the effects of catecholamines on intermediary metabolism are the very opposite of those of insulin.[59] Physiologic concentrations of epinephrine stimulate muscle glycogenolysis, adipocyte lipolysis, and hepatic gluconeogenesis and glycogenolysis.[60] These effects cause an increase in the net glucose production rate. In addition, catecholamines stimulate glucagon secretion.[59]

At pathologic levels, the effects of catecholamines on glucose disposal are more profound than those on glucose production. Catecholamines affect glucose utilization largely at the level of

insulin secretion,[53] and, to a lesser extent, at the level of peripheral glucose uptake.[59] Studies in vitro of rabbit pancreas,[61] as well as studies in vivo of normal humans,[62] have shown that insulin secretion in response to various secretagogues is inhibited by epinephrine and norepinephrine, and this is reversed by the α-adrenergic blocker phentolamine. Epinephrine directly interferes with exocytosis of insulin from pancreatic B cells,[63] and does so at a step distal to the membrane depolarization–induced increase in intracellular calcium.[64] On the other hand, insulin secretion also may be stimulated by the β-adrenergic effects of catecholamines[65] (see Chap. 134). Although patients with pheochromocytoma and impaired glucose tolerance usually have reduced insulin secretion,[66–68] hyperinsulinemia has been reported in this setting.[69] These observations suggest that although α-adrenergic effects on insulin secretion usually predominate in the setting of catecholamine excess, β-adrenergic effects may be obvious under certain clinical pathologic circumstances.

In contrast, the effects of catecholamines on the insulin target tissues, liver, muscle, and fat, are mediated primarily through cAMP-dependent, β-adrenergic receptor mechanisms. However, α-adrenergic receptors may participate in hepatic glycogenolysis.[70] Specifically, catecholamines impair insulin sensitivity, particularly in skeletal muscle,[71] by inhibiting both insulin-stimulated glucose transport[72] and insulin-mediated muscle glycogenesis.[73] Catecholamines, especially epinephrine, increase the net glucose production rate by direct effects on liver glycogenolysis and gluconeogenesis, muscle glycogenolysis, and fat lipolysis. Given the different affinities of epinephrine and norepinephrine for α- and β-adrenergic receptors, the overproduction ratio of these two catecholamines in any individual patient may determine whether the α-inhibitory or β-stimulatory effects on both glucose production and glucose utilization, particularly via insulin secretion, are predominant.

### CLINICAL FEATURES

The incidence of glucose intolerance in patients with pheochromocytoma ranges from 25% to 75%.[67,74,75] Most often, the fasting plasma glucose concentration is normal. The impaired glucose tolerance is associated with a blunted total insulin secretion and a delay in the time of peaking.[76,77] In these patients, the lack of ketoacidosis probably arises from the somewhat paradoxical enhancement of fatty acid reesterification observed with hyperglycemia.[75] The administration of α-adrenergic blockers, such as phentolamine, often restores insulin secretion and glucose tolerance to normal.[76] Likewise, successful resection of the tumor restores glucose homeostasis.[67,74,75] This response may not be immediate, however, and can occur up to 4 weeks or more postoperatively. During this period, insulin secretion is restored but glucose tolerance remains subnormal.[75] This suggests that some degree of reduced insulin sensitivity persists, even after circulating catecholamine levels return to normal.

## OTHER ENDOCRINE DISORDERS ASSOCIATED WITH IMPAIRED GLUCOSE TOLERANCE

Several other endocrine disorders are found in which overproduction of a hormone may cause impaired glucose tolerance (Table 139-2; see also Table 139-1). These include hyperthyroidism, hyperprolactinemia, primary hyperaldosteronism, and the carcinoid syndrome. The degree of the defect in these cases is almost always mild, with normal fasting plasma glucose levels, and requires no treatment. Whereas primary hyperaldosteronism and carcinoid syndrome reduce glucose tolerance through effects on insulin secretion, the effects of hyperthyroidism and hyperprolactinemia on glucose homeostasis are more complex.

### HYPERTHYROIDISM

Thyroid hormones directly alter the activity of several glycometabolic enzymes such as hepatic[78] and muscle[79] glycogen syn-

TABLE 139-2.
**Mechanisms of Glucose Intolerance in Diseases of Hormone Overproduction**

| Endocrine Disorder | Hormone Overproduced | Effects on Glucose Production | | Effects on Glucose Utilization | |
|---|---|---|---|---|---|
| | | *Glycogenolysis* | *Gluconeogenesis* | *Insulin Secretion* | *Insulin Action* |
| ACROMEGALY | Growth hormone | − | − | − | + |
| CUSHING SYNDROME | Glucocorticoids | + | + | + | + |
| GLUCAGONOMA | Glucagon | + | + | + | − |
| PHEOCHROMOCYTOMA | Catecholamines | + | + | + | − |
| HYPERTHYROIDISM | Thyroxine, triiodothyronine | + | + | + | + |
| PRIMARY HYPERALDOSTERONISM | Aldosterone | − | − | + | − |
| CARCINOID TUMOR | Serotonin | − | − | + | − |
| PROLACTINOMA | Prolactin | − | − | − | + |

thase, and also impair insulin-mediated suppression of hepatic glycogenolysis and gluconeogenesis.[80] In addition to their direct effects on glucose production, excess thyroid hormones also may impair glucose-induced GH suppression,[81] adding another factor favoring the development of glucose intolerance. Glucose disposal, particularly in adipocytes, also is affected by thyrotoxicosis. Insulin-stimulated glucose transport is minimally increased,[82] and this effect is associated with an increase in the appearance of GLUT4 glucose transporters in the plasma membrane of adipocytes.[83] More importantly, hyperthyroidism increases basal lipolysis, augments the maximal response of lipolysis to norepinephrine stimulation, and blunts the sensitivity of norepinephrine-stimulated lipolysis to suppression by insulin.[82] Clinically, these effects on glucose tolerance and insulin sensitivity appear to be more pronounced in obese than in nonobese hyperthyroid women,[84] perhaps because the decrease in nonoxidative glucose metabolism caused by hyperthyroidism cannot be adequately compensated for in the presence of the impaired oxidative glucose metabolism of obesity.[85]

### HYPERPROLACTINEMIA

Moderate chronic hyperprolactinemia is associated with reduced thresholds for basal and glucose-stimulated insulin release[86] and pancreatic B-cell proliferation,[87] mediated, perhaps, by altered expression of glucokinase, hexokinase, and GLUT2 glucose transporter in islet cells.[88] Prolactin also has effects, however, on extramammary tissue insulin resistance and glucose tolerance.[89] Studies in hyperprolactinemic, pituitary-grafted mice[90] and rats[91] suggest that the effects of prolactin on hepatic insulin action, unlike its gender-neutral effects on insulin secretion, may require estrogen for full expression. The molecular basis for prolactin's effects on insulin action in the presence and absence of estrogen has not been elucidated, and well-controlled studies testing this hypothesis in hyperprolactinemic men and women have not been performed.

## PANCREOPRIVIC DIABETES

### PANCREATECTOMY

#### CLINICAL FEATURES

Subtotal or total pancreatectomy may be performed for the removal of pancreatic neoplasms or cysts or as therapy for relapsing pancreatitis. Pancreatic exocrine and endocrine deficiency rarely result unless >75% of the pancreas is removed or destroyed. Endocrine secretion from all islet-cell types is reduced, resulting not only in insulin deficiency under basal and/or stimulated conditions, but also in diminished pancreatic glucagon, somatostatin, and pancreatic polypeptide (PP) secretion. Despite preserved secretion of glucagon-like substances of duodenal origin in patients who have not undergone pancreatoduodenectomy, reduced levels of pancreatic glucagon

account for the relative resistance of these patients to ketoacidosis, notwithstanding their insulin deficiency. In addition, average daily insulin requirements are lower in pancreatectomized diabetic patients than in matched patients with type 1 diabetes.[92,93] Hypoglycemic events, however, occur with increased frequency in pancreatectomized patients,[94,95] and their response to spontaneous or induced hypoglycemia is delayed compared to that of patients with both type 1 and type 2 diabetes.[95,96]

#### PATHOPHYSIOLOGY

A marked decrease in insulin secretion is the major factor underlying postpancreatectomy diabetes. Plasma glucagon may be low, normal, or even high.[97] This is partly due to cross-reactivity of the antibodies used in the immunoassay with glucagon-like substances of gastrointestinal origin, the levels of which may be elevated after pancreatectomy. The absence of a glucagon response to arginine stimulation and the very low levels of 3500-Da glucagon indicate deficient A-cell function.[92] The low levels of pancreatic glucagon are responsible for the relative resistance to ketosis characteristic of this group of patients. This, along with increased cellular insulin binding and enhanced hepatic and extrahepatic sensitivity to exogenous insulin,[94] is also responsible for the high frequency of hypoglycemic episodes. Pancreatectomized subjects also display subnormal epinephrine responses to insulin-induced hypoglycemia, which are significantly more severe than those seen in patients with type 1 diabetes matched for autonomic neuropathy or for the level of C peptide.[96] Because free insulin levels are not significantly different in pancreatectomized patients from those in other insulin-requiring diabetic patients, the absence of spontaneous glucose recovery seen in these patients is probably secondary to the combined defects in glucagon and epinephrine response.

### PANCREATITIS

#### CLINICAL FEATURES

Glucose intolerance may be part of the clinical picture in both acute and chronic pancreatitis. Hyperglycemia is often transient in acute pancreatitis, and may be severe. Abnormalities may persist in 3% to 5% of patients.[98] Chronic pancreatitis may be associated with diabetes in up to 60% of patients, with the incidence varying with the geographic location. This reflects the fact that alcoholic pancreatitis, the most common cause of chronic pancreatitis in the United States, is relatively infrequently associated with diabetes, whereas diabetes occurs frequently with fibrocalcific pancreatitis, especially in the tropical regions of the world. This has led to the use of the terms "tropical diabetes"[99] and "J-type diabetes" ("J" is for Jamaica). These forms of secondary diabetes often include degrees of both pancreatic exocrine and endocrine dysfunction. Diabetes secondary to pancreatitis differs somewhat from diabetes secondary to pancreatectomy, with a reduced frequency of hypoglycemic events, a higher incidence of development of ketosis, and, generally, a greater requirement for insulin.

## PATHOPHYSIOLOGY

Patients with pancreatitis exhibit variable decreases in the plasma insulin level. This decrease correlates with increased pancreatic enzyme release in acute pancreatitis and decreased pancreatic exocrine function in chronic cases. Carbohydrate intolerance usually has been attributed to the diminished insulin secretion[98]; however, patients with chronic pancreatitis often have normal basal plasma insulin levels but decreased insulin responses to glucose, arginine, and glucagon challenge.[98,100] Studies in the canine pancreatic duct ligation model of chronic pancreatitis[101] suggest that abnormal islet responsiveness with resultant circulating insulin deficiency may be associated with pancreatic acinar fibrosis, whereas the islets of Langerhans remain histologically and ultrastructurally intact.

Insulin deficiency alone may not be the only factor responsible for the development of secondary diabetes in the setting of pancreatitis. Hepatic resistance to insulin, accompanied by loss of sensitivity to insulin-induced hepatic glucose suppression, is a prominent feature of canine and rodent chronic pancreatitis.[102] Deficiency of PP has been implicated as a factor in this resistance, and infusion of bovine PP ameliorates glucose intolerance and restores suppression of hepatic glucose output by insulin in PP-deficient animals[103,104] and patients with chronic pancreatitis.[105] In addition, the basal pancreatic glucagon level is significantly higher in patients than in controls,[106] and it is increased further after oral glucose and arginine infusion.[100] Evidence exists that "pancreatic" glucagon may also be secreted by the duodenal mucosa[107] and that this may be the source of the elevated glucagon levels found in patients with pancreatitis and B-cell secretory deficiency. In contrast, because the duodenum is often removed along with the pancreas during pancreatectomy, duodenal glucagon may not be available in pancreatectomized patients.

# HEMOCHROMATOSIS

## CLINICAL FEATURES

Hemochromatosis includes various clinical conditions in which cirrhosis is accompanied by a markedly increased hepatic iron content, as well as by variable amounts of iron deposition in other tissues (see Chap. 131). Hemochromatosis may be a primary (idiopathic) familial disorder or secondary to iron overload. The latter form of hemochromatosis occurs in some patients with chronic hemolytic anemia or thalassemia, in patients receiving multiple transfusions, or in persons ingesting large amounts of iron, such as the Bantus, who drink excessive amounts of Kaffir beer. Clinical diabetes or impaired glucose tolerance occurs in 75% to 90% of patients with primary hemochromatosis and up to 65% of patients with hemochromatosis secondary to hemolytic anemia, multiple transfusions, or iron ingestion, and usually precedes other manifestations of the disease.[108–110] The diabetes of both primary and secondary hemochromatosis often requires insulin administration, and ketosis can occur.

## PATHOPHYSIOLOGY

Three factors contribute to the abnormal glucose tolerance in hemochromatosis: cirrhosis, pancreatic iron deposition, and the coexistence of primary diabetes mellitus. Although the presence of cirrhosis increases the likelihood of abnormal glucose metabolism, hepatic iron content, serum ferritin levels, or the extent of liver damage correlate poorly with the presence of impaired glucose homeostasis. A positive family history of diabetes may, perhaps, be the best predictor of glucose intolerance, at least among patients with primary, hereditary hemochromatosis.[111] Hepatic insulin resistance clearly plays an important role in patients with both varieties of hemochromatosis.[112,113] Defective first-phase insulin secretion is also observed, however, even in the absence of significant degrees of islet iron dep-

**TABLE 139-3.**
**Diabetogenic Pharmacologic Agents**

**DRUGS THAT AFFECT INSULIN SECRETION**
*Anticonvulsant*
  Phenytoin sodium
*Diuretics*
  Thiazides
  Furosemide
  Ethacrynic acid
*Cations*
  Barium
  Cadmium
  Lithium
  Potassium
  Zinc
*Hormones*
  Somatostatin
*Pesticides*
  DDT
  Fluoride
  Pyriminil (Vacor)
*Anthelminthics*
  Pentamidine isethionate
*Antineoplastics*
  L-Asparaginase
  Mithramycin
**DRUGS THAT AFFECT INSULIN ACTION**
*Hormones*
  Calcium
  Glucagon
  Glucocorticoids
  Growth hormone
**DRUGS THAT AFFECT BOTH INSULIN SECRETION AND**
**    INSULIN ACTION**
*Adrenergic Compounds*
  Epinephrine
  Norepinephrine
*Antihypertensive*
  Clonidine hydrochloride
  Diazoxide
  Prazosin hydrochloride
*Blocking Agents*
  β-Adrenergic blockers
  Calcium-channel blockers
  Histaminergic blockers
*Psychopharmacologic Agents*
  Benzodiazepines
  Ethanol
  Opiates
  Phenothiazines

osition. Glucose- and insulin-tolerance testing and euglycemic clamp studies[109,110,113] suggest that the defect in insulin secretion is more important than is insulin resistance in this syndrome. This diminished insulin secretion, however, may be preceded by insulin resistance and increased insulin secretion,[110] a pattern reminiscent of the natural history of type 2 diabetes mellitus. Overall, however, the relative contributions of genetic factors versus iron overload to the pathophysiology of diabetes secondary to hemochromatosis are not yet clear.

# DRUG-INDUCED DIABETES

A wide variety of pharmacologic agents can induce glucose intolerance (Table 139-3). Individual drugs may affect glucose homeostasis by interfering with insulin secretion, insulin action, or both. Whether its effect is primarily on insulin secretion or insulin action, a drug itself may mediate the effect directly or indirectly through balance of insulin counterregulatory hormones or cations (e.g., $K^+$) critical to the mechanisms that control insulin release. Glucohomeostatic effects of supraphysiologic levels of GH, glucocorticoids, and catecholamines best illustrate the direct and indirect consequences of pharmacologically altered insulin action. As the links between altered insulin sensitivity and altered insulin secretion tighten, assigning a drug an effect based solely on insulin action becomes more and more difficult. Clinically, these agents may uncover previously silent insulin-secretory defects or insulin resistance and consequently induce glucose intolerance in a previously undiagnosed patient or worsen the diabetic state when administered to patients with antecedent diabetes mellitus.

## IMPAIRED INSULIN SECRETION (DIRECT EFFECT)—PROTOTYPE: PHENYTOIN SODIUM

The diabetogenic effect of phenytoin sodium in humans and animals has been known for many years.[114] Early studies in the isolated perfused rat pancreas showed that high concentrations of this drug completely inhibited both first and second phases of insulin release.[115] Phenytoin sodium has been shown to reversibly inhibit calcium inflow into the B cell through voltage-dependent calcium channels.[116] When given orally to normal subjects in doses sufficient to achieve therapeutic blood levels, the drug produces a significant decrease in both early and late insulin responses to intravenous glucose, accompanied by a significant rise in plasma glucose level.[117]

Another pharmacologic agent in this category that deserves special mention is pentamidine isethionate, a drug used in the treatment of trypanosomiasis and leishmaniasis and now extensively used to treat *Pneumocystis carinii* pneumonia. Given the wide use of this drug in the management of patients with acquired immunodeficiency syndrome, its effects on glucose homeostasis are being noted with increasing frequency.[118] The chemical structure of pentamidine isethionate is somewhat similar to that of the diabetogenic rodenticide pyriminil (Vacor).[119] When pentamidine isethionate is incubated in vitro with islet cells, an initial passive release of insulin occurs, followed by a significant decrease in B-cell response to glucose and theophylline. The proposed mechanism of pentamidine toxicity, therefore, is an early cytolytic release of insulin followed by B-cell exhaustion and insulin deficiency.

## IMPAIRED INSULIN SECRETION (INDIRECT EFFECT)—PROTOTYPE: THIAZIDE DIURETICS

The incidence of glucose intolerance in patients taking thiazide diuretics varies between 10% and 40%, depending on the duration of administration of the drug.[120] Thiazides were thought to adversely affect insulin secretion and promote glucose intolerance indirectly through production of hypokalemia,[121] in a manner similar to that proposed for primary hyperaldosteronism. Although prevention or correction of hypokalemia does ameliorate thiazide-induced glucose intolerance, direct effects of thiazides themselves on pancreatic B-cell secretion have been described. Unlike the structurally related compound diazoxide, thiazides do not hyperpolarize B cells by opening the adenosine triphosphate (ATP)–sensitive potassium channels closed by the sulfonylureas.[122] Instead, they, like diphenylhydantoin, may affect stimulus-secretion coupling in the B cell by inhibiting calcium uptake.[123] Similarly, the loop diuretics, thought to share with the thiazides an indirect effect on B-cell secretion mediated through hypokalemia, also directly affect insulin secretion by inhibiting chloride pump function in the B-cell membrane.[124]

## IMPAIRED INSULIN ACTION—PROTOTYPE: GLUCOCORTICOIDS

The mechanism of glucocorticoid-induced glucose intolerance has been presented earlier. Like the catecholamines, glucocorticoids increase glucose production as well as decrease insulin secretion and insulin-stimulated glucose utilization (see Table 139-2). Although glucocorticoid administration was used formerly as a diagnostic maneuver in an attempt to precipitate abnormal glucose tolerance in individuals with a family history of diabetes, this test has proved unreliable because all individuals are prone to the diabetogenic actions of these drugs.

## IMPAIRED INSULIN SECRETION AND IMPAIRED INSULIN ACTION—PROTOTYPE: β-ADRENERGIC BLOCKERS

The effects of β-adrenergic blocking agents on intermediary metabolism can be deduced from a knowledge of the adrenergic control of insulin secretion, glucose production, and glucose utilization. Generally, nonselective β-blockade decreases pancreatic insulin secretion. Glycogenolysis and gluconeogenesis also may be impaired, but the clinical effect of these may be offset by the reduction in insulin secretion. Consequently, a worsening of glucose tolerance in patients receiving β-blockers is not unusual.[125] The occurrence of hypoglycemia in these patients is somewhat less common.[126] The α-adrenergic contribution to hepatic glycogenolysis may be the reason for the low frequency of this finding. Relatively selective β-blockade (e.g., with drugs such as atenolol) would be expected to have a smaller effect on insulin secretion and on recovery from insulin-induced hypoglycemia, because the stimulatory pancreatic α-adrenoreceptor is $\alpha_2$ in subtype and the hepatic β-adrenoreceptor is $\beta_2$ in subtype (see Chap. 85).

The opiates also fall into this category of pharmacologic agents. The hyperglycemic effect of morphine has been well described,[127] and heroin addicts have elevated basal plasma insulin levels but markedly reduced plasma insulin responses to intravenous glucose in comparison with age-, gender-, and weight-matched controls.[128] Beta-endorphin can be found in human pancreatic tissue.[129] This observation raises the question of a possible role for endogenous opioids in the intrapancreatic control of insulin secretion.

# GENETIC SYNDROMES ASSOCIATED WITH IMPAIRED GLUCOSE TOLERANCE

The list of genetic syndromes that include glucose intolerance as part of their profile is extensive and growing (see Table 139-1). Among members of this list, relatively pure defects in insulin secretion are represented by diseases such as cystic fibrosis, whereas leprechaunism may be regarded as a prototypical syndrome of insulin resistance. However, multiple pathophysiologic mechanisms that affect both glucose production and glucose utilization combine, in most cases, to produce the full-blown syndromes and the glucose intolerance that characterizes them. Advances in the molecular genetics and molecular pathophysiology of these syndromes likely will shed light not only on the dysregulated glucose handling in these syndromes but also on mechanisms of altered glucose homeostasis common to secondary as well as to primary forms of diabetes.

# COMPLICATIONS OF SECONDARY DIABETES

Over the past 20 years, the question of whether the vascular complications of diabetes are a direct consequence of the metabolic abnormalities present in the diabetic patient or are secondary to another genetic lesion has remained controversial. The results of the Diabetes Control and Complications Trial provide compelling evidence that strict control of plasma glucose levels in patients with type 1 diabetes can retard the progression of microangiopathic changes in the eye, kidney, and nerves.[130] Whether such therapy can actually prevent these complications is still unknown. This question has been difficult to answer for at least two reasons: first, there is a lack of information about a possible underlying genetic defect in diabetes. Second, it is not known whether hyperglycemia itself or some other factor in the diabetic milieu (insulin, IGF-I, other growth factors) initiates the sequence of events leading to microangiopathy. Even less is known about the relationship of these factors, if any, to macrovascular changes.

Patients with glucose intolerance secondary to one of the diseases of hormone overproduction have a notable lack of microangiopathic complications. This is not surprising because frank diabetes is relatively uncommon in this group (affecting <20%), and for the disease to persist untreated for 20 years or more is unusual. Abnormal glucose tolerance may be present in as many as 75% to 90% of patients in each category, and some do have disease for prolonged periods. Retinal, renal, and neurologic sequelae do appear in these patients and increase with the increasing duration of disease.[131–133]

Retinopathy occurs in patients with pancreatic diabetes. Among patients with pancreatitis and those who have had pancreatectomy, fluorescein angiography discloses retinopathy in 7% to 30%.[132] Retinopathy is usually of the background type; proliferative retinopathy is extremely rare in this group (see Chap. 151).

In patients with hemochromatosis and diabetes, retinopathy also occurs in 20% to 30%.[108,109] Although the therapeutic depletion of iron stores is associated with an improvement in carbohydrate tolerance in up to 40% of these patients,[108] whether iron load has an independent effect on the development of microvascular disease is unknown. As in the patients with pancreatitis or pancreatectomy, the relationship of a positive family history for primary diabetes to the risk of diabetic microvascular disease is unclear.

## THERAPY FOR SECONDARY DIABETES

The therapy for secondary diabetes centers on the correction of the underlying disturbance. Until this is accomplished, or if this cannot be accomplished, patients with fasting hyperglycemia should be treated with an understanding of the pathophysiologic basis of their diabetes. Therapy with diet or oral hypoglycemic agents may be successful in patients with acromegaly and Cushing syndrome who have preserved insulin secretion. Nevertheless, some may require insulin therapy to achieve normoglycemia. Frequently, those with pheochromocytoma or glucagonoma who have prominent impairment of insulin secretion require insulin therapy to normalize plasma glucose concentration. Little correlation appears to exist between the need for insulin therapy during the period of the secondary diabetes and the likelihood that abnormal glucose tolerance will persist after treatment of the underlying disease.

## REFERENCES

1. Glick SM, Roth J, Yalow RS, Berson SA. The regulation of growth hormone secretion. Recent Prog Horm Res 1965; 21:241.
2. Merimee TJ, Felig P, Marliss E, et al. Glucose and lipid homeostasis in the absence of human growth hormone. J Clin Invest 1971; 50:574.
3. Gerich JR, Lorenzi M, Bier DM, et al. Effects of physiologic levels of glucagon and growth hormone on human carbohydrate and lipid metabolism studies involving administration of exogenous hormone during suppression of endogenous hormone secretion with somatostatin. J Clin Invest 1976; 57:875.
4. Tai TY, Pek S. Direct stimulation by growth hormone of glucagon and insulin release from isolated rat pancreas. Endocrinology 1976; 99:669.
5. Goodman HM. Growth hormone and the metabolism of carbohydrate and lipid in adipose tissue. Ann N Y Acad Sci 1968; 148:419.
6. Daughaday WH, Kipnis DM. The growth promoting and anti-insulin action of somatotropin. Recent Prog Horm Res 1966; 22:49.
7. Argetsinger L, Carter-Su C. Mechanism of signaling by growth hormone receptor. Physiol Rev 1996; 76:1089.
8. Fineberg SE, Merimee TJ, Rabinowitz D, Edgar PJ. Insulin secretion in acromegaly. J Clin Endocrinol Metab 1970; 30:288.
9. Sonksen PH, Greenwood FC, Ellis JP, et al. Changes in carbohydrate tolerance in acromegaly with progress of the disease and in response to treatment. J Clin Endocrinol Metab 1967; 27:1418.
9a. Kasayamu S, Otsuki M, Takagi M, et al. Impaired beta-cell function in the presence of reduced insulin sensitivity determines glucose tolerance status in acromegalic patients. Clin Endocrinol (Oxf) 2000; 52:549.
10. Kahn CR, Goldfine ID, Neville DM Jr, DeMeyts P. Alterations in insulin binding induced by change in vivo in the levels of glucocorticoids and growth hormone. Endocrinology 1978; 103:1054.
11. Muggeo M, Bar RS, Roth J, et al. The insulin resistance of acromegaly: evidence for two alterations in the insulin receptor on circulating monocytes. J Clin Endocrinol Metab 1979; 48:17.
12. Sugimoto M, Takeda N, Nakashima K, et al. Effects of troglitazone on hepatic and peripheral insulin resistance induced by growth hormone excess in rats. Metabolism 1998; 47:783.
13. Orskov L, Schmitz O, Jorgensen JOL, et al. Influence of growth hormone on glucose-induced glucose uptake in normal men as assessed by the hyperglycemic clamp technique. J Clin Endocrinol Metab 1989; 68:276.
14. Thirone ACP, Carvalho CRO, Brenelli SL, et al. Effect of chronic growth hormone treatment on insulin signal transduction in rat tissues. Mol Cell Endocrinol 1997; 130:33.
15. Foss MC, Saad MJ, Paccola BM, et al. Peripheral glucose metabolism in acromegaly. J Clin Endocrinol Metab 1991; 72:1048.
16. Eastman RC, Gorden P, Roth J. Conventional supervoltage irradiation is an effective treatment for acromegaly. J Clin Endocrinol Metab 1979; 48:931.
17. Roelfsema F, Frolich M. Glucose tolerance and plasma immunoreactive insulin levels in acromegalics before and after selective transsphenoidal surgery. Clin Endocrinol (Oxf) 1985; 22:531.
18. Ezzat S, Ren SG, Braunstein GD, Melmed S. Octreotide stimulates insulin-like growth factor binding protein-1: a pituitary-independent mechanism for drug action. J Clin Endocrinol Metab 1992; 75:1459.
19. Koop BL, Harris AG, Ezzat S. Effect of octreotide on glucose tolerance in acromegaly. Eur J Endocrinol 1994; 130:581.
20. Mischke WJ, Ebers S, Boisch KH, Tamm J. The influence of intravenously administered cortisol with and without the addition of insulin or pre-treatment with propranolol on various parameters of fat and carbohydrate metabolism in blood plasma of human beings. Acta Endocrinol (Copenh) 1974; 75(suppl 186):1.
21. Imai E, Stromstedt PE, Quinn PG, et al. Characterization of a complex glucocorticoid response unit in the phosphoenolpyruvate carboxykinase gene. Mol Cell Biol 1990; 10:4712.
22. Valera A, Pujol A, Pelegrin M, Bosch F. Transgenic mice overexpressing phosphoenolpyruvate carboxykinase develop non-insulin dependent diabetes. Proc Natl Acad Sci U S A 1994; 91:9151.
23. Nyirenda MJ, Lindsay RS, Kenyon CJ, et al. Glucocorticoid exposure in late gestation permanently programs rat hepatic phosphoenolpyruvate carboxykinase and glucocorticoid receptor expression and causes glucose intolerance in adult offspring. J Clin Invest 1998; 101:2174.
24. O'Brien RM, Granner DK. Regulation of gene expression by insulin. Biochem J 1991; 278:609.
25. Muggeo M, Saviolakis GA, Wachslicht-Rodbard H, Roth J. Effects of chronic glucocorticoid excess in man on insulin binding to circulating cells: differences between endogenous and exogenous hypercortisolism. J Clin Endocrinol Metab 1983; 56:1169.
26. Fantus G, Ryan J, Hizuka N, Gorden P. The effect of glucocorticoids on the insulin receptor: an in vivo and in vitro study. J Clin Endocrinol Metab 1981; 52:953.
27. Ishizuka T, Nagashima T, Kajita K, et al. Effect of glucocorticoid receptor antagonist RU 38486 on acute glucocorticoid-induced insulin resistance in rat adipocytes. Metabolism 1997; 46:997.
28. Weinstein SP, Paquin T, Pritsker A, Haber RS. Glucocorticoid-induced insulin resistance: dexamethasone inhibits the activation of glucose transport in rat skeletal muscle by both insulin- and non-insulin-related stimuli. Diabetes 1995; 44:441.
29. Dimitriadis G, Leighton B, Parry-Billings M, et al. Effects of glucocorticoid excess on the sensitivity of glucose transport and metabolism to insulin in rat skeletal muscle. Biochem J 1997; 321:707.
30. Saad MJA, Folli F, Kahn JA, Kahn CR. Modulation of insulin receptor, insulin receptor substrate-1, and phosphatidylinositol 3-kinase in liver and muscle of dexamethasone-treated rats. J Clin Invest 1993; 92:2065.
31. Delaunay F, Khan A, Cintra A, et al. Pancreatic β cells are important targets for the diabetogenic effects of glucocorticoids. J Clin Invest 1997; 100:2094.
32. Gremlich S, Roduit R, Thorens B. Dexamethasone induces posttranslational degradation of GLUT2 and inhibition of insulin secretion in isolated pancreatic β cells. J Biol Chem 1997; 272:3216.
33. Lambillotte C, Gilon P, Henquin JC. Direct glucocorticoid inhibition of insulin secretion. J Clin Invest 1997; 99:414.
34. Perley N, Kipnis DM. Effect of glucocorticoids on plasma insulin. N Engl J Med 1966; 274:1237.
35. Wajchenberg BL, Leme CE, Lerario AC, et al. Insulin resistance in Cushing's disease evaluation by studies of insulin binding to erythrocytes. Diabetes 1984; 33:455.
36. Woods JE, Zincke H, Palumbo PJ, et al. Hyperosmolar non-ketotic syndrome and steroid diabetes: occurrence after renal transplantation. JAMA 1975; 231:1261.
37. Arner P, Gunnarsson R, Blomdahl S, Groth C. Some characteristics of steroid diabetes: a study in renal-transplant patients receiving high-dose corticosteroid therapy. Diabetes Care 1983; 6:23.

38. Lohr KM. Precipitation of hyperosmolar non-ketotic diabetes on alternate day corticosteroid therapy. JAMA 1984; 252:628.

39. Etxabe J, Vazquez JA. Morbidity and mortality in Cushings disease. An epidemiological approach. Clin Endocrinol 1994; 40:479.

40. McGavian MH, Unger RH, Recant L, et al. A glucagon-secreting α cell carcinoma of the pancreas. N Engl J Med 1966; 271:1408.

41. Mallinson CN, Bloom SR, Warin AP, et al. A glucagonoma syndrome. Lancet 1974; 2:1.

42. Binnick AN, Spencer SK, Dennison WL, Horton ES. Glucagonoma syndrome: report of two cases and literature review. Arch Dermatol 1977; 113:749.

43. Liljenquist JE, Meuller GL, Cherrington AD, et al. Evidence for an important role of glucagon in the regulation of hepatic glucose production in normal man. J Clin Invest 1977; 59:369.

44. Wahren J, Efendic S, Luft R, et al. Influence of somatostatin on splanchnic glucose metabolism in post-absorptive and 60 hour fasted humans. J Clin Invest 1977; 59:299.

45. Unger RH. α and β Cell interrelationship in health and disease. Metabolism 1974; 23:581.

46. Marliss EB, Aoki TT, Unger RH, et al. Glucagon levels and metabolic effects in prolonged fasted man. J Clin Invest 1970; 49:2256.

47. Unger RJ, Okneda A, Aguilar-Parada E, Eisentraut AM. The role of aminogenic glucagon secretion in blood glucose homeostasis. J Clin Invest 1969; 48:810.

48. Jaspan JB, Rubinstein AH. Circulating glucagon: plasma profiles and metabolism in health and disease. Diabetes 1977; 26:887.

49. Vassilopoulou-Sellin R, Ajani J. Islet cell tumors of the pancreas. Endocrinol Metab Clin North Am 1994; 23:53.

50. Aoki TT, Muller WA, Brennan MF, Cahill GF Jr. Effect of glucagon on amino acid and nitrogen metabolism in fasting man. Metabolism 1974; 23:805.

51. Norton JA, Kahn CR, Schiebinger R, et al. Amino acid deficiency and the skin rash associated with glucagonoma. Ann Intern Med 1979; 91:213.

52. Unger RH. Glugacon physiology and pathophysiology. N Engl J Med 1971; 285:443.

53. Porte DL Jr. A receptor mechanism for inhibition of insulin release. J Clin Invest 1966; 46:86.

54. Bani D, Biliotti G, Sacchi TB. Morphological changes in the human endocrine pancreas induced by chronic excess of endogenous glucagon. Virchows Arch B Cell Pathol 1991; 60:199.

55. Lightman SL, Bloom SR. Cure of insulin-dependent diabetes mellitus by removal of a glucagonoma. BMJ 1974; 1:367.

56. Danforth DN, Triche T, Doppman JC, et al. Elevated plasma proglucagon-like component with a glucagon secreting tumor: effects of streptozotocin. N Engl J Med 1976; 295:242.

57. Long RG, Adrian TE, Brown MR, et al. Suppression of pancreatic endocrine tumor secretion by long-acting somatostatin analogue. Lancet 1979; 2:764.

58. Manger WM, Gifford RW. Pheochromocytoma. New York: Springer-Verlag, 1977.

59. Himms-Hagen J. Sympathetic regulation of metabolism. Pharmacol Rev 1967; 19:367.

60. Rizza RA, Cryer PE, Haymond MW, Gerich JE. Adrenergic mechanisms for the effects of epinephrine on glucose production and clearance in man. J Clin Invest 1980; 65:682.

61. Coore RG, Randle PJ. Regulation of insulin secretion studied with pieces of rabbit pancreas incubated in vitro. Biochem J 1964; 93:66.

62. Porte D Jr, Williams RH. Inhibition of insulin release by norepinephrine. Science 1966; 152:1248.

63. Lehr S, Herbst M, Kampermann J, et al. Adrenaline inhibits depolarization-induced increases in capacitance in the presence of elevated intracellular calcium concentration in insulin secreting cells. FEBS Lett 1997; 415:1.

64. Renstrom E, Ding WG, Bokvist K, Rorsman P. Neurotransmitter-induced inhibition of exocytosis in insulin-secreting β cells by activation of calcineurin. Neuron 1996; 17:513.

65. Smith PH, Porte D Jr. Neuropharmacology of the pancreatic islets. Annu Rev Pharmacol Toxicol 1976; 16:269.

66. Wilber JF, Turtle JR, Crane NA. Inhibition of insulin secretion by phaeochromocytoma. Lancet 1966; 2:733.

67. Turnbull DM, Johnston DG, Alberti KGMM, Hall R. Hormonal and metabolic studies in a patient with a pheochromocytoma. J Clin Endocrinol Metab 1980; 51:930.

68. Isles CG, Johnson JK. Phaeochromocytoma and diabetes mellitus: further evidence that α2 receptors inhibit insulin release in man. Clin Endocrinol (Oxf) 1983; 18:37.

69. Renata L, Daniela L, Valeria C, Francesca S. Letter to editors. Clin Endocrinol (Oxf) 1983; 19:275.

70. Exton JH, Harper SC. Role of cyclic AMP in the actions of catecholamines on hepatic carbohydrate metabolism. Adv Cyclic Nucleotide Res 1975; 5:519.

71. Capaldo B, Napoli R, Di Marino L, Sacca L. Epinephrine directly antagonizes insulin-mediated activation of glucose uptake and inhibition of free fatty acid release in forearm tissues. Metab Clin Exp 1992; 41:1146.

72. Laakso M, Edelman SV, Brechtel G, Baron AD. Effects of epinephrine on insulin-mediated glucose uptake in whole body and leg muscle in humans: role in blood flow. Am J Physiol 1992; 263:E199.

73. Raz I, Katz A, Spencer MK. Epinephrine inhibits insulin-mediated glycogenesis but enhances glycolysis in human skeletal muscle. Am J Physiol 1991; 260:E430.

74. Modlin IM, Farndom JR, Shepherd A, et al. Phaeochromocytoma in 72 patients: clinical and diagnostic features, treatment, and long-term results. Br J Surg 1979; 66:456.

75. Stenström G, Sjöström L, Smith U. Diabetes mellitus in phaeochromocytoma: fasting blood glucose levels before and after surgery in 60 patients with phaeochromocytoma. Acta Endocrinol (Copenh) 1984; 106:511.

76. Spergel G, Bleicher SJ, Estel NH. Carbohydrate and fat metabolism in patients with pheochromocytoma. N Engl J Med 1968; 278:803.

77. Vance JE, Buchanan KD, O'Hara D, et al. Insulin and glucagon responses in subjects with pheochromocytoma: effect of α adrenergic blockade. J Clin Endocrinol Metab 1969; 29:911.

78. Malbon CC, Campbell R. Thyroid hormones regulate hepatic glycogen synthase. Endocrinology 1984; 115:681.

79. Dimitriadis GD, Leighton B, Vlachonikolis IG, et al. Effects of hyperthyroidism on the sensitivity of glycolysis and glycogen synthesis to insulin in the soleus muscle of the rat. Biochem J 1988; 253:87.

80. Holness MJ, Sugden MC. Hepatic carbon flux after re-feeding: hyperthyroidism blocks glycogen synthesis and the suppression of glucose output observed in response to carbohydrate refeeding. Biochem J 1987; 247:627.

81. Tosi F, Moghetti P, Castello R, et al. Early changes in plasma glucagon and growth hormone response to oral glucose in experimental hyperthyroidism. Metabolism 1996; 45:1029.

82. Fryer LG, Holness MJ, Sugden MC. Selective modification of insulin action in adipose tissue by hyperthyroidism. J Endocrinol 1997; 154:513.

83. Matthei S, Trost B, Hamann A, et al. Effect of in vivo thyroid hormone status on insulin signalling and GLUT1 and GLUT4 glucose transport systems in rat adipocytes. J Endocrinol 1995; 144:347.

84. Gonzalo MA, Grant C, Moreno I, et al. Glucose tolerance, insulin secretion, insulin sensitivity and glucose effectiveness in normal and overweight hyperthyroid women. Clin Endocrinol 1996; 45:689.

85. Bonadonna RC, DeFronzo RA. Glucose metabolism in obesity and type II diabetes. In: Bjorntorp P, Brodoff BN, eds. Obesity. Philadelphia: JB Lippincott; 1992:474.

86. Sorenson RL, Brejle TC, Hegre OD, et al. Prolactin (in vitro) decreases the glucose stimulation threshold, enhances insulin secretion, and increases dye coupling among islet B cells. Endocrinology 1987; 121:1447.

87. Brejle TC, Parsons JA, Sorenson RL. Regulation of islet β-cell proliferation by prolactin in rat islets. Endocrinology 1994; 43:263.

88. Weinhaus AJ, Stout LE, Sorenson RL. Glucokinase, hexokinase, glucose transporter 2, and glucose metabolism in islets during pregnancy and prolactin-treated islets in vitro: mechanisms for long term up-regulation of islets. Endocrinology 1996; 137:1640.

89. Wade GN, Schneider JE. Metabolic fuels and reproduction in female mammals. Neurosci Biobehav Rev 1992; 16:235.

90. Matsuda M, Mori T. Effect of estrogen on hyperprolactinemia-induced glucose intolerance in SHN mice. Proc Soc Exp Biol Med 1996; 212:243.

91. Reis FM, Reis AM, Coimbra CC. Effects of hyperprolactinaemia on glucose tolerance and insulin release in male and female rats. J Endocrinol 1997; 153:423.

92. Del Prato S, Fiengo A, Baccaglini U, et al. Effect of insulin replacement on intermediary metabolism in diabetes secondary to pancreatectomy. Diabetologia 1983; 25:252.

93. Barnes AJ, Bloom SR, Alberti KGMM, et al. Ketoacidosis in pancreatectomized man. N Engl J Med 1977; 296:1250.

94. Nosadini R, Del Prato S, Fiengo A, et al. Insulin sensitivity, binding, and kinetics in pancreatogenic and type I diabetes. Diabetes 1982; 31:346.

95. Joffe BI, Bank S, Marks IN. Hypoglycemia in pancreatitis. Lancet 1968; 2:1038.

96. Polonsky KS, Herold KC, Gilden JL, et al. Glucose counterregulation in patients after pancreatectomy. Diabetes 1984; 33:1112.

97. Muller WA, Berger M, Suter P, et al. Glucagon immunoreactivities and amino acid profile in plasma of duodenopancreatectomized patients. J Clin Invest 1979; 83:620.

98. Joffe BI, Bank S, Jackson WPU, et al. Insulin reserve in patients with chronic pancreatitis. Lancet 1968; 11:890.

99. Mohan V, Snehalatha C, Ahmed MR, et al. Exocrine pancreatic function in tropical fibrocalculous pancreatic diabetes. Diabetes Care 1989; 12:145.

100. Kalk WJ, Vinik AI, Bank S, et al. Glucagon response to arginine in chronic pancreatitis. Diabetes 1974; 23:257.

101. Yeo CJ, Bastidas JA, Schmieg RE Jr, et al. Pancreatic structure and glucose tolerance in a longitudinal study of experimental pancreatitis-induced diabetes. Ann Surg 1989; 210:150.

102. Seymour NE, Turk JB, Laster MK, et al. In vitro hepatic insulin resistance in chronic pancreatitis in the rat. J Surg Res 1989; 46:450.

103. Sun YS, Brunicardi FC, Druck P, et al. Reversal of abnormal glucose metabolism in chronic pancreatitis by administration of pancreatic polypeptide. Am J Surg 1986; 151:130.

104. Goldstein JA, Kirwin JD, Seymour NE, et al. Reversal of in vitro hepatic insulin resistance in chronic pancreatitis by pancreatic polypeptide in the rat. Surgery 1989; 106:1128.

105. Brunicardi FC, Chaiken RL, Ryan AS, et al. Pancreatic polypeptide administration improves abnormal glucose metabolism in patients with chronic pancreatitis. J Clin Endocrinol Metab 1996; 81:3566.

106. Unger RH, Dobbs RC, Orci L. Insulin, glucagon, and somatostatin secretion in the regulation of metabolism. Annu Rev Physiol 1978; 40:307.

107. Donowitz M, Hendler R, Spiro HM, et al. Glucagon secretion in acute and chronic pancreatitis. Ann Intern Med 1975; 83:778.

108. Dymock IW, Cassai J, Pyke DA, et al. Observations on the pathogenesis, complications and treatment of diabetes in 115 cases of hemochromatosis. Am J Med 1972; 52:203.

109. Rowe JW, Wands JR, Mezey E, et al. Familial hemochromatosis: characteristics of the pre-cirrhotic stage in a large kindred. Medicine 1977; 56:197.
110. Merkel PA, Simonson DC, Amiel SA, et al. Insulin resistance and hyperinsulinemia in patients with thalassemia major treated by hypertransfusion. N Engl J Med 1988; 318:809.
111. Hramiak IM, Finegood DT, Adams PC. Factors affecting glucose tolerance in hereditary hemochromatosis 1. Clin Invest 1997; 20:110.
112. Stremmel W, Niederau C, Berger M, et al. Abnormalities in estrogen, androgens, and insulin metabolism in hereditary hemochromatosis. Ann N Y Acad Sci 1988; 526:209.
113. Bierens de Haan B, Scherrer JR, Stauffseker W, Pometta D. Iron excess, early glucose intolerance and impaired insulin secretion in idiopathic hemochromatosis. Eur J Clin Invest 1973; 3:179.
114. Goldberg EM, Sanbar SS. Hyperglycemic, nonketotic coma following administration of Dilantin (diphenylhydantoin). Diabetes 1969; 18:101.
115. Levin SR, Booker J, Smith DF, et al. Inhibition of insulin secretion by diphenylhydantoin in the isolated perfused pancreas. J Clin Endocrinol Metab 1970; 30:400.
116. Siegel EG, Janjic D, Wollheim CB. Phenytoin inhibition of insulin release. Studies on the involvement of $Ca^{2+}$ fluxes in rat pancreatic islets. Diabetes 1982; 31:265.
117. Malherbe C, Burrill KC, Levin SR, et al. Effect of diphenylhydantoin on insulin secretion in man. N Engl J Med 1972; 286:339.
118. Shen M, Orwoll ES, Conte JE Jr, et al. Pentamidine-induced pancreatic β-cell dysfunction. Am J Med 1989; 86:726.
119. Karam JH, Prosser PR, Lewitt PA. Islet-cell surface antibodies in a patient with diabetes mellitus after rodenticide ingestion. N Engl J Med 1978; 299:1191.
120. Murphy MB, Kohner E, Lewis PJ, et al. Glucose intolerance in hypertensive patients treated with diuretics: a fourteen-year follow-up. Lancet 1982; 2:1293.
121. Helderman JH, Eelaahi D, Andersen DK, et al. Prevention of glucose intolerance of thiazide diuretics by maintenance of body potassium. Diabetes 1983; 32:106.
122. Tucker SJ, Gribble FM, Zhao C, et al. Truncation of Kir6.2 produces ATP-sensitive $K^+$ channels in the absence of the sulphonylurea receptor. Nature 1997; 387:179.
123. Sandstrom PE. Inhibition by hydrochlorothiazide of insulin release and calcium influx in mouse pancreatic β cells. Br J Pharmacol 1993; 110:1359.
124. Sandstrom PE. Bumetanide reduces insulin release by a direct effect on the pancreatic β cells. Eur J Pharmacol 1990; 187:377.
125. Podolsky S, Pattavina CG. Hyperosmolar non-ketotic diabetic coma: a complication of propranolol therapy. Metabolism 1973; 22:685.
126. Kotler MN, Berman L, Rubenstein AH. Hypoglycemia precipitated by propranolol. Lancet 1966; 2:1389.
127. Feldberg VS, Shaligram SV. The hyperglycemic effect of morphine. Br J Pharmacol 1972; 46:602.
128. Passariello N, Grisgliano D, Quatraro A, et al. Glucose tolerance and hormonal responses in heroin addicts: a possible role for endogenous opiates in the pathogenesis of non-insulin-dependent diabetes. Metabolism 1983; 32:1163.
129. Bruni JF, Watkins WE, Yen SSC. β-Endorphins: the human pancreas. J Clin Endocrinol Metab 1980; 49:649.
130. The Diabetes Control and Complications Trial Research Group. The effect of intensive treatment of diabetes on the development and progression of long-term complications in insulin-dependent diabetes mellitus. N Engl J Med 1993; 329:977.
131. Merimee TJ, Fineberg SE, Hollander W. Vascular disease in the chronic HGH-deficient state. Diabetes 1973; 22:813.
132. Verdonk CA, Palumbo PJ, Gharib H, Bartholomew LG. Diabetic microangiopathy in patients with pancreatic diabetes mellitus. Diabetologia 1975; 11:395.
133. Tiengo A, Segato T, Briani G, et al. The presence of retinopathy in patients with secondary diabetes following pancreatectomy or chronic pancreatitis. Diabetes Care 1983; 6:570.

# CHAPTER 140

# EVALUATION OF METABOLIC CONTROL IN DIABETES

ALLISON B. GOLDFINE

Since the introduction of insulin therapy in 1921, controversy has existed over whether improvement in glycemic control is associated with a decrease in the complications of diabetes, including retinopathy, nephropathy, neuropathy, and macrovascular disease, or whether these complications represent associated genetic manifestations of the disease. For years, much of the evidence indicating the importance of glycemic control came from animal studies, such as those showing that islet cell transplantation or insulin treatment can reduce retinopathy and nephropathy in rats and dogs with chemically induced diabetes.[1,2] The fact that autoimmune type 1, insulin-resistant type 2, and secondary diabetes mellitus (e.g., associated with chronic pancreatitis, surgical pancreatectomy, acromegaly, hemochromatosis) are conditions with widely different pathophysiologic bases that have similar complications also suggests that hyperglycemia plays an important role in the development of complications.

The most compelling evidence that hyperglycemia is associated with diabetic complications was obtained from several major human studies. The Diabetes Control and Complications Trial (DCCT) demonstrated that, in patients with type 1 diabetes, intensive insulin therapy with the goal of near-normalization of blood glucose levels could delay the onset or slow the progression of clinically important retinopathy, nephropathy, and neuropathy by 35% to 70%.[3] Any improvement in glycemia that was achieved was associated with a decreased risk of complications, and no glycemic target could be demonstrated below which no additional benefit to the patient resulted. This intensive insulin treatment, however, was associated with approximately a three-fold increase in the risk of significant hypoglycemia, defined as hypoglycemia in which assistance was required for treatment and included coma and seizures.[4] Comparable results have been demonstrated in important smaller studies and in metaanalyses of the effects of intensive blood glucose control on the development of complications.[5,6] The applicability of these results to the many individuals who have type 2 diabetes has been demonstrated in the United Kingdom Prospective Diabetes Study (UKPDS), in which the intensive control cohort demonstrated a 10% to 12% lower risk for combined diabetes-related end points or diabetes-related death.[7] As seen in other studies, most risk reduction was found in microvascular end points.[7,8] Thus, a clear rationale exists for the intensive treatment of patients with diabetes, with the goal of normalization or near-normalization of blood glucose levels. To determine safe glycemic ranges for individual patients, physicians must consider their age, coexisting medical problems, degree of hypoglycemia awareness, and ability to follow a labor-intensive treatment program.

## HOME BLOOD GLUCOSE MONITORING

To achieve near-normalization of blood glucose levels, each patient requires a different regimen, including multiple daily injections of insulin, use of subcutaneous insulin pumps, use of oral hypoglycemic or insulin-sensitizing agents, exercise, and/or control of diet. To ensure patient safety, frequent measurements of the blood glucose level are necessary to determine the 24-hour glucose profile and allow adjustments to be made in the treatment regimen. Several companies market small meter devices that accurately measure blood glucose levels. These can be carried in a purse or wallet-sized case. A 2 to 20 μL blood sample is obtained from a fingertip puncture and placed on a reagent strip. The most common method of measuring the glucose level involves the conversion of glucose to gluconic acid and hydrogen peroxide by glucose oxidase impregnated in the meter's reagent strip. The hydrogen peroxide is a substrate for a chromogen that also is present on the strip and generates the color change. After the blood is wiped off the strip, the meter reads the intensity of the color change and provides a digital readout of the blood glucose level. Some chemical strips also can be read visually by comparing them to a standardized chart. Systems that use electrochemical reactions instead of colorimetric reactions have become widely used because they do not require attention to timing or wiping of the reagent strip, and the older systems are becoming obsolete. These systems make it easier for patients to perform the analysis but provide no visual means of assessing the accuracy of the reading. Essentially all the available meters are reliable, with little variability in accuracy and precision when used appropriately, but patient education in correct use is important and technique should be checked occasionally. Common causes of erroneous values include insufficient blood on the test strip, touching of the sample application area, improper capping of vials (allowing exposure of the reagent strip to moisture), inadequate cleaning of the optical window, poor environmental operating conditions (such as extremes of light, altitude, humidity, or temperature), and failure to coordinate the meter to the lot number of the test strips. Biologic variables that could affect accuracy include abnormal hematocrit or triglyceride levels. Machine calibration can best be evaluated by running a sample on the meter and simultaneously sending a sample to the laboratory for comparison; however, capillary whole blood glucose values may be 12% lower than those of venous plasma. Some meters are calibrated to whole blood and others to plasma. In addition, meters requiring 2 to 5 µL blood samples tend to report lower values than meters requiring larger blood samples.

Products are now available to minimize the discomfort of obtaining capillary blood, such as laser finger perforators and meter devices that sample from the forearm and thigh, which contain fewer nerve endings than the fingertip. Minimally invasive devices, which are currently under development, use a soft catheter (inserted for several days into the subcutaneous tissue to sample interstitial fluid) that is connected to a small external meter to evaluate glucose by electroenzymatic or microdialysis methods. These monitors can evaluate glucose on a continuous basis, and prototypes are equipped with alarms to signal high and low glucose values. If glucose levels are changing rapidly, glucose sensor measurements in subcutaneous tissue may precede or follow those in the blood. The first noninvasive device uses infrared absorption through cutaneous tissue. Although averaged glucose results correlate well with blood measurements, the variation of an individual determination is large, and the system cannot be used for intensive management. Other noninvasive devices are under development.

For any of these devices to be useful to either patients or physicians, patients must chart their blood glucose measurements carefully in an organized manner. Data collection forms are available from many of the meter companies, or individualized forms can be made that include space in which to note the time of day, the blood glucose value, the relationship of the measurement to meals, the insulin dose, and any unusual physical activity or symptoms. Some meters have an internal memory and can be connected directly to a personal computer to generate a printout of the glucose data and averages of blood glucose determinations or to a modem to transmit the information to the physician. These applications have not yet been used extensively by patients, but their value may increase as personal computers become more widely available.

Home blood glucose monitoring should be considered mandatory for pregnant patients with diabetes, as well as for all patients who are attempting to achieve near-normalization of blood glucose levels. Home monitoring also is helpful for confirming the clinical diagnosis of hypoglycemia in patients who have equivocal symptoms or hypoglycemic awareness. Many patients are relieved by the ability to obtain accurate home blood glucose determinations because it provides them with greater control over their disease and gives them the freedom to live a more active and normal life. The optimum number of times per day that patients should measure their blood glucose levels has not been extensively evaluated. Studies show that, of all patients who use home blood glucose monitoring, only 28% obtain a measurement more than once per day; 10% do so less than once per week.[9] In contrast, subjects in the intensive treatment group of the

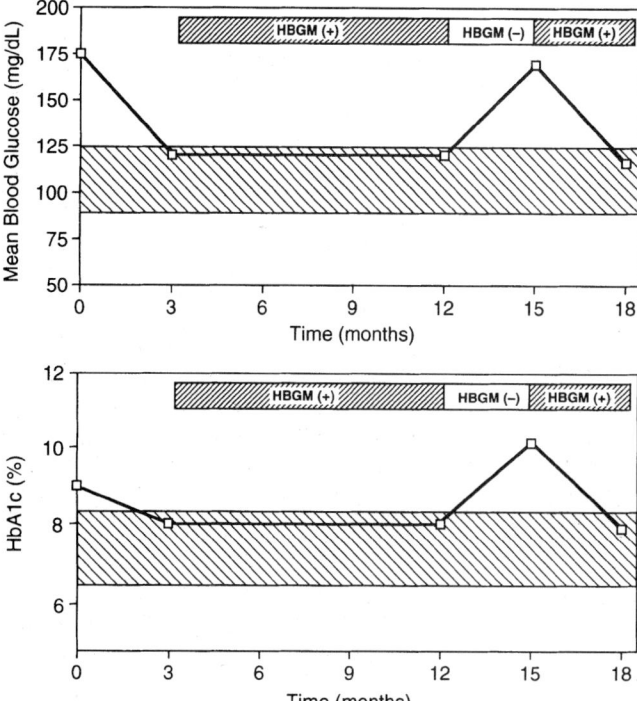

**FIGURE 140-1.** Mean blood glucose and hemoglobin $A_{1c}$ ($HbA_{1c}$) levels in subjects with type 1 diabetes mellitus with and without home blood glucose monitoring. With multiple home glucose determinations performed at least four to seven times daily [$HBGM(+)$], subjects were able to normalize their mean blood glucose and $HbA_{1c}$ levels. When the frequency of monitoring decreased to twice daily [$HBGM(-)$], however, both mean blood glucose and $HbA_{1c}$ levels increased above normal. These indices of glycemic control improved again when the frequency of monitoring was increased. (Adapted from Shiffrin A, Belmonte M. Multiple daily glucose monitoring. Diabetes Care 1982; 5:479.)

DCCT performed four to seven measurements daily. In other studies of subjects with type 1 diabetes who were treated with continuous subcutaneous insulin infusion or multiple subcutaneous insulin injections, the pattern of insulin requirements varied sufficiently in each patient that optimal glucose control could not be maintained when frequent self-monitoring was interrupted. When glucose determinations were performed at least four to seven times per day, subjects were able to maintain mean blood glucose levels of 118 mg/dL and hemoglobin (Hb) $A_1$ levels within the normal range (8.3%). When the frequency of capillary glucose level determinations was decreased to twice per day, mean blood glucose levels increased to 162 mg/dL and $HbA_1$ levels increased to above normal (10.1%). When an increased monitoring frequency was resumed, mean blood glucose and $HbA_1$ levels returned toward normal. Importantly, however, the glucose determinations were used to adjust insulin doses each day[10] (Fig. 140-1). Multiple daily testing does not improve glucose control if the insulin dose remains fixed. If patients are not able or willing to perform multiple daily measurements, less frequent home blood glucose determinations can be useful to assess the therapeutic regimen, especially if glucose is sampled at different times of the day on a regular basis throughout the week or month. In addition, controversy exists over whether patients should check their blood glucose levels before or after meals. Preprandial glucose levels should be at the lower end of a target range and postprandial levels should be at the upper end. Specific recommendations for individual patients are determined by clinical factors, such as the ability to sense a low blood glucose level. Measurement of postprandial values generally is recommended in prenatal care.

The only disadvantages of home blood glucose monitoring are the local discomfort from the finger stick and the cost of the reagent strips, which is not universally reimbursed by insurance companies despite the major health advantages for patients derived from improved glycemic control.

## URINE TESTING

### GLUCOSE

Urinary glucose measurements are not the best means of monitoring glycemic control; however, some patients with diabetes are unwilling or unable to perform home blood glucose determinations but will comply with urine glucose testing. Much like the reagent strips used in blood glucose monitoring, the urine reagent strips are impregnated with glucose oxidase and generate characteristic color changes in the presence of urine glucose. Blood and urine reagent strips are not interchangeable. Urine testing, even when performed correctly, gives only a crude estimate of plasma glucose levels. The renal threshold for glucose varies among individuals. In most individuals, however, when plasma glucose levels exceed ~180 mg/dL, glycosuria occurs. Unfortunately, this threshold is not fixed for an individual and can change under the influence of physiologic states such as pregnancy, which decreases the threshold, or aging, which increases it. It also is important to remember that urine collected in the bladder reflects plasma glucose levels over the time interval since the last void, so that testing the first morning void might represent glucose levels since the patient went to bed the night before. To assess morning plasma glucose levels more closely, patients should be instructed to perform a double void, in which the bladder is emptied and the urine is discarded, then the patient voids again after a 15- to 20-minute interval and tests this second sample for glucose. This technique can be used before meals and at bedtime. If it is done accurately, it can provide some assessment of glycemic stability and facilitate tailoring of a therapeutic regimen. With the advent of home capillary blood glucose monitoring, however, this method is no longer optimal.

### KETONES

Urine ketones should be measured in patients with type 1 diabetes who have hyperglycemia with glucose levels higher than 250 mg/dL. This test allows physicians and patients to recognize and respond to the development of early diabetic ketoacidosis. It reveals the degree of insulin deficiency, which helps physicians determine how much insulin should be delivered as an additional "booster" to treat hyperglycemia. Booster shots generally consist of 5% to 25% of a patient's total daily insulin dose, given in the form of regular or short-acting insulin. Measurement of urine ketones also is useful clinically to assess the response to therapy in both the inpatient and outpatient settings, and can be performed conveniently with the use of reagent strips such as Ketostix. These products generally detect ketone bodies (acetoacetic acid and acetone) but not β-hydroxybutyric acid. Freshly voided urine contains ~10 times more acetoacetic acid than acetone. Over time, however, acetoacetic acid spontaneously degrades, leaving a greater proportion of acetone. Ketones may be absent from the urine in individuals with uremia. Similarly, urine and serum ketone levels can be falsely low if the keto acid equilibrium is shifted toward the reduced state (predominantly β-hydroxybutyrate), such as when the redox potential of the patient is high (as in alcoholic ketoacidosis). After the initiation of therapy for diabetic ketoacidosis, an apparent worsening of ketone levels can be observed; as the redox potential of the patient shifts, β-hydroxybutyrate clears through conversion to acetoacetate and acetone, which are measured by the standard assays. Ferric chloride (Gerhardt) and sodium nitroprusside (Rothera) tests also can be performed in the clinical laboratory, but are more labor intensive and time consuming, and do not yield great advantage. Like urine glucose levels, urine ketone levels represent the metabolic status of the patient since the time of the last void. Similarly, however, when ketones have been cleared from the bloodstream, test results for urine ketones become negative, making this a rapid and inexpensive way to monitor the evolution of diabetic ketoacidosis at the bedside.

Other causes of ketoaciduria include alcoholic ketoacidosis, starvation (which is accelerated in late pregnancy and lactation), severely hypocaloric diets, and fasting ketosis. In alcoholic ketoacidosis, an underlying nutritional deficiency and an exaggerated response to fasting are present. Unlike diabetic ketoacidosis, this condition often resolves with the administration of glucose alone and can be differentiated on the basis of history and, sometimes, positive blood alcohol levels. In starvation and pregnancy, hyperglycemia and glycosuria usually are absent. In fasting, urine ketones are rarely above trace levels and total serum ketones rarely exceed 4 to 6 mmol/L.[11]

## GLYCATED HEMOGLOBIN

Measurements of glycated Hb are of major clinical value for objective monitoring of glucose control in patients with diabetes and have been correlated with long-term complications of diabetes and with fetal outcome in pregnant patients with diabetes. Unfortunately, glycated Hb measurements cannot discriminate impaired glucose tolerance or mild diabetes from normal glucose tolerance, and are inadequate as a screening test in the diagnosis of gestational diabetes because of the high rate of false-negative results. Glycated Hb measurements provide only an estimate of the average blood glucose level over the preceding interim and indicate nothing about the variability of the glucose level (i.e., the patient's brittleness) during that period (Fig. 140-2). Adult Hb consists of ~97% HbA ($\alpha_2\beta_2$), 2.5% HbA$_2$ ($\alpha_2\gamma_2$), and 0.5% HbF ($\alpha_2\delta_2$). Also found are several minor species, HbA$_{1a}$, HbA$_{1b}$, and HbA$_{1c}$, which are collectively known as glycated Hb. Glycohemoglobin is formed continuously in erythrocytes as the product of a nonenzymatic reaction between Hb and glucose, first forming the labile Schiff base, or pre-A$_{1c}$, then the more stable Amadori product (Fig. 140-3). HbA$_{1c}$ specifically refers to the Amadori product of the N-terminal valine of each β chain of HbA with glucose, whereas HbA$_{1a}$ and HbA$_{1b}$ have the carbohydrate moiety attached to other amino acids. HbA$_{1c}$ makes up ~80% of the glycated HbA$_1$

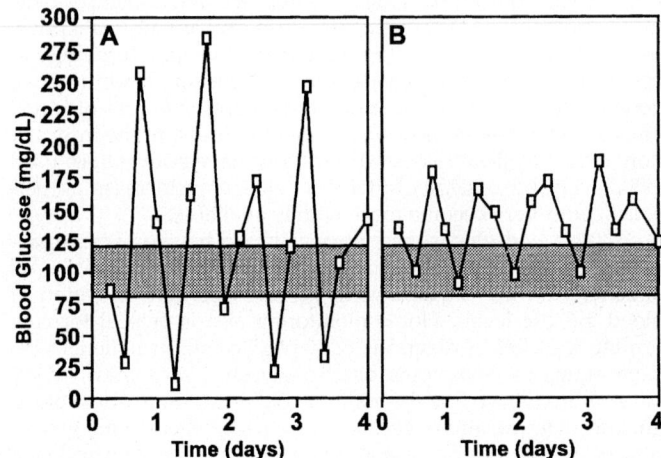

**FIGURE 140-2.** Blood glucose determinations in patients with diabetes mellitus. Home blood glucose analysis shows both mean blood glucose levels and the variation, or lability, of these values in a patient. Both patients represented here have mean glucose levels of 140 mg/dL; however, the patient in panel **A** would be considered more brittle than the patient in panel **B**.

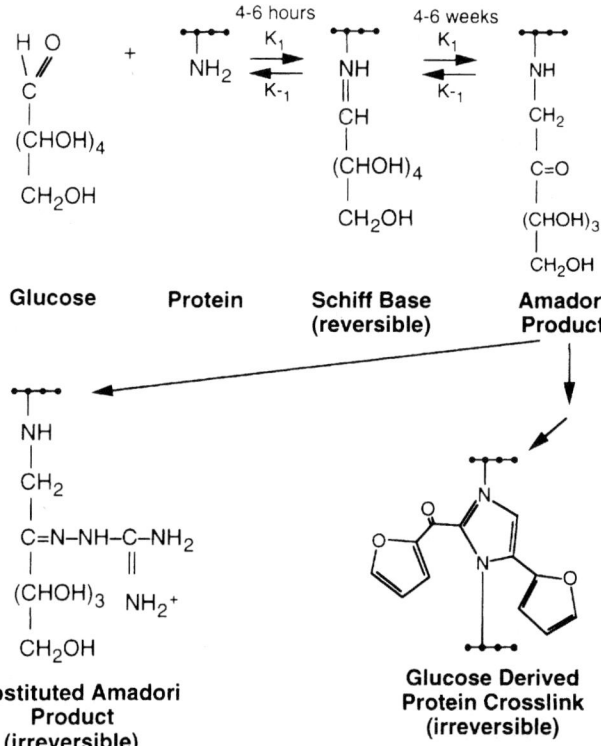

**FIGURE 140-3.** Protein glycation is shown as the nonenzymatic reaction between the protein (often measured as hemoglobin) and glucose, first forming the reversible, labile Schiff base, and then the more stable Amadori product, which can go on to form irreversible substitutions and cross-linking.

and is the fraction that best reflects average blood glucose concentrations. Other carbohydrate moieties, such as fructose-1,6-diphosphate and glucose-6-phosphate, can react with the Hb molecules to form other glycated hemoglobins, such as $HbA_{1a1}$ and $HbA_{1a2}$, respectively. Glycohemoglobin measurements can serve as a reliable index of average blood glucose concentrations over the preceding 6 to 8 weeks because of the long half-life of red blood cells.

Methods of measuring glycohemoglobin fall into two main categories, depending on the manner in which the glycated and nonglycated Hbs are separated. Some methods are based on charge separation (e.g., ion-exchange chromatography or electrophoresis and high-performance liquid chromatography), and some methods are based on structural characteristics of the glycation group on the Hb (e.g., affinity chromatography and immunoassay).[12] Glycated Hb results are method and laboratory specific. $HbA_1$ results tend to be higher than $HbA_{1c}$ results. The numerous techniques used in different laboratories make it difficult to compare an individual patient's results across laboratories.[12] In addition, these techniques are associated with different false elevations and suppressions, such as those caused by Hb structural variants like HbS, HbC, or HbE; Hb synthesis variants such as β-thalassemia; and posttranslational modifications of Hb such as the Schiff base and carbamylated Hb or acetylated Hb.[13] Carbamylated Hb, which increases with renal failure, is least affected by chromatography or immunoassay techniques. Any condition that leads to increased red blood cell turnover and shortened exposure to glucose leads to decreased glycosylated Hb levels by all assay methods. Likewise, processes that lengthen red blood cell survival, such as iron deficiency anemias, increase glycohemoglobin measurements. Other leading causes of falsely elevated or suppressed measurements include the presence of HbS, which would reduce the relative amount of HbA and, therefore, decrease the measured $HbA_{1c}$ by all methods except

affinity chromatography; and the persistence of HbF, which coelutes with $HbA_{1c}$ in methods based on charge separation and, thus, could increase these readings. (See refs. 14 and 15.)

## FRUCTOSAMINE

Many clinical situations exist in which it would be helpful to have an objective measurement of glucose control over a shorter time span than that provided by measurements of glycohemoglobin. These occasions arise most often when sudden changes occur in a patient's degree of control, such as with the initiation of new therapy for hyperglycemia, during the planning period for a pregnancy or at the time of conception, during a superimposed medical illness, or with the addition of a new medication that may alter insulin sensitivity. Because serum proteins other than Hb become glycated in the presence of hyperglycemia, these may be used as alternatives to $HbA_{1c}$. The best characterized of these proteins is albumin, with a half-life of 2 to 3 weeks, which reflects glycemic control over this shorter interval.

Nitroblue tetrazolium colorimetric methods have been used to measure glycated serum proteins, particularly albumin, and are known as the fructosamine assay. These methods are limited by the nonspecific nature of the reaction. Uric acid, bilirubin, and lipids all interfere with the assay. In addition, changes in albumin concentration, such as occur with alterations in nutritional status or with liver or kidney disease, can affect the measurements. Assay standardization also has been less reliable in early versions of this test compared with the synthetic deoxymorpholinofructose standard.[16] Thus, although the test has been available for more than a decade, it has not been favored clinically. Second-generation assays have been introduced that incorporate uricase in the reagent to eliminate the interference with uric acid and use nonionic surfactants to eliminate the protein-matrix effects and the interference from lipemia. These assays also are standardized against glycated polylysine standards, which are more physiologic.[17,18] Further improvements in assay technique are being developed and should lead to more widespread use of these measurements. Fructosamine levels can now be determined by the patient on a portable meter device.

Although both fructosamine and glycohemoglobin levels correlate well with outpatient measurements of capillary blood glucose concentrations, no absolute correlation exists between fructosamine and glycohemoglobin levels, because the value for each assay depends on the half-lives of the major proteins measured and the average glycemic control for the different intervals preceding the blood collection.[18,19]

## REFERENCES

1. Engerman R, Bloodworth JMB Jr, Nelson S. Relationship of microvascular disease in diabetes to metabolic control. Diabetes 1977; 26:760.
2. Mauer SM, Steffes MW, Brown DM. The kidney in diabetes. Am J Med 1981; 70:603.
3. Diabetes Control and Complication Research Group. The effect of intensive treatment of diabetes on the development and progression of long-term complications in insulin-dependent diabetes mellitus. N Engl J Med 1993; 329:977.
4. Diabetes Control and Complication Research Group. Epidemiology of severe hypoglycemia in the Diabetes Control and Complication Trial. Am J Med 1991; 90:450.
5. Reichard P, Nilsson BY, Rosenqvist U. The effect of long-term intensified insulin treatment on the development of microvascular complications of diabetes mellitus. N Engl J Med 1993; 329:304.
6. Wang PH, Lau J, Chalmers TC. Meta-analysis of effects of intensive blood-glucose control on late complications of type I diabetes. Lancet 1993; 341:1306.
7. United Kingdom Prospective Diabetes Study Group. Intensive blood glucose control with sulphonylureas or insulin compared with conventional treatment and risk of complications in patients with type 2 diabetes (UKPDS-33). Lancet 1998; 352:837.
8. Brownlee M. Glycation products and the pathogenesis of diabetic complications. Diabetes Care 1992; 15:1835.
9. 1993 Diabetes Tracking Study. New York: Crossley Surveys, 1993.

10. Schiffrin A, Belmonte M. Multiple daily self-glucose monitoring: its essential role in long-term glucose control in insulin-dependent diabetic patients treated with pump and multiple subcutaneous injections. Diabetes Care 1982; 5:479.
11. Cahill GF, Herrerra MG, Morgan AP, et al. Hormone-fuel interrelationships during fasting. J Clin Invest 1966; 45:1751.
12. Little FF, Wiedmeyer HM, England JD, et al. Interlaboratory comparison of glycohemoglobin results: College of American Pathologists survey data. Clin Chem 1991; 37:1725.
13. Weykamp CW, Penders TJ, Muskiet FAJ, Van Der Slik W. Influence of hemoglobin variants and derivatives on glycohemoglobin determinations as investigated by 102 laboratories using 16 methods. Clin Chem 1993; 39:1717.
14. Thomas A. Standardization of HbAic measurement—the issues. Diabetic Med 2000; 17:2.
15. McKenzie PT, Sugarman JR. Implications for clinical performance measurement of interlaboratory variability in methods for glycosylated hemoglobin testing. Am J Med Qual 2000; 15:62.
16. Vogt BW. Development of an improved fructosamine test. In: Workshop report, fructosamine. Mannheim, Germany: Boehringer Mannheim GmbH, 1989:21.
17. Baker J, Metcalf P, Scragg R, Johnson R. Fructosamine test-plus, a modified fructosamine assay evaluated. Clin Chem 1991; 37:552.
18. Cefalu WT, Bell-Farrow AD, Petty M, et al. Clinical validation of a second-generation fructosamine assay. Clin Chem 1991; 37:1252.
19. Shield JP, Poyser K, Hunt L, Pennock CA. Fructosamine and glycated hemoglobin in the assessment of long term glycaemic control in diabetics. Arch Dis Child 1994; 71:443.

# CHAPTER 141

# DIET AND EXERCISE IN DIABETES

OM P. GANDA

Diet and exercise are two of the most important modalities in the therapy of diabetes and have been considered in its management for centuries. Previously, however, most of the recommendations for diet and exercise given to the diabetic patient were based on speculation; only recently have they been subjected to rigorous scientific scrutiny. Considerable controversy exists, particularly regarding dietary therapy in diabetes,[1–3] although everyone agrees that careful attention to diet is an essential component in the management of diabetes.

As early as the eighteenth century, diet modification was advocated to control glycosuria. In the preinsulin era, Allen initiated diet therapy, consisting of periods of starvation to prevent ketoacidosis in young diabetics, and diet regimens calling for high intake of fat (up to 60–80% of total calories) and low intake of carbohydrates in adult diabetics.[2,4] Subsequently, during most of the twentieth century, a tradition of a low-carbohydrate, high-fat diet evolved as a general principle. In the past two decades, however, serious questions have arisen about the rationale for such regimens. Diabetologists now agree that the fat intake in the diabetic diet has been much too liberal and should be curtailed in an effort to prevent long-term vascular complications. However, the idea of a more liberal allowance of carbohydrate in the diabetic patient's diet is not novel. As early as 1927, Joslin[5] suggested that the increased prevalence of atherosclerosis in older diabetics was secondary to obesity and high fat intake. In 1935, a relatively high carbohydrate diet was shown to improve glucose tolerance as well as to improve insulin sensitivity in nondiabetic persons and in patients with "impaired" glucose tolerance.[6] Thus, the idea emerged that a more liberal intake of carbohydrate may not worsen and may actually improve diabetes control.

The current interest in diet therapy lies in the systematic investigation of the mechanisms by which various diet components affect metabolic control in diabetics and of the variable effects of various types of carbohydrates in the treatment, and possibly in

the prevention, of diabetes. Interest is also great in the role of fiber and the role of specific dietary factors in the lipid abnormalities that are frequently observed, particularly in type 2 diabetes.

## PRINCIPLES OF DIET THERAPY IN DIABETES

Because of the heterogeneity of diabetic syndromes, no single diabetic diet exists, even for a given type of diabetes.[1,7] The diet for a diabetic individual must be planned according to age; nutritional status; severity of metabolic disorder; level of physical activity; educational, social, cultural, and economic factors; and the presence of any associated problems such as hyperlipidemia, hypertension, or renal disease. In children and adolescents with type 1 diabetes, the main objective is to provide adequate calories, distributed in a balanced proportion of all food exchanges (milk, vegetables, fruit, bread, meat, and fat) to achieve optimal growth and development. In most patients with type 2 diabetes and associated obesity, the primary goal is to achieve compliance with a hypocaloric, yet practical, meal plan to succeed in weight reduction. Even modest weight reduction can improve various aspects of type 2 diabetes (e.g., glucose control, insulin secretion, insulin action) and improve hypertension and hyperlipidemia, which frequently coexist in such patients.[8–10] Unfortunately, long-term success in maintaining a lowered weight level is often limited and is dependent largely on factors such as patient motivation, success in behavior modification, and frequent contact with health care professionals (see Chap. 126).[11] Severely restricted (<800 calories), protein-supplemented starvation diets are usually ineffective in the long term and sometimes are associated with serious cardiovascular complications.[12] Such approaches should be followed only under strict medical supervision.

### CARBOHYDRATE CONTROVERSY AND THE ROLE OF FIBER

Controversy continues over several aspects of diet composition, including (a) carbohydrate content, (b) the source of carbohydrate (simple vs. complex), (c) the relative glycemic potential of different carbohydrates within simple and complex carbohydrates, and (d) the role of fiber in the diet.

The advice to increase the carbohydrate content of the diabetic diet to 55% to 60% of total calories was promulgated by the American Diabetes Association in 1986.[13] However, revised guidelines recommend a more individualized approach.[7] The addition of sucrose, added to account for 15% to 20% of calories in a mixed meal, does not appear to aggravate the postprandial hyperglycemic response in well-controlled type 1 or type 2 diabetes.[14] In some patients, however, sucrose or fructose may aggravate hypertriglyceridemia. Although no epidemiologic or experimental studies are available on the effect of variations of carbohydrate content on the long-term complications in patients with diabetes, such dietary modification does allow a decrease in the fat content of the diet (30–35% of total calories). The latter may be of considerable benefit. Several large, prospective, multicenter trials have shown that the lowering of LDL cholesterol is associated with a significant decrease in the development and progression of macrovascular disease in nondiabetic as well as diabetic individuals (see Chap. 164).

Traditionally, recommendations have included limiting the intake of simple carbohydrates considerably.[15,16] When the postprandial serum glucose response to white bread is used as a reference (100%), the *glycemic index*[15] of various simple carbohydrates is variable (e.g., glucose, 140%; sucrose, 85%; lactose [as milk or yogurt], 50%; and fructose, 30%). Similarly, a marked variation exists among complex carbohydrates (e.g., breakfast cereals, 70–110%; spaghetti, 60%; dried legumes [lentils, beans, peas], 40–60% [with soybeans having a glycemic index as low as 20%]. In patients with both type 1 and type 2 diabetes, however, equivalent amounts of glucose, fructose, potato, or wheat produced similar glycemic responses and, in those with type 2 diabetes, similar insulin responses.[17] Similarly, when foods are consumed as mixed meals, the different glycemic indices of the individual foods do not always reflect postprandial glycemic excursion accurately.[18,19] Nevertheless, at least in some situations, consumption of meals with a high glycemic index might promote higher insulin levels, increased energy intake, and greater weight gain.[20]

Several factors that affect the glycemic response to the carbohydrate include other nutritional components (fat, protein) in the mixed meal, the physical state of a food item (e.g., whole grain vs. ground rice; the effect of cooking), the content of *antinutrients* in legumes (phytates, lectins, saponins, tannins, enzyme inhibitors), and, perhaps most important, the fiber content of a meal.[21,22] Dietary fiber is generally defined as the complex polysaccharides that are not digested by the small intestine and that lack caloric value. Various fibers are known, including cellulose, hemicellulose, pectins, lignins, gums, and mucilages. The high fiber content of foods such as lentils and beans in some way accounts for their low glycemic index by virtue of the slow absorption of such foods—hence the term *lente* carbohydrates.[15] The mechanisms of the proposed beneficial effects of fiber on glucose control and circulating lipid levels[3,15,21,22] remain unclear, but they include delayed gastric emptying, altered transit time in the small intestine, insulation of carbohydrate from digestive enzymes, and digestive enzyme inhibition. Soluble, viscous plant fiber, such as gums and pectin, significantly decreases postprandial hyperglycemia and may lower serum lipid levels.[21,22,22a] The effects of fiber in some patients are quite modest,[21] however, and they are not infrequently associated with significant gastrointestinal side effects. Lack of palatability also leads to poor long-term compliance. The possible effects of high-fiber diets in inducing mineral or vitamin deficiency because of bile acid interaction need to be further studied. In patients with autonomic neuropathy and delayed gastric emptying, high-fiber diets are of little benefit, and in a few such patients such diets have led to gastric bezoar.

The clinical relevance of the quantity and type of carbohydrates (simple vs. complex; high vs. low glycemic index) and the fiber content of the diet can be best assessed only by long-term randomized or case-control studies, but such evidence is lacking. Long-term observational studies of large numbers of men (>40,000)[23] and women (>60,000),[24] however, have indicated that intake of foods with a high glycemic index or low fiber, particularly cereal fiber, is independently associated with increased risk of developing diabetes. Multivariate analyses in these studies revealed a greater than two-fold increased risk of diabetes. In another large, cross-sectional study, the glycemic index of the diet, but not total carbohydrate or fat intake, was found to be a strong inverse correlate of high-density lipoprotein (HDL) cholesterol level, particularly in women.[25] However, factors other than lipid effects alone probably contribute to the potential protective effects of increased fiber intake on coronary heart disease.[26]

## FAT IN THE DIABETIC DIET

With an increased proportion of carbohydrate in the diet, dietary fat can be reduced, and a strong case for a lower fat content can be made because of the very high prevalence of atherosclerosis in persons with diabetes. Several epidemiologic studies have established that patients with diabetes have a two- to four-fold higher incidence of coronary artery disease even when the low-density lipoprotein (LDL) cholesterol is within the normal range. The current dietary approach, which recommends a fat intake of <30% of calories, with saturated fat accounting for ≤10% of calories and a cholesterol intake of 200 to 300 mg/day, is the most important step to implement before considering drug therapy for hypercholesterolemia.[7,27] This

approach is particularly relevant for diabetic patients with other risk factors for macrovascular disease (hypertension, proteinuria, and obesity). Diets high in saturated fat have also been shown to impair insulin action, probably by alterations in cell membrane phospholipids and glucose transport.[28,29] Long-chain, polyunsaturated fatty acids in skeletal muscle phospholipids, on the other hand, are associated with improved insulin sensitivity.[28] Some evidence from various studies, however, suggests that increasing dietary carbohydrates to allow a reduction in fat content can result in a significant increase in triglyceride levels, a lowering of HDL cholesterol, and sometimes a worsening of glycemic control.[30,31] This is of particular concern in patients with type 2 diabetes, who frequently manifest hypertriglyceridemia and low levels of HDL cholesterol. Studies in which monounsaturated fatty acids are substituted for carbohydrates in the diet, albeit short term, have shown that such a dietary modification may allow a better lipid profile without adversely affecting glycemic control in patients with type 2 diabetes.[32-35] Such diets may also decrease the susceptibility of LDL to oxidation, an important step in atherogenesis.[36] An important consideration in the fat content of the diet is the adverse effects of *trans* fatty acids, *hydrogenated* by-products of treated vegetable oils. A number of studies have demonstrated their greater LDL-raising and HDL-lowering effects, compared with *unhydrogenated*, unsaturated fats.[37,38] Estimates indicate that *trans* fatty acids may raise the ratio of LDL to HDL cholesterol more than do saturated fatty acids.[38] This may at least partly explain the epidemiologic evidence for the increased risk of coronary disease events with consumption of *trans* fats, compared with all other types of fats.[38,39] The long-term effectiveness, difficulty of compliance, and practicability of a diet high in monounsaturated fat, however, remain to be established.

Unlike ω-6 polyunsaturated fatty acids (e.g., linoleic acid), the ω-3 polyunsaturated fatty acids present in fish (e.g., *eicosapentaenoic acid*, or *EPA*, and *docosahexaenoic acid*, or *DHA*) have multiple protective effects against atherothrombosis. These include effects on prostaglandins, on platelet aggregation, on nitric oxide synthesis in the endothelium, and on cytokine, growth factor, and very low density lipoprotein (VLDL) synthesis.[40] These effects may explain the inverse relationship between fish consumption and mortality from coronary heart disease in epidemiologic studies (see Chap. 164).[41] The effects of ω-3 fatty acids in patients with diabetes may be more complex, however, and requires further evaluation.[42] For example, fish oil supplements may impair endogenous insulin secretion and may raise LDL cholesterol in some patients in a dose-dependent manner.[42,43]

For patients with triglyceride levels of >1000 mg/dL, caused by chylomicron accumulation,[44] a marked reduction in the total fat intake (<30–40 g per day) is necessary to minimize the risk of acute pancreatitis and the abdominal pain syndrome caused by hyperchylomicronemia. In this situation, abstinence from alcohol, weight reduction, and meticulous control of hyperglycemia are critical to the prevention of severe hypertriglyceridemia and pancreatitis.

## MEAL PLANNING AND DIET PRESCRIPTION

A diabetic meal plan should be tailored for each individual patient, depending on his or her *nutritional status* (i.e., presence or absence of obesity), *level of physical activity* (i.e., energy expenditure), *socioeconomic background*, as well as ethnic, cultural, and personal *dietary preference*. These are common sense but critical factors in achieving good compliance.

The average daily total caloric requirement can be calculated by the simple formula 25 × desirable weight (kg) for sedentary individuals. To this, up to 10 to 20 cal/kg should be added for individuals engaged in various grades of physical activity. For children and adolescents, further appropriate modifications are necessary, and individual requirements should be reassessed frequently on the basis of growth chart patterns.

The specific diet should distribute approximately 20%, 20% to 25%, and 30% to 35% of the total daily caloric requirement into breakfast, lunch, and dinner, respectively, with the remaining 20% to 30% of calories in the form of two or three snacks. Current recommendations for nutrient intake are that the proportion of carbohydrates, protein, and saturated fat in the diet should be 50% to 60%, 10% to 20%, and <10% of calories, respectively, and that fiber intake should be 20 to 35 g per day, with a balanced disbursement of all food exchanges (meat, bread, fat, milk, fruit, and vegetables). Items containing *trans* fatty acids should be avoided. In patients with hypertriglyceridemia, a reduction in total carbohydrates and increase in monounsaturated fat may be considered. The food-exchange concept makes it convenient for patients to select and to interchange food items with equivalent caloric value within specific categories, thus allowing greater flexibility and participation in meal planning. Finally, patients should be educated to be prudent in the use of alcohol, which contains additional calories in addition to having potentially harmful metabolic effects. Patients with preexisting hypertriglyceridemia may be particularly susceptible to the hyperlipidemic effects of alcohol.

## EXERCISE AND DIABETES

Exercise is a useful adjunct to diabetes therapy. Its effects on intermediary metabolism are complex and depend on a number of important variables, including nutritional status, cardiorespiratory condition, previous activity level (i.e., sedentary vs. athletic), and state of diabetes control before exercise. Its long-term effects can be beneficial from the viewpoint of blood glucose control, lipoprotein metabolism, body composition, and cardiovascular conditioning (see Chap. 132).

### EXERCISE AND DIABETES CONTROL

Exercise potentiates the effects of insulin but, in the absence of adequate insulin reserve, it can cause a deterioration of diabetes control and even ketoacidosis. In fairly well-controlled, nonketotic diabetic subjects, an intensive exercise period may variably reduce the blood glucose level or result in clinical hypoglycemia.[45] In patients with type 1 diabetes whose disease is optimally controlled with a continuous, subcutaneous insulin infusion regimen, mild to moderate exercise in the postprandial state is generally not associated with severe hypoglycemia.[46] In fact, acute bouts of intense exercise (~80% maximum oxygen consumption [$VO_{2max}$]) may occasionally be followed by a period of sustained hyperglycemia.[47] In some patients, however, hypoglycemia may develop several hours after strenuous exercise, reflecting an increased muscle glucose uptake to replenish glycogen stores, as well as an enhanced insulin sensitivity.[48] The extent of glucoregulation during exercise depends on the intensity of exercise, insulin availability, and the level of sympathetic activation and counterregulatory hormones.[49] Exercise also increases insulin binding to circulating erythrocytes and monocytes,[50] and presumably to muscle cells, as in normal persons. Insulin and exercise, however, appear to facilitate different signaling pathways in skeletal muscle. Whereas insulin-stimulated GLUT4 translocation to the plasma membrane is reduced in type 2 diabetes,[51] normally it is augmented by an acute bout of exercise.[52] Exercise also increases the rate of insulin absorption from subcutaneous sites.[53] Given the potential benefits of exercise training on long-term glycemic control, as well as on the cardiovascular system, an exercise program should be a part of the treatment for all patients with diabetes, with appropriate cautions regarding exercise type and intensity in those with certain preexisting clinical complications.[54]

## THERAPEUTIC EFFECTS OF PHYSICAL TRAINING IN DIABETES TREATMENT

In nondiabetic, nonobese or obese persons, endurance training is associated with significantly lowered serum insulin levels and enhanced insulin sensitivity[55]; however, glucose tolerance may or may not be improved, depending on diet, weight status, and other factors.[56,57] In trained athletes, serum levels of triglycerides and LDL cholesterol are generally lower, and levels of HDL cholesterol are higher.[54,57] Exercise potentiates the lipid-lowering effects achieved by diet alone in both men and women.[58] The adipose tissue and muscle lipoprotein lipase activity is stimulated by long-term physical conditioning and may, at least partly, account for these effects on circulating lipids. In nondiabetic as well as mildly diabetic individuals, *even moderate, nonvigorous activities* (intensity of 50–60% $VO_{2max}$, or <6.0 metabolic equivalents [METs], three to five times a week for 30–60 minutes) are associated with beneficial effects.[54,55]

In patients with type 1 diabetes, prospective studies indicate that a 6-week moderate-exercise training program normalizes peripheral glucose disposal, as assessed by the euglycemic insulin clamp technique.[59] The overall insulin requirement decreased only modestly, however, and hemoglobin $A_{1c}$ levels remained unchanged. In patients with type 2 diabetes (which is frequently associated with obesity and insulin resistance), physical training for 6 weeks to 6 months may moderately improve the oral glucose tolerance in some patients[60,61] but only minimally improves it in others.[57] Any beneficial effects of physical training on glucose tolerance and insulin sensitivity are evanescent, indicating the need for *persistent, regular exercise* to sustain the improvement.[54,57] Even in trained athletes, detraining over a period of a few days reverses the increased insulin sensitivity and decreases insulin receptor concentrations on erythrocytes.[62]

### ROLE OF DIET AND EXERCISE PROGRAMS IN THE PREVENTION OF DIABETES AND CARDIOVASCULAR DISEASE

Physical inactivity as well as obesity are undoubtedly major contributors to diabetes and cardiovascular disease in our society. Estimates are that physical inactivity accounts for 24% of the total risk for type 2 diabetes. This is a matter of great concern, particularly in minority populations.[63] Over the past decade, a number of large, prospective epidemiologic studies have shown a substantial inverse relationship between regular, moderately intense physical activity or cardiorespiratory fitness and the risk of type 2 diabetes.[64-68] The odds ratios for diabetes in men and women in these studies were as low as 0.3 to 0.5 after adjustments for other risk factors for diabetes. The benefits of diet and exercise may be especially striking and sustainable in relatively young individuals with visceral obesity (with or without increased body mass index), insulin resistance, and increased risk for diabetes.[69,70] Thus far, two long-term trials of diet and exercise involving subjects with impaired glucose tolerance have reported a 30% to 50% reduction in the progression to diabetes.[71,72] Only one of these studies, done in China,[72] was a randomized trial. Currently, a large prospective trial, the Diabetes Prevention Program (DPP), is under way, and >3000 subjects with impaired glucose tolerance have been randomized to different treatment groups, including an intensive lifestyle intervention arm.[73]

The potential health benefits of diet and exercise programs extend *far beyond* the realm of diabetes. Cardiorespiratory fitness and regular physical activity predict cardiovascular as well as total mortality in long-term observational studies in nondiabetic populations,[74-79] as well as in the elderly[76-79] and in diabetic subgroups,[78,79] after adjustments for a number of other known cardiovascular risk factors. Risk reductions of ≥50% have been reported in these analyses in individuals engaging in moderate-intensity, habitual physical activities. Randomized

16- to 24-week trials, with up to 2 years of maintenance programs, have shown the success of lifestyle interventions to be comparable to that of structured exercise programs in improving physical fitness and cardiovascular risk factors (e.g., blood pressure and lipids) in overweight men and women.[80,81] The DPP will also assess the impact of lifestyle intervention on cardiovascular end points.[73]

# REFERENCES

1. Franz MJ, Horton ES, Bantle JP, et al. Nutrition principles for the management of diabetes and related complications. Diabetes Care 1994; 17:490.
2. Nuttall FQ. Diet and the diabetic patient. Diabetes Care 1983; 6:197.
3. Vinik A, Wing RR. Nutritional management of the person with diabetes. In: Ellenberg M, Rifkin H, eds. Diabetes mellitus: theory and practice, 4th ed. New York: Elsevier, 1990:464.
4. Fitz R. The treatment of diabetes mellitus. Med Clin North Am 1923; 7:649.
5. Joslin EP. Arteriosclerosis and diabetes. Ann Clin Med 1927; 5:1061.
6. Himsworth HP. The dietetic factor determining the glucose tolerance and sensitivity to insulin in healthy men. Clin Sci 1935; 2:67.
7. Position statement. Nutrition recommendations and principles for people with diabetes mellitus. Diabetes Care 1994; 17:519.
8. Hughes TA, Gwynne JT, Switzer BR, et al. Effects of caloric restriction and weight loss on glycemic control, insulin release and resistance, and atherosclerotic risk in obese patients with type II diabetes mellitus. Am J Med 1984; 77:7.
9. Markovic TP, Jenkins AB, Campbell LV, et al. The determinants of glycemic responses to diet restriction and weight loss in obesity and NIDDM. Diabetes Care 1998; 21:687.
10. Pi-Sunyer FX, Maggio CA, McCarron DA. Multi-center, randomized trial of a comprehensive prepared meal program in type 2 diabetes. Diabetes Care 1999; 22:191.
11. Clinical guidelines on the identification, evaluation and treatment of overweight and obesity in adults—the evidence report. Obes Res 1998; 6(Suppl 2):51S.
12. Wadden TA, Stunkard AJ, Brownell KD. Very low calorie diets: their efficacy, safety and future. Ann Intern Med 1983; 99:675.
13. American Diabetes Association. Nutritional recommendations and principles for individuals with diabetes mellitus. Diabetes Care 1987; 10:176.
14. Slama G, Haardt MJ, Jean-Joseph P, et al. Sucrose taken during mixed meal has no additional hyperglycaemic action over isocaloric amounts of starch in well-controlled diabetics. Lancet 1984; 2:122.
15. Jenkins DJA, Wolever TMS, Jenkins AL, et al. The glycemic index of foods tested in diabetic patients: a new basis for carbohydrate exchange favoring the use of legumes. Diabetologia 1983; 24:257.
16. Wolever TMS. The glycemic index: flogging a dead horse? Diabetes Care 1997; 20:452.
17. Bantle JP, Laine DC, Castle GW, et al. Postprandial glucose and insulin responses to meals containing different carbohydrates in normal and diabetic subjects. N Engl J Med 1983; 309:7.
18. Laine DC, Thomas W, Levitt MD, Bantle JP. Comparison of predictive capabilities of diabetic exchange lists and glycemic index of foods. Diabetes Care 1987; 10:387.
19. Coulston AM, Hollenbeck CB, Swislock ALM, Reaven CM. Effect of source of dietary carbohydrate on plasma glucose and insulin responses to mixed meals in subjects with NIDDM. Diabetes Care 1987; 10:395.
20. Ludwig DS, Majzoub JA, Al-Zahrani A, et al. High glycemic index foods, overeating, and obesity. Pediatrics 1999; 103:26.
21. Nuttall FQ. Dietary fiber in the management of diabetes. Diabetes 1993; 42:503.
22. Wursh P, Pi-Sunyer FX. The role of viscous soluable fiber in the metabolic control of diabetes. A review with special emphasis on cereals rich in B-glucan. Diabetes Care 1997; 20:1774.
22a. Chandalia M, Garg A, Lutjohann D, et al. Beneficial effects of luten dietary fiber intake in patients with type 2 diabetes mellitus. N Engl Med 2000; 342:1392.
23. Salmeron J, Ascherio A, Rimm EB. Dietary fiber, glycemic load and risk of NIDDM in men. Diabetes Care 1997; 20:545.
24. Salmeron J, Manson JE, Stampfer MJ, et al. Dietary fiber, glycemic load and risk of NIDDM in women. JAMA 1997; 277:472.
25. Frost G, Leeds AA, Dore CJ. Glycemic index as a determinant of serum HDL-cholesterol concentration. Lancet 1999; 353:1045.
26. Wolk A, Manson JE, Stampfer M, et al. Long-term intake of dietary fiber and decreased risk of coronary heart disease among women. JAMA 1999; 281:1998.
27. American Diabetes Association. Detection and management of lipid disorders in diabetes. Diabetes Care 1993; 16:828.
28. Storlein LH, Baur LA, Kriketos AD, et al. Dietary fats and insulin action. Diabetologia 1996; 39:621.
29. Zierath JR, Houseknecht KL, Gnudi L, Kahn BB. High fat feeding impairs insulin stimulated GLUT4 recruitment via an early insulin-signaling defect. Diabetes 1997; 46:215.
30. O'Brien T, Nguyen TT, Buithieu J, Kottke BA. Lipoprotein compositional changes in the fasting and postprandial state on a high-carbohydrate low

31. Chen YD, Coulston AM, Zhou MY, et al. Why do low-fat high-carbohydrate diets accentuate postprandial lipemia in patients with NIDDM? Diabetes Care 1995 Jan; 18(1):10.
32. Garg A, Bantle JP, Henry RR, et al. Effects of varying carbohydrate content of diet in patients with non-insulin dependent diabetes mellitus. JAMA 1994; 271:1421.
33. Rasmussen OW, Vesterlund M, Thomsen C, et al. Effects on blood pressure, glucose, and lipid levels of a high-monounsaturated fat diet compared with a high-carbohydrate diet in NIDDM subjects. Diabetes Care 1993; 16:1565.
34. Campbell LV, Marmot PE, Dyer JA, et al. The high-monounsaturated fat diet as a practical alternative for NIDDM. Diabetes Care 1994; 17:177.
35. Lerman-Garber I, Ichazo-Cerro S, Zamora-Gonzales J. Effect of a high-monounsaturated fat diet enriched with avocado in NIDDM patients. Diabetes Care 1994; 17:311.
36. Gumbiner B, Low CC, Reaven PD. Effects of a monounsaturated-fatty-acid-enriched hypocaloric diet on cardiovascular risk factors in obese patients with type 2 diabetes. Diabetes Care 1998; 21:9.
37. Lichtenstein AH, Ausman LM, Jalbert SM, Schaefer EJ. Effects of different forms of dietary hydrogenated fats on serum lipoprotein cholesterol levels. N Engl J Med 1999; 340:1933.
38. Ascherio A, Katan M, Zock PL, et al. Trans fatty acids and coronary heart disease. N Engl J Med 1999; 340:1994.
39. Hu FB, Stampfer M, Manson JE. Dietary fat intake and the risk of coronary heart disease in women. N Engl J Med 1997; 337:1491.
40. Connor SL, Connor WE. Are fish oils beneficial in the prevention and treatment of coronary artery disease? Am J Clin Nutr 1997; 66(Suppl):1020S.
41. Kromhout D, Bosschieter EB, Coulander CD. The inverse relation between fish consumption and 20-year mortality from coronary heart disease. N Engl J Med 1985; 312:1205.
42. Friedberg CE, Janssen MJEM, Heine RJ, Grobbe DE. Fish oil and glycemic control in diabetes. A meta-analysis. Diabetes Care 1998; 21:494.
43. Malasanos TH, Stacpoole PW. Biological effects of Ω-3 fatty acids in diabetes mellitus. Diabetes Care 1991; 14:1160.
44. Santamarina-Fojo S. The familial chylomicronemia syndrome. Endocrinol Metab Clin North Am 1998; 27:551.
45. Bjorkman O. Fuel metabolism during exercise in normal and diabetic man. Diabetes Metab Rev 1986; 2:319.
46. Trovati M, Carta Q, Cavalot F, et al. Continuous subcutaneous insulin infusion and postprandial exercise in tightly controlled type I (insulin-dependent) diabetic patients. Diabetes Care 1984; 7:327.
47. Mitchell TH, Abraham G, Schiffrin A, et al. Hyperglycemia after intense exercise in IDDM subjects during continuous subcutaneous insulin infusion. Diabetes Care 1988; 11:311.
48. Ruderman NB, Balon T, Zorzano A, Goodman M. The post-exercise state: altered effects of insulin on skeletal muscle and their physiological relevance. Diabetes Metab Rev 1986; 2:425.
49. Hoelzer DR, Dalsky GP, Clutter WE, et al. Glucoregulation during exercise: hypoglycemia is prevented by redundant glucoregulatory systems, sympathochromaffin activation, and changes in islet hormone secretion. J Clin Invest 1986; 77:212.
50. Pedersen O, Beck-Nielsen H, Heding L. Increased insulin receptors after exercise in patients with insulin-dependent diabetes mellitus. N Engl J Med 1980; 302:886.
51. Garvey WT, Maianu L, Zhu JH, et al. Evidence for defects in the trafficking and translocation of GLUT4 glucose transporters in skeletal muscle as a cause of human insulin resistance. J Clin Invest 1998; 101:2377.
52. Kennedy JW, Hirshman MF, Gervino EV, et al. Acute exercise induces GLUT4 translocation in skeletal muscle of normal human subjects and subjects with type 2 diabetes. Diabetes 1999; 48:1192.
53. Berger M, Halban PA, Assal JP, et al. Pharmacokinetics of subcutaneously injected tritiated insulin: effects of exercise. Diabetes 1979; 28(Suppl 1):53.
54. American Diabetes Association. Diabetes mellitus and exercise. Position statement. Diabetes Care 1997; 20:1908.
55. Mayer-Davis EJ, D'Agostino R, Karter AJ, et al. Intensity and amount of physical activity in relation to insulin sensitivity. The Insulin Resistance Atherosclerosis Study. JAMA 1998; 279:669.
56. Björntorp P, Sjöström L. Carbohydrate storage in man: speculations and some quantitative considerations. Metabolism 1978; 27(Suppl 2):1853.
57. Ruderman NB, Schneider SH. Diabetes, exercise, and atherosclerosis. Diabetes Care 1992; 15(Suppl 4):1787.
58. Wood PD, Stefanick ML, Williams PT, Haskell WL. The effects on plasma lipoproteins of a prudent weight-reducing diet, with or without exercise, in overweight men and women. N Engl J Med 1991; 325:461.
59. Yki-Jarvinen H, Defronzo RA, Koivisto VA. Normalization of insulin sensitivity in type 1 diabetic subjects by physical training during insulin pump therapy. Diabetes Care 1984; 7:525.
60. Trovati M, Carta Q, Cavalot F, et al. Influence of physical training on blood glucose control, glucose tolerance, insulin secretion, and insulin action in non-insulin-dependent diabetic patients. Diabetes Care 1984; 7:416.
61. Reitman JS, Vasquez B, Klimes I, Nagulesparan M. Improvement of glucose homeostasis after exercise training in non-insulin-dependent diabetes. Diabetes Care 1984; 7:434.
62. Burstein R, Polychronakos C, Toews CJ, et al. Acute reversal of the enhanced insulin action in trained athletes: association with insulin receptor changes. Diabetes 1985; 34:756.

63. Clark DO. Physical activity efficacy and effectiveness among older adults and minorities. Diabetes Care 1997; 20:1176.

64. Helmrich SP, Ragland DR, Leung RW, Paffenberger RS. Physical activity and reduced occurrence of non-insulin dependent diabetes mellitus. N Engl J Med 1991; 325:147.

65. Manson JE, Rimm EB, Stampfer MJ, et al. Physical activity and incidence of non–insulin-dependent diabetes mellitus in women. Lancet 1991; 338:774.

66. Manson JE, Nathan DM, Krolewski AS, et al. A prospective study of exercise and incidence of diabetes among US male physicians. JAMA 1992; 268:63.

67. Lynch J, Helmrich SP, Lakka TA, et al. Moderately intense physical activities and high levels of cardiorespiratory fitness reduce the risk of non-insulin-dependent diabetes mellitus in middle-aged men. Arch Intern Med 1996; 156:1307.

68. Wei M, Gibbons LW, Mitchell, et al. The association between cardiorespiratory fitness and impaired fasting glucose and type 2 diabetes mellitus in men. Ann Intern Med 1999; 130:89.

69. Ruderman N, Chisholm D, Pisunyer X, Schneider S. The metabolically obese individual revisited. Diabetes 1998; 47:699.

70. Goodpaster BH, Kelley DE, Wing RR, et al. Effects of weight loss on regional fat distribution and insulin sensitivity in obesity. Diabetes 1999; 48:839.

71. Eriksson KF, Lindgarde F. Prevention of type 2 diabetes (non-insulin-dependent) diabetes mellitus. The 6-year Malmö feasibility study. Diabetologia 1991; 34:89.

72. Pan XR, Li GW, Hu YH, et al. Effects of diet and exercise in preventing NIDDM in people with impaired glucose tolerance. The Da Quing IGT and diabetes study. Diabetes Care 1997; 20:537.

73. The Diabetes Prevention Program Research Group. The Diabetes Prevention Program. Design and methods for a clinical trial in the prevention of type 2 diabetes. Diabetes Care 1999; 22:623.

74. Blair SN, Kampert JB, Kohl HW III, et al. Influences of cardiovascular fitness and other precursors on cardiovascular disease and all-cause mortality in men and women. JAMA 1996; 276:205.

75. Erikssen G, Liestol K, Bjornholt J, et al. Changes in physical fitness and changes in mortality. Lancet 1998; 352:759.

76. Bijnen FCH, Caspersen LT, Feskens EJM, et al. Physical activity and 10 year mortality from cardiovascular diseases and all causes. The Zutphen Elderly Study. Arch Intern Med 1998; 158:1499.

77. Hakim AA, Petrovitch H, Burchfiel CM, et al. Effects of walking on mortality among non-smoking retired men. N Engl J Med 1998; 338:94.

78. Leon A, Connett J, Jacobs DR, Rauramaa R. Leisure-time physical activity levels and risk of coronary heart disease and death: the multiple risk factor intervention trial. JAMA 1987; 258:2388.

79. Kohl HW, Villegas JA, Gordon NF, Blair SN. Cardiorespiratory fitness, glycemic status, and mortality risk in men. Diabetes Care 1992; 15:184.

80. Dunn AL, Marcus BH, Kampert JB, et al. Comparison of lifestyle and structural interventions to increase physical activity and cardiorespiratory fitness: a randomized trial. JAMA 1999; 281:327.

81. Andersen RE, Wadden TA, Bartlett SJ, et al. Effects of lifestyle activity vs. structured aerobic exercise in obese women. A randomized trial. JAMA 1999; 281:335.

# CHAPTER 142

# ORAL AGENTS FOR THE TREATMENT OF TYPE 2 DIABETES MELLITUS

ALLISON B. GOLDFINE AND
ELEFTHERIA MARATOS-FLIER

Initially, *sulfonylureas* were the only class of oral agent available in the United States for the treatment of type 2 diabetes mellitus (non–insulin-dependent diabetes mellitus) refractory to diet and exercise. Subsequently, *biguanides, α-glucosidase inhibitors, meglitinides,* and most recently *thiazolidinediones* have become available. The United Kingdom Prospective Diabetes Study (UKPDS) compared the impact of intensive and conventional blood glucose control with sulfonylureas, biguanides, or insulin on the risk of complications in patients with type 2 diabetes.[1] In the intensive treatment arm, the risk reduction was 10% for diabetes-related death and 12% for any diabetes-related end point—largely due to a 25% reduction in occurrence of microvascular end points. No significant reduction in mac-

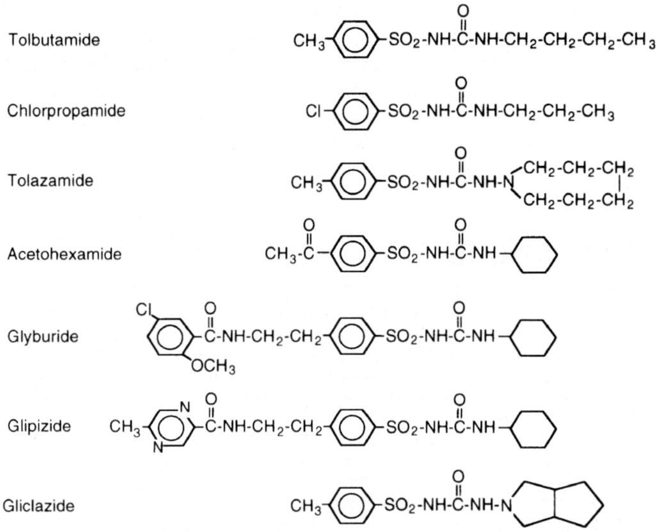

**FIGURE 142-1.** Structure of first- and second-generation sulfonylureas.

rovascular disease was seen. The risk of hypoglycemic events increased 2- to 2.5-fold, and weight gain was greater in the intensive treatment group.

Goals of glycemic treatment must take into account the patient's age and comorbid medical conditions. A good response to oral therapy in a younger patient is the achievement of a fasting plasma glucose level of <100 to 120 mg/dL and a 2-hour postprandial glucose level of <120 to 140 mg/dL, as well as a glycohemoglobin ($HbA_{1c}$) level of ≤7%.

## SULFONYLUREAS

Sulfonylureas are related to sulfonamide drugs. They all contain a sulfonylurea moiety, with different side chains attached (Fig. 142-1). The hypoglycemic action of sulfonylureas was noted serendipitously in 1942,[2] and first-generation sulfonylureas became available in 1955. First-generation agents include *chlorpropamide, tolbutamide, tolazamide,* and *acetohexamide.* Two second-generation agents, *glyburide* and *glipizide,* and later *glimepiride,* became available. Another agent, *gliclazide,* is available only in Europe. The sulfonylureas have similar effects and mechanisms of action, although the second-generation agents have 100-fold greater intrinsic activity.[3,4] The maximal therapeutic benefits are similar for both first- and second-generation agents, except for tolbutamide, which has a lower therapeutic efficacy.[3,5] The major advantage of the second-generation agents is that maximal benefit can be achieved at lower dosages.

Approximately 50% of the sulfonylurea dose is rapidly absorbed; levels can be detected in serum 1 hour after administration.[4] Ninety percent to 99% of the drug is bound to plasma proteins, especially albumin.[6] Binding of second-generation agents is limited to nonionic sites; hence, they are less likely to interact with other medications than are first-generation agents. The drugs are detectable in the serum within 1 hour of ingestion. For most agents, peak levels are achieved within 2 to 4 hours. Half-lives of first-generation agents vary from 7 hours for acetohexamide to 24 to 48 hours for chlorpropamide; half-lives of second-generation sulfonylureas are short (3–5 hours); however, for unexplained reasons, the hypoglycemic effects of these drugs are evident for 12 to 24 hours. Table 142-1 provides a summary. (A micronized version of glyburide is also available. This version has improved bioavailability, and a higher serum concentration can be achieved with a lower dose. For most patients, a 3-mg tablet of this newer formulation is equivalent to a 5-mg tablet of the original glyburide.[7])

**TABLE 142-1.**
**Pharmacologic Features of Sulfonylureas**

| Drug | Plasma $T_{1/2}$ (h)* | Duration of Action (h)* | No. Daily Doses | Starting Dosage (mg/day)* | Maximum Dosage (mg/day) |
|---|---|---|---|---|---|
| **FIRST-GENERATION** | | | | | |
| Tolbutamide | 3–7 | 6–12 | 2–3 | 1000–2000 | 3000 |
| Acetohexamide | 6–8 | 8–12 | 2 | 250–1500 | 1500 |
| Tolazamide | 7 | 12–18 | 1–2 | 100–250 | 1000 |
| Chlorpropamide | 25–45 | 40–60 | 1 | 250 | 500 |
| **SECOND-GENERATION** | | | | | |
| Glipizide | 3–5 | 12–18 | 1–2 | 5 | 40 |
| Glyburide (glibenclamide) | 3–5 | 16–24 | 1–2 | 2.5–5 | 20 |
| Glyburide (micronized) | 3–5 | 16–24 | 1–2 | 1.5–3 | 12 |

$T_{1/2}$, half-life.
*The starting dosage and maximum dosage may need to be lower in patients with liver disease, renal disease, or malnutrition, or in geriatric patients.

Increasingly, second-generation drugs such as glipizide and glyburide are the agents of choice in the treatment of type 2 diabetes because the therapeutic index of these medications is higher than that of the first-generation agents, the total effective dosage is significantly lower, and side effects are less frequent (see Table 142-1 for dosage). The dosage of these drugs can be increased every 2 to 3 days, depending on the glycemic response. At dosages of >20 mg per day, glipizide should be given as a split dose. Glyburide, even at its maximum dosage, needs to be given only once a day.

The major mode of inactivation of sulfonylureas is metabolism in the liver, where they may be completely or partially metabolized to inactive metabolites. First-generation agents and their metabolites are largely excreted by the kidney, whereas second-generation agents are excreted both by the kidney and in bile in varying proportions. In general, hepatic insufficiency is a contraindication to the use of sulfonylureas, because their metabolism is impaired. Moreover, in such cases, an inability to respond to counterregulatory hormones and to recover from hypoglycemia may be present. In patients with renal insufficiency, glipizide is the agent of choice because its metabolites are inactive.

Sulfonylureas improve diabetes control through their insulinotropic effects. Insulin secretion from the islet is stimulated in a biphasic fashion,[8] perhaps by increasing B-cell sensitivity to glucose. The effect is probably mediated by a receptor on the B cell, because the bioactivity of sulfonylureas appears to correlate with their binding capacity.[9,10] This receptor is linked to an adenosine triphosphate (ATP)–sensitive $K^+$ channel that is closed by the sulfonylureas, leading to membrane depolarization.[11] This results in the opening of a voltage-dependent $Ca^{2+}$ channel and an intracellular influx of calcium. The rise in cytosolic calcium stimulates insulin release. Accordingly, this insulinotropic action is associated with an increase in circulating insulin levels in patients with type 2 diabetes,[12–14] leading to an improvement in metabolic control. When glucose and insulin are measured at frequent intervals over the course of a day, patients treated with glyburide or glipizide have a smaller area under the glucose curve and a significantly greater area under the insulin curve than do placebo-treated patients.[15] Treatment with sulfonylureas does not prevent progression of insulin resistance over a 15-month period because glycohemoglobin, glucose, and insulin levels all rise over time.[14] Sulfonylureas may affect glucagon and somatostatin release; however, the nature, degree, and importance of such effects remain uncertain.[16–19] Potential extrapancreatic effects of sulfonylureas continue to be debated.[8] The absence of any effect of sulfonylureas in reducing glucose levels in animals or humans who have undergone pancreatectomy argues against a major extrapancreatic role.[20]

Studies showing effects of these agents on hepatic glucose production did not take into account peripheral and hepatic insulin resistance caused by chronic hyperglycemia.[8,21] Studies of the effects of sulfonylureas on insulin-receptor number also have been inconsistent, with some studies showing increased binding in treated patients[22,23] and others showing no effect.[24]

## INDICATIONS FOR USE

Diet and exercise represent the first line of therapy for patients with type 2 diabetes. However, few patients achieve adequate control of blood glucose levels using this approach alone. The use of sulfonylureas may be considered in patients who are obese or of normal weight, are older than 30 years, and are not considering pregnancy. The reported rate of *primary failure* of sulfonylurea therapy (i.e., the inability to achieve a good or adequate glucose response) varies from 5% to 30%.[25–27] These studies antedate the use of glycosylated hemoglobin measurements as an index of glycemic control; also, different levels of glucose control were used as target goals, making it difficult to evaluate them fully. Furthermore, these studies may have included some patients with late-onset autoimmune diabetes. Factoring in the contribution of inadequate dietary compliance to primary failure also is difficult. Patients who are older than 40 years and have had diabetes for <5 years are more likely to respond to therapy. The degree of glycemia and glycohemoglobin value are not particularly useful in excluding patients from a trial of sulfonylurea therapy, because rare patients with glucose levels of >400 mg/dL and glycohemoglobin values of >15% achieve a good response.

The rate of *secondary failure* in patients who have an initial response to treatment with sulfonylureas ranges from 5% to 10% each year; after 10 years, only 50% have satisfactory control.[4] The causes of secondary failure include B-cell exhaustion and dietary noncompliance. Numerous drugs (e.g., niacin, thiazide diuretics, β-blockers, corticosteroids) reduce insulin sensitivity and, thus, decrease the clinical efficacy of sulfonylureas, and their use may lead to deteriorating glycemic control. Potential alternatives to these drugs that do not worsen insulin resistance should be considered if continued sulfonylurea therapy is desirable.

## MEGLITINIDES

Meglitinides are oral hypoglycemic agents derived from benzoic acid and chemically unrelated to the sulfonylurea agents. Repaglinide, the first meglitinide to receive Food and Drug Administration approval, lowers blood glucose by stimulating the release of insulin from the pancreas. Thus, it requires functioning B cells and is ineffective in type 1 diabetes. Repaglinide, which is rapidly absorbed after oral administration, reaches peak plasma levels within 1 hour and is rapidly eliminated by oxidation and conjugation with glucuronic acid (with a half-life of ~1 hr). The cytochrome P450 enzyme system, specifically 3A4, is involved in further metabolism; however, metabolites do not contribute to the glucose-lowering effect of the drug. Tablets are available in 0.5-, 1-, and 2-mg strengths. Recommended dosage is from 0.5 to 4 mg taken with meals 2 to 4 times daily, with a maximum dosage of 16 mg per day. This dosage may need adjustment in liver disease. Patients who skip (or add) extra meals should skip (or add) a dose for that meal. Repaglinide is effective with metformin; however, it should *not* be used in conjunction with the sulfonylureas.

Stimulation of insulin secretion occurs by processes both similar to and distinct from those of the sulfonylureas. Like sulfonylureas, repaglinide binds to a site on the B-cell membrane; however, the affinity of the binding sites appears different for meglitinide and glipizide.[28] Binding closes ATP-dependent $K^+$ channels. The consequent $K^+$ channel blockade, in turn, leads to depolarization of the B cell by the opening of the $Ca^{2+}$ channels, resulting in calcium influx which induces insulin secretion. The ion-channel binding is highly tissue specific; low-affinity binding is seen in cardiac and skeletal muscle tissues.

## BIGUANIDES

Three derivatives of guanidine—phenformin, metformin, and buformin—have glucose-lowering effects.[29] Of these, only metformin, which is available in the United States, is used clinically, because phenformin and buformin use is associated with the development of lactic acidosis.[30] This also has been observed with metformin use, but almost all affected patients had impaired renal function. When metformin is used appropriately, the incidence of lactic acidosis is rare. In 56,000 patient-years of use in Canada, no cases of lactic acidosis were reported.[31]

Metformin is partially absorbed from the gastrointestinal tract and has a bioavailability of 50% to 60%. The drug is stable, does not bind to plasma proteins, and is not metabolized. It is excreted in the urine and has a plasma half-life of 1.7 to 4.5 hours. Of a given dose, 90% is cleared within 12 hours.[32]

Metformin does not have a hypoglycemic effect, but acts as an "antihyperglycemic."[33] It lowers blood glucose levels in hyperglycemic patients with type 2 diabetes but has no effect on glucose levels in normal subjects. The mechanism of action remains unclear. Metformin reduces absorption of glucose from the gastrointestinal tract, probably due to inhibition of glucose uptake at the mucosal surface.[34] Metformin also inhibits hepatic glucose production[35] and increases insulin-stimulated glucose uptake at the periphery[36,37] by stimulating the GLUT4 glucose transporter.[38]

Unlike therapy with insulin or sulfonylureas, therapy with metformin does not lead to weight gain and may be associated with modest weight loss because of a slight anorectic effect of the drug.[39] In addition, patients with hypertriglyceridemia may experience reductions in triglyceride levels of as much as 50%.[40,41]

Starting dosages of metformin range from 1.0 to 2.0 g per day in divided doses of 500 mg or 850 mg. The maximum dosage is 3 g, usually given in three divided doses. Primary failure rates of 5% to 20% have been reported. Secondary failure rates range from 5% to 10% per year. Metformin has been used successfully in combination with sulfonylureas, especially in patients older than 60 years.[42,43] Contraindications to metformin therapy include impaired creatinine clearance, liver disease, heart failure, chronic obstructive lung disease, and alcohol abuse. Side effects are mainly gastrointestinal; abdominal discomfort, diarrhea, and nausea and vomiting have been reported.

## CARBOHYDRASE INHIBITORS

The group of agents known as carbohydrase inhibitors includes acarbose[44]; miglitol is still in clinical trials. The mechanism of action of both drugs is inhibition of the α-glucosidases in the intestinal brush border, leading to a delay in carbohydrate absorption. Clinical studies with these agents have demonstrated a reduction in postprandial glucose elevations in both types 1 and 2 diabetes mellitus.[45–49] Doses of the carbohydrase inhibitors must be titrated to balance the decreased glycemic response against malabsorption and other gastrointestinal side effects. For both agents, the therapeutic dose is between 50 and 100 mg; higher doses lead to abdominal distention, flatulence, malabsorption, and diarrhea. Both these agents have also been used in combination with sulfonylureas.[50,51] The use of these agents has generally been associated with only modest improvements in glycosylated hemoglobin measurements but may moderate the weight gain seen with the sulfonylureas.

## THIAZOLIDINEDIONES

In contrast to sulfonylureas and meglitinides, which are oral hypoglycemic agents, thiazolidinediones act to enhance insulin sensitivity. These agents have been studied extensively in obese, insulin-resistant rodent models, including kk, db/db, and ob/ob mice, and the Zucker rat. Two drugs in this category are currently marketed in the United States: *rosiglitazone* and *pioglitazone*.

*Rosiglitazone* is dosed at 2 or 4 mg twice daily or 8 mg once daily, and studies show that effectiveness is decreased little with once daily dosing. This product may not have a favorable effect on lipid profiles: total cholesterol and low-density lipoproteins (LDL) are slightly increased. Triglycerides are unaffected, although high-density lipoproteins (HDL) may be increased. In premarketing studies, rosiglitazone was not associated with drug-induced hepatotoxicity or elevation of the liver enzyme alanine transaminase. Although rare reports of hepatic toxicity have appeared, one occurring two weeks after commencement of therapy,[52] these cases are not clearly attributable to the use of this agent. The drug has been approved for type 2 diabetes as monotherapy and in combination with sulfonylureas or with metformin, but not with insulin.

*Pioglitazone* is the most recent thiazolidinedione to be marketed. The initial dosage is 15 to 30 mg once daily, without relationship to meals. The maximum dose is 45 mg. The lipid effects may be beneficial: triglycerides are decreased, HDL is increased; total cholesterol and LDL are unaffected.[53] In vitro, the drug inhibits the growth of cultured vascular smooth muscle cells (VSMC). In vivo studies of stroke-prone spontaneously hypertensive rats, which are subjected to endothelial injury, reveal a protective effect against both acute and chronic vascular injury via inhibition of VSMC proliferation.[54] In patients, pioglitazone did not increase hepatic enzymes compared with controls, and, to date, hepatotoxicity has not been encountered. Pioglitazone is approved in type 2 diabetes as monotherapy and in combination with sulfonylureas, metformin, or insulin, but not for triple combination therapy.

All of the thiazolidinediones are associated with a statistically increased incidence of edema and weight gain when compared with placebo. When edema occurs, it tends to be mild or moderate. The thiazolidinediones should not be used in patients with congestive heart failure. The drugs are associated with an increase of plasma fluid volume and may result in mild, dilutional-related decreases in hemoglobin, hematocrit, and white cell count. In some studies, the weight gain was thought to correlate with the improvement in hyperglycemia. Also, weight gain is a known occurrence in many longitudinal studies of patients with type 2 diabetes in general.

With rosiglitazone or pioglitazone, therapy should not be commenced if the plasma aspartate transaminase exceeds 2.5

times the upper limit of normal. Liver enzymes should be measured before therapy, then perhaps every 2 months for a year, and periodically thereafter. Women taking these drugs who have polycystic disease or who are taking oral contraceptives may ovulate; hence, alternative forms of contraception should be suggested.

Oral doses of thiazolidinediones lower blood glucose levels and decrease insulin levels. An increase in the insulin content of pancreatic islets is also noted.[55,56] No hypoglycemia is seen when the drugs are administered to nondiabetic animals. The mechanism of action of the thiazolidinediones is not completely understood. Initial steps include binding to a member of the nuclear receptor *peroxisome proliferator-activated receptor* (PPAR) family to regulate the transcription of a number of insulin-responsive genes.[57] They may also stimulate uncoupling proteins, although less evidence exists for this. Binding is specific to the PPAR-γ isoform that is present mainly in adipose tissue. However, because thiazolidinediones influence metabolism in liver, pancreas, and skeletal muscle—if the drugs work solely through this receptor—either all of these tissues must contain sufficient levels of this PPAR isoform, or in vivo and in vitro isoform binding may differ. PPARs exist as heterodimers with another nuclear receptor, the retinoid X receptor (RXR). In addition, the drug effects are dependent on the presence of insulin, perhaps through separate insulin-regulated transcription factors. Nuclear-receptor binding is linked to an increased rate of the transcription of PPAR-γ responsive genes, including glucose transporters, critical for the control of glucose metabolism. In addition, some studies suggest improved vascular function through increased expression of plasminogen activator inhibitor type 1 (PAI-1) in endothelial cells[58] and inhibition of angiogenesis.[59] The mechanisms of action of oral agents are compared in Table 142-2.

## OTHER STRATEGIES FOR DRUG THERAPY

Several other strategies for treating type 2 diabetes are under investigation. New approaches include products that antagonize glucagon action to suppress hepatic glucose production (e.g., glucagon analogs that antagonize the action of glucagon and glucagon-receptor antagonists[60,61]) and oxidation inhibitors that might interdict the actions of fatty acids in stimulating hepatic gluconeogenesis and in attenuating glucose disposal in muscle, as well as in diminishing the rates of ketone, cholesterol, and triglyceride synthesis.[62] Another strategy involves modulators of the RXR, which interact with the PPAR nuclear receptors to improve insulin sensitivity. In addition, peptides with insulinotropic effects, such as glucagon-like peptides, are under investigation.[62a] New methods to target comorbid conditions that worsen insulin resistance are also under study, such as β$_3$-receptor agonists for the treatment of obesity and neuropeptides to suppress appetite. The ideal therapy for type 2 diabetes probably will not be achieved until the fundamental pathogenesis of the disease is better understood, and then therapies likely will be tailored to specific molecular defects.

Weight loss to improve insulin sensitivity and glucose control as well as lipid abnormalities should also be strongly considered in obese patients with type 2 diabetes.[63,64] Currently, approved agents for weight loss are limited. *Sibutramine* acts to suppress appetite by inhibiting reuptake of serotonin, norepinephrine, and dopamine.[65,66] It is available in 5-, 10-, and 15-mg tablets that are administered once daily and is metabolized into active metabolites in the liver by the cytochrome P450 enzymes. It is contraindicated in patients with coronary artery disease (because it may increase the heart rate and blood pressure) and in those requiring monoamine oxidase inhibitors. *Orlistat*, a lipase inhibitor, prevents the gastrointestinal absorption of ~30% of dietary fat and may lower the glucose level, the cholesterol level, and blood pressure.[67] It is given at a dosage of 120

**TABLE 142-2.**

**Mechanisms of Action of Oral Agents Used to Treat Type 2 Diabetes Mellitus**

| Class | Example | Action |
|---|---|---|
| Sulfonylureas | Glyburide | Insulinotropic, increases circulating insulin |
| Meglitinides | Repaglinide | Insulinotropic, increases circulating insulin |
| Biguanides | Metformin | Increases insulin-stimulated glucose uptake, reduces hepatic glucose production |
| Carbohydrase inhibitors | Acarbose | Delays carbohydrate absorption |
| Thiazolidinediones | Pioglitazone | Increases insulin sensitivity |

mg three times daily with meals. The drug may cause gastrointestinal discomfort. One should emphasize that weight loss is modest with both of these agents, and as both are new, *no* data exist on long-term safety or efficacy for either compound. Finally, the role of gastric bypass surgery to manage weight and glucose intolerance should be considered in the morbidly obese diabetic patient, with attention to the benefits as well as the limitations and risks of this procedure.[68]

## REFERENCES

1. United Kingdom Prospective Diabetes Study (UKPDS) Group. Intensive blood-glucose control with sulphonylureas or insulin compared with conventional treatment and risk of complications in patients with type 2 diabetes (UKPDS 33). Lancet 1998; 352:837.
2. Loubatieres A. The hypoglycemic sulfonamides: history and development of the problem from 1942–1945. Ann N Y Acad Sci 1957; 71:4.
3. Melander A, Bitzen P-O, Faber O, Groop L. Sulphonylurea antidiabetic drugs: an update of their clinical pharmacology and rational therapeutic use. Drugs 1989; 37:58.
4. Skillman TG, Feldman JM. The pharmacology of sulfonylureas. Am J Med 1981; 70:361.
5. Gerich JE. Oral hypoglycemic agents. N Engl J Med 1989; 321:1231.
6. Kahn CR, Schecte Y. Oral hypoglycemic agents. In: Gilman AG, Rall TW, Nies AS, Taylor P, eds. The pharmacologic basis of therapeutics. New York: McGraw-Hill, 1993:1485.
7. Carlson RF, Isley WL, Ogrine FG, Klobucar TR. Efficacy and safety of reformulated, micronized glyburide tablets in patients with non-insulin-dependent diabetes mellitus: a multicenter, double blind, randomized trial. Clin Ther 1993; 15:788.
8. Groop L, Luzi L, Melander A, et al. Different effects of glyburide and glipizide on insulin secretion and hepatic glucose production in normal and NIDDM subjects. Diabetes 1987; 36:1320.
9. Shmid-Antomarchi H, DeWeille J, Fosset M, Lazdunski M. The receptor for the antidiabetic sulfonylureas controls the activity of the ATP-modulated K$^+$ in insulin secreting cells. J Biol Chem 1987; 262:15840.
10. Siconolfi-Baez L, Banerji MA, Lebovitz HE. Characterization and significance of sulfonylurea receptors. Diabetes Care 1990; 13:2.
11. Boyd AE III. Sulfonylurea receptors, ion channels and fruit flies. Diabetes 1988; 37:847.
12. Feldman JM, Lebovitz HE. Endocrine and metabolic effects of glibenclamide. Diabetes 1971; 20:745.
13. Kolterman OG, Olefsky JM. The impact of sulfonylurea treatment upon the mechanisms responsible for the insulin resistance in type II diabetes. Diabetes Care 1984; 7:81.
14. Birkeland KI, Furuseth K, Melander A, et al. Long-term randomized placebo-controlled double-blind therapeutic comparison of glipizide and glyburide: glycemic control and insulin secretion during 15 months. Diabetes Care 1994; 17:43.
15. Groop L, Groop P-H, Stenman S, et al. Comparison of pharmacokinetics, metabolic effects and mechanisms of action of glyburide and glipizide during long term treatment. Diabetes Care 1987; 10:671.
16. Tsalikian E, Dunphy TW, Bohannon NV, et al. The effect of chronic oral antidiabetic therapy on insulin and glucagon responses to a meal. Diabetes 1977; 26:314.
17. Pfeifer MA, Beard JC, Halter JB, et al. Suppression of glucagon secretion during a tolbutamide infusion in normal and noninsulin-dependent diabetic subjects. J Clin Endocrinol Metab 1983; 56:586.
18. Pek S, Fajans SS, Floyd JC Jr, et al. Failure of sulfonylureas to suppress plasma glucagon in man. Diabetes 1972; 21:216.
19. Efendic S, Enzmann F, Nylen A, et al. Effect of glucose/sulfonylurea interaction on release of insulin, glucagon and somatostatin from isolated perfused rat pancreas. Proc Natl Acad Sci U S A 1979; 76:5901.

20. Beck-Nielsen H, Hother-Nielsen O, Pedersen O. Mechanism of action of sulphonylureas with special reference to the extrapancreatic effect: an overview. Diabet Med 1988; 5:613.
21. Rossetti L, Smith D, Shulman GI, et al. Correction of hyperglycemia with phlorizin normalizes tissue sensitivity to insulin in diabetic rats. J Clin Invest 1987; 79:1510.
22. Olefsky JM, Reaven GM. Effects of sulfonylurea therapy on insulin binding in mononuclear leukocytes of diabetic patients. Am J Med 1976; 60:89.
23. Beck-Nielsen H, Pedersen O, Lindskov HO. Increased insulin sensitivity and cellular insulin binding in obese diabetics following treatment with glibenclamide. Acta Endocrinol (Copenh) 1979; 90:451.
24. Grunberger G, Ruan J, Gorder P. Sulfonylureas do not affect insulin binding or glycemic control in insulin-dependent diabetics. Diabetes 1982; 31:890.
25. Bernhard H. Long-term observations on oral hypoglycemic agents in diabetes. The effect of carbutamide and tolbutamide. Diabetes 1965; 14:59.
26. Balodimos MC, Camerini-Davalos RA, Marble A. Nine years' experience with tolbutamide in the treatment of diabetes. Metabolism 1966; 11:957.
27. Lebovitz HE. Clinical utility of oral hypoglycemic agents in the management of patients with noninsulin-dependent diabetes mellitus. Am J Med 1983; 75: 94.
28. Fuhlendorff J, Rorsman P, Kofod H, et al. Stimulation of insulin release by repaglinide and glibenclamide involves both common and distinct processes. Diabetes 1998; 47:345.
29. Bailey CJ. Biguanides and NIDDM. Diabetes Care 1992; 15:755.
30. Williams RH, Palmer JP. Farewell to phenformin for treating diabetes mellitus. Ann Intern Med 1975; 83:567.
31. Lucis OJ. The status of metformin in Canada. Can Med Assoc J 1983; 128:24.
32. Hermann LS. Metformin: a review of its pharmacologic properties and therapeutic use. Diabetes Metab Rev 1979; 5:233.
33. Bailey CJ. Metformin revisited: its actions and indications for use. Diabet Med 1988; 5:315.
34. Caspary WF, Creutzfeldt W. Analysis of the inhibitory effect of biguanides on glucose absorption: inhibition of sugar transport. Diabetologia 1971; 7:379.
35. Inzucchi SE, Maggs DG, Spollett GR, et al. Efficacy and metabolic effects of metformin and troglitazone in type II diabetes mellitus. N Engl J Med 1998; 338: 867.
36. Rossetti L, DeFronzo RA, Gherzi R, et al. Effect of metformin treatment on insulin action in diabetic rats: in vivo and in vitro correlations. Metabolism 1990; 39:425.
37. Schernthaner G. Improvement in insulin action is an important part of the antidiabetic effect of metformin. Horm Metab Res Suppl 1985; 15:116.
38. Klip A, Leiter LA. Cellular mechanisms of action of metformin. Diabetes Care 1990; 13:696.
39. Clarke BF, Duncan LJP. Comparison of chlorpropamide and metformin treatment on weight and blood glucose response of uncontrolled obese diabetics. Lancet 1968; 1:123.
40. Wu MS, Johnston P, Sheu WH, et al. Effect of metformin on carbohydrate and lipoprotein metabolism in NIDDM patients. Diabetes Care 1990; 13:1.
41. Schneider J, Erren T, Zofel P, Kaffarnik H. Metformin induced changes in serum lipids, lipoproteins and apoproteins in non-insulin dependent diabetes mellitus. Atherosclerosis 1990; 82:97.
42. Clarke BF, Duncan LJP. Biguanide treatment in the management of insulin independent (maturity-onset) diabetes: clinical experience with metformin. Res Clin Forums 1979; 1:52.
43. Nattrass M, Hinks L, Smythe P. Metabolic effects of combined sulphonylurea and metformin therapy in maturity-onset diabetics. Horm Metab Res 1979; 11:332.
44. Lindström J, Tuomilehto J, Spenglert M. Acarbose treatment does not change the habitual diet of patients with type 2 diabetes mellitus. Diabet Med 2000; 17:20.
45. Vierhapper H, Bratusch-Marrain A, Waldhause W. α-Glucosidase hydrolase inhibition in diabetes. Lancet 1978; 2:1386.
46. Hanefeld M, Fischer S, Schulze J. Therapeutic potentials of acarbose as first-line drug in NIDDM insufficiently treated with diet alone. Diabetes Care 1991; 14:732.
47. Walton RJ, Sherif IT, Noy GA, Alberti KGGM. Improved metabolic profiles in insulin-treated diabetic patients given an α-glucosidehydrolase inhibitor. BMJ 1979; 1:220.
48. Dimitriadis G, Hatziagelaki E, Ladas S, et al. Effects of prolonged administration of two new α-glucosidase inhibitors on blood glucose control, insulin requirements and breath hydrogen excretion in patients with insulin-dependent diabetes mellitus. Eur J Clin Invest 1988; 18:33.
49. Arends J, Wilms BH. Smoothening effect of a new α-glucosidase inhibitor, BAY m 1099, on blood glucose profiles of sulfonylurea-treated type II diabetic patients. Horm Metab Res 1986; 18:761.
50. Reaven GM, Lardinois CK, Greenfield MS, et al. Effect of acarbose on carbohydrate and lipid metabolism in NIDDM patients poorly controlled by sulfonylureas. Diabetes Care 1990; 13:32.
51. Johnston PS, Coniff FR, Hoogwerf BJ, et al. Effects of the carbohydrase inhibitor miglitol in sulfonylurea-treated NIDDM patients. Diabetes Care 1994; 17:20.
52. Al-Salman J, Arjomand H, Kemp DG, Mittal M. Hepatocellular injury in a patient receiving rosiglitazone. Ann Intern Med 2000; 132:121.
53. Yamasaki Y, Kawamori R, Wasada T, et al. Pioglitazone (AD-4833) ameliorates insulin resistance in patients with NIDDM. AD-4833 glucose clamp study group, Japan. Tohoku J Exp Med 1997; 183:173.
54. Yoshimoto T, Naruse M, Shizume H, et al. Vasculo-protective effect of insulin sensitizing agent pioglitazone in neointimal thickening and hypertensive vascular hypertrophy. Atherosclerosis 1999; 145:333.
55. Colca JR, Wyse BM, Sawada G, et al. Ciglitazone, a hypoglycemic agent: early effects on the pancreatic islets of ob/ob mice. Metabolism 1988; 37:276.
56. Fujiwara T, Wada M, Fukuda K, et al. Characterization of CS-045, a new oral antidiabetic agent, II. Effects on glycemic control and pancreatic islet structure at a late stage of the diabetic syndrome in c57BL/KsJ-db/db mice. Metabolism 1991;40:1213.
57. Krebs EG. Historical perspectives on protein phosphorylation and a classification system for protein kinases. Philos Trans R Soc Lond Biol Sci 1983; 302:3.
58. Krebs EG. The enzymology of control by phosphorylation. In: Boyer PD, Krebs EG, eds. The enzymes, 3rd ed. Orlando, FL: Academic Press, 1986:3.
59. Xin X, Yang S, Kowalski J, Gerritsen ME. Peroxisome proliferator-activated receptor gamma ligands are potent inhibitors of angiogenesis in vitro and in vivo. J Biol Chem 1999; 274:9116.
60. Unson XG, MacDonald D, Ray K, et al. Position 9 replacement analogs of glucagon uncouple biological activity and receptor binding. J Biol Chem 1991; 266:2763.
61. Madsen P, Brand CL, Holst JJ, Knudsen B. Advances in non-peptide glucagon receptor antagonists. Curr Pharm Des 1999; 5:683.
62. Foley JE. Rationale and application of fatty acid oxidation inhibitors in treatment of diabetes mellitus. Diabetes Care 1992; 15:773.
62a. Vella A, Shah P, Basu R, et al. Effect of glucagon-like peptide 1 (7–36) amide on glucose effectiveness and insulin action in people with type 2 diabetes. Diabetes 2000; 49:611.
63. Kelley DE, Goodpaster B, Wing RR, Sinoneau JA. Skeletal muscle fatty acid metabolism in association with insulin resistance, obesity, and weight loss. Am J Physiol 1999; 277:E1130.
64. Purnell JQ, Kahn SE, Albers JJ, et al. Effect of weight loss with reduction of intra-abdominal fat on lipid metabolism in older men. J Clin Endocrinol Metab 2000; 85:977.
65. Lean ME. Sibutramine—a review of clinical efficacy. Int J Obes 1997; 21:S30.
66. Cuellar GE, Ruiz AM, Monsalve MC, et al. A six-month treatment of obesity with sibutramine 15 mg; a double-blind, placebo-controlled monocenter clinical trial in a Hispanic population. Obes Res 2000; 8:71.
67. Rossner S, Sjostrom L, Noack R, et al. Weight loss, weight maintenance, and improved cardiovascular risk factors after 2 years treatment with orlistat for obesity. Obes Res 2000; 8:49.
68. Sjostrom CD, Lissner L, Wedel H, Sjostrom L. Reduction in incidence of diabetes, hypertension and lipid disturbances after intentional weight loss induced by bariatric surgery: the SOS intervention study. Obes Res 1999; 7:477.

# CHAPTER 143

# INSULIN THERAPY AND ITS COMPLICATIONS

GORDON C. WEIR

Insulin is the mainstay of therapy for all patients with type 1 diabetes and for many of those with type 2 diabetes. Subcutaneous insulin therapy attempts to mimic normal physiologic insulin secretion and regulation of fuel metabolism.[1] It is subject to many variables that can be controlled only partially in everyday life. Insulin therapy differs from physiologic insulin secretion in at least two major ways. First, insulin secretion in normal persons is an exquisitely regulated process that rapidly responds to changes in the circulating concentrations of glucose, amino acids, other fuels, gut hormones, and the autonomic nervous system. Second, insulin normally is secreted into the portal circulation, where it acts on hepatic metabolic processes before entering the peripheral circulation. With injection of insulin, a constant problem exists of matching fuel flux with appropriate insulin levels. Nonetheless, considerable success can be achieved with this imperfect therapy.

## INSULIN PURITY AND SOURCES

The insulin market in most nations is now dominated by human insulin preparations; pork insulin and beef-pork mixtures may soon be completely discontinued by the major

**TABLE 143-1.**
**Characteristics of the Most Widely Available Insulins in the United States**

| Type and Preparation | Constituents | Action Profile (Hours)* | | | Special Considerations |
|---|---|---|---|---|---|
| | | *Onset* | *Peak* | *Duration* | |
| **SHORT-ACTING** | | | | | |
| **Regular (human)** | Solution of unmodified zinc insulin crystals | 0.5–1.0 | 2–3 | 6–8 | For intravenous, intraperitoneal, and pump use |
| **Lispro** | Analog | 0.2 | 0.5–1.5 | 2–3 | |
| **U500** | Concentrated, unmodified | 1–3 | 6–12 | 12–18 | This is a purified pork preparation |
| | | | | | For use only in cases of insulin resistance with requirements >200 U per day |
| **INTERMEDIATE-ACTING** | | | | | |
| **NPH (human)** | Protamine zinc, phosphate buffer | 1.5 | 5–8 | 18–24 | Premixing with delay before injection may result in loss of regular insulin action |
| **Lente (human)** | Amorphous, acetate buffer | 2.5 | 6–12 | 18–28 | |
| **LONG-ACTING** | | | | | |
| **Ultralente (human)** | Amorphous and crystalline mix | 3–4 | 9–15 | 22–26 | |
| **MIXTURES** | | | | | |
| **NPH/regular** | NPH 70%, regular 30% | 0.5–1.0 | 3–8 | 18–24 | Biphasic action, not suitable when frequent dose adjustments are required |
| | NPH 50%, regular 50% | 0.5–1.0 | 3–8 | 18–24 | |

*NPH*, neutral protamine Hagedorn insulin.
*Onset, peak, and duration of action of insulins are approximations, because they vary according to injection technique, site, presence of insulin antibodies, and other variables that affect insulin pharmacokinetics.

manufacturers. Beef insulin is the most immunogenic of these, whereas pork insulin is only slightly more immunogenic than human insulin.[1,2] This is consistent with the fact that beef insulin differs from human insulin by three amino acids, whereas pork insulin differs from human insulin by only one amino acid. Previously, insulin preparations contained trace amounts of proinsulin-like intermediates, desaminoinsulin, glucagon, pancreatic polypeptide, somatostatin, and other contaminants of islet and exocrine tissue. Antibodies to many of these substances were found in the plasma of patients treated with these older insulin preparations. Modern purified insulins are much "cleaner" than those used 20 years ago, and the contaminants are usually present at levels of <20 ppm.[1]

## HUMAN INSULIN

Biosynthetic human insulin was introduced commercially in 1982 and, since then, several improvements have been made in the manufacturing process. One approach is to use an *Escherichia coli* fermentation to produce proinsulin, which then is enzymatically cleaved to C peptide and insulin, with subsequent purification. The preparations are extremely pure, and proinsulin contamination is <1 ppm.[3] Moreover, no immune responses to contaminating *E. coli* proteins have been identified. The other major approach is to produce a nonhuman proinsulin precursor protein in yeast (*Saccharomyces cerevisiae*), which is then secreted into the media, cleaved to human insulin, and purified.

Human regular insulin, perhaps because it is slightly more hydrophobic, is absorbed more rapidly than is pork insulin.[4] A widely publicized report suggested that the use of human insulin was associated with more serious hypoglycemia than was the use of animal insulins.[5] This concern has been evaluated extensively in several thorough studies, which concluded that the risk of more dangerous hypoglycemia from human insulin than from pork insulin is either nonexistent or trivial.[6] Although human insulin preparations are not appreciably superior to the purified pork insulin, probably they eventually will completely replace animal insulins.

Biosynthetic proinsulin has a potency that is 5% to 10% that of insulin, and at one point was thought to have therapeutic potential. Because of concerns about possible adverse effects on

vascular disease, however, plans for its therapeutic use have been abandoned.[7]

## INSULIN CONCENTRATIONS AND PREPARATIONS

Worldwide, insulin usually is provided in a concentration of 100 U/mL (U100). Other concentrations can still be found in various parts of the world, so clinicians should be alert to unexpected concentrations used by international patients. Less concentrated preparations can be useful for administering lower doses to children; these can be made up using a commercially available dilution fluid. Regular insulin is available in a U500 strength for use in patients with high requirements (>200 U per day). The three most widely used insulin preparations are short-acting, intermediate-acting, and long-acting insulins (Table 143-1; see Chap. 236).

### SHORT-ACTING INSULINS

Lispro insulin is more rapid-acting and has a shorter duration of action than regular insulin.[8–10] This is a human insulin analog in which the amino acids at positions 28 and 29 on the B chain are reversed, thus giving Lys (B28), Pro (B29). Lispro insulin is equipotent to regular insulin. The chemical modification produces faster dissociation from hexamers to monomers, however, thus allowing more rapid absorption from subcutaneous depots. Peak levels are seen 30 to 90 minutes after injection, and duration of action is at most 3 hours, unless it is held in the circulation by antibodies. It is particularly useful for providing metabolic control for meals and for rapidly bringing high glucose levels under control. Lispro insulin usually is most conveniently given just before a meal, although in some circumstances it might be given 15 minutes before a meal or even 15 minutes after the initiation of a meal if delayed gastric emptying is a concern or if the meal is expected to be prolonged.[10] For routine treatment regimens, it is used effectively in combination with an intermediate- or a long-acting preparation.[11] Patients who take lispro insulin before dinner usually do not require a bedtime snack, even for glucose values in the range of 90 to 110 mg/dL, whereas those who take regular insulin—which can have a duration of action extending well past 6 hours—must consume a snack for protection against hypoglycemia.[12] The frequency of hypoglycemia is less with lispro than with regular insulin.[13] The administration of lispro insulin by a pen device is becoming a popular option; lispro insulin also is becoming the preferred choice of insulin for continuous subcutaneous insulin infusion (CSII) therapy.[14] Lispro insulin can be used intravenously for the treatment of diabetic ketoacidosis, hyperosmolar nonketotic coma, or shock, during surgery, and in other unstable metabolic settings, although in these situations it has no advantage over regular insulin.

Regular (crystalline zinc) insulin is contained in a clear neutral pH buffer and for years was the standard rapid-acting insulin. Now, however, its role is often displaced by lispro insulin. When administered subcutaneously, its onset of action is 30 to 45 minutes, depending on the site of injection and local blood flow. Its action peaks at 2 to 3 hours and lasts ~6 hours, although it can exert effects for as long as 12 hours. For optimal efficacy, regular insulin is best taken 30 to 45 minutes before meals. In spite of the growing popularity of lispro insulin, the longer duration of action of regular insulin can be very useful in some circumstances, such as maintaining good control when a long time elapses between meals. For a metabolically unstable patient in a hospital setting, "sliding scales" with regular insulin given subcutaneously every 6 hours can be very effective. A sliding scale using lispro insulin would require injection every 3 to 4 hours, which would make it less convenient.

### INTERMEDIATE-ACTING INSULINS

Neutral protamine Hagedorn (NPH) insulin and Lente insulin are the most frequently used intermediate-acting preparations. NPH insulin is complexed with zinc and protamine in a phosphate buffer. Lente insulin is a mixture of crystallized and amorphous insulin in an acetate buffer that gradually is released in the subcutaneous tissues. Lente insulin and NPH insulin have slightly different time-action profiles.[4,15] NPH insulin has a more rapid onset of action, which begins ~1 hour after injection and peaks between 5 and 8 hours; usually, virtually all of its activity is lost considerably before 24 hours. Lente insulin, which has a slower onset of action (~2.5 hours) and peaks slightly later than NPH, also usually will not last for 24 hours. Intermediate-acting insulins generally are given once or twice a day. Some clinicians, however, are finding benefits from giving small doses of NPH with short-acting insulin before breakfast, lunch, and supper, and giving NPH alone at bedtime.[9,16] Sometimes NPH and Lente insulins can have effects for >24 hours, causing early morning hypoglycemia; for some patients, this may be due to circulating antibodies that were generated by previous use of less purified insulins. Care must be taken to ensure that "frosting" of NPH (precipitation on the walls of the vial that leads to loss of insulin potency) does not occur.[17] This phenomenon can be due to freezing or overheating of the vials. Patients should be taught to routinely examine the vials carefully before injection.

### LONG-ACTING INSULINS

Manufacture of the first long-acting insulin preparation, protamine zinc insulin, has been discontinued. The only currently available long-acting preparation is human Ultralente. It acts like a slow NPH, with an onset of action at 3 to 4 hours, a broad peak at 9 to 15 hours, and a duration that may not reach 24 hours.[4,18] Ultralente is usually given twice a day, most commonly before breakfast and before supper.

## INSULIN PHARMACOKINETICS

After intravenous injection, the half-life of circulating insulin appears to be 5 to 10 minutes in normal persons and patients with diabetes who do not have insulin antibodies.[19] The disappearance curve is explained best by a multiexponential model.[19] The distribution space has been estimated to approximate the extracellular space, which is ~16% of body weight. The apparent distribution space is increased in the presence of antibodies[19] but otherwise appears to be similar in normal persons and patients with insulin-treated diabetes.[20]

The liver is the major site of insulin clearance, accounting for ~50% of the total; the kidney accounts for ~30%, and skeletal muscle accounts for most of the rest.[22] The metabolic clearance rate of insulin is 700 to 800 mL/m$^2$ per minute.[21] At supraphysiologic concentrations of insulin, hepatic clearance may become saturated, but this does not seem to occur in the kidney.[23] Reduced insulin clearance has been found in obese persons.[22] Renal function also is an important determinant of circulating insulin levels. Insulin doses usually must be lowered as renal function deteriorates.

Insulin pharmacokinetics are complicated further by the many factors that alter insulin absorption from the subcutaneous site.[24] These may cause much more variability in insulin action than is generally appreciated, both from one individual to another and from day to day in a given individual.[25] Circulating insulin antibodies have important effects on insulin pharmacokinetics, delaying the onset of action of rapid-acting insulin and increasing the duration of action of both short- and longer-acting insulins.[26] Today, they rarely cause insulin resistance.

Factors that tend to produce relatively *increased insulin absorption* include low doses of insulin, dilute insulin solution, increased subcutaneous blood flow (exercise, massage, heat), local tissue injury, abdominal injection, and intramuscular injection. Factors that tend to produce relatively *decreased insulin absorption* include high doses of insulin, concentrated insulin solution, decreased subcutaneous blood flow (shock, cold, standing), lipohypertrophy, intradermal injection, and injection into limbs (at rest). The insulin absorption rate is inversely proportional to the volume and concentration of the injected insulin.[24] Thus, even U500 regular insulin, when given in large volumes, may have a duration of action similar to that of smaller volumes of intermediate-acting insulin.

### SITE OF INJECTION

Insulin conventionally is injected into the subcutaneous tissues of the abdomen, buttock, anterior thigh, and dorsal arm. In unusual circumstances, insulin also may be injected intramuscularly to achieve more rapid uptake. Prolonged intramuscular insulin therapy, besides being painful, causes tissue scarring. Insulin is absorbed more rapidly from the abdominal subcutaneous tissue than from the thigh or upper limb. If the limb is exercised, absorption is more rapid than expected because of increased blood flow. Traditionally, rotation of insulin injection sites has been advocated to prevent lipohypertrophy or lipoatrophy. The increased purity of insulin preparations has greatly reduced the incidence of lipoatrophy, but hypertrophy still occurs if insulin is repetitively injected into the same site. The injection patterns should be consistent; for example, abdominal sites might be used in the morning and thigh sites at night.

### SUBCUTANEOUS BLOOD FLOW

With upright posture, subcutaneous blood flow diminishes considerably in the lower limbs (and to a lesser extent in the abdominal wall), decreasing the absorption rate of insulin.[27] Conversely, massage, increased ambient temperature (including hot baths and showers), and exercise increase the rate of absorption. Insulin reactions seem to occur more often during heat waves.

### MIXTURE OF INSULINS

When regular (and probably lispro) insulin is mixed in the same syringe with Lente insulin, some of the rapid-acting component can be lost in just a few minutes, so the mixture must be injected immediately.[28] The problem is potentially even more severe if regular insulin is mixed with Ultralente insulin.[4,29,30] No difficulty is found when regular or lispro insulin is mixed with NPH insulin.[11,24] Premixed insulin preparations are widely used. A mixture of 70% NPH and 30% regular insulin is the most common, but a mixture of 50% NPH and 50% regular insulin is also available. Mixtures of lispro insulin and intermediate-acting insulin are under study.[31]

## INDICATIONS FOR INSULIN THERAPY

Virtually all patients with type 1 diabetes should be treated with insulin. Although some patients with very early type 1 diabetes can be kept in control with sulfonylureas, the theoretical potential of insulin to slow the process of autoimmune destruction[32] makes the use of insulin advisable. Also, patients with gestational diabetes who have a fasting glucose level of >120 mg/dL should be treated with insulin. Insulin is indicated in patients with type 2 diabetes who fail to respond to an adequate trial of diet and oral hypoglycemic agents.[1,33]

## DIABETES CONTROL AND COMPLICATIONS TRIAL

The 9.5-year Diabetes Control and Complications Trial (DCCT) was carried out in 29 centers and included 1441 patients with type 1 diabetes.[34] The study had two arms, a group with no complications and a group with "very mild to moderate" nonproliferative retinopathy. A mean hemoglobin $A_{1c}$ of ~7% was achieved in the intensive therapy group compared with a level of ~9% in the standard therapy group. The efficacy of intensive treatment was dramatic. In the primary prevention group, the risk of developing retinopathy was reduced by 76%, and in the secondary intervention cohort, the risk of progression was reduced by 54%. The risk of developing microalbuminuria was reduced by 34% and 56%, respectively. The risk of developing neuropathy was reduced by 57% and 69%, respectively. A tendency was seen for a reduction in the number of major cardiovascular and peripheral vascular events that had borderline statistical significance. Questions remain about the existence of a threshold for glycemic control that must be reached before benefits occur. The data suggest a continuum of beneficial effect such that any improvement in glycemic control should be expected to help. This is an important and practical concept for those patients who are not able make a full commitment to a DCCT-style regimen.

With regard to adverse effects, the incidence of severe hypoglycemia (reactions needing assistance) was increased three-fold in the intensive therapy group. Intensive therapy also was associated with weight gain, which was 4.6 kg more than in the conventional group after 5 years. Although concern exists regarding how many patients will be able to follow this difficult regimen, the DCCT sets a new standard of care for persons with type 1 diabetes. Caution must be used in applying a DCCT level of care to children younger than 13 years, persons with hypoglycemic unawareness, and patients with advanced complications.

## UNITED KINGDOM PROSPECTIVE DIABETES STUDY

Much debate existed about whether the DCCT results could be extrapolated to patients with type 2 diabetes. This question has been largely answered by the United Kingdom Prospective Diabetes Study (UKPDS).[35,36] In this study, 5102 patients were followed for an average of 10 years. Treatment was with insulin, sulfonylureas, or metformin. Although the statistical power for the group receiving insulin was insufficient to allow separate

analysis, evaluation of all groups revealed that lowering of the hemoglobin $A_{1c}$ from 7.9% to 7.0% produced a 25% reduction in microvascular complications. Moreover, a continuous relationship was found between risk of microvascular complications and glycemia, and no evidence was seen for a threshold for the development of complications above a hemoglobin $A_{1c}$ of 6.2%. *These data support the hypothesis that hyperglycemia causes or is the major contributor to these complications.* These results were not surprising because of the similarity in the progression and character of the complications of type 1 and type 2 diabetes.[37]

Various arguments have been raised about whether insulin treatment, by raising plasma insulin concentrations, might worsen macrovascular disease.[38] The UKPDS did not unequivocally answer this question, but for the combined treatment groups, a 16% reduction was seen in combined fatal or nonfatal myocardial infarctions and sudden death ($p = 0.052$). For the group receiving insulin, *no* evidence was found of an increase in macrovascular disease or death rate, even though this group showed higher fasting plasma insulin levels than were found in the other treatment groups. More weight gain occurred in the patients treated with insulin and sulfonylureas than in those treated with metformin. *The results of the UKPDS are very helpful for countering the anxiety about the potential cardiovascular risks of insulin therapy.*

## SETTING GOALS OF THERAPY

Although normalization of all aspects of metabolism is the ideal in the treatment of type 1 and type 2 diabetes, this goal rarely is attainable with current forms of therapy. Nevertheless, near-normal glycemia can be achieved in selected patients and, ideally, should be the goal of therapy for all, with recognition that this goal must be modified for many individuals. The American Diabetes Association (ADA) has set forth goals of obtaining preprandial glucose values of between 80 and 120 mg/dL and bedtime glucose levels of 100 to 140 mg/dL.[39] The goal for hemoglobin $A_{1c}$ is <7%. The DCCT goals for the experimental group were to achieve fasting glucose levels of between 70 and 120 mg/dL, but because so much hypoglycemia was seen in the study, the ADA has recommended a higher lower bound of 80 mg/dL. Some value is seen in monitoring 2-hour postprandial blood glucose levels to optimize premeal doses of short-acting insulin, but no specific goals were established, although keeping glycemic excursions below 160 mg/dL would be a reasonable objective. Many variables prevent patients from meeting these goals, so the physician must individualize. One of the main limiting factors preventing individuals from obtaining such excellent control is hypoglycemia, which is debilitating and life-threatening. Some patients have very unstable diabetes—the pathophysiology of which is still not well understood—and must accept glucose levels that otherwise would be considered much too high. Other patients have defective counterregulatory hormone responses and/or hypoglycemia unawareness, which puts them at particular risk.[6,40] Many patients are unwilling or unable to follow the demanding regimens required for success, too, so they, too, may need modified goals.

Achieving optimal control is often easier in patients with type 2 diabetes because glucose fluctuations are less marked, and these patients are less prone to severe hypoglycemia. In spite of this more favorable pathophysiology, which probably is due largely to residual insulin secretion, the UKPDS suggests that even very motivated physicians have difficulty keeping patients with type 2 diabetes under recommended control.[35,36]

## PRINCIPLES OF INSULIN THERAPY

Now that general agreement exists that good glycemic control with near-normal glycemia can prevent or slow the development of complications, what used to be called intensive therapy is becoming the standard of care.[39] This approach demands intensive monitoring of blood glucose, careful attention to diet, an insulin regimen that mimics the normal diurnal and post-prandial insulin excursions, and frequent adjustment of the insulin dosage to match changing circumstances. The two approaches include multiple injections (intensive conventional therapy) or CSII (pump therapy). Provided the guidelines are followed, both approaches can provide sustained improvements in metabolic control.

## BENEFITS AND RISKS

Any improvement in control can be expected to have a beneficial influence on the development of complications. Moreover, with very good control, one can expect to achieve near-normalization of plasma glucose values, lipid levels, and amino-acid concentrations; also, glucagon and growth hormone diurnal profiles may approach a more normal pattern. The potential benefits of intensive therapy must be weighed carefully against the risks. Any intensive therapy regimen increases the risk of hypoglycemia, the danger of which must not be underestimated.[6,40] Patients who have hypoglycemic reactions without warning should not undertake intensive therapy with the objective of achieving normoglycemia.

## INITIATION OF TREATMENT FOR TYPE 1 DIABETES

Once initial instability is controlled with a combination of short- and intermediate-acting insulins, treatment of type 1 diabetes is best begun by giving intermediate-acting insulin twice a day, before breakfast as well as at bedtime or before supper at a dosage of 0.2 to 0.3 U/kg per day. This dosage is increased gradually with or without the use of short-acting insulin given before breakfast and supper while the blood glucose profile is observed.

## DAILY REQUIREMENTS

Daily insulin production in normal persons usually is 24 to 36 U; however, this is secreted into the portal circulation. Patients with type 1 diabetes who have no endogenous insulin secretion, as evidenced by the absence of circulating C peptide, generally require between 0.5 and 1.0 U/kg per day. Requirements may be divided into basal and prandial needs. The basal requirement is necessary for suppression of hepatic glucose output, and usually constitutes 40% to 60% of the daily dose. The remaining amount is necessary for nutrient disposal after meals.[1] These considerations are applied most easily using the CSII approach.

Insulin requirements in thin patients with type 2 diabetes usually are similar to those of patients with type 1 diabetes. Obese patients generally require more insulin, with requirements sometimes as high as 2.0 U/kg per day.

Patients who require <0.5 U/kg per day may have some endogenous insulin production or may be insulin sensitive because of vigorous physical conditioning or diminished food intake. Renal failure or a counterregulatory hormone defect, such as adrenocortical or pituitary failure, also should be considered. Nonobese patients whose disease remains poorly controlled on >1.0 U/kg per day should be evaluated carefully for compliance failure or for occult causes of insulin resistance.

## INSULIN TREATMENT OF TYPE 2 DIABETES

In view of the confirmed benefits of glycemic control for people with type 2 diabetes, more reason exists to be aggressive with whatever combination of diet, oral agents, and insulin provides the recommended control. Clearly insulin treatment alone can be very successful.[33] In general, achieving smooth control is easier in type 2 diabetes because of the beneficial

influence of persistent endogenous insulin secretion. Patients are also more likely to have better counterregulatory defense mechanisms than patients with type 1 diabetes, which can protect them against hypoglycemia. A variety of insulin regimens can provide excellent control; debate exists about which ones are preferable.[31,33,41,42] Oral agents may be combined with insulin. Nevertheless, when insulin is used alone, in some cases only one injection of NPH or Lente in the morning can provide acceptable control. Because these insulins rarely have meaningful effect at 24 hours, however, two injections usually must be given. Many patients find it convenient to take the second one at bedtime. Sometimes a single injection of Ultralente in the morning can provide adequate coverage, particularly in patients who have a difficult time with multiple injections. Often, the addition of short-acting insulin before meals is not necessary, but this can help when added before breakfast and supper. Many patients have trouble mixing insulins, so premixed NPH and regular insulin (70% NPH and 30% regular) can be very useful. Generally ~60% is given before breakfast and 40% before supper. Some patients with type 2 diabetes have a less stable pattern and may require a more complex regimen similar to that used in type 1 diabetes. Many clinicians are reluctant to use insulin for treatment of type 2 diabetes because of concern about weight gain. Some weight gain can be documented, but the UKPDS found that weight gain under insulin treatment was *not* very different from weight gain under treatment with sulfonylureas alone.[35,36]

## COMBINED USE OF INSULIN AND ORAL AGENTS

Interest has been growing in the use of oral agents and insulin together for the treatment of type 2 diabetes.[43] The various rationales have included cost reduction, minimization of patient effort, limitation of weight gain, reduction of number of injections, and the hope of minimizing plasma insulin concentrations. One of the most popular is the *BIDS* regimen of *bedtime insulin and daytime sulfonylureas.* This regimen is usually initiated when sulfonylurea failure begins, and intermediate-acting insulin is used at bedtime. Sometimes use of a mixture of short-acting and intermediate-acting insulins before supper, even in the form of a premixed preparation such as 70/30 insulin, is advantageous. Metformin may be added to an insulin regimen, with the hope of limiting weight gain and reducing the dosage of insulin. Sometimes metformin can even be combined with a single injection of insulin at bedtime.[42] The use of metformin instead of a sulfonylurea combined with NPH at bedtime may lead to less weight gain.[42] However, care must be taken to avoid metformin when a variety of severe coexisting diseases are present. Acarbose has been used along with insulin to control postprandial insulin excursions, and it may limit weight gain more effectively than sulfonylureas. Thiazolidinediones (e.g., pioglitazone) have been added to insulin regimens to improve control and lower insulin dosage. The benefits obtained from reducing insulin dosages in this way remain to be established. In spite of these oral options, insulin alone can be very effective when given without an oral agent.

## SELECTION OF A REGIMEN FOR TREATMENT OF TYPE 1 DIABETES

Although proving that CSII provides better control than multiple injections is difficult, most clinicians have the strong impression that it gives superior results with less hypoglycemia.[44] The alternative approach of using multiple injections with attention to all of the other details of management is usually very effective, however, and is much less expensive. If the physician's experience and support team for CSII management

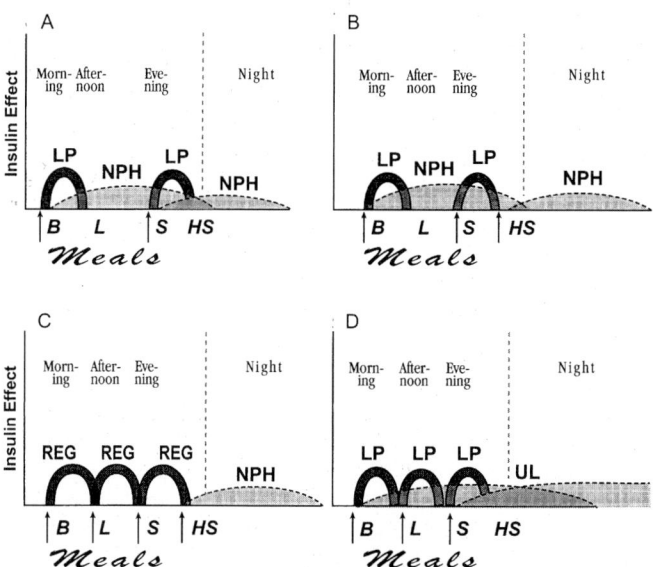

**FIGURE 143-1.** Regimens commonly used for insulin therapy (see text for discussion). (*B, L, S,* and *HS,* refer to breakfast, lunch, supper, and bedtime, respectively; *LP* refers to lispro insulin; *REG* refers to regular insulin; *NPH* refers to neutral protamine Hagedorn insulin; and *UL* refers to Ultralente insulin.) **A,** Traditional split-mix regimen, which can use either NPH or Lente as the intermediate-acting insulin and either lispro or regular insulin as the fast-acting preparation. **B,** A commonly used three-shots-per-day regimen. **C,** Patients on this regimen should usually use regular insulin rather than lispro because of its longer action, thus compensating for the lack of NPH coverage during the day. **D,** This regimen uses Ultralente twice a day with either lispro or regular insulin given before meals.

is limited, intensive conventional therapy probably is preferable. Patients who choose pump therapy are often those who adhere to the disciplines of diabetes treatment with a multiple-injection approach but fail to reach their therapeutic goals. Some patients prefer the pump because of the greater flexibility it provides with meal timing and because it reduces the need for snacks, which is an important consideration for patients with demanding occupations. The pump may help to prevent the adverse effect of unpredictable peaking of intermediate-acting insulin that is seen in some patients with conventional therapy. Before starting CSII, *testing the patient's response to intensive conventional therapy* is useful, because this provides the physician with an idea of patient compliance and psychological adaptability. Despite intensive encouragement, many patients are not motivated to perform the necessary monitoring four to six times each day, to ensure regular meal timing, and to take additional snacks. With pump therapy, considerable attention to detail is required; for example, infusion lines must be changed regularly and managed meticulously, batteries must be changed, and the pump must be protected from water and must undergo periodic maintenance. If the patient can achieve excellent control with conventional therapy, a change to a pump is unlikely to provide additional benefits.

Among drug improvements in recent years, lispro insulin is usually the preferred insulin for premeal injections because its pharmacokinetics better match food absorption profiles. The approach to premeal insulin administration has become much more rigorous as sliding scales coupled with carbohydrate counting have become more frequently used.[45]

Four regimens of intensive conventional therapy are commonly used (Fig. 143-1). Regimen A, commonly called a *split mix,* is a frequently used approach in patients who are not undergoing intensive therapy. In conjunction with careful caloric control, exercise, and more frequent monitoring, however, it can yield a blood glucose profile and glycohemoglobin level that are nearly as good as those obtained with more com-

**TABLE 143-2.**

**Goals of Insulin Therapy and Guide for Adjusting Conventional or Pump Therapy**

| Time | Blood Glucose Goal | | Therapy Requiring Adjustment | |
| --- | --- | --- | --- | --- |
| | *(mg/dL)* | *(mmol/L)* | *Conventional* | *Pump* |
| Fasting (pre-breakfast) | 80–120 | 4.4–6.6 | Ultralente or intermediate | Basal rate |
| Before meals | 80–120 | 4.4–6.6 | Check meal and snack timing and profile of intermediate-acting insulin | |
| 2 hours after meals | ≤160 | ≤9.0 | Premeal injection | Bolus dose |
| 2 a.m. to 4 a.m. | 80–120 | 4.4–6.6 | Intermediate or Ultralente | Basal rate |

plex regimens. Regimens B, C, and D involve three or more injections per day. These regimens may have a greater potential for suppressing fasting hepatic glucose output before breakfast. Postprandial glucose excursions can be controlled by lispro insulin given immediately before meals or regular insulin injections given 30 minutes before meals according to a sliding scale.

Although regimen A (split mix) is the simplest regimen, it has the greatest potential for causing nocturnal hypoglycemia because of the peaking of intermediate-acting insulin during the early hours of the morning. Regimens B and C may reduce the chance of nocturnal hypoglycemia and also are more likely to suppress the dawn rise in blood glucose. With a variation of regimen B, some are finding benefit from combining NPH and lispro not only before breakfast but also before lunch and supper, with a last injection of NPH given at bedtime.[9,16] This repetitive use of NPH is thought to provide better basal coverage. For regimen C in which intermediate-acting insulin is given only at bedtime, regular insulin rather than lispro insulin should be used; the duration of action of lispro insulin is not long enough to cover the period between meals.[8]

Regimen D, an Ultralente program in which the Ultralente is given twice a day, attempts to mimic the continuous basal insulin delivery achieved with a pump. The basal Ultralente insulin doses are given as 40% to 60% of total daily requirements, typically administered before breakfast and then before either supper or bedtime.[18] In all four regimens, the fasting blood glucose level guides the choice of dosage for the intermediate- and long-acting insulins. Blood glucose should be checked intermittently at 2:00 to 3:00 a.m. to document possible nocturnal hypoglycemia. Generally, with intensive conventional therapy, the insulin dosage exceeds that required for CSII by 20%. The goal of therapy (Table 143-2) should be a premeal blood glucose level of between 80 and 120 mg/dL, and a 1- to 2-hour postprandial peak of <160 mg/dL. Total daily dosage requirements usually are between 0.5 and 1.0 U/kg. The premeal short-acting insulin doses are based on a sliding scale, often combined with carbohydrate counting.[45] The doses for the sliding scale are, therefore, determined by the premeal glucose level and the amount of carbohydrate expected in the meal, with much of the fine tuning being determined by trial and error. The prebreakfast insulin dose often is greater than that needed for the evening meal. Delivery of short-acting insulins may be facilitated by a pen delivery device.

## CONTINUOUS SUBCUTANEOUS INSULIN INFUSION REGIMENS

Various pumps for CSII delivery are available that provide more flexibility in delivery rates, additional safety features, and greater portability than earlier models.[46] Lispro insulin is rapidly becoming the preferred insulin for CSII.[47] The basal dose usually is 40% to 60% of the total daily dose[1] and can be delivered at variable rates depending on the time of day. Typically the basal rate required for the early morning hours is twice that needed in the early evening. The fasting and postprandial blood glucose goals are the same as for conventional insulin therapy, and the premeal dose also is based on a sliding scale determined from a trial-and-error approach, which often is coupled with carbohydrate counting. The premeal bolus should be delivered 30 minutes before meals, as with conventional therapy. Ketoacidosis can occur in patients receiving CSII if pump failure occurs (particularly in the early hours of sleeping), which results in virtually complete insulin deficiency. Potential causes of interruption include mechanical failure, accidental kinking of the infusion catheter, dislodgment of the needle, and insulin aggregation in the infusion line. These mishaps may be compounded by failure of the patient to take appropriate corrective action, such as restarting conventional therapy promptly. The risk of diabetic ketoacidosis appears to be falling as experience with CSII grows. The use of CSII may cause subcutaneous abscesses and cellulitis. Staphylococcal infections of the skin are a contraindication to CSII because of the danger of septicemia and endocarditis. Patients with psychiatric disturbances, alcoholism, poor comprehension, and multiple advanced complications generally are not suitable candidates for intensive therapy. Intensive therapy is a demanding and expensive undertaking, especially with the pump devices, and many patients who start these programs are unable to continue for a prolonged period.

## BRITTLE DIABETES

*Brittle diabetes* has been variously defined.[48] Some reserve the term for describing patients with type 1 diabetes in whom diabetic ketoacidosis frequently develops. Others include a broader group of patients with diabetes who have severe glycemic excursions for which an obvious explanation is not apparent. Brittle diabetes is a heterogeneous entity. For some patients, no obvious explanation can fully explain their instability. A mixture of contributing factors (e.g., erratic gastric emptying, defective counterregulation, and autonomic neuropathy) may be present, but often their apparent intrinsic brittleness remains poorly understood. In other patients, the metabolic instability has its main origins in the inability of patients to follow the demands of the regimen; frequently, psychological and social problems need to be resolved before control can be improved. Occasionally, patients may be labeled as having a subcutaneous insulin degradation syndrome, but this phenomenon has been well documented in only a few patients[24,49,50] and is extremely rare.

The management of brittle diabetes begins with the taking of a *detailed history*. The circumstances and details of previous hospitalizations must be examined carefully. To fully understand the problem, *frequent blood glucose sampling* should be performed (on at least six occasions over 24 hours, preferably with two samples at night [e.g., 2:00 a.m. and 6:00 a.m.] to detect possible nocturnal hypoglycemia [between 2:00 a.m. and 3:00 a.m.] and the "dawn phenomenon" [6:00 a.m.]). It may also be helpful to *interview members of the patient's family*. In those severe cases that result in hospitalization, the patient's activities should be supervised carefully, particularly the *dietary intake* and *level of activity*, and the patient should not be allowed to leave the ward unsupervised. Under certain circumstances, all insulin injections should be administered by the nursing staff, and the patient should not have access to needles or syringes. Psychological and social support for both the patient and the family is necessary in most cases of brittle diabetes.

Patients who are *overinsulinized* with resultant frequent hypoglycemia and rebound hyperglycemia should be identified, because improvement will occur with a reduction of the insulin dose. With psychological testing, some patients may be

found to have a *learning disorder*; in these cases, special teaching may be required. Some patients with chaotic blood glucose patterns may have *gastroparesis* caused by diabetic autonomic neuropathy, which can be diagnosed by history or a gastric emptying study (see Chap. 149).

## TREATMENT IN CHILDHOOD AND ADOLESCENCE

The general principles of insulin treatment already outlined also are applicable to children.[51] In young children, unpredictable food intake and activity increase the likelihood of hypoglycemia and marked glucose excursion. Low-dose insulin syringes should be used. Sometimes, insulin doses of 2 U and less may be required, so that the insulin must be diluted. Insulin administration should be performed by parents until children are 5 or 6 years old. After that, injections may be given by children, usually under supervision until the age of 10 to 12 years. Nocturnal hypoglycemia is a common occurrence with conventional insulin therapy, and may present as seizures. These patients, who may have a low seizure threshold, should have their nocturnal blood glucose measured periodically, receive a bedtime snack routinely, and usually should be given their second injection of intermediate-acting insulin before bedtime.

Adolescents face many temptations to reject the disciplines necessary for adequate diabetes management[52]; therefore, brittle diabetes is commonly seen in this age group. During the growth spurt, insulin requirements generally increase substantially and should be reviewed regularly (see Chap. 157). Now that the importance of good glycemic control has been accepted, more children and adolescents are able to follow an intensive regimen.[12]

## TREATMENT IN PREGNANCY

The benefits of good diabetes control have been demonstrated most impressively for pregnant patients with diabetes[53,54] (see Chap. 156). These patients generally are highly motivated to carry out the disciplines of intensive insulin therapy. Insulin requirements may drop slightly in the first trimester, then gradually increase in the second trimester, and finally peak in the third trimester. Immediately after delivery, requirements drop precipitously and return to prepregnancy levels.

## TREATMENT IN OLD AGE

The prospects for leading a vigorous life in old age continue to improve, so attention to diabetes control for the purpose of limiting complications is often appropriate for individuals in their 70s and 80s. When disabilities develop in people of any age, however, the goals of therapy must often be modified, with emphasis on symptomatic relief, prevention of diabetic ketoacidosis, halting of unwanted weight loss, and prevention of hypoglycemia. The last is an important consideration in socially isolated patients, and a visiting nurse may provide valuable assistance. Major concern arises when patients are unreliable about glucose testing, injection technique, and maintenance of regular eating schedules, and have a lack of exercise. Premixed insulins such as 70/30 insulin (70% NPH and 30% regular insulin) given before breakfast and supper have proved to be especially useful. More tailor-made mixtures might be prepared by a pharmacist or family member. Although most older patients have stable diabetes, some may have labile diabetes that is extremely difficult to manage.

## REMISSION FROM TYPE 1 DIABETES

A few weeks or sometimes months after the onset of type 1 diabetes, a remission frequently is observed that is manifested as a rapidly diminishing insulin requirement (the *honeymoon period*).[1,55] Sometimes, insulin therapy can be discontinued for a few weeks or even for months. The need to continue monitoring must be emphasized, because an abrupt decompensation may occur with the development of an intercurrent illness. Meticulous control does not seem to preserve residual function in the long term.[56]

## SURGERY AND ACUTE ILLNESS

Patients with diabetes are likely to undergo surgery at some time in their lives, and they often are at increased risk because of heart disease, sepsis, impaired wound healing, negative nitrogen balance, electrolyte disturbances, and renal failure. Meticulous anesthetic and metabolic care should be provided. Diabetes may present for the first time during an acute illness; thus, if possible, the metabolic state should be stabilized before embarking on surgery.

General anesthesia, surgery, and even the expectation of an operation may greatly increase the secretion of counterregulatory hormones, such as cortisol, catecholamines, glucagon, and growth hormone; this has an adverse effect on blood glucose levels. During general anesthesia, the patient is fasting and unconscious; therefore, particular care must be taken to prevent hypoglycemia. Fewer problems are seen with spinal or local anesthesia.

The specific metabolic aims in the surgical patient with diabetes are prevention of hypoglycemia and excess hyperglycemia (>250 mg/dL). The regimen should be easily understood and executed, with awareness that the surgical and nursing teams may have many other critical concerns during and after the operation. Surgery should be elective whenever possible, so that good preoperative diabetic control can be achieved. Ideally, the patient's operation should be scheduled at an early hour to facilitate the careful monitoring that is necessary after surgery.

Many insulin regimens have been advocated for management during the perioperative period. An easy and generally reliable regimen is to give half the total dosage as intermediate-acting insulin subcutaneously on the morning of the operation. In addition, the best course is to reduce the dose of intermediate insulin taken the night before surgery by 20% to 30% to prevent early morning hypoglycemia that might otherwise occur in these fasting patients. Infusing 5% dextrose at the rate of 100 mL per hour during the procedure is advisable. The major alternative is to give regular insulin by continuous infusion at a rate of 0.5 to 2.0 U per hour, with adjustments as needed. A disadvantage of insulin infusion is that, if the intravenous line is turned off inadvertently, ketosis may develop rapidly because of the short half-life of intravenous insulin. Insulin may stick to tubing, reducing its bioavailability; this problem may be overcome by running 50 mL of the infusate through the line before starting the infusion. Intravenous insulin therapy may be particularly useful with surgery that entails cardiopulmonary bypass, because requirements may increase suddenly during hypothermia and again during rewarming. In the postoperative period, the patient's ability to eat is a major determinant of the subsequent insulin requirement.

## RENAL FAILURE

Normally, the kidney is responsible for ~30% of insulin clearance.[57] In patients with diabetes, advanced nephropathy (creatinine clearance of <20 mL per minute) is accompanied by a reduction in insulin requirements resulting from reduced insulin clearance.[57] Insulin requirements may fall by 50% or more and, occasionally, patients can discontinue insulin therapy because residual insulin production is sufficient to achieve acceptable glycemic control. Insulin requirements also fall with acute renal failure in patients with diabetes, and the institution of dialysis often leads to an increase in insulin requirements, suggesting that some circulating substance is present in renal failure that facilitates insulin action or diminishes clearance.[58] In

**TABLE 143-3.**

**Causes of Hypoglycemia in Diabetic Patients Receiving Insulin Treatment**

| Causes of Hypoglycemia | Circumstances |
|---|---|
| ERRATIC NUTRIENT INTAKE | Missed meals and snacks; gastroparesis; malabsorption |
| ERRATIC INSULIN ABSORPTION | Changes in subcutaneous blood flow (e.g., exercise, heat, massage) |
| ENHANCED INSULIN AVAILABILITY | Renal failure, hypothyroidism |
| EXERCISE | Facilitates glucose disposal (glycogen repletion), increased insulin absorption |
| COUNTERREGULATORY HORMONE FAILURE | Addison disease, hypopituitarism |
| ALTERED GLUCONEO-GENESIS | Alcohol excess, β-adrenergic blockade, advanced liver disease |
| BEHAVIORAL DISORDER | Injection mistakes, psychological problems, learning disorder, factitious causes |
| OVERINSULINIZATION | Remission from type 1 diabetes, recovery from period of insulin resistance, marked reduction in caloric intake |

patients undergoing peritoneal dialysis, insulin can be given intraperitoneally; this yields satisfactory control, although substantial dosages (60–200 U per day) may be needed.[59]

## SIDE EFFECTS OF INSULIN TREATMENT

### HYPOGLYCEMIA

Hypoglycemia is the most frequently occurring side effect of insulin treatment. The common causes of hypoglycemia include missed meals or erratic meal timing, excessive insulin dosage, and unplanned exercise (Table 143-3). Other causes include failure to reduce insulin dosage after temporary periods of increased requirements during illness and pregnancy. Renal failure, alcohol excess, and remission from diabetes also must be considered. Rare causes include Addison disease, hypopituitarism, hypothyroidism, and intentional overdosage, which may be factitious or suicidal. Although these factors should be considered, occasionally hypoglycemia may occur with no demonstrable cause. With the increased emphasis on tight metabolic control, the incidence of hypoglycemia increases, as has been well demonstrated by the DCCT.[34] Considerable attention has been paid to the concept of hypoglycemia unawareness.[6,40] Repetitive episodes of even mild hypoglycemia reduce sympathetic responses to hypoglycemia and possibly even the threshold for neuroglycopenic symptoms. This phenomenon can be reversed by avoiding hypoglycemic episodes,[59a] but often this is accomplished at the expense of good glycemic control. In addition to the reversible reduction in epinephrine responses due to hypoglycemic episodes, concurrent permanent autonomic neuropathy can cause problems with both the release and potency of catecholamines.[60,61] This and other causes of hypoglycemia unawareness not only continue to be life-threatening but also are the major limiting factors to achievement of ideal control.

### POSTHYPOGLYCEMIC HYPERGLYCEMIA

Many years ago, Somogyi[62] postulated that overtreatment with insulin produces hypoglycemia, which is followed by hyperglycemia caused by activation of counterregulatory hormones. As the relative contributions of glucagon, epinephrine, cortisol, and growth hormone to the counteraction of hypoglycemia became better understood, a solid pathophysiologic basis seemed to exist for this putative *Somogyi phenomenon*. Studies in persons without diabetes have shown that, when glucose levels fall to ≤55 mg/dL, increased plasma glucagon and epinephrine levels have important stimulatory effects on hepatic glucose output.[63,64] Cortisol and growth hormone secretion also are stimulated by hypoglycemia, but do not contribute as much to the glucose rise that occurs after hypoglycemia. Persons with normal B-cell function do not become hyperglycemic after experimental insulin-induced hypoglycemia because the glucose rise is limited by increased insulin secretion. The situation is different in those with type 1 diabetes. For reasons that are unclear, glucagon responses are lost once B-cell function is markedly reduced; then epinephrine assumes the dominant protective role against hypoglycemia.[63] Because increasing glucose levels after hypoglycemia cannot be restrained by compensatory insulin secretion in individuals with type 1 diabetes, extremely high glucose responses, a *rebound*, might reasonably be expected. However, serious questions have been raised about how often such a rebound actually occurs.

The assumption that high glucose levels, particularly in the morning, result from the Somogyi phenomenon (rebound) had become a convenient and popular explanation for part of the instability commonly seen in type 1 diabetes. When careful studies were performed to determine how often this phenomenon actually occurred, nocturnal hypoglycemia was found to be followed only infrequently by morning hyperglycemia. These studies examined persons with documented low blood glucose levels in the middle of the night and found that, if anything, this hypoglycemia was followed by low glucose values before breakfast and even later in the day.[65,66] The best explanation is that when enough insulin is present to cause hypoglycemia at night, enough persisting insulin effect is usually also present from the subcutaneous insulin to limit whatever rebound might occur.

## UNEXPLAINED MORNING HYPERGLYCEMIA

Patients with type 1 diabetes often have high glucose levels in the morning that are difficult to explain. Although rebound can occur, it appears to be infrequent, and alternative explanations should be considered. The dawn phenomenon occurs in persons with and without diabetes.[67,68] In the early morning hours, a transient state of insulin resistance occurs that may be partially due to nocturnal secretion of growth hormone and cortisol.[40,69] In persons without diabetes, this early morning insulin resistance is limited by compensatory insulin secretion, but in patients with type 1 diabetes, troublesome hyperglycemia can occur. Patients with type 1 diabetes who use insulin pumps often set their pumps to provide increased basal insulin secretion in the early morning hours to counter this dawn phenomenon. The consistency of the dawn phenomenon in diabetes has not been well defined, but variability in growth hormone secretion may contribute to difficult-to-understand differences in morning glucose levels.

In patients with diabetes (both type 1 and type 2), administration of intermediate-acting insulin at dinnertime can create problems in controlling high prebreakfast glucose levels. The NPH or Lente can peak as early as midnight and often at 2 a.m. to 3 a.m., causing hypoglycemia that can be associated with rebound. In addition, the efficacy of the intermediate-acting insulin is often essentially gone by 7 a.m. to 8 a.m., exacerbating the problem. Moving the second injection of intermediate-acting insulin to bedtime can be very helpful. Other factors that frequently are responsible for morning hyperglycemia are consumption of large evening meals or late snacks.

## INSULIN EDEMA

Frank edema occurs in some patients with diabetes after treatment of uncontrolled diabetes is instituted, and mild sodium and fluid retention is a common occurrence even without edema.[70] Patients can be frustrated to find that improved diabetes control often is associated with transient weight gain from fluid retention in spite of decreased caloric intake. For patients with troublesome edema, the judicious use of diuretics can be helpful. Insulin's sodium-retaining effect on the kidney could be the best explanation for this phenomenon. Another contributor could be glucagon, which is known to have a natriuretic effect. Plasma glucagon levels are increased in uncontrolled diabetes, and a fall in glucagon with insulin treatment could contribute to the sodium retention. An inverse phenomenon probably accounts for the natriuresis and fluid loss that accompanies caloric restriction, which is associated with decreased plasma insulin and increased glucagon levels. Another contributor to the edema of insulin treatment may be the increased capillary permeability that is associated with poor metabolic control.[71,72]

## LIPOATROPHY

Lipoatrophy is characterized by a loss of subcutaneous fat at insulin injection sites that can be severe enough to be disfiguring.[2,15] Now that purified insulin is used, this phenomenon is seen infrequently. The cause of this complication is unknown but is suspected to be immunologic. Biopsies of affected areas reveal the presence of immunologic mediators such as immunoglobulin (Ig) M, IgE, and C3.[73] Perhaps a lipolytic cytokine is released during an immune reaction. When unpurified insulins were the culprit, the atrophy could be reversed by injecting the affected area with purified insulin, resulting in restoration of the subcutaneous fat in a few months.

Lipohypertrophy is a nonimmune phenomenon, consisting of a localized hypertrophy of subcutaneous fat that develops from repeated injections of insulin into a highly circumscribed area. The skin over the area tends to become less sensitive; patients, particularly children, use these sites repeatedly to avoid the discomfort of using new injection sites. Insulin absorption may be delayed at these sites,[74] which can lead to problems with glycemic control. The hypertrophy is assumed to be the result of repeated local stimulation of adipocyte hypertrophy by insulin. Lipohypertrophy resolves spontaneously with the use of other insulin injection sites.

## ORTHOSTATIC HYPOTENSION

Normally, insulin stimulates the cardiovascular sympathetic nervous system.[75] In the presence of autonomic neuropathy, however, insulin has a direct vasodilator effect on the vascular bed that can lead to hypotension.[76] These episodes sometimes are manifest as atypical "hypoglycemia," because the patient may experience sweating, tremor, and excitement as a result of the cardiovascular activation of adrenomedullary catecholamines. Neuroglycopenia may be mimicked by the fall in cerebral perfusion from the orthostatic hypotension.[76]

## INSULIN ALLERGY

Shortly after the introduction of insulin treatment in the 1920s, allergic reactions were noted to occur frequently. In retrospect, this is not surprising, because the preparations were impure and contained insulin fragments, insulin multimers, proinsulin, proinsulin intermediates, and whole or fragmented C peptide. In addition, many other peptides were included in the preparations. For example, patients could be found to have circulating antibodies against glucagon, somatostatin, and pancreatic polypeptide.[77] The problem of insulin allergy has been greatly reduced by the purification of animal insulins and by the introduction and widespread use of human insulin.[2,15]

The immunogenicity of insulin has undergone extensive study and is receiving renewed attention because insulin may serve as an important B-cell antigen in the pathogenesis of autoimmune diabetes.[32] A genetic predisposition to insulin allergy has been found, such that insulin antibodies are more likely to develop in persons with the human leukocyte antigen haplotypes B15 and DR4 than in those with the haplotypes B8 and DR3.[78,79] Moreover, the combination of BW44 and DR7 makes a person particularly susceptible to antibody formation. The species of insulin used also makes a difference: beef insulin, which differs from human insulin by three amino-acid residues, is more immunogenic than is pork insulin, which has only one amino-acid difference. Interestingly, human insulin also is immunogenic, with low titers of antibodies developing in most patients. The tertiary structure of human insulin probably is slightly altered in the manufacturing process or in subcutaneous sites, so that new antigenic epitopes can be presented. The immunogenicity of insulin preparations is not limited to insulin itself; both protamine and zinc occasionally can elicit allergic reactions.[80,81]

## INFLUENCE OF INSULIN ANTIBODIES ON INSULIN REQUIREMENTS AND PHARMACOKINETICS

When antibodies develop against a particular species of insulin, such as beef, cross-reactivity is almost always found with other insulins, such as pig and human, even though this reactivity usually is weaker.[2,15] This has important clinical ramifications, because a typical patient treated with beef-pork insulin may have some increase in insulin requirements as a result of insulin binding by antibodies in plasma. These antibodies could be less reactive with human insulin, so that switching to a human preparation might lead to insulin reactions and a need for a reduction in dosage. On the other hand, the difference in reactivity could be minimal and necessitate no meaningful change in dosage. Discontinuing insulin therapy used to be feared because of concern that an amnestic antibody response might occur when therapy was restarted[2]; however, now that highly purified human insulin is so widely used, insulin administration can be discontinued during remissions without worry.

The effect of insulin antibodies on insulin pharmacokinetics may be important but has been difficult to study. The presence of binding IgG antibodies in serum can delay the time needed to reach peak levels of free insulin and also can cause a prolongation of insulin effect.[82,83] This binding theoretically should alter the peak actions of rapid-, intermediate-, and long-acting insulins. The effects on regular or lispro insulin should be adverse, because the desired fast action for meals would be altered. Some prolongation of the peak effects of NPH or Lente insulins potentially could even be beneficial for some patients, except that such an antibody effect could not be expected to be consistent. Measurement of antibody titers is rarely of any clinical help. The experience with the DCCT suggests that good to excellent control can be achieved with similar approaches in most patients with type 1 diabetes, indicating that differences in insulin antibodies usually are not clinically important. Nonetheless, clinicians should be aware of the potential influence of insulin antibodies in certain situations, such as in the commonly encountered patient who has problems with insulin reactions 22 to 24 hours or more after the administration of NPH or Lente insulin.

### IMMUNE INSULIN RESISTANCE

Immune insulin resistance is a rare problem today. When impure insulin was used, such resistance was more common and usually was defined as high titers of antibodies and insulin requirements of >200 U per day.[15,84] The plasma of patients with immune insulin resistance can bind >50 U of insulin per liter, which means that the amount introduced by subcutaneous injections is a small proportion of the total amount of bound insulin. Sometimes

these patients were extremely difficult to treat because they had poor control even when given thousands of units of insulin per day. Such patients have no meaningful peak of whatever insulin they are given and sometimes are best treated with U500 regular insulin administered twice a day. A species switch to human insulin sometimes leads to a reduction in the dosage requirement, and even lispro insulin has helped when antibodies are strongly directed against human insulin.[85] Another strategy has been to give corticosteroids to reduce antibody production. (Some success also has been obtained with sulfated insulin, which is not as well bound by antibodies because epitopes are hidden by the added sulfate groups.[84] However, sulfated insulin is no longer routinely made by any companies.)

## LOCALIZED REACTIONS TO INSULIN

Localized reactions to insulin used to be seen commonly with the initiation of insulin treatment, but with the introduction of purified insulin, they are now rarely significant. Reactions used to be noted in as many as 50% of patients but now are found in <2%.[2,15] They usually occur after 10 days of treatment and within the first few months of therapy. They can subside spontaneously within a few days, but often persist for weeks.

Several types of immune reactions have been defined. *Immediate hypersensitivity reactions* (type I, IgE-mediated reactions) have been the most common. These occur minutes after injection and consist of local swelling, itching, erythema, and even wheal and flare responses, with dissipation usually occurring in a few hours. Less commonly seen are *delayed reactions* (type IV, T-cell mediated). Inflammation can start 8 to 12 hours after the injection, with a peak at 24 to 48 hours. These reactions typically consist of swelling, erythema, and induration. The least commonly seen reaction is the *intermediate reaction* (type III or Arthus reaction caused by immune complexes). These begin 4 to 8 hours after injection and peak at ~12 hours. The reaction consists of induration, itching, and pain. These different reactions can overlap, so that clinical identification of the specific type often is not possible. Because the reactions often are self-limited and cause little discomfort, treatment rarely is needed. Use of oral antihistamines can be helpful for those with reactions having a significant IgE component. Cell-mediated reactions can be eased by injecting a small amount of glucocorticoid along with the insulin (0.1 mg or less of dexamethasone should suffice).

## SYSTEMIC REACTIONS TO INSULIN

Systemic reactions to insulin occur infrequently, particularly now that purified insulins are so widely used.[15] Nonetheless, they are frightening and often difficult to treat. The reactions usually are IgE mediated, with generalized urticaria, pruritus, flushing, and wheezing. Anaphylactic shock with circulatory collapse occurs rarely. These patients have high circulating levels of IgE, which reacts with beef, pork, and human insulin and shows similar cross-reactivity to that seen with IgG. Skin testing usually elicits wheal and flare reactions to all three of these insulins and can be useful to identify the least antigenic insulin. Skin testing is important for confirming that the reactions can be linked with insulin and not some other immunogen. Testing also should be carried out with zinc and protamine, which can cause allergic responses; these can be obtained from Eli Lilly Company. Intradermal skin testing should be initiated with an insulin dose of 0.001 U in a volume of 0.02 mL. If no reaction occurs, 0.1 U should be used, and then 1.0 U should be tried, as a negative reaction to this larger dose makes it unlikely that insulin allergy is responsible. Other systemic reactions that have been attributed to insulin allergy include thrombocytopenic purpura, serum sickness, and Coombs-positive hemolytic anemia. High levels of IgG sometimes are seen in these patients.

TABLE 143-4.
**Insulin Allergy Desensitization Schedule**

| Time (hours) | Dose (U/0.1 mL) |
|---|---|
| 0 | 0.001 id |
| 0.5 | 0.002 id |
| 1 | 0.004 sc |
| 1.5 | 0.01 sc |
| 2 | 0.02 sc |
| 2.5 | 0.04 sc |
| 3 | 0.1 sc |
| 3.5 | 0.2 sc |
| 4 | 0.4 sc |
| 4.5 | 1 sc |
| 5 | 2 sc |
| 5.5 | 4 sc |
| 6 | 8 sc |

*id*, intradermal; *sc*, subcutaneous.
(From Van Haeften TW, Gerich JE. Complications of insulin therapy. In: Becker KL, ed. Principles and practice of endocrinology and metabolism, 1st ed. Philadelphia: Lippincott, 1990:112.)

For severe systemic reactions, the patient should be desensitized in a hospital setting. Desensitization kits can be obtained from the Eli Lilly Company. Human insulin should be used for the process, and the starting dose should be 0.001 U given intradermally. The dose then should be increased at 30-minute intervals, as shown in Table 143-4. If a reaction occurs, the next injection should be dropped back by two dilutions. During the procedure, epinephrine, oxygen, antihistamines, and corticosteroids should be available, and medical personnel should be ready to perform cardiopulmonary resuscitation. Most patients can be desensitized within 10 hours, and the procedure has been found to be successful in 94% of cases in one large series.[15] Pork insulin was used in this series, but human insulin can be expected to do as well. To maintain the desensitization, administering insulin at least twice a day is probably best. The small number of patients who continue to have some allergic manifestations often are treated with antihistamines and, sometimes, corticosteroids.

The mechanism for the desensitization still is not well understood. Perhaps the most attractive explanation is that the continuing administration of antigen keeps mast cells and basophils depleted of mediators such as histamine. Another hypothesis is that antigen stimulates IgG formation, which can block the ability of antigen to reach IgE sites. In addition, for unclear reasons, IgE levels seem to fall during desensitization.

# EXPERIMENTAL FORMS OF INSULIN THERAPY

Experimental approaches to insulin therapy include the use of new insulin analogs, nasal insulin, implantable insulin pumps, "closed-loop" insulin delivery systems, and pancreas and islet transplantation.

Thanks to the power of recombinant DNA technology, the fast-acting analog lispro insulin is now in widespread use.[8,85,85a] Other analogs are being evaluated in clinical trials. Insulin aspart is an analog designed to reduce multimer formation, so that, like lispro insulin, it has a rapid entrance into the circulation.[86] Work is being done to develop insulin preparations with a longer duration of action than NPH and Lente that may have some advantages over Ultralente, which usually will not last a full 24 hours. Glargine is Gly (A31), Arg (B31), Arg (B32) insulin that has a higher isoelectric point than human insulin.[87] Moreover, when mixed with small amounts of zinc, it forms more stable hexamers, which helps to retard its absorption. HOE 901 is injected as a clear solution and has a lag time before reaching a plateau that lasts for >24 hours. Another approach to prolonging the action of insulin is to couple a fatty acid chain to Lys (B29), a modification that prolongs insulin's action because the fatty acid binds to albumin.[88]

Recombinant human insulin-like growth factor-I (IGF-I) combined with insulin has been given by injection on an experimental basis to patients with type 1 diabetes and has resulted in some improvement in control.[89] The long-term influence of IGF-I on the micro- and macrovascular complications of diabetes remains to be determined.

The administration of insulin by the nasal route has been studied by several groups, but problems with nasal irritation and variable absorption have made it problematic.[90] The use of inhaled insulin may be more promising.[91] The absorption of this form of insulin is very rapid and could be very useful when given before meals.

Variable-rate insulin pumps implanted in the abdominal wall with delivery of insulin into the peritoneal space have received considerable attention in the past few years as potential treatment options for patients with both type 1 and type 2 diabetes.[92] Some patients have been treated successfully with these devices for >5 years. Intraperitoneal insulin delivery is attractive because of the theoretic advantages of portal insulin delivery, including the possibility of reducing systemic hyperinsulinemia and better regulating intermediary metabolism. The devices are "open-loop" systems that rely on self-monitoring of the glucose level. A "closed-loop" system, in which a monitor capable of continuous glucose sensing is linked to an intraperitoneal pump, would be a major advance. A large and complex closed-loop artificial pancreas has been available for hospitalized patients for some time, but it is impractical for home use and rarely is used now, even in hospitals. Progress in development of glucose sensors has been slow, but some advances have been made with a noninvasive approach in which absorbance spectra are measured using light spectroscopy in the near infrared range.[93] Another approach has been to use a glucose oxidase–sensing system on the tip of a needle, which could provide a constant readout of subcutaneous glucose levels for a period of several days.

Whole pancreas transplantation is now being offered by many medical centers but is largely restricted to patients who also are receiving kidney transplants with immunosuppression (see Chap. 144). Islet transplantation with human islet allografts is being studied as an experimental procedure in a small number of centers; results are improving but still are not equal to those obtained with whole pancreas transplants (see Chap. 144).

# REFERENCES

1. Rosenzweig JL. Principles of insulin therapy. In: Kahn CR, Weir GC, eds. Joslin's diabetes mellitus, 13th ed. Philadelphia: Lea & Febiger, 1994:460.
2. Schernthaner G. Immunogenicity and allergenic potential of animal and human biosynthetic human insulin. Diabetes Care 1993; 16(Suppl 3):133.
3. Chance RE, Frank BH. Research, development, production, and safety of biosynthetic human insulin. Diabetes Care 1993; 16(Suppl 3):133.
4. Heinemann L, Richter B. Clinical pharmacology of human insulin. Diabetes Care 1993; 16(Suppl 3):90.
5. Berger W, Keller U, Honegger B, Jaeggi E. Warning symptoms of hypoglycemia during treatment with human and porcine insulin in diabetes mellitus. Lancet 1989; 1:1041.
6. Cryer PE. Hypoglycemia unawareness in IDDM. Diabetes Care 1993; 16(Suppl 3):40.
7. Galloway JA, Kooper SA, Spradlin CT, et al. Biosynthetic human proinsulin: review of chemistry, in vitro and in vivo receptor binding, animal and human pharmacology studies, and clinical experience. Diabetes Care 1992; 14:666.
8. Holleman F, Hoekstra JBL. Insulin lispro. N Engl J Med 1997; 337:176.
9. Lalli C, Ciofetta M, Del Sindaco P, et al. Long-term intensive treatment of type 1 diabetes with the short-acting insulin analog lispro in variable combination with NPH insulin at mealtime. Diabetes Care 1999; 22:468.
10. Rassam AG, Zeise TM, Burge MR, et al. Optimal administration of lispro insulin in hyperglycemic type 1 diabetes. Diabetes Care 1999; 22:133.

11. Joseph SE, Korzon-Burakowska A, Woodworth JR, et al. The action profile of lispro is not blunted by mixing in the syringe with NPH insulin. Diabetes Care 1999; 21:2098.

12. Mohn A, Ross KM, Matyka KA, et al. Lispro of regular insulin for multiple injection therapy in adolescence: differences in free insulin and glucose levels overnight. Diabetes Care 1999; 22:27.

13. Brunell RL, Llewelyn J, Anderson Jr JH, et al. Meta-analysis of the effect of insulin lispro on severe hypoglycemia in patients with type 1 diabetes. Diabetes Care 1998; 21:1726.

14. Melki V, Renard E, Lassmann-Vague V, et al. Improvement of HbA$_{1C}$ and blood glucose stability in IDDM patients treated with lispro insulin analog in external pumps. Diabetes Care 1999; 21:977.

15. Galloway JA, de Shazo RD. Insulin chemistry, pharmacology, dosage algorithms and the complications of insulin treatment. In: Rifkin H, Porte D Jr, eds. Ellenberg and Rifkin's diabetes mellitus theory and practice, 4th ed. New York: Elsevier, 1990:497.

16. Ahmed ABE, Home PD. Optimal provision of daytime NPH insulin in patients using the insulin analog lispro. Diabetes Care 1998; 21:1707.

17. Anderson JH, Massey EH. Flocculated humulin N insulin. (Letter). N Engl J Med 1987; 316:1027.

18. Zinman B, Ross S, Campos RV, et al. Effectiveness of human Ultralente versus NPH insulin in providing basal insulin replacement for an insulin lispro multiple daily injection regimen. Diabetes Care 1999; 22:603.

19. Sherwin RS, Kramer KJ, Tobin JD, et al. A model of the kinetics of insulin. J Clin Invest 1974; 53:1481.

20. Stimmler L. Disappearance of immunoreactive insulin in normal and adult onset subjects. Diabetes 1967; 16:652.

21. Navelesi R, Pilo A, Ferrannini E. Kinetic analysis of plasma disappearance in non-ketotic diabetic patients and in normal subjects. J Clin Invest 1978; 61:197.

22. Polonsky KS, Given BD, Hirsch L, et al. Quantitative study of insulin secretion and clearance in normal and obese subjects. J Clin Invest 1988; 81:435.

23. Ferrannini E, Wahren J, Faber OK, et al. Splanchnic and renal metabolism of insulin in human subjects: a dose response study. Am J Physiol 1983; 244:E517.

24. Binder C, Lauritzen T, Faber O, Prammer S. Insulin pharmacokinetics. Diabetes Care 1984; 7:188.

25. Galloway JA, Spradlin CT, Howey DC, Dupre J. Intrasubject differences in pharmacokinetic and pharmacodynamic responses: the immutable problem of present day treatment? In: Serrano-Rio M, Lefebvre PJ, eds. Diabetes 1985, New York: Elsevier, 1986:877.

26. Kurtz AB, Nabarro JDN. Circulating insulin-binding antibodies. Diabetologia 1980; 19:329.

27. Hildebrant P, Birch K, Sestoft O, Nielson ST. Orthostatic changes in subcutaneous blood flow and insulin absorption. Diabetes Res 1985; 2:187.

28. Heine RJ, Bilo HJG, Fonk T, et al. Absorption kinetics and action profiles of mixtures of short- and intermediate-acting insulins. Diabetologia 1984; 27:558.

29. Colagiuri S, Villalobos S. Assessing effect of mixing insulins by glucose-clamp technique in subjects with diabetes mellitus. Diabetes Care 1986; 9:579.

30. Galloway JA, Spradlon T, Jackson RL, et al. Mixtures of intermediate acting insulin: an update. In: Skyler JS, ed. Insulin update: 1982. Amsterdam: Excerpta Medica, 1982:111.

31. Koivisto VA, Tuominen JA, Ebeling P. Lispro Mix25 insulin as premeal therapy in type 2 diabetic patients. Diabetes Care 1999; 22:459.

32. Simone EA, Wegmann DR, Eisenbarth GS. Immunologic "vaccination" for the prevention of autoimmune diabetes (type 1A). Diabetes Care 1999; 22(Suppl 2):B7.

33. Berger M, Jorgens V, Muhihauser I. Rationale for the use of insulin therapy alone as the pharmacological treatment of type 2 diabetes. Diabetes Care 1999; 22(Suppl 3):C71.

34. The Diabetes Control and Complications Trial Research Group. The effects of intensive treatment of diabetes on the development and progression of long-term complications in insulin-dependent diabetes mellitus. N Engl J Med 1993; 329:977.

35. Intensive blood-glucose control with sulfonylureas or insulin compared with conventional treatment and risk of complications in patients with type 2 diabetes (UKPDS 33). United Kingdom Prospective Diabetes Study Group. Lancet 1998; 352:837.

36. Effect of intensive blood-glucose control with metformin on complications in overweight patients with type 2 diabetes (UKPDS 34). United Kingdom Prospective Diabetes Study Group. Lancet 1998; 352:854.

37. Nathan DM. Long-term complications of diabetes mellitus. N Engl J Med 1993; 328:1676.

38. Boyne MS, Saudek CD. Effect of insulin therapy on macrovascular risk factors in type 2 diabetes. Diabetes Care 1999; 22(Suppl 3):C45.

39. American Diabetes Association. Standards of medical care for patients with diabetes mellitus. Diabetes Care 1999; 22(Suppl 1):S32.

40. Bolli GB. How to ameliorate the problem of hypoglycemia in intensive as well as nonintensive treatment of type 1 diabetes. Diabetes Care 1999; 22(Suppl 2):B43.

41. Yki-Jarvinen H, Kauppila M, Kujansuu E, et al. Comparison of insulin regimens in patients with NIDDM. N Engl J Med 1992; 327:1426.

42. Yki-Jarvinen H, Ryysy L, Nikkila K, et al. Comparison of bedtime insulin regimens in patients with type 2 diabetes mellitus: a randomized trial. Ann Intern Med 1999; 130:389.

43. Buse JB. Overview of current therapeutic options in type 2 diabetes. Diabetes Care 1999; 22:C65.

44. Bode BW, Steed RD, Davidson PC. Reduction in severe hypoglycemia with long-term continuous subcutaneous insulin infusion in type 1 diabetes. Diabetes Care 1996; 19:324.

45. Gillespie SA, Kulkarni KD, Daly AE. Using carbohydrate counting in diabetes clinical practice. J Am Diet Assoc 1998; 98:897.

46. Farkas-Hirsch R, Hirsch IB. Continuous subcutaneous insulin infusion: a review of the past and its implementation for the future. Diabetes Spectrum 1994; 7:80.

47. Zinman B, Tildesley H, Chaisson JL, et al. Insulin lispro in CSII: results of a double-blind crossover study. Diabetes 1997; 46:440.

48. Gill GV, Walford S, Alberti KGMM. Brittle diabetes. Present concepts. Diabetologia 1985; 28:579.

49. Paulsen EP, Courtney GW, Duckworth WC. Insulin resistance caused by massive degradation of subcutaneous insulin. Diabetes 1979; 28:640.

50. Home PD, Massi-Benedetti M, Gill GV, et al. Impaired subcutaneous absorption of insulin in "brittle" diabetes. Acta Endocrinol (Copenh) 1982; 101:414.

51. Wolfsdorf JI, Anderson BJ, Pasquarello C. Treatment of the child with diabetes. In: Kahn CR, Weir GC, eds. Joslin's diabetes mellitus, 13th ed. Philadelphia: Lea & Febiger, 1994:530.

52. Tattersall RB, Lowe J. Diabetes and adolescence. Diabetologia 1981; 20:517.

53. Kitzmiller JL. Sweet success with diabetes: the development of insulin therapy and glycemic control for pregnancy. Diabetes Care 1993; 16(Suppl 3):107.

54. Hadden DR. How to improve prognosis in type 1 diabetic pregnancy: old problems, new concepts. Diabetes Care 1999; 22(Suppl 2):B104.

55. Agner T, Damni P, Binder C. Remission in IDDM: prospective study of basal C-peptide and insulin dose in 265 consecutive patients. Diabetes Care 1987; 10:164.

56. Perlman K, Erlich RM, Filler RM, Albisser AM. Sustained normoglycemia in newly diagnosed type I diabetic subjects: short term effects and one year followup. Diabetes 1984; 33:995.

57. Rabkin R, Simon NM, Steiner S, Colwell JA. Effect of renal disease on renal uptake and excretion of insulin in man. N Engl J Med 1970; 282:182.

58. Rabkin R, Ryan MP, Duckworth WC. The renal metabolism of insulin. Diabetologia 1984; 27:35.

59. Amair P, Khanna R, Leibel B, et al. Continuous ambulatory dialysis in diabetics with end-stage renal disease. N Engl J Med 1982; 306:625.

59a. Fritsche A, Stumvoll M, Häring HU, Gerich JE. Reversal of hypoglycemia unawareness in a long-term type 1 diabetic patient by improvement of β-adrenergic sensitivity after prevention of hypoglycemia. J Clin Endocrinol Metab 2000; 85:523.

60. Korytkowski MT, Mokan M, Veneman TF, et al. Reduced β-adrenergic sensitivity in patients with type 1 diabetes and hypoglycemia unawareness. Diabetes Care 1998; 21:1939.

61. Meyer C, Grosmann R, Mitrakou A, et al. Effects of autonomic neuropathy on counterregulation and awareness of hypoglycemia in type 1 diabetic patients. Diabetes Care 1998; 21:1960.

62. Somogyi M. Insulin as a cause of extreme hyperglycemia and instability. Bull St Louis Med Soc 1938; 32:498.

63. Gerich JE, Campbell PJ. Overview of counterregulation and its abnormalities in diabetes mellitus and other conditions. Diabetes Metab Rev 1988; 4:93.

64. Clutter WE, Rizza RA, Gerich JE, Cryer PE. Regulation of glucose metabolism by sympathochromaffin catecholamines. Diabetes Metab Rev 1988; 4:1.

65. Lerman IG, Wolfsdorf JI. Relationship of nocturnal hypoglycemia to daytime glycemia in IDDM. Diabetes Care 1988; 11:636.

66. Hirsch IB, Smith LJ, Havlin CE, et al. Failure of nocturnal hypoglycemia to cause daytime hyperglycemia in patients with IDDM. Diabetes Care 1990; 13:133.

67. Gerich JE. Glucose counterregulation and its impact on diabetes mellitus. Diabetes 1988; 37:1608.

68. Bolli G, Fanelli CG, Perrielbo G, De Feo P. Nocturnal blood glucose control in type 1 diabetes mellitus. Diabetes Care 1993; 16(Suppl 3):71.

69. Campbell P, Bolli G, Cryer P, Gerich J. Pathogenesis of the dawn phenomenon in patients with insulin-dependent diabetes mellitus. N Engl J Med 1985; 312:1473.

70. Evans DJ, Pritchard-Jones K, Trotman-Dickenson B. Insulin oedema. Postgrad Med J 1986; 62:665.

71. O'Hare JA, Ferriss JB, Twomey B, O'Sullivan DJ. Poor metabolic control, hypertension and microangiopathy independently increase the transcapillary escape rate of albumin in diabetes. Diabetologia 1983; 25:260.

72. Wheatly T, Edwards OM. Insulin edema and its clinical significance: metabolic studies in three cases. Diabet Med 1985; 2:400.

73. Reeves W, Allen B, Tattersell R. Insulin-induced lipoatrophy: evidence for an immune pathogenesis. Br Med J 1980; 280:1500.

74. Young RJ, Hannan W, Frier B, et al. Diabetic lipohypertrophy delays insulin absorption. Diabetes Care 1984; 7:479.

75. Rowe JW, Young JB, Minaker KM, et al. Effect of insulin and glucose infusions on sympathetic nervous system activity in normal man. Diabetes 1981; 30:219.

76. Page MM, Watkins PJ. Provocation of postural hypotension by insulin in diabetic autonomic neuropathy. Diabetes 1976; 25:90.

77. Chance R, Root M, Galloway J. The immunogenicity of insulin preparations. Acta Endocrinol (Copenh) 1976; 83(Suppl 205):185.

78. Kahn C, Mann D, Rosenthal A, et al. The immune response to insulin in man: interaction of HLA alloantigens and the development of the immune response. Diabetes 1982; 31:716.

79. Kahn C, Rosenthal A. Immunologic reactions to insulin: insulin allergy, insulin resistance and the autoimmune insulin syndrome. Diabetes Care 1979; 2:283.

80. Stewart W, McSweeney S, Kellett M, et al. Increased risk of severe protamine reactions in NPH-insulin-dependent diabetics undergoing cardiac catheterization. Circulation 1984; 70:788.

81. Feinglos M, Jegasothy B. "Insulin" allergy due to zinc. Lancet 1979; 1:122.
82. Waldhäusl W, Bratusch-Marrain P, Kruse V, et al. Effect of insulin antibodies on insulin pharmacokinetics and glucose utilization in insulin-dependent diabetic patients. Diabetes 1985; 34:166.
83. Van Haeften T, Bolli G, Dimitriadis G, et al. Effect of insulin antibodies and their kinetic characteristics on plasma free insulin dynamics in patients with diabetes mellitus. Metabolism 1986; 35:1649.
84. Davidson J, DeBra D. Immunologic insulin resistance. Diabetes 1978; 27:307.
85. Uahtela JT, Antonen J, Knip M, et al. Severe insulin-mediated human insulin resistance: successful treatment with the insulin analog lispro. Diabetes Care 1997; 20:71.
85a. Gale EA. A randomized, controlled trial comparing insulin lispro with human soluble insulin in patients with Type 1 diabetes on intensified insulin therapy. The UK trial group. Diabet Med 2000; 17:209.
86. Home PD, Lindholm A, Hylleberg B, et al. Improved glycemic control with insulin aspart. Diabetes Care 1999; 21:1904.
87. Gillies PS, Figgitt DP, Lamb HM. Insulin glargine. Drugs 2000; 59:253.
88. Markussen J, Havelund S, Kurtzhals P, et al. Soluble fatty acid acylated insulins bind to albumin and show protracted action in pigs. Diabetologia 1996; 39:281.
89. Thrailkill KM, Quattrin T, Baker U, et al. Cotherapy with recombinant human insulin-like growth factor I and insulin improves glycemic control in type 1 diabetes. Diabetes Care 1999; 22:585.
90. Salzman R, Manson JE, Griffing GT, et al. Intranasal aerosolized insulin: mixed meal studies and long-term use in type I diabetes. N Engl J Med 1985; 312:1078.
91. Gelfand R, Sherwyn L, Schwartz L, et al. Pharmacological reproducibility of inhaled human insulin pre-meal dosing in patients with type 2 diabetes. Diabetes 1998; 47(Suppl 1):A99.
92. Saudek CD. Future developments in insulin delivery systems. Diabetes Care 1993; 16(Suppl 3):122.
93. Gough DA, Armour JC, Baker DA. Advances and prospects in glucose assay technology. Diabetologia 1997; 40(Suppl 2):102.

# CHAPTER 144

# PANCREAS AND ISLET TRANSPLANTATION

GORDON C. WEIR

Although insulin was discovered many years ago, the complications of diabetes still produce devastating consequences. The link between high blood-glucose levels and the complications of retinopathy, nephropathy, and neuropathy is now established beyond doubt.[1] Although we know more than ever about insulin therapy, largely thanks to self blood-glucose monitoring, only a small proportion of people with type 1 diabetes obtain good enough glycemic control to avoid complications (see Chaps. 136, 138, and 143). And even for those, the cost in terms of lifestyle change and monetary expense is substantial. Type 2 diabetes, being greater than ten times more common than type 1 diabetes, causes even more problems in terms of health outcomes, economic cost, and personal tragedy; yet this, too, has proved difficult to control (see Chaps. 137 and 139).

Although solutions to the problem of diabetes could come from various unknown sources, an obvious path is some form of B-cell replacement therapy. This is an accepted goal for type 1 diabetes, but even type 2 diabetes could be greatly helped by such a therapy. Major contributing factors to the development of type 2 diabetes are the Western way of life, with its obesity and sedentary lifestyle, and strong genetic factors that work together to cause insulin resistance (see Chaps. 141, 145, and 146). Diabetes only develops when the pancreatic B cells (beta cells) can no longer compensate. Relative B-cell failure is a critical factor that could be remedied by B-cell replacement therapy. There are two potential routes for B-cell replacement, one being some form of B-cell transplantation in the form of a pancreas transplant or as insulin-producing cells; the other is a mechanical B cell, a path that continues to be elusive.

## PANCREAS TRANSPLANTATION

The first pancreas transplants were performed in the 1960s, but the procedure was not widely applied until the mid-1980s.[2–5] Since 1978, >9000 pancreas transplants have been performed, and currently >1000 are done yearly, ~70% of these in the United States. The most common transplants are simultaneous kidney/pancreas (SKP) transplants, given to type 1 diabetic patients with advanced nephropathy who need a kidney transplant. Much less common are pancreas transplants done after a kidney allograft (pancreas after kidney; PAK), which usually require more immunosuppression, and even fewer receive a pancreas transplant alone (PTA), although a single center has reported 225 cases of PTA.[6] In making decisions, patients with failing kidneys are often urged to accept a kidney from a living related or unrelated donor because of the benefits obtained from receiving a kidney alone, rather than waiting for an SKP from a cadaver donor. Some patients are judged to have so much trouble with their diabetes (with problems such as hypoglycemia unawareness) that a PTA is recommended. Some centers have experience with living related donors who provide the distal portion of their pancreases, but there continues to be uncertainty about the overall benefit of this approach, because the donors can experience dangerous surgical complications and often have glucose intolerance after the procedure, with some developing diabetes.[7]

The best results are obtained when a kidney and pancreas are transplanted simultaneously (SKP), with experienced centers finding that ~85% of the pancreases maintain perfect control 1 year after the transplant, and ~50% of the transplants are still working well after 5 years. Fewer good results are reported for PAK and PTA, but with more aggressive immunosuppression better results are being obtained.

Although the first experimental transplants used enteric drainage, for a period of ~10 years the favored approach was to place the pancreas with the duodenum attached in the right lower pelvis, with pancreatic juices draining through the duodenum into the anastomosed bladder. Because many patients have had problems with acidosis, dehydration, and a variety of bladder problems, many centers have now switched back to enteric drainage.[8] The most commonly used immunosuppression in the past has been triple therapy with cyclosporine, azathioprine, and prednisone, but now many centers are switching to tacrolimus (FK-506) and mycophenolate mofetil, and continuing with prednisone.[9] Antibodies against thymocytes and the interleukin-2 (IL-2) receptor are also used. In general, higher doses of immunosuppression are used for pancreas transplants than for kidney transplants alone, which is worrisome because of the increased incidence of infection and malignancy. The immunosuppression is required, not only for allograft rejection but also for autoimmunity. An interesting set of pancreas/kidney transplants was performed between identical twins, who were not given immunosuppressive medication. As expected there was no rejection of the exocrine pancreas or liver, but diabetes recurred with immune destruction of the islet demonstrated by biopsy, no doubt mediated by the autoimmunity that caused the diabetes in the first place.[10] The extra surgery of a pancreas transplant is accompanied by considerable morbidity. Patients often have long hospitalizations and readmissions for such problems as intraabdominal infection and vascular thrombosis. There is even a report showing a modest increase in mortality, which is not surprising considering the major surgery being performed in patients with advanced diabetic complications.[11]

Successful pancreas transplants render recipients normoglycemic and insulin-independent, such that they have normal glucose levels around the clock, normal glycohemoglobin levels, and no dietary restrictions.[11a] This occurs even though patients may be taking medications such as cyclosporine or tacrolimus that can inhibit insulin secretion,[12] and glucocorticoids with their separate diabetogenic effects. Questions have been raised about whether there is more reactive hypoglycemia than in normal subjects, but such episodes are uncommon and rarely significant.

Debate continues about how much benefit is provided from pancreas transplants. Most of the recipients already have established complications, so it is not surprising that improvement of these has been modest at best. Various studies have found that there may be some stabilization of retinopathy and improvement in nerve conduction velocity, but these small changes seem to have little clinical impact. Protection of the transplanted kidney from the characteristic histologic lesions of diabetic nephropathy has been demonstrated. It was reported that when the kidneys of patients with PTA were biopsied 5 years after the pancreas transplant, no benefit was seen, but after a biopsy at 10 years there was impressive reversion of histology toward normal.[13] A provocative study suggests that patients with autonomic neuropathy before a pancreas transplant have better survival 7 years later than those with failed grafts[14]; although encouraging, this finding needs to be confirmed. The most obvious benefit of pancreas transplants is that patients believe that their quality of life is improved, particularly with freedom from insulin injections, hypoglycemic episodes, and food restrictions. However, quality of life has proved to be a very difficult parameter to evaluate.[2,15] Indeed, it has been difficult to show that patients' lives are truly improved using such standard parameters as whether they are more active or have better performance at work. The most striking finding is that patients are very happy to be free of their diabetes, but it is difficult to know what value to place on this psychological benefit.

With pancreas transplantation providing benefits that are counterbalanced by substantial risk and cost, active debate continues about overall value and about how to handle the financial burdens, which are typically more than $100,000 per patient.[15] Although there has been a call for controlled clinical trials to answer some of these questions, it will be difficult to organize such large trials; thus, research will probably be restricted to small studies. In the meantime, patients will continue to want pancreas transplants in spite of the risks. The psychological desire for such transplants will continue to be strong, and some patients will benefit from being relieved of the devastating impact of hypoglycemia unawareness. Important questions are being asked about the potential benefits of pancreas transplants alone for patients with early proteinuria, which still has a poor prognosis. Pancreas transplants usually provide truly normal glucose levels, which is considerably better than the control achieved by the Diabetes Control and Complications Trial (DCCT), which had strong protective effects on diabetic complications.[1] Until islet transplantation becomes successful and accessible, the potential benefits of pancreas transplantation will continue to be explored.

# ISLET TRANSPLANTATION

There was great excitement in the early 1970s when the first successful islet transplants were performed in rodents, because many expected that successful routine transplants for patients were only a few years away. Sadly, more than 25 years later, only a very small number of patients have received any benefit from B-cell replacement therapy. Because of the high expectations, the issue has been emotionally charged, but, in spite of many missteps, substantial progress has been made. Moreover, there are different potential approaches that are emerging, some of which should lead to progress and eventual success. There are many political as well as strategic issues about how to approach the problem, which have been discussed elsewhere.[16]

## HUMAN ISLET ALLOGRAFTS

After much work with small and large animal models, it finally became possible in the late 1980s to start human islet allografts in immunosuppressed patients with kidney transplants.[17–22] Some of these early transplants used islets obtained from as many as five donor pancreases, with most being cryopreserved and some being fresh. These islets are injected into the portal vein, whereupon they wedge in the hepatic sinusoids and engraft, receiving their vascular supply from host vessels growing into the islets. Islet allografts have few complications because islets can be delivered to the liver via the portal vein, either with a relatively simple transhepatic angiographic procedure or a more direct approach to the portal vein with dissection along the umbilical vein. Portal hypertension has only rarely been a problem. In spite of the excitement of a few early successes with some recipients who were insulin-free for more than 2 years, the initial results were disappointing. Data from the International Islet Transplantation Registry show that by the end of 1995, of 270 islet allografts, only 27 (10%) of the recipients remained insulin-free for more than a week.[23] Some recipients even lost circulating C-peptide levels within a few days, a phenomenon called *primary nonfunction*, which may be secondary to rapid autoimmune destruction.

The reasons for this apparent lack of success are not yet understood, but closer examination of the data indicates that many of the recipients who remained hyperglycemic have benefited from partial graft function, which has led to lower insulin requirements, smoother control, excellent glycohemoglobin levels, and often many fewer problems with hypoglycemia.[24] Nonetheless, the lack of success is striking when compared to pancreas transplantation, with which there is often 85% graft function with insulin independence at 1 year. This suggests that the islets contained in one pancreas are sufficient, and that both transplant rejection and autoimmunity can be controlled by conventional immunosuppression. Somehow, the islets contained in their normal home in the pancreas must be less vulnerable to immune injury. It is also possible that the ability of the pancreas to generate new islets from ducts may be helpful. Over the past few years, a more rigorous approach to islet allografts seems to have led to better results in some centers.[25] Some of this improvement is likely due to meticulous attention to detail. For example, the pancreas should have cold-ischemia-time of <8 hours before islet isolation; usually > 6000 islet equivalents per kilogram should be given, and every effort should be made to maintain euglycemia with insulin therapy in the early posttransplant period.[25a] There is some evidence that the use of antithymocyte globulin is beneficial. Because of these encouraging results and the development of some attractive new approaches to immunosuppression, an increasing number of human allografts are expected to be performed in the next few years.

## ALLOGRAFTS IN THE ABSENCE OF AUTOIMMUNITY

Cluster operations for abdominal cancer have been performed in which liver, pancreas, and other organs are removed; then a liver from a cadaver donor is transplanted with islets isolated from the pancreas of the same donor injected into the portal vein.[23] These transplants more often produced normoglycemia than allograft islets given to patients with type 1 diabetes, with patients becoming insulin-independent 60% of the time, and one patient being off insulin for 5 years. Although transplantation of the liver may have had some beneficial modulating influence on the immune system, the absence of autoimmunity is suspected to be the major reason for the success.

## AUTOGRAFTS

People with painful pancreatitis sometimes undergo pancreatectomy with resultant insulin-dependent diabetes. There has been

**TABLE 144-1.**
**Potential Sources of Insulin-Producing Cells for Islet Transplantation**

**HUMAN SOURCES**
    Live donors (probably not an option)
    Cadaver pancreases
    Fetal pancreases
    Expansion of human B cells in vitro or in vivo
    New islet development from precursor duct cells in vitro or in vivo
    Cell lines
**XENOGRAFT SOURCES**
    Pigs, cows, rodents, rabbits, fish, other
    Cell lines
    Transgenic pigs (or other species)

some experience in isolating islets from these pancreases and injecting them back into the portal vein. These patients do remarkably well, with ~75% being insulin independent at 1 year.[23] Sometimes, even <200,000 islets can be successful, which is considerably less than what is usually required for successful allografts.[26,27] The most obvious explanation for success is that there are no problems with either allorejection or autoimmunity, but it must also be remembered that the removal of glucagon by the pancreatectomy and the tendency of these patients to be thin could make them relatively insulin sensitive.

## THE TWO MAJOR BARRIERS TO SUCCESSFUL ISLET TRANSPLANTATION

In the simplest possible terms, the problems facing B-cell replacement are, first, how to find a satisfactory source of insulin-producing cells, and, second, how to prevent these cells from being destroyed by the immune system, through the processes of transplant rejection and autoimmunity.

## WHAT SOURCES OF INSULIN-PRODUCING TISSUE ARE AVAILABLE?

Although living donors have sometimes given a segment of their pancreas to a diabetic recipient, human insulin-producing cells almost always come from cadaver donors. The supply of human pancreatic tissue is woefully inadequate. In the United States, it would be a major challenge to obtain 3000 usable cadaver pancreases per year, yet the incidence of type 1 diabetes is ~30,000 cases per year,[28] and more than ten times as many people develop type 2 diabetes. Some encouraging results have come from using islets from a single cadaver pancreas for a recipient, but many patients are likely to need more than one donor pancreas, particularly if the recipient has a high insulin requirement. There has been much discussion about the possibility of using human fetal tissue, but in spite of some important advances this is proving to be a difficult road.[29,30] Presently, we do not know how to exploit the growth potential of fetal pancreases, and in addition, many ethical and practical issues cloud the future of this approach.

## XENOTRANSPLANTATION

With the limitation of human tissue, many are exploring the possibility of using tissue from other species as xenotransplants (Table 144-1). A variety of potential species have been proposed—including pigs, cows, rabbits, rodents, and even fish. Pigs have had particular appeal, in part because human and pig insulin are almost identical, as well as the similarity between porcine and human blood-glucose levels. Because pigs are part of the food chain, people tend to be comfortable with the prospect of using this source. It is not easy to work with pig islet tissue. It continues to be difficult to generate high-quality islets

from adult pigs.[31,32] Much work is now being done to develop ways to use either fetal or neonatal islet tissue, both of which are attractive sources because of their growth potential.[33–35] One of the problems with this tissue is that the cells are immature, which means they are less efficient in normalizing glucose levels rapidly in recipients. Another potential problem is that porcine tissue contains retroviruses that can be transferred to human cells in tissue culture.[36] There is considerable uncertainty about whether this represents a health threat, but in the United States, transplants using porcine tissue for the treatment of neurologic disease have been allowed to proceed cautiously.

## EFFORTS TO EXPAND B CELLS AND TO CREATE INSULIN-PRODUCING CELLS WITH GENETIC ENGINEERING

Although B cells have the capacity for some replication, and new B cells can develop from precursor pancreatic duct cells even in adults, it has not been possible to expand B cells in a meaningful way in the laboratory. A great deal of work is now being done to better understand the mechanisms of B-cell growth and development in the hope that with some fairly simple maneuver, B-cell populations can be expanded. Efforts are also under way to create B-cell lines that might be useful for transplantation.[37,38] It has been possible to transform rodent insulin-producing cells that have some potential for transplantation, but it has proved to be difficult to create a comparable human cell line. Thanks to dramatic advances in molecular and cell biology, it is now feasible to manipulate the differentiation of cells through genetic engineering; therefore, they might be useful for transplantation. For example, the insulin gene can be expressed in cells that normally do not make insulin, with the result that these cells not only can make insulin, but also can store and secrete it in response to a variety of stimuli. By adding additional genes that influence glucose metabolism, it is even possible to manipulate these cells so they secrete insulin when exposed to glucose.[39,40] In spite of these encouraging preliminary results, it is becoming clear that normal B cells are remarkably complicated, which means it may be difficult to create near normal B cells by altering a few genes. On the other hand, as more is learned about the master switches that control the differentiation of cells, more promising approaches may emerge.

## IMMUNE ATTACK ON TRANSPLANTED ISLETS

Islets given to recipients with type 1 diabetes are faced with two types of immune assault, transplant rejection and autoimmunity (Table 144-2). The first is a rejection process that, in the case of transplanted human islets, is called *allograft rejection*. This is a complicated process that is dependent on T cells. When tissues from other species are used, the process is called *xenograft rejection* and is even more complex.[41,42] There is an early attack called *hyperacute rejection* that is mediated by antibodies and complement and can occur within minutes. These preformed, largely immunoglobulin M (IgM) antibodies recognize a glycoprotein called the Gal-alpha(1,3)Gal epitope (Gal epitope), which is heavily expressed on the surface of endothelial cells. There are, however, some indications that adult pig islet cells do not have this Gal epitope; therefore, these cellular transplants, in contrast to organs, may not face this destructive mechanism. With time, xenografted tissue is also subjected to T-cell–mediated damage, which seems to be similar to allorejection, and to other insults such as infiltration with eosinophils.[41,43]

Type 1 diabetes is caused by autoimmunity, a process whereby an individual's own lymphocytes destroy B cells. Even though patients may have lost most of their B cells decades before a transplant, the process of autoimmunity can still be activated. It is not surprising that such a process would attack human allografted islets, but there is even some evidence

**TABLE 144-2.**
**Immunologic Challenges to Transplanted Islets**

**ALLOREJECTION**
 T cells, macrophages, natural killer cells
**AUTOIMMUNITY**
 Acute: primary nonfunction
 Chronic: T cell–dependent
**XENOREJECTION**
 Hyperacute rejection: preformed antibody and complement
 Acute rejection: activation of endothelial cells
 Semiacute rejection: T cells, macrophages, natural killer cells, eosinophils

**TABLE 144-3.**
**Approaches to Tolerance Induction**

**GRAFT-BASED TOLERANCE INDUCTION**
 Major histocompatibility complex (*MHC*) knock-outs (class I or II MHC antigens)
 Remove donor APCs (passenger lymphocytes)
 Masking of class I MHC antigens by antibodies
 Privileged sites (brain, testes, thymus, anterior chamber, other)
 Gene transfer to islets (CTLA4Ig, interleukin-4, transforming growth factor-β, etc.)
**HOST RESPONSE-BASED TOLERANCE INDUCTION**
 Central tolerance
  Clonal deletion: thymic injection of antigen
  Clonal inactivation: thymic irradiation
 Peripheral tolerance
  Anergy
  Immune deviation: from $T_H1$ to $T_H2$
  Inhibition of costimulation (CTLA4Ig, anti-CD40 ligand)
  Peptide-based therapy (parenteral or oral for autoimmunity)
  Immunosuppression
  Donor-specific transfusion (*DST*)
  Peripheral cell suppression (CD4 subsets)
  Clonal deletion of peripheral T cells
  Chimerism

(Adapted from Rossini AA, Greiner DL, Mordes JP. Induction of immunologic tolerance for transplantation. Physiol Rev 1999; 79:99.)

that xenografted islets might be susceptible to autoimmunity (see also Chap. 136).

## THERAPEUTIC APPROACHES OF REJECTION AND AUTOIMMUNITY

Current organ transplants are successful because of immunosuppression, which, although more effective than ever, continues to be associated with notable toxicity, with the main threats being reduced capacity to combat infection and the development of neoplasia.[44] Clearly, there is great reluctance to use such toxic drugs on people with type 1 diabetes who might otherwise have a good prognosis. Tremendous progress is being made in the field of immunology, which is already leading to the development of safer and more effective immunosuppressive drugs. With successful pancreas transplants and islet allografts, the immunosuppressive regimens are able to control both the rejection process and autoimmunity. However, as more is learned about the differences between rejection and autoimmunity, different approaches can be expected to be used for each process. Different drugs might be used for xenograft rejection, that work through separate mechanisms. One of the most promising new approaches is to block costimulation by using antibodies against CD40 ligand on T cells, inhibiting their activation by antigen-presenting cells. This new agent has produced excellent results in monkey islet allograft experiments, with normalization of glucose levels and seemingly minimal toxicity.[22] Immunologists are also learning more about immunoprivileged sites such as the testes, brain, thymus, and anterior chamber of the eye, which may provide insights into new strategies.[45]

One of the dreams of transplantation is *to induce tolerance*, which means that treatment given only at the time of transplantation will somehow trick recipients into accepting transplanted foreign tissue as their own (Table 144-3). Tolerance to transplanted tissue has been induced in a number of experimental models by a variety of techniques,[46] but many scientific and safety hurdles must be overcome before such approaches can be used in humans. A separate major challenge in diabetes research is to control the process of autoimmunity, which not only will provide a way to prevent type 1 diabetes but also should be very helpful for islet transplantation, whether by allografts or xenografts.

## IMMUNOBARRIER TECHNOLOGY

One attractive approach is to use an immunobarrier to prevent destructive lymphocytes from killing transplanted islet tissue[47,48] (Fig. 144-1). For this purpose, a semipermeable membrane is used, with the holes being large enough for glucose, oxygen, and nutrients to reach islets contained inside the membrane and for insulin to be released through the membrane to enter the bloodstream. On the other hand, the holes are small enough so that lymphocytes cannot penetrate the membrane and reach the islet cells. The reason why there is so much hope

about the immunobarriers is that, if they were to succeed, it might be possible to avoid the use of immunosuppressive medication altogether. The two major approaches are *macroencapsulation* and *microencapsulation*. Macroencapsulation uses devices such as hollow fibers or flat sheets sealed at the edges, in which many islets are contained within a single device.[49] One of the

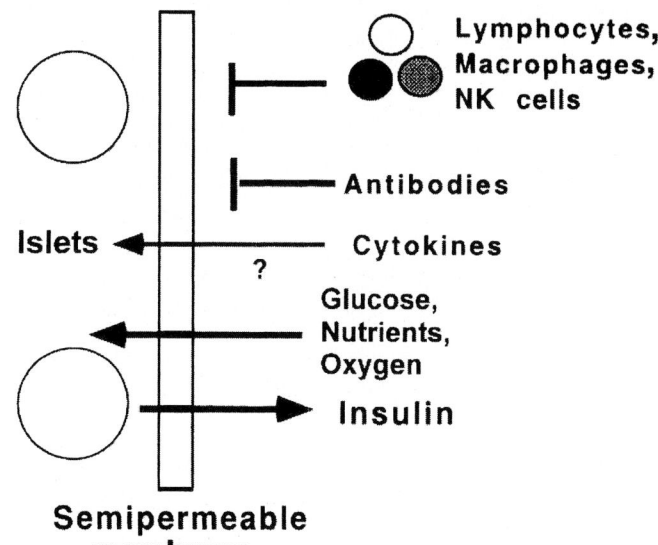

**FIGURE 144-1.** Principle of immunobarrier protection. Islets are protected from immune destruction by a semipermeable membrane, which contains islets in the configuration of microencapsulation, most commonly small beads of alginate covered by polylysine, or macroencapsulation in the form of hollow tubes or planar sheets. The membrane will prevent penetration by cells and limit the entrance of antibodies. A typical exclusion limit might be 60 kDa, so that cytokines may enter, but whether the concentrations would be high enough to cause damage is unclear. The membrane must be permeable enough to allow passage of glucose, nutrients, and oxygen to the islets, and to allow insulin to diffuse out into small vessels. (*NK*, natural killer.)

major advantages of such an approach is that the devices could be implanted in a variety of locations and yet still be retrievable or reloadable. At present it has been difficult to achieve a practical packing density, which means that too much surface area is required to support the contained islet tissue. Moreover, there are still some questions about whether insulin will be released quickly enough to control blood-glucose levels adequately. There are a variety of tissue-engineering approaches that might be able to improve the potential of macrodevices.

Microencapsulation is an approach in which either single or a small number of islets are contained within a membrane. The most commonly used method uses alginate obtained from seaweed that can form a gel after exposure to calcium or barium in solution.[50–54a] Thus, islets can be captured in a small gel bead <1 mm in diameter that can be coated with a material such as polylysine, which interacts with the alginate to create an immune barrier. Another promising approach is to use a polyethylene glycol coating.[55] For a human transplant, more than 300,000 islets will probably need to be encapsulated and placed into the peritoneal cavity. An intermediate approach that is gaining some attention is to use a macrobead or slab, whereby a material such as alginate or a mixture of agarose and collagen is used to enclose many islets. Although a variety of apparently successful experiments have been performed in both large and small animal models, the feasibility and reproducibility of this approach has not yet been established.

## GENE-TRANSFER TECHNOLOGY TO PROTECT ISLETS

An increasing number of ways are being found to transfer genes into cells.[56,57] This means that the transferred genes can be expressed so as to make proteins not normally made by the cells, or to make more of a given protein than normal. The genes are introduced into cells with vectors that might be either viral or lipid carriers, or electroporation. The goal is to transfer genes so that they are permanently expressed in all of the insulin-producing cells of an islet. Adenoviral vectors are now available that can transfer genes into islets on a temporary basis, thus allowing investigators to start to learn which genes might be helpful in protecting transplanted islets. The new vectors that seem to hold the most promise for efficient gene transfer are lentiviruses, adenoassociated viruses, and synthetic lipid carriers. In addition, it may be possible to introduce genes into porcine B cells by using an insulin promoter construct to make transgenic pigs.

There are many ways in which islets might be protected from either transplant rejection or autoimmune attack. For example, some of the proteins on the outside of a cell, such as class I major histocompatibility complex (MHC) antigens, might be deleted or changed, so that the B cells appear to be different and escape recognition by the immune system. Another approach is to introduce proteins that might be secreted by the cells and serve as missiles to disable invading lymphocytes. It has already been shown that islets engineered to secrete the small protein CTLA4Ig are more resistant to transplant rejection. There are a number of cytokines, such as IL-4, IL-10, or transforming growth factor-β (TGF-β), which might exert different kinds of inhibitory influences on attacking lymphocytes. Still another way to improve survival might be to bolster the B cells' internal defense mechanisms. Cells have proteins that protect them against oxidant injury and a process called *apoptosis*, which is a pathway of cell death. Thus, one could introduce a gene to make B cells overexpress catalase or superoxide dismutase, which are enzymes that protect against oxidant injury. Alternatively, one could add either A20 or Bcl2, which are antiapoptotic genes. Still other genes could provide protection against injury from a combined attack by antibody and complement, a phenomenon that occurs in the early stages of xenograft rejection.

## PREDICTING THE FUTURE

For the field of islet transplantation, predicting the future has proved hazardous. Many unexpected obstacles have emerged in the past; considering the difficulty of the task, one should not predict anything different for the future. It seems likely that success will occur in small increments. The results obtained with human allografts should continue to improve as new methods for immunosuppression and the induction of tolerance emerge, with the result that more people without kidney transplants should be able to receive islets. Although many questions remain about using porcine islets as xenografts, it seems probable that they will be used increasingly. When first tried, it may be necessary to use some immunobarrier mechanism combined with immunosuppressive drugs and even some modification of the porcine islet cells with gene transfer methodology. Perhaps someone will achieve a breakthrough in the expansion of human B cells that would solve the supply problem for transplantable insulin-producing cells. Considerable effort is being expended on creating new B cells with genetic engineering or making an insulin-producing cell line that could be used for transplantation. These, too, are very difficult challenges that should eventually be overcome.

## REFERENCES

1. The Diabetes Control and Complications Trial Research Group. The effect of intensive treatment of diabetes on the development and progression of long-term complications in insulin-dependent diabetes mellitus. N Engl J Med 1993; 329:977.
2. Holohan TV. Simultaneous pancreas-kidney and sequential pancreas-after-kidney transplantation. Health Technol Assess Rep 1995; 4:1.
3. Stratta RJ, Weide LG, Sindhi R, et al. Solitary pancreas transplantation. Diabetes Care 1997; 20:362.
4. Sutherland DE. Pancreas and pancreas-kidney transplantation. Curr Opin Nephrol Hypertens 1998; 7:317.
5. Sollinger HW, Odorico JS, Knechtle SJ, et al. Experience with 500 simultaneous pancreas-kidney transplants. Ann Surg 1998; 228:284.
6. Gruessner RW, Sutherland DE, Najarian JS, et al. Solitary pancreas transplantation for nonuremic patients with labile insulin-dependent diabetes mellitus. Transplantation 1997; 64:1572.
7. Kendall DM, Sutherland DER, Najarian JS, et al. Effects of hemipancreatectomy on insulin secretion and glucose tolerance in healthy humans. N Engl J Med 1990; 322:898.
8. Bloom RD, Olivares M, Rehman L, et al. Long-term pancreas allograft outcome in simultaneous pancreas-kidney transplantation: a comparison of enteric and bladder drainage. Transplantation 1997; 64:1689.
9. Gruessner RW. Tacrolimus in pancreas transplantation: a multicenter analysis. Tacrolimus pancreas transplant study group. Clin Transplant 1997; 11:299.
10. Sutherland DER, Goetz FC, Sibley RK. Recurrence of disease in pancreas transplants. Diabetes 1989; 38:85.
11. Manske CL, Wang Y, Thomas W. Mortality of cadaveric kidney transplantation versus combined kidney-pancreas transplantation in diabetic patients. Lancet 1995; 346:1658.
11a. Robertson RP, Sutherland DER, Lanz KJ. Normoglycemia and preserved insulin secretory reserve in diabetic patients 10–18 years after pancreas transplantation. Diabetes 1999; 48:1737.
12. Herold KC, Nagamatsu S, Buse JB, et al. Inhibition of glucose-stimulated insulin release from bTEC3 cells and rodent islets by an analog of FK506. Transplantation 1993; 55:186.
13. Fioretto P, Steffes MW, Sutherland DER, et al. Reversal of lesions of diabetic nephropathy after pancreas transplantation. N Engl J Med 1998; 339:69.
14. Navvaro X, Kennedy WR, Sutherland DER. Autonomic neuropathy and survival in diabetes mellitus: effects of pancreas transplantation. Diabetologia 1991; 34:S108.
15. Robertson RP, Holohan TV, Genuth S. Therapeutic controversy: pancreas transplantation for type I diabetes. J Clin Endocrinol Metab 1998; 83:1868.
16. Weir GC, Bonner-Weir S. Scientific and political impediments to successful islet transplantation. Diabetes 1997; 46:1247.
17. Scharp DW, Lacy PE, Santiago JV, et al. Results of our first nine intraportal islet allografts in type 1, insulin dependent diabetic patients. Transplantation 1991; 51:76.
18. Socci C, Falqui L, Davalli AM, et al. Fresh human islet transplantation to replace pancreatic endocrine function in type I diabetic patients. Acta Diabetol 1991; 28:151.
19. Warnock G, Kneteman NM, Ryan EA, et al. Long-term follow-up after transplantation of insulin-producing pancreatic islets into patients with type I (insulin-dependent) diabetes mellitus. Diabetologia 1992; 35:89.
20. Ricordi C, Tzakis AG, Carroll PB, et al. Human islet isolation and allotransplantation transplantation in 22 consecutive cases. Transplantation 1992; 53:407.

21. Tzakis AG, Ricordi C, Alejandro R, et al. Pancreatic islet transplantation after upper abdominal exenteration and liver replacements. Lancet 1990; 336:402.
22. Hering BJ, Ricordi C. Islet transplantation for patients with type 1 diabetes. Graft 1999; 2:12.
23. Hering BJ. Insulin independence following islet transplantation in man: a comparison of different recipient categories. Int Islet Transpl Registry 1996; 6:5.
24. Alejandro R, Lehmann R, Ricordi C, et al. Long-term function (6 years) of islet allografts in type 1 diabetes. Diabetes 1997; 46:1983.
25. Hering BJ, Ernst W, Eckhard M, et al. Improved survival of single donor islet allografts in IDDM recipients by refined peritransplant management (Abstract). Diabetes 1997; 46:251.
25a. Merino JF, Nacher V, Raurell M, et al. Optimal insulin treatment in syngeneic islet transplantation. Cell Transplant 2000; 9:11.
26. Sutherland DER, Gores PF, Hering BJ, et al. Islet transplantation: an update. Diabetes Metab Rev 1996; 12:137.
27. Pyzdrowski KL, Kendall DM, Halter JB, et al. Preserved insulin secretion and insulin independence in recipients of islet autografts. N Engl J Med 1992; 327:220.
28. LaPort RE, Matsushima M, Chang Y-F. Prevalence and incidence of insulin-dependent diabetes. In: Diabetes in America, 2nd ed. NIH, 1995:37.
29. Beattie GM, Otonkoski T, Lopez AD, et al. Functional B-cell mass after transplantation of human fetal pancreatic cells. Diabetes 1997; 46:244.
30. Tuch BE, Simpson AM. Experimental fetal islet transplantation. In: Ricordi C, ed. Pancreatic islet cell transplantation. Pittsburgh: R.G. Landes, 1992:279.
31. Davalli A, Ogawa Y, Scaglia L, et al. Function, mass and replication of porcine and rat islets transplanted into diabetic nude mice. Diabetes 1995; 44:104.
32. Weir GC, Davalli AM, Ogawa Y, et al. Transplantation of porcine islets in nude mice: implications for islet replacement therapy in humans. Xenotransplantation 1995; 2:201.
33. Mandel TE, Koulmanda M, Kovarik J, et al. Transplantation of organ cultured fetal pig pancreas in non-obese diabetic (NOD) mice and primates (*Macaca fascicularis*). Xenotransplantation 1996; 2:128.
34. Korsgren O, Andersson A, Sandler S. Pretreatment of fetal porcine pancreas in culture with nicotinamide accelerates reversal of diabetes after transplantation to nude mice. Surgery 1993; 113:205.
35. Korbutt GS, Elliott JF, Ao Z, et al. Large scale isolation, growth, and function of neonatal porcine islets. J Clin Invest 1996; 97:2119.
36. Patience C, Takeuchi Y, Weiss RA. Infection of human cells by an endogenous retrovirus of pigs. Nat Med 1997; 3:282.
37. Knaack D, Fiore DM, Surana M, et al. Clonal insulinoma cell line that stably maintains correct glucose responsiveness. Diabetes 1994; 43:1413.
38. Asfari M, Janjic D, Meda P, et al. Establishment of 2-mercaptoethanol-dependent differentiated insulin-secreting cell lines. Endocrinology 1992; 130:167.
39. Clark SA, Quaade C, Constandy H, et al. Novel insulinoma cell lines produced by iterative engineering of GLUT2, glucokinase, and human insulin expression. Diabetes 1997; 46:958.
40. Hohmeier HE, BeltrandelRio H, Clark SA, et al. Regulation of insulin secretion from novel engineered insulinoma cell lines. Diabetes 1997; 46:968.
41. Bach FH, Winkler H, Ferran C, et al. Delayed xenograft rejection. Immunol Today 1996; 17:379.
42. Dorling A, Riesbeck K, Warrens A, et al. Clinical xenotransplantation of solid organs. Lancet 1997; 349:867.
43. Bach FH, Auchincloss H Jr, Robson SC. Xenotransplantation. In: Bach FH, Auchincloss H Jr, eds. Transplantation immunology. New York: Wiley-Liss, 1995:305.
44. London NJ, Farmery SM, Will EJ, et al. Risk of neoplasia in renal transplant patients. Lancet 1995; 346:714.
45. Selawry HP. Islet transplantation to immunoprivileged sites. In: Lanza RP, Chick WL, eds. Pancreatic islet transplantation. Pittsburgh: R.G. Landes, 1994:75.
46. Rossini AA, Greiner DL, Mordes JP. Induction of immunologic tolerance for transplantation. Physiol Rev 1999; 79:99.
47. Colton CK. Implantable biohybrid artificial organs. Cell Transplant 1995; 4:415.
48. Lacy PE. Treating diabetes with transplanted cells. Sci Am 1995; 273:54.
49. Suzuki K, Bonner-Weir S, Trivedi N, et al. Function and survival of macroencapsulated syngeneic islets transplanted into streptozocin-diabetic mice. Transplantation 1998; 66:21.
50. Sun Y, Ma X, Zhou D, et al. Normalization of diabetes in spontaneously diabetic cynomolgus monkeys by xenografts of microencapsulated porcine islets without immunosuppression. J Clin Invest 1996; 98:1417.
51. De Vos P, De Haan BJ, Wolters GHJ, et al. Improved biocompatibility but limited graft survival after purification of alginate for microencapsulation of pancreatic islets. Diabetologia 1997; 40:262.
52. Soon-Shiong P, Heintz RE, Merideth N, et al. Insulin independence in type 1 diabetic patients after encapsulated islet transplantation. Lancet 1994; 343:950.
53. Lanza RP, Chick WL. Transplantation of encapsulated cells and tissues. Surgery 1997; 121:1.
54. Calafiore R. Perspectives in pancreatic and islet cell transplantation for the therapy of IDDM. Diabetes Care 1997; 20:889.
54a. Charles R, Harland RC, Ching D, Opara EC. Storage and microencapsulation of islets for transplantation. Cell Transplant 2000; 9:33.
55. Brissova M, Petro M, Lacik I, et al. Evaluation of microcapsule permeability via inverse size exclusion chromatography. Anal Biochem 1996; 242:104.
56. Mulligan RC. The basic science of gene therapy. Science 1993; 260:926.
57. Saldeen J, Curiel DT, Eizirik DL, et al. Efficient gene transfer to dispersed human pancreatic islet cells in vitro using adenovirus-polylysine/DNA complexes or polycationic liposomes. Diabetes 1996; 45:1197.

# CHAPTER 145

# SYNDROME X

GERALD M. REAVEN

That resistance to insulin-mediated glucose disposal is characteristic of patients with type 2 diabetes mellitus and that fasting hyperglycemia supervenes when such individuals are no longer able to sustain the degree of compensatory hyperinsulinemia necessary to overcome the defect in cellular insulin action has been apparent for some time.[1–3] Less well appreciated, however, was the fact that insulin-resistant subjects able to sustain the degree of compensatory hyperinsulinemia necessary to maintain near-normal glucose homeostasis were at risk to develop a cluster of additional abnormalities, including some impairment of glucose tolerance, a high plasma triglyceride (TG) level and low concentration of high-density lipoprotein (HDL) cholesterol, and hypertension.[3] In 1988, the relationship between insulin resistance and this cluster of related abnormalities, all of which increase risk of coronary heart disease (CHD), was identified and designated as syndrome X.[3] This formulation has received considerable support since its introduction, and the list of abnormalities associated with insulin resistance and compensatory hyperinsulinemia has grown considerably. The goal of this chapter is to summarize the evidence linking insulin resistance and compensatory hyperinsulinemia to all the abnormalities now presumed to comprise syndrome X, as illustrated in Figure 145-1.

## INSULIN RESISTANCE AND COMPENSATORY HYPERINSULINEMIA

The central defect in syndrome X is postulated to be insulin resistance and compensatory hyperinsulinemia, and it is this combination that differentiates syndrome X from type 2 diabetes. As depicted in Figure 145-1, insulin resistance is influenced by both lifestyle and genetic background. Because the genes

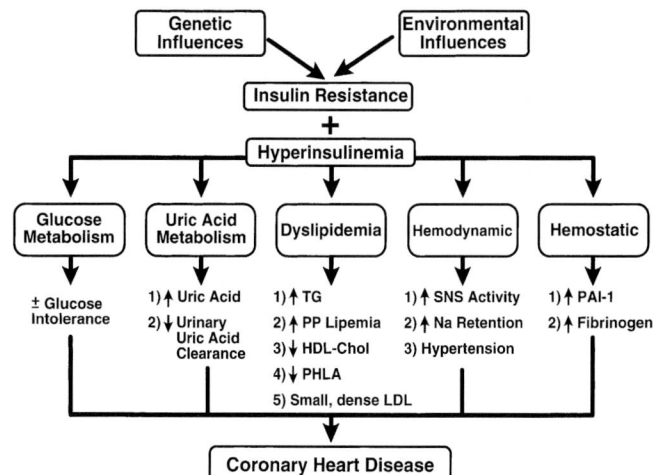

**FIGURE 145-1.** A diagrammatic representation of the relationship between insulin resistance plus compensatory hyperinsulinemia and the cluster of abnormalities that comprise syndrome X. (*TG*, triglyceride; *PP*, postprandial; *HDL-Chol*, high-density lipoprotein cholesterol; *PHLA*, plasma post–heparin lipolytic activity; *LDL*, low-density lipoprotein; *SNS*, sympathetic nervous system; *PAI-1*, plasminogen activator inhibitor-1.)

responsible for differences in insulin resistance are unknown, their influence cannot be evaluated directly. However, data indicate that obesity and physical inactivity, the two most important lifestyle variables that decrease insulin action, each explain ~25% of the differences in insulin action from person to person.[4] By inference, then, one can argue that differences in genetic background account for the remaining 50% of the variability in insulin resistance. The crucial point is that variations in body weight and level of physical activity are modulators of insulin action; they are not the primary cause of insulin resistance.

## ABNORMALITIES RELATED TO INSULIN RESISTANCE AND COMPENSATORY HYPERINSULINEMIA

### GLUCOSE METABOLISM

The earliest recognizable defect in prediabetic individuals is insulin resistance (see Chap. 146).[5] The majority of insulin-resistant individuals are able to maintain normal glucose tolerance by secreting large amounts of insulin. Indeed, within the population of individuals with absolutely normal glucose tolerance, the greater their degree of insulin resistance, the higher their plasma glucose concentration.[6] In some insulin-resistant individuals, the degree of compensatory hyperinsulinemia is not sufficient to maintain normal glucose tolerance, and such individuals are classified as having impaired glucose tolerance.[7] In an even smaller subset of insulin-resistant individuals, insulin-secretory function fails sufficiently to permit manifest hyperglycemia to develop.[5] Such individuals have type 2 diabetes (see Chap. 137) and should be differentiated from individuals with syndrome X; the latter term is used to describe insulin-resistant individuals who, although they may even develop impaired glucose tolerance, are not diabetic. Syndrome X and type 2 diabetes share insulin resistance, but *the designation of syndrome X should be limited to individuals who have maintained sufficient insulin secretory function to remain nondiabetic.*

### URIC ACID METABOLISM

An association between serum uric acid concentration and CHD was demonstrated almost 50 years ago (see Chap. 192).[8] In addition, hyperuricemia is commonly seen in individuals with glucose intolerance, dyslipidemia, and hypertension[9]—the central characteristics of syndrome X. An explanation for these various relationships has evolved from the results of several studies. Specifically, studies of normal, healthy volunteers have shown that significant correlations exist between serum uric acid concentration and both insulin resistance and the plasma insulin response to an oral glucose challenge.[10] Subsequently, healthy volunteers with asymptomatic hyperuricemia have been demonstrated to have higher plasma insulin responses to oral glucose, higher plasma TG, lower HDL cholesterol concentrations, and higher blood pressure compared with a well-matched group of volunteers with normal serum uric acid concentrations.[11]

Evidence presented in these earlier studies suggested that the association between insulin resistance, hyperinsulinemia, and serum uric acid concentration was related to a decrease in urinary clearance of uric acid, a finding which raised the possibility that the link between insulin metabolism and hyperuricemia was the renal handling of uric acid. The hypothesis that insulin acts on the kidney to decrease renal clearance of uric acid has subsequently been supported by results of studies of both normotensive and hypertensive subjects.[12,13]

Based on these data, the association between CHD and uric acid concentration seems most likely to be an epiphenomenon. Thus, insulin-resistant individuals try to secrete increased

### TABLE 145-1.
**Abnormalities of Lipoprotein Metabolism Associated with Insulin Resistance, Compensatory Hyperinsulinemia, and Hypertriglyceridemia**

Increased postprandial concentration of triglyceride-rich lipoproteins

Decreased high-density lipoprotein cholesterol concentration

Relative failure to increase adipose tissue lipoprotein lipase (*LPL*) mRNA and plasma post-heparin LPL activity

Decrease in low-density lipoprotein particle diameter

amounts of insulin in an effort to prevent the development of type 2 diabetes. If successful, they are likely to develop the characteristics of syndrome X,[3] and to be at increased risk of CHD.

## DYSLIPIDEMIA

### PLASMA TRIGLYCERIDE CONCENTRATION

Reports published ~30 years ago documented a significant relationship between plasma insulin and triglyceride concentrations (see Chaps. 163 and 166).[14] Subsequently, a significant, direct relationship was shown to exist between resistance to insulin-mediated glucose disposal, compensatory hyperinsulinemia, and plasma TG concentration in both hypertriglyceridemic and normotriglyceridemic subjects.[15,16] Because kinetic measurements of hepatic synthesis and secretion of very low-density lipoprotein (VLDL) and TG were shown to be correlated with plasma VLDL-TG concentrations, the conclusion was drawn that, the more insulin resistant an individual and the higher the resultant plasma insulin concentration, the greater would be the increase in hepatic VLDL-TG synthesis and secretion, and the more elevated the plasma TG concentration. Once the plasma TG concentration begins to increase, another series of changes in lipoprotein metabolism takes place, as outlined in Table 145-1.

### POSTPRANDIAL LIPEMIA

The higher the fasting TG concentration, the greater the postprandial accumulation of TG-rich lipoproteins.[17] In addition, the magnitude of postprandial lipemia is greater in patients with type 2 diabetes than in a control population when subjects are matched for fasting plasma TG concentrations.[18] The postprandial increase in TG-rich lipoproteins is significantly correlated with the postprandial insulin concentrations, and both insulin resistance and compensatory hyperinsulinemia are also significantly related to the postprandial accumulation of TG-rich lipoproteins in nondiabetic individuals.[19] Thus, elevations in postprandial lipemia appear to be highly correlated with insulin resistance and compensatory hyperinsulinemia—both directly, by mechanisms as yet unknown, and indirectly, by virtue of the role played by insulin resistance and/or compensatory hyperinsulinemia in stimulating hepatic VLDL-TG secretion and in increasing the fasting TG-pool size.

### HIGH-DENSITY LIPOPROTEIN CHOLESTEROL

The fact that low levels of HDL cholesterol often accompany hypertriglyceridemia may, at least in part, reflect the movement of cholesterol from HDL to VLDL, catalyzed by cholesteryl ester transfer protein (see Chap. 163).[20] The higher the VLDL pool size, the greater the transfer rate of cholesterol ester from HDL to VLDL, and the lower the ensuing HDL cholesterol concentration. In addition, evidence has been found that the fractional catabolic rate (FCR) of apoprotein A-I is increased in patients with endogenous hypertriglyceridemia,[21] hypertension,[22] and type 2 diabetes.[23] In the latter case, the higher the insulin level, the lower the HDL cholesterol concentration. Given evidence that the higher the apoprotein A-I FCR, the lower the HDL cholesterol concentration,[24] insulin resistance and hyperinsulinemia are likely to contribute indirectly to a low concentration of HDL cholesterol by being responsible for the increase in VLDL pool size, and to contribute directly by increasing the FCR of apoprotein A-I.

## LIPOPROTEIN LIPASE

Lipoprotein lipase (LPL) plays a key role in the catabolism of TG-rich lipoproteins, and the activity of this enzyme is generally thought to be decreased in insulin-deficient states.[25] If LPL were to increase to a sufficient degree in subjects who were insulin resistant and hyperinsulinemic, the increase in hepatic VLDL-TG synthesis present in these individuals would not necessarily lead to higher plasma TG concentrations. The fact that hypertriglyceridemia does occur in this situation is consistent with the view that at least a relative failure of LPL to maintain TG homeostasis is present in patients with syndrome X. To test this hypothesis, the relationship between insulin-mediated glucose disposal; fasting insulin and TG concentrations; plasma post-heparin lipoprotein lipase (PH-LPL) activity and mass; and adipose tissue LPL activity, mass, and mRNA content in nondiabetic men has been defined.[26] The degree of insulin resistance was significantly correlated with fasting TG concentrations, plasma PH-LPL activity and mass, and adipose tissue LPL mRNA content. Thus, the more insulin resistant an individual, the lower the level of plasma PH-LPL activity and mass, and the higher the plasma TG concentration. Concentrations of adipose tissue LPL mRNA were also correlated directly with plasma PH-LPL mass and inversely with both plasma TG concentration and insulin resistance. These results support the view that failure of insulin to appropriately stimulate LPL activity in insulin-resistant and hyperinsulinemic individuals accentuates the magnitude of hypertriglyceridemia that develops in association with the increase in hepatic TG synthesis and secretion that characterizes insulin-resistant individuals.

## LOW-DENSITY LIPOPROTEIN PARTICLE DIAMETER

Analysis of low-density lipoprotein (LDL) particle size distribution by nondenaturing gradient gel electrophoresis[27] has identified multiple distinct LDL subclasses and has shown that in most individuals LDL can be characterized by a predominance of either larger LDL particles (diameter of >255 Å, pattern A) or smaller LDL particles (diameter of ≤255 Å, pattern B). Individuals with pattern B have higher plasma TG and lower HDL cholesterol concentrations and are at increased risk of CHD.[27] Because similar changes in plasma TG and HDL cholesterol concentrations are associated with resistance to insulin-mediated glucose uptake and/or hyperinsulinemia,[28] pattern B is also probably associated with insulin resistance. Evidence has now been published demonstrating that healthy volunteers with small, dense LDL particles (pattern B) are relatively insulin resistant, glucose intolerant, hyperinsulinemic, hypertensive, and hypertriglyceridemic, and have a lower HDL cholesterol concentration.[29] Thus, this change in LDL composition should be added to the cluster of abnormalities constituting syndrome X.

## HEMODYNAMICS

### SYMPATHETIC NERVOUS SYSTEM ACTIVITY

Not only is the resting heart rate higher in patients with high blood pressure (HBP), but it also is a predictor of hypertension.[30] Moreover, patients with HBP demonstrate resistance to insulin-mediated glucose disposal and/or compensatory hyperinsulinemia compared with normotensive individuals,[5] and these changes can also be seen in normotensive first-degree relatives of patients with hypertension.[31] A review article has summarized evidence that insulin resistance and compensatory hyperinsulinemia can predispose individuals to develop hypertension via stimulation of the sympathetic nervous system (SNS).[32] Thus, the association between hypertension and increased heart rate could be secondary to enhanced SNS activity in insulin-resistant subjects. Evidence in support of this view has come from a study of normotensive, nondiabetic individuals in whom both insulin resistance and the plasma insulin response to glucose were significantly correlated with heart rate.[33] Cross-sectional data do not provide proof of causal relationships, but the suggestion that SNS activity is increased in insulin-resistant individuals seems reasonable. This finding may explain why both resistance to insulin-mediated glucose disposal (or hyperinsulinemia) and an increase in heart rate have been shown to predict development of hypertension.

## SODIUM RETENTION

The acute infusion of insulin increases renal sodium retention in both normal individuals and patients with HBP.[12,13] Importantly, the ability of insulin to enhance renal sodium absorption was discerned in patients whose muscles are resistant to insulin-mediated glucose disposal.[12,13] This represents another instance in which renal sensitivity to an action of insulin is maintained despite a loss of muscle insulin sensitivity, similar to the situation described with regard to renal uric acid clearance. Indeed, these two effects of insulin on the kidney seem to be related, in that the increase in sodium retention is associated with the decrease in uric acid clearance. If insulin enhances renal sodium retention in insulin-resistant subjects, one might predict that such individuals would also be salt sensitive. Although this issue has not been definitively settled, evidence has been found in both normotensive and hypertensive individuals that the blood pressure is sensitive to salt in insulin-resistant individuals.[34] Irrespective of the role played by insulin resistance and/or compensatory hyperinsulinemia in the pathogenesis of salt-sensitive hypertension, however, enhanced renal tubular sodium reabsorption appears to be part of syndrome X.

## HYPERTENSION

Insulin-resistant and hyperinsulinemic individuals are at increased risk of developing HBP[34a] (see Chap. 82). The considerable evidence in support of this view[5,31,32] can be summarized as follows: (a) cross-sectional studies have repeatedly shown that patients with HBP are insulin resistant and hyperinsulinemic compared with well-matched groups of normotensive individuals; (b) patients with secondary forms of hypertension are not insulin resistant, and effective drug treatment of patients with HBP does not restore insulin sensitivity to normal in insulin-resistant patients with hypertension; (c) normotensive first-degree relatives of patients with HBP are insulin resistant and hyperinsulinemic compared with normotensive subjects without a family history of hypertension; and (d) hyperinsulinemia predicts the development of hypertension in prospective studies.

On the other hand, probably no more than half of patients with HBP are insulin resistant and hyperinsulinemic,[35] and insulin-resistant and hyperinsulinemic individuals with normal blood pressure certainly exist. Thus, any effort to define a causal relationship between insulin resistance, hyperinsulinemia, and hypertension must take into account the fact that the defects in insulin metabolism can only be relevant to the development of hypertension in the subset of patients with HBP. Furthermore, even if insulin resistance and hyperinsulinemia are related to the pathogenesis of hypertension, they most likely play a permissive role, increasing the risk of an individual's developing hypertension. A good deal remains to be learned about the relationship between insulin resistance, hyperinsulinemia, and hypertension, but no doubt remains that an association between these variables exists. Therefore, the inclusion of hypertension in Figure 145-1 is certainly warranted.

## HEMOSTASIS

Concentrations of plasminogen activator inhibitor-1 (PAI-1) are higher in patients with hypertriglyceridemia, hypertension, and CHD.[36–38] Given the association between PAI-1, CHD, and the other features of syndrome X, PAI-1 concentrations possibly are related to insulin resistance and/or compensatory hyperinsulinemia.[39,40] Perhaps the most compelling evidence comes from the European Concerted Action on Thrombosis and Disabilities Angina Pectoris Study,[38] in which PAI-1 concentrations were found to be significantly associated with hyperinsulinemia, hypertriglyceridemia, and hypertension in 1500 patients with angina pectoris.[38] The evidence that elevated fibrinogen levels are also part of syndrome X is not as strong. Although insulin resistance and fibrinogen levels have been shown to be correlated, the argument has been made that the relationship in this case is not an independent one but is the manifestation of an acute-phase reaction in patients with CHD.

## CONCLUSION

The ability of insulin to stimulate glucose uptake varies widely from person to person. In an effort to maintain the ambient plasma glucose concentration between ~80 and 140 mg/dL, the pancreatic B cell attempts to secrete whatever amount of insulin is required to accomplish this goal (see Chap. 135). The more resistant a normal individual is to insulin-mediated glucose disposal, the greater must be the degree of compensatory hyperinsulinemia. If the B cell cannot sustain this effort, type 2 diabetes ensues.

Although hyperinsulinemia may prevent the development of type 2 diabetes, the ability of insulin-resistant individuals to maintain normal or near-normal glucose tolerance by secreting large amounts of insulin is hardly benign. Specifically, the combination of insulin resistance and compensatory hyperinsulinemia appears to lead to the cluster of abnormalities that make up the current version of syndrome X, as shown in Figure 145-1. In this formulation, resistance to insulin-mediated glucose disposal and compensatory hyperinsulinemia are viewed as the central defects. Arguments may continue regarding the relative importance of nature versus nurture in the genesis of insulin resistance, but general agreement exists that insulin resistance leads to an effort on the part of the B cell to secrete more insulin to prevent decompensation of glucose homeostasis. Normal, or near-normal, glucose tolerance can be maintained if insulin-resistant individuals are able to maintain a state of chronic hyperinsulinemia. Unfortunately, the consequences of this "victory" put an individual at greatly increased risk to develop all of the abnormalities shown in Figure 145-1. More to the point, all of the various facets of syndrome X are involved to a substantial degree in the cause and clinical course of CHD.

On the basis of the previous considerations, one might suggest that resistance to insulin-mediated glucose disposal, and the manner in which the organism responds to this defect, play major roles in the pathogenesis and clinical course of what are often referred to as diseases of Western civilization.

## REFERENCES

1. Ginsberg H, Kimmerling G, Olefsky JM, Reaven GM. Demonstration of insulin resistance in untreated adult onset diabetic subjects with fasting hyperglycemia. J Clin Invest 1975; 55:454.
2. Reaven GM. Insulin resistance in noninsulin-dependent diabetes mellitus: does it exist and can it be measured? Am J Med 1983; 74(Suppl 1A):3.
3. Reaven GM. Role of insulin resistance in human disease. Diabetes 1988; 37:1595.
4. Bogardus C, Lillioja S, Mott DM, et al. Relationship between degree of obesity and *in vivo* insulin action in man. Am J Physiol 1985; 248(3 Pt 1):E286.
5. Lillioja SD, Mott DM, Spraul M, et al. Insulin resistance and insulin secretory dysfunction as precursors of non-insulin-dependent diabetes mellitus. N Engl J Med 1993; 329:1988.
6. Reaven GM, Brand RJ, Chen Y-DI, et al. Insulin resistance and insulin secretion are determinants of oral glucose tolerance in normal individuals. Diabetes 1993; 42:1324.
7. Reaven GM, Miller RG. An attempt to define the nature of chemical diabetes using a multidimensional analysis. Diabetologia 1979; 16:17.
8. Gertler MM, Garn SM, Levine SA. Serum uric acid in relation to age and physique in health and coronary heart disease. Am J Med 1951; 34:1421.
9. Wyngaarden JB, Kelley WN. Gout. In: Metabolic basis of inherited disease, 5th ed. New York: McGraw-Hill, 1983:1043.
10. Facchini F, Chen Y-DI, Hollenbeck CB, Reaven GM. Relationship between resistance to insulin-mediated glucose uptake, urinary uric acid clearance, and plasma uric acid concentration. JAMA 1991; 266:3008.
11. Zavaroni I, Vazza S, Fantuzzi M, et al. Changes in insulin and lipid metabolism in males with asymptomatic hyperuricemia. J Intern Med 1993; 234:24.
12. Quinones GA, Natali A, Baldi S, et al. Effect of insulin on uric acid excretion in humans. Am J Physiol 1995; 268:E1.
13. Muscelli E, Natali A, Bianchi S, et al. Effect of insulin on renal sodium and uric acid handling in essential hypertension. Am J Hypertens 1996; 9:746.
14. Reaven GM, Lerner RL, Stern MP, Farquhar JW. Role of insulin in endogenous hypertriglyceridemia. J Clin Invest 1967; 46:1756.
15. Olefsky JM, Farquhar JW, Reaven GM. Reappraisal of the role of insulin in hypertriglyceridemia. Am J Med 1974; 57:551.
16. Tobey TA, Greenfield M, Kraemer F, Reaven GM. Relationship between insulin resistance, insulin secretion, very low density lipoprotein kinetics, and plasma triglyceride levels in normotriglyceridemic man. Metabolism 1981; 30:165.
17. Wilson DE, Chan I-F, Buchi KN, Horton SC. Postchallenge plasma lipoprotein retinoids: chylomicron remnants in endogenous hypertriglyceridemia. Metabolism 1985; 34:551.
18. Chen Y-DI, Swami S, Skowronski R, et al. Differences in postprandial lipemia between patients with normal glucose tolerance and noninsulin-dependent diabetes mellitus. J Clin Endocrinol Metab 1993; 76:172.
19. Jeppesen J, Hollenbeck CB, Zhou M-Y, et al. Relation between insulin resistance, hyperinsulinemia, postheparin plasma lipoprotein lipase activity, and postprandial lipemia. Arterioscler Thromb Vasc Biol 1995; 15:320.
20. Swenson TL. The role of the cholesteryl ester transfer protein in lipoprotein metabolism. Diabetes Metab Rev 1991; 7:139.
21. Fidge N, Nestel P, Toshitsugu I, et al. Turnover of apoproteins A-I and A-II of high density lipoprotein and the relationship to other lipoproteins in normal and hyperlipidemic individuals. Metabolism 1980; 29:643.
22. Chen Y-DI, Sheu WH-H, Swislocki ALM, Reaven GM. High density lipoprotein turnover in patients with hypertension. Hypertension 1991; 17:386.
23. Golay A, Zech L, Shi M-Z, et al. High density lipoprotein (HDL) metabolism in noninsulin-dependent diabetes mellitus: measurement of HDL turnover using tritiated HDL. J Clin Endocrinol Metab 1987; 65:512.
24. Brinton EA, Eisenberg S, Breslow JL. Human HDL cholesterol levels are determined by apoA-I fractional catabolic rate, which correlates inversely with estimates of HDL particle size. Effects of gender, hepatic and lipoprotein lipases, triglyceride and insulin levels, and body fat distribution. Arterioscler Thromb 1994; 14:707.
25. Eckel RH. Lipoprotein lipase: a multifunctional enzyme relevant to common metabolic diseases. N Engl J Med 1989; 320:1060.
26. Maheux P, Azhar S, Kern PA, et al. Relationship between insulin-mediated glucose disposal and regulation of plasma and adipose tissue lipoprotein lipase. Diabetologia 1997; 40:850.
27. Austin MA, Breslow JL, Hennekens CH, et al. Low-density lipoprotein subclass patterns and risk of myocardial infarction. JAMA 1988; 260:1917.
28. Reaven GM, Chen Y-DI, Jeppesen J, et al. Insulin resistance and hyperinsulinemia in individuals with small, dense, low density lipoprotein particles. J Clin Invest 1993; 92:141.
29. Laws A, Reaven GM. Evidence for an independent relationship between insulin resistance and fasting plasma HDL-cholesterol, triglyceride and insulin concentrations. J Intern Med 1992; 231:25.
30. Selby JV, Friedman GD, Quesenberry CP. Precursors of essential hypertension: pulmonary function, heart rate, uric acid, serum cholesterol and other serum chemistries. Am J Epidemiol 1990; 131:1017.
31. Reaven GM. Hypertension in diabetes. London: Martin Dunitz, 1999; in press.
32. Reaven GM, Lithell H, Landsberg L. Hypertension and associated metabolic abnormalities—the role of insulin resistance and the sympathoadrenal system. N Engl J Med 1996; 334:374.
33. Facchini FS, Stoohs RA, Reaven GM. Enhanced sympathetic nervous system activity—the linchpin between insulin resistance, hyperinsulinemia, and heart rate. Am J Hypertens 1996; 9:1013.
34. Zavaroni I, Coruzzi P, Bonini L, et al. Association between salt sensitivity and insulin concentrations in patients with hypertension. Am J Hypertens 1995; 8:855.
34a. Weston PJ. Insulin resistance and hypertension: is impaired arterial baroreceptor sensitivity the missing link? Clin Science 2000; 98:125
35. Zavaroni I, Mazza S, Dall'Aglio E, et al. Prevalence of hyperinsulinaemia in patients with high blood pressure. J Intern Med 1992; 231:235.
36. Landin K, Tengvory L, Smith U. Elevated fibrinogen and plasminogen activator (PAI-1) in hypertension are related to metabolic risk factors for cardiovascular disease. J Intern Med 1990; 227:273.
37. Juhan-Vague I, Alessi MC, Vague P. Increased plasma plasminogen activator inhibitor 1 levels. A possible link between insulin resistance and atherothrombosis. Diabetologia 1991; 34:457.
38. Juhan-Vague I, Thompson SG, Jespersen J, on behalf of the ECAT Angina Pectoris Study Group. Involvement of the hemostatic system in the insulin resistance syndrome. Arterioscler Thromb 1993; 13:1865.

39. Valle M, Gascon F, Martas R, et al. Infantile obesity: a situation of athero-thrombotic risk? Metabolism 2000; 49:672.

40. Meige JB, Mittleman MA, Nathan DM, et al. Hyperinsulinemia, hyperglycemia, and impaired hemostasis: the Framingham Offspring Study. JAMA 2000; 283:221.

# CHAPTER 146

# SYNDROMES OF EXTREME INSULIN RESISTANCE

JEFFREY S. FLIER AND CHRISTOS S. MANTZOROS

This chapter considers a group of syndromes that have in common severe *tissue resistance to the actions of insulin*. Insulin resistance that occurs in association with a variety of common states (e.g., obesity, noninsulin-dependent diabetes mellitus [type 2], polycystic ovary syndrome [PCOS], hypertension, and syndrome X[1–3]) is not addressed. The insulin resistance that is due to antiinsulin antibodies, as occurs in patients receiving insulin therapy for diabetes, is considered in Chapter 143. In this review of syndromes characterized by severe insulin resistance, the authors discuss the tools and criteria for diagnosis, current knowledge of pathophysiologic mechanisms, clinical phenotypes[3,4] (Table 146-1), and current therapeutic approaches.

## INSULIN RECEPTORS AND INSULIN ACTION

Although insulin is best known for its ability to promote glucose metabolism, this hormone exerts a wide variety of effects at the cellular level. In addition to stimulating glucose and amino-acid transport, insulin also can activate or inactivate cytoplasmic and membrane enzymes, alter the rate of synthesis and degradation of various proteins and specific mRNAs, and influence the processes of cell growth and differentiation.[1–3] These multiple effects vary widely from tissue to tissue and in dose-response and time course. Some effects, such as the stimulation of glucose transport activity, occur within seconds at very low insulin concentrations. At the other extreme, actions to pro-

**TABLE 146-1.**
**Clinical Syndromes of Extreme Insulin Resistance**

---

**INHERITED (PRIMARY) CELLULAR DEFECTS IN INSULIN ACTION**
*Classic type A syndrome of insulin resistance with acanthosis nigricans*
*Variants of type A syndrome with*
 Muscle cramps
 Acral hypertrophy, pseudoacromegaly
 Lipodystrophy
*Pediatric syndromes with severe insulin resistance*
 Leprechaunism (abnormal facies, growth retardation)
 Rabson-Mendenhall syndrome (dental dysplasia, dystrophic nails, precocious puberty)
*Pseudoacromegaly*
*Other complex syndromes with severe insulin resistance* (see text)
**ACQUIRED INSULIN RESISTANCE**
*Autoantibodies to the insulin receptor (type B)*
*Accelerated insulin degradation*

---

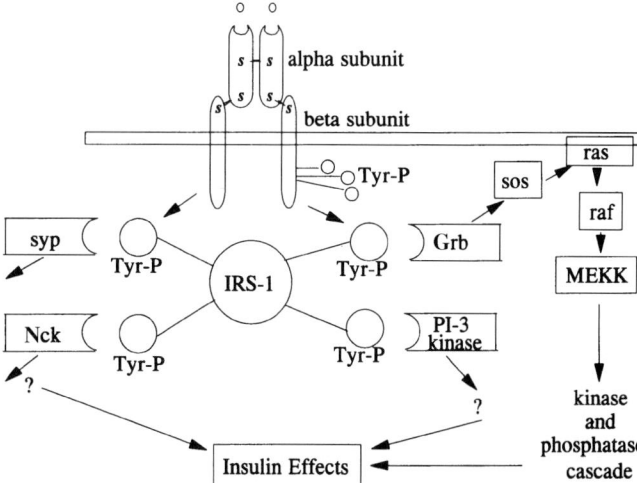

**FIGURE 146-1.** Schematic representation of the insulin receptor and insulin signal transduction. The binding of insulin to the α subunit activates autophosphorylation of tyrosine residues on the β subunit, leading to activation of the intrinsic tyrosine kinase of the receptor. The major known substrate of the insulin receptor tyrosine kinase is IRS-1. Tyrosine phosphorylation of specific tyrosines on IRS-1 causes interaction with molecules such as syp, Nck, phosphatidyl inositol-3 (*PI-3*) kinase, and Grb through specific domains on these molecules (see text; see also Chap. 135).

mote cell growth in certain cells require hours and generally involve higher concentrations of the hormone. Further complicating the study of insulin action is the relationship between insulin and the so-called insulin-like growth factors (IGFs; see Chaps. 12 and 173). These peptides (IGF-I and IGF-II) have major structural homologies with insulin, but they have little or no immunologic cross-reactivity with the hormone. Both IGF-I and IGF-II have distinct receptors to which insulin also can bind, but with reduced affinity.[5] The IGF-I receptor can mediate many of the same acute metabolic events that are regulated by the insulin receptor. Generally, however, the IGFs, acting through the IGF-I receptor, have more potent effects on cell growth than does insulin, acting through the insulin receptor (IR). Some of the actions of insulin that are seen at very high concentrations appear to be exerted through binding to and activation of IGF receptors (rather than IRs).

### INSULIN RECEPTORS

The IR is a glycoprotein composed of two distinct subunits, referred to as α and β, with molecular masses of 135,000 and 95,000 daltons, respectively.[6] These two subunits are held together by disulfide bonds and arise from a common precursor proreceptor molecule that is encoded by a single gene. The number of receptors expressed per cell varies considerably, from several hundred per mature erythrocyte to several hundred thousand per adipocyte.

Insulin binds to the extracellular subunits of its heterotetrameric receptor and activates the intracellular tyrosine kinase of the transmembrane β subunits[6] (Fig. 146-1). This results in IR autophosphorylation and subsequent tyrosine phosphorylation of critical intracellular signaling intermediates. These include IR substrates (IRS-1, IRS-2), Shc, and Gab1.[6,7] These molecules bind to and activate other downstream molecules, including the adapter proteins Grb2 and Nck, the tyrosine phosphatase Syp, and the phosphoinositide 3-kinase, which amplify and diversify the initial signal generated by insulin binding to its receptor.[6] Several signaling pathways are subsequently activated, including the *ras* (Grb2-mSOS-Ras)-mitogen–activated protein kinase pathway, the pp70 kinase, the PKB/Akt (protein kinase B), and possibly other unidentified pathways. Activation

**TABLE 146-2.**
**Diseases and Clinical States with Insulin Resistance in Which Insulin Receptor Expression or Function May Be Altered**

**INSULIN-RESISTANT STATES**

Obesity

Metabolic syndrome (syndrome X)

Type 2 diabetes

Diabetic ketoacidosis

Endocrinopathies (e.g., acromegaly, glucocorticoid excess, pheochromocytoma, thyrotoxicosis, insulinoma, or other hyperinsulinemic states)

Uremia

Cirrhosis of liver

Viral infection

Stress (e.g., trauma, sepsis)

Genetic syndromes

   (Type A syndrome of insulin resistance with acanthosis nigricans, leprechaunism, Rabson-Mendenhall syndrome, ataxia telangiectasia, myotonic dystrophy, etc.)

Antiinsulin receptor antibodies

Other factors (cytokines, free fatty acids)

**INSULIN-SENSITIVE STATES**

Growth hormone deficiency

Glucocorticoid deficiency

Anorexia nervosa

---

of these molecules results in the well-documented insulin effects, such as stimulation of cellular glucose and amino-acid uptake, glycogen synthesis, lipogenesis, and mitogenesis.[6] The complexity of this downstream cascade, which is far greater than was previously anticipated, is reviewed in more detail in Chapter 135.

### RECEPTOR REGULATION

IRs are not static components of the cellular machinery; rather, they have a half-life measured in hours. A major factor regulating the concentration of IRs is insulin itself. Thus, when cells are cultured in a medium containing insulin, they exhibit a time- and temperature-dependent decrease in the concentration of IRs, a phenomenon termed *down-regulation*.[8] The mechanism for this may be complex, but typically appears to involve an insulin-induced acceleration of receptor degradation, and the number of IRs on cells has correlated inversely with the concentration of insulin to which the cells are tonically exposed in vivo.

Many other modulators of receptor concentration or affinity have been described through in vivo or in vitro studies. These include various *physiologic states* (e.g., age, diurnal variation, diet, exercise, menstrual cycle, and pregnancy) and *drugs* (e.g., oral hypoglycemic agents, such as sulfonylureas and the biguanides, and corticosteroids). Other modulators are dietary maneuvers such as fasting or high-carbohydrate feeding, exercise, and the level of specific molecules that can influence receptor expression, such as hormones (cortisol, growth hormone [GH]), nucleotides, ketones, and autoantibodies against the receptor.[9] In many diseases, one or more of these receptor modulators may be responsible for insulin receptor alterations and partially responsible for the clinical resistance to insulin (Table 146-2).

## INSULIN RESISTANCE: GENERAL CONSIDERATIONS

### DEFINITIONS AND IN VIVO ASSESSMENT OF INSULIN RESISTANCE

Insulin resistance has been broadly defined as "a state (of a cell, tissue, or organism) in which a greater than normal amount of

insulin is required to elicit a quantitatively normal response."[3] Usually, this brings to mind the image of an insulin-treated diabetic patient who remains hyperglycemic despite large doses of exogenous insulin. Although such a patient certainly is insulin resistant, this clinical situation represents only one of many clinical presentations of the insulin-resistant disorders. However, insulin resistance can be selective (i.e., involving only certain aspects of insulin action).[1,3]

Patients with insulin resistance thus span a broad spectrum of glucose homeostasis: At one end, these patients may be grossly diabetic despite large doses of insulin; at the other end, they may be normoglycemic despite severe insulin resistance, which is overcome by the compensatory hypersecretion of endogenous insulin. Clinical assessment of insulin resistance relies on several tests, which, in order of increasing complexity, include (a) the determination of insulin levels in either the fasted state or after oral glucose-tolerance testing (OGTT), the results of which must be interpreted in the context of plasma glucose levels[10]; (b) the calculation of the homeostasis (HOMA) index; (c) the assessment of sequential plasma glucose levels after the intravenous administration of insulin (insulin tolerance test)[10]; (d) the estimation of an index of insulin sensitivity (Si), by applying the minimal model technique to data obtained from the frequently sampled intravenous glucose-tolerance test (FSIVGTT)[11]; and (e) the measurement of in vivo insulin-mediated glucose disposal by the euglycemic hyperinsulinemic clamp procedure.[12]

## BIOCHEMICAL BASIS FOR CLINICAL HETEROGENEITY IN INSULIN-RESISTANT STATES

The diverse cellular actions of insulin result from at least two factors: the generation of multiple distinct effects on postreceptor signaling pathways within target cells and the ability of insulin to bind to and act through the IGF-I receptor as well as through the classic IR. As one consequence of these complex signaling mechanisms, resistance to one action of insulin (e.g., its glucose-lowering effect) need not necessarily be associated with equally severe resistance to other important actions of insulin (e.g., antilipolysis, amino-acid uptake, or growth stimulation). It is likely that heterogeneity in the degree to which insulin action on various cellular pathways is impaired plays a central role in determining the clinical specificity of these heterogeneous disorders.

## PATHOGENETIC MECHANISMS RESPONSIBLE FOR SEVERE INSULIN RESISTANCE

Several different classifications for the pathogenesis of insulin resistance have been proposed. One useful classification divides these disorders into those in which there is "primary" target cell resistance to insulin and those in which insulin resistance is caused by factors apart from the target cell.

### PRIMARY TARGET CELL DEFECTS

Primary target cell defects can be due to defects in the IR itself, or to defects in signaling components apart from the IR (Table 146-3). Disorders at the level of the IR gene have been defined over the past few years.[13,14] These may present as a marked reduction in the number of (functionally normal) IRs, due to multiple biochemical defects, including mutations in the receptor gene or its promoter, causing reduced ability to synthesize receptor mRNA, or to mutations in the receptor gene, causing impaired ability of the mature receptor protein to insert into or remain within the membrane. Alternatively, qualitative abnormalities of receptor function have been seen, also resulting from multiple gene defects. These have included receptor structural mutations causing reduced affinity of hormone binding, altered function of the receptor as a hormone-activated kinase, and impaired interaction of an activated receptor with other signaling components.

## AUTOANTIBODIES

Severe insulin resistance also can be caused by several mechanisms apart from primary defects in cellular responsiveness. One well-described mechanism involves the spontaneous development of circulating autoantibodies that recognize determinants in the IR molecule. Anti-IR antibodies occur presumably as a result of either loss of immune tolerance or generation of an immune response to an exogenous antigen and autoantibody formation through molecular mimicry.[3] These antibodies can lead to insulin resistance by sterically interfering with insulin binding,[3] although some anti-IR antibodies appear to lead to IR activation, explaining the fasting hypoglycemia that may occur in these patients.[1,3–5,15,16]

## ACCELERATED DEGRADATION

The biochemical basis for insulin degradation in vivo is imperfectly understood. It is known that the in vivo clearance and subsequent degradation of circulating insulin are, to a large degree, a process that is mediated through the IR.[17,18] Several proteolytic enzymes that may be responsible for hormonal degradation subsequent to receptor binding have been identified.[17] Whether subcutaneously administered insulin is excessively degraded by extracellular enzymes in some patients is uncertain, and the enzymes responsible for such an activity have not been identified.

## OTHER POTENTIAL MECHANISMS

Theoretically, a mutation in the insulin molecule might produce a molecule that would have characteristics of a competitive antagonist. Mutant insulins have been described,[19] but these have been weak agonists that have reduced receptor affinity, without the properties of a competitive antagonist (i.e., they have full bioactivity for any amount of receptor occupancy). However, because these species bind to receptors with low affinity and are poorly cleared from the circulation, these mutant insulins circulate at high concentrations, and an insulin-

resistant state can be mistakenly diagnosed. Unlike patients with true insulin-resistant states, patients with such mutant insulins are normally sensitive to exogenous insulin. The second potential mechanism would be a, heretofore undescribed, paracrine or circulating factor (hormonal, metabolic) that might induce a state of insulin resistance. The observation that tumor necrosis factor may be overproduced by adipocytes in obesity and may be capable of inducing insulin resistance is an example of such a mechanism.[20] Current evidence indicates that the presence of a dominant negative mutation in human PPARγ is associated with severe insulin resistance, diabetes mellitus, and hypertension, indicating that this nuclear receptor (which is responsible for adipocyte differentiation) is important in the control of insulin sensitivity, glucose homeostasis, and blood pressure in humans.[21]

# NATURE AND PATHOGENETIC BASIS FOR CLINICAL FEATURES COMMONLY ASSOCIATED WITH SEVERE INSULIN RESISTANCE

Many patients with extreme target tissue resistance to insulin do not have overt diabetes. However, nearly all such patients do manifest one or more of a group of characteristic clinical features that suggest the existence of severe insulin resistance. These features include the skin lesion acanthosis nigricans, ovarian hyperandrogenism, accelerated or impaired linear growth, lipoatrophy/lipohypertrophy, and a variety of others (see Table 146-1). All patients with syndromes of severe insulin resistance share a number of laboratory findings. Among these, hyperinsulinemia, resulting from increased insulin secretion to compensate for the peripheral insulin resistance is by far the most consistent finding.[1,3,4] Additionally, impaired glucose tolerance or frank diabetes mellitus commonly, but not universally, occurs at a later stage.[1,3,4] These manifestations depend on the ability of the pancreas to compensate for the peripheral insulin resistance by increasing insulin secretion.[1,3,4]

The molecular basis for the association of these features with severe tissue resistance to insulin is only partially understood, but the clinical importance of these associations is clear.

## ACANTHOSIS NIGRICANS

### THE LESION

Acanthosis nigricans is a skin lesion characterized by brown, velvety, hyperkeratotic plaques, most often found in the axillae, the back of the neck, and other flexural areas[22] (Fig. 146-2A). The condition ranges in severity from minimal cases with mild discoloration of limited areas to extreme cases in which the entire surface of the skin may be heavily involved. The pathologic changes are found primarily in the epidermis. There is a complex folding (papillomatosis) of an overgrown epidermis that, although only slightly thickened, has an increased number of cells per unit surface area (Fig. 146-2B). Other changes noted are hyperkeratosis and an increase in the number of melanocytes, the latter contributing to the darkened appearance (see Chaps. 153 and 218).

### CLINICAL ASSOCIATIONS

The clinical associations of acanthosis nigricans fall into two main groups: malignant neoplasms and insulin-resistant states. No feature of the skin lesion itself (i.e., the site or histologic appearance) differentiates between these two groups. Acanthosis nigricans associated with insulin resistance appears to be more common than the form associated with internal malignancy. The lesion is found in all clinical conditions that are characterized by markedly reduced insulin action at the cellular

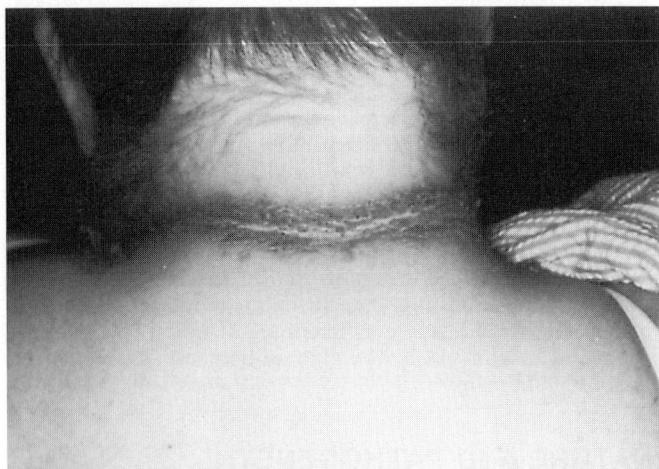
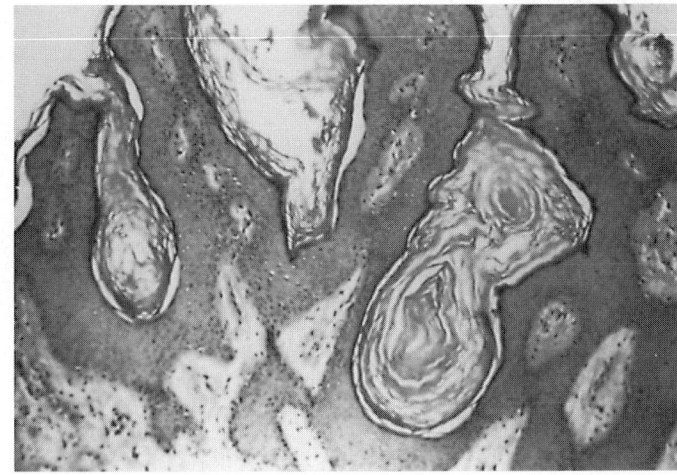

**FIGURE 146-2. A,** Clinical appearance of acanthosis nigricans on the back of the neck. **B,** Photomicrograph of acanthotic skin, revealing papillomatosis, increased keratin, and thickening of epidermis.

level. These include genetic defects in insulin action, antireceptor antibody-induced insulin resistance, and the more common, and pathogenetically less well-defined, insulin-resistant states, such as those associated with obesity.[1–4] The acanthosis that occasionally is present in various endocrinopathies (e.g., Cushing syndrome, acromegaly) also may reflect the insulin resistance that is commonly present in these disorders.[22,23]

### CELLULAR MECHANISMS

The precise mechanism responsible for the association between tissue insulin resistance and acanthosis nigricans is unknown. Perhaps the skin lesions are caused by high levels of circulating insulin acting through receptors for IGF in the skin.[22] Given the fact that various growth factors are produced by tumors,[24] this hypothesis also could account for malignancy-associated acanthosis, if tumor oncogene products were able to activate IGF receptors in the skin.

### CLINICAL IMPLICATIONS

Because of an increased awareness of the association between acanthosis and insulin resistance, this skin condition is being recognized more often by internists, endocrinologists, and gynecologists; it is not as uncommon as previously thought. For example, it has been detected in as many as 10% of women being evaluated for polycystic ovary disease, none of whom had overt diabetes.[25] Because multiple molecular defects, ranging from autoimmune receptor antibodies to genetic abnormalities of receptor molecules and obesity, may be responsible for this lesion, the referral of patients with acanthosis nigricans for metabolic evaluation should be considered. The possibility of a malignant tumor always should be raised, especially when the condition develops rapidly in an adult, although experience suggests that it is much less often a sign of a malignant neoplasm (see Chap. 219) than of an insulin-resistant state. The extent of a metabolic evaluation should depend on the clinical context, including the presence or absence of other clinical features of insulin resistance. The measurement of plasma glucose and insulin levels constitutes the minimum evaluation to determine the presence of insulin resistance in patients with acanthosis nigricans; if the glucose and insulin levels are normal, an insulin-resistant state can be ruled out. Hyperinsulinemia, with or without hyperglycemia, is consistent with insulin resistance, and this finding should prompt further studies, such as attempts to detect circulating anti-IR antibodies or studies of IR expression and function using receptors expressed on circulating blood cells or cultured skin fibroblasts.

## OVARIAN DYSFUNCTION

Evidence from various sources suggests that insulin and IGFs are important regulators of ovarian function. Clinically, there is an association between hyperinsulinemic states of tissue insulin resistance and ovarian hyperandrogenism. Ovarian hyperandrogenism has been seen in a wide range of insulin-resistant states, including genetic disorders of tissue resistance to insulin,[26] autoimmune IR deficiency,[26] a subset of patients with obesity and polycystic ovary disease in whom insulin resistance may have both genetic and nutritional components,[25–27] and a much larger group of patients with typical polycystic ovary disease in whom a correlation between ambient insulin levels and the degree of hyperandrogenism has been defined.[1–4,28] The breadth of this clinical association suggests that insulin may play a surprisingly pervasive role in the pathogenesis of these ovarian disorders.[29,30] In further support of this notion, in vitro studies demonstrate that insulin and IGF both have specific receptors in human ovarian cells[31,32] and exert multiple effects on ovarian growth and steroidogenesis[33–35] (see Chaps. 94, 96, and 101).

### MECHANISM FOR THE ASSOCIATION

There are two major hypotheses for the association of ovarian hyperandrogenism and insulin resistance in these patient groups. The first views insulin as exerting its actions through IGF receptors in the ovary, a result of the extremely high circulating levels of insulin. This explanation requires that IGF receptor pathways are normal, or at least less impaired than IR pathways. Alternatively, as has been observed for other metabolic pathways (e.g., persistent antilipolysis, and the absence of ketosis despite marked hyperglycemia in patients with both genetic and immune-mediated insulin resistance), the action of insulin to promote events in the ovary through IRs may be maintained despite the loss of action on pathways related to glucose homeostasis. Additionally, excessive IR serine phosphorylation has been implicated as a potential mechanism for insulin resistance in a subset of PCOS patients.[2]

### PATHOLOGIC FINDINGS

Pathologic findings in the ovary are nonspecific, and range from typical findings of polycystic ovary disease to extreme cases of ovarian hyperthecosis. The latter is more prevalent in those patients with the greatest degrees of androgen overproduction. Testosterone levels in some of these patients are sufficiently high (>200 ng/mL) to strongly suggest the existence of an androgen-producing tumor. In such situations, the documentation of insulin resistance should serve to diminish this possibility markedly.

# SPECIFIC SYNDROMES OF EXTREME INSULIN RESISTANCE

## CLINICAL PHENOTYPES

Unique features associated with each syndrome, which have been recognized as a result of extensive studies, have led to the classification of patients with severe insulin resistance into several distinct phenotypes.

## SYNDROME OF INSULIN RESISTANCE CAUSED BY AUTOANTIBODIES TO THE INSULIN RECEPTOR (TYPE B INSULIN RESISTANCE)

The existence of IR autoantibodies was first documented during the evaluation of three patients who exhibited extremely insulin-resistant diabetes and acanthosis nigricans.[26] At least 50 additional patients have been described since. As is often found in autoimmune disease, the condition is more common in women. Cases have been recorded in various ethnic groups, including Japanese and Mexican, but most cases have been among blacks. The mean age of first diagnosis is between 30 and 40 years, but the diagnosis has been made as early as 12 years and as late as 78 years. Acanthosis nigricans is a characteristic feature, but the skin lesion occasionally has been absent.

The most common clinical presentation is symptomatic diabetes, marked by symptoms of polyuria, polydipsia, and weight loss. Although plasma glucose values have varied, levels >300 mg/dL have been common. However, ketoacidosis is generally absent or mild. Resistance to exogenous insulin therapy is the hallmark of the disease, and this typically is noted to be present at the time of initial insulin use (unlike the insulin resistance caused by autoantibodies to insulin). The extent of the insulin resistance is indicated by the marked endogenous hyperinsulinemia, and by the fact that individual patients have failed to respond to insulin in dosages as high as 100,000 U per day. In these circumstances, patients may not derive any benefit from continued insulin therapy. A few patients have only mild glucose intolerance and, in a small subgroup, preexisting insulin-resistant diabetes may be followed by a phase of severe hypoglycemia.[36] In other patients, in whom diabetes or glucose intolerance never developed, autoantibodies to the IR have caused hypoglycemia.[37]

### CLINICAL COURSE AND THERAPY

Over several years of follow-up, patients with this syndrome have had various outcomes. The spontaneous remission of insulin resistance with disappearance of receptor antibodies has been documented in a few patients.[36] In another group, diabetes and severe insulin resistance have persisted for several years, and insulin therapy apparently has been of little or no benefit. Patients with marked hyperglycemia and refractory severe insulin resistance have been treated with various experimental regimens. These have included glucocorticoids,[36] antimetabolites, and plasma exchange.[38] Given the fluctuating course in the absence of therapy, and the few patients studied, it has been difficult to obtain a strong indication of the degree to which these therapies have been effective. At least 3 of 30 reported patients have died while experiencing spontaneous hypoglycemia after a prior diabetic phase, and although the pathogenetic basis for this transition has not been elucidated, there appears to be a significant risk for the development of hypoglycemia among those who have this condition.

## AUTOIMMUNE FEATURES

Patients with autoantibodies to the IR characteristically also have symptoms or laboratory test results indicative of more widespread autoimmune disease (e.g., leukopenia [>80%], antinuclear antibodies [>80%], elevated sedimentation rate [>80%], elevated serum immunoglobulin G [IgG >80%], proteinuria [50%], alopecia [36%], nephritis [30%], hypocomplementemia [29%], arthritis [20%], and vitiligo [14%]).[39] Prominent among these are alopecia, vitiligo, arthralgias and arthritis, Raynaud phenomenon, enlarged salivary glands, elevated sedimentation rate, leukopenia, hypergammaglobulinemia, and a positive antinuclear antibody test result. Approximately one-third of patients meet the established criteria for systemic lupus erythematosus, Sjögren syndrome, or some other distinct autoimmune entity. Among those patients with systemic lupus, lupus nephritis has been seen. Premenopausal women with IR autoantibodies may have ovarian hyperandrogenism of a type similar to that observed in patients with other syndromes of extreme tissue resistance to insulin.

## CHARACTERISTICS OF ANTIBODIES TO THE INSULIN RECEPTOR

The extent of insulin binding to receptors on circulating monocytes of these individuals is markedly reduced and of low affinity, and sera from affected patients can reproduce these findings when exposed to normal IRs in vitro.[40] The inhibitory capacity of these sera is due to antibodies, predominantly IgG,[41] that bind to the IR molecule and sterically hinder insulin binding. The antibodies also can precipitate IRs from solution. Titers vary over a wide range and have been extremely high in some individuals, typically those with the greatest insulin resistance. Antibodies from these patients inhibit insulin binding to IRs from a wide variety of target tissues and a broad range of animal species, suggesting interaction with a highly conserved region of the receptor molecule. Indeed, a conserved epitope in the IR α subunit has been identified as the site of antibody binding in most cases.[42] The antibodies have been polyclonal, and individual populations of antibodies in some sera may show some degree of specificity for receptors on a given target tissue. Essentially all sera from affected patients have proved capable of inhibiting insulin binding to the IR, although sensitive assays based on the ability to precipitate receptors from solution have not been designed. The existence of precipitating antibodies that do not inhibit binding is reported to occur,[43] as seen in myasthenia gravis, in which antibodies to acetylcholine receptors of this type are the predominant antibody species. Antibodies from some patients also can inhibit IGF-I binding to its closely related receptor, although the functional significance of these antibodies is unknown.

The ability of antibodies to bind to the IR and inhibit insulin binding provides an explanation for the reduced insulin binding and the observed insulin resistance. However, studies of the bioactivity of these antibodies in vitro are more complex. Sudden exposure of cells to antireceptor immunoglobulins elicits a wide range of insulin-like effects.[44] This finding raises a potential paradox between in vitro and in vivo observations. A partial resolution of this paradox has come from in vitro studies in which the insulin-mimetic effects are seen to be transient, followed by insulin resistance. The latter is due to postreceptor desensitization of some step that is subsequent to insulin binding, as well as to an enhanced rate of receptor degradation.[45] A persistent insulin-like action of these antibodies may account for the hypoglycemia that occurs during the course of the illness in some of these patients, but so far, in vitro examination of the antibodies from hyperglycemic or hypoglycemic patients has not provided an explanation for these differences. The passive transfer of antibodies obtained from one patient to rabbits has caused an insulin-resistant phenotype with postprandial hyperglycemia.[46] However, animals so treated also have a tendency to fasting hypoglycemia, and this probably is a reflection of persistent insulin-like properties of the antibodies.

## TYPE A SYNDROME OF INSULIN RESISTANCE AND ITS VARIANTS

### CLINICAL FEATURES

The initial description of the type A syndrome of insulin resistance involved three peripubertal, thin women with carbohydrate intolerance or overt diabetes, hyperandrogenism, acanthosis nigricans, and severe target cell resistance to insulin.[26] Usually, patients are first seen for evaluation of signs and symptoms of marked hyperandrogenism, acanthosis nigricans, or both. Typically, glucose tolerance in these patients is mildly impaired or even normal. Although patients typically are first seen at about the age of expected puberty, some cases have been discovered much later in life, and when younger siblings of affected patients have been evaluated, insulin resistance has been found at substantially younger ages. Insulin resistance has been observed in a brother of an affected female proband, indicating that the disorder can occur in men, and that androgen excess is not required for the development of insulin resistance.[47] However, the apparent absence of hyperandrogenism in affected men removes one of the major presenting complaints in this disorder, and an accurate prevalence in both men and women is unknown.

**Habitus.**  The body habitus of these patients is noteworthy. Some patients are thin and others are remarkably muscular. Excessive muscular development may be due in part to hyperandrogenism, but it also may be due to the effects of high plasma concentrations of insulin, possibly acting through IGF-I receptors in muscle. Some patients have had acral enlargement, most notably involving the hands, as well as coarsening of the facial features (Fig. 146-3). A role for insulin, acting through both insulin and IGF-I receptors that are unable to signal increased glucose uptake, but are capable of stimulating other pathways, has been suggested as a cause of this "pseudoacromegaly" in one well-studied patient.[48] The acanthosis nigricans has ranged from mild to moderately severe, and usually does not develop before the age of 7 to 10 years. Ovarian hyperandrogenism ranges from moderate to severe, and has tended to be refractory to all the usual therapeutic modalities. Pathologic examination of ovarian tissue in a few individuals has shown ovarian hyperthecosis and stromal hyperplasia.[49] In one patient, complete ovariectomy with a resultant fall in androgen levels did not yield any change in insulin sensitivity or IR status. The relationship of this disorder to the more common clinical group with obesity and hyperandrogenism was discussed earlier.

### CLINICAL PHYSIOLOGY

Relatively little information is available on the clinical physiologic function of these patients. The use of euglycemic insulin clamps in several patients has disclosed a severely impaired ability of insulin to promote glucose utilization as well as a marked defect in insulin clearance.[18] The latter probably arises because receptor-mediated pathways play an important role in the clearance of insulin.

### INSULIN ACTION AT THE CELLULAR LEVEL

Insulin action at the cellular level has been studied intensively in a few patients with these syndromes. Although it was anticipated that the clinical phenotypes seen in individual patients with distinct insulin-resistant syndromes each would be associated with a unique abnormality at the level of the target cell, the current molecular understanding of these syndromes has not yet provided such a correlation. Three patients with distinct insulin-resistant syndromes have been shown to have different mutations in the IR gene.[50–52]

Studies of insulin action have involved IR binding on various cell types, studies of the IR kinase, and studies of insulin action on classic biochemical pathways. Insulin-binding studies can be divided into two types: those performed with freshly obtained cells (most commonly monocytes[53] and red cells,[54] but occasionally adipocytes) and those performed with cultured cells. Studies with fresh cells most closely reflect the in vivo milieu, and studies with cultured skin fibroblasts[55,56] or Epstein-Barr virus–transformed lymphoblasts[57] permit an assessment of the genetic component of the defect. At the level of IR binding, three categories of abnormalities have been observed: a markedly reduced number of IRs that are otherwise normal in affinity, receptors that bind insulin with altered affinity, and receptors that are normal in both number and affinity of insulin binding. The latter group may be the most common variety.

With the discovery that the IR is a tyrosine protein kinase that is autophosphorylated when insulin binds, the kinase function of the IR in these patients became the subject of intense scrutiny. Studies have been performed in circulating monocytes and erythrocytes,[54] as well as in cultured fibroblasts[56] and Epstein-Barr virus–transformed lymphoblasts.[58] As expected, patients with markedly decreased binding have decreased kinase activity. More interesting is that several patients with normal binding have reduced kinase activity, consistent with a

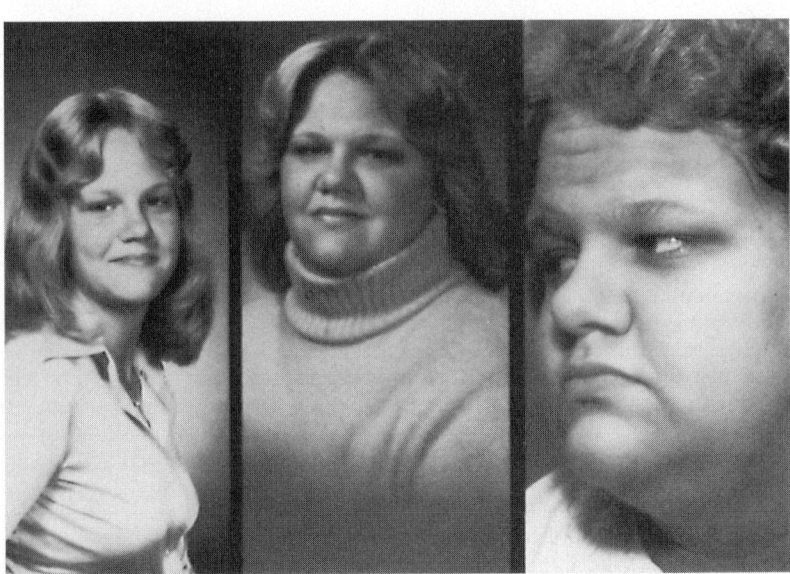

**FIGURE 146-3.** Progressive coarsening of facial features over a 5-year period in a patient with severe insulin resistance and "pseudoacromegaly."

role for this biochemical function in transduction of the insulin signal.[56,59,60] The normalcy of insulin binding and kinase activity in other patients is consistent with a defect that is truly beyond the level of the IR.

Studies of insulin action in freshly isolated adipocytes or cultured fibroblasts of these patients are limited. Defects in insulin-stimulated glucose transport or utilization have been demonstrated,[61] but limited data are available on other pathways of insulin or of IGF action.

Family studies indicate an autosomal dominant or autosomal recessive pattern of transmission of the type A syndrome, with variable penetrance.[1,3,4] Genetic studies have revealed that many patients with the type A syndrome have mutations at the IR gene locus that typically alter the expression or function of one allele.[13,14] Although several IR mutations have been previously associated with the type A syndrome,[7,62] it currently appears that most patients with this syndrome do not possess such mutations, implying the presence of other critical primary defects in insulin signaling,[60–63] as seems to be the case in patients with type 2 diabetes.[64] In addition, a transmembrane glycoprotein named *PC-1*, which interacts with the α subunit of the IR and subsequently inhibits IR function, has been implicated in the pathogenesis of the type A syndrome and type 2 diabetes.[7,65,66] However, its significance remains to be conclusively demonstrated.[7]

## RABSON-MENDENHALL SYNDROME

Another very rare syndrome associated with severe insulin resistance (initially described by Mendenhall)[3,67] is currently known as the *Rabson-Mendenhall syndrome*. These patients present in childhood with severe insulin resistance and diabetes mellitus (commonly refractory to large doses of insulin), acanthosis nigricans, abnormal nails and dentition, short stature, protruberant abdomen, precocious pseudopuberty, and, ostensibly, pineal hyperplasia.[3,67] Prognosis is generally poor, mainly due to the development of severe microvascular complications of diabetes.[3]

## LEPRECHAUNISM

Leprechaunism is a rare inherited disease characterized by an unusual facial appearance (Fig. 146-4), intrauterine and postnatal growth retardation, sparse subcutaneous fat, hirsutism, clitoromegaly, and early death.[68] Patients have abnormalities of glucose homeostasis as well as fasting hypoglycemia associated with B-cell hypertrophy and marked endogenous hyperinsulinemia. Additionally, affected female infants commonly have hirsutism and clitoromegaly, whereas affected boys commonly present with penile enlargement.[3,68] Other features of this syndrome include dysmorphic lungs, renal disease, and breast hyperplasia.[3] Few of these infants live beyond the first year of life, although some may survive until adolescence.[3,68]

Cultured cells from several patients have shown heterogeneous abnormalities of insulin action,[69] IR binding,[70] and IR function, as well as defects in IGF-I receptor pathways.[69] All patients studied to date have had mutations affecting the expression or function of both alleles of the IR gene,[14] and patients with no functional IRs have been described.

## LIPODYSTROPHIC STATES

The lipodystrophic states are a phenotypically diverse group of syndromes characterized by either complete or partial lack of adipose tissue, often severe abnormalities of carbohydrate and lipid metabolism, and various associated somatic features. The disorders are considered here because of their frequent coexistence with severe tissue resistance to insulin, as well as a spectrum of clinical features that overlap with those seen in other syndromes of severe insulin resistance.

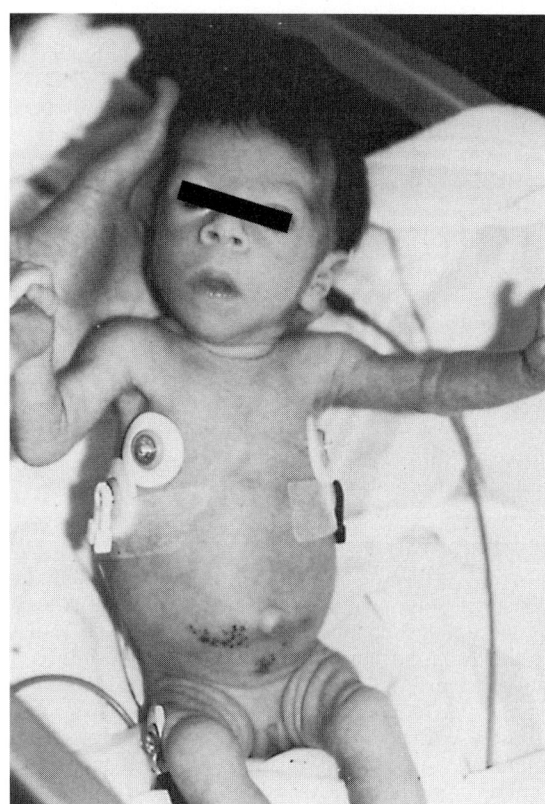

**FIGURE 146-4.** Neonate with leprechaunism, displaying characteristic facies and muscle wasting.

## CLINICAL FEATURES

The lipodystrophy syndromes represent a diverse group of disorders characterized by severe insulin resistance and associated with severe hypertriglyceridemia, which lead to pancreatitis and fatty infiltration of the liver, thereby eventuating with cirrhosis.[3,10] The extent of fat loss predicts the severity of metabolic complications. These syndromes have been conveniently subclassified according to the extent and location of the lipodystrophy and the age of onset[3,10] (Table 146-4).

**Congenital Forms of Total Lipodystrophy.** In its congenital form, the lipoatrophy may be generalized (transmitted as an autosomal recessive trait) or partial (transmitted as an autosomal dominant trait). More than 40 cases of the congenital total lipoatrophy syndrome (also known as the *Berardinelli-Seip syndrome*) have been described.[71] The locus for one gene associated

**TABLE 146-4.**
**Classification of Lipodystrophic Disorders**

**CONGENITAL LIPODYSTROPHY**
  Total lipoatrophy (Berardinelli-Seip syndrome)
  Partial lipoatrophy
    Dunningan variety
    Kobberling variety
    Other types
**ACQUIRED LIPODYSTROPHY**
  Total lipoatrophy (Lawrence syndrome)
  Partial lipoatrophy
    Upper atrophy–lower hypertrophy
    Dermatome pattern
  Human immunodeficiency virus (HIV-1) protease inhibitor-induced lipodystrophy
  Localized lipodystrophies

**TABLE 146-5.**
**Clinical Features of Patients with Lipodystrophic Disorders**

Lipodystrophy
Metabolic dysfunction
    Altered glucose homeostasis: hyperglycemia, no ketosis
    Insulin resistance: endogenous, exogenous
    Hypertriglyceridemia
    Hypermetabolism: increased metabolic rate
Acanthosis nigricans
Accelerated linear growth, acromegaloid features
Muscle hypertrophy, phlebomegaly, genital hypertrophy
Hepatomegaly: fatty liver, cirrhosis
Hypertrichosis, hirsutism
Cardiomegaly: idiopathic hypertrophic subaortic stenosis (IHSS), also
    termed asymmetric septal hypertrophy (ASH)
Miscellaneous
    Mental retardation, central nervous system dysfunction
    Cystic angiomatosis of bone

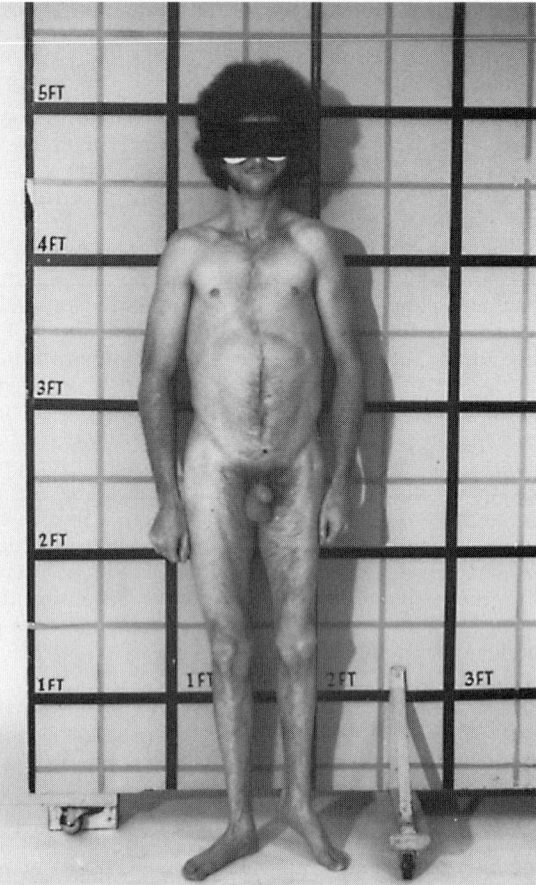

**FIGURE 146-5.** A patient with acquired total lipoatrophy, accompanied by muscular hypertrophy, cirrhosis, and characteristic curly hair.

with this syndrome was found to map to human chromosome 9q34.[72] Parental consanguinity is high in these patients, in whom the disease occurs equally in boys and girls; it usually is diagnosed at birth or within the first 2 years of life. Newborns or infants with congenital generalized lipodystrophy (Berardinelli-Seip syndrome) lack adipose tissue completely in both subcutaneous and visceral locations but have normal adipose tissue in areas of mechanical adipose tissue, such as the orbits, hands, palms, and so forth.[3] Patients have accelerated linear growth, accelerated genital maturation, muscle hypertrophy, and various other congenital defects but no structural brain abnormalities (Table 146-5). Insulin resistance, as assessed by elevated fasting insulin levels, develops or becomes manifest between the ages of 6 and 9 years, preceding the development of diabetes by several years. Hepatosplenomegaly, hypertriglyceridemia, and decreased low-density lipoprotein (LDL) are common, whereas high-density lipoprotein (HDL) is usually normal. Hepatic cirrhosis, which develops in the context of fatty liver, is a major cause of morbidity and mortality.

    **Acquired Forms of Total Lipodystrophy.** Lipoatrophy also can be either total or partial. Acquired total lipoatrophy is not known to be inherited, and can first develop in childhood or adulthood (Fig. 146-5). In contrast to the Berardinelli-Seip syndrome, patients with acquired total lipoatrophy (*Lawrence syndrome*) appear normal at birth, but develop lipoatrophy over days to weeks, sometimes after an infectious prodrome.[3] Histologic evidence of panniculitis has suggested an inflammatory etiology for this syndrome, although this remains to be demonstrated.[3] Although alterations in linear growth rate usually are not found in this disorder, the other associated features typical of congenital lipoatrophy are commonly seen, including insulin-resistant diabetes, acanthosis nigricans, muscle hypertrophy, hepatic cirrhosis, and an increased metabolic rate.

    **Congenital and Acquired Forms of Partial Lipodystrophy.** In addition to the above variants of generalized lipodystrophy, several forms of partial lipodystrophy have been recognized and affect specific body areas (Fig. 146-6). Thus, face-sparing lipodystrophy (*Dunningan variety*), initially reported as an X-linked but increasingly reported as an autosomal dominant condition, spares the face, which is typically full, in contrast to the lipoatrophic trunk and extremities.[3,73] The gene for the autosomal dominant form of this syndrome is located on chromosome 1q21–22,[74] and mutations of the LMNA gene encoding nuclear lamins A and C have been proposed to mediate this degenerative disorder of adipose tissue.[75] Patients develop hypertriglyceridemia and hyperchylomicronemia that can result in pancreatitis. Another variety of the familial partial lipodystrophies is *Kobberling syndrome*, in which the loss of adi-

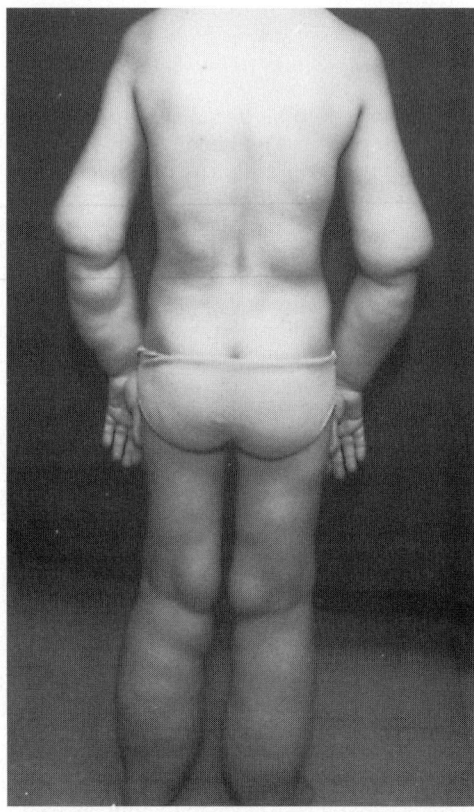

**FIGURE 146-6.** Posterior view of a patient with distal extremity lipohypertrophy and proximal extremity and truncal lipodystrophy.

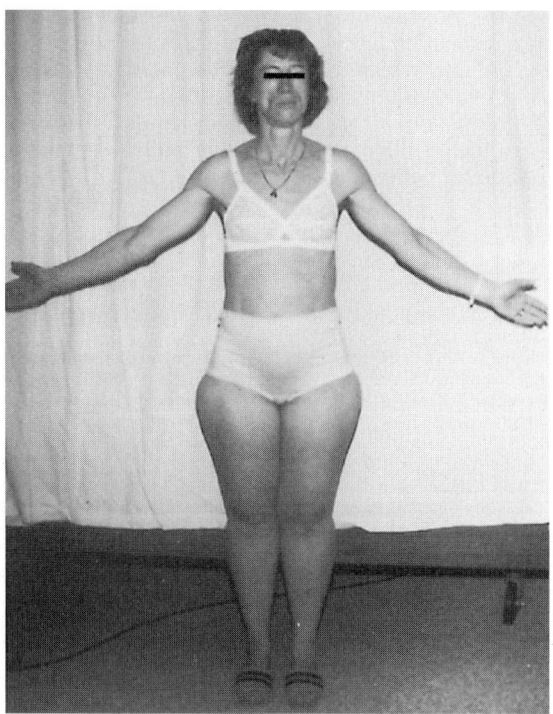

**FIGURE 146-7.** Patient with acquired partial (face and upper extremity) lipoatrophy with hypocomplementemic nephritis.

pose tissue is restricted to the extremities. Patients may have normal amounts of visceral fat and may even have excessive amounts of subcutaneous truncal fat. Another form of partial lipodystrophy, which occurs in association with mandibuloacral dysplasia and joint contractures, is termed *lipodystrophy with other dysmorphic features*.[3] Additionally, a sporadic form of partial lipodystrophy, named *cephalothoracic lipodystrophy*, which has been described predominantly in women, occurs in association with mesangiocapillary glomerulonephritis, presumably as a result of complement activation[3] (Fig. 146-7). Several of these patients have autoimmune abnormalities (including a distinct alteration in complement metabolism), with accelerated catabolism of $C_3$ as well as a serum IgG called C3NeF in ~90% of patients. The mechanistic link between this defect and the lipoatrophy remains an enigma. Patients infected with human immunodeficiency virus (HIV) being treated with the highly effective HIV-1 protease inhibitors develop lipodystrophy characterized by loss of subcutaneous adipose tissue from the extremities and face and deposition of excess fat in the neck and trunk. These patients have insulin resistance and develop hyperglycemia and hyperlipidemia sooner and more frequently than do patients who are on other regimens for HIV.[76] The mechanism underlying the development of lipodystrophy and insulin resistance remains to be elucidated.

**Localized Lipodystrophies.** Finally, localized lipodystrophies are characterized by a loss of subcutaneous adipose tissue from small areas or from small parts of a limb, but these patients do not develop insulin resistance or metabolic abnormalities. Drug-induced lipodystrophy was a frequent complication before the availability of purified human insulin, but is rather uncommon today. Other rare causes of localized lipodystrophy are due to repeated pressure and panniculitis or as part of a rare syndrome called *lipodystrophia centrifugalis abdominalis infantilis*.

### INSULIN RESISTANCE IN LIPODYSTROPHIC STATES

The pathogenesis of the insulin resistance in lipoatrophic diabetes is poorly understood, and efforts to define it are complicated by the marked heterogeneity within this group of disorders. As

in the type A and B syndromes of insulin resistance, initial efforts to understand the lipodystrophic states have focused on the IR or postreceptor molecules. Although an autosomal recessive mode of transmission has been suggested for the Berardinelli-Seip syndrome,[3,10] the pathogenesis of associated insulin resistance is poorly understood, and it remains unclear whether insulin resistance is primary or occurs secondary to lipodystrophy. Linkage analysis in ten families with congenital lipodystrophy failed to implicate 14 candidate genes (including the IR, IRS-1, and IGF-I genes).[77] Studies of cultured fibroblasts obtained from patients with congenital total lipoatrophy reveal either a modest reduction in insulin binding or normal insulin-binding characteristics.[78,79] Likewise, studies of IRs on circulating monocytes and erythrocytes have yielded heterogeneous results, including normal binding, decreased binding associated with a reduced number of receptors, and reductions in receptor affinity.[80] To further complicate our understanding, affected persons within the same family have different patterns of insulin binding, suggesting that the observed receptor abnormalities may be secondary to other unknown abnormalities.

### PSEUDOACROMEGALY

Another rare syndrome of severe insulin resistance is associated with acromegaloidism.[48] In addition to severe insulin resistance, these patients have features reminiscent of acromegaly, including coarse facies and bone thickening, despite a GH–IGF-I axis that appears to be normal.[3,48] However, whether these physical findings result from high insulin levels signaling through the IGF-I receptor or, alternatively, the IR gene per se remains to be established.[3,48] Selective impairment of insulin-stimulated phosphoinositide 3-kinase activity has been demonstrated in three patients with severe insulin resistance and pseudoacromegaly.[81]

### OTHER COMPLEX SYNDROMES OF INSULIN RESISTANCE

Finally, a number of rare genetic syndromes are associated with severe insulin resistance.[82] Among them, *Alstrom syndrome*, an autosomal recessive disorder, which presents with retinitis pigmentosa, sensorineural deafness, hypogonadism, and obesity, is commonly associated with severe insulin resistance and acanthosis nigricans.[3] *Myotonic dystrophy*, an autosomal dominant condition that presents with progressive muscular dystrophy, myotonia, mild mental retardation, baldness, cataracts, and postpubertal testicular atrophy, has been associated with severe insulin resistance.[3,82a] *Werner syndrome*, a progeria syndrome, presents with bird-like facies, gray hair, cataract formation, slender extremities, and severe insulin resistance.[83,83a]

### SUBCUTANEOUS INSULIN DEGRADATION SYNDROME

Among insulin-treated diabetics, a subgroup has been described in whom the subcutaneous administration of insulin in high doses is ineffective, whereas insulin administered by the intravenous route produces a normal response.[84] A role for subcutaneous insulin-degrading activity in the etiology of this syndrome is suggested both by direct assay of such activity in subcutaneous tissue and by the therapeutic response observed when insulin is coinjected with the protease inhibitor aprotinin (Trasylol). Other causes for insulin resistance have been excluded in such patients, some of whom apparently have required prolonged administration of insulin by the intravenous route. The course is one of spontaneous exacerbations and remissions. The initial patient with this syndrome was extremely well documented. However, in a follow-up study of 20 patients referred for evaluation of this entity, subcutaneous insulin degradation could not be documented.[17,85] Instead, these patients had problems with compliance or other emotional problems responsible for their difficulty with insulin therapy. Thus, such problems should be evaluated carefully in patients referred for evaluation of resistance to subcutaneous insulin with sensitivity to intravenous insulin.

## TREATMENT

Since the pathogenesis of the syndromes of severe insulin resistance is incompletely understood, available therapies are nonspecific. Diet, which is the first-line treatment option for diabetes mellitus,[86] was not effective in a small study of women with severe insulin resistance.[86] Additionally, it is unknown whether exercise has a beneficial effect. Thus, the roles of diet and exercise in these syndromes need further study. Although it appears unlikely that the commonly lean, insulin-resistant individuals will significantly benefit from caloric restriction and exercise, it is prudent to recommend long-term caloric restriction to patients with obesity and polycystic ovary disease, in whom the insulin resistance probably is multifactorial and less severe. In several cases, this has caused improvement in the insulin resistance as well as the acanthosis nigricans and hyperandrogenism.[25]

Drugs for patients with severe insulin resistance syndromes are limited. Insulin, administered in very high doses, usually fails to provide adequate control.[3,86] Similarly, administration of sulfonylureas to patients with severe insulin resistance does not result in significant benefits.[86] Metformin, an insulin sensitizer biguanide that suppresses hepatic glucose output and increases insulin-mediated glucose disposal, improved glycemia in patients with the type B syndrome or lipoatrophic diabetes, but did not improve the insulin resistance in patients with myotonic dystrophy.[86] In addition, insulin sensitizers (i.e., metformin and thiazolidinediones) are effective treatments for the insulin resistance associated with polycystic ovarian disease.[86–88] Administration of IGF-I, which acts either through the IGF-I receptor or through a functioning IR, in patients with the type A or B syndromes, the Rabson-Mendenhall syndrome, leprechaunism, and lipodystrophy, has led to improvement in glycemic control and a decrease in fasting insulin levels in short-term studies.[86,89,90] Some of these effects were not maintained in a 10-week trial, however.[89] IGF-I administration is infrequently associated with acute side effects (e.g., fluid retention, carpal tunnel syndrome, jaw pain) and may exacerbate the development of microvascular complications (particularly retinopathy)[86]; increased endogenous IGF-I levels have been associated with several common malignancies (i.e., colon, breast, and prostate cancer).[91–96] Thus, the efficacy-safety profile of IGF-I requires further study in patients with severe insulin resistance.

Thiazolidinediones, which improve insulin resistance in patients with Werner syndrome,[97] are being studied in individuals with other syndromes of severe insulin resistance. Administration of vanadate or vanadium salts to patients with type 2 diabetes has had beneficial effects in insulin resistance,[86,98] but their roles in patients with severe insulin resistance remain unclear. Limited data suggest an improvement in insulin sensitivity in response to administration of phenytoin to patients with the type A syndrome,[86] and in response to administration of bezafibrate[99] or dietary supplementation with n-3 fatty acid–rich fish oil[86] in patients with lipodystrophy. Finally, immunosuppressants and plasmapheresis have been tried with good results in patients with the type B syndrome.[3] In addition, in patients with ovarian hyperandrogenism and insulin resistance caused by anti-IR antibodies, the ovarian lesion remits when antireceptor antibodies disappear, whether spontaneously or because of immunosuppressive therapy.

Surgical treatment has been recommended for certain patients with insulin-resistant disorders. Women with clearly genetic syndromes of insulin resistance, in whom ovarian hyperandrogenism is often the most severe clinical complaint, have not responded to the usual therapies for polycystic ovary disease, but may respond to wedge resection. In a few patients, complete ovariectomy has been required, with a consequent marked reduction in androgen levels and, as expected, no change in the insulin action defect.[100] Finally, cosmetic surgery is an option for patients with lipodystrophy.[74]

## REFERENCES

1. Moller DE, Flier JS. Insulin resistance: mechanisms, syndromes, and implications. N Engl J Med 1991; 325:938.
2. Dunaif A, Xia J, Book CB, et al. Excessive insulin receptor serine phosphorylation in cultured fibroblasts and in skeletal muscle. A potential mechanism for insulin resistance in the polycystic ovary syndrome. J Clin Invest 1995; 96:801.
3. Mantzoros CS, Flier JS. Insulin resistance: the clinical spectrum. In: Mazzaferi E, ed. Advances in endocrinology and metabolism, vol 6. St. Louis: Mosby–Year Book, 1995:193.
4. Kahn CR, Flier JS, Bar RS, et al. The syndromes of insulin resistance and acanthosis nigricans: insulin receptor disorders in man. N Engl J Med 1976; 294:739.
5. Rechler MM, Nissley SP. The nature and regulation of the receptors for insulin-like growth factors. Annu Rev Med 1985; 47:425.
6. Cheatham B, Kahn CR. Insulin action and the insulin signaling network. Endocr Rev 1995; 16:117.
7. Baynes KCR, Whitehead J, Krook A, O'Rahilly S. Molecular mechanisms of inherited insulin resistance. Q J Med 1997; 90:557.
8. Gavin JR III, Roth J, Neville DM Jr. Insulin dependent regulation of insulin receptor concentrations: a direct demonstration in cell culture. Proc Natl Acad Sci U S A 1974; 71:84.
9. Grunberger G, Taylor SI, Doris RF, Gorden P. Insulin receptors in normal and disease states. J Clin Endocrinol Metab 1983; 12:191.
10. Vidal-Puig A, Moller DE. Insulin resistance: classification, prevalence, clinical manifestations, and diagnosis. In: Azziz R, Nestler JE, Dewailly D, eds. Androgen excess disorders in women. Philadelphia: Lippincott–Raven, 1997:227.
11. Bergman RN. Toward physiological understanding of glucose tolerance: minimal model approach. Diabetes 1989; 38:1512.
12. Bergman RN, Prager R, Volund A, Olefsky JM. Equivalence of the insulin sensitivity model method and the euglycemic glucose clamp. J Clin Invest 1987; 79:790.
13. Flier JS. Syndromes in insulin resistance: mechanisms, syndromes and implications. N Engl J Med 1991; 325:935.
14. Taylor SI. Lilly Lecture: molecular mechanisms of insulin resistance. Lessons from patients with mutations in the insulin-receptor gene. Diabetes 1992; 41:1473.
15. O'Brien TD, Rizza RA, Carney JA, Butler PC. Islet amyloidosis in a patient with chronic massive insulin resistance due to antiinsulin receptor antibodies. J Clin Endocrinol Metab 1994; 79:290.
16. Taylor SI, Grunberger G, Marcus-Samuels B, et al. Hypoglycemia associated with antibodies to the insulin receptor. N Engl J Med 1982; 307:1422.
17. Duckworth WC, Bennett RG, Hamel FG. Insulin degradation: progress and potential. Endocr Rev 1998; 19(5):608.
18. Flier JS, Minaker KL, Landsberg L, et al. Impaired in vivo insulin clearance in patients with target cell resistance to insulin. Diabetes 1982; 31:132.
19. Haneda M, Polonsky KS, Tager HS, et al. Familial hyperinsulinemia due to a structurally abnormal insulin: definition of an emerging new clinical syndrome. N Engl J Med 1984; 310:1288.
20. Hotamisligil GS, Shargill NS, Spiegelman BM. Adipose expression of tumor necrosis factor-alpha: direct role in obesity-linked insulin resistance. Science 1993; 259:87.
21. Barosso I, Gurnell M, Crowley VEF, et al. Dominant negative mutations in human PPARγ associated with severe insulin resistance, diabetes mellitus and hypertension. Nature 1999; 402:880.
22. Flier JS. The metabolic importance of acanthosis nigricans. Arch Dermatol 1985; 121:193.
23. Ober KP. Acanthosis nigricans and insulin resistance associated with hypothyroidism. Arch Dermatol 1985; 121:229.
24. Bishop JM. The molecular genetics of cancer. Science 1987; 235:305.
25. Flier JS, Eastman RC, Minaker KL, et al. Acanthosis nigricans in obese women with hyperandrogenism: characterization of an insulin-resistant state distinct from the type A and type B syndromes. Diabetes 1985; 34:101.
26. Kahn CR, Flier JS, Bar RS, et al. The syndromes of insulin resistance and acanthosis nigricans: insulin receptor disorders in man. N Engl J Med 1976; 294:739.
27. Peters EJ, Stuart CA, Prince MJ. Acanthosis nigricans and obesity: acquired and intrinsic defects in insulin action. Metabolism 1986; 35:807.
28. Poretsky L, Kalin MF. The gonadotropic function of insulin. Endocr Rev 1987; 8:132.
29. Poretsky L. On the paradox of insulin-induced hyperandrogenism in insulin resistant states. Endocr Rev 1991; 12:3.
30. Dunaif A. Insulin resistance and ovarian dysfunction in insulin resistance. In: Moller D, ed. Insulin resistance. New York: John Wiley and Sons, 1993:301.
31. Poretsky L, Grigorescu F, Seibel M, et al. Distribution and characterization of insulin and insulin-like growth factor I (IGF-I) receptors in normal human ovary. J Clin Endocrinol Metab 1985; 61:728.

32. Adashi EY, Resnick CE, Hernandez ER, et al. Characterization and regulation of a specific cell membrane receptor for somatomedin-C insulin-like growth factor I in cultured rat granulosa cells. Endocrinology 1988; 122:194.

33. Veldhuis JD, Kolp LA, Toaff ME, et al. Mechanisms subserving the trophic actions of insulin on ovarian cells. J Clin Invest 1983; 72:1046.

34. Veldhuis JD, Nestler JE, Strauss JF III. The insulin-like growth factor, somatomedin-C, modulates low density lipoprotein metabolism by swine granulosa cells. J Endocrinol 1987; 113:21.

35. Veldhuis JD, Rodgers RJ. Mechanisms subserving the steroidogenic synergism between follicle-stimulating hormone and insulin-like growth factor I (somatomedin C). Alterations in cellular sterol metabolism in swine granulosa cells. J Biol Chem 1987; 262:7658.

36. Flier JS, Bar RS, Muggeo M, et al. The evolving clinical course of patients with insulin receptor antibodies: spontaneous remission or receptor proliferation with hypoglycemia. J Clin Endocrinol Metab 1978; 47:985.

37. Taylor SI, Grunberger G, Marcus-Samuels B. Hypoglycemia associated with antibodies to the insulin receptor. N Engl J Med 1982; 307:1422.

38. Muggeo M, Flier JS, Abrams RA, et al. Treatment by plasma exchange of a patient with autoantibodies to the insulin receptor. N Engl J Med 1979; 300:477.

39. Tsokos GC, Gorden P, Antonovych T, et al. Lupus nephritis and other autoimmune features in patients with diabetes mellitus due to autoantibody to insulin receptors. Ann Intern Med 1985; 102:176.

40. Flier JS, Kahn CR, Roth J, Bar RS. Antibodies that impair insulin receptor binding in an unusual diabetic syndrome with severe insulin resistance. Science 1975; 190:63.

41. Flier JS, Kahn CR, Jarrett DB, Roth J. Characterization of antibodies to the insulin receptor: a cause of insulin resistant diabetes in man. J Clin Invest 1976; 58:1442.

42. Zhang B, Roth RA. A region of the insulin receptor important for ligand binding (residues 450–601) is recognized by patients' autoimmune antibodies and inhibitory monoclonal antibodies. Proc Natl Acad Sci U S A 1991; 88:9858.

43. Bloise W, Wajchenberg BL, Moncada VY, et al. Atypical antiinsulin antibodies in a patient with type B insulin resistance and scleroderma. J Clin Endocrinol Metab 1989; 68:227.

44. Kahn CR, Baird KL, Flier JS, Jarrett DB. Effect of anti-insulin receptor antibodies on isolated adipocytes. J Clin Invest 1977; 60:1094.

45. Taylor SI, Marcus-Samuels B. Anti-receptor antibodies mimic the effect of insulin to down regulate insulin receptors in cultured human lymphoblastoid cells. J Clin Endocrinol Metab 1984; 58:182.

46. Dons RF, Havlik R, Taylor SI. Clinical disorders associated with autoantibodies to the insulin receptor. Stimulation by passive transfer of immunoglobulins to rats. J Clin Invest 1983; 72:1072.

47. Flier JS, Young JB, Landsberg L. Familial insulin resistance with acanthosis nigricans, acral hypertrophy and muscle cramps: a new syndrome. N Engl J Med 1980; 390:970.

48. Flier JS, Moller DE, Moses AC, et al. Insulin-mediated pseudoacromegaly: clinical and biochemical characterization of a syndrome of selective insulin resistance. J Clin Endocrinol Metab 1993; 76:1533.

49. Flier JS. Virilization and hyperpigmentation in a 15 year old girl. N Engl J Med 1982; 306:1537.

50. Kadowski T, Bevins CL, Cama A, et al. Two mutant alleles of the insulin receptor gene in a patient with extreme insulin resistance. Science 1988; 240:787.

51. Yoshimasa Y, Seino S, Whittaker J, et al. Insulin-resistant diabetes due to a point mutation that prevents proreceptor processing. Science 1988; 240:784.

52. Moller DE, Flier JS. Detection of an alteration in the insulin-receptor gene in a patient with insulin resistance, acanthosis nigricans, and the polycystic ovary syndrome. N Engl J Med 1988; 319:1526.

53. Bar RS, Muggeo M, Kahn CR, et al. Characterization of the insulin receptor in patients with syndromes of insulin resistance and acanthosis nigricans. Diabetologia 1980; 18:209.

54. Grigorescu F, Flier JS, Kahn CR. Characterization of binding and phosphorylation defects of insulin receptors in the type A syndrome of insulin resistance. Diabetes 1986; 35:127.

55. Podskalny JM, Kahn CR. Cell culture studies on patients with extreme insulin resistance. I. Receptor defects on cultured fibroblasts. J Clin Endocrinol Metab 1982; 54:261.

56. Grigorescu F, Flier JS, Kahn CR. Defect in insulin receptor phosphorylation in erythrocytes and fibroblasts associated with severe insulin resistance. J Biol Chem 1984; 259:15003.

57. Taylor SI, Samuels B, Roth J. Decreased insulin binding in cultured lymphocytes from two patients with extreme insulin resistance. J Clin Endocrinol Metab 1982; 54:919.

58. Whittaker J, Zick Y, Roth J, Taylor SI. Insulin-stimulated receptor phosphorylation appears normal in cultured Epstein-Barr virus-transformed lymphocyte cell lines derived from patients with extreme insulin resistance. J Clin Endocrinol Metab 1985; 60:381.

59. Grunberger G, Zick Y, Gorden P. Defect in phosphorylation of insulin receptors in cells from an insulin-resistant patient with normal insulin binding. Science 1984; 223:932.

60. Moller DE, Cohen O, Yamaguchi Y, et al. Prevalence of mutations, in the insulin receptor gene in subjects with features of the type A syndrome of insulin resistance. Diabetes 1994; 43:247.

61. Podskalny JM, Kahn CR. Cell culture studies on patients with extreme insulin resistance. II. Abnormal biological responses in cultured fibroblasts. J Clin Endocrinol Metab 1982; 54:269.

62. Moller DE, Cohen O, Yamaguchi Y, et al. Prevalence of mutations of the insulin receptor gene in subjects with features of the type A syndrome of insulin resistance. Diabetes 1994; 43:247.

63. Krook A, Kumar S, Laing I, et al. Molecular scanning of the insulin receptor gene in syndromes of insulin resistance. Diabetes 1994; 43:357.

64. Krook A, O'Rahilly S. Mutant receptors in syndromes of insulin resistance. Clin Endocrinol Metab 1996; 10:97.

65. Maddux BA, Goldfine ID. Membrane glycoprotein PC-1 inhibition of insulin receptor function occurs via direct interaction with the receptor alpha-subunit. Diabetes 2000; 49(1):13.

66. Sbraccia P, Goodman PA, Maddux BA, et al. Production of an inhibitor of insulin receptor tyrosine kinase in fibroblasts from a patient with insulin resistance and NIDDM. Diabetes 1991; 40:295.

67. Mendenhall EN. Tumor of the pineal gland with high insulin resistance. J Indiana State Med Assoc 1950; 43:32.

68. Donohue WL, Uchida I. Leprechaunism: a euphemism for a rare familial disorder. J Pediatr 1954; 45:505.

69. Knight AB, Rechler MM, Romanus JA, et al. Stimulation of glucose incorporation and amino acid transport by insulin and an insulin-like growth factor in fibroblasts with defective insulin receptors cultured from a patient with leprechaunism. Proc Natl Acad Sci U S A 1981; 78:2554.

70. Taylor SI, Roth J, Blizzard RM, Elders MJ. Qualitative abnormalities in insulin binding in a patient with extreme insulin resistance: decreased sensitivity to alterations in temperature and pH. Proc Natl Acad Sci U S A 1981; 76:7157.

71. Berardinelli W. An undiagnosed endocrinometabolic syndrome: report of 2 cases. J Clin Endocrinol Metab 1954; 14:193.

72. Garg A, Wilson R, Barnes R, et al. A gene for congenital generalized lipodystrophy maps to human chromosome 9q34. J Clin Endocrinol Metab 1999; 84(9):3390.

73. Kobberling J, Dunningan MG. Familial partial lipodystrophy: two types of an X linked dominant syndrome, lethal in the hemizygous state. J Med Genet 1986; 23:120.

74. Peters JM, Barnes R, Bennett L, et al. Localization of the gene for familial partial lipodystrophy (Dunningan variety) to chromosome 1q21–22. Nat Genet 1998; 18:292.

75. Cao H, Hegele RA. Nuclear lamin A/C R482Q mutation in Canadian kindreds with Dunningan-type familial partial lipodystrophy. Hum Molec Genet 2000; 9:109.

76. Tsiodras S, Mantzoros C, Hammer S, Samore M. Effects of protease inhibitors on hyperglycemia, hyperlipidemia and lipodystrophy. A five-year cohort study. Arch Intern Med 2000; (in press).

77. Vigouroux C, Khallouf E, Bourut C, et al. Genetic exclusion of 14 candidate genes in lipoatrophic diabetes using linkage analysis in 10 consanguineous families. J Clin Endocrinol Metab 1997; 82:3438.

78. Oseid S. Decreased binding of insulin to its receptor in patients with congenital generalized lipodystrophy. N Engl J Med 1977; 296:245.

79. Rosenbloom AL. Normal insulin binding to cultured fibroblasts from patients with lipoatrophic diabetes. J Clin Endocrinol Metab 1977; 44:803.

80. Wachslicht-Rodbard H, Muggeo M, Kahn CR, et al. Heterogeneity of the insulin-receptor interaction in lipoatrophic diabetes. J Clin Endocrinol Metab 1981; 52:416.

81. Dib K, Whitehead JP, Humphreys PJ, et al. Impaired activation of phosphoinositide 3 kinase by insulin in fibroblasts from patients with severe insulin resistance and pseudoacromegaly. J Clin Invest 1998; 101:1111.

82. Tritos NA, Mantzoros CS. Clinical review 97: syndromes of severe insulin resistance. J Clin Endocrinol Metab 1998; 83:3025.

82a. Marchini C, Lonigro R, Verriello L, et al. Correlations between individual clinical manifestations and CTG repeat amplification in myotonic dystrophy. Clin Genet 2000; 57:74.

83. Uotani S, Yamaguchi Y, Yokota A, et al. Molecular analysis of insulin receptor gene in Werner's syndrome. Diabetes Res Clin Pract 1994; 26:175.

83a. Abe T, Yamaguchi Y, Izumino K, et al. Evaluation of insulin response in glucose tolerance test in a patient with Werner's syndrome: a 16-year follow-up study. Diabetes Nutr Metab 2000; 13:113.

84. Freidenberg GR, White N, Cataland S, et al. Diabetes response to intravenous but not subcutaneous effectiveness of aprotinin. N Engl J Med 1981; 305:363.

85. Schade DS, Duckworth WC. In search of the subcutaneous-insulin-resistance syndrome. N Engl J Med 1986; 315:147.

86. Mantzoros CS, Moses AC. Treatment of severe insulin resistance. In: Azziz R, Nestler JE, Dewailly D, eds. Androgen excess disorders in women. Philadelphia: Lippincott–Raven, 1997:247.

87. Dunaif A, Scott D, Finegood D, et al. The insulin-sensitizing agent troglitazone improves metabolic and reproductive abnormalities in the polycystic ovary syndrome. J Clin Endocrinol Metab 1996; 81(9):3299.

88. Ehrmann DA. Insulin-lowering therapeutic modalities for polycystic ovary syndrome. Endocrinol Metab Clin North Am 1999; 28(2):423.

89. Vestergaard H, Rossen M, Urhammer SA, et al. Short and long-term metabolic effects of recombinant human IGF-I treatment in patients with severe insulin resistance and diabetes mellitus. Eur J Endocrinol 1997; 136:475.

90. Nakae J, Kato M, Murashita M, et al. Long-term effect of recombinant human IGF-I on metabolic and growth control in a patient with leprechaunism. J Clin Endocrinol Metab 1998; 83:542.

91. Mantzoros CS, Tzonou A, Signorello LB, et al. Insulin-like growth factor 1 in relation to prostate cancer and benign prostatic hyperplasia. Br J Cancer 1997; 76:1115.

92. Shaneyfelt T, Husein R, Bubley G, Mantzoros C. Hormonal predictors of prostate cancer. A meta-analysis. J Clin Oncol 2000; 18:847.
93. Wolk A, Mantzoros CS, Andersson SO, et al. Insulin-like growth factor 1 and prostate cancer risk: a population-based, case-control study. J Natl Cancer Inst 1998; 17;90(12):911.
94. Bohlke K, Cramer DW, Trichopoulos D, Mantzoros CS. Insulin-like growth factor-I in relation to premenopausal ductal carcinoma in situ of the breast. Epidemiology 1998; 9(5):570.
95. Manousos O, Souglakos J, Bosetti C, et al. IGF-I and IGF-II in relation to colorectal cancer. Int J Cancer 1999; 24;83(1):15.
96. Chan JM, Stampfer MJ, Giovannucci E, et al. Plasma insulin-like growth factor-I and prostate cancer risk: a prospective study. Science 1998; 23;279(5350):563.
97. Izumino K, Sakamaki H, Ishibashi M, et al. Troglitazone ameliorates insulin resistance in patients with Werner's syndrome. J Clin Endocrinol Metab 1997; 82:2391.
98. Goldfine AB, Simonson DC, Folli F, et al. Metabolic effects of sodium metavanadate in humans with insulin-dependent and noninsulin-dependent diabetes mellitus: in vivo and in vitro studies. J Clin Endocrinol Metab 1995; 80:3311.
99. Panz VR, Wing JR, Raal FJ, et al. Improved glucose tolerance after effective lipid-lowering therapy with bezafibrate in a patient with lipoatrophic diabetes mellitus: a putative role for Randle's cycle in its pathogenesis? Clin Endocrinol (Oxf) 1997; 46:365.
100. Mantzoros CS, Lawrence WD, Levy J. Insulin resistance in a patient with ovarian stromal hyperthecosis and the hyperandrogenism, insulin resistance and acanthosis nigricans syndrome. Report of a case with a possible endogenous ovarian factor. J Reprod Med 1995; 40(6):491.

# CHAPTER 147

# CARDIOVASCULAR COMPLICATIONS OF DIABETES MELLITUS

KARIN HEHENBERGER AND GEORGE L. KING

Diabetes mellitus often causes many chronic complications, including cardiovascular disease, retinopathy, nephropathy, neuropathy, and chronic foot ulcers involving both micro- and macrovessels.[1,2] The presence and severity of these microangiopathies and cardiovascular diseases are associated with the duration, the severity of metabolic disturbances, and modulation by genetic factors (Fig. 147-1). Due to these vascular diseases, diabetes is a major contributor to cardiovascular morbidity and mortality, to blindness, and to renal failure. The increase in cardiovascular mortality results from the acceleration of atherosclerosis of coronary and peripheral arteries, cardiomyopathy, and cardiac neuropathy. In addition, diabetes is associated with an unusual

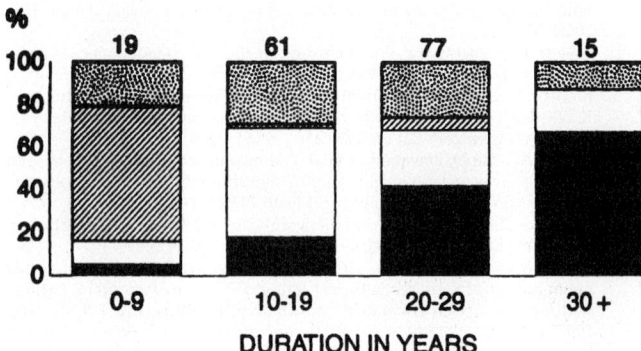

**FIGURE 147-1.** Causes of death in insulin-dependent (type 1) diabetic patients. (■, cardiovascular; ▢, renal; ▨, other diabetes related; ▦, nondiabetes related.) (From Orchard TJ. From diagnosis and classification to complications and therapy. Diabetes Care 1994; 17:326.)

vascular sclerosis arising from calcification of the media of large arteries (termed *Monckeberg sclerosis*), which rarely occurs in the nondiabetic population.[3] Many studies have suggested that the increased cardiovascular risks in diabetic patients are due to multiple factors, with alterations in many vascular cell functions. Among these factors are insulin resistance, hyperlipidemia, endothelial dysfunction, hypertension, hypercoagulation, and hyperglycemia.[4–8] Prospective studies have demonstrated that lipid-lowering drugs and antihypertensive agents in combination with glycemic control can clearly decrease the mortality of diabetes patients due to cardiovascular diseases.[8]

This chapter reviews the pathology of the various cardiovascular diseases previously stated and describes the possible mechanisms. Current treatment regimens are outlined at the end of the chapter.

## EPIDEMIOLOGY

An excess of coronary artery disease (CAD) in patients with insulin-dependent diabetes mellitus (type 1) is usually observed in patients older than 30 years of age.[4–6] The cardiovascular risk in the diabetic population has been assessed by many studies[5,6,8,9]; among these, the Framingham Study (a longitudinal survey of >5000 patients with a follow-up of 18 years) demonstrated that the incidence of the major clinical manifestations of coronary disease was higher in diabetic patients.[9] Type 1 diabetics followed for 20 to 40 years had a 33% incidence of death due to CAD between the ages of 30 and 55, whereas for nondiabetics in the same age group, the incidence of death due to CAD was only 8% among men and 4% among women.[5] There was not only an excess of mortality among these patients, but also an excess of symptomatic and asymptomatic CAD among survivors. Among women, there was a significant twofold increase in incidence of the major clinical manifestations of coronary disease. The risks of CAD in men and women with type 1 diabetes are similar and increase at the same rate after age 30 regardless of whether the onset of diabetes was in early childhood or in late adolescence.

In noninsulin-dependent diabetes (type 2), the prevalence of CAD is also increased. Furthermore, CAD and type 2 diabetes frequently cluster in families.[5–9] Hyperinsulinemia and insulin resistance, which often precede type 2 diabetes, are also independent predictors of the development of elevated blood pressure and lipid abnormalities.[7,10–14] In the presence of type 2 diabetes, risk factors for CAD become more prevalent and more intense.

In the Framingham Study, it was found that the risk of CAD increases with duration; this reflects the effect of the aging process. In contrast, in patients with diabetes, the increased risk may reflect the combined effects of aging and duration of diabetes.[9] More than 50% of mortality in diabetic patients is related to cardiovascular diseases—the risk for developing cardiac or cerebrovascular disease is two to four times higher in diabetic patients than in the general population. The effect of diabetes on CAD risk may be greater for women than for men (five-fold increase in women compared to a two-fold increase in men). Several studies have shown that type 2 diabetics treated with insulin have a higher risk of CAD than do noninsulin-treated type 2 diabetics, indicating that the severity of the disease, the loss of islet cell functions, or exogenous insulin treatment may have a greater impact on CAD.[7,10,11]

Diabetes also has a significant adverse impact on peripheral vascular disease and congestive heart failure. For CAD, not only is diabetes synergistic with other risk factors (age, hypercholesterolemia, hypertension, and smoking), but it also is an independent risk factor.[9,12–22] The extent and complexity of coronary artery lesions in diabetic patients are greater than those in the general population. (It is not certain whether atherosclerosis is more diffuse within the coronary vasculature in diabetic patients as compared with the general population. If so, this could be clinically important, because diffuse coronary lesions limit the ability to treat coronary disease by surgical means.)

Hyperinsulinemia may be an important risk factor for ischemic heart disease. Among >2000 men who did not have ischemic heart disease, those persons who eventually experienced a coronary event had higher fasting insulin levels, even after controlling for lipid levels. High fasting insulin concentrations appeared to be an independent predictor of ischemic heart disease in men.[7]

Myocardial infarction is the leading cause of death in both type 1 and 2 diabetic patients.[5,6,9,14,17] This results not only from the higher incidence of CAD, but also from the higher acute and long-term mortality in diabetic patients who have had a myocardial infarction.[23,24,27] Several prospective studies have been performed to determine whether a more intensive insulin treatment protocol can decrease the morbidity and mortality due to cardiovascular events in diabetic patients. In the University Group Diabetes Program (UGDP), a more intensive insulin strategy was not associated with a change in cardiovascular event rates when compared to standard insulin or diet therapy.[25] Intensive insulin therapy in newly diagnosed nonobese, insulin-sensitive, type 2 diabetic Japanese patients slowed the progression of retinopathy, nephropathy, and neuropathy, but had too few cardiovascular events to detect the effect of intensive glucose management.[26] A Swedish study comparing intensive insulin with standard antidiabetic therapy in patients with a recent myocardial infarction[23,24] showed that the very high death rates in the first 3.4 years after myocardial infarction in diabetes (44%) can be significantly lowered by early intensive insulin management (33%). Most of these patients (82%) had type 2 diabetes. This effect was observed within a few months after infarction, and may have been the result of the action of insulin on platelet function, thrombosis, or myocardial dysfunction after coronary occlusion, rather than of an effect on long-term atherosclerotic disease. In fact, the risk of myocardial infarction in diabetic patients without a history of myocardial infarction is equal to that of nondiabetic patients with a history of myocardial infarction.[27]

The United Kingdom Prospective Diabetes Study (UKPDS) in newly diagnosed type 2 diabetic patients examined the issue of glycemic control and complications.[8] This study showed that intensive glucose control is associated with a 12% reduction in the risk of pooled macrovascular and microvascular events. However, the effect is primarily due to the slowing of progression of microvascular rather than macrovascular events.

## PATHOLOGY

### ATHEROSCLEROSIS

In general, the atherosclerotic lesions in diabetic patients are similar, but they appear earlier and in greater number as compared to the nondiabetic population.

The earliest lesions are fatty streaks in focal areas of the intima, characterized microscopically by the presence of macrophages, lipid deposits, and smooth muscle cells. Later lesions include fibrofatty plaques. The latest, complicated lesions are characterized by fibrosis, calcium deposits, plaque fissuring, hemorrhage, and thrombosis.[12–22a]

### CARDIAC PATHOLOGY

Histologic abnormalities in the hearts of diabetic patients can occur at all levels of the myocardium, extending from the basement membrane to major intramural arteries.[13,14,28–30] Specifically, the thickness of the capillary basement membrane is increased in the myocardium, as it is in all tissues. In addition,

small capillaries and venules exhibit aneurysmal formation and, occasionally, intense vasospasm, which can lead to a state of transient myocardial ischemia. The arterial vasculature also exhibits changes, consisting of medial hypertrophy, endothelial thickening, and a thickened extracellular matrix of the intramural arterioles. Autonomic nerve pathologies can be found in diabetic patients with reduced myelinated fiber density, degeneration and regeneration of unmyelinated fibers, and capillary basement membrane thickening.[30] In the myocardium, fibrosis, hypertrophy, and increased extracellular matrix are commonly observed.[28]

Changes in cardiac function and histology also occur in animal models of diabetes. There is an impairment in the development of left ventricular pressure and a delay in the rate of muscle relaxation.[31] However, some differences have been reported between type 1 and type 2 diabetic animal models. First, the heart of the type 1 animal has a greater impairment in generating tension against an elevated preload. Second, the hearts of type 2 animals exhibit a greater decrease in cardiac compliance than do those of type 1 diabetic animals; these findings have been observed in diabetic patients as well.[31–35]

Increases in fatty acids and triglycerides have been noted in the cardiac tissues of diabetic animals, possibly as a result of elevated plasma levels. Increases in fatty acid metabolism elevate the accumulation of citric acid cycle intermediates, which are potent inhibitors of phosphofructokinase, a rate-limiting enzyme of glycolysis. Glycolysis and glucose oxidation are hindered further by decreases in glucose uptake and in activities of pyruvate dehydrogenase, which are regulated by insulin.[36] These changes in carbohydrate metabolism may be partly responsible for the dysfunction in the heart under stress. Besides abnormal glucose metabolism, abnormalities of calcium transport between the sarcolemma and the sarcoplasmic reticulum have also been reported.[37,38] Since $Ca^{2+}$ fluxes are important for cardiac contractility, the decrease in the $Ca^{2+}$ pool may be responsible for some of the reduction of the contractility observed in the cardiac muscles of diabetic animals and humans. The decreases in contractility in the heart could also be due to changes of the predominant active form of myosin adenosine triphosphatase (ATPase) in the heart to a less active type.[38] The $a_1$-adrenoceptor is decreased in diabetic rats; this change could be the result of protein kinase C (PKC) activation.[38,39] Furthermore, other changes (e.g., cardiac lipoprotein lipase abnormalities, altered G-protein actions, increased NADPH/NADP [nicotinamide adenine dinucleotide phosphate] ratio, increased type IV collagen, and decreased [$\gamma$-2-$(Na^+)$-$K^+$-ATPase] activities) have all been reported.[40–42]

At the molecular level, the expression of multiple genes in the heart is altered by diabetes. *Glucose transporter* (GLUT4), which is expressed mostly in insulin-sensitive tissue (e.g., muscle, fat, and the heart), is reduced in diabetic rats, leading to the hypothesis that the decrease in glucose transport could be partially responsible for the decrease in cardiac work. The expression of cardiac myosin heavy chain shifts from predominantly $\alpha$ to predominantly $\beta$, with the onset of diabetes; this effect is reversed by insulin administration. The expression of $Ca^{2+}$ ATPase mRNA is reduced in diabetic as well as in insulin-resistant obese mice, providing an explanation for the delay in diastolic relaxation.[41,42] The expression of *core 2 transferase*, an enzyme involved in O-linked glycosylation, is increased in the myocardium of diabetic animals. This finding could explain the increased enzymatic glycosylation observed in the hearts of diabetic patients.[43]

Thus, cardiac dysfunction in diabetic patients can be due to atherosclerotic changes in the coronary macrovessels or due to metabolic alterations of the myocardium resulting from exposure to the abnormal metabolic milieu of diabetic patients. Although glycemic control may be able to reverse the latter changes, the data are not clear concerning any beneficial effects in preventing or reversing atherosclerotic pathologies.

## ENDOTHELIAL CELLS

Endothelial cells have an active role in maintaining vascular function involving anticoagulation, contractility, leukocyte trafficking, and vascular permeability. Endothelial cells can produce large numbers of vasoactive agents (e.g., platelet-derived growth factor [PDGF], endothelin, prostaglandins, and various other cytokines; see Chap. 173) that have significant effects on the metabolism and proliferation of vascular cells. Moreover, large polypeptides (e.g., insulin-like growth factors [IGFs] and low-density lipoproteins [LDL]) have receptors on the endothelial cells, and may be transported across the cells in a receptor-mediated transcytosis pathway.[44,45] Injury to the endothelium can result in alteration of its many functions, thereby decreasing its nonthrombogenic surfaces and releasing factors that affect smooth muscle cells.[18–20,46,47] In the diabetic environment, many factors, such as hyperglycemia, insulin resistance, increased plasma LDL, decreased high-density lipoproteins (HDL), abnormal rheologic factors, platelet aggregation, and coagulation, can contribute to endothelial cell injury.[13–22,47–49] Much interest has been focused on insulin's effects on endothelial cells, especially the blunting of insulin's vasodilatory effects in insulin-resistant states.[50] Infusion of insulin can cause vasodilation in several local vascular beds (e.g., leg, arm, and retina). However, insulin does not appear to induce any acute systemic vascular changes (i.e., consistent changes in blood pressure or pulse rates have not been observed). The vasodilatory effect of insulin is mediated by increases in nitric oxide (NO) production, either by activating or by enhancing the expression of NO synthase.[50,51] The physiologic importance of insulin's acute vasodilatory effect is unclear; it is minor in comparison to other vasodilators, such as acetylcholine. Chronically, insulin may modulate the level of endothelial nitric oxide (eNO) and regulate endothelial functions. Hyperglycemia alters endothelial functions (e.g., increased production of oxidants, increased production of adhesion molecules, and decreased production of NO). As a result of these factors, many functions mediated by the endothelium are abnormal in the diabetic state, leading to conditions favoring atherosclerosis.[52,52a]

## SMOOTH MUSCLE CELLS

Smooth muscle cells, which play a major role in the development of atherosclerosis, are found in fibrous plaques and fatty streaks, together with macrophages and monocytes. In general, smooth muscle cells can incorporate a variety of lipid particles, migrate into the intima, and proliferate. Among the many growth factors that have been implicated in this process are PDGF, IGFs, angiotensin, growth hormone (GH), and endothelin. The most-studied of these factors in diabetic conditions is insulin, because multiple epidemiologic studies have suggested a connection between hyperinsulinemia, insulin resistance, and atherosclerosis.[7,10,51–54] Since insulin can enhance the migration and proliferation of smooth muscle cells, it has been postulated that the hyperinsulinemia observed in insulin resistance states may enhance the atherosclerotic process. However, the mitogenic effects of insulin on smooth muscle cells are relatively weak and require insulin concentrations 10 to 50 times above the physiologic levels. Nonetheless, insulin resistance appears to be consistently associated with an increased risk of atherosclerosis. Thus, it is likely that insulin has antiatherosclerotic effects, such as the activation of eNO activity. In insulin-resistant states, insulin's effects are decreased, thereby accelerating atherosclerosis.[51–54] Studies on insulin's direct effects on the vasculature of insulin-resistant animals have shown that there is a selective inhibition of insulin's acute actions (e.g., on NO production), but its chronic effects are not impaired.[55]

## HEMATOGENOUS FACTORS

In the blood, platelets and macrophages play important roles in the development of atherosclerosis. They secrete vasoactive factors, including PDGF, fibroblast growth factor (FGF), tumor necrosis factor (TNF), and other cytokines.[56–60] Abnormalities in the platelet function of diabetic patients[13] include increased sensitivity to aggregation and augmented synthesis of prothrombotic prostaglandins such as thromboxane $A_2$.[60] These abnormalities enhance the release of growth factors and other cytokines both in platelets and vascular cells.

The plasma of diabetics also contains another group of atherogenic components, namely abnormal lipids and lipoproteins (see Chap. 166). In more than half of diabetic patients, especially type 2 diabetic patients, a decrease in HDL cholesterol and hypertriglyceridemia occurs.[12,61,62]

LDLs are the main carrier of cholesterol to tissues. Elevation of LDL levels is associated with an early onset of atherosclerosis. In type 2 diabetics and in poorly controlled type 1 diabetics, LDL cholesterol levels are reported to be elevated. Furthermore, LDLs are modified in diabetes; hyperglycemia can increase levels of glycated or oxidized LDL,[63,64] which are internalized less and, hence, less degraded. The LDLs of diabetic patients may also be enriched in triglycerides, thus increasing the modified or small dense LDLs that are known to be more atherogenic.[65] These altered LDLs can bind to circulating macrophages, which can then interact with the vascular cell wall, releasing vasoactive factors and becoming foam cells.

The most common lipid abnormality in diabetic patients is hypertriglyceridemia.[65–68] This is likely due to a decrease in the lipoprotein lipase (LPL) activity, which is necessary for the breakdown of chylomicrons and triglycerides.[66] Thus, the plasma levels of chylomicrons and very low-density lipoproteins (VLDL) are elevated.[65–68] The elevation of triglycerides has been reported mainly in type 2 diabetic patients, since insulin is a major regulator of LPL activity.[69] Increases of VLDL levels accelerate the atherosclerotic process in a number of ways: (a) VLDL may be toxic for the metabolism and growth of endothelial cells,[70] and (b) VLDL from diabetic animals may deposit more lipids in macrophages, which can be precursors of foam cells in the arterial walls.[13–20]

Plasma HDL levels may also be decreased in diabetic patients,[67,68] especially those with insulin resistance. The role of HDL is to remove cholesterol from peripheral tissue; hence, a low HDL level is associated with the premature onset of atherosclerosis. HDL levels can be elevated by improved plasma glucose control, by using either insulin or by decreasing insulin resistance.[55] The decrease in HDL is probably due to the diminution of insulin-sensitive LPL, which indirectly causes a decrease in the transfer of phospholipids and proteins from VLDL and chylomicrons to $HDL_3$, resulting in a decrease of $HDL_{2A}$, which is important for transferring cholesterol. HDL catabolism may be accelerated because of the increased nonenzymatic glycosylation of HDL.[64] Some reports indicate that this decrease in HDL levels is much greater in women than in men, perhaps explaining the increased risk of cardiovascular events in women with diabetes.

## METABOLIC FACTORS THAT CONTRIBUTE TO THE DEVELOPMENT OF CARDIOVASCULAR DISEASE

### HYPERGLYCEMIA

Hyperglycemia has been postulated to have a major role in the development of complications in diabetic patients.[8,71] In both type 1 and type 2 diabetic patients, strict metabolic control can reduce cardiovascular and microvascular complications.[8] Sev-

**TABLE 147-1.**
**Possible Mechanisms of Hyperglycemia's Adverse Effects**

Sorbitol-myoinositol changes (via aldose reductase pathway)
Oxidant-redox potential alterations
Nonenzymatic glycation reactions
Activation of protein kinase C (PKC)
Diacylglycerol (DAG) pathway

eral theories have been proposed to explain the adverse effects of hyperglycemia on vascular cells (Table 147-1). One theory is based on the finding that intracellular levels of sorbitol are increased, due to an augmented conversion via aldose reductase within the cells.[72,73] The high concentrations of sorbitol may alter cellular functions by osmotic changes or by altering levels of myoinositol and other enzymes, such as $Na^+$-$K^+$-ATPase (see Chap. 148). The metabolism of sorbitol may also alter the NAD/NADH ratio, thus potentially altering vascular cellular metabolism.

A second theory suggests that in patients with poorly controlled diabetes, hyperglycemia may interact with primary amines of proteins to form nonenzymatic glycation products with cellular and matrix proteins.[74,75] Glycated proteins (e.g., albumin or LDL) may interact differently with vascular cells to cause injury to endothelial cells and to increase the proliferation of smooth muscle cells.[63,64] In addition, the degradation products of cross-linked proteins may interact with specific receptors on macrophages, which then release vasoactive substances (e.g., PDGF or TNF). Possibly, hyperglycemia may also enhance the effects of other risk factors (e.g., lipoproteins). Nonenzymatic glycation of proteins can also lead to increased formation of oxidative products that can react with lipids and proteins to cause vascular changes and damage.[74-76]

Another likely candidate for causing the adverse effects of hyperglycemia is an increased production of oxidants. As stated previously, hyperglycemia can increase oxidant production in at least two ways: by the nonenzymatic glycation process and by enhanced production of $H_2O_2$ via an increase in the mitochondrial flux.[76,77] Evidence in support of an increase in oxidative stress can be observed in vascular tissues, as measured by elevations in lipid peroxidation and levels of antioxidative enzymes. Treatment with antioxidants, such as vitamins E and C, has been reported to prevent early changes in the cardiovascular system in diabetic animals, although the plasma levels of these vitamins are probably not significantly reduced in diabetes.[78,79]

Lastly, changes in signal transduction of the vascular cells induced by hyperglycemia can also cause cardiovascular complications. One of the best-documented changes in vascular tissues is the activation of PKC.[80-84] The activation of PKC appears to regulate a number of vascular and hematologic functions, including vascular permeability, contractility, cellular proliferation, basement membrane synthesis, platelet aggregation, macrophage activation, and signaling mechanisms for various cytokines and hormones.[85,86] Since the vascular pathologies of diabetes mellitus and atherosclerosis exhibit changes in all of these properties, activation of PKC is likely to play a role.

Elevated levels of glucose in diabetes mellitus can activate PKC by increasing the formation of diacylglycerol (DAG), one of two physiologic regulators of PKC (calcium is the other). In animals with chemically or genetically induced diabetes, intracellular DAG levels and PKC activity are elevated in many vascular tissues (i.e., the retina, aorta, heart, and renal glomeruli[80-84]), as well as in noncardiovascular tissues (i.e., the liver[87]; Fig. 147-2). Elevated PKC has been reported in monocytes, platelets, and (possibly) the myocardium of diabetic patients. Oxidants and glycation products have also been reported to activate PKC in

vascular cells, suggesting that alteration in signal transduction in the vascular cells could be the common downstream mechanism by which hyperglycemia causes many of its adverse effects.[88,89]

Functional abnormalities in diabetes, such as changes in blood flow and contractility, can be observed in many organs (e.g., retina, kidney, skin, large vessels, and microvessels of peripheral nerves) of diabetic patients and animals. In animal models of diabetes, decreases in neuronal and retinal blood flow can be normalized by intravitreous injection of an isoform-specific PKC inhibitor (LY333531).[81,82-90] In the kidney, an elevated glomerular filtration rate is a common finding in patients with short-term diabetes mellitus[91] and in experimental animal models of diabetes.[92] This may be the result of hyperglycemia-induced decreases in afferent arteriolar resistance.[91,92] Transgenic mice overexpressing the $PKC\beta$ isoform specifically in the myocardium develop cardiac hypertrophy and fibrosis, which are likewise observed in diabetic cardiomyopathy.[93]

## HORMONES

The levels of many hormones are altered in the plasma of diabetic patients; some of these substances have been reported to be vasoactive or trophic. Those that have been associated with an increased risk of cardiovascular disease are described briefly.

Elevated plasma insulin levels (either in fasting states as may occur in type 2 diabetes or in patients treated with exogenous insulin) may enhance the proliferation of arterial smooth muscle cells, especially in the presence of other growth factors.[56-59] Hyperinsulinemia and insulin resistance have been associated with the development of hypertension and an increased risk of macrovascular diseases in diabetic or insulin-resistant patients. However, only insulin resistance appears to be consistently associated across all ethnic groups. The molecular explanation of how insulin resistance can cause acceleration of atherosclerosis has been studied intensively without any clear conclusion. To summarize briefly, insulin has multiple effects on the endothelial and smooth muscle cells, including activation of NO, protein synthesis, expression of cytokines and extracellular proteins, and growth. In general, there appears to be a selective resistance to insulin's actions in the vascular tissue. For example, insulin's vasodilation effect, as mediated by increasing NO production, is blunted in the insulin-resistant state and in type 2 diabetes.[50,51] Yet, insulin's mitogenic effect on smooth muscle cells appears to be unaffected (Fig. 147-2). These findings indicate that insulin's physiologic effects (e.g., on NO production) are mainly antiatherogenic. The loss of

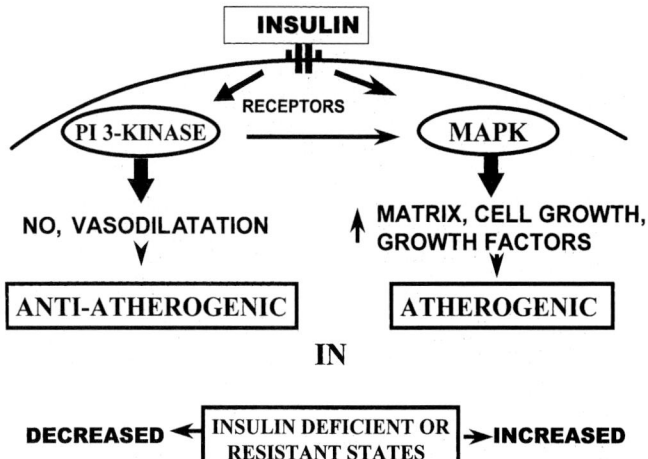

**FIGURE 147-2.** Schematic description of insulin's potential vascular actions in physiologic and insulin-deficient or resistant state. (*MAPK,* mitogen-activated protein kinase; *NO,* nitric oxide.)

these effects in insulin-resistant states creates conditions that can enhance atherosclerosis without the requirement for hyperinsulinemia. If hyperinsulinemia is present, then the migration and growth of smooth muscle cells may also be enhanced. However, it is unclear whether insulin's growth-promoting effects have any physiologic significance, since this would require plasma insulin concentrations that are 10 to 100 times above the levels normally encountered.

IGF-I, IGF-II, and GH also increase the synthesis of DNA and induce cellular proliferation of smooth muscle cells.[94,95] However, these growth factors probably do not have a major role in initiating atherosclerosis, because in conditions in which GH and IGF-I levels are elevated (e.g., acromegaly), the prevalence of atherosclerosis is not significantly increased. Some reports indicate that GH replacement therapy may decrease atherosclerosis in GH-deficient individuals. Levels of counter-regulatory hormones (e.g., cortisol and catecholamines) are also elevated. In this regard, there is some suggestive evidence that CAD is increased in Cushing syndrome and in patients treated with prednisone.[96]

Increased angiotensin actions have also been suggested, since treatment with angiotensin-converting enzyme inhibitors can decrease the risk of nephropathy and possible cardiovascular events in diabetic patients. However, angiotensin levels are not demonstrably elevated in the plasma or vascular tissues of diabetic patients.[97]

## CARDIOLOGIC DISEASES IN DIABETES

Cardiomyopathy without significant CAD has also been described in diabetics, including up to 20% of diabetics who have congestive heart failure. In addition, autonomic neuropathy can cause cardiac arrhythmia.

### CARDIOMYOPATHY

Although the causes of diabetic cardiomyopathy may be multiple, it is clear that the acute metabolic derangements that occur in diabetes can produce alterations in cardiac myofibrillar performance. Numerous studies examining the myocardium of experimental animals and of diabetic patients have demonstrated that altered glucose and free fatty acid metabolism results in a derangement of myocardial performance.[36,41] Tissue culture studies have shown a decrease in the velocity of contraction of myocardial cells when exposed to a high glucose environment. In addition, in the presence of high glucose concentrations, alterations are often found in the relaxation pattern of myocardial cells. Normalization of the glucose concentrations results in restoration of normal contractile relaxation indices.[98]

Diabetic cardiomyopathy has been reported for both type 1 and type 2 diabetics.[31–33] With the use of gated-blood pool studies after vigorous exercise, both type 1 and type 2 diabetic patients have demonstrated an abnormal ejection fraction response. In catheterization studies, consistent abnormalities of cardiac function have been demonstrated in diabetic patients, even those with no or minimal evidence of CAD. These abnormalities have included elevated left ventricular and diastolic pressures, decreased ejection fractions, and increased ventricular wall stiffness. Hemodynamic functional abnormalities, including lower cardiac output and lower left ventricular compliance, have also been found in newly diagnosed diabetic patients under the stress of exercise.

Studies of systolic time intervals and M-mode echocardiography in asymptomatic diabetic patients have revealed an increase of the pre-ejection period (PEP)/left ventricular ejection time (LVET), which is an index of decreased left ventricular contractility and compliance. Other evidence suggests that myocardial dysfunction is related to metabolic control. In one

study, 3 months of intensive insulin therapy reversed the previously noted abnormalities.[33,99]

Despite a preponderance of theoretical evidence, it has been difficult to make a specific diagnosis of diabetic cardiomyopathy, because of other potential etiologies that can lead to poor cardiac function in diabetic patients. In addition, the prevalence of CAD in diabetics could contribute significantly to the systolic or diastolic cardiac impairment. Another confounding factor in diabetics is a history of hypertension, which, by itself, can lead to the development of cardiac abnormalities. Other factors (e.g., renal failure with resultant anemia, hypertension, and volume overload) can impose additional stress on the myocardium, unmasking an underlying diabetic myopathic state. Thus, diabetic cardiomyopathy is frequently the silent partner of a more clinically obvious form of diabetic heart disease. Its effect may influence both the presenting clinical symptoms and the response to therapy.

## CORONARY ARTERY DISEASE IN DIABETES

Multiple large population-based studies have demonstrated that the major clinical complication of long-standing diabetes is atherosclerotic cardiovascular disease.[4–6] The Framingham Study demonstrated a marked prevalence of CAD in both men and women with diabetes.[9] Diabetic men have a two-fold greater risk of dying of ischemic heart disease than do nondiabetic controls. Female diabetic patients are particularly vulnerable to the effects of atherosclerotic heart disease; their incidence of ischemic heart disease is five-fold that of the nondiabetic female population.[9,14]

A review of the coronary angiograms of cardiac patients revealed a higher incidence of atherosclerosis in diabetic patients; they also had had a more diffuse pattern than did nondiabetic patients.[100] Similar conclusions were reached in an angiographic study of patients with juvenile-onset type 1 diabetes. In addition, female juvenile diabetic patients were particularly prone to have a diffuse pattern of coronary artery involvement.

Although classic manifestations of CAD are often observed in the diabetic patient, there may be a discrepancy between the clinical symptoms and the severity of underlying heart disease. Not uncommonly, rather mild symptoms are associated with marked, and potentially life-threatening, coronary artery lesions. Although this phenomenon occurs in many nondiabetic patients with ischemic heart disease, it appears to be more prevalent in people with diabetes. Not uncommonly, diabetic patients with ischemic heart disease may not experience chest pain; they may complain of nonspecific or ambiguous findings such as exertional dyspnea, mild diaphoresis, nausea, and vomiting, or generalized weakness. Thus, in assessing the diabetic patient with CAD, it is important to have a high index of suspicion of underlying atherosclerotic cardiovascular disease and not to be misled by what appear to be mild or stable clinical symptoms.[100]

Because of the subtlety of presentation and the difficulty in relying on symptomatology to assess the clinical severity of coronary atherosclerosis, an objective evaluation using some modality of exercise testing to assess both the presence and the severity of CAD should be performed. Indications for coronary angiography are the same for diabetic and nondiabetic patients. The outcome of coronary bypass graft surgery in diabetic patients is excellent in terms of survival and symptomatic relief.[100] The hazards of angiography per se in diabetic patients are increased only in those patients with abnormal renal function, due to an increased risk of compromising renal function when using radiographic dyes. This risk can be normalized by reducing the dose of the dye, by hydrating the patients, and by the possible use of mannitol to augment urine output and to avoid hypotension. On the day of the procedure, good glucose control should be maintained—either by continuous insulin pump or by splitting the morning dose of insulin (half before the procedure and the remaining half afterward). The blood glucose value should be checked frequently during the patient procedure. A cautionary note should be raised in the care of insulin-taking diabetic patients who are scheduled to undergo cardiac surgery after angiography. There is an increased danger of anaphylaxis after the injection of protamine, which is used to neutralize the actions of administered heparin. The increased rate of reaction is probably due to previous exposure to protamine in the neutral protamine Hagedorn (NPH) insulin used by diabetic patients.[84]

## MYOCARDIAL INFARCTION

In a previous review of morbidity and mortality in diabetics after myocardial infarction,[5,100] an overall mortality of 30% was found; there was a high frequency of congestive heart failure. In addition, 30% of the diabetic patients presenting to the coronary care unit had no pain, compared with <10% of the nondiabetic population. The 1-year mortality was markedly increased (40%) compared with the generally expected mortality of 15% to 20% in the nondiabetic population. A review of the Joslin Diabetes Center experience has confirmed the continuing high mortality in diabetic patients having either an initial or subsequent myocardial infarction.[5] Interestingly, female diabetic patients had a particularly poor prognosis, both for their initial infarct and during the 1 year of follow-up.[5,100]

In a large, multicenter study that examined the 1-year mortality after a myocardial infarction, diabetic patients emerged as a subgroup with a particularly poor prognosis. Although the nondiabetic counterparts experienced only a 10% mortality, the diabetic population had >20% mortality within 2 years.[5,23,28,100] Analysis of multiple cardiovascular parameters did not elucidate the cause of the increased mortality in the diabetic group. Specifically, the extent of myocardial infarction as assessed by global left ventricular function (quantitated by radionuclide ventriculogram) failed to explain the marked discrepancy found between diabetic and nondiabetic patients. In addition, the results of baseline Holter monitoring and low-grade exercise tolerance tests before discharge from the hospital were not statistically different between the two groups. The mode of death in the diabetic group usually consisted of progressive congestive heart failure or sudden death.

Although the underlying cause for the increased mortality is not definitely known, the unique characteristics of diabetic heart disease may be important factors. For example, there is an increased propensity for lethal ventricular arrhythmias, presumably caused by more extensive fibrosis and, hence, less responsiveness to antiarrhythmic agents. In addition, the cardiomyopathic changes unique to diabetes may result in more dramatic abnormalities because of the altered diastolic compliance of the left ventricle. Although indices of systolic performance may be comparable in diabetic and nondiabetic groups, increased stiffness of the diabetic ventricle may aggravate hemodynamic changes and thereby lead to more severe and progressive congestive heart failure.[25] Autonomic neuropathy, particularly the loss of parasympathetic innervation, may predispose to a more vulnerable ventricular myocardium in terms of arrhythmia potential.[101] There is a greater propensity for coronary vasoconstriction to occur in diabetic patients with parasympathetic denervation. Although speculative, some or all of these unique characteristics of diabetic heart disease may be responsible for the increased initial and first-year mortality found in diabetics with acute myocardial infarction.

In the Diabetes Insulin-Glucose in Acute Myocardial Infarction (DIGAMI) study, it was found that intensive metabolic treatment of diabetic patients with acute myocardial infarction with insulin-glucose infusion followed by multidose insulin treatment improved the prognosis.[23,24] The effect was most apparent in patients who had not previously received insulin

treatment and who were at low cardiovascular risk. The overall mortality after 1 year was 19% in the insulin group compared to 26% among controls. The most frequent cause of death in all patients was congestive heart failure, but cardiovascular mortality tended to be decreased in insulin-treated patients.[23,24]

## AUTONOMIC NEUROPATHY

Abnormalities in cardiac innervation have been associated with two types of cardiac dysfunctions, involving both sensory and autonomic nerve fibers. Injury to sensory fibers could result in the phenomenon of silent, painless infarctions.

Various abnormalities in heart rate occur in the diabetic population. These include persistent tachycardia, absence of a rate variation with Valsalva maneuver, and a blunting of the normal variation of the heart rate that occurs during deep breathing.[101–103] These abnormalities are mainly due to dysfunctions of the vagus nerve, although sympathetic activity in the heart may also be altered in patients with severe autonomic neuropathy. Loss of sympathetic modulation may be important during exercise, when maximizing heart rate may be functionally significant.[101–103]

An evaluation of the parasympathetic regulation of the heart rate can be clinically useful. Several methods have been used to evaluate cardiac parasympathetic function, including heart rate or RR interval variation during deep breathing, heart rate response to Valsalva maneuver, and heart rate response to standing. The sensitivity for detecting a clinically relevant abnormality is increased if two of these tests are used together.

The principle behind these assays is to measure the vagal regulation of the heart rate, which is reflected in the RR intervals.[103a] The variation in the heart rate change depends on the blood flow back to the heart. The tachycardia normally observed during the Valsalva maneuver is induced by the lack of vagal tone, whereas the bradycardia that occurs after the maneuver is due mainly to an increase of vagal tone. Thus, a deficiency of vagal activity will lead to a decrease in the variation of heart rate during these maneuvers. In one study, the variation in heart rate during one deep breath was reduced significantly in 62 of 64 diabetic patients with other autonomic symptoms, and in 30% of diabetic patients who had peripheral neuropathy but no autonomic symptomatology.[101–103] Prolonged follow-up of up to 5 years did not show any improvement and, in some patients, demonstrated deterioration. Indeed, the rate of mortality differed remarkably between diabetic patients with and without abnormal cardiovascular reflex tests. In a study of 73 diabetic patients, the mortality in those with abnormal cardioreflex testing was three- to four-fold higher; in 20%, the death was sudden, suggesting cardiac arrhythmia as a possible cause.[102] Similar findings of a decrease in respiratory variations of the electrocardiographic RR interval in diabetic patients have also been reported; however, these differences are not as marked as the heart rate variation. The high rate of mortality is mostly due to other serious illnesses. Nevertheless, diabetic patients with severe cardiac autonomic dysfunction should be carefully followed, cardiac dysfunction should be treated appropriately, and blood glucose should be strictly controlled.[103b]

## MANAGEMENT OF DIABETIC ISCHEMIC HEART DISEASE

### MEDICAL MANAGEMENT

#### DIET PLAN

The diet plan is one of the most important aspects of therapy for both type 1 and type 2 diabetic patients. First, with proper diet and weight loss the peripheral sensitivity, insulin secretion, or both, can be improved in type 2 diabetes. This improvement in blood-glucose control can reduce some of the risk factors by lowering LDL and increasing HDL levels. Second, it is important for patients on insulin to consume similar amounts of calories during the same time period every day, since this will require fewer changes in insulin dose. The initial goal in the diet plan is to construct a diet that will enable the diabetic patient, if obese, to lose weight. Without unusual physical activity, patients who are taking in 35 kcal/kg will, in general, maintain their weight. Because a deficit of 3500 kcal is needed to lose 1 lb, in patients with normal physical activity, a diet program allowing 1200 kcal per day will result in a loss of 1 to 2 lb per week. Although this may not appear to be particularly significant, many obese diabetic patients have a clear improvement in insulin sensitivity after losing only a few pounds. An increase in fiber content of the diet also may be helpful for this, owing to its effect in delaying enteric absorption (see Chaps. 124 and 141).

The second goal of the diet plan is to attempt to decrease risk factors such as hyperlipidemia, hypertension, and nephropathy—all of which will accelerate the rate of atherosclerosis. Thus, a diet low in saturated fat should be strictly followed. Other factors that can accentuate the lipid abnormalities, such as alcoholic beverages, should be avoided, although moderate intake of red wine has been suggested to decrease cardiovascular risk by increasing HDL in both diabetic and nondiabetic populations. In addition, familial hyperlipidemia, which will greatly accentuate the lipid abnormalities (especially the elevation of plasma triglyceride levels), may be found.[20,104–107] Drug treatment with triglyceride- and cholesterol-lowering agents may be required (see Chap. 164). However, glycemic control should be tried first since this can significantly lower both plasma VLDL and LDL levels and decrease the adverse effects of hyperglycemia.

The frequency of hypertension is also increased in the diabetic population even before the development of clinical renal disease. Hypertension is a strong risk factor for the development and progression of diabetic, cardiac, renal, retinal, and peripheral vascular complications[108]; therefore, it should be treated vigorously. A low-salt diet in combination with drug therapy is often required. Also, animal studies suggest that a low-protein diet along with plasma glucose control in diabetic patients may improve or stabilize deteriorating renal function, although the effect in humans may not be as significant. It should be emphasized that cigarette smoking in diabetic patients must be strongly discouraged because the increase of risk for cardiovascular morbidity and mortality is enhanced in a multiple fashion (see Chap. 234).

### EXERCISE

Exercise in diabetic patients can be helpful in several ways. First, moderate exercise has been demonstrated to improve insulin sensitivity and glucose tolerance, even in the absence of weight loss. Second, in combination with a proper diet program, exercise can be helpful in promoting weight loss and thereby lead to reduced cardiovascular risks. Exercise may also reduce the risk of vascular complications, not only by improving plasma glucose control but by increasing plasma HDL, which can lessen the risk of cardiovascular disease. In addition, risk factors for macrovascular disease in diabetic patients, such as the levels of LDL, VLDL, and fasting insulin levels, may also be lowered.

Although the advantages of an exercise program can be substantial for diabetic patients, it should not be initiated without proper planning since there are potential risks. The occurrence of hypoglycemia may be increased in patients taking oral hypoglycemia agents because of an augmented sensitivity to insulin or an increased absorption of exogenously administered insulin. Exercise, which may increase retinal intravascular pressure, such as that associated with straining (e.g., in weight lifting), should also be limited. Patients who experience severe sensory neuropathy have an increased risk of injuring their lower extremities.

For type 2 diabetic patients, who are generally older than type 1 diabetics, care should be taken to avoid precipitating cardiac ischemia, which may lead to arrhythmia and myocardial infarction. Also, the high prevalence of peripheral vascular involvement in diabetic patients may result in easily bruised skin, which could lead to abscess formation and osteomyelitis. Nevertheless, a supervised and planned exercise program can usually avoid these potential hazards[109] (see Chaps. 132 and 141).

**Exercise Regimen.** In the initial medical evaluation, a detailed examination of the cardiac and vascular systems, in addition to ophthalmoscopic studies, is necessary to rule out cardiac lesions or proliferative retinopathy, which may be exacerbated by strenuous exercise programs. Laboratory evaluations are necessary to evaluate the control of plasma glucose levels and to determine the patient's working capacity. Evaluation of cardiac and working capacities should include resting and exercise electrocardiograms in the patient older than 40 or with a history of cardiac symptoms.

Endurance-type exercise, such as walking, cycling, jogging, and aerobic workouts, is generally recommended over strength building (e.g., weight lifting) because of the increased potential of the latter to raise blood pressure transiently. The exercise plan usually begins with a short warm-up period with stretching routines, followed by 10 to 30 minutes of endurance-building activities. These exercises should stimulate the heart rate to 50% to 75% of the maximal rate, depending on the persistence in the exercise program. These exercise plans need to be performed at least three times a week to achieve beneficial effects, such as lower cardiovascular risks and decreased insulin resistance.

### DRUG THERAPY

Specific pharmacologic therapy for cardiac dysfunctions among the diabetic and nondiabetic populations do not differ greatly. However, several general points should be stressed. As discussed previously, in patients with type 1 and 2 diabetes, normalized glucose excursions can prevent or delay the development of cardiovascular and myocardiovascular complications.[8,26]

Questions have been raised concerning the safety of the sulfonylureas in diabetic patients with a history of cardiac disease, as a result of the findings of the UGDP, which concluded that there was an increase of cardiovascular deaths in the tolbutamide-treated group compared with the insulin-treated group.[25] These differences became significant after 3.5 years. However, the UKPDS has laid these fears to rest since intensive treatment with sulfonylurea, insulin, or metformin was equally effective in reducing fasting plasma glucose concentrations in type 2 diabetic patients.[8] They also found that intensive glucose control with metformin appears to reduce the risk of diabetes-related cardiovascular end points in overweight diabetic patients as compared to insulin or sulfonylurea groups. Moreover, treatment with metformin is associated with less weight gain and fewer hypoglycemic attacks than are either insulin or sulfonylureas, suggesting that it may be the first-line pharmacologic therapy of choice in these patients.

Even after starting oral hypoglycemic agents, diet and weight-control programs should be continued. These drugs should be discontinued if further weight reduction alone can result in satisfactory control of plasma glucose. The insulin-sensitizing agents, thiazolidinediones, exert direct effects on the PPARγ receptors, resulting in improved insulin action and reduced hyperinsulinemia. These glitazone compounds can improve insulin action and reduce glycemia and insulin requirements in type 2 diabetics.[110] Other symptoms such as dyslipidemia and hypertension could also improve following a decrease in insulin resistance. In addition to the novel mechanism of action through binding and activation of PPARγs, the glitazones are potent antioxidants since it contains vitamin E within its structure. However, the side effect of liver damage can be severe (even if uncommon) and has led to the development of alternative drugs. Additionally, these compounds are less suitable for obese patients, since there is a weight gain of up to 5 kg during treatment. Thiazolidinedione compounds provide an important additional resource for the health care provider in the management of type 2 diabetes and other aspects of the insulin resistance syndrome.[110]

The drug therapy of angina pectoris in diabetic patients differs slightly from that of the nondiabetic population. This primarily pertains to the use of β-adrenergic blocking agents. Although β-blockers are effective in diabetic patients without risk factors (e.g., hypoglycemia unawareness[111]), long-standing diabetics with impaired autonomic function often have a poor sympathetic response to hypoglycemia for which some of the warning signs may be blunted. In addition, nonselective β-adrenergic blockers inhibit gluconeogenesis, thereby prolonging the hypoglycemia recovery phase because of the requirement for mobilization of glucose from the liver. Clinically, these problems are best dealt with by warning diabetic patients that their symptoms of hypoglycemia may be more subtle. When the symptoms of hypoglycemia are finally perceived, the patients will have a shorter time to respond before unconsciousness may occur. The complete absence of symptoms when hypoglycemia occurs usually constitutes a contraindication to the use of β-adrenergic blocking drugs. The advantage of a selective β-blocker is limited to a faster recovery phase from hypoglycemia; it would appear that this minor advantage may be clinically worthwhile.

Another problem encountered with the use of β-adrenergic blocking drugs in diabetic patients is the lack of efficacy among those patients with significant autonomic neuropathy. A major benefit of β-adrenergic blockers is the slowing of heart rate and a subsequent decrease of myocardial oxygen requirements, thereby minimizing the possibility of myocardial ischemia. However, in autonomic neuropathy, the parasympathetic control of heart rate is often lost. Consequently, the resting heart rate is higher than in those persons with a normally functioning vagus nerve. Patients with parasympathetic denervation do not experience the same magnitude of decrease in heart rate after full β-adrenergic blocking doses. This is due to the relatively greater importance of the parasympathetic tone, which results in only minor changes in heart rate response and, therefore, only minor improvement of myocardial oxygen requirements. Combined with the propensity of β-adrenergic blockers to aggravate hypoglycemic episodes, this narrows the therapeutic/toxic ratio of these agents. In individuals with autonomic dysfunction, it is sometimes best to select a calcium-channel antagonist as a primary mode of therapy, since these drugs cause a decrease in heart rate by a direct nonadrenergic-mediated depression of sinus mode function. Frequently, calcium-channel antagonists can result in a more impressive negative chronotropic response than do β-adrenergic blockers, especially when there is substantial autonomic dysfunction.

Lastly, angiotensin-converting enzyme inhibitors (ACEI) are widely used for treatment of hypertension in diabetes since multiple studies have shown that they may delay the onset of diabetic nephropathy and decrease cardiac mortality in diabetic patients.[112–114] It is likely that angiotensin receptor antagonists will have effects similar to ACEI. In nondiabetic patients (and most likely in diabetic patients), ACEI have cardiac protective effects in addition to antihypertensive effects.

Hyperlipidemia is very common in both type 1 and 2 diabetics, and, as stated previously, diet and glycemic control can decrease both cholesterol and triglyceride levels. Hypercholesterolemia is a condition that occurs more often in diabetic patients than in the general population. The targeted level of cholesterol for diabetic patients should be lower than that of the general population (e.g., ideally to the range of 150 mg/dL). In the randomized trial of cholesterol lowering in patients with coronary heart disease, the Scandinavian Simvastatin Survival Study (4S) showed that long-term treatment with simvastatin, an HMG-reductase (hydroxymethylglutaryl-CoA reductase) inhibitor, is safe and improves survival in patients with coronary heart

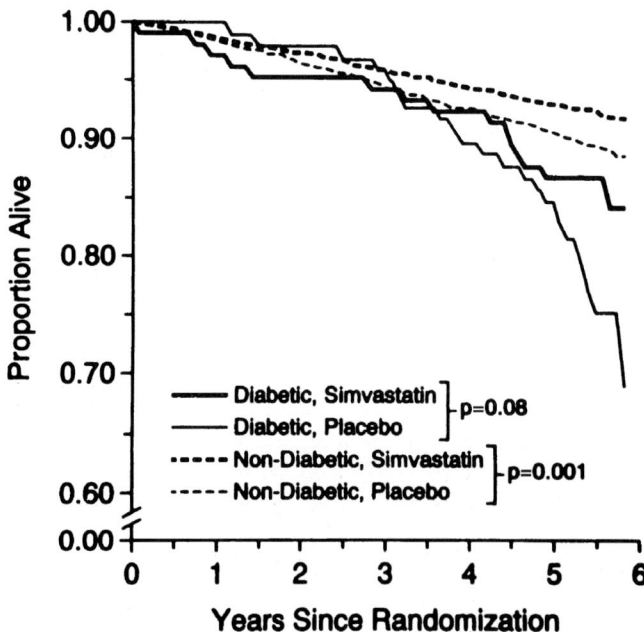

**FIGURE 147-3.** Proportion alive of diabetic and nondiabetic patients treated with placebo or simvastatin in the Scandinavian Simvastatin Survival Study (4S). (From Pyorala K, Pedersen TR, Kjekshus J, et al. Cholesterol lowering with simvastatin improves prognosis of diabetic patients with coronary heart disease. A subgroup analysis of the Scandinavian Simvastatin Survival Study [4S]. Diabetes Care 1997; 20[4]:614.)

disease (Fig. 147-3).[115] Over the 5.4-year median follow-up period, simvastatin produced mean changes in total cholesterol, LDL cholesterol, and HDL cholesterol of –25%, –35%, and +8%, respectively. There were fewer adverse effects among the diabetic patients in the simvastatin group (8% died, compared with 12% in the placebo group; Fig. 147-3). There were 111 coronary deaths in the simvastatin group and 189 in the placebo group (relative risk 0.58, 95% cumulative index [CI] 0.46–0.73), while noncardiovascular causes accounted for 46 and 49 deaths, respectively. One or more major coronary events occurred in 622 patients in the placebo group (28%) and in 431 patients in the simvastatin group (19%). The relative risk was 0.66 (95% CI 0.59–0.75, $p$ <.00001), and the probabilities of escaping such events were 70.5% and 79.6%, respectively. This risk was also significantly reduced in subgroups consisting of women and patients of both sexes 60 years of age or older. Other benefits of treatment included a 37% reduction ($p$ <.00001) in the risk of undergoing myocardial revascularization procedures.

The most common lipid abnormality in type 1 and type 2 diabetes is an increase in circulating VLDL. Insulin deficiency or resistance accelerates the release of VLDL from the liver. However, the susceptibility to vascular disease observed among diabetic patients may be the result of the increased levels of IDL produced when VLDL is metabolized to LDL. In addition, the HDL cholesterol levels are often decreased in type 2 diabetics (women exhibiting a greater decrease than men). Lipid-lowering drugs, particularly the fibrates, may be needed for treating diabetic patients, since they lower both cholesterol and triglycerides and raise HDL levels. Fibrates are the drugs of choice for the correction of hypertriglyceridemia.[104–107]

## SURGICAL APPROACHES

### BALLOON ANGIOPLASTY

Coronary artery balloon angioplasty has been used extensively in both diabetic and nondiabetic populations. The results have shown that hospital death is very low, ~0.2% in some centers, and restenosis rates are <30% to 40% in 6 months. However, diabetes, along with male sex, unstable angina, and pathologic findings of long or near total lesions, are risk factors that result in higher mortality and higher rates of restenosis.

The Bypass Angioplasty Revascularization Investigation (BARI) trial indicated that the 5-year cardiac mortality in diabetic patients with multivessel disease on drug therapy was significantly greater after initial treatment with coronary balloon angioplasty than with coronary artery bypass graft (CABG) alone.[116] The better survival rate with CABG was due to reduced cardiac mortality (5.8% vs. 20.6%, $p = .0003$), which was confined to those receiving at least one internal mammary artery graft. Long-term internal mammary artery graft patency may contribute to this improved outcome by reducing the fatality from follow-up myocardial infarction. Stents may improve patency rates; further large studies like the BARI trial are needed to evaluate the benefit of using stents in diabetic patients.

### CORONARY ARTERY BYPASS SURGERY

Numerous studies have demonstrated the effectiveness of coronary artery bypass surgery, when feasible, in both type 1 and type 2 diabetes.[81–83] However, patients with type 1 diabetes represent a unique population in whom CAD is more extensive and diffuse; hence, they have been considered to be high-risk candidates for bypass surgery.[117–119a]

A small group of type 1 diabetics were followed after having coronary artery bypass surgery. At the time of the operation, the patients had a mean age of 44 years and mean duration of diabetes of 30 years. Retinopathy and neuropathy were noted in all patients. All except one of these patients were classified as functional class IV by the criteria of the New York Heart Association. Because of the frequent occurrence of angina, in spite of maximal medical therapy, the patients underwent coronary angiography and surgery. Angiographic findings showed that eight patients had more than one vessel with ≥70% narrowing. Two of 13 patients had left main coronary artery stenosis. More than 70% of the patients had focal narrowing. Left ventricle function studies revealed an ejection fraction >50% in all patients. All the nondiffuse vessels were bypassed and no perioperative mortality was reported. Clinical evaluation for up to 8 years showed an initial symptomatic improvement in all of the patients after 1 year, and 60% of the treated patients remained minimally symptomatic after 5 years. Repeat angiograms found that progression of disease occurred mainly in previously nongrafted vessels. Thus, in this study, type 1 diabetics with CAD could be treated with CABGs with good results.

With type 2 diabetics, the results of CABG have also been quite favorable, both for symptomatic relief and survival. Compared with the nondiabetic patients, as a group, the adult-onset diabetics included a higher percentage of females, a higher prevalence of hypertension, and an increased prevalence of ventricular hypertrophy. Angiographic studies have suggested that coronary arteries from diabetic patients have more diffuse disease, resulting in a greater number of grafts performed. Perioperative morbidity, involving infection, wound healing, and renal failure, was also greater in the diabetic group. Also, long-term survival appears to be lower than in the nondiabetic population.

In spite of increased perioperative complications, a better survival rate in diabetic patients with bypass grafts compared with medical management alone has been reported.[120] The perioperative morbidity can be minimized by regulating precisely the patient's glucose levels with strict euglycemic control, using an insulin pump or with multiple insulin injections and frequent blood-glucose monitoring. In addition, hydration needs to be carefully monitored to avoid renal dysfunction during cardiac catheterization or surgery.

## DIABETIC PERIPHERAL VASCULAR DISEASE

The increased incidences of peripheral vascular disease, gangrene, and subsequent amputation in diabetic patients have been documented in many studies.[1,14,120–122] In one report, 5% of patients had symptoms of peripheral vascular disease within 1 year of diagnosis of their diabetes; after 12 years of follow-up, this increased to 23%. In the Framingham Study, 12.6% of the male diabetic patients had intermittent claudication, as opposed to only 3.3% of the control group.[9]

Although peripheral vascular disease is more common in nondiabetic men than in nondiabetic women, the incidence between the sexes in diabetic patients is almost equal. Also, peripheral vascular disease occurs more commonly below the knees in diabetics, whereas in the nondiabetic it is more likely to be situated in the aortic, iliac, and femoral vessels. Because atherosclerosis of large vessels, small vessels, or arterioles does not progress at the same rate, it is possible to have more severe disease in small vessels than in large vessels, leading to small patchy areas of gangrene of the foot or the toes in the presence of a palpable dorsal pedal or posterior tibial pulse.[1,14,120–124] In addition, collateral circulation may develop poorly in diabetic patients.

Not to be confused with the atherosclerosis process is focal calcification of the media, particularly in the medium-sized muscular arteries (Monckeberg sclerosis); this is also increased in diabetic patients. This process involves degeneration of smooth muscle cells, followed by calcium deposition. Its characteristic radiographic appearance consists of regular, concentric calcifications that are seen prominently in the pelvic and femoral vessels. These medial changes alone do not cause narrowing of the lumen and have little clinical significance, unless they are associated with atherosclerosis, in which case an arterial occlusion may occur.

### SIGNS AND SYMPTOMS

The earliest symptom of peripheral vascular disease is intermittent claudication, which is characterized by pain on walking and is relieved by stopping. This usually begins in the calf and may involve various muscle groups, depending on the location of the occlusion.[120–124] A more serious symptom is rest pain, which is usually worse at night and may require narcotics for relief. Because rest pain is often relieved by sitting with the feet dependent, edema of the legs may occur in those patients who sleep in a chair.

Cold feet are a common complaint in patients with peripheral arterial insufficiency. The cold feet are what prompt the diabetic patients to use heating pads, often resulting in burns to their relatively insensitive feet. The presence of diabetic neuropathy is the main and primary cause of foot lesions. Because of sensory deficiency, diabetic patients may repeatedly injure their feet, which then may heal poorly because of the compromised vasculature. The poor blood supply results in malnutrition of the foot, leading to thickened nails, diminished subcutaneous fat, and loss of hair. Frequently, there is associated fungal infection (see Chaps. 148, 153, and 154).

Examination of the patient with peripheral vascular disease often reveals diminished or absent pulses, depending on the areas of involvement. Similarly to nondiabetic patients, there is a high occurrence of atherosclerotic occlusion of the femoral and popliteal arteries. However, there is a strikingly increased involvement of the tibial and peroneal arteries. Therefore, it is common to find the presence of femoral pulses in a patient with an ischemic foot. Pallor of the foot on elevation is an important sign of ischemia. If the patient sits with the legs dependent, venous and capillary filling times are usually less than 20 seconds if collateral circulation to the foot is satisfactory; this may be prolonged to minutes if the extremity is ischemic. Also, a bright or dusky red color may develop on dependency if the circulation is inadequate.

Neuropathy affects the sensory nerves first, leading to paresthesias and pain. In later stages, the patient has less tactile and pain sensation, increasing the risks of injury and chronic wounds. The motor nerves are not severely involved except in mononeuropathy, which can result in muscle atrophy. The muscle atrophy can also affect the lower leg, predisposing to venous ulcers. Autonomic neuropathy decreases perspiration, giving rise to thin and vulnerable skin that can be easily bruised; painful cracks are common on the dry foot. Regulation of the circulation to the foot is affected, leading to increased arteriovenous shunting of blood.[121–124]

## LABORATORY TESTS

Two of the most widely used noninvasive tests include segmental blood pressures in the leg and pulse volume recordings (with the Doppler flowmeter). Segmental systolic pressures are used to identify the area or level of the obstruction. By consecutively inflating the cuffs, which are placed below the knee and above the ankle, segmental pressures can be obtained. All pressure gradients should demonstrate a drop of less than 30 mm Hg. Diabetic patients frequently have elevated systolic pressures at all levels; this is thought to be due to medial calcification of the peripheral vessels.

Pulse volume recordings are used to measure the instantaneous variations of arterial volume in a specific limb segment during each cardiac cycle. Specially designed cuffs are used for digital tracing; this is particularly important in diabetic patients, who are prone to develop disease of the small arteries.

An exercise test or reactive hyperemia test may also be valuable when patients experience claudication, even though the resting pressure and volume index may be normal. These patients may have small vessel disease. However, clinical judgment is often more valuable than noninvasive tests in determining the level of occlusion and the likelihood of success.

## THERAPY FOR PERIPHERAL VASCULAR DISEASE

The treatment of peripheral vascular disease requires multiple approaches, including meticulous control of the plasma glucose level, weight reduction, cessation of smoking, and avoidance of injury. None of the vasodilator drugs available can help this condition; indeed, they may be contraindicated because of their effect in lowering systemic pressure, leading to decreased collateral blood flow.

The main objective of medical treatment is to educate the patients to take good care of their feet; this can markedly reduce the rate of amputation. Such measures involve a daily inspection of the feet and the use of correctly fitted shoes. Nails and calluses should be regularly examined by a podiatrist. The feet should be kept warm, dry, and clean. If any infection or lesion is found, hospitalization and antibiotics are indicated. Besides good foot care, the cessation of cigarette smoking is also extremely important and effective in decreasing symptoms and amputation rates. Exercise programs, such as walking, can improve the symptoms in most patients.

Various drug treatments have been tried with inconclusive results. Pentoxifylline, a drug that appears to increase the flexibility of red blood cells, is being used for improving the symptoms of intermittent claudication.[125] However, the reported results have not been encouraging. Aspirin has also been used because of its possible beneficial effect in diminishing the ability of platelets to adhere to one another. However, no prospective trials of its effect on peripheral vessels have been reported,

although it may be helpful in preventing coronary and cerebral events. Vasodilators are not effective for intermittent claudication, probably because of such factors as sclerosis of the vessel, abnormalities of autonomic control, and vessels that may already be dilated.

Therapy of the wound may be nonsurgical or surgical. The nonsurgical treatment (following early diagnosis by clinical investigation, distal blood pressure measurement, radiography, and determination of the partial pressure of tissue oxygen) includes the removal of edema by diuretics and compression, metabolic control by more aggressive insulin treatment, prohibition of smoking, diminishing pressure on the wound by orthopedic shoes and plasters, local wound treatment by debridement and zinc applications, and, if needed, the administration of broad-spectrum antibiotics.[126] Surgical treatment is necessary when ischemic pain develops; normally, angiography must be performed before intervention. Vascular surgery, thromboendarterectomy, bypass operation, and balloon dilatation are the three most common procedures. If vascular surgery fails, amputation is the last resort. Hyperbaric treatment has been shown to decrease the number of amputations in diabetic patients with hypoxic, neuropathic wounds.[127]

Vascular surgery is the definitive procedure for improving blood flow in peripheral vascular disease. Indications for arterial surgery include rest pain, claudication that interferes with work, or an area of gangrene. Before surgery, the location and extent of involvement, as well as the feasibility of improvement, must be ascertained by cautious angiography.

Operations to restore blood flow to the ischemic limb include angioplasty and bypass surgery. In angioplasty, a small balloon catheter, carefully put into place and distended under fluoroscopy, may push the diseased areas into the arterial wall, relieving the obstruction. In the diabetic patient, multisegmental artery disease is often present and involvement of small vessels may render this method less useful. In addition, the resistance is much greater, further decreasing the success of this procedure.

Saphenous vein grafts or other graft materials such as Dacron tubes or glutaraldehyde-treated umbilical veins can be used to bypass the obstructing arterial lesions. The results of bypass surgery have been relatively good. Because the vessels frequently involved are tibial and peroneal arteries, vein graft from the popliteal to either the dorsalis pedis or posterior tibial artery can be performed successfully.[128,129] By using the bypass to the dorsalis pedis artery from the popliteal artery, the rate of limb salvage has been increased to 91%, but this technique can be used in only ~30% of all cases.[130] The long-term results of arterial reconstruction using this procedure are almost identical between diabetic and nondiabetic patients.[128,129]

## REFERENCES

1. Cudworth E. Diabetes and its late complications. London: John Libbey & Co, 1982.
2. Orchard TJ. From diagnosis and classification to complications and therapy. Diabetes Care 1994; 17:326.
3. Niskamen L, Siltonen O, Suhonen M, Uusitupa MI. Medial artery calcification predicts cardiovascular mortality in patients with NIDDM. Diabetes Care 1994; 17:1252.
4. Knuiman MW, Welborn TA, McCann VJ. Prevalence of diabetic complications in relation to risk factors. Diabetes 1986; 35:1332.
5. Krolewski AS, Kosinski EJ, Warram JH, et al. Magnitude and determinants of coronary artery disease in juvenile-onset, insulin dependent diabetes mellitus. Am J Cardiol 1987; 59:750.
6. Kessler II. Mortality experience of diabetic patients—a twenty-six year follow-up study. Am J Med 1971;51:715.
7. Despres JP, Lamarche B, Mauriege P, et al. Hyperinsulinemia as an independent risk factor for ischemic heart disease. N Engl J Med 1996; 334:952.
8. Adler AI, Neil HA, Manley SE, et al. Hyperglycemia and hyperinsulinemia at diagnosis of diabetes and their association with subsequent cardiovascular disease in the United Kingdom Prospective Diabetes Study (UKPDS 47). Am Heart J 1999; 138(5 Pt 1):353.

9. Kannel WB, McGee DL. Diabetes and cardiovascular disease: the Framingham Study. JAMA 1979; 241:2035.

10. Jarrett RJ. Is insulin atherogenic? Diabetologia 1988; 31:71.

11. Janka HU, Ziegler AG, Standl E, Mehnert H. Daily insulin dose as a predictor of macrovascular disease in insulin treatment of non-insulin-dependent diabetics. Diabetes Metab 1987; 13:359.

12. Steiner G. Atherosclerosis, the major complication of diabetes. Adv Exp Med Biol 1985; 189:277.

13. Colwell JA, Lopes-Virella M, Halushka PV. Pathogenesis of atherosclerosis in diabetes mellitus. Diabetes Care 1981; 4:121.

14. Ruderman NB, Haudenschild C. Diabetes as an atherogenic factor. Prog Cardiovasc Dis 1984; 26:373.

15. Ross R. The pathogenesis of atherosclerosis—an update. N Engl J Med 1986; 314:488.

16. Stamler J. Atherosclerotic coronary heart disease etiology and pathogenesis: the epidemiologic findings. In: Stamler J, ed. Lectures on preventive cardiology. New York: Grune & Stratton, 1967.

17. Moss SE, Klein R, Klein DE. Cause-specific mortality in a population-based study of diabetes. Am J Public Health 1991; 81:1158.

18. Watts HF. Basic aspects of the pathogenesis of atherosclerosis. Hum Pathol 1971; 2:31.

19. Benditt EP. Implications of the monoclonal characteristic of human atherosclerotic plaque. Am J Pathol 1977; 86:693.

20. Steinberg D. Lipoproteins and atherosclerosis, a look back and a look ahead. Arteriosclerosis 1983; 3:283.

21. Geer JC. Fine structure of human aortic intimal thickening and fatty streaks. Lab Invest 1963; 141:1764.

22. McGill HC Jr, ed. The geographic pathology of atherosclerosis. Baltimore: Williams & Wilkins, 1968.

22a. Shechter M, Noel Bairy Merz C, Paul-Labrador MJ, Kaul S. Blood glucose and platelet-dependent thrombosis in patients with coronary artery disease. J Am Coll Cardiol 2000; 35:300.

23. Malmberg K. Prospective randomised study of intensive insulin treatment on long-term survival after acute myocardial infarction in patients with diabetes mellitus. DIGAMI (Diabetes Mellitus, Insulin Glucose Infusion in Acute Myocardial Infarction) Study Group. Br Med J 1997; 314:1512.

24. Malmberg K, Ryden L, Hamsten A, et al. Effects of insulin treatment on cause-specific one-year mortality and morbidity in diabetic patients with acute myocardial infarction. DIGAMI Study Group. Diabetes insulin-glucose in acute myocardial infarction. Eur Heart J 1996; 17:1337.

25. Genuth S. Exogenous insulin administration and cardiovascular risk in non-insulin-dependent and insulin-dependent diabetes mellitus. Ann Intern Med 1996; 1;124(1 Pt 2):104.

26. Ohkubo Y, Kishikawa H, Araki E, et al. Intensive insulin therapy prevents the progression of diabetic microvascular complications in Japanese patients with non-insulin-dependent diabetes mellitus: a randomized prospective 6-year study. Diabetes Res Clin Pract 1995; 28(2):103.

27. Haffner SM, Lehto S, Ronnemaa T, et al. Mortality from coronary heart disease in subjects with type 2 diabetes and in nondiabetic subjects with and without prior myocardial infarction. N Engl J Med 1998; 339(4):229.

28. Fein FS, Sonnenblick EH. Diabetic cardiomyopathy. Prog Cardiovasc Dis 1985; 27:255.

29. Factor SM, Okun EM, Minase T. Capillary microaneurysms in the human diabetic heart. N Engl J Med 1980; 302:384.

30. Britland ST, Young RJ, Sharma AK, et al. Vagus nerve morphology in diabetic gastropathy. Diabetes Med 1990; 7:780.

31. Shimoni Y, Ewart HS, Severson D. Type I and II models of diabetes produce different modifications of K currents in rat heart: role of insulin. J Physiol 1998; 507:485.

32. Charlstrom S, Karlefors T. Haemodynamic studies on newly diagnosed diabetics before and after adequate insulin treatment. Br Heart J 1970; 32:355.

33. Rubler S, Dlugash J, Yuceoglu YZ, et al. New type of cardiomyopathy associated with diabetic glomerulosclerosis. Am J Cardiol 1972; 30:599.

34. Schaffer SW, Artman MF, Wilson GL. Properties of insulin-dependent and non–insulin-dependent diabetic cardiomyopathies. In: Kawai C, Abelmann WH, eds. Pathogenesis of myocarditis and cardiomyopathy. Tokyo: University of Tokyo Press, 1987:149.

35. Leland OS, Makie PC. Heart disease and diabetes. In: Marble A, Krall LP, Bradley RF, et al., eds. Joslin's diabetes mellitus. Philadelphia: Lea & Febiger, 1985:553.

36. Kerby AL, Radcliffe PM, Rundle JR. Diabetes and the control of pyruvate dehydrogenase in rat heart mitochondria by concentration ratios of adenosine triphosphate/adenosine diphosphate of reduced/oxidized nicotinamide-adenine dinucleotide and of acetyl-coenzyme $A_1$ coenzyme A. Biochem J 1977; 164:504.

37. Pierce GN, Kutrsyk MJB, Dhalla NS. Alteration in $Ca^{2+}$-binding by and composition of the cardiac sacrolemmal membrane in chronic diabetes. Proc Natl Acad Sci U S A 1983; 80:5412.

38. Dillmann WH. Methylpalmoxrate increases $Ca^{2+}$-myosin ATPase activity and changes myosin isoenzyme distribution in the diabetic rat heart. Am J Physiol 1985; 248:E602.

39. Tanaka Y, Kashiwagi A, Saeki Y, Takagi Y. Effects of verapamil on the cardiac alpha 1-adrenoceptor signaling system in diabetic rats. Eur J Pharmacol 1993; 244:105.

40. Aronstam RS. Insulin prevention of altered muscarinic receptor-G protein coupling in diabetic rat atria. Diabetes 1989; 38:1611.

41. Gravey WT, Hardin D, Juhaszova M, Doninguez JH. Effects of diabetes on myocardial glucose transport system in rats: implications for diabetic cardiomyopathy. Am J Physiol 1993; 264:H387.

42. Dillmann WH, Barrieux A, Shanker R. Influence of thyroid hormone on myosin heavy chain mRNA and other messenger RNAs in the rat heart. Endocrine Res 1989;15:565.

43. Nishio Y, Warren CE, Buczek-Thomas JA, et al. Identification and characterization of a gene regulating enzymatic glycosylation which is induced by diabetes and hyperglycemia specifically in rat cardiac tissue. J Clin Invest 1995; 96:1759.

44. King GL, Johnson SM. Receptor-mediated transport of insulin across endothelial cells. Science 1985; 1583.

45. Navab M, Hough GD, Berliner JA, et al. Rabbit beta-migrating very low density lipoprotein increases endothelial macromolecular transport without altering electrical resistance. J Clin Invest 1986; 78:389.

46. Moncada S, Herman AG, Higgs EA, Vane JR. Differential formation of prostacyclin (PGX or PGI2) by layers of the arterial wall: an explanation for the anti-thrombotic properties of the vascular endothelium. Thromb Res 1977; 11:323.

47. Davies PF, Dewey CF, Bussolari SR, et al. Influence of hemodynamic forces on vascular endothelial function in in vitro studies of shear stress and pinocytosis in bovine aortic cells. J Clin Invest 1984; 73:11121.

48. Lorenzi M, Mortisano DF, Toledo S, Barrieux A. High glucose induces DNA damage in cultured human endothelial cells. J Clin Invest 1986; 77:322.

49. McMillan DE. Effects of insulin on physical factors: atherosclerosis in diabetes mellitus. Metabolism 1985; 34(Suppl):70.

50. Baron AD. Insulin and the vasculature—old actors, new roles. J Investig Med 1996; 44:406.

51. Feener EP, King GL. Vascular dysfunction in diabetes mellitus. Lancet 1997; 350(Suppl)1:S19.

52. King GL. The role of hyperglycemia and hyperinsulinaemia in causing vascular dysfunction in diabetes. Ann Med 1996; 28:427.

52a. Vallejo S, Angulo J, Peiró C, et al. Highly glycated oxyhaemoglobin impairs nitric oxide relaxations in human mesenteric microvessels. Diabetologia 2000; 43:83.

53. Stout RW. The role of insulin in atherosclerosis in diabetics and non-diabetics, a review. Diabetes 1981; 30(Suppl 2):54.

54. King GL. Cell biology as an approach to the study of the vascular complications of diabetes. Metabolism 1985; 34(Suppl 1):17.

55. Jiang ZY, Lin YW, Clemont A, et al. Characterization of selective resistance to insulin signaling in the vasculature of obese Zucker (fa/fa) rats. J Clin Invest 1999; 104:447.

56. Hamet P, Sugimoto H, Umeda F, et al. Abnormalities of platelet-derived growth factors in insulin-dependent diabetes mellitus. Metabolism 1985; 34(Suppl 1):25.

57. Beutler B, Cerami A. Cachectin: more than a tumor necrosis factor. N Engl J Med 1987; 316:379.

58. Assoian RK, Grotendorst GR, Miller DM, et al. Cellular transformation by coordinated action of three peptide growth factors from human platelets. Nature 1984; 309:804.

59. Anayeva NM, Tjurmin AV, Berliner JA, et al. Oxidized LDL mediates the release of fibroblast growth factor-1. Arterioscler Thromb Vasc Biol 1997; 17(3):445.

60. Prisco D, Rogasi PG, Paniccia R, et al. Altered membrane fatty acid composition and increased thromboxane A2 generation in platelets from patients with diabetes. Prostaglandins Leukot Essent Fatty Acids 1989; 35:15.

61. Nikkila EA. High density lipoproteins in diabetes. Diabetes 1981; 30(Suppl 2):82.

62. Schonfeld G. Diabetes, lipoprotein and atherosclerosis. Metabolism 1985; 34(Suppl 1):41.

63. Gomen B, Baenziger J, Schonfeld G, et al. Non-enzymatic glycosylation of low density lipoprotein in vitro: effects on cell interactive properties. Diabetes 1981; 30:871.

64. Witzum JL, Fisher M, Tiziana P, et al. Non-enzymatic glycosylation of high density lipoproteins accelerates its catabolism in guinea pigs. Diabetes 1982; 31:1023.

65. Ginsberg H, Grundy SM. Very low density lipoprotein metabolism in non-ketotic diabetes mellitus: effect of dietary restrictions. Diabetologia 1982; 23:421.

66. Taskinen MR, Beltz WF, Harper I, et al. Effect of NIDDM on very low density lipoprotein triglyceride and apolipoprotein B metabolism: studies before and after sulfonylurea therapy. Diabetes 1986; 35:1268.

67. Miller GJ. High density lipoprotein and atherosclerosis. Ann Rev Med 1980; 31:97.

68. Kaplan RM, Wilson DK, Hartwell SC, et al. Prospective evaluation of HDL cholesterol changes after diet and physical conditioning programs for patients with type II diabetes mellitus. Diabetes Care 1985; 8:343.

69. Bagdede JD, Kelley DE, Henry RR, et al. Effects of multiple daily insulin injections and intraperitoneal insulin therapy on cholesteryl ester transfer and lipoprotein lipase activities in NIDDM. Diabetes 1997; 46(3):414.

70. Tauber JP, Cheng J, Gaspodarowicz D. Effect of high low-density lipoproteins in proliferation of cultured bovine vascular endothelial cells. J Clin Invest 1980; 66:696.

71. The Diabetes Control and Complications (DCCT) Research Group. Effect of intensive therapy on the development and progression of diabetic nephropathy in the Diabetes Control and Complications Trial. Kidney Int 1995; 47:1703.

72. Pfeifer MA, Schumer MP, Gelber DA. Aldose reductase inhibitors: the end of an era or the need for different trial designs? Diabetes 1997; 46(Suppl 2):S82.

73. Ramasamy R, Oates PJ, Schaefer S. Aldose reductase inhibition protects diabetic and nondiabetic rat hearts from ischemic injury. Diabetes 1997; 46(2):292.

74. Schmidt AM, Yan SD, Wautier JL, Stern D. Activation of receptor for advanced glycation end products: a mechanism for chronic vascular dysfunction in diabetic vasculopathy and atherosclerosis. Circ Res 1999; 84(5):489.

75. Brownlee M. Lilly Lecture 1993. Glycation and diabetic complications. Diabetes 1994; 43(6):836.

76. Monnier VM, Glomb M, Elgawish A, Sell DR. The mechanism of collagen cross-linking in diabetes: a puzzle nearing resolution. Diabetes 1996; 45(7 Suppl 3):S67.

77. Baynes JW, Thorpe SR. Role of oxidative stress in diabetic complications: a new perspective on an old paradigm. Diabetes 1999; 48(1):1.

78. Bursell SE, Clermont AC, Aiello LP, et al. High-dose vitamin E supplementation normalizes retinal blood flow and creatinine clearance in patients with type 1 diabetes. Diabetes Care 1999; 22(8):1235.

79. Timimi FK, Ting HH, Haley EA, et al. Vitamin C improves endothelium-dependent vasodilation in patients with insulin-dependent diabetes mellitus. J Am Coll Cardiol 1998; 31(3):552.

80. Shiba T, Inoguchi T, Sportsman JR, et al. Correlation of diacylglycerol level and protein kinase C activity in rat retina to retinal circulation. Am J Physiol 1993; 265:E783.

81. Ishii H, Jirousek MR, Koya D, et al. Amelioration of vascular dysfunctions in diabetic rats by an oral PKC beta inhibitor. Science 1996; 272:728.

82. Koya D, King GL. Protein kinase C activation and the development of diabetic complications. Diabetes 1998; 47:859.

83. Inoguchi T, Battan R, Handler E, et al. Preferential elevation of protein kinase C isoform beta II and diacylglycerol levels in the aorta and heart of diabetic rats: differential reversibility to glycemic control by islet cell transplantation. Proc Natl Acad Sci U S A 1992; 89:11059.

84. Derubertis FR, Craven PA. Activation of protein kinase C in glomerular cells in diabetes. Mechanisms and potential links to the pathogenesis of diabetic glomerulopathy. Diabetes 1994; 43(1):1.

85. Mellor H, Parker PJ. The extended protein kinase C superfamily. Biochem J 1998; 332(Pt 2):281.

86. Nishizuka Y. Protein kinase C and lipid signaling for sustained cellular responses. FASEB J 1995; 9(7):484.

87. Considine RV, Nyce MR, Allen LE, et al. Protein kinase C is increased in the liver of humans and rats with non-insulin-dependent diabetes mellitus: an alteration not due to hyperglycemia. J Clin Invest 1995; 95:2938.

88. Ha H, Kim KH. Pathogenesis of diabetic nephropathy: the role of oxidative stress and protein kinase C. Diabetes Res Clin Pract 1999; 45(2–3):147.

89. Li PF, Maasch C, Haller H, et al. Requirement for protein kinase C in reactive oxygen species-induced apoptosis of vascular smooth muscle cells. Circulation 1999; 31:100(9):967.

90. Nakamura J, Kato K, Hamada Y, et al. A protein kinase C-beta-selective inhibitor ameliorates neural dysfunction in streptozotocin-induced diabetic rats. Diabetes 1999; 48(10):2090.

91. Viberti GC. Early functional and morphological changes in diabetic nephropathy. Clin Nephrol 1979; 12:41.

92. Hostetter TH, Troy JL, Brenner BM. Glomerular hemodynamics in experimental diabetes mellitus. Kidney Int 1981; 20:451.

93. Wakasaki H, Kova D, Schoen FJ, et al. Targeted overexpression of protein kinase C beta2 isoform in myocardium causes cardiomyopathy. Proc Natl Acad Sci U S A 1998; 94(17):9320.

94. Grant MB, Wargovich TJ, Bush DM, et al. Expression of IGF-1, IGF-1 receptor and TGF-beta following balloon angioplasty in atherosclerotic and normal rabbit iliac arteries: an immunocytochemical study. Regul Pept 1999; 79(1):47.

95. Bengtsson BA, Johannsson G. Effect of growth-hormone therapy on early atherosclerotic changes in GH-deficient adults. Lancet 1999; 5:35(9168):1898.

96. Colao A, Pivonello R, Spiezia S, et al. Persistence of increased cardiovascular risk in patients with Cushing's disease after five years of successful cure. J Clin Endocrinol Metab 1999; 84(8):2664.

97. Kleinert S. HOPE for cardiovascular disease prevention with ACE-inhibitor ramipril. Heart Outcomes Prevention Evaluation. Lancet 1999; 4:354(9181):841.

98. Malhotra A, Sanghi V. Regulation of contractile proteins in diabetic heart. Cardiovasc Res 1997; 34(1):34.

99. Joffe II, Travers KE, Perreault-Micale CL, et al. Abnormal cardiac function in the streptozotocin-induced non-insulin-dependent diabetic rat: noninvasive assessment with Doppler echocardiography and contribution of the nitric oxide pathway. J Am Coll Cardiol 1999; 34(7):2111.

100. Raman M, Nesto RW. Heart disease in diabetes mellitus. Endocrinol Metab Clin North Am 1996; 25(2):425.

101. Stein PK, Kleiger RE. Insights from the study of heart rate variability. Annu Rev Med 1999; 50:249.

102. Ewing DJ. Diabetic autonomic neuropathy and the heart. Diabetes Res Clin Pract 1996; 30(Suppl):31.

103. Watkins PJ, MacKay JD. Cardiac denervation in diabetic neuropathy. Ann Intern Med 1980; 92:304.

103a. Guo N, Luz Z, Xue X, et al. Assessment of autonomic function in patients with acute myocardial infarction or diabetes mellitus by heart rate variability, ventricular late potential and QT dispersion. Hypertens Res 2000; 23:367.

103b. Isotani H, Fukumoto Y. Reversibility of autonomic nerve function in relation to rapid improvement of glycemic control. Horm Metab Res 2000; 32:115.

104. Howard BV. Insulin resistance and lipid metabolism. Am J Cardiol 1999; 8;84(1A):28J.

105. Taskinen MR. Broader metabolic control in diabetes management. Diabetes Metab Rev 1998; 14(Suppl 1):S39.

106. Garg A. Dyslipoproteinemia and diabetes. Endocrinol Metab Clin North Am 1998; 27(3):613.

107. Steiner G. Clinical trial assessment of lipid-acting drugs in diabetic patients. Am J Cardiol 1998; 23;81(8A):58F.

108. Guzman CB, Sowers JR. Special considerations in the therapy of diabetic hypertension. Prog Cardiovasc Dis 1999; 41(6):461.

109. Blair SN, Horton E, Leon AS, et al. Physical activity, nutrition, and chronic disease. Med Sci Sports Exerc 1996; 28(3):335.

110. Henry RR. Thiazolidinediones. Endocrinol Metab Clin North Am 1997; 26(3):553.

111. Majumdar SR. Beta-blockers for the treatment of hypertension in patients with diabetes: exploring the contraindication myth. Cardiovasc Drugs Ther 1999; 13(5):435.

112. MacDonald TM, Butler R, Newton RW, Morris AD. Which drugs benefit diabetic patients for secondary prevention of myocardial infarction? DARTS/MEMO Collaboration. Diabet Med 1998; 15(4):282.

113. Poulsen PL, Ebbehoj E, Hansen KW, Mogensen CE. High normo- or low microalbuminuria: basis for intervention in insulin-dependent diabetes mellitus. Kidney Int Suppl 1997; 63:S15.

114. Lewis EJ, Hunsicker LG, Bain RP, Rohde RO. The effect of angiotensin-converting enzyme inhibition on diabetic nephropathy. N Engl J Med 1993; 329:1456.

115. Pyorala K, Pedersen TR, Kjekshus J, et al. Cholesterol lowering with simvastatin improves prognosis of diabetic patients with coronary heart disease. A subgroup analysis of the Scandinavian Simvastatin Survival Study (4S). Diabetes Care 1997; 20(4):614.

116. Detre KM, Guo P, Holubkov R, et al. Coronary revascularization in diabetic patients: a comparison of the randomized and observational components of the Bypass Angioplasty Revascularization Investigation (BARI). Circulation 1999; 99(5):633.

117. Salomon NW, Page US, Okies JE, et al. Diabetes mellitus and coronary artery bypass. J Thorac Cardiovasc Surg 1983; 85:264.

118. Johnson WD, Pedraza PM, Kayser KL. Coronary artery surgery in diabetes: 261 consecutive patients followed four to seven years. Am Heart J 1982; 104:823.

119. Batist G, Blaker M, Kosinski EJ, et al. Coronary bypass surgery in juvenile onset diabetes. Am Heart J 1983; 106:51.

119a. Kornowski R, Lansky AJ. Current perspectives on interventional treatment strategies in diabetic patients with coronary artery disease. Catheter Cardiovasc Interv 2000; 50:245.

120. Blackshear JL, O'Callaghun WG, Califf RM. Medical approaches to the prevention of restenosis after coronary angioplasty. J Am Coll Cardiol 1987; 9:834.

121. Strandness DE Jr, Priest RE, Gibbons GE. Combined clinical and pathologic study of diabetic and nondiabetic peripheral arterial disease. Diabetes 1964; 13:366.

122. Wheelock FC Jr, Gibbons GW, Marble A. Surgery in diabetes. In: Marble A, Krall LP, Bradley RF, et al., eds. Joslin's diabetes mellitus. Philadelphia: Lea & Febiger, 1985:712.

123. LoGerfo FW. Vascular disease, matrix abnormalities and neuropathy: implications for limb salvage in diabetes mellitus. J Vasc Surg 1987; 5:793.

124. Lithner F. The diabetic gangrene: research and clinical practice. Acta Med Scand 1984; (Suppl):687.

125. Green R, McNamara J. The effect of pentoxifylline on patients with intermittent claudication. J Vasc Surg 1988; 7:356.

126. Apelquist J, Ragnarsson-Tennwall G, Larsson J. Topical treatment of diabetic foot ulcers; an economic analysis of treatment alternatives and strategies. Diabet Med 1995; 12:123.

127. Williams RL. Hyperbaric oxygen therapy and the diabetic foot. J Am Podiatr Med Assoc 1997; 87(6):279.

128. Akbari CM, LoGerfo FW. Diabetes and peripheral vascular disease. J Vasc Surg 1999; 30(2):373.

129. LoGerfo FW, Gibbons GW. Vascular disease of the lower extremities in diabetes mellitus. Endocrinol Metab Clin North Am 1996; 25(2):439.

130. Estes JM, Pomposelli FB Jr. Lower extremity arterial reconstruction in patients with diabetes mellitus. Diabet Med 1996; 13(Suppl 1):S43.

# CHAPTER 148

# DIABETIC NEUROPATHY

EVA L. FELDMAN, MARTIN J. STEVENS, JAMES W. RUSSELL, AND DOUGLAS A. GREENE

Peripheral neuropathy is probably the most common, and certainly one of the most troubling, of the chronic complications of diabetes.[1] Although first described as a clinical entity almost 200 years ago, diabetic neuropathy was recognized relatively recently as a sequela rather than a cause of diabetes,[2] and its pathogenesis and therapy remain controversial.[1,3–5] Advances in our understanding of nerve metabolism have provided a rationale for definitive therapeutic approaches that now are undergoing clinical trials.[6]

**TABLE 148-1.**
**Classification of Diabetic Neuropathy**

I. **Distal symmetric polyneuropathy**
  A. Sensory neuropathy
  B. Sensorimotor neuropathy
    1. Predominantly large-fiber involvement
    2. Predominantly small-fiber involvement
    3. Diffuse (large and small) fiber involvement
II. **Focal and multifocal neuropathies**
  A. Cranial mononeuropathy
  B. Somatic mononeuropathy
    1. Entrapment mononeuropathy (median, ulnar, radial, peroneal)
    2. Other mononeuropathies (femoral)
III. **Radiculopathy and plexopathy**
  A. Lumbar roots (asymmetric motor neuropathy)
  B. Thoracic roots (intercostal neuropathy)
IV. **Autonomic neuropathy**

## DEFINITION AND PREVALENCE

Diabetic neuropathy is characterized as *clinical* or *subclinical* based on clinical signs and symptoms, and as *distal symmetric polyneuropathy, focal* or *multifocal neuropathy,* and *autonomic neuropathy,* depending on its distribution (Table 148-1). In both insulin-dependent (type 1) and non–insulin-dependent (type 2) diabetes mellitus, the prevalence of neuropathy varies with the duration and severity of hyperglycemia.[1,2] Clinical neuropathy is rarely reported within the first 5 years of diabetes, except in patients with type 2 disease, in whom preexisting asymptomatic hyperglycemia is difficult to exclude. In a 25-year prospective study of 4400 unselected diabetics, neuropathy, defined clinically as the loss of Achilles or patellar reflexes, or both, plus diminished vibratory sensation, with or without other clinical signs and symptoms of peripheral neuropathy, was detected in 12% of patients at diagnosis, primarily older, presumably type 2 diabetics.[7] Thereafter, prevalence increased linearly with the duration of diabetes, reaching 50% after 25 years. The duration-corrected prevalence and incidence rates of neuropathy did not differ substantially with age, suggesting that neuropathy occurs similarly in types 1 and 2 diabetes. Of 8757 diabetic patients examined in Italy, 32% had diabetic neuropathy, and the presence and severity of neuropathy correlated with the duration of diabetes.[8] These estimates agree with a study from the United Kingdom in which 44% of patients with diabetes had neuropathy by age 70.[9] In two population-based studies (the Pittsburgh Epidemiology of Diabetes Study and the Rochester Diabetic Neuropathy Study), 58% and 45%, respectively, of type 1 diabetic patients older than 30 years of age had neuropathy.[10,11] Of longitudinally examined type 2 diabetic patients, 54% had neuropathy.[10] Neuropathy also complicates secondary forms of diabetes (pancreatectomy, nonalcoholic pancreatitis, and hemochromatosis); therefore, it reflects the duration and severity, rather than the underlying pathogenesis, of diabetes.[1,2]

## PATHOLOGY OF DIABETIC NEUROPATHY

In diabetic neuropathy, the numbers of larger nerve fibers are reduced and smaller fibers increased, suggesting either sprouting of smaller, or shrinkage of larger, fibers. Demyelination and remyelination are mild except in rare cases with associated, prominent proliferation of Schwann cells. Axonal loss and atrophy account for most clinical and functional impairment in diabetic polyneuropathy. Endoneurial fibrosis, connective tissue proliferation and thickening, and reduplication of endoneurial capillary and perineurial basement membranes all parallel the nerve fiber damage; however, none are pathognomonic for dia-

betes. Programmed cell death of sensory neurons and Schwann cells also contributes to the damage of the peripheral nervous system in diabetics.[12]

## ELECTROPHYSIOLOGY

Nerve conduction velocities vary inversely with the duration and severity of hyperglycemia[1]; however, the predictive value of conduction slowing in subclinical neuropathy for the subsequent clinical development or the course of neuropathy is uncertain. Because maximum conduction velocity primarily reflects large rapidly conducting fibers, small-fiber neuropathy may not reveal itself in standard electrodiagnostic studies.

In clinically overt neuropathy, most slowing of nerve conduction is attributable to the loss of large-diameter nerve fibers, with a small, additional component for which there is no structural explanation and which possibly reflects persistent direct metabolic effects. Conversely, in acutely diabetic animals, the marked but reversible conduction slowing is unaccompanied by any segmental demyelination or axonal degeneration. Thus, conduction slowing in diabetes reflects a dynamic combination of altered structure and metabolism in a diabetic nerve that cannot be easily differentiated electrophysiologically.[1]

## CLINICAL SYNDROMES OF DIABETIC NEUROPATHY

Clinical diabetic neuropathy is categorized into distinct syndromes according to the distribution of the neurologic deficit, each syndrome having a characteristic presentation and course (see Table 148-1). However, in many cases, the occurrence of overlap syndromes precludes a straightforward classification.

### DISTAL SYMMETRIC POLYNEUROPATHY

Distal symmetric polyneuropathy is the most commonly recognized peripheral neurologic complication of diabetes.[1] The symptoms and signs begin distally and spread proximally in a symmetric, fiber-length–dependent fashion, ultimately involving all sensorimotor modalities, but with an initial propensity for sensory over motor involvement. Neurologic impairment usually begins in the feet or toes and may progress proximally up both the upper and lower extremities. With continued progression, a coexisting verticoanterior chest band of sensory deficit may develop as the tips of the shorter truncal nerves become involved (Fig. 148-1). Histologic and nerve conduction studies suggest that nerve damage occurs in virtually all peripheral nerve trunks, with a propensity for sensory over motor and for distal over proximal. Thus, the generalized motor and sensory conduction slowing and the axonal degeneration and demyelination that are characteristic of chronic diabetes are exaggerated in patients with distal symmetric polyneuropathy; nerve conduction slowing closely parallels the histologic fiber loss.[1,13]

The distal symmetric pattern seen in diabetes mellitus, and shared with other "metabolic" neuropathies (including uremic and various nutritional neuropathies), is attributed to selective damage to the most distal parts of the axon (a "dying-back" neuropathy), to the cumulative effect of randomly distributed vascular lesions along nerve trunks that accumulate in greater numbers along longer axons, and to programmed cell death of sensory and motor neurons and supporting Schwann cells.[6] Clinically detectable neurologic deficits evolve only when diffuse peripheral nerve damage outstrips compensatory collateral reinnervation, usually as a late stage in a chronic underlying process. Because the signs and symptoms of diabetic distal symmetric polyneuropathy are identical with those that occur in other distal symmetric neuropathies, the clinical diagnosis is one of exclusion (Table 148-2).

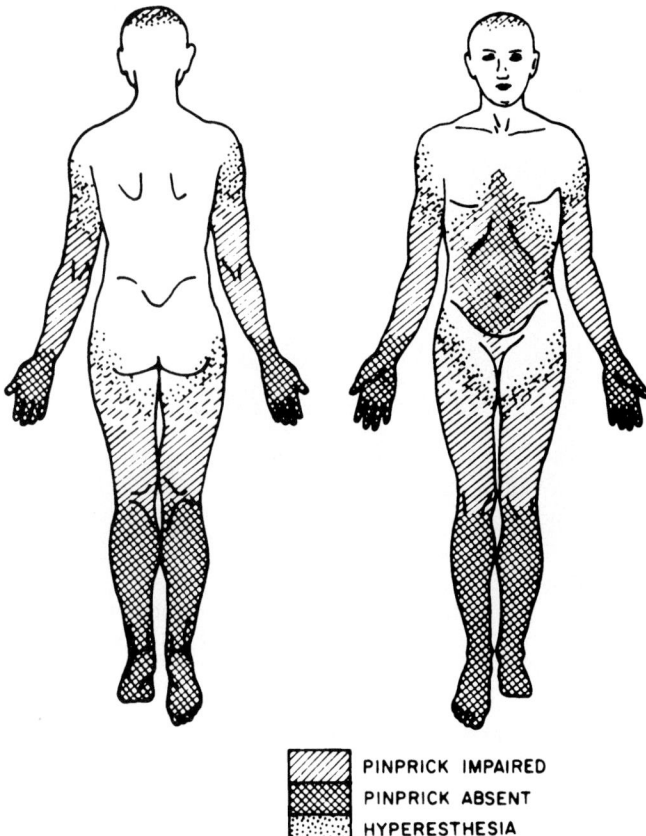

| | |
|---|---|
| ▨ | PINPRICK IMPAIRED |
| ▤ | PINPRICK ABSENT |
| ▦ | HYPERESTHESIA |

**FIGURE 148-1.** Sensory deficits in distal symmetric polyneuropathy. (Reprinted from Sabin TD, et al. In: Waxman SG, ed. Physiology and pathobiology of axons. New York: Raven Press, 1978:431.)

**Sensorimotor and Autonomic ("Mixed") Neuropathy.** Sensorimotor neuropathy is the most common form of distal symmetric polyneuropathy; it is characterized by diffuse fiber damage with a predominance of sensory over motor involvement. The destruction of large sensory fibers diminishes position and light-touch sensation, whereas small-fiber damage impairs pain and temperature sensation and produces paresthesias; mixed neuropathy contains symptoms referable to both large and small fibers. Motor weakness is usually minimal until the neuropathy is far advanced, involving primarily the most distal intrinsic muscles of the hands and feet (Fig. 148-2). Diminished deep tendon reflexes, especially the Achilles tendon reflex, are often early features.

**Neuropathy: Predominantly Large-Fiber Involvement.** Selective large-fiber sensory neuropathy impairs balance, diminishes proprioception and position sense, and reduces vibration sensation, usually in the absence of subjective pain, paresthesias, or numbness. Therefore, this neuropathy may be detected by routine physical examination or may present with secondary neuropathic complications. In its most severe form, sensory ataxia resembling that of posterior column disease is referred to as pseudotabetic diabetic neuropathy. Nerve conduction slowing is usually marked, because of the selective involvement of the large, rapidly conducting fiber population.[1]

**Sensory Neuropathy: Predominantly Small-Fiber Involvement.** Small-fiber sensory neuropathy, which damages the fibers responsible for pain and temperature sensation, often, but not always, is marked by early subjective symptoms of numb, cold, or "dead" feet; spontaneous paresthesias; and pain. The latter include typical neuropathic distal *paresthesias* (spontaneously occurring uncomfortable sensations) or *dysesthesias* (contact paresthesias), whereas some patients complain

**TABLE 148-2.**
**Differential Diagnosis of Diabetic Neuropathy**

**DISTAL SYMMETRIC POLYNEUROPATHY**
*Metabolic*
  Diabetes mellitus
  Uremia
  Folic acid/cyanocobalamin deficiency
  Hypothyroidism
  Acute intermittent porphyria
*Toxic*
  Alcohol
  Heavy metals (lead, mercury, arsenic)
  Industrial hydrocarbons
  Various drugs
*Infectious or Inflammatory*
  Sarcoidosis
  Leprosy
  Periarteritis nodosa
  Other connective tissue diseases (e.g., systemic lupus erythematosus)
*Other*
  Dysproteinemias and paraproteinemias
  Paraneoplastic syndrome
  Leukemias and lymphomas
  Amyloidosis
  Hereditary neuropathies
**PAINS AND PARESTHESIAS WITHOUT NEUROLOGIC DEFICIT**
  Early small-fiber sensory neuropathy
  Psychophysiologic disorder (e.g., severe depression, hysteria)
**AUTONOMIC NEUROPATHY WITHOUT SOMATIC COMPONENT**
  Shy-Drager syndrome (progressive autonomic failure)
  Diabetic neuropathy with mild somatic involvement
  Riley-Day syndrome
  Idiopathic orthostatic hypotension
**DIFFUSE MOTOR NEUROPATHY WITHOUT SENSORY DEFICIT**
  Guillain-Barré syndrome
  Primary myopathies
  Myasthenia gravis
  Heavy-metal toxicity
**FEMORAL NEUROPATHY (SACRAL PLEXOPATHY)**
  Degenerative spinal-disk disease (e.g., Paget disease of the spine)
  Intrinsic spinal-cord-mass lesion
  Equina cauda lesions
  Coagulopathies
**CRANIAL NEUROPATHY**
  Carotid aneurysm
  Intracranial mass
  Elevated intracranial pressure
**MONONEUROPATHY MULTIPLEX**
  Vasculitis
  Amyloidosis
  Hypothyroidism
  Acromegaly
  Coagulopathies

of exquisite cutaneous contact hypersensitivity to light touch, superficial burning or stabbing pain, or bone-deep, aching, or tearing pain. These symptoms are more noticeable at night, producing associated insomnia. Pain may become the overriding feature of small-fiber sensory diabetic neuropathy, yet conduction velocity may not be dramatically impaired, vibration sensation may be intact, and motor weakness may be absent. If the patient's symptoms bring him or her to the physician's attention early in the course of the disease, the sensory loss may not be striking. With further progression, marked deficits in pain and temperature sensation predispose to undetected trauma of

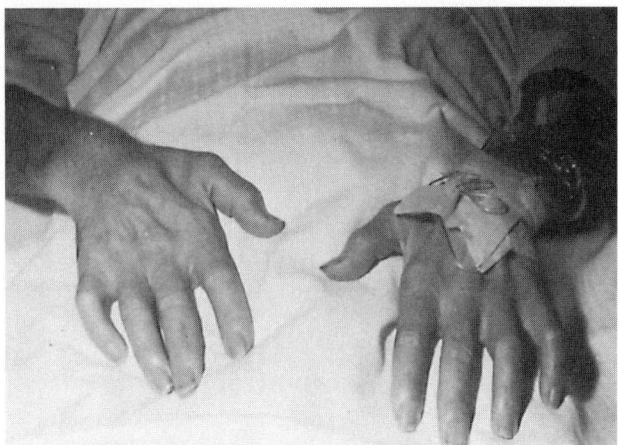

**FIGURE 148-2.** Type 1 diabetic with severe, bilateral atrophy of the interosseous muscles (between the metacarpal bones). There was also loss of the thenar and hypothenar eminences and atrophy of the forearm muscle flexors.

the extremities, such as cigarette burns of the hand (Fig. 148-3), bath-water burns of the feet, or acute foot ulcerations from unnoticed foreign objects retained inside the shoe or from ill-fitting footwear.[1]

Commonly, one encounters *diffuse* involvement, affecting both large and small fibers.

**Distal Motor Neuropathy.**    Distal motor neuropathy rarely occurs in diabetes and should suggest another etiology such as Guillain-Barré syndrome (see Table 148-2). A primary motor neuropathy has been described in psychiatric patients who have been treated by insulin induction of hypoglycemia and also in patients with insulin-secreting tumors; hence, recurrent insulin-related hypoglycemia should be considered in any diabetic presenting primarily with a distal motor neuropathy.[1]

### COMPLICATIONS OF DISTAL SYMMETRIC POLYNEUROPATHY

The mechanical and traumatic consequences of sensory or motor denervation pose a critical potential risk to neuropathic patients; this is almost completely avoidable with patient and physician education—particularly that dealing with foot care and hygiene (see Chap. 154). Even high-risk diabetic patients in a specialty clinic frequently did not have examinations or instructions directed to the early detection and prevention of foot problems.[10]

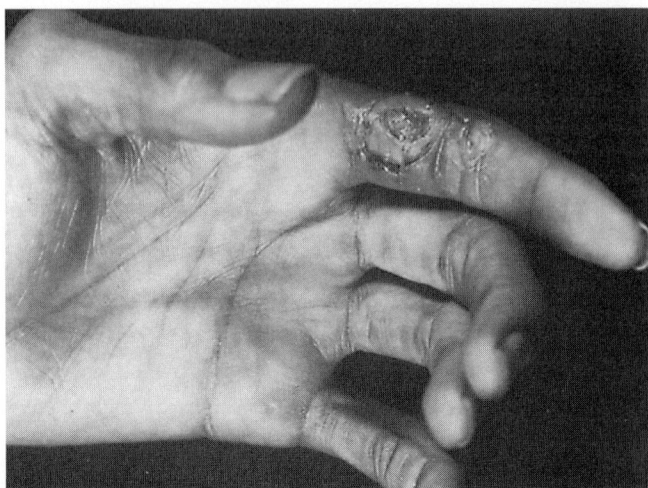

**FIGURE 148-3.** Painless cigarette burn on the finger of a diabetic with diminished skin sensation.

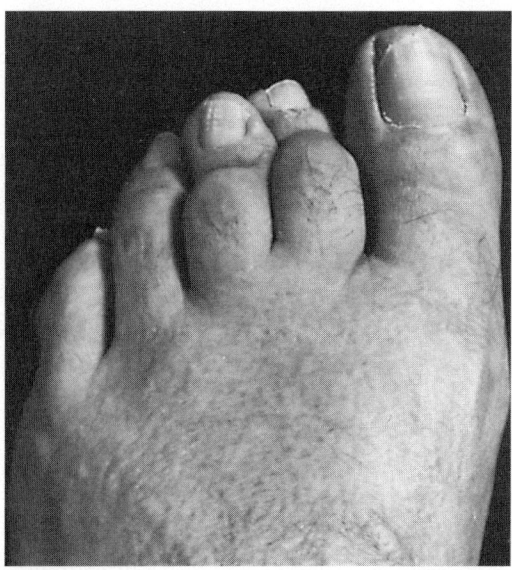

**FIGURE 148-4.** Claw toe (hammertoe) deformity in a diabetic. There is neuropathic loss of the distal motor fibers innervating the intrinsic muscles of the toes. The resulting dominance of the long flexors and extensors results in a flexion contraction at the proximal interphalangeal joints. Often, this causes pressure and friction of the shoes on the dorsal surface of these joints, resulting in abrasions and ulcerations. (This can be avoided by the wearing of extra-depth shoes.) In addition, the flexed toes result in a transfer of weight-bearing to the metatarsal heads, leading to ulceration. (Courtesy of Dr. Charles J. Shuman.)

**Neuropathic Foot Ulceration.**    Neuropathic foot ulceration occurs with great frequency in sensory neuropathies and may reflect unnoticed traumatic damage to the skin and soft tissues of the foot; however, diminished proprioception and muscle strength, as well as vascular factors, also may play contributing roles. In the classic plantar ulcer, neurogenic atrophy of the intrinsic foot muscles that normally counterbalance the more proximal foot flexors and extensors produces chronic flexion of the metatarsophalangeal joints, thereby drawing the toes into a cocked-up position (claw toe deformity; Fig. 148-4). Weight-bearing is thereby redistributed to the now-uncovered metatarsal heads, leading to thinning and atrophy of the normal fat pad; thick callus formation further shifts weight-bearing to the metatarsal heads and, subsequently, leads to breakdown of the callus with ulcer formation. In the absence of pain sensation, this may remain unnoticed, even when secondary infection develops. Neuropathic foot ulceration at other than weight-bearing sites usually reflects undetected incidental trauma that becomes secondarily infected. In neuropathic patients, the generally thin dorsal dermis of the foot may be abraded within hours by ill-fitting footwear or foreign bodies trapped within the shoe. Frequent self-examinations are required when wearing new footwear or with prolonged weight-bearing. Ischemia has also been invoked as a factor, since proximal occlusive vascular disease delays healing of neuropathic foot ulcers. However, the neuropathic ulcerated foot is generally warm, with easily palpable dorsalis pedis pulses. Studies suggest that increased blood flow results from abnormal local arteriovenous shunting in the neuropathic foot that, paradoxically, may decrease oxygen delivery to the tissues (Fig. 148-5). Thus, changes in autonomic nervous system vascular function may affect oxygen delivery to the skin and theoretically contribute to the development of diabetic foot ulcers.

The treatment of diabetic foot ulcers attempts to eliminate further traumatic injury by readjusting weight-bearing using appropriate orthopedic devices and by callus debridement, as well as by partial elimination of weight-bearing through decreased ambulation, non–weight-bearing casts, and special orthoses or nearly complete cessation of weight-bearing with a

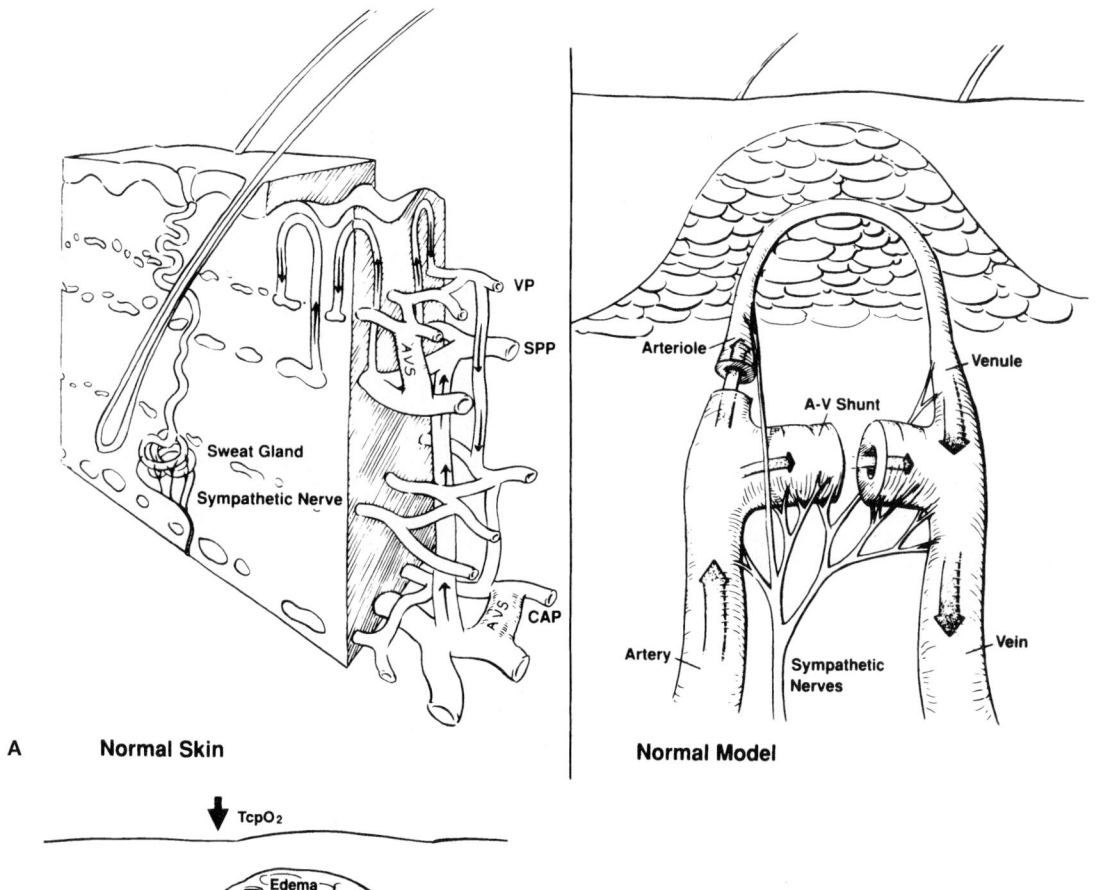

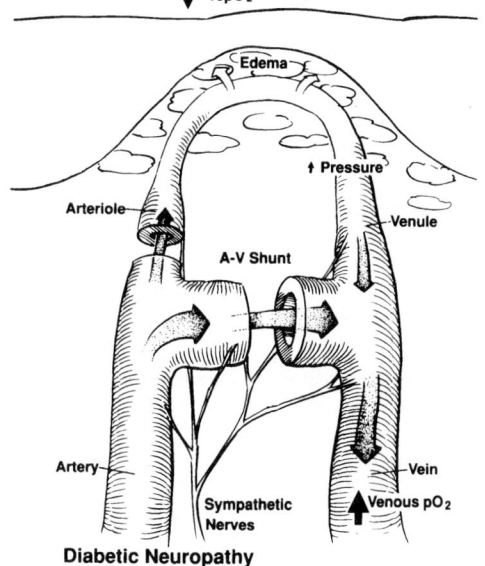

**FIGURE 148-5. A,** Microvasculature of the normal foot. Small subcutaneous arteries penetrate the dermis and anastomose in the cutaneous arterial plexus (*CAP*). Arterioles arise from this plexus and ascend to form the subpapillary plexus (*SPP*). Arteriovenous anastomoses (AV shunts; *AVS*) are richly innervated, are under rigid sympathetic control, and connect small arteries and arterioles to small veins and venules. (*VP*, venous plexus.) **B,** Proposed mechanism of AV shunting in diabetic neuropathy. A decrease in sympathetic innervation of the richly innervated AV shunt and less innervated arterioles results in relatively greater dilatation of the AV shunt and only a modest dilatation of the arteriole. This leads to a shunting of blood away from the capillary dermal papillae loops, a decrease in transcutaneous oxygen tension at the skin, an increase in foot venous oxygen tension, and low skin temperature.

wheelchair or enforced bed rest. Good foot hygiene and adequate oxygenation should be established. Complicating infection should be treated vigorously.[3]

**Neuroarthropathy ("Charcot Joint").** Charcot joint complicates any neurologic disease that impairs sensation but spares motor function (see Chap. 211). Syphilitic neuroarthropathy classically involves the large weight-bearing joints, whereas diabetic neuroarthropathy primarily involves distal joints of the foot (tarsometatarsal or metatarsophalangeal) or ankle. Diabetic neuroarthropathy generally presents as painless swelling and redness of the foot, without fever or leukocytosis; it may resemble cellulitis or osteomyelitis, depending on the extent of bony destruction. Unhealed painless fractures are often visible radiographically, and a history of recent painless trauma is sometimes elicited. Gross architectural distortion of the foot, with shortening and widening of the joint, may occur with repeated injury. In its most advanced stage, multiple painless fractures are accompanied by extensive bone demineralization and reabsorption, so that the foot resembles "a bag of bones." Therapy is directed at removal of continued trauma by decreasing ambulation or redistributing weight-bearing (e.g., use of a cane, crutches, or wheelchair).[3,14]

**Diabetic Neuropathic Cachexia.** Occasionally, a painful neuropathy is seen, typically in elderly men, and is associated with depression, consequent anorexia, and undernutrition. This has been termed *diabetic neuropathic cachexia*.

### TREATMENT OF DISTAL SYMMETRIC DIABETIC POLYNEUROPATHY

It has previously been debated whether improving glycemic control would slow the progression of diabetic neuropathy. In the Diabetes Control and Complication Trial (DCCT), an intensive insulin regimen of either four injections of insulin per day

**TABLE 148-3.**
**Drugs Used in the Treatment of Painful Diabetic Neuropathy**

**NONSTEROIDAL ANTI-INFLAMMATORY DRUGS**
  Ibuprofen, 600 mg qid
  Sulindac, 200 mg bid
**ANTIDEPRESSANT DRUGS**
  Amitriptyline, 50–150 mg at night
  Nortriptyline, 50–150 mg at night
  Imipramine, 100 mg qhs
  Paroxetine, 40 mg qd
**NEURALEPTICS**
  Carbamazepine, 200 mg qid
  Gabapentin, 900 mg tid
**OTHERS**
  Capsaicin, 0.075% qid (topical)
  Fluphenazine, 1 mg tid
  Mexiletine, 150–450 mg qid
  Transcutaneous nerve stimulation

  (Adapted from Feldman EL, Stevens MJ, Greene DA. Treatment of diabetic neuropathy. In: Mazzaferri EL, Bar RS, Kreisberg RA, eds. Advances in endocrinology and metabolism, vol 5. St. Louis: Mosby, 1994:393.)

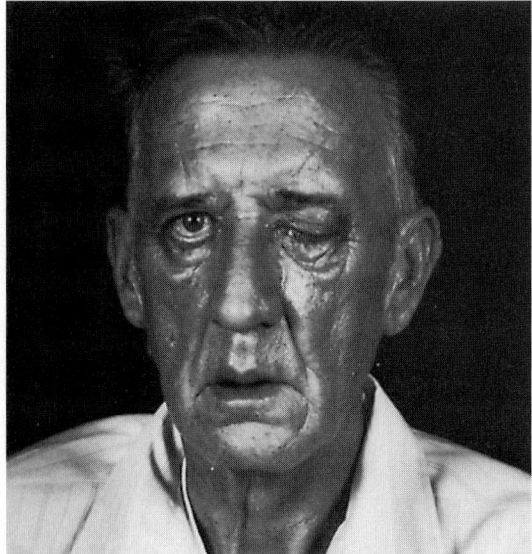

**FIGURE 148-6.** Diabetic patient with acute paralysis of the facial muscles on the right owing to involvement of the facial (seventh) nerve at the level of the brainstem nucleus. This painless condition is characterized by a sagging of the facial muscles and, in particular, the lower lid. There is flattening of the nasolabial fold. The patient is attempting to close his eyes; instead, the right eyeball deviates upward (Bell phenomenon).

or insulin pump resulted in a 60% reduction in the risk of neuropathy and a delay in the progression of neuropathy.[2]

The clinical importance of asymptomatic sensory deficits revolves around the patient's proneness to secondary complications. Hence, management of these disorders primarily involves prophylactic patient education. Symptomatic paresthesias and dysesthesias are usually well tolerated by those patients who are informed of their possible reparative significance. Even debilitating neuropathic pain often improves spontaneously within months. Thus, patient education and optimistic support are key elements in the management of this disorder.

However, when neuropathic pain is unremitting, this can be an extremely difficult and frustrating problem to treat. Chronic use of narcotics should be avoided because of the abuse potential and development of tolerance. There have been multiple trials evaluating single agents in the treatment of neuropathic pain, with variable results. One study found that treating patients based on the categorization of their neuropathic pain by symptoms and pathogenesis resulted in improvement in more than 87% of subjects.[15] Superficial pain, often described as "burning" or "sunburn-like tingling," responds well to topical agents, such as capsaicin cream (0.25–0.75%) applied four times a day to the dysesthetic areas.[16] Deep pain, described as "pins and needles" or "sharp and stabbing," generally responds well to gabapentin or tricyclic medications (especially imipramine, amitriptyline, and desipramine).[3] In refractory cases, tricyclic drugs may be combined with oral mexiletine[3] or a local anesthetic (e.g., lidocaine).[3] Muscular pain, or cramps, generally responds to skeletal muscle relaxants, nonsteroidal antiinflammatory medications, and passive muscle stretching. (Table 148-3 lists commonly used medications.[3])

## FOCAL AND MULTIFOCAL NEUROPATHIES

Focal and multifocal neuropathies are characterized by neurologic deficits in the distribution of single or multiple peripheral nerves (*mononeuropathy*), nerve roots (*radiculopathy*), or brachial or lumbosacral plexuses (*plexopathy*). Their abrupt onset and complete or partial remission suggest a vascular or traumatic etiology, although some reports suggest an inflammatory component.

### CRANIAL NEUROPATHY

Cranial neuropathies are common in diabetic patients, especially in the elderly, but they also occasionally occur in diabetic children, usually in the absence of generalized diabetic neuropathy.[1] The cranial palsies may be recurrent or bilateral. The third cranial nerve is most commonly involved, producing unilateral ophthalmoplegia that spares lateral eye movement and pupillary function. There may be headache that, typically, is intense and referred above or behind the eye. Histologically, the presumed vascular basis of focal diabetic neuropathy is demonstrated most convincingly for isolated third nerve palsy. Other cranial nerves less commonly involved in diabetic neuropathy include the sixth, the fourth (usually in combination with other cranial nerves), and the seventh, presumably also on a vascular basis (Fig. 148-6). Most cases of diabetic neuropathy resolve spontaneously in several weeks to months.

### MONONEUROPATHY

Clinical or electrophysiologic evidence of superimposed focal injury at common sites for *nerve entrapment* (e.g., median nerve at the wrist and palm, radial nerve in the upper arm, ulnar nerve at the elbow, lateral cutaneous nerve of the thigh [meralgia paresthetica], and peroneal nerve at the fibular head) is found in more than one-third of diabetic patients with diffuse neuropathy, suggesting that diffuse diabetic neuropathy predisposes to entrapment neuropathy.[1] Nerves not commonly exposed to compression or entrapment damage also occasionally demonstrate focal impairment in patients with diabetes; this may occur coincidentally.

### RADICULOPATHY AND PLEXOPATHY

*Diabetic polyradiculopathy* of the high lumbar spine occurs spontaneously in diabetics (also known as *femoral neuropathy, diabetic amyotrophy,* or *asymmetric proximal motor neuropathy*). Disabling weakness of thigh flexion and knee extension accompany pain in the anterior thigh and medial calf; sensory loss is usually less marked. The pain may extend from the hip to the anterior and lateral surface of the thigh, radiate into the foot, or originate in the sacroiliac region and extend down the leg dorsally. The pain, which may develop gradually, is often worse at night. The muscle weakness most often affects the iliopsoas, quadriceps, and adductor muscles; hip extensors; and hamstrings. The anterolateral muscles in the calf may be involved, mimicking an

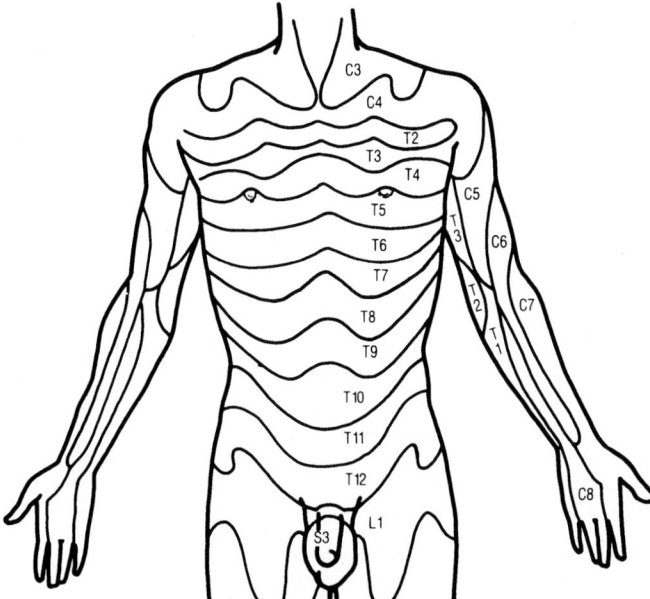

**FIGURE 148-7.** Diabetic radiculopathy is frequently misdiagnosed as an acute intrathoracic or intraabdominal emergency (e.g., myocardial infarction, cholecystitis, peptic ulcer, or appendicitis), as is easily understood from a knowledge of the anterior distribution of the thoracic nerves shown here. Cutaneous hypesthesia in a root distribution is a useful physical finding. When there is doubt, electromyographic studies may help to verify the diagnosis. (Adapted from Ellenberg M. Diabetic truncal mononeuropathy: a new clinical syndrome. Diabetes Care 1978; 1:10.)

"anterior tibial compartment syndrome." Detailed histopathologic study of an autopsy case of diabetic polyradiculopathy has shown multiple, necrotic-appearing lesions in the roots, the lumbosacral plexus, and the femoral, obturator, lateral femoral cutaneous, sciatic, common peroneal, and posterior tibial nerves; there was both distal wallerian degeneration and segmental demyelination in the setting of diffuse atherosclerosis. Because of the similarities between the diabetic and nondiabetic polyradiculopathy, diabetic polyradiculopathy remains a diagnosis of exclusion. When radiculopathy is bilateral and associated with advanced distal symmetric neuropathy with a motor component, it sometimes is referred to as *diabetic polyradiculoneuropathy.*

Nearly complete recovery is very common, although not universal; the syndrome may persist or may recur. Treatment is supportive, pending spontaneous recovery.

Diabetic radiculopathy of thoracic roots (*intercostal neuropathy*) presents with acute dermatomal pain and the diminution of cutaneous sensation, subsequently followed by hypesthesia or paresthesia in the same distribution. Although radiculopathy is often mistakenly attributed to nerve root compression, results of radiographic studies and myelography in this condition are negative. When the pain is prominent and the hypesthesia is subtle, truncal radiculopathy (Fig. 148-7) is frequently misdiagnosed as being an acute intrathoracic or intraabdominal emergency (e.g., myocardial infarction, cholecystitis, peptic ulcer, or appendicitis). Electrophysiologic studies of the paraspinal muscles are usually diagnostic. Subtle signs of diffuse distal symmetric polyneuropathy are often present. Spontaneous resolution of both symptoms and signs is the rule.[1]

## AUTONOMIC NEUROPATHY

Autonomic neuropathy is frequently unnoticed by both the patient and the physician, because of its characteristically multiorgan involvement and its insidious onset. Conversely, symp-

toms of autonomic neuropathy confined to a single organ system may become the subject of intense evaluation, only to be misdiagnosed and treated as another medical condition. Consequently, the prevalence of diabetic autonomic neuropathy, although thought to be very high, is difficult to quantitate. Functional tests of autonomic competence may provide identification of patients with autonomic neuropathy. Studies of autonomic neuropathy are complicated by their complex reflex arcs, dual innervation, and the anatomic dispersion of the autonomic nervous system.

### CLINICAL CHARACTERISTICS OF AUTONOMIC NEUROPATHY

Autonomic neuropathy is classified by its organ system involvement.

**Sudomotor Dysfunction.**   Sudomotor dysfunction produces distal anhidrosis, causing diminished thermoregulatory reserve that is manifested as excessive compensatory truncal and facial sweating and heat intolerance.[1,3] *Diabetic cystopathy* (autonomic neuropathy of the bladder) initially blocks bladder afferents without impairing motor function, leading only to reduced urinary frequency and increased bladder volume. Late in the course, efferent involvement leads to complaints of incomplete or difficult bladder emptying, dribbling, overflow incontinence, residual volumes >150 mL, and recurrent urinary tract infections. Management of diabetic cystopathy emphasizes the facilitation of bladder emptying and the treatment of urinary incontinence. The Credé method and intraabdominal straining (Valsalva technique) increase intravesicular pressure and may allow for passive voiding in milder cases. Medications, including cholinergic stimulants (e.g., bethanechol chloride), which facilitate bladder contractions, and α-adrenergic agonists (e.g., phenoxybenzamine, prazosin, and terazosin), which relax the internal sphincter, may help facilitate bladder emptying. In advanced conditions, chronic catheterization may be necessary. If incontinence develops because of an incomplete sphincter, placement of an artificial urinary sphincter bladder, bladder neck reconstruction, or a fascial sling bladder neck suspension may be of benefit.[1,3] *Neuropathic sexual dysfunction* affects 50% of diabetic men, producing impotence or retrograde ejaculation. *Erectile impotence* must be distinguished from psychogenic impotence and organic impotence of other causes by a detailed sexual history and appropriate laboratory tests. Yohimbine, an $\alpha_2$-adrenergic blocker, may help increase penile rigidity by increasing blood flow to the corpus of the penis. Other vasoactive medications, including phentolamine, papaverine, or prostaglandins, may be injected directly into the corpora cavernosa. Several mechanical devices are available that help produce erections by creating a vacuum to draw blood into the penis. If these treatments are ineffective, a penile prosthesis may be efficacious.[1,3] *Retrograde ejaculation,* caused by the uncoordinated closure of the internal vesicle sphincter and relaxation of the external vesicle sphincter, is diagnosed by an absent ejaculate plus the recovery of live, mobile sperm in the postcoital urine (see Chaps. 117 and 118). Anatomic, nondiabetic causes of retrograde ejaculation must be excluded. Artificial insemination of sperm recovered from fresh urine samples may circumvent the resulting infertility.[1,3] The *blunted epinephrine response to hypoglycemia* produces hypoglycemic unawareness that greatly complicates intensive insulin treatment; it is ascribed to autonomic neuropathy of the adrenal medulla, although it may occur in patients without apparent neuropathy.

**Gastrointestinal Neuropathy.**   Gastrointestinal neuropathy, which can involve the entire gastrointestinal tract, probably explains the high frequency of complaints involving this system in diabetics[1,3] (see Chap. 149). *Esophageal motility disorders,* although usually asymptomatic, are common in long-standing diabetes.[1,3] Diabetic *gastropathy* diminishes gastric acid secretion and motility, explaining both the reduced frequency of duodenal ulceration in diabetics and the presence of anorexia, nausea, vomiting, postprandial fullness, and early satiety in the absence of demonstrable intrinsic lesions. Delayed gastric emptying may complicate diabetic control because of retarded postprandial caloric absorption. Gastric emptying may be improved by erythromycin, which increases gastric motility through simulating the action of motilin; by bethanechol, which increases gastric contractibility through stimulation of muscarinic receptors; or by metoclopramide, which inhibits central and peripheral dopaminergic pathways and allow endogenous parasympathetic tone to act uninhibited.[1,3] In refractory cases of gastroparesis, surgical procedures including jejunostomy, pyloroplasty, or partial gastrectomy may be beneficial. *Diabetic diarrhea* may reflect intestinal hypermotility from decreased sympathetic inhibition, hypomotility with consequent bacterial overgrowth, bile salt malabsorption, diabetic "sprue" (steatorrhea with mucosal histology resembling gluten sensitivity), and pancreatic insufficiency.[1,3]

**Cardiovascular Autonomic Neuropathy.** Cardiovascular autonomic neuropathy (see Chap. 147) produces *exercise intolerance* and *orthostatic hypotension*, the former from reduced augmentation of cardiac output and impaired constriction of the visceral vascular bed and the latter from an impaired sympathetically mediated compensatory increase in peripheral vascular resistance.[1,3] Initial treatment of symptomatic orthostatic hypotension includes the use of waist-high compressive stockings, keeping the head of the bed elevated at night, and use of salt supplements, all of which act to increase blood volume and cardiac filling. If nonpharmacologic measures are ineffective, medications including fludrocortisone or short-acting pressor agents (e.g., ephedrine, midodrine, yohimbine, ergotamine, clonidine, and phenylephrine hydrochloride [used as an atomized nasal spray]) may be of benefit.[1,3] Some studies suggest that erythropoietin may increase standing blood pressure in diabetic patients with orthostatic hypotension. Octreotide has also been used with some success. *Cardiac denervation* is marked by an invariant pulse of 80 to 90 beats per minute that is unresponsive to stress, exercise, or sleep; it is associated with painless myocardial infarction, coronary artery spasm, and sudden cardiac death.[1,3]

# PATHOGENESIS AND THERAPEUTIC IMPLICATIONS OF DIABETIC NEUROPATHY

A pathogenetic role for the metabolic alterations resulting from insulin deficiency is now generally accepted for diabetic neuropathy; however, the nature, extent, and importance of that role remain controversial.[6] There is an array of interrelated metabolic alterations in diabetic nerves resulting from elevated ambient glucose concentrations (Fig. 148-8), several of which appear to interact, in a self-reinforcing or synergistic fashion, with a negative impact on nerve function. These changes include (a) increased activity of the polyol pathway leading to accumulation of sorbitol and fructose and imbalances in nicotinamide adenine dinucleotide phosphate (NADP)/NADPH,[17–19] (b) formation of reactive oxygen species via glucose autooxidation,[20,20a] (c) nonenzymatic glycation of proteins resulting in production of "advanced glycation end products" (AGEs),[18,19,19a] and (d) inappropriate activation of protein kinase C.[18,19] One unifying mode of injury among these different metabolic impairments lies in the production and decreased scavenging of reactive oxygen species, thereby promoting cellular oxidative stress and mitochondrial dysfunction that can lead to programmed cell death of nervous system tissues.[12,17–24]

## POLYOL PATHWAY

The polyol pathway refers to the enzymatic conversion of glucose to sorbitol and then to fructose. Because this reaction is dependent on the concentration of glucose, sorbitol and fructose are formed

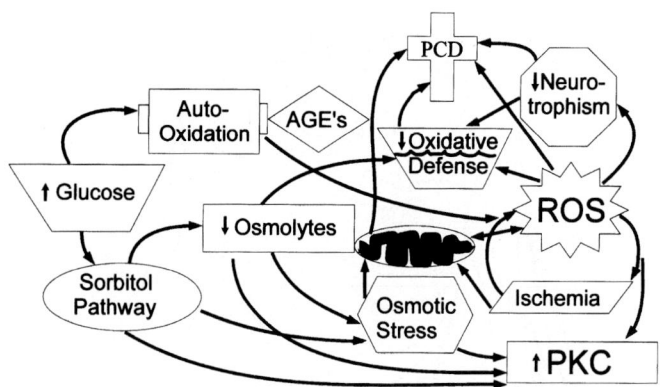

**FIGURE 148-8.** Increased glucose is thought to initiate a cascade of putatively cytotoxic metabolic events through autooxidation, glycation, and formation of advanced glycation end products (*AGEs*), and through increased sorbitol pathway activity. Autooxidation and/or AGEs are thought to promote the generation of toxic free radicals, including a variety of reactive oxygen species (*ROS*). Sorbitol production produces compensatory depletion of other organic osmolytes such as *myo*-inositol and taurine, and endogenous antioxidant, with resulting attenuation of oxidative defense. Sorbitol accumulation and/or reciprocal osmolyte depletion also produce osmotic stress, which may damage mitochondria and stimulate protein kinase C (*PKC*). PKC may also be activated by shifts in triose phosphates toward diacylglycerol production as a result of increased sorbitol pathway activity. Both ROS and PKC activation have been implicated in microvascular dysfunction in peripheral nerve and retina, producing tissue ischemia. Ischemia impairs mitochondrial function and generates additional ROS. Mitochondrial dysfunction and ROS further impair oxidative defense mechanisms. Neurotrophic support through nerve growth factor (NGF) and perhaps other neurotrophins that regulate oxidative defense mechanisms may be impaired by ROS. Mitochondrial damage is thought to lead to the release of cytochromes, activation of caspases, and induction of apoptosis or programmed cell death (*PCD*).

in high concentrations in many tissues of the diabetic, including nerves. Conversion of glucose to sorbitol is dependent on aldose reductase, while sorbitol is converted to fructose via sorbitol dehydrogenase. Both reactions change the oxidation/reduction state of the cell, decreasing NADPH/NADP+ and NADH/NAD+ ratios, respectively. This alters the normal redox potential of the cell and not only decreases the ability of the cell to detoxify reactive oxygen species but also promotes nerve ischemia and free radical injury of mitochondria.[17–20,23,24] Mitochondrial dysfunction further impairs the cell's ability to function in the presence of unchecked reactive oxygen species by decreasing the available adenosine triphosphate (ATP), which is needed for the de novo synthesis of free radical scavengers.[25] Left unchecked, reactive oxygen species produce (a) lipid, DNA, and protein peroxidation[17–20]; (b) further ischemia and reduced nerve blood flow[21–24]; and (c) cellular apoptosis.[12,26] These collective metabolic and vascular impairments result in peripheral nervous system injury and clinical neuropathy. Animal studies have revealed that indicators of oxidative stress parallel neuropathy, and antioxidants that block formation of reactive oxygen species prevent neuropathy.[6] In addition, insulin and aldose reductase inhibitors (which block the accumulation of sorbitol) prevent formation of reactive oxygen species and experimental diabetic neuropathy.[17–24]

## AUTOOXIDATION OF GLUCOSE AND ADVANCED GLYCATED END PRODUCT FORMATION

During diabetes, trace amounts of *free transition metals* (e.g., iron and copper) promote autooxidation of glucose, leading to further formation of reactive oxygen species.[17–19,23] In experimental diabetes, metal-chelating agents preserve both nerve function and blood flow. Reactive oxygen species also may link autooxidation and AGE formation. High ambient glucose results in glycation of proteins and oxidation by reactive oxygen species, with the final end products known as *AGEs*. *Reactive oxygen species* enhance AGE formation, which, in turn, further accelerates *reactive oxygen species (ROS)* formation (a process known as *autooxidative glycosylation*). AGE accumulation correlates with endothelial dysfunction, impaired nerve blood flow, and ischemia.[17–19,23]

## NERVE GROWTH FACTORS

Once diabetic neuropathy becomes clinically evident, structural and functional abnormalities within the peripheral nervous system presumably are widespread and of long standing. To what degree these structural abnormalities are reversible is unclear; however, the studies described earlier have shown greater improvement after treatment in patients with early neuropathy. This suggests that interventions should be introduced as early as possible and should be geared toward slowing the progression of neuropathy rather than reversing the clinical signs and symptoms. Studies evaluating other neurotropic growth factors, which induce axonal sprouting in injured neurons, and may be a means to overcome some of the structural damage in diabetic neuropathy, are either planned or are under way.[27.]

## REFERENCES

1. Greene DA, Feldman EL, Stevens MJ, et al. Diabetic neuropathy. In: Porte D Jr, Sherwin R, eds. Diabetes mellitus. East Norwalk, CT: Appleton & Lange, 1997:1009.
2. DCCT Research Group. The effect of intensive treatment of diabetes on the development and progression of long-term complications in insulin-dependent diabetes mellitus. N Engl J Med 1993; 329:977.
3. Feldman EL, Stevens JJ, Greene DA. Clinical management of diabetic neuropathy. In: Veves A, ed. Clinical management of diabetic neuropathy. Totowa: Humana Press, 1998:89.
4. Salpeter MM, Spanton S, Holley K, Podleski TR. Brain extract causes acetylcholine receptor redistribution which mimics some early events at developing neuromuscular junctions. J Cell Biol 1982; 93:417.
5. Stevens MJ, Feldman EL, Thomas T, Greene DA. Pathogenesis of diabetic neuropathy. In: Veves A, ed. Clinical management of diabetic neuropathy. Totowa: Humana Press, 1998:13.
6. Feldman EL, Russell JW, Sullivan KA, Golovoy D. New insights into the pathogenesis of diabetic neuropathy. Curr Opin Neurol 1999; 12:553.
7. Pirart J. Diabetes mellitus and its degenerative complications; a prospective study of 4,400 patients observed between 1947 and 1973. Diabetes Care 1978; 1:168.
8. Fedele D, Comi G, Coscelli C, et al. A multicenter study on the prevalence of diabetic neuropathy in Italy. Diabetes Care 1997; 20:836.
9. Young MJ, Boulton AJM, Macleod AF, et al. A multicentre study of the prevalence of diabetic peripheral neuropathy in the United Kingdom hospital clinic population. Diabetologia 1993; 36:150.
10. Dyck PJ, Kratz KM, Karnes JL, et al. The prevalence by staged severity of various types of diabetic neuropathy, retinopathy, and nephropathy in a population-based cohort: the Rochester Diabetic Neuropathy Study. Neurology 1993; 43:817.
11. Maser RE, Steenkiste AR, Dorman JS, et al. Epidemiological correlates of diabetic neuropathy. Report from Pittsburgh Epidemiology of Diabetes Complications Study. Diabetes 1989; 38:1456.
12. Russell JW, Sullivan KA, Windebank AJ, et al. Neurons undergo apoptosis in animal and cell culture models of diabetes. Neurobiol Dis 1999; 6:347.
13. Stevens MJ, Feldman EL, Greene DA. Diabetic peripheral neuropathy. In: DeFronzo RA, ed. Current therapy of diabetes mellitus. St. Louis: Mosby–Year Book, 1997:160.
14. Greene DA, Feldman EL, Stevens MJ. Neuropathy in the diabetic foot: new concepts in etiology and treatment. In: Levin M, O'Neal L, eds. The diabetic foot. St. Louis: Mosby, 1993:135.
15. Pfeifer MA, Ross DR, Schrage JP, et al. A highly successful and novel model for treatment of chronic painful diabetic peripheral neuropathy. Diabetes Care 1993; 16:1103.
16. The Capsaicin Study Group. Treatment of painful diabetic neuropathy with topical capsaicin: a multicenter, double-blind, vehicle controlled study. Arch Intern Med 1991; 151:2225.
17. Feldman EL, Stevens MJ, Greene DA. Pathogenesis of diabetic neuropathy. Clin Neurosci 1997; 4:365.
18. Greene DA, Stevens MJ, Obrosova I, Feldman EL. Glucose-induced oxidative stress and programmed cell death in diabetic neuropathy. Eur J Pharmacol 1999; 375:217.
19. Greene DA, Obrosova IG, Stevens MJ, Feldman EL. Pathways of glucose-mediated oxidative stress in diabetic neuropathy. In: Packer L, Tritschler

HJ, King GL, Azzi A, eds. Antioxidants in diabetes management. New York: Marcel Dekker, Inc., 2000: 111.
19a. Rahbar S, Hadler JL. A new rapid method to detect inhibition of Amador; product generated by delta-gluonolactone. Clin Chim Acta 1999; 287:123.
20. van Dam PS, Bravenboer B. Oxidative stress and antioxidant treatment in diabetic neuropathy. Neurosci Res Commun 1997; 21:41.
20a. Stevens MJ, Obrosova I, Cao X, et al. Effects of DL–alpha–lipoic acid on peripheral nerve conduction, blood flow, energy metabolism, and oxidative stress in experimental diabetic neuropathy. Diabetes 2000; 49:1006.
21. Low PA, Nickander KK, Tritschler HJ. The roles of oxidative stress and antioxidant treatment in experimental diabetic neuropathy. Diabetes 1997; 46(Suppl 2):S38.
22. Tomlinson DR. Future prevention and treatment of diabetic neuropathy. Diabetes Metab 1998; 24(Suppl 3):79.
23. Zochodne DW. Diabetic neuropathies: features and mechanisms. Brain Pathol 1999; 9:369.
24. Cameron NE, Cotter MA. Metabolic and vascular factors in the pathogenesis of diabetic neuropathy. Diabetes 1997; 46(Suppl 2):S31.
25. Heiden MG, Chandel NS, Schumacker PT, Thompson CB. Bcl-xL prevents cell death following growth factor withdrawal by facilitating mitochondrial ATP/ADP exchange. Mol Cell 1999; 3:159.
26. Anderson KM, Seed T, Ou D, Harris JE. Free radicals and reactive oxygen species in programmed cell death [In Process Citation]. Med Hypotheses 1999; 52:451.
27. Feldman EL, Windebank AJ. Growth factors and peripheral neuropathy. In: Dyck PJ, Thomas PK, eds. Diabetic neuropathy. Philadelphia: WB Saunders, 1998:377.

# C H A P T E R  1 4 9

# GASTROINTESTINAL COMPLICATIONS OF DIABETES

FREDERIC D. GORDON AND KENNETH R. FALCHUK

Diabetes mellitus can affect many organs in the gastrointestinal tract. The metabolic derangements caused by diabetes can have a significant impact on the function of the digestive and hepatobiliary systems. Rundles, in 1945, was the first to draw attention to the effects of diabetes on the gut.[1] Subsequently, others have confirmed the observation of altered motility in diabetics with autonomic neuropathy. Dysphagia, nausea, vomiting, diarrhea, constipation, and fecal incontinence are common complaints among these patients. Differentiating the various causes of these symptoms can be difficult and should not necessarily be attributed to diabetes alone. Recent developments have led to a better understanding of the pathophysiology of diabetic gastroenteropathy. These advances have broadened the therapeutic options. In this chapter the focus is on the pathophysiology, clinical features, diagnosis, and treatment of the common gastrointestinal complications of diabetes.

## PATHOGENESIS

Despite recent scientific advances, the pathogenetic mechanisms causing diabetic gastrointestinal symptoms remain poorly understood. The most widely accepted theory is that an autonomic visceral neuropathy plays an important role in the development of symptoms. This is supported by the observation that diabetics with impaired gastric emptying have the same clinical constellation and radiographic findings as postvagotomy patients.[2] The delay in gastric emptying may result from impaired myogenic contraction and altered cholinergic pathways. Nitric oxide may play a critical role in mediating gastric wall tone and compliance. In diabetic animal models, nitric oxide synthase activity is decreased, resulting in gastrointestinal motor dysfunction.[3] In addition, electron microscopic studies have demonstrated a decreased density of unmyelinated axons in the vagus nerve of diabetics with gastroparesis.[4] Furthermore, additional manifestations of autonomic neuropathy such as orthostatic hypotension, urinary bladder dysfunction, and impotence are often present in these patients. Other mechanisms have also been proposed. Hyperglycemia and electrolyte imbalance (e.g., hyperkalemia, hypokalemia) may affect nerve function and delay gut motility.[5] Diabetics may also have altered production of various hormones such as motilin, pancreatic polypeptide, somatostatin, vasoactive intestinal peptide, calcitonin gene-related peptide, glucagon, and gastrin, which are known to influence gastrointestinal tract motility, absorption, and secretion.[6,7] Finally, diabetic microangiopathy may play a causal role in the development of gastrointestinal tract complications.[8] Surprisingly, none of the abnormalities caused by these proposed mechanisms correlate with the duration of diabetes, the severity of the neuropathy, the degree of blood sugar control, the presence of other diabetic complications, or the age or sex of the patient.[9]

## ESOPHAGUS

Although diabetics rarely complain of symptoms referable to the esophagus, the most typical symptoms are heartburn, and less frequently dysphagia and chest pain. Esophageal motor dysfunction in diabetics has been extensively studied using various techniques, including barium studies, nuclear radiographic methods, and manometry. Delayed esophageal transit and emptying have been demonstrated in up to 35% of both type 1 and type 2 diabetics.[10–12] Esophageal manometry can reveal multiple aberrant motor patterns, including reduced or absent peristalsis, tertiary contractions, and decreased lower esophageal sphincter pressures.[13] The correlation between investigative studies and clinical symptoms is inconsistent.

Diabetics with dysphagia warrant complete investigation to rule out gastroesophageal reflux, benign or malignant esophageal strictures, and infectious esophagitis. Endoscopy is the preferred method of evaluation. Biopsy samples can be obtained and therapeutic maneuvers can be performed. Gastroesophageal reflux disease can be treated with $H_2$-receptor antagonists or proton pump inhibitors alone or in combination with a prokinetic agent. If esophageal biopsy samples document candidal esophagitis, antifungal therapy can be instituted.

## STOMACH

The most common gastric disorder of diabetes is gastroparesis, which is manifested by postprandial fullness, vague epigastric pain, nausea, vomiting, heartburn, and anorexia. The onset of symptoms is usually insidious, but symptoms may arise acutely, especially in association with ketoacidosis. There is a strong correlation between the onset of gastroparesis and the development of other diabetic complications, such as peripheral neuropathy, retinopathy, and nephropathy. It is important to exclude other causes of impaired gastric emptying such as gastric outlet obstruction, peptic ulcer disease, side effects of pharmacologic agents, and uremia.

Barium studies in patients with gastroparesis can demonstrate an elongated stomach with sluggish, ineffective, or absent peristalsis. At times, solid residue can be found in the stomach of these patients (Fig. 149-1). Because gastric emptying of liquids is usually normal, barium contrast studies are insensitive in assessing gastric dysmotility. By using solid, nondigestible radiopaque markers, the gastric emptying of nondigestible solids is found to be more prolonged than the

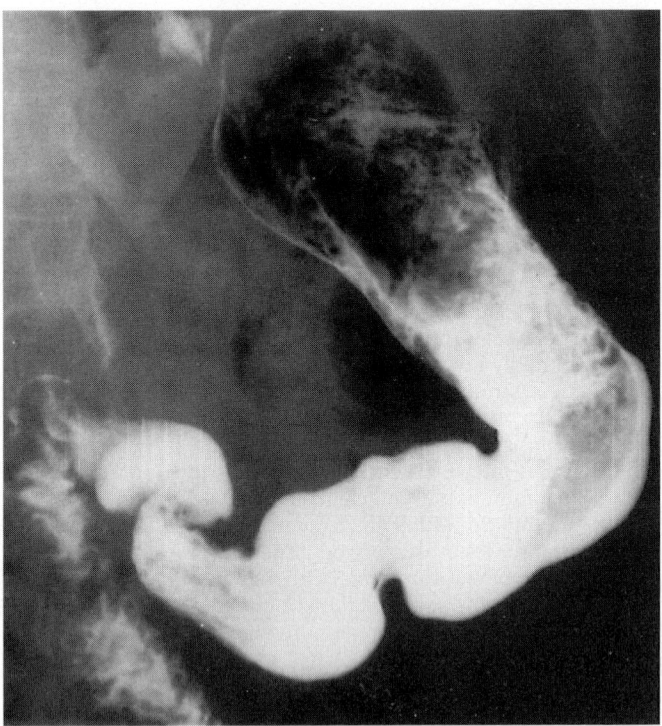

**FIGURE 149-1.** Barium upper gastrointestinal radiograph in a patient with diabetic gastroparesis. The stomach is elongated and filled with food debris.

emptying of digestible solids.[14] Results of radioisotope gastric-emptying studies are more accurate because both liquid- and solid-phase motility are assessed.[15] Because of the impaired gastric emptying, these patients are predisposed to the formation of bezoars, consisting of nondigestible foods. Gastroparesis leads to the irregular emptying of solids into the small intestine, resulting in erratic serum glucose control that may, in turn, worsen gastric emptying. To break this cycle, frequent small meals and close monitoring of the serum glucose concentration are advised.

Should symptoms persist, various antiemetic and prokinetic agents can be used (Table 149-1). Metoclopramide is an antidopaminergic drug that inhibits dopamine-induced gastric smooth muscle relaxation.[16] It also has cholinergic activity that probably acts by increasing the release of acetylcholine from postganglionic neurons or by enhancing acetylcholine receptor sensitivity in the gastric wall.[17] In addition to its cholinergic effects, metoclopramide binds to medullary chemoreceptors in the brain, preventing emesis. As a result of its ability to penetrate the blood–brain barrier, side effects such

**TABLE 149-1.**

**Prokinetic Agents Commonly Used for the Treatment of Diabetic Gastroparesis: Their Mechanisms of Action and Side Effects**

| Drug | Mechanisms of Action | Side Effects |
|------|---------------------|--------------|
| Metoclopramide | Dopamine antagonist | Hyperprolactinemia |
| | Cholinergic agonist | Diarrhea, cramps, tremor |
| | | Tardive dyskinesia |
| | Central antiemetic effect | Anxiety, depression |
| Domperidone | Dopamine antagonist | Hyperprolactinemia |
| | Central antiemetic effect | |
| Erythromycin | Motilin receptor agonist | Diarrhea, cramps, nausea |

as sedation, tremulousness, headache, galactorrhea, and amenorrhea due to hyperprolactinemia can occur. Several studies have shown that while metoclopramide is effective with short-term use, tachyphylaxis may develop.[18] Domperidone is a potent dopamine antagonist lacking cholinergic activity. It enhances gastric emptying and has central antiemetic properties. Side effects of domperidone are infrequent because of its limited penetration of the blood–brain barrier, although hyperprolactinemia can occur. It is beneficial for long-term treatment and has an excellent safety profile.[19,20] Erythromycin is another drug that is effective in relieving symptoms of gastroparesis. It is a macrolide antibiotic that has prokinetic properties attributed to its ability to bind to motilin receptors in the antrum and duodenum. Numerous studies have shown improvement in gastric emptying.[21,22]

Gastroparesis can be a difficult disorder to manage; symptoms may persist despite aggressive medical treatment. Patients who have failed prokinetic therapy may benefit from a percutaneous endoscopic gastrostomy and jejunostomy that allows gastric decompression and adequate nutritional support. This nonpharmacologic approach is well tolerated.[23]

Gastric pacing has been shown to improve gastric emptying. This technique entrains and improves gastric slow-wave activity and enhances slow-wave amplitude. This leads to a normalization of gastric dysmotility.[24]

## SMALL INTESTINE

The incidence of diarrhea in the diabetic population is ~22%, occurring primarily in patients with poorly controlled diabetes.[25] The clinical features are nonspecific, consisting of chronic intermittent diarrhea alternating with normal bowel movements or constipation. Despite the chronicity, weight loss is distinctly uncommon and should elicit a search for other causes of diarrhea.

The etiology of diarrhea in diabetes is multifactorial. Autonomic dysfunction plays a role in diabetic diarrhea. Specifically, $\alpha_2$-adrenergic receptors in enterocytes of the small and large intestines stimulate absorption of sodium chloride and inhibit bicarbonate secretion, resulting in a net influx of fluids and ions into the gut.[26] A second cause may be bacterial overgrowth. Up to 4% of diabetics have achlorhydria,[27] and many have delayed gastric and small bowel transit. These features alone or in combination can allow overgrowth of *Escherichia coli*, enterococci, and staphylococci. These bacteria deconjugate bile salts, preventing micelle formation and resulting in the development of fat malabsorption. There is also evidence that pancreatic insufficiency is a contributing factor.[28]

The evaluation of diabetics with diarrhea should be directed by their clinical presentation. Stool output should be quantified to separate true diarrhea from fecal incontinence. Stool cultures for enteric pathogens and 72-hour fecal fat studies should be performed. Patients with documented steatorrhea need to be evaluated for exocrine pancreatic insufficiency, bacterial overgrowth, or a primary malabsorptive disorder such as celiac disease. Pancreatic insufficiency can be diagnosed by a secretin/cholecystokinin stimulation test or a clinical response to a trial of pancreatic enzyme replacement. Bacterial overgrowth can be diagnosed by various methods, including breath tests and quantitative small bowel bacterial cultures. Alternatively, a response to a 2-week trial of antibiotics, such as tetracycline, can assist in the evaluation of this condition. Malabsorptive processes often require biopsy of the small bowel for diagnosis. Patients without steatorrhea or evidence of enteric infection fall into the category of "idiopathic diabetic diarrhea" and may benefit from a trial of clonidine, conventional antidiarrheal agents (loperamide, diphenoxylate, codeine), anticholinergic agents, or psyllium.

## CELIAC DISEASE

Celiac disease has been reported to occur in diabetics with greater frequency than in the general population.[29,30] The histocompatibility antigens HLA-DR3 and HLA-DQB1*0201 have been linked to celiac disease and type 1 diabetes, suggesting a genetic predisposition to both conditions. The clinical manifestations of celiac disease and diabetic diarrhea are similar, although celiac disease may be distinguished by the absence of peripheral neuropathy, the onset of diarrhea before the initial diagnosis of diabetes, and steatorrhea, which is rare in diabetic diarrhea. In these patients, biopsy of the small bowel is essential. A presumptive diagnosis of celiac disease can be made if the biopsy shows flattened villi and increased cellularity in the lamina propria. A gluten-free diet will improve both the symptoms and histology and thus confirm the diagnosis. Serum immunoglobulin A (IgA) antiendomysial and IgA antigliadin antibodies may also be useful in diagnosing and monitoring patients with celiac disease. Several studies have shown 80% to 100% sensitivity and specificity of these antibodies for celiac disease, although their use cannot substitute for a histologic diagnosis.[31,32] With successful treatment, titers of these antibodies decrease or even disappear and can, therefore, be used to monitor compliance with a gluten-free diet.

## LARGE INTESTINE

The most common gastrointestinal complaint among diabetics is chronic constipation, occurring in 20% to 60% of patients.[24,33] The pathogenesis is poorly understood, although neurogenic dysfunction is thought to be the primary cause. Diminished or delayed postprandial myoelectric colonic activity is observed in diabetics without constipation, and absent activity is observed in those with constipation.[34] Pharmacologic challenge with neostigmine or metoclopramide induces a return of the myoelectric response.

The evaluation of chronic constipation in the diabetic should be guided by the patient's age, associated symptoms, and family history. In patients with rectal bleeding, occult blood in the stool, age older than 40, or a family history of colon cancer, malignancy should be ruled out by appropriate studies such as flexible sigmoidoscopy, barium enema, or colonoscopy. Treatment of constipation should include dietary fiber, stool softeners, and rarely laxatives.

Fecal incontinence is common and often coincides with the onset of diarrhea.[34a] There is a strong association of incontinence with autonomic neuropathy. The pathogenesis is complex and incompletely understood. Initially it was thought that diminished rectal sensation with intact anal sphincter function allowed incontinent passage of stool.[35] Later, anorectal manometry was used to demonstrate that fecal incontinence is caused by aberrant sphincter function; however, it is unclear whether autonomic neuropathy or abnormal intrinsic sphincter smooth muscle underlies the manometric findings.[36] Therapy for fecal incontinence is difficult but responds to the control of diarrhea. If this fails, biofeedback and sphincter tone improving techniques can be used, although the results are not always successful.

## GALLBLADDER DISEASE

The management of gallstones in diabetics is a controversial subject because of the vast number of studies and the opposing conclusions reached. In autopsy studies, diabetics have approximately twice the incidence of gallstones as compared with the nondiabetic population.[36a,37] Although no specific cause has been determined, factors that may predispose to cholelithiasis include impaired gallbladder emptying, altered glucose metabolism, hyperinsulinemia, and supersaturation of gallbladder bile levels with decreased bile acid concentrations.[38] Other studies, however, indicate that comorbid conditions, such as obesity and hyperlipidemia, are confounding variables and that diabetics are not at increased risk of gallstone formation.[39] Asymptomatic gallstones in the general population rarely lead to life-threatening complications.[40] It is not clear whether this applies to diabetic patients. Several studies in diabetics have shown that when gallstones become symptomatic, morbidity and mortality are increased, primarily due to infectious complications.[41] Previously, emergency cholecystectomy in the diabetic population was reported to have a five- to ten-fold increase in mortality when compared with the nondiabetic population.[42] It has been demonstrated that diabetes itself does not increase morbidity and mortality, but rather its associated conditions (e.g., renal failure, vascular disease) are responsible.[43] Additionally, complication rates have decreased significantly because of the early detection of gallstones and cholecystitis by ultrasonography, the more effective use of antibiotics, and improved intraoperative hemodynamic monitoring.[44]

Because diabetics often have comorbid conditions, patients with biliary colic or cholecystitis should be advised to undergo cholecystectomy as soon as possible. In the past, it has been recommended that diabetics with asymptomatic gallstones also have surgery to reduce the chance of potential morbidity in the future. This concept has been carefully reevaluated in the past 10 years. Expectant management of diabetics with asymptomatic gallstones has been shown to be safer and less costly than prophylactic cholecystectomy.[44,45] The introduction of laparoscopic cholecystectomy, while potentially less invasive than conventional surgery, should not influence the decision to operate on a patient with asymptomatic cholelithiasis until this concept is studied in more detail.

## LIVER DISEASE

The incidence of liver dysfunction in diabetics ranges from 28% to 39%.[46] Viral hepatitis is seen in diabetics two to four times more frequently than in the general population.[47] Previously, this was thought to be due to needle sticks; however, the association remains constant even in the era of disposable needles. More likely, it is caused by increased nosocomial exposures or diminished resistance to infection.[48]

Many of the medications used to treat diabetes and its complications can cause liver function test abnormalities. These drugs include the oral hypoglycemic sulfonylureas, many antihypertensive agents, and antibiotics. Both transaminase elevations and cholestatic jaundice can be seen as side effects of medication. Rarely does the side effect manifest clinically, and stopping the offending agent usually leads to a clinical and biochemical resolution.

Increased glycogen deposition is the most common hepatic disorder found in diabetics. Excessive glycogen stores have been documented in up to 80% of persons with type 1 and 2 diabetes and is thought to be stimulated by exogenous hyperinsulinemia.[47]

A second liver lesion associated with diabetes is *nonalcoholic steatohepatitis* (NASH).[49] This condition must be distinguished from hepatic steatosis, a noninflammatory process, which occurs in up to 50% of type 2 diabetics. The diagnosis of NASH requires a liver biopsy showing moderate to gross macrovesicular steatosis in association with inflammation. Additionally, there must be negligible alcohol consumption and absence of active viral infection. The mechanism of fat accumulation in type 1 diabetics is thought to be due to chronic hyperglycemia coupled with inadequate insulin levels that stimulate the release of fatty acids from adipose tissue. These fatty acids are then transported to the liver, where they are deposited into the hepatocyte. Fat accumulates because of increased hepatocellular triglyceride production and diminished secretion in the form of very low-density lipoprotein. In type 2 diabetes the mechanism of fat deposition is different and probably accounts for the increased incidence of NASH when compared with type 1 diabetes. In the type 2 diabetic population, obesity rather than hyperglycemia and hypoinsulinemia seems to be the critical factor. Intake of excessive dietary fats and carbohydrates leads to high levels of free fatty acids that are stored in hepatocytes.[46] Accumulation of fatty acids may be responsible for hepatic inflammation because they are highly reactive and can damage biomembranes. Physical examination of the diabetic patient with NASH can be normal or reveal an enlarged, tender liver. The alkaline phosphatase value is typically normal or slightly elevated. Serum transaminase levels can be slightly elevated, but more significant elevations should prompt an evaluation of other etiologies of hepatitis (e.g., infections, drugs). Radiologic evaluation may be normal or show evidence of fatty infiltration of the liver. The diagnosis of NASH, however, can be confirmed only by liver biopsy.

The course of NASH is typically indolent, but nearly 50% of patients develop hepatic fibrosis and up to 15% will develop cirrhosis. There is no proven therapy for NASH although gradual and sustained weight loss is recommended.[50]

## REFERENCES

1. Rundles RW. Diabetic neuropathy. Medicine 1945; 24:111.
2. Zitomer BR, Gramm HF, Kozak GP. Gastric neuropathy in diabetes mellitus: radiologic observations. Metabolism 1968; 17:199.
3. Takahashi T, Nakamura K, Itoh H, et al. Impaired nitric oxide synthase in the gastric myenteric plexus of spontaneously diabetic rats. Gastroenterology 1997; 113:1535.
4. Guy R, Dawson J, Garrett J, et al. Diabetic gastroparesis from autonomic neuropathy: surgical considerations and changes in vagus nerve morphology. J Neurol Neurosurg Psychiatry 1984; 47:686.
5. DeBoer SY, Masclee AAM, Lamers CBHW. Effect of hyperglycemia on gastrointestinal and gallbladder motility. Scand J Gastroenterol 1992; 27(Suppl 194):13.
6. Hilsted J. Pathophysiology in diabetic autonomic neuropathy: cardiovascular, hormonal, and metabolic studies. Diabetes 1982; 31:730.
7. Belai A, Lincoln J, Burnstock G. Lack of vasoactive intestinal polypeptide and calcitonin gene-related peptide during electrical stimulation of enteric nerves in streptozotocin diabetic rats. Gastroenterology 1987; 93:1034.
8. Liberski S, Koch K, Atnip R, et al. Ischemic gastroparesis: resolution after revascularization. Gastroenterology 1990; 99:252.
9. Keshavarzian A, Iber F, Nasrallah S. Radionuclide esophageal emptying and manometric studies in diabetes mellitus. Am J Gastroenterol 1987; 82:625.
10. Westin L, Lilja B. Oesophageal scintigraphy in patients with diabetes mellitus. Scand J Gastroenterol 1986; 21:1200.
11. Borgstrom P, Olsson R, Sundkvist G, et al. Pharyngeal and oesophageal function in patients with diabetes mellitus and swallowing complaints. Br J Radiol 1988; 61:817.
12. Horowitz M, Harding P, Maddox A, et. al. Gastric and oesophageal emptying in patients with type 2 diabetes mellitus. Diabetologia 1989; 32:151.
13. Mandelstam P, Lieber A. Esophageal dysfunction in diabetic neuropathy gastroenteropathy. JAMA 1967; 201:88.14.Feldman M, Smith H, Simon T. Gastric emptying of solid radiopaque markers: studies in healthy subjects and diabetic patients. Gastroenterology 1984; 87:895.
15. Siegel JA, Urbain JL, Adler LP, et al. Biphasic nature of gastric emptying. Gut 1988; 29:85.
16. Peringer E, Jenner P, Donaldson JM, et al. Metoclopramide and dopamine receptor blockade. Neuropharmacology 1976; 15:463.
17. Hay AM, Man WK. Effect of metoclopramide on guinea pig stomach: critical dependence on intrinsic stores of acetylcholine. Gastroenterology 1979; 76:492.
18. Schade RR, Dugas MC, Lhostky DM, et al. Effect of metoclopramide on gastric liquid emptying in patients with diabetic gastroparesis. Dig Dis Sci 1985; 30:10.
19. Soykan I, Sarosiek I, McCallum RW. The effect of oral domperidone therapy on gastrointestinal symptoms, gastric emptying, and quality of liver in patients with gastroparesis. Am J Gastroenterol 1997; 92(6):976.
20. Silvers D, Kipnes M, Broadstone V, et al. Domperidone in the management of symptoms of diabetic gastroparesis. Clin Ther 1998; 20:438.

21. Altomare DF, Rubini D, Pilot M-A, et al. Oral erythromycin improves gastrointestinal motility and transit after subtotal but not total gastrectomy for cancer. Br J Surg 1997; 84:1017.
22. Janssens J, Peeters TL, Vantrappen G, et al. Erythromycin improves delayed gastric emptying in diabetic gastroparesis. N Engl J Med 1990; 322:1028.
23. Kim CH, Nelson DK. Venting percutaneous gastrostomy in the treatment of refractory idiopathic gastroparesis. Gastrointest Endosc 1998; 47(1):67.
24. McCallum RW, Chen JDZ, Lin Z, et al. Gastric pacing improves emptying and symptoms in patients with gastroparesis. Gastroenterology 1998; 114:456.
25. Feldman M, Schiller L. Disorders of gastrointestinal motility associated with diabetes mellitus. Ann Intern Med 1983; 98:378.
26. Ogbonnaya K, Arem R. Diabetic diarrhea: pathophysiology, diagnosis, and management. Arch Intern Med 1990; 150:262.
27. Ungar B, Stocks AE, Martin FIR, et al. Intrinsic-factor antibody, parietal-cell antibody, and latent pernicious anemia in diabetes mellitus. Lancet 1968; 2:415.
28. Newihi H, Dooley C, Saad C, et al. Impaired exocrine pancreatic function in diabetics with diarrhea and peripheral neuropathy. Dig Dis Sci 1988; 33:705.
29. Walsh CH, Cooper BT, Wright AD, et al. Diabetes mellitus and celiac disease: a clinical study. Q J Med 1978; 47:89.
30. Rensch MJ, Merenich JA, Lieberman M, et al. Gluten-sensitive enteropathy in patients with insulin-dependent diabetes mellitus. Ann Intern Med 1996; 124(6):564.
31. Corroccio A, Iacono G, Montalto G, et al. Immunologic and absorptive tests in celiac disease: can they replace intestinal biopsy? Scand J Gastroenterol 1993; 28:673.
32. McMillan SA, Haughton DJ, Biggart JD, et al. Predictive value for coeliac disease of antibody to gliadin, endomysium, and jejunum in patients attending for jejunal biopsy. Br Med J 1991; 303:1163.
33. Goyal RK, Spiro HM. Gastrointestinal manifestations of diabetes mellitus. Med Clin North Am 1971; 55:1031.
34. Battle WM, Snaper WJ Jr, Alavi A, et al. Colonic dysfunction in diabetes mellitus. Gastroenterology 1980; 79:1217.
34a. Folnaczny C, Riepl R, Tschop M, Landgraf R. Gastrointestinal involvement in patients with diabetes mellitus: part I. Epidemiology, pathophysiology, clinical findings. Z Gastroenterol 1999; 37:803.
35. Katz LA, Kaufman HJ, Spiro HM. Anal sphincter pressure characteristics. Gastroenterology 1967; 52:513.
36. Schiller LR, Santa Ana CA, Schmulen AC, et al. Pathogenesis of fecal incontinence in diabetes mellitus. N Engl J Med 1982; 307:1666.
36a. Ruhl CE, Everhart JE. Association of diabetes, serum insulin and C-peptide with gallbladder disease. Hepatology 2000; 31:299.
37. Lieber MM. The incidence of gallstones and their correlation with other diseases. Ann Surg 1952; 135:394.
38. DeSantis A, Attili AF, Corradini SG, et al. Gallstones and diabetes: a case-control study in a free-living population sample. Hepatology 1997;25:787.
39. Persson GE, Thulin AJG. Prevalence of gallstone disease in patients with diabetes mellitus: a case-control study. Eur J Surg 1991; 157:579.
40. Gracie WA, Ransohoff DF. The natural history of silent gallstones. N Engl J Med 1982; 307:798.
41. Hickman MS, Schwesinger WH, Page CP. Acute cholecystitis in the diabetic. Arch Surg 1988; 123:409.
42. Pellegrini C. Asymptomatic gallstones: does diabetes mellitus make a difference? Gastroenterology 1986; 91:245.
43. Haff RC, Butcher HR, Ballinger WF. Factors influencing morbidity in biliary tract operations. Surg Gynecol Obstet 1971; 132:195.
44. Friedman LS, Roberts MS, Brett AS, et al. Management of asymptomatic gallstones in the diabetic patient. Ann Intern Med 1988; 109:913.
45. Ransohoff DF, Gracie MD, Wolfenson LB, et al. Prophylactic cholecystectomy or expectant management for silent gallstones. Ann Intern Med 1983; 99:199.
46. Falchuk KR, Fiske S, Haggitt R, et al. Pericentral hepatic fibrosis and intracellular hyalin in diabetes mellitus. Gastroenterology 1980; 78:535.
47. Stone B, Van Thiel D. Diabetes mellitus and liver disease. Semin Liver Dis 1985; 5:8.
48. Khuri KG, Shamma MH, Abourizk N. Hepatitis B virus markers in diabetes mellitus. Diabetes Care 1985; 8:250.
49. Luyckx FH, Lefebvre PJ, Scheen AJ. Non-alcoholic steatohepatitis: association with obesity and insulin resistance, and influence of weight loss. Diabetes Metab 2000; 26:98.
50. Sheth SG, Gordon FD, Chopra S. Nonalcoholic steatohepatitis. Ann Intern Med 1997; 126(2):137.

# CHAPTER 150

# DIABETIC NEPHROPATHY

RALPH A. DEFRONZO

Of the ~1 million people with type 1 (previously called *insulin-dependent*) diabetes mellitus in the United States, 30% to 40% eventually develop end-stage renal failure,[1] and there is little evidence that the incidence of diabetic nephropathy in type 1 diabetics has changed within the last decade.[2] Type 2 (previously called *non–insulin-dependent*) diabetes mellitus is much more common, affecting some 15 million people.[3] Among type 2 diabetic patients, the incidence of renal disease is lower (~5–10%).[4,5] However, the incidence of nephropathy in type 2 diabetics varies considerably among ethnic groups, being three to four times higher in blacks and Hispanics and seven times higher in Native Americans when compared to whites.[6–8] Nevertheless, in absolute terms, more type 2 than type 1 diabetic patients eventually progress to renal insufficiency. The magnitude of the problem can be readily appreciated when it is realized that every third person who is started on dialysis is diabetic,[9] and that the Medicare payment for diabetics is ~$51,000 per year per patient.[10]

## DIABETIC NEPHROPATHY

Since the original description of diabetic nephropathy by Kimmelstiel and Wilson[11] in 1936, numerous studies have reported the renal histologic changes and the clinical course, which is characterized by hypertension, edema, heavy albuminuria, and varying degrees of renal insufficiency.[5] Three major histopathologic alterations have been described in the diabetic kidney: glomerulosclerosis, vascular involvement, and tubulointerstitial disease.[12–14]

### GLOMERULOSCLEROSIS

Glomerular involvement is the most characteristic feature of diabetic nephropathy and includes three distinctive lesions: diffuse intercapillary glomerulosclerosis, nodular glomerulosclerosis, and glomerular basement membrane (GBM) thickening (Fig. 150-1).

#### DIFFUSE AND NODULAR LESIONS

Diffuse intercapillary glomerulosclerosis, the most frequent histologic abnormality, is characterized by increased, periodic acid–Schiff–positive, eosinophilic material within the mesangial region (see Fig. 150-1A). The process is diffuse, involving the entire glomerulus, and generalized, affecting all glomeruli throughout the kidney. The earliest change is a widening of the mesangial matrix. With time, this mesangial material expands and coalesces, encroaching on adjacent capillary lumina. As this process progresses, entire glomeruli may become hyalinized. There is no increase in mesangial cell number, but mesangial cell volume is increased.[15] In 40% to 50% of patients, the increase in mesangial matrix forms large acellular nodules at the center of peripheral glomerular lobules (see Fig. 150-1B). This nodular lesion is invariably associated with the diffuse lesion and is pathognomonic of diabetes mellitus. The nodular lesion correlates poorly with the severity of clinical renal disease; the best predictor of clinical renal disease is the diffuse lesion.[13,15]

Immunofluorescent staining reveals diffuse linear deposition of immunoglobulin G (IgG) along the GBM. Although this

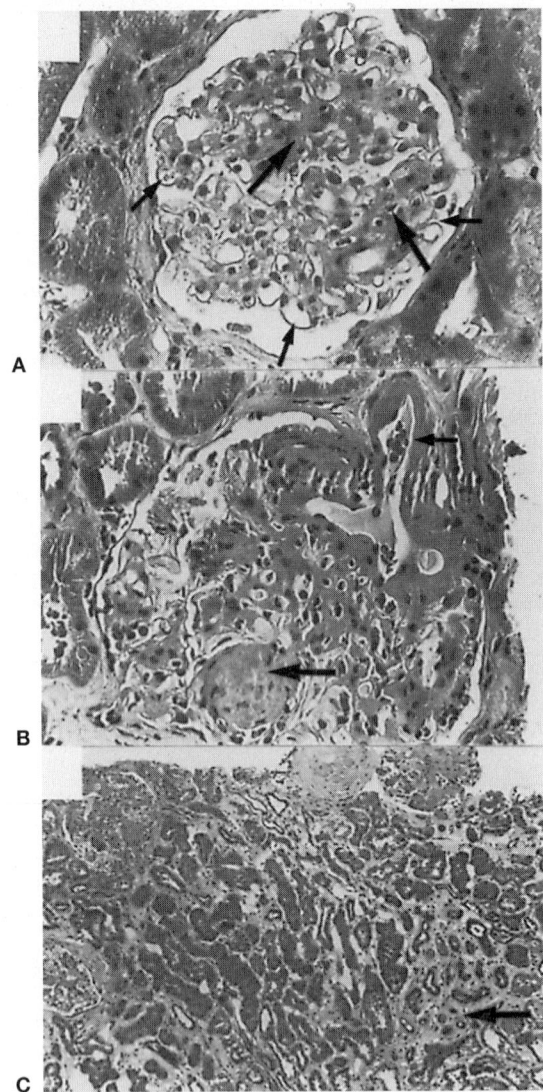

**FIGURE 150-1.** **A,** Diffuse diabetic glomerulosclerosis with marked mesangial matrix hyperplasia (*thick arrows*) and thickened glomerular basement membranes (*thin arrows*). No hypercellularity is evident. **B,** Nodules (*thick arrow*) usually are observed in the peripheral capillary loops and rarely are seen without the diffuse lesion. Note the prominent arteriolosclerosis in the efferent and afferent arterioles. **C,** Interstitial fibrosis, tubular atrophy (*thick arrow*), and thickening of the tubular basement membranes. (From DeFronzo RA. Diabetes and the kidney: an update. In: Olefsky JM, Sherwin RS, eds. Diabetes mellitus: management and complications. New York: Churchill Livingstone, 1985:161.)

linear pattern of immunoglobulin deposition is reminiscent of anti-GBM nephritis, eluted IgG has no affinity for the GBM and most likely represents nonspecific trapping of filtered proteins.

### BASEMENT MEMBRANE THICKENING

Thickening of the GBM is an early and characteristic change of diabetic glomerulosclerosis (see Fig. 150-1*A*). Basement membrane thickening is not limited to the glomerulus but can be observed in capillaries throughout the body, including muscle, skin, and retina.

The GBM is a collagen-like protein that is synthesized by visceral epithelium of the glomerulus.[12] The integrity of the GBM is maintained by the continuous addition of new material from the epithelial aspect and by the simultaneous removal from the endothelial side by mesangial cells. The half-life of the GBM is ~100 days. Both increased epithelial synthesis and impaired removal by mesangial cells contribute to the basement membrane thickening.

Biochemical analysis of the normal GBM has demonstrated significant differences in the collagen and protein content compared with basement membranes from nonrenal tissues.[16] These differences in chemical composition account for the high glomerular filtration coefficient, which permits a water flux that is 50 to 100 times greater than in other capillaries, yet totally restricts the passage of serum proteins. The ability to restrict proteins selectively also is related to the strong negative charge provided by heparin sulfate and sialic acid residues within the GBM.

A number of biochemical alterations in the composition of the GBM occur in diabetic nephropathy.[16,17] Moreover, studies in alloxan diabetic rats have demonstrated increased activity of glucosyltransferase, the enzyme involved in the assembly of hydroxylysine-linked carbohydrate units. The restoration of normoglycemia with insulin normalized the activity of this enzyme. These results suggest that the accelerated synthesis of hydroxylysine-glucose-galactose subunits contributes to the GBM thickening; other investigators have been unable to demonstrate a significant alteration in amino acid or glucosylgalactose content in diabetic GBM. A polyantigenic expansion, involving all of the intrinsic components of the GBM and mesangium, has been demonstrated.[18] This suggests an overall increase in the synthetic rate of normal basement membrane or a decrease in the rate of degradation. In diabetics with advanced nephropathy, the sialic acid and heparin sulfate proteoglycan content of the GBM is uniformly diminished. This decrease in anionic charge contributes to the increased clearance of negatively charged macromolecules, such as albumin.[19] In vitro studies using isolated glomeruli have shown that glucose stimulates its own incorporation into capillary basement membrane in a dose-dependent fashion. Excessive glycosylation of the GBM may render collagen more resistant to degradation and contribute to the GBM thickening.

### VASCULAR INVOLVEMENT

Accelerated renal arteriosclerosis and arteriolosclerosis are more characteristic of the diabetic than the nondiabetic kidney (see Fig. 150-1*B*). In the larger arteries, atheromatous changes are often advanced and may contribute to renal failure by causing ischemic parenchymal atrophy. In the smaller renal arterioles, hyaline thickening involves the afferent and efferent vessels. Although arteriosclerosis and arteriolosclerosis may be extensive, neither process correlates with the severity of glomerular change.

### TUBULOINTERSTITIAL DISEASE

Although not usually appreciated, tubulointerstitial changes (see Fig. 150-1*C*) are common in the diabetic kidney, and in advanced cases, there is marked tubular atrophy, thickening of the tubular basement membrane, and interstitial fibrosis.[14,20,21] Such changes are typically observed with renal ischemia, but in the diabetic, the tubular changes correlate poorly with the degree of vascular involvement and may be seen in their absence. The involved tubules often show thickening of the tubular basement membrane, and immunofluorescent studies have demonstrated deposition of IgG along the tubular basement membrane. The interstitial area surrounding the involved tubules is fibrotic and may contain a cellular infiltrate of lymphocytes and plasma cells. These changes progress with increasing duration of the diabetes.[13,14]

The interstitial reaction does not imply infection, such as pyelonephritis, although asymptomatic bacteriuria and pyelonephritis are twice as common in diabetics, particularly women, than in nondiabetics.[22] This propensity to urinary tract infection probably results from various factors, including impaired renal blood flow, bladder dysfunction, interstitial scarring, impaired polymorphonuclear leukocyte function, defective leukocyte chemotaxis, and glucosuria, which enhance bacterial growth. It has been difficult

**TABLE 150-1.**
**Metabolic and Genetic Theories of Diabetic Nephropathy**

**METABOLIC/HEMODYNAMIC (ACQUIRED) THEORY**

Renal involvement is absent when diabetes first is diagnosed. Basement membrane thickening and mesangial changes do not become manifest until 2–3 years later.

Typical changes of diabetic nephropathy have been observed in pancreatic diabetes (hemochromatosis, chronic pancreatitis, pancreatectomy, and cystic fibrosis).

In the dog, monkey, rat, and mouse, lesions similar to those observed in human diabetic nephropathy have been documented after the induction of diabetes.

Tight regulation with insulin prevents the development of renal lesions in all diabetic animal models.

Transplantation of kidneys from diabetic into normal rats cures the renal disease.

Tight glycemic control before or during the phase of microalbuminuria can prevent or halt the progression of microalbuminuria.

Normal human kidneys, transplanted into diabetic patients, develop changes of diabetic nephropathy within 2–5 years. Transplantation of diabetic kidneys into nondiabetic patients leads to a resolution of the diabetic renal lesion.

Pancreatic transplantation reverses established lesions of diabetic nephropathy.

**GENETIC THEORY**

Marked variation in the incidence of nephropathy among type 2 diabetes mellitus patients from different ethnic groups.

Poor correlation exists between diabetic glomerulosclerosis and the degree of diabetic control as judged by blood-glucose levels.

Excellent glucose control with the insulin pump (artificial pancreas) for 1–2 years has failed to reverse clinically overt proteinuria, and most diabetics have experienced progressive proteinuria and azotemia.

Only a minority of pancreatic diabetics develop glomerulosclerosis.

Diabetic nephropathy has been reported early in the course of diabetes, in the prediabetic state, and occasionally in patients with normal glucose tolerance.

Diabetic nephropathy clusters within families in individuals with both type 1 and type 2 diabetes mellitus.

Sib-pair linkage studies have shown an association between diabetic nephropathy and specific chromosomal regions, although no specific genes have yet been identified.

(Adapted from DeFronzo RA. In: Olefsky JM, Sherwin RS, eds. Diabetes mellitus: management and complications. New York: Churchill Livingstone, 1985:166.)

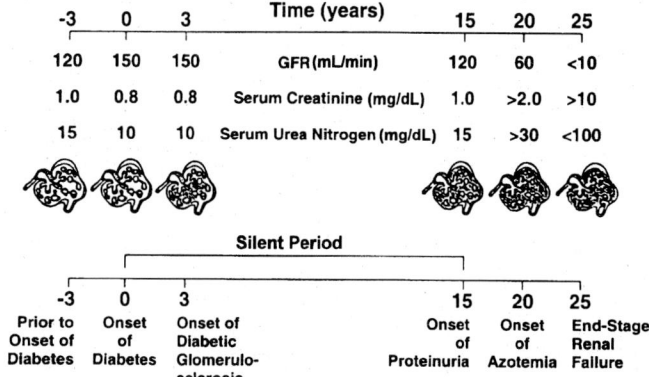

**FIGURE 150-2.** Natural course of diabetic nephropathy. At the initial diagnosis, renal function and glomerular histology are normal. Within 2 to 3 years, increased mesangial matrix and basement membrane thickening are observed. Renal function remains normal until ~15 years, when proteinuria develops. This is an ominous sign and usually indicates advanced diabetic glomerulosclerosis. Within 5 years after the onset of proteinuria, elevation of the serum urea nitrogen and creatinine levels is observed, and within 3 to 5 years after the development of azotemia, half of the patients have advanced to end-stage renal insufficiency. (*GFR,* glomerular filtration rate.) (Modified from DeFronzo RA. Diabetes and the kidney: an update. In: Olefsky JM, Sherwin RS, eds. Diabetes mellitus: management and complications. New York: Churchill Livingstone, 1985:169.)

renal changes are caused by a combination of metabolic and hemodynamic changes that result from a lack of insulin. The second argues that genetic factors are responsible for the alterations in renal structure and function.

## ACQUIRED (METABOLIC/HEMODYNAMIC) THEORY

A large body of data now indicates that diabetic nephropathy is acquired. First, renal involvement is absent in newly diagnosed diabetics (Fig. 150-2). Basement membrane thickening, expansion of the mesangium, and vascular changes do not become evident until 2 to 3 years after the onset of diabetes.[12,13,25] Second, typical changes of diabetic nephropathy occur in patients with pancreatic diabetes (e.g., hemochromatosis, chronic pancreatitis, pancreatectomy).[26] Third, diabetic nephropathy can be produced in various animal models, including the rat, mouse, dog, and monkey, irrespective of the means of induction of diabetes. Fourth, transplantation of pancreatic islets into diabetic rats prevents the development of renal lesions. Fifth, when diabetic rat kidneys are transplanted into nondiabetic rats, the renal lesions resolve. Conversely, when normal kidneys are transplanted into diabetic rats, diabetic nephropathy ensues. Sixth, when kidneys from nondiabetic persons are transplanted into diabetics, all of the typical histologic changes of diabetic nephropathy develop within 2 to 5 years.[25] The Diabetes Control and Complications Trial (DCCT), a study carried out in 1441 type 1 diabetics, has conclusively shown that intensive insulin therapy can prevent the development of nephropathy.[27] Tight glycemic control reduced the occurrence of microalbuminuria (40–300 mg per day) and of overt albuminuria (>300 mg per day) by 39% and 54%, respectively. Intensified insulin therapy was effective both in primary and secondary prevention of nephropathy[27] (Fig. 150-3).

The importance of the metabolic and hemodynamic environment is underscored by a case report, in which kidneys were transplanted from a type 1 diabetic with established proteinuria and biopsy-proven diabetic nephropathy into two nondiabetic patients.[28] After 7 months, renal function in both recipients was normal, proteinuria had disappeared, and renal biopsy showed resolution of the diffuse diabetic glomerulosclerosis. Similarly, others have demonstrated the regression of established diabetic

to demonstrate any relationship between the frequency or severity of interstitial changes and urinary tract infection, and patients whose bacteriuria was not eradicated fared no worse than those in whom the bacteriuria was cured.[23] The interstitial changes likely represent a direct representation of the diabetic state. The only tubular lesion that is characteristic of the diabetic state is the *Armanni-Ebstein lesion*, a vacuolization of the proximal tubular cells of the pars recta. These vacuoles contain glycogen and are most often observed in poorly controlled diabetics.

*Papillary necrosis*, a special type of interstitial lesion, is observed in diabetics; indeed, diabetes mellitus accounts for over half of all cases.[24] This is the result of ischemic damage to the inner medulla with eventual infarction and sloughing of part or all of the papilla. These patients may present with an acute fulminant illness, with fever, shock, flank pain, gross hematuria, pyuria, oliguria, and renal failure, or they may have a more subacute form characterized by microscopic hematuria, pyuria, and indolent renal failure. Urinary tract obstruction and pyelonephritis often complicate the diabetes and cause renal papillary necrosis. Because phenacetin has commonly been associated with papillary necrosis, chronic use of this analgesic should be avoided in the diabetic population.

## PATHOGENESIS OF DIABETIC GLOMERULOSCLEROSIS

Two theories have been proposed to explain the development of diabetic renal disease (Table 150-1). The first states that the

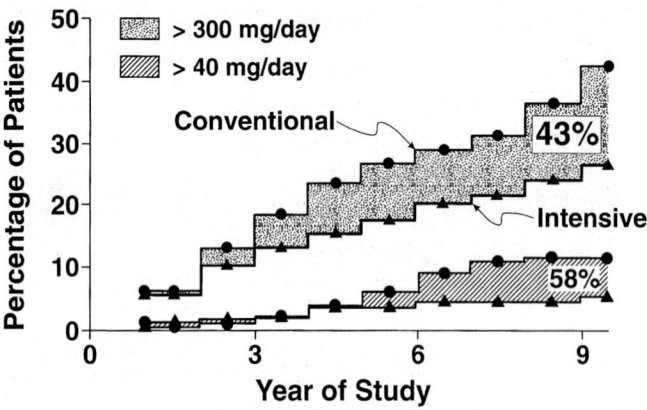

**FIGURE 150-3.** Effect of intensive versus conventional glycemic control with insulin on the albumin excretion rate in type 1 diabetics. Tight glycemic control significantly reduced the risk of developing microalbuminuria and macroalbuminuria in normoalbuminuria patients. (Reproduced from DCCT Research Group. The effect of intensive treatment of diabetes on the development and progression of long-term complications in insulin-dependent diabetes mellitus. N Engl J Med 1993; 329:977.)

nephropathy in diabetic patients after pancreatic transplantation. Lastly, pancreatic transplantation has reversed established lesions of diabetic nephropathy.[29]

### GENETIC THEORY

Proponents of the genetic theory cite the poor correlation between diabetic glomerulosclerosis and the degree of diabetic control. Evidence is available to support or to negate the role of metabolic control in the pathogenesis of diabetic complications.

In short-term studies with a follow-up of 1 to 2 years, the achievement of good metabolic control has failed to reverse or to ameliorate established nephropathy or to prevent the emergence of new cases of diabetic renal disease.[30–32] This information has been offered in favor of inheritance as the primary determinant of diabetic nephropathy. However, the follow-up period was <2 years, and insulin pump therapy was not instituted until after patients had had their diabetes for many years.[30–32] Major renal hemodynamic and structural changes occur within the initial 2 to 3 years after the diagnosis of diabetes, and, if allowed to persist, may lead to fixed, irreversible alterations that may be responsible for the relentless progression to renal insufficiency. One study[33] suggests that, if blood pressure is well controlled, improved glycemic control may slow the progression of established diabetic nephropathy, and after 5 to 10 years of successful pancreatic transplantation, improvement in renal structure and function has been demonstrated.[29]

The development of diabetic glomerulosclerosis only in a minority of patients with secondary causes of diabetes (i.e., hemochromatosis, etc.), in occasional cases of diabetic nephropathy early in the course of diabetes, or in the prediabetic state, plus the finding of typical diabetic glomerulosclerosis in patients without glucose intolerance—all suggest a genetic etiology.[26,34] A genetic component to the GBM thickening is supported by the finding of muscle capillary basement membrane thickening in adult type 1 diabetics at the time of diagnosis.[35] However, this observation has been refuted by others.[36]

More direct evidence for a genetic etiology of diabetic nephropathy in both type 1 and type 2 diabetics includes (a) the familial clustering of diabetic nephropathy and increased albumin excretion rates and hypertension in nondiabetic family members[37–41] and (b) results of studies of glomerular structure in type 1 diabetic sibling pairs.[42] Sib-pair linkage analysis has demonstrated that several chromosomal regions are associated with diabetic nephropathy in Pima Indians,[43] a population

group that has the highest documented incidence of diabetic renal disease in the world. A number of candidate genes have been proposed and reviewed.[44,44a]

Clearly, metabolic and hemodynamic disturbances play a major role in the development of diabetic nephropathy. However, it would appear that these metabolic derangements operate on a genetic background that predisposes the kidney to the development of diabetic glomerulosclerosis. The marked difference in renal disease among different racial groups[6–8,45] also emphasizes the important role of genetic factors in the etiology of diabetic renal disease.

## CLINICAL COURSE

Epidemiologic studies from a number of large diabetes centers have documented that fewer than half of all type 1 diabetics who have had their disease for 20 to 30 years develop clinically significant renal disease.[1,2,46,47] At the time of diagnosis, there are no clinical or laboratory findings that predict which patients will progress to end-stage renal failure.[47,48] Although it is often stated that the incidence of glomerulosclerosis is more common in type 1 (30–40%) than in type 2 (5–10%) diabetics, type 2 diabetic Pima Indians have the highest known incidence of diabetic nephropathy.[49,50] Furthermore, some studies suggest that the incidence of renal disease may be similar in type 1 and type 2 diabetics.[51,52] The dramatic rise in the incidence of renal disease in type 2 diabetes may result from enhanced awareness and improved treatment of hypertension and dyslipidemia, which allows them to live longer, thereby exposing them to a greater burden of hyperglycemia.

### EARLY CHANGES IN RENAL FUNCTION

The glomerular filtration rate (GFR) is characteristically increased early in the course of diabetes (see Fig. 150-2) and correlates with increased kidney weight and size, increased glomerular volume, and increased capillary luminal area per glomerulus.[47–49,53] At this time, increased mesangial matrix and basement membrane thickening are present. Short-term blood-glucose control normalizes the GFR without any reduction in renal size.[54] This latter observation suggests that the augmented GFR is not causally related to the renal hypertrophy. However, within 6 weeks after the start of intensive insulin therapy, a significant reduction in kidney size can be demonstrated in type 1 diabetic patients.[55] Experimental diabetes in the rat also is associated with an augmented GFR, which correlates with increased glomerular volume and glomerular capillary length and diameter. All of these changes are reversible with insulin treatment or islet cell transplantation.[47]

In early diabetes, no consistent change in renal plasma flow (RPF) has been observed. Although an increase in RPF has been reported by some investigators, most have found blood flow to the kidney to be normal. In all studies, the filtration fraction (GFR/RPF) was elevated.[47]

### LATE CHANGES IN RENAL FUNCTION

In diabetics destined to develop renal insufficiency, a predictable sequence of events ensues[13,47–49] (see Fig. 150-2). There is a long (15–18 years) silent period, during which there is no laboratory evidence of renal dysfunction. However, renal biopsy demonstrates a progressive, widespread increase in mesangial matrix material, capillary GBM thickening, interstitial fibrosis, and arteriolosclerosis. Diabetics with clinical nephropathy have more mesangial matrix material and fewer open glomerular capillaries than do diabetic subjects without clinical nephropathy. An inverse correlation is found between the increase in mesangial matrix and the area of open capillary loops. These observations suggest that in the advanced stages of diabetic nephropathy,

**TABLE 150-2.**
**Definition of Microalbuminuria***

|  | Urinary AER (mg per 24 h) | Urinary AER (µg per min) | Urine Albumin/ Creatinine Ratio (mg/mg) |
|---|---|---|---|
| Normoalbuminuria† | <30 | <20 | <0.02 |
| Microalbuminuria | 30–300 | 20–200 | 0.02–0.20 |
| Macroalbuminuria | >300 | >200 | >0.20 |

*See text for a more detailed discussion.
†The mean value for urinary albumin excretion rate (*AER*) in normal individuals is 10 ± 3 mg per day or 7 ± 2 µg per minute.

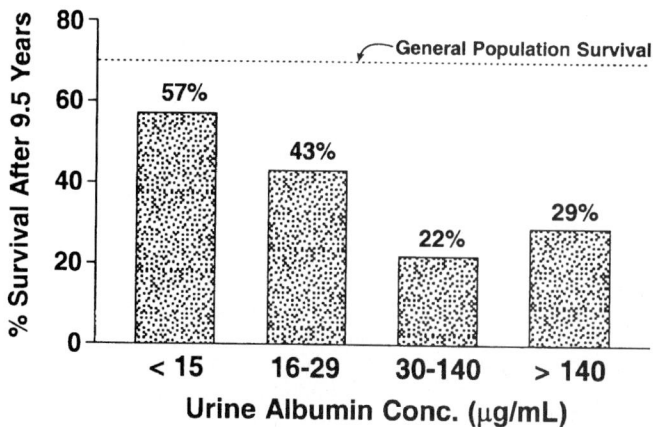

**FIGURE 150-4.** Overall survival in 76 type 2 diabetic patients with varying degrees of microalbuminuria based on the urinary albumin concentration. Patients with microalbuminuria in the moderate to high range (*two right columns*) demonstrated a markedly shortened survival compared to an age-matched control population. (From Morgensen CE. Microalbuminuria predicts clinical proteinuria and early mortality in maturity-onset diabetes. N Engl J Med 1984; 311:89.)

encroachment of capillary lumina by the expanding mesangial matrix material contributes to the decline in GFR. However, nonhistologic factors must be important to the diminution of renal function, because the severity of diabetic glomerulosclerosis in patients without clinically evident renal disease often is as severe as in patients with advanced renal insufficiency.[56,57]

## STAGING OF DIABETIC NEPHROPATHY

Many studies have demonstrated that microalbuminuria is the earliest detectable stage of diabetic nephropathy,[58–60] and diabetics with microalbuminuria are said to have *incipient diabetic nephropathy.*[47–49,52] In healthy persons, albumin excretion ranges from 2.5 to 25.0 mg per day, with a mean of ~10 mg per day[58] (Table 150-2). The Albustix reaction does not become positive until the albumin excretion rate exceeds 300 mg per day. Obviously, there is a wide subclinical range (30–300 mg per day) in which urinary albumin excretion is increased, but cannot be detected by routine laboratory methods. Sensitive radioimmunoassay techniques have been developed for accurate measurement of albumin excretion at these lower, yet elevated, rates.[47,61] Diabetics, in whom the urinary albumin excretion rate is in the range of 30 to 300 mg per day, are defined as having microalbuminuria (see Table 150-2), and they have a 20-fold increased likelihood of developing clinical proteinuria (>300 mg per day of albumin) or a diminished GFR within a period of 10 years.[58–60] Patients with high-grade microalbuminuria (>100 mg per day) are at particularly high risk of developing renal impairment.[47–49] Microalbuminuria also predicts the development of diabetic nephropathy in type 2 diabetics,[47–49,52,62–64] although it is not as strong a predictor for these patients as it is for type 1 diabetics. In both type 1 and type 2 diabetics, microalbuminuria is a very strong predictor of macrovascular complications (i.e., heart attacks, stroke)[48,62,65–67] (Fig. 150-4).

Some caution must be exercised concerning the clinical interpretation of microalbuminuria. The upper limit of normal should not be considered as absolute, and common sense must be used in judging borderline cases. A number of factors (e.g., exercise, high blood pressure, urinary tract infection, and very poor diabetic control) elevate the urinary albumin excretion rate. Obviously, if such confounding factors are present, the finding of microalbuminuria does not necessarily imply incipient diabetic nephropathy. Although several authors have suggested that exercise-induced microalbuminuria is a harbinger of diabetic renal disease, there are few experimental data to support this. Another concern about the clinical interpretation of microalbuminuria centers on its development during the first 5 years in type 1 diabetics. In these patients, microalbuminuria is unlikely to have the same ominous prognostic significance as microalbuminuria that occurs 10 to 15 years after the onset of diabetes. This statement is not applicable to type 2 diabetics, who may have had their disease for many years before the diagnosis of diabetes was established. The interpretation of microalbuminuria in white type 2 diabetics is further complicated by the observation that ~25% of such patients have microalbuminuria, yet the incidence of renal disease in this

population is only 5% to 10%.[48,62–64,67] Although microalbuminuria predicts the development of renal disease in type 2 diabetics, it is not as strong a predictor as in type 1 diabetics. Thus, type 2 diabetics with microalbuminuria have a five-fold (compared to 20-fold in type 1 diabetics) increased risk of developing proteinuria over a 10-year period. However, in certain ethnic populations with a high incidence of diabetic nephropathy, including Native Americans, Mexican-Americans, and blacks, microalbuminuria is a very strong predictor of proteinuria and impaired renal function.[6,49,66,68]

From the routine laboratory standpoint, the earliest detectable manifestation of diabetic glomerulosclerosis is Albustix-positive proteinuria (see Fig. 150-2), which begins ~15 to 18 years after the diagnosis of diabetes.[47,49,52,58–60,62,66] At this time, the GFR may still be normal or even elevated, but within a mean of 5 years after the onset of overt proteinuria, the GFR begins to decline, and the serum urea nitrogen and creatinine concentrations increase. Within 3 to 5 years after the first elevation of serum creatinine concentration, approximately half of the patients have progressed to end-stage renal insufficiency. Heavy proteinuria (>3 g per day) and the nephrotic syndrome are common, occurring in more than half of those who progress to end-stage renal failure.

## LABORATORY ABNORMALITIES

### PROTEINURIA

Proteinuria is the earliest laboratory manifestation of diabetic renal disease. When the urine albumin excretion exceeds 300 mg per day (corresponding to a urine protein excretion >500 mg per day), the subject is said to have *overt diabetic nephropathy.* Using fractional dextran clearances and urinary albumin and IgG excretion, the increased transglomerular flux of proteins has been shown to result from an augmented transglomerular ultrafiltration pressure gradient and an alteration in the molecular charge of the glomerular barrier that results from the loss of anionic charges (i.e., heparin sulfate and sialic acid residues) from the GBM.[63,66,69–72] Neither the number of pores in the GBM nor the pore size is altered early in the course of diabetic nephropathy. At this stage, loss of barrier charge selectivity, without alteration of pore-size diameter, appears to be the primary factor that allows the escape of albumin without change in the clearance of other macromolecules, and improved glycemic control with intensive insulin therapy decreases the albumin excretion rate.[73] With progressive proteinuria and the development of impaired renal function, glomerular charge and size selectivity is lost, there is an increase in pore size with the appearance of large molecular weight proteins in the urine, and enhanced transglomerular passage of plasma proteins contributes to progressive kidney damage.

## GLOMERULAR FILTRATION RATE

Early in the natural history of diabetic nephropathy, before the onset of microalbuminuria, the GFR is increased[47–49,62–67,70,72,74,75]; this is believed to result from increased intraglomerular pressure and increased glomerular capillary surface area.[47,48,70,72] The GFR often remains elevated, although marked renal histologic changes are present. Thus, a decline in GFR from elevated to normal values without an improvement in metabolic control represents an ominous finding. The most widely used laboratory tests for GFR are the serum creatinine and the serum urea nitrogen concentrations. However, both are influenced by prerenal (i.e., extracellular fluid volume depletion) and postrenal (i.e., urinary tract obstruction) factors. More importantly, the GFR may decline by 40% to 50% before either test increases into the abnormal range. Therefore, many authors have advocated serial determinations of the creatinine clearance. In patients with renal failure of diverse causes, a plot of the reciprocal of the serum creatinine concentration as a function of time is useful in following the progression of renal disease. Pragmatically, the author advocates following the creatinine clearance in diabetic patients with normal serum creatinine levels. Once the serum creatinine concentration becomes elevated, either the reciprocal of the serum creatinine or the creatinine clearance can be followed.

The GFR is determined by two factors: the net transmembrane ultrafiltration pressure and the glomerular ultrafiltration coefficient. The ultrafiltration pressure is governed by the balance between the transmembrane hydraulic pressure, which increases GFR, and the intraglomerular oncotic pressure, which decreases GFR. In animals and in humans, experimental diabetes elevates the transmembrane ultrafiltration pressure.[63,70] Because the glomerular capillary oncotic pressure is normal or reduced in patients with diabetic nephropathy, this factor cannot explain the decrease in GFR. By exclusion, therefore, it has been concluded that the glomerular ultrafiltration coefficient must be reduced. The ultrafiltration coefficient is determined by the surface area available for filtration and the hydraulic permeability. Changes in the latter term have not been evaluated. Early in the course of type 1 diabetes mellitus, the total glomerular capillary surface area is increased and contributes to the glomerular hyperfiltration. However, in diabetics with clinically manifest renal disease, the mesangial matrix is greatly expanded, with obliteration of many capillary lumina. Anatomically, this reduction in surface area for filtration plays a significant role in the decline in GFR in patients with advanced diabetic nephropathy.

## GLUCOSURIA

In normal persons, the maximum tubular reabsorptive capacity for glucose ($Tm_G$) varies inversely with the GFR, and similar observations have been made in recent-onset, type 2 diabetics.[76] However, in long-term diabetics with reduced GFR and diabetic glomerulosclerosis, the $Tm_G$ is raised and glucose in the urine becomes an unreliable means of monitoring the adequacy of diabetic control. Even in diabetic patients without renal disease, glucosuria correlates poorly with the plasma glucose concentration.

## HYPERKALEMIA

Normally, potassium homeostasis depends on both renal and extrarenal mechanisms.[77] Many factors predispose the diabetic to the development of hyperkalemia. The primary hormones that regulate the distribution of potassium between intracellular and extracellular compartments are insulin, epinephrine, and aldosterone. Because all of these hormones may be deficient, it is not surprising that hyperkalemia is so prevalent in the diabetic population.[77] Furthermore, as the plasma glucose concentration rises, the increased tonicity causes an osmotic shift of fluid and electrolytes, primarily potassium, out of cells. Metabolic acidemia, common in diabetic patients, also predisposes to hyperkalemia. During the development of metabolic acidemia, about half of a hydrogen ion load is buffered within cells; this occurs in exchange for potassium ions.[77]

Renal mechanisms also contribute to the development of hyperkalemia in the diabetic patient. When the GFR falls to less than 15 to 20 mL per minute, the ability of the kidney to excrete potassium may become impaired.[77] Many diabetic patients demonstrate a marked interstitial nephritis with prominent tubular atrophy and tubular basement membrane thickening.[14,20,21] Because most urinary potassium is derived from distal and collecting tubular cell secretion, renal potassium excretion becomes impaired.

Hypoaldosteronism is common in diabetics, particularly in those with evidence of impaired renal function.[77,78] Most patients with hypoaldosteronism have no clinical symptoms and are diagnosed on routine laboratory screening or during evaluation for some other, unassociated illness. The baseline plasma aldosterone concentration is low and fails to increase normally after volume contraction. In most patients, the plasma renin level also is reduced and accounts for the hypoaldosteronism. However, in ~20% of patients with hypoaldosteronism, normal basal renin values have been reported.[77–79] Moreover, all patients with the syndrome of hyporeninemic hypoaldosteronism have clinically significant hyperkalemia, which is the most potent stimulus to aldosterone secretion. This suggests that, along with hyporeninemia, there may be a primary adrenal defect in aldosterone secretion. This hypothesis is supported by the observation that the aldosterone response to angiotensin II and adrenocorticotropic hormone, agents that directly stimulate aldosterone secretion by the zona glomerulosa, is markedly impaired in persons with hypoaldosteronism.[77,79]

The cause of the defect in aldosterone secretion is unknown. A number of mechanisms have been suggested. Hyporeninemia could result from damage to the juxtaglomerulosa apparatus, impaired conversion of the biologically inactive renin precursor ("big renin") to renin, decreased circulating catecholamine levels or autonomic neuropathy, diminished circulating prostaglandin levels, or chronic extracellular fluid volume expansion secondary to hyperglycemia and sodium retention. However, none of these explanations can satisfactorily account for the development of hyporeninemia in most diabetics. Impaired aldosterone secretion may be caused by intracellular potassium depletion within the zona glomerulosa of the adrenal gland secondary to insulin deficiency or insulin resistance.[77,78] Several enzymatic steps involved in aldosterone biosynthesis are potassium dependent.[77] A disruption of normal tubuloglomerular feedback mechanisms may also suppress aldosterone secretion.[77] In diabetic patients with fasting plasma glucose levels in excess of 180 mg/dL, there is a large increase in the filtered load of glucose. The resultant osmotic diuresis would be expected to impair sodium and chloride reabsorption by all segments of the nephron, disrupting the normal tubuloglomerular feedback control mechanism and leading to suppression of renin and aldosterone secretion.

The complexity of the alterations in the renin-aldosterone axis in the diabetic is underscored by a report in which the aldosterone axis was characterized in 59 normokalemic diabetics with normal GFR.[80] In half of the patients, both the renin and aldosterone responses were normal; 10% demonstrated diminished aldosterone secretion despite a normal renin response, 20% had impaired renin release with a normal aldosterone response, and 20% manifested impaired secretion of both renin and aldosterone. These results suggest that there are multiple defects in the renin-aldosterone axis and that the origin of hyperkalemia is multifactorial.

Many drugs impair aldosterone secretion,[77] and, if used in the diabetic, the plasma potassium concentration should be closely monitored. Of these, the β-blockers are the most widely known. Captopril, a converting enzyme inhibitor, has been advocated for the treatment of diabetic nephropathy. This agent infrequently causes hyperkalemia, and this complication should be monitored closely at the start of therapy.[77] Another widely used class of drugs, the nonsteroidal antiinflammatory prostaglandin inhibitors, causes hyporeninemic hypoaldosteronism and hyperkalemia.[77] The diuretic agents (e.g., spironolactone, triamterene, and amiloride) block potassium secretion by the renal tubular cell.[77]

## METABOLIC ACIDOSIS

Metabolic acidosis commonly is observed in diabetic patients.[77,78,81] Metabolic acidosis can be divided into two broad categories: *anion gap* and *nonanion gap* or *hyperchloremic*. The anion gap is calculated by subtracting the concentrations of the major anions (chloride plus bicarbonate) from the major cation (sodium). The difference should not exceed 12 ± 2 mEq/L. If the value is >14 mEq/L, an anion gap acidosis is present.

In the diabetic, there are three causes of an *anion gap acidosis*: renal insufficiency, ketoacidosis, and lactic acidosis. The latter two are discussed in Chapter 155. In diabetic nephropathy, as in other causes of chronic renal disease, when the GFR declines to 20 to 25 mL per minute, the ability of the kidney to excrete titratable acid becomes impaired, and the laboratory manifestation is an anion gap acidosis.

The causes of an anion gap acidosis are well known to the clinician. Less well recognized is the frequent occurrence of a *hyperchloremic* (or *nonanion gap*) *metabolic acidosis*. The syndrome of hypoaldosteronism is commonly observed in diabetic patients, particularly those with renal impairment.[77–79] Aldosterone is an important regulator of ammonia production and hydrogen ion secretion by the distal nephron, and more than half of the reported cases of hyporeninemic hypoaldosteronism present with a hyperchloremic metabolic acidosis.[77–79] Because aldosterone does not affect urinary acidification, urine pH remains acidic (pH <5.4). Some diabetic patients have a primary renal tubular defect in hydrogen secretion and present with true distal renal tubular acidosis, that is, an inability to acidify the urine (pH >5.4) despite systemic acidosis. This defect may be related to the prominent interstitial nephritis, to the tubular basement membrane thickening, or to an intracellular abnormality in any of the steps involved in hydrogen ion secretion. Other diabetics may present with a hyperchloremic metabolic acidosis due to widespread chronic interstitial nephritis with decreased ammonia production. Their urine pH is maximally acidic, indicating that the ability of the distal tubule and collecting duct to generate a steep pH gradient is intact. In these patients, the primary problem is impaired ammonia production, leading to a decrease in the total amount of hydrogen ion that can be excreted. In the absence of ammonia, which is one of the major urinary buffers, the urine pH is maximally acidic. Hyperkalemia also may cause a hyperchloremic metabolic acidosis by inhibiting ammonia synthesis by the renal tubular cell.

## CLINICAL CORRELATIONS

It often is stated that diabetic nephropathy is unusual in the absence of retinopathy, neuropathy, and hypertension. These associations were first popularized by Root and colleagues,[82] who referred to the triopathy of diabetes: nephropathy, retinopathy, and neuropathy. The occurrence of this triad was supported by other studies.[83] However, the validity of this association has been challenged,[84] and several reviews[85–87] suggest a more variable association between the three microvascular complications. Diabetic patients with nephropathy invariably have retinopathy; thus, the diagnosis of diabetic nephropathy should not be made in the absence of retinopathy. This association has been referred to as the *retinal syndrome*. However, fewer than half of diabetic patients with retinopathy have clinically evident renal disease. The associations between diabetic neuropathy and retinopathy/ nephropathy are even more variable.

## DIABETIC RETINOPATHY

Diabetic retinopathy (e.g., hemorrhages, exudates, proliferative retinopathy) is present in most diabetic patients with end-stage renal failure who are admitted into dialysis or transplantation programs.[87,88] However, when diabetic nephropathy is first diagnosed (i.e., documentation of persistent proteinuria or elevation of the serum creatinine concentration), 30% to 40% of patients do not have evidence of diabetic retinopathy by routine ophthalmologic examination,[83,84,87,89] even though fluorescein angiography will demonstrate typical diabetic abnormalities in essentially 100% of patients. As the renal disease progresses, however, diabetic retinopathy appears to accelerate.[86–88] In one study, evidence of retinopathy was noted in only 61 of 150 diabetic patients when nephropathy was first diagnosed, but retinal involvement developed in another 42 during the follow-up.[89] In diabetic patients placed on hemodialysis, a rapid progression of diabetic retinopathy often ensues. A dissociation between retinopathy and nephropathy is evident if one examines diabetic patients with established retinopathy. After 15 to 20 years, >80% of diabetic patients have evidence of retinopathy, but as many as 30% to 50% have no laboratory evidence of renal disease.

## DIABETIC NEUROPATHY

The association between diabetic nephropathy and neuropathy is much less impressive than between diabetic nephropathy and retinopathy. In patients who have had diabetes for 20 years, approximately one-half have some evidence of neuropathic involvement.[87,90–92] In diabetics with end-stage renal failure, the incidence of neuropathy varies from 50% to 90%, depending on how carefully one looks for evidence of diabetic neuropathic involvement. Peripheral neuropathy is more common than autonomic neuropathy. In one study, symptomatic diabetic gastroparesis was observed in ~50% of diabetic patients treated with dialysis.[93] However, the specificity of these neuropathologic abnormalities, especially those relating to peripheral neuropathy, must be questioned because dialysis and transplantation often lead to reversal of the abnormalities,[94] suggesting a uremic etiology. As with retinopathy, uremia appears to exacerbate the progression of diabetic neuropathy. When diabetic nephropathy is first diagnosed, fewer than half of patients have clinically evident diabetic neuropathy.

## HYPERTENSION

The incidence of hypertension, as well as the relationship between hypertension and renal disease, are very different in type 1 and type 2 diabetes mellitus. In newly diagnosed type 2 diabetics, ~50% to 60% have hypertension, whereas <10% of type 1 diabetic patients have hypertension at the time of initial diagnosis.[47,48,52,95–97] In type 1 diabetes, the development of hypertension occurs at or slightly after the onset of microalbuminuria.[47,48,95–97] In both type 1 and type 2 diabetics, the incidence and severity of hypertension progress as the proteinuria becomes more severe. When end-stage renal failure ensues, 70% to 80% of diabetics are hypertensive. Patients with heavy proteinuria are particularly prone to develop hypertension. In most patients, the hypertension is volume-dependent and

**TABLE 150-3.**
**Treatment of Diabetic Nephropathy**

1. **Hypertension**—the single most important factor shown to accelerate the progression of renal failure.
   a. Converting enzyme inhibitors (CEI) and calcium-channel blockers are efficacious, relatively free of side effects, and appear to have a specific renal protective effect. Hyperkalemia and decreased glomerular filtration rate (GFR) may occur with CEI.
   b. Because of the development of dyslipidemia and insulin resistance, diuretics should not be considered as first-line agents unless used in very low doses; they are, however, indicated in hypertensive patients with evidence of excessive sodium retention, i.e., edema.

   Avoid propranolol and other nonspecific β-adrenergic blockers (hyperkalemia, hypoglycemia, hyperglycemia).

2. **Urinary tract infection**—increased incidence, frequent cultures.

3. **Neurogenic bladder**—parasympathetic/adrenergic drugs, voiding maneuvers.

4. **Intravenous pyelography**—increased incidence of acute renal failure, particularly if heavy proteinuria and renal impairment are present.

5. **Blood glucose control**
   a. Tight blood glucose control, if instituted before or during the phase of microalbuminuria, prevents the development of overt proteinuria and progressive renal failure.
   b. There is little evidence that tight metabolic control prevents or ameliorates the progression of established renal disease (albumin excretion rate >300–500 mg per day or elevated serum creatinine).
   c. Uremia is associated with insulin resistance and increased insulin requirements.
   d. With advanced uremia (GFR <15–20 mL per minute), decreased insulin requirements may be observed because the kidney removal of secreted insulin is impaired and hepatic degradation of insulin is inhibited by uremia.

   After the institution of dialysis, the situation is complex. Insulin sensitivity improves (→hypoglycemia), but the degradation of insulin is enhanced (→hyperglycemia); however, most insulin-treated diabetics who are started on dialysis experience an increase in their daily insulin requirement.

6. **Dialysis**
   a. One in every 3 patients beginning dialysis in the United States is diabetic.
   b. Diabetics do significantly worse on dialysis than do nondiabetics.
   c. The increased mortality in diabetics treated with dialysis is largely due to cardiovascular deaths resulting from myocardial infarction and stroke. Other complications include peripheral vascular disease, infections, psychiatric problems, and progressive retinopathy and neuropathy.
   d. Diabetic patients treated with peritoneal dialysis appear to do as well as those treated with hemodialysis.

7. **Transplantation**
   a. If a well-matched, living, related donor can be found, renal transplantation is the preferable mode of therapy in most diabetics.

8. **Protein restriction**
   a. There are good data in animals that show that a low-protein diet slows the progression of diabetic renal disease.
   b. In small, uncontrolled studies in humans, a low-protein diet has been shown to slow the progression of established diabetic renal disease.
   c. In a large, well-controlled, prospective study, a low-protein diet did not alter the rate of decline in GFR. In this study, the majority of patients were on an antihypertensive agent (CEI or calcium-channel blocker). It is likely that a low-protein diet has no added beneficial effect beyond that afforded by the angiotensin-converting enzyme (ACE) inhibitor or a calcium-channel blocker.

(Modified from DeFronzo RA. Diabetes and the kidney. In: Olefsky JM, Sherwin RS, eds. Diabetes mellitus: management and complications. New York: Churchill Livingstone, 1985:189.)

becomes relatively easy to control after dialysis is started and dry weight is attained.[98,99]

### EDEMA

The full-blown Kimmelstiel-Wilson syndrome includes edema, hypertension, proteinuria, and azotemia. In patients without

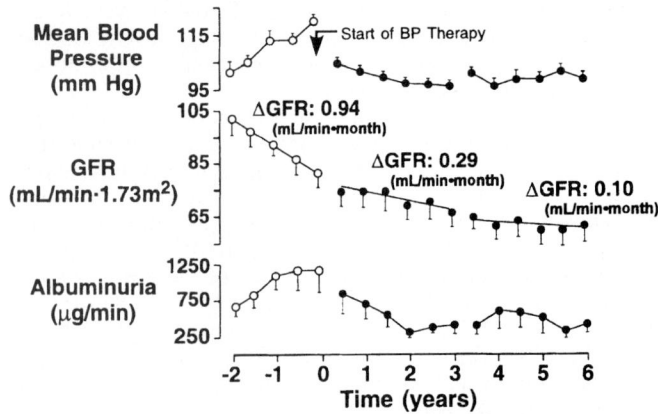

**FIGURE 150-5.** Effect of antihypertensive treatment (*solid circles*) on blood pressure (*BP*), glomerular filtration rate (*GFR*), and albuminuria in type 1 diabetic patients. The rate of decline in GFR and the rate of rise in albuminuria before and after the start of antihypertensive therapy (*open circles*) were markedly slowed by effective reduction of the arterial blood pressure. (From Parving HH, Andersen AR, Smidt UM, et al. Effect of antihypertensive treatment on kidney function in diabetic nephropathy. Br Med J 1987; 294:1443.)

renal disease or in those with early proteinuria (<0.5–1.0 g per day) and a normal GFR, edema is uncommon. However, when the urinary albumin excretion exceeds 1 to 2 g per day, and especially when the GFR begins to decline, the incidence of edema increases precipitously. This is caused by decreased oncotic pressure secondary to hypoalbuminemia and sodium retention secondary to renal disease. When end-stage renal failure ensues, >50% to 75% of patients have some evidence of edema.[89,100]

## TREATMENT OF DIABETIC NEPHROPATHY

The treatment of diabetic nephropathy is largely preventive (Table 150-3). If end-stage renal failure ensues, two options are available: dialysis or transplantation.

### HYPERTENSION

Hypertension is associated with decreased survival in nondiabetic individuals; this effect is magnified in diabetics.[101] Hypertension is the most important factor that accelerates the progression of diabetic renal disease; treatment of the hypertension, regardless of the agent used, markedly slows the progression of renal insufficiency in diabetics with established renal disease.[47,101]

In 1976, it was first demonstrated that antihypertensive therapy reduced albuminuria and slowed the rate of decline in GFR in type 1 diabetics with established nephropathy,[102] and this initial observation has been consistently confirmed[47,48,72,103–105] (Fig. 150-5). In a long-term, randomized, double-blind, prospective study of 409 type 1 diabetics with established nephropathy,[106] it was demonstrated that antihypertensive therapy with captopril decreased the doubling time of serum creatinine by 48% and reduced by 50% the combined end points of death, dialysis, and renal transplantation.

Simple clinical observations have emphasized the importance of hemodynamic factors in the development of diabetic nephropathy. In type 1 diabetics with renal artery stenosis, extensive diabetic glomerulosclerosis occurs in the unprotected kidney, but the kidney behind the stenosis displays only mild diabetic changes.[107] Similar observations have been reported in diabetic rats with Goldblatt kidney hypertension. Furthermore, in diabetic rats, dogs, and humans with a unilateral kidney, there is a marked acceleration of diabetic nephropathy in the remaining kidney, even though systemic hypertension does not develop.[108] These latter observations emphasize the role of intrarenal hemodynamic factors in the initiation and progression of diabetic glomerulopathy.[47,70] In both type 1 and type 2 diabetics, genetic factors also play an important role in the development of hypertension.[109,110] Hypertension and microalbuminuria also occur as part of the insulin-resistance syndrome.[47,111]

Because of the deleterious effects of hypertension on renal function, it is essential that all diabetic patients have their blood pressure normalized. Even mild hypertension (130/90 mm Hg) should not be tolerated in diabetics. The sixth report of the Joint National Committee recommends a blood pressure goal of 130/85 mm Hg in diabetic patients.[112] This is consistent with the recommendation of the American Diabetes Association. The Hypertension Optimal Treatment (HOT) trial, which compared the achievement of a diastolic blood pressure <80 versus <85 versus <90 mm Hg, concluded that the optimal blood pressure in diabetic patients to prevent macrovascular complications should be <120/80 to 130/80 mm Hg.[113] It is the author's opinion that the goal of antihypertensive therapy should be to reduce the blood pressure to what the patient's level was before the onset of hypertension or renal disease. In some cases, this may be <120/80 mm Hg. If the patient's blood pressure before the onset of hypertension or renal impairment is not known, then the standard textbook value of 120/80 mm Hg is appropriate. However, special care should be taken in normalizing the blood pressure in elderly patients, especially those with underlying cardiovascular disease. Because the hypertension in diabetic patients is very volume-dependent, a low-sodium diet should be used to initiate therapy.[114,115] The characteristics of the ideal antihypertensive drug in diabetes mellitus are shown in Table 150-4. Because of the important role of sodium in the hypertensive diabetic, diuretics would appear to be a logical first-line choice. However, this class of drugs worsens insulin resistance, impairs insulin secretion, and causes dyslipidemia.[116,117] Because of these adverse effects on glucose tolerance and plasma lipid levels, if thiazide diuretics are to be used as first-line agents in the treatment of the hypertensive diabetic, they should be used in low doses of <25 mg per day.[109,112,116,117] In diabetic patients with edema or renal insufficiency, a diuretic usually is required to normalize the blood pressure. Moreover, when the serum creatinine concentration is >2 mg/dL, a more potent loop diuretic is needed. β-Adrenergic antagonists, especially nonspecific β-blockers, are contraindicated in diabetic patients. They impair insulin secretion and worsen glucose tolerance in type 2 diabetics. In type 1 diabetic patients, β-blockers cause hypoglycemia by inhibiting hepatic glucose production, impair the counterregulatory hormone response to hypoglycemia, and mask the clinical symptoms of hypoglycemia. They also cause a worsening of the plasma lipid profile and may aggravate peripheral vascular disease in both type 1 and type 2 diabetics. Despite these concerns, the United Kingdom Prospective Diabetes Study (UKPDS)[118] demonstrated that after 9 years of treatment, atenolol, a selective β[1] antagonist, was as effective as captopril in reducing overall mortality, macrovascular complications (i.e., myocardial infarction, stroke, peripheral vascular disease), and microvascular complications (i.e., primarily retinopathy). Dyslipidemia and glycemic control were not aggravated by atenolol. It is likely that the failure to observe any adverse metabolic effects of atenolol is related to its β[1] selectivity.

Because of their ability to reduce the elevated intraglomerular pressure that characterizes the diabetic kidney,[70] the angiotensin-converting enzyme (ACE) inhibitors have gained widespread acceptance as drugs of choice in the treatment of the hypertensive diabetic, especially if proteinuria or renal insufficiency is present.[47,48,52,72,104–106,114,115,119] ACE inhibitors also have been shown to be effective in halting the progression of albuminuria and the decline in GFR in both type 1 and type 2 diabetics with microalbuminuria[47,48,52,96,104,106,114,115,119–126,126a,126b]

**TABLE 150-4.**
**The Ideal Antihypertensive Drug in Diabetes Mellitus**

**Is metabolically "neutral" and does not inhibit**
  Insulin secretion
  Insulin action
  Hepatic glucose production
  Counterregulatory hormone release
**Does not**
  Cause or mask symptoms of hypoglycemia
  Aggravate dyslipidemia
  Promote orthostatic hypotension
  Aggravate coronary/peripheral vascular disease
**Does**
  Specifically preserve renal function

(Fig. 150-6). Importantly, a sustained protective effect of captopril has been demonstrated in type 1 diabetics over a follow-up period of 10 years.[20] In short-term studies, the antiproteinuric effect of the angiotensin II receptor blockers and ACE inhibitors was similar in diabetic and nondiabetic patients with renal disease,[127] but there are no long-term studies that have examined the effect of the angiotensin II receptor blockers on the progression of renal failure. An added advantage of the ACE inhibitors is that they improve insulin sensitivity and may have a beneficial effect on the plasma lipid profile.[116,117,126] The calcium-channel blockers and postsynaptic α[1]-adrenergic blockers also effectively lower blood pressure in diabetic patients and have a beneficial effect on renal function in diabetic patients with proteinuria.[47,113,114,128–134] Some evidence suggests that an ACE inhibitor plus a calcium-channel blocker may provide an additive effect in preventing the progression of renal disease.[135–137] The calcium-channel blockers have no adverse effects on either glucose or lipid metabolism, while the α-blockers increase insulin sensitivity and promote a less atherogenic plasma lipid profile.[128,129] In summary, the ACE inhibitors, along with the calcium-channel antagonists and the α-blockers, should be considered the agents of choice in treating the hypertensive diabetic patient. It is the author's opinion that treatment of hypertension is the single most important factor in preventing the progression of diabetic nephropathy,[47] and that the ACE

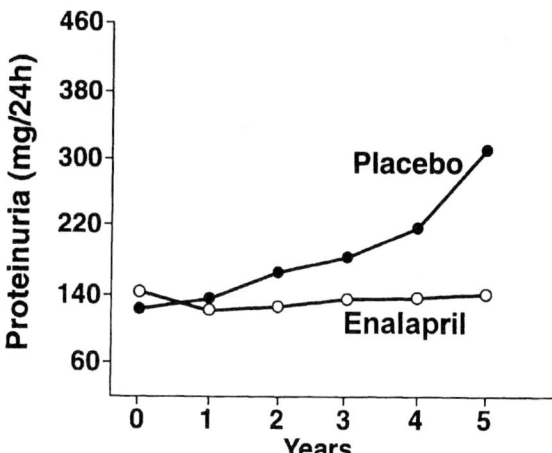

**FIGURE 150-6.** Effect of enalapril treatment on the progression of microalbuminuria in normotensive type 2 diabetic patients. (From Ravid M, Savin H, Jutrin I, et al. Long-term stabilizing effect of angiotensin-converting enzyme inhibition on proteinuria in normotensive type II diabetic patients. Ann Intern Med 1993; 188:577.)

**TABLE 150-5.**
**Recommended Levels of Glycemic Control in Diabetic Individuals**

|  | Normal | Type 1 Diabetes-Intensive Control | Type 1 Diabetes-Acceptable Control | Type 2 Diabetes-Intensive Control | Type 2 Diabetes-Acceptable Control |
|---|---|---|---|---|---|
| Mean premeal blood glucose (mg/dL) | ~90 | 80–120 | <140–160 | <110 | 126 |
| Hemoglobin $A_{1c}$ (%) | 4.0–6.0 | <6.0 | <7.0 | <6.0 | <7.0 |

inhibitors provide a modest additional benefit beyond their antihypertensive action by their effect on intrarenal hemodynamics[70] and nonhemodynamic mechanisms.[138]

## URINARY TRACT INFECTION

Diabetics have an increased incidence of urinary tract infection. Therefore, it is important that a urinalysis be performed on each clinic visit. If white blood cells or bacteriuria are noted, a urine culture should be done. Periodic urine cultures should be obtained, and positive cultures should be treated with an appropriate bactericidal antibiotic.

## NEUROGENIC BLADDER

The clinician caring for the diabetic patient must have a high index of suspicion to establish the diagnosis of neurogenic bladder. In addition to the history, repeated bouts of urinary tract infection should provide a clue to the diagnosis. If the presence of a neurogenic bladder is confirmed by cystometrogram, the patient should receive instruction in the Credé manual voiding maneuver, which should be performed every 6 to 8 hours. Agents such as bethanechol also may be tried. In some diabetics, adrenergic drugs (i.e., phenoxybenzamine) have proved useful. The success of these various medical interventions can be evaluated by determining the postvoid residual volume. If medical therapy proves unsuccessful, intermittent, straight catheterization should be performed at least two to three times a day.

## INTRAVENOUS PYELOGRAPHY

Diabetic patients are at increased risk to develop acute renal failure after radiocontrast procedures (e.g., arteriography, cholangiography, intravenous and retrograde pyelography, computed tomographic scanning).[139] Patients with impaired renal function (i.e., serum creatinine >2 mg/dL) or heavy proteinuria are at greatest risk. With the judicious use of ultrasound, radionuclide studies, and computed tomographic scanning without contrast, most of the information necessary to ensure adequate diagnosis and treatment can be obtained. If diabetic patients must receive radiocontrast dye, hydration with normal saline should be started 12 to 24 hours before the procedure.[140]

## BLOOD GLUCOSE CONTROL

### GLYCEMIC CONTROL (TABLE 150-5)

Diabetic nephropathy and other microvascular complications (retinopathy and neuropathy) do not occur in the absence of poor glycemic control. The product of the mean day-long blood glucose concentration (as reflected by the hemoglobin $A_{1c}$ [$HbA_{1c}$]) and the duration of diabetes provide the total hyperglycemic burden and are the best predictors of microvascular complications.[87,141] Poor glycemic control is a major risk factor for diabetic nephropathy in both type 1 and type 2 diabetics,[47,87,119,141–143] and diabetic nephropathy is uncommon when the glycosylated hemoglobin is maintained at <7.0%.[144,145] In the Diabetes Control and Complications Trial,[27,146,146a] intensive glycemic control with insulin in type 1 diabetics markedly decreased the risk of microvascular complications. In type 2 diabetics,

intensive glycemic control with insulin[147,148] or oral agents[148,149] was equally effective in decreasing the risk of microalbuminuria, as well as other microvascular complications. A similar conclusion was reached from the metaanalysis of several smaller studies.[150] Animal models of diabetes have conclusively established the important role of good glycemic control in preventing diabetic nephropathy.[151] Similarly, in humans, combined pancreatic and renal transplantation prevents the recurrence of diabetic nephropathy in the transplanted kidney as long as the pancreatic transplant functions normally.[152,153] Conversely, the transplantation of kidneys with established diabetic nephropathy into nondiabetic patients leads to a reversal of the renal disease.[28] Nonetheless, despite the encouraging results observed from diabetic animal models and human transplantation, the initiation of tight glycemic control after the onset of overt proteinuria (>300 mg per day of albumin) or renal insufficiency has uniformly been ineffective in halting the relentless progression to end-stage renal failure in type 1 diabetes.[47,89,154–157] These findings suggest that *intensive insulin therapy in humans is most effective when started early*, that is, before or during the phase of microalbuminuria (30–300 mg per day; see Fig. 150-2), before the advanced lesions of diabetic nephropathy have become manifest. From the available evidence, it is recommended that the $HbA_{1c}$ in diabetic patients with microalbuminuria and without microalbuminuria be maintained at <7% and ideally <6%. In diabetic patients with renal insufficiency (serum creatinine ≥2.0 mg%), an $HbA_{1c}$ between 7% and 8% is appropriate. In diabetics with normal serum creatinine and albumin excretion rates >300 mg/dL, strict glycemic control ($HbA_{1c}$ <7.0%) is recommended, because it has not been established at what level of albuminuria intensified glycemic control no longer is capable of preventing the progression of renal disease, and progression of retinopathy and neuropathy still remains a concern.

## CHANGES IN INSULIN DEGRADATION AND INSULIN SENSITIVITY: IMPLICATIONS FOR THERAPY IN DIABETIC PATIENTS WITH CHRONIC RENAL FAILURE

Nondiabetic patients with renal insufficiency are characterized by moderate to severe insulin resistance, which resides in peripheral tissues, primarily muscle.[158] Therefore, in both type 1 and type 2 diabetics, it is not uncommon to observe a deterioration of glucose control with the advent of renal insufficiency. However, when the GFR declines to 15 to 20 mL per minute, both the renal (loss of nephron mass) and hepatic clearance of insulin (uremia inhibits insulin degradation by the liver) become markedly reduced. At this stage, it is common to observe an improvement in glucose tolerance because of the prolonged half-life of insulin, and some diabetics may even cease to require insulin. After the institution of hemodialysis therapy, a complex situation ensues. Dialysis enhances tissue sensitivity to insulin, decreasing insulin requirements.[159] However, dialysis also returns insulin degradation toward normal, increasing the need for insulin.[159] Moreover, the stress of dialysis may increase insulin requirements. In any given uremic diabetic who is started on dialysis, it is difficult to predict what will happen to the insulin requirements. Either an increase or a decrease in the daily insulin dose may be required. In general, most diabetic patients experience an increase in insulin requirements when dialysis is initiated because of the release of insulin antagonistic hormones in response to fluid shifts.

Based on the previous considerations, it is obvious that the physician must be careful in selecting oral hypoglycemic agents for the treatment of diabetics with impaired renal function.[160] The ideal oral agent should not enhance insulin secretion, and the metabolism of the oral agent should not be influenced by diminished kidney function. Theoretically, insulin sensitizers, such as thiazolidinediones (rosiglitazone and pioglitazone) appear to be ideal candidates, but there are no published data with this class of drugs in patients with chronic renal failure (CRF). Pioglitazone has the advantage of having a significant hypolipidemic effect.[161] Because metformin is excreted via the kidneys, it should not be used if the serum creatinine is >1.4 mg/dL in women or 1.5 mg/dL in men, corresponding to a GFR of ~70 mL per minute.[162] Retention of the biguanide may lead to lactic acidosis. Of the sulfonylureas, the only truly short-acting agent is gliclazide, which is not available in the United States. Glipizide is almost entirely metabolized by the liver, and its metabolites are inactive.[163] Therefore, it is well suited for use in diabetics with CRF. Glimeperide also can be used in CRF patients.[164] Glyburide should be avoided because it has a long half-life and because its metabolites have hypoglycemic activity and are excreted in the urine.[163] Because all sulfonylureas stimulate insulin secretion, titration should be slow (every 2 weeks or longer) in patients with CRF. Repaglinide is a nonsulfonylurea insulin secretagogue that belongs to the meglitinide class of drugs.[165] It is a very short-acting agent that must be given three times per day before meals and undergoes hepatic metabolism to inactive products that are excreted in the bile. Because of these characteristics, it is well suited for use in diabetic patients with CRF. Acarbose is not approved for use in diabetics with an elevated serum creatinine. Insulin therapy always remains an option in the treatment of diabetics with CRF, but the physician must be aware of the alterations in insulin metabolism discussed previously. Although $HbA_{1c}$ levels may be slightly reduced in CRF patients because of shortened red blood cell survival, it remains the best tool for assessing glycemic control in diabetics with CRF.[166]

## HYPOGLYCEMIA IN CHRONIC RENAL FAILURE AND DIALYSIS PATIENTS

Spontaneous hypoglycemia occurs not infrequently in both diabetic and nondiabetic patients with CRF. However, the pathogenic mechanisms responsible for the hypoglycemia have not been elucidated. In type 1 diabetics, the low blood sugar level most likely results from diminished insulin degradation by the kidneys and the liver. However, in type 2 diabetics (who are not on insulin or an oral agent) and in nondiabetic CRF patients, plasma insulin levels usually are normal or only slightly elevated. It is likely that these patients have a defect in hepatic glucose production. Decreased hepatic glucose production, secondary to diminished alanine availability for gluconeogenesis, has been documented in a single uremic diabetic patient with spontaneous hypoglycemia.[167] However, the frequency with which decreased alanine turnover contributes to spontaneous hypoglycemia is unclear. Severe hypoglycemia has been reported in nondiabetic patients on chronic maintenance hemodialysis[168] in the absence of malnourishment or elevated plasma insulin levels. All patients were on propranolol, and this agent was implicated in the pathogenesis of the hypoglycemia. Although propranolol causes hypoglycemia by inhibiting hepatic glucose production, the author frequently has observed symptomatic hypoglycemia in hemodialysis patients who were not taking β-adrenergic blocking agents.

## PERITONEAL DIALYSIS, GLUCOSE ABSORPTION, AND INSULIN REQUIREMENTS

Standard hemodialysate solutions contain no glucose. However, there has been considerable interest in *continuous ambula-* *tory peritoneal dialysis* (CAPD), especially in diabetic patients. Because dialysis is performed continuously, glucose absorption is considerable. In nondiabetic patients, plasma glucose levels in excess of 160 to 180 mg/dL are uncommon. However, in diabetics, severe hyperglycemia presents a significant problem with this mode of therapy. To circumvent this problem, insulin has been added to the dialysis fluid, and intraperitoneal insulin administration has been used effectively to achieve excellent glucose control. However, insulin requirements usually are increased two-fold to four-fold with this modality of therapy. In addition to the increased glucose load, obesity and loss of endogenous insulin secretion (which is related to the duration of diabetes) correlate closely with the increased insulin requirements in CAPD patients.[169] It is best to start patients on CAPD in the hospital setting so that optimal glucose control can be achieved within the shortest time and without hypoglycemic or hyperglycemic complications.

## PROTEIN RESTRICTION

Clinicians have had a long-standing interest in the use of low-protein diets to prevent the progression of CRF.[170] The use of protein-restricted diets is based on two assumptions: (a) The adaptive increases in glomerular pressures and renal blood flow that occur after a reduction in renal mass are responsible for the progressive injury to remaining nephrons, and (b) the adaptive increases in renal hemodynamics can be prevented by restricting the dietary protein intake, thereby protecting renal function.

In rats, when renal mass is reduced by any one of a number of experimental maneuvers, there is an initial stabilization of renal function due to increases in single-nephron glomerular plasma flow and intraglomerular pressure, which combine to augment the single-nephron GFR.[171] Eventually, however, these adaptive changes are followed by a progressive decline in GFR secondary to the chronic elevation in intraglomerular pressure, and this leads to severe glomerular sclerosis and heavy proteinuria. When rats with a remnant kidney are placed on a protein-restricted diet, the rise in single-nephron GFR, glomerular plasma flow, and transcapillary hydraulic pressure are prevented, glomerular histology is markedly improved, and kidney survival is significantly prolonged. Based on the results obtained in animals, a number of studies have examined whether a low-protein diet in humans also will have a palliative effect on the progression of renal failure.[172–174] Most of these studies have been retrospective and uncontrolled and have involved small numbers of patients, few of whom were diabetic. Nonetheless, the results consistently demonstrated that a low-protein diet slows the decline in GFR in patients with advanced renal failure. Although of great interest, the validity of these studies has been undermined by a well-controlled prospective study involving 840 patients with renal disease of diverse etiology[175,176] (Fig. 150-7). Insulin-requiring diabetics were excluded from the study, and diet-treated and sulfonylurea-treated diabetics were not analyzed separately. At the end of the 3-year follow-up period, no difference in the rate of decline in GFR was observed between the patients receiving the low-protein diet (0.58 g/kg) and those maintained on a normal-protein intake (1.3 g/kg). The failure of this large prospective study[175,176] to demonstrate any beneficial effect of a low-protein diet stands in contrast to many previously published studies with smaller numbers of patients.[172–174] It is likely that any beneficial effect of the low-protein diet in this large prospective study was obscured by the concomitant use of antihypertensives, which were taken by 80% of participants; 44% were taking ACE inhibitors, which have a specific renal protective effect in diabetics. Based on these results, it seems prudent to recommend modest protein restriction (~1.0 g/kg per day) in diabetic patients who are taking an ACE inhibitor or calcium-channel blocker, while reserving more severe protein restriction (0.6 g/kg per day) for patients who are not taking any antihyperten-

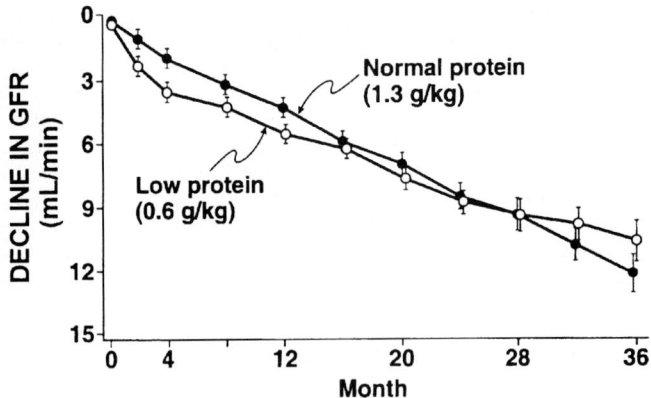

**FIGURE 150-7.** Effect of low-protein diet on the rate of decline in glomerular filtration rate (*GFR*) in patients with chronic renal disease of diverse etiology, including type 2 diabetes mellitus. (From Klahr S, Levey AS, Beck GJ, et al. The effects of dietary protein restriction and blood pressure control on the progression of chronic renal disease. N Engl J Med 1994; 330:877.)

sive medications. If a very low-protein diet is used, this can lead to negative nitrogen balance, acceleration of muscle protein breakdown, and the development of clinically manifest myopathy. Therefore, such patients require very close nutritional monitoring. Lastly, it should be noted that compliance with these very low-protein diets is difficult.

## DYSLIPIDEMIA

Diabetic patients with normal renal function commonly have dyslipidemia, characterized by hypertriglyceridemia, reduced high-density lipoprotein (HDL) cholesterol, small dense low-density lipoprotein (LDL), and postprandial hyperlipidemia.[111] With the onset of renal insufficiency, the dyslipidemia is aggravated, and in diabetics with heavy proteinuria, elevated LDL cholesterol is commonly observed.[177] When diabetics are started on dialysis, the dyslipidemia usually worsens.[177] Diabetics with impaired renal function are at extremely high risk to develop heart attacks and stroke,[62,64,65,178] and dyslipidemia represents a major risk factor for cardiovascular disease.[179,180] In addition, hyperlipidemia has been implicated as a causative factor in the progression of diabetic nephropathy.[181–183] Most diabetic patients on dialysis have some form of dyslipidemia, and cardiovascular disease is epidemic in this group.[8,184–188] Therefore, it is imperative that all diabetic patients, whether they have normal renal function, impaired renal function, or are on dialysis, receive aggressive dietary and pharmacologic therapy. The goal of antilipidemia therapy is to reduce the LDL cholesterol and triglycerides to <100 mg/dL and <200 mg/dL, respectively. This can be achieved with hydroxymethyl glutaryl-coenzyme A (HMG-CoA) reductase inhibitors and fibric acid derivatives.[177,183] The HDL cholesterol should be increased to at least 45 mg/dL, but this often is difficult to achieve with pharmacologic therapy.

## DIALYSIS

Once end-stage renal failure ensues, the patient and physician must choose from one of three options: *hemodialysis, peritoneal dialysis,* or *continuous ambulatory peritoneal dialysis.*[88]

One of the most important questions that the physician faces is when to initiate dialysis in the diabetic patient with advanced renal insufficiency. Vascular access and dialysis should be instituted earlier in diabetic than in nondiabetic patients for many reasons. After the serum creatinine concentration has risen to 3 to 4 mg/dL, there is a rapid deterioration in renal function, and most diabetics require dialysis within 6 to 12 months, if not

sooner. Generally, diabetics tolerate uremia more poorly than nondiabetic uremic patients; in particular, there is a marked acceleration of diabetic retinopathy and neuropathy. Diabetic control becomes more difficult, and negative nitrogen balance, protein wasting, and myopathy become significant management problems with advancing uremia. Hypertension becomes more difficult to control. All of these complications are easier to manage if dialysis is instituted early.[88] A reasonable approach is to establish vascular access when the serum creatinine reaches 4 to 5 mg/dL and to initiate dialysis at creatinine levels of 6 to 8 mg/dL. Although hemodialysis is the most frequently used form of dialysis therapy in diabetic and nondiabetic patients with end-stage renal failure, it does not appear to be superior to any other dialysis technique. Morbidity and mortality statistics are similar with intermittent peritoneal and chronic ambulatory peritoneal dialysis.[8,9,185] Regardless of the type of dialysis that is chosen, survival in diabetics is much worse than in nondiabetics.[184,185]

Nutritional management of the diabetic patient on dialysis represents a major problem. Many patients are malnourished before starting dialysis, and achieving a positive nitrogen balance is difficult. Diabetic patients should receive 37.5 to 40.0 calories/kg ideal body weight, with approximately one-half of the calories given as carbohydrates, primarily complex. To achieve a positive nitrogen balance, at least 1.5 g/kg high biologic value protein is needed. With this intake, most insulin-requiring diabetic patients on dialysis require a split, mixed insulin regimen to achieve adequate glucose control. A morning and evening injection of long-acting insulin (i.e., neutral protamine Hagedorn [NPH]) is usually required, and this should be administered with sufficient quantities of regular insulin to cover the postprandial glucose excursions. Importantly, once dialysis is started, the total daily insulin requirement usually increases by 50% to 100%.[189] Because of frequent, unpredictable fluctuations in glucose control, it is advisable for the diabetic patient to perform home glucose monitoring.

## RENAL TRANSPLANTATION

The results from the United States Renal Data System[184,187] indicate that diabetics who are treated by kidney transplantation, especially if the kidney is received from a living donor, have a much better survival than do those who are placed on dialysis. If a human leukocyte antigen (HLA)–identical donor can be found, the chances of long-term patient and graft survival are far superior to dialysis. HLA-nonidentical recipients also do better than diabetic patients treated with dialysis. Long-term survival with cadaveric renal transplantation is slightly better than with dialysis. Therefore, in the absence of an HLA-related donor, the choice between dialysis and transplantation must be individualized for each diabetic patient. Combined pancreatic/kidney transplantation is at an early stage but may be beneficial in preventing the recurrence of diabetic nephropathy in the transplanted kidney.[29] Newer immunosuppressive regimens may bring further improvements in patient survival after cadaveric renal transplantation.

## PATHOGENESIS OF DIABETIC NEPHROPATHY

Two major causal factors have been implicated in the development of diabetic nephropathy: metabolic and hemodynamic[47,70,72,119,155,156] (Fig. 150-8). In the absence of hyperglycemia, renal disease does not occur, and correction of hyperglycemia prevents the development of diabetic nephropathy.[27,144–150] Hyperglycemia has a direct toxic effect on renal cells and leads to the formation of advanced glycosylation end products, activation of protein kinase C, increased growth factors, and production of cytokines; these collectively cause an increase in extracellular matrix formation.[47] Of the cytokines, transforming growth factor-$\beta_1$ has been the most extensively studied.[47,72,190] It

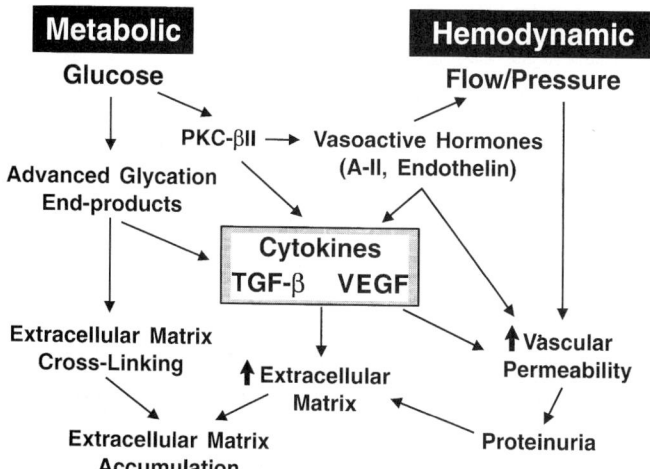

**FIGURE 150-8.** Pathogenic schema depicting the contribution of metabolic and hemodynamic factors to the development of diabetic nephropathy. (*PKC*, protein kinase C; *TGF-β*, transforming growth factor-β; *VEGF*, vascular endothelial growth factor.) (From Cooper ME. Pathogenesis, prevention, and treatment of diabetic nephropathy. Lancet 1998; 352:213.)

is expressed in all glomerular cells, and its production is markedly accelerated in both human and animal models of diabetic nephropathy in response to hyperglycemia, angiotensin II, and advanced glycosylation end products. Hyperglycemia also directly glycosylates proteins in the kidney, and advanced glycosylation end products in the circulation accumulate in the kidney.[191,192] Protein kinase C, which is activated by hyperglycemia, increases endothelial cell permeability to albumin, stimulates matrix-protein synthesis by mesangial cells, and increases the production of vasodilatory prostaglandins, all of which may contribute to early renal hyperperfusion and hyperfiltration.[47,70,72] Increased glucose flux through the aldose-reductase pathway leads to the accumulation of a variety of polyols and intracellular depletion of myoinositol, which can lead to the activation of protein kinase C. In various animal models of diabetes, inhibition of the βII isoform of protein kinase C prevents the development of hyperfiltration and albuminuria[193]; protein kinase C inhibitors currently are undergoing clinical testing in humans.

Both systemic and local renal hemodynamic factors play an important role in the development of diabetic nephropathy (see Fig. 150-8).[47,70,72] (The contribution of systemic hypertension was discussed previously.) In animal models of diabetes mellitus, there is a marked increase in single-nephron GFR, RPF, and intraglomerular pressure. The increase in intraglomerular pressure results from enhanced sensitivity of the efferent arteriole to angiotensin II. These changes in renal hemodynamics occur after the induction of experimental diabetes in the rat, are reversed by insulin therapy, and are similar to those observed in the remnant kidney model of renal insufficiency. An increased transglomerular passage of albumin, owing to the elevated intraglomerular pressure, has been demonstrated during the early phase of diabetes in humans and in animals. The increase in single-nephron RPF and glomerular transcapillary hydraulic pressure, whether due to intrinsic renal disease or diabetes mellitus, if sustained over a prolonged period, leads to cellular injury, proliferation of mesangial matrix material, and glomerulosclerosis. The elevation in glomerular plasma flow and transcapillary hydraulic pressure leads to increased transcapillary protein flux, which may further exacerbate the mesangial-cell injury and the proliferation of mesangial-matrix material. With progressive renal injury, permselectivity changes in the glomerular barrier occur and further exacerbate the proteinuria. Consistent with this pathogenesis, in diabetic animal models, ACE inhibitors decrease intraglomerular pressure, lower GFR and RPF, reduce proteinuria, and prevent the histologic changes of diabetic nephropathy. Improved renal

function also has been observed in both type 1 and type 2 diabetic humans who are treated with ACE inhibitors. It should be noted, however, that angiotensin II has a number of nonhemodynamic actions,[138] which would be expected to exacerbate diabetic nephropathy. Angiotensin II is a potent growth factor that directly stimulates mesangial-matrix proliferation, stimulates collagen and fibronectin synthesis, causes renal hypertrophy, and potentiates the effects of a variety of growth factors on the kidney.

Thus, hyperglycemia sets into play a number of hemodynamic and metabolic abnormalities that eventuate in the typical histologic and clinical picture that is seen in patients with diabetic nephropathy.

## REFERENCES

1. Krolewski AS, Warram JH, Rand LI, Kahn CR. Epidemiologic approach to the etiology of type I diabetes mellitus and its complications. N Engl J Med 1987; 317:1390.
2. Krolewski M, Eggers PW, Warram JH. Magnitude of end-stage renal disease in IDDM: a 35 year follow-up study. Kidney Int 1996; 50:2041.
3. Harris MI, Flegal KM, Cowie CC, et al. Prevalence of diabetes, impaired fasting glucose, and impaired glucose tolerance in U.S. adults. The Third National Health and Nutrition Examination Survey, 1988–1994. Diabetes Care 1998; 21:518.
4. Ballard DJ, Humphrey LL, Nelton LJ, et al. Epidemiology of persistent proteinuria in type II diabetes mellitus: population-based study in Rochester, Minnesota. Diabetes 1988; 37:405.
5. Teutsch S, Newman J, Eggers P. The problem of diabetic renal failure in the United States: an overview. Am J Kidney Dis 1989; 13:11.
6. Pugh JA, Stem MP, Haffner SM, et al. Incidence of end-stage renal disease secondary to diabetes mellitus in Mexican-Americans and non-Hispanic whites. Am J Epidemiol 1987; 127:135.
7. Hawthorne V, Hamman R, Keen H, et al. Preventing the kidney disease of diabetes mellitus. Am J Kidney Dis 1989; 13:2.
8. Agodoa LY, Jones CA, Held PJ. End-stage renal disease in the USA: data from the United States renal data system. Am J Nephrol 1996; 16:7.
9. United States Renal Data System. USRDS 1998 Annual Data Report. National Institutes of Health, National Institutes of Diabetes and Digestive and Kidney Diseases, Bethesda, MD, 1998. Am J Kidney Dis 1998; 32(Suppl 1):S1.
10. USRDS 1999 Annual Data Report. The economic cost of ESRD and Medicare spending for alternative modalities of treatment. Am J Kidney Dis 1999; 34(Suppl 1):S124.
11. Kimmelstiel P, Wilson C. Intercapillary lesions in glomeruli of kidney. Am J Pathol 1936; 12:83.
12. Osterby R, Gundersen HJG, Horlyck A, et al. Diabetic glomerulopathy: structural characteristics of the early and advanced stages. Diabetes 1983; 32:79.
13. Fioretto P, Steffes MW, Sutherland DER, Mauer M. Sequential renal biopsies in insulin dependent diabetic patients: structural factors associated with clinical progression. Kidney Int 1995; 48:1929.
14. Ziyadeh FN. The extracellular matrix in diabetic nephropathy. Am J Kidney Dis 1993; 22:736.
15. Steffes MW, Bilous RW, Sutherland DER, Mauer SM. Cell and matrix components of the glomerular mesangium in type I diabetes. Diabetes 1992; 41:679.
16. Spiro RG. Biochemistry of the renal glomerular basement membrane and its alteration in diabetes mellitus. N Engl J Med 1973; 288:1337.
17. Wahl P, Depperman D, Hasslacher C. Biochemistry of glomerular basement membrane of the normal and diabetic human. Kidney Int 1982; 21:744.
18. Falk RJ, Scheinman JI, Mauer SM, Michael AF. Polyantigenic expansion of basement membrane constituents in diabetic nephropathy. Diabetes 1983; 32:34.
19. Scandling JD, Myers BD. Glomerular size-selectivity and microalbuminuria in early diabetic glomerular disease. Kidney Int 1992; 41:840.
20. Lane PH, Steffes MS, Fioretto P, Mauer SM. Renal interstitial expansion in insulin-dependent diabetes mellitus. Kidney Int 1993; 43:661.
21. Brito PL, Fioretto P, Drummond, et al. Proximal-tubular basement membrane width in insulin-dependent diabetes mellitus. Kidney Int 1998; 53:754.
22. Vejlsgaard R. Studies on urinary tract infection in diabetics. Acta Med Scand 1966; 179:173.
23. Batalla MA, Balodimos MC, Bradley RF. Bacteriuria in diabetes mellitus. Diabetologia 1971; 7:297.
24. Lauler DP, Schreiner GE, David A. Renal medullary necrosis. Am J Med 1960; 29:132.
25. Mauer SM, Steffes MW, Connett J, et al. The development of lesions in the glomerular basement membrane and mesangium after transplantation of normal kidneys to diabetic patients. Diabetes 1983; 32:948.
26. Becker D, Miller M. Presence of diabetic glomerulosclerosis in patients with hemochromatosis. N Engl J Med 1960; 263:367.

27. The Diabetes Control and Complications Trial Research Group. The effect of intensive treatment of diabetes on the development and progression of long-term complications in insulin-dependent diabetes mellitus. N Engl J Med 1993; 329:977.

28. Abouna GM, Kremer GD, Daddah SK, et al. Reversal of diabetic nephropathy in human cadaveric kidneys after transplantation into non-diabetic recipients. Lancet 1983; 2:1274.

29. Fioretto P, Steffes MW, Sutherland DER, et al. Reversal of lesions of diabetic nephropathy after pancreas transplantation. N Engl J Med 1998; 339:69.

30. KROC Collaborative Study. Blood glucose control and the evaluation of diabetic retinopathy and albuminuria. N Engl J Med 1984; 311:365.

31. Viberti GC, Bilous RW, Mackintosh D, et al. Long-term correction of hyperglycaemia and progression of renal failure in insulin dependent diabetics. Br Med J 1983; 286:598.

32. Steno Study Group. Effect of six months of strict metabolic control on eye and kidney function in insulin-dependent diabetics with background retinopathy. Lancet 1982; 1:121.

33. Alaveras AE, Thomas SM, Sagriotis A, Viberti GC. Promoters of progression of diabetic nephropathy: the relative roles of blood glucose and blood pressure control. Nephrol Dial Transplant 1997; 2:71.

34. Linner E, Svanborg A, Zelander T. Retinal and renal lesions of diabetic type, without obvious disturbances in glucose metabolism, in a patient with family history of diabetes. Am J Med 1971; 39:298.

35. Siperstein MD, Unger RH, Madison LL. Studies of muscle capillary basement membranes in normal subjects, diabetic and prediabetic patients. J Clin Invest 1968; 47:1973.

36. Williamson JR, Kilo C. A common sense approach resolves the basement membrane controversy and the NIH Pima Indian study. Diabetologia 1979; 17:129.

37. Seaquist ER, Goetz FC, Rich SS, Barbosa J. Familial clustering of diabetic kidney disease: evidence for genetic susceptibility to diabetic nephropathy. N Engl J Med 1989; 320:1161.

38. DCCT Research Group. Clustering of long-term complications in families with diabetes in the Diabetes Control and Complications Trial. Diabetes 1997; 46:1829.

39. Pettitt DJ, Saad MF, Bennett PH, et al. Familial predisposition to renal disease in two generations of Pima Indians with type 2 (non-insulin-dependent) diabetes mellitus. Diabetologia 1990; 33:438.

40. Faronato PP, Maioli M, Tonolo G, et al. Clustering of albumin excretion rate abnormalities in Caucasian patients with NIDDM. The Italian NIDDM nephropathy study group. Diabetologia 1997; 40:816.

41. Viberti GC, Keen H, Wiseman MJ. Raised arterial pressure in parents of proteinuric insulin-dependent diabetics. Br Med J 1987; 295:515.

42. Fioretto P, Steffes MW, Barbosa J, et al. Is diabetic nephropathy inherited? Studies of glomerular structure in type 1 diabetic sibling pairs. Diabetes 1999; 48:865.

43. Imperatore G, Hanson RL, Pettitt DJ, et al. Sib-pair linkage analysis for susceptibility genes for microvascular complications among Pima Indians with type 2 diabetes mellitus. Diabetes 1998; 47:821.

44. Krolewski AS. Genetics of diabetic nephropathy: evidence for major and minor gene effects. Kidney Int 1999; 55:1582.

44a. Bain SC, Chowdhury TA. Genetics of diabetic nephropathy and microalbuminuria. J R Soc Med 2000; 93:62.

45. Cowie CC, Port FK, Wolfe RA, et al. Disparities in incidence of diabetic end-stage renal disease according to race and type of diabetes. N Engl J Med 1989; 321:1074.

46. Borch-Johnsen K, Nissen H, Henriksen E, et al. The natural history of insulin-dependent diabetes mellitus in Denmark. 1. Long term survival with and without late diabetic complications. Diabetic Med 1987; 4:201.

47. DeFronzo RA. Diabetic nephropathy: etiologic and therapeutic considerations. Diabetes Rev 1995; 3:510.

48. Mogensen CE. Microalbuminuria, blood pressure and diabetic renal disease: origin and development of ideas. Diabetologia 1999; 42:263.

49. Nelson RG, Bennett PH, Beck GJ, et al, for the Diabetic Renal Disease Study Group. Development and progression of renal disease in Pima Indians with non-insulin-dependent diabetes mellitus. N Engl J Med 1996; 335:1636.

50. Knowler WC, Bennett PH, Hamman RF, Miller M. Diabetes incidence and prevalence in Pima Indians: a 19-fold greater incidence than in Rochester, Minnesota. Am J Epidemiol 1978; 108:497.

51. Hasslacher C, Ritz E, Wahl P, Michael C. Similar risk of nephropathy in patients with type I or type II diabetes mellitus. Nephrol Dial Transplant 1989; 4:859.

52. Ritz E, Orth SR. Nephropathy in patients with type 2 diabetes mellitus. N Engl J Med 1999; 341:1127.

53. Mogensen CE, Osterby R, Gundersen HJG. Early functional and morphologic vascular renal consequences of the diabetic state. Diabetologia 1979; 17:71.

54. Wiseman MJ, Saunders AJ, Keen H, Viberti GC. Effect of blood glucose control on increased glomerular filtration rate and kidney size in insulin-dependent diabetes. N Engl J Med 1985; 312:617.

55. Tuttle KR, Bruton JL, Perusek MC, et al. Effects of strict glycemic control on basal and insulin stimulated renal hemodynamic and kidney size in insulin-dependent diabetes mellitus. N Engl J Med 1991; 324:1626.

56. Thomsen OF, Andersen AR, Christiansen JS, Deckert T. Renal changes in long-term type I (insulin-dependent) diabetic patients with and without clinical nephropathy: a light microscopic, morphometric study of autopsy material. Diabetologia 1984; 26:361.

57. Deckert T, Parving HH, Thomsen OF, et al. Renal structure and function in type I (insulin-dependent) diabetic patients: a study of 44 kidney biopsies. Diabetic Nephropathy 1985; 4:163.

58. Viberti GC, Wiseman M, Radmond RS. Microalbuminuria: its history and potential for prevention of clinical nephropathy in diabetes mellitus. Diabetic Nephropathy 1984; 3:79.

59. Parving HH, Oxenboll B, Svendsen PA, et al. Early detection of patients at risk of developing diabetic nephropathy: a longitudinal study of urinary albumin excretion. Acta Endocrinol (Copenh) 1982; 100:550.

60. Mogensen CE, Christensen CK. Predicting diabetic nephropathy in insulin-dependent patients. N Engl J Med 1984; 311:89.

61. Mogensen CE, Viberti GC, Preheim E, et al. Multicenter evaluation of the micral-test II test strip, an immunologic rapid test for the detection of microalbuminuria. Diabetes Care 1997; 20:1642.

62. Mogensen CE. Microalbuminuria predicts clinical proteinuria and early mortality in maturity-onset diabetes. N Engl J Med 1984; 310:356.

63. Ruggenenti P, Remuzzi G. Nephropathy of type-2 diabetes mellitus. J Am Soc Nephrol 1998; 9:2157.

64. Gall MA, Rossing P, Skott P, et al. Prevalence of micro- and macroalbuminuria, arterial hypertension, retinopathy and large vessel disease in European type 2 (non-insulin-dependent) diabetic patients. Diabetologia 1991; 34:655.

65. Mattock MB, Morrish NJ, Viberti G, et al. Prospective study of microalbuminuria as predictor of mortality in NIDDM. Diabetes 1992; 41:736.

66. Nelson RG, Meyer TW, Myers BD, Bennett PH. Clinical and pathological course of renal disease in non-insulin-dependent diabetes mellitus: the Pima Indians experience. Semin Nephrol 1997; 17:124.

67. Schmitz A, Vaeth M. Microalbuminuria: a major risk factor in non-insulin dependent diabetes: a 10-year follow-up study of 503 patients. Diabetic Med 1988; 5:126.

68. Consensus statement. Am J Kidney Dis 1989; 13:2.

69. Friedman S, Jones HW, Golbetz HV, et al. Mechanisms of proteinuria in diabetic nephropathy. II. A study of the size selective glomerular filtration barriers. Diabetes 1983; 32:40.

70. Hostetter TH. Mechanisms of diabetic nephropathy. Am J Kidney Dis 1994; 23:188.

71. Deckert T, Kofoed-Enevoldsen A, Vidal P. Size and charge selectivity of glomerular filtration in type 1 (insulin-dependent) diabetic patients with and without albuminuria. Diabetologia 1993; 36:244.

72. Cooper ME. Pathogenesis, prevention, and treatment of diabetic nephropathy. Lancet 1998; 352:213.

73. Bangstad H-J, Kofoed-Enevoldsen A, Dahl-Jorgensen K, Hanssen KF. Glomerular charge selectivity and the influence of improved blood glucose control in type 1 (insulin-dependent) diabetic patients with microalbuminuria. Diabetologia 1992; 35:1165.

74. Mogensen CE. Glomerular hyperfiltration in human diabetes. Diabetes Care 1994; 17:770.

75. Rudberg S, Persson B, Dahlquist G. Increased glomerular filtration rate as a predictor of diabetic nephropathy: results from an 8-year prospective study. Kidney Int 1992; 41:822.

76. Mogensen CE. Maximum tubular reabsorption capacity for glucose and renal hemodynamics during rapid hypertonic glucose infusion in normal and diabetic men. Scand J Clin Lab Invest 1971; 28:101.

77. DeFronzo RA, Smith JD. Disorders of potassium metabolism: hyperkalemia. In: Arieff A, DeFronzo RA, eds. Fluid, electrolyte and acid-base disorders. New York: Churchill Livingstone, 1995:319.

78. DeFronzo RA. Hyperkalemia and hyporeninemic hypoaldosteronism. Kidney Int 1980; 17:118.

79. Schambelan M, Sebastian A, Biglieri E. Prevalence, pathogenesis, and functional significance of aldosterone deficiency in hyperkalemic patients with chronic renal insufficiency. Kidney Int 1980; 17:89.

80. deChatel R, Weidmann P, Flammer J, et al. Sodium, renin, aldosterone, catecholamines and blood pressure in diabetes mellitus. Kidney Int 1977; 12:412.

81. Halperin ML, Bear RA, Hannaford MC, Goldstein MB. Selected aspects of the pathophysiology of metabolic acidosis in diabetes mellitus. Diabetes 1981; 30:781.

82. Root HF, Porte WH, Frehner H. Triopathy of diabetes: sequence of neuropathy, retinopathy, and nephropathy. Arch Intern Med 1984; 94:931.

83. Pirart J. Diabetes mellitus and its degenerative complications: a prospective study of 4,400 patients observed between 1944 and 1973. Diabetes Care 1978; 1:168.

84. Bilous RW, Viberti GC, Christiansen JS, et al. Dissociation of diabetic complications in insulin-dependent diabetics: a clinical report. Diabetic Nephropathy 1985; 4:73.

85. Chahal PS, Kohner EM. The relationship between diabetic retinopathy and diabetic nephropathy. Diabetic Nephropathy 1983; 2:4.

86. Strowig SM, Raskin P. Glycemic control and the complications of diabetes. Diabetes Rev 1995; 3:237.

87. Hamman RF. Epidemiology of microvascular complications. In: Alberti KGMM, Zimmet P, DeFronzo RA, eds. International textbook of diabetes mellitus. New York: John Wiley and Sons, 1997:1293.

88. Friedlander MA, Hricik DE. Optimizing end-stage renal disease therapy for the patient with diabetes mellitus. Semin Nephrol 1997; 17:331.

89. Goldstein DA, Massry SG. Diabetic nephropathy: clinical course and effect of hemodialysis. Nephron 1978; 20:286.

90. McCrary RF, Pitts TO, Puschett JB. Diabetic nephropathy: natural course, survivorship, and therapy. Am J Nephrol 1981; 1:206.

91. Orchard TJ, Dorman JS, Maser RE, et al. Prevalence of complications in IDDM by sex and duration. Pittsburgh Epidemiology of Diabetes Complications Study. Diabetes 1990; 39:1116.

92. Sima AAF, Thomas PF, Ishil D, Vinik A. Diabetic neuropathies. Diabetologia 1997; 40:B74.

93. Eisenberg B, Murata G, Tzamaloukas A, et al. Gastroparesis in diabetics on chronic dialysis: clinical and laboratory associations and predictive features. Nephrology 1995; 70:296.

94. Najarian JS, Sutherland DER, Simmons RL, et al. Kidney transplantation for the uremic diabetic patient. Surg Gynecol Obstet 1977; 144:682.

95. Mogensen CE. Prediction of clinical diabetic nephropathy in IDDM patients. Alternatives to microalbuminuria? Diabetes 1990; 39:761.

96. Mathiesen ER. Prevention of diabetic nephropathy. Microalbuminuria and perspectives for intervention in insulin-dependent diabetes. Dan Med Bull 1993; 40:273.

97. Nosadini R, Fioretto P, Trevisan R, Crepaldi G. Insulin-dependent diabetes mellitus and hypertension. Diabetes Care 1991; 14:210.

98. Markell MS, Friedman EA. Care of the diabetic patients with end-stage renal disease. Semin Nephrol 1990; 10:274.

99. Venkatesan J, Henrich WL. Anemia, hypertension, and myocardial dysfunction in end-stage renal disease. Semin Nephrol 1997; 17:257.

100. Kjellstrand CM, Whitley K, Comty CM, Shapiro FL. Dialysis in patients with diabetes mellitus. Diabetic Nephropathy 1983; 2:5.

101. Elving LD, Wetzels JFM, van Lier HJJ, et al. Captopril and atenolol are equally effective in retarding progression of diabetic nephropathy. Results of a 2-year prospective, randomized study. Diabetologia 1994; 37:604.

102. Mogensen CE. Progression of nephropathy in long-term diabetics with proteinuria and effect of initial anti-hypertensive treatment. Scand J Clin Lab Invest 1976; 36:383.

103. Parving H-H. Impact of blood pressure and antihypertensive treatment on incipient and overt nephropathy, retinopathy, and endothelial permeability in diabetes mellitus. Diabetes Care 1991; 14:260.

104. Mogensen CE. Long-term antihypertensive treatment inhibiting progression of diabetic nephropathy. Br Med J 1982; 285:685.

105. Parving H-H, Andersen AR, Smidt UM, et al. Effect of antihypertensive treatment on kidney function in diabetic nephropathy. Br Med J 1987; 294:1443.

106. Lewis EJ, Hunsicker LG, Bain RP, Rohde RD. The effect of angiotensin-converting-enzyme inhibition on diabetic nephropathy. N Engl J Med 1993; 329:1456.

107. Berkman J, Rifkin H. Unilateral nodular diabetic glomerulosclerosis (Kimmelstiel-Wilson): report of a case. Metabolism 1973; 22:175.

108. Steffes MW, Buchwald H, Wigness BD, et al. Diabetic nephropathy in the uninephrectomized dog: microscopic lesions after one year. Kidney Int 1982; 21:721.

109. Barbosa J, Steffes MW, Sutherland DE, et al. Effects of glycemic control on early diabetic renal lesions: a 5-year randomized controlled trial of insulin-dependent diabetic kidney transplant recipients. JAMA 1994; 272:600.

110. Krolewski AS, Canessa M, Warram JH, et al. Predisposition to hypertension and susceptibility to renal disease in insulin-dependent diabetes mellitus. N Engl J Med 1988; 318:140.

111. DeFronzo RA, Ferrannini E. Insulin resistance: a multifaceted syndrome responsible for NIDDM, obesity, hypertension, dyslipidemia, and ASCVD. Diabetes Care-Reviews 1991; 14:173.

112. The Sixth Report of the Joint National Committee on Prevention, Detection, Evaluation, and Treatment of High Blood Pressure. Arch Intern Med 1997; 157:2413.

113. Hansson L, Zanchetti A, Carruthers SG, et al. For the HOT Study Group. Effects of intensive blood-pressure lowering and low-dose aspirin in patients with hypertension: principal results of the Hypertension Optimal Treatment (HOT) randomised trial. Lancet 1998; 351:1755.

114. Bakris GL. Pathogenesis of hypertension in diabetes. Diabetes Rev 1995; 3:460.

115. Ismail N, Becker B, Strzelcyzyk P, Ritz E. Renal disease and hypertension in non-insulin-dependent diabetes mellitus. Kidney Int 1999; 55:1.

116. Elliott WJ, Stein PP, Black HR. Drug treatment of hypertension in patients with diabetes. Diabetes Rev 1995; 3:477.

117. Bressler P, DeFronzo RA. Drugs and diabetes. Diabetes Rev 1994; 2:53.

118. UK Prospective Diabetes Study Group. Tight blood pressure control and risk of macrovascular and microvascular complications in type 2 diabetes. UKPDS 38. Br Med J 1998; 317:703.

119. Tuttle KR, DeFronzo RA, Stein JH. Treatment of diabetic nephropathy: a rational approach based on its pathophysiology. Semin Nephrol 1991; 11:220.

120. Ravid M, Savin H, Jutrin I, et al. Long-term stabilizing effect of angiotensin-converting enzyme inhibition on proteinuria in normotensive type II diabetic patients. Ann Intern Med 1993; 188:577.

121. Ravid M, Brosh D, Levi Z, et al. Use of enalapril to attenuate decline in renal function in normotensive, normoalbuminuric patients with type 2 diabetes mellitus. A randomized, controlled trial. Ann Intern Med 1998; 128:982.

122. Mogensen CE. Microalbuminuria, early blood pressure elevation, and diabetic renal disease. Curr Opin Endocrinol Diab 1994; 4:239.

123. Viberti G, Chaturvedi N. Angiotensin converting enzyme inhibitors in diabetic patients with microalbuminuria or normoalbuminuria. Kidney Int 1997; 52(Suppl 63):S32.

124. The Microalbuminuria Captopril Study Group. Captopril reduces the risk of nephropathy in IDDM patients with microalbuminuria. Diabetologia 1996; 39:587.

125. Nielsen FS, Rossing P, Gall M-A, et al. Long-term effect of lisinopril and atenolol on kidney function in hypertensive NIDDM subjects with diabetic nephropathy. Diabetes 1997; 46:1182.

126. Lithell HOL. Effect of antihypertensive drugs on insulin, glucose, and lipid metabolism. Diabetes Care 1991; 14:203.

126a. Heart Outcome Prevention Evaluation. Effects of ramipril on cardiovascular and microvascular outcomes in people with diabetes mellitus: results of the HOPE study and micro-HOPE substudy. Lancet 2000; 355:253.

126b. Chan JCN, Ko GTC, Leung DHY, et al. Long-term effects of angiotensin-converting enzyme inhibition and metabolic control in hypertensive type 2 diabetic patients. Kidney Int 2000; 57:590.

127. Ganesvoort RT, de Zeeuw D, de Jong PE. Is the antiproteinuric effect of ACE inhibition mediated by interference in the renin-angiotensin system? Kidney Int 1994; 45:861.

128. Giordano M, Matsuda M, Canessa ML, DeFronzo RA. The effects of ACE inhibitors, calcium channel antagonists, and alpha adrenergic blockers on glucose and lipid metabolism in type II diabetic patients with hypertension. Diabetes 1995; 44:665.

129. Giordano M, Sanders LR, Castellino P, et al. Effect of alpha-adrenergic blockers, ACE inhibitors, and calcium channel antagonists on renal function in non-insulin dependent diabetic patients. Nephron 1996; 72:447.

130. Bakris GL, Copley JB, Vicknair N, et al. Calcium channel blockers versus other antihypertensive therapies on progression of NIDDM associated nephropathy. Kidney Int 1996; 50:1641.

131. Zucchelli P, Zuccala A, Borghi M, et al. Long-term comparison between captopril and nifedipine in the progression of renal insufficiency. Kidney Int 1992; 42:452.

132. Kloke HJ, Branten AJ, Huysmans FT, Wetzels JF. Antihypertensive treatment of patients with proteinuric renal diseases: risks or benefits of calcium channel blockers? Kidney Int 1998; 53:1559.

133. Velussi M, Brocco E, Frigato F, et al. Effects of cilazapril and amlodipine on kidney function in hypertensive NIDDM patients. Diabetes 1996; 45:216.

134. Bakris GL, Copley JB, Vicknair N, et al. Calcium channel blockers versus other antihypertensive therapies on progression of NIDDM associated nephropathy. Kidney Int 1996; 50:1641.

135. Munter K, Hergenroder S, Jochims K, Kirchengast M. Individual and combined effects of verapamil or trandolapril on attenuating hypertensive glomerulopathic changes in the stroke-prone rat. J Am Soc Nephrol 1996; 7:681.

136. Bakris GL, Weir MR, DeQuattro V, McMahaon FG. Effects of an ACE inhibitor/calcium antagonist combination on proteinuria in diabetic nephropathy. Kidney Int 1998; 54:1283.

137. Stefanski A, Amann K, Ritz E. To prevent progression: ACE inhibitors, calcium antagonists or both? Nephrol Dial Transplant 1995; 10:151.

138. Wolf G, Ziyadeh FN. The role of angiotensin II in diabetic nephropathy: emphasis on nonhemodynamic mechanisms. Am J Kidney Dis 1997; 29:153.

139. Bryd L, Sherman RL. Radio-contrast-induced renal failure: a clinical and pathophysiologic review. Medicine 1979; 58:270.

140. Solomon R, Werner C, Mann D, et al. Effects of saline, mannitol, and furosemide to prevent acute decreases in renal function induced by radiocontrast agents. N Engl J Med 1994; 331:1416.

141. Klein R. Hyperglycemia and microvascular and macrovascular disease in diabetes. Diabetes Care 1995; 18:258.

142. Ballard DJ, Humphrey LL, Melton LJ, et al. Epidemiology of persistent proteinuria in type II diabetes mellitus: population-based study in Rochester, Minnesota. Diabetes 1988; 37:405.

143. Microalbuminuria Collaborative Study Group. Microalbuminuria in type I diabetic patients. Diabetes Care 1992; 15:495.

144. Norgaard K, Storm B, Graae M, Feldt-Rasmussen B. Elevated albumin excretion and retinal changes in children with type I diabetes are related to long-term poor blood glucose control. Diabetic Med 1989; 6:325.

145. Torffvit O, Agardh E, Agardh CD. Albuminuria and associated medical risk factors: a cross-sectional study in 476 type 1 (insulin-dependent) diabetic patients (Pt I). J Diab Compl 1991; 5:23.

146. The absence of a glycemic threshold for the development of long-term complications: the perspective of the Diabetes Control and Complications Trial. Diabetes 1996; 45:1289.

146a. Diabetes Control and Complications Trial. Retinopathy and nephropathy in patients with type 1 diabetes four years after a trial of intensive therapy. N Engl J Med 2000; 342:381.

147. Ohkubo Y, Kishikawa H, Araki E, et al. Intensive insulin therapy prevents the progression of diabetic microvascular complications in Japanese patients with non-insulin-dependent diabetes mellitus: a randomized prospective 6-year study. Diabetes Res Clin Pract 1995; 28:103.

148. UK Prospective Diabetes Study Group. Intensive blood glucose control with sulphonylureas or insulin compared with conventional treatment and risk of complications in patients with type 2 diabetes (UKPDS 33). Lancet 1998; 352:837.

149. UK Prospective Diabetes Study Group. Effect of intensive blood glucose control with metformin on complications in overweight patients with type 2 diabetes (UKPDS 34). Lancet 1998; 352:854.

150. Wang PH, Lau J, Chalmers TC. Meta-analysis of effects of intensive blood glucose control on late complications of type I diabetes. Lancet 1993; 341:1306.

151. Rasch R. Prevention of diabetic glomerulopathy in streptozotocin diabetic rats by insulin treatment. Diabetologia 1979; 16:125.

152. Bilous RW, Mauer SM, Sutherland DER, et al. The effects of pancreas transplantation on the glomerular structure of renal allografts in patients with insulin-dependent diabetes. N Engl J Med 1989; 321:80.

153. Fioretto P, Mauer SM, Bilous RW, et al. Effects of pancreas transplantation on glomerular structure in insulin-dependent diabetic patients with their own kidneys. Lancet 1993; 342:1193.

154. Feldt-Rasmussen B. Microalbuminuria and clinical nephropathy in type I (insulin-dependent) diabetes mellitus: pathophysiological mechanisms and intervention studies. Danish Med Bull 1989; 36:405.

155. Viberti GC, Walker JD. Diabetic nephropathy: etiology and prevention. Diabetes Metab Rev 1988; 4:147.

156. Mogensen CE. Prevention and treatment of renal disease in insulin-dependent diabetes mellitus. Semin Nephrol 1990; 10:260.

157. The Kroc Collaborative Study Group. Blood glucose control and the evolution of diabetic retinopathy and albuminuria: a preliminary multicenter trial. N Engl J Med 1984; 311:365.

158. DeFronzo RA, Alvestrand A, Smith D, et al. Insulin resistance in uremia. J Clin Invest 1981; 67:563.

159. DeFronzo RA, Tobin JD, Rowe JW, Andres R. Glucose intolerance in uremia: quantification of pancreatic beta cell sensitivity to glucose and tissue sensitivity to insulin. J Clin Invest 1978; 62:425.

160. DeFronzo RA. Pharmacologic therapy for type 2 diabetes mellitus. Ann Intern Med 1999; 131:281.

161. Yamasaki Y, Kawamori R, Wasada T, et al. Pioglitazone (AD-4833) ameliorates insulin resistance in patients with NIDDM. AD-4833 glucose clamp study group. Tohoku J Exp Med 1997; 183:173.

162. Sambol NC, Chiang J, Lin ET, et al. Kidney function and age are both predictors of pharmacokinetics of metformin. J Clin Pharmacol 1995; 35:1094.

163. Prendergast BD. Glyburide and glipizide, second-generation oral sulfonylurea hypoglycemic agents. Clin Pharmacol 1984; 3:473.

164. Rosenkranz B. Pharmacokinetic basis for the safety of glimepiride in risk groups of NIDDM patients. Horm Metab Res 1996; 28:434.

165. Marbury T, Huang W-C, Strange P, Lebovitz H. Repaglinide versus glyburide: a one-year comparison trial. Diab Res Clin Pract 1999; 43:155.

166. Tzamaloukas AH. Interpreting glycosylated hemoglobin in diabetic patients on peritonal dialysis. Adv Peritoneal Dialysis 1996; 12:171.

167. Garber AJ, Bier D, Cryer PE, Pagliara AS. Hypoglycemia in compensated chronic renal insufficiency: substrate limitation of gluconeogenesis. Diabetes 1974; 23:982.

168. Grajower M, Walter L, Albin J. Hypoglycemia in chronic hemodialysis patients: association with propranolol use. Nephron 1980; 26:126.

169. Wong TY-H, Chan JCN, Szeto CC, et al. Clinical and biochemical characteristics of type 2 diabetic patients on continuous ambulatory peritoneal dialysis: relationships with insulin requirement. Am J Kidney Dis 1999; 34:514.

170. Giordano C. Protein restriction in chronic renal failure. Kidney Int 1982; 22:401.

171. Brenner BM, Meyer TW, Hostetter TH. Dietary protein intake and the progressive nature of kidney disease. N Engl J Med 1982; 307:652.

172. Zeller KR, Whittaker E, Sullivan L, et al. Effect of restricting dietary protein on the progression of renal failure in patients with insulin-dependent diabetes mellitus. N Engl J Med 1991; 324:78.

173. Pedrini MT, Levey AS, Lau J, et al. The effect of dietary protein restriction on the progression of diabetic and nondiabetic renal diseases: a meta-analysis. Ann Intern Med 1996; 124:627.

174. Walker JD, Dodds RA, Murrells TJ, et al. Restriction of dietary protein and progression of renal failure in diabetic nephropathy. Lancet 1989; 2:1411.

175. Klahr S, Levey AS, Beck GJ, et al. The effects of dietary protein restriction and blood-pressure control on the progression of chronic renal disease. N Engl J Med 1990; 330:877.

176. Modification of Diet in Renal Disease Study Group. Effects of dietary protein restriction on the progression of moderate renal disease in the modification of diet in renal disease study. J Am Soc Nephrol 1996; 7:2616.

177. Kasiske BL. Hyperlipidemia in patients with chronic renal disease. Am J Kidney Dis 1998; 32:S142.

178. Deckert T, Feldt-Rasmussen B, Borch-Johnsen, et al. Albuminuria reflects widespread vascular damage. The Steno hypothesis. Diabetologia 1989; 32:219.

179. Wilson PWF, Culleton BF. Cardiovascular disease in the general population. Epidemiology of cardiovascular disease in the United States. Am J Kidney Dis 1998; 32(Suppl 3):S56.

180. Wilson PWF. Diabetes mellitus and coronary heart disease. Am J Kidney Dis 1998; 32(Suppl 3):S89.

181. Keane WF. Lipids and progressive renal disease: the cardio-renal link. Am J Kidney Dis 1999; 34:xliii.

182. Krolewski AS, Warram JH, Christlieb AR. Hypercholesterolemia: a determinant of renal function loss and deaths of IDDM patients with nephropathy. Kidney Int 1994; 45(Suppl 45):S125.

183. Oda H, Keane WF. Recent advances in statins and the kidney. Kidney Int 1999; 56(Suppl 71):S2.

184. USRDS 1999 Annual Data Report. V. Patient mortality and survival. Am J Kidney Dis 1999; 34(Suppl 1):S74.

185. USRDS 1999 Annual Data Report. VI. Causes of death. Am J Kidney Dis 1999; 34(Suppl 1):S87.

186. Herzog CA, Ma JZ, Collins AJ. Long-term outcome of dialysis patients in the United States with coronary revascularization procedures. Kidney Int 1999; 56:324.

187. USRDS 1999 Annual Data Report. VII. Renal transplantation: access and outcomes. Am J Kidney Dis 1999; 34(Suppl 1):S95.

188. Herzog CA. Acute myocardial infarction in patients with end-stage renal disease. Kidney Int 1999; 56(Suppl 71):S130.

189. Comty CM, Leonard A, Shapiro FL. Nutritional and metabolic problems in dialyzed patients with diabetes mellitus. Kidney Int 1974; 6:S51.

190. Riser BL, Cortes P, Yee J, et al. Mechanical strain- and high glucose-induced alterations in mesangial cell collagen metabolism: role of TGF-β. J Am Soc Nephrol 1998; 9:827.

191. Makita Z, Bucala R, Rayfield EJ, et al. Reactive glycosylation endproducts in diabetic uraemia and treatment of renal failure. Lancet 1994; 343:1519.

192. Makita Z, Radoff S, Rayfield E, et al. Advanced glycosylation end products in patients with diabetic nephropathy. N Engl J Med 1991; 325:836.

193. Ishi H, Jirousek MR, Koya D, et al. Amelioration of vascular dysfunctions in diabetic rats by an oral PKC beta inhibitor. Science 1996; 272:728.

# CHAPTER 151

# DIABETES AND THE EYE

LAWRENCE I. RAND

Diabetes is a leading cause of blindness and vision disability in the nations in which nutritional and infectious diseases have, for the most part, been controlled.[1,2] The improved quality of medical care in these countries has allowed diabetic individuals to survive the 20 to 40 years necessary for severe eye complications to develop. During the past 15 years, knowledge of the natural history of diabetic eye disease has greatly increased, and equally impressive advances have been made in its treatment. Knowledge about the determinants of this disease has improved but is still rudimentary. However, clinical management guidelines can now be established that should reduce dramatically the occurrence of severe vision disability and blindness.

## DIABETIC RETINOPATHY

The principal cause of blindness among diabetic patients is disease of the retina. Those who are particularly interested in the cause and treatment of diabetic retinopathy commonly use several abbreviations, which are listed in Table 151-1.

### EPIDEMIOLOGY

#### DISTRIBUTION

Epidemiology is the study of the distribution and determinants of disease. Knowledge of when and how often diabetic eye disease develops has been advanced by studies using standardized photographic evaluations of the fundus to detect early retinopathy.[3,4]

Although older studies had suggested that retinopathy was uncommon before 10 years' duration of type 1 diabetes mellitus, new studies indicate that >50% of patients develop retinopathy within that time. A large population study indicated that more

**TABLE 151-1.**
**Abbreviations Used to Describe Diabetic Retinopathy and Its Study**

| OPHTHALMOLOGIC TERMS | |
| --- | --- |
| BDR | Background diabetic retinopathy |
| DR | Diabetic retinopathy |
| HMA | Hemorrhages and microaneurysms |
| HRC | High-risk characteristics |
| Type 1 | Insulin-dependent diabetes mellitus |
| ILM | Internal limiting membrane |
| IRMA | Intraretinal microvascular abnormalities |
| Type 2 | Non–insulin-dependent diabetes mellitus |
| NPDR | Nonproliferative diabetic retinopathy |
| NVD | New blood vessels on the optic disc |
| NVE | New blood vessels elsewhere |
| PDR | Proliferative diabetic retinopathy |
| PPDR | Preproliferative diabetic retinopathy |
| TDR | Transitional diabetic retinopathy |
| **EPIDEMIOLOGIC AND PATHOPHYSIOLOGIC STUDIES** | |
| DCCT | Diabetes Control and Complications Trial |
| DRS | Diabetic Retinopathy Study |
| DRVS | Diabetic Retinopathy Vitrectomy Study |
| ETDRS | Early Treatment Diabetic Retinopathy Study |

**TABLE 151-2.**
**Classification of Diabetic Retinopathy**

| Nonproliferative | | | Proliferative |
|---|---|---|---|
| *Background* | *Transitional* | *Preproliferative* | |
| Microaneurysm alone or with occasional blotch hemorrhage or fleck of hard exudate | Significant blotch hemorrhages (STD2A) or intraretinal microvascular abnormalities (IRMAs) or soft exudates or venous abnormalities | Three or more of the transitional lesions present in multiple fields or large amounts of any one lesion in the presence of others | New blood vessels on the optic disc (NVD); new blood vessels elsewhere (NVE); fibrous proliferation; preretinal hemorrhage; vitreous hemorrhage |

than 60% of patients showed retinopathy by 10 years, and the prevalence approached 100% after 15 years.[5] This investigation also identified proliferative diabetic retinopathy (PDR), the most sight-threatening type, in 40% to 60% of patients who had had diabetes for 20 years or more. This high prevalence had been suggested 20 years earlier, but the figure was at variance with the findings of other research of the time.[6] In a study of patients with type 1 diabetes who were followed from the onset of their diabetes, a 60% cumulative incidence of PDR was found by 40 years.[7]

In type 1 disease, background diabetic retinopathy (BDR) commonly develops after 5 years of diabetes and is ubiquitous by 15 to 20 years. PDR is uncommon in disease of <10 years' duration, develops during the second decade of the disease, and becomes very common after 20 years. Very young patients are relatively immune from developing significant eye disease until after puberty.

Data on older patients (who have primarily type 2 or non–insulin-dependent diabetes mellitus) show two major differences: retinopathy is present in ~20% of patients at the onset of diabetes, probably reflecting the uncertainty in dating the actual onset, and the percentage of patients developing any retinopathy or PDR is lower (i.e., 60–80% develop retinopathy; 10–20% develop PDR).[8] Patients who are older at disease onset who do develop PDR do so after shorter durations of diabetes than do their younger cohorts.[9]

### DETERMINANTS

Many risk factors for diabetic retinopathy have been noted, but the evidence for most of these is inconclusive. The duration of diabetes has been uniformly accepted as an important factor, but it may be a surrogate variable representing increasing exposure to one or more components of the diabetic syndrome. The most thoroughly investigated of these is the level of plasma glucose, and most studies have supported an association between lower plasma glucose levels and a lower incidence of retinopathy.[10–14a]

The largest and most definitive of these studies was the Diabetes Control and Complications Trial (DCCT), which randomly assigned 1441 Type 1 patients, who were 13 to 39 years of age, to either standard diabetes therapy or an intensive therapy aimed at keeping blood sugars as close to normal as possible. After an average of >6 years of follow-up, intensively treated patients who had no retinopathy at baseline showed a 27% reduction in the development of first microaneurysms and a 76% reduction in the occurrence of a sustained three-step change in retinopathy level from baseline. Among those who already had some retinopathy, intensively treated patients showed a 54% reduction in the sustained three-step end point and a 47% reduction in the development of PDR. The risks of worsening albuminuria and of neuropathy were also reduced.[15] This study established intensive therapy aimed at achieving near-normal glycemia as the treatment of choice in type 1 diabetes. Whether patients with type 2 diabetes would benefit similarly was not addressed by the DCCT, but many physicians in the diabetes community have drawn that conclusion.[16] The major adverse effects of intensive therapy were a three-fold increase in episodes of severe hypoglycemia and weight gain.

Other factors in addition to hyperglycemia probably influence retinopathy, the balance of which determines an individual's risk of developing severe retinopathy. Some factors are metabolic and are related to plasma glucose levels; others may be systemic but not necessarily diabetes specific; and yet others may be localized within the eye.[17] Evidence exists that HLA-associated factors may influence risk of retinopathy (see Chap. 194).

Hypertension has been suggested as an important predictor of retinopathy.[18,19] Because hypertension in these patients most often is associated with renal disease, it may be part of the diabetic syndrome.[20] Only ~50% of patients who develop PDR have or ultimately develop nephropathy. This group has hypertension and a high mortality (i.e., 60% 5-year survival). The other 50% are nonhypertensive and have almost normal long-term survival.[21] Hypertension may increase extravasation of intravascular fluid and large molecules, and an association with lipid deposits in the retina has been found. The balance between intravascular and extravascular (i.e., intraocular) pressure, however, may have the greatest influence on this process. Although cigarette smoking is not a major risk factor for retinopathy, it should be avoided[22] (see Chap. 234). Increased plasma homocysteine is a risk factor for retinal vascular occlusive disease.[22a]

After significant retinopathy develops, local factors within the eye related to the type and severity of retinopathy are the best predictors of long-term vision outcome.[23] The most important of these is the presence of *neovascularization on the optic disc (NVD)*, along with vitreous or preretinal hemorrhage, severe intraretinal hemorrhages and microaneurysms (HMA), and venous beading. Among systemic factors, only proteinuria is an important predictor of severe vision loss.

### CLASSIFICATION

Pathologists have divided *diabetic retinopathy* into two categories, *nonproliferative diabetic retinopathy* (NPDR) and *PDR*, based on the absence or presence of preretinal new blood vessels or other fibroproliferative tissue. Previously, the term BDR had been used synonymously with NPDR. A clinically useful classification scheme is shown in Table 151-2. NPDR is divided into three stages: *BDR*, now used in a more restricted way; *transitional diabetic retinopathy*; and *preproliferative diabetic retinopathy*.

#### NONPROLIFERATIVE DIABETIC RETINOPATHY

**Background Diabetic Retinopathy.**  BDR is the earliest ophthalmoscopically visible stage of retinopathy (Fig. 151-1) and includes the first microaneurysms, along with an occasional dot or blot hemorrhage or a hard exudate. Most diabetic patients develop this degree of retinopathy, and it is of limited prognostic importance unless it develops before puberty or after a very short duration of diabetes. It is the "noise" or "background" in the system.

Patients who develop these changes may not progress any further, at least not for many years. The lesions may come and go, probably explaining the small group of patients who have no apparent retinopathy despite long-duration diabetes. For an eye to have >10 microaneurysms without having at least one small intraretinal hemorrhage or fleck of exudate is unusual. However, an eye may have several dozen microaneurysms

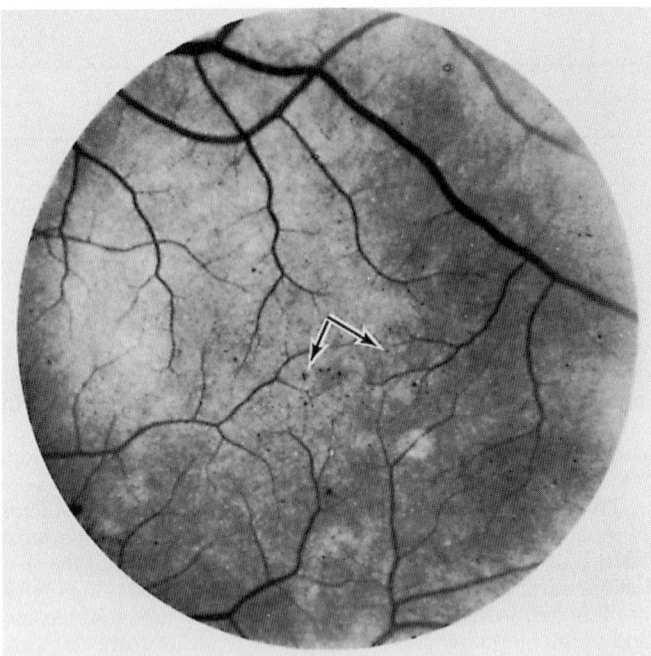

**FIGURE 151-1.** Scattered microaneurysms (*arrows*) and occasional blotch hemorrhages in background diabetic retinopathy. These are more apparent on this black and white photograph than they would be in the fundus (i.e., red against an orange background). (Courtesy of Fundus Photo Reading Center, Madison, WI.)

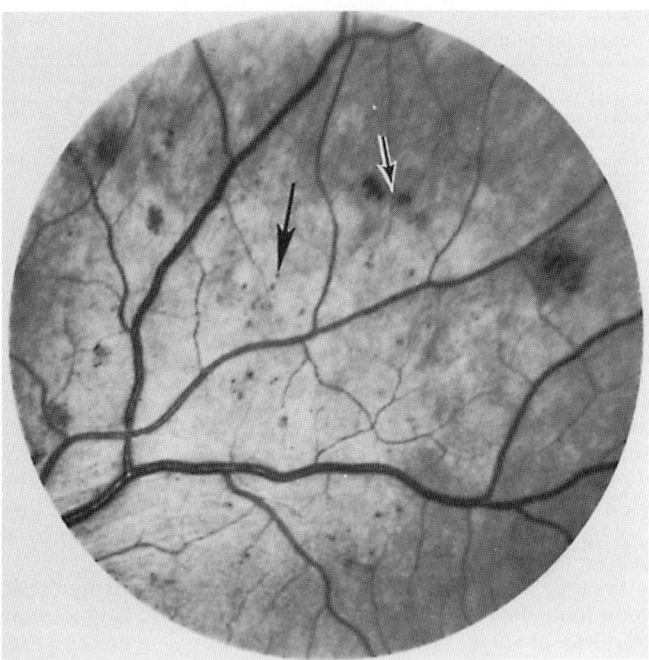

**FIGURE 151-2.** Diabetic Retinopathy Study Standard Photo 2A shows moderate hemorrhages (*thin arrow*) and microaneurysms (*thick arrow*). (Courtesy of Fundus Photo Reading Center, Madison, WI.)

without having any other lesions and still be considered to show BDR. This early stage of retinopathy is characterized pathophysiologically by predominantly intravascular and perivascular abnormalities: basement membrane thickening, pericyte loss, capillary dilation, and microaneurysm formation.[24,25] These processes antecede the first visibly detectable lesions and may be caused directly by the metabolic abnormalities of diabetes or secondarily by retinal hyperperfusion.[26]

**Transitional Diabetic Retinopathy.** The development of soft exudates (i.e., cotton wool spots), venous-caliber abnormalities, *intraretinal microvascular abnormalities* (IRMAs), or more extensive amounts of HMA moves an eye to a "transitional" stage of retinopathy[27] (Fig. 151-2). In these conditions, the pathologic processes extend from the capillary and its wall to involve larger blood vessels and areas of nonvascular neural retina. Soft exudates are infarcts in the nerve fiber layer of the retina; microscopically, they show swollen areas of axonal debris. These are the lesions that were reported to progress early in the course, after the rapid normalization of plasma glucose levels.

Hemorrhages are predominantly extravasated blood in the retinal substance; the various shapes are determined by the location of the blood: dot and blot, deep, flame-shaped, superficial lesions. IRMAs and venous abnormalities are caused by different responses to intraretinal vascular occlusive phenomena. IRMAs probably are dilated capillaries remaining in areas where parts of the capillary bed have closed down. The early-occurring venous abnormalities are localized irregularities in vessel caliber related to local hemodynamic factors. Some eyes may remain stable for many years and may even appear to revert to BDR as soft exudates resolve and blood resorbs. Other eyes rapidly progress to more advanced stages. Only regular follow-up, at 6-month intervals, can differentiate these groups.

**Preproliferative Diabetic Retinopathy.** The presence of large numbers and combinations of lesions advance the status of an eye to the preproliferative stage. Retinal ischemia progresses from being focal and limited to being the dominant process. Most of these eyes advance to PDR after several years and should be closely followed at 4-month intervals. Severely affected eyes in

this group show large areas of avascular retina along with severe venous beading and can develop severe NVD and hemorrhage and loss of vision in a few months. They are probably at greater risk for severe vision loss than eyes with mild PDR that have only small, nonelevated patches of *new vessels elsewhere*.

## PROLIFERATIVE DIABETIC RETINOPATHY

PDR is considered to be the most ominous stage of retinopathy. In the past, it was associated with vision loss. It is characterized by the growth of abnormal new blood vessels through the internal limiting membrane of the retina and onto the retinal surface. These vessels frequently attach to the posterior surface of the vitreous. When this gel liquefies and contracts, as it is prone to do in diabetics, the vessels are pulled forward toward the center of the eye. Tension is exerted along the attachments of these vessels to the retina and vitreous, and these fragile vessels bleed, causing various degrees of vision loss.

Not all PDR rapidly leads to blindness. Patches of new blood vessels >1 disc diameter from the optic disc that are <0.5 disc area in size and are not associated with vitreous or preretinal hemorrhage do not place the eye at great risk of severe vision loss (7% 2-year risk). These eyes may remain stable for many years without treatment, and in >10% of cases the condition actually may regress. When the patches become large and grow densely along an elevated posterior vitreous face, they can bleed and lead to retinal detachment and severe vision loss (25% 2-year risk).

NVDs are associated with the worst vision prognosis. New blood vessels frequently are located near the optic disc, partly because the internal limiting membrane is absent in this area, but also because it is the natural path of egress of substances from the eye, including a putative neovascular factor.[28,29] Hemodynamic factors may also contribute to the location of blood vessels on or near the optic disc. Small amounts of NVDs are associated with a 10% 2-year risk of severe vision loss unless vitreous or preretinal hemorrhage is present, in which case the risk increases to 26%. When NVDs alone cover one-third or more of the surface of the disc (Fig. 151-3), they are also associated with a 26% 2-year risk of severe vision loss. NVDs of this extent associated with vitreous or preretinal hemorrhages carry a 37% 2-year risk of severe vision loss.

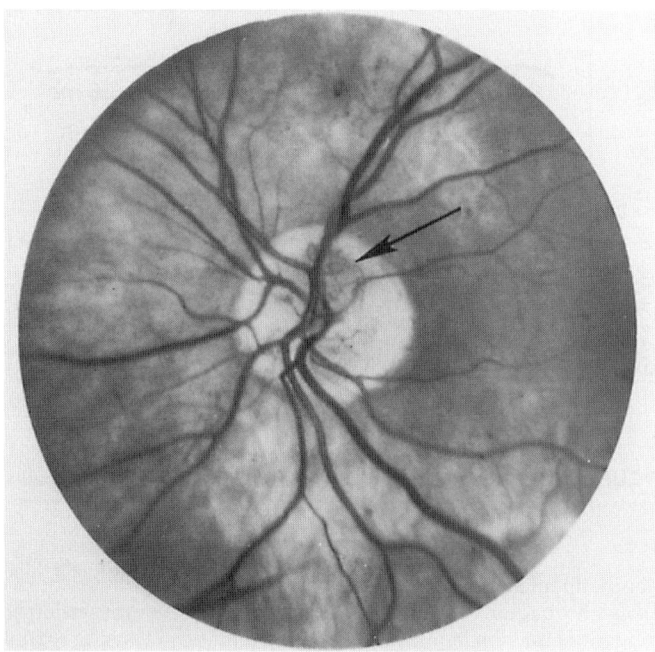

**FIGURE 151-3.** Diabetic Retinopathy Study Standard Photo 10A shows moderate neovascularization of the optic disc (*arrow*). The extent of new vessel formation often causes severe vision loss. (Courtesy of Fundus Photo Reading Center, Madison, WI.)

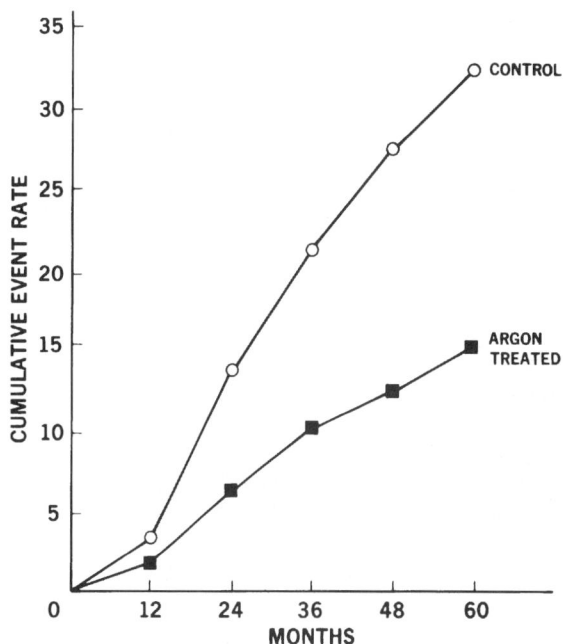

**FIGURE 151-4.** Cumulative event rates of severe vision loss (acuity <5/200 at two consecutive visits 4 months apart). Data are shown for panretinal argon laser treatment.

Those characteristics of PDR that carry a 25% or greater 2-year risk of severe vision loss have been designated as *high-risk characteristics* and mandate immediate consideration of panretinal photocoagulation.[30,31] Eyes with high-risk characteristics and eyes with significant areas of retinal ischemia are at risk of developing *rubeosis iridis* and *neovascular glaucoma.* In rubeosis, new blood vessels develop on the surface of the iris, frequently starting at the pupillary margin. These must be differentiated from dilated capillaries on the sphincter, referred to as microrubeosis, which are less ominous. Rubeosis can progress rapidly to cover large areas of the iris surface and, more importantly, to cover the filtration angle responsible for the egress of fluid from the eye. When this occurs, the eye is considered to have impending neovascular glaucoma. Immediate panretinal photocoagulation is indicated for these eyes, along with goniophotocoagulation (i.e., direct photocoagulation of blood vessels on the surface of the angle) as a stop-gap measure in some instances. After the filtration angle is closed, neovascular glaucoma develops, and the eye has an extremely poor vision prognosis.

### DIABETIC MACULOPATHY

Diabetic maculopathy, which encompasses the lesions of diabetic retinopathy (e.g., hemorrhages, microaneurysms, hard exudates, IRMAs) and is associated with retinal edema and its sequelae, is located in the macular region of the retina.[32] It is the major vision-threatening component of diabetic retinopathy. It may occur in any stage. It is most common and is the primary problem in patients with adult-onset diabetes. In these patients, most of the retina may be spared, aside from a thickening of the retina with edema and deposition of lipid rings and plaques in the outer retinal layers near the center of vision. In younger patients, the edema is associated more with areas of nonperfusion and diffuse capillary leakage and less with deposition of exudates. In these eyes, maculopathy is associated with proliferative disease. The 3-year risk of vision loss (i.e., doubling of minimum discriminable vision angle from an acuity of 20/20 to 20/40) in a large, heterogeneous group of maculopathy patients with good vision was 24%.[33]

*Optic disc edema* is accumulation of fluid around the optic nerve head, which frequently is asymptomatic. It is usually unilateral and may be detected on a routine ophthalmoscopic examination. It appears as a congested and swollen nerve head and must be differentiated from papilledema, NVD, and ischemic optic neuropathy. Visual acuity is normal or only slightly decreased. The blind spot is enlarged without characteristic visual field defects. Laboratory workup and neurologic evaluation to rule out other causes of a congested optic nerve are negative. The edema resolves spontaneously over several months, but these eyes must be watched closely for the development of NVD.

Most eyes with diabetic retinopathy go into remission. In patients who never develop severe changes, it may appear as if no retinopathy were ever present. Macular edema dries up, leaving a mottled pigment epithelium, and new blood vessels shrink and are replaced by fibrous tissue. This fibrous tissue can lead to further vision problems if it exerts traction on the retina. Anteroposterior traction can lead to traction retinal detachment, and tangential traction can lead to retinal wrinkling. Remission often comes too late, and many eyes are left quiescent but with poor vision function. The condition of these eyes, with pale optic nerve heads, wispy fibrous strands, and attenuated retinal vessels, has been called *involutional diabetic retinopathy.* With panretinal photocoagulation and vitrectomy, vision function can be preserved or restored in many cases.

### MANAGEMENT

#### PHOTOCOAGULATION

Photocoagulation refers to the use of light to destroy tissue. In diabetes, the tissue being destroyed is the retina, and the modalities used are xenon arc white light and argon or krypton laser. Both xenon arc and argon laser panretinal photocoagulation were proven effective in treating PDR by the Diabetic Retinopathy Study (DRS) (Fig. 151-4). A 60% reduction in severe vision loss (i.e., vision <5/200 at two consecutive visits) in treated eyes was documented at 2 years and was maintained at

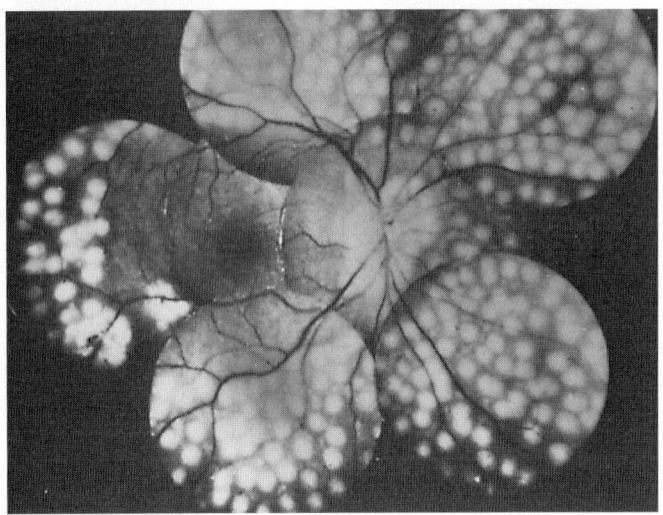

**FIGURE 151-5.** Retina at 24 hours after argon laser panretinal photocoagulation for a patient in the Diabetic Retinopathy Study. (Courtesy of Fundus Photo Reading Center, Madison, WI.)

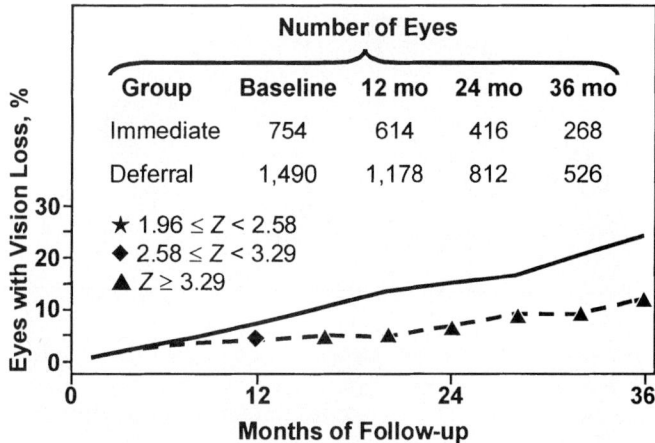

| | Number of Eyes | | | |
|---|---|---|---|---|
| Group | Baseline | 12 mo | 24 mo | 36 mo |
| Immediate | 754 | 614 | 416 | 268 |
| Deferral | 1,490 | 1,178 | 812 | 526 |

★ $1.96 \leq Z < 2.58$
◆ $2.58 \leq Z < 3.29$
▲ $Z \geq 3.29$

**FIGURE 151-6.** Results of the Early Treatment Diabetic Retinopathy Study show a 50% reduction in vision loss (from 24% to 12%) at 3 years.

5 years. In most modern treatments, an argon laser is used, primarily because of its ease of application and low incidence of side effects. The krypton laser, a new red laser that penetrates blood, has been used to treat eyes when adequate argon photocoagulation is not possible because of vitreous hemorrhage or other opacities. It should not be substituted routinely for argon laser in clear-media cases, because its use is more painful.

Photocoagulation is routinely applied to eyes with high-risk characteristics. In these eyes, the DRS study showed that the 2-year risk of severe vision loss was reduced from 24% to 12%. Treatment consists of the application of 1200 to 2000 or more 500-μm burns placed 0.5 burn diameters apart, avoiding the macula, papillomacular bundle, optic disc, and major vessels and extending out to the equator (Fig. 151-5). The application of only 100 to 200 burns is not panretinal photocoagulation; it probably is not effective and should not be considered acceptable therapy unless extenuating circumstances are present. Treatment is usually applied in two to four sessions and may require retrobulbar anesthesia. Eyes with less severe proliferative retinopathy than those showing high-risk characteristics frequently are treated, but the 5-year risk of severe vision loss is 3.7% in these eyes. Early treatment reduces the risk to 2.6%.[31]

Focal treatment of macular edema has been proven effective by the Early Treatment Diabetic Retinopathy Study (ETDRS) (Fig. 151-6). The 3-year rate of doubling of the minimum discriminable vision angle was reduced from 24% to 12%.[34,35] Treatment involves considerably fewer burn applications than panretinal photocoagulation, perhaps only 5 or 10, most commonly 50 to 200, and in rare cases as many as 500. Burns are smaller (50–100 μm), more focused, and confined to the macular region. They are aimed at focal leakage points seen on a fluorescein angiogram or are delivered in a grid-like pattern to areas of diffuse leakage or capillary nonperfusion.[36] The treatable lesions are those which the ETDRS has decided warrant photocoagulation if clinically significant macular edema is present. They include discrete points of retinal hyperfluorescence or leakage (most are microaneurysms), areas of diffuse leakage within the retina (e.g., microaneurysms, intraretinal microvascular abnormalities, diffusely leaking retinal capillary bed), and retinal avascular zones.

### VITRECTOMY

When photocoagulation fails to stem the course of retinopathy, and recurrent vitreous hemorrhage or a traction detachment of the macula develops, vitrectomy surgery may become necessary.[37] Surgery is rarely performed unless hemorrhage has been present for several months or detachment involves or immi-

nently threatens the fovea. The goals of vitrectomy surgery are to clear an opaque vitreous and to release any anteroposterior or tangential traction being exerted on the retina and causing retinal detachment or distortion. The lens often must be removed during surgery, but this increases the risk of postoperative neovascular glaucoma and is done only when lens opacities interfere with the surgeon's ability to perform an adequate vitrectomy.[38]

The Diabetic Retinopathy Vitrectomy Study group has shown that performing early vitrectomy for nonclearing vitreous hemorrhage is preferable to waiting a year or more, particularly in patients with juvenile-onset diabetes.[39] The study group also reported benefit from vitrectomy in some eyes before hemorrhage or detachment occurs.[40]

Numerous instruments are available to perform the surgery, each with its own advantage. It is difficult surgery, and results are not uniformly good. With the increasing use of timely photocoagulation, vitrectomy is being performed on fewer diabetic eyes than 5 years ago.

### GUIDELINES FOR FOLLOW-UP

Diabetic patients should have regular eye examinations for diabetic retinopathy. Yearly examinations should begin after 5 years in patients with juvenile-onset type 1 diabetes and at the onset of diabetes in patients with the adult-onset type. Examinations should be through a dilated pupil or a nonmydriatic fundus camera should be used for screening people without known disease. After significant retinopathy develops, an ophthalmologist should examine the eyes every 4 to 6 months.[41] Following these simple guidelines enables timely treatment of patients with retinopathy and markedly reduces the development of vision loss in diabetic patients.

## OTHER EYE DISORDERS IN DIABETES

### DIABETIC CATARACT

Opacification of the crystalline lens or cataract is an important ocular manifestation of diabetes.[42] Three types of cataracts have been documented: the metabolic or "snowflake" cataract, the senile cataract, and secondary cataract or cataract "complicata."[43]

*Metabolic cataracts* are seen primarily in young diabetic patients with uncontrolled diabetes.[44] The snowflake appellation derives from their flocculent appearance, which starts in the subcapsular regions of the lens. They may progress rapidly, and rarely, total opacification of the lens can occur over a period of days, resulting in a mature cataract. The institution of adequate diabetic control stops or reverses these lens opacities if they are discovered in their incipient stages. Metabolic cataract develops in most animal models of diabetes.

Investigation of this cataract led to the discovery of the sorbitol pathway, an alternative route for glucose metabolism requiring the enzyme aldose reductase, in which sorbitol, a sugar alcohol, is the by-product (see Chap. 148). Inhibition of sorbitol production by the use of an aldose reductase inhibitor prevents the development of cataract in experimental animals with diabetes or galactosemia. The possible role of sugar alcohol accumulation as an underlying factor in other diabetic complications, such as neuropathy and retinopathy, has received much attention. Aldose reductase inhibitors are under investigation, but their clinical efficacy is still uncertain.[45] Hyperlipidemia may favor the onset of metabolic cataracts.[46]

*Senile cataract* is the most common form of cataract seen in diabetic patients, and it cannot be differentiated from the senile cataract seen in nondiabetic individuals. However, the senile changes of nuclear sclerosis and cortical and subcapsular opacification develop at an earlier age in diabetic patients than in nondiabetic persons: they are found in 59% of diabetic patients with adult-onset diabetes who are between 35 and 54 years of age, compared with 12% in nondiabetic patients of similar age.[42] These cataracts may progress to a vision-impairing level more rapidly, necessitating cataract extraction.

*Cataract complicata,* which is associated with other ocular diseases such as iridocyclitis, chorioretinitis, high myopia, or retinal detachment, was seen in 6% of a large group of diabetic patients, a rate that is not significantly different from the rate among nondiabetic individuals.[43]

The indications for cataract surgery and intraocular lens (IOL) insertion have changed over time. Initially, the insertion of IOLs was not recommended in diabetic patients, particularly in cases complicated by retinopathy. This was because of poor visibility of the fundus, with iris clip and anterior chamber lenses precluding good laser treatment. With the development of posterior chamber lenses and yttrium-aluminum-garnet (YAG) laser capsulotomy, however, these problems were overcome, and diabetic patients, even those with significant retinopathy, can benefit from this revolutionary advance in vision rehabilitation after cataract surgery. Nevertheless, the vision outcome is not as good in diabetic patients as in nondiabetic patients, primarily because of worsening maculopathy after surgery, particularly after YAG laser capsulotomy. Although the visual acuities usually improve postoperatively, the criteria for surgery probably should be more stringent for diabetic patients than for nondiabetic patients. Laser treatment of all leaking microaneurysms in or near the macula should be performed before surgery, if possible. The incidence of rubeosis iridis and neovascular glaucoma in these eyes after cataract extraction is significant.[44]

## DIABETIC OPHTHALMOPLEGIA

Paralysis of ocular movement due to cranial nerve palsies is an uncommon (0.4% of cases) but dramatic complication of diabetes.[47] The third nerve is most commonly affected, followed by the sixth nerve. Infrequently, the fourth nerve may be involved alone or in combination with one of the other nerves. Usually, the presenting complaint is diplopia; it may be associated with ipsilateral headache or eye pain, which can precede the onset of diplopia. Bilateral nerve palsies are not rare. Multiple simultaneous cranial neuropathies may occur.[48]

Complete recovery of function usually occurs in 1 to 9 months. The condition may recur, but aberrant regeneration of the nerve is not seen. Particularly important in third-nerve palsies of diabetic origin is the sparing of the pupillary fibers; this sparing differentiates these palsies from those due to intracranial aneurysms and tumors, which affect the pupil in 80% to 90% of patients. Nevertheless, the occurrence of ocular palsies in a diabetic patient should prompt a thorough medical and neurologic evaluation, because 42% of palsies seen in diabetic patients in one study series were of

nondiabetic origin.[47] Other diagnoses to consider include myasthenia gravis, Graves disease, herpes zoster, demyelinating disease, primary and metastatic brain tumors, and hypoglycemia.

The treatment of ophthalmoplegia is symptomatic and is aimed at relieving the diplopia. It usually consists of temporary occlusion of one eye and administration of a mild analgesic, if needed. Severe pain is not characteristic, and the need for strong analgesics may indicate an intracranial aneurysm.

## GLAUCOMA

Primary open-angle glaucoma is more common among individuals with diabetes (4.0%) than it is among those without this disease (1.8%). Moreover, diabetes is more common among glaucoma patients (4–18%) than in the general population (2%).[49] Glaucoma (i.e., elevated intraocular pressure) has been proposed to protect an eye from developing severe diabetic retinopathy, based on studies of patients with diabetes and unilateral glaucoma, however, this is controversial.[50] Because the intraocular pressure is the main component of tissue pressure in the eye and retinal venous pressure usually just barely exceeds intraocular pressure, alterations in the regulation of intraocular pressure and its relationship with vascular resistance may play roles in the pathogenesis of diabetic retinopathy.

The treatment of open-angle glaucoma in diabetic patients must be influenced by their general medical conditions. Some caution must be exercised in the use of topical β-blockers, which can mask hypoglycemic symptoms or affect frequently coexistent cardiovascular disease. Application of punctal pressure after instillation of drops can reduce the systemic effects of these medications. Acetazolamide (Diamox) or other carbonic anhydrase inhibitors may be used if needed, but because they can cause a metabolic acidosis, more frequent electrolyte monitoring is required. Renal disease may influence how these and other pressure-lowering drugs may be used, and close cooperation between the ophthalmologist and internist is important.

## REFERENCES

1. Kahn HA, Hiller R. Blindness caused by diabetic retinopathy. Am J Ophthalmol 1974; 78:58.
2. Caird FI, Pirie A, Ramsell TG. Diabetes and the eye. Oxford: Blackwell Scientific Publications, 1969.
3. Rand LI. Recent advances in diabetic retinopathy. Am J Med 1981; 70:595.
4. Krolewski AS, Warram JH, Rand LI, Kahn CR. Epidemiologic approach to the etiology of type I diabetes mellitus and its complications. N Engl J Med 1987; 317:22.
5. Klein R, Klein BEK, Moss SE, et al. The Wisconsin epidemiologic study of diabetic retinopathy. II. Prevalence and risk of diabetic retinopathy when age at diagnosis is less than 30 years. Arch Ophthalmol 1984; 102:520.
6. White P. Childhood diabetes. Diabetes 1960; 9:345.
7. Krolewski AS, Warram JH, Rand LI, et al. Risk of proliferative diabetic retinopathy in juvenile-onset type I diabetes—a 40-year follow-up study. Diabetes Care 1986; 9:443.
8. Klein R, Klein BEK, Moss SE, et al. The Wisconsin epidemiologic study of diabetic retinopathy. III. Prevalence and risk of diabetic retinopathy when age at diagnosis is 30 or more years. Arch Ophthalmol 1984; 102:527.
9. Aiello LM, Rand LI, Briones JC, et al. Diabetic retinopathy in Joslin Clinic patients with adult-onset diabetes. Ophthalmology 1981; 88:619.
10. Knowles HC Jr. The control of diabetes mellitus and the progression of retinopathy. In: Goldberg MF, Fine SL, eds. Treatment of diabetic retinopathy. Warrenton, VA: Airlie House, 1968:115.
11. Canny CLB, Kohner EM, Trautman J, et al. Comparison of stereo fundus photographs for patients with insulin-dependent diabetes during conventional insulin treatment or continuous subcutaneous insulin infusion. Diabetes 1985; 34(Suppl):50.
12. Lauritzen T, Frost-Larsen K, Laresen HW, et al. Effect of 1 year of near-normal blood glucose levels on retinopathy in insulin-dependent diabetics. Lancet 1983; 1:200.
13. Dahl-Jorgensen K, Hanssen KF, Brinchmann-Hansen O, et al. Near-normoglycemia retards the progression of early retinopathy and neuropathy in IDDM. Three year results from the Oslo Study. Diabetes 1986; 35:41A.
14. Ramsay RC, Goetz FC, Sutherland DER, et al. Progression of diabetic retinopathy after pancreas transplantation for insulin-dependent diabetes mellitus. N Engl J Med 1988; 318:208.

14a. Roy MS. Diabetic retinopathy in African Americans with type 1 diabetes: the New Jersey 725. II. Risk factors. Arch Ophthalmal 2000; 118:105.

15. The Diabetes Control and Complications Trial Research Group. The effect of intensive treatment of diabetes on the development and progression of long-term complications in insulin-dependent diabetes mellitus. N Engl J Med 1993; 329:977.

16. Effects of intensive diabetes treatment on development and progression of long-term complication in adolescents with insulin dependent diabetes mellitus: Diabetes Control and Complications Trial. The Diabetes Control Complications Trial Research Group. J Pediatr 1994; 125:177.

17. Rand LI, Krolewski AS, Aiello LM, et al. Multiple factors in the prediction of risk of proliferative diabetic retinopathy. N Engl J Med 1985; 313:1433.

18. Knowler WC, Bennett PH, Ballintine EJ. Increased incidence of diabetic retinopathy with elevated blood pressure. N Engl J Med 1980; 302:645.

19. Janka HU, Warram JH, Rand LI, Krolewski AS. Risk factors for progression of background retinopathy in long-standing IDDM. Diabetes 1989; 38:460.

20. Krolewski AS, Canessa M, Warram JH, et al. Predisposition to hypertension and susceptibility to renal disease in insulin-dependent diabetes mellitus. N Engl J Med 1988; 318:140.

21. Rand LI, Krolewski AS, Warram JH. Late complications: the critical period. In: Friedman EA, L'Esperance FA Jr, eds. Diabetes renal-retinal syndrome. Prevention and management. New York: Grune & Stratton, 1985:297.

22. Christiansen JS. Cigarette smoking and prevalence of microangiopathy in juvenile-onset insulin-dependent diabetes mellitus. Diabetes Care 1978; 1:146.

22a. Cahill M, Karabatzaki M, Meleady R, et al. Raised plasma homocysteine as a risk factor for retinal vascular occlusive disease. Br J Ophthalmol 2000; 84:154.

23. Rand LI, Prud'homme JG, Ederer F, et al. Factors influencing the development of visual loss in advanced diabetic retinopathy. Diabetic Retinopathy Study report no. 10. Invest Ophthalmol 1985; 26:983.

24. Cogan DG, Kuwabara T. The Mural cell in perspective. Arch Ophthalmol 1967; 78:133.

25. Ashton N. Vascular basement membrane changes in diabetic retinopathy. Br J Ophthalmol 1974; 58:344.

26. Soeldner JS, Christacopoulos PD, Gleason RE. Mean retinal circulation time as determined by fluorescein angiography in normal, prediabetic, and chemical diabetic subjects. Diabetes 1976; 25:903.

27. The Diabetic Retinopathy Study Research Group. A modification of the Airlie House Classification of Diabetic Retinopathy. Diabetic Retinopathy Study (DRS) report no. 7. Invest Ophthalmol 1981; 21:210.

28. D'Amore P, Thompson RW. Mechanisms of angiogenesis. Annu Rev Physiol 1987; 49:453.

29. Aiello LP, Avery RL, Arrigg PG, et al. Vascular endothelial growth factors in ocular fluid of patients with diabetic retinopathy and other retinal disorders. N Engl J Med 1994; 331:1480.

30. The Diabetic Retinopathy Study Research Group. Four risk factors for severe visual loss in diabetic retinopathy. The third report from the Diabetic Retinopathy Group. Arch Ophthalmol 1979; 97:654.

31. The Diabetic Retinopathy Study Research Group. Preliminary report on effects of photocoagulation therapy. Am J Ophthalmol 1976; 81:1.

32. Barrie T. Progress in diabetic maculopathy. Br J Ophthalmol 1999; 83:3.

33. Early Treatment Diabetic Retinopathy Study Research Group. Photocoagulation for diabetic macular edema. Early Treatment Diabetic Retinopathy Study report no. 1. Arch Ophthalmol 1985; 103:1796.

34. Early Treatment Diabetic Retinopathy Study Research Group. Early photocoagulation for diabetic retinopathy. ETDRS report number 9. Ophthalmology 1991; 98(Suppl):766.

35. Fong DS, Ferris FL 3rd, Davis MD, Chew EY. Causes of severe visual loss in the early treatment diabetic retinopathy study: ETDRS report no. 24. Early Treatment Diabetic Retinopathy Study Research Group. Am J Ophthalmol 1999; 127:137.

36. Rand LI, Davis MD, Hubbard LD, et al. Color photography vs. fluorescein angiography in the detection of diabetic retinopathy in the Diabetes Control and Complications Trial. Arch Ophthalmol 1987; 105:1344.

37. Arrigg PG, Cavallerano J. The role of vitrectomy for diabetic retinopathy. J Am Optom Assoc 1998; 69:733.

38. Rice TA, Michels RG, Maguire MG, Rice EF. The effect of lensectomy on the incidence of iris neovascularization and neovascular glaucoma after vitrectomy for diabetic retinopathy. Am J Ophthalmol 1983; 95:1.

39. The Diabetic Retinopathy Vitrectomy Study Research Group. Early vitrectomy for severe vitreous hemorrhage in diabetic retinopathy. Two-year results of a randomized trial. Diabetic Retinopathy Vitrectomy Study report no. 2. Arch Ophthalmol 1985; 103:1644.

40. The Diabetic Retinopathy Vitrectomy Study Research Group. Early vitrectomy for severe proliferative diabetic retinopathy in eyes with useful vision. Clinical application of results of a randomized trial. Diabetic Retinopathy Vitrectomy Study report no. 4. Ophthalmology 1988; 95:1321.

41. Grunwald JE, Riva CE, Sinclair SH, et al. Laser Doppler velocimetry study of the retinal circulation in diabetes mellitus. Arch Ophthalmol 1986; 104:991.

42. Klein BEK, Klein R, Moss S. Prevalence of cataracts in a population based study of persons with diabetes mellitus. Ophthalmology 1985; 92:1191.

43. Waite JH, Beetham WP. Visual mechanism in diabetes mellitus. Comparative study of 2002 diabetics and 457 non-diabetics for control. N Engl J Med 1935; 212:367.

44. Aiello LM, Rand LI, Weiss JN, et al. The eyes and diabetes. In: Marble A, Krall L, Bradley RF, et al., eds. Joslin's diabetes mellitus, 12th ed. Philadelphia: Lea & Febiger, 1985:600.

45. Costantino L, Rastell G, Vianello P, et al. Diabetes complications and their

46. Tsutsumi K, Inoue Y, Yeshida C. Acceleration of development of diabetic cataract by hyperlipidemia and low high-density lipoprotein in rats. Biol Pharm Bull 1999; 22:37.

47. Zorrilla C, Kozak GP. Ophthalmoplegia in diabetes mellitus. Ann Intern Med 1967; 67:968.

48. Eshbaugh CG, Siatkowski RM, Smith JL, Kline LB. Simultaneous, multiple cranial neuropathies in diabetes mellitus. J Neuroophthalmol 1995; 15:219.

49. Armstrong JR, Daily RK, Dobson HL, Gerard LJ. The incidence of glaucoma in diabetes mellitus. A comparison with the incidence in the general population. Am J Ophthalmol 1960; 50:55.

50. McKay R, McCarty CA, Taylor HR. Diabetic retinopathy in Victoria, Australia: the Visual Impairment Project. Br J Opthalmol 2000; 84:865.

potential prevention: aldose reductase inhibition and other approaches. Med Res Rev 1999; 19:3.

# CHAPTER 152

# DIABETES AND INFECTION

GEORGE M. ELIOPOULOS

Previously, infection was a major cause of death in patients with diabetes mellitus. Thus, considerable attention has been focused on the impact of various infections in diabetic patients.[1,1a] With the development of effective antibiotics and the recognition of the importance of glucose regulation, uncontrolled sepsis has become an uncommon primary cause of mortality in diabetes.[2] Nevertheless, infection is still responsible for serious morbidity in this disease. Diabetic patients do appear to be predisposed to certain infections; some infections occur almost exclusively in diabetic individuals or in immunocompromised patients (e.g., malignant external otitis, rhinocerebral mucormycosis); some occur predominantly in patients with diabetes mellitus (e.g., emphysematous cystitis, emphysematous pyelonephritis, emphysematous cholecystitis, acute necrotizing fasciitis); and some are increased in incidence in diabetic patients (e.g., tuberculosis, urinary tract infection [in women], gram-negative pneumonia). Once established, many infections are tolerated poorly in this population, and the stress of infection often complicates glucose control.

Although great strides have been made against diseases such as tuberculosis, which had affected diabetic patients disproportionately, medical progress actually has broadened the spectrum of infections encountered today. For example, treatment of end-stage diabetic nephropathy with hemodialysis, peritoneal dialysis, or renal transplantation subjects many diabetics to the infectious complications associated with these therapeutic modalities. Currently, optimal treatment regimens for other serious medical conditions (e.g., immunosuppressive agents, HIV protease inhibitors) may themselves precipitate diabetes mellitus.[3,4]

Usually, infections encountered in diabetic patients are not unique to this group. Although the clinician must be aware of the unusual disorders to which the diabetic patient is subject, perhaps even more important is familiarity with measures for the aggressive diagnosis and treatment of the more common infections that may manifest in an unusual manner or with greater severity in the patient with diabetes mellitus.

## HOST FACTORS PREDISPOSING TO INFECTION

### PRIMARY BARRIERS TO INFECTION

The integrity of the skin and mucosal defenses is the primary barrier to local or systemic infection. Breaks in the skin, whether they are minor fissures in dystrophic areas or frank ulcerations due to neuropathic trauma, provide an opportunity for bacterial invasion. Most common in the diabetic foot (see Chap. 154), such infections are increasingly encountered in the hands[5] and also arise in the perineum or elsewhere. Vascular punctures for hemodialysis and indwelling catheters for peritoneal dialysis obviously disrupt these natural barriers and pose a risk of infection. Patients with diabetes undergoing major cardiothoracic or abdominal surgery also appear to be at greater risk for postoperative wound infection,[6–9] which may be exacerbated by hyperglycemia in the immediate postoperative period.[7,9]

Factors that determine microbial colonization of skin and mucosal surfaces are poorly understood. Carriage rates of *Staphylococcus aureus* and pharyngeal colonization with gram-negative bacilli may be increased in diabetics.[10,11] Because colonization with a microorganism frequently precedes infection, these observations may explain the frequent occurrence of staphylococcal infections and the increased risk of gram-negative pneumonia in diabetics.[12,13]

## DEFENSES AGAINST MICROBIAL INVASION

### PHAGOCYTES

Evidence suggests that abnormalities in phagocytic cell function contribute to the susceptibility of diabetic patients to infection or to the increased severity of some infections. Reported defects include decrease of mobilization, chemotaxis, adherence, phagocytosis, and killing by polymorphonuclear leukocytes; also noted have been reductions in levels of leukotriene $B_4$, prostaglandin E, and thromboxane $B_2$.[14–21] In monocytes, phagocytosis is decreased.[22] Expression of monocyte carbohydrate-binding receptors (which would be expected to recognize components of bacterial cell walls) was reduced in patients recovering from ketoacidosis.[23]

Studies of phagocytosis of microbes by polymorphonuclear leukocytes give variable results, which may be due to methodologic factors or the particular organism examined. Phagocytosis of *Candida guilliermondii* by leukocytes obtained from diabetic patients is abnormal.[17] Both leukocytes and plasma in diabetic patients contribute to this defect, but neither blood glucose concentration nor levels of glycosylated hemoglobin correlate with functional abnormalities. Patients with type 2 diabetes mellitus were found to have polymorphonuclear leukocytes with impaired phagocytic activity (for lipopolysaccharide-coated oil droplets), elevated basal levels of cytosolic calcium, and reduced levels of adenosine triphosphate,[24] all of which improved after 3 months of treatment with glyburide. Defects in phagocytosis of staphylococci by polymorphonuclear leukocytes have also been reported in diabetes.

Impairment of microbial killing by leukocytes of diabetic patients has been documented more consistently. A detailed study of bactericidal activity against *S. aureus* found defective killing in patients with poorly controlled diabetes but not in patients with well-controlled type 1 diabetes.[18] However, increased levels of bactericidal activity occurred in leukocytes from nondiabetic patients with acute infections but not in leukocytes from acutely infected patients with well-controlled diabetes. Controlled insulin withdrawal, causing mild ketoacidosis, induced defective leukocyte killing, which was reversed by in vitro incubation of cells with insulin. Experimental evidence suggests that inhibition of aldose reductase mitigates reductions of superoxide production and intracellular killing by leukocytes from diabetic subjects when these cells are incubated in glucose in vitro.[25,26] Administration of an aldose reductase inhibitor to patients with diabetes also resulted in improved generation of oxygen-derived free radicals.[27] Diminished killing of bacteria by polymorphonuclear leukocytes from diabetic patients correlated with impairment of oxygen-dependent microbicidal systems; however, the direct relevance of these findings to the risk of infection in diabetes is not clear.[28]

Evidence for defective control of fungi by monocytes from diabetic patients is supported by animal studies.[22]

### LYMPHOCYTES

Defects in cell-mediated immunity have been described in diabetic patients, but malnutrition and chronic debilitation probably contribute to clinically significant abnormalities.[2] Impaired mitogenic response to phytohemagglutinin has been demonstrated inconsistently.[29,30] Abnormal responses to phytohemagglutinin and to staphylococcal lysate are not correlated with glucose levels.[29,30] Release of the lymphokine "migration inhibition factor" was abnormal in cells obtained from patients with maturity-onset diabetes and nonhyperglycemic obese individuals but not from ketosis-prone patients with well-controlled diabetes.[31] Defective responses correlated inversely with fasting insulin levels but not with levels of plasma glucose.

### ANTIBACTERIAL PROTEINS

The antibacterial proteins lactoferrin and lysozyme are inactivated by specific binding to glucose-modified serum and tissue proteins found in diabetic patients.[32] Impairment of the activity of these substances may increase the susceptibility of such patients to infection.

## BACTERIAL INFECTIONS

### STAPHYLOCOCCAL INFECTIONS

Infections due to *S. aureus* are common in patients with diabetes, but little evidence of increased risk is found. Early experience suggested a higher mortality rate in diabetics with staphylococcal bacteremia, particularly in patients with cardiovascular disease or ketoacidosis. A study in which diabetic and nondiabetic patients with bacteremia were stratified by severity of underlying illness, however, found no increase in mortality in the diabetic group.[33] Nevertheless, among patients with an identifiable source of infection, significantly more diabetic patients developed endocarditis. Patients with chronically infected foci (e.g., chronic foot ulcers) who become bacteremic with *S. aureus* probably represent a group at risk for infective endocarditis.[12]

### PNEUMONIA

Diabetic patients are not at significantly increased risk of developing pneumococcal pneumonia in the absence of complicating illness, but bacteremia is more likely and is associated with higher mortality.[13] Antibody response to pneumococcal polysaccharide vaccine is not impaired by diabetes, and the protective efficacy of pneumococcal vaccine has been demonstrated in diabetic patients.[34] Immunization rates remain low, however.[34a]

Pharyngeal colonization with gram-negative bacteria is more common in diabetic patients, and diabetes is a risk factor for the development of gram-negative pneumonia.[11,13]

### TUBERCULOSIS

Before the availability of effective antimycobacterial chemotherapy, tuberculosis was up to 16 times more common in diabetic than in nondiabetic patients.[2] Today, diabetes remains a risk factor for tuberculosis in the United States, as in other parts of the world.[35,36]

### MALIGNANT EXTERNAL OTITIS

Malignant external otitis due to *Pseudomonas aeruginosa* is an aggressive, locally invasive (hence "malignant") infection, which occurs almost exclusively in diabetics.[37] Infection begins in the external ear canal, where pain, purulent drainage, and granulations are characteristically present. Tenderness and swelling may extend to the pinna and periauricular tissues. Fever and leukocytosis are uncommon. Spread to deeper tissues causes osteomyelitis of the temporal bone and cranial neuropathies. Neurologic complications other than isolated facial nerve palsy adversely affect prognosis. In the past, treatment consisted of administration of an antipseudomonal penicillin plus an aminoglycoside for a minimum of 4 weeks. Both ceftazidime and ciprofloxacin have been used as single agents with high success rates in the treatment of this entity.[38–40] Radiologic demonstration of osteomyelitis may necessitate surgical debridement and an extended course of antibiotics in some patients (see Chap. 216).

## NECROTIZING SOFT TISSUE INFECTION

Necrotizing infections of the skin and soft tissues are fortunately rare, but frequently progress rapidly to cause death or serious morbidity.[41] Necrotizing fasciitis primarily involves the fascia and subcutaneous tissues. Originally described in connection with group A streptococci (i.e., streptococcal gangrene), necrotizing fasciitis may also arise as a synergistic process involving streptococci, gram-negative bacilli, and anaerobes. Twenty percent or more of cases occur in diabetic individuals. Commonly involving the leg or perineum, these infections develop after surgery or minor trauma, or they may spread from perianal infections. Systemic toxicity and pain are usually prominent, and gas may be present. The term *necrotizing cellulitis* is applied if the process extends to involve muscle. *Fournier gangrene* is a form of necrotizing fasciitis or cellulitis affecting the male genitalia and perineum; an analogous situation is seen in women with involvement of the vulva and perineum. Treatment requires wide surgical debridement and administration of antibiotics. In mixed infections, empiric therapy is directed against streptococci, Enterobacteriaceae, and anaerobes, including *Bacteroides fragilis*. Diabetes remains a risk factor for invasive group A streptococcal infections today.[42]

## URINARY TRACT INFECTION

Several studies have reported an increased incidence of bacteriuria in diabetic women.[43,43a] The frequency of asymptomatic bacteriuria is not significantly increased in diabetic schoolgirls, nor is urinary tract infection in males.[44,45] Emphysematous cystitis is an uncommon manifestation of bladder infection seen largely in diabetic patients (>50% of cases). Gas in the bladder wall is produced by bacterial fermentation. Gross hematuria occurs in approximately half of the cases. In most patients the infection responds to appropriate antibiotic therapy.[46]

Autopsy studies from the 1930s indicated that pyelonephritis was more common in diabetic patients than in the general population. Pyelonephritis may be complicated in rare cases by renal papillary necrosis, and the sloughed papillae may subsequently obstruct urine outflow. A rare, severe form of renal parenchymal infection, emphysematous pyelonephritis, occurs more frequently in diabetic patients (Fig. 152-1).[47] Gas is seen in the renal tissue, and the kidney may be completely destroyed. Infection is most often caused by *Escherichia coli* or *Klebsiella*. Failure to respond to appropriate antibiotic therapy may necessitate nephrectomy. Even after nephrectomy, mortality in these severely ill patients remains high. At least one-third of patients with perinephric abscesses have diabetes. The advent of computed tomography has facilitated delineation of such processes (Fig. 152-2).

Although the development of a neurogenic bladder is a frequent complication of diabetes, ascribing any increased tendency toward urinary infections to this condition has been difficult except as related to the need for instrumentation.[48] Additional factors such as nonneurogenic bladder outlet disorders probably contribute to the risk of infection. Animal studies suggest that osmotic diuresis, as seen in uncontrolled diabetes,

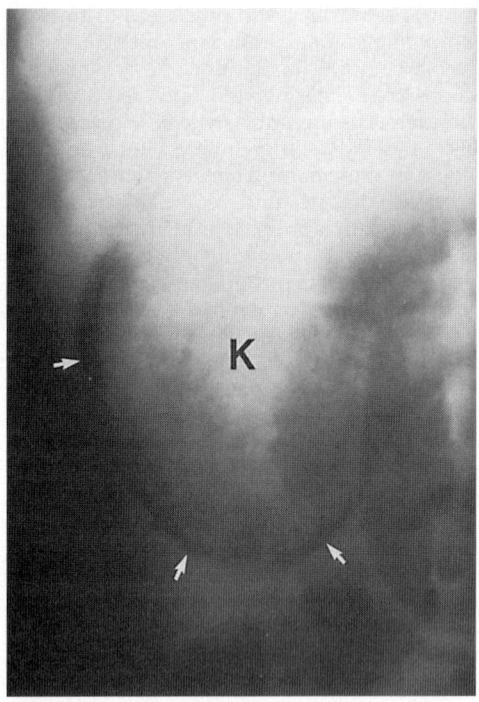

**FIGURE 152-1.** A middle-aged diabetic woman presented with fever and gross pyuria. A coned-down anteroposterior radiograph of the right kidney shows gas within the parenchyma of the kidney (*K*) and subcapsular gas (*arrows*). A nephrectomy was performed within 24 hours. The kidney was diffusely involved with multiple small, gas-filled microabscesses. (Courtesy of Dr. Michael Hill.)

predisposes to ascending infections, possibly because of vesicoureteral reflux or dilution of urinary bacteriostatic activity.[49]

## EMPHYSEMATOUS CHOLECYSTITIS

Diabetes is present in approximately one-third of cases of emphysematous cholecystitis, in which gas is found within the gallbladder lumen, gallbladder wall, or pericholecystic tissues.[50] Organisms recovered at surgery include streptococci, clostridia, and gram-negative bacilli. In contrast to the more common form of cholecystitis, this type of cholecystitis occurs more often in men, and gangrene of the gallbladder is more frequent.

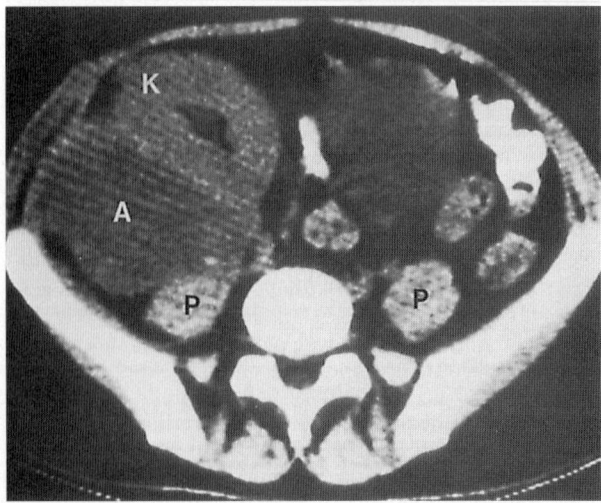

**FIGURE 152-2.** Computed tomographic demonstration of a perinephric abscess (*A*) arising from a transplanted kidney (*K*). (*P*, psoas muscle.)

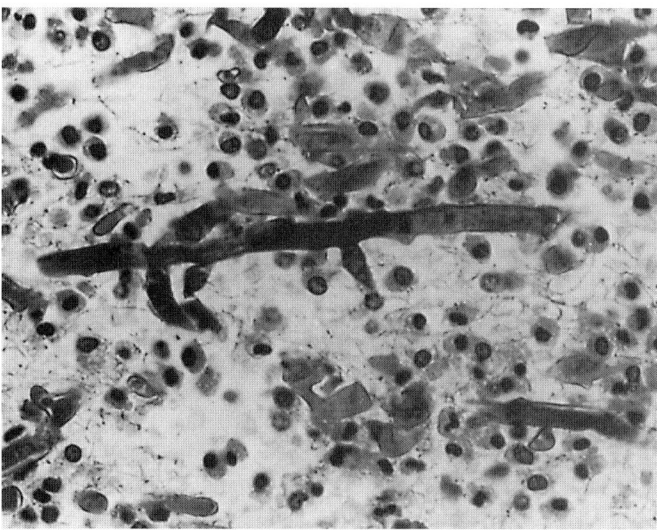

**FIGURE 152-3.** Broad, nonseptate hyphae with right-angle branching seen in mucormycosis.

## FUNGAL INFECTIONS

### RHINOCEREBRAL MUCORMYCOSIS

Diabetic ketoacidosis is a major predisposing factor in rhinocerebral mucormycosis, a rare infection caused by fungi of the order Mucorales (e.g., *Mucor, Rhizopus,* and *Absidia*).[51] The process begins on the palate or in the nasal passages, where a black eschar may be seen. Infection spreads to the paranasal sinuses, orbits, or brain. Necrosis is prominent because of blood vessel invasion. Fever, lethargy, headache, and facial swelling are often present. Orbital invasion causes proptosis, decreased ocular motion, and vision loss. Thrombosis of the venous sinuses or carotid system may occur. Diagnosis is made by biopsy of affected tissues. Broad, nonseptate hyphae that tend to branch at right angles are characteristic (Fig. 152-3).

Treatment requires prompt control of diabetes and correction of acidosis, aggressive surgical debridement of infected tissues, and the systemic administration of amphotericin B aggressively. Studies suggest that diabetic ketoacidosis induces a defect in the ability of macrophages to inhibit spore germination and impairs both leukocyte chemotaxis to fungal products and leukocyte-mediated hyphal injury. These organisms may also cause a fungal pneumonia in patients with diabetes mellitus, which is associated with high fatality rates.[13]

### FUNGAL URINARY TRACT INFECTION

Funguria with *Candida* species is common in diabetic patients, particularly with urethral catheterization, with the prior use of antibiotics, and in the presence of glucosuria.[52] Yeast infections may be asymptomatic or may produce symptoms that are indistinguishable from those of bacterial infection. Occasionally, such infections ascend to the renal parenchyma, cause ureteral obstruction, or disseminate hematogenously.[53] Systemic therapy is required with upper tract disease.[54] Candida may even cause emphysematous pyelonephritis.[51a]

## REFERENCES

1. Sentochnik DE, Eliopoulos GM. Infection and diabetes. In: Kahn CR, Weir GC, eds. Joslin's diabetes mellitus, 13th ed. Philadelphia: Lea & Febiger, 1994:867.
1a. Joshi N, Caputo GM, Weitekamp MR, Karchmer AW. Infections in patients with diabetes mellitus. N Engl J Med 1999; 341:1906.
2. Coopan R. Infection and diabetes. In: Marble A, Krall LP, Bradley RF, et al., eds. Joslin's diabetes mellitus, 12th ed. Philadelphia: Lea & Febiger, 1985:737.
3. Margarit C, Rimola A, Gonzalez-Pinto I, et al. Efficacy and safety of oral low-dose tacrolimus treatment in liver transplantation. Transpl Int 1998;11 Suppl 1:S260.
4. Walli R, Herfort O, Michl GM, et al. Treatment with protease inhibitors associated with peripheral insulin resistance and impaired oral glucose tolerance in HIV-1 infected patients. AIDS 1998; 12(15):F167.
5. Gunther SF, Gunther SB. Diabetic hand infections. Hand Clin 1998; 14(4):647.
6. Borger MA, Rao V, Weisel RD, et al. Deep sternal wound infection: risk factors and outcomes. Ann Thorac Surg 1998; 65(4):1050.
7. Pomposelli JJ, Baxter JK 3rd, Babineau TJ, et al. Early postoperative glucose control predicts nosocomial infection rate in diabetic patients. J Parenter Enteral Nutr 1998; 22(2):77.
8. Babineau TJ, Bothe A Jr. General surgery considerations in the diabetic patient. Infect Dis Clin North Am 1995; 9(1):183.
9. Zerr KJ, Furnary AP, Grunkemeier GL, et al. Glucose control lowers the risk of wound infection in diabetics after open heart operations. Ann Thorac Surg 1997; 63(2):356.
10. Chandler PI, Chandler SD. Pathogenic carrier rate in diabetes mellitus. Am J Med Sci 1977; 273:259.
11. Mackowiak PA, Martin RM, Jones SR, Smith JW. Pharyngeal colonization by gram-negative bacilli in aspiration-prone persons. Arch Intern Med 1978; 138:1224.
12. Breen JD, Karchmer AW. *Staphylococcus aureus* infections in diabetic patients. Infect Dis Clin North Am 1995; 9(1):11.
13. Koziel H, Koziel MJ. Pulmonary complications of diabetes mellitus. Infect Dis Clin North Am 1995; 9(1):65.
14. Brayton RG, Stokes PE, Schwartz MS, Louria DB. Effect of alcohol and various diseases on leukocyte mobilization, phagocytosis, and intracellular bacterial killing. N Engl J Med 1970; 282:123.
15. Molenaar DM, Palumbo PJ, Wilson WR, Ritts RE Jr. Leukocyte chemotaxis in diabetic patients and their non-diabetic first-degree relatives. Diabetes 1976; 25:880.
16. Bagdade JD, Stewart M, Walters E. Impaired granulocyte adherence: a reversible defect in host defense in patients with poorly controlled diabetes. Diabetes 1978; 27:677.
17. Davidson NJ, Sowden JM, Fletcher J. Defective phagocytosis in insulin controlled diabetics: evidence for a reaction between glucose and opsonising proteins. J Clin Pathol 1984; 37:783.
18. Repine JE, Clawson CC, Goetz FC. Bactericidal function of neutrophils from patients with acute bacterial infections and from diabetics. J Infect Dis 1980; 142:869.
19. Jubiz W, Draper RE, Gale J, Nolan G. Decreased leukotriene B$_4$ synthesis by polymorphonuclear leukocytes from male patients with diabetes mellitus. Prostaglandins Leukot Med 1984; 14:305.
20. Qvist R, Larkins RG. Diminished production of thromboxane B$_2$ and prostaglandin E by stimulated polymorphonuclear leukocytes from insulin-treated subjects. Diabetes 1983; 32:622.
21. Delamaire M, Maugendre D, Moreno M, et al. Impaired leucocyte functions in diabetic patients. Diabet Med 1997; 14(1):29.
22. Geisler C, Almdal T, Bennedsen J, et al. Monocyte functions in diabetes mellitus. Acta Pathol Microbiol Immunol Scand 1982; 90:33.
23. Stewart J, Collier A, Patrick AW, et al. Alterations in monocyte receptor function in type 1 diabetic patients with ketoacidosis. Diabetic Med 1991; 8:213.
24. Alexiewicz JM, Kumar D, Smogorzewski M, et al. Polymorphonuclear leukocytes in non-insulin dependent diabetes mellitus: abnormalities in metabolism and function. Ann Intern Med 1995; 123:919.
25. Tebbs SE, Lumbwe CM, Tesfaye S, et al. The influence of aldose reductase on the oxidative burst in diabetic neutrophils. Diabetes Res Clin Pract 1992; 15:121.
26. Tebbs SE, Gonzales AM, Wilson RM, et al. The role of aldose reductase inhibition in diabetic neutrophil phagocytosis and killing. Clin Exp Immunol 1991; 84:482.
27. Sato N, Kashima K, Uehara Y, et al. Epalrestat, an aldose reductase inhibitor, improves an impaired generation of oxygen-derived free radicals by neutrophils from poorly controlled NIDDM patients. Diabetes Care 1997; 20(6):995.
28. Wykretowicz A, Wierusz-Wysocka B, Wysocki J, et al. Impairment of the oxygen-dependent microbicidal mechanisms of polymorphonuclear neutrophils in patients with type 2 diabetes is not associated with increased susceptibility to infection. Diabetes Res Clin Pract 1993; 19:195.
29. Speert DP, Silva J Jr. Abnormalities of in vitro lymphocyte response to mitogens in diabetic children during acute ketoacidosis. Am J Dis Child 1978; 132:1014.
30. Casey J, Strum C Jr. Impaired response of lymphocytes from non–insulin-dependent diabetics to staphage lysate and tetanus antigen. J Clin Microbiol 1982; 15:109.
31. Kolterman OG, Olefsky JM, Kurahara C, Taylor K. A defect in cell-mediated immune function in insulin-resistant diabetic and obese subjects. J Lab Clin Med 1980; 96:535.
32. Li YM. Glycation ligand binding motif in lactoferrin. Implications in diabetic infection. Adv Exp Med Biol 1998; 443:57.
33. Cooper G, Platt R. *Staphylococcus aureus* bacteremia in diabetic patients: endocarditis and mortality. Am J Med 1982; 73:658.
34. Butler JC, Breiman RF, Campbell JF, et al. Pneumococcal polysaccharide vaccine efficacy. An evaluation of current recommendations. JAMA 1993; 270(15):1826.
34a. Centers for Disease Control and Prevention. Influenza and pneumococcal vaccination rates among persons with diabetes mellitus—United States, 1997. MMWR Morb Mort Wkly Rep 1999; 48:961.
35. Pablos-Mendez A, Blustein J, Knirsch CA. The role of diabetes mellitus in

the higher prevalence of tuberculosis among Hispanics. Am J Public Health 1997; 87(4):574.

36. Olmos P, Donoso J, Rojas N, et al. Tuberculosis and diabetes mellitus: a longitudinal retrospective study in a teaching hospital. Rev Med Chile 1989; 117:979.

37. Doroghazi RM, Nadol JB Jr, Hyslop NE Jr, et al. Invasive external otitis: report of 21 cases and review of the literature. Am J Med 1981; 71:603.

38. Johnson MP, Ramphal R. Malignant external otitis: report on therapy with ceftazidime and review of therapy and prognosis. Rev Infect Dis 1990; 12:173.

39. Lang R, Goshen S, Kitzes-Cohen R, et al. Successful treatment of malignant external otitis with ciprofloxacin: report of experience with 23 patients. J Infect Dis 1990; 161:537.

40. Giamarellou H. Malignant otitis externa: the therapeutic evolution of a lethal infection. J Antimicrob Chemother 1992; 30:745.

41. LeFrock JL, Mulavi A. Necrotizing skin and subcutaneous infections. J Antimicrob Chemother 1982; 9:183.

42. Davies HD, McGeer A, Schwartz B, et al. Invasive group A streptococcal infections in Ontario, Canada. Ontario Group A Streptococcal Study Group. N Engl J Med 1996; 335(8):547.

43. Patterson JE, Andriole VT. Bacterial urinary tract infections in diabetes. Infect Dis Clin North Am 1995; 9(1):25.

43a. Geerlings SE, Stolk RP, Camps MJ, et al. Asymptomatic bacteriuria may be considered a complication in women with diabetes. Diabetes Care 2000; 23:744.

44. Pometta D, Rees SB, Younger D, Kass EH. Asymptomatic bacteriuria in diabetes mellitus. N Engl J Med 1967; 276:1118.

45. Lindberg U, Bergström AL, Carlsson E, et al. Urinary tract infection in children with type I diabetes. Acta Paediatr Scand 1985; 74:85.

46. Lee JB. Cystitis emphysematosa. Arch Intern Med 1960; 105:150.

47. Evanoff GV, Thompson CS, Foley R, Weinman EJ. Spectrum of gas within the kidney: emphysematous pyelonephritis and emphysematous pyelitis. Am J Med 1987; 83:149.

48. Sobel JD. Pathogenesis of urinary tract infections. Infect Dis Clin North Am 1987; 1:751.

49. Levison ME, Pitsakis PG. Effect of insulin treatment on the susceptibility of the diabetic rat to *Escherichia coli*-induced pyelonephritis. J Infect Dis 1984; 150:554.

50. Sarmiento RV. Emphysematous cholecystitis. Arch Surg 1966; 93:1009.

51. Nussbaum ES, Hall WA. Rhinocerebral mucormycosis: changing patterns of disease. Surg Neurol 1994; 41:152.

52. Kauffman CA, Vasquez JA, Sobel JA, et al. Prospective multicenter surveillance study of funguria in hospitalized patients. Clin Infect Dis 2000; 30:14.

53. Hildebrand TS, Nibbe L, Frei U, Schindler R. Bilateral emphysematous pyelonephritis caused by Candida infection. Am J Kidney Dis 1999; 33:E10.

54. Vazquez JA, Sobel JD. Fungal infections in diabetes. Infect Dis Clin North Am 1995; 9(1):97.

# CHAPTER 153

# DIABETES AND THE SKIN

ROBERT J. TANENBERG AND RICHARD C. EASTMAN

The skin of the patient with diabetes may manifest various abnormalities and is prone to the development of certain infections.[1,2] Additionally, the injection or infusion of insulin and the administration of oral hypoglycemic agents may lead to cutaneous reactions. Occasionally, skin and soft tissue changes may alert the clinician to the presence of diabetes.

## NONINFECTIOUS COMPLICATIONS OF DIABETES

Various noninfectious skin diseases may occur in the patient with diabetes. Some conditions, such as xanthomas in patients with hypertriglyceridemia, carotenoderma, and reduced skin elasticity, are directly related to metabolic abnormalities, while other conditions, such as diabetic dermopathy, necrobiosis lipoidica diabeticorum, granuloma annulare, and bullosis diabeticorum, are of uncertain etiology and may occur in nondiabetics, in patients with impaired glucose tolerance, and in patients with overt diabetes. In these conditions, subtle metabolic factors, environmental factors, or genetic factors probably influence the development of the skin abnormality. The relationship between metabolic control and these cutaneous manifestations is not clear.[1,3]

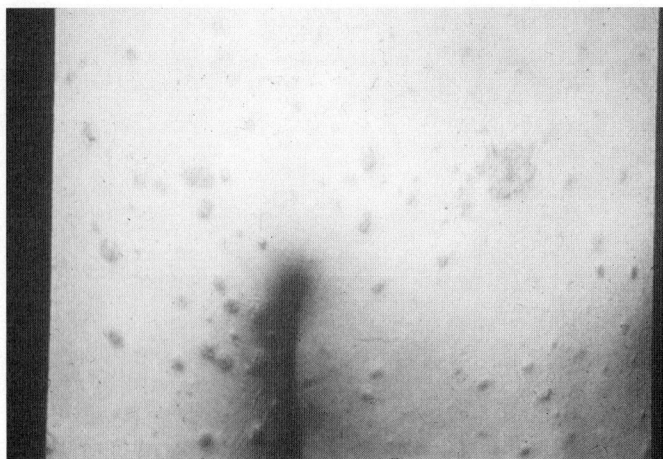

**FIGURE 153-1.** Eruptive xanthomas on the buttocks of a patient with hypertriglyceridemia and uncontrolled diabetes mellitus.

## XANTHOMAS

Xanthomas due to hypertriglyceridemia may occur in the uncontrolled diabetic. Triglyceride levels are usually >1000 mg/dL when xanthomas are present. Concomitant lipemia retinalis is usually noted on funduscopic examination. Eruptive xanthomas characteristic of hypertriglyceridemia occur in clusters primarily on the extensor surfaces of the extremities and over the buttocks. They manifest as red-yellow, 2- to 5-mm maculopapular lesions (Fig. 153-1). A red inflammatory border is characteristic. Initially, the lesions contain more triglycerides and free fatty acids than cholesterol; later, as the xanthomas begin to resolve, cholesterol predominates.[4]

Eruptive xanthomas secondary to uncontrolled diabetes usually clear with improved metabolic control. Patients with familial dyslipidemias may require therapy with drugs to reduce triglyceride levels to a satisfactory range (see Chap. 164).

## SCLEREDEMA

Scleredema (also known as *scleredema diabeticorum*) is asymmetric nonpitting induration of the skin on the posterolateral aspects of the neck, shoulders, and upper back.[5,6] Although the condition is often preceded by a streptococcal infection in the nondiabetic, this is rarely the case in the patient with diabetes.[1,3,5] Males with diabetes are four times more likely to develop this lesion than are diabetic females. Patients are frequently obese and often have microvascular and macrovascular complications of diabetes. Spontaneous resolution in 6 months to 2 years is common in the nondiabetic, but rarely occurs in patients with diabetes.[5] There is no known treatment.

## WAXY SKIN AND REDUCED JOINT MOBILITY

Reduced skin elasticity in patients with diabetes has long been recognized; it has a "hidebound" quality, resembling the skin of patients with scleroderma.[5] The condition is associated with limited joint mobility and with poor metabolic control. The correlation of these abnormalities with concentrations of glycosylated hemoglobin suggests that metabolic factors influence the development of the skin and joint changes. Improvement may occur with improved metabolic control[5] (see Chap. 211). This condition is distinct from Dupuytren contracture of the palmar fascia, which, although increased in incidence in diabetic individuals, is extremely common in the nondiabetic population.

## PERFORATING DERMATOSES

Kyrle disease, perforating folliculitis, and reactive perforating collagenosis are disorders that may be more common in patients with diabetes, particularly in those with chronic renal failure.[1] In a review of acquired reactive perforating collagenosis, 72% of the patients had diabetes with micro- or macrovascular complications.[7] These disorders are characterized by papules with a central plug that extrudes keratin or collagen. Patients typically complain of pruritus, which may be severe. Lesions have a predilection for the extensor surfaces of the upper and lower extremities, trunk, and buttocks. The lesions are often refractory to therapy, although retinoic acid with or without ultraviolet light may improve some cases.[7]

## YELLOW SKIN

The elastic tissue of patients with diabetes may demonstrate yellow discoloration possibly secondary to deposition of carotenoids, which are pigments present in green and yellow vegetables. The frequency may be as high as 10% in patients with diabetes.[1,3] Blood carotene levels are usually elevated. Hypothyroidism, hypogonadism, hypopituitarism, bulimia, and anorexia nervosa are also associated with carotenoderma and should be considered in the differential diagnosis. Brown discoloration of the nail fold due to advanced glycosylation end products also may occur in patients with diabetes.[3]

## DIABETIC DERMOPATHY

Dermopathy is a common complication of diabetes, occurring twice as often in males.[1,3] The occurrence of the lesions in patients without diabetes is evidence that factors other than hyperglycemia are causative. The high frequency of other complications of diabetes in affected patients suggests that microangiopathy is an important factor in the pathogenesis. Half of the patients have concurrent retinopathy, neuropathy, and nephropathy. Basement membrane thickening is found in areas of dermopathy, yet adjacent areas of unaffected skin show similar changes. The predominant occurrence of the lesions on the lower extremities implicates trauma, neuropathy, and basement membrane thickening. However, the lesions are not reliably reproduced by trauma. Heat or cold traumatization of the extremities in diabetics of more than 10 years' duration may induce lesions that resemble those of dermopathy.[8]

Although the lesions occur mostly on the lower extremities ("shin spots"), they also may occur on the arms, thighs, trunk, and scalp; they begin as dull red macules or papules, which are 5 to 12 mm in diameter.[3] Crops of four to five lesions may appear over a period of a week and then persist or slowly resolve (Fig. 153-2). As the lesions evolve, they become shallow, depressed, hyperpigmented scars. The lesions are asymptomatic and require no treatment.

## NECROBIOSIS LIPOIDICA DIABETICORUM

Necrobiosis (degeneration of collagen) is an uncommon complication of diabetes of unknown etiology. Although it occurs in only 0.3% of all patients with diabetes, 65% of the patients presenting with this lesion have diabetes. Of the remaining patients, many have impaired glucose intolerance or a positive family history of diabetes. It is three times more common in women. A review of the literature concluded that "necrobiosis lipoidica diabeticorum is usually associated with poor glucose control and that tighter glucose control, as currently practiced, might improve or prevent the disorder."[9]

Pathologically the lesions show degeneration of collagen, granulomatous inflammation of subcutaneous tissues and of blood vessels, capillary basement membrane thickening, and obliteration of vessel lumina. The yellow color in the central

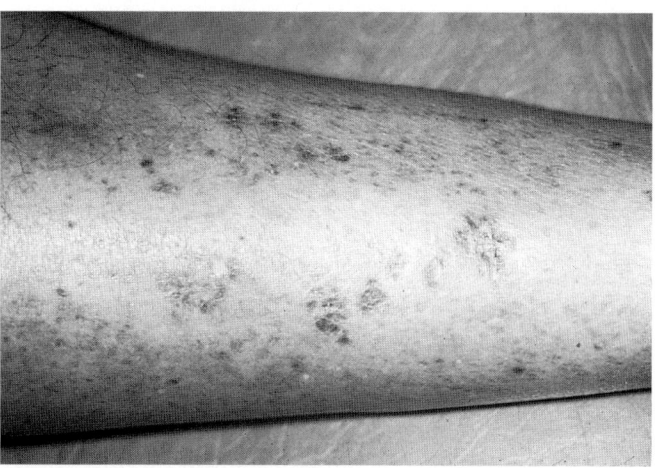

**FIGURE 153-2.** Diabetic dermopathy on the anterior tibial surfaces. The lesions are pigmented and slightly depressed below the surrounding skin.

area of the lesions is most likely secondary to thinning of the dermis, making subcutaneous fat more visible.

The lesions of necrobiosis occur most commonly in the pretibial areas and are bilateral in 75% of the cases. They begin as red-brown papules that enlarge and coalesce to form irregular lesions, which may be several centimeters in diameter (Fig. 153-3). The lesions ulcerate in 35% of the cases; although usually painless, they may be painful and become infected when ulcerated. For this reason, trauma to the anterior tibial area should be avoided. As the lesions evolve, they appear as atrophic plaques with a thin, translucent surface manifesting a "porcelain-like sheen."

Various therapies have been used: fluorinated corticosteroids (applied topically, under occlusive dressings, or injected into the lesion), salicylates with dipyridamole, pentoxifylline, systemic corticosteroids, nicotinamide, clofazimine, and ticlopidine.[10] Topical benzoyl peroxide, seaweed-based alginate dressings, and hydrocolloid occlusive dressings may be helpful.[3] Grafting of ulcerated areas may occasionally be necessary, although recurrences are common. Spontaneous resolution of necrobiosis occurs infrequently, but the lesions may fade in appearance.

## GRANULOMA ANNULARE

Granuloma annulare is a dermatitis with histologic similarities to necrobiosis lipoidica diabeticorum. Clinically, these lesions

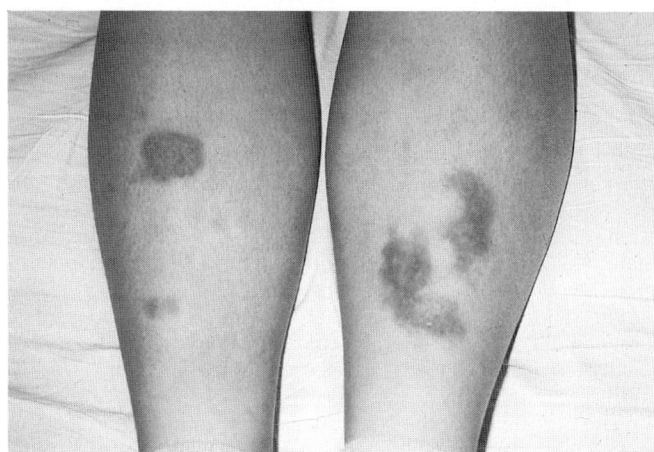

**FIGURE 153-3.** Necrobiosis lipoidica diabeticorum. These typical lesions were initially noted in this 9-year-old girl several months before the diagnosis of type 1 diabetes. (Courtesy of Dr. William Burke.)

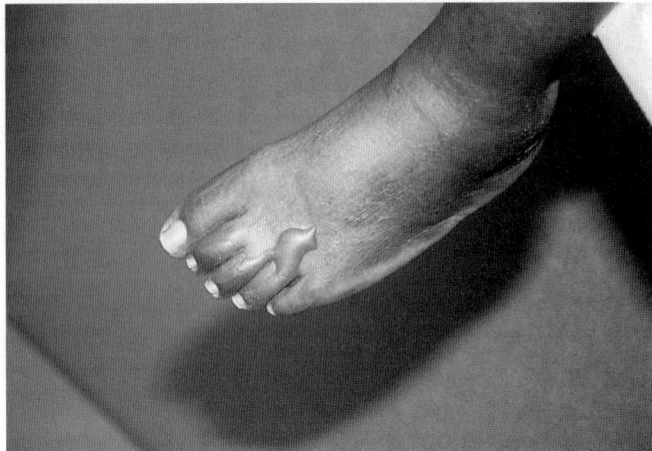

**FIGURE 153-4.** Bullosis diabeticorum. The lesion was noted in a 48-year-old black man with a 28-year history of type 1 diabetes, complicated by severe neuropathy and end-stage renal disease. (Courtesy of Dr. Michael Pfeifer.)

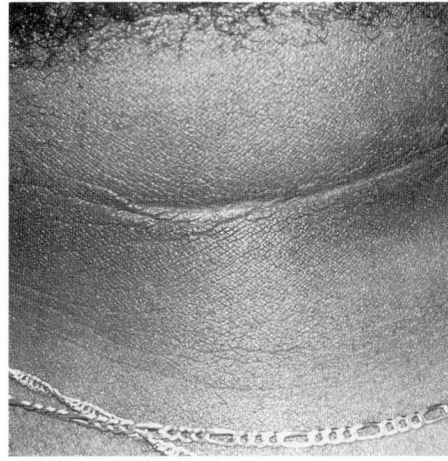

**FIGURE 153-5.** Acanthosis nigricans. Typical lesion on the back of the neck in a young obese black woman with type 2 diabetes.

may initially have a similar appearance; subsequently, as they enlarge, differences become apparent. Granuloma annulare lesions do not develop the yellow color and rarely ulcerate or form permanent scar tissue.

Patients with the generalized type of granuloma annulare are more likely to demonstrate impaired glucose tolerance or overt diabetes.[2] The lesions occur predominantly on the upper extremities and manifest as flesh-colored plaques with a raised border. Resolution in the patient with diabetes may occur spontaneously over several years.[1] Treatment with photochemotherapy has been used successfully for this condition.[11]

## BULLOSIS DIABETICORUM

Tense bullae of the feet and hands are rare but distinctive manifestations of diabetes. The lesions are of uncertain cause, although trauma, microangiopathy, and vasculitis have been implicated.[1,3] Differential diagnosis includes bullous impetigo, bullous pemphigoid, and bullous erythema mulitiforme secondary to drugs. The blisters may develop in patients during bed rest, indicating that factors other than trauma are involved. The plantar surfaces and margins of the feet are the most common sites of occurrence (Fig. 153-4). The lesions develop acutely, are asymptomatic, and manifest as tense, 0.5- to 3.0-cm bullae without surrounding inflammation. Healing without scarring occurs over a period of 2 to 4 weeks. Rupture of the lesions should be avoided to prevent superinfection. Drainage and topical antibiotics may be required for large lesions to prevent secondary infection.[1]

## ACANTHOSIS NIGRICANS

Acanthosis nigricans is an important skin lesion most commonly associated with type 2 diabetes mellitus, which is considered a marker for hyperinsulinemia. There may be a genetic basis for this association.[11a] Benign acanthosis nigricans is also associated with obesity, lipodystrophic diabetes, and hyperandrogenic states (e.g., polycystic ovary syndrome); it is less frequently associated with acromegaly, Cushing syndrome, other endocrine disorders, and multiple nonfamilial congenital syndromes (e.g., Prader-Willi).[12] In addition, hormonal therapy (e.g., the use of methyltestosterone in a hypogonadal patient) has been known to induce acanthosis nigricans.

The prevalence of the benign form of acanthosis nigricans in the general population varies with race. One study of adolescents noted incidences of this lesion in 0.5% of whites, 5% of Hispanic Americans, and 13% of blacks.[13] This same study noted a 27% incidence in moderately obese (120% of ideal body weight) adolescents and a 66% incidence in the same age group with severe obesity (200% of ideal body weight).

The term *acanthosis nigricans* literally means blackish thorn, which is an apt description of the characteristic velvet-like epidermal thickening associated with hyperpigmentation. The lesions have a predilection for the back and sides of the neck, axillae, and other skinfolds (Fig. 153-5).

The pathogenesis of acanthosis nigricans is theorized to result from excess insulin binding to insulin-like growth factor receptors in the epidermis.[14]

It is important to identify this skin lesion in younger patients who may have hyperinsulinemia and be at high risk to develop type 2 diabetes mellitus. Hyperinsulinemia, even without diabetes, is a known risk factor for cardiovascular disease. Weight loss has been shown to lead to complete regression of the skin lesion,[12] presumably secondary to the reduction of hyperinsulinemia. Whether oral agents such as metformin and the thiazolidinediones, which reduce hyperinsulinemia, will reverse this skin lesion is yet to be determined.

Patients are occasionally bothered by the acanthosis lesions and may unsuccessfully attempt to scrub them off. The use of keratolytic agents such as salicylic acid has been reported to improve the cosmetic appearance. In addition, the use of omega-3 fatty acid as found in dietary fish oil supplements has also been reported to improve the skin lesions.[15]

Clinicians should keep in mind that acanthosis nigricans may also be the sign of an occult malignancy, most commonly a gastrointestinal adenocarcinoma. In the elderly, nonobese patient with diabetes, new onset of acanthosis nigricans warrants a thorough evaluation to exclude a malignancy.[12]

## ACROCHORDONS

More than 20 years ago, acrochordons (skin tags) were found to be associated with diabetes.[16] More recent studies have confirmed this association: It appears that 66% to 75% of all patients with skin tags have diabetes.[17] These soft fibromas have a predilection for the eyelids, neck, and axillae and increase in frequency with age (Fig. 153-6). Skin tags may be associated with acanthosis nigricans and may also be related to an excess of insulin-like growth factors. These lesions, although only a cosmetic problem, may be yet another marker for type 2 diabetes mellitus.[17]

## NECROLYTIC MIGRATORY ERYTHEMA

Necrolytic migratory erythema is a unique skin rash associated with A-cell tumors of the pancreas, that is, glucagonoma. The glucagonoma syndrome includes the clinical triad of diabetes mellitus, weight loss, and necrolytic migratory erythema. The

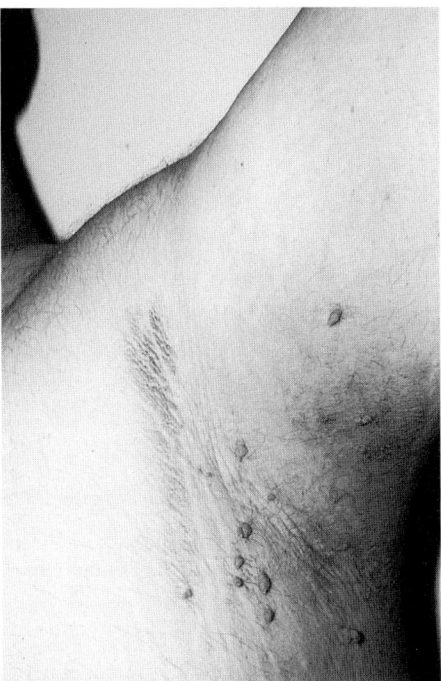

**FIGURE 153-6.** Acrochordons with acanthosis nigricans. Axillary lesions noted in a middle-aged white man with type 2 diabetes.

diagnosis is confirmed by elevated glucagon levels and pancreatic islet cell neoplasm.[18] These rare tumors are most frequently found in the tail of the pancreas, which has the highest concentration of glucagon-producing A cells.

The rash of necrolytic migratory erythema is distinctive with erythema, vesicles, bullae, pustules, and erosions with a predilection for the face, groin, and other intertriginous areas (Fig. 153-7). This rash may be present for years before the correct diagnosis is made. It is often confused with *Candida* or misdiagnosed as psoriasis or chronic eczema.[19] Clues to the diagnosis include associated glossitis, stomatitis, and angular cheilitis. These findings with a similar rash may also be found in acrodermatitis enteropathica, which is associated with zinc deficiency.

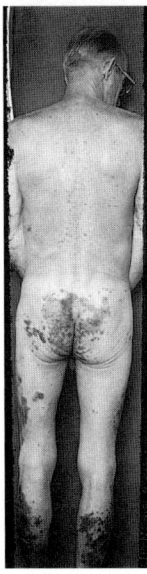

**FIGURE 153-7.** Necrolytic migratory erythema. A 72-year-old white man with metastatic islet cell tumor and a glucagon level of 11,496 pg/mL. Eruptions were noted on the scrotum, buttocks, and lower extremities. (Courtesy of Dr. George Lawrence.)

The patient with necrolytic migratory erythema usually presents with mild type 2 diabetes, anorexia, weight loss, anemia, and often gastrointestinal ulcerations. The rash is considered to be secondary to excessive catabolism of amino acids. The resultant amino-acid deficiency, which is similar to pellagra, has a toxic effect on keratinocytes. Patients typically present with glucagon levels >1000 pg/mL, although tumors may occur in patients whose glucagon levels are <600 pg/mL.[20]

The tumors are usually localized by computed tomographic (CT) scan or arteriography. In rare cases, selective glucagon sampling may be needed for localization. These tumors are usually treated with a partial pancreatectomy, with resection of the tail and body of the gland. Successful surgery will lead to normalization of glucagon levels and resolution of the rash but the diabetes may persist. Recurrent and unresectable glucagonomas are usually responsive to chemotherapy. Patients with diabetes and a chronic unexplained dermatologic disorder should be screened with a serum glucagon level.[20]

## OTHER ASSOCIATED DERMATOSES

Other conditions in which an association with diabetes has been reported are lichen planus, lichen sclerosus et atrophicus, psoriasis, bullous pemphigoid, pyoderma gangrenosum, and Kaposi sarcoma.[21–23] Vitiligo may be present in patients with autoimmune diseases associated with diabetes.[3] Patients with diabetes may also manifest changes of the fingernails due to infections (with *Pseudomonas aeruginosa*, *Staphylococcus aureus*, *Proteus mirabilis*, or *Candida albicans*) or to vascular insufficiency (hypertrophic changes, pterygium, yellow discoloration).[24] Controlled studies have not shown an increased prevalence of epidermophytosis or of generalized pruritus in patients with diabetes.[25]

## INFECTIONS OF THE SKIN AND SOFT TISSUES

Various factors have been identified that may predispose the diabetic patient to infectious diseases[26] (see Chap. 152). Persons with uncontrolled diabetes may be immunocompromised and susceptible to the development of certain infections of the skin and soft tissues.[26–29] Patients with diabetes, especially those with poor glycemic control, may have an increased rate of colonization as well as infections of the skin with *C. albicans*, *Staphylococcus*, and *Streptococcus*.[26,30] Intertriginous areas in obese and, less often, nonobese patients with diabetes are frequently infected with these organisms. Glucosuria predisposes to recurrent candidal vulvovaginitis in females (Fig. 153-8). *Balanitis diabetica* refers to inflammation of the glans penis from gluco-

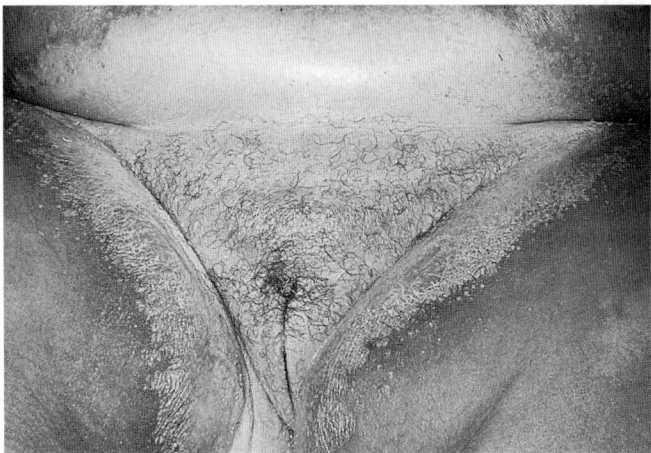

**FIGURE 153-8.** Candidal vulvovaginitis. Typical eruption noted in a black female with uncontrolled type 2 diabetes.

suria usually associated with candidiasis. These male patients frequently have coexisting phimosis and poor glycemic control of their diabetes. Deterioration of metabolic control in susceptible individuals may be accompanied by recurrent infection. Surgical wounds or minor abrasions are more likely to become infected. Certain cutaneous infections are particularly likely to appear in the diabetic patient and deserve special consideration. Prompt diagnosis and appropriate treatment of some infections at an early stage are essential to avoid serious, even life-threatening, complications.

## NECROTIZING FASCIITIS

Patients with uncontrolled diabetes may develop necrotizing fasciitis, an uncommon but potentially lethal skin and soft tissue infection.[31,32] Eighty percent of the cases of necrotizing fasciitis occur as an extension of an often trivial skin lesion (e.g., boil, insect bite, or from an injection site).[33] The infection may be monomicrobial or polymicrobial with both aerobic and anaerobic bacteria cultured. The most common offending organisms include *Streptococcus pyogenes, Staphylococcus aureus,* anaerobic streptococci, and *Bacteroides.*[33] Decubitus ulcers, the skin of the perineum, and the extremities are often the sites of initiation of the infection. Infections beginning in the scrotum or perineum (*Fournier gangrene*) have a mortality rate as high as 40% despite appropriate antibiotics and surgical therapy.[33,33a] At the time of diagnosis, the infection has usually spread laterally, dissecting along fascia planes. The infection is limited to the subcutaneous tissues, sparing the underlying muscle.[31]

The early symptoms may be misleadingly benign, suggesting musculoskeletal pain. Careful physical examination and a high index of suspicion are necessary to make the diagnosis. On examination, there is tenderness in response to palpation over the infected area. Subcutaneous gas occasionally may be noted by palpation but is detected more reliably by radiographs. Hypalgesia or anesthesia may be present, owing to involvement of cutaneous nerves. A thin, gray-brown exudate with a feculent odor is characteristic. Systemic toxicity is manifested by fever, tachycardia, and elevated white blood cell count out of proportion to the local manifestations; ketoacidosis and coma have also been reported.[26,31,34]

Debridement, at times radical, of necrotic tissue is necessary for the patient to survive. Antibiotics should be started empirically after appropriate cultures of tissue and blood are obtained. A combination of clindamycin and an aminoglycoside will provide the necessary coverage for *Staphylococcus,* anaerobes, and gram-negative rods and should be continued until the patient is out of danger. Even with optimal surgical and medical treatment, this condition has an overall mortality of 20% to 30%.[33]

## MALIGNANT EXTERNAL OTITIS

Malignant external otitis occurs in patients who are immunocompromised and may complicate diabetes.[33,35–37] Microangiopathy of the ear canal resulting in poor local perfusion has been implicated in the pathogenesis of the infection.[35] The infection may begin indolently with ear pain and drainage and, if untreated, may extend to the periaural soft tissues, to the cells of the mastoid process, and to the meninges, brain substance, and sinuses. Thrombosis of the intracranial veins may occur. On examination, the pinna and adjacent soft tissue may be tender. The external auditory canal is usually swollen and contains a purulent discharge.[33] Granulation tissue can be visualized at the juncture of the cartilaginous and bony portions of the canal in most cases.[35] The tympanic membrane may be intact, perforated, or obscured by debris, edema, or granulation tissue.[33] Culture of the drainage typically yields *P. aeruginosa.*[37]

The ear canal should be irrigated, drained, and debrided, if indicated. Consultation with an otolaryngologist is advisable. Systemic antibiotic therapy with an aminoglycoside and a semi-

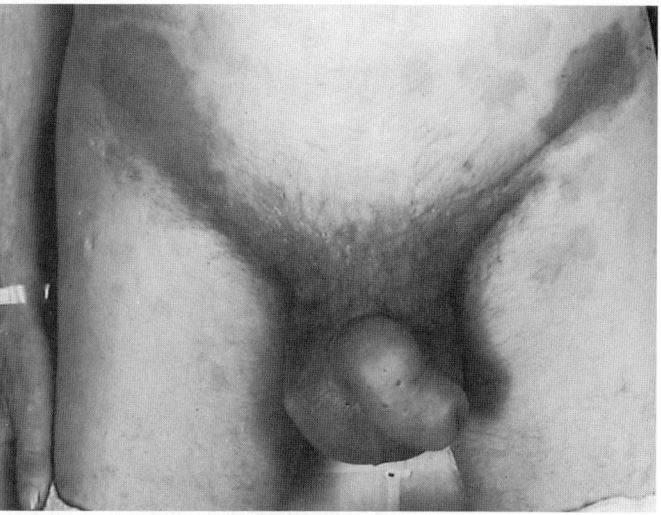

**FIGURE 153-9.** Erythrasma in a male with type 1 diabetes and nephrotic syndrome. Note the swollen genitalia. The borders of the lesions are sharply defined and irregular.

synthetic penicillin, such as ticarcillin, piperacillin, or carbenicillin, is the treatment of choice. Monotherapy with intravenous (iv) ceftazadime or oral ciprofloxacin compares successfully with combination therapy in moderate infections.[33,38]

## RHINOCEREBRAL MUCORMYCOSIS

Mucormycosis is a rare, but life-threatening, complication of diabetes.[26,33,39] It may be a presenting manifestation of diabetes in elderly patients, may occur with or without the presence of ketoacidosis, and may occur in patients with well-controlled diabetes.[40] The infection begins with invasion through the nasal mucosa by fungi of the genus *Mucor, Rhizopus,* or *Absidia.* There is early spread to the soft tissues of the face, orbit, and sinuses. Thrombosis of the vascular supply may produce necrosis of the palate and septum.

The patient characteristically presents with facial cellulitis and orbital swelling and may manifest an orbital apex syndrome with oculomotor palsies and loss of vision. There is a black nasal discharge and black eschar of the nasal mucosa. Gram stain of the discharge will show broad, nonseptate hyphae, and culture usually yields the organism.

Amphotericin B is the treatment of choice. Surgical debridement is essential, because the organism may persist in devitalized tissue.

## ERYTHRASMA

Erythrasma is a common, often-recognized, superficial skin infection occurring in patients with diabetes.[3,26] It begins as a pruritic, red-brown patch in the axillae or groin (Fig. 153-9). Involvement may be extensive. The lesions manifest a characteristic coral-red fluorescence under a Wood light. Gram stain shows a small, gram-positive bacillus, and aerobic culture of the material will grow *Corynebacterium minutissimum.* Treatment with oral erythromycin is effective.

# DERMATOLOGIC COMPLICATIONS OF THE TREATMENT OF DIABETES

## IMMUNOLOGIC REACTIONS TO INSULIN

Hypersensitivity reactions to insulin preparations occurred commonly in the past, before the application of improved puri-

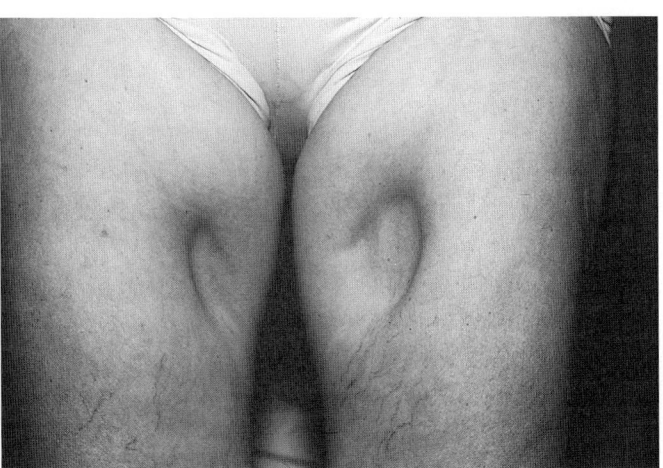

**FIGURE 153-10.** Focal lipoatrophy of the thighs in a woman with type 1 diabetes using beef-pork insulin. The lipoatrophy cleared with injection of human insulin into the affected areas.

fication techniques for commercial insulins and before the availability of monospecies pork and human insulins.[25] Although less common, hypersensitivity reactions may occur in patients on the new insulins and may pose difficult management problems (see Chap. 143).

Focal lipoatrophy, or loss of subcutaneous fat in areas of insulin injection, most likely represents an immunologic reaction to impurities in the insulin preparation and is less common in patients using the purer forms of insulin (Fig. 153-10). In contrast, focal lipohypertrophy at areas of insulin injections is most likely due to inhibition of lipolysis by high local concentrations of insulin (see Chap. 143). For unknown reasons, females are more likely to develop atrophy, whereas lipohypertrophy is more common in males. In both disorders, patients often give a history of repeated injections into the same site. Lipohypertrophy will often improve by simply avoiding the affected area and using alternative sites for injection. Lipoatrophy usually improves with injection of human insulin directly into the affected area.

## COMPLICATIONS OF CONTINUOUS SUBCUTANEOUS INSULIN ADMINISTRATION

Local infection, allergy to tape and tubing materials, and hard subcutaneous nodules are uncommon complications of external insulin pump therapy (also known as *continuous subcutaneous insulin infusion*).[41] In the Diabetes Control and Complications Trial (DCCT), the incidence of skin infections in patients continuously using insulin pumps ranges from one event every 8 to 14 years.[42] Localized areas of cellulitis and abscess formation may infrequently occur in patients treated by continuous subcutaneous insulin infusion (external insulin pump). Leaving the catheter or needle in place for more than 72 hours increases the risk of infection. Deterioration in the degree of glycemic control may be the first sign of problems at the infusion site, before overt signs of infection or inflammation are present. When there is an unexplained deterioration in blood glucose control, the needle and catheter should be changed. Local abscesses are treated with warm compresses, incision and drainage if necessary, and antibiotic therapy.

Infrequently, patients on continuous subcutaneous insulin infusion may develop tender nodules with a rock-hard consistency at the sites of needle insertion.[41] Local trauma from prolonged contact of needles left under the skin, multiple injections into the same site, or local hematoma formation from the movement of needles under the skin may explain the development of these nodules. Since most local complications of insulin pump therapy begin with irritation and inflammation at the insertion site, plastic cannulas have provided a mechanism for reducing accidental trauma to the skin. Newer infusion sets with soft Teflon cannulas also have an antibacterial dressing designed to retard the growth of bacteria at the infusion site. Nonetheless, sterile technique and adequate attention to site preparation should be mandatory. Frequent site changes will minimize both infection and inflammatory sequelae of continuous subcutaneous insulin infusion.[43]

## REACTIONS TO ORAL ANTIDIABETIC AGENTS

Oral hypoglycemic agents for diabetes include sulfonylureas that are structurally related to the sulfonamides. Sulfonylureas have been reported to cause allergic skin reactions, including pruritus, erythemas (multiforme and nodosum), urticaria, morbilliform rash, and lichenoid eruptions.[44] These side effects may be transient and may resolve despite continued use of the drug. Less common skin reactions to sulfonylureas include granuloma annulare, exfoliative dermatitis, and Stevens-Johnson syndrome.[45] Jaundice may occur secondary to reversible intrahepatic cholestasis induced by sulfonylureas, most typically chloropropamide. (This drug caused 8 of 53 cases of drug-induced acute liver disease in a Jamaican hospital over a 15-year period.[46] Of these eight cases, five were diagnosed with intrahepatic cholestasis and three with diffuse hepatic necrosis.)

Chloropropamide is the most likely of the sulfonylureas to induce alcohol flushing similar to that caused by disulfiram. This reaction has been reported in 10% to 15% of patients receiving chloropropamide.[47] The second-generation sulfonylurea agents glipizide and glyburide do not cause this troublesome reaction (see Chap. 142).

Photosensitivity is another dermatologic side effect of sulfonylureas. These drugs induce a photoallergic reaction when the skin is exposed to ultraviolet B radiation (290–320 nm). A 24- to 48-hour latent period after exposure is required for sensitization to occur. In contradistinction to phototoxic reactions, the photoallergic reaction caused by sulfonylureas is not related to the dose of the drug.[45] The eruptions typically occur on the face, hands, and the "V" of the neck, and other sites exposed to the sun.

Other oral antidiabetic agents include the biguanides (e.g., metformin), thiazolidinediones, alpha glucosidase inhibitors (e.g., acarbose), and the meglitinides (e.g., repaglinide). Metformin monotherapy has no greater incidence of dermatologic side effects than placebo. Likewise, no dermatologic side effects have been reported with acarbose or repaglinide. In the North American clinical trials, 20 of 2510 patients developed liver function test abnormalities.[48] Two of the 20 patients developed reversible jaundice. It is not yet known whether the newer thiazolidinediones will cause similar idiosyncratic reactions.

## DERMATOLOGIC FINDINGS IN SECONDARY DIABETES

Skin problems, such as excessive sweating in patients with acromegaly, plethora or hirsutism in the patient with Cushing syndrome, or pallor and sweating due to pheochromocytoma, may initially bring the patient to medical attention. All of these endocrine disorders may be associated with secondary diabetes mellitus. Glucose intolerance or secondary diabetes mellitus also occurs in several uncommon syndromes, such as hemochromatosis and porphyria cutanea tarda. Many of these patients also have characteristic dermatologic manifestations, which are summarized in Table 153-1.

**TABLE 153-1.**
**Dermatologic Findings in Syndromes or Diseases Associated with Diabetes**

| | |
|---|---|
| Polyglandular failure | Vitiligo, premature graying, addisonian hyperpigmentation, chronic mucocutaneous candidiasis |
| Hemochromatosis | Gray, brown, or intermediate shades of hyperpigmentation; alopecia |
| Porphyria cutanea tarda | Bullous eruption in sun-exposed areas, hypertrichosis, milia |
| Syndromes of insulin resistance and acanthosis nigricans: | |
|   Type A | Acanthosis nigricans, hirsutism, accelerated growth, clitoromegaly |
|   Type B | Acanthosis nigricans, alopecia |
| Polycystic ovary syndrome | Hirsutism, acne, alopecia, acanthosis nigricans |
| Total lipoatrophy (Lawrence-Seip syndrome) | Absent subcutaneous fat, acanthosis nigricans, hyperhidrosis, masculinization |
| Leprechaunism | Acanthosis nigricans, premature aging of the skin |
| Ataxia-telangiectasia | Telangiectasia |
| Progressive lipodystrophy | Hyperhidrosis, absent subcutaneous fat |

## REFERENCES

1. Jelinek JE. The skin and diabetes. Philadelphia: Lea & Febiger, 1986.
2. Perez MI, Kohn SR. Cutaneous manifestations of diabetes. J Am Acad Dermatol 1994; 30:519.
3. Jelinek JE. The skin in diabetes. Diabet Med 1993; 10:201.
4. Parker F, Bagdade JD, Odland GF, Bierman EL. Evidence for the chylomicron origin of lipids accumulating in diabetic eruptive xanthomas: a correlative lipid biochemical, histochemical, and electron microscopic study. Clin Invest 1970; 49:2172.
5. Brik R, Berant M, Vardi P. The scleroderma-like syndrome of insulin-dependent diabetes mellitus. Diabetes Metab Rev 1991; 7:121.
6. Iwasaki T, Kohama T, Houjou S, et al. Diabetic scleredema-like changes in a patient with maturity onset type diabetes of young people. Dermatology 1994; 188:228.
7. Faver IR, Daoud MS, Su WP. Acquired reactive perforating collagenosis. Report of six cases and review of the literature. J Am Acad Dermatol 1994; 30:575.
8. Lithner F. Cutaneous reactions of the extremities of diabetics to local thermal trauma. Acta Med Scand 1975; 198:319.
9. Cohen O, Yaniv R, Karasik A, Trau H. Necrobiosis lipoidica and diabetic control revisited. Med Hypotheses 1996; 46:348.
10. Lowitt MH, Dover JS. Necrobiosis lipoidica. J Am Acad Dermatol 1991; 25:735.
11. Kerker BJ, Huang CP, Morison WL. Photochemotherapy of generalized granuloma annulare. Arch Dermatol 1990; 126: 359.
11a. Burke JP, Puggirla R, Hale DE, et al. Genetic basis of acanthosis nigricans in Mexican Americans and its association with phenotypes related to type 2 diabetes. Hum Genet 2000; 106:467.
12. Rogers DL. Acanthosis nigricans. Semin Dermatol 1991; 10:160.
13. Stuart CA, Pate CJ, Peters EJ. Prevalence of acanthosis nigricans in an unselected population. Am J Med 1989; 87:269.
14. Cruz PD, Hud JA. Excess inulin binding to insulin-like growth factor receptors: proposed mechanism for acanthosis nigricans. J Invest Dermatol 1992; 98(Suppl): 82S.
15. Sherertz EF. Improved acanthosis nigricans with lipodystrophic diabetes during dietary fish oil supplementation. Arch Dermatol 1988; 124:1094.
16. Margolis J, Margolis LS. Skin tags—a frequent sign of diabetes mellitus. N Engl J Med 1976; 294:1184.
17. Thappa DM. Skin tags as markers of diabetes mellitus: an epidemiological study in India. J Dermatol 1995; 22:729.
18. Mallinson CN, Bloom SR, Warin AP, et al. A glucagonoma syndrome. Lancet 1974; 2:1.
19. Montenegro F, Lawrence GD, Macon W, Pass C. Metastatic glucagonoma: improvement after surgical debulking. Am J Surg 1980; 139:424.
20. Edney JA, Hofmann S, Thompson JS, Kessinger A. Glucagonoma syndrome is an underdiagnosed clinical entity. Am J Surg 1990; 160: 625.
21. Garcia-Bravo B, Sanchez-Pedreno P, Rodriguez-Pichardo A, Camacho F. Lichen sclerosus et atrophicus: a study of 76 cases and their relation to diabetes. J Am Acad Dermatol 1988; 19:482.
22. Goodfield MJ, Millard LC. The skin in diabetes mellitus. Diabetologia 1989; 31:567.
23. Dahl MV. Bullous pemphigoid: associated diseases. Clin Dermatol 1987; 5:64.
24. Greene RA, Scher RK. Nail changes associated with diabetes mellitus. J Am Acad Dermatol 1987; 16:1015.
25. Feingold KR, Elias PM. Endocrine-skin interactions: cutaneous manifesta-

26. Murphy DP, Tan JS, File TM. Infectious complications in diabetic patients. Primary Care 1981; 8:695.
27. Repine JE, Clauson CC, Goetz FC. Leucocytes and host defense: bactericidal functions of neutrophils from patients with acute bacterial infections and from diabetes. J Infect Dis 1980; 142:869.
28. Rayfield EJ, Ault MJ, Keusch GT, et al. Infection and diabetes: the case for glucose control. Am J Med 1982; 72:439.
29. Wilson RM. Neutrophil function in diabetes. Diabetic Med 1986; 3:509.
30. Bartholomew G, Roden B, Bell DAH. Oral candidiasis in IDDM. Diabetes 1985; 34:103A.
31. Addison WA, Livengood CH, Hill GB, et al. Necrotizing fasciitis of vulvar origin in diabetic patients. Obstet Gynecol 1984; 63:473.
32. Farrell LD, Karl SR, Davis PK, et al. Postoperative necrotizing fasciitis in children. Pediatrics 1988; 82:874.
33. Gorbach SL, Bartlett JG, Blacklow NR. Infectious diseases, 2nd ed. Philadelphia: WB Saunders, 1998.
33a. Eke N. Fournier's gangrene: a review of 1726 cases. Br J Surg 2000; 87:718.
34. Hautekeefe ML, Nagler JM, Mertens AH, et al. Necrotizing fasciitis precipitating diabetic ketoacidotic coma. Intensive Care Med 1986; 12:383.
35. Doroghazi RM, Nadol JB, Hyslop NE, et al. Invasive external otitis. Am J Med 1981; 71:603.
36. Cohen D, Friedman P. The diagnostic criteria of malignant external otitis. J Laryngol Otol 1987; 101:216.
37. Scherbeuske JM, Winton GB, James WD. Acute *Pseudomonas* infection of the external ear (malignant external otitis). J Dermatol Surg Oncol 1988; 14:165.
38. Myers BR, Mendelson MH, Parisier SC, Hirschman SF. Malignant external otitis: comparison of monotherapy vs. combination therapy. Arch Otolaryngol Head Neck Surg 1987; 113:974.
39. Kilpatrick CJ, Speer AG, Tress BM, King JO. Rhinocerebral mucormycosis. Med J Aust 1983; 1:308.
40. Sandler R, Tallman CB, Keamy DG, Irving WR. Successfully treated rhinocerebral phycomycosis in well-controlled diabetes. N Engl J Med 1971; 285:1180.
41. Levandoski LA, White NH, Santiago JV. Localized skin reactions to insulin: insulin lipodystrophies and skin reactions to pumped subcutaneous insulin therapy. Diabetes Care 1982; 5:6.
42. Diabetes Control and Complications Trial Research Group. Implementation of treatment protocols in the Diabetes Control and Complications Trial. Diabetes Care 1995; 18:361.
43. American Diabetes Association. Continuous subcutaneous insulin infusion. Position statement. Diabetes Care 1999; 22:S87.
44. Division of Drugs and Toxicology. Drug evaluations: annual 1995. Chicago: American Medical Association, 1995.
45. Litt JZ, Pawlak WA. Drug eruption reference manual. New York: Parthenon Publishing Group, 1997.
46. Reynolds JEF (ed). Martindale: the extra pharmacopoeia, 31st ed. London: Royal Pharmaceutical Society, 1996.
47. Hardman JG. Goodman and Gilman's the pharmacological basis of therapeutics, 9th ed. New York: McGraw-Hill, 1996.
48. Physicians' desk reference, 53rd ed. Montvale, NJ: Medical Economics Co, 1999.

---

# CHAPTER 154

# THE DIABETIC FOOT

GARY W. GIBBONS

## PREVALENCE

Foot problems and diabetes are almost synonymous. Approximately 25% of diabetics will eventually consult a clinician, surgeon, or podiatrist for diabetes-related problems of the lower extremities. Because diabetics are 17 times more likely to develop gangrene (a word to avoid using in front of the patient), it is not surprising that 66% of the major amputations performed in the United States are performed on diabetics. The American Diabetes Association and Healthy People 2000 (the health objectives of the U.S. Public Health Service) have a goal to reduce this major amputation rate.[1] Despite the tremendous advances that have been made in the knowledge, technology, and treatment of diabetes, diabetic foot problems continue to be a major health concern, causing serious morbidity, mortality, and economic consequences. Many of these tragic conse-

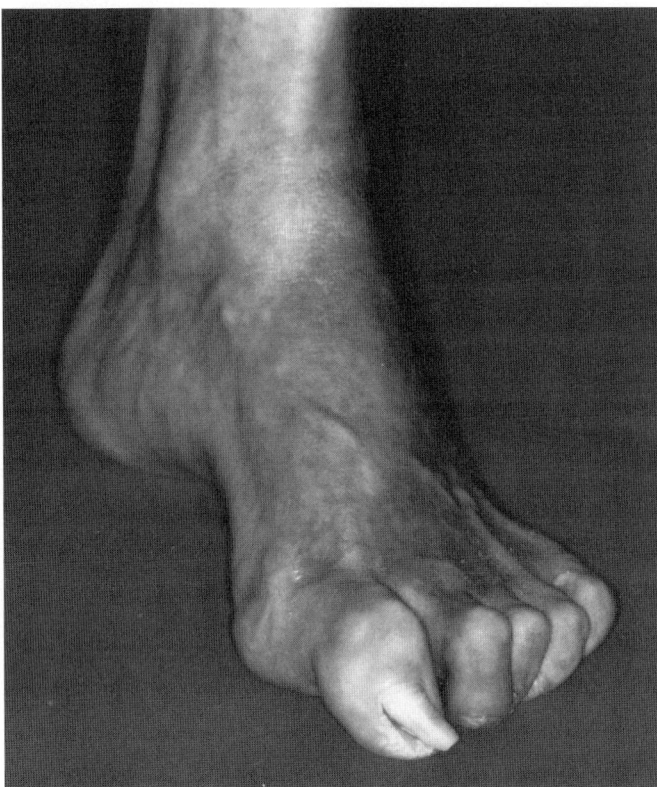

**FIGURE 154-1.** Diabetic man with clawing of all of his toes (hammertoes). There is hyperextension of the metatarsal joints and flexion of the proximal interphalangeal joints. The loss of innervation of the intrinsic muscles of the feet results in imbalance, and a resultant pull by the flexor digitorum longus. This may result in abnormal weight-bearing, pressure against the top of the shoe, and resultant ulcerations.

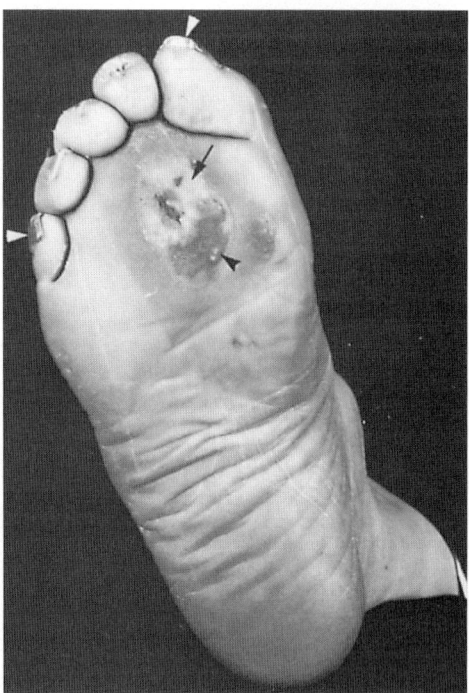

**FIGURE 154-2.** Plantar neuropathic ulcer in a diabetic patient. There is a nonhealing, painless, circular, punched-out ulceration surrounded by a callus (*dark arrow and arrowhead*) overlying the metatarsal head. These ulcers, which are due to the combined effects of neuropathy and ischemia, occur at sites of greatest pressure. The anesthesia and anhidrosis predispose to their formation. If improperly treated, these ulcers progress to osteomyelitis and gangrene. Therapy includes debridement, trimming of the callus, rest, redistribution of weight with custom-molded inserts, and appropriate education in foot care. Note the onychomycosis of the toenails (*arrowheads*), a condition to which diabetics are predisposed.

quences could be avoided by better patient education and understanding and by eliminating misconceptions of many health care professionals regarding the treatment of diabetic foot problems.

## PATHOPHYSIOLOGY

Although careful control of diabetes and avoidance of smoking may postpone the development of foot problems, it will not prevent them. Three primary pathologic situations occur in the diabetic, which singly or in combination are responsible for the development of foot problems: neuropathy, arterial insufficiency, and infection.

### NEUROPATHY

The diabetic neuropathic foot may look healthy, but it has altered proprioception, making the patient less aware of the position of his or her foot, and diminished touch and pain, causing an insensitive foot. Moreover, peripheral neuropathy affects the intrinsic and skeletal muscles of the foot and leg, causing atrophy and deformity. The result of this motor neuropathy is a muscle-wasted foot with prominent metatarsal heads, clawed toes, and limited joint mobility (Fig. 154-1). The resulting deformities create high foot pressures with subsequent callus formation and ulceration if repetitive moderate stress (as in walking) continues. The patient is unaware of these stresses because of an insensitive foot. The autonomic system is adversely affected by neuropathy, often causing autosympathectomy in the lower extremities; the feet become anhidrotic, and the skin is dried and cracks easily. The overall result is a

limb that is highly susceptible to minor trauma and a patient who is unaware of an existing problem until it has become a serious limb-threatening infection (Figs. 154-2 and 154-3; see Chap. 148).

## ISCHEMIA

Although the severity of diabetes is not crucial to the development of vascular disease, peripheral vascular disease is estimated to be 20 times more common in the diabetic population

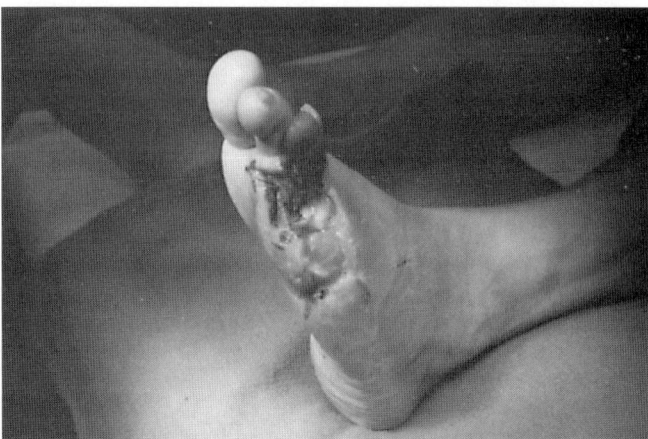

**FIGURE 154-3.** Severe ulceration and gangrene of the foot of a diabetic patient, requiring amputation. Many of these tragic complications can be avoided by education of patients and of health care professionals.

TABLE 154-1.
**Patient Education and Responsibility**

---

**DAILY FOOT INSPECTION BY PATIENT AND FAMILY**
  Red or ecchymotic areas
  Calluses
  Blisters
  Open sores or dry fissures
  Fungus infections
**GOOD HYGIENE**
  No heat or soaks in any form
  Wash and dry carefully
  No astringents
  Antifungal medication as needed
  Lanolin preparation or petroleum jelly as needed
  No bathroom surgery
  Proper nail, corn, and callus treatment
**FITTED FOOTWEAR**
  No barefoot walking
  No crowding from the toes to the heel
  Podiatric appliances, such as molded insoles
  Keep feet and shoes dry
  Break in new shoes slowly
  Inspect footwear for foreign bodies or wear
**AVOID POTENTIALLY INJURIOUS OBJECTS AND SITUATIONS;
  KEEP NIGHT-LIGHT IN BATHROOM AND BEDROOM**
**EARLY AND PROMPT REPORTING OF ANY CHANGES OR CONCERNS**

---

(see Chap. 147). It appears at a younger age, there is an almost equal affinity for men and women, and bilateral involvement is usual. The pathology of atherosclerosis resembles that of the nondiabetic, with three main distinctions. There is a predilection for the more distal tibial/peroneal vessels of the lower leg, as demonstrated by the fact that 40% of diabetics presenting with gangrene will have a palpable popliteal pulse. The foot arteries, especially the dorsalis pedis and its branches, are usually spared. There is no occlusive microvascular lesion affecting the foot arteries that precludes revascularization, and this myth must be eliminated to reduce the frequency of major amputation.[2,3] Diabetics also tend to have poor collateral circulation, with much more atherosclerotic involvement of the distal zones of the profunda femoral artery and the infragenicular arteries.[4] Further, the atherosclerotic plaque and media of diabetic arteries frequently contain extensive calcium (medial calcinosis), making the artery rigid and noncompressible. These peculiarities may explain the interpretive results of standard noninvasive tests, which are often incorrect or misleading when applied to the diabetic lower extremity.[5] Ischemia may complicate up to 60% of nonhealing diabetic foot ulcers.

## INFECTION

Diabetic patients tolerate infection poorly. Infection prevents diabetic control, and uncontrolled diabetes affects infection. Defects in the host defense mechanism of many diabetics predispose them to infection and certainly alter their response to infections. Chemotaxis, phagocytosis, and the bactericidal function of diabetic neutrophils are diminished, particularly in patients with hyperglycemia or ketoacidosis (see Chap. 152). Systemic signs and symptoms (such as fever or elevation of the white blood cell count) of a septic process often occur late, making unexplained and uncontrolled hyperglycemia the only reliable sign of a potentially limb-threatening infection.[6,7] Patients with a foot ulcer should not be sent home just because they are afebrile or have a normal white blood cell count.

More commonly, it is a combination of the three primary pathologic situations that interact to cause the problem.[8,8a] The unprotected neuropathic foot is particularly prone to breakdown and ulcerations. Vascular compromise in the traumatized area delays an already compromised host response to infection, the delivery of antimicrobial agents to the area, and proper wound healing.

## MANAGEMENT

### IMPORTANCE OF PREVENTION

The most successful management of diabetic foot problems begins with prevention. The level of patient education and understanding correlates inversely with the development of foot problems. The same must be said for the physician who elects to care for these patients. Both must realize that any traumatic lesion or ulcer on the lower extremity is important and must be attended to immediately.

The patient should be educated to understand his or her responsibilities as outlined in Table 154-1. Patients and their families need to establish a routine that begins with daily inspection of the feet and legs. Because the loss of visual acuity is common in many diabetic patients, a family member or friend may help look for calluses, fissures, red or ecchymotic areas, fungal infections, and open sores or blisters. Proper hygiene includes washing and drying the feet carefully and avoiding the use of all astringents. Heat or soaks in any form are to be avoided. Lanolin preparations or petroleum jelly must be used on dry areas, and antifungal medication should be used as needed. "Bathroom surgery" must be avoided, especially for the nails, corns, or calluses. When nails are trimmed, a slight rounding of the edges is preferred.

Proper footwear is essential because the diabetic will not tolerate crowding in any area of the foot. Podiatric appliances such as inserts and spacers are often needed to protect sensitive, high-risk areas. Extra-depth shoes may be helpful, but simply changing shoes periodically during the day suffices for most patients. The diabetic should never go barefoot and should avoid situations likely to cause problems. There should be a night-light in the bedroom. All footwear must be inspected daily for foreign bodies or wear, and new shoes must be broken in slowly. Although these principles sound simple, it must be remembered that it is patient understanding and adherence to proper care that play a primary role in avoidance of foot problems.[8]

### THERAPY FOR A FOOT ULCER

The course of treatment for a foot ulcer depends on its severity[9,10] (Table 154-2). The first major decision is whether the patient needs to be admitted to the hospital or treated at home. The severity of tissue destruction may not be totally apparent to the patient from just looking at the ulcer or infected callus, especially in those who continue to bear weight on a painless area or do not have the visual acuity to recognize a problem. It is imperative for the physician to unroof all encrusted areas and inspect the wound to determine the extent of any deep tissue destruction and the presence of any possible bone and/or joint involvement. The physician must emphasize to the patient and family the importance of debridement and inspection so that the patient understands that the debridement did not cause the problem.

Early superficial ulcers may be treated at home provided that cellulitis, if present, is only minimal; that there is no evidence of any systemic toxicity; and that the patient is compliant and reliable, and has a vigilant support system. The injured foot must be put to complete rest; neuropathy includes sensory and proprioceptor loss, so that partial

**TABLE 154-2.**
**Diabetic Foot Ulcer**

| Mild | Limb Threatening |
|---|---|
| Superficial | Deep ulcer |
| Minimal or no cellulitis | ±Bone involvement |
| No bone involvement | >2-cm cellulitis |
| No systemic toxicity | Threatened limb loss |
| | ±Systemic toxicity |
| $R_x$ | $R_x$ |
| Rest injured part | Immediate admission |
| Culture and sensitivities | Control blood glucose |
| Initial broad-spectrum oral anti- | Culture and sensitivities |
| biotic (change based on sensi- | Initial broad-spectrum intravenous anti- |
| tivities and response) | biotics; specific antibiotics based on |
| Careful debridement | sensitivities and response |
| Local dressings | Early surgical debridement, dependent |
| Podiatric appliances and special | drainage and open amputation |
| shoes | Local dressings |
| Careful follow-up | Later selected revascularization and con- |
| | servative amputations or revisions |
| | Podiatric appliances and special shoes |
| | Careful follow-up |

weight-bearing as perceived by the patient actually may be full weight-bearing. If infection is present, cultures are taken and initially a broad-spectrum oral antibiotic is started and changed, pending subsequent sensitivity reports and the response of the wound. *Staphylococcus aureus* and *Streptococcus* species are most often cultured, and antibiotic therapy should at least effectively cover these organisms. Dressings must be kept simple, such as plain gauze sponges moistened with diluted isotonic antiseptic solutions applied to the open areas one to two times a day. Quarter-strength povidone-iodine (Betadine) or plain saline is frequently used. Dry cracks or fissures respond to antibiotic ointments or lanolin-based creams. Dressings can easily be done by the patient, a family member, or a friend; this will become even more important with increasing cost constraints on all treatment programs. Whirlpools, heat, or soaks in any form are to be avoided, as is the use of enzymatic debriding agents or astringents. If an ulcer is infected and if there is no significant improvement within 48 hours, hospitalization is advised.

Once healing is achieved under careful surveillance, graduated weight-bearing is begun, with podiatric appliances and modifications of footwear a prerequisite for sensitive, high-risk areas of the foot. A Charcot joint may develop if weight-bearing progresses too rapidly. Its presentation may be strikingly similar to that of an acute infection, with warmth, redness, and swelling.[11] With an early Charcot joint, there is usually no open area and an antecedent history of some minor trauma initiating the process. The radiographic picture may be misinterpreted as osteomyelitis, but the experienced clinician can usually make the diagnosis, especially if it is included early in the differential diagnosis.

## LIMB-THREATENING INFECTIONS

Limb-threatening infections (see Table 154-2) require immediate admission to the hospital, with the patient placed on complete bed rest. Because hyperglycemia must be brought under control rapidly, insulin (not oral agents) is most often required. Although the patient's condition must be stabilized medically, this should not delay necessary surgical intervention. The essentials for limb salvage include proper surgical

wound care and antibiotic therapy. Frequently, systemic toxicity or shock will not be reversed until the septic process is debrided and drained. It is a fallacy to think that antibiotics alone will solve the problem. In the author's experience, 6-week courses of antibiotics alone to treat deeply infected wounds and osteomyelitis frequently result in failure and a higher amputation level.

The choice of an initial antibiotic regimen is influenced by several variables, including likely pathogens, Gram staining of the purulent material, local bacterial resistance patterns, prior antibiotic therapy, preexisting renal or hepatic dysfunction, and the severity of the infection. A review of diabetic patients with serious limb-threatening infections has emphasized the importance of mixed and multiple organisms (3.2 isolates per ulcer).[12] Aerobic gram-positive cocci (93%) and gram-negative bacilli (50%) are prevalent in a similar manner, whether systemic toxicity is present or not. Anaerobic cultures are positive in 69% of patients. Certainly, any wound that has crepitance; a foul, fetid odor; or gas evident on radiography is harboring anaerobes. As soon as deep cultures are obtained, broad-spectrum intravenous antibiotics are administered to ensure adequate serum levels. Later, changes are made depending on sensitivity reports and the response of the infection, provided that proper wound care has been achieved.

Proper surgical wound care is essential to the successful management of any limb-threatening infection.[7,9] This requires immediate surgical debridement of all necrotic tissue and drainage of pus. This must be done even in a patient with compromised circulation. Vascular reconstruction in a patient with an ongoing limb-threatening infection is contraindicated. The severity of tissue destruction and sepsis may not be totally apparent from looking at the ulcer or infected callus. Diabetics do not tolerate undrained infection; adequate debridement cannot be achieved in a deep necrotic diabetic wound using small stab wounds or drains. The debridement and drainage must be such that all necrotic material is removed and dependent drainage is adequate to prevent any pooling of pus.

Dressings are initiated with the initial surgical procedure. The purpose of the dressing is to provide a moistened wound environment, most conducive to healing. The dressing should protect the wound, absorb excess exudate, and also protect the wound and other high-risk areas. The most effective dressings are plain gauze sponges moistened with isotonic antiseptic solutions or saline and applied to the open wound two to three times a day. Whirlpools, soaks, or hot compresses are avoided because they may lead to more complications. Enzymatic debriding ointments and other astringents, especially full-strength solutions, are also to be avoided, because they are injurious to already compromised tissues.

Topical growth factors may hold promise for the future, but they are expensive for routine use and further clinical trials are needed. There is no indication for hyperbaric oxygen limb chambers and little evidence supporting immersion chambers for routine treatment of infected diabetic ulcers.

Other important measures are to control edema and to ensure adequate nutritional support and blood sugar control. Physical therapy and conditioning exercises are extremely important throughout the course of treatment.

## OSTEOMYELITIS

Inadequate diagnosis and treatment of osteomyelitis increase the risk of major amputation. All of the reports recommending one or more combinations of any of the current radiologic imaging techniques are flawed, and these tests are expensive. A sterile probe hitting the bone or joint is equal in sensitivity and specificity to any of these tests. A plain radiograph is recommended on admission, but special scans are reserved for complicated cases where probing is equivocal. Prolonged courses of antibiotics rarely cure osteomyelitis, especially cases with associated deep infection, gangrene, ischemia, and bacteremia. Dead necrotic infected bone should be removed for the reasons mentioned previously.

## ROLE OF VASCULAR RECONSTRUCTION

Once the situation is fully stabilized, arteriographic visualization of the foot vessels and vascular reconstruction can be undertaken in selected patients with vascular insufficiency who are suitable candidates.[13,13a] The results of inflow and outflow procedures in diabetics compare favorably with those dealing primarily with nondiabetic patients, in whom most of the procedures are done for claudication and not for limb salvage.[14,15,15a] The major difference is that ~33% of the diabetics are dead at 5 years from other complications. Advances in arteriography, microscopic loops, fine arterial sutures, needles, and instruments now allow for routine successful revascularization of the pedal arteries of ischemic diabetic feet.[16]

In diabetic patients with extensive foot tissue loss, maximizing arterial flow by restoring a pulse to the foot achieves the most rapid and durable healing. The dorsalis pedis bypass constitutes > 25% of the author's distal vascular reconstructions, with a 5-year patency of 82% and limb salvage of 88% in > 500 patients who otherwise faced a major amputation.

If successful revascularization is accomplished, more conservative reconstructive foot surgery, distal amputations, or revisions can be carried out to achieve healing and limb salvage.[17] Gradual and progressive weight-bearing under careful surveillance is mandatory and often requires special orthotics and/or shoes to keep these high-risk areas healed and pressure free.

## CONCLUSION

The fear of gangrene or amputation is one of the overwhelming concerns of diabetic patients who experience the many complications of their disease. Neuropathy, ischemia, and an altered host defense mechanism make these patients particularly prone to developing foot ulcers, which often become infected. Occasionally, it is only the complications of odor, hyperglycemia, or systemic symptoms that bring the patient to the hospital with a septic foot.

Preventing limb-threatening ulcers or infections begins with patient education and understanding. Early recognition of any foot problem and its prompt treatment are essential. Treating serious limb-threatening conditions requires considerable experience. Diabetics generally have greater risk factors (usually cardiac), and diabetic arteries require the maximum skill and experience of the operating surgeon. A team approach is the most cost-effective method to salvage the diabetic foot.[18] In the past decade, the amputation rate at all levels of the diabetic lower extremity has been reduced by utilizing the concepts outlined in this chapter.[19] An aggressive approach to limb salvage is less expensive than resorting to major amputation, and the benefits to the patient and society are unquestionably superior.[20]

## REFERENCES

1. US Department of Health and Human Services. Healthy People 2000—national health promotion and disease prevention objectives. Washington, DC: US Government Printing Office, 1991:73.
2. LoGerfo FW, Coffman JD. Vascular and microvascular disease in the diabetic foot: implications for foot care. N Engl J Med 1984; 311:1615.
3. Berceli SA, Chan AK, Pomposelli FB Jr. Efficacy of dorsal pedal artery bypass in limb salvage for ischemic heel ulcers. J Vasc Surg 1999; 30:499.
4. King TA, DePalma RG, Rhodes RS. Diabetes mellitus and atherosclerosis involvement of the profunda femoris artery. Surg Gynecol Obstet 1984; 159:553.
5. Gibbons GW, Wheelock FC Jr. Problems in the noninvasive evaluation of the peripheral circulation in the diabetic. Prac Cardiol 1982; 8:115.
6. Gibbons GW, Freeman DV. Diabetic foot infections. In: Howard RJ, Simmons RL, eds. Surgical infectious diseases. Norwalk, CT: Appleton & Lange, 1988:585.
7. Gibbons GW. Diabetic foot sepsis. In: Brewster D, ed. Common problems in vascular surgery. Chicago: Year Book, 1989:412.
8. Delbridge L, Appleberg M, Reeve TS. Factors associated with development of foot lesions in the diabetic. Surgery 1983; 93:78.
8a. Benotmane A, Mohammedi F, Ayed F, et al. Diabetic foot lesions: etiologic and prognostic factors. Diabetes Metab 2000; 26:113.
9. Gibbons GW, Wheelock FC Jr. Cutaneous ulcers of the diabetic foot. In: Ernest CB, Stanley JC, eds. Current therapy in vascular surgery. Philadelphia: BC Decker, 1987:233.
10. Gibbons GW. Diabetic foot sepsis. Semin Vasc Surg 1992; 5(4):1.
11. Sinha S, Frykberg RG, Kozak GP. Neuroarthropathy in the diabetic foot. In: Kozak G, ed. Clinical diabetes mellitus. Philadelphia: WB Saunders, 1983:415.
12. Gibbons GW, Eliopoulos GM. Infection of the diabetic foot. In: Kozak GP, Hoar CS, Rowbotham JL, et al., eds. Management of the diabetic foot problem. Joslin Clinic and New England Deaconess Hospital. Philadelphia: WB Saunders, 1984:97.
13. Gibbons GW, Freeman DV. Vascular evaluation and treatment of the diabetic. Clin Podiatr Med Surg 1987; 4:337.
13a. Feinglass J, Kaushik S, Handel D, et al. Peripheral bypass surgery and amputation: northern Illinois demographics. Arch Surg 2000; 135:75.
14. Hoar CS, Campbell DR. Aorto-iliac reconstruction. In: Kozak GP, Hoar CS, Rowbotham JL, et al., eds. Management of the diabetic foot problem. Joslin Clinic and New England Deaconess Hospital. Philadelphia: WB Saunders, 1984:159.
15. Wheelock FC, Gibbons GW. Arterial reconstruction: femoral, popliteal, tibial. In: Kozak GP, Hoar CS, Rowbotham JL, et al., eds. Management of the diabetic foot problem. Joslin Clinic and New England Deaconess Hospital. Philadelphia: WB Saunders, 1984:173.
15a. Akbari CM, Pomposelli FB Jr, Gibbons GW, et al. Lower extremity revascularization in diabetes: late observations. Arch Surg 2000; 135:452.
16. Pomposelli FB, Jepson SJ, Gibbons GW, et al. A flexible approach to infrapopliteal vein grafts in patients with diabetes mellitus. Arch Surg 1991; 126:724.
17. LoGerfo FW, Gibbons GW, Pomposelli FB, et al. Trends in the care of the diabetic foot. Arch Surg 1992; 127:617.
18. Caputo GM, Cavanagh PR, Ulbrecht JS, et al. Current concepts: assessment and management of foot disease in patients with diabetes. N Engl J Med 1994; 13:854.
19. Gibbons GW, Maracaccio EJ, Burgess AM, et al. Improved quality of diabetic foot care, 1984 vs. 1990: reduced length of stay and costs, insufficient reimbursement. Arch Surg 1993; 1283:576.
20. Gibbons GW, Burgess AM, Guadagnoli E, et al. Return to well-being and function after infrainguinal revascularization. J Vasc Surg 1995;21:35.

# CHAPTER 155

# DIABETIC ACIDOSIS, HYPEROSMOLAR COMA, AND LACTIC ACIDOSIS

K. GEORGE M. M. ALBERTI

The diabetic acidoses and comas remain a significant cause of mortality and morbidity, much of it unnecessary. Many of the problems encountered could be avoided by the education of patients, health care professionals, and physicians in appropriate preventive measures and by the use of systematic, logical therapy. Several reviews are recommended for further reading.[1-9]

## DIABETIC KETOACIDOSIS

Diabetic ketoacidosis (DKA) may be defined as a state of uncontrolled diabetes mellitus in which there is hyperglycemia (usually >300 mg/dL or 16.7 mmol/L) with a significant lowering of arterial blood pH (<7.3) and an elevation of total blood ketone body concentration (β-hydroxybutyrate [3-hydroxybutyrate] plus acetoacetate; >5 mmol/L). The cutoff between DKA and hyperosmolar hyperglycemic nonketotic coma (HONK) is somewhat arbitrary, although hyperglycemia tends to be much more severe in the latter, with ketone body levels lower.

## EPIDEMIOLOGY

There are few good data available on the incidence of DKA. In a survey in Rhode Island, DKA accounted for 1.6% of all admissions to the hospital, with previously undiagnosed diabetes accounting for 20% of these. The annual incidence was 14 per 100,000 people.[10] In Denmark an annual incidence of 4.5% was reported, with highest risk in female adolescents.[11] The best data have been compiled by the National Diabetes Group in the United States, who report an annual incidence of three to eight episodes per 1000 diabetic patients, with 20% to 30% occurring in new diabetics.[12] Higher figures have been reported by the Centers for Disease Control and Prevention[13] at 26 to 38 per 100,000 population and an annual incidence of 1.0% to 1.5% of all diabetics in the period 1980 to 1987. Rates were three-fold higher in black men than in white men. There is increasing recognition of DKA in type 2 diabetic patients, particularly nonwhites such as American Indians,[14] Japanese,[15] blacks,[16] and Asian Indians.[17]

Mortality for established DKA is relatively high, accounting for 10% of all diabetes-related deaths in the United States between 1970 and 1978.[18] Rates were highest in nonwhites and in the older than 65-year-old age group (59% of all DKA deaths). In most published series, mortality lies between 4% and 10%, although 0% has been reported in one large series in the United States.[19] A report from Birmingham, United Kingdom, showed a rate of 3.9% in 929 episodes over a 21-year period, with <2% in those younger than 70 years of age.[20] In nonspecialized centers, rates increase to 20% or 25%, with even higher rates in the elderly. Poor prognostic factors include age, low pH, hypotension, high plasma urea and glucose, and severe associated disease. Many of the deaths, particularly metabolic deaths in younger patients, are avoidable.[21]

## PATHOPHYSIOLOGY

DKA results from absolute or relative insulin deficiency.[1–4] In the former, there is a total lack of insulin, as found in a newly presenting, young patient with insulin-dependent (type 1) diabetes mellitus. In relative insulin deficiency, circulating insulin is present, but there is excessive secretion of the counterregulatory hormones (e.g., glucagon, catecholamines, cortisol, growth hormone), and insulin secretion cannot increase sufficiently to counter their actions.

Normally, metabolic homeostasis is maintained by a fine balance between the actions of insulin and the actions of the counterregulatory hormones. Insulin has anabolic and anticatabolic actions; the other hormones are primarily catabolic, with the exception of growth hormone, which has both anabolic (i.e., protein metabolism) and catabolic (i.e., carbohydrate and lipid metabolism) effects. The normal control of metabolism by insulin and the catabolic hormones is reviewed in Chapters 129 and 134 and is outlined here only briefly.

### FAT METABOLISM

In the fed state in healthy persons, the high circulating insulin levels inhibit adipose tissue lipolysis and stimulate reesterification through the provision of glycerol 3-phosphate from glucose, which is actively transported into the cell. Endothelial cell lipoprotein lipase activity in adipose tissue is also stimulated, releasing fatty acids from triglycerides, which diffuse into the adipocyte and are esterified to form triglyceride (Fig. 155-1). In the fasted state, the lower insulin levels are adequate to reduce but not prevent lipolysis, reesterification is low, and fatty acids (and glycerol) diffuse into the circulation. Lipolysis is maintained through the actions of the catecholamines and cortisol.

The increased circulating fatty acids are taken up by the liver and activated to fatty acyl-coenzyme A (CoA). In the fed state, these would be mainly esterified to triglyceride. At the same time, insulin stimulates de novo synthesis of fatty acids from

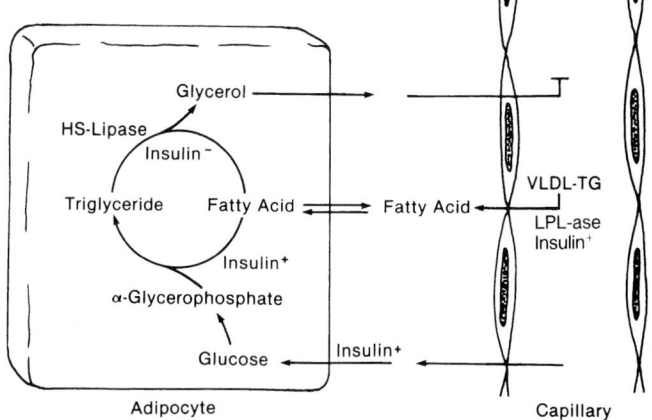

**FIGURE 155-1.** Adipose tissue fatty acid metabolism. (*HS-Lipase*, hormone-sensitive lipase; *LPL-ase*, lipoprotein lipase; *Insulin+*, stimulated by insulin; *Insulin−*, inhibited by insulin; *VLDL-TG*, very-low-density lipoprotein triglyceride.)

glucose, which follows the same route. In the fasted state, the actions of glucagon predominate, with fatty acyl-CoA entering the mitochondria via the carnitine shuttle (Fig. 155-2). This is the key regulatory step through modulation of the enzyme carnitine acyl transferase I situated on the outer membrane of the mitochondrion. Lack of insulin causes direct stimulation of enzyme activity, and a decrease in the levels of malonyl-CoA has the same effect. Malonyl-CoA is a key intermediate early in the fatty acid synthetic pathway. This pathway is stimulated by insulin and inhibited by glucagon by direct actions on acetyl-CoA carboxylase; in the fasted state, the high glucagon and low insulin levels result in low activity and low malonyl-CoA levels. Glucagon also increases the amount of carnitine available for the shuttle, probably by enhancing hepatic uptake of carnitine, with activation of the shuttle through a mass action effect.

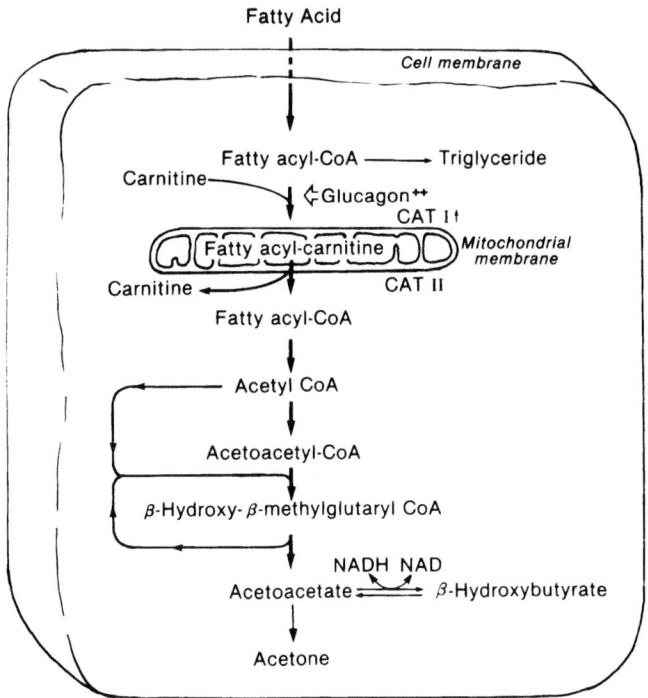

**FIGURE 155-2.** Ketone body formation in liver cells in insulin deficiency. (*CAT I* and *CAT II*, carnitine acyl transferases I and II; *CoA*, coenzyme A; *NAD*, nicotinamide adenine dinucleotide; *NADH*, nicotinamide adenine dinucleotide [reduced form].)

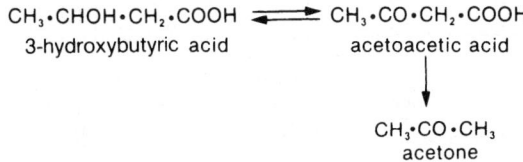

$$CH_3 \cdot CHOH \cdot CH_2 \cdot COOH \rightleftharpoons CH_3 \cdot CO \cdot CH_2 \cdot COOH$$

3-hydroxybutyric acid          acetoacetic acid

$$\downarrow$$

$$CH_3 \cdot CO \cdot CH_3$$
acetone

**FIGURE 155-3.** Ketone bodies. Note that 3-hydroxybutyric acid is not chemically a ketone, but it is referred to as a ketone body.

The net result is an increase in fatty acid oxidation, with the formation of increased quantities of acetyl-CoA and the formation of acetoacetyl-CoA through 3-hydroxy-3-methylglutaryl-CoA. Some acetyl-CoA condenses with oxaloacetate to form citrate, which enters the tricarboxylic acid cycle, but the capacity for this is limited and oxaloacetate levels are decreased in severe insulin deficiency. Acetoacetyl-CoA is converted to acetoacetate and 3-hydroxybutyrate, with some spontaneous decarboxylation of the former to yield acetone (Fig. 155-3). Acetone levels may approach those of acetoacetate in insulin deficiency. The ketone bodies cannot be used in the liver because the enzyme thiolase is lacking. They diffuse into the circulation and are used as fuels by many tissues after being converted to acetoacetyl-CoA and acetyl-CoA.

In starvation, there is controlled release of ketone bodies into the circulation, with levels reaching a plateau at 4 to 6 mmol/L after several days, as utilization matches production, although there are some urinary losses. There is sufficient insulin available to balance the effects of glucagon and the other catabolic hormones. In severe insulin deficiency, absolute or relative, the key factors are a large increase in fatty acid supply to the liver and unrestrained β-oxidation and ketone body production. Indeed, the former may be sufficient to saturate the mitochondrial uptake mechanisms, and there is spillover into triglyceride production, with resultant fatty liver and hypertriglyceridemia. There is diminished extrahepatic ketone body use because insulin is lacking.

Ketone bodies accumulate in the circulation and levels may reach concentrations of 30 mmol/L. The two major ketone bodies are weak acids, and they dissociate completely at normal pH. This creates a major hydrogen ion load that soon exceeds normal buffering mechanisms. Hyperventilation eliminates some of the acid, and there is a loss of hydrogen ions in the urine buffered by phosphate and ammonia. Some ketone bodies are lost in the urine, with sodium as the accompanying cation.

The excess hydrogen ions have pathophysiologic consequences. They have a negative inotropic effect and cause peripheral vasodilatation, resulting in lower blood pressure (BP). The peripheral vasodilatation also explains both the warm periphery displayed by most patients, even when they are hypotensive and dehydrated, and the low or normal body temperature during infection. If pH levels fall below 7.0, there may be inhibition of the central nervous system. One reflection of this is inhibition of the respiratory center, causing a paradoxically normal respiratory rate. Insulin resistance also occurs, exacerbating the ketoacidotic state. This is not, however, a major problem during therapy. Hydrogen ion excess also displaces potassium from within cells. There is some dispute about whether this occurs with organic acidemias, but plasma $K^+$ levels rise with acute ketoacidosis in humans.[22]

## CARBOHYDRATE METABOLISM

In normal persons in the fasted state, there is a controlled supply of glucose from the liver, maintaining blood-glucose levels between approximately 54 and 90 mg/dL (3–5 mmol/L; see Chap. 205). Gluconeogenesis is promoted by glucagon, cortisol, and catecholamines, and glycogenolysis is fostered by glucagon and catecholamines. Insulin exerts an anticatabolic effect by decreasing these processes. In extrahepatic tissues, there is

insufficient insulin to enhance glucose uptake, particularly in muscle and adipose tissue. Catecholamines, cortisol, and growth hormone also inhibit glucose uptake. Fatty acids and ketone bodies become major oxidative fuels. There is an increase in the flow of the gluconeogenic substrates, lactate, pyruvate, glycerol, and alanine to the liver, with increased hepatic extraction. Glucagon enhances alanine uptake, and cortisol induces several transaminases, increasing the carbon skeletons available for gluconeogenesis.

In the liver, the key regulatory step for glycogenolysis and for gluconeogenesis is as follows:

phosphofructokinase

FRUCTOSE 6-PHOSPHATE ⇌ FRUCTOSE 1,6-BISPHOSPHATE

fructose 1,6-bisphosphatase

This step is finely regulated by fructose 2,6-bisphosphate, which stimulates phosphofructokinase and inhibits fructose 1,6-bisphosphatase, increasing flux down the glycolytic pathway. Glucagon, and to a lesser extent epinephrine, inhibits fructose 2,6-bisphosphate formation. Thus, in the fasted state, there is an increased flow of carbon toward gluconeogenesis. The effects of glucagon on this process are sustained, but glucagon has shorter effects on glycogenolysis. This makes teleologic sense in that supplies of glycogen are limited.

In the fed state, glycogenolysis and gluconeogenesis are inhibited. Insulin levels are high, and glycogen synthesis from glucose 6-phosphate is stimulated through activation of glycogen synthase. The amount of dietary glucose passing directly to glycogen is small. Instead, glucose is broken down to lactate and pyruvate in the intestinal mucosa, and these intermediates pass directly to the liver by the portal vein for incorporation into glycogen. Similarly, some lactate and pyruvate from peripheral tissues follow the same route (Fig. 155-4). At the same time, hepatic glycolysis is stimulated by insulin. These two processes (gluconeogenesis and glycolysis) probably occur in different cell types in the liver. At first, this looks like a catabolic process, but it is the route for de novo fatty acid synthesis

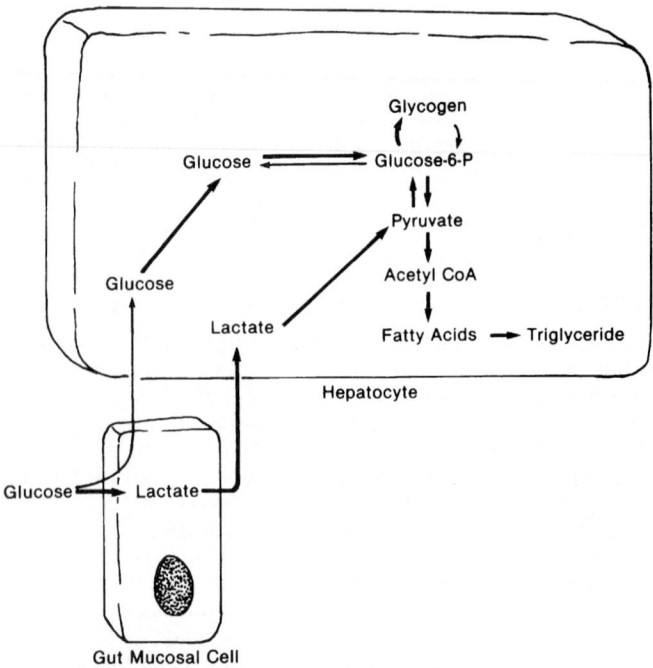

**FIGURE 155-4.** Hepatic glucose metabolism in the fed state. (*CoA*, coenzyme A; *glucose-6-P*, glucose-6-phosphate.)

from glucose and allows for the storage of excess dietary carbohydrate as fat. Insulin stimulates pyruvate dehydrogenase, yielding acetyl-CoA and then malonyl-CoA through the action of acetyl-CoA carboxylase at the beginning of the fatty acid synthetic pathway. The fatty acids are then esterified and transported to adipose tissue as very low-density lipoproteins. There is a paradox in that both glycolysis and upward flow of three-carbon units must be happening simultaneously. This probably is achieved by heterogeneity of function within the hepatocyte population. In extrahepatic tissues, primarily muscle and adipose tissue, insulin enhances glucose uptake through mobilization of glucose transporters. In muscle, glycogen reserves are replenished, and glucose is used as an oxidative fuel, with lipid metabolism decreased. In adipose tissue, there is increased glycerol 3-phosphate ($\alpha$-glycerophosphate) formation and reesterification of fatty acids from lipolysis and from circulating very low-density lipoproteins.

In insulin deficiency, absolute or relative, there is accentuation of the processes seen in the fasted state. Thus, hepatic glucose production rapidly increases, doubling within 2 hours of insulin deprivation of insulin-treated diabetic patients.[23] There is a small mass action effect of glucose tending to inhibit glucose production, but this is insufficient to make a significant impact. In the fed state, hepatic glucose production remains unabated, peripheral glucose uptake and metabolism are diminished, and hyperglycemia is greatly accentuated. Experimentally, insulin deficiency is associated with a failure to mobilize and synthesize GLUT4, the insulin-sensitive glucose transporter.[24] For more severe hyperglycemia to occur, the catabolic hormones are critical. Glucagon levels increase early in insulin deprivation, with cortisol levels increasing later. In pancreatectomized patients, insulin deprivation results in a much diminished and sluggish rise in plasma glucose levels and very little increase in ketogenesis. In pure insulin deficiency, there is a long prodromal period before very high glucose levels are found. This may be related to the developing acidemia, with the stimulating effects of the increased production of reducing equivalents from $\beta$-oxidation. In most cases of DKA, precipitating factors cause a rapid rise in catabolic hormone secretion, which will cause rapidly accelerated glucose production. Experimental insulin deficiency is also accompanied by a fall in free insulin-like growth factor-I (IGF-I) levels that will further compound the hyperglycemia.[25] In established DKA, secretion of all the counterregulatory hormones is markedly increased, leading to a vicious metabolic circle.

The hyperglycemia is associated with glycosuria as the renal threshold for glucose is exceeded. If sustained, this causes an osmotic diuresis, with considerable loss of fluid and electrolytes. In severe DKA, the following deficits, expressed per kilogram of body weight, are encountered: water, 50 to 100 mL; sodium, 7 to 10 mmol; potassium, 3 to 12 mmol; chloride, 4 to 7 mmol; phosphate, 0.5 to 1.5 mmol; magnesium, 0.25 to 0.75 mmol; and calcium, 0.25 to 0.75 mmol. The loss is hypotonic with respect to saline, which has implications for replacement therapy. There is progressive dehydration, with loss of intracellular fluids and electrolytes into the extracellular fluid, with the water and potassium lost into the urine. Eventually, there is hypovolemia with hypotension and tachycardia, which are worsened by the acidemia.

### PROTEIN METABOLISM

In the fed state, insulin stimulates amino-acid uptake by tissues such as muscle and increases protein synthesis. This effect is balanced by cortisol, which promotes protein degradation. In the fasted state, if insulin levels are low, there is controlled degradation of protein, enabling amino acids to be used for gluconeogenesis. The plasma levels of branched chain amino acids are increased, and alanine levels tend to fall. There is a clear reciprocal relationship between alanine and ketone body levels, which tends to conserve amino acids when ketone body levels are high.

Insulin deficiency leads to increased protein degradation and decreased protein synthesis, with the increase in amino-acid availability providing the substrate for gluconeogenesis. Clinically, this protein catabolism is reflected as muscle wasting, with visceral proteins tending to be spared. Wasting is apparent, however, only if there has been a prolonged prodromal period.

### PRECIPITATING FACTORS

Infection is by far the most common of the precipitating factors for DKA, causing >50% of identified causes in nearly all series. This may occur in established type 1 diabetics or in previously undiagnosed patients, who form 20% to 30% of the total admissions. Infections may be minor, such as urinary tract infection, skin lesions, or bacterial throat infections, or more severe. Infection causes a marked increase in secretion of cortisol and glucagon. Established type 1 diabetics with infections often diminish their food intake and may mistakenly decrease their insulin doses, whereas these should be increased based on the results of home blood glucose monitoring. Urine ketones should also be checked routinely in ill type 1 diabetics with increased insulin doses if ketones are more than trace positive.

Other precipitating factors include omission of insulin doses in known type 1 diabetics, a well-known phenomenon in many "brittle" diabetics and in any young type 1 diabetic with recurrent episodes of DKA. In a large study in Scotland, young people admitted in DKA were less likely to have taken their prescribed doses of insulin,[26] and in New Zealand, 61% of DKA patients were found to have made errors in insulin self-administration.[27] Children with DKA have a greater risk of associated psychopathology[28] and are more likely to come from disadvantaged backgrounds.[29] Children presenting for the first time in DKA tend to be those with the lowest C-peptide (i.e., insulin) reserves.[30] Another cause of "pure" insulin deficiency is the malfunction of insulin infusion devices, with very high occurrence rates in some centers, in particular because of catheter failure, with a rate of 0.14 per patient-year in one large series.[31]

Other established precipitating factors include cerebrovascular accidents, acute myocardial infarction, and trauma. Each of these is accompanied by increased secretion of catecholamines, glucagon, and cortisol, with predictable metabolic consequences if insulin doses are not increased. Rarer causes include *Fourier gangrene* (sudden, severe gangrene of the scrotum), infusion of $\beta$-sympathomimetic agents, pheochromocytoma, and treatment with the antipsychotic drugs clozapine and olanzapine.[32]

### SIGNS AND SYMPTOMS

The classic clinical presentation of severe DKA includes Kussmaul respiration (i.e., deep, sighing hyperventilation), dehydration, hypotension, tachycardia, warm skin, normal or low temperature, and altered state of consciousness. Only ~10% are totally unconscious, and even this figure has diminished recently. Often, the breath smells of acetone, and there may be oliguria in the later stages. Preceding symptoms include nausea and vomiting, thirst, and polyuria in nearly all cases, and, less commonly, leg cramps and abdominal pain.

There may also be no bowel sounds, with gastric stasis and pooling of fluid. Occasionally, the patient may present with an acute abdomen (pain and rigidity). If this occurs in young patients, virtually all cases resolve with conservative treatment; in older patients, there may be intraabdominal disease.[33] It is sensible to treat the metabolic disturbance first. If there is no resolution or there is worsening of the abdominal state during

TABLE 155-1.
Signs and Symptoms of Diabetic Ketoacidosis

| Symptoms, Signs | Cause |
|---|---|
| Polyuria, polydipsia | Osmotic diuresis |
| Anorexia, fatigue | ? |
| Nausea, vomiting | ?Ketosis |
| Weight loss | Protein, fat catabolism |
| Abdominal pain | ?$K^+$ depletion, fluid pooling |
| Leg cramps | ?$K^+$ depletion |
| Dehydration | Osmotic diuresis |
| Hypotension | Dehydration, acidemia |
| Tachycardia | Dehydration, acidemia |
| Hyperventilation | Acidemia |
| Gastric stasis | ?$K^+$ depletion |
| Hypothermia | Peripheral vasodilation, acidemia |
| Impaired consciousness | Hyperosmolality |

the first 3 to 4 hours of treatment, diagnostic reevaluation should be considered.

Nearly all the signs and symptoms of DKA can be ascribed to different aspects of the metabolic disturbance (Table 155-1). Thus, the dehydration, polyuria, and thirst are secondary to the osmotic diuresis. The hypotension and tachycardia are caused by the fluid loss and the acidemia. Acidemia also causes the hyperventilation. The inappropriately low body temperature and warm skin are the result of the vasodilatation caused by the acidemia. The vomiting and nausea are probably the consequence of hyperketonemia, and the leg cramps and gastric stasis may be secondary to intracellular potassium depletion. The impaired consciousness correlates only with plasma osmolality, implying that intracellular fluid loss from cerebral cells is involved, although impaired cerebral circulation caused by hypotension may also contribute. Hypovolemia and hypotension cause prerenal failure with consequent oliguria.

## DIAGNOSIS

In most cases, the rapid diagnosis of DKA should be possible at the bedside (Table 155-2). The clinical history usually is helpful. Clinical examination and bedside measurement of blood glucose and plasma ketones (using a test strip) should complete the diagnosis. Emergency room staff should be instructed in test-strip glucose measurement. The condition of "euglycemic" ketoacidosis should also be noted, in which blood glucose levels are not very elevated despite severe ketoacidosis,[34] although if this is defined as a blood glucose level of ≤180 mg/dL, it is rare, occurring in only 1% of cases.[35] This has been found in patients who have been on insulin pump therapy, in those who have fasted for long periods before admission, and in pregnancy.[36] One study has confirmed that insulin deficiency in the fasted state is associated

with a more rapid rise in hydrogen ion concentration but a slower rise in blood glucose than in the fed state, although glucose levels still were not strictly "euglycemic."[37]

Ketone bodies in plasma are tested for, using either test strips or tablets. For tablets, plasma should be diluted and a positive result at a dilution of 1 in 8 or above is significant. For the test strips, 1-plus or more is significant. These nitroprusside-based tests respond only to acetoacetate and, to a lesser extent, acetone. If the 3-hydroxybutyrate:acetoacetate ratio is greatly elevated, which occasionally occurs in severe acidemia or anoxia, a false-negative finding may result. A sensitive whole blood β-hydroxybutyrate test strip has been developed, which should be helpful although it is not yet widely used.[38]

Using Table 155-2, it should be possible to distinguish clearly between the different diabetic comas. If there is doubt as to the presence of hypoglycemia, 20 mL of 50% glucose can be given intravenously (iv). The other diagnostic difficulty may be the distinction between severe DKA and lactic acidosis, because there is always some excess ketosis in the latter. Usually, blood glucose levels are much more elevated in DKA, but laboratory measurement may be necessary to distinguish between these two acidoses.

## INITIAL LABORATORY INVESTIGATIONS

At the same time as the diagnosis is being made at the bedside, various tests should be ordered (Table 155-3). The most urgent of these is arterial blood pH, because the extent of acidemia will influence treatment. If there is a problem obtaining arterial blood, capillary and venous measurements give remarkably similar results.[39] Generally, $PCO_2$ and $PO_2$ are estimated at the same time, the former helping if there is a mixed respiratory and metabolic acid-base disturbance.[40] Usually, the $PO_2$ is normal or high but, paradoxically, may be low in a significant number of older patients, presumably owing to pulmonary arteriovenous shunting.

Formal measurement of plasma glucose is required to confirm the diagnosis. Plasma urea, creatinine, and electrolyte levels also are essential. Creatinine gives an indication of dehydration and prerenal failure; plasma urea may indicate the extent of protein catabolism. The measurement of the four major electrolytes allows calculation of the anion gap. This usually is increased (>12), but patients can present with a normal anion gap and a hyperchloremic acidosis.[40] There are other causes of an acidosis with an increased anion gap, including lactic acidosis, uremia, and ingestion of agents such as methanol and salicylates; therefore, plasma ketones must be checked as well.[6] Plasma sodium levels usually are low despite the total body deficit of hypotonic saline. This is because the hyperglycemia draws fluid from the intracellular space, diluting the plasma. It can be calculated that for every 100-mg/dL elevation in plasma glucose, plasma sodium is decreased by 2.4 mmol/L; a plasma glucose of 750 mg/dL with a plasma sodium of 128 mmol/L implies a "true" sodium of 144 mmol/L.[41] Pseudohy-

TABLE 155-2.
Bedside Differential Diagnosis of Coma

| Diagnosis | Blood Glucose* (mg/dL) | Plasma Ketones* | Hyperventilation | Dehydration | Blood Pressure | Skin |
|---|---|---|---|---|---|---|
| Diabetic ketoacidosis | >300 | + to +++ | ++ | ++ | Low to normal | Warm |
| Hyperosmolar, hyperglycemic, nonketotic coma | >500 | 0 to + | 0 | +++ | Low to normal | Normal |
| Hypoglycemic coma | <50 | 0 | 0 | 0 | Normal | Cold, clammy |
| Lactic acidosis | 20–200 | Tr to + | +++ | 0 | Low | Warm |
| Nonmetabolic comas | Normal or raised | 0 to Tr | 0 to + | 0 to + | Variable | Normal |

*Tr*, trace; +, mild; ++, moderate; +++, severe.
*Using test strips.

**TABLE 155-3.**
**Initial Investigation for the Diagnosis and Management of Diabetic Ketoacidosis**

| Bedside | Laboratory |
|---|---|
| 1. Blood glucose (using test strips) | 1. Blood glucose |
| 2. Plasma ketones (test strips or tablets) | 2. Plasma urea and electrolytes |
| 3. Plasma potassium* | 3. Arterial blood pH, $P_{CO_2}$, $P_{O_2}$† |
| 4. Plasma creatinine* | 4. Microscopy and culture of urine |
| 5. Plasma urea* | 5. Blood culture |
| 6. Electrocardiogram | 6. Throat swab culture |
| 7. Chest radiograph | 7. Hemoglobin |

*These are available in certain centers as "dry chemistry" bedside methods using machines such as the Reflotron, Seralyser, or Ektachem.
†Capillary pH and blood gases may be measured instead.

ponatremia occasionally is found in DKA patients with severe hyperlipidemia.[42] The laboratory often informs the clinician of the problem, because the blood sample may have caused blockage of the laboratory autoanalyzers.

Plasma potassium levels can be high, normal, or low. High levels usually are indicative of very acute onset of DKA, with urinary excretion not having kept pace with intracellular losses. They also may be found in the "sick-cell syndrome" or in acute anuria occurring simultaneously with DKA. Normal plasma levels generally are associated with a significant total body potassium deficit. Low plasma potassium levels are an indication of a very large total body deficit. They occur either in an insidious onset of DKA or in patients presenting with DKA who have been taking diuretics without adequate oral replacement.

Serum bicarbonate levels are less helpful. In any significant metabolic acidosis, bicarbonate levels are very low, and the pH and $P_{CO_2}$ give more useful information. Chloride levels do not help, except in occasional cases of hyperchloremic acidosis.

Plasma osmolality is a useful guide to the severity of the metabolic state. It can be calculated easily using the following equation:

$$2(\text{plasma Na}^+ + \text{K}^+)(\text{mmol/L}) + \frac{\text{plasma glucose(mg/dL)}}{18}$$

$$+ \frac{\text{blood urea nitrogen (mg/dL)}}{2.8} = \frac{\text{plasma osmolality}}{\text{in mOsmol/L}}$$

In those centers using Systeme Internationale units, the equation becomes

$$2(\text{Na}^+ + \text{K}^+)(\text{mmol/L}) + \text{glucose(mmol/L)}$$

$$+ \text{plasma urea (mmol/L)} = \text{osmolality in mOsmol/L}$$

This gives results that agree closely with measured osmolality, except in occasional situations, such as alcohol overdose.

Other tests that should be carried out routinely include sending urine and blood samples for culture and sensitivity and a throat swab, if indicated. Because infection is a common precipitating factor, antibiotics frequently will be used. Samples for culture should be sent before antibiotic therapy begins. Blood for hemoglobin (Hb), hematocrit, and white blood cell count (WBC) tends to be sent routinely as well. These tests are less helpful. The hematocrit indicates hemoconcentration, but so does creatinine. The WBC is singularly unhelpful and can be misleading. There is almost always a leukocytosis in severe DKA, but this correlates with blood ketone body levels and *not* with the presence of infection.[43] The two main signs of infection—pyrexia and leukocytosis—are either absent or misleading in DKA.

An electrocardiogram should be performed in the emergency room. This may give information on ischemic heart disease or myocardial infarction. More important, it provides a yardstick

for subsequent acute changes in plasma potassium levels, which should be followed by electrocardiographic monitoring. The baseline electrocardiogram is necessary because acidemia itself can produce changes, some of which can mimic ischemia, and a pseudoinfarction pattern has been described.[44,45] A chest radiograph is often done routinely. This is probably reasonable, in case of subsequent iatrogenic disorders, such as the adult respiratory distress syndrome or infection.

## TREATMENT

There are five main elements of treatment: fluid, insulin, potassium, alkali, and "other" measures. These are discussed in turn (see Appendix 1).

### FLUID

The first priority of treatment is fluid replacement. Insulin therapy is effective only if fluid is given rapidly in the early stages. The total water deficit ranges from 50 to 100 mL/kg body weight, with a sodium deficit of 7 to 10 mmol/kg. Several tailored replacement fluids that were relatively hypotonic were previously recommended. Now, it is agreed that isotonic saline (0.154 mol/L; 0.9%) is the appropriate initial replacement fluid. Concerns have been expressed about overzealous rates of fluid replacement. The author's current practice is to give 1 L in the first hour, then 1 L in 2 hours, and then 1 L every 4 hours until the patient is well hydrated (see Appendix 1). This routine should be varied according to the fluid status of the patient. In patients with cardiovascular disease or in elderly or shocked patients, who are at increased risk for development of heart failure,[46] a central venous pressure (CVP) line should be inserted and the rate of fluid administration guided by CVP measurement.

The exception to the use of isotonic saline is the presence or development of hypernatremia (measured plasma sodium >150–155 mmol/L). In this case, half-normal (0.45%) saline should be used, but infused more slowly. When saline is used, plasma sodium levels inevitably rise, partly because the infused fluid has a higher sodium content than the extracellular fluid in DKA patients, partly because water without sodium will be moving into cells, and partly because glucose levels will be falling. This rise in sodium levels is helpful, however, in that it prevents plasma osmolality from falling too quickly. This may be beneficial in preventing cerebral edema. Hyperchloremia almost invariably develops late in treatment, but there is little evidence to suggest that it is harmful.

Most DKA patients who are hypotensive on presentation respond with a rise in BP to the first 1 to 2 L saline. If systolic BP remains below 90 mm Hg, 1 to 2 U blood or plasma expanders should be given. If this fails, 100 mg hydrocortisone sodium succinate may be given iv, with an appropriate increase in subsequent insulin therapy.

Once blood glucose levels have fallen to 250 mg/dL (13.8 mmol/L), 10% glucose is substituted for saline. If this occurs before the patient is adequately rehydrated, saline should be continued simultaneously.

The importance of adequate early rehydration cannot be overemphasized. Simple rehydration alone lowers blood glucose levels by improving the renal excretion of glucose, with hemodilution accounting for as much as a 23% fall in blood glucose. Tissue perfusion is also improved, allowing the small amounts of insulin present to begin to act. Rehydration, even without insulin, decreases counterregulatory hormone secretion.

### INSULIN

Before 1973, large doses of insulin (i.e., hundreds of units) were routinely used in DKA. Then it was shown that relatively small amounts of insulin given intramuscularly (im) or as a continuous iv infusion were just as effective in lowering blood glucose, and had several advantages.[46,47] Among the advantages of the low-dose regimens are decreased problems with hypokalemia during therapy, a lower occurrence of late hypoglycemia, and a more predictable response to therapy. There is also an adequate but somewhat slower rate of fall of blood glucose levels, which is less likely to cause osmotic disequilibrium.

**Insulin Resistance.** The major concern in the use of low doses of insulin has been insulin resistance. It has been shown that fractional glucose turnover and the rate of fall of blood glucose levels in DKA patients are decreased up to ten-fold compared with nonketotic, well-controlled diabetics. Similarly, in animals and humans, insulin binding by adipocytes is decreased, as is postreceptor insulin action. This is accompanied, in ketoacidotic rats, by a marked diminution in total body insulin responsiveness. These changes correlate with the degree of acidemia, which is most severe when the pH is <7.0, and can be reproduced by $NH_4Cl$ administration, suggesting that it is the acidemia per se that is responsible.

Despite these experimental findings, major insulin resistance only rarely is a clinical problem. There is a somewhat slower rate of fall of glucose in patients with infections, but the response usually is adequate. There are several reasons for this. First, the initial response to therapy is primarily the result of rehydration. Second, the circulating insulin levels produced with low-dose regimens are high physiologically. An infusion of 10 U of insulin per hour produces peripheral insulin levels of >150 µU/mL, well above those found in normal persons. Similarly, with standard im regimens, levels of >80 µU/mL are engendered. These levels are sufficient, even in the face of insulin resistance, to inhibit lipolysis, thereby cutting off the supply of substrate for ketogenesis, restraining hepatic gluconeogenesis and helping to decrease glucagon levels. There is little impact on peripheral glucose uptake initially, but there are adequate circulating fuels, and ketone body use steadily increases; the insulin influence on potassium transport into cells is also submaximal, which may be an advantage.

**Intravenous Insulin Regimens.** Several insulin regimens have been proposed, with doses ranging from 2 to 10 U per hour as a continuous infusion. Good results have been reported with 1.4 to 1.6 U per hour after an initial small bolus.[19] The author's routine is to give 6 U per hour in saline, using an infusion pump and a separate line (see Appendix 1). In children, a dosage of 0.1 U/kg per hour is used. Because insulin has a circulating half-life of 4 to 5 minutes and a biologic half-life of no more than 30 minutes, it is critical that the insulin be given continuously. If the infusion stops for any reason, the effects will rapidly disappear. Insulin adsorbs to plastic and glass; therefore, some physicians recommend making the insulin solution in polygeline or albumin or drawing back 1 mL of the patient's blood into the syringe. In practice, adsorption is not a problem.

Blood glucose levels should be checked after the first 2 hours. If there has not been a significant fall (50–100 mg/dL or 2.8–5.7 mmol/L), then the infusion pump and line, the rehydration scheme, and the BP should be checked, and the insulin infusion rate should be doubled if these are satisfactory. This should be repeated every 2 hours until blood glucose levels are falling satisfactorily. When blood glucose levels have fallen to 250 µg/dL and 10% dextrose has been substituted for saline (100 mL per hour), the insulin dose should be decreased to 4 U per hour, and subsequently modified according to hourly bedside blood glucose readings.

**Intramuscular Regimen.** Hourly im insulin provides an alternative to continuous iv insulin and is particularly useful in centers where reliable infusion pumps are not available or where nursing care is inadequate. In this case, a loading dose of insulin should be given as either 20 U im or 10 U im plus 10 U iv in hypotensive or very dehydrated patients. Thereafter, 5 to 6 U should be given hourly as deep im injections. In children, a loading dose of 0.25 U/kg is given, followed by 0.1 U/kg hourly. Adequate rehydration is critical for im insulin to be effective. If, after 2 hours, there is not a significant response, the im regimen should be substituted with continuous iv insulin, having first checked that rehydration is progressing satisfactorily. When blood glucose reaches 250 mg/dL and iv glucose is commenced, the insulin dose should be decreased to 5 to 6 U every 2 hours (see Appendix 1).

## POTASSIUM

More iatrogenic deaths during the treatment of DKA have been caused by changes in plasma potassium than by any other factor. There is usually a large deficit of intracellular total body potassium (3–12 mmol/kg body weight). Despite this, as many as 33% of DKA patients may have elevated plasma $K^+$ levels initially. This loss of intracellular potassium into the extracellular space, which occurs in all cases, has been attributed to the acidemia, intracellular volume depletion, and lack of insulin. The role of acidemia has been questioned, however. Additional factors include a direct effect of hyperglycemia and hyperglucagonemia. In a careful analysis, glucose, pH (negatively), and the anion gap were independent, significant determinants of plasma $K^+$ on presentation.[48] Once treatment commences, plasma $K^+$ levels inevitably fall, except in those presenting with the sick-cell syndrome. The fall is the result of intracellular volume repletion, hemodilution, reversal of the acidemia, loss of $K^+$ in the urine as urine flow is reestablished, and a direct effect of insulin on intracellular $K^+$ transport. Thus, hypokalemia is inevitable unless potassium is replaced.

There are arguments about when potassium replacement should begin. Some recommend waiting until plasma potassium levels are known, levels are low normal or low, and urine flow has been reestablished; probably, this is too late. The author's practice is to start cautious replacement at 20 mmol KCl per hour in the saline infusion from the time of the first dose of insulin, then to modify the amount infused according to subsequent plasma values (see Appendix 1). It has been suggested that potassium should be given as phosphate or half as phosphate and half as chloride. However, phosphate requirements are very different from those for potassium, so it is probably sensible to replace them separately, if at all, and to use KCl.

Electrocardiographic monitoring is an invaluable guide to rapid changes in plasma potassium, and all patients should be monitored at least in the early stages of therapy. For as long as iv therapy is continued, iv potassium replacement should be continued. Thereafter, oral potassium replacement should be continued for several days, because much of the potassium administered iv will be lost in the urine, and the total body deficit will be only partly replenished. If alkali is given, additional potassium should be given (20 mmol/100 mmol sodium bicarbonate).

## OTHER ELECTROLYTES

There is a deficiency of magnesium, calcium, and phosphate, as well as of sodium and potassium in DKA patients. It is arguable, however, whether these need to be replaced immediately. Most debate has concerned phosphate.

During treatment of DKA, plasma phosphate levels fall, sometimes to undetectable levels. Red cell 2,3-diphosphoglycerate levels are also very low and take 4 to 48 hours to return to normal. This may cause impaired oxygen delivery to tissues when the acidemia is corrected. It has been argued that the low phosphate levels impede recovery of 2,3-diphosphoglycerate. Several trials of phosphate replacement have been carried out. None of the more recent trials has shown benefit, and in all cases, biochemical hypocalcemia was found in the treated group.[49] It is possible that phosphate changes are less with the use of low-dose insulin than they were previously. It is not the author's practice to replace phosphate. Similarly, although magnesium levels are low during therapy, no convincing evidence shows that replacement is beneficial.

**TABLE 155-4.**
**General Therapy for Diabetic Ketoacidosis**

Search for and treat any precipitating factors
Nasogastric suction
Catheterization
Intravenous furosemide for oliguria
Whole blood or plasma expanders for hypotension
Central venous pressure monitoring
Electrocardiographic monitoring
Antibiotics
Low-dose heparinization

## ALKALI

There is still no universal agreement about correcting the acidemia of severe DKA. The acidemia has certain pathophysiologic consequences, including negative inotropism, peripheral vasodilatation, central nervous system depression, and insulin resistance. On the other hand, vigorous alkalinization has deleterious consequences, including hypokalemia, a paradoxical fall in cerebrospinal fluid pH, impaired oxyhemoglobin dissociation, and rebound alkalosis.[50] Human data suggest that bicarbonate either has no benefit or, indeed, may slow clearance of ketones and metabolic normalization.[51–53]

Despite this, it is usually considered advisable to give moderate amounts of bicarbonate when the pH is <6.95; 100 mmol containing 20 mmol KCl should be given over 45 minutes. This should be repeated until the pH is above 7.0. It also may be helpful to give 50-mmol bicarbonate containing 10 mmol KCl to those patients distressed by hyperventilation.

## OTHER MEASURES

Clinical therapy for DKA patients should not be forgotten (Table 155-4). On admission, an assiduous search should be made for precipitating factors. This is most likely to be infection, but careful clinical examination is required, and appropriate therapy should be instituted. If there is any hint of infection or if major invasive measures are used, broad-spectrum antibiotics should be given once appropriate cultures have been taken. Because signs of infection may be missing or misleading and phagocyte function is impaired in uncontrolled diabetes, antibiotics should be used less cautiously than is usual.

In many patients, there is considerable pooling of fluid in the gastrointestinal tract; often, there is vomiting. Because aspiration of vomit is a known cause of morbidity and mortality in DKA patients, nasogastric suction should be instituted early in the semiconscious or unconscious patient.

The use of CVP and electrocardiographic monitoring has been discussed. Urine output is another guide to progress. If no urine has been passed in the first 4 hours, the bladder should be catheterized (with simultaneous antibiotics). If there is oliguria or anuria, 40 mg furosemide given iv may reinstitute adequate urine flow. If oliguria or anuria persists, potassium replacement should be stopped. Fluid should be replaced less aggressively unless the patient is still very dehydrated with a low CVP and BP.

There is an increased risk of thromboembolic episodes, particularly in the elderly, the unconscious, and those with very hyperosmolar conditions. In these patients, heparin (500 U every 4–6 hours given subcutaneously) should be used. Some patients become extremely agitated and may harm valuable iv lines. A small dose of iv lorazapam can help, and it does not have any deleterious metabolic effects.

## MONITORING OF THERAPY

A guide to the monitoring of therapy is given in Table 155-5. This includes both biochemical and clinical monitoring essen-

**TABLE 155-5.**
**Monitoring Therapy for Diabetic Ketoacidosis**

| Parameter | Action |
|---|---|
| **CLINICAL** | |
| Pulse, BP | Every half hour for 4 h, every hour for 4 h, then every 2–4 h |
| Temperature | At 0, 2, 4, 6 h, then every 6 h |
| Urine flow | Hourly for 6 h, then every 4 h with fluid balance chart |
| Conscious state | Every hour |
| CVP | Every hour in those with CVP line |
| **BIOCHEMICAL** | |
| Plasma glucose | Hourly by test strip until BG <250 mg/dL, then every 2 h. Confirm in laboratory at 0, 2, 6 h, and then every 4 h. |
| Plasma $K^+$, $Na^+$ | Monitor $K^+$ continuously with electrocardiogram. Obtain laboratory determinations at 0, 2, 6 h, and then every 4 h. |
| Plasma creatinine | Obtain laboratory determinations at 0, 2, 6, 24 h. |
| pH and $P_{CO_2}$ | If pH >7.0: obtain at 0 and 4–6 h. If pH <7.0: obtain at 0 and after each bicarbonate infusion until >7.0, then 4 h later. |
| Plasma ketones | At 0, 6, and 12 h |
| Urine glucose | Every 4 h |

*BP*, blood pressure; *BG*, blood glucose; *CVP*, central venous pressure.

tial to the successful outcome of treatment. The guidelines will require modification according to the individual needs of patients. Temperature measurement may be helpful because an infection-induced pyrexia may be revealed after 4 to 6 hours of treatment. Charts should be prepared for standard use to prevent omissions. Caution should be exercised in interpreting urine or plasma ketones. These will diminish but may remain positive for as long as 48 hours; however, this is not caused by continued ketogenesis. Rather, because acetone is extremely lipid soluble, it will continue to diffuse out of structural lipid for many hours. In contrast, blood 3-hydroxybutyrate will fall rapidly, although this is not measured by the usual tablet or test-strip procedures.

## SECONDARY PHASE OF TREATMENT

Even if blood glucose levels have fallen toward normal, continued vigilance and care are required. Ketoacidosis may recur. Saline should be replaced with 10% dextrose containing 20 mmol KCl/500 mL, given at 100 mL per hour. This is used in preference to 5% dextrose because it provides more calories in the catabolic patients, and it has been shown that the ketosis and acidemia clear more rapidly with the higher carbohydrate load.[38,54] Insulin doses should be modified as described earlier. Intravenous therapy should be continued until the first meal, when subcutaneous short-acting insulin should be given. If iv insulin has been used, the insulin infusion should be continued until at least 1 hour after the subcutaneous insulin is given to allow time for absorption of the latter.

## COMPLICATIONS OF THERAPY

There are several well-recognized complications that can occur during the treatment of DKA.

### HYPOGLYCEMIA

Hypoglycemia was common as a late sequel to the treatment of DKA when larger doses of insulin were used, particularly with im or subcutaneous regimens. It is less common now but still occurs if monitoring is not adequate or if the results of monitoring are not acted on. An alarmingly high rate has been reported from three private hospitals.[55]

## HYPERKALEMIA AND HYPOKALEMIA

Hyperkalemia and hypokalemia were discussed in detail elsewhere[48] and earlier. Hypokalemia is more common. It is unnecessary and does not occur if potassium replacement is commenced soon enough and if monitoring is adequate. It is more likely to occur in those with initially low or low-normal plasma potassium levels, in those previously treated with potassium-losing diuretics, and in those with a long period of poor control preceding the episode of DKA.

## FLUID OVERLOAD AND HYPERNATREMIA

Fluid overload occurs if rehydration is too rapid, particularly in those with cardiovascular disease or with impaired renal function. This may be caused by the use of crystalloid infusions rather than colloids, but it is rare if there is proper monitoring. Hypernatremia may occur with the use of saline for rehydration. It is unlikely to cause problems below a plasma sodium level of 160 mmol/L, but can cause cerebral irritation and coma. It should be suspected (as should cerebral edema) if a patient's conscious state worsens during treatment. It is unlikely to occur if plasma sodium levels are being monitored and acted on. The appropriate treatment is the replacement of the saline infusion with 5% dextrose and an increase in the insulin dose. This effectively provides free water, and levels will slowly fall.

## CEREBRAL EDEMA

Cerebral edema has long been recognized as a complication of treatment, particularly in children, and the outcome is poor. It is a rare event, but subclinical cerebral edema is probably more common. Studies have shown many cases of DKA to have a decrease in cerebroventricular volume during therapy.[56,57]

Several reasons have been advanced to explain the occurrences of this complication. One group postulated the buildup of "idiogenic" osmoles in cerebral cells during severe hyperglycemia.[58] When the osmolality of the extracellular fluid falls rapidly with treatment, these trapped osmoles draw fluid into the cerebral cells. In animals, it also was shown that if blood glucose was not allowed to fall below 200 mg/dL, cerebral edema did not occur. Another group has suggested that the phenomenon is caused by activation of the sodium-hydrogen countertransport system in the brain, which is more active because of diffusion into brain cells of undissociated organic acids (3-hydroxybutyric acid and acetoacetic acids), which release protons.[59] Both of these hypotheses require proof.

A feature common to most reported cases is the use of hypotonic rehydration fluids (e.g., hypotonic saline or glucose) that yield free water.[60] This leads to a more rapid fall in extracellular fluid osmolality than occurs with isotonic saline infusion. Indeed, an association with hyponatremia has been reported.[61] This could cause an imbalance between brain intracellular osmolality and the extracellular fluid, with resultant intracellular movement of water.

In practical terms, cerebral edema is rarely, if ever, seen if isotonic saline is used as the primary rehydration solution and if blood glucose concentration is not allowed to fall below 250 mg/dL (13.8 mmol/L). Nonetheless subclinical brain dysfunction may be common during treatment of DKA.[62] (See also refs. 62a and 62b.)

## ADULT RESPIRATORY DISTRESS SYNDROME

The adult respiratory distress syndrome is now recognized as a rare but real complication of the treatment of DKA.[63] The mortality is close to 100%, and it occurs at all ages, including childhood. The mechanism is unclear. Some researchers suggest that it is the result of a rapid fall in oncotic pressure, caused by crystalloid infusions. Others have suggested that it is caused by an alveocapillary permeability defect induced by acidosis and hyperventilation. Most cases (as with cerebral edema) have been in patients rehydrated with hypotonic fluids. It is noteworthy that intestinal pulmonary edema may be relatively common in children with DKA even before treatment is commenced,[64] suggesting that there is indeed an alveocapillary defect.

## THROMBOEMBOLIC EPISODES

Careful examination shows that most DKA patients have platelet hyperaggregability, elevation of clotting factors, increases in circulating fibrin degradation products, or combinations of all these. Disseminated intravascular coagulopathy occurs in DKA patients during therapy, and there is an increase in late thromboembolic phenomena in those who are elderly or very hyperosmolar. These increased risks certainly warrant the use of routine anticoagulation in the more severely affected patients.

## OTHER COMPLICATIONS

Inhalation pneumonia and shock have been described. Mucormycosis and rhabdomyolysis are rare complications (see Chap. 152).

## MORTALITY

Deaths in DKA can be subdivided into avoidable and unavoidable. In the unavoidable category are overwhelming infection, massive myocardial infarction, or terminal carcinoma, in which DKA is a secondary event. The avoidable category includes the many different iatrogenic causes. In a survey of deaths in DKA in patients younger than 50 years of age, most were deemed avoidable; hypokalemia, uncontrolled sepsis, inhalation pneumonia, cerebral edema, and clotting disorders comprise the bulk of such causes. In another study, thromboembolic events, bronchopneumonia, and cardiac failure were the main causes.[20] Some problems are undoubtedly due to poor adherence to guidelines; up to 70% failed to do so in one series.[65]

## PREVENTION

Because the mortality of severe DKA ranges from 5% to 20%, prevention is extremely important. This implies proper education of the patient and primary health care personnel. The patient should have clear information on how to respond to illness and to periods of poor control. All patients should be given "sick-day rules" (see Appendix 2). The primary health care physician or nurse should be quick to respond to impending ketosis with, for example, one to two insulin injections every hour and with instructions to increase fluid intake. This should be combined with the instruction that, as soon as vomiting commences, medical help should be sought because it indicates the need for iv fluids. Such guidance should decrease the incidence of severe DKA.

# HYPEROSMOLAR HYPERGLYCEMIC NONKETOTIC COMA

HONK occurs at approximately a tenth of the frequency of classic DKA; however, it carries a much higher mortality.[66] This is consistent with the finding that most patients are older than 50 years of age, although it can occur in children.[67] It usually occurs in patients with type 2 diabetes mellitus and often is the first indication that the patient has diabetes.

## PATHOPHYSIOLOGY

The cause of HONK is unclear.[4] There is undoubtedly insulin deficiency, albeit relative, with marked hypersecretion of the counterregulatory hormones. However, presumably there is enough insulin to suppress lipolysis or ketogenesis. Perhaps the following occurs: Patients with type 2 diabetes mellitus have insulin insensitivity. Hepatic glucose production is accelerated and hyperglycemia occurs. If there is an increase in counterregulatory hormone secretion, it further increases hepatic glucose output and decreases extrahepatic glucose use. There is then increasing hyperglycemia, which is exacerbated by oral carbohydrate ingestion, because the extra glucose load cannot be metabolized. There is still sufficient insulin, however, to prevent accelerated lipolysis. The hyperglycemia leads to intracellular fluid loss and osmotic diuresis with dehydration, hemoconcentration, and further worsening of the hyperglycemia. Potassium is lost from cells and excreted in the urine. The loss of potassium conceivably may further inhibit insulin secretion. Many of the patients are elderly and are taking diuretics, which accelerate dehydration. At the same time, thirst mechanisms are defective in the elderly, increasing the rate at which dehydration occurs. Patients sometimes consume large volumes of soft drinks with high sugar content in response to thirst, worsening the hyperglycemia.

None of these theories explains the lack of ketoacidosis. Usually, ketone body levels are elevated, but less than in DKA patients, suggesting a continuum rather than two totally separate conditions. Levels of counterregulatory hormones and of insulin do not clearly separate DKA from HONK patients.

The hyperosmolality is caused partly by glucose, the levels of which are higher on average in HONK than in DKA patients. HONK patients also tend to have higher plasma urea levels, although the latter diffuses freely into most cells and does not contribute substantially to altered osmotic gradients. At least half of HONK patients, however, also have high normal or high plasma sodium levels. If glucose levels are allowed for, then, there is marked, "real" hypernatremia in most cases.[68] The cause of this is unknown, except for the dehydration being more severe, but plasma sodium often makes a major contribution to the hyperosmolality.

## PRECIPITATING FACTORS

The precipitating factors for HONK are multiple and many case reports have appeared of rare causes.[7] Infection is the single most important factor, with presumed counterregulatory hormone hypersecretion as the cause of the metabolic disturbance. Cardiovascular emergencies, such as a cerebrovascular accident and myocardial infarction, are the other major factors. The cerebrovascular accident is particularly important because it can cause severe hyperglycemia, or "piqûre" diabetes. This may be associated with an inability to drink, and hyperosmolality can ensue. Drugs such as corticosteroids and thiazides also precipitate HONK.

## PRESENTATION

Usually, patients with HONK are older than those with DKA, although HONK can occur in youth, and the history of poorly controlled diabetes (e.g., polyuria, polydipsia, anorexia, some weight loss, fatigue) may extend back for several weeks.[60] There is often recent infection. Focal neurologic signs may be present, and there almost always is impaired consciousness, with 20% or more being in coma.[69,70] Presentation with seizures has also been reported.[71] On examination, there is severe dehydration and hypotension, with or without shock.

## DIAGNOSIS

The history and initial clinical examination often suggest the diagnosis; there is an obvious lack of hyperventilation. However, in the comatose patient not previously known to be diabetic, severe dehydration may be the only clue. Bedside diagnosis with glucose test strips will give a firmer guide, together with plasma ketones, which are negative or only trace positive (see Table 155-2). Initial therapy can be commenced

while waiting for laboratory results. Laboratory investigations are the same as for DKA (see Table 155-3). These reveal a very high blood glucose (600–2500 mg/dL; 33.3–138.0 mmol/L), often hypernatremia, a normal or low potassium, and a grossly elevated blood urea. Calculated osmolality is >350 mOsmol/L and often is >400 mOsmol/L. Arterial pH is >7.2; $PO_2$ is often decreased, but the anion gap paradoxically tends to be increased. A review of the literature[7] has shown a mean glucose of 1166 mg/dL compared with 475 mg/dL in DKA, Na$^+$ higher at 143 compared to 131 mEq/L, and free fatty acids lower at 0.73 to 0.96 mmol/L compared to >2 mmol/L. Glucagon levels, however, were higher. Osmolality also was much higher, 384 versus 309 mOsmol/kg.

## TREATMENT

The general principles of treatment are similar to those outlined for DKA.

### FLUIDS

The priority in treatment is rehydration. The average fluid deficit is ~9 L. Until laboratory results are available, isotonic saline may be given, giving 1 L in 15 to 30 minutes, and a second liter during 1 to 2 hours. If the patient is normonatremic or hypernatremic (>145 mmol/L), half-normal saline should be used, giving 1 L every 2 hours for 6 hours, then 1 L every 4 hours. CVP monitoring should be used routinely to provide rapid rehydration. If sodium levels remain very high, 5% dextrose can be used for rehydration. HONK patients usually are insulin sensitive, and the extra glucose load can be coped with easily. Shock or hypotension is often a problem on admission or during therapy, and the use of 1 to 2 L of a plasma expander or of albumin can be invaluable. Although plasma osmolality tends to fall rapidly, cerebral edema is less of a problem in patients with HONK than with DKA. When blood glucose levels approach 250 mg/dL (13.8 mmol/L), 10% dextrose should be commenced. It may be necessary to continue hypotonic saline infusion simultaneously.

### INSULIN

Patients with HONK are sensitive to low doses of insulin. The same routine can be used for these patients as for those with DKA. Thus, 6 U per hour should be given iv (or 6 U im hourly). If the rate of fall of glucose exceeds 150 to 200 mg/dL per hour, the rate of insulin administration can be halved. As with DKA, if the blood-glucose diminution is unsatisfactory, the rehydration schedule should be reexamined, and the iv dose increased, or if im insulin is being used, the iv route should be substituted. When the glucose infusion is commenced, the insulin administration rate should be decreased by a third and further doses dictated by bedside blood glucose monitoring.

### POTASSIUM

Despite no significant acidemia, there is usually a large total body potassium deficit (5–12 mmol/kg). This is caused by the long prodromal period, intracellular fluid depletion, urinary loss, decreased insulin action, and hyperglycemia. Levels may fall precipitously after fluid and insulin therapy is instituted, and severe hypokalemia is a major risk. This can have catastrophic cardiovascular effects on a group of patients already in circulatory collapse and often with preexisting cardiac disease. Electrocardiographic monitoring is mandatory. The same regimen should be used as with DKA, starting with 20 mmol KCl per hour (see Appendix 1).

### OTHER MEASURES

Many treatment measures are as described for DKA. Antibiotics and plasma volume support are important. Anuria or oli-

**TABLE 155-6.**
**Classification of Lactic Acidosis**

| Type | Description |
| --- | --- |
| **Type A** | Hypoxic, poor tissue perfusion, shock |
| **Type B1** | Associated with common disorders: diabetes mellitus, renal failure, liver failure, infection, leukemia |
| **Type B2** | Due to drugs or toxins: phenformin, metformin, buformin, ethanol, salicylates, fructose, methanol |
| **Type B3** | Hereditary forms: glucose 6-phosphatase deficiency, infantile lactic acidosis |
| **Type B4** | Miscellaneous |

(From Cohen RD, Woods HF. Clinical and biochemical aspects of lactic acidosis. Oxford: Blackwell, 1976:42.)

guria is more likely to be present because of both prerenal failure and preexisting renal disease. Equally important are thromboembolic phenomena, which are common in HONK, in which hyperosmolality, age, hyperglycemia, and unconsciousness contribute.[72] Thromboembolic complications, circulatory collapse, and preexisting severe disease are often causes of death in these patients, and anticoagulation is indicated.

HONK is a serious, often lethal, form of diabetic coma. As with DKA, it is often preventable by early diagnosis of type 2 diabetes mellitus and by careful attention to education of patients about infections. Many HONK patients do not require insulin after the acute episode, and a trial without insulin should be carried out before the patient leaves the hospital.

# LACTIC ACIDOSIS

Lactic acidosis occurs when the metabolism of pyruvate and lactate is blocked.[73] It is a condition in which blood lactate levels are >5 mmol/L, and there is a significant decrease in arterial blood pH (<7.2).

## PATHOPHYSIOLOGY

There are many different causes of lactic acidosis, and these are summarized in Table 155-6. *Type A lactic acidosis* is by far the most common form and is the result of tissue hypoxia. It occurs in shock or any condition in which there is a major decrease in tissue perfusion. It occurs in both diabetics and nondiabetics.

*Type B lactic acidosis* is further subdivided into four groups. Of relevance to diabetes are *types B1* and *B2*.[73] There have been sporadic reports of lactic acidosis occurring in diabetic patients without specific drug therapy (type B2). The reasons for this are unclear. In stable type 1 diabetics, blood lactate levels are consistently elevated, but at levels between 1 and 2 mmol/L (normal range, 0.4–1.0 mmol/L), rather than the higher levels required for lactic acidosis. In DKA, however, 10% to 15% of patients may have blood lactate concentrations >5 mmol/L. This presumably is caused by hypotension and impaired liver and tissue perfusion, as well as by epinephrine and cortisol, both of which cause an increase in blood lactate. In addition, 3-hydroxybutyrate inhibits the lactate transporter in hepatocytes; therefore, it impairs lactate clearance.[9] Thus, lactic acidosis secondary to DKA is probably common, but it responds rapidly to normal DKA therapy. Liver disease is also a precipitating factor, because the liver is critical for the clearance of lactate produced by other tissues.

Type B2 (drug-induced) lactic acidosis is more relevant to diabetes. It has been found particularly in patients taking biguanides. It is more common with phenformin than with buformin, with the lowest incidence occurring with metformin.[74] Biguanides act through interference with proton transport across hepatic mitochondrial membranes. Therapeutically, they exert a hypoglycemic effect by inhibiting hepatic gluconeogenesis, by inhibiting glucose transport across the small intestine, and, more questionably, by stimulating glycolysis in peripheral tissues. In all cases, blood lactate and pyruvate levels rise, presumably owing to the hepatic effect. This effect is greater with phenformin than with metformin. If there is overdosage, hepatic damage, or impaired renal excretion of the drugs, lactic acidosis will develop. The greater incidence with phenformin probably reflects the fact that phenformin is concentrated in and metabolized by the liver, but metformin is excreted unchanged by the kidneys. Virtually all the cases of lactic acidosis associated with metformin have occurred in patients with acute anuria or severely impaired renal function. Lactic acidosis is more likely to develop in patients with hypotension or shock who also are taking biguanides.

The incidence of lactic acidosis has decreased sharply since its association with phenformin (and buformin) usage became well known. Metformin is now the only biguanide that is widely available; the incidence of lactic acidosis associated with its use is five to ten per 100,000 patient-years, only marginally above the rate in non-metformin users.[75–77] Renal function should be monitored at every visit to the physician, and the drug should be stopped if there is any deterioration of renal function or any hypoxic state.

## DIAGNOSIS AND PRESENTATION

Patients with lactic acidosis probably will be hypotensive, obviously ill, and hyperventilating. They are likely to be oliguric or anuric. There will be a history of metformin use or of cardiovascular disease, and there may be a recent cerebrovascular accident or myocardial infarction. This information should be sought. Diagnosis is aided by the scheme shown in Table 155-2. Blood glucose is likely to be low or normal, the patient will be clinically acidotic (hyperventilating), and ketone bodies usually will be trace positive or positive. Blood should be sent immediately for measurements of arterial pH, $PO_2$, $PCO_2$, serum creatinine, and electrolytes. There will be evidence of a more severe acidemia than indicated by ketone body measurement (pH <7.0), low $PCO_2$, low $PO_2$, and high plasma creatinine levels. DKA patients frequently have raised lactate levels with high levels of ketone bodies, high glucose levels, and dehydration. Definitive diagnosis requires a blood lactate measurement, which is available only in a few hospitals. However, the diagnosis can be made on the basis of exclusion.

## TREATMENT

Treatment of lactic acidosis is unsatisfactory, with a mortality of ~50% in biguanide-associated cases and 60% to 80% in others.

The first priority is vascular support and reversal of hypotension, without which treatment is unsuccessful. Any cause should be treated (e.g., stopping the administration of biguanides). Equally important is reversal of the acidemia. As long as pH remains below 7.0, the liver produces, rather than clears, lactate and is not able to generate hydroxyl ions through the oxidation of lactate. A vicious cycle then develops. Sodium bicarbonate should be given iv in large amounts, 250 mmol over 1 hour initially, with repeated similar doses until the pH is >7.1. In some patients, as much as 2500 mmol has been given with success. Mortality is reportedly lower in those given large amounts of alkali.[74,78] This amount of bicarbonate carries with it a large sodium load, the equivalent of 17 L isotonic saline. Almost inevitably, patients require hemodialysis or peritoneal dialysis. This also may help remove the hydrogen ion load and any responsible drugs. Arrangements for dialysis should be made as soon as the diagnosis of severe lactic acidosis is made.

Other measures have been used with mixed success. Some physicians recommend the use of insulin and glucose, the

1. $CH_3 \cdot CH_2OH + NAD^+ \longrightarrow CH_3 \cdot CHO + NADH$
   Ethanol                              Acetaldehyde

2. $CH_3 \cdot CO \cdot COOH + NADH \longrightarrow CH_3 \cdot CHOH + NAD^+$
   Pyruvate                            Lactate

3. $Oxaloacetate + NADH \longrightarrow Malate + NAD^+$

**FIGURE 155-5.** Metabolism of ethanol. Nicotinamide adenine dinucleotide (*NADH*) is formed in large amounts and causes a shift in the pyruvate/lactate and oxaloacetate/malate equilibria toward lactate and malate.

hypothesis being that this may clear lactate through activation of pyruvate dehydrogenase. This has not been substantiated but probably does little harm because many of the patients have poorly regulated diabetes, and it may help diminish the associated ketosis. Dichloroacetate has been used successfully, acting through activation of pyruvate dehydrogenase, but it is not freely available.[79] It has toxic effects when used chronically, but this is irrelevant in treating an acute condition with high mortality. Other agents, such as the buffer tromethamine and the oxidizing agent methylene blue, have been tried but probably do not help.

It is obvious that the most effective treatment is prevention. If lactic acidosis does occur, treatment should include vigorous alkalinization (with careful watch on plasma potassium and calcium levels), circulatory support, treatment of the cause, and dialysis as necessary to accommodate the inevitable sodium load.

## ALCOHOLIC KETOACIDOSIS

Alcoholic ketoacidosis is associated with alcohol abuse in fasting individuals; it probably is more common in diabetic than in nondiabetic persons.[80,81] The pathogenesis is somewhat obscure. It occurs after heavy drinking that is followed by severe, prolonged vomiting. It is often associated with hypoglycemia due to rapid consumption of nicotinamide adenine dinucleotide (NAD) for metabolizing alcohol to acetate with a high ratio of NADH to NAD. Consequently, pyruvate is diverted to lactate (Figs. 155-5 and 155-6; see Chap. 205). The formation of excess ketone bodies is probably the result of starvation but may also reflect direct conversion of acetate to ketone bodies. Lipolysis is accelerated, partly by starvation and partly by increased catecholamine secretion when insulin levels are low. This provides more substrate for ketogenesis.

Patients present with an acutely ill appearance or may be unconscious. Hyperventilation is obvious. Often, plasma ketones are negative or only trace positive because the β-hydroxybutyrate/acetoacetate ratio is very high. However, the history should make the diagnosis obvious after acidemia is diagnosed. Lactic acidosis, however, can also develop in patients with alco-

holic poisoning. Alcoholic ketoacidosis responds rapidly to a trial glucose infusion. If there is no response, a definitive assay for blood lactate and β-hydroxybutyrate is required.[82]

## APPENDIX 1. GUIDELINES TO THE MANAGEMENT OF DIABETIC KETOACIDOSIS

These principles should be followed in treating the patient with DKA.[83]

### INITIAL MEASURES

1. Clinical examination: BP, pulse, ventilatory rate, skin turgor, and temperature; search for infection; conscious state
2. Blood for bedside measurement of glucose (test strips) and plasma ketones (test strips or tablets)
3. Blood to laboratory for tests: glucose, creatinine, urea, electrolytes; arterial pH, $PO_2$, $PCO_2$; Hb, WBC, differential
4. Blood, urine, throat swab for cultures
5. If diagnosis suggested by bedside examination, start fluid and insulin

### TREATMENT

1. *Fluid.* One liter isotonic (0.9%) saline in 1 hour, 1 L in 2 hours, 2 L in 8 hours, and then 0.5 L every 4 hours. Check CVP if cardiovascular disease. If sodium rises above 155 mmol/L, change to half-normal (0.45%) saline. N.B. More slowly in the elderly.
2. *Insulin.* iv regimen: Infuse 6 to 8 U per hour as 1 U/mL solution in saline, using infusion pump. im regimen: Give 20 U im (or 10 U iv plus 10 U im if patient is hypotensive) initially; then, 6 U per hour. In children, give 0.1 U/kg per hour as continuous iv infusion or 0.25 U/kg im loading dose followed by 0.1 U/kg per hour im.
3. *Potassium* (chloride or phosphate). Start at 20 mmol per hour in the saline infusion from time of first insulin administration. Stop if laboratory $K^+$ >6 mmol/L. Maintain $K^+$ between 4 and 5 mmol/L. If $K^+$ <3 mmol/L, increase to 40 mmol per hour; if $K^+$ is 3 to 4 mmol/L, increase to 30 mmol per hour; if $K^+$ is 5 to 6 mmol/L, decrease to 10 mmol per hour. Monitor with electrocardiogram.
4. *Sodium bicarbonate.* If pH <6.95, give 100 mmol with 20 mmol KCl over 45 minutes as isotonic solution. Check pH 15 to 30 minutes later. Repeat until pH >7.0. For distressing hyperventilation with pH >7.0, give 50 mmol containing 10 mmol KCl.
5. *Continued treatment.*
   A. Monitor glucose with test strip at bedside hourly and in laboratory at hours 2 and 6, then every 4 hours.
   B. Monitor $K^+$ in laboratory at hours 2 and 6, then every 6 hours.
   C. Laboratory measurements of creatinine and electrolytes at hours 3, 6, and 24.
   D. Frequent monitoring of pulse, BP, temperature (see Table 155-5).
   E. When blood glucose <250 mg/dL, change to 10% dextrose, 500 mL every 4 hours. Continue saline if patient still dehydrated. Change insulin to 4 U per hour iv or 6 U im every 2 hours. Modify according to bedside glucose estimations. Maintain blood glucose between 150 and 250 mg/dL.
   F. When patient is ready to eat, reinstitute short-acting, subcutaneous insulin therapy. If on iv insulin regimen, continue for 1 hour after subcutaneous insulin is given.
   G. Continue oral $K^+$ replacement for 1 week.

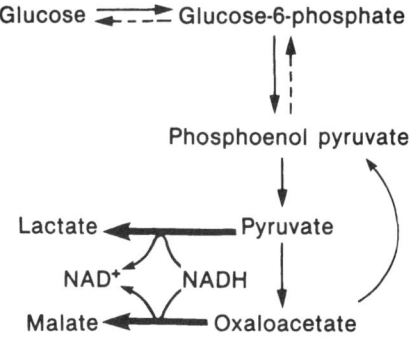

**FIGURE 155-6.** Effect of ethanol-induced nicotinamide adenine dinucleotide (*NADH*) accumulation on gluconeogenesis.

6. *Other measures.*
    A. If no urine passed by hour 4, catheterize.
    B. Give 40 mg furosemide if oliguric.
    C. Give antibiotics if infection suspected or invasive procedures used.
    D. Institute nasogastric suction if patient is comatose or semiconscious.
    E. Give oxygen if $PO_2$ <80 mm Hg.
    F. Heparinize (500 U subcutaneously every 4 hours) if patient is comatose or very hyperosmolar (>360 mOsmol/L).
    G. Give blood or plasma expander (2 U) if systolic BP <80 mm Hg at hour 2.

## APPENDIX 2. SICK-DAY RULES FOR TYPE 1 PATIENTS

1. Insulin should *never* be omitted.
2. If food is not taken, the carbohydrate equivalent should be taken as milk or sugar-containing fluids.
3. Blood glucose levels should be self-monitored before each meal and at bedtime.
4. If blood glucose <234 mg/dL (13 mmol/L), continue usual insulin. If blood glucose >234 mg/dL (13 mmol/L) but <400 mg/dL (22.2 mmol/L), take 4 U extra of regular insulin. If blood glucose >400 mg/dL (22.2 mmol/L), take 8 U extra of regular insulin.
5. Test urine for ketones two to three times each day.
6. If vomiting occurs or blood glucose >400 mg/dL for 24 hours, or if urine ketones are 2 plus, call a physician or go to the nearest emergency room.

## REFERENCES

1. Genuth SM. Diabetic ketoacidosis and hyperglycemic hyperosmolar coma. Curr Ther Endocrinol Metab 1997; 6:438.
2. Klekamp J, Churchwell KB. Diabetic ketoacidosis in children: initial clinical assessment and treatment. Pediatr Ann 1996; 25:387.
3. Ennis ED, Stahl EJvB, Kreisberg RA. Diabetic ketoacidosis. In: Porte D, Sherwin RS, eds. Ellenberg and Rifkin's diabetes mellitus, 5th ed. Stamford: Appleton & Lange, 1997:827.
4. Umpierrez GE, Khajavi M, Kitabchi AE. Diabetic ketoacidosis and hyperglycemic hyperosmolar non-ketotic syndrome. Am J Med Sci 1996; 311:225.
5. Schreiber M, Kamel KS, Cheema-Dhadli S, Halperin ML. Ketoacidosis: emphasis on acid-base aspects. Diabetes Reviews 1994; 2:98.
6. Marshall SM, Walker M, Alberti KGMM. Diabetic ketoacidosis and hyperglycaemic non-ketotic coma. In: Alberti KGMM, DeFronza RA, eds. International textbook of diabetes mellitus, 2nd ed. Chichester: John Wiley, 1997:1215.
7. Ennis ED, Stahl EJvB, Kreisberg RA. The hyperosmolar hyperglycemic syndrome. Diabetes Reviews 1994; 2:115.
8. Lorber D. Nonketotic hypertonicity in diabetes mellitus. Med Clin North Am 1996; 79:39.
9. Cohen RD. Lactic acidosis: new perspectives on origins and treatment. Diabetes Reviews 1994; 2:86.
10. Faich GA, Fishbein HA, Ellis SE. The epidemiology of diabetic acidosis: a population-based study. Am J Epidemiol 1983; 117:551.
11. Snorgaard O, Eskildsen PC, Vadstrup S, Nerup J. Diabetic ketoacidosis in Denmark: epidemiology, incidence rates, precipitating factors and mortality rates. J Int Med 1989; 226:223.
12. Fishbein HA. Diabetic ketoacidosis, hyperosmolar nonketotic coma, lactic acidosis and hypoglycemia. In: Harris MI, Hamman RF, eds. Diabetes in America. Washington, DC: US Department of Health and Human Services, 1985:XII.
13. Division of Diabetes Translation. In: Diabetes Surveillance 1980–1987. Atlanta: US Department of Health and Human Services, Centers for Disease Control, 1990:27.
14. Wilson C, Krakoff J, Gohdes D. Ketoacidosis in Apache Indians with non-insulin-dependent diabetes mellitus. Arch Intern Med 1997; 157:2098.
15. Yamada K, Nonaka K. Diabetic ketoacidosis in young obese Japanese men. Diabetes Care 1996; 19:671.
16. Pinhas-Hamiel O, Dolan LM, Zeitler PS. Diabetic ketoacidosis among obese African-American adolescents with NIDDM. Diabetes Care 1997; 20:484.
17. Adhikari PM, Mohammed N, Pereira P. Changing profile of diabetic ketosis. J Indian Med Assoc 1997; 95:540.
18. Holman RC, Herron CA, Sinnock P. Epidemiologic characteristics of mortality from diabetes with acidosis or coma, United States 1970–78. Am J Public Health 1983;73:1169.
19. Wagner A, Risse A, Brill H-L, et al. Therapy of severe diabetic ketoacidosis. Zero-mortality under very-low-dose insulin application. Diabetes Care 1999; 22:674.
20. Basu A, Close CF, Jenkins D, et al. Persisting mortality in diabetic ketoacidosis. Diabet Med 1993;10:282.
21. Tunbridge WMG. Deaths due to diabetic ketoacidosis. Q J Med 1981; 50:502.
22. Oster JR, Perez GO, Vaamonde CA. Relationship between blood pH and potassium and phosphorus during acute metabolic acidosis. Am J Physiol 1978; 235:F345.
23. Miles JM, Gerich JE. Glucose and ketone body kinetics in diabetic ketoacidosis. Clin Endocrinol Metab 1983; 12:303.
24. Sivitz WI, DeSautel SL, Kayano T, et al. Regulation of glucose transporter messenger RNA in insulin-deficient states. Nature 1989; 340:72.
25. Attia N, Caprio S, Jones TW, et al. Changes in free insulin-like growth factor-1 and leptin concentrations during acute metabolic decompensation in insulin withdrawn patients with type 1 diabetes. J Clin Endocrinol Metab 1999; 84: 2324.
26. Morris AD, Boyle DI, McMahon AD, et al. Adherence to insulin treatment, glycaemic control and ketoacidosis in insulin-dependent diabetes mellitus. The DARTS/MEMO Collaboration. Lancet 1997; 351:674.
27. Bagg W, Sathu A, Streat S, Braatvedt GD. Diabetic ketoacidosis in adults at Auckland Hospital. Aust NZ J Med 1998; 28:604.
28. Liss DS, Waller DA, Kennard BD, et al. Psychiatric illness and family support in children and adolescents with diabetic ketoacidosis: a controlled study. J Am Acad Child Adolesc Psychiatry 1998; 37:536.
29. Smith CP, Firth D, Bennett S, et al. Ketoacidosis occurring in newly diagnosed and established diabetic children. Acta Paediatr 1998; 87:537.
30. Komulainen J, Lounamaa R, Knip M, et al. Ketoacidosis at the diagnosis of type 1 (insulin dependent) diabetes mellitus is related to poor residual beta cell function. Arch Dis Child 1996; 75:410.
31. Chantelau E, Spraul M, Muhlhauser I, et al. Longterm safety, efficacy and side-effects of continuous subcutaneous insulin infusion treatment for type I (insulin-dependent) diabetes mellitus: a one centre experience. Diabetologia 1989; 32:421.
32. Gatta B, Rigalleau V, Gin H. Diabetic ketoacidosis with olanzapine treatment. Diabetes Care 1999; 22:1002.
33. Campbell IW, Duncan LJP, Innes JA, et al. Abdominal pain in diabetic metabolic decompensation: clinical significance. JAMA 1975; 233:166.
34. Munro JF, Campbell IW, McCuish AC, Duncan LJP. Euglycemic diabetic ketoacidosis. Br Med J 1973; 2:578.
35. Jenkins D, Close CF, Krentz AJ, et al. Euglycaemic diabetic ketoacidosis: does it exist? Acta Diabetol 1993; 30:251.
36. Cullen MT, Reece EA, Hamko CJ, Sivan E. The changing presentation of diabetic ketoacidosis during pregnancy. Am J Perinatol 1996; 13:449.
37. Burge MR, Hardy KJ, Schade DS. Short term fasting is a mechanism for the development of euglycemic ketoacidosis during periods of insulin deficiency. J Clin Endocrinol Metab 1993; 76:1192.
38. Wiggam MI, O'Kane MJ, Harper R, et al. Treatment of diabetic ketoacidosis using normalization of blood 3-hydroxybutyrate concentration as the end-point of emergency management. Diabetes Care 1997; 20:1347.
39. Brandenburg MA, Dire DJ. Comparison of arterial and venous blood gas values in the initial emergency department evaluation of patients with diabetic ketoacidosis. Ann Emerg Med 1998; 31:459.
40. Adrogue HJ, Wilson H, Boyd AE, et al. Plasma acid-base patterns in diabetic ketoacidosis. N Engl J Med 1982; 307:1603.
41. Hillier TA, Abbott RD, Barrett EJ. Hyponatremia: evaluating the correction factor for hyperglycemia. Am J Med 1999; 106:399.
42. Kaminska ES, Pourmotabbed G. Spurious laboratory values in diabetic ketoacidosis and hyperlipidemia. Am J Emerg Med 1993; 11:77.
43. Alberti KGMM, Hockaday TDR. Diabetic coma: a reappraisal after five years. Clin Endocrinol Metab 1977; 6:421.
44. Kamimura M, Hancock EW. Acute MI pattern in diabetic ketoacidosis. Hosp Pract 1992; 15:28.
45. Sweterlitsch EM, Murphy GW. Acute electrocardiographic pseudoinfarction pattern in the setting of diabetic ketoacidosis and severe hyperkalemia. Am Heart J 1996; 132:1086.
46. Alberti KGMM, Hockaday TDR, Turner RC. Small doses of intramuscular insulin in the treatment of diabetic coma. Lancet 1973; 2:515.
47. Page MM, Alberti KGMM, Greenwood R, et al. Treatment of diabetic coma with continuous low-dose intravenous insulin. Br Med J 1974; 2:687.
48. Adrogue HJ, Lederer ED, Suki WN, Eknoyan G. Determinants of plasma potassium levels in diabetic ketoacidosis. Medicine (Baltimore) 1986; 65:163.
49. Wilson HK, Keuer SP, Lea AS, et al. Phosphate therapy in diabetic ketoacidosis. Arch Intern Med 1982; 142:517.
50. Oster JR, Alpert HC, Rodriguez GR, Vaamonde CA. Effect of acute reversal of experimentally induced ketoacidosis with sodium bicarbonate on the plasma concentrations of phosphorus and potassium. Life Sci 1988; 42:811.
51. Green SM, Rothrock SG, Ho JD, et al. Failure of adjunctive bicarbonate to improve outcome in severe pediatric diabetic ketoacidosis. Ann Emerg Med 1998; 31:41.
52. Okunda Y, Adrogue HJ, Field JB, et al. Counterproductive effects of sodium bicarbonate in diabetic ketoacidosis. J Clin Endocrinol Metab 1996; 81:314.
53. Gamba G, Oseguera J, Castrejon M, et al. Bicarbonate therapy in severe diabetic ketoacidosis: a double blind, randomised placebo controlled trial. Rev Invest Clin 1991; 43:234.
54. Mincu I, Ionescu-Tiigoviste C, Cheta D, Babes E. Le rôle de l'apport de glucose dans le traitement de la cétoacidose diabétique sevère. Gazette Med France 1979; 86:1665.

55. Malone NL, Klos SE, Gennis VM, Goodwin JS. Frequent hypoglycemic episodes in the treatment of patients with diabetic ketoacidosis. Arch Intern Med 1992; 152:2472.
56. Fein IA, Rackow EC, Sprung CL, Grodman R. Relation of colloid osmotic pressure to arterial hypoxemia and cerebral edema during crystalloid volume loading of patients with diabetic ketoacidosis. Ann Intern Med 1982; 96:570.
57. Krane EJ, Rockoff MA, Wallman JK, Wolfsdorf JI. Subclinical brain swelling in children during treatment of diabetic ketoacidosis. N Engl J Med 1985; 312:1147.
58. Arieff AI, Kleeman CR. Studies of mechanisms of cerebral edema in diabetic comas: effects of hyperglycemia and rapid lowering of plasma glucose in normal rabbits. J Clin Invest 1973; 52:571.
59. Van der Meulen JA, Klip A, Grinstein S. Possible mechanism for cerebral oedema in diabetic ketoacidosis. Lancet 1987; 2:306.
60. Edge JA, Dunger DB. Variations in the management of diabetic ketoacidosis in children. Diabet Med 1994; 11:981.
61. Hale PM, Rozvani I, Braunstein AW, et al. Factors predicting cerebral edema in young children with diabetic ketoacidosis and new onset type 1 diabetes. Acta Paediatr 1997; 86:626.
62. Eisenhuber E, Madl C, Kramer L, Grimm G. Subclinical brain dysfunction in patients with diabetic ketoacidosis. Diabetes Care 1996; 19:1455.
62a. Rosenbloom AL. Cerebral edema in diabetic ketoacidosis. J Clin Endocrinol Metab 2000; 85:507.
62b. Finberg L. Appropriate therapy can prevent cerebral swelling in diabetic ketoacidosis. J Clin Endocrinol Metab 2000; 85:508.
63. Carroll P, Matz R. Adult respiratory distress syndrome complicating severe uncontrolled diabetes mellitus: report of 9 cases and a review of the literature. Diabetes Care 1982; 5:574.
64. Hoffman WH, Locksmith JP, Burton EM, et al. Interstitial pulmonary edema in children and adolescents with diabetic ketoacidosis. J Diab Comp 1998; 12:314.
65. Singh RK, Perros P, Frier BM. Hospital management of diabetic ketoacidosis: are clinical guidelines implemented effectively? Diabet Med 1997; 14:482.
66. Khardori R, Soler NG. Hyperosmolar hyperglycemic nonketotic syndrome: report of 22 cases and a brief review. Am J Med 1984; 77:899.
67. Gottschalk ME, Ros SP, Zeller WP. The emergency management of hyperglycemic-hyperosmolar nonketotic coma in the pediatric patient. Pediatr Emerg Care 1996; 12:48.
68. Van der Meulen JA, Klip A, Grinstein S. Possible mechanism for cerebral oedema in diabetic ketoacidosis. Lancet 1987; 2:306.
69. Wachtel TJ, Silliman RA, Lamberton P. Predisposing factors for the diabetic hyperosmolar state. Arch Intern Med 1988; 147:499.
70. Press GA, Barshop BA, Haas RH, et al. Abnormalities of the brain in nonketotic hyperglycemia: MR manifestations. AJNR 1989; 10:315.
71. Nagaraja D, Taly AB, Rao TV, Joshy EV. Non-ketotic hyperglycemia and recurrent seizures. Nimhans J 1996; 14:9.
72. Whelton MJ, Walde D, Havard CWH. Hyperosmolar nonketotic diabetic coma: with particular reference to vascular complications. Br Med J 1971; 1:85.
73. Cohen RD, Woods HF. Lactic acidosis revisited. Diabetes 1984; 32:181.
74. Luft D, Schmulling RM, Eggstein M. Lactic acidosis in biguanide treatment of diabetics. Diabetologia 1978; 14:75.
75. Stang MR, Wysowski DK, Butler-Jones D. Incidence of lactic acidosis in metformin users. Diabetes Care 1999; 22:925.
76. Brown JB, Pedula K, Barzilay J, et al. Lactic acidosis rates in type 2 diabetes. Diabetes Care 1998; 21:1659.
77. Chan NN, Brain HP, Feher MD. Metformin-associated lactic acidosis: a rare or very rare clinical entity. Diabet Med 1999; 16:273.
78. Cohen RD, Woods HF. Clinical and biochemical aspects of lactic acidosis. Oxford: Blackwell, 1976.
79. Stacpoole PW, Lorenz AC, Thomas RG, Harman EM. Dichloroacetate in the treatment of lactic acidosis. Ann Intern Med 1988; 108:58.
80. Fulop M, Hoberman HD. Alcoholic ketosis. Diabetes 1975; 24:785.
81. Fulop M. Alcoholism, ketoacidosis, and lactic acidosis. Diabetes Metab Rev 1989; 5:365.
82. Iten PX, Meier M. Beta-hydroxybutyric acid—an indicator for an alcoholic ketoacidosis as cause of death in deceased alcohol abusers. J Forensic Sci 2000; 45:624.
83. Marshall SM. Hyperglycaemic emergencies. J R Coll Phys Edinb 1995; 25:105.

# CHAPTER 156

# DIABETES MELLITUS AND PREGNANCY

LOIS JOVANOVIC

Before the advent of insulin, few young diabetic women lived to childbearing age. Before 1922, fewer than 100 pregnancies in diabetic women were reported, with a >90% infant mortality rate and a 30% maternal mortality rate.[1] In the mid-1970s, physicians were

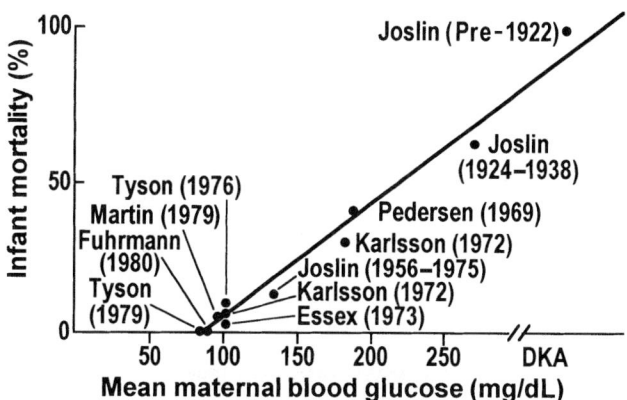

**FIGURE 156-1.** The relationship between mean maternal glucose level and infant mortality over the years. (*DKA*, diabetic ketoacidosis.)

still counseling diabetic women to avoid pregnancy.[2] This viewpoint was justified because of the poor obstetric history in 30% to 50% of diabetic women. Infant mortality rates finally improved when treatment strategies stressed better control of maternal plasma glucose levels. As the pathophysiology of pregnancy complicated by diabetes has been elucidated and as management programs have achieved and maintained normoglycemia throughout pregnancy, perinatal mortality rates have decreased to levels seen in the general population (Fig. 156-1).[3]

## DIABETOGENIC FACTORS OF PREGNANCY

### PLASMA GLUCOSE DURING PREGNANCY

The fetal demise associated with pregnancy complicated by diabetes seems to arise from glucose.[4] Elevated maternal plasma glucose levels should always be avoided. To achieve normoglycemia, a clear understanding of "normal" carbohydrate metabolism in pregnancy is paramount.[4a]

Glucose is transported to the fetus by facilitated diffusion, whereas amino acids are actively transported across the placenta. Moreover, alanine is siphoned selectively to the fetus.[5] The maternal serum glucose concentration drops below nonpregnancy (between 55 and 65 mg/dL in the fasting state).[6] Simultaneously, plasma ketone concentrations are several times higher and free fatty acids are elevated after an overnight fast.[7,8] Thus, pregnancy simulates a state of "accelerated starvation" in which alternative fuels are used for maternal metabolism, while glucose is spared for fetal consumption (Fig. 156-2).[9]

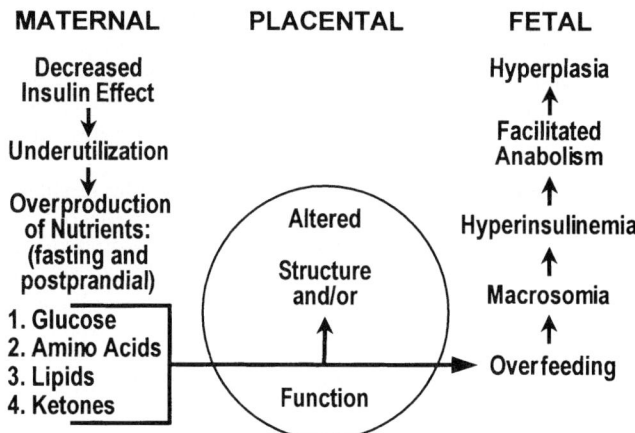

**FIGURE 156-2.** Schematic representation of nutrient fluxes across the placenta.

## DIABETOGENIC HORMONES OF THE PLACENTA

The second half of pregnancy is characterized by a further lowering of plasma glucose levels. Although maternal glucose levels remain below levels during nonpregnancy, insulin levels increase markedly, partly because of increasing antiinsulin hormonal activity. The major diabetogenic hormones of the placenta are human somatomammotropin (hCS), previously referred to as human placental lactogen (hPL), estrogen, and progesterone. Also, serum maternal cortisol levels (both bound and free) are increased. At the elevated levels seen during gestation, prolactin has a diabetogenic effect.[10]

### HUMAN CHORIONIC SOMATOMAMMOTROPIN

The strongest insulin antagonist of pregnancy is hCS. This placental hormone appears in increasing concentration beginning at 10 weeks of gestation (see Chap. 108). By 20 weeks of gestation, plasma hCS levels are increased 300-fold, and by term, the turnover rate is ~1000 mg per day.[11] The mechanism of action whereby hCS raises plasma glucose levels is unclear but probably originates from its growth hormone–like properties. The hCS also promotes free fatty acid production by stimulating lipolysis, which promotes peripheral resistance to insulin.

### CORTISOL

Most of the marked rise of serum cortisol during pregnancy can be attributed to the increase of cortisol-binding globulin induced by estrogen. However, free cortisol levels are also increased.[12] Thus, the rising cortisol levels may unmask diabetes in a predisposed individual.

### PROGESTERONE

When progesterone is administered to normal nonpregnant fasting women, the serum insulin concentration rises and the glucose concentration remains unchanged. In monkeys, progesterone increases both early and total insulin responses to glucose.

### PROLACTIN

The rise in pituitary prolactin early in pregnancy is triggered by the rising estrogen levels. The structure of prolactin is similar to that of growth hormone, and at concentrations reached by the second trimester (>200 ng/mL) prolactin can affect glucose metabolism. Although no studies have examined the role of prolactin alone as an insulin antagonist, indirect evidence exists that suppressing prolactin in gestational diabetic women with large doses of pyridoxine improves glucose tolerance.

## INSULIN DEGRADATION DURING PREGNANCY

Degradation of insulin is increased in pregnancy. This degradation is caused by placental enzymes comparable to liver insulinases. The placenta also has membrane-associated insulin-degrading activity.[13]

Concomitant with the hormonally induced insulin resistance and increase in insulin degradation, the rate of disposal of insulin slows. The normal pancreas can adapt to these factors by potentiation of insulin secretion. If the pancreas fails to respond adequately to these alterations, or if the clearance of glucose is defective, then gestational diabetes results.

## EFFECT OF HYPERGLYCEMIA ON THE PREGNANCY AND THE FETUS

If the mother has hyperglycemia, the fetus will be exposed to either sustained hyperglycemia or intermittent pulses of hyperglycemia. Both situations prematurely stimulate fetal insulin secretion. The Pedersen hypothesis links maternal hyperglycemia-induced fetal hyperinsulinemia to morbidity of the infant.[4] Fetal hyperinsulinemia may cause increased fetal body fat (macrosomia) and, therefore, a difficult delivery, or may cause inhibition of pulmonary maturation of surfactant and, therefore, respiratory distress of the neonate. The fetus may also have decreased serum potassium levels caused by the elevated insulin and glucose levels and may therefore have cardiac arrhythmias. Neonatal hypoglycemia may cause permanent neurologic damage. Hyperglycemia in the mother may lead to maternal complications, such as polyhydramnios, hypertension, urinary tract infections, candidal vaginitis, recurrent spontaneous abortions, and infertility. Thus, a vigorous effort should be made to diagnose diabetes early and to achieve and maintain normoglycemia throughout pregnancy. As mentioned earlier, improved treatment protocols have lowered maternal plasma glucose levels, and the infant mortality rate has dropped (see Fig. 156-1). Treatment protocols should be designed to establish normoglycemia before conception (Table 156-1).

## GESTATIONAL DIABETES

The literal meaning of *gestational diabetes mellitus* is pregnancy-related diabetes, which usually refers to diabetes that occurs during pregnancy and disappears after the pregnancy is over. This label may be applied to any pregnant woman who is diagnosed with a high blood glucose level during pregnancy, even if she has developed type 1 or type 2 diabetes during pregnancy. The accepted definition is *glucose intolerance of variable degree with onset or first recognition during pregnancy*.[14] Usually, gestational diabetes occurs during the second half of pregnancy in those who are overweight, unfit, or aging, and who have a family history of diabetes. The report from the Fourth International Gestational Diabetes Workshop-Conference[15] suggests that women who are at *any risk* of an elevated blood glucose should be screened for gestational diabetes at some time during their 24th to 28th week of gestation. The definition of *any risk* is the presence of one or more of the following: patient is older than 25 years; ethnic background is Asian, black, Hispanic, and/or Native American (up to 12% prevalence in these groups)[14]; patient has a family history of type 2 diabetes; patient has a body mass index of 27 (i.e., even mildly overweight). In programs in which large populations of pregnant women are screened, screening only women who have one or more of these risk factors is most cost effective; nonetheless, 10% of women found to have gestational diabetes have none of the risk factors. Women from a low-risk group still have been reported to have a 2.8% prevalence rate.[16] These women had pregnancy outcomes similar to those of other women with gestational diabetes. The authors of this study concluded that the recommendation not to test women from low-risk groups requires further evaluation in different populations before it can be endorsed. An editorial based on this study[17] suggested that "until more data are available to support the new American Diabetes Association recommendations, the health of children will best be served by making every effort to determine the presence and degree of glucose intolerance in every pregnancy." The California Diabetes and Pregnancy Sweet Success Guidelines for care have continued to recommend screening of all pregnant women between 24 and 28 weeks of gestation.[18] The diabetogenic stimuli during these weeks are sufficient to manifest diabetes in at least 75% of women with gestational diabetes. If the screening is delayed until the 32nd week of gestation, 100% of women with gesta-

**TABLE 156-1.**
**Flow Chart for Management of Diabetes (Type 1) and Pregnancy**

| Week of Gestation | Test | Treatment |
|---|---|---|
| –6 | Glycosylated hemoglobin (GHb) level | Normalization of GHb levels |
| | Self blood glucose monitoring (SBGM) daily* | |
| –2 | GHb | Recheck of GHb to assure normality before conception |
| | SBGM daily* | Instruction in basal temperature checking |
| +2 | GHb | Reinforcement of insulin and diet plan |
| | SBGM daily* | Insulin: 0.7 U/kg/24 hours |
| | Thyroid function | Diet: 25 kcal/kg/24 hours |
| | Kidney function | |
| | Eye examination | |
| | Physical examination | |
| | Routine prenatal care | |
| +8–18 | GHb every 2 weeks | Increase in diet up to 30 kcal/kg/24 hours and insulin as needed |
| | SBGM daily* | |
| | Sonogram at 8 and 12 weeks | |
| +18–20 | GHb every 2 weeks | Increase in diet as needed |
| | SBGM daily* | Increase in insulin to 0.8 U/kg/24 hours |
| | Kidney function at 22 weeks | |
| | Eye examination at 22 weeks | |
| | Thyroid function at 22 weeks | |
| | Physical examination at 22 weeks | |
| | Sonogram at 22 weeks | |
| +30–36 | GHb every 2 weeks | Increase in insulin and diet as needed |
| | SBGM daily* | Admission for bed rest if blood pressure is rising |
| | Repeat kidney, eye, and physical examination at 32–34 weeks | |
| +36–41 | Obstetric surveillance protocol established to assess uterine growth, fetal well-being, GHb every 2 weeks | Increase in diet as needed |
| | SBGM daily* | Increase in insulin to 0.9–1.0 U/kg/24 hours |
| | | Delivery if fetal distress |

*For women with type 1 diabetes, perform 6–8 times daily and check the reflectance meter weekly for accuracy.

**TABLE 156-2.**
**Diagnosis of Gestational Diabetes Mellitus**

| | mg/dL | mmol/L |
|---|---|---|
| **100-g ORAL GLUCOSE LOAD*** | | |
| Fasting | 95 | 5.3 |
| 1 hour | 180 | 10.0 |
| 2 hour | 155 | 8.6 |
| 3 hour | 140 | 7.8 |
| **75-g ORAL GLUCOSE LOAD*** | | |
| Fasting | 95 | 5.3 |
| 1 hour | 180 | 10.0 |
| 2 hour | 155 | 8.6 |
| **CLASSIFICATION** | | |
| DIET-CONTROLLED GESTATIONAL DIABETES | Fasting capillary whole-blood glucose <90 mg/dL (5.30 mmol/L). | |
| TREATMENT | Trial of diet. Initiate insulin if normoglycemia† is not maintained on diet alone. | |
| INSULIN REQUIREMENT | If the fasting capillary whole-blood glucose level is >90 mg/dL and/or postprandial glucose levels are >120 mg/dL (6.7 mmol/L), then insulin should be prescribed immediately. | |

*Two or more of the venous plasma concentrations must be met or exceeded for a positive diagnosis.

†Normoglycemia = fasting glucose level of <90 mg/dL and level 1 hour after meal of <120 mg/dL.

betes. If her plasma glucose level is >140 mg/dL (>7.8 mmol/L), a glucose-tolerance test is indicated.

In the summary of the Fourth International Gestational Diabetes Mellitus Workshop-Conference,[15] the recommendations for the diagnostic oral glucose-tolerance test allow the clinician to choose between a 100-g glucose drink[20] and a 75-g glucose drink.[21] Table 156-2 describes these tests. Either glucose load should be administered after a minimum of 8 hours of fasting. A fasting plasma glucose blood sample should be drawn no later than 9:00 a.m. In the case of the 100-g load, plasma glucose levels should be obtained 1, 2, and 3 hours after the glucose load. In the case of the 75-g glucose load, testing is really necessary only at the 0-, 1-, and 2-hour time points.

The glucose level should be determined on venous plasma using the hexokinase method, and not on capillary blood using glucose oxidase–impregnated test strips, which are less accurate for this purpose. Once the diagnosis of gestational diabetes is made, however, these strips become the mainstay of treatment strategies.

## DIAGNOSTIC STRATEGIES

The diagnostic criteria for gestational diabetes are based on the oral glucose-tolerance test (see Table 156-2).[20] These criteria correctly identify women at risk for a stillbirth. They do not identify women at risk of delivering a macrosomic infant. Other tests and cutoffs need to be used to identify the macrosomic fetus.[22] Blood glucose values at 4 and 5 hours after glucose load have no diagnostic significance. Measurement of glycosylated hemoglobin levels, which is a test of long-term plasma glucose control in type 1 and type 2 diabetes mellitus, is not sensitive enough to diagnose gestational diabetes.[19]

Use of a single diagnostic test, rather than the two-step method used in most of the United States, greatly simplifies the procedure. A single 75-g glucose load[21] is all that is necessary; gestational impaired glucose tolerance is defined as a 2-hour postload glucose concentration of >140 mg/dL (7.8 mmol/L). This constitutes a diagnosis of gestational diabetes and warrants treatment.

tional diabetes will be detected, but by then, after 4 to 6 weeks of sustained hyperglycemia, 75% of the infants may already have developed fetopathy.[19]

If the suspicion exists that a pregnant woman in her first trimester may have preexisting, undiagnosed diabetes, then the screening should be performed at the first visit. If the testing is negative in the first trimester and at the usual examination between 24 and 28 weeks, the woman may be among the 25% of women with gestational diabetes who develop diabetes in the third trimester. These women tend to be older than 33 years of age and are >120% of ideal body weight.[19]

The screening test consists of oral administration of 50 g of glucose and a plasma glucose determination at 1 hour, and it may be given regardless of the time of the last meal. If the plasma glucose concentration 1 hour after the oral load is <140 mg/dL (7.8 mmol/L), the woman does not have gestational dia-

TABLE 156-3.
Diet Calculation for Women 80% to 120% of Ideal Body Weight

| Time | Meal | Fraction (kcal/24 hours) | % of Daily Carbo-hydrate Allowed |
|------|------|--------------------------|----------------------------------|
| 8:00 a.m. | Breakfast | 2/18 | 10 |
| 10:30 a.m. | Snack | 1/18 | 5 |
| 12:00 noon | Lunch | 5/18 | 30 |
| 3:00 p.m. | Snack | 2/18 | 10 |
| 5:00 p.m. | Dinner | 5/18 | 30 |
| 8:00 p.m. | Snack | 2/18 | 5 |
| 11:00 p.m. | Snack | 1/18 | 10 |

TABLE 156-4.
Initial Calculation of Insulin Therapy for Four Injections a Day*

| Time | Fraction of Total Insulin Dose | |
|------|------|------|
| | *NPH* | *Regular* |
| Prebreakfast | 5/18 | 2/9 |
| Prelunch | — | 1/6 |
| Predinner | — | 1/6 |
| Bedtime | 1/6 | — |

*NPH*, neutral protamine Hagedorn insulin.
*Total insulin = 0.7 U/kg for weeks 6–18; 0.8 U/kg for weeks 18–26; 0.9 U/kg for weeks 26–36; 1.0 U/kg for weeks 36–40.

## TREATMENT OF GESTATIONAL DIABETES

The goal of management of gestational diabetes is to maintain normoglycemia. Most pregnant women never exceed 120 mg/dL of plasma glucose, even at 1 hour after a meal, despite the ingestion of large quantities of carbohydrate. If the peak post-prandial glucose value is >120 mg/dL, the risk of macrosomia rises exponentially.[23] Because a nutritious meal for the mother and her unborn child necessitates at least a 40 mg/dL increase of plasma glucose, if the woman's fasting glucose level is much greater than 90 mg/dL (whole-blood capillary glucose), she will be unable to maintain her postprandial levels at <120 mg/dL. Therefore, any woman whose fasting whole-blood capillary glu-cose level is elevated above 90 mg/dL requires insulin to allow for the postprandial excursions resulting from the minimal nutritional requirements of pregnancy. Both the fasting and the 1-hour postprandial glucose levels need to be monitored, even in a woman with diet-controlled gestational diabetes.

### DIET

If the woman's fasting whole-blood capillary glucose level is <90 mg/dL, then a trial of dietary therapy is possible. The diet in pregnancy of a diabetic woman who is 80% to 120% of ideal body weight is the same as for a nondiabetic pregnant woman, or 30 kcal/kg per 24 hours. Less than 40% of the calories should be consumed in the form of carbohydrate, because carbohy-drate is the main contributor to the peak postprandial glucose level.[24,25]

The breakfast meal must be small, and the carbohydrate por-tion of this meal minimal. The dietary plan of frequent, small feedings is designed to avoid postprandial hyperglycemia and preprandial starvation ketosis (Table 156-3). In the obese dia-betic woman (>120% of ideal body weight), fewer calories per kilogram of total pregnant weight need be given, because these women have a larger percentage of body weight in the form of adipose tissue; 24 kcal/kg per 24 hours or less often allows the patient to maintain euglycemia and remain ketosis free.[26]

### INSULIN

If a woman does need insulin because her plasma glucose levels exceed the criteria for normoglycemia or her blood glucose level can be normalized only by starvation,[27] a four-injection-per-day regimen is prescribed, similar to the one outlined later for women with type 1 insulin-dependent diabetes (Table 156-4). In a massively obese woman, the initial doses of insulin may need to be increased to 1.5 to 2.0 U/kg to overcome the combined insulin resistance of pregnancy and obesity.[27]

### EXERCISE

Arm exercises performed in a seated position are safe and facil-itate the maintenance of normoglycemia.[28,29]

## PREGESTATIONAL DIABETES: TYPE 1 AND TYPE 2

### CLASSIFICATION

Classifications of pregestational diabetes have emerged to help the physician predict the outcome of pregnancy for both the mother and child. The White classification categorized diabetic women based on the mode of therapy, duration, and age at onset of diabetes, and the degree of vascular compromise of each patient at the beginning of the pregnancy.[1] This classification led to confusion, because the "B" determination was given to both women with pregnancy-related diabetes (gestational diabetes) that necessitated insulin, and to pregestational women who had undergone fewer than 10 years of insulin therapy. As the evi-dence mounts that maternal normoglycemia is necessary at the time of conception, during fetal organogenesis, and throughout gestation, however, a new classification has been developed that places more emphasis on the maternal plasma glucose level. This classification should include a statement about the control of the patient's diabetes, with the category of either pregestational or gestational. The criteria for "good" diabetic control should be plasma glucose levels equal to those of nondiabetic pregnant women. This should include a fasting blood glucose concentra-tion of 55 to 65 mg/dL, average blood glucose level of 84 mg/dL, and 1-hour postprandial blood glucose value of <120 mg/dL.[23]

### RISK FACTORS

Plasma glucose levels are the major predictors of outcome in preg-nancies complicated by diabetes.[30] The outcome for the mother or the fetus need not be influenced by retinopathy, peripheral vascu-lar disease, or nephropathy.[31,32] Moreover, kidney function seems to improve if normal plasma glucose levels are maintained, despite decreased function before pregnancy.[31] Hypertension, however, confers an independent and worrisome risk. Type 1 dia-betes commencing during gestation (generally presenting with maternal ketoacidosis) also implies a poor prognosis.

Several medical conditions of concern frequently coexist in the diabetic patient. The paramount goal in the treatment of coexisting medical problems is to avoid harming the fetus while helping the mother.

### HYPERTENSION

In the case of preexisting hypertension, all medication ideally should be discontinued before fetal organogenesis. The safest antihypertensive protocol, as far as the fetus is concerned, is restriction of salt and water intake: 2 to 3 g of sodium each day and <2 L of oral fluid intake every 24 hours. If this regimen does not control blood pressure, methyldopa or hydralazine can be used, because these agents do not appear to interfere with organogenesis. Angiotensin-converting inhibitors are contraindicated because they are associated with congenital defects. If blood pressure rises despite these suggestions, then advising against pregnancy should be considered rather than adding toxic medications that would endanger the fetus.

### INFECTION

Special considerations in pregnancy include urinary tract infections, which are reported in as many as 20% of pregnant women with diabetes (see Chap. 152).[33] Infection may lead to exaggerated hyperglycemia, which should be normalized to protect the fetus. The diabetic patient is also subject to the adverse effects of maternal infection with rubella, toxoplasmosis, syphilis, and other infections associated with fetal morbidity and mortality. Antibiotic therapy should be used sparingly, because the fetal serum levels could be significant. Antibiotics usually considered safe in pregnancy include penicillin and erythromycin. Tetracycline and sulfa drugs should be avoided because of their effects on tooth coloration and bilirubin metabolism, respectively.

### THYROID DYSFUNCTION

Forty percent of patients with type 1 diabetes may have coexisting thyroid dysfunction.[34,35] Because the stress of pregnancy may unmask this predisposition to thyroid disease, a radioimmunoassay for thyroid hormone, paired with a serum thyroid-stimulating hormone level, should be determined once pregnancy has been diagnosed and at least twice more during pregnancy. Hypothyroidism should be treated with L-thyroxine ($T_4$) in a dose titrated according to the level of plasma $T_4$ that is desired. Because pregnancy raises the thyroid-binding globulin level, a normal thyroxine level is ~20% above the standard in nonpregnancy.

Hyperthyroidism diagnosed during pregnancy should be treated medically until delivery, after which time definitive treatment can be given in the form of radioactive iodine therapy or surgery (see Chap. 42).

### RETINOPATHY

Retinopathy is not a contraindication for pregnancy, but a retinal specialist should examine the patient before a planned pregnancy and follow the patient closely, perhaps monthly, throughout pregnancy. Treatment with laser therapy is possible if neovascularization occurs.[32]

In the author's experience, patients without retinopathy do not develop retinopathy during pregnancy. However, existent retinopathy may progress during pregnancy.[36] This progression seems to be potentiated by rapid normalization of the plasma glucose level, long duration of diabetes, and presence of hypertension, nephropathy, and retinopathy in the first trimester.[36] Because urgent normalization is necessary during pregnancy for the sake of fetal well-being, the best treatment strategy for the diabetic woman with retinopathy is to begin a program of normalization of plasma glucose concentrations before pregnancy. This should progress slowly over 3 to 6 months, while a retinal specialist follows the retinal status. Once the plasma glucose is stabilized within or near the normal range and is well maintained for another 3 to 6 months, pregnancy can be safely undertaken.

### NEPHROPATHY

Nephropathy and proteinuria are not contraindications for pregnancy. Kidney disease does not necessarily complicate the pregnancy unless superimposed hypertension intervenes.[31] Kidney function should be assessed by a formal creatinine clearance measurement. Most experts suggest that a creatinine clearance of <50 mL per minute is a contraindication to pregnancy because of the risk of pregnancy-associated hypertension in these women. A creatinine clearance >50 mL per minute in normotensive women did not have an effect on the mother or the infant in a group of 22 women studied by the author. In fact, in these women, a normal increase in glomerular filtration rate was seen as pregnancy progressed.

Pregnancy does predispose to urinary tract infections. Fifteen percent of all the author's patients had bacteriuria. Therefore, urine culture should be performed monthly and infections treated vigorously to prevent ascending pyelonephritis.

Women with proteinuria before pregnancy are predisposed to increasing proteinuria during pregnancy. Despite the massive proteinuria that may develop, as long as normoglycemia is sustained, the postpartum proteinuria should return to baseline levels. When the syndrome is associated with hypertension, avoidance of pregnancy probably is wise because of the untoward effects on the mother and fetus.

## TREATMENT OF THE PREGNANT DIABETIC WOMAN

### DIET PRESCRIPTION AND MONITORING

The goal of dietary management for women with type 1 diabetes, like that of women with gestational diabetes, is to maintain normoglycemia.[37] Moreover, in either women with insulin-requiring gestational diabetes or women with type 1 diabetes, the food and the insulin must match. The diet shown in Table 156-3 of frequent, small feedings is designed to avoid postprandial hyperglycemia and preprandial starvation ketosis and to promote an average weight gain of 12.5 kg in accord with the recommendations of the Committee on Maternal Nutrition.[38] In obese women with type 1 diabetes (>120% of ideal body weight), as in obese women with gestational diabetes, fewer calories per kilogram of total pregnant weight are needed to prevent ketosis yet provide sufficient nutrition for the fetus and mother (~24 kcal/kg/24 hours). Reports have indicated that when ketone production is completely suppressed in pregnant women by overfeeding, the risk of macrosomia is increased.[39]

For each woman with gestational or pregestational diabetes, a diet should be prescribed and the monitoring protocol explained at the same visit.

### IMPLEMENTATION OF THERAPY

No matter how educated the pregestational woman is about managing her diabetes, metabolism is affected so greatly by pregnancy that reinforcement is necessary. Ideally, education to achieve and maintain normoglycemia should be instituted before conception or as soon as the diagnosis of pregnancy is made. Usually, 5 to 7 days are required to teach the patient the requisite goals and skills to normalize plasma glucose level throughout gestation through the use of insulin adjustments. The training process is best achieved in centers specialized for education of diabetes self-care.

### STEPS IN A NORMALIZATION PROGRAM

The first step in the self-care program is to teach home blood glucose monitoring and to ensure, through a quality-control program, that the values are accurate to within 10% of a laboratory standard. Most women prefer systems using reflectance meters because of the perceived increased accuracy over visually readable reagent strips. A woman with diet-controlled gestational diabetes must monitor her blood glucose level four times a day (fasting and 1 hour after each meal). A diabetic woman who requires insulin must monitor her blood glucose level six times a day (before and 1 hour after each meal).[23]

The diet is maintained as described earlier, and insulin is administered to mimic normal pancreatic function. The normal

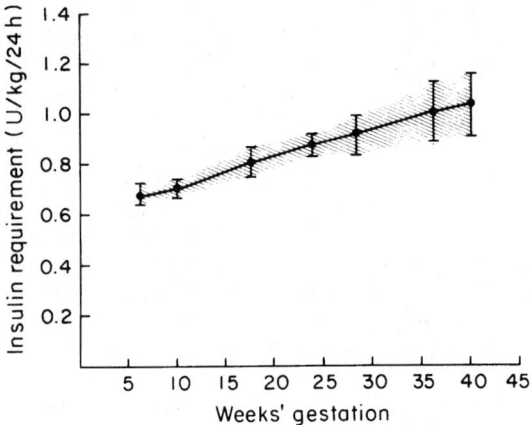

**FIGURE 156-3.** Pregnancy increases insulin requirements. The *bars* indicate ±1 standard deviation from the mean.

pancreas secretes 50% of the insulin as mealtime boluses. This delivery may be mimicked by four injections a day of combinations of neutral protamine Hagedorn (NPH) and regular insulin (see Table 156-4); however, the number of injections can be decreased to three a day if the patient is willing to time her lunch to coincide with the preprogrammed insulin midday peak. The total daily dose of insulin is based on the gestational week and the woman's current pregnant body weight (Fig. 156-3). After the initial insulin calculation, the dose is adjusted for each woman until all the blood glucose levels before and after each meal are normal. Six or more glucose measurements each day may be required to optimize therapy.

The titration of insulin needs to blood glucose levels is based on frequent monitoring and ensures a smooth increase of insulin as the pregnancy progresses to a higher insulin requirement of up to 1.0 U/kg per 24 hours at term (see Fig. 156-3). Twin gestations cause an approximate doubling of the insulin requirement throughout pregnancy. Each patient must also be taught her personal lag time between the insulin injection and the initiation of the meal. The simultaneous injection of insulin and ingestion of glucose cause "brittle diabetes": the simple sugars in food raise the blood glucose level before the action of the subcutaneous insulin peaks, and the quickly metabolized glucose is gone when the insulin levels are at their maximum. To correct this problem, the insulin should be injected at least 30 to 45 minutes before the meal to allow the insulin and the food effects to peak together.

### FOLLOW-UP VISITS

The outpatient visits should be frequent enough to provide the needed consultation, guidance, and emotional support to facilitate compliance. Moreover, tests and therapy should be appropriate for gestational age (see Table 156-1). The health care delivery team should put forth an extra effort during pregnancy. Each patient should have telephone access to the team on a 24-hour basis for questions concerning therapy, and visits should be frequent (i.e., 2 weeks apart). Measurement of glycosylated hemoglobin (hemoglobin $A_{1c}$) on blood samples drawn at monthly intervals helps to confirm that the home blood glucose diary reflects the real maternal blood glucose control (see Table 156-1).

### GLYCOSYLATED HEMOGLOBIN LEVELS IN PREGNANCY

Glycosylated hemoglobin levels are not sensitive enough to detect minor elevations of glucose and cannot be used as a

screening tool for gestational diabetes; however, the glycosylated hemoglobin levels can be used to monitor diabetic control.[37,40] As noted earlier, serial determinations (once every 2 weeks [see Table 156-1]) can reinforce the patient's records and also are useful to enable the patient to see her own trends compared with her starting glycosylated hemoglobin level. Treatment decisions should be based solely on the self-monitored glucose levels, with double-checking of this value against a laboratory standard.

The best way to use glycosylated hemoglobin levels in pregnancy is to create "pregnancy norms." Because the mean plasma glucose level is ~20% lower in pregnancy, the glycosylated hemoglobin levels in normal pregnancy are ~20% lower than levels in nonpregnancy. When a glycosylated hemoglobin level is markedly elevated above the mean for a nondiabetic woman in the first 8 weeks of pregnancy, then the risk of a congenital anomaly in the infant is as high as 25%.[41,42] Achieving a glycosylated hemoglobin level within 6 standard deviations above the mean of nondiabetic women decreases the rates of retinopathy progression,[36] spontaneous abortion, and birth defects to near that of the general population.[36,43–45] Therefore, optimal therapy demands that normoglycemia be achieved before conception, because most of fetal organogenesis is complete by the seventh or eighth week of gestation.[46]

### PREVENTION OF REBOUND HYPERGLYCEMIA

Each patient should be taught to respond to symptoms of hypoglycemia (e.g., tingling sensations, diaphoresis, palpitations) by first checking her blood glucose level. If the level is <70 mg/dL, the patient should be instructed to drink 240 mL (8 oz) of milk and to recheck her blood glucose level 15 minutes later. This protocol is designed to normalize glucose without rebound hyperglycemia.

Patients and their families should be taught to inject glucagon subcutaneously to treat insulin reactions that cannot be corrected with food. During times of morning sickness or vomiting, the judicious use of glucagon can prevent hypoglycemia. Generally, 0.15 mg of glucagon injected subcutaneously raise blood glucose values 30 mg/dL within 15 minutes and maintains the levels for ~3 hours.

### RATIONALE FOR THE USE OF HUMAN INSULIN IN PREGNANCY

Maternal antiinsulin antibodies may contribute to hyperinsulinemia in utero and thus potentiate the metabolic aberrancy. Although insulin does not cross the placenta, antibodies to insulin do, and may bind fetal insulin; this necessitates the increased production of free insulin to reestablish normoglycemia. Thus, the antiinsulin antibodies may potentiate the effect of maternal hyperglycemia to produce fetal hyperinsulinemia. Human and highly purified insulins are significantly less immunogenic than mixed beef-pork insulins.[47] Use of human insulin treatment has been reported to improve pregnancy and infant outcome compared with use of highly purified animal insulins.[48] The insulin analog lispro (the amino-acid sequence in the β chain is reversed at positions B28 and B29) has been reported to be more efficacious than human regular insulin in normalizing the blood glucose levels in women with gestational diabetes. Use of this insulin lowered the postprandial glucose levels, thereby decreasing the glycosylated hemoglobin levels, and resulted in fewer hypoglycemic episodes and no increase the antiinsulin antibody levels.[49] The safety and efficacy of lispro insulin in the treatment of type 1 and type 2 diabetic women throughout the first 8 weeks of pregnancy, the period of organogenesis, is not yet known.

# DELIVERY

## TIMING OF DELIVERY

When pregnancy is complicated by hyperglycemia, the risk of stillbirth increases as term approaches.[50] In an attempt to decrease these losses, obstetricians have delivered such pregnancies electively between 35 and 38 weeks of gestation. This approach may have caused significant neonatal morbidity, however, due to prematurity and hyaline membrane disease.[51]

Neonatal morbidity can be markedly reduced if delivery is delayed until pulmonary maturity is documented.[51] Eighty percent of preterm infants have some form of morbidity, compared with 40% of term infants.[52] Therefore, watchful waiting is warranted after the 36th week of gestation and should be continued as long as maternal normoglycemia is maintained and as long as the fetus remains stable, as documented by antepartum heart rate testing every 2 to 3 days and fetal movement records, which are made on a daily basis (see Table 156-1). Because programs of normoglycemia are relatively new and because tools for fetal surveillance are improving rapidly, a protocol for optimal fetal surveillance remains to be worked out. Taking at least two sonograms during pregnancy (at 22 weeks and 32 weeks) is useful to document gestational age and to diagnose defects.[53]

In pregnancies in which glucose control has been less than optimal, the lecithin/sphingomyelin (L/S) ratio of the amniotic fluid should be assessed at 36 or 37 weeks' gestation. Patients with documented good control do not need early delivery, and amniocentesis is not needed.[50] The presence of phosphatidylglycerol in the fluid indicates pulmonary maturity.[51,54] The fetus with documented pulmonary maturity and poor results on fetal surveillance protocols should be delivered immediately. In pregnancies in which glucose control is documented to be normal by six daily blood glucose self-determinations and monthly normal glycosylated hemoglobin tests, women should be allowed to go to term, as long as the fetal surveillance tests are normal (see Table 156-1).

## LABOR AND DELIVERY

With improvement in antenatal care, intrapartum events play an increasingly crucial role in the outcome of pregnancy.[52,55] The artificial B cell may be used to maintain normoglycemia during labor and delivery, but normoglycemia can be maintained easily by subcutaneous injections.[54,56] Before active labor, insulin is required, and glucose infusion is not necessary to maintain a blood glucose level of 70 to 90 mg/dL. With the onset of active labor, insulin requirements decrease to zero and glucose requirements are relatively consistent at 2.5 mg/kg per minute. From these data, a protocol for supplying the glucose needs of labor has been developed.

The goal is to maintain maternal plasma glucose between 70 and 90 mg/dL. In cases of the onset of active spontaneous labor, insulin is withheld and an intravenous dextrose infusion is begun at a rate of 2.55 mg/kg per minute. If labor is latent, normal saline is usually sufficient to maintain normoglycemia until active labor begins, at which time dextrose is infused at 2.55 mg/kg per minute. Blood glucose is then monitored hourly, and if it is below 60 mg/dL, the infusion rate is doubled for the subsequent hour. If the blood glucose rises to >120 mg/dL, 2 to 4 U of regular insulin is given subcutaneously each hour until the blood glucose level is 70 to 80 mg/dL and is titrated to the target infusion rate of 2.55 mg/kg per minute as active labor is achieved. In the case of an elective cesarean section, the bedtime dose of NPH insulin is repeated at 8 a.m. on the day of surgery and every 8

hours if the surgery is delayed. A 10% dextrose infusion may be started if the plasma glucose level falls below 60 mg/dL.

## POSTPARTUM MANAGEMENT

### DECREASED MATERNAL INSULIN REQUIREMENTS

Maternal insulin requirements usually drop precipitously postpartum; therefore, women with gestational diabetes may not require further insulin.

On the other hand, women with pregestational diabetes require the resumption of insulin therapy, but these requirements may be decreased for 48 to 96 hours postpartum. Insulin requirements should be recalculated at 0.6 U/kg based on the postpartum weight and should be started when the 1-hour postprandial plasma glucose value is >150 mg/dL or the fasting glucose level is >100 mg/dL. The postpartum caloric requirements are 25 kcal/kg per day, based on postpartum weight. For women who wish to breast-feed, the calculation is 27 kcal/kg per day and insulin requirements are 0.6 U/kg per day. The insulin requirement during the night drops dramatically during lactation, owing to siphoning of glucose into the breast milk. Thus, the majority of the insulin requirement is needed during the daytime to cover the increased caloric needs of breast-feeding. Normoglycemia should especially be prescribed for nursing diabetic women, because hyperglycemia elevates milk glucose levels.[57]

### POSTPARTUM COURSE OF GESTATIONAL DIABETES

Almost 98% of all women with gestational diabetes revert to normoglycemia postpartum. A glucose-tolerance test should be performed 6 weeks postpartum, or when breast-feeding is stopped, to ensure that the diabetes has disappeared. Women should be warned that the probability that diabetes will recur in each subsequent pregnancy is ~90%. Therefore, women should be screened during each pregnancy. Moreover, if a woman remains overweight, she has a 60% chance of manifesting overt diabetes within 20 years. Therefore, the postpartum period is an important time in which to initiate the process of weight loss. The second goal of management of pregnancies complicated by gestational diabetes is to prevent obesity-induced diabetes in the future.

## NEONATAL CARE

If the blood glucose concentration is normalized throughout pregnancy in a woman with diabetes, no evidence exists that excess attention need be paid to her offspring. If the normal blood glucose level has not been documented throughout pregnancy, however, the wise course is to monitor the neonate in an intensive care situation for at least 24 hours postpartum. Blood glucose levels should be monitored hourly for 6 hours. If the neonate shows no signs of respiratory distress, hypocalcemia, or hyperbilirubinemia at 24 hours after delivery, he or she can be safely discharged to the normal nursery.[58]

## PERINATAL OUTCOME

With the advent of tools and techniques to maintain normoglycemia before, during, and between all pregnancies complicated by diabetes, infants of diabetic mothers now have the same chances of good health as infants born to nondiabetic women.

Animal and human studies clearly implicate glucose as the teratogen.[58a] In a Boston study, hyperglycemia in the first trimester was associated with a 23% incidence of major malformations; in an East Germany study, the malformation rate associated with elevated glycohemoglobin during the first trimester was

15.8%.[41,42] In the latter study, when the glucose level was normalized before conception, the malformation rate dropped to 1.6%. These studies and others emphasize the need for preconceptional programs to achieve and maintain normoglycemia.[44,59]

The morbidity and subsequent development of the infant of the diabetic mother is associated with hyperglycemia.[60] Neonatal macrosomia, hyperinsulinism, and hypoglycemia improve after maternal glucose is normalized. In one study series, all 53 infants born to 52 women with type 1 diabetes who maintained normoglycemia were normal.[58]

Therefore, the goal for all pregnancies complicated by diabetes is to achieve and maintain normoglycemia.

# REFERENCES

1. White P. Pregnancy and diabetes. In: Marble A, White P, Bradley RF, Krall LP, eds. Joslin's diabetes mellitus, 11th ed. Philadelphia: Lea & Febiger, 1971:50.
2. Pedersen J. The pregnant diabetic and her newborn: problems and management. Baltimore: Williams & Wilkins, 1967.
3. Jovanovic L, Peterson CM, Fuhrmann K, eds. Diabetes and pregnancy: teratology, toxicology and treatment. Philadelphia: Praeger, 1985.
4. Pedersen J, Pedersen LM. Diabetes mellitus and pregnancy: the hyperglycemia, hyperinsulinemia theory and the weight of the newborn baby. In: Rodriguez RR, Vallance-Owen J, eds. Proceedings of the 7th Congress of the International Diabetes Federation. Amsterdam: Excerpta Medica, 1971:678.
4a. Butte NF. Carbohydrate and lipid metabolism in pregnancy: normal compared with gestational diabetes mellitus. Am J Clin Nutr 2000; 71(5 Suppl):1256S.
5. Herrera E, Knopp RH, Freinkel N. Plasma fuels, insulin liver composition, gluconeogenesis and nitrogen metabolism during late gestation in the fed and fasted rat. J Clin Invest 1969; 48:2260.
6. Gillmer MDG, Beard RW, Brooke FM, Oakley NW. Carbohydrate metabolism in pregnancy. II. Diurnal plasma glucose profile in normal and diabetic women. BMJ 1975; 3:399.
7. Felig P. Maternal and fetal fuel homeostasis in human pregnancy. Am J Clin Nutr 1973; 26:998.
8. Bleicher SG, Sullivan JB, Freinkel N. Carbohydrate metabolism in pregnancy: the interrelationships among glucose, insulin and free fatty acids in late pregnancy and postpartum. N Engl J Med 1964; 271:866.
9. Freinkel N. Effects of the conceptus on maternal metabolism during pregnancy. In: Leibel BS, Wrenshall GA, eds. On the nature and treatment of diabetes. Amsterdam: Excerpta Medica, 1965:679.
10. Klopper A. The assessment of placental function in clinical practice. In: Klopper A, Diczfalusy E, eds. Foetus and placenta. Oxford: Blackwell Scientific Publications, 1969:471.
11. Josimovich JB. Placental lactogenic hormone. In: Endocrinology of pregnancy. New York: Harper & Row, 1971:184.
12. Doe RP, Dickinson P, Zinneman HH, Seal US. Elevated non–protein-bound cortisol in pregnancy, during estrogen administration and in carcinoma of the prostate. J Clin Endocrinol 1983; 29:757.
13. Freinkel N, Goodner CJ. Carbohydrate metabolism in pregnancy: the metabolism of insulin by human placental tissue. J Clin Invest 1960; 39:116.
14. Hadden DR. Geographic, ethnic and racial variations in the incidence of gestational diabetes mellitus. Diabetes 1985; 34:8.
15. Metzger BE, Coustan DR, and the Organizing Committee. Summary and recommendations of the Fourth International Workshop-Conference on Gestational Diabetes Mellitus. Diabetes Care 1998; 21:B161.
16. Moses RG, Moses J, Davis WS. Gestational diabetes: do lean young Caucasian women need to be tested? Diabetes Care 1998; 21:1803.
17. Pettitt DJ. Gestational diabetes mellitus. Who to test. How to test. Diabetes Care 1998; 21:1789.
18. Sweet success guidelines for care. State program guide. Sacramento: California Diabetes & Pregnancy Program, Maternal & Child Health Branch, California Department of Health Services, 1998.
19. Jovanovic L, Peterson CM. Screening for gestational diabetes: optimal timing and criteria for retesting diabetes. Diabetes 1985; 34:21.
20. O'Sullivan JB, Mahan CB. Criteria for the oral glucose tolerance test in pregnancy. Diabetes 1964; 13:278.
21. Moses RG, Moses M, Russell KG, Schier GM. The 75-g glucose tolerance test in pregnancy. A reference range determined on a low-risk population and related to selected pregnancy outcomes. Diabetes Care 1998; 21:1807.
22. Jovanovic-Peterson L, Crues J, Durak E, Peterson CM. Magnetic resonance imaging in pregnancies complicated by gestational diabetes predicts infant birth weight ratio and neonatal morbidity. Am J Perinatol 1994; 10:432.
23. Jovanovic-Peterson L, Peterson CM, Reed G, et al. Postprandial blood glucose levels predict birthweight: the Diabetes in Early Pregnancy Study. Am J Obstet Gynecol 1991; 164:103.
24. Jovanovic-Peterson L, Peterson CM. Dietary manipulation as a primary treatment strategy for pregnancies complicated by diabetes. J Am Coll Nutr 1990; 9:320.
25. Peterson CM, Jovanovic-Peterson L. Percentage of carbohydrate and glycemia response to breakfast, lunch, and dinner in women with gestational diabetes. Diabetes 1991; 40(Suppl 2):172.
26. Jovanovic-Peterson L, Peterson CM. Nutritional management of the obese gestational diabetic woman. (Guest editorial). J Am Coll Nutr 1992; 11:246.
27. Jovanovic-Peterson L, Peterson CM. Sweet success, but an acid aftertaste? (Editorial). N Engl J Med 1991; 325:959.
28. Jovanovic-Peterson L, Durak EP, Peterson CM. Randomized trial of diet versus diet plus cardiovascular conditioning on glucose levels in gestational diabetes. Am J Obstet Gynecol 1989; 161:415.
29. Jovanovic-Peterson L, Peterson CM. Is exercise safe or useful for gestational diabetic women? Diabetes 1991; 40(Suppl 2):179.
30. Jovanovic L, Peterson CM, Saxena BB, et al. Feasibility of maintaining normal glucose profiles in insulin-dependent pregnant women. Am J Med 1980; 68:105.
31. Jovanovic L, Peterson CM. Is pregnancy contraindicated in women with diabetes mellitus. Diabetic Nephrop 1984; 3:36.
32. Jovanovic-Peterson L, Peterson CM. Diabetic retinopathy. In: Coustan DR, guest ed; Pitkin RM, Scott JR, eds. Clinical obstetrics and gynecology: diabetes and pregnancy. Philadelphia: JB Lippincott, 1991:516.
33. Fuhrmann K. Outcome of normoglycemic diabetic pregnancies in Karlsburg. In: Jovanovic L, Peterson CM, Fuhrmann K, eds. Diabetes and pregnancy: teratology, toxicology and treatment. Philadelphia: Praeger, 1985:168.
34. Mestman JH. Autoimmune diseases associated with diabetic pregnancies. In: Jovanovic L, Peterson CM, Fuhrmann K, eds. Diabetes and pregnancy: teratology, toxicology and treatment. Philadelphia: Praeger, 1985:32.
35. Jovanovic-Peterson L, Peterson CM. De novo hypothyroidism in pregnancies complicated by type I diabetes, subclinical hypothyroidism, and proteinuria: a new syndrome. Am J Obstet Gynecol 1988; 159:442.
36. Chew EY, Mills JL, Metzger BE, et al. Metabolic control and progression of retinopathy. The Diabetes in Early Pregnancy Study. National Institute of Child Health and Human Development Diabetes in Early Pregnancy Study. Diabetes Care 1995; 18:631.
37. Jovanovic L, Peterson CM, eds. Contemporary issues in nutrition: diabetes mellitus. New York: Alan R Liss, 1985.
38. Committee of Nutrition. Nutrition in maternal health care. Chicago: American College of Obstetricians and Gynecologists, 1974.
39. Jovanovic L, Metzger BE, Knopp RH, et al. The Diabetes in Early Pregnancy Study: beta-hydroxybutyrate levels in type 1 diabetic pregnancy compared with normal pregnancy. National Institute of Child Health and Human Development Diabetes in Early Pregnancy Study Group. Diabetes Care 1998; 21:1978.
40. Jovanovic L, Peterson CM. The clinical utility of glycosylated hemoglobin. Am J Med 1981; 70:331.
41. Miller E, Hare JW, Clogerty JP, et al. Elevated maternal hemoglobin A1c in early pregnancy and major congenital anomalies in infants of diabetic mothers. N Engl J Med 1981; 304:1331.
42. Fuhrmann K, Ruher H, Semmler K, et al. Prevention of congenital malformations in infants of insulin dependent diabetic mothers. Diabetes Care 1983; 6:219.
43. Mills JL, Simpson JL, Driscoll SG, et al. Incidence of spontaneous abortion among normal women and insulin dependent diabetic women whose pregnancies were identified within 21 days of conception. National Institutes of Child Health and Human Development Diabetes in Early Pregnancy Study. N Engl J Med 1988; 319:1617.
44. Mills JL, Knopp RH, Simpson JL, et al. Lack of relation of increased malformation roles in infants of diabetic mothers to glycemic control during organogenesis. N Engl J Med 1988; 318:671.
45. Kitzmiller JL, Gavin LA, Gin GD, et al. Preconceptional care of diabetes: glycemic control prevents congenital anomalies. JAMA 1991; 265:731.
46. Mills JL, Baker L, Goldman A. Malformations in infants of diabetic mothers occur before the seventh gestational week: implications for treatment. Diabetes 1979; 23:292.
47. Jovanovic L, Mills JL, Peterson CM. The rationale for the use of human insulin in pregnancy. In: Jovanovic L, Peterson CM, Fuhrmann K, eds. Diabetes mellitus: teratology, toxicology and treatment. Philadelphia: Praeger, 1985:157.
48. Jovanovic-Peterson L, Kitzmiller JL, Peterson CM. Randomized trial of human versus animal species insulin in pregnancies complicated by diabetes. Am J Obstet Gynecol 1992; 167:1325.
49. Jovanovic L, Ilic S, Pettitt DJ, et al. Metabolic and immunologic effects of insulin lispro in gestational diabetes. Diabetes Care 1999; 22(9):1422.
50. Gabbe SG, Lowenson RI, Wu PY, Guerra G. Current patterns of neonatal morbidity and mortality in infants of diabetic mothers. Diabetes Care 1978; 1:335.
51. Driscoll SG, Benirshke K, Curtis GW. Neonatal deaths among infants of diabetic mothers. Am J Dis Child 1961; 100:818.
52. Kenny JD, Adams JM, Corbet AJ, Rudolph AJ. The role of acidosis at birth in the development of hyaline membrane disease. Pediatrics 1976; 58:181.
53. Buchanan TA, Kjos SL, Montoro MN, et al. Use of fetal ultrasound to select metabolic therapy for pregnancies complicated by mild gestational diabetes. Diabetes Care 1994; 17:275.
54. Freeman RK. Obstetric management of the diabetic patients. Contemp Obstet Gynecol 1976; 1:51.
55. Gurson CT, Etili L, Soyak S. Relation between endogenous lipoprotein lipase activity, free fatty acids, and glucose in plasma of women in labor and of their newborns. Arch Dis Child 1968; 43:679.
56. Jovanovic L, Peterson CM. Glucose and insulin requirements during labor in insulin-dependent pregnant diabetic women. Am J Med 1983; 75:607.
57. Jovanovic-Peterson L, Fuhrmann K, Hedden K, Walker L, Peterson CM. Maternal milk and plasma glucose and insulin levels: studies in normal and diabetic subjects. Am J Nutr 1989; 8:125.
58. Jovanovic L, Druzin M, Peterson CM. Effect of euglycemia on the outcome of pregnancy in insulin-dependent diabetic women as compared with normal control subjects. Am J Med 1981; 71:921.

58a. Suhonen L, Hiilesmaa V, Teramo K. Glycaemic control during early pregnancy and fetal malformations in women with type 1 diabetes mellitus. Diabetologia 2000; 43:79.
59. Jovanovic L, Peterson CM, Fuhrmann K, eds. Diabetes in pregnancy: teratology, toxicology and treatment. Philadelphia: Praeger, 1985.
60. Petersen M, Pedersen SA, Greisen G, et al. Early growth delay in diabetic pregnancy: relation to psychomotor development at age 4. BMJ 1988; 296:598.

# CHAPTER 157

# DIABETES MELLITUS IN THE INFANT AND CHILD

DOROTHY J. BECKER AND ALLAN L. DRASH

Diabetes mellitus can present very different medical and psychosocial issues in the child from those found in the adult. Even among childhood cases, manifestations, goals of therapy, clinical course, and susceptibility to a variety of acute, intermediate, and chronic complications vary with age.

## MAGNITUDE OF THE PROBLEM

Insulin-dependent diabetes mellitus (IDDM) is one of the most common serious chronic diseases of childhood. The majority of cases are classified as type 1 diabetes, which usually is due to autoimmune destruction of the B cells of the islets of Langerhans. In the United States, an apparent increase is occurring in the frequency of "atypical type 1 diabetes," which is seen mostly in black adolescents but also in Hispanics and whites. Such patients typically are obese with acanthosis nigricans, and present with episodes of ketosis or ketoacidosis; although they initially require insulin therapy, they later become non–insulin dependent.[1]

Type 1 diabetes in the neonate may be transient, in which case it is often related to intrauterine growth retardation. Cases of permanent neonatal diabetes that is nonautoimmune and usually familial have also been described, with some patients showing agenesis of the pancreas or islet cells. Interestingly, classic type 2 (non–insulin dependent) diabetes is being seen with increasing frequency by pediatricians. It occurs primarily in obese black and Hispanic patients and is seen more commonly in girls than in boys.[2] Another form of nonautoimmune type 1 diabetes being recognized more often in childhood is *maturity-onset diabetes of youth (MODY)*. MODY patients eventually require insulin; often they are initially treated with oral agents, and usually they are not obese. Their insulin-secretory deficits are due to genetic mutations of the glucokinase gene and of a number of transcription factors (MODY 1-5).[3] *Secondary diabetes* is being seen with increasing frequency in patients with cystic fibrosis, who are living longer, and also in patients receiving immunosuppressive agents for organ transplantation, which now is more common.

### TYPE 1 DIABETES

Among children, type 1 diabetes remains the most prevalent form of the disease in the United States. This disorder occurs with an annual incidence of 17 to 18 cases per 100,000 persons younger than 19 years.[4] The prevalence is increasing because the incidence is rising and mortality rates are decreasing. One of the more intriguing aspects of the study of the epidemiology of type 1 diabetes is the remarkable variation in prevalence and incidence in various parts of the world. Incidence figures are lowest in Asia; Japan, Korea, and China report approximately one case per 100,000 population each year. Rates are highest in the Scandinavian countries, especially Finland, and in Sardinia, with incidence rates approaching 40 cases per 100,000 children and adolescents per year.[5] The explanation for these geographic differences is still unclear. Although the frequency of genetic susceptibility haplotypes probably plays a major role among the different races, other populations have very similar gene frequencies. Thus, geographic variations and the rising incidence of type 1 diabetes around the world point to the role of yet-to-be-determined environmental factors in precipitating insulin deficiency.[5–8]

Approximately 10% of the 10,000,000 Americans with known diabetes have type 1 diabetes. Although a large proportion of these patients (probably >50%), acquire the disease before the age of 20, recognition is increasing that type 1 diabetes may present in adulthood, either with a typical acute onset, or with an indolent course, and is often misdiagnosed as type 2 diabetes. In childhood, the mean age of onset is ~8 years. A peak is seen in adolescence, which occurs somewhat earlier in girls than in boys. A rise in incidence has been reported among children younger than 5 years.[9] No significant difference is seen in sex distribution of diabetes during childhood.[10]

Mortality is higher in diabetic children and adolescents than in age- and sex-matched nondiabetic American children.[11,12] On the other hand, although no recent analyses have been published of mortality due to diabetes in childhood, the general impression is that these rates are decreasing. Death occurring at the onset, however, often related to a missed diagnosis, continues to occur. Death related to the *chronic* complications of type 1 diabetes is *almost never* seen in adolescents today. *The single most important diabetes-related cause of death during childhood is diabetic ketoacidosis (DKA).*[13] This occurs both at presentation and later during the course of type 1 diabetes and accounts for >40% of pediatric deaths. In the authors' experience, ~40% of patients with newly diagnosed type 1 diabetes present in DKA. The mortality due to DKA at the authors' institution over the past 30 years is <0.5%, and the rate has declined significantly over the past two decades.

## ETIOLOGY OF TYPE 1 DIABETES MELLITUS

Type 1 diabetes is caused by the autoimmune destruction of the B cells of the pancreas.[14] Greater than 90% of the total B-cell mass and insulin secretory capacity must be destroyed or incapacitated before overt diabetes appears. The fact that susceptibility to the development of type 1 diabetes has a *significant genetic component* has long been known. However, type 1 diabetes per se is not inherited.[15,16] The most clearly identified genetic risk factors are located on chromosome 6, within the major histocompatibility antigens (*IDDM1*).[17] Early studies documented the very high frequency of HLA-DR3 and HLA-DR4 in the development of type 1 diabetes among whites.[18] Later studies focused their attention on the HLA-DQ region of chromosome 6, with initial emphasis on the role of a single amino-acid substitution at position 57 of the β chain (non-Asp 57), and the presence of an arginine at position 52 on the α chain, which confer a markedly increased risk for the eventual development of type 1 diabetes.[19] Following current nomenclature, the highest risk DQ haplotypes around the world are HLA-DQ A1 0301-DQβ 1 0302, and DQ A1 0501-DQβ2 0201, with the former HLA genes associated with earlier onset of type 1 diabetes. Non-HLA genes may modulate the progression of the autoimmune process or play a role in susceptibility to the disorder in non–HLA-DR3/DR4 subjects.[20] A number of candidate genetic markers have been described (*IDDM2–IDDM14*), with none playing a major role, but polymorphisms in the promoter of the insulin gene (*IDDM2*) are the most prominent.[17]

Data showing that clinical diabetes per se is not inherited come from research in identical twins.[21] Despite the fact that they have identical genotypes, among twin pairs in which one twin has type 1 diabetes, only 30% to 40% of the second twins will develop the disease, although many more have evidence of autoimmunity against the B cells. This indicates an important role for the *environment* in precipitating insulin deficiency.

The autoimmune character of type 1 diabetes is demonstrated by the lymphocytic infiltration of the islets seen in both humans and rodents at clinical onset.[22] The specific initiator of this autoimmune attack remains an enigma. The amino-acid structure of the HLA region appears to be important in determining the presentation of specific antigens by the macrophage to the T-lymphocyte receptor, resulting in cytokine release and the initiation of the autoimmune cascade.[19] Both B-cell and T-cell autoimmune markers have been demonstrated before and at the onset of type 1 diabetes. B-cell autoimmunity was the first to be discovered following the development of *islet cell antibody (ICA)* assays in the 1970s.[23] These antibodies are seen in ~90% of patients with type 1 diabetes at the time of diagnosis, although lower frequencies are found in some populations.[24] Prospective surveillance of family members and of people with type 1 diabetes, as well as of the general population, show the development of ICAs many years (up to 20) before the overt development of type 1 diabetes.[25,26] In general, the higher the titer of the ICA, the greater the risk of development of type 1 diabetes during the period of observation. Because a number of individuals do not progress to overt insulin deficiency, an extensive search has been made for more specific markers that might predict the development of clinical disease. *Insulin antibodies* were the first to be identified and are seen particularly in younger patients at onset and younger individuals converting to type 1 diabetes, who have been followed from autoimmunity to clinical disease.[27] The next antigen to be identified was *glutamic acid decarboxylase (GAD)*. Antibodies to this enzyme were detected in 60% to 90% of new-onset cases.[24,28,29] Subsequently, antibodies to a *tyrosine phosphatase*, IA-2 (ICA512), have been shown to occur in 60% to 80% of new-onset cases; their presence confers high risk for the development of clinical disease in prospectively followed cohorts.[24,30] Arguments continue as to whether any one antibody is the first to present, although IA-2 antibodies appear later in most studies. Antibodies to a number of other intracellular B-cell antigens have been demonstrated at disease onset, suggesting that all these are markers of destruction of the cell, mediated by $T_H1$ lymphocytes. T-lymphocyte proliferative responses that are specific to intra–islet cell antigens and some environmental antigens may be seen both in patients at disease onset and in first-degree relatives without clinical type 1 diabetes.[31,31a] Although controversial, these studies support the animal research, which shows the important role of T cells and their cytokines in the destruction of the B cell in genetically susceptible mouse and rat strains. If the pathogenesis of human type 1 diabetes is similar to that in rodent models of spontaneous diabetes, then an *initial accumulation of dendritic cells and T lymphocytes around the periphery of the islet* may be anticipated. This is followed by *islet invasion and ultimate destruction of the B cells.*[32] Resistant strains of nonobese diabetic (NOD) mice show perinsulitis for prolonged periods, until something triggers the invasion. In human diabetes, this trigger is thought to be an environmental insult. In diabetes-prone NOD mice and bio-

breeding (BB) rats, numerous experimental manipulations have been shown to prevent or delay the manifestation of insulin deficiency; they fail to prevent perinsulitis but do halt its progression to invasion. Whether these manipulations can delay or prevent the onset of type 1 diabetes in humans remains to be proven. These animal studies are the basis for two ongoing large (and many smaller) intervention studies in high-risk first-degree relatives and general-population research volunteers. The largest of these studies are the European Nicotinamide Diabetes Intervention Trial (ENDIT) nicotinamide intervention studies currently ongoing in Europe, Canada, and Texas[33] and the North American parenteral and oral insulin intervention study Diabetes Prevention Trial-I (DPT-I) in first-degree relatives.[34]

Critical remaining questions are: What antigen or antigens initiate this autoimmune destructive process? What is the role of environmental factors in provoking both initial B-cell damage and in precipitating progression to insulin deficiency? Older research has described associations between viral infections and type 1 diabetes in both animals and humans, with case reports of small series invoking congenital rubella and B4 coxsackieviruses.[35] Immunization against the former has essentially eliminated this causal agent. Initial case-control studies of antibodies to coxsackievirus and other enteroviruses were disappointing.[36] Epidemiologic data, however, suggest that these may play a role as initiators of B-cell damage, even as early as during pregnancy. Whether this is a direct insult or operates via possible molecular mimicry of the GAD molecule is currently controversial.[37,38] Other environmental factors that have been implicated over the years include toxins and food components. Currently, interest has been rekindled in the role of early exposure to cow's milk protein in susceptible infants as an important risk factor for the later development of type 1 diabetes.[39] The epidemiologic data supporting this concept have shown an increased relative risk for the development of type 1 diabetes in certain populations exposed to cow's milk early in infancy, but these results have not been confirmed in some other studies.[40] A pilot randomized study of the avoidance of cow's milk protein in the first 6 months of life in high-risk neonatal first-degree relatives of patients with type 1 diabetes has produced some preliminary data showing a dramatically decreased incidence of islet cell autoantibodies in the intervention group fed with a hydrolyzed formula, compared with the control group.[39,41] A large full-scale study will be required for ultimate confirmation. Abnormal immune responses have been reported to a number of different cow's milk proteins by different research groups. One of the earliest studies reported antibodies to bovine serum albumin in 100% of Finnish children newly diagnosed with type 1 diabetes but in <2% of controls.[42] The epitope to which this autoimmunity was directed, known as ABBOS, has molecular similarities to an islet cell antigen known as ICA69.[43] Subsequent documentation of autoimmunity to lactoglobulin and casein makes the interpretation of these studies somewhat difficult.[43a,43b] In addition, in experimental animals other dietary components such as soy and wheat have been reported to accelerate the onset of type 1 diabetes in animals.[44] A large amount of further research is required before any particular nutritional element can be indicted in the pathogenesis of type 1 diabetes.

## CLINICAL PRESENTATION

Most children with diabetes present with the classic "3 P's": polyuria, polydipsia, and polyphagia. Additional symptoms include weight loss, fatigue, and blurred vision. In very young children, these symptoms may not be as clear, and *irritability* and *excess hunger* may be the first manifestations. If the diagnosis is not made at this stage, further deterioration of energy homeostasis occurs, with the development of DKA. Symptoms may progress to include anorexia, nausea, vomiting, central nervous system (CNS) depression, and eventually coma. In countries where urine screening is routine, the diagnosis may be made in totally asymptomatic children (the ideal situation).

Although, in its full-blown form, diabetes is readily diagnosed, the diagnosis is all too frequently missed at earlier stages, increasing the likelihood of later progression to DKA and coma. This is particularly true in infants, toddlers, and preschoolers, in whom the diagnosis is rarely considered because of the previous infrequency of the disease in these age groups. Symptoms in these younger children may be less sharply defined, not because the functional abnormality is different, but because of the problems of communication and the child's relative immobility, which limits access to fluids. Polyuria may go unobserved, and polydipsia may be misconstrued as irritability. As symptoms are frequently precipitated by intercurrent illnesses, their association with diabetes is often missed. If an upper respiratory tract infection is present, the development of Kussmaul respiration may be misinterpreted as bronchitis, pneumonia, or even asthma. Increased urinary frequency, initially often missed in the diaper-wearing toddler, may be misinterpreted as a urinary tract infection. The recurrence of enuresis in the toilet-trained child is frequently an initial sign of polyuria and should not be misconstrued as a psychological issue. Vomiting associated with DKA may be misdiagnosed as gastroenteritis, and abdominal pain due to ketosis is often initially investigated as an acute abdomen.

Usually, the duration of diabetes-related symptoms before diagnosis is relatively short. Ninety percent of patients have a clinical history of <3 weeks' duration. In contrast, adolescents with type 2 diabetes have a much longer prodrome. Generally, the younger the child, the shorter the period of symptoms and the more severe the metabolic derangements at diagnosis. Conversely, the older teenager frequently has a more indolent clinical history, with milder symptoms and less extreme metabolic changes. In any age group, however, variations in both duration and severity of clinical symptoms and biochemical alterations may be seen. These variations range from the case of an asymptomatic 6-year-old whose disease is detected on routine urinalysis as part of a physical examination, to that of an 11-year-old who presents with mild ketosis and a 2-year history of urinary frequency associated with the absence of both linear growth and weight gain, to that of a 14-year-old male athlete who successfully participated in competitive swimming until 5 days before presentation in DKA and coma. In the 1980s, 55% of new patients at the authors' center presented in DKA; of these, 12% had evidence of CNS depression, although <1% presented in coma (see Chap. 155). The frequency of severe DKA and CNS depression is decreasing in white children (by 40%). However, the frequency of both DKA and hyperosmolar hyperglycemia (with or without coma) has remained steady in African American children.[44a] A great worldwide variability is seen in the reported frequency with which DKA is present as part of the initial complex in the child with newly diagnosed diabetes. DKA appears to be less frequent in Israel and southern Europe and is found more frequently in northern Europe, particularly in the Scandinavian countries. In the United States the rate varies from 5% to 50%, whereas in Japan, where diabetes is uncommon in children, DKA occurs with a frequency similar to that in Pittsburgh (based on data collected in the 1980s).[45] Obviously, the frequency of DKA, as well as its concomitant morbidity, mortality, and health care expense, could be significantly reduced if diabetes mellitus were diagnosed at an earlier stage. The routine use of urinalysis by the private physician, hospital clinic, and emergency room personnel for all patients with nonspe-cific as well as potentially diabetes-related complaints would dramatically reduce DKA-related problems in patients newly diagnosed with the disease.

## ANTECEDENT EVENTS

Because a flu-like illness is seen in ~60% of children during the 2 to 3 months before diagnosis (with positive immunoglobulin M [IgM] titers to enteroviruses in 89%[46]), viral infections have been implicated in the precipitation of clinical type 1 diabetes in many cases, but have been "proven" to be the cause of few.[37,46a] Perhaps a viral infection, acting as a superantigen, might precipitate the final destructive process.[47] On the other hand, the possibility is great that, when such an event does occur, it happens far earlier in the prodrome of the disorder, with the more recent viral infection increasing the insulin requirement and, thus, the demand on the very limited insulin secretory capacity of the damaged B cell. Stress is also thought to precipitate the presentation of some cases of type 1 diabetes as well as some other autoimmune disorders, such as thyrotoxicosis. Several reports show that serious emotional trauma—including parental separation, divorce, death, or alcoholism, or child abuse—has occurred before the onset of diabetes in a significant number of children.[48,49] The potential mechanisms by which stress may mediate manifest insulin deficiency are by altering immunologic response mechanisms or by increasing the secretion of counter-regulatory hormones, particularly epinephrine and cortisol.

## EARLY CLINICAL COURSE

The natural history of diabetes in the child can be viewed from the perspective of B-cell functional capacity as a transition through four phases: (a) clinical presentation, (b) remission, (c) relapse, and (d) total diabetes.

### CLINICAL PRESENTATION

At the time of diagnosis, the B-cell secretory capacity as measured by both serum insulin levels and C-peptide concentration is usually low, but rarely absent.[10] As insulin deficiency at onset may be absolute or relative to the insulin secretory needs in the face of insulin resistance, significant amounts of insulin or C peptide, even amounts within the normal range, may be measurable. This is particularly true when fasting levels are measured in very early onset cases, in which the damaged islet cells secrete an increased proportion of proinsulin, measured as high postabsorptive insulin levels.[50] Despite this, probably >90% of the pancreatic B-cell mass is nonfunctional at this time. Many of these cells are probably irreversibly destroyed, but a significant number appear to have some capacity for recovery. Currently, debate exists as to whether the recovery is related to insulin secretory capacity, cell number, or both.

### REMISSION

The remission phase represents both a return toward secretory normality of the remaining B cells and a decrease in factors that have resulted in insulin resistance.[51] The clinical remission may be partial or complete. *Partial remission* usually is defined as a period of near metabolic normality, sustained by an insulin requirement of <0.5 U/kg per day. The increasing C-peptide levels, both basal and stimulated, suggest that a rise in insulin secretory capacity is the major mechanism of improved control. Approximately 65% of children and adolescents experience partial remission during the first several months after diagnosis. Although this phenomenon was rarely seen in children younger than age 5 years,[52] even toddlers now can undergo significant partial remissions, possibly associated with the tighter metabolic control achievable with frequent blood glucose monitoring.

*Total remission* is the spontaneous or induced return to metabolic normality documented by normal glycated hemoglobin measurements, without a requirement for exogenous insulin. Before the availability of glycated hemoglobin assays, the authors documented that 3% of patients went through a period of complete insulin withdrawal lasting for 1 month to more than 2 years. It is now clear that very few of these patients had true remissions, however, as glycated hemoglobin levels were abnormally high, despite blood glucose levels that were reported to be normal. All these patients eventually returned to an insulin-requiring state, necessitating dosages comparable to those in patients who did not sustain a remission.[52] The newly emerging syndrome of "atypical diabetes" shows a very different clinical picture. In patients with this syndrome, the disease very often can be controlled with oral agents or diet alone after recovery from the initial ketotic episode. Patients may have perfectly normal glycated hemoglobin levels but may experience recurrent DKA or hyperglycemia during periods of stress or infection.

### RELAPSE

The irreversible loss of insulin secretory capacity in patients with remission is usually gradual. Insulin requirements, as expressed per kilogram of body weight, may not reach a plateau for 2 to 6 years after diagnosis. Intercurrent infections or other stress-related problems, however, may be associated with an acute loss of insulin secretory capacity and an abrupt increase in insulin requirements. Unless patients are monitoring regularly and accurately, a marked deterioration in glycemic control often occurs during this period, as insulin doses are not increased rapidly enough.

### TOTAL DIABETES

*Total diabetes* refers to the metabolic state that results from complete B-cell destruction, with minimal or no capacity for endogenous insulin synthesis or release. Patients with total diabetes are completely dependent on administered insulin for metabolic control. Although this is the expected consequence of type 1 diabetes, particularly that occurring in the younger child, some patients may retain B-cell function for many years.[53] Various small studies have been reported showing varying success in preserving C-peptide secretion for short periods of time. These have included treatment with corticosteroids, interferon, plasmapheresis, a combination of insulin and sulfonylurea, and nicotinamide. A number of studies have suggested that initiation of nicotinamide treatment at the onset of diabetes in adults may result in prolonged B-cell secretion, but this strategy has not been shown to be effective in children.[54] Several studies administering cyclosporine to patients with newly diagnosed type 1 diabetes documented that immune suppression was associated with a more complete and more prolonged clinical remission based on preservation of B-cell function, particularly in older patients and those treated early after onset.[55] Continued immunosuppression beyond 1 year after diagnosis was almost invariably associated with loss of effectiveness and a progressive decline in insulin secretory capacity, with a need to return to full insulin therapy by 2 years after diagnosis.[56] In addition, effective doses of immunosuppressants frequently result in renal damage.[57]

## MANAGEMENT OF TYPE 1 DIABETES MELLITUS IN THE CHILD

The basic components of diabetes therapy—insulin administration, diet, exercise, and emotional support—are the same for the child as for the adult with diabetes. The development of specific therapeutic goals and the strategies necessary to implement them, however, may be vastly different.

Of all the serious, chronic diseases of childhood, such as congenital cardiac defects, chronic renal disease, asthma, epilepsy, inflammatory bowel disease, cystic fibrosis (without diabetes), cancer, and leukemia, diabetes is unique in the number and intensity of the therapeutic demands placed on both the patient and the family. The basis for diabetes management is education. The patient and family must obtain a broad knowledge of the disease and its acute and chronic clinical manifestations, as well as a detailed knowledge of the day-to-day management procedures. This knowledge must be translated into specific skills, such as insulin injection techniques, monitoring of urine and blood glucose levels, selection of appropriate foods and timing of consumption, and integration of exercise, dietary intake, and insulin therapy into an acceptable lifestyle.

Barriers to the success of diabetes management in the child and adolescent are many.[58] These vary with the age of the child. The preschooler, especially the toddler, has great variability in daily blood glucose levels. Severe hypoglycemia is more frequent in this age group and carries an increased likelihood of CNS damage with measurable decreases in mental efficiency.[59] Although parental control of the treatment regimen is highest at this age, it is frequently offset by an unwillingness to enforce treatment restrictions and to consistently carry out unpleasant or painful procedures, especially insulin injections. In addition, at this age, food intake is highly variable and timing of consumption is sometimes difficult to control.

The period from 5 to 11 years of age, the latency years, is thought to be critical for personality development. Although this is usually an interval of reasonably good metabolic control, growth, and development, with improved consistency in eating, greater variability in energy expenditure is now seen, which requires insulin and food adjustment. At this stage, the demands of the therapeutic regimen may begin to cause rebelliousness, falsification of monitoring records, and manipulation of the family around issues of food and activity. Parental skills are especially needed to provide a consistent, warm, loving environment in which the medical demands of the disease are balanced against the emotional developmental demands of the growing child.

Adolescence is a demanding time for all. It is the interval during which the child must begin to grow away from the protective and dependent relationship with the parents and other adults, and establish increasingly important relationships with peers. Value systems and role models begin to change. The teenager is highly vulnerable to emotional trauma related to issues of body image, peer group acceptance, and dependent-independent relationships. The superimposition of diabetes and its regimented lifestyle on this critical developmental stage frequently causes behaviors characterized by belligerence, antisocial acts, refusal to participate in the management responsibilities of diabetes, withdrawal, or depression. A high frequency of depression and eating disorders has been reported in adolescents with diabetes. Both of these psychopathologic disorders are related to an increased prevalence of subsequent microvascular complications. Their prevention and detection are, thus, extremely important.[60,61] Clearly, the features of psychosocial development during adolescence collide with the requirements of diabetes treatment regimens, usually to the detriment of both.[62–65]

The physician who attempts to manage the diabetic child without an appreciation of the impact of the disorder on the entire family and without a knowledge and understanding of the developmental aspects of childhood, as well as the possible adverse effects of emotional stress on the system, is unlikely either to achieve metabolic goals or to assist the patient in moving with confidence and emotional stability toward a productive adult life. Not only is an understanding of the psychosocial and educational aspect of diabetes important, but the physician also needs sufficient time to be able to address these aspects.

## THERAPEUTIC TEAM

The complexity of diabetes and the multiple demands it generates make it exceedingly difficult for any physician to provide total care for the diabetic patient and the family. The emergence and current acceptance of the diabetes therapy team represent one of the most significant advances in diabetes management over the past two decades. The importance of the diabetes therapeutic team, in which specific responsibilities are assigned to team members who have unique skills, was substantiated in the multicenter Diabetes Control and Complications Trial (DCCT).[66] The physician must establish the overall management guidelines tailored to each individual patient and integrate the contributions of the various team members to ensure that a coordinated approach to management is achieved.

## THERAPEUTIC GOALS

The DCCT was a 10-year multicenter North American study of the effect of metabolic control on microvascular complications of type 1 diabetes.[66] The results unequivocally documented that intensive diabetes management directed toward achieving metabolic control close to normal was associated with a significant decrease in the development and rate of progression of diabetic retinopathy, nephropathy, and neuropathy.[66] The number of events was insufficient to show a statistically significant effect with regard to macrovascular complications. Intensively treated adult patients achieved a mean hemoglobin $A_{1c}$ ($HbA_{1c}$) value of 7.2% (upper limit of normal, 6.05%) compared with mean values of 8.8% to 9.0% in the conventionally treated patients. Mean blood glucose levels were ~50 mg/dL lower in the intensively treated group. Two adverse complications were associated with intensive insulin therapy. The major one, hypoglycemia, occurred three times as often in the intensively treated patients than in the conventionally treated patients. The frequency of hypoglycemia was inversely related to $HbA_{1c}$ concentrations. The second major complication was excessive weight gain, which also was more common in the intensively treated patients.[66]

The DCCT patient population included highly screened and selected patients with type 1 diabetes who were between 13 and 39 years of age at entry. Approximately 15% of the subjects were adolescents at the time of recruitment. Subgroup analyses of these patients documented that the effectiveness of intensive diabetes therapy is comparable in teenagers and adults. However, average $HbA_{1c}$ was higher in both the intensively treated (~8%) and conventionally treated adolescent patients. In addition, severe hypoglycemia was more common in both groups of adolescent patients, so that the risk ratio for the development of this complication was the same as in the adult group.[67]

The DCCT results demonstrate unequivocally the beneficial effects of intensive diabetes therapy on the development and progression of the microvascular complications in a very large group of adolescents and adults with type 1 diabetes. Both the beneficial effects and increased frequency of severe hypoglycemia confirm the results of the Swedish Intensive Therapy Intervention Study.[68] The beneficial effects on microvascular complications were related to the intensive therapy regimen rather than the $HbA_{1c}$[68a] and persisted for 4 years following the end of the intervention.[68b] These results reaffirm the essential need for a therapeutic team and mandate increasing efforts to achieve the best possible metabolic control in adolescents with

type 1 diabetes.[69] This has been shown to require more frequent interaction of the diabetes team, continued education of the patients and their families, routine use of dietary expertise in management issues, and great flexibility in tailoring therapeutic activities to each individual patient. Concurrently, major emphasis should be placed on the prevention of hypoglycemia and excessive weight gain.

Because none of the DCCT patients were younger than age 13, translating these results to the management of younger children should be approached with considerable caution.[70] Of particular concern are the increasing frequency of hypoglycemia in both younger children and those with better glycated hemoglobin levels, and the high level of stress associated with this therapeutic modality. An attempt should be made to achieve the best glycosylated hemoglobin levels possible in all pediatric patients without causing severe hypoglycemia. This entails the development of an individualized therapeutic plan with the aim of assisting the patients and their families in achieving and sustaining a metabolic state as normal as is reasonable, given the capabilities of the families and their ability to avoid both severe hypoglycemia and frequent mild hypoglycemia, which could progress to the *hypoglycemia unawareness syndrome*. This requires daily monitoring of blood glucose a minimum of four and often more times per day, with appropriate adjustments in insulin, diet, and exercise to meet changing requirements of growth and activity. Urine should be checked for both glucose and ketones at least once daily, preferably in the morning, to detect ketonuria produced by either nocturnal hypoglycemia or the waning effect of nocturnal basal insulin delivery. The goal is to achieve fasting morning and preprandial blood glucose values of between 80 and 120 mg/dL, although a goal of up to 140 mg/dL is often more practical. If meters are calibrated to serum, the lower limits should be increased by 10% to avoid hypoglycemia. Postprandial levels should be between 120 and 180 mg/dL. If the patient's blood glucose values are constantly high, an assessment should be made as to whether this is due to excessive or constant eating or whether insulin adjustments are appropriate. Careful history-taking and assessment of growth and weight gain are used to make this decision.

Because of the greater concern for the possible detrimental effects of hypoglycemia on cognitive function in the preschool-age child, blood glucose goals are slightly higher, and are even higher in the toddler. Preprandial goals should be between 100 and 180 mg/dL and postprandial levels should be up to 220 mg/dL.

The determination of a glycosylated hemoglobin level at least every 3 months, and ideally every 6 weeks, is critical to properly assess glycemic control and allow appropriate therapeutic adjustments. The physician should be able to relate the local laboratory methodology to results obtained in the DCCT across the whole spectrum of $HbA_{1c}$ levels. This requires more than knowledge of the local normal range, because the relationship between $HbA_{1c}$ and mean blood glucose values varies markedly among different laboratory techniques, even if the normal ranges are similar.[71] International standardization of $HbA_{1c}$ assays is imminent.[71a]

## INSULIN THERAPY

Some confusion often exists regarding the relationship between *intensive diabetes therapy* and *intensive insulin therapy*. The former includes an increased level and frequency of attention directed toward all aspects of diabetes care and monitoring of glycosylated hemoglobin levels, and usually, but not necessarily, entails an increased frequency of insulin injections or insulin delivery by subcutaneous insulin infusion pump. Intensified insulin therapy should not be equated with intensified diabetes therapy (i.e., the mere increase in number of injections per day, without the other components of therapy, is unlikely to result in improvement of metabolic control). Observational studies in adolescents have shown no difference in HbA$_{1c}$ levels among patients treated with two, three, or four injections per day.[72] The insulin regimen must be individualized for each patient and tailored to lifestyle, school and sports schedule, and independence. The results of the DCCT have encouraged pediatric diabetologists to treat most adolescents with multiple insulin injections, and interest has grown in the use of constant subcutaneous insulin infusion using insulin pumps. In the United States, because the school systems allow only a very short lunch period, a lunchtime injection, although providing more flexibility, is not always practical; therefore, a regimen of four injections per day is sometimes difficult to maintain. A convenient starting insulin delivery regimen for adolescents is the use of an intermediate-acting insulin such as neutral protamine Hagedorn (NPH) or Lente at breakfast and before a bedtime snack, and the use of a short-acting insulin (either regular or lispro) at breakfast, dinner, and often also to cover an evening snack—especially in growing boys. A number of adolescents who eat a large midafternoon snack after school cover this with a small amount of lispro. Although in the DCCT adults in the intensive treatment group were treated successfully with an insulin regimen in which human Ultralente insulin was used once or twice daily and regular insulin was used before each meal, the experience with children has been somewhat less successful because the larger doses that are required result in prolongation and some overlap of hypoglycemic effect. Also, marked variability in absorption is seen. The use of insulin pens that contain either regular or lispro insulin has become increasingly accepted among the U.S. pediatric and adolescent population. The majority of children and adolescents, however, prefer to use a syringe to deliver a combination of intermediate and short-acting insulins, rather than take two injections with a pen, as in some adult populations. The development of the ultra-short-acting insulin analog lispro has provided a much more convenient regimen for patients, because after their insulin injection they do not need to wait 30 minutes before eating.[73] The disadvantage of this short-acting insulin is that it results in hyperglycemia before the following meal. This is a problem especially in patients who eat dinner relatively early and have a 4- to 6-hour interval before taking their nighttime insulin dose. The use of the longer-acting pork NPH in the morning appears to ameliorate this problem somewhat, although its efficacy has not been investigated in a clinical trial. Another strategy is the addition of either regular or NPH insulin at dinnertime, but this requires a syringe or two injections with a pen.[74]

Continuous subcutaneous insulin infusion (CSII) is the most nearly physiologic of the currently available insulin-delivery systems, but the peripheral rather than portal entry of insulin into the circulation still makes this method nonphysiologic. The use of insulin infusion pumps in the pediatric and adolescent population has both advantages and disadvantages. Early experience with CSII led to the conclusion (by a majority of diabetologists) that few adolescents have the maturity or desire to effectively adjust their lifestyles to the rigors of insulin infusion therapy. However, the improvement in currently available pumps (in terms of size, convenience, and safety) has led to a resurgence of interest in CSII for adolescents.[74a] For the motivated, mature, and intelligent patient, the insulin infusion pump provides a greater degree of flexibility in determining both the basal rate of insulin delivery and timing of meals than does any other regimen. The disadvantages are that the new found flexibility in meal timing and content is often difficult to handle, and glycosylated hemoglobin levels may deteriorate in patients whose disease was previously well controlled. In contrast, in a number of adolescents, the novelty of this new system can sometimes result in improved control. CSII should be attempted only when an experienced diabetes team is available and the family is highly motivated.

The insulin requirement varies over time and circumstances during childhood and adolescence. The best single indicator of a patient's potential insulin dose requirement is body weight. The preadolescent patient generally needs <1 U/kg, whereas the adolescent patient generally requires >1 U/kg per day and often up to 1.8 U/kg per day. Major variations are found in insulin requirements based on the time since the diagnosis (partial remissions may occur during the first weeks and may last for many months up to years after diagnosis), level of physical activity and physical fitness, food intake, emotional stress, and other factors. The highest doses are needed in patients with insulin resistance due to glucose toxicity[51] or in patients undergoing periods of very rapid growth (particularly boys). After completion of growth at the end of adolescence, patients generally find that insulin requirements decline significantly, and variations decrease with the assumption of a more consistent lifestyle as patients move toward adulthood. The authors' group continues to prefer pork to human NPH insulin, particularly in the younger child and also in patients using lispro insulin, because of the longer duration of pork insulin action. As the production of genetically engineered insulin becomes more cost effective for insulin manufacturers, there is constant discussion and concern that all animal insulin may be withdrawn from the market. Hopefully this will not occur until insulin analogs are available that prolong the action of intermediate human insulin (human Ultralente has proved not to be a good substitute).[75,75a]

Insulin regimens for the toddler and young child should be determined according to the patient's and family's response to insulin injections. Because patients at this age have a fairly regimented lifestyle and go to bed relatively early, they can be managed on two injections a day of mixed intermediate and short-acting insulin. If they eat a lot in the middle of the day, however, adding a lunch injection is preferable, as an increase in morning NPH carries over to the night and often results in nocturnal hypoglycemia. Decreases in the evening dose of intermediate-acting insulin do not resolve this problem. The advantage of using lispro insulin in a toddler with a very variable appetite is the ability to give the injection immediately after a meal according to the food consumed, without excessively compromising glycemic control. (Nevertheless, giving the insulin before the child starts to eat is always preferable.)

## NUTRITIONAL MANAGEMENT

Chapters 124, 125, and 141 contain detailed discussions of the nutritional principles and dietary aspects of diabetes management. Nutritional therapy is certainly important in the child with diabetes, as it is in the adult. In many ways, it is harder in the child, particularly the adolescent, because of the restrictions on spontaneous eating that are contrary to modern lifestyles. The major difference between nutritional management for children and that for adults is the need to ensure that the child or adolescent has completely adequate calories and protein for normal growth and development. The calories consumed should be distributed throughout the waking hours both to minimize hyperglycemia and to avoid very large insulin requirements and hypoglycemia (although ultra-short-acting lispro has made coverage of large meals easier). The very young child almost always requires a program that includes three meals and three between-meal snacks: at midmorning, midafternoon, and bedtime. Many older children and adolescents do not need a morning snack unless they are active. General nutritional recommendations continue to be provision of a diet containing ~55% of the total calories from carbohydrates, preferably with most from complex starches and the remainder from disaccharides. Total fat content should make up ~30% of the total calories, with a polyunsaturated/saturated fat ratio of ≥1 and a cholesterol content of <250 mg per day. The protein intake should be no more than 15% to 20% of the calories each day, because of the continued concern that excess protein intake may overload the kidneys and accelerate nephropathy. However, a direct relationship between protein in the diet and microalbuminuria has not yet been clearly demonstrated in humans, although suggestive data have been obtained in small studies. Specific calorie recommendations are tailored to age and activity, with recognition that the appetite of the younger child and growing boy is often a better guide to caloric requirements than a predetermined calorie estimation. In contrast, patients who are gaining excess weight (most commonly adolescent girls) do require dietary restriction to prevent obesity. Caloric intake should be constantly monitored along with weight gain and growth, and appropriate changes should be made as needed.[76]

Interest has grown in the use of "carbohydrate counting" to allow more liberal consumption of carbohydrates, especially free sugar (usually the extra calories are exchanged for carbohydrate in that meal or 1 U of insulin is added for every 10 to 15 g of excess carbohydrates eaten). The advantages of this dietary approach are that the patient can be more flexible with meal planning and can eat some sweets that are covered with ultra-short-acting insulin without inducing unacceptable hyperglycemia.[77] This approach should be used with caution, however, because the effects of the carbohydrates clearly vary depending on the amount of fat in the meal, which influences gastric emptying. Thus, the protein and fat exchanges should be fairly stable, particularly at night, in children and adolescents, as protein is needed to prevent nocturnal hypoglycemia. The therapist should also remember that insulin is required for protein and fat metabolism as well as metabolism of carbohydrates. Currently the authors monitor only glucose excursions and have no way to measure the effects of protein or fat excess on a short-term basis.

The required focus on food in the treatment of the diabetic patient is the probable reason for the increased frequency of eating disorders in adolescents with type 1 diabetes compared with the normal population. These disorders are usually related to very poor control, leading to an excess of microvascular complications; thus, the diagnosis should be made and aggressive intervention initiated as soon as possible.[61]

### EXERCISE

Physical fitness is generally accepted to be an important component of diabetes management (see Chap. 141). The fit, competitive athlete with diabetes frequently has a lower insulin requirement and better metabolic control than nonathletic peers. Also, the improvement of body image associated with athletic participation is an important factor in management. Patients must learn how to balance their physical activity requirements with insulin and diet to prevent hypoglycemia. One should also be aware that vigorous exercise in a patient with poorly controlled, under-insulinized diabetes may induce DKA because of the increase in stress associated with glucagon, catecholamine, and cortisol secretion. Exercise, therefore, should not be recommended for the purpose of lowering elevated blood glucose values and clearing ketonuria; these patients need appropriate insulin and dietary therapy.

### EMOTIONAL SUPPORT

One of the most difficult aspects of diabetes management in children and adolescents is the emotional disequilibrium resulting from both the disease, with its known complications, and the demands of therapy. An evaluation of the psychological strengths and weaknesses of the family soon after the diagnosis of diabetes may be exceedingly helpful in developing therapeutic strategies that allow appropriate emotional support as needed to prevent a serious breakdown of family dynamics and important interpersonal relationships. This is particularly true for adolescents, who are at especially high risk of developing psychiatric disturbances as a concomitant or consequence of diabetes mellitus. The prevalence of depression is particularly high among patients with diabetes and occurs most commonly among high-risk individuals.[60] Inclusion of a behavioral scientist consultant on the therapy team is important to provide guidance and therapy for such families.[78–80]

## TYPE 2 DIABETES IN THE CHILD

Over the past few years, diabetologists in the United States have noted a rising frequency of type 2 diabetes in the pediatric population, particularly among adolescents but also occasionally in preadolescent children.[2,80a] The increased frequency is notable particularly (but not exclusively) among black and Hispanic populations. The disease is almost always associated with obesity, and its rising incidence in younger patients is probably associated with the increasing obesity in this age group in the United States.[80b] These patients very often have associated acanthosis nigricans, which indicates the importance of insulin resistance in the pathogenesis of their hyperglycemia. What proportion of these patients present with ketosis or ketoacidosis (i.e., the atypical type 1 diabetes described previously[1]) is not yet clear.

The majority of these patients should be treated with insulin at presentation, unless their diabetes is very mild. This allows the rapid reversal of glucose toxicity,[51] after which time treatment with oral agents is more likely to be successful in maintaining euglycemia. Because the major mechanism inducing diabetes in these subjects is insulin resistance, metformin is probably the drug of choice; it is currently being tested for use in children in the United States. Initiating therapy with this drug at very low doses and gradually building up to the desired amount (usually ~1000 mg twice a day) avoids the frequent side effect of abdominal discomfort. Obviously, a calorie-restricted diet is imperative for the successful control of hyperglycemia in these patients. If significant weight loss is accomplished, these patients often can be treated with diet therapy alone.

## COMPLICATIONS OF DIABETES MELLITUS

Both acute and chronic complications of type 1 diabetes are discussed elsewhere in this book. However, some related issues are specific to the pediatric age group.

### DIABETIC KETOACIDOSIS

As described earlier, children and adolescents still frequently present with DKA at diagnosis. Five percent to 10% of children and adolescents require a hospital admission for DKA during the course of their disease after onset, and a small percentage of these patients have recurrent DKA. In the authors' experience, when circulating free insulin levels are measured at presentation in the emergency room, they are almost always extremely low. This corroborates the results of a Scottish study showing that patients in poor control and those with recurrent DKA do not use the amount of insulin prescribed.[81] Less frequently, an episode of DKA is associated with illness when the increased insulin requirements have not been recognized. The major cause of mortality and morbidity related to DKA in pediatric and adolescent patients is cerebral edema. This complication is rare in adults with DKA, and the reason for the difference in susceptibility according to age group is unknown. In contrast, cerebral thrombosis is rare in the pediatric group. Thus, the treatment approach in pediatric patients with regard to correction of dehydration and fluid therapy is different from that in adults. Rehydration should be slow, with correction over 24 to 48 hours. Normal saline should be used over the first 2 hours, at a maximum of 20 mL/kg per hour during the first hour and decreasing to 10 mL/kg per hour during the second hour. Fluid replacement should be calculated to half correct the deficit over the first 8 to 10 hours. Patients should be monitored with extreme care for signs and symptoms of impending *cerebral edema* (e.g., headache, change of behavior, or enuresis). A danger signal is a rapid drop in osmolarity or a decrease in serum sodium concentrations to <130 mEq/L, while the blood glucose concentrations are falling. Mannitol should be available at the bedside and should be administered immediately if cerebral edema occurs.

## HYPOGLYCEMIA

The most feared complication of type 1 diabetes in childhood is hypoglycemia. The possibility of a severe hypoglycemic episode with unconsciousness and/or a seizure is the major concern of parents of children and adolescents with diabetes. If such an episode should occur, the psychological distress increases. The resultant fear of hypoglycemia often leads families to allow unacceptably high glycemic control with deterioration of $HbA_{1c}$ levels. Although in the DCCT study, episodes of severe hypoglycemia were not shown to result in long-term neuropsychological deficits in adolescents and adults, some controversy exists as to whether permanent brain damage does occur in adults.[82,83] However, little controversy exists regarding the vulnerability of younger children, particularly those younger than 6 years of age, to the effects of diabetes, with neuropsychological complications and cognitive deficits being demonstrated in both retrospective and prospective studies in this age group that are correlated with the frequency of hypoglycemia.[59,84,85] In addition, children diagnosed before 5 years of age are more likely to show a variety of electroencephalographic abnormalities, and these are more common in those who have had one or more previous episodes of severe hypoglycemia.[86] Both retrospective and prospective studies have shown that children in this vulnerable age group also have the highest risk of experiencing frequent severe hypoglycemic episodes.[87] Because children in this age group are less likely to recognize hypoglycemic warning symptoms, even mild hypoglycemia is more frequent and probably leads to the *hypoglycemic unawareness syndrome* and *failure of counterregulation* as has also been demonstrated in adults.[88] Thus, even mild or moderate hypoglycemia should be avoided in children of this age. Severe hypoglycemia is also more common in adolescents than it is in adults, irrespective of whether they are receiving intensive therapy.[67] Most diabetologists believe that this is related to their very erratic lifestyles and energy expenditures. Although the majority of these episodes occur at night during sleep, the danger that a severe hypoglycemic event might occur while the patient is driving makes frequent glucose monitoring even more important in this age group. Even mild hypoglycemia (60 mg/dL) has been shown to cause transient deterioration in mental efficiency.[89] If such episodes should occur repeatedly at school, they could interfere with learning abilities and could partially explain deterioration of intellectual ability and academic performance over time.[90]

## MICROVASCULAR COMPLICATIONS

Retinopathy, nephropathy, and neuropathy are discussed elsewhere in this book (see Chaps. 148, 150, and 151). Although overt microvascular complications are becoming less and less frequent in childhood and adolescence in Western countries, no doubt exists that the subclinical manifestations of background retinopathy, microalbuminuria, and abnormalities of nerve conduction may already occur in this age group. Careful fundus photography showed that the prevalence of retinopathy was 25% among patients younger than 18 years (varying from 14% to 30%); extremely rare cases of preproliferative or proliferative retinopathy are still being reported.[91-94] The first retinal changes usually can be detected after a median diabetes duration of ~9 years[92]; however, both before and after puberty, they may be observed as early as 5 years after onset, related to poor glycemic control.[91] Even in childhood, other factors such as blood pressure and lipid abnormalities appear to play a role.[91,95] Some controversy has existed regarding the effect of puberty on the timing of the onset of mild background retinopathy,[91,96–99] but all studies agree that the degree of glycemic control has an important influence on its prevalence. These data suggest that the development of early background retinopathy is unaffected by pubertal status; however, progression to severe retinopathy is accelerated after puberty.

The prevalence of microalbuminuria is usually somewhat lower: 5% to 37% of adolescents. There is some agreement that it usually appears after the onset of puberty.[91] Microalbuminuria does *not* always progress to overt diabetic nephropathy as was claimed in the early 1980s. Regression has been reported to occur in 32% of adolescents who experience initial microalbuminuria (in most cases levels return to the normal range); progression to overt proteinuria occurs in 18% and is largely influenced by the quality of metabolic control.[100] In the authors' experience, overt nephropathy (proteinuria) is becoming increasingly uncommon. Supporting data from Sweden show a decrease in the prevalence of proteinuria over three decades.[101] Diabetes-induced renal failure is virtually never seen in adolescents.

Sensory neuropathy has also been well described in the pediatric age group. Prevalence rates of 10% to 23% are reported. Like nephropathy, it is seen mostly in those with poor metabolic control and after puberty.[91,93,102] The prevalence rates of abnormalities of motor nerve conduction are much higher, with rates of 50% to 72% being reported.[91] In contrast, on careful examination, only 3% of the adolescent population studied by the authors were found to have clinical distal neuropathy (only minimal).[91] Overt clinical neuropathy is extremely rare in the pediatric group.

Brainstem evoked potentials to both visual and auditory stimuli have been reported to be impaired in 37% of children with type 1 diabetes. Correlates of these electrophysiologic abnormalities include longer duration of diabetes, younger age of onset as well as a history of severe hypoglycemia, and poorer metabolic control.[91,103]

## FUTURE FOR THE CHILD WITH DIABETES MELLITUS

In the last decade, important research advances have been made in patient management. One of the most significant in terms of convenience for the patient with diabetes, particularly the school-age child and adolescent, is the availability of lispro insulin.[73] Use of this type of insulin eliminates the 30-minute waiting period to eat following the insulin injection. It also allows some spontaneous eating between meals, which can be covered with an extra injection of small amounts of lispro insulin. Lispro has also been very valuable in treating the toddler with erratic food intake, as it can be given safely after a meal. In addition, the use of lispro in insulin infusion pumps has now been shown to give better control because it produces less postprandial hyperglycemia than is attainable with regular insulin.[104]

New smaller glucose-monitoring meters are becoming available. The health care provider needs to be aware that many of these are calibrated somewhat differently, and they cannot be used interchangeably. Although transplantation research in adults is documenting longer-term successes with whole pancreas transplantations, usually associated with kidney transplantation, similar successes have not been obtained with islet cell transplantation.[105] Nevertheless, advances are being made in techniques that might protect B cells from both rejection and continued autoimmune attacks; this approach provides some hope for the future. Assays available for screening susceptible populations for diabetes are improving, and these will allow more accurate prediction of the future development of clinical type 1 diabetes, although the time of onset is not yet predictable. Progress in this field will provide the basis for further studies on the causes and triggers of type 1 diabetes and allow the design of new intervention studies.

The DCCT results unequivocally documented that sustained metabolic improvement in diabetes control is associated with highly significant reductions in the frequency, severity, and rate of progression of the serious microvascular complications. The challenge to society is to deliver intensive diabetes therapy to type 1 diabetic patients at large, in a cost-effective manner, by teams with the appropriate expertise. Although much controversy continues regarding the funding of this therapeutic approach, there is optimism that adequate diabetes care will become available to all children and adolescents with diabetes, so that they can enter adult life with confidence that the complications of this disease have been delayed or even prevented.

# REFERENCES

1. Winter WE, Maclaren NK, Riley WJ, et al. Maturity-onset diabetes of youth in black Americans. N Engl J Med 1987; 316:285.
2. Rosenbloom AL, Joe JR, Young RS, Winter WE. Emerging epidemic of type 2 diabetes in youth. Diabetes Care 1999; 22:345.
3. Freugel P, Velho G. Molecular genetics of maturity-onset diabetes of the young. Trends Endocrinol Metab 1999; 10:142.
4. Libman IM, LaPorte RE, Becker D, et al. Was there an epidemic of diabetes in nonwhite adolescents in Allegheny County, Pennsylvania? Diabetes Care 1998; 21:1278.
5. Karvonen M, Tuomilehto J, Libman I, LaPorte R. A review of the recent epidemiological data on the worldwide incidence of type 1 (insulin-dependent) diabetes mellitus. World Health Organization DIAMOND Project Group. Diabetologia 1993; 36:883.
6. Diabetes Epidemiology Research International Group. Geographic patterns of childhood insulin-dependent diabetes mellitus. Diabetes 1988; 37:1113.
7. Dahlquist G. Etiological aspects of insulin-dependent diabetes mellitus: an epidemiological perspective. Autoimmunity 1993; 15:61.
8. Trucco M. To be or not to be ASP 57, that is the question. Diabetes Care 1992; 15:712.
9. Dokheel TM. An epidemic of childhood diabetes in the United States? Evidence from Allegheny County, Pennsylvania. Pittsburgh Diabetes Epidemiology Research Group. Diabetes Care 1993; 16:1606.
10. Drash AL. Clinical care of the diabetic child. Chicago: Year Book Medical Publishers, 1987.
11. Dorman JS, LaPorte RE, Kuller LH, et al. The Pittsburgh insulin-dependent diabetes mellitus morbidity and mortality study: mortality results. Diabetes 1984; 33:271.
12. Dorman JS, Tajima N, LaPorte RE, et al. The Pittsburgh IDDM morbidity and mortality study: case-control analyses of risk factors for mortality. Diabetes Care 1985; 8(Suppl 1):54.
13. Scibillia J, Finegold D, Dorman J, et al. Why do children with diabetes die? Acta Endocrinol (Copenh) 1986; 121(Suppl 279):326.
14. Eisenbarth GS. Type I diabetes mellitus: an autoimmune disease. N Engl J Med 1986; 314:1360.
15. Orchard TJ, Dorman JS, LaPorte RE, et al. Host and environmental interactions in diabetes mellitus. J Chronic Dis 1986; 39:979.
16. Bottazzo GF. Death of a beta cell: homicide or suicide? Diabetic Medicine 1986; 3:119.
17. Todd JA. Genetic analysis of type 1 diabetes using whole genome approaches. Proc Natl Acad Sci U S A 1995; 29:8560.
18. Nerup J, Mandrup-Poulsen T, Molvig J. The HLA-IDDM association: implications for etiology and pathogenesis of IDDM. Diabetes Metab Rev 1987; 3:779.
19. Trucco M. Immunogenetics of insulin-dependent diabetes mellitus: the 2nd event hypothesis. Curr Top Diabetes Res (Series: Frontiers in Diabetes) 1993; 12:135.
20. Van der Auwera B, Schuit F, Lyaruu I, et al. Genetic susceptibility for insulin-dependent diabetes mellitus in Caucasians revisited: the importance of diabetes registries in disclosing interactions between HLA-DQ- and insulin gene-linked risk. Belgian Diabetes Registry. J Clin Endocrinol Metab 1995; 80:2567.
21. Rowe RE, Leslie RD. Twin studies in insulin dependent diabetes and other autoimmune diseases. Diabetes Metab Rev 1995; 11:121.
22. Eisenbarth GS. Mouse or man: is GAD the cause of type I diabetes? Diabetes Care 1994; 17:605.
23. Wilkin TJ. Antibody markers for type I diabetes: the issues. Trends Endocrinol Metab 1990; 1:204.
24. Libman IM, Pietropaolo M, Trucco M, et al. Islet cell autoimmunity in white and black children and adolescents with IDDM. Diabetes Care 1998; 21:1824.
25. Lipton RB, Atchison J, Dorman JS, et al. Genetic, immunological, and metabolic determinants of risk for type 1 diabetes mellitus in families. Diabetic Med 1992; 9:224.
26. Knip M, Vähäsälo P, Karjaleinen J, et al. Natural history of preclinical IDDM in high risk siblings. The Childhood Diabetes in Finland Study Group. Diabetologia 1994; 37:388.
27. Palmer JP. Insulin antibodies: their role in the pathogenesis of IDDM. Diabetes Metab Rev 1987; 3:1005.
28. Baekkeskov S, Aanstoot HJ, Christgau S, et al. Identification of the 64K autoantigen in insulin-dependent diabetes as the GABA-synthesizing enzyme glutamic acid decarboxylase. Nature 1990; 13:151.
29. Sabbah E, Savola K, Kulmala P, et al. Disease associated autoantibodies and HLA-DQB1 genotypes in children with newly diagnosed insulin-dependent diabetes mellitus (IDDM). The Childhood Diabetes in Finland Study Group. Clin Exp Immunol 1999; 116:78.
30. Savola K, Bonifacio E, Sabbah E, et al. IA-2 antibodies—a sensitive marker of IDDM with clinical onset in childhood and adolescence. Childhood Diabetes in Finland Study Group. Diabetologia 1998; 41:424.
31. Roep BO. T-cell responses to autoantigens in IDDM. The search for the holy grail. Diabetes 1996; 9:1147.
31a. Dosch HM, Cheung RK, Karges W, et al. Persistent T Cell energy in human type 1 diabetes. J Immunol 1999; 163:6933.
32. Fox CJ, Danska JS. Independent genetic regulation of T-cell and antigen presenting cell participation in autoimmune islet inflammation. Diabetes 1998; 47:331.
33. Gale BA. Theory and practice of nicotinamide trials in pre-type 1 diabetes. J Pediatr Endocrinol Metab 1996; 9:375.
34. Schatz DA, Rogers DG, Brouhard BH. Prevention of insulin-dependent diabetes mellitus: an overview of three trials. Cleve Clin J Med 1996; 270.
35. Yoon JW. Viruses in the pathogenesis of type I diabetes. Curr Probl Clin Biochem 1983; 12:11.
36. Drash AL, Cavender D, Atchison B, et al. The Pittsburgh diabetes mellitus study: studies on the etiology of insulin-dependent diabetes with special reference to viral infections. Behring Inst Mitt 1984; 1:58.
37. Yoon JW. A new look at viruses in type 1 diabetes. Diabetes Metab Rev 1995; 11:83.
38. Oldstone MB. Molecular mimicry and immune-mediated diseases. FASEB J 1998; 12:1255.
39. Akerblom HK, Knip M. Putative environmental factors in type 1 diabetes. Diabetes Metab Rev 1998; 14:31.
40. Gerstein HC. Cow's milk exposure and type I diabetes mellitus: a critical overview of the clinical literature. Diabetes Care 1994; 17:13.
41. Akerblom HK, Virtanen SM, Hamalainen A, et al. Emergence of diabetes associated autoantibodies in the nutritional prevention of IDDM (TRIGR) project. Diabetes 1999; 48:A45.
42. Karjalainen J, Martin JM, Knip M, et al. A bovine albumin peptide as a possible trigger of insulin-dependent diabetes mellitus. N Engl J Med 1992; 327:302.
43. Miyazaki I, Gaedigk R, Hui MF, et al. Cloning of human and rat p69, a candidate autoimmune target in type 1 diabetes. Biochim Biophys Acta 1994; 1227:101.
43a. Vaarala O, Klemetti P, Savilahti E, et al. Cellular immune response to cow's milk beta-lactoglobulin in patients with newly diagnosed IDDM. Diabetes 1996; 45:178.
43b. Cavallo MG, Fava D, Monetini L, et al. Cell-mediated immune response to betacasein in recent-onset insulin-dependent diabetes: implication for disease pathogenesis. Lancet 1996; 348:926.
44. Scott FW. Food-induced type 1 diabetes in the BB rat. Diabetes Metab Rev 1996; 12:341.
44a. Nitadori Y. Personal communication. 2000.
45. Diabetes Epidemiology Research International Mortality Study Group. International evaluation of cause specific mortality and IDDM. Diabetes Care 1990; 14:55.
46. Helfand RF, Gary HE, Freeman CY, Anderson LJ, Pallansch MA. Serologic evidence of an association between entero viruses and the onset of type 1 diabetes mellitus. Pittsburgh Diabetes Research Group. J Infect Dis 1995; 172:1206.
46a. Lonnrot NI, Salminen K, Knip M, et al. Enterovirus RNA in serum is a risk factor for beta-cell autoimmunity and clinical type 1 diabetes: a prospective study. J Med Virol 2000; 61:214.

47. Conrad B, Trucco M. Superantigens as etiopathogenetic factors in the development of insulin-dependent diabetes mellitus. Diabetes Metab Rev 1994; 10:309.

48. Leaverton DR, White SA, McCormick CR, et al. Parental loss antecedent to childhood diabetes mellitus. J Am Acad Child Psychiatry 1980; 19:678.

49. Tarnow JD, Silverman SW. The psychophysiologic aspects of stress in juvenile diabetes mellitus. J Psychiatr Med 1981; 11:25.

50. Hartling SG, Knip M, Roder ME, et al. Longitudinal study of fasting proinsulin in 148 siblings of patients with insulin-dependent diabetes mellitus. Study Group on Childhood Diabetes in Finland. Eur J Endocrinol 1997; 137:490.

51. Yki-Jarvinen H. Glucose toxicity. Endocr Rev 1992; 13:415.

52. Drash AL. Clinical characteristics: presentation and initial clinical course. In: Drash AL, ed. Clinical care of the diabetic child. Chicago: Year Book Medical Publishers, 1987:33.

53. The Diabetes Control and Complications Trial Research Group. Effect of intensive therapy on residual β-cell function in patients with type 1 diabetes in the Diabetes Control and Complications Trial. A randomized, controlled trial. Ann Intern Med 1998; 128:517.

54. Pozzilli P, Browne PD, Kolb H. Meta-analysis of nicotinamide treatment in patients with recent-onset IDDM. The Nicotinamide Trial Lists. Diabetes Care 1996; 19:1357.

55. The Canadian-European Randomized Control Trial Group. Cyclosporin-induced remission of IDDM after early intervention: association of 1 yr of cyclosporin treatment with enhanced insulin secretion. Diabetes 1988; 37:1574.

56. DeFilippo G, Carel JC, Boitard C, Bougneres PF. Long-term results of early cyclosporine therapy in juvenile IDDM. Diabetes 1996; 45:101.

57. Mahon JL, Dupre J, Stiller CR, et al. Immunosuppression in IDDM: rationale, risks, benefits and strategies. (Comment). Diabetes Care 1990; 13:806.

58. Fonagy P, Moran GS, Lindsay MK, et al. Psychological adjustment and diabetic control. Arch Dis Child 1987; 62:1009.

59. Ryan C, Vega A, Drash A. Cognitive deficits in adolescents who developed diabetes early in life. Pediatrics 1985; 75:921.

60. Kovacs M, Obrosky DS, Goldston D, Drash A. Major depressive disorder in youths with IDDM. A controlled prospective study of course and outcome. Diabetes Care 1997; 20:45.

61. Rydall AC, Rodin GM, Olmsted MP, et al. Disordered eating behavior and microvascular complications in young women with insulin-dependent diabetes mellitus. N Engl J Med 1997; 336:1849.

62. Anderson DJ, Auslander WF. Research on diabetes management and the family: a critique. Diabetes Care 1980; 6:696.

63. Johnson SB. Psychosocial factors in juvenile diabetes: a review. J Behav Med 1980; 3:95.

64. White K, Kollman ML, Wexler P, et al. Unstable diabetes and unstable families: a psychosocial evaluation of diabetic children with recurrent ketoacidosis. Pediatrics 1984; 73:749.

65. Gustafsson PA, Cederblad M, Ludvigsson J, Lundin B. Family interaction and metabolic balance in juvenile diabetes mellitus: a prospective study. Diabetes Res Clin Pract 1987; 4:7.

66. The Diabetes Control and Complications Trial Research Group. The effect of intensive treatment of diabetes on the development and progression of long-term complications in insulin-dependent diabetes mellitus. N Engl J Med 1993; 329:977.

67. The Diabetes Control and Complications Trial Research Group. Effect of intensive diabetes treatment on the development and progression of long-term complications in adolescents with insulin-dependent diabetes mellitus: Diabetes Control and Complications Trial. J Pediatr 1994; 125:177.

68. Reichard P, Nilsson BY, Rosenqvist U. The effect of long-term intensified insulin treatment on the development of microvascular complications of diabetes mellitus. N Engl J Med 1993; 329:304.

68a. The relationship of glycemic exposure "HbA1c" to the risk of development and progression of retinopathy in the diabetes control and complications trial. Diabetes 1995; 44:968.

68b. The Diabetes Control and Complications Trial/Epidemiology of Diabetes Interventions and Complications Research Group. Retinopathy and nephropathy in patients with type 1 diabetes four years after a trial of intensive therapy. N Engl J Med 2000; 10:381.

69. Position statement of the American Diabetes Association. Implications of the Diabetes Control and Complications Trial. Diabetes Care 1993; 16:1517.

70. Becker DJ, Ryan CM. Intensive diabetes therapy in childhood: Is it achievable? Is it desirable? Is it safe? J Pediatr 1999; 134:392.

71. Santiago JV. Lesson from the Diabetes Control and Complications Trial. Diabetes 1993; 42:1549.

72. Mortensen HB, Robertson KJ, Aanstoot HJ, et al. Insulin management and metabolic control of type 1 diabetes mellitus in childhood and adolescence in 18 countries. Hvidore Study Group on Childhood Diabetes. Diabet Med 1998; 15:752.

73. Holleman F, Hoekstra JB. Insulin lispro. N Engl J Med 1997; 337:176.

74. Ciofetta M, Lalli C, Del Sindaco P, et al. Contribution of postprandial versus interprandial blood glucose to HbA1c in type 1 diabetes on physiologic intensive therapy with lispro insulin at mealtime. Diabetes Care 1999; 22:795.

74a. Boland EA, Grey M, Oesterel A, et al. Continous subcutaneous insulin infusion. A new way to lower risk of severe hypoglycemia, improve metabolic control, and enhance coping in adolescents with type 1 diabetes. Diabetes Care 1999; 22:1779.

75. Barnett AH, Owens DR. Insulin analogs. Lancet 1997; 349:47.

75a. Ratner RE, Hirsch IB, Neifing JL, et al. Less hypoglycemia with insulin glargine in intensive insulin therapy for type 1 diabetes. US Study group of insulin glargine in Type 1 diabetes. Diabetes Care 2000; 23:639.

76. Drash AL, Becker DJ. Nutritional considerations in the therapy of the child with diabetes mellitus. In: Suskind RM, Lewinter-Suskind L, eds. Textbook of pediatric nutrition. New York: Raven Press, 1992:309.

77. American Diabetes Association. Nutrition recommendations and principles for people with diabetes mellitus. Diabetes Care 1998; 21(Suppl 1):S32.

78. Drash AL, Becker DJ. Behavioral issues in patients with diabetes mellitus with special emphasis on the child and adolescent. In: Rifkin H, Porte D, eds. Ellenberg and Rifkin's diabetes mellitus: theory and practice, 4th ed. New York: Elsevier Science, 1989:922.

79. Hanson CL, Henggelen SW, Burghen GA. Social competence and parental support as mediators of the link between stress and metabolic control in adolescents with insulin-dependent diabetes mellitus. J Consult Clin Psychol 1987; 55:529.

80. Pegnot MF, McMung JF. Stress buffering and glycemic control: the role of coping styles. Diabetes Care 1992; 15:842.

80a. Fagot-Campagna A, Pettitt DJ, Engelgau MM, et al. Type 2 diabetes among North American children and adolescents: an epidemiologic review and a public health perspective. Pediatr 2000; 136:664.

80b. Young TK, Dean HJ, Flett B, Wood-Steiman P. Childhood obesity in a population at high risk for type 2 diabetes. J Pediatr 2000; 136:365.

81. Morris AD, Boyle DI, McMahon AD, et al. Adherence to insulin treatment, glycaemic control, and ketoacidosis in insulin-dependent diabetes mellitus. The DARTS/MEMO Collaboration. Diabetes Audit and Research in Tayside Scotland. Medicines Monitoring Unit. Lancet 1997; 350(9090):1505.

81a. Rosenbloom AL, Schatz DA, Krischer JP, et al. Prevention and treatment of diabetes in children. J Clin Endocrinol and Metab 2000; 85:494.

82. Diabetes Control and Complications Trial Research Group. Effects of intensive diabetes therapy on neuropsychological function in adults in the Diabetes Control and Complications Trial. Ann Intern Med 1996; 124:379.

83. Deary IJ, Frier BM. Severe hypoglycaemia and cognitive impairment in diabetes: link not proven. BMJ 1996; 313:767.

84. Rovet JF, Ehrlich RM, Hoppe MG. Specific intellectual deficits associated with the early onset of insulin-dependent diabetes mellitus in children. Diabetes Care 1987; 10:510.

85. Northam EA, Anderson PJ, Werther GA, et al. Neuropsychological complications of IDDM in children 2 years after disease onset. Diabetes Care 1998; 21:379.

86. Soltesz G, Acsadi G. Association between diabetes, severe hypoglycemia and electroencephalographic abnormalities. Arch Dis Child 1989; 64:992.

87. Davis EA, Keating B, Byrne GC, et al. Hypoglycemia: incidence and clinical predictors in a large population-based sample of children and adolescents with IDDM. Diabetes Care 1997; 20:22.

88. Cryer PE. Iatrogenic hypoglycemia as a cause of hypoglycemia-associated autonomic failure. A vicious cycle. Diabetes 1992; 41:255.

89. Ryan CM, Atchison J, Puczynski S, et al. Mild hypoglycemia associated with deterioration of mental efficiency in children with insulin dependent diabetes mellitus. J Pediatr 1990; 117:32.

90. Kovacs M, Goldston D, Iyengar S. Intellectual development and academic performance of children with insulin dependent diabetes mellitus: a longitudinal study. Dev Psychol 1992; 28:676.

91. Becker DJ, Orchard TJ, Lloyd CE. Control and outcome: clinical and epidemiologic aspects in children and adolescent diabetes. In: Kelnar C, ed. Childhood and adolescent diabetes. New York: Chapman & Hall, 1995:519.

92. Danne T, Kordonouri O, Hovener G, Weber B. Diabetic angiopathy in children. Diabet Med 1997; 14:1012.

93. Bognetti E, Calori G, Meschi F, et al. Prevalence and correlations of early microvascular complications in young type I diabetic patients: role of puberty. J Pediatr Endocrinol Metab 1997; 10:587.

94. Kernell A, Dedorsson I, Johansson B, et al. Prevalence of diabetic retinopathy in children and adolescents with IDDM. A population-based multicentre study. Diabetologia 1997; 40:307.

95. Danne T, Kordonouri O, Enders I, et al. Factor modifying the effect of hyperglycemia on the development of retinopathy in adolescents with diabetes. Results of the Berlin Retinopathy Study. Horm Res 1998; 50 (Suppl 1):28.

96. Kostraba NJ, Dorman JS, Orchard TJ, et al. Contribution of diabetes duration before puberty to development of microvascular disease in insulin dependent diabetes subjects. Diabetes Care 1989; 12:686.

97. Holl RW, Lang GE, Grabert M, et al. Diabetic retinopathy in pediatric patients with type-1 diabetes: effect of diabetes duration, prepubertal and pubertal onset of diabetes, and metabolic control. J Pediatr 1998; 132:790.

98. Donaghue KC, Fung AT, Hing S, et al. The effect of prepubertal diabetes duration on diabetes. Microvascular complications in early and late adolescence. Diabetes Care 1997; 20:77.

99. Murphy RP, Nanda M, Plotnick L, et al. The relationship of puberty to diabetic retinopathy. Arch Ophthalmol 1990; 108:215.

100. Gorman D, Sochett E, Daneman D. The natural history of microalbuminuria in adolescents with type 1 diabetes. J Pediatr 1999; 134:333.

101. Bojestig M, Arnqvist HJ, Hermansson G, et al. Declining incidence of nephropathy in insulin-dependent diabetes mellitus. N Engl J Med 1994; 330(1):15.

102. Barkai L, Kempler P, Vamosi I, et al. Peripheral sensory nerve dysfunction in children and adolescents with type 1 diabetes mellitus. Diabet Med 1998; 15:228.

103. Seidl R, Birnbacher R, Hauser E, et al. Brainstem auditory evoked potentials and visually evoked potentials in young patients with IDDM. Diabetes Care 1996; 19:1220.

104. Zinman B, Tildesley H, Chiasson JL, et al. Insulin lispro in CSII: results of a double-blind crossover study. Diabetes 1997; 46(3):440.

105. Manske CL. Risks and benefits of kidney and pancreas transplantation for diabetic patients. Diabetes Care 1999; 22(Suppl 2):B114.

# SECTION C

# HYPOGLYCEMIA

## CHAPTER 158

## HYPOGLYCEMIC DISORDERS IN THE ADULT

RICHARD J. COMI AND PHILLIP GORDEN

### DEFINITION OF HYPOGLYCEMIA

The patient equates hypoglycemia with a symptom complex of weakness, malaise, sweating, tremulousness, and anxiety that can be relieved by food ingestion. These symptoms, however, are neither unique to nor specific for hypoglycemia. For the physician, hypoglycemia is defined by a minimum set of criteria: symptoms of confusion, aberrant behavior, lightheadedness, loss of consciousness, or seizure; plasma glucose concentration of <40 mg/dL concomitant with these symptoms; and relief from the symptoms with the administration of glucose.[1,2] The physician must first establish that the patient has a pathologic reduction in the plasma glucose level before seeking a specific cause. No formal studies have been made of the test characteristics of fasting glucose concentrations in the diagnosis of hypoglycemia. Although a plasma fasting glucose value below 50 mg/dL (2.8 mmol/L) should raise the suspicion of a hypoglycemic disorder, most authorities rely on values below 40 mg/dL (2.2 mmol/L) as diagnostic.[3,4]

### PHYSIOLOGY OF FED AND FASTED STATES

The plasma glucose concentration in the fasting and postprandial states (Fig. 158-1) is maintained at 60 to 150 mg/dL (3.3–8.6 mmol/L). This provides a steady source of fuel to the central nervous system (CNS). The concentration of circulating glucose is monitored and adjusted by the interplay of two pancreatic hormones: insulin and glucagon. Within the normal range of plasma glucose levels, insulin is the dominant regulatory hormone. Insulin is released initially into the splanchnic circulation in response to a nutrient load and then distributes to the periphery. Insulin suppresses hepatic glucose production and encourages peripheral glucose (fat and muscle) use, except in the CNS.[5] Postprandially, the hepatic extraction of circulating glucose is quantitatively increased, but at the same efficiency as in the fasting state. The hepatic and peripheral effects of insulin, plus the quantitative increase in hepatic glucose uptake, maintain the plasma glucose within a narrow range despite nutrient loading.

In the fasting state, the liver is the sole supplier of circulating glucose. Hepatic breakdown of glycogen and gluconeogenesis supply glucose to the circulation.[6] Insulin secretion and plasma insulin levels fall during fasting, removing insulin's suppressive effects and allowing a gradual increase in hepatic glucose production. In prolonged fasting, gluconeogenesis alone supplies circulating glucose and depends on the supply of precursors from muscle and adipose tissue.[7]

The role of glucagon in the maintenance of normal plasma glucose levels is more subtle, and it probably acts as a modulator of insulin action on the liver. Glucagon release is less sensitive to variations of glucose within the normal range of plasma concentrations than to excursions outside the normal range.[8]

### PHYSIOLOGY OF THE NORMAL RESPONSE TO HYPOGLYCEMIA

Insulin-induced hypoglycemia is an excellent model of the response of homeostatic mechanisms to falling plasma glucose levels (Table 158-1; see Fig. 158-1). The physiologic response to insulin-induced hypoglycemia involves several reinforcing hormonal responses that center on hepatic glucose production and, to a lesser extent, on decreased insulin release and decreased glucose use. Human experiments featuring stepped reductions in glycemia, using the glucose clamp technique, demonstrate the initiation of increased release of epinephrine, norepinephrine, glucagon, and growth hormone at blood glucose concentrations of 60 to 66 mg/dL (3.3–3.6 mmol/L)[9] (Fig. 158-2). The catecholamines are the hormonal cause of the early symptom complex (tremulousness, tachycardia) and stimulate glycogenolysis; however, glucagon is the dominant physiologically effective hormone for rapid response to hypoglycemia, because it stimulates glycogenolysis and gluconeogenesis and antagonizes insulin action in the periphery.[10] In the absence of the glucagon response, the combined effects of catecholamine-mediated glycogenolysis and insulin antagonism, growth hormone, and cortisol lead to

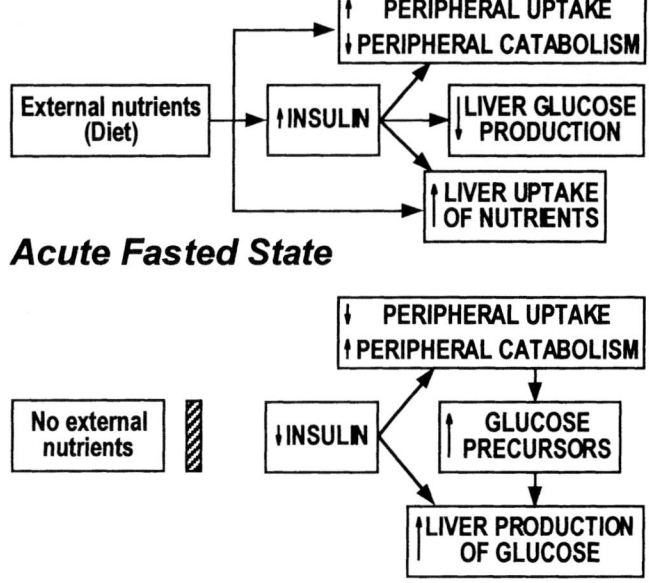

**FIGURE 158-1.** Physiology of fed and fasted states.

**TABLE 158-1.**
Physiologic Response to Hypoglycemia

| Hormone | Response | Time Course for Effect | Effect | Relative Importance in Restoring Euglycemia |
|---|---|---|---|---|
| Glucagon | Increase | Rapid (min) | ↑ Glycogenolysis | Major |
| | | Rapid (<1 h) | ↑ Gluconeogenesis | Major |
| | | Rapid (min) | Antagonizes hepatic effects of insulin | Major |
| Insulin | Decrease | Rapid (min) | ↑ Gluconeogenesis | Major |
| Catecholamines (norepinephrine and epinephrine) | Increase | Rapid (min) | ↑ Glycogenolysis | Minor |
| | | | ↑ Gluconeogenesis | Minor |
| | | | Antagonizes peripheral insulin effects | Minor |
| Growth hormone | Increase | Rapid (min) | Antagonizes all insulin effects | Minor |
| Corticosteroids | Increase | Slow (h) | ↑ Gluconeogenesis | Minor |
| | | | Antagonizes insulin effects | Minor |
| | | | ↓ Glucose use | Minor |

recovery from hypoglycemia, but over a longer span of time (Table 158-2).

## SYMPTOMS OF HYPOGLYCEMIA AND PATIENT HISTORY

True hypoglycemia causes symptoms that are characteristic but nonspecific. The automatic responses to falling plasma glucose concentrations are sensitive indicators of hypoglycemia. Epinephrine release from the adrenal medulla causes tachycardia, pallor, anxiety, and tremulousness by stimulating β-adrenergic receptors (i.e., noradrenergic symptoms). Sweating is a prominent symptom of hypoglycemia and probably has a cholinergic cause. All of these symptoms may be attenuated or absent in the setting of β-blockade, autonomic neuropathy, or chronic hypoglycemia, and the subjective sensation of hypoglycemia varies among individuals. Although some patients have symptoms when the plasma glucose is only moderately decreased, others may tolerate very low levels with a paucity of symptoms.

Neurologic symptoms, such as confusion, lightheadedness, headache, aberrant behavior, blurred vision, loss of consciousness, or seizure, are called *neuroglycopenic symptoms* if they are relieved by food ingestion or the administration of glucose. Such symptoms, especially if recurrent, are more specific and indicate a pathologic cause of hypoglycemia. These symptoms are usually gradual in onset and progressive unless treated with nutrients. The hypoglycemic individual may not notice them if onset is slow, and interviewing acquaintances or family members can help to determine the symptoms' timing and frequency.[11,12]

The history of hypoglycemia should be carefully assessed for any temporal association of the symptoms with meals or medica-

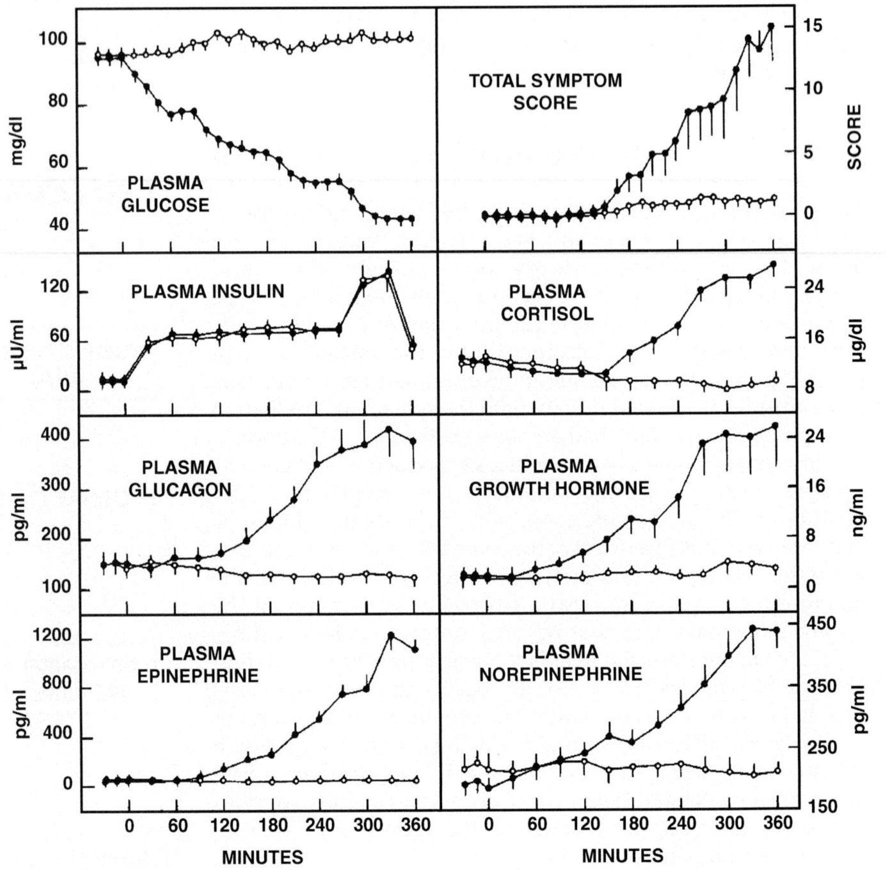

**FIGURE 158-2.** Physiology and symptoms of hypoglycemia. Plasma levels of glucose, insulin, and counterregulatory hormones and total symptom score (i.e., adrenergic and neuroglycopenic) during glucose clamp–induced hypoglycemia (*filled circles*) and euglycemia (*open circles*) in 10 nonobese, nondiabetic individuals. Total symptom score and hormonal responses rise when glucose is below 66 mg/dL (after 165–180 minutes); the exception was cortisol secretion, which required a lower plasma glucose level to become activated. (From Mitrakou A, Ryan C, Veneman T, et al. Hierarchy of glycemic thresholds for counterregulatory hormone secretion, symptoms and cerebral dysfunction. Am J Physiol 1991; 260:E67.)

**TABLE 158-2.**
**Differential Diagnosis of Acute Hypoglycemia**

**MEDICATION OR TOXIN INDUCED**
Excessive insulin effect
  Insulin
  Sulfonylureas
  Rodenticides (e.g., Vacor)
Diffuse hepatic dysfunction
  Ethanol
  Nonselective β-blocking agents
  Other medications
**FASTING HYPOGLYCEMIA**
Excessive insulin effects
  Insulinoma
  Surreptitious insulin injection
  Surreptitious sulfonylurea ingestion
  Insulin-receptor autoantibodies
  Antiidiotypic antibodies to antiinsulin antibodies
  Humoral tumor-associated hypoglycemia
Diffuse hepatic dysfunction
  Congestive heart failure
  Septic shock syndrome
  Combined endocrine deficiency states
Limitation of substrate for gluconeogenesis
  Uremia
Excessive glucose consumption
  Large sarcomas (?)
**POSTPRANDIAL HYPOGLYCEMIA**
Excessive insulin effect
  After gastric surgery
  Reactive hypoglycemia
Hepatic dysfunction
  Hypoglycin ingestion (i.e., Jamaican vomiting illness)

tions (see Table 158-2). Preprandial recurrent symptoms are more suggestive of pathologic hypoglycemia, which requires elaborate evaluation and invasive intervention, than are postprandial symptoms (i.e., within 4 to 5 hours of eating). A dietary history, including snacking and recent changes in eating patterns, is important, because many patients with true hypoglycemic disorders change their dietary patterns to prevent hypoglycemic episodes. The longest regular fast of the day, usually bedtime to breakfast, should be identified and scrutinized for symptoms. The use of insulin, sulfonylureas, alcohol, or other medications should be considered as the possible cause of hypoglycemia, particularly in the setting of poor or erratic nutrition.

## CAUSES OF HYPOGLYCEMIA

### INSULIN-INDUCED HYPOGLYCEMIA IN THE TREATMENT OF DIABETES

The most common cause of hypoglycemia in adults is insulin treatment in the management of diabetes.[13,14] The emphasis on aggressive attempts to maintain plasma glucose values in the normal range has increased the risk of episodes of hypoglycemia. The administration of a depot of subcutaneous insulin that is then slowly released into the circulation is an inflexible delivery of insulin, independent of dietary modifications. Erratic dietary and exercise patterns, which are typical of many individuals, can lead to hypoglycemic episodes. In the management of the diabetic patient with frequent episodes of hypoglycemia, meals, exercise, and the dose and duration of action of the insulin must be considered.[13,14]

Patients with diabetes may be less aware of hypoglycemia because of the use of other medications such as β-blockers, a change in the usual symptom complex after switching from animal to human insulins, or autonomic neuropathy and loss of the catecholamine-mediated symptoms. In virtually all patients with type 1 diabetes, the glucagon response to hypoglycemia is lost after 2 to 3 years of diabetes, rendering them more susceptible to prolonged episodes of hypoglycemia. Concern exists that patients who switch from animal to human insulins become insensitive to hypoglycemia. The loss of hypoglycemic symptoms after initiation of human insulin therapy has not been verified in randomized controlled trials, but patients should be counseled that the subjective warning signs of hypoglycemia may change when they switch from animal to human insulins because of improved glycemic control or more gradual diminution in blood glucose under a new insulin regimen.[15,16]

Another common manifestation of hypoglycemia in insulin-treated diabetics is the "Somogyi effect," in which fasting glucose concentrations seem to increase in response to increasing doses of insulin (see Chap. 143). This is the result of episodes of marked hypoglycemia at hours when patients are not testing their glucose concentrations (2:00 to 3:00 a.m.). It is followed by secretion of counterregulatory hormones, which in turn produces high levels of serum glucose at a later time when patients are testing their glucose concentrations (6:00 to 8:00 a.m.).

The treatment of acute episodes of hypoglycemia, insulin-induced or otherwise, is the administration of a nutrient and monitoring of plasma glucose over the next 1 to 2 hours. In episodes of severe hypoglycemia (i.e., confusion, loss of consciousness, seizures), intravenous glucose (50 mL of 50% glucose) should be administered to reverse the situation rapidly. In milder episodes, a small amount (15 g) of simple carbohydrates followed by nutrients with slower gastrointestinal absorption (e.g., whole milk, cheese) may be used. The response to administered nutrients should be immediate. Prolonged or delayed resolution of symptoms (>10 minutes) suggests inadequate treatment or another cause of the symptoms. Prolonged or repeated hypoglycemia can cause permanent neurologic injury.[17]

## FASTING HYPOGLYCEMIA

### EVALUATION

The evaluation of fasting hypoglycemia (Fig. 158-3) is essentially the workup for possible insulinoma.[18,18a] The investigation of insulinoma entails invasive testing, and the treatment is primarily surgical. Fasting hypoglycemia and an inappropriate hyperinsulinemia at the time of hypoglycemia must be documented before any further tests are performed. The single most useful test is the in-hospital monitored fast lasting for up to 48 hours. The insulin that is released by insulinomas usually is not suppressed by declining plasma glucose levels. Fasting individuals with insulinomas become hypoglycemic because the fasting plasma glucose level depends on the hepatic output of glucose. In contrast, normal individuals rarely develop plasma glucose concentrations <40 mg/dL during a 48-hour fast, and almost never develop neuroglycopenic symptoms in this setting.[3,4]

The observed fast is the most important test in evaluating fasting hypoglycemia, and it should be carefully performed, with attention to the collection of appropriate data. The intent is to demonstrate pathologic hypoglycemia, and this is best accomplished by demonstrating spontaneous hypoglycemia with neuroglycopenic symptoms. The fast must be conducted in the hospital and with provision for careful observation. The patient must not be allowed to leave the room, and frequent assessment by medical staff is essential. A secure intravenous line, preferably with a running infusion without glucose, must

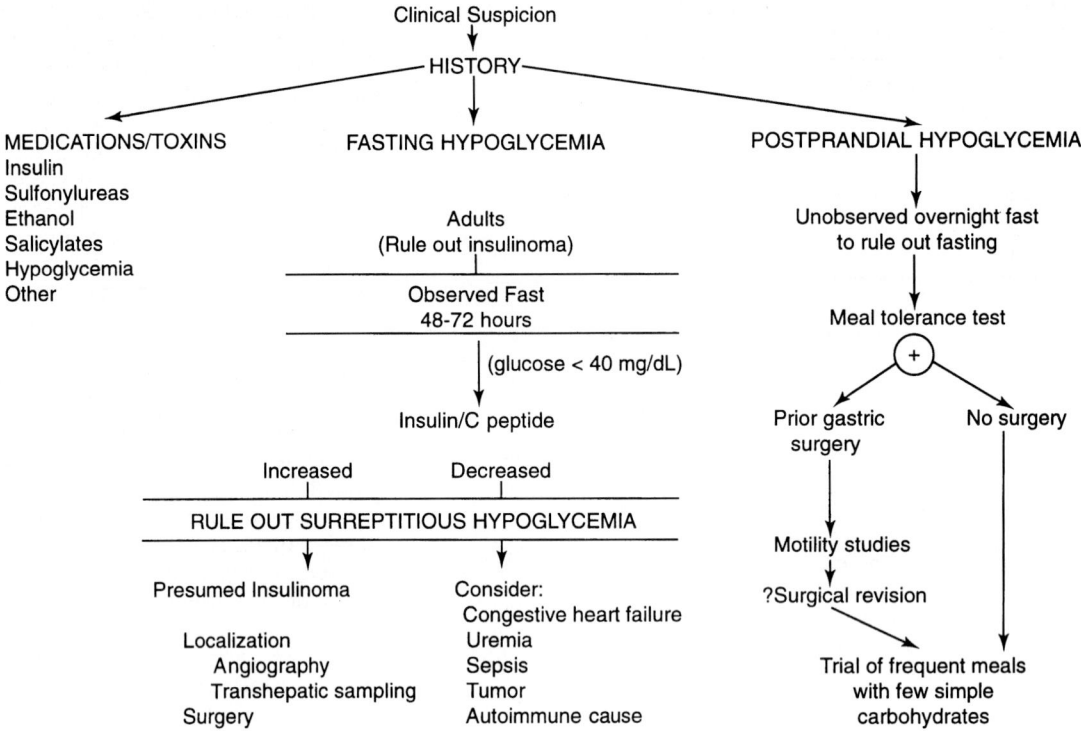

**FIGURE 158-3.** Algorithm for the evaluation of hypoglycemia.

be present, and an ampule of 50% glucose solution for rapid administration should be available. Access to glucagon usually is unnecessary. Before initiation of the fast, a simple neurologic examination stressing coordination, recent memory, and calculations should be performed to provide a baseline.

The time of initiating the fast is determined by a careful history to elicit a reasonable estimate of the patient's tolerance for fasting. Timing the hypoglycemia to occur midday with adequate staffing present is best. Fasts often are begun at midnight or after breakfast, depending on whether symptoms occur only after skipping meals or usually occur before breakfast, and depending on the severity of the symptoms. During the fast, patients may ingest noncaloric foods such as black coffee or artificially sweetened noncaloric beverages. Simultaneous insulin and glucose samples are obtained at the beginning of the fast and every 4 hours thereafter. Glucose levels should be determined by the glucose oxidase method in the clinical laboratory and not solely by a bedside glucose meter, because the latter often is inaccurate at glucose levels of <60 mg/dL. When the blood glucose has fallen below 50 mg/dL, insulin and glucose samples should be obtained every hour and bedside glucose meter determinations should be made every 30 minutes or with changes in clinical status (e.g., sweating).

These procedures are continued until the blood glucose falls below 40 mg/dL. This is significant hypoglycemia, and the patient should be assessed for neuroglycopenia frequently thereafter. Specimens for insulin and glucose values usually are drawn every 15 minutes. At the termination of the fast, a C-peptide level is also obtained to independently verify endogenous inappropriate insulin secretion. The fast should be terminated only when true neuroglycopenia appears and not because of signs of catecholamine excess, such as sweating or tremor. At the least, to rule out laboratory error, two or more blood glucose levels below 40 mg/dL should be obtained before the fast is concluded.

Although neuroglycopenic symptoms may be subtle in some patients, the 48-hour fast should provide all the necessary diagnostic information.[18b] An analysis of the pattern of insulin and glucose levels during the fast is helpful. Insulin levels should fall progressively with prolonged fasting. Failure of suppression of insulin and C-peptide levels despite prolonged fasting indicates inappropriate insulin secretion.

For a blood glucose value of <40 mg/dL (2.2 mmol/L), the appropriate concentration of insulin in the serum is <6 μU/mL (36 pmol/L). Insulin levels above the limits of detectability in such well-supervised insulin assays suggest an insulinoma, especially if confirmed by detectable levels of C peptide. The combination of fasting hypoglycemia values of <40 mg/dL, neuroglycopenia, and the failure to suppress insulin secretion are diagnostic of an insulinoma. Plotting all the insulin and glucose values obtained during the fast also is useful. Ketonuria after 12 or more hours of fasting indicates normal suppression of insulin during a fast and is not observed in patients with insulinomas.

In some centers, calculation of the ratio of insulin (in μU/mL) to glucose (in mg/dL) is used to analyze data from a fast. In cases of insulinoma, the insulin/glucose ratio exceeds 0.3 during the fast. This analysis usually is unnecessary, and false-positive results are observed in obese individuals with moderate insulin resistance. The authors prefer to evaluate absolute end points to avoid these false-positive results.

Several important caveats should be noted regarding the observed fast. First, women have lower plasma concentrations of glucose during a fast than men, and normal women occasionally have values below 40 mg/dL in the second 24 hours.[4] These women, however, are asymptomatic and have insulin concentrations that are normally suppressed. Second, some insulinomas suppress their insulin release in response to hypoglycemia. Third, false elevations can occur in serum insulin measurements

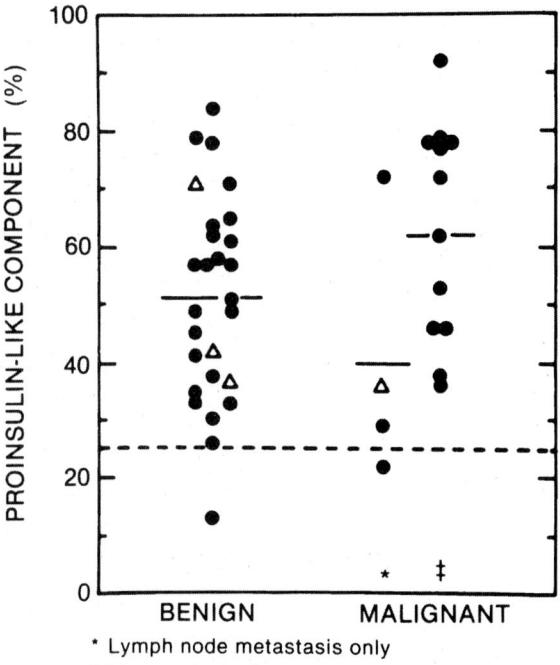

**FIGURE 158-4.** Proinsulin-like component in insulinoma patients. The normal amount of immunoreactive insulin that migrates with proinsulin on gel filtration is <25%, as indicated by the dotted line. In >90% of the patients with benign or malignant insulinomas, the plasma contains much more proinsulin than normal. Although the average percentage of proinsulin (*horizontal bars*) is higher for patients with malignant insulinoma than for those with benign tumors, because of an overlap of values, this difference cannot allow discrimination of benign from malignant tumors. The triangles denote patients with MEN1.

because of the presence of antiinsulin antibodies. To avoid these pitfalls, the fast should be continued under close supervision until mild but definite neuroglycopenic symptoms are documented. The appearance of symptomatic hypoglycemia is pathologic and, in the presence of inappropriate hyperinsulinemia, is diagnostic for insulinoma.[18b]

The diagnosis of insulinoma in these patients is further supported by the finding that a high percentage (>25%) of circulating fasting immunoreactive insulin is actually proinsulin, suggesting poor processing of the peptide by the tumor (Fig. 158-4). The determination of the percentage of insulin that is the proinsulin-like component (PLC) is based on measurements using an insulin standard for the insulin and PLC. The PLC is elevated in patients with type 2 diabetes and familial hyperproinsulinemia, but these are hyperglycemic, not hypoglycemic, conditions. In a review of 25 patients with documented insulinoma, an analysis of samples drawn at the termination of a fast and in the presence of hypoglycemia showed that an elevated percentage of proinsulin had a sensitivity of 84%. Although PLC measurement is an experimental test, the direct measurement of proinsulin yields similar results.[18–20]

Other tests to detect insulinomas can be divided in two types. One type relies on the demonstration of increased insulin secretory capacity. The best standardized example is the tolbutamide test, although calcium and glucagon challenges have been used.[21] These tests rely on good characterization of a normal range, established at the test center. The second type demonstrates the inability to suppress insulin secretion. The C-peptide level in plasma is measured before and after an infusion of exogenous insulin. The response is blunted or absent in insulinoma patients. Because this test does not rely on external controls, it may be very useful and is appealing in its simplicity.[22] Whether

it will supplant the observed fast cannot yet be determined. Both tests of insulin secretory capacity and tests of insulin suppression can be useful in difficult cases for which the routine fasting results are equivocal.

## MANAGEMENT

The only effective treatment of insulinoma is surgical extirpation. Insulinomas usually are discrete, single nodules (<2 cm in diameter), which are evenly distributed throughout the pancreas. Pancreatic surgery is fraught with morbidity, particularly if the pancreatic duct is injured. The preoperative localization of insulinomas is extremely important and should be pursued aggressively (see Chap. 159).

For the localization of insulinomas, abdominal ultrasonography and computerized tomography (CT) with or without bolus contrast enhancement have sensitivities of 30% to 50%.[18] CT scans may be useful to document metastatic disease and are commonly performed in the evaluation of insulinoma. Although the experience with magnetic resonance imaging (MRI) is limited, it is more sensitive for identifying metastases and may be more sensitive for identifying the primary pancreatic tumor. The octreotide scan, which uses intravenous injection of the somatostatin analog octreotide labeled with an indium radionucleotide, when correlated with CT or MRI images, is less useful for insulinomas than for other tumors.[23]

When available, the best test for insulinoma localization is angiography with subselective injections to visualize the entire pancreatic vascular bed. The success rate with this technique is 30% to 50% for primary tumors and >90% for metastatic disease.[18] In cases not identified by subselective arteriography, localization is accomplished by demonstrating excessive insulin secretion from a region of the pancreas. One of two techniques is calcium infusion in the arterial branches of the celiac plexus, with immediate sampling for stimulation of insulin release into the hepatic vein. This technique can identify vascular beds that harbor insulinomas by demonstrating exaggerated responsiveness to calcium. Experience suggests that this may be the method of choice because of a high sensitivity (e.g., positive results for 10 of 11 patients studied) and low risk of complications.[18] Percutaneous transhepatic venous sampling of the pancreatic venous drainage is also successful in identifying 70% of occult insulinomas by demonstrating a "step-up" in insulin secretion from a region of the pancreas. This technique, however, is associated with greater morbidity.

Multiple insulinomas occur in ~10% of cases, particularly in the setting of familial type 1 multiple endocrine neoplasia (MEN1), and excessive secretion by one of several nodules may impede demonstration of the multiplicity of the tumors. Patients with MEN1 may have several tumors, only some of which secrete insulin. These patients may present with symptoms referable to another hormone secreted in excess and may incidentally be found to have an insulinoma (see Chap. 188). For example, patients with the MEN1 syndrome may present with symptoms referable to hyperparathyroidism or the Zollinger-Ellison syndrome, but an incidental insulinoma is found by careful history-taking, screening tests, or surgery. Determination of insulin levels and the percentage of proinsulin may be used to screen for insulinoma. Preoperative localization does not obviate careful palpation of the entire pancreas, especially when the nodule is localized by venous sampling alone. Intraoperative ultrasonography may facilitate the exploration of the pancreas, particularly by identifying the depth of the nodule within the substance of the pancreas.

Rarely, excessive insulin secretion is caused by diffuse lesions of the pancreas, such as multiple adenomatosis or *nesidioblastosis*. Nesidioblastosis probably is a congenital lesion of the pan-

TABLE 158-3.

**Insulinoma: Insulin-Suppressing Agents and Chemotherapy for Metastatic Disease**

| Agent | Trade Name | Dosage | Complete or Partial Response | Excretion | Toxicity |
|---|---|---|---|---|---|
| **INSULIN-SUPPRESSING AGENTS USED IN INSULINOMA THERAPY** | | | | | |
| Diazoxide | Proglycem | 200–600 mg po daily | 50% | Renal | Gastrointestinal intolerance; edema; hirsutism |
| Somatostatin analog | Octreotide acetate, Sandostatin | Experimental, sc | Anecdotal | | Abdominal cramps, possible gall-stones |
| Verapamil | Isoptin, Calan | Experimental, iv | Anecdotal | Liver | Heart block; hypotension |
| Phenytoin | Dilantin | 300–400 mg po daily | Anecdotal | Liver | CNS effects; hepatotoxicity; skin rash; thrombocytopenia, leukopenia |
| **CHEMOTHERAPEUTIC AGENTS TO TREAT METASTATIC INSULINOMA** | | | | | |
| Streptozocin | Same | 500 mg/m² iv daily for 5 days of Rx; cycled every 6 wk | 35–50% | Liver > renal | Nephrotoxicity; bone marrow effects; hepatotoxicity |
| Streptozocin plus 5-FU | Same + fluorouracil | Same as above plus 5-FU, 400 mg/m² iv, both daily for 5 days of Rx; cycled every 6 wk | 60% | See above, plus liver for 5-FU | Same as above; diarrhea; mucositis; hepatotoxicity (5-FU) |
| Doxorubicin | Adriamycin | 60 mg/m² iv; cycled every 2–3 wk; limit: 450 mg/m² | Under study | Liver | Myelosuppression; cardiotoxicity; alopecia |
| Dacarbazine | DTIC-Dome | 250 mg/m² iv daily for 5 days; cycled monthly | Anecdotal | Renal > liver | Myelosuppression; thrombo-cytopenia |

*po*, by mouth; *sc*, subcutaneously; *iv*, intravenously; *CNS*, central nervous system; *5-FU*, 5-fluorouracil.
(From Comi RJ, Gorden P, Doppman JL. Insulinoma. In: Go VL, Di Magno E, Gardner J, et al., eds. The pancreas: biology, pathobiology and diseases. New York: Raven Press, 1993:979.)

creas and is a common cause of hypoglycemia in infants. It is extremely rare and should be carefully verified before being accepted as a cause of hypoglycemia in adults (see Chap. 161).[24] Familial hyperinsulinism has also been described as a rare cause of noninsulinoma pancreatogenous hypoglycemia. Whether these lesions actually harbor small adenomas is controversial; however, the lack of increased serum proinsulin and lack of a family history of MEN1 syndrome, added to the histologic finding of a diffuse increase in insulin-containing islet cells, indicates that this is a separate entity.[25] Finally, increased insulin secretion from diffuse islet cell proliferation in the setting of pancreatic fibrosis has been described.[26]

Surgical removal of an insulinoma (see Chap. 160) is curative in >80% of the cases.[27] Distal tail lesions may require concomitant splenectomy, and preoperative pneumococcal vaccination is advisable. The exploration of lymph nodes in the region is important in assessing the nature of the tumor. Insulinoma histology does not correlate well with tumor behavior. Ten percent of all insulinomas are malignant, and these are recognized solely by the presence of hepatic metastases.[18] Occasionally, only local lymph node spread is found at surgery. In the absence of hepatic disease, the resection of involved nodes is often curative, and surgical debulking of malignant tissue can be of great benefit. Islet cell tumor metastases may be nonsecretory or may secrete a hormone different from that of the primary tumor. Isolated metastases to tissues outside the abdomen have not been reported.

Medicinal therapy to diminish insulin release from the tumor is limited (Table 158-3). Diazoxide suppresses insulin release in ~50% of all insulinoma lesions, and the response to this agent may be inversely correlated with the elevation of the percentage of proinsulin.[28] In responsive cases, diazoxide, in dosages of 400 to 600 mg per day, can be extremely useful in preoperative or long-term management. Side effects include salt retention and gastrointestinal intolerance. These can be minimized by gradual escalation from small doses to effective amounts. The long-acting somatostatin analog octreotide acetate is the second-line agent and has variable effectiveness (see Chap. 169).[29] Other agents of occasional use are calcium channel–blocking agents and phenytoin sodium (Dilantin), which can reduce insulin release in a few cases.

In difficult cases of severe hypoglycemia with nonresectable metastatic tumors, some success has been reported with alternative therapies, such as catheterization and occlusion of the vascular supply to the tumor.[30] These approaches have limited applicability, however, because of the presence of multiple vessels supplying blood to the tumor and the difficulty in selectively damaging the tumor without affecting normal tissue.

Metastatic insulinoma requires careful evaluation for proper management. Large, rapidly expanding liver metastases or hyperinsulinism and hypoglycemia are clear indications for chemotherapeutic intervention. The progression of metastases may be slow, and small amounts of nonfunctional metastatic disease may not require intervention, particularly in elderly patients. In cases requiring therapy, the most effective regimen is a combination of streptozocin and 5-fluorouracil, which achieves partial or complete response in 60% of patients (see Table 158-3). The main side effect of this therapy is the nephrotoxicity of the streptozocin, which can cause permanent renal damage and necessitates the cessation of therapy. Doxorubicin (Adriamycin) has been added to the combination regimen in some trials. Assay of tumor markers is particularly helpful in following the course of metastatic insulinomas. These markers include insulin, the percentage of PLC, and α human chorionic gonadotropin (α-hCG). Elevated levels of these markers can precede the detection of increased tumor burden, and an increase in serum hCG or its α subunit occurs in ~50% of cases of malignant insulinoma. Chemotherapy is not curative; the goal of therapy is the relief of symptoms.

## HYPOGLYCEMIA ASSOCIATED WITH NONINSULINOMA TUMORS

Certain tumors have been associated with profound fasting hypoglycemia (Table 158-4; see Chap. 219).[31] The hypoglycemic syndrome caused by these noninsulinoma tumors is clinically indistinguishable from that resulting from insulinoma, but the lesions are easily differentiated by the absence of inappropriate hyperinsulinemia. Hypoglycemia is most commonly a late manifestation of these tumors, appearing when they are quite large (400 g to 1 kg). Mesenchymal tumors, particularly those com-

**TABLE 158-4.**
**Noninsulinoma Tumor–Associated Hypoglycemia**

**TUMOR TYPE (IN ORDER OF FREQUENCY)**

| | |
|---|---|
| Mesenchymal | Benign tumor or sarcoma of muscle, mesothelial cell and neurofibroma, hemangiopericytoma, fibrosarcoma |
| Hepatoma | |
| Adrenocortical tumor | Usually carcinoma, often left-sided |
| Gastrointestinal tumors | Epithelial tumors from all regions of gastrointestinal tract |
| Lymphoma | |
| Other | Teratoma, genitourinary epithelial tumors |

**COMMON FEATURES OF HYPOGLYCEMIA-ASSOCIATED NONINSULINOMA TUMORS**

| | |
|---|---|
| Large size | >500 g, 5 cm in diameter |
| Localization | Abdominal more than thoracic (50% retroperitoneal) |
| Age at presentation | Usually older than 30 years |
| Local invasion | Occasionally metastatic or multicentric |

**TABLE 158-5.**
**Features That Differentiate Hypoglycemia Due to Insulinoma from Factitious Hypoglycemia**

| Test | Insulinoma | Surreptitious Administration or Ingestion | |
|---|---|---|---|
| | | *Insulin* | *Sulfonylurea* |
| **Antibodies to insulin** | Not present | *Present** | Not present |
| **Sulfonylurea (blood or urine)** | Not present | Not present | *Present* |
| **Immunoreactive insulin** | Normal or elevated | Normal or elevated | Normal or elevated |
| **C peptide** | Normal or elevated | *Decreased* | Normal or elevated |
| **Proinsulin** | *Usually increased* | Normal or decreased | Normal |

*Italics indicate the most diagnostic test in each situation.

posed of spindle cells, are the most common types associated with hypoglycemia. Other tumors that may cause hypoglycemia include sarcomas, hepatocellular tumors, and carcinoid-like tumors.[21] Mesenchymal tumors associated with hypoglycemia can be benign or malignant. The absence of inappropriate circulating insulin is a hallmark of patients with these tumors. Interestingly, ectopic insulin production is extremely rare.

Hypoglycemia associated with mesenchymal tumors is caused by excessive production of a poorly processed and O-glycosylated form of insulin-like growth factor-II (IGF-II). Most "big IGF-II" associates with IGF-binding protein-2 in a highly bioavailable complex, which in turn suppresses secretion of growth hormone, insulin, and normal IGF-II. Because it suppresses normal IGF-II concentrations, total IGF-II concentrations in standard assays may be normal or only slightly elevated; however, excessive big IGF-II levels in these patients may be identified with an assay for a unique peptide in big IGF-II. Big IGF-II has been shown to cause hypoglycemia by markedly increasing glucose disposal into muscle, while preventing a compensatory increase in hepatic glucose output.[31–33]

These tumors, because of their large size, are usually easily detected by radiologic investigations of the thoracic, abdominal, or retroperitoneal cavities. Treatment is primarily surgical, although radiation therapy sometimes has been effective. Generally, they are unresponsive to antitumor agents. Table 158-4 summarizes typical tumor types and features observed in noninsulinoma tumor–associated hypoglycemia.

In rare cases, tumor consumption of glucose, perhaps in an autocrine response to its own production of big IGF-II, or extensive hepatic destruction by metastatic disease may result in tumor-associated hypoglycemia.

## FACTITIOUS HYPOGLYCEMIA

Surreptitious, self-induced (i.e., factitious) hypoglycemia is difficult to document, even when suspected, and it is extremely difficult to discover if unsuspected. It is not rare; factitious hypoglycemia should be an early and seriously considered diagnosis for all patients with hypoglycemia.[18,34] Individuals with access to insulin, such as medical personnel or relatives of diabetics, are especially suspect. These persons rigorously deny self-induced hypoglycemia and may permit invasive testing and even unnecessary surgery (Table 158-5). A search of the patient's possessions or room usually is unrewarding.

The single most important diagnostic maneuver is the measurement of C peptide in the blood at the time of hypoglycemia. The C

peptide is cleaved out of proinsulin in the insulin secretion granule and is released into the circulation with endogenous insulin. Circulating C-peptide concentrations are suppressed during the hypoglycemia that is induced by the hyperinsulinemia of exogenous insulin administration. Hypoglycemia due to sulfonylurea use, however, is associated with normal to high C-peptide levels because endogenous insulin secretion is increased by these agents; therefore, urinary measurement of sulfonylureas is also useful.

Measurement of antibodies to insulin may also be helpful.[34] The presence of these antibodies is indicative of prior exogenous insulin administration, particularly of bovine and porcine insulins. Because the titers of this antibody may be low, a concentrating technique or gel filtration may be necessary for their detection. The increased use of human insulins from recombinant sources, however, makes antibody testing less useful than in the past. Although insulin antibodies may be present in rare, autoimmune forms of hypoglycemia, factitious disease must be specifically excluded in these patients.

## AUTOIMMUNE CAUSES OF HYPOGLYCEMIA

The first and best characterized autoimmune disease associated with hypoglycemia is the syndrome of *type B extreme insulin resistance,* in which circulating antibodies to the insulin receptor are present[35] (see Chap. 146). Persons with this syndrome usually demonstrate the skin lesion acanthosis nigricans and various nonspecific autoimmune features, including anemia, thrombocytopenia, nephritis, and an elevated sedimentation rate. Typically, these persons are insulin resistant and hyperglycemic; rarely, they manifest severe fasting hypoglycemia from an insulinomimetic effect. In some of these patients, alternating episodes of hyperglycemia and hypoglycemia may occur. Because the degradation of insulin normally is mediated by the receptor, circulating insulin levels may be paradoxically elevated at times of hypoglycemia, mimicking the features of insulinoma. Plasma PLC levels and insulin response to secretagogues are normal, and the demonstration of anti–insulin receptor antibodies confirms the diagnosis.

The *spontaneous autoimmune antiinsulin antibody syndrome* is also associated with hypoglycemic episodes. This syndrome is extremely rare, with most reported cases occurring in Japan and in association with treatment with propylthiouracil for autoimmune thyroid disease.[36,37] The disease is difficult to document in sporadic cases, and prior insulin use must be carefully excluded. The mechanism of hypoglycemia in this disorder is not understood, but it is postulated to involve the production of antiidiotypic antibodies to the antiinsulin antibodies, which interact with the insulin receptor to mimic insulin at its receptor.

Finally, multiple myeloma has been reported to produce insulin-binding immunoglobulin G that binds insulin secreted normally in association with meal consumption and prolongs its presence in the serum. This results in hyperglycemia immediately after a meal, and severe hypoglycemia before the next meal.[38]

## ALCOHOL-INDUCED HYPOGLYCEMIA

The liver is the central organ in normal glucose homeostasis (see Fig. 158-1). Hepatic disease can impair the ability of the liver to store or to produce glucose. The glycogen storage diseases and other enzymatic deficiencies that impair hepatic glucose metabolism are usually discovered early in life.[39] Rarely, a mild form of these disorders occurs in adolescence, but ordinarily, genetic enzymatic deficiencies are not a consideration in adult hypoglycemia (see Chap. 161). Diffuse acquired liver disease, such as cirrhosis, fulminant hepatitis, and even hepatic congestion caused by congestive heart failure, can result in impaired hepatic gluconeogenesis, although very late in the course of these diseases.[40] Focal liver diseases, including extensive hepatic metastases, rarely cause hypoglycemia (see Chap. 205).[39] An acute glucagon challenge test has been used to determine if the liver has adequate glycogen stores to support serum glucose levels in cases of hypoglycemia associated with metastatic liver disease.[41]

Most commonly, fasting hypoglycemia of hepatic origin derives from acute, acquired impairment of hepatic glucose output, primarily by hepatic toxins.[42] The most common circumstance is hypoglycemic coma in those with chronic alcoholism. The patient usually has a history of extremely poor nutrition for several days, followed by acute alcohol ingestion. The metabolism of alcohol and the production of glucose from precursors require oxidative steps using nicotinamide-adenine dinucleotide (NAD) as a proton receptor. Acute alcohol administration depletes the liver of NAD, and gluconeogenesis ceases.[43] This causes profound hypoglycemia and neuroglycopenia, manifested as coma. These individuals are treated with administration of glucose and thiamine. The latter is required for CNS glucose metabolism, and administration of glucose alone may precipitate another deficiency state with neurologic sequelae. Hypoglycemia in sepsis probably is of hepatic origin; hepatic gluconeogenesis is presumably impaired by a toxin.

## HYPOGLYCEMIA ASSOCIATED WITH HORMONAL DEFICIENCY SYNDROMES

Endocrinopathies can affect circulating glucose levels by impairing gluconeogenesis.[44,45,45a] Deficiencies of corticotropin, cortisol, growth hormone, or thyroxine can diminish the amounts and activities of the enzymes involved in gluconeogenesis and diminish the hepatic capacity for glucose output. These hormonal deficiencies alone rarely produce hypoglycemia, but they can compound other hypoglycemic stresses, such as use of certain medications.[45b] Combined deficiencies, such as of cortisol and growth hormone, can cause spontaneous hypoglycemia. Deficiencies of other hormones such as glucagon, catecholamines, or other pituitary hormones are not associated with hypoglycemic syndromes.

## POSTPRANDIAL HYPOGLYCEMIA

Postprandial hypoglycemia (see Fig. 158-3) or *reactive hypoglycemia* is better designated as a *postprandial syndrome*. This diagnosis is controversial. A few patients experience symptomatic hypoglycemia 2 to 4 hours after a meal. In one study of 116 patients referred for evaluation of reactive hypoglycemia, 16 developed symptoms at the time of their lowest glucose level during oral glucose-tolerance testing, but 14 of these developed the same symptoms after receiving a placebo without caloric value in a blinded fashion.[46] No consistent relationship was found between blood glucose concentrations and symptoms in a study using well-standardized home glucose monitoring in a large number of patients with postprandial syndromes.[47] Only 8 of 132 measurements obtained at the time of symptoms showed a glucose level of <50 mg/dL (2.8 mmol/L).

Patients complaining of neuroglycopenic symptoms 1.5 to 5 hours after meals should be investigated by means of a mixed meal tolerance test, in which a standardized meal of normal composition is ingested, and then the plasma glucose concentration is monitored every 30 minutes for 5 hours while the patient is observed for symptoms. Patients who develop symptoms simultaneously with true hypoglycemia may be considered to have postprandial hypoglycemia. The treatment is a trial of a low-carbohydrate diet, which is effective in many cases. Ingestion of more frequent, but smaller, meals also may be effective. The diagnosis should not be evaluated by means of an oral glucose-tolerance test, because careful studies have shown an incidence of hypoglycemia in as many as 16% of normal persons after the ingestion of large amounts of simple carbohydrates, and the low blood sugar levels in such instances are an irrelevant artifact of the unusually large ingestion of simple carbohydrate. A limited number of trials have been performed of the medication acarbose, which slows the absorption of carbohydrates in the small intestine by competitively inhibiting the disaccharidases.[48] Administration of this agent may become a useful approach in refractory cases.

An important subgroup of patients with a postprandial syndrome are patients who have undergone gastric outlet surgery, particularly for peptic ulcer.[49] In these patients, postprandial hypoglycemia does occur, probably because of rapid transit of large amounts of nutrients, especially carbohydrates, from the gastric remnant to the small bowel. Although the process is not well understood, this is thought to cause the elaboration of large amounts of local gut factors that result in a hypersecretion of insulin from the pancreas. This phenomenon is distinct from the dumping syndrome, in which the rapid transit of a large osmotic load through the gut causes a rapid fluid shift and a marked autonomic response without an associated hypoglycemia. The treatment of postsurgical postprandial hypoglycemia usually consists of instituting a regimen of small meals; if this fails, surgical intervention may be required. Figure 158-3 summarizes the approach to the postprandial syndrome.

## OTHER CAUSES OF HYPOGLYCEMIA

True pseudohypoglycemia can be observed in unrefrigerated samples of blood containing large numbers of granulocytes. The granulocytes actively consume the serum glucose in the time between phlebotomy and laboratory assay. This is most likely to occur in leukemoid reactions, leukemia, or after the administration of colony-stimulating factors such as granulocyte colony-stimulating factor (G-CSF), in samples where the granulocyte count may exceed 40,000 cells per cubic millimeter.[50]

Several pharmacologic agents cause hypoglycemia as a side effect.[42] The most common offenders after the insulins are the sulfonylureas. These include pentamidine, which is used in the treatment of *Pneumocystis carinii* infections,[51] antiarrhythmic agents such as disopyramide, and some antimalarial drugs. The acute ingestion of hepatic toxins, such as large doses of acetaminophen, also causes hypoglycemia as a result of fulminant liver failure. Hypoglycemia may be caused by ingestion of the Caribbean fruit ackee, from which a substance called *hypoglycin* has been isolated (see Chap. 235).[52] In any evaluation of hypoglycemia, a careful drug and ingestion history is required.

Plasma glucose levels of <50 mg/dL (2.8 mmol/L) may occur after prolonged strenuous exercise, such as running a marathon. Although seizures attributed to hypoglycemia have occasionally been reported, symptomatic hypoglycemia is unusual in these individuals, and symptoms of exhaustion have not been shown to be caused by hypoglycemia.[53]

Uremia also has been associated with hypoglycemia. The fasting hypoglycemia occurring in this condition is attributed to a failure to produce substrate from the peripheral tissues (notably alanine) for hepatic glyconeogenesis. However, this complication of uremia is rare.[54]

## REFERENCES

1. Whipple AO. The surgical therapy of hyperinsulinism. J Int Chir 1938; 3:237.
2. Service FJ. Hypoglycemic disorders. Endocrinol Metab Clin North Am 1999; 28:467.
3. Marks V. Recognition and differential diagnosis of spontaneous hypoglycaemia. Clin Endocrinol 1992; 37:309.
4. Merimee T, Tyson JE. Hypoglycemia in man. Diabetes 1977; 26:161.
5. Katz LD, Glickman MG, Rapoport S, et al. Splanchnic and peripheral disposal of oral glucose in man. Diabetes 1983; 32:675.
6. Cahill GF Jr. Starvation in man. N Engl J Med 1970; 282:668.
7. Felig P, Marliss E, Owen E, Cahill GF Jr. Role of substrate in the regulation of hepatic gluconeogenesis in man. Adv Enzyme Regul 1969; 7:41.
8. Felig P, Wahrin J, Sherwin R, Hendler R. Insulin and glucose in normal physiology and diabetes. Diabetes 1976; 25:1091.
9. Mitrakou A, Ryan C, Veneman T, et al. Hierarchy of glycemic thresholds for counterregulatory hormone secretion, symptoms and cerebral dysfunction. Am J Physiol 1991; 260:E67.
10. Rizza RA, Cryer PE, Gerich JE. Role of glucagon, catecholamines, and growth hormone in human glucose counterregulation: effects of somatostatin and combined α- and β-adrenergic blockade on plasma glucose recovery and glucose flux rates following insulin-induced hypoglycemia. J Clin Invest 1978; 64:62.
11. Field JB. Hypoglycemia. Endocrinol Metab Clin North Am 1989; 18:27.
12. Blackman JD, Towle VL, Lewis GF, et al. Hypoglycemic threshold for cognitive dysfunction in humans. Diabetes 1990; 39:828.
13. Diabetes Complications and Control Trial Research Group. Hypoglycemia in the Diabetes Complications and Control Trial. Diabetes 1997; 46: 271.
14. Cryer P, Gerich J. Glucose counterregulation, hypoglycemia and intensive insulin therapy in diabetes mellitus. N Engl J Med 1985; 313:232.
15. Gerich JE, Mokaw M, Veneman T, et al. Hypoglycemia unawareness. Endocr Rev 1991; 12:356.
16. Comi RJ. Approach to adult hypoglycemia. Endocrinol Metab Clin North Am 1993; 22:247.
17. Malouf R, Brust JCM. Hypoglycemia: causes, neurological manifestations and outcome. Ann Neurol 1985; 17:421.
18. Comi RJ, Gorden P, Doppman JL. Insulinoma. In: Go VL, Di Magno E, Gardner J, et al., eds. The pancreas: biology, pathobiology and diseases. New York: Raven Press, 1993;979.
18a. Gorden P, Skarulis MC, Roach P, et al. Plasma proinsulin-like component in insulinoma: a 25 year experience. J Clin Endocrinol Metab 1995; 80:2884.
18b. Hirshberg B, Livi A, Bartlett DL, et al. 48 hr fast: the diagnostic test for insulinoma. J Clin Endocrinol Metab 2000; 85:In Press.
19. Rao PC, Taylor RL, Service FJ. Proinsulin by immunochemicoluminometric assay for the diagnosis of insulinoma. J Clin Endocrinol Metab 1994; 76:1048.
20. Doherty GM, Doppman JL, Shawker TH, et al. Results of a prospective strategy to diagnose, localize and resect insulinoma. Surgery 1991; 110:989.
21. McMahon MM, O'Brien PC, Service FJ. Diagnostic interpretation of the intravenous tolbutamide test for insulinoma. Mayo Clin Proc 1989; 64:1481.
22. Service FJ, O'Brien PC, Yao OP, Young WF. C peptide stimulation test: effects of gender, age, and body mass index; implications for the diagnosis of insulinoma. J Clin Endocrinol Metab 1992; 74:204.
23. Krausz Y, Bar Ziu J, de Jong RB, et al. Somatostatin receptor scintography in the management of gastroenteropancreatic tumors. Am J Gastroenterol 1998; 93: 66.
24. Fuller PF, Erlich AR, Susil B, Zeimer H. Insulin gene expression in adult onset nesidioblastosis. Clin Endocrinol 1997; 47:245.
25. Burnam W, McDermott MT, Borneman M. Familial hyperinsulihism presenting in adults. Arch Intern Med 1992; 152:2125.
26. Sangueza O, Wei J, Isales CM. Pancreatic fibrosis with islet cell paraneoplastic hyperplastic proliferation as a cause of hypoglycemia. Ann Intern Med 1997; 127:1042.
27. Norton JA, Doherty GM, Fraker DL. Surgery for endocrine tumors of the pancreas. In: Go VL, Di Magno E, Gardner J, et al., eds. The pancreas: biology, pathobiology and diseases. New York: Raven Press, 1993:997.
28. Berger M, Bordi C, Cuppers HJ, et al. Functional and morphological characterization of human insulinomas. Diabetes 1983; 32:921.
29. Kvols LK, Buck M, Moertel CG, et al. Treatment of metastatic islet cell carcinoma with a somatostatin analogue SMS201995. Ann Intern Med 1987; 107:162.
30. Moore TJ, Peterson LM, Harrington DP, Smith RJ. Successful arterial embolization of an insulinoma. JAMA 1982; 248:1353.
31. Daughaday WH, Emanuelle MA, Brooks MH, et al. Synthesis and secretion of insulin-like growth factor II by a leiomyosarcoma with associated hypoglycemia. N Engl J Med 1988; 319:1434.
31a. Seckl MJ, Mulholland PJ, Bishop AE, et al. Hypoglycemia due to an insulin-secreting small-cell carcinoma of the cervix. N Engl J Med 1999; 341:733.

32. Zapf J, Futo E, Froesch ER. Can "big" insulinlike growth factor II in serum of tumor patients account for the development of extrapancreatic tumor hypoglycemia? J Clin Invest 1992; 90:2574.
33. Chung J, Henry RR. Mechanisms of tumor induced hypoglycemia with intraabdominal hemangiopericytoma. J Clin Endocrinol Metab 1996; 81:919.
34. Grunberger G, Weiner JL, Silverman R, et al. Factitious hypoglycemia due to surreptitious administration of insulin: diagnosis, treatment, and long-term follow-up. Ann Intern Med 1988; 108:252.
35. Taylor SI, Barbetti F, Accili D, et al. Syndromes of autoimmunity and hypoglycemia. Autoantibodies directed against insulin and its receptor. Endocrinol Metab Clin North Am 1989; 18:123.
36. Ichihara K, Shima K, Sarto Y, et al. Mechanism of hypoglycemia observed in a patient with insulin autoimmune syndrome. Diabetes 1977; 26:500.
37. Benson EA, Ho P, Wang C, et al. Insulin autoimmunity as a source of hypoglycemia. Arch Intern Med 1984; 144:2351.
38. Redmon B, Pyzdrowski KL, Elson MK, et al. Hypoglycemia due to an insulin binding monoclonal antibody in multiple myeloma. N Engl J Med 1992; 326:994.
39. Greene HL, Ghishan FK, Brown B, et al. Hypoglycemia in type IV glycogenesis: hepatic improvement in two patients with nutritional management. J Pediatr 1988; 112:55.
40. Felig P, Brown WV, Levine RA, Klatskin G. Glucose homeostasis in viral hepatitis. N Engl J Med 1970; 283:1436.
41. Hoff AO, Vassilopoulou-Sellin R. The role of glucagon administration in the diagnosis and treatment of patients with tumor hypoglycemia. Cancer 1998; 82:1585.
42. Seltzer H. Drug induced hypoglycemia. Endocrinol Metab Clin North Am 1989; 18:163.
43. Kreisberg RA, Siegel AM, Owen CW. Glucose-lactate interrelationship: effect of ethanol. J Clin Invest 1971; 50:175.
44. Wajchenberg BL, Pereira VG, Pupo AA, et al. On the mechanism of insulin hypersensitivity in adrenocortical deficiency. Diabetes 1964; 13:169.
45. Hochberg Z, Hardoff D, Atias D, Spindel A. Isolated ACTH deficiency with transitory GH deficiency. J Endocrinol Invest 1985; 8:67.
45a. McAulay V, Frier BM. Addison's disease in type 1 diabetes presenting with recurrent hypoglycaemia. Postgrad Med J 2000; 76:230.
45b. Féry F, Plat L, van de Borne, et al. Impaired counterregulation of glucose in a patient with hypothalamic sarcoidosis. New Engl J Med 1999; 340:852.
46. Lev-Ran A, Anderson RW. The diagnosis of postprandial hypoglycemia. Diabetes 1981; 30:996.
47. Palardy J, Havrankova J, Lepage R, et al. Blood glucose measurements during symptomatic episodes in patients with suspected postprandial hypoglycemia. N Engl J Med 1989; 321:1421.
48. Lefebre PJ, Scheen AJ. The use of acarbose in the prevention and treatment of hypoglycemia. Eur J Clin Invest 1994; 24(Suppl 3):40.
49. Andreasen JJ, Orskov C, Holet JJ. Secretion of glucagonlike peptide-1 and reactive hypoglycemia after partial gastrectomy. Digestion 1994; 55:221.
50. Astles JR, Petros WP, Peters WP, Sedor FA. Artifactual hypoglycemia associated with hematopoietic cytokines. Arch Pathol Lab Med 1995; 119:713.
51. Sweeney BJ, Edgecombe J, Churchill DR, et al. Choreoathetosis/bullismus associated with pentamidine-induced hypoglycemia in a patient with the acquired immunodeficiency syndrome. Arch Neurol 1994; 51:723.
52. McTague JA, Forney R Jr. Jamaican vomiting sickness in Toledo, Ohio. Ann Emerg Med 1994; 23:116.
53. Felig P, Cherif A, Minagawa A, et al. Hypoglycemia during prolonged exercise in normal men. N Engl J Med 1982; 306:895.
54. Garber AJ, Bier DM, Cryer PE, Pagliara AS. Hypoglycemia in compensated chronic renal insufficiency: substrate limitation of gluconeogenesis. Diabetes 1974; 23:982.

## CHAPTER 159

# LOCALIZATION OF ISLET CELL TUMORS

DONALD L. MILLER

Approximately one-third of all islet cell tumors are *clinically silent* (nonfunctioning) and of little interest to the endocrinologist. Localization of these tumors is trivial because they are virtually always large at presentation. In general, this is also true of the less common functioning islet cell tumors, including glucagonomas, VIPomas, and the rarer functioning tumors.[1] Unfortunately, insulinomas and gastrinomas, which are much more common than all other functioning islet cell tumors combined, are also much smaller at presentation. Patients with these

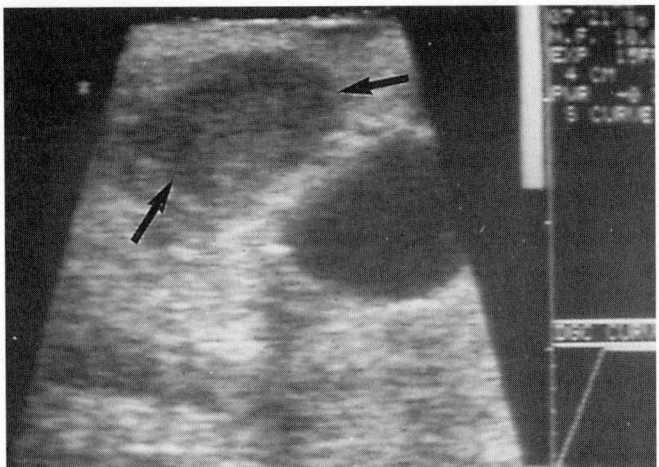

**FIGURE 159-1.** Intraoperative ultrasonography of the pancreatic head in the transverse plane. The insulinoma is a 10 × 16 mm sonolucent mass (*arrows*) adjacent to the superior mesenteric vein. Visualization of intrapancreatic structures, such as the superior mesenteric vein and the pancreatic duct, is very helpful as a guide for the surgeon. The tumor was successfully enucleated.

lesions present the endocrinologist, radiologist, and surgeon with the challenging problem of tumor localization, an essential prerequisite to effective surgical therapy.[2-6]

Differences between insulinomas and gastrinomas affect the sensitivity of individual localization procedures. The localization of insulinomas is of greater importance clinically, because no effective medical therapy exists for hyperinsulinism. Insulinomas, which are solitary (90%), benign (90%), intrapancreatic (99.5%), and tend to be distributed uniformly throughout the pancreas, are more easily located than are gastrinomas, 80% of which are multifocal and 30% of which are located outside the pancreas.[1,6,7] Most of these are in the "gastrinoma triangle."[8] Approximately 5% of gastrinomas are ectopic; that is, they are located outside the pancreas, duodenum, and adjacent lymph nodes.[9] Reported sites include the liver, omentum, jejunum, stomach, ovary, and heart.[9,10] (Also see Chap. 160.)

Localization efforts should not begin until an endocrine diagnosis has been established. The diagnosis of an insulinoma or gastrinoma does not depend on the radiologic demonstration of a tumor. Attempts at localization in the absence of a firm diagnosis may confuse matters if imaging procedures yield false-positive or equivocal results. Furthermore, the failure to locate a tumor does not mean that the diagnosis is incorrect. The tumor may be too small to image. The cardinal rule of endocrine radiology is *diagnosis first, localization second.*

## IMAGING MODALITIES FOR ISLET CELL TUMOR LOCALIZATION

A number of imaging studies are available to the endocrine radiologist for localizing islet cell tumors. Broadly speaking, the available imaging modalities may be classified as *noninvasive* or *invasive.* Newer modalities, including endoscopic ultrasonography (EUS), somatostatin-receptor scintigraphy (SRS), and arterial stimulation and venous sampling (ASVS), have shown greater sensitivity than conventional cross-sectional imaging studies.

These techniques tend to be complementary. The use of more than one in a patient with an insulinoma or gastrinoma is often helpful, but applying all of them is inappropriate and economically irresponsible. The remainder of this chapter reviews the available imaging studies and suggests algorithms for localization of insulinomas and gastrinomas.

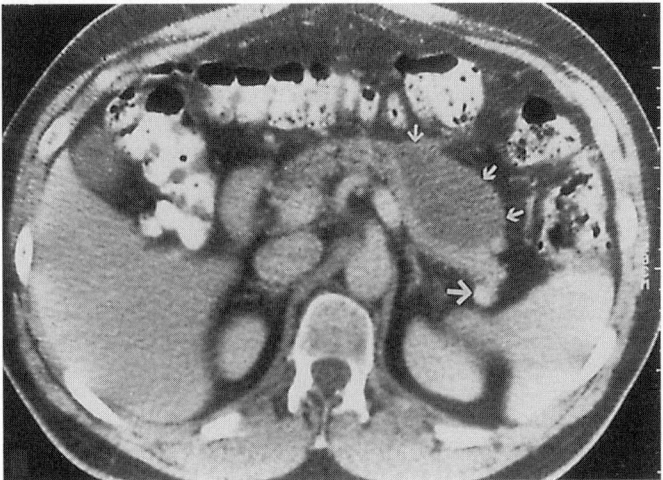

**FIGURE 159-2.** Computed tomography image of a 45-year-old man demonstrated a 12-mm insulinoma (*large arrow*) adjacent to the tail of the pancreas. The pseudocyst (*small arrows*) along the anterior margin of the pancreatic body resulted from a previous unsuccessful operation.

## NONINVASIVE STUDIES

### ULTRASONOGRAPHY

Standard abdominal ultrasonography is most helpful when the patient is thin and the tumor is large. Anatomic factors and the presence of gas in overlying bowel usually prevent examination of the entire pancreas. The sensitivity of ultrasonography for detection of primary insulinomas varies by an order of magnitude in published studies, from 7% to 79%.[11-13] This reflects its extreme dependence on operator expertise. Sensitivity is 30% or less in most series.[2,4,14,15]

On ultrasonographic examinations, islet cell tumors are well defined, smoothly marginated, round or oval lesions that are usually hypoechoic compared with the surrounding pancreas (Fig. 159-1). They may have a thin hyperechoic rim. The appearance is the same on all types of ultrasonographic examinations, including standard abdominal ultrasonography, EUS, and intraoperative ultrasonography (IOUS, discussed later).[1,16]

### COMPUTED TOMOGRAPHY

Small islet cell tumors may be difficult to identify on conventional CT. These tumors are seen as well defined, round or oval, enhancing masses (Fig. 159-2). The degree of enhancement is variable. A contour abnormality may be the only CT indication of the tumor.[1] Rare cases of nonenhancing small islet cell tumors have been reported.[1]

As endocrine diagnostic methods improve, patients present with ever smaller tumors, and CT sensitivity has decreased. The National Institutes of Health experience is that only 25% to 30% of primary gastrinomas and insulinomas are detected by CT.[2,4] In one series of 120 patients with insulinomas, CT had a sensitivity of only 24%.[14] Newer CT techniques, particularly dynamic spiral CT with two-dimensional and three-dimensional reconstruction, may improve these results.[17,18] In a series of seven patients studied using these methods, the islet cell tumor was identified in all.[17]

### MAGNETIC RESONANCE IMAGING

Magnetic resonance imaging (MRI) is not ideal for the examination of the pancreas because long scanning times, peristalsis, and respiratory and cardiac motion induce significant noise in images of the upper abdomen, and fluid-filled loops of bowel create difficulties in interpretation. Islet cell tumors demonstrate

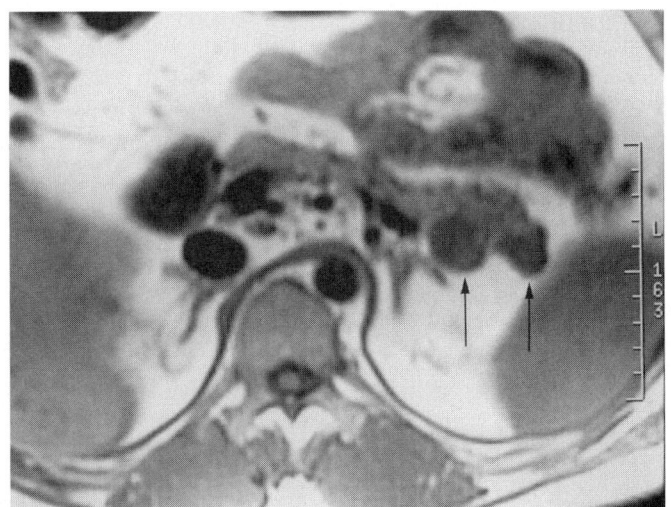

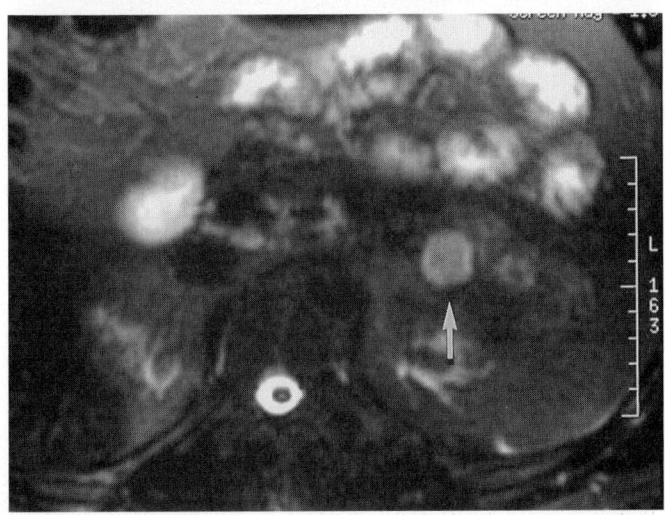

**FIGURE 159-3.** Magnetic resonance images taken of a 27-year-old man with multiple endocrine neoplasia type 1 and hyperinsulinism demonstrates two islet cell tumors in the tail of the pancreas. **A,** On a T1-weighted spin-echo image, the tumors (*arrows*) are dark (low signal intensity). **B,** On a T2-weighted spin-echo image, one tumor is bright (*arrow*), whereas the other is poorly seen.

high signal intensity on T2-weighted spin-echo images and short $T_1$ inversion recovery (STIR) fat suppression images (Fig. 159-3). Increased amounts of collagen in the tumor result in lower signal intensity on STIR images.[19]

The reported sensitivity for detection of insulinoma and primary gastrinoma ranges from 30% to 75%.[4,12,20,20a] MRI is more sensitive for the detection of liver metastases, identifying 71% of such lesions compared with 42% detected with CT in a series of 24 patients with gastrinomas and liver metastases.[20] (Also see ref. 20b.)

### SOMATOSTATIN-RECEPTOR SCINTIGRAPHY

More than 90% of gastrinomas contain somatostatin receptors.[7] Five subtypes of somatostatin receptor have been identified. The receptor subtype in gastrinomas has a high affinity for octreotide.[21] Administration of [[111]In-DTPA-D-Phe[1]]octreotide (OctreoScan, Mallinckrodt Medical), a radiolabeled somatostatin analog, permits scintigraphic detection of some of these tumors (Fig. 159-4). As with CT, MRI, and ultrasonography, tumor size affects the sensitivity of SRS.[2,3,22] Overall, the sensitivity of SRS for detection of primary gastrinomas is 55% to 60%.[20,22] SRS is more sensitive than ultrasonography, CT, or MRI[20,23] but still fails to permit detection of at least 20% of gas-

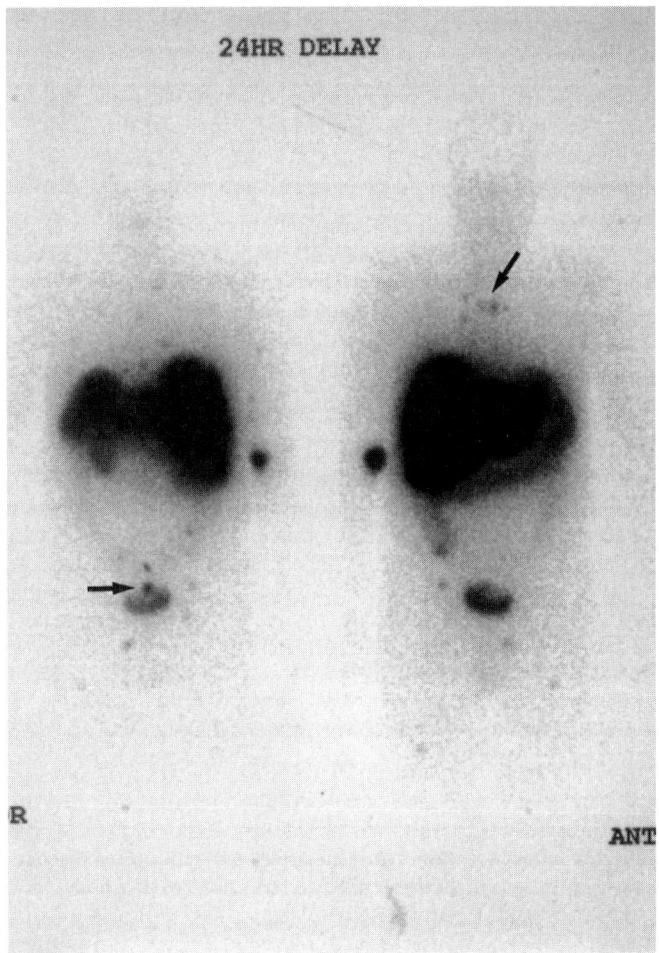

**FIGURE 159-4.** Somatostatin-receptor scintigraphy (*left*, posterior view; *right*, anterior view) in a 40-year-old man with multiple endocrine neoplasia type 1 and Zollinger-Ellison syndrome demonstrates multiple focal areas of uptake in the abdomen, pelvis, and chest, some of which are indicated by *arrows*. In addition, numerous discrete foci of uptake are present in the liver, but difficult to appreciate on this image. All of these represent metastases.

trinomas.[20] In two series, preoperative use of SRS altered management in 25% to 47% of gastrinoma patients.[3,23]

Insulinomas appear to have a different somatostatin-receptor subtype, with a lower affinity for octreotide.[21,24] Thus, although as many as 70% of insulinomas contain somatostatin receptors,[25] SRS is rarely helpful in these cases.[4] In one series, SRS results were negative in six of six patients with insulinomas.[26] (Also see Chap. 169.)

### INVASIVE PROCEDURES

#### ENDOSCOPIC ULTRASONOGRAPHY

EUS, performed with a special endoscope containing an ultrasonic transducer at its tip, allows the placement of the transducer closer to the pancreas. In turn, this permits the use of higher frequency transducers, typically 7.5 or 12 MHz, resulting in greater spatial resolution and improved sensitivity compared with standard abdominal ultrasonography.[11,13,26a] In a series of 37 patients with 39 islet cell tumors, none of which had been detected with standard ultrasonography or CT, EUS enabled the localization of 32 tumors (82% sensitivity) with no incorrect localizations.[27]

The technique is most sensitive for the detection of tumors in the pancreatic head and body, and less sensitive for the detection of tumors in the pancreatic tail, the duodenum, and other extra-pancreatic locations.[15,22,28] In patients with gastrinomas, EUS and SRS are complementary. In a series of 21 patients, each technique had a sensitivity of 58%, but the combined use of the two studies had a sensitivity of 90% for detection of primary gastrinomas.[22]

## ANGIOGRAPHY

Since the introduction of SRS and EUS, angiography is no longer a first-line procedure for islet cell tumor localization. It is currently performed only when ASVS (see later) is needed.[5–7] For the detection of primary islet cell tumors, the reported sensitivity of angiography ranges from 10% to 65%.[2,4,13–15]

Pancreatic arteriography for islet cell tumor localization should include selective arteriography of the proper or common hepatic artery (and any accessory hepatic arteries), the gastroduodenal artery, the splenic artery, the superior mesenteric artery, and, if possible, the dorsal pancreatic artery.[1]

On arteriograms, small islet cell tumors appear as rounded or oval, well-marginated lesions with smooth borders and homogeneous intense staining that persists into the late arterial and capillary phases. The stain results from the filling of vessels that are too small to be individually resolved, so neovascularity and discrete vessels are not seen within the tumor.[1] Hypovascular islet cell tumors exist but are rare.

## ARTERIAL STIMULATION AND VENOUS SAMPLING

ASVS was originally introduced for the localization of gastrinomas and has since been refined for the localization of both gastrinomas and insulinomas.[29,30] During angiography, a secretagogue is injected into one of the arteries that supplies the pancreas and liver (secretin is used to stimulate gastrinomas, and calcium is used to stimulate insulinomas). Venous blood samples are obtained from a catheter placed in a hepatic vein. These samples reflect the hormone concentration in portal venous blood. The process is then repeated for each of the other arteries supplying the pancreas and liver.

The hepatic vein samples are assayed for either gastrin or insulin, as appropriate. An increase of 100% in hormone concentration over baseline levels permits a localization to the arterial territory supplied by the injected artery. In this manner, the tumor can be localized to the head or tail of the pancreas (Fig. 159-5), although the exact site cannot be determined unless the arteriogram also demonstrates the lesion. The sensitivity of this technique ranges from 93% to 100% in various series.[4,13,14,31] In a series of seven patients with insulinomas and negative ultrasonographic, CT, MRI, and EUS results, ASVS was positive in all seven.[32]

In patients with a presumed insulinoma, a negative ASVS study should lead one to question the diagnosis. One patient in each of two separate series had a negative ASVS study.[31,33] Subsequently, one of these two patients had a negative result on repeated testing after a 72-hour fast, and the other was diagnosed with intermittent sulfonylurea abuse. All of the other patients in these two series had insulinomas.

## INTRAOPERATIVE ULTRASONOGRAPHY

IOUS, the ultimate invasive study, permits the transducer to be placed directly on intraabdominal structures. No gas or bone intervenes to impede sound transmission, and the spatial resolution is much higher than that achievable with conventional ultrasonography (see Fig. 159-1 and Chap. 160).

For insulinomas, which are almost always within the pancreas, the reported sensitivity rate of IOUS ranges from 85% to 100%, with false-positive results being relatively uncommon.[4,14,34,35] In studies in which IOUS has been compared with other modalities, it is usually superior to all of them.[1,4,14]

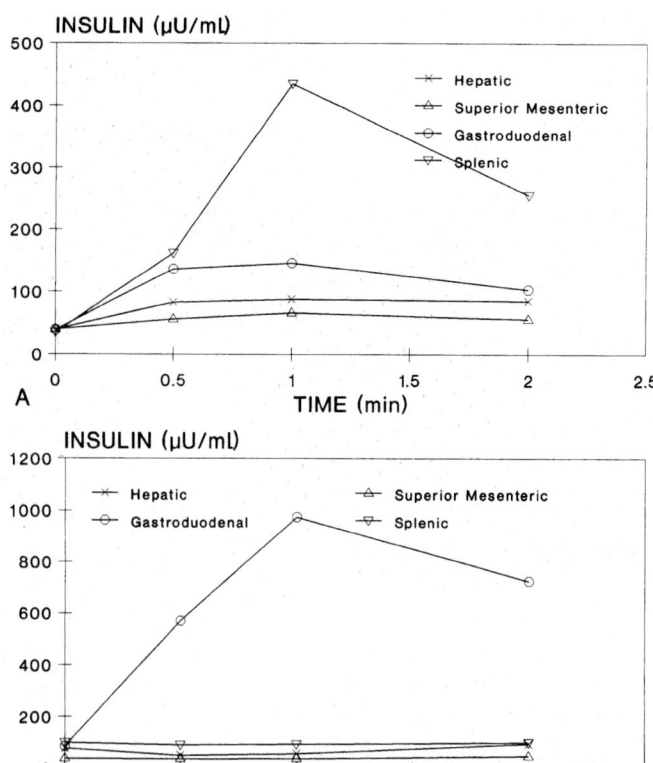

**FIGURE 159-5.** Two typical examples of the results of arterial stimulation and venous sampling for the localization of insulinomas. **A,** A brisk rise in insulin from right hepatic vein samples is seen after the injection of calcium into the gastroduodenal artery. The insulin levels were not affected by similar calcium injection into the superior mesenteric and splenic arteries. This result localizes the tumor to the pancreatic head. The arteriography result was negative, and an 8-mm tumor was resected from deep within the head of the pancreas using intraoperative ultrasonography. **B,** The elevation of insulin levels follows the injection of calcium into the splenic vein. In this patient, the arteriography result also was negative. A 13-mm tumor was removed from the proximal pancreatic tail.

Because of the difficulty of detecting extrapancreatic primary lesions, this technique is less effective for the localization of gastrinomas, although sensitivities of >90% have been achieved.[7,15]

## SCREENING FOR METASTATIC DISEASE

Malignant islet cell tumors metastasize to peripancreatic lymph nodes and to the liver. Spread to local-regional nodes is not considered a contraindication to attempts at curative surgery.[15,36]

All of the cross-sectional imaging techniques (ultrasonography, CT, MRI) are effective for evaluation of the liver, but MRI is probably the best of these techniques.[20] MRI has superseded angiography, which had been considered the most sensitive technique for the detection of hepatic metastases for these tumors. Newer MRI contrast agents may further enhance the sensitivity of this modality.[37,38]

In patients with gastrinomas, SRS is clearly the procedure of choice for the detection of liver metastases (see Fig. 159-4).[3,20,23,39] ASVS has a high specificity for the detection of liver metastases in these patients, but its sensitivity is low.[40]

Bone metastases occur in 7% of all patients with gastrinoma and in 31% of gastrinoma patients with liver metastases.[41] SRS is the best method for the detection of bone metastases in patients with gastrinomas (see Fig. 159-4).[41,42] MRI is recommended for patients with malignant insulinoma, given the poor sensitivity of SRS in these patients and the effectiveness of MRI for the detection of bone metastases in gastrinoma patients.[41]

## RADIOLOGIC APPROACH TO ISLET CELL TUMOR LOCALIZATION

Because of the different biology and clinical characteristics of insulinomas and gastrinomas, the radiologic approach to localization differs for the two lesions. The algorithms presented in the following sections are not rigid. The choice of procedures is highly dependent on the skill and experience of the radiologist (and for EUS, the gastroenterologist) who performs them. The patient may best be served by referral to a center where larger numbers of these patients are seen.[43]

### INSULINOMA

Given the nearly 100% rate of intraoperative tumor localization using IOUS and surgical palpation,[6,14,35] a reasonable question is whether any preoperative localizing procedures are warranted in patients with insulinomas. The surgeons at the Mayo Clinic use conventional abdominal ultrasonography as the only preoperative localizing procedure.[6] Some also believe that preoperative localization is unnecessary.[43a] This minimalist approach to localization requires that radiologists and surgeons be highly skilled and experienced.

Most surgeons prefer a more extensive series of preoperative localization procedures.[43–45] A reasonable first step would be either CT with dynamic spiral technique or MRI. These noninvasive procedures are used to search for a primary tumor as well as to evaluate the liver for possible metastatic disease. If noninvasive imaging is negative, EUS should be performed next, as the first invasive imaging study. If EUS is also negative, many surgeons proceed to arteriography with ASVS.[44,45] ASVS may draw attention to tumors that would otherwise be missed by IOUS and palpation.[4] Finally, IOUS must be available during surgical exploration.

### GASTRINOMA

Gastrinomas are frequently extrapancreatic and multiple. In addition, duodenal gastrinomas may be extremely small.[22,46] Because the sensitivities of all of the imaging studies used for islet cell tumor localization are proportional to tumor size, and because detection of extrapancreatic primary lesions is more difficult than detection of lesions within the pancreas, preoperative localization of gastrinomas is more difficult than localization of insulinomas, and frequently fails.

SRS should be the first localization procedure. It is a useful technique for detection of both primary gastrinomas and metastases. Although SRS fails to identify 20% to 33% of gastrinomas,[2,20] it is still the most sensitive noninvasive imaging method for these tumors. The addition of SRS information to the findings of other imaging procedures has been shown to change surgical treatment strategy and patient management.[3,23] SRS has poor spatial resolution, which makes CT a useful additional noninvasive study. Some surgeons prefer CT as the initial localization study.[5,15]

Some authors recommend proceeding directly to surgery if no metastases have been demonstrated with these procedures, even if the primary tumor has not been located.[2,15] Others suggest that, if previous localization studies were negative, EUS should be performed next.[5] ASVS may occasionally be useful if all other imaging studies have been unrevealing.[5] ASVS is usu-

ally not worthwhile in patients with gastrinomas, however, because it cannot distinguish among pancreatic, duodenal, and peripancreatic nodal disease, any or all of which may be present.

As with surgery for insulinomas, IOUS must be available in the operating room and should be part of a thorough surgical exploration of the pancreas and gastrinoma triangle.

## MULTIPLE ENDOCRINE NEOPLASIA TYPE 1

Gastrinomas and insulinomas may occur sporadically or as part of the multiple endocrine neoplasia type 1 (MEN1) syndrome. The syndrome is a genetic disorder, inherited in an autosomal dominant fashion and characterized by mutations of the *MEN1* tumor-suppressor gene on chromosome band 11q13.[47] Gastrinomas are the most common functioning islet cell tumors in patients with MEN1, and MEN1 is present in 20% to 38% of all patients with gastrinomas.[48] Patients with MEN1 are more likely to have multiple islet cell tumors—gastrinomas, insulinomas, and clinically nonfunctioning tumors (see Fig. 159-3). Gastrinomas in these patients are more likely to be multiple and to be located in the duodenum.[48,49] (Also see Chap. 188.)

In general, surgical exploration in MEN1 patients with gastrinomas is not recommended.[49a] MEN1 patients with hyperinsulinism and multiple pancreatic tumors may benefit from ASVS, which can aid in determining which lesion is the insulin source.[50]

## REFERENCES

1. Miller DL. Islet cell tumors of the pancreas: diagnosis and localization. In: Freeny PC, Stevenson GW, eds. Margulis and Burhenne's alimentary tract radiology, 5th ed. St. Louis: CV Mosby, 1994:1167.
2. Alexander HR, Fraker DL, Norton JA, et al. Prospective study of somatostatin receptor scintigraphy and its effect on operative outcome in patients with Zollinger-Ellison syndrome. Ann Surg 1998; 228:228.
3. Lebtahi R, Cadiot G, Sarda L, et al. Clinical impact of somatostatin receptor scintigraphy in the management of patients with neuroendocrine gastroenteropancreatic tumors. J Nucl Med 1997; 38:853.
4. Brown CK, Bartlett DL, Doppman JL, et al. Intraarterial calcium stimulation and intraoperative ultrasonography in the localization and resection of insulinomas. Surgery 1997; 122:1189.
5. Prinz RA. Localization of gastrinomas. Int J Pancreatol 1996; 19:79.
6. Grant CS. Insulinoma. Baillières Clin Gastroenterol 1996; 10:645.
7. Jensen RT. Gastrin-producing tumors. Cancer Treat Res 1997; 89:293.
8. Passaro E Jr, Howard TJ, Sawicki MP, et al. The origin of sporadic gastrinomas within the gastrinoma triangle: a theory. Arch Surg 1998; 133:13.
9. Wu PC, Alexander HR, Bartlett DL, et al. A prospective analysis of the frequency, location, and curability of ectopic (nonpancreaticoduodenal, nonnodal) gastrinoma. Surgery 1997; 122:1176.
10. Gibril F, Curtis LT, Termanini B, et al. Primary cardiac gastrinoma causing Zollinger-Ellison syndrome. Gastroenterology 1997; 112:567.
11. Zimmer T, Stölzel U, Bäder M, et al. Endoscopic ultrasonography and somatostatin receptor scintigraphy in the preoperative localisation of insulinomas and gastrinomas. Gut 1996; 39:562.
12. Angeli E, Vanzulli A, Castrucci M, et al. Value of abdominal sonography and MR imaging at 0.5 T in preoperative detection of pancreatic insulinoma: a comparison with dynamic CT and angiography. Abdom Imaging 1997; 22:295.
13. Soga J, Yakuwa Y. The gastrinoma/Zollinger-Ellison syndrome: statistical evaluation of a Japanese series of 359 cases. J Hepatobiliary Pancreat Surg 1998; 5:77.
14. Kuzin NM, Egorov AV, Kondrashin SA, et al. Preoperative and intraoperative topographic diagnosis of insulinomas. World J Surg 1998; 22:593.
15. Kisker O, Bastian D, Bartsch D, et al. Localization, malignant potential, and surgical management of gastrinomas. World J Surg 1998; 22:651.
16. Hayashi Y, Nakazawa S, Kimoto E, et al. Clinicopathologic analysis of endoscopic ultrasonograms in pancreatic mass lesions. Endoscopy 1989; 21:121.
17. Chung MJ, Choi BI, Han JK, et al. Functioning islet cell tumor of the pancreas: localization with dynamic spiral CT. Acta Radiol 1997; 38:135.
18. King AD, Ko GTC, Yeung VTF, et al. Dual phase spiral CT in the detection of small insulinomas of the pancreas. Br J Radiol 1998; 71:20.
19. Mori M, Fukuda T, Nagayoshi K, et al. Insulinoma: correlation of short-TI inversion-recovery (STIR) imaging and histopathologic findings. Abdom Imaging 1996; 21:337.
20. Gibril F, Reynolds JC, Doppman JL, et al. Somatostatin receptor scintigraphy: its sensitivity compared with that of other imaging methods in detecting primary and metastatic gastrinomas. A prospective study. Ann Intern Med 1996; 125:26.

20a. Thoeni RF, Mueller-Lisse UG, Chen R, et al. Detection of small, functional islet cell tumors in the pancreas: selection of MR imaging sequences for optimal sensitivity. Radiology 2000; 214:483.

20b. Semelka RC, Custodio CM, Cem Balci N, Woosley JT. Neuroendocrine tumors of the pancreas: spectrum of appearances on MRI. J Magn Reson Imaging 2000; 11:141.

21. Tang C, Biemond I, Verspaget HW, et al. Expression of somatostatin receptors in human pancreatic tumor. Pancreas 1998; 17:80.

22. Cadiot G, Lebtahi R, Sarda L, et al. Preoperative detection of duodenal gastrinomas and peripancreatic lymph nodes by somatostatin receptor scintigraphy. Gastroenterology 1996; 111:845.

23. Termanini B, Gibril F, Reynolds JC, et al. Value of somatostatin receptor scintigraphy: a prospective study in gastrinoma of its effect on clinical management. Gastroenterology 1997; 112:335.

24. Lamberts SWJ, Krenning EP, Reubi J-C. The role of somatostatin and its analogs in the diagnosis and treatment of tumors. Endocr Rev 1991; 12:450.

25. Van Eyck CHJ, Bruining HA, Reubi J-C, et al. Use of isotope-labeled somatostatin analogs for visualization of islet cell tumors. World J Surg 1993; 17:444.

26. Kisker O, Bartsch D, Weinel RJ, et al. The value of somatostatin-receptor scintigraphy in newly diagnosed endocrine gastroenteropancreatic tumors. J Am Coll Surgeons 1997; 184:487.

26a. Ardengh JC, Rosenbaum P, Ganc AJ, et al. Role of EUS in the preoperative localization of insulinomas compared with spiral CT. Gastrointest Endosc 2000; 51:552.

27. Rüsch T, Lightdale CJ, Botet JF, et al. Localization of pancreatic endocrine tumors by endoscopic ultrasonography. N Engl J Med 1992; 326:1721.

28. Schumacher B, Lübke HJ, Frieling T, et al. Prospective study on the detection of insulinomas by endoscopic ultrasonography. Endoscopy 1996; 28:273.

29. Doppman JL, Miller DL, Chang R, et al. Insulinomas: localization with selective intraarterial injection of calcium. Radiology 1991; 178:237.

30. Doppman JL, Miller DL, Chang R, et al. Gastrinomas: localization by means of selective intraarterial injection of secretin. Radiology 1990; 174:25.

31. O'Shea D, Rohrer-Theurs AW, Lynn JA, et al. Localization of insulinomas by selective intraarterial calcium injection. J Clin Endocrinol Metab 1996; 81:1623.

32. Pereira PL, Roche AJ, Maier GW, et al. Insulinoma and islet cell hyperplasia: value of the calcium intraarterial stimulation test when findings of other preoperative studies are negative. Radiology 1998; 206:703.

33. Defreyne L, König K, Lerch MM, et al. Modified intra-arterial calcium stimulation with venous sampling test for preoperative localization of insulinomas. Abdom Imaging 1998; 23:322.

34. Correnti S, Liverani A, Antonini G, et al. Intraoperative ultrasonography for pancreatic insulinomas. Hepatogastroenterology 1996; 43:207.

35. Huai J-C, Zhang W, Niu H-O, et al. Localization and surgical treatment of pancreatic insulinomas guided by intraoperative ultrasound. Am J Surg 1998; 175:18.

36. Thompson NW. Current concepts in the surgical management of multiple endocrine neoplasia type 1 pancreatic-duodenal disease. Results in the treatment of 40 patients with Zollinger-Ellison syndrome, hypoglycaemia or both. J Intern Med 1998; 243:495.

37. Vandevenne JE, Deckers F, Mana F, et al. Insulinoma associated with liver lesions: value of MR imaging. Am J Gastroenterol 1998; 93:1559.

38. Wang C, Ahlström H, Eriksson B, et al. Uptake of mangafodipir trisodium in liver metastases from endocrine tumors. J Magn Reson Imaging 1998; 8:682.

39. Termanini B, Gibril F, Doppman JL, et al. Distinguishing small hepatic hemangiomas from vascular liver metastases in gastrinoma: use of a somatostatin-receptor scintigraphic agent. Radiology 1997; 202:151.

40. Gibril F, Doppman JL, Chang R, et al. Metastatic gastrinomas: localization with selective arterial injection of secretin. Radiology 1996; 198:77.

41. Gibril F, Doppman JL, Reynolds JC, et al. Bone metastases in patients with gastrinomas: a prospective study of bone scanning, somatostatin receptor scanning, and magnetic resonance image in their detection, frequency, location, and effect of their detection on management. J Clin Oncol 1998; 16:1040.

42. Cadiot G, Bonnaud G, Lebtahi R, et al. Usefulness of somatostatin receptor scintigraphy in the management of patients with Zollinger-Ellison syndrome. Gut 1997; 41:107.

43. Lo C-Y, Lam KYL, Kung AWC, et al. Pancreatic insulinomas: a 15-year experience. Arch Surg 1997; 132:926.

43a. Hashimoto, Walsh RM. Preoperative localization of insulinomas is not necessary. J Am Coll Surg 1999; 189:368.

44. Bliss RD, Carter PB, Lennard TWJ. Insulinoma: a review of current management. Surg Oncol 1997; 6:49.

45. Wiersema MJ. Insulinoma: finding the needle in a haystack. Endoscopy 1996; 28:310.

46. Schröder W, Hölscher AH, Beckurts T, et al. Duodenal microgastrinomas associated with Zollinger-Ellison syndrome. Hepatogastroenterology 1996; 43:1465.

47. Zhuang Z, Vortmeyer AO, Pack S, et al. Somatic mutations of the MEN1 tumor suppressor gene in sporadic gastrinomas and insulinomas. Cancer Res 1997; 57:4682.

48. Jensen RT. Management of the Zollinger-Ellison syndrome in patients with multiple endocrine neoplasia type 1. J Intern Med 1998; 243:477.

49. Mignon M, Cadiot G. Diagnostic and therapeutic criteria in patients with Zollinger-Ellison syndrome and multiple endocrine neoplasia type 1. J Intern Med 1998; 243:489.

49a. Norton JA, Fraker DL, Alexander HR, et al. Surgery to cure the Zollinger-Ellison syndrome. N Engl J Med 1999; 341:635.

50. Doppman JL. Problems in endocrinologic imaging. Endocrinol Metab Clin North Am 1998; 26:973.

# CHAPTER 160

# SURGERY OF THE ENDOCRINE PANCREAS

JON C. WHITE

Surgery for tumors of the pancreas often is considered futile because of the predominance of exocrine tumors of this organ, which are usually malignant, often unresectable, and rarely curable.[1] Indeed, pancreatic cancer is the fifth leading cause of cancer death in the United States,[2] with a 2-year survival rate of 8%.[3] Five percent to 15% of all pancreatic neoplasms are nonductal, and 50% of these tumors are of endocrine origin.[4] Although approximately one-half of pancreatic endocrine tumors are reported to be benign,[5] this figure varies across series because there are no histologic features that distinguish benign from malignant lesions.[6] Quantitative DNA analysis has demonstrated that the DNA content of endocrine tumors has an influence on long-term survival, with hypertriploid tumors having a significantly worse prognosis than diploid, monoploid, or triploid tumors. Nevertheless, neither molecular nor cellular techniques can draw a distinct difference between benign and malignant neoplasms.[7] Malignancy may be reliably determined only by the presence of distant metastases or local tumor invasion.[8] When these tumors are determined to be benign, they can be resected and cured. Even malignant tumors may be resected, resulting in significant palliation or even cure.

The first successful resection of an insulinoma took place in 1929, although the insulinoma syndrome was not described by Whipple until 1935. Since then, many different islet cell tumors and syndromes have been recognized, including gastrinomas, vasoactive intestinal polypeptide tumors (VIPomas), glucagonomas, somatostatinomas, and other lesions that produce a variety of humoral products, such as pancreatic polypeptide (PP), adrenocorticotropic hormone (ACTH), parathyroid hormone–related protein, and serotonin. Clinically, these tumors are differentiated by the syndromes they induce or by the biochemical profiles they produce.

The surgical approach to each of these pancreatic endocrine neoplasms varies according to the end organs affected by its secreted products, its malignant potential, its solitary or multiple nature, and the ease with which it can be localized (Tables 160-1 and 160-2). The surgical procedures used to cure or palliate pancreatic endocrine tumors are more varied than are those used for pancreatic exocrine tumors.

As many as 19 different gastroenteropancreatic neuroendocrine cells have been identified that elaborate up to 40 different humoral products.[9] Some of these humoral products are associated with clinical endocrine manifestations (e.g., insulin, gastrin, glucagon, somatostatin, ACTH, corticotropin-releasing hormone [CRH], parathyroid hormone–related protein [PTHrP], growth hormone–releasing hormone [GHRH]). Others are not associated with any known syndromes but may have an important role as a tumor marker for diagnosing or following the clinical progress of the neoplasm (e.g., PP, neurotensin, calcitonin, α human chorionic gonadotropin[10–13]). The tumors associated with the most clinically relevant hormones are considered in the next section.

## FUNCTIONAL ISLET CELL TUMORS

### INSULINOMA

Insulinomas are the most common functional islet cell tumors, with an incidence of one case per million population per year.[14]

**TABLE 160-1.**
**Characteristics of Functional Pancreatic Endocrine Tumors**

| Tumor | Rate of Malignancy (%) | Incidence | Associated Clinical Syndrome |
|---|---|---|---|
| Insulinoma | 10[99] | 1.0/MPY[29] | Hypoglycemia and hyperinsulinemia |
| Gastrinoma | 60–70[99] | 0.1–0.4/ MPY[29] | Zollinger-Ellison syndrome |
| Glucagonoma | 60–70[99] | 0.06/MPY[100] | Dermatitis, diabetes, anemia, deep venous thrombosis |
| VIPoma | 60–70[99] | 0.13/ MPY[100] | Watery diarrhea, hypokalemia, achlorhydria |
| Somatostatinoma | 90[99] | <0.06/MPY[100] | Cholelithiasis, diabetes, steatorrhea |
| Miscellaneous ACTH CRH GHRH PTHrP | Insufficient data | Rare | ACTH, CRH: Cushing syndrome; GHRH: acromegaly; PTHrP: hypercalcemia |

*MPY*, per million population per year; *ACTH*, adrenocorticotropic hormone; *CRH*, corticotropin-releasing hormone; *GHRH*, growth hormone–releasing hormone; *PTHrP*, parathyroid hormone–related protein; *VIPoma*, vasoactive intestinal polypeptide tumor.

Most are solitary and benign (75%), but a few are malignant (10% to 15%) or multifocal (10% to 15%).[15] These tumors may be extremely small or they may present as hyperplasia. Because of variability in their size and appearance, they can be difficult to localize. Despite the fact that most of these lesions are benign, the hyperinsulinemia they cause can be dangerous, so that complete resection or maximal cytoreduction is desirable and often necessary (see Chap. 158).

Localization of insulinomas, which can be accomplished with computed tomography (CT), magnetic resonance imaging (MRI), mesenteric angiography, or portal venous sampling, should be attempted before surgery. CT and angiography usually are performed first and are most useful in detecting larger lesions (see Chap. 159).[16] Although these techniques are relatively specific, they are not very sensitive. Their accuracy generally is reported to be ~80%. If a tumor cannot be identified with CT or angiography, either portal venous sampling or injection of the mesenteric artery with calcium to stimulate insulin secretion may allow localization of the neoplasm to a particular region. Portal venous sampling is the most sensitive preoperative localization technique, with a reported sensitivity of 70% to 100%.[17] Radiolabeled octreotide[18,19] and provocative angiographic studies using calcium stimulation[20] also have been used to improve the accuracy of preoperative localization. Both endoscopic ultrasonography (EUS) and intraductal ultrasonography (IDUS)[21] have been used to localize tumors as small as 5 mm. Some surgeons, however, believe that extensive preoperative localization is neither indicated nor cost effective. They contend that intraoperative localization by ultrasonography, endoscopic transillumination, and palpation are more sensitive than preoperative techniques.[22,23]

When all attempts to localize a tumor at surgery are unsuccessful, some surgeons perform a blind distal pancreatectomy in the hope of excising an occult tumor. If the hyperinsulinemia is responsive to diazoxide, another approach is to perform a biopsy of the pancreas to rule out hyperplasia and then to institute medical therapy.[24] On occasion, patients can be maintained on diazoxide until their tumors grow to a detectable size and can be localized and resected. If diazoxide therapy is ineffective before surgery, an 80% pancreatectomy may be required to control the hyperinsulinemia.[24]

If the insulinoma has been localized and is small and benign, enucleation or local excision is the preferred approach. If the

**TABLE 160-2.**
**Surgical Aspects of Pancreatic Endocrine Tumors**

| Type | Size | Location | Surgical Approach |
|---|---|---|---|
| **FUNCTIONAL TUMORS** | | | |
| Insulinoma | Often small, but can be large[16] | Distributed throughout pancreas[16] | Preoperative and intraoperative localization can be challenging. Resection of benign or malignant disease should be aggressive. When hyperplasia or occult tumors cause significant symptoms, a subtotal pancreatectomy may be required. The objective of surgery should be to extirpate the neoplasm completely or to control the hyperinsulinemia. |
| Gastrinoma | Often small, but can be large | Pancreatic head, duodenum[34] | Tumors usually are found in the "gastrinoma triangle" but can be difficult to locate. Symptoms can be controlled with medical or surgical treatment of the end organ (stomach), but resection of tumor can improve long-term survival and sometimes is curative. |
| Glucagonoma | Large[16] | Pancreatic body and tail[58] | Glucagonomas usually are found in the body and tail of the pancreas, so that distal pancreatectomy is the most commonly performed resection. Most tumors are large when first seen and are not amenable to curative resection, but may be debulked. |
| VIPoma | Large[62] | 75% pancreatic body and tail,[62] retroperitoneum, adrenal gland, lung | VIPomas usually are found in the body and tail of the pancreas but may be found in other pancreatic and extrapancreatic locations, making localization important. Pancreatic tumors in the body and tail may be resected by distal pancreatectomy. |
| Somatostatinoma | Small to large | Pancreatic head and tail, duodenum | Somatostatinomas produce a mild and nonspecific clinical syndrome and often are found incidentally during routine surgical exploration. Tumors are distributed throughout the pancreas and duodenum. Despite the mild symptomatology of the syndrome, an aggressive surgical approach to pancreatic and extrapancreatic tumors is warranted. |
| **MISCELLANEOUS TUMORS** | | | |
| ACTH, CRH, GHRH, PTHrP | Often small, but can be large | Variable | Surgical ablation of these tumors results in regression of the associated humoral syndromes and should be considered the primary treatment modality. |
| **NONFUNCTIONAL TUMORS** | | | |
| | Large[88] | Pancreatic head[88] | Nonfunctional tumors are detected late, when mass effects from large tumors cause symptoms. When they can be extirpated completely, resection is indicated. Debulking is controversial. |

*ACTH*, adrenocorticotropic hormone; *CRH*, corticotropin-releasing hormone; *GHRH*, growth hormone–releasing hormone; *PTHrP*, parathyroid hormone–related protein; *VIPoma*, vasoactive intestinal polypeptide tumor.

tumor is large or malignant, a formal pancreatic resection, including pancreaticoduodenectomy,[25] or tumor debulking may be needed to resect the tumor completely and control the hyperinsulinemia. Although enucleation is appealing because of the greater conservation of pancreatic tissue, the incidence of pancreatic fistula is higher than after pancreatectomy.[26] The results of surgery with all procedures tend to be excellent, with 70% to 90% of patients experiencing relief of symptoms or complete cure.

During surgical intervention, a thorough exploration of the abdominal cavity should be performed to look for metastases, with focus on the liver and regional lymph nodes. Any extrapancreatic spread of tumor indicates malignancy, and the lesions should be removed at the time of the pancreatic resection.

When the surgical localization or extirpation of an insulinoma is not possible, streptozocin, especially in combination with 5-fluorouracil, can be administered to destroy the B cells.[15] Evidence also exists that the somatostatin analog octreotide may effectively suppress insulin release and reduce the morbidity and mortality of the persistent hyperinsulinemia (see Chap. 169).[27] Although this drug has been less effective for treating insulinomas than for treating other pancreatic tumors, a therapeutic trial is warranted.[28]

Most cases of insulinoma are nonfamilial and sporadic, but 10% are associated with the multiple endocrine neoplasia type 1 (MEN1) syndrome (see Chap. 188). Patients with insulinoma and MEN1 often have multiple pancreatic tumors. Consequently, surgical extirpation is not as effective in these patients as it is in patients with sporadic tumors. The principal objective of surgery in patients with hyperinsulinemia and MEN1 is to resect the primary tumor, which is likely to be secreting most of the insulin. When a single tumor has been identified and enucleated, a blind distal pancreatectomy is recommended to remove occult tumors, which are inevitably present.[29] Although hyperinsulinemia can be controlled using this approach, these patients must be observed carefully for recurrent disease.

## GASTRINOMA

Gastrinomas are a type of ectopic islet cell tumor[30] and are the most common malignant functional endocrine tumors of the pancreas (see Chap. 220). Although 60% of gastrinomas are malignant, long-term survival can be achieved by resection or by appropriate treatment of the end-organ symptomatology. Islet cell tumors are present in 65% to 80% of patients with the MEN1 syndrome, and gastrinoma is the most common type.[31] When gastrinomas occur in MEN1, the pancreatic tumors always are multiple and are not amenable to surgical resection. No case of MEN1 has ever been reported in which the local resection of a tumor has normalized serum gastrin levels, although aggressive subtotal resection has been reported to provide symptomatic relief.[32]

Gastrinoma is most noted for its endocrine effects. In 1955, Zollinger and Ellison[33] described two patients with ulcers in the jejunum and outlined a syndrome in which pancreatic tumors were associated with aggressive peptic ulcer disease. Because Zollinger-Ellison syndrome is being recognized and diagnosed earlier, the associated ulcers often are less virulent and tend to be routine ulcers of the duodenum. The presence of gastrinoma is suggested by a serum gastrin level of >500 pg/mL and is confirmed with a secretin test.

Both gastrinomas and insulinomas differ from other pancreatic endocrine tumors in that they often are small and difficult to localize. Insulinomas are distributed equally throughout the pancreas, but most gastrinomas are found in the *gastrinoma triangle,* which is bordered by the cystic and common bile ducts

superiorly, the junction of the second and third portions of the duodenum inferiorly, and the junction of the neck and body of the pancreas medially.[34] Most intraabdominal gastrinomas also are found on the right side of the abdomen.[35] A smaller number are found to the left of the superior mesenteric artery. Tumors in different locations do not exhibit the same biologic behavior, suggesting that they may have different causes.[36] CT, MRI, sonography, arteriography, and percutaneous transhepatic venous sampling are used for preoperative localization of gastrinoma in the same manner as for insulinoma. Secretin is the agent used to stimulate gastrin secretion during provocative angiography.[37] In vivo imaging with a gamma camera after injection of radiolabeled octreotide[37a] has been reported to localize nearly 100% of gastrinomas.[38]

Although most gastrinomas can be localized before surgery using these techniques, intraoperative exploration may be the most direct and sensitive means of detecting occult tumors.[5] These neoplasms are being found increasingly often in the duodenum, and occasionally can be located by preoperative duodenal endoscopy, intraoperative endoscopy with transillumination, or intraoperative duodenotomy with exploration.[39] Duodenal tumors are located most often in the proximal duodenum just distal to the pylorus. Small duodenal tumors also can be located with the help of intraarterial methylene blue injection during surgical exploration. This is usually done through the same catheter used for preoperative angiographic secretin stimulation.[40] Despite the variety of preoperative and intraoperative techniques available for localizing these tumors, many are never located and successfully resected. Often, metastases are discovered in lymph nodes but the primary tumor cannot be found.

Zollinger and Ellison performed total gastrectomies on their initial two patients to treat their fulminant ulcer disease. Now the view is that tumor localization should be attempted in all patients. Patients other than those with widespread liver metastases should undergo surgical exploration and extirpation of the tumor. If preoperative localization is successful and resection is feasible, as much of the gastrinoma should be removed as possible.[41,42] This can involve enucleation or a formal resection, which achieves cure rates approaching 35%.[43] If a curative resection is not possible, tumor debulking may offer significant palliation. Pancreaticoduodenectomy is seldom necessary[14] but may be used for both duodenal and pancreatic tumors if they are large or have multiple foci.[44–46] If the tumor cannot be localized or resected, symptoms may be relieved by treating the ulcer disease medically with $H_2$-receptor blockers or $H^+$-$K^+$ proton pump inhibitors. In fact, the introduction of proton pump inhibitors has almost eliminated the need for gastrectomy in these patients.[45] Vagotomy has been used to reduce medication requirements, with mixed results.[47] These procedures have played a smaller role since effective medications to inhibit gastric acid secretion have become available. Patients with malignant tumors treated either medically or with ulcer operations ultimately succumb to metastatic disease. The complete resection of all grossly evident tumor seems to provide the greatest long-term survival[48] and should be the primary surgical goal in all patients without metastatic disease or the MEN1 syndrome. Surgical exploration not only provides the only chance for cure but also is helpful in identifying prognostic features associated with long-term survival, such as small tumor size, an extrapancreatic primary tumor, and the absence of tumor metastases.[49]

Patients with MEN1 and gastrinomas represent a special case, because their tumors are multifocal, difficult to localize, and may have less malignant behavior than sporadic tumors.[50] Some surgeons advocate an aggressive approach, similar to that pursued with other gastrinomas, whereas others recommend that patients with MEN1 not undergo exploration at all.

Formerly, the removal of metastatic lymph nodes in addition to gastrectomy was believed to result in regression of the primary tumor in some patients with gastrinoma. It now seems more likely that most of these apparent "regressions" resulted from the serendipitous removal of small duodenal tumors during gastrectomy,[51] and little support exists for the concept of gastrinoma regression.

All patients should receive long-term postoperative follow-up, because recurrent disease can present many years after apparently curative resection. Calcium or secretin provocative tests may be helpful for detecting recurrent disease early or for predicting whether a patient will remain free of symptoms.[52] Even after apparently curative resection, some patients with gastrinoma retain a slightly hypersecretory state and require low doses of antisecretory drugs.[53]

When resection of a gastrinoma is not possible or the tumor cannot be found at surgical exploration, streptozocin and 5-fluorouracil can be used for palliation, as they are in insulinoma. These chemotherapeutics have no positive effect on survival. $H_2$ receptors or $H^+$-$K^+$ proton pump blockers can be used to control the ulcer disease. Octreotide may reduce symptoms and occasionally controls tumor growth.[54] Lipidol-transcatheter arterial embolization has been used for unresectable hepatic metastases.[54a]

## GLUCAGONOMA

Although glucagonomas are the third most frequently encountered functional tumor, only 400 cases have been reported in the world literature.[55] The first glucagon-producing tumor associated with a cutaneous rash was reported in 1942,[56] but the "glucagonoma syndrome" was not fully described until 1966.[57] Although 60% of these tumors are malignant, most are solitary; hence, surgical resection can be curative.[58] The most characteristic and debilitating clinical finding in patients with glucagonoma is a necrolytic migratory rash. This skin lesion results from an amino-acid deficiency[59] and, when seen in association with diabetes and weight loss, should suggest the diagnosis. Elevated serum immunoreactive glucagon levels should instigate a search for the tumor (see Chap. 220). These tumors, which tend to be large and located in the body and tail of the pancreas, are usually easy to detect. If a glucagonoma cannot be seen on routine imaging studies, mesenteric arteriography or selective venous sampling with radioimmunoassay for glucagon may be required.[60]

If the diagnosis is made early and the tumor is localized to the body or tail of the pancreas, a distal pancreatectomy can be curative. This operation, which does not require concomitant duodenectomy with reanastomosis of the pancreatic duct, common bile duct, and gastrointestinal tract, has minimal morbidity. Tumors in the head of the pancreas require pancreaticoduodenectomy for complete excision. Aggressive cytoreduction of large, unresectable tumors is indicated before the use of chemotherapy. When resection is complete (no metastases), 10-year survival is better than 60%.[29]

Chemotherapy for glucagonoma has been disappointing. Streptozocin has been used in combination with 5-fluorouracil and octreotide to alleviate symptoms in patients with unresectable disease,[29a] but has met with limited success. Because the tumor grows slowly, patients who are not candidates for curative resection still can enjoy prolonged symptom-free survival.[58]

## VIPOMA

VIPomas are extremely rare tumors that elaborate vasoactive intestinal peptide (VIP), producing a syndrome characterized by *watery diarrhea, hypokalemia, and achlorhydria (WDHA syndrome)* or *pancreatic cholera* (see Chap. 220). VIPomas typically secrete a range of peptides, of which VIP is the most clinically relevant. Diagnosing these neoplasms on the basis of basal serum VIP levels can be difficult,[61] but the use of pentagastrin as a provocative agent has been helpful.[11] Similar to glucagonomas, VIPomas usually are large and easy to locate. Although 80% are located in the pancreas, others can be found in the retroperitoneum, the adrenal gland, or the lung,[62] making preoperative localization helpful. These tumors are located predominantly in the body and tail of the pancreas. CT and angiography are the primary radiographic techniques used when localization is required. VIPomas have also been localized by technetium-99m sestamibi scanning.[63]

Because the VIPoma syndrome can be caused by a malignant tumor (50%) or by hyperplasia (20%), the surgical approach varies widely, depending on the results of the preoperative evaluation. As with all tumors of the endocrine pancreas, complete resection is desirable, but aggressive cytoreduction helps to control the clinical syndrome when total extirpation is not possible. Tumors located in the body and tail of the pancreas usually can be resected by distal pancreatectomy. When tumors are not found in the pancreas, an extensive exploration may be necessary. When the lesions still cannot be located after careful exploration of the abdomen, including the retroperitoneum, some surgeons advocate distal pancreatectomy. Patients whose disease is not controlled with distal pancreatectomy may require total pancreatectomy to alleviate their symptoms.[62] Resolution of symptoms has been reported even with resection of recurrent metastatic disease.[64]

When surgery fails to control the WDHA syndrome, octreotide administration has been shown to inhibit the release of VIP from human VIPoma cells and, rarely, to shrink metastases.[65]

## SOMATOSTATINOMA

Somatostatinomas are among the more recently described pancreatic endocrine tumors. They are usually found in the pancreas or duodenum, with the pancreatic tumors carrying a worse prognosis.[66] Most pancreatic or duodenal tumors reported have been solitary, malignant, and virulent.[62,67–69] Overproduction of somatostatin, an inhibitory hormone acting on the endocrine system and digestive organs, leads to vague clinical symptoms (see Chap. 220). The true incidence of somatostatinoma may not be known, because the symptom complex of diabetes, cholelithiasis, and steatorrhea is nonspecific and usually not very severe.[70] Somatostatin inhibits the release of glucagon as well as insulin, so the diabetes produced is mild and often is not insulin-dependent. A finding of increased serum levels of somatostatin and depressed plasma concentrations of both immunoreactive insulin and glucagon can be used to establish the diagnosis of somatostatinoma.[30] These tumors have been discovered in the head and tail of the pancreas and in the duodenum.[71] Most somatostatinomas located in the duodenum cause only symptoms related to local disease, such as obstructive jaundice.[72]

Because humoral manifestations of the somatostatinoma syndrome are vague, these tumors often present with local symptoms. Most are detected as incidental findings on surgical exploration or abdominal radiography, so the need to localize occult somatostatinomas is unusual. When localization is required, CT and arteriography are useful. When the results of hormonal studies raise suspicion for somatostatinoma, endoscopy or contrast radiography are helpful in localizing the tumor because of the frequent occurrence of duodenal neoplasms. Somatostatin analog (octreotide) scintigraphy has been used to localize lesions, and, subsequently, the drug has been used to treat symptoms of patients with somatostatinoma.[73]

As with other functional pancreatic endocrine tumors, surgical excision of somatostatinomas should be attempted when possible. Somatostatinomas in the head of the pancreas usually require pancreaticoduodenectomy. In addition, distal pancreatectomy and enucleation have been reported for treatment of pancreatic tumors.[30] Masses in the periampullary region of the duodenum cause jaundice and may require pancreaticoduodenectomy, whereas other duodenal tumors can be excised by segmental duodenal resection. When metastatic disease is encountered, an aggressive approach to the primary disease as well as tumor debulking is warranted.

## MISCELLANEOUS FUNCTIONAL ISLET CELL TUMORS

### PANCREATIC POLYPEPTIDE

Pancreatic polypeptide (PP) is a pancreatic hormone whose function is not completely understood. Because it is secreted by many pancreatic endocrine tumors, >50% of the cells of a neoplasm must secrete PP for it to be considered a PPoma.[9] A fasting PP level of >300 pmol/mL is the best diagnostic parameter because clinical symptomatology is not well established.[74] These tumors are usually large, making wide resection necessary.[75] In the case of an unresectable tumor, debulking is appropriate.

### PARATHYROID HORMONE–RELATED PROTEIN

PTHrP-producing tumors of the pancreas are of particular interest because this hormone can cause hypercalcemia (see Chaps. 52 and 219). Although not all PTHrP-secreting tumors produce elevated levels of calcium,[76] some are associated with life-threatening hypercalcemia.[77] These lesions can be mistaken for a MEN1 syndrome with associated parathyroid hyperplasia, but the two entities can be differentiated by measuring PTH and PTHrP levels.[78] Tumor resection results in resolution of the hypercalcemia.

### GROWTH HORMONE–RELEASING HORMONE

GHRH, which usually is secreted by the hypothalamus, can be produced and secreted by a pancreatic islet cell tumor. The resulting acromegaly can be treated by resection of the pancreatic tumor, which corrects the biochemical abnormalities (see Chap. 219).[79] Recurrent tumor causes a relapse of the endocrine disorder, demonstrating that the optimal therapy is complete extirpation of the neoplasm.

### ADRENOCORTICOTROPIC HORMONE AND CORTICOTROPIN-RELEASING HORMONE

ACTH or CRH can be secreted by pancreatic tumors.[80,81] CRH is commonly produced by pancreatic endocrine tumors but is only rarely associated with elevated levels of ACTH or manifestations of Cushing syndrome.[81] When large pancreatic tumors secrete ACTH, however, they can cause severe hypercortisolism, with asthenia, muscle weakness, hypertension, hypokalemic alkalosis, and carbohydrate intolerance. When tumors producing ACTH or CRH can be located, they should be resected (see Chaps. 75 and 219). When Cushing syndrome is produced, bilateral adrenalectomy may be helpful.[82]

## NONFUNCTIONAL ISLET CELL TUMORS

Once thought to be rare, nonfunctioning islet cell tumors account for ~50% the endocrine tumors of the pancreas reported in some series.[5,83] This increased incidence is due to the widespread use of abdominal CT and MRI, which can detect small and previously occult lesions. Although some of these masses may represent functional tumors that are discovered before they become clinically significant, many nonfunctional tumors grow large, calcific, cystic, or necrotic and do not produce any recognized hormonal syndromes.[84] They are often said to present at a later stage when resectability is less likely, although this concept has been challenged.[85] These clinically silent tumors usually demonstrate neurosecretory granules that contain immunoreactive peptides on immunohistochemical staining.[86] This suggests that these nonfunctional tumors secrete peptide products that are not bioactive or are secreted in amounts too small to be clinically relevant. The presence in the serum of clinically silent secretory products can be useful to detect recurrence of these nonfunctional tumors after resection. PP, neurotensin, calcitonin, and α human chorionic gonadotropin can be used as markers for some nonfunctional pancreatic endocrine tumors.[10–13]

Because nonfunctional tumors do not induce any characteristic clinical syndromes, their presentation is similar to that of adenocarcinoma of the pancreas. Nonfunctional islet cell and ductal tumors usually cause symptoms from their mass effects, which lead to biliary and gastrointestinal obstruction, back pain, and weight loss. Because small tumors cause no symptoms, they are not discovered except as an incidental finding during abdominal exploration or imaging. Localization of occult nonfunctional tumors usually is not required.

In one large series investigating nonfunctioning pancreatic masses, nonductal neoplasms represented >8% of all the pancreatic tumors evaluated.[87] Because the prognosis and treatment of nonductal tumors is different from that of the more commonly encountered ductal neoplasms, a histopathologic diagnosis should be established for all pancreatic masses before a treatment plan is formulated.

Nonfunctional tumors are predominantly malignant (90%)[88] and are found most often in the head of the pancreas. Despite their size and location, 40% are resectable at the time of discovery.[15] Because they do not produce debilitating syndromes related to the elaboration of humoral products, the risks and benefits of resective surgery should be weighed carefully. If a formal pancreatic resection can extirpate the entire tumor, most surgeons would agree that this is the preferred approach.[89] Although some surgeons advocate tumor debulking,[90] others question the advisability of any resection short of curative extirpation in patients without humorally related disease. Biliary bypass, gastrointestinal bypass, and chemical splanchnicectomy are used to relieve symptoms created by the mass effects of the tumor in patients with adenocarcinoma of the pancreas. These also are appropriate operations in patients with nonfunctional endocrine tumors of the pancreas, who often have symptoms related to local disease. Nonoperative percutaneous or endoscopic biliary bypass also can be helpful in selected cases when the risks of surgery are prohibitive.

Unlike patients with adenocarcinoma of the pancreas, patients with nonfunctional endocrine tumors can have long-term survival, and this should be taken into account when considering palliative procedures. Specifically, if an operation is performed for biliary obstruction, a concomitant gastrointestinal bypass should be considered, because enteric obstruction becomes more likely with prolonged survival. Long-term survival after gastrojejunostomy also makes peristomal jejunal ulceration more likely. For this reason, vagotomy should be performed or appropriate $H_2$-receptor–blocker prophylaxis initiated.

Elevated plasma levels of α-fetoprotein have been measured in metastatic nonfunctioning endocrine tumors of the pancreas.[91] Alpha-fetoprotein is, most likely, a tumor marker for all metastatic islet cell malignancies and may be used to track the progress of metastatic disease. This feature would make it particularly helpful in following nonfunctioning tumors that do not elaborate other measurable hormones or peptide markers.

# SURGICAL ASPECTS OF PANCREATIC ENDOCRINE TUMORS

## EXOCRINE TUMORS VERSUS ENDOCRINE TUMORS

Adenocarcinoma of the pancreas is the fifth leading cause of cancer death in the United States. Approximately 20,000 new cases are diagnosed each year, and 5-year survival is ~2% regardless of therapy.[92] By comparison, 200 to 1000 endocrine tumors of the pancreas are found in the United States each year,[29,93] and 5-year survival after surgery is nearly 100% for benign tumors and >40% for malignant tumors.[94] Another advantage of operating on endocrine tumors is the significant symptomatic relief from hormonal syndromes that can be obtained by curative resection or tumor cytoreduction.

## SURGICAL PROCEDURES

Like ductal tumors, islet cell tumors of the pancreas may be solid or cystic.[95] The treatment of cystic endocrine tumors, whether benign, malignant, functional, or nonfunctional, is similar to that of solid endocrine tumors. Operations performed for endocrine tumors of the pancreas include enucleation, segmental resection, distal pancreatectomy, pancreaticoduodenectomy, total and near-total pancreatectomy, tumor cytoreduction, bypass procedures, and surgery on other involved organs such as the stomach, duodenum, and liver (see Table 160-2). Multiple cases of laparoscopic (minimally invasive) resections of islet cell tumors of the distal pancreas have been reported.[96] Some centers have performed total hepatectomy with orthotopic liver transplantation for patients with metastases confined to the liver.[97]

One unusual feature of endocrine tumors of the pancreas not shared by nonendocrine tumors is the *response to tumor debulking*. With some of these tumors, surgical reduction of the size of the lesion alone can significantly improve long-term survival.[98] In contrast, surgery for adenocarcinoma of the pancreas is limited mainly to total resection by pancreaticoduodenectomy or palliation with bypass.

## INTRAOPERATIVE LOCALIZATION

Tumor localization is important and sometimes difficult for endocrine neoplasms, which can be small but clinically symptomatic. On occasion, tumors cannot be localized before surgery and must be found at surgery. Surgeons performing these operations should be familiar with intraoperative ultrasonography, duodenotomy, intraarterial methylene blue administration, and other intraoperative localizing techniques, as well as with the indications for biopsy or blind resection.

Any physician evaluating patients with pancreatic masses must understand the possibility and significance of finding an endocrine tumor. Also, any surgeon operating on patients with pancreatic endocrine tumors must be thoroughly familiar with the evaluation and localization of these lesions, with the intraoperative decision-making process, and with the wide range of ablative procedures used for these unusual neoplasms.

## REFERENCES

1. Warshaw AL, Swanson RS. What's new in general surgery: pancreatic cancer in 1988. Ann Surg 1988; 208:541.
2. Gold EB. Epidemiology of and risk factors for pancreatic cancer. Surg Clin North Am 1995; 75:819.
3. National Institutes of Health, National Cancer Institute. SEER Cancer Statistics Review, 1973–1990. Bethesda, MD: National Institutes of Health, 1993. NIH publication 93-2789.
4. De Jong SA, Pickleman J, Rainsford K. Nocturnal tumors of the pancreas. Arch Surg 1993; 128:730.
5. Yeo CJ, Wang BH, Anthone GJ, Cameron JL. Surgical experience with pancreatic islet-cell tumors. Arch Surg 1993; 128:1143.
6. Capella C, Heitz PH, Hofler H, et al. Revised classification of neuroendocrine tumors of the lung, pancreas and gut. Virchows Arch 1995; 425:547.
7. Bottger TH, Seidl C, Seifert JK, et al. Value of quantitative DNA analysis in endocrine tumors of the pancreas. Oncology 1997; 54:318.
8. Grant CS. Surgical management of malignant islet cell tumors. World J Surg 1993; 17:498.
9. Delcore R, Friesen SR. Gastrointestinal neuroendocrine tumors. J Am Coll Surg 1994; 178:187.
10. Strodel WE, Vinik AI, Lloyd RV, et al. Pancreatic polypeptide-producing tumors. Silent lesions of the pancreas? Arch Surg 1984; 119:508.
11. Brunt LM, Mazoujian G, O'Dorisio TM, Wells SA. Stimulation of vasoactive intestinal peptide and neurotensin secretion by pentagastrin in a patient with VIPoma syndrome. Surgery 1994; 115:362.
12. McCleod MK, Vinik AI. Calcitonin immunoreactivity and hypercalcitoninemia in two patients with sporadic, nonfamilial, gastroenteropancreatic neuroendocrine tumors. Surgery 1992; 111:484.
13. Perkins PL, McLeod MK, Jin L, et al. Analysis of gastrinomas by immunohistochemistry and in situ hybridization histochemistry. Diagn Mol Pathol 1992; 1:155.
14. Bieligk S, Jaffe BM. Islet cell tumors of the pancreas. Surg Clin North Am 1995; 75:1025.
15. Modlin IM, Lewis JJ, Ahlman H, et al. Management of unresectable malignant endocrine tumors of the pancreas. Surg Gynecol Obstet 1993; 176:507.
16. Hammond PJ, Jackson JA, Bloom SR. Localization of pancreatic endocrine tumors. Clin Endocrinol (Oxf) 1994; 40:3.
17. Vinik AI, Delbridge L, Moattari R, et al. Transhepatic portal vein catheterization for localization of insulinomas: a ten year experience. Surgery 1991; 109:1.
18. Van Eijck CH, Brunning HA, Reubi JC, et al. Use of isotope-labeled somatostatin analogs for visualization of islet-cell tumors. World J Surg 1993; 17:444.
19. Van Eijck CH, Lamberts SW, Lemaire LC, et al. The use of somatostatin receptor scintigraphy in the differential diagnosis of pancreatic duct cancers and islet cell tumors. Ann Surg 1996; 224:119.
20. Doppman JL, Miller DL, Chang R, et al. Intraarterial calcium stimulation test for detection of insulinomas. World J Surg 1993; 17:439.
21. Ariyama J, Suyama M, Satoh K, Wakabayashi K. Endoscopic ultrasound and intraductal ultrasound in the diagnosis of small pancreatic tumors. Abdom Imaging 1998; 23:380.
22. Bottger TC, Junginger T. Is preoperative radiographic localization of islet cell tumors in patients with insulinomas necessary? World J Surg 1993; 17:427.
23. Norton JA, Cromack DT, Shawker TH, et al. Intraoperative ultrasonographic localization of islet cell tumors. Ann Surg 1988; 207:160.
24. Joffe SN. Pancreatic islet cell tumor. In: Cameron JL, ed. Current surgical therapy, 2nd ed. St. Louis: CV Mosby, 1986:285.
25. Udelsman R, Yeo CJ, Hruban RH, et al. Pancreaticoduodenectomy for selected pancreatic endocrine tumors. Surg Gynecol Obstet 1993; 177:269.
26. Menegaux F, Schmitt G, Mercadier M, Chigot JP. Pancreatic insulinomas. Am J Surg 1993; 165:243.
27. Von Eyben FE, Grodum E, Gjessing HJ, et al. Metabolic remission with octreotide in patients with insulinoma. J Intern Med 1994; 235:245.
28. Buchanan KD. Effects of somatostatin on neuroendocrine tumors of the gastrointestinal system. Recent Results Cancer Res 1993; 129:45.
29. Lo CY, Lam KY, Fan ST. Surgical strategy for insulinomas in multiple endocrine neoplasia type I. Am J Surg 1998; 175:305.
29a. Tomassetti P, Migliori M, Corinaldesi R, Gullo L. Treatment of gastroenteropancreatic neuroendocrine tumors with octreotide LAR. Aliment Pharmacol Ther 2000; 14:557.
30. Friesen SR. Tumors of the endocrine pancreas. N Engl J Med 1982; 306:580.
31. Shepard JJ, Challis DR, Davies PF, et al. Multiple endocrine neoplasia, type 1. Arch Surg 1993; 128:1133.
32. Cherner JA, Sawyers JL. Benefit of resection of metastatic gastrinoma in multiple endocrine neoplasia type 1. Gastroenterology 1992; 102:109.
33. Zollinger RM, Ellison EH. Primary peptic ulcerations of the jejunum associated with islet cell tumors of the pancreas. Ann Surg 1955; 142:709.
34. Stabile BE, Morrow DJ, Passaro E. The gastrinoma triangle: operative implications. Am J Surg 1984; 147:25.
35. Sawicki MP, Howard TJ, Dalton M, et al. The dichotomous distribution of gastrinomas. Arch Surg 1990; 125:1584.
36. Howard TJ, Sawicki MP, Stabile BE, et al. Biologic behavior of sporadic gastrinoma located to the right and left of the superior mesenteric artery. Am J Surg 1993; 165:101.
37. Imamura M, Takahashi K. Use of selective arterial secretin injection test to guide surgery in patients with Zollinger Ellison syndrome. World J Surg 1993; 17:433.
37a. Jensen RT, Gibril F. Somatostatin receptor scintigraphy in gastrinomas. Ital J Gastroenterol Hepatol 1999; 31(Suppl 2):S179.
38. Kvols L, Brown M, O'Connor L, et al. Evaluation of radiolabeled somatostatin analog (e.g., [123]I-octreotide) in the detection and localization of carcinoid and islet cell tumors. Radiology 1993; 187:129.
39. Thompson NW, Pasieka J, Fukuuchi A. Duodenal gastrinomas, duodenotomy, and duodenal exploration in the surgical management of Zollinger-Ellison syndrome. World J Surg 1993; 17:455.
40. Ko TC, Flisak M, Prinz RA. Selective intra-arterial methylene blue injection: a novel method of localizing gastrinoma. Gastroenterology 1992; 102:1062.

41. Harmon JW, Norton JA, Collin MJ, et al. Removal of gastrinomas for control of Zollinger-Ellison syndrome. Ann Surg 1984; 200:396.

42. Norton JA, Doppman JL, Jensen RT. Curative resection in Zollinger-Ellison syndrome: results of a 10-year prospective study. Ann Surg 1992; 215:8.

43. Howard T, Zinner M, Stabile B, et al. Gastrinoma excision for cure. Ann Surg 1990; 211:9.

44. Delcore R, Friesen SR. Role of pancreatoduodenectomy in the management of primary duodenal wall gastrinomas in patients with Zollinger-Ellison syndrome. Surgery 1992; 112:1016.

45. Orloff SL, Debas HT. Advances in the management of patients with Zollinger-Ellison syndrome. Surg Clin North Am 1995; 75:511.

46. Phan GQ, Yeo CJ, Cameron JL, et al. Pancreaticoduodenectomy for selected periampullary neuroendocrine tumors: fifty patients. Surgery 1997; 122:989.

47. Richardson CT, Feldman M, McClelland RN, et al. Effect of vagotomy in Zollinger-Ellison syndrome. Gastroenterology 1979; 77:682.

48. Zollinger RM, Ellison EC, Fabri PJ, et al. Primary peptic ulcerations of the jejunum associated with islet cell tumors: twenty five year evaluation. Ann Surg 1980; 192:422.

49. Farley DR, van Heerden JA, Grant CS. The Zollinger-Ellison syndrome: a collective surgical experience. Ann Surg 1992; 215:561.

50. Sheppard B, Norton J, Doppman J, et al. Management of islet cell tumors in patients with multiple endocrine neoplasia: a prospective study. Surgery 1989; 106:1108.

51. Delcore R, Friesen SR. Zollinger-Ellison syndrome. Arch Surg 1991; 126:556.

52. Fishbeyn VA, Norton JA, Benya RV, et al. Assessment and prediction of long-term cure in patients with the Zollinger-Ellison syndrome: the best approach. Ann Intern Med 1993; 119:199.

53. Pisegna JR, Norton JA, Slimak GG, et al. Effects of curative gastrinoma resection on gastric secretory function and antisecretory drug requirement in the Zollinger-Ellison syndrome. Gastroenterology 1992; 102:767.

54. Arnold R, Neuhaus C, Benning R, et al. Somatostatin analog Sandostatin and inhibition of tumor growth in patients with metastatic endocrine gastroenteropancreatic tumors. World J Surg 1993; 17:511.

54a. Sato T, Konishi K, Kimura H, et al. Strategy for pancreatic endocrine tumors. Hepatogastroenterology 2000; 47:537.

55. Soga J, Yakuwa Y. Glucagonomas/diabetico-dermatogenic syndrome (DDS): a statistical evaluation of 407 reported cases. J Hepatobiliary Pancreat Surg 1998; 5:312.

56. Becker SW, Kahn D, Rothman S. Cutaneous manifestations of internal malignant tumors. Arch Dermatol Syph 1942; 45:1069.

57. McGavran MH, Unger RH, Recant L, et al. A glucagon-secreting alpha-cell carcinoma of the pancreas. N Engl J Med 1966; 274:1408.

58. Higgins GA, Recant L, Fischman AB. The glucagonoma syndrome: surgically curable diabetes. Am J Surg 1979; 137:142.

59. Norton JA, Kahn CR, Shiebinger R, et al. Amino acid deficiency and the skin rash associated with glucagonoma. Ann Intern Med 1979; 91:213.

60. Ingemansson S, Holst J, Larsson LI, Lunderquist A. Localization of glucagonomas by catheterization of the pancreatic veins and with glucagon assay. Surg Gynecol Obstet 1977; 145:509.

61. Park S, O'Dorisio M, O'Dorisio T. Vasoactive intestinal polypeptide-secreting tumours: biology and therapy. Baillières Clin Gastroenterol 1996; 10:673.

62. Jaffe BM. Surgery for gut hormone-producing tumors. Am J Med 1987; 82:68.

63. Cesani F, Ernst R, Walser E, Villanueva-Meyer J. Tc-99m sestamibi imaging of a pancreatic VIPoma and parathyroid adenoma in a patient with multiple type I endocrine neoplasia. Clin Nucl Med 1994; 19:532.

64. Nagorney DM, Bloom SR, Polak JM, Blumgart LH. Resolution of recurrent Verner-Morrison syndrome by resection of metastatic vipoma. Surgery 1983; 93:348.

65. Kraenzlin ME, Ch'ng JLC, Wood SM, et al. Long-term treatment of a VIPoma with somatostatin analogue resulting in remission of symptoms and possible shrinkage of metastases. Gastroenterology 1985; 88:185.

66. Mathoulin-Portier MP, Payan MJ, Monges G, et al. Pancreatic and duodenal somatostatinoma. Two clinico-pathologic entities. Ann Pathol 1996; 16:299.

67. Larsson LI, Holst JJ, Kuhl C, et al. Pancreatic somatostatinoma: clinical features and physiologic implications. Lancet 1977; 1:666.

68. Sakazaki S, Umeyama K, Nakagawa H, et al. Pancreatic somatostatinoma. Am J Surg 1983; 146:674.

69. Kelly TR. Pancreatic somatostatinoma. Am J Surg 1983; 146:671.

70. Krejs GJ, Orci L, Conlon JM, et al. Somatostatinoma syndrome: biochemical, morphologic and clinical features. N Engl J Med 1979; 301:285.

71. Kaneko H, Yanaihara N, Ito S, et al. Somatostatinoma of the duodenum. Cancer 1979; 44:2273.

72. O'Brien TD, Chejfec G, Prinz RA. Clinical features of duodenal somatostatinomas. Surgery 1993; 114:1144.

73. Angeletti S, Corleto VD, Schillaci O, et al. Use of the somatostatin analogue octreotide to localise and manage somatostatin-producing tumours. Gut 1998; 42:792.

74. Adrian T, Uttenthal L, Williams S, et al. Secretion of pancreatic polypeptide in patients with pancreatic endocrine tumors. N Engl J Med 1986; 315:287.

75. Mozell E, Stenzell P, Woltering E, et al. Functional endocrine tumors of the pancreas: clinical presentation, diagnosis, and treatment. Curr Probl Surg 1990; 27:303.

76. Miraliakbari BA, Asa L, Boudreau SF. Parathyroid hormone–like peptide in pancreatic endocrine carcinoma and adenocarcinoma associated with hypercalcemia. Hum Pathol 1992; 23:884.

77. Tarver DS, Birch SJ. Case report: life-threatening hypercalcemia secondary to pancreatic tumor secreting parathyroid hormone–related protein—successful control by hepatic arterial embolization. Clin Radiol 1992; 46:204.

78. Mitlak BH, Hutchinson JS, Kaufman SD, Nussbaum SR. Parathyroid hormone–related peptide mediates hypercalcemia in an islet cell tumor of the pancreas. Horm Metab Res 1991; 23:344.

79. Price DE, Absalom SR, Davidson K, et al. A case of multiple endocrine neoplasia: hyperparathyroidism, insulinoma, GRF-oma, hypercalcitoninemia and intractable peptic ulceration. Clin Endocrinol (Oxf) 1992; 37:187.

80. Gullo L, De Giorgio R, D'Errico A, et al. Pancreatic exocrine carcinoma producing adrenocorticotropic hormone. Pancreas 1992; 7:172.

81. Tsuchihashi T, Yamaguchi K, Abe K, et al. Production of immunoreactive corticotropin-releasing hormone in various neuroendocrine tumors. Jpn J Clin Oncol 1992; 22:232.

82. Amikura K, Alexander HR, Norton JA, et al. Role of surgery in management of adrenocorticotropic hormone–producing islet cell tumors of the pancreas. Surgery 1995; 118:1125.

83. Venkatesh S, Ordonez NG, Ajani J, et al. Islet cell carcinoma of the pancreas. Cancer 1990; 65:354.

84. Buetow PC, Miller DL, Parrino TV, Buck JL. Islet cell tumors of the pancreas: clinical, radiologic, and pathologic correlation in diagnosis and localization. Radiographics 1997; 17:453.

85. White TJ, Edney JA, Thompson JS, et al. Is there a prognostic difference between functional and nonfunctional islet cell tumors? Am J Surg 1994: 168:627.

86. Heitz PU, Kasper M, Polak JM, et al. Pancreatic endocrine tumors. Hum Pathol 1982; 13:263.

87. De Jong SA, Pickleman J, Rainsford K. Nonductal tumors of the pancreas. The importance of laparotomy. Arch Surg 1993; 128:730.

88. Kent RB, van Heerden JA, Weiland LH. Nonfunctioning islet cell tumors. Ann Surg 1981; 193:185.

89. Evans DB, Skibber JM, Lee JE, et al. Nonfunctioning islet cell carcinoma of the pancreas. Surgery 1993; 114:1175.

90. Eckhauser FE, Cheung PS, Vinik AI, et al. Nonfunctioning malignant neuroendocrine tumors of the pancreas. Surgery 1986; 100:978.

91. Lesur G, Bergemer AM, Turner L, et al. Increases in alpha-fetoprotein in pancreatic endocrine tumors with hepatic metastases. Gastroenterol Clin Biol 1996; 20:204.

92. Gordis L, Gold EB. Epidemiology of pancreatic cancer. World J Surg 1984; 8:808.

93. Brennan MF, MacDonald JS. The endocrine pancreas. In: DeVita V, Hellman S, Rosenberg SA, eds. Principles and practice of oncology, 2nd ed. Philadelphia: JB Lippincott, 1985:1206.

94. Thompson GB, van Heerden JA, Grant CS, et al. Islet cell carcinoma of the pancreas: a twenty-year experience. Surgery 1988; 104:1011.

95. Schwartz RW, Munfakh NA, Zweng T, et al. Nonfunctioning cystic neuroendocrine neoplasms of the pancreas. Surgery 1994; 115:645.

96. Vezakis A, Davides D, Larvin M, McMahan MJ. Laparoscopic surgery combined with preservation of the spleen for distal pancreatic tumors. Surg Endosc 1999; 13:26.

97. Dousset B, Houssin D, Soubrane O, et al. Metastatic endocrine tumors: is there a place for liver transplantation? Liver Transpl Surg 1995; 1:111.

98. Danforth DN, Gorden P, Brennan MF. Metastatic insulin-secreting carcinoma of the pancreas: clinical course and the role of surgery. Surgery 1984; 96:1027.

99. Debas HT, Mulvihill SJ. Neuroendocrine gut neoplasms: important lessons from uncommon tumors. Arch Surg 1994; 129:965.

100. Buchanan KD, Johnston CF, O'Hare MMT, et al. Neuroendocrine tumors: a European view. Am J Surg 1986; 81:14.

# CHAPTER 161

# HYPOGLYCEMIA OF INFANCY AND CHILDHOOD

JOSEPH I. WOLFSDORF AND MARK KORSON

Glucose is the predominant metabolic fuel utilized by the brain. Because the brain cannot synthesize glucose or store more than a few minutes' supply as glycogen, survival of the brain requires a continuous supply of glucose.[1] Recurrent hypoglycemia during the period of rapid brain growth and differentiation in infancy can result in long-term neurologic sequelae and psychomotor retardation. Therefore, prevention of hypoglycemia and expeditious diagnosis and vigorous treatment when it occurs are essential to prevent the potentially devastating consequences of hypoglycemia on the brain.

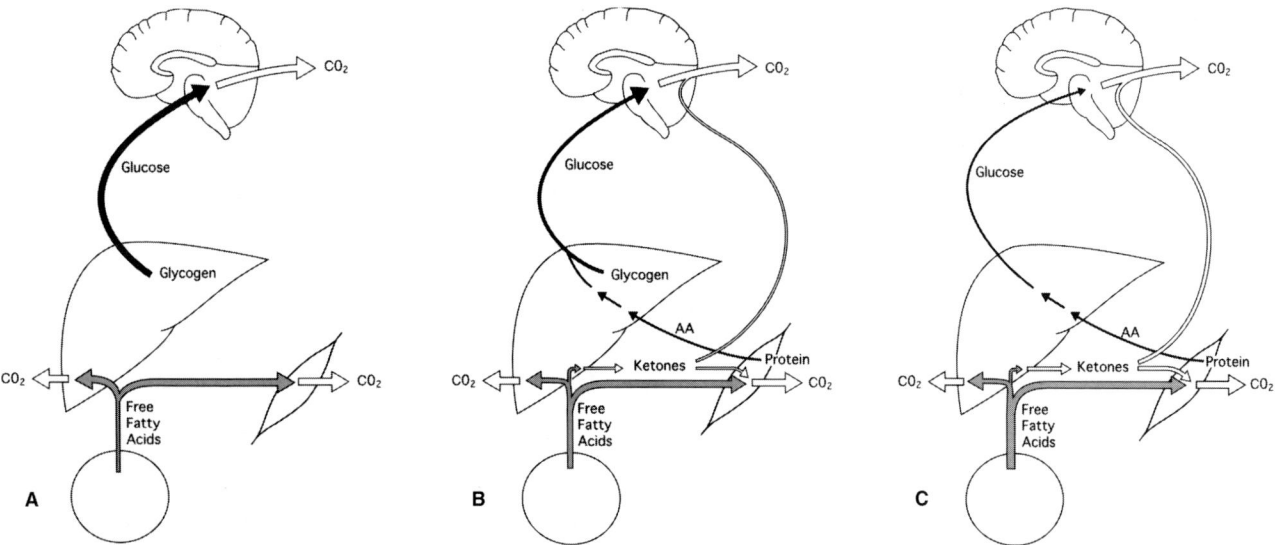

**FIGURE 161-1.** Transition from the fed to the fasted state. **A,** Between meals: Glucose is derived from hepatic glycogenolysis; free fatty acids are an important fuel for muscle. **B,** Overnight fast (postabsorptive state): Liver glycogen becomes depleted; gluconeogenesis becomes the principal source of glucose. Hepatic ketone production increases, providing an alternative fuel for brain and muscle. **C,** Prolonged fasting: Fatty acids and ketones are the principal metabolic substrates. Brain utilization of ketones increases. Glucose is derived from gluconeogenesis.

## INCREASED SUSCEPTIBILITY OF THE INFANT AND CHILD TO HYPOGLYCEMIA

Hypoglycemia is most common in the newborn period. During infancy and childhood, it occurs most frequently when nighttime feeding is discontinued and when intercurrent illness interrupts the normal feeding pattern, causing periods of relative starvation. Basal energy needs during infancy are high. A full-term newborn baby, for example, has a ratio of surface area to body mass that is more than twice that of an average adult, necessitating a high rate of energy expenditure to maintain body temperature. Also, the infant brain is large relative to body mass and its energy requirement is mainly derived from the oxidation of circulating glucose. To meet the high demand for glucose, the rate of glucose production in infants and young children is two to three times that of older children and mature adults.[2] Although the demand for glucose is high, the activity of several liver enzymes involved in energy production is low in the newborn compared to that of older children and adults. Consequently, until feeding is well established, maintenance of glucose homeostasis in the newborn period is more precarious than it is later in childhood.

In the postabsorptive state, the rate of glucose turnover in adults is ~2 mg/kg per minute (8–10 g per hour), whereas the average basal (4–6 hours after feeding) rate of glucose turnover is 6 mg/kg per minute in newborns, approximately three times the adult rate. During prolonged fasting, infants and children cannot sustain this high rate of glucose production. Normal children, 18 months to 9 years of age, fasted for 24 hours, have a mean blood glucose concentration of $52 \pm 14$ (standard deviation [SD]) mg/dL. Indeed, 22% have blood glucose concentrations <40 mg/dL and glucose values conform to a Gaussian pattern of distribution.[3] For these reasons, infants and young children are more prone than adolescents and adults to develop hypoglycemia when normal feeding patterns are disturbed by intercurrent illness.

## AN OVERVIEW OF FUEL METABOLISM

The physiologic mechanisms that normally prevent hypoglycemia ensure that the brain receives a continuous supply of glu-

cose.[4] Blood-to-brain glucose transport is a function of the arterial plasma glucose concentration. The brain, therefore, is dependent on the precise regulation of systemic glucose balance that maintains the arterial plasma glucose concentration above the critical level that becomes limiting to brain glucose metabolism. None of the glucoregulatory factors, including insulin, modifies glucose uptake into the brain.

Glucose is derived from intestinal absorption following digestion of dietary carbohydrate (exogenous glucose delivery) or from endogenous glucose production (*glycogenolysis and gluconeogenesis*). Gluconeogenesis refers to the formation of glucose from three carbon precursors including lactate, pyruvate, amino acids (especially alanine and glutamine), and glycerol. The integrated regulatory effects of hormones, neural pathways, and metabolic substrates normally result in the precise matching of glucose utilization and the sum of exogenous glucose delivery and endogenous glucose production. The key glucoregulatory factors are insulin, glucagon, and epinephrine. Additional factors, including growth hormone (GH) and cortisol, modify the effectiveness of these glucoregulatory hormones.

After feeding, exogenous glucose delivery increases at a rate largely determined by the carbohydrate content of the ingested food and the rate of gastric emptying. The increase in circulating glucose concentration stimulates the secretion of insulin, which enhances glucose entry into fat, muscle, and liver cells. Liver and muscle, but not kidney or brain, express glycogen synthase at high levels and can store appreciable quantities of glucose as glycogen. In the liver, glucose is also converted to fat, which can be stored in the liver or transported to other tissues in the form of very low-density lipoproteins. Endogenous glucose production is suppressed by high postprandial plasma insulin concentrations.

Despite a substantial increase in glucose influx into the circulation, the increase in plasma glucose concentration is relatively small after a meal, and plasma glucose and insulin concentrations return to basal levels within a few hours. The transition from endogenous glucose production to exogenous glucose delivery shortly after a meal and the later transition from exogenous glucose delivery back to endogenous glucose production are finely regulated. Hypoglycemia normally does not occur in the interval between meals, and glucose delivery to the brain continues unabated (Fig. 161-1A).

The amount of glycogen stored in the liver is modest—~5% of the wet weight of the liver. For example, the liver of a 10-year-old child weighing 30 kg contains ~45 g glycogen. This could, theoretically, satisfy the basal requirement for glucose (~9 g per hour) for only 5 to 6 hours. Thus, gluconeogenesis soon plays the major part in maintaining normal blood glucose concentrations (Fig. 161-1B). Although muscle can store glucose as glycogen, it lacks the enzyme glucose-6-phosphatase and, therefore, cannot release free glucose. In muscle, glucose is metabolized via glycolysis to pyruvate, which can be reduced to lactate, transaminated to form alanine, or undergo oxidation. Lactate and pyruvate released from muscle are transported to the liver, where they serve as a gluconeogenic precursor (the Cori or glucose-lactate-glucose cycle). Alanine, glutamine, and other amino acids also flow from muscle to the liver and serve as gluconeogenic precursors. Circulating alanine carbon is largely derived from glucose (glucose-alanine-glucose cycle). Glutamine, the other major amino-acid precursor for new glucose formation, is also partially derived from glucose (glucose-glutamine cycle).[5]

Liver and kidney express the critical gluconeogenic enzymes: pyruvate carboxylase, phosphoenolpyruvate carboxykinase, fructose-1,6-bisphosphatase, and glucose-6-phosphatase. These organs can form free glucose that can be released into the circulation. In the postabsorptive state, hepatic gluconeogenesis soon plays the major role in maintaining normal blood glucose concentrations (see Fig. 161-1B). The oxidation of fatty acids produces the energy, reducing equivalents, and metabolic intermediates required to sustain the high rate of hepatic gluconeogenesis that occurs during fasting. Free fatty acids are released from adipose tissue stores (lipolysis) and normally are abundant during fasting.[6,7] Free fatty acids also provide many tissues (including cardiac and skeletal muscle) with a substrate that can be readily used to provide energy. A fraction of the free fatty acids undergoes β-oxidation in the liver to form ketone bodies (acetoacetate and β-hydroxybutyrate) (Figs. 161-1B and C). High rates of ketone body production are reached during fasting in children. After 20 to 22 hours of fasting, the ketone body turnover rate in young children is comparable to that achieved by adults after fasting for several days.[8] Fasting ketonemia provides the brain, which cannot utilize free fatty acids, and other tissues with an alternative source of energy.[9,10] Because the brain can oxidize ketones, it is not solely dependent on glucose as an energy substrate. Normally, the large amounts of ketones generated during fasting results in a decrease in the brain's rate of glucose consumption, and glucose is thereby conserved.

These metabolic responses to fasting (increased gluconeogenesis, lipolysis, and ketogenesis) are finely regulated by changes in the circulating concentrations of hormones. This includes a fasting decrease in insulin secretion and increased plasma concentrations of glucagon, epinephrine, GH, and cortisol, the latter collectively referred to as the counterregulatory hormones.

Red cells lack mitochondria; consequently, glycolysis stops with the formation of lactate. In other cells, glucose can be completely oxidized to carbon dioxide and water. During a fast, muscle can oxidize fatty acids to meet its energy needs and substantially reduce its glucose uptake. Proteolysis in muscle provides the liver with amino acids for gluconeogenesis. Whether complete oxidation of glucose occurs depends on the activity of the enzyme pyruvate dehydrogenase, which is inactivated by products of fatty acid oxidation. The availability of other fuels for oxidation, fatty acids or ketones, affects the activity of pyruvate dehydrogenase and determines whether glucose is completely oxidized to carbon dioxide and water, or is conserved via recycling of lactate, pyruvate, and alanine back to glucose in the liver (glucose-lactate-glucose and glucose-alanine-glucose cycles).

In summary, the adaptation to fasting involves a major change in the body's fuel economy. As fasting is prolonged, there is decreased dependence on glucose and increased reliance on the products of fat as the primary sources of fuel for energy metabolism (see Fig. 161-1C). A failure to oxidize fatty acids or to synthesize or utilize ketones results in greater utilization of glucose, impaired gluconeogenesis, and inability to conserve glucose, which leads to hypoglycemia.

## DEFINITION OF HYPOGLYCEMIA

The definition of hypoglycemia, especially in neonates, has been controversial[11–13]; opinions range from 25 to 30 mg/dL (1.4–1.7 mmol/L) up to 60 to 70 mg/dL (3.3–3.9 mmol/L).[14,14a] In 1976, Cornblath and Schwartz[15] defined hypoglycemia in the newborn as a whole blood glucose level of <30 mg/dL (<1.7 mmol/L) in term infants and <20 mg/dL (1.1 mmol/L) in premature infants. This definition, based on statistical analysis of the distribution of blood glucose concentrations in a newborn nursery, was obtained at a time when it was common practice to withhold feeds for at least 12 hours in healthy newborn babies and for 24 hours in low-birth-weight babies.[16] The definition has been modified as changes have occurred in the treatment of mothers in labor and delivery and of newborn infants. Furthermore, most laboratories now measure glucose in serum or plasma, in which the concentration is 10% to 15% higher than in whole blood. More recent studies have defined hypoglycemia in term infants as a serum glucose concentration <40 to 45 mg/dL (<2.2–2.5 mmol/L) after the first 24 hours of life.[17,18] However, even this is unsatisfactory because it is a definition based on statistics rather than the physiologic variable of importance, namely, the correlation of plasma glucose concentrations with central nervous system (CNS) function and neurodevelopmental outcomes.[19]

There is no empiric evidence that blood glucose levels in infants should be different from those of older children or adults. There are, also, no data showing that glucose extraction across the blood–brain barrier in newborns is greater than in adults. Brain glucose uptake is dependent on the circulating arterial glucose concentration.

During acute insulin-induced hypoglycemia in normal adults, symptoms appear at plasma glucose levels (measured in arterialized venous blood) of ~60 mg/dL (3.3 mmol/L) and impairment of brain function occurs at ~50 mg/dL (2.8 mmol/L).[20–22] Comparable levels in venous blood are ~3 mg/dL lower.[23] In children, functional changes in the CNS (brainstem auditory and somatosensory evoked potentials) occur when the plasma glucose concentration falls below 47 mg/dL (2.6 mmol/L).[19] These facts suggest that the physiologic threshold is a plasma glucose concentration in the range of 50 to 60 mg/dL (2.8–3.3 mmol/L). Therefore, one should regard a plasma glucose concentration of 60 mg/dL (3.3 mmol/L) or greater as normoglycemia and plasma glucose levels below 50 mg/dL (2.8 mmol/L) as hypoglycemia. At plasma glucose levels from 50 to 60 mg/dL (2.8–3.3 mmol/L), the infant should be fed and glucose levels carefully monitored.

## CLINICAL MANIFESTATIONS OF HYPOGLYCEMIA

The symptoms of hypoglycemia are not specific. Therefore, when a patient's symptoms are suspected to be due to hypoglycemia, it is essential to measure the blood glucose concentration and confirm that it is low and demonstrate that administration of glucose relieves the symptoms.

**TABLE 161-1.**
**Signs and Symptoms of Hypoglycemia**

| Autonomic | Neuroglycopenic |
|---|---|
| Sweating | Warmth |
| Hunger | Fatigue |
| Paresthesias (tingling, numbness) | Weakness |
| Tremors | Dizziness |
| Pallor | Headache |
| Anxiety | Inability to concentrate |
| Nausea | Drowsiness |
| Palpitations | Blurred vision |
| | Difficulty speaking |
| | Confusion |
| | Bizarre behavior |
| | Loss of coordination |
| | Difficulty walking |
| | Coma |
| | Seizures |

The symptoms of hypoglycemia (Table 161-1) can be classified into two major groups based on the mechanism responsible for their generation: Autonomic symptoms result from activation of the autonomic nervous system (both sympathetic and parasympathetic divisions), while neuroglycopenic symptoms result from the effects of brain glucose deprivation. The symptoms of hypoglycemia in children are similar to those in adults. In newborns and infants, hypoglycemia typically manifests as irritability, tremors, feeding difficulty, lethargy, hypotonia, tachypnea, cyanosis, or apnea (see Table 161-1).

## NEONATAL HYPOGLYCEMIA

The fetus relies on a continuous supply of glucose from the maternal circulation. From the moment the umbilical cord is severed, the newborn infant is totally dependent on its own resources to maintain its fuel supply until regular feeding commences. Thus, at birth, the newborn baby must make an abrupt transition to endogenous glucose production.[24] The initial counterregulatory response is glycogenolysis. However, the hepatic glycogen store that can be mobilized to provide circulating glucose is limited, and the availability of milk during nursing is initially inadequate. Consequently, the newborn baby rapidly becomes critically dependent on gluconeogenesis to prevent hypoglycemia. The regulatory signals involved in this metabolic adaptation are decreased serum insulin and increased glucagon, epinephrine, GH, and cortisol levels.

Transient hypoglycemia is almost universal in all newborn mammals after birth. However, in human infants, even if enteral feeds are withheld, the blood glucose concentration rises spontaneously. Beyond the first 2 postnatal hours, blood glucose concentrations <47 mg/dL (<2.6 mmol/L) may recur in many healthy babies, particularly in those who are fed on demand, with long intervals between feeds, and in babies who are breast-fed.[25] A marked ketogenic response to low blood glucose concentrations occurs in these infants and is presumed to be protective of neurologic function, as ketone bodies are important glucose-sparing cerebral fuels.

Although hepatic glycogen deposition begins in the first trimester, large amounts of glycogen do not accumulate in the liver until late in the third trimester. Consequently, when babies are born prematurely, before the period of maximal glycogen accumulation, they have minimal glycogen stores and are susceptible to hypoglycemia. Because the fetal liver is capable of glycogenolysis, which is activated when fetal substrate delivery is inadequate, conditions associated with prolonged fetal substrate deprivation (e.g., various causes of intrauterine growth

**TABLE 161-2.**
**Conditions Associated with Neonatal Hypoglycemia**

**FAILURE TO STORE GLYCOGEN IN PREMATURE NEONATES**
**DEPLETION OF GLYCOGEN STORES**
  Small-for-gestational age (SGA) infants
  Postmaturity
  Sepsis
  Hypothermia
  Hypoxia
  Adrenal hemorrhage
**HYPERINSULINEMIA**
  Infants of mothers with diabetes mellitus or gestational diabetes
  Exposure to maternal drugs (sulfonylureas, β2-adrenergic agonists [terbutaline])
  Persistent hereditary hyperinsulinemia of infancy (PHHI)
  Beckwith-Wiedemann syndrome
  Iatrogenic (insulin added to parenteral nutrition solution)
  Blood group alloimmunization
**INBORN ERRORS OF CARBOHYDRATE, FAT, AND PROTEIN METABOLISM** (see Table 161-4)
**HORMONE DEFICIENCY**
  Congenital hypopituitarism
  Growth hormone (GH) deficiency
  Adrenocorticotropic hormone (ACTH) deficiency
  Cortisol deficiency

retardation, decline in placental function in postterm babies) may exhaust hepatic glycogen stores. These babies are also at increased risk of neonatal hypoglycemia.

Transient neonatal hypoglycemia is relatively common in premature neonates and in various perinatal conditions that deplete hepatic glycogen (Table 161-2). It is particularly common in developing countries because of common risk factors such as low birth weight, hyperthermia, and delays in breastfeeding.[25a] Recurrent or persistent hypoglycemia (>72 hours of life) is considerably less common, occurring in neonates with inborn errors of metabolism that impair glycogenolysis, gluconeogenesis, and production or utilization of alternative substrates. Likewise, recurrent or persistent hypoglycemia occurs in babies with dysregulated insulin secretion (hyperinsulinemia) or deficiency of counterregulatory hormones.

Recommendations for treatment of neonatal hypoglycemia are summarized in Table 161-3.

## CAUSES OF HYPOGLYCEMIA IN INFANCY AND CHILDHOOD

The clinical syndrome of hypoglycemia has numerous causes and diverse clinical manifestations (see Table 161-1). Almost all

**TABLE 161-3.**
**Recommendations for Treatment of Neonatal Hypoglycemia[85]**

**ASYMPTOMATIC OTHERWISE HEALTHY FULL-TERM NEONATE**
  5% dextrose in water, 30–60 mL orally
  Measure glucose levels every 15–30 min
  Start iv therapy if baby becomes symptomatic or hypoglycemia persists
**SYMPTOMATIC OR PRETERM NEONATES**
  10% dextrose in water, 2 mL/kg iv bolus
  Continuous iv infusion at 8 mg/kg per min
  Measure glucose levels every 15–30 min
  If hypoglycemia persists or recurs, repeat 10% dextrose in water, 2 mL/kg iv bolus, and increase continuous iv infusion by 2 mg/kg per min
  If hypoglycemia persists despite continuous administration of 12–5 mg/kg per min, consider hyperinsulinism and manage accordingly

**TABLE 161-4.**
**Causes of Hypoglycemia in Infancy and Childhood**

**ACCELERATED STARVATION (KETOTIC HYPOGLYCEMIA)**
**HYPERINSULINISM**
  Infant of diabetic mother
  Maternal drugs (sulfonylureas, $\beta_2$-adrenergic agonist)
  Persistent hereditary hyperinsulinemia of infancy (PHHI)
  Insulinoma
  Rh and ABO incompatibility
  Beckwith-Wiedemann syndrome
  Sulfonylurea ingestion
  Factitious
**HORMONE DEFICIENCY**
  Adrenocorticotropic hormone (ACTH)/cortisol
  Growth hormone (GH)
  Hypopituitarism (ACTH/cortisol and GH)
**METABOLIC DEFECTS**
  *Defects In Carbohydrate Metabolism*
  Glycogen synthetase deficiency
  Glycogen storage disease
  Glucose-6-phosphatase deficiency (type I)
  Amylo-1,6-glucosidase deficiency (type III)
  Phosphorylase deficiency (type VI)
  Phosphorylase kinase deficiency (type IX)
  Galactose-1-phosphate uridyltransferase deficiency (galactosemia)
  Fructose-1-phosphate aldolase deficiency (fructose intolerance)
  Defects in gluconeogenesis
  Pyruvate carboxylase deficiency
  Phosphoenolpyruvate carboxykinase deficiency
  Fructose-1,6-bisphosphatase deficiency
  *Defects In Fatty Acid Oxidation*
  Carnitine transport and metabolism
  $\beta$-Oxidation cycle
  Electron transfer
  Hydroxymethylglutaryl coenzyme A (CoA) lyase deficiency
  *Defects In Protein Metabolism*
  Branched-chain ketoacid decarboxylase deficiency (maple syrup urine disease)
  Methylmalonic acidemia
**MISCELLANEOUS**
  Nonpancreatic tumor hypoglycemia (insulin-like growth factor-II [IGF-II])
  Salicylate intoxication
  Ethanol intoxication
  Malaria
  Diarrhea
  Malnutrition
  Propionic acidemia
  Reactive hypoglycemia (dumping syndrome)

**TABLE 161-5.**
**Differential Diagnosis of Ketotic Hypoglycemia**

**LIVER LARGE**
  Glycogen storage diseases (types I, III, VI, IX)
  Disorders of gluconeogenesis (e.g., fructose-1,6-bisphosphatase)
**LIVER NORMAL SIZE**
  Accelerated starvation (ketotic hypoglycemia)
  Cortisol/adrenocorticotropic hormone (ACTH) deficiency
  Growth hormone (GH) deficiency
  Panhypopituitarism
  Glycogen synthetase deficiency
  Organic acidemias (e.g., maple syrup urine disease; methylmalonic, propionic acidemias)

cases of hypoglycemia fall into one of the five categories shown in Table 161-4.

## ACCELERATED STARVATION (KETOTIC HYPOGLYCEMIA; TRANSIENT INTOLERANCE OF FASTING)

Accelerated starvation is the most common cause of hypoglycemia in children beyond infancy. Hypoglycemia typically first occurs between 18 months and 5 years of age and remits spontaneously by 8 or 9 years of age. Many children with accelerated starvation are small and thin for their age and have decreased muscle mass. Many were born small for gestational age and may have had transient neonatal hypoglycemia. Hypoglycemia typically occurs during periods of intercurrent illness when food intake is limited by anorexia or vomiting,

includes neurologic symptoms ranging from lethargy to seizures and coma, and usually occurs in the morning before breakfast. Sometimes, hypoglycemia occurs in the morning after unusually intense physical exertion on the previous day and/or after the child has eaten poorly or completely omitted an evening meal.

The precise pathophysiologic cause of accelerated starvation is unclear. Children with ketotic hypoglycemia have low serum alanine levels. The gluconeogenic pathway is intact, and the serum glucose concentration increases appropriately when alanine is infused at the time of hypoglycemia. Hypoglycemia may result from decreased glucose production because of deficient availability of gluconeogenic substrate, especially alanine from muscle.[26] However, the cause of the hypoalaninemia is controversial. An alternative explanation is that it is a consequence of decreased muscle glucose uptake, which would affect flux through the glucose-alanine-glucose cycle.[27] Alternatively, it may be the result of a specific defect in protein catabolism or reflect decreased muscle mass. The plasma epinephrine response to hypoglycemia is reduced in about half the patients with ketotic hypoglycemia.[28] It has been suggested, therefore, that these children may have a deficient catecholamine response to hypoglycemia that results in increased glucose utilization.

After 8 to 16 hours, children with accelerated starvation show the same metabolic pattern as normal healthy children fasted for 24 to 36 hours. In many instances, the differentiation between accelerated starvation and the normal response to fasting is indistinct. Because healthy children can become hypoglycemic after a fast of 24 to 36 hours,[3,29] accelerated starvation may be one end of the normal spectrum of children's response to starvation rather than a distinct syndrome.[30,31]

### DIAGNOSIS

Because ketosis is a normal response to a falling plasma glucose concentration, ketotic hypoglycemia should not be regarded as a specific diagnosis. The differential diagnosis of the hypoglycemic child with an appropriately suppressed serum insulin concentration and ketosis is shown in Table 161-5. Accelerated starvation should only be diagnosed when the other causes of ketotic hypoglycemia have been ruled out.

Children with accelerated starvation typically become hypoglycemic in 12 to 24 hours and have a normal metabolic and hormonal response to fasting. At the time of hypoglycemia, blood ketone body concentrations are raised, there is ketonuria, plasma alanine is low, and blood lactate and pyruvate levels are normal.[32] Plasma insulin levels are appropriately suppressed and the concentrations of counterregulatory hormones are increased. The glycemic response to glucagon is normal in the fed state, but blunted at the time of hypoglycemia.

**TABLE 161-6.**
**Clinical and Biochemical Features of Hyperinsulinemic Hypoglycemia**

Usually younger than 12 mo of age at time of presentation

Hypoglycemia soon after feeding (0–5.5 h, average ~2 h)

Urinary ketones negative, trace, or small

Serum insulin $\geq 2\,\mu U/mL$ (15 pmol/L) with plasma glucose <45 mg/dL (2.5 mmol/L)

Plasma ketone (β-OH-butyrate and acetoacetate) concentrations inappropriately low

Brisk glycemic response to glucagon >30 mg/dL (>1.7 mmol/L)

Parenteral glucose required to maintain normoglycemia is 2- to 4-fold greater than glucose production rate (~6 mg/kg per min)

Decreased plasma branched-chain amino acids (valine, leucine, isoleucine)

Decreased insulin-like growth factor–binding protein-1 (IGFBP-1); all other endocrinologic and metabolic abnormalities with fasting hypoglycemia are associated with decreased insulin secretion and increased IGFBP-1 levels

Leucine and/or tolbutamide cause an exaggerated hyperinsulinemic response

Growth hormone (GH), cortisol concentrations usually normal but may be inappropriately low if hypoglycemia develops gradually or is recurrent (blunted counterregulatory hormone responses)

## TREATMENT

Treatment consists of educating parents to ensure that the child avoids prolonged periods of fasting. A bedtime snack consisting of both carbohydrate and protein prevents further episodes of hypoglycemia. During intercurrent illness, providing carbohydrate-rich drinks at frequent intervals during both the day and night can prevent hypoglycemia. Parents are instructed to test urine for ketones during intercurrent illnesses. The appearance of ketonuria precedes the onset of hypoglycemia by several hours. If the child cannot tolerate oral carbohydrate, intravenous glucose will be necessary to avert the development of hypoglycemia.

## HYPERINSULINISM

Hyperinsulinism caused by generalized B-cell dysfunction is the most common cause of persistent hypoglycemia in infancy. Islet cell adenomas are rare in children younger than 1 year of age. Hyperinsulinism that presents in an older child is more likely to be caused by an insulinoma or exogenous insulin administration (factitious hypoglycemia).

Several distinct genetic forms of congenital hyperinsulinism have been described. The most common variety is an autosomal recessive defect[33,33a] either due to homozygous mutations in the B-cell sulfonylurea-receptor (SUR1) gene[34] or due to mutations in the inward-rectifying potassium channel (Kir6.2) gene,[35,36] which are adjacent on chromosome 11p15.1. Both genes encode components of $K_{ATP}$ channels involved in glucose-regulated insulin release. These mutations result in uncoupling of insulin secretion from glucose metabolism.

The clinical features of autosomal dominant hyperinsulinism are usually milder than those of the recessive form. Affected individuals may not have symptomatic hypoglycemia until later in childhood or in adult life and hypoglycemia is usually more easily controlled with either diet alone or with diazoxide.[37] An activating mutation of B-cell glucokinase causing increased affinity of the enzyme for glucose has been found in one family with autosomal dominant hyperinsulinism.[38]

A distinct form of hyperinsulinism is associated with persistent mild hyperammonemia. Blood ammonium levels are in the range of 100 to 200 μmol/L, three to six times normal.[39–41] The hyperammonemia is asymptomatic and is not associated with any of the abnormalities of amino acids or organic acids found in the urea cycle enzyme defects. The syndrome is caused by a gain of function mutation of glutamate dehydrogenase resulting in excessive glutamate oxidation in the B cell, which increases the adenosine triphosphate/adenosine diphosphate (ATP/ADP) ratio, resulting in unregulated release of insulin. In the liver, excessive glutamate oxidation results in decreased levels of glutamate, which is required for the production of *n*-acetyl-glutamate, an allosteric activator of ureagenesis.[41]

## DIAGNOSIS

The clinical and biochemical features of hyperinsulinemic hypoglycemia are summarized in Table 161-6 (see Chap. 158). Reliable methods are still not widely available to distinguish between a focal lesion adenoma and a diffuse B-cell functional disorder in neonates and infants. Sonographic and computed tomography (CT) are insensitive (20–66% sensitivity) imaging modalities. Intraabdominal sonography is more sensitive (up to 84%) in localizing focal pancreatic lesions, but depends on the experience of the operator. In adults, pancreatic venous sampling is useful for defining focal lesions, but is technically difficult in infants and young children because of the small size of the vessels.[41a] Serum insulin measurements in hepatic vein samples after intraarterial injection of calcium may be the best technique currently available for defining focal lesions in children. However, the sensitivity and specificity of this procedure have not yet been clearly defined.

Hypoglycemia due to malicious insulin administration should be suspected if severe hypoglycemia is associated with very high serum insulin (>100 μU/mL) and is confirmed by finding concomitantly low or suppressed serum C-peptide levels.

## TREATMENT

The goal of therapy of the hyperinsulinemic hypoglycemia of infancy is to prevent hypoglycemia to protect the developing brain from possible damage, using a regimen that can be safely and effectively implemented at home. Successful treatment is defined by the following criteria: maintaining plasma glucose concentrations >60 mg/dL (>3.3 mmol/L) without intravenous infusions of glucose or glucagon, a feeding schedule appropriate for the age of the infant, and a fasting tolerance of 6 to 8 hours in the newborn infant, 12 hours in infants up to 1 year of age, or 16 hours or more in older children. Prompt effective treatment is necessary to minimize the risk of long-term adverse neurologic sequelae.[42] Initially, this requires a glucose infusion at two- to four-fold (average 14.5 ± 1.7 mg/kg per minute[43]) the basal rate of glucose production, and occasionally reaches 25 mg/kg per minute. Placement of a central venous line is usually necessary to be able to infuse hypertonic glucose solutions. Treatment with oral diazoxide, which opens normal $K_{ATP}$ channels and thereby suppresses insulin secretion, should be given a trial (15–25 mg/kg per day in 3 doses at 8-hour intervals). Its effect may be potentiated by the addition of a thiazide diuretic. Diazoxide is ineffective in infants whose hyperinsulinism is caused by mutations of the $K_{ATP}$ channel. A long-acting somatostatin analog (octreotide) may be successful in maintaining normoglycemia in up to 50% of cases of congenital hyperinsulinism. Octreotide inhibits insulin secretion by decreasing the influx of calcium ions into B cells and through a direct effect on secretory granules. The starting dose is 5 μg/kg every 6 to 8 hours. If glucose is not maintained (≥60 mg/dL), the dosage of octreotide is increased up to a maximum of 40 to 60 μg/kg per day, divided into three to six doses. Because of the marked variability of response to octreotide, the therapeutic regimen has to be adapted for each individual patient, and its effects closely monitored.[44] Many infants fail to respond to medical therapy and require a 95% subtotal pancreatectomy to restore normoglycemia.[45,45a]

## HORMONE DEFICIENCY

### ADRENOCORTICOTROPIC HORMONE/CORTISOL DEFICIENCY

Cortisol limits glucose utilization in several tissues, including skeletal muscle, by directly opposing the action of insulin and, secondarily, by promoting lipolysis. It stimulates protein breakdown and increases release of gluconeogenic precursors from muscle and fat. Cortisol stimulates hepatic gluconeogenesis and glycogen synthesis and exerts permissive influences on the gluconeogenic and glycogenolytic effects of glucagon and epinephrine. By all these effects, cortisol tends to raise plasma glucose concentrations.

Adrenocortical insufficiency should be considered in the differential diagnosis of patients who present with hypoglycemia and ketosis. In infancy, adrenocortical insufficiency may be secondary to congenital adrenal hyperplasia or congenital adrenal hypoplasia. In older children, adrenocortical insufficiency is more likely to be caused by Addison disease. Adrenocorticotropic hormone (ACTH) deficiency or panhypopituitarism can present with hypoglycemia in infancy or in later childhood.

**Diagnosis.** A serum cortisol concentration <10 μg/dL at the time of hypoglycemia should suggest the diagnosis. The diagnosis is confirmed by definitive tests that evaluate the hypothalamic–pituitary–adrenal axis.

**Treatment.** Treatment consists of physiologic replacement of cortisol; mineralocorticoid replacement is required in patients with salt wasting.

### HYPOPITUITARISM

GH decreases sensitivity to insulin, stimulates lipolysis, decreases glucose utilization, and supports glucose production. Congenital hypopituitarism often presents in the newborn period with hypoglycemia, persistent hyperbilirubinemia, and a microphallus. Approximately 20% of children with isolated GH deficiency or multiple anterior pituitary hormone deficiencies present with fasting hypoglycemia and ketosis. The occurrence of hypoglycemia in children with GH deficiency is inversely related to age.[46]

**Diagnosis.** Low serum GH and cortisol concentrations at the time of hypoglycemia suggest hypopituitarism. However, serum GH levels during spontaneous hypoglycemia do not correlate well with GH levels obtained by stimulation tests of pituitary GH secretory reserve. Therefore, a single low serum GH concentration cannot be relied on to make the diagnosis of GH deficiency.[47] Pituitary GH secretory reserve should be formally tested if there is any suspicion of GH insufficiency.

**Treatment.** Treatment of panhypopituitarism is with replacement of thyroxine, cortisol, and GH.

## DISORDERS OF GLYCOGEN SYNTHESIS, GLYCOGEN DEGRADATION, AND GLUCONEOGENESIS

### GLYCOGEN SYNTHETASE DEFICIENCY

Glycogen synthetase deficiency is a rare autosomal recessive disorder caused by mutations in the human liver glycogen synthase (GYS2) gene[48] on chromosome 12p12.2 resulting in lack of glycogen synthase activity in the liver. Because dietary carbohydrate cannot be stored as glycogen, glucose is preferentially converted to lactate. Severe fasting hypoglycemia and hyperketonemia characterize the disorder before breakfast, alternating with daytime hyperglycemia and hyperlactacidemia after meals. The glycogen content of the liver is markedly diminished; the liver is not enlarged. The disorder should be considered in children who have hypoglycemia and ketonuria before the first meal of the day[49] (Table 161-5).

The goal of treatment is to prevent periods of starvation with frequent feedings of a diet containing increased amounts of protein and correspondingly less carbohydrate during the day,[50] the former to provide substrate for gluconeogenesis and reduce the carbohydrate load, which causes hyperglycemia and hyperlactacidemia. At night, hypoglycemia is prevented by nighttime feedings of a suspension of uncooked cornstarch.[49]

### GLUCOSE-6-PHOSPHATASE DEFICIENCY

Glucose-6-phosphatase deficiency (type Ia glycogen storage disease) is an autosomal recessive disease that results from lack of glucose-6-phosphatase activity, the enzyme that catalyzes the final step in the production of glucose from glucose-6-phosphate.[51] Glucose production both from glycogenolysis and gluconeogenesis is severely impaired, resulting in postprandial hypoglycemia and increased production of lactic acid, uric acid, free fatty acids, and triglycerides. Glycogen and fat accumulate in the liver, resulting in hepatomegaly and a protuberant abdomen (Fig. 161-2). Infants occasionally develop symptomatic hypoglycemia soon after birth; however, most are asymptomatic as long as they receive frequent feedings containing sufficient glucose to prevent hypoglycemia. Symptoms of hypoglycemia usually appear when the interval between feedings gradually increases and the infant begins to sleep through the night. Later in infancy, untreated patients tend to have a characteristic physical appearance due to a progressive decrease in linear growth, muscle wasting, delayed motor development, and the development of a cushingoid appearance. The kidneys are enlarged; renal tubular dysfunction and glomerular hyperfiltration are common in childhood. Increased urinary albumin excretion may be observed in adolescents. More severe renal injury (proteinuria, hypertension, decreased creatinine clearance) due to focal segmental glomerulosclerosis and interstitial fibrosis is common in young adults. Inadequate therapy causes pronounced retardation of physical growth and delay in the onset of puberty. Hepatic adenomas usually develop in the second and third decades of life, and may undergo malignant degeneration or hemorrhage. Patients with type Ib glycogen storage disease (caused by deficiency of the translocase function required to move glucose-6-phosphate across the microsomal membrane, where it is exposed to the hydrolytic function of the glucose-6-phosphatase enzyme system) have similar symptoms. In addition, they have either constant or cyclic neutropenia with an increased frequency of staphylococcal and candidal infections. Neutropenia is a consequence of disturbed myeloid maturation and is accompanied by functional defects of circulating neutrophils and monocytes. Some patients develop an inflammatory bowel disease resembling Crohn disease.

**Diagnosis.** In infancy, severe hypoglycemia accompanied by marked hyperlactacidemia develops 3 to 4 hours after a feed. The serum is often cloudy or milky with very high triglyceride and moderately increased levels of cholesterol. Serum uric acid is increased and serum aspartate aminotransferase (AST) and alanine aminotransferase (ALT) levels are moderately elevated. Glucagon causes either no increase or only a small increase in blood glucose, whereas the already elevated blood lactate level increases further. Assay of glucose-6-phosphatase on a frozen liver biopsy specimen confirms the enzyme abnormality causing type I glycogen storage disease. Mutational analysis can be used to confirm the diagnosis in a high proportion of patients.

**Treatment.** Treatment consists of providing a continuous dietary source of glucose at a rate that maintains the blood glucose level above the threshold for activating glucose counterregulation, ~70 mg/dL. The amount of glucose required varies

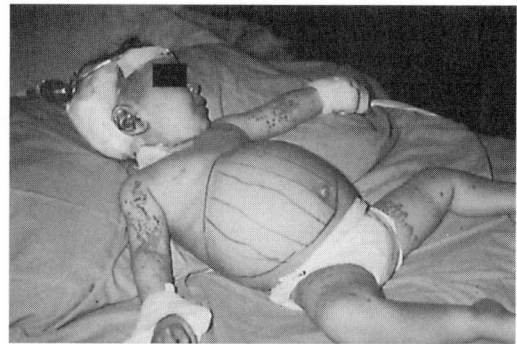

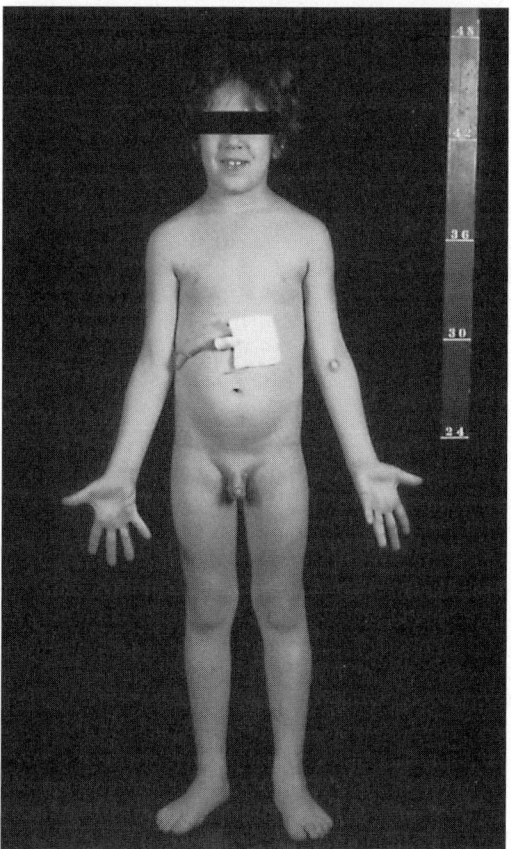

**FIGURE 161-2. A,** A child age 25 months with untreated type Ia glycogen storage disease with failure to thrive (length and weight <3rd percentile), a markedly protuberant abdomen with hepatomegaly, and eruptive xanthomas (serum triglycerides 12,300 mg/dL) on the arms and legs. **B,** The same child at age 7.5 years after nearly 3 years of continuous glucose therapy (frequent feeds supplemented with oral glucose at 2- to 3-hour intervals during the day and overnight intragastric glucose infusion via a gastrostomy). Growth is normal (height and weight >50th percentile); liver size has decreased, abdomen is less protuberant, and serum triglyceride concentration is reduced to within the normal range.

among patients, but can be approximated, initially, by using the formula for calculating basal glucose production rate: $y = 0.0014x^3 - 0.214x^2 + 10.411x - 9.084$, where y = mg glucose per minute, and x = body weight in kg.[2] Glucose itself or glucose-containing polymers can be given intermittently during the day and continuously (via a nasogastric tube or gastrostomy) at night. Alternatively, after 6 to 8 months of age, intermittent feedings of uncooked cornstarch can be used as the source of continuous glucose administration. Orally administered uncooked or raw cornstarch appears to act as an intestinal reservoir of glucose that is slowly absorbed into the circulation. It is given in a

slurry of water or artificially flavored drink (or in milk or formula for infants) at 3- to 5-hour intervals during the day and 4- or 5-hour intervals overnight.[52,53]

## AMYLO-1,6-GLUCOSIDASE DEFICIENCY (TYPE III GLYCOGEN STORAGE DISEASE; GLYCOGEN DEBRANCHER ENZYME DEFICIENCY)

The glycogen debrancher enzyme (GDE) gene is on chromosome 1p21.[54] The disorder is transmitted as an autosomal recessive trait. In the absence of GDE activity, breakdown of glycogen can only proceed until the outermost branch points are reached. Approximately 80% of patients with GSD III lack GDE activity (deficiency of transferase and glucosidase activities) in both liver and muscle (GSD IIIa)[55] and show clinical evidence of hepatic dysfunction and myopathy. Approximately 15% of patients have GDE deficiency only in the liver (GSD IIIb).[55] In rare cases, selective loss of only one of the two GDE activities (glucosidase [type IIIc], or transferase [type IIId]) has been demonstrated.[56,57] GSD types IIIa and IIIb have different prognoses and outcomes. Myopathy and cardiomyopathy are common in GSD IIIa and can lead to early death or debilitation in adult life. Muscle involvement can be inferred from very high levels of plasma creatine kinase (CK). Definitive subtyping of GSD III requires both liver and muscle biopsy.

Several distinct clinical features distinguish type III from type I GSD. Because glucose can be produced from 1,4 segments beyond the outermost branch points and from gluconeogenesis, patients with GDE deficiency are able to tolerate longer periods of fasting and develop less severe hypoglycemia than patients with glucose-6-phosphatase deficiency. Infants who are fed frequently may not have symptoms. Fasting causes hypoglycemia with ketosis (as a result of an accelerated transition to the starving state),[58] mild hypercholesterolemia, and hypertriglyceridemia, without elevation of blood lactate and serum uric acid levels. Liver enzymes (AST, ALT, alkaline phosphatase, lactic acid dehydrogenase [LDH]) are consistently elevated in children, but decline at puberty concomitant with a decrease in liver size[59] and may be normal in adults. Often, the presenting clinical finding is growth failure and hepatomegaly, which may be associated with an enlarged spleen that develops at 4 to 6 years of age in patients who have hepatic fibrosis. The kidneys are not enlarged; renal dysfunction does not occur. Untreated infants and children have a decreased rate of linear growth and puberty is delayed. Although muscle is involved in ~85% of patients with GSD III, weakness is usually not clinically significant. A subset of patients primarily manifest myopathic symptoms, and myopathy may be progressive. Abnormal glycogen (limit dextrin) may also accumulate in the heart.[60] Subclinical evidence of cardiac involvement is seen in the form of ventricular hypertrophy on electrocardiography (ECG), and abnormal echocardiographic findings are common.[61] Some patients develop a cardiomyopathy similar to hypertrophic obstructive cardiomyopathy. Hepatic adenomas occur less frequently in GSD III than in GSD I, and the transformation of an adenoma into a hepatocellular carcinoma is rare. With the exception of myopathy, symptoms and signs characteristically ameliorate with increasing age. The size of the liver tends to decrease to normal during puberty; however, most patients show hepatic fibrosis on biopsy, and some adult patients develop cirrhosis and its complications.[62]

**Diagnosis.** Administration of glucagon after an overnight fast does not cause the low blood glucose or normal blood lactate levels to increase. When glucagon is given 2 hours after a high-carbohydrate meal, which lengthens the outer branches of glycogen, a glycemic response occurs. Definitive diagnosis is obtained by enzyme assay on liver and muscle (if serum CK is abnormally increased).

**Treatment.**    As in type I GSD, continuous provision of an adequate amount of glucose, using uncooked cornstarch, combined with a normal intake of total calories, protein, and other nutrients, corrects the clinical and biochemical disorder and restores normal growth.[63,64] Raw cornstarch has been used both as initial treatment and in subjects previously treated by other means.[63] A dose of 1.75 g/kg at 6-hour intervals maintains normoglycemia, increases growth velocity, and decreases serum aminotransferase concentrations.[64]

For type III patients who have significant growth retardation and myopathy, continuous nocturnal feeding of a nutrient mixture composed of glucose, glucose oligosaccharides, and amino acids (Vivonex) and intermittent daytime feedings high in protein may result in clinical improvement.[65] The composition of the diet should be ~55% to 60% carbohydrate, 15% to 20% protein, and 20% to 30% fat. Milk products and fruits can be allowed without restriction, as galactose and fructose can be normally converted into glucose.

## HEPATIC GLYCOGEN PHOSPHORYLASE DEFICIENCY

The GSDs associated with a reduction in liver phosphorylase activity are a heterogeneous group of disorders that include autosomal recessive liver glycogen phosphorylase deficiency (type VI or Hers disease), an autosomal recessive phosphorylase kinase (PHK) b deficiency (type VIII), and X-linked phosphorylase kinase deficiency (type IX). They are all mild forms of hepatomegalic glycogenosis without hyperlactacidemia or hyperuricemia.

These disorders present in infancy or early childhood and are characterized by mild to moderate hypoglycemia, ketosis, growth retardation, and prominent hepatomegaly. Blood levels of lactic acid and uric acid are normal. The heart and skeletal muscles are not affected. The clinical course is benign. Symptoms remit and hepatomegaly decreases at puberty. The prognosis is excellent.

## PHOSPHORYLASE KINASE DEFICIENCY

PHK deficiency accounts for ~25% of all cases of GSD and occurs with a frequency of ~1 in 100,000 births.[51,66] X-linked liver glycogenosis (XLG) is the most common type of PHK deficiency and usually is a mild disease. Patients seldom have symptomatic hypoglycemia during infancy unless they fast for a prolonged period of time. Fasting can cause hyperketosis similar to, but usually milder than, that seen in type III GSD. Metabolic acidosis is rare. The disorder is usually discovered in early childhood when an enlarged liver and protuberant abdomen are noted during a physical examination. Physical growth may be retarded, and motor development may be delayed as a consequence of muscular hypotonia in the rare case with reduced enzyme activity in muscle as well as liver. Hypoglycemia is unusual and the blood lactate and uric acid levels are normal. Mild hypertriglyceridemia, hypercholesterolemia, and elevated serum AST and ALT levels may be present. Functional tests are not especially useful in evaluating these patients. The administration of glucagon after an overnight fast usually elicits a brisk glycemic response without a rise in the blood lactate level. The glycemic response to glucagon cannot be used to distinguish between phosphorylase kinase deficiency and lack of phosphorylase itself. With increasing age, clinical and biochemical abnormalities gradually disappear, and most adult patients are asymptomatic despite persistent PHK deficiency.

**Diagnosis.**    Liver phosphorylase deficiency can be difficult to diagnose biochemically and difficult to differentiate from the more common deficiency of the activating enzyme, phosphorylase kinase. Mutation analysis may aid in the laboratory diagnosis of deficiencies of the liver phosphorylase system. Definitive diagnosis of PHK b deficiency requires demonstration of the enzymatic defect in affected tissues.

**Treatment.**    Most patients do not require treatment. For the minority of patients prone to fasting hypoglycemia during childhood, a late-night snack usually will suffice to prevent morning hypoglycemia. The enlarged liver regresses when patients reach puberty. Uncooked cornstarch given at night has been beneficial in preventing hypoglycemia and ketosis in the unusual patient who experiences overnight hypoglycemia and ketosis.[67]

## DEFECTS IN GLUCONEOGENESIS

Deficiency of any of the key gluconeogenic enzymes, pyruvate carboxylase, phosphoenolpyruvate carboxykinase, fructose-1,6-bisphosphatase, and glucose-6-phosphatase severely impairs gluconeogenesis and causes hypoglycemia accompanied by hyperlactacidemia.

The biochemical abnormalities caused by fructose-1,6-bisphosphatase deficiency are similar to those for glucose-6-phosphatase deficiency. Hypoglycemia occurs during fasting and is associated with ketosis, hypertriglyceridemia, and hyperuricemia. Hepatomegaly is caused by fatty infiltration of the liver.

**Diagnosis.**    Diagnosis is based on demonstrating decreased enzyme activity in the liver.

**Treatment.**    Treatment consists of eliminating dietary fructose and sucrose and avoiding prolonged fasts. During intercurrent illness, intravenous glucose must be given to arrest catabolism.

## GALACTOSEMIA

Galactosemia is caused by deficiency of galactose-1-phosphate uridyl transferase. Hypoglycemia occurs following ingestion of galactose (contained in milk). Hypoglycemia has been attributed to inhibition of glycogenolysis.[68] Patients may present with neonatal sepsis, diarrhea, vomiting, failure to thrive, hepatomegaly, jaundice, ascites, cataracts, and mental retardation. The urine contains a reducing substance that is not glucose.

**Diagnosis.**    Diagnosis is confirmed by identifying a marked increase in blood levels of galactose and galactose-1-phosphate and near-absent galactose-1-phosphate uridyl transferase activity in red blood cells.

**Treatment.**    Treatment consists of eliminating galactose from the diet.

## HEREDITARY FRUCTOSE INTOLERANCE

Hereditary fructose intolerance is caused by deficiency of fructose-1-phosphate aldolase. It usually presents after the introduction of a commercial formula containing sucrose (e.g., Isomil) or at the time of weaning after ingestion of fructose or sucrose for the first time. Fructose causes vomiting, diarrhea, and hypoglycemia. Chronic exposure to fructose causes hepatomegaly, jaundice, failure to thrive, and renal tubular dysfunction with aminoaciduria. Fructose-1-phosphate accumulates in the liver and acutely inhibits glycogenolysis and gluconeogenesis.[69,69a]

**Diagnosis.**    The diagnosis is suggested by fructosuria after meals; a fructose tolerance test results in hypoglycemia.

**Treatment.**    Treatment consists of eliminating fructose from the diet.

## DEFECTS OF CARNITINE METABOLISM AND FATTY ACID β-OXIDATION

Disorders of carnitine metabolism and fatty acid β-oxidation are characterized by impaired ability to metabolize free fatty acids to acetyl coenzyme A (CoA) in various tissues and to synthesize ketones in the liver (Fig. 161-3). Their clinical manifesta-

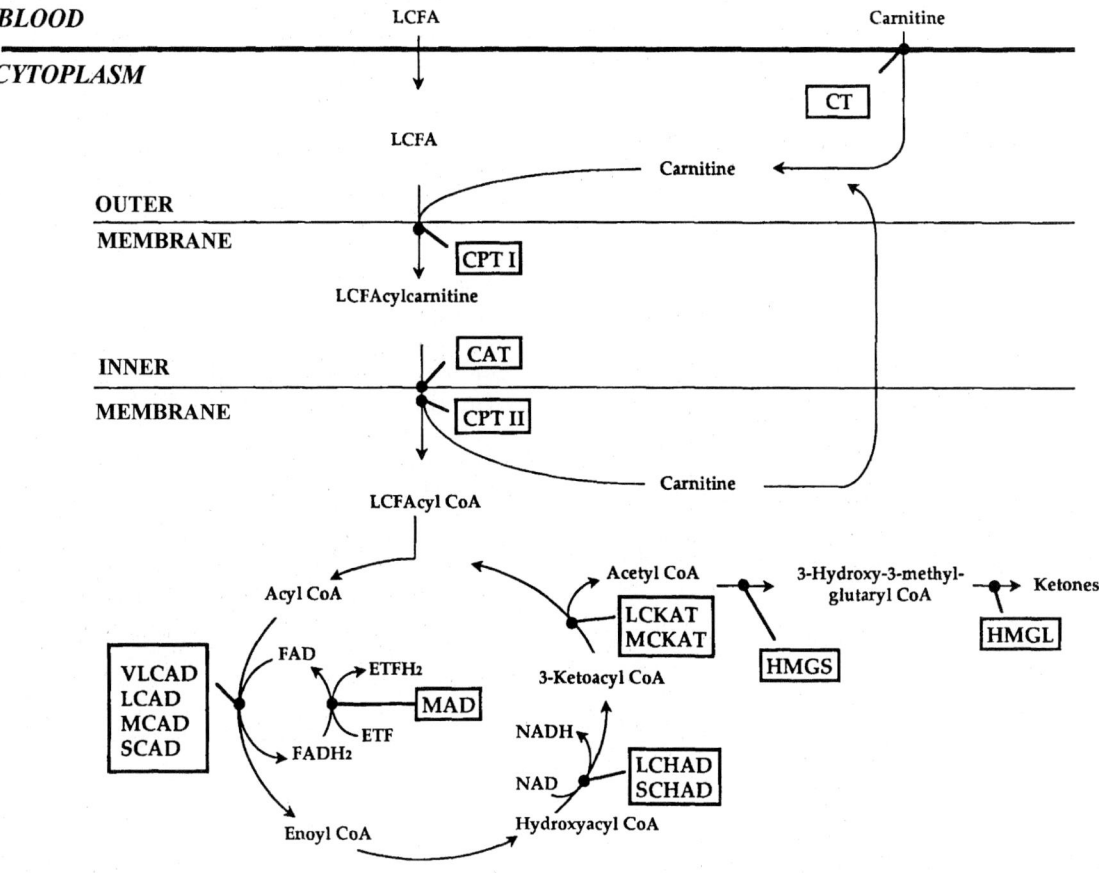

## MITOCHONDRION

**FIGURE 161-3.** Carnitine metabolism and fatty acid β-oxidation with reactions associated with known metabolic defects highlighted. (*LCFA*, long-chain fatty acid; *CT*, carnitine transporter; *CPT I*, carnitine palmitoyltransferase I; *CAT*, carnitine-acylcarnitine translocase; *CPT II*, carnitine palmitoyltransferase II; *MAD*, multiple acyl coenzyme A [CoA] dehydrogenase; *VLCAD*, very long-chain acyl CoA dehydrogenase; *LCAD*, long-chain acyl CoA dehydrogenase; *MCAD*, medium-chain acyl CoA dehydrogenase; *SCAD*, short-chain acyl CoA dehydrogenase; *LCHAD*, long-chain hydroxyacyl CoA dehydrogenase; *SCHAD*, short-chain hydroxyacyl CoA dehydrogenase; *LCKAT*, long-chain 3-ketoacyl CoA thiolase; *MCKAT*, medium-chain 3-ketoacyl CoA thiolase; *HMGS*, 3-hydroxy-3-methylglutaryl CoA synthetase; *HMGL*, 3-hydroxy-3-methylglutaryl CoA lyase; *NAD*, nicotinamide adenine dinucleotide; *NADH*, nicotinamide adenine dinucleotide [reduced form]; *FAD*, flavin adenine dinucleotide, *ETF*, electron transfer flavoprotein.)

tions typically appear during periods of catabolic stress and/or reduced calorie consumption such as occurs during an intercurrent illness.[70] The clinical features of these disorders are summarized in Tables 161-7 and 161-8. Symptoms of an acute metabolic crisis include nausea and/or vomiting, lethargy or frank coma, seizures, or sudden death.[70,71] Symptoms may appear gradually as the patient becomes increasingly dependent on fat as a source of energy. Alternatively, a crisis may be more dramatic, as when a child cannot be roused from sleep. In disorders associated with hyperammonemia, the presentation may resemble Reye syndrome.

Presentation as an acute encephalopathy is common in all the disorders that present in infancy and childhood.[71] The adult myopathic presentations of carnitine palmitoyltransferase (CPT) II, very long-chain acyl CoA dehydrogenase (VLCAD), and long-chain hydroxyacyl CoA dehydrogenase (LCHAD) deficiency usually do not manifest as alterations in mental status.

Hepatomegaly and liver dysfunction are common during episodes of acute decompensation.[70,71] The micro- and macrovesicular steatosis of the liver and other tissues (muscle, heart, and kidney) can resemble the fat accumulation in the liver that is characteristic of Reye syndrome. Mitochondria may be abnormal in shape and size in both disorders. In fatty acid oxidation defects electron microscopy reveals dense condensation of mitochondria with inclusion bodies, in contrast to the mitochondrial swelling seen in Reye syndrome.[72]

Patients with defects in carnitine transport and metabolism (other than CPT I deficiency) or in the oxidation of longer-chain fatty acids (long-chain acyl CoA dehydrogenase [LCAD], VLCAD, LCHAD, multiple acyl CoA dehydrogenase [MAD] deficiency) may have hypertrophic or dilated cardiomyopathy.[70,71,73] Symptoms are generally those of congestive heart failure or cardiovascular arrest. Arrhythmias have also been described.

The most severe cases present in the neonatal period. Neonatal MAD deficiency (glutaric acidemia type II) and CPT II deficiency may have dysmorphic features, developmental malformations of the brain (defects in neuronal migration), renal cysts, severe liver dysfunction or even cirrhosis, metabolic acidosis, hyperammonemia, and hypoglycemia. Severely affected infants usually die within days after birth.[74,75]

Patients who present at an older age with CPT II, VLCAD, and LCHAD deficiency may have rhabdomyolysis with severe muscle pain and myoglobinuria after strenuous activity. Chronic muscle weakness is less common.

**TABLE 161-7.**
**Disorders of Carnitine Metabolism**[70,71]

| Enzyme Deficiency | CT | CAT | CPT I | CPT II |
|---|---|---|---|---|
| **CLINICAL** | | | | |
| Fasting intolerance | + | + | + | + |
| Acute episodes | + | + | + | + |
| Coma/seizures | + | + | + | + |
| Muscle weakness/ myopathy | + | + | | +A |
| Muscle pain/myoglo- binuria | | | | +A |
| Cardiomyopathy/ arrhythmia | + | + | | + |
| Hepatopathy | + | + | + | + |
| Nephropathy | | | + | |
| Congenital anomalies | | | | + |
| **BIOCHEMICAL** | | | | |
| Hypoglycemia* | + | + | + | + |
| Ketones | Low | Low | Low | Low |
| Ammonia* | High | High | High | High |
| AST, ALT* | Abnl. | Abnl. | Abnl. | Abnl. |
| Plasma carnitine* | Very low | Low/ normal | High/ normal | Low/nor- mal |
| Dicarboxylic aciduria | No | +/− | No | No |
| Other abnormal organic acids | No | No | No | No |

*CT*, carnitine transporter; *CAT*, carnitine-acylcarnitine translocase; *CPT I*, carnitine palmitoyltransferase I; *CPT II*, carnitine palmitoyltransferase II; *+A*, adult presentation; *AST*, aspartate aminotransferase; *ALT*, alanine aminotransferase; *Abnl.*, abnormal.
*May be normal.

Approximately 5% of cases of sudden infant death syndrome (SIDS) are believed to be caused by defects in carnitine transport and/or fatty acid oxidation, including deficiencies of medium-chain acyl CoA dehydrogenase (MCAD), VLCAD, LCHAD, MAD.[76]

The characteristic biochemical features of disorders of carnitine metabolism and fatty acid oxidation are summarized in Tables 161-7 and 161-8. Acute metabolic crises are frequently, but not invariably, associated with hypoglycemia and metabolic acidosis. Hypoglycemia results from increased utilization of glucose in the absence of an alternative energy source and impaired gluconeogenesis. Metabolic acidosis is accompanied by an increased anion gap. Mild to marked hyperammonemia may occur as a result of secondary inhibition of *n*-acetylglutamate synthesis in the urea cycle. Hepatic dysfunction generally manifests with increases in serum AST and ALT concentrations, and when muscle is affected—especially in the older-onset cases of deficiencies of CPT II, VLCAD, and LCHAD—serum CK increases during symptomatic episodes. The cause of the increased serum uric acid level is unclear.

Urinalysis shows an inappropriately low level of ketonuria relative to the duration of fasting and/or degree of hypoglycemia. Ketones are rarely completely absent from the urine. Note, however, that ketonuria is abundant in patients with defects limited to the oxidation of short-chain fatty acids (short-chain acyl CoA dehydrogenase [SCAD] and short-chain hydroxyacyl CoA dehydrogenase [SCHAD] deficiency). In these disorders, most of the long-chain fatty acid is oxidized to ketones without difficulty. Only the metabolism of the short-chain remnants is impaired.

Quantitative assays of the plasma carnitine concentration measure total carnitine as well as free carnitine and bound (or esterified) carnitine. Normally, the free fraction comprises ~80% of the total. Primary carnitine deficiency (carnitine transport defect) is rare. It is characterized by extremely low total and free carnitine levels in blood and urine (generally <10 μmol/L). Carnitine loading (e.g., 100 mg/kg) raises blood levels of carnitine but produces an inappropriate carnitinuria. Secondary carnitine deficiency is much more common. A low level of total plasma carnitine is usually the result of dietary carnitine deficiency in which the ratio of the free and esterified fractions to total carnitine generally remains normal. A low free/total carnitine ratio can occur as a result of physiologic ketosis (when acetyl CoA binds free carnitine to form acetylcarnitine) and with certain

**TABLE 161-8.**
**Disorders of Fatty Acid Oxidation**[70,71,75,86,87]

| Enzyme Deficiency | MAD | V/LCAD | MCAD | SCAD | LCHAD | SCHAD | KAT | HMGL |
|---|---|---|---|---|---|---|---|---|
| **CLINICAL** | | | | | | | | |
| Fasting intolerance | + | + | + | + | + | + | + | + |
| Acute episodes | + | + | + | + | + | + | + | + |
| Coma/seizures | + | + | + | + | + | + | + | + |
| Myopathy/weakness | + | +A | | +A | + | + | + | |
| Myoglobinuria/pain | | +A | | | + | + | | |
| Neuropathy | | + | | | + | | | |
| Retinopathy | | | | | + | | | |
| Cardiomyopathy | + | + | | | + | + | + | |
| Hepatopathy | + | + | + | + | + | + | + | + |
| Nephropathy | | + | | | | | | |
| Congenital anomalies | + | | | | | | | |
| **BIOCHEMICAL** | | | | | | | | |
| Hypoglycemia* | + | + | + | + | + | + | + | + |
| Ketones | Low | Low | Low | High | Low | High | Low | Low |
| Ammonia* | High | High | High | High | High | | High | High |
| AST, ALT* | Abnl. | Abnl. | Abnl. | Abnl. | Abnl. | Abnl. | Abnl. | Abnl. |
| Plasma carnitine* | Low | Low | Low | Low | Low | Low | Low | Low |
| Dicarboxylic aciduria | Yes | Yes | Yes | Yes | Yes | Yes | Yes | No |
| Other abnormal organic acids | Yes | Yes | Yes | Yes | Yes | Yes | Yes | Yes |

*+A*, adult presentation; *MAD*, multiple acyl coenzyme A (CoA) dehydrogenase; *V/LCAD*, very long/long-chain acyl CoA dehydrogenase; *MCAD*, medium-chain acyl CoA dehydrogenase; *SCAD*, short-chain acyl CoA dehydrogenase; *LCHAD*, long-chain hydroxyacyl CoA dehydrogenase; *SCHAD*, short-chain hydroxyacyl CoA dehydrogenase; *KAT*, 3-ketoacyl CoA thiolase; *HMGL*, 3-hydroxy-3-methylglutaryl CoA lyase; *Abnl.*, abnormal; *AST*, aspartate aminotransferase; *ALT*, alanine aminotransferase.
*May be normal.

medications (e.g., valproate binds carnitine to form valproylcarnitine). In disorders of fatty acid oxidation, carnitine binds with intermediate compounds in the pathway (e.g., octanoylcarnitine) resulting in decreased total and free carnitine and increased esterified fractions.

**Diagnosis.**    Analysis of urine organic acids by gas chromatography/mass spectrometry reveals the biochemical abnormalities most useful for diagnosis. The urinary excretion of ketones is reduced (except in SCAD and SCHAD deficiencies). In all defects characterized by impaired β-oxidation of fatty acids, intermediate compounds accumulate and undergo ω-oxidation, resulting in the production of dicarboxylic acids (adipic, suberic, and sebacic acids, corresponding to the saturated fatty acids hexanoate, octanoate, and decanoate, respectively). The excretion of dicarboxylic acids is not necessarily pathologic. This may occur to a limited degree during physiologic ketosis. Also, patients receiving medium-chain triglycerides (MCT) have dicarboxylic aciduria. Defects in carnitine transport and metabolism do not directly disrupt β-oxidation and are not generally associated with dicarboxylic aciduria. In 3-hydroxy-3-methyl-glutaryl CoA lyase deficiency, only adipic acid is found in urine during a metabolic crisis. Other metabolites in the organic acid analysis can help to identify the site of the metabolic block.

Glycine and carnitine are normal cellular constituents that displace CoA from organic acyl and fatty acyl intermediates, producing acylglycines and acylcarnitines, respectively. The former is analyzed in urine, the latter in plasma or in blood filter paper specimens. Certain compounds have a higher affinity for glycine, others for carnitine. The specific pattern of unusual compounds identified by these techniques, in concert with the urine organic acid findings, increases the likelihood of making a diagnosis. Quantitative free fatty acid profiles allow direct analysis of all fatty acid intermediates and may ultimately provide a more specific screen than the analysis of acylcarnitines and acylglycines. The importance of obtaining diagnostic specimens during the acute catabolic phase of an illness cannot be overstated. Once treatment is begun with oral and/or intravenous glucose, fatty acid flux through the defective pathway decreases and the characteristic biochemical abnormalities may not be evident by the time urine and blood samples are obtained.

There are several options for investigating the asymptomatic patient suspected of having a defect in carnitine metabolism or fatty acid oxidation: (a) Arrangements can be made for diagnostic blood and urine specimens to be obtained when the patient is under catabolic stress (e.g., during a fever or intercurrent illness); (b) the patient can be admitted to the hospital for a monitored fast[7,77]; (c) a supervised oral fat load is a useful test to identify defects involving longer-chain fatty acid metabolism[78]; (d) in all cases of suspected carnitine transport and fatty acid oxidation defects, but especially in very young patients or when it would be inappropriate for a patient to undergo a fast or a provocative study, skin fibroblasts may be obtained for fatty acid oxidation studies and direct enzyme analysis; and (e) mutational analysis can be performed for diseases with common mutations, for example, MCAD and LCHAD deficiency.

Several states in the United States and regions in Europe are using tandem mass spectrometry to screen for fatty acid oxidation disorders on filter paper blood specimens obtained during the newborn period.[79]

**Treatment.**    The specific treatment of diseases of carnitine metabolism and defects of fatty acid oxidation depends on the individual defect. For all disorders of fatty acid oxidation, the primary recommendation is to avoid prolonged fasting and ensure a regular feeding regimen when patients are at risk for acute decompensation. Provision of a continuous exogenous source of carbohydrate obviates dependence on fatty acids and ketones for energy. During intercurrent illnesses, or when calorie intake decreases for any reason, patients should be fed every 4 hours around the clock until a normal diet is resumed and symptoms of the illness abate. When nausea and vomiting prevent adequate consumption of food or fluids, a 10% glucose solution must be given intravenously at ~1.5 times the hepatic glucose production rate to stimulate insulin secretion and inhibit glucose counterregulation.

Dietary therapy for defects of fatty acid oxidation is controversial. For the well child older than 1 year of age, raw cornstarch (1–2 g/kg) at bedtime decreases the need for fatty acids as a source of energy. Restriction of fat has been used, but excessive restriction may lead to deficiencies of essential fatty acids. Supplemental dietary MCT allows ketone synthesis to occur in defects of long-chain fat oxidation. The availability of MCT as a substrate for energy may be beneficial even during an acute metabolic crisis.

Carnitine supplementation (100 mg/kg per day) is indicated for carnitine transport defects; however, it is unclear whether carnitine supplementation is beneficial for other defects of fatty acid oxidation. It is postulated that carnitine displaces CoA bound to toxic intermediates. The liberated CoA is free to participate in other metabolic reactions, allowing excretion of the acyl-carnitines. Long-chain acylcarnitines may be toxic.[71]

Patients with later-onset MAD deficiency (i.e., glutaric acidemia type II) may respond to high-dose (100–200 mg per day) riboflavin supplementation.

Because defects in carnitine metabolism and fatty acid oxidation may be asymptomatic, the siblings of probands should be screened and parents should be counseled regarding the autosomal recessive pattern of inheritance of these diseases. Prenatal diagnosis may be available depending on the specific disorder under consideration.

### DEFECTS IN AMINO-ACID METABOLISM

Hypoglycemia associated with ketoacidosis occurs in maple syrup urine disease (branched-chain ketoaciduria), which is caused by deficiency of the branched-chain ketoacid dehydrogenase complex. The levels of the branched-chain amino acids (leucine, isoleucine, and valine), particularly leucine, are elevated in plasma, and the urine contains large amounts of branched-chain ketoacids that impart the odor of maple syrup.[80] The odor is also particularly noticeable in cerumen. Gluconeogenesis is also impaired in methylmalonic acidemia, a defect in the intermediary metabolism of methionine, threonine, isoleucine, valine, and odd-chain fatty acids caused by deficiency of methylmalonyl-CoA mutase.[81] Hypoglycemia is also observed in infants with propionic acidemia and 3-methylcrotonyl CoA carboxylase deficiency, defects in amino-acid intermediary metabolism.

**Treatment.**    Treatment consists of a diet restricted in the precursors to the enzyme defect, avoidance of and aggressive treatment of catabolic states, and supplementation with carnitine and vitamin cofactors.

## DETERMINING THE CAUSE

The cause of hypoglycemia is often readily apparent, for example, in the child with type 1 diabetes mellitus treated with insulin or when hypoglycemia occurs in a child with fulminant hepatitis or Reye syndrome. When the cause of hypoglycemia is not obvious, following the diagnostic approach outlined below will usually lead to the specific etiology. Determining the cause begins with a detailed history and physical examination. Important features of the history and physical examination are shown in Tables 161-9 and 161-10. Hypoglycemia within the first few

**TABLE 161-9.**
**History**

Birth weight, gestational age, maternal health and medications
Symptoms of hypoglycemia at birth or during neonatal period
Prolonged neonatal jaundice
Age at onset of symptoms
Family history of hypoglycemia
History of consanguinity
Frequency of hypoglycemia
Temporal relationship to feedings
    <4 h suggests a defect in glycogenolysis or hyperinsulinism
    10–12 h suggests a defect in gluconeogenesis or fatty acid β-oxidation
Specific content of feedings and relationship to onset of symptoms
Food intolerance or aversion
Unexplained infant deaths or sudden infant death syndrome (SIDS) in family; Reye syndrome, cardiomyopathy, myopathy
Potential drug exposure (oral hypoglycemic agents, insulin)
Hypoglycemia after an adult party ?alcohol ingestion
Recurrent "pneumonia"—episodes of hyperventilation from metabolic acidosis
Unusual odors, especially when sick

hours of life is usually seen in small-for-gestational-age infants and with transient hyperinsulinism caused by maternal diabetes mellitus. Hypoglycemia that presents shortly after birth and persists beyond 72 hours of life is characteristic of the persistent hyperinsulinemic hypoglycemia of infancy. Infants with hyperinsulinism who do not present in the newborn period usually present within the first 6 to 12 months of life. Hyperinsulinism

**TABLE 161-10.**
**Physical Examination**

| Examination | Possible etiology |
|---|---|
| Short stature; growth failure | GH deficiency, hypopituitarism |
| Microphallus | GH deficiency, hypopituitarism |
| Midline facial defects | GH deficiency, hypopituitarism |
|   Cleft lip and palate | |
|   Single central incisor | |
|   Optic nerve hypoplasia | |
| Abnormal skin pigmentation | Addison disease |
| Large liver | Glycogen storage disease |
| | Disorder of gluconeogenesis |
| | Galactosemia |
| | Disorder of fatty acid β-oxidation |
| | Disorder of carnitine metabolism |
| | Tyrosinemia type I |
| Macrosomia | Beckwith-Wiedemann syndrome |
|   Large tongue | |
|   Omphalocele/umbilical hernia | |
|   Visceromegaly | |
|   Horizontal grooves on ear lobes | |
| Hyperventilation | Metabolic acidosis, hyperammonemia |
| Odor | Maple syrup urine disease, isovaleric acidemia, 3-methylcrotonyl CoA carboxylase deficiency, multiple acyl CoA dehydrogenase deficiency (glutaric acidemia type II) |
| Heart | Disorder of fatty acid β-oxidation |
|   Gallop or murmur | Disorder of carnitine transport or metabolism |
|   Cardiomyopathy | |

*GH,* growth hormone; *CoA,* coenzyme A.

rarely presents for the first time in childhood or adolescence. When it does, one should suspect an islet cell adenoma (often part of multiple endocrine neoplasia type 1). GH and/or cortisol deficiency usually presents in the newborn period or in early childhood. Accelerated starvation usually presents at 18 months to 5 years old. Hepatomegaly, ketosis, and metabolic acidosis suggest an inborn error of metabolism, which may present either in the neonatal period or later in infancy, usually precipitated by cessation of overnight feeding or an infection that interrupts the child's normal feeding pattern and causes catabolic stress. A hypoketotic response to hypoglycemia indicates either a hyperinsulinemic state in which lipolysis and ketogenesis are inhibited or a defect in carnitine metabolism or fatty acid β-oxidation. In the latter, liberation of free fatty acids is unimpaired but ketone formation is disrupted.

## EVALUATION OF RESPONSE TO THERAPY AND LABORATORY EVALUATION

Glucose meters are widely used in newborn nurseries and in emergency departments to screen for hypoglycemia. These instruments are not consistently reliable at low blood glucose concentrations; therefore, any value <3.3 mmol/L (60 mg/dL) should be confirmed by a laboratory measurement of the plasma glucose concentration.[82] In addition, a simultaneous "critical" blood sample should be obtained for the measurement of hormones, metabolic substrates, and serum chemistries (Table 161-11). Immediately after the "critical" blood sample has been obtained, 0.3 g/kg glucose is injected intravenously over 10 minutes to restore a normal plasma glucose concentration. A continuous infusion of 10% dextrose solution at a rate of ~6 to 8 mg/kg per minute is given to maintain normoglycemia. This rate of glucose infusion is usually sufficient to reverse catabolism. The plasma glucose concentration is monitored and the infusion rate adjusted to maintain a level of ~80 mg/dL (4.5 mmol/L). Valuable diagnostic information can be obtained from the response to treatment. Infants and children with hyperinsulinism characteristically require considerably higher rates (14.5 ± 1.7 mg/kg per minute) of glucose infusion to prevent hypoglycemia.[43] In disorders of fatty acid oxidation, administration of glucose at ~1.5 times basal glucose production (10 mg/kg/minute) stimulates insulin secretion, inhibits lipolysis, and

**TABLE 161-11.**
**Laboratory Investigation of Unexplained Hypoglycemia**

| Blood | | | | |
|---|---|---|---|---|
| *Metabolites* | *Insulin Secretion* | *Counter-regulation* | *Fatty Acid Oxidation* | *Urine* |
| Glucose | Insulin | Growth hormone | Free fatty acids | Ketones |
| Lactate/pyruvate | C-peptide | Cortisol | Fatty acid profile | Reducing sugars |
| Amino acids (alanine) | Proinsulin | Glucagon | β-OHB | Organic acids |
| Uric acid | | Epinephrine | AcAc | Acylglycine |
| Serum electrolytes (anion gap) | | | Carnitine | |
| pH, bicarbonate | | | Acylcarnitines | |
| AST, ALT, CK | | | | |

*β-OHB,* β-hydroxybutyrate; *AcAc,* acetoacetate; *AST,* aspartate aminotransferase; *ALT,* alanine aminotransferase; *CK,* creatine kinase.

reverses the acute metabolic disorder and leads to a decrease in liver size to normal over several days.

The first urine sample obtained after the episode of hypoglycemia should be tested for the presence of ketones (ketotic vs. nonketotic hypoglycemia), reducing sugars (suggest galactosemia or fructose intolerance), and glucose (using a glucose-specific method). An aliquot should be saved and frozen for possible later analysis of amino acids, organic acids, and acylglycines after the initial laboratory investigations have been completed.

The initial laboratory evaluation should include measurement of serum insulin to determine whether the hypoglycemia is associated with a normal (suppressed) or an inappropriately increased serum insulin concentration, and measurement of urinary ketones to determine if the hypoglycemia is associated with ketosis. Absence of urinary ketones or their presence in only trace or small amounts, that is, nonketotic or hypoketotic hypoglycemia, is characteristic of hyperinsulinism and disorders of carnitine metabolism and fatty acid oxidation and/or ketogenesis. The serum C-peptide concentration is low or undetectable when hyperinsulinism is caused by exogenous insulin administration. If the serum insulin concentration is appropriately suppressed ($<2 \mu U/mL$ with a highly sensitive insulin assay), the diagnosis is likely to be a disorder of fatty acid oxidation. Encephalopathy is common at the time of acute metabolic decompensation; the liver may be moderately enlarged from acute fatty infiltration (microvesicular steatosis), and liver enzymes (AST, ALT) and plasma ammonia levels are increased during acute episodes of catabolic stress.[70] If a disorder of fatty acid oxidation is suspected, plasma total and esterified carnitine, plasma (or filter paper) acylcarnitines,[83] and plasma free fatty acids should be measured, and urine analyzed for organic acids and acylglycines.[84]

Ketosis with hypoglycemia is a normal physiologic response to a falling blood glucose concentration. The differential diagnosis of the hypoglycemic child with an appropriately suppressed serum insulin concentration and ketosis (see Table 161-5) can be further delineated depending on whether the liver is large. Elevated levels of GH and cortisol exclude deficiency of these counterregulatory hormones and obviate the need for further testing. On the other hand, random values that appear to be inappropriately low during a spontaneous episode of hypoglycemia do not constitute definitive evidence of deficient secretion. Specific testing must be performed.

A large liver suggests a GSD or disorder of gluconeogenesis (e.g., fructose-1,6-bisphosphatase deficiency). The liver size is normal in patients with accelerated starvation, cortisol deficiency, GH deficiency, glycogen synthetase deficiency, maple syrup urine disease, and the other conditions listed in Table 161-5. Transient enlargement of the liver during an acute metabolic crisis can occur in organic acidemia, fatty acid oxidation defects, and disorders of carnitine metabolism; it results from acute fatty deposition in the cytosol associated with impaired mitochondrial function.

A specific diagnosis of the cause of the hypoglycemia usually is evident from the analysis of the results of the "critical" blood sample obtained at the time of hypoglycemia (see Table 161-11) and application of the diagnostic algorithm shown in Figure 161-4. However, if the laboratory data required to make a diagnosis are not available, it may be necessary to perform a comprehensive evaluation of intermediary metabolism by reproducing the conditions that caused the hypoglycemia. This involves measurement of hormones and metabolic substrates that reflect carbohydrate, fat, and amino-acid metabolism during a monitored fast of specified duration depending on the age of the child.[7,77] Fasting may be hazardous and can even be lethal in patients with a disorder of fatty acid oxidation. Before subjecting any child to a monitored fast, one should attempt to rule out a disorder of fatty acid oxidation by measuring nonfasting plasma acylcarnitines (by tandem mass spectrometry if available)[83] and urinary acylglycines.[84]

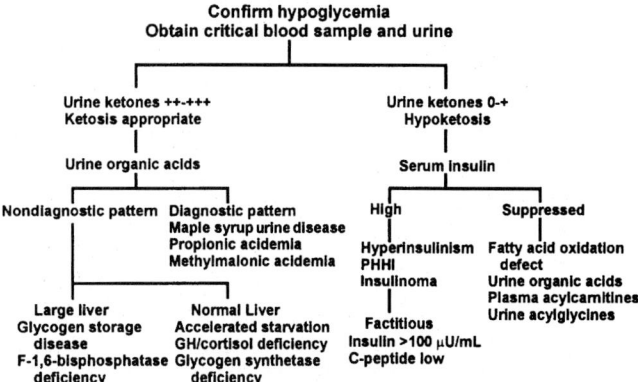

**FIGURE 161-4.** Algorithm for the evaluation of hypoglycemia. (*F-1,6-bisphosphatase*, fructose-1,6-bisphosphatase; *GH*, growth hormone; *PHHI*, persistent hereditary hyperinsulinemia of infancy.)

## REFERENCES

1. Sokoloff L. Circulation and energy metabolism of the brain. In: Siegel G, Agranoff B, Albers R, Molinoff P, eds. Basic neurochemistry. New York: Raven Press, 1989:565.
2. Bier DM, Leake RD, Haymond MW, et al. Measurement of "true" glucose production rates in infancy and childhood with 6,6-dideuteroglucose. Diabetes 1977; 26:1016.
3. Chaussain J. Glycemic response to 24 hour fast in normal children and children with ketotic hypoglycemia. J Pediatr 1973; 82:438.
4. Cryer P. Glucose metabolism and systemic glucose balance. In: Cryer P, ed. Hypoglycemia: pathophysiology, diagnosis, and management. New York: Oxford University Press, 1997:11.
5. Perriello G, Jorde R, Nurjhan N, et al. Estimation of glucose-alanine-lactate-glutamine cycles in postabsorptive humans: role of skeletal muscle. Am J Physiol 1995; 269:E443.
6. Wolfsdorf J, Sadeghi-Nejad A, Senior B. Fat derived fuels during a 24 hour fast in children. Eur J Pediatr 1982; 138:141.
7. Bonnefont J, Specola N, Vassault A, et al. The fasting test in paediatrics: application to the diagnosis of pathological hypo- and hyperketotic states. Eur J Pediatr 1990; 150:80.
8. Bougneres PF, Ferre P. Study of ketone body kinetics in children by a combined perfusion of 13C and 2H3 tracers. Am J Physiol 1987; 253:E496.
9. Settergren G, Lindblad B, Persson B. Cerebral blood flow and exchange of oxygen, glucose, ketone bodies, lactate, pyruvate, and amino acids in infants. Acta Paediatr Scand 1976; 65:343.
10. Hasselbalch SG, Knudsen GM, Jakobsen J, et al. Blood-brain barrier permeability of glucose and ketone bodies during short-term starvation in humans. Am J Physiol 1995; 268:E1161.
11. Cornblath M, Schwartz R, Aynsley-Green A, Lloyd J. Hypoglycemia in infancy: the need for a rational definition. Pediatrics 1990; 85:834.
12. Gregory J, Aynsley-Green A. The definition of hypoglycaemia. Baillière's Clin Endocrinol Metab 1993; 7:587.
13. Halamek L, Benaron D, Stevenson D. Neonatal hypoglycemia (Pt I): background and definition. Clin Pediatr 1997; 36:675.
14. Koh T, Eyre J, Aynsley-Green A. Neonatal hypoglycaemia—the controversy regarding definition. Arch Dis Child 1988; 63:1386.
14a. Cornblath M, Hawdon JM, Williams AF, et al. Controversies regarding definition of neonatal hypoglycemia: suggested operational thresholds. Pediatrics 2000; 105:1141.
15. Cornblath M, Schwartz R. Disorders of carbohydrate metabolism in infancy, 2nd ed. Philadelphia: WB Saunders, 1976.
16. Cornblath M, Reisner S. Blood glucose in the neonate and its clinical significance. N Engl J Med 1965; 273:378.
17. Srinivasan G, Pildes R, Cattamanachi G, et al. Plasma glucose values in normal neonates: a new look. J Pediatr 1986; 109:114.
18. Heck L, Erenberg A. Serum glucose levels in term neonates during the first 48 hours of life. J Pediatr 1987; 110:119.
19. Koh T, Aynsley-Green A, Tarbit M, Eyre J. Neural dysfunction during hypoglycaemia. Arch Dis Child 1988; 63:1353.
20. Schwartz N, Clutter W, Shah S, Cryer P. Glycemic thresholds for activation of glucose counterregulatory systems are higher than the threshold for symptoms. J Clin Invest 1987; 79:777.
21. Mitrakou A, Ryan C, Veneman T, et al. Hierarchy of glycemic thresholds for counterregulatory hormone secretion, symptoms, and cerebral dysfunction. Am J Physiol 1991; 260:E67.
22. Cryer P. Glucose counterregulation: the physiological mechanisms that prevent or correct hypoglycaemia. In: Frier B, Fisher B, eds. Hypoglycaemia and diabetes: clinical and physiological aspects. London: Edward Arnold, 1993:34.
23. Liu D, Moberg E, Kollind M, et al. Arterial, arterialized venous, venous and capillary blood glucose measurements in normal man during hyperinsulinemic euglycemia and hypoglycemia. Diabetologia 1992; 35:287.

24. Sperling M, Ganguli S, Leslie N, Landt K. Fetal-perinatal catecholamine secretion: role in perinatal glucose homeostasis. Am J Physiol 1984; 247:E69-74.

25. Hawdon J, Ward Platt M, Aynsley-Green A. Patterns of metabolic adaptation for preterm and term neonates in the first postnatal week. Arch Dis Child 1992; 67:357.

25a. Pal DK, Manandhar DS, Rajbhandari S, et al. Neonatal hypoglycemia in Nepal 1. Prevalence and risk factors. Arch Dis Child Fetal Neonatal Ed 2000; 82:F46.

26. Haymond MW, Pagliara AS. Ketotic hypoglycaemia. Clin Endocrinol Metab 1983; 12:447.

27. Wolfsdorf J, Sadeghi-Nejad A, Senior B. Hypoalaninemia and ketotic hypoglycemia: cause or consequence? Eur J Paediatr 1982; 138:28.

28. Hansen IL, Levy MM, Kerr DS. The 2-deoxyglucose test as a supplement to fasting for detection of childhood hypoglycemia. Pediatr Res 1984; 18:490.

29. Chaussain J, Georges P, Olive G, Job J. Glycemic response to a 24-hour fast in normal children and children with ketotic hypoglycemia. II. Hormonal and metabolic changes. J Pediatr 1974; 85:776.

30. Senior B. Ketotic hypoglycemia. J Pediatr 1973; 82:555.

31. Dahlquist G, Gentz J, Hagenfeldt L, et al. Ketotic hypoglycemia of childhood—a clinical trial of several unifying etiological hypotheses. Acta Paediatr Scand 1979; 68:649.

32. Pagliara A, Karl I, DeVivo D, et al. Hypoalaninemia: a concomitant of ketotic hypoglycemia. J Clin Invest 1972; 51:1440.

33. Thornton P, Sumner A, Ruchelli E, et al. Familial and sporadic hyperinsulinism: histopathology and segregation analysis support a single autosomal recessive disorder. J Pediatr 1991; 119:721.

33a. Glaser B, Thornton P, Otonkoski T, Junien C. Genetics of neonatal hyperinsulinism. Arch Dis Child Fetal Neonatal Ed 2000; 82:F79.

34. Thomas P, Cote G, Wohlik N, et al. Mutations in the sulfonylurea receptor gene in familial persistent hyperinsulinemic hypoglycemia of infancy. Science 1995; 268:426.

35. Thomas P, Ye Y, Lightner E. Mutations of the pancreatic islet inward rectifier Kir6.2 also lead to familial persistent hyperinsulinemic hypoglycemia of infancy. Hum Mol Genet 1996; 5:1809.

36. Dunne M, Kane C, Shepherd R, et al. Familial persistent hyperinsulinemic hypoglycemia of infancy and mutations in the sulfonylurea receptor. N Engl J Med 1997; 336:703.

37. Thornton PS, Satin-Smith MS, Herold K, et al. Familial hyperinsulinism with apparent autosomal dominant inheritance: clinical and genetic differences from the autosomal recessive variant. J Pediatr 1998; 132:9.

38. Glaser B, Kesavan P, Heyman M, et al. Familial hyperinsulinism caused by an activating glucokinase mutation. N Engl J Med 1998; 338:226.

39. Weinzimer S, Stanley C, Berry G, et al. A syndrome of congenital hyperinsulinism and hyperammonemia. J Pediatr 1997; 130:661-4.

40. Zammarchi E, Filippi L, Novembre E, Donati M. Biochemical evaluation of a patient with a familial form of leucine-sensitive hypoglycemia and concomitant hyperammonemia. Metabolism 1996; 45:957.

41. Stanley CA, Lieu YK, Hsu BY, et al. Hyperinsulinism and hyperammonemia in infants with regulatory mutations of the glutamate dehydrogenase gene. N Engl J Med 1998; 338:1352.

41a. de Lonlay-Debeney P, Poggi-Travert F, Fournet JC, et al. Clinical features of 52 neonates with hyperinsulinism. N Engl J Med 1999; 340:1169.

42. Aynsley-Green A, Polak J, Bloom S, et al. Nesidioblastosis of the pancreas: definition of the syndrome and the management of severe neonatal hyperinsulinemic hypoglycaemia. Arch Dis Child 1981; 56:496.

43. Antunes JD, Geffner ME, Lippe BM, Landaw EM. Childhood hypoglycemia: differentiating hyperinsulinemic from nonhyperinsulinemic causes. J Pediatr 1990; 116:105.

44. Thornton P, Alter C, Levitt Katz L, et al. Short- and long-term use of octreotide in the treatment of congenital hyperinsulinism. J Pediatr 1993; 123:637.

45. Spitz L, Bhargava RK, Grant DB, Leonard JV. Surgical treatment of hyperinsulinaemic hypoglycaemia in infancy and childhood. Arch Dis Child 1992; 67:201.

45a. Aynsley-Green A, Hussain K, Hall J, et al. Practical management of hyperinsulinism in infancy. Arch Dis Child Fetal Neonatal Ed 2000; 82:F98.

46. Wolfsdorf J, Sadeghi-Nejad A, Senior B. Hypoketonemia and age-related fasting hypoglycemia in growth hormone deficiency. Metabolism 1983; 32:457.

47. Aynsley-Green A, McGann A, Deshpande S. Control of intermediary metabolism in childhood with special reference to hypoglycaemia and growth hormone. Acta Paediatr Scand Suppl 1991; 377:43.

48. Orho M, Bosshard N, Buist N, et al. Mutations in the liver glycogen synthase gene in children with hypoglycemia due to glycogen storage disease type 0. J Clin Invest 1998; 102:507.

49. Gitzelmann R, Spycher M, Feil G, et al. Liver glycogen synthase deficiency: a rarely diagnosed entity. Eur J Pediatr 1996; 155:561.

50. Aynsley-Green A, Williamson DH, Gitzelmann R. The dietary treatment of hepatic glycogen synthetase deficiency. Helv Paediatr Acta 1977; 32:71.

51. Chen Y-T, Burchell A. Glycogen storage diseases. In: Scriver C, Beaudet A, Sly W, Valle D, eds. The metabolic and molecular bases of inherited disease, 7th ed. New York: McGraw-Hill; 1995:935.

52. Wolfsdorf JI, Plotkin RA, Laffel LMB, Crigler JF Jr. Continuous glucose for treatment of patients with type I glycogen-storage disease: comparison of the effects of dextrose and uncooked cornstarch on biochemical variables. Am J Clin Nutr 1990; 52:1043.

53. Wolfsdorf JI, Ehrlich S, Landy HS, Crigler JF Jr. Optimal daytime feeding regimen to prevent postprandial hypoglycemia in type 1 glycogen storage disease. Am J Clin Nutr 1992; 56:587.

54. Yang-Feng TL, Zheng K, Yu J, et al. Assignment of the human glycogen debrancher gene to chromosome 1p21. Genomics 1992; 13:931.

55. Brown B, Brown D. Glycogen storage diseases: types I, III, IV, V, VII and unclassified glycogenoses. In: Dickens F, Randle P, Whelan W, eds. Carbohydrate metabolism and its disorders. New York: Academic Press; 1968:123.

56. Ding JH, de Barsy T, Brown BI, et al. Immunoblot analyses of glycogen debranching enzyme in different subtypes of glycogen storage disease type III. J Pediatr 1990; 116:95.

57. Van Hoof F, Hers H. The subgroups of type III glycogenosis. Eur J Biochem 1967; 2:265.

58. Fernandes J, Pikaar NA. Ketosis in hepatic glycogenosis. Arch Dis Child 1972; 47:41.

59. Coleman RA, Winter HS, Wolf B, Chen YT. Glycogen debranching enzyme deficiency: long-term study of serum enzyme activities and clinical features. J Inherit Metab Dis 1992; 15:869.

60. DiMauro S, Hartwig GB, Hays A, et al. Debrancher deficiency: neuromuscular disorder in 5 adults. Ann Neurol 1979; 5:422.

61. Moses S, Wanderman K, Myroz A, Frydman M. Cardiac involvement in glycogen storage disease type III. Eur J Pediatr 1989; 148:764.

62. Markowitz AJ, Chen YT, Muenzer J, et al. A man with type III glycogenosis associated with cirrhosis and portal hypertension. Gastroenterology 1993; 105:1882.

63. Borowitz SM, Greene HL. Cornstarch therapy in a patient with type III glycogen storage disease. J Pediatr Gastroenterol Nutr 1987; 6:631.

64. Gremse DA, Bucuvalas JC, Balistreri WF. Efficacy of cornstarch therapy in type III glycogen storage disease. Am J Clin Nutr 1990; 52:671.

65. Slonim A, Weisberg C, Benke P, et al. Reversal of debrancher deficiency myopathy by the use of high-protein nutrition. Ann Neurol 1982; 11:420.

66. Kiliman MW. Glycogen storage disease due to phosphorylase kinase deficiency. In: Swallow DM, Edwards YH, eds. Protein dysfunction in human genetic disease. Oxford: BIOS Scientific, 1997:57.

67. Nakai A, Shigematsu Y, Takano T, et al. Uncooked cornstarch treatment for hepatic phosphorylase kinase deficiency. Eur J Pediatr 1994; 153:581.

68. Segal S, Berry G. Disorders of galactose metabolism. In: Scriver C, Beaudet A, Sly W, Valle D, eds. The metabolic and molecular basis of inherited disease, 7th ed. New York: McGraw-Hill, 1995:967.

69. Gitzelmann R, Steinmann B, Van den Berghe G. Disorders of fructose metabolism. In: Scriver C, Beaudet A, Sly W, Valle D, eds. The metabolic and molecular basis of inherited disease, 7th ed. New York: McGraw-Hill, 1995:905.

69a. Hillebrand G, Schneppenheim R, Oldigs HD, Santer R. Hereditary fructose intolerance and alpha (1) antitrypsin deficiency. Arch Dis Child 2000; 83:72.

70. Hale D, Bennett M. Fatty acid oxidation disorders: a new class of metabolic diseases. J Pediatr 1992; 121:1.

71. Roe C, Coates P. Mitochondrial fatty acid oxidation disorders. In: Scriver C, Beaudet A, Sly W, Valle D, eds. The metabolic and molecular bases of inherited disease, 7th ed. New York: McGraw-Hill; 1995:1501.

72. Treem WR, Witzleben CA, Piccoli DA, et al. Medium-chain and long-chain acyl CoA dehydrogenase deficiency: clinical, pathologic and ultrastructural differentiation from Reye's syndrome. Hepatology 1986; 6:1270.

73. Stanley C, DeLeeuw S, Coates P, et al. Chronic cardiomyopathy and weakness or acute coma in children with a defect in carnitine uptake. Ann Neurol 1991; 30:709.

74. North KN, Hoppel CL, De Girolami U, et al. Lethal neonatal deficiency of carnitine palmitoyltransferase II associated with dysgenesis of the brain and kidneys. J Pediatr 1995; 127:414.

75. Frerman F, Goodman S. Nuclear-encoded defects of the mitochondrial respiratory chain, including glutaric acidemia type II. In: Scriver C, Beaudet A, Sly W, Valle D, eds. The metabolic and molecular bases of inherited disease, 7th ed. New York: McGraw-Hill; 1995:1611.

76. Boles RG, Buck EA, Blitzer MG, et al. Retrospective biochemical screening of fatty acid oxidation disorders in postmortem livers of 418 cases of sudden death in the first year of life. J Pediatr 1998; 132:924.

77. Morris A, Thekekara A, Wilks Z, et al. Evaluation of fasts for investigating hypoglycaemia or suspected metabolic disease. Arch Dis Child 1996; 75:115.

78. Parini R, Garavaglia B, Saudubray JM, et al. Clinical diagnosis of long-chain acyl-coenzyme A-dehydrogenase deficiency: use of stress and fat-loading tests. J Pediatr 1991; 119:77.

79. Seymour CA, Thomason MJ, Chalmers RA, et al. Newborn screening for inborn errors of metabolism: a systematic review. Health Technol Assess 1997; 1:1.

80. Chuang D, Shih V. Disorders of branch chain amino acid and ketoacid metabolism. In: Scriver C, Beaudet A, Sly W, Valle D, eds. The metabolic and molecular basis of inherited disease, 7th ed. New York: McGraw-Hill; 1995:1239.

81. Haymond M, Ben-Galim E, Strobel K. Glucose and alanine metabolism in children with maple syrup urine disease. J Clin Invest 1978; 62:398.

82. Holtrop P, Madison K, Kiechle F, et al. A comparison of chromogen test strip (Chemstrip bG) and serum glucose values in newborns. Am J Dis Child 1990; 144:183.

83. Van Hove J, Zhang W, Kahler SG, et al. Medium-chain acyl-CoA dehydrogenase (MCAD) deficiency: diagnosis by acylcarnitine analysis in blood. Am J Hum Genet 1993; 52:958.

84. Rinaldo P, O'Shea J, Coates P, et al. Medium-chain acyl-CoA dehydrogenase deficiency. Diagnosis by stable isotope dilution measurement of urinary $n$-hexanoylglycine and 3-phenylpropionylglycine. N Engl J Med 1988; 319:1308.

85. Halamek L, Stevenson D. Neonatal hypoglycemia (Pt II): pathophysiology and therapy. Clin Pediatr 1997; 37:11.

86. Bennett MJ, Sherwood WG. 3-Hydroxydicarboxylic and 3-ketodicarboxylic aciduria in three patients: evidence for a new defect in fatty acid oxidation at the level of 3-ketoacyl-CoA thiolase. Clin Chem 1993; 39:897.

87. Kamijo T, Indo Y, Souri M, et al. Medium chain 3-ketoacyl-coenzyme A thiolase deficiency: a new disorder of mitochondrial fatty acid beta-oxidation. Pediatr Res 1997; 42:569.

# SECTION D

# LIPID METABOLISM

## CHAPTER 162

# BIOCHEMISTRY AND PHYSIOLOGY OF LIPID AND LIPOPROTEIN METABOLISM

ROBERT W. MAHLEY

## LIPIDS, LIPOPROTEINS, AND LIPID TRANSPORT

An efficient system for lipid transport is a prerequisite for normal metabolism in vertebrates. Most lipids are found in membranes, which maintain the integrity of cells and allow compartmentalization of the cytoplasm into specific organelles. Lipids also function as a major form of stored nutrients (e.g., triglycerides), as precursors for steroid hormones and bile acids (e.g., cholesterol), and as intracellular and intercellular messengers (e.g., prostaglandins, phosphatidylinositol).

Lipids are organic molecules that are insoluble or minimally soluble in water because of their hydrophobic nature. One class of lipids is fatty acids. There are numerous types of fatty acids, which differ in length and in the number and position of their double bonds. Fatty acids that lack double bonds are called *saturated*, and those with one or more double bonds are *unsaturated* or *polyunsaturated*. The most abundant saturated fatty acids are 16 and 18 carbons long and are referred to as *palmitic* and *stearic acids*, respectively. The common unsaturated fatty acids have one to three double bonds and are typically 16 to 20 carbons long. Linoleic acid, for example, has two double bonds and 18 carbons; linolenic acid has three double bonds and 18 carbons. Fatty acids are free (i.e., nonesterified) or esterified to other organic molecules. Free fatty acids are transported in the plasma bound to albumin and serve as a readily available form of energy or as a substrate for complex lipid biosynthesis.

There are three major classes of complex lipids: *triglycerides*, *cholesterol*, and *phospholipids*. The most abundant complex lipid is triglyceride (i.e., triacylglycerol), which serves as a storage form of fatty acids. Triglycerides consist of three fatty acid molecules esterified to one glycerol molecule. Glycerol esters containing one or two fatty acid molecules are called *monoglycerides* and *diglycerides*, respectively. Cholesterol, composed of a four-ring hydrocarbon and an eight-carbon side chain, is an important class of lipids that serves in membrane structure and as a precursor to steroid hormones and bile acids. In the blood, approximately two-thirds of the cholesterol is esterified to a fatty acid through the hydroxyl group at residue 3 of the cholesterol molecule to form cholesteryl ester. Phospholipids contain two fatty acids esterified to two of the three hydroxyl groups on glycerol. The third hydroxyl group is esterified to phosphate; this complex lipid is referred to as phosphatidic acid. Typically, in mammalian tissue, the phosphatidic acid is esterified to the hydroxyl group of a hydrophilic molecule, such as choline,

serine, or ethanolamine, forming phosphatidylcholine, phosphatidylserine, and phosphatidylethanolamine, respectively. The combination of hydrophobic and hydrophilic molecules in phospholipids allows them to function at water-lipid interfaces, making them ideal components of membranes and of surface coats of plasma lipoproteins.

Disorders in lipid transport, often reflected in changes in the quantity and structure of plasma lipoproteins, cause metabolic derangements that lead to several diseases. An understanding of the cause and treatment of these disorders requires a knowledge of the metabolism of the various plasma lipoproteins.

The principal sites of synthesis of plasma lipoproteins are the liver and the intestine. The plasma lipoproteins are water-soluble macromolecular complexes (i.e., pseudomicellar particles) of lipids (e.g., triglycerides, cholesterol, phospholipids) and one or more specific proteins, referred to as *apolipoproteins* or *apoproteins (apo)*. The apoprotein component of these complexes determines the fate of the various lipoproteins by targeting their delivery of lipid to specific cells. Generally, the nonpolar lipids (i.e., triglycerides and cholesteryl esters) are found in the center of the particles, surrounded by the more polar lipids (i.e., phospholipids and free cholesterol) and apoproteins.

Human plasma lipoproteins are commonly divided into six major classes, differentiated primarily by the *density* at which they float during ultracentrifugation. They are defined further on the basis of *particle size, electrophoretic mobility*, and *apoprotein content*. The major classes of lipoproteins and their roles in metabolism are listed in Table 162-1.[1,2]

## PLASMA LIPOPROTEINS: AN OVERVIEW

### CHYLOMICRONS AND CHYLOMICRON REMNANTS

Chylomicrons (density <0.95 g/mL) are synthesized by the small intestine to transport dietary triglyceride and cholesterol from the site of absorption by the intestinal epithelium to various cells of the body (Fig. 162-1). They are normally absent from the plasma after fasting overnight (12 hours). The triglycerides of these particles are hydrolyzed within the plasma compartment by the action of *lipoprotein lipase* (LPL), which is attached to the endothelial surfaces of capillaries, especially in adipose tissue, the heart, and skeletal muscle. The lipoprotein particles generated by the action of LPL on chylomicrons are referred to as *chylomicron remnants*. They are enriched in cholesterol (by virtue of the loss of triglyceride) and, under normal conditions, are rapidly cleared by the liver.

Chylomicron remnants, which accumulate in the plasma of animals whose diets are high in fat and cholesterol and in the plasma of patients with type III hyperlipoproteinemia (dysbetalipoproteinemia), have been linked to the development of accelerated atherosclerosis.[3,3a]

### VERY-LOW-DENSITY LIPOPROTEINS

Very-low-density lipoproteins (VLDL; density <1.006 g/mL) are synthesized by the liver to transport triglycerides and choles-

**TABLE 162-1.**
**Characterization of Plasma Lipoproteins**

| Class | Density of Flotation (g/mL) | Major Lipids | Major Apoproteins | Origins | Functions |
|---|---|---|---|---|---|
| **MAJOR CLASSES OF PLASMA LIPOPROTEINS** | | | | | |
| Chylomicrons | $d < 0.95$ | Triglyceride | B-48, A-I, A-IV (E and Cs by transfer from HDL) | Synthesized by small intestine | Transport of dietary triglyceride and cholesterol from the intestine to other tissues |
| Chylomicron remnants | $d < 0.95$ | Triglyceride, cholesterol | B-48, E | Derived from chylomicrons by lipase hydrolysis of triglyceride | Delivery of cholesterol to the liver; represent atherogenic lipoproteins |
| Very-low-density lipoproteins (VLDL) | $d < 1.006$ | Triglyceride | B-100, E, Cs | Synthesized by liver | Transport of triglyceride to peripheral tissues; free fatty acids liberated by lipase hydrolysis |
| Intermediate-density lipoproteins (IDL) | $d = 1.006–1.019$ | Triglyceride, cholesterol | B-100, E | Derived from VLDL by lipase hydrolysis of triglyceride | Precursor of LDL; a fraction is taken up by the liver |
| Low-density lipoproteins (LDL) | $d = 1.019–1.063$ | Cholesterol | B-100 | Derived from VLDL and IDL by lipase hydrolysis of triglyceride | Major carrier of cholesterol, which is utilized by peripheral tissue via LDL receptor–mediated uptake; correlates directly with accelerated coronary artery disease |
| High-density lipoproteins (HDL) | $d = 1.063–1.21$ | Phospholipid, cholesterol | A-I, A-II, Cs | Synthesized by liver and intestine; also derived from surface of chylomicrons and VLDL during lipolysis | Facilitate removal of cholesterol from peripheral tissues; redistribute cholesterol to other tissues and to the liver; HDL cholesterol correlates inversely with coronary artery disease |
| **SPECIALIZED CLASSES OF PLASMA LIPOPROTEINS** | | | | | |
| Lipoprotein (a) [Lp(a)] | $d = 1.05–1.12$ | Cholesterol | B-100, apo (a) | Apo (a) from the liver complexes with LDL | Concentration correlates directly with accelerated coronary artery disease |
| β-Very-low-density lipoproteins (β-VLDL) | | | | | |
| Fraction I | $d < 1.006$ | Triglyceride, cholesterol | B-48, E | Intestine | Chylomicron remnants; atherogenic lipoproteins |
| Fraction II | $d < 1.006$ | Triglyceride, cholesterol | B-100, E | Liver | VLDL remnants; atherogenic lipoproteins |

*Apo*, apolipoprotein.

terol from the hepatocytes to various tissues of the body (see Fig. 162-1). Within the plasma compartment, the triglycerides of VLDL are hydrolyzed by LPL and hepatic LPL, generating a series of smaller, cholesterol-enriched lipoproteins: *intermediate-density lipoproteins* (IDL; density = 1.006–1.019 g/mL) and *low-density lipoproteins* (LDL; density = 1.019–1.063 g/mL). Smaller

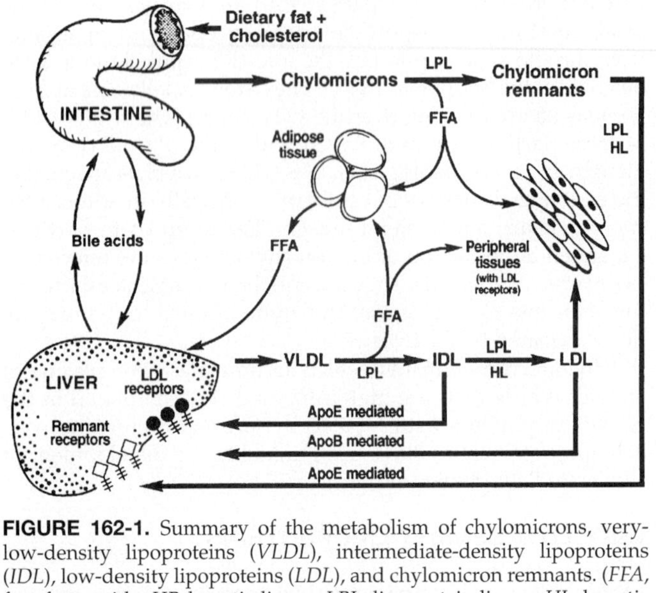

**FIGURE 162-1.** Summary of the metabolism of chylomicrons, very-low-density lipoproteins (*VLDL*), intermediate-density lipoproteins (*IDL*), low-density lipoproteins (*LDL*), and chylomicron remnants. (*FFA*, free fatty acids; *HP*, hepatic lipase; *LPL*, lipoprotein lipase; *HL*, hepatic lipase; *Apo*, apolipoprotein.)

VLDL and IDL, referred to as VLDL remnants, appear to be atherogenic lipoproteins.[3]

## LOW-DENSITY LIPOPROTEINS

LDL represent the end product of VLDL catabolism and are the major cholesterol-transporting lipoproteins in the plasma. Because of defective or absent LDL receptors in patients with familial hypercholesterolemia or defective apo B-100 in patients with familial defective apo B-100, LDL accumulate in the plasma at levels that correlate directly with the existence of accelerated coronary artery disease.[3–5]

## HIGH-DENSITY LIPOPROTEINS

High-density lipoproteins (HDL; density = 1.063–1.21 g/mL) originate from several sources: the liver, the intestine, and within the plasma compartment during lipolytic processing of chylomicrons and VLDL. The HDL participate in a process referred to as *reverse cholesterol transport*, a postulated pathway whereby HDL acquire cholesterol from peripheral tissues and transport the cholesterol, directly or indirectly, to the liver for excretion[1,1a] (Fig. 162-2). Observations suggesting an inverse correlation between HDL levels and atherosclerotic vascular disease in humans (i.e., low HDL levels associated with increased coronary artery disease) have focused attention on this lipoprotein class and its role in cholesterol metabolism. In humans, much of the cholesteryl ester present in the lipoproteins appears to be formed in plasma in association with HDL by the enzyme *lecithin:cholesterol acyltransferase* (LCAT).[6] This enzyme catalyzes the transfer of a fatty acid from phospholipid (i.e., lecithin) to the 3β-hydroxy position of cholesterol, forming

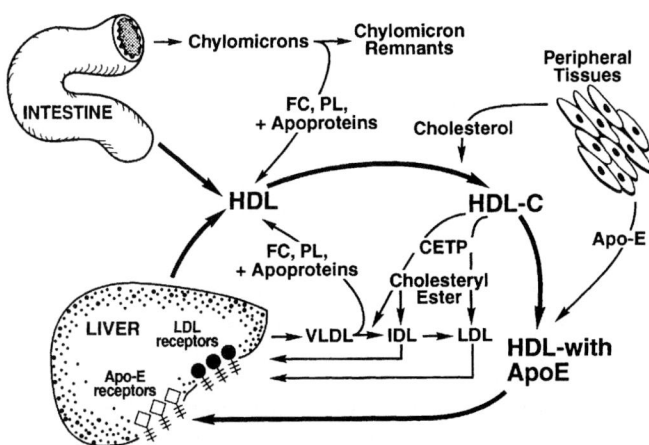

**FIGURE 162-2.** Summary of the metabolism of high-density lipoproteins (*HDL*). The HDL are formed by the intestine and liver and by the transfer of free cholesterol (*FC*), phospholipid (*PL*), and apoproteins from chylomicrons and very-low-density lipoproteins (*VLDL*) during lipolysis. The HDL can acquire cholesterol from various tissues possessing excess cholesterol (*HDL-C*). The E apoprotein produced by various cells in peripheral tissues is added to the HDL-C to form HDL with apo E. (*IDL*, intermediate-density lipoproteins; *LDL*, low-density lipoproteins; *CETP*, cholesteryl ester transfer proteins; *Apo*, apolipoprotein.)

a cholesteryl ester. The cholesteryl esters formed by this reaction are transferred to other lipoproteins by the cholesteryl ester transfer protein (CETP).[7]

## APOPROTEINS

The metabolism of the various plasma lipoproteins is regulated and directed by the presence of specific apoproteins that characterize each of the major lipoprotein classes. The characterization of the major apoproteins is listed in Table 162-2. To understand lipoprotein metabolism and the disease states associated with lipid abnormalities, it is necessary to consider functions that have been ascribed to specific apoproteins.

## TRANSPORT AND REDISTRIBUTION OF LIPIDS AMONG CELLS

### APOPROTEINS B AND E

Apo B-100 and E are the major proteins responsible for recognition of lipoproteins by specific cell-surface receptors that mediate uptake of lipoprotein cholesterol by cells.[1,2,8–10] Apo B-48 lacks the receptor-binding domain and does not bind to the LDL receptor. The major lipoprotein receptors are members of the LDL receptor gene family. The two principal receptors regulating lipoprotein metabolism are the LDL receptor and the LDL receptor–related protein, which serves as the chylomicron (apo E) remnant receptor.[1,8,11–13] In addition, it is now known that cell-surface heparan sulfate proteoglycans play a major role in combination with the LDL receptor–related protein (the heparan sulfate proteoglycan/LDL receptor–related protein pathway) or alone (for review, see ref. 13).

**Low-Density Lipoprotein Receptor.** The LDL receptor, sometimes referred to as the *apo B-100,E receptor*, is on the surface of most extrahepatic cells and hepatic parenchymal cells.[4] This receptor participates in the delivery of cholesterol to various cells, where it is used in membrane biosynthesis, or to steroid-producing cells, where it acts as a precursor for hormone production. In the liver, the LDL receptor functions in the removal and catabolism of LDL and a fraction (approximately one-half) of the VLDL and IDL.

The LDL receptors bind apo B-100– and apo E-containing lipoproteins; once bound, the lipoproteins are internalized by endocytosis of the receptors in coated pits and are degraded within the lysosomes of the cells. Before the complex enters the lysosome, the receptors dissociate from the lipoprotein in an endosomal compartment of the cell and recycle to the surface of the cell, where they can again participate in lipoprotein binding and uptake. The receptors have a half-life ($t_{1/2}$) of ~20 hours.

The cholesterol liberated from the degraded lipoproteins participates in three ways in the regulation of intracellular cholesterol metabolism. First, the delivery of lipoprotein cholesterol to the cell suppresses cholesterol synthesis by regulating the activity of *3-hydroxy-3-methylglutaryl–coenzyme A reductase (HMG-CoA reductase)*, the rate-limiting enzyme involved in intracellular cho-

**TABLE 162-2.**
**Characterization of the Major Apoproteins**

| Apoprotein | Plasma Concentration (mg/dL) | Molecular Mass (daltons) | Major Sites of Synthesis | Functions |
|---|---|---|---|---|
| B-100 | 80–100 | ~513,000 | Liver | Intracellular formation of VLDL; ligand for the LDL receptor; structural protein for VLDL, IDL, and LDL |
| B-48 | <5 | ~246,000 | Intestine | Intracellular formation of chylomicrons; structural protein for chylomicrons and their remnants |
| E | 3–6 | 34,200 | Liver, macrophages in various organs, astrocytes in the brain, keratinocytes in the skin | Ligand for the LDL and apo E receptors; mediates uptake of chylomicron remnants, certain VLDL, IDL, and HDL with apo E (HDL$_1$, HDL$_c$) |
| A-I | 100–150 | 28,100 | Intestine, liver | LCAT activation; structural protein of HDL |
| A-II | 30–50 | 17,400 | Liver | Structural protein of HDL |
| A-IV | 15 | 43,000 | Intestine | LCAT activation; associated with triglyceride transport in chylomicrons |
| C-I | ~6 | 6600 | Liver | LCAT activation, modulation of receptor-mediated uptake of triglyceride-rich remnant lipoproteins |
| C-II | 3–8 | 8800 | Liver | LPL activation |
| C-III | 8–15 | 8750 | Liver | Modulation of receptor-mediated uptake of triglyceride-rich remnant lipoproteins (possibly by displacing or masking apo E) |

*apo E*, apolipoprotein E; *HDL*, high-density lipoproteins; *IDL*, intermediate-density lipoproteins; *LCAT*, lecithin:cholesterol acyltransferase; *LDL*, low-density lipoproteins; *LPL*, lipoprotein lipase; *VLDL*, very-low-density lipoprotein.

### Absence of Sterol: Generation of Active SREBP

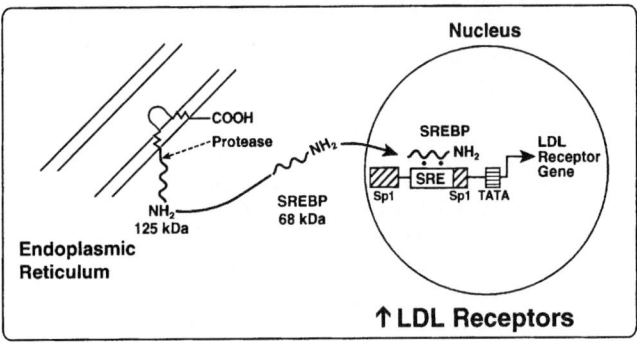

↑ LDL Receptors

### Presence of Sterol: No Generation of Active SREBP

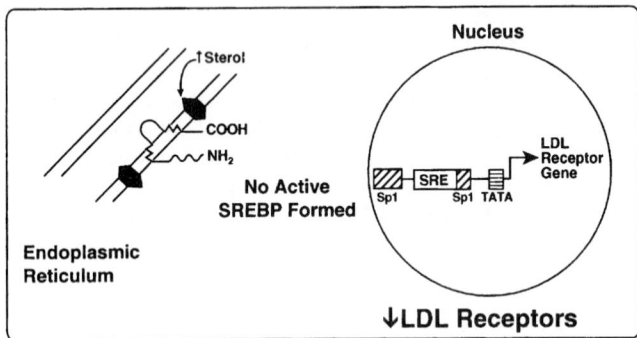

↓ LDL Receptors

**FIGURE 162-3.** Low-density lipoprotein (*LDL*) receptor gene regulation. In the absence of sufficient levels of intracellular cholesterol for the maintenance of cellular processes, the sterol regulating element-binding protein (*SREBP*) is hydrolyzed by a specific enzyme and the active amino-terminal region is translocated from the endoplasmic reticulum to the nucleus. In the nucleus, the SREBP interacts with the sterol regulatory element (*SRE*) of the LDL receptor gene and stimulates LDL receptor expression. The presence of adequate intracellular cholesterol down-regulates expression of the LDL receptor. (From Mahley RW, Weisgraber KH, Farese RV Jr. Disorders of lipid metabolism. In: Wilson JD, Foster DW, Kronenberg HM, Larsen PR, eds. Williams textbook of endocrinology, 9th ed. Philadelphia: WB Saunders, 1998:1099.)

lesterol biosynthesis from mevalonate. Second, intracellular lipoprotein cholesterol stimulates the activity of *acyl-CoA:cholesterol acyltransferase (ACAT)*. This causes the reesterification of excess cholesterol so that it can be stored, usually in small quantities, within the cell as cholesteryl ester. Third, the delivery of lipoprotein cholesterol by receptor-mediated uptake in quantities exceeding cellular needs causes down-regulation of the expression of the LDL receptor on the cell surface. Conversely, a deficiency of cholesterol causes an increase in the number of receptors. This regulation of expression also appears to function in vivo, in that dietary saturated fat and cholesterol consumption decrease the expression of hepatic LDL receptors, but treatment with the bile acid sequestrant cholestyramine or suppression of HMG-CoA reductase with a statin increases the expression of hepatic LDL receptors. Delivery of lipoprotein cholesterol to the cell follows a tightly regulated pathway that functions in the maintenance of intracellular cholesterol homeostasis.[1,2,8–10]

The control of LDL receptor expression has been elucidated[14–16]: Transcription factors, called *sterol regulatory element-binding proteins (SREBP-1 and SREBP-2)*, regulate the level of LDL receptors. The intact 125-kDa SREBP is an integral membrane protein containing two membrane-spanning regions (Fig. 162-3). The full-length protein is localized in the nuclear membrane and endoplasmic reticulum, not within the nucleus as was expected. To become an active transcription factor and to be

translocated into the nucleus where it interacts with the sterol regulatory element of the LDL receptor gene, the intact SREBP must be cleaved by a protease to liberate an ~68-kDa fragment representing the amino-terminal active one-half of the protein. The carboxyl-terminal domain of the SREBP remains membrane-bound. It is postulated that, when sterols are present in the cells, the SREBP assumes a conformation within the membrane that prevents the protease from releasing the active component of the SREBP. On the other hand, an absence or deficiency of sterols may allow the SREBP to be present in a conformation that allows proteolysis and the liberation of the active component, which is transported to the nucleus, where it induces LDL receptor expression as well as the genes involved in cholesterol biosynthesis.

The LDL receptor pathway is regulated similarly by apo B- or apo E-containing lipoproteins.[1,8–10] However, there is one major difference between these two ligands: Apo E–containing lipoproteins bind to the receptor with a much higher affinity (20- to 25-fold) than do apo B–containing LDL. Analysis of the structure of the LDL receptor reveals several cysteine-rich repeats that also possess critical negatively charged glutamic acid and aspartic acid residues involved in the binding of apo B-100– or apo E–containing lipoproteins.[4] The physiologic importance of the high binding affinity of apo E-containing lipoproteins lies in the very rapid rate of plasma clearance of these lipoproteins (in minutes), compared with the much slower clearance of apo B–containing LDL (2–3 days). Apo E is the protein determinant responsible for mediating the uptake of chylomicron remnants, certain VLDL, IDL, and HDL with apo E.[1,9,10]

Much has been learned about normal and abnormal lipid metabolism by the elucidation of the receptor-binding domain of apo E that governs its binding to the LDL receptor.[1,3,9,10,17,18,18a] Initial studies highlighted the importance of arginine and lysine as key residues in apo E binding. Selective chemical modification of arginine or lysine residues of apo E prevents the interaction of this apoprotein with the receptor. Likewise, modification of these same amino acids in apo B-100 abolishes the binding of LDL to the LDL receptor. Similarly, in vivo plasma clearance of apo E– and apo B–containing lipoproteins was inhibited after arginine or lysine modification.

Studies of the naturally occurring mutants of apo E in patients with type III hyperlipoproteinemia (*dysbetalipoproteinemia*) helped to localize the receptor-binding domain to key arginine and lysine residues near the middle of the apo E molecule.[1,9,17,18] The genetic defect responsible for the hypercholesterolemia and hypertriglyceridemia in type III hyperlipoproteinemia is secondary to the presence of apo E variants that are defective in the ability to bind to lipoprotein receptors. The most informative mutations, involving neutral amino acids interchanged for the normally occurring arginine or lysine residues, occurred at residues 136, 142, 145, 146, and 158 (Table 162-3). These observations, in addition to those obtained with monoclonal antibodies and fragments of apo E, localized the receptor-binding domain to the amino acids in the vicinity of residues 140 to 160. The determination of the three-dimensional structure of the amino-terminal region of apo E, which contains the receptor-binding domain, has further suggested that critical arginine or lysine residues in the 136 to 150 region interact directly with the LDL receptor,[10,19] but the arginine at residue 158 is involved indirectly in receptor binding. The substitution of cysteine for arginine at 158, the most common variant responsible for type III hyperlipoproteinemia, disrupts receptor binding by altering the conformation of the 136 to 150 region of the apo E molecule.

The postulated ligand-binding sites of the LDL receptor are enriched in the acidic amino acids aspartate and glutamate.[4] An ionic interaction between the acidic residues of the receptor and

## TABLE 162-3.
### Human Apolipoprotein E Variants

| Isoelectric Focusing Position | Charge Relative to Apo E-3* | Substitutions | Defective in Receptor Binding |
|---|---|---|---|
| E-4 | +1 | Cys$_{112}$→Arg | No |
| E-2† | −1 | Arg$_{158}$→Cys | Yes |
| E-2† | −1 | Arg$_{145}$→Cys | Yes |
| E-2† | −1 | Lys$_{146}$→Gln | Yes |
| E-3† | 0 | Cys$_{112}$→Arg, Arg$_{142}$→Cys | Yes |
| E-1† | −2 | Gly$_{127}$→Asp, Arg$_{158}$→Cys | Yes |
| E-2† | −1 | Arg$_{136}$→Ser | Yes |
| E-1† | −2 | Lys$_{146}$→Glu | Yes |
| E-3† | 0 | 7–amino-acid tandem insertion (residues 121–127) | Yes |

*Cys*, cystene; *Arg*, arginine; *Lys*, lysine; *Gly*, glycene; *Asp*, aspartic acid; *Ser*, serine; *Gln*, glutamine; *Glu*, glutamic acid.

*The electrophoretic charge, structure, and low-density lipoprotein receptor–binding activity of the variants are compared with those of normal apo E-3, the most frequently occurring apo E structure.[3,17,18]

†The defect is associated with type III hyperlipoproteinemia (i.e., presence of β–very-low-density lipoproteins in the plasma).

the basic amino acids of apo E appears to mediate the binding. The receptor-binding region in the carboxyl-terminal domain of apo B-100 has also been shown to be enriched in arginine and lysine residues and to encompass amino-acid residues 3359 to 3369.[20] The importance of the carboxyl terminus of apo B in mediating receptor binding was highlighted by the identification of a naturally occurring mutation in apo B-100 that prevents the normal interaction of LDL with the LDL receptor. The mutation, responsible for causing increased plasma LDL and the disorder referred to as *familial defective apo B-100*, involves a glutamine substituted for arginine at residue 3500.[5]

Examination of the sequence of the LDL receptor (a protein of 839 amino acids) has identified five structural domains within the molecule.[4,11] The ligand-binding sites are located in the amino-terminal one-third of the receptor (292 amino acids). The second domain lies in the midportion of the molecule (composed of ~400 amino acids) and contains a sequence homologous to that of the epidermal growth factor (EGF) precursor. A third domain that is rich in the amino acids serine and threonine represents a region of extensive glycosylation (18 serine or threonine residues out of 58 amino acids). A portion of the receptor molecule that consists of 22 hydrophobic amino acids (i.e., fourth domain) spans the plasma membrane and anchors the receptor in the bimolecular leaflet. On the cytoplasmic side of the membrane is the carboxyl-terminal region (i.e., fifth domain), composed of 50 amino acids. This region is involved in clustering the receptors in coated pits and in mediating internalization of the ligand-receptor complex. The carboxyl-terminal amino acids may interact with clathrin or other proteins found in the coated pits.

Five classes of mutations of the LDL receptor that disrupt receptor function have been identified.[4] These receptor mutants lead to the accumulation of LDL in the plasma and are responsible for familial hypercholesterolemia.[11,21]

**Low-Density Lipoprotein Receptor–Related Protein.**  Over the years several observations had suggested the existence of a separate chylomicron remnant (apo E) receptor. The postulated remnant receptor is the LDL receptor–related protein and it, along with the LDL receptor, can mediate the internalization of remnant lipoproteins.[12,13] However, chylomicron remnant clearance from the plasma involves several steps.[13] The initial rapid clearance of remnants from the plasma involves sequestration of these lipoproteins within the space of Disse, between the sinusoidal endothelial cells and hepatic parenchymal cells. This sequestration

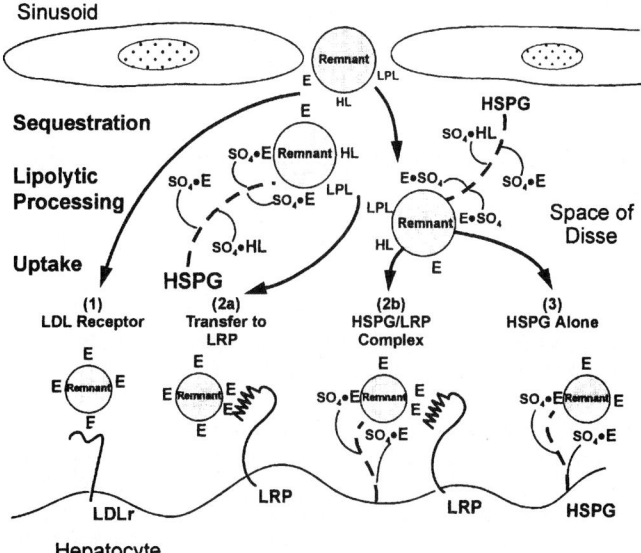

**FIGURE 162-4.** Summary of remnant lipoprotein uptake by the low-density lipoprotein (*LDL*) receptor, heparan sulfate proteoglycan/LDL receptor–related protein (*HSPG/LRP*) pathway, and HSPG alone. HSPG are abundant in the space of Disse and on the surface of hepatocytes. Apolipoprotein E (*E*) and hepatic lipase (*HL*), secreted by the hepatocytes, appear to bind to the HSPG and to be available to enrich the remnant lipoproteins. The HSPG/apo E appear to fulfill a critical role in the sequestration or capture of the remnants. Three major pathways for internalization are illustrated: (1) direct uptake by LDL receptor; (2) HSPG/LRP pathway (2a) remnants transferred to the LRP for uptake or (2b) HSPG/LRP complex internalized; and (3) HSPG alone mediating direct uptake. (*LPL*, lipoprotein lipase.) (From Mahley RW, Ji Z-S. Remnant lipoprotein metabolism: key pathways involving cell-surface heparan sulfate proteoglycans and apolipoprotein. E J Lipid Res 1999; 40:1.)

appears to be mediated by the binding of apo E-enriched remnant lipoproteins to heparan sulfate proteoglycans in the space of Disse.[22] A second step appears to involve further lipolytic processing of the particles before uptake by the hepatocytes. LPL has been implicated in this process, and hepatic lipase enhances the binding of remnants to cell-surface heparan sulfate proteoglycans and may participate, along with LPL, in further processing and in the sequestration of the remnants before uptake. The final step, internalization of the lipoprotein particles by hepatocytes, is mediated at least in part by the LDL receptor and the LDL receptor–related protein. In addition, cell-surface heparan sulfate proteoglycans play a critical role in remnant uptake, not only in the initial sequestration or capture step, but also as an essential component of the heparan sulfate proteoglycan/LDL receptor–related protein pathway. The heparan sulfate proteoglycans can also function alone as a receptor to mediate uptake of remnant lipoproteins.[13] These pathways are illustrated in Figure 162-4.

### APOPROTEIN A-I AND HIGH-DENSITY LIPOPROTEINS

HDL, possessing primarily apo A-I, readily accept cholesterol from cells.[23–26] Two mechanisms may be responsible for the efficient transfer of cholesterol to the HDL. Free cholesterol can traverse the aqueous layer around the cell and be incorporated into the HDL. This mechanism does not require contact between the HDL and the cell surface for cholesterol efflux to occur. However, the HDL actually may bind to the cell surface, creating a second mechanism that may facilitate cholesterol transfer. One such receptor has been identified and is known as the *SR-BI receptor*.[27] In addition, it has been suggested, at least for macrophages, that the HDL are internalized into an endosomal compartment, where the HDL acquire the cholesterol. The cholesterol-loaded HDL are then returned to the surface of the cell by retroendocytosis and released. It appears that apo E synthesized by the macrophages may also be acquired by the HDL during this process.

## COFACTORS FOR ENZYMES OF LIPID METABOLISM

### APOPROTEIN A-I AND LECITHIN:CHOLESTEROL ACYLTRANSFERASE

Cholesteryl esters associated with lipoproteins are formed in the plasma primarily by the action of the enzyme LCAT.[1,6,26,28,29,29a] The LCAT circulates in the plasma as a complex with components of HDL. It catalyzes the transfer of a fatty acid (usually linoleic acid) from the β position of phosphatidylcholine (i.e., lecithin) to the 3β-hydroxy position of cholesterol.

Apo A-I appears to be required for LCAT activity in vitro. There is no such requirement for LCAT activity in vivo, but it appears that other apoproteins (i.e., apo C-I, apo A-IV) can serve as cofactors for LCAT. Model peptides possessing amphipathic helical structures (including those lacking sequence homology with apo A-I) can serve as LCAT activators.

### APOPROTEIN C-II AND LIPOPROTEIN LIPASE

LPL is the enzyme responsible for the hydrolysis of the triglycerides of chylomicrons and VLDL.[1,30–32] It catalyzes the hydrolysis of the ester bond of the triglyceride, releasing free fatty acid. The free fatty acids are bound to albumin and transported in the plasma to various cells or are taken up directly by nearby cells. Moreover, LPL displays enzymatic activity capable of hydrolyzing phospholipids on the surface of lipoproteins.

LPL is located on the luminal surface of vascular endothelial cells, primarily those in adipose tissue, skeletal muscle, myocardium, mammary gland, and lung. The LPL is synthesized by underlying parenchymal cells and transferred to the vascular endothelial cells. It is bound to the endothelial cell surface through its interaction with cell-surface proteoglycans (apparently heparan sulfate). Under normal conditions, very little LPL circulates free in the plasma; however, it can be released from endothelial cells by an intravenous injection of heparin (a procedure used to quantitate LPL in patients with hypertriglyceridemia).

The primary role of LPL is the removal of triglycerides from plasma chylomicrons and VLDL, a key step in the catabolism of these two lipoproteins, initiating the release of surface components (e.g., apo A-I, phospholipids) and resulting in the formation of HDL and the production of IDL and LDL. The free fatty acids liberated are transferred to various tissues for oxidation as a source of energy (e.g., myocardium, skeletal muscle), for storage in the form of triglyceride droplets (e.g., adipose tissue), or for reutilization in triglyceride secretion (e.g., mammary gland and liver).

The initial step in the hydrolysis of chylomicron and VLDL triglyceride is the attachment of the lipoproteins to the endothelial cells by direct binding to the lipase or to sites on the endothelial cell surface that recognize one of the apoproteins (e.g., apo E may mediate binding to heparan sulfate or a cell receptor adjacent to the LPL). Chylomicrons attached to endothelial cells are enveloped by finger-like processes of the cells, bringing the lipoproteins into close contact with a large area of the surface membranes. It has been postulated that the free fatty acid generated is taken up directly by the plasma membranes of the cell and is transferred into the cells by lateral diffusion within the membranes. Conversely, it appears that VLDL may interact with LPL and be released, only to be rebound to the LPL and undergo stepwise hydrolysis of the triglyceride.

Apo C-II is a protein on the surface of chylomicrons and VLDL that serves as a cofactor to enhance the activity of LPL many fold. The enhancement of LPL activity appears to involve a direct protein-protein interaction between the LPL and apo C-II. The precise mechanism responsible for the cofactor activity of apo C-II is imprecisely understood.

Triglyceride accumulation in the plasma may arise from primary (genetic) or secondary defects.[30–33] The primary defects responsible for hypertriglyceridemia are an absence or deficiency of LPL synthesis or the presence of defective LPL. Patients with an absence or deficiency of apo C-II or the presence of structurally abnormal apo C-II have been described (see Chap. 163). Secondary hypertriglyceridemia can occur in uncontrolled juvenile or adult-onset diabetes, pancreatitis, or severe alcoholism; LPL activity can be low in these conditions.

### HEPATIC LIPASE

A lipase with properties distinct from those of LPL has been localized primarily to the liver, bound to heparan sulfate proteoglycans on sinusoidal endothelial cells and the microvillus surface of hepatocytes.[1,30–32,34] This lipase is released into the circulation after an intravenous injection of heparin. However, its activity could be differentiated from that of LPL. LPL activity is inhibited by a high salt concentration and protamine sulfate and requires apo C-II as a cofactor, but hepatic lipase activity is not sensitive to salt concentration or protamine sulfate and does not require apo C-II. Apo E appears to facilitate the hydrolysis catalyzed by hepatic lipase.[35]

LPL is most active in chylomicron triglyceride hydrolysis, and hepatic lipase is more active in VLDL and IDL lipolysis. In patients with LPL absence or deficiency, chylomicron triglyceride accumulation accounts for most of the hypertriglyceridemia, and VLDL do not accumulate markedly. One reason for this observation is that, in the absence of LPL, the hepatic lipase may possess sufficient activity to prevent VLDL triglyceride accumulation. Hepatic lipase is also involved in the conversion of larger HDL (HDL$_2$) to smaller HDL (HDL$_3$). This results in the regeneration of HDL$_3$ that is capable of acquiring more cholesterol from cells during the process of *reverse cholesterol transport*.[36]

## MAINTENANCE OF LIPOPROTEIN STRUCTURE BY FORMATION OF WATER-SOLUBLE LIPID PSEUDOMICELLES

The lipoproteins transport water-insoluble lipids in a soluble form in the plasma. Generally, the nonpolar lipids—triglycerides and cholesteryl esters—occupy the central core of the lipoproteins, and the more polar lipids—phospholipids and free cholesterol—are found on the surface with the apoproteins. All of the apoproteins bind to lipid, presumably to phospholipids on the particle surface. The lipid-binding affinities vary among the different apoproteins; certain apoproteins are more loosely associated with the particles and can exchange or transfer from one lipoprotein or lipoprotein class to another.[1,2] This is particularly true for the C apoproteins (i.e., C-I, C-II, and C-III) and apo E. For example, the C apoproteins are rapidly transferred from HDL to chylomicrons and VLDL when the chylomicrons and VLDL enter the lymph and plasma in an apo C-deficient form. Apo C-II is required by these triglyceride-rich lipoproteins to serve as an important cofactor for LPL. During triglyceride hydrolysis of these lipoproteins, the C apoproteins (including apo C-II) redistribute back to HDL; from there, they can be reused when another load of triglyceride-rich lipoproteins reaches the plasma. The relative content of the C apoproteins on the surface of triglyceride-rich lipoproteins modulates the binding of chylomicron and VLDL remnants to the LDL receptor and to the LDL receptor–related protein.[12,13] The content of the C apoproteins, especially apo C-I and apo C-III, may mask or sterically inhibit the ability of apo E, which is on the surface of these particles, to mediate lipoprotein binding and uptake by the receptors or may actually displace the apo E from the surface of the lipoproteins. The interchange of apoproteins participates in maintaining lipoprotein structure and in modulating the stepwise metabolism of the lipoproteins.

Lipid binding of most apoproteins has been ascribed to amphipathic $\alpha$-helical segments.[37] An amphipathic helix is characterized by an alignment of hydrophilic and hydrophobic amino acids on opposite faces of an $\alpha$-helical region of the protein. It is postulated that the fatty acid side chains of the phospholipids interact with the hydrophobic face of the helix. Comparison of the structure of several of the apoproteins (i.e., apo A-I, apo A-IV, and apo E) has revealed a series of tandemly repeated 22–amino-acid segments with amphipathic helical potential. There is a striking homology displayed among these proteins in the repeated regions.[38] These regions may be important in lipid binding.

The structure responsible for the lipid binding of apo B-100 does not appear to be an amphipathic helical region. Apo B-100, the exclusive protein constituent of LDL and a major protein of VLDL, is unique among apoproteins in other regards as well.[39,40] It is the largest of the apoproteins, ~500,000 Da, and is not exchanged from one lipoprotein to another; it appears to behave like an integral membrane protein inserted into the lipid surface of the particle. Moreover, the region in apo B that may be responsible for lipid binding appears to possess a $\beta$-pleated sheet, not an $\alpha$-helical structure. These regions are enriched in proline residues and have alternating hydrophilic and hydrophobic amino-acid residues, such that the hydrophilic side chains are on one face of the $\beta$-sheet and the hydrophobic side chains are on the other. These regions may represent amphipathic $\beta$-sheets that are analogous to the amphipathic $\alpha$-helices seen in other apoproteins.

# LIPOPROTEIN STRUCTURE AND METABOLIC FUNCTION

## CHYLOMICRONS

### CHARACTERISTICS

Chylomicrons are the largest of the plasma lipoproteins (>100 nm in diameter) and readily float by ultracentrifugation (density <0.95 g/mL). They are composed of ~98% to 99% lipid (~90% of the lipid is triglyceride) and 1% to 2% protein. Chylomicrons are present in postprandial plasma (but absent after an overnight fast) and possess several apoproteins (i.e., B-48, A-I, A-IV, E, and Cs) as they circulate in the plasma. The distinctive apoprotein is apo B-48, a form of apo B that has an apparent molecular mass approximately one-half that of apo B-100. It is the form of apo B synthesized by the intestine and is a marker for lipoproteins produced by the intestinal epithelium.[1,39–41] Apo B-48 is formed in the intestine by a unique process that edits the mRNA, resulting in the formation of a shortened form of apo B that is synthesized by these cells.[40,41] Apo B-48 does not possess the LDL receptor–binding region and, thus, does not interact with LDL receptors.

### ORIGIN

Chylomicrons are produced by the epithelial cells, particularly those of the proximal jejunum. Their synthesis is induced when dietary fat and cholesterol are presented to the brush border of the epithelial cell membranes. Triglycerides are synthesized

within the smooth endoplasmic reticulum in the apical region of the cells from the absorbed fatty acids and monoglycerides. Phospholipids and cholesterol (absorbed or synthesized by the intestinal cells) are used in the formation of the large chylomicron particles. The chylomicrons accumulate in the Golgi apparatus and are secreted into the space along the lateral border of the intestinal cells. From here, they enter the mesenteric lymph, proceeding to the thoracic duct lymph and finally entering the general circulation. Newly synthesized chylomicrons possess apo B-48, apo A-I, and apo A-IV (intestinally synthesized apoproteins) and acquire the apo Cs and apo E from lipoproteins in the lymph and blood (primarily from HDL).

### METABOLIC FATE

Chylomicrons are acted on by LPL, which catalyzes the release of free fatty acids and converts the chylomicrons into triglyceride-poor, cholesterol-enriched chylomicron remnants (see Fig. 162-1). The free fatty acids are taken up by various tissues to be stored as triglyceride, oxidized as an energy source, or reused in lipoprotein and triglyceride synthesis. The chylomicron remnants are cleared from the plasma by the lipoprotein receptors and are ultimately taken up and degraded by hepatic parenchymal cells (see Fig. 162-4). Plasma clearance includes sequestration within the space of Disse by heparan sulfate proteoglycans, the involvement of lipases in further processing and cell-surface binding, and internalization mediated by the heparan sulfate proteoglycan/LDL receptor–related protein pathway and the LDL receptors.[9,13,22]

The apoprotein that mediates the uptake of the chylomicron remnants is apo E. Remnants, referred to as $\beta$-VLDL, accumulate in the plasma of patients with type III hyperlipoproteinemia because of a structurally abnormal form of apo E, a site-specific mutation that disrupts the ability of apo E to bind to the lipoprotein receptor.[9,13,17,18] $\beta$-VLDL remnants accumulate in the plasma of animals (and presumably humans) after a high-fat, high-cholesterol meal is consumed. Their accumulation in this condition is caused by the downregulation in expression of the LDL receptors and an overproduction by the intestine and liver secondary to the excessive consumption of fat and cholesterol.

Chylomicron remnants, a subclass of $\beta$-VLDL induced in type III hyperlipoproteinemia or by dietary fat and cholesterol consumption, are atherogenic lipoproteins.[3,18] These lipoproteins have a high propensity to deliver excessive quantities of cholesterol to macrophages, converting these cells in vitro to cholesteryl ester–loaded foam cells. The macrophage is one of the major cell types responsible for cholesteryl ester accumulation in the atherosclerotic lesion.

## VERY-LOW-DENSITY LIPOPROTEINS

### CHARACTERISTICS

The VLDL are particles 30 to 70 nm in diameter that float by ultracentrifugation at a density <1.006 g/mL. They are composed of 85% to 90% lipid (~55% triglyceride, ~20% cholesterol, ~15% phospholipid) and 10% to 15% protein. Their distinctive apoprotein constituent is apo B-100, the hepatic form of apo B. Moreover, the VLDL contain apo E and apo Cs. The VLDL have pre-$\beta$- or $\alpha_2$-electrophoretic mobility and were once referred to as pre-$\beta$-lipoproteins.

### ORIGIN

The VLDL are synthesized by the liver, and their production can be stimulated by an increased availability of free fatty acid delivered to the hepatocytes. Synthesis of triglyceride and phospholipid to be used in the formation of VLDL occurs in the rough and smooth endoplasmic reticulum. The VLDL cholesterol may be synthesized de novo or reused from cholesterol acquired by the liver during lipoprotein catabolism (e.g., from LDL cholesterol). Electron microscopy has shown that the VLDL particles first appear in the cell at the rough endoplasmic reticulum–smooth endoplasmic reticulum junction (i.e., transitional elements) before they enter the Golgi apparatus. Large Golgi apparatus secretory vesicles appear to fuse with the luminal surface of hepatocytes and to release the VLDL particles into the space of Disse, from which they enter the plasma. The major protein constituents of the newly synthesized VLDL are apo B-100, apo E, and small amounts of the apo Cs. Within the plasma, the VLDL acquire additional C apoproteins, primarily from HDL.

### METABOLIC FATE

The VLDL triglycerides are hydrolyzed by the action of LPL and, to a lesser extent, by hepatic lipase (see Fig. 162-1). The VLDL are progressively converted to smaller and smaller particles that become increasingly cholesterol rich. The products of VLDL catabolism are referred to as IDL (density = 1.006–1.019 g/mL) and LDL (density = 1.019–1.063 g/mL). Approximately 50% of the VLDL is removed directly from the plasma by the liver before the VLDL molecules are converted to either IDL or LDL. The percentage of VLDL converted to LDL appears to depend partially on the number of LDL receptors expressed by the liver. For example, in Watanabe heritable hyperlipidemic rabbits, which have defective receptors, there is a marked increase in the conversion of VLDL to LDL, compared with normal rabbits (i.e., a decreased hepatic uptake of VLDL secondary to decreased numbers of LDL receptors and an increased conversion of VLDL to LDL).[42]

The receptor-mediated uptake of VLDL (and partially lipolyzed VLDL) depends primarily on the presence of apo E on these particles, and the receptor responsible for their uptake appears to be the LDL receptor. In cholesterol-fed animals, in which the LDL receptors are markedly down-regulated, the partially lipolyzed VLDL are not readily cleared, but are largely converted to LDL in a much higher percentage than is observed in normal animals.

### INTERMEDIATE-DENSITY LIPOPROTEINS

#### CHARACTERISTICS

The IDL (density = 1.006–1.019 g/mL) are normally present in very low concentrations in the plasma and are intermediate in size and composition between VLDL and LDL. Their primary protein constituents are apo B-100 and apo E.

#### ORIGIN

The IDL are metabolic products of VLDL catabolism and precursors of LDL generated in the plasma by the action of lipases.

#### METABOLIC FATE

As shown in Figure 162-1, the IDL may be further processed by the action of LPL and hepatic lipase or removed from the plasma by the LDL receptor. These lipoproteins are considered to be atherogenic and constitute a component of VLDL remnant particles that float at a density of 1.006 to 1.019 g/mL.

### LOW-DENSITY LIPOPROTEINS

#### CHARACTERISTICS

The LDL (density = 1.019–1.063 g/mL) are the major cholesterol-carrying lipoproteins in the plasma; ~70% of the total plasma

cholesterol is in LDL. They are ~20 nm in diameter and are composed of ~75% lipid (~35% cholesteryl ester, ~10% free cholesterol, ~10% triglyceride, ~20% phospholipid) and 25% protein. The apo B-100 is essentially the only protein present in these particles. The LDL have β-electrophoretic mobility and were once referred to as β-lipoproteins.

#### ORIGIN

The LDL represent the end products of lipase-mediated hydrolysis of VLDL. Moreover, as the triglyceride-rich core of the larger VLDL particles is removed, the surface lipids and proteins are remodeled with the transfer of excess surface constituents to HDL. The result is the formation of a cholesterol-rich small particle devoid of almost all apoproteins, except apo B-100.

#### METABOLIC FATE

The LDL are removed from the plasma at a relatively slow rate ($t_{1/2}$ of 2–3 days) through interaction with LDL receptors in the liver hepatocytes and extrahepatic tissues (see Fig. 162-1). Apo B-100 is the protein moiety that mediates their uptake by the receptors. It appears that more than two-thirds of LDL are actually cleared from the plasma by receptors in the liver. The LDL are degraded in the hepatocytes, and the cholesterol is reused for lipoprotein (VLDL) biosynthesis and membrane synthesis or becomes a precursor for the biosynthesis of bile acids. The bile acids and free cholesterol are delivered to the bile. It is through this latter mechanism that cholesterol is eliminated from the body.

The LDL are recognized as major atherogenic lipoproteins. This is demonstrated most clearly in patients with familial hypercholesterolemia.[8,11] These individuals lack LDL receptors or have defective receptors, incapable of mediating normal binding or uptake of LDL. Individuals homozygous for such defects have markedly elevated LDL concentrations (>500 mg/dL) and usually die of coronary artery disease as teenagers. The LDL also accumulate in the plasma of patients with familial defective apo B-100.[5,43] This disorder is caused by a single amino-acid substitution of glutamine for arginine at residue 3500 in the apo B-100, which prevents the interaction of the LDL with the LDL receptor.

### HIGH-DENSITY LIPOPROTEINS

#### CHARACTERISTICS

The HDL are smaller particles (8–13 nm) and float by ultracentrifugation at a density of 1.063 to 1.21 g/mL. They contain ~50% lipid (~25% phospholipid, ~15% cholesteryl esters, ~5% free cholesterol, ~5% triglyceride) and 50% protein. Their major apoproteins are apo A-I, apo A-II, and apo Cs. The HDL migrate in the $\alpha_1$ position on electrophoresis and were once referred to as α-lipoproteins. The HDL can be further subdivided into HDL$_2$ (density = 1.063–1.125 g/mL) and HDL$_3$ (density = 1.125–1.21 g/mL). They can also be subdivided on the basis of their apoprotein content: apo A-I alone or apo A-I/A-II particles.

#### ORIGIN

The different forms of HDL are synthesized by the liver and intestine (see Fig. 162-2); however, the intracellular sites of synthesis and secretion of these particles remain poorly defined. Apo A-I–containing disks (pre-β$_1$ HDL) are produced by the intestine and liver and generated from the surface of remnant lipoproteins during lipolysis. It appears that these precursors of HDL are converted to spherical particles by the action of LCAT on the cholesterol acquired by the HDL. Cholesteryl ester formation catalyzed by LCAT enriches the core of the disk with cholesteryl esters, causing conversion of the disks to spherical particles.

By ultracentrifugation, HDL are subdivided commonly into $HDL_2$ (i.e., larger, more lipid-rich HDL) and $HDL_3$ (i.e., smaller HDL particles). Metabolic interconversions between $HDL_2$ and $HDL_3$ have also been described. For example, the smaller $HDL_3$ acquire phospholipid and cholesterol during chylomicron and VLDL lipolysis or acquire cholesterol from cells, converting them to the larger $HDL_2$. The CETP transfers cholesterol from the $HDL_2$ to lower-density lipoproteins (e.g., VLDL, IDL) and the $HDL_2$ become enriched in triglycerides. Hepatic lipase catalyzes the hydrolysis of the triglycerides and surface phospholipids from the $HDL_2$, regenerating the $HDL_3$ from the $HDL_2$ particles. The HDL have received considerable attention because it is the change in their concentration that correlates inversely with coronary artery disease.

The $HDL_2$ and $HDL_3$ have been further fractionated into numerous subfractions; there are distinct subclasses within $HDL_2$ and $HDL_3$ that differ biochemically and metabolically. For example, within the $HDL_2$ subclass, there are HDL that contain apo E along with apo A-I. The presence of the apo E has significant metabolic consequences; these particles can be recognized by the LDL receptor, but HDL that lack apo E cannot. This subclass, characterized by being more enriched in cholesterol and containing apo E, is referred to as $HDL_1$ or $HDL_c$. The $HDL_1$ (HDL with apo E) are present as a minor subclass in the plasma of humans, but they are more abundant in the plasma of many animals that lack or are deficient in CETP.

The HDL participate in a process of redistribution of cholesterol among cells, a process referred to as *reverse cholesterol transport*. Cholesterol from peripheral cells is transferred to the liver for excretion from the body[1,36] (see Fig. 162-2). The HDL (primarily $HDL_3$, but also $HDL_2$) can acquire cholesterol from cells possessing excess cholesterol. The cholesterol can be esterified by the action of LCAT, increasing the cholesteryl ester content of the particles. In humans, most cholesteryl esters are transferred by CETP to VLDL, IDL, or LDL, and the cholesteryl esters of HDL are indirectly delivered to the liver for excretion from the body through the LDL pathway (Fig. 162-5, ①). During the process of cholesterol loading of the HDL, some of the cholesterol-enriched HDL also acquire apo E. By virtue of the presence of apo E, these HDL are then recognized by the lipoprotein receptors on various cells. Cholesterol transport to the liver may occur directly by the interaction between HDL with apo E and the hepatic lipoprotein receptors and by the subsequent uptake of the cholesterol. Furthermore, there may be an HDL receptor that recognizes one of the other apoproteins, such as apo A-I or apo A-II, and mediates uptake of the whole HDL particle (Fig. 162-5, ③). In addition, it has been demonstrated that HDL cholesteryl esters can be selectively removed from the HDL particle,[27] presumably by the HDL binding to SR-BI on the surface of hepatocytes. After selective uptake of cholesteryl esters, the HDL particle is released back into the plasma (Fig. 162-5, ②). The three pathways mediating reverse cholesterol transport involving HDL are illustrated in Figure 162-5. These mechanisms may represent the process whereby HDL exert their protective effect in retarding or reversing coronary artery disease.

## METABOLIC FATE

In addition to the complex series of interconversions (as described previously), HDL are catabolized primarily in the liver. The whole HDL particle is eventually cleared from the plasma.

## OTHER SPECIALIZED LIPOPROTEINS

### LIPOPROTEIN(a)

**Characteristics.** The density of flotation of lipoprotein(a) (Lp[a]; density = 1.05–1.12 g/mL) is between that of LDL and HDL. The Lp(a) particles closely resemble LDL in lipid composition and

represent apo B-100–containing LDL that acquire apo (a).[44–46] The Lp(a) particles migrate with $\alpha_2$ mobility on electrophoresis.

Apo B-100 is a major protein constituent of Lp(a); however, unlike the apo B-100 of LDL, the apo B-100 of Lp(a) is disulfide-linked to another protein referred to as the Lp(a) antigen, or apo (a).[44–46] The apo B-100 and apo (a) are present in the Lp(a) at a ratio of 1:1. The apo (a) is highly glycosylated and exists in multiple forms. There may be more than 30 allelic forms of apo (a) in the human population, with molecular weights from ~400,000 to 800,000.[46] The concentration of Lp(a) in the plasma varies indirectly with the molecular size, ranging from barely detectable to as much as 100 mg lipoprotein per deciliter. Most consider values of <30 mg/dL for Lp(a) to be desirable, and high levels appear to be correlated with an increased risk of coronary artery disease.

The sequence of apo (a) has been determined, and it has a remarkable homology to plasminogen. Apo (a) has numerous repeats of a sequence homologous to kringle 4 of plasminogen.[44–46] Apo (a) has been shown to bind to plasminogen receptors; it may interfere with fibrinolysis by disrupting the conversion of plasminogen to plasmin. Apo (a), although homologous to plasminogen, possesses no enzymatic activity.

**Origin.** The origin of Lp(a) is poorly understood. Although apo (a) is synthesized by the liver, it is unclear whether it associates with LDL-like particles within the liver and is secreted into the plasma as a complex. It is possible to assemble the complex in vitro, and it has been established that apo (a) secreted from the liver of transgenic mice forms the Lp(a) complex in the plasma when human LDL are injected into transgenic mice expressing apo (a)[47] or when human apo B–producing mice are crossed with those expressing apo (a).[48]

**Metabolic Fate.** Little is known about the metabolism of Lp(a).[49] Plasma levels of this lipoprotein do not correlate with age, sex, total cholesterol, triglyceride, or apo B.[50] With some

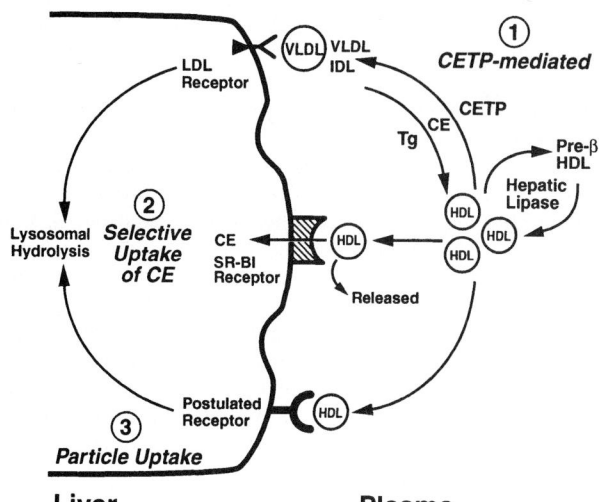

**FIGURE 162-5.** Reverse cholesterol transport involving high-density lipoprotein (*HDL*). HDL deliver cholesterol to the liver via several mechanisms. 1: The majority of HDL cholesteryl ester is transferred from HDL particles to lower-density lipoproteins by the action of cholesteryl ester transfer protein (*CETP*). The lower-density lipoproteins (remnants, very-low-density lipoprotein [*VLDL*], intermediate-density lipoprotein [*IDL*], and low-density lipoprotein [*LDL*]) are then taken up by the liver. Thus, indirectly the HDL particle delivers its cholesteryl ester to the liver. 2: HDL may bind to the SR-BI receptor, which facilitates the direct removal of cholesteryl ester from the particle for selective uptake of HDL cholesteryl ester by the liver. The cholesteryl ester–depleted particle is released from the cell surface. 3: There is a postulated hepatocyte receptor that could interact with the HDL particle and remove it from the plasma. If apolipoprotein E is associated with the HDL, then the receptor would be the LDL receptor. (*CE*, cholestryl ester; *Tg*, triglyceride.)

exceptions, Lp(a) levels are rather refractory to pharmacologic and dietary manipulation.[50] There is a correlation between high levels of Lp(a) and accelerated coronary artery disease in some studies, but not others.[50,51] Apo (a) has been detected immunochemically within atherosclerotic lesions.[52]

## β–VERY LOW-DENSITY (REMNANT) LIPOPROTEINS

**Characteristics and Origin.** The β-VLDL are β-migrating, cholesterol-enriched plasma lipoproteins that float at a density of <1.006 g/mL. They are induced by fat and cholesterol feeding and are present in the plasma of patients with type III hyperlipoproteinemia.[3,17,18] There are two major subclasses of β-VLDL. Fraction I, which is of intestinal origin, consists of chylomicron remnants that accumulate in the plasma and contains predominantly apo B-48 and apo E. Fraction II, which is of hepatic origin, consists of VLDL remnants that contain predominantly apo B-100 and apo E. Both fractions are composed primarily of triglyceride and cholesterol and are more cholesterol rich than chylomicrons or VLDL.

The fraction I and fraction II β-VLDL accumulate in the plasma in response to diets high in fat and cholesterol. It appears that their accumulation is secondary to excessive consumption of dietary fat and cholesterol and to a decrease in the expression of hepatic LDL receptors that are down-regulated by the increased delivery of dietary cholesterol to the liver.[3]

Fraction I and fraction II β-VLDL accumulate in type III hyperlipoproteinemia and are responsible for the hypertriglyceridemia and hypercholesterolemia seen in patients with this disorder. Their accumulation is partially a result of the occurrence of genetic variants of apo E (usually apo E-2) that are defective in their ability to bind to the lipoprotein receptors[3,17,18] (see Table 162-2).

**Metabolic Fate.** The normal metabolic fates of chylomicron remnants and VLDL were described earlier. In both conditions in which β-VLDL accumulate, the normal processes are impaired.[3,17,18] The accumulation of fraction I β-VLDL (i.e., cholesterol-enriched chylomicron remnants) is secondary to impaired hepatic clearance and overproduction of these particles. Fraction II β-VLDL (i.e., VLDL remnants) accumulate because of impaired hepatic uptake and retarded conversion to LDL.

Under the abnormal condition of β-VLDL accumulation, it appears that these lipoproteins are cleared by alternative mechanisms, which may account for their apparent atherogenicity. Accelerated atherosclerosis in many animals fed diets high in fat and cholesterol and in patients with type III hyperlipoproteinemia correlates with the occurrence of β-VLDL in the plasma. These β-VLDL are unique in their ability to cause marked cholesteryl ester accumulation in macrophages, which they can convert in vitro to foam cells.[3,17,18] Macrophages are one of the major cell types responsible for cholesterol accumulation in atherosclerosis.

## REFERENCES

1. Mahley RW, Weisgraber KH, Farese RV Jr. Disorders of lipid metabolism. In: Wilson JD, Foster DW, Kronenberg HM, Larsen PR, eds. Williams textbook of endocrinology, 9th ed. Philadelphia: WB Saunders, 1998:1099.
1a. Silver DL, Jiang XC, Arai T, et al. Receptors and lipid transfer proteins in HDL metabolism. Ann NY Acad Sci 2000; 102:103.
2. Havel RJ, Kane JP. Introduction: structure and metabolism of plasma lipoproteins. In: Scriver CR, Beaudet AL, Sly WS, Valle D, eds. The metabolic and molecular bases of inherited disease, 7th ed, vol 2. New York: McGraw-Hill, 1995:1841.
3. Mahley RW, Weisgraber KH, Innerarity TL, Rall SC Jr. Genetic defects in lipoprotein metabolism: elevation of atherogenic lipoproteins caused by impaired catabolism. JAMA 1991; 265:78.
3a. Goldberg IJ, Kako Y, Lutz EP. Responses to eating: lipoproteins, lipolytic products and atherosclerosis. Curropin Lipidol 2000; 11:235.
4. Hobbs HH, Russell DW, Brown MS, Goldstein JL. The LDL receptor locus in familial hypercholesterolemia: mutational analysis of a membrane protein. Annu Rev Genet 1990; 24:133.
5. Innerarity TL, Mahley RW, Weisgraber KH, et al. Familial defective apolipoprotein B100: a mutation of apolipoprotein B that causes hypercholesterolemia. J Lipid Res 1990; 31:1337.
6. Assmann G, von Eckardstein A, Funke H. Lecithin:cholesterol acyltransferase deficiency and fish-eye disease. Curr Opin Lipidol 1991; 2:110.
7. Tall A. Plasma lipid transfer proteins. Annu Rev Biochem 1995; 64:235.
8. Brown MS, Goldstein JL. A receptor-mediated pathway for cholesterol homeostasis. Science 1986; 232:34.
9. Mahley RW. Apolipoprotein E: cholesterol transport protein with expanding role in cell biology. Science 1988; 240:622.
10. Mahley RW, Huang Y. Apolipoprotein E: from atherosclerosis to Alzheimer's disease and beyond. Curr Opin Lipidol 1999; 10:207.
11. Goldstein JL, Hobbs HH, Brown MS. Familial hypercholesterolemia. In: Scriver CR, Beaudet AL, Sly WS, Valle D, eds. The metabolic and molecular bases of inherited disease, 7th ed, vol 2. New York: McGraw-Hill, 1995:1981.
12. Herz J, Willnow TE. Lipoprotein and receptor interactions in vivo. Curr Opin Lipidol 1995; 6:97.
13. Mahley RW, Ji Z-S. Remnant lipoprotein metabolism: key pathways involving cell-surface heparan sulfate proteoglycans and apolipoprotein. E J Lipid Res 1999; 40:1.
14. Sato R, Yang J, Wang X, et al. Assignment of the membrane attachment, DNA binding, and transcriptional activation domains of sterol regulatory element-binding protein-1 (SREBP-1). J Biol Chem 1994; 269:17267.
15. Hua X, Sakai J, Ho YK, et al. Hairpin orientation of sterol regulatory element-binding protein-2 in cell membranes as determined by protease protection. J Biol Chem 1995; 270:29422.
16. Brown MS, Goldstein JL. The SREBP pathway: regulation of cholesterol metabolism by proteolysis of a membrane-bound transcription factor. Cell 1997; 89:331.
17. Mahley RW, Rall SC Jr. Type III hyperlipoproteinemia (dysbetalipoproteinemia): the role of apolipoprotein E in normal and abnormal lipoprotein metabolism. In: Scriver CR, Beaudet AL, Sly WS, Valle D, eds. The metabolic and molecular bases of inherited disease, 7th ed. New York: McGraw-Hill, 1995:1953.
18. Mahley RW, Huang Y, Rall SC Jr. Pathogenesis of type III hyperlipoproteinemia (dysbetalipoproteinemia). Questions, quandaries, and paradoxes. J Lipid Res 1999; 40:1933.
18a. Curtiss LK, Boisvert WA. Apolipoprotein E and atherosclerosis. Curr Opiri Lipidol 2000; 11:243.
19. Fielding CJ. Reverse cholesterol transport. Curr Opin Lipidol 1991; 2:376.
20. Breslow JL. Familial disorders of high-density lipoprotein metabolism. In: Scriver CR, Beaudet AL, Sly WS, Valle D, eds. The metabolic and molecular bases of inherited disease, 7th ed, vol 2. New York: McGraw-Hill, 1995:2031.
21. Hobbs HH, Brown MS, Goldstein JL. Molecular genetics of the LDL receptor gene in familial hypercholesterolemia. Hum Mutat 1992; 1:445.
22. Ji Z-S, Fazio S, Lee Y-L, Mahley RW. Secretion-capture role for apolipoprotein E in remnant lipoprotein metabolism involving cell surface heparan sulfate proteoglycans. J Biol Chem 1994; 269:2764.
23. Wilson C, Wardell MR, Weisgraber KH, et al. Three-dimensional structure of the LDL receptor-binding domain of human apolipoprotein E. Science 1991; 252:1817.
24. Borén J, Lee I, Zhu W, et al. Identification of the low density lipoprotein receptor–binding site in apolipoprotein B100 and the modulation of its binding activity by the carboxyl terminus in familial defective apo-B100. J Clin Invest 1998; 101:1084.
25. Tall AR, Breslow JL. Plasma high-density lipoproteins and atherogenesis. In: Fuster V, Ross R, Topol EJ, eds. Atherosclerosis and coronary artery disease, vol 1. Philadelphia: Lippincott-Raven, 1996:105.
26. Rader DJ, Ikewaki K. Unravelling high density lipoprotein–apolipoprotein metabolism in human mutants and animal models. Curr Opin Lipidol 1996; 7:117.
27. Acton S, Rigotti A, Landschulz KT, et al. Identification of scavenger receptor SR-BI as a high density lipoprotein receptor. Science 1996; 271:518.
28. Barter PJ. Enzymes involved in lipid and lipoprotein metabolism. Curr Opin Lipidol 1990; 1:518.
29. Brown ML, Hesler C, Tall AR. Plasma enzymes and transfer proteins in cholesterol metabolism. Curr Opin Lipidol 1990; 1:122.
29a. Peelman F, Vandekerckhore J, Rosseneu M. Structure and function of lecithin cholesterol acyl transferase: new insights from structural predictions and animal models. Curr Opin Lipidol 2000; 11:155.
30. Hayden MR, Ma Y, Brunzell J, Henderson HE. Genetic variants affecting human lipoprotein and hepatic lipases. Curr Opin Lipidol 1991; 2:104.
31. Kern PA. Lipoprotein lipase and hepatic lipase. Curr Opin Lipidol 1991; 2:162.
32. Olivecrona T, Bengtsson-Olivecrona G. Lipases involved in lipoprotein metabolism. Curr Opin Lipidol 1990; 1:116.
33. Brunzell JD. Familial lipoprotein lipase deficiency and other causes of the chylomicronemia syndrome. In: Scriver CR, Beaudet AL, Sly WS, Valle D, eds. The metabolic and molecular bases of inherited disease, 7th ed, vol 2. New York: McGraw-Hill, 1995:1913.
34. Bensadoun A, Berryman DE. Genetics and molecular biology of hepatic lipase. Curr Opin Lipidol 1996; 7:77.
35. Thuren T, Wilcox RW, Sisson P, Waite M. Hepatic lipase hydrolysis of lipid monolayers. Regulation by apolipoproteins. J Biol Chem 1991; 266:4853.
36. Barter PJ, Rye K-A. Molecular mechanisms of reverse cholesterol transport. Curr Opin Lipidol 1996; 7:82.
37. Segrest JP, Jackson RL, Morrisett JD, Gotto AM Jr. A molecular theory of lipid–protein interactions in the plasma lipoproteins. FEBS Lett 1974; 38:247.
38. Breslow JL. Genetic basis of lipoprotein disorders. J Clin Invest 1989; 84:373.
39. Mahley RW, Young SG. Hyperlipidemia: molecular defects of apolipoproteins B and E responsible for elevated blood lipids. In: Mockrin SC, ed.

Molecular genetics and gene therapy of cardiovascular disease. New York: Marcel Dekker Inc, 1996:173.

40. Young SG. Recent progress in understanding apolipoprotein B. Circulation 1990; 82:1574.

41. Scott J. Regulation of the biosynthesis of apolipoprotein B$_{100}$ and apolipoprotein B$_{48}$. Curr Opin Lipidol 1990; 1:96.

42. Bilheimer DW, Watanabe Y, Kita T. Impaired receptor-mediated catabolism of low density lipoprotein in the WHHL rabbit, an animal model of familial hypercholesterolemia. Proc Natl Acad Sci U S A 1982; 79:3305.

43. Innerarity TL. Familial hypobetalipoproteinemia and familial defective apolipoprotein B$_{100}$: genetic disorders associated with apolipoprotein B. Curr Opin Lipidol 1990; 1:104.

44. Utermann G. The mysteries of lipoprotein(a). Science 1989; 246:904.

45. Utermann G. Lipoprotein (a): a genetic risk factor for premature coronary heart disease. Curr Opin Lipidol 1990; 1:404.

46. Lackner C, Boerwinkle E, Leffert CC, et al. Molecular basis of apolipoprotein (a) isoform size heterogeneity as revealed by pulsed-field gel electrophoresis. J Clin Invest 1991; 87:2153.

47. Chiesa G, Hobbs HH, Koschinsky ML, et al. Reconstitution of lipoprotein(a) by infusion of human low density lipoprotein into transgenic mice expressing human apolipoprotein(a). J Biol Chem 1992; 267:24369.

48. Linton MF, Farese RV Jr., Chiesa G, et al. Transgenic mice expressing high plasma concentrations of human apolipoprotein B100 and lipoprotein(a). J Clin Invest 1993; 92:3029.

49. Rader DJ, Cain W, Ikewaki K, et al. The inverse association of plasma lipoprotein(a) concentrations with apolipoprotein(a) isoform size is not due to differences in Lp(a) catabolism but to differences in production rate. J Clin Invest 1994; 93:2758.

50. Spinler SA, Cziraky MJ. Lipoprotein(a): physiologic function, association with atherosclerosis, and effects of lipid-lowering drug therapy. Ann Pharmacother 1994; 28:343.

51. Daida H, Lee YJ, Yokoi H, et al. Prevention of restenosis after percutaneous transluminal coronary angioplasty by reducing lipoprotein (a) levels with low-density lipoprotein apheresis. Am J Cardiol 1994; 73:1037.

52. Beisiegel U. Lipoprotein (a) in the arterial wall. Curr Opin Lipidol 1991; 2:317.

# CHAPTER 163

# LIPOPROTEIN DISORDERS

ERNST J. SCHAEFER

## HYPERLIPIDEMIA AND CORONARY ARTERY DISEASE

Coronary heart disease (CHD) is a major cause of death in the United States.[1] Although the CHD age-adjusted mortality is declining, this illness nevertheless kills ~500,000 Americans annually.[1] It is estimated that almost 70% of all Americans have some degree of atherosclerotic narrowing of their coronary arteries.[1] Approximately 12 million Americans experience CHD, and one-third of these have limited activity as a result.[1] Each year, ~1.1 million Americans have a myocardial infarction, ~1.2 million undergo cardiac catheterization, 600,000 receive coronary artery bypass grafts, 350,000 have an angioplasty procedure performed, and about the same number die from CHD.[1]

A primary contributing factor to CHD is an elevated blood cholesterol level due to an increased level of low-density lipoprotein (LDL) cholesterol.[1-4] Approximately 50% of all U.S. adults (i.e., 100 million persons) have serum cholesterol levels >200 mg/dL, and ~40 million adults have values >240 mg/dL. Approximately 60 million are candidates for medical advice and intervention.[4]

Elevated LDL cholesterol is a significant risk factor for CHD, and lowering LDL cholesterol decreases this risk.[1-6] Severely elevated triglycerides (>1000 mg/dL or 11.3 mmol/L) are associated with an increased risk of pancreatitis, and lowering these levels reduces this risk.[5,6]

Serum or plasma LDL cholesterol levels are increased by diets high in saturated fat and cholesterol, mainly because of decreased LDL receptor–mediated catabolism.[7,8] Human populations on high-saturated-fat and high-cholesterol diets have elevated LDL cholesterol levels and a significantly higher rate of CHD due to atherosclerosis than do populations on low-saturated-fat and low-cholesterol diets.[3,4,9] Elevated LDL cholesterol levels and decreased high-density lipoprotein (HDL) cholesterol levels are independent risk factors for premature CHD in Western society.[3,4,9-12] A decreased HDL cholesterol of <35 mg/dL confers a 50% increased CHD risk in men and a 100% increased risk in women, compared with those with average risk.[12] Women have higher HDL cholesterol levels and a lower age-adjusted risk of CHD than do men.[9-11]

Prospective studies indicate that dietary treatment or diet and drug therapy that lower total serum cholesterol or LDL cholesterol can reduce subsequent CHD morbidity and mortality.[13-35] In patients with established CHD, it is clearly more optimal to lower LDL cholesterol to <100 mg/dL than to <130 mg/dL.[28,34,35] Many large trials, including the Coronary Primary Prevention Trial, the West of Scotland Study, CARE, AFCAPS/TexCAPS, and LIPID, have documented that significant reductions in LDL cholesterol levels lead to significant decreases of 22% to 37% in the incidence of CHD.[27-35] Moreover, 3-hydroxy-3-methylglutaryl–coenzyme A (HMG-CoA) reductase inhibition has now been documented to reduce CHD risk in both men and women (with or without CHD, among the elderly, among diabetics, and among smokers).[27-35]

Some studies also indicate a benefit in CHD risk reduction from increasing HDL cholesterol.[22-26,36,37] In CHD patients, it now appears to be prudent to raise HDL cholesterol to >35 mg/dL with either a fibric acid derivative or niacin.[22-26,37] Moreover, aggressive lipid modification can result in stabilization of existing coronary atherosclerosis and some regression of this process.[38-47]

### EPIDEMIOLOGIC EVIDENCE

A large body of epidemiologic evidence supports a direct relationship between the serum levels of total and LDL cholesterol and the risk of CHD. This association is continuous throughout the range of cholesterol levels in the population.[2-4,9-11] According to results from the third National Health and Nutrition Examination Survey, the average LDL cholesterol level of U.S. adults is 130 mg/dL.[4] At higher levels of total and LDL cholesterol, the direct relationship between CHD risk and cholesterol levels becomes particularly strong; for persons with cholesterol values in the top 10% of the population distribution, the risk of CHD mortality is four times as high as the risk in the bottom 10% of the population.[9-12] An LDL cholesterol level >160 mg/dL confers about a 70% increase in CHD risk as compared to a value <130 mg/dL in both men and women.[12] An HDL cholesterol <35 mg/dL confers about a 50% increased risk in men and a 100% increased risk in women compared to subjects with values >35 mg/dL.[12]

### GENETIC AND PHYSIOLOGIC EVIDENCE

Premature CHD can result from high LDL cholesterol levels even in the absence of other risk factors. This is most clearly demonstrated in children with the rare homozygous familial hypercholesterolemia, characterized by the absence of specific cell-surface receptors that normally remove LDL cholesterol from the circulatory system. LDL cholesterol levels can be as high as 1000 mg/dL (26 mmol/L), and severe atherosclerosis and CHD often develop before 20 years of age.[5,7,48,49] Patients with the more common heterozygous form of familial hypercholesterolemia and partial deficiencies of LDL-receptor function generally develop premature CHD in the middle decades of life.[5,7,50]

## ANIMAL MODEL EVIDENCE

Animal models have demonstrated a direct relationship between LDL cholesterol and atherosclerosis. Animals consuming diets high in saturated fat and cholesterol develop LDL cholesterol elevation and atherosclerosis.[51] Such diets also increase HDL cholesterol, an effect that may be compensatory. These hypercholesterolemic animals develop intimal lesions that progress from fatty streaks to ulcerated plaques, resembling those of human atherosclerosis. In laboratory trials, severe atherosclerosis in monkeys regresses when blood cholesterol is lowered through diet or drug therapy. Such studies support a causal relationship between LDL cholesterol and atherosclerosis and suggest reversibility of the process with the reduction of the serum LDL cholesterol level.[51]

The combined findings of these studies support the concept that lowering total and LDL cholesterol levels can reduce the incidence of CHD events and the death rate due to myocardial infarction.[13–48] Moreover, the pooled analysis of clinical trial findings suggests that intervention is as effective in preventing recurrent myocardial infarction and mortality in patients experiencing a recurrent attack as it is in primary prevention. The complete set of evidence strongly supports the concept that reducing total and LDL cholesterol levels can reduce CHD risk in younger and older men, in women, and in individuals with moderate elevations of cholesterol.[4]

It is important to recognize the magnitude of CHD reduction associated with lowering serum cholesterol levels. For persons with serum cholesterol levels initially in the range of 250 to 300 mg/dL (6.5–7.8 mmol/L), each 1% reduction in serum cholesterol level yields approximately a 1% to 2% reduction in CHD rates.[9] A 30% reduction in the LDL cholesterol level will reduce CHD risk by as much as 50%.[13–47] Moreover, studies indicate that aggressive lipid modification can result in stabilization of existing coronary atherosclerosis and some degree of regression.[19,38–47]

## PATIENT EVALUATION

The Adult Treatment Panel of the National Cholesterol Education Program (NCEP) has recommended that individuals at risk for CHD should be identified by total serum cholesterol and HDL cholesterol levels, and that, if indicated, they should be further classified for treatment based on LDL cholesterol levels.[3,4,52]

The NCEP's continuing mandate is to develop guidelines for the detection of hypercholesterolemia and therapeutic guidelines that affect its treatment. The NCEP also enlists participation by and contributions from interested national, state, and local organizations. Its purpose is to educate physicians, other health professionals, and the general public about the significance of elevated blood cholesterol levels and the importance of treatment.

### TOTAL CHOLESTEROL AND HIGH-DENSITY LIPOPROTEIN CHOLESTEROL

The classification system begins with the measurement of total cholesterol and HDL cholesterol levels for screening the general population in the fasting or nonfasting state. In the author's view, it is not unreasonable to get a screening triglyceride value at that time. Accurate fingerstick methods are available for cholesterol and HDL cholesterol screening in the office setting.[53] An accurate home cholesterol test that can be self-administered by the patient has become available.[54] Total cholesterol levels <200 mg/dL (5.2 mmol/L) have been classified as desirable, those between 200 and 239 mg/dL (5.2–6.2 mmol/L) have been classified as borderline-high, and those ≥240 mg/dL (6.2 mmol/L) have been classified as high risk. Levels of HDL cholesterol <35 mg/dL (0.9 mmol/L) have been classified as low.[3,4] Fasting triglyceride levels ≥400 mg/dL (4.5 mmol/L) have been classified as elevated.[3,4]

Approximately 25% of the adult population (>40 million persons) in the United States who are 20 years of age or older fall into the high-risk blood cholesterol classification, and another 54 million people have borderline-high blood cholesterol levels.[4] Approximately 20% of males and 5% of females have low HDL cholesterol levels, and fewer than 5% of men and women have elevated triglyceride levels.

All patients who are screened should receive information about an NCEP or American Heart Association step 1 diet and CHD risk factors. According to the NCEP Adult Treatment Panel guidelines, patients who have desirable total cholesterol and normal HDL cholesterol values should have their values checked again within 5 years.[3,4,52] If the patient has a borderline-high value, information about other CHD risk factors should be obtained[3,4] (Table 163-1).

If the patient has a cholesterol value in the borderline-risk category and a normal HDL cholesterol level, in the absence of CHD (i.e., prior myocardial infarction or angina) or two or more CHD risk factors (see Table 163-1), dietary information should be provided and the cholesterol value checked within the next year.

If the patient has a borderline-high value and a history of CHD or two or more CHD risk factors, or the patient has a high-risk total cholesterol value or has a low HDL cholesterol value, LDL cholesterol levels should be assessed so that an appropriate treatment regimen can be determined.[3,4] LDL cholesterol is routinely calculated after measuring serum total cholesterol, triglyceride, and HDL cholesterol after an overnight fast. The normal ranges for total cholesterol, triglyceride, very-low-density lipoprotein (VLDL) cholesterol, LDL cholesterol, and HDL cholesterol are provided in Table 163-1, and options for measuring LDL cholesterol are discussed later.

Another issue is whether apoliprotein (apo) A-I, apo B, Lp(a), or LDL size should be measured for assessing CHD risk. In prospective studies, only Lp(a) among these parameters has been shown to be an independent risk factor, after smoking, blood pressure, diabetes, LDL cholesterol, and HDL cholesterol were taken into account.[55–115] In the author's view, direct measurements of LDL cholesterol, HDL cholesterol, remnant lipoprotein cholesterol, and Lp(a) cholesterol will become the method of choice for lipoprotein assessment in the future. A remnant lipoprotein cholesterol >10 mg/dL confers a 100% increased risk in women, and a substantially increased risk in men.[70–74] Similarly, an Lp(a) cholesterol >10 mg/dL confers a 100% increased CHD risk, especially in men.[98] An Lp(a) cholesterol and remnant lipoprotein cholesterol should be part of CHD risk assessment.[74,98,112–115] Measurement of other parameters cannot be recommended at this time.

### NATIONAL CHOLESTEROL EDUCATION PROGRAM GUIDELINES

The NCEP Adult Treatment Panel has developed guidelines for the diagnosis and treatment of individuals older than 20 years of age with elevated blood cholesterol levels associated with an increase in LDL cholesterol levels.[3,4] The goals of therapy and the particular level of LDL cholesterol requiring the initiation of diet and drug therapy depend on the presence or absence of CHD or two or more CHD risk factors (Table 163-2). The pres-

**TABLE 163-1.**
**Normal Values for Plasma Lipid and Lipoprotein Cholesterol Concentrations***

| Age (yr) | Plasma Cholesterol (mg/dL) | | | | | Plasma Triglyceride (mg/dL) | | | VLDL Cholesterol (mg/dL) | | | LDL Cholesterol (mg/dL) | | | | | HDL Cholesterol (mg/dL) | | | | | HDL/Cholesterol Ratio | | |
|---|---|---|---|---|---|---|---|---|---|---|---|---|---|---|---|---|---|---|---|---|---|---|---|---|
| *Percentiles* | 10 | 25 | 50 | 75 | 90 | 10 | 50 | 90 | 10 | 50 | 90 | 10 | 25 | 50 | 75 | 90 | 10 | 25 | 50 | 75 | 90 | 10 | 50 | 90 |
| **MALES** | | | | | | | | | | | | | | | | | | | | | | | | |
| 0–4 | 125 | 137 | 151 | 171 | 186 | 33 | 51 | 84 | † | | | | | | | | | | | | | | | |
| 5–9 | 130 | 143 | 159 | 175 | 191 | 33 | 51 | 85 | 2 | 7 | 15 | 69 | 80 | 90 | 103 | 117 | 42 | 49 | 54 | | 70 | 0.27 | 0.36 | 0.44 |
| 10–14 | 127 | 140 | 155 | 173 | 190 | 37 | 59 | 102 | 2 | 9 | 18 | 72 | 81 | 94 | 109 | 122 | 40 | 49 | 55 | | 71 | 0.26 | 0.34 | 0.43 |
| 15–19 | 120 | 132 | 146 | 165 | 183 | 43 | 69 | 120 | 3 | 12 | 23 | 68 | 80 | 93 | 109 | 123 | 34 | 39 | 46 | | 59 | 0.21 | 0.30 | 0.41 |
| 20–24 | 130 | 146 | 165 | 186 | 204 | 50 | 86 | 165 | 5 | 12 | 24 | 73 | 85 | 101 | 118 | 138 | 32 | 38 | 45 | | 57 | 0.19 | 0.28 | 0.39 |
| 25–29 | 143 | 159 | 178 | 202 | 227 | 54 | 95 | 199 | 6 | 15 | 31 | 75 | 96 | 116 | 138 | 157 | 32 | 37 | 44 | | 58 | 0.17 | 0.25 | 0.37 |
| 30–34 | 148 | 167 | 190 | 213 | 239 | 58 | 104 | 213 | 8 | 18 | 36 | 88 | 107 | 124 | 144 | 166 | 32 | 38 | 45 | | 59 | 0.16 | 0.24 | 0.34 |
| 35–39 | 157 | 176 | 197 | 223 | 249 | 62 | 113 | 251 | 7 | 19 | 46 | 92 | 110 | 131 | 154 | 176 | 31 | 36 | 43 | | 58 | 0.15 | 0.21 | 0.30 |
| 40–44 | 163 | 182 | 203 | 228 | 250 | 64 | 122 | 248 | 8 | 21 | 43 | 98 | 115 | 135 | 157 | 173 | 31 | 36 | 43 | | 60 | 0.15 | 0.21 | 0.30 |
| 45–49 | 169 | 188 | 210 | 234 | 258 | 68 | 154 | 253 | 8 | 20 | 40 | 106 | 120 | 141 | 163 | 186 | 33 | 38 | 45 | | 60 | 0.15 | 0.21 | 0.29 |
| 50–54 | 169 | 187 | 210 | 235 | 261 | 68 | 124 | 250 | 10 | 23 | 49 | 102 | 118 | 143 | 162 | 185 | 31 | 36 | 44 | | 58 | 0.14 | 0.21 | 0.28 |
| 55–59 | 167 | 189 | 212 | 235 | 262 | 67 | 119 | 235 | 6 | 19 | 39 | 103 | 126 | 145 | 168 | 191 | 31 | 38 | 46 | | 64 | 0.15 | 0.22 | 0.34 |
| 60–64 | 171 | 188 | 210 | 235 | 259 | 68 | 119 | 235 | 4 | 16 | 35 | 106 | 121 | 143 | 165 | 188 | 34 | 41 | 49 | | 69 | 0.16 | 0.24 | 0.33 |
| 65–69 | 170 | 190 | 210 | 233 | 258 | 64 | 112 | 208 | 6 | 16 | 40 | 104 | 125 | 146 | 170 | 199 | 33 | 39 | 49 | | 74 | 0.15 | 0.23 | 0.34 |
| 70+ | 162 | 182 | 205 | 229 | 252 | 67 | 111 | 212 | 3 | 15 | 31 | 100 | 119 | 142 | 164 | 182 | 33 | 40 | 48 | | 70 | 0.16 | 0.24 | 0.34 |
| **FEMALES** | | | | | | | | | | | | | | | | | | | | | | | | |
| 0–4 | 120 | 139 | 156 | 172 | 189 | 38 | 59 | 96 | † | | | | | | | | | | | | | | | |
| 5–9 | 134 | 146 | 163 | 179 | 195 | 36 | 55 | 90 | 1 | 9 | 19 | 73 | 88 | 98 | 115 | 125 | 38 | 47 | 52 | | 67 | 0.24 | 0.32 | 0.43 |
| 10–14 | 131 | 144 | 158 | 174 | 190 | 44 | 70 | 114 | 3 | 10 | 20 | 73 | 81 | 94 | 110 | 126 | 40 | 45 | 52 | | 64 | 0.25 | 0.33 | 0.42 |
| 15–19 | 126 | 139 | 154 | 171 | 190 | 44 | 66 | 107 | 4 | 11 | 20 | 67 | 78 | 93 | 110 | 127 | 38 | 43 | 51 | | 68 | 0.24 | 0.33 | 0.44 |
| 20–24 | 130 | 143 | 160 | 182 | 203 | 41 | 64 | 112 | 3 | 10 | 22 | 62 | 80 | 98 | 113 | 136 | 37 | 43 | 50 | | 68 | 0.22 | 0.32 | 0.42 |
| 25–29 | 136 | 151 | 168 | 187 | 209 | 42 | 65 | 116 | 4 | 11 | 22 | 73 | 87 | 103 | 122 | 141 | 40 | 47 | 55 | | 73 | 0.22 | 0.33 | 0.43 |
| 30–34 | 139 | 154 | 172 | 193 | 213 | 44 | 69 | 123 | 2 | 9 | 20 | 73 | 89 | 108 | 126 | 142 | 40 | 46 | 55 | | 71 | 0.22 | 0.32 | 0.42 |
| 35–39 | 147 | 163 | 182 | 202 | 225 | 46 | 73 | 137 | 3 | 13 | 26 | 81 | 96 | 116 | 139 | 161 | 38 | 44 | 52 | | 74 | 0.19 | 0.30 | 0.43 |
| 40–44 | 154 | 170 | 191 | 214 | 235 | 51 | 82 | 155 | 5 | 12 | 26 | 89 | 105 | 120 | 145 | 164 | 39 | 48 | 55 | | 78 | 0.19 | 0.28 | 0.41 |
| 45–49 | 161 | 177 | 199 | 224 | 247 | 53 | 87 | 171 | 4 | 14 | 32 | 90 | 105 | 127 | 150 | 173 | 39 | 46 | 56 | | 78 | 0.19 | 0.28 | 0.39 |
| 50–54 | 172 | 192 | 215 | 241 | 268 | 59 | 97 | 186 | 4 | 14 | 32 | 102 | 118 | 141 | 169 | 192 | 40 | 49 | 59 | | 77 | 0.15 | 0.26 | 0.35 |
| 55–59 | 183 | 204 | 228 | 253 | 282 | 63 | 106 | 204 | 4 | 18 | 40 | 103 | 126 | 148 | 176 | 204 | 39 | 47 | 58 | | 82 | 0.17 | 0.26 | 0.36 |
| 60–64 | 186 | 203 | 228 | 254 | 280 | 64 | 105 | 202 | 3 | 13 | 30 | 105 | 130 | 151 | 172 | 201 | 43 | 49 | 60 | | 85 | 0.14 | 0.25 | 0.36 |
| 65–69 | 183 | 208 | 229 | 256 | 280 | 66 | 112 | 204 | 3 | 15 | 36 | 104 | 128 | 156 | 189 | 208 | 38 | 46 | 60 | | 79 | 0.14 | 0.25 | 0.38 |
| 70+ | 180 | 200 | 226 | 256 | 278 | 69 | 111 | 204 | 0 | 13 | 34 | 107 | 126 | 146 | 170 | 189 | 37 | 48 | 60 | | 82 | 0.16 | 0.26 | 0.37 |

*HDL*, high-density lipoprotein; *LDL*, low-density lipoprotein; *VLDL*, very-low-density lipoprotein.
*Based on Lipid Research Clinics population studies in the United States and Canada for white males and females (non–sex hormone users) as derived from National Institutes of Health publication No. 80-1527, 1980. All subjects were samples in the fasting state.
†No data because there were fewer than 100 subjects in a cell.

ence of secondary causes of elevated LDL cholesterol levels (>160 mg/dL or 4.1 mmol/L) must be ruled out. These include hypothyroidism, obstructive liver disease, and nephrotic syndrome. LDL cholesterol decision points for initiating diet and drug therapy are given in Table 163-3. The NCEP guidelines have been accepted by all major U.S. medical organizations, including the American College of Physicians, the American Heart Association, and the American Medical Association.[4] Guidelines for the general population and children and adolescents have also been developed.[116,117]

**TABLE 163-2.**
**National Cholesterol Education Program Major Coronary Heart Disease Risk Factors in Addition to Low-Density Lipoprotein Cholesterol**

High-density lipoprotein (HDL) cholesterol <35 mg/dL (0.9 mmol/L)
Hypertension
Cigarette smoking
Diabetes
Family history of myocardial infarction or sudden death before age 55 in a male parent or sibling or age 65 in a female parent or sibling
Male 45 years of age or older
Female 55 years of age or older or premature menopause who is not on hormone replacement therapy
Subtract one risk factor if HDL cholesterol ≥60 mg/dL (1.6 mmol/L)

**TABLE 163-3.**
**National Cholesterol Education Program Adult Treatment Panel II Treatment Guidelines**

| Therapy | Low-Density Lipoprotein Cholesterol Values (mg/dL [mmol/L]) | | |
|---|---|---|---|
| | ≥130 (3.4) | ≥160 (4.2) | ≥190 (5.0) |
| **DIET*** | Yes, if CHD is present | Yes, if 2 or more CHD risk factors are present | Yes |
| **DRUGS (AFTER DIET*)** | Yes, if CHD is present | Yes, if 2 or more CHD risk factors are present | Yes |

*CHD*, coronary heart disease.
*The goal of diet therapy is reading the initiation value, and the goal of drug therapy is 30 mg/dL or 0.8 mmol/L below the initiation value. CHD risk factors are listed in Table 163-2. All CHD patients should be placed on a National Cholesterol Education Program step 2 diet.

The recommendation that LDL cholesterol values be used as the primary criterion for treatment decisions for patients with elevated cholesterol levels makes accurate measurement a national public health imperative as reviewed by the NCEP Laboratory Standardization Panel.[118]

If a patient has an LDL cholesterol level of 160 mg/dL (4.1 mmol/L), it represents approximately the 75th percentile for middle-aged Americans (see Table 163-1). It is important to confirm any abnormalities by repeat determinations. Hospitalization or acute illness can affect lipid values, and lipid determinations should generally be carried out in the free-living state.[119] An elevated or borderline-high triglyceride level (200 mg/dL or 2.3 mmol/L) has not clearly been shown to be an independent risk factor for premature heart disease. However, an elevated triglyceride level is inversely associated with a low level of HDL cholesterol, which has been shown to be a significant risk factor for CHD. Common secondary causes of elevated LDL cholesterol and triglyceride values and of decreased HDL cholesterol include diabetes, hypothyroidism, obstructive liver disease, kidney disease, excess alcohol intake, and the use of corticosteroids, anabolic steroids, estrogens, β-blocking agents, and thiazide diuretics.[4] If possible, these factors should be screened for and treated before diet or drug therapy for lipid disorders is initiated. Screening should include an evaluation of glucose, albumin, liver transaminases, alkaline phosphatase, creatinine, and thyroid-stimulating hormone, and the patient should be asked about alcohol intake and the use of β-blockers, estrogens, corticosteroids, anabolic steroids, and thiazides.

## LOW-DENSITY LIPOPROTEIN CHOLESTEROL MEASUREMENT

Unlike total cholesterol quantitation, there is no consensus-approved and validated reference method for the direct measurement of LDL cholesterol. The accurate measurement of LDL cholesterol depends on the separation of LDL particles in serum from other lipoproteins: chylomicrons, VLDL, and HDL. Traditionally, LDL has been defined as all lipoproteins within the density range of 1.019 to 1.063 g/mL. However, in common practice, the definition has been broadened to include intermediate-density lipoprotein (IDL; 1.006–1.019 g/mL). Using this definition, LDL is composed of LDL + IDL + Lp(a). This definition serves as the basis for the cut-points defined by the NCEP Adult Treatment Panel. The options for measuring LDL cholesterol include ultracentrifugation, the Friedewald calculation for estimating LDL cholesterol levels, and a direct method for measuring LDL cholesterol that uses immunoseparation of lipoproteins by their respective apolipoprotein content.

Ultracentrifugation involves the separation of lipoproteins based on their density differences after an 18-hour spin at 109,000 × g. The VLDL and chylomicrons float to the top and are separated using a tube slicing technique from the 1.006-g/mL infranatant (i.e., "1.006 bottom"). This infranatant fraction contains LDL and HDL. A heparin-manganese precipitation reagent is added to the 1.006 bottom to precipitate LDL, leaving HDL in the supernatant. The cholesterol concentrations of the 1.006 g/mL of infranatant and the HDL cholesterol supernatant are measured using the Abell-Kendall cholesterol reference method: LDL cholesterol = infranatant cholesterol − HDL cholesterol.

This procedure has been adopted by the Centers for Disease Control and Prevention and the Reference Network Laboratories for Standardizations as a means of directly measuring LDL cholesterol in the research setting and serves as the standard.[118] However, ultracentrifugation is poorly suited to the routine, clinical laboratory for several reasons. It requires cumbersome procedures; it is extremely labor intensive and technique dependent; it requires expensive instrumentation; and although it is the accepted reference method, it is an indirect measurement.

Most clinical laboratories use the equation known as the *Friedewald formula*[119] to estimate a patient's LDL cholesterol concentration: estimation of LDL cholesterol = total cholesterol − HDL cholesterol − VLDL cholesterol. The estimation of VLDL cholesterol equals the triglyceride level divided by five.[119]

The Friedewald formula estimates the LDL cholesterol concentration by subtracting the cholesterol associated with the other classes of lipoproteins from total cholesterol. This involves three independent lipid analyses, each contributing a potential source of error. It also involves a potentially inaccurate estimate of VLDL cholesterol. Because no direct VLDL cholesterol assay is available, it is calculated from the triglyceride value divided by a factor of five. This divisor can also add error to all LDL cholesterol estimates, but it is especially inappropriate for individuals with elevated triglyceride levels. Clinical laboratories use automated enzymatic analyses for cholesterol and triglyceride within serum or plasma, and HDL cholesterol is measured after precipitation of other lipoproteins in serum or plasma with heparin manganese chloride, dextran magnesium sulfate, or phosphotungstic acid.[118] On-line direct assays of HDL cholesterol are now available. The drawbacks of using the Friedewald formula for determining levels of LDL cholesterol are that it is estimated by calculation; it requires multiple assays and multiple steps, each adding a potential source of error; it is increasingly inaccurate as triglyceride levels increase; it requires that patients fast for 12 to 14 hours before specimen collection to avoid a triglyceride bias; and it is not standardized.[118,119] Moreover, LDL cholesterol concentrations cannot be reported for individuals with elevated triglyceride levels (>400 mg/dL or 4.5 mmol/L) or in the nonfasting state.[119,120] It has been reported that the formula becomes increasingly inaccurate in calculating true LDL cholesterol levels at borderline triglyceride levels (200–400 mg/dL or 2.3–4.5 mmol/L).[112–115]

The inadequacies of the methods for measuring LDL cholesterol necessitated the development of a direct method by which clinical laboratories may accurately and practically assess LDL cholesterol concentrations in patient samples. In 1990, the Laboratory Standardization Panel of the NCEP recommended the development of a direct LDL cholesterol measurement method.[118] The direct method for measuring serum or plasma LDL cholesterol concentration that was introduced was suitable for routine use in the clinical laboratory. This immunoseparation technology uses affinity-purified goat polyclonal antisera to human apo A-I and apo E, which are coated on latex particles; this facilitates the removal of chylomicrons, VLDL, and HDL in nonfasting or fasting specimens. After incubation and centrifugation, LDL cholesterol remains in the filtrate solution. The LDL cholesterol concentration is obtained by performing an enzymatic cholesterol assay on the filtrate solution.

The *direct LDL cholesterol immunoseparation method* allows for the direct quantitation of LDL cholesterol from one measurement, the use of fasting and nonfasting samples, and an LDL cholesterol measurement regardless of elevated triglyceride levels. When the direct LDL cholesterol assay was carried out on serum obtained from 115 subjects, who were fasting or nonfasting and were normal or hyperlipidemic, and was compared with those obtained by ultracentrifugation analysis, the correlation was 0.97, with a small negative bias of 2.9%. Subjects with LDL cholesterol levels ≥160 mg/dL, as obtained by ultracentrifugation, were correctly classified 93.8% of the time. In a similar study carried out on serum obtained from 177 subjects with normal or elevated lipid levels, the correlation between the direct LDL cholesterol and the value obtained by ultracentrifugation was 0.98, with between-run and within-run coefficients of variation <3%. The direct LDL cholesterol assay was found to be accurate using nonfasting and hypertriglyceridemic samples in the author's laboratory. This direct LDL cholesterol assay has been approved by the Food and Drug Administration and is commercially available to laboratories.[113,114] Moreover, the on-line direct LDL cholesterol assays now available also have high accuracy and precision.

# TREATMENT

## TREATMENT GUIDELINES FOR ELEVATED LOW-DENSITY LIPOPROTEIN CHOLESTEROL

### DIET THERAPY

LDL cholesterol levels requiring dietary intervention are shown in Table 163-3. The cornerstone of the treatment of lipid disorders is diet therapy requiring the *restriction of total fat* to 30% or less of calories, saturated fat to 10% (step 1 diet) or <7% (step 2 diet); and *restriction of cholesterol* to <300 mg per day (step 1 diet) or <200 mg per day (step 2 diet).[2-4] Approximately 50% of saturated fat and 70% of cholesterol in the U.S. diet come from hamburgers, cheeseburgers, meatloaf, beef steaks, and roasts; eggs; whole milk, cheese, and other dairy products, including ice cream; hot dogs, ham, and lunch meat; and doughnuts, cookies, and cake. These foods should be restricted, and they should be substituted with poultry (white meat) without skin, fish, skimmed or low-fat milk, nonfat or low-fat yogurt, and low-fat cheeses. The use of fruits, vegetables, and grains is encouraged. Oils that can be used are unsaturated vegetable oils containing polyunsaturated fat and monounsaturated fatty acids, such as canola, soybean, olive, or corn oil. However, such oils should only be used in moderation. The consumption of hydrogenated vegetable oils rich in *trans*-fatty acids, such as stick margarine, should be kept to a minimum. The consumption of a plant stanol ester-containing spread appears to be effective in reducing LDL cholesterol levels.[120a]

Excellent patient dietary pamphlets are available from the American Heart Association as well as the NCEP on the step 1 and step 2 diets. The step 1 diet is recommended for the entire U.S. population, and for patients with elevated LDL cholesterol; the step 2 diet is used if an inadequate response to the step 1 diet is achieved. Patients who are unable to achieve an adequate response with diet after receiving pamphlets and counseling by the physician and office nurse should be referred to a registered dietitian for instruction on following the step 2 diet. In most cases, diet therapy should be tried for at least 6 months before drug therapy is initiated, and a regular exercise program and control of other risk factors should be encouraged. Dietary modification can lower total serum cholesterol and LDL cholesterol by ~15% and significantly lower CHD risk.[15-21,121-128] However, compliance remains a major issue.[128] Dietary fat restriction (<30% of calories) along with exercise appears to be essential in preventing the age-related weight gain and obesity that often are associated with hyperlipidemia in society.[124] Such restriction is important in hypertriglyceridemic subjects to promote weight loss (see Chap. 164).

Responsiveness to dietary therapy is related to compliance and specific genetic factors (e.g., apo E and apo A-IV isoforms), and compliance and success should be monitored using LDL cholesterol levels.[125,126]

### DRUG THERAPY

Levels of LDL cholesterol requiring drug therapy after diet treatment are shown in Table 163-3. Lipid-lowering medications can be divided into two general classes: drugs effective in lowering LDL cholesterol (>15% reduction) and drugs effective in lowering triglyceride levels (>15% reduction). There are three classes of agents that meet the LDL cholesterol–lowering criteria: HMG-CoA reductase inhibitors (e.g., lovastatin, pravastatin, simvastatin, fluvastatin, atorvastatin, and cerivastatin), anion exchange resins (e.g., cholestyramine, colestipol), and niacin. Of these three types of drugs, patient compliance with resins and niacin is often poor, but with the HMG-CoA reductase inhibitors, it is generally excellent, as is their efficacy (20–60% LDL-C reduction). Moreover, long-term safety and efficacy in CHD risk reduction in large-scale, long-term, placebo-controlled trials have now been documented with the "statins."[27-35] Angiographic studies also indicate safety, efficacy, and significant benefit with respect to coronary atherosclerosis and CHD risk reduction.[38-47] The resins and niacin are now second-line drugs for lowering LDL cholesterol. HMG-CoA reductase inhibitors are currently the drugs of choice.

There are five agents that can lower triglyceride levels by >15%: niacin, gemfibrozil, fenofibrate, fish oil capsules, and the HMG-CoA reductase inhibitors. All of these agents generally also lower LDL cholesterol levels and raise HDL cholesterol levels. Niacin, gemfibrozil, and the HMG-CoA reductase inhibitors have all been shown to lower CHD risk prospectively[22-37] (see Chap. 164).

## TREATMENT OF VARIOUS LIPID ABNORMALITIES

### PATIENTS WITH ONLY ELEVATED LOW-DENSITY LIPOPROTEIN CHOLESTEROL

For all patients with increased LDL cholesterol, the drugs of choice are now HMG-CoA reductase inhibitors. If patients cannot tolerate these agents, niacin or a combination of resins and niacin should be used. The combinations of an HMG-CoA reductase inhibitor or niacin with an anion exchange resin are also effective.[129,130] For postmenopausal women who have had a hysterectomy, estrogen replacement is modestly effective in lowering LDL cholesterol and raising HDL cholesterol, but estrogens should not be used in patients with hypertriglyceridemia.[131-134] In some cases, the estrogen patch can be used and the hypertriglyceridemia treated with other medications. In women with an intact uterus, estrogen must be given together with progesterone to prevent uterine cancer. Estrogen use has been associated with a significant reduction in CHD mortality in postmenopausal women.[132,133] However, in a large trial (2763 postmenopausal women with established CHD), *no* significant risk reduction was noted in women randomized to the combination of conjugated equine estrogen (0.625 mg per day), and progesterone (2.5 mg per day) versus placebo over a 4-year period.[135] Therefore, *in men and women (with or without CHD), the HMG-CoA reductase inhibitors are the drugs of choice for LDL lowering and CHD risk reduction.*

### PATIENTS WITH ELEVATED LOW-DENSITY LIPOPROTEIN CHOLESTEROL AND ELEVATED TRIGLYCERIDES

For patients with elevations in LDL cholesterol and triglycerides (>200 mg/dL or 2.3 mmol/L), the drugs of choice are now HMG-CoA reductase inhibitors, especially atorvastatin. For patients who cannot tolerate these agents, niacin can be used. A combination of an HMG-CoA reductase inhibitor and a fibric acid derivative can also be used. This latter combination is generally well tolerated, but patients should be monitored for the possible development of myositis. The combination of an HMG-CoA reductase inhibitor with niacin or fish oil can also be tried.

### PATIENTS WITH HYPERTRIGLYCERIDEMIA AND NORMAL LOW-DENSITY LIPOPROTEIN CHOLESTEROL

For patients with hypertriglyceridemia only (>200 mg/dL or 2.3 mmol/L) and normal LDL cholesterol levels, there are no clear medication guidelines.[3,4] However, diet and exercise are encouraged, as well as the elimination of secondary causes of elevated triglycerides, such as lack of exercise, obesity, diabetes, alcohol, estrogens, and β-blockers. If the patient has a fasting triglyceride level >1000 mg/dL (11.3 mmol/L) while on a restricted diet, medication to reduce the risk of pancreatitis is recommended. However, before taking this step, the physician should make sure that these patients are not taking estrogens, thiazides, or β-blockers; are not using alcohol; or do not have uncontrolled diabetes mellitus. Caloric and fat restriction (<20% of calories) is also important in these patients. The drugs of choice in such individuals are generally gemfibrozil or fenofibrate because most have glucose intolerance. In the absence of glucose intolerance, niacin can be tried. In patients in whom these agents are not effective or if additional triglyceride reduction is needed, fish oil capsules (1 g) at a dosage of three to five capsules twice a day are effective in lowering triglycerides.

## PATIENTS WITH MODERATE HYPERTRIGLYCERIDEMIA OR LOW HIGH-DENSITY LIPOPROTEIN CHOLESTEROL

In patients with moderate hypertriglyceridemia, especially in those with HDL cholesterol deficiency, lifestyle changes including weight reduction and an exercise program are very helpful, as are the cessation of smoking and β-blockers. If patients have established heart disease, the use of niacin, gemfibrozil, or reductase inhibitors should be considered to normalize their lipid levels. The goal of therapy in CHD patients is to achieve an LDL cholesterol <100 mg/dL (2.6 mmol/L).[3,4] Some experts also recommend reduction of triglycerides to <200 mg/dL (2.3 mmol/L), and efforts to increase the HDL cholesterol to >35 mg/dL (0.9 mmol/L) if possible, and attempts to decrease the total cholesterol/HDL cholesterol ratio to <5.0. The goal of raising HDL cholesterol to >35 mg/dL can now be justified in CHD patients, based on the results of the Veterans Affairs High-Density Lipoprotein Intervention Trial (HIT), which used gemfibrozil in men with low HDL and CHD.[37] In the absence of heart disease, only lifestyle modification (i.e., diet and exercise) can be recommended to patients with moderate hypertriglyceridemia or HDL cholesterol deficiency.

## LIPID-LOWERING DRUGS

### ANION EXCHANGE RESINS

Cholestyramine and colestipol are anion exchange resins that bind bile acids, increase conversion of liver cholesterol to bile acids, and up-regulate LDL receptors in the liver.[2–6] These processes result in an increase in LDL catabolism and a decrease in plasma LDL cholesterol by ~20%. Side effects include bloating and constipation, elevation of triglycerides, and interference with the absorption of digoxin, tetracycline, thyroxine, phenylbutazone, and warfarin (Coumadin); these drugs should be given 1 hour earlier or 4 hours after the resin. Cholestyramine (4-g resin in packets, or scoops of powder) or colestipol (5-g packets or scoops of granules) can be started at one packet or scoop twice a day and gradually increased to two scoops twice a day or two scoops three times a day; the scoops are half the price of the packets. Cholestyramine tablets (1 g) were taken off the market because of difficulties with swallowing. Colestipol tablets (1 g) are available (2–16 g per day once or in divided doses; swallow tablets whole, one at a time; take with ample fluid). The constipation caused by the anion exchange resins may require treatment. Cholestyramine (6 scoops per day) has been shown to lower LDL cholesterol by 12% and reduce CHD risk prospectively by 19% over 7 years in middle-aged, asymptomatic, hypercholesterolemic men.[13,14] These agents are now second-line drugs, and are only first-line agents in children and adolescents with marked hypercholesterolemia.

### NIACIN

Niacin decreases triglycerides and VLDL cholesterol by 40%, decreases LDL cholesterol by 20%, and raises HDL cholesterol values by 20%. Niacin should be started at a dosage of 100 mg, taken orally twice a day with meals, and gradually increased to 1 g, taken orally twice or three times a day with meals (some authorities recommend higher doses up to 9 g per day). Side effects include flushing, gastric irritation, and elevations of uric acid, glucose, and liver enzymes in some patients. Niacin should not be used in patients with liver disease or a history of an ulcer or used by diabetic patients not on insulin. Long-acting niacin causes less flushing and can be used initially, but it results in excess gastrointestinal toxicity. A sustained-release formulation, Niaspan, which has now become available, is very well tolerated and is given once a day, starting at 375 mg per day and titrating up to 2 g per day. Niacin should be discontinued if liver enzymes increase to over three times the upper normal limit. Regular niacin was shown to lower total cholesterol levels by 10% and to reduce the recurrence of myocardial infarction by 20% after a 5-year period of administration in men with CHD.[136] The use of niacin was also associated with an 11% reduction in all-cause mortality 10 years after the cessation of niacin.[26] Niacin in combination with clofibrate has been shown to reduce mortality in CHD patients compared with usual care.[22] Niacin has the benefit of having favorable effects on all lipoproteins because it significantly lowers LDL cholesterol, triglycerides, remnant lipoproteins, and Lp(a), and raises HDL cholesterol. Nevertheless, because of its unfavorable side-effect profile, it should not be used in diabetic subjects, and remains a second-line lipid-lowering agent.

### FIBRIC ACID DERIVATIVES

**Gemfibrozil.**    Gemfibrozil is given at a dose of 600 mg, taken orally twice a day before meals, and it is generally well tolerated. The drug is effective in lowering triglycerides and VLDL cholesterol by 35% by enhancing the breakdown of VLDL triglyceride. The drug usually lowers LDL cholesterol by 5% to 15% and increases HDL cholesterol by 5% to 15%. Rarely, patients may get gastrointestinal symptoms, muscle cramps, or intermittent indigestion. The drug should not be used by patients with renal insufficiency, and it is also known to potentiate the action of warfarin. The drug may raise LDL cholesterol levels in hypertriglyceridemic patients. Gemfibrozil has been found to reduce CHD prospectively by 34% over 5 years in middle-aged, asymptomatic, hypercholesterolemic men, and by 22% in male CHD patients with LDL cholesterol levels <140 mg/dL and HDL cholesterol levels <40 mg/dL.[23–25,37] Because of this latter trial, gemfibrozil is the drug of choice in CHD patients with LDL cholesterol levels <130 mg/dL and HDL cholesterol levels <35 mg/dL. It is also the drug of choice in patients with severe hypertriglyceridemia.

**Fenofibrate.**    Fenofibrate is a new fibric acid derivative on the U.S. market that has been used in Europe for many years. It is as effective in lowering triglycerides as gemfibrozil, and appears to be slightly more effective in LDL cholesterol lowering (~15%).

### 3-HYDROXY-3-METHYLGLUTARYL–COENZYME A REDUCTASE INHIBITORS

The HMG-CoA reductase inhibitors, which are now the drugs of choice for LDL lowering, should be started at a low dose and gradually titrated upward, because the effect may be maximal at 20 mg per day with any of these agents (instead of 40–80 mg per day). These drugs are generally well tolerated, but occasionally may cause liver enzyme elevation (1–2%); significant creatine phosphokinase (CPK) elevation with myalgias and myositis (0.1%), especially in combination with gemfibrozil or cyclosporine; and can have gastrointestinal side effects.[137] Carefully controlled studies indicate that these agents do not cause cataracts, sleep problems, or daytime performance disturbances. Pravastatin use may be associated with less myositis and should be considered in patients who have developed this problem with other statins. Fluvastatin is the least expensive of these compounds, but only 25% reductions in LDL cholesterol occur at a dose of 40 mg per day.[138] Atorvastatin is the most potent, with a 60% reduction in LDL cholesterol achieved at a dosage of 80 mg per day.[139] Moreover, this agent is very effective in lowering triglyceride levels. These drugs inhibit HMG-CoA reductase, the rate-limiting enzyme in cholesterol biosynthesis, causing a decrease in the secretion of apo B-containing lipoproteins, and in some cases also causing up-regulation of LDL receptors, enhancing LDL catabolism. At maximal dosages, the four agents decrease plasma LDL cholesterol by 25% to 60%.[139,140] These agents decrease plasma triglycerides and cholesterol and increase HDL cholesterol levels moderately.[139,140]

Long-term safety and efficacy in CHD and stroke and mortality risk reduction have been established.[27–35] These agents are now the drugs of choice in patients with elevations of LDL cholesterol alone, or in combination with hypertriglyceridemia (triglycerides >200 mg/dL).

**Lovastatin.** Lovastatin is a fungal metabolite and is produced by fermentation. The drug is usually started at a dose of 10 to 20 mg, taken orally every day at supper, and it can be increased to 40 mg, taken orally every day; 20 mg, taken orally twice a day; or even 40 mg, taken orally twice a day. In the Post-CABG Study, the need for revascularization was decreased by 29% in post-bypass patients randomized to aggressive LDL lowering to 94 mg/dL (with lovastatin and, if necessary, resins), versus 134 mg/dL (low-dose lovastatin alone) over a 5-year period.[34] In the AFCAPS/TexCAPS Study, lovastatin (20–40 mg/dL) versus placebo lowered LDL cholesterol 25% and CHD prospectively by 37% (in 6605 men and women without CHD, with LDL cholesterol of 130–190 mg/dL, and with HDL cholesterol <50 mg/dL) over a 5-year period.[32]

**Pravastatin.** Pravastatin is usually started at 10 or 20 mg, taken orally each day at bedtime, and it can be increased to 40 mg, taken orally each day at bedtime. Its structure is similar to that of lovastatin, except that it is in the open acid form and has a hydroxyl group attached to it, making it a more polar compound; consequently, this drug has greater liver selectivity and less penetration into other tissues. In the West of Scotland Study, pravastatin (40 mg per day) lowered LDL cholesterol by 26% and CHD risk by 31% (in 6595 hypercholesterolemic men without CHD) over 5 years.[30] In CARE, pravastatin (40 mg per day) versus placebo lowered LDL cholesterol by 26% and CHD risk by 24% (in 4159 CHD patients with LDL cholesterol of 115–174 mg/dL) over 5 years.[31] In LIPID, pravastatin (40 mg per day) versus placebo lowered LDL cholesterol by 25%, CHD risk by 29%, CHD death by 24%, and stroke death by 19%, over 6.1 years (in 9014 patients with CHD and initial total cholesterol levels of 155–271 mg/dL).[33]

**Simvastatin.** Simvastatin is usually started at a dose of 10 mg, taken orally each day at supper, and it can be increased to 20 or 40 mg, taken orally daily. Its structure is similar to that of lovastatin, except that it has an additional methyl group. In the Scandinavian Simvastatin Survival Study (4S), simvastatin (20–40 mg per day) versus placebo lowered LDL cholesterol by 35%, CHD risk by 34%, stroke by 37%, CHD mortality by 42%, and the need for angioplasty or bypass surgery by 37% (in 4444 men and women with CHD and total cholesterol between 200 and 300 mg/dL) over a 5-year period.[27,28]

**Fluvastatin.** Fluvastatin is structurally different from the other agents and was the first synthetic HMG-CoA reductase inhibitor. It is usually started at a dose of 20 mg, taken orally each day, and it can be increased to 40 mg, taken orally once a day. At this latter dose it lowers LDL cholesterol by 25%. Fluva-

statin has been shown to decrease coronary artery atherosclerosis progression as compared to placebo when assessed angiographically in CHD patients.[138]

**Atorvastatin.** Atorvastatin (a very potent statin that is available in 10-, 20-, and 40-mg tablets) causes reductions in LDL cholesterol of 39%, 43%, and 50%, respectively.[139] The starting dose is 10 mg per day and the maximal dose is 80 mg per day, with LDL cholesterol reductions of 61% and triglyceride reductions of up to 40%.[139,140] It is very effective in hypertriglyceridemic patients.[140] In the AVERT Study (in 341 CHD patients), atorvastatin (80 mg per day) versus angioplasty and usual care (mean LDL cholesterol 118 mg/dL) decreased CHD end points by 36% and lowered LDL cholesterol to 77 mg/dL over a 1.5-year period.[35]

**Cerivastatin.** Cerivastatin is a synthetic statin that lowers LDL cholesterol by 35% at the maximal dose of 0.4 mg per day.

### PROBUCOL

Probucol is an antioxidant, given at a dose of 500 mg that is taken orally twice a day. It is a second-line drug that lowers LDL cholesterol 10% to 15%. It can be used in treating familial hypercholesterolemia for increasing nonreceptor LDL catabolism; it may cause gastrointestinal side effects. The drug also lowers HDL cholesterol by 15% to 25% by decreasing its production. The long-term safety and efficacy in CHD risk reduction have not been established. A femoral artery angiographic study did not demonstrate any significant benefit with probucol.[141] Therefore, this agent cannot be recommended, even though it is very potent in preventing LDL from being oxidized.[141a]

### FISH OIL CAPSULES

Fish oil capsules are rich in eicosapentaenoic acid (20:5n3) and docosahexaenoic acid (22:6n3). These capsules lower triglyceride significantly (20–25%) by shunting fatty acid production into phospholipids and away from triglycerides. Moreover, these agents may be very useful for maintenance of fluidity and preventing cardiac arrhythmias and sudden death. In the Diet and Reinfarction Trial (DART; in >2000 men with CHD), an increased fish intake or two 500-mg fish oil capsules per day reduced CHD death by 29%.[142]

### COMBINATION DRUG THERAPIES

Niacin and resins together are very effective, as are reductase inhibitors and niacin, in lowering LDL cholesterol. The combination of fibric acid derivatives and reductase inhibitors should be used with caution because the myositis incidence is increased.[137,143] If this combination is used, the CPK levels should be monitored.[141] Niacin and reductase inhibitors are also effective, but because the incidence of significant liver enzyme elevation is ~10%, this combination should be used with caution. Gemfibrozil with fish oil capsules or with niacin can be used to lower triglycerides. The response to drug therapy should be monitored by measuring LDL cholesterol, HDL cholesterol, and triglyceride levels. Also, toxicity should be checked by measuring liver enzymes and CPK levels.

## FAMILIAL LIPOPROTEIN DISORDERS

### FAMILIAL HYPERCHOLESTEROLEMIA WITH XANTHOMAS

Familial hypercholesterolemia with xanthomas was originally recognized in the 1930s, and its autosomal codominant mode of inheritance was subsequently documented.[144–146] With the

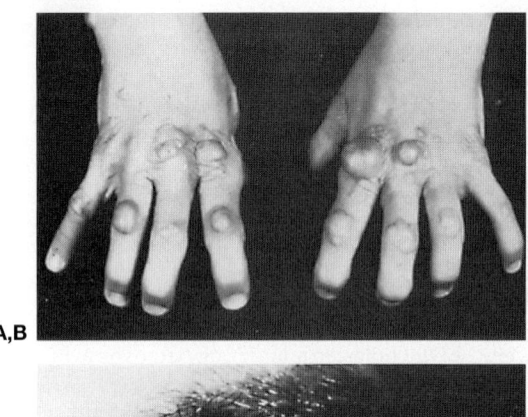
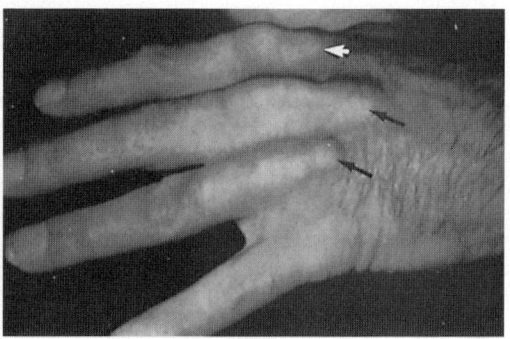

**A,B**

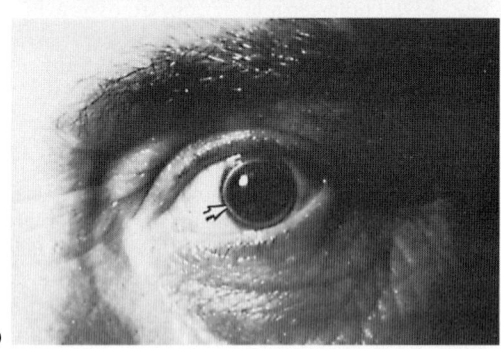
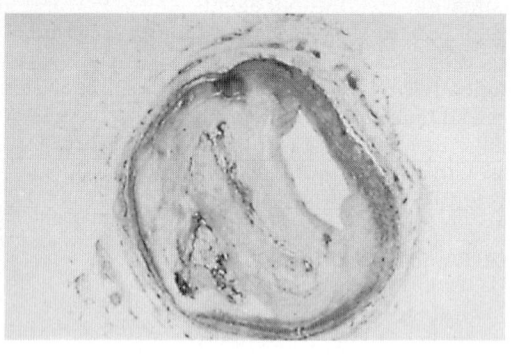

**C,D**

**FIGURE 163-1. A** and **B,** Tuberous xanthomas in a patient with homozygous familial hypercholesterolemia (i.e., low-density lipoprotein receptor negative) and tendinous xanthomas (*arrows*). **C** and **D,** Circus corneae (*arrow*) and severe coronary atherosclerosis in patients with heterozygous familial hypercholesterolemia.

advent of the classification of lipoprotein disorders in the 1960s, it was recognized that this condition was associated with marked elevations in LDL, with other lipoprotein fractions being reasonably normal (i.e., type IIA hyperlipoproteinemia).[5]

It was later documented that ~30% of 500 male survivors of myocardial infarction younger than 60 years of age had serum cholesterol or triglyceride levels above the 95th percentile.[147,148] Moreover, it was shown that of 176 families of these hyperlipidemic myocardial infarction survivors, 15 families or 3% of the total group of 500 subjects had familial hypercholesterolemia and that five kindreds or 1% had familial hypercholesterolemia that was associated with tendinous xanthomas.[148] Phenotype analysis revealed increased LDL or β-lipoproteins in these kindreds.[149] In the author's studies of 102 kindreds in whom the proband had documented coronary atherosclerosis by angiography before 60 years of age, 3% of the kindreds had isolated LDL cholesterol levels above the 90th percentile, with 1% of the kindreds having familial hypercholesterolemia with tendinous xanthomas and an LDL-receptor mutation.[150] A few patients have tendinous xanthomas and normal cholesterol levels. These patients are discussed in the sections on cerebrotendinous xanthomatosis (CTX) or β-sitosterolemia.

Patients with heterozygous familial hypercholesterolemia have been documented to have delayed clearance of LDL apo B.[151] Patients with familial hypercholesterolemia were shown to have various mutations at the LDL-receptor gene locus, resulting in a lack of expression or expression of defective LDL receptors.[7,152–154,154a] Many different mutations at this locus have been described.[152–154] The estimated prevalence of this disorder in the heterozygous state is 1 of 500 persons in the general population, although large-scale population studies have not been performed. Some patients with phenotypic familial hypercholesterolemia have a defect within apo B-100, resulting in defective binding of LDL to the LDL receptor.[155,156,156a]

In adults with heterozygous familial hypercholesterolemia, LDL cholesterol levels are usually >250 mg/dL, but triglyceride and HDL cholesterol levels are generally normal.[50] Clinically, these patients usually develop arcus senilis and tendinous xanthomas. The clinical diagnosis, in the author's view, is established by an LDL cholesterol level above the 90th percentile in two or more family members and the presence of tendinous xan-

thomas within the kindred (Fig. 163-1). The average age of onset of CHD is ~45 years for men and 55 years for women with untreated heterozygous familial hypercholesterolemia.[50] These patients may also have a higher than normal prevalence of calcific aortic stenosis.

Treatment consists of an NCEP step 2 diet low in saturated fat (<7% of calories) and cholesterol (<200 mg per day) and, in most cases, combined drug therapy. Dietary treatment alone usually results in only small reductions in LDL cholesterol in these patients, and the initial drug of choice is an HMG-CoA reductase inhibitor, which can be combined with resin or niacin.[3,4,27,35,157,158] The most effective therapy for heterozygotes is atorvastatin, 80 mg per day, as monotherapy, or, if necessary, in combination with an anion exchange resin.

Some homozygotes may respond modestly to medications, but these patients generally require selective pheresis to remove LDL every 1 to 2 weeks for effective control and CHD prevention.[159–161] Portacaval shunting, liver transplantation, and gene therapy remain experimental.[162] Familial hypercholesterolemia homozygotes often have LDL cholesterol levels >500 mg/dL, and they frequently have decreased HDL cholesterol levels. In addition to having tendinous xanthomas, these patients often develop tuberous xanthomas and aortic stenosis secondary to cholesterol deposits on the valve leaflets[49] (see Fig. 163-1). The average onset of CHD is ~10 years of age for receptor-negative homozygotes and 20 years for receptor-defective homozygotes. LDL-lowering therapy is mandatory for CHD prevention in these patients. Selective LDL apheresis weekly or biweekly is now approved in the United States for patients on maximal diet and drug therapy who have LDL cholesterol >300 mg/dL and total cholesterol >400 mg/dL.

## POLYGENIC FAMILIAL HYPERCHOLESTEROLEMIA WITHOUT XANTHOMAS

Among the 3% of CHD patients who have familial hypercholesterolemia, only one-third have tendinous xanthomas and are truly heterozygous for familial hypercholesterolemia with potential LDL receptor defects.[147–149] Other CHD kindreds with familial hypercholesterolemia have more modest LDL cholesterol elevations (>190 mg/dL) without xanthomas.

These kindreds have been classified as *polygenic familial hypercholesterolemia*; no clear defect has been found. Having the apo E-4 allele is known to be associated with elevations in LDL cholesterol levels, and these patients may be more likely to be heterozygous or homozygous for apo E-4.[115,163,164] The clinical diagnosis of this disorder is established by the presence of LDL cholesterol values greater than the 90th percentile in two or more family members and a lack of xanthomas in the family. The treatment of these patients includes implementation of an NCEP step 2 diet and the use of cholesterol-lowering medications, such as HMG-CoA reductase inhibitors, resins, or niacin.

## FAMILIAL COMBINED HYPERLIPIDEMIA

Familial combined hyperlipidemia was initially characterized by the finding of hypercholesterolemia and hypertriglyceridemia within the same kindred and by relatives having one or both of these abnormalities.[147–149,165] This disorder was found in ~10% of myocardial infarction survivors younger than 60 years of age. Using 95th percentile criteria for serum cholesterol and triglyceride levels, affected subjects were shown to have elevations in VLDL, LDL, or both on phenotyping analysis.[148,149] In the author's series, ~14% of kindreds with premature CHD had familial combined hyperlipidemia.

The clinical diagnosis of familial combined hyperlipidemia is established by the finding of serum or plasma LDL cholesterol or triglyceride levels above the 90th percentile (usually LDL cholesterol >190 mg/dL or triglyceride >50 mg/dL) within the family and in at least two family members, with both abnormalities occurring within the kindred.[150] Most patients with familial combined hyperlipidemia also have HDL cholesterol values below the tenth percentile.[150] It has been reported that patients with familial combined hyperlipidemia have overproduction of apo B-100, but the precise defect is unknown.[166–168] Data indicate that hepatic apo B-100 secretion is largely substrate driven.[169] Patients with familial combined hyperlipidemia often are overweight and hypertensive, and they may also be diabetic and have gout. Treatment with diet, an exercise program, and, if necessary, the use of an HMG-CoA reductase inhibitor is important for CHD prevention. Niacin is an alternative form of therapy in this condition.

## FAMILIAL HYPERAPOBETALIPOPROTEINEMIA

Familial hyperapobetalipoproteinemia is characterized by apo B values above the 90th percentile in the absence of other lipid abnormalities in the kindred with at least two affected family members, using age- and gender-adjusted norms.[169–172] This disorder occurred in 5% of CHD kindreds in the author's series; it is thought to be a variant of familial combined hyperlipidemia. It also is associated with overproduction of apo B-100.[150]

## FAMILIAL DYSLIPIDEMIA

Familial hypertriglyceridemia is a common familial lipid disorder in which at least two kindred members have fasting triglyceride levels greater than the 90th percentile of normal. Approximately 5% of myocardial infarction survivors younger than 60 years of age were found to have this disorder, using the 95th percentile as the standard.[147–149] In the author's studies, using the 90th percentile, ~15% of CHD kindreds had this disorder.[150] In the author's series, all kindreds except one had HDL cholesterol deficiency within the family as well. The author and colleagues have named this disorder *familial dyslipidemia*. Hypertriglyceridemia and HDL cholesterol levels must be less than the tenth percentile in the kindred for the family to have this condition.[150] These patients are frequently overweight and

may have male-pattern obesity, insulin resistance, type II diabetes, and hypertension. The precise defect is unknown, but the patients have increased hepatic triglyceride secretion and enhanced HDL apo A-I fractional catabolism.[166–168,173–176]

No clear therapeutic guidelines have been formulated, other than treatment of other CHD risk factors, a diet and exercise program, and optimization of LDL cholesterol levels. However, in CHD patients with this disorder and LDL cholesterol <130 mg/dL, gemfibrozil therapy can be recommended if their HDL cholesterols are <35 mg/dL, based on the recent Veterans Affairs HIT Study.[37]

## FAMILIAL HYPOALPHALIPOPROTEINEMIA

Severe HDL deficiency (HDL cholesterol < 10 mg/dL) is rare and can be caused by Tangier disease, the apo A-I deficiency states, apo A-I variants, lecithin:cholesterol acyltransferase (LCAT) deficiency, or fish eye disease.[177–198] CHD is less associated with these disorders if LCAT activity is impaired than if it is not impaired. In the case of the apo A-I deficiency states, apo A-I synthesis is reduced, but in Tangier disease and LCAT deficiency, HDL apo A-I fractional catabolism is enhanced.[174–176,178,183–188,196] The apo A-I deficiency states are caused by deletions, rearrangements, or point mutations within the apo A-I/C-III/A-IV gene complex, resulting in lack of expression of all three proteins, of apo A-I and apo C-III, or only of apo A-I.[186,189–192] These rare disorders are discussed later in this chapter.

Familial hypoalphalipoproteinemia is relatively common. It is characterized by HDL cholesterol levels that are less than the tenth percentile of normal in two or more kindred members, and it is observed in ~4% of kindreds with premature CHD.[150,199,200] These patients have decreased HDL apo A-I production or enhanced HDL apo A-I fractional catabolism.[174–176,201] The precise molecular defects are being studied.[201a] Familial combined hyperlipidemia, familial hyperapobetalipoproteinemia, familial dyslipidemia, and familial hypoalphalipoproteinemia may be variants of the same disorder, characterized by a genetic predisposition in populations on atherogenic diets, especially in those with male-pattern obesity; the condition is associated with oversecretion of apo B-containing lipoproteins and enhanced catabolism of apo A-I–containing lipoproteins. These derangements are common, are clearly not monogenic, and result in an accumulation of LpB:E and LpB and in decreases in LpA-I and LpA-I/A-II particles.[202,203]

Treatment consists of a step 2 diet and efforts to optimize HDL cholesterol, triglyceride, and LDL cholesterol levels with niacin, gemfibrozil, or a statin, or combinations thereof. Based on the Veterans Affairs HIT Study, gemfibrozil can be recommended in CHD patients with HDL cholesterol <35 mg/dL.[37]

## FAMILIAL DYSBETALIPOPROTEINEMIA

Familial dysbetalipoproteinemia was originally named type III hyperlipoproteinemia.[5] These patients accumulate VLDL (density <1.006 g/mL) that are cholesterol ester rich and have beta mobility on lipoprotein electrophoresis.[5] The disorder was estimated to be present in 0.5% of kindreds with premature CHD, and these patients were reported to have a mean VLDL cholesterol/triglyceride ratio of more than 0.3 (normal, 0.2) based on quantification of VLDL cholesterol levels after ultracentrifugation.[5,149,204,205] With the aid of the remnant lipoprotein cholesterol and triglyceride assay, the diagnosis can now be made without ultracentrifugation of plasma.[70–74] The disease is a result of the apo E-2/2 phenotype or, rarely, an apo E deficiency.[204–212] Apo E-2 has defective binding to the B:E or LDL receptor compared with apo E-3, and this isoform usually results from a cysteine for arginine substitution at residue 158 within the apo E sequence.[209] Apo E is necessary for the normal receptor-mediated uptake of chylo-

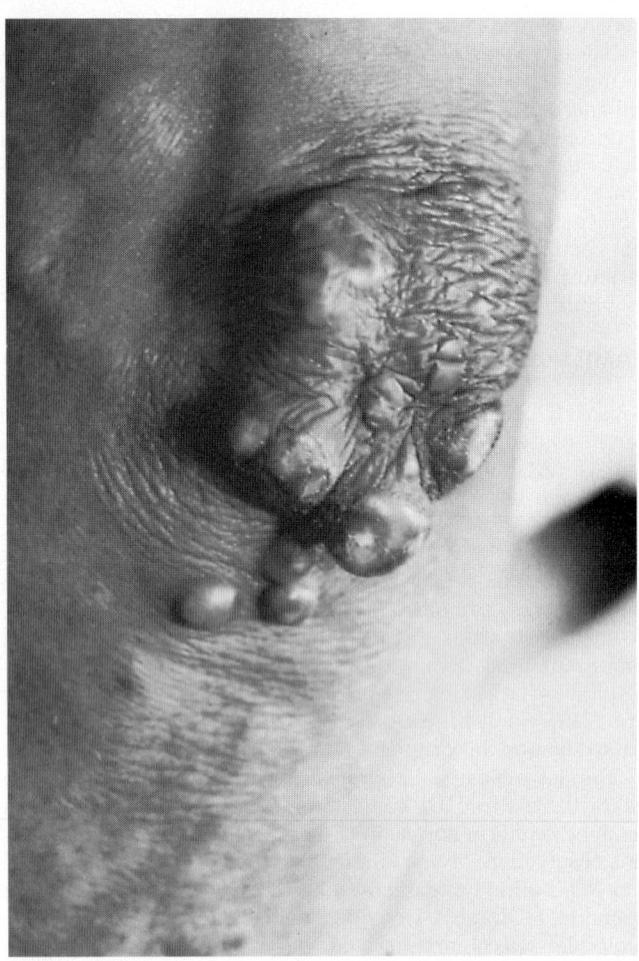

**FIGURE 163-2.** Tuboeruptive xanthomas on the elbow of a patient with dysbetalipoproteinemia or type III hyperlipoproteinemia associated with apolipoprotein E deficiency.

micron and VLDL remnants, and persons with dysbetalipoproteinemia have delayed catabolism of these lipoproteins.[208–211] These patients may have tuberous and planar xanthomas, and they commonly are obese, diabetic, hypertensive, and hyperuricemic.[213] (Figs. 163-2 and 163-3). These patients may have the apo E-2/2 phenotype and may have another common familial disorder, such as familial combined hyperlipidemia or a full-blown dysbetalipoproteinemia, because many apo E-2/2 homozygotes in the population do not have hyperlipidemia.[163,164]

Treatment consists of an NCEP step 2 diet and niacin, a fibric acid derivative, or an HMG-CoA reductase inhibitor. If the patients are diabetic, niacin should not be prescribed.

## FAMILIAL LIPOPROTEIN(a) EXCESS

Lp(a) is a lipoprotein particle similar to LDL, except that it is attached to a molecule of apo (a).[75–77] Elevated Lp(a) is a highly heritable trait.[75–79] A value greater than the 90th percentile of normal is considered elevated (>40 mg/dL, using assays that assess the level of the entire particle).[92–97] Elevated levels of Lp(a) are associated with premature CHD.[83–98] Approximately 15% of patients with premature CHD have familial Lp(a) excess.[150] These patients do not have xanthomas. Lp(a) appears to promote atherosclerosis and atherothrombosis by two mechanisms: deposition in the arterial wall and inhibition of fibrinolysis.[80–82]

Assays for the measurement of Lp(a) are commercially available, and an Lp(a) cholesterol assay has been developed as well.[98] Isoproteins of apo (a) differ in their molecular weights. Decreased apo (a) molecular weight is associated with increased Lp(a) levels.[77–79] Apo (a) has been shown to contain multiple repeats of a protein domain that is highly homologous to the kringle 4 domain of plasminogen and one repeat of a protein domain highly homologous to the kringle 5 domain of plasminogen.[78] The variability in apo (a) molecular weight appears to be related to a decreased number of kringle 4–like repeats.[78] Elevated levels of Lp(a) are also observed in patients with heterozygous familial hypercholesterolemia.[214]

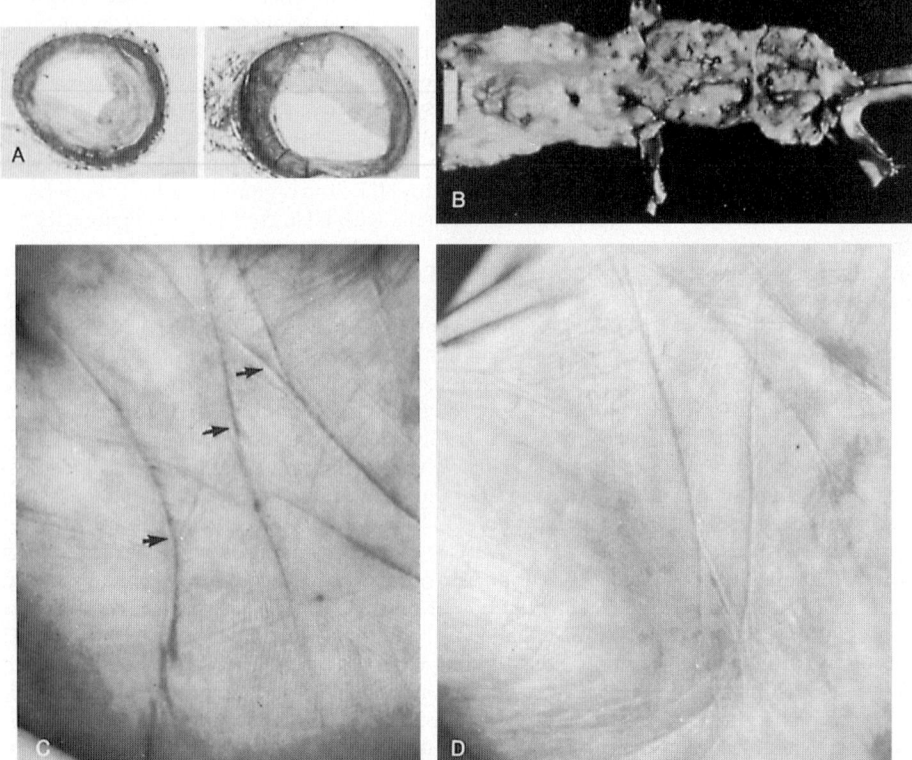

**FIGURE 163-3.** Cross sections of coronary artery (low-power microscopy), showing atherosclerosis (**A**), aortic and iliac atherosclerosis (**B**), and palmar xanthomas (**C**), compared with normal palm (**D**), in patients with dysbetalipoproteinemia or type III hyperlipoproteinemia associated with apolipoprotein E-2 homozygosity.

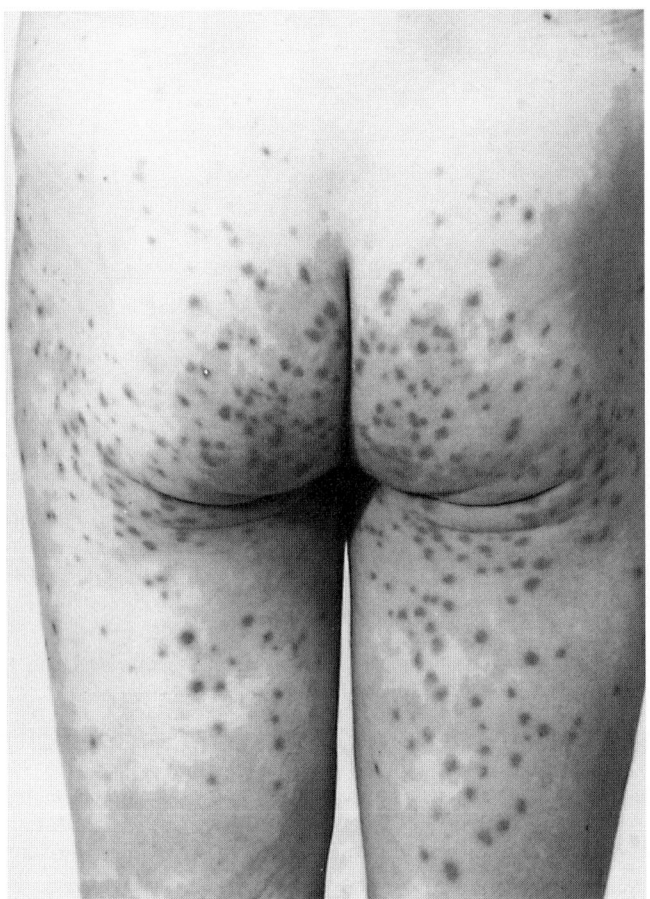

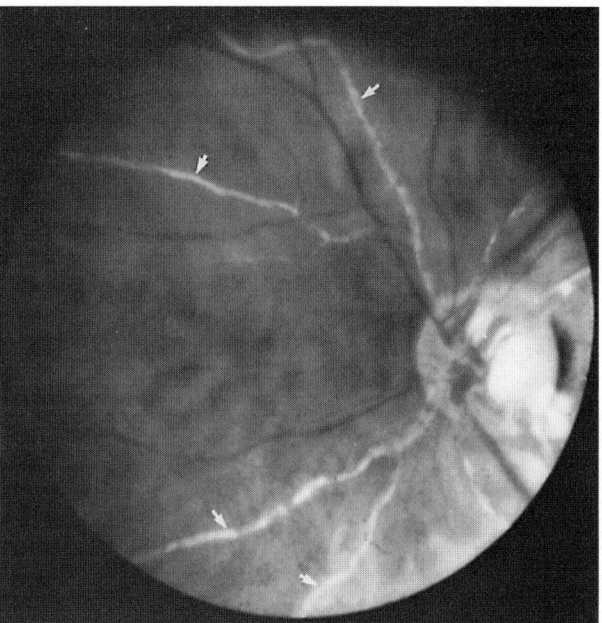

**FIGURE 163-6.** Lipemia retinalis in the veins of the retina in a patient with severe hypertriglyceridemia associated with lipoprotein lipase deficiency. The patient had marked hypertriglyceridemia (>2000 mg/dL). There is a nonuniform, white, mottled appearance of the veins (*arrows*).

**FIGURE 163-4.** Eruptive xanthomas on the buttocks of a patient with severe hypertriglyceridemia and diabetes mellitus.

Diets and medications (e.g., resin, HMG-CoA reductase inhibitors) that lower LDL levels have no effect on Lp(a), but niacin and estrogen administration have been reported to decrease Lp(a) levels.[134,215] No guidelines for the treatment of Lp(a) excess have been formulated, but treatment with niacin of such patients is warranted if they have established CHD,

because such therapy has been shown to decrease morbidity and mortality in unselected CHD patients.[26,136]

## SEVERE HYPERTRIGLYCERIDEMIA

Severe hypertriglyceridemia (triglyceride values >1000 mg/dL or 11.3 mmol/L) occasionally is observed in middle-aged or elderly individuals who are obese and have glucose intolerance and hyperuricemia.[5,6] They usually have familial hypertriglyceridemia or familial combined hyperlipidemia that is exacerbated by other factors such as obesity and diabetes mellitus. These patients usually have HDL cholesterol deficiency and may develop lipemia retinalis and eruptive xanthomas (Figs. 163-4 through 163-6). They are

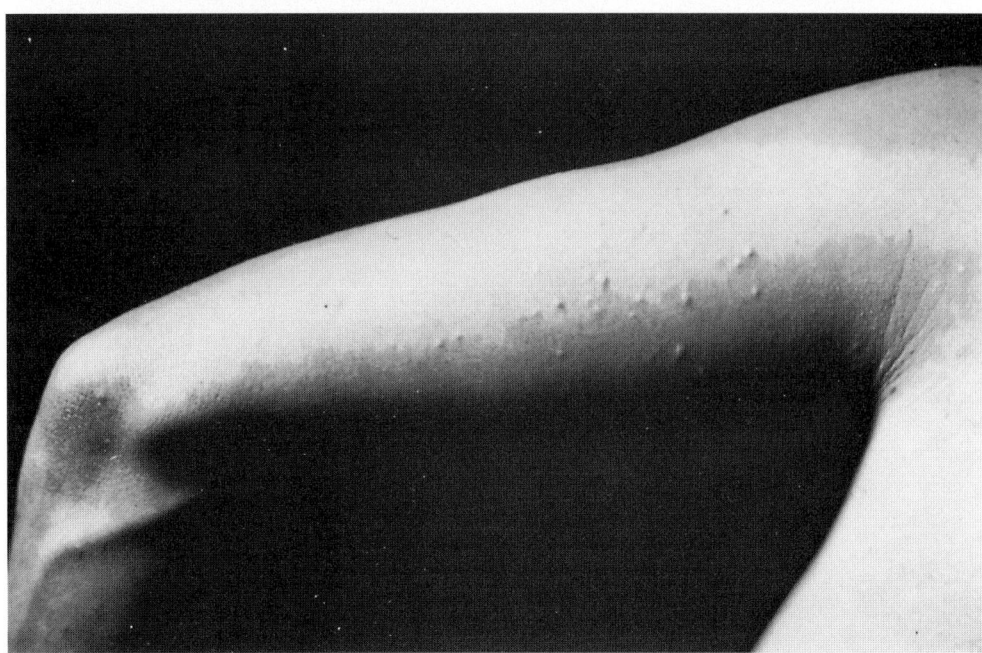

**FIGURE 163-5.** Eruptive xanthomas in a patient with severe hypertriglyceridemia associated with lipoprotein lipase deficiency. The xanthomas are filled with lipid-laden macrophages.

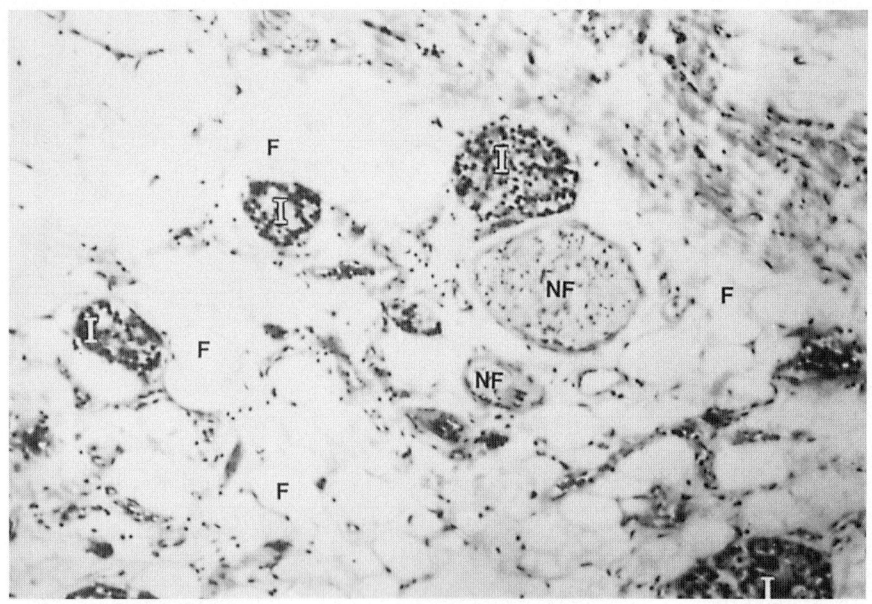

**FIGURE 163-7.** Section of pancreatic tissue from a patient with chronic recurrent pancreatitis secondary to severe hypertriglyceridemia associated with lipoprotein lipase deficiency. Notice the replacement of acinar cells with fat (*F*) and the presence of intact islets of Langerhans (dark-staining cells; *I*), and nerve fibers (*NF*; lighter-staining cells in round cluster within sheath).

at increased risk for developing pancreatitis due to triglyceride deposition in the pancreas and in the liver (Figs. 163-7 and 163-8) and may have paresthesias and emotional lability. They often have delayed chylomicron and VLDL cholesterol clearance and excess VLDL production.

Treatment consists of a calorie-restricted step 2 diet. For patients with diabetes mellitus, it is crucial to control the blood glucose as well as possible. Medications that are effective in lowering the triglycerides to <1000 mg/dL (11.3 mmol/L) to reduce the risk of pancreatitis include gemfibrozil and fish oil capsules (6–10 capsules per day).[216]

Patients who have severe hypertriglyceridemia in childhood or early adulthood and who are not obese often have a deficiency of the enzyme lipoprotein lipase or its activator protein (apo C-II), resulting in markedly impaired removal of triglyceride. They have a defect in chylomicron and VLDL catabolism. These patients are at increased risk for recurrent pancreatitis; it is important to restrict their dietary fat to <20% of calories. Niacin or gemfibrozil is generally ineffective. However, fish oil capsules (6–10 per day) may help certain patients to keep their

triglyceride levels below 1000 mg/dL (11.3 mmol/L) and to minimize the risk of pancreatitis.[216]

## SEVERE HIGH-DENSITY LIPOPROTEIN DEFICIENCIES

Severe HDL deficiencies are rare disorders that are characterized by HDL cholesterol levels below 10 mg/dL in the absence of liver disease or severe hypertriglyceridemia, and some have been associated with premature CHD.

### APOLIPOPROTEIN A-I, C-III, AND A-IV DEFICIENCY

The proband in the kindred with apo A-I, apo C-III, and apo A-IV deficiencies died of severe diffuse coronary atherosclerosis at 45 years of age. She had marked HDL deficiency, decreased triglyceride levels, and normal LDL cholesterol values.[183–186] She had mild corneal opacification but no planar xanthomas. There also has been evidence of fat malabsorption (i.e., vitamin E, vitamin K, and essential fatty acid deficiency). Plasma apo A-I and apo C-III were undetectable.[184] Heterozygotes had levels of HDL cholesterol, apo A-I, apo C-III, and apo A-IV that were 50% of nor-

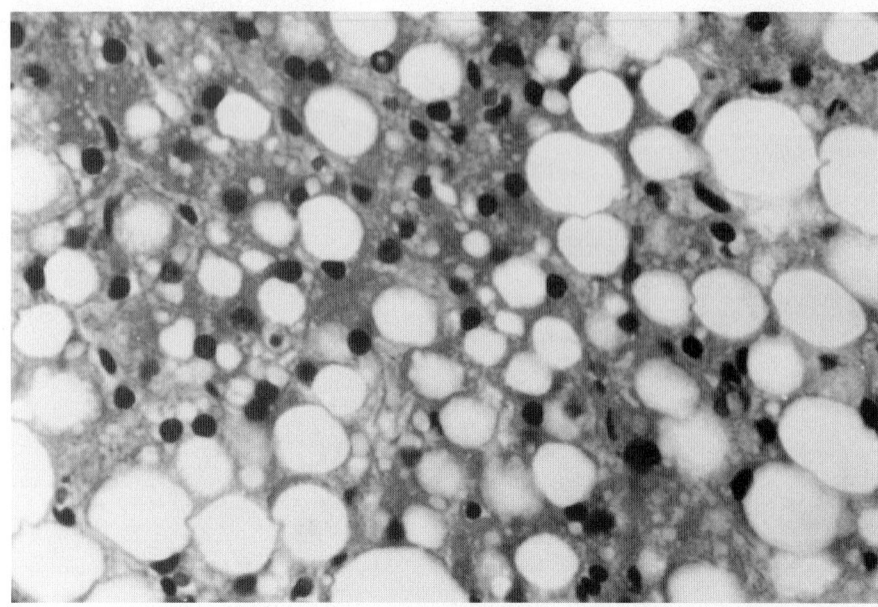

**FIGURE 163-8.** Diffuse triglyceride deposition in the liver parenchyma of a patient with severe hypertriglyceridemia associated with lipoprotein lipase deficiency.

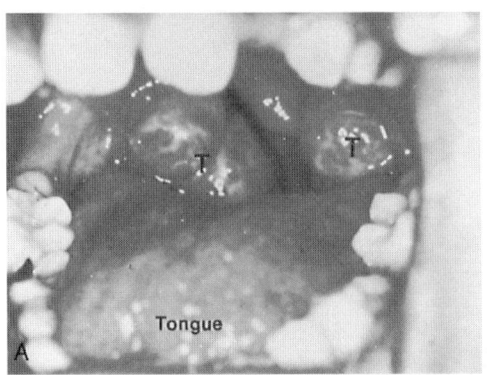 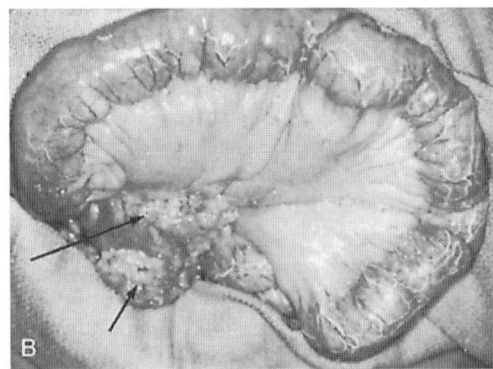 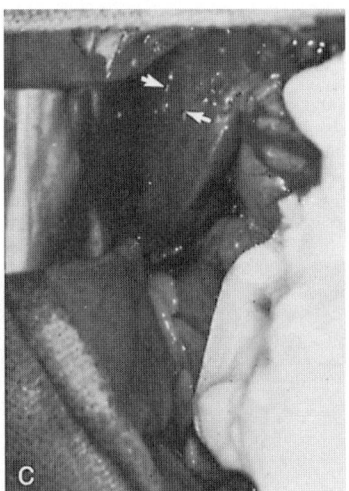

**FIGURE 163-9.** Enlarged orange tonsils (*T*) (**A**); omental lipid deposition (*arrows*), at the base of the mesentery (**B**); and stippled liver with lipid deposition (*arrows*) (**C**), in a patient with homozygous Tangier disease undergoing surgical exploration. The lipid deposition is characterized by cholesterol ester–laden macrophages. The patient also had mild corneal opacification. (From Schaefer EJ, Triche TJ, Zech LA, et al. Massive omental reticuloendothelial cell lipid uptake in Tangier disease after splenectomy. Am J Med 1983; 75:521.)

mal.[186] The defect is a deletion of the entire apo A-I/C-III/A-IV gene complex.[186] Treatment should consist of optimization of other risk factors, including LDL cholesterol levels.

### APOLIPOPROTEIN A-I AND C-III DEFICIENCY

A kindred has been reported in which two sisters presented in their late twenties with CHD, planar xanthomas, and mild corneal opacification with marked HDL deficiency, normal LDL cholesterol values, and decreased triglycerides. No evidence of fat malabsorption was found.[187,188] Plasma apo A-I and apo C-III were not detectable in these homozygotes, and the defect was shown to be a DNA rearrangement affecting the adjacent apo A-I and apo C-III genes.[189] Heterozygotes in this kindred had HDL cholesterol, apo A-I, and apo C-III values that were ~50% of normal. Treatment is to optimize other CHD risk factors.

### APOLIPOPROTEIN A-I DEFICIENCY

Several kindreds have been reported in which the homozygous proband had HDL deficiency, planar xanthomas, and undetectable plasma levels of apo A-I.[190,191] The defect has been shown to be due to various point mutations, resulting in lack of apo A-I gene expression. No evidence of fat malabsorption was noted. Treatment is to optimize other CHD risk factors.

### APOLIPOPROTEIN A-I VARIANTS

Studies examining apo A-I isoforms by isoelectric focusing have led to the discovery of 18 different mutations within the apo A-I sequence. The mutations are at residues 3 (Pro, 2 mutations), 4 (Pro), 89 (Asp), 103 (Asp), 107 (Lys, 2 mutations), 136 (Glu), 139 (Glu), 143 (Pro), 147 (Glu), 158 (Ala), 165 (Pro), 169 (Glu), 173 (Arg), 177 (Arg), 198 (Glu), and 213 (Asp) within the 243-residue apo A-I sequence.[192–195] All diagnosed persons have been heterozygotes. The residue 173 mutation (Arg-Cys) is known as *apo A-I Milano* and is associated with mild hypertriglyceridemia and markedly decreased HDL cholesterol levels and no evidence of premature CHD.[193] The residue 165 mutation (Pro-Arg) has also been associated with decreased HDL cholesterol and apo A-I levels, as has the 143 mutation (Pro-Arg).[194] The latter mutation results in decreased ability of apo A-I to activate the enzyme LCAT. Other mutations have not been associated with

decreased HDL cholesterol, but the mutations at residue 3 (Pro-His or Pro-Arg) result in an increased pro-apo A-I/apo A-I ratio in plasma, suggesting reduced conversion of pro-apo A-I to mature apo A-I in these persons.[194] The incidence of apo A-I variants is rare, occurring in 1 of 1000 normal persons as well as in myocardial infarction survivors.[194]

### TANGIER DISEASE

Tangier disease was named after the Chesapeake Bay island home of the original kindred. Homozygotes with this disorder have marked HDL deficiency, mild hypertriglyceridemia, and decreased LDL cholesterol values.[177–179] Apo A-I levels are 1% of normal, but apo C-III and apo A-IV values are within normal limits. These patients have lipid-laden macrophages resulting in enlarged orange tonsils, hepatosplenomegaly, and lymphadenopathy[179] (Fig. 163-9). These patients have hypercatabolism of HDL constituents, but the primary structures of apo A-I and apo A-II are normal.[177,178] Heterozygotes have HDL cholesterol and apo A-I values that are 50% of normal. Homozygotes often develop premature CHD and peripheral neuropathy.[179] The defect is caused by defective cellular cholesterol efflux due to various mutations in the adenosine triphosphate (ATP)–binding cassette protein gene (ABC 1).[180–182] This defect results in lack of normal HDL formation and hypercatabolism. Treatment consists of optimization of CHD risk factors.

### LECITHIN:CHOLESTEROL ACYLTRANSFERASE DEFICIENCY

The enzyme LCAT is responsible for cholesterol esterification in plasma. Patients with LCAT deficiency have a very high proportion of plasma cholesterol in the unesterified form, marked HDL cholesterol deficiency, hypertriglyceridemia, and increased amounts of free cholesterol–rich VLDL and LDL. They develop marked corneal opacification, anemia, proteinuria, renal insufficiency, and atherosclerosis. Treatment consists of dietary saturated fat and cholesterol restriction, and renal dialysis and transplantation if necessary.[196]

### FISH EYE DISEASE

Fish eye disease is associated with mild hypertriglyceridemia and significant HDL deficiency. Patients with fish eye disease

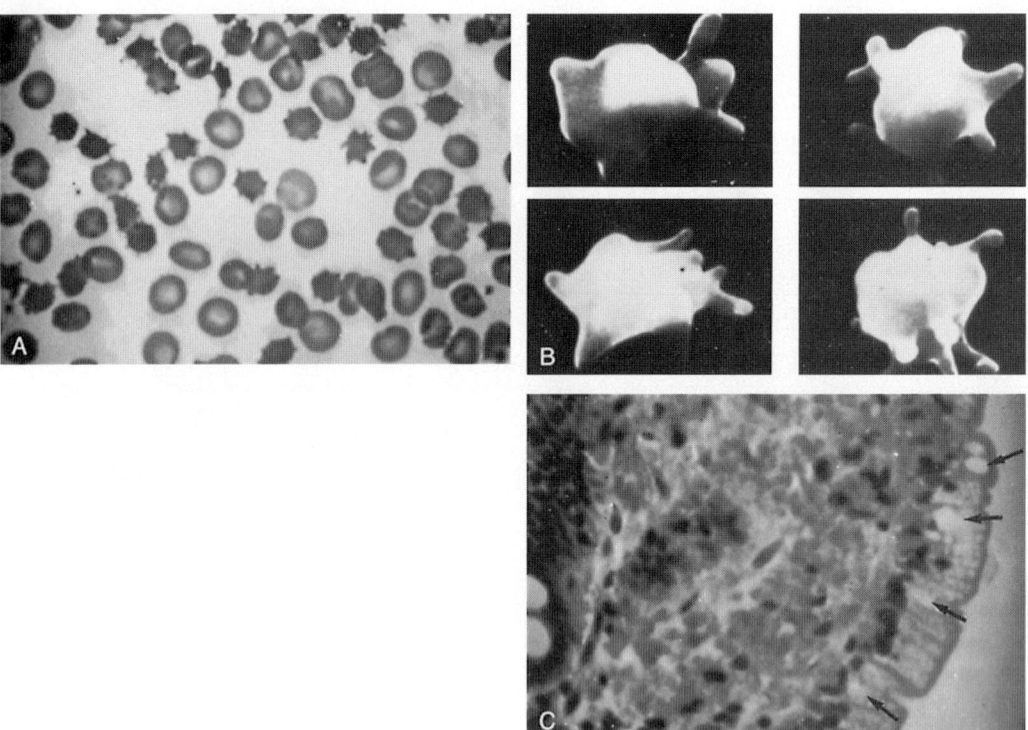

**FIGURE 163-10.** Light microscopy and scanning electron microscopy of acanthocytes (**A** and **B**) and lipid-laden intestinal epithelial cells (*arrows* in **C**) in a patient with abetalipoproteinemia.

develop striking corneal opacification, but they have not been reported to develop premature CHD. These patients have a deficiency of α-LCAT, which differs from β-LCAT in that it acts only on HDL; β-LCAT acts on VLDL and LDL. This disorder appears to be a milder variant of LCAT deficiency.[197,198]

## DEFICIENCIES OF VERY-LOW-DENSITY LIPOPROTEIN AND LOW-DENSITY LIPOPROTEIN

### ABETALIPOPROTEINEMIA

Abetalipoproteinemic patients often present in childhood with diarrhea, fat malabsorption, and failure to gain weight normally. Intestinal biopsy reveals lipid-laden epithelial cells (Fig. 163-10). Untreated, these patients develop spinocerebellar ataxia and retinitis pigmentosa in their teens and twenties. Laboratory analysis reveals plasma cholesterol values of ~40 mg/dL, triglyceride levels of 20 mg/dL, and HDL cholesterol of ~40 mg/dL.[217,218] The diagnosis is confirmed by undetectable plasma apo B. The defect is an inability to secrete apo B-containing lipoproteins (e.g., chylomicrons, VLDL, LDL).[218] Intestinal apo B mRNA levels are increased. Patients also have acanthocytosis and deficiencies of fat-soluble vitamins and essential fatty acids.[218] (see Fig. 163-10).

Supplementation with vitamin A and E is recommended.[219–222] Vitamin E replacement appears to prevent the onset of neuropathy.[219–222] Obligate heterozygotes (parents) have normal lipoprotein profiles. Restriction of dietary fat may be necessary to minimize diarrhea. It is not known whether these patients should be supplemented with the essential fatty acids linoleic acid and α-linolenic acid. The defect is due to mutations in the microsomal transfer protein (MTP) gene, resulting in lack of apo B secretion.[223]

### HYPOBETALIPOPROTEINEMIA

The clinical and laboratory picture is the same for hypobetalipoproteinemic patients as for those with abetalipoproteinemia.[224–227] However, obligate heterozygotes in these kindreds have LDL cholesterol and apo B values that are 50% of normal. The defect is an inability to synthesize normal amounts of apo B protein, and intestinal apo B mRNA levels are decreased.[227] The treatment is the same as in abetalipoproteinemia and is only indicated for homozygotes.

### NORMOTRIGLYCERIDEMIC ABETALIPOPROTEINEMIA

Some persons have normal chylomicron formation but lack plasma apo B-100 and LDL in plasma. One patient had serum cholesterol levels of 25 mg/dL and a triglyceride level that increased from 30 mg/dL to 250 mg/dL with fat feeding. She had mental retardation, marked vitamin E deficiency, and ataxia, which improved with vitamin E supplementation. These patients have apo B-48 in their plasma and have been classified as having normotriglyceridemic abetalipoproteinemia.[228]

### HYPOBETALIPOPROTEINEMIA WITH ABNORMAL APOLIPOPROTEIN B MOLECULAR WEIGHT

Another variant of these disorders, hypobetalipoproteinemia with abnormal apo B molecular weight, is associated with abnormal apo B molecular weight. These subjects have marked deficiencies of VLDL and LDL and very low plasma apo B levels. The apo B is of abnormal molecular weight as assessed by polyacrylamide gels.[229–232] This disorder has been called *hypobetalipoproteinemia with truncated apo B*. Cholesterol levels are ~40 mg/dL, but triglyceride levels can be as high as 100 mg/dL.

### CHYLOMICRON RETENTION DISEASE

Another group of patients with fat malabsorption, diarrhea, and deficiency of fat-soluble vitamins, and lipid-laden intestine epithelial cells, has been described. LDL cholesterol and apo B levels are ~50% of normal, and after fat feeding, no significant increase in triglyceride levels occurs.[233,234] The defect is an inability to secrete apo B-48–containing lipoprotein from the intestine. Only apo B-100 is present in plasma; no apo B-48 is found. Treatment is similar to that of abetalipoproteinemia. This disorder has been designated as chylomicron retention disease or Anderson disease.[233]

## XANTHOMAS WITH NORMAL LIPOPROTEIN LEVELS

### CEREBROTENDINOUS XANTHOMATOSIS

CTX is a rare familial sterol storage disorder with accumulations of cholestanol and cholesterol in most tissues, particularly in xanthomas and the brain. Clinically, this disorder is characterized by dementia, spinocerebellar ataxia, tuberous and tendinous xanthomas, early atherosclerosis, and cataracts. The defect in CTX is a lack of the hepatic mitochondrial 26-hydroxylase enzyme involved in the normal biosynthesis in bile lipids and bile acids. Patients with CTX have normal plasma lipoprotein levels, except for reduced plasma HDL cholesterol. The diagnosis should be suspected in a patient with tendinous xanthomas and a normal cholesterol level. It can be established by documentation of elevated plasma cholestanol levels by gas chromatography. If the diagnosis is made reasonably early, treatment with chenodeoxycholate at a dosage of 250 mg three times a day reduces cholestanol levels to normal and apparently halts the progression of the disease.[235]

### PHYTOSTEROLEMIA

Phytosterolemia is a rare, inherited sterol storage disorder characterized by tendinous and tuberous xanthomas and by a strong predisposition to premature coronary atherosclerosis.[235] Increased amounts of phytosterols such as sitosterol and campesterol are found in plasma and in various tissues. Increased serum cholesterol and cholestanol levels have also been found in some patients. The basic biochemical defect has not been elucidated. Unlike normal persons, these patients absorb plant sterols from the intestine. Phytosterolemia should be suspected in patients who develop xanthomas in early childhood despite normal or only moderately elevated serum cholesterol levels. The diagnosis can easily be established by an analysis of plasma sterols.

Treatment consists of a diet containing the lowest possible amount of plant sterols, with the elimination of all sources of vegetable fats and all plant foods with a high fat content. Such a diet should not contain vegetable oil, shortening, or margarine, nor should it contain nuts, seeds, chocolate, olives, or avocados. Cholestyramine should be used in addition to restricted diets, because it causes significant reductions in serum phytosterols, cholesterol, and cholestanol. Such treatment presumably can reduce the risk of subsequent atherosclerosis in these patients.[235]

### WOLMAN DISEASE

Wolman disease appears in the first few weeks of life, with persistent vomiting and diarrhea, hepatosplenomegaly, xanthomatosis, and adrenal calcification. Usually, anemia is evident by the sixth week of life. These patients have fat malabsorption and steatorrhea, and they develop liver enzyme abnormalities. They have decreased adrenal responsiveness to adrenocorticotropic hormone (ACTH) stimulation. Plasma lipid levels are generally normal or decreased. Cholesterol ester and triglyceride deposition occurs in the lysosomes of liver parenchymal and Kupffer cells and in macrophages of the adrenal gland, lymph nodes, intestinal mucosa, spleen, testes, thyroid, ovaries, and other tissues. Patients with Wolman disease have a complete absence of enzyme A of lysosome acid lipase (enzymes B and C are present), which can be demonstrated by Cellogel electrophoresis of the enzyme obtained from circulating lymphocytes or fibroblasts. The condition is usually fatal by 6 months of age.

## CHOLESTEROL ESTER STORAGE DISEASE

Patients with cholesterol ester storage disease are first seen in the first or second decade of life with hepatomegaly. The liver disease may progress to hepatic fibrosis, causing esophageal varices. Malabsorption is not a feature. Lysosomal cholesterol ester deposition in macrophages in liver, intestine, spleen, lymph nodes, and aorta has been documented. Usually, these patients have type IIa or type IIb hyperlipoproteinemia, and occasionally also have HDL deficiency. They have a marked deficiency of isoenzyme A of lysosomal acid lipase, as assessed in fibroblasts or circulating lymphocytes. The disease differs from Wolman disease in its severity, its lack of intestinal malabsorption, the lipoprotein abnormalities, and the predominantly lysosomal cholesterol ester deposition instead of cholesterol ester and triglyceride accumulation. Patients with cholesterol ester storage disease may develop strikingly premature coronary artery atherosclerosis. Heterozygotes exist for acid lipase deficiency (i.e., Wolman disease or cholesterol ester storage disease), and they appear to be at increased risk for premature CHD.

## CONCLUSION

The routine measurement of apolipoproteins is not recommended because of a lack of standardization in available assays and the lack of prospective data documenting that the assays are superior to standard lipid measurements in CHD risk assessment. Lp(a) may be the exception. Direct measurements of the cholesterol (C) content of serum lipoproteins for the detection of high-risk LDL C (>160 mg/dL), remnant lipoprotein C (>10 mg/dL), and Lp(a) C (>10 mg/dL) and decreased HDL C (<35 mg/dL) are important contributions; they facilitate the diagnosis and management of lipid disorders. The availability of the HMG-CoA reductase inhibitors has had a profound effect on the management of lipid disorders, and their use has achieved significantly decreased age-adjusted CHD rates.[27-35] Very effective agents are now available that can reduce LDL C by 50% or more. More emphasis should be placed on diet and exercise programs. Fibric acid derivatives (e.g., gemfibrozil and fenofibrate), as well as niacin products, increase HDL C and decrease remnant lipoprotein C. Thus, their use can now be recommended in CHD patients with normal LDL C and low HDL C.[22-26,37] In the future more efficacious and better-tolerated HDL raising agents will be marketed.

## REFERENCES

1. American Heart Association. 1999. Heart and stroke statistical update supplement. Dallas: American Heart Association, 1999:1.
2. The Expert Panel. Report of the national cholesterol education program expert panel on detection, evaluation, and treatment of high blood cholesterol in adults. Arch Intern Med 1988; 148:36.
3. The Expert Panel. Summary of the second report of the national cholesterol education program (NCEP) expert panel on detection, evaluation, and treatment of high blood cholesterol in adults (Adult Treatment Panel II). JAMA 1993; 269:3015.
4. The Expert Panel. Second report of the expert panel on detection, evaluation, and treatment of high blood cholesterol in adults. National Institutes of Health Publication No. 93-3095. Bethesda, MD: US Department of Health and Human Services, 1993.
5. Fredrickson DS, Levy RI, Lees RS. Fat transport in lipoproteins—an integrated approach to mechanisms and disorders. N Engl J Med 1967; 276:34.
6. Schaefer EJ, Levy RI. The pathogenesis and management of lipoprotein disorders. N Engl J Med 1985; 312:1300.
7. Brown MS, Goldstein JL. The LDL receptor concept: clinical and therapeutic implications. In: Stokes J III, Mancini M, eds. Hypercholesterolemia: clinical and therapeutic implications, vol 18. Atherosclerosis reviews, 1987. New York: Raven Press, 1988:85.
8. Nicolosi RJ, Stucchi AF, Kowala MC, et al. Effect of dietary fat saturation and cholesterol on low density lipoprotein composition and metabolism. I.

In vivo studies of receptor and non-receptor mediated catabolism of LDL in Cebus monkeys. Arteriosclerosis 1990; 10:119.

9. Stamler J, Wentworth D, Neaton JD. Is the relationship between serum cholesterol and risk of premature death from coronary heart disease continuous and graded? Findings in 356,222 primary screenees of the Multiple Risk Factor Intervention Trial (MRFIT). JAMA 1986; 256:2823.

10. Kannel WB, Castelli WP. Cholesterol in the prediction of atherosclerotic disease: new perspectives based on the Framingham Study. Ann Intern Med 1979; 90:85.

11. Anderson KM, Wilson PWF, Odell PM, Kannel WB. An updated coronary risk profile. A statement for health professionals. AHA medical/scientific statement science advisory. Circulation 1991; 83:356.

12. Wilson PWF, D'Agostino RB, Levy D, et al. Prediction of coronary heart disease using risk factor categories. Circulation 1998; 87:1837.

13. The Lipid Research Clinics Program. The Lipid Research Clinics Coronary Primary Prevention Trial I. Reduction in incidence of coronary heart disease. JAMA 1984; 251:351.

14. The Lipid Research Clinics Program. The Lipid Research Clinics Coronary Primary Prevention Trial II. The relationship of reduction in incidence of coronary heart disease to cholesterol lowering. JAMA 1984; 251:365.

15. Dayton S, Pearce ML, Hashimoto S, et al. A controlled clinical trial of a diet high in unsaturated fat in preventing complications of atherosclerosis. Circulation 1969; 40(Suppl II):11.

16. Hjermann I, Holme I, Byre KV, Leren P. Effect of diet and smoking intervention on the incidence of coronary heart disease. Lancet 1981; 2:1303.

17. Holme I, Hjermann I, Helgelend A, Leren P. The Oslo Study: diet and anti-smoking advice: additional results from a 5 year primary prevention trial in middle aged men. Prev Med 1985; 14:279.

18. Miettinen M, Karvonen MJ, Turpeiner O, et al. Effect of cholesterol lowering diet on mortality from coronary heart disease and other causes. A twelve year clinical trial in men and women. Lancet 1972; 2:835.

19. Ornish D, Brown SK, Scherwitz LW, et al. Can life-style changes reverse coronary heart disease? Lancet 1990; 326:129.

20. Leren P. The effect of plasma cholesterol lowering diet in male survivors of myocardial infarction. Acta Med Scand 1966; 466(Suppl):92.

21. DeLorgeril M, Renaud S, Mamelle N, et al. Mediterranean alpha-linolenic acid-rich diet in secondary prevention of coronary heart disease. Lancet 1994; 343:1454.

22. Carlson LA, Rosenhamer G. Reduction of mortality in the Stockholm Ischemic Heart Disease Study by combined treatment with clofibrate and nicotinic acid. Acta Med Scand 1988; 223:405.

23. Frick MH, Elo O, Haapa K, et al. Helsinki Heart Study: primary prevention trial with gemfibrozil in middle-aged men with dyslipidemia. N Engl J Med 1987; 317:1237.

24. Manninen V, Elo O, Frick MH, et al. Lipid alterations and decline in the incidence of coronary heart disease in the Helsinki Heart Study. JAMA 1988; 260:641.

25. Manninen V, Tenkanen L, Koskinen P, et al. Joint effects of triglyceride, LDL cholesterol, and HDL cholesterol concentrations on coronary heart disease risk in the Helsinki Heart Study. Implication for treatment. Circulation 1992; 85:37.

26. Canner PL, Berge KG, Wenger NK, et al. Fifteen-year mortality in Coronary Drug Project patients: long-term benefit with niacin. J Am Coll Cardiol 1986; 8:1245.

27. Scandinavian Simvastatin Survival Study Group. Randomized trial of cholesterol lowering in 4444 patients with coronary heart disease: the Scandinavian Simvastatin Survival Study (4S). Lancet 1994; 344:383.

28. Pedersen TR, Kjekshus J, Berg K, et al. Cholesterol lowering and the use of healthcare resources: results of the Scandinavian Simvastatin Survival Study. Circulation 1996; 93:1796.

29. Byington RP, Jukema JA, Salonen JT, et al. Reduction in cardiovascular events during pravastatin therapy. Pooled analysis of clinical events of the Pravastatin Atherosclerosis Intervention Program. Circulation 1995; 92:2419.

30. Shepherd J, Cobbe SM, Ford I, et al. Prevention of coronary heart disease with pravastatin in men with hypercholesterolemia: West of Scotland Coronary Prevention Study Group. N Engl J Med 1995; 333:1301.

31. Sacks FM, Pfeffer MA, Moye LA, et al. The effect of pravastatin on coronary events after myocardial infarction in patients with average cholesterol levels: Cholesterol and Recurrent Events Trial investigators. N Engl J Med 1996; 335:1001.

32. Downs JR, Clearfield M, Weis S, et al. Primary prevention of acute coronary events with lovastatin in men and women with average cholesterol levels. Results of AFCAPS/TexCAPS. JAMA 1998; 279:1615.

33. The Long-Term Intervention with Pravastatin in Ischemic Disease (LIPID) Study Group. Prevention of cardiovascular events and death with pravastatin in patients with coronary heart disease and a broad range of initial cholesterol levels. N Engl J Med 1998; 339:1349.

34. Post CABG Coordinating Center. The effect of aggressive lowering of low-density lipoprotein cholesterol and low-dose anticoagulation on obstructive changes in saphenous vein coronary artery bypass grafts. N Engl J Med 1997; 337:1859.

35. Pitt B, Waters D, Brown WV, et al. Aggressive lipid-lowering therapy compared with angioplasty in stable coronary artery disease. Atorvasatatin versus Revascularization Treatment Investigators. N Engl J Med 1999; 341:70.

36. Gordon DJ, Knoke J, Probstfeld JL, et al. High density lipoprotein cholesterol and coronary heart disease in hypercholesterolemic men: the Lipid Research Clinics Coronary Primary Prevention Trial. Circulation 1986; 74:1217.

37. Rubins HB, Robins SJ, Collins D, et al. Gemfibrozil for the secondary prevention of coronary heart disease in men with low levels of high-density lipoprotein cholesterol. N Engl J Med 1999;342:410.

38. Alderman E, Haskell WL, Fain JM, et al. Beneficial angiographic and clinical response to multifactor modification in the Stanford Coronary Risk Intervention Project (SCRIP). Circulation 1991; 84:11.

39. Blankenhorn DH, Nessim SA, Johnson RL, et al. Beneficial effects of combined colestipol-niacin therapy on coronary atherosclerosis and coronary venous bypass grafts. JAMA 1987; 257:3233.

40. Blankenhorn DH, Azen SP, Kramsch DM, et al. Coronary angiographic changes with lovastatin therapy. The Monitored Atherosclerosis Regression Study (MARS). Ann Intern Med 1993; 1119:969.

41. Brensike JF, Levy RI, Kelsey SF, et al. Effects of therapy with cholestyramine on progression of coronary atherosclerosis. Results of the NHLBI type II coronary intervention study. Circulation 1984; 69:313.

42. Brown BG, Zhao XQ, Sacco DE, Albers JJ. Lipid lowering and plaque regression. New insights into prevention of plaque disruption and clinical events in coronary disease. Circulation 1993; 87:1781.

43. Brown BG, Albers JJ, Fisher LD, et al. Regression of coronary artery disease as a result of intensive lipid-lowering therapy in men with high levels of apolipoprotein B. N Engl J Med 1990; 323:1289.

44. Buchwald H, Varco, Matts JP, et al. Effect of partial ileal bypass on mortality and morbidity from coronary heart disease in patients with hypercholesterolemia. Report of the Program on Surgical Control of the Hyperlipidemias (POSCH). N Engl J Med 1990; 323:946.

45. Kane JP, Malloy MJ, Ports TA, et al. Regression of coronary atherosclerosis during treatment of familial hypercholesterolemia with combined drug regimens. JAMA 1990; 264:3007.

46. Watts GF, Lewis B, Brunt JNH, et al. Effects on coronary artery disease of lipid lowering diet, a diet plus cholestyramine in the St. Thomas Atherosclerosis Regression Study (STARS). Lancet 1992; 339:563.

47. Schuler G, Hambrecht R, Schlierf G, et al. Regular exercise and low fat diet: effects on progression of coronary artery disease. Circulation 1992; 86:1.

48. NIH Consensus Conference. Lowering blood cholesterol to prevent heart disease. JAMA 1985; 253:2080.

49. Sprecher DL, Schaefer EJ, Kent KM, et al. Cardiovascular features of homozygous familial hypercholesterolemia: analysis of 16 patients. Am J Cardiol 1984; 54:20.

50. Stone NJ, Levy RI, Fredrickson DS, Verter J. Coronary artery disease in 116 kindreds with familial type II hyperlipoproteinemia. Circulation 1974; 49:476.

51. Ross R. Update on atherosclerosis. Nature 1993; 362:801.

52. NIH Consensus Conference. Triglycerides, HDL cholesterol, and coronary heart disease. JAMA 1993; 269:505.

53. Kaufman HW, McNamara JR, Anderson KM, et al. How reliably can compact analyzers measure lipids? JAMA 1990; 263:1245.

54. McNamara JR, Warnick GR, Leary ET, et al. A multi-center evaluation of a patient-administered test for blood cholesterol measurement. Prev Med 1996; 25:583.

55. Rosengren A, Wihelmsen L, Eriksson E, et al. Lipoprotein (a) and coronary heart disease: a prospective case-control study in the general population sample of middle aged men. Br Med J 1990; 301:1248.

56. Sigurdsson G, Baldursdottir A, Sigvalderson H, et al. Predictive value of apolipoproteins in a prospective survey of coronary artery disease in men. Am J Cardiol 1992; 69:1251.

57. Jauhiainen M, Koskinen P, Ehnholm C, et al. Lipoprotein (a) and coronary heart disease risk: a nested case-control study of the Helsinki Heart Study participants. Atherosclerosis 1991; 89:59.

58. Ridker PM, Hennekens CH, Stampfer MJ. A prospective study of lipoprotein (a) and the risk of myocardial infarction. JAMA 1993; 270:2195.

59. Schaefer EJ, Lamon-Fava S, Jenner JL, et al. Lipoprotein (a) levels and risk of coronary heart disease in men. The Lipid Research Clinics Coronary Primary Prevention Trial. JAMA 1994; 271:999.

60. Cremer P, Nagel D, Labrot B, et al. Lipoprotein (a) as predictor of myocardial infarction in comparison to fibrinogen, LDL cholesterol, and other risk factors: results from the prospective Gottingen Risk Incidence and Prevalence Study (GRIPS). Eur J Clin Invest 1994; 24:444.

61. Ishikawa T, Fidge N, Thelle DS, et al. The Tromso Heart Study: serum apolipoprotein A-I concentration in relation to future coronary heart disease. Eur J Clin Invest 1978; 8:179.

62. Salonen JT, Salonen R, Penttila I, et al. Serum fatty acids apolipoproteins, selenium and vitamin antioxidants and the risk of death from coronary artery disease. Am J Cardiol 1985; 56:226.

63. Cremer P, Muche R. The Gottingen Risk, Incidence and Prevalence Study (GRIPS). Recommendations for the prevention of coronary heart disease. Ther Umsch 1990; 47:482.

64. Stampfer MJ, Sacks FM, Salvini S, et al. A prospective study of cholesterol, apolipoproteins, and the risk of myocardial infarction. N Engl J Med 1991; 325:373.

65. Coleman MP, Key TJ, Wang DY, et al. A prospective study of obesity, lipids, apolipoproteins, and ischemic heart disease in women. Atherosclerosis 1992; 92:177.

66. Campos H, Genest JJ, Blijlevens E, et al. Low density lipoprotein particle size and coronary artery disease. Arterioscler Thromb 1992; 12:187.

67. Schaefer EJ, Lamon-Fava S, Ordovas JM, et al. Factors associated with low and elevated plasma high density lipoprotein cholesterol and apolipoprotein A-I levels in the Framingham Offspring Study. J Lipid Res 1994; 35:871.

68. Schaefer EJ, Lamon-Fava S, Cohn SD, et al. Effects of age, gender and menopausal status on plasma low density lipoprotein cholesterol and apolipoprotein B levels in the Framingham Offspring Study. J Lipid Res 1994; 35:779.

69. Seman LJ, Jenner JL, McNamara JR, Schaefer EJ. Quantitation of plasma lipoprotein (a) by cholesterol assay of lectin bound lipoprotein (a). Clin Chem 1994; 40:400.

70. Nakajima K, Saito T, Tamura A, et al. Cholesterol in remnant-like lipoproteins in human serum using monoclonal anti apo B-100 and anti apo A-I immunoaffinity mixed gels. Clin Chim Acta 1993; 223:53.

71. McNamara JR, Shah PK, Nakajima K, et al. Remnant lipoprotein cholesterol and triglyceride: reference ranges from the Framingham Heart Study. Clin Chem 1998; 44:1224.

72. Takeichi S, Yukawa N, Nakajima Y, et al. Association of plasma triglyceride-rich lipoprotein remnants with coronary atherosclerosis in cases of sudden cardiac death. Atherosclerosis 1999;142:309.

73. Kugiyama K, Doi H, Takazoe K, et al. Remnant lipoprotein levels in fasting serum predict coronary events in patients with coronary artery disease. Circulation 1999; 99:2858.

74. Gianturco SH, Bradley WA. Pathophysiology of triglyceride-rich lipoproteins in atherothrombosis: cellular aspects. Clin Cardiol 1999; 22(Suppl):7.

75. Berg K. A new serum type system in man: the Lp system. Acta Pathol Microbiol Scand 1963; 59:369.

76. McLean JW, Tomlinson JE, Kuang WJ, et al. cDNA sequence of human apolipoprotein (a) is homologous to plasminogen. Nature 1987; 330:132.

77. Utermann G. The mysteries of lipoprotein(a). Science 1989; 246:904.

78. Lackner C, Boerwinkle E, Leffert CC, et al. Molecular basis of apolipoprotein(a) isoform heterogeneity as revealed by pulsed-field gel electrophoresis. J Clin Invest 1991; 87:2153.

79. Boerwinkle E, Leffert CC, Lin J, et al. Apolipoprotein(a) gene accounts for greater than 90% of the variation in plasma lipoprotein(a) concentrations. J Clin Invest 1992; 90:52.

80. Loscalzo J, Weinfeld M, Fless GM, Scanu AM. Lipoprotein (a), fibrin binding, and plasminogen activation. Arteriosclerosis 1990; 10:240.

81. Miles LA, Fless GM, Levin EG, et al. A potential basis of the thrombotic risks associated with lipoprotein (a). Nature 1989; 339:301.

82. Hajjar KA, Gavish D, Breslow JL, Nachman RL. Lipoprotein (a) modulation of endothelial cell surface fibrinolysis and its potential role in atherosclerosis. Nature 1989; 339:303.

83. Dahlen GH, Guyton JR, Altar M, et al. Association of levels of lipoprotein (a), plasma lipids, and other lipoproteins with coronary artery disease documented by angiography. Circulation 1986; 74:758.

84. Armstrong VW, Cremer P, Eberle E, et al. The association between serum Lp(a) concentrations and angiographically assessed coronary atherosclerosis. Atherosclerosis 1986; 62:249.

85. Zenker G, Költringer P, Bone G, et al. Lipoprotein(a) as a strong indicator for cerebrovascular disease. Stroke 1986; 17:942.

86. Murai A, Miyahara T, Fujimoto N, et al. Lp(a) lipoprotein as a risk factor for coronary heart disease and cerebral infarction. Atherosclerosis 1986; 59:199.

87. Hoefler G, Harnoncourt F, Paschke E, et al. Lipoprotein Lp(a): a risk factor for myocardial infarction. Arteriosclerosis 1988; 8:398.

88. Sandkamp M, Funke H, Schulte H, et al. Lipoprotein (a) is an independent risk factor for myocardial infarction at a young age. Clin Chem 1990; 36:20.

89. Genest J Jr, Jenner JL, McNamara JR, et al. Prevalence of lipoprotein (a) [Lp(a)] excess in coronary artery disease. Am J Cardiol 1991; 67:1039.

90. Genest JJ Jr, McNamara JR, Ordovas JM, et al. Lipoprotein cholesterol, apolipoprotein A-I and B and lipoprotein(a) abnormalities in men with premature coronary artery disease. J Am Coll Cardiol 1992; 19:792.

91. Genest JJ Jr, Martin-Munley SS, McNamara JR, et al. Familial lipoprotein disorders in patients with premature coronary artery disease. Circulation 1992; 85:2025.

92. Jenner JL, Ordovas JM, Lamon-Fava S, et al. Effects of age, sex, and menopausal status on plasma lipoprotein (a) levels. The Framingham Offspring Study. Circulation 1993; 87:1135.

93. Rosengren A, Wihelmsen L, Eriksson E, et al. Lipoprotein (a) and coronary heart disease: a prospective case-control study in the general population sample of middle aged men. Br Med J 1990; 301:1248.

94. Cantin B, Moorjani S, Despres J-P, et al. Lp(a) in ischemic heart disease: the Quebec Cardiovascular Study. JACC 1994; 23:482A.

95. Bostom AG, Gagnon DR, Cupples LA, et al. A prospective investigation of elevated lipoprotein(a) detected by electrophoresis and cardiovascular disease in women. The Framingham Heart Study. Circulation 1994; 90:1688.

96. Assman G, Schulte H, von Eckardstein A. Hypertriglyceridemia and elevated lipoprotein(a) are risk factors for major coronary events in middle aged men. Am J Cardiol 1996; 77:1179.

97. Bostom AG, Cupples LA, Jenner JL, et al. Elevated lipoprotein(a) and coronary heart disease in men aged 55 years and younger. JAMA 1996; 276:544.

98. Seman LJ, DeLuca C, Jenner JL, et al. Lipoprotein(a)-cholesterol and coronary heart disease in the Framingham Heart Study. Clin Chem 1999; 45:1039.

99. Avogaro P, Bittolo Bon G, Cazzolato G, Quinci GB. Are apolipoproteins better discriminators than lipids for atherosclerosis? Lancet 1979; 1:901.

100. Sniderman A, Shapiro S, Marpole D, et al. Association of coronary atherosclerosis with hyperapobetalipoproteinemia (increased protein but normal cholesterol levels in human plasma low density lipoproteins). Proc Natl Acad Sci U S A 1980; 77:604.

101. Whayne TF, Alaupovic P, Curry MD, et al. Plasma apolipoprotein B and VLDL-, LDL-, and HDL-cholesterol as risk factors in the development of coronary artery disease in male patients examined by angiography. Atherosclerosis 1981; 39:411.

102. Kwiterovich PO Jr, Bachorik PS, Smith HH, et al. Hyperapobetalipoproteinaemia in two families with xanthomas and phytosterolaemia. Lancet 1981; 1:466.

103. Maciejko JJ, Holmes DR, Kottke BA, et al. Apolipoprotein A-I as a marker of angiographically assessed coronary artery disease. N Engl J Med 1983; 309:385.

104. Stampfer MJ, Krauss RM, Ma J, et al. A prospective study of triglyceride level, low density lipoprotein particle diameter, and risk of myocardial infarction. JAMA 1996; 276:882.

105. Wald NJ, Law M, Watt HC, et al. Apolipoproteins and ischaemic heart disease: implications for screening. Lancet 1994; 343:75.

106. Lamarche B, Despres JP, Moorjani S, et al. Prevalence of dyslipidemic phenotypes in ischemic heart disease (prospective results from the Quebec Cardiovascular Study). Am J Cardiol 1995; 75:1189.

107. Marcovina SM, Albers JJ, Henderson LO, Hannon WH. International Federation of Clinical Chemistry standardization project for measurements of apolipoproteins A-I and B. III. Comparability of apolipoprotein A-I values by use of international reference material. Clin Chem 1993; 39:773.

108. Marcovina SM, Albers JJ, Kennedy H, et al. International Federation of Clinical Chemistry standardization project for measurements of apolipoproteins A-I and B. IV. Comparability of apolipoprotein B values by use of international reference material. Clin Chem 1994; 40:586.

109. Contois JH, McNamara JR, Lammi-Keefe CJ, et al. Reference intervals for plasma apolipoprotein A-I as determined with a commercially available immunoturbidometric assay: results from the Framingham Offspring Study. Clin Chem 1996; 42:507.

110. Contois JH, McNamara JR, Lammi-Keefe CJ, et al. Reference intervals for plasma apolipoprotein B as determined with a commercially available immunoturbidometric assay: results from the Framingham Offspring Study. Clin Chem 1996; 42:515.

111. Alfthan G, Pekkanen J, Juuhiainen M, et al. Relation of serum homocysteine and lipoprotein(a) concentrations to atherosclerotic disease in a prospective Finnish population based study. Atherosclerosis 1994; 106:9.

112. McNamara JR, Cohn JS, Wilson PWF, Schaefer EJ. Calculated values for low density lipoprotein cholesterol in the assessment of lipid abnormalities and coronary disease risk. Clin Chem 1990; 36:36.

113. McNamara JR, Cole TG, Contois JH, et al. Immunoseparation method for measuring low-density lipoprotein cholesterol directly from serum evaluated. Clin Chem 1995; 41(2):232.

114. Pisani T, Gebski CP, Leary ET, et al. Accurate direct determination of low-density lipoprotein cholesterol using an immunoseparation reagent and enzymatic cholesterol assay. Arch Pathol Lab Med 1995; 119(12):1127.

115. Schaefer EJ, Lamon-Fava S, Johnson S, et al. Effects of gender and menopausal status on the association of apolipoprotein E phenotype with plasma lipoprotein levels. Results from the Framingham Offspring Study. Arterioscler Thromb 1994; 14:1105.

116. Expert Panel. Blood cholesterol levels in children and adolescents. National Institutes of Health Publication No. 91-2732, 1-119. Washington, DC: US Government Printing Office, 1990.

117. Expert Panel. Population strategies for blood cholesterol reduction. National Institutes of Health Publication No. 90-3046, I-39. Washington, DC: US Government Printing Office, 1990.

118. Laboratory Standardization Panel. Recommendations for improving cholesterol measurements. National Institutes of Health Publication No. 90-2964, 1-64. Washington DC: US Government Printing Office, 1990.

119. Friedewald WT, Levy RI, Fredrickson DS. Estimation of the concentration of low density lipoproteins separated by three different methods. Clin Chem 1972; 18:499.

120. Cohn JS, McNamara JR, Schaefer EJ. Lipoprotein concentrations in plasma of human subjects as measured in the fed and fasted states. Clin Chem 1988; 34:2456.

120a. Blair SN, Capuzzi DM, Gottlieb SO, et al. Incremental reduction of serum total cholesterol and low-density lipoprotein cholesterol with the addition of plant ester-containing spread to statin therapy. Am J Cardiol 2000; 86:46.

121. Schaefer EJ, Lichtenstein AH, Lamon-Fava S, et al. Efficacy of a National Cholesterol Education Program step 2 diet in normolipidemic and hyperlipidemic middle aged and elderly men and women. Arterioscler Thromb Vasc Biol 1995; 15:1079.

122. Schaefer EJ, Lichtenstein AH, Lamon-Fava S, et al. Effects of National Cholesterol Education Program step 2 diets relatively high or relatively low in fish-derived fatty acids on plasma lipoproteins in middle-aged and elderly subjects. Am J Clin Nutr 1996; 63:234.

123. Lichtenstein AH, Ausman LM, Schaefer EJ. Effects of canola, corn, and olive oils on fasting and postprandial plasma lipoproteins in humans as part of a National Cholesterol Education Program step 2 diet. Arterioscler Thromb 1993; 13:1533.

124. Schaefer EJ, Lichtenstein AH, Lamon-Fava S, et al. Body weight and low density lipoprotein cholesterol changes after consumption of a low fat ad libitum diet. JAMA 1995; 274:1450.

125. Mata P, Ordovas JM, Lopez-Miranda J, et al. ApoA-IV phenotype affects diet induced plasma LDL cholesterol lowering. Arterioscler Thromb 1994; 14:884.

126. Lopez-Miranda J, Ordovas JM, Mata P, et al. Effect of apolipoprotein E phenotype on diet-induced lowering of plasma low density lipoprotein cholesterol. J Lipid Res 1994; 35(11):1965.

127. Krauss RM, Deckelbaum RJ, Ernst N, et al. Dietary guideline for healthy American adults: a statement for health professionals from the Nutrition Committee, American Heart Association. Circulation 1996; 94:1795.

128. Hunninghake DB, Stein FA, Dujorne CA, et al. The efficacy of intensive dietary therapy alone or combined with lovastatin in outpatients with hypercholesterolemia. N Engl J Med 1993; 328:1213.

129. Kane JP, Malloy MJ, Tun P, et al. Normalization of low density lipoprotein levels in heterozygous familial hypercholesterolemia with a combined drug regimen. N Engl J Med 1981; 304:251.

130. Mabuchi H, Sakai T, Sakai Y. Reduction of serum cholesterol in heterozygous patients with familial hypercholesterolemia. Additive effects of compactin and cholestyramine. N Engl J Med 1983; 308:609.

131. Granfone A, Campos H, McNamara JR, et al. Effects of estrogen replacement on plasma lipoproteins and apolipoproteins in dyslipidemic postmenopausal women. Metabolism 1992; 41:1193.

132. Barrett-Connor E, Bush TL. Estrogen and coronary heart disease in women. JAMA 1991; 265:1861.

133. Stampfer ME, Colditz GA. Estrogen replacement therapy and coronary heart disease: a quantitative assessment of the epidemiologic evidence. Prev Med 1991; 20:47.

134. Kim CJ, Jang HC, Min YK. Effect of hormone replacement therapy on lipoprotein(a) and lipids in post-menopausal women. Arterioscler Thromb 1994; 14:275.

135. Hulley S, Grady D, Bush T, et al. Randomized trial of estrogen plus progestin for secondary prevention of coronary heart disease in postmenopausal women. Heart and Estrogen/progestin Replacement Study (HERS) Research Group. JAMA 1998; 280:605.

136. Coronary Drug Project Research Group. Clofibrate and niacin in coronary heart disease. JAMA 1975; 231:360.

137. Pierce LR, Wysowski DK, Gross TP. Myopathy and rhabdomyolysis associated with lovastatin-gemfibrozil combination therapy. JAMA 1990; 264:71.

138. Herd JL, Ballantyne CM, Farmer JA, et al. Effects of fluvastatin on atherosclerosis in patients with mild to moderate cholesterol elevations (Lipoprotein and Coronary Atherosclerosis Study [LCAS]). Am J Cardiol 1997; 80:278.

139. Nawrocki JW, Weiss SR, Davidson MH, et al. Reduction of LDL cholesterol by 25% to 60% in patients with primary hypercholesterolemia by atorvastatin, a new HMG CoA reductase inhibitor. Arterioscler Thromb Vasc Biol 1995; 15:67S.

140. Bakker-Arkema RG, Davidson MH, Goldstein RJ, et al. Efficacy and safety of a new HMG CoA reductase inhibitor–atorvastatin, in patients with hypertriglyceridemia. JAMA 1996; 275:128.

141. Walldius G, Regnstrom J, Nilsson J, et al. The effect of probucol on femoral atherosclerosis: the Probucol Quantitative Regression Swedish Trial. Am J Cardiol 1994; 74:875.

141a. Azevedo LC, Pedro MA, Souza LC, et al. Oxidative stress as a signaling mechanism of the vascular response to injury. The redox hypothesis of restenosis. Cardiovasc Res 2000; 47:436.

142. Burr ML, Fehily AM, Gilbert JF, et al. Effect of changes in fat, fish, and fibre intakes on death and myocardial infarction: diet and reinfarction trial (DART). Lancet 1989; 2:757.

143. Wiklund O, Angelin B, Bergman M, et al. Pravastatin and gemfibrozil alone and in combination for the treatment of hypercholesterolemia. Am J Med 1993; 94:13.

144. Muller C. Xanthomata, hypercholesterolemia, angina pectoris. Acta Med Scand 1938; 89(Suppl):75.

145. Thannhauser SJ, Magendantz H. The different clinical groups of xanthomatous diseases: a clinical physiological study of 22 cases. Ann Intern Med 1938; 11:1662.

146. Khachadurian AK. The inheritance of essential familial hypercholesterolemia. Am J Med 1964; 37:402.

147. Goldstein JL, Hazzard WR, Schrott HG, et al. Hyperlipidemia in coronary heart disease: I. Lipid levels in 500 survivors of myocardial infarction. J Clin Invest 1973; 52:1533.

148. Goldstein JL, Schrott HG, Hazzard WR, et al. Hyperlipidemia in coronary heart disease: II. Genetic analysis of lipid levels in 176 families and delineation of a new inherited disorder, combined hyperlipidemia. J Clin Invest 1973; 52:1544.

149. Hazzard WR, Goldstein JL, Schrott MG, et al. Hyperlipidemia in coronary heart disease. 3. Evaluation of lipoprotein phenotypes of 156 genetically defined survivors of myocardial infarction. J Clin Invest 1973; 52(7):1569.

150. Genest JJ, Martin-Munley S, McNamara JR, et al. Prevalence of familial lipoprotein disorders in patients with premature coronary artery disease. Circulation 1992; 85:2025.

151. Langer T, Stober W, Levy RI. The metabolism of LDL in familial type II hyperlipoproteinemia. J Clin Invest 1972; 51:1528.

152. Goldstein JL, Brown MS. Progress in understanding the LDL receptor and HMG-CoA reductase, two membrane proteins that regulate plasma cholesterol. J Lipid Res 1984; 25:1450.

153. Russell DW, Esser V, Hobbs HH. Molecular basis of familial hypercholesterolemia. Arteriosclerosis 1989; 9:1.

154. Goldstein JL, Brown MS. The LDL receptor defect in familial hypercholesterolemia—implications for pathogenesis and therapy. Med Clin North Am 1982; 66:335.

154a. Bertolini S, Cantafora A, Averna M, et al. Clinical expression of familial hypercholesterolemia in clusters of mutations of the LDL receptor gene that cause a receptor–defective or receptor–negative phenotype. Arterioscler Thromb Vasc Biol 2000; 20:E41.

155. Vega GL, Grundy S. In vivo evidence for reduced binding of low density lipoproteins to receptors as a cause of primary moderate hypercholesterolemia. J Clin Invest 1986; 78:1410.

156. Innerarity TL, Weisgraber KH, Arnold KS, et al. Familial defective apolipoprotein B-100: low density lipoproteins with abnormal receptor binding. Proc Natl Acad Sci U S A 1987; 84:6919.

156a. Ceska R, Vrablik M, Horinek A. Familial defective apolipoprotein B–100: a lesson from homozygous and heterozygous patients. Physiol Res 2000; 49(Suppl 1):S125.

157. Hashim SA, Van Itallie TB. Cholestyramine resin therapy for hypercholesterolemia. JAMA 1965; 192:289.

158. Illingworth DR. Mevinolin plus colestipol in therapy for severe heterozygous familial hypercholesterolemia. Ann Intern Med 1984; 101:598.

159. Thompson GR, Lowenthal R, Myant NB. Plasma exchange in the management of homozygous familial hypercholesterolaemia. Lancet 1975; 1:1208.

160. Yokoyama S, Hayashi R, Satani M, Yamamoto A. Selective removal of low density lipoprotein by plasmapheresis in familial hypercholesterolemia. Arteriosclerosis 1985; 5:613.

161. Eisenhauer T, Armstrong VW, Wieland H, et al. Selective removal of low density lipoproteins (LDL) by precipitation at low pH: first clinical application of the HELP system. Klin Wochenschr 1987; 65:161.

162. Starzl TE, Chase HP, Ahrens EH Jr, et al. Portacaval shunt in patients with familial hypercholesterolemia. Ann Surg 1983; 198:273.

163. Sing CF, Davignon J. Role of the apolipoprotein E polymorphism in determining normal plasma lipid and lipoprotein variation. Am J Hum Genet 1985; 37:268.

164. Ordovas JM, Litwack-Klein LE, Schaefer MM, et al. Apolipoprotein E isoform phenotyping methodology and population frequency with identification of apo E1 and apo E5 isoforms. J Lipid Res 1987; 28:371.

165. Rose HG, Kranz P, Weinstock M, Juliano J, Haft JI. Inheritance of combined hyperlipoproteinemia: evidence for a new lipoprotein phenotype. Am J Med 1973; 54:148.

166. Chait A, Albers JJ, Brunzell JD. Very low density lipoprotein overproduction in genetic forms of hypertriglyceridaemia. Eur J Clin Invest 1980; 10:17.

167. Kissebah AH, Alfarsi S, Adams PW. Integrated regulation of very low density lipoprotein triglyceride and apolipoprotein-B kinetics in man: normolipemic subjects, familial hypertriglyceridemia and familial combined hyperlipidemia. Metab Clin Exp 1981; 30:856.

168. Janus ED, Nicoll AM, Turner PR, et al. Kinetic bases of the primary hyperlipidaemias: studies of apolipoprotein B turnover in genetically defined subjects. Eur J Clin Invest 1980; 10:161.

169. Sniderman A, Cianflone K. Substrate delivery as a determinant of hepatic apoB secretion. Arterioscler Thromb 1993; 13:629.

170. Sniderman A, Teng B, Genest J, et al. Familial aggregation and early expression of hyperapobetalipoproteinemia. Am J Cardiol 1985; 55:291.

171. Sniderman AD, Wolfson C, Teng B, et al. Association of hyperapobetalipoproteinemia with endogenous hypertriglyceridemia and atherosclerosis. Ann Intern Med 1982; 97:833.

172. Teng B, Thompson GR, Sniderman AD, et al. Composition and distribution of low density lipoprotein fractions in hyperapobetalipoproteinemia, normolipidemia, and familial hypercholesterolemia. Proc Natl Acad Sci U S A 1983; 80:6662.

173. Genest J, Sniderman A, Cianflone K, et al. Hyperapobetalipoproteinemia: plasma lipoprotein responses to oral fat load. Arteriosclerosis 1986; 6:297.

174. Schaefer EJ, Zech LA, Jenkins LJ, et al. Human apolipoprotein A-I and A-II metabolism. J Lipid Res 1982; 23:850.

175. Schaefer EJ, Ordovas, JM. Metabolism of the apolipoproteins A-I, A-II, and A-IV. In: Segrest J, Albers J, eds. Methods in enzymology, plasma lipoproteins (Pt B): characterization, cell biology and metabolism. New York: Academic Press, 1986:420.

176. Brinton EA, Eisenberg S, Breslow JL. Increased apo A-I and apo A-II fractional catabolic rate in patients with low high density lipoprotein-cholesterol levels with or without hypertriglyceridemia. J Clin Invest 1991; 87:536.

177. Fredrickson DS, Altrocchi PH, Avioli LC. Tangier disease: combined clinical staff conference at the National Institutes of Health. Ann Intern Med 1961; 55:1016.

178. Schaefer EJ, Blum CB, Levy RI, et al. Metabolism of high density lipoproteins apolipoproteins in Tangier disease. N Engl J Med 1978; 299:905.

179. Serfaty-Lacrosniere C, Lanzberg A, Civeira F, et al. Homozygous Tangier disease and cardiovascular disease. Atherosclerosis 1994; 107:85.

180. Bodzioch M, Orso E, Kluchben J, et al. The gene encoding ATP binding cassette transporter 1 is mutated in Tangier disease. Nat Genet 1999; 22:347.

181. Brooks-Wilson A, Marcil M, Clee SM, et al. Mutations in ABC1 in Tangier disease and familial high density lipoprotein deficiency. Nat Genet 1999; 22:336.

182. Rust S, Rosier M, Funke H, et al. Tangier disease is caused by mutations in the gene encoding ATP binding cassette transporter 1. Nat Genet 1999; 22:352.

183. Schaefer EJ, Heaton WH, Wetzel MG, Brewer HB Jr. Plasma apolipoprotein A-I absence associated with a marked reduction of high density lipoproteins and premature coronary artery disease. Arteriosclerosis 1982; 2:16.

184. Schaefer EJ. Clinical, biochemical, and genetic features in familial disorders of high density lipoproteins. Arteriosclerosis 1984; 4:303.

185. Schaefer EJ, Ordovas JM, Law S, et al. Familial apolipoprotein A-I and C-III deficiency, variant II. J Lipid Res 1985; 26:1089.

186. Ordovas JM, Cassidy DK, Civeira F, et al. Familial apolipoprotein A-I, C-III and A-IV deficiency and premature atherosclerosis due to deletion of a gene complex on chromosome 11. J Biol Chem 1989; 264:16339.

187. Norum RA, Lakier JB, Goldstein S, et al. Familial deficiency of apolipoprotein A-I and C-III and precocious coronary artery disease. N Engl J Med 1982; 306:1513.

188. Norum RA, Forte TM, Alaupovic P, Ginsberg HN. Clinical syndrome and lipid metabolism in hereditary deficiency of apolipoproteins A-I and C-III, variant I. Adv Exp Med Biol 1986; 201:137.

189. Karathanasis SK, Ferris E, Haddad IA. DNA inversion within the apolipo-proteins AI/CIII/AIV-encoding gene cluster of certain patients with pre-mature atherosclerosis. Proc Natl Acad Sci U S A 1987; 84:7198.

190. Matsunaga T, Hiasa Y, Yanagi H, et al. Apolipoprotein A-I deficiency due to a codon 84 nonsense mutation of the apolipoprotein A-I gene. Proc Natl Acad Sci U S A 1991; 88:2793.

191. Deeb SS, Cheung MC, Peng R, et al. A mutation in the human apolipopro-tein A-I gene: dominant effect on the level and characteristics of plasma high density lipoproteins. J Biol Chem 1991; 266:13654.

192. Funke H, Von Eckardstein A, Pritchard PH, et al. A frameshift mutation in the human apolipoprotein A-I gene causes high density lipoprotein defi-ciency, partial lecithin:cholesterol acyltransferase deficiency, and corneal opacities. J Clin Invest 1991; 87:371.

193. Weisgraber KH, Bersot TP, Mahley RW, et al. A-I Milano apoprotein: isola-tion and characterization of a cysteine-containing variant of the A-I apopro-tein from human high density lipoproteins. J Clin Invest 1980; 66:901.

194. Von Eckardstein A, Funke H, Walter M, et al. Structural analysis of human apolipoprotein A-I variants. J Biol Chem 1990; 265:8610.

195. Von Eckardstein A, Holz H, Sandkamp M, et al. Apolipoprotein C-III (Lys58-Glu). J Clin Invest 1991; 87:1724.

196. Glomset JA, Norum KR, Gjone E. Familial lecithin: cholesterol acyltransferase deficiency. In: Stanbury JB, Wyngaarden JB, Fredrickson DS, et al., eds. The metabolic basis of inherited disease. New York: McGraw-Hill, 1983:643.

197. Carlson LA. Fish-eye disease: a new familial condition with massive corneal opacities and dyslipoproteinemia. Eur J Clin Invest 1982; 12:41.

198. Carlson LA, Holmquist L. Evidence for deficiency of high density lipopro-tein lecithin:cholesterol acyltransferase activity (LCAT) in fish-eye disease. Acta Med Scand 1985; 218:189.

199. Vergani C, Bettale A. Familial hypoalphalipoproteinemia. Clin Chim Acta 1981; 114:45.

200. Third JLHC, Montag J, Flynn M, et al. Primary and familial hypoalphalipo-proteinemia. Metabolism 1984; 33:136.

201. Le AN, Ginsberg HN. Heterogeneity of apolipoprotein A-I turnover with reduced concentrations of plasma high density lipoprotein cholesterol. Metabolism 1988; 37:614.

201a. Mott S, Yu L, Marcil M, et al. Decreased cellular cholesterol efflux is a com-mon cause of familial hypoalphalipoproteinemia: role of the ABCA1 gene mutations. Atherosclerosis 2000; 152:457.

202. Genest JJ, Bard JM, Fruchart JC, et al. Plasma apolipoproteins (a), A-I, A-II, B, E, and C-III containing particles in men with premature coronary artery disease. Atherosclerosis 1991; 90:149.

203. Genest JJ Jr, Bard JM, Fruchart JC, et al. Familial hypoalphalipoproteinemia in premature coronary disease. Arterioscler Thromb 1993; 13:1728.

204. Morganroth J, Levy RI, Fredrickson DS. The biochemical, clinical and genetic features of type III hyperlipoproteinemia. Ann Intern Med 1975; 82:158.

205. Utermann G, Hees M, Steinmetz A. Polymorphism of apolipoprotein E and occurrence of dysbetalipoproteinaemia in man. Nature 1977; 269:604.

206. Zannis VI, Breslow JL. Human very low density lipoprotein apolipoprotein E isoprotein polymorphism is explained by genetic variation and posttrans-lational modification. Biochemistry 1981; 20:1033.

207. Hazzard WR, O'Donnell TF, Lee YL. Broad-beta disease (type III hyperlipo-proteinemia) in a large kindred. Evidence for a monogenic mechanism. Ann Intern Med 1975; 92:141.

208. Weisgraber KH, Rall SC Jr, Mahley RW. Human apolipoprotein E isoprotein subclasses are genetically determined. Am J Hum Genet 1981; 33:11.

209. Rall SC Jr, Weisgraber KH, Innerarity TL, et al. Identical structural and receptor binding defects in apolipoprotein E2 in hypo-, normo- and hyper-cholesterolemic dysbetalipoproteinemia. J Clin Invest 1983; 71:1023.

210. Ghiselli G, Schaefer EJ, Gascon P, Brewer HB Jr. Type III hyperlipoproteine-mia associated with apolipoprotein E deficiency. Science 1981; 214:1239.

211. Schaefer EJ, Gregg RE, Ghiselli G, et al. Familial apolipoprotein E deficiency. J Clin Invest 1986; 78:1206.

212. Cladaras C, Hadzopoulou-Cladaras M, Felber B, et al. The molecular basis of a familial apo E deficiency: an acceptor splice site mutation in the third intron of the deficient apo E gene. J Biol Chem 1987; 262:2310.

213. Schaefer EJ. Dietary and drug treatment. In: Brewer HB Jr, ed. Moderator, type III hyperlipoproteinemia: diagnosis, molecular defects, pathology and treatment. Ann Intern Med 1983; 93:623.

214. Seed M, Hoppichler F, Reaveley D, et al. Relation of serum lipoprotein (a) concentration and apolipoprotein (a) phenotype to coronary heart disease in patients with familial hypercholesterolemia. N Engl J Med 1990; 322:1494.

215. Carlson LA, Hamsten A, Asplund A. Pronounced lowering of serum levels of lipoprotein (a) in hyperlipidaemic subjects treated with nicotinic acid. J Intern Med 1989; 226:271.

216. Schaefer EJ. Hyperlipoproteinemia. In: Rakel RE, ed. Conn's current ther-apy. Philadelphia: WB Saunders, 1991:515.

217. Bassen FA, Kornzweig AL. Malformation of the erythrocytes in a case of atypical retinitis pigmentosa. Blood 1950; 5:381.

218. Gotto AM, Levy RI, John K, Fredrickson DS. On the nature of the protein defect in abetalipoproteinemia. N Engl J Med 1971; 284:813.

219. Muller DPR, Lloyd JK, Bird AC. Long-term management of abetalipopro-teinemia. Arch Dis Child 1977; 52:209.

220. Muller DPR, Lloyd JK, Wolff OH. Vitamin E and neurological function. Lan-cet 1983; 1:225.

221. Hegele RA, Angel A. Arrest of neuropathy and myopathy in abetalipopro-teinemia with high dose vitamin E therapy. Can Med Assoc J 1985; 12:41.

222. Kayden HJ, Traber MG. Clinical, nutritional, and biochemical consequences of apolipoprotein B deficiency. Adv Exp Med Biol 1986; 201:67.

223. Wetterau JR, Aggerbeck LP, Bouma ME, et al. Absence of microsomal tri-glyceride transfer protein in individuals with abetalipoproteinemia. Science 1992; 258:999.

224. Levy RI, Langer T, Gotto AM, Fredrickson DS. Familial hypobetalipopro-teinemia, a defect in lipoprotein synthesis. Clin Res 1970; 18:539.

225. Cottrill C, Glueck CJ, Leuba V, et al. Familial homozygous hypobetalipopro-teinemia. Metabolism 1974; 23:779.

226. Berger GMB, Brown G, Henderson HE, Bonnici F. Apolipoprotein B detected in the plasma of a patient with homozygous hypobetalipopro-teinemia: implications for aetiology. J Med Genet 1983; 20:189.

227. Ross RS, Gregg RE, Law SW, et al. Homozygous hypobetalipoproteinemia: a disease distinct from abetalipoproteinemia at the molecular level. J Clin Invest 1988; 81:590.

228. Malloy MJ, Kane JP, Hardman DA, et al. Normotriglyceridemic abetalipo-proteinemia: absence of the B-100 apolipoprotein. J Clin Invest 1981; 67:1441.

229. Steinberg D, Grundy SM, Mok HY, et al. Metabolic studies in an unusual case of asymptomatic familial hypobetalipoproteinemia and fasting chylo-micronemia. J Clin Invest 1979; 64:292.

230. Young SG, Northey ST, McCarthy BJ. Low plasma cholesterol levels caused by a short deletion in the apoB gene. Science 1988; 241:591.

231. Witzum JL. Lipoprotein B37, a naturally occurring lipoprotein containing the amino-terminal portion of apolipoprotein B-100, does not bind to the apolipo-protein B, E (low-density lipoprotein) receptor. J Biol Chem 1987; 262:16604.

232. Collins DR, Knott TJ, Pease RJ, et al. Truncated variants of apolipoprotein B cause hypobetalipoproteinemia. Nucleic Acids Res 1988; 16:8361.

233. Anderson CM, Townley RRW, Freeman JP. Unusual causes of steatorrhea in infancy and childhood. Med J Aust 1961; 11:617.

234. Levy E, Marcel Y, Deckelbaum RJ, et al. Intestinal apo B synthesis, lipids, and lipoproteins in chylomicron retention disease. J Lipid Res 1987; 28:1263.

235. Bjorkem I, Skrede S. Familial diseases with storage of sterols other than cho-lesterol: cerebrotendinous xanthomatosis and phytosterolemia. In: Scriver CR, Beaudet AL, Sly WS, Valle D, eds. Metabolic basis of inherited disease. New York: McGraw-Hill, 1989:1283.

# CHAPTER 164

# TREATMENT OF THE HYPERLIPOPROTEINEMIAS

JOHN C. LAROSA

## RATIONALE FOR THERAPY

The treatment of hyperlipoproteinemia involves both diet and drug therapy and, in rare patients for whom these are inade-quate, more invasive interventions.

Clinical trials with end points of both coronary heart disease (CHD) mortality and morbidity as well as trials using serial angiography[1,2] have demonstrated that the lowering of plasma low-density lipoprotein (LDL) cholesterol levels slows the pro-gression of coronary atherosclerosis and lowers the risk of coro-nary events.

High levels (>55 mg/dL) of high-density lipoprotein (HDL) cholesterol are a powerful negative predictor of coronary risk. Clinical trials have not yet demonstrated clearly the indepen-dent value of raising HDL levels.[3]

Elevated triglyceride levels are often associated with elevated cholesterol and frequently are a marker for familial disorders in which atherogenic lipoproteins, such as intermediate-density lipoprotein (IDL) and chylomicron remnants, accumulate. Plasma triglyceride levels of >150 mg/dL (1.6 mmol/L), more-over, are associated with the appearance of a triglyceride-rich, small, dense form of LDL, which is thought to be particularly atherogenic. In addition, triglyceride levels of >1000 mg/dL (11.4 mmol/L) indicate chylomicronemia, a condition that, if left untreated, may cause pancreatitis.[4]

TABLE 164-1.
**Summary of National Cholesterol Education Program (NCEP) Guidelines**

|  | *For Screening,* Use Total Cholesterol | *For Therapeutic Decisions,* Use LDL |
|---|---|---|
| **High** | ≥240 mg/dL (6.2 mmol/L) | >160 mg/dL (4.1 mmol/L) |
| **Borderline high** | 200–239 mg/dL (5.2–6.2 mmol/L) | 130–159 mg/dL (3.4–4.1 mmol/L) |
| **Desirable** | <200 mg/dL (5.2 mmol/L) | <130 mg/dL (3.4 mmol/L) |
|  |  | **Threshold for Dietary Intervention** |
| **LDL** |  | >130 mg/dL (3.4 mmol/L) |
| **LDL if CHD is present** |  | >100 (2.6 mmol/L) |
|  | **Threshold for Drug Intervention (After Diet Trial)** | **Targets for Therapy** |
| **LDL if no other risk factors*** | ≥190 mg/dL (4.9 mmol/L) |  |
| **LDL if no CHD is present** | ≥160 mg/dL (4.1 mmol/L) | <130 mg/dL (3.4 mmol/L) |
| **LDL if CHD is present** | ≥130 mg/dL (3.4 mmol/L) | <100 mg/dL (2.6 mmol/L) |
|  |  | **Triglycerides** |
| **High** |  | >400 mg/dL (4.5 mmol/L) |
| **Borderline high** |  | 200–399 mg/dL (2.3–4.5 mmol/L) |
| **Normal** |  | <200 mg/dL (2.3 mmol/L) |

*LDL,* low-density lipoprotein; *CHD,* coronary heart disease.

*\*NCEP risk factors:* age (years), male 45 years or older; female 55 years or older, or postmenopausal; family history of premature CHD; current cigarette smoker; hypertension (blood pressure ≥140/90 mm Hg or taking antihypertensive medication); low high-density lipoprotein (HDL) cholesterol (<35 mg/dL [0.9 mmol/L]); diabetes mellitus. *Negative risk factor:* high HDL cholesterol (≥60 mg/dL [1.6 mmol/L]).

## GOALS OF THERAPY

### CHOLESTEROL

The goal of therapy in hyperlipoproteinemia is the prevention of its complications. For most patients, these are vascular. The National Cholesterol Education Program (NCEP), coordinated by the National Institutes of Health (NIH), has issued guidelines for detection and treatment of hypercholesterolemia (Table 164-1).[5] A detailed description of these guidelines is beyond the scope of this chapter. In general, however, patients with cholesterol levels in excess of 240 mg/dL (6.2 mmol/L) are candidates for diet and perhaps drug therapy if their LDL levels are 160 mg/dL (4.1 mmol/L) or greater. Therapeutic targets are to lower LDL cholesterol levels below 130 mg/dL (3.4 mmol/L) and even below 100 mg/dL (2.6 mmol/L) if the patient already has CHD.

Support for actively treating cholesterol elevations in adults is now well established.[1,2] Dyslipoproteinemia is less common in children than in adults; when it does occur, it is more likely to be related to a genetic abnormality. As with adults, diet therapy should always be attempted first. In children, drugs should be used more sparingly and only in the most resistant cases. Guidelines for detection and treatment of hypercholesterolemia in children have also been developed by the NCEP.[6]

The value of therapy in elderly patients is somewhat less certain. Epidemiologic evidence indicates that total cholesterol levels continue to predict coronary risk in elderly patients. Clinical trials have now demonstrated that cholesterol-lowering benefits are demonstrable in those older than age 65.[7] Less is known about its value in the "older" elderly, that is, those older than 75 years of age. Older patients, moreover, are more likely to have advanced atherosclerosis. Prudence dictates that particular attention be paid to the overall nutritional adequacy of the diet and the possibility that older patients may be more susceptible to the side effects of drugs.

## TRIGLYCERIDE

Triglyceride levels higher than 1000 mg/dL (11.4 mmol/L) are associated with high levels of circulating chylomicrons and may lead to pancreatitis. In such cases, severe restriction of all dietary fat is necessary. Chylomicronemia is affected only marginally and unpredictably by drugs.

Elevated triglyceride levels are often associated with low HDL levels.[3] In addition, elevated triglyceride may also be a marker for dyslipoproteinemias, which are associated with increased cardiovascular risk. Some patients with high triglyceride levels have familial combined hyperlipidemia. A few patients with hypertriglyceridemia have type III dyslipoproteinemia, that is, accumulation of IDL and chylomicron remnants. Both of these groups are at increased risk for development of atherosclerosis and should be treated.

An NIH consensus panel recommended that persons with triglyceride levels of >200 mg/dL (2.3 mmol/L) be considered candidates for therapy if they have a concomitant increase in LDL cholesterol levels, a low HDL cholesterol level, or a family history of CHD that might be indicative of a genetic abnormality of lipoprotein metabolism.[8]

### HIGH-DENSITY LIPOPROTEIN

As yet, clinical trials provide no definitive evidence that changing HDL levels retards atherogenesis or lowers coronary risk. However, data from the National Health, Lung, and Blood Institute Type II Intervention Study,[9] the Lipid Research Clinic Coronary Primary Prevention Trial,[10] the Helsinki Study,[11] and the Veterans Administration HDL Study[12] suggest an independent benefit.

Although dietary factors can affect HDL levels, diet does not seem to be a prominent determinant of HDL cholesterol, which is more closely related to body weight and body fat distribution, exercise status, and gender.

NCEP guidelines for cholesterol management do not specify therapeutic targets for HDL. An HDL level below 35 mg/dL (0.9 mmol/L) is considered a CHD risk factor. In the NCEP guidelines, it is used to identify those requiring additional screening and therapy. An HDL level of >60 mg/dL (1.6 mmol/L), on the other hand, is considered a negative risk factor.

## THERAPEUTIC APPROACH TO PATIENTS WITH DYSLIPOPROTEINEMIA

The precise determination of the genetic or acquired cause of hyperlipoproteinemia is difficult. Most practicing physicians have available to them findings from the history and physical examination and laboratory measurements of total cholesterol, total triglycerides, and HDL cholesterol. Sampling of family members to define genetic abnormalities often is somewhat difficult, although it should be done whenever possible because it is an efficient means of identifying others whose lipoprotein abnormalities require attention. The NCEP guidelines do not emphasize diagnoses of genetic abnormalities, but instead recognize that an elevated LDL level, whatever its cause, is a CHD risk factor requiring medical attention.

### DIETARY TREATMENT OF HYPERLIPOPROTEINEMIA

Several dietary factors influence lipoprotein levels and should be considered in prescribing a diet[13] (Table 164-2).

**TABLE 164-2.**
**Effect of Major Dietary Components on Plasma Lipoproteins**

| | Chylo-microns | VLDL | LDL | IDL | HDL |
|---|---|---|---|---|---|
| Calories | ↑ | ↑ | ↑ | ↑ | ↓ |
| Cholesterol | ↑ | ↑ | ↑ | ↑ | ↑ |
| Saturated fat | ↑ | ↑ | ↑ | ↑ | ↑ |
| Polyunsaturated fat (plants and vegetables) | ↑ | ↓ | ↓ | ↓ | ↓ |
| Polyunsaturated fat (fish oils) | ↑ | ↓ | ↑ | ↓ | ↑ |
| Monounsaturated fat | ↑ | ? | ↓ | ? | N |
| Carbohydrates | N | ↑ | ↓ | ↑ | ↓ |
| Alcohol* | ↑ | ↑ | N or ↑ | ↑ | ↑ |
| Soluble fiber | N | N | ↓ | ? | N |

↑, increased; ↓, decreased; *N*, no effect; *VLDL*, very-low-density lipoproteins; *LDL*, low-density lipoproteins; *IDL*, intermediate-density lipoproteins; *HDL*, high-density lipoproteins.

*Alcohol raises HDL cholesterol levels in most people without much effect on triglycerides; in some, however, it may raise triglyceride and lower HDL levels.

## CALORIES

In overweight patients, the value of weight reduction should not be overlooked. Very-low-density lipoprotein (VLDL) levels often can be dramatically reduced. Weight reduction may also be of benefit in reducing LDL, IDL, and chylomicron levels. The HDL levels can be increased by weight loss, particularly in persons with VLDL elevations. Weight loss can also enhance the decline in LDL levels in response to a diet low in saturated fat.[14]

In some persons, particularly those with modest elevations of VLDL, weight reduction may be associated with a temporary increase in LDL cholesterol levels because of increased VLDL-to-LDL conversion. The same effect is sometimes seen with drug therapy in such patients. Because thin individuals have lower LDL levels than their heavier peers, weight loss–related LDL elevations probably are transient.

## CHOLESTEROL

The ingestion of cholesterol leads to elevations of VLDL, LDL, and HDL cholesterol levels. In both animals and humans, cholesterol feeding also causes an appearance of lipoproteins with large amounts of apoprotein E, or β-VLDL.[15] These lipoproteins are atherogenic in animals. Their appearance is not always associated with increases in plasma cholesterol levels, indicating that the atherogenic potential of a diet may not be reflected in its effect on total cholesterol levels.

Dietary cholesterol is first presented to the liver in the form of chylomicron remnants. Remnants not only inhibit hepatic cholesterol synthesis and increase bile acid excretion, but also increase VLDL production and secretion and inhibit LDL-receptor formation.[16] The net effect in most persons is a rise in total cholesterol levels.

## FATTY ACIDS

The effect of dietary cholesterol is also influenced by the fatty acid composition of the diet (Fig. 164-1). As dietary polyunsaturated fat levels increase, the ability of a given dietary cholesterol load to increase blood cholesterol levels is dramatically decreased. Saturated fats have the opposite effect.[17] Quantitatively, saturated fat has twice the power to raise cholesterol levels as polyunsaturated ones have to lower them.

All saturated fats, however, are not equivalent. Studies have indicated that stearic acid, a saturated fat that is converted to a monounsaturate after absorption, does not raise cholesterol levels.[18]

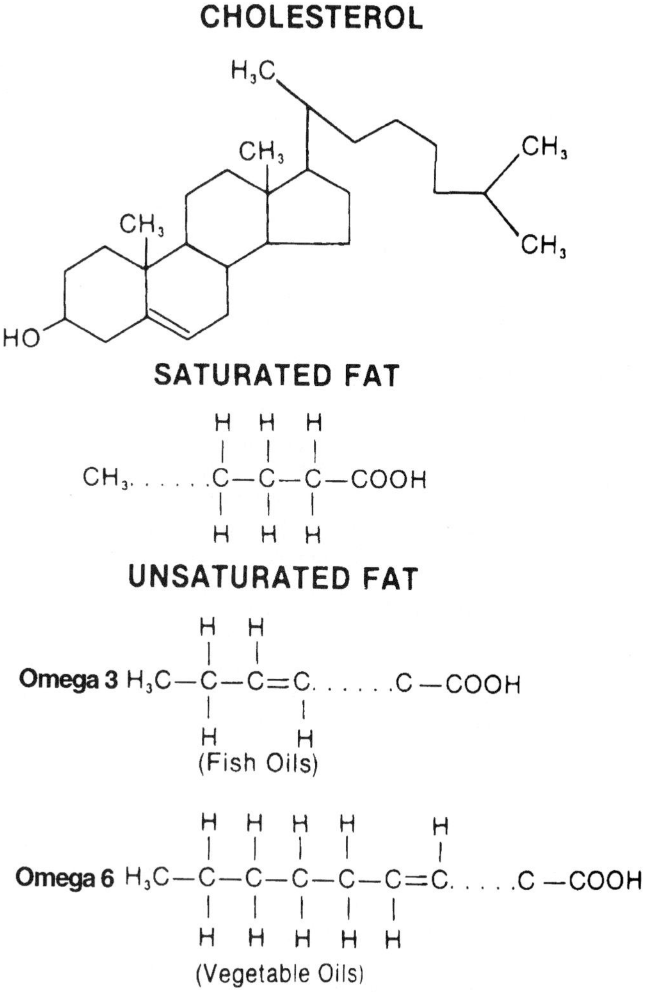

**FIGURE 164-1.** *Saturated fats* are triglycerides with fatty acids containing no carbon–carbon double bonds. *Polyunsaturated fats* contain two or more double bonds; they are of two types, depending on their fatty acid content: *fish oils* contain omega-3 fatty acids with the first carbon–carbon double bond at carbon 3. *Vegetable oils* contain omega-6 fatty acids, with the first carbon–carbon double bond at carbon 6.

Despite considerable research, the differential effects of polyunsaturated and saturated fats are poorly understood. Polyunsaturated fats increase cholesterol excretion in bile. They also may alter the structure of lipoproteins, making them more susceptible to clearance from the plasma.

Polyunsaturated fats can be subdivided into two groups. The omega-6 fatty acids (the first unsaturated carbon is the sixth from the methyl end of the molecule) are most commonly found in vegetable oils. Omega-3 polyunsaturated fatty acids are found both in vegetables and in fish oils. Omega-3 fatty acids found in fish oils can effectively lower plasma VLDL levels, but affect LDL and HDL levels weakly and variably.[19] The ingestion of high levels of fish oil has been associated with lower rates of death from cardiovascular disease,[20] and fish oil ingestion has been shown to lower restenosis rates after angioplasty.[21]

The use of polyunsaturates is not entirely without hazard. They increase cholesterol in bile and may lead to gallstones. The use of omega-3 fish oils in the diet may lead to decreased platelet adhesiveness and prolonged bleeding times. Also, because all fats are very calorie-dense foods (9 calories/g compared to 4 calories/g for carbohydrates and protein), the ingestion of polyunsaturated, as well as saturated, fat may interfere with attempts to control body weight.[13]

Monounsaturated fats, found in large quantities in olive oil (oleic acid), are neutral in terms of their effects on total plasma cholesterol. Studies have demonstrated that both polyunsaturated and monounsaturated fat can lower LDL levels while sparing HDL.[22] LDL-containing oleic acid, moreover, is resistant to oxidation, and may, therefore, be less atherogenic.[23] All monounsaturates are not equivalent. Elaidic acid is formed when omega-3 fatty acids are commercially hydrogenated. Unlike oleic acid (a *cis* fatty acid), this *trans* fatty acid behaves like a saturated fat, raising LDL levels.[24] *Trans* fatty acids also raise levels of lipoprotein(a) [Lp(a)][25] and have been associated, in population studies, with increased cardiovascular risk.[13,26]

## CARBOHYDRATES

In most lipid-lowering diets, carbohydrates can adequately replace fat as a source of calories. The NCEP guidelines, for example, recommend that total fat be reduced to 30% of calories and that complex carbohydrates be substituted.[5] Transient increases in triglyceride levels are less likely to occur with complex carbohydrates than with sucrose. The suggestion has been made that, because of the possibility of carbohydrate-induced hypertriglyceridemia and hyperinsulinemia, monounsaturated fat, as found in olive oil, might be a better substitute for saturated fat than carbohydrates (the "Mediterranean" diet). Because this would not result in any decline in caloric intake, however, this issue is unsettled at present.[13]

## ALCOHOL

Like consumption of fish oils, alcohol ingestion is associated with a decline in CHD rates in both men and women.[26a] In fact, the "French paradox" (high levels of saturated fat in the French diet are, paradoxically, not associated with high rates of coronary risk) is largely explained by the high alcohol content of the French diet.[27] Alcohol, like estrogen and bile sequestrants, simultaneously raises HDL and triglycerides. In addition, it has other effects that may inhibit atherogenesis, including decreasing LDL oxidation, decreasing platelet stickiness, and decreasing fibrinogen levels.[28] Alcohol, of course, is an addicting drug that has a direct deleterious effect on myocardium, so that only in moderation can its ingestion be considered useful for the prevention of atherogenesis.

## ANTIOXIDANTS

Dietary antioxidant vitamins do not appreciably alter levels of circulating lipoproteins. The atherogenicity of LDL, however, is thought to be directly related to its level of oxidation. It is oxidized LDL that is taken up by macrophages, which convert it to foam cells. On the other hand, preliminary evidence suggests that reverse cholesterol transport may be enhanced when HDL is oxidized.[29]

The net effect of antioxidants seems to be the inhibition of atherogenesis. For example, oleic acid from olive oil, when incorporated into LDL, makes it more resistant to oxidation and less likely to be taken up by macrophages,[22] thereby contributing to the protective value of the "Mediterranean" diet.

Observational studies of the intake of both β-carotene and vitamin E (α-tocopherol), either as dietary constituents or dietary supplements, have shown a trend toward lower relative risk of vascular disease, although with wide variation.[30] Trials of β-carotene supplementation, on the other hand, have also demonstrated potential harm in promoting malignancies, particularly in smokers.[31,32] A report on >22,000 male physicians (largely nonsmokers) demonstrated no effect of β-carotene supplementation on malignant neoplasms, cardiovascular events, or death from all causes.[33] A small clinical trial in a subset from that same study, however, did demonstrate a substantial 44% decline in recurrent coronary events.[34]

A clinical trial of vitamin E supplementation demonstrated a 47% decline in cardiovascular events, although during the period of observation in the study a slight excess mortality from cardiovascular disease was seen in the vitamin E group.[35] At this point, the evidence that antioxidants are of benefit in controlling atherogenesis is mixed. The evidence is somewhat better for vitamin E than for β-carotene.

## OTHER DIETARY COMPONENTS

Vegetable fiber has independent lipid-lowering effects. A number of human trials indicate that soluble fiber, such as found in oat bran and psyllium seeds, can lower LDL levels 5% to 10%.[36]

Other dietary constituents have also been implicated in the prevention of atherosclerosis. Diets high in soy, containing antioxidant flavonoids and phytoestrogens, have been demonstrated in cynomolgus monkeys to raise HDL and to lower LDL levels.[37] Similar effects have been reported in humans consuming soy-containing diets, although whether this effect is related to phytoestrogens or some other component of soy, such as antioxidant flavonoids, has not been determined.[38] Estrogens, including (presumably) phytoestrogens, have antiatherogenic effects, among them, favorable changes in circulating lipoproteins, inhibition of arterial wall LDL uptake, inhibition of platelet stickiness, and prevention of paradoxical vascular contraction in response to acetylcholine.[39]

Over the years, the effect of coffee on cardiovascular disease has been widely debated. Although coffee has little effect on circulating lipoproteins, some studies indicate that excessive coffee intake is associated with the progression of coronary disease. That concern has now been put to rest. In a large observational study in men, even coffee consumption of >4 cups per day did not appear to increase the relative risk of coronary disease.[40]

Finally, increased consumption of nuts, particularly walnuts, which contain high levels of polyunsaturated fat, has been associated with reduced risk of CHD.[41] In similar fashion, metaanalysis of studies of garlic consumption and coronary artery disease also indicates a favorable effect on circulating total cholesterol levels.[42] A clinical trial, however, did not demonstrate any effect of ingestion of 300-mg garlic tablets (three tablets per day) on levels of circulating lipoproteins.[43]

## DIETS FOR HYPERLIPOPROTEINEMIA

Most patients with hyperlipoproteinemia have elevations of either LDL or VLDL. Diets low in cholesterol and saturated fat, relatively higher in polyunsaturated fat and carbohydrates, and with calories sufficient to maintain, but not exceed, ideal body weight, are likely to be most effective in controlling elevated lipoprotein levels.

Low-cholesterol, low-fat diets are recommended by the NCEP (Table 164-3). These diets progressively lower both dietary cholesterol and fat intake, substituting carbohydrate for lost calories. Step 2 of the diet, with a cholesterol content of <200 mg per day (5.2 mmol/L per day) and only 7% of calories coming from saturated fat is, of course, a substantial departure from the current American diet.

Patients in whom chylomicron levels are elevated need diets that are even lower in total fat. Such a patient may be required to lower total fat intake to fewer than 10% of calories and substitute medium-chain triglycerides, which are not formed into chylomicrons, for dietary fat.

## DRUG TREATMENT

In patients without clinical coronary disease, drug therapy usually should not be instituted until an adequate trial of dietary therapy has been completed. This may take 3 to 6 months. The diet trial should last long enough to allow the patient to adopt

**TABLE 164-3.**
**Diet Composition***

| | "Usual" American Diet (For a 40-Year-Old Man) | NCEP Diet | |
| | | Step 1 | Step 2 |
|---|---|---|---|
| Protein | 15 | 15 | 15 |
| Carbohydrate† | 40 | 55 | 60 |
| Fat | 40 | | |
|   Saturated | 15 | 10 | <7 |
|   Monounsaturated | 16 | Up to 15% of total calories | |
|   Polyunsaturated | 7 | Up to 10% of total calories | |
| Cholesterol‡ | 500 | <300 | <200 |

NCEP, National Cholesterol Education Program.
*Expressed as percentage of total calories (except as noted).
†Alcohol may make up as much as 5% of total calories in the "usual" American diet.
‡Expressed in mg per day.

**TABLE 164-4.**
**Effects of Lipid-Lowering Drugs***

| Lipoprotein | Nicotinic Acid | Bile Acid Sequestrants | HMG-CoA-Reductase Inhibitors | Gem-fibrozil |
|---|---|---|---|---|
| Chylomicrons | ?↓ | ? | N | ?↓ |
| VLDL | ↓ | N or ↑ | N?↓ | ↓ |
| IDL | ↓ | N or ↑ | ?↓ | ↓ |
| LDL | ↓ | ↓ | ↓↓ | N or ↑ |
| HDL | ↑ | N or ↑ | N or ↑ | N or ↑ |

↑, increased; ↓, decreased; N, no effect; HMG-CoA, 3-hydroxy-3-methylglutaryl coenzyme A; VLDL, very-low-density lipoprotein; IDL, intermediate-density lipoprotein; LDL, low-density lipoprotein; HDL, high-density lipoprotein.
*Lipoprotein effects of currently used hypolipidemic agents are listed. Doses are approximate and should be tailored to the individual patient.

new dietary tastes and habits. In patients with severe genetic lipid abnormalities or with clinical coronary disease in whom LDL targets of <100 mg/dL (<2.6 mmol/L) are anticipated, on the other hand, drug therapy may be instituted immediately or after 2 to 3 weeks of diet trial. This is because such patients are unlikely to be adequately treated with diet alone.

Lipid-lowering agents can be conveniently divided into those that lower total cholesterol and LDL levels and those that lower total levels of triglycerides and the triglyceride-carrying lipoproteins, VLDL, chylomicrons, and their remnants. All should be used prudently, with attention to the lowest dose necessary to reach the therapeutic goal. Tables 164-1, 164-4, and 164-5 summarize some useful clinical information about these agents.

## CHOLESTEROL-LOWERING DRUGS

**Nicotinic Acid.** Nicotinic acid (niacin) is a B vitamin ($B_3$) that, when given in pharmacologic doses, has profound lipid-lowering effects.[44] Its mechanism of action is wide ranging, including stimulation of lipoprotein lipase activity and the inhibition of VLDL synthesis and secretion in the liver. Lower LDL levels also result, because LDL is formed as a product of VLDL catabolism. HDL levels rise, perhaps because of increased VLDL catabolism. LDL lowering requires higher doses in general than lowering of triglyceride (and HDL increases). Nicotinic acid is the only commonly used lipid-lowering agent that can lower levels of Lp(a).[45]

In a long-term trial of the effect of nicotinic acid administration in the secondary prevention of coronary disease, the incidence of nonfatal myocardial infarction was reduced. Furthermore, long-term follow-up of patients in the trial for several years after drug therapy was discontinued indicated a lower mortality among those who had taken the drug.[46]

Nicotinic acid has some troublesome side effects that balance its remarkably beneficial effects on lipoprotein levels. The most common is cutaneous vasodilation and flushing, which occur an hour or two after ingestion of the drug. Tolerance to this effect develops over time. Because it is prostaglandin mediated, flushing may be decreased by ingestion of an aspirin tablet before taking nicotinic acid. Nicotinic acid may also cause acanthosis nigricans and skin rashes.

Gastrointestinal side effects, such as cramping, nausea, and abdominal discomfort, can be partially diminished by taking the drug with meals or antacids. The most serious side effect is liver toxicity, particularly with the sustained-release form.[45] Other effects of nicotinic acid include decreased glucose tolerance and hyperuricemia, so its use is contraindicated in diabetes and gout. In some patients, abnormal liver function test results may occur. Finally, nicotinic acid has been associated with an increase in atrial arrhythmias and is contraindicated in patients with a history of such arrhythmias.

These side effects often lead to poor patient compliance. In a study of the use of a combination of neomycin and niacin in the treatment of patients with type II hyperlipoproteinemia, fewer than half of the patients given nicotinic acid were able to tolerate it for >6 months.[47] Nicotinic acid commonly is administered at an initial dosage of 100 mg three times daily and increased gradually, as tolerated, to doses as high as 2 g twice a day.

**Bile Acid Sequestrants.** Bile acid sequestrants, cholestyramine and colestipol, are anion-exchange polymers with positively charged amine groups capable of binding bile salts and interrupting their enterohepatic circulation.[48] This, in turn, stimulates the liver to synthesize increased numbers of LDL receptors to obtain additional LDL cholesterol for bile synthesis. The result is a fall in plasma LDL cholesterol levels. In patients with borderline triglyceride elevations, bile acid sequestrants may increase triglyceride levels even while decreasing LDL cholesterol levels. For unknown reasons, these drugs also are associated with a slight increase in HDL cholesterol levels. These effects can be demonstrated even in persons with heterozygous familial hypercholesterolemia, who are deficient in LDL receptors under basal conditions.

**TABLE 164-5.**
**Side Effects of Lipid-Lowering Drugs**

| Nicotinic Acid | Bile Acid Sequestrants | HMG-CoA Reductase Inhibitors | Gemfibrozil |
|---|---|---|---|
| Flushing; rash; acanthosis nigricans; gastrointestinal cramping, nausea, abdominal pain; abnormal liver function tests; ↓ glucose tolerance; ↑ uric acid; ↑ atrial arrhythmias | Bloating; constipation; binding of vitamins and medications; hyperchloremic acidosis (in children) | Drug-induced hepatitis (<1% of patients); rhabdomyolysis (0.05%) | Rare drug-induced hepatitis; ? myopathy; ? cholelithiasis |

↑, increased; ↓, decreased; HMG-CoA, 3-hydroxy-3-methylglutaryl coenzyme A.

Bile acid sequestrants are supplied as nonabsorbable powders, taken in gram quantities after being suspended in water or other clear liquids. Their major side effects are gastrointestinal. Patients may complain of bloating and nausea, and even abdominal pain shortly after taking the drug. These side effects may be diminished by antacids, and are usually transient. A full dose of 24 to 30 g per day is frequently accompanied by constipation, which may be helped by stool softeners, bulk laxatives, or an increase in dietary fiber. Over a period of months, gastrointestinal side effects usually decline. Nevertheless, as with nicotinic acid, bile acid sequestrants pose formidable compliance problems for some patients.

In some children, the chloride ion released when bile is bound to the drug may be absorbed and cause hyperchloremic acidosis. This usually is not a problem in adults.

Bile acid sequestrants also bind fat-soluble vitamins and various medications, including digitalis compounds, thiazides, anticoagulants, and thyroxine. Vitamin deficiency has not been a clinical problem; nevertheless, the ingestion of one multivitamin tablet a day is a useful precaution. The decreased absorption of drugs can be minimized by separating sequestrant ingestion from ingestion of other drugs by ~2 hours. For maximum effect, bile acid sequestrants should be given at least twice a day, ~1 hour before meals.

Many patients with moderate elevations of LDL cholesterol (type II hyperlipoproteinemia) who do not respond satisfactorily to a diet regimen can be treated with small doses of bile acid sequestrants with a minimum of side effects. Bile acid sequestrants also are effective in combination with drugs such as nicotinic acid or statins (see later).

**3-Hydroxy-3-Methylglutaryl Coenzyme A Reductase Inhibitors.**   Six agents, lovastatin,[49] pravastatin,[50] simvastatin,[51] fluvastatin,[52] atorvastatin,[53] and cerivastatin,[54] are available that inhibit the action of 3-hydroxy-3-methylglutaryl coenzyme A reductase (HMG-CoA reductase), the rate-limiting enzyme in cholesterol biosynthesis. By inhibiting intracellular cholesterol biosynthesis in the liver, these agents stimulate proliferation of LDL receptors, increase binding of LDL, and decrease plasma cholesterol levels.

Thus far, these drugs seem comparatively free of serious side effects. Less than 2% of patients have had significant elevations of liver enzymes necessitating cessation of therapy. Rhabdomyolysis develops in a very small number (0.05%), which may lead to elevated creatine phosphokinase (CPK) levels, myoglobinemia, myoglobinuria, and even acute renal failure. The incidence of this complication may be considered higher when certain of these drugs (all but pravastatin and fluvastatin) are used in combination with drugs like inhibitors of the cytochrome CYP344 (including erythromycin, ketoconazole, or mibefradil).[55] This side effect is also increased with concurrent use of gemfibrozil, niacin, or cyclosporine. Patients therefore must be instructed to stop medication if any unusual muscle pain develops. Risk of hepatic or muscular toxicity is not increased when these drugs are combined with bile acid sequestrants.

The efficacy of reductase inhibitors is impressive. They lower LDL levels up to 60%.[56] Unlike bile acid sequestrants, they are conveniently given in pill form, have few immediate side effects, and pose few compliance problems.

### TRIGLYCERIDE-LOWERING DRUGS

**Nicotinic Acid.**   Because of its influence on VLDL levels, nicotinic acid is an effective drug for lowering levels of triglycerides as well as cholesterol. Its actions and side effects have been reviewed previously.

**Fibric Acid Derivatives.**   A series of drugs derived from fibric acid, including clofibrate, gemfibrozil, bezafibrate, and fenofibrate, have found use as triglyceride-lowering agents.[57,58] These drugs primarily act to stimulate VLDL lipolysis by lipoprotein lipase. They are most useful in patients who accumulate IDL and chylomicron remnants (type III hyperlipoproteinemia). In such patients, the fall in triglyceride and cholesterol levels may be quite substantial. They are also effective in patients with elevated VLDL (type IV hyperlipoproteinemia). They are variably effective in patients with chylomicronemia (niacin is a better treatment for this disorder). With these drugs, LDL or HDL elevations may accompany VLDL declines.

Side effects include an increase in lithogenic bile, leading to cholelithiasis, rhabdomyolysis with elevated plasma CPK levels, and the enhancement of warfarin anticoagulant effects.

Clofibrate was the subject of study in two major clinical trials. In the Coronary Drug Project, its use reduced triglyceride levels by 22% and plasma cholesterol levels by 6%. The number of nonfatal myocardial infarctions declined, but no overall decline in cardiovascular mortality was seen.[59] In a clinical trial sponsored by the World Health Organization, clofibrate therapy was associated with an excess mortality from gastrointestinal disease, including cancer.[60] This led to a dramatic reduction in its use. Today, clofibrate is rarely prescribed. On the other hand, the Helsinki Study, a long-term trial with gemfibrozil, demonstrated no increase in noncardiovascular mortality and did show a significant decrease in coronary events.

**Combination Drug Therapy.**   Combination drug therapy may be useful to maximize efficacy (i.e., LDL lowering), to obtain multiple effects (i.e., LDL lowering as well as triglyceride lowering or HDL rise), or to minimize dosage and side effects of any one drug.[61] Bile acid sequestrants may be combined with any single "systemic" drug without concern about increased toxicity. Combining two systemic drugs, however (for example, a "statin" drug and gemfibrozil, or niacin and a statin drug), increases the risk of both hepatic toxicity and rhabdomyolysis.[62] Therefore, if such a combination is used, alanine aminotransferase levels should be measured every 2 to 3 months. Rhabdomyolysis is first manifested by pain *before* CPK levels rise. Therefore, patients must be carefully instructed to report muscle pain and stop medications if it occurs. Rhabdomyolysis can be confirmed by measuring CPK levels.

**Estrogen.**   Both natural and synthetic estrogen have favorable effects on lipoproteins, lowering LDL 5% to 15% and raising HDL 5% to 10%.[63] Newer synthetic estrogen substitutes (selective estrogen-receptor modulators, or SERMS), including tamoxifen and raloxifene, may have similar effects on LDL.[64] Observational studies of coronary disease have indicated beneficial effects of estrogen replacement therapy on coronary disease, although the effect could not be demonstrated in the only clinical trial to examine this issue.[65] Until this issue is clarified, hormone replacement should not be used in place of cholesterol lowering in women at risk of coronary disease.

### LOW-DENSITY LIPOPROTEIN APHERESIS

Techniques that use antibodies or heparin-bound inert materials can remove LDL from circulating plasma in a procedure similar to hemodialysis.[66] The procedure must be performed 1 to 2 times per week to maintain low LDL. It not only removes LDL but also removes other atherogenic lipoproteins, as well as fibrinogen. Studies involving serial angiograms have suggested that prolonged LDL lowering by this technique is associated with regression of atherosclerosis.[67] This technique may eventually find application in the treatment of those with severe hypercholesterolemia that is unresponsive to conventional diet and drug therapy.

## CONCLUSION

Knowledge of the patient's total cholesterol, total triglycerides, and HDL cholesterol levels, measurements that are available from most clinical laboratories, can provide a framework to guide the selection of appropriate diet and drugs. Many patients with hyperlipoproteinemia can be effectively treated with diet. In many cases, however, diet regimens are insufficient to bring lipoprotein levels to within acceptable limits. Nevertheless, in most patients drug therapy should be instituted only after a trial of diet therapy.

The treatment of elevated cholesterol has now been unequivocally proven to be of benefit in the prevention of atherosclerosis progression and in lowering coronary risk. Therapy should be aimed at reducing total cholesterol levels to between 160 and 200 mg/dL (4.9 and 5.2 mmol/L). Although this goal may not be achievable in every patient, evidence indicates a linear relationship between LDL cholesterol and coronary risk. Thus, cholesterol lowering short of this ideal is still likely to be of substantial benefit.

# REFERENCES

1. Gould AL, Roussouw JE, Santanello NC, et al. Cholesterol reduction yields clinical benefit. Impact of statin trials. Circulation 1998; 97:946.
2. Ballantyne CM. Low-density lipoproteins and risk for coronary artery disease. Am J Cardiol 1998; 82:3Q.
3. Kwiterovich PO, Jr. The antiatherogenic role of high density lipoprotein cholesterol. Am J Cardiol 1998; 82:13Q.
4. Santamarina-Fojo S. The familial chylomicronemia syndrome. Med Clin North Amer 1998; 27:551.
5. National Cholesterol Education Program Expert Panel. Summary of the second report of the National Cholesterol Education Program (NCEP) Expert Panel on Detection, Evaluation, and Treatment of High Blood Cholesterol in Adults (Adult Treatment Panel II). JAMA 1993; 269:3015.
6. Expert Panel on Blood Cholesterol Levels in Children and Adolescents. National Cholesterol Education Program: highlights of the report of the Expert Panel on Blood Cholesterol Levels in Children and Adolescents. Pediatrics 1992; 89:495.
7. LaRosa JC. Cholesterol management in women and the elderly. J Intern Med 1997; 241:307.
8. National Institutes of Health Consensus Development Panel. Triglyceride, high-density lipoprotein, and coronary heart disease. February 26–28, 1992, Bethesda, Maryland. JAMA 1993; 269:505.
9. Levy RI, Brensike JF, Epstein SE, et al. The influence of changes in lipid values induced by cholestyramine and diet progression of coronary artery disease: results of the National Heart, Lung and Blood Institute Type II Coronary Intervention Study. Circulation 1984; 69:325.
10. Lipid Research Clinics Program. The Lipid Research Clinic Coronary Primary Prevention Trial Results: I. reduction in the incidence of coronary heart disease. JAMA 1984; 251:351.
11. Frick MH, Elo O, Haapa K, et al. Helsinki Heart Study: primary-prevention trial with gemfibrozil in middle-aged men with dyslipidemia. Safety of treatment, changes in risk factors, and incidence of coronary heart disease. N Engl J Med 1987; 317:1237.
12. Late-breaking lipid trials. Conference Coverage. American Heart Association Annual Scientific Sessions; November 8–11, 1998; Dallas. TX. Intern Med Alert 1998; 20:185.
13. LaRosa JC. Diet and cardiovascular disease. Prev Cardiol 1998; 1:40.
14. Hannah JS, Heiser CC, Jablonski KA, et al. Effects of obesity on the response to a low fat diet. (Abstract). Circulation 1994; 90(4, pt 2):I-236.
15. Mahley RW. Cholesterol feeding: effects on lipoprotein structure and metabolism. In: Gotto AM, Smith LC, Allen B, eds. Atherosclerosis. New York: Springer-Verlag, 1980:641.
16. Mustad VA, Ellsworth J, Cooper AD, et al. Dietary linoleic acid increases and palmitic acid decreases hepatic LDL receptor protein and mRNA abundance in young pigs. J Lipid Res 1996; 37:2310.
17. Schonfeld G, Patsch W, Rudel LL, et al. Effects of dietary cholesterol and fatty acids on plasma lipoproteins. J Clin Invest 1982; 69:1072.
18. Bonanome A, Grundy SM. Effect of dietary stearic acid on plasma cholesterol and lipoprotein levels. N Engl J Med 1988; 318:1244.
19. Schmidt EB, Dyerberg J. Omega-3 fatty acids. Current status in cardiovascular medicine. Drugs 1994; 47:405.
20. Kromhout D, Bosschieter EB, Coulander CL. The inverse relation between fish consumption and 20-year mortality from coronary heart disease. N Engl J Med 1985; 312:1205.
21. Gapinski JP, Van Ruiswyk JV, Heudebert GR, et al. Preventing restenosis with fish oils following coronary angioplasty. Arch Intern Med 1993; 153:1595.
22. Mattson FH, Grundy SM. Comparison of effects of dietary saturated, monounsaturated, and polyunsaturated fatty acids on plasma lipids and lipoproteins in man. J Lipid Res 1985; 26:194.
23. Parthasarathy S, Khoo JC, Miller E, et al. Low density lipoprotein rich in oleic acid is protected against oxidative modification: implications for dietary prevention of atherosclerosis. Proc Natl Acad Sci U S A 1990; 87:3894.
24. Gardner CD, Kraemer HC. Monounsaturated versus polyunsaturated dietary fat and serum lipids: a meta-analysis. Arterioscler Thromb Vasc Biol 1995; 15:1917.
25. Mensink RP, Zock PL, Katan MB, et al. Effect of dietary cis and trans fatty acids on serum lipoprotein(a) levels in humans. J Lipid Res 1992; 33:1493.
26. Kromhout D, Menotti A, Bloemberg B, et al. Dietary saturated and trans fatty acids and cholesterol and 25-year mortality from coronary heart disease: the Seven Countries Study. Prev Med 1995; 24:308.
26a. Nanchahal K, Ashton WP, Wood DA. Alcohol consumption, metabolic cardiovascular risk factors and hypertension in women. Int J Epidemiol 2000; 29:57.
27. Hegsted DM, Ausman LM. Diet, alcohol and coronary heart disease. J Nutr 1988; 118:1184.
28. Suh I, Shaten BJ, Cutler JA, Kuller LH. Alcohol use and mortality from coronary heart disease: the role of high-density lipoprotein cholesterol. The Multiple Risk Factor Intervention Trial Research Group. Ann Intern Med 1992; 116:881.
29. Berliner JA, Heinecke JW. The role of oxidized lipoproteins in atherogenesis. Free Radic Biol Med 1996; 20:707.
30. Rexode KM, Manson JE. Antioxidants and coronary heart disease: observational studies. J Cardiovasc Res 1996; 3:363.
31. Albanes D, Heinonen OP, Taylor PR, et al. Alpha-tocopherol and beta-carotene supplements and lung cancer incidence in the Alpha-Tocopherol, Beta-Carotene Cancer Prevention Study: effects of base-line characteristics and study compliance. J Natl Cancer Inst 1996; 88:1560.
32. Omenn GS, Goodman GE, Thornquist MD, et al. Effects of a combination of beta-carotene and vitamin A on lung cancer and cardiovascular disease. N Engl J Med 1996; 334:1150.
33. Hennekens CH, Buring JE, Manson JE, et al. Lack of effect of long term supplementation with beta carotene on the incidence of malignant neoplasms and cardiovascular disease. N Engl J Med 1996; 334:1145.
34. Gaziano JM, Manson JE, Ridker PM, et al. Beta carotene therapy for chronic stable angina. Circulation 1991; 82(Suppl 3):201.
35. Stephens NG, Parsons A, Schofield PM, et al. Randomised controlled trial of vitamin E in patients with coronary disease: Cambridge Heart Antioxidant Study (CHAOS). Lancet 1996; 347:781.
36. Kestin M, Moss R, Clifton PM, et al. Comparative effects of three cereal brans on plasma lipids, blood pressure, and glucose metabolism in mildly hypercholesterolemic men. Am J Clin Nutr 1990; 52:661.
37. Anthony MS, Clarkson TB, Bulock BC. Soy protein versus soy phytoestrogens (isoflavones) in the prevention of coronary artery atherosclerosis of cynomolgus monkeys. (Abstract). Circulation 1996; 94:I-265.
38. Hertog MGL, Kromhout D, Aravanis C, et al. Flavonoid intake and long term risk of coronary heart disease and cancer in the Seven Countries Study. Arch Intern Med 1995; 4:588.
39. LaRosa JC. Estrogen: risk versus benefit for the prevention of coronary artery disease. Coron Artery Dis 1993; 4:588.
40. Grobbee DE, Rimm EB, Giovannucci E, et al. Coffee, caffeine, and cardiovascular disease in men. N Engl J Med 1990; 323:1026.
41. Sabate J, Fraser GD. Nuts: a new protective food against coronary heart disease. Curr Opin Lipidol 1994; 119:599.
42. Warshafsky S, Kamer RS, Sivak SL. Effect of garlic on total serum cholesterol. Ann Intern Med 1993; 119:599.
43. Niel HAW, Cilagy CA, Lancaster T, et al. Garlic powder in the treatment of moderate hyperlipidaemia: a controlled trial and meta-analysis. J R Coll Physicians Lond 1996; 30:329.
44. Ginsberg HN. Nicotinic acid. In: LaRosa JC, ed. Practical management of lipid disorders. Fort Lee, NJ: Health Care Communications, 1992:49.
45. Goldberg A, Alagona P Jr, Capuzzi DM, et al. Multiple-dose efficacy and safety of an extended-release form of niacin in the management of hyperlipidemia. Am J Cardiol 2000; 85:1100.
46. Canner PL. Mortality in coronary drug project patients during a nine-year post-treatment period. J Am Coll Cardiol 1985; 5:442.
47. Hoeg JM, Maher MB, Bou E, et al. Normalization of plasma lipoprotein concentrations in patients with type II hyperlipoproteinemia by combined use of neomycin and niacin. Circulation 1984; 70:1004.
48. Gordon DJ. Bile acid sequestrants. In: LaRosa JC, ed. Practical management of lipid disorders. Fort Lee, NJ: Health Care Communications, 1992:37.
49. Illingworth DR, Stein EA, Mitchel YB, et al. Comparative effects of lovastatin and niacin in primary hypercholesterolemia. A prospective trial. Arch Intern Med 1994; 154:1586.
50. Santinga JT, Rosman HS, Rubenfire M, et al. Efficacy and safety of pravastatin in the long-term treatment of elderly patients with hypercholesterolemia. Am J Med 1994; 96:509.
51. Keech A, Collins R, McMahon S, et al. Three-year follow-up of the Oxford Cholesterol Study: assessment of the efficacy and safety of simvastatin in preparation for a large mortality study. Eur Heart J 1994; 15:255.
52. Banga JD, Jacotot B, Pfister P, Mehra M. Long-term treatment of hypercholesterolemia with fluvastatin: a 52-week multicenter safety and efficacy study. French-Dutch Fluvastatin Study Group. Am J Med 1994; 96(6A):87S.
53. Nawrocki JW, Weiss SR, Davidson MH, et al. Reduction of LDL cholesterol by 25% to 60% in patients with primary hypercholesterolemia by atorvastatin, a new HMG-CoA reductase inhibitor. Arterioscler Thromb Vasc Biol 1995; 15:678.
54. Stein E, Sprecher D, Allenby KS, et al. Cerivastatin, a new potent synthetic HMG Co-A reductase inhibitor: effect of 0.2 mg daily in subjects with primary hypercholesterolemia. J Cardiovasc Pharmacol Therapeut 1997; 2:7.
55. Transon C, Leemann T, Dayer P. In vitro comparative inhibition profiles of major human drug metabolising cytochrome P450 isozymes (CYP2C9, CYP2D6 and CYP3A4) by HMG-CoA reductase inhibitors. Eur J Clin Pharmacol 1996; 50:209.

56. Jones P, Kafonek S, Laurora I, Hunninghake D, for the CURVES Investigators. Comparative dose efficacy study of atorvastatin versus simvastatin, pravastatin, lovastatin, and fluvastatin in patients with hypercholesterolemia (The CURVES Study). Am J Cardiol 1998; 81:582.

57. Brown WV. The fibric acid derivatives. In: LaRosa JC, ed. Practical management of lipid disorders. Fort Lee, NJ: Health Care Communications, 1992:61.

58. Packard CJ. Overview of fenofibrate. Eur Heart J 1998; (Suppl A):A62.

59. Coronary Drug Project Research Group. Clofibrate and niacin in coronary heart disease. JAMA 1975; 231:360.

60. World Health Organization European Collaborative Group. Multifactorial trial in the prevention of coronary heart disease: incidence and mortality rates. Eur Heart J 1983; 4:141.

61. Blum CB. Drug combination therapy for lipid disorders. In: LaRosa JC, ed. Practical management of lipid disorders. Fort Lee, NJ: Health Care Communications, 1992:115.

62. Bermingham RP, Whitsitt TB, Smart ML, et al. Rhabdomyolysis in a patient receiving the combination of cerivastatin and gem fibrozil. Am J Health Syst Pharm 2000; 57:461.

63. LaRosa JC. Women, dyslipoproteinemia, and estrogens. Endocrinol Metab Clin North Am 1998; 27:61.

64. Delmas PD, Bjarnason NH, et al. Effects of raloxifene on bone mineral density, serum cholesterol concentrations, and uterine endometrium in postmenopausal women. N Engl J Med 1997; 337:1641.

65. Herrington DM, Fong J, Sempos CT, et al., for the HERS Study Group. Comparison of the Heart and Estrogen/Progestin Replacement Study (HERS) cohort with women with coronary disease from the National Health and Nutrition Examination Survey III (NHANES III). Am Heart J 1998; 136:115.

66. Schaumann D, Welch-Wichary A, Schmidt VH, Olbricht CJ. Prospective crossover comparisons of three low-density lipoprotein (LDL)-apheresis methods in patients with familial hypercholesterolaemia. Eur J Clin Invest 1996; 26:1033.

67. Kroon AA, Aengevaeren WRM, van der Werf Tjeerd, et al. LDL-Apheresis Atherosclerosis Regression Study (LAARS). Effect of aggressive versus conventional lipid lowering treatment on coronary atherosclerosis. Circulation 1996; 93:1826.

# CHAPTER 165

# ENDOCRINE EFFECTS ON LIPIDS

HENRY N. GINSBERG, IRA J. GOLDBERG, AND CATHERINE TUCK

Many interactions can occur between aberrant hormone physiology and lipoprotein metabolism. This chapter focuses on areas that have significant clinical impact, particularly the effects of thyroid hormones, growth hormone (GH), glucocorticoids, and sex hormones. The impact of abnormal glucose metabolism and diabetes mellitus on lipid and lipoprotein metabolism are covered in Chapter 166.

## LIPOPROTEIN STRUCTURE AND COMPOSITION

The major neutral lipids transported through the bloodstream, *triglycerides* and *cholesteryl esters*, are insoluble in aqueous solutions

and, therefore, must be protected from plasma by a coating of amphipathic (both hydrophobic and hydrophilic) molecules (see Chap. 162). *Lipoproteins* are macromolecular complexes carrying various lipids and proteins in plasma that provide just such protection to triglycerides and cholesteryl esters. The hydrophobic triglyceride and cholesteryl ester molecules comprise the core of the lipoproteins and are enveloped by an amphipathic monolayer of phospholipids, free cholesterol, and proteins. The proteins, called *apoproteins* (apos) or apolipoproteins, are critical regulators of lipid transport. Several major classes of lipoproteins have been defined by their physical-chemical characteristics: *chylomicrons, very-low-density lipoproteins* (VLDL), *intermediate-density lipoproteins* (IDL), *low-density lipoproteins* (LDL), and *high-density lipoproteins* (HDL). The physical-chemical characteristics of the major lipoprotein classes are presented in Table 165-1. Apos, found on the surface of lipoproteins, provide structural stability to the lipoproteins and/or play critical roles in regulating lipoprotein metabolism. Some apos act as cofactors for plasma lipid-modifying enzymes. The structure and function of each apoprotein and the major lipid enzymes are described in Chapter 162, but a brief review is presented.[1]

*Apolipoprotein B-100* (hereafter referred to as either *apo B-100* or simply *apo B*) is synthesized mainly in the liver. It is the major apo of VLDL, IDL, and LDL, comprising ~30%, 60%, and 95% of the protein in these respective lipoproteins. Apo B is necessary for the initial assembly and secretion of VLDL by the liver. In the plasma, via interaction with the LDL receptor, apo B plays a crucial role in the catabolism of LDL, and probably of VLDL and IDL as well. Apolipoprotein B-48 (apo B-48) is the result of alteration of apo B-100 messenger RNA in the small intestine. Found on chylomicrons, it is necessary for intestinal assembly and secretion of these lipoproteins.

*Apolipoprotein C-I (apo C-I), apolipoprotein C-II (apo C-II)*, and *apolipoprotein C-III (apo C-III)* are synthesized in the liver. Apo C-I (a minor component of chylomicrons, VLDL, IDL, and HDL) blocks uptake of lipoproteins by the liver. Apo C-II (found on chylomicrons, VLDL, IDL, and HDL) is a necessary activator of *lipoprotein lipase* (LpL). Severe hypertriglyceridemia with chylomicronemia is present in individuals lacking apo C-II. Apo C-III is a major component of VLDL, in which it accounts for ~40% of the protein. It is also present on chylomicrons, IDL, and HDL. In vitro and in vivo studies indicate that apo C-III inhibits both LPL action and hepatic uptake of chylomicron and VLDL remnants.

*Apolipoprotein E (apo E)* is synthesized in the liver and is found on all the lipoproteins except LDL. Apo E plays a critical role in the removal of remnant lipoproteins from plasma by interacting with several receptors in the liver, including the LDL receptor and the *LDL receptor–related protein* (LRP). Apo E has three major alleles—apo E-1, apo E-2, and apo E-4. Apo E-2 cannot bind to the LDL receptor, and its presence (particularly in the homozygous state) can be associated with the accumulation of cholesteryl-ester enriched VLDL remnants.

The major protein present on HDL is *apoprotein A-I (apo A-I)*, which comprises 70% to 80% of the protein mass. It is synthe-

**TABLE 165-1.**
**Physiochemical Characteristics of the Major Lipoprotein Classes**

| Lipoprotein | Density (g/dL) | Molecular Mass (Da) | Diameter (nm) | Triglycerides (%)* | Cholesterol (%)* | PL (% Total Lipid) |
|---|---|---|---|---|---|---|
| Chylomicrons | 0.95 | $400 \times 10^6$ | 75–1200 | 80–95 | 2–7 | 3–9 |
| VLDL | 0.95–1.006 | $10–80 \times 10^6$ | 30–80 | 55–80 | 5–15 | 10–20 |
| IDL | 1.006–1.019 | $5–10 \times 10^6$ | 25–35 | 20–50 | 20–40 | 15–25 |
| LDL | 1.019–1.063 | $2.3 \times 10^6$ | 18–25 | 5–15 | 40–50 | 20–25 |
| HDL | 1.063–1.21 | $1.7–3.6 \times 10^5$ | 5–12 | 5–10 | 15–25 | 20–30 |

*PL*, phospholipid; *VLDL*, very-low-density lipoprotein; *IDL*, intermediate-density lipoprotein; *LDL* low-density lipoprotein; *HDL*, high-density lipoprotein.
*Percent composition of lipids; apolipoproteins make up the rest.

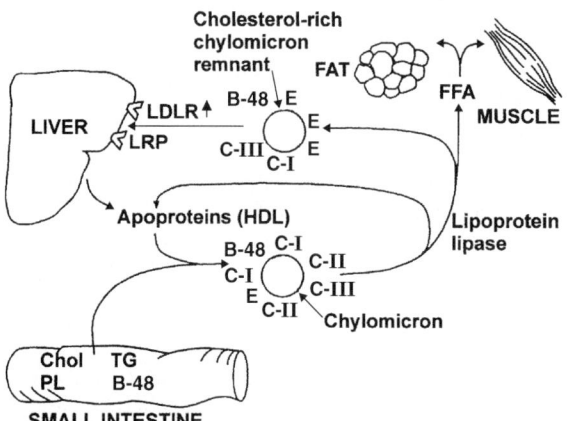

**FIGURE 165-1.** Transport of chylomicron and chylomicron remnants. The key steps in the transport of dietary nutrients take place when the chylomicron interacts with lipoprotein lipase in adipose and muscle tissue and when the chylomicron remnant is removed from the circulation via receptor–mediated pathways in the liver. (*LDLR*, low-density lipoprotein receptor; *B-48*, apoprotein B-48; *E*, apoprotein E; *FFA*, free fatty acids; *LRP*, LDLR-related protein; *C-III*, apoprotein C-III; *C-I*, apoprotein C-I; *HDL*, high-density lipoprotein; *C-II*, apoprotein C-II; *Chol*, cholesterol; *TG*, triglycerides; *PL*, phospholipid.)

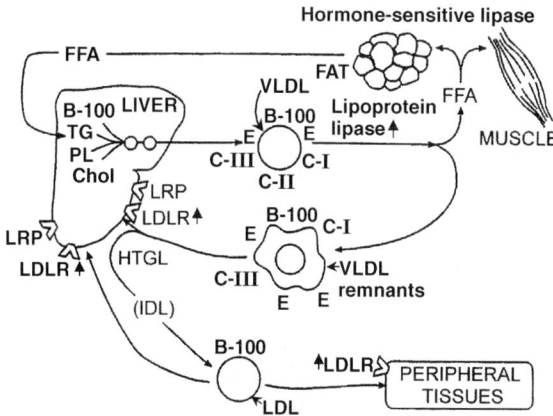

**FIGURE 165-2.** Transport of very-low-density lipoprotein (*VLDL*), intermediate-density lipoprotein (*IDL*), and low-density lipoprotein (*LDL*). The availability of core lipids, triglycerides (*TG*) and cholesterol (*Chol*), in the liver stimulates the assembly and secretion of VLDL, which then interacts with LDL in adipose and muscle tissue. The VLDL remnant (IDL) can then be removed via receptor-mediated pathways in the liver or be converted to LDL. LDL removal by the liver and peripheral tissues is mainly via the LDL receptor pathway. (*FFA*, free fatty acids; *B-100*, apoprotein B-100; *E*, apoprotein E; *PL*, phospholipid; *C-III*, apoprotein C-III; *C-II*, apoprotein C-II; *C-I*, apoprotein C-I; *LRP*, LDL receptor–related protein; *LDLR*, LDL receptor; *HTGL*, hepatic triglyceride lipase.)

sized in both the liver and the small intestine. It is secreted from the intestine on nascent chylomicrons but quickly transfers to HDL during lipolysis of the chylomicron-triglyceride. Apo A-I plays a critical role in "reverse cholesterol transport," possibly as a ligand for the *scavenger receptor B1* (SRB-1) at which HDL cholesteryl ester is delivered to cells. Subjects without apo A-I have essentially no HDL cholesterol. The exact role of *apoprotein A-II (apo A-II)* in lipoprotein physiology remains to be determined. No definite function has been attributed to the mostly lipoprotein-free *apoprotein A-IV (apo A-IV)*, which is a minor component of HDL and chylomicrons.

## PLASMA LIPASES

LPL converts lipoprotein-triglyceride into free fatty acids and mono- and diglycerides, allowing uptake of fatty acids by peripheral tissues. LPL is synthesized in adipose tissue and muscle but is active after secretion and binding to the luminal surface of capillary endothelial cells. Patients lacking LPL have severe hypertriglyceridemia. A number of relatively common polymorphisms and mutations in LPL have been identified that appear to predispose individuals to moderate hypertriglyceridemia.

*Hepatic lipase* (HL) functions as a triglyceride hydrolase and phospholipase. HL is synthesized in the liver and binds to the luminal surface of endothelial cells in hepatic sinusoids. Its major physiologic actions are to remove triglycerides and phospholipids from chylomicron remnants and VLDL remnants, and possibly to augment chylomicron remnant uptake by the liver. It may also play a role in the conversion of VLDL to LDL and in LDL subfraction patterns. Individuals lacking HL accumulate VLDL remnants but have normal or elevated levels of HDL despite having hypertriglyceridemia.

## TRANSPORT OF EXOGENOUS (DIETARY) LIPIDS

Chylomicrons are the lipoproteins that transport dietary fats, cholesterol, and fat-soluble nutrients (Fig. 165-1). The core is

~90% triglyceride by weight; therefore, the density of this lipoprotein is less than that of plasma. After entry into plasma from the intestinal lymph, chylomicrons acquire apo C-I, apo C-II, apo C-III, and apo E from the surface of HDL and then interact with LPL at the surface of capillary endothelial cells in fat and muscle. This initiates core triglyceride hydrolysis. Apo C-II is needed for this step, and apo C-III may modulate lipolysis by its ability to inhibit the interaction of lipoproteins with the endothelial cell surface and/or LPL. LPL-mediated triglyceride hydrolysis results in the generation of cholesteryl ester and apo E–enriched remnant particles, which can interact with receptors on hepatocytes and be removed rapidly from the circulation. Individuals lacking apo E, or having only the LDL receptor–binding-defective apo E-2 isoform, may accumulate chylomicron remnants in plasma.

## TRANSPORT OF ENDOGENOUS LIPIDS

The liver assembles and secretes apo B–containing lipoproteins, mainly VLDL (Fig. 165-2). The availability of the major lipoprotein-lipids, triglycerides, cholesteryl esters, and phospholipids determines whether nascent apo B is degraded or secreted. *Microsomal triglyceride transfer protein* (MTP) is necessary for the assembly and secretion of apo B–containing lipoproteins from both the intestine and the liver, and the human disorder abetalipoproteinemia results from mutations in the gene for the MTP large subunit.

Increased fatty acid flux from peripheral tissues to the liver is a major stimulus for both lipid synthesis and VLDL secretion. The association of physiologic or pathophysiologic states in which fatty acid flux is increased with increased rates of VLDL apo B secretion are numerous; obesity and diabetes mellitus are two well-defined examples. The link between insulin resistance and increased levels of plasma VLDL appears to derive from the increased plasma free fatty acid levels. Indeed, the targeting of newly synthesized apo B for secretion by hepatic fatty acids may be a major determinant of common lipoprotein disorders characterized by increased apo B secretion, such as familial combined hyperlipidemia and hyperapobetalipoproteinemia.

VLDL catabolism is characterized by several key branch points, and the outcome depends on which path individual particles take along the route. Interaction with LPL on endothelial cell surfaces initiates VLDL catabolism. As lipolysis proceeds, VLDL become smaller and denser, and are converted to IDL (also called *VLDL remnants*). These particles are either removed from plasma as a remnant akin to the chylomicron remnant, or converted to LDL. Currently no method exists to clearly identify and isolate VLDL that are destined for one or the other fates. However, apo E, LpL, HL, and several components of the hepatic pathway for remnant removal, including the LRP, all play roles at this branch point.

Once LDL is formed, its clearance from plasma is determined mainly by the availability (or "activity") of LDL receptors. After LDL apo B (or lipoproteins containing apo E) has interacted with the LDL receptor, these lipoproteins are internalized and degraded by lysosomes. The lysosomes release free cholesterol into the cytoplasm, where intracellular cholesterol and fatty acid metabolism are regulated via a pathway linked to activation of a transcription factor, sterol regulatory element–binding protein. In normal individuals, 60% to 80% of LDL can be cleared from plasma by LDL receptor–mediated pathways, with the remainder cleared via "nonreceptor" pathways. Lack of LDL receptors results in unregulated cellular cholesterol metabolism and markedly increased levels of plasma LDL cholesterol. The homozygous form of familial hypercholesterolemia is the paradigm for this abnormal state.

## HIGH-DENSITY LIPOPROTEIN METABOLISM

HDL comprises an extremely complex lipoprotein class of subclasses varying in size, density, and lipid composition. The scheme for HDL metabolism presented here focuses on the transport of cholesterol through HDL—the "reverse cholesterol transport" system (see Chap. 162, Fig. 162-2).

Most mature HDL are formed by the apparent coalescence of individual phospholipid-apoprotein discs containing apo A-I, apo A-II, and possibly apo E. Both the intestine and the liver appear to secrete individual apos with a small amount of phospholipid. These small, cholesterol-poor HDL can adsorb free cholesterol from cell membranes and become nascent $HDL_3$ particles. A protein member of the ABC family (see "Tangier Disease" in Chap. 163) has been identified as the plasma membrane channel through which cellular cholesterol effluxes to apoprotein acceptors. $HDL_3$-free cholesterol can be esterified to cholesteryl ester, allowing $HDL_3$ to accept more free cholesterol. $HDL_3$ particles enlarge and can now accommodate apo C-II and apo C-III, as well as more phospholipid, on their surfaces. The result of these processes is the formation of $HDL_2$. The fate of $HDL_2$ is very complicated as well, but can be divided into two major categories—transfer of the cholesterol components of $HDL_2$ to other lipoproteins (via cholesteryl ester transfer protein [CETP]) and to cells (via SRB-1), and metabolism (with removal from plasma) of the $HDL_2$ apoproteins. The relationship of these two pathways of HDL metabolism to the antiatherogenic properties of this lipoprotein class needs to be clarified.

## THYROID HORMONES AND LIPOPROTEIN METABOLISM

Numerous studies have documented that thyroid hormone has important effects on lipid and lipoprotein metabolism at several key points.[2] These points include fatty acid and triglyceride metabolism, cholesterol metabolism, apoprotein synthesis, and lipoprotein catabolism.[3] Thyroid hormone has the unique effect of increasing both the synthesis and the oxidation of fatty acids. Overall, this results in a reduction in the quantity of hepatic fatty acids available for incorporation into triglyceride. On the other hand, elevated levels of thyroid hormone result in increased lipolysis of triglycerides in adipose tissue and increased plasma levels of free fatty acids. Efficient hepatic extraction of plasma free fatty acids, unaffected by thyroid hormone status, results in an actual increase in the delivery of fatty acids to hepatocytes. Low thyroid hormone levels produce the opposite effects—decreased fatty acid synthesis and oxidation in the liver with more triglyceride formation and decreased fatty acid delivery from adipose tissue. Thus, the overall effect of thyroid hormone status depends on the delivery of adipose tissue–derived fatty acids, synthesis of fatty acids in the liver, and the rate of fatty acid oxidation. Thyroid hormone effects on cholesterol metabolism are also wide ranging. Thyroid hormone stimulates synthesis of the LDL receptor at the level of gene expression. Bile acid formation and biliary cholesterol secretion are stimulated by thyroid hormone, which also stimulates LDL receptors. Thyroid hormone also amplifies apo B gene expression in cultured hepatocytes, increasing the potential for assembly and secretion of cholesterol-carrying lipoproteins.

## LIPID AND LIPOPROTEIN METABOLISM IN THE HYPOTHYROID STATE

Early studies of cholesterol removal from plasma showed that it was decreased in hypothyroid patients. Subsequently, studies demonstrating increased levels of LDL cholesterol in hypothyroid subjects were published, and these were paralleled by the demonstration that thyroid replacement therapy lowered LDL cholesterol levels. Later investigations showed that the fractional clearance of LDL was reduced in hypothyroidism.[4] Indeed, in one study, LDL fractional clearance was as low as that seen in homozygous familial hypercholesterolemia and was normalized by thyroid replacement.[5] These data were complemented by studies showing that LDL-receptor levels were regulated, in part, by thyroid hormone in both tissue culture and animal studies. Contemporary studies of cholesterol synthesis, bile acid formation, and sterol excretion were not as enlightening. Although early studies suggested reductions in cholesterol synthesis and in bile formation and excretion, later studies did not confirm these abnormalities. Studies of apo B metabolism in hypothyroidism and the effects of replacement therapy indicate major effects on the conversion of VLDL remnants to LDL and improved fractional clearance of LDL.[6] Overall, increased LDL cholesterol levels in hypothyroid patients appear to be the result of decreased LDL-receptor function and concomitant defective clearance of LDL cholesterol from plasma.

Of interest is the finding in humans that the hypercholesterolemia of hypothyroidism is associated not only with increased LDL cholesterol concentrations but also with an increase in HDL cholesterol levels. Although agreement in this area is not universal, the majority of investigators have observed elevated levels of HDL cholesterol in hypothyroid patients and reductions in those levels after restoration to the euthyroid state. The rise in HDL cholesterol levels appears to be due mainly to increases in $HDL_2$ and in the Apo A-I–only fractions of HDL. Apo A-I levels are increased in hypothyroidism. This may be due to a direct effect on apo A-I synthesis, although data from humans are lacking, and results from studies of the apo A-I gene in rats indicate that thyroid hormone can both inhibit and stimulate expression. Other factors that would influence HDL cholesterol levels are CETP and HL activities. CETP activity appears to be decreased in hypothyroid patients, although this may not be due to decreased levels of CETP but rather to ineffective interaction with HDL particles. HL activity is clearly decreased in hypothyroidism.[7] Both of these changes would result in increased levels of HDL cholesterol. Treatment of hypothyroidism is associated with lowering of HDL cholesterol levels and normalization of CETP and HL activities.

Although general agreement exists that hypercholesterolemia is associated with hypothyroidism, the relationship observed between low thyroid hormone levels and levels of blood triglycerides has been more variable. This is probably due to the greater complexity of the role that thyroid hormone plays in triglyceride synthesis, secretion, and catabolism from blood.[3] As noted earlier, thyroid deficiency is associated with both less fatty acid delivery to the liver from adipose tissue and greater fatty acid synthesis in the hepatocyte. Thus, the rate of triglyceride synthesis, a key stimulus for VLDL secretion, would depend on the balance of these two opposing effects of thyroid hormone deficiency. Other factors known to affect plasma triglyceride levels, such as increases in hepatic triglyceride secretion due to obesity, appear to be more important determinants of plasma triglyceride levels in hypothyroid patients than is the deficiency in the hormone itself.[7] Obese hypothyroid patients have elevations in their plasma triglyceride levels, which are reduced by therapy. Nonobese individuals are not significantly affected, in terms of triglyceride metabolism, by thyroid hormone deficiency.

Several studies have linked hypothyroidism with elevations in plasma levels of *lipoprotein(a)* [Lp(a)]—lipoprotein comprised of an LDL particle on which a second protein, apoprotein(a) [Ap(a)], is covalently linked to LDL apo B.[8,9] Lp(a) levels fall after treatment with thyroid hormones.

As in overt hypothyroidism, patients with subclinical hypothyroidism have elevated cholesterol. Treatment with thyroid replacement decreases cholesterol by ~6%, with inconsistent changes in HDL.[10]

## LIPID AND LIPOPROTEIN METABOLISM IN THE HYPERTHYROID STATE

As expected, plasma cholesterol levels are reduced in patients with hyperthyroidism. This is due in large part to decreased levels of LDL cholesterol. Studies have documented increased fractional removal rates of LDL particles in patients with excess thyroid hormone.[4] This abnormality is reversed by ablation of the thyroid or treatment with antithyroid medications. Total body cholesterol synthesis appears to be slightly increased in hyperthyroid states, and this is balanced by slight increases in sterol excretion.

HDL cholesterol is reduced in most patients with hyperthyroidism and HDL levels rise when treated patients become euthyroid. The reductions in HDL are associated with increases in CETP and HL activities in blood. Levels of apo A-I also decrease in the presence of excess thyroid hormone and increase after treatment. Of interest, apo A-II levels are normal in the hyperthyroid state and are unchanged by treatment.

As was the case with thyroid hormone deficiency, the relationship between plasma triglyceride levels and thyroid hormone excess is less clear than the relationship between hormone levels and cholesterol metabolism. In most patients, excess fatty acid release from adipose tissue appears to have a greater impact on hepatic triglyceride synthesis than does the increase in fatty acid oxidation and reduction in fatty acid synthesis in the liver. As a result, hyperthyroid patients assemble and secrete slightly more VLDL than do euthyroid individuals.[7] Because of increased lipolysis of VLDL triglycerides in the bloodstream, however, plasma triglyceride concentrations are normal or slightly lower in hyperthyroid patients. One possible explanation for the improved lipolysis of triglyceride is the

finding that apo C-III gene expression is decreased in rats who are regularly given thyroid hormone.[11] If these finding extend to humans, less apo C-III could be present in blood and, therefore, the interaction between VLDL and lipoprotein lipase could be more efficient. As noted earlier, hyperthyroidism has been associated with increased HL but has not been associated with changes in LPL.[7]

# GROWTH HORMONE AND LIPOPROTEIN METABOLISM

GH is a key anabolic hormone that spares protein catabolism by stimulating utilization of fat for energy. GH deficiency can occur in children due to genetic causes or in children and adults secondary to pituitary neoplasms and hypopituitarism. Although for many years replacement therapy has been standard for children with GH deficiency, replacement of GH was not thought to be important in adults. In the past decade, however, research has shown that the absence of GH can have long-term detrimental effects in adults, including an increased risk for developing atherosclerotic cardiovascular disease.[12,13] In addition, the observation that GH secretion decreases with increasing age has led to suggestions that "physiologic" GH deficiency might play a role in atherosclerosis in the general population. At the other end of the spectrum, acromegaly is also associated with increased risk for atherosclerotic cardiovascular disease. Central to both of these relationships is the effect of GH on plasma lipid levels and lipoprotein metabolism.

## EFFECTS OF GROWTH HORMONE ON PLASMA LIPIDS AND LIPOPROTEINS

GH has the potential to exert major effects on both triglyceride and LDL cholesterol levels. It stimulates lipolysis of triglycerides and, therefore, release of fatty acids from adipose tissue. Increased fatty acid uptake by the liver stimulates the synthesis of triglyceride, which in turn, stimulates the assembly and secretion of VLDL. This sequence of events has been demonstrated in both perfused livers and cultured liver cells.[14,15] GH also plays a key role in regulating the number of LDL receptors in the liver, probably through stimulation of gene transcription.[16] GH also appears to be required for the increase of LDL receptors associated with estrogen treatment. Administration of GH significantly increases levels of plasma Lp(a) by undefined mechanisms.

## LIPID AND LIPOPROTEIN METABOLISM IN GROWTH HORMONE DEFICIENCY

The lipid profile associated with GH deficiency is one of elevated plasma levels of VLDL triglycerides and LDL cholesterol.[17] The latter is expected, based on the role of GH in regulating LDL receptors; the former is unexpected, because GH deficiency would be anticipated to result in lower free fatty acid delivery to the liver and, therefore, lower VLDL secretion. A study using stable isotope tracer methods, however, has demonstrated increased VLDL secretion in patients with GH deficiency.[18] The latter finding cannot easily be integrated into a metabolic scheme in which decreased GH would be expected to be associated with lower triglyceride concentrations. One possibility is that the increased adiposity that accompanies GH deficiency is an overriding stimulus for increased VLDL secretion. In addition, increased insulin resistance has been reported in adults. HDL cholesterol levels are lower in GH deficient patients; the cause of this is unclear, although it may simply be a concomitant of higher levels of plasma triglycerides and greater adiposity.

The most uniform effect of GH replacement therapy is a lowering of LDL cholesterol levels.[19,20] This effect is evident by 6 months of therapy, but the literature is conflicting regarding the long-term effects of GH replacement; some studies suggest return of LDL cholesterol levels to baseline by 12 or 36 months. The effects of GH on the LDL-receptor number seem to be at the level of gene transcription.[16] Effects of GH therapy on plasma triglyceride levels are variable, with some studies showing no change and others showing increased levels of VLDL triglycerides. This latter finding is consistent with the lipolytic effects of GH, but as noted above, the finding of increased triglycerides in states of GH deficiency means that the actions of GH on triglyceride metabolism are complex. GH treatment can also increase HDL cholesterol concentrations.[21]

GH is used as a "treatment" for short stature in otherwise normal children. In one study, both triglycerides and LDL cholesterol increased (within the normal range) after 6 months of treatment but returned to baseline by 1 year.

Lp(a) concentrations increase when GH is used to treat either GH deficiency or short stature.[19-21] The effect can be significant (~25%), although the impact on atherosclerosis risk is unclear. The basis for this is undefined at the molecular level, although the fact that insulin-like growth factor-I (IGF-I) is not the final messenger of the effects of GH is known. In fact, in studies in which IGF-I has been used to treat osteoporosis, Lp(a) levels have fallen.

## LIPID AND LIPOPROTEIN METABOLISM IN ACROMEGALY

Acromegaly is associated with increased levels of plasma triglycerides and lower concentrations of HDL cholesterol.[22,23] Consistent with this lipid profile, an increase in small, dense LDL is found in acromegalic patients. Treatment using surgical[22,23] or medical[24] approaches results in reductions in triglyceride concentrations, no change in LDL cholesterol, and variable changes in HDL cholesterol. Lp(a) levels fall, but may remain higher than normal.[22,23,23a]

# SEX HORMONES AND LIPOPROTEIN METABOLISM

Sex hormones have important effects on lipoprotein metabolism, and their effects may differ somewhat between men and women. Differences in sex hormone levels probably explain why women have an average HDL level 10 mg/dL higher than do men, and why LDL levels rise and HDL levels fall somewhat after menopause, when estrogen production by the ovary ceases.

## SEX HORMONE LEVELS AND LIPIDS IN POSTMENOPAUSAL WOMEN

Among premenopausal women, estrogen and progesterone levels are high, rising and falling in cyclic fashion during the menstrual cycle. After menopause, estrogen and progestin production by the ovary ceases, although androgen production by the adrenals and ovary continues, and small amounts of estrogen are present due to aromatization of androgen precursors. Among normal women undergoing menopause, LDL levels rise by ~0.31 mmol/L and HDL levels fall by ~0.09 mmol/L.[25]

Hormone replacement therapy for postmenopausal women may affect lipid levels differently, depending on whether estrogen alone or combined estrogen and progestin therapy is used,

and also on whether an oral or transdermal route of delivery is used. In the Postmenopausal Estrogen/Progestin Interventions (PEPI) Trial, use of oral estrogen alone led to a 10% decrease in LDL levels, a 10% increase in HDL levels, and an 8% increase in triglyceride levels.[26] Careful metabolic turnover studies have shown that oral estrogen increases large VLDL apo B and triglyceride levels by ~30%, due to an 80% increase in large VLDL secreted by the liver.[27] Most of the additional large VLDL secreted by the liver is not converted to small VLDL or to LDL, however, because the clearance of the large VLDL fraction also increases by 140%. Apo E production and LDL-receptor activity are both known to increase in response to estrogen. This could explain the improved clearance of large VLDL particles by the liver. LDL apo B and cholesterol levels are lowered by estrogen, due to a 36% increase in LDL catabolism, which overcomes an increase of 21% in LDL production. Although LDL levels are lower, triglyceride enrichment of the LDL is present, and other studies have shown increased presence of small, dense LDL in response to oral estrogen, probably due to increased triglyceride levels. Estrogen increases $HDL_2$ levels more than $HDL_3$ levels, and the increase is due entirely to an increased production of apo A-I, with unchanged apo A-I catabolism. Transdermal estrogen has no effects on lipid metabolism, despite similarly raised plasma estradiol levels, implying that oral estrogen works mainly via a first-pass effect on the liver. Oral estrogen also decreases Lp(a) levels by ~20% and is one of only a few pharmacologic agents found to affect Lp(a) levels.

The *selective estrogen-receptor modulator* (SERM) drugs mimic the estrogen lowering effect on LDL, Lp(a), and apo B in postmenopausal women but do not appear to affect HDL or triglycerides.[28]

The effects of progesterone, given along with estrogen for postmenopausal hormone replacement therapy, differ depending on the kind of progesterone used. Natural progesterone, given cyclically as a micronized preparation in the PEPI Trial, did not interfere with estrogen's beneficial lipid effects, and the lipid profiles were similar to those produced by oral estrogen alone. Synthetic progestins, however, which have been used because natural progesterone is poorly absorbed without micronization, tend to lower HDL levels in a dose-dependent fashion, with more androgenic progestins causing even more HDL lowering. The mechanism appears to involve an increase in HL activity. Progestins also decrease triglycerides and modestly lower LDL levels, due to decreased production of VLDL apo B.[29]

## LIPID LEVELS IN HYPOGONADAL WOMEN

Women with ovariectomy or with Turner syndrome represent a somewhat different model from typical hypogonadal postmenopausal women, because they no longer have significant androgen or estrogen production by their ovaries. Older girls with Turner syndrome, when compared with age-matched controls, have higher total cholesterol levels, higher LDL levels; and also higher HDL levels, despite being more obese than the control population. Amenorrheic athletes have higher levels of plasma cholesterol, triglyceride, LDL, and HDL cholesterol than do eumenorrheic athletes, implying that estrogen deficiency leads to increased LDL cholesterol levels but that the vigorous athletic activity keeps the HDL levels from falling.[30]

## LIPID EFFECTS OF ANDROGENS IN WOMEN

The effects of androgens on lipid levels in normal women are not well studied. Women with endogenous hyperandrogenism related to the polycystic ovary syndrome (PCOS) often have low HDL cholesterol and high triglycerides and LDL cholesterol, associated with insulin resistance and obesity. Lowering of androgen levels in such women by administration of oral contraceptives often results in improvement in HDL levels, but whether this is due to increased estrogen levels or to decreased androgen levels is not clear. Partial androgen suppression in women with PCOS by administration of a gonadotropin-releasing hormone (GnRH) agonist for 3 months results in no change in insulin resistance or lipoprotein levels, indicating that the lipoprotein abnormalities are due to insulin resistance and not to the androgen levels.[31] However, use of flutamide, an androgen-receptor blocker, does not improve lipid levels in women with PCOS, suggesting that some of the lipid effects may be due to hyperandrogenism. When testosterone is given parenterally to normal women, such as to transsexuals undergoing sex change procedures, LDL cholesterol and triglyceride levels do not change, but HDL cholesterol levels fall by ~15%.[32] Anabolic steroids—modified forms of testosterone (given orally) that are not aromatized to estrogen—cause decreases in HDL levels (~30%) and increases in LDL levels (30–40%).[33] Anabolic steroids also decrease triglyceride levels and can decrease Lp(a) levels by as much as 80%. The mechanism for the profound HDL changes is thought to be increased HL activity.

## SEX HORMONE LEVELS AND LIPIDS IN MEN

The effects of androgens on serum lipids in males are complex. Boys experience a drop in HDL cholesterol as they go through puberty. Also, when normal men are given a GnRH antagonist and made acutely hypogonadal, their HDL levels increase by 30%.[34] Both of these results imply that testosterone in men lowers HDL levels, probably by increasing HL activity. Among populations of normal men, however, increased levels of testosterone are associated with higher HDL levels rather than lower HDL levels.[35] Among normal men, higher testosterone levels are also associated with better insulin sensitivity and lower triglyceride levels. Testosterone levels in men decrease with increasing obesity, and prospective studies have shown that low testosterone levels predict subsequent central adiposity. When testosterone is given to men with central obesity, beneficial changes in waist-hip ratio and insulin sensitivity are observed. Thus, among normal men, higher rather than lower androgen levels are associated with a more beneficial metabolic profile, and this may be due in part to the associations between central obesity, insulin resistance, and lower testosterone levels.

## LIPID EFFECTS OF ANDROGENS IN HYPOGONADAL MEN

Hypogonadal men have higher LDL levels, triglyceride levels, and cholesterol/HDL ratios than eugonadal men, although HDL levels are not significantly different from those of eugonadal men. When testosterone replacement is given to hypogonadal men, lipid effects have been variable; LDL and total cholesterol levels increased, decreased, or remained the same.[36] These conflicting results may be due to differences in hormone replacement regimens and time of sampling, because testosterone is usually given intermittently as intramuscular injections. Effects of testosterone replacement on HDL, triglycerides, and Lp(a) have been minimal in studies so far, although increased HL activity after testosterone replacement has been clearly documented.

## GLUCOCORTICOIDS AND LIPOPROTEIN METABOLISM

Glucocorticoids are essential steroid hormones produced exclusively by the adrenal cortex. In humans the major hormone of

this group is cortisol. Glucocorticoids are required for maintenance of blood pressure, operating via a permissive action to allow a normal response to catecholamines (see Chap. 78). In addition, they are required for hepatic gluconeogenesis.

Neither endogenous overproduction of glucocorticoids (Cushing syndrome) nor glucocorticoid deficiency (Addison disease) is particularly associated with alterations in risk of cardiovascular disease. In contrast, prolonged pharmacologic use of glucocorticoids in diseases such as lupus erythematosus leads to a greater incidence of vascular disease.[37]

Lipoproteins have been assessed after short- and long-term exposure to glucocorticoids. The effects differ *depending on length of administration*. In metabolic studies of healthy volunteers, short courses of glucocorticoids primarily lead to increased HDL levels.[38,39] In contrast, long-term use of high-dose corticosteroids also increases plasma LDL, sometimes dramatically. This is most commonly seen in patients receiving immunosuppressive dosages after organ transplantation.[40,41] In vitro data suggest that the pathophysiology is a reduction in LDL receptors, a decrease that is exacerbated when both corticosteroids and cyclosporine are administered together. Decreased fraction removal of LDL particles from the plasma, a finding consistent with a reduction in LDL receptors, has been found in corticosteroid-treated monkeys.[42]

In patients with Cushing syndrome, triglyceride elevations are often noted. This is associated with insulin resistance and leads to a picture similar to that of the metabolic syndrome X (see Chap. 145).[43] The cause of these changes is not totally clear. Hepatic triglyceride production is increased by glucocorticoids. Studies of LpL activity have not been consistent.

## CATECHOLAMINES AND LIPIDS

Catecholamines stimulate the release of free fatty acids from adipocytes, and epinephrine excretion correlates with HDL levels. The β-receptor blockers raise triglyceride levels and lower HDL levels, whereas α-receptor blockers can raise HDL levels. Although the catecholamines have only a modest effect on lipids, the overall impact on cardiovascular risk may be very significant.

## REFERENCES

1. Ginsberg HN. Lipoprotein physiology. Endocrinol Metab Clin North Am 1998; 27(3):503.
2. Ginsberg HN, Goldberg IJ. Dyslipoproteinemias in thyroid disease. In: Fruchart JC, Shepherd J, eds. Clinical biochemistry: principles, methods, applications, vol 3. Human plasma lipoproteins. Berlin: Walter deGruyter, 1989.
3. Heimberg M, Olubadewo JO, Wilcox HG. Plasma lipoproteins and regulation of hepatic metabolism of fatty acids in altered thyroid states. Endocr Rev 1985; 6:590.
4. Walton KW, Scott PJ, Dykes PW, Davies JWL. Alterations of the metabolism and turnover of 131-I-low density lipoproteins in hypothyroidism and thyrotoxicosis. Clin Sci 1965; 29:217.
5. Thompson GR, Soutar AK, Spengel FA, et al. Defects of receptor-mediated low density lipoprotein catabolism in homozygous familial hypercholesterolemia and hypothyroidism in vivo. Proc Natl Acad Sci U S A 1981; 78:2591.
6. Packard CJ, Shepherd J, Lindsay GM, et al. Thyroid replacement therapy and its influence on postheparin plasma lipases and apolipoprotein B metabolism in hypothyroidism. J Clin Endocrinol Metab 1993; 76:1209.
7. Abrams JJ, Grundy SM, Ginsberg H. Metabolism of plasma triglycerides in hypothyroidism and hyperthyroidism in man. J Lipid Res 1981; 22:307.
8. Martinez-Triguero ML, Hernandez-Mijares A, Nguyen TT, et al. Effect of thyroid hormone replacement on lipoprotein (a), lipids, and apolipoproteins in subjects with hypothyroidism. Mayo Clin Proc 1998; 73:837.
9. Dullaart RP, van Doormaal JJ, Hoogenberg K, Sluiter WJ. Triiodothyronine rapidly lowers plasma lipoprotein (a) in hypothyroid subjects. Neth J Med 1995; 46:179.
10. Tanis BC, Westendorp RGJ, Smelt AHM. Effect of thyroid substitution on hypercholesterolemia in patients with subclinical hypothyroidism. Clin Endocrinol 1996; 44:643.

11. Lin-Lee YC, Strobl W, Soyal S, et al. Role of thyroid hormones in the expression of apolipoprotein A-IV and C-III genes in rat liver. J Lipid Res 1993; 34:249.

12. Rosen T, Bengtsson BA. Premature mortality due to cardiovascular disease in hypopituitarism. Lancet 1990; 336:285.

13. Markussis V, Beshyah SA, Fisher C, et al. Detection of premature atherosclerosis by high-resolution ultrasonography in symptom-free hypopituitary adults. Lancet 1992; 340:1188.

14. Elam MB, Wilcox HG, Solomon SS, Heimberg M. In vivo growth hormone treatment stimulates secretion of very low density lipoprotein by the isolated perfused rat liver. Endocrinology 1992; 131:2717.

15. Sjoberg A, Oscarsson J, Boren J, et al. Mode of growth hormone administration influences triacylglycerol synthesis and assembly of apolipoprotein B-containing lipoproteins in cultured rat hepatocytes. J Lipid Res 1996; 37:275.

16. Angelin B, Rudling M. Growth hormone and hepatic lipoprotein metabolism. Curr Opin Lipidol 1994; 5:160.

17. Al-Shoumer KA, Cox KH, Hughes CL, et al. Fasting and postprandial lipid abnormalities in hypopituitary women receiving conventional replacement therapy. J Clin Endocrinol Metab 1997; 82:2653.

18. Cummings MH, Christ E, Umpleby AM, et al. Abnormalities of very low density lipoprotein apolipoprotein B-100 metabolism contribute to the dyslipidemia of adult growth hormone deficiency. J Clin Endocrinol Metab 1997; 82:2010.

19. Garry P, Collins P, Devlin JG. An open 36-month study of lipid changes with growth hormone in adults: lipid changes following replacement of growth hormone in adult acquired growth hormone deficiency. Eur J Endocrinol 1996; 134:61.

20. Webster JM, Stewart M, al-Maskari, et al. The effect of growth hormone replacement therapy for up to 12 months on lipoprotein composition and lipoprotein (a) in growth hormone deficient adults. Atherosclerosis 1997; 133:115.

21. Eden S, Wiklund O, Oscarsson J, et al. Growth hormone treatment of growth hormone deficient adults results in a marked increase in Lp(a) and HDL cholesterol concentrations. Arterioscler Thromb 1993; 13:296.

22. Oscarsson J, Wiklund O, Jakobsson KE, et al. Serum lipoproteins in acromegaly before and 6–15 months after transsphenoidal adenomectomy. Clin Endocrinol (Oxf) 1994; 41:603.

23. Tsuchiya H, Onishi T, Mogami H, Iida M. Lipid metabolism in acromegalic patients before and after selective pituitary adenomectomy. Endocrinol Jpn 1990; 37:797.

23a. Maldonado Castro GF, Escobar-Morreale HF, Ortega H, et al. Effects of normalization of GH hypersecretion on lipoprotein (a) and other lipoprotein serum levels in acromegaly. Clin Endocrinol 2000; 53:313.

24. James RA, Moller N, Chatterjee S, et al. Carbohydrate tolerance and serum lipids in acromegaly before and during treatment with high dose octreotide. Diabet Med 1991; 8:517.

25. Matthews KA, Meilahn E, Kuller LH, et al. Menopause and risk factors for coronary heart disease. N Engl J Med 1989; 321:641.

26. Writing Group for the PEPI Trial. Effects of estrogen or estrogen/progestin regimens on heart disease risk factors in postmenopausal women: The Postmenopausal Estrogen/Progestin Interventions (PEPI) Trial. JAMA 1995; 273:199.

27. Walsh BM, Schiff I, Rosner B, et al. Effects of postmenopausal estrogen replacement on the concentration and metabolism of plasma lipoproteins. N Engl J Med 1991; 3225:11996.

28. Walsk BW, Kuller LH, Wild RA, et al. The effect of raloxifene on markers of cardiovascular risk in healthy, post-menopausal women. JAMA 1998; 279:1445.

29. Wolfe BM, Huff MW. Effect of low dosage progestin-only administration upon plasma triglycerides and lipoprotein metabolism in postmenopausal women. J Clin Invest 1993; 92:456.

30. Friday KE, Drinkwater BL, Bruemmer B, et al. Elevated plasma low-density lipoprotein and high density lipoprotein cholesterol levels in amenorrheic athletes: effects of endogenous hormone status and nutrient intake. J Clin Endocrinol Metab 1993; 77:1605.

31. Wild RA, Alaupovic P, Parker IJ. Lipid and apolipoprotein abnormalities in hirsute women 1. The association with insulin resistance. Am J Obstet Gynecol 1992; 166:1191.

32. Asscheman H, Gooren LJG, Megens JAJ, et al. Serum testosterone level is the major determinant of the male-female differences in serum levels of high-density lipoprotein (HDL) cholesterol and HDL$_2$ cholesterol. Metabolism 1994; 43:935.

33. Bagatell CJ, Bremner WJ. Androgen and progestogen effects on plasma lipids. Prog Cardiovasc Disease 1995; 38:255.

34. Bagatell CJ, Knopp RH, Vale WW, et al. Physiologic testosterone levels in normal men suppress high-density lipoprotein cholesterol levels. Ann Intern Med 1992; 116:967.

35. Haffner SM, Mykkanen L, Valdez RA, Katz MS. Relationship of sex hormones to lipids and lipoproteins in nondiabetic men. J Clin Endocrinol Metab 1993; 77:1610.

36. Snyder PJ, Peachey H, Berlin JA, et al. Effects of testosterone replacement in hypogonadal men. J Clin Endocrinol Metab 2000; 85:2670.

37. Petri M, Perez-Gutthann S, Spence D, Hochberg MC. Risk factors for coronary artery disease in patients with systemic lupus erythematosus. Am J Med 1992; 93:513.

38. Taskinen MR, Kuusi T, Yki-Jarvinen H, Nikkila EA. Short-term effects of prednisone on serum lipids and high density lipoprotein subfractions in normolipidemic healthy men. J Clin Endocrinol Metab 1988; 67:291.

39. Donahoo WT, Kosmiski LA, Eckel RH. Drugs causing dyslipoproteinemia Endocrinol Metab Clin North Am 1998; 27:677.

40. Fernandez-Miranda C, Guijarro C, de la Calle A, et al. Lipoid abnormalities in stable liver transplant recipients—effects of cyclosporin, tacrolimus and steroids. Transpl Int 1998; 11:137.

41. Hilbrands LB, Demacker PN, Hoitsma AJ, et al. The effects of cyclosporine and prednisone on serum lipid and apolipoprotein levels in renal transplant recipients. J Am Soc Nephrol 1995; 5:2073.

42. Ettinger WH, Dysko RC, Clarkson TB. Prednisone increases low density lipoprotein in cynomolgus monkeys fed saturated fat and cholesterol. Arteriosclerosis 1989; 9:848.

43. Friedman TC, Mastorakos G, Newman TD, et al. Carbohydrate and lipid metabolism in endogenous hypercortisolism: shared features with metabolic syndrome X and NIDDM. Endocrinol J 1996; 43:645.

# CHAPTER 166

# LIPID ABNORMALITIES IN DIABETES MELLITUS

ROBERT E. RATNER, BARBARA V. HOWARD, AND WILLIAM JAMES HOWARD

Atherosclerosis, as manifested by cardiovascular, cerebrovascular, and peripheral vascular disease, occurs more commonly and results in greater morbidity and mortality in persons with diabetes. In diabetic patients, cardiovascular disease alone accounts for 69.7% of deaths.[1] Although typically associated with type 2 diabetes mellitus and frequently a part of the insulin resistance–hyperinsulinemia syndrome, cardiovascular disease also accounts for 25% to 50% of deaths in persons older than 30 years of age with type 1 diabetes mellitus. One of the most important contributing factors is the alteration in lipoproteins associated with diabetes.[2] Although lipoprotein changes are an intrinsic part of the disease, such alterations also are induced by diabetes-associated complications such as obesity and renal disease, and are sometimes exacerbated by therapeutic regimens.

Reports by the National Cholesterol Education Program (NCEP) focused attention on the necessity for managing lipid disorders.[3,4] Several additional issues must be considered, however, including the relationship between glycemic control and lipoproteins and the potential for a different response by individuals with diabetes to lipid-lowering agents. (See the reviews published by American Diabetes Association [ADA].[5,6]) Understanding the etiology of dyslipidemia in diabetes is important in developing strategies for its control.

## LIPOPROTEIN METABOLISM

### STRUCTURE AND CLASSIFICATION

Lipoproteins are spherical particles composed of lipids (cholesterol, cholesterol ester, triglyceride, and phospholipid) and proteins (apoproteins). Their function is to transport non–water-soluble cholesterol and triglycerides in plasma. The central core of nonpolar lipids (primarily triglycerides and cholesterol ester) is surrounded by a surface monolayer of phospholipids and apoproteins. Free cholesterol is present primarily in the surface monolayer. Five major lipoprotein classes are distinguished on the basis of composition, size, density, and function (see Chaps. 162 and 163).[7–10]

The metabolism and production of all lipoproteins are controlled primarily by the apoproteins. All of these apoproteins have been sequenced and their genes localized.[11] Most are hydrophobic proteins and serve as ligands for specific receptors involved in the metabolism of the various lipoproteins and as cofactors for enzymatic activities involved in lipoprotein metabolism. Several other proteins and enzymes play key roles in plasma lipoprotein transport, including *lipoprotein lipase* (LpL) and *hepatic lipase,* which catalyze the delipidation of triglyceride-rich particles; *lecithin-cholesterol acyltransferase,* which is responsible for the synthesis of virtually all cholesterol esters in plasma lipoproteins; and *cholesterol ester transfer protein,* which facilitates the transfer of cholesterol and cholesterol ester between lipoproteins during their metabolism.

Chylomicrons, particles that are primarily triglyceride bearing, are produced by the intestine after exogenous fat undergoes digestion. Intermediate-density lipoproteins (IDL) are remnants of the metabolism of triglyceride-rich lipoproteins and are also intermediates in the conversion of very-low-density lipoproteins (VLDL) to low-density lipoproteins (LDL). LDL are the major cholesterol-bearing lipoproteins and are most strongly related to the occurrence of cardiovascular disease. LDL particles occur over a range of size and density. The presence of small, dense LDL has been shown in multiple studies to be correlated with coronary heart disease.[12] Most individuals can be segregated into two LDL subclass patterns, A and B, and this pattern is determined by a major dominant gene. Lipoprotein(a) is a subclass of the LDL fraction that consists of LDL complexed to a large glycoprotein resembling plasminogen; this complex has also been associated with atherosclerosis.[13] High-density lipoproteins (HDL) are the smallest and densest of the lipoproteins. Although HDL also transport substantial amounts of cholesterol, they are inversely associated with cardiovascular disease. HDL can be divided into subfractions, the most abundant of which are $HDL_2$ (with densities between 1.063 and 1.125) and $HDL_3$ (with densities between 1.125 and 1.210).[14]

## LIPOPROTEIN ALTERATIONS IN TYPE 1 DIABETES

Dyslipidemia in type 1 diabetes has been found with a prevalence as high as 40%. In 205 men and women with type 1 diabetes, 27% were found to have hypercholesterolemia (serum cholesterol levels of >6.5 mmol/L [250 mg/dL]) and 31% had hypertriglyceridemia (serum triglyceride levels of >2.25 mmol/L [199 mg/dL]). These findings are supported by Finnish studies of patients with type 1 diabetes in which 40% of the men and 26% of the women were found to be hypercholesterolemic,[15] as well as other studies.[16]

In general, dyslipidemia is associated with the degree of glycemic control obtained in type 1 diabetes. The Diabetes Control and Complications Trial, which examined 1569 patients with type 1 diabetes, found that good metabolic control, as measured by glycohemoglobin level and body weight, correlated negatively with total cholesterol, LDL cholesterol, and triglyceride levels.[17] Because the level of glycemic control is the major determinant of lipoprotein abnormalities, type 1 diabetic patients with poor glycemic control tend to have the most marked changes. Diabetic ketoacidosis is associated with chylomicronemia and marked hypertriglyceridemia.[18] Increased hepatic VLDL production is seen, and plasma VLDL levels are further elevated by deficient LpL activity, resulting in reduced VLDL clearance. Insulin therapy decreases triglyceride levels to normal in most patients within 24 hours.[19]

Poorly controlled type 1 diabetes, short of diabetic ketoacidosis, is also associated with moderate increases in cholesterol, triglycerides, and LDL cholesterol. Initiation of insulin therapy results in a fall in elevated triglyceride levels, together with a decrease in total and LDL cholesterol levels and a significant increase in HDL cholesterol levels.[20] Insulin reduces hepatic synthesis of VLDL and increases LpL-mediated triglyceride metabolism, resulting in an increase in HDL cholesterol levels.[21] Although production and clearance of VLDL triglyceride are normalized with insulin therapy, composition of the VLDL particle shows enrichment with cholesterol and apolipoprotein B (apo B) in diabetic patients as compared with normolipidemic, nondiabetic patients.[22] This smaller, denser VLDL particle is thought to be more atherogenic and fails to respond to glycemic control.

In the Diabetes Control and Complications Trial, LDL cholesterol levels were lower in patients with type 1 diabetes who were younger than 25 years and were similar to the mean values found by the Lipid Research Center for patients with type 1 diabetes who were older than 25 years.[17] Despite the finding of normal LDL concentrations, multiple abnormalities of LDL metabolism may still be noted in association with type 1 diabetes. Modifications of the LDL particle by virtue of nonenzymatic glycation with subsequent impairment in clearance have been noted.[23] In addition, decreased LDL clearance by means of the LDL receptor occurs, and may relate to deficiencies in insulin-stimulated LDL receptor activity.

Secondary causes of hyperlipidemia also occur in the setting of diabetes. Proteinuria accompanying diabetic nephropathy is associated with higher levels of triglycerides, VLDL cholesterol, LDL cholesterol, and apo B.[24] Obesity also adversely affects lipoproteins in patients with type 1 diabetes, although not as severely as in type 2 diabetes.[25] Other well-known causes of secondary hyperlipidemia, such as hypothyroidism and the effects of drugs such as diuretics and β-adrenergic blockers, occur in the setting of type 1 diabetes.

## LIPOPROTEIN ALTERATIONS IN TYPE 2 DIABETES

Table 166-1 summarizes the commonly observed lipoprotein abnormalities in patients with type 2 diabetes and their possible metabolic determinants.

### TRIGLYCERIDES AND VERY-LOW-DENSITY LIPOPROTEINS

Patients with type 2 diabetes have a 50% to 100% elevation in plasma levels of total and VLDL triglycerides compared with

**TABLE 166-1.**
**Lipoprotein Abnormalities in Type 2 Diabetes Mellitus**

| Lipoprotein | Alteration |
|---|---|
| VLDL (↑) | Increased production of TG and apo B |
| | Decreased clearance of TG and apo B |
| | Enriched in remnants |
| | Increased induction of cellular lipid accumulation |
| LDL (↑ or N) | Increased production of apo B |
| | Decreased receptor-mediated clearance |
| | Smaller size; more dense |
| | TG enrichment |
| | Glycation |
| | Oxidation |
| | Immunogenicity |
| HDL (↓) | Increased clearance of apo A |
| | Decreased proportion of $HDL_2$ |
| | TG enrichment |
| | Glycation |
| | Diminished reverse cholesterol transport |

*VLDL,* very-low-density lipoprotein; ↑, increased; *TG,* triglycerides; *apo,* apoprotein; *N,* no change; *LDL,* low-density lipoprotein; *HDL,* high-density lipoprotein; ↓, decreased.

nondiabetic persons. Individuals with type 2 diabetes who have concentrations of total triglycerides of >350 to 400 mg/dL probably also have primary genetic defects in lipoprotein metabolism.[26]

Overproduction of VLDL triglyceride, resulting from increased hepatic influx of substrates such as glucose and free fatty acids, appears to be the most likely explanation for the hypertriglyceridemia.[27] It is further exacerbated by defects in the clearance of VLDL triglycerides that parallel hyperglycemia.[28] Impaired LpL activity seen in type 2 diabetes may play a critical role in the hypertriglyceridemia associated with insulin resistance and insulin deficiency.[29]

Whether hyperinsulinemia or insulin resistance is the cause of the VLDL overproduction in type 2 diabetes is unclear. Insulin may have a permissive effect on VLDL production, in that some insulin is necessary for protein synthesis; however, VLDL production is inhibited when insulin concentrations are raised, and insulin stimulates apo B degradation in hepatocytes, thus inhibiting VLDL secretion. In studies using euglycemic clamp techniques, significant correlations have been noted between VLDL and insulin resistance independent of insulin concentrations. Thus, insulin resistance may be the predominant determinant of VLDL overproduction in type 2 diabetes because it is associated with increased glucose and free fatty acid flux in the liver.

Observations of abnormal in vitro metabolism of VLDL obtained from persons with type 2 diabetes suggest compositional alterations: VLDL isolated from normotriglyceridemic patients with type 2 diabetes produced a greater cellular accumulation of lipids in mouse peritoneal macrophages than did VLDL isolated from either normotriglyceridemic or hypertriglyceridemic nondiabetic control subjects.[30] The alteration in VLDL particles may have implications for the increased propensity for atherosclerosis among individuals with type 2 diabetes, because cholesterol-enriched VLDL or VLDL remnants may be atherogenic.[28,31]

### LOW-DENSITY LIPOPROTEINS

Elevated LDL cholesterol (>160 mg/dL) occurs more often in patients with type 2 diabetes than in nondiabetic control subjects.[32] Ethnic differences may exist, because no changes in LDL cholesterol levels are noted in patients with type 2 diabetes from either the Native American or Mexican American populations.[33] Defects in LDL clearance occur in type 2 diabetes and may be related to insulin resistance.[28]

A number of potentially atherogenic changes in LDL composition may occur in type 2 diabetes. Subjects with elevated triglycerides and insulin resistance appear to have a high proportion of small, dense LDL particles consistent with subclass pattern B.[34] Compositional changes in LDL are noted disproportionately in women with diabetes and appear to be related to the degree of glycemic control.[35] Small LDL particles accompany type 2 diabetes, independent of plasma lipid concentrations.[36]

As with other body proteins, nonenzymatic glycation of 2% to 5% of the apo B component of LDL occurs in patients with moderately controlled type 2 diabetes.[37] This structural modification of the molecule decreases LDL catabolism in vivo by 5% to 25%.[38] In addition, glycated LDL enhances cholesterol ester synthesis in human macrophages with altered endothelial response, perhaps providing a mechanism to explain the increased atherogenesis seen in type 2 diabetes.[39]

Another effect of glycation may be to confer increased susceptibility of the LDL to oxidation in diabetics.[40] Oxidative modification of LDL renders the molecule highly atherogenic by virtue of its rapid uptake by macrophages and subsequent foam cell formation. Together, glycation and oxidation render LDL more immunogenic, with formation of antibody–antigen complexes stimulating macrophage accumulation and further foam

cell formation.[41] Thus, independent of LDL concentrations, persons with type 2 diabetes have a more atherogenic molecule that could theoretically accelerate atherogenesis.

### HIGH-DENSITY LIPOPROTEINS

Lower HDL concentrations are as prevalent as increased triglycerides in patients with type 2 diabetes.[42] This could result from the impaired VLDL clearance and lower LpL activity previously described, which lead to diminished HDL accumulation. In addition, HDL clearance appears to be elevated in patients with type 2 diabetes, resulting in net lower HDL plasma concentrations.[43] Decreased HDL levels in type 2 diabetes typically reflect decreases in the $HDL_2$ subfraction, with a higher proportion of triglycerides in the particle. Significant negative relationships between plasma concentrations of insulin and HDL have been observed in patients with type 2 diabetes, as well as a negative relationship between insulin resistance and HDL cholesterol that is independent of VLDL concentrations.

As with LDL, nonenzymatic glycation of HDL occurs in type 2 diabetes and may interfere with HDL receptor binding.[44] Thus, lower concentrations of HDL together with altered composition may impair cellular cholesterol efflux, resulting in abnormal cholesterol transport and transfer and potentially inhibiting the reverse cholesterol transfer process.

### LIPOPROTEIN(A)

Probably, lipoprotein(a) is unchanged in individuals with type 2 diabetes.[45]

## RATIONALE AND GOALS FOR TREATMENT OF LIPID ABNORMALITIES IN DIABETES

### RATIONALE FOR THERAPY

The concern about lipid abnormalities in patients with diabetes is a response to the increasing body of data implicating abnormal lipids as significant risk factors for arteriosclerotic vascular disease.[46] The accumulation of evidence that modification of risk factors can lower mortality related to cardiovascular disease in the general population[47,48] has brought with it an increased mandate for managing all the cardiovascular risk factors in persons with diabetes, as well as controlling their blood glucose levels. Thus, total risk management in the patient with diabetes must include attention to the lipid abnormalities.

Lowering serum lipids reduces the risk of cardiovascular disease.[49] In addition, the prognosis for people with preexisting cardiovascular disease can be significantly improved by lipid-lowering therapy. Results from both primary and secondary intervention studies (Air Force Coronary Atherosclerosis Prevention Study/Texas Coronary Atherosclerosis Prevention Study [AFCAPS/TexCAPS] and the Cholesterol and Recurrent Events [CARE] trial) confirm that lipid lowering in nondiabetic individuals with average lipid levels reduces the risk of coronary events.[50,51] In the CARE study, results for patients with diabetes did not differ significantly from those for nondiabetic participants.[51]

Primary prevention trials of lipid-lowering therapy in diabetic individuals with normal cholesterol levels are currently under way, but such patients' increased probability of having a first cardiac event and their subsequent poor outcome would support a more aggressive therapeutic approach than in the nondiabetic population.[6,52,53]

In diabetic subjects with known coronary disease, aggressive LDL-cholesterol lowering has been long advocated. This conclusion was supported by data from the Scandinavian Simvastatin

**TABLE 166-2.**
**Risk Factors for Atherosclerosis**

| Classification | LDL Cholesterol | Triglycerides | HDL Cholesterol |
|---|---|---|---|
| **Risk** | | | |
| **Higher** | >130 (>100 if CAD) | ≥400 | <35 |
| **Borderline** | 100–129 | 200–399 | 35–45 |
| **Lower** | <100 | | |
| Male gender | | | |
| Family history of premature CAD | | | |
| Cigarette smoking (>10 cigarettes per day) | | | |
| Hypertension | | | |
| Glucose intolerance/diabetes mellitus | | | |
| HDL cholesterol <35 mg/dL | | | |
| History of other arteriosclerotic vascular diseases | | | |
| Significant obesity (>30% overweight) | | | |

*LDL*, low-density lipoprotein; *HDL*, high-density lipoprotein; *CAD*, coronary artery disease. (Adapted from American Diabetes Association. Position statement: management of dyslipidemia in adults with diabetes. Diabetes Care 1998; 21:179; and from National Cholesterol Education Program. Summary of the second report of the National Cholesterol Education Program [NCEP] Expert Panel on Detection, Evaluation and Treatment of High Blood Cholesterol in Adults [Adult Treatment Panel II]. JAMA 1993; 269:3015.)

Survival Study (4S), which found that cholesterol lowering in diabetic patients with coronary heart disease significantly lowered their risk of recurrent coronary disease and atherosclerotic events.[54]

In patients with diabetes, lipid abnormalities other than elevations of LDL cholesterol also must be considered potentially atherogenic. For patients with diabetes, unlike the general population, hypertriglyceridemia has been implicated as an important contributor to atherosclerotic vascular disease. Epidemiologic studies show an inverse relationship between the concentration of HDL cholesterol and atherosclerotic vascular disease.[55] Interventions that produce increases in HDL reduce the incidence of atherosclerotic vascular disease, and possibly slow or reverse the progression of established atherosclerotic vascular disease. The frequent occurrence of low HDL levels in persons with diabetes is probably also a contributing factor in the increased frequency and severity of atherosclerotic vascular disease in these patients.[56]

## GOALS OF THERAPY

The Adult Treatment Panel II of the NCEP Expert Panel released its revised recommendations concerning the diagnosis and management of hyperlipidemia in adults in the United States.[4] This group recommended that serum total cholesterol be measured in all adults 20 years of age and older at least once every 5 years, and that HDL cholesterol be measured at the same time if appropriate laboratory support is available. In people free of atherosclerotic disease, total cholesterol levels <200 mg/dL are classified as "desirable blood cholesterol," levels of 200 to 239 mg/dL as "borderline/high blood cholesterol," and levels ≥240 mg/dL as "high blood cholesterol." An HDL cholesterol level <35 mg/dL is defined as "low" and constitutes an atherosclerotic risk factor (Table 166-2). In the absence of atherosclerotic disease, initial classification is based on these values. The presence of an HDL cholesterol level of at least 35 mg/dL together with a total cholesterol concentration of <200 mg/dL constitutes an acceptable range, and only general educational materials are provided. Repeat lipid measurements are recommended in 5 years. Those persons with total cholesterol levels of >200 mg/dL together with an HDL cholesterol of <35 mg/dL should proceed to lipoprotein analysis, as should those with a total cholesterol level of >240 mg/dL. This lipoprotein analysis should be obtained after a 12-hour fast and consists of measurements of

total cholesterol, HDL cholesterol, and triglycerides, with a calculation of the LDL cholesterol. All further therapeutic decisions are then based on the LDL cholesterol value.

These recommendations are grounded in studies of the general population. Although the NCEP acknowledges the high risk for coronary artery disease in the setting of diabetes, in the absence of primary prevention trials to prove that cholesterol lowering reduces such risk in diabetic patients, a definitive recommendation to reduce LDL cholesterol levels to a lower threshold could not be made. Nonetheless, given the NCEP guidelines for high-risk persons, a more aggressive position on intervention is entertained when two or more risk factors for coronary artery disease are present (see Table 166-2) or established coronary artery disease is present. Thus, all men with diabetes automatically fall within the high-risk category. In addition, women with diabetes are considered to be at high risk in the presence of concomitant obesity, hypertension, cigarette smoking, or family history of atherosclerosis.

Notwithstanding the original publication of the NCEP report in 1988,[3] and despite a growing awareness of the importance of atherosclerosis in the morbidity and mortality of diabetes, little attention seems to be paid to the management of hyperlipidemia in diabetic patients.[57,58]

Thus, the ADA position statement[6] endeavors to increase the frequency of detection of lipid disorders in patients with diabetes and improve their management. An aggressive lowering of LDL cholesterol is recommended in both men and women with diabetes, similar to that recommended for patients with established coronary disease (see Table 166-2). The ADA recommends optimal cholesterol and triglyceride levels for diabetic patients of <100 mg/dL (2.60 mmol/L) for LDL, ≥45 mg/dL (1.15 mmol/L) for HDL, and <200 mg/dL (2.30 mmol/L) for triglycerides. Treatment priorities are, in order, (a) LDL cholesterol lowering, (b) HDL cholesterol raising, (c) triglyceride lowering, and (d) combined lipid therapy. LDL lowering was listed as the top priority because moderately high LDL cholesterol levels (130–160 mg/dL) in diabetic individuals appear to be equivalent to much higher levels in nondiabetic subjects in terms of promotion of coronary heart disease.

## NONPHARMACOLOGIC THERAPY OF DIABETIC DYSLIPIDEMIA

The ADA strongly emphasizes the role of nonpharmacologic strategies in treating dyslipidemia in diabetes.[6] These include dietary modification, with weight loss if required, increased physical activity, and successful glycemic control. These strategies are interrelated, with the first two contributing to glycemic control, and glycemic control in turn often contributing to the improvement in the dyslipidemia.

### DIET THERAPY

Caloric restriction resulting in weight reduction decreases insulin resistance and hyperinsulinemia, with subsequent beneficial effects on both hyperglycemia and dyslipidemia.[59] Weight reduction in type 2 diabetes results in lowering of triglyceride concentrations, increase in HDL cholesterol, and, in some studies, a lowering of LDL cholesterol.[60] Although the nutrition principles released by the ADA in 1994 have resulted in more controversy than clarification with regard to dietary prescriptions,[61] previous ADA guidelines[62] for treatment of diabetic patients had been consistent with dietary recommendations by the NCEP.[4] These include reduction in the amount of total fat to <30% of total calories and of saturated fat to <10% (preferably to 7%) of total calories. Saturated fat should be replaced by polyunsaturated fat up to 10% of total calories, and the remainder should be monounsaturated fat. Cholesterol intake should be reduced to <300 mg per day, and the rest of the diet should consist of ~15% of calories from protein and the remaining 50% to 60% from complex carbohydrates. The increase in the amount of complex carbohydrates results in a concomitant increase in fiber, particularly soluble fiber. Intake of up to 40 g per day of fiber has been recommended for patients with type 2 diabetes. This is important to prevent the increase in triglycerides sometimes induced by high-carbohydrate diets.[63] The ADA position statement suggested that normal-weight diabetic patients replace the saturated fat in their diets with carbohydrate or monounsaturated fat, and that, in obese patients, a high-fat diet may impede weight loss.[5]

Most studies of patients with type 2 diabetes found that replacing foods high in saturated fats with foods containing predominantly complex carbohydrates and high fiber lowers both total and LDL cholesterol.[63] Decreases in HDL cholesterol concentrations have been observed in some studies of type 2 diabetes in which complex carbohydrates replaced saturated fat; decreases in HDL concentration appear to be less pronounced in those diabetic patients with lower initial HDL concentrations. Significant increases in fasting triglyceride concentrations have not been seen in most studies of type 2 diabetes patients consuming solid-food, high-carbohydrate diets that contain adequate soluble fiber. Studies measuring postprandial triglyceride concentrations also found no changes.[64] An additional advantage of diets high in complex carbohydrates is that they are lower in calories per comparable portion size, possibly promoting weight reduction. On the other hand, a metaanalysis concluded that consumption of diets high in monounsaturated fats by diabetic patients reduced plasma triglycerides by 19% and VLDL cholesterol by 22%, and caused a small increase in HDL cholesterol without raising LDL cholesterol levels.[65]

Few data are available regarding the effect of following nutrition guidelines on lipid profiles in individuals with type 2 diabetes in free-living situations.[66] A flexible approach should be adopted in medical nutrition therapy that considers the patient's weight and specific lipid abnormalities. For many, a diet high in complex carbohydrates can improve lipid levels and induce weight loss.

A final dietary approach suggested for patients with diabetes is increasing the amount of omega-3 polyunsaturated fatty acids. These fatty acids, which are found predominantly in fish oils, have a hypotriglyceridemic action, and fish oil supplements have been shown to reduce serum triglyceride levels in some studies of patients with type 2 diabetes.[67] Increases in LDL cholesterol, however, may occur in hypertriglyceridemic subjects given fish oil. Thus, this approach may need to be used in combination with other LDL-lowering strategies. In addition, in some patients the use of fish oil supplements may adversely affect glycemic control.

### EXERCISE

Regular physical exercise is a first-line recommendation that can have beneficial effects on glucose levels, insulin sensitivity, and dyslipidemia.[68] Exercise can also complement dietary regimens for weight control. Before beginning an exercise program, all patients with diabetes should be carefully screened for preexisting coronary disease and for previously undiagnosed hypertension, neuropathy, retinopathy, nephropathy, and other complications. To maintain beneficial effects on insulin sensitivity, exercise is recommended three times per week for 20 to 45 minutes at 50% to 70% of maximum capacity. If weight loss is the goal, patients should exercise five to seven times per week. Regular physical exercise favorably influences the lipid profile in patients with diabetes, leading to a significant reduction in total and LDL cholesterol and a concomitant increase in HDL.

Exercise has also been shown to lower triglyceride levels in persons with type 2 diabetes.

## PHARMACOLOGIC THERAPY FOR TYPE 1 DIABETES AND ITS RELATION TO DYSLIPIDEMIA

In type 1 diabetic patients with diabetic dyslipidemia (i.e., patients who do not have underlying primary abnormalities of lipid metabolism in addition to type 1 diabetes), adequate insulin therapy often completely corrects all of the diabetes-associated lipid abnormalities.[69] In patients with poorly controlled type 1 diabetes, the clearance of both chylomicrons and LDL is accelerated by the stimulatory effect of insulin therapy on LpL activity, with a resulting resolution of hypertriglyceridemia within several days. Overproduction of VLDL and the subsequent abnormal composition of VLDL, VLDL remnants, and LDL often respond to adequate control of glucose with insulin therapy. Finally, HDL levels are often increased to normal or even supranormal levels with insulin therapy.

The degree of glucose control has a direct effect on the normalization of lipids. When standard insulin therapy is unsuccessful, tight control with multiple subcutaneous insulin injections or with subcutaneous insulin infusion by means of an insulin pump often results in near-normalization of glucose levels and in significant improvement in the diabetic dyslipidemia.[70] The concern as to whether the insulin therapy might contribute to atherogenesis has been somewhat mitigated by the trend toward a lower frequency of macrovascular complications in the intensively treated group of the Diabetes Control and Complications Trial.[70] The effect of differential routes of insulin administration is also being investigated, and preliminary data suggest that intraperitoneal delivery may normalize VLDL composition independent of glycemic control.

## PHARMACOLOGIC THERAPY FOR TYPE 2 DIABETES AND ITS RELATION TO DYSLIPIDEMIA

When diet and exercise are insufficient to control plasma glucose in type 2 diabetes, other glucose-lowering therapeutic regimens may be used that also have a beneficial effect on dyslipidemia. When sulfonylurea, repaglinide, or metformin therapy is instituted to lower glucose levels, concomitant hyperlipidemia is often significantly reduced as well. The effects of thiazolidinediones remain problematic and drug specific. Some lower triglyceride levels, whereas others may be neutral or may raise triglyceride levels, depending on the peroxisome proliferator activated receptor γ (PPARγ) activity of the agent. Improved glycemic control in type 2 diabetes with sulfonylurea therapy is usually accompanied by decreases in plasma cholesterol, triglyceride, and apo B.[71] The effects of control with sulfonylurea therapy on HDL levels are variable, with some studies showing no change and others demonstrating a moderate increase.

Insulin therapy in type 2 diabetic patients with significant dyslipidemia often helps control the accompanying lipid disorders. When blood glucose is effectively controlled with insulin, many patients with type 2 diabetes experience a normalization of their triglyceride concentrations and a decrease in total and LDL cholesterol. HDL often increases but may not return to a desirable range.[69] When significant doses of insulin are required, it should be administered in multiple-dose regimens using mixtures of short-acting and intermediate-acting insulin, just as in type 1 diabetes.

## DRUG THERAPY FOR DYSLIPIDEMIA

The ADA recognizes that if 3 to 6 months of nonpharmacologic therapy, including dietary modification, physical activity, and

**TABLE 166-3.**
**Drugs Used in the Treatment of Dyslipidemia**

| Drug | LDL | VLDL | HDL | Glucose Levels | Special Considerations in Diabetes Mellitus |
|---|---|---|---|---|---|
| Fibric acid derivative | Variable | ↓ | ↑ | N or ↓ | May elevate LDL |
| Gemfibrozil 1.2 g | ↓ | | | | May increase bile lithogenicity |
| Micronized fenofibrate 67–201 mg | ↓ | | ↑ | | Lowers triglyceride levels |
| HMG-CoA reductase inhibitors | ↓ | N or ↓ | N or ↑ | N | |
| Lovastatin 10–80 mg | | | | | |
| Simvastatin 20–80 mg | | | | | |
| Pravastatin 10–40 mg | | | | | |
| Fluvastatin 20–40 mg | | | | | |
| Atorvastatin 10–80 mg | | | | | Lowers triglyceride levels |
| Cerivastatin 0.3–0.8 mg | | | | | Lowers triglyceride levels |
| Bile acid sequestrants | ↓ | ↑ | N or ↑ | N | May elevate TG |
| Cholestyramine 8–24 g | | | | | May interfere with drug absorption |
| Colestipol 5–30 g | | | | | |
| Nicotinic acid 1–6 g | ↓ | ↓ | ↑ | ↑ | May precipitate gout; liver toxicity |
| Niacin 1–6 g | | | | | ↑ Insulin resistance |
| Niacin extended-release 2 g | | | | | ↑ Glucose |
| Probucol 500–1000 mg | ↓ | N | ↓ | N | Lowers HDL; may inhibit LDL oxidation |

↑, increased; ↓, decreased; N, no change; *LDL*, low-density lipoprotein; *VLDL*, very-low-density lipoprotein; *HDL*, high-density lipoprotein; *HMG-CoA*, 3-hydroxy-3-methylglutaryl coenzyme A; *TG*, triglyceride.

successful glycemic control, fail to improve lipid levels, drug therapy may be warranted.[5] Drugs from five pharmacologic classes have been recommended to control dyslipidemia in diabetic patients (Table 166-3).

### FIBRIC ACID DERIVATIVES

Gemfibrozil and fenofibrate are the two drugs in this class that are available in the United States. These drugs increase LpL activity, increase the clearance of VLDL triglycerides, and sometimes enhance LDL clearance. A significant increase in HDL cholesterol also occurs, the mechanism of which is unknown. A transient increase in LDL cholesterol may occur in some patients with hypertriglyceridemia, and the increase may be sustained in others. The mechanism of this increase in LDL is unclear. Micronized fenofibrate, a new formulation of the fibric acid derivative fenofibrate, is more easily absorbed than its predecessor. It was as effective as simvastatin and pravastatin in reducing total and LDL cholesterol levels, but produced greater improvements in HDL and triglyceride levels.[72]

In patients with diabetic dyslipidemia, fibrates result in no apparent increase in insulin resistance or deterioration of glucose control. In the largest study of gemfibrozil involving 400 patients with type 2 diabetes,[73] it lowered total, LDL, and VLDL cholesterol and triglycerides, and increased HDL cholesterol. The ratio of HDL to total cholesterol also improved significantly. These agents are the only ones shown to reduce the proportion of small, dense LDL. The effects of gemfibrozil therapy were also assessed in 134 diabetic men in the Helsinki Heart Study,[74] a 5-year primary prevention trial. After 5 years, changes in levels of lipids and lipoproteins were similar in diabetic and nondiabetic subjects. The incidence of cardiac events in patients with type 2 diabetes was lower in the gemfibrozil-treated group, although the difference did not reach statistical significance.

Side effects of fibric acid derivatives are gastrointestinal symptoms, rash, and cholelithiasis. These agents are contraindicated in patients with hepatic or renal disease or cholelithiasis. The combination of gemfibrozil and 3-hydroxy-3-methylglutaryl coenzyme A (HMG-CoA) reductase inhibitors may cause myositis.

### 3-HYDROXY-3-METHYLGLUTARYL COENZYME A REDUCTASE INHIBITORS

The statin drugs are safe and effective in lowering LDL cholesterol levels. Lovastatin, simvastatin, pravastatin, fluvastatin, atorvastatin, and cerivastatin are inhibitors of the rate-limiting enzyme of cholesterol synthesis. These agents lower serum total and LDL cholesterol by increasing the LDL receptor–mediated metabolism of LDL cholesterol.[74a] In addition, conversion of VLDL remnants to LDL is significantly decreased in patients treated with these agents. These drugs are the most effective single agents in reducing LDL cholesterol, and they produce moderate decreases in triglycerides and increases in HDL as well. No adverse effects on glucose tolerance have been observed with lovastatin use during clinical trials. Lovastatin was administered to 52 patients with type 2 diabetes and significant hypercholesterolemia for 24 weeks.[75] Total, LDL, and VLDL cholesterol were significantly reduced, and HDL cholesterol increased. Lovastatin therapy was also assessed in a 4-week, double-blind, placebo-controlled study of 16 patients with type 2 diabetes.[75a] Use of the drug produced lower levels of total cholesterol, VLDL, and triglycerides than a placebo. No significant change in HDL cholesterol was noted. The use of simvastatin[76] and pravastatin[76a] in diabetic patients has also been evaluated with similar outcomes. Rhabdomyolysis with acute renal failure has been reported with the combined use of lovastatin and cyclosporine; consequently, the combination of an HMG-CoA reductase inhibitor and cyclosporine should be approached with extreme caution. Although the risk of myositis appears to be increased when lovastatin and a fibric acid derivative are used together, the low frequency of this complication allows this drug combination to be attempted with careful monitoring in patients who are at very high risk for cardiovascular disease and have significant hyperlipidemia.[77]

Atorvastatin, a highly effective, wide-spectrum agent, has been shown to effectively lower LDL cholesterol levels, especially when combined with a resin. It appears to be as effective as simvastatin, pravastatin, lovastatin, and fluvastatin in lowering LDL cholesterol, and was shown to be more effective than these other agents in lowering total cholesterol.[78] Further, the ability of atorvastatin to lower triglyceride levels suggests that combined hyperlipidemia, previously treatable only with combination therapy, may now be treated with a single drug. Cerivastatin, another synthetic HMG-CoA reductase inhibitor, lowers triglyceride levels as well as total and LDL cholesterol at doses 1% to 3% of those required for other statin drugs.[79]

## BILE ACID SEQUESTRANTS

Bile acid sequestrants (cholestyramine and colestipol) are not absorbed and act primarily in the intestinal tract to bind bile acids. By interfering with the enterohepatic circulation, they force the liver to increase the synthesis of bile acid from stored cholesterol, resulting in an up-regulation of LDL receptors and increased LDL clearance.[72] A major limiting factor in the use of bile acid sequestrants in diabetes is the observed increase in triglyceride levels after initiation of therapy in patients with preexisting hypertriglyceridemia. In the few studies assessing the effect of bile acid sequestrants in diabetic patients, serum cholesterol levels were lowered but triglyceride levels were raised during treatment.[79a] As a result, the ADA recommends their use in the diabetic patient only with caution.[53] In individuals with desirable triglyceride levels or those in whom triglycerides have been controlled pharmacologically, however, bile acid sequestrants can be safely combined with either fibric acid derivatives or HMG-CoA reductase inhibitors to increase LDL reduction. The addition of a bile acid sequestrant is frequently required in patients with diabetes when initial hypertriglyceridemia is controlled by monotherapy with gemfibrozil with a resulting undesirable increase in LDL cholesterol, as described earlier. Side effects of these agents include constipation in 10% to 20% of patients and gastric distress in an additional significant number. Side effects may be minimized by slowly increasing the dose and by administering these drugs with fluids, fiber, and agents to reduce intestinal gas.

## NICOTINIC ACID

Nicotinic acid is a cofactor for intermediary metabolism, but at pharmacologic doses (1000 mg per day or greater) it has profound lipid-lowering effects. It decreases hepatic synthesis of VLDL, reduces plasma concentrations of triglyceride and LDL cholesterol, and significantly raises HDL cholesterol. It initially acts to inhibit lipolysis, but this is not thought to be a primary mechanism of cholesterol lowering.

Nicotinic acid is the most economic of hypolipidemic drugs. In studies of nicotinic acid therapy in patients with type 2 diabetes, total and LDL cholesterol was reduced, VLDL triglycerides and cholesterol were reduced, and HDL was elevated.[80]

The clinical utility of nicotinic acid has been diminished by the frequent occurrence of side effects, including flushing, gastrointestinal symptoms, itching, and rash. Hepatic dysfunction is another potentially serious side effect. Some of these adverse effects can be avoided or minimized by initiating therapy at low doses and by administering with aspirin. The worsening of glycemic control often observed with nicotinic acid is thought to be a result of its action to increase insulin resistance. For all these reasons, the ADA noted that nicotinic acid is not recommended as first-line therapy and should be used only in diabetic patients with refractory dyslipidemia and only with careful follow-up evaluations.[6]

## PROBUCOL

Probucol is an antioxidant that reduces total and LDL cholesterol. It also reduces HDL cholesterol levels by ~25%. The hypolipidemic action of probucol has been demonstrated in patients with type 2 diabetes[81] and includes modest decreases in cholesterol and triglycerides. Side effects include mild gastrointestinal reactions, but it has also been shown to prolong QT intervals and is therefore contraindicated in patients with arrhythmias. Interest has focused on probucol because of its antioxidant action, which potentially might be beneficial in inhibiting the atherosclerotic process.[82] This agent is no longer marketed in the United States.

# CONCLUSION

Although mortality related to cardiovascular disease has decreased in the general population in the United States since the late 1960s, that same decrease has not been demonstrated in patients with diabetes. Dyslipidemia is one of the most important contributors to the accelerated arteriosclerosis observed in diabetes. Other risk factors also may be lipid related. An understanding of the pathophysiology and treatment of diabetic dyslipidemia is essential for successful management. NCEP and ADA guidelines have provided a framework for the detection of dyslipidemia, establishment of goals, and management of diabetic patients with these disorders.

# REFERENCES

1. Gu K, Cowie CC, Harris MI. Mortality in adults with and without diabetes in a national cohort of the U.S. population, 1971–1993. Diabetes Care 1998; 21:1138.
2. Bierman EL. Atherogenesis in diabetes. Arterioscler Thromb 1992; 12:647.
3. The Expert Panel. Report of the National Cholesterol Education Program Expert Panel on Detection, Evaluation, and Treatment of High Blood Cholesterol in Adults. Arch Intern Med 1988; 148:36.
4. National Cholesterol Education Program. Summary of the second report of the National Cholesterol Education Program (NCEP) Expert Panel on Detection, Evaluation and Treatment of High Blood Cholesterol in Adults (Adult Treatment Panel II). JAMA 1993; 269:3015.
5. Haffner SM. Management of dyslipidemia in adults with diabetes. Diabetes Care 1998; 21:160.
6. American Diabetes Association. Position statement: management of dyslipidemia in adults with diabetes. Diabetes Care 1998; 21:179.
7. Havel RJ, Kane JP. Introduction: structure and metabolism of plasma lipoproteins. In: Scriver CR, Beaudet AL, Sly WS, Valle D, eds. The metabolic basis of inherited disease, 6th ed. New York: McGraw-Hill, 1989:1129.
8. Kane JP, Havel RJ. Disorders of the biogenesis and secretion of lipoproteins containing the B apolipoproteins. In: Scriver CR, Beaudet AL, Sly WS, Valle D, eds. The metabolic basis of inherited disease, 6th ed. New York: McGraw-Hill, 1989:1164.
9. Goldstein JL, Brown MS. Familial hypercholesterolemia. In: Scriver CR, Beaudet AL, Sly WS, Valle D, eds. The metabolic basis of inherited disease, 6th ed. New York: McGraw-Hill, 1989:1250.
10. Grundy SM. Cholesterol and atherosclerosis: diagnosis and treatment. Philadelphia: JB Lippincott, 1990.
11. Brewer HB Jr, Santamarine-Fojo S, Hoeg JM. Molecular biology of lipoproteins, their receptors, and lipoprotein lipase: primary hyperlipidemias. In: Jeffers D, ed. Primary hyperlipidemias, vol 3. New York: McGraw-Hill, 1991:74.
12. Campos H, Genest JJ, Blijlevens E, et al. Low density lipoprotein particle size and coronary artery disease. Arteriosclerosis 1992; 12:187.
13. Scanu AM, Fles GM. Lipoprotein (a): heterogeneity and biological relevance. J Clin Invest 1990; 85:1709.
14. Eisenberg S. High density lipoprotein metabolism. J Lipid Res 1984; 25:1017.
15. Taskinen M-R. Quantitative and qualitative lipoprotein abnormalities in diabetes mellitus. Diabetes 1992; 41(Suppl 2):12.
16. Orchard TJ. Dyslipoproteinemia in diabetes. Endocrinol Metab Clin North Am 1990; 19:361.
17. Diabetes Control and Complications Trial Research Group. Lipid and lipoprotein levels in patients with IDDM: Diabetes Control and Complications Trial experience. Diabetes Care 1992; 15:886.
18. Weidman SW, Ragland JB, Fisher JN, et al. Effects of insulin on plasma lipoproteins in diabetic ketoacidosis: evidence for a change in high density lipoprotein composition during treatment. J Lipid Res 1982; 23:171.
19. Dunn FL. Management of hyperlipidemia in diabetes mellitus. Endocrinol Metab Clin North Am 1992; 21:395.
20. Falko JM, O'Dorisio TM, Cataland S. Improvement of high density lipoprotein cholesterol levels: ambulatory type I diabetes treated with subcutaneous insulin pump. JAMA 1982; 247:37.
21. Nikkila EA, Hormila P. Serum lipids and lipoproteins in insulin-treated diabetes: demonstration of increased high-density lipoprotein concentrations. Diabetes 1987; 27:1078.

22. Rivellese A, Riccardi G, Romano G, et al. Presence of very low density lipoprotein compositional abnormalities in type I diabetic patients: effects of blood glucose optimization. Diabetologia 1988; 31:884.
23. Witztum JL, Mahoney EM, Branks MJ, et al. Non-enzymatic glycosylation of low density lipoprotein alters its biological activity. Diabetes 1982; 31:283.
24. Winocour PH, Durington PN, Ishola M, et al. Influence of proteinuria on vascular disease, blood pressure, and lipoproteins in insulin-dependent diabetes mellitus. BMJ 1987; 294:1648.
25. Laakso M, Pyorala K. Adverse effect of obesity on lipid and lipoprotein levels in insulin dependent and non-insulin dependent diabetes. Metabolism 1990; 39:117.
26. Brunzell JD, Hazzard WR, Motulsky AG, Bierman EL. Evidence for diabetes mellitus in genetic forms of hypertriglyceridemia as independent entities. Metabolism 1975; 24:1115.
27. Abrams JJ, Ginsberg H, Grundy SM. Metabolism of cholesterol and plasma triglycerides in non-ketotic diabetes mellitus. Diabetes 1982; 31:903.
28. Howard BV, Abbott WGH, Beltz WF, et al. Integrated study of low density lipoprotein metabolism and very low density lipoprotein metabolism in non-insulin dependent diabetes. Metabolism 1987; 36:870.
29. Taskinen MR. Lipoprotein lipase in diabetes. Diabetes Metab Rev 1987; 3:551.
30. Klein RL, Lyons TJ, Lopes-Virella MF. Metabolism of very low and low-density lipoproteins isolated from normolipidemic type II (non-insulin-dependent) diabetic patients by human monocyte-derived macrophages. Diabetologia 1990; 33:299.
31. Patti L, Swinburn B, Riccardi G, et al. Alterations in very-low-density lipoprotein subfractions in normotriglyceridemic non-insulin-dependent diabetics. Atherosclerosis 1991; 91:15.
32. Harris MI. Hypercholesterolemia in individuals with diabetes and glucose intolerance in the U.S. population. Diabetes Care 1991; 14:366.
33. Howard BV, Knowler WC, Vasquez B, et al. Plasma and lipoprotein cholesterol and triglyceride in the Pima Indian population. Comparison of diabetics and nondiabetics. Arteriosclerosis 1984; 4:462.
34. Feingold KR, Grunfeld C, Pang M, et al. LDL subclass phenotypes and triglyceride metabolism in non-insulin-dependent diabetes. Arterioscler Thromb 1992; 12:1496.
35. Haffner SM, Mykkanen L, Stern MP, et al. Greater effect of diabetes on LDL size in women than men. Diabetes Care 1994; 17:1164.
36. Okumura K, Matsui H, Kawakami K, et al. Low density lipoprotein particle size is associated with glycosylated hemoglobin levels regardless of plasma lipid levels. Intern Med 1998; 37:273.
37. Kim HJ, Kurup IV. Nonenzymatic glycosylation of human plasma low density lipoprotein: evidence for in vitro and in vivo glycosylation. Metabolism 1982; 31:348.
38. Steinbrecher UP, Witztum JL. Glucosylation of low-density lipoproteins to an extent comparable to that seen in diabetes slows their catabolism. Diabetes 1984; 33:130.
39. Lorenzi M, Cagliero E, Markey B, et al. Interaction of human endothelial cells with elevated glucose concentrations and native and glycosylated low density lipoproteins. Diabetologia 1984; 26:218.
40. Bowie A, Owens D, Collins P, et al. Glycosylated low density lipoprotein is more sensitive to oxidation: implications for the diabetic patient? Atherosclerosis 1993; 102:63.
41. Witzum JL, Steinberg D. Role of oxidized low density lipoprotein in atherogenesis. J Clin Invest 1991; 88:1785.
42. Ginsberg HN. Lipoprotein physiology in nondiabetic and diabetic states: relationship to atherogenesis. Diabetes Care 1991; 14:839.
43. Golay A, Zech L, Shi MZ, et al. High density lipoprotein (HDL) metabolism in non-insulin dependent diabetes mellitus: measurement of HDL turnover using tritiated HDL. J Clin Endocrinol Metab 1987; 65:512.
44. Duell PB, Bierman EL. Diabetic HDL has reduced capacity to promote HDL receptor-mediated cholesterol efflux. (Abstract). Circulation 1990; 82(Suppl III):1298.
45. Haffner SM. Lipoprotein (a) in diabetes: an update. Diabetes Care 1993; 16:835.
46. Gotto AM Jr, LaRosa JC, Hunninghake D, et al. The cholesterol facts: a summary of the evidence relating dietary fats, serum cholesterol, and coronary heart disease: a joint statement by the American Heart Association and the National Heart, Lung and Blood Institute. Circulation 1988; 81:1721.
47. Sytkowski PA, Kannel WB, D'Agostino RB. Changes in risk factors and the decline in mortality from cardiovascular disease: The Framingham Heart Study. N Engl J Med 1990; 322:1635.
48. Eisenberg DA. Cholesterol lowering in the management of coronary artery disease: the clinical implications of recent trials. Am J Med 1998; 104(2A):2s.
49. Pearson TA. Primary and secondary prevention of coronary artery disease: trials of lipid lowering with statins. Am J Cardiol 1998; 82(10A):28S.
50. Downs JR, Clearfield M, Weis S, et al. Primary prevention of acute coronary events with lovastatin in men and women with average cholesterol levels: results of AFCAPS/TexCAPS. Air Force/Texas Coronary Atherosclerosis Prevention Study. JAMA 1998; 279:1615.
51. Sacks FM, Moye LA, Davis BR, et al. Relationship between plasma LDL concentrations during treatment with pravastatin and recurrent coronary events in the Cholesterol and Recurrent Events Trial. Circulation 1998; 97:1446.
52. Haffner SM, Lehto S, Ronnemaa T, et al. Mortality from coronary heart disease in subjects with type 2 diabetes and in nondiabetic subjects with and without prior myocardial infarction. N Engl J Med 1998; 339:229.
53. Miettinen H, Lehto S, Salomaa VV, et al. Impact of diabetes on mortality after the first myocardial infarction. Diabetes Care 1998; 21:69.
54. Pyorala K, Pedersen TR, Kjekshus J, et al. Cholesterol lowering with simvastatin improves prognosis of diabetic patients with coronary heart dis-
55. Abbott RD, Wilson PWF, Kannel WB, Castelli WP. High density lipoprotein cholesterol, total cholesterol screening, and myocardial infarction: The Framingham Study. Arteriosclerosis 1988; 8:207.
56. Karhapaa P, Malkki M, Laakso M. Isolated low HDL cholesterol: an insulin resistant state. Diabetes 1994; 43:411.
57. Stern MP, Patterson JK, Haffner SM, et al. Lack of awareness and treatment of hyperlipidemia in type II diabetes in a community survey. JAMA 1989; 262:360.
58. Streja DA, Rabkin SW. Factors associated with implementation of preventive measures in patients with diabetes. Arch Intern Med 1999; 159:294.
59. National Institutes of Health. Consensus development conference on diet and exercise in non-insulin-dependent diabetes mellitus. Diabetes Care 1987; 10:639.
60. Ginsberg H, Grundy SM. Very low density lipoprotein metabolism in non-ketotic diabetes mellitus: effect of dietary restriction. Diabetologia 1982; 25:421.
61. Franz MJ, Horton ES, Bantle JP, et al. Nutrition principles for the management of diabetes and related complications. Diabetes Care 1994; 17:490.
62. American Diabetes Association. Position statement: nutritional recommendations and principles for individuals with diabetes mellitus. Diabetes Care 1987; 10:126.
63. Howard BV, Abbott WGH, Swinburn BA. Evaluation of metabolic effects of substitution of complex carbohydrates for saturated fat in individuals with obesity and NIDDM. Diabetes Care 1991; 14:786.
64. Ullmann D, Connor WE, Hatcher LA. Will a high-carbohydrate, low-fat diet lower plasma lipids and lipoproteins without producing hypertriglyceridemia? Arterioscler Thromb 1991; 11:1059.
65. Garg A. High-monounsaturated-fat diets for patients with diabetes mellitus: a meta-analysis. Am J Clin Nutr 1998; 67(Suppl):577S.
66. Milne RM, Mann JI, Chisholm AW, Williams SM. Long-term comparison of three dietary prescriptions in the treatment of NIDDM. Diabetes Care 1994; 17:74.
67. Kasim SE. Dietary marine fish oils and insulin action in type II diabetes. Ann N Y Acad Sci 1993; 683:250.
68. American Diabetes Association. Diabetes mellitus and exercise: position statement. Diabetes Care 1999; 22(Suppl 1):S49.
69. Lopes-Virella MF, Wohltmann HJ, Mayfield RK, et al. Effect of metabolic control on lipid, lipoprotein, and apolipoprotein levels in 55 insulin-dependent diabetic patients: a longitudinal study. Diabetes 1983; 32:20.
70. The Diabetes Control and Complications Trial Research Group. The effect of intensive treatment of diabetes on the development and progression of long-term complications in insulin-dependent diabetes mellitus. N Engl J Med 1993; 329:977.
71. Taskinen MR, Bekltz WF, Harper I, et al. Effects of NIDDM on very low density lipoprotein triglyceride and apolipoprotein B metabolism: studies before and after sulfonylurea therapy. Diabetes 1986; 35:1268.
72. Adkins JC, Faulds D. Micronised fenofibrate: a review of its pharmacodynamic properties and clinical efficacy in the management of dyslipidemia. Drugs 1997; 54:615.
73. Vinik AL, Colwell JA, and the Hyperlipidemia in Diabetes investigators. Effects of gemfibrozil on triglyceride levels in patients with NIDDM. Diabetes Care 1993; 16:37.
74. Frick MH, Elo O, Haapa K, et al. Helsinki Heart Study: primary-prevention trial with gemfibrozil in middle-aged men with dyslipidemia. Safety of treatment, changes in risk factors, and incidence of coronary heart disease. N Engl J Med 1987; 317:1237.
74a. Grundy SM. HMG-CoA reductase inhibitors for treatment of hypercholesterolemia. N Engl J Med 1988; 319:24.
75. Goldberg R, La Belle P, Zupkis R, Ropnca P. Comparison of the effects of lovastatin and gemfibrozil on lipids and glucose control in non-insulin-dependent mellitus. Am J Cardiol 1990; 66:16B.
75a. Garg A, Grundy SM. Lovastatin for lowering cholesterol levels in non-insulin-dependent diabetes mellitus. N Engl J Med 1988; 318:81.
76. Bach L, Wirth A, O'Brien RC, et al. Cholesterol lowering effects of simvastatin in patients with non-insulin dependent diabetes mellitus. Diabetes Nutr Metab 1991; 4:123.
76a. Yoshino G, Kazumi T, Iwai M. Long-term treatment of hypercholesterolemic non-insulin dependent diabetes (NIDDM) with pravastatin (CS-514). Atherosclerosis 1989; 75:67.
77. Garg A, Grundy SM. Gemfibrozil alone and in combination with lovastatin for treatment of hypertriglyceridemia in NIDDM. Diabetes 1989; 38:364.
78. Jones P, Kafonek S, Laurora I, Hunninghake D. Comparative dose efficacy study of atorvastatin versus simvastatin, pravastatin, lovastatin, and fluvastatin in patients with hypercholesterolemia (the CURVES study). Am J Cardiol 1998; 81:582.
79. Stein E. Cerivastatin in primary hyperlipidemia: a multicenter analysis of efficacy and safety. Am J Cardiol 1998; 82(4B):40J.
79a. Duntsch G. Langzeittherapie der Hypercholesterinamie bein Diabetiker mit Colestipol. Fortschr Med 1981; 99:73.
80. Garg A, Grundy SM. Nicotinic acid as therapy for dyslipidemia in non-insulin-dependent diabetes mellitus. JAMA 1990; 264:723.
81. Lane JT, Subbaiah PV, Otto ME, Bagdade JD. Lipoprotein composition and HDL particle size distribution in women with non-insulin dependent diabetes mellitus and the effects of probucol treatment. J Lab Clin Med 1991; 118:120.
82. Tardif JC. Insights into oxidative stress and atherosclerosis. Can J Cardiol 2000; 16(Suppl D):2D.

# PART X

# DIFFUSE HORMONAL SECRETION

ERIC S. NYLÉN, EDITOR

# CHAPTER 167

# GENERAL CHARACTERISTICS OF DIFFUSE PEPTIDE HORMONE SYSTEMS

JENS F. REHFELD

Endocrinology was born in the darkness of the gut when, in 1902, Bayliss and Starling[1] reported that blood-borne messengers from the intestine stimulated bicarbonate secretion from the pancreas. The bicarbonate secretagogue was named *secretin*, a natural designation for the first hormone. Bayliss and Starling realized that secretin represented a new concept but had difficulties finding a general designation for such blood-borne substances. Hardy, a linguist from Cambridge, England, then proposed the Greek name *hormoa* or *hormone* ("I arouse to activity"), which Starling[2] introduced in 1905 as the general designation for blood-borne chemical messengers. Hence, endocrinology became the science dealing with blood-borne control of the body.

In the last two decades, the concept of peptide hormones has been enormously expanded because of several fundamental discoveries. First, known peptide hormones are often also transmitters within the nervous system. Moreover, peptide transmitters in the brain are often expressed in peripheral tissues and may be blood-borne (*hemocrine*) messengers[3] (see Chap. 1). Second, peptides acting through the blood or nerves may also act on their immediate environment through *paracrine* secretion.[4] They may even act through exocrine secretion from the skin and mammary glands. Third, in addition to their acute metabolic actions, peptide hormones also may function as long-acting growth factors (see Chap. 173). Fourth, several cell types other than neurons and classic endocrine cells express and release peptides that may influence body functions (see Chap. 175). For instance, cancer cells may stimulate their own growth by expression of both growth-stimulating peptide hormones and the corresponding membrane receptors (*autocrine* secretion).[4a] (Also see Chap. 1.) Thus, potent, phylogenetically well preserved, hormonal peptides seem to be universal coordinators of cell functions.[5]

A suitable general designation for intercellular peptide coordinators has not been established or accepted. Terms like "regulatory," "neurohormonal," or "biologically active" have been proposed to describe these peptides. Certainly, the word "hormone" should itself be liberated from its narrow blood-bound meaning and should be used in its original broad sense, that is, "arousing to activity," and applied as a general designation for the active, universal body system of chemical messengers (see Chap. 1).

An understanding of the individual peptide hormone systems described in the following chapters, as well as in other chapters of this text, requires insight into several molecular and cellular features of hormonal peptides. Therefore, five general characteristics of diffuse peptide hormone systems are discussed.[5]

## HOMOLOGY OF PEPTIDE HORMONES AND THEIR GENES

Most peptide hormones and peptide hormone genes display structural homology with other hormones and genes. The homology often encompasses structures that are essential for conformation and bioactivity, so that the homology has both functional and clinical implications. Homologous hormones can be grouped into families (Table 167-1), the origin of which may

**TABLE 167-1.**
**Examples of Peptide Hormone Families**

**INSULIN FAMILY**
 Proinsulin
 Insulin-like growth factor-I (IGF-I)
 Insulin-like growth factor-II (IGF-II)
 Relaxin
**OPIOID PEPTIDE FAMILY**
 Proopiomelanocortin (POMC)
 Preproenkephalin
 Preprodynorphin
**OXYTOCIN FAMILY**
 Oxytocin
 Vasopressin
**SECRETIN FAMILY**
 Secretin
 Glucagon
 Vasoactive intestinal peptide (VIP)
 Gastric inhibitory peptide (GIP)
**SOMATOSTATIN FAMILY**
 Corticostatin
 Somatostatin
**SOMATOTROPIN FAMILY**
 Somatotropin (growth hormone [GH])
 Somatomammotropin
 Prolactin
**TACHYKININ FAMILY**
 Substance P
 Substance K
 Physalaemin
 Eledoisin
**THYROTROPIN FAMILY**
 Thyrotropin (thyroid-stimulating hormone [TSH])
 Follicle-stimulating hormone (FSH)
 Luteinizing hormone (LH)
 Chorionic gonadotropin

be traced to the evolution of genes. From a single ancestral gene, several hormones may develop by *duplication* and subsequent somatic mutations. Sometimes, DNA sequences encoding several homologous peptides are preserved within the transcriptional unit of a single gene. Well-known examples are α-, β-, and γ-melanocyte–stimulating hormone in the proopiomelanocortin gene; methionine and leucine enkephalin in the proenkephalin gene; vasoactive intestinal peptide (VIP) and peptide histidyl isoleucine (PHI) in the VIP gene; glucagon and the two glucagon-like peptides (GLP-1 and GLP-2), and several others. Other homologous peptides are encoded by separate genes as, for example, insulin, insulin-like growth factors (IGF-I and IGF-II), and relaxin; secretin, glucagon, and VIP; cholecystokinin and gastrin; oxytocin and vasopressin; and others. Occasionally, the evolution of homologous genes from one ancestral gene is reflected in gene clusters at the same chromosomal location, as in the case of human growth hormone and human chorionic somatomammotropin (human placental lactogen).[6]

Clinically, owing to overlap of function, the abnormal overproduction of one hormone may mimic the overproduction of another family member.[7] Such a situation may be difficult to diagnose unless the assays are specific for the portion of the structure that is nonhomologous.

## MOLECULAR HETEROGENEITY

All peptide hormones mature to bioactive forms by processing of the primary translation product, the *preprohormone*. The

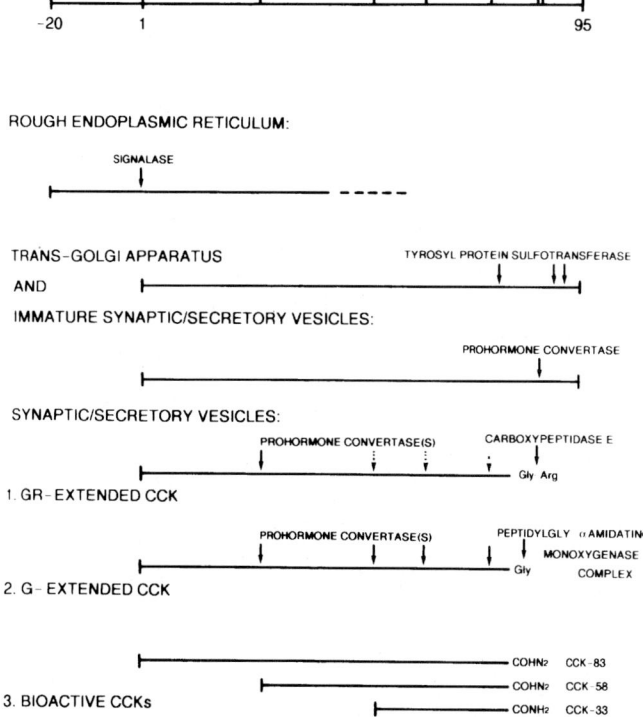

**FIGURE 167-1.** Schematic illustration of the posttranslational processing of preprocholecystokinin in cerebral neurons and the I cells of the small intestine. (*CCK*, cholecystokinin; *G*, glycine; *GR*, glycine-arginine.)

co- and posttranslational processing comprises two sorts of covalent modifications: cleavage of peptide bonds (often at the carboxyl end of single or double basic amino-acid residues),[8-10] and amino-acid derivations (acetylations, amidations, glycosylations, methylations, sulfations, and the like). The degree of processing varies considerably. Sometimes the preprohormones are processed through a few steps to a single active form, as for insulin. Other preprohormones undergo multiple modifications to yield several bioactive forms, as illustrated for cholecystokinin in Figure 167-1.

Because prohormone maturation is governed by the activity of processing enzymes, much effort has been devoted to characterization of these enzymes. So far, a number of essential enzymes have been identified. Of central significance is a family of *subtilisin-related endoproteases*, which cleave the dibasic Arg-Arg and Lys-Arg sites. These prohormone convertases are all structurally related, calcium-dependent, serine proteases. The enzyme family contains nine or more dibasic-specific endoproteases, but prohormone convertases 1 (PC1/3) and 2 (PC2) appear most important for prohormone processing in mammals.[8,9] Also, an *aspartyl endoprotease* that cleaves prohormones at monobasic sites has been identified.[10] Because the biologic activity of half of the diffuse peptide hormone systems depends on α-amidation of the C-terminal acid group, much interest has accompanied the identification of the amidation enzyme complex. Carboxyamidation requires two sequentially acting enzymes that use glycine as the amide donor. The first enzyme is a copper- and ascorbate-dependent *peptidyl-glycine α-hydroxylating monooxygenase* (PHM), derived from the N-terminal part of the amidation enzyme precursor. The second enzyme is a separate *peptidyl-α-hydroxyglycine α-amidating lyase* (PAL), derived from the remaining intragranular region of the same amidation enzyme precursor.[11,12] Although proteolysis at dibasic or monobasic sites and carboxyamidation are fundamental in the maturation of most prohormones, the vast number of different posttranslational modifications indicates that more processing enzymes are to be found. The full extent to which defective processing enzymes can explain endocrine diseases remains to be shown; however, *fat/fat* mice experience obesity and slow-onset diabetes mellitus due to carboxypeptidase-E deficiency,[13] and mutations in the gene encoding PC1 may be associated with obesity, mild diabetes mellitus, and hypogonadotropic hypogonadism in humans.[14]

Although endocrine cells or neurons may contain several bioactive products of the preprohormone, these cells frequently release only a few active forms in significant amounts. The released forms may then undergo postsecretory enzymatic modifications in the blood or, alternatively, at the target site. One such enzyme, *neutral endopeptidase*, which belongs to the neprilysin family,[15] is anchored in the plasma membrane and actively cleaves peptides in the immediate vicinity. Poorly and/or inappropriately processed prohormones in the synthesizing tissue are, accordingly, intermediate precursors or degradation fragments. Their clinical significance relates to hypersecretion by endocrine tumors, which often release incompletely processed intermediates of variable bioactivity; sometimes, a tumor secretes normal amounts of the principal mature peptide but also releases into the blood increased amounts of intermediate products.

Molecular heterogeneity of a peptide system may not be attributable only to multiple steps in the posttranslational phase of its biosynthesis. Differences in posttranscriptional processing (*alternative splicing*) may also produce different molecular forms of the same hormone, as illustrated by the 22- and 20-kDa forms of human growth hormone.[6] Finally, heterogeneity may result when multiple genes encode the same peptide hormone with only a few amino-acid substitutions. These substitutions may have no effect on bioactivity, as, for example, in the two forms of insulin that occur in the rat. On the other hand, they may have considerable pathogenetic implications, as in the case of the mutant insulins found in some families with diabetes mellitus. Regardless of whether the molecular heterogeneity is caused by multiple posttranslational or postsecretory modifications, by multiple genes or gene transcripts, the phenomenon may merit considerable biochemical investigation and sophisticated diagnostic assays before the clinical implications can be dealt with appropriately.

## WIDESPREAD EXPRESSION

All cells in the body (except haploid sex cells) have all of the genes for all hormonal peptides. In principle, therefore, all cells could conceivably synthesize all hormones. Endocrine cells and neurons are highly differentiated, however, so at one time the assumption was that one endocrine cell type could express the gene for only one peptide system. The names assigned to endocrine cells and neurons reflected this unambiguous concept: the secretin cell, the insulin cell, the oxytocin neuron, among others. Studies have revealed a system for regulating gene activation that is considerably more complex, however. Most hormonal peptides are synthesized in several different cell types in different regions of the body (see Chap. 175). This "diffuse" synthesis varies greatly at different ontogenic and phylogenic stages. Thus, in adult mammals, somatostatin is synthesized in and released from endocrine cells in the thyroid (C cells), the pancreas (D cells), endocrine and paracrine cells in the upper gut, and various neurons in both the central and peripheral nervous systems. Cholecystokinin is synthesized in large amounts in all regions of the brain, in various pituitary neurons, in peripheral neurons in the distal part of the gut, as well as in endocrine cells in the gut (I cells), adrenal medulla, and pituitary.[5,16]

The phenomenon of widespread expression casts doubt on the concept that hormone production by tumors is really "ectopic." Perhaps hormone-secreting tumors always originate from cells that have been tailored to synthesize the hormones that are subsequently released from that particular tumor. Such synthesis may occur at a low level, or it may follow a cell-specific type of processing. Therefore, this may not be detected until the transformation of the cells has increased the rate of synthesis to an extent sufficient to cause symptoms (see Chap. 219).

## CELL-SPECIFIC PROCESSING

To some extent, widespread peptide gene expression is differentiated. Thus, although a gene for a hormone may be expressed at the translational level in different cell types, the processing of the prohormone may vary in different cells. For instance, the single gastrin gene is expressed in three different endocrine cells in mammals: the antral G cells, the pituitary corticotropes, and the endocrine cells dispersed in the exocrine pancreas.[5,16] The posttranslational processing in these cells differs greatly. The antral cells contain a mixture of large and small gastrins in tyrosine-O-sulfated, as well as nonsulfated, forms. The end product in the pituitary is exclusively nonsulfated large gastrins, whereas the pancreas synthesizes only completely sulfated gastrin-17. Similar cell specificity of the posttranslational processing has been found for cholecystokinin, glucagon, somatostatin, the opioid peptides, the tachykinins, and other peptide systems.

Such cell specificity occurs not only at the posttranslational level, however. For example, the calcitonin gene and other hormone genes can be processed at the posttranscriptional level to completely different mRNAs through alternative splicing.[17] Thus, whereas the calcitonin gene in the thyroid C cells is expressed as the well-known hormone calcitonin, the same gene in hypothalamic and other neurons is expressed as a structurally unrelated peptide, calcitonin gene–related peptide (see Chaps. 3 and 53).

Cell-specific processing, therefore, economizes with genes, so that a single gene may be expressed in a number of different peptides with different bioactivities. That the differentiation may occur during both the posttranscriptional and posttranslational phases only emphasizes the versatility of gene expression mechanisms. Again, the transformed cells in hormone-secreting tumors do not respect the normal cell-specific differentiation, and the hormone genes may be expressed as many kinds of peptides. The diagnosis and, perhaps, the therapeutic control of such tumors may depend on an understanding of these possible variations in both posttranscriptional and posttranslational processing.

## COSYNTHESIS

A final characteristic of the diffuse peptide hormonal endocrine system is that many cells known to synthesize a given peptide hormone or transmitter also synthesize other hormones or transmitters.[18] These may be amines, but often they are genetically and structurally unrelated peptide systems. When assayed using the immunocytochemical methods that predominate (with the inaccuracies inherent in these techniques at the molecular level), this cosynthesis may appear to be haphazard. However, more in-depth examinations using more accurate biochemical methods have indicated that some order exists to peptide cosynthesis. For instance, endocrine cells and neurons that produce peptides belonging to the opioid family (products of the proopiomelanocortin, proenkephalin, and prodynorphin genes) often contain peptides belonging to the gastrin-cholecystokinin family. When adrenocorticotropic hormone or opioid peptides, or both, are the main products of the cell, however (as, for example, with corticotropes and melanotropes), the gastrin-cholecystokinin peptide concentration is low and the peptide processing is directed toward inactive molecular forms.[19] Conversely, antral gastrin cells contain low amounts of opioid peptides that occur in forms that differ from the known active peptides. Although the cosynthesis of peptides in normal cells may seem to be regulated in a

sophisticated manner, this process may appear to be chaotic in the case of hormone-secreting tumors.

## REFERENCES

1. Bayliss WM, Starling EH. On the causation of the so-called "peripheral reflex secretion" of the pancreas. Proc R Soc Lond 1902; 69:352.
2. Starling EH. The chemical correlation of the functions of the body: the chemical control of the functions of the body. Croonian Lecture I. Lancet 1905; 2:338.
3. Krieger D. Brain peptides: what, where and why? Science 1983; 222:975.
4. Larsson LI, Goltermann N, de Magistris L, et al. Somatostatin cell processes as pathway for paracrine secretion. Science 1979; 205:1395.
4a. Carlevaro MF, Cermelli S, Cancedda R, et al. Vascular endothelial growth factor (VEGF) in cartilage neovascularization and chondrocyte differentiation: autoparacrine role during endochondral bone formation. J Cell Sci 2000; 113:59.
5. Rehfeld JF. The new biology of gastrointestinal hormones. Physiol Rev 1998; 78:1087.
6. Seeburg PH. The human growth hormone locus: the genes and their products. In: Håkanson R, Thorell J, eds. Biogenetics of neurohormonal peptides. London: Academic Press, 1985:83.
7. Fradkin JE, Eastman RC, Lesniak MA, Roth J. Specificity spillover at the hormone receptor: exploring its role in human disease. N Engl J Med 1989; 320:640.
8. Steiner DF. The proprotein convertases. Curr Opin Chem Biol 1998; 2:31.
9. Nakayama K. Furin: a mammalian subtilisin/Kex2p-like endoprotease involved in processing of a wide variety of precursor proteins. Biochem J 1997; 327:625.
10. Bourbonnais Y, Ash J, Daigle M, Thomas DY. Isolation and characterization of S. cerevisiae mutants defective in somatostatin expression: cloning and functional role of a yeast gene encoding an aspartyl protease in precursor processing at monobasic cleavage sites. EMBO J 1993; 12:285.
11. Mains RE, Milgram SL, Keutmann HT, Eipper BA. The NH2 terminal proregion of peptidylglycine α-amidating monooxygenase facilitates the secretion of soluble proteins. Mol Endocrinol 1995; 9:3.
12. Eipper BA, Stoffers DA, Mains RE. The biosynthesis of neuropeptides: peptide γ-amidation. Ann Rev Neurosci 1992; 15:57.
13. Naggert JK, Fricker LD, Varlamov O, et al. Hyperinsulinemia in fat/fat mice associated with a carboxypeptidase E mutation which reduces enzyme activity. Nat Genet 1995; 10:135.
14. Jackson RS, Creemers JWM, Ihagi S, et al. Obesity and impaired prohormone processing associated with mutations in the human prohormone convertase 1 gene. Nat Genet 1997; 16:303.
15. Turner AJ, Brown CD, Carson JA, Barnes K. The neprilysin family in health and disease. Adv Exp Med Biol 2000; 477:229.
16. Rehfeld JF, Solinge WW. The tumor biology of gastrin and cholecystokinin. Adv Cancer Res 1994; 63:295.
17. Amara SG, Jonas V, Rosenfeld MG, et al. Alternative RNA processing in calcitonin gene expression. Nature 1982; 298:240.
18. Cuello AC, ed. Co-transmission. London: Macmillan, 1985.
19. Rehfeld JF. Accumulation of nonamidated products of preprogastrin and preprocholecystokinin in pituitary corticotrophs: evidence for posttranslational control of cell differentiation. J Biol Chem 1986; 261:5841.

# CHAPTER 168

# ENDOGENOUS OPIOID PEPTIDES

BRIAN M. COX AND GREGORY P. MUELLER

## CHEMISTRY

Three families of endogenous opioid peptides have been identified: *endorphins*, *enkephalins*, and *dynorphins* (Figs. 168-1 and 168-2). The simplest of the opioid peptides—methionine and leucine enkephalin (ME and LE, respectively)—were isolated from extracts of porcine brain.[1] Subsequently, the ME sequence was recognized to be contained in the 31-amino-acid C-terminal fragment of a previously isolated pituitary peptide, β-lipotropin (β-LPH). This fragment was shown to have a high affinity for opioid receptors, and it became known as β-*endorphin* (β-END). Another pituitary opioid, dynorphin A (DYN A), is a C-

**Enkephalin family**

|  | 1 | 5 |  | 1 | 5 |
|---|---|---|---|---|---|
| **ME** | Tyr-Gly-Gly-Phe-Met | | **ME-RF** | Tyr-Gly-Gly-Phe-Met-Arg-Phe | |
| **LE** | Tyr-Gly-Gly-Phe-Leu | | **ME-RGL** | Tyr-Gly-Gly-Phe-Met-Arg-Arg-Val-NH$_2$ | |

**β-endorphin family**

|  | 1 | 5 | 10 | 15 | 20 | 25 | 30 |
|---|---|---|---|---|---|---|---|
| **β-END** | Tyr-Gly-Gly-Phe-Met-Thr-Ser-Glu-Lys-Ser-Gln-Thr-Pro-Leu-Val-Thr-Leu-Phe-Lys-Asn-Ala-Ile-Ile-Lys-Asn-Ala-Tyr-Lys-Lys-Gly-Glu |
| **α-END** | β-END$_{1-16}$ |
| **γ-END** | β-END$_{1-17}$ |

**Dynorphin family**

|  | 1 | 5 | 10 | 15 |
|---|---|---|---|---|
| **DYN A** | Tyr-Gly-Gly-Phe-Leu-Arg-Arg-Ile-Arg-Pro-Lys-Leu-Lys-Trp-Asp-Asn-Gln |
| **DYN B** | Tyr-Gly-Gly-Phe-Leu-Arg-Arg-Gln-Phe-Lys-Val-Val-Thr |
| **α-neo-END** | Tyr-Gly-Gly-Phe-Leu-Arg-Lys-Tyr-Pro-Lys |

**Endomorphins/Exomorphin\***

|  | 1 | 5 |  | 1 | 5 |
|---|---|---|---|---|---|
| **Endo-1** | Tyr-Pro-Trp-Gly-NH$_2$ | | **Endo-2** | Tyr-Pro-Phe-Phe-NH$_2$ | |
| **ß-casomorphin** | Tyr-Pro-Phe-Pro-Gly-Pro-Ile | | **gluten exorphin A5** | Gly-Tyr-Tyr-Pro-Thr | |

**Nociceptin/orphanin FQ**

|  | 1 | 5 | 10 | 15 |
|---|---|---|---|---|
| **N/OFQ** | Phe-Gly-Gly-Phe-Thr-Gly-Ala-Arg-Lys-Ser-Ala-Arg-Lys-Leu-Ala-Asn-Gln |

**FIGURE 168-1.** Structure of major endogenous opioids and exorphins. (*ME*, [Met⁵]enkephalin; *ME-RF*, [Met⁵]enkephalyl-Arg-Phe; *LE*, leucine enkephalin; *ME-RGL*, [Met⁵]enkephalyl-Arg-Gly-Leu; *END*, endorphin; *DYN*, dynorphin; *neo-END*, neoendorphin; *Endo*, endomorphin; *N/OFQ*, nociceptin/orphanin FQ.)

terminal–extended LE.[2] At least three different genes direct the synthesis of endogenous opioid peptides: one for the enkephalins, one for β-END, and one for dynorphins (see later). These genes are expressed in cells of the nervous, endocrine, and immune systems. Related peptides are found in the hydrolysis products of casein and wheat gluten (see Fig. 168-1).

The first four amino acids of the enkephalin sequence (Tyr-Gly-Gly-Phe) represent the minimum sequence for activation of opioid receptors, although this tetrapeptide has weak activity and does not occur naturally in significant concentrations. C-terminal extensions of this peptide, such as Met⁵ or Leu⁵ in the enkephalins, Met⁵-Glu³¹ in β-END, and Leu⁵-Gln¹⁷ in DYN A, increase affinity at one or more of the various types of opioid receptor. They provide some specificity in the actions of each peptide. The Tyr¹ residue must have a free α-amino group for opioid activity. Thus, N-terminal–extended peptides, as found in precursors, have a negligible affinity for opioid receptors. Many analogs of the naturally occurring peptides have been synthesized. Some of these have increased resistance to degradation by peptidases and increased specificity for particular opioid-receptor types.

After the cloning of three major types of opioid receptor, another mRNA coding for a related receptor-like protein was identified by homology cloning. This receptor, designated ORL-1 (*opioid receptor–like clone 1*)[3] has high sequence homology with the other opioid receptors but, when expressed, does not bind any of the peptides noted earlier or most opiate drugs. Screening of brain extracts for peptides that would bind to the expressed ORL-1 receptor yielded a novel peptide with high sequence homology to DYN A, with the important exception that the Tyr¹ of DYN A was replaced by a Phe¹ residue. This novel peptide was called *nociceptin*[4] and *orphanin FQ*[5] by the two groups that independently isolated the peptide; here it is identified as *N/OFQ*, because no consensus name for this peptide yet exists. Subsequent studies have shown that N/OFQ and ORL-1 are normally expressed in the nervous system and elsewhere. N/OFQ has no effect

at the three major types of opioid receptor. Similarly, the enkephalins, dynorphin and B-endorphin do not interact with ORL-1 receptors. The high sequence homology of N/OFQ to DYN A, and of ORL-1 to the κ-type opioid receptor, indicate that the N/OFQ and its receptor, ORL-1, have evolved from or in paralled with the other endogenous opioid systems. Functional studies also suggest that N/OFQ is involved in regulation of function in many systems regulated in part by the classic opioid peptides, although the effects of N/OFQ often differ from those of the other opioids.[6] N/OFQ may also serve other functions not served by enkephalins or other opioids.

## ANATOMIC DISTRIBUTION AS A REFLECTION OF BIOLOGIC FUNCTION

The anatomic distribution of endogenous opioid peptides provides an important insight into their biologic functions.[3] The presence of high concentrations of β-END in the pituitary gland and of enkephalins in the adrenal medulla, and their release into blood, together point to potential endocrine functions of these peptides. In the central nervous system (CNS), endorphin, enkephalin, and dynorphin peptides exist in neuronal systems of arborizing axons and terminal networks with numerous varicosities that resemble classic monoamine neurons. In vitro studies that have demonstrated the presence of brain opioid receptors and have shown that the release of the peptides is calcium dependent have also provided additional evidence for the role of endogenous opioid peptides as brain neurotransmitters. These peptides are also produced by discrete, specialized cells in several peripheral organs and, in some cases, are localized in peripheral neurons (e.g., ME in the myenteric plexuses of the gastrointestinal tract). In other instances, such as endorphin peptides in pancreatic D cells, peptides derived from opioid peptide genes in testicular Leydig cells,[7] and enkephalins in some gastrin-containing cells of the stom-

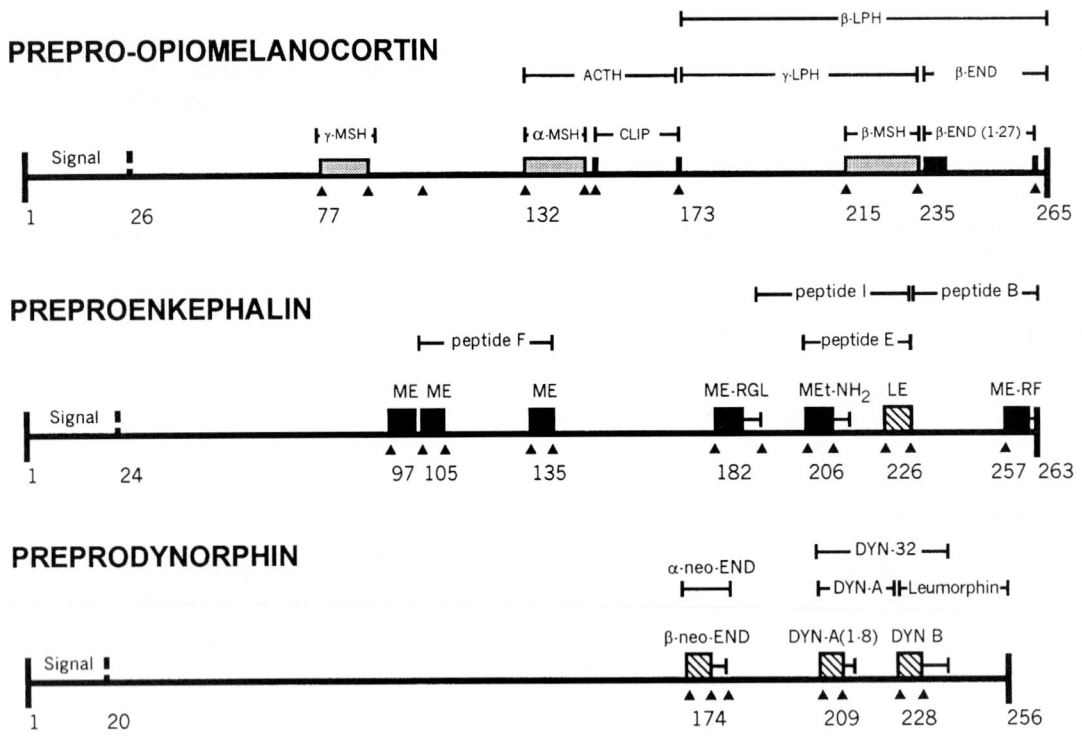

## PREPROENKEPHALIN

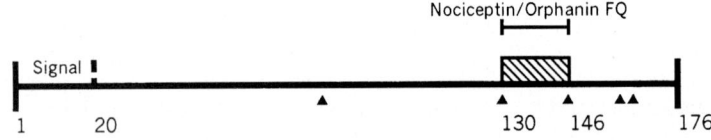

**FIGURE 168-2.** Comparison of the structures of preproopiomelanocortin, preproenkephalin, prepro-dynorphin, and prepronociceptin. The N terminus of each peptide is to the left. The positions of paired basic amino-acid residues, signals for cleavage by processing enzymes, are indicated by the black triangles. The horizontal bars indicate the positions of identified peptides from each precursor. (*LPH*, lipotropin; *ACTH*, adrenocorticotropic hormone; *END*, endorphin; *MSH*, melanocyte-stimulating hormone; *CLIP*, corticotropin-like intermediate lobe peptide; *ME*, [Met5]enkephalin; *ME-RGL*, [Met5]enkephalyl-Arg-Gly-Leu; *Met-NH2*, metorphamide; *LE*, [Leu5]enkephalin; *ME-RF*, [Met5]enkephalyl-Arg-Phe; *neo-END*, neoendorphin; *DYN*, dynorphin.) Numbers refer to amino-acid positions in the precursor peptides.

ach, endogenous opioid peptides are produced by peripheral endocrine cells and presumably have a role in paracrine regulation. Nociceptin is most highly expressed in the brain and spinal cord and only weakly in the ovary.[7] Anatomical and functional evidence for roles of endogenous opioid peptides is steadily growing. Cells of the immune system express both opioid peptides and receptors and may, thus, coordinate immune functions via opioid signaling as discussed in greater detail later.

## SYNTHESIS AND PROCESSING

### SYNTHESIS

The genes that encode for the endorphin, enkephalin, dynorphin, and N/OFQ precursor proteins have been elucidated, and the mechanisms through which their expression is regulated is under active investigation.[8-10] The large, inactive precursors are synthesized on membrane-bound ribosomes and undergo a series of posttranslational modifications en route through the

Golgi apparatus and during maturation in secretory granules. Paired, dibasic residues (Arg-Lys, Lys-Arg, Lys-Lys, or Arg-Arg) are recognition sites for the action of the trypsin-like proprotein convertase (PC) enzymes that cleave the precursors. These calcium-dependent enzymes constitute a family of five endoproteinases that are expressed in a tissue-specific manner and process a wide variety of secretory precursor proteins, including those of the endogenous opioid peptides.[11] Carboxypeptidase E (CPE) trims the C terminals of the peptide intermediates, after which α-amidation may ensue, as occurs for metorphamide. Gene disruption studies and investigation of naturally occurring mutations have clearly demonstrated the essential roles of the PCs and CPE in mediating the formation of peptide messengers. For example, loss of either proprotein convertase 1 (PC1) or CPE by mutation in humans results in defective prohormone processing, elevated plasma concentrations of unprocessed prohormone, hypogonadism, hypocortisolism, and obesity.[12,13] Mutational and knock-out analyses of the amidating enzyme, peptidylglycine α-amidating monooxygenase (PAM)[14] have yet to be conducted. Other posttranslational modifications include glycosylation, phosphorylation, and tyrosine sulfation.

Both propiomelanocortin (POMC) and proenkephalin A are subject to glycosylation on asparagine residues, and POMC is phosphorylated as well. Although these modifications to the precursors do not show up in the final opioid peptide products, they are necessary for guiding their movement in the secretory pathway.[15,16] N-acetylation of β-END occurs in the pituitary neurointermediate lobe and to a small extent in the brain. Although this modification completely eliminates opioid activity, it generates yet another class of chemical messengers having possible actions on immune cells and other targets. With the cloning of the posttranslational processing enzymes (PC1, PC2, PC3, PC4, PC5, CPE, and PAM), the molecular mechanisms that coordinate the expression of opioid peptide precursors with the activity of their respective processing enzymes can now be investigated. Findings indicate that processing enzymes are themselves regulated and may, therefore, represent therapeutic targets for drug actions.[15–17]

## PATTERNS OF PRECURSOR PROCESSING

### PROOPIOMELANOCORTIN

The pattern of precursor processing differs among various cell types.[11] In corticotropes of the anterior pituitary, POMC is processed primarily to adrenocorticotropic hormone (ACTH), β-LPH, and γ-endorphin (γ-END). In the melanotropes of the intermediate lobe, these products are processed further to yield primarily α-melanocyte–stimulating hormone (α-MSH), β-LPH, and shortened and acetylated forms of endorphin that are inactive at opioid receptors. The processing of POMC in the brain resembles a hybrid of the two patterns that occur in the pituitary gland. POMC-ergic neurons mainly express β-END$_{1-31}$ and smaller amounts of the shortened and acetylated forms of β-END, ACTH, and α-MSH. Tissue-specific processing of POMC is rigidly sustained under extreme conditions. For example, intermediate pituitary tumors induced by a POMC-simian virus large T-antigen transgene are faithful in their processing of POMC according to the pattern that exists in normal melanotropes.[18]

### PROENKEPHALIN, PRODYNORPHIN, AND PRONOCICEPTIN

Regional differences in the processing of proenkephalin and prodynorphin also exist. The adrenal glands of some species (e.g., bovine) are especially rich in enkephalins and provide a model for studying proenkephalin processing; the posterior pituitary is used in the study of prodynorphin processing. Proenkephalin contains six copies of ME and one of LE; however, as predicted by the positioning of paired dibasic amino acids, two of the ME sequences occur in two C-terminal–extended forms—ME-Arg-Gly-Leu and ME-Arg-Phe—which are stored and secreted intact. In adrenal glands, ME and LE account for only 20% of the total enkephalin peptides. The remainder consist of the larger, ME-containing peptides: peptide F, peptide I, peptide E, and peptide B.[13] This is in marked contrast to the brain, in which the immunoreactive enkephalins are largely ME, LE, ME-Arg-Phe, and ME-Arg-Gly-Leu. The gene for preprodynorphin encodes for three sequences of LE, multiple forms of dynorphin, and two neoendorphins, but not ME or β-END. Three LE sequences in prodynorphin form the N termini of α-neoendorphin, DYN A, and dynorphin B (DYN B). In some tissues, these peptides may be processed further to α-neoendorphin, DYN A$_{1-8}$, or LE. In the brain, levels of LE and DYN A$_{1-8}$ are considerably higher than those of longer prodynorphin products. Pronociceptin contains only one copy of N/OFQ in addition to at least one other peptide whose sequence is conserved across rodent and human species.[4,5,10] Although potential roles of N/OFQ in pain perception and anxiety are being revealed by genetic studies in mice lacking the nociceptin receptor,[19,20] functions of other products of pronociceptin remain to be determined.

## RECEPTORS FOR ENDOGENOUS OPIOIDS

Endogenous opioids serve as neuronal and endocrine cell regulators by interacting with opioid receptors. Four major types of opioid receptors are found, which have been given the following designations: μ, with preferential affinity for morphine and related drugs; δ, with preferential affinity for ME and LE; κ, with preferential affinity for DYN A and related peptides; and ORL-1, highly selective for N/OFQ. The mRNAs for each type of opioid receptor have been cloned and their amino-acid sequences determined.[21,22] Opioid-receptor mRNAs have been detected in brain and several peripheral tissues. The size of mRNA forms expressed in different tissues is variable.[21] Each receptor is composed of a single protein chain with seven putative transmembrane domains, placing these receptors in the large group of plasma membrane receptors whose effects are transduced by interactions with guanine nucleotide binding proteins (G proteins). Overall homology in the amino-acid sequences of μ, δ, κ, and ORL-1 receptors is greater than that between opioid receptors and other G protein–coupled receptors.[22]

The structural features necessary for binding or activation of each type of opioid receptor have been extensively studied, and subtypes of each of the major forms have been proposed.[23,24] The molecular basis for this apparent heterogeneity remains uncertain, however; the reported heterogeneity in mRNAs for each receptor type does not fully explain the functional evidence for receptor subtypes, raising the possibility that additional genes for the subtypes await identification. Receptors responding specifically to β-END (termed ε receptors) have also been proposed,[25] but these have not yet been cloned. The nature of proposed receptors in immune cells (mainly lymphocytes) with selectivity for β-END, β-LPH, and extended enkephalin-containing products of proenkephalin is also unknown.

## OPIOID RECEPTOR–EFFECTOR SYSTEMS

Opioid receptors are expressed in the plasma membranes of selected neuronal, endocrine, and immune system cells. Opioid-receptor protein can be observed in intracellular membrane fractions and presumably reflects newly synthesized receptor protein moving to the plasma membrane or internalized receptors destined for degradation or recycling back to the plasma membrane. Plasma membrane–bound opioid receptors regulate G proteins of the G$_i$ or G$_o$ type. Agonist activation of μ, δ, κ, or ORL-1 receptors facilitates the dissociation of guanosine diphosphate from the α subunits of the receptor-associated G protein. This allows guanosine triphosphate (GTP) to bind to the α subunit, triggering dissociation of the α subunit from the β and γ subunits. The liberated α subunit can now interact with effector proteins; as the effector is activated, the G protein α subunit hydrolyzes bound GTP to guanosine diphosphate (GDP). The βγ subunit complex may also play a role in opioid-receptor signal transduction. After hydrolysis of GDP, reassociation of the α and βγ subunits occurs. Thus, GTP is essential for opioid-receptor activation of effector systems.[26] Cellular effector systems regulated by opioid receptors are listed in Table 168-1. Opening of K$^+$ channels results in membrane hyperpolarization; closing of N-type Ca$^{2+}$ channels reduces neurotransmitter release.[26,27] Regulation of adenylate cyclases, activation of L-type Ca$^{2+}$ channels, or activation of mitogen-activated protein kinase may be involved in opioid-mediated regulation of gene expression and cell proliferation in some cell types.[28]

## LONG-TERM OPIOID TREATMENT: TOLERANCE AND DEPENDENCE

Long-term treatment with opiate drugs or opioid peptides may cause a state of tolerance; the opioid becomes less effec-

**TABLE 168-1.**
**Opioid Receptor Transduction Systems**

| Effector System | Opioid-Receptor Type | Effects of Opioid-Receptor Activation | G-Protein Transducer |
|---|---|---|---|
| Adenylate cyclase (type V)[52] | μ, δ, κ, and ORL-1 | Inhibition | αi |
| Adenylate cyclase (type II)[52] | μ, δ | Activation | βγ |
| Phospholipase C[53] | μ, δ | Activation | α, via $Ca^{2+}$ influx; possibly βγ |
| MAPK[28] | μ, δ, ORL-1 | Activation | Probably βγ |
| $K^+$ channels[26] | μ, δ, κ, and ORL-1 | Channel opening; in many cell types | Both α and βγ |
| $Ca^{2+}$ channels (N-type)[26] | μ, δ, κ, and ORL-1 | Channel closing; in neurons | Both α and βγ |
| $Ca^{2+}$ channels (L-type)[53] | μ, δ, κ | Channel opening; in neurons and nonneuronal cells | αi, other? |

*ORL-1*, opioid receptor–like clone 1; *MAPK*, mitogen-activated protein kinase.

tive in inducing a biologic response. In some systems, a state of dependence on the presence of opioid can also arise. In these systems, normal function requires the continued presence of opioid agonist. Dependence probably develops as a result of a compensatory increase in the activity of enzymes (e.g., adenylate cyclase) and other regulatory proteins whose activity is depressed during the acute phase of opioid action. Such enhanced activity may result from an increased rate of synthesis of the effector protein to compensate for the level of inhibition induced by the presence of opioid. If the opiate drug is removed, either by discontinuation of administration or by competition for the receptor sites by an antagonist opiate (e.g., naloxone), the increased level of effector protein results in a hyperactivity of the opioid-regulated pathway, which is manifest as the opiate withdrawal syndrome.[26] Enhanced activity of opioid-regulated effector systems also contributes to the tolerance to opioid action that occurs during long-term opiate drug treatment, but other factors may also play a part in tolerance. Long-term opioid treatment reduces the extent of coupling between opioid receptors and the G proteins, thereby mediating their effects and making receptor activation less effective. High concentrations of opioids may also induce a reduction in the number of receptors available to be activated. These adaptive changes in opioid effect, resulting from long-term opioid exposure, affect the activity of endogenous opioid peptides as well as opiate drugs. Receptor

sensitivity may recover quickly after discontinuation of opiate drug exposure, but changes in effector system activity, which may involve altered expression of certain proteins, can persist for days or even weeks.[26,27]

## DISTRIBUTION OF RECEPTORS

Opioid receptors of all types are distributed widely throughout the CNS and peripheral autonomic nervous system. Some correlation is seen between the distribution of receptors and that of endogenous opioid peptides. The correlation in distribution is not perfect, however, because the peptides are often synthesized in neural cell somata for secretion from axon terminals at a distant site. Considerable differences exist among species in the distribution of both endogenous opioids and their receptors (Table 168-2).

## RELATIONSHIP BETWEEN PHYSIOLOGIC FUNCTION AND RECEPTOR TYPE IN THE NERVOUS SYSTEM

Endogenous opioids play a modulatory role in the regulation of neural function. Complete blockade of opioid receptors with a nonselective antagonist like naltrexone does not produce a catastrophic disruption of function. A unique association of one endogenous opioid and one opioid-receptor type with a specific neural system also seldom is found.

**TABLE 168-2.**
**Properties of Receptors for Endogenous Opioids**

| Receptor Type | μ Receptors | δ Receptors | κ Receptors | ORL-1 Receptors |
|---|---|---|---|---|
| **SELECTIVE ENDOGENOUS OPIOIDS** | Endomorphins 1 and 2; β-casomorphin (low affinity) | Unknown | DYN A; DYN B; α-neo-END | N/OFQ |
| **ENDOGENOUS OPIOIDS WITH HIGH, BUT NONSELECTIVE, AFFINITY** | β-END; ME; LE; metorphamide; DYN $A_{1-8}$ | β-END; ME; LE; DYN $A_{1-8}$ | DYN $A_{1-8}$; β-neo-END | None |
| **SELECTIVE OPIATE DRUGS** | Morphine | | Ethylketocyclazocine*; U69593† | None |
| **ANTAGONISTS (NONSELECTIVE DRUGS APPEAR IN PARENTHESES)** | Naloxone‡; naltrexone‡ | ICI 174864¶ (naloxone‡) | Nor-binaltorphimine (naloxone‡) | None |
| **REGULATION OF AGONIST AFFINITY BY $Na^+$ AND GUANOSINE TRIPHOSPHATE** | Yes | Yes | Yes (weak) | Yes |
| **STRUCTURES WITH HIGH RECEPTOR CONCENTRATIONS IN CENTRAL NERVOUS SYSTEM** | Thalamus; pons–medulla; dorsal horn (spinal cord) | Limbic system; striatum; globus pallidus | Cortex; cerebellum (some species); dorsal horn (spinal cord) | Hypothalamus; amygdala; anterior olfactory nucleus; periaqueductal gray; brainstem |
| **PERIPHERAL TISSUES** | Myenteric plexus (gastrointestinal tract) | Vas deferens (mouse, hamster) | Myenteric plexus; vas deferens (rabbit); placenta (human) | Gastrointestinal tract; vas deferens; liver; spleen |

*ORL-1*, opioid receptor–like clone 1; *DYN*, dynorphin; *N/OFQ*, nociceptin/orphanin FQ; *neo-END*, neoendorphin; *END*, endorphin; *ME*, methionine enkephalin; *LE*, leucine enkephalin.
*Ethylketocyclazocine shows κ activity in pharmacologic assays and is an antagonist at μ receptors.
†U69593 is a selective agonist at κ receptors. The structure is (5a, 7a, 8b)-(-)-N-Met-N-(7-[1-pyrrolidinyl]-1-oxaspiron[4,5]-dec-8-yl)benzenacetamide.
‡Naloxone and naltrexone have preferential affinity for μ receptors, but at high concentrations they antagonize agonist effects at δ, κ, and ε receptors.
¶ICI 174864 is a selective antagonist at δ receptors. Its structure is N,N-diallyl-Tyr-Aib-Aib-Phe-Leu (Aib is α-amino isobutyric acid).

The roles of specific receptor types or specific opioid peptide gene products have been evaluated by examining changes in phenotype associated with specific gene deletions (Table 168-3). These studies confirm previous work indicating that natural opiates (such as morphine) and synthetic analog drugs (such as methadone or fentanyl) produce analgesia exclusively through μ receptors, the receptor type for which they have highest affinity. Receptors of the μ type are located at critical points in the major afferent sensory pathway from periphery to brain (e.g., in the dorsal horn of spinal cord and in several thalamic nuclei), as well as at critical points in descending pain control pathways (e.g., periaqueductal gray matter, ventral medulla), which serve to modulate activity in the afferent pain pathways. Endogenous opioid peptides and receptors of the δ, κ, and ORL-1 types are also present at several of these sites, suggesting that endogenous opioids and each of the major opioid-receptor types probably play a physiologic role in the regulation of pain sensitivity.[29,30]

Endogenous opioids also play a role in neural reinforcement pathways and motor control mechanisms. Dopamine release in the nigrostriatal, mesolimbic, and mesocortical systems is activated (indirectly) by μ and δ agonists, and inhibited by κ agonists acting directly on the dopamine neurons. Cells containing γ-aminobutyric acid (GABA) in the regions innervated by these dopamine-containing neurons also carry μ and δ receptors. These systems, in which endogenous opioids are also present in relatively high concentration, are primary locations for opiate-induced reinforcement and modulation of behaviors.

Hypothalamic β-END acts on μ receptors to decrease the pulsatile release of gonadotropin-releasing hormone, apparently by inhibiting nitric oxide–expressing interneurons involved in the activation and release of the hormone.[31,32] In the case of stress,[33] this mechanism is initiated through the local release of corticotropin-releasing hormone. Endogenous opioids also exert a reciprocal inhibitory tone over the secretion of corticotropin-releasing hormone; however, this regulation is complex, involving more than one opioid peptide and receptor subtype.[34]

Intracerebroventricular administration of N/OFQ exerts potent anxiogenic effects.[19] Because this peptide and its receptor, ORL-1, are present in relatively high concentrations in the amygdala, N/OFQ likely plays a physiologic role in anxiety and fear responses. Mice with deletion of the ORL-1 gene surprisingly showed enhanced learning abilities relative to controls (see Table 168-3), suggesting that the anxiogenic actions of endogenous N/OFQ might lead to some impairment of learning in complex environments.[20]

# HEMOCRINE AND PARACRINE FUNCTIONS

## PITUITARY PROOPIOMELANOCORTIN

### SYNTHESIS AND CONCENTRATIONS

Beta-END is cosynthesized and secreted with ACTH and β-LPH from the anterior pituitary. The intermediate lobe, present in most mammals but not in adult humans, contains higher concentrations of total endorphins (together with α-MSH), but 90% of this material consists of shorter, acetylated forms of β-END that are not active on conventional opioid receptors. In the anterior and intermediate lobes of pituitary, β-END synthesis is regulated by different mechanisms (Fig. 168-3).[35]

Normal circulating levels of peptides derived from POMC are as follows: β-END, 5 to 20 fmol/mL; β-LPH, 10 to 35 fmol/mL. In chronic pain, these values are 230 fmol/mL and 440 fmol/mL, respectively. After adrenalectomy, the levels increase markedly (β-END, 1700 fmol/mL; β-LPH, 7600 fmol/mL.

### PHYSIOLOGIC TARGETS

Physiologic targets for the POMC-derived peptides of the pituitary gland include the adrenal gland, melanophores, and, possibly, peripheral nerves carrying pain signals, cells of the gastrointestinal tract, and lymphocytes. Pituitary β-END and other pituitary peptides may exert some actions directly on the CNS, but firm evidence to support this hypothesis is lacking. Some evidence suggests that, in addition to ACTH, β-LPH may also act on the adrenal cortex, enhancing secretion of aldosterone. Primary afferent nociceptor neurons (PAN) respond with increasing firing frequency to intense mechanical, thermal, or chemical stimuli. These changes in firing rate, which ultimately result in the interneuronal release of substance P and the perception of pain, are modulated by endogenous opioid peptides. The μ receptors located on peripheral terminals of PAN decrease firing rate through a G protein–coupled mechanism. This response underlies the physiologic means for alteration of the perception of pain by circulating opioid peptides. These peripheral opioid receptors also respond to endogenous opioids secreted by immune cells infiltrating inflamed tissues,[36] in addition to those released by the pituitary and adrenal glands. The δ and κ receptor subtypes, present on central terminals of PAN, also reduce the release of substance P from PAN. In contrast, very low doses of N/OFQ, acting at ORL-1 receptors, facilitate release of substance P from the peripheral terminals of PAN. Second-order nociresponsive neurons in the dorsal horn express all four opioid-receptor subtypes, allowing endogenous and exogenous opioids to control directly the flow of information in

**TABLE 168-3.**
**Phenotypic Consequences of Deletions of Selected Opioid Peptide or Receptor Genes in Mice**

| Gene Deletion | Phenotype—Physiology | Phenotype—Pharmacology |
|---|---|---|
| μ Receptor[54] | Unchanged nociceptive threshold | Loss of morphine analgesia, respiratory depression, and behavioral reinforcement (reward) |
|  | Unchanged levels of δ and κ receptors | Impairment of immune function |
|  | Increased cell proliferation during hematopoiesis | Unchanged analgesic effects of κ-receptor agonists |
|  | Reduced sperm counts and impaired mating function in males | Reduced analgesic and respiratory depressant effects of some δ-receptor agonists |
| ORL-1 receptor[20] | Unchanged nociceptive threshold and locomotor activity | Loss of inhibition of locomotor activity by N/OFQ |
|  | Impaired adaptation to auditory stimuli |  |
|  | Facilitation of long-term potentiation and memory |  |
| Proenkephalin[55] | Unchanged levels of β-endorphin and dynorphin | (Not reported) |
|  | Unchanged stress-induced analgesic responses |  |
|  | Increased anxiety and aggressiveness |  |
|  | Hypersensitivity to noxious stimuli |  |

*ORL-1*, opioid receptor–like clone 1; *N/OFQ*, nociceptin/orphanin FQ.

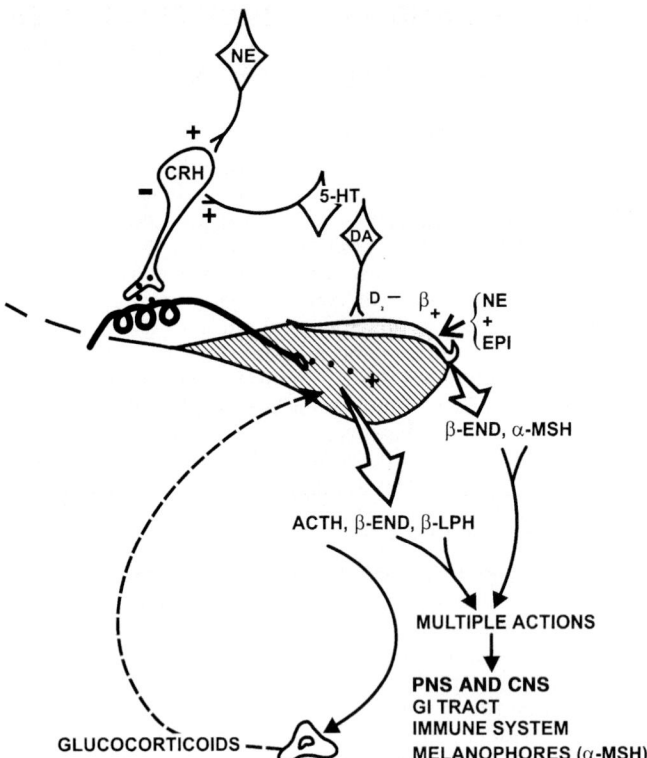

**FIGURE 168-3.** Pathway for secretion and regulation of pituitary opioid peptides. Brain norepinephrine (*NE*) and serotonin (*5-HT*) neurons evoke the release of corticotropin-releasing hormone (*CRH*) into hypophysial portal blood. In the anterior lobe, CRH stimulates corticotropes to release adrenocorticotropic hormone (*ACTH*), β-endorphin (*β-END*), and β-lipotropin (*β-LPH*) into the general circulation. ACTH enhances the secretion of adrenal cortisol, which, in turn, acts at the level of the hypothalamus to inhibit CRH release and at the level of the pituitary to inhibit CRH action. Release of β-END and melanotrope peptides from the intermediate lobe is stimulated directly by circulating NE and epinephrine (*EPI*) via a β-adrenergic receptor (*β*). By contrast, hypothalamic dopamine (*DA*) neurons innervate and tonically inhibit melanotrope secretion via a dopamine 2 (*D₂*)–receptor mechanism. (*α-MSH*, α-melanocyte-stimulating hormone; *PNS*, peripheral nervous system; *CNS*, central nervous system; *GI*, gastrointestinal.)

ascending pain pathways.[37] Neuronal release of opioid peptides also exerts control over nociception at sites within the central nervous system.

Lymphocytes express the conventional opiate receptors as well as receptors for both ACTH and β-END.[38–40] Speculation is that pituitary ACTH and β-END play a role in marshaling immune responses. The β-END–binding sites recognize the middle and C-terminal regions of β-END. This is in marked contrast to the classic opioid receptors, which require the N-terminal regions of opiate peptides. Lymphocytes express the POMC gene and store γ-END. Thus, to consider that lymphocytes themselves may be targets for the endorphin peptides they elaborate is not unreasonable. Endorphin peptides alter several functions of the immune system, including increasing T-cell blastogenesis, natural killer cell cytotoxicity, and tumor resistance. Evidence that the lymphokine interleukin-1 activates the release of POMC peptides from the pituitary gland indicates that the interaction between the neural and endocrine systems is bidirectional.[39,41] The mRNA for μ-type opioid receptors is also expressed in lymphocytes, and long-term morphine treatment is known to suppress immune system function. Immune cell death induced by Fas (a receptor on the cell surface that triggers cell death by apoptosis when activated by its ligand, FasL) is promoted by morphine treatment.[41]

## ENKEPHALIN AND DYNORPHIN IN THE PARS NERVOSA OF THE PITUITARY

Immunocytochemical studies have shown that ME, LE, DYN A, and DYN B are all present in the magnocellular neuronal perikaryon in the supraoptic and paraventricular nuclei of the hypothalamus,[42,43] and that they are cosequestered with vasopressin and oxytocin in the same neurosecretory vesicles of the pars nervosa. These peptides are probably coreleased in response to appropriate stimuli. Parallel changes in the levels of vasopressin and dynorphins in the pars nervosa after dehydration or hemorrhage have been reported.

The functions of opioids in the pars nervosa are only partially understood. The κ-type receptors are found in this structure. Because the molar ratio of vasopressin to DYN A in the rat pars nervosa is >500:1, the primary target of released dynorphin probably is within the pituitary itself. A paracrine role for secretory regulation of the neurohypophysial peptides seems likely, because opioid-induced modulation of vasopressin and oxytocin secretion from isolated neural lobes of rat pituitary has been reported. Also κ-selective agonists induce a profound diuresis,[44] whereas the opiate antagonist naloxone potentiates the stimulated release of vasopressin and oxytocin. Thus, evidence exists for opioid regulation of neurohypophysial peptide secretion.

## ENDOGENOUS OPIOIDS IN THE ADRENAL MEDULLA

Proenkephalin products are present in relatively high concentrations in the adrenal medulla of most species. In some species, including humans, opioids derived from prodynorphin and POMC are also present. The enkephalins are stored together with catecholamines in secretory vesicles of adrenal chromaffin cells and are secreted into adrenal venous blood after treatments that stimulate catecholamine secretion.[45] Studies have also revealed the presence of opioid receptors in adrenal medulla, a finding that suggests a local mechanism for controlling the release of adrenal catecholamines. Enkephalin-containing peptides are secreted into the circulation after splanchnic nerve stimulation to exert effects in other tissues. Although pentapeptide enkephalins are hydrolyzed very rapidly in circulating blood, a role for enkephalins secreted from the adrenal medulla in modulating the function of circulating cells of the immune system is likely. Finally, the colocalization of enkephalins with catecholamines, as well as the nature of some of the potential target sites for adrenal enkephalins, suggest that they may have a role that is complementary to that of the catecholamines in the physiologic response to stress.

## ENDOGENOUS OPIOIDS AND THE GASTROINTESTINAL TRACT

Both enkephalins and dynorphins are present in the neurons that innervate the gastrointestinal tract.[46,47] Enkephalins and dynorphins are present in many myenteric plexus neurons and a few neurons of the submucous plexus throughout the gastrointestinal tract. These neurons innervate sphincters, circular muscle, and longitudinal muscle of the stomach and intestine. The release of dynorphin-like material into the vascular perfusate of guinea pig intestine during peristalsis has been reported. The presence of μ, δ, and κ opioid receptors throughout the digestive tract[48] suggests that endogenous opioid peptides act locally in this system.

Gastrointestinal motility is substantially modified by opioids, but the effects often vary widely among species. In humans, opioids increase the tone of sphincters and the frequency of segmenting, nonpropulsive contractions of circular muscle. This action has been ascribed to the increased local release of serotonin by opioids. A reduction in nitric oxide–dependent neurotransmission may also be involved.[49] Concomitantly, the peristaltic reflex is depressed, and the contractions of longitudinal muscle are decreased as a result of a reduction in acetylcholine secretion. Enkephalins reduce secretions, both in the stomach and in the intestine. Thus, the propulsion of gastrointestinal contents is decreased, and water content is reduced. Opioids, therefore, provide symptomatic relief of diarrhea. These actions are all reversed by naloxone. Hydrolysis of the milk protein β-casein yields a peptide–β-casomorphin that has some activity at μ receptors.[50] In breast-fed neonates, this peptide may be produced locally in sufficient concentrations to reduce gastrointestinal activity.[51]

# REFERENCES

1. Hughes J, Smith TW, Kosterlitz HW, et al. Identification of two related pentapeptides from the brain with potent opiate agonist activity. Nature 1975; 258:577.
2. Cox BM. Endogenous opioid peptides: a guide to structures and terminology. Life Sci 1982; 31:1645.
3. Mollereau C, Parmentier M, Mailleux P, et al. ORL-1, a novel member of the opioid receptor family—cloning, functional expression and localization. FEBS Lett 1994; 341:33.
4. Meunier JC, Mollereau C, Toll L, et al. Isolation and structure of the endogenous agonist of opioid receptor-like ORL-1 receptor. Nature 1995; 377:532.
5. Reinscheid RK, Nothacker H-P, Bourson A, et al. Orphanin FQ: a neuropeptide that activates an opioidlike G protein-coupled receptor. Science 1995; 270:792.
6. Calo G, Guerrini R, Rizzi A, et al. Pharmacology of nociceptin and its receptor: a novel therapeutic target. Br J Pharmacol 2000; 129:1261.
7. Douglass J, Cox BM, Quinn B, et al. Expression of the prodynorphin gene in male and female mammalian reproductive tissues. Endocrinology 1987; 120:707.
8. Herbert E, Seasholtz A, Comb M, et al. Study of the regulation of expression of neuropeptide genes by gene transfer methods. In: Meltzer HY, ed. Psychopharmacology: the third generation of progress. New York: Raven Press 1987:373.
9. Leslie FM, Chen Y, Winzer-Serhan UH. Opioid receptor and peptide mRNA expression in proliferative zones of fetal rat central nervous system. Can J Physiol Pharmacol 1998; 76:284.
10. Mollereau C, Simons MJ, Soularue P, et al. Structure, tissue distribution, and chromosomal localization of the prenociceptin gene. Proc Natl Acad Sci U S A 1996; 93:8666.
11. Steiner DF. The proprotein convertases. Curr Opin Chem Biol 1998; 2:31.
12. Jackson RS, Creemers JW, Ohagi S, et al. Obesity and impaired prohormone processing associated with mutations in the human prohormone convertase 1 gene. Nat Genet 1997; 16:218.
13. Asteria C. Genetic alterations of enzymes involved in prohormone processing as common molecular mechanisms of human and rodent obesity. Eur J Endocrinol 1998; 139:150.
14. Prigge ST, Kolhekar AS, Eipper BA, et al. Amidation of bioactive peptides: the structure of peptidylglycine alpha-hydroxylating monooxygenase. Science 1997; 278:1300.
15. Bennett HPJ, Bradbury AF, Huttner WB, Smyth DG. Processing of propeptides: glycosylation, phosphorylation, sulfation, acetylation and amidation. In: Loh YP, ed. Mechanisms of intracellular trafficking and processing of proproteins. Boca Raton, FL: CRC Press, 1993:251.
16. Dickerson IM, Noül G. Tissue-specific peptide processing. In: Fricker LD, ed. Peptide biosynthesis and processing. Boca Raton, FL: CRC Press 1991:71.
17. Eipper BA, Bloomquist BT, Husten, et al. Peptidylglycine α-amidating monooxygenase and other processing enzymes in the neurointermediate pituitary. Ann N Y Acad Sci 1993; 689:147.
18. Low MJ, Liu B, Hammer GD, et al. Post-translational processing of proopiomelanocortin (POMC) in mouse pituitary melanotrope tumors induced by a POMC-simian virus 40 large T antigen transgene. J Biol Chem 1993; 268:24967.
19. Jenck G, Moreau JL, Martin JR, et al. Orphanin FQ acts as an anxiolytic to attenuate behavioral responses to stress. Proc Natl Acad Sci U S A 1997; 94:14854.
20. Manabe T, Noda Y, Mamiya T, et al. Facilitation of long-term potentiation and memory in mice lacking nociceptin receptors. Nature 1998; 394:577.
21. Evans CF, Keith DE Jr, Morrison H, et al. Cloning of a delta opioid receptor by functional expression. Science 1992; 258:1952.
22. Blake AD, Bot G, Reisine T. Structure-function analysis of the cloned opiate receptors: peptide and small molecule interactions. Chem Biol 1996; 3:967.
23. Jiang Q, Takemori AE, Sultana M, et al. Differential antagonism of opioid delta antinociception by [D-Ala², Leu⁵, Cys⁶]enkephalin and naltrindole 5′-isothiocyanate: evidence for delta receptor subtypes. J Pharmacol Exp Ther 1991; 257:1069.
24. Kim K-W, Cox BM. Inhibition of norepinephrine release from rat cortex slices by opioids: differences among agonists in sensitivities to antagonists suggest receptor heterogeneity. J Pharmacol Exp Ther 1993; 267:1153.
25. Schulz R, Wüster M, Herz A. Pharmacological characterization of the ε-opiate receptors. J Pharmacol Exp Ther 1981; 216:604.
26. Cox BM. Opioid receptor–G protein interactions: acute and chronic effects of opioids. In: Herz A, ed. Handbook of experimental pharmacology, vol 104/I. Opioids I. Berlin: Springer-Verlag, 1993:145.
27. Nestler EJ, Hope BT, Widnell KL. Drug addiction: a model for the molecular basis of neural plasticity. Neuron 1993; 11:995.
28. Ignatova EG, Belcheva MM, Bohn LM, et al. Requirement of receptor internalization for opioid stimulation of mitogen-activated kinase: biochemical and immunofluorescence confocal microscopic evidence. Neuroscience 1999; 19:56.
29. Fields HL. Brainstem mechanisms of pain modulation: anatomy and physiology. In: Hertz A, ed. Handbook of experimental pharmacology, Vol 104/II. Opioids II. Berlin: Springer-Verlag, 1993:3.
30. Aicher SA, Punnoose A, and Goldberg A. Mu-opioid receptors often colocalize with the substance P receptor (NK1) in the trigeminal dorsal horn. J Neurosci 2000; 20:4325.
31. Ferin M. Neuropeptides, the stress response, and the hypothalamic–pituitary–gonadal axis in the female rhesus monkey. Ann N Y Acad Sci 1993; 697:106.
32. Faletti AG, Mastronardi CA, Lomnuczi A, et al. β-Endorphin blocks luteinizing hormone releasing hormone release by inhibiting the nitricoxidergic pathway controlling its release. Proc Natl Acad Sci U S A 1999; 96:1722.
33. Rivest S, Plotsky PM, Rivier C. CRF alters the infundibular LHRH secretory system from the medial preoptic area of female rats: possible involvement of opioid receptors. Neuroendocrinology 1993; 57:236.
34. Pechnick RN. Effects of opioids on the hypothalamic-pituitary-adrenal axis. Annu Rev Pharmacol Toxicol 1993; 32:353.
35. Vale W, Rivier J, Guillemin R, Rivier C. Effects of purified CRF and other substances on the secretion of beta-endorphin-like immunoreactivities by cultured anterior or neurointermediate pituitary cells. In: Collu R, Barbeau A, Ducharme JR, Rochefort J-G, eds. Central nervous system effects of hypothalamic hormones and other peptides. New York: Raven Press, 1979:163.
36. Schäfer M, Carter L, Stein C. Interleukin 1β and corticotrophin-releasing factor inhibit pain by releasing opioids from immune cells in inflamed tissue. Proc Natl Acad Sci U S A 1994; 91:4219.
37. Levine JD, Fields HL, Basbaum AI. Peptides and the primary afferent nociceptor. J Neurosci 1993; 13:2273.
38. Peterson PK, Molitor TW, Chao CC. The opioid-cytokine connection. J Neuroimmunol 1998: 83:63.
39. Sapolsky R, Rivier C, Yamamoto G, et al. Interleukin-1 stimulates the secretion of hypothalamic corticotropin-releasing factor. Science 1987; 238:522.
40. Blalock JE. Proopiomelamoncortin and the immune-neuroendocrine connection. Ann NY Acad Sci 1999: 885:161.
41. Yin D, Mufson RA, Wang R, Shi Y. Fas-mediated cell death promoted by opioids. Nature 1999; 397:218.
42. Martin R, Geis R, Holl R, et al. Co-existence of unrelated peptides in oxytocin and vasopressin terminals of rat neurohypophyses: immunoreactive methionine⁵-enkephalin-, leucine⁵-enkephalin-, and cholecystokinin-like substances. Neuroscience 1983; 8:213.
43. Eriksson M, Ceccatelli S, Uvnas-Moberg K, et al. Expression of Fos-related antigens, oxytocin, dynorphin and galanin in the paraventricular and supraoptic nuclei of lactating rats. Neuroendocrinology 1996; 63:356.
44. Leander JD. A kappa opioid effect: increased urination in the rat. J Pharmacol Exp Ther 1983; 224:89.
45. Chaminade M, Foutz AS, Rossier J. Co-release of enkephalins and precursors with catecholamines from perfused cat adrenal gland in situ. J Physiol 1984; 353:157.
46. Yuferov VP, Culpepper-Morgan JA, La Forge KS, et al. Regional quantitation of preprodynorphin mRNA in guinea pig gastrointestinal tract. Neurochem Res 1998; 23:505.
47. Kromer W. Endogenous and exogenous opioids in the control of gastrointestinal motility and secretion. Pharmacol Rev 1989; 40:121.
48. Wittert G, Hope P, Pyle D. Tissue distribution of opioid receptor gene expression in the rat. Biochem Biophys Res Commun 1996; 218:877.
49. Bayguinov O, Sanders KM. Regulation of neural responses in the canine pyloric sphincter by opioids. Br J Pharmacol 1993; 108:1024.
50. Brantl V, Teschemacher H, Blasig J, et al. Opioid activities of beta-casomorphins. Life Sci 1981; 28:1903.
51. Froetschel MA. Bioactive peptides in digesta that regulate gastrointestinal function and intake. J Anim Sci 1999; 74:2500.
52. Avidor-Reiss T, Nevo I, Saya D, et al. Opiate-induced adenylyl cyclase superactivation is isozyme-specific. J Biol Chem 1997; 272:5040.
53. Smart D, Hirst RA, Hirota K, et al. The effects of recombinant rat μ-opioid receptor activation in CHO cells on phospholipase C, [Ca²⁺]i and adenylyl cyclase. Br J Pharmacol 1997; 120:1165.
54. Matthes HWD, Maldonaldo R, Simonin F, et al. Loss of morphine-induced analgesia, reward effect and withdrawal symptoms in mice lacking the μ-opioid-receptor gene. Nature 1996; 383:819.
55. König M, Zimmer AM, Steiner H, et al. Pain responses, anxiety and aggression in mice deficient in pre-proenkephalin. Nature 1996; 383:535.

# CHAPTER 169

# SOMATOSTATIN

YOGESH C. PATEL

Somatostatin (SST) was first found in the mammalian hypothalamus as a tetradecapeptide (SST-14), which inhibited the release of growth hormone (GH). It has since come to be known as a multifunctional hormone that is also produced throughout the central nervous system and in most peripheral organs. Somatostatin acts on a diverse array of endocrine, exocrine, neuronal, and immune cell targets to inhibit secretion, to modulate neurotransmission, and to regulate cell growth. These actions are mediated by a family of G protein–coupled receptors with five distinct subtypes (termed SSTR1 through SSTR5). SST is best regarded as an endogenous inhibitory regulator of the secretory and proliferative responses of many different target cells. In addition, the peptide may be of importance in the pathophysiology of several diseases such as neoplasia, inflammation, Alzheimer and Huntington diseases, and acquired immunodeficiency syndrome (AIDS), and has found a number of clinical applications in the diagnosis and treatment of neuroendocrine tumors and various gastrointestinal disorders.[1-8]

## SOMATOSTATIN GENES AND GENE PRODUCTS

Like other protein hormones, somatostatin is synthesized as part of a large precursor protein (proSST) that is processed to generate two bioactive forms, SST-14 and SST-28 (Fig. 169-1). In humans only one somatostatin gene is found, located on the long arm of chromosome 3, which encodes for both SST-14 and SST-28, whereas lower vertebrates (e.g., fish) have two somatostatin genes that separately encode for SST-14 or SST-28.[2,4,8] The

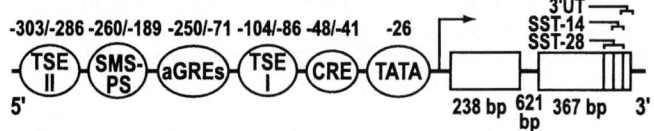

**FIGURE 169-2.** Schematic depiction of the rat somatostatin gene and its regulatory domains. The mRNA coding region consists of two exons of 238 and 367 base pairs (*bp*) separated by an intron of 621 bp. Located upstream (i.e., 5′ end) from the start site of mRNA transcription (*arrow*) are the regulatory elements TATA, cyclic adenosine monophosphate response element (*CRE*), atypical glucocorticoid response element (*aGRE*), and somatostatin promoter silence element (*SMS-PS*). Tissue-specific elements (*TSE*) consisting of TATA motifs that operate in concert with CRE to provide high-level constitutive activity are shown. (*3′UT*, 3′ untranslated region; *SST-14*, somatostatin-14; *SST-28*, somatostatin-28.)

transcriptional unit of the rat SST gene consists of exons of 238 and 367 base pairs (bp) separated by an intron of 621 bp (Fig. 169-2). The 5′-upstream region contains a number of regulatory elements for tissue-specific and extracellular signals, including a cyclic adenosine monophosphate (cAMP) response element (CRE) and two nonconsensus glucocorticoid response elements (GREs).[2,4] The SST-14 sequence has been totally conserved throughout vertebrate evolution, whereas the amino-acid structure of SST-28 has changed ~30% during evolution from fish to humans.[2,4,8] A novel second SST-like gene, *cortistatin (CST)*, which has been described in humans, yields two cleavage products, CST-17 and CST-29, which are comparable to SST-14 and SST-28 (see Fig. 169-1).[9] The CST peptides interact with all five SSTRs, but unlike somatostatin, expression of cortistatin is restricted to the cerebral cortex and its biofunction(s) remains unknown.[3,9]

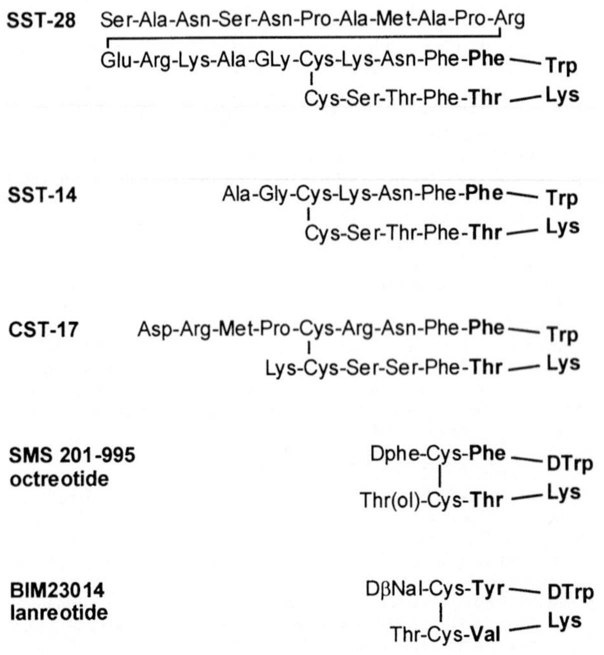

## ANATOMIC DISTRIBUTION OF SOMATOSTATIN CELLS

Somatostatin-producing cells occur in high densities throughout the central and peripheral nervous systems, and in the endocrine pancreas and gut. They occur in smaller numbers in the thyroid, adrenal medulla, testes, prostate, submandibular gland, kidneys, and placenta[1,8,10] (Table 169-1). The typical morphologic appearance of an SST cell is that of a neuron with multiple branching processes, or of a secretory cell, often with short cytoplasmic extensions (D cells). In the brain, the highest concentrations of SST are found in the hypothalamus, neocortex, and basal ganglia, throughout the limbic system, and at all levels of the major sensory systems.[1,8,10,11] The approximate relative amounts of SST in the major regions of the brain are as follows: cerebral cortex, 49%; spinal cord, 30%; brainstem, 12%; hypothalamus, 7%; olfactory lobe, 1%; and cerebellum, 1%.[11]

SST cells in the pancreas are almost exclusively islet D cells and account for 2% to 3% of the total adult islet cell population.[12] Gut SST cells are of two types: D cells in the mucosa and neurons that are intrinsic to the submucous and myenteric plexuses.[13] In the thyroid, SST coexists with calcitonin in a subpopulation of C cells.[1] In addition to these typical SST-producing neuroendocrine cells, which secrete large amounts of the peptide from storage pools, inflammatory and immune cells also produce SST, usually in small amounts on activation.[14,15] In the rat, the gut accounts for ~65% of total body SST, whereas lesser amounts occur in the brain (25%), the pancreas (5%), and the remaining organs (5%).

The relative proportions of SST-14 and SST-28 synthesized and secreted vary considerably in different tissues.[4] SST-14 is the predominant form in the brain, pancreas, upper gut, and enteric neurons, whereas SST-28 is an important constituent of brain and is the predominant molecular form in the intestinal mucosa.

**SST-28**    Ser-Ala-Asn-Ser-Asn-Pro-Ala-Met-Ala-Pro-Arg
Glu-Arg-Lys-Ala-GLy-Cys-Lys-Asn-Phe-**Phe** — **Trp**
Cys-Ser-Thr-Phe-**Thr** — **Lys**

**SST-14**    Ala-Gly-Cys-Lys-Asn-Phe-**Phe** — **Trp**
Cys-Ser-Thr-Phe-**Thr** — **Lys**

**CST-17**    Asp-Arg-Met-Pro-Cys-Arg-Asn-Phe-**Phe** — **Trp**
Lys-Cys-Ser-Ser-Phe-**Thr** — **Lys**

**SMS 201-995 octreotide**    Dphe-Cys-**Phe** — **DTrp**
Thr(ol)-Cys-**Thr** — **Lys**

**BIM23014 lanreotide**    DβNal-Cys-**Tyr** — **DTrp**
Thr-Cys-**Val** — **Lys**

**FIGURE 169-1.** Structure of naturally occurring somatostatin peptides. (*SST-28*, somatostatin-28; *SST-14*, somatostatin-14; *CST-17*, human cortistatin-17.) Amino-acid residues necessary for bioactivity are shown in bold. Octreotide and lanreotide are synthetic somatostatin analogs.

**TABLE 169-1.**
**Localization of Somatostatin**

| Body Region | Type of Cells | Locale |
|---|---|---|
| **MAJOR SITES** | | |
| Nervous system | Neurons | Hypothalamus |
| | | Cerebral cortex |
| | | Limbic system |
| | | Basal ganglia |
| | | Major sensory systems |
| | | Spinal cord |
| | | Dorsal root ganglia |
| | | Autonomic ganglia |
| Pancreas | D cells | Islets |
| Gut | D cells | Mucosal glands |
| | Neurons | Submucous and myenteric plexuses |
| **MINOR SITES** | | |
| Adrenal | — | Scattered medullary cells |
| Placenta | — | Cytotrophoblasts in chorionic villi |
| Reproductive organs | — | Testis, epididymis, prostate |
| Submandibular gland | D cells | Scattered ductal cells |
| Thyroid | C cells | Scattered parafollicular cells (coexisting with calcitonin) |
| Urinary system | — | Scattered cells in renal glomerulus and collecting ducts |

## SOMATOSTATIN IN THE PLASMA AND OTHER BODY FLUIDS

Both SST-14 and SST-28 are released readily from tissues and are detected in blood.[1,4,8,16] The main source of circulating SST is the gastrointestinal tract.[17] Circulating SST is inactivated rapidly by the liver and kidneys. The plasma half-life of SST-14 is 2 to 3 minutes, whereas that of SST-28 is slightly longer.[4] Fasting plasma concentrations of SST-like immunoreactivity (SST-LI) range from 5 to 18 pmol/L. These levels double in response to the ingestion of a mixed meal.[4] The bioactive circulating forms consist of SST-14, des-Ala[1] SST-14 (a postsecretory conversion product of SST-14), and SST-28.[16] With few exceptions, fluctuations in peripheral plasma levels of SST-LI are small. The main clinical utility of plasma measurements is in the diagnosis of SST-producing tumors, which are associated with marked hypersomatostatinemia.

SST is secreted into the cerebrospinal fluid (CSF), probably from all parts of the brain.[18,19] It is stable in this medium and attains a concentration that is approximately twice that in the general circulation. Significant amounts are also excreted in the urine (4–6 pmol/L). Semen contains high levels of SST-LI, 200-fold greater than those in plasma. Amniotic fluid is rich in SST-LI originating from the fetus.

## REGULATION OF SOMATOSTATIN SECRETION AND GENE EXPRESSION

Because SST cells are so widely distributed and interact with many different body systems, the fact that the secretion of SST can be influenced by a broad array of secretagogues, ranging from ions and nutrients to neuropeptides, neurotransmitters, classic hormones, and growth factors, is not surprising.[1,2,4,8] Glucagon, GH-releasing hormone (GHRH), neurotensin, corticotropin-releasing hormone (CRH), calcitonin gene–related peptide (CGRP), and bombesin are potent stimulators of SST release, whereas opioids and γ-aminobutyric acid (GABA) generally inhibit SST secretion.[1,4,8] Of the various hormones studied, thyroid hormones enhance SST secretion from the hypothalamus; their effect on secretion from other tissues has not been ade-

quately investigated.[4,8] Glucocorticoids exert a dose-dependent biphasic effect on SST secretion; low doses are stimulatory and high doses are inhibitory.[4] Insulin stimulates hypothalamic SST release but has an inhibitory effect on the release of SST from islet and gut.[4] Finally, members of the growth factor–cytokine family such as GH, insulin-like growth factor-I (IGF-I), interleukin-1 (IL-1), tumor necrosis factor-α (TNF-α), and interleukin-6 (IL-6) are capable of stimulating SST secretion from brain cells.[2]

Many of the agents that influence SST secretion also regulate SST gene expression.[2,4,8] Steady-state SST mRNA levels are stimulated by growth factors and cytokines (e.g., GH, IGF-I, IGF-II, IL-1, TNF-α, IL-6, interferon-γ, and interleukin-10), glucocorticoids, testosterone, estradiol, and N-methyl-D-aspartate–receptor agonists; and are inhibited by insulin, leptin, and transforming growth factor-β (TGF-β). Among the intracellular mediators known to modulate SST gene expression are $Ca^{2+}$, cAMP, cyclic guanosine monophosphate (cGMP), and nitric oxide (NO).[2,4,8] Activation of the adenylate cyclase–cAMP pathway plays an important role in the stimulation of SST secretion and gene transcription.[20] Cyclic AMP–dependent transcriptional enhancement is mediated by the nuclear protein *cAMP response element–binding protein (CREB)*, which binds to the cAMP response element on the SST gene.[20] $Ca^{2+}$-dependent induction of the SST gene occurs through phosphorylation of CREB by the $Ca^{2+}$-dependent protein kinase I and protein kinase II. GH, IGF-I, IGF-II, and glucocorticoids have all been shown to induce the SST gene by direct interaction with its promoter.[4] The molecular mechanisms underlying the effects of estrogens, testosterone, cGMP, and NO on SST mRNA levels remain to be determined.[4]

## ACTIONS OF SOMATOSTATIN

SST not only has wide anatomic distribution, but also acts on multiple targets, including the brain, pituitary, endocrine and exocrine pancreas, gut, kidney, adrenal, thyroid, and immune cells[1,2,7,8] (Fig. 169-3). Its actions include inhibition of virtually every known endocrine and exocrine secretion, and of various neurotransmitters; behavioral and autonomic effects if centrally administered; and effects on gastrointestinal and biliary motility, vascular smooth muscle tone, and intestinal absorption of nutrients and ions. SST also blocks the release of growth factors (e.g., IGF-I, epidermal growth factor [EGF], and platelet-derived growth factor [PDGF]) and cytokines (e.g., IL-6, interferon-γ), and inhibits the proliferation of lymphocytes and of inflammatory, intestinal mucosal, and cartilage and bone precursor cells.[2] All of these diverse effects of SST can be explained by its inhibition of two key cellular processes, secretion and cell proliferation.

## SOMATOSTATIN RECEPTORS, RECEPTOR SUBTYPES, AND SIGNAL TRANSDUCTION

Somatostatin acts through high-affinity plasma membrane receptors that are pharmacologically heterogeneous and feature several different isoforms.[2,3,5,6,21] Molecular cloning has revealed a family of five structurally related SSTR subtype genes that encode for seven transmembrane domain, G protein–coupled receptor proteins that display distinct agonist-binding profiles for natural and synthetic SST peptides[2,3,21] (Table 169-2). Receptor types 1 through 4 bind SST-14 and SST-28 approximately equally, whereas the type 5 receptor displays relative selectivity for binding of SST-28.[2,3,21] Four of the genes (the exception is SSTR2) appear to have no introns. Each of the receptor genes is located on a separate chromosome. The mRNA for individual human SSTR subtypes is widely expressed in brain, pituitary, pancreatic islets, stomach, jejunum, colon, lung, kidney, and liver, with a characteristic tissue-specific pattern for each receptor.[2,3,21,22] Typically, more than one subtype occurs in a given tar-

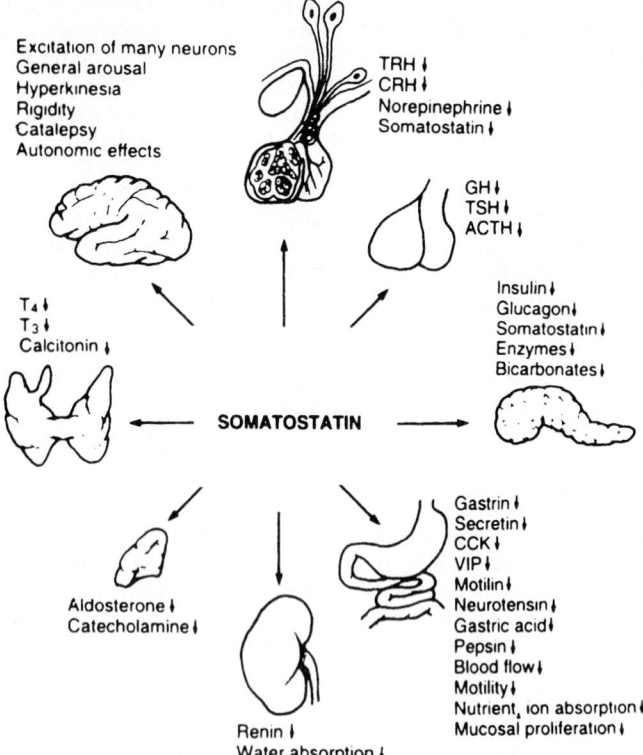

**FIGURE 169-3.** Principal actions of somatostatin. Somatostatin inhibits the release of dopamine from the midbrain and of norepinephrine, thyrotropin-releasing hormone (*TRH*), corticotropin-releasing hormone (*CRH*), and endogenous somatostatin from the hypothalamus. It also inhibits both the basal and the stimulated secretion of growth hormone (*GH*), thyroid-stimulating hormone (*TSH*), and islet hormones. It has no effect on luteinizing hormone (*LH*), follicle-stimulating hormone (*FSH*), prolactin, or adrenocorticotropic hormone (*ACTH*) in normal subjects. It does, however, suppress elevated ACTH levels in Addison disease and in ACTH-producing tumors. In addition, it inhibits the basal and the TRH-stimulated release of prolactin in vitro and diminishes elevated prolactin levels in acromegaly. In the gastrointestinal tract, somatostatin inhibits the release of virtually every gut hormone that has been tested. It has a generalized inhibitory effect on gut exocrine secretion (gastric acid, pepsin, bile, colonic fluid) and suppresses motor activity generally, through inhibition of gastric emptying, gallbladder contraction, and small intestine segmentation. Somatostatin, however, stimulates migrating motor complex activity. The effects of somatostatin on the thyroid include inhibition of the TSH-stimulated release of thyroxine ($T_4$) and triiodothyronine ($T_3$). The adrenal effects consist of the inhibition of angiotensin II–stimulated aldosterone secretion and the inhibition of acetylcholine-stimulated medullary catecholamine secretion. In the kidneys, somatostatin inhibits the release of renin stimulated by hypovolemia and inhibits antidiuretic hormone (*ADH*)–mediated water absorption. (*CCK*, cholecystokinin; *VIP*, vasoactive intestinal peptide.) (Modified from Patel YC. General aspects of the biology and function of somatostatin. In: Weil C, Muller EE, Thorner MO, eds. Somatostatin. Basic and clinical aspects of neuroscience series, vol 4. Berlin: Springer-Verlag, 1992:1.)

get tissue (e.g., SSTR1 through SSTR5 in the brain, stomach, pancreatic islets, and aorta; SSTR1, SSTR2, SSTR3, and SSTR5 in the pituitary). SSTR2 is the most abundantly expressed subtype, in terms of both the number of tissues that express this receptor and the level of expression. It is preferentially expressed by islet A cells and immune cells. SSTR1 and SSTR5 are the main subtypes expressed by islet B cells.[23] SSTR2 and SSTR5 are the principal subtypes found in somatotropes.

SST receptors elicit their cellular responses through G protein–linked modulation of multiple second messenger systems (Fig. 169-4), including (a) receptor coupling to adenylate cyclase, (b) receptor coupling to K+ channels, (c) receptor coupling to Ca2+ channels, (d) receptor coupling to exocytotic vesicles, (e) receptor

**TABLE 169-2.**
**Characteristics of Cloned Human Somatostatin Receptor (hSSTR), Types 1–5**

| | hSSTR1 | hSSTR2 | hSSTR3 | hSSTR4 | hSSTR5 |
|---|---|---|---|---|---|
| Amino acids | 391 | 369 | 418 | 388 | 363 |
| Chromosomal location | 14 | 17 | 22 | 20 | 16 |
| Agonist binding* | | | | | |
| SST-14 | ++ | ++ | ++ | ++ | ++ |
| SST-28 | ++ | ++ | ++ | ++ | +++ |
| Octreotide | – | ++ | + | – | ++ |
| Lanreotide | – | ++ | + | – | ++ |
| G-protein coupling | Yes | Yes | Yes | Yes | Yes |
| Effector coupling | | | | | |
| Adenylate cyclase activity | ↓ | ↓ | ↓ | ↓ | ↓ |
| Tyrosine phosphatase activity | ↑ | ↑ | ↑ | ↑ | ↑ |
| MAPK activity | ↑ | ↓ | ↓↑ | ↑ | ↓ |
| Tissue distribution+ | | | | | |
| Brain | Yes | Yes | Yes | Yes | Yes |
| Pituitary | Yes | Yes | Yes | | Yes |
| Islet | Yes | Yes | Yes | Yes | Yes |
| Stomach | Yes | Yes | Yes | Yes | Yes |
| Liver | Yes | | | | |
| Lungs | | | | Yes | |
| Kidneys | Yes | Yes | | | |
| Placenta | | | | Yes | |

↑, increased; ↓, decreased; *SST-14*, somatostatin-14; *SST-28*, somatostatin-28; *MAPK*, mitogen-activated protein kinase.

*Binding potency shown is based on the concentration required for half maximal inhibition of binding ($IC_{50}$) value for each agonist: –, $IC_{50}$ 150–1000 nM; +, $IC_{50}$ 10–20 nM; ++, $IC_{50}$ 1–10 nM; +++, $IC_{50}$ <1 nM.

+Not all tissues have been tested simultaneously.

(Data from Patel YC. Somatostatin and its receptor family. Frontiers Neuroendocrinol 1999; 20:157; Patel YC. Molecular pharmacology of somatostatin receptor subtypes. J Endocrinol Invest 1997; 20:348; Lamberts SWJ, Van Der Lely A-J, de Herder WW. Drug therapy: octreotide. N Engl J Med 1996; 334:246; and Reisine T, Bell GI. Molecular biology of somatostatin receptors. Endocr Rev 1995; 16:427.)

coupling to phosphotyrosyl protein phosphatase (PTP), and (f) receptor coupling to the mitogen-activated protein kinase (MAPK) pathway.[2,3,21] The five receptors share common signaling pathways, such as the inhibition of adenylate cyclase, activation of PTP, and modulation of MAPK[2] (see Table 169-2). SSTR2, SSTR3, SSTR4, and SSTR5 are coupled to K+ channels; SSTR1 and SSTR2, to voltage-dependent Ca2+ channels; SSTR2 and SSTR5, to phospholipase C; and SSTR1, to a Na+/H+ exchanger.[2]

## SOMATOSTATIN RECEPTOR–MEDIATED INHIBITION OF SECRETION AND CELL PROLIFERATION

The pronounced ability of SST to block regulated secretion from many different cells is due in part to receptor-induced inhibition of two key intracellular mediators, cAMP and Ca2+, because of receptor-linked effects on adenylate cyclase and on K+ and Ca2+ ion channels[2] (see Fig. 169-4). In addition, SST inhibits secretion stimulated by cAMP, Ca2+ ions, or any other known second messenger through a distal effect, which is targeted directly to secretory granules and is dependent on activation of the protein phosphatase cal-

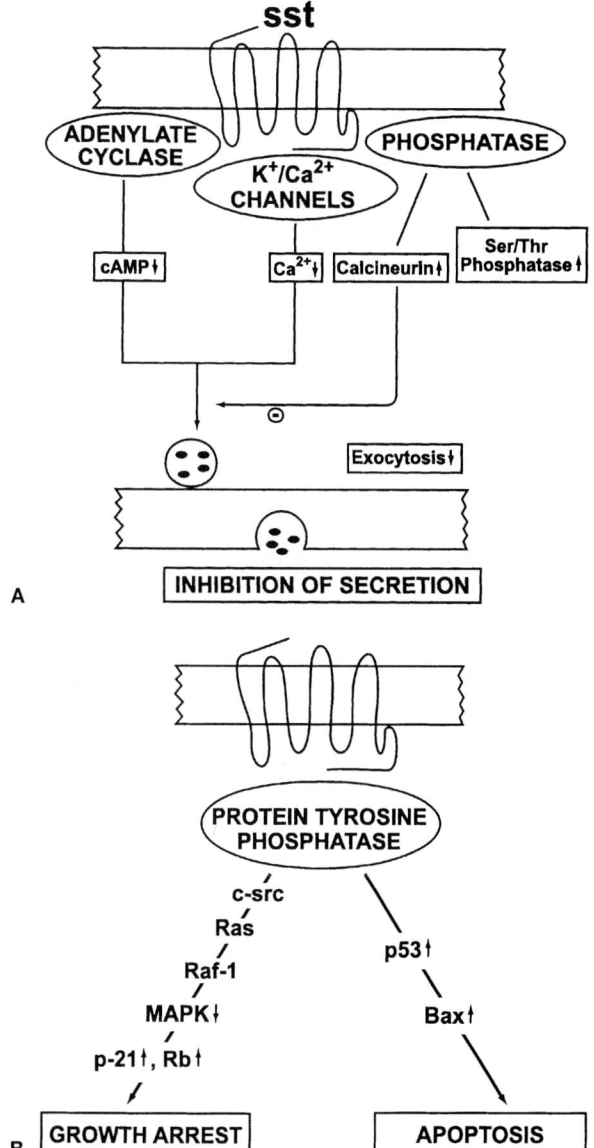

**A**

**B**

**FIGURE 169-4.** Schematic depiction of somatostatin-receptor (*SSTR*)–signaling pathways leading to inhibition of secretion (**A**) and to cell proliferation and induction of apoptosis (**B**). Receptor activation leads to a fall in intracellular cyclic adenosine monophosphate (*cAMP*) (due to inhibition of adenylate cyclase), a fall in Ca²⁺ influx (due to activation of K⁺ and Ca²⁺ ion channels), and stimulation of phosphatases such as *calcineurin*, which inhibits exocytosis, and *serine threonine (Ser/Thr) phosphatases*, which dephosphorylate and activate Ca²⁺ and K⁺ channel proteins. Blockade of secretion by somatostatin (*SST*) is in part mediated through inhibition of Ca²⁺ and cAMP (proximal effect) and through a more potent distant effect involving direct inhibition of exocytosis via SST-dependent activation of calcineurin. Induction of protein tyrosine phosphatase by SST plays a key role in mediating cell growth arrest (via SSTR1, SSTR2, SSTR4, SSTR5), or apoptosis (via SSTR3). Cell growth arrest is dependent on activation of the mitogen-activated protein kinase (*MAPK*) pathway and induction of *Rb (retinoblastoma tumor-suppressor protein)*, and *p21 (cyclin-dependent kinase inhibitor)*. C-src, which associates with both the activated receptor and phosphotyrosyl protein phosphatase (*PTP*), may provide the link between the receptor, PTP, and the mitogenic signaling complex. Induction of apoptosis is associated with dephosphorylation-dependent activation of the tumor-suppressor protein p53 and the proapoptotic protein Bax. (From Patel YC. Somatostatin and its receptor family. Frontiers Neuroendocrinol 1999; 20:157.)

cineurin.[2,3,7] The antiproliferative effects of SST were recognized through the use of long-acting analogs (i.e., octreotide) for the treatment of hormone hypersecretion from pancreatic, intestinal, and pituitary tumors. SST not only blocked hormone hypersecre-

tion from these tumors but also caused variable tumor shrinkage through an additional antiproliferative effect. The antiproliferative effects of SST have since been demonstrated in normal dividing cells (e.g., intestinal mucosal cells), in activated lymphocytes, and in inflammatory cells as well as in vivo in solid tumors and various cultured tumor cell lines.[2] These effects involve cytostatic (growth arrest) and cytotoxic (apoptotic) actions. SST acts directly (via SSTRs present on tumor cells) and indirectly (via SSTRs present on nontumor cell targets) to inhibit the secretion of hormones and growth factors that support angiogenesis and promote tumor growth. Several SSTR subtypes and signal-transduction pathways have been implicated[2,3,21] (see Fig. 169-4). Most interest is focused on protein phosphatases that dephosphorylate receptor tyrosine kinases or modulate the MAPK-signaling cascade, thereby attenuating mitogenic signal transduction.[24,25] Four of the receptors (SSTR1, SSTR2, SSTR4, SSTR5) induce cell-cycle arrest via PTP-dependent modulation of MAPK associated with induction of the retinoblastoma tumor-suppressor protein and p21.[2] In contrast, SSTR3 uniquely triggers PTP-dependent apoptosis accompanied by activation of p53 and the proapoptotic protein Bax.[26]

## PHYSIOLOGIC SIGNIFICANCE OF SOMATOSTATIN

Evidence is growing, both direct and indirect, that SST modulates the physiologic function of various target cells.[1,2,4,5,8] It subserves mainly local regulatory functions, acting as either a neurotransmitter or neuromodulator; a neurosecretory substance (i.e., one released directly from nerve axons into the bloodstream as in the median eminence); or a paracrine-autocrine regulator (local cell-to-cell interaction or self-regulation). In addition, SST may act via the circulation as a true endocrine substance to influence distant targets.

Direct evidence exists of a physiologic role for hypothalamic SST in the regulation of GH and thyroid-stimulating hormone (TSH) secretion by the pituitary.[1,8,27] A variety of physiologic GH responses are orchestrated by SST, acting either alone or in concert with GHRH.[1,8,27] SST participates in the genesis of the normal pulsatile pattern of GH secretion and in GH regulatory responses to physiologic stimuli such as stress, glucose administration, or food deprivation. GHRH and SST neurons in the hypothalamus are anatomically coupled and influence each other reciprocally.[8,27] SST inhibits GH secretion both by a direct action on the pituitary, and indirectly through suppression of GHRH release (Fig. 169-5). The secretion of SST in turn is stimulated by GHRH and is subject to positive feedback regulation by GH (*short loop*) and by IGF-I produced by GH action on the liver (*long loop*). Because of the extensive extrahypothalamic brain distribution of SST, its effects on the spontaneous electrical activity of neurons, its release from nerve endings in response to depolarization, and its behavioral effects, this peptide has been postulated to serve as a central neurotransmitter or neuromodulator.[1,5] Given the high concentration of both SST neuronal elements and SSTRs in limbic, neocortical, striatal, and sensory areas, SST appears to be particularly important in modulating functions in these regions. Within the pancreatic islets, the close anatomic proximity of SST cells to the A and B cells, the demonstration that insulin and glucagon are exquisitely sensitive to inhibition by low concentrations of SST, and the finding that inactivation of islet D-cell function augments insulin and glucagon output, all provide evidence for the possible modulation of pancreatic islet A- and B-cell function by SST[4,8] (Fig. 169-6). The suggestion has been made that islet D cells, which produce predominantly SST-14 and only negligible amounts of SST-28, regulate A cells by local action, whereas SST-28 released in the circulation from the gut in response to food ingestion modulates nutrient-stimulated insulin release by a hemocrine mechanism.[28] The diffuse distribution of SST throughout the gut, together with its pleiotropic effects and the complex regulation

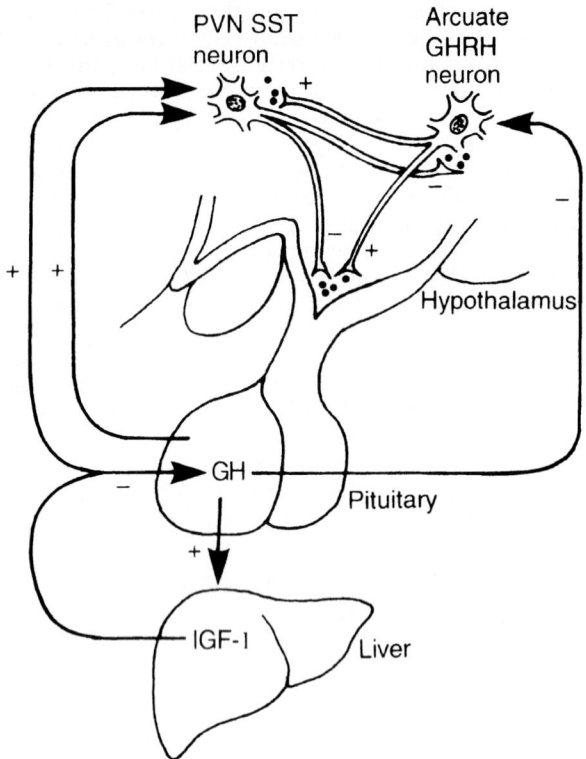

**FIGURE 169-5.** Schematic representation of the interaction between soma-tostatin (*SST*), growth hormone–releasing hormone (*GHRH*), growth hormone (*GH*), and insulin-like growth factor-I (*IGF-I*) in regulating GH secretion. GH release is stimulated by GHRH (produced by GHRH neurons in the arcuate nucleus) and inhibited by SST (produced by soma-tostatinergic neurons in the anterior hypothalamic periventricular nucleus [*PVN*]). SST inhibits GH secretion both by direct action at the pituitary level and indirectly through suppression of GHRH release. GHRH, in turn, stimulates SST secretion. GH exerts negative feedback on its own secretion by inhibiting GHRH release, stimulating SST release, and potentiating the release of IGF-I from the liver. IGF-I, in turn, stimulates SST release and inhibits GH secretion by a direct action on the pituitary. (Modified from Patel YC. General aspects of the biology and function of somatostatin. In: Weil C, Muller EE, Thorner MO, eds. Somatostatin. Basic and clinical aspects of neuroscience series, vol 4. Berlin: Springer-Verlag, 1992:1.)

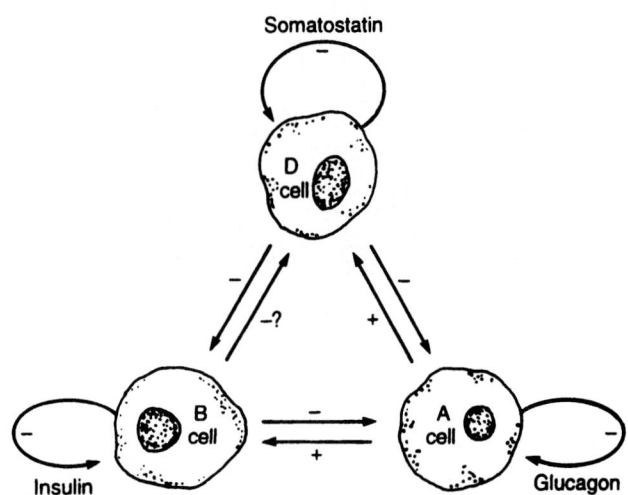

**FIGURE 169-6.** Effects of endogenous or exogenous somatostatin (*SST*), insulin, and glucagon on the function of pancreatic islet cells. SST inhibits insulin and glucagon release, glucagon stimulates insulin and SST release, and insulin inhibits the release of glucagon and possibly of SST. In addition, all three islet hormones inhibit their own secretion by an autocrine mechanism. Physiologically, intraislet insulin and glucagon regulate the secretion of SST, and intraislet insulin regulates glucagon release. The precise physiologic role of intraislet SST remains unclear (see text for details). (Modified from Patel YC. General aspects of the biology and function of somatostatin. In: Weil C, Muller EE, Thorner MO, eds. Somatostatin. Basic and clinical aspects of neuroscience series, vol 4. Berlin: Springer-Verlag, 1992:1.)

of its secretion, suggests that SST exerts control over many discrete cell systems involved in gastrointestinal, pancreatic, and biliary functions. SST regulates acid secretion both directly through the circulation to inhibit parietal cells and through a paracrine mechanism to suppress gastrin release.[29] Circulating SST is also a physiologic regulator of pancreatic exocrine secretion.[30] Elsewhere in the gut, evidence exists to suggest that SST controls the rate of absorption of nutrients and participates in the regulation of gut hormone secretion, gastrointestinal motor tone, blood flow, and mucosal cell proliferation.[31] Although acute changes in tissue or circulating levels of SST are accompanied by alterations in the function of target organs (e.g., the pituitary or gut), an interesting finding is that SST deficiency from birth (as in the SST knock-out mouse) does not produce any developmental defect or growth abnormality in young animals.[32] This means either that the SST gene is redundant or, more likely, that adaptive responses occur from other genes (e.g., *cortistatin*), which compensate for the loss of the SST gene.

## SUBTYPE-SELECTIVE BIOACTIONS OF SOMATOSTATIN RECEPTORS

Because SST exerts its numerous bioeffects through five receptors, the question arises whether a given response is selective for

one subtype or whether multiple subtypes are involved. The marked overlap in the cellular pattern of expression of the different SSTR pathways, coupled with the finding that individual target cells typically express multiple SSTR subtypes and often all five isoforms in the same cell, suggests that SSTRs may operate in concert rather than as individual members. Nonetheless, evidence exists for relative subtype selectivity for some SSTR effects. At the level of cell secretion and cell proliferation, the two general cellular effects modulated by SST, four of the subtypes (SSTR1, SSTR2, SSTR4, SSTR5) are capable of arresting cell growth, whereas SSTR3 is uniquely cytotoxic. In contrast to the case for cell proliferation, surprisingly little is known about subtype selectivity, if any, for cell secretion. Immune, inflammatory, and neoplastic cells are important targets for SST action.[2,14,15] Unlike the classic SST-producing neuroendocrine cells (e.g., in the hypothalamus or islets), which release large quantities of the peptide acutely from storage pools, SST and SST receptors in inflammatory cells (e.g., macrophages and lymphocytes) are coinduced, probably by growth factors and cytokines, as part of a general mechanism for activating the endogenous SST system for paracrine-autocrine modulation of the proliferative and hormonal responses associated with inflammatory and immune reactions. SSTR2, the main isotype expressed in lymphocytes and inflammatory cells, appears to be the functional SSTR responsible for modulating the proliferative and secretory responses of these cells.[15] Based on the pattern of SSTR subtype expression as well as the effects of selective nonpeptide agonists, SSTR2 and SSTR5 are the subtypes involved in regulating GH and TSH secretion from the human pituitary.[2,33] Similar studies in the case of islet hormones suggest a preferential effect of SSTR2 on glucagon release and of SSTR5 and possibly SSTR1 on insulin secretion.[23,34] Despite the pharmacologic evidence for the involvement of SSTR2 in pituitary GH secretion, an SSTR2-deficient mouse shows only subtle abnormalities of neuroendocrine GH feedback control. The animals grow normally both in utero and postnatally, a finding that suggests maintenance of overall GH secretion.[35] These animals display high basal gastric acid secretion in the face of normal gastrin levels, indicating that SSTR2 is the subtype responsible for SST suppression of endogenous gastric acid.

## SOMATOSTATIN IN DISEASE

Given the wide distribution of SST cells in the body, the fact that only a single disease—the *somatostatinoma syndrome*—has been attributed directly to SST dysfunction is surprising (see Chap. 220). No functional mutations of either SST or its receptor genes have been identified. Even in this syndrome, the associated profound hypersomatostatinemia is accompanied by relatively minor symptoms (*cholelithiasis, steatorrhea*, and *mild diabetes*).[36] This probably is due to tachyphylaxis and to the fact that many of the target cells on which SST normally acts locally are not accessible to circulating SST. Most somatostatinomas are actively secreting, malignant islet cell tumors that are associated with high plasma levels of SST-LI (600–15,000 pmol/L).[36] Lesser degrees of hypersomatostatinemia have been observed in nonpancreatic SST-producing tumors, such as duodenal somatostatinoma, medullary thyroid carcinoma, pheochromocytoma, extraadrenal paraganglioma, and small cell cancer of the lung. The serial measurement of plasma SST-LI values has proved useful as a tumor marker in the follow-up of these patients.

In several diseases, disordered SST function occurs probably as a secondary feature. Foremost among these is *Alzheimer disease*, in which a decrease in the levels of SST in the cerebral cortex and CSF is seen.[5,19] The reduction in cortical SST correlates with the number of senile plaques and neurofibrillary tangles, and although its pathophysiologic significance is unclear, it has become an important biochemical marker for the disease. Cerebrocortical SST, CSF SST, or both are also decreased in *other neuropsychiatric disorders* such as depression, Parkinson disease, and multiple sclerosis.[19] Whereas the reduction in brain or CSF SST in Alzheimer disease appears to be secondary to neurodegeneration, the SST changes that occur in depression and multiple sclerosis fluctuate with disease activity and reflect functional alterations in peptide production. In contrast to the loss of SST in Alzheimer disease, SST neurons in the striatum in *Huntington disease* are selectively resistant to neurodegeneration and show up-regulated function. Selective survival and up-regulation of SST gene expression in response to neuronal injury has also been demonstrated in the striatum in animal models of *hypoxia-ischemia* and in the cortex of monkeys and human patients with *AIDS encephalopathy*.

Plasma SST levels are elevated significantly in *hepatic cirrhosis* and in *chronic renal failure*, an elevation that reflects impaired metabolism. In experimental hyperinsulinemic diabetes and in human *type 2 diabetes*, release of gut SST in response to *meal ingestion* is impaired. Patients with *duodenal ulcers* have reduced antral SST-LI levels, implicating local deficiency of SST in the pathogenesis of this disorder. Despite the large amounts of SST present in the gut, primary gastrointestinal disease generally is not associated with alterations in circulating SST concentrations.

## CLINICAL APPLICATIONS OF SOMATOSTATIN AND ITS ANALOGS

The potent pharmacologic properties of SST have attracted much interest in the use of this substance as a therapeutic agent for the treatment of various diseases. The naturally occurring forms proved unsuitable, however, because their short half-lives made continuous intravenous administration necessary. The specificity of endogenous SST derives from the fact that it is produced mainly at local sites of action and is rapidly inactivated after release by peptidases in tissue and blood,

so that unwanted systemic effects are minimized. Injections of synthetic SST, on the other hand, produce a wide array of effects due to simultaneous activation of multiple target sites. Thus, for effective pharmacotherapy with SST, analogs must be designed that have *more selective actions* and *greater metabolic stability* than the naturally occurring peptides. Early observations that the SST-14 molecule was amenable to a wide range of chemical modifications allowed the synthesis of structural analogs with enhanced metabolic stability. One such analog is the long-acting cyclic octapeptide, *octreotide acetate*[6,37] (Sandostatin; see Fig. 169-1). Virtually 100% of this drug is absorbed after subcutaneous administration, and it is eliminated from plasma with a half-life of 70 to 113 min.[37] The bioresponse is maintained for 8 or more hours after a single injection. Octreotide thus has therapeutic efficacy with two to three daily subcutaneous (sc) injections and has emerged as the first SST analog suitable for long-term treatment.[38] Long-acting slow-release formulations of both octreotide (Sandostatin LAR [long-acting release]) and a second octapeptide analog *lanreotide* (BIM23014, Somatuline) have become available.[37,39–42] *Sandostatin LAR* incorporates octreotide into microspheres of a biodegradable polymer (polyDL-lactide-co-glycolide glucose), allowing slow release of the drug by cleavage of the polymer ester linkage through hydrolysis in tissues.[37,39] It is administered as a once-a-month intramuscular (im) depot injection and, after a lag period of 7 to 10 days, produces stable blood octreotide concentrations comparable to that of continuous infusion.[39] Lanreotide is available only as the slow-release formulation, and because of its comparatively shorter duration of action (10–14 days), it must be injected two to three times per month.[40,41] Both analogs are at least as effective as sc octreotide in blocking the excessive production of hormones from neuroendocrine tumors of the gastrointestinal tract, pancreatic islets, and pituitary.[37–42] Furthermore, they have a safety profile similar to that of the sc injections, and, because of better patient compliance, are likely to become the drugs of choice for SST pharmacotherapy. Both the subcutaneous and LAR forms of octreotide are approved by the Food and Drug Administration for the treatment of carcinoid tumors, VIPomas, and acromegaly. Lanreotide should shortly be available in North America. Octreotide and lanreotide bind to only three of the five SSTRs (types 2, 3, and 5) (see Table 169-2), displaying high affinity for subtypes 2 and 5, moderate affinity for subtype 3, and no binding to types 1 and 4.[2,3,6,21] The binding affinity of these analogs for subtypes 2 and 5 is comparable to that of SST-14, indicating that they are neither selective for these subtypes nor more potent than endogenous SST. A series of high-affinity *nonpeptide agonists* have been identified for several of the human SSTRs. These should facilitate the development of orally active subtype-selective therapeutic compounds.[34]

## TREATMENT OF NEUROENDOCRINE AND NONNEUROENDOCRINE TUMORS

Octreotide provides potent palliative therapy for hormone-producing neuroendocrine tumors (Table 169-3). It acts in two ways to *combat the effects of hormone hypersecretion*: (a) directly on tumor cells to *inhibit secretion*, and (b) indirectly to *block the action* of the hypersecreted hormone at its target site. In addition, octreotide may cause *tumor shrinkage* or *stabilization of tumor growth* in some instances by shrinkage of tumor-cell volume through long-term inhibition of secretion (comparable to the shrinkage of prolactinomas induced by dopamine agonists) and inhibition of tumor growth via cytostatic and cytotoxic (apoptotic) effects (see Fig. 169-4).

Binding studies have shown that neuroendocrine as well as common solid nonneuroendocrine tumors are rich in SSTRs (Table 169-4).[3,38] Currently available binding analyses, however, cannot distinguish the individual SSTR subtypes because of the lack of subtype-selective radioligands. Accordingly, investiga-

**TABLE 169-3.**
**Proven and Potential Clinical Applications of Somatostatin Analogs**

| Disorder | Indication |
|---|---|
| **HORMONE-PRODUCING TUMORS** | |
| *Gastroenteropancreatic* | |
| Carcinoid | Definite |
| VIPoma | Definite |
| Glucagonoma | Definite |
| Insulinoma | Probable |
| Gastrinoma | Possible |
| Somatostatinoma | Possible |
| GHRH-producing tumors | Possible |
| *Pituitary* | |
| Acromegaly | Definite |
| TSH-producing adenoma | Definite |
| Nelson syndrome | Probable |
| *Others* | |
| Paraneoplastic ACTH-producing tumors | Possible |
| Medullary carcinoma of thyroid | Possible |
| **GASTROINTESTINAL APPLICATIONS** | |
| Variceal bleeding | Probable |
| Pancreatic fistula | Probable |
| Secretory diarrhea | Probable |
| AIDS-related diarrhea | Probable |
| Postgastrectomy dumping | Possible |
| Scleroderma | Possible |
| **ORTHOSTATIC HYPOTENSION** | Possible |
| **DIABETES** | Possible |

*VIP,* vasoactive intestinal peptide; *GHRH,* growth hormone releasing hormone; *TSH,* thyroid-stimulating hormone; *ACTH,* adrenocorticotropic hormone; *AIDS,* acquired immunodeficiency syndrome.

tors have resorted to mRNA analysis and receptor immunocytochemical analysis with *subtype-selective antibodies* to characterize the pattern of expression of the five SSTR subtypes. Investigation of mRNA expression for the five SSTRs in >100 pituitary tumors, both secretory (producing GH, TSH, prolactin, or ACTH) and nonsecretory (i.e., chromophobe adenomas), and in 32 gastroenteropancreatic tumors (i.e., carcinoid, insulinoma, glucagonoma) has revealed multiple SSTR genes in most tumors.[3,43–45] SSTR1 and SSTR2 appear to be the predominant forms in all tumors. Pituitary adenomas are also rich in the expression of SSTR5. Many nonneuroendocrine tumors (e.g., breast and renal carcinomas) are also SSTR positive.[43,45] The extent of malignant disease as well as differential tumor expression of SSTRs may account for the variable clinical response observed with different tumor types. The presence of octreotide-sensitive subtypes, such as SSTR2 and SSTR5, in the majority of neuroendocrine tumors correlates with the responsiveness of these tumors to treatment with the analog.

Treatment is indicated in patients with severe symptoms and resultant metabolic derangements that require control before surgery or other therapy; in patients with residual tumor or metastatic end-stage disease who have had relapse after standard therapeutic modalities (e.g., surgery, chemotherapy, and hepatic artery embolization); and as prophylaxis against acute crises resulting from sudden discharge of tumor products, such as in carcinoid crisis. In these instances, octreotide administration has produced extended and useful symptomatic remissions. The initial dosage may be 50 to 100 µg of sc octreotide twice daily or 10 mg im of octreotide LAR per month. The dosage may be increased gradually over 6 to 12 months (or as required) to 500 µg three times daily of sc octreotide and 30 mg per month of the LAR preparation. Generally, clinical improvement parallels a reduction in the plasma level of the hormone being hypersecreted by the tumor.

**TABLE 169-4.**
**Expression of Somatostatin Receptors (SSTRs) in Tumors In Vitro and In Vivo**

| | | Incidence of Somatostatin Receptors | | | | | |
|---|---|---|---|---|---|---|---|
| | | In Vitro % Positive for SSTR mRNA | | | | | In Vivo Number Positive by Receptor Scan |
| Tumor | *n* | SSTR1 | SSTR2 | SSTR3 | SSTR4 | SSTR5 | |
| **GASTROENTEROPANCREATIC TUMORS** | | | | | | | |
| Carcinoid | 26 | 77 | 81 | 35 | 40 | 45 | 37/39 (95%) |
| Insulinomas | 4 | 100 | 75 | 50 | 100 | 0 | 5/8 (63%) |
| Glucagonomas | 2 | 100 | 100 | 100 | 100 | 0 | |
| Gastrinomas | | | | | | | 10/10 (100%) |
| **PITUITARY ADENOMAS** | | | | | | | |
| GH* | 38–41 | 53 | 90 | 47 | 5 | 85 | 12/15 (80%) |
| TSH | | | | | | | 2/2 (100%) |
| PRL* | 17–19 | 84 | 63 | 35 | 6 | 71 | |
| ACTH* | 7–9 | 56 | 67 | 25 | 0 | 86 | |
| Nonfunctioning* | 35–36 | 31 | 61 | 46 | 13 | 49 | 6/8 (75%) |
| **OTHER TUMORS** | | | | | | | |
| Pheochromocytoma | 11 | 100 | 100 | 73 | 73 | 73 | 2/3 (67%) |
| Medullary thyroid carcinoma | 14 | 29 | 79 | 36 | 0 | 64 | 11/17 (65%) |
| Breast carcinoma | 100 | 39 | 98 | 40 | 24 | 35 | 39/52 (75%) |
| Renal carcinoma | 13 | 85 | 100 | 0 | 46 | NT | |
| Meningioma | 14 | 86 | 100 | 54 | 50 | 71 | 11/11 (100%) |
| Glioma | 7 | 100 | 100 | 66 | 71 | 57 | |

*GH,* growth hormone; *TSH,* thyroid-stimulating hormone; *PRL,* prolactin; *ACTH,* adrenocorticotropic hormone; *NT,* not tested.
*The number of tumors analyzed for each of the different subtypes varied slightly in the pooled data shown.
(Data from Patel YC. Molecular pharmacology of somatostatin receptor subtypes. J Endocrinol Invest 1997; 20:348; Lamberts SWJ, Krenning EP, Reubi JC. The role of somatostatin and its analogs in the diagnosis and treatment of tumors. Endocr Rev 1991; 12:450; Vikic-Topic S, Raisch KP, Kvols LK, Vuk-Pavlovic S. Expression of somatostatin receptor subtypes in breast carcinoma, carcinoid tumor, and renal cell carcinoma. J Clin Endocrinol Metab 1995; 80:2974; Schaer J-C, Waser B, Mengod G, Reubi JC. Somatostatin receptor subtypes sst₁, sst₂, sst₃ and sst₅ expression in human pituitary, gastroentero-pancreatic and mammary tumors: comparison of mRNA analysis with receptor autoradiography. Int J Cancer 1997; 70:530; and Evans AA, Cook T, Laws SAM, et al. Analysis of somatostatin receptor subtype mRNA expression in human breast cancer. Br J Cancer 1997; 75:798.)

# GASTROENTEROPANCREATIC TUMORS

## CARCINOID TUMORS

SST analogs play a central role in the management of symptoms of metastatic carcinoid disease. More than 200 cases of metastatic carcinoid tumors and carcinoid syndrome treated with octreotide have now been reported.[6,38,42,46–49] The drug is highly effective in this condition and produces a marked clinical and biochemical improvement. Flushing and diarrhea, the two most prominent symptoms, are rapidly relieved in >90% of patients. The clinical improvement is paralleled by a reduction in urinary 5-hydroxyindoleacetic acid (5-HIAA) levels, which drop by >50% in 70% of treated patients *without, however, being completely normalized in any patient*. A *small proportion* of patients (~14%) show *measurable regression of hepatic and lymph node metastases*.[46,49] In 80 patients treated with octreotide, median survival from the diagnosis of metastatic disease was 8.8 years compared with 1.8 years in historical controls. The average dose required for symptomatic and biochemical control ranges from 100 to 150 μg sc every 8 hours. Because of the dual actions of SST in blocking both the secretion and the action of hormones overproduced by tumors, the dose required to control symptoms such as diarrhea may be lower than that necessary for reducing urine 5-HIAA levels. *Resistance* to therapy eventually occurs with an increase in tumor bulk. Such resistance may be due to down-regulation of SST receptors or, more likely, to the emergence of receptor-negative or more virulent clones. Recurrence of disease on therapy may be controlled in some but not all patients by increasing the dose. Doses as high as 1 to 2 mg sc every 8 hours have been administered in this disease and appear to be well tolerated. A study comparing sc and long-acting formulations of octreotide found that monthly injections of octreotide LAR were as effective as sc octreotide in controlling the symptoms and in suppressing urinary 5-HIAA levels in 79 patients.[42] The recommended average dose is 20 mg octreotide LAR, increasing to 30 to 60 mg in some patients with resistant or advanced disease. Lanreotide 30 mg im every 10 to 14 days is also effective.[41] In addition to its application in long-term treatment of metastatic carcinoid disease, octreotide is very useful in preventing carcinoid crisis when administered intravenously in susceptible patients immediately before and for 7 to 10 days after surgery, chemotherapy, or hepatic artery embolization.

## VIPOMAS

Like carcinoid tumors, VIPomas tend to be malignant, with extensive metastatic disease from the outset. Octreotide has become the *first-line drug* for the symptomatic control of this disease. Of 25 patients with VIPoma treated with octreotide for 15 months, 85% showed improvement in or resolution of diarrhea, which was associated with a reduction in plasma levels of vasoactive intestinal peptide in 60%.[47–49] The effect of octreotide is usually rapid and occurs with relatively low doses, 50 to 100 μg every 8 to 12 hours. With time, efficacy is lost in some patients and high-dose regimens are required. Reduction in tumor size has been reported in as many as 40% of patients treated with octreotide for 2 months or longer.[49]

## GLUCAGONOMAS

Approximately 10 patients with glucagonomas who have been treated with octreotide have been described.[47–49] Glucagonomas are slowly growing, malignant tumors associated with severe constitutional symptoms as well as a characteristic rash (see Chap. 220). Therapy with octreotide resolves the rash in a few days and improves other symptoms such as weight loss, anorexia, abdominal pain, and diarrhea. Because no other form of therapy exists for the systemic manifestations of glucagonoma, especially its dermatologic complication, octreotide has assumed a primary role in the medical treatment of this disorder. Usually little effect is seen on the size of the tumor.

## INSULINOMAS

Unlike non–B-cell tumors, 90% of insulinomas are benign and can be cured by surgical resection. Octreotide suppresses insulin levels by >50%, elevates blood glucose levels, and prevents hypoglycemic attacks in many patients.[47–49] Thus, it is effective in the *preoperative treatment of patients with benign insulinoma*. Diazoxide, however, also lowers insulin levels effectively in this setting. It remains to be determined whether octreotide offers any specific advantage. In most patients with *malignant insulinoma*, octreotide is effective in *preventing hypoglycemic attacks*. Loss of efficacy is common, however, and it may be overcome by increasing the dosage. Of greater concern is the *worsening* of hypoglycemia in some patients as a result of the greater suppression by octreotide of the counterregulatory hormones (GH and glucagon) than of insulin. In view of this possibility, plasma glucose levels should be monitored carefully at the initiation of octreotide therapy.

## GASTRINOMAS

Gastrinomas are commonly malignant islet cell tumors that have metastasized at the time of diagnosis. In the >50 reported cases treated with octreotide, the response has been variable, with only modest reductions in gastrin levels.[47–49] Furthermore, tumor growth may progress during octreotide treatment. Because the clinical manifestations of gastrinoma result from the hypersecretion of gastric acid, which can be controlled effectively by oral medications such as $H_2$-receptor antagonists or the $Na^+/H^+$ adenosine triphosphatase inhibitor omeprazole, octreotide serves only an adjunctive role in treatment of this disorder.

## TUMORS PRODUCING GROWTH HORMONE–RELEASING HORMONE

Several patients with GHRH-producing tumors (bronchial carcinoid tumors or metastatic islet cell tumors) who received treatment with octreotide showed good symptomatic and biochemical response.[49] Octreotide reduced plasma concentrations of GHRH and GH, probably through a dual effect on tumor cells and pituitary somatotropes.

# TREATMENT OF PITUITARY TUMORS

## ACROMEGALY

SST analogs significantly reduce GH secretion and IGF-I levels in patients with acromegaly and have become *effective agents in the treatment of this disorder*.[6,37–40,47,49–52] Their use is indicated in the treatment of patients with a macroadenoma who have persistent disease after transsphenoidal surgery, as interim treatment in patients awaiting the full effects of external irradiation, and as preoperative treatment for 2 to 3 months to improve the medical condition of patients with severe disease. They can also be offered as primary therapy to patients who refuse surgery or those with severe medical problems that preclude surgery. Octreotide has been proposed as primary therapy for patients with invasive macroadenomas not causing chiasmatic compression, who are unlikely to be cured surgically.[51] This is an attractive idea, especially with the availability of slow-release preparations; it needs to be further assessed in prospective studies comparing the relative efficacy and cost effectiveness of primary SST analog therapy versus surgery for treatment of acromegaly.[51] With sc injections of 100 μg octreotide three times daily (mean optimal efficacious dosage), a prompt reduction in plasma GH levels occurs, followed by a decline in circulating IGF-I levels during the first week.[50,52] This is accompanied by immediate relief of many of the clinical symptoms of acromegaly, including fatigue, headache, excessive perspiration, arthralgia, and soft-tissue swelling.[50,52] Relief of headache is often seen immediately after the injections are started and before serum GH levels have declined, perhaps as a result of a vascular or analgesic action of the drug. Improvement in facial coarsening and acral enlargement occurs after longer periods of treatment. Sustained improvement with minimal side effects has been noted with treatment for 10 or more years. Drug resistance may develop during long-term treatment, necessitating increased dosages. In a double-blind, randomized, multicenter study of 115 patients with acromegaly,[52] administration of octreotide at a dosage of 100 µg three times a day for 6 months was effective in reducing GH levels in 71% of patients and IGF-I levels in 93%. Mean integrated GH levels were reduced 70% from $40 \pm 13$ µg/L to $12 \pm 4$ µg/L, and mean integrated IGF-I levels were suppressed 60% from $4800 \pm 354$ U/L to $1900 \pm 200$ U/L. Normalization of GH secretion, defined as a reduction of integrated mean GH levels to <5 µg/L, occurred in 53% of patients, whereas IGF-I levels normalized in 68%. A decrease in pituitary tumor size (25–50%) has been observed in 20% to 47% of patients with acromegaly receiving long-term octreotide therapy.[50-53] Tumor shrinkage may be dose dependent, as it is greater with larger doses of octreotide. Preoperative treatment for 8 to 12 weeks shrinks invasive somatotrope macroadenomas by ~40%, but whether such shrinkage affects the surgical outcome remains controversial.[53] Early results with the slow-release SST preparations suggest that administration of octreotide LAR (20–30 mg per month) and lanreotide (30–60 mg two to three times per month) is as effective as multiple daily sc injections of octreotide in controlling GH hypersecretion.[39,40] In most patients with acromegaly, SST analogs are more effective in lowering GH levels than the dopamine agonists bromocriptine or cabergoline.[51] Occasionally, however, patients (typically those with mixed GH/prolactin-producing tumors) exhibit greater sensitivity to dopamine receptor agonists. In addition, use of a combination of SST analogs and dopamine-receptor agonists is of value in some patients who do not respond to either drug alone.

### THYROTROPIN-SECRETING PITUITARY ADENOMAS

*Most TSH-secreting tumors are sensitive to octreotide treatment.*[6,47,49,54] In 73 such tumor cases, octreotide (50–750 µg sc two to three times daily) reduced TSH secretion in 92% of cases and α-subunit secretion in 93%, with normalization of TSH in 79% and restoration of the euthyroid state in the majority.[54] In 52% of patients, clear evidence of tumor shrinkage was found. Treatment is indicated for residual tumor after surgery and/or radiotherapy. The place of SST analogs as primary therapy for these tumors remains to be established.

### ADRENOCORTICOTROPIC HORMONE–SECRETING PITUITARY ADENOMAS

Although SST receptors have been identified in corticotrope adenomas, these tumors generally show *poor* responsiveness to octreotide. A *few* patients with invasive corticotrope adenomas associated with Nelson syndrome have responded to octreotide therapy with a decrease in ACTH secretion as well as a possible reduction in tumor size.[6] Likewise, some cases of *paraneoplastic ACTH secretion from bronchial and thymic carcinoids* can be controlled by octreotide.

### NONFUNCTIONING PITUITARY ADENOMAS

Many nonfunctioning pituitary adenomas express SST receptors, with a preponderance of the octreotide-sensitive SSTR2 and SSTR5 subtypes (see Table 169-4). These tumors secrete low levels of gonadotropins, but generally show *little* change in tumor size with octreotide therapy despite inhibition of glycoprotein hormone and subunit release in some instances.[6,49]

### POSSIBLE ONCOLOGIC APPLICATIONS

Although for many years neuroendocrine tumors have been known to possess SSTRs and to be amenable to treatment with SST analogs, the more recent realization that common solid tumors such as breast, colon, and prostate cancers are also rich in SSTRs has led to mounting interest in the more general oncologic usefulness of SST analogs.[2,3,6,43,45] Any effect of SST on these tumors appears to be quite variable, however, probably due to patient selection (e.g., early vs. end-stage disease); the absence of appropriate SSTRs in the tumors being treated (e.g., tumors expressing SSTR1 and SSTR4 do not respond to octreotide; SSTR3 expression is required for inducing apoptosis); the presence of mutated p53 gene, which abrogates the apoptotic effect of SST; and the dose and duration of treatment. Most current interest is focused on breast cancer because (a) the incidence of SSTR expression is high,[43,45] (b) SST analogs inhibit the growth of breast cancer cells in vivo and in vitro by inducing cell growth arrest and apoptosis,[2,55] (c) octreotide potentiates the antineoplastic effects of tamoxifen in experimental mammary carcinoma in the rat,[56] and (d) sc octreotide treatment for 6 weeks to 6 years in combination with norprolac (a dopamine-receptor agonist to inhibit prolactin secretion) enhanced the effectiveness of tamoxifen therapy in 22 patients with advanced breast cancer.[57] These findings have generated interest in SST as *adjuvant therapy for breast cancer* and have led to several multicenter North American clinical trials involving >3000 patients. These currently ongoing studies will look at the effect of high-dose octreotide given alone as a monthly injection for 2 years or in combination with tamoxifen to women with estrogen receptor–positive stage I and stage II breast cancer.

## GASTROINTESTINAL APPLICATIONS

Short- or long-term octreotide administration is useful in treating numerous gastrointestinal disorders (see Table 169-3). These conditions are more common than neuroendocrine tumors and account for much of the hospital-based usage of octreotide. SST is a potent constrictor of the splanchnic circulation and is effective in controlling variceal bleeding. In a randomized, double-blind, placebo-controlled trial of 120 patients, infusion of SST-14 at a dosage of 250 µg per hour for 5 days controlled bleeding and reduced transfusion requirements.[58] In a study of 100 patients, octreotide given intravenously for 48 hours was as effective as emergency sclerotherapy in the treatment of acute variceal hemorrhage.[6] The antisecretory effects of SST on the pancreas have led to the successful use of octreotide in the treatment of pancreatic fistulas. More than 60 patients so treated have been described.[59] Most reports indicate a closure rate of pancreatic fistulas approximating 70% within a week. In addition to the diarrhea that occurs with hormone-secreting tumors, other forms of secretory diarrhea such as that associated with high-output ileostomy, diabetic diarrhea, AIDS diarrhea, chemotherapy-induced diarrhea, and diarrhea associated with amyloidosis all have been reported to be variably controlled with octreotide.[47] In these diarrheal states, octreotide acts by blocking the normal production of gastric and pancreatic exocrine secretion destined for reabsorption in the distal bowel, and by directly inhibiting intestinal fluid and electrolyte secretion. In a randomized double-blind trial involving 10 patients with severe postgastrectomy dumping syndrome, the administration of octreotide 100 µg 30 minutes before eating prevented the development of vasomotor symptoms (early dumping) as well as the hypoglycemia and diarrhea characteristic of late dumping.[60] Finally, in patients with scleroderma and intestinal dysmotility, the short-term administration of octreotide improved intestinal motility by stimulating the frequency of intestinal migrating motor complexes and reducing bacterial overgrowth, leading to an improvement in abdominal symptoms such as nausea, bloating, and pain.[61]

## ORTHOSTATIC HYPOTENSION

Postprandial and orthostatic hypotension in patients with autonomic neuropathy is abolished by low dosages of octreotide (0.2–0.4 µg/kg). In these cases, the drug acts as a potent pressor agent and has emerged as a new form of therapy for this condition as well as for other types of postprandial hypotension, such as that which occurs in the elderly.[62]

## SIDE EFFECTS

Although the acute administration of SST produces a large number of inhibitory effects, continued exposure results in an *escape from the acute effects of the peptide*.[2,6] This may be due to up-regulation of some of the receptor subtypes, which compensates for the desensitized responses of others and thereby maintains normal overall SST responsiveness. Side effects associated with the long-term administration of octreotide for up to 2 years have been remarkably few.[6,37,39–42,49,50–52] Most patients complain of pain at the injection site, and abdominal cramps and mild steatorrhea to which they become tolerant after 10 to 14 days. No nutritional deficiency has been reported with long-term octreotide therapy. Patients also adapt rapidly to some of the other effects of SST (e.g., inhibition of insulin and TSH secretion). A mild impairment of glucose tolerance may occur, consisting of a minimal increase in postprandial glucose levels only, with maintenance of normal fasting glucose levels. Normal thyroid function is maintained and hypothyroidism is rare. Some effects, however, do persist; for example, inhibition of gallbladder emptying causes a significant increase in the incidence of biliary sludge and cholesterol gallstones in 20% to 30% of patients after 1 to 2 years of treatment.[6] Those receiving long-term treatment warrant initial ultrasonographic evaluation, and subsequently evaluation as necessary, depending on symptoms. The incidence of adverse effects with the slow-release preparations of SST is comparable to that with the subcutaneous injections.[37,39,40–42] Interestingly, the persistent steatorrhea and mild diabetes mellitus that are associated with the chronic hypersomatostatinemia in patients with SST-producing tumors[36] are not observed in patients during long-term treatment with the slow-release forms of the SST analogs, despite the sustained high blood levels of the drugs. This no doubt reflects the narrower binding specificity of the synthetic SST analogs, which bind to only three of the SSTR subtypes, compared with SST-14 and SST-28, which are typically produced by somatostatinomas and bind to all five SSTRs (see Table 169-2). Although normal tissues adapt to the long-term effects of octreotide, hormone-producing tumors continue to respond to octreotide injections with persistent suppression of hormone secretion, frequently for several years. This suggests a *differential regulation of SSTRs in normal tissues and in tumors*. Tumors express a higher density of SSTRs than do surrounding normal tissues. Conceivably, SSTRs in tumors behave differently due to a loss of normal receptor regulatory function, due to an alteration in the pattern and composition of the various subtypes expressed, or due to abnormal receptor signaling.

## SOMATOSTATIN-RECEPTOR SCANS

A method for the in vivo imaging of SSTR-positive tumors and their metastases has been developed using as radionuclides [[123]I]Tyr[3] octreotide or an indium-labeled octreotide preparation that is now available commercially ([111]In-diethylenetriamine pentaacetic acid[DTPA]-D-Phe-1-octreotide).[37,38,63,64] The rationale for the method lies in the demonstration that most endocrine tumors that respond to octreotide therapy do so because they are rich in SSTRs. Direct binding studies of surgically removed specimens have revealed a higher density of receptors in tumor tissue than in the surrounding healthy tissue.[38] After intravenous administration, the radioligand binds to SSTRs on primary and metastatic tumor cells, which then can be visualized by computerized γ-scintigraphy. Unbound radioactive material is rapidly degraded in the liver and excreted in the bile, or eliminated through the kidneys. The technique is relatively simple and effective. Among 59 patients with metastatic carcinoid disease or pancreatic endocrine tumors, primary tumors and their metastases were successfully localized in all but five cases (see Table 169-4). Particularly impressive is the ability of the receptor-scanning technique to visualize many unsuspected metastases that escape detection by clinical examination and conventional imaging techniques such as computed tomographic scanning and magnetic resonance imaging.[38,63] Overall, the specificity of the method is high as judged by the close correlation among the in vivo tumor receptor scans, the inhibitory effect of octreotide on the secretion of hormone by the tumor, and the presence of SSTRs as demonstrated by direct in vitro binding studies of surgically removed tumor samples.[38,63] SSTR scanning offers several distinct advantages over the currently used standard imaging methods. The first is its high power of resolution for tumors as small as 1 cm in diameter, which are difficult to visualize with conventional scanning techniques.[63] Second, because the whole body is imaged, abnormalities in areas not under clinical suspicion can be detected, and the full extent of metastatic disease accurately mapped. Third, this method provides a functional index of the SSTR status of tumor cells that could be useful in tumor management. For instance, positivity for receptors can predict tumor responsiveness to SST therapy and may serve as a prognostic index of a favorable outcome for some tumors. The technique has some limitations. The first is that secretory tumors that do not express SSTRs are not amenable to analysis with this method. Second, because octreotide does not bind to two of the SSTR subtypes (types 1 and 4), those tumors that uniquely express these receptor isoforms will escape detection. SST-receptor scans are now available at most major centers and are widely used in the *assessment of carcinoid and islet cell tumors, paragangliomas, pheochromocytomas*, and *medullary thyroid carcinoma*.[38] They are of *little value in the imaging of pituitary tumors*, which are better defined by conventional techniques. Because of the rich expression of the type 2 SSTR in immune and inflammatory cells, lesions of several *granulomatous, inflammatory, and immune disorders* have been successfully imaged by SSTR scintigraphy, for example, rheumatoid joints, sarcoid lesions, Hodgkin and non-Hodgkin lymphomas, and thyroid eye disease. The value of SST-receptor scan in the routine assessment of these disorders, however, remains to be determined.

## SOMATOSTATIN RECEPTOR–TARGETED RADIOABLATION OF TUMORS

The property of rich SSTR expression by tumors which allows their visualization by the receptor-imaging approach can be further applied to achieve receptor-targeted ablation of the tumors. Binding of radioligand to SSTRs on the cell surface triggers their internalization.[2] Specifically, SSTR subtypes 2, 3, and 5, which bind octreotide, all undergo agonist-dependent internalization, suggesting that the use of octreotide-based ligands coupled to α- or β-emitting radioisotopes could provide a method for delivering targeted radiation to the interior of the cell. Preliminary results with [111]In-DTPA-D-Phe-1-octreotide in several patients with inoperable metastatic islet and carcinoid tumors suggest partial tumor responses as determined by radiographic tumor shrinkage.[65] A second analog of octreotide labeled with yttrium-90 ([90]Y-DOTA-D-Phe[1]-Tyr[3] octreotide), in which the DTPA molecule is replaced by another chelator, DOTA (tetraazacyclododecane tetraacetic acid), which is a more potent β-emitting isotope that has been reported to be highly effective in inducing radionecrosis of human small cell lung tumor transplanted into nude mice, is undergoing clinical trials.[37] Because SSTRs are expressed in many normal cells that would undoubtedly take up the radioligands, the question of whether significant damage to organs (e.g., the pituitary, islets, and gut) occurs with this type of treatment remains to be determined. Nonetheless, this is a promising new approach that could be applied not just to neuroendocrine tumors but also to all SSTR-rich tumors, and it awaits further study.

# REFERENCES

1. Reichlin S. Somatostatin. N Engl J Med 1983; 309:1495.
2. Patel YC. Somatostatin and its receptor family. Frontiers Neuroendocrinol 1999; 20:157.
3. Patel YC. Molecular pharmacology of somatostatin receptor subtypes. J Endocrinol Invest 1997; 20:348.
4. Patel YC, Liu JL, Galanopoulou AS, Papachristou DN. Production, action, and degradation of somatostatin. In: Jefferson LS, Cherrington AD, eds. The handbook of physiology: the endocrine pancreas and regulation of metabolism. New York: Oxford University Press, 2000.
5. Epelbaum J, Dournaud P, Fodor M, Viollet C. The neurobiology of somatostatin. Crit Rev Neurobiol 1994; 8:25.
6. Lamberts SWJ, Van Der Lely A-J, de Herder WW. Drug therapy: octreotide. N Engl J Med 1996; 334:246.
7. Patel YC, Tannenbaum GS, eds. Somatostatin: basic and clinical aspects. Metabolism 1990; 39(Suppl 2).
8. Patel YC. General aspects of the biology and function of somatostatin. In: Weil C, Muller EE, Thorner MO, eds. Somatostatin. Basic and clinical aspects of neuroscience series, vol 4. Berlin: Springer-Verlag, 1992:1.
9. De Lecea L, Criado JR, Prospero-Garcia O, et al. A cortical neuropeptide with neuronal depressant and sleep-modulating properties. Nature 1996; 381:242.
10. Hokfelt T, Efendic S, Hellerstrom C, et al. Cellular localization of somatostatin in endocrine-like cells and neurons of the rat with special reference to the A$_1$-cells of the pancreatic islets and to the hypothalamus. Acta Endocrinol (Copenh) 1975; 80 (Suppl 200):5.
11. Patel YC, Reichlin S. Somatostatin in hypothalamus, extrahypothalamic brain and peripheral tissues of the rat. Endocrinology 1978; 102:523.
12. Baetens D, Malaisse-Lagae F, Perrelet A, et al. Endocrine pancreas: three dimensional reconstruction shows two types of islets of Langerhans. Science 1979; 206:1323.
13. Larsson LI. Distribution and morphology of somatostatin cells. Adv Exp Biol Med 1985; 188:383.
14. Aguila MC, Dees WL, Haensly WE, McCann SM. Evidence that somatostatin is localized and synthesized in lymphoid organs. Proc Natl Acad Sci U S A 1991; 88:11485.
15. Elliott DE, Blum AM, Li J, et al. Preprosomatostatin messenger RNA is expressed by inflammatory cells and induced by inflammatory mediators and cytokines. J Immunol 1998; 160:3997.
16. Shoelson SE, Polonsky KS, Nakabayashi T, et al. Circulating forms of somatostatin-like immunoreactivity in human plasma. Am J Physiol 1986; 250:E428.
17. Taborsky GT Jr, Ensinck JW. Contribution of the pancreas to circulating somatostatin-like immunoreactivity in the normal dog. J Clin Invest 1984; 73:216.
18. Patel YC, Rao K, Reichlin S. Somatostatin in human cerebrospinal fluid. N Engl J Med 1977; 296:529.
19. Rubinow DR, Davis CL, Post RM. Somatostatin in neuropsychiatric disorders. In: Weil C, Muller EE, Thorner MO, eds. Somatostatin. Basic and clinical aspects of neuroscience series, vol 4. Berlin: Springer-Verlag, 1992:29.
20. Montminy M, Brindle P, Arias J, et al. Regulation of somatostatin gene transcription by cAMP. In: Somatostatin and its receptors. Ciba Foundation Symposium 190. West Sussex: John Wiley and Sons, 1995:7.
21. Reisine T, Bell GI. Molecular biology of somatostatin receptors. Endocr Rev 1995; 16:427.
22. Bruno JF, Yun XU, Song J, et al. Tissue distribution of somatostatin receptor subtype messenger ribonucleic acid in the rat. Endocrinology 1993; 133:2561.
23. Kumar U, Sasi R, Suresh S, et al. Subtype-selective expression of the five somatostatin receptors (hSSTR1-5) in human pancreatic islet cells: a quantitative double-label immunohistochemical analysis. Diabetes 1999; 48:77.
24. Pan MG, Florio T, Stork PJC. G protein activation of a hormone-stimulated phosphatase in human tumor cells. Science 1992; 256:1215.
25. Reardon DB, Dent P, Wood SL, et al. Activation in vitro of somatostatin receptor subtypes 2, 3, or 4 stimulates protein tyrosine phosphatase activity in membranes from transfected Ras-transformed NIH 3T3 cells: coexpression with catalytically inactive SHP-2 blocks responsiveness. Mol Endocrinol 1997; 11:1062.
26. Sharma K, Patel YC, Srikant CB. Subtype selective induction of p53-dependent apoptosis but not cell cycle arrest by human somatostatin receptor 3. Mol Endocrinol 1996; 10:1688.
27. Tannenbaum GS, Epelbaum J. Somatostatin. In: Costio JL, ed. Handbook of physiology, vol 5. Hormonal control of growth. Sect vii, The endocrine system. New York: Oxford, 1999:221.
28. D'Alessio DA, Sieber C, Beglinger C, et al. A physiologic role for somatostatin-28 as a regulator of insulin secretion. J Clin Invest 1989; 84:857.
29. Colturi TJ, Unger RH, Feldman M. Role of circulating somatostatin in regulation of gastric acid secretion, gastrin release and islet cell function. Studies in healthy subjects and duodenal ulcer patients. J Clin Invest 1984; 74:417.
30. Gyr K, Beglinger C, Kohler E, et al. Circulating somatostatin: physiological regulator of pancreatic function? J Clin Invest 1987; 79:1595.
31. Yamada T. Gut somatostatin. In: Reichlin S, ed. Somatostatin: basic and clinical status. New York: Plenum, 1987:221.
32. Juarez RA, Rubinstein M, Chan EC, et al. Increased growth following normal development in middle aged somatostatin deficient mice. In: Program of the Annual Meeting of the Society for Neuroscience; October 1997; New Orleans. Abstract 659.10:1684.
33. Shimon I, Taylor JE, Dong JZ, et al. Somatostatin receptor subtype specificity in human fetal pituitary culture. J Clin Invest 1997; 99:789.
34. Rohrer SP, Birzin ET, Mosley RT, et al. Rapid identification of subtype-selective agonists of the somatostatin receptor through combinatorial chemistry. Science 1998; 282:737.
35. Zheng H, Bailey A, Jiang MH, et al. Somatostatin receptor subtype 2 knockout mice are refractory to growth hormone, negative feedback on arcuate neurons. Mol Endocrinol 1997; 11:1709.
36. Krejs GJ, Orci L, Conlon JM, et al. Somatostatinoma syndrome: biochemical, morphological and clinical features. N Engl J Med 1979; 301:285.
37. Marbach P, Bauer W, Bodmer D, et al. Discovery and development of somatostatin agonists. Pharm Biotechnol 1998; 11:183.
38. Lamberts SWJ, Krenning EP, Reubi JC. The role of somatostatin and its analogs in the diagnosis and treatment of tumors. Endocr Rev 1991; 12:450.
39. Lancranjan L, Bruns C, Grass P, et al. Sandostatin LAR: pharmacokinetics, pharmacodynamics, efficacy, and tolerability in acromegalic patients. Metabolism 1995; 44:18.
40. Giusti M, Gussoni G, Cuttica CM, et al. Effectiveness and tolerability of slow release lanreotide treatment in active acromegaly: six-month report on an Italian multicenter study. J Clin Endocrinol Metab 1996; 81:2089.
41. Tomassetti P, Migliori M, Gullo L. Slow-release lanreotide treatment in endocrine gastrointestinal tumors. Am J Gastroenterol 1998; 93:1468.
42. Rubin J, Ajani J, Schirmer W, et al. Octreotide acetate long-acting formulation versus open-label subcutaneous octreotide acetate in malignant carcinoid syndrome. J Clin Oncol 1999; 17:600.
43. Vikic-Topic S, Raisch KP, Kvols LK, Vuk-Pavlovic S. Expression of somatostatin receptor subtypes in breast carcinoma, carcinoid tumor, and renal cell carcinoma. J Clin Endocrinol Metab 1995; 80:2974.
44. Schaer J-C, Waser B, Mengod G, Reubi JC. Somatostatin receptor subtypes sst$_1$, sst$_2$, sst$_3$ and sst$_5$ expression in human pituitary, gastroentero-pancreatic and mammary tumors: comparison of mRNA analysis with receptor autoradiography. Int J Cancer 1997; 70:530.
45. Evans AA, Cook T, Laws SAM, et al. Analysis of somatostatin receptor subtype mRNA expression in human breast cancer. Br J Cancer 1997; 75:798.
46. Kvols LK, Moertal OG, O'Connell MJ, et al. Treatment of the malignant carcinoid syndrome: evaluation of a long-acting somatostatin analogue. N Engl J Med 1986; 315:663.
47. Gorden P, Comi RJ, Maton PN, et al. Somatostatin and somatostatin analog (SMS 201-995) in treatment of hormone secreting tumors of the pituitary and gastrointestinal tract and nonneoplastic diseases of the gut. Ann Int Med 1989; 110:35.
48. Wynick D, Bloom SR. The use of the long-acting somatostatin analog octreotide in the treatment of gut neuroendocrine tumors. J Clin Endocrinol Metab 1991; 73:1.
49. Maton PN, Avaraki RF. Therapeutic use of somatostatin and octreotide acetate in neuroendocrine tumors. In: Weil C, Muller EE, Thorner MO, eds. Somatostatin. Basic and clinical aspects of neuroscience series, vol 4. Berlin: Springer-Verlag, 1992:55.
50. Sassolas G, Harris AG, James-Deidier A, et al. Long-term effect of incremental doses of the somatostatin analog SMS 201-995 in 58 acromegalic patients. J Clin Endocrinol Metab 1990; 71:391.
51. Melmed S, Jackson I, Kleinberg D, Klibanski A. Current treatment guidelines for acromegaly. J Clin Endocrinol Metab 1998; 83:2646.
52. Ezzat S, Snyder PJ, Young WF, et al. Octreotide treatment of acromegaly. Ann Intern Med 1992; 117:711.
53. Barkan AL, Lloyd RV, Chandler WF, et al. Preoperative treatment of acromegaly with long-acting somatostatin analog SMS 201-995: shrinkage of invasive pituitary macroadenomas and improved surgical remission rate. J Clin Endocrinol Metab 1988; 67:1040.
54. Beck-Peccoz P, Brucker-Davis F, Persani L, et al. Thyrotropin-secreting pituitary tumors. Endocr Rev 1996; 17:610.
55. Sharma K, Srikant CB. Induction of wild type p53, bax and acidic endonuclease during somatostatin signaled apoptosis in MCF-7 human breast cancer cells. Int J Cancer 1998; 76:259.
56. Weckbecker G, Tolcsvai L, Stolz B, et al. Somatostatin analogue octreotide enhances the antineoplastic effect of tamoxifen and ovariectomy on 7, 12-dimethylbenz(a)anthracene-induced rat mammary carcinomas. Cancer Res 1994; 54:6334.
57. Bontenbal M, Foekens JA, Lamberts SWJ, et al. Feasibility, endocrine and anti-tumor effects of a triple endocrine therapy with tamoxifen, a somatostatin analogue and an antiprolactin in post-menopausal breast cancer: a randomized study with long-term follow-up. Br J Cancer 1998; 77:115.
58. Burroughs AK, McCormick PA, Hughes MD, et al. Randomized double blind placebo controlled trial of somatostatin for variceal bleeding. Gastroenterology 1990; 99:1388.
59. Torres A, Landa J, Moreno-Azcoita M, et al. Somatostatin in the management of gastrointestinal fistulas. Arch Surg 1992; 127:97.

60. Geer RJ, Richards WO, O'Dorisio TM, et al. Efficacy of octreotide acetate in treatment of severe postgastrectomy dumping syndrome. Ann Surg 1990; 212:678.
61. Soudah HC, Hasler WL, Owyang C. Effect of octreotide on intestinal motility and bacterial overgrowth in scleroderma. N Engl J Med 1991; 325:1461.
62. Hoeldtke RD, Israel BC. Treatment of orthostatic hypotension with octreotide. J Clin Endocrinol Metab 1989; 68:1051.
63. Lamberts SWJ, Bakker WH, Reubi J-C, et al. Somatostatin receptor imaging in the localization of endocrine tumors. N Engl J Med 1990; 323:1246.
64. Hofland LJ, Breeman WAP, Krenning EP, et al. Internalization of [DOTA⁰, ¹²⁵I-Tyr³] octreotide by somatostatin receptor-positive cells in vitro and in vivo: implications for somatostatin receptor-targeted radioguided surgery. Proc Assoc Am Phys 1999; 111:63.
65. McCarthy KE, Woltering EA, Espenan GD, et al. In situ radiotherapy with ¹¹¹In-pentetreotide: initial observations and future directions. Cancer J Sci Amer 1998; 4:94.

# CHAPTER 170

# KININS

DOMENICO C. REGOLI

## THE KALLIKREIN–KININ SYSTEM

### CHEMISTRY

The kinins are potent vasodilator peptides that are contained in large precursors (*kininogens*), from which they are released into the blood and biologic fluids through the action of proteolytic enzymes (*kallikreins*). In contrast to neuropeptides and many other endogenous hormonal agents that are synthesized and stored in nerve and endocrine cells, kinins are generated in the blood and tissues.[1] The kallikreins, which are responsible for the formation of kinins, originate from the liver (*plasma kallikreins*), from exocrine glands (*glandular kallikreins*),[2] from the kidney, and from other organs and tissues.[3] The kallikreins exist in blood and tissues as precursors (prekallikreins) that are activated by various chemical and physical factors. Among the endogenous activators are the Hageman factor, several enzymes (trypsin, plasmin, factor XI), and, in vitro, glass surfaces, kaolin, collagen, and other charged substances, such as cellulose sulfate.[4,5] Plasma prekallikrein (with a molecular mass of 130,000 daltons) is the precursor of kallikrein (95,000–100,000 daltons), which interacts with the high-molecular-mass kininogen (88,000–114,000 daltons) to release the nonapeptide *bradykinin*[5] (Fig. 170-1). Glandular kallikreins are acidic glycoproteins (27,000–43,000 daltons) that release the decapeptide kallidin (see Fig. 170-1) from kininogens of low molecular mass (48,000–70,000 daltons).[2,3,6] Kallikreins and kininogens have been cloned: Sequence structures of the enzymes and the substrates are known (see comprehensive review[7,8]).

### INACTIVATION

Kinins are rapidly inactivated by several proteolytic enzymes present in plasma and tissues that act either at the amino or at the carboxyl end of the kinins (see Fig. 170-1). The metabolic products of kinins are inactive except for the bradykinin that is released from kallidin by the aminopeptidase, and the desArg⁹ bradykinin or desArg¹⁰ kallidin that is released from bradykinin and kallidin by *kininase I*.[9,10] The most efficient system for inactivating kinins and activating angiotensin I to angiotensin II is *kininase II*, a carboxydipeptidase that is widely distributed in plasma, endothelial cells, and various organs, such as the lung and the kidney.[9]

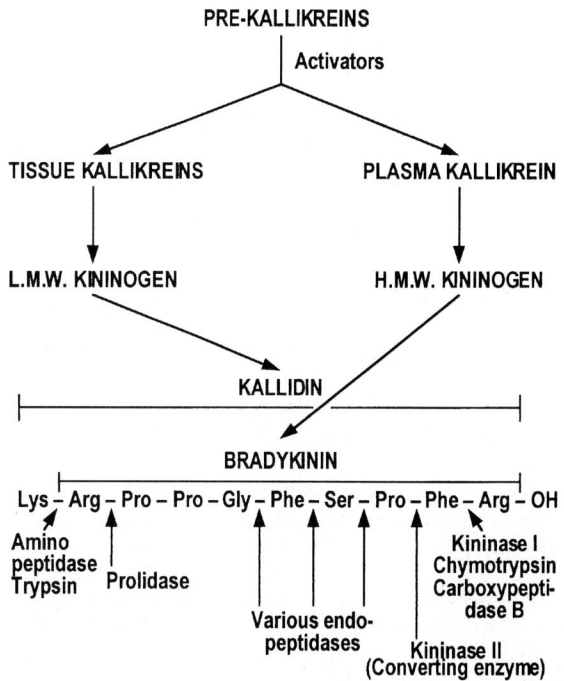

**FIGURE 170-1.** Formation and degradation of kinins. (*LMW,* low molecular weight; *HMW,* high molecular weight.) (From Regoli D. Polypeptides et antagonistes. In: Giroud J-P, Mathé G, Meyniel G, eds. Pharmacologie clinique: bases de la thérapeutique, 2nd ed. Paris: Expansion Scientifique Française, 1988:691.)

Kininase II is particularly active in the pulmonary vascular bed: 80% to 95% of kinins are eliminated during the short time in which the blood passes through the pulmonary circulation.[11] Because of their rapid inactivation in the lung and in other tissues, the biologic half-lives of bradykinin and kallidin in the dog are 0.27 and 0.32 minutes, respectively. Thus, as a result of the balance between the simultaneous processes of production and inactivation, kinins circulate at very low concentrations.

### MEASUREMENT IN BLOOD

#### BLOOD LEVELS IN HEALTHY SUBJECTS

Various investigators have reported extreme variations (from 0.07–5.0 ng/mL) in circulating kinin concentrations in healthy volunteers, using either bioassays or radioimmunoassays.[10] One group has reported a concentration of 0.025 ng/mL, a value 100 to 200 times lower than any previously reported.[12] Such discrepancies are attributable largely to the fact that prekallikreins in blood are rapidly activated by contact with glass surfaces and by numerous other physical and chemical factors.[1] Therefore, most of the data on the blood concentration of kinins reported since the 1970s reflect figures that are much too high compared to more recent results obtained with sensitive radioimmunoassays.[4]

When both types of assays have been used for the same plasmas, radioimmunoassay has yielded values two to six times higher than those derived from bioassay, probably because antibodies that are directed against the C-terminal part of the kinin molecules measure both the biologically active kinins and some inactive metabolites.[4,10]

#### BLOOD LEVELS IN DISEASE

An increase of bradykinin-like material (measured by bioassay or radioimmunoassay) has been reported in the blood of patients affected by the dumping syndrome, postgastrectomy with or without dumping, dengue fever and shock, bronchial asthma, or hyperbradykininism, as well as in the synovial fluid of patients with rheumatoid and psoriatic arthritis.[4,10] Again, the levels of circulating kinins reported by several of these authors are too high. More sensitive and specific radioimmuno-assays[13] and better-controlled experimental conditions for blood collection are needed to demonstrate significant changes of circulating kinins in pathophysiology.

Alternatively, the activity of the kallikrein–kinin system can be evaluated by relating the activity of kallikreins to the rate of generation of kinins in vitro, in a manner similar to that used to estimate renin. Several researchers have used this approach to measure urinary kallikreins in an attempt to evaluate the possible role of renal kallikreins in human and experimental hypertension.[14]

## KININ RECEPTORS

Naturally occurring kinins and their potentially active metabolites exert various biologic actions and have different metabolic and pharmacologic features.[10] Pharmacologic studies suggest that kinins may exert their numerous biologic effects by activating two different types of receptors.[4,10] Differentiation between the two receptors has been accomplished by using classic criteria,[15] and other modern criteria[16] in relation to the $B_1$ receptor. Thus, rabbit aorta, which contains the $B_1$ receptor, is particularly sensitive to desArg[9] bradykinin and desArg[10] kallidin, the metabolites of bradykinin and kallidin released by kininase I. Conversely, the receptor of the rabbit jugular vein is much more sensitive to kallidin and bradykinin than to their metabolites. The discovery of specific and competitive antagonists for the $B_1$ receptor, such as [Leu[9]]desArg[10] kallidin and other similar compounds,[10] as well as the finding that [Thi[5,8],Phe[7]] bradykinin acts as a specific antagonist of $B_2$ receptors,[17] confirms the existence of two receptor types for the kinins. In fact, [Leu[9]]desArg[10] kallidin is active on the $B_1$ receptor and inactive on the $B_2$ receptor, whereas [Thi[5,8],Phe[7]] bradykinin is active on the $B_2$ receptor. A selective $B_2$-receptor antagonist, HOE 140 (D-Arg[Hyp[3],Thi[5],D-Tic[7],Oic[8]]BK) has been reported[18] and shown to be resistant to degradation and to have prolonged effects in vivo. The human $B_1$ and $B_2$ receptors have been cloned and shown to be rhodopsin-like proteins linked to G proteins.[19,20] Two $B_2$-receptor subtypes have been identified and characterized.[21,22]

Kininase II, the enzyme that releases desPhe[8],desArg[9] bradykinin from bradykinin, and desPhe[9] and desArg[10] kallidin from kallidin, is indeed the most efficient inactivating system, because the metabolites are practically inactive in both preparations and, therefore, on both receptor types.

## BIOACTIVITIES OF KININS

### VASCULAR EFFECTS

The kallikreins and kinins were discovered mainly because of their potent cardiovascular effects.[1,23] One of their prominent actions is the dilatation of peripheral vessels, resulting from the activation of $B_2$ receptors on the vascular endothelium.[24,24a] Similar to other agents, kinins may release a potent endogenous vasodilator from the endothelium that reduces the arterial smooth muscle tone, thereby increasing the blood flow to most of the peripheral organs and reducing the systemic blood pressure.[25] Kinins also influence other blood vessels: They increase capillary permeability, probably by diminishing the size (possibly through contraction) of the endothelial cells[10]; they stimulate the veins; and they also modulate the functions of a variety of blood and tissue cells.

### INFLAMMATION

Kinins are among the most potent activators of the arachidonic acid cascade,[26] and they promote the release of prosta-

glandins, prostacyclins, and other similar compounds from various cells (see Chap. 172). Kinins also stimulate the release of histamine and, possibly, of 5-hydroxytryptamine from mast cells. Moreover, they modulate the motility and the function of leukocytes, macrophages, fibroblasts, and other cells.[4,26] Kinins have also been implicated in the pathogenesis of inflammation, of tissue reactions to injury, and of tissue repair. In this context, two biologic effects of kinins are particularly important: the stimulation of the mitosis of T lymphocytes[27] and the activation of protein formation and cell division (by both bradykinin and desArg[9] bradykinin) in human lung fibroblasts.[28] Collagen formation also appears to be stimulated by the kinins. The involvement of $B_2$ and especially $B_1$ receptors in acute or chronic pain and inflammation has been discussed.[16,29]

### ALGOGENIC EFFECT

Kinins are the most active natural substances that are algogenic (producing pain). When injected intraarterially or applied on a cutaneous "blister base," these peptides evoke pain in both human subjects and animals. It is still uncertain whether kinins produce the pain by direct stimulation of the nerve endings or through the release of prostaglandins, which strongly potentiate kinin algogenic actions.[26,29]

Most of the effects mentioned earlier, including pain, are mediated by $B_2$ receptors, which are constitutive: In pathologic conditions, the inducible (e.g., by interleukin-1$\beta$[16]) $B_1$ receptors sustain the acute effects initiated by the $B_2$.[16,29]

### OTHER ENDOCRINE AND EXOCRINE EFFECTS

Kinins increase the release of both catecholamines from the adrenal glands and renin from the kidney. The physiologic significance of such effects is uncertain, considering the high concentrations ($10^{-6}$ M) of kinins that are needed to stimulate the hormonal release. Kinins also promote the secretion of exocrine glands, such as the pancreas and the salivary glands, which have a very high kallikrein content.[8,10]

### OTHER POSSIBLE PHYSIOLOGIC EFFECTS

Receptors for kinins, generally of the $B_2$ type, are found in various smooth muscles in the gastrointestinal and urinary tracts, the tracheobronchial tree, and the uterus. Except for the bronchi, the physiologic significance of such stimulatory effects of the kinins in all of these organs remains to be established. Through a complex mechanism involving the prostaglandins, angiotensin, and histamine, and also through direct effects on several types of renal cells (vascular, parenchymatous, interstitial), kinins act on the kidney to induce natriuresis and diuresis. They also antagonize the effect of vasopressin on water excretion.[30,31]

In the pancreas and the kidney, glandular kallikreins may act as activators of proinsulin and prorenin; such observations are interesting because they suggest that kallikreins may be involved in the conversion of prohormones to hormones. Moreover, these enzymes and their peptide products have other effects,[32] since they promote sperm motility and cell proliferation. Furthermore, the $\beta$-nerve growth factor, endopeptidase, appears to be a kallikrein.[33] Surveys of the many possible biologic roles of kallikreins and an overview of kallikrein and kininogens in general have been published.[6,8]

## PATHOPHYSIOLOGIC ASPECTS OF KININS

### KININ ACTIVATION

Apparently, kinins and kallikreins are hormones that are activated or generated by noxious stimuli to participate in the processes of tissue defense and repair. Probably the first of these processes is blood clotting and fibrinolysis. Both plasma kallikrein and the Hageman factor (kallikrein activator) promote clotting; deficiencies of these factors are the major causes of the Fitzgerald, the Williams, the Flanjeac, and also the Fugiwara traits. The interactions between the various factors involved have been summarized as follows.

Contact with negatively charged surfaces converts Hageman factor (clotting factor XII) to its active form (XIIa). The active enzyme XIIa then initiates intrinsic and extrinsic blood clotting, fibrinolysis, and plasma kinin formation, by activating clotting factors VII and XI, prekallikrein, and plasminogen activator, respectively. The active factor XIa, plasmin, and plasma-kallikrein then convert more factor XII to XIIa. High-molecular-weight kininogen facilitates the interaction between XIIa and kallikrein, and also serves as a kinin-yielding substrate. Prekallikrein is also activated by plasmin.[34]

Such activations may occur in several pathologic states. According to one investigator,[34] "significant activation may be produced by urate and pyrophosphate crystals in gout and pseudogout, by collagen in vascular injury, by glomerular basement membrane in some forms of glomerulonephritis, and by lipopolysaccharides in gram-negative infections."

Kinins contribute to the basic vascular and cellular events that occur in inflammation.[35] Local activation of kallikrein and an increased production of kinins have been found in various inflammatory lesions produced experimentally, for example, by carrageenan, urate crystals, heat, and other noxious manipulations.[10] The decrease of pH in inflamed tissues may activate kallikreins and reduce the degradation of kinins, thereby maintaining fairly high concentrations of these peptides during the acute and chronic phases of inflammation. In experimental shock, the kallikrein–kinin system is activated.[36] Kinins contribute not only to rubor, dolor, calor, and tumor, but to tissue defense and repair by the activation of cell (polymorphonucleocytes, leukocytes) migration. Kallikrein may also influence the renal response to sepsis.[37]

## KALLIKREIN–KININS AND HYPERTENSION

The findings that high concentrations of kallikreins and traces of kinins are present in the urine of healthy people, and that kallikreins are decreased in some forms of hypertension, have caused great interest. Kallikreins are synthesized in the distal tubule, possibly to control water and electrolyte excretion. They have a functional link with the renin-angiotensin system.[38] By diffusing to the juxtaglomerular apparatus, kallikreins promote the conversion of prorenin to renin.[3] The urinary kallikreins are influenced by variations in sodium and mineralocorticoids; they are increased in patients consuming a low-sodium diet and in those with primary aldosteronism, Bartter syndrome, or hyponatremia. They are reduced in essential hypertension and after the administration of spironolactone.[39] This decrease in kallikrein excretion is found in both human and experimental hypertension, and it has been suggested that a decreased activity level of the kallikrein–kinin system in the kidney might generate favorable conditions for the development and maintenance of high blood pressure.[12] Other implications of the kinins and their receptors in pathophysiology have been reviewed.[16,40]

## REFERENCES

1. Rocha e Silva M. Kinin hormones. Springfield, IL: Charles C Thomas Publisher, 1970.
2. Pisano JJ. Chemistry and biology of the kallikrein-kinin system. In: Reich E, Rifkin DB, Shaw E, eds. Proteases and biological control, vol 2. Cold Spring Harbor, NY: Cold Spring Harbor Laboratory, 1975:199.
3. Levinsky NG. The renal kallikrein-kinin system. Circ Res 1979; 44:441.
4. Marceau F, Lussier A, Regoli D, Giroud J-P. Pharmacology of kinins:

their relevance to tissue injury and inflammation. Gen Pharmacol 1983; 14:209.
5. Colman RW. Formation of human plasma kinin. N Engl J Med 1974; 291:509.
6. Schachter M. Kallikreins (kininogenases): a group of serine proteases with bioregulatory actions. Pharmacol Rev 1980; 31:1.
7. Hall JM. Bradykinin receptors: pharmacological properties and biological roles. Pharmacol Ther 1992; 56:131.
8. Bhoola KD, Figneroa CD, Worthy K. Bioregulation of kinins: kallikreins, kininogens and kininases. Pharmacol Rev 1992; 44:1.
9. Erdüs EG. Kininases. Handbook Exp Pharmacol 1979; 25(Suppl):427.
10. Regoli D, Barabé J. Pharmacology of bradykinin and related kinins. Pharmacol Rev 1980; 32:1.
11. Ferreira SH, Vane JR. The detection and estimation of bradykinin in the circulating blood. Br J Pharmacol 1967; 29:367.
12. Carretero OA, Scicli AG. Possible role of kinins in circulatory homeostasis. Hypertension 1981; 3:1.
13. Shimamoto K, Ando T, Tanaka S, et al. An improved method for the determination of human blood kinin levels by sensitive kinin radioimmunoassay. Endocrinol Jpn 1982; 29:487.
14. Carretero OA, Scicli AG. The renal kallikrein–kinin system. Am J Physiol 1980; 238:F247.
15. Schild HO. Receptor classification with special reference to beta adrenergic receptors. In: Rang HP, ed. Drug receptors. Baltimore: University Park Press, 1973:29.
16. Marceau F, Hess JF, Bachvarov DR. The B$_1$ receptor for kinins. Pharmacol Rev 1998;50:357.
17. Vavrek RJ, Stewart JM. Competitive antagonists of bradykinin. Peptides 1985; 6:161.
18. Wirth K, Hock FJ, Albus U, et al. HOE 140, a new potent and long-acting bradykinin antagonist: in vivo studies. Br J Pharmacol 1991; 102:774.
19. Hess JF, Borkowski JA, Young GS, et al. Cloning and pharmacological characterization of a human bradykinin (BK-2) receptor. Biochem Biophys Res Commun 1992; 184:260.
20. Menke JG, Borkowski JA, Bierilo KK, et al. Expression cloning of a human B$_1$ bradykinin receptor. J Biol Chem 1994; 269:21583.
21. Regoli D, Jukic D, Rhaleb NE, Gobeil F. Receptors for bradykinin and related kinins. A critical analysis. Can J Physiol Pharmacol 1993; 71:556.
22. Regoli D, Gobeil F, Nguyen OT, et al. Bradykinin receptor types and subtypes. Life Sci 1994; 55:735.
23. Werle E, Berek U. Zur Kenntnis des Kallikreins. Z Angew Chemie 1948; 60A:53.
24. D'Orléans-Juste P, Dion S, Mizrahi J, Regoli D. Effects of peptides and non-peptides on isolated arterial smooth muscles: role of endothelium. Eur J Pharmacol 1985; 114:9.
24a. Halle S, Gobeil F Jr, Ouellette J, et al. In vivo and in vitro effects of kinin B(1) and B(2) receptor agonists and antagonists in inbred control and cardiomyopathic hamsters. Br J Pharmacol 2000; 129:1641.
25. Thorgeirsson G. Endothelial autacoids. Acta Med Scand 1985; 217:453.
26. Nasjletti A, Malik KU. Relationships between the kallikrein–kinin and prostaglandin systems. Life Sci 1979; 25:99.
27. Perris AO, Whitfield JF. The mitogenic action of bradykinin on thymic lymphocytes and its dependence on calcium. Proc Soc Exp Biol Med 1969; 62:1198.
28. Goldstein RH, Wall M. Activation of protein formation and cell division by bradykinin and desArg$^9$-bradykinin. J Biol Chem 1984; 259:9263.
29. Dray A, Perkins M. Bradykinin and inflammatory pain. Trends Neurosci 1993; 16:99.
30. Abe K, Irokawa N, Yasujima M, et al. The kallikrein–kinin system and prostaglandins in the kidney. Circ Res 1978; 43:254.
31. Yamada K, Hasunuma K, Shiina T, et al. Inter-relationship between urinary kallikrein–kinins and arginine vasopressin in man. Clin Sci 1989; 76:13.
32. Jauch KW, Hartl WH, Georgieff M, et al. Low-dose bradykinin infusion reduces endogenous glucose production in surgical patients. Metabolism 1988; 37:185.
33. Bothwell MA, Wilson WH, Shooter EM. The relationship between glandular kallikrein and growth factor-processing proteases of mouse submaxillary gland. J Biol Chem 1979; 254:7287.
34. Eisen V. Kinins in physiology and pathology. Trends Pharmacol Sci 1980; 1:212.
35. Garcia-Leme J. Bradykinin system. Handbook Exp Pharmacol 1979; 50:464.
36. Christopher TA, Xin-Liang MA, Gouthier TW, Lefer AM. Beneficial actions of CP-0127, a novel bradykinin receptor antagonist, in murine traumatic shock. Am J Physiol 1994; 266:H867.
37. Cumming AD, Driedger AA, McDonald JW, et al. Vasoactive hormones in the renal response to systemic sepsis. Am J Kidney Dis 1988; 11:23.
38. Cumming AD, Jeffrey S, Lambic AT, Robson JS. The kallikrein–kinin and renin–angiotensin systems in nephrotic syndrome. Nephron 1989; 51:185.
39. Mills IH. Kallikrein, kininogen and kinins in control of blood pressure. Nephron 1979; 23:61.
40. Stewart JM, Gera L, Chan DC, et al. Potent, long-acting bradykinin antagonists for a wide range of applications. Can J Physiol Pharmacol 1997; 75:719.

# CHAPTER 171

# SUBSTANCE P AND THE TACHYKININS

NEIL ARONIN

Substance P, which is an 11–amino-acid peptide formed by cleavage of a larger precursor molecule, has a widespread and heterogeneous distribution in the central and peripheral nervous systems, the gastrointestinal tract, and the endocrine tissues.[1–5] Consistent with its presence in multiple tissues, this peptide has diverse actions, stimulating or enhancing activity in some cells, while inhibiting activity in others. For example, in the dorsal horn of the spinal cord, substance P acts as an excitatory neurotransmitter in primary afferents conveying pain, whereas in the ventral horn of the spinal cord, substance P inhibits Renshaw cell activity. Detailed reviews on the discovery, localization, and physiologic role of substance P in the neural and gastrointestinal systems are available.[3–5,5a] Current research on substance P (and the related peptides, tachykinins) centers on their contributions to inflammation. The availability of tachykinin-specific receptor antagonists and knock-out mice has provided useful tools to study the potential role of substance P and tachykinins in the pathogenesis and treatment of a variety of diseases.

## TACHYKININS

Substance P shares a common carboxyl-terminus (C-terminus) sequence with other peptides. Together, these related peptides with common hypotensive properties are known as *tachykinins* (Fig. 171-1). A number of laboratories contributed to the discovery and naming of the tachykinin family of peptides. A uniform nomenclature has now been adopted. Substance P, neurokinin A, neuropeptide K, and neuropeptide γ are all found in mammalian tissues. In general, substance P is the tachykinin of highest abundance. Physalaemin, which may be found in small amounts in mammalian brain, was first isolated from the skin of a South American amphibian. Eledoisin was discovered in extracts from cephalopod salivary glands. Neurokinin A (heretofore, substance K) was discovered in a prohormone that also contains substance P.[6,7] Neuropeptide K (previously called *neuromedin K*) resembles other tachykinins structurally and shares some of their biologic effects, but is generated from a different tachykinin precursor.[8] Many of the biologic activities of the tachykinins reside in the amidated C terminus.

## BIOSYNTHESIS OF SUBSTANCE P

Three protein precursors to substance P have been identified: α-, β-, and γ-preprotachykinin A. The primary structures of these precursors have been derived from mammalian brain

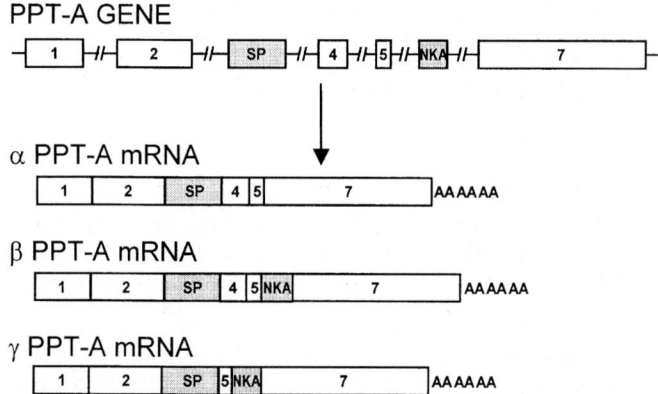

**FIGURE 171-2.** The preprotachykinin-A (*PPT-A*) gene and alternatively spliced *mRNA* structures: α-, β-, γ-preprotachykinin A mRNAs. Different tissues may have a preference for expressing one of the mRNAs. The unamidated substance P (*SP*), neurokinin A (*NKA*), and N terminally extended forms of NKA, neuropeptide K (β-PPT-A mRNA), and neuropeptide γ (γ-PPT-A mRNA) would then be cleaved enzymatically from the precursor protein and amidated to form bioactive peptides. (Reprinted from Nawa H, Kotani H, Nakanishi S. Tissue-specific generation to two preprotachykinin mRNAs from one gene by alternative RNA splicing. Nature 1984; 312:733, copyright 1984, Macmillan Journals Limited.)

cDNA sequences.[4,6,7,9] These tachykinin precursors are nearly homologous (Fig. 171-2) and differ in the inclusion (or exclusion) of specific exons in the cDNAs. Both substance P and neurokinin A are present in β- and γ-preprotachykinin A. Only substance P is found in α-preprotachykinin A. All three preprotachykinin mRNAs originate from a single gene, preprotachykinin A, and are subsequently generated by alternative RNA splicing.[6,9] A separate gene, preprotachykinin B, leads to the synthesis of the protein precursor to neurokinin B.[8] A cDNA encoding β-preprotachykinin A has been isolated in a human carcinoid tumor containing a large amount of immunoreactive substance P.[10] The human cDNA for β-preprotachykinin A has extensive sequence overlap with bovine cDNA β-preprotachykinin A.

The relative distribution of mRNAs for α-, β-, and γ-preprotachykinin A varies in neural and nonneural tissues; their peptide products also vary.[4,7] The finding of several, structurally related tachykinins in the same brain regions and peripheral tissues suggests that these peptides may interact on their target cells. There is little information on putative interactions, however. Substance P and neurokinin A share properties of the tachykinin family, but differ in potency.[11] Clues to cellular effects of the tachykinins may be emerging from advances on tachykinin receptors. Until now, the designation of tachykinin receptors was based on relative affinities to physalaemin, eledoisin, and substance K (neurokinin A). It is now known that tachykinin receptors (to date, NK1, NK2, NK3) are each encoded by a separate gene. NK1 has highest affinity to substance P; NK2 to neurokinin A; NK3 to neurokinin B.[12,13] However, each NK-receptor subtype binds other tachykinin peptides.[13] The receptors couple to G protein (possibly through a pertussis toxin-insensitive G protein) and appear to participate in the regulation of intracellular $Ca^{2+}$ by affecting phosphoinositide hydrolysis.[13,14] Specific actions of the receptor subtypes are under intense investigation, especially with use of newly developed pharmacologic tools such as peptide and nonpeptide tachykinin receptor agonists and antagonists.[15]

## DISTRIBUTION AND ACTIONS OF SUBSTANCE P IN ENDOCRINE GLANDS

Substance P–like immunoreactivity is measurable in most endocrine tissues by radioimmunoassay and immunohisto-

| | |
|---|---|
| **Substance P** | Arg-Pro-Lys-Pro-Gln-Gln-Phe-Phe-Gly-Leu-Met-NH₂ |
| **Neurokinin A** | His-Lys-Thr-Asp-Ser-Phe-Val-Gly-Leu-Met-NH₂ |
| **Neuropeptide K** | β-PPT(72-97)-His-Lys-Thr-Asp-Ser-Phe-Val-Gly-Leu-Met-NH₂ |
| **Neuropeptide γ** | γ-PPT(72-82)-His-Lys-Thr-Asp-Ser-Phe-Val-Gly-Leu-Met-NH₂ |
| **Neurokinin B** | Asp-Met-His-Asp-Phe-Phe-Val-Gly-Leu-Met-NH₂ |
| **Physalaemin** | pGlu-Ala-Asp-Pro-Asn-Lys-Phe-Tyr-Gly-Leu-Met-NH₂ |
| **Eledoisin** | pGlu-Pro-Ser-Lys-Asp-Ala-Phe-Ile-Gly-Leu-Met-NH₂ |

**FIGURE 171-1.** Structures of substance P and some related peptides. (*pGlu*, pyroglutamic acid; *PPT*, preprotachykinin.)

chemistry. However, despite studies suggesting that it may influence the release of various hormones, specific roles for substance P in endocrine tissues have not yet been elucidated.[16,17] Most of these studies examined effects of substance P, rather than the related tachykinins; the results can be attributed to substance P primarily.

## ANTERIOR PITUITARY

Substance P may gain access to the regulation of the anterior pituitary at many sites along the hypothalamic-hypophysial axis. Substance P is detected in neural afferents to the hypothalamus, neuroendocrine cells of the hypothalamus, hypothalamic interneurons, the median eminence, neural fibers in the anterior pituitary, and cells composing the anterior pituitary.[16,18–20] It is probably not surprising that effects of substance P on hormone release appear to depend (at least in part) on the route of administration. Thus, the substance P–induced increase in prolactin secretion is usually consistent, whether the tachykinin is administered intravenously or intracerebroventricularly, or in vitro. However, the substance P effects on growth hormone, luteinizing hormone, corticotropin, and thyroid-stimulating hormone secretion are less consistent and vary according to route of peptide administration, use of antipeptide antisera, overall hormonal state of the animal, and maturation of the animal. Results of intravenous injection of substance P on pituitary hormone release in human subjects do not necessarily correspond to findings in other experimental animals.[17,21]

There is, nonetheless, some enthusiasm for a paracrine role for substance P (or other tachykinins) in the anterior pituitary gland. Substance P is measurable in anterior pituitary extracts, its pituitary concentrations are regulated by thyroid hormone and gonadal steroids, and it is located primarily in somatotropes in male rats and more frequently in thyrotropes in female rats.[19,22–24] Substance P is synthesized in the anterior pituitary (including human), and the pituitary concentrations of several preprotachykinin A mRNAs are regulated by thyroid hormone and gonadal steroids.[25] Direct effects of substance P on secretion of hormones in the anterior pituitary have been demonstrated.[16,17,26]

## THYROID

Substance P immunoreactivity in the thyroid has been demonstrated in neural fibers surrounding blood vessels and follicles. No effect of substance P on iodothyronine release has been observed, but in the rat, substance P is known to stimulate calcitonin secretion.[27]

## ADRENAL GLAND, OVARY, AND TESTIS

The substance P that is found in the adrenal medulla appears to be localized to nerve fibers that originate from the splanchnic nerve and terminate adjacent to chromaffin cells. Many studies have supported the concept of a modulatory role for substance P in catecholamine release; alone, this peptide has little or no direct influence on catecholamine secretion. There is evidence that substance P enhances catecholamine release after splanchnic nerve stimulation, by facilitating acetylcholine release presynaptically and postsynaptically to protect against nicotinic receptor desensitization.[28,29] Substance P may also influence cortisol secretion from adrenocortical cells. In vitro, substance P increased cortisol release in a $Ca^{2+}$-dependent manner in the adrenal cortex (where adrenocorticotropic hormone acts primarily through cyclic adenosine monophosphate–dependent signal transduction).[30] A physiologic role for substance P in adrenal cortical control remains speculative. Likewise, substance P and neurokinin A mRNAs and tachykinin receptors are detectable in testis, albeit in low abundance.[31] Substance P is distributed in nerve fibers in the ovary and also may be pro-

duced in both granulosa and luteal cells in culture, where it inhibits androstenedione and progesterone release, but stimulates estradiol secretion.[32] The studies are few, however, and the results unconfirmed.

## PANCREAS

In the pancreas, substance P is found in neural fibers; it influences secretion from the exocrine and endocrine pancreas. Arterial infusion of substance P increases total pancreatic outflow, and, therefore, secretion of bicarbonate and amylase.[33] During meals or secretin administration, substance P inhibits amylase secretion. There is evidence that it promotes hyperglycemia, but direct effects on insulin and glucagon secretion (either enhancing or diminishing) are inconsistent. Because substance P and calcitonin gene-related peptide (CGRP) are localized in pancreatic nervous tissue, neural stimulation in the pancreas may be attributable to one or both of these chemical messengers.[34] Different responses also probably depend on differences in study designs.

## SUBSTANCE P IN THE BLOOD

Substance P has been measured by radioimmunoassay in plasma extracts. In humans, reported normal values for immunoreactive substance P vary from 30 to more than 600 fmol/mL.[35–37] As with many small peptides, plasma measurements are likely to be influenced by the method of extraction, as well as by nonspecific factors that alter antibody-peptide binding in the radioimmunoassay. Much of the circulating substance P appears to be derived from the intestine because the portal venous blood contains four times the concentration of the peptide in peripheral areas. The physiologic role of circulating substance P remains unknown.

## SUBSTANCE P IN CLINICAL MEDICINE

Carcinoid tumors contain peptides, along with serotonin or its metabolites. Substance P immunoreactivity has been detected in carcinoid tumors originating in the midgut region, as well as in less common sites of origin, such as the testicle and ovary. High circulating levels of substance P have been found in patients with carcinoid tumors.[38,39] This finding suggests that substance P may be a useful marker for the localization of these tumors. In one report in which selective catheterization and measurement of plasma serotonin failed to localize an ovarian carcinoid tumor, selective intraoperative blood sampling and measurement of substance P from the ovarian venous drainage revealed an increase in plasma concentrations of substance P.[40] Occasionally, increased plasma concentrations of substance P have been found in patients with carcinoid tumors when simultaneous measurements of serotonin or serotonin metabolite levels were negative.[33] These observations must be confirmed prospectively to determine whether plasma substance P can be used for diagnosing carcinoid, for precisely localizing the tumor, and for judging efficacy of treatment.

Because substance P can mediate many vascular changes, including enhancement of vascular permeability and vasodilation, as well as increase intestinal motility, a role for substance P in the carcinoid diathesis has been postulated.[33] In dogs, the arterial infusion of substance P in amounts sufficient to equal the plasma concentrations of substance P found in patients with carcinoid tumors reduced systemic vascular resistance, increased cardiac output, and enhanced the redistribution of blood flow to the muscular layers of the gastrointestinal tract.[41]

There are a few reports of the presence of substance P in other types of cancers. In some cases of medullary carcinoma of the thyroid, substance P immunoreactivity has been documented in the tumor, and increased levels have been detected in plasma extracts.[32] Antagonists directed to tachykinin receptors were shown to inhibit the growth of small cell lung cancer transplanted in nude mice.[42] Because antagonists to substance P receptors can have broad effects against other neuropeptide receptors (bombesin, gastrin-releasing peptide, vasopressin), a specific growth-promoting role for tachykinins in this experimental paradigm remains unsettled.

A number of investigations support a role for tachykinins in the pathogenesis of diseases involving inflammation. There is evidence that the substance P that is released from peripheral nerve terminals may contribute to the development of rheumatoid arthritis. When incubated with substance P, synoviocytes from patients with rheumatoid arthritis were found to increase the generation of prostaglandin $E_2$ and the release of collagenase.[43] These effects may be observed with as little as $10^{-9}$ M of substance P, and are inhibited by a substance P antagonist. Furthermore, it has been proposed that substance P may mediate neural effects on the initiation or maintenance of the inflammatory process in the arthritic joint.[43] Substance P, in partnership with proinflammatory cytokines, increases the expression of the adhesion molecule, vascular cell adhesion molecule-1 (VCAM-1), in fibroblast-like synoviocytes, thus promoting inflammation of the synovium.[44]

Tachykinins, especially substance P, may contribute to the pulmonary inflammation and airway hyperactivity found in experimental asthma.[45–47] Agents that cause tachykinin release from nerve endings, such as capsaicin, can result in contraction of isolated tracheal smooth muscle, an effect mediated by NK1 and NK2 receptors. Pretreatment with capsaicin, which probably depletes neuropeptides from autonomic nerve endings, markedly attenuates carbachol-induced hyperactivity in mice that manifest tracheal hyperactivity.[47] Altogether, tachykinins may modulate immune function and reactions by effects on cellular mediators of inflammation (mast cells, macrophages, T cells), by stimulating contractility of smooth muscle (bronchoconstriction), and by affecting proliferation of smooth muscle cells, endothelial cells, and fibroblasts.[45,47]

Use of NK1 knock-out mice has confirmed a role for substance P in pulmonary inflammation. The expected proinflammatory response to immune complex was abrogated in mice lacking NK1 receptors.[48–50] Non-peptide tachykinin antagonists offer promise of reducing tachykinin-dependent plasma extravasation or bronchoconstriction after a variety of chemical challenges to the airway.[51] To date, the efficacy of tachykinin antagonists in human pulmonary disease remains unknown.

The original extracts in which substance P was found included intestinal tissues.[1] Substance P and tachykinins are expressed throughout the gut—primarily in the enteric and extrinsic primary afferent nervous systems, but also in endocrine cells in the epithelium, immune cells, and endothelial cells.[52] Diseases affecting the enteric or primary afferent nervous system in the intestines are associated with substance P reduction. These diseases include Hirschsprung disease and megacolon in patients with myotonic dystrophy. Increases in substance P receptor expression or sensitivity are reported in inflammatory bowel disease, implicating actions of tachykinins in their inflammatory and vascular abnormalities.

Substance P may also prove useful in the early detection of diabetic sensory neuropathy of the skin. Exposure to noxious agents stimulates the release of transmitters from primary sensory neurons innervating skin. This release is followed by immediate vasodilatation, an increase in vascular permeability, and the release of histamine from local mast cells that causes a visible cutaneous "flare" and wheal. The phenomenon, which is called the *axon response* or *triple response of Lewis*, is thought to be mediated by a number of components, including substance P found in a subpopulation of primary sensory neurons. Diabetic patients with clinical sensory neuropathy exhibit a reduced flare response after the intradermal injection of substance P, as compared to that of healthy subjects or diabetics without clinical evidence of neuropathy.[53] Also, the impaired responses in diabetics have been found to occur in medial forearm skin, where sensory function is often normal by clinical examination (see Chap. 148). Thus, the substance P–provoked flare response may be a sensitive indicator of both the presence of cutaneous sensory neuropathy in diabetic patients and changes in sensory neural function after therapy. There is also clinical evidence that depletion of substance P (or other effects on the C fiber) after daily application of dilute capsaicin to the skin has salutary effects in the treatment of painful diabetic neuropathy.[54] Not all sensory modalities may be improved, but it appears that up to half of diabetic patients with uncontrolled, painful neuropathy may benefit from this therapy. Long-term side effects of this treatment are not known.

Continued use of the noncommittal term "substance P" seems appropriate. This hormone may have multiple roles in the endocrine system—as a neurotransmitter, neuromodulator, or paracrine agent—in keeping with its presence in neural inputs to endocrine glands, as well as its expression in endocrine cells. Substance P and its related tachykinins also serve as mediators at neural and immune junctions. Advances in the knowledge of tachykinin receptors and the availability of peptide and nonpeptide receptor antagonists offer considerable possibilities in the treatment of a wide variety of clinical disorders in which the tachykinins are implicated to play an important role.

# REFERENCES

1. von Euler US, Gaddum JH. An unidentified depressor substance in certain tissue extracts. J Physiol 1931; 72:74.
2. Chang MM, Leeman SE, Niall HD. Amino acid sequence of substance P. Nature 1971; 232:86.
3. Aronin N, DiFiglia M, Leeman SE. Substance P. In: Krieger DT, Brownstein MJ, Martin JB, eds. Brain peptides. New York: John Wiley and Sons, 1983:783.
4. Krause JE, MacDonald MR, Takeda Y. The polyprotein nature of substance P precursors. Bioessays 1989; 10:62.
5. Otsuka M, Yoshioka K. Neurotransmitter functions of mammalian tachykinins. Physiol Rev 1993; 73:229.
5a. Hokfelt T, Broberger C, Xu ZQ, et al. Neuropeptides—an overview. Neuropharmacol 2000; 39:1337.
6. Nawa H, Hirose T, Takashima H, et al. Nucleotide sequences of cloned cDNAs for two types of bovine brain. Nature 1983; 306:32.
7. Nawa H, Kotani H, Nakanishi S. Tissue-specific generation to two preprotachykinin mRNAs from one gene by alternative RNA splicing. Nature 1984; 312:729.
8. Kotani H, Hoshimaru M, Nawa H, Nakanishi S. Structure and gene organization of bovine neuromedin K precursor. Proc Natl Acad Sci U S A 1986; 83:7074.
9. Krause JE, Chirgwin JM, Caarter MS, et al. Three rat preprotachykinin mRNAs encode the neuropeptides substance P and neurokinin A. Proc Natl Acad Sci U S A 1987; 84:881.
10. Harmer AJ, Armstrong A, Pascall JC, et al. cDNA sequence of human β-preprotachykinin, the common precursor to substance P and neurokinin A. FEBS Lett 1986; 208:67.
11. Nawa H, Doteuchi M, Igano K, et al. Substance K: a novel mammalian tachykinin that differs from substance P in its pharmacological profile. Life Sci 1984; 34:1153.
12. Masu Y, Nakayama K, Tamaki H, et al. cDNA cloning of bovine substance-K receptor through oocyte expression system. Nature 1987; 329,836.
13. Watson S, Girdleston D. Receptor and ion channel nomenclature supplement. Trends Pharmacol Sci 1994; 15:40.
14. Kwatra MM, Schwinn DA, Schreurs J, et al. The substance P receptor, which couples to $G_{q/11}$, is a substrate of β-adrenergic receptor kinase 1 and 2. J Biol Chem 1993; 268:9161.
15. Watling KJ, Krause J. The rising sun shines on substance P and related peptides. Trends Pharmacol Sci 1993; 14:81.
16. Aronin N, Coslovsky R, Leeman SE. Substance P and neurotensin: their roles in the regulation of anterior pituitary function. Annu Rev Physiol 1985; 48:537.
17. Jessop DS, Chowdrey HS, Larsen PJ, Lightman SL. Substance P: multifunctional peptide in the hypothalamo-pituitary system? J Endocrinol 1992; 132:331.
18. Larsen PJ. Distribution of substance P-immunoreactive elements in the preoptic area and the hypothalamus of the rat. J Comp Neurol 1992; 316:287.
19. Brown ER, Roth KA, Krause JE. Sexually dimorphic distribution of substance P in specific anterior pituitary cell populations. Proc Natl Acad Sci U S A 1991; 88:1222.
20. Ju G, Liu S-J, Ma D. Calcitonin gene-related peptide- and substance P-like immunoreactivity innervation of the anterior pituitary in the rat. Neuroscience 1993; 54:981.

21. Coiro V, Capretti L, Volpi R, et al. Stimulation of ACTH/cortisol by intravenously infused substance P in normal men: inhibition by sodium valproate. Neuroendocrinology 1992; 56:459.

22. Aronin N, Morency K, Leeman SE, et al. Regulation by thyroid hormone of the concentration of substance P in the rat anterior pituitary. Endocrinology 1984; 114:2138.

23. Coslovsky R, Evans RW, Leeman SE, et al. The effects of gonadal steroids on the content of substance P in the rat anterior pituitary. Endocrinology 1984; 115:2285.

24. Aronin N, Coslovsky R, Chase K. Hypothyroidism increases substance P concentrations in the heterotopic anterior pituitary. Endocrinology 1988; 122:2911.

25. Jonassen JA, Mullikin-Kilpatrick D, McAdam A, Leeman SE. Thyroid hormone status regulates preprotachykinin-A gene expression in male rat anterior pituitary. Endocrinology 1987; 121:1555.

26. Shamgochiam MD, Leeman SE. Substance P stimulates luteinizing hormone secretion from anterior pituitary cells in culture. Endocrinology 1992; 131:871.

27. Ahren B, Grundiz T, Ekman R, et al. Neuropeptides in the thyroid gland: distribution of substance P and gastrin/cholecystokinin and their effects on the secretion of iodothyronine and calcitonin. Endocrinology 1983; 113:379.

28. Livett BG, Kozousek V, Mizobe F, Dean RM. Substance P inhibits nicotinic activation of chromaffin cells. Nature 1979; 278:256.

29. Zhou X-F, Livett BG. Substance P increases catecholamine secretion from perfused rat adrenal glands evoked by prolonged field stimulation. J Physiol 1990; 425:321.

30. Yoshida T, Mio M, Tasaka K. Cortisol secretion induced by substance P from bovine adrenocortical cells and its inhibition by calmodulin inhibitors. Biochem Pharmacol 1992; 43:513.

31. Chiwakata C, Brackmann B, Hunt N, et al. Tachykinin (substance-P) gene expression in Leydig cells of the human and mouse testis. Endocrinology 1991; 128:2441.

32. Pitzel L, Jarry H, Wuttke W. Effects of substance-P and neuropeptide-Y on in vitro steroid release by porcine granulosa and luteal cells. Endocrinology 1991; 129:1059.

33. Pernow B. Substance P. Pharmacol Rev 1983; 35:85.

34. Carlsson P-O, Sandler S, Jansson L. Influence of the neurotoxin capsaicin on rat pancreatic islets in culture, and on the pancreatic islet blood flow of rats. Eur J Pharmacol 1996; 312:75.

35. Nilsson G, Pernow B, Fisher GH, Folkers K. Presence of substance P-like immunoreactivity in plasma from man and dog. Acta Physiol Scand 1975; 94:542.

36. Powell D, Skrabanek P, Cannon D, Balfe A. Substance P in human plasma. In: Marsan CA, Traczyk WX, eds. Neuropeptides and neural transmission. New York: Raven Press, 1980:105.

37. Skrabanek P, Cannon D, Kirrane J, et al. Circulating immunoreactive substance P in man. Ir J Med Sci 1976; 145:399.

38. Hakanson R, Bengmark S, Brodin E. Substance P-like immunoreactivity in intestinal carcinoid tumors. In: von Euler US, Pernow B, eds. Substance P (Nobel symposium). New York: Raven Press, 1977:55.

39. Emson PC, Gilbert RFT, Martensson H, Nobin A. Elevated concentrations of substance P and 5-HT in plasma in patients with carcinoid tumors. Cancer 1984; 54:714.

40. Strodel WE, Vinik AI, Jaffe BM, et al. Substance P in the localization of a carcinoid tumor. J Surg Oncol 1984; 27:106.

41. Zinner MJ, Yeo CJ, Jaffe BM. The effect of carcinoid levels of serotonin and substance P on hemodynamics. Ann Surg 1984; 199:197.

42. Langdon S, Sethi T, Ritchie A, et al. Broad spectrum neuropeptide antagonists inhibit the growth of small cell lung cancer in vivo. Cancer Res 1992; 52:4554.

43. Lotz M, Carson DA, Vaughan JH. Substance P activation of rheumatoid synoviocytes: neural pathway in pathogenesis of arthritis. Science 1987; 235:893.

44. Lambert N, Lescoulie PL, Yassine-Diab B, et al. Substance P enhances cytokine-induced vascular cell adhesion molecule-1 (VCAM-1) expression on cultured rheumatoid fibroblast-like synoviocytes. Clin Exp Immunol 1998; 113:269.

45. Payan DG. Neuropeptides and inflammation: the role of substance P. Annu Rev Med 1989; 40:341.

46. Ellis JL, Undem BJ. Inhibition by capsazepine of resiniferatoxin- and capsaicin-induced contractions of guinea pig trachea. J Pharmacol Exp Ther 1994; 268:85.

47. Joos GF, Germonpre PR, Pauwels RA. Neural mechanism in asthma. Clin Exp Allergy 2000; 30:605.

48. Colten HR, Krause JE. Pulmonary inflammation—a balancing act. N Engl J Med 1997; 336:1094.

49. Reynolds PN, Holmes MD, Scicchitano R. Role of tachykinins in bronchial hyper-responsiveness. Clin Exp Pharmacol Physiol 1997; 24:273.

50. Bozic CR, Lu B, Hopken UE, et al. Neurogenic amplification of immune complex inflammation. Science 1996; 273:1722.

51. Bertrand C, Geppetti P. Tachykinin and kinin receptor antagonists: therapeutic perspectives in allergic airway disease. TIPS 1996; 17:255.

52. Holzer P, Holzer-Petsche U. Tachykinins in the gut. Part II. Roles in neural excitation, secretion and inflammation. Pharmacol Ther 1997; 73:219.

53. Aronin N, Leeman SE, Clements RS Jr. Diminished flare response in neuropathic diabetic patients: comparison of effects of substance P, histamine, and capsaicin. Diabetes 1987; 36:1139.

54. Chad DA, Aronin N, Lundstrom R, et al. Does capsaicin relieve the pain of diabetic neuropathy? Pain 1990; 42:387.

# CHAPTER 172

# PROSTAGLANDINS, THROMBOXANES, AND LEUKOTRIENES

R. PAUL ROBERTSON

Few scientific areas have surpassed the field of arachidonic acid metabolism in the accumulation of new biologic information over the past three decades. Arachidonic acid and one or more of its *products—prostaglandins* (PG), *thromboxanes* (TX), and *leukotrienes* (LT)—have been investigated as regulators or counterregulators of virtually every organ and tissue in the mammalian body. Moreover, roles for these fatty acids have emerged and continue to be discovered for many endocrine organs and their target tissues.

PG, TX, and LT are not blood-borne hormones in the classic sense. Although it is true that they have many hormone-like effects, there is no evidence that they have hemocrine characteristics. Rather, they are paracrine hormones, or autacoids, that are synthesized by the tissue in which they act and primarily provide fine modulation of ongoing cellular activity.

## ARACHIDONIC ACID METABOLISM

PGs were the first arachidonic acid metabolites to be discovered and were so named because they were originally identified in seminal fluid and thought to be secreted by the prostate. Arachidonic acid is stored in the membranes of cells as part of phospholipids. Phospholipase $A_2$ activation is the mechanism for cleavage of arachidonic acid from phospholipid and initiation of the arachidonic acid cascade. A phospholipase-activating protein termed *PLAP* has been identified in some cells. An alternate mechanism involves phosphatidylinositol and three enzymes: phospholipase C, a diacylglycerol lipase, and a monoglyceride lipase.

The *cyclooxygenase* and the *lipoxygenase* pathways are two major routes by which arachidonic acid is oxygenated. Products of the cyclooxygenase pathway include all of the *PG* and *TX*. The lipoxygenase pathway generates the *LT* and other substances such as *hydroxyeicosatetraenoic acids* (HETE). Several lipoxygenase pathways, including 5-lipoxygenase and 12-lipoxygenase, are important to human physiology.

The first product of the cyclooxygenase pathway is the cyclic endoperoxide prostaglandin $G_2$ ($PGG_2$), which is converted to prostaglandin $H_2$ ($PGH_2$). $PGG_2$ and $PGH_2$ are the key intermediates in the formation of physiologically active prostaglandins ($PGD_2$, $PGE_2$, $PGF_{2\alpha}$, and $PGI_2$) and thromboxane $A_2$ ($TXA_2$). The first product of the 5-lipoxygenase pathway is 5-hydroperoxyeicosatetraenoic acid (5-HPETE), which is an intermediate in the formation of 5-hydroxyeicosatetraenoic acid (5-HETE) and the leukotrienes ($LTA_4$, $LTB_4$, $LTC_4$, $LTD_4$, and $LTE_4$).

All metabolites of arachidonic acid, collectively, are called *eicosanoids*. Arachidonic acid metabolites in the cyclooxygenase pathway carry the subscript 2; LT derivatives in the lipoxygenase pathway carry the subscript 4. These subscripts designate the number of double bonds between carbon atoms in the chains. Eicosanoids are not stored within cells; they are synthesized rapidly according to the needs of the tissue in which they originate. Fish oils contain omega-3 fatty acids, which can decrease production of some arachidonate metabolites and increase levels of prostanoids (cyclooxygenase derivatives) with the subscript 3.

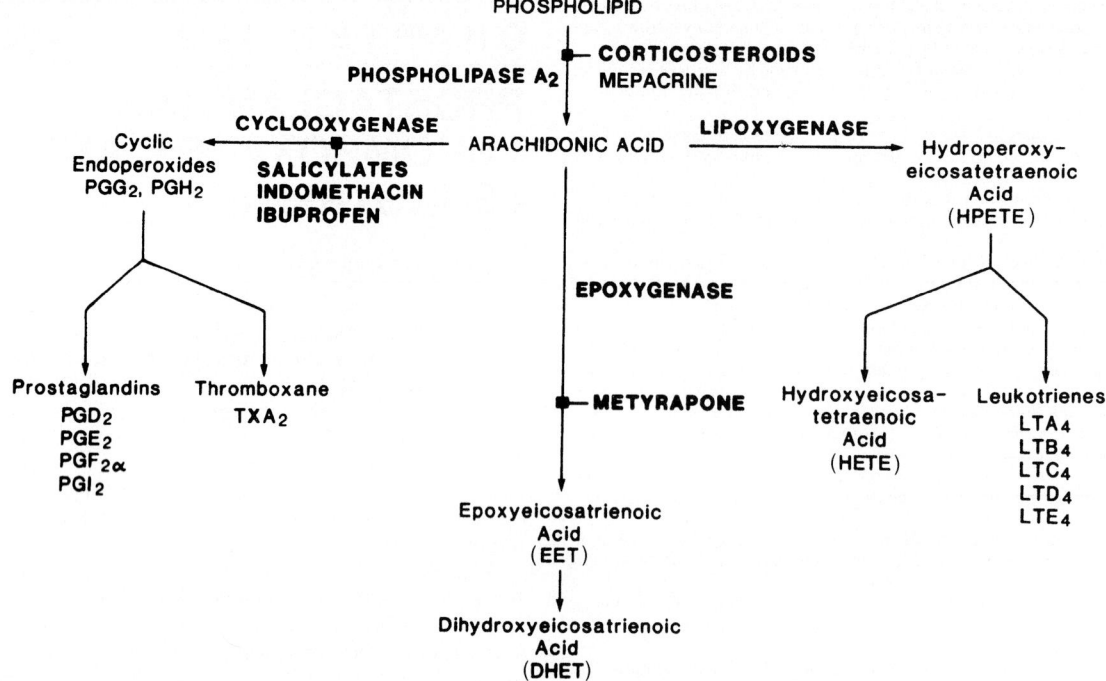

**FIGURE 172-1.** Arachidonic acid metabolism. In this scheme, arachidonic acid is cleaved from phospholipid by phospholipase $A_2$ and subsequently oxygenated predominantly by cyclooxygenase or lipoxygenase. Active metabolites of the former pathway include the prostaglandins (*PG*) and thromboxane $A_2$ (*TXA$_2$*), whereas active metabolites of the latter pathway include the leukotrienes (*LT*) and hydroxyeicosatetraenoic acid (*HETE*). Phospholipase-activating protein (*PLAP*) and 5-lipoxygenase-activating protein (*FLAP*) are found in some cells and activate, respectively, phospholipase and 5-lipoxygenase.

## INFLUENCE OF DRUGS

Several groups of drugs in clinical practice, including *corticosteroids* and *nonsteroidal antiinflammatory* drugs (NSAIDs), inhibit the arachidonic acid cascade (Fig. 172-1). Although these drugs have important clinical uses and historically were of key importance to understanding the relevance of arachidonic acid metabolism to mammalian physiology, none of them specifically inhibits the synthesis of single eicosanoids. The sites of action of these drugs occur early in the arachidonic acid cascade; consequently, they influence the production of many eicosanoids simultaneously. Therefore, it is difficult to ascribe the clinical effect of any of these drugs to the absence of a particular eicosanoid. Another major limitation to full elucidation of the roles of arachidonic acid metabolites has been the paucity of drugs available to serve as specific eicosanoid receptor antagonists.

There are two forms of cyclooxygenase.[1-3] *COX-1*, a basal or constitutive form, generally plays a role in modulating physiologic activities in tissues (Fig. 172-2). The other form, *COX-2*, is a regulated or inducible form of the enzyme that responds to specific stimuli and is usually associated with inflammatory or noxious events in tissues. NSAIDs, as a class, were found to affect the two enzymes with differing potencies,[4] and some of these drugs affect the posttranscriptional mechanisms that form the enzymes as well as their enzymatic activities (Fig. 172-2, Table 172-1). These observations provide new insight into the sites of action for these drugs. For example, aspirin and sodium salicylate can decrease the mass of COX-2 protein as well as inhibit its activity. Drugs such as aspirin, indomethacin, ibuprofen, acetaminophen, and sodium salicylate are more potent in inhibiting COX-1 than COX-2, whereas diclofenac and naproxen are more potent in inhibiting COX-2 than COX-1. Newer, more specific inhibitors of COX-2 include rofecoxib and celecoxib with improved gastrointestinal safety profile.[4a,4b] Thus, the undesirable side effects of NSAIDs are due to interference with normal physiologic processes dependent on COX-1, and specific COX-2 inhibitors may offer more specific treatment of inflammatory processes with

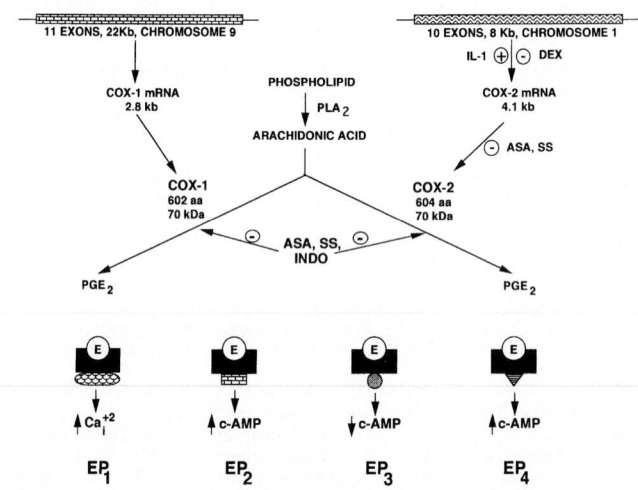

**FIGURE 172-2.** Molecular regulation of prostaglandin synthesis. The COX-1 and COX-2 genes control synthesis of the COX-1 and COX-2 enzymes, respectively. The two genes are located on separate chromosomes and give rise to mRNAs of different sizes. The two enzymes are approximately the same size but have ~60% homology. Both enzymes use arachidonic acid as substrate to generate biologically active prostanoids (PGD$_2$, PGE$_2$, PGF$_{2\alpha}$, PGI$_2$, and TXA$_2$), here represented by PGE$_2$. Once PGE$_2$ is formed, it can interact with any one subtype or all four subtypes of EP receptors. Cytokines, such as interleukin-1 (*IL-1*), and epinephrine (*EPI*) increase gene expression of COX-2 mRNA but do not affect COX-1 mRNA levels. Dexamethasone (*DEX*) diminishes the induction of COX-2 gene expression. Acetylsalicylic acid (*ASA*) and sodium salicylate (*SS*) decrease the mass of COX-2 enzyme translated and processed. These two nonsteroidal antiinflammatory drugs (*NSAIDs*) and others, represented by indomethacin (*INDO*), also inhibit activation of the COX-1 and COX-2 enzymes. None of the NSAIDs affect expression of the COX-1 gene or translation and processing of the COX-1 enzyme. (*c-AMP*, cyclic adenosine monophosphate.) (Adapted from Robertson RP. Molecular regulation of prostaglandin synthesis: implications for endocrine systems. TEM 1995; 6:293.)

**TABLE 172-1.**
IC$_{50}$ Values ($\mu$g/mL) for Nonsteroidal Antiinflammatory Drugs on COX-1 and COX-2 Activity

| NSAID | COX-1 | COX-2 | Ratio |
|---|---|---|---|
| Aspirin | $0.3 \pm 0.2$ | $50 \pm 10$ | 166 |
| Indomethacin | $0.01 \pm 0.001$ | $0.6 \pm 0.08$ | 60 |
| Ibuprofen | $1.0 \pm 0.07$ | $15 \pm 5.3$ | 15 |
| Acetaminophen | $2.7 \pm 2.0$ | $20 \pm 12$ | 7.4 |
| Sodium salicylate | $35 \pm 11$ | $100 \pm 16$ | 2.8 |
| Diclofenac | $0.5 \pm 0.2$ | $0.35 \pm 0.15$ | 0.7 |
| Naproxen | $2.2 \pm 0.9$ | $1.3 \pm 0.8$ | 0.6 |

*cAMP*, cyclic adenosine monophosphate.
(From Mitchell JA, Akarasereenont P, Thiemermann C, et al. Selectivity of nonsteroidal antiinflammatory drugs as inhibitors of constitutive and inducible cyclooxygenase. Proc Natl Acad Sci U S A 1994; 90:11,693.)

**TABLE 172-2.**
Nomenclature for Receptor Subtypes of Cyclooxygenase-Derived Prostanoids and Their Mechanisms of Action

| Receptor Subtype | Mechanisms of Action |
|---|---|
| DP | Stimulation of adenylate cyclase and increased cAMP levels via G$_s$ |
| EP | |
| EP$_1$ | Stimulation of phosphatidylinositol turnover and elevation of intracellular free Ca$^{2+}$ via G$_q$ |
| EP$_2$ | Stimulation of adenylate cyclase and increased cAMP levels via G$_s$ |
| EP$_3$ | Inhibition of adenylate cyclase and decreased cAMP levels via G$_{i/o}$ |
| EP$_4$ | Stimulation of adenylate cyclase and increased cAMP levels via G$_s$ |
| FP | Stimulation of phosphatidylinositol turnover and elevation of intracellular free Ca$^{2+}$ via G$_q$ |
| IP | Stimulation of adenylate cyclase and increased cAMP levels via G$_s$ |
| TP | Stimulation of phosphatidylinositol turnover and elevation of intracellular free Ca$^{2+}$ via G$_q$ |

fewer side effects. Sodium salicylate, specifically, may have yet another mechanism of action involving the transcription factor nuclear factor-kappaB (NF-$\kappa$B), which induces the expression of many genes involved in inflammation and infection. Sodium salicylate and aspirin inhibit the activation of NF-$\kappa$B,[5] which may be involved in the molecular regulation of PG synthesis through its binding site on the COX-2 gene promoter.

## CATABOLISM

Eicosanoids are catabolized rapidly in vivo. Prostaglandin E (PGE) and prostaglandin F (PGF) are degraded almost completely during a single passage through the liver or the lung. Nonmetabolized PGE$_2$ in the urine reflects renal and seminal vesicle production, whereas urinary PGE$_2$ metabolites represent total body synthesis. Both PGI$_2$ and TXA$_2$ are also rapidly catabolized in vivo, as are the LTs. However, most of the eicosanoids have much longer chemical half-lives when stored under proper laboratory conditions.

## ASSAY

Six methods are available to measure eicosanoids in physiologic fluids: bioassay, radioimmunoassay, chromatography, receptor assay, enzyme-linked immunoassay, and mass spectrometry. Special precautions should be taken in handling samples because eicosanoid synthesis may be stimulated during the collection procedure. For example, PGE$_2$ and TXA$_2$ may be generated if blood is allowed to clot or if platelets are not carefully separated from plasma. This problem can be minimized by using an inhibitor of eicosanoid synthesis in the collection tube. Measurements of inactive metabolites of PGE$_2$, PGI$_2$, and TXA$_2$ (e.g., 13,14-dihydro-15-keto-PGE$_2$, 6-keto-PGF$_{1\alpha}$, and TXB$_2$, respectively) are commonly used for physiologic fluids because the parent substances are so short-lived in vivo. Native eicosanoids can be reliably measured in studies using in vitro experiments, such as organ incubations or cell culture.

## MECHANISM OF ACTION

Tissues and cells with receptors for eicosanoids include adipocytes, hepatocytes, pancreatic B cells, adrenal cortex and medulla, corpus luteum, uterus, kidney, stomach, ileum, thymus, skin, brain (including pineal gland), lung, platelets, red blood cells, neutrophils, macrophages, and monocytes. These receptors are found in the plasma membrane and the nucleus and are specific for a given type of eicosanoid. Receptor density can decrease or increase in response to local increases or decreases, respectively, of the ligand for that receptor with corresponding postreceptor effects.[6,7]

Current nomenclature refers to eicosanoid receptors as P receptors; a preceding letter indicates the prostanoid to which

each receptor is most sensitive.[3] Thus, the terms DP, EP, FP, IP, and TP are used. The EP$_1$, EP$_2$, EP$_3$, and EP$_4$ receptors are coupled to transduction systems that alter phosphoinositide hydrolysis or adenylate cyclase activity (Table 172-2). Current research is focused on identification and characterization of the various types and subtypes of prostanoid receptors in tissues throughout the human body. This should help to explain how a given PG might have opposite effects on enzymatic activity, such as for adenylate cyclase in the same or different tissues under differing physiologic or pathophysiologic conditions.

## PHYSIOLOGY AND PATHOPHYSIOLOGY RELEVANT TO THE ENDOCRINE SYSTEM

The areas of endocrinology and metabolism in which eicosanoids have been investigated most intensely include carbohydrate metabolism, lipolysis, bone resorption, and reproductive physiology. However, effects of eicosanoids and drugs that prevent their synthesis have also been investigated in several other endocrine and metabolic tissues.

### CARBOHYDRATE METABOLISM AND DIABETES MELLITUS

Reports of the involvement of PGs in carbohydrate metabolism appeared as early as the later nineteenth century. Sodium salicylate was used in the late 1800s to decrease glycosuria in diabetic patients. Very little significance was attributed to this therapy, especially because insulin was discovered in the 1920s. However, the situation changed with the discovery that NSAIDs inhibit cyclooxygenase.[8] Concomitantly, it was found that PGs of the E series inhibit glucose-induced insulin secretion.[9–11] This PGE effect is mediated by G proteins. It is associated with stimulation of GTPase[12] and a decreased production of cyclic adenosine monophosphate (AMP) that is preventable by pertussis toxin,[13] an agent that inhibits G$_1$ and G$_0$ activity. This inhibitory effect is specific for glucose because the insulin response to other secretagogues is not influenced by PGE$_2$.

The pancreatic islet is an exception to the current dogma about the two cyclooxygenases. Only one COX mRNA has been identified in various nonstimulated and stimulated preparations of pancreatic islets and transformed B-cell lines.[14] The single form is COX-2, which is expressed both basally and under stimulated conditions. COX-2 mRNA is appropriately decreased with dexamethasone, and a COX-2–specific inhibitor blocks all PG synthesis by islets. This COX-2 dominance is associated with high levels of NF-1L6, a transcription factor that stimulates the promoter region of the COX-2 gene. Thus, it appears that under physiologic conditions, the islet tonically synthesizes $PGE_2$, a process known to be stimulated by glucose. Since $PGE_2$ inhibits glucose-induced insulin secretion, this high basal activity of COX-2 might serve to modulate insulin release during physiologic stimulation with glucose.

Type 2 diabetics characteristically lack first-phase insulin responses to intravenous glucose, but retain responsiveness to other secretagogues. Exogenous $PGE_2$ inhibits first-phase insulin responses to glucose stimulation.[9,10] In addition, all NSAIDs (except indomethacin) consistently enhance glucose-induced insulin secretion.[15] Intravenous sodium salicylate infusion doubles the basal insulin level, partially restores defective first- and second-phase insulin responses to intravenous glucose, and accelerates glucose disappearance rates after intravenous glucose challenges in type 2 diabetes.[10] Exogenous $PGE_2$ reverses the augmentation of glucose-induced insulin secretion by NSAIDs.[16] Consequently, it has been hypothesized that PGs of the E series may contribute to abnormal glucose-induced insulin secretion in diabetes mellitus.[17]

Conflicting reports fall into two categories. The first involves studies of the effects of $PGE_2$ itself, rather than effects of $PGE_2$ on glucose stimulation of insulin secretion. Sometimes, $PGE_2$ behaves as a weak stimulator of insulin secretion if glucose concentrations are held constant. This effect appears to depend on activation of islet adenylate cyclase.[18] The second category involves the use of indomethacin as an inhibitor of islet cyclooxygenase. Indomethacin not only fails to augment insulin secretion, but usually inhibits it. Although indomethacin inhibits islet cyclooxygenase, it also affects other enzyme systems and calcium flux across membranes. This multiplicity of indomethacin's effects may explain why it is discordant with other structurally unrelated inhibitors of cyclooxygenase that augment glucose-induced insulin secretion.

Increased circulating levels of $PGE_2$ and $PGI_2$ have been reported in patients in diabetic ketoacidosis[19,20] and in animals made diabetic experimentally. Consequently, it has been hypothesized that increased $PGE_2$ production may represent the host's attempt to counterregulate the accelerated lipolysis present in ketoacidosis, and that both $PGE_2$ and $PGI_2$ may play roles in the decreased vascular resistance and hypotension sometimes observed in diabetic ketoacidosis.

### LIPOXYGENASE PRODUCTS

There has been much work examining the effect of lipoxygenase products on insulin secretion.[21,22] Generally, drugs that inhibit lipoxygenase inhibit glucose-induced insulin secretion. 12-HETE appears to be the major lipoxygenase product in the pancreatic islet. 12-Hydroperoxyeicosatetraenoic acid (12-HPETE), the precursor to 12-HETE, augments glucose-induced insulin secretion, whereas many other lipoxygenase products, including 12-HETE, do not. Few clinical studies that assess the effects of lipoxygenase products or inhibitors on human insulin secretion are available.

### DUAL ACTION OF ARACHIDONIC ACID METABOLITES

The prevailing hypothesis is that arachidonic acid pathways can exert both negative and positive modulatory effects on glucose-induced insulin secretion.[17] The negative modulatory effect appears to be mediated by $PGE_2$, whereas the positive modulatory effect appears to be mediated by 12-HPETE (Fig. 172-3). It is not yet established under what physiologic or pathophysiologic conditions one or the other of these two pathways dominate to cause net negative or net positive modulatory effects.

### EFFECTS ON HEPATIC GLUCOSE PRODUCTION

Eicosanoids also have been implicated in the regulation of glucose production by the liver, a major component of carbohy-

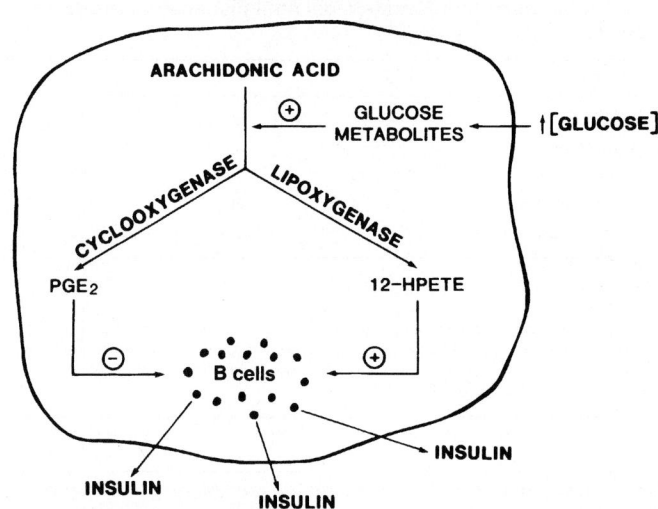

**FIGURE 172-3.** Hypothetical relationship between arachidonic acid metabolites and glucose-induced insulin secretion in the pancreatic islet. The cyclooxygenase pathway is shown to have a prostaglandin $E_2$ ($PGE_2$)–mediated negative modulatory effect on insulin secretion, whereas the lipoxygenase pathway has a 12-hydroxyperoxyeicosatetraenoic acid ($HPETE$)–mediated positive modulatory effect on insulin secretion. Which physiologic and pathophysiologic conditions regulate the cyclooxygenase and lipoxygenase pathways, respectively, to yield net negative and net positive modulation of glucose-induced insulin secretion are unknown.

drate homeostasis. Hepatocytes contain receptors that are specific for PGE, and down-regulation of these receptors is associated with heterologous desensitization of hepatocyte adenylate cyclase.[23] Exogenous $PGE_2$ inhibits glucagon-induced glucose production,[24] although it also has been suggested that PGE exerts a positive modulatory role on glycogenolysis.[25] Little information is available about the effects of lipoxygenase products on hepatic glucose production.

### LIPOLYSIS

The ability of $PGE_2$ to inhibit hormone-stimulated lipolysis was one of the first physiologic actions of PGs to be discovered[26]: $PGE_2$ is as potent as insulin in this regard. Also, PGE receptors were first demonstrated in fat cells.[27] An early hypothesis,[28,29] still being evaluated, is that fat cells synthesize $PGE_2$ intracellularly in response to incoming hormonal signals to provide local counterregulation of hormone-induced lipolysis (Fig. 172-4). Although the inhibitory effect of $PGE_2$ on lipolysis is easily reproduced in vitro, inconsistent effects of NSAIDs on lipolysis have raised doubts about this hypothesis. Most of the drugs used in these older studies were not specific inhibitors of $PGE_2$ synthesis, and how effectively many of these agents inhibit cyclooxygenase in fat cells has not been assessed.

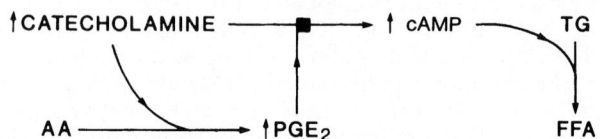

**FIGURE 172-4.** Hypothetical sequence of events in fat cells in which a hormone stimulates the formation of cyclic adenosine monophosphate ($cAMP$) and lipolysis but, at the same time, stimulates synthesis of prostaglandin $E_2$ ($PGE_2$), which then produces negative feedback on adenylate cyclase to counterregulate the generation of cAMP and lipolysis. ($AA$, arachidonic acid; $FFA$, free fatty acid; $TG$, triglyceride.)

## BONE RESORPTION AND THE HYPERCALCEMIA OF MALIGNANCY

$PGE_2$ is equipotent to parathyroid hormone (PTH) as a stimulator of bone resorption.[30] After this bone-resorptive effect of $PGE_2$ had been demonstrated, two extensive series of experiments in two different animal models[31,32] were conducted. They convincingly demonstrated that tumor-bearing animals had increased synthesis of $PGE_2$, and that treatment of the animals with corticosteroids and NSAIDs decreased both $PGE_2$ synthesis and circulating levels of calcium. These experiments led to the hypothesis that hypercalcemia associated with certain malignancies in humans might be explained by increased levels of $PGE_2$. Initially, it was thought that ectopic (paraneoplastic) production of PTH explained most of these cases. It has become apparent, however, that this is a rare phenomenon (see Chap. 59). Greater interest in $PGE_2$ arose when it was observed that urinary levels of PGE metabolites were elevated in hypercalcemic patients who had solid malignancies, a finding not observed in normocalcemic patients with malignancies or in hypercalcemic patients with parathyroid adenomas.[31] The suggestion that tumor-associated increased synthesis of $PGE_2$ might account for the hypercalcemia was strengthened by observations that NSAIDs could lower elevated calcium levels in patients with malignancies.[33] However, it has become evident that most subjects with hypercalcemia and malignancies do not respond to these drugs.[34] Nevertheless, it appears that the responders were the patients with independent evidence for elevated $PGE_2$ levels.[35] Evidence now indicates that parathyroid hormone–related protein (PTHrP) is the most common mediator of hypercalcemia in malignancy (see Chap. 52).

The source of the excess $PGE_2$ levels is not clear. One possibility is that in the presence of lung metastases, venous drainage from the tumor containing $PGE_2$ arrives at bone through the arterial circulation without first passing through lung and liver tissue, where PGE would be degraded. Another explanation is metastatic seeding of bone. That tumor cells can synthesize $PGE_2$ in culture suggests that metastatic tumor cells in bone could synthesize $PGE_2$, which could act locally to resorb bone. Although hypercalcemia in malignancy can occur in the absence of demonstrable bone metastases, radioisotope scans may not be sensitive enough to detect multiple, small metastases. Alternatively, circulating white cells that collect at metastatic sites may be involved in increased $PGE_2$ production. It is possible that there is a linkage among PTHrP, cytokines, and $PGE_2$. Evidence for this linkage includes the following: Cytokines, including interleukin-1 (IL-1), which is known to induce bone resorption, increase PTHrP levels; IL-2 increases PTHrP production and secretion by human T-cell leukemia virus–infected T cells[36]; several cytokines (epidermal growth factor, transforming growth factor-α, platelet-derived growth factor) increase $PGE_2$ synthesis and bone resorption in vivo and in vitro[37,38]; and indomethacin inhibits epidermal growth factor (EGF)–induced hypercalcemia in mice. These observations suggest that $PGE_2$ may play a role in cytokine-induced hypercalcemia. In this regard, $PGE_1$ increases PTHrP mRNA levels and PTHrP secretion in the human T-cell leukemia virus–infected T-cell line.[39]

## REPRODUCTIVE PHYSIOLOGY

### LUTEOLYSIS

Hysterectomy in sheep during the luteal phase is associated with luteal maintenance, suggesting that the uterus produces a luteolytic substance. $PGF_{2\alpha}$ can cause luteal regression. Consequently, experiments were designed[40] to assess whether $PGF_{2\alpha}$ in uterine venous drainage might reach the ovary without passing through the systemic and pulmonary circulations, where it would be degraded. After the infusion of radiolabeled $PGF_{2\alpha}$ into the uterine vein of sheep, the amount of radioactivity was many times higher in the ovarian arterial plasma than in the iliac arterial plasma. Consequently, a countercurrent phenome-

**TABLE 172-3.**

**Stimulatory and Inhibitory Actions of Eicosanoids on Endocrine Organ Function***

| Organ/Function | Stimulator | Inhibitor |
|---|---|---|
| **PANCREAS** | | |
| Glucose-stimulated insulin secretion | 12-HPETE | $PGE_2$ |
| Glucagon secretion | $PGD_2$, $PGE_2$ | |
| **LIVER** | | |
| Glucagon-stimulated glucose production | | $PGE_2$ |
| **FAT** | | |
| Hormone-stimulated lipolysis | | $PGE_2$ |
| **BONE** | | |
| Resorption | $PGE_2$, PGE-m, 6-K-$PGE_1$ $PGF_{1\alpha}$, $PGI_2$ | |
| **UTERUS** | | |
| Contraction | $PGE_2$, $PGF_{2\alpha}$ | |
| **OVARIES** | | |
| Progesterone | | $PGF_{2\alpha}$ |
| **PITUITARY** | | |
| Prolactin | $PGE_1$ | |
| LH | $PGE_1$, $PGE_2$, 5-HETE | |
| TSH | $PGA_1$, $PGB_1$, $PGE_1$, $PGE_{1\alpha}$ | |
| GH | $PGE_1$ | |
| **PARATHYROID** | | |
| PTH | $PGE_2$ | $PGF_{2\alpha}$ |

*GH*, growth hormone; *HETE*, hydroxyeicosatetraenoic acid; *HPETE*, hydroperoxyeicosatetraenoic acid; *LH*, luteinizing hormone; *PG*, prostaglandin; *PTH*, parathyroid hormone; *TSH*, thyroid-stimulating hormone.

*General trends of literature reports; based on experiments in which exogenous eicosanoids have been studied directly.

non between the uterine vein and ovarian artery may allow $PGF_{2\alpha}$ from the uterus to reach the ovary and induce luteolysis.

### UTERINE EFFECTS: DYSMENORRHEA

PGs of the E and F series are synthesized by human endometrium. These PGs stimulate uterine contractions; therefore, their administration by intravenous infusion or tablet form has been used to initiate labor.[41] The hypothesis that PGE or PGF, or both, may participate in dysmenorrhea follows from the clinical observation that women have successfully used NSAIDs to treat the discomfort associated with this syndrome. Moreover, it has been observed that PGF and PGE levels in menstrual blood are decreased in patients taking drugs that inhibit PG synthesis. In controlled trials comparing PG synthesis inhibitors with placebo in women with dysmenorrhea, symptomatic improvement has been greater after therapy with these drugs.[42]

### OTHER ENDOCRINE GLANDS

Eicosanoids have been implicated in the control of hormone secretion by several other endocrine glands (Table 172-3). For example, a number of eicosanoids stimulate hormone release[43-47] from the pituitary gland (see Table 172-3). Other studies assessing the effects of NSAIDs on the secretion of these hormones have been performed. Research in these areas is insufficient to determine to what extent eicosanoids might be important modulators of pituitary gland function or might be pathophysiologic agents in pituitary disease states.

The observations that $PGE_2$ decreases[48] and $PGF_{2\alpha}$ increases[49] PTH secretion remain uncontested. Somewhat more work has been done on the potential roles of eicosanoids as regulators of adrenal cortex function.[50,51] However, this area also needs substantially more work before many of the conflicting reports can be satisfactorily resolved.

# PHYSIOLOGY AND PATHOPHYSIOLOGY RELEVANT TO OTHER BODY SYSTEMS[52,53]

## PLATELETS

It has been proposed that a balance between $PGI_2$ and $TXA_2$ levels modulates platelet aggregation.[54] Platelets synthesize $TXA_2$, which is a potent stimulator of aggregation. $PGI_2$ is synthesized by endothelial cells of blood vessels, and it potently antagonizes platelet aggregation. It is thought that $TXA_2$ and $PGI_2$ exert their opposing effects by decreasing and increasing, respectively, platelet generation of cyclic AMP. It follows that endothelial damage, and a concomitant decrease in $PGI_2$ synthesis, may allow unbridled platelet aggregation at the site of vessel wall damage. It has been hypothesized that this situation would favor the eventual development of atherosclerosis. These considerations have led to the therapeutic use of aspirin to suppress platelet aggregation. Cyclooxygenase inhibition by a single dose of aspirin is of longer duration in platelets than in other tissues because the platelet, in contrast to nucleated cells that can synthesize new proteins, does not have the nuclear machinery to form new cyclooxygenase. Consequently, the effect of aspirin persists until newly formed platelets have been released from bone marrow. On the other hand, endothelial cells rapidly recover cyclooxygenase activity after aspirin ingestion, thereby restoring $PGI_2$ production.

## INFLUENCE ON DUCTUS ARTERIOSUS

Many eicosanoids are vasoactive substances. $PGE_2$ and $PGI_2$ are vasodilators, whereas $PGF_{2\alpha}$, $TXA_2$, and $LTC_4$, $LTD_4$, and $LTE_4$ are vasoconstrictors in most vascular beds. $PGE_2$ has been postulated to be a primary factor in the maintenance of physiologic patency of the ductus arteriosus in the fetus. Trials with NSAIDs have been undertaken in newborn human infants with patent ductus arteriosus that caused closure of this vessel.[55] Infants younger than 35 weeks of age are most likely to respond, and some individuals require a second course of therapy.

## RENAL EFFECTS

### GENERAL EFFECTS

Arachidonic acid metabolites influence both the renin-angiotensin–aldosterone system and the vasopressin system[56,57] (see Chaps. 25 and 183). Both $PGE_2$ and $PGI_2$ stimulate renin secretion. They also decrease renal vascular resistance and increase blood flow. The NSAIDs decrease total renal blood flow and can lead to acute renal vasoconstriction and decreased renal function in some circumstances, such as in volume depletion, in edematous states, and in older patients. Indomethacin increases sensitivity to exogenous vasopressin, and, conversely, $PGE_2$ decreases vasopressin-stimulated water transport.

### BARTTER SYNDROME

Bartter syndrome is characterized by increased levels of plasma renin, aldosterone, and bradykinin; resistance to the pressor effect of angiotensin infusion; hypokalemic alkalosis; and renal potassium wasting in the presence of normal blood pressure (see Chap. 80). It has been postulated that excessive $PGE_2$ or $PGI_2$ synthesis plays a role in this syndrome.[58] Both $PGE_2$ and $PGI_2$ stimulate the release of renin and blunt the pressor effects of angiotensin. Elevated levels of $PGE_2$ and $PGI_2$ metabolites have been found in the urine of patients with this syndrome. Therapeutic trials with NSAIDs have reversed virtually all of these clinical abnormalities except hypokalemia. Consequently, it has been concluded that a PG, presumably $PGE_2$ or $PGI_2$, may be responsible for mediating many of the manifestations of Bartter syndrome, although excessive PG levels themselves are not the primary defect.

## GASTROINTESTINAL EFFECTS

PGE, taken orally, protects the gastrointestinal mucosa from several forms of injury by a direct, cytoprotective effect.[59] It also inhibits gastric acid secretion. Because gastric acid secretion is excessive in patients with peptic ulcer disease, analogs of $PGE_2$ have been used as therapeutic agents.[54] These agents are more effective than placebo in relieving pain and decreasing gastric acid secretion in patients with peptic ulcer disease. The healing of ulcer craters is accelerated in patients treated with these analogs compared with placebo-treated patients.[60]

## PULMONARY EFFECTS

Arachidonic acid metabolites may play a role in the clinical manifestations of allergic and drug-associated asthma.[61] Many arachidonic acid metabolites can be formed by lung tissue. $PGF_{2\alpha}$, $TXA_2$, $LTC_4$, $LTD_4$, and $LTE_4$ are potent bronchoconstrictors, whereas $PGE_2$ is a potent bronchodilator. The effect of $PGF_{2\alpha}$ is antagonized by $PGE_2$ and by catecholamines, but not by atropine, antihistamines, serotonin antagonists, or $\alpha$-adrenergic antagonists.

An interesting subset of asthmatic patients have symptoms precipitated by drugs such as aspirin and indomethacin—the syndrome of *aspirin-sensitive asthma*. If arachidonic acid metabolites play a role in this particular syndrome, it might involve the inhibition of cyclooxygenase and shunting of substrate to the LT pathway, thereby inducing formation of large amounts of bronchoconstrictor substances.

## IMMUNOREGULATION AND INFLAMMATION

### INFLAMMATORY RESPONSE

Much information about potential roles of eicosanoids in the immune response continues to accumulate.[62] It has been recognized that small amounts of $PGE_2$ suppress stimulation of human lymphocytes by mitogens. Moreover, the inflammatory response usually is associated with the local release of arachidonic acid metabolites. This has led to the hypothesis that eicosanoids act as negative modulators of lymphocyte function. Release of PGE by mitogen-stimulated lymphocytes is envisioned as a negative-feedback control mechanism by which lymphocyte activity is regulated. Indomethacin augments lymphocyte responsiveness to mitogens.

Several lines of evidence support a relationship between inflammation and the generation of arachidonic acid metabolites. Inflammatory stimuli, such as histamine and bradykinin, release PGs. $LTC_4$, $LTD_4$, and $LTE_4$ are more potent than histamine as bronchoconstrictors. $PGE_2$ and $LTD_4$ are commonly present in areas of inflammation. During phagocytosis, polymorphonuclear cells release eicosanoids that are chemotactic for leukocytes. Vasodilatation induced by PGE is not abolished by antagonists of known mediators of the inflammatory response such as atropine, propranolol, methysergide, or antihistamines. Thus, it has been postulated that PGE and other eicosanoids may have direct inflammatory effects, and other mediators of inflammation may act by influencing eicosanoid release.

Mastocytosis and other disorders related to mast cell activation (see Chap. 181) have been related to excessive production of $PGD_2$.[63] Symptoms in these syndromes include flushing, tachycardia, hypotension, abdominal cramping, diarrhea, chest pain, headache, dyspnea, and itching. Use of NSAIDs in combination with antihistaminic drugs has been reported to be effective therapy for mastocytosis. However, a small subset of patients have attacks that are provoked by aspirin.

### RHEUMATOID ARTHRITIS

The inflammatory response and bone resorption that accompany rheumatoid arthritis may depend, to some degree, on the local generation of eicosanoids. Rheumatoid synovia synthesize $PGE_2$

in tissue culture, and media from these cultures promote bone resorption. The inclusion of indomethacin in the culture medium blocks this bone-resorptive capacity, but does not prevent bone resorption caused by exogenous $PGE_2$. Hence, it has been postulated that $PGE_2$ produced by the synovia may be responsible for the bone resorption seen in patients with rheumatoid arthritis.[64] A site of action for glucocorticoids has been identified in experiments using synovial tissue from patients with rheumatoid arthritis; that is, COX-2 mRNA and COX-2 protein are markedly suppressed by dexamethasone.[65] This observation is important because previously glucocorticoids were thought to act on arachidonic acid metabolism exclusively by inhibiting phospholipase $A_2$ activity.

## PLATELET-ACTIVATING FACTOR

A related compound to arachidonic acid is platelet-activating factor (PAF). PAF is a phospholipid synthesized by the hydrolysis of arachidonic acid. This phospholipid autacoid has a wide range of physiologic actions, including platelet activation, increased vascular permeability, uterine contraction, and several effects on reproductive function.[66]

## CONCLUSION

Arachidonic acid metabolites are important modulators of physiologic activity in many tissues, and eicosanoids may play a role in the pathogenesis of human disease. These metabolites and their inhibitors may have important therapeutic applications (e.g., *metabolites* [peptic ulcer disease, ductus-dependent congenital heart disease, hypertension,[67] induction of labor, excessive lipolysis] and *inhibitors* [rheumatoid arthritis, hypercalcemia of cancer, inflammation, fever, dysmenorrhea, Bartter syndrome, type 2 diabetes mellitus, anticoagulation, patent ductus arteriosus]). The development and use of drugs that specifically and selectively inhibit the synthesis of single eicosanoids and that selectively antagonize receptors for specific eicosanoids are beginning to yield new and important physiologic and pathophysiologic information.

## REFERENCES

1. Robertson RP. Molecular regulation of prostaglandin synthesis: implications for endocrine systems. TEM 1995; 6:293.
2. Smith WL, Dewitt DL. Prostaglandin endoperoxide H synthases-1 and 2. Adv Immunol 1966; 62:167.
3. Coleman RA, Smith WL, Narumiya S. VIII. International union of pharmacology classification of prostanoid receptors: properties, distribution, and structure of the receptors and their subtypes. Pharmacol Rev 1994; 46:205.
4. Mitchell JA, Akarasereenont P, Thiemermann C, et al. Selectivity of nonsteroidal antiinflammatory drugs as inhibitors of constitutive and inducible cyclooxygenase. Proc Natl Acad Sci U S A 1994; 90:11,693.
4a. Clemett D, Goa KL. Celecoxib: a review of its use in osteoarthritis, rheumatoid arthritis, and acute pain. Drugs 2000; 59:957.
4b. Cannon GW, Caldwell JR, Holt P, et al. Rofecoxib, a specific inhibitor of cyclooxygenase–2. Arthritis Rheum 2000; 43:978.
5. Kopp E, Ghosh S. Inhibition of NF-kB by sodium salicylate and aspirin. Science 1994; 265:956.
6. Robertson RP, Westcott KR, Storm DR, Rice MG. Down-regulation in vivo of prostaglandin E receptors and adenylate cyclase stimulation in rat liver plasma membranes. Am J Physiol 1980; 239:E75.
7. Robertson RP, Little SA. Down-regulation of prostaglandin E receptors and homologous desensitization of isolated adipocytes. Endocrinology 1983; 113:1732.
8. Vane JR. Inhibition of prostaglandin synthesis as a mechanism of action for aspirin-like drugs. Nature 1971; 231:232.
9. Robertson RP, Gavareski DJ, Porte D Jr, Bierman EL. Inhibition of in vivo insulin secretion by prostaglandin $E_1$. J Clin Invest 1974; 54:310.
10. Robertson RP, Chen M. A role for prostaglandin E (PGE) in defective insulin secretion and carbohydrate intolerance in diabetes mellitus. J Clin Invest 1977; 60:747.
11. Burr IM, Sharp R. Effects of prostaglandin $E_1$ and of epinephrine on the dynamics of insulin release in vitro. Endocrinology 1974; 94:835.
12. Kowluru A, Metz SA. Stimulation of prostaglandin $E_2$ of a high-affinity GTPase in the secretory granules of normal rat and human pancreatic islets. Biochem J 1994; 297:399.
13. Robertson RP, Tsai P, Little SA, et al. Receptor-mediated adenylate cyclase-coupled mechanism for $PGE_2$ inhibition of insulin secretion in HIT cells. Diabetes 1987; 36:1047.
14. Sorli CH, Zhang H-J, Armstrong MB, et al. Basal expression of cyclooxygenase-2 and NIF-1L6 are dominant and coordinately regulated by IL-1 in the pancreatic islet. Proc Natl Acad Sci U S A 1998; 95:1788.
15. Robertson RP. Arachidonic acid metabolite regulation of insulin secretion. Diabetes Metab Rev 1986; 2:261.
16. Metz SA, Robertson RP, Fujimoto WF. Inhibition of prostaglandin E synthesis augments glucose-induced insulin secretion in cultured pancreas. Diabetes 1981; 30:551.
17. Robertson RP. Eicosanoids as pluripotential modulators of pancreatic islet function. Diabetes 1988; 37:367.
18. Johnson DG, Fujimoto WY, Williams RH. Enhanced release of insulin by prostaglandins in isolated pancreatic islets. Diabetes 1973; 22:658.
19. McRae JR. Day RP, Metz SA, et al. Prostaglandin E2 metabolite levels during diabetic ketoacidosis. Diabetes 1985; 34:761.
20. Axelrod L, Shulman GI, Blackshear PJ, Bomstein W, et al. Plasma level of 13, 14-dihydro-15-keto-PGE2 in patients with diabetic ketoacidosis and in normal fasting subjects. Diabetes 1986; 35:1004.
21. Metz S, VanRollins M, Strife R, et al. Lipoxygenase pathway in islet endocrine cells. J Clin Invest 1983; 71:1191.
22. Yamamoto S, Nakadate T, Nakaki T, et al. Prevention of glucose-induced insulin secretion by lipoxygenase inhibitor. Eur J Pharmacol 1982; 78:225.
23. Garrity MJ, Andreason TJ, Storm DR, Robertson RP. PGE-induced heterologous desensitization of hepatic adenylate cyclase: consequences on the guanyl nucleotide regulatory complex. J Biol Chem 1983; 258:8692.
24. Brass EP, Garrity MJ, Robertson RP. Inhibition of glucagon-stimulated hepatic glycogenolysis by E-series prostaglandins. FEBS Lett 1984; 169:293.
25. Ganguli S, Sperling MA, Frame E, Christensen R. Inhibition of glucagon-induced hepatic glucose production by indomethacin. Am J Physiol 1979; 236:E58.
26. Steinberg D, Vaughn M, Nestel PJ, et al. Effects of the prostaglandins on hormone-induced mobilization of free fatty acids. J Clin Invest 1964; 43:1533.
27. Kuehl FA, Humes JL. Direct evidence for a prostaglandin receptor and its application to prostaglandin measurements. Proc Natl Acad Sci U S A 1972; 69:480.
28. Shaw JE, Ramwell PW. Release of prostaglandin from rat epididymal fat pad on nervous and hormonal stimulation. J Biol Chem 1968; 243:1498.
29. Christ EJ, Nugteren DH. The biosynthesis and possible function of prostaglandins in adipose tissue. Biochim Biophys Acta 1970; 218:296.
30. Klein DC, Raisz LG. Prostaglandins: stimulation of bone resorption in tissue culture. Endocrinology 1970; 86:1436.
31. Tashjian AH Jr, Voelkel EF, Levine L, Goldhaber P. Evidence that the bone resorption-stimulating factor produced by mouse fibrosarcoma cells is prostaglandin $E_2$: a new model for the hypercalcemia of cancer. J Exp Med 1972; 136:1329.
32. Voelkel EF, Tashjian AH Jr, Franklin R, et al. Hypercalcemia and tumor prostaglandins: the $VX_2$ carcinoma model in the rabbit. Metabolism 1975; 24:973.
33. Seyberth HW, Segre GV, Morgan JL, et al. Prostaglandins as mediators of hypercalcemia associated with certain types of cancer. N Engl J Med 1975; 293:1278.
34. Robertson RP, Baylink DJ, Metz SA, Cummings KB. Plasma prostaglandin E in patients with cancer with and without hypercalcemia. J Clin Endocrinol Metab 1976; 43:1330.
35. Metz SA, McRae JR, Robertson RP. Prostaglandins as mediators of paraneoplastic syndromes: review and up-date. Metabolism 1981; 30:299.
36. Ikeda K, Okazaki R, Inoue D, et al. Interleukin-2 increases production and secretion of parathyroid hormone-related peptide by human T cell leukemia virus type-I-infected T cells: possible role in hypercalcemia associated with adult T cell leukemia. Endocrinology 1993b; 132:2551.
37. Tashjian AH Jr, Hohmann EL, Antoniades HN, Levine L. Platelet-derived growth factor stimulates bone resorption via a prostaglandin-mediated mechanism. Endocrinology 1982; 111:118.
38. Tashjian AH Jr, Voelkel EF, Lloyd W, et al. Actions of growth factors on plasma calcium: epidermal growth factor and human transforming growth factor-alpha cause elevation of plasma calcium in mice. J Clin Invest 1986; 78:1405.
39. Ikeda K, Okazaki R, Inoue D, et al. Transcription of the gene for parathyroid hormone-related peptide from the human is activated through a cAMP-dependent pathway by prostaglandin $E_1$ in HTLV-I-infected T cells. J Biol Chem 1993a; 268:1174.
40. McCracken JA, Baird DT, Goding JR. Factors affecting the secretion of steroids from the transplanted ovary in the sheep. Recent Prog Horm Res 1971; 27:537.
41. Casey C, Kehoe J, Mylotte MJ. Vaginal prostaglandins for the ripe cervix. Int J Gynaecol Obstet 1994; 44:21.
42. Budoff PW. Zomspirac sodium in the treatment of primary dysmenorrhea syndrome. N Engl J Med 1982; 307:714.
43. Ojeda SR, Harms PG, McCann SM. Central effect of prostaglandin $E_1$ ($PGE_1$) on prolactin release. Endocrinology 1974; 95:613.
44. Naor Z, Vanderhoek JY, Lindner HR, Catt KJ. Arachidonic acid products as possible mediators of the action of gonadotropin-releasing hormone. Adv Prostaglandin Thromboxane Leukotriene Res 1983; 12:259.
45. Brown MR, Hedge GA. In vivo effects of prostaglandins on TRH-induced TSH secretion. Endocrinology 1974; 95:1392.
46. Drouin J, Labrie F. Specificity of the stimulatory effect of prostaglandins on hormone release in rat anterior pituitary cells in culture. Prostaglandins 1976; 11:355.

47. Hedge GA. Hypothalamic and pituitary effects of prostaglandins on ACTH secretion. Prostaglandins 1976; 11:293.
48. Gardner DG, Brown EM, Windeck R, Aurbach GD. Prostaglandin E$_2$ stimulation of adenosine 3',5'-monophosphate accumulation and parathyroid hormone release in dispersed bovine parathyroid cells. Endocrinology 1978; 103:577.
49. Gardner DG, Brown EM, Windeck R, Aurbach GD. Prostaglandin F$_{2\alpha}$ inhibits 3',5'-adenosine monophosphate accumulation and parathyroid hormone release from dispersed bovine parathyroid cells. Endocrinology 1979; 104:1.
50. Matsuoka H, Tan SY, Mulrow PJ. Effects of prostaglandins on adrenal steroidogenesis in the rat. Prostaglandins 1980; 19:291.
51. Carchman RA, Shen JC, Bilgin S, Rubin RP. Diverse effects of Ca$^{2+}$ on the prostacyclin and corticotropin modulation of adenosine 3',5'-monophosphate and steroid production in normal cat and mouse tumor cells of the adrenal cortex. Biochem Pharmacol 1980; 29:2213.
52. Robertson RP, ed. Symposium on prostaglandins in health and disease. Med Clin North Am 1981; 65:711.
53. Zipser RD, Laffi G. Prostaglandins, thromboxanes and leukotrienes in clinical medicine. West J Med 1985; 143:485.
54. Moncada S, Vane JR. Arachidonic acid metabolites and the interactions between platelets and blood vessel walls. N Engl J Med 1979; 300:1142.
55. Van Overmeire B, Smets K, Lecoutere D, et al. A comparison of ibuprofen and indomethacin for closure of patent ductus arteriosus. N Engl J Med 2000; 343:674.
56. Ferris TF. Prostaglandins and the kidney. Am J Nephrol 1983; 13:139.
57. Orloff J, Handler JS, Bergstrom S. Effect of prostaglandin (PGE$_1$) on the permeability response of the toad bladder to vasopressin, theophylline and adenosine 3',5'-monophosphate. Nature 1965; 205:397.
58. Gill JR. Frolich JC, Bowden RE, et al. Bartter's syndrome: a disorder characterized by high urinary prostaglandins and a dependence of hyperreninemia on prostaglandin synthesis. Am J Med 1976; 61:43.
59. Redfern JS, Feldman M. Role of endogenous prostaglandins in preventing gastrointestinal ulceration: induction of ulcers by antibodies to prostaglandins. Gastroenterology 1989; 96:596.
60. Vantrappen G, Janssens J, Popiela T, et al. Effect of 15(R)-15-methylprostaglandin E$_2$ (arbaprostil) on the healing of duodenal ulcer. Gastroenterology 1982; 83:357.
61. Hyman AL, Mathe AA, Lippton HL, Kadowitz PJ. Prostaglandins and the lung. Med Clin North Am 1981; 65:789.
62. Goetzl E, Scott WA, eds. Regulation of cellular activities by leukotrienes. J Allergy Clin Immunol 1984; 74:309.
63. Roberts LJ 2d. Carcinoid syndrome and disorders of systemic mast-cell activation including systemic mastocytosis. Endocrinol Metab Clin North Am 1988; 17:415.
64. Robinson DR, Tashjian AH, Levine L. Prostaglandin-stimulated bone resorption by rheumatoid synovia. J Clin Invest 1975; 56:1181.
65. Crofford LJ, Wilder RL, Ristimaki AP, et al. Cyclooxygenase-1 and -2 expression in rheumatoid synovial tissues: effects of interleukin-1β, phorbol ester, and corticosteroids. J Clin Invest 1994; 93:1095.
66. Venable ME, Zimmerman GA, MacIntyre TM, Prescott SM. Platelet-activating factor: a phospholipid autocoid with diverse actions. J Lipid Res 1993; 34:691.
67. Hoeper MM, Schwarze M, Ehlerding S, et al. Long-term treatment of primary pulmonary hypertension with aerosolized iloprost; a prostacyclin analogue. N Engl J Med 2000; 342:1866.

# CHAPTER 173

# GROWTH FACTORS AND CYTOKINES

DEREK LEROITH AND VICKY A. BLAKESLEY

## INSULIN-LIKE GROWTH FACTOR SYSTEM

This chapter on growth factors begins with a discussion of the insulin-like growth factors (IGFs), their receptors and binding proteins. This format reflects the authors' belief that the IGF system represents an excellent paradigm for both growth factors and cytokines, and, furthermore, is one of the more clinically relevant growth factor families for the academic and practicing endocrinologist. Descriptions are given of structural and functional aspects of the ligands, receptors, and binding proteins, followed by examples of clinically relevant aspects of the IGF system.[1] Subsequently, other growth factors and cytokines are discussed, with emphasis

**TABLE 173-1.**
**Growth Factor Families**

| | |
|---|---|
| Insulin-like growth factor (IGF) family | IGF-I, IGF-II, insulin |
| Vascular endothelial growth factor (VEGF) | |
| Nerve growth factor (NGF) family | NGF, bone-derived growth factor, neurotropins (NT-3, -4, and -5) |
| Platelet-derived growth factors (PDGFs) | PDGF-AA, PDGF-BB, PDGF-AB |
| Epidermal growth factor (EGF) family | EGF, transforming growth factor-α (TGF-α), amphiregulin, heparin-binding EGF |
| Transforming growth factor-β (TGF-β) family | TGF-β 1–6; inhibin A and B; activin A, B, and C; müllerian inhibitory substance |
| Fibroblast growth factor (FGF) family | Acidic and basic FGF, keratinocyte growth factor |

on their potential roles in clinically related disorders. A list of the families of growth factors is presented in Table 173-1. A more complete list of the cytokine families can be found in Chapter 174.

## INSULIN-LIKE GROWTH FACTORS

IGF-I and IGF-II are small (~70 amino acids) secreted peptides that are structurally related to proinsulin. In mammals they are encoded by large, complex, single-copy genes, homologues of which are found in all vertebrate species.[2] As with most secreted proteins, they are synthesized as precursors containing N- and C-terminal extensions. The N-terminal signal peptide directs the IGFs to the constitutive secretory pathway, and the C-terminal E-peptide moiety of the prohormone is cleaved during transit through the Golgi network to yield the mature molecule. The mature IGF-I peptide consists of B and A domains, of which the amino-acid sequences are homologous to the B and A chains of insulin, linked by a short C domain. IGFs also contain a short, C-terminal D domain for which no analogy exists in the mature insulin molecule. Most circulating IGFs occur in the fully processed form, without the E peptide. Under certain conditions, the prohormone can be detected in the serum with the E peptide as part of the IGF molecule (Fig. 173-1A).

IGF-I and IGF-II messenger ribonucleic acid (mRNA) or protein can be detected at some developmental stage in every tissue examined. In rodents, the expression of the IGF-II gene is highest prenatally, with expression decreasing dramatically postnatally. IGF-I gene expression, while present in fetal tissues, tends to increase dramatically postnatally, especially during the peripubertal period when growth hormone (GH) responsiveness develops.[3] In humans, however, circulating IGF-II levels remain high even in adults. These distinct patterns of expression suggest that IGF-I and IGF-II serve unique functions during development.

In humans, GH exerts a major influence on IGF-I gene expression, particularly in the liver, consistent with a classic endocrine pathway. The production of IGF-I and IGF-II by most tissues is consistent with their roles as autocrine/paracrine growth factors, in addition to their obvious roles as classic endocrine agents. In support of this view, IGF-I gene expression is also modulated by numerous hormones, nutrients, and molecules.

The control of IGF-II gene expression is similarly complex, with various mRNA species differentially expressed at different stages of development and in different tissues. The IGF-II promoter is imprinted, with only one allele normally being expressed. It is also controlled by tumor-suppressor gene products (e.g., Wilms tumor WT1) and the adjacent H19 gene. Dysregulation of these control mechanisms may explain its frequent overexpression by multiple tumors. Both IGF-I and IGF-II gene expression are subject to complex control mechanisms consistent with their postulated roles of fetal and postnatal growth factors.[4]

The importance of the IGFs in normal growth and development has been addressed by an elegant series of gene-targeting

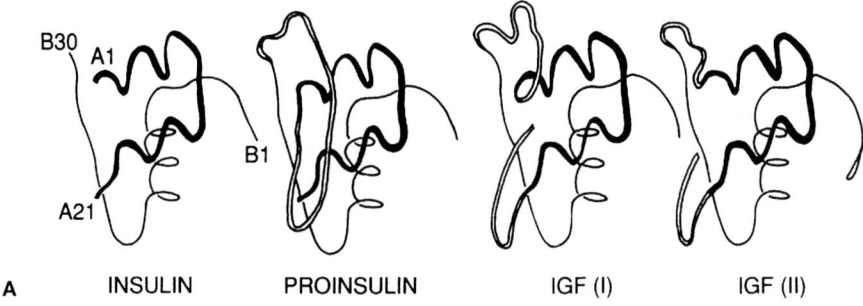

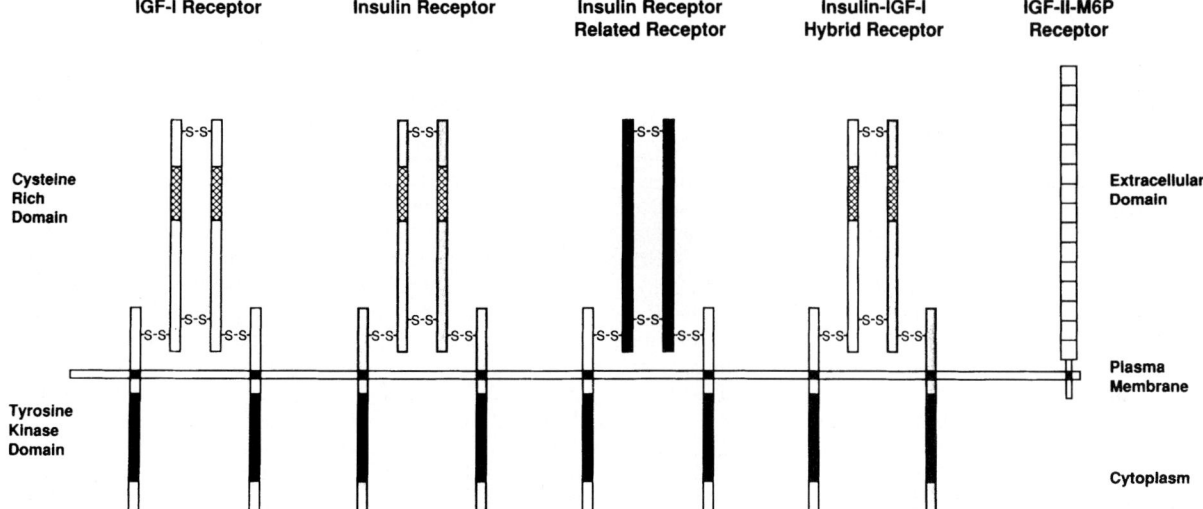

**FIGURE 173-1. A,** The insulin-like growth factor (*IGF*) family of peptides. Insulin, IGF-I, and IGF-II are processed from precursor molecules. In the case of insulin, the C peptide is removed, whereas the IGF-I and IGF-II molecules retain the C peptide and, in addition, contain a D extension at the carboxyl terminal ends of their A chains. The E peptide found in the proIGF-I and proIGF-II molecules is cleaved during processing. A chains are in bold, C peptides and D extensions are shown in double lines, and the B chain is represented as a single line. **B,** The insulin-like growth factor receptors. Schematic representation of the IGF-I receptor. The IGF-I receptor is a heterotetrameric transmembrane tyrosine kinase receptor. Each hemireceptor is comprised of an α and a β subunit covalently bound by disulfide bonds. A doublet of hemireceptors constitutes the active IGF-I receptor. The α subunit is entirely extracellular and contains the ligand (IGF-I or -II)–binding domain. The β subunit spans the membrane and is divided into the extracellular, transmembrane, juxtamembrane, tyrosine kinase, and C-terminal domains. The essential adenosine triphosphate (*ATP*)–binding site is at lysine 1003 within the tyrosine kinase domain. Also within the catalytic domain is a triple tyrosine cluster (tyrosines 1131, 1135, and 1136).

studies in which the IGF-I and IGF-II genes, singly and in combination, have been inactivated.[5] Homozygous IGF-I– and IGF-II–deficient mice exhibited a 30% reduction in body growth during embryonic development.[6] While the IGF-II–deficient mice continued to grow at this reduced level postnatally, IGF-I–deficient mice died immediately after birth. Double mutants (generated by crossing) exhibited an additive 60% decrease in growth. Both IGF-I and IGF-II appear to be necessary for full growth potential. As demonstrated by more recent models of IGF-I–deficient mice, IGF-I also plays an important role for specific tissue function. These IGF-I–deficient mice show improved postnatal survival but lack the normal peripubertal growth spurt due to absent responsiveness to GH-induced IGF-I production. The mice are also infertile. These in vivo models show that the IGFs are important growth regulators for which synthesis is subject to complex control mechanisms.

## INSULIN-LIKE GROWTH FACTOR RECEPTORS

The actions of the IGFs require their interaction with specific cell-surface receptors. The family of receptors involved in the bioactions of the IGFs include the insulin receptor, the IGF-I receptor (type I IGF receptor), the IGF-II/mannose-6-phosphate receptor (type II IGF receptor), the insulin-receptor–related receptor (IRR),

and hybrid receptors (consisting of an insulin α and β subunit and an IGF-I receptor α and β subunit).[7] The relative binding affinities of these receptors for their potential ligands are delineated in Table 173-2.

The IGF-I and insulin receptors are structurally similar molecules encoded by distinct genes.[8] Both consist of two extracellular glycosylated α subunits containing cysteine-rich regions. These cysteine-rich regions in the IGF-I receptor are primarily responsible for IGF binding, but ligand binding to the insulin receptor requires regions flanking the cysteine-rich domain. The α subunits are joined to each other and to the transmem-

**TABLE 173-2.**
**Relative Affinities of Insulin-Like Growth Factor Ligands for Their Receptors**

| Receptor | Relative Ligand Affinities |
|---|---|
| **IGF-I receptor** | IGF-I > IGF-II > insulin |
| **IGF-II receptor** | IGF-II >> IGF-I > insulin |
| **Insulin receptor** | Insulin >> IGF-II > IGF-I |
| **Hybrid receptor** | IGF-I >> insulin |

IGF, insulin-like growth factor.

brane β subunits by disulfide bonds that are formed after proteolytic cleavage of the prorereceptor into α and β subunits in the Golgi apparatus. The β subunit consists of a short extracellular domain, a transmembrane region, a cytoplasmic juxtamembrane region in which tyrosine-containing motifs important for receptor internalization and interaction with endogenous substrates occur, a tyrosine kinase domain that includes an adenosine triphosphate (ATP)–binding motif, a cluster of tyrosine residues subject to autophosphorylation, and a C-terminal domain containing several tyrosine residues that are also autophosphorylated following activation of the receptor. The tyrosine kinase domain is the most highly conserved (~87%), while the C-terminal domain is the least conserved between the IGF-I and insulin receptors. The IGF-I and insulin receptor are members of a receptor tyrosine kinase family that includes the epidermal growth factor (EGF) and platelet-derived growth factor (PDGF) receptors, but they are atypical in that they occur in a heterotetrameric structure and are considered to be "pre-dimerized," unlike the other receptors of this family that require ligand binding for dimerization and activation (Fig. 173-1*B*).

The IGF-II/mannose-6-phosphate receptor is unrelated structurally to the IGF-I and insulin receptors, because it contains a long extracellular domain consisting of numerous repeats of a short amino-acid sequence, a transmembrane domain, and a short cytoplasmic tail.[9] The extracellular domain contains binding sites for IGF-II and mannose-6-phosphate, and ligand binding at one site influences ligand binding at the other. This receptor is important in the uptake and intracellular trafficking of mannose-6-phosphate–containing lysosomal enzymes and may play a role in the clearance of IGF-II from the circulation. The cytoplasmic tail lacks any obvious catalytic activity or classic binding sites for known endogenous substrates and—in the absence of any convincing evidence to the contrary—has generally been considered to lack signaling properties. Proteolytic cleavage of the extracellular domain releases a circulating form of the receptor, which may then act as a binding protein for IGF-II. Since the IGF-I receptor is considered to mediate the actions of the IGFs, functional aspects of this receptor are dealt with in more detail in the following section.

### INSULIN-LIKE GROWTH FACTOR-I RECEPTOR

The IGF-I receptor gene is expressed ubiquitously in most tissues.[10] The gene contains 21 exons, and two mRNA species can be found in human tissues, one of ~11 kilobases (kb) and a second of ~7 kb.[11] The mRNA contains an ~1-kb 5' untranslated (UT) region, a coding region of ~5 kb, and a 3' UT region of ~5 kb. Both the 5' UT and 5' flanking regions of the gene are enriched in GC sequences, and the expression is regulated by SP1 and WT1 transcription factors that bind specifically to these GC-rich boxes in the promoter region.[12] This region is also responsible for the regulation of the IGF-I receptor gene by growth factors.[13,14] EGF, PDGF, and bFGF up-regulate gene expression, whereas IGF-I down-regulates its own receptor at the transcriptional level.[15,16] The 3' UT region most likely is involved in the stability of the mRNA.

The sequence of events initiated by ligand binding to receptor tyrosine kinases has been elucidated for a number of these receptors.[17] In the case of the IGF-I receptor, ligand binding to the α subunit alters the conformation of the extracellular and transmembrane portions of the receptor, leading to a change in the cytoplasmic domain, which in turn results in activation of the tyrosine kinase and phosphorylation of a cluster of three tyrosine residues in the kinase domain itself.[18,19] Subsequently, tyrosines in the juxtamembrane and C-terminal domains are phosphorylated along with other substrates.[20] The insulin receptor substrate (IRS) family of proteins, of which four have been characterized together with the protein Shc, represent the most well studied of the substrates involved in IGF-I and insulin-receptor signal transduction.[21] Their primary site of interaction is the phosphorylated tyrosine at residue 960 within the juxtamembrane domain of the IGF-I receptor. IGF-I–receptor activation results in tyrosine phosphorylation of

IRS (1–4) and Shc.[22–24] Phosphorylated tyrosine residues on the IRS molecules are found in consensus sequences for the binding of Src homology domain (SH2) domains of several proteins of the signal transduction pathways.[25] These include the p85 subunit of phosphoinositide-3'kinase (PI3'K), growth factor receptor bound protein-2 (Grb-2), the tyrosine phosphatase Syp, Crk adapter proteins, and Nck[26] (Fig. 173-2). PI3'K activation leads to pathways involved in preventing apoptosis (via protein kinase B/Akt), signaling to focal adhesion sites and even mitogenesis.[27] Grb-2 is an adapter protein that interacts via its SH2 domain with both tyrosine phosphorylated IRS and Shc.[28] Bound Grb-2 then interacts via its SH3 domain with the mammalian homologue of son-of-sevenless (mSOS), which contains the appropriate proline-rich region required for SH3 domain interaction.[29,30] This interaction recruits mSOS to the plasma membrane where mSOS, a guanine nucleotide exchange factor, activates p21ras by facilitating the displacement of guanine diphosphate (GDP) from the guanine nucleotide-binding site of p21ras and its replacement with guanine triphosphate (GTP). GTP-p21ras interacts with raf proteins and thereby activates the mitogen-activated protein (MAP) kinase/Erk pathway. The final result is the transport of active molecules into the nucleus and enhancement of specific gene transcription, leading to increased mitogenic signals and cellular proliferation. These major pathways are the ones that have been most clearly characterized for IGF-I–receptor signaling. Additionally, a host of other substrates and pathways have been delineated.

The Crk family of adapter proteins, CrkI and II and CrkL, while lacking catalytic activity, play important roles in the signal transduction pathways of growth factor receptors including the IGF-I receptor.[31,32] IGF-I–receptor activation results in tyrosine phosphorylation of both CrkII and CrkL, which probably occurs by the association of these molecules with members of the IRS family of proteins. CrkII is involved in the differentiated function of the IGF-I receptor, whereas CrkL results in the more transforming phenotype.[33–35] Examples of recently described substrates involved in IGF-I receptor-signaling cascades include the *vav* protooncogene in hematopoietic cells, two isoforms of the 14-3-3 family of proteins that interact directly with the IGF-I receptor, protein kinase C isoforms (i.e., PKC α), the G protein Gβγ, focal adhesion kinase, Janus kinase 1 (JAK1), signal transducers and activators of transcription (Stat) 3, and suppressor of cytokine signaling (SOCS-2). IGF-I–receptor activation also results in enhanced expression of a large number of genes. These include *vascular endothelial growth factor* (VEGF), elastin, myogenin, cyclin D1, c-*myc*, c-*fos*, c-*jun*, tubulin, and neurofilament. The wide array of genes affected by IGF-I–receptor signaling attests to the pleiotropic responses to this receptor, which range from cell-cycle progression and cellular proliferation to differentiated functions in specialized tissues.

### INSULIN-LIKE GROWTH FACTOR–BINDING PROTEINS

A third, yet important, component of the IGF system is the family of IGF-binding proteins (IGFBPs).[36,37] IGFBPs-1 through -6 are encoded by a gene family and are characterized by cysteine-rich N and C termini with less-conserved central regions.[38] IGFBPs are produced by a variety of biologic tissues and are found in serum and other biologic fluids.[39] Some of the general characteristics are shown in Table 173-3.[40]

### REGULATION

The production of IGFBPs is regulated by several factors. All of the IGFBPs are developmentally regulated from fetal levels through the aging process. IGFBP-1 gene expression and circulating levels are regulated by nutritional status, insulin, and glucocorticoids. GH, on the other hand, increases the levels of both IGFBP-3 and the acid-labile subunit (ALS), both of which form the major serum complex that binds the majority of circulating IGFs. The effect of GH on IGFBP-3 is probably mediated by IGF-I

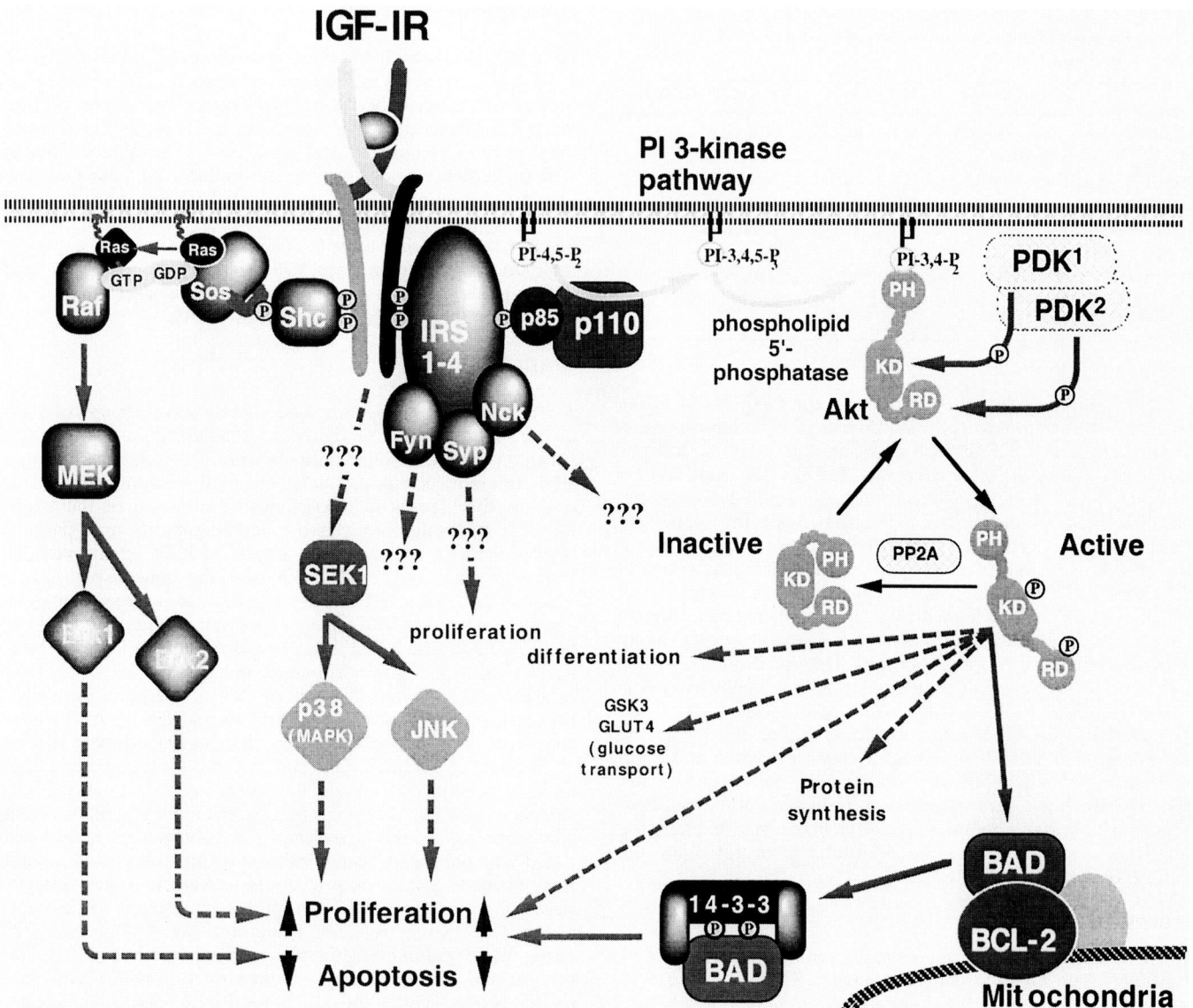

**FIGURE 173-2.** Signal transduction by the activated insulin-like growth factor-I (*IGF-I*) receptor. Similar to most tyrosine kinase transmembrane receptors, the IGF-I receptor has multiple substrates and pathways via which it mediates its cellular responses. Important substrates include SHC and the insulin receptor substrate (*IRS*) family of proteins. These interact with downstream substrates to result eventually in cellular proliferation and/or inhibition of apoptosis. *Akt*, a serine/threonine kinase, also known as *PKB* (protein kinase B); *Fyn*, an adapter protein encoded by c-fyn oncogene; *IGF-IR*, insulin-like growth factor-I receptor; *IRS 1-4*, insulin receptor substrates 1-4; *GDP*, guanosine diphosphate; *GLUT4*, glucose transporter 4; *GSK3*, glycogen synthase kinase 3; *GTP*, guanosine triphosphate; *JNK*, c-Jun NH2-terminal kinase, also known as *SAPK1* (stess-activated protein kinase 1); *MAPK*, mitogen-activated protein kinase; *MEK* or *MAPK/Erk 1*, MAPK/extracellular signal-regulated protein kinase 1; *Nck*, a SH2- and SH3-containing adapter protein; *p38 MAPK*, p38 mitogen-activated protein kinase, also known as *SAPK2* (stess-activated protein kinase 2); *PDK1 and 2*, phosphatidylinositol-dependent kinase 1 and 2; *PI3-kinase*, phosphoinositide 3-kinase; *PI-3,4-P2*, phosphatidylinositol-3,4-bisphosphate; *PI-3,4,5-P3*, phosphatidylinositol-3,4,5-trisphosphate; *PI-4,5-P2*, phosphatidylinositol-4,5-bisphosphate; *PP2A*, protein phosphatase 2A; *Raf*, a serine/threonine kinase encoded by c-raf oncogene; *Ras*, a guanine nucleotide binding protein encoded by H-ras oncogene; *SEK1*, stress signaling kinase 1, also known as *MKK4* (MAP kinase kinase 4); *Shc*, src homology/collagen protein; *Syp*, a SH2-containing protein tyrosine phosphatase, also known as *SH-PTP2* or *PTP1D* (src homology 2-binding tyrosine phosphatase 1D); *SOS*, a guanylnucleotide exchange factor that is the mammalian homologue of son-of-sevenless.

itself. At the tissue level, the IGFBPs are also regulated by other hormones, including retinoic acid and cytokines, and intracellular messengers such as cyclic adenosine monophosphate (AMP).

Several IGFBPs are subject to phosphorylation and glycosylation. Most IGFBPs are present in soluble and cell-associated forms via the Arg-Gly-Asp (RGD) sequences that may interact with integrins.[41] Most IGFBPs are subject to proteolytic cleavage by specific proteases, which themselves are subject to regulation.[42] Thus, the production and activity of the IGFBPs are controlled at multiple levels, including synthesis, degradation, posttranslational modification, and cell association.

### FUNCTIONS

In human serum, the major pool of IGFs circulate as an ~150-kDa (IGFBP-3/ALS) complex, a smaller pool as an ~50-kDa complex, and ~1% as free IGF. Bound IGFs in the serum have a half-life of up to 15 hours when bound to the IGFBP-3/ALS complex, but

TABLE 173-3.
**Characteristics of the Human Insulin-Like Growth Factor–Binding Proteins**

|  | Specific Features | IGF Affinity | Effect on IGF Action |
|---|---|---|---|
| **IGFBP-1** | Arg-Gly-Asp (RGD sequence) | IGF-I = IGF-II | Inhibit/potentiate |
| **IGFBP-2** | RGD sequence | IGF-II > IGF-I | Inhibition |
| **IGFBP-3** | N-glycosylation | IGF-I = IGF-II | Inhibit/potentiate |
| **IGFBP-4** | Extra cysteines | IGF-I = IGF-II | Inhibition |
| **IGFBP-5** |  | IGF-II > IGF-I | Potentiate |
| **IGFBP-6** | O-glycosylation | IGF-II > IGF-I | Inhibition |

*IGF,* insulin-like growth factor.

only ~20 minutes when they circulate in the free form or in the smaller 50-kDa complex. The 150-kDa complex can serve as a reservoir from which IGFs can be dissociated into the free form or transferred directly to other circulating IGFBPs. The small 50-kDa complex can leave the bloodstream and deliver IGF-I to target tissues. The major bound form of IGFs also prevents the hypoglycemia that would occur if the high concentrations of IGFs were in the free form and able to bind, albeit with a low affinity, to insulin receptors in muscle and liver.[43] Locally produced IGFBPs affect the interaction of the IGFs with the target tissues. Under certain circumstances, IGFBPs may enhance IGF action by effectively increasing the local concentration of IGF, by presentation of IGF to the receptor, or possibly by triggering IGF-independent events that contribute to IGF action at a postreceptor level.

Generally, the IGFBPs demonstrate a higher affinity for the IGFs compared to the IGF-I receptor, especially when in the soluble form or matrix-bound.[44] This affinity falls dramatically when cleaved by proteases, phosphorylated, or partitioned, that is, cell-surface bound.[45] These changes may explain the ability of certain IGFBPs either to inhibit or to potentiate the actions of the IGFs at the target.[46]

### INDEPENDENT ACTION

Current evidence strongly suggests that some of the IGFBPs may function in an IGF-independent manner.[47] IGFBP-1 and -2 both contain RGD sequences that may enable them to bind to integrins and promote cellular migration and possibly proliferation. IGFBP-3 binds to the cell surface by an undetermined mechanism. Furthermore, IGFBP-3 has been shown to inhibit proliferation and even induce apoptosis via an IGF-I receptor–independent mechanism.[48] Binding of IGFBP-3 to the cell surface may be the signal for this antiproliferative effect. No specific receptor for IGFBP-3 (or for any IGFBP) has been described; thus, the exact mechanisms whereby the IGFBPs affect cellular processes remain to be determined.

## INSULIN-LIKE GROWTH FACTORS IN HEALTH AND DISEASE

### NORMAL GROWTH AND DEVELOPMENT

The IGFs are essential for normal growth and development. The ligands, receptors, and certain IGFBPs are expressed in the prenatal stage.[49,50] When individual genes encoding certain members of the IGF system are inactivated by mutation or by homologous recombinant gene-targeting techniques, the consequences for fetal development are extremely serious.[51,52] Loss of the IGF-II/mannose-6-phosphate receptor due to the Tme-deletion mutant results in fetal death, whereas homologous deletion of IGF-I, IGF-II, or the IGF-I–receptor genes results in overall growth retardation of the fetus, generalized retardation in organ development, and, in the case of IGF-I and the IGF-I receptor gene deletion, in perinatal lethality.

## GROWTH DISORDERS

GH-deficient dwarfs have reduced circulating IGF-I levels. Serum IGF-I levels return to normal on replacement with recombinant human GH. Laron-type dwarfs have similar reductions in circulating IGF-I levels despite elevated serum GH levels, due to mutations in the GH receptor and resultant GH resistance. Patients with malnutrition and/or poorly controlled type 1 diabetes have lowered circulating IGF-I levels due partly to lower insulin levels and partly to postreceptor abnormalities in the tissues, leading to GH resistance. To date there has been only one report of a growth-retarded male patient with an IGF-I–gene deletion. Growth retardation is also seen in rare patients with deletion of the IGF-I receptor due to a ring form of chromosome 15.

## DIABETES

The IGF system has been implicated in the development of many of the complications of diabetes. A delayed pubertal growth spurt in poorly controlled patients with type 1 diabetes is associated with reduced circulating levels of IGF-I secondary to insulinopenia that causes GH resistance at the level of the liver.[53] Diabetic microangiopathy and macroangiopathy may partially be the result of the mitogenic effects of IGFs on the vascular smooth muscle cells. IGF-I enhances the gene expression of VEGF in these cells. IGF-I appears to have an indirect angiogenic effect by increasing VEGF gene expression. Retinal pigment epithelial cells release VEGF into the culture media in response to IGF-I with a resultant stimulation of capillary endothelial cell proliferation in mixed cultures of RPE and endothelial cells.[54] Enlargement of the kidneys at early stages of diabetes is associated with increased hemodynamic changes secondary to IGF-I.

Recombinant human IGF-I (rhIGF-I) has been tested in diabetics in an attempt to overcome the severe insulin resistance.[55] Subcutaneous injection of rhIGF-I reduces the requirement for insulin administration in both types 1 and 2 diabetic patients and is associated with enhanced insulin-induced disposal of glucose, inhibition of hepatic glucose output, and improvement in the metabolic status of these patients. Systemically administered rhIGF-I suppresses GH (thereby reducing insulin resistance), suppresses glucagon (thereby abrogating the glucagon-enhanced hepatic glucose output), and, in the case of type 2 diabetics, suppresses insulin levels (thereby preventing the "down-regulation" of insulin receptors on peripheral target cells that occurs in response to elevated insulin levels).[56] These effects of administered rhIGF-I may explain the improvement in the glucose homeostasis of these patients. It remains to be determined if rhIGF-I therapy will become a viable treatment for diabetic patients.[56a]

## CANCER

Many components of the IGF system appear to play important roles in cancer.[57,58,58a] Numerous tumors express high levels of IGFs, both types of IGF receptors, and many of the IGFBPs in various combinations.[59] IGF-II is commonly expressed at high levels in many tumors due to loss of imprinting, or mutations of tumor-suppressor gene products, such as WT1, which normally control its expression.[60] In the case of the IGF-II gene (chromosome 11p15), studies have shown that the maternal allele, which is imprinted in normal tissue, may be expressed in Wilms tumors without *loss of heterozygosity* (LOH).[61] This *loss of imprinting* (LOI) results in the expression of both maternal and paternal IGF-II alleles. Similar LOI can be seen with various lung, breast, and colon cancers. LOI is also associated with *microsatellite instability* (MSI). Imprinting has been ascribed to methylation of the gene. Hypermethylation appears to favor imprinting and it is postulated that hypomethylation is associated with expression of the gene. Expression of the IGF-II gene may also be due to hypomethylation of the neighboring inhibitory H19 gene.

Many nonislet cell tumors, primarily of mesenchymal origin, overexpress an incompletely processed prohormone form of IGF-II (termed "big IGF-II"), which leads to clinically apparent hypoglycemia.[62] Big IGF-II is incompletely neutralized by the 150-kDa IGFBP-3 complex and associates preferentially with the smaller 50-kDa IGFBP-2 complex.[63,64] This complex rapidly transfers the ligand out of the circulation and delivers it to the target tissues, thereby inducing hypoglycemia.[65]

The IGF-I receptor has intrinsic tyrosine kinase activity and mediates cell proliferation.[66] It is commonly overexpressed in tumors, thereby enhancing tumor growth, presumably by increasing responsiveness to the IGFs.[67] Circulating levels of IGF-I are increased in patients with prostatic, colon, breast, and lung cancer.[68] Results of prospective studies suggest an increased risk for the development of these and other cancers in the setting of elevated IGF-I levels. Elevated IGF-I levels have also been measured in cancer patients in case-controlled studies. Whether the increased IGF-I levels are merely markers for cancer development or intimately involved in the development of tumor growth remains to be answered. Further study is also needed to determine the origin(s) of these increased IGF-I levels in the circulation.

### NERVOUS SYSTEM

The IGF system is involved in the growth and development of the nervous system. IGFs acting through the IGF-I receptor modulate growth and differentiation of neurons and glial cells. IGFs stimulate neurite outgrowth, synaptogenesis in sympathetic precursors, and commitment of progenitors to the oligodendrocytic lineage. The important role of the IGFs in adult nervous tissue centers primarily on the control of apoptosis. During development, apoptosis is essential to the removal of excess neurons, whereas, in adult tissue, antiapoptosis is essential to prevent the loss of neurons after certain injuries and neurodegenerative diseases. IGFs signaling via the IGF-I receptor are powerful antiapoptotic agents. The major signaling pathways impacting apoptosis have been elucidated in cell culture systems. Activation of the PI3'K system in turn activates protein kinase B/Akt. In some specific cell types, the MAP kinase pathways are also involved in control of apoptosis. In vivo models of hypoxic brain injury corroborate the importance of IGF-I in the control of apoptosis. Hypoxic/ischemic brain infarction is associated with a large area of apoptosis, which occurs in the surrounding tissue and may lead to a greater degree of cerebral dysfunction than the ischemic region itself. Local injection of rhIGF-I immediately after the infarction greatly reduces the neuronal loss and preserves function.[69,70]

### IMMUNE SYSTEM

Differentiation of T cells, induction of granulocytic differentiation by granulocyte and macrophage colony-stimulating factor (GM-CSF), and differentiation of hematopoietic progenitors by erythropoietin (EPO) are associated with local production of IGF-I, which acts through the IGF-I receptors that are widely expressed on all myeloid and lymphoid cells. In addition to stimulating proliferation and differentiation of these cells, IGF-I exerts chemoattractant effects on T-cell progenitors migrating from hematopoietic tissues to the thymus, where they are further differentiated by cytokines.[71] At sites of inflammation, macrophage-derived IGF-I, together with interleukin-1 (IL-1), enhances migration of T lymphocytes to the site. These cytokine-activated T cells undergo clonal expansion in response to IGF-I.[72]

In nonhuman primates, administration of rhIGF-I alone, or with rhGH, increases T cells in the spleen with a concomitant increase in the CD4/CD8 ratio.[73] The potential use of IGF-I as a therapy for immunodeficiency states requires further study.

### REPRODUCTIVE SYSTEM

Delayed puberty is commonly associated with GH deficiency and is assumed to be the result of reduced IGF-I levels, which play an important role in ovarian, uterine, and testicular physiology.[74] Gonadotropins and sex steroids enhance local IGF-I production and IGF-I–receptor expression. Conversely, IGF-I modulates follicle-stimulating hormone (FSH) action on the ovary and enhances steroidogenesis in the ovary and testes.[75] Patients undergoing hormonal manipulation for in vitro fertilization show an improved response when GH is administered systemically, presumably by enhancing hemocrine and local IGF-I production. Estrogen enhances uterine IGF-I expression, which in turn affects endometrial physiology; moreover, IGF-I may also be important for embryo implantation in the uterus.[76]

### BONE

The pubertal growth spurt is mediated by IGF-I, either from the circulation or more likely from local autocrine/paracrine IGF-I production.[77] Osteoblasts produce IGF-I, and this expression is enhanced by parathyroid hormone, prostaglandin $E_2$ ($PGE_2$), and estrogen.[78,79] In cooperation with other growth factors, IGFs affect proliferation and differentiation of bone cells. These actions may be extremely important in callus formation after a fracture and may be therapeutically relevant in cases of osteoporosis. IGFBPs are also expressed by osteoblasts, and the level of IGFBP-4 that inhibits IGF-I action on proliferation and differentiation is increased by $1,25(OH)_2$ vitamin $D_3$. IGFBP-5 enhances IGF-I effects on bone cells; IGF-I enhances formation of multinucleated osteoclastic cells, thereby coupling bone formation and resorption.[80]

### POTENTIAL CLINICAL USES

Recombinant human IGF-I has been extremely useful clinically in reversing the negative nitrogen balance in several catabolic states and reducing insulin resistance in types 1 and 2 diabetes.[81] It induces growth in Laron-type dwarfism, for which it has been approved.[82] Other potential uses include treatment for diabetic neuropathy, amyotrophic lateral sclerosis, bony fractures, osteoporosis, and wound healing. It also may be useful in reactivating the immune response in acquired immunodeficiency syndrome (AIDS). Its usefulness may be enhanced by the coadministration of IGFBP-3. Yet to be confirmed are its potential long-term side effects, including enhanced mitogenesis and tumor growth.[83]

## OTHER GROWTH FACTORS

### VASCULAR ENDOTHELIAL GROWTH FACTOR

Angiogenesis, a process of new blood vessel formation, is a fundamental requirement for organ development and differentiation during embryogenesis. This has been confirmed by homologous recombination null mutants for VEGF and its receptors that are invariably fatal during embryogenesis due to a failure of blood vessel development.[84] It is also implicated in numerous pathologic processes, including tumor growth, metastases, and diabetic retinopathy.[85] Although there are a number of angiogenic factors, including the fibroblast growth factors (FGFs), tumor necrosis factor $\alpha$ (TNF-$\alpha$), transforming growth factor-$\alpha$ and -$\beta$ (TGF-$\alpha$ and -$\beta$), and leptin,[86] the most powerful known regulator of normal and tumor angiogenesis is VEGF. There are a number of VEGF isoforms, each with a different pattern of secretion. Some isoforms are retained on cell surfaces, and others are sequestered in the extracellular matrix by heparan sulfate proteoglycans. The larger VEGF family of peptides includes placenta-derived growth factor, and VEGF A, B, and C. These three, well-characterized, transmembrane VEGF receptors are expressed almost exclusively by vascular endothelial cells and contain extracellular immunoglobulin repeats and a split tyrosine kinase domain in the cytoplasmic portion of the molecule. Activation of the receptor kinase leads to signaling via phospholipase C-$\gamma$ (PLC-$\gamma$), PI3'K, and ras

GTPase-activating protein (GAP), Fyn and Yes (Src family of proteins). VEGF is expressed by a variety of tumors, and the degree of vascularization of the malignancy correlates with the level of VEGF mRNA. Antibodies to VEGF can inhibit tumor growth, suggesting an important role in tumor progression and supporting the theory that there may indeed be a role for an antagonist to VEGF in treating tumors and restenosis after angioplasty.[87]

## NERVE GROWTH FACTOR FAMILY

Nerve growth factor (NGF) is part of a family of neurotropins that includes brain-derived neurotropic factor (BDNF), neurotropin-3 (NT-3), NT-4, and NT-5. NGF is a highly conserved, 118–amino-acid protein exhibiting more than 70% homology across all vertebrate species. The various members of the family (i.e., NGF, BDNF, and the NTs) are also conserved in certain regions and also have similar predicted tertiary structures.

### RECEPTORS

Initial studies demonstrated the existence of low-affinity receptors that bound NGF, BDNF, and NT-3, and high-affinity receptors were found that were specific for NGF or BDNF. The low-affinity receptor was shown to be a 75-kDa intrinsic membrane protein (p75). A 140-kDa tyrosine kinase receptor encoded by the protooncogene *Trk* (or TRK-A) binds NGF with high affinity and mediates NGF effects. TRK-B is a TRK-related gene product that binds BDNF and NT-3, and TRK-C binds NT-3 with high affinity. TRK-A, TRK-B, and TRK-C contain tyrosine kinase activity, but p75 does not. A model for the functional interaction of the NGF-related peptides and functional receptors suggests that p75, TRK-A, and TRK-B individually are low-affinity receptors, and the association of p75 with TRK-A or TRK-B generates a high-affinity, functional receptor. The TRK-A tyrosine kinase receptor is responsible for mediating NGF signaling. The signaling pathways include PLC-$\gamma$, PI3'K, ras GAP, Shc, and the MAP kinase/Erk1 pathways.[88]

### FUNCTIONS

NGF-related peptides stimulate survival and differentiation of a range of target neurons. TRK-B expression is widespread throughout the central nervous system, serving more general functions. TRK and p75 are colocalized to the medial septal nucleus and the nucleus of the Broca diagonal band, which contains the NGF-responsive magnocellular cholinergic neurons projecting to the hippocampus and cerebral cortex.

NGF is the prototypic growth factor that controls cell survival. Neurons that project to an inappropriate target are automatically eliminated, because they fail to be stimulated by neurotropic factors, but neurons projecting to the appropriate target cell are innervated accordingly. The other members of the family have similar functions but act on different subsets of neurons.

Selective degeneration of magnocellular cholinergic neurons in the nucleus basalis of Meynert is seen in patients with Alzheimer disease. Clinical trials have begun using NGF directly intraventricularly in patients with Alzheimer dementia or to support transplanted adrenal medullary tissue in Parkinson disease.

## PLATELET-DERIVED GROWTH FACTORS

### STRUCTURE

PDGFs are a family of proteins consisting of disulfide-bonded dimers of A and B chains.[89] The A and B chains are encoded by separate genes that apparently arose by gene duplication and divergence. They have retained ~60% similarity in their amino-acid sequences, and their eight cysteine residues are perfectly conserved. The major form of PDGF in humans is the AB heterodimer, which is expressed primarily by platelets in adults. The BB homodimer (homologous to the viral *sis* oncogene) is

found in other species, and the AA homodimer is expressed by certain tissues and various tumors (i.e., osteosarcomas, melanomas, and glioblastomas). PDGFs are also produced by macrophages, mesangial cells, placental cytotrophoblasts, smooth muscle cells, endothelial cells, fibroblasts, neurons, glial cells, and embryonic cells.

PDGF receptors are expressed by vascular smooth muscle cells, fibroblasts, and glial cells, but the receptors are not expressed by most hematopoietic, epithelial, or endothelial cells. Two subtypes have been identified. The $\alpha$ receptor binds all three PDGF isoforms (i.e., AA, AB, and BB), and the $\beta$ receptor binds only PDGF-BB with high affinity. Both receptor subtypes contain five immunoglobulin-like domains, a single transmembrane sequence, and an intracellular protein tyrosine kinase region that is split by a kinase insert region. Ligand binding leads to receptor dimerization, activation of the kinase, and subsequent association and activation of numerous endogenous substrates. These include phospholipase $A_2$, PLC-$\gamma$, PI3'K, and ras GAP. These substrates interact directly with phosphotyrosine residues on the PDGF receptor by means of their SH2 domains.

### FUNCTIONS

PDGF induces cell proliferation in mesenchymal cells, including fibroblasts, osteoblasts, arterial smooth muscle cells, and brain glial cells. PDGF is a competence factor, allowing cells to enter the $G_0/G_1$ phase of the cell cycle, but further progression is the function of other growth factors.

**Wound Healing.** PDGF is synthesized and released at the site of injury by platelets, vascular cells, monocyte-macrophages, fibroblasts, and skin epithelial cells. PDGF, by means of a paracrine mechanism, induces proliferation and chemotaxis of connective tissue cells and production of extracellular matrix, thereby enhancing healing.

**Osteogenesis.** PDGF plays an important role in bone formation and metabolism by stimulating DNA synthesis and collagen synthesis by osteoblasts. In addition to normal bone development, PDGF is potentially capable of enhancing new bone formation after fractures.

**Atherosclerosis.** Atherosclerosis is an abnormal proliferation of arterial smooth muscle cells, increased number of macrophages, and excessive deposition of connective tissue. In addition to platelet-derived PDGF, vascular endothelial cells and activated macrophages express PDGF. PDGF-receptor expression is increased in the cells proximal to the macrophages, the intimal smooth muscle cells. PDGF is one of the most important growth factors involved in atherogenesis.

The restenosis that follows balloon angioplasty is also associated with increased PDGF and receptor expression, particularly by neointimal smooth muscle cells.

**Fibrosis.** PDGF and receptors play a role in many fibrotic diseases, including myelofibrosis, scleroderma, and pulmonary fibrosis, by stimulating connective tissue cell proliferation, chemotaxis, and collagen synthesis, which are all pathognomonic features of these diseases.

**Neoplasia.** The acutely transforming simian sarcoma virus genome contains a retroviral homologue of the cellular gene encoding PDGF-B. This finding led to speculation that the cell-cycle competence factor PDGF may be involved in tumor cell growth. Tumors such as gliomas, sarcomas, melanomas, mesotheliomas, carcinomas, and hematopoietic cell-derived tumors overexpress PDGF. Many tumors express PDGF receptors that may be activated in the absence of the ligand. Transforming effects of v-*sis* may occur by this mechanism. Furthermore, chronic myelomonocytic leukemia is associated with a fusion protein produced by chromosomal translocation. This fusion protein consists of the PDGF kinase domain fused to an *ets*-like gene product. The fusion product serves to autodimerize the receptor, thereby activating it in the absence of ligand.[90]

Although PDGF may be involved in pathologic states, its value therapeutically in treating wounds and bone fractures, to name a few examples, remains to be explored.

## EPIDERMAL GROWTH FACTOR FAMILY

The EGF family of growth factors includes EGF, TGF-α, amphiregulin, heparin-binding EGF, schwannoma-derived growth factor, and the vaccinia virus growth factor.[91] They are each synthesized as a much larger membrane-bound glycosylated precursor before being processed into a smaller mature peptide.

### EPIDERMAL GROWTH FACTOR

The 1217–amino-acid, membrane-bound EGF precursor (PreproEGF) and the 53–amino-acid mature peptide are capable of interacting with cell-surface EGF receptors. This interaction causes dimerization of the single-chain EGF receptors, activation of the cytoplasmic tyrosine kinase domain, and subsequent biologic responses.

EGF is a potent stimulator of cell multiplication, and it modulates the differentiation and specialized functions of various cells. EGF's effects on development include eyelid opening, teeth eruption, lung maturation, and skin development. In keeping with its initial isolation from salivary glands, EGF has been shown to protect the gastric mucosa by inhibiting gastric acid secretion.

In addition to its angiogenic and proliferative ability, EGF displays a chemotactic activity for inducing migration of fibroblasts into the wound area.[92] The overexpression of EGF and the EGF receptor occurs in certain carcinomas. The EGF receptor (c-*erb*1) is homologous to the avian viral oncogene v-*erb*B, strongly supporting the notion that overexpression may be involved in tumorigenesis. A correlation has been demonstrated between amplification of the EGF-receptor gene and poor prognosis in breast, lung, and bladder cancers.

### TRANSFORMING GROWTH FACTOR-α

TGF-α resembles EGF structurally and functionally. It is synthesized as part of a 160–amino-acid cell-surface precursor, and the mature 50–amino-acid TGF-α is proteolytically cleaved and released from the extracellular domain. It is a potent mitogen, acting through the EGF receptor. It is expressed in preimplantation embryos and the fetus and is essential in normal development. In adults, it is expressed by the anterior pituitary, brain, decidual cells, skin keratinocytes, bronchus, kidney, and genital tract and has been implicated in wound healing and inflammation, angiogenesis, and bone resorption. TGF-α is overexpressed in many cancers, in which it is implicated, along with the EGF receptor, as being tumorigenic.[93]

### TRANSFORMING GROWTH FACTOR-β FAMILY

TGF-β1 is a disulfide-linked dimer of two identical chains of 112 amino acids. The chains are synthesized as 390–amino-acid precursor molecules. The cleaved proregion remains associated with the mature TGF-β1 dimer forming a biologically latent complex, which becomes active on disassembly of this complex. This family of growth factors in humans includes TGF-β, the activin-inhibin family, and müllerian inhibitory hormone.

### BIOSYNTHESIS

The TGF-β peptides represent three separate gene products expressed by many normal cells and tissues. Expression is active throughout embryonic development and into adulthood. Gene expression is regulated by multiple factors at the level of transcription, and except in the case of platelets, in which TGF-β is stored in α-granules, the TGF-βs are released from cells through a constitutive pathway. TGF-β1 released from cells is in the "latent" form and the proregion contains mannose-6-phosphate, which binds to IGF-II/mannose-6-phosphate receptors, and an RGD

sequence, which may be important for its interaction with integrin receptors. The role of these residues in regulating the release of active TGF-β remains undefined; however, proteases play a definitive role in conversion from the latent to the active form.

### RECEPTORS

There are at least two distinct receptors that mediate the effects of TGF-β. The type I receptor is expressed only by hematopoietic cells that are growth-inhibited by TGF-β and is expressed with the type II receptor by many different cells and tissues in which growth inhibition, extracellular matrix protein synthesis, and differentiation are the major responses. In addition to these two classic receptors, betaglycan (the type III TGF-β receptor), an abundant membrane proteoglycan, also binds TGF-β. A soluble form of betaglycan is found in the extracellular matrix. Betaglycan binding of TGF-β has been invoked as important in the storage of TGF-β in the matrix, presentation of the ligand to the receptor, and even clearance of TGF-β, whereby the membrane form internalizes with the ligand. Type V TGF-β receptor contains an amino-acid sequence that shows homology to the type II TGF-β receptor.[94] This receptor also appears to play a role in internalizing the ligand.

Type I, II, and V TGF-β receptors are members of the family of transmembrane serine-threonine kinases. Members of this family include receptors for activin and müllerian inhibiting substance. Type I TGF-β receptors cannot bind ligand independently. Type I, II, III, and V receptors undergo autophosphorylation.[95]

One of the most important effects of TGF-β is its inhibitory effect on cell proliferation. Inhibition of phosphorylation of the retinoblastoma gene product is apparently the mechanism whereby TGF-β inhibits cell-cycle progression.

### ACTIONS

The bioactions of TGF-β are extensive and varied. TGF-β can inhibit or stimulate proliferation, depending on the culture conditions. In the presence of mitogen-rich medium, TGF-β inhibits; in the presence of mitogen-free medium, TGF-β can enhance proliferation by inducing PDGF.[96]

TGF-β causes enhanced cell-cell adhesion in mesenchymal and epithelial cells and various cell lines. This process is accompanied by increased extracellular matrix production and expression of cell-adhesion receptors. These effects explain, at least in part, the role of TGF-β in wound healing, tissue repair, and angiogenesis. TGF-β is expressed by activated macrocytes and macrophages at sites of wound healing or inflammation and is a chemoattractant for these cells. Bone remodeling is enhanced by locally produced TGF-β.

TGF-β has also been invoked as a causative mediator in diseases, including acute mesangial proliferative glomerulosclerosis, fibrotic diseases such as lung fibrosis, liver cirrhosis, arterial restenosis after angioplasty, and myelofibrosis. Because TGF-β forms have antiproliferative effects on T- and B-lymphocytes, they have potent immunosuppressive effects in vivo. The elevated TGF-β expression in lymphocytes may be one explanation for the general immunosuppressive effects of the AIDS virus despite the limited number of lymphocytes that are actually infected. The potential benefits of the antiinflammatory and immunosuppressive effects of TGF-β in systemic disease, such as rheumatoid arthritis, await further experimentation. As a suppressor of cell proliferation, the absence of TGF-β or its receptor may result in oncogenesis. Only retinoblastoma cells have been reported to be devoid of TGF-β receptors, which may enable increased oncogenic potential.

## INHIBIN, ACTIVIN, AND MÜLLERIAN-INHIBITING HORMONE

Inhibins and activins are dimeric polypeptides composed of similar subunits (see Chaps. 16, 113, and 114). Inhibins inhibit production of FSH in pituitary cells, sex steroid in the gonads, and many placental hormones. The activins stimulate the production of all these hormones. Activins also induce differentiation of erythroleukemia cells.

Müllerian-inhibiting substance (MIH) induces müllerian duct regression, inhibits oocyte maturation, and is capable of inhibiting production of desaturated phosphatidylcholine, a component of surfactant.[97]

## FIBROBLAST GROWTH FACTOR FAMILY

Seven members of the FGF family are known.[98] Acidic FGF (FGF-α) and basic FGF (FGF-β) have different tissue preferences for expression and function. The family includes a newly described member: keratinocyte growth factor (KGF). The FGFs support the survival of neural cells and stimulate proliferation of many types of cells, including fibroblasts, endothelial cells, smooth muscle cells, hepatocytes, and skeletal myoblasts. Moreover, mesoderm induction is FGF dependent.

Two classes of FGF-binding sites have been characterized. The low-affinity, high-capacity receptors are cell-surface proteoglycans containing heparan sulfate side chains. The high-affinity tyrosine kinase receptors are important for transducing the signals. These high-affinity receptors represent a family of gene products. The extracellular domains have three immunoglobulin-like loops, which are involved in ligand binding and are highly conserved.

The high- and low-affinity receptors collaborate in FGF binding. The low-affinity, heparan sulfate–containing receptors bind the FGF molecule, allowing it to dimerize so that it can bind to the high-affinity receptors. This results in activation of tyrosine kinase activity and activation of phospholipase Cγ 1, one of the major receptor substrates in the signal transduction pathway.

# CYTOKINES

The cytokine family contains a diverse collection of proteins that, by activation of specific cell-surface receptors, regulate many cellular processes, including the immune and inflammatory systems (see Chap. 227), and differentiation processes such as hematopoiesis and leukopoiesis. This family includes the interleukins (IL), the tumor necrosis factors (TNF-α and -β), the interferons (IFN-α, -β, and -γ), the macrophage and granulocyte colony-stimulating factors (M-CSF/CSF-1, G-CSF, and GM-CSF), and several other molecules. In this section, the major subgroups of this family are discussed, including the ILs, TNFs, IFNs, and CSFs.

Cytokines are closely allied with growth factors because they are often synthesized by multiple cell types. Exceptions to this are IL-2 through IL-5 and IFN-γ, which are produced specifically by lymphoid cells. IL-3, for example, is predominantly produced by activated T cells. Also similar to many growth factors, cytokines modulate the activity of several types of cells rather than just one specific target cell.

## INTERLEUKINS

### INTERLEUKIN-1

IL-1α and IL-1β are encoded by similar but distinct genes. Both proteins are synthesized as part of larger precursor proteins. IL-1 is produced by many cell types, including monocytes and macrophages, neutrophils, astrocytes and microglia, endothelial cells, fibroblasts, T and B lymphocytes, and platelets. IL-1 is one of the most pleiotropic interleukins in that it induces the widest array of responses. IL-1β is involved in the immune and inflammatory responses, and in hematopoiesis. It has been shown to be cytotoxic for isolated pancreatic cells and may play a causative role in the development of autoimmune or type 1 diabetes. IL-1β induces the apoptotic response of many cells by activating the caspase cascade of events. Almost all of the effects of IL-1 are seen with TNF, and synergy with TNF can be demonstrated in many cases.

### INTERLEUKIN-2

IL-2 is an important component in the immune response.[99] It is produced by antigen-induced T cells, and its subsequent interaction with IL-2 receptors, which are also antigen induced, leads to clonal expansion of effector T-cell populations. In addition to proliferative effects, IL-2 stimulates differentiation, inducing the production of IFN-γ and IL-4 by T cells. IL-2 also affects B cells, natural killer cells (NK), lymphokine-activated killer (LAK) cells, monocytes, macrophages, and oligodendrocytes. The T-cell–activating capacity has promoted its consideration as a form of immune replacement therapy in immunodeficient (AIDS) or immunocompromised patients. Its effect on LAK cell function has led to its use as a possible antitumor therapy (IL-2/LAK) in patients with renal carcinoma and malignant melanoma.[100]

The major dose-limiting toxicity of IL-2 is due to extravasation of fluid and protein into the interstitium.[101] This toxicity seems to be due to activation of the endothelium subsequent to the IL-2–induced release of IL-1, TNF-α, and interferon; it may be reduced by depletion of NK cells. Pharmacologically, this side effect may be reduced by concomitant steroid therapy and lymphocyte depletion, but these modalities reduce the antitumor efficacy of the primary treatment. Endocrine toxicity of IL-2 therapy includes hypothyroidism, associated with the development of antimicrosomal and antithyroglobulin antibodies. In rare instances, adrenal insufficiency occurs after IL-2 therapy.

### INTERLEUKIN-3

IL-3 is produced primarily by activated T lymphocytes. Its major function is in the hematopoietic system, where it stimulates the growth of bone marrow stem cells and the differentiation of myeloid stem cells into many different lineages, including platelets, mast cells, eosinophils, basophils, and erythroid cells. Thus, it links the lymphoid system with the hematopoietic system. It has been proposed that IL-3 may be important in the recovery after myelotoxicity especially of the platelets. However, IL-3 may be involved in allergy production by enhancing mast cell production. Thus, its potential use in enhancing hematopoietic cell differentiation will need further evaluation given its effect on the allergic system.[102]

### INTERLEUKIN-4

IL-4 is produced by T cells, primarily T$_H$2 as well as NK cells, and leads to a preferential stimulation of humoral immunity by its effect on B-cell development.[103] IL-4 enhances the antigen-presenting capacity of B cells toward T cells. It induces activated B cells to produce IL-6 and TNF cytokines, which play an important role in the activation and clonal expansion of activated T cells. Thus, IL-4 favors T-B cell interactions. IL-4 inhibits the production of IFN-γ by activated T cells and, in doing so, favors the generation of T cells of the T$_H$2 type. Blood mononuclear cells from atopic patients display an increased capacity to produce IL-4. The deregulated immunoglobulin E (IgE) synthesis by cells from atopic patients can be inhibited by anti–IL-4 antibodies. In patients with severe atopic dermatitis, circulating and skin-derived T cells produce higher levels of IL-4 and less IFN-γ. IL-4 is a potent antitumor agent in mice. When expressed by plasmacytoma cell lines, IL-4 inhibits growth; this is reversed by anti–IL-4 antibodies. IL-4 has been tested in humans with melanoma and renal cell cancer.[104] Nasal congestion and gastritis due to histamine release are specific side effects. When used with IL-2, some remission has been shown (e.g., spleen and lymph node reductions in patients with low-grade lymphoma; even complete remission in cases of Hodgkin lymphoma). Complete remission of pulmonary metastases in cases of renal carcinoma has been seen. Similarly to IL-3, while it may have an antitumor effect, it also is involved in allergy development.[105]

## INTERLEUKIN-5

IL-5 is produced by leukocytes. Within the lymphocyte lineage, T helper cells produce IL-5, whereas among the myeloid lineages, mast cells and eosinophils are the major producers of IL-5.

IL-5—as well as being an antiapoptotic agent for B cells that, thus, enlarges the B-cell population—affects B-cell differentiation and causes B cells to produce antibodies.[106] IL-5 also enhances eosinophil development and activation, as well as basophil histamine release. Thus, IL-5 may be involved in the pathogenesis of inflammation in allergies (e.g., the chronic asthmatic response). It has been implicated in the eosinophilic response to helminth infections in which IL-5–mediated eosinophilia may evoke an immunologic protection against helminthes. IL-5 injection in murine models of sarcoma and lymphoma led to an eosinophilic infiltration of the malignancy and tumor rejection. Eosinophilic infiltration of allografts is associated with increased expression of IL-5 by the allograft-infiltrating cells and may result in allograft rejection.[107]

## INTERLEUKIN-6

IL-6 is a multifunctional cytokine with a broad range of biologic actions. IL-6 inclusion with IL-1 and glucocorticoids is primarily responsible for the liver induction of the acute-response proteins after severe injury and inflammation. IL-6 also affects the hypothalamic–pituitary–adrenal axis by increasing the production and release of corticotropin-releasing hormone (CRH), which causes increased adrenocorticotropic hormone (ACTH) and glucocorticoid release in response to stress (see Chap. 229). The major source of IL-6 in the bone marrow is macrophages, where it synergistically, with other cytokines, stimulates proliferation of progenitor hematopoietic cells. Activated B cells express IL-6 receptors that respond with enhanced antibody production. IL-6 activates NK cells, but simultaneously enhances plasmacytoma and myeloma growth. Circulating levels of IL-6 are elevated in autoimmune diseases (i.e., systemic lupus erythematosus [SLE], rheumatoid arthritis, and AIDS), implicating IL-6 in these diseases. IL-6 induces the differentiation of numerous nervous system cell lineages and stimulates the secretion of prolactin (PRL), GH, and luteinizing hormone (LH) from the pituitary gland. IL-6, which normally is produced by osteoblasts, is overproduced in ovariectomized mice, leading to enhanced osteoclast development, suggesting a role for IL-6 in the production of postmenopausal osteoporosis, as well as its putative roles in cancer and inflammatory/immune diseases.[108]

## INTERLEUKIN-7

In addition to its traditional role in promotion of growth of B-cell progenitors, IL-7 affects thymopoiesis, myelopoiesis, and neuronal cell survival. In addition, it has profound immunomodulatory effects ranging from augmentation of immunotherapeutically effective T-cell responses to tumor antigens—such as its ability to enhance the generation of cytolytic T lymphocytes (CTL) and to enhance immune responses to virally mediated pathologic conditions (e.g., influenza A). Moreover, IL-7 improves immune responses to parasitic infections. For example, IL-7 treatment of murine macrophages, which are infected with *Leishmania* major, reduces the number of infected cells by 50% and reduces the parasite burden per cell.[109]

## INTERLEUKIN-8

More than 15 chemokines, chemoattractants for inflammatory cells, have been discovered thus far. Structurally, they are divided into two major subgroups, C-X-C and C-C chemokines, depending on the presence of one amino acid between the first two cysteine residues. Intradermal injection of IL-8 induces massive local neutrophil infiltration; both lymphocytes and eosinophils infiltrate in response to IL-8. Since many diseases are associated with neutrophil infiltration, it is not surprising that IL-8 may be responsible. Thus, it may play a role in neutrophil infiltration into the synovial fluids of rheumatoid arthritis, osteoarthritis, and gout.[110] In acute respiratory distress syndrome, increased concentrations of IL-8 are found in bronchial lavage specimens. Urinary IL-8 levels are increased in cases of glomerulonephritis, IgA nephropathy, lupus nephritis, and so forth.

## INTERLEUKIN-9

IL-9 functions as a growth factor for helper T cells and as an erythroid colony stimulating factor (CSF). Its lymphocytic activity appears to be specific since it is active with CD4T cells but is inactive with cytotoxic CD8T cells.

## INTERLEUKIN-10

IL-10 was initially identified as a "cytokine synthesis inhibitory factor," but, in fact, it demonstrates both inhibitory and stimulatory effects, depending on the local context in which it is produced. IL-10 is produced by $T_H2$ lymphocytes and by B cells, macrophages, and keratinocytes. IL-10, when secreted by $T_H2$ cells, inhibits $T_H1$-cell cytokine synthesis. Parasitic infections (e.g., *Schistosoma mansoni* infection) result in a strong $T_H2$ response with concomitant suppression of the $T_H1$ response. The reduction in IFN-γ allows the infection to occur, and this effect can be blocked with the administration of anti–IL-10 monoclonal antibodies. In addition, nitric oxide production by macrophages and subsequent killing of parasites is inhibited by IL-10. Similar results were noted with mycobacterial infections. On the other hand, in SLE, glomerulonephritis can be prevented by anti–IL-10 monoclonal antibody administration, probably via elevated TNF-α levels. IL-10 has also been shown to function in B-cell growth and differentiation into immunoglobulin-secreting cells.[111] In the skin, ultraviolet (UV) radiation causes increased IL-10, which may mediate the immune tolerance after UV radiation and participate in the development of tumors.[112]

## INTERLEUKIN-18

IL-18 induces IFN-γ; it is structurally related to IL-1 and demonstrates bioactions shared with IL-1 and IL-12. The IL-18 receptor signals via NFκB and the ras/raf/MAP kinase pathways. It shows some anticancer effects when administered with IL-12. Aberrant regulation of IL-18 may account for the $T_H1$-dependent autoimmunity seen in the NOD mice that develop diabetes; furthermore, one genomic locus associated with type 1 diabetes in NOD mice (namely, *Idd*2) maps in close proximity to the IL-18 gene.[113–115]

## TUMOR NECROSIS FACTOR AND LYMPHOTOXIN

TNF-α (cachectin) and TNF-β (lymphotoxin) are potent cytokines encoded by genes that are near each other within the major histocompatibility complex on human chromosome 17.[116] TNF-α is produced by monocytes, neutrophils, fibroblasts, NK cells, vascular endothelial cells, mast cells, glial cells, astrocytes, smooth muscle cells, and certain cancers. TNF has extremely powerful cytotoxic effects. The effect on cellular killing may be either via apoptosis or via necrosis, depending on the cell type. Apoptosis is mediated via a mechanism similar to Fas ligand and FAS activation.[117] Crucial for the immunomodulatory effects of TNF is its ability to alter cell-surface proteins (e.g., human leukocyte antigen [HLA] class I and II antigen, intercellular adhesion molecule [ICAM], E-selectin, and vascular adhesion molecule [VCAM]), to alter production of cytokines (e.g., IL-6 and IL-1), and to alter production of receptors (e.g., EGF and IL-2). TNF is a costimulator for immune cells (e.g., T and B cells), macrophages, and monocytes; its effect on osteoblasts and osteoclasts leads to reduced bone formation and increased bone resorption, thus promoting osteoporosis. TNF was originally described as a cachectic factor after infections. TNF may down-regulate lipoprotein lipase at the transcriptional level and may up-regulate lipolytic and glycogenolytic pathways in muscle.[118] Lipopolysaccharide (LPS) stimulates the production of TNF, which synergistically along with the other cytokines is responsible for the septic shock syndrome. Many viral infections induce TNF production by macrophages and monocytes; in turn, TNF is an antiviral agent. However, some evidence indicates that TNF, like some other cytokines, may stimulate the proliferation of viruses (i.e., human immunodeficiency virus [HIV]). In multiple sclerosis, the intracranial injection of anti-TNF antibodies has shown some promise in controlling the disease; in rheumatoid arthritis, systemic anti-TNF antibody injections have shown efficacy.[119] TNF has been tested as an anticancer therapy; alone it has had no beneficial effect; however, in some tumors (i.e., sarcomas and melanomas), when used with cytostatics or IFN-γ, some benefit has been achieved. Generally, its initial promise as an anticancer agent has not been realized; its greatest limitation lies in its systemic toxicity effects.[120]

Unlike TNF, the cellular production of lymphotoxin is limited to the B-lymphocyte lineage. IL-1, IL-2, IL-4, and IL-6, as well as viruses, can induce the production and release of lymphotoxin. While lymphotoxin exerts its physiologic actions through the same receptor as TNF, its effects differ. Although it is unknown how these cytokines exert similar but distinct functions, it is possible that this occurs because of different binding affinities and domains for the same receptor.

Missense mutations of the 55-kDa TNF receptor (TNFR1) have been demonstrated in six of seven families with autosomal dominant periodic fever. These mutations, found in the transmembrane domain, result in reduced cleavage and impaired down-regulation of membrane TNFR1. Thus, the periodic syndrome(s) may be due to constitutively activated receptors.[121]

Lymphotoxin is antiproliferative for certain tumors, acts as a growth factor for normal B cells and B-cell lymphomas, and induces proliferation and differentiation of hematopoietic cells. Thus, it causes differentiation of human myeloid leukemic cells without any cytotoxic effect. Like TNF it interacts with neutrophils and activates them for antibody-dependent cell-mediated cytotoxicity. It modulates endothelial cell function, including increased permeability, and activates fibroblasts to produce GM-CSF, M-CSF, and IL-6. It is cytotoxic to keratinocytes and causes bone resorption. It can kill virally infected cells and, like TNF, induces lipolysis in adipocytes. In addition, it also acts as an antitumor agent.

Lymphotoxin may also play a role in autoimmune diseases (e.g., the insulinitis seen in type 1 diabetes).

## INTERFERONS

IFNs are a family of proteins that are related by their ability to protect cells from viral infections.[122] Based on their physical properties and source, the IFNs were subsequently divided into type I or type II. Type I IFNs include IFN-α (originally known as *leukocyte IFN*) and IFN-β (originally known as *fibroblast IFN*). IFN-γ, known as *type II IFN* or "immune" IFN, is produced only by T lymphocytes and NK cells. IFN-α and -β are very powerful antiviral agents, whereas IFN-γ is less potent as an antiviral agent and more potent as an immunomodulator.[123,124]

Differential effects are seen with IFN-α and IFN-β. For example, certain tumor-derived cell lines are inhibited by one and not the other. On the other hand, their antiviral and immune effects are mediated similarly.

In general, IFN-β is produced by fibroblasts and epithelial cells, whereas IFN-α is produced by blood leukocytes. IFNs have been biosynthesized by recombinant technology; however, when administered they have a number of side effects. Acute effects are flulike, whereas chronic administration results in neurologic (depression) and cardiac toxicity, autoimmune thyroiditis, and hematologic suppression. The development of antibodies after repeated use may limit its usefulness. Clinical trials in multiple sclerosis (MS) patients have not been particularly successful. Condylomas, cervical neoplasia, and herpes simplex skin lesions have proved more responsive. Acute and chronic hepatitis C and B have been treated with IFNs, and the response of some tumors seems promising.

Transgenic mice expressing IFN-α within the pancreatic islets develop diabetes, and IFN-α expression increases in the islets of mice with streptozotocin-induced diabetes and in the pancreases of patients with type 1 diabetes. On the other hand, IFN-α administration to NOD mice, which usually develop diabetes, prevents the development of the disease. This paradoxic response may be due to a dose- and time-response effect. IFN-α can augment or suppress cellular and humoral immunity; its effect depends on the time course of the disease. Similarly, IL-1 and IL-12 can either prevent or accelerate diabetes in NOD mice. The inhibition of diabetes is associated with the absence of insulinitis.

IFN-γ is produced by all CD8 and subsets of CD4 T lymphocytes. The primary physiologic stimulus is an antigen in the context of either major histocompatibility complex (MHC) class II for CD4 cells, or MHC class I for CD8 cells. NK-stimulatory factor or IL-12, a product of B cells, can induce IFN-γ production and together with TNF-α can induce production of IFN-γ in NK cells. This latter effect is important in the early response to microbial infections, as the IFN-γ can rapidly activate macrophage populations until T-cell–dependent sterilizing immunity can be generated. IFN-γ regulates MHC class I and class II protein expression in a variety of immunologically important cell types (especially macrophage/monocytes), thereby promoting antigen presentation during the inductive phase of immune responses.

IFN-γ appears to be necessary for $T_H1$ cell development, leading to cell-mediated immune responses. When IL-10 inhibits IFN-γ production, $T_H2$ cells develop to initiate a humoral response. IFN-γ is the major physiologic macrophage-activating factor and as such is the major cytokine responsible for inducing nonspecific cell-mediated mechanisms of host defense. It plays an important role in promoting inflammatory reactions and increases TNF-α and TNF-receptor expression, thereby enhancing the LPS-mediated tissue damage. The action of IL-12 as an antitumor agent is mediated by IFN-γ. One possible mechanism for this is that IFN-γ up-regulates the presentation of tumor antigens to CD4 and CD8 cells, resulting in tumor-cell recognition and regression.

## CYTOKINE RECEPTORS

The cytokine/hematopoietin receptor superfamily includes receptors for EPO, granulocyte-CSF, GM-CSF, ciliary neurotrophic factor (CNTF), IL-2, IL-3, IL-4, IL-5, IL-6, IL-7, IL-9, IL-10, IL-11, IL-12, thrombopoietin, interferons, leptin, GH, and PRL.[86,125,126]

The signaling cascade is activated after binding of the ligand to the extracellular domain of one of the receptor subunits, followed by heterodimerization, recruitment, and activation of a member of the *Janus family of tyrosine kinases (JAKs)*.[127] JAKs phosphorylate a family of transcription factors (*Stats*) that translocate to the nucleus and induce gene expression.[128] In addition, many other cascades of events are activated by the various cytokine receptors.

## REFERENCES

1. LeRoith D. Insulin-like growth factors. N Engl J Med 1997; 336:633.
2. Daughaday WH, Rotwein P. Insulin-like growth factors I and II. Peptide, messenger ribonucleic acid and gene structures, serum, and tissue concentrations. Endocr Rev 1989; 10:68
3. Mathews LS, Norstedt G, Palmiter RD. Regulation of insulin-like growth factor I gene expression by growth hormone. Proc Natl Acad Sci U S A 1986; 83:9343.
4. Pao CI, Farmer PK, Begovic S, et al. Expression of hepatic insulin-like growth factor-I and insulin-like growth factor-binding protein-1 genes is transcriptionally regulated in streptozotocin-diabetic rats. Mol Endocrinol 1992; 6:969.
5. Baker J, Liu JP, Robertson EJ, Efstratiadis A. Role of insulin-like growth factors in embryonic and postnatal growth. Cell 1993; 75:73.

6. Powell-Braxton L, Hollingshead P, Warburton C, et al. IGF-I is required for normal embryonic growth in mice. Genes Dev 1993; 7:2609.

7. Treadway JL, Morrison BD, Goldfine ID, Pessin JE. Assembly of insulin/insulin-like growth factor-1 hybrid receptors in vitro. J Biol Chem 1989; 264:21450.

8. Ullrich A, Gray A, Tam AW, et al. Insulin-like growth factor I receptor primary structure: comparison with insulin receptor suggests structural determinants that define functional specificity. Embo J 1986; 5:2503.

9. Morgan DO, Edman JC, Standring DN, et al. Insulin-like growth factor II receptor as a multifunctional binding protein [published erratum appears in Nature 1988; 20(7):442]. Nature 1987; 329:301.

10. Lowe WL Jr, Adamo M, Werner H, et al. Regulation by fasting of rat insulin-like growth factor I and its receptor. Effects on gene expression and binding. J Clin Invest 1989; 84:619.

11. Abbott AM, Bueno R, Pedrini MT, et al. Insulin-like growth factor I receptor gene structure. J Biol Chem 1992; 267:10759.

12. Werner H, Re GG, Drummond AI, et al. Increased expression of the insulin-like growth factor I receptor gene, IGF1R, in Wilms tumor is correlated with modulation of IGF1R promoter activity by the WT1 Wilms tumor gene product. Proc Natl Acad Sci U S A 1993; 90:5828.

13. Werner H, Bach MA, Stannard B, et al. Structural and functional analysis of the insulin-like growth factor I receptor gene promoter. Mol Endocrinol 1992; 6:1545.

14. Werner H, Woloschak M, Adamo M, et al. Developmental regulation of the rat insulin-like growth factor I receptor gene. Proc Natl Acad Sci U S A 1989; 86:7451.

15. Hernandez-Sanchez C, Werner H, Roberts CT, et al. Differential regulation of insulin-like growth factor-I (IGF-I) receptor gene expression by IGF-I and basic fibroblastic growth factor. J Biol Chem 1997; 272:4663.

16. Rubini M, Werner H, Gandini E, et al. Platelet-derived growth factor increases the activity of the promoter of the insulin-like growth factor-1 (IGF-1) receptor gene. Exp Cell Res 1994; 211:374.

17. Cheatham B, Kahn CR. Insulin action and the insulin signaling network. Endocr Rev 1995; 16:117.

18. Kato H, Faria TN, Stannard B, et al. Essential role of tyrosine residues 1131:1135, and 1136 of the insulin-like growth factor-I (IGF-I) receptor in IGF-I action. Mol Endocrinol 1994; 8:40.

19. Garrett TP, McKern NM, Lou M, et al. Crystal structure of the first three domains of the type-1 insulin-like growth factor receptor. Nature 1998; 394:395.

20. LeRoith D, Werner H, Beitner-Johnson D, Roberts CT Jr. Molecular and cellular aspects of the insulin-like growth factor I receptor. Endocr Rev 1995; 16:143.

21. Bruning JC, Winnay J, Cheatham B, Kahn CR. Differential signaling by insulin receptor substrate 1 (IRS-1) and IRS-2 in IRS-1-deficient cells. Mol Cell Biol 1997; 17:1513.

22. Lavan BE, Fantin VR, Chang ET, et al. A novel 160-kDa phosphotyrosine protein in insulin-treated embryonic kidney cells is a new member of the insulin receptor substrate family. J Biol Chem 1997; 272:21403.

23. Lavan BE, Lane WS, Lienhard GE. The 60-kDa phosphotyrosine protein in insulin-treated adipocytes is a new member of the insulin receptor substrate family. J Biol Chem 1997; 272:11439.

24. Isakoff SJ, Yu YP, Su YC, et al. Interaction between the phosphotyrosine binding domain of Shc and the insulin receptor is required for Shc phosphorylation by insulin in vivo. J Biol Chem 1996; 271:3959.

25. Patti ME, Sun XJ, Bruening JC, et al. 4PS/insulin receptor substrate (IRS)-2 is the alternative substrate of the insulin receptor in IRS-1-deficient mice. J Biol Chem 1995; 270:24670.

26. Kuhne MR, Pawson T, Lienhard GE, Feng GS. The insulin receptor substrate 1 associates with the SH2-containing phosphotyrosine phosphatase Syp. J Biol Chem 1993; 268:11479.

27. Parrizas M, Saltiel AR, LeRoith D. Insulin-like growth factor 1 inhibits apoptosis using the phosphatidylinositol 3'-kinase and mitogen-activated protein kinase pathways. J Biol Chem 1997; 272:154.

28. Pronk GJ, McGlade J, Pelicci G, et al. Insulin-induced phosphorylation of the 46- and 52-kDa Shc proteins. J Biol Chem 1993; 268:5748.

29. Skolnik EY, Lee CH, Batzer A, et al. The SH2/SH3 domain-containing protein GRB2 interacts with tyrosine-phosphorylated IRS1 and Shc: implications for insulin control of ras signalling. Embo J 1993; 12:1929.

30. Skolnik EY, Batzer A, Li N, et al. The function of GRB2 in linking the insulin receptor to Ras signaling pathways. Science 1993; 260:1953.

31. Beitner-Johnson D, Blakesley VA, Shen-Orr Z, et al. The proto-oncogene product c-Crk associates with insulin receptor substrate-1 and 4PS. Modulation by insulin growth factor-I (IGF) and enhanced IGF-I signaling. J Biol Chem 1996; 271:9287.

32. Beitner-Johnson D, LeRoith D. Insulin-like growth factor-I stimulates tyrosine phosphorylation of endogenous c-Crk. J Biol Chem 1995; 270:5187.

33. ten Hoeve J, Morris C, Heisterkamp N, Groffen J. Isolation and chromosomal localization of CRKL, a human crk-like gene. Oncogene 1993; 8:2469.

34. Koval AP, Karas M, Zick Y, LeRoith D. Interplay of the proto-oncogene proteins CrkL and CrkII in insulin-like growth factor-I receptor-mediated signal transduction. J Biol Chem 1998; 273:14780.

35. Koval AP, Blakesley VA, Roberts CT Jr, et al. Interaction in vitro of the product of the c-Crk-II proto-oncogene with the insulin-like growth factor I receptor. Biochem J 1998; 330:923.

36. Lamson G, Giudice LC, Rosenfeld RG. Insulin-like growth factor binding proteins: structural and molecular relationships. Growth Factors 1991; 5:19.

37. Jones JI, Clemmons DR. Insulin-like growth factors and their binding proteins: biological actions. Endocr Rev 1995; 16:3.

38. Rajaram S, Baylink DJ, Mohan S. Insulin-like growth factor-binding proteins in serum and other biological fluids: regulation and functions. Endocr Rev 1997; 18:801.

39. Jones JI, Gockerman A, Busby WH Jr, et al. Extracellular matrix contains insulin-like growth factor binding protein-5: potentiation of the effects of IGF-I. J Cell Biol 1993; 121:679.

40. Rechler MM. Insulin-like growth factor binding proteins. Vitam Horm 1993; 47:1.

41. Jones JI, Gockerman A, Busby WH Jr, et al. Insulin-like growth factor binding protein 1 stimulates cell migration and binds to the α 5 β 1 integrin by means of its Arg-Gly-Asp sequence. Proc Natl Acad Sci U S A 1993; 90:10553.

42. Maile LA, Xu S, Cwyfan-Hughes S, et al. Active and inhibitory components of the insulin-like growth factor binding protein-3 protease system in adult serum, interstitial, and synovial fluid. Endocrinology 1998; 139:4772.

43. Zapf J. Physiological role of the insulin-like growth factor binding proteins. Eur J Endocrinol 1995; 132:645.

44. Collett-Solberg PF, Cohen P. The role of the insulin-like growth factor binding proteins and the IGFBP proteases in modulating IGF action. Endocrinol Metab Clin North Am 1996; 25:591.

45. Giudice LC. IGF binding protein-3 protease regulation: how sweet it is! J Clin Endocrinol Metab 1995; 80:2279.

46. De Mellow JS, Baxter RC. Growth hormone-dependent insulin-like growth factor (IGF) binding protein both inhibits and potentiates IGF-I-stimulated DNA synthesis in human skin fibroblasts. Biochem Biophys Res Commun 1988; 156:199.

47. Oh Y, Muller HL, Lamson G, Rosenfeld RG. Insulin-like growth factor (IGF)-independent action of IGF-binding protein-3 in Hs578T human breast cancer cells. Cell surface binding and growth inhibition. J Biol Chem 1993; 268:14964.

48. Cohen P, Lamson G, Okajima T, Rosenfeld RG. Transfection of the human insulin-like growth factor binding protein-3 gene into Balb/c fibroblasts inhibits cellular growth. Mol Endocrinol 1993; 7:380.

49. Bondy CA, Werner H, Roberts CT Jr, LeRoith D. Cellular pattern of insulin-like growth factor-I (IGF-I) and type I IGF receptor gene expression in early organogenesis: comparison with IGF-II gene expression. Mol Endocrinol 1990; 4:1386.

50. Bondy C, Werner H, Roberts CT Jr, LeRoith D. Cellular pattern of type-I insulin-like growth factor receptor gene expression during maturation of the rat brain: comparison with insulin-like growth factors I and II. Neuroscience 1992; 46:909.

51. Liu JL, Grinberg A, Westphal H, et al. Insulin-like growth factor-I affects perinatal lethality and postnatal development in a gene dosage-dependent manner: manipulation using the Cre/loxP system in transgenic mice. Mol Endocrinol 1998; 12:1452.

52. Liu JP, Baker J, Perkins AS, et al. Mice carrying null mutations of the genes encoding insulin-like growth factor I (Igf-1) and type 1 IGF receptor (Igf1r). Cell 1993; 75:59.

53. LeRoith D, Clemmons D, Nissley P, Rechler MM. NIH conference. Insulin-like growth factors in health and disease. Ann Intern Med 1992; 116:854.

54. Punglia RS, Lu M, Hsu J, et al. Regulation of vascular endothelial growth factor expression by insulin-like growth factor I. Diabetes 1997; 46:1619.

55. Schoenle EJ, Zenobi PD, Torresani T, et al. Recombinant human insulin-like growth factor I (rhIGF I) reduces hyperglycaemia in patients with extreme insulin resistance. Diabetologia 1991; 34:675.

56. Moses AC, Young SC, Morrow LA, et al. Recombinant human insulin-like growth factor I increases insulin sensitivity and improves glycemic control in type II diabetes. Diabetes 1996; 45:91.

56a. Clemmons DR, Moses AC, McKay MJ, et al. The combination of insulin-like growth factor I and insulin-like growth factor-binding protein-3 reduces insulin requirements in insulin-dependent type 1 diabetes: evidence for in vivo biological activity. J Clin Endocrinol Metab 2000; 85(4):1518.

57. Aaronson SA. Growth factors and cancer. Science 1991; 254:1146.

58. Macaulay VM. Insulin-like growth factors and cancer. Br J Cancer 1992; 65:311.

58a. Khandwala HM, McCutcheon IE, Flyvbjerg A, Friend KE. The effects of insulin-like growth factors on tumorigenesis and neoplastic growth. Endocr Rev 2000; 21(3):215.

59. LeRoith D, Baserga R, Helman L, Roberts CT Jr. Insulin-like growth factors and cancer [see comments]. Ann Intern Med 1995; 122:54.

60. Drummond IA, Madden SL, Rohwer-Nutter P, et al. Repression of the insulin-like growth factor II gene by the Wilms tumor suppressor WT1. Science 1992; 257:674.

61. DeChiara TM, Robertson EJ, Efstratiadis A. Parental imprinting of the mouse insulin-like growth factor II gene. Cell 1991; 64:849.

62. Lowe WL Jr, Roberts CT, LeRoith D, et al. Insulin-like growth factor-II in nonislet cell tumors associated with hypoglycemia: increased levels of messenger ribonucleic acid. J Clin Endocrinol Metab 1989; 69:1153.

63. Zapf J. Role of insulin-like growth factor (IGF) II and IGF binding proteins in extrapancreatic tumour hypoglycaemia. J Intern Med 1993; 234:543.

64. Baxter RC, Daughaday WH. Impaired formation of the ternary insulin-like growth factor-binding protein complex in patients with hypoglycemia due to nonislet cell tumors. J Clin Endocrinol Metab 1991; 73:696.

65. Eastman RC, Carson RE, Orloff DG, et al. Glucose utilization in a patient with hepatoma and hypoglycemia. Assessment by a positron emission tomography. J Clin Invest 1992; 89:1958.

66. Werner H, LeRoith D. The insulin-like growth factor-I receptor signaling pathways are important for tumorigenesis and inhibition of apoptosis. Crit Rev Oncog 1997; 8:71.

67. Werner H, Karnieli E, Rauscher FJ, LeRoith D. Wild-type and mutant p53 differentially regulate transcription of the insulin-like growth factor I receptor gene. Proc Natl Acad Sci U S A 1996; 93:8318.

68. Chan JM, Stampfer MJ, Giovannucci E, et al. Plasma insulin-like growth factor-I and prostate cancer risk: a prospective study. Science 1998; 279:563.

69. Gluckman P, Klempt N, Guan J, et al. A role for IGF-1 in the rescue of CNS neurons following hypoxic-ischemic injury. Biochem Biophys Res Commun 1992; 182:593.

70. Guan J, Williams C, Gunning M, et al. The effects of IGF-1 treatment after hypoxic-ischemic brain injury in adult rats. J Cereb Blood Flow Metab 1993; 13:609.

71. Landreth KS, Narayanan R, Dorshkind K. Insulin-like growth factor-I regulates pro-B cell differentiation. Blood 1992; 80:1207.

72. Fu YK, Arkins S, Wang BS, Kelley KW. A novel role of growth hormone and insulin-like growth factor-I. Priming neutrophils for superoxide anion secretion. J Immunol 1991; 146:1602.

73. LeRoith D, Yanowski J, Kaldjian EP, et al. The effects of growth hormone and insulin-like growth factor I on the immune system of aged female monkeys. Endocrinology 1996; 137:1071.

74. Levy MJ, Hernandez ER, Adashi EY, et al. Expression of the insulin-like growth factor (IGF)-I and -II and the IGF-I and -II receptor genes during postnatal development of the rat ovary. Endocrinology 1992; 131:1202.

75. Adashi EY, Resnick CE, Svoboda ME, Van Wyk JJ. Somatomedin-C enhances induction of luteinizing hormone receptors by follicle-stimulating hormone in cultured rat granulosa cells. Endocrinology 1985; 116:2369.

76. Kapur S, Tamada H, Dey SK, Andrews GK. Expression of insulin-like growth factor-I (IGF-I) and its receptor in the peri-implantation mouse uterus, and cell-specific regulation of IGF-I gene expression by estradiol and progesterone. Biol Reprod 1992; 46:208.

77. Okazaki R, Riggs BL, Conover CA. Glucocorticoid regulation of insulin-like growth factor-binding protein expression in normal human osteoblast-like cells. Endocrinology 1994; 134:126.

78. McCarthy TL, Ji C, Shu H, et al. 17β-estradiol potently suppresses cAMP-induced insulin-like growth factor-I gene activation in primary rat osteoblast cultures. J Biol Chem 1997; 272:18132.

79. Ernst M, Rodan GA. Estradiol regulation of insulin-like growth factor-I expression in osteoblastic cells: evidence for transcriptional control. Mol Endocrinol 1991; 5:1081.

80. Birnbaum RS, Wiren KM. Changes in insulin-like growth factor-binding protein expression and secretion during the proliferation, differentiation, and mineralization of primary cultures of rat osteoblasts. Endocrinology 1994; 135:223.

81. Dunger DB, Cheetham TD, Crowne EC. Insulin-like growth factors (IGFs) and IGF-I treatment in the adolescent with insulin-dependent diabetes mellitus. Metabolism 1995; 44:119.

82. Backeljauw PF, Underwood LE. Prolonged treatment with recombinant insulin-like growth factor-I in children with growth hormone insensitivity syndrome—a clinical research center study. GHIS Collaborative Group. J Clin Endocrinol Metab 1996; 81:3312.

83. Butler AA, Blakesley VA, Tsokos M, et al. Stimulation of tumor growth by recombinant human insulin-like growth factor-I (IGF-I) is dependent on the dose and the level of IGF-I receptor expression. Cancer Res 1998; 58:3021.

84. Dumont DJ, Jussila L, Taipale J, et al. Cardiovascular failure in mouse embryos deficient in VEGF receptor-3. Science 1998; 282:946.

85. Ferrara N, Davis-Smyth T. The biology of vascular endothelial growth factor. Endocr Rev 1997; 18:4.

86. Sierra-Honigmann MR, Nath AK, Murakami C, et al. Biological action of leptin as an angiogenic factor. Science 1998; 281:1683.

87. Klagsbrun M, D'Amore PA. Vascular endothelial growth factor and its receptors. Cytokine and Growth Factor Reviews 1996; 7:259.

88. Kaplan DR, Stephens RM. Neurotrophin signal transduction by the Trk receptor. J Neurobiol 1994; 25:1404.

89. Heldin CH. Structural and functional studies on platelet-derived growth factor. Embo J 1992; 11:4251.

90. Golub TR, Barker GF, Lovett M, Gilliland DG. Fusion of PDGF receptor β to a novel ets-like gene, tel, in chronic myelomonocytic leukemia with t(5;12) chromosomal translocation. Cell 1994; 77:307.

91. Massague J, Czech MP, Iwata K, et al. Affinity labeling of a transforming growth factor receptor that does not interact with epidermal growth factor. Proc Natl Acad Sci U S A 1982; 79:6822.

92. Buckley-Sturock A, Wodward SC, Senior RM, et al. Differential stimulation of collagenase and chemotactic activity in fibroblasts derived from rat wound repair tissue and human skin by growth factors. J Cell Physiol 1989; 138:70.

93. de Larco JE, Todaro GJ. Growth factors from murine sarcoma virus-transformed cells. Proc Natl Acad Sci U S A 1978; 75:4001.

94. O'Grady P, Liu Q, Huang SS, Huang JS. Transforming growth factor β (TGF-β) type V receptor has a TGF-β-stimulated serine/threonine-specific autophosphorylation activity. J Biol Chem 1992; 267:21033.

95. O'Grady P, Kuo MD, Baldassare JJ, et al. Purification of a new type high molecular weight receptor (type V receptor) of transforming growth factor beta (TGF-beta) from bovine liver. Identification of the type V TGF-beta receptor in cultured cells. J Biol Chem 1991; 266:8583.

96. Laiho M, DeCaprio JA, Ludlow JW, et al. Growth inhibition by TGF-β linked to suppression of retinoblastoma protein phosphorylation. Cell 1990; 62:175.

97. Behringer RR, Finegold MJ, Cate RL. Müllerian-inhibiting substance function during mammalian sexual development. Cell 1994; 79:415.

98. Rosenthal SM, Brown EJ, Brunetti A, Goldfine ID. Fibroblast growth factor inhibits insulin-like growth factor-II (IGF-II) gene expression and increases IGF-I receptor abundance in BC3H-1 muscle cells. Mol Endocrinol 1991; 5:678.

99. Weil-Hillman G, Schell K, Segal DM, et al. Activation of human T cells obtained pre- and post-interleukin-2 (IL-2) therapy by anti-CD3 monoclonal antibody plus IL-2: implications for combined in vivo treatment. J Immunother 1991; 10:267.

100. Lotze MT, Chang AE, Seipp CA, et al. High-dose recombinant interleukin 2 in the treatment of patients with disseminated cancer. Responses, treatment-related morbidity, and histologic findings. JAMA 1986; 256:3117.

101. Rosenstein M, Ettinghausen SE, Rosenberg SA. Extravasation of intravascular fluid mediated by the systemic administration of recombinant interleukin 2. J Immunol 1986; 137:1735.

102. Donahue RE, Seehra J, Metzger M, et al. Human IL-3 and GM-CSF act synergistically in stimulating hematopoiesis in primates. Science 1988; 241:1820.

103. Banchereau J, de Paoli P, Valle A, et al. Long-term human B cell lines dependent on interleukin-4 and antibody to CD40. Science 1991; 251:70.

104. Parronchi P, De Carli M, Manetti R, et al. Aberrant interleukin (IL)-4 and IL-5 production in vitro by CD4+ helper T cells from atopic subjects. Eur J Immunol 1992; 22:1615.

105. Obiri NI, Hillman GG, Haas GP, et al. Expression of high affinity interleukin-4 receptors on human renal cell carcinoma cells and inhibition of tumor cell growth in vitro by interleukin-4. J Clin Invest 1993; 91:88.

106. Huston MM, Moore JP, Mettes HJ, et al. Human B cells express IL-5 receptor messenger ribonucleic acid and respond to IL-5 with enhanced IgM production after mitogenic stimulation with Moraxella catarrhalis. J Immunol 1996; 156:1392.

107. Martinez OM, Ascher NL, Ferrell L, et al. Evidence for a nonclassical pathway of graft rejection involving interleukin 5 and eosinophils. Transplantation 1993; 55:909.

108. Black K, Garrett IR, Mundy GR. Chinese hamster ovarian cells transfected with the murine interleukin-6 gene cause hypercalcemia as well as cachexia, leukocytosis and thrombocytosis in tumor-bearing nude mice. Endocrinology 1991; 128:2657.

109. Lynch DH, Miller RE. Interleukin 7 promotes long-term in vitro growth of antitumor cytotoxic T lymphocytes with immunotherapeutic efficacy in vivo. J Exp Med 1994; 179:31.

110. Endo H, Akahoshi T, Takagishi K, et al. Elevation of interleukin-8 (IL-8) levels in joint fluids of patients with rheumatoid arthritis and the induction by IL-8 of leukocyte infiltration and synovitis in rabbit joints. Lymphokine Cytokine Res 1991; 10:245.

111. Katsikis PD, Chu CQ, Brennan FM, et al. Immunoregulatory role of interleukin 10 in rheumatoid arthritis. J Exp Med 1994; 179:1517.

112. Enk AH, Angeloni VL, Udey MC, Katz SI. Inhibition of Langerhans cell antigen-presenting function by IL-10. A role for IL-10 in induction of tolerance. J Immunol 1993; 151:2390.

113. Okamura H, Tsutsi H, Komatsu T, et al. Cloning of a new cytokine that induces IFN-γ production by T cells. Nature 1995; 378:88.

114. Parnet P, Garka KE, Bonnert TP, et al. IL-1Rrp is a novel receptor-like molecule similar to the type I interleukin-1 receptor and its homologues T1/ST2 and IL-1R AcP. J Biol Chem 1996; 271:3967.

115. Rothe H, Jenkins NA, Copeland NG, Kolb H. Active stage of autoimmune diabetes is associated with the expression of a novel cytokine, IGIF, which is located near Idd2. J Clin Invest 1997; 99:469.

116. Scheurich P, Thoma B, Ucer U, Pfizenmaier K. Immunoregulatory activity of recombinant human tumor necrosis factor (TNF)-α: induction of TNF receptors on human T cells and TNF-α-mediated enhancement of T cell responses. J Immunol 1987; 138:1786.

117. Aggarwal BB, Graff K, Samal B, et al. Regulation of two forms of the TNF receptors by phorbol ester and dibutyryl cyclic adenosine 3',5'-monophosphate in human histiocytic lymphoma cell line U-937. Lymphokine Cytokine Res 1993; 12:149.

118. Grell M, Scheurich P, Meager A, Pfizenmaier K. TR60 and TR80 tumor necrosis factor (TNF)-receptors can independently mediate cytolysis. Lymphokine Cytokine Res 1993; 12:143.

119. Aderka D, Wysenbeek A, Engelmann H, et al. Correlation between serum levels of soluble tumor necrosis factor receptor and disease activity in systemic lupus erythematosus. Arthritis Rheum 1993; 36:1111.

120. Fuchs P, Strehl S, Dworzak M, et al. Structure of the human TNF receptor 1 (p60) gene (TNFR1) and localization to chromosome 12p13 [published erratum appears in Genomics 1992; 13(4):1384]. Genomics 1992; 13:219.

121. McDermott MF, Aksentijevich I, Galon J, et al. Germline mutations in the extracellular domains of the 55-kDa TNF receptor, TNFR1, define a family of dominantly inherited autoinflammatory syndromes. Cell 1999; 97:133.

122. Sen GC, Lengyel P. The interferon system. A bird's eye view of its biochemistry. J Biol Chem 1992; 267:5017.

123. Uze G, Lutfalla G, Bandu MT, et al. Behavior of a cloned murine interferon α/β receptor expressed in homospecific or heterospecific background. Proc Natl Acad Sci U S A 1992; 89:4774.

124. Uze G, Lutfalla G, Gresser I. Genetic transfer of a functional human interferon α receptor into mouse cells: cloning and expression of its cDNA. Cell 1990; 60:225.

125. Bazan JF. Structural design and molecular evolution of a cytokine receptor superfamily. Proc Natl Acad Sci U S A 1990; 87:6934.

126. Bazan JF. A novel family of growth factor receptors: a common binding domain in the growth hormone, prolactin, erythropoietin and IL-6 receptors, and the p75 IL-2 receptor β-chain. Biochem Biophys Res Commun 1989; 164:788.

127. Hunter T. Signal transduction. Cytokine connections. Nature 1993; 366:114.

128. Stahl N, Farruggella TJ, Boulton TG, et al. Choice of STATs and other substrates specified by modular tyrosine-based motifs in cytokine receptors. Science 1995; 267:1349.

# CHAPTER 174

# COMPENDIUM OF GROWTH FACTORS AND CYTOKINES

BHARAT B. AGGARWAL

## GENERAL FEATURES OF CYTOKINES

Cytokines are polypeptide hormones, which, when secreted by a cell, affect the growth and metabolism of either the same (autocrine) or a neighboring cell (paracrine). Growth factors, which are also peptide hormones, induce cellular proliferation. The appellations, cytokines and growth factors, have been used interchangeably. Although the hormones produced by endocrine organs are not considered cytokines, extensive research has revealed no definitive criteria that can distinguish between cytokines, growth factors, and endocrine hormones, except that not all endocrine hormones are polypeptides. Perhaps the first cytokine to be discovered was interferon (IFN)—found in 1957 by Issacs and Lindenmann as a soluble factor produced by cells after exposure to heat-inactivated influenza virus. Among the growth factors, the nerve growth factor (NGF) and epidermal growth factor (EGF) were the first to be identified. Within the last two decades, an avalanche of novel cytokines and growth factors have been reported, and several monographs and reviews have been written on this subject.[1-28] In this chapter, the author provides a compendium of cytokines and growth factors, with most information summarized in tables. For original

references, the reader should consult the monographs listed at the end of the chapter (see also Chaps. 173, 180, and 212).

Within the last two decades, as many as 200 cytokines have been identified, and each year more are added to the list. This rapid development is most likely due to the availability of the human genome sequence, which allows searches for structurally homologous genes. Some of the general features of most cytokines are given in Table 174-1. Although it was initially believed that most cytokines are secreted, it now appears that several of them are transmembrane proteins. For instance, of the 17 known members of the tumor necrosis factor (TNF) superfamily, all except lymphotoxin (also called TNF-β) are type II transmembrane proteins (i.e., its carboxyl terminus is extracellular as opposed to the amino terminus in type I). Why cytokines exist in transmembrane form is not clear, but one reason might be the localized action of the cytokine. Once secreted by proteolytic cleavage, the cytokine could have pathologic effects. Thus, the secretion of cytokines appears to be a highly regulated process.

Although cytokines and growth factors were initially thought to be produced by specific cell types, sensitive methods of detection have now revealed that most cell types have the potential to express the gene for the various cytokines. Table 174-2 lists some

## TABLE 174-1.
### Common Features of Most Cytokines

1. Cytokines are simple polypeptides or glycoproteins with a molecular mass of <30 kDa (some cytokines form higher molecular mass oligomers). Only one known cytokine, interleukin-12 (IL-12), is a heterodimer. They generally have acidic isoelectric points. Cytokines are often stable at room temperature.

2. The gene size for cytokines may range from 1–100 kb. The mRNA for most cytokines is <10 kb. Most cytokines have AU-rich sequences in the 3' untranslated region, which correlates with the unstable nature of the mRNA.

3. Production is regulated by various inducing stimuli at the level of transcription or translation; constitutive production of cytokines is usually low or absent. Most cytokines are products of the immune system, but some are highly ubiquitous. Production of cytokines is modulated by a wide variety of diverse stimuli including other cytokines, viruses, bacteria, parasites, and tumor cells. Most cytokines are produced in trace amounts (picogram to nanogram range).

4. Cytokines are produced transiently and act locally in a combined autocrine and paracrine rather than hemocrine manner.

5. Cytokines regulate the amplitude and duration of biologic response. Cytokines are extremely potent at even picomolar concentration. They act by binding to specific high-affinity cell-surface receptors.

6. Their cell-surface binding leads to induction of different genes, resulting in intracellular changes.

7. Several different cytokines may exhibit overlapping and sometimes redundant actions.

8. The response is dependent on local concentration, cell types, and regulatory factors to which they are exposed.

9. They interact in a network by inducing or suppressing the expression of each other. They are capable of transmodulating their own or another cytokine cell-surface receptor.

10. Different cytokines may exhibit synergistic, additive, and antagonistic interaction on cell function. Most cytokines display multipotential activities.

11. Biologic activities of cytokines in vitro do not always indicate their action in vivo. The effects of most cytokines are modulated by other cytokines. Autocrine production of cytokines or their receptors can lead to desensitization.

## TABLE 174-2.
### Cytokine Production by Different Cell Types

| Cell Type | Cytokine |
|---|---|
| **Endocrine organs** | |
| Placental cells | IL-1, IL-2, IL-6, IFN-α, IFN-β, TNF |
| Anterior pituitary cells | IL-6, MIF |
| Granulosa cells | TNF |
| Oocytes | IL-1, IL-6, CSF-1 |
| **Immune system** | |
| T lymphocytes | |
| $T_H1$ | IL-1, IL-2, IL-9, IL-17, IFN-γ, LT, G-CSF, M-CSF, GM-CSF |
| $T_H2$ | IL-3, IL-4, IL-5, IL-6, IL-10, IL-13, IL-14, MIP-1α, MIP-1β, RANTES, TNF, LT, LIF, OSM |
| CTL | TNF, LT, IFN-γ, IL-2 |
| NK | TNF, LT, IFN-γ, IL-3, G-CSF, M-CSF, GM-CSF |
| B lymphocytes | IL-1, IL-5, IL-6, LT, TNF, GM-CSF, IFN-γ, IFN-α |
| Macrophages | IL-1α, IL-1β, IL-5, IL-6, IL-8, IL-10, IL-12, IFN-α, TNF, LIF, OSM, PDGF, MIF, MCAF, bFGF, FAF, TGF-α, TGF-β, GRO-α, MIP-1α, MIP-1β, EPO, thymosine-α1, GM-CSF, G-CSF, M-CSF, β-endorphin, ACTH, NGF, VEGF, HB-EGF |
| Neutrophils | IL-1α, IL-1β, IL-3, IL-6, IL-8, G-CSF, M-CSF, GM-CSF, IL-1RA, IFN-α, GRO-α |
| Mast cells | IL-1, IL-3, IL-4, IL-5, IL-6, IL-8, MIP-1α, MIP-1β, TNF, GM-CSF |
| Eosinophils | IL-3, IL-5, IL-1α, IL-6, TNF, MIP-1α, GM-CSF, TGF-α, TGF-β |
| Platelets | PDGF, TGF-β, EGF, RANTES, IL-1, HGF, GRO-α, PD-ECGF |
| **Others** | |
| Endothelial cells | GM-CSF, IL-1, IL-6, PDGF, VEGI, TNF |
| Smooth muscle cells | IL-1α, IL-1β, TNF |
| Fibroblasts | bFGF, IL-6, IL-1β, G-CSF |
| Astrocytes | IL-1, TNF |

*IL*, interleukin; *IFN*, interferon; *TNF*, tumor necrosis factor; *MIF*, macrophage migration inhibitory factor; *CSF*, colony-stimulating factor; *LT*, lymphotoxin; *G-CSF*, granulocyte colony-stimulating factor; *M-CSF*, macrophage colony-stimulating factor; *GM-CSF*, granulocyte and macrophage colony-stimulating factor; *MIP*, monocyte chemotactic inhibitory protein; *RANTES*, regulated on activation, normal T expressed and secreted; *LIF*, leukemia inhibitory factor; *OSM*, oncostatin M; *PDGF*, platelet-derived growth factor; *MCAF*, macrophage-derived cartilage activating factor; *bFGF*, basic fibroblast growth factor; *FAF*, fibroblast activating factor; *TGF*, transforming growth factor; *GRO*, growth factor; *EPO*, erythropoietin; *ACTH*, adrenocorticotropic hormone; *NGF*, nerve growth factor; *VEGF*, vascular endothelial cell growth factor; *HB-EGF*, heparin-binding epidermal growth factor; *IL-1RA*, interleukin-1 receptor antagonist; *HGF*, hepatocyte growth factor; *PD-ECGF*, platelet-derived endothelial cell growth factor; *VEGI*, vascular endothelial cell growth inhibitor.

**TABLE 174-3.**
**Cytokines with Multiple Biologic Responses**

| Cytokine* | Abbreviation | MW (kDa) | mRNA (kb) | Carbohydrate† |
|---|---|---|---|---|
| **GROWTH ENHANCERS** | | | | |
| Platelet-derived growth factor | (PDGF) | 28§§ | 2.8 & 3.5 | + |
| Fibroblast growth factor (basic) | (bFGF) | 16 | 7.0ʲʲ | − |
| Fibroblast growth factor (acidic) | (aFGF) | 16 | 4.2 | − |
| Epidermal growth factor | (EGF) | 6.4 | 4.9 | − |
| Transforming growth factor-α | (TGF-α) | 5–20¶¶ | 4.5–4.8 | + |
| Betacellulin | (BTC) | 32 | 3.0 | + |
| Insulin-like growth factor | (IGF-I & II) | 6.0 | 7.6 & 6.0 | − |
| Hepatocyte growth factor | (HGF) | 82*** | 6.0 | + |
| Autocrine motility factor | (AMF) | 55 | NA | − |
| Androgen-induced growth factor | (AIGF) | 28–32 | 1.0–1.2 | + |
| Heregulin | (erbB2/HER2 ligand) | 45 | 6.6 | + |
| Glia activating factor | (GAF) | 25–30 | NA | + |
| Glia maturation factor | (GMF) | 16–17 | 3.7 | − |
| ACh receptor-inducing activity | (ARIA) | 42 | 7.3, 3.0 | + |
| Pleiotrophin/midkine | (PTN/MK) | 18 | 1.5 | − |
| Osteogenic protein-2 | (OP) | 32–36 | 1.8–5.0 | − |
| Bone morphogenic proteins | (BMP) | 30 | 2.8–4.0 | − |
| Vascular endothelial cell growth factor | (VEGF) | 46§§§ | 1.6 | + |
| Ciliary neurotrophic factor | (CNTF) | 23 | 1.2 | − |
| flt3/flk-2 ligand | | 24 | 0.82 | + |
| Cardiotropin-1 | (CT-1) | 21.5 | 1.4 kb | + |
| Epiregulin | | 5.4 | | |
| A proliferation-inducing ligand | (APRIL) | 28 | 1.5–2.0 | + |
| **T-CELL GROWTH FACTORS** | | | | |
| Interleukin-2 | (IL-2) | 15–17.2 | 0.9 | + |
| Interleukin-4 | (IL-4) | 15–20 | 0.9 | + |
| Interleukin-7 | (IL-7) | 22–28 | 1.8, 2.4 | + |
| Interleukin-9 | (IL-9) | 37–40 | 0.7 | + |
| Interleukin-12 | (IL-12) | 75ʲ | 2.4 & 1.4 | + |
| **HEMATOPOIETIC FACTORS** | | | | |
| Interleukin-3 | (IL-3) | 15–17 | 1.0 | + |
| Interleukin-11 | (IL-11) | 23 | 2.5 | − |
| Macrophage colony-stimulating factor | (M-CSF) | 45–90 | 4.2¶ | + |
| Granulocyte colony-stimulating factor | (G-CSF) | 19.6 | 1.6 | + |
| Granulocyte & macrophage colony-stimulating factor | (GM-CSF) | 18–32 | 0.7 | + |
| Leukemia inhibitory factor | (LIF) | 32–45 | 4.2 | + |
| Stem cell factor | (SCF) | 36 | 6.0 | + |
| Erythropoietin | (EPO) | 34–36 | 1.6 | + |
| Thrombopoietin | (TPO) | 35–70 | 10 | + |
| Erythroid differentiation factor | (EDF) | 14 | 7.2 | + |
| CD27 ligand | (CD 27L) | 50 | 1.2 | + |
| CD30 ligand | (CD 30L) | | | |
| CD40 ligand | (CD 40L) | 39 | 2.3 | |
| 4-1BB ligand | (4-1BBL) | 50–60 | | − |
| OX40 ligand | (OX40L) | | | |
| Interleukin-16 | (IL-16) | 13.5–28.0 | | |
| Interleukin-17 | (IL-17) | 17–21 | | + |
| **B-CELL GROWTH FACTORS** | | | | |
| B-cell growth factor | (BCGF) | 12 | 1.0, 1.7 | + |
| Interleukin-4 | (IL-4) | 15–20 | 0.9 | + |
| Interleukin-5 | (IL-5) | 18 | 0.9 | + |
| Interleukin-6 | (IL-6) | 21–26 | 1.3 | + |
| TNF-related activation protein | (TRAP/CD40 ligand) | 29 | 2.3 | + |
| Interleukin-14 | (IL-14; HMW-BCGF) | 53 | 1.8 | + |
| **GROWTH INHIBITORS§** | | | | |
| Tumor necrosis factor | (TNF) | 17 | 1.7 | − |
| Lymphotoxin | (LT) | 20–25 | 1.3 | + |
| Amphiregulin | (AR) | 9.0–9.8 | 1.4 | + |
| Oncostatin M | (OM) | 20–36 | 2.0 | + |
| Müllerian inhibiting substance | (MIS) | 140** | 2.1 | + |
| Fas ligand | (FasL) | 38–42 | 2.0 | + |
| TNF-related apoptosis-inducing ligand | (TRAIL) | 26 | 2.2 | + |
| TNF-weak homologue | (TWEAK) | | | |
| **ANGIOGENIC FACTORS** | | | | |
| Fibroblast growth factor | (FGF) | | | |
| Vascular endothelial cell growth factor | (VEGF) | | | |
| Platelet-derived growth factor | (PDGF) | | | |
| Tumor necrosis factor | (TNF) | | | |
| Angiogenin | | 14 | 0.9 | |
| **ANGIOSTATIC FACTORS** | | | | |
| Endostatin (collagen XVIII fragment) | | 20 | | |
| Angiostatin (plasminogen fragment) | | 38 | | |
| Vascular endothelial cell growth inhibitor | (VEGI) | 22 | 2.6 | + |
| **ANTIVIRAL** | | | | |
| Interferon-α | (IFN-α) | 19–29 | 1–2 | + |
| Interferon-β | (IFN-β) | 20 | 0.7 | + |
| Interferon-γ | (IFN-γ) | 20–25 | 1.2 | + |
| Interferon-Ω | (IFN-Ω) | 24.5 | 1 | + |
| **INFLAMMATION** | | | | |
| Interleukin-1α | (IL-1α) | 17.5 | 2.1 | − |
| Interleukin-1β | (IL-1β) | 17.5 | 1.6 | − |
| Interleukin-1 receptor antagonist | (IL-1RA) | 25 | 1.8 | + |
| Interleukin-6 | (IL-6) | 21–26 | 1.3 | + |
| Interleukin-8 | (IL-8) | 8 | 1.8 | − |
| Tumor necrosis factor | (TNF) | 17 | 1.7 | − |
| Lymphotoxin | (LT) | 20–25 | 1.3 | + |
| Interleukin-17 | (IL-17) | 16 | | + |
| Interleukin-18 | (IL-18) | 18.3 | | |
| **CHEMOTACTIC FACTORS** | | | | |
| Interleukin-8 | (IL-8) | 8 | 1.8 | − |
| Monocyte chemotactic protein-1 | (MCP-1) | 15 | 0.7 | + |
| Growth factor inducible chemokine | (FIC) | 11 | 0.6 | + |
| Macrophage inflammatory protein-1 | (MIP-1α) | 8 | 0.8 | − |
| | (MIP-1β) | 8 | 0.8 | − |
| Regulated on activation, normal T expressed and secreted | (RANTES) | 8 | 1.1 | |
| Melanoma growth stimulatory activity | (MGSA) | 13–16 | 1.1–1.2 | + |
| Macrophage migration inhibitory factor | (MIF) | 12 | 0.7 | + |
| **SUPPRESSOR MOLECULES** | | | | |
| Interleukin-4 | (IL-4) | 15–20 | 0.9 | + |
| Interleukin-10 | (IL-10) | 17–21 | 1.0–1.5 | + |
| Interleukin-13 | (IL-13) | 9 & 17 | 1.4 | + |
| Transforming growth factor-β | (TGF-β) | 11.5–12.5 | 5.8 | + |
| **OTHERS** | | | | |
| Lymphotoxin-β | (LT-β) | 25–26 | 0.9–1.0 | + |
| Interleukin-16 | (IL-16) | 13.5 | | |

MW, molecular weight; NA, not available.

*Space limitation permits only commonly used names and abbreviations of cytokines.

†+, glycosylated; −, no glycosylation.

§TGF-β, IL-1, IL-4, and IL-6 also display growth inhibitory effects on certain cells.

ʲDisulfide-linked heterodimer of 40-kDa and 35-kDa subunits.

¶Due to alternative splicing, mRNA of 1.6, 2.2, and 2.5 kb sizes have been reported.

**Disulfide linked homodimer of 72-kDa subunit.

§§Disulfide linked homo- and heterodimer of A and B chain.

ʲʲIn addition to major mRNA species, minor mRNAs of 1.5, 2.5, 3.7, and 4.5 kb for bFGF and 0.8, 1.2, 2.7, and 3.2 kb for aFGF are also found.

¶¶Molecular weights of secreted forms are indicated.

***Heterodimer of α (Mr, 69 kDa) and β (Mr, 34 kDa). An mRNA of 6.0 kb gives rise to a preprotein, which after processing generates α and β subunits.

§§§Dimer of 23- and 18-kDa subunits.

of the known examples, indicating that the same cytokine can be produced by a wide variety of different cell types. For example, TNF—once thought to be produced only by macrophages—later was found to be expressed by a wide variety of cells, tissues, and organs. Why a cytokine should be produced by so many different cell types is unclear, but the diversity may explain the multipotential activities assigned to this cytokine.

Various observations indicate that biologic systems are highly redundant and overlapping; this may serve the purpose of protection against system-wide failure in the event that an individual component fails. Table 174-3 lists cytokines that have antiviral, inflammatory, growth modulatory, chemotactic, angiogenic, and antiangiogenic activities. At least four different gene products, referred to as IFN, have been reported to have antiviral activities. Why several cytokines exhibit similar activities is unclear, but perhaps this is a mechanism developed by nature to ensure the normality of the function in case a given cytokine gene is deleted or mutated.

The physicochemical characteristics of most cytokines are very similar. As listed in Table 174-3, the genes for most cytokines have mRNA of ~1 to 2 kb encoding a protein with molecular mass <30 kDa. Several of them undergo posttranslational glycosylation. During the last few years, the three-dimensional structures of several of these cytokines have been elucidated (Table 174-4). Knowledge of the crystal structure of cytokines has allowed researchers to engineer the agonist and antagonist to the native molecule by recombinant DNA methods. It has also made possible the synthesis, using the peptidomimetics technique, of small molecules that can mimic cytokines. These are, thus, more effective drugs, having improved delivery and pharmacokinetics in patients.

Cytokines regulate biologic responses in multiple directions. A list of cellular and physiologic responses mediated by different cytokines is outlined in Table 174-5. It appears that several

### TABLE 174-5.
### Major Cellular and Physiologic Roles of Cytokines

Control of cell proliferation
Control of cell differentiation and phenotype
Regulation of hematopoiesis
Regulation of immune responses
Control of host defenses against bacterial, viral, and parasitic infections
Regulation of inflammatory responses and fever
Control of cytotoxic and phagocytic cells
Wound healing, tissue remodeling, and bone formation
Modulation of cellular metabolism and control of nitrogen balance

cytokines together form a cascade leading to an end response. The presence of cytokines early in development suggests their possible role both in embryologic growth and in differentiation. For instance, TNF, colony-stimulating factor-1 (CSF-1), interleukin-1 (IL-1), and interleukin-6 (IL-6) are present in oocytes before fertilization. Their levels increase after fertilization and during embryo cleavage from zygote to the eight-cell stage. Leukemia inhibitory factor (LIF) has been demonstrated to play an important role during development of the mouse. It inhibits the differentiation of embryonic stem cells and maintains them in a pluripotent state. LIF has been detected in preimplantation blastocysts and in extraembryonic tissue and placenta.

In vivo, several cytokines and their receptors are secreted and found in serum, synovial fluid, cerebrospinal fluid, ovarian ascites, and urine. Very few cytokines are present in the urine of healthy subjects although EGF was first isolated from human urine. Some of the conditions that lead to excretion of cytokines in the urine are listed in Table 174-6. It is only during fever, bacterial or viral infection, or cancer that these cytokines are secreted, indicating their pathologic role.

Perhaps the best evidence that cytokines play roles in growth, development, and normal survival has come from the gene knock-out mouse.[29] Gene knock-out mice are made by

### TABLE 174-4.
### Cytokines with Known Three-Dimensional Structures

| Cytokine | Characteristics |
|---|---|
| **MAINLY α-HELICAL STRUCTURES** | |
| hIL-2 | Left-handed 4-α-helix bundles |
| hIL-4 | Left-handed 4-α-helix bundle + a short 2-stranded β-sheet |
| mIFN-β | Left-handed 4-α-helix bundle + 1 long α-helix |
| hIFN-γ | Dimer of mutually interlocked subunits composed of 5-α-helices |
| hGM-CSF | Left-handed 4-α-helix bundle + a short 2-stranded β-sheet |
| hM-CSF | Two GM-CSF–like 4-α-helix bundles connected by a disulfide bond |
| G-CSF | Antiparallel 4-α-helix bundle with up-up-down-down connectivity |
| **MAINLY β-SHEET STRUCTURES** | |
| hTNF | Trimeric molecule |
| | Each subunit consists of an antiparallel B-sandwich |
| | Remarkable similarity to the "jellyroll" motif found in viral coat proteins |
| hLT | Trimeric molecules "jellyroll": β-sheet sandwich |
| hIL-1β | Capped β-barrel consisting of 12 antiparallel β-strands; no α-helices |
| hIL-1α | Similar to IL-1β |
| bFGF | Similar to IL-1β |
| hIL-8 | Dimeric molecule; each subunit consists of 3 antiparallel β-strands and 1 α-helix |

IL, interleukin; IFN, interferon; GM-CSF, granulocyte and macrophage colony-stimulating factor; hTNF, human tumor necrosis factor; hLT, human lymphotoxin; bFGF, basic fibroblast growth factor.

### TABLE 174-6.
### Cytokines and Their Receptors in Human Urine

| Cytokine/Receptor | Condition |
|---|---|
| **CYTOKINE** | |
| Interleukin-1 | Normal individuals |
| Interleukin-2 | BCG therapy |
| Interleukin-6 | BCG therapy |
| | Renal transplant recipient |
| TNF | BCG therapy |
| IFN-γ | BCG therapy |
| M-CSF | Normal individuals |
| EPO | Aplastic anemia |
| AMF | Bladder cancer |
| bFGF | Bladder cancer |
| | Kidney cancer |
| EGF (β-urogastrone) | Normal individuals |
| TGF-α | Breast cancer |
| **CYTOKINE RECEPTORS** | |
| IL-2R | Normal individuals |
| IL-6R | Normal individuals |
| TNFR | Normal individuals |
| | Regular hemodialysis treatment |
| | Febrile patients |
| IFN-γR | Normal individuals |

BCG, Bacillus Calmetti Gurrien; TNF, tumor necrosis factor; IFN, interferon; M-CSF, macrophage colony-stimulating factor; EPO, erythropoietin; AMF, autocrine motility factor; bFGF, basic fibroblast growth factor; EGF, epidermal growth factor; TGF, transforming growth factor; IL, interleukin; TNFR, TNF receptor.

**TABLE 174-7.**
**Effect of Deletion of Cytokine and Cytokine Receptors on Growth and Development**

| Cytokine/Receptor | Defect |
| --- | --- |
| **CYTOKINES** | |
| IL-2 | Animals display normal T- and B-cell development |
| | Poor T-cell response to Con A or anti-CD3 |
| | 50% of animals die from 4–6 months |
| | Develop ulcerative colitis |
| IL-4 | Normal T- and B-cell development |
| | Reduced serum IgG1 and IgE levels |
| | No dominance of IgG1, is T-cell dependent |
| | No IgE response to nematode infection |
| | Reduced production of IL-3, IL-5, and IL-10 |
| | Resistance to retrovirus-induced immunodeficiency syndrome |
| IL-10 | Animals are growth retarded and anemic, and suffer from chronic enterocolitis |
| TGF-β | Excessive inflammatory response |
| | 20 days after birth there is a rapid wasting syndrome and tissue necrosis, leading to organ failure and early death |
| α-Inhibin | Animals develop mixed or incompletely differentiated gonadal stromal tumors either unilaterally or bilaterally |
| IFN-γ | Impaired production of macrophage antimicrobial products |
| | Reduced expression of macrophage MHC-II |
| | Animals are killed by *Mycobacterium bovis* |
| | Uncontrolled proliferation of splenocytes |
| SCF* | Encodes membrane stem cell factor or c-*kit* ligand |
| | Leads to *Steel-Dickie* mutation |
| | Pleiotropic defects similar to those caused by mutations at the W locus |
| | Animals are sterile, anemic, and black-eyed white |
| Fas ligand* | Mice carrying *gld* mutation develop lymphadenopathy and systemic autoimmunity similar to that in *lpr/lpr* mice |
| M-CSF* | Deficiency of osteoclasts, monocytes |
| | Osteopetrosis *(op)* due to osteoclast defect |
| | Defective in production of M-CSF |
| LIF | Females are fertile but their blastocysts fail to implant and, thus, do not develop |
| TGF-α | Abnormalities in hair follicles and eyes |
| CD40L* | X-linked hyper-IgM *(HIGM)* syndrome |
| | Elevated levels of serum IgM |
| | Low or no IgG, IgA, and IgE |
| TNF | Sensitive to *Listeria monocytogenes* infection |
| LT | No lymph nodes |
| **RECEPTORS** | |
| TNF-R (p55) | Resistance to endotoxin |
| | Sensitive to *L. monocytogenes* infection |
| TNF-R (p75) | Hypersensitive to TNF |
| IFN-γR | Defective natural resistance |
| | Increased susceptibility to infection by *L. monocytogenes*, vaccinia virus, and *Mycobacterium tuberculosis* |
| Fas* | Mice with *lpr/lpr* develop massive lymphadenopathy associated with proliferation of aberrant T cells |
| | Systemic autoimmunity |

*IL*, interleukin; *Ig*, immunoglobulin; *TGF*, transforming growth factor; *IFN*, interferon; *MHC*, major histocompatibility complex; *SCF*, stem cell factor; *M-CSF*, macrophage colony-stimulating factor; *LIF*, leukemia inhibitory factor; *TNF*, tumor necrosis factor; *LT*, lymphotoxin.
*Abnormalities based on natural mutation of the gene.

cloning a particular gene, disrupting it by introducing a short DNA sequence, and inserting it into a mouse stem cell. The disrupted gene replaces the normal gene by a process called *homologous recombination*. These cells are injected into the mouse embryo, yielding mice that are then bred to produce a strain in which all cells lack the gene (i.e., the gene is knocked out). By these techniques, the function of the missing gene product can be ascertained. The deletion of genes for specific cytokines has resulted in defective development in the embryo. For instance, deletion of LIF leads to retardation of blastocyst development due to the lack of its implantation. A deletion of the interleukin-10 (IL-10) gene in most animals leads to growth retardation and anemia, whereas animals lacking the interleukin-2 (IL-2) gene develop normally during the first 3 to 4 weeks of age, some dying later, between 4 and 9 weeks after birth. The defects that result from deletion of other cytokine genes are outlined in Table 174-7. It clearly documents the importance of various cytokines during early development, growth, and survival.

## CONCLUSION

Cytokines, a new class of molecules discovered within the last two decades, play an important role in both the pathogenesis and treatment of disease. Cytokines have already made the transition from concept to clinic and have attracted the attention of many scientists both in academic and industrial settings during the last few years. Because of their importance to homeostasis and therapy, the multiplicity of their interactions, and the complexity of their modulation, it is certain that studies of cytokines will continue to expand. Several cytokines have been approved by the Food and Drug Administration for human use in the United States, including interferon-α, -β, and -γ (IFN-α, IFN-β, IFN-γ); granulocyte colony-stimulating factor (G-CSF); granulocyte and macrophage colony-stimulating factor (GM-CSF); erythropoietin (EPO); IL-2; and interleukin-11 (IL-11). In addition, anti-TNF antibodies for Crohn disease and a soluble form of human TNF receptor for rheumatoid arthritis have also been approved.[30] However, due to complex interactions between different cytokines and other soluble factors, our knowledge is very much incomplete. We know too little about their roles in several diseases or even in physiologic processes, especially the important interaction between cytokines and extracellular matrix components. Exploration of these mechanisms will probably lead to great progress in the understanding of cellular biology and management of diseases.

## REFERENCES

1. Oppenheim JJ, Cohen S, eds. Interleukins, lymphokines and cytokines. New York: Academic Press, 1983:1.
2. Goldstein AL. Thymic hormones and lymphokine. New York: Plenum Publishing, 1984:235.
3. Sorg C, Schimpl A, eds. Cellular and molecular biology of lymphokines. New York: Academic Press, 1985:1.
4. Webb DR, Goeddel DV, eds. Lymphokines: molecular cloning and analysis of lymphokines. New York: Academic Press, 1987:1.
5. Sporn MB, Roberts AB. Peptide growth factors are multifunctional. Nature 1988; 332:217.
6. Balkwill FR. Cytokines in cancer therapy. Oxford: Oxford University Press, 1989; 297:1.
7. Melli M, Parente L, eds. Cytokines and lipocortins in inflammation and differentiation. New York: Wiley-Liss, 1990:1.
8. Clemens MJ. Cytokines. Oxford: BIOS Scientific Publishers, 1991:1.
9. Balkwill FR. Cytokines: practical approach. Oxford: Oxford University Press, 1991:1.
10. Nathan C, Sporn M. Cytokines in context. J Cell Biol 1991; 113:981.
11. Aggarwal BB, Vilcek J, eds. Tumor necrosis factor: structure, function and mechanism of action. New York: Marcel Dekker Inc, 1992:1.
12. Aggarwal BB, Gutterman JU, eds. Human cytokines: a handbook for basic and clinical researchers, vol I. Boston: Blackwell Science, 1992:1.
13. Aggarwal BB, Pocsik E. Cytokines: from clone to clinic. Arch Biochem Biophys 1992; 292:335.
14. Galvani DW, Cawley JC, eds. Cytokine therapy. London: Cambridge Press, 1992:1.
15. Kroemer G, Alboran M, Gonzalo JA, Martinez C. Immunoregulation by cytokines. Crit Rev Immunol 1993; 13:163.

16. Elsasser-Beile U, Von Kleist S. Cytokines as therapeutic and diagnostic agents. Tumor Biol 1993; 14:69.
17. Nicola NA. Hematopoietic growth factors and their receptors. In: Thomas ED, ed. Applications of basic science to hematopoiesis and treatment of disease. New York: Raven Press, 1993, 261.
18. Nicola NA, ed. Cytokines and their receptors. Oxford: Sambrook and Tooze Publication, Oxford University Press, 1994:1.
19. Callard R, Gearing A, eds. The cytokine fact book. New York: Academic Press, 1994:1.
20. Thompson A, ed. The cytokine handbook. New York: Academic Press, 1994:1.
21. Aggarwal BB, Puri RK, eds. Human cytokines: their role in disease and therapy. Boston: Blackwell Science, 1995:1.
22. Aggarwal BB, Gutterman JU, eds. Human cytokines: a handbook for basic and clinical researchers, vol II. Boston: Blackwell Science, 1996:1.
23. Aggarwal BB, Natarajan K. Tumor necrosis factors: developments during last decade. Eur Cytokine Network 1996; 7:93.
24. Darnay B, Aggarwal BB. Human cytokines. In: Bittar EE, Bittar N, eds. Advances in oncobiology, vol 1. Greenwich, CT: JAI Press, 1996:179.
25. Le Roith D, Bondy C. Growth factor and cytokines in health and disease, vol 2B. Greenwich, CT: JAI Press, 1997:727.
26. Aggarwal BB, ed. Human cytokines: a handbook for basic and clinical researchers, vol III. Boston: Blackwell Science, 1997:1.
27. Darnay BG, Aggarwal BB. Early events in TNF signaling: a story of associations and dissociations. J Leukocyte Biol 1997; 61:559.
28. Shrivastava A, Aggarwal BB. Cytokines as biological regulators of homeostasis. J Biol Regulators and Homeostatic Agents 1998; 12:1.
29. Durum SC, Muegge K. Cytokine knockouts. Totowa, NJ: Humana Press, 1998.
30. O'Reilly MS, Boehm T, Shing Y, et al. Endostatin: an endogenous inhibitor of angiogenesis and tumor growth. Cell 1997; 88:277.

# CHAPTER 175

# THE DIFFUSE NEUROENDOCRINE SYSTEM

ERIC S. NYLÉN AND KENNETH L. BECKER

The diffuse neuroendocrine system (DNES) comprises a widespread system of endocrine cells that are scattered throughout many organs and tissues (Table 175-1). Many of these cells constitute an important part of several large "classic" glands, such as the hypothalamus, pituitary, thyroid, parathyroid, pancreas, and adrenal medulla. As in the glandular-based cells, the dispersed cells also contain characteristic secretion granules and produce and secrete certain bioactive peptide hormones that have local and distal functions. Frequently, there is independent secretion of the same peptide hormones in different regions of the body, where these substances may have different functions. These endocrine cells and their peptide hormones combine many aspects of the "traditional" nervous and endocrine systems.

## THE NERVOUS ENDOCRINE OVERLAP

Previously, although involved in homeostatic regulation, nervous and endocrine cells were regarded as distinct anatomic and functional entities. Conceptually, neurons were considered to be ectodermal, often possessing a characteristically elongated shape, and controlling other cells by synaptic neurocrine release (see Chap. 1). Conversely, endocrine cells previously were thought to be quite different cells that release hormones into the blood to control distal sites. Furthermore, it was postulated that the evolutionary development of nervous and endocrine cells occurred at different times.

This concept of distinct nervous and endocrine systems has been shown to be oversimplified and, more importantly, inaccurate. These two major regulatory systems are known to share

**TABLE 175-1.**

**Distribution and Classification of Some of the Peptide- and Amine-Containing Cells of the Diffuse Neuroendocrine System***

| Tissue | Cell Types | Peptides | Biogenic Amines |
|---|---|---|---|
| **Thyroid** | C cell | CT, PDN-21 | 5-HT |
| | C cell | CGRP, BLP, SN | |
| **Lung** | PNE or K cell | CT, BLP | 5-HT |
| | PNE or K cell | Leu-Enk | |
| | PNE or K cell | CGRP, CCK, Endo | |
| **Stomach** | G | Gastrin, Enk | |
| | D | SN | |
| | EC | | 5-HT |
| | ECL | | H |
| **Intestine** | D | SN | |
| | S | Secretin | |
| | EC$_1$ | SP, SK | |
| | EC$_2$(M) | Motilin | 5-HT |
| | I(CCK) | CCK | |
| | G | Gastrin | |
| | K(GIP) | GIP | |
| | L | GFP, PYY | |
| | N | NT | |
| **Pancreas** | A | Glucagon, CRH | 5-HT |
| | B | Insulin | 5-HT |
| | D | SN | DA |
| | G | Gastrin | |
| | PP | PP, CRH | |
| **Adrenal** | A | Enk, NPY | E |
| | NA | Dynorphin, BLP | NE |
| **Sympathetic ganglia** | SIF | Enk | DA, 5-HT |
| **Paraganglia** | Main | Enk | NE, DA |
| **Carotid** | I cell | SP | NE, DA |
| | | Met- and Leu-Enk | |
| **Skin** | Merkel | CT, BLP, Met-Enk, VIP | H |
| **Genitourinary** | | CT, BLP, SN | 5-HT |

*BLP*, bombesin-like peptides; *CCK*, cholecystokinin; *CGRP*, calcitonin gene-related peptide; *CRH*, corticotropin-releasing hormone; *CT*, calcitonin; *DA*, dopamine; *E*, epinephrine; *EC*, enterochromaffin; *ECL*, enterochromaffin-like; *Endo*, endothelin; *Enk*, enkephalin; *GFP*, glucagon family peptides (including enteroglucagon); *GIP*, gastric inhibitory peptide (glucose-dependent insulinotropic peptide); *5-HT*, serotonin; *H*, histamine; *Leu-Enk*, leu-enkephalin; *Met-Enk*, met-enkephalin; *NE*, norepinephrine; *NPY*, neuropeptide Y; *NT*, neurotensin; *PDN-21*, katacalcin; *PP*, pancreatic polypeptide; *PYY*, peptide YY; *SIF*, small intensely fluorescent cells; *SK*, substance K; *SN*, somatostatin; *SP*, substance P; *VIP*, vasoactive intestinal peptide.

*This listing is a composite of several classifications. It is undergoing continuous modifications and updating, and is shown for illustrative purposes only.

(Data from Pearse AGE, Takor-Takor T. Embryology of the diffuse neuroendocrine system and its relationship to the common peptides. Fed Proc 1979; 38;2288; di Sant'Agnese PA, deMesy Jensen KL. Endocrine-paracrine [APUD] cells of the human female urethra and paraurethral ducts. J Urol 1987; 7:1250; and Solicia E, et al. Experientia 1987; 43:839.)

features of genetic programming,[1,2] messenger transduction, and physiologic function that derive from ancient unicellular development. Even in specialized multicellular organisms, these shared features render any facile distinction between neurons and endocrine cells difficult to impossible.

The adrenal chromaffin cell was one of the first noted exceptions to the traditional dichotomy between neurons and endocrine cells. These medullary cells release large amounts of catecholamines into the circulation, acting on distal tissues; however, embryologically, they originate from the neural crest, and histologically, they have the appearance of nerve cells (see Chaps. 71 and 85). Another inconsistency is the hypothalamus: a "gland" that consists of neurons that produce oxytocin and vasopressin; after storage in the posterior pituitary, these hormones are released systemically (see Chaps. 8 and 25). Additionally, cells of the gastrointestinal tract were described as early as 1870 and, thereafter, were considered to constitute part of a diffuse endocrine system possessing a paracrine function. Subsequently, remarkable similarities have been demonstrated between these latter epithelial cells and the nervous system.

## HISTORICAL BACKGROUND

The existence of a diffuse system of endocrine cells was first suggested by work on the intestinal mucosa by Haidenhain.[3] Subsequently, this concept was extended by several investigators, including Pearse and co-workers,[4-6] who pointed out that although these cells occur in different anatomic sites, they share certain similar morphologic and functional properties. Because of their cytochemical characteristics, these cells were grouped under the acronym APUD (*amine precursor uptake and subsequent decarboxylation*). This system of classification, which also included the gastrointestinal endocrine cells, was considered to correspond to the diffuse endocrine system that had been proposed previously in 1969 by Feyrter.[7]

On the basis of the observation that the autonomic neurons, the thyroidal C cells, and the adrenal chromaffin cells are derived from the neural crest, Pearse and co-workers further suggested that the APUD cells share a common embryologic origin; partly based on this presumed common embryogenesis, they used the categorical term *neuroendocrine*. Subsequently, several studies have shown that neural-like APUD characteristics do not necessitate either a neural crest or ectodermal origin. Although some of these cells are, indeed, derived from the neural crest, a series of allograft experiments have shown, for example, that the so-called gastroenteropancreatic axis of endocrine cells is derived from endoderm.[8]

As information has evolved, it appears best to reserve the term APUD to indicate the aforementioned histochemical characteristics. The term *neuroendocrine cell* refers to shared phenotypic expression involving established neuronal and endocrine features such as morphology and genetic programming.

## DISTRIBUTION OF THE DIFFUSE NEUROENDOCRINE SYSTEM CELLS

The DNES consists of specialized endocrine cells that mostly are intraepithelial and typically are scattered in several luminal tissues. All are characterized by the presence of hormonal peptides and amines stored within cytoplasmic secretory granules. Pearse and co-workers have included at least 40 individual cell types in the DNES. Accordingly, the system has a *central division*, which comprises the neuroendocrine cells of the hypothalamic-pituitary axis and the pineal gland, and a *peripheral division* (see Table 175-1), which includes the neuroendocrine cells of the gastroenteropancreatic axis, lung, parathyroid, adrenal medulla, sympathetic ganglia, skin, and thyroid C cells. Additional neuroendocrine cells of the breast, endometrium, prostate, urethra, and testicular Leydig cells also have been included.[9-12] Because of the diminishing distinctions between neurons and endocrine cells and the absence of a strict definition of a DNES cell, it is not surprising that this classification is controversial and that it is modified as new peptides and related marker proteins are discovered. Nevertheless, despite such incertitudes of classification, the concept of the DNES is both creative and practical.

## HISTOLOGY AND MORPHOLOGY

Historically, the silver stains, which demonstrate either *argentaffin* staining (uptake and deposition of silver on secretion granules) or *argyrophilic* staining (positive silver staining after

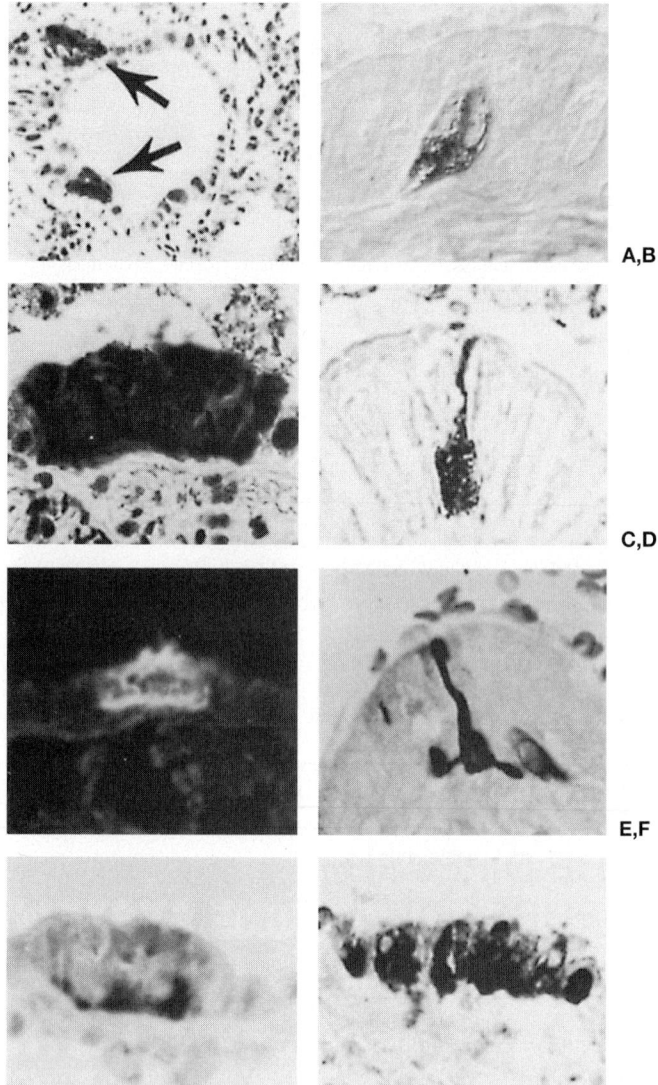

**FIGURE 175-1.** The pulmonary neuroendocrine cells (*PNECs*) and neuroepithelial bodies (*NEBs*). The photomicrographs on the *left* (**A, C, E, G**) illustrate NEBs in adult hamster lungs after exposure to a systemic carcinogen, diethylnitrosamine, whereas the *right-hand panel* shows DNES cells of human bronchial epithelium. In these photomicrographs, the cells have been visualized by using special staining techniques. **A,** A small bronchus with two NEBs (Grimelius silver impregnation, magnification ×130). **B,** Two PNECs with chromogranin A immunoreactivity. Notice the overlying ciliated epithelium (Nomarski optics, ×570). **C,** Strongly argyrophilic, large NEB (Grimelius silver impregnation, ×330). **D,** Classic, flask-shaped PNEC reaching the bronchial lumen (Leu-7 immunoreactivity, ×840). **E,** Formaldehyde-induced fluorescence of serotonin in a NEB. Notice the surrounding bronchial epithelium and alveoli, which are negatively stained (×260). **F,** A solitary PNEC with characteristic cell processes that extend from the basal membrane to the bronchial lumen. The adjacent PNEC demonstrates an unstained nucleus (serotonin immunoreactivity, ×660). **G,** A NEB with basally located calcitonin immunoreactivity (×340). **H,** Hyperplastic PNECs along the bronchial epithelium demonstrating bombesin immunoreactivity (×410). The general techniques and markers such as silver impregnation, formaldehyde-induced fluorescence, chromogranin A, and Leu-7 allow a universal identification of dispersed endocrine cells in various organs, whereas the specific hormonal products such as serotonin, calcitonin, and bombesin characterize selected subpopulations of cells. (Courtesy of Dr. R. Ilona Linnoila, NCI, Bethesda, MD.)

the addition of a mild reducing agent), were the commonly used stains for identifying many of the DNES cells (Fig. 175-1).

Because of the APUD properties of the DNES cells, they often show a characteristic fluorescence of their biogenic

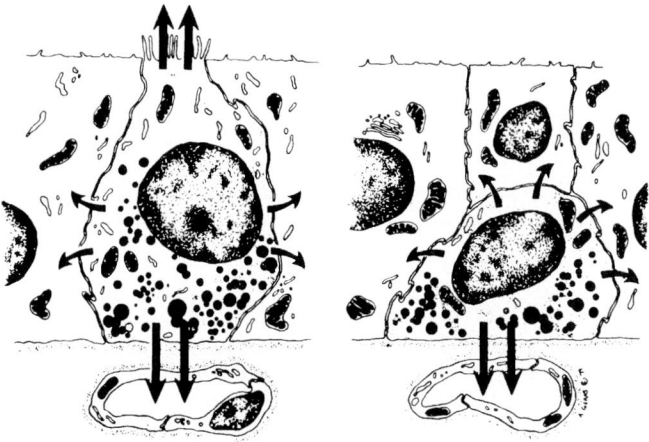

**FIGURE 175-2.** Schematic representation of flask-shaped neuroendocrine cells of the "open" (*left*) and "closed" (*right*) types. Both cell types can release hormonal substances into the circulation (hemocrine) and to neighboring cells (paracrine). The open-cell type can, in addition, release its content into the luminal aspect (solinocrine). (Modified from Track NS, et al. In: Glass BJ, ed. Gastrointestinal hormones. New York: Raven Press, 1980:75.)

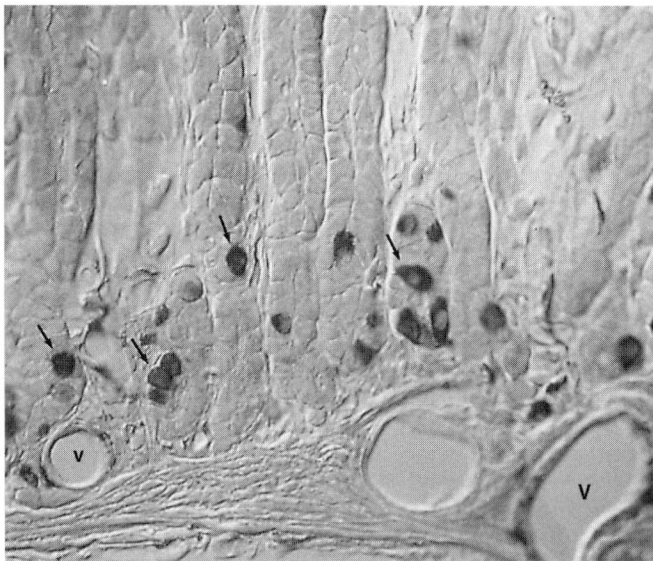

**FIGURE 175-3.** By use of Nomarski optics, synaptophysin (p38) immunoreactivity is seen localized to the mucosa of the rat fundus. Endocrine cells staining positive for p38 (*arrow*) are scattered among glands. The exocrine cells of the gastric glands do not stain for p38. (*v*, blood vessels surrounded by immunoreactive en passant varicose terminals.) (Courtesy of Drs. F. Navone, R. Jahn, P. Greengard, P. DeCamilli, University of Milano, Italy.)

amines when exposed to formaldehyde vapor (see Fig. 175-1). Additionally, the DNES cells stain avidly for certain enzymes, including glycerophosphate dehydrogenase, nonspecific esterases, and cholinesterase.

The most recently developed techniques for the localization of DNES cells involve immunohistochemistry; these methods rely on a specific antigen-antibody reaction linked to a well-visualized probe such as a fluorochrome or enzyme[13] (see Fig. 175-1). In hybridization histochemistry, a labeled, cloned complementary DNA (or RNA) probe is hybridized to the intracellular DNA or RNA of a peptide and subsequently localized by autoradiography or peroxidase staining.[14] This method, in contrast to immunocytochemistry, reveals the genetic expression.

Morphologically, most of the epithelial DNES cells reach the luminal aspect of the epithelium; often, there is a striking polarity of orientation into a pyramidally shaped structure, with a narrow apical portion (see Fig. 175-1) that often possesses microvillus extensions. In the gut, where most anatomic studies have been performed, those cells reaching the lumen are termed *open*, whereas those without luminal contact are termed *closed* (Fig. 175-2). The DNES cells may form organoid clusters, such as in the lung (neuroepithelial bodies), or in the carotid body.

## ULTRASTRUCTURE

The DNES cell possesses all of the ultrastructural characteristics of an actively secreting cell, with well-developed endoplasmic reticulum and Golgi apparatus, and an abundant microfilament and microtubular system. Electron microscopic and immunohistochemical analyses have revealed that certain DNES cells and their malignant counterparts contain cytoskeletal intermediate filaments, termed *neurofilaments*, which previously were thought to be associated exclusively with neurons.[15]

The most distinctive feature shared by neurons and DNES cells is the presence of cytoplasmic secretory granules, with an electron-dense core of variable density and appearance, and a single, limiting outer membrane. The size of these secretion granules varies from 50 to 400 nm in diameter. Often, there is a relative homogeneity of size or appearance for granules of a given peptide population. These secretion granules are highly complex structures[16] that store hormonal peptides and their precursors, as well as biogenic amines, high-energy phosphate compounds, ions, polyamines,[17] and chromogranins. Studies with colloidal

gold conjugated to immunoglobulins[18] have disclosed that secretion granules in some cells contain more than one peptide.[19] Generally, the secretion of the intragranular peptide hormones of the DNES occurs by exocytosis and is discontinuous: There is a preliminary accumulation and storage of the hormone, which is discharged in response to specific local stimuli.

Brain neurons contain, along with secretion granules, an abundance of small synaptic vesicles (40–60 nm diameter) that are thought to be the storage sites of "classic" neurotransmitters. These small synaptic vesicles, in contrast with the dense-core secretion granules, undergo local regeneration and contain certain characteristic intrinsic membrane proteins including *synaptophysin* (p38).[20] Interestingly, this acidic glycosylated protein (~38,000 daltons) also has been localized to many DNES cells (e.g., adrenal medulla, carotid body, pituitary gland, pancreatic islets, gastric mucosa, thyroid, skin, and lung) and DNES tumors.[21] This finding emphasizes that small synaptic vesicles and dense-core granules constitute different secretory organelles and that there are common and distinctive endomembranous systems that are shared by both neurons and many endocrine cells (Figs. 175-3 and 175-4).

## NEUROENDOCRINE MARKERS

The DNES cells display certain distinctive features that serve as useful markers, such as the presence of large concentrations of a highly acidic glycolytic enolase isoenzyme (2-phospho-D-glycerate hydroxylase) called *neuron-specific enolase*.[22] This enolase enzyme (EC 4.2.1.11) consists of two subunits giving rise to three isoenzymes: $\alpha$, $\beta$, and $\gamma$. Immunostaining of the 78,000-dalton $\gamma$ subunit of this cytoplasmic enzyme has shown that it is not exclusive to mature neurons, but that it is also present in DNES cells as either the $\gamma\gamma$ or $\alpha\gamma$ isomers, thus providing a vehicle for mapping the distribution of the DNES. This "neuronal" glycolytic enzyme is also found within the derivative neoplasms of the DNES and can be detected in the circulation.[23]

Another marker is the Leu-7 (HNK-1) antigen, which initially was shown to react with natural killer cells. This 110,000-dalton glycoprotein is associated with myelinated nerves in the

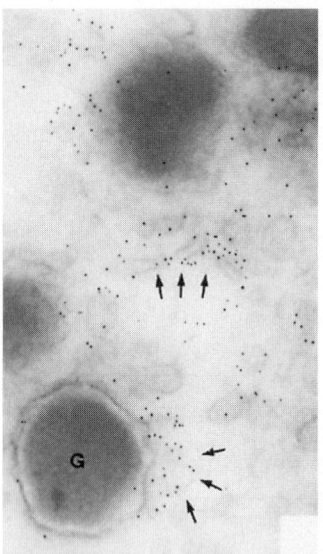
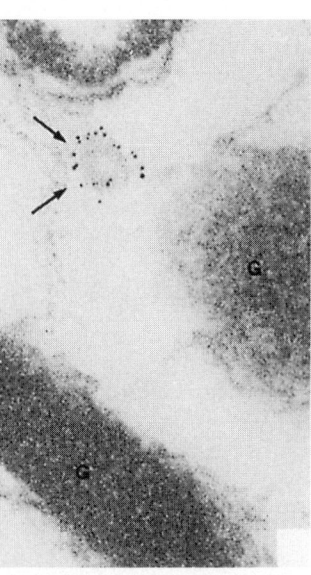

**A,B**

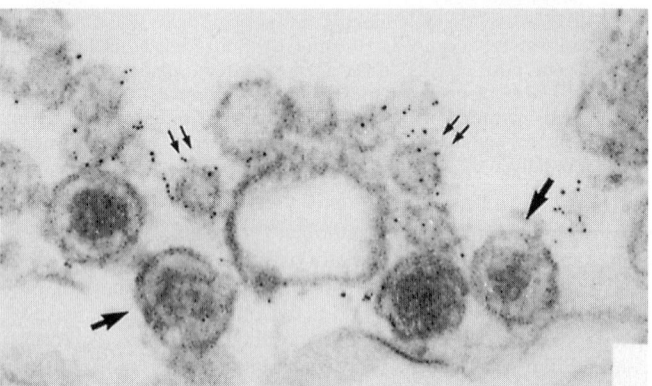

**C**

**FIGURE 175-4.** Electron micrographs using immunogold labeling. **A,** Anterior pituitary: ultrathin frozen sections showing most of the gold particles associated with small vesicular profiles with clear content (*arrows*). These are interspersed among secretory granules (G) and, sometimes, in close proximity to them (calibration bar = 150 nm). **B,** Adrenal medulla: agarose-embedded subcellular particles of the adrenal medulla showing a small, round vesicle immunoreactive for p38 (*arrows*). Membranes of secretory granules (G) are unlabeled (calibration bar = 100 nm). **C,** Immunogold particles are selectively localized on the cytoplasmic surface of small synaptic vesicles (*pairs of small arrows*). Large dense-core vesicles (*large arrows*) are unlabeled (calibration bar = 100 nm). (From Navone F, Jahn R, DiGioia G, et al. Protein p38: an integral membrane protein specific for small vesicles of neurons and neuroendocrine cells. J Cell Biol 1986; 103:2511.)

central nervous system (CNS) and peripheral nervous system (PNS), as well as endocrine cells in the gut, pancreas, and lung.[24] Additionally, certain neuroendocrine tumors such as neuroblastoma, melanoma, and small cell lung cancer also react with Leu-7 antisera. Interestingly, this antigen also is found in macrophages, and it has been suggested that these two different cell types (small cell lung cancer and macrophages) share a common hematopoietic origin.[25] However, it has been argued that the presence of shared antigens does not prove a common ancestral lineage.[24]

Chromogranin originally was found to be stored within the cells of the adrenal medulla and to be secreted along with catecholamines during the exocytosis of their secretion granules.[26] The chromogranins have been separated into three classes: A, B, and C. They all have similar properties and tissue distribution and are cosecreted with bioactive peptides. They are acidic proteins, with a high glutamic acid content. Chromogranin A (~48,000 daltons) is a structural protein often present in neurons (CNS and PNS), neuroendocrine cells, and tumors of the

**TABLE 175-2.**
**Potential Physiologic Roles of Chromogranin A**

Catecholamine binding

Modulation of intravascular hormone processing

Glucocorticoid-responsive autocrine inhibition of proopiomelanocortin secretion

Production of bioactive peptides such as pancreastatin and chromostatin

neuroendocrine cells; it is not found in secretion granules of exocrine glands.[27] Staining for chromogranin A has suggested additional cellular DNES candidates, including cells within the lobular ductules of the breast and cells in lymphoid tissues such as the spleen, the lymph nodes, the lamina propria, and the human fetal liver.[28] A portion of the chromogranin A structure gives rise to the peptide pancreastatin, which exerts inhibitory influences on insulin, gastric acid, and exocrine secretion.[27,29] Another portion of chromogranin A gives rise to an additional peptide: chromostatin (Table 175-2).

Several other features are characteristic of the DNES. Because of its APUD nature, these cells and their related tumors commonly express the biogenic amine enzyme levodopa (L-dopa) decarboxylase[30] and characteristic vesicular monoamine transporters.[31] Other characteristics include the presence of the brain creatine kinase BB enzymes and aldolase C.[32,33] Protein gene product 9.5, with a molecular mass of 25 kDa, is present in the CNS and the PNS. It has been demonstrated in the DNES, except for the gastrointestinal tract. It is a cytoplasmic protein with a wider distribution than neuron-specific enolase. Its name derives from its 9.5-cm mobility on polyacrylamide gel electrophoresis.[34-36] Additional markers include neural-adhesion molecule (N-CAM),[37] and 7B2. The latter is a secretory protein that is found in multiple DNES sites.[38]

## PEPTIDE CONTENT

More than 35 physiologically active peptides have been identified as DNES products (see Table 175-1). Occasionally, the same peptide hormone has been found in different constituent DNES cells: Calcitonin is found in the hypothalamus, in the pituitary gland, in C cells of the thyroid, and in the pulmonary neuroendocrine cell; oxytocin is found in the hypothalamus and in the ovary; and somatostatin is found in the hypothalamus, the D cells of the stomach, intestine, and pancreas, and in thyroid C cells. Many of the cells of the DNES, as well as many neurons, produce more than one peptide; for example, the pulmonary neuroendocrine cells produce bombesin, calcitonin, calcitonin gene-related peptide, Leu-enkephalin, endothelin, cholecystokinin, and perhaps somatostatin[39] (see Chap. 177). Many of these coexpressed peptides also can be costored in the same secretion granule.[19]

Most of the peptides of the DNES are shared with the somatic and autonomic nervous system (e.g., endorphins, somatostatin, calcitonin, vasoactive intestinal peptide [VIP], gastrin, cholecystokinin, and insulin). Importantly, the synthetic steps in the neurons and in the DNES cells that lead to the production and eventual secretion of these peptides and amines are similar (Fig. 175-5). Neurons of the CNS and PNS containing peptides have been termed *peptidergic*. These peptides typically are involved in neurocrine transmission or neuromodulation, or both. This multifaceted function has led to the use of the term *regulatory* peptides.

## BIOGENIC AMINES

At some time during their development, all DNES cells synthesize biogenic amines. However, at any one time, only a few

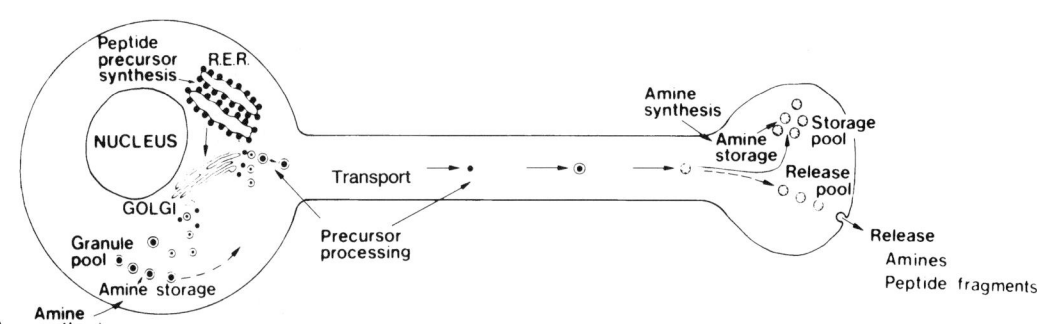

**FIGURE 175-5. A,** The localization of the process of peptide and amine synthesis in a neuroendocrine cell is depicted. Peptide production is initiated with *mRNA* transcription followed by accumulation and processing in the rough endoplasmic reticulum (*RER*) and Golgi apparatus. Dense-core vesicles produced from the latter site further process and store the peptide, followed by transport to terminal sites and subsequent release by exocytosis. Small synaptic vesicles are found in the terminals where they undergo local regeneration. (From Hakanson R, Sundler F. The design of the neuroendocrine system: a unifying concept and its consequences. Trends Pharmacol Sci 1983; 4:41.) **B,** The enzyme L-dopa decarboxylase (*DDC*) plays a key role in the production of serotonin and catecholamines in neuroendocrine cells.

mature DNES cells store these amines. Typically, biogenic amine synthesis is demonstrated by preincubation with the amine precursors L-dopa or 5-hydroxytryptophan. The synthesis of dopamine and serotonin from their respective amino-acid precursors requires L-dopa decarboxylase (see Fig. 175-5). The endogenous amines of the DNES include dopamine, serotonin, norepinephrine, epinephrine, and histamine (see Table 175-1). Although amines are present along with peptides within the secretory granules, little is known about the role of amines in the synthesis or secretion of the coexistent peptides. The relative proportions of these different substances vary considerably, depending on the particular cell type. For example, the adrenal medullary cells predominantly produce and secrete biogenic amines, whereas the pancreatic islet cells principally produce and secrete peptides.

# CLINICAL RELEVANCE OF THE DIFFUSE NEUROENDOCRINE SYSTEM

## PHYSIOLOGY

### PARACRINE SECRETION

The aforementioned presence of several features that classically had been associated with only neurons has validated the concept of a DNES. It is difficult to obtain experimental physiologic information from a system of scattered cells; diffuse surgical extirpation is impossible, and studies of the release of small amounts of hormone by one or several cells are difficult. As initially suggested by Feyrter[7] these cells exert local regulatory influences through *paracrine* secretion. This form of secretory transport represents one of the first means of cell-to-cell regulation; it occurs early in the evolutionary record within coelenterates, organisms that lack a circulatory system. Paracrine secretion has been retained in mammals, for which an important role for this form of communication and control is gradually being uncovered. With the recognition of the ubiquitous distribution of peptide-containing cells, the existence of a para-

crine cell-to-cell transfer of information is seen to provide a means by which such communication can be regulated locally, precisely, and with relevance to local needs. The paracrine response to local stimulation may be highly specific, similar to the initiation of follicular maturation by ovarian androgens,[40] or more generalized, as in epithelial growth.[41] Paracrine secretion can occur through discrete anatomic delivery systems, which involve long cytoplasmic processes that also include terminal swellings adjacent to target cells—a structuring that is reminiscent of neurons. Furthermore, the message is delivered in a highly concentrated form. Interestingly, DNES cells in culture can display neuron-like processes. In keeping with their neuroendocrine characteristics, these cultured cells generate depolarizing currents that reach a threshold and produce an all-or-nothing action potential—a phenomenon that previously had been seen only in nerve and muscle.[42,43] These properties are observed in normal as well as in tumor cells and can be enhanced by nerve growth factor.

The copresence of several amines and peptides and the highly structural cellular specialization of DNES cells provide an increased plasticity to the possible informational content of the paracrine messages from any single cell.

### THE DIFFUSE NEUROENDOCRINE SYSTEM AND THE GUT

The gut exemplifies an extraordinary functional convergence of the nervous and endocrine systems. Subsequent to substance P being detected in the gut and in the brain,[44] many endocrine peptides found within the gut also have been found in the CNS and vice versa; this has prompted the concept of a "brain-gut" axis. Also, functionally, portions of the autonomic nervous system (including, in particular, the gastrointestinal tract, as well as the urogenital, respiratory, and cardiovascular systems) are regarded as components of a nonadrenergic noncholinergic effector system.[45] In many of these tissues, the DNES cells, and these local peptide-containing neuronal cells and ganglia, together coordinate local neuroendocrine regulatory functions.[46] This is particularly prominent in the gut, which possesses an autonomous "enteric nervous system"[47] (see Chap. 182).

## CHEMORECEPTION

Many of the DNES cells of the gut (open type; see Fig. 175-2), and DNES cells elsewhere, have morphologic and functional characteristics of specialized *chemoreceptive* cells. These cells maintain the basic architecture of primitive neurons, with an apical receptive site containing microvilli or cilia and a basal secretory portion; the cells appear to perform sensory stimulus reception and conduction tasks. Their receptive sites are activated by various stimuli, which include dissolved (or ambient) oxygen tension and other undefined chemicals in the different luminal milieux.[48] Many of the DNES cells that have this configuration are primary sensory cells, such as taste buds, hair cells of the inner ear, and olfactory cells; in an expanded concept, these latter sensory cells, as well as DNES cells, have been grouped by some investigators into a system of *paraneurons*.[49]

The chemoreceptive neuroendocrine cells, such as the type 1 glomus cell of the carotid body, the pulmonary neuroendocrine cell, and the gastric and pancreatic islet cells, often are associated with, and influenced by, the presence of autonomic nerves. Regarding the carotid body and pulmonary neuroendocrine cells, there is evidence for a complex synaptic interaction.[50,51] The type 1 glomus cell, which is involved in the sensing of oxygen dissolved in the blood, can directly modulate the firing rate of the local afferents by the release of its dopamine content. Thus, the DNES and the local "enteric nervous system" represent additional functional arms of the autonomic nervous system. In this context, the abnormally elevated calcitonin precursor level (a DNES-derived peptide) often associated with severe illnesses, such as burns and sepsis, may be viewed as a marker of the regulatory systemic activity of the DNES[52] (see Chaps. 53 and 228).

## CONTROL OF CELLULAR GROWTH

Several of the peptides produced and secreted by the DNES possess a trophic growth activity that is exerted via autocrine or paracrine means. Thus, bombesin-like peptide has an important regulatory role on the maturation and proliferation of cells in the lung and gut (see Chap. 182). Bombesin-like peptides and other DNES peptides, such as calcitonin gene-related peptide, calcitonin, and endothelin have a broad repertoire of growth-stimulatory and inhibitory activity on a variety of cells. Refinements in the preparation and cell culture of the DNES should provide further insights into this important area of cell physiology.[53]

## DYSREGULATED GROWTH AND CANCER

Hyperplasia, dysplasia, and neoplasia (neuroendocrinomas or neuroendocrine tumors) involving the DNES are well-established phenomena. Indeed, often there is a gradual progression from the hyperplastic phase to overt neoplasia (e.g., familial medullary thyroid cancer), and the tumor growth is characteristically slow. Many of the features of the normal DNES cells are either maintained or frankly overexpressed in these abnormal cells; this has significant clinical impact on diagnosis and therapy. Thus, a wide range of DNES hyperplasias and tumors produce and secrete constituents that give rise to hormonal syndromes of paraneoplastic nature (e.g., lung cancer and the adrenocorticotropic hormone [ACTH]–induced Cushing syndrome; see Chap. 219). Furthermore, the measurement of the particular hormone can be used as an aid in the diagnosis and in following the therapeutic impact of treatment. An advance in the area of neuroendocrine oncology has been the introduction of diagnostic ligands to receptors on DNES cells. Thus, a wide variety of tumors can be visualized by means of octreotide scintigraphy that can visualize somatostatin-binding sites.[54] Many of these tumors that have somatostatin receptors also respond to administration of this somatostatin analog by decreased peptide secretion and diminished growth (see Chap. 169). Another

radioactive ligand being similarly investigated is VIP, which appears to bind selectively to a different class of DNES tumor receptors from those occupied by octreotide.[55] In view of the abundance of peptide receptors on DNES tumors, various synthetic receptor ligands should prove to be extremely useful in both the diagnostic exploration for tumors and the therapeutic delivery of tumoricidal substances to receptor-bearing tumors.[56]

## CONCLUSION

The DNES is a vast entity that comprises cells that are dispersed throughout many organs and tissues. These cells possess distinctive "neuronal" characteristics, including the presence of dense-core secretion granules that contain regulatory peptides and biogenic amines. They also possess several enzymatic and physicochemical features found in neurons. Some DNES cells display chemoreceptive features. By means of locally released peptides and amines, the DNES cells, in parallel with local neurons and ganglia, constitute a functional homeostatic system that is concerned with precise regulatory adjustments that reflect local tissue requirements, but that also may respond to nervous or humoral stimulation from distant regions of the body. The increased knowledge concerning the DNES[1] and the improved techniques of selective gene removal (i.e., knock-out) have, in addition, broadened our ability to investigate further this vast system of cells.[57]

## REFERENCES

1. Borges M, Linnoila RI, van de Velde HJK, et al. An achaete-scute homologue essential for neuroendocrine differentiation in the lung. Nature 1997; 386:852.
2. Anderson DJ. Cellular and molecular biology of neural crest cell lineage determination. Trends Genet 1997; 13:7.
3. Haidenhain R. Untersuchungen uber den Bau der Labdrusen. Arch Mikrosk Anat 1870; 6:368.
4. Pearse AGE. Common cytochemical properties of cells producing polypeptide hormones, with particular reference to calcitonin and the thyroid C cells. Vet Rec 1966; 79:587.
5. Pearse AGE, Takor-Takor T. Embryology of the diffuse neuroendocrine system and its relationship to the common peptides. Fed Proc 1979; 38:2288.
6. Pearse AGE. Neuroendocrine system, dispersed: APUD. In: Adelman G, ed. Encyclopedia of neuroscience, vol 2. Boston: Birkhauser, 1987:777.
7. Feyrter F. Die Periheren endokrinen (parakrinen), Drusen. Lehrbuchder speziellen pathologischen anatomie, vol 11–12. Berlin: De Gruyter, 1969.
8. Fontaine J, LeDouarin NM. Analysis of endoderm formation in the avian blastoderm by the use of quail chick chimeras: the problem of the neuroectodermal origin of the cells of the APUD series. J Embryol Exp Morphol 1977; 41:209.
9. Winkelmann RK. The Merkel cell and comparison between it and the neurosecretory or APUD cell system. J Invest Dermatol 1977; 69:41.
10. Cohen RJ, Glezerson G, Taylor LF, et al. The neuroendocrine cell population of the human prostate gland. J Urol 1993; 150:365.
11. di Sant'Agnese PA, de Mesy Jensen KL. Endocrine-paracrine (APUD) cells of the human female urethra and paraurethral ducts. J Urol 1987; 137:1250.
12. Davidoff MS, Schulze W, Middendorff R, Holstein AF. The Leydig cell of the human testis: a new member of the diffuse neuroendocrine system. Cell Tissue Res 1993; 271:429.
13. Sternberger B. Immunocytochemistry. New York: John Wiley and Sons, 1979.
14. Peuschow JD, Haralambidis J, Darling PE, et al. Hybridization histochemistry. Experientia 1987; 43:741.
15. Torikata C, Mukai M, Kawakita H, Kageyama K. Neurofilaments of the Kulschitsky cells in human lung. Acta Pathol Jpn 1986; 36:93.
16. Njus D, Kelley PM, Harnadek GJ. The chromaffin vesicle: a model secretory organelle. Physiologist 1985; 28:235.
17. Hougard DM, Larsson L-I. Localization and possible function of polyamines in protein and peptide secreting cells. Med Biol 1986; 64:89.
18. Varnelli IM, Tapia FJ, Probert L, et al. Immunogold staining procedure for the localization of regulatory peptides. Peptides 1982; 3:259.
19. Stahlman MT, Gray ME. Colocalization of peptide hormones in neuroendocrine cells of human fetal and newborn lungs: an electron microscopic study. Anat Rec 1993; 236:206.
20. Navone F, Jahn R, DiGioia G, et al. Protein p38: an integral membrane protein specific for small vesicles of neurons and neuroendocrine cells. J Cell Biol 1986; 103:2511.
21. Buffa R, Guido V, Sessa F, et al. Synaptophysin immunoreactivity and small clear vesicles in neuroendocrine cells and related tumours. Mol Cell Probes 1988; 2:367.

22. Bishop AE, Polak JM, Facer P, et al. Neuron specific enolase: a common marker for the endocrine cells and innervation of the gut and pancreas. Gastroenterology 1982; 83:902.
23. Printz RA, Marangos PJ. Use of neuron-specific enolase as a serum marker for neuroendocrine neoplasms. Surgery 1982; 92:887.
24. Bunn PA Jr, Linnoila RI, Minna JD, et al. Small cell lung cancer, endocrine cells of the fetal bronchus, and other neuroendocrine cells express the Leu-7 antigenic determinant present on natural killer cells. Blood 1985; 65:764.
25. Ruff MR, Pert CB. Small cell carcinoma of the lung: macrophage-specific antigens suggest hematopoietic origin. Science 1984; 225:1034.
26. Blaschko H, Courline RS, Schneider FH, et al. Secretion of a chromaffin granule protein, chromogranin, from the adrenal gland after splanchnic stimulation. Nature 1967; 215:58.
27. Angeletti RH. Chromogranins and neuroendocrine secretion. Lab Invest 1986; 55:387.
28. Hagn C, Schmidt KW, Fischer-Colbrie R. Chromogranin A, B, and C in human adrenal medulla and endocrine tissues. Lab Invest 1986; 55:405.
29. Garcia GE, Gabbai FB, O'Connor DT, et al. Does chromostatin influence catecholamine release or blood pressure in vivo? Peptides 1994; 15:195.
30. Lauweryns JM, Van Ranst L. Immunocytochemical localization of aromatic L-amino acid decarboxylase in human, rat, and mouse broncho-pulmonary and gastrointestinal cells. J Histochem Cytochem 1988; 36:1181.
31. Erickson JD, Schafer MK, Bonner TI, et al. Distinct pharmacological properties and distribution in neurons and endocrine cells of two isoforms of the human vesicular monoamine transporter. Proc Natl Acad Sci U S A 1996; 93:166.
32. Griffiths JC. Creatine kinase isoenzyme 1. Clin Lab Med 1982; 2:493.
33. Inagaki H, Haimoto H, Hosoda S, Kato K. Aldolase C is localized in neuroendocrine cells. Experientia 1988; 44:749.
34. Jackson P, Thomson VM, Thompson RJ. A comparison of the evolutionary distribution of the two neuroendocrine markers, neurone-specific enolase and protein gene product 9.5. J Neurochem 1985; 45:185.
35. Lauweryns JM, Van Ranst L. Protein gene product 9.5 expression in the lungs of humans and other mammals: immunocytochemical detection in neuroepithelial bodies, neuroendocrine cells, and nerves. Neurosci Lett 1988; 85:311.
36. Lauweryns JM, Seldeslagh KA. Immunochemical expression of protein gene product 9.5 in the cat bronchopulmonary neuroendocrine cells and nerves. Anat Rec 1993; 236:191.
37. Seldeslagh KA, Lauweryns JM. NCAM expression in the pulmonary neural and diffuse neuroendocrine cell system. Microsc Res Tech 1997; 37:69.
38. Seldeslagh KA, Lauweryns JM. Spatial and temporal distribution of 7B2 in the pulmonary diffuse neuroendocrine system in the cat. Neurosci Lett 1995; 188:85.
39. Cutz E, Chan W, Track NS. Bombesin, calcitonin, and Leu-enkephalin immunoreactivity in endocrine cells of human lung. Experientia 1981; 37:765.
40. Franchimont P. Paracrine control. Clin Endocrinol Metab 1986; 15:1.
41. Goodland RA, Wright NA. Peptides and epithelial growth regulation. Experientia 1987; 43:780.
42. Ozawa S, Sand O. Electrophysiology of excitable endocrine cells. Physiol Rev 1986; 66:887.
43. Johansson S, Rydqvist B, Swerup C, et al. Action potential of cultured human oat cells: whole-cell measurement with the patch-clamp technique. Acta Physiol Scand 1989; 135:573.
44. Von Euler US, Gaddum JH. An unidentified substance in certain tissue extracts. J Physiol 1931; 72:74.
45. Burnstock G. The non-adrenergic non-cholinergic neuron systems. Arch Int Pharmacodyn Ther 1986; 280:1.
46. Hakanson R, Sundler F. The design of the neuroendocrine system: a unifying concept and its consequences. Trends Pharmacol Sci 1983; 4:41.
47. Wood JD. Physiology of the enteric nervous system. In: Johnson LR, ed. Physiology of the gastrointestinal tract. New York: Raven Press, 1987:67.
48. Ito T, Ohyama K, Kusano T, et al. Pulmonary endocrine cell hyperplasia and papilloma in rats induced by intratracheal injections of extract from particulate air pollutants. Exp Toxicol Pathol 1997; 49:65.
49. Fujita T, Kobayashi S. Current views on the paraneurone concept. Trends Neurosci 1979; 2:27.
50. Biscoe TJ. Carotid body: structure and function. Physiol Rev 1971; 51:437.
51. Lauweryns JM, von Lommel AT, Dom RJ. Innervation of rabbit intrapulmonary neuroepithelial bodies: quantitative and qualitative study after vagotomy. J Neurol Sci 1985; 67:81.
52. Whang KT, Steinwald PM, White JC, et al. Serum calcitonin precursors in sepsis and systemic inflammation. J Clin Endocrinol Metab 1998; 83:3296.
53. Linnoila IR. Pulmonary endocrine cells in vivo and in vitro. In: Kaliner MA, Barnes PJ, Kunkel G, Baraniuk, eds. Neuropeptides in the respiratory tract. New York: Marcel Dekker Inc, 1994:197.
54. Krenning EP, Kwekkeboom DJ, Reubi JC, et al. [111]Inoctreotide scintigraphy in oncology. Metabolism 1992; 41:83.
55. Virgolini I, Raderer M, Kurtaran A, et al. Vasoactive intestinal peptide-receptor imaging for the localization of intestinal adenocarcinomas and endocrine tumors. N Engl J Med 1994; 331:1116.
56. Seregni E, Chiti A, Bombardieri E. Radionuclide imaging of neuroendocrine tumours: biological basis and diagnostic results. Eur J Nucl Med 1998; 25:639.
57. Douglas AJ, Ludwig M. Quo vadis neurohypophysial hormone research? Exp Physiol 2000; 85:267S.

# CHAPTER 176

# THE ENDOCRINE BRAIN

ABBA J. KASTIN, WEIHONG PAN, JAMES E. ZADINA, AND WILLIAM A. BANKS

Considerable communication exists between peripheral hormones and the brain, both direct and indirect. This can involve selective saturable transport systems in the *blood–brain barrier* (BBB), which facilitate penetration of substances from blood to brain and from brain to blood in addition to communication by simple diffusion.

Peripheral production of hormones does not arise exclusively in ductless "endocrine" organs. The word *hormone* originated with a gastrointestinal hormone—secretin—discovered almost a hundred years ago[1] followed shortly thereafter by discovery of the second hormone, gastrin (see Chap. 167). More recently, the confining definition of hormone was expanded by the finding that a substance produced in fat cells—leptin—is saturably transported into the brain to reach its receptors in the hypothalamus.[2]

The endocrine brain includes peptides and polypeptides, such as leptin and cytokines, and steroids, such as dehydroepiandrosterone.[3] Receptors for many other substances, including steroids, are located in selected areas throughout the brain, and these areas are not necessarily involved in synthesis. Such recent findings reinforce the older concept of the extraendocrine effects of hormones in the classic sense and emphasize the importance of the endocrine brain.[4]

## MECHANISMS OF INTERACTIONS (TABLE 176-1)

The brain acts as both a major target for hormones and as a source of secretion of regulatory substances into the blood. Interactions between brain and blood are complicated because of the presence of the BBB, which is composed of a monolayer of cells between the central nervous system (CNS) and blood.[5] The vascular component of the BBB exists because the endothelial cells comprising the brain capillaries and lining the arterioles and venules are modified to limit the unregulated influx of substances into the CNS. The major modification is the existence of tight junctions between adjacent endothelial cells, which effectively eliminates interendothelial gaps and therefore the production of a plasma ultrafiltrate. The choroid plexus forms the "blood–CSF barrier," consisting of epithelial cells that also are joined by tight junctions, so that functionally there are similarities in these barriers. Humorally mediated communication between the CNS and peripheral tissues must negotiate these arms of the BBB for effective endocrine-like communication to occur.

Blood-borne substances can affect brain function through at least five broad categories of mechanisms. First, hormones can affect afferent neural transmission as exemplified by some actions of cholecystokinin (CCK) on feeding and of cytokines on some aspects of sickness behavior.[6,7] Second, they can modify the blood levels of another substance that crosses the BBB to affect brain function directly, as exemplified by insulin-induced coma mediated through hypoglycemia or by adrenocorticotropic hormone (ACTH) release of glucocorticoids. Third, they can act at the circumventricular organs (CVOs), areas of the CNS that are deficient in classic BBB function but have their own barriers, with subsequent relay of information to the rest of the CNS. Some of the effects of angiotensin on thirst are mediated through this mechanism.[8] Fourth, hor-

**TABLE 176-1.**
**Central Nervous System Effects of Peptides**

| Peptide | Examples of Central Nervous System Effects* | Peptide | Examples of Central Nervous System Effects* |
|---|---|---|---|
| ACTH | Modulates stress-related effects; decreases food ingestion and GI motility; increases grooming and vocalization; neuroprotective | MCH | Increases feeding |
| | | MIF-1 | Endogenous opiate antagonist; decreases aggression; facilitates maturation of EEG spectra |
| Adreno-medullin | Decreases food ingestion | Melanocortin | Decreases feeding and fever; enhances learning and memory (especially attention); influences neuronal differentiation; neuroprotective |
| Amylin | Decreases food ingestion and locomotor activity | | |
| ANP | Affects cardiovascular system and salt/water balance | Morphiceptin | Analgesic |
| AgRP | Increases food ingestion | Motilin | Decreases anxiety; increases food ingestion |
| ATII | Modulates cerebral circulation; induces water drinking; inhibits long-term potentiation | MPF | Neuronal protection |
| | | Neo-kyotor-phin | Analgesic |
| Bombesin | Increases α and β waves and decreases slow waves in EEG; reduces food and salt ingestion and gastric acid secretion | Neuromedin | Increases aggression; increases self-stimulation reward; decreases food ingestion |
| Calcitonin | Analgesic; decreases food ingestion, gastric acid secretion, and intestinal motility | NEI | Increases exploration; stimulates antinociception; decreases osmoregulation |
| CART | Decreases food ingestion | NPFF | Antiopiate; decreases food ingestion |
| β-Casomor-phin | Analgesic; increases fat ingestion | NPY | Increases food ingestion; decreases spontaneous activity; affects phase shifts of circadian rhythm; decreases social stress; thermoregulation |
| CCK | Decreases food ingestion; opiate antagonist; may decrease or enhance memory | | |
| CGRP | Pain transmitter; decreases food ingestion | Neurotensin | Decreases GI motility, locomotor activity, and food ingestion; analgesic; hypothermic; potentiates reward; affects sensory transmission and cardiovascular system |
| CLIP | Increases paradoxical sleep | | |
| CNP | Cardiovascular pressor response; vasodilation | | |
| CRH | Modulates stress-related effects; possibly increases depression and anxiety; decreases food ingestion, gastric acid secretion, and GI motility; increases temperature | Nociceptin | Opiate agonist and antagonist |
| | | ODN | Induces anxiety |
| | | Orexin | Increases feeding; deficiency related to narcolepsy |
| | | Oxytocin | Facilitates reproductive, maternal, and social behavior |
| Cyclo(His-Pro) | Decreases food ingestion; hyperthermia | PACAP | Increases heart rate; decreases water drinking and feeding; neuroprotective |
| Deltorphin | Analgesic | | |
| Dermorphin | Analgesic; hypothermia in cold; hyperthermia in heat | Pancreastatin | Enhances memory |
| DSIP | Increases growth hormone release; may increase sleep; enhances hypothermia | PP | Cardiovascular effects; decreases food ingestion |
| | | Peptide T | Neuroprotective |
| Dynorphin | Analgesic; decreases activity and food ingestion | PYY | Induces emesis; vasoconstriction of cerebral blood vessels; increases food intake |
| EGF | Decreases activity and water drinking; increases temperature | | |
| Eledoisin | Decreases blood pressure | Sauvagine | Decreases aggression; decreases feeding and social behavior |
| β-Endorphin | Analgesic; involved in seizures, sexual behavior, and neuronal differentiation; thermoregulative changes | SRIF | Increases REM sleep; analgesic; modulates taste/nutrient preference |
| Endomor-phins | Analgesic; highly selective for μ opiate receptor | Substance P | Pain transmitter; attenuates seizures; increases grooming |
| Endothelin | Increases blood pressure and heart rate | Tachykinin | Inhibits alcohol and water intake; increases salivation |
| Enkephalin | Analgesic; decreases water drinking and feeding | Thermal peptide | Enhances memory |
| Enterostatin | Decreases fat intake and weight | | |
| FMRFamide | Opiate antagonist | TRH | Arousal effects; increases temperature, ventilation, and vocalization |
| Galanin | Decreases food ingestion; improves memory | | |
| GHRH | Increases slow wave sleep and food ingestion | Tyr-MIF-1 | Opiate agonist and antagonist; decreases aggression |
| GHRPs | Regulate circadian rhythm; stimulate growth hormone secretion | Tyr-W-MIF-1 | Opiate agonist and antagonist |
| | | Urocortin | Effects similar to CRH, including appetite suppression and vasodilation |
| GLP-1 | Decreases food ingestion | | |
| Glucagon | Decreases food ingestion | Urotensin | Effects similar to CRH |
| GRP | Stimulates gastrin release | Vasopressin | Enhances attention, cognition, learning, emotion, and grooming; decreases water drinking; hypothermic |
| Hemorphin | Analgesic | | |
| Kassinin | Decreases water ingestion | Vasotocin | Increases blood pressure |
| Kentsin | Analgesic; decreases GI motility | VIP | Decreases activity, mean arterial pressure, and memory; increases heart rate, cardiac output, and electrical discharge; induces sleep |
| Leptin | Decreases feeding | | |
| LHRH | Increases mating behavior | | |

*ACTH*, adrenocorticotropic hormone (corticotropin); *ANP*, atrial natriuretic peptide; *AgRP*, agouti-related protein; *ATII*, angiotensin II; *CART*, cocaine- and amphetamine-related transcript; *CCK*, cholecystokinin; *CGRP*, calcitonin gene-related peptide; *CLIP*, corticotropin-like intermediate lobe peptide; *CNP*, C-type natriuretic peptide; *CNS*, central nervous system; *CRH*, corticotropin-releasing hormone; *DSIP*, delta sleep-inducing peptide; *EGF*, epidermal growth factor; *FMRFamide*, Phe-Met-Arg-Phe-NH$_2$; *GHRH*, growth hormone–releasing hormone; *GHRP*, growth hormone–releasing peptide; *GLP*, glucagon-like peptide; *GRP*, gastrin-releasing peptide; *LHRH*, luteinizing hormone–releasing hormone; *MCH*, melanin-concentrating hormone; *MIF-1*, melanocyte-stimulating hormone release-inhibiting factor-1; *MPF*, melanotropin-potentiating factor; *NEI*, neuropeptide E-I; *NPFF*, neuropeptide FF; *NPY*, neuropeptide Y; *ODN*, octadecaneuropeptide; *PACAP*, pituitary adenylate cyclase–activating polypeptide; *PP*, pancreatic polypeptide; *PYY*, peptide YY; *SRIF*, somatotropin release-inhibiting factor (somatostatin); *TRH*, thyrotropin-releasing hormone; *Tyr-MIF-1*, Tyr-Pro-Leu-Gly-NH$_2$; *Tyr-W-MIF-1*, Tyr-Pro-Trp-Gly-NH$_2$; *VIP*, vasoactive intestinal peptide.

*Based mainly on compilation from Pan W, Kastin AJ, Banks WA, Zadina JE. Effects of peptides: a cross-listing of peptides and their central actions published in the journal Peptides from 1994 through 1998. Peptides 1999; 20:1127.

mones can alter the permeability of the BBB to other substances, as exemplified by the ability of arginine vasopressin (AVP) and amylin to change amino-acid transport into the CNS.[9,10] Fifth, some hormones, including peptides (<100 amino acids), polypeptides (100–200 amino acids), and even small proteins (>200 amino acids), can directly cross the BBB in amounts sufficient to affect CNS functioning. Such direct passage can occur by diffusion through the endothelial and epithelial cell membranes that compose the BBB, as in the case of steroid hormones such as testosterone and cortisol, or by specific saturable transport systems, as in the case of thyroid hormones[11,12] and many peptides and polypeptides.[13,14]

Secretion of hormones in the opposite direction, from brain into blood, also can be classified into broad categories. The best defined is that of secretion into the hypothalamic-pituitary portal circulation. A second mechanism occurs by the bulk flow that characterizes the reabsorption of cerebrospinal fluid (CSF) into the blood. Any substance found in the CSF will enter the blood in this manner and, when CSF levels are high and the peripheral pharmacokinetics are favorable, this can lead to high sustained levels in blood. The best examples of this mechanism are provided by cytokines, which can be expressed at very high levels by CNS tissue during infection.[15] A third mechanism is drainage of CSF via the primitive lymphatics in the brain, which provides a direct route from brain to the cervical lymph nodes. This mechanism has been associated with CNS immunization, a phenomenon by which peripheral immune responses are greatly modified by the administration of antigens directly into the CNS.[16] Fourth, substances can cross the elements of the BBB in the CNS-to-blood direction by either saturable or nonsaturable mechanisms. As much as 50% of plasma methionine enkephalin may be derived from the brain by this mechanism, and corticotropin-releasing hormone (CRH) is secreted directly from brain into blood in amounts that can alter splenic production of β-endorphin.[17,18]

These pathways, including the saturable transport systems for hormones found at the BBB, can be modified by endocrine disease and by disease that affects the endocrine system. In other situations, as illustrated by obesity, disease may be explained by the dysfunction of these mechanisms or interactions.

## INGESTION

Ingestion is a complex of behaviors that includes seeking, acquisition, selection, regulation of rate and amount of ingestion (oral metering), and integration with other behaviors, such as social interactions, storage, and defecation. Food selection and aspects of oral metering are of particular interest to endocrinologists because of their role in the control of body weight (see Chap. 125). However, dysregulation of thirst, cravings, and other aspects of ingestion also are encountered in endocrine diseases.

An increasing emphasis is being placed on the ability of hormones, especially peptides, polypeptides, and small proteins, to control ingestion by acting on the CNS. For example, cytokines, such as tumor necrosis factor-α (TNF-α), are implicated in the anorexia of infection and cancer. CCK, thyrotropin-releasing hormone (TRH), somatostatin, and glucagon probably affect feelings of satiety, hunger, and food selection through interactions at the vagus nerve and CVOs. AVP, angiotensin II, and aldosterone affect drinking, probably by acting at CVOs. Angiotensin II, tachykinins, testosterone, and aldosterone may affect the craving for salt, natriuresis, and atrial natriuretic peptide release through CNS-mediated mechanisms.[19] Alcohol ingestion is inversely related to brain levels of methionine enkephalin and serotonin.

Recent attention has focused on insulin, leptin, agouti-related protein (AgRP), CART (cocaine- and amphetamine-regulated transcript), and, to a lesser extent, pancreatic polypeptide to modulate feeding. These substances may act within the CNS to alter levels of neuropeptides and neurotransmitters that stimulate feeding (e.g., opiates, galanin, norepinephrine, peptide YY, motilin, and especially neuropeptide Y[19a]). Although receptors and degradative enzymes for insulin, leptin, and pancreatic polypeptide are found throughout the CNS, these substances do not seem to be synthesized within the CNS. Instead, their source is in peripheral tissues, so that these substances must cross the BBB to exert their effects.

Leptin is secreted by fat cells and crosses the BBB by a saturable transport mechanism to inhibit CNS-mediated feeding (see Chaps. 125 and 186). A direct correlation exists between the amount of body fat and serum leptin levels. In humans, obesity is associated with high concentrations of leptin in the serum but low concentrations in the CSF and, therefore, is thought to represent a leptin-resistant state. Evidence suggests that this resistance may be explained by a decreased ability of leptin to cross the BBB.

## NEUROIMMUNOENDOCRINOLOGY

Modulation of the neuroimmune axis by hormones is increasingly recognized. Classic studies have shown that steroid hormones and peptides such as α-MSH (melanocyte-stimulating hormone) and the endogenous opiates affect immune cell function. At least some of the effects on the CNS are likely mediated by cytokines derived from blood.[13] Cytokines, CRH, and the enkephalins produced by brain can modulate peripheral immune events after their secretion into blood and may underlie the phenomenon of CNS immunization. Cytokines secreted from immune cells or by brain have been shown to affect fever, feeding, and aspects of sickness behavior (see Chap. 173). These substances also may affect CNS events under conditions in which infection is absent, as exemplified by the effects of TNF and granulocyte and macrophage colony-stimulating factor (GM-CSF) on physiologic sleep.

## SLEEP

Among the CNS processes not well understood, sleep is probably the most obvious, since we spend approximately one-third of our life sleeping. Although theories abound, the purpose of sleep is still not known. Moreover, it also is not clear what substance(s) are primarily involved in causing sleep.

The substances for which sleep-promoting properties have been well studied include delta sleep-inducing peptide (DSIP), phosphorylated DSIP, factor S, muramyl peptides, sleep-promoting substance, cytokines (such as TNF, interleukin-1, and interferon), and oxidized glutathione. Most recently, GM-CSF and macrophage-CSF have been shown to induce rapid eye movement (REM) as well as non-REM sleep without the co-occurrence of pyrogenic responses.

Evidence also exists that sleep can be induced by several of the classic hormones, the best established being growth hormone (GH), growth hormone–releasing hormone (GHRH), and prolactin. Since postprandial satiety can induce sleepiness, there are reports that satiety-inducing peptides such as CCK and bombesin can induce sleep, as can acidic fibroblast growth factor (aFGF) and vasoactive intestinal peptide (VIP).

The sleep substances illustrate several principles involved in many aspects of the endocrine brain. These include the multiple actions of peptides,[20] the misleading nature of constrictive nomenclature,[21] and the inverted U-shaped dose-response curve.[22]

## LEARNING

The major hormones involved in investigations of learning have been AVP and MSH. Although much work was done with AVP, the early results were confounded by its cardiovascular and endocrine effects. The use of the AVP analog 1-desamino-D-arginine vasopressin (DDAVP) obviated the confounding effects, but the results are still inconclusive, although there appears to be a modest facilitation of memory.[23] The related posterior pituitary hormone oxytocin may also affect the recognition aspect of learning.[24]

It was the early studies with MSH that showed peptide hormones can affect attention, the processing of information before it becomes memory. Unlike most experimental situations, this was shown in humans[25] before it was confirmed in several animal studies.[20]

Learning provides another good example of the endocrine brain, where a renin-angiotensin system also exists. Not only are all the enzymes and peptides necessary for angiotensin II present in the brain, but also specific angiotensin II receptors are found in the amygdala and hippocampus. Angiotensin II blocks long-term potentiation (LTP), a neuronal model of learning.[26,27]

## DEVELOPMENT OF THE BRAIN

Circulating hormones play a critical role in normal brain development. One of the most dramatic examples of this phenomenon is the role of gonadal steroid hormones. In adult animals, androgens and estrogens activate neural and endocrine events leading to successful reproduction. At critically timed periods in development, these steroids can change neural structures in ways that dramatically affect their later responsiveness to the steroids.[28] This critical period occurs around the time of birth in the rat, and between the fourth and seventh month of fetal life in the human. Stress during this period can interfere with development.

Genetic programs induce differentiation of primordial gonadal tissue into either testes or ovaries. Subsequent hormonal secretions, especially androgen from the testes, determine whether neural structures regulating endocrine and behavioral functions will become male or female. Genetically female rats injected with androgen during the critical period show an adult pattern of luteinizing hormone–releasing hormone (LHRH) secretion that is tonic (normal male pattern) rather than cyclic (normal female pattern). As a consequence, the female is no longer able to ovulate, and androgen in adulthood induces male reproductive behavioral patterns.

Conversely, for male rats castrated during the critical period, the pattern of LHRH release shifts from tonic to cyclic. Ovaries implanted in these animals as adults show female-typical cycles, and their reproductive behavior in response to estrogen is the stereotypical female pattern. Manipulation of the androgen levels at a time other than the critical period does not produce these dramatic results. Thus, neural mechanisms for both the control of LHRH release and complex reproductive behaviors are profoundly affected by the hormonal milieu present in a specific, critical period of development of the nervous system.

Although usually not as dramatic as steroid effects, many peptides administered to developing animals also have been shown to affect brain development and later function. These include TRH (which causes emotionality in later life); fragments and analogs of MSH and ACTH that affect various tasks related to leaning, memory, and attention in later life; and opiate peptides.[29–31] The administration of β-endorphin to rats at about the time of birth alters sensitivity to heat-induced pain, brain opiate receptors, social and sexual behavior, attention, learning, and activity. CRH given to neonatal rats dramatically changes growth and eye opening as well as plasma and adrenal corticosterone concentrations seen in later development. As adults, these animals show altered behavior in an open field. Injections of substance P to neonatal rats produce a long-term increase in the sensitivity of the animals to pain,[32] and neonatal AVP induces a long-lasting deficit in the ability of the kidney to respond to AVP.[33]

Thus, the concentrations of hormonal steroids and peptides during development can permanently affect the responsiveness to them in adulthood. It appears that a delicate balance of these molecules during the formative period of the CNS can have profound and long-lasting effects on brain development.

## REPRODUCTION

There is probably no area of behavioral physiology in which hormones play so commanding a role as in reproductive behavior. In addition to the well-established effects of gonadal hormones on animal reproductive behavior, brain-derived peptides normally associated with regulation of gonadal hormones also have been implicated in direct actions on behavior. LHRH, a hypothalamic peptide that regulates pituitary control of gonadal steroids, can directly induce the stereotypic mating posture called *lordosis* in female rats. This was shown in animals given estrogen in doses too low to induce the posture, and in animals with pituitaries removed, indicating that the effect of LHRH occurred directly on the brain rather than through the pituitary-gonadal axis.[34,35] The regulation of both behavioral and gonadal function by LHRH is normally synchronized for successful reproduction. The independence of the mechanisms of these actions, however, was demonstrated with some analogs of LHRH. Although most analogs have either agonist or antagonist effects for both gonadal and behavioral functions, some analogs could block ovulation while enhancing behavior, and for others, the opposite is true.[36] This indicates separate as well as concerted actions at the brain and pituitary.

Other peptides also are involved in mating and reproductive function. Opiate peptides, for example, can inhibit or abolish elements of male copulatory behavior.[31,37] CRH, acting at least in part through an opiate mechanism, can inhibit lordosis.[37] MSH and ACTH also affect lordosis. Thus, even with behaviors for which the requirements for steroid hormones have been extensively documented, a new understanding of hormonal influences on brain function is being discovered in parallel with the ongoing discovery of new peptides in the endocrine brain.

## PAIN

Pain normally serves a protective function by warning of tissue damage. Anecdotal experience from wars, childbirth, and dental operations, however, indicates that the perception of pain can be dramatically altered by situational variables. In addition, many pathologic states can produce chronic pain that persists beyond the duration of tissue damage, negating its protective function. There is considerable plasticity and complexity in the neural mechanisms that modulate the perception and emotional reaction to pain.

Peptide transmitters and hormones play a critical role in the perception of pain. Peptides with excitatory effects on cells, such as substance P and calcitonin gene–related peptide (CGRP), are involved in the transmission of nociceptive signals that, at higher centers, are perceived as pain. Like the plant alkaloid morphine, however, endogenous opiate peptides inhibit the excitability of neurons that mediate pain perception. Endogenous opiate peptides consist of three families of peptides that have been known for ~20 years (enkephalins, dynorphins, and β-endorphin)[38] and the more recently discovered endomorphins[39] (see Chap. 168). Three known receptors, cloned in the early 1990s, mediate the effects of these peptides. Enkephalin, the first discovered opiate peptide, preferentially binds to the δ receptor, and dynorphin is considered the natural agonist for the κ receptor. β-Endorphin, the major blood-borne opiate, binds equally well to the μ (morphine) and δ receptors. The endomorphins are highly selective for the μ receptor, the receptor most involved in modulating pain.

Several areas in the CNS contain high concentrations of opiate peptides and their receptors, and are sensitive to exogenously administered opiates. Electrical stimulation of some of these areas produces a suppression of nociceptive dorsal horn neurons and, consequently, causes analgesia. The ability to block this analgesia with an opiate antagonist provided one of the early indications that opiates are present endogenously. In the brainstem, these areas include the periaqueductal gray and the rostral ventromedial medulla. Primary afferent neurons that transmit pain signals from the periphery to the CNS have their first synapse in the outer layers of the dorsal horn of the spinal cord. This area is rich in μ opiate receptors and is an important site for the analgesic actions of morphine. This area also is rich in endomorphin, which may naturally modulate pain perception at this early stage in neural processing. Nerve injury and inflammation lead to extensive plasticity in the expression of many peptides in this area, often leading to hyperexcitability of neurons and chronic pain.[40]

Many peptides have been shown to have bidirectional effects on pain or to modulate or antagonize the effects of morphine or stress on pain responses. First shown with melanocyte-stimulating hormone release-inhibiting factor-1 (MIF-1; Pro-Leu-Gly-NH₂), these peptides include Tyr-MIF-1 (Tyr-Pro-Leu-Gly-NH₂), Tyr-W-MIF-1 (Tyr-Pro-Trp-Gly-NH₂), CCK-8, MSH, FMRF-NH₂, neuropeptide FF, β-endorphin when cleaved to its 1-27 fragment, and orphanin FQ/nociceptin. This last peptide is the endogenous ligand for a receptor (ORL) that was cloned based on homology to the opiate receptors. Most of these peptides exert their opiate antagonist properties by acting at sites other than the opiate receptor, regulating signaling pathways that counteract the effects of opiates.[40a] Others, including Tyr-MIF-1 and Tyr-W-MIF-1, can act at the opiate receptor and, depending on the state of the tissue (e.g., opiate naive or opiate tolerant), can act as agonists or antagonists.[41] Antiopiate peptides could, therefore, play a role in opiate tolerance and dependence by at least two mechanisms: (a) occupancy of opiate receptors with less efficacy than morphine (partial agonist), or (b) action at non-opiate sites with cellular effects that counteract opiates.[42] These processes, alone or in combination, could provide a dynamic, wide range for control of pain perception, emphasizing the influence of peptides and hormones on the functioning of the endocrine brain.

## REFERENCES

1. Bayliss VM, Starling EH. The mechanism of pancreatic secretion. J Physiol 1902; 28:325.
2. Banks WA, Kastin AJ, Huang W, et al. Leptin enters the brain by a saturable system independent of insulin. Peptides 1996; 17:305.
3. Zwain IH, Yen SC. Dehydroepiandrosterone: biosynthesis and metabolism in the brain. J Clin Metab Endocrinol 1999; 140:880.
4. Kastin AJ, Plotnikoff NP, Nair RMG, et al. MIF: its pituitary and extra-pituitary effects. In: Gual C, Rosemberg E, eds. Hypothalamic hypophysiotropic hormones: clinical and physiological studies. Amsterdam: Excerpt Med Int Congr Series no. 263, 1972:159.
5. Davson H, Segal MB. Morphological aspects of the barriers. In: Physiology of the CSF and blood-brain barriers. Boca Raton, FL: CRC Press, 1996:93.
6. Dantzer R, Kelley KW. Stress and immunity: an integrated view of relationships between the brain and the immune system. Life Sci 1989; 44:1995.
7. Smith GP, Gibbs J, Jerome C, et al. The satiety effect of cholecystokinin: a progress report. Peptides 1981; 2(Suppl 2):57.
8. Johnson AK, Gross PM. Sensory circumventricular organs and brain homeostatic pathways. FASEB J 1993; 7:678.
9. Brust P. Changes in regional blood-brain transfer of L-leucine elicited by arginine-vasopressin. J Neurochem 1986; 46:534.
10. Chance WT, Balasubramaniam A, Thomas I, Fischer JE. Amylin increases transport of tyrosine and tryptophan into the brain. Brain Res 1992; 593:20.
11. Davson H, Segal MB. Special aspects of the blood-brain barrier. In: Physiology of the CSF and blood-brain barriers. Boca Raton: CRC Press, 1996:303.
12. Nilsson C, Lindvall-Axelsson M, Owman C. Neuroendocrine regulatory mechanisms in the choroid plexus-cerebrospinal fluid system. Brain Res Rev 1992; 17:109.
13. Banks WA, Kastin AJ, Broadwell RD. Passage of cytokines across the blood-brain barrier. Neuroimmunomodulation 1995; 2:241.
14. Banks WA, Kastin AJ. Passage of peptides across the blood-brain barrier: pathophysiological perspectives. Life Sci 1996; 59:1923.
15. Romero LI, Ildiko K, Lechan RM, Reichlin S. Interleukin-6 (IL-6) is secreted from the brain after intracerebroventricular injection of IL-1 beta in rats. Am J Physiol 1996; 270:R518.
16. Cserr HF, Knopf PM. Cervical lymphatics, the blood-brain barrier and the immunoreactivity of the brain: a new view. Immunol Today 1992; 13:507.
17. Banks WA, Kastin AJ. The role of the blood-brain barrier transporter PTS-1 in regulating concentrations of methionine enkephalin in blood and brain. Alcohol 1997; 14:237.
18. Martins JM, Banks WA, Kastin AJ. Transport of CRH from mouse brain directly affects peripheral production of β-endorphin by the spleen. Am J Physiol 1997; 273:E1083.
19. Epstein AN. Neurohormonal control of salt intake in the rat. Brain Res Bull 1991; 27:315.
19a. Polidoni C, Ciccocioppo R, Regoli D, Massi M. Neuropeptide Y receptor(s) mediating feeding in the rat: characterization with antagonists. Peptides 2000; 21:29.
20. Kastin AJ, Olson RD, Sandman CA, et al. Multiple independent actions of neuropeptides on behavior. In: Martinez JL, Jensen RA, Messing RB, et al., eds. Endogenous peptides and learning memory processes. New York: Academic Press, 1981:563.
21. Kastin AJ, Banks WA, Zadina JE, Graf MV. Brain peptides: the dangers of constricted nomenclatures. Life Sci 1983; 32:295.
22. Kastin AJ, Banks WA, Olson RD, Zadina JE. Novel concepts from novel peptides. Ann NY Acad Sci 1994; 739:1.
23. Beckwith BE, Petros TV, Bergloff PJ, et al. Failure of posttrial administration of vasopressin analogue (DDAVP) to influence memory in healthy, young, male volunteers. Peptides 1995; 16:1327.
24. Dluzen DE, Muraoka S, Engelmann M, Landgraf R. The effects of infusion of arginine vasopressin, oxytocin, or their antagonists into the olfactory bulb upon social recognition responses in male rats. Peptides 1998; 19:999.
25. Kastin AJ, Miller LH, Gonzalez-Barcena D, et al. Psycho-physiological correlates of MSH activity in man. Physiol Behav 1971; 7:893.
26. Armstrong DL, Garcia EA, Ma T, et al. Angiotensin-II blockade of long-term potentiation at the perforant path-granule cell synapse in-vitro. Peptides 1996; 17:689.
27. von Bohlen und Halbach O, Albrecht D. Angiotensin II inhibits long-term potentiation within the lateral nucleus of the amygdala through AT$_1$ receptors. Peptides 1998; 19:1031.
28. Goy RJ, McEwen BS. Sexual differentiation of the brain. Cambridge, MA: MIT Press, 1980.
29. Sandman CA, Kastin AJ. The influence of fragments of the LPH chains on learning, memory and attention in animals and man. Pharmacol Ther 1981; 13:39.
30. Zadina JE, Kastin AJ, Coy DH, Adinoff BA. Developmental, behavioral, and opiate receptor changes after prenatal or postnatal β-endorphin, CRF, or Tyr-MIF-1. Psychoneuroendocrinology 1985; 10:367.
31. Meyerson BJ. Influence of early β-endorphin treatment on the behavior and reaction to β-endorphin in the adult male rat. Psychoneuroendocrinology 1985; 10:135.
32. Handelmann GE, Selsky JH, Helke CJ. Substance P administration to neonatal rats increases adult sensitivity to substance P. Physiol Behav 1984; 33:297.
33. Handelmann GE, Russell JT, Gainer H, et al. Vasopressin administration to neonatal rats reduces antidiuretic response to adult kidneys. Peptides 1983; 4:827.
34. Moss RL, McCann SM. Induction of mating behavior in rats by luteinizing hormone-releasing factor. Science 1973; 181:177.
35. Pfaff DW. Luteinizing hormone-releasing factor potentiates lordosis behavior in hypophysectomized ovariectomized female rats. Science 1973; 182:1148.
36. Zadina JE, Kastin AJ. Multi-independent actions of peptides in the brain: LHRH, MIF-1 and CRF. Am Zool 1986; 26:951.
37. Sirinathsinghji DJS. Modulation of lordosis behavior in the female rat by corticotropin releasing factor, β-endorphin and gonadotropin releasing hormone in the mesencephalic central gray. Brain Res 1985; 336:45.
38. Terenius L. The endogenous opioids and other central peptides. In: Melzack R, Wall PD, eds. Textbook of pain. New York: Churchill Livingstone, 1984:133.
39. Zadina JE, Hackler L, Ge L-J, Kastin AJ. A potent and selective endogenous agonist for the μ-opiate receptor. Nature 1997; 386:499.
40. Dubner R, Basbaum AI. Spinal dorsal horn plasticity following tissue or nerve injury. In: Wall PD, Melzack R, Edinburgh R, eds. Textbook of pain, 3rd ed. New York: Churchill Livingstone, 1994:225.
40a. Calo G, Guerrini R, Rizzi A. Pharmacology of nociceptin and its receptor: a novel therapeutic target. Br J Pharmacol 2000; 129:1261.
41. Zadina JE, Kastin AJ, Kersh D, Wyatt A. Tyr-MIF-1 and hemorphin can act as opiate agonists as well as antagonists in the guinea pig ileum. Life Sci 1992; 51:869.
42. Harrison LM, Kastin AJ, Zadina JE. Opiate tolerance and dependence: receptors, G-proteins, and antiopiates. Peptides 1998; 19:1603.

# CHAPTER 177

# THE ENDOCRINE LUNG

KENNETH L. BECKER

## ANATOMY AND PHYSIOLOGY

The lungs have unique topographic, anatomic, and metabolic characteristics.[1,2] They possess a huge interface between the outside environment and the body, facilitating their function as organs of gaseous exchange that are responsible for the oxygenation of all body tissues. The enormous, distensible, low-resistance vasculature of the lungs receives the entire systemic venous output of the body by the pulmonary artery and bears the responsibility for its arterialization. The hepatic venous blood joins the inferior vena cava near the right side of the heart, bringing hepatic metabolic products directly to the lungs. The thoracic duct carries gastrointestinal chylomicrons to the superior vena cava, to the heart, and to the lungs. Innumerable changes in pleural pressure subject the lungs to expansion and relaxation to draw air into the bronchial tree and to facilitate the systemic inflow of venous blood into the heart. A great diversity of cell types accomplishes these physiologic functions. Finally, the left side of the heart pumps the oxygenated blood from the lungs to all tissues throughout the body.

## METABOLIC ACTIVITIES

The lungs are enormous endocrine organs.[3] Metabolically, the lungs degrade, modify, or activate many substances that arrive from the systemic venous circulation. The vast surface area of the pulmonary endothelium provides the enzymatic machinery required to inactivate some of the prostaglandins and other arachidonic acid metabolites. Other bioactive hormonal substances, such as serotonin, norepinephrine, and bradykinin, are metabolized intracellularly by the lungs. Moreover, the relatively inactive substance, angiotensin I, which is formed within the blood by the action of renin on angiotensinogen, is hydrolyzed within the pulmonary endothelium to form the active angiotensin II. Other metabolic functions of the lung include steroid transformations and lipolysis.

## ENDOCRINE ACTIVITIES

The lungs generate many hormones that act on cells and tissues within the lung and that also influence other tissues.[3,4] These pulmonary hormones, none of which is unique to the lungs, include the *biogenic amines,* the *arachidonic acid and other cell membrane phospholipid metabolites,* and *peptides.* Depending on the hormone and its site, the stimuli that induce the release of these various chemical messengers may be intraluminal stimuli (e.g., inspired air), mechanical stimuli (e.g., inhaled dusts), neural stimuli (e.g., vagal or sympathetic nerves), chemical perturbation of adjacent tissues (e.g., acidosis), or blood-borne hormonal stimuli from distant tissues (e.g., catecholamines). These released hormones may stimulate, inhibit, modulate, or integrate their effector cells. Within the lungs, they may alter regional blood flow, dilate or contract bronchial smooth muscle, influence mucous gland activity, change vascular permeability, modify the metabolism of adjacent pulmonary cells, or influence cellular secretion or cellular proliferation.

### BIOGENIC AMINES

Biogenic amines include serotonin, dopamine, norepinephrine, epinephrine, and histamine. Two related substances are acetylcholine and γ-aminobutyric acid (Fig. 177-1). Most of these sub-

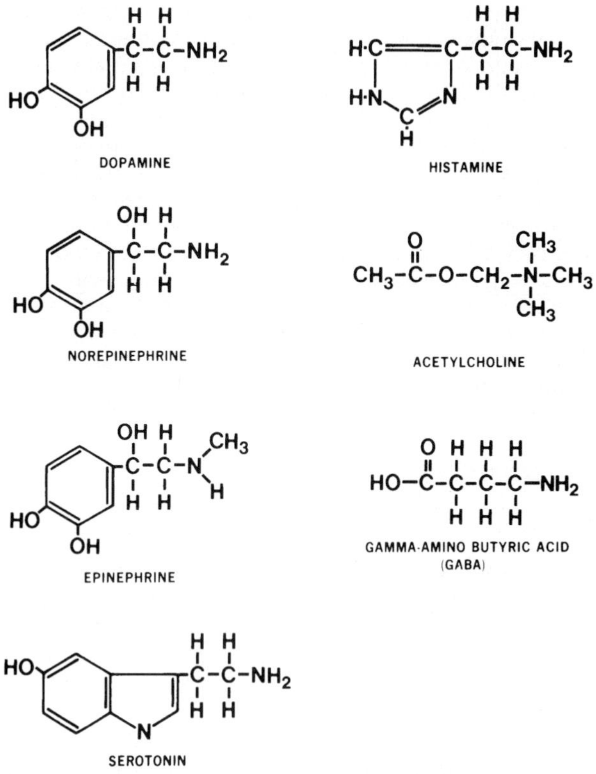

**FIGURE 177-1.** Structure of several of the nonpeptide neurotransmitters and bioactive derivatives. (From Becker KL. The endocrine lung. In: Becker KL, Gazdar AF, eds. The endocrine lung in health and disease. Philadelphia: WB Saunders, 1984:5.)

stances can act as neurotransmitters (Fig. 177-2), and some also are contained within the synaptosomes of neurons and within the secretion granules of endocrine cells. The biogenic amines may be detectable in the peripheral blood of normal persons, and their levels are increased in various pathologic conditions. Within the lung, the biogenic amines function as potent paracrine or hemocrine hormones.

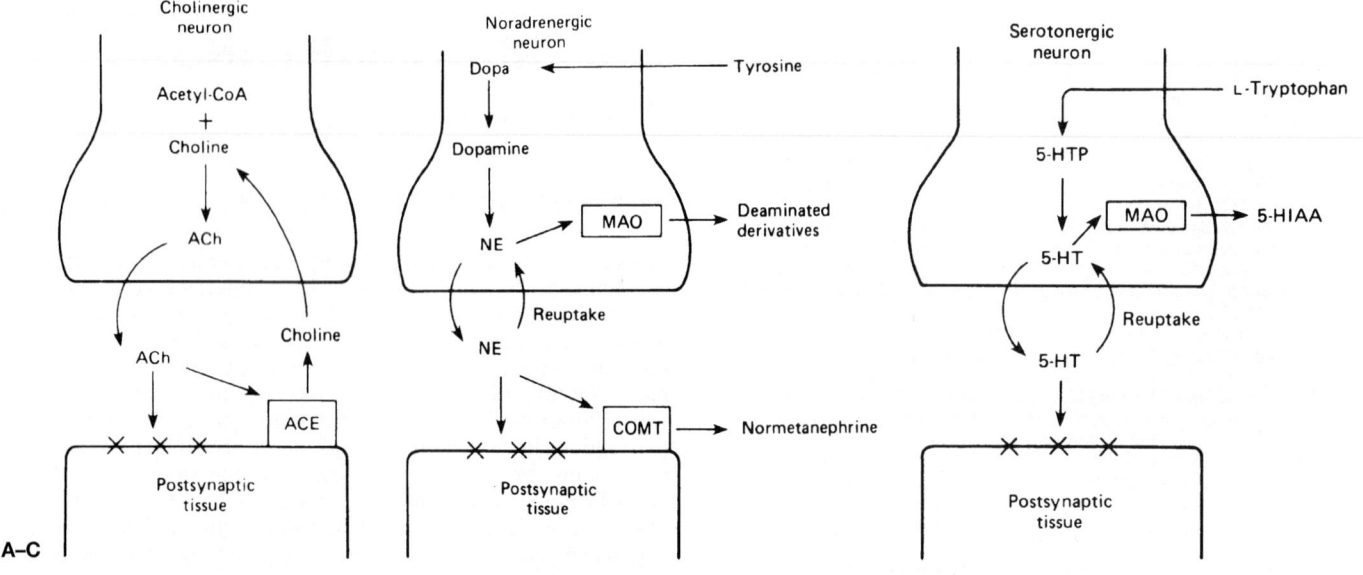

**FIGURE 177-2.** Biochemical events occurring at synapses that involve some of the biogenic amines. **A,** Cholinergic neuron. **B,** Noradrenergic neuron. **C,** Serotonergic neuron. (*CoA,* coenzyme A; *ACh,* acetylcholine; *ACE,* acetylcholinesterase; *x,* receptor; *NE,* norepinephrine; *MAO,* monoamine oxidase; *COMT,* catechol-*O*-methyltransferase; *5-HTP,* 5-hydroxytryptophan; *5-HT,* 5-hydroxytryptamine [serotonin]; *5-HIAA,* 5-hydroxyindoleacetic acid.) (From Ganong WF. Review of medical physiology. Norwalk, CT: Appleton & Lange, 1987.)

The principal pulmonary source of histamine is the pulmonary mast cell (see Chap. 181). These cells, which are numerous near pulmonary blood vessels, in the respiratory epithelium, and also free within the bronchial lumen, produce histamine and many other hormonal mediators, including prostaglandins. Important intrapulmonary sources of several biogenic amines (e.g., serotonin, norepinephrine, and perhaps dopamine) are the pulmonary neuroendocrine (PNE) cells.

## PULMONARY NEUROENDOCRINE CELLS

The PNE cells (also called *Feyrter cells* or *Kulchitsky cells*) are distinctive, scattered cells found within the bronchial epithelium of humans, other mammals, birds, amphibians, and reptiles.[5] These cells, which stain with silver, may form intramucosal clusters called neuroepithelial bodies (see Fig. 175-1 in Chap. 175).

PNE cells are situated near the basement membrane of the epithelium of the entire respiratory airway. They occur in the larynx, trachea, bronchi, bronchioles, alveoli, and ducts of the peribronchial glands. In particular, they are found at bifurcations of the bronchial tree. In humans, they are seen as early as the eighth week of gestation.[6] The PNE cells are far more numerous in the developing fetus and newborn than in the adult, in whom they are sparse. The neuroepithelial bodies are rare in the adult.

In common with the widespread diffuse neuroendocrine system of peptide-secreting cells of the anterior pituitary gland, thyroid C cells, pancreatic islets, and gastrointestinal tract, the PNE cells fluoresce when exposed to formaldehyde vapor, either spontaneously or after exposure to 5-hydroxytryptophan or dihydroxyphenylalanine (L-dopa); this indicates the presence of the intracellular enzyme L-dopa decarboxylase (see Chap. 175). Further, this broad group of cells contains an enzyme of the brain and peripheral nervous system, neuron-specific enolase[7] (see Chap. 175).

By electron microscopy, the PNE cells, which often have pseudopod-like cytoplasmic processes that interdigitate with other cells, contain rounded or ovoid membrane-bound secretion granules, which are situated principally at the basal pole of the cell and are extruded by exocytosis. The PNE cells may abut on the airway lumen; the neuroepithelial bodies protrude into the lumen in a spherical fashion. No consistent, immediately adjacent vascular supply is found to either the PNE cells or the neuroepithelial bodies. Although the PNE cells are seldom individually and directly associated with nerve endings, the neuroepithelial bodies often are innervated and respond to neurocrine stimuli.[8] The intraluminal protrusion of the neuroepithelial bodies and their nervous connections suggest that these organoid structures might function as sensing elements, responding to local airway changes, such as humidity, temperature, pH, inspired air content, particulate matter, or various irritants.[9]

Several peptide hormones occur within the secretion granules of the PNE cells. Presumably, along with acting on adjacent cells in a paracrine manner, the biogenic amines play a role in the synthesis, storage, or secretion of these peptide hormones with which they coexist.

The large number of PNE cells in the fetus and newborn suggests a role in pulmonary development and in postnatal circulatory adjustments. Experimentally, the PNE cells discharge their granules when exposed to acute or chronic hypoxia, hypercapnia, irritant gases like nitrous oxide, and various drugs like nicotine, reserpine, or calcium ionophores. Some of these agents also may exert prenatal influences on the PNE cells.[10] The PNE cells also probably exert important effects in disease states. Hyperplasia of the PNE cells occurs in laboratory animals after the chronic inhalation of asbestos and after the administration of the pulmonary carcinogen diethylnitrosamine.[11,12] Also, the antenatal exposure of maternal monkeys to dexamethasone increases the number of neuroepithelial bodies in their newborn.[13] A marked PNE cell hyperplasia occurs in patients with acute pneumonitis and chronic obstructive lung

disease; in heavy smokers; in patients with intrinsic, nonimmunologic bronchial asthma; and in infants with chronic bronchopulmonary dysplasia.

Often, chronic PNE cell hyperplasia is associated with the appearance of increased peripheral blood levels of one or more of their hormonal products. In addition, acute pulmonary stimulation, such as occurs in hamsters exposed to cigarette smoke, in humans with acute pneumonitis, or in those who inhale noxious fumes in a fire, releases PNE cell hormones into the blood.[14,15]

## PULMONARY PROSTAGLANDINS AND OTHER ARACHIDONIC ACID AND CELL MEMBRANE PHOSPHOLIPID METABOLITES

The physiologically active prostaglandins and other arachidonic acid metabolites produced within the lungs include platelet-activating factor (PAF), the prostaglandins (e.g., $PGE_2$, $PGF_{2\alpha}$, $PGD_2$, and prostacyclin), thromboxane, and the leukotrienes (e.g., $LTB_4$, $LTC_4$, $LTD_4$, and $LTE_4$).[16–18] These hormones are not stored in the lungs but are newly synthesized by various pulmonary cellular constituents, such as the mast cells, smooth muscle, fibroblasts, endothelium (prostacyclin in particular), alveolar macrophages, type II alveolar epithelial cells, polymorphonucleocytes, basophils, and platelets. Most of the active arachidonic acid metabolites are biosynthesized by the cyclooxygenase pathway; the lipoxygenase pathway leads to the formation of the leukotrienes (see Chap. 172). PAF is a metabolite of cell membrane phospholipid, which plays an important role in inflammatory pulmonary conditions and other lung disorders.[19]

These pulmonary metabolites produce effects that differ according to the site of the pulmonary effector cells or tissues, the prior functional state of the cells or tissues, and the presence or absence of other pulmonary hormones. Pharmacologically, the pulmonary action often differs according to the route of administration, the species studied, and the experimental design. Their release can be induced by several other pulmonary hormones (e.g., serotonin, histamine, angiotensin II, endothelin-1, and bradykinin). These potent, evanescent compounds are also released in various pathologic pulmonary conditions, such as asthma, pulmonary edema, or asbestosis. Arachidonic acid and other cell membrane phospholipid metabolites are important in both normal pulmonary physiology and in disease processes involving the lungs. Some of their pharmacologic and physiologic pulmonary effects are summarized in Table 177-1.

## PEPTIDE HORMONES

The pulmonary peptide hormones originate mostly from four sources: the PNE cell (e.g., calcitonin, calcitonin gene–related peptide [CGRP], bombesin-like peptide, cholecystokinin, somatostatin, and leu-enkephalin),[20] peptidergic nerves (e.g., CGRP, vasoactive intestinal peptide [VIP], and substance P), the pulmonary endothelial cell (e.g., angiotensin II, and endothelin-1), and the blood of the pulmonary vasculature (e.g., bradykinin, which is produced in the blood from kininogen by the action of the enzyme kallikrein) (see Chaps. 79 and 170). Undoubtedly, several other pulmonary cells produce peptide hormonal products. Some of the pharmacologic and physiologic effects of the pulmonary peptides and biogenic amines are shown in Table 177-2. Sometimes, a hormone is produced by more than one cell type; potentially functions as a neurocrine, an autocrine, a paracrine, a solinocrine, or a hemocrine messenger (see Chap. 1); and exerts effects that vary according to its site of production.

## GROWTH FACTORS AND CYTOKINES

Although they are peptides, the many humoral growth factors and cytokines often are discussed under a category separate from that of the other peptide hormones. Many cells of the lung

TABLE 177-1.
**Pharmacologic and Physiologic Actions of Pulmonary Arachidonic Acid Metabolites and Other Derivatives of Membrane Phospholipids Synthesized in the Lung***

| Metabolite | Effect on Bronchi | Effect on Pulmonary Vessels | Other Pertinent Effects | Comments |
|---|---|---|---|---|
| PAF | Constriction | Constriction | A proinflammatory peptide. Induces leukocyte recruitment. Releases mediators from inflammatory and epithelial cells. Increases thromboxane and histamine release. | Plays an important role in pathogenesis of several pulmonary inflammatory diseases; increased mRNA expression in asthmatic patients; participates in the development of allergic reactions; induces bronchial hyperreactivity; induces airway microvascular leakage and may cause lung edema; induces aggregation of platelets; stimulates neutrophil adhesion to endothelial cells; plays a role in neonatal respiratory disease syndrome. |
| $PGE_2$ | Dilation | Variable (often vasodilation but can constrict) | Induces systemic vasodilation. Decreases mucus secretion. Inhibits platelet aggregation. Maintains patency of ductus arteriosus in fetus. Potentiates vasoconstriction by histamine. Decreases postinjury leak from vasculature. Decreases postinjury neutrophil recruitment. Regulates fetal lung fluid transport. Ameliorates the hypoxia of ischemic lung injury. Inhibits production of tumor necrosis factor $\alpha$. | Rapidly inactivated by lung endothelium. |
| $PGF_{2\alpha}$ | Constriction | Constriction (potent) | Variably induces systemic vasoconstriction. Increases mucus secretion. Antagonizes $TXA_2$-induced platelet aggregation. Stimulates rapidly adapting receptors, which may play a role in reflex bronchoconstriction of anaphylaxis. Regulates fetal lung fluid transport. | Rapidly inactivated by lung endothelium. |
| $PGD_2$ | Constriction | Constriction | Induces slight systemic vasodilation. Increases mucus secretion. Inhibits platelet aggregation. | Pulmonary vasodilation in fetal goats. |
| $PGI_2$ | Dilation | Dilation (potent) | Induces systemic vasodilation (potent). Inhibits platelet aggregation (potent). Disaggregates platelets. Antithrombotic effect may protect against atherosclerosis. Exerts membrane-stabilizing effect. Maintains patency of ductus arteriosus in fetus. Inhibits release of leukotrienes. | Synthesized by endothelial cells; short-lived, but not appreciably metabolized by lungs. Degraded to 6-keto-$PGF_{1\alpha}$; pulmonary vasodilating effects may facilitate newborn adaptation to extrauterine life; reverses physiologic dead space and shunting associated with pulmonary embolism; inhibits leukocyte aggregation; protects lungs against the pulmonary hypertension and increased permeability caused by endotoxin injury; protects pulmonary circulation from excess vasoconstriction. |
| $TXA_2$ | Constriction | Constriction (potent) | Stimulates platelet aggregation (potent). Enhances leukocyte adhesiveness. Inhibits release of leukotrienes. | Active and short lived; contained within platelets. An ingredient of RCS; inhibits adenylate cyclase activity in platelets; degraded to the inactive $TXB_2$; mediator of hypoxic vasoconstriction. |
| Leukotrienes | Constriction | Variable | Increases capillary permeability. Increases mucus release. Chemotactic for polymorphonuclear cells ($LTB_4$). Decreases tracheal mucus velocity. Releases $TXA_2$ and prostaglandins from lung. | $LTB_4$ attracts alveolar macrophages. $LTC_4$ and $LTD_4$ are ingredients of SRS-A. Pulmonary vasoconstriction of $LTD_4$ is mediated by cyclooxygenase metabolites. Pulmonary vasodilation of $LTE_4$ is mediated by prostaglandins. Direct effect of $LTE_4$ may be pulmonary vasoconstriction. Leukotrienes mediate allergen-induced bronchoconstriction. |

*PAF*, platelet-activating factor; *PGE_2*, prostaglandin E_2; *PGF_{2α}*, prostaglandin F_{2α}; *TXA_2*, thromboxane A_2; *PGD_2*, prostaglandin D_2; *PGI_2*, prostaglandin GI_2; *PGF_{1α}*, prostaglandin F_{1α}; *RCS*, rabbit aorta-contracting substances; *LTB_4*, leukotriene B_4; *LTC_4*, leukotriene C_4; *LTD_4*, leukotriene D_4; *SRS-A*, slow-reacting substance of anaphylaxis; *LTE_4*, leukotriene E_4.
*Some of these effects vary with the species studied, the dosage, the route of administration, and the experimental design.
(Modified from Becker KL. The endocrine lung. In: Becker KL, Gazdar AF, eds. The endocrine lung in health and disease. Philadelphia: WB Saunders, 1984.)

give rise to various forms of these substances, which may be secreted in physiologic circumstances (e.g., by alveolar macrophages, leukocytes, mast cells, smooth muscle cells, bronchial epithelium, and type II cells). In pathologic circumstances, the growth factors and cytokines exert important effects. These actions, which may be helpful or harmful, depend on the circumstances, the presence of other humoral substances, and the amount of the agents that are secreted. Some of their pharmacologic and physiologic effects are shown in Table 177-3.

## FUNCTIONS OF PULMONARY HORMONES

Both the secretion and the action of most of the pulmonary hormones depend on or are modulated by the presence or absence of other hormones: adrenocorticotropic hormone (ACTH) noncompetitively inhibits the pulmonary synthesis of angiotensin II; bradykinin competitively inhibits the synthesis of angiotensin II; angiotensin II releases prostacyclin; substance P releases mast cell histamine; histamine releases pulmonary arachidonic acid metabolites; endothelin-1 induces the release of PAF; calcitonin and CGRP block bombesin- and substance P–induced increases in airway tone[20]; and VIP counteracts the vasoconstrictor and bronchoconstrictor effects of $LTD_4$.

## PHYSIOLOGIC ROLE AT BIRTH

Pulmonary hormones play an important role in pulmonary adaptations that occur at birth. After aeration of the lungs, the pulmonary vasoconstriction of the fetus reverts to dilatation.[21] This change is essential. It permits gas exchange and allows the right ventricle to perfuse the pulmonary circulation with little effort. This vasodilation likely results from the diffuse intrapulmonary release of prostacyclin.[22] The therapeutic administra-

**TABLE 177-2.**
**Some Pharmacologic and Physiologic Effects of Pulmonary Pertinence Caused by Known or Suspected Hormones within the Lung**

| Hormone | Location within Lung | Effects |
|---|---|---|
| Angiotensin II | Endothelium | Causes pulmonary vasoconstriction; releases pulmonary prostaglandins, including prostacyclin; might play a role in hypoxic vasoconstriction. |
| Atrial natriuretic peptide | Alveolar cells, muscle of pulmonary veins, PNE cells | Causes vasodilation, bronchodilation, and decrease in pulmonary artery pressure; stimulates surfactant production; increases blood flow perfusing poorly ventilated regions. |
| Bombesin-like peptides | PNE cells, alveolar macrophages | Causes constriction of pulmonary artery; causes bronchoconstriction that cannot be inhibited by antagonists of acetylcholine, histamine, or serotonin; releases serotonin and histamine from mast cells; enhances growth of bronchial epithelial cells; induces mitosis in PNE cells; stimulates surfactant biosynthesis; induces mucus secretion. Centrally, it can increase pulmonary tidal volume and can cause apneusis-like alterations in the breathing pattern. The high levels during the fetal–neonatal period suggest a role in intrauterine life or in neonatal adaptation; increases lung branching in embryogenesis. |
| Bradykinin | Plasma of lung vasculature | Causes pulmonary vasodilation or contraction; causes bronchoconstriction, either directly or through prostaglandin release; stimulates pulmonary release of prostaglandins, prostacyclin, and thromboxane; releases histamine from mast cells; competitively inhibits enzymic conversion of angiotensin I to II; may play a role in the physiologic pulmonary vasodilation at birth; may contract the ductus arteriosus; increases permeability of pulmonary endothelium. |
| Calcitonin | PNE cells | Promotes growth of cartilage; increases endothelial prostacyclin synthesis; inhibits synthesis of prostaglandins and thromboxane within the lungs; centrally, can increase tidal volume; antagonizes the bronchoconstrictor effects of bombesin-like peptide and of substance P; may control local immune reactions by influencing multinuclear alveolar macrophages. Precursor peptides (e.g., procalcitonin) are produced as a result of the inflammatory cytokine cascade and may play a role in the pulmonary response to injury or sepsis. |
| Calcitonin gene–related peptide | PNE cells, nerves | Causes vasodilation and bronchodilation; blocks the bombesin-related peptide–induced and substance P–induced increase in airway tone; increases ciliary beat frequency; induces eosinophilic chemotaxis; induces proliferation of bronchial epithelium; inhibits degradation of tachykinin. Its peptidergic neurotransmitter role may mediate receptor functions of the respiratory epithelium. |
| Cholecystokinin | Nerves? PNE cells | Possibly has a peptidergic function in the lung; may cause bronchoconstriction; increases pulmonary blood flow. |
| CRH | Unknown | Unknown. |
| Endothelin | Endothelium of vasculature, bronchiolar epithelium, submucosal glands, PNE cells, type II alveolar pneumocytes | Causes bronchoconstriction and vasoconstriction; can be vasodilatory, depending on $K^+$ channel; influences airway mucosal blood flow; enhances vascular permeability; stimulates pulmonary arachidonate 15-lipoxygenase activity; induces release of thromboxane, histamine, and prostacyclin in the lung; may be involved in airway differentiation during embryogenesis; stimulates surfactant secretion from alveolar type II cells; stimulates surfactant secretion from alveolar type II cells; influences neuronal transmission; may function as a proinflammatory peptide, being locally produced at sites of pulmonary injury, and may play a role in causation of the adult respiratory distress syndrome. Increased levels in congestive heart failure may protect the lung from pulmonary edema. |
| Galanin | Nerves | Possibly has peptidergic effects; possibly is antagonist of substance P. |
| Histamine | Mast cells, PNE cells? | Causes vasoconstriction of pulmonary arteries; may cause vasodilation; may play a role in the local regulation of pulmonary blood flow and in hypoxic vasoconstriction; increases vascular permeability; usually causes bronchoconstriction but may cause bronchodilation; releases prostaglandins, thromboxane, and leukotrienes from lung; stimulates bronchial glandular secretion. |
| Neurokinin A (NKA) | Nerves? | Causes vasodilation and possibly bronchoconstriction; increases mucus secretion; increases pulmonary vascular permeability. |
| Neuropeptide K (NPK) | Nerves? | Possibly causes bronchoconstriction. |
| Neuropeptide Y (NPY) | Nerves | Possibly has peptidergic function; potentiates catecholamine-induced vasoconstriction. |
| Neurotensin | Nerves? PNE cells? | Possibly has peptidergic function; causes bronchoconstriction; degranulates mast cells and releases histamine; increases vascular permeability; induces leukocyte chemotaxis; enhances phagocytosis; inhibits cholinergic and noncholinergic neurotransmission. |
| Opioid peptides | PNE cells, nerves | β-Endorphin and met- and leu-enkephalins competitively inhibit angiotensin-converting enzyme. Intravenously, leu-enkephalin increases respiratory rate and can affect pulmonary artery pressure; intraarterially, it causes pulmonary vasoconstriction. Enkephalin may stimulate pulmonary J receptors, with consequent apnea, bradycardia, and hypotension. Endogenous opiates may minimize the stress of chronic airway obstruction. Opioids may function as neurotransmitters in PNE cell–sensory nerve interaction. They inhibit release of endogenous acetylcholine from postganglionic parasympathetic pulmonary neurons; depress the contractile response of tracheal smooth muscle, which is induced by field stimulation and hence may have a role in bronchodilation; and may play a role in immune–inflammatory reactions. |
| Peptide histidine isoleucine (PHI) | Nerves | Possibly has a peptidergic function in the lung. |
| Peptide histidine methionine (PHM) | Nerves | Possibly causes bronchodilation. |
| Serotonin | Platelets, PNE cells | Causes pulmonary vasoconstriction and, in some species, pulmonary venodilation; causes bronchoconstriction; stimulates synthesis of prostaglandins within the lungs; promotes platelet aggregation. |
| Somatostatin | Nerves, PNE cells | Possibly has peptidergic function in the lung; intravenously, increases pulmonary artery pressure; releases serotonin and histamine from mast cells; down-regulates β-adrenergic function of airway smooth muscle. |
| Substance P | Nerves | Possibly has peptidergic function in the lung; causes tracheobronchoconstriction, increased pulmonary vascular permeability, and possibly vasodilation; stimulates synthesis and release of tracheobronchial mucus; releases histamine from mast cells. |
| Vasoactive intestinal peptide (VIP) | Nerves | Possibly has peptidergic function in the lung; suppresses acetylcholine release from vagus nerve terminals; enhances ventilation and causes bronchoconstriction; decreases thromboxane release; protects against histamine and $PGF_{2\alpha}$- and leukotriene $D_4$–induced bronchoconstriction; dilates pulmonary vessels that have previously been constricted by prostaglandin or leukotriene; inhibits basal bronchial mucus production; increases ciliary beat frequency. |

*PNE*, pulmonary neuroendocrine; *CRH*, corticotropin-releasing hormone; *$PGF_{2\alpha}$*, prostaglandin $F_{2\alpha}$.
(Modified from Becker KL. The endocrine lung. In: Becker KL, Gazdar AF, eds. The endocrine lung in health and disease. Philadelphia: WB Saunders, 1984.)

**TABLE 177-3.**
**Pharmacologic and Physiologic Actions of Some of the Growth Factors and Cytokines within the Lung***

| Growth Factor/ Cytokine | Pharmacologic and Physiologic Effects |
| --- | --- |
| Basic fibroblast growth factor | Decreases elastin production by neonatal lung fibroblasts; stimulates growth of fibroblasts and endothelial cells; may play a role in fibroproliferation after acute lung injury. |
| Epidermal growth factor | Plays a role in the differentiation of pulmonary epithelium; increases synthesis and secretion of surfactant; enhances pulmonary functional maturation in utero. |
| Fibroblast growth factor | Has mitogenic effect for fibroblasts and possibly for vascular smooth muscle. |
| Granulocyte/ macrophage colony-stimulating factor | Increases proliferation of neutrophil precursors; prolongs the survival of neutrophils and increases their bactericidal activity; facilitates IgA–mediated phagocytosis. |
| Interferon-γ | Activates alveolar macrophages and increases their ability to express IgG Fc receptors and class II histocompatibility antigens; augments neutrophil recruitment and enhances their microbial activity; stimulates release of tumor necrosis factor α; increases release of oxygen radicals; induces synthesis of phospholipase $A_2$ and third component of complement; inhibits growth of fibroblasts and collagen synthesis. |
| Interleukins | Exert a vast number of effects on the lung. For example: *IL-1* is proinflammatory. It induces leakage of proteins from the vasculature, increases accumulation of neutrophils, increases cellular antimicrobial activity, and augments antibody formation. It activates fibroblasts and induces their production of IL-6 and also induces granulocyte/macrophage colony-stimulating factor release from the bronchial epithelium. It interacts with tumor necrosis factor α in mediating septic shock. *IL-3* damages vascular endothelium and predisposes to pulmonary edema. It augments production of IL-6. *IL-6* is a proinflammatory cytokine that is involved in the tissue immune response. It also may serve as a marker for lung injury. It is an important mediator of the sepsis syndrome. *IL-12* enhances the cytologic activity of lymphocytes and induces production of tumor necrosis factor α. It inhibits the development of pulmonary fibrosis via suppression of the synthesis of collagen. In some models, interferon-γ inhibits the inflammatory response and diminishes protective immunity in the host. |
| Keratinocyte growth factor | Stimulates growth of type II pneumocytes. |
| Platelet-derived growth factor | Increases growth of lung fibroblasts and may play a role in maintaining normal lung structure and repairing injury. |
| Tumor necrosis factor α | Potent mediator of the inflammatory cascade; produced in response to many pathogens; stimulates macrophages and polymorphonuclear chemotaxis and activates their antimicrobial activity; stimulates neutrophil adhesion to endothelial cells; induces vascular proliferation and collagen synthesis; inhibits the synthesis of protein and, at higher levels, causes breakdown of protein; stimulates production of other cytokines. |

*IgA,* immunoglobulin A; *IgG,* immunoglobulin G; *IL-1,* interleukin-1; *IL-6,* interleukin-6; *IL-3,* interleukin-3; *IL-12,* interleukin-12.

*This is a partial list of the growth factors and cytokines that are secreted in the lungs. These substances are multifunctional and have important roles in both normal homeostasis and in the pathogenesis of lung disease. Their effects vary according to their level of secretion, the presence of other humoral agents, and the overall clinical setting.

tion of prostacyclin into the pulmonary artery of a human neonate has successfully ameliorated the refractory hypoxemia resulting from the syndrome of persistent fetal circulation. The initial oxygenation of the newborn releases bradykinin, which causes pulmonary vasodilation and assists in constricting the ductus arteriosus. This blood vessel, which connects the pulmonary artery and aorta, allows blood to bypass the vasoconstricted fetal pulmonary bed and decreases the workload of the heart. During fetal development, it is the secretion of $PGE_2$ and,

perhaps, the local endothelial production of prostacyclin that maintains the patency of the ductus arteriosus. This effect wanes just before birth, possibly because of an increased degradation of $PGE_2$. At birth, exposure to atmospheric oxygen probably promotes the synthesis of $PGF_{2\alpha}$, which may effect the closure of the ductus arteriosus. Pulmonary hormones also appear to play a role in postnatal lung development.[23]

## PULMONARY HORMONES IN LUNG DISEASE

Not only do pulmonary hormones have normal physiologic effects, but also the increased levels of these hormones in lung disease influence the symptomatology, course, and outcome of the illness. For example, asthma, a condition characterized by paroxysmal wheezing resulting from narrowing of the bronchial airways, is associated with the release of several bronchoconstrictive hormones: histamine, PAF, $PGF_{2\alpha}$, the leukotrienes, thromboxane $A_2$, substance P, serotonin, and endothelin.[24–26] A similar panoply of bronchoconstrictive hormonal agents is released during systemic anaphylaxis (i.e., extreme hypersensitivity to a substance manifested by a diffuse bronchoconstriction and perivascular congestion that can cause fatal respiratory failure).[27] In this condition, the secretion of $PGF_{2\alpha}$ probably facilitates the release of histamine and leukotrienes. The release of prostacyclin may blunt this bronchoconstriction.

In localized hypoxia within the lung, pulmonary blood must be diverted away from the hypoxic alveoli to improve the perfusion-ventilation balance (i.e., hypoxic vasoconstrictor response).[28] This local pulmonary vasoconstriction probably is mediated by one or more of the hormones released in hypoxia (e.g., angiotensin II, endothelin-1, serotonin, and histamine).[29] Alternatively, an excessive secretion of these hormones during hypoxia can be harmful (e.g., angiotensin II can cause ultrastructural lesions of the alveolar epithelium). Bradykinin, which is released in local lung hypoxia, is thought to modulate the vasoconstrictor reflex. In severe acute hypoxia, VIP and prostacyclin are secreted, both of which may cause a protective pulmonary vasodilation in nonhypoxic areas of the lungs and may enhance the vascular perfusion of the myocardium and the brain. In this respect, the vasorelaxant properties of nitric oxide clearly exert a protective function in pulmonary vascular beds.[29]

The excess oxygenation of the lungs (i.e., hyperoxia) can be harmful, leading to pulmonary congestion, endothelial necrosis, and edema.[30] In this condition, pulmonary serotonin is increased, partly because of poor degradation. This leads to obstruction of the vasculature by platelet aggregation. Also, the potent vasoconstrictor thromboxane $A_2$ is increased in hyperoxia because of inhibition of its inactivating enzyme, 15-hydroxyprostaglandin dehydrogenase. Chronic hyperoxia also causes significant PNE cell hyperplasia.

In pulmonary embolism, the local acute obstruction of blood supply leads to physiologic shunting, perhaps mediated by release of serotonin, $PGF_{2\alpha}$, and $PGD_2$, but the vasodilatory effect of the secreted prostacyclin ameliorates the severity of the acute pulmonary hypertension, decreases obstruction by diminishing platelet aggregation, and facilitates the eventual reversal of the vascular shunting.[3,31] Excess levels of bradykinin and subsequent pulmonary endothelial permeability can lead to the pulmonary edema seen in the acute respiratory failure of pulmonary embolism.

Various pulmonary hormones are increased locally or peripherally in other conditions involving the lung, such as hypoxia, mechanical ventilation, environmental injury from irritant gases or inorganic dusts, and acute or chronic cigarette smoking.[32] Increased production of fibroblast-promoting growth factors by the alveolar macrophage may play a role in the abnormal type III procollagen metabolism in patients with idiopathic pulmonary fibrosis.[33] In asthma, VIP is absent from nerve fibers of the lung, lung levels of endothelin-1 are increased,[34–36] and secretion of tumor necrosis factor α, granulocyte/macrophage colony-stimulating factor, and the interleukins (e.g., IL-1, IL-2, IL-3, IL-4, IL-5, IL-6, and IL-8) are increased.[37,38] Other bronchoconstricting peptides, such as neurokinin A and substance P, also may play a role in asthma,[39,40] and the increased levels of urinary cyclooxygenase metabolites of arachidonic acid bear witness to the important role of mast-cell hormones in both allergic and exercise-induced asthma.[41]

## PULMONARY HORMONES IN PERIPHERAL BLOOD

To what extent is the local increase of a pulmonary hormone accompanied by an increased level in the peripheral blood? Experimentally, when PNE cell hyperplasia is induced in hamsters by the administration of nitrosamines, a progressive increase in pulmonary calcitonin is paralleled by an increase in blood levels of this hormone.[42] In patients with acute bacterial or viral pneumonitis and in burn patients with acute lung injury from irritant gases, serum levels of several peptides including calcitonin (especially calcitonin precursors) are increased.[43–45,45a] Serum calcitonin precursor levels often are high in pulmonary tuberculosis and in patients with chronic lung disease from cystic fibrosis.[46,47] Chronic smokers have increased levels of bombesin-like peptides in their bronchial tree and urine.[48] Serum calcitonin precursors and ACTH precursors, as well as atrial natriuretic peptide, are increased in chronic obstructive pulmonary disease.[46,49] It is mostly the procalcitonin component of the *CALC-1* gene that is increased in many of these conditions (see Chap. 53). Interestingly, in this regard, serum calcitonin precursor levels are high in the systemic inflammatory response syndrome (SIRS), because of either infectious or noninfectious injury.[50,51] Indeed, such levels may be used as a measure of the severity of the condition. Although the source of the calcitonin precursors in this condition is uncertain, much of it may be from the lung, because adult respiratory distress syndrome (ARDS) is commonly a component of SIRS.[51] Serum angiotensin II levels are increased in rodents with thiourea- or paraquat-induced lung damage after an increase in angiotensin-converting enzyme activity. Similar increases occur in patients with pulmonary sarcoidosis, pulmonary embolism, or anaphylaxis, and in oxygenation of the fetus.[52] Blood bradykinin levels are increased in the respiratory distress syndrome of the neonate and in endotoxic shock. Blood endorphins, perhaps of pulmonary origin, are increased in hypoxic sheep and also in humans with high-altitude pulmonary edema, as well as in patients showing the pulmonary changes accompanying endotoxic shock.[53] Blood VIP levels are increased in animals with anaphylaxis, acute hypoxia, or acute respiratory acidosis.

## PULMONARY HORMONES IN LUNG CANCER

Peripheral blood levels of some of the pulmonary hormones are increased in some varieties of lung cancer. The hormones that are commonly increased in patients with the relatively benign pulmonary carcinoid or the malignant small cell lung cancer (SCLC) often are the hormones known or suspected to be produced by the normal or the dysplastic PNE cell (e.g., calcitonin, CGRP, mammalian bombesin, ACTH, and somatostatin).[54] Increased blood levels of VIP, a hormone found in pulmonary nerves and ganglia, usually are associated with types of lung malignancy other than SCLC.[55] The study of the carcinoid tumor and SCLC (see Chap. 221) offers important insights into the nature of their putative cells of origin, the PNE cells.[56]

Some of the peptide hormones that commonly are increased in the blood of SCLC patients frequently are increased in patients with other varieties of lung cancer. Perhaps this is because of a heterogeneity of cell types within the tumor. Alternatively, the high levels of some of the hormones encountered in the blood of patients with cancer of the lung other than SCLC may reflect their smoking-related PNE cell hyperplasia.[57] In this respect, some studies of long-term cell cultures of lung cancer demonstrate that bombesin-like peptides and calcitonin occur almost exclusively in SCLC cultures.[58] Somatostatin and ACTH are found frequently, but not exclusively, in these cell lines.[59]

Of course, one or more of the PNE cell–associated peptides are found in the endocrine cells of many other tissues (e.g., anterior pituitary gland, thyroid C cells, gastrointestinal endocrine cells, and pancreatic islets), and tumors involving nonendocrine tissues are commonly associated with increased hormonal peptide blood levels.

In health and in disease, the lung is a complex endocrine organ that produces a host of hormones that act locally or diffusely within the lung and that affect extrapulmonary tissues. The pulmonary effects of most of these hormones vary according to the concurrent physiobiochemical status of their environment. Some of these effects are beneficial and some are not.

Other hormones that are pathophysiologically important must be present within the lung. Some of them may be peptide portions of the larger precursors from which most active peptides are synthesized, and some may be products of alternative posttranslational processing steps. As is the case with the known pulmonary hormones, they also will be found within other tissues and will act on different effectors.

## REFERENCES

1. Fishman AP. The diverse functions of the lung. In: Becker KL, Gazdar AF, eds. The endocrine lung in health and disease. Philadelphia: WB Saunders, 1984:47.
2. Said SI. Metabolic functions of the pulmonary circulation. Circ Res 1982; 50:325.
3. Becker KL. The endocrine lung. In: Becker KL, Gazdar AF, eds. The endocrine lung in health and disease. Philadelphia: WB Saunders, 1984:3.
4. Becker KL. The coming of age of a bronchial epithelial cell. Am J Respir Crit Care Med 1994; 149:183.
5. Becker KL, Gazdar A. The pulmonary endocrine cell and the tumors to which it gives rise. In: Reznick-Schuller HM, ed. Comparative respiratory tract carcinogenesis, vol 2. Boca Raton, FL: CRC Press, 1984:161.
6. Cutz E, Conen PE. Endocrine-like cells in human fetal lungs: an electron microscopic study. Anat Rec 1972; 173:115.
7. Schmechel DE, Marangos PJ, Brightman MW. Neuron-specific enolase is a marker for peripheral and central neuroendocrine cells. Nature 1979; 276:834.
8. Nylen ES, Becker KL, Snider RH, et al. Cholinergic-nicotinic control of growth and secretion of cultured pulmonary neuroendocrine cells. Anat Rec 1993; 236:129.
9. Lauweryns JM, Goddeeris P. Neuroepithelial bodies in the human child and adult lung. Am Rev Respir Dis 1975; 111:469.
10. Nylén ES, Linnoila RI, Becker KL. Prenatal cholinergic stimulation of pulmonary neuroendocrine cells by nicotine. Acta Physiol Scand 1988; 132:117.
11. Johnson NF, Wagner JC, Wills HA. Endocrine cell proliferation in the rat lung following asbestos inhalation. Lung 1980; 158:221.
12. Reznick-Schuller H. Proliferation of endocrine (APUD-type) cells during early DEN-induced lung carcinogenesis in hamsters. Cancer Lett 1971; 1:255.
13. Dayer AM, Kapanci Y, Rademakers A, et al. Increased numbers of neuroepithelial bodies (NEB) in lungs of fetal Rhesus monkeys following maternal dexamethasone treatment. Cell Tissue Res 1985; 239:703.
14. Tabassian AR, Nylén ES, Giron AE, et al. Evidence for cigarette smoke-induced calcitonin secretion from lungs of man and hamster. Life Sci 1988; 42:2323.
15. Tabassian AR, Snider RH Jr, Nylén ES, et al. Heterogeneity studies of hamster calcitonin following acute exposure to cigarette smoke: evidence for monomeric secretion. Anat Rec 1993; 236:253.
16. Greally P, Cook AJ, Sampson AP, et al. Atopic children with cystic fibrosis have increased urinary leukotriene E4 concentrations and more severe pulmonary disease. J Allergy Clin Immunol 1994; 93:100.
17. Trochtenberg DS, Lefferts PL, King GA, et al. Effects of thromboxane synthase and cyclooxygenase inhibition on PAF-induced changes in lung function and arachidonic acid metabolism. Prostaglandins 1992; 44:555.
18. Boichot E, Lagente V, Mencia-Huerta M, Braquet P. Bronchopulmonary responses to endothelin-1 in sensitized and challenged guinea pigs: role of cyclooxygenase metabolites and platelet-activating factor. Fundam Clin Pharmacol 1993; 7:281.
19. Chung KF. Platelet-activating factor in inflammation and pulmonary disorders. Clin Sci 1992; 83:127.
20. Polak JM, Becker KL, Cutz E, et al. Lung endocrine cell markers, peptides and amines. Anat Rec 1993; 236:169.
21. Assali NS, Morris JA. Circulatory and metabolic adjustments of the fetus at birth. Biol Neonate 1964; 7:141.

22. Leffler CW, Hessler JR. Perinatal pulmonary prostaglandin production. Am J Physiol 1981; 241:H756.

23. Motoyama EK, Brody JS, Colten HR, Warshaw JB. Postnatal lung development in health and disease. Am Rev Respir Dis 1988; 137:742.

24. Rothenburg ME, Zimmerman N, Mishra A, et al. Chemokines and chemokine receptors: their role in allergic airway disease. J Clin Immunol 1999; 19:250.

25. Busse WW, McGill KH, Horwitz RJ. Leukotriene pathway inhibitors in asthma and chronic obstructive pulmonary disease. Clin Exp Allergy 1999; 29(Suppl 2):110.

26. Shimizu T. The future potential of eicosanoids and their inhibitors in paediatric practice. Drugs 1998; 56:169.

27. Schulman ES, Newball HH, Demers LM, et al. Anaphylactic release of thromboxane A$_2$, prostaglandin D$_2$, and prostacyclin from human lung parenchyma. Am Rev Respir Dis 1981; 124:402.

28. Fishman AP. Vasomotor regulation of the pulmonary circulation. Annu Rev Physiol 1980; 42:211.

29. Rubino A, Loesch A, Burnstock G. Nitric oxide and endothelin-1 in coronary and pulmonary circulation. Int Rev Cytol 1999; 189:59.

30. Clark JM, Lambertsen CJ. Pulmonary oxygen toxicity: a review. Pharmacol Rev 1971; 23:37.

31. Malik AB, Johnson A, Tahamont MV. Mechanisms of lung vascular injury after intravascular coagulation. Ann N Y Acad Sci 1982; 384:213.

32. Tabassian AR, Nylén ES, Linnoila RI, et al. Stimulation of pulmonary neuroendocrine cells and associated peptides following repeated exposure to cigarette smoke in hamsters. Am Rev Respir Dis 1989; 140:436.

33. Cantin AM, Boilcau R, Begin R. Increased procollagen III, aminoterminal peptide-related antigens and fibroblast growth signals in the lungs of patients with idiopathic pulmonary fibrosis. Am Rev Respir Dis 1988; 137:572.

34. Ollerenshaw S, Jarvis D, Woolcock A, et al. Absence of immunoreactive vasoactive intestinal polypeptide in tissue from the lungs of patients with asthma. N Engl J Med 1989; 320:1244.

35. Goldie RG. Endothelins in health and disease: an overview. Clin Exp Pharmacol Physiol 1999; 26:145.

36. Hay DW. Putative mediator role of endothelin-1 in asthma and other lung diseases. Clin Exp Pharmacol Physiol 1999; 26:168.

37. Marini M, Vittori E, Hollenberg J, Mattoli S. Expression of the potent inflammatory cytokines, granulocyte-macrophage–colony-stimulating factor and interleukin-6 and interleukin-8, in bronchial epithelial cells of patients with asthma. J Allergy Clin Immunol 1992; 89:1001.

38. Bradding P, Roberto JA, Montefort S, et al. Interleukin-4, -5, and -6 and tumor necrosis factor-alpha in normal and asthmatic airways: evidence for the human mast cell as a source of these cytokines. Am J Respir Cell Mol Biol 1994; 10:471.

39. Choi DC, Kwon OJ. Neuropeptides and asthma. Curr Opin Pulm Med 1998; 4:16.

40. Proud D. The kinin system in rhinitis and asthma. Clin Rev Allergy Immunol 1998; 16:351.

41. O'Sullivan S. On the role of PGD$_2$ metabolites as markers of mast cell activation in asthma. Acta Physiol Scand Suppl 1999; 644:1.

42. Linnoila RI, Becker KL, Silva OL, et al. Calcitonin as a marker for diethylnitrosamine-induced pulmonary endocrine cell hyperplasia in hamsters. Lab Invest 1984; 51:39.

43. Becker KL, O'Neil WJ, Snider RH Jr, et al. Hypercalcitonemia in inhalation burn injury: a response of the pulmonary neuroendocrine cell? Anat Rec 1993; 236:136.

44. Nylén ES, Jeng J, Jordan MH, et al. Late pulmonary sequela following burns: persistence of hyperprocalcitonemia using a 1–57 amino acid N-terminal flaking peptide assay. Respir Med 1995; 89:41.

45. Nylén ES, Snider RH Jr, Thompson KA, et al. Pneumonitis-associated hyperprocalcitoninemia. Am J Med Sci 1996 312(1):12.

45a. Onuoha GN, Alpar EK, Gowar J. Plasma levels of atrial natriuretic peptide in severe burn injury. Burns 2000; 26:449.

46. Becker KL, Nash DR, Silva OL, et al. Increased serum and urinary calcitonin levels in patients with pulmonary disease. Chest 1981; 79:211.

47. Becker KL, Silva OL, Snider RH, et al. The pathophysiology of pulmonary calcitonin. In: Becker KL, Gazdar AF, eds. The endocrine lung in health and disease. Philadelphia: WB Saunders, 1984:277.

48. Aguayo SM, Kane MA, King T, et al. Increased level of bombesin-like peptides in the lower respiratory tract of asymptomatic cigarette smokers. J Clin Invest 1989; 84:1105.

49. Ayvazian LF, Schneider B, Gewirtz G, Yalow RS. Ectopic production of big ACTH in carcinoma of the lung. Am Rev Respir Dis 1975; 3:279.

50. Assicot M, Gendrel D, Carsin H, et al. High serum procalcitonin concentrations in patients with sepsis and infection. Lancet 1993; 1:515.

51. Bone RC, Balk RA, Cerra FB, et al. Definitions for sepsis and organ failure and guidelines for the use of innovative therapies in sepsis. Chest 1992; 101:1644.

52. Lieberman J, Nosal A, Schlessner LA, Sastre-Foken A. Serum angiotensin-converting enzyme for diagnosis and therapeutic evaluation of sarcoidosis. Am Rev Respir Dis 1979; 120:329.

53. Bar-or D, Marx JA, Good JT Jr. Naloxone, beta endorphins, and high-altitude pulmonary edema. Ann Intern Med 1982; 96:684.

54. Horton KM, Fishman EK. Cushing syndrome due to a pulmonary carcinoid tumor: multimodality imaging and diagnosis. J Comput Assist Tomogr 1998; 22:804.

55. Said SI, Faloona GR. Elevated plasma and tissue levels of vasoactive intestinal polypeptide in the watery-diarrhea syndrome due to pancreatic, bronchogenic and other tumors. N Engl J Med 1975; 293:155.

56. Becker KL, Nylén ES, Cassidy MM, Tabassian AR. The normal and abnormal pulmonary endocrine cell. In: Kaiser HE, ed. Progressive stages of malignant neoplastic growth. Netherlands: Martinus Nijhoff, 1988.

57. Kelley MJ, Becker KL, Rushin JM, et al. Calcitonin elevation in small cell lung cancer without ectopic production. Am J Respir Crit Care Med 1994; 149:183.

58. Novak J, Escobedo-Morse A, Kelley K, et al. Nicotine effects on proliferation and the bombesin-like peptide system in human small cell lung carcinoma SHP77 cells in culture. Lung Cancer 2000; 29:1.

59. Gazdar AF, Carney DN, Becker KL, et al. Expression of peptide and other markers in lung cancer cell lines. Recent Results Cancer Res 1985; 99:167.

# CHAPTER 178

# THE ENDOCRINE HEART

MIRIAM T. RADEMAKER AND ERIC A. ESPINER

A role for the heart as an endocrine organ was suspected as early as 1956, when secretory-like granules were detected in atrial myocytes (Fig. 178-1).[1] The view that the heart may be able to sense the fullness of the circulation and signal this to the kidney was supported by the finding that balloon dilatation of the left atrium increased urine volume.[2] Some 25 years later, a peptide factor that possessed strong natriuretic and vasodepressor activity was discovered in rat atrial muscle. This led to the recognition of a novel hormonal system based in the heart and capable of affecting all tissues involved in sodium and blood pressure homeostasis.[3] The amino-acid structure of this "atrial factor" was subsequently identified and it was designated *atrial natriuretic peptide* (ANP) (also known as *atrial natriuretic factor*, *atrial natriuretic hormone*, *atrin*, *atriopeptin*, *auriculin*, *cardiodilatin*, and *cardionatrin*).[4] The identification of other structurally and functionally related peptides followed; among these were *brain natriuretic peptide* (BNP; also known as *B-type natriuretic peptide*)[5]; and *C-type natriuretic peptide* (CNP).[6] These three peptides, present in many species, constitute a family of natriuretic peptides of which the signature is a characteristic 17-amino-acid ring structure within the bioactive portion of the prohormone. Although the term "natriuretic peptides" may be historically correct, it underrepresents the wide range of activi-

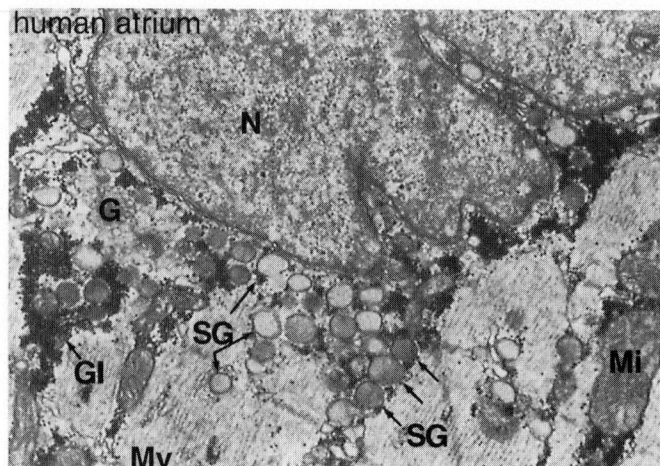

**FIGURE 178-1.** Myoendocrine cell from human right atrium showing secretory granules (*SG*), nucleus (*N*), mitochondria (*Mi*), myofibrils (*My*), glycogen (*Gl*), and Golgi apparatus (*G*). ×20,000 (From Forssmann, Hock D, Lottspeich F, et al. The right auricle of the heart is an endocrine organ. Anat Histol Embryol 1983; 168:307.)

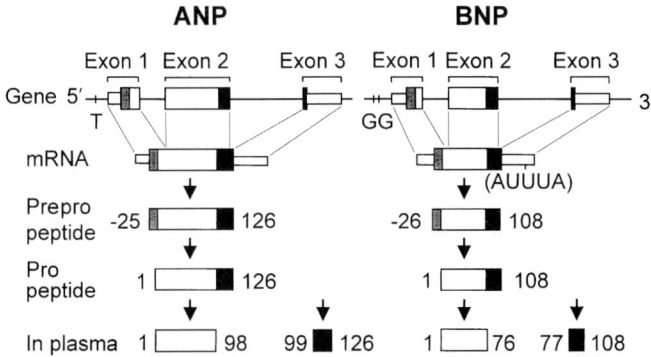

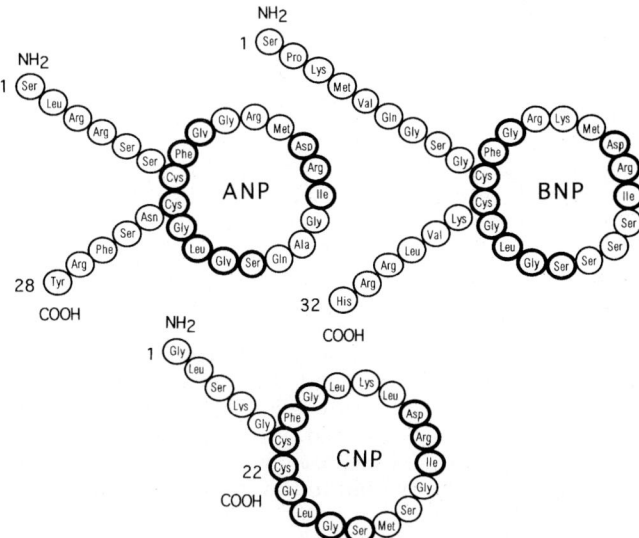

**FIGURE 178-2.** Structure of human atrial natriuretic peptide (*ANP*) and brain natriuretic peptide (*BNP*) genes (located on chromosome 1 in region p36) and subsequent steps to the mature processed products found in plasma. *Solid black sections* are those that ultimately constitute the mature active peptides. *Stippled areas* are those from which the amino-terminal fragments are derived. *Striped sections* represent the region coding for the signal peptide and the signal peptide itself. *T* indicates the location of the TATAAA sequence upstream from the transcription initiation site of ANP, whereas *GG* is the location of the two GATAAA sequences (potential TATAAA sequences) on the BNP gene. (Modified from Nakao K, Ogawa Y, Suga S, Imura H. Molecular biology and biochemistry of the natriuretic peptide system. I: Natriuretic peptides. J Hypertens 1992; 10:907.)

**FIGURE 178-3.** Mature forms of human atrial natriuretic peptide (*ANP*), brain natriuretic peptide (*BNP*), and C-type natriuretic peptide (*CNP*). *Bold circles* are amino acids common to the three human hormones. The mature forms shown are ANP, BNP-32, and CNP-22. (Modified from Nakao K, Ogawa Y, Suga S, Imura H. Molecular biology and biochemistry of the natriuretic peptide system. I: Natriuretic peptides. J Hypertens 1992; 10:907.)

ties of these peptides, which embraces antiproliferative effects and vascular remodeling.

Both ANP and BNP are true circulating hormones secreted predominantly by the atria and ventricles of the heart, respectively. CNP, in contrast, is not primarily a product of cardiac secretion. Originally isolated in porcine brain, where it is the most abundant of the three natriuretic peptides, CNP gene transcripts and specific CNP receptors are found outside the central nervous system (CNS), most notably in vascular endothelial and smooth muscle tissue, but also in the heart and kidney.[7] Although elevated levels in blood occur in septic shock[8] and chronic renal failure,[9] no change in plasma CNP levels occur in patients with hypertension or heart failure—in sharp contrast to ANP and BNP.[10] Most likely, CNP is a paracrine factor, possibly interdigitating with the other (circulating) natriuretic peptides[7] in a vascular CNP system[11] concerned with the regulation of local vasomotor tone and vascular cell growth. Other hormones, such as the renin-angiotensin system[12]—endothelin,[13] adrenomedullin,[14] and parathyroid hormone–related protein[15]—are found in cardiac tissues, but evidence for their possible endocrine roles is scant.

## NATRIURETIC PEPTIDE GENES

Two distinct, single-copy genes encode ANP and BNP. Both genes are similar in organization and structure (Fig. 178-2). In humans, they are organized in tandem (BNP–ANP in the 5' to 3' orientation ~8 kb apart) on the short arm of chromosome 1.[16] Each gene consists of three exons separated by two introns with regulatory elements upstream (5') of the encoding sequence. Exon 1 encodes the signal peptide and the first portion of the propeptide, whereas the second exon codes for the bulk of the prepropeptide. Immediately upstream from the transcription initiation site in the ANP gene is a TATAAA sequence that is homologous to the consensus promoter sequence for mRNA transcription. In the BNP gene, however, some species (including humans) have no TATAAA sequence but have two GATAAA sequences, which may fulfill this function. In other species, both sequences are present.[17] A feature distinguishing the ANP gene from the BNP gene is the conserved repetitive ATTA sequences (AUUUA in mRNA) in the 3'-untranslated region of the BNP gene in all species studied (see Fig. 178-2).[17]

This repeated sequence destabilizes the mRNA, suggesting that the expression of BNP is regulated at the level of transcription differently from that of ANP.

## PEPTIDE SYNTHESIS AND STRUCTURE

The transcription of the ANP gene yields preproANP, which contains 151 amino acids in humans. Each preproANP molecule contains a short (N-terminal) hydrophobic signal segment, involved in the cotranslational transport of the peptide across the membrane of the endoplasmic reticulum. This signal peptide is cleaved at the C terminus by an endoprotease during the transport to produce the 126-amino-acid prohormone that is the predominant storage form observed in atrial cardiocyte granules[18] (see Fig. 178-1). The amino-acid sequence of proANP is highly homologous (~74%) in mammals.[7,17] Final processing of the stored proANP by proteolytic cleavage of the Arg98-Ser99 bond takes place during its release into the circulation, yielding the 28-amino-acid bioactive peptide ANP99-126 (or ANP-28) (Fig. 178-3) and the N-terminal fragment ANP1-98. Constitutive secretion of the mature ANP peptide (i.e., ANP99-126) may occur from the ventricle,[19] although cultured ventricular myocytes possess at least some characteristics of regulated secretion.[20] The mature ANP hormone is conserved across all mammalian species thus far studied with the exception of rodents and rabbits, in which isoleucine replaces methionine at position 110. As shown in Figure 178-3, ANP-28 contains the characteristic 17-amino-acid ring structure in which an intramolecular cysteine-to-cysteine disulfide bond connects residues 105 and 121. Disruption of this ring by proteolytic cleavage or reduction of the disulfide bridge leads to loss of bioactivity.[21] Transcription of the BNP gene yields the precursor preproBNP, which contains between 121 and 134 amino acids, depending on the species (134 amino acids in humans) and is molecularly similar to preproANP. Removal of the hydrophobic signal peptide gives rise to the proBNP peptide, which consists of 108 amino acids in humans.[17] As with ANP, the bioactive sequence of BNP resides in the C-terminal portion of the prohormone. Compared with ANP precursors, however, BNP sequence homology among species is lower and is confined largely to the C-terminal region. Processing of proBNP to the mature peptide also differs from that of ANP in that cleavage occurs after the Arg-X-X-Arg sequence, consistent with the action of a furin protease.[17] Because the processing site itself is not highly conserved, the mature peptide differs appreciably across species. These differences may account for the observed species-specific receptor selectivity[22] and variations in bioactivity among BNP forms.[23] In humans, the circulating forms of BNP include the mature 32-amino-acid peptide BNP77-108 (or BNP-32) (see Fig. 178-3), the N-terminal fragment BNP1-76, and a higher molecular weight component, probably proBNP1-108.[24] The mature form of BNP in humans shows strong sequence homology with mature ANP (~70 %) and retains the 17-residue ring structure. At least two mature forms of CNP (CNP82-103 [CNP-22] and CNP51-103 [CNP-53]) have been isolated, each with similar bioactivity, but their proportions in different tissues need to be clarified. The structure of CNP-22 (see Fig. 178-3) appears to be identical in all mammals.[17] CNP also has a 17-amino-acid ring but differs in having no C-terminal extension.

Whereas the stored form of ANP within the atria is the prohormone (ANP1-126) in all species studied, BNP forms extracted from atrial tissue differ across species. In humans and rats, the main component is the mature peptide, indicating that posttranslational processing of the BNP precursor occurs in the heart and not during secretion, as in the case of ANP. In pigs and sheep, the dominant form in atrial tissue extracts is proBNP.[17] Thus, atrial granules in the rat, and probably in humans, may contain unprocessed proANP as well as smaller amounts of mature BNP, indicating different processing pathways for the peptides in the atria leading to common storage and regulated secretion. In the ventricle, BNP appears to be secreted mostly from the myocytes as the mature peptide via the constitutive pathway,[25] although regulated secretion may also occur.[20]

## TISSUE DISTRIBUTION AND GENE EXPRESSION

The tissue distribution of natriuretic peptides also exhibits significant variations. ANP gene expression is highest in the cardiac atria, which produce ~95% of the total cardiac secretion of this peptide.[26] ANP mRNA is also present in the ventricles, although at only 1% of atrial mRNA concentrations. Gene expression in the ventricle, however, may increase markedly in pathologic states such as ventricular hypertrophy and congestive heart failure (CHF).[27] ANP gene expression is also observed (but at much lower levels) in noncardiac tissues, including vascular tissue, kidney, adrenal medulla, lung, thymus, gastrointestinal tract, and eye. The expression of the ANP gene in the kidney is likely to be the source of an aminoterminal extended form of ANP (urodilatin, i.e., ANP95-126) generated from proANP by alternative gene splicing.[28] ANP transcripts are also found at low levels within the CNS where, as part of a brain natriuretic peptide system, they may participate in the neuroregulation of cardiovascular and body fluid homeostasis.[27] The low levels of transcripts in extracardiac sites (<1% of atrial levels) make it unlikely that they contribute substantially to circulating levels of ANP.

Although BNP was first identified in porcine brain (hence, its name), the main site of synthesis and secretion is the heart. As with ANP, the highest levels are found in atrial tissue, albeit at 5% of ANP levels, where it is costored with ANP in certain types of granules.[29] Small amounts of BNP are present in the ventricle (1% of atrial BNP levels), consistent with its constitutive secretion from ventricular myocytes.[25] The ratio of ventricular to atrial BNP mRNA (~1:2) is much higher than that for ANP, suggesting that the ventricle is the major source of BNP

secretion[26,30] (i.e., 60–80% of cardiac BNP secretion arises from the ventricles).[25,26,30] As in the case of ANP, BNP transcripts are markedly elevated in the ventricles of subjects with CHF and cardiac hypertrophy,[25,30,31] with BNP increasing more than ANP.

Extracardiac BNP synthesis occurs in the adrenal medulla (at levels greater than the synthesis of ANP) and in the kidney, thyroid, lung, spleen, and amnion tissue.[7] BNP transcripts have also been found in human brain, porcine brain (where mRNA levels are ten-fold those of ANP), and bovine brain but are almost undetectable in murine and rat brain.[5,7]

## REGULATION

The secretion of ANP is determined largely by *increases in atrial transmural pressure or stretch*.[32] In humans, for each 1 mm Hg rise in atrial pressure, an associated rise of 10 to 14 pmol/L occurs in peripheral venous plasma ANP levels. Similarly, *acute reduction of atrial pressure reduces ANP secretion*. Discrepancies between atrial pressure and ANP release can occur, as has been observed during cardiac tamponade and after intravenous volume loading.[7] A direct autocrine inhibitory effect of ANP has also been described.[33] The mechanism whereby increased stretch of the cardiocyte is coupled to secretion remains unclear, but it is likely to involve protein phosphokinase activation and increased intracellular calcium concentrations.[27] A number of chemical factors also may be involved in the regulation of ANP secretion from the heart, including endothelin-1, angiotensin II (Ang II), vasopressin, catecholamines, prostaglandins, glucocorticoids, growth factors, and thrombin.[27] Locally produced secretagogues, especially Ang II and endothelin-1, mediate the ANP response to an acute volume load.[34]

Numerous factors affect ANP secretion, including increased sodium intake, supine posture, water immersion, exercise, tachycardia, volume expansion, hypoxia, myocardial ischemia, and hypertrophy.[7] Many of these can be related wholly, or in part, to changes in atrial transmural pressure. Increased heart rate, particularly the frequency of atrial contraction, is also a potent stimulus for ANP secretion. Controversy exists over a possible regulatory role of the CNS in cardiac ANP secretion.[7]

During embryonic development, the ANP gene is expressed in both atrial and ventricular tissues. After birth, ANP gene expression in the ventricle, in contrast to BNP gene expression, is rapidly down-regulated and remains suppressed.[35] Ventricular hypertrophy reactivates ANP gene expression, so that the ventricle becomes a major source of ANP secretion in states of cardiac overload, including that of established heart failure.[27]

Less attention has been focused on the mechanisms of BNP release, largely because species-specific antisera are required. Nonetheless, several studies suggest that both ANP and BNP respond *similarly* in many circumstances. Plasma BNP has been shown to be elevated with increasing age[36] and in states of volume overload (e.g., chronic renal failure[37] and chronic dietary sodium loading).[38] Usually, the increase in plasma BNP parallels that of ANP. In rat atrial myocytes, both ANP and BNP release are enhanced by endothelin,[39] whereas in the isolated perfused ventricular myocardium both peptides are released similarly in response to hypoxia[40] and stretch.[41] Therefore, the fact that both peptides are elevated after myocardial infarction and in states of chronic cardiac overload (e.g., hypertension and CHF) is not surprising.[25,42–44] On the other hand, BNP is less responsive to acute changes in intracardiac pressure, as may occur during changes in posture,[43] exercise,[45] and acute saline loading.[46] These differences presumably reflect the lower content of BNP in readily releasable stores within the atrial granules. Greater increases in plasma BNP levels (compared with ANP levels) occur after acute myocardial infarction,[47] in hypertrophic cardiomyopathy,[48] and in CHF,[25] consistent with the

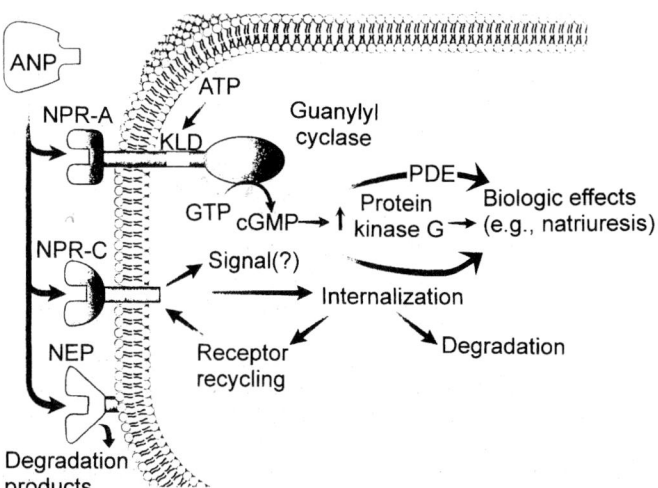

**FIGURE 178-4.** Action of atrial natriuretic peptide (*ANP*) at the target cell. ANP (and brain natriuretic peptide [*BNP*]) bind to natriuretic peptide receptor A (*NPR-A*) and, in an adenosine triphosphate (*ATP*)–dependent fashion, which requires the kinase-like domain (*KLD*), stimulate the intrinsic guanylate cyclase activity of the receptor. Cyclic guanosine monophosphate (*cGMP*) exerts its bioeffects indirectly through cGMP-dependent protein kinase G or one or more phosphodiesterases (*PDEs*). Natriuretic peptide receptor B (*NPR-B*; not shown) is activated in a similar fashion by C-type natriuretic peptide. ANP (and BNP) also bind to the natriuretic peptide receptor C (*NPR-C*), after which they are internalized and degraded. The NPR-C receptors may also have independent signaling functions. ANP (and BNP) may be degraded by extracellular neutral endopeptidase E.C. 24.11 (*NEP*). (*GTP*, guanosine triphosphate.) (Modified from Levin ER, Gardner DG, Samson WK. Natriuretic peptides. N Engl J Med 1998; 339:321.)

markedly augmented gene expression of BNP compared with ANP expression in overloaded ventricles.[49] Predictably, the responses of ANP and BNP in heart failure differ according to the underlying cardiac disorder affecting the distribution of increased pressure within the heart.[50] Evidence also is found of differential regulation of BNP secretion from atrial and ventricular tissues. Cannulation studies in patients with heart failure[51] indicate that the chronically overloaded ventricle has the ability to augment BNP production, whereas atrial BNP mRNA and BNP secretion remain relatively unchanged. A possible role of the CNS in the regulation of BNP secretion from the heart remains to be defined. Although little is known of the cellular mechanisms governing the synthesis of BNP, evidence exists that (as with ANP) BNP mRNA expression is increased by protein kinase C activation and by $\alpha_1$-adrenergic agonists.[52] Stretch-induced increases in BNP transcripts appear to be mediated by locally generated Ang II and endothelin-1.[53] Compared with the ANP mRNA response, these increases in BNP gene expression are much more rapid[52] and raise the possibility that BNP also may have some unique paracrine function within the heart itself.

## RECEPTORS

Three different subtypes of *natriuretic peptide receptors* (NPR) have been identified (Fig. 178-4). Two of them, *NPR-A* and *NPR-B*, contain an intracellular kinase-like domain and a guanylate cyclase (GC) catalytic domain, which appear to mediate most of the bioactions of the natriuretic peptides.[54] In the absence of ligand, the kinase-like domain represses the activity of GC. Binding of the peptide to the extracellular portion of the receptor activates the GC moiety, leading to the generation of the intracellular second messenger, cyclic guanosine monophosphate (cGMP). This event is accompanied by loss of receptor

affinity, resulting in rapid receptor-ligand dissociation. Newly generated cGMP stimulates cGMP-dependent protein kinases responsible for phosphorylation of a large number of intracellular proteins. In addition, under some conditions, cGMP suppresses cyclic adenosine monophosphate (cAMP) concentrations by augmenting phosphodiesterase activity.[55] The third receptor subtype, *NPR-C*, differs in that it has no kinase-like or GC domains, retaining only the extracellular ligand-binding domain connected to a short intracytoplasmic tail (see Fig. 178-4). Further, compared with NPR-A and NPR-B, it has a broad specificity, binding all three natriuretic peptides and other related analogs with relatively high affinity. The NPR-C receptor is thought to function largely as a clearance receptor, regulating the uptake, internalization, and intracellular (lysosomal) degradation of the peptides.[54] After delivery of the peptide to the lysosome, the internalized receptor is recycled to the cell surface. Some evidence exists that the NPR-C receptor may serve functions in addition to that of clearance, because occupancy by ANP (and BNP) or other NPR-C ligands (such as the truncated bioinactive peptide C-ANP4-23) may activate the phosphoinositol pathway and inhibit cAMP production.[56] A number of studies,[57] but not all,[58] suggest that NPR-C receptors mediate the antimitogenic effects of the natriuretic peptides, as well as some neuromodulatory actions within the CNS.

As with the mature hormones, all three natriuretic peptide receptors exhibit strong homology across species. At the amino-acid level, the extracellular domains of NPR-A and NPR-B are 44% identical to each other and 30% identical to those of NPR-C. The rank order of selectivity of the peptides for NPR-A is ANP > BNP >> CNP; for NPR-B it is CNP > ANP > BNP; and for NPR-C it is ANP > CNP > BNP.[22] These findings suggest that ANP and BNP act through the NPR-A receptor, whereas CNP acts through the NPR-B receptor.[54] Notably, none of these receptors is preferentially activated by BNP and, as yet, no specific receptor for either BNP or ANP has been identified. All three peptides appear to bind with almost equal and high affinity to the NPR-C receptor. An exception is the relatively low binding affinity exhibited by human BNP for the human NPR-C receptor. Whereas ANP binds similarly to both the rat and human NPR-C, the affinity of human BNP for human NPR-C is ten-fold lower than the affinity of human BNP for the rat NPR-C.[22,59] This difference in binding affinity appears to be determined by amino acid 188 of the NPR-C receptor, because the substitution of alanine for isoleucine at this residue of the human NPR-C achieves the high-affinity state of human BNP evident for rat NPR-C.[59] This observation may explain in part the differences in plasma half-life of BNP (prolonged in the human) across species.

The NPR-A receptor is most abundantly expressed in kidney, adrenal glands, heart, vascular smooth muscle, lung, adipose tissue, and brain.[60] In the bovine kidney, mRNA expression of the NPR-A is concentrated in the glomerulus and inner medullary collecting duct,[61] a finding that points to the dominant functional role of the natriuretic peptides at these sites. The overall distribution of this receptor overlaps to some extent with sites of NPR-B expression. The NPR-C receptors comprise the majority of the natriuretic peptide receptors (~80%), at least in the rat, and are located in many tissues, including vascular endothelial and smooth muscle cells, heart, adrenal glands, and kidney.[7,17,60] In rat aorta, NPR-A predominates, whereas in the inferior vena cava the major receptor is NPR-C.[62]

The number and expression of receptors probably are regulated by a variety of other factors including hormones. Heterologous down-regulation of receptor levels occurs on the surface of target cells after treatment with cGMP,[63] Ang II,[64] and endothelin.[65] The up-regulation of NPR-A receptors by bradykinin has also been reported in hypertensive rats,[66] whereas dehydration has been shown to increase the density of NPR-C receptors in rat glomeruli.[67] Many of these findings remain controversial, however, as the response to regulatory stimuli may be tissue specific. Further complicating interpretation is the change in receptor phenotype during cell culture.[68] Nonetheless, the net activity of the natriuretic peptide system is determined not only by circulating levels of the individual peptides and the phenotypic profile of receptors available to them, but also by the relative activities of the individual regulatory factors that control receptor function. So far, there is little to indicate down-regulation of NPR-C by high circulating levels of hormone. Whether the expression of NPR-A is reduced in states of sustained and high hormone secretion (e.g., chronic heart failure) remains controversial.

## METABOLISM

The metabolism of both ANP and BNP involves at least two major pathways: enzymatic cleavage by neutral endopeptidase E.C. 24.11 (NEP) (see later) and binding to the specific (high-capacity) clearance receptors, NPR-C (see Fig. 178-4). Renal excretion is relatively unimportant. Clearance sites include the kidney, lung, liver/splanchnic vascular beds, and large muscles. Human studies using ANP labeled with iodine-125 show a very high extraction ratio (50%) across a wide range of peripheral tissue.[69] The half-life of human BNP in humans (22 minutes) is much prolonged compared to that of ANP (3 minutes) due to the uniquely low affinity of human BNP for the (human) NPR-C and NEP. Despite this, the metabolic clearance rate (MCR) of human ANP and BNP is similar in humans (2–4 L per minute),[7] indicating a markedly different volume of distribution of the two peptides (greater for BNP). The concept of shared degradative pathways for ANP and BNP suggests potentially important interactions between the two hormones—support for which is provided by the finding that the addition of one hormone raises the steady-state level of the other,[70,71] presumably through competitive interaction in their metabolic/clearance pathways. These findings, however, are difficult to reconcile with other studies in which ANP clearance was not saturable at hormone concentrations three- to five-fold the basal concentration.[72]

NEP is a membrane-bound zinc metalloprotease present in many epithelial tissues, particularly the luminal proximal tubular membrane of the nephron (see Fig. 178-4). A soluble form is also detectable in human plasma.[17,73] NEP exhibits a broad specificity, acting not only on the natriuretic peptides but also on other vasoactive hormones, including bradykinin, angiotensin I (Ang I), Ang II, and endothelin. By cleaving the ring structure, the enzyme renders the hormone bioinactive. In humans, CNP is the preferred substrate for the enzyme, followed by ANP and, to a much lesser degree, BNP.[17] Addition of endopeptidase inhibitors delays clearance of exogenous peptide[74] and raises endogenous levels in healthy humans[75] as well as in patients with hypertension or heart failure.[76] These findings support the view that NEP plays a significant role in natriuretic peptide metabolism. In addition, some evidence exists that the enzyme itself may be subject to regulation, because plasma NEP levels have been shown to be significantly increased in volume-loaded states such as end-stage renal failure[73] and hypertension.[77]

The second major pathway for the clearance is receptor-mediated endocytosis by the NPR-C receptors (see Fig. 178-4). As noted, NPR-C receptors appear to comprise the majority of the natriuretic peptide receptors (at least in the rat) and are located in a wide variety of tissues.[7,60] Reflecting the high density of NPR-C and the high affinity for ANP, uptake of ANP by NPR-C appears to be a fast and effective mechanism for its removal from the circulation.[54] The NPR-C receptor may play a dominant role when receptor occupancy is low (<5%).[60] On the other hand, when endogenous ANP and BNP levels are much increased, NEP may become more important. In pacing-induced heart failure, however, NPR-C blockade significantly

elevates plasma natriuretic peptide levels. Thus, enzymatic and receptor clearance contribute equally to the clearance of ANP and BNP,[78] although this may not be true in humans.

## BIOACTIONS

The identification and localization of specific receptors for the natriuretic peptides in many tissues, including the heart, point to a vast range of bioactions—most of which appear to be concerned with *blood pressure and volume homeostasis and opposing those of the renin-angiotensin system*. Most of these effects appear to be mediated by GC receptors and a concentration-dependent increase of the intracellular second messenger, cGMP (see Fig. 178-4).[54] Details of the precise intracellular mechanisms are both complex and tissue specific but, as noted previously, are likely to involve protein kinase activation, phosphorylation of intracellular proteins, and associated changes in cytosolic ionized calcium.[79] However, the *ultimate effects of ANP and BNP in vivo are influenced by a variety of physiologic variables, including resting arterial pressure, sodium status, the degree of neurohormonal activation, and age.* In addition to ANP itself, the N-terminal proANP peptide and its putative fragments (proANP1-30, proANP31-67, and proANP79-98) are reported to have bioactivity in humans: natriuresis, diuresis, vasodilation, and stimulation of cGMP[80] (however, these findings could not be confirmed in rats,[81] and their significance remains to be clarified). The possible bioactivity of N-terminal proBNP and its fragments is unknown.

### RENAL EFFECTS

The first and best-known function of ANP is its *action on the kidney to facilitate the excretion of sodium and water*.[3] The diuretic and natriuretic effects of ANP result from complex interactions on renal hemodynamics, tubular sodium handling, and reabsorption, and modulation of a number of hormones and intrarenal paracrine factors, the influence of which varies according to volume status. Single-bolus or short-term administration of ANP in normovolemic states induces a prompt natriuresis and diuresis, and smaller increases in divalent ion and phosphate excretion without significantly increasing potassium excretion.[82] These effects are due to both renal hemodynamic and direct tubular actions. Glomerular filtration rate (GFR) is increased by ANP to dilate the afferent and constrict the efferent renal arteriole. The glomerular permeability coefficient is also enhanced through relaxation of mesangial cells, thereby increasing the area of filtration.[83] Smaller increases in ANP levels need not affect GFR to promote natriuresis but do increase the filtration fraction and, by its actions on sodium transport in the inner medullary collecting duct, increase fractional sodium excretion.[83] Most, if not all, of these actions are mediated by the NPR-A receptors and are directly related to intrarenal actions of cGMP. Other renal actions of ANP include inhibition of Ang II–induced antinatriuresis (at the level of the proximal tubule) as well as inhibition of the tubular actions of arginine vasopressin (AVP) and aldosterone.[83] ANP has also been shown to redistribute blood flow to the deeper nephrons with less sodium reabsorptive capacity. Some of the renal actions currently attributed to the circulating natriuretic peptide system could in fact be mediated by an intrarenal (paracrine) factor, *urodilatin*,[28] which has been isolated from human urine.

The natriuretic potency and mode of action of BNP in humans are likely to be *similar* to those of ANP.[70] When small equimolar doses of ANP and BNP were compared directly in normal humans, however, the renal effects were similar, yet the BNP-induced increase in plasma cGMP was less than half that induced by ANP,[84] results which raise the possibility of different mechanism(s) of action by BNP. When both hormones were administered together, the effects were additive rather than synergistic.[70,84]

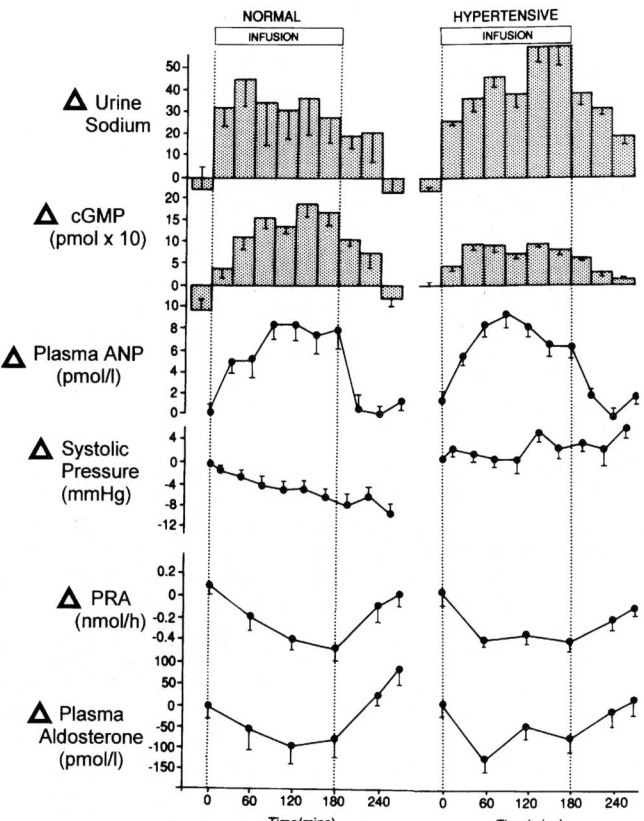

**FIGURE 178-5.** Response to intravenous administration of atrial natriuretic peptide (*ANP*) (2.25 ng/kg per minute for 180 minutes) in six normotensive subjects (*left panel*) and six hypertensive subjects (*right panel*) equilibrated on a daily sodium intake of 150 mmol. Values (mean and standard error of the mean) are plotted as change (Δ) from time-matched levels on the control day. Change in urine sodium excretion is expressed as percent change from baseline (mean of first three collection periods before infusion = 100%). Change in systolic blood pressure is shown relative to values integrated for 30 minutes immediately before infusion. (*cGMP*, cyclic guanosine monophosphate; *PRA*, plasma renin activity.) (Modified from Espiner EA, Richards AM. Atrial natriuretic peptide. An important factor in sodium and pressure regulation. Lancet 1989; 1[8640]:707; copyright The Lancet Ltd.)

The natriuretic response to ANP is critically dependent on baseline volume sodium status and renal arterial perfusion pressure, or a closely related variable. In health, increasing ANP secretion in response to small increases in atrial pressure (as occurs with increasing sodium intake or volume-expanding maneuvers) acts to increase natriuresis and restore normal intracardiac pressure. Exactly the opposite occurs when central volume is reduced: ANP secretion decreases and the renal response to the hormone is attenuated, so that sodium is conserved. A characteristic effect of prolonged (vasodepressor) infusions of ANP is an initial transient natriuresis (negative sodium balance) followed by a return to a new steady state (i.e., sodium balance is again achieved, but at a lower level of arterial perfusion pressure).[85] In other words, the familiar pressure-natriuresis curve is shifted to the left, and *the kidney can continue to excrete sodium at a lower level of blood pressure* (unless activation of the renin-angiotensin axis supervenes).[86] On the other hand, increased renal perfusion pressure, as may occur in volume-expanded states accompanying some forms of hypertension, augments the natriuretic effect of ANP (Fig. 178-5). Whether this increased responsiveness is also a reflection of a relatively depressed sympathetic nervous system (SNS) and/or low local (intrarenal) renin-Ang II activation is still unclear. In contrast to normotensive and hypertensive states, the renal response (especially natriuresis) to ANP in moderate or severe CHF

appears blunted.[87] In this setting, extracellular fluid (ECF) volume expansion is associated with reduced cardiac output, reduced renal perfusion pressure, and, therefore, reduced renal responsiveness to ANP (although plasma levels may be greatly increased). In addition to abnormal renal hemodynamics, the reduced responsiveness in heart failure is likely to be affected by enhanced activity of antinatriuretic systems (e.g., the renin-angiotensin system, SNS, and AVP), enhanced proximal tubular endopeptidase activity, and/or enhanced (cGMP) phosphodiesterase.[88] The importance of the renin-angiotensin system in this setting is demonstrated in experimental models of heart failure in which the natriuretic effect of ANP is restored by factors reducing intrarenal Ang II.[89] In contrast, angiotensin inhibition in sodium-replete normal humans has no effect on the natriuretic response to infused ANP.[90]

The natriuretic potency of BNP exceeds that of ANP in patients with heart failure.[71] As with ANP, however, the natriuretic response to exogenous BNP is impaired in patients with CHF.[91] Further work is required before one can conclude that the renal actions of BNP differ from those of ANP in sodium-retaining states such as CHF.

## HEMODYNAMIC EFFECTS

A wide range of hemodynamic actions attributable to the natriuretic peptides has been documented. Debate still exists, however, regarding the vasomotor role of the circulating hormones ANP and BNP, and their precise hemodynamic effects in health and in arterial pressure regulation. The possible vasodepressor actions of atrial extract[3] received early support from in vitro studies showing that ANP relaxed preconstricted aortic ring preparations.[92] Further, very large bolus doses of ANP lowered blood pressure acutely and also induced peripheral vasodilation.[93,94] Other studies of the short-term effects of ANP, however, have failed to show peripheral vascular relaxation. In fact, more often, peripheral vascular resistance is increased.[95] General agreement now exists that the early vasodepressor action of ANP is largely due to a fall in cardiac output dependent on reduction in cardiac filling pressure (preload). Multiple factors contribute to this effect, including dilation of capacitance veins, increased resistance to venous return, and perhaps most importantly, a shift of intravascular fluid into the interstitial space.[7] A prompt increase in venous hematocrit is a predictable and sensitive marker of this action of both ANP and BNP in humans and other species and presumably reflects both increased hydraulic pressure in the capillary bed and an increase in permeability of the vascular endothelium (Fig. 178-6). In the lung, this action of the natriuretic peptides is likely to have a protective effect against edema, because an increase in permeability in the low-pressure lung capillaries favors fluid resorption rather than filtration.[83] Other well-documented acute actions of natriuretic peptides affecting hemodynamics include early natriuresis, inhibition of renin secretion, inhibition of aldosterone secretion, and inhibition of the vasopressor response to Ang II and endothelin. ANP also reduces sympathetic tone in the peripheral vasculature by a direct inhibitory effect on sympathetic nerve outflow[96] in addition to sensitizing vagal afferent input, so that reflex tachycardia and the vasoconstrictor response to falls in preload are reduced.[97] Whereas these investigations show a wide range of hemodynamic actions in the short term, study of small changes in plasma ANP or BNP induced by constant infusion for several days in the physiologic range demonstrate significant reductions in arterial pressure (chiefly systolic) and reduced plasma volume and central filling pressure, followed later by a sustained fall in peripheral vascular resistance without any increase in renin-angiotensin-aldosterone or SNS activity.[98] Similar trends were observed in studies using long-term (4-day) infusions of ovine BNP in normotensive sheep.[99] These long-term hypotensive effects of the natriuretic peptides are not dependent on an intact vascular endothelium.[100]

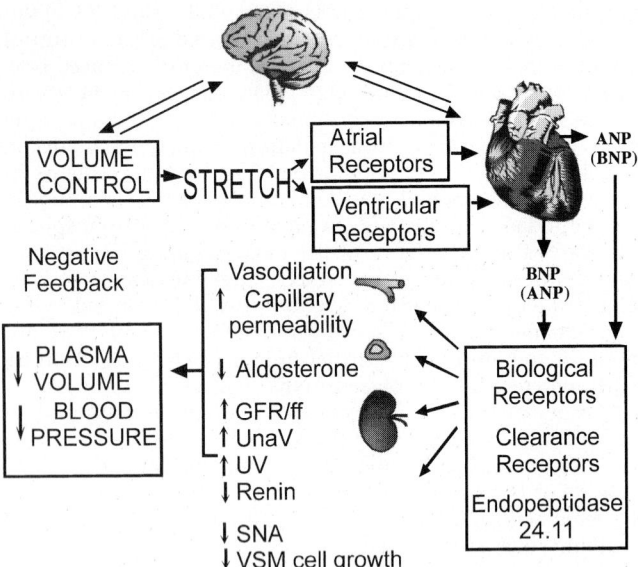

**FIGURE 178-6.** Schematic diagram showing the regulation and integrated actions of atrial natriuretic peptide (*ANP*) and brain natriuretic peptide (*BNP*). Paracrine actions of the natriuretic peptides (also C-type natriuretic peptide) on vessel wall, kidney, etc., are omitted for reasons of clarity. (*GFR*, glomerular filtration rate; *ff*, filtration fraction; *UnaV*, urine sodium excretion; *UV*, urine volume; *SNA*, sympathetic nervous activity; *VSM*, vascular smooth muscle.) (Modified from Espiner EA. Physiology of natriuretic peptides. J Intern Med 1994; 235:527; with permission of Blackwell Science, Ltd.)

The hemodynamic effects of the natriuretic peptides in pathologic states have been the subject of extensive study. In general, the response to supraphysiologic doses in the hypertensive state is similar to that in the normotensive state, although the fall in blood pressure is greater and more consistent.[101] In experimental models of volume-dependent hypertension, ANP-induced falls in blood pressure appear to be due mainly to a decrease in blood volume and cardiac output, whereas in renin-dependent models of hypertension, ANP decreases arterial pressure mainly by counteracting vasoconstriction, and cardiac output may even increase.[102] In hypertensive humans, 5-day, low-dose infusions of ANP (doubling basal plasma ANP levels) induced a prolonged hypotensive effect, first evident at 24 hours without any change in plasma renin-angiotensin but associated with a significant fall in plasma volume.[103] More unanimity is found concerning the effects of ANP and BNP infusions in heart failure. Large infusions consistently lowered preload, mean arterial pressure, and peripheral resistance, and increased cardiac output without changing the heart rate or SNS activity.[71,87,104] These beneficial hemodynamic effects are largely due to peripheral vasodilation (possibly a result of inhibition of Ang II-induced vasoconstriction), which in heart failure may fail to evoke a normal neurohumoral response.

## ANTIPROLIFERATIVE EFFECTS

All three natriuretic peptides have antiproliferative (antimitogenic) effects in a variety of tissues, including vascular smooth muscle, adrenal gland, kidney, brain, myocardiocytes, and endothelial cells.[105] ANP, acting via the NPR-A receptor,[106] induces apoptosis in neonatal rat heart cardiac myocytes. ANP and BNP have also been shown to inhibit both endothelin-1–stimulated and Ang II–stimulated incorporation of [3H]thymidine into cardiac fibroblasts.[107] This raises the possibility that natriuretic peptides regulate cell growth within the cardiac and vascular system, influencing remodeling and possibly vessel wall changes accompanying atheroma or other trauma. In this context, speculation exists that CNP, as an endothelium-

derived factor, might also play an important antimitogenic role in the prevention of vascular and cardiac remodeling.[11] Not only is CNP mRNA expression markedly enhanced in endothelial cells by cytokines and transforming growth factor-β,[108,109] but prolonged infusions of CNP in rats have been shown to significantly reduce lumen constriction (restenosis) after injury to the arterial vessel wall.[110] How the circulating hormones, ANP and BNP, interact with the vascular (paracrine) natriuretic peptide system and their relative roles as antimitogenic factors remain to be determined. However, striking ventricular overgrowth together with perivascular fibrosis occur in transgenic mice lacking a functional NPR-A receptor[111]—findings that support the view that natriuretic peptides have important roles in regulating ventricular cell growth.

## ENDOCRINE EFFECTS

Many if not all the actions of the natriuretic peptides *oppose those of the circulating and tissue renin-angiotensin system.* Although no unifying theory exists, presumably these differences ultimately depend on differential effects on intracellular movements of ionized calcium. In humans, renin is itself inhibited by small increases in either ANP or BNP within the physiologic range (see Fig. 178-6).[71,112] Inhibition is likely to be mediated by enhanced delivery of sodium and chloride to the macula densa, although evidence also exists of a direct inhibitory action of ANP on the juxtaglomerular cells.[113] Aldosterone secretion is also inhibited by ANP and BNP (see Fig. 178-6). In humans, small increases in ANP levels inhibit the effects of most aldosterone secretagogues (including potassium, adrenocorticotropin hormone [ACTH] and metoclopramide), but the stimulating effect of Ang II is most affected. In a direct comparative study of equimolar doses of ANP and BNP in normal humans, ANP significantly inhibited the plasma aldosterone response to stepped infusions of Ang II, whereas BNP did not.[84] These differences occurred despite comparable natriuresis, plasma volume contraction, and inhibition of renin. Early work showed that the mechanism of ANP's inhibitory effect on the adrenal glomerulosa involved actions to inhibit the uptake of cholesterol into the mitochondria. Specifically, ANP inhibits *steroidogenic acute regulatory (StAR) protein* gene expression, which regulates the transfer of cholesterol from the outer to the inner mitochondrial membrane.[114] Many of these findings relate to short-term effects (hours) of the natriuretic peptides. Longer-term inhibitory effects on renin-aldosterone are less well defined.[115] In fact, evidence from studies of the transgenic hypotensive mouse that overexpresses the ANP gene[116] indicates that renin-aldosterone activity is increased. These observations are consistent with findings in cases of severe heart failure in which the inhibitory effect of ANP (at least on renin secretion) is attenuated.[117] Taken together, these findings suggest that the *endocrine effects of the natriuretic peptides are more readily overridden than are the vascular vasodepressor actions.*

Numerous other endocrine actions of ANP (and BNP) have been reported in animal studies. These include inhibition of ACTH, AVP, and prolactin secretion.[7] However, none of these actions has been confirmed unequivocally in humans. Similarly, the relevance of a stimulatory effect in vitro of natriuretic peptides on testosterone secretion in Leydig cells[118] and progesterone secretion in granulosa cells[119] remains to be clarified. Natriuretic peptides, especially CNP, increase the growth of osteoblasts in vitro.[120] Further, markedly increased skeletal overgrowth occurs in the transgenic mouse that overexpresses the BNP gene,[121] suggesting that natriuretic peptides may act as paracrine factors that regulate bone formation and/or endochondral ossification.

## CENTRAL NERVOUS SYSTEM EFFECTS

Although ANP and BNP do not cross the blood–brain barrier, the finding of NPR-A receptors in subfornical and circumventricular tissues suggests that circulating ANP and BNP may affect central neural tissues regulating blood pressure and fluid homeostasis.[122] Direct central administration of ANP and BNP has been shown to reduce systemic blood pressure; to attenuate the pressor action of central Ang II; to reduce heart rate; to suppress basal, dehydration-induced, and Ang II-induced drinking; to inhibit sodium appetite; and in some circumstances to induce natriuresis and diuresis.[7,122] Thus, circulating hormone levels, acting via central NPR-A receptors, probably complement the physiologic role of systemic hormones. The presence of all three receptors as well as ANP mRNA, BNP mRNA, and especially CNP mRNA in discrete and diverse regions of the brain and spinal cord suggests the existence of an *additional brain natriuretic peptide system acting inside the blood–brain barrier.* As yet, no unified role has emerged for this complex system, and how it interdigitates, if at all, with the systemic hormonal system and blood pressure and fluid regulation remains to be seen.

## ROLE OF NATRIURETIC PEPTIDE IN PHYSIOLOGY AND PATHOPHYSIOLOGY

The diverse actions of natriuretic peptides, which affect almost all tissues concerned with the regulation of blood pressure and fluid homeostasis, provide strong circumstantial evidence that these cardiac hormones have a fundamentally important role. The foregoing clearly indicates that *ANP and BNP together constitute a dual hormonal system* (largely responsive to increases in atrial and ventricular pressure, respectively) *that serves to prevent ECF volume expansion by promoting natriuresis and vascular relaxation while concomitantly inhibiting the action of vasoconstrictor peptides and SNS activity* (see Fig. 178-6).

Nonetheless, the role and function of the natriuretic peptides have been questioned for several reasons, including lack of potency when used at physiologic concentrations for short-term periods and lack of any consistent relationship between the hormone level in blood and the natriuretic effect.[123] A number of studies have demonstrated the importance of the natriuretic peptide system, however, by examining the consequences of deficient peptide production. For example, the total removal of the heart in calves, with replacement by an artificial pump, markedly lowered plasma ANP levels and was associated with increasing edema and renin-aldosterone and AVP stimulation. In control studies, calves with artificial ventricles of comparable function, but with intact atria and normal ANP production, failed to exhibit such signs of cardiac decompensation.[124] Similarly, in comparative studies of two types of experimental heart failure in dogs, one that increases plasma ANP (rapid ventricular pacing) and one that does not (thoracic inferior vena cava constriction), much greater sodium retention and renin-angiotensin-aldosterone activation are found in the latter model despite comparable depression of cardiac output and arterial pressure.[125] If plasma ANP levels were restored in the low-ANP model, sodium retention and renin-angiotensin-aldosterone activation did not occur. Other approaches to defining the importance of sustained secretion of cardiac natriuretic peptides include the use of specific inhibitors of hormone production or action. Acute administration of HS-142-1, an inhibitor of the GC-coupled receptor, reduces sodium excretion, GFR, ventricular relaxation, and coronary blood flow, and increases blood pressure and plasma levels of renin-aldosterone, endothelin, and norepinephrine.[126–129] Other animal studies have shown that blockade of circulating ANP impairs the organism's defense against the development of hypertension[130] and/or heart failure.[128] Transgenic mice that overexpress the ANP[131] or BNP[132] gene demonstrate elevated plasma natriuretic peptide and cGMP concentrations in association with a marked and lifelong hypotension compared with wild-type controls. Mice lacking the NPR-C receptor gene (and therefore exhibiting reduced clearance of the natriuretic peptides) tend

to be volume depleted and hypotensive.[132a] Conversely, mice with a disruption of the ANP gene show no circulating ANP in conjunction with elevated blood pressures.[133] In another study, mice were generated with one, two, three, or four copies of the gene coding for the bioactive receptor, NPR-A. These animals exhibited natriuretic peptide-dependent GC activity ranging progressively from ~50% of normal in one-copy animals to twice normal in four-copy animals; corresponding blood pressures ranged from above to below normal, respectively.[134] Furthermore, mice entirely lacking a functional gene encoding NPR-A (and, therefore, largely unable to respond to either ANP or BNP) exhibit not only increased blood pressure but also marked cardiac hypertrophy and dilatation as well as (particularly in males) an increased incidence of sudden death.[111] Taken together, these studies provide strong support for the view that cardiac natriuretic peptides play a critical role in circulatory homeostasis.

## CIRCULATING LEVELS OF NATRIURETIC PEPTIDES IN HUMANS

### ASSAYS AND CLINICAL USE

The plasma venous concentration of immunoreactive ANP approximates 5 to 25 pmol/L and shows little if any evidence of pulsatile secretion or intrinsic diurnal rhythmicity. Levels increase with age and are higher in sodium-loaded or volume expanded states. A change from supine to upright posture decreases plasma ANP levels. In keeping with high tissue extraction, the arteriovenous ratio is ~2:1 across the lower limb, kidney, and liver.[135] In contrast, plasma immunoreactive BNP levels in normal subjects are lower (0.3–10 pmol/L) than those of ANP. Variations in levels reported by different laboratories may relate to the choice of antiserum (monoclonal or polyclonal) and/or method of extraction (if any), which may affect the ability to detect the high-molecular-weight forms (proBNP) that circulate in human plasma.[17,24] Like ANP, BNP levels increase in the elderly and rise with increasing dietary sodium intake but show less fluctuation than ANP with posture, exercise, and so on, in keeping with a lower atrial content and lower affinity of human BNP for NPR-C and NEP 24.11,[22,59] and the longer half-life in plasma (seven-fold to that of ANP). The arteriovenous BNP ratio is lower than that of ANP.[44]

In keeping with changes in the intracardiac pressure, plasma ANP and BNP levels are elevated in a wide range of pathologic disorders. The most striking increases occur in CHF (Fig. 178-7), with both ANP and BNP secreted according to the severity of ventricular dysfunction[25] (see later). Plasma BNP appears to be uniquely elevated in hypertrophic obstructive cardiomyopathy.[136] Whereas the proportion of proBNP in normal plasma (~66% of total immunoreactive BNP) does not change as heart failure supervenes,[36] the proportion of high-molecular-weight ANP (and the secretion of β–ANP, an antiparallel dimer with reduced bioactivity)[137] increases with the severity of cardiac decompensation. These changes in molecular forms of plasma ANP are presumably related to the increase in (constitutive) ANP secretion from the ventricle.[17] As shown in Figure 178-7, plasma levels of both ANP and BNP are also increased soon after myocardial infarction even in the absence of clinical cardiac decompensation, although overall levels do reflect infarct size and the increase in cardiac filling pressure.[42] The increased concentrations of ANP and BNP in chronic renal failure may also reflect volume overload,[138] particularly as levels fall after dialysis (ANP > BNP; see Fig. 178-7). Raised levels of both hormones are also observed in pulmonary hypertension (reflecting right ventricular dysfunction),[139] in acute lung injury,[140] and in a variety of other noncardiac edematous states—including nephrosis and cirrhosis, in which the central blood volume may be increased.[141] Significant but smaller increases in both ANP

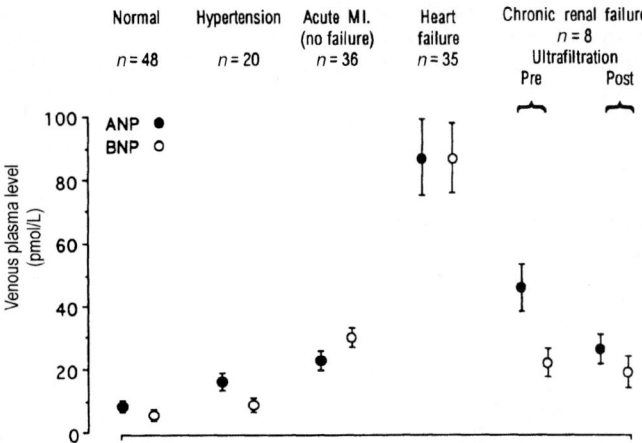

**FIGURE 178-7.** Venous plasma atrial natriuretic peptide (*ANP*) levels (*filled circles*) and concurrent brain natriuretic peptide (*BNP*) levels (*open circles*) in normal subjects and patients with circulatory disorders (mean ± standard error of the mean; *n* = number of subjects in each group). All samples were assayed in the same laboratory using previously published techniques. Hypertensive patients showed no evidence of significant end-organ disease. Patients with acute (uncomplicated) myocardial infarction (*MI*) had blood drawn within 24 hours of admission. Heart failure was of recent onset, New York Heart Association functional class II–IV. In patients with chronic renal failure, blood was drawn before and after acute volume depletion by ultrafiltration. (Data for hypertensive patients from Richards AM, Crozier IG, Espiner EA, et al. Plasma brain natriuretic peptide and endopeptidase 24.11 inhibition in hypertension. Hypertension 1993; 22:231; and from Pidgeon BG, Richards AM, Nicholls MG, et al. Differing metabolism and bioactivity of atrial and brain natriuretic peptides in essential hypertension. Hypertension 1996; 27:906. Data for patients with acute MI from Foy SG, Crozier IG, Richards AM, et al. Neurohormonal changes after acute myocardial infarction: relationships with haemodynamic indices and effects of ACE inhibition. Eur Heart J 1995; 16:770. Data for normal patients and those with heart failure from Yandle TG, Richards AM, Gilbert A, et al. Assay of brain natriuretic peptide [BNP] in human plasma: evidence for high molecular weight BNP as a major plasma component in heart failure. J Clin Endocrinol Metab 1993 76:832. Data for patients with chronic renal failure from Corboy JC, Walker RJ, Simmonds MB, et al. Plasma natriuretic peptides and cardiac volume during acute changes in intravascular volume in haemodialysis patients. Clin Sci [Colch] 1994 87[6]:679.)

and BNP levels occur in hypertension (see Fig. 178-7) and correlate with left ventricular hypertrophy.[101] Consistent with the effect of atrial or ventricular pacing in experimental heart failure, a variety of tachyarrhythmias may markedly increase plasma hormone levels (ANP > BNP in humans).[142] Rapid supraventricular tachycardia may initiate a polyuric syndrome with natriuresis, as described 20 years before the discovery of the natriuretic peptides.[143] The possibility that increases in circulating natriuretic peptides may underlie syndromes of cerebral salt wasting[144] has received support from studies of patients with subarachnoid hemorrhage.[145] Although one study reports a uniquely increased secretion of BNP (ten-fold the basal level, with ANP unchanged),[145] comparable studies in the authors' laboratory show that both ANP and BNP are similarly increased after the acute insult. Further work is required to determine the mechanism of this increase and its significance in the pathogenesis of hyponatremic syndromes accompanying acute brain injury.

Thus, altered levels of circulating hormones, ANP and BNP, are *largely secondary to changes in the intracardiac pressure and/or altered myocardial work*. Few, if any, reports have been published of primary disorders of natriuretic peptide secretion or action that resulted in disease, with the possible exception of cases of

familial open-angle glaucoma.[146] The findings in transgenic animal studies[111,133,134] suggest that, conceivably, polymorphism in the NPR-A or other genes may contribute to some forms of essential hypertension[147,147a] or predispose to the onset of early heart failure after myocardial injury in humans. Excessive production of ANP has been reported[148]; however, proof of a gradient across the tumor and restoration of normal levels after resection of the tumor has yet to be shown. Even if plasma hormone assays have yet to prove themselves in the diagnosis of primary disorders of blood pressure or volume status, a large body of evidence now supports their use as markers of cardiac function. For example, raised levels of ANP or BNP, or their N-terminal peptides (which have slower clearance rates and, hence, higher plasma concentrations) are indicators of symptomless left ventricular dysfunction[149,150] and predict subsequent deterioration in hemodynamic function or the development of frank heart failure.[151,152] In patients presenting with acute dyspnea, raised plasma concentrations of BNP give strong support to a diagnosis of cardiac failure, as opposed to primary lung disease,[153] whereas in patients with essential hypertension, elevated levels of circulating natriuretic peptides may reflect increased left ventricular mass.[154] The prognosis for patients who experience acute myocardial infarction,[152,155,156] or those with established heart failure,[157] is also predicted by levels of the cardiac natriuretic peptides. BNP in particular (due to its predominantly ventricular origin, more rapid induction, and slower clearance rate), and its N-terminal fragment (NT-BNP),[158] may be especially useful in clinical diagnosis and in determining prognosis, as these hormones correlate better with severity and indicators of cardiac dysfunction than do ANP and NT-ANP (Fig. 178-8).[25,44,156]

Thus, a relatively cheap and rapid blood test may ultimately be a *guide for the introduction or intensification of cardiac treatment*. Further, patients with possible ventricular dysfunction may be *screened* using plasma BNP assays, permitting selection of patients for more detailed (and costly) investiga-

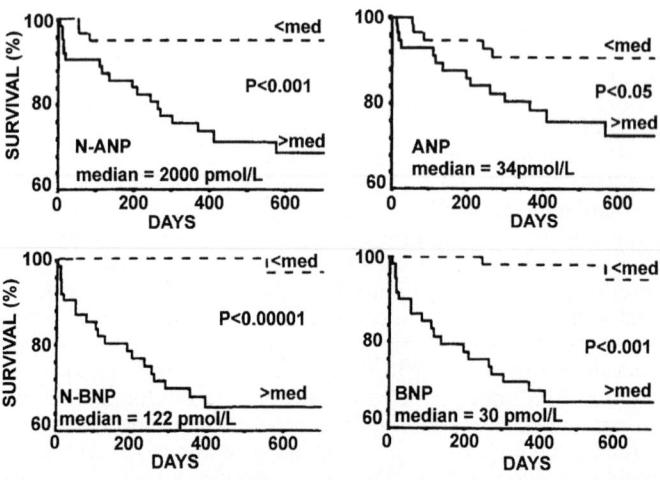

**FIGURE 178-8.** Kaplan-Meier survival curves for 121 patients with myocardial infarction. Patients were divided into two subgroups with early postinfarction plasma natriuretic peptide concentrations (atrial natriuretic peptide [ANP] and its N-terminal fragment [N-ANP], brain natriuretic peptide [BNP] and its N-terminal fragment [N-BNP]) that were above (*solid line*) and below (*dashed line*) the group median (med). Venous blood was drawn between 24 and 96 hours after the onset of symptoms. Inclusion criteria were age younger than 80 years of age, absence of cardiogenic shock, and survival for at least 24 hours after myocardial infarction. *p* Values refer to significance values for the differences between the two groups. (From Richards AM, Nicholls MG, Yandle TG, et al. Plasma N-terminal pro-brain natriuretic peptide and adrenomedullin: new neurohormonal predictors of left ventricular function and prognosis after myocardial infarction. Circulation 1998; 97:1921.)

tions, such as echocardiography. Indeed, the levels of cardiac peptides appear to be *superior to time-honored indicators (such as ejection fraction) in detecting heart failure based on diastolic dysfunction, which comprises one-third of all clinical heart failure.*[159] Further, a study has shown that the use of plasma NT-proBNP measurements to guide treatment for heart failure (compared to standardized clinical assessment) both reduced total cardiovascular events and delayed the time of the first event.[159a] The same hormone measurements may provide *prognostic insights after myocardial infarction*[155,156] and *in heart failure*[10] *that are independent of ejection fraction.* How useful the cardiac natriuretic peptides become in everyday clinical decision making involving patients at risk for heart disease remains to be seen. Again, whether the measurement of natriuretic peptide levels will eventually help clinicians to assess volume status in noncardiac disorders is unclear. Plasma ANP (which increases) is more responsive to salt loading than plasma renin activity (which decreases),[160] a finding that has led to the use of ANP assays in *assessing the adequacy of mineralocorticoid replacement in patients with Addison disease.*[161] Similarly, the possibility exists that, along with aldosterone and renin, measurement of plasma natriuretic peptides (e.g., NT-BNP) may prove to be a useful marker of the *hyperexpanded state associated with primary hyperaldosteronism.*[162]

## THERAPEUTIC IMPLICATIONS

Due to the vasodilator, natriuretic/diuretic, renin-angiotensin-aldosterone–inhibitory and antimitogenic actions of these peptides, any maneuver that increases their circulating and tissue levels is likely to be helpful in the treatment of a variety of cardiovascular and volume-overload disorders. As mentioned previously, the short-term intravenous administration of exogenous ANP and BNP in various doses has been shown to have beneficial hemodynamic and renal effects in patients with hypertension or heart failure.[71,104,163] Natriuretic peptide administration may also be a beneficial adjunctive component of reperfusion therapy for patients with acute myocardial infarction, as ANP is reported to inhibit reperfusion-induced ventricular arrhythmias and preserve ATP content in the ischemic myocardium.[164] The infusion of ANP has been shown to reduce anginal symptoms,[165] whereas BNP is reported to suppress hyperventilation-induced attacks in patients with variant angina by reducing coronary artery spasm.[166] Furthermore, ANP gene therapy, by direct intraluminal delivery via the affected vessel, is already a prospect.[167] In patients with acute renal failure, large doses of ANP significantly improve glomerular function and reduce the need for dialysis.[168] Although the peptidic nature (requiring intravenous administration) and relatively short half-lives of ANP and BNP in plasma limit their clinical application, the routine infusion of ANP is currently approved in Japanese hospitals for patients with fluid-overload states.

An alternative approach is to *enhance levels of the endogenous peptides through inhibition of their enzymatic breakdown by NEP 24.11.* This approach appears to have a number of advantages, including availability of oral inhibitors and a relatively prolonged effect in enhancing circulating levels of the cardiac natriuretic peptides (ANP more than BNP in humans). The beneficial hemodynamic, hormonal, and renal effects of short-term NEP inhibition in hypertension and heart failure are well documented and mimic those of exogenous ANP and BNP.[43,169,170] A major advantage of NEP inhibition (compared with exogenous natriuretic peptide administration) is the increased protection of the peptides from degradation within the kidney, thus increasing the local hormone concentration and enhancing natriuresis. Indeed, NEP administration in heart failure is associated with an increased natriuresis and diuresis[170] in contrast with the blunted renal response observed with exogenous ANP infusion alone.[87] Long-term use of NEP inhibitors has also been

shown to reduce intraocular pressure and may have a place in the management of glaucoma.[171] Another potential approach increases endogenous natriuretic peptide levels by blocking the clearance receptor, NPR-C.[78] The blockade of both degradative pathways, as shown in sheep with experimental heart failure, induces greater than additive increments in plasma ANP, BNP, and cGMP concentrations and enhances the beneficial hemodynamic and renal effects (compared with blocking enzyme or receptor alone).[78] The long-term use of compounds that potentiate circulating levels of the natriuretic peptides and their actions may also promote the antiproliferative effects of these peptides and may impede the detrimental consequences of cardiac and vascular smooth muscle hypertrophy and endothelial proliferation.[172]

## FUTURE PROSPECTS AND CONCLUSIONS

A wealth of information exists on the molecular biology, physiology, and pathophysiology of the cardiac natriuretic peptides. They have a well-established role in pressure and volume homeostasis. A number of questions remain unanswered, however. Do ANP and BNP simply duplicate one another's roles, or do they have distinct functions? Differences listed in Table 178-1 suggest that distinct functions are highly probable. If so, do specific receptors exist for either ANP or BNP? Do the amino-terminal forms (NT-ANP, NT-BNP) perform any role in health or disease? The picture is complicated by the identification of multiple natriuretic hormones—some circulating, others largely confined to tissues—with the potential to interact, as observed in other vasoactive hormonal systems such as the renin-angiotensin system. Untangling the individual roles of these hormones will be difficult and will require specific antagonists and/or use of transgenic models. Results from BNP knock-out, disruption of NPR-B and NPR-C receptors, or combinations of these are awaited with interest. Finally, how hormones of the natriuretic peptide system interact with other local vasoactive (nonangiotensin) systems—

**TABLE 178-1.**

**Comparative Physiology of Atrial Natriuretic Peptide (ANP) and Brain Natriuretic Peptide (BNP) in Humans**

|  | ANP | BNP |
|---|---|---|
| **Major site of synthesis** | Cardiac atrium | Cardiac ventricle |
| **Cardiac mRNA content:** | | |
| Normal | Ventricle << atrium | Ventricle > atrium |
| Heart failure | Ventricle > atrium | Ventricle >> atrium |
| Induction | Slow | Rapid |
| mRNA turnover | Slow | Rapid |
| **Major stimulus to synthesis** | Atrial transmural pressure | Ventricular wall tension |
| **Major type of secretion** | Regulated | Constitutive |
| **Major storage form in atria** | Prohormone (ANP1-126) | Mature hormone (BNP-32) |
| **Major plasma form** | Mature hormone (ANP-28) | Prohormone (BNP1-108) |
| **Normal plasma levels** | 5–20 pmol/L | 0.6–9.0 pmol/L |
| **Plasma half-life** | 3 min | 22 min |
| **C-receptor affinity** | High | Lower than ANP |
| **Affinity for NEP** | High | Lower than ANP |
| **Bioreceptor type** | NPR-A (other?) | NPR-A (other?) |
| **Dissimilar bioactivity** | | Less cGMP generation? |
| | | Less inhibition of aldosterone? |

*NEP,* neutral endopeptidase; *NPR-A,* natriuretic peptide receptor A; *GMP,* guanosine monophosphate.

such as nitric oxide, endothelin, and adrenomedullin—is largely unexplored.

# REFERENCES

1. Kisch B. Electron microscopy of the atrium of the heart. Exp Med Surg 1956; 14:99.
2. Henry JP, Gauer ON, Reeves JL. Evidence on the atrial location of receptors influencing urine flow. Circ Res 1956; 5:85.
3. De Bold AJ, Borenstein HB, Veress AT, Sonnenberg H. A rapid and potent natriuretic response to intravenous injection of atrial myocardial extracts in rats. Life Sci 1981; 28:89.
4. Kangawa H, Marsuo H. Purification and complete amino acid sequence of alpha human atrial natriuretic polypeptide (alpha-h ANP). Biochem Biophys Res Commun 1984; 18:131.
5. Sudoh T, Kangawa K, Minamino N, Matsuo H. A new natriuretic peptide in porcine brain. Nature 1988; 332:78.
6. Sudoh T, Minamino N, Kangawa K, Matsuo H. C-type natriuretic peptide (CNP): a new member of natriuretic peptide family identified in porcine brain. Biochem Biophys Res Commun 1990; 168:863.
7. Espiner EA, Richards AM, Yandle TG, Nicholls MG. Natriuretic hormones. Endocrinol Metab Clin North Am 1995; 24:481.
8. Hama N, Itoh H, Shirakami G, et al. Detection of C-type natriuretic peptide in human circulation and marked increase of plasma CNP levels in septic shock patients. Biochem Biophys Res Commun 1994; 198:1177.
9. Totsune K, Takahashi K, Murakami O, et al. Elevated plasma C-type natriuretic peptide concentrations in patients with chronic renal failure. Clin Sci 1994; 87:319.
10. Wei CM, Heublein DM, Perrella MA, et al. Natriuretic peptide system in human heart failure. Circulation 1993; 88:1004.
11. Itoh H, Suga S, Ogawa Y, et al. Cellular and molecular aspects of C-type natriuretic peptide (CNP). In: Samson WK, Levin ER, eds. Contemporary endocrinology: natriuretic peptides in health and disease. Totowa, NJ: Humana Press, 1997:Chapter 7.
12. Lindpaintner K, Ganten D. The cardiac renin angiotensin system. An appraisal of present experimental and clinical evidence. Circ Res 1991; 68:905.
13. Colucci WS. Myocardial endothelin. Does it play a role in myocardial failure? Circulation 1996; 93:1069.
14. Jougasaki M, Wei CM, Heublein DM, et al. Immunohistochemical localization of adrenomedullin in canine heart and aorta. Peptides 1995; 16:773.
15. Bui TD, Shallal A, Malik AN, et al. Parathyroid hormone related peptide gene expression in human fetal and adult heart. Cardiovasc Res 1993; 27:1204.
16. Tamura N, Ogawa Y, Yasoda A, et al. Two cardiac natriuretic peptide genes (atrial natriuretic peptide and brain natriuretic peptide) are organized in tandem in the mouse and human genomes. J Mol Cell Cardiol 1996; 28:1811.
17. Yandle TG. Biochemistry of natriuretic peptides. J Intern Med 1994; 235:561.
18. Klein RM, Kelly KB, Meriskoliversidge EM. A clathrin-coated vesicle-mediated pathway in atrial natriuretic peptide (ANP) secretion. J Mol Cell Cardiol 1993; 25:437.
19. Bloch KD, Seidman JG, Naftilan JD, et al. Neonatal atria and ventricles secrete atrial natriuretic factor via tissue-specific secretory pathways. Cell 1986; 47:695.
20. Irons CE, Sei CA, Glembotski CC. Regulated secretion of atrial natriuretic factor from cultured ventricular myocytes. Am J Physiol 1993; 264:H282.
21. Misono KS, Grammer RT, Fukumi H, Inagami T. Rat atrial natriuretic factor: isolation, structure and biological activities of four major peptides. Biochem Biophys Res Commun 1984; 123:444.
22. Suga S, Nakao K, Hosoda M, et al. Receptor selectivity of natriuretic peptide family, atrial natriuretic peptide, brain natriuretic peptide, and C-type natriuretic peptide. Endocrinology 1992; 130:229.
23. Kambayashi Y, Nakao K, Kumura H, et al. Biological characterization of human brain natriuretic peptide (BNP) and rat BNP: species-specific actions of BNP. Biochem Biophys Res Commun 1990; 173:599.
24. Hunt PJ, Yandle TG, Nicholls MG, et al. The amino-terminal portion of pro-brain natriuretic peptide (Pro-BNP) circulates in human plasma. Biochem Biophys Res Commun 1995; 214:1175.
25. Mukoyama M, Nakao K, Hosoda K, et al. Brain natriuretic peptide as a novel cardiac hormone in humans. Evidence for an exquisite dual natriuretic peptide system, atrial natriuretic peptide and brain natriuretic peptide. J Clin Invest 1991; 87:1402.
26. Ogawa Y, Nakao K, Mukoyama M, et al. Natriuretic peptides as cardiac hormones in normotensive and spontaneously hypertensive rats. The ventricle is a major site of synthesis and secretion of brain natriuretic peptide. Circ Res 1991; 69:491.
27. Ruskoaho H. Atrial natriuretic peptide: synthesis, release, and metabolism. Pharmacol Rev 1992; 44:479.
28. Forssmann W-G. Urodilatin (ularitide, INN): a renal natriuretic peptide. Molecular biology and clinical importance. Nephron 1995; 69:211.
29. Nakamura S, Naruse M, Naruse K, et al. Atrial natriuretic peptide and brain natriuretic peptide coexist in the secretory granules of human cardiac myocytes. Am J Hypertens 1991; 4:909.
30. Hosoda K, Nakao K, Mukoyama M, et al. Expression of brain natriuretic peptide gene in human heart. Hypertension 1991; 17:1152.
31. Tanaka M, Hiroe M, Nishikawa T, et al. Cellular localization and structural characterization of natriuretic peptide-expressing ventricular myocytes from patients with dilated cardiomyopathy. J Histochem Cytochem 1994; 42:1207.
32. Ledsome JR, Wilson N, Courneya CA, Rankin AJ. Release of atrial natriuretic peptide by atrial distention. Can J Physiol Pharmacol 1985; 63:739.
33. Leskinen H, Vuolteenaho O, Toth M, Ruskoaho H. Atrial natriuretic peptide (ANP) inhibits its own secretion via ANPA receptors: altered effect in experimental hypertension. Endocrinology 1997; 138:1893.
34. Leskinen H, Vuolteenaho O, Toth M, Ruskoaho H. Combined inhibition of endothelin and angiotensin II receptors blocks volume load induced cardiac hormone release. Circ Res 1997; 80:114.
35. Cameron VA, Aitken GD, Ellmers LJ, et al. The sites of gene expression of atrial, brain and C-type natriuretic peptides in mouse fetal development: temporal changes in embryos and placentas. Endocrinology 1996; 137:817.
36. Yandle TG, Richards AM, Gilbert A, et al. Assay of brain natriuretic peptide (BNP) in human plasma: evidence for high molecular weight BNP as a major plasma component in heart failure. J Clin Endocrinol Metab 1993; 6:832.
37. Buckley MG, Sethi D, Markandu ND, et al. Plasma concentrations and comparisons of brain natriuretic peptide and atrial natriuretic peptide in normal subjects, cardiac transplant recipients and patients with dialysis-independent or dialysis-dependent chronic renal failure. Clin Sci 1992; 83:437.
38. Lang CC, Coutie WJ, Khong TK, et al. Dietary sodium loading increases plasma brain natriuretic peptide levels in man. J Hypertens 1991; 9:779.
39. Thibault G, Doubell AF, Garcia R, et al. Endothelin-stimulated secretion of natriuretic peptides by rat atrial myocytes is mediated by endothelin A receptors. Circ Res 1994; 74:460.
40. Toth M, Vuorinen KH, Vuolteenaho O, et al. Hypoxia stimulates release of ANP and BNP from perfused rat ventricular myocardium. Am J Physiol 1994; 266:H1572.
41. Kinnunen P, Vuolteenaho O, Ruskoaho H. Mechanisms of atrial and brain natriuretic peptide release from rat ventricular myocardium: effect of stretching. Endocrinology 1993; 132:1961.
42. Nicholls MG. The natriuretic peptides in heart failure. J Intern Med 1994; 235:515.
43. Richards AM, Crozier IG, Espiner EA, et al. Plasma brain natriuretic peptide and endopeptidase 24.11 inhibition in hypertension. Hypertension 1993; 22:231.
44. Richards AM, Crozier IG, Yandle TG, et al. Brain natriuretic factor: regional plasma concentrations and correlations with haemodynamic state in cardiac disease. Br Heart J 1993; 69:414.
45. Nicholson S, Richards M, Espiner E, et al. Atrial and brain natriuretic peptide response to exercise in patients with ischaemic heart disease. Clin Exp Pharmacol Physiol 1993; 20:535.
46. Lang CC, Choy AMJ, Turner K, et al. The effect of intravenous saline loading on plasma levels of brain natriuretic peptide in man. J Hypertens 1993; 11:737.
47. Morita E, Yasue H, Yoshimura M, et al. Increased plasma levels of brain natriuretic peptide in patients with acute myocardial infarction. Circulation 1993; 88:82.
48. Yoshibayashi M, Kamiya T, Saito Y, Matsuo H. Increased plasma levels of brain natriuretic peptide in hypertrophic cardiomyopathy. N Engl J Med 1993; 329:433.
49. Shimoike H, Iwai N, Kinoshita M. Differential regulation of natriuretic peptide genes in infarcted rat hearts. Clin Exp Pharmacol Physiol 1997; 24:23.
50. Yoshimura M, Yasue H, Okumura K, et al. Different secretion patterns of atrial natriuretic peptide and brain natriuretic peptide in patients with congestive heart failure. Circulation 1993; 87:464.
51. Yasue H, Yoshimura M, Sumida H, et al. Localisation and mechanism of secretion of B-type natriuretic peptide in comparison with those of A-type natriuretic peptide in normal subjects and patients with heart failure. Circulation 1994; 90:195.
52. Hanford DS, Thuerauf DJ, Murray SF, Glembotski CC. Brain natriuretic peptide is induced by α1-adrenergic agonists as a primary response gene in cultured rat cardiac myocytes. J Biol Chem 1994; 269:26227.
53. Liang F, Gardener DG. Autocrine/paracrine determinants of strain-activated brain natriuretic peptide gene expression in cultured cardiac myocytes. J Biol Chem 1998; 273:14612.
54. Maack T, Nikonova LN, Friedman O, Cohen D. Functional properties and dynamics of natriuretic factor receptors. Proc Soc Exp Biol Med 1996; 213:109.
55. Kishi Y, Ashikaga T, Watanabe R, Numano F. Atrial natriuretic peptide reduces cyclic AMP by activating cyclic GMP-stimulated phosphodiesterase in vascular endothelial cells. J Cardiovasc Pharmacol 1994; 24:351.
56. Anand-Srivastava MB, Sehl PD, Lowe DG. Cytoplasmic domain of natriuretic peptide receptor-C inhibits adenylyl cyclase. Involvement of a pertussis toxin-sensitive G protein. J Biol Chem 1996; 271:19324.
57. Levin ER. Natriuretic peptide C-receptor: more than a clearance receptor. Am J Physiol 1993; 264:E483.
58. Hutchinson HG, Trindade PT, Cunanan DB, et al. Mechanisms of natriuretic-peptide-induced growth inhibition of vascular smooth muscle cells. Cardiovasc Res 1997; 35:158.
59. Engel AM, Schoenfeld JR, Lowe DG. A single residue determines the distinct pharmacology of rat and human natriuretic peptide receptor-C. J Biol Chem 1994; 269:17005.

60. Nakao K, Ogawa Y, Suga S, Imura H. Molecular biology and biochemistry of the natriuretic peptide system. II: Natriuretic peptide receptors. J Hypertens 1992; 10:1111.

61. Yamamoto T, Feng L, Mizuno T, et al. Expression of mRNA for natriuretic peptide receptor subtypes in bovine kidney. Am J Physiol 1994; 267:F318.

62. Yoshimoto T, Naruse M, Naruse K, et al. Differential gene expression of vascular natriuretic peptide receptor subtype in artery and vein. Biochem Biophys Res Commun 1995; 216:535.

63. Kato J, Lanier-Smith KL, Currie MG. Cyclic GMP down-regulates atrial natriuretic peptide receptors on cultured vascular endothelial cells. J Biol Chem 1991; 266:14681.

64. Yoshimoto T, Naruse M, Naruse K, et al. Angiotensin II-dependent down-regulation of vascular natriuretic peptide type C receptor gene expression in hypertensive rats. Endocrinology 1996; 137:1102.

65. Jaiswal RK. Endothelin inhibits the atrial natriuretic factor stimulated cGMP production by activating the protein kinase C in rat aortic smooth muscle cells. Biochem Biophys Res Commun 1992; 182:395.

66. Yoshimoto T, Naruse K, Shionoya K, et al. Angiotensin converting enzyme inhibitor normalizes vascular natriuretic peptide type A receptor gene expression via bradykinin-dependent mechanism in hypertensive rats. Biochem Biophys Res Commun 1996; 218:50.

67. Kollenda MC, Vollmar AM, McEnroe GA, Gerbes AL. Dehydration increases the density of C receptors for ANF on rat glomerular membranes. Am J Physiol 1990; 256:R1084.

68. Suga S, Nakao K, Kishimoto I, et al. Phenotype-related alteration in expression of natriuretic peptide receptor in aortic smooth muscle cells. Circ Res 1992; 71:34.

69. Pilo A, Iervasi G, Clerico A, et al. Circulatory models in metabolic studies of rapidly renewed hormones: application to ANP kinetics. Am J Physiol 1998; 274:E560.

70. Florkowski CM, Richards AM, Espiner EA, et al. Renal, endocrine, and hemodynamic interactions of atrial and brain natriuretic peptides in normal man. Am J Physiol 1994; 266:R1244.

71. Yoshimura M, Yasue H, Morita E, et al. Hemodynamic, renal, and hormonal responses to brain natriuretic peptide in patients with congestive heart failure. Circulation 1991; 84:1581.

72. Iervasi G, Clerico A, Pilo A, et al. Evidence that atrial natriuretic peptide tissue extraction is not changed by large increases in its plasma levels induced by pacing in humans. J Clin Endocrinol Metab 1997; 82:884.

73. Deschodt-Lanckman M, Micheaux F, De Prez E, et al. Increased serum levels of endopeptidase 24.11 ("enkephalinase") in patients with end-stage renal failure. Life Sci 1989; 45:133.

74. Richards AM, Wittert G, Espiner EA, et al. EC 24.11 inhibition in man alters clearance of atrial natriuretic peptide. J Clin Endocrinol Metab 1991; 72:1317.

75. Richards M, Espiner E, Frampton C, et al. Inhibition of endopeptidase EC 24.11 in humans—renal and endocrine effects. Hypertension 1990; 16:269.

76. Schwartz J-C, Gros C, Lecomte J-M, Bralet J. Enkephalinase (EC 3.4.24.11) inhibitors: protection of endogenous ANF against inactivation and potential therapeutic applications. Life Sci 1990; 47:1279.

77. Yandle T, Richards AM, Smith MW, et al. Assay of endopeptidase.11 (EC3.4.24.11) activity in human plasma. Application to in vivo studies of endopeptidase inhibitors. Clin Chem 1992; 38:1785.

78. Rademaker MT, Charles CJ, Kosoglou T, et al. Clearance receptors and endopeptidase: equal role in natriuretic peptide metabolism in heart failure. Am J Physiol 1997; 273:H2372.

79. Anand-Srivastava MB, Trachte GJ. Atrial natriuretic factor receptors and signal transduction mechanisms. Pharmacol Reviews 1993; 45:455.

80. Vesely DL, Douglass MA, Dietz JR, et al. Three peptides from the atrial natriuretic factor prohormone amino terminus lower blood pressure and produce diuresis, natriuresis, and/or kaliuresis in humans. Circulation 1994; 90:1129.

81. Weir ML, Honrath U, Flynn TG, Sonnenberg H. Lack of biological activity or specific binding of amino-terminal pro-ANP segments in the rat. Regul Pept 1994; 53:111.

82. Richards AM, McDonald D, Fitzpatrick MA, et al. Atrial natriuretic hormone has biological effects in man at physiological plasma concentrations. J Clin Endocrinol Metab 1988; 67:1134.

83. Maack T. Role of atrial natriuretic factor in volume control. Kidney Int 1996; 49:1732.

84. Hunt P, Espiner EA, Nicholls MG, et al. Differing biological effects of equimolar atrial and brain natriuretic peptide infusions in normal man. J Clin Endocrinol Metab 1996; 81:3871.

85. Hildebrandt DA, Mizelle HL, Brands MW, et al. Intrarenal natriuretic peptide infusion lowers arterial pressure chronically. Am J Physiol 1990; 259:R585.

86. Lohmeier TE, Shin Y, Reinhart GA, Hester RL. Angiotensin and ANP secretion during chronically controlled increments in atrial pressure. Am J Physiol 1994; 266:R989.

87. Cody RJ, Atlas SA, Laragh JH, et al. Atrial natriuretic factor in normal subjects and heart failure patients. Plasma levels and renal, hormonal and hemodynamic responses to peptide infusion. J Clin Invest 1986; 78:1362.

88. Lee EY, Humphreys MH. Phosphodiesterase activity as a mediator of renal resistance to ANP in pathological salt retention. Am J Physiol 1996; 271:F3.

89. Lohmeier TE, Mizelle HL, Reinhart GA, et al. Atrial natriuretic peptide and sodium homeostasis in compensated heart failure. Am J Physiol 1996; 271:R1353.

90. Richards AM, Rao G, Espiner EA, Yandle TG. Interaction of angiotensin converting enzyme and atrial natriuretic factor. Hypertension 1989; 13:193.

91. Jensen KT, Eiskjaer H, Carstens J, Pederson EB. Renal effects of brain natriuretic peptide in patients with congestive heart failure. Clin Sci 1999; 96:5.

92. Winquist RJ, Faison EP, Nutt RF. Vasodilator profile of synthetic atrial natriuretic factor. Eur J Pharmacol 1984; 102:169.

93. Richards AM. Atrial natriuretic factor administration to humans: 1984. J Cardiovasc Pharmacol 1989; 13:S69.

94. Shen Y-T, Graham RM, Vatner SF. Effects of atrial natriuretic factor on blood flow distribution and vascular resistance in conscious dogs. Am J Physiol 1991; 260:H1893.

95. Woods RL. Vasoconstrictor actions of atrial natriuretic peptide in the splanchnic circulation of anesthetized dogs. Am J Physiol 1998; 275:R1822.

96. Floras JS. Sympathoinhibitory effects of atrial natriuretic factor in normal humans. Circulation 1990; 81:1860.

97. Volpe M. Atrial natriuretic peptide and baroreflex control of circulation. Am J Hypertens 1992; 5:488.

98. Charles CJ, Espiner EA, Richards AM. Cardiovascular actions of ANF: contributions of renal, neurohumoral and hemodynamic factors in sheep. Am J Physiol 1993; 264:R533.

99. Charles CJ, Espiner EA, Richards AM, et al. Chronic infusions of brain natriuretic peptide in conscious sheep: bioactivity at low physiological levels. Clin Sci 1998; 95:701.

100. Melo LG, Veress AT, Ackermann U, Sonnenberg H. Chronic regulation of arterial blood pressure by ANP: role of endogenous vasoactive endothelial factors. Am J Physiol 1998; 275:H1826.

101. Richards AM. The natriuretic peptides and hypertension. J Intern Med 1994; 235:543.

102. Atlas SA, Maack T. Atrial natriuretic factor. In: Windhager EE, ed. Handbook of physiology: renal physiology. New York: Oxford University Press, 1992:1577.

103. Janssen MT, de Zeeuw D, van der Hem GK, de Jong PE. Antihypertensive effect of a 5-day infusion of atrial natriuretic peptide in man. Hypertension 1989; 13:640.

104. Marcus LS, Hart D, Packer M, et al. Hemodynamic and renal excretory effects of human brain natriuretic peptide infusion in patients with congestive heart failure. Circulation 1996; 94:3184.

105. Appel RG. Growth-regulatory properties of atrial natriuretic factor. Am J Physiol 1992; 262:F911.

106. Wu CF, Bishopric NH, Pratt RE. Atrial natriuretic peptide induces apoptosis in neonate rat cardiac myocytes. J Biol Chem 1997; 272:14860.

107. Fujisaki H, Ito H, Hirata Y, et al. Natriuretic peptides inhibit angiotensin II-induced proliferation of rat cardiac fibroblasts by blocking endothelin-1 gene expression. J Clin Invest 1995; 96:1059.

108. Suga S, Nakao K, Itoh H, et al. Endothelial production of C-type natriuretic peptide and its marked augmentation by transforming growth factor β. Possible existence of "vascular natriuretic peptide system." J Clin Invest 1992; 90:1145.

109. Suga S, Itoh H, Komatsu Y, et al. Endothelial production of C-type natriuretic peptide—evidence for cytokine regulation. (Abstract). Circulation 1993; 88:I-621.

110. Furuya M, Aiska K, Miyazaki T, et al. C-type natriuretic peptide inhibits intimal thickening after vascular injury. Biochem Biophys Res Commun 1993; 193:248.

111. Oliver PM, Fox JE, Kim R, et al. Hypertension, hypertrophy, and sudden death in mice lacking natriuretic peptide receptor A. Proc Natl Acad Sci U S A 1997; 94:14730.

112. Florkowski CM, Richards AM, Espiner EA, et al. Low-dose brain natriuretic peptide infusion in normal men and the influence of endopeptidase inhibition. Clin Sci 1997; 92:255.

113. Kurtz A, Bruna RD, Pfeilschifter J, et al. Atrial natriuretic peptide inhibits renin release from juxtaglomerular cells by a cGMP-mediated process. Proc Natl Acad Sci U S A 1986; 83:4769.

114. Cherradi N, Brandenburger Y, Rossier MF, et al. Atrial natriuretic peptide inhibits calcium-induced steroidogenic acute regulatory protein gene transcription in adrenal glomerulosa cells. Mol Endocrinol 1998; 12:962.

115. Beland B, Tuchelt H, Bahr V, Oelkers W. The role of atrial natriuretic factor[α-human A NF(996)] in the hormonal and renal adaptation to sodium deficiency. J Clin Endocrinol Metab 1994; 79:183.

116. Lichardus B, Veress AT, Field LJ, Sonnenberg H. Blood pressure regulation in ANF-transgenic mice: role of angiotensin and vasopressin. Physiol Res 1994; 43:145.

117. Kanamori T, Wada A, Tsutamoto T, Kinoshita M. Possible regulation of renin release by ANP in dogs with heart failure. Am J Physiol 1995; 269:H2281.

118. Khurana ML, Pandey KN. Receptor-mediated stimulatory effect of atrial natriuretic factor, brain natriuretic peptide, and C-type natriuretic peptide on testosterone production in purified mouse Leydig cells: activation of cholesterol side-chain cleavage enzyme. Endocrinology 1993; 133:2141.

119. Johnson KM, Hughes FM, Fong YY, et al. Effects of atrial natriuretic peptide on rat ovarian granulosa cell steroidogenesis in vitro. Am J Reprod Immunol 1994; 31:163.

120. Hagiwara H, Inoue A, Yamaguchi A, et al. cGMP produced in response to ANP and CNP regulates proliferation and differentiation of osteoblastic cells. Am J Physiol 1996; 270:C1311.

121. Suda M, Ogawa Y, Tanaka K, et al. Skeletal overgrowth in transgenic mice that overexpresses brain natriuretic peptide. Proc Natl Acad Sci U S A 1998; 95:2337.

122. Imura H, Nakao K, Itoh H. The natriuretic peptide system in the brain: implications in the central control of cardiovascular and neuroendocrine functions. Frontiers Neuroendocrinol 1992; 13:217.

123. Goetz KL. Evidence that atriopeptin is not a physiological regulator of sodium excretion. Hypertension 1990; 15:9.

124. Westenfelder C, Birth FM, Baranowski RL, et al. Volume homeostasis in calves with artificial atria and ventricles. Am J Physiol 1990; 258:F1005.

125. Lee ME, Miller WL, Edwards BS, Burnett JC. Role of endogenous atrial natriuretic factor in acute congestive heart failure. J Clin Invest 1989; 84:1962.

126. Hirata Y, Matsuoka H, Suzuki E, et al. Role of endogenous atrial natriuretic peptide in DOCA-salt hypertensive rats. Effects of a novel antagonist for atrial natriuretic peptide receptor. Circulation 1993; 87:554.

127. Yamamoto K, Burnett JC, Redfield MM. Effect of endogenous natriuretic peptide system on ventricular and coronary function in failing heart. Am J Physiol 1997; 273:H2406.

128. Wada A, Tsutamoto T, Matsuda Y, Kinoshita M. Cardiorenal and neurohumoral effects of endogenous atrial natriuretic peptide in dogs with severe congestive heart failure using a specific antagonist for guanylate cyclase-coupled receptors. Circulation 1994; 9:2232.

129. Wada A, Tsutamoto T, Maeda Y, et al. Endogenous atrial natriuretic peptide inhibits endothelin-1 secretion in dogs with severe congestive heart failure. Am J Physiol 1996; 270:H1819.

130. Itoh H, Nakao K, Mukoyama M, et al. Chronic blockade of endogenous atrial natriuretic polypeptide (ANP) by monoclonal antibody against ANP accelerates the development of hypertension in spontaneously hypertensive and deoxycorticosterone acetate-salt-hypertensive rats. J Clin Invest 1989; 84:145.

131. Barbee RW, Perry BD, Re RN, et al. Hemodynamics in transgenic mice with overexpression of atrial natriuretic factor. Circ Res 1994; 74:747.

132. Ogawa Y, Itoh H, Tamura N, et al. Molecular cloning of the cDNA and gene that encode mouse brain natriuretic peptide gene and generation of transgenic mice that overexpress the brain natriuretic peptide gene. J Clin Invest 1994; 93:1911.

132a. Matsukawa N, Grzesik WJ, Takahashi N, et al. The natriuretic peptide clearance receptor locally modulates the physiological effects of the natriuretic peptide system. Proc Nat Acad Sci U S A 1999; 96:7403.

133. John SW, Krege JH, Oliver PM, et al. Genetic decreases in atrial natriuretic peptide and salt-sensitive hypertension. Science 1995; 267:679.

134. Oliver PM, John SW, Purdy KE, et al. Natriuretic peptide receptor 1 expression influences blood pressures of mice in a dose-dependent manner. Proc Natl Acad Sci U S A 1998; 95:2547.

135. Crozier IG, Nicholls MG, Ikram H, et al. Atrial natriuretic peptide in humans: production and clearance by various tissues. Hypertension 1986; 8:II-11.

136. Nishigaki K, Tomita M, Kagawa K, et al. Marked expression of plasma brain natriuretic peptide is a special feature of hypertrophic obstructive cardiomyopathy. J Am Coll Cardiol 1996; 28:1234.

137. Ando K, Hirata Y, Emori T, et al. Circulating forms of atrial natriuretic peptide in patients with congestive heart failure. J Clin Endocrinol Metab 1990; 70:1603.

138. Shemin D, Dworkin LD. Sodium balance in renal failure. Curr Opin Nephrol Hypertens 1997; 6:128.

139. Nagaya N, Nishikimi T, Okano Y, et al. Plasma brain natriuretic peptide levels increase in proportion to the extent of right ventricular dysfunction in pulmonary hypertension. J Am Coll Cardiol 1998; 31:202.

140. Mitaka C, Hirata Y, Nagura T, et al. Increased plasma concentrations of brain natriuretic peptide in patients with acute lung injury. J Crit Care 1997; 12:66.

141. Wong F, Blendis F. Pathophysiology of sodium retention and ascites formation in cirrhosis: role of atrial natriuretic factor. Semin Liver Dis 1994; 14:59.

142. La Villa G, Padeletti L, Lazzeri C, et al. Plasma levels of natriuretic peptides during ventricular pacing in patients with a dual chamber pacemaker. Pacing Clin Electrophysiol 1994; 17:953.

143. Wood P. Polyuria in paroxysmal tachycardiac and paroxysmal atrial flutter and fibrillation. Br Heart J 1963; 25:273.

144. Cort JH. Cerebral salt wasting. Lancet 1954; i:752.

145. Berendes E, Walter M, Cullen P, et al. Secretion of brain natriuretic peptide in patients with aneurysmal subarachnoid haemorrhage. Lancet 1997; 349:245.

146. Tunny TJ, Richardson KA, Clark CV, Gordon RD. The atrial natriuretic peptide gene in patients with familial primary open-angle glaucoma. Biochem Biophys Res Commun 1996; 223:221.

147. Rutledge DR, Sun Y, Ross EA. Polymorphisms within the atrial natriuretic peptide gene in essential hypertension. J Hypertens 1995; 13:953.

147a. Sarzani R, Dessi-Fulgheri P, Salvi F, et al. A novel promoter variant of the natriuretic peptide clearance receptor gene is associated with lower atrial natriuretic peptide and higher blood pressure in obese hypertensives. J Hypertens 1999; 17:1301.

148. Shimizu K, Nakano S, Nakano Y, et al. Ectopic atrial natriuretic peptide production in small cell lung cancer with the syndrome of inappropriate antidiuretic hormone secretion. Cancer 1991; 68:2284.

149. Francis GS, Benedict C, Johnstone DE, et al. Comparison of neuroendocrine activation in patients with left ventricular dysfunction with and without congestive heart failure: a substudy of the Studies of Left Ventricular Dysfunction (SOLVD). Circulation 1990; 82:1724.

150. Lerman A, Gibbons RJ, Rodeheffer RJ, et al. Circulating N-terminal atrial natriuretic peptide as a marker for symptomless left-ventricular dysfunction. Lancet 1993; 341:1105.

151. Foy SG, Crozier IG, Richards AM, et al. Neurohormonal changes after acute myocardial infarction: relationships with haemodynamic indices and effects of ACE inhibition. Eur Heart J 1995; 16:770.

152. Rouleau JL, Packer M, Moye L, et al. Prognostic value of neurohumoral activation in patients with acute myocardial infarction: effect of captopril. J Am Coll Cardiol 1994; 24:583.

153. Davis M, Espiner E, Richards G, et al. Plasma brain natriuretic peptide in assessment of acute dyspnoea. Lancet 1994; 343:440.

154. Takeda T, Kohno M. Brain natriuretic peptide in hypertension. Hypertens Res 1995; 18:259.

155. Omland T, Aakvaag A, Bonarjee VVS, et al. Plasma brain natriuretic peptide as an indicator of left ventricular systolic function and long-term survival after acute myocardial infarction: comparison with plasma atrial natriuretic peptide and N-terminal proatrial natriuretic peptide. Circulation 1996; 93:1963.

156. Richards AM, Nicholls MG, Yandle TG, et al. Plasma N-terminal pro-brain natriuretic peptide and adrenomedullin: new neurohormonal predictors of left ventricular function and prognosis after myocardial infarction. Circulation 1998; 97:1921.

157. Swedberg K, Eneroth P, Kjekshus J, Wilhelmsen L. Hormones regulating cardiovascular function in patients with severe congestive heart failure and their relation to mortality. Circulation 1990; 82:1730.

158. Hunt PJ, Richards AM, Nicholls MG, et al. Immunoreactive amino-terminal pro-brain natriuretic peptide (NT-proBNP): a new marker of cardiac impairment. Clin Endocrinol 1997; 47:287.

159. Lainchbury JG, Nicholls MG, Espiner EA, et al. Cardiac hormones. Auckland, New Zealand: The National Heart Foundation of New Zealand, 1997. Technical report no. 72.

159a. Troughton RW, Frampton CM, Yandle TG, et al. Treatment of heart failure guided by plasma aminoterminal brain natriuretic peptide (N-BNP) concentrations. Lancet 2000; 355:1126.

160. Espiner EA, Nicholls MG. Human atrial natriuretic peptide. Clin Endocrinol 1987; 26:637.

161. Cohen N, Gilbert R, Wirth A, et al. Atrial natriuretic peptide and plasma renin levels in assessment of mineralcorticoid replacement in Addison's disease. J Clin Endocrinol Metab 1996; 81:1411.

162. Naruse M, Takeyama Y, Tanabe A, et al. Atrial and brain natriuretic peptides in cardiovascular diseases. Hypertension 1994; 23:I-231.

163. Pidgeon BG, Richards AM, Nicholls MG, et al. Differing metabolism and bioactivity of atrial and brain natriuretic peptides in essential hypertension. Hypertension 1996; 27:906.

164. Takata Y, Hirayama Y, Kiyomi S, et al. The beneficial effects of atrial natriuretic peptide on arrhythmias and myocardial high-energy phosphates after reperfusion. Cardiovasc Res 1996; 32:286.

165. Lai CP, Egashira K, Tashiro H, et al. Beneficial effects of atrial natriuretic peptide on exercise induced myocardial ischaemia in patients with stable angina pectoris. Circulation 1993; 87:144.

166. Kato H, Yasue H, Yoshimura M, et al. Suppression of hyperventilation-induced attacks with infusion of B-type (brain) natriuretic peptide in patients with variant angina. Am Heart J 1994; 128:1098.

167. Isner JM, Feldman LJ. Gene therapy for arterial disease. Lancet 1994; 344:1653.

168. Rahman SN, Kim GE, Mathew AS, et al. Effects of atrial natriuretic peptide in clinical acute renal failure. Kidney Int 1994; 45:1731.

169. Kimmelstiel CD, Perrone R, Kilcoyne L, et al. Effects of renal neutral endopeptidase inhibition on sodium excretion, renal hemodynamics and neuro-hormonal activation in patients with congestive heart failure. Cardiology 1996; 87:46.

170. Rademaker MT, Charles CJ, Espiner EA, et al. Neutral endopeptidase inhibition: augmented atrial and brain natriuretic peptide, haemodynamic and natriuretic responses in ovine heart failure. Clin Sci 1996; 91:283.

171. Wolfensberger TJ, Singer DRJ, Freegard T, et al. Evidence for a new role for natriuretic peptides: control of intraocular pressure. Br J Ophthalmol 1994; 78:446.

172. Thompson JS, Sheedy W, Morice A. Effects of the neutral endopeptidase inhibitor SCH 41495, on the cardiovascular remodelling secondary to chronic hypoxia in rats. Clin Sci 1994; 87:109.

# CHAPTER 179

# THE ENDOCRINE ENDOTHELIUM

FRANCESCO COSENTINO AND THOMAS F. LÜSCHER

In addition to the cells of the "classic" endocrine glands that secrete hormones, several other cells, such as the vascular endothelium, are capable of generating substances that can circulate and affect neighboring smooth muscle cells and blood cells. Hence, the endothelium acts as an important regulatory organ within the circulation by generating vasoactive substances that act in a paracrine, autocrine, solinocrine, and, under certain conditions, hemocrine fashion (see Chap. 1).

TABLE 179-1.
**Angiogenic and Antiangiogenic Factors**

| Angiogenic Factors | Antiangiogenic Factors |
|---|---|
| Vascular endothelial growth factor (VEGF) | Angiostatin |
| Basic fibroblast growth factor (bFGF) | Endostatin |
| Epidermal growth factor (EGF) | Transforming growth factor-$\beta$ |
| Transforming growth factor-$\beta$ (TGF-$\beta$) | (TGF-$\beta$) |
| Angiopoietin-1 | Angiopoietin-2 |
| Angiogenin | Interferon-$\gamma$ |
| | Platelet factor-4 fragment |
| | Lymphotoxin |
| | Thrombospondin |

TABLE 179-2.
**Cardiovascular Diseases Associated with Elevated Endothelin Levels**

Acute myocardial infarction
Atherosclerosis
Cardiogenic shock
Cerebral/myocardial vasospasm
Congestive heart failure
Diabetes
Endotoxic shock
Hypertension
Pulmonary hypertension
Raynaud phenomenon

Critically located as a barrier between smooth muscle cells and the blood, the endothelium plays a pivotal functional role in maintaining the homeostasis of the normal vessel by generating substances that modulate vascular tone as well as growth, coagulation, platelet function, and the release of circulating hormones.[1] Furthermore, the endothelium is a target organ in cardiovascular disease (Tables 179-1 and 179-2).

Endothelial cells produce and release a variety of vasoactive substances[1] (Fig. 179-1): (a) endothelium-derived relaxing factors (EDRFs), such as nitric oxide (NO), endothelium-derived hyperpolarizing factor, and prostacyclin (prostaglandin $I_2$ [$PGI_2$]), as well as other prostaglandins; and (b) endothelium-derived contracting factors, including cyclooxygenase-derived contracting factors, endothelin, and angiotensin II.

# ENDOTHELIUM-DERIVED RELAXING FACTORS

## ENDOTHELIUM-DERIVED NITRIC OXIDE

In the presence of endothelium, acetylcholine induces relaxation. This relaxation cannot be prevented by the use of inhibitors of cyclooxygenase (which blocks $PGI_2$ production), suggesting that a different EDRF must be involved.[2] Endothelium-dependent relaxations have been demonstrated in large (conduit) arteries and in resistance vessels of most mammalian species, including humans.[1,3,4] The release of EDRF can be demonstrated under basal conditions: in response to mechanical forces such as shear

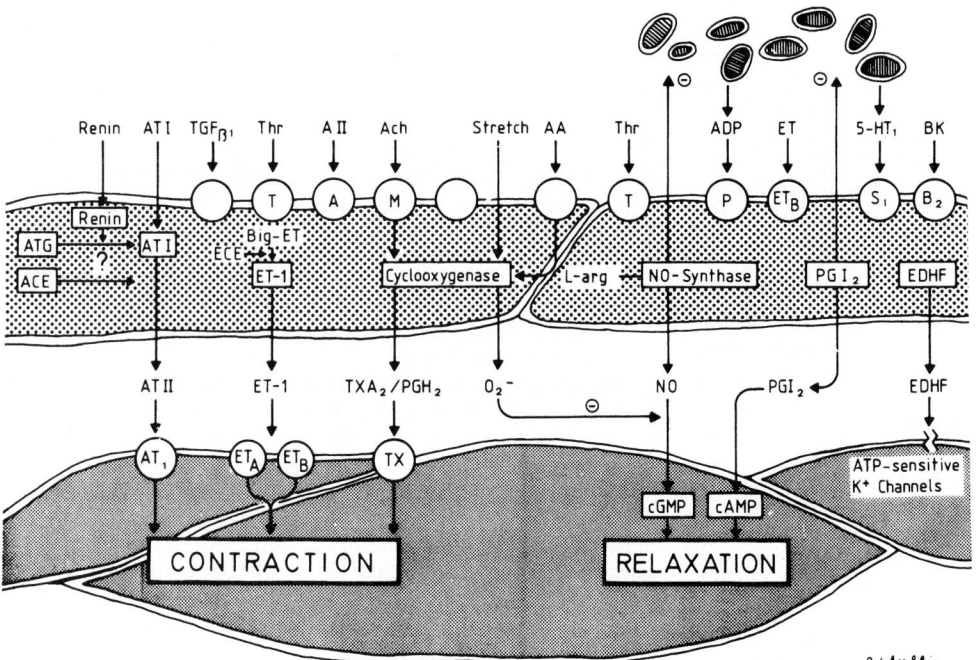

**FIGURE 179-1.** Endothelium-derived vasoactive substances. The endothelium releases relaxing factors (*right*) and contracting factors (*left*). The relaxing factors include nitric oxide (*NO*), prostacyclin (*PGI₂*), and endothelium-derived hyperpolarizing factor (*EDHF*). NO and PGI₂ cause not only relaxation but also inhibition (Θ) of platelet function. The contracting factors include the local vascular renin-angiotensin system, endothelin (*ET*), and cyclooxygenase-derived contracting factors such as thromboxane A₂ (*TXA₂*) and prostaglandin H₂ (*PGH₂*). In addition, the cyclooxygenase pathway is a source of oxygen-derived free radicals (O₂⁻). *Circles* represent receptors. (*ATI*, angiotensin I; *TGF-β₁*, transforming growth factor-β₁; *Thr*, thrombin; *AII*, angiotensin II; *Ach*, acetylcholine; *AA*, arachidonic acid; *ADP*, adenosine diphosphate; *5-HT*, serotonin; *BK*, bradykinin; *T*, thrombin receptor; *A*, angiotensin receptor; *M*, muscarinic receptor; *P*, phosphate; ET_B, endothelin-receptor subtype; *S₁*, serotonergic receptor; *B₂*, bradykinin receptor; *ATG*, angiotensinogen; *ACE*, angiotensin-converting enzyme; *ECE*, endothelin-converting enzyme; *ET-1*, endothelin-1; *L-Arg*, L-arginine; *NOS*, nitric oxide synthase; *ATII*, angiotensin II; *AT₁*, angiotensin subtype 1 receptor; *ET_A*, endothelin-receptor subtype; *TX*, thromboxane receptor; *cGMP*, cyclic guanosine monophosphate; *cAMP*, cyclic adenosine monophosphate; *ATP*, adenosine triphosphate.) (From Lüscher TF, Boulanger CM, Dohi Y, Yang Z. Endothelium-derived contracting factors. Hypertension 1992; 19:117.)

stress (exerted by the circulating blood)[5,6] and after activation of receptor-operated mechanisms by acetylcholine, neurotransmitters, various local and circulating hormones, and substances derived from platelets and the coagulation system[3,4] (see Fig. 179-1). The EDRF is a diffusible substance with a half-life of a few seconds that has been identified as NO.[7,8]

Relaxation of smooth muscle cells by endothelium-derived NO (EDNO) is associated with activation of soluble guanylate cyclase (GC) and an increase in intracellular cyclic 3'5'-guanosine monophosphate (cGMP) in vascular smooth muscle[9] (see Fig. 179-1). An inhibitor of soluble GC, methylene blue, prevents the production of cGMP and inhibits endothelium-dependent relaxations. Soluble GC is also present in platelets and is activated by EDNO[10] (see Fig. 179-1). Increased levels of cGMP in platelets are associated with reduced adhesion and aggregation. Therefore, EDNO causes both vasodilatation and platelet deactivation and, thereby, represents an important antispastic and antithrombotic feature of the endothelium.

EDNO is formed from L-arginine by oxidation of its guanidino-nitrogen terminal[11] (see Fig. 179-1) by NO synthase, which has been cloned.[12] NO synthase is primarily a cytosolic enzyme requiring calmodulin, $Ca^{2+}$, β-nicotinamide-adenine dinucleotide hydrogen phosphate (NADPH), and tetrahydrobiopterin, and has similarities with cytochrome P450 enzymes.[13] Several isoforms of the enzyme occur in endothelial cells, as well as in platelets, macrophages, vascular smooth muscle cells, and the brain.

Analogs of L-arginine, such as NG-monomethyl L-arginine (L-NMMA), or L-nitroarginine methyl ester (L-NAME), inhibit endothelium-dependent relaxations to serotonin in porcine coronary arteries, an effect that is restored by L-arginine but not by D-arginine.[14] In quiescent arteries, L-NMMA causes endothelium-dependent contractions.[15] In intact organs, L-NAME markedly decreases local blood flow.[16] When infused in rabbits, L-arginine methyl ester induces long-lasting increases in blood pressure that are reversed by L-arginine.[17] This demonstrates that the vasculature is in a constant state of vasodilation because of the continuous basal release of NO from the endothelium. Of particular pathophysiologic interest is the discovery of an endogenous inhibitor of the L-arginine–NO pathway known as *asymmetric dimethyl-arginine*,[18] which is also produced by cultured endothelial cells. This indicates that endogenously produced substances can regulate the activity of this pathway both locally and systemically (it is also detected in plasma). Hence, increased production or elimination of this endogenous inhibitor can profoundly affect the function of the cardiovascular system.[19]

### ENDOTHELIUM-DERIVED HYPERPOLARIZING FACTORS

In the porcine coronary circulation, L-NMMA inhibits relaxations to serotonin but only slightly inhibits those to bradykinin.[12,14] Other inhibitors of the action of EDNO, such as hemoglobin and methylene blue, as well as inhibitors of cyclooxygenase, also are ineffective. Thus, endothelial cells appear to release a relaxing factor distinct from NO and $PGI_2$. Acetylcholine causes not only endothelium-dependent relaxation but also endothelium-dependent hyperpolarization of vascular smooth muscle.[20] An endothelium-dependent hyperpolarizing factor (see Fig. 179-1) distinct from NO could explain these responses, although NO also has been shown to have hyperpolarizing properties under certain conditions. The endothelium-derived hyperpolarizing factor appears to activate adenosine triphosphate–sensitive $K^+$ channels,[19] but its chemical nature remains elusive.

### PROSTACYCLIN

Endothelial cells are an important source of $PGI_2$, which is synthesized within the vasculature in response to shear stress, hypoxia, and several mediators also leading to the formation of EDNO[22] (see Fig. 179-1 and Chap. 172). Prostacyclin causes

relaxation by increasing cyclic 3',5'-adenosine monophosphate (cAMP) in smooth muscle and platelets,[23] where it also inhibits platelet aggregation, particularly together with NO.

## ENDOTHELIUM-DERIVED CONTRACTING FACTORS

### CYCLOOXYGENASE-DEPENDENT ENDOTHELIUM-DERIVED CONTRACTING FACTOR

Exogenous arachidonic acid can evoke endothelium-dependent contractions that can be prevented by indomethacin (an inhibitor of cyclooxygenase), suggesting that cyclooxygenase products, besides $PGI_2$, can produce vasoconstriction.[1,24] In the human saphenous vein, acetylcholine and histamine evoke endothelium-dependent contractions; in the presence of indomethacin, however, endothelium-dependent relaxations are unmasked.[25] The products of cyclooxygenase-mediated contractions are thromboxane $A_2$ ($TXA_2$), in the case of acetylcholine, and endoperoxides (prostaglandin $H_2$ [$PGH_2$]), in the case of histamine.[25] $TXA_2$ and endoperoxide activate both vascular smooth muscle and platelets, thereby counteracting the protective effects of NO and $PGI_2$ in the blood vessel wall (see Fig. 179-1).

The cyclooxygenase pathway is also the source of superoxide anions that can mediate endothelium-dependent contractions either by enhancing the breakdown of NO or by directly affecting vascular smooth muscle.[1,26] Thus, the cyclooxygenase pathway produces various potentially contracting factors. Their release appears particularly prominent in veins and in the cerebral and ophthalmic circulation (see Chap. 172). The use of more specific inhibitors than indomethacin (such as the $TXA_2/PGH_2$ receptor antagonists and the superoxide anion scavengers) is allowing their importance in vascular function to be characterized. Such a selective pharmacologic approach has emphasized the important role of superoxide anions in the balance between endothelium-dependent contractions and relaxations.[27]

### ENDOTHELIN

Endothelial cells produce the 21-amino-acid peptide endothelin[28] (Fig. 179-2). Of the three peptides endothelin-1, endothelin-2, and endothelin-3, endothelial cells appear to produce exclusively endothelin-1.

The translation of mRNA generates preproendothelin, which is converted to big endothelin. Conversion of the latter to endothelin-1 by endothelin-converting enzyme (ECE) is necessary for the development of full vascular activity.[28] The expression of mRNA and the release of the peptide are stimulated by thrombin, transforming growth factor-β, interleukin-1, epinephrine, angiotensin II, arginine vasopressin, calcium ionophore, and phorbol ester (Fig. 179-3).[28–31] In addition, hypoxia stimulates the release of endothelin in isolated vessels.[32]

Endothelin-1 is a potent vasoconstrictor both in vitro and in vivo.[28,33] In the human heart, eye, and forearm, endothelin causes vasodilation at lower concentrations and marked con-

Endothelin-1:     CSCSSLM DKECVYFCHLDIIW

Endothelin-2:     CSCSSWL DKECVYFCHLDIIW

Endothelin-3:     CTCFTYK DKECVYYCHLDIIW

**FIGURE 179-2.** The structures of the three 21-amino-acid human endothelins. Complete sequence homologies between the three peptides are underlined. Amino acids are designated by standard one-letter abbreviations (see Chap. 94, Fig. 94-23 for the key to these amino-acid abbreviations).

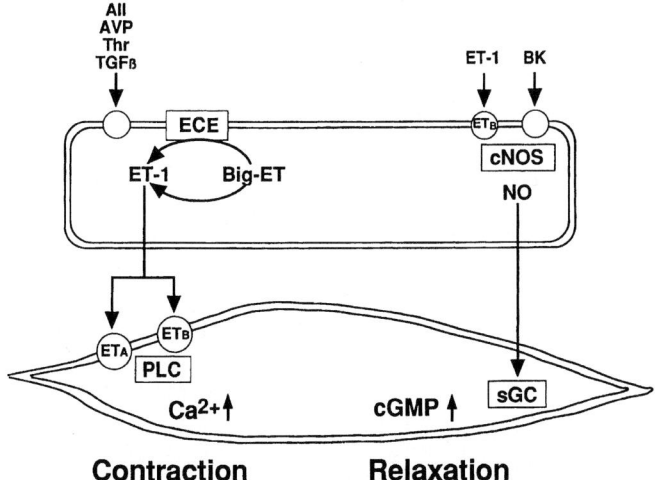

**FIGURE 179-3.** The vascular endothelin system and its interactions with the L-arginine–nitric oxide pathway. (*AII*, angiotensin II; *AVP*, arginine vasopressin; *Thr*, thrombin; *TGF-β*, transforming growth factor-β; *ET-1*, endothelin-1; *BK*, bradykinin; *ECE*, endothelin converting enzyme; *ET_B*, endothelin-receptor subtype; *cNOS*, constitutive nitric oxide synthase; *NO*, nitric oxide; *ET_A*, endothelin-receptor subtype; *PLC*, phospholipase C; *cGMP*, cyclic guanosine monophosphate; *sGC*, soluble guanylate cyclase.)

tractions at higher concentrations.[1,16,34] In the heart, this may lead to ischemia, arrhythmias, and death.

Circulating levels of endothelin-1 are low,[28] suggesting that little of the peptide is formed under physiologic conditions because of the absence of stimuli or the presence of potent inhibitory mechanisms. Alternatively, it may be released preferentially toward smooth muscle cells.[23,28] Possible pathways involved in regulating the mechanism of endothelin production are (a) a cGMP-dependent pathway,[30,35] (b) a cAMP-dependent pathway,[36] and (c) a pathway involving an inhibitory factor produced by vascular smooth muscle cells.[37] Furthermore, endothelin can release NO and prostacyclin from endothelial cells, possibly representing a negative-feedback mechanism.[38] EDNO also modulates the actions of endothelin at the level of vascular smooth muscle. The contractions in response to endothelin are enhanced after endothelial removal, indicating that basal production of EDNO reduces its response.[33] Stimulation of the formation of EDNO by acetylcholine reverses endothelin-induced contractions in most blood vessels, although this mechanism appears to be less potent in veins.[33]

Three distinct endothelin receptors have been cloned: the ET_A, ET_B, and ET_C receptors.[39–41] Endothelial cells express ET_B receptors linked to the formation of NO and PGI_2, possibly explaining the transient vasodilator effects of endothelin when it is infused into intact organs or organisms. In vascular smooth muscle, ET_A and, partly, ET_B receptors mediate contraction and proliferation (see Fig. 179-3). ET_B receptors bind endothelin-1 and endothelin-3 equally, whereas ET_A receptors preferentially bind endothelin-1. Several endothelin antagonists lower blood pressure, suggesting that endothelin may contribute to blood pressure regulation.[42]

## ANGIOTENSINS

Angiotensin II is a vasoactive octapeptide formed from its inactive decapeptide precursor, angiotensin I, by the action of a dipeptidyl carboxypeptidase, angiotensin-converting enzyme (ACE), which also is present on endothelial cells[43] (see Fig. 179-1 and Chap. 79). Possible local angiotensin II synthesis in the vascular wall is of special interest in view of the multiple vascular actions of angiotensin II.

Angiotensin II not only exerts a direct vasoconstrictor effect but also enhances sympathetic noradrenergic transmission,[44]

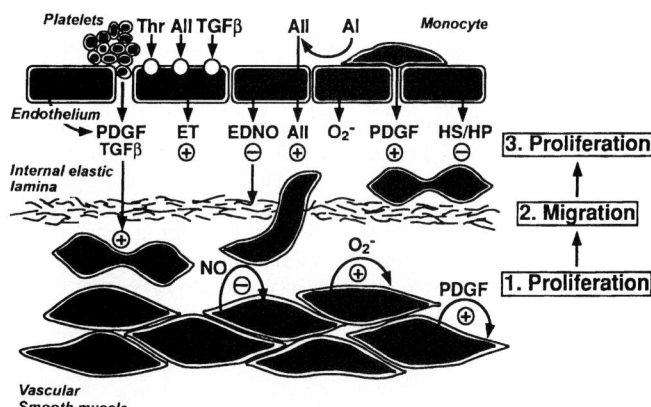

**FIGURE 179-4.** Endothelium-derived vasoactive factors and vascular growth. The endothelium produces growth inhibitors such as heparin (*HP*), heparan sulfate (*HS*), and nitric oxide (*EDNO*). It releases endothelium-derived growth promoters such as platelet-derived growth factor (*PDGF*), basic fibroblast growth factor (*bFGF*), transforming growth factor-β (*TGF-β*), and endothelin (*ET*). At sites of damaged endothelium, the production of EDNO and prostacyclin (*PGI_2*) is diminished, favoring monocyte adhesion and platelet aggregation. Growth factors are released by these cells as well as the endothelium and lead to proliferation as well as migration of vascular smooth muscle cells into the intima. (*Thr*, thrombin; *AII*, angiotensin II; *AI*, angiotensin I; *O_2^-*, oxygen-derived free radicals; *NO*, nitric oxide.) (From Lüscher TF, Noll G. In: Braunwald E, ed. Heart disease. Philadelphia: WB Saunders, 1996.)

exhibits mitogenic and trophic actions in the vasculature,[45] and induces endothelin synthesis.[31] Hence, vascular or endothelial ACE activity may play an important role in regulating normal vascular function.

## REGULATION OF VASCULAR STRUCTURE AND ANGIOGENESIS

### VASCULAR STRUCTURE

The endothelium produces several factors that regulate the proliferation and migration of underlying smooth muscle cells[46,47] (Fig. 179-4). Denudation of endothelial cells is followed by platelet adhesion and aggregation, resulting in the release of platelet-derived growth factor (PDGF) and other mitogens. These events lead to the migration and proliferation of vascular smooth muscle cells and strongly suggest that the endothelium normally has a net inhibitory influence on these responses (see Fig. 179-4). The endothelium synthesizes substances, including heparan sulfate, NO, and prostaglandins, that inhibit the growth of smooth muscle cells; this may explain why vascular structure normally remains stable[46–49] (see Fig. 179-4). Under certain conditions, the endothelium can generate substances such as PDGF, basic fibroblast growth factor, insulin-like growth factor-I, colony-stimulating factor I, endothelin-1, transforming growth factor-β, interleukin-1, and tumor necrosis factor-α that can either induce proliferation by themselves or stimulate growth factor gene expression in smooth muscle cells.[46,47,50] In addition, endothelial dysfunction is associated with adhesion of circulating blood cells, such as platelets and monocytes, which also are an important source of growth factors.

Endothelial dysfunction in certain disease states could markedly alter the effects of endothelial cells on the behavior of smooth muscle cells and contribute to changes in vascular structure. Structural abnormalities of the media of large conduit and resistance arteries are involved in the pathophysiology of hypertension. In large conduit arteries, intimal thickening and atherosclerosis are important consequences of hypertension and other cardiovascular risk factors, which are responsible for cardiovascular complications such as myocardial infarction and stroke (see later). Hypertensive resistance arteries exhibit an increased media/lumen ratio, which primarily involves the migration and rearrangement of vascular smooth muscle cells within the media (i.e., remodeling). This contributes to the increase in peripheral vascular resistance in hypertension. Although not observed, an imbalance in the production of endogenous inhibitors of migration and proliferation, and of promoters of these responses by endothelial cells could partially explain these structural vascular changes occurring in hypertension.

## ANGIOGENESIS

Normal organ growth and development as well as the maintenance of homeostasis rely on precise control of the blood supply by the circulatory system. This system delivers oxygen and nutrients to each organ. Indeed, during the development of the fetus the circulatory system is the earliest organ system to develop. Once the rudimentary system of the early embryo has been formed, further growth of blood vessels (angiogenesis) occurs by proliferation of existing vascular endothelial cells in response to factors secreted by surrounding tissues. Quiescent endothelium responds to vascular endothelial growth factor or basic fibroblast growth factor by entering the cell cycle. Angiogenesis, similar to all tissue growth, is under multiple positive and negative regulatory controls. The fact that a growing tumor secretes factors that induce blood vessel growth in order to support its own growth and survival is well known.

Consequently, angiogenesis is an attractive target for anticancer therapies. This therapeutic approach has been shown to be promising by the discovery of angiostatin[51] and endostatin,[52] strong and specific inhibitors of the proliferation of endothelial cells. Sequence analysis of these two polypeptides revealed that they are proteolytic fragments of plasminogen and collagen XVIII, respectively. They can inhibit angiogenesis in both in vivo and in vitro assay systems and block the growth of metastases as well as of several primary tumors. The first step toward using such inhibitors for human therapy, however, is to determine the most effective delivery system (i.e., systemic injection of purified or recombinant protein, or the gene delivery system). Currently, antiangiogenic therapy is a promising form of cancer therapy.[53] As shown in Table 179-1, however, a growing number of factors are known to regulate angiogenesis, underscoring the need for more extensive studies to better characterize the basic molecular mechanisms of blood vessel formation.

## ENDOCRINE EFFECTS OF ENDOTHELIAL MEDIATORS

The endothelium-derived mediators can affect the production of circulating hormones and, at least in certain disease states, increased production of these substances allows them to act as humoral factors (Fig. 179-5).

### RENIN-ANGIOTENSIN SYSTEM

In isolated renal tissue, NO, released either from isolated canine blood vessels or from cultured porcine endothelial cells, inhibits renin production.[54] Considering that NO is released in response to shear stress, this mechanism could regulate renin secretion in response to changes in local hemodynamics and, hence, act as an intrarenal baroreceptor.[1] Endothelin inhibits renin production in vitro[55] in isolated glomeruli of the rat[55] but augments renin production markedly in vivo because of the pronounced renal vasoconstriction.[56] Angiotensin II, however, which is the final product of the renin-angiotensin system,

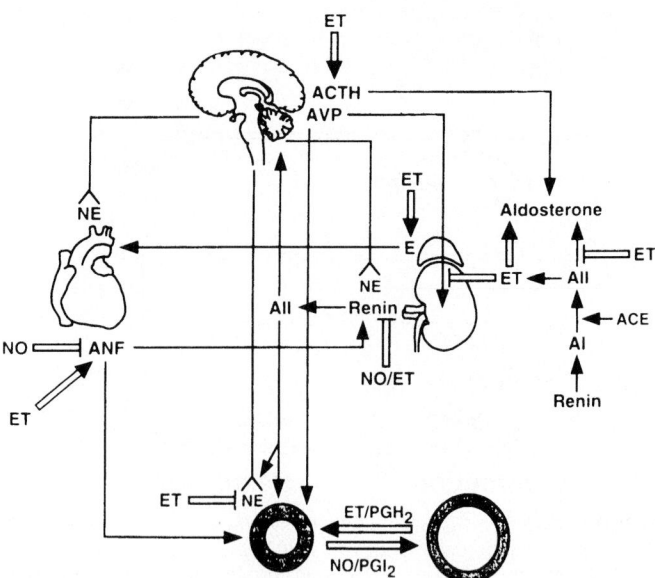

**FIGURE 179-5.** Endocrine actions of endothelium-derived mediators. Nitric oxide (*NO*) and endothelin (*ET*) can affect various endocrine regulators of the cardiovascular system, such as the renin-angiotensin system, atrial natriuretic peptide/factor (*ANF*), the hypophysis, and the adrenal glands. (*ACTH*, adrenocorticotropic hormone; *AVP*, arginine vasopressin; *NE*, norepinephrine; *E*, epinephrine; *AII*, angiotensin II; *ACE*, angiotensin-converting enzyme; *AI*, angiotensin I; *PGH₂*, prostaglandin $H_2$; *PGI₂*, prostacyclin.)

stimulates endothelin production in endothelial cells in culture,[29] as well as in intact blood vessels.[31]

### ATRIAL NATRIURETIC PEPTIDE

In the atrium of the rat, removal of the endocardium augments the basal release of atrial natriuretic peptide[57] (ANH; see Chap. 178). A similar effect can be obtained with inhibitors of EDNO, suggesting that the endothelium acts as an inhibitor of the myocardial production of ANH. Endothelin-1, however, is a potent secretagogue for ANH in cultured rat atrial myocytes.[58] ANH released from myocytes can increase cGMP in the endothelium and, in turn, inhibit the release of endothelin-1 and, possibly, of NO.[35]

### PITUITARY HORMONES

Endothelin is produced by neuronal cells and also is found in human cerebrospinal fluid, findings which suggest that it acts as an important mediator in the central nervous system. In humans, intravenous administration of endothelin-1 increases basal plasma concentrations of corticotropin, whereas levels of prolactin, thyrotropin, luteinizing hormone, follicle-stimulating hormone, and growth hormone remain unchanged.[59] Stimulated serum concentrations of luteinizing hormone and follicle-stimulating hormone tend to be higher in the presence of endothelin infusion, however, whereas the peptide exerts a suppressive action on stimulated plasma concentrations of prolactin and growth hormone. In addition, endothelin-1 reduces the antidiuretic effects of arginine vasopressin in vivo.

### CATECHOLAMINES

The addition of endothelin-1 to primary cultures of bovine adrenal chromaffin cells augments the efflux of norepinephrine and epinephrine.[60] In contrast, endothelin inhibits adrenergic neurotransmission in the guinea pig femoral artery.[61] In adrenocortical glomerulosa cells, endothelin-1 stimulates aldosterone release.[62]

# ENDOTHELIUM DYSFUNCTION IN HYPERTENSION

Abnormal vascular tone and growth are important in the pathophysiology of hypertension and atherosclerosis.[1] The endothelium is critically involved in this process because several endothelium-derived vasoactive factors influence these features in an autocrine or paracrine fashion. In hypertension, certain morphologic and functional alterations of the endothelium occur.[1] Endothelial cells of hypertensive vessels have an increased volume and bulge into the lumen, and the subintimal space exhibits structural changes, with increased fibrin and cell deposition. Furthermore, the interaction of platelets and monocytes with the endothelium is greater than in normotensive control subjects.

## ENDOTHELIUM-DEPENDENT RELAXATION

Endothelium-dependent relaxation in response to acetylcholine is reduced in the aortic, cerebral, and peripheral microcirculations of most experimental models of hypertension.[63–65] Similarly, the vasodilator effects of acetylcholine in the human forearm of hypertensive subjects have been found to be blunted in most studies.[66–71] In the coronary circulation of the spontaneously hypertensive rat (SHR), little endothelial dysfunction occurs.[72] In the human coronary circulation, however, endothelium-dependent responses are impaired in epicardial vessels and microvessels in patients with hypertension, particularly in the presence of left ventricular hypertrophy.[73] The response to the direct vasodilator sodium nitroprusside remains preserved, and the impaired responses to acetylcholine must be related to alterations in endothelial function.

In experimental animals, the degree of impairment of endothelium-dependent responses is positively correlated with the level of blood pressure and seems to increase as a function of the severity and duration of hypertension.[74] This suggests that most of the endothelial dysfunction in hypertension is a consequence rather than a cause of the high blood pressure. As in perfused mesenteric resistance arteries of the SHR, endothelium-dependent relaxation is reduced by intraluminal but not by extraluminal application of acetylcholine.[75]

The mechanisms responsible for impaired endothelium-dependent responses in hypertension (Fig. 179-6) include (a) decreased release or increased inactivation of EDNO; (b) decreased release of other endothelium-derived vasodilator substances, such as endothelium-dependent hyperpolarizing factor or $PGI_2$; (c) impaired diffusion of these substances from the endothelium to the vascular smooth muscle cells; (d) decreased responsiveness of the vascular smooth muscle cells to vasodilator substances; and (e) augmented release of endothelium-derived contracting factors.

## FORMATION OF NITRIC OXIDE

Although endothelium-dependent relaxation is either diminished or normal in spontaneous hypertension, the production of NO seems to be increased. The release of NO from isolated coronary vessels is augmented in the SHR.[76] The activity of constitutive nitric oxide synthase (cNOS) is also enhanced in the SHR.[77] These data suggest that, in the rat, blood pressure per se is a stimulus for NOS activation. This interpretation is reinforced by the fact that cNOS activity is normal in the prehypertensive 4-week old SHR.[77] In spite of an increased activity of the L-arginine pathway, however, the bioavailability of NO probably is diminished due to its increased inactivation.[75] Nevertheless, NO production and inactivation might be heterogeneously affected in different forms of hypertension. Indeed, in Dahl salt-sensitive rats, endothelium-dependent relaxation is impaired, without an involvement of the cyclooxygenase-dependent pathway (see later). This suggests that the decreased NO production could contribute to the pathogenesis of this form of hypertension (see Fig. 179-6).

# Genetic Hypertension

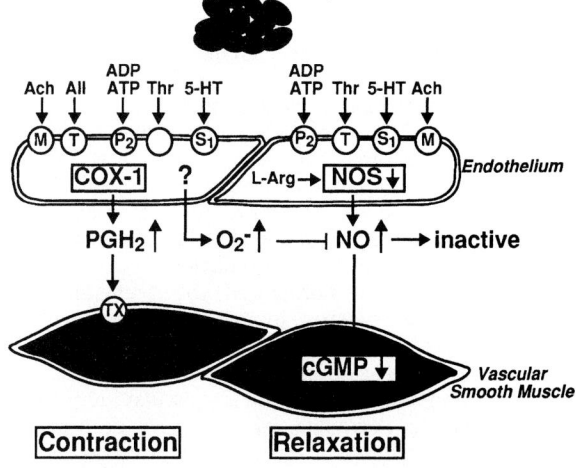

# Salt-induced Hypertension

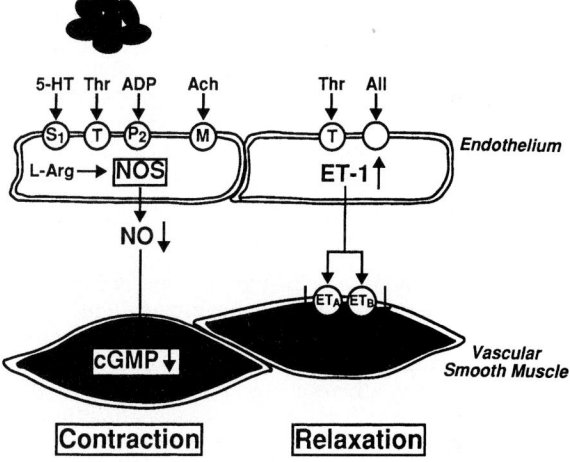

**FIGURE 179-6.** Heterogeneity of endothelial dysfunction in spontaneous and salt-induced hypertension. Although the L-arginine–nitric oxide (*NO*) pathway is overactive in the former, NO seems to be inactivated by oxygen-derived free radicals ($O_2^-$) in the latter. In addition, a vasoconstrictor prostanoid (prostaglandin $H_2$ [$PGH_2$]) is formed (*top panel*). In contrast, in the Dahl rats, a deficient production of NO is most likely (*bottom panel*). *Circles* represent receptors. (*ADP*, adenosine diphosphate; *Ach*, acetylcholine; *AII*, angiotensin II; *ATP*, adenosine triphosphate; *Thr*, thrombin; *5-HT*, serotonin; *M*, muscarinic receptor; *T*, thrombin receptor; $P_2$, purinergic receptor; $S_1$, serotonergic receptor; *COX-1*, cyclooxygenase-1; *L-Arg*, L-arginine; *NOS*, nitric oxide synthase; *Tx*, thromboxane receptor; *cGMP*, cyclic guanosine monophosphate; *ET-1*, endothelin-1; $ET_A$, endothelin-receptor subtype; $ET_B$, endothelin-receptor subtype.) (From Moreau P, Nava E, Takase H, Luscher TF. Handbook of hypertension, vol 17. Pathophysiology of hypertension. Zanchetti A, Mancia G, eds. Amsterdam: Elsevier Science, 1997.)

Pharmacologic experiments in humans have provided indirect evidence for a diminished basal and stimulated NO production. Most studies have found a reduced endothelium-dependent vasodilation in patients with primary or secondary hypertension.[69] In patients with hypertension, the endothelium-dependent vasodilation in response to acetylcholine is improved after treatment with a cyclooxygenase inhibitor.[69] Because inhibition of cyclooxygenase-derived contracting factors does not fully normalize endothelium-dependent vasodilation in hypertensive subjects, however, an additional defect that involves the L-arginine–NO pathway is implicated. In patients with essential hypertension, treatment with L-arginine does not affect the response to acetylcholine,[78] suggesting that this defect involves either the uptake of the precursor of NO or another pathway (i.e., endothelium-dependent hyperpolarizing factor; see earlier).

## ENDOTHELIUM-DEPENDENT CONTRACTIONS

Although the assumption is commonly made that impaired endothelium-dependent relaxations are primarily related to reduced activity of NO, they may also be caused by increased production of endothelium-derived contracting factors (EDCF)[63] (see Fig. 179-6). In the SHR, the reduced response to acetylcholine in the aorta is related to the production of $PGH_2$. In the circulation of the human forearm, impaired vasodilation to acetylcholine is improved (although not normalized) by pretreatment with indomethacin (a cyclooxygenase inhibitor) in patients with essential hypertension,[78] suggesting that increased production of $PGH_2$ or another cyclooxygenase-derived contracting factor contributes to impaired endothelium-dependent vascular regulation in human hypertension. A similar observation has been made in a new model in which hypertension was produced by long-term administration of L-NAME; in these animals, increased endothelium-dependent contractions mediated by $TXA_2/PGH_2$ were seen in the aorta.[79] This finding does not seem to be limited to the use of acetylcholine, because adenosine diphosphate–adenosine triphosphate and serotonin also triggered an enhanced production of EDCF in the cerebral and coronary microcirculation of the SHR. Platelet-derived substances may, therefore, produce more contraction when aggregating in damaged vessels of hypertensive animals or individuals via a cyclooxygenase-dependent pathway, thus contributing to the complications of hypertension (i.e., stroke, myocardial infarction).[64]

## ENDOTHELIN

Circulating levels of endothelin typically are not increased in experimental hypertensive models or humans with hypertension.[28] This suggests that at least the luminal release of the peptide into the circulation is unaltered except in the presence of vascular disease (i.e., atherosclerosis) or renal failure. Because more than twice as much endothelin is released abluminally,[23] however, measurement of circulating endothelin levels may not be appropriate to determine local vascular endothelin production. In mesenteric resistance arteries of DOCA (desoxycorticosterone acetate)–salt hypertensive rats, but not in SHRs, increased production of endothelin occurs even in the presence of normal circulating levels of the peptide (see Fig. 179-6).

In contrast to the direct contractile responses to endothelin, the potentiating properties of low and threshold concentrations of endothelin are increased with aging and hypertension,[28,31] indicating that this indirect amplifying effect of endothelin could contribute to increased vascular contractility as pressure rises and the blood vessel wall ages.

The use of endothelin-receptor antagonists, which are becoming increasingly available, will help to determine the role of endothelin in health and disease. In hypertension the picture is still unclear. In DOCA-salt hypertensive rats, endothelin seems to be implicated in the maintenance of hypertension and in vascular hypertrophy.[80] In SHRs, however, the effect does not seem consistent, as two studies reported conflicting effects of BQ-123, a selective $ET_A$-receptor antagonist.[81,82] Studies of human hypertension using the first approved antagonists are elucidating the contribution of endothelin in hypertension.[83]

## ENDOTHELIUM-DEPENDENT RESPONSES IN ATHEROSCLEROSIS

### HYPERLIPIDEMIA

Morphologically, the endothelium remains intact in preatherogenesis to the early stage of atherogenesis.[85] Functional alter-

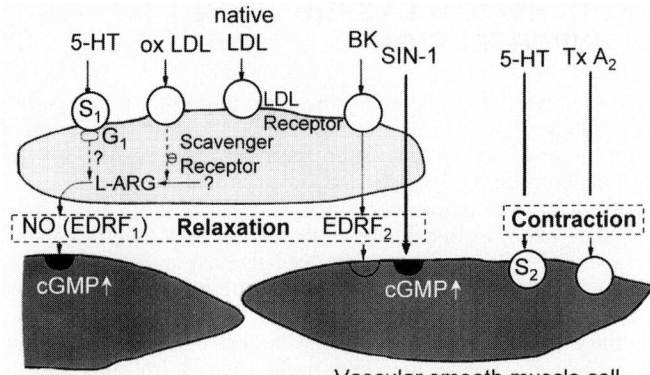

**FIGURE 179-7.** Schematic representation of the effects of low-density lipoproteins (*LDL*) in the blood vessel wall. Most likely, oxidation of LDL is an important step in the dysfunction of the endothelium in hyperlipidemia and atherosclerosis. Oxidized low-density lipoproteins (*OX-LDL*) may interact with the intracellular availability of L-arginine (*L-Arg*) and the G protein ($G_i$) of the serotonergic receptor ($S_1$), and they may also inactivate nitric oxide (*NO*). In addition, OX-LDL can increase the endothelial production of endothelin-1 by protein kinase C. (*5-HT*, serotonin; *BK*, bradykinin; *SIN-1*, molsidomine [nitric acid donor]; *TXA_2*, thromboxane $A_2$; *EDRF_1*, endothelium-derived relaxing factor 1; *cGMP*, cyclic guanosine monophosphate; $S_2$, 5-HT_2 [5-hydroxytryptamine] serotonergic receptor.)

ations occur, however, possibly due to the presence of oxidized low-density lipoproteins (OX-LDLs).[86]

In isolated porcine coronary arteries, endothelium-dependent relaxation to platelets, serotonin, and thrombin is inhibited by OX-LDLs.[87,88] In contrast, relaxation to the NO-donor linsidomine is maintained, excluding reduced responsiveness of smooth muscle to EDNO. This inhibition is specific for OX-LDLs because it is not induced by comparable concentrations of native LDL.[87] The inhibitor of NO production, L-NMMA, exerts an inhibitory effect on endothelium-dependent relaxation similar to that of the modified lipoproteins, suggesting that OX-LDLs interfere with the L-arginine pathway. The activity of NO synthase appears to remain unaffected, because L-arginine evokes full relaxation in vessels treated with OX-LDLs. Pretreatment of isolated vessels with L-arginine improves the reduced endothelium-dependent responses to serotonin.[89] Thus, OX-LDLs may interact with the intracellular signal transduction mechanisms (e.g., the function of $G_i$ proteins)[90] or the availability of L-arginine[87] (Fig. 179-7). Similarly, in hypercholesterolemic pigs, in vivo inhibition of endothelium-dependent relaxation in response to serotonin occurs in coronary arteries exposed to OX-LDLs.[91] Furthermore, in humans with hypercholesterolemia, L-arginine infusion augments the blunted increase in local blood flow in response to acetylcholine.[92] In addition to their effect on the L-arginine pathway, OX-LDLs inactivate NO and cause endothelium-dependent,[89] as well as endothelium-independent, contractions.[93]

OX-LDLs induce endothelin-1 mRNA expression and endothelin-1 release[94] (see Fig. 179-7). Threshold and low concentrations of endothelin potentiate contractions induced by serotonin in the human coronary artery. Similarly, endothelin-1 potentiates norepinephrine- and serotonin-induced contractions in the human internal mammary artery. Thus, even small increases in local endothelin levels may be important.[95]

### ATHEROSCLEROSIS

Atherosclerosis is associated with severe morphologic changes of the intima of large arteries (i.e., intimal thickening, proliferation of smooth muscle cells, accumulation of lipid-containing macrophages).[85] Endothelial denudation does not occur, however, except at late stages.

In porcine coronary arteries, established atherosclerosis severely impairs endothelium-dependent relaxation to serotonin and also reduces endothelium-dependent relaxation to bradykinin in the presence of hypercholesterolemia.[91] Endothelium-independent relaxation to nitrovasodilators remains preserved, however, except in severely atherosclerotic arteries. Similarly, in atherosclerotic human coronary arteries, endothelium-dependent relaxation to substance P, bradykinin, aggregating platelets, and calcium ionophores is attenuated,[96] and in vivo acetylcholine causes paradoxical vasoconstriction.

In vivo, the activity of the L-arginine/NO pathway is a balance between the synthesis and the breakdown of NO.[97] Controversy exists regarding the mechanism responsible for the marked impairment or loss of endothelium-dependent relaxation in atherosclerosis. EDRF release as measured by bioassay experiments in porcine coronary arteries with hypercholesterolemia and atherosclerosis have shown that the release of bioactive NO is reduced.[91] Direct measurements of NO in the rabbit aorta, however, suggest increased formation of NO with concomitant massive breakdown of the endogenous nitrovasodilator (to the bioinactive nitrite and nitrate).[98] This observation suggests that increased formation of superoxide radicals and other products in the endothelium inactivates NO, possibly as a result of decreased activity of superoxide dismutase in the atherosclerotic blood vessel wall.

Increased circulating levels of endothelin are associated with human atherosclerosis,[99] and the increase in endothelin levels correlates positively with the degree of atherosclerotic disease and the number of vascular beds involved. The increased endothelin production is derived not only from endothelial cells of atherosclerotic blood vessels, but also from vascular smooth muscle cells migrating into the intima. Increased local levels of endothelin may contribute to the known vasoconstrictor responses of atherosclerotic blood vessels and, because of the proliferative properties of endothelin,[50] to the atherosclerotic process itself.

## DIABETES

Micro- and macrovascular damage are hallmark abnormalities associated with diabetes (see Chap. 147). Endothelial dysfunction, including abnormal expression of NO and endothelin, is noted in type 1 and type 2 diabetes mellitus and in the earliest stages, including in impaired glucose tolerance, and in first-degree relatives.[100,101]

## REFERENCES

1. Lüscher TF, Vanhoutte PM. The endothelium: modulator of cardiovascular function. Boca Raton, FL: CRC Press, 1990:1.
2. Furchgott RF, Zawadzki JV. The obligatory role of endothelial cells in the relaxation of arterial smooth muscle by acetylcholine. Nature 1980; 299:373.
3. Yang Z, Stulz P, von Segesser L, et al. Different interactions of platelets with arterial and venous coronary bypass vessels. Lancet 1991; 337:939.
4. Lüscher TF, Diederich D, Siebenmann R, et al. Difference between endothelium-dependent relaxations in arterial and in venous coronary bypass grafts. N Engl J Med 1991; 319:462.
5. Rubanyi GM, Romero JC, Vanhoutte PM. Flow-induced release of endothelium-derived relaxing factor. Am J Physiol 1986; 250:H1145.
6. Pohl U, Holtz J, Busse R, Bassenge E. Crucial role of endothelium in the vasodilator response to increased flow in vivo. Hypertension 1986; 8:37.
7. Palmer RMJ, Ferrige AG, Moncada S. Nitric oxide release accounts for the biological activity of endothelium-derived relaxing factor. Nature 1987; 327:524.
8. Feelisch M, te Poel M, Zamora R, et al. Understanding the controversy over the identity of EDRF. Nature 1994; 368:62.
9. Rapoport RM, Draznin MB, Murad F. Endothelium-dependent relaxation in rat aorta may be mediated through cyclic GMP-dependent protein phosphorylation. Nature 1983; 306:174.
10. Radomski MW, Palmer RMJ, Moncada S. Comparative pharmacology of endothelium-derived relaxing factor, nitric oxide and prostacyclin in platelets. Br J Pharmacol 1987; 92:181.
11. Palmer RMJ, Ashton DS, Moncada S. Vascular endothelial cells synthesize nitric oxide from L-arginine. Nature 1988; 333:664.
12. Bredt DS, Hwang PM, Glatt CE, et al. Cloned and expressed nitric oxide synthase structurally resembles cytochrome P-450 reductase. Nature 1991; 351:714.
13. Cosentino F, Luscher TF. Tetrahydrobiopterin and endothelial function. Eur Heart J 1998; suppl G:G3.
14. Richard V, Tschudi MR, Lüscher TF. Differential activation of the endothelial L-arginine pathway by bradykinin, serotonin and clonidine in porcine coronary arteries. Am J Physiol 1990; 259:H-1433.
15. Tschudi M, Richard V, Bühler FR, Lüscher TF. Importance of endothelium-derived nitric oxide in intramyocardial porcine coronary arteries. Am J Physiol 1990; 260:H13.
16. Meyer P, Flammer J, Lüscher TF. Endothelium-dependent regulation of the ophthalmic microcirculation in the perfused porcine eye. Role of nitric oxide and endothelins. Invest Ophthalmol Vis Sci 1993; 34:3614.
17. Rees DD, Palmer RMJ, Moncada S. The role of endothelium-derived nitric oxide in the regulation of blood pressure. Proc Natl Acad Sci U S A 1989; 86:3375.
18. Vallance P, Leone A, Colver A, et al. Accumulation of an endogenous inhibitor of nitric acid synthesis in chronic renal failure. Lancet 1992; 339:572.
19. Boger RH, Bode-Boger SM, Szuba A, et al. Asymmetric dimethylarginine (ADMA): a novel risk factor for endothelial dysfunction. Its role in hypercholesterolemia. Circulation 1998; 98:1842.
20. Feletou M, Vanhoutte PM. Endothelium-dependent hyperpolarization of canine coronary smooth muscle. Br J Pharmacol 1988; 93:515.
21. Standen NB, Quayle JM, Davies NW, et al. Hyperpolarizing vasodilators activate ATP-sensitive K+-channels in arterial smooth muscle. Science 1989; 245:177.
22. Moncada S, Vane JR. Pharmacology and endogenous roles of prostaglandin endoperoxides, thromboxane A2 and prostacyclin. Pharmacol Rev 1979; 30:293.
23. Wagner O, Christ G, Wojta J, et al. Polar secretion of endothelin-1 by cultured endothelial cells. J Biomed Chem 1992; 267:16066.
24. De Mey JG, Claeys M, Vanhoutte PM. Endothelium-dependent inhibitory effects of acetylcholine, adenosine diphosphate, thrombin and arachidonic acid in the canine femoral artery. J Pharmacol Exp Ther 1982; 222:166.
25. Yang Z, von Segesser L, Bauer E, et al. Differential activation of the endothelial L-arginine and cyclooxygenase pathway in the human internal mammary artery and saphenous vein. Circ Res 1991; 68:52.
26. Katusic ZS, Vanhoutte PM. Superoxide anion is an endothelium-derived contracting factor. Am J Physiol 1989; 257:H33.
27. Cosentino F, Katusic ZS. Role of superoxide anion in mediation of endothelium-dependent contractions. Hypertension 1994; 23:229.
28. Lüscher TF, Boulanger CM, Dohi Y, Yang Z. Endothelium-derived contracting factors. (Brief review). Hypertension 1992; 19:117.
29. Kohno M, Yasunari K, Yokokawa K, et al. Inhibition by atrial and brain natriuretic peptide of endothelin. A secretion after stimulation with angiotensin II and thrombin of cultured human endothelial cells. J Clin Invest 1991; 87:1999.
30. Boulanger C, Lüscher TF. Release of endothelin from the porcine aorta: inhibition by endothelium-derived nitric oxide. J Clin Invest 1990; 85:587.
31. Dohi Y, Hahn AWA, Boulanger CM, et al. Endothelin stimulated by angiotensin II augments vascular contractility of hypertensive resistance arteries. Hypertension 1992; 19:131.
32. Kourembanas S, Marsden PA, McQullan LP, Faller DV. Hypoxia induces endothelin gene expression and secretion in cultured human endothelium. J Clin Invest 1991; 88:1054.
33. Lüscher TF, Yang Z, Tschudi M, et al. Interaction between endothelin-1 and endothelium-derived relaxing factor in human arteries and veins. Circ Res 1990; 66:1088.
34. Kiowski W, Lüscher TF, Linder L, Bühler FR. Endothelin-1-induced vasoconstriction in man: reversal by calcium channel blockade but not by nitrovasodilators or endothelium-derived relaxing factor. Circulation 1991; 83:469.
35. Saijonmaa O, Ristimäki A, Fyhrquist F. Atrial natriuretic peptide, nitroglycerine, and nitroprusside reduce basal and stimulated endothelin production from cultured endothelial cells. Biochem Biophys Res Commun 1990; 173:514.
36. Yokokawa K, Kohno M, Yasunari K, et al. Endothelin-3 regulates endothelin-1 production in cultured human endothelial cells. Hypertension 1991; 18:304.
37. Stewart DJ, Langleben D, Cernacek P, Cianflone K. Endothelin release is inhibited by coculture of endothelial cells with cells of vascular media. Am J Physiol 1990; 259:H1928.
38. Warner TD, Mitchell JA, de Nucci G, Vane JR. Endothelin-1 and endothelin-3 release EDRF from isolated perfused arterial vessels of the rat and rabbit. J Cardiovasc Pharmacol 1989; 13(Suppl 5):85.
39. Arai H, Hori S, Aramori I, et al. Cloning and expression of a cDNA encoding an endothelin receptor. Nature 1990; 348:730.
40. Sakurai T, Yanagisawa M, Takuwa Y. Cloning of a cDNA encoding a non-isopeptide-selective subtype of the endothelin receptor. Nature 1990; 348:732.
41. Emori T, Hirata Y, Marumo F. Specific receptors for endothelin-3 in cultured bovine endothelial cells and its cellular mechanism of action. FEBS Lett 1990; 263:261.
42. Lüscher TF. Do we need endothelin antagonists? Cardiovasc Res 1993; 27:2089.
43. Shai S-Y, Fishel RS, Martin BM, et al. Bovine angiotensin converting enzyme cDNA cloning and regulation. Increased expression during endothelial cell growth arrest. Circ Res 1992; 70:1274.
44. Severs WB, Daniels-Severs AE. Effects of angiotensin on the central nervous system. Pharmacol Rev 1973; 25:415.
45. Dubey RK, Roy A, Overbeck HW. Culture of renal arteriolar smooth muscle cells: mitogenic responses to Ang II. Circ Res 1992; 71:1143.
46. Lüscher TF, Tanner FC. Endothelial regulation of vascular tone and growth. Am J Hypertens 1993; 6:283S.
47. Dzau VJ, Gibbons GH. Vascular remodelling: mechanisms and implications. J Cardiovasc Pharmacol 1993; 21(Suppl I):S1.
48. Garg UC, Hassid A. Nitric-oxide generating vasodilators and 8-bromo-cyclic guanosine monophosphate inhibit mitogenesis and proliferation of cultured rat vascular SMCs. J Clin Invest 1989; 83:1774.

49. Dubey RK, Ganten D, Lüscher TF. Enhanced migration of smooth muscle cells from Ren-2 transgenic rats in response to angiotensin II: inhibition by nitric oxide. Hypertension 1993; 22:412.
50. Hirata Y, Takagi Y, Fukuda Y, Marumo F. Endothelin is a potent mitogen for rat vascular smooth muscle cells. Atherosclerosis 1989; 78:225.
51. O'Reilly MS, Holmgren L, Shing Y, et al. Angiostatin: a novel angiogenesis inhibitor that mediates the suppression of metastases by Lewis lung carcinoma. Cell 1994; 79:315.
52. O'Reilly MS, Boehm T, Shin Y, et al. Endostatin: an endogenous inhibitor of angiogenesis and tumor growth. Cell 1997; 88:277.
53. Harris AL. Are angiostatin and endostatin cures for cancer? Lancet 1998; 351:1598.
54. Vidal-Ragout MJ, Romero JC, Vanhoutte PM. Endothelium-derived relaxing factor inhibits renin release. Eur J Pharmacol 1988; 149:401.
55. Matsumura Y, Nakase K, Ikegawa R, et al. The endothelium-derived vasoconstrictor peptide endothelin inhibits renin release in vitro. Life Sci 1989; 44:149.
56. Miller WL, Redfield MM, Burnett JC Jr. Integrated cardiac, renal, and endocrine actions of endothelin. J Clin Invest 1989; 83:317.
57. Lorenz RR, Sanchez-Ferrer CF, Burnett JC, Vanhoutte PM. Influence of endocardial derived factor(s) on the release of atrial natriuretic factor. (Abstract). FASEB J 1988; 2:1293.
58. Fukuda Y, Hirata Y, Yoshimi H, et al. Endothelin is a potent secretagogue for atrial natriuretic peptide in cultured rat atrial myocytes. Biochem Biophys Res Commun 1988; 155:167.
59. Vierhapper H, Wagner O, Nowotny P, Waldhäusl W. Effect of endothelin-1 in man. Circulation 1990; 81:1415.
60. Boarder MR, Marriott DB. Characterization of endothelin-1 stimulation of catecholamine release from adrenal chromaffin cells. J Cardiovasc Pharmacol 1989; 13(Suppl 5):223.
61. Wiklundin NP, Oehlen A, Cederqvist B. Inhibition of adrenergic neuroeffector transmission by endothelin in the guinea-pig femoral artery. Acta Physiol Scand 1988; 134:311.
62. Gomez-Sanchez CE, Foecking MF, Chiou S. Endothelin binding to cultured calf adrenal zona glomerulosa cells and stimulation of aldosterone secretion. J Clin Invest 1989; 84:1032.
63. Lüscher TF, Vanhoutte PM. Endothelium-dependent contractions to acetylcholine in the aorta of the spontaneously hypertensive rat. Hypertension 1986; 8:344.
64. Lüscher TF, Vanhoutte PM. Endothelium-dependent responses to aggregating platelets and serotonin in spontaneously hypertensive rats. Hypertension 1986; 8(Suppl II):55.
65. Mayhan WG, Faraci FM, Heistad DD. Impairment of endothelium-dependent responses of cerebral arterioles in chronic hypertension. Am J Physiol 1987; 253:H1435.
66. Linder L, Kiowski W, Bühler FR, Lüscher TF. Indirect evidence for release of endothelium-derived relaxing factor in human forearm circulation in vivo: blunted response in essential hypertension. Circulation 1990; 81:1762.
67. Panza JA, Quyyumi AA, Brush JE Jr, Epstein SE. Abnormal vascular endothelium-dependent vascular relaxation in patients with essential hypertension. N Engl J Med 1990; 323:22.
68. Creager MA, Roddy M-A, Coleman SM, Dzau VJ. The effect of ACE inhibition on endothelium-dependent vasodilation in hypertension. J Vasc Res 1992; 29:97.
69. Taddei S, Virdis A, Mattei P, Salvetti A. Vasodilation to acetylcholine in primary and secondary forms of human hypertension. Hypertension 1993; 21:929.
70. Lüscher TF. The endothelium and cardiovascular disease—a complex relation. N Engl J Med 1994; 330:1081.
71. Cockcroft J, Chowienczyk PJ, Benjamin N, Ritter JM. Preserved endothelium-dependent vasodilation in patients with essential hypertension. N Engl J Med 1994; 330:1036.
72. Tschudi MR, Criscione L, Lüscher TF. Effect of aging and hypertension on endothelial function of rat coronary arteries. J Hypertens 1991; 9(Suppl 6):164.
73. Treasure CB, Manoukian SV, Klein JL, et al. Epicardial coronary artery responses to acetylcholine are impaired in hypertensive patients. Circ Res 1992; 71:776.
74. Lüscher TF, Vanhoutte PM, Raij L. Antihypertensive therapy normalizes endothelium-dependent relaxations in salt-induced hypertension of the rat. Hypertension 1987; 9(Suppl III):193.
75. Dohi Y, Thiel M, Bühler FR, Lüscher TF. Activation of the endothelial L-arginine pathway in pressurized mesenteric resistance arteries: effect of age and hypertension. Hypertension 1990; 15:170.
76. Kelm M, Feelisch M, Krebber T, et al. The role of nitric oxide in the regulation of coronary vascular resistance in arterial hypertension: comparison of normotensive and spontaneously hypertensive rats. J Cardiovasc Pharmacol 1992; 20:183.
77. Nava E, Noll G, Luscher TF. Increased activity of constitutive nitric oxide synthase in cardiac endothelium in spontaneous hypertension. Circulation 1995; 91:2310.
78. Panza JA, Casino PR, Badar DM, Quyyumi AA. Effect of increased availability of endothelium-derived nitric oxide on endothelium-dependent vascular relaxation in normals and in patients with essential hypertension. Circulation 1993; 87:1475.
79. Kung CF, Moreau P, Takase H, Luscher TF. L-NAME-induced hypertension impairs endothelial function in rat aorta: reversal by trandolapril and verapamil. Hypertension 1995; 26(5):744.
80. Li JS, Lariviere R, Schiffrin EL. Effect of a nonselective endothelin antagonist on vascular remodeling in deoxycorticosterone acetate salt hyperten-sive rats: evidence for a role of endothelin in vascular hypertrophy. Hypertension 1994; 24:183.
81. Bank N, Aynedijan HS, Khan GA. Mechanism of vasoconstriction induced by chronic inhibition of nitric oxide in rats. Hypertension 1994; 24:322.
82. Nishikibe M, Ikada M, Tsuchida S, et al. Antihypertensive effect of a newly synthesized endothelin antagonist, BQ-123, in genetic hypertension models. J Hypertens 1992; 10(Suppl 4):53.
83. Krum H, Viskoper RJ, Lacourciere Y, et al. The effect of an endothelin-receptor antagonist, bosentan, on blood pressure in patients with essential hypertension. N Engl J Med 1998; 338:784.
84. Hayzer PJ, Cicila G, Cockerham C, et al. Endothelin A and B receptors are downregulated in the hearts of hypertensive rats. Am J Med Sci 1994; 307:222.
85. Ross R. The pathogenesis of atherosclerosis—an update. N Engl J Med 1986; 314:488.
86. Ylä-Herttuala S, Palinski W, Rosenfeld ME, et al. Evidence for the presence of oxidatively modified low-density lipoproteins in atherosclerotic lesions of rabbit and man. J Clin Invest 1989; 84:1086.
87. Tanner FC, Noll G, Boulanger CM, Lüscher TF. Oxidized low-density lipoproteins inhibit relaxations of porcine coronary arteries: role of scavenger receptor and endothelium-derived nitric oxide. Circulation 1991; 83:2012.
88. Kugiyama K, Kerns SA, Morrisett JD, et al. Impairment of endothelium-dependent arterial relaxation by lysolecithin in modified low-density lipoproteins. Nature 1990; 344:160.
89. Simon BC, Cunningham LD, Cohen RA. Oxidized low density lipoproteins cause contraction and inhibit endothelium-dependent relaxation in the pig coronary artery. J Clin Invest 1990; 86:75.
90. Flavahan NA. Atherosclerosis or lipoprotein-induced endothelial dysfunction: potential mechanisms underlying reduction in dysfunction in EDRF/nitric oxide activity. Circulation 1992; 85:1927.
91. Shimokawa H, Vanhoutte PM. Impaired endothelium-dependent relaxation to aggregating platelets and related vasoactive substances in porcine coronary arteries in hypercholesterolemia and atherosclerosis. Circ Res 1989; 64:900.
92. Creager MA, Gallagher SH, Girerd XJ, et al. L-arginine improves endothelium-dependent vasodilation in hypercholesterolemic humans. J Clin Invest 1992; 90:1248.
93. Galle J, Bassenge E, Busse R. Oxidized low-density lipoproteins potentiate vasoconstrictions to various agonists by direct interaction with vascular smooth muscle. Circ Res 1990; 66:1287.
94. Boulanger CM, Tanner FC, Hahn AWA, et al. Oxidized low-density lipoproteins induce mRNA expression and release of endothelin from human and porcine endothelium. Circ Res 1992; 70:1191.
95. Yang Z, Richard V, von Segesser L, et al. Threshold concentrations of endothelin-1 potentiate contractions to norepinephrine and serotonin in human arteries: a new mechanism of vasospasm? Circulation 1990; 82:188.
96. Förstermann U, Mügge A, Alheid U, et al. Selective attenuation of endothelium-mediated vasodilation in atherosclerotic human coronary arteries. Circ Res 1988; 62:185.
97. Wever RMF, Luscher TF, Cosentino F, Rabelink TJ. Atherosclerosis and the two faces of endothelial nitric oxide synthase. Circulation 1998; 97:108.
98. Minor RL, Myers RR Jr, Guerra R Jr, et al. Diet-induced atherosclerosis increases the release of nitrogen oxides from rabbit aorta. J Clin Invest 1990; 86:2109.
99. Lerman A, Edwards BS, Hallett JW, et al. Circulating and tissue endothelin immunoreactivity in advanced atherosclerosis. N Engl J Med 1991; 325:997.
100. De Vriese AS, Verbeuren TJ, Van de Voorde J, et al. Endothelial dysfunction in diabetes. Br J Pharmacol 2000; 130:963.
101. Balletshoffer BM, Rittig K, Enderle MD, et al. Endothelial dysfunction is detectable in young normotensive first-degree relatives of subjects with type 2 DM associated with insulin resistance. Circ 2000; 101:1780.

# CHAPTER 180

# THE ENDOCRINE BLOOD CELLS

HARISH P. G. DAVE AND BEAT MÜLLER

## FLOATING ENDOCRINE SYSTEM

Blood cells play a critical role in tissue oxygenation as well as in hemostasis and immune function. Besides these well-established and accepted roles of blood cells, recognition is emerging of the ability of these cells to elaborate a variety of substances (e.g., cytokines, regulatory peptides, and glycoproteins) that

**TABLE 180-1.**
**Hormones Produced by Blood Cells**

---

**LYMPHOCYTES**

IL-1, IL-2, IL-3, IL-4, IL-5, IL-6, IL-9, IL-10, IL-13, IL-14, G-CSF, GM-CSF, M-CSF, interferons, TNF, RANTES, TNF, LIF, NGF, CGRP, MIF, ACTH, TSH, GH and IGF-I, PTHrP, VIP, prolactin, vasopressin, enkephalin, preprotachykinin, GnRH, CRH, TRH

**MONOCYTES/MACROPHAGES/DENDRITIC CELLS**

IL-1, IL-5, IL-6, IL-8, IL-10, IL-12, G-CSF, GM-CSF, M-CSF, interferons, TNF, LIF, MIF, TGF, FGF, MIP, NGF, VEGF, ACTH, preprotachykinin, proglucagon, prosomatostatin, propancreatic polypeptide, preproinsulin, VIP, TSH, ?GnRH

**NEUTROPHILS**

IL-1, IL-3, IL-6, IL-8, G-CSF, GM-CSF, M-CSF, interferons

**EOSINOPHILS**

IL-1, IL-3, IL-5, IL-6, GM-CSF, TNF, MIP, TGF

**BASOPHILS/MAST CELLS**

IL-1, IL-3, IL-4, IL-5, IL-6, IL-8, GM-CSF, MIP, TNF, LIF

**PLATELETS**

IL-1, PDGF, TGF, EGF, RANTES

---

See text for abbreviation nomenclature.

---

have autocrine, paracrine, juxtacrine, and hemocrine effects. They also secrete classic hormones of the endocrine system. With this plurality of hormonal effects, blood cells constitute a *floating endocrine system*.

## ENDOCRINE BLOOD CELLS

Blood cells consist of lymphocytes, neutrophils, monocytes, eosinophils, and basophils—all subsets of leukocytes (white cells)—as well as thrombocytes (platelets) and erythrocytes (red cells).[1] All of these cell types, except for the mature circulating erythrocytes, produce hormones. The red cell loses its nucleus before emerging from the bone marrow and does not directly elaborate hormones. The hormones produced by these various blood cell types are summarized in Table 180-1.

### MONOCYTES

Monocytes are bone marrow–derived cells that represent from 1% to 6% of leukocytes in the adult. After a short stay in the circulation, they enter the tissues and are recognizable there as *macrophages*, which are longer-lived cells. Tissue macrophages may also replenish themselves by cell division depending on local factors and are not wholly dependent on the blood monocyte pool. They have three main functions[2]: as *phagocytic* cells, they engulf microbes and other foreign particles, and, together with monocytes and polymorphonuclear granulocytes, form the phagocytic system of the body; as *antigen-presenting cells*, they take up, process, and present antigen to T and B lymphocytes; finally, as *immunomodulators*, they produce and release various cytokines (also called *monokines*).

Macrophages produce an array of secretory chemicals that are important regulators of inflammation. The lymphocyte activation that occurs from antigen presentation results in the secretion of additional factors that further activate the macrophage. The secretory products include polypeptide hormones, cytokines, inhibitors of cytokines, bioactive oligopeptides and lipids, sterol hormones, reactive oxygen and its intermediaries, and reactive nitrogen intermediaries.[3]

Macrophages are strategically positioned to provide a defense against organisms entering the body via the respiratory tract (alveolar macrophages), gastrointestinal tract (Kupffer cells of the liver and peritoneal macrophages), bloodstream (splenic macrophages), skin (Langerhans cells), and lymphatics (lymph node macrophages). In addition, they are present in all other organs and tissues in a large variety of phenotypes, extending from microglial cells of the brain, synovial A cells of the synovial cavity of joints, and mesangial phagocytes in the kidney, to the multinucleated osteoclasts of the bone. Kupffer cells in the liver contribute up to 90% of all the macrophages in the body and up to 15% of all cells in the liver. The phagocytic tissue macrophages, together with endothelial cells, constitute what was previously called the "reticuloendothelial system" (RES).

Through phagocytosis, tissue macrophages play an important role in the clearing of microbes and the removal of damaged or effete tissue cells or of extracellular matrix. Specific receptors on the cell surface of macrophages mediate the phagocytic function: receptors for the Fc portion of immunoglobulin G antibody recognize antibody-coated microbes; CR1 and CR3 receptors recognize complement; and CD40 receptors recognize lipopolysaccharide found in the cell wall of gram-negative bacteria, among others.

Specialized macrophages, also known as interdigitating *dendritic cells*, are typical antigen-presenting cells. These cells are able to initiate a specific immune response against a microbial antigen. Dendritic cells ingest a microbial or tumor antigen and process it. After migrating into secondary lymphoid tissue, they present the processed antigen (on the surface in association with the major histocompatibility complex [MHC] class II) to other cells of the immune system (i.e., T cells).[4] Dendritic cells are highly mobile cells, and the sequential migration of these cells into and out of tissues is accompanied by phenotypical as well as functional changes that are instrumental to their role as sentinels of the immune system.[5–7] Dendritic cells can be of macrophage or lymphocyte origin. The cytokine expression pattern and behavior differ between dendritic cells that are morphologically and immunophenotypically related to macrophages, between those that are classified as immature or mature dendritic cells, and also between those that are related to B or to T lymphocytes. A detailed list of the cytokines that these cells produce is likely to be incomplete, because newer subsets are in the process of being defined and tested under various experimental conditions. At a minimum, most dendritic cells produce a number of interleukins (i.e., IL-1β, IL-6, IL-10, IL-12, and IL-18) and tumor necrosis factor-α (TNF-α).[8–13] Determining the precise cellular origin of interferons has been difficult due to the rapid apoptosis of these cells; nonetheless, evidence indicates that the dendritic cells are the source of these cytokines, which play an important role in the antiviral immune response. Intriguing evidence also exists for the expression of preproinsulin by murine thymic dendritic cells. Dendritic cells also produce macrophage inflammatory protein-1γ (MIP-1γ), macrophage inflammatory protein-1α (MIP-1α), and macrophage inflammatory protein-2 (MIP-2).[8] Nitric oxide, a potent regulator of disparate cellular processes, is also elaborated by dendritic cells.[14] Dendritic cell–derived nitric oxide promotes apoptosis[15] of autoreactive T cells and may therefore play a role in autoimmunity.

**Cytokines.** Macrophages produce and secrete a wide array of substances (termed *cytokines* or *monokines*) ranging in molecular mass from 32 Da (superoxide anion) to almost 500,000 kDa (fibronectin), and ranging in bioactivity from induction of cell growth to cell death.[16] TNF-α and several interleukins (e.g., IL-1 and IL-6) are the classic mediators of these cells; however, the nitric oxide that is also produced by macrophages may differentially affect vascular tone in different vascular beds. Macrophage migration inhibitory factor

(MIF) is released by macrophages and T cells in response to glucocorticoids as well as to various proinflammatory stimuli. Once secreted, the MIF "overrides" the immunosuppressive effects of glucocorticoids on macrophages and T cells. MIF is also produced by many other cell types, which in turn can trap and also respond to these cytokines via cognate receptors.[2]

Cytokines are *acutely synthesized and secreted in response to stimuli*, unlike most classic hormones, which are *preformed and stored within cell granules before a suitable stimulus is received*. Similar to most classic hormones, most cytokines (with the notable exceptions of IL-1 and TNF-α) are synthesized in the form of precursors and have an amino-terminal leader sequence directing their transport to the Golgi apparatus in preparation for subsequent secretion. Most of the monokines have potent and diverse systemic effects in addition to their effects on immune function. The effects of different cytokines are often pleiotropic and overlapping; they can be synergistic or antagonistic, depending on the experimental system. A subset of monokines with known interactions with the endocrine system is listed in Table 180-2.

Reports of the production of classic hormones by macrophages (detected at the mRNA or protein level) have also appeared. These include preprotachykinin in human mononuclear phagocytes and lymphocytes, as well as preproinsulin, proglucagon, propancreatic polypeptide, and prosomatostatin within the human and murine thymus.[17] Hormone expression is enriched in the antigen-presenting cell population, which is presumed to be a mixture of macrophages and dendritic cells. Autoimmunity and self-reactivity are prevented by the deletion of lymphocyte clones reactive to self-antigens. The close association of hormone-producing cells and dendritic cells in the thymus could lead to the development of a self-reactive lymphocyte clone that is subsequently deleted, thereby reducing the likelihood that hormones and other proteins expressed at low levels will incite an autoimmune reaction. Thus, the presence of these pancreatic hormones (i.e., preproinsulin, proglucagon, propancreatic polypeptide, and prosomatostatin) at low levels in the thymus may be critical in inducing central tolerance to proteins of restricted expression. This would suggest that other self-antigens will also be found in the thymus. Indeed, the presence of albumin, insulin, glucagon, thyroid peroxidase, glutamic acid peroxidase, thyroglobulin, myelin basic protein, and retinal S antigen has been demonstrated by reverse transcription polymerase chain reaction in the human thymus at ages from 8 days to 13 years.[18] (This study did not exclude the presence of some of these substances in thymic epithelial cells.) Vasoactive intestinal peptide (VIP) and VIP-1 receptor have been detected in rat macrophages.[19]

**Monocytes.** Although monocytes are less well studied, they have a pattern of cytokine production similar to that of macrophages. Besides the various cytokines, these cells also synthesize prostaglandins and leukotrienes. Transforming growth factor-β (TGF-β) is an autocrine hormone for these cells, and its production is further stimulated by 1,25 dihydroxyvitamin $D_3$ and retinoids.[20] Interestingly, monocytes in culture can be stimulated by thyrotropin-releasing hormone (TRH) to release thyroid-stimulating hormone (TSH), an effect that can be totally blocked by adding triiodothyronine to the cultured cells.[21] Thus, these cells exhibit the same type of control as the hypothalamic–pituitary–thyroid axis. They also display receptors for various peptide hormones and, as with lymphocytes, undergo an increase in receptor number on activation. Activation of monocytes by growth hormone (GH) results in an increase in interferon-γ (IFN-γ) secretion,[22] which, in turn, has additional effects on the surrounding immune cells.

## LYMPHOCYTES

Lymphocytes are mononuclear cells that represent 20% to 50% of leukocytes. They are further characterized by a cluster of differentiation (CD) antigens. Broadly, they can be categorized as B, T, and natural killer (NK) lymphocytes, although clearly, the CD expression pattern can lead to much more refined subtyping. The majority of lymphocytes are long-lived cells that play a critical role in the humoral and cellular immune response; they are the repositories of immune memory.

Like the macrophages and dendritic cells, the lymphocytes are metabolically active cells. They produce a multitude of interleukins (IL-1, IL-2, IL-3, IL-4, IL-5, IL-6, IL-9, IL-10, IL-13, IL-14), colony-stimulating factors (granulocyte colony-stimulating factor [G-CSF], granulocyte-macrophage colony-stimulating factor [GM-CSF], and macrophage colony-stimulating factor [M-CSF]), interferons (IFN-α, IFN-γ), and other factors such as MIP-1, RANTES (regulated on activation, normal T-expressed and secreted), TNF-α, leukemia inhibitory factor (LIF), and nerve growth factor (NGF).[1,23] They are also well endowed with receptors for many of the interleukins and interferons, so that the cells can be affected in both an autocrine and paracrine fashion. In addition, lymphocytes express receptors for many bioactive peptides such as adrenocorticotropic hormone (ACTH), calcitonin, endorphins, enkephalins, vasopressin, oxytocin, thyrotropin, GH, somatostatin, substance P, and VIP.[3] In general, the density of peptide hormone receptors increases markedly after activation of the cells, implying a role for classic hormones as well as the various interleukins in lymphocyte regulation.

Just as hormone receptors have been identified on these cells, so has the ability to produce some of their cognate hormones. Concanavalin A–stimulated human lymphocyte cultures produce detectable levels of prolactin, luteinizing hormone (LH) and follicle-stimulating hormone (FSH).[24] Prolactin production, which can also follow T-cell stimulation of B cells,[25] in turn, enhances NK cell function, activates the interferon-regulated factor-1 (IRF-1) transcription factor, and interacts with or generates IL-2 and IFN-γ.[26] The suggestion has also been made that lymphocytes may have an endocrine role in infertility: lower levels of these hormones are produced by the lymphocytes of infertile women. Unstimulated lymphocytes secrete GH.[27] However, unlike the situation with TSH in monocytes, this GH secretion is not subject to the same regulatory mechanisms as GH production by pituitary cells. Incubation of lymphocytes in media containing growth hormone–releasing hormone (GHRH) and somatostatin has no effect on GH release.[28] Acromegaly has been reported in a patient with a non-Hodgkin lymphoma whose tumor cells secreted GH.[28a] In addition, pituitary GH deficiency has not been associated with immunodeficiency in humans.

Lymphocytes also express the proopiomelanocortin (POMC) gene, leading to the detection of β-endorphin, enkephalin, and ACTH in these cells.[29,30] Human immunodeficiency virus (HIV) infection of lymphocytes leads to the production of ACTH, which has the same bioactivity as ACTH produced by the pituitary.[31] The mechanism for this is unclear, but it may reflect part of the pleiotropic effects of TAT protein produced by the virus. The *trans*-activation of the enkephalin gene by HTLV-I TAX protein, which is closely analogous to TAT, has been demonstrated.[32] This ACTH production may lead to further immunosuppression in HIV-infected individuals.

Macrophage MIF is released by macrophages and T cells in response to glucocorticoids as well as in response to stimulation by various proinflammatory stimuli.[33] MIF has also been isolated from anterior pituitary cells.[33]

Calcitonin gene–related peptide (CGRP), vasopressin, and VIP have been detected in certain subsets of lymphocytes, but their roles in lymphocyte development and immune function are unclear.[19,34,35]

**TABLE 180-2.**
**Some Cytokines/Monokines Released by Blood Cells and Their Relationship to the Endocrine System***

| Cytokine | Major Immune Functions | Endocrine Effects and Clinical Implications |
|---|---|---|
| **INTERLEUKINS (ILs)** | | |
| IL-1 ($\alpha$ and $\beta$ form) | Prototypic "multifunctional" monokine; affects nearly every cell type, often in concert with other cytokines; mediates acute-phase inflammatory response; cofactor for immune and endothelial cell proliferation and activation; enhances production of tumor necrosis factor (TNF), IL-1, interferon (IFN), and colony-stimulating factors. | Stimulates hypothalamic–pituitary–adrenocortical (HPA) axis, including corticotropin-releasing hormone secretion; inhibits gonadotropin-releasing hormone secretion; inhibits thyroid cell function. |
| IL-1 receptor antagonist (IL-1ra) | Binds to IL-1 receptor; fails to transduce signal, thereby antagonizing effects of IL-1. | Antagonizes IL-1 effects. |
| IL-6 | Mediates inflammatory response by stimulating the production of acute-phase proteins in hepatocytes; activates hematopoietic progenitor cells and shortens their $G_0$ period; induces growth and/or differentiation of T cells, B cells, hepatocytes, keratinocytes, and nerve cells; enhances B-cell differentiation to immunoglobulin-secreting plasma cells; induces maturation of megakaryocytes, thereby increasing the number of platelets. | Stimulates HPA axis, gonadotropin, vasopressin, and growth hormone secretion. Suppresses thyroid axis and serum lipid levels; regulates osteoclast proliferation and recruitment. Raised levels found in Paget disease, estrogen deficiency, and hyperthyroidism. |
| IL-10 | Produced by antigen-presenting cells to modulate T-helper cell immune response ($T_H1$ and $T_H2$); potent immunosuppressant of macrophage function by down-regulation of major histocompatibility complex (MHC) class II expression, and cytokine synthesis; enhances B-cell growth and secretion of immunoglobulin; cofactor for mast cell growth. | Glucocorticoids favor the development of a $T_H2$ immune response, possibly by stimulation of IL-10 and suppression of IL-12 production in antigen-presenting cells. |
| IL-12 | Initiates cell-mediated immunity by inducing the differentiation of $T_H1$ cells from uncommitted T cells; stimulates the growth and functional activity of T cells and natural killer cells, induces IFN-$\gamma$ production. | Injection of IL-12 in cancer patients increased the serum levels of cortisol, prolactin, and estradiol. IL-12 is expressed in cultured thyroid cells, especially after stimulation with thyroid-stimulating hormone, IL-1, or IFN-$\gamma$. |
| **TUMOR NECROSIS FACTORS (TNFs)** | | |
| TNF-$\alpha$ (and -$\beta$) | Together with IL-1 is the principal mediator of tissue destruction in many immune-inflammatory diseases. Important mediator of inflammation; vital in keeping infections localized and for the maturation and function of the immune system; induces fever, endothelial cell activation, and angiogenesis; cofactor for macrophage activation and for B-cell and T-cell proliferation; enhances expression of adhesion molecules on leukocytes; induces catabolic state; membrane form mediates cytotoxicity. | Stimulates secretion of luteinizing hormone, prolactin, and adrenocorticotropic hormone from the pituitary; mediator in the pathogenesis of autoimmune type 1 diabetes. TNF-$\alpha$ plays a role in the state of insulin resistance associated with obesity and type 2 diabetes. Thiazolidinediones specifically block TNF-$\alpha$-induced insulin resistance, contributing to their antidiabetic action. |
| **INTERFERON (IFN)** | Initially characterized for their ability to "interfere" with viral replication. | |
| IFN-$\alpha$ | Interferes with viral replication; increases expression of MHC class I; enhances natural killer cell function. | Directly stimulates adrenal glucocorticoid production; participates in the regulation of various endocrine systems; modulates temperature, glucose sensitivity, feeding pattern, and opiate activity. |
| IFN-$\gamma$ | Produced mainly by T cells; same biologic functions as IFN-$\alpha$; in addition, increases MHC class II expression; activates macrophages; inhibits IgE production; inhibits proliferation of $T_H2$ cells. | Possible pathophysiologic role in the autoimmune insulitis of type 1 diabetes. |
| **CHEMOKINES** | Chemotactic cytokines. | |
| $\alpha$-Family (e.g., IL-8, macrophage inflammatory protein [MIP]-2) | Chemoattractants for neutrophil granulocytes. | IL-8 is secreted from primary follicular thyroid cell cultures, indicating a possible link with autoimmune thyroiditis. |
| $\beta$-Family (e.g., monocyte chemoattractant protein [MCP]-1, MIP-1$\alpha$ and MIP-1$\beta$) | Chemoattractants and activators for lymphocytes, monocytes, eosinophil granulocytes, and basophil granulocytes; stimulate production of other inflammatory mediators such as IL-1, TNF-$\alpha$, and histamine. | MCP-1 expressed in thyroid cells with possible link to autoimmune thyroiditis; correlation between prolactin and MIP-1$\alpha$ in patients with rheumatoid arthritis. |
| **COLONY-STIMULATING FACTORS** | | |
| Macrophage colony-stimulating factor (M-CSF), granulocyte colony-stimulating factor (G-CSF), granulocyte-macrophage colony-stimulating factor (GM-CSF) | Stimulates growth of mononuclear phagocytes (M-CSF) and granulocytes (G-CSF) and enhances their function. | M-CSF, together with transforming growth factor-$\beta$, is important for the growth and differentiation of the peri-implantation embryo. GM-CSF increases serum levels of cortisol and growth hormone in cancer patients. |
| **"HORMONE-LIKE" SUBSTANCES** | | |
| Macrophage migration inhibitory factor (MIF) | Released from macrophages and T lymphocytes that have been stimulated by glucocorticoids; inhibits random migration of macrophages. | Glucocorticoid counterregulator; overcomes the inhibitory effects of glucocorticoids on cytokine production. |
| 1,25-Dihydroxyvitamin $D_3$ | Behaves as a paracrine factor in the immune system; produced by monocytes and macrophages; has potent actions on immune cells; pathophysiologic roles in sarcoidosis and autoimmune diseases such as type 1 diabetes. | Important mediator in bone metabolism and calcium homeostasis. |
| Calcitonin precursors (CTpr) | Reliable sepsis marker; novel mediator and potential therapeutic target in sepsis; increases cytokine production in peripheral blood mononuclear cells. Stimulated macrophages are, at least in part, responsible for the CTpr production in parenchymatous tissues such as liver, lung, kidney, spleen, and others. | Mature calcitonin, which is not elevated in sepsis, plays a role in calcium homeostasis and bone metabolism. Endocrine functions of calcitonin precursors not yet known. |
| Adrenomedullin (ADM) | Inhibits secretion of cytokine-induced neutrophil chemoattractant, a member of the IL-8 family, from activated rat alveolar macrophages in vitro. Endometrial macrophages of women receiving tamoxifen strongly express ADM, and the angiogenesis capabilities of ADM might play a role in tamoxifen-induced endometrial hyperplasia. | Discovered in extracts of human pheochromocytoma but also produced in many other tissues. Very potent vasodilator and has potential role in septic shock. Elevated in patients with primary hypertension, and in patients with Graves disease. |

*Most of these substances are produced by a variety of cell types and have many additional effects not mentioned in this table. The complexity of the system is necessarily oversimplified for didactic purposes.

## NEUTROPHILS

Polymorphonuclear neutrophils (PMNs) are phagocytic cells for which the primary function is the ingestion and destruction of invading microorganisms. Biochemically, they are highly active cells. The primary granules contain digestive and hydrolytic enzymes that are used in the phagosomes. The secondary and tertiary granules, which are released by exocytosis in response to external stimuli, are crucial to mobilizing mediators of inflammation.

Neutrophils are subject to the effects of G-CSF and GM-CSF during their maturation and secrete certain interleukins (e.g., IL-1, IL-3, IL-6, IL-8, IL-10).[1,3,36] TNF-α and its receptors are also produced by neutrophils. Soluble TNF-receptor production increases whereas a concomitant decrease occurs in the cell-surface receptor.[37] Thus, neutrophils can decrease the inflammatory response by altering the cellular effect of TNF-α via modulation of levels of both cell-surface and soluble TNF receptors. Lactoferrin released from these granules can inhibit the release of GM-CSF activity from macrophages, thereby attenuating granulopoiesis.

Proenkephalin has been demonstrated in neutrophils, as well as in lymphocytes and neuronal cells. Prolactin receptors are present on neutrophils, although no evidence exists of prolactin production per se by these cells.

Less is known about neutrophils than about monocytes, macrophages, and lymphocytes because of the difficulty of isolating them without activating them and thereby causing changes in the granule content and composition. Isolating mRNA from these enzyme-rich cells is difficult, further hindering molecular studies. Neutrophils are likely to have as rich an array of hormone receptors as do the mononuclear cells and to be influenced by the neuro–immuno–endocrine axis.

## EOSINOPHILS

Eosinophils are relatively uncommon polymorphonuclear leukocytes. They are notable for their strikingly large eosinophilic granules. The number of these cells is low in the nonallergic adult, usually $<0.45 \times 10^9$/L. A marked diurnal variation is found in eosinophil numbers, with the highest numbers seen in the morning. Acute infections, glucocorticoids, ACTH, prostaglandins, and epinephrine decrease eosinophil numbers. Eosinophils develop in the bone marrow under the influence of colony-stimulating factors such as GM-CSF and of certain interleukins (i.e., IL-1, IL-5, and IL-6). Glucocorticoids and ACTH reduce the numbers of circulating eosinophils.

The eosinopenia that is noted within hours of glucocorticoid exposure may result from the sequestration of eosinophils in the reticuloendothelial and vascular systems. This eosinopenia is unlikely to result from a direct toxicity of glucocorticoids, because exposure to corticosteroids in vitro does not result in lysis. Chronic exposure to glucocorticoids decreases the marrow production and release of eosinophils. This may occur indirectly by the stabilization of basophil and mast cell membranes with a resultant decrease in histamine levels. Histamine, which is a chemotactic agent for eosinophils, may stimulate the production and release of eosinophils from the bone marrow.[1,3]

Cytokines (e.g., NGF,[38] TNF-α, TGF-β, and MIP) have been found in eosinophils. The role of these cytokines in eosinophil function remains to be elucidated.

## BASOPHILS AND MAST CELLS

Basophils are the rarest of circulating leukocytes, comprising ~0.5% of circulating white blood cells. The function of basophils is poorly understood, as are alterations in their numbers. Mast cells reside in the connective tissue, especially beneath epithelial surfaces and near blood vessels. They are long-lived cells and are not found in the peripheral blood (see Chap. 181).[1,3]

Basophils and mast cells, which are rich in granules that contain proteoglycans, are the body's major source of histamine. In addition to histamine, other substances that can influence the course of inflammatory reactions are also present in these cells. These include proteases, proteoglycans, leukotrienes, and platelet-activating factor. These cells can also secrete IL-1, IL-3, IL-4, IL-5, IL-6, and IL-10, as well as other cytokines such as MIP, TNF, and LIF. The central location of mast cells near blood vessels and beneath the epithelial surface, as well as their intimate association with nerve endings, imply a pivotal role for the mast cell in the neuro–immuno–endocrine system.

## PLATELETS

Platelets are generated from multinucleated megakaryocytes and are critical for hemostasis. These granule-rich anuclear cells circulate in the bloodstream, are highly active metabolically, and accumulate at sites of vessel damage, where they form a platelet clot. The platelets are rich in platelet-specific proteins (e.g., platelet factor-4 and thromboglobulin), coagulation factors, and growth factors (e.g., platelet-derived growth factor [PDGF], TGF-β, connective tissue–activating peptide [CTAP], epidermal growth factor [EGF], RANTES, and IL-1). Platelets also contain amino acids and nucleotides that are important in platelet activation.[1,3]

PDGF exerts a growth-stimulating effect by binding to its cognate receptor on target cells. The PDGF receptor is also present on platelets, where its stimulation causes an inhibition of platelet activation. TGF-β is released when a clot is formed; it exerts pleiotropic effects (including stimulation of bone growth) in the early stages. This may be physiologically relevant in wound healing and general bone development. CTAP stimulates a number of metabolic activities (e.g., DNA and glycosoaminoglycan synthesis) in connective tissue cells.

Platelet membranes contain receptors for platelet-activating and inactivating agonists. Vasopressin binds to a $V_1$ receptor, controlling platelet activation and inhibition of adenylate cyclase. Serotonin also binds to a specific receptor that is associated with platelet activation. Platelets are sensitive to the effects of prostanoids via specific receptors, which either activate platelets or inhibit platelet responses through adenylate cyclase.[1,3]

## ERYTHROCYTES

Erythrocytes are abundant, long-lived circulating cells that shed their nuclei before entering the circulation. The red cell interior contains the metabolic machinery needed to maintain hemoglobin function. Identifiable erythroid precursors in the marrow express the erythropoietin receptor, which facilitates the orderly maturation of the cell that occurs under the influence of erythropoietin. Earlier erythrocyte stages probably are susceptible to growth factors such as stem cell factor and IL-3. The mature erythrocytes, however, do not express cytokines or hormones, nor do they respond to them. Nevertheless, these erythroid cells are not hormonally inert: they play a major role in removing nitric oxide from the circulation, thereby influencing vascular tone. Nitric oxide is a potent endogenous vascular-relaxing agent produced by the vascular endothelium and macrophages (see Chap. 179). The erythrocytes rapidly inactivate circulating nitric oxide. These cells are present in large numbers and, via the vascular system, are distributed widely in the body, thus occupying a central role in the tight regulation of nitric oxide activity. Evidence is emerging that hemoglobin may also deliver nitric oxide to areas of hypoxia. Both oxygen and nitric oxide can be subsequently unloaded in areas of low oxygen tension.[39–41] The ensuing vasodilation ensures that blood flow increases to an involved area, with a consequent improvement in the local metabolic state. The ability to bind and inactivate nitric oxide also limits

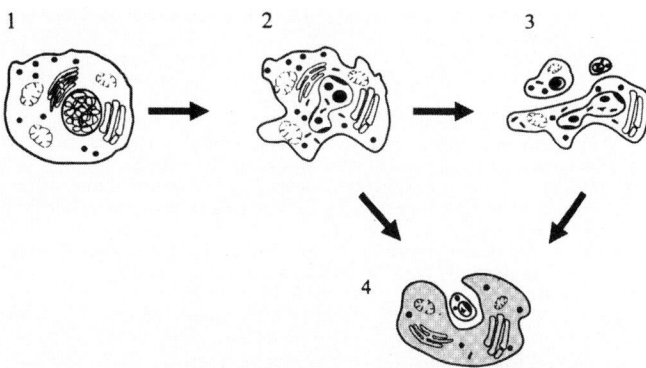

**FIGURE 180-1.** The morphologic changes associated with apoptosis. **1,** Normal cell. **2,** Initial apoptotic changes, including blebbing of the plasma membrane, chromatin condensation, and DNA fragmentation. **3,** Chromatic dense apoptotic bodies. **4,** Engulfment of apoptotic structures by phagocytes. (Adapted from Trudeau JD, Dutz JP, Arany E, et al. Neonatal β-cell apoptosis: a trigger for autoimmune diabetes? Diabetes 2000; 49:1.)

**TABLE 180-3.**
**Some of the Signaling Factors Involved in Apoptosis**

| Antiapoptosis | Proapoptosis |
|---|---|
| Protein kinase C | TNFR-1 |
| Protein kinase B/AKT | CD95/Fas antigen |
| NF-κB | Oxidative stress |
| Bcl* | Calcium |
| Bcl-x$_L$* | Low cellular pH |
| Bcl-w* | cAMP |
| Mcl-1* | Ceramide |
| A1* | MAP kinases |
| BHRF-1* | Bax* |
| IGF-I | Bak* |
| | Bad* |
| | Bok* |
| | Bik* |
| | Bid* |
| | Nitric oxide |
| | Glucocorticoids |

*Members of the *bcl*-2 family.
*TNFR-I,* tumor necrosis factor receptor-1; *NF-κB,* nuclear factor-kappa B; *IGF-I,* insulin-like growth factor-I.

the use of hemoglobin-based blood substitutes, because the binding of nitric oxide by these substitutes leads to increased vascular tone and hypertension.

# NEURO–IMMUNO–ENDOCRINE INTERACTIONS

Evidence is increasing of links among the cells of the nervous, immune, and endocrine systems (see Table 180-2). The earlier conventional distinctions between "classic" hormones (e.g., those produced by the pituitary, thyroid, parathyroids, pancreas, and adrenals) and cytokines, CSFs, prostanoids, and various active endogenous chemicals such as nitric oxide are no longer valid. These agents are capable of autocrine and paracrine effects and sometimes effects that are far removed from the site of production. In addition, an intimate connection is seen to the nervous system by influences on the hypothalamus and the pituitary and also by the close proximity of nerve endings to many hematopoietic cells and blood cells. That the production of the "classic" hormones is not the exclusive province of the "classic" endocrine glands is also increasingly clear. As discussed, the nervous, immune, and endocrine systems share many ligands and receptors, resulting in constant and important bidirectional communication. For example, immunostimulatory hormones include estrogens, prolactin, dehydroepiandrosterone sulfate (DHEAS), GH, and insulin-like growth factor-I (IGF-I), whereas immunoinhibitory hormones include glucocorticoids, ACTH, and testosterone. The immune system is subject to nervous system and endocrine regulation. Conversely, substances produced by the immune and nervous systems may cause responses in the endocrine system.

# APOPTOSIS

The process of *apoptosis* (regulated cell death) plays a vital role in a multitude of cellular responses that are particularly prominent during blood cell development, neoplasia, embryogenesis, thymic development, and neoplasia. Apoptotic cell death is an active, energy-requiring process that follows a stereotypical pattern regardless of the initiating mechanism (Fig. 180-1). The cytoplasm shrinks, the plasma membrane forms blebs and vesicles, and phosphatidylserine redistributes to the cell surface. A

characteristic process of chromatin condensation occurs, with DNA fragmentation into high-molecular-weight and oligonucleosomal pieces.[42] This is in contrast to *cell necrosis,* in which the cell swells and bursts with the consequent release of cellular material. *Caspase proteinases* play a central role in the initiation and propagation of the apoptotic signal, activating other components of the apoptotic machinery.[42] Table 180-3 lists some common *proapoptotic and antiapoptotic* signals.

In certain estrogen-sensitive tissues, the hormone that appears to potentiate cell growth may not necessarily be a mitogen but may act only to *prevent* cell death, thereby resulting in an increased number of cells—the same effect that would have occurred had the hormone been a mitogen.[43] A classic example is the role of erythropoietin in erythrocyte development. The withdrawal of erythropoietin from erythroid progenitors results in orchestrated cellular changes that ultimately result in DNA fragmentation and cell death through apoptosis.[44] The presence of erythropoietin greatly reduces apoptosis, which, in erythroid cells, is mediated by *Bcl-2* and *Bcl-x$_L$*.[45] This role as a survival factor has also been demonstrated for other cytokines (e.g., GM-CSF, G-CSF and IL-3); when these cytokines are withdrawn from a cytokine-dependent cell line, apoptosis results. The effect of IL-3 withdrawal can be ameliorated by overexpression of *Bcl-2* in these cells.

Apoptosis is critically important in many types of neoplasia. Normal B cells of the lymphoid follicle respond to T cell–dependent antigens by generating high-affinity antibody. Cells that do not receive a sufficient signal are deleted by apoptosis. In contrast, follicular B-cell lymphoma cells express high levels of *Bcl-2,* resulting in increased cellular longevity and an increase in tumor cell burden. Apoptosis can be triggered in these and other tumor types by various stimuli, including chemotherapeutic agents, monoclonal antibodies, and such physical techniques as exposure to ionizing radiation. Glucocorticoids may kill certain tumor types by triggering apoptosis in sensitive cells in multiple myeloma and acute lymphoblastic leukemia.

Apoptosis also plays a critical role in CD4+ and CD8+ depletion in HIV infection.[46] The binding of HIV-1 recombinant envelope glycoprotein activates caspases and increases the rates of apoptosis seen in primary CD4+ T cells.[47] The administration of highly active antiretroviral therapy (HAART) results in a decrease in the viral copy number and apoptotic rate along with a concomitant rise in CD4+ T cells. This effect can be augmented by the administration of low doses of IL-2.[48]

## CONCLUSION

A broader definition of what constitutes a hormone is clearly desirable. The present heuristic barriers discourage cross-fertilization between the fields of hematology and endocrinology to the detriment of both. Once a broader definition of hormones is accepted, the question arises as to why blood cells need to produce hormones and to express their complementary receptors. Two hypotheses, which are not mutually exclusive, can be proposed to answer this question. First, recognition of the effects of the central nervous system on both endocrine gland function and immune function is increasing. Conceivably, the bidirectional communication that occurs between the endocrine, nervous, and hematopoietic systems may be mediated by the expression of hormones and hormone receptors in these cell types. Second, the expression of peptide hormones by lymphocytes, macrophages, and dendritic cells is somewhat more easily explained by the concept of induction of immune tolerance. Low-level expression of these hormones in cells that traffic to the thymus results in the apoptosis of self-reactive clones.

## REFERENCES

1. Lee GR, Foerster J, Lukens J, Wintrobe MM. Wintrobe's clinical hematology, 10th ed. Baltimore: Williams & Wilkins, 1999.
2. Cavaillon JM. Cytokines and macrophages. Biomed Pharmacother 1994; 48:445.
3. Williams WJ, Beutler E, Erslev AJ, Lichtman, MA. Hematology, 5th ed. New York: McGraw-Hill, 1994.
4. Akira S, Kishimoto T. Role of interleukin-6 in macrophage function. Curr Opin Hematol 1996; 3:87.
5. Reid CD. The biology and clinical applications of dendritic cells. Transfus Med 1998; 8:77.
6. Lindhout E, Figdor CG, Adema GJ. Dendritic cells: migratory cells that are attractive. Cell Adhes Commun 1998; 6:117.
7. Robinson SP, Saraya K, Reid CD. Developmental aspects of dendritic cells in vitro and in vivo. Leuk Lymphoma 1998; 29:477.
8. Heufler C, Topar G, Koch F, et al. Cytokine gene expression in murine epidermal cell suspensions: interleukin 1β and macrophage inflammatory protein 1α are selectively expressed in Langerhans cells but differentially regulated in culture. J Exp Med 1992; 176:1221.
9. Heufler C, Koch F, Stanzl U, et al. Interleukin-12 is produced by dendritic cells and mediates T helper I development as well as interferon-gamma production by T helper I cells. Eur J Immunol 1996; 26:659.
10. Cumberbatch M, Dearman RJ, Kimber I. Constitutive and inducible expression of interleukin-6 by Langerhans cells and lymph node dendritic cells. Immunology 1996; 87:513.
11. Thurnher M, Ramoner R, Gastl G, et al. Bacillus Calmette-Guerin mycobacteria stimulate human dendritic cells. Int J Cancer 1997; 70:128.
12. Cella M, Scheidegger D, Palmer-Lehmann K, et al. Ligation of CD40 on dendritic cells triggers production of high levels of interleukin-12 and enhances T-cell stimulatory capacity: T-T help via APC activation. J Exp Med 1996; 184:747.
13. de Saint-Vis B, Fugier-Vivier I, Massacrier C, et al. The cytokine profile expressed by human dendritic cells is dependent on cell subtype and mode of activation. J Immunol 1998; 160:1666.
14. Bonham CA, Lu L, Hoffman RA, et al. Generation of nitric oxide by mouse dendritic cells and its implications for immune response regulation. Adv Exp Med Biol 1997; 417:283.
15. Lu L, Bonham CA, Chambers FG, et al. Induction of nitric oxide synthase in mouse dendritic cells by IFN-gamma, endotoxin, and interaction with allogeneic T cells: nitric oxide production is associated with dendritic cell apoptosis. J Immunol 1996; 157:3577.
16. Nathan CF. Secretory products of macrophages. J Clin Invest 1987; 79:319.
17. Throsby M, Pleau J, Dardenne M, Homo-Delarche F. Thymic expression of the pancreatic endocrine hormones. Neuroimmunomodulation 1999; 6:108.
18. Sospedra M, Ferrer-Francesch X, Dominguez O, et al. Transcription of a broad range of self-antigens in human thymus suggests a role for central mechanisms in tolerance toward peripheral antigens. J Immunol 1998; 161:5918.
19. Delgado M, Pozo D, Martinez C, et al. Characterization of gene expression of VIP and VIP1-receptor in rat peritoneal lymphocytes and macrophages. Regul Pept 1996; 62:161.
20. Defacque H, Piquemal D, Baset A, et al. Transforming growth factor-beta 1 is an autocrine mediator of U937 cell growth arrest and differentiation induced by vitamin D3 and retinoids. J Cell Physiol 1999; 178:109.
21. Komorowski J, Stepien H, Pawlikowski M. The evidence of thyroliberin/triiodothyronine control of TSH secretory response from human peripheral blood monocytes cultured in vitro. Neuropeptides 1993; 25:31.
22. Mustafa A, Nyberg F, Mustafa M, et al. Growth hormone stimulates production of interferon-gamma by human peripheral mononuclear cells. Horm Res 1997; 48:11.
23. Towle MF, Mondragon-Escorpizo M, Norin A, Fukada K. Deprivation of leukemia inhibitory factor by its function-blocking antibodies augments T cell activation. J Interferon Cytokine Res 1998; 18:387.
24. Shahani SK, Gupta SM, Meherji PK. Lymphocytes—their possible endocrine role in the regulation of fertility. Am J Reprod Immunol 1996; 35:1.
25. Matera L. Endocrine, paracrine and autocrine actions of prolactin on immune cells. Life Sci 1996; 59:599.
26. Matera L. Action of lymphocyte and pituitary prolactin. Neuroimmunomodulation 1997; 4:171.
27. de Mello-Coelho V, Gagnerault MC, Souberbielle JC, et al. Growth hormone and its receptor are expressed in human thymic cells. Endocrinology 1998; 139:3837.
28. Hattori N, Ikekubo K, Ishihara T, et al. Spontaneous growth hormone (GH) secretion by unstimulated lymphocytes and the effects of GH-releasing hormone and somatostatin. J Clin Endocrinol Metab 1994; 79:1678.
28a. Beuschlein F, Strasburger CJ, Siegerstetter V, et al. Acromegaly caused by secretion of growth hormone by a non-Hodgkin's lymphoma. N Engl J Med 2000; 342:1871.
29. Lyons PD, Blalock JE. Pro-opiomelanocortin gene expression and protein processing in rat mononuclear leukocytes. J Neuroimmunol 1997; 78:47.
30. Joshi JB, Dave HPG. Activation of enkephalin gene promoter in lymphocytes. Unpublished data, 2000.
31. Hashemi FB, Hughes TK, Smith EM. Human immunodeficiency virus induction of corticotropin in lymphoid cells. J Clin Endocrinol Metab 1998; 83:4373.
32. Joshi JB, Dave HPG. Transactivation of the proenkephalin gene promoter by the Tax1 protein of human T-cell lymphotropic virus type I. Proc Natl Acad Sci U S A 1992; 89:1006.
33. Bucala R. Neuroimmunomodulation by macrophage migration inhibitory factor (MIF). Ann N Y Acad Sci 1998; 840:74.
34. Jessop DS, Chowdrey HS, Lightman SL, Larsen PJ. Vasopressin is located within lymphocytes in the rat spleen. J Neuroimmunol 1995; 56:219.
35. Xing L, Guo J, Tang J, et al. Morphological evidence for the location of calcitonin gene-related peptide (CGRP) immunoreactivity in rat lymphocytes. Cell Vis 1998; 5:8.
36. Shimonkevitz R, Bar-Or D, Harris L, et al. Granulocytes, including neutrophils, synthesize IL-10 after traumatic pancreatitis. J Trauma 2000; 48:165.
37. Jalonska E, Jablonski J, Holownia A. Role of neutrophils in release of some cytokines and their soluble receptors. Immunol Lett 1999; 70:191.
38. Aloe L, Bracci-Laudiero L, Bonini S, Manni L. The expanding role of nerve growth factor: from neurotropic activity to immunologic diseases. Allergy 1997; 52:883.
39. Jia L, Bonaventura C, Bonaventura J, Stamler JS. S-nitrosohemoglobin: a dynamic activity of blood involved in vascular control. Nature 1996; 380:221.
40. Stamler JS, Jia L, Eu JP, et al. Blood flow regulation by S-nitrosohemoglobin in the physiologic oxygen gradient. Science 1997; 276:2034.
41. Gow AJ, Stamler JS. Reactions between nitric oxide and hemoglobin under physiological conditions. Nature 1998; 391:169.
42. Wolf BB, Green DR. Suicidal tendencies: apoptotic cell death by caspase family proteinases. J Biol Chem 1999; 274:20049.
43. Soto A, Sonnenschein C. Cell proliferation of estrogen-sensitive cells: the case for negative control. Endocr Rev 1987; 8:44.
44. Koury MJ, Bondurant MC. Erythropoietin retards DNA breakdown and prevents programmed cell death in erythroid progenitor cells. Science 1990; 248:378.
45. Silva M, Grillot D, Benito A, et al. Erythropoietin can promote erythroid progenitor survival by repressing apoptosis through Bcl-XL and Bcl. Blood 1996; 88:1576.
46. Gougeon ML, Montagnier L. Programmed cell death as a mechanism of CD4 and CD8 T cell depletion in AIDS. Molecular control and effect of highly active anti-retroviral therapy. Ann N Y Acad Sci 1999; 887:199.
47. Cicala C, Arthos J, Rubbert A, et al. HIV-1 envelope induces activation of caspase-3 and cleavage of focal adhesion kinase in primary CD4(+) T cells. Proc Natl Acad Sci U S A 1997; 97:1178.
48. Pandolfi F, Pierdominici M, Marziali M, et al. Low dose IL-2 reduces lymphocyte apoptosis and increases naive CD4 cells in HIV-1 patients treated with HAART. Clin Immunol 2000; 94:153.

# CHAPTER 181

# THE ENDOCRINE MAST CELL

STEPHEN I. WASSERMAN

The mast cell—by virtue of its distribution throughout the body, its content of potent biologic mediators, and its ability to release these mediators as well as to generate, on appropriate stimulation, new, unstored, mediators and cytokines, each with a variety of effects—functions as a hemocrine, paracrine, and autocrine cell. This chapter focuses on the development of mast cells, the mediators that mast cells contain or generate, the mechanisms by which mast cells are activated, and the relevance of these cells and their mediators to clinical medicine.

## GROWTH, DIFFERENTIATION, AND LOCALIZATION OF MAST CELLS

Mast cells (Fig. 181-1) are found in virtually all parts of the body, but they are especially prominent in perivascular locations of loose connective tissue and at sites of the host–environment interface, such as the upper and lower respiratory tract (epithelium, lamina propria, and free within the bronchial lumen), the gastrointestinal tract (epithelium, lamina propria), and skin (superficial and deeper dermis). The number of mast cells in the lungs, skin, and gut is ~20,000/mm$^3$, and this number is increased in areas of inflammatory and immune reactions.[1] Mast cells normally do not circulate in peripheral blood. Two classes of mast cells are found: the *connective tissue* type and the *mucosal* type. Both types of mast cells develop from CD34$^+$ precursors found initially in the bone marrow.[2] Their maturation is dependent on the action of stem cell factor (SCF) on the c-*kit* receptor, a tyrosine kinase, on the mast cell surface.[3] Interestingly, SCF exists in a soluble

form that acts on mast cells at a distance, and also in a form bound to fibroblast, endothelial, and stromal cell membranes—where it presumably acts on mast cells in a cognate fashion to stimulate their growth and development. In the mouse, the first committed mast cell precursor that can be identified is marked by Thy-1$^{lo}$ c-*kit*$^{hi}$.[4]

The connective tissue mast cell is distinguished by its content of heparin, its prominent intracellular granules, its unique array of generated mediators, its intense metachromasia, and its content of both tryptic and chymotryptic proteases.[2,5] The mucosal mast cells most prominent in the gastrointestinal tract of the rodent are distinguished from the connective tissue form by their content of oversulfated chondroitin sulfates, their less intense metachromasia, and their unique array of generated mediators. In the human, this population of mast cells appears to predominate over the connective tissue type, and it lacks the chymotryptic protease (chymase).

The implications of these differing morphologies are uncertain and remain speculative.

## MAST CELL PHYSIOLOGY

### ACTIVATION OF MAST CELLS

The activation of mast cells for the purposes of generating unstored mediators and releasing their granular constituents occurs in a noncytolytic process. Various stimuli can activate mast cells. Most prominent among these are the immunoglobulin E (IgE)–mediated signals. Mast cells possess 50,000 to 250,000 high-affinity membrane receptors for the crystallizable fragment portion of IgE. This receptor is comprised of three components, an α chain that binds the Fc portion of IgE, a β chain that augments signaling, and two γ chains that signal the mast cell interior.[6] Interestingly, the number of IgE receptors is increased in the presence of IgE,[7] whereas the FcγRII receptor negatively regulates IgE-mediated signaling via the FcεRI receptor.[8] Cross linking of adjacent, cell-bound IgE molecules by specific antigen conveys to the cell a signal that leads to the generation of new mediators, the extrusion of granular constituents, and the synthesis and later release of several cytokines. The following phenomena are associated temporally with cell activation: increases in Ca$^{2+}$ influx and efflux and in total intracellular free Ca$^{2+}$, tyrosine phosphorylation, generation of diacylglycerol and inositol phosphates, increases in cyclic adenosine monophosphate (cAMP), and utilization of protein kinases,[9,10] such as lyn and syk. Along with IgE-mediated signals, several other signals can activate mast cells: fragments of complement (C3a, C5a), highly charged molecules (eosinophil major basic protein), ionophores, enzymes (chymotrypsin, phospholipase), and opiates and neuropeptides, including substance P. In addition, SCF can both directly activate and prime mast cells for enhanced response to IgE-mediated signals.[11] Although it does not directly activate mast cells, the nucleoside adenosine markedly potentiates the release of mast cell granule contents induced by other stimuli.[12]

### PRODUCTS OF MAST CELLS

The products that are generated and released by mast cells comprise a disparate group of amines, peptides, lipids, proteins, proteoglycans, and nucleosides that collectively are termed *mediators*.[13] These molecules possess a wide range of bioeffects that can be categorized as *vasoactive-spasmogenic, chemotactic,* and *enzymatic* (Table 181-1). A family of cytokines also is synthesized and released by mast cells.

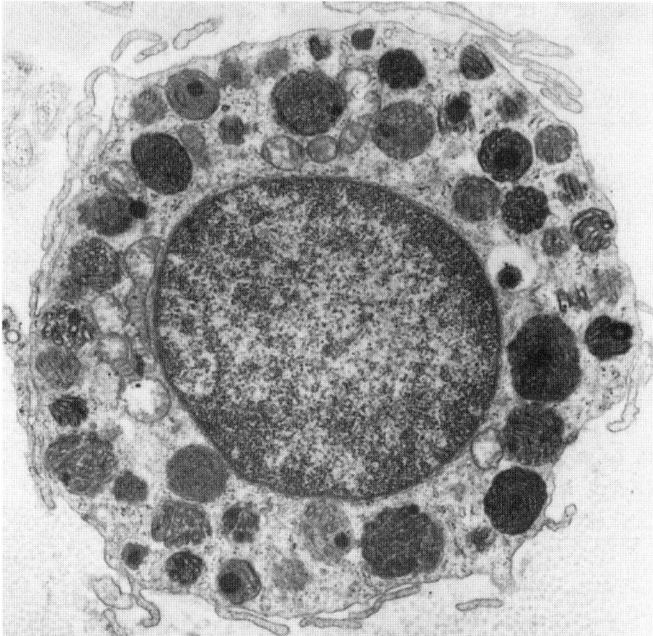

**FIGURE 181-1.** Electron micrograph of a human mast cell. Note the mononuclear nucleus and numerous cytoplasmic granules. (Courtesy of Dr. H. Powell, Department of Pathology, University of California, San Diego.)

**TABLE 181-1.**
**Mast Cell–Dependent Hormonal Mediators**

**VASOACTIVE**
  Histamine
  PAF
  $PGD_2$
  Leukotrienes ($C_4$, $D_4$, and $E_4$)
  Adenosine
**CHEMOTACTIC**
  Selective
    High-molecular-weight neutrophil chemotactic factor
    ECF of anaphylaxis
    ECF peptides
  Nonselective
    PAF
    Histamine
    Monohydroxy and dihydroxy fatty acids
    $PGD_2$
**ENZYMATIC**
  Tryptase
  Chymase
  Lysosomal hydrolases
**CYTOKINE**
  Tumor necrosis factor α
  IL-3
  IL-4
  IL-5
  IL-6
  MIP-1α

*PAF,* platelet-activating factor; *PGD₂,* prostaglandin D₂; *ECF,* eosinophil chemotactic factor; *IL-3,* interleukin-3; *IL-4,* interleukin-4; *IL-5,* interleukin-5; *IL-6,* interleukin-6; *MIP-1α,* macrophage inflammatory peptide-1α.

## VASOACTIVE-SPASMOGENIC MEDIATORS

**Histamine.** Histamine is the only preformed vasoactive-spasmogenic mediator in the human mast cell.[13] It is generated by decarboxylation of the amino acid histidine (Fig. 181-2) and is stored (in amounts of 1 to 5 μg/10⁶ cells) in the granules bound to the proteoglycan-protein core. When the granule core is exposed to extracellular fluid, histamine is eluted by exchange with $Na^+$. Released histamine is inactivated rapidly by oxidative deamination or by methylation via the enzymes diamine oxidase and histamine methyltransferase, respectively. Histamine circulates in plasma at concentrations of ~300 pg/mL, with peak levels occurring in the early morning hours. Nearly 10 μg is excreted in the urine daily. Increased levels of blood histamine are found in patients with various forms of urticaria, asthma, anaphylaxis, and mastocytosis. This amine exerts its effects by interacting with specific membrane receptors on target tissues termed $H_1$, $H_2$, and $H_3$ (Table 181-2).

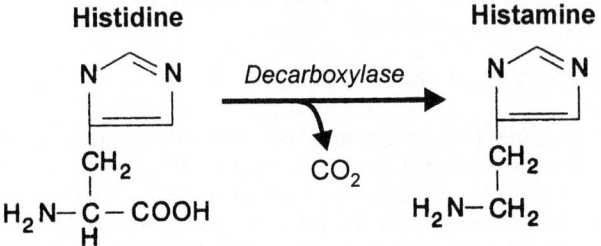

**FIGURE 181-2.** Histamine is formed by decarboxylation of the amino acid histidine.

**TABLE 181-2.**
**Actions of Histamine**

**$H_1$-MEDIATED**
  Bronchoconstriction
  Mucus secretion
  Prostaglandin generation
  Pulmonary vasoconstriction
  Suppression of cardiac atrioventricular node
  Increased cyclic guanosine monophosphate levels
**$H_2$-MEDIATED**
  Gastric acid secretion
  Mucus secretion
  Activation of suppressor lymphocytes
  Increased cyclic adenosine monophosphate levels
  Bronchodilation
  Induction of idioventricular responses
  Inhibition of basophilic mediator release
**$H_1$- AND $H_2$-MEDIATED**
  Pruritus
  Increased vascular permeability
  Ventricular fibrillation
**$H_3$-MEDIATED**
  Central nervous system histamine synthesis

The *$H_1$ receptor* mediates histamine-induced smooth muscle contraction, vasopermeability, wheal and flare responses, augmentation of mucus release, alterations in cardiac rhythm, and the secondary generation of prostaglandins by nonmast cells. These actions of histamine are prevented by the classic antihistaminic drugs. The *$H_2$ receptor*–mediated actions of histamine include lesser degrees of augmentation of vascular permeability, increased mucus secretion, stimulation of gastric acid secretion, increases in cellular cyclic adenosine monophosphate (cAMP) content, alterations in cardiac rhythm, and stimulation of suppressor lymphocyte function. These actions are inhibited by cimetidine and ranitidine. The full expression of pruritus, wheal and flare responses, and cardiac rhythmic changes requires both $H_1$- and $H_2$-receptor occupancy. An $H_3$ receptor capable of regulating histamine synthesis has been identified in the brain.

**Platelet-Activating Factor.** Whereas all of the other mast cell vasoactive-spasmogenic mediators are generated only after cell stimulation, the phospholipid mediator *platelet-activating factor* (PAF; 1-0-alkyl-2-0-acetyl, 3 phosphocholine) is generated by mast cells on IgE-dependent activation. Although it is called PAF, the actions of this lipid are largely independent of platelets.[14] The structural integrity of PAF is essential for its bioactivity; it is rapidly inactivated by an acid-labile plasma enzyme termed *acetylhydrolase*. PAF is an extraordinarily potent mediator, with effects at $10^{-10}$ or $10^{-11}$ mol/L. The actions of PAF include wheal and flare vasopermeability responses, bronchoconstriction, tachypnea, hypotension, cardiac depression, and aggregation and activation of platelets and neutrophils. It is also the most potent lipid eosinophil chemoattractant yet identified.

**Arachidonic Acid Metabolites.** Several metabolites of arachidonic acid are produced by activated mast cells. Human mast cells are capable of generating large quantities of the cyclooxygenase product *prostaglandin $D_2$* ($PGD_2$) and the lipoxygenase metabolite *leukotriene $C_4$* ($LTC_4$).[15,15a] Generation of $PGD_2$, like that of prostaglandins in general, is inhibited by nonsteroidal antiinflammatory agents. This compound is a potent bronchoconstrictor. It induces wheal and flare vasopermeability responses and, by increasing cAMP concentrations, inhibits platelet activation. It is preferentially produced by cutaneous mast cells. $LTC_4$ is a glutathione adduct of oxygenated arachidonic acid that can be metabolized further to the bioactive *leukotriene D₄* (LTD$_4$) and *leukotriene E₄* (LTE$_4$) by removal of the terminal glutamine and glycine residues, respectively. LTC$_4$, LTD$_4$, and LTE$_4$ comprise what was once termed *slow-reacting substance of anaphylaxis*. These sulfidopeptide leukotrienes are potent inducers of wheal and flare vasopermeability responses and, in addition, cause gastrointestinal and respiratory smooth muscle contraction, lower blood pressure, increase airway mucus secretion, depress cardiac function, and inhibit lymphocyte functions. LTC$_4$ is generated predominantly by lung and gut mast cells. Leukotriene degradation is accomplished by oxidation.

**Adenosine.** The nucleoside adenosine is generated from adenosine triphosphate during mast cell activation. Adenosine not only can augment mast cell mediator release by acting on specific membrane A$_2$ receptors to activate protein kinase C, but it also potently mediates vasopermeability and bronchospasm in asthmatic persons and can induce Cl⁻ flux across epithelial barriers in the gut and lungs. The receptor-mediated actions of adenosine are prevented by therapeutic concentrations of xanthines.[12]

### CHEMOTACTIC MEDIATORS

Several compounds capable of altering directed and random mobility of leukocytes are generated because of mast cell activation.[16] Some of these, including histamine, PGD$_2$, PAF, and hydroxylated derivatives of arachidonic acid, are not cell specific and act on various leukocyte populations. On the other hand, several mast cell products have restricted target cell specificity.

A unique neutral, isoelectric point protein, high-molecular-weight *neutrophil chemotactic factor* (HMW-NCF), has been identified in blood after mast cell activation in patients with antigen-induced bronchospasm or physical urticaria. Generation of HMW-NCF is prevented by pretreatment of patients with mast cell–inhibitory drugs, such as cromolyn. Moreover, at least three low-molecular-weight *eosinophil chemotactic materials*, differing in their charge and hydrophobicity, can be identified in blood after mast cell activation. Uncharacterized mast cell factors capable of attracting lymphocytes, mononuclear leukocytes, and basophils have also been reported.

### ENZYMES AND PROTEOGLYCANS

A wide variety of mediators with enzymatic activity have been identified in extracts of mast cells, and several are released from the mast cell granule by IgE-mediated processes.[16a] These mediators include β-hexosaminidase, β-glucuronidase, arylsulfatase B, superoxide dismutase, myeloperoxidase, and carboxypeptidase.

The most prominent human mast cell enzyme, however, is a tryptic neutral protease termed *tryptase*.[17] This tetramer, with a molecular mass of 134 kDa, constitutes half of the protein of the mast cell granule and is found in all human mast cells. It is capable of cleaving kininogen to generate bradykinin; it can also generate C3a from the complement component C3, in addition to hydrolyzing fibrinogen; and it degrades a variety of bronchodilator peptides but is inactive against the bronchoconstrictor substance P.[18] It most likely is responsible for other proteolytic events that depend on mast cells, such as activation of Hageman factor and prekallikrein. Tryptase also sensitizes bronchial smooth muscle to contractile stimuli.[19] Tryptase actions, and its stability, are promoted by its binding to heparin, and it is not known to be inhibited by plasma antiproteases. A second neutral protease, *chymase*, is present in a subset of human mast cells that are most prominent in the skin and deeper connective tissue. This enzyme can cleave angiotensinogen, type IV collagen, and substance P, and can stimulate mucous glands.[20]

Proteoglycans form the structural backbone of mast cell granules, provide them with their characteristic metachromatic staining properties, and serve as binding sites for histamine and various peptides and proteins. In the rodent, the proteoglycan of connective tissue mast cells is *heparin*, whereas oversulfated chondroitin sulfates are found in mucosal mast cells. Heparin is present in all human mast cells,[21] and small amounts of chondroitin sulfate E are present in the human mucosal form. The heparin proteoglycan not only binds to tryptase and alters its function but is also an anticoagulant and a potent factor in angiogenesis and bone remodeling. It can also inhibit complement activation.

### CYTOKINES

Mast cells have been shown to be prominent sources of the inflammatory cytokines tumor necrosis factor α (TNF-α)[22] and interleukin-4 (IL-4), interleukin-5 (IL-5), and interleukin-6 (IL-6).[23,24] TNF-α increases bronchial reactivity,[25] is a chemoattractant for mononuclear leukocytes and neutrophils, and is vasoactive. It is an important factor in up-regulating the leukocyte adhesion molecules VCAM-1 and ICAM-1.[26] Mast cell–derived TNF-α has also been implicated in a host defense role of the innate immune system in an animal model in which mast cell deficiency is associated with failure to resist bacterial infection.[27]

IL-4 is a centrally important proallergic, proinflammatory cytokine that is synthesized and released by mast cells. It induces and enhances IgE production,[28] stimulates VCAM-1 expression[29] (essential to eosinophil, basophil, and T-lymphocyte recruitment to inflammatory sites via adhesion to VLA$_4$), and favors the production of T$_H$2 memory T lymphocytes,[30] which are also known to be major sources of IL-4 and IL-5.

IL-5 is the major eosinophilopoietic factor that drives eosinophil growth, differentiation, and activation[31,32] and inhibits their apoptosis. IL-5 primes eosinophils to release LTC$_4$ and to degranulate, enhances their adherence to endothelia, and fosters their chemotactic responses.

IL-6 enhances IgE synthesis (driven by IL-4) and is a major acute-phase reactant.

Taken together, these cytokines are capable of engendering a unique, allergic-type of inflammation that is dominated by eosinophils, basophils, and T lymphocytes.

### MEDIATOR ACTIONS

The best idea as to how mast cell products work in vivo has been derived from studies of human skin and airways. In skin,[33] the IgE antigen–mediated activation of mast cells causes rapid onset (within 1 to 5 minutes) of a relatively short-lived (30- to 60-minute) pruritic wheal and flare response that, histologically, is represented by mast cell degranulation, tissue edema, and endothelial cell activation (*early phase*). Frequently, this early reaction is followed, after 4 to 6 hours, by a second, more prolonged, cutaneous response manifested by painful erythematous induration (*late phase*). Histologic assessment of the late-phase response demonstrates perivascular leukocytic infiltration, hemorrhage, and fibrin deposition, which often is of sufficient severity to warrant the diagnosis of vasculitis. In the lung, IgE antigen–mediated early- and late-phase bronchospastic responses also occur. Direct bronchoscopic visualization of the airway, complemented by bronchoalveolar lavage, has shown the early phase to be associated with edema, erythema, and mucus release, whereas the later response has been shown to be characterized first by neutrophilic and then by eosinophilic influx.

Although the precise mediators responsible for these early and late phases are uncertain, vasoactive-spasmogenic mediators probably account for much of the early response, whereas enzymes, chemotactic mediators, and cytokines may mediate the late phase. The late phase is particularly important because its occurrence is associated with the development of heightened nonspecific airway reactivity, the sine qua non of asthma.

# MAST CELLS AND DISEASE

The pathophysiologic role of mast cells has been defined on the basis of the known triggers of the cell, the actions of its mediators, and the effect of pharmacologic inhibitors of mast cell activation or of mediator action. Moreover, the clinical findings observed in the spectrum of disorders known collectively as *mastocytosis*, and characterized by an increased number of mast cells, also have been applied to the understanding of mast cell function.

## MASTOCYTOSIS

Mastocytosis, the abnormal accumulation of mast cells, may occur primarily in the skin (*urticaria pigmentosa*) or it may be *systemic*, involving the liver, spleen, bone marrow, gastrointestinal tract, or bone.[34] *Malignant mastocytosis* occurs rarely. In some patients, a point mutation in the catalytic domain of c-*kit* has been deemed causative of mast cell proliferation. The clinical features of mastocytosis reflect the body burden of mast cells and the specific tissues involved, and the diagnosis is based on the histologic confirmation of increased numbers of normal-appearing mast cells in tissue. Organomegaly and skin nodules reflect specific organ infiltration with mast cells. Proliferation in bone may be accompanied by local pain and is best identified by radionuclide bone scan. Malabsorption may be a consequence of extensive gut infiltration. Cutaneous signs and symptoms of systemic mastocytosis include dermatographism, pruritus, urtication, and flushing, all of which may be attributed to the action of histamine. Hypotensive episodes may occur through the action of $PGD_2$. Acute episodes, which may be triggered by alcoholic beverages or foods or may occur spontaneously, commonly mimic anaphylaxis because they are marked by hypotension, nausea, diarrhea, abdominal cramping, and flushing. Less common symptoms include rhinorrhea and intestinal bleeding (perhaps aggravated by mast cell heparin). Nonspecific symptoms, such as headache, palpitations, and tachycardia, are thought to reflect the marked elevation in blood histamine levels (2 to 20 times higher than normal) that occurs during attacks. Peripheral blood eosinophilia (reflecting mast cell chemotactic factors) and altered coagulation tests and blood lipids (both perhaps caused by heparin) also are seen. Peptic ulcers are common (owing to the $H_2$ action of histamine).

Treatment of mastocytosis has included use of combined $H_1$ and $H_2$ antagonists, nonsteroidal antiinflammatory drugs (to prevent $PGD_2$ generation), and oral cromolyn (to prevent mast cell activation). Decreased tissue histamine levels and clinical improvement have been reported in patients whose urticaria pigmentosa has been treated with topical corticosteroids.[35]

## ASTHMA

In asthma, mast cells are prominent in the airway, particularly in the periphery, and their numbers increase after immunization by the inhaled route. In patients dying of asthma, hypogranulation of mast cells is associated with mucus plugging, sloughing of epithelium, and tissue eosinophilia. In allergic asthma, chemotactic factors, cytokines, and histamine are found in blood and alveolar lavage fluids, indicating mast cell participation in this disorder.[36] In nonallergic asthma, the role of the mast cell is less certain; however, evidence linking mast cell–mediated inflammation to bronchial hyperactivity suggests such a role.[37] Furthermore, mast cell–dependent chemotactic mediators have been identified in blood in models of nonallergic asthma. The ability of mast cell mediators to induce bronchospasm, enhance mucus release, and mediate tissue eosinophilia further supports the role of mast cells in this disorder.[38]

## URTICARIA AND ANGIOEDEMA

A common feature in urticaria—whether caused by IgE-mediated processes, physical factors (i.e., heat or cold), immune complexes, or unknown causes—is the histologic evidence of degranulating mast cells. Experimentally induced and idiopathic urticaria and angioedema also are associated with the appearance of histamine in blood or local tissue fluid, or both, often accompanied by other mast cell–dependent mediators, such as chemotactic factors and PAF. Because histamine, PAF, $PGD_2$, adenosine, and leukotrienes all can induce pruritic wheal and flare responses, the relevance of mast cell activation to this clinical condition is clearly apparent. Current evidence suggests that a significant minority of patients with chronic urticaria express a circulating IgE antibody to the mast cell FcεRI receptor. Moreover, this antibody can induce a wheal and flare reaction in vivo and can cause histamine release from mast cells in vitro.[39] The beneficial effect but incomplete efficacy of antihistaminic drugs further supports the role of the mast cell and the participation of mediators other than histamine in the full expression of the disorder.

## ANAPHYLAXIS

Anaphylaxis is a syndrome involving acute onset of *cutaneous* (urticaria/angioedema), *respiratory* (laryngeal edema, asthma), *gastrointestinal* (nausea, vomiting, abdominal pain, diarrhea), and *cardiovascular* (hypotension, dysrhythmia, collapse, death) signs and symptoms that occur singly or in combination. Most commonly, anaphylaxis is attributable to IgE-dependent mechanisms, but immune complex–dependent, complement-mediated, and idiopathic forms also exist. Anaphylaxis usually is of abrupt onset, with manifestations often occurring within seconds of the host's encounter with an eliciting stimulus; rarely do initial signs and symptoms begin after an interval of 1 to 2 hours. Histamine and tryptase have been identified in biologic fluids of patients experiencing anaphylaxis. Although cogent arguments can be made for the participation of other vasoactive mediators in human anaphylaxis, their role in this syndrome has yet to be demonstrated. See also ref. 39a.

## ALLERGIC RHINITIS

Mast cells, basophils, and eosinophils are found in increased numbers in the superficial nasal epithelium and in nasal secretions of patients with allergic rhinitis. When persons with this disorder encounter antigen, increased nasal mucus and fluid secretion occurs, accompanied by nasal pruritus, nasal airway obstruction, and sneezing. In some patients, a late-phase nasal response also occurs, which is associated with infiltration of the nasal tissues with eosinophils and basophils. Analysis of secreted nasal fluid reveals, acutely, the presence of histamine, an enzyme with tryptic specificity, $LTC_4$, and $PGD_2$; in the late phase, all but $PGD_2$ are identified. The ability of oral antihistamines, topical cromolyn, and topical corticosteroids to alleviate allergic rhinitis lends further support to mast cell participation in this disease.[40] Antihistamines prevent the end-organ response to histamine, whereas cromolyn appears to prevent mast cell mediator release, and corticosteroids act to prevent accumulation of basophils and eosinophils.

## OTHER DISORDERS RELATED TO MAST CELLS

Other disorders in which increased numbers of mast cells have been identified include inflammatory bowel and bladder disease, parasitic infestation, lymphoreticular malignant disease, inflammatory arthritis, atherosclerosis, and osteoporosis.[41–44] Intestinal mast cell accumulation and mediator release are related temporally to worm expulsion and worm death in animals and rejection of ectoparasites.[45,46] In addition, heparin is important in vascular endothelial growth and bone remodeling; therefore, it is implicated in osteoporosis, in the bony remodeling seen in rheumatoid arthritis, and, by its ability to bind endothelial growth factors, in regulation of neovascularization in malignant disease.

## REFERENCES

1. Metcalfe DD. Effector cell heterogeneity in immediate hypersensitivity reactions. Clin Rev Allergy 1983; 1:311.
2. Kirschenbaum AS, Goff JP, Kessler SW, et al. Effect of IL-3 and stem cell factor on the appearance of human basophil and mast cells from CD34+ pleuripotent progenitor cells. J Immunol 1992; 148:772.
3. Galli SJ, Zsebo KM, Geissler EN. The kit ligand, stem cell factor. Adv Immunol 1994; 55:1.
4. Rodewald H-R, Dessing M, Dvorak AM, et al. Identification of a committed precursor for the mast cell lineage. Science 1996; 271:818.
5. Irani AM, Schechter NM, Craig S, et al. Two human mast cell subsets with different neutral protease composition. J Allergy Clin Immunol 1986; 76:18.
6. Beaven MA, Metzger H. Signal transduction by Fc receptors. Immunol Today 1993; 14:222.
7. Yamaguchi M, Lantz CS, Oettgen HC, et al. IgE enhances mouse mast cell FcεRI expression in vitro and in vivo. J Exp Med 1997; 185:663.
8. Takai T, Ono M, Hikida M, et al. Augmented hormonal and anaphylactic responses in FcγRII deficient mice. Nature 1996; 379:346.
9. White JR, Pluznik DM, Ishizaka K, Ishizaka T. Antigen-induced increase in protein kinase C activity in plasma membrane of mast cells. Proc Natl Acad Sci U S A 1985; 82:8193.
10. Takei M, Urashima H, Endo K, Muramatu M. Role of calcium in histamine release from mast cells activated by various secretagogues: intracellular calcium mobilization correlates with histamine release. Biol Chem Hoppe Seyler 1989; 370:1.
11. Takaishi T, Morita Y, Hirai K, et al. Effect of cytokines on mediator release from human dispersed lung mast cells. Allergy 1994; 49:837.
12. Marquardt DL, Walker LL, Wasserman SI. Adenosine receptors on mouse bone marrow-derived mast cells: functional significance and regulation by aminophylline. J Immunol 1984; 133:923.
13. Wasserman SI. Mediators of immediate hypersensitivity. J Allergy Clin Immunol 1983; 72:101.
14. Wasserman SI. Platelet-activating factor as a mediator of bronchial asthma. Hosp Pract 1988; 23:49.
15. MacGlashan DW Jr, Scheimer RP, Peters SP, et al. Generation of leukotrienes by purified human lung mast cells. J Clin Invest 1982; 70:747.
15a. Pearse JF, Austen KF. The biochemical, molecular, and genomic aspect of leukotriene C4 synthesis. Proc Assoc Am Phys 1999; 111:537.
16. Atkins PC, Wasserman SI. Chemotactic mediators. Clin Rev Allergy 1983; 1:385.
16a. Marquardt DL, Walker LL. Dependence of mast cell IgE-mediated cytokine production on nuclear factor-κB activity. J Allergy Clin Immunol 2000; 105:500.
17. Schwartz LB, Lewis RA, Austen KF. Tryptase from human pulmonary mast cells: purification and characterization. J Biol Chem 1981; 256:11939.
18. Tam EK, Caughey GH. Degradation of airway neuropeptides by human lung tryptase. Am J Respir Cell Mol Biol 1990; 3:27.
19. Sekizawa K, Caughey GH, Lazarus SC, et al. Mast cell tryptase causes airway smooth muscle hyperresponsiveness in dogs. J Clin Invest 1989; 83:175.
20. Church MK, Bradding P, Walls AF, et al. Human mast cells and basophils. In: Kay AB, ed. Allergy and allergic diseases. Oxford: Blackwell Science, 1997:149.
21. Metcalfe DD, Lewis RA, Silbert JE, et al. Isolation and characterization of heparin from human lung. J Clin Invest 1979; 64:1537.
22. Walsh LJ, Trinichieri G, Waldorf HA, et al. Human dermal mast cells contain and release tumor necrosis factor α, which induces endothelial leukocyte adhesion molecule. Proc Natl Acad Sci U S A 1991; 88:4220.
23. Bradding P, Feather IH, Howarth PH, et al. Interleukin 4 is localized to and released by human mast cells. J Exp Med 1992; 126:1381.
24. Bradding P, Feather IH, Wilson S, et al. Immunolocalization of cytokines in the nasal mucosa of normal and perennial rhinitic subject: the mast cell as a source of IL-4, IL-5 and IL-6 in human allergic mucosal inflammation. J Immunol 1993; 51:3853.
25. Kips JC, Tavernier J, Pauwels RA. Tumor necrosis factor causes bronchial hyperresponsiveness in rats. Am Rev Respir Dis 1992; 145:332.
26. Bevilaqua MP. Endothelial-leukocyte adhesion molecules. Annu Rev Immunol 1993; 11:767.
27. Galli SJ, Wershil BK. The two faces of the mast cell. Nature 1996; 381:21.
28. Del Prete G, Maggi E, Parronchi P. IL-4 is an essential co-factor for the IgE synthesis induced in vitro by human T cell clones and their supernatants. J Immunol 1988; 140:4193.
29. Schleimer RP, Sterbinsky SA, Kaiser J, et al. Il-4 induces adherence of human eosinophils and basophils but not neutrophils to endothelium: association with egression of VCAM-1. J Immunol 1992; 148:1086.
30. LeGros G, Ben Sasson SZ, Seder R, et al. Generation of interleukin 4 (IL-4) producing cells in vivo and in vitro generation of IL-4 producing cells. J Exp Med 1990; 172:921.
31. Sedgwick JB, Quan SF, Calhoun WJ, et al. Effect of interleukin-5 and granulocyte-macrophage colony stimulating factor on in vitro eosinophil function: comparison with airway eosinophils. J Allergy Clin Immunol 1995; 96:375.
32. Gleick GJ, Adolphson CR, Leiferman KM. The biology of the eosinophilic leukocyte. Annu Rev Med 1993; 44:85.
33. Solley GO, Gleich GJ, Jordan RE, Schroeter AL. The late phase of the immediate wheal-and-flare skin reaction: its dependence upon IgE antibodies. J Clin Invest 1976; 58:408.
34. Topar G, Standacher C, Geisin F, et al. Urticaria pigmentosa: a clinical, hematopathological and serologic study of 30 adults. Am J Pathol 1998; 109:229.
35. Lauker RM, Schechter NM, Guzzo C, Lazarus GS. Aggressive topical corticosteroid therapy: a novel approach to mast-cell-dependent cutaneous disorders. Dermatologica 1987; 175:213.
36. Wasserman SI. The regulation of inflammatory mediator production by mast cell products. Am Rev Respir Dis 1987; 135:546.
37. Cockcroft DW, Ruffin RE, Dolovich J, Hargreaves FE. Allergen-induced increase in nonallergic bronchial hyperreactivity. Clin Allergy 1977; 7:503.
38. Wasserman SI. Basic mechanisms in asthma. Ann Allergy 1988; 60:477.
39. Sabroe RA, Greaves MW. The pathogenesis of chronic idiopathic urticaria. Arch Dermatol 1997; 133:1003.
39a. Williams CMM, Golli SJ. The diverse potential effector and immunoregulatory roles of mast cells in allergic disease. J Allergy Clin Immunol 2000; 105:847.
40. Pipkorn U, Enerbück L. Nasal mucosal mast cells and histamine in hay fever: effect of topical glucocorticoid treatment. Int Arch Allergy Appl Immunol 1987; 84:123.
41. McKenna MJ, Frame B. The mast cell and bone. Clin Orthop 1985; 200:226.
42. Matzsch T, Bergqvist D, Hedner U, et al. Heparin-induced osteoporosis in rats. Thromb Haemost 1986; 56:293.
43. Atkinson JB, Harlan CW, Harlan GC, Virmani R. The association of mast cells and atherosclerosis: a morphological study of early atherosclerotic lesions in young people. Hum Pathol 1994; 25:154.
44. Sant GR, Theoharides TC. The role of the mast cell in interstitial cystitis. Urol Clin North Am 1994; 21:41.
45. Reed ND. Function and regulation of mast cells in parasite infections. In: Galli SJ, Austen KF, eds. Mast cell and basophil differentiation and function in health and disease. New York: Raven Press, 1989:205.
46. Matssuda H, Watanabe K, Kiso Y, et al. Necessity of IgE antibodies and mast cells for manifestation of resistance against larval *Haemaphysalis longicornis* ticks in mice. J Immunol 1990; 144:259.

---

# CHAPTER 182

# THE ENDOCRINE ENTERIC SYSTEM

JENS J. HOLST

Phylogenetically, the gut is the oldest endocrine organ in the body. Endocrine cells developed 1 billion years ago in structures such as the hydra, a primitive animal that mainly consists of two cell layers forming a primitive gastrointestinal (GI) tract. It is also the largest endocrine organ. Endocrine cells are found throughout the mucosa of the GI tract, outnumbering those in any other endocrine organ. However, in contrast to other organs, the endocrine cells are typically scattered among other cell types, and many are found all the way from the upper small intestine to the rectal mucosa. Thus, it has been relatively difficult to identify the discrete endocrine functions of the gut; lesions or surgical removal of parts of the gut rarely cause complete hormone deficiency, and total removal of the gut is incompatible with survival. Although tumors producing GI hormones have provided important clues as to the functions of the individual hormones, such tumors are rare (see Chap. 220). The syndromes associated with these tumors failed to be recognized and/or characterized for many years, and full comprehension of the pathogenic mechanisms involved had to await chemical identification of the causative agents.

Today, the secretory products of the GI tract endocrine cells are well known, facilitating detailed characterization of the endocrine functions of the gut. Moreover, the rate at which new peptides are being isolated from the gut (exponential in the 1970s and 1980s) has plateaued. Nonetheless, new peptides are still being identified. Many endocrine cells may produce more than a single peptide; therefore, localization of a given peptide to a specific gut endocrine cell does not preclude the production of other peptides by that cell.

Many of the concepts associated with peptides originated from the study of GI hormones. The surprising localization of gut peptides (believed to be GI hormones), to neurons and paracrine cells, led to the concept of the *diffuse neuroendocrine system* (see Chap. 175). The gut remains a rich source for peptides: The *enteric nervous system* harbors approximately the same number of neurons as the spinal cord.

## HISTORICAL STUDIES OF ENDOCRINE SECRETION

With the discovery of the first endocrine mechanism of the gut came the discovery of the first hormone. In 1902, Bayliss and Starling discovered what they called a chemical reflex.[1] When they found that careful denervation of a segment of the upper small intestine to which they applied dilute HCl did not abrogate the effect of this HCl on pancreatic exocrine secretion, they realized that this was a "chemical" rather than a neural reflex. An extract from the mucosa of this segment (the first hormonal preparation) was injected into a cervical vein, and the pancreas again responded with secretion. Thus, it was apparent that a stimulatory, chemical agent had been transported from the gut mucosa to the pancreas via the bloodstream. The active agent was named *secretin*, and the regulatory principle was given the designation *hormone* (Greek for "arouse to activity"). What they had discovered was not a specific hormone (their crude extract of the mucosa contained thousands of active agents), but the principle that pancreatic secretion could be regulated via an endocrine route. In this experiment, they had denervated the endocrine secretory organ (i.e., the gut) to identify the endocrine mechanism. In further physiologic studies, the general approach has been to denervate the target organ to define endocrine regulation (e.g., the Heidenhain pouches are denervated pouches of the gastric wall, widely used in the study of endocrine regulation of gastric secretion). Transplantation or autotransplantation experiments have also been used to provide complete denervation (e.g., autotransplanted segments of the pancreas to demonstrate unequivocally endocrine regulation of pancreatic enzyme[2]). Cross-circulation experiments in which the circulation of one animal is fused with that of another animal have been used to prove the endocrine regulation of gallbladder emptying: Fat solutions introduced into the duodenum of one animal cause contraction of the gallbladder in the other animal.[3] Thus, it is possible to determine which functions are mainly regulated by GI hormones. In general, the endocrine regulatory functions of GI hormones are confined to the GI tract itself (Table 182-1), appetite regulation being an important exception.

## ENDOCRINE TERMINOLOGY

Investigators traditionally have assigned new names for the observed endocrine peptides or functions. Thus, while the agent responsible for the endocrine regulation of pancreatic secretion of fluid and bicarbonate was called "secretin," the agent responsible for endocrine regulation of gallbladder emptying was called "cholecystokinin" (CCK; Greek for "moving the gallblad-

**TABLE 182-1.**

**Some Physiologic/Pharmacologic Actions of Gastrointestinal Regulatory Peptides**

| PEPTIDE | ACTION |
|---|---|
| Cholecystokinin | Stimulates pancreatic enzyme secretion; stimulates gallbladder contraction; stimulates SS secretion |
| Galanin | Inhibits SS, insulin, PP, NT; potentiates the effects of norepinephrine |
| Gastrin | Stimulates gastric acid secretion; stimulates growth of corpus; modulates SS secretion |
| Gastrin-releasing peptide | Stimulates gastrin release and gallbladder contraction |
| GIP | Stimulates insulin release; modulates SS secretion |
| GLP-1 | Stimulates insulin synthesis and release; inhibits glucagon release; modulates SS secretion; inhibits gastric acid secretion and gastric emptying |
| GLP-2 | Inhibits upper GI motility and secretion; trophic effects on intestinal epithelium |
| Motilin | Initiates gastric MMC activity; possible acceleration of gastric emptying |
| Neurokinin A | Smooth muscle contraction; vasodilation |
| Neuropeptide Y | Potentiates actions of norepinephrine vasoconstrictor |
| Neurotensin | Inhibits gastric secretion (i.e., enterogastrone); stimulates pancreatic secretion and intestinal growth; transmitter in the central nervous system |
| Peptide YY | Inhibits gastric acid secretion (i.e., enterogastrone); inhibits motility and pancreatic enzyme secretion |
| Secretin | Stimulates pancreatic bicarbonate secretion; inhibits gastric acid secretion (i.e., enterogastrone) |
| SS | Inhibits gastrin release; inhibits insulin and glucagon |
| Substance P | Nociception, vasodilation |
| VIP | Relaxation of lower esophageal sphincter; relaxation of gastric fundus; inhibits gastric secretion; modulates gut motility; stimulates intestinal secretion; relaxation of anal sphincter |

*GI*, gastrointestinal; *GIP*, gastric inhibitory polypeptide; *GLP-1*, glucagon-like peptide-1; *GLP-2*, glucagon-like peptide-2; *PP*, pancreatic polypeptide; *NT*, neurotensin; *SS*, somatostatin; *MMC*, migrating motor complex; *VIP*, vasoactive intestinal peptide.

der"), and the agent responsible for pancreatic secretion of enzymes was called "pancreozymin."[4] When the endocrine regulatory actions were first[5] discovered, however, the responsible hormone could not always be established. Subsequently, the GI hormones have been isolated and their structures determined, allowing for synthetic preparations to be made. For example, synthetic secretin,[6] which has been shown to be structurally related to pancreatic glucagon, is as effective in eliciting pancreatic secretion as is natural secretin isolated from intestinal extracts. Thus, this hormone has been correctly identified. During the isolation of CCK, it was found that the specific activity of the preparation increased in parallel with the specific activity of a stimulant of pancreatic enzyme secretion, and as the compound was further purified to homogeneity, it retained a maximal specific activity with respect to both gallbladder emptying and pancreatic secretion.[6] Thus, it was concluded that CCK and pancreozymin were the same hormone.

The list of peptides that could be isolated from the gut mucosa grew quickly; new additions were gastric inhibitory polypeptide (GIP),[7] motilin,[8] and somatostatin-28, a longer analog of the hypothalamic peptide.[9]

## PHYSIOLOGIC STUDIES

As new hormones became available in synthetic form and radioimmunoassays were developed for determining plasma levels, it became possible to answer the question, could the secretion of the hormone explain the physiologically defined function? That is, was secretion of the hormone (e.g., secretin) really responsible for the regulatory actions (e.g., the pancreatic secretion of fluid and bicarbonate)? Initial experiments were promising; introduction of dilute HCl into the duodenum increased plasma levels of secretin in parallel with increased pancreatic bicarbonate secretion.[10] The next question was whether introduction of HCl into the duodenum was really a physiologic stimulus. Some investigators questioned not only this but also whether secretin was really secreted.[11] While duodenal pH was rarely <4, at this pH there was no measurable secretion of secretin. Moreover, whereas intraduodenal acidification was a reliable stimulus for secretin secretion, the ingestion of mixed meals did not result in consistent changes in plasma levels of secretin; indeed, decreases were sometimes observed. These results are explained by an inadequate analysis of the intraduodenal pH. Recorded continuously, the duodenal pH fluctuates markedly with average values from 4 to 6, but with short-lasting dips to as low as 1 to 2 at varying intervals. These fluctuations reflect the emptying and rapid passage of boluses of gastric chyme.[12] Small intraduodenal boluses of HCl followed by neutralization with bicarbonate accurately mimicked the spontaneously occurring pulses, eliciting significant elevations of plasma secretin. Furthermore, similar elevations of plasma secretin, achieved by intravenous infusion of exogenous secretin, caused the same level of bicarbonate secretion as that elicited by the HCl boluses. Finally, secretin responses to meal ingestion were shown to depend on the duodenal pH pulses: Reduction of these pulses (achieved with histamine $H_2$-receptor blockade) reduced the secretin response accordingly.[13] Also, the decreases in plasma secretin sometimes observed after meal ingestion are related to the buffering capacity of the meal; indeed, the plasma secretin response clearly correlates with the duodenal delivery of acid, which, during ingestion of particularly buffering meals, could decrease considerably.[14] Thus, these studies established that secretin has the expected actions and is secreted in parallel with the gastric emptying of acid into the duodenum. It may be more important for neutralizing gastric chyme in the fasting state than after meal ingestion, depending on the buffering capacity of the meal. This analysis of the physiologic functions of secretin was accomplished by infusion of exogenous hormone, and by determination of the serum levels of the endogenous hormone, a method called *mimicry*.

Initially, mimicry was used extensively in attempts to establish the functions of new hormones, but soon it became clear that many hormones had overlapping activities and that many functions were regulated by more than one hormone. In addition, mimicry could not *prove* that an actual response was caused by the hormone in question; it merely established the possibility. A particularly powerful method is *immunoneutralization*, in which blocking antibodies are administered to experimental animals. Thus, the administration of a potent antiserum against secretin dramatically reduces meal-induced pancreatic bicarbonate secretion, thus *proving* the importance of secretin for this response.[15] Immunoneutralization continues to be an important tool in endocrine physiology, because of the often extreme specificity of antibodies for their ligands (which often far exceeds the specificity of receptor antagonists). However, it may be difficult to develop antibodies with sufficient affinity to compete with the typically high affinity of the hormone receptors and to bind sufficient amounts of the hormones at the extremely low concentrations at which they occur in the circulation. In addition, antibodies are confined mainly to the circulation and are available to antagonize peptide-receptor interactions in the extravascular compartments only to a limited extent.

# MOLECULAR APPROACHES

Advances in molecular biology have made it possible not only to characterize the *genes* producing the GI hormones (thus defining the molecular heterogeneity that characterizes many of the peptides), but also to characterize their *receptors*. Nearly all of the receptors for the GI peptides have been cloned. Transfection of cloned receptors into suitable cell lines is possible, allowing for the development and characterization of *receptor agonists* and *antagonists*. The development of such agents, although performed mainly in the search for new pharmaceuticals, has been instrumental not only in the classification of the *receptor subtypes* (which can often be distinguished because of their differential interaction with the various antagonists or agonists), but also in delineating the physiologic functions of hormones and their receptors. For example, specific CCK-receptor antagonists have made it possible to dissect, in detail, the role of CCK in regulating gallbladder emptying and pancreatic secretion. Thus, specific antagonists for the CCK-A receptor unambiguously demonstrated that the gallbladder wall was essential for meal-induced emptying of the gallbladder.[16] In contrast, by use of specific antagonists it was shown that the role of CCK in the regulation of pancreatic enzyme secretion is more complex. For many other peptidergic systems, antagonists have not become available. However, molecular-targeting techniques have provided an extremely potent tool in physiology; thus, experimental deletion of the genes that encode the peptides and/or their receptors has become a standard technique. For example, a knock-out of the CCK-A receptor is clearly associated with disturbances of gallbladder emptying and subsequent formation of gallstones (whereas signs of pancreatic dysfunction are not evident).[17] Nonetheless, hormone gene deletions cause a lifelong chronic deficiency of a given hormone or receptor, and the effects of such deficiencies may be concealed when compensatory mechanisms are induced. This may occur for many of the functions regulated by gut peptides, which characteristically exhibit a *great redundancy of regulatory systems*. The advent of techniques that allow inducible gene deletions (e.g., the Cre-Lox technique wherein genetic modification is engineered into the genome, using a Cre site-specific bacteriophage DNA recombinase that accomplishes directed nucleotide recombination at so-called Lox sites) may circumvent this problem.

# THE GASTROINTESTINAL HORMONES

## GASTRIN

Gastrin, a 17-amino-acid polypeptide (Table 182-2) secreted from the antral G cells (Fig. 182-1), is essential for gastric acid secretion and growth.[18,19]

**Secretion and Bioaction.** Gastric acid secretion is regulated in a complex interplay between endocrine, neural, and paracrine factors. Physiologic experiments using neutralizing antibodies against gastrin have been used to gauge the relative importance of this hormone in meal-induced acid secretion.[20] While species differences may exist, the results are in concert with previous studies comparing plasma gastrin responses to meal ingestion in humans and with the results of infusions of gastrin to achieve similar plasma levels (i.e., *mimicry*). Thus, these studies indicate that gastrin is responsible for a large part of the secretory response to meal ingestion. Both gastrin knock-out experiments and CCK-B receptor (gastrin receptor) knock-out confirm the importance of gastrin for acid secretion[21,22] and its trophic effects on parietal and enterochromaffin-like cells (ECL cells) (Fig. 182-2). Other regulatory functions were not apparent in these knock-out mice, for which the phenotype,

**TABLE 182-2.**
**Structures of Some Gastrointestinal Regulatory Peptides**

| | |
|---|---|
| Cholecysto-kinin-33 | KAPSGRMSIVKNLQNLDPSHRISDRDY(SO₄)MGW MDF |
| Galanin | GWTLNSAGYLLGPHAVGNHRSFSDKNGLTS |
| Gastrin-34 | QLGPQGPPHLVADPSKKQGPWLEEEEEAY(SO₄)GW MDF |
| GIP | YAEGTFISDYSIAMDKIHQQDFVNWLLAQKGKKN DWKHNITQ |
| GLP-1 | HAEGTFTSDVSSYLEGQAAKEFIAWLVKGR |
| GLP-2 | HADGSFSDEMNTILDNLAARDFINWLIQTKITDR |
| Glucagon | HSQGTFTSDYSKYLDSRRAQDFVQWLMNT |
| GRP | VPLPAGGGTVLTKMYPRGNHWAVGHLM |
| Motilin | FVPIFTYGELQRMQEKERNKGQ |
| Neurokinin A | HKTDSFVGLM |
| Neuropeptide Y | YPSKPDNPGEDAPAEDMARYYSALRHYINLITRQRY |
| Neurotensin | QLYENKPRRPYIL |
| PACAP | HSDGIFTDSYSRYRKQMAVKKYLAAVLGKRYKQR VKNK |
| Peptide YY | YPIKPEAPGEDASPEELNRYYASLRHYLNLVTTRQRY |
| Secretin | HSDGTFTSELSRLREGARLQRLLQGLV |
| Somatostatin-28 | SANSNPAMAPRERKAGCKNFFWKTFTSC |
| Substance P | RPKPQQFFGLM |
| VIP | HSDAVFTDNYTRLRKQMAVKKYLNSILN |

*A*, alanine; *B*, asparagine or aspartic acid; *C*, cysteine; *D*, aspartic acid; *E*, glutamic acid; *F*, phenylalanine; *G*, glycine; *H*, histidine; *I*, isoleucine; *K*, lysine; *L*, leucine; *M*, methionine; *N*, asparagine; *P*, proline; *Q*, glutamine; *R*, arginine; *S*, serine; *T*, threonine; *V*, valine; *W*, tryptophan; *Y*, tyrosine; *Z*, glutamine or glutamic acid.

*PACAP*, pituitary adenylate cyclase–activating peptide; *GRP*, gastrin-releasing peptide; *VIP*, vasoactive intestinal polypeptide; *GIP*, gastric inhibitory polypeptide; *GLP-1*, glucagon-like peptide-1; *GLP-2*, glucagon-like peptide-2.

apart from the gastric changes, was unremarkable. The importance of gastrin for the secretion of pepsinogen has been less rigorously studied, but it is clear that the chief cells express a different set of receptors from those of the parietal cells and that their rate of secretion is differently regulated. The CCK-B receptor has been cloned from a canine parietal cell library[23]; however, there is general agreement that, in most species, the primary target for gastrin is likely to be the histamine-producing ECL cells.[24] Thus, gastrin activates the parietal cells indirectly via histamine release from the ECL cells,[25] explaining the extreme efficiency of histamine H₂-receptor antagonists in inhibiting acid secretion.

**Growth.** The trophic effects of gastrin, which in the parietal cells may be mediated by heparin-binding epidermal growth factor,[26] are evident in transgenic mice,[27,28] and also occur in patients

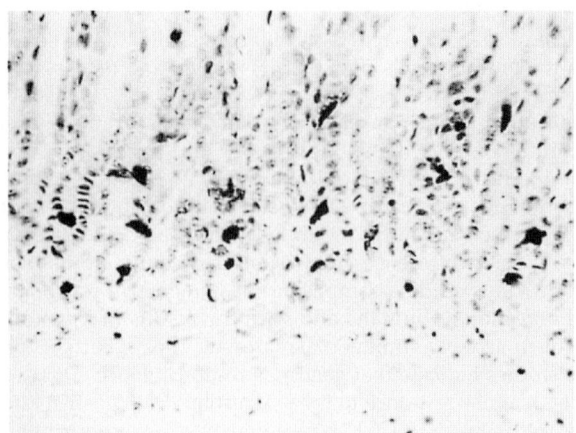

**FIGURE 182-1.** Normal human antrum immunostained for gastrin. Numerous G cells can be seen in the mucosa. ×125 (Courtesy of S. R. Bloom and J. M. Polak.)

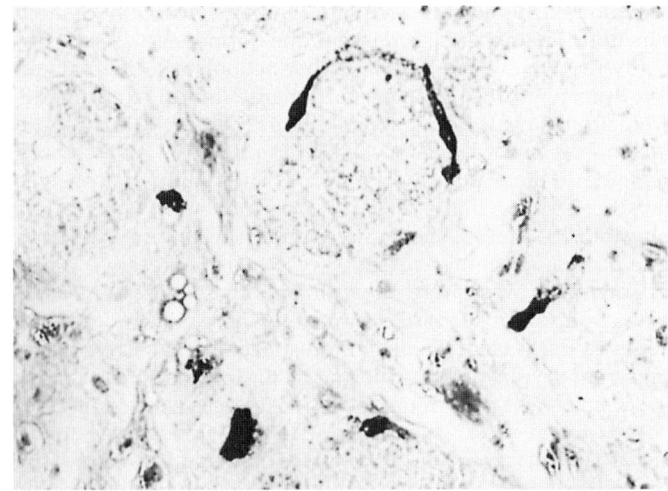

**FIGURE 182-2.** Enterochromaffin-like cells lying against the basement membrane of human fundic mucosa. (Bouins fixed tissue, Servier and Munger silver impregnation technique.) ×500 (Courtesy of S. R. Bloom and J. M. Polak.)

with gastrin-producing tumors, in whom the gastric mucosa exhibit gross hyperplasia (see Chap. 220). It has been contended that gastrin also might act as a trophic factor for the intestinal epithelium; whether it has a role in the development of colonic and other GI cancers is controversial.[29,30] Endogenous hypergastrinemia does not have trophic effects on colonic mucosa in rats and does not promote the growth of transplantable colon adenocarcinoma[31]; however, antisense oligonucleotides to gastrin inhibit the growth of human pancreatic cancer.[32]

**Pathophysiology.** Gastrin is considered a key hormone in the development of duodenal ulcers, in which infection with *Helicobacter pylori* causes hypersecretion of gastrin.[33] Its key role in the pathogenesis of the Zollinger-Ellison syndrome has been clearly established[34] (see Chap. 220). There has been speculation over the extent to which gastrin influences pancreatic exocrine and endocrine secretion. The original identification of the CCK-A receptors (CCK preferring) in the pancreas would seem incompatible with a major role for gastrin in this respect, but the pattern of receptor expression may vary between species. Thus, in humans[35,36] and pigs[37,38] the CCK-B receptor is also expressed in the pancreas, possibly explaining the significant secretory effects of gastrin in these species.

## CHOLECYSTOKININ

CCK, secreted from the I cells of the small intestinal mucosa,[39] like gastrin, has a pronounced molecular heterogeneity, and there has been considerable disagreement about which molecular form is the most abundant or important. As for gastrin, the different molecular forms arise by proteolytic cleavage of a large precursor molecule.[40] All of the bioactivity apparently resides in a sulfated and amidated carboxyl-terminal octapeptide, localized near the carboxyl terminus of the precursor; this fragment is also the most potent (see Table 182-2). The amino terminally elongated form, CCK-33 (33 amino acids), which was isolated first,[41] is also highly active; the two together along with another elongated form, consisting of 22 amino acids, constitute the principal circulating forms.[42] Plasma also contains a very large form, CCK-58.

**Secretion.** CCK is produced both in the I cells and in numerous neurons, particularly in the central nervous system (CNS), where the peptide (mainly CCK-8) seems to function as a neurotransmitter. Some of the peripheral actions also seem to involve neural mechanisms, making precise elucidation of its physiologic actions difficult.[39] It is secreted from the intestinal mucosa in response to the luminal micellar fat and protein digests, particularly during acidic conditions.[43] Studies of CCK-secreting cell lines suggest that fatty acids may directly stimulate secretion via a $Ca^{2+}$-dependent mechanism.[44] A chain length of at least 12 carbon atoms is required both for stimulation and to elicit CCK-mediated effects (e.g., on gastric motility).[45] Because luminal administration of trypsin inhibitors may increase CCK secretion, it is assumed that secretion may be regulated in an autocrine manner. There are two CCK-releasing peptides (i.e., the monitor peptide and the luminal CCK-releasing factor[46]). Their physiologic significance remains uncertain, particularly in humans who respond with pancreatic enzyme secretion after administration of trypsin inhibitors but not with CCK secretion.

**Receptors.** CCK shares its receptors with gastrin but interacts with the CCK-A receptor with 1000-fold higher potency than does gastrin.[47] Specific agonists and antagonists for the CCK-A and B receptors[48,49] have helped to characterize the physiologic functions of these receptors, and studies involving targeted disruptions of these receptors have also provided important information.[21,50,51] In addition, it seems that the so-called Otsukyu Long-Evans Tokushima fatty rats (OLETF rats) may be a useful rat model for CCK-A–receptor deficiency, harboring a non-sense mutation of the receptor gene.[52,53]

**Bioaction.** Knock-out and antagonist studies all indicate a major role for CCK in the regulation of gallbladder and bile-duct motility.[17,54,55] Thus, potent CCK-A–receptor antagonists completely block meal-induced gallbladder emptying,[16] and the knock-out mice develop gallstones. The gallbladder smooth muscles are equipped with CCK-A receptors, perhaps accounting for the endocrine effect of CCK. However, since gallbladder function is also neurally regulated, some of its actions may depend on neural interactions.

With respect to the pancreas, intravenous infusions of CCK stimulate the secretion of proteins (i.e., enzymes). The pancreatic secretory response to meal stimulation (duodenal instillation of nutrient solutions), on the other hand, is only partially or weakly antagonized by specific CCK-A antagonists, whereas muscarinic antagonists may completely inhibit the response.[56,57] This suggests that, physiologically, the actions of CCK may depend on interaction with autonomic cholinergic neurons. Studies suggest that CCK interacts with afferent nerve fibers localized in the duodenal mucosa and elsewhere,[58] which in turn reflexively activate efferent neurons that innervate the pancreas. However, the human pancreas has both CCK-A and CCK-B receptors,[36] a fact that may explain part of the inefficiency of the CCK-A–receptor antagonists in inhibiting meal-induced secretory responses.[55,56] Another important action of CCK (counteracted by antagonists) is pancreatic growth. This action suggested the possible use of CCK-A antagonists to treat pancreatic cancer; however, successful treatment has not yet been reported (side effects include disturbed motility of the biliary system). Antagonist studies also indicate that CCK has a role in the regulation of gastric motility,[54] which is enhanced by CCK-A antagonists. The antagonists have also provided insight into the role of CCK in the regulation of acid secretion. CCK would be expected to interact as well as gastrin with the CCK-B receptors of parietal and ECL cells of the gastric mucosa and, therefore, to act as a full agonist for acid secretion. However, CCK is a weak and partial agonist for acid secretion, particularly in higher doses, because CCK activates CCK-A receptors on D cells located in the vicinity of the parietal cells, releasing somatostatin, which inhibits parietal cell secretion. Because of the extreme inhibitory potency of somatostatin on acid secretion, inhibition predominates.[59] Antagonist studies indicate that CCK may also influence lower esophageal sphincter function in humans.[60]

**Appetite.** CCK seems to play an important role in the regulation of food intake (see Chap. 125), acting as a meal-related satiety signal to terminate ingestion.[61] This concept has not been supported in knock-out mice, which develop normally and do not become obese.[51] These studies confirm that intact CCK-A but not CCK-B receptors are required to elicit the anorectic effects of CCK. However, it is generally conceded that knock-out of one of the many factors regulating food intake cannot be expected to result in a striking phenotype; the regulatory function of the deficient factor is taken over by other mechanisms. CCK administration reliably inhibits food intake, and in some studies the administration of an antagonist has resulted in increased food intake.[62] Moreover, the OLETF rats do develop obesity.[63] Again, the inhibitory mechanism seems to involve afferent sensory nerve fibers. A CCK-B receptor antagonist increased food intake in rats.[64]

**Glucose Homeostasis.** CCK has been included among the *incretin hormones* (i.e., the insulinotropic hormones that enhance and potentiate meal-related, substrate-induced insulin secretion) because it stimulates insulin secretion in rodents. In humans, however, it is without effect,[65] and rats with CCK receptor deletions are normoglycemic.[51]

**Anxiety.** As a cerebral transmitter, CCK is also involved in anxiety-, panic-, and stress-related behavior that is transmitted via the CCK-B receptor[66]; CCK-B receptor antagonists have been suggested for the treatment of anxiety-related disorders.[67] However, all of the cerebral effects seem to depend critically on organismic and procedural variables[68]; thus, caution has to be exercised before these findings are extrapolated to human physiology.

## SECRETIN

The physiologic importance of secretin is well worked out using mimicry[13,69] and immunoneutralization studies.[15] The secretin receptor has been cloned and its localization conforms with the expected targets of secretin action.[70]

**Secretion.** Like CCK, secretin circulates in extremely low concentrations (a few pmol/L), but the physiologic variations are sufficient to influence pancreatic bicarbonate secretion. Initially, it was unclear why plasma secretin concentrations do not exhibit a clear relationship to meal ingestion. Subsequent studies revealed that secretion closely follows the concentration of hydrogen ions in the chyme that enters the duodenum.[14] During ingestion of meals with a high-buffering capacity, the gastric pH increases, and the chyme that enters the duodenum may have a pH too high to stimulate secretin secretion (for which a pH of ~2–3 is required). In contrast, in the fasting state, the boluses of chyme that enter the duodenum may have a low pH, and may cause secretion of short pulses of secretin. If the frequency of chyme expulsion from the stomach is low, a low-average secretin concentration in plasma will be the result. As the postprandial gastric chyme eventually becomes acidified, a more frequent (because of the meal) emptying of acidic chyme may cause a more sustained increase in plasma secretin.[14] The cellular mechanism whereby the low pH of the duodenal contents stimulates secretin secretion is not known; a high tension of carbon dioxide has no influence on secretion, indicating that the hydrogen ions themselves, rather than changes in intracellular pH, trigger secretion. Although there is evidence for secretin-releasing peptides in analogy to the CCK-releasing peptides, their physiologic relevance has not been established.[71]

**Bioaction.** Secretin acts on the ductular epithelium of the pancreas to increase secretion of bicarbonate and water. Despite progress (e.g., the involvement of the cystic fibrosis transmembrane conductance regulator [CFTR] protein, which plays an important role for the exchange of $Cl^-$ and $HCO_3^-$ between the lumen and the interstitium), the secretory mechanism is still unclear.[72] Secretin has no effect on pancreatic protein secretion. The secretory actions of secretin on one hand, and cholinergic agonists and CCK on the other, exhibit strong potentiating synergism.[73] Thus, combinations of small or even subthreshold amounts of these factors may cause considerable pancreatic secretion of fluid as well as protein and bicarbonate, illustrating the importance of neuroendocrine regulation of the pancreas.[74] In addition to its pancreatic actions, secretin is thought to play a role as a choleretic agent,[75,76] and it acts in cholangiocytes by stimulating translocation of aquaporin-1 water channels from an intracellular vesicular pool to the cholangiocyte plasma membrane.[77] Immunoneutralization studies suggest that secretin may be a physiologic inhibitor of gastric acid secretion in dogs, but this has not been confirmed in humans.[78] On the other hand, physiologic elevations of plasma secretin inhibit gastric emptying, and this effect (which was also evident in the immunoneutralization studies) may be physiologically relevant. However, as an enterogastrone (i.e., intestinal hormonal inhibitor of gastric functions), secretin may be much more potent in dogs[79,80] than in humans.

**Central Nervous System Effects.** A family of *hypocretins*, which are hypothalamus-specific peptides with neuroexcitatory activity and strong amino-acid homology with secretin, have been uncovered.[81] These peptides cause an increased food intake when administered into the cerebral ventricles, and are, therefore, also designated as *orexins*[82] (see Chap. 125). This discovery may explain the occasional reports of immunoreactive secretin in neurons of the brain. Surprisingly, injection of secretin into the cerebral ventricles influences pancreatic secretion.[83]

## MOTILIN

Motilin is a 22-amino-acid peptide produced in endocrine cells of the upper intestinal mucosa[84] (see Table 182-2). It also seems to be produced in certain regions of the brain, where motilin-binding sites are found, but little is known about its importance as a brain peptide.[85,86] Motilin is encoded by a gene from chromosome 6; its precursor is a peptide of 114 amino acids.[87] Nothing is known about the possible functions of the nonmotilin parts of the precursor.

**Secretion and Bioaction.** Motilin is secreted in response to intraluminal changes in pH and the presence of bile.[88] However, important differences between species seem to exist. In humans, its secretion parallels the occurrence of the *migrating motor complexes* (MMCs) in the fasting state, and its functions seem to be related to the regulation of GI motility. Thus, infusion of motilin can induce premature MMCs, and immunoneutralization[89] disrupts the spontaneous (fasting) motility pattern in the upper gut. However, the cyclic variations in secretion of motilin could also reflect cyclic neural interdigestive activity, which is also reflected in periodic bursts of GI secretion and emptying of the gallbladder.[90]

Motilin receptors have not been cloned, and there are no currently available antagonists. Binding studies have revealed different pharmacologic characteristics for receptors (binding sites) occurring in the antrum and the duodenum.[91] It is generally assumed that high concentrations of motilin activate smooth muscles directly. At lower concentrations, motilin seems to activate cholinergic neural networks, and it appears that the cyclic changes in plasma motilin can initiate cyclic changes in parasympathetic efferent activity.[92] However, its ability to induce premature MMCs does not seem to be dependent on the extrinsic innervation, and CNS input is not necessary for cyclic interdigestive activity or cyclic release of motilin.[93] Erythromycin and related macrolide antibiotics are

potent agonists, and the stimulation of GI motor activity that can be elicited with erythromycin is thought to reflect its interaction with motilin receptors.[84,94,95] Moreover, infusions of motilin (as norLeu-13-motilin, which is more stable) and erythromycin and related substances have beneficial effects in patients with impaired motility (e.g., diabetic gastroparesis; see Chap. 149).[96] Disturbed secretion of motilin has not been implicated in the pathogenesis of disease.

## GASTRIC INHIBITORY POLYPEPTIDE OR GLUCOSE-DEPENDENT INSULINOTROPIC PEPTIDE (GIP)

GIP is a peptide of 42 amino acids belonging to the glucagon-secretin family of peptides. The sequence homology is particularly strong in the amino-terminal part. It is processed from a precursor of 153 amino acids,[97] but specific functions for other fragments of the precursor have not been identified. Most antisera raised against GIP cross-react with a larger molecule (GIP 8000); the relationship of this molecule to GIP is not known.[98] It does not seem to be a product of the GIP precursor. In some instances, GIP 8000 may have originated from the related peptide glicentin, which may cross-react with some GIP antisera. Preferably, GIP assays should not cross-react with GIP 8000. The GIP receptor, which has been cloned, is related to the receptors for the other members of the glucagon-secretin family of peptides. It is expressed in the pancreatic islets and also in the gut, adipose tissue, heart, pituitary, adrenal cortex, and several regions of the brain.[99]

**Secretion.** GIP is secreted from the so-called K cells, which exhibit their highest density in the duodenum, although GIP cells are found in the entire small intestinal mucosa. Secretion is stimulated by absorbable carbohydrates and by lipids. GIP secretion is, therefore, greatly increased in response to meal ingestion, resulting in 10- to 20-fold elevations.[100]

**Bioaction.** Interaction of GIP with its receptor on the pancreatic B cells increases cyclic adenosine monophosphate (cAMP) levels, which in turn increase the intracellular calcium concentration and enhance the exocytosis of insulin-containing granules.[101] Thus, GIP is considered one of the incretin hormones. The incretin function of GIP has been probed in immunoneutralization studies,[102] and in studies employing a fragment, GIP$_{7-30}$amide, which is a GIP receptor antagonist.[103] Both treatments reduce insulin responses to oral glucose and impaired glucose tolerance. Mice with a targeted deletion of the GIP receptor gene become glucose intolerant.[104]

GIP has been reported to influence lipid metabolism.[105] In particular, the hormone enhances lipoprotein lipase activity, inhibits lipolysis, and promotes synthesis of triglycerides, all of which would be expected to promote the postprandial clearance of dietary lipids. Furthermore, functional receptors on adipocytes generate cAMP after activation by GIP.[106,107]

As suggested from its name, GIP was isolated as an inhibitor of acid secretion. In humans, however, its activity is weak and it also seems to have little effect on GI motility.[108]

**Pathophysiology.** GIP is implicated in postprandial Cushing syndrome.[109] The adrenal either overexpresses and/or has increased sensitivity of its GIP receptors, with subsequent hypersecretion of adrenal corticosteroids in relation to meal ingestion, when GIP levels are high.[110] Patients with type 2 diabetes mellitus have been reported to hypersecrete GIP, but this is noted only with certain assays. Nonetheless, in these patients, there is a weak or absent incretin function, and exogenous GIP has little or no insulinotropic effect.[111] Thus, type 2 diabetes seems to be characterized by defective functioning of the pancreatic GIP receptor, a finding that could be of great pathophysiologic significance. Detected polymorphisms in the coding region of the GIP-receptor gene are not associated with diabetes,[112] or with defective signaling.[113] Disturbances of GIP secretion or action in other metabolic diseases, notably in obesity, have not been established, but the deranged lipid metabolism in type 2 diabetes and other dyslipidemic disorders could represent another target.[114]

## SOMATOSTATIN

Somatostatin is a 14-amino-acid peptide (SS14) originally isolated as the growth hormone (GH) release-inhibiting factor from the hypothalamus (see Chap. 169). The single somatostatin gene is also expressed in many endocrine cells in the GI system, including the mucosa and the pancreatic islets, and in many neurons of the enteric nervous system. In the intestinal mucosa, however, the 92-amino-acid precursor is processed to release a 28-amino-acid peptide (SS28) of which SS14 occupies the carboxyl-terminal 14 amino acids[108,115] (see Table 182-2). Thus, upon appropriate stimulation, it is SS28, rather than SS14, that is released from the gut.[116] Its half-life in the circulation is considerably greater than that of SS14, in keeping with the notion that SS28 functions as a circulating hormone, whereas the SS14 functions in local regulation, either as a neurotransmitter or as a paracrine mediator.

**Receptors.** The somatostatins act through five different, but related, receptors.[117] The fifth receptor (SST-5) seems to prefer SS28, whereas the others have similar affinities for both SS14 and SS28. The receptor subtype composition characteristically varies between the different somatostatin-responsive tissues. Generally, in the GI tract, the SST-2 and SST-3 isoforms predominate. All receptors seem to inhibit cell function, mostly through inhibition of adenylate cyclase via an inhibitory G protein, but other signaling pathways may also be activated (e.g., tyrosine phosphatases, which could transmit the inhibitory effects on growth in certain tissues).

**Secretion.** Somatostatin 28 is released in response to meal ingestion. A low pH in the upper intestine may be the proper stimulus, but the increases are small. Somatostatin released from nerves or paracrine cells (SS14) is usually not detectable in the peripheral blood and, therefore, probably does not play a role in hemocrine regulation.

**Bioaction.** To the extent that the arterial concentration of somatostatin reaches sufficient levels, it could affect the functions of virtually any organ, because it is capable of inhibiting the secretion of most hormones including the GI hormones. It may also inhibit exocrine secretion from the entire GI tract and has effects on blood flow, absorption, and growth. Finally, it has variable but highly significant effects on GI motility. SS28 acting as a hormone has at least the potential to inhibit pancreatic exocrine secretion[118]; however, the extent to which it exerts such regulatory functions is unknown. Clearly, the diversity of its receptors and functions makes it very difficult to analyze the effects of any gene knock-outs; potent and selective antagonists have generally not been available, although more or less subtype-specific antagonists are being developed.[119–121] Immunoneutralization studies suggest, however, that circulating somatostatin may play a role as an enterogastrone hormone, mediating the inhibition of upper GI functions that are elicited by lipids or acid in the small intestine.[122] SST-2 knock-out mice have a high basal gastric acid secretion that is mediated by gastrin.[123] Possibly, somatostatin also participates in the regulation of absorption, but whether this is a local effect or is due to circulating SS28 is not known.[124]

**Cortistatin.** Another member of the somatostatin family of peptides, the 17-amino-acid brain peptide cortistatin, is a product of a separate gene, but has structural similarities to somatostatin and binds to and activates all five somatostatin receptors.[125,126] It may have both similar and dissimilar effects on cerebral functions.[127]

**Pathophysiology.** Clinical conditions associated with a deficiency of somatostatin secretion have not been described (although conditions with decreased paracrine function may exist), but several patients have had disorders associated with somatostatin-secreting tumors,[128] some in the pancreas and others in the duodenum. These patients exhibit, to a variable degree, disturbances that are related to the actions of somatostatin. Impaired biliary function with gallstone formation seems to be one of the most frequent features, and most patients have some degree of diabetes mellitus. A metabolically stable form of somatostatin, octreotide,[129] is commonly used to treat endocrine tumors (GI and pituitary), and patients on constant octreotide therapy may develop diarrhea and steatorrhea. Scintigraphy after injection of radioactively labeled octreotide is a very useful tool in the diagnosis of neuroendocrine tumors, which often express a high density of somatostatin receptors.[130] *H. pylori* infection causes hypersecretion of acid because of relative hypergastrinemia. There is evidence that the infection decreases the density of somatostatin cells in the antrum, thus causing hypergastrinemia.[131] Thus, eradication of the infection is associated with normalization of somatostatin cell density and gastrin concentrations.[132]

## THE DISTAL GUT HORMONES

### THE PROGLUCAGON-DERIVED PEPTIDES

The glucagon gene is expressed not only in the pancreatic A cells but also in the so-called L cells of the intestinal mucosa, which have their highest density in the lower small intestine. Here, the primary translation product is proglucagon (ProG, 160 amino acids; Fig. 182-3). Proglucagon is not cleaved into glucagon and the fragment corresponding to ProG sequences 33–61 and 78–158, respectively, as occurs in the pancreas. Rather, it is released to form glicentin (i.e., enteroglucagon), corresponding to $ProG_{1-69}$ and the two glucagon-like peptides contained in the major ProG fragment: glucagon-like peptides-1 (i.e., $ProG_{78-107}$amide) and -2 (i.e., $ProG_{126-158}$) or glucagon-like peptides-1 and -2 (GLP-1 and -2), respectively[133] (see Table 182-2). The major ProG fragment from the pancreas and glicentin both seem to be bioinactive. Thus, in the pancreas the specific gut products (GLP-1 and -2) are inactivated via incorporation into the major ProG fragment, while in the gut, glucagon is inactivated by being incorporated into glicentin. In vivo, small amounts of glicentin may be cleaved to release oxyntomodulin (i.e., $ProG_{33-69}$), which shares some of the activities of glucagon (because of their common amino terminus), but generally with low potency.

**Secretion.** Glicentin, GLP-1, and GLP-2 are secreted in response to meal ingestion. Carbohydrates and fat in the gut lumen seem to be the appropriate stimulus for the L cells (which are of the open type). Because the meal response is rapid, it has been speculated that neuroendocrine regulation may also play a role. Because the three peptides are secreted in parallel, the results of older studies of enteroglucagon secretion do, to some extent, apply to the glucagon-like peptides.[133]

**Glucagon-Like Peptide-1 Receptors.** GLP-1, a 30-amino-acid peptide having 50% homology with glucagon, interacts with a single receptor, which belongs to the glucagon-secretin family.[134] The main site of expression is in the pancreatic islets, but receptors are also present in the lungs, the stomach, and the brain.

**Glucagon-Like Peptide-1 Bioaction.** Activation of the B-cell receptor causes a stimulation of insulin secretion similar to that elicited by GIP. GLP-1, therefore, is considered to be the more distal incretin hormone, playing a role when not only the

## PROGLUCAGON

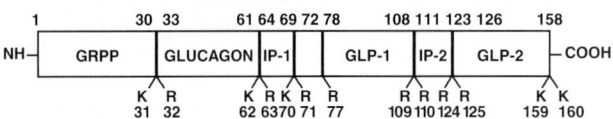

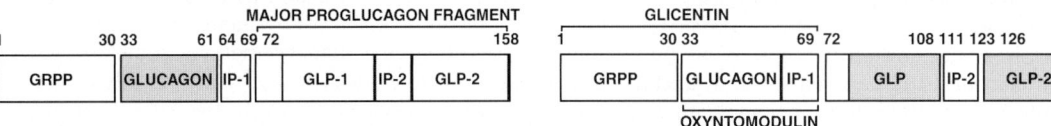

**FIGURE 182-3.** Alternative posttranslational processing of proglucagon in pancreas, intestine, and the brain. Enzymatic cleavage at specific pairs of basic amino acids (K, lysine; R, arginine) produces numerous peptides. (*GLP-1*, glucagon-like peptide-1; *GLP-2*, glucagon-like peptide-2; *GRPP*, glicentin-related pancreatic peptide; *IP-1* and *IP-2*, intervening peptides.) (Adapted from Fig. 8B [only], Kieffer TJ, Habener JF. The glucagon-like peptides. Endocr Rev 1999; 20:885.)

upper but also the lower small intestine is exposed to nutrients, mainly carbohydrates (but also lipids). Unlike GIP secretion, which is either "on" or "off," GLP-1 secretion reflects the size of the meal and/or the rate of gastric emptying. Its function as an incretin hormone has been probed with both receptor antagonists and receptor knock-out studies. A truncated form of exendin-4, a lizard peptide, interacts specifically with the GLP-1 receptor, and administration of this antagonist along with oral glucose impairs insulin responses and glucose tolerance.[135] Mice with a targeted disruption of the GLP-1–receptor gene[136] are glucose intolerant, and the males have fasting hyperglycemia (i.e., they are diabetic). Unlike GIP, the incretin effect of GLP-1 is completely preserved in type 2 diabetes mellitus,[137] and infusions of small amounts of GLP-1 completely normalize the blood glucose levels of patients with long-standing diabetes.[138] Part of the efficacy of GLP-1 is due to its inhibitory effect on glucagon secretion (which is not shared by GIP). GLP-1 efficiently lowers the hepatic glucose production, which is elevated in these patients. Considerable efforts are being made to develop a clinically useful therapy with this metabolically unstable peptide.[139,139a,139b] Physiologically, the GI actions of GLP-1 may be more important,[133] as it strongly inhibits upper GI secretion and motility.[140] If it is infused together with a meal, the meal-induced insulin secretion actually decreases.[141] This is because GLP-1 slows motility and absorption so that the nutrient-induced insulin secretion (and, thereby, the GLP-1–potentiated response) decreases. This inhibitory mechanism (a part of the so-called *ileal brake mechanism*[142]) seems to involve activation of afferent sensory nerve fibers that reflexively inhibit the cephalic parasympathetic outflow, and functions that are regulated by the vagus nerves.[143] Surprisingly, GLP-1 is rapidly inactivated by a local enzyme (dipeptidyl peptidase IV, DPP-IV), such that about half of the GLP-1 that leaves the gut is already bioinactive.[144] This suggests that, physiologically, GLP-1 interacts with local afferent nerve fibers immediately on its release, before being degraded.

**Central Nervous System Effects of Glucagon-Like Peptide-1.** GLP-1 inhibits appetite and food intake[145] and may represent one of the meal-related intestinal satiety signals that terminate food intake.[61] GLP-1 receptors are also expressed in the brain, particularly in the hypothalamus,[146] where they seem to be targets for GLP-1 produced in neurons of the brainstem. Injected into the cerebral ventricles, GLP-1 strongly inhibits food intake,[147] but this mechanism seems to be unrelated to the satiating effects of peripheral GLP-1. Similar to the CCK receptor

knock-outs, mice with a GLP-1 receptor knock-out do not become obese.

**Secretion and Bioaction of Glucagon-Like Peptide-2.** GLP-2 is released in parallel with GLP-1 and shares with it inhibitory effects on upper GI motility and secretion.[148] It has attracted more interest because of its growth-promoting effects.[149] Although its physiologic role in intestinal growth is unknown, infusions or injections of GLP-2 into rodents cause a marked growth of the entire intestine, with the most notable effects being on the small intestine. Both the length and weight of the gut increase as well as the crypt depth and villus height; thus, GLP-2 has been proposed to be the endocrine factor that induces adaptive growth (e.g., in relation to intestinal transposition or resection studies). Enteroglucagon was thought to be involved in this mechanism because of a striking relationship between its plasma levels and adaptive growth; however,[150] GLP-2 secretion is likely to show the same correlation because the two peptides are secreted in parallel. Of clinical interest is the demonstration that the intestinal atrophy that accompanies total parenteral nutrition can be completely prevented by GLP-2 infusion.[151] A GLP-2 receptor, which has been cloned, is closely related to the GLP-1 receptor.[152]

### NEUROTENSIN

Neurotensin (NT) is a 13-amino-acid peptide produced in the N cells, the distribution of which resembles that of the L cell.[153] The NT gene encodes a precursor of 170-amino acids, in which NT is located near the carboxyl terminus.[154] Adjacent to the amino terminus of NT is the sequence of neuromedin N, another bioactive peptide. Neuromedin N, however, is not released from the precursor in the N cells, but is released from the many peripheral neurons (particularly in the CNS) that express the NT gene. While there is little doubt that NT plays an important role as a neurotransmitter in the CNS (e.g., in nociceptive and neuroendocrine systems[155]), its function as a hormone is much less clear.

**Receptors.** NT may interact with two receptors (high affinity[156] and low affinity[157]), both of which are expressed in numerous neural tissues. In the periphery, receptors (high affinity) are mainly localized in the colon, followed by the liver, the duodenum, and the pancreas.[158]

**Bioaction.** NT secretion is stimulated by luminal lipids, but the plasma concentration increases by only a few pmol/L. The peptide seems to be cleaved almost immediately after secretion into the inactive (peripherally) 1–8 fragment. When reproduced by infusion, the low circulating concentrations of NT have little effect,[159] whereas higher concentrations have marked inhibitory effects on gastric function and stimulatory effects on pancreatic secretion.[160] The effects seem to require an intact vagal innervation, and it seems possible that NT, like GLP-1, could act locally on sensory afferent nerve fibers before it is degraded. A similar mechanism may apply to peptide YY (PYY) and may, thus, characterize the entire ileal brake mechanism. In addition to its regulatory actions with respect to organ function, NT is thought to act as a growth factor for the large bowel, the pancreas, and the stomach.[153] High-affinity receptor antagonists are now available,[161] but have not been applied to studies of its functions as a GI hormone.

**Pathophysiology.** Results from using a nonpeptide antagonist for the high-affinity receptor (i.e., SR 48692) suggest that NT could play an essential role in mediating the colonic inflammation induced by toxin A of *Clostridium difficile*.[162] Furthermore, using SR 48692,[163] evidence was found that the growth of colon cancers may depend on blood-borne NT, suggesting that therapeutics based on this antagonist's structure could be useful.

## PEPTIDE YY

PYY is a peptide of 36-amino acids that belongs to a family of peptides (the PP-fold family, having a common, characteristic molecular configuration) comprising, in addition, neuropeptide Y (NPY) and pancreatic polypeptide (PP). All contain 36-amino acids, exhibit a high degree of sequence homology, and have one or two terminal tyrosine residues (hence the Ys).

**Secretion.** Whereas NPY (phylogenetically the oldest) is an obligatory neuropeptide, PYY and PP are hormones; PP is secreted from cells of the pancreatic islets, and PYY is secreted from endocrine cells of the distal intestinal mucosa,[164] some of which also produce the proglucagon-derived peptides. Under some experimental conditions the secretion of PYY and GLP-1 parallel each other. Like GLP-1, PYY is metabolized by the enzyme DPP-IV. Whereas all stored GLP-1 is intact, part of PYY is stored and secreted as the metabolite, $PYY_{3-36}$. PYY is secreted in response to meal ingestion, but lipids seem to be particularly effective as stimulants.[165] There may be a stimulatory loop from the upper to the distal gut with CCK or gastrin stimulating PYY secretion, which in turn may inhibit gastrin and CCK secretion.[166]

**Receptors.** The PP family operates via a family of receptors comprising six members, the $Y_{1-6}$ receptors, all of which (except for $Y_3$) have been cloned.[167–169] Of these, $Y_4$ has the highest affinity for PP, whereas the others can be distinguished not only on the basis of structural differences, but also by their interactions with various analogs and fragments of the PP family of peptides. With NPY being the most widely distributed member, it is perhaps not surprising that the receptors are also expressed in neural tissues, central as well as peripheral. NPY and PYY both activate the $Y_1$ and $Y_2$ receptors, whereas carboxyl-terminal fragments of PYY, including $PYY_{3-36}$, interact only with the $Y_2$ receptor. Since the tissue distribution of the two receptor types is markedly distinct, it follows that the conversion of PYY by the enzyme DPP-IV has important functional consequences. PYY does not immediately cross the blood–brain barrier; therefore, it is not capable of interacting with the Y receptors of the CNS. Whereas NPY may reach high local concentrations at neuroeffector junctions on activation of the nerves, the plasma concentrations of PYY are in the low pM range, and circulating PYY, therefore, activates only accessible, high-affinity receptors. This probably limits the physiologic actions of PYY.

**Physiology.** PYY operates as an inhibitor of many GI functions, including upper GI secretion and motility, but it also inhibits intestinal secretion and promotes absorption.[170] It is possible that its effect on intestinal secretion may be exerted locally (i.e., it acts as a paracrine regulator). As is the case for GLP-1, its inhibitory effects on gastric and pancreatic function

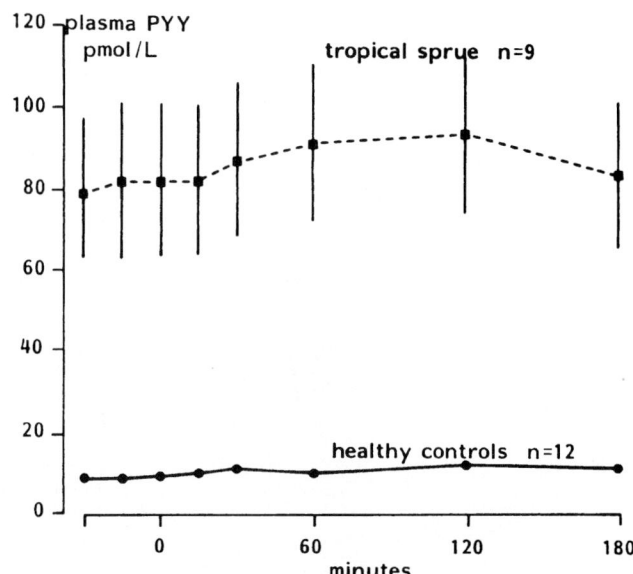

**FIGURE 182-4.** Plasma peptide YY (*PYY*) concentrations in nine patients with severe tropical sprue and 12 age-matched and sex-matched healthy controls after eating a 530-kcal test breakfast at time zero. (From Adrian TE, Savage AP, Bacarese-Hamilton AJ, et al. Peptide YY abnormalities in gastrointestinal diseases. Gastroenterology 1986; 90:374.)

seem to involve the parasympathetic nervous system,[171] and the two peptides may act in very similar ways.[172] As inhibitors of gastric secretion, the two peptides have additive effects and strongly inhibit acid secretion at very low concentrations.[173] In dogs, PYY may be the most important peptide of the ileal brake mechanism,[80] whereas in humans, GLP-1 may be more significant. PYY is secreted in response to the luminal presence of fiber and short chain fatty acids, but in humans, both GLP-1 and PYY are unaffected by colonic carbohydrate fermentation.[174] Both are released in response to luminal bile and bile salts. There have been no reported knock-outs of the Y receptors or PYY (a knockout of NPY had mainly cerebral effects[175]). Selective agonist and antagonist studies have failed to elucidate the physiology of PYY; one immunoneutralization study[176] confirmed that the fat-induced ileal brake effects in dogs depend on the actions of PYY, whereas in another study antibodies against PYY had little effect on lipid-induced inhibition of acid secretion. A CCK-A–receptor antagonist reversed this inhibition.[177]

**Pathophysiology.** A pathology specifically related to PYY secretion has not been identified. The endocrine functions of PP are largely unknown, but it may act as an inhibitor of the motility and secretion of the biliary system.[178] Elevated plasma PYY has been reported in tropical sprue (Fig. 182-4).

## HORMONES OF THE COLON

All of the hormones from the distal small intestine are also produced in the numerous endocrine cells of the colon and rectal mucosa (Fig. 182-5). However, very little is known about the functional role of these endocrine cells,[179] and it is not known whether regulation of colon secretion differs from that of the ileum. Resection studies have not been informative.

## PARACRINE REGULATION OF THE GASTROINTESTINAL TRACT

The most prominent examples of paracrine regulation are related to gastric acid secretion, although it appears likely that paracrine mechanisms regulate function throughout the GI

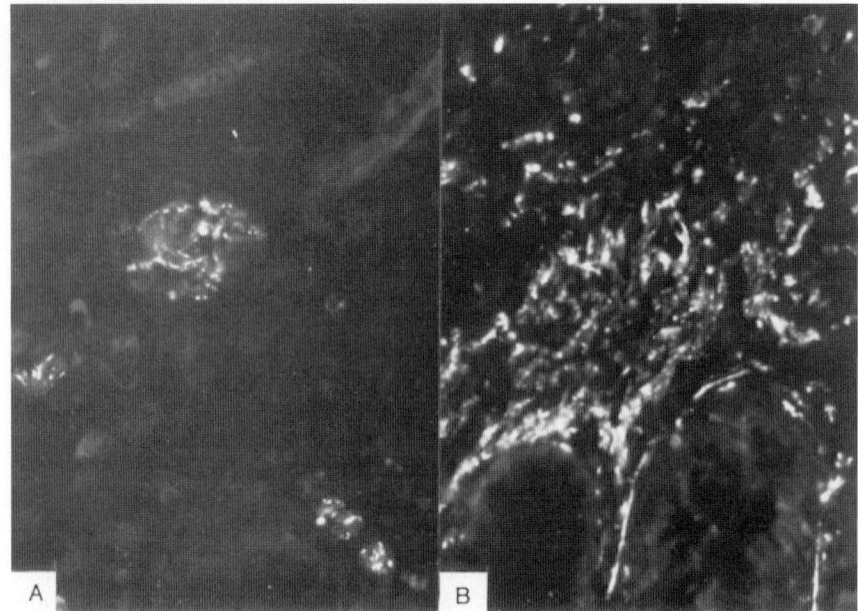

**FIGURE 182-5. A,** Submucosa of normal human colon showing bundles of vasoactive intestinal peptide immunoreactive fibers. ×350 **B,** Submucosa and base of mucosa of colon from a patient with Crohn colitis. ×350 (Courtesy of S. R. Bloom and J. M. Polak.)

tract. One paracrine regulator is histamine secreted from the ECL cells of the gastric mucosa. Studies have suggested that a local histamine release from these cells, with histamine subsequently diffusing toward the parietal cell for interaction with $H_2$ receptors, represents one of the most important stimulatory pathways for acid secretion. Histamine release from the ECL cell, in turn, is regulated by gastrin secretion and by neural or paracrine mechanisms. The other prominent paracrine transmitter is somatostatin. In the gastric mucosa, somatostatin is produced in the D cells, which, in the corpus and fundus, are mainly endocrine cells of the closed type (i.e., no luminal contact). In the antral glands they appear characteristically open. The somatostatin cells may send out dendrite-like cytoplasmic processes, which seem to establish close contact with neighboring cells, leading to the hypothesis that gastric somatostatin might act as a paracrine rather than an endocrine transmitter.[180] The activity of paracrine cells is not likely to be reflected in the concentrations of the transmitter in the peripheral plasma, but a spillover of the transmitter after activation of the paracrine cells may be detected in the local veins draining the region. For somatostatin in the antrum, the main target seems to be the gastrin cells, and the main stimulus to the D cells seems to be the luminal pH. Thus, a high acidity in the antral lumen stimulates paracrine somatostatin release, which in turn inhibits gastrin secretin, thus creating a feedback loop.[181,182] Antral somatostatin secretion is also regulated by neural and hormonal (i.e., CCK) factors. In the corpus region, the parietal and/or the ECL cells are the targets for D-cell secretion, and somatostatin is an exceedingly potent inhibitor of acid secretion, acting via receptors located on the parietal (or ECL) cells. Neural stimuli seem to regulate D-cell secretion, with inhibitory cholinergic influences probably being the most important.[183] Activation of vagal cholinergic fibers may, therefore, stimulate acid secretion, partly by interacting with stimulatory cholinergic receptors on the parietal cells, and partly by inhibiting tonically inhibitory paracrine D cells. The D cells have CCK-A receptors, which may be activated by CCK from the duodenum.[184,185] This probably explains why CCK—which is a full agonist for the CCK-B receptors on ECL cells and parietal cells and, therefore, should be a full agonist for acid secretion—is in fact a partial agonist and may actually inhibit gastrin-stimulated secretion, mainly by stimulation of the paracrine, inhibitory D cells.[59] Interestingly, the antral para-

crine regulation of gastrin secretion seems to be one of the targets of *H. pylori* infection.[33]

## NEUROPEPTIDES OF THE GUT

**Innervation.**   The innervation of the gut may be divided into *intrinsic* and *extrinsic systems*.[186] The extrinsic system comprises efferent and afferent sympathetic and parasympathetic pathways, the cell bodies from which are located outside the gut. The intrinsic system contains the numerous (more than $10^8$ cell bodies) neurons of the *enteric nervous system* that remain intact after extrinsic denervation. These cell bodies are mainly located in the plexuses of the gut (myenteric and the submucous plexuses). The enteric nervous system comprises sensory neurons and a large number of interneurons and effector neurons, and is, thus, able to create full reflex loops without involving the spinal cord.

**Neuropeptides.**   Both the intrinsic and the extrinsic systems are sources of numerous neuropeptides,[187,188] which may coexist with each other and with nonpeptide transmitters (e.g., acetylcholine, noradrenaline, and serotonin). The system is incredibly diverse; it is extremely difficult to assign specific functions to the individual peptides. An indication of the importance of the neuropeptides for gut function is provided by hypersecretion of the peptides in neuroendocrine tumors. Thus, hyperproduction of vasoactive intestinal polypeptide (VIP) is the pathogenetic mechanism behind the watery diarrhea, hypokalemia, and achlorhydria syndrome (Verner Morrison syndrome), with its dramatic secretory diarrhea. Importantly, the intestinal neuropeptides, although in many cases isolated from and identified for the first time in the gut, are widely distributed throughout the entire organism, and have numerous important functions beyond the gut.

**Vasoactive Intestinal Polypeptides.**   VIP is one of the most abundant neuropeptides, and regulates both motility and secretion. It is a peptide of 27-amino acids and belongs to the glucagon-secretin family (see Table 182-2). Upstream in the VIP precursor is found the homologous peptide PHI or PHM (peptide histidine isoleucine in pigs and methionine in humans), which is liberated along with VIP during the processing of the precursor.[189] It shares many of the actions of VIP and seems to be an example of amplification of a neural signal by duplication of the transmitter in the precursor. *Pituitary adenylate cyclase–activating polypeptide* (PACAP), which is closely related to VIP, is a peptide of 38-amino acids originally isolated from the hypothalamus. VIP/PACAP operate via at least three receptors that are structurally related to the other receptors of this peptide family. However, one receptor is PACAP preferring (has the highest affinity for PACAP), while the remaining receptors are activated equally well by both peptides.[190] Again, because of the complexity of the peptide and receptor distribution patterns, the precise functions of these peptides are difficult to unravel, and antagonist studies have not been informative. Nonetheless, VIP seems to function in the descending relaxation of the circular muscles of the gut that constitute part of peristalsis. All three receptors typically activate adenylate cyclase via cAMP, to cause relaxation of the smooth muscles. Activation of nitric oxide synthase, leading to a production of the inhibitory transmitter nitric oxide (which activates the guanylate cyclase of the smooth muscles; see Chap. 179), also seems to play a role. Stimulation of intestinal secretion of electrolytes and water may be another important effect of the VIPergic neurons, and it is well established that the VIPergic fibers, by their relaxing effect on the smooth muscles of the vascular walls, play an important role in the regulation of blood flow in the intestine as well as elsewhere in the body.

**Neuropeptide Y.** NPY is another abundant neuropeptide in the gut, which is found both in intrinsic neurons and in extrinsic sympathetic nerve fibers, where it coexists with noradrenaline, the actions of which it seems to potentiate. The intrinsic NPY neurons may function mainly in the regulation of secretion and absorption.

**Tachykinins.** Tachykinins, the most important of which are substance P and neurokinin A, emerge by differential processing of the mRNA as well as the peptide precursors resulting from expression of the preprotachykinin gene[191]; this explains why they coexist in most tissues and nerve fibers (see Chap. 171). They activate a group of receptors, designated neurokinin 1–3 ($NK_{1-3}$),[192] which are expressed in several structures of the gut, including smooth muscles and other neurons. Importantly, the tachykinins seem to coexist with acetylcholine in excitatory motor neurons. The functions of the tachykinins have been probed with specific receptor antagonists, and, although the cholinergic activation of muscles predominates, there is little doubt that the tachykinins support or enhance reflexively stimulated intestinal contractions, and may, therefore, play an important role in generating the ascending contractions of peristalsis.[193] Substance P is also found in extrinsic sensory nerve fibers, thought to transmit nociceptive information to the dorsal horns of the spinal cord. The importance of the tachykinins for nociception and inflammation was demonstrated in mice with deletion of either the preprotachykinin or the NK1-receptor genes.[194,195] In these sensory fibers, substance P coexists with the *calcitonin gene–related polypeptide* (CGRP), a product of calcitonin gene expression (see Chap. 53). When expressed in neural tissue, the calcitonin part is excised as an intron, while the neuropeptide sequence is transcribed—another example of differential RNA precursor splicing.[196] CGRP, however, is also found in intrinsic neurons, presumably interneurons that seem to activate cholinergic motor neurons. CGRP-containing fibers are often associated with blood vessels and may help regulate blood flow, causing pronounced vasodilatation. The tachykinins are often produced in large amounts in carcinoids[197] (see Chap. 221)—the neuroendocrine tumors of the gut; here, excessive concentrations of tachykinins, together with an overproduction of serotonin, may cause flushing and diarrhea, particularly when metastases are present in the liver, which otherwise efficiently clears the plasma of the substances that cause the syndrome.

**Opioid Peptides.** Enkephalins, dynorphin, and related products are also widely distributed in the enteric nervous system (see Chap. 168). Acting via opioid receptors, their specific functions have been evaluated using specific agonists and antagonists of these receptors; however, the results have been confusing. Possibly, their main effect is to modulate neural transmission via presynaptic inhibition, as is observed in other parts of the nervous system.

**Gastrin-Releasing Peptide.** Gastrin-releasing peptide (GRP, mammalian bombesin; see Table 182-2) and the truncated form, neuromedin C, constituting the carboxyl-terminal decapeptide of GRP, are best known for their effects on gastrin secretion; however, GRP fibers are scattered throughout the GI tract. In general, GRP has a stimulatory or excitatory effect on motility as well as on exocrine or endocrine secretion. Four receptors have been cloned, and effective antagonists are available.[198,199] Mice with a knock-out of the high-affinity GRP-receptor gene should prove helpful in evaluating the receptor functions.[200] Interestingly, mice with a null mutation of the low-affinity GRP receptor (bombesin receptor subtype-3) develop obesity, hypertension, and impairment of glucose metabolism, all features that characterize the "metabolic syndrome" or "syndrome X"[201] (see Chap. 145). Finally, GRP is considered to be an autocrine growth factor (e.g., small cell lung cancers)[202] (see Chap. 219).

**Galanin and Somatostatin.** Galanin (see Table 182-2) and somatostatin are also widespread neuropeptides.[203,204] Both peptides may affect gut motility, galanin being predominantly inhibitory[205] and somatostatin being mostly excitatory. The latter is surprising in view of the generally inhibitory responses elicited by somatostatin in other tissues. In agreement with this, somatostatin profoundly inhibits neural transmission in the ganglia, and it is thought that its motor effects may be due to inhibition of an inhibitory neuron.

# REFERENCES

1. Bayliss WM, Starling EH. The mechanisms of pancreatic secretion. J Physiol 1902; 28:330.
2. Wang CC, Grossman MI. Physiological determination of release of secretin and pancreazymin from intestine of dogs with transplanted pancreas. Am J Physiol 1951; 164:527.
3. Ivy AC, Oldberg E. Hormone mechanism for gallbladder contraction and evacuation. Am J Physiol 1928; 85:599.
4. Harper AA, Raper HS. Pancreozymin, a stimulant of the secretion of pancreatic enzymes in extracts of the small intestine. J Physiol 1943; 102:115.
5. Jorpes JE, Mutt V, eds. Secretin, cholecystokinin, pancreozymin, and gastrin. New York: Springer-Verlag 1973:1.
6. Mutt V, Jorpes JE, Magnusson S. Structure of porcine secretin. The amino acid sequence. Eur J Biochem 1970;15:513.
7. Brown JC, Dryburgh JR, Frost JL, et al. Physiology and pathophysiology of GIP. Adv Exp Med Biol 1978; 106:169.
8. Brown JC, Cook MA, Dryburgh JR. Motilin, a gastric motor activity-stimulating polypeptide: final purification, amino acid composition, and C-terminal residues. Gastroenterology 1972; 62:401.
9. Pradayrol L, Chayvialle J, Mutt V. Pig duodenal somatostatin: extraction and purification. Metabolism 1978; 27:1197.
10. Fahrenkrug J, Schaffalitzky OB, Rune SJ. pH threshold for release of secretin in normal subjects and in patients with duodenal ulcer and patients with chronic pancreatitis. Scand J Gastroenterol 1978; 13:177.
11. Wormsley KG. Progress report. Is secretin secreted? Gut 1973; 14:743.
12. Schaffalitzky OB. Secretin and pancreatic bicarbonate secretion in man. Scand J Gastroenterol 1980; 61(Suppl):1.
13. Schaffalitzky OB, Fahrenkrug J, Matzen P, et al. Physiological significance of secretin in the pancreatic bicarbonate secretion. II. Pancreatic bicarbonate response to a physiological increase in plasma secretin concentration. Scand J Gastroenterol 1979; 14:85.
14. Schaffalitzky OB, Fahrenkrug J, Nielsen J, et al. Meal-stimulated secretin release in man: effect of acid and bile. Scand J Gastroenterol 1981; 16:981.
15. Chey WY, Kim MS, Lee KY, Chang TM. Effect of rabbit antisecretin serum on postprandial pancreatic secretion in dogs. Gastroenterology 1979; 77:1268.
16. Liddle RA, Gertz BJ, Kanayama S, et al. Effects of a novel cholecystokinin (CCK) receptor antagonist, MK-329, on gallbladder contraction and gastric emptying in humans. Implications for the physiology of CCK. J Clin Invest 1989; 84:1220.

17. Kopin AS, Nguyen M, Chiu M, et al. CCK-A receptor deficient mice develop gallstones and lack of CCK mediated inhibition of food intake. Regul Pept 1996; 64:97.
18. Sawada M, Dickinson CJ. The G cell. Annu Rev Physiol 1997; 59:273.
19. Walsh JH, ed. Gastrin. New York: Raven Press, 1993:1.
20. Kovacs TO, Walsh JH, Maxwell V, et al. Gastrin is a major mediator of the gastric phase of acid secretion in dogs: proof by monoclonal antibody neutralization. Gastroenterology 1989; 97:1406.
21. Friis-Hansen L, Sundler F, Li Y, et al. Impaired gastric acid secretion in gastrin-deficient mice. Am J Physiol 1998; 274:G561.
22. Langhans N, Rindi G, Chiu M, et al. Abnormal gastric histology and decreased acid production in cholecystokinin-B/gastrin receptor-deficient mice. Gastroenterology 1997; 112:280.
23. Kopin AS, Lee YM, McBride EW, et al. Expression cloning and characterization of the canine parietal cell gastrin receptor. Proc Natl Acad Sci U S A 1992; 89:3605.
24. Håkanson R, Chen D, Sundler F. The ECL cells. In: Johnson LR, ed. Handbook of gastrointestinal physiology. New York: Raven Press, 1994:1171.
25. Gantz I, Schaffer M, DelValle J, et al. Molecular cloning of a gene encoding the histamine H2 receptor [published erratum appears in Proc Natl Acad Sci U S A 1991; 88(13):5937]. Proc Natl Acad Sci U S A 1991; 88:429.
26. Miyazaki Y, Shinomura Y, Tsutsui S, et al. Gastrin induces heparin-binding epidermal growth factor-like growth factor in rat gastric epithelial cells transfected with gastrin receptor. Gastroenterology 1999; 116:78.
27. Nagata A, Ito M, Iwata N, et al. G protein-coupled cholecystokinin-B/gastrin receptors are responsible for physiological cell growth of the stomach mucosa in vivo. Proc Natl Acad Sci U S A 1996; 93:11825.
28. Wang TC, Koh TJ, Varro A, et al. Processing and proliferative effects of human progastrin in transgenic mice. J Clin Invest 1996; 98:1918.
29. Baldwin GS, Whitehead RH. Gut hormones, growth and malignancy. Baillière's Clin Endocrinol Metab 1994; 8:185.
30. Joshi SN, Gardner JD. Gastrin and colon cancer: a unifying hypothesis. Dig Dis 1996; 14:334.
31. Chen D, Destree M, Hakanson R, Willems G. Endogenous hypergastrinaemia does not promote growth of colonic mucosa or of a transplanted colon adenocarcinoma in rats. Eur J Gastroenterol Hepatol 1998; 10:293.
32. Smith JP, Verderame MF, Zagon IS. Antisense oligonucleotides to gastrin inhibit growth of human pancreatic cancer. Cancer Lett 1999; 135:107.
33. Calam J, Gibbons A, Healey ZV, et al. How does Helicobacter pylori cause mucosal damage? Its effect on acid and gastrin physiology. Gastroenterology 1997; 113:S43.
34. Vinayek R, Frucht H, Chiang HC, et al. Zollinger-Ellison syndrome. Recent advances in the management of the gastrinoma. Gastroenterol Clin North Am 1990; 19:197.
35. Monstein HJ, Nylander AG, Salehi A, et al. Cholecystokinin-A and cholecystokinin-B/gastrin receptor mRNA expression in the gastrointestinal tract and pancreas of the rat and man. A polymerase chain reaction study. Scand J Gastroenterol 1996; 31:383.
36. Nishimori I, Kamakura M, Fujikawa-Adachi K, et al. Cholecystokinin A and B receptor mRNA expression in human pancreas. Pancreas 1999; 19:109.
37. Morisset J, Levenez F, Corring T, et al. Pig pancreatic acinar cells possess predominantly the CCK-B receptor subtype. Am J Physiol 1996; 271:E397.
38. Philippe C, Lhoste EF, Dufresne M, et al. Pharmacological and biochemical evidence for the simultaneous expression of CCKB/gastrin and CCKA receptors in the pig pancreas. Br J Pharmacol 1997; 120:447.
39. Liddle RA. Cholecystokinin cells [published erratum appears in Annu Rev Physiol 1998; 60:XII]. Annu Rev Physiol 1997; 59:221.
40. Takahashi Y, Kato K, Hayashizaki Y, et al. Molecular cloning of the human cholecystokinin gene by use of a synthetic probe containing deoxyinosine. Proc Natl Acad Sci U S A 1985; 82:1931.
41. Mutt V, Jorpes JE. Structure of porcine cholecystokinin-pancreozymin. 1. Cleavage with thrombin and with trypsin. Eur J Biochem 1968; 6:156.
42. Rehfeld JF. Accurate measurement of cholecystokinin in plasma. Clin Chem 1998; 44:991.
43. Rehfeld JF, Holst JJ, Jensen SL. The molecular nature of vascularly released cholecystokinin from the isolated perfused porcine duodenum. Regul Pept 1982; 3:15.
44. McLaughlin JT, Lomax RB, Hall L, et al. Fatty acids stimulate cholecystokinin secretion via an acyl chain length-specific, $Ca^{2+}$-dependent mechanism in the enteroendocrine cell line STC-1. J Physiol 1998; 513 (Pt 1):11.
45. McLaughlin J, Grazia LM, Jones MN, et al. Fatty acid chain length determines cholecystokinin secretion and effect on human gastric motility. Gastroenterology 1999; 116:46.
46. Miyasaka K, Funakoshi A. Luminal feedback regulation, monitor peptide, CCK-releasing peptide, and CCK receptors. Pancreas 1998; 16:277.
47. Wank SA, Pisegna JR, de Weerth A. Brain and gastrointestinal cholecystokinin receptor family: structure and functional expression. Proc Natl Acad Sci U S A 1992; 89:8691.
48. Jensen RT. CCKB/gastrin receptor antagonists: recent advances and potential uses in gastric secretory disorders. Yale J Biol Med 1996; 69:245.
49. Dunlop J. CCK receptor antagonists. Gen Pharmacol 1998; 31:519.
50. Samuelson LC, Gillespie PJ, May JM, et al. Generation of a CCK loss of function mutation in the mouse by homologous recombination in the ES cells. Regul Pept 1996; 64:166.
51. Kopin AS, Mathes WF, McBride EW, et al. The cholecystokinin-A receptor mediates inhibition of food intake yet is not essential for the maintenance of body weight [published erratum appears in J Clin Invest 1999; 103(5):759]. J Clin Invest 1999; 103:383.
52. Takiguchi S, Takata Y, Funakoshi A, et al. Disrupted cholecystokinin type-A receptor (CCKAR) gene in OLETF rats. Gene 1997; 197:169.
53. Nakamura H, Kihara Y, Tashiro M, et al. Defects of cholecystokinin (CCK)-A receptor gene expression and CCK-A receptor-mediated biological functions in Otsuka Long-Evans Tokushima Fatty (OLETF) rats. J Gastroenterol 1998; 33:702.
54. Schmidt WE, Creutzfeldt W, Schleser A, et al. Role of CCK in regulation of pancreaticobiliary functions and GI motility in humans: effects of loxiglumide. Am J Physiol 1991; 260:G197.
55. Cantor P, Mortensen PE, Myhre J, et al. The effect of the cholecystokinin receptor antagonist MK-329 on meal-stimulated pancreaticobiliary output in humans. Gastroenterology 1992; 102:1742.
56. Adler G, Beglinger C, Braun U, et al. Interaction of the cholinergic system and cholecystokinin in the regulation of endogenous and exogenous stimulation of pancreatic secretion in humans. Gastroenterology 1991; 100:537.
57. Adler G, Nelson DK, Katschinski M, Beglinger C. Neurohormonal control of human pancreatic exocrine secretion. Pancreas 1995; 10:1.
58. Hillsley K, Grundy D. Serotonin and cholecystokinin activate different populations of rat mesenteric vagal afferents. Neurosci Lett 1998; 255:63.
59. Schmidt WE, Schenk S, Nustede R, et al. Cholecystokinin is a negative regulator of gastric acid secretion and postprandial release of gastrin in humans. Gastroenterology 1994; 107:1610.
60. Zerbib F, Bruley des Varannes S, Scarpignato C, et al. Endogenous cholecystokinin in postprandial lower esophageal sphincter function and fundic tone in humans. Am J Physiol 1998; 275:G1266.
61. Read N, French S, Cunningham K. The role of the gut in regulating food intake in man. Nutr Rev 1994; 52:1.
62. Rose C, Vargas F, Facchinetti P, et al. Characterization and inhibition of a cholecystokinin-inactivating serine peptidase. Nature 1996; 380:403.
63. Moran TH, Katz LF, Plata-Salaman CR, Schwartz GJ. Disordered food intake and obesity in rats lacking cholecystokinin A receptors. Am J Physiol 1998; 274:R618.
64. Dorre D, Smith GP. Cholecystokinin B receptor antagonist increases food intake in rats. Physiol Behav 1998; 65:11.
65. Fieseler P, Bridenbaugh S, Nustede R, et al. Physiological augmentation of amino acid-induced insulin secretion by GIP and GLP-I but not by CCK-8. Am J Physiol 1995; 268:E949.
66. Dauge V, Lena I. CCK in anxiety and cognitive processes. Neurosci Biobehav Rev 1998; 22:815.
67. Revel L, Mennuni L, Garofalo P, Makovec F. CR 2945: a novel CCKB receptor antagonist with anxiolytic-like activity. Behav Pharmacol 1998; 9:183.
68. Fink H, Rex A, Voits M, Voigt JP. Major biological actions of CCK—a critical evaluation of research findings. Exp Brain Res 1998; 123:77.
69. Schaffalitzky OB, Fahrenkrug J, Rune SJ. Physiological significance of secretin in the pancreatic bicarbonate secretion. I. Responsiveness of the secretin-releasing system in the upper duodenum. Scand J Gastroenterol 1979; 14:79.
70. Ulrich CD, Holtmann M, Miller LJ. Secretin and vasoactive intestinal peptide receptors: members of a unique family of G protein-coupled receptors. Gastroenterology 1998; 114:382.
71. Herzig KH. Cholecystokinin- and secretin-releasing peptides in the intestine—a new regulatory interendocrine mechanism in the gastrointestinal tract. Regul Pept 1998; 73:89.
72. Argent BE, Case RM. Pancreatic ducts: cellular mechanism and control of bicarbonate secretion. In: Johnson LR, ed. Handbook of gastrointestinal physiology. New York: Raven Press, 1994;1473.
73. Park HS, Lee YL, Kwon HY, et al. Significant cholinergic role in secretin-stimulated exocrine secretion in isolated rat pancreas. Am J Physiol 1998; 274:G413.
74. Holst JJ, Schaffalitzky de Muckadell OB, Fahrenkrug J. Nervous control of pancreatic exocrine secretion in pigs. Acta Physiol Scand 1979; 105:33.
75. Erlinger S. New insights into the mechanisms of hepatic transport and bile secretion. J Gastroenterol Hepatol 1996; 11:575.
76. Marinelli RA, Pham L, Agre P, LaRusso NF. Secretin promotes osmotic water transport in rat cholangiocytes by increasing aquaporin-1 water channels in plasma membrane. Evidence for a secretin-induced vesicular translocation of aquaporin-1. J Biol Chem 1997; 272:12984.
77. Marinelli RA, Tietz PS, Pham LD, et al. Secretin induces the apical insertion of aquaporin-1 water channels in rat cholangiocytes. Am J Physiol 1999; 276:G280.
78. Kleibeuker JH, Eysselein VE, Maxwell VE, Walsh JH. Role of endogenous secretin in acid-induced inhibition of human gastric function. J Clin Invest 1984; 73:526.
79. Chey WY, Kim MS, Lee KY, Chang TM. Secretin is an enterogastrone in the dog. Am J Physiol 1981; 240:G239.
80. Lloyd KC, Amirmoazzami S, Friedik F, et al. Candidate canine enterogastrones: acid inhibition before and after vagotomy. Am J Physiol 1997; 272:G1236.
81. de Lecea L, Kilduff TS, Peyron C, et al. The hypocretins: hypothalamus-specific peptides with neuroexcitatory activity. Proc Natl Acad Sci U S A 1998; 95:322.
82. Sakurai T, Amemiya A, Ishii M, et al. Orexins and orexin receptors: a family of hypothalamic neuropeptides and G protein-coupled receptors that regulate feeding behavior. Cell 1998; 92:573.
83. Conter RL, Hughes MT, Kauffman GLJ. Intracerebroventricular secretin enhances pancreatic volume and bicarbonate response in rats. Surgery 1996; 119:208.

84. Itoh Z. Motilin and clinical application. Peptides 1997; 18:593.

85. Depoortere I, Van Assche G, Peeters TL. Distribution and subcellular localization of motilin binding sites in the rabbit brain. Brain Res 1997; 777:103.

86. Depoortere I, De Clercq P, Svoboda M, et al. Identification of motilin mRNA in the brain of man and rabbit. Conservation of polymorphism of the motilin gene across species. Peptides 1997; 18:1497.

87. Seino Y, Tanaka K, Takeda J, et al. Sequence of an intestinal cDNA encoding human motilin precursor. FEBS Lett 1987; 223:74.

88. Goll R, Nielsen SH, Holst JJ. Regulation of motilin release from isolated perfused pig duodenum. Digestion 1996; 57:341.

89. Poitras P. Motilin is a digestive hormone in the dog. Gastroenterology 1984; 87:909.

90. Qvist N, Oster-Jorgensen E, Pedersen SA, et al. Increases in plasma motilin follow each episode of gallbladder emptying during the interdigestive period, and changes in serum bile acid concentration correlate to plasma motilin. Scand J Gastroenterol 1995; 30:122.

91. Poitras P, Miller P, Dickner M, et al. Heterogeneity of motilin receptors in the gastrointestinal tract of the rabbit. Peptides 1996; 17:701.

92. Boivin M, Pinelo LR, St.-Pierre S, Poitras P. Neural mediation of the motilin motor effect on the human antrum. Am J Physiol 1997; 272:G71.

93. Siadati M, Sarr MG. Role of extrinsic innervation in release of motilin and patterns of upper gut canine motility. J Gastrointest Surg 1998; 2:363.

94. Peeters TL. Erythromycin and other macrolides as prokinetic agents. Gastroenterology 1993; 105:1886.

95. Peeters TL, Depoortere I. Motilin receptor: a model for development of prokinetics. Dig Dis Sci 1994; 39:76S.

96. Ishii M, Nakamura T, Kasai F, et al. Erythromycin derivative improves gastric emptying and insulin requirement in diabetic patients with gastroparesis. Diabetes Care 1997; 20:1134.

97. Takeda J, Seino Y, Tanaka K, et al. Sequence of an intestinal cDNA encoding human gastric inhibitory polypeptide precursor. Proc Natl Acad Sci U S A 1987; 84:7005.

98. Krarup T. Immunoreactive gastric inhibitory polypeptide. Endocr Rev 1988; 9:122.

99. Usdin TB, Mezey E, Button DC, et al. Gastric inhibitory polypeptide receptor, a member of the secretin-vasoactive intestinal peptide receptor family, is widely distributed in peripheral organs and the brain. Endocrinology 1993; 133:2861.

100. Pederson RA. Gastric inhibitory polypeptide. In: Walsh JH, Dockray GJ, eds. Gut peptides. New York: Raven Press, 1994:217.

101. Ding WG, Renstrom E, Rorsman P, et al. Glucagon-like peptide I and glucose-dependent insulinotropic polypeptide stimulate $Ca^{2+}$-induced secretion in rat alpha-cells by a protein kinase A-mediated mechanism. Diabetes 1997; 46:792.

102. Lauritsen KB, Holst JJ, Moody AJ. Depression of insulin release by anti-GIP serum after oral glucose in rats. Scand J Gastroenterol 1981; 16:417.

103. Tseng CC, Kieffer TJ, Jarboe LA, et al. Postprandial stimulation of insulin release by glucose-dependent insulinotropic polypeptide (GIP). Effect of a specific glucose-dependent insulinotropic polypeptide receptor antagonist in the rat. J Clin Invest 1996; 98:2440.

104. Miyawaki K, Yamada Y, Ihara Y, et al. Glucose intolerance in mice with disruption of the gastric inhibitory polypeptide receptor gene. Proc Natl Acad Sci U S A 1999; 96:14843.

105. Morgan LM. The role of gastrointestinal hormones in carbohydrate and lipid metabolism and homeostasis: effects of gastric inhibitory polypeptide and glucagon-like peptide-1. Biochem Soc Trans 1998; 26:216.

106. Yip RG, Boylan MO, Kieffer TJ, Wolfe MM. Functional GIP receptors are present on adipocytes. Endocrinology 1998; 139:4004.

107. McIntosh CH, Bremsak I, Lynn FC, et al. Glucose-dependent insulinotropic polypeptide stimulation of lipolysis in differentiated 3T3-L1 cells: wortmannin-sensitive inhibition by insulin. Endocrinology 1999; 140:398.

108. Walsh JH. Gastrointestinal hormones. In: Johnson LR, ed. Handbook of gastrointestinal physiology. New York: Raven Press, 1994:1.

109. de Herder WW, Hofland LJ, Usdin TB, et al. Food-dependent Cushing's syndrome resulting from abundant expression of gastric inhibitory polypeptide receptors in adrenal adenoma cells. J Clin Endocrinol Metab 1996; 81:3168.

110. Lebrethon MC, Avallet O, Reznik Y, et al. Food-dependent Cushing's syndrome: characterization and functional role of gastric inhibitory polypeptide receptor in the adrenals of three patients. J Clin Endocrinol Metab 1998; 83:4514.

111. Holst JJ, Gromada J, Nauck MA. The pathogenesis of NIDDM involves a defective expression of the GIP receptor. Diabetologia 1997; 40:984.

112. Kubota A, Yamada Y, Hayami T, et al. Identification of two missense mutations in the GIP receptor gene: a functional study and association analysis with NIDDM: no evidence of association with Japanese NIDDM subjects. Diabetes 1996; 45:1701.

113. Almind K, Ambye L, Urhammer SA, et al. Discovery of amino acid variants in the human glucose-dependent insulinotropic polypeptide (GIP) receptor: the impact on the pancreatic beta cell responses and functional expression studies in Chinese hamster fibroblast cells. Diabetologia 1998; 41:1194.

114. Gama R, Norris F, Morgan L, et al. Elevated postprandial gastric inhibitory polypeptide concentrations in hypertriglyceridaemic subjects. Clin Sci (Colch) 1997; 93:343.

115. Chiba T, Yamada T. Gut somatostatin. In: Walsh JH, Dockray GJ, eds. Gut peptides. New York: Raven Press, 1994:123.

116. Baldissera FG, Nielsen OV, Holst JJ. The intestinal mucosa preferentially releases somatostatin-28 in pigs. Regul Pept 1985; 11:251.

117. Bell GI, Reisine T. Molecular biology of somatostatin receptors. Trends Neurosci 1993; 16:34.

118. Hildebrand P, Ensinck JW, Gyr K, et al. Evidence for hormonal inhibition of exocrine pancreatic function by somatostatin 28 in humans. Gastroenterology 1992; 103:240.

119. Baumbach WR, Carrick TA, Pausch MH, et al. A linear hexapeptide somatostatin antagonist blocks somatostatin activity in vitro and influences growth hormone release in rats. Mol Pharmacol 1998; 54:864.

120. Liu S, Tang C, Ho B, et al. Nonpeptide somatostatin agonists with sst4 selectivity: synthesis and structure-activity relationships of thioureas. J Med Chem 1998; 41:4693.

121. Rossowski WJ, Cheng BL, Jiang NY, Coy DH. Examination of somatostatin involvement in the inhibitory action of GIP, GLP-1, amylin and adrenomedullin on gastric acid release using a new SRIF antagonist analogue. Br J Pharmacol 1998; 125:1081.

122. Orloff SL, Bunnett NW, Walsh JH, Debas HT. Intestinal acid inhibits gastric acid secretion by neural and hormonal mechanisms in rats. Am J Physiol 1992; 262:G165.

123. Martinez V, Curi AP, Torkian B, et al. High basal gastric acid secretion in somatostatin receptor subtype 2 knockout mice. Gastroenterology 1998; 114:1125.

124. Schusdziarra V, Zyznar E, Rouiller D, et al. Splanchnic somatostatin: a hormonal regulator of nutrient homeostasis. Science 1980; 207:530.

125. de Lecea L, Criado JR, Prospero-Garcia O, et al. A cortical neuropeptide with neuronal depressant and sleep-modulating properties. Nature 1996; 381:242.

126. Fukusumi S, Kitada C, Takekawa S, et al. Identification and characterization of a novel human cortistatin-like peptide. Biochem Biophys Res Commun 1997; 232:157.

127. Vasilaki A, Lanneau C, Dournaud P, et al. Cortistatin affects glutamate sensitivity in mouse hypothalamic neurons through activation of sst2 somatostatin receptor subtype. Neuroscience 1999; 88:359.

128. Service FJ. Insulinoma and other islet-cell tumors. Cancer Treat Res 1997; 89:335.

129. Arnold R, Frank M. Control of growth in neuroendocrine gastroenteropancreatic tumours. Digestion 1996; 57(S1):69.

130. Reubi JC. Regulatory peptide receptors as molecular targets for cancer diagnosis and therapy. Q J Nucl Med 1997; 41:63.

131. Calam J. Helicobacter pylori and somatostatin cells. Eur J Gastroenterol Hepatol 1998; 10:281.

132. Tham TC, Chen L, Dennison N, et al. Effect of Helicobacter pylori eradication on antral somatostatin cell density in humans. Eur J Gastroenterol Hepatol 1998; 10:289.

133. Holst JJ. Enteroglucagon. Annu Rev Physiol 1997; 59:257.

134. Thorens B, Porret A, Buhler L, et al. Cloning and functional expression of the human islet GLP-1 receptor. Demonstration that exendin-4 is an agonist and exendin-(9–39) an antagonist of the receptor. Diabetes 1993; 42:1678.

135. Kolligs F, Fehmann HC, Goke R, Goke B. Reduction of the incretin effect in rats by the glucagon-like peptide 1 receptor antagonist exendin (9-39) amide. Diabetes 1995; 44:16.

136. Scrocchi LA, Brown TJ, MaClusky N, et al. Glucose intolerance but normal satiety in mice with a null mutation in the glucagon-like peptide 1 receptor gene. Nat Med 1996; 2:1254.

137. Nauck MA, Heimesaat MM, Orskov C, et al. Preserved incretin activity of glucagon-like peptide 1 [7–36 amide] but not of synthetic human gastric inhibitory polypeptide in patients with type-2 diabetes mellitus. J Clin Invest 1993; 91:301.

138. Nauck MA, Kleine N, Orskov C, et al. Normalization of fasting hyperglycaemia by exogenous glucagon-like peptide 1 (7-36 amide) in type 2 (non-insulin-dependent) diabetic patients. Diabetologia 1993; 36:741.

139. Holst JJ. Treatment of type 2 diabetes with glucagonlike peptide 1. Curr Opin Endocrinol Diabetes 1998; 5:108.

139a. Vella A, Shah P, Basu R, et al. Effect of glucagon-like peptide-1 (7–36) in people with type 2 diabetes. Diabetes 2000; 49:611.

139b. Vilsboll T, Toft-Nielsen MB, Krarup T. Evaluation of beta-cell secretory capacity using glucagon-like peptide-1. Diab Care 2000; 23:807.

140. Wettergren A, Schjoldager B, Mortensen PE, et al. Truncated GLP-1 (proglucagon 78–107-amide) inhibits gastric and pancreatic functions in man. Dig Dis Sci 1993; 38:665.

141. Nauck MA, Niedereichholz U, Ettler R, et al. Glucagon-like peptide 1 inhibition of gastric emptying outweighs its insulinotropic effects in healthy humans. Am J Physiol 1997; 273:E981.

142. MacFarlane A, Kinsman R, Read NW. The ileal brake: ileal fat slows small bowel transit and gastric emptying in man. Gut 1983; 24:471.

143. Wettergren A, Wojdemann M, Holst JJ. Glucagon-like peptide-1 inhibits gastropancreatic function by inhibiting central parasympathetic outflow. Am J Physiol 1998; 275:G984.

144. Holst JJ, Deacon CF. Inhibition of the activity of dipeptidyl-peptidase IV as a treatment for type 2 diabetes. Diabetes 1998; 47:1663.

145. Flint A, Raben A, Astrup A, Holst JJ. Glucagon-like peptide 1 promotes satiety and suppresses energy intake in humans. J Clin Invest 1998; 101:515.

146. Wei Y, Mojsov S. Tissue-specific expression of the human receptor for glucagon-like peptide-I: brain, heart and pancreatic forms have the same deduced amino acid sequences. FEBS Lett 1995; 358:219.

147. Turton MD, O'Shea D, Gunn I, et al. A role for glucagon-like peptide-1 in the central regulation of feeding. Nature 1996; 379:69.

148. Wojdemann M, Wettergren A, Hartmann B, et al. Inhibition of sham feeding-stimulated human gastric acid secretion by glucagon-like peptide-2. J Clin Endocrinol Metab 1999; 84:2513.

149. Drucker DJ, Erlich P, Asa SL, Brubaker PL. Induction of intestinal epithelial proliferation by glucagon-like peptide 2. Proc Natl Acad Sci U S A 1996; 93:7911.

150. Bloom SR. Gut hormones in adaptation. Gut 1987; 28(Suppl):31.

151. Chance WT, Foley-Nelson T, Thomas I, Balasubramaniam A. Prevention of parenteral nutrition-induced gut hypoplasia by coinfusion of glucagon-like peptide-2. Am J Physiol 1997; 273:G559.

152. Munroe DG, Gupta AK, Kooshesh F, et al. Prototypic G protein-coupled receptor for the intestinotrophic factor glucagon-like peptide 2. Proc Natl Acad Sci U S A 1999; 96:1569.

153. Shulkes A. Neurotensin. In: Walsh JH, Dockray GJ, eds. Gut peptides. New York: Raven Press, 1994:371.

154. Dobner PR, Barber DL, Villa-Komaroff L, McKiernan C. Cloning and sequence analysis of cDNA for the canine neurotensin/neuromedin N precursor. Proc Natl Acad Sci U S A 1987; 84:3516.

155. Rostene WH, Alexander MJ. Neurotensin and neuroendocrine regulation. Front Neuroendocrinol 1997; 18:115.

156. Tanaka K, Masu M, Nakanishi S. Structure and functional expression of the cloned rat neurotensin receptor. Neuron 1990; 4:847.

157. Yamada M, Lombet A, Forgez P, Rostene W. Distinct functional characteristics of levocabastine sensitive rat neurotensin NT2 receptor expressed in Chinese hamster ovary cells. Life Sci 1998; 62:(PL) 375.

158. Mendez M, Souaze F, Nagano M, et al. High affinity neurotensin receptor mRNA distribution in rat brain and peripheral tissues. Analysis by quantitative RT-PCR. J Mol Neurosci 1997; 9:93.

159. Mogard MH, Maxwell V, Sytnik B, Walsh JH. Regulation of gastric acid secretion by neurotensin in man. Evidence against a hormonal role. J Clin Invest 1987; 80:1064.

160. Gullo L, De Giorgio R, Corinaldesi R, Barbara L. Neurotensin: a physiological regulator of exocrine pancreatic secretion? Ital J Gastroenterol 1992; 24:347.

161. Gully D, Lespy L, Canton M, et al. Effect of the neurotensin receptor antagonist SR48692 on rat blood pressure modulation by neurotensin. Life Sci 1996; 58:665.

162. Castagliuolo I, Wang CC, Valenick L, et al. Neurotensin is a proinflammatory neuropeptide in colonic inflammation. J Clin Invest 1999; 103:843.

163. Maoret JJ, Anini Y, Rouyer-Fessard C, et al. Neurotensin and a non-peptide neurotensin receptor antagonist control human colon cancer cell growth in cell culture and in cells xenografted into nude mice. Int J Cancer 1999; 80:448.

164. Larhammar D. Evolution of neuropeptide Y, peptide YY and pancreatic polypeptide. Regul Pept 1996; 62:1.

165. Mass MI, Hopman WP, Katan MB, Jansen JB. Release of peptide YY and inhibition of gastric acid secretion by long-chain and medium-chain triglycerides but not by sucrose polyester in men. Eur J Clin Invest 1998; 28:123.

166. Liu CD, Hines OJ, Newton TR, et al. Cholecystokinin mediation of colonic absorption via peptide YY: foregut-hindgut axis. World J Surg 1996; 20:221.

167. Larhammar D. Structural diversity of receptors for neuropeptide Y, peptide YY and pancreatic polypeptide. Regul Pept 1996; 65:165.

168. Widdowson PS, Upton R, Henderson L, et al. Reciprocal regional changes in brain NPY receptor density during dietary restriction and dietary-induced obesity in the rat. Brain Res 1997; 774:1.

169. Inui A. Neuropeptide Y feeding receptors: are multiple subtypes involved? Trends Pharmacol Sci 1999; 20:43.

170. Nakanishi T, Kanayama S, Kiyohara T, et al. Peptide YY-induced alteration of colonic electrolyte transport in the rat. Regul Pept 1996; 61:149.

171. Chen CH, Rogers RC. Central inhibitory action of peptide YY on gastric motility in rats. Am J Physiol 1995;269:R787.

172. Wettergren A, Petersen H, Orskov C, et al. Glucagon-like peptide-1 7–36 amide and peptide YY from the L-cell of the ileal mucosa are potent inhibitors of vagally induced gastric acid secretion in man. Scand J Gastroenterol 1994; 29:501.

173. Wettergren A, Maina P, Boesby S, Holst JJ. Glucagon-like peptide-1 7–36 amide and peptide YY have additive inhibitory effect on gastric acid secretion in man. Scand J Gastroenterol 1997; 32:552.

174. Ropert A, Cherbut C, Roze C, et al. Colonic fermentation and proximal gastric tone in humans. Gastroenterology 1996; 111:289.

175. Erickson JC, Clegg KE, Palmiter RD. Sensitivity to leptin and susceptibility to seizures of mice lacking neuropeptide Y. Nature 1996; 381:415.

176. Lin HC, Zhao XT, Wang L, Wong H. Fat-induced ileal brake in the dog depends on peptide YY. Gastroenterology 1996; 110:1491.

177. Zhao XT, Walsh JH, Wong H, et al. Intestinal fat-induced inhibition of meal-stimulated gastric acid secretion depends on CCK but not peptide YY. Am J Physiol 1999; 276:G550.

178. Adrian TE, Mitchenere P, Sagor G, Bloom SR. Effect of pancreatic polypeptide on gallbladder pressure and hepatic bile secretion. Am J Physiol 1982; 243:G204.

179. Christiansen J, Lorentzen M, Holst J. Influence of peptides on anorectal function. Ann Med 1990; 22:413.

180. Larsson LI, Goltermann N, de Magistris L, et al. Somatostatin cell processes as pathways for paracrine secretion. Science 1979; 205:1393.

181. Holst JJ, Jorgensen PN, Rasmussen TN, Schmidt P. Somatostatin restraint of gastrin secretion in pigs revealed by monoclonal antibody immunoneutralization. Am J Physiol 1992; 263:G908.

182. Holst JJ, Orskov C, Seier-Poulsen S. Somatostatin is an essential paracrine link in acid inhibition of gastrin secretion. Digestion 1992; 51:95.

183. Holst JJ, Skak-Nielsen T, Orskov C, Seier-Poulsen S. Vagal control of the release of somatostatin, vasoactive intestinal polypeptide, gastrin-releasing peptide, and HCl from porcine non-antral stomach. Scand J Gastroenterol 1992; 27:677.

184. Park J, Chiba T, Yakabi K, Yamada T. Cholecystokinin (CCK) stimulates somatostatin release from isolated canine D-cells via both gastrin and CCK-selective receptors. Gastroenterology 1987; 92:1566.

185. Beglinger C, Hildebrand P, Meier R, et al. A physiological role for cholecystokinin as a regulator of gastrin secretion. Gastroenterology 1992; 103:490.

186. Furness JB, Costa M. The enteric nervous system. Edinburgh: Churchill Livingstone, 1987:1.

187. Daniel EE. Neuropeptide function in the gastrointestinal tract. Boca Raton, FL: CRC Press, 1990:1.

188. Furness JB, Bornstein JC, Murphy R, Pompolo S. Roles of peptides in transmission in the enteric nervous system. Trends Neurosci 1992; 15:66.

189. Itoh N, Obata K, Yanaihara N, Okamoto H. Human preprovasoactive intestinal polypeptide contains a novel PHI-27-like peptide, PHM. Nature 1983; 304:547.

190. Arimura A. Perspectives on pituitary adenylate cyclase activating polypeptide (PACAP) in the neuroendocrine, endocrine, and nervous systems. Jpn J Physiol 1998; 48:301.

191. Nakanishi S. Substance P precursor and kininogen: their structures, gene organizations, and regulation. Physiol Rev 1987; 67:1117.

192. Nakanishi S. Mammalian tachykinin receptors. Annu Rev Neurosci 1991; 14:123.

193. Schmidt PT, Holst JJ. Use of antagonists to define tachykininergic control of intestinal motility in pigs. Peptides 1997; 18:373.

194. Cao YQ, Mantyh PW, Carlson EJ, et al. Primary afferent tachykinins are required to experience moderate to intense pain. Nature 1998; 392:390.

195. De Felipe C, Herrero JF, O'Brien JA, et al. Altered nociception, analgesia and aggression in mice lacking the receptor for substance P. Nature 1998; 392:394.

196. Rosenfeld MG, Mermod JJ, Amara SG, et al. Production of a novel neuropeptide encoded by the calcitonin gene via tissue-specific RNA processing. Nature 1983; 304:129.

197. Mertz HR, Walsh JH. Gastrointestinal neuroendocrine tumours. In: Walsh JH, Dockray GJ, eds. Gut peptides. New York: Raven Press, 1994:785.

198. Milusheva EA, Kortezova NI, Mizhorkova ZN, et al. Role of different bombesin receptor subtypes mediating contractile activity in cat upper gastrointestinal tract. Peptides 1998; 19:549.

199. Pradhan TK, Katsuno T, Taylor JE, et al. Identification of a unique ligand which has high affinity for all four bombesin receptor subtypes. Eur J Pharmacol 1998; 343:275.

200. Wada E, Watase K, Yamada K, et al. Generation and characterization of mice lacking gastrin-releasing peptide receptor. Biochem Biophys Res Commun 1997; 239:28.

201. Ohki-Hamazaki H, Watase K, Yamamoto K, et al. Mice lacking bombesin receptor subtype-3 develop metabolic defects and obesity. Nature 1997; 390:165.

202. Siegfried JM, Han YH, DeMichele MA, et al. Production of gastrin-releasing peptide by a non-small cell lung carcinoma cell line adapted to serum-free and growth factor-free conditions. J Biol Chem 1994; 269:8596.

203. Harling H, Messell T, Poulsen SS, et al. Galanin and vasoactive intestinal polypeptide: coexistence and corelease from the vascularly perfused pig ileum during distension and chemical stimulation of the mucosa. Digestion 1991; 50:61.

204. Skak-Nielsen T, Holst JJ, Baldissera FG, Poulsen SS. Localization in the gastrointestinal tract of immunoreactive prosomatostatin. Regul Pept 1987; 19:183.

205. Rattan S. Role of galanin in the gut. Gastroenterology 1991; 100:1762.

# C H A P T E R   1 8 3

# THE ENDOCRINE KIDNEY

ALAN DUBROW AND LUCA DESIMONE

The kidney, in addition to playing a major role in volume homeostasis, also functions as part of the endocrine system. The components of the endocrine kidney include the renin-angiotensin system (RAS), prostaglandins, the kallikrein-kinin system, vitamin D, erythropoietin, and endothelin.

## RENIN-ANGIOTENSIN SYSTEM

The interrelationship of structure and function is evident in the juxtaglomerular apparatus in the juxtaposition of the macula

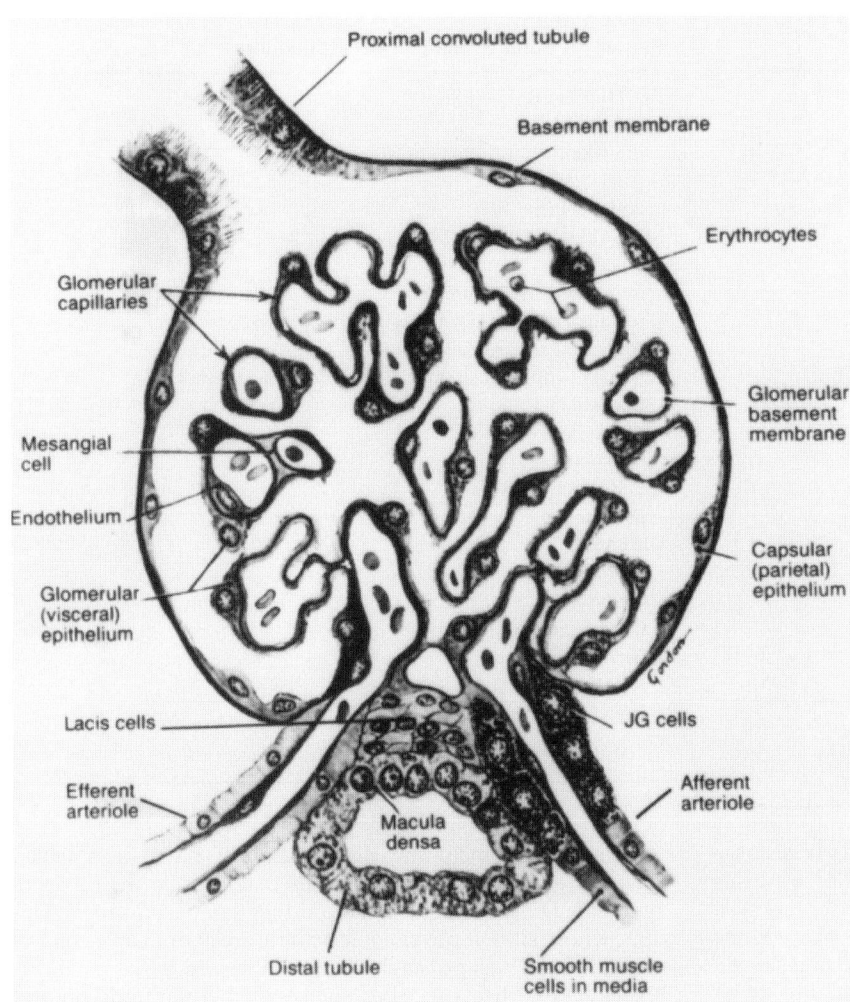

**FIGURE 183-1.** The juxtaglomerular (*JG*) apparatus is a triangular-shaped formation situated at the hilus of the glomerulus. It comprises the macula densa, consisting of modified small, cuboidal epithelial cells at the commencement of the distal renal convoluted tubule, which are immediately adjacent to the afferent arteriole. The granular cells (myoepithelioid, epithelioid, or JG cells) are located within the media of the distal region of the afferent arteriole at its junction with the glomerulus. These are modified smooth muscle cells possessing secretory granules that contain renin. The extraglomerular mesangial cells (agranular, lacis, or Goormaghtigh cells) lie adjacent to the macula densa, filling the space between the arterioles and the distal tubular cells. They possess contractile myofibrils and also appear to contain renin. Renin is found principally in cells near the distal afferent arteriole and is released by conditions that decrease extracellular fluid volume or blood pressure (decreased effective intravascular volume) or that augment sympathetic output. The specific mechanisms of renin release from the JG apparatus are not agreed on, although it is stimulated by intracellular cyclic adenosine monophosphate and inhibited by calcium. The baroreceptor concept postulates that decreased renal arteriolar pressure is sensed by the granular cells, which then increase renin output. The macula densa concept postulates the presence of receptors sensitive to the decreased transport or concentration of sodium and chloride in the distal tubules, which then increase renin output. Additional influences include direct stimulation of renin release by sympathetic discharge and by humoral factors such as angiotensin II, endothelin, vasopressin, and adenosine, all of which are inhibitory. (Modified from Ham AW. Histology. Philadelphia: JB Lippincott, 1969.)

densa segment of the early distal convoluted tubule with the glomerular vascular pole (Fig. 183-1). From this structural delineation, the concept of affector and effector limbs of the RAS was postulated.[1] This complex system operates at three levels: through the systemic circulation, within the vasculature itself, and by direct renal effects.

Renin is a proteolytic enzyme with relative specificity for the Leu-Leu bond or $NH_2$-terminal fragment of angiotensinogen. It is synthesized and stored primarily within the juxtaglomerular apparatus, in the distal portion near the afferent arteriole, although it also is found in salivary glands and the central nervous system.[2] Renin, consisting of two peptide chains linked by disulfide bridges, also exists as a prorenin (an inactive zymogen) that is activated by proteolytic enzymes. It is bound to renin-binding protein and may be stabilized by an endogenous renin inhibitor. Angiotensinogen is a large $\alpha_2$-globulin that primarily is synthesized by the liver but also is found in the kidney.[3] The action of renin on angiotensinogen generates *angiotensin I,* a ten-amino-acid peptide with little physiologic effect. Angiotensin-converting enzyme (ACE), a nonspecific COOH-terminal dipeptidase, forms the physiologically active *angiotensin II* by the clearing of His-Leu. The enzyme is diffusely located in lung, brain, kidney, and endothelial surfaces.[4] The location of angiotensin within the kidney and in the renal lymph, along with the intrarenal demonstration of angiotensin II receptors, complete the elements necessary for an intrarenal and extrarenal RAS.[5]

The control of RAS activity, ranging from renin synthesis and release through angiotensinogen concentration and ACE activity, involves multiple factors (see Chap. 79). The RAS is designed to regulate arterial pressure, organ perfusion, and extracellular fluid volume status through modulation of both sodium chloride and water homeostasis; moreover, it can be modulated by pressure, volume status, and vasoactive hormones, as well as by the sympathetic nervous system.[6,7]

Angiotensin II acts systemically—both as a vasoconstrictor and as a stimulus to the adrenal zona glomerulosa—to produce *aldosterone,* the major volume-regulating hormone.

## INTRARENAL RENIN-ANGIOTENSIN SYSTEM

Within the kidney, the RAS has a significant role in regulating both glomerular filtration rate (GFR) and renal blood flow (RBF), major determinants of renal function that influence systemic pressure and volume homeostasis. The system is set to protect against any excessive reductions of GFR, in response to either hypotension or volume depletion, that could impair renal excretion of metabolic products, acids, or toxins. A reduction in renal perfusion stimulates renin synthesis and release, angiotensin generation and conversion, and angiotensin II–enhanced efferent glomerular tone through the angiotensin I receptor, maintaining the GFR despite a reduction in renal perfusion.[8] This system operates with other systems regulating GFR and in concert with other vasoactive modulators, such as vasopressin, endothelin, and adenosine.[8,9]

If released angiotensin II had the effect on afferent glomerular arterioles that it does on efferent glomerular arterioles, GFR would decline. The sustained GFR that occurs with renal hypoperfusion may represent the intrarenal net effect of the RAS activity interacting with other vasoactive regulators (e.g., vasodilatation caused by prostaglandins or kinins). Perhaps, the occurrence of

**TABLE 183-1.**
**Modulators of Renin-Angiotensin System Activity**

**PROSTAGLANDINS**

| | |
|---|---|
| Stimulation: | Prostaglandin E$_2$ |
| | Prostacyclin (6-keto-F$_2\alpha$) |
| Modulation: | Macula densa |
| Inhibition: | Nonsteroidal antiinflammatory drugs |

**SYMPATHETIC NERVOUS SYSTEM**

| | |
|---|---|
| Stimulation: | β-Agonists |
| Inhibition: | β-Antagonists |
| | α-Agonists |

**IONS**

| | |
|---|---|
| Stimulation: | Diminished serum ionized calcium |
| | Diminished serum [K$^+$] |
| Inhibition: | Increased serum ionized calcium |
| | Increased serum [K$^+$] |

**MISCELLANEOUS**

| | |
|---|---|
| Stimulation: | Kallikrein/kinins |
| | Glucagon |
| | Parathyroid hormone |
| | Nitric oxide |
| | Endothelin |
| | Adenosine |
| Inhibition: | Vasopressin |
| | Angiotensin II |
| | Somatostatin |
| | Caffeine |

**TABLE 183-2.**
**Stimuli for Renal Prostaglandin Production**

**PEPTIDE HORMONES**
 Vasopressin
 Bradykinin
 Angiotensin II
 Endothelin-1

**MISCELLANEOUS STIMULI**
 Calcium
 Intravenous loop diuretics
 α-Adrenergic catecholamines
 Adenosine triphosphate
 Dietary supplementation with arachidonic acid precursors
 Interleukin-1α
 Tumor necrosis factor α
 Serotonin
 Endotoxin
 Estradiol

**DISEASES**
 Glomerulonephritis
 Cirrhosis
 Congestive heart failure
 Bartter syndrome
 Renal ischemia
 Ureteral obstruction

(Modified from Dunn MJ. Renal endocrinology. Baltimore: Williams & Wilkins, 1983:4.)

---

increased efferent resistance without increased afferent resistance serves a second purpose, by permitting the excretion of toxins and metabolic products while enhancing the conservation of sodium chloride and water, which induces extracellular volume expansion and improves renal perfusion. Local renal angiotensin II formation can enhance renal tubular reabsorption directly by acting on the proximal tubular epithelium and through renal hemodynamic changes (e.g., efferent constriction, diminished peritubular capillary hydrostatic pressure, and increased capillary colloid oncotic pressure).[10]

Angiotensin I derived outside the kidney can be converted to angiotensin II within the kidney. Thus, distinguishing the source of the RAS affecting renal function can be difficult. Moreover, caution must be exercised in extrapolating from study results derived from the use of ACE inhibitors and in extrapolating from pathologic states to normal physiologic events. The interdependence of the various vasoactive and volume-control systems further increases the difficulty in assessing the physiologic effect of changes in one parameter without measuring any parameters of the other systems that may have been altered (Table 183-1). Nevertheless, a disproportionate increase in RAS activity seems to occur in experimentally induced diabetes.[11] Renal renin gene production also is altered in pathophysiologic states such as salt depletion, ureteral obstruction, Bartter syndrome, and high-protein feeding.

# PROSTAGLANDINS

The oxygenation of arachidonic acid through either the cyclooxygenase or the lipoxygenase pathway leads to the formation of various biologically important compounds known collectively as *eicosanoids* (see Chap. 172). Included are prostaglandins, thromboxanes, leukotrienes, and hydroxy fatty acids. Before its conversion to eicosanoids, arachidonic acid must be released from membrane-bound phospholipids by the action of phospholipases. In the kidney, various chemical and hormonal stimuli serve to activate phospholipase (Table 183-2).

Eicosanoids, including prostaglandins, have been called *autacoids*. Autacoids are compounds that act near their sites of synthesis. Different regions of the kidney synthesize prostaglandins, whose sites of physiologic activity are at or near their sites of synthesis. Thus, prostaglandins synthesized in the renal cortex regulate cortical processes, such as glomerular filtration, and prostaglandins synthesized in the medulla exert their effects on medullary sodium and water metabolism and on medullary blood flow.[12,13] In addition, several prostaglandin receptor subtypes are found that have distinct cellular localization as well as second messenger responses. The prostaglandin E (PGE) receptor, for example, consists of three subtypes that confer multiple functions in different segments of the nephron.[14]

The loci of renal prostaglandin synthesis are the glomeruli, arterioles, collecting ducts, and medullary interstitial cells. In humans, *prostacyclin* (prostaglandin I$_2$, or PGI$_2$) is the principal prostaglandin synthesized by the glomeruli, where it participates in the regulation of GFR. PGI$_2$ also is the major prostaglandin synthesized by arterioles, acting to regulate RBF by modulating vascular resistance. The medullary collecting duct and medullary interstitial cells, in contrast, synthesize predominantly prostaglandin E$_2$ (PGE$_2$) and virtually no PGI$_2$.[15]

The nonsteroidal antiinflammatory drugs (NSAIDs; e.g., aspirin and indomethacin) inhibit cyclooxygenase activity in vivo by 75% to 90%, as assessed by measurements of urinary prostaglandins.[16] This is a reasonable index of renal prostaglandin production, because prostaglandins synthesized by other organs are not excreted in the urine.[12]

The major renal effects of prostaglandins are control of renal vascular resistance, regulation of glomerular filtration, stimulation of renin secretion, enhancement of water excretion, increase of sodium chloride excretion, and stimulation of erythropoietin release.

PGE$_2$ and PGI$_2$ are vasodilators and increase RBF, but they have little effect on glomerular filtration under physiologic conditions.[17,18] In any clinical setting characterized by effective intravascular volume depletion (e.g., diuretic-induced or dietary sodium restriction, congestive heart failure, cirrhosis, or nephrotic syndrome), the RAS is activated, and prostaglandins assume a critical role in offsetting vasoconstriction and preserving GFR. Probably, vasodilative prostaglandins relax the glomerular mesangium and blood vessels, thereby augmenting the filtration surface area and the ultrafiltration coefficient.[15]

The renal vasculature and glomeruli are sensitive to the vasoconstrictor peptides angiotensin II and vasopressin. Both these hormones stimulate the release of $PGI_2$ and $PGE_2$, which modulate the constrictor response. NSAID inhibition of prostaglandin synthesis leads to an augmentation of the vasoconstrictor effects and can cause significant reductions in both RBF and GFR. In healthy animals and humans, however, vasodilative prostaglandins appear to exert little control over RBF or GFR. The acute administration of NSAIDs does not reduce renal function unless they are given in a setting of increased vasoconstriction. In that circumstance, vasodilative prostaglandins would be expected to serve a counterbalancing effect to the vasoconstriction.[19,20]

$PGE_2$ is the principal eicosanoid participating in the regulation of tubular reabsorption of sodium and water. Sodium chloride reabsorption is enhanced in the medullary thick ascending limb of the loop of Henle and in the cortical and medullary collecting ducts when $PGE_2$ is inhibited. The major sites of inhibition of vasopressin-mediated water reabsorption are in the cortical and medullary collecting ducts.[17] These effects appear to be largely independent of RBF, representing instead direct actions on renal tubular cells. The inhibition of prostaglandin synthesis with indomethacin reduces the urinary sodium chloride concentration, interferes with the effects of diuretic agents, decreases urinary osmolarity, and, in certain clinical settings, can induce a net positive sodium balance and edema.[12,17,19]

A complex system of negative-feedback relationships preserves the GFR. Stimuli that induce renal vasoconstriction stimulate the synthesis of vasodilative $PGI_2$ and $PGE_2$. These prostaglandins, in turn, may modulate their own actions by stimulating renin secretion. The danger of NSAID administration under circumstances of stimulated renin or vasopressin release cannot be overemphasized.

## RENAL KALLIKREIN-KININ SYSTEM

The renal kallikrein-kinin system, the activity of which appears to be interrelated with the RAS and prostaglandins, may participate in the control of RBF and function by altering the tone of renal and extrarenal blood vessels, and by directly regulating intrarenal sodium and water excretion. The role of the kallikrein-kinin system in normal and pathologic processes will be clarified further with the information forthcoming from molecular cloning of the kallikrein genes[21] (see Chap. 170).

*Kallikreins* are serine proteases that release *kinins* from plasma substrates, known as *kininogens*. Renal kallikrein appears to favor low-molecular-weight kininogen, forming a compound known as Lys-bradykinin or *kallidin*. The kinins formed are inactivated rapidly by enzymes called *kininases,* which are found in blood and other tissues. The two major kininases are *kininase I* and *kininase II.* Kininase II, a peptidyl dipeptidase, also is known as *ACE.*

The activity of the renal kallikrein-kinin system usually is studied by measuring urinary kallikrein. Methodologic problems have been posed, however, by the lack of specificity of some of the methods used to measure kallikrein.[22] Urinary kallikrein is synthesized by the kidney; 90% of renal kallikrein is found in the cortex, with little in the medulla or papilla.[23] The granular portions of the distal convoluted and cortical collecting tubules form a single segment known as the *collecting tubule,* which is the site of kallikrein synthesis. The discrete tubular localization of kallikrein suggests a specific role of renal kallikrein at this site.[24]

Micropuncture evidence has confirmed that renal kallikreins are secreted into the urine at the level of the distal tubule and that urinary kinins are formed.[23,25] Kininase II and other peptidases in the proximal tubular lumen prevent filtered kinins from reaching distal nephron segments. Urinary kinins appear to be formed from low-molecular-weight kininogen, and the kidney may produce its own kininogen.

Numerous complex interactions occur among the kallikrein-kinin, renin-angiotensin-aldosterone, vasopressin, and prostaglandin systems of the kidney. Urinary kallikrein converts inactive renin (or prorenin) to active renin in vitro, and the in vivo activation of renin by kallikrein has been suggested.[26] Converting enzyme (kininase II), which is found in high concentrations in vascular endothelial cells of the lung, has the concurrent functions of converting angiotensin I to angiotensin II and inactivating kinins, which promote vasoconstriction. More than 90% of kinins found in the venous circulation are inactivated in a single passage through the lung, suggesting that kinins formed within the kidney act in a paracrine manner, mediating intrarenal vasodilatation and perhaps regulating blood flow to specific regions of the kidney.

The administration of mineralocorticoids, as well as angiotensin II and vasopressin, appears to stimulate renal kallikrein excretion.[27-29] Moreover, kinins infused into the renal artery stimulate the synthesis of $PGE_2$ in the collecting duct and medulla and of $PGI_2$ in the arterioles.[30] Prostaglandins stimulate, and prostaglandin synthesis inhibitors suppress, the renal release of kallikreins, completing the negative-feedback circuit.[31] The physiologic role played by these interactions remains speculative, however. An isolated increase in the activity of the RAS would produce both peripheral and renal vasoconstriction, which could impair RBF. Angiotensin II and aldosterone, however, stimulate the release of renal kallikrein and prostaglandins, which would augment RBF and offset vasoconstrictor influences.

Studies using both ACE inhibitors and aprotinin, an inhibitor of kallikrein, suggest that kinins released within the kidney cause natriuresis, diuresis, and the release of prostaglandins. Whether these effects are due to a direct effect of kinins on distal nephron sodium transport, to changes in RBF and distribution, or to both, is unclear.

## VITAMIN D

The kidney has a primary role in calcium homeostasis, acting both as a target organ for parathyroid hormone (PTH) and as the source of 1,25-dihydroxyvitamin $D_3$ [$1,25(OH)_2D_3$].

PTH in the kidney reduces proximal tubular phosphate reabsorption, causing enhanced excretion, and also increases the serum phosphate level by its effect on bone metabolism and intestinal absorption. In a patient with intact renal function, the excretion effect is predominant; therefore, PTH ultimately decreases the serum phosphate level.

Vitamin $D_3$, or cholecalciferol, functions both as a vitamin and as a steroid prohormone, which is converted to an active form, $1,25(OH)_2D_3$ (see Chap. 54). The kidney, as the major site of this final and most closely regulated step of synthesis, is the principal regulator of vitamin $D_3$ action.[32,33]

The sterol 7-dehydrocholesterol, derived from cholesterol in the skin, is converted by ultraviolet irradiation to previtamin $D_3$, and then, when thermal conditions are appropriate, to vitamin $D_3$ (see Chaps. 54 and 185). This endogenous vitamin $D_3$, as well as vitamin $D_3$ or $D_2$ ingested from dietary sources, is bound to vitamin D–binding protein and transported to the liver. Hydroxylation of vitamin $D_3$ in the liver forms 25-hydroxycholecalciferol ($25[OH]D_3$), which is bound to vitamin D–binding protein for transport to the kidney. Although $25(OH)D_3$ is the predominant circulating form of vitamin $D_3$ in the plasma, only 1% to 2% of vitamin D–binding protein is saturated with this substance.

The $25(OH)D_3$ is converted in the kidney to $1,25(OH)_2D_3$ by the enzyme $1\alpha$-hydroxylase. This enzyme has been localized to renal proximal tubule mitochondria and is substrate specific.[34] It is a closely regulated enzyme and can be affected by several factors. Parathyroid hormone, hypocalcemia, and hypophosphatemia all stimulate hydroxylation, whereas vitamin $D_3$ and $1,25(OH)_2D_3$ inhibit activity. Other hormonal changes can affect $1,25(OH)_2D_3$ synthesis: increased levels of calcitonin, sex hormones (e.g., in pregnancy), prolactin, or growth hormone stimulate enzyme activity, whereas exogenous glucocorticoids suppress it. Some of the hormonal effects occur via gene regulation.[35] Many sites of action of $1,25(OH)_2D_3$ are found. The intestinal absorption of both calcium and phosphorus is enhanced. The absorption of calcium by active transport in the duodenum is exquisitely sensitive to this hormone.[36] The skeletal effect of the vitamin D family of compounds also is important, albeit less well understood. Calcium and phosphorus supplementation heals rickets only when vitamin D or its metabolites are administered concomitantly. In addition, $1,25(OH)_2D_3$ exerts a permissive effect on PTH-mediated bone resorption.

The effects of the vitamin D metabolites on renal transport are unclear and may depend on the vitamin D and PTH status.[37] The acute administration of $1,25(OH)_2D_3$ exerts an antiphosphaturic effect when renal cyclic adenosine monophosphate (cAMP) is stimulated concomitantly by phosphaturic agents. The calcitriol receptor is localized to the distal tubule, the collecting duct, the proximal tubule, and the parietal epithelial cells of the glomerulus.[38]

The abnormalities of vitamin D metabolism in patients with advanced renal failure are caused by impaired production of $1,25(OH)_2D_3$. Decrements of glomerular filtration of up to 40 mL per minute usually are not associated with vitamin D deficiency and disordered calcium homeostasis. Below that level, the characteristic osteodystrophy of renal disease may supervene (see Chap. 61).

# ERYTHROPOIETIN

Erythropoietin is the primary regulator of erythrocyte production (see Chap. 212). It is a nondialyzable glycoprotein with a molecular mass of 39,000 Da, containing carbohydrates (notably sialic acid) that are essential for biologic function. Measurement by various methods, including the polycythemic mouse bioassay, in vitro marrow culture, and radioimmunoassay, have estimated human serum levels at ~15 mU/mL.[39]

The role of the kidney in erythropoietin production was established with the demonstration that rats without kidneys (but not those with comparable uremia but intact kidneys) failed to show an increase in plasma erythropoietic activity in response to hypoxia.[40] Until recently, bioassays of renal tissue failed to detect erythropoietic activity, which sparked several hypotheses to explain the kidney's role in erythropoietin production.

The proposal was made that the kidneys release an enzyme, erythrogenin, that converts a circulating erythropoietinogen into active erythropoietin.[41] Alternatively, the suggestion was put forward that the kidneys produce an erythropoietin "proform" that is activated in plasma, or that the hormone is produced in the kidneys but is protected from inhibitors by a plasma factor. Studies have negated these theories by isolating significant amounts of active erythropoietin from kidney tissue.[42] The postulated enzyme "erythrogenin" has not been isolated.

The intrarenal site of erythropoietin production remains controversial. Evidence suggesting cortical glomerular synthesis of the hormone is derived principally from studies that demonstrate erythropoietin activity in supernatant cultures of cortical glomeruli, localization of fluorescein-labeled globulins to glomerular tufts, and localization of horseradish peroxidase–labeled antibodies to epithelial foot processes of glomerular cells.[43] The glomerular basement membrane, however, may nonspecifically trap antigen-antibody complexes, and the significance of these findings has been questioned.

The juxtaglomerular apparatus also has been considered as a site for erythropoietin synthesis, because changes in juxtaglomerular cell granularity have been correlated with tissue oxygen tension. Others attribute these changes to alterations in blood volume, rather than to any control mechanisms related to erythrocyte production.[44,45]

With in situ hybridization, localization of erythropoietin mRNA was noted in cortical cells of anemic rat kidneys, which suggested interstitial or capillary endothelial cells as the site.[46] Extrarenal sources probably account for <10% of erythropoietin in adults but may contribute significant amounts in nephrectomized animals. The liver and possibly the reticuloendothelial system are the major proposed extrarenal sites of erythropoietin production.[43]

Erythropoietin is produced in response to renal tissue hypoxia, as determined by the balance between renal oxygen supply and consumption. Because the kidney's arterial-venous oxygen difference is relatively small, renal tissue oxygen content reflects the systemic oxygen supply.[43] Serum levels of the hormone are increased in response to systemic hypoxia, such as that caused by high altitude and altered oxygen dissociation. Changes in RBF produce tissue hypoxia and stimulate erythropoietin production. Polycythemia can occur when significant renal artery stenosis is present, after transplantation with alterations in renal vasculature, and in the presence of renal cysts compressing surrounding renal parenchyma.

A proposed mechanism by which hypoxic stimuli induce erythropoietin production states that hypoxia may allow increased calcium entry into the glomerular cell, activating phospholipase and triggering the synthesis of prostaglandins, including $PGL_2$.[39] $PGL_2$ or its metabolite 6-keto-prostaglandin $F_{2\alpha}$, subsequently activates adenylate cyclase, increasing renal cAMP and initiating or enhancing erythropoietin production. Oxygen-sensing and erythropoietin gene regulation may occur by several means.[47]

Erythropoietin, which is considered a cytokine, acts on several steps in the production of erythrocytes.[44] Erythroid colony-forming units are exquisitely sensitive to erythropoietin and may be the principal sites of regulation of erythrocytes by this hormone. Moreover, erythropoietin causes the early release of large "stress" reticulocytes, accelerates bone marrow transit time, and increases the hemoglobin concentration of individual red blood cells. Thus, the erythroid marrow can increase production to six to ten times basal rates in response to prolonged stimulation.[44]

The anemia of chronic renal failure has many causes.[48] Serum levels of erythropoietin are lower in patients with chronic renal failure than in patients with comparable anemia but normal renal function. Shortened red blood cell survival times and the presence of inhibitors of erythropoiesis have been demonstrated. Red blood cell survival can be improved by dialysis, resulting in a lessening of the anemia.[49] Studies of patients receiving maintenance hemodialysis have demonstrated the correction of anemia with administration of recombinant human erythropoietin,[50,51] and this form of therapy is a mainstay for such patients, improving quality of life and dramatically reducing the need for blood transfusions. The synthetic hormone appears to be equally effective in correcting the anemia of patients with chronic renal insufficiency that has not progressed to end-stage renal failure.

Other effects of erythropoietin include antinatriuresis through the production of renal angiotensin II and stimulation of endothelin production.[52,53]

## ENDOTHELIN

Endothelins are among the most potent renal peptides, regulating renal homeostasis by several actions (see Chap. 179).[54] Endothelin-1 (ET-1) and the highly homologous isoforms endothelin-2 (ET-2) and endothelin-3 (ET-3) have direct vasoconstrictive and tubular transport actions that affect the control of RBF, GFR, and sodium and water excretion. These peptides are synthesized and released by endothelial cells in the lung, gut, and multiple renal sites. They act predominantly in a paracrine and autocrine fashion. Two receptors have been identified—type $ET_A$ and type $ET_B$. $ET_A$ receptors are mostly involved in smooth muscle cell proliferation and vasoconstriction, whereas $ET_B$ receptors influence vasopressin-induced cAMP formation, thereby affecting water balance. The effect on renal sodium excretion is highly complex and not elucidated fully; however, renal natriuretic effects include decreased renin secretion and inhibition of $Na^+$-$K^+$ adenosine triphosphatase. Antinatriuretic effects include effects on GFR and direct effects on $Na^+$ reabsorption. Endothelin has been implicated in the pathogenesis of cyclosporine nephrotoxicity, essential hypertension, pregnancy-induced hypertension, atherosclerosis, cerebral and myocardial vasospasm, acute renal failure due to radiocontrast agents, and chronic progressive nephropathies.[55–57]

## NITRIC OXIDE

All three major isoforms of nitric oxide synthase are expressed in the kidney in a cell-specific pattern. Nitric oxide has multiple renal effects, including proximal tubular activity, renin release, and cyclooxygenase expression.[57a–57c] Studies using nitric oxide synthase inhibitors show increased renal vascular resistance, decreased renal plasma flow and GFR, antinatriuresis, and antidiuresis.[58]

## REFERENCES

1. Goormaghtigh N. Existence of an endocrine gland in the media of the renal arterioles. Proc Soc Exp Biol Med 1939; 42:688.
2. Cantin M, Gutowska J, Lacasse J, et al. Ultrastructural immunocytochemical localization of renin and angiotensin II in the juxtaglomerular cells of the ischemic kidney in experimental renal hypertension. Am J Pathol 1984; 115:212.
3. Morris B, Johnston CI. Renin substrate in granules from rat kidney cortex. Biochem J 1976; 154:625.
4. Hall ER, Kato J, Erdos EG, et al. Angiotensin I-converting enzyme in the nephron. Life Sci 1976; 18:1299.
5. Burns KD, Homma T, Harris RC. The intrarenal renin-angiotensin system. Semin Nephrol 1993; 101:169.
6. Di Bona GF. Neural regulation of renal tubular sodium reabsorption and renin secretion: integrative aspects. Clin Exp Hypertens [A] 1987; 9:1515.
7. Osborn JL, Johns EJ. Renal neurogenic control of renin and prostaglandin release. Miner Electrolyte Metab 1989; 15:51.
8. Hall JE. Regulation of renal hemodynamics. Int Rev Physiol 1982; 26:243.
9. Navar LG. Renal autoregulation: perspectives from whole kidney and single nephron studies. Am J Physiol 1978; 234:F357.
10. Schuster VL, Kokko JP, Jacobson HR. Angiotensin II directly stimulates transport in rabbit proximal convoluted tubules. J Clin Invest 1984; 73:507.
11. Anderson S, Tung FF, Jugelfinger JR. Renal renin-angiotensin system in diabetes: functional, immunohistochemical, and molecular biological correlations. Am J Physiol 1993; 265:F477.
12. Dunn MJ. Renal prostaglandins. In: Dunn MJ, ed. Renal endocrinology. Baltimore: Williams & Wilkins, 1983:1.
13. Levenson DJ, Simmons CE Jr, Brenner BM. Arachidonic acid metabolism, prostaglandins and the kidney. Am J Med 1982; 72:354.
14. Sugimoto Y, Namba T, Shigemoto R, et al. Distinct cellular localization of mRNAs for three subtypes of prostaglandin E receptor in kidney. Am J Physiol 1994; 266:F823.
15. Scharschmidt LA, Lianos E, Dunn MJ. Arachidonate metabolites and the control of glomerular function. Fed Proc 1983; 42:3058.
16. Dunn MJ, Zambraski EJ. Renal effects of drugs that inhibit prostaglandin synthesis. Kidney Int 1980; 18:609.
17. Anderson RJ, Berl T, McDonald KM, Schrier RW. Prostaglandins: effects on blood pressure, renal blood flow, sodium and water excretion. Kidney Int 1976; 10:205.
18. Gerber JG, Nies AS, Friesinger GL, et al. The effect of $PGI_2$ on canine renal function and hemodynamics. Prostaglandins 1978; 16:519.
19. Dunn MJ. Nonsteroidal anti-inflammatory drugs and renal function. Annu Rev Med 1984; 35:411.
20. Terragno NA, Terragno DA, McGiff JC. Contribution of prostaglandins to the renal circulation in conscious, anesthetized and laparotomized dogs. Circ Res 1977; 40:590.
21. Lin FK, Lin CH, Chou CC, et al. Molecular cloning and sequence analysis of the monkey and human tissue kallikrein genes. Biochim Biophys Acta 1993; 1173:325.
22. Marin-Grez M, Carretero OA. A method for measurement of urinary kallikrein. J Appl Physiol 1972; 32:428.
23. Scieli AG, Carretero OA, Oza NB. Distribution of kidney kininogenases. Proc Soc Exp Biol Med 1976; 151:57.
24. Beasley D, Oza NB, Levinsky NG. Micropuncture localization of kallikrein secretion in the rat nephron. Kidney Int 1987; 32:26.
25. Imai M. The connecting tubule: a functional subdivision of the rabbit distal nephron segments. Kidney Int 1979; 15:346.
26. Sealey JE, Atlas SA, Laragh JH. Linking the kallikrein and renin system via activation of inactive renin. Am J Med 1978; 65:994.
27. Mills IH. Kallikrein, kininogen and kinins in control of blood pressure. Nephron 1979; 23:61.
28. Margolius HS, Horowitz D, Pisano JJ, Keiser HR. Urinary kallikrein excretion in normal man. Relationships to sodium intake and sodium-retaining steroids. Circ Res 1974; 35:812.
29. Fejes-Toch G, Zahajszky T, Filep J. Effect of vasopressin on renal kallikrein excretion. Am J Physiol 1980; 239:F388.
30. Terragno NA, Lonigro AJ, Malik KU, McGiff JC. The relationship of the renal vasodilator action of bradykinin to the release of prostaglandin E-like substances. Experientia 1972; 28:437.
31. Nasjletti A, Malik KU. Relationships between the kallikrein-kinin and prostaglandin system. Life Sci 1979; 25:99.
32. Coburn JW, Slatopolsky E. Vitamin D, parathyroid hormone and renal osteodystrophy. In: Brenner B, Rector F, eds. The kidney. Philadelphia: WB Saunders, 1985:1657.
33. Reichel H, Koeffler HP, Norman AW. The role of the vitamin D endocrine system in health and disease. N Engl J Med 1989; 320:980.
34. Slatopolsky E. Renal regulation of extrarenal function: bone. In: Seldin DW, Giebisch G, eds. The kidney: physiology and pathophysiology. New York: Raven Press, 1985:823.
35. Murayama A. Positive and negative regulations of the renal 25-hydroxyvitamin $D_3$ 1$\alpha$-hydroxylase gene by parathyroid hormone, calcitonin, and 1$\alpha$,25-$(OH)_2D_3$ in intact animals. Endocrinology 1999; 140:2224.
36. Lemman J Jr, Gray RW. Vitamin D metabolism and the kidney. In: Dunn NJ, ed. Renal endocrinology. Baltimore: Williams & Wilkins, 1983:114.
37. Norman AW. Vitamin D metabolites 1,25$(OH)_2D$ and 24,25$(OH)_2D$. In: Massry SG, Glassock RJ, eds. Textbook of nephrology. Baltimore: Williams & Wilkins, 1980:2.
38. Kumar R, Schaefer J, Grande JP, Roche PC. Immunolocalization of calcitriol receptor, 24-hydroxylase cytochrome P-450, and calbindin D28K in human kidney. Am J Physiol 1994; 266:F477.
39. Fischer JW, Nelson PK, Beckman B, Burdowski A. Kidney control of erythropoietin production. In: Dunn MJ, ed. Renal endocrinology. Baltimore: Williams & Wilkins, 1983:142.
40. Jacobsen LO, Goldwasser E, Fried W, Pezak L. Role of the kidney in erythropoiesis. Nature 1957; 179:633.
41. Gordon AS, Cooper GW, Zanjani ED. The kidney and erythropoiesis. Semin Hematol 1967; 4:337.
42. Fried W, Barone-Vazelas J, Berman M. Detection of high EP titers in renal extracts of hypoxic rats. J Lab Clin Med 1981; 97:82.
43. Powell JS, Adameon JW. Hematopoiesis and the kidney. In: Seldon DW, Giebisch G, eds. The kidney: physiology and pathophysiology. New York: Raven Press, 1985.
44. Spivak JL. The mechanism of action of erythropoietin. Int J Cell Cloning 1986; 4:139.
45. Erslev AJ. Production of erythrocytes. In: Williams WJ, Beutler E, Erslev AJ, Lichtman MA, eds. Hematology. New York: McGraw Hill, 1983:142.
46. Koury ST, Bondurant MC, Koury MJ. Localization of erythropoietin synthesizing cells in murine kidneys by in situ hybridization. Blood 1988; 71:524.
47. Daghman NA, McHale CM, Savage GM, et al. Regulation of erythropoietin gene expression depends on two different oxygen-sensing mechanisms. Mol Genet Metab 1999; 67:113.
48. Paganini EP, Garcia J, Abdulhadi M, et al. The anemia of chronic renal failure. Overview and early erythropoietin experience. Cleve Clin J Med 1989; 56:79.
49. Anagnostou A, Kurtzman NA. Hematological consequences of renal failure in the kidney. In: Brenner BM, Rector FC, eds. Philadelphia: WB Saunders, 1986:1631.
50. Bommer J, Alexiou C, Meuller-Beuhl U, et al. Recombinant human erythropoietin therapy in haemodialysis patients—dose determination and clinical experience. Nephrol Dial Transplant 1987; 2:238.
51. Eschbach JW, Kelly MR, Haley NR, et al. Treatment of the anemia of progressive renal failure with recombinant human erythropoietin. N Engl J Med 1989; 321:158.

52. Brier ME, Bunke CM, Lathon PV, Aronoff GR. Erythropoietin-induced antinatriuresis mediated by angiotensin II in perfused kidneys. J Am Soc Nephrol 1993; 3:1583.

53. Carlini R, Dusso A, Obialo C, et al. Recombinant human erythropoietin does not regulate the expression of endothelin-1 release by endothelial cells. Kidney Int 1993; 43:1010.

54. Kohan D. Endothelins in the normal and diseased kidney. Am J Kidney Dis 1997; 29:2.

55. Simonson MS. Endothelins: multifunctional renal peptides. Physiol Rev 1993; 73:375.

56. Remuzzi G, Benigni A. Endothelins in the control of cardiovascular and renal function. Lancet 1993; 342:589.

57. Perico N, Remuzzi G. Role of endothelin in glomerular injury. Kidney Int Suppl 1993; 39:S76.

57a. Liang M, Knox FG. Production and functional roles of nitric oxide in the proximal tubule. Am J Physiol Regul Integr Comp Physiol 2000; 278:R1117.

57b. Persson AE, Gutierrez A, Pittner J, et al. Renal NO production and the development of hypertension. Acta Physiol Scand 2000; 168:169.

57c. Cheng HF, Wang JL, Zhang MZ, et al. Nitric oxide regulates renal cortical cyclooxygenase expression. Am J Physiol Renal Physiol 2000; 279:F122.

58. Gabbai FB, Blantz RC. Role of nitric oxide in renal hemodynamics. Semin Nephrol 1999; 19:242.

# CHAPTER 184

# THE ENDOCRINE GENITOURINARY TRACT

JAN FAHRENKRUG AND SØREN GRÄS

The intrinsic control of some functions in the genitourinary tract cannot be attributed to cholinergic and adrenergic nerves. The demonstration of prostaglandins, regulatory peptides, and nitric oxide (NO) in urogenital tissues suggests that these substances may account for these local, noncholinergic, nonadrenergic physiologic events.

Several peptides have been found in the urogenital tract (Table 184-1). With the exception of relaxin, all peptides originally were isolated from extragenital sources.

## PEPTIDE HORMONES OF THE GENITOURINARY TRACT

Information concerning the different peptides in the genitourinary tract varies considerably, from the mere demonstration of immunoreactivity in tissue extracts to detailed studies on cellular localization and function.

## SUBSTANCE P

Substance P (see Chap. 171) is found in nerve fibers of the smooth muscle layers of the fallopian tube and uterus and around blood vessels in the vagina.[1] Substance P–containing nerve terminals, which probably represent primary sensory neurons, are found in the vaginal epithelium and clitoris. In the male genital tract, substance P–containing nerves are concentrated mainly in a group of fibers in the corpuscular receptors underneath the epithelium of the glans penis.[2] In the urinary tract, similar nerve fibers are encountered in the lamina propria and the muscle layer, especially in the detrusor muscles.[3]

## CALCITONIN GENE–RELATED PEPTIDE

Afferent nerves immunoreactive for calcitonin gene–related peptide (CGRP) (see Chap. 53) occur in the female genital tract,

**TABLE 184-1.**
**Hormonal Substances in the Female and Male Genitourinary Tracts**

**GUT-BRAIN HORMONES**
Substance P
Vasoactive intestinal peptide
Neuropeptide Y
Enkephalins
Gastrin-releasing peptide/bombesin-like peptides
**HYPOTHALAMIC HORMONES**
Somatostatin
**NEUROHYPOPHYSIAL HORMONES**
Oxytocin
**PITUITARY HORMONES**
β-Endorphin
Prolactin
**VASOACTIVE HORMONES**
Renin
Endothelin
Atrial natriuretic peptide
Nitric oxide
**OTHERS**
Calcitonin gene–related peptide
Galanin
Pituitary adenylate cyclase–activating peptide
Relaxin

mainly associated with blood vessels, nonvascular smooth muscle, squamous epithelium, and uterine and cervical glands.[4] In men CGRP nerves are prevalent in the penis.[5]

## VASOACTIVE INTESTINAL PEPTIDE

Vasoactive intestinal peptide (VIP; see Chap. 182) is localized in nerve fibers throughout the female genital tract.[6] This peptide occurs in large, electron-dense granules in nerve terminals that seem to innervate epithelial cells, blood vessels, and smooth muscle cells. A particularly rich supply of fibers is found in the cervical os and the isthmic part of the fallopian tube. The VIP nerves in the female genital tract are intrinsic, originating mainly from local ganglia in the paracervical tissue. In the male genital tract, VIP nerves are abundant in the erectile tissue of the corpus cavernosum and around arteries and arterioles.[2,6] The nonvascular smooth muscle and glands in the prostate and seminal vesicles are also associated with VIP nerves. In the urinary tract, VIP-immunoreactive nerves are distributed widely in all regions but are particularly dense in the bladder, mainly beneath the epithelium and the muscle layer of the trigone.[3,6]

## NEUROPEPTIDE Y

Neuropeptide Y (NPY) has a widespread distribution in both the male and female genital tracts and is found in the nerve fibers associated with vascular and nonvascular smooth musculature.[2,7,8] In the urinary tract, NPY nerves are seen in the muscle layer, particularly in the trigonal area.[3]

## GALANIN

Galanin-immunoreactive nerve fibers (see Chap. 182) are found in the female and male genital tracts, with the exception of ovary and testis. Galanin nerve fibers are found within smooth muscle and in close relationship to arteries and veins.[9] Galanin fibers are most abundant in the female paracervical tissue, however, where they surround ganglion cells.[10]

## ENKEPHALINS

In the female genital tract, the two enkephalin pentapeptides (see Chap. 168) are present in nerve fibers within the smooth muscle layers of the uterine cervix and in local ganglia surrounding nonimmunoreactive cell bodies.[11] The latter localization is interesting in view of their suspected neuromodulatory role. In the urinary tract, a few single fibers are found along bundles of smooth muscle cells.

## GASTRIN-RELEASING PEPTIDE

Gastrin-releasing peptide (bombesin-like peptides; see Chap. 182) is found throughout nerve fibers scattered in the smooth musculature of the male and female genital tracts. In men, it is found mainly in the musculature of the seminal vesicles, urethra, and vas deferens. In the urinary bladder, gastrin-releasing peptide has a diffuse distribution, in contrast to VIP, substance P, and NPY, which are concentrated in the trigone of the bladder.

## PITUITARY ADENYLATE CYCLASE–ACTIVATING PEPTIDE

Pituitary adenylate cyclase–activating polypeptide (PACAP) is localized in nerve fibers throughout the human and rat female genitourinary tracts innervating epithelium, smooth muscle cells, and blood vessels.[12,13] In the ovary PACAP is transiently expressed during the periovulatory period in steroidogenic cells.[14] In these cells, PACAP may be involved in the local regulation of acute periovulatory progesterone production and subsequent luteinization.[14a,14b] In the rat testis, PACAP is stage-specifically expressed in the spermatogenic epithelium.[15]

## SOMATOSTATIN

Nerve fibers containing somatostatin (see Chap. 169) are distributed sparsely in the genital tract, occurring mainly in the smooth musculature.[2]

## OXYTOCIN

Immunoreactivity to oxytocin (see Chap. 25) and to oxytocin mRNA is found in corpora lutea of the human and nonhuman primate ovary, localized primarily to luteal cells.[16,17] The oxytocin receptor is also present in the human ovary; thus, the peptide may be involved in the local regulation of luteal function. Furthermore, oxytocin immunoreactivity, oxytocin mRNA, and oxytocin-receptor immunoreactivity are present in Leydig cells from the human testis, where the peptide has been implicated in the local regulation of steroidogenesis.[18]

## β-ENDORPHIN

Positive immunostaining for β-endorphin (see Chap. 168) is seen in the cytoplasm of Leydig cells and in the epithelium of the epididymis, seminal vesicles, and vas deferens of rats.[19]

## PROLACTIN

Prolactin, structurally identical to pituitary prolactin (see Chap. 13), is produced de novo in decidual and myometrial cells of the human uterus. Its role remains unknown; however, the production increases during pregnancy, and large concentrations of the hormone are found in amniotic fluid.[20]

## RENIN

Locally produced renin (see Chaps. 79 and 183) and all other components of the renin-angiotensin system (tissue RAS) are present in human endometrial and decidual cells and in myometrial perivascular cells. Tissue RAS is also present in the ovary, primarily confined to follicular cells and the corpora lutea. In men, RAS components are found in Leydig cells and in the epididymal epithelium. Tissue RAS in the genital tract has been implicated in the local regulation of such diverse functions as uterine contraction, blood flow and epithelial secretion, ovarian steroid production, oocyte maturation and ovulation, and testicular testosterone production.[21]

## ENDOTHELIN

The potent vasoconstrictor endothelin-1 (see Chap. 179) is expressed in endometrial cells and the glandular epithelium of the human uterus, and its expression is regulated during the menstrual cycle.[22] In the human testis, endothelin-1 is expressed primarily in Sertoli cells of the seminiferous tubules. The endothelin receptor is found on both Leydig cells and germ cells, suggesting multiple roles for the peptide.[23]

## ATRIAL NATRIURETIC PEPTIDE

Atrial natriuretic peptide (ANP; see Chap. 178) is expressed in the human testis, prostate, uterus, and ovary.[24] ANP expression is particularly high in the ovary, where ANP binding sites have been described.[25]

## NITRIC OXIDE

During the past decade, the gaseous signalling molecule NO (see Chap. 179) has been discovered to be an important component in the local regulation of a variety of physiologic events. NO is produced by nitric oxide synthase (NOS), which exists in at least three different isoforms. The various isoforms of NOS have been found throughout the male and female genitourinary tracts within nerves, vascular endothelial cells, smooth muscle cells, epithelial cells, glandular cells, and immunologic cells. In many nerves, NOS is colocalized with regulatory peptides.[26–28] (Also see Chap. 179.)

## RELAXIN

Relaxin originally was isolated from the corpus luteum of pregnant sows.[29] Relaxin immunoreactivity is found in both the nongestational and gestational corpus luteum and in the secretory endometrium of nonpregnant women. The suggestion has been made that relaxin is involved in the maintenance of uterine quiescence and in the softening of the uterine cervix.

# GENITOURINARY FUNCTIONS OF LOCAL HORMONES

The mechanism whereby communication occurs between the hormone-producing cells and their target cells is not fully understood. In autocrine or paracrine secretion, the hormone acts on the cell of origin or on neighboring cells by extracellular fluid transport systems. Any effects mediated by autocrine or paracrine secretion may be either quick or prolonged, and may include trophic effects and influences on cell differentiation.

The final mode of communication used by peptides or NO confined to nerve fibers (i.e., neurocrine) is synaptic transmission. The targets of this communication are mainly vascular cells

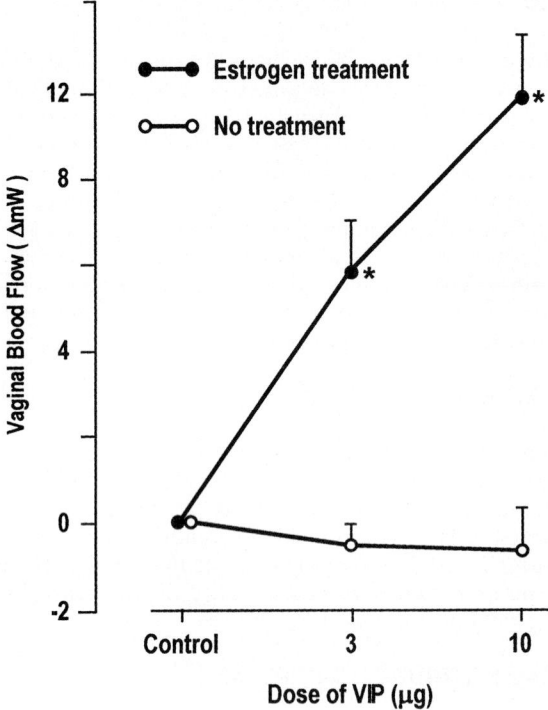

**FIGURE 184-1.** Effect of vasoactive intestinal peptide (*VIP*) on vaginal blood flow in postmenopausal women receiving no medication (*open circles*) and in those receiving hormone-replacement therapy (*closed circles*). Values are means of six experiments with standard error of the mean. Infusion of saline solution did not change vaginal blood flow (not shown). Asterisks indicate significant difference from before VIP injection, $p < .05$.

and nonvascular muscle cells, and the purpose is to effect control of blood flow and smooth muscle activity.

## LOCAL NONADRENERGIC NONCHOLINERGIC CONTROL OF BLOOD FLOW

VIP and substance P cause uterine vasodilation by directly affecting vascular smooth muscle.[6] VIP also increases vaginal blood flow.[6] Strong evidence exists that this peptide participates as the noncholinergic vasodilatory transmitter in the control of uterine blood flow and is responsible for the increase in vaginal blood flow and vaginal lubrication evoked by sexual excitement.[6] VIP loses its ability to increase vaginal blood flow after menopause, but the vasodilatory response can be restored by hormone-replacement therapy (Fig. 184-1), indicating that the milieu of sex steroids can influence VIP function.[30] In humans, VIP is a possible mediator of erection: intracavernous VIP injection causes erection, and during visually induced erection, a local release of this peptide occurs (Fig. 184-2).[31] An abundance of evidence now indicates that the local production of NO and the subsequent stimulation of intracellular cyclic guanosine monophosphate (cGMP) in penile vasculature is a major pathway controlling penile erection.[26–28] A suggested contribution by CGRP remains to be clarified.[32]

## LOCAL NONADRENERGIC NONCHOLINERGIC CONTROL OF SMOOTH MUSCLE ACTIVITY

The activity of genital smooth musculature seems to be under dual peptidergic control by excitatory substance P nerves and inhibitory VIP nerves and NPY nerves.[6,33] Moreover, VIP is able to abolish both spontaneous and oxytocin- and prostaglandin $F_{2\alpha}$–induced mechanical and myoelectrical activity in the uterus.[6] VIP is also an inhibitory neurotransmitter in the urinary

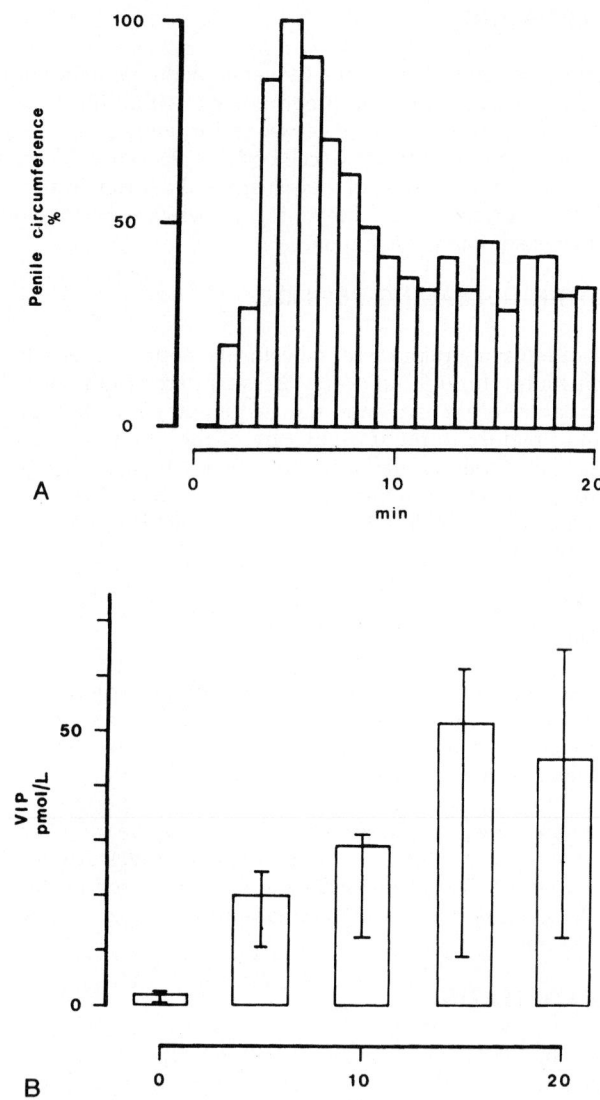

**FIGURE 184-2. A,** Effect of intracavernous injection of vasoactive intestinal peptide (*VIP*) (200 pmol) on penile erection in healthy men, expressed as the increase in penile circumference measured with a strain gauge (full erection = 100%; flaccidity = 0%). **B,** Concentration of VIP in corpus cavernosum blood during erection and tumescence. Stimulation was started at 0 minutes; tumescence or erection was obtained after 2 to 4 minutes and remained unchanged during the observation period. Values are medians and interquartile ranges of 11 experiments.

tract.[34] In the bladder, VIP seems to decrease the muscular tone during passive filling, thus maintaining normal compliance until micturition occurs. Micturition involves cholinergic detrusor contraction and a VIP-induced trigone relaxation.

## PATHOPHYSIOLOGIC IMPLICATIONS

Abnormalities in the peptidergic nerves of the genitourinary tract are known to occur in two disease states, both of them involving VIP. Healthy people can inhibit bladder detrusor contractions until they are ready to urinate. Patients with bladder instability cannot, and may manifest symptoms such as increased frequency, nocturia, urgency, incontinence, and enuresis. In patients with urodynamically proven idiopathic detrusor instability (i.e., no evidence of outflow obstruction, neuropathy, or structural lesions), the number of VIP nerves is greatly decreased in all layers, but particularly in the muscle.[34] In the penile tissue of impotent diabetics with autonomic neuropathy, the number of VIP nerves is decreased.[35] In many patients with erectile failure, VIP alone is not sufficient to induce full erection, but in combination with a small dose of the α-adrenoceptor–blocking drug, phentolamine, VIP is now successfully used as self-injection therapy for male impotence.[36] Decreased penile NOS activity has also been associated with erectile dysfunction. The local application of the NO donor linsidomine[27,28] has been used to correct erection disorders in men. The new oral drug sildenafil exploits another component of the NO pathway by increasing intracellular levels of cGMP in penile tissue. Undoubtedly, as the physiologic roles of local regulators in the genitourinary tract are deciphered, many more clinical examples of pathologic dysfunction will be found.

## REFERENCES

1. Skrabanek P, Powell D. Substance P in obstetrics and gynecology. Obstet Gynecol 1983; 61:641.
2. Gu J, Polak JM, Probert L, et al. Peptidergic innervation of the human male genital tract. J Urol 1983; 130:386.
3. Gu J, Blank MA, Huang WM, et al. Peptide-containing nerves in human urinary bladder. Urology 1984; 24:353.
4. Inyama CO, Wharton J, Su HC, et al. CGRP-immunoreactive nerves in the genitalia of the female rat originate from dorsal root ganglia $T_{11}$-$L_3$ and $L_6$-$S_1$: a combined immunocytochemical and retrograde tracing study. Neurosci Lett 1986; 69:13.
5. McNeill DL, Papka RE, Harris CH. CGRP immunoreactivity and NADPH-diaphorase in afferent nerves of the rat penis. Peptides 1992; 13:1239.
6. Ottesen B, Fahrenkrug J. Vasoactive intestinal polypeptide and other pre-provasoactive intestinal polypeptide–derived peptides in the female and male genital tract: localization, biosynthesis, and functional and clinical significance. Am J Obstet Gynecol 1995; 172:1615.
7. Stjernquist M, Emson P, Owman C, et al. Neuropeptide Y in the female reproductive tract of the rat: distribution of nerve fibers and motor effects. Neurosci Lett 1983; 39:279.
8. Fallgren B, Edvinsson L, Ekblad E, Ekman R. Involvement of perivascular neuropeptide Y nerve fibers in uterine arterial vasoconstriction in conjunction with pregnancy. Regul Pept 1989; 24:119.
9. Bauer FE, Christofides ND, Hacker GW, et al. Distribution of galanin immunoreactivity in the genitourinary tract of man and rat. Peptides 1986; 7:5.
10. Stjernquist M, Ekblad E, Owman C, et al. Immunocytochemical localization of galanin in the rat male and female genital tracts and motor effects in vitro. Regul Pept 1988; 20:335.
11. Alm P, Alumets J, Håkanson R, et al. Enkephalin-immunoreactive nerve fibers in the feline genito-urinary tract. Histochemistry 1981; 72:351.
12. Steenstrup BR, Alm P, Hannibal J, et al. Pituitary adenylate cyclase–activating polypeptide: occurrence and relaxant effect in female genital tract. Am J Physiol Endocrinol Metab 1995; 32:E108.
13. Fahrenkrug J, Hannibal J. Pituitary adenylate cyclase activating polypeptide immunoreactivity in capsaicin-sensitive nerve fibres supplying the rat urinary tract. Neuroscience 1998; 83:1261.
14. Gräs S, Hannibal J, Georg B, Fahrenkrug J. Transient periovulatory expression of pituitary adenylate cyclase activating peptide in rat ovarian cells. Endocrinology 1996; 137:4779.
14a. Gräs S, Hannibal J, Fahrenkrug J. Pituitary adenylate cyclase-activating polypeptide is an auto/paracrine stimulator of acute progesterone accumulation and subsequent luteinization in cultured periovulatory granulosa cells. Endocrinology 1999; 140:2199.
14b. Gräs S, Hedetoft C, Pedersen SH, Fahrenkrug J. Pituitary adenylate cyclase activating peptide stimulates acute progesterone production in rat granulosa/lutein cells via two receptor subtypes. Biol Reprod 2000; 63:206.
15. Shioda S, Legradi G, Leung W-C, et al. Localization of pituitary adenylate cyclase-activating polypeptide and its messenger ribonucleic acid in the rat testis by light and electron microscopic immunocytochemistry and in situ hybridization. Endocrinology 1994; 135:818.
16. Ivell R, Kenichi F, Brackmann B, et al. Expression of the oxytocin and vasopressin genes in human and baboon tissues. Endocrinology 1990; 127:2990.
17. Einspanner A, Ivell R, Rune G, et al. Oxytocin gene expression and oxytocin immunoreactivity in the ovary of the common marmoset monkey (callithrix jacchus). Biol Reprod 1994; 50:1216.
18. Frayne J, Nicholson HD. Localization of oxytocin receptors in the human and macaque monkey male reproductive tracts: evidence for a physiological role of oxytocin in the male. Mol Hum Reprod 1998; 14:527.
19. Sharp B, Pekary AE, Meyer NV, Hershman JM. β-endorphin in male rat reproductive organs. Biochem Biophys Res Commun 1980; 95:618.
20. Ben-Jonathan N, Mershon JL, Allen DL, Steinmetz RW. Extrapituitary prolactin: distribution, regulation, functions, and clinical aspects. Endocrine Rev 1996; 17:639.
21. Vinsen GP, Saridogan E, Puddefoot JR, Djahanbakch O. Tissue renin-angiotensin system and reproduction. Hum Reprod 1997; 12:651.

22. Economos K, MacDonald PC, Casy ML. Endothelin-1 gene expression and protein biosynthesis in human endometrium: potential modulator of endometrial blood flow. J Clin Endocrinol Metab 1992; 74:14.
23. Maggi M, Barni T, Orlando C, et al. Endothelin-1 and its receptors in human testis. J Androl 1995; 16:213.
24. Gerbes AL, Dagnino L, Nguyen T, Nemer M. Transcription of brain natriuretic peptide and atrial natriuretic peptide genes in human tissues. J Clin Endocrinol Metab 1994; 78:1306.
25. Gutkowska J, Tremblay J, Antakly T, et al. The atrial natriuretic peptide system in rat ovaries. Endocrinology 1993; 132:693.
26. Rajfer J, Aronson WK, Bush PA, et al. Nitric oxide as a mediator of relaxation of the corpus cavernosum in response to nonadrenergic, noncholinergic neurotransmission. N Engl J Med 1992; 326:90.
27. Burnett AL. Nitric oxide control of lower genitourinary tract functions: a review. Urology 1995; 45:1071.
28. Roselli M, Keller PJ, Dubey RK. Role of nitric oxide in the biology, physiology, and pathophysiology of reproduction. Hum Reprod 1998; 4:3.
29. Blankenship T, Stewart DR, Benirschke K, et al. Immunocytochemical localization of nonluteal ovarian relaxin. J Reprod Med 1994; 39:235.
30. Palle C, Bredkjaer HE, Fahrenkrug J, et al. Vasoactive intestinal polypeptide loses its ability to increase vaginal blood flow after menopause. Am J Obstet Gynecol 1991; 164:556.
31. Ottesen B, Wagner G, Virag R, Fahrenkrug J. Penile erection: possible role for vasoactive intestinal polypeptide as a neurotransmitter. Br Med J 1984; 16:1.
32. Djamilian M, Stief CG, Kuczyk M, Jonas U. Followup results of a combination of calcitonin gene-related peptide and prostaglandin $E_1$ in the treatment of erectile dysfunction. J Urol 1993; 149:1296.
33. Tenmoku S, Ottesen B, O'Hare MMT, et al. Interaction of NPY and VIP in regulation of myometrial blood flow and mechanical activity. Peptides 1988; 9:269.
34. Gu J, Restorick JM, Blank MA, et al. Vasoactive intestinal polypeptide in the normal and unstable bladder. Br J Urol 1983; 55:645.
35. Gu J, Polak JM, Lazarides M, et al. Decrease of vasoactive intestinal polypeptide (VIP) in the penises from impotent men. Lancet 1984; 2:315.
36. Gerstenberg T, Metz P, Ottesen B, et al. Intracavernous self-injection with vasoactive intestinal polypeptide and phentolamine in the management of erectile failure. J Urol 1992; 147:1277.

# CHAPTER 185
# THE ENDOCRINE SKIN

MARK R. PITTELKOW

The skin serves as a unique endocrine organ. While performing its function as a barrier to physical, chemical, and biologic adversities, the skin is poised to sense and transmit innumerable signals from the external environment. Thermal and pressure stimuli can initiate homeostatic endocrine responses. Exogenous chemicals directly absorbed through the skin or metabolized en route by cutaneous tissues can regulate or alter other endocrine organ responses. Also, one region of the electromagnetic spectrum, ultraviolet radiation, participates in the generation of vitamin D hormone precursors.

Numerous hormones that have been purified and characterized from classic endocrine tissues have their counterparts in the skin. Some of these hormones may function locally within the skin or merely represent trivial, vestigial, or nonfunctional remnants of evolutionary change. Nevertheless, the number of hormones synthesized and secreted or metabolized by the skin indicates that this tissue should be regarded as an integral part of the endocrine system.

The anatomy and cellular composition of the skin are reviewed briefly because there are several diverse and important resident and transient cell populations that constitute the integument. The *epidermis* and *dermis* are easily recognized in a histologic section of normal skin (Fig. 185-1). They are separated but attached by a *basement membrane* that provides cellular integrity and tissue interactions while limiting the unrestricted passage of cells and mediators between compartments.

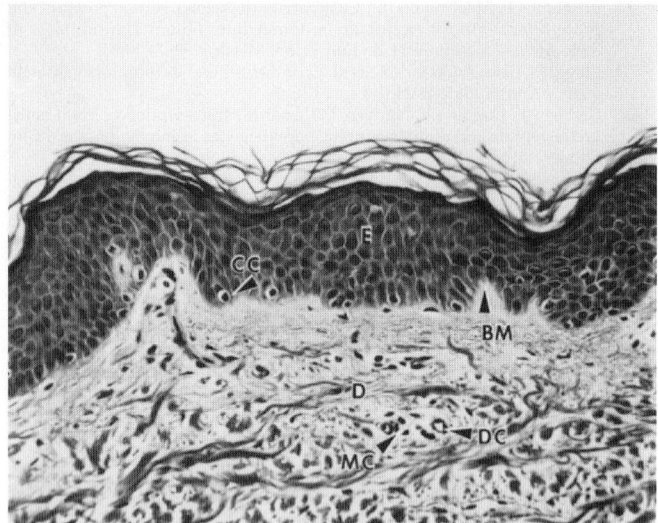

**FIGURE 185-1.** Human arm skin. The epidermis (*E*) is composed predominantly of darkly stained keratinocytes and a few "clear" cells (*CC*). Also shown is the basement membrane (*BM*) of the dermal-epidermal junction. The dermis (*D*) contains dermal capillary (*DC*) and perivascular mononuclear cells (*MC*) within the connective tissue (hematoxylineosin). ×250

## THE EPIDERMIS

### KERATINOCYTES

The epidermis mainly consists of stratified epithelial cells or keratinocytes.[1] Skin, a stratified epithelium, undergoes differentiation or *keratinization*. Keratinization is a complex, coordinated process of regulated gene expression, protein and macromolecule synthesis, and eventual nuclear dissolution that causes the formation of the *stratum corneum*, the outermost epidermal layer. The *stratum basale* or basal layer is the epithelial germinative compartment. The sebaceous gland and associated hair follicle and apocrine and eccrine sweat glands are specialized *epithelial appendages* (Fig. 185-2). Appendageal or epithelial glandular structures likely are capable of selected endocrine function not possessed by the other skin structures.

## MELANOCYTES AND LANGERHANS CELLS

Other cells comprising the epidermal resident population are the *melanocyte*, *Langerhans cell*, and *Merkel cell*. The melanocyte and Langerhans cells are distinctive, early embryonic migrants to the epidermis that associate with keratinocytes. The melanocyte arises from neuroectoderm and produces the pigment melanin by the enzymatic action of tyrosinase on tyrosine. Melanin is transferred to keratinocytes and functions as a natural photoprotective substance that screens skin from excessive, harmful ultraviolet radiation. The Langerhans cell originates from the bone marrow. It is a dendritic, immunocompetent cell (see Chap. 180) capable of antigen presentation. This capability is shared with other tissue-localized cells of monocyte-macrophage lineage. The melanocyte and Langerhans cells are recognized by light microscopy as basally located cells that possess a lightly stained cytoplasm, hence the term "clear cells" (see Fig. 185-1). They can be readily distinguished by histochemical, immunochemical, and ultrastructural markers.

### MERKEL CELLS

The Merkel cell is of ectodermal origin and is first identifiable during middle or late embryonic development. Unlike the Langerhans cell or melanocyte, the Merkel cell has desmosomal connections to surrounding basal keratinocytes. Merkel cells are associated with subepithelial nerve endings and occasionally cluster about hair to form discrete structures in animal skin known as "touch discs" or "haarsheiben." Merkel cells appear as clear cells on routine histologic examination, but ultrastructurally, they possess distinctive cytoplasmic organelles known as *neurosecretory granules* (Fig. 185-3). The Merkel cell can be recognized by specific histochemical or immunochemical staining procedures.

### TRANSIENT CELL CONSTITUENTS

The main cell types of the epidermis and their identifying markers are summarized in Table 185-1. Other cell lineages transiently occupy the epidermis. These include *mast cells*, *lymphocytes*, *granulocytes*, and *histiocytic cells*. In certain diseases, these cells appear to possess a proclivity to migrate to skin and enter the epidermis.

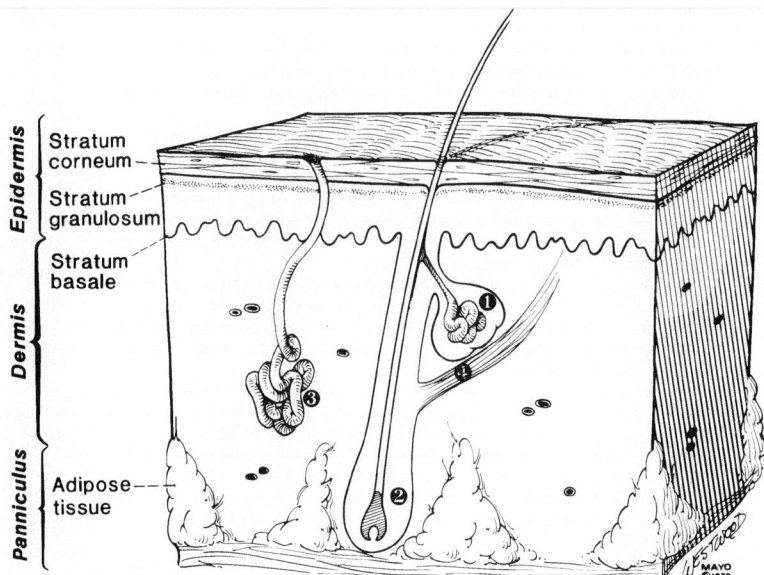

**FIGURE 185-2.** Cross section of human skin depicting sebaceous or apocrine gland (1), hair follicle (2), eccrine gland (3), and arrectores pilorum muscle (4) situated in the dermis. Dermis overlies adipose tissue.

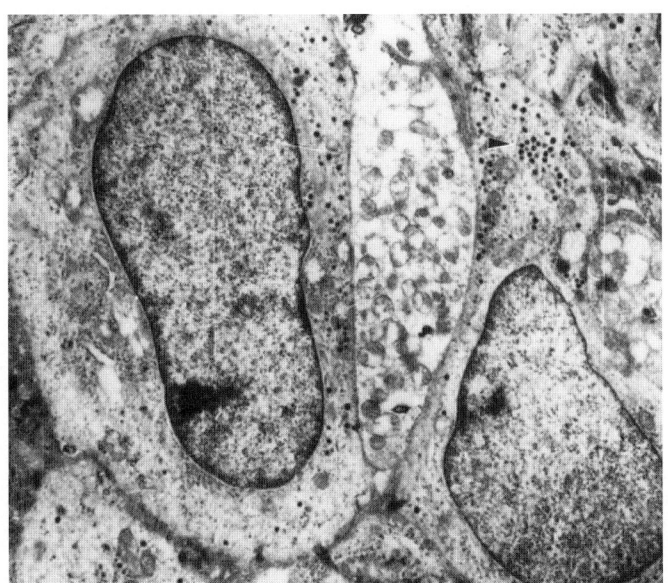

**FIGURE 185-3.** Epidermal Merkel cells. Note intracytoplasmic, membrane-bound, dense-core granules or neurosecretory granules (*arrow*) (electron micrograph; ×10,000). (Courtesy of R. K. Winkelmann.)

## THE DERMIS

Although the dermis is largely composed of collagen and other connective tissue elements, many cells of ectodermal, mesenchymal, and bone marrow origin occupy this compartment of the skin.[1] Organized structures include vascular and lymphatic vessels, and nerves and smooth muscle that constitute the arrectores pilorum apparatus. Dermal inhabitant cells include the *mast cell, lymphocyte, granulocyte, histiocyte-macrophage,* and *fibroblast.*

## CUTANEOUS BIOTRANSFORMATIONS OF HORMONES

In the context of cutaneous endocrine cooperation, several important biotransformations occur in the skin. Occasionally,

metabolic reactions can be localized to selected tissues or cells of the skin.

### METABOLISM OF TESTOSTERONE

The major conversion step for testosterone is its metabolism to 5α-dihydroxytestosterone (5α-DHT). It is performed within the skin by the enzyme 5α-reductase (see Chaps. 90 and 101). Other weak androgens, dehydroepiandrosterone and androstenedione, are converted to 5α-DHT (Fig. 185-4). 5α-Reductase activity appears to be localized mainly to the appendageal structures, especially the sebaceous and apocrine glands, although the epidermis and dermis also contain reductase activity. Isozymes of 5α-reductase have been identified, and human scalp contains predominantly 5α-reductase 1, which is distinct from the 5α-reductase 2 that predominates in prostate. 5α-Reductase activity may play an important role in development of androgenetic alopecia[2] (see Chap. 101). Testosterone metabolism may be a cooperative effort among several glandular epithelial cells at various stages of differentiation.[3] Hydroxysteroid oxidoreductases may also be localized in these glands. Epidermal keratinocytes can metabolize testosterone to 5α-DHT. 17β-Hydroxysteroid oxidoreductase and 3β-hydroxysteroid oxidoreductase also have been isolated from cultured keratinocytes.[4] It is likely that 5α-DHT is not the only active androgen. The androgen receptor for testosterone and 5α-DHT appears to be the same, although the receptor has increased affinity for 5α-DHT. The receptor does not appear to be modulated by androgens, because similar levels are seen in the skin of normal persons and patients with hirsutism. The androgen receptor is expressed by keratinocytes of epidermis and fibroblasts and vascular endothelial cells of dermis as well as eccrine glands, sebocytes, hair follicle root sheath, and papilla cells.[5] Human genital skin fibroblasts express both a complete 110-kDa isoform (type B) and an 87-kDa truncated (type A) form of androgen receptor that may differentially regulate androgen responsiveness of target tissues.[6] Aging may decrease androgen receptors.

### ABNORMALITIES OF ANDROGEN BIOTRANSFORMATION

Several studies have delineated abnormalities of androgen biotransformation. Pubic skin fibroblasts from patients with

**TABLE 185-1.**
**Epidermal Cell Populations**

| Cell | Ontogeny | Histochemistry | Immunochemistry | Ultrastructural Markers |
|---|---|---|---|---|
| **KERATINOCYTE** | Ectoderm | Keratin stains | Keratins | Keratin tonofilament |
| | | Acid phosphatase | Desmosomal proteins | Desmosomes |
| | | Succinic dehydrogenase | Lectin binding | Keratohyalin |
| | | Indoxyl-esterase | Epithelial differentiation antibodies | |
| **MELANOCYTE** | Neuroectoderm | Dihydroxyphenylalanine (DOPA) | Vimentin | Melanosomes |
| | | | S100 CD57 | |
| | | Silver stains | Tyrosinase and melanosome-specific antibodies | |
| **LANGERHANS CELL** | Bone marrow | Gold chloride | CD1, CD4, CD23, CD45, CD83 | Birbeck or Langerhans cell granules |
| | | Heavy metal ions | Class II MHC antigens (HLA-DR) | |
| | | Adenosine triphosphatase (ATPase) | FcIgG | |
| | | | C3 receptor | |
| | | | Vimentin | |
| | | | S100 | |
| **MERKEL CELL** | Ectoderm | Cholinesterase (neurite complex) | Keratin | Neurosecretory granules |
| | | Grimelius (argyrophilic) stain | Neuron-specific enolase | Cytoplasmic rodlet |
| | | Quinacrine | Neuropeptides | Perinuclear whorls |

*Fc,* fragment of crystallization; *HLA-DR,* human leukocyte antigen DR; *MHC,* major histocompatibility complex.

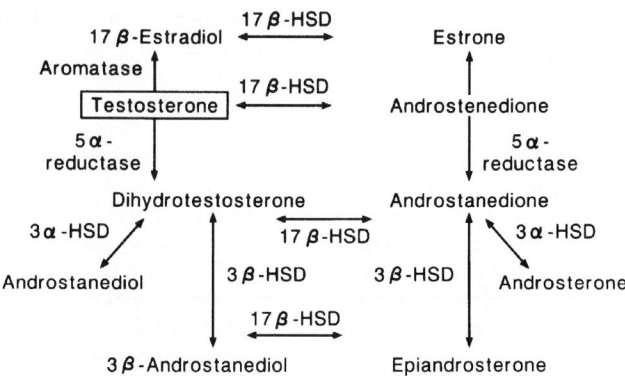

**FIGURE 185-4.** Cutaneous androgen metabolism. Androgens can be metabolized to estradiol by aromatase. (*HSD*, hydroxysteroid dehydrogenases or hydroxysteroid oxidoreductases.)

"idiopathic" hirsutism exhibit increased 5α-reductase levels.[7] In hirsute patients with polycystic ovary syndrome (see Chap. 96), a serum metabolite, androstanediol glucuronide, is elevated markedly.[8] Although not the cause of hirsutism, this metabolite may serve as a marker of increased androgen formation in peripheral tissues at the level of the pilosebaceous gland. Patients with late-onset adrenal hyperplasia and hirsutism do not have increased 5α-reductase activity[9] (see Chap. 77). In these cases, hirsutism results from the overproduction of androgens, especially androstenedione, which can be detected because of the high levels of 3α-androstanediol excreted in the urine. In this condition, hirsutism probably depends on the capacity of the skin to use circulating androgens. Conversely, rare forms of male pseudohermaphroditism arise from deficiency of 5α-reductase activity that prevents the production of the active tissue metabolite, 5α-DHT, or from androgen insensitivity. Skin and its appendages, including hair development, fail to respond normally during sexual development (see Chap. 90).

## SYNTHESIS OF ESTROGEN

The synthesis of estrogen in peripheral tissues from circulating androgen is a major pathway for estrogen formation. It accounts for virtually all estrogen production in men and postmenopausal women. Human hair follicle tissue has the capacity for the aromatization of androstenedione[10] (see Fig. 185-4). Reports have documented rare instances of massive extraglandular aromatization of androstenedione in prepubertal boys that cause feminization.[11] However, in normal adults, aromatase activity is low in all tissues, including skin.

## GLUCOCORTICOID RECEPTORS

Human skin fibroblasts and keratinocytes contain macromolecules that bind glucocorticoids with high affinity. Glucocorticoid receptors occur in epidermis and dermis. However, negligible biosynthesis of glucocorticoids occurs in skin, although these sterols undergo biotransformation and metabolism in skin.

## CARBOHYDRATE METABOLISM OF THE SKIN

Glucose serves as a metabolic energy source and a substrate for the biosynthesis of glycogen, glycoproteins, glycolipids, mucopolysaccharides, and nucleic acids. Compared with other tissues, skin does not differ significantly in pathways of glycolysis and oxidation. Circulating glucose appears to diffuse readily into the dermis and epidermis, where glucose appears to cross the epidermal cell membrane, accounting for its apparent excess in extracellular fluid. Rates of glucose metabolism are comparable to those in other active tissues, such as muscle. Within the epidermis, it is likely that the various stages of differentiation influence glucose use. Less glucose is used in more-keratinized layers. In certain proliferative states and epidermal diseases with increased metabolic demand, glucose metabolism is increased. Anagen hair follicles (see Chap. 101) metabolize twice the glucose of resting follicles. Healing epidermis and psoriatic epidermis also demonstrate enhanced glucose uptake. Conversely, the glucose use of dermis is much lower.

Insulin appears to regulate glucose metabolism in skin, and epidermis in culture possesses receptors for insulin. Untreated diabetics have been shown to have reduced lipogenic activity in skin that is corrected by insulin administration.

Glucose metabolism by the skin occurs readily because all enzymes of the glycolytic pathway and tricarboxylic acid cycle are found in skin. In addition, the hexose monophosphate pathway appears to be active in the epidermis and is increased in epidermal proliferative states such as psoriasis, neoplasia, and hyperplasia.

Products of glucose metabolism include glycogen, which occurs preferentially in epidermis and is quantitatively altered by various diseases or by physical, chemical, and environmental factors. Glycoproteins, glycolipids, and glycosaminoglycans are synthesized in skin from glucose metabolites. They are integral components of a number of skin-related organelles or functions involved in keratinization and differentiation.[12,13]

## MISCELLANEOUS HORMONE BIOTRANSFORMATIONS

### MONODEIODINATION OF THYROXINE

Thyroxine ($T_4$) is metabolized largely by either outer ring monodeiodination to active triiodothyronine ($T_3$) or by inner ring monodeiodination to the inactive form, reverse $T_3$ ($rT_3$; see Chap. 30).[14,15] Cultured human keratinocytes convert $T_4$ to $T_3$ by an outer ring deiodinase.[16] There are several distinct iodothyronine 5'-deiodinases (types I, Ia, II, and III); type II is the active enzyme in cultured keratinocytes.[16]

Monodeiodination of $T_4$ contributes ~80% of the serum $T_3$ and almost 95% of the $rT_3$ produced daily in humans. Until relatively recently, the organs or tissues that metabolized $T_4$ to $rT_3$ were unknown. Skin appears to be several times more active in inner ring monodeiodination than brain, both tissues possessing many times more activity than other organs.[14] No difference in deiodinating activity is seen with skin from various anatomic sites. The activity is predominantly isolated from the microsomal fraction of skin and appears to be enzymatic. It is inactivated by heating and inhibited by $T_3$ and 3,5-diiodothyronine, but not by inhibitors of $T_4$ outer ring (5') deiodinase, such as propylthiouracil. During pregnancy, the skin production of $rT_3$ is decreased and placental monodeiodination is increased. Apparently, skin contributes significantly to the conversion of $T_4$ to $rT_3$, and this reaction may be physiologically regulated. The effects of $rT_3$ have yet to be elucidated.

### PEPTIDE BIOTRANSFORMATION

Human skin contains a chymotrypsin-like proteinase, as well as several other proteases that may participate in peptide biotransformations. One such biotransformation is the conversion of angiotensin I to angiotensin II, in which cleavage of the Phe[8]-His[9] bond from the decapeptide precursor occurs by angiotensin-converting enzyme (ACE). Human skin chymotrypsin-like proteinase can perform this enzymatic function, with kinetic constants that are physiologically relevant.[17] Other proteinases, such as human leukocyte cathepsin $G_1$, can convert angiotensinogen to angiotensin II in the absence of renin or ACE. The tissue microenvironment, especially skin, may provide enzymatic activity for angiotensin II production by ACE-independent pathways. Neutral endopeptidase is another peptidase localized to keratinocytes, hair follicles, and eccrine and sebaceous glands. Localized near nerve endings, this membrane-associated peptidase can inactivate proinflammatory and mitogenically active neuropeptides.[18]

## CUTANEOUS VITAMIN D BIOSYNTHESIS

Of all the hormones synthesized in the skin, perhaps the best-known and characterized hormone has been vitamin D (see Chap. 54). The early biosynthetic steps of vitamin D have been defined.[19–21] Although early clinical observations in the seventeenth to nineteenth centuries suggested a relationship between sunlight and the cure and prevention of rickets, it was not until the early 1900s that vitamin D from dietary sources was shown to be the same as that made in mammalian skin from exposure to the ultraviolet radiation (UVR) of sunlight. Only in the past decade have the intricacies of the production and regulation of previtamin $D_3$ by the skin been unraveled. Vitamin $D_3$ does not fulfill the strict requirements for a vitamin, because skin, in conjunction with UVR, has the capacity to synthesize this sterol.

### PHOTOCONVERSION

7-Dehydrocholesterol (provitamin $D_3$) in skin is converted to previtamin $D_3$ by UVR that cleaves the bond at $C_9$-$C_{10}$ (Fig. 185-5). Using skin slices and selective separation techniques, this reaction is found to occur mainly throughout the epidermis and only to a small extent in the dermis. Owing to the proximity to the circulating blood pool, most of the synthetic activity is localized to the stratum basale and midepidermal layers. Photoconversion occurs over a fairly wide absorption spectrum, with a peak at 295

to 300 nm. Narrow-band irradiation of skin produces significantly greater amounts of previtamin $D_3$ than does simulated sunlight exposure. This is because of the fact that during prolonged exposure and longer-band irradiation, previtamin $D_3$ is photolyzed to the inactive product, lumisterol, and in lesser amounts to tachysterol. These photoisomers are generated by wider-band UVR. After 8 hours of exposure, almost 50% of 7-dehydrocholesterol is converted to lumisterol in light-skinned persons. The synthesis of previtamin $D_3$ reaches a plateau of 10% to 15% of the original cutaneous 7-dehydrocholesterol concentration. The inactive photoisomers, lumisterol and tachysterol, have little affinity for vitamin D–binding proteins and likely are sloughed off during the natural turnover of skin. The conversion of previtamin $D_3$ to inactive photoisomers is reversible, so that if vitamin $D_3$ is depleted, more previtamin $D_3$ is converted from lumisterol.

The subsequent conversion of previtamin $D_3$ to vitamin $D_3$ occurs by simple thermal isomerization. Approximately 50% of previtamin $D_3$ in rat skin is isomerized in vivo to vitamin $D_3$ in 18 hours. By 3 days, 95% of the remaining material is present as vitamin $D_3$. Skin specimens subjected to temperatures of 0°C formed virtually no vitamin $D_3$.

Mammalian skin had been assumed to produce only a single vitamin D. However, studies have demonstrated at least one other provitamin D, namely, 24-dehydroprovitamin $D_3$.[22] It is detected not only in human skin, but in the skin of rats, reptiles, amphibians, and birds. As shown in Figure 185-5, 24-dehydroprovitamin $D_3$ can be photoconverted to 24-dehydroprevitamin $D_3$ and isomerized to dehydrovitamin $D_3$. Approximately 20% of the total provitamin D in skin occurs as the 24-dehydro form. The physiologic function is not known, although it has been suggested that 24-dehydrovitamin $D_3$ is bioactive, albeit to a lesser degree than is vitamin $D_3$.

Studies have shown that cultured human keratinocytes and perfused pig skin also synthesize 1,25-dihydroxyvitamin $D_3$ [$1,25(OH)_2D_3$] from 25-hydroxyvitamin $D_3$ [$25(OH)D_3$].[23] Furthermore, $1,25(OH)_2D_3$ inhibits its own production in cultured keratinocytes and induces $24,25(OH)_2D_3$ and $1,24,25(OH)_3D_3$. These findings indicate that human keratinocytes possess 1α-hydroxylase and 24α-hydroxylase activity. Anephric patients have very low levels of $1,25(OH)_2D_3$, because the major conver-

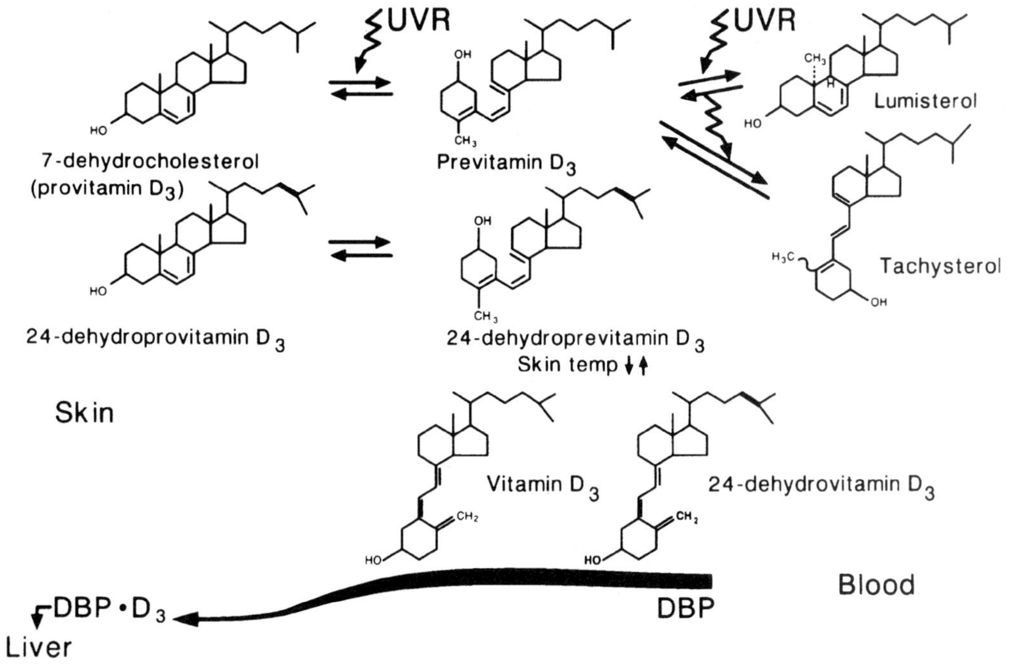

**FIGURE 185-5.** Cutaneous vitamin D biosynthesis. Diagrammatic representation of photoconversion of 7-dehydrocholesterol or 24-dehydroprovitamin $D_3$ in skin and transfer of vitamin $D_3$ or 24-dehydrovitamin $D_3$ to vitamin D–binding protein (*DBP*) in blood. (*UVR*, ultraviolet radiation.) (Modified from Holick MF. The cutaneous photosynthesis of previtamin $D_3$: a unique photoendocrine system. J Invest Dermatol 1981; 76:51.)

sion of 25(OH)D$_3$ by 1α-hydroxylase occurs in the kidney. However, local production, utilization, and metabolism of 1,25(OH)$_2$D$_3$ occurs in epidermis.

## TRANSLOCATION TO THE BLOOD

Vitamin D$_3$ is preferentially removed from the skin into the circulation by vitamin D–binding protein, where it is carried to liver and kidney for further hydroxylation. The translocation from skin to blood provides for efficient and selective removal of the product, vitamin D$_3$, which, in turn, shifts the thermal isomerization equilibrium from previtamin D$_3$ to vitamin D$_3$. The advantage of this regulatory pathway to the organism is that a short exposure to sunlight can readily convert provitamin D$_3$ to previtamin D$_3$, which is stored in skin. The thermal isomerization of previtamin D$_3$ to vitamin D$_3$ is slow and allows D$_3$ release into the circulation for several days after exposure to light.

## PATHOPHYSIOLOGIC INFLUENCES

Correlative studies have demonstrated effects of skin pigmentation, seasonal exposure to sunlight, aging, and vitamin D deficiency on the regulation of cutaneous vitamin D$_3$ biosynthesis. For example, after whole body exposure to UVR, vitamin D–deficient individuals had significant increases in serum 1,25(OH)$_2$D$_3$ concentrations, compared with otherwise healthy persons.[24] Skin from elderly persons possesses less than half the biosynthetic activity for vitamin D$_3$ that is found in the skin of young people.[25] Equal doses of UVR produce significantly greater concentrations of serum vitamin D in lightly pigmented whites than are produced in heavily pigmented black persons.[26] Only with much greater doses of UVR do serum vitamin D concentrations increase for the skin of blacks. It appears that melanized skin competes with 7-dehydrocholesterol for photon energy from UVR. This may explain the occurrence of rickets among black infants in cities of the northeastern United States.

Intriguing regulatory functions are continually being established for vitamin D synthesis in the skin.[27,28] The hydroxylated vitamin, 1,25(OH)$_2$D$_3$, active in target tissues, is concentrated in skin. Administration of 1,25(OH)$_2$D$_3$ to vitamin-deficient animals increases the concentration of 7-dehydrocholesterol in skin. This likely occurs through the stimulation of 7-dehydrocholesterol biosynthesis from mevalonate. Patients with vitamin D–dependent rickets (type II) who possess a defective cytosolic receptor for 1,25(OH)$_2$D$_3$ fail to demonstrate this positive-feedback activity (see Chaps. 54 and 63).

# EICOSANOIDS

The resident and transient populations of skin cells are capable of synthesizing arachidonic acid metabolites, collectively named *eicosanoids* (see Chap. 172). Major groups of the eicosanoids include the prostaglandins (PG), hydroxyeicosatetraenoic acids (HETE), leukotrienes (LT), thromboxanes, and lipoxins.

The major substrate for eicosanoid production is arachidonic acid. Arachidonic acid is present in most cell membranes esterified to glycerophospholipids and is enzymatically cleaved to the free acid by phospholipase A$_2$ or phospholipase C and diglyceride lipase. Arachidonic acid is a substrate for two categories of enzymes that generate the eicosanoids. Cyclooxygenase catalyzes the synthesis of the PGs and thromboxanes, and the lipoxygenases generate the various HETEs and LTs. Many tissues and cell types synthesize arachidonic acid products, including the skin. Initial studies demonstrating PG production

by a variety of tissues led to the concept that there was minimal specificity for the generation of these compounds. However, as the complexity of the eicosanoid synthetic pathways became known and purified cell populations were assayed for selected enzymatic activities and for the synthesized products, it became apparent that a unique profile of eicosanoid production existed for each cell type and that certain tissues did not possess particular enzymatic capabilities.

## CYCLOOXYGENASE PATHWAY OF THE EPIDERMIS

In the early 1970s, it was shown that human skin was able to synthesize PGs.[29,30] PGE$_2$, PGF$_{2\alpha}$, and PGD$_2$ are produced by the cyclooxygenase pathway of skin, involving the two isoenzymes COX-1 and COX-2.[31] 12-HETE is the major HETE metabolite.[32] Epidermal cells, in short-term culture, produce PGE$_2$, which can be inhibited by indomethacin and aspirin.[33] PGE$_2$ can be extracted from human sweat, implying that glandular (e.g., eccrine) epithelium may be capable of eicosanoid production.

Although 90% to 95% of the epidermal cell population is composed of keratinocytes, the small percentage of Langerhans cells, melanocytes, or other migrant cells may produce significant quantities of eicosanoid products that differ from keratinocyte products. Long-term cultures of purified keratinocytes have shown that PGE$_2$ and PGF$_{2\alpha}$ are synthesized by keratinocytes.[34] Calcium appears to modulate arachidonic acid metabolism at a number of regulatory points.

## LIPOXYGENASE PATHWAY OF THE EPIDERMIS

Because lipoxygenase products are among the most potent chemoattractants for granulocytes and monocytes, and because they increase vascular permeability, these phlogistic substances have been implicated in the etiopathogenesis of a variety of inflammatory skin diseases. Several reports have demonstrated that LT-like substances are extractable from pathologic scale or epidermis of psoriasis and other inflammatory dermatoses, or can be generated when keratinocytes are cultured.[35-37]

LTB$_4$ material has been isolated from psoriatic scale; however, leukocytes within the epidermis may be responsible for this finding. A novel stereoisomer, 12(R)-HETE, has been shown to be a major lipoxygenase product along with authentic LTB$_4$ in psoriatic scale.[38] The rare but distinctive glucagonoma syndrome presents with the cutaneous finding of necrolytic migratory erythema. The epithelial toxic reaction may be the result of arachidonic acid metabolites generated in skin that are induced by elevated glucagon levels.[39]

Other studies have failed to demonstrate eicosanoid production from melanoma cells, although normal melanocytes may produce these mediators. Because Langerhans cell purification and culture are limited, no definitive evidence for the production of eicosanoids has appeared. Langerhans cells, however, probably possess capabilities for the generation of arachidonic acid metabolites similar to those of other bone marrow–derived, immunocompetent cells.

## DERMAL EICOSANOIDS

Dermal resident cells, particularly fibroblasts, are known to synthesize a variety of eicosanoids; also, the hematopoietic-derived dermal cells (i.e., lymphocytes, granulocytes, mast cells, and histiocytes) contribute significantly to eicosanoids generated in the dermis. Endothelial cells lining blood and lymphatic capillaries have been shown to produce PGs, including prostacyclin (PGI$_2$). Thromboxanes are generated by platelets and may participate in local tissue reactions if platelets accumulate in dermal capillaries. Macrophages also produce thromboxanes and pathway-related derivatives that are chemotactic for human eosinophils and neutrophils.

## PATHOPHYSIOLOGIC FUNCTIONS OF THE EICOSANOIDS

In addition to their chemoattractant and proinflammatory properties, the eicosanoids have been implicated in the regulation of several other cutaneous functions. PGs may regulate keratinocyte proliferation. $PGE_2$ injected into skin increases the mitotic index of epidermal basal cells, but $PGF_{2\alpha}$ has no effect. This may occur through activation of cyclic adenosine monophosphate (cAMP). Proliferating cultures of keratinocytes synthesize increased quantities of $PGE_2$, and indomethacin inhibits the proliferative rate.[40] Similar activities have been demonstrated for $LTB_4$, $C_4$, and $D_4$, although the mechanism of induction is unknown. Eicosanoids applied to the skin, injected intradermally, or released locally in the skin by various stimuli, such as histamine, anthralin, or UVR, can produce erythema and neutrophil accumulation with intraepidermal pustule formation.[41] $PGE_2$ functions as a vasodilator, and $PGF_{2\alpha}$ is a vasoconstrictor. $LTC_4$, $D_4$, and $E_4$ can induce vascular leakage, and topically applied $LTB_4$ causes neutrophil adherence to endothelium and exocytosis into the epidermis, forming micropustules.

Inhibitors of eicosanoid production include the nonsteroidal antiinflammatory drugs, such as aspirin and indomethacin, which inhibit cyclooxygenase and prostanoid production. Arachidonic acid production can be significantly decreased by corticosteroids. Corticosteroid activity is mediated by lipocortin-like proteins that form a family of steroid-induced inhibitors of phospholipase activity. These proteins are found in diverse cell types, including fibroblasts and epithelial cells.[42] Although these inhibitors decrease inflammation and improve skin diseases in which eicosanoid production is abnormal (e.g., psoriasis), it would be presumptuous to state that eicosanoids represent the central defect in these skin disorders. However, skin has the potential to synthesize a wide spectrum of eicosanoids, which probably contribute significantly to the physiologic regulation and pathologic disorders of skin and other target tissues.

## CATECHOLAMINES AND CHOLINERGIC MEDIATORS

The skin has been identified as a source for catecholamine synthesis, because epidermis and human keratinocytes express biopterin-dependent tyrosine hydroxylase as well as phenylethanolamine-N-methyl transferase[43] (see Chap. 85). Tyrosine is a central substrate in human epidermis for the biosynthesis of melanins in melanocytes and catecholamines by keratinocytes. Melanocytes and melanoma cells exhibit catechol-O-methyltransferase activity for catecholamine removal,[44] and skin also appears to be a source of monoamine oxidase activity.

Both keratinocytes and melanocytes of epidermis and dermal fibroblasts express $\beta_2$-adrenoceptors and, therefore, also respond to locally expressed catecholamines. Expression of $\beta_2$-adrenoreceptors in epidermis appear to be regulated by differentiation and also may mediate cellular calcium regulation.[45]

The dual expression of catecholamines and adrenergic receptors in skin, appendageal glands, and cutaneous neurovascular structures allows local mediation of responses within this tissue (see Chap. 85). The essential cofactor for phenylalanine hydroxylase, which converts phenylalanine to tyrosine, is 5,6,7,8-tetrahydrobiopterin. Regulation of melanin biosynthesis as well

as development of a disorder of pigmentation, vitiligo, may be exerted through these cofactors and metabolic pathways.[46]

The nonneuronal cholinergic transmitter system is active in skin, whereas keratinocytes express muscarinic receptors and also exhibit enzymatic activities capable of synthesizing, secreting, and degrading acetylcholine.[47,48] This transmitter system may function in epidermis to regulate various physiologic responses, including reepithelialization as well as cell-cell adhesion. Its role in mediating dyshesive, acantholytic diseases such as pemphigus or other skin diseases is under investigation.

## PEPTIDE HORMONES, CYTOKINES, AND GROWTH FACTORS

An array of peptide hormones has been isolated from human and animal skin (Table 185-2). Amphibian skin actively synthesizes and stores thyrotropin-releasing hormone and many other hormones, such as bombesin, vasoactive intestinal peptide (VIP), tachykinins (substance P–like), opioid peptides, xanopsin (neurotensin-like), and cerulein (cholecystokinin-like).[49,50] Indeed, the localization and possible function of these hormones in various mammalian tissues follow early investigations characterizing similar peptides isolated from amphibian skin. These biologically active peptides appear to function in the mammalian central nervous system as neurotransmitters or neuromodulators, and in specific, responsive tissues that possess receptors for these hormones. The functional significance of the occurrence of high levels of these peptide hormones in dermal glands of amphibian skin is unknown. Their occurrence in mammalian skin often is restricted to nerves, although equivalent hormones have been demonstrated in the gastrointestinal tract, brain, and peripheral tissues.

The proopiomelanocortin products, $\alpha$ melanocyte–stimulating hormone ($\alpha$-MSH) and adrenocorticotropin (ACTH), are synthesized in skin, and both are active at the melanocortin-1 receptor found on melanocytes, keratinocytes, dermal fibroblasts, hair follicles, and sweat glands.[51] MSH appears to regulate pigmentation via synthesis of *eumelanin* and to modulate inflammatory and immune processes via effects on nuclear factor-κB (NF-κB).[52]

## PARATHYROID HORMONE–LIKE AND PHOSPHATURIC FACTORS IN SKIN

Peptide hormones secreted by diverse endocrine tissues have been localized within human skin or synthesized and secreted by cultured epithelial or mesenchymal skin cells. In this regard, parathyroid hormone (PTH)–like factors have been found in extracts of squamous epithelial tumors (see Chaps. 52, 59, and 219).[53,54] These tumors are associated with the humoral hypercalcemia of malignancy. Human keratinocytes in culture synthesize a PTH-like molecule that binds to the PTH receptor and stimulates cAMP production.[55] The molecular masses of the PTH-like material vary from 6 to 17 kDa. The gene for PTH-related protein (PTHrP) has been sequenced and shown to be expressed in normal epidermal keratinocytes, other epithelial tissues (e.g., lactating mammary epithelium), and a variety of carcinomas.[56] The physiologic significance of PRP expression in normal epithelium remains to be defined. Normal expression of PRP may regulate differentiation of epidermis and epithelial appendages, because inhibition of expression inhibits keratinocyte differentiation, and overexpression in transgenic animals disrupts normal hair follicle formation.[57] This may involve regulation of keratinocyte growth factor.[58]

**TABLE 185-2.**
**Peptide Hormones of Skin of Humans and Other Mammals**

**KERATINOCYTES**
  Parathyroid-hormone–related protein
  Osteoclast-activating factor–like polypeptide
  Thymic peptide hormones
    Thymulin
    Thymopoietin
    Thymosin$_4$
  Proopiomelanocortin-melanocyte–stimulating hormone
  Interleukins
    Epidermal thymocyte-activating factor/IL-1
    IL-3
    IL-7
    IL-8
    IL-10
  Colony-stimulating factors
    Granulocyte-macrophage colony-stimulating factor
    Granulocyte colony-stimulating factor
    Macrophage colony-stimulating factor
  Growth factors/growth regulators
    Transforming growth factor-α
    Amphiregulin
    Heparin-binding epidermal growth factor
    Fibroblast growth factors
    Mast-cell growth factor (c-*kit* ligand)
    Nerve growth factor
    Platelet-derived growth factor
    Tumor necrosis factor
    Transforming growth factor-β
**LANGERHANS CELL AND NERVES**
  Neuropeptides
    Calcitonin gene–related peptide
  IL-12
**MELANOCYTES**
  Interleukins
    IL-1α, IL-1β
    IL-3
    IL-6
    IL-8
  Granulocyte-macrophage colony-stimulating factor
  Tumor necrosis factor
  Macrophage chemotactic and activating factor
  Transforming growth factor-β
**MERKEL CELLS (NEUROENDOCRINE CELLS) AND NERVES**
  Neuropeptides
  Substance P
  Vasoactive intestinal peptide
  Bombesin-like peptides
  Somatostatin*
  Serotonin*
  Calcitonin*
  Adrenocorticotropic hormone
  Leu-met-enkephalin*
**FIBROBLASTS**
  Insulin-like growth factor-I/somatomedin C
  Fibroblast growth factor, keratinocyte growth factor
  IL-6

*IL*, interleukin.
*Found in neuroendocrine tumors.

Another cytokine, osteoclast-activating factor, is released from T lymphocytes. Osteoclast-mediated bone resorption can be stimulated by a soluble factor from cultured keratinocytes. Clinically, however, primary hypoparathyroid states or the sur-

gical extirpation of parathyroid glands cause a hormonal deficiency that is not ameliorated by other extraglandular sources, such as skin. The significance of skin-related calcitropic hormones and the PTH-like activity purified from selected malignant tissues is poorly understood.

Factors stimulating phosphaturia that lead to a vitamin D–resistant rickets have been identified in tumorous skin and subcutaneous lesions, and the condition has been designated oncogenic osteomalacia.[59] Angiofibromatous dermal lesions from rare cases of epidermal nevus syndrome exhibiting osteomalacia contain a phosphaturic substance.[60] A peptide factor has been isolated from a subcutaneous sclerosing hemangioma and shown to inhibit phosphate transport without increasing cellular concentrations of cAMP.[61] Further characterization is in progress; this factor may represent a novel peptide hormone, "phosphatonin," that is expressed by various cutaneous and subcutaneous vascular or mesenchymal tumors and causes oncogenic osteomalacia.[62]

## IMMUNE-RELATED PEPTIDES

The skin can produce several distinct, immune-related peptides that have traditionally been isolated from the thymus gland or lymphoid cells (i.e., lymphocytes and macrophages). Skin and thymic epithelium bear distinct morphologic resemblance. Both tissues are composed of keratinizing epithelium and share expression of surface and cytoplasmic antigens.[63,64] Several thymic hormones have been isolated from skin. Cultured human keratinocytes produce thymopoietin and antibodies to thymulin (formerly *facteur thymique serique*), bind to skin, and appear to localize to intracellular, intermediate-sized filaments.[65,66]

Thymosin B$_4$, originally isolated from thymus and purified from cruder fractions designated thymosin and thymosin fraction 5, is detected by immunoreactive assays in a variety of tissues and organs, including skin. Thymosin B$_4$ induces expression of terminal deoxynucleotidyl transferase, an early marker of T-lymphocyte differentiation. Supernatants from epidermal cell cultures are able to induce human T cells to express terminal deoxynucleotidyl transferase.[67] These thymic preparations and purified peptide hormones are effective in regulating immune function by enhancing T-cell differentiation of prothymocytes and specific subclasses of T lymphocytes. Although the functions of numerous thymic peptides are still being classified, the thymus gland has assumed the status of an endocrine organ (see Chap. 193). The skin, possessing the ability to secrete selected thymic hormones, may be a potential site for the extrathymic maturation of T lymphocytes.

## INTERLEUKINS, CHEMOKINES, COLONY-STIMULATING FACTORS, AND OTHER CYTOKINES

Soluble, immunoregulatory hormones secreted by lymphoid cells and termed *lymphokines* or *interleukins*, are also produced by the skin (see Chap. 195). Interleukin-1 (IL-1), a product initially isolated from macrophages, enhances the growth of thymocytes. A chemically and biologically similar polypeptide is secreted by cultured human epidermal cells and is designated epidermal thymocyte-activating factor (ETAF).[68–70] It is synthesized by keratinocytes and can be augmented by UVR in vitro or in vivo.[71] Purified populations of Langerhans cells also appear to synthesize IL-1.[72] ETAF possesses biologic properties similar to IL-1. ETAF is a chemoattractant for neutrophils and lymphocytes and can induce fever when administered systemically. Nuclear hybridization studies suggest that ETAF is homologous to IL-1. Substantial amounts of ETAF and IL-1 are present in normal stratum corneum.[73] This hormone may serve as an early inflammatory mediator to signal disruption of epithelial integrity. The stratum corneum may function as a physiologic receptacle, and with desquamation, excessively produced hormone is conveniently removed. As a proinflammatory substance and thymocyte activator, ETAF or IL-1 may participate in the development of a variety of inflammatory dermatoses and cutaneous lymphoproliferative disorders (e.g., cutaneous T-cell lymphoma or mycosis fungoides) in which malignant T cells preferentially migrate and localize in skin.[74,75]

IL-1–receptor antagonists and IL-1 receptors are also expressed within the epidermis and skin and, together, they regulate IL-1 activities and inflammatory responses in healthy skin and in disease.[76]

Other interleukins, including IL-3, IL-6, IL-7, IL-8, IL-10, and IL-12, also appear to be expressed in skin and its specific component cell types. The molecular interactions of these factors on immune and nonimmune cells are complex, but their bioactivities suggest they may exert significant effects on the regulation of normal immunologic function in skin as well as in immunologic or malignant diseases such as allergic dermatitis and cutaneous T-cell lymphoma.[77] Additional cytokines expressed by skin, epidermis, cultured keratinocytes, Langerhans cells, or melanocytes include the colony-stimulating factors (CSF), specifically granulocyte CSF, macrophage CSF, and granulocyte-macrophage CSF.[78–80]

Immunoeffector molecules such as tumor necrosis factor (cachectin), which is primarily secreted by activated macrophages, have been localized to epidermis after selected stimuli.[81] As with thymic hormones, however, the biologic significance of these cytokines in normal and abnormal cutaneous immunoregulation remains to be defined (see Chap. 173).

Another family of novel small cytokines related to IL-8 is the chemokines. These peptide factors number at least 16 and contain four conserved cysteines that form disulfide bonds. The arrangement of cysteines, either adjacent (C-C) or separated by one amino acid (C-X-C), constitutes two subfamilies of the chemokines. Chemokines, including monocyte chemotactic protein-1, macrophage inflammatory protein, RANTES (regulated on activation, normal T expressed and secreted), neutrophil-activating protein-2, and the GRO-related proteins, participate in recruiting and activating leukocytic cells and regulating the inflammatory response.[82,82a] Several of these family members and their receptors have been identified in skin, and their roles in locally mediated endocrine responses and allergic inflammation are being elaborated.

## NEUROPEPTIDES

Neuropeptides have been isolated from the skin of humans and other mammals. Neurotensin, substance P, and VIP are immunocytochemically localized to subepithelial nerves, dermal papillae, epidermis, Meissner corpuscles, and nerves closely connected to sweat ducts and blood vessels.[83,84] Bombesin-like peptides and somatostatin have been detected in cat and pig skin, and preliminary reports indicate their presence in human skin, although localization to specific structures has been unsuccessful.

Calcitonin gene–related peptide (CGRP) is a neuropeptide and vasodilatory factor that localizes to cutaneous nerves, and CGRP nerve endings have been shown to impinge on Langerhans cells in epidermis. CGRP inhibits Langerhans cell antigen presentation and appears to exert immunomodulatory effects in vivo.[85] Neuroimmunologic networks, therefore, are active in the skin and regulate cutaneous immune function among other biologic responses.

Substance P appears to play an important role in neurogenic inflammation of peripheral tissues.[86] When injected, it causes vasodilation and plasma extravasation, producing wheal-and-flare responses. The wheal response is directly related to substance P; the flare is caused by the release of histamine from skin mast cells (see Chap. 181). Substance P transmits nociceptive signals and elicits a cutaneous itch sensation.

VIP may be important in regulating skin blood flow and secretion. An abnormality of VIP innervation is seen in cystic fibrosis.[87] Skin biopsy specimens from patients with cystic fibrosis show a marked deficiency of VIP-immunoreactive nerve fibers around sweat glands and ducts.

## BRADYKININ

Bradykinin is a small peptide hormone representative of a class of widely distributed neuropeptides called *kinins* (see Chap. 170). Kinins are formed by activation of larger precursor molecules, kininogens. The enzymes that activate kininogens are proteases, designated kallikreins, that are found in liver, kidney, and exocrine glands. Bradykinin is a nonapeptide, and a related homologue is lys-bradykinin (or kallidin), which differs by an additional lysine at the amino terminus of the peptide. The half-lives of these molecules are very short. They exert their influence by binding to the cell-surface receptor, which releases other chemical mediators, such as VIP, substance P, or PG. Bradykinin is increased in inflammatory skin diseases and can be isolated from sweat glands.[88] Local proteases, such as the chymotrypsin-like protease or the kallikrein-like enzyme from human skin, may be tissue-localized enzymes for activation of kininogens in skin.[89]

## NEUROENDOCRINE ASPECTS OF THE MERKEL CELL

The Merkel cell is the sole epidermal resident that demonstrates VIP immunoreactivity in the skin of various mammals, including humans.[90,91] In rodents, met-enkephalin reactivity also is detected, but is not present in human, cat, or dog Merkel cells. Neuron-specific enolase, an enzyme present in neural tissues, exists in Merkel cells.[92] Ultrastructural studies reveal distinct neurosecretory granules in the cytoplasm of Merkel cells. Coupled with their immunohistochemical reactivity, Merkel cells are designated as neuroendocrine cells. However, additional, anticipated biochemical properties of neural and neuroendocrine (or APUD–amine precursor uptake and decarboxylation) cells are not possessed by Merkel cells. They were suspected to contain catecholamines, but attempts to demonstrate biogenic amines have been unsuccessful. Merkel cells represent a small, identifiable population of cells in the dermis. They are similar to their epidermal counterparts, possessing intermediate filaments that stain with appropriate keratin antibodies, and they have cytoplasmic neurosecretory granules.

Merkel cells of the skin can proliferate, causing hyperplasia.[93] Primary neuroendocrine carcinoma of the skin is a distinct neoplastic tumor.[94] The relationship of the Merkel cell to neuroendocrine carcinoma is controversial. It is likely that neuroendocrine stem cell populations in the dermis account for the histogenesis of this uncommon malignancy. Although the two cell types are similar, it is not likely that resident Merkel cells of the epidermis are the tumorigenic precursors.

Chronic skin irritation can cause neuroendocrine cell hyperplasias. Merkel cells become more abundant and more widely distributed throughout the epidermis. VIP, ACTH, leu-enkephalin, bombesin-like peptides, and serotonin are expressed. Neuroendocrine carcinoma of skin has displayed immunoreactivity for these hormones, and occasionally contains calcitonin, somatostatin, and gastrin. Only rarely have overt paraneoplastic syndromes resulted from neuroendocrine carcinoma of the skin (see Chap. 219).

## GROWTH FACTORS

Growth factors represent a distinct class of peptide hormones, and are produced by various tissues and organs (see Chap. 173). A number of families of growth factors that have been identified are expressed in skin, including the epidermal growth factor (EGF) family, the fibroblast growth factor (FGF) family, the platelet-derived growth factor (PDGF) family, and several others.[95,96] The skin is a target organ for growth factor activities as well as a source of production of various growth factors.[97] The epidermis expresses several members of the EGF family, including transforming growth factor-α, amphiregulin, and heparin-binding EGF. The family of human EGF receptors (HER) that mediate responses to the EGF-related growth factors include HER-1, 2, 3, and 4. Several of these receptors are expressed in skin and epidermis and coordinately regulate proliferation, differentiation, and other biologic responses that are exerted by these EGF-related factors. Overexpression of EGF-related ligands or altered activation of HERs appears to participate in hyperproliferative skin diseases such as psoriasis and in the development of cutaneous carcinoma.[97–100]

Several members of the FGF family are expressed in skin and appear to act in a paracrine manner.[95] Keratinocyte growth factor is produced by dermal fibroblasts but exerts its major activity on epidermal keratinocytes as a mitogenic and differentiation-regulating factor. Wounding markedly increases dermal expression of keratinocyte growth factor. Acidic and basic FGF (FGF1 and 2) also are expressed in dermis, and mediate biologic responses of proliferation and neovascular regeneration in skin.

PDGF isoforms are produced by injured epithelium and act predominantly in dermal tissues. Another member of the PDGF family, vascular endothelial growth factor, is induced in wounded and diseased epidermis and selectively affects vascular endothelial cells of the dermis.

Insulin-like growth factors I and II are mesenchymally derived trophic factors that act on dermal and epidermal cell types in skin to regulate gene expression, cell proliferation, and differentiation. Transforming growth factor-β and related members of this family, including the bone morphogenic proteins (e.g., BMP-6), are potent negative growth regulatory and differentiation-regulating proteins expressed by epidermis and dermal tissues of skin.[95] Selected transforming growth factor-β superfamily members also mediate biologic activities of matrix molecule expression, morphogenesis, and wound repair through autocrine and paracrine regulatory loops. This family of growth factors also appears to function in suppression of carcinogenetic events and malignant progression in skin. Increased expression of activin, a transforming growth factor member, is seen in repair processes. Sustained enhanced levels may contribute to fibrotic reactions.[101]

New growth factors, cytokines, and other trophic peptide hormones expressed in skin continue to be identified and characterized. For example, mast-cell growth factor (c-*kit* ligand) appears to be expressed by keratinocytes, and its expression and distribution in epidermis and dermis are altered in cutaneous mastocytosis (urticaria pigmentosa).[102]

The hemocrine, paracrine, and autocrine activities exhibited by these and other growth factors undoubtedly signify their importance in integrating the function of diverse cell populations within the skin and other tissues.

## REFERENCES

1. Holbrook KA, Wolff K. The structure and development of skin. In: Fitzpatrick TB, Eisen A, Wolff K, et al., eds. Dermatology in general medicine, 4th ed. New York: McGraw-Hill, 1993:97.
2. Harris G, Azzolina B, Baginsky W, et al. Identification and selective inhibition of an isozyme of steroid 5 alpha-reductase in human scalp. Proc Natl Acad Sci U S A 1992; 89:10787.
3. Goos CMA, Wirtz P, Vermorken AJM, Mauvais-Jarvis P. Androgenic effect of testosterone and some of its metabolites in relation to their biotransformation in the skin. Br J Dermatol 1982; 107:549.
4. Milewich L, Kaimal V, Shaw CB, Sontheimer RD. Epidermal keratinocytes: a source of 5-dihydrotestosterone production in human skin. J Clin Endocrinol Metab 1986; 62:739.
5. Liang T, Hoyer S, Yu R, et al. Immunocytochemical localization of androgen receptors in human skin using monoclonal antibodies against the androgen receptor. J Invest Dermatol 1993; 100:663.
6. Wilson CM, McPhaul MJ. A and B forms of the androgen receptor are present in human genital skin fibroblasts. Proc Natl Acad Sci U S A 1994; 91:1234.
7. Serafini MD, Lobo RA. Increased 5α-reductase activity in idiopathic hirsutism. Fertil Steril 1985; 43:74.
8. Lobo RA, Goebelsmann U, Horton R. Evidence for the importance of peripheral tissue events in the development of hirsutism in polycystic ovary syndrome. J Clin Endocrinol Metab 1983; 57:393.
9. Kuttenn F, Couillin P, Girard F, et al. Late-onset adrenal hyperplasia in hirsuitism. N Engl J Med 1985; 313:224.
10. Schweikert HU, Milewich L, Wilson JD. Aromatization of androstenedione by isolated human hairs. J Clin Endocrinol Metab 1975; 40:413.
11. Hemsell DL, Edman CD, Marks JF, et al. Massive extraglandular aromatization of plasma androstenedione resulting in feminization of a prepubertal boy. J Clin Invest 1977; 60:455.
12. Johnson JA, Fusaro RM. The role of the skin in carbohydrate metabolism. In: Levine R, Luft R, eds. Advances in metabolic disorders, vol 6. New York: Academic Press, 1972:1.
13. Freinkel R. Carbohydrate metabolism of epidermis. In: Goldsmith L, ed. Physiology, biochemistry and molecular biology of the skin, 2nd ed, vol I. New York: Oxford University Press, 1991:452.
14. Huang T-S, Chopra IJ, Beredo A, et al. Skin is an active site for the inner ring monodeiodination of thyroxine to 3,3',5'-triiodothyronine. Endocrinology 1985; 117:2106.
15. Kaplan M, Gordon P, Pan C, et al. Keratinocytes convert thyroxine to triiodothyronine. Ann NY Acad Sci 1988; 548:56.
16. Kaplan MM, Pan C, Gordon PR, et al. Human epidermal keratinocytes in culture convert thyroxine to 3,5',3'-triiodothyronine by type II iodothyronine deiodination: a novel endocrine function of the skin. J Clin Endocrinol Metab 1988; 66:815.
17. Wintroub BU, Schechter NB, Lazarus GS, et al. Angiotensin I conversion by human and rat chymotryptic proteinases. J Invest Dermatol 1984; 83:336.
18. Olerud JE, Usui ML, Seckin D, et al. Neutral endopeptidase expression and distribution in human skin and wounds. J Invest Dermatol 1999; 112:873.
19. Holick MF. The photobiology of vitamin D and its consequences for humans. Ann N Y Acad Sci 1985; 453:1.
20. Holick MF. The cutaneous photosynthesis of previtamin $D_3$: a unique photoendocrine system. J Invest Dermatol 1981; 76:51.
21. Smith EL, Holick MF. The skin: the site of vitamin $D_3$ synthesis and a target tissue for its metabolite 1,25-dihydroxy vitamin $D_3$. Steroids 1987; 49:103.
22. Holick SA, St. Lezin M, Young D, et al. Isolation and identification of 24-dehydroprovitamin $D_3$ and its photolysis to 24-dehydroprevitamin $D_3$ in mammalian skin. J Biol Chem 1985; 260:12181.
23. Bikle DD, Halloran BP, Riviere JE. Production of 1,25 dihydroxyvitamin $D_3$ by perfused pig skin. J Invest Dermatol 1994; 102:796.
24. Adams JS, Clemens TL, Parrish JA, Holick MF. Vitamin-D synthesis and metabolism after ultraviolet irradiation of normal and vitamin-D-deficient subjects. N Engl J Med 1982; 306:722.
25. MacLaughlin J, Holick MF. Aging decreases the capacity of human skin to produce vitamin $D_3$. J Clin Invest 1985; 76:1536.
26. Clemens TL, Henderson SL, Adams JS, Holick MF. Increased skin pigment reduces the capacity of skin to synthesize vitamin $D_3$. Lancet 1982; 1:74.
27. Reichel H, Koeffler HP, Norman AW. The role of vitamin D endocrine system in health and disease. N Engl J Med 1989; 989:320.
28. Morimoto S, Yoshikawa K. Psoriasis and vitamin $D_3$. Arch Dermatol 1989; 125:231.
29. Kassis V. The prostaglandin system in human skin. Dan Med Bull 1983; 30:320.
30. Ziboh VA. Prostaglandins, leukotrienes, and hydroxy fatty acids in epidermis. Semin Dermatol 1992; 11:114.
31. Leong J, Hughes-Felford M, Rakhlin N. Cyclooxygenase in human and mouse skin in cultured keratinocytes: association of COX-2 with human keratinocyte differentiation. Exp Cell Res 1996; 224:79.
32. Hammarström S, Hamberg M, Samuelsson B. Increased concentrations of nonesterified arachidonic acid, 12-L-hydroxy-5,8,10,14-eicosatetraenoic acid, prostaglandin $E_2$ and prostaglandin $F_{2\alpha}$ in epidermis of psoriasis. Proc Natl Acad Sci U S A 1975; 72:5130.
33. Forstrom L, Goldyne ME, Winkelmann RK. Prostaglandin production by human epidermal cells in vitro: a model for studying pharmacologic inhibition of prostaglandin synthesis. Prostaglandins 1974; 8:107.
34. Fairley JA, Weiss J, Marcelo CL. Increased prostaglandin synthesis by low calcium-regulated keratinocytes. J Invest Dermatol 1986; 86:173.
35. Brain S, Camp R, Derm FF, et al. The release of leukotriene $B_4$-like material in biologically active amounts from the lesional skin of patients with psoriasis. J Invest Dermatol 1984; 83:70.

36. Brain SD, Camp RDR, Cunningham FM, et al. Leukotriene B$_4$-like material in scale of psoriatic skin lesions. Br J Pharmacol 1984; 83:313.

37. Grabbe J, Czarnetzki BM, Mardin M. Release of lipoxygenase products of arachidonic acid from freshly isolated human keratinocytes. Arch Dermatol Res 1984; 276:128.

38. Woolard P. Novel stereoisomer of 12-hydroxy-5,8,10,14-eicosatetraenoic acid in psoriasis. Adv Prostaglandin Thromboxane Leukotriene Res 1987; 17:627.

39. Peterson LL, Shaw JC, Acott KM, et al. Glucagonoma syndrome: in vitro evidence that glucagon increases epidermal arachidonic acid. J Am Acad Dermatol 1984; 11:468.

40. Pentland AP, Needleman P. Modulation of keratinocyte proliferation in vitro by endogenous prostaglandin synthesis. J Clin Invest 1986; 77:246.

41. Sondergaard J, Bisgaard H, Thorsen S. Eicosanoids in skin UV inflammation. Photodermatology 1985; 2:359.

42. Pepinsky RB, Sinclair LK, Browning JL, et al. Purification and partial sequence analysis of a 37-kDa protein that inhibits phospholipase A$_2$ activity from rat peritoneal exudates. J Biol Chem 1986; 261:4239.

43. Schallreuter KU, Wood JM, Lemke R, et al. Production of catecholamines in the human epidermis. Biochem Biophys Res Commun 1992; 189:72.

44. Smit NPM, Pavel S, Kammeyer A, Westerhof W. Determination of catechol O-methyltransferase activity in relation to melanin metabolism using high-performance liquid chromatography with fluorimetric detection. Anal Biochem 1990; 190:286.

45. Schallreuter KU, Wood JM, Pittelkow MR, et al. Increased in vitro expression of beta$_2$-adrenoceptors in differentiating lesional keratinocytes of vitiligo patients. Arch Dermatol Res 1993; 285:216.

46. Schallreuter KU, Wood JM, Pittelkow MR, et al. Regulation of melanin biosynthesis in the human epidermis by tetrahydrobiopterin. Science 1994; 263:1444.

47. Grando SA, Kist DA, Qi M, Dahl MV. Human keratinocytes synthesize, secrete, and degrade acetylcholine. J Invest Dermatol 1993; 101:32.

48. Grando SA, Crosby AM, Zelickson BD, Dahl MV. Agarose gel keratinocyte outgrowth system as a model of skin re-epithelialization: requirement of endogenous acetylcholine for outgrowth initiation. J Invest Dermatol 1993; 101:804.

49. Mueller GP, Alpert S, Reichlin S, Jackson IMD. Thyrotropin-releasing hormone and serotonin secretion from frog skin are stimulated by norepinephrine. Endocrinology 1980; 106:1.

50. Bloom SR, Polak JM. Regulatory peptides and the skin. Clin Exp Dermatol 1983; 8:3.

51. Wakamatsu K, Graham A, Cook P, Thody AJ. Characterization of ACTH peptides in human skin and their activation of the melanocortin-1 receptor. Pigment Cell Res 1997; 10:288.

52. Haycock JW, Wagner M, Moradini R, et al. Alpha melanocyte stimulating hormone inhibits NF-kappa B activation in human melanocytes and melanoma cells. J Invest Dermatol 1999; 113:560.

53. Strewler GJ, Williams RD, Nissenson RA. Human renal carcinoma cells produce hypercalcemia in the nude mouse and a novel protein recognized by parathyroid hormone receptors. J Clin Invest 1983; 71:769.

54. Rabbani SA, Mitchell J, Roy DR, et al. Purification of peptides with parathyroid hormone-like bioactivity from human and rat malignancies associated with hypercalcemia. Endocrinology 1986; 118:1200.

55. Merendino JJ Jr, Insogna KL, Milstone LM, et al. A parathyroid hormone-like protein from cultured human keratinocytes. Science 1986; 231:388.

56. Suva L, Winslow R, Wettenhall R, et al. A parathyroid hormone-related protein implicated in malignant hypercalcemia: cloning and expression. Science 1987; 237:893.

57. Wysolmerski JJ, Broadus AE, Zhou J, et al. Overexpression of parathyroid hormone-related protein in the skin of transgenic mice interferes with hair follicle development. Proc Natl Acad Sci U S A 1994; 91:1133.

58. Blomme EA, Sugimoto Y, Lin YC, et al. PTHrP is a positive regulator of keratinocyte growth factor expression by normal dermal fibroblasts. Mol Cell Endocrinol 1999; 152:189.

59. Salassa RM, Jowsey J, Phil D, Arnaud CD. Hypophosphatemic osteomalacia associated with nonendocrine tumors. N Engl J Med 1970; 283:65.

60. Aschinberg LC, Solomon LM, Zeis PM, et al. Vitamin D-resistant rickets associated with epidermal nevus syndrome: demonstration of a phosphaturic substance in the dermal lesions. J Pediatr 1977; 91:56.

61. Cai Q, Hodgson SF, Kao PC, et al. Brief report: inhibition of renal phosphate transport by a tumor product in a patient with oncogenic osteomalacia. N Engl J Med 1994; 330:1645.

62. Econs MJ, Dretner MK. Tumor-induced osteomalacia: unveiling a new hormone. N Engl J Med 1994; 330:1679.

63. von Gaudecker B, Schmale E-M. Similarities between Hassall's corpuscles of the human thymus and the epidermis. Cell Tissue Res 1974; 347:348.

64. Singer KH, Harden EA, Robertson AL, et al. Expression of antigens by cultured epithelial cells: comparison of epidermis and thymic epithelium. J Invest Dermatol 1985; 85:67s.

65. Chu AC, Patterson JAK, Goldstein G, et al. Thymopoietin-like substance in human skin. J Invest Dermatol 1983; 81:194.

66. Kato K, Ikeyama S, Takaoki M, et al. Epithelial cell components, immunoreactant with anti-serum to thymic factor (FTS): possible association with intermediate-sized filaments. Cell 1981; 24:885.

67. Rubenfield MR, Silverstone AE, Knowles DE, et al. Induction of lymphocyte differentiation by epidermal cultures. J Invest Dermatol 1981; 77:221.

68. Luger TA, Stadler BM, Katz SI, Oppenheim JJ. Epidermal cell (keratinocyte)-derived thymocyte-activating factor (ETAF). J Immunol 1981; 127:1493.

69. Luger TA, Stadler BM, Luger BM, et al. Characteristics of an epidermal cell thymocyte-activating factor (ETAF) produced by human epidermal cells and a human squamous cell carcinoma cell line. J Invest Dermatol 1983; 81:187.

70. Sauder DN. Biologic properties of epidermal cell thymocyte-activating factor (ETAF). J Invest Dermatol 1985; 85:176s.

71. Ansel JC, Luger TA, Green I. The effect of in vitro and in vivo UV irradiation on the production of ETAF activity by human and murine keratinocytes. J Invest Dermatol 1983; 81:519.

72. Sauder DN, Dinarello CA, Morhenn VB. Langerhans cell production of interleukin-1. J Invest Dermatol 1984; 82:605.

73. Gahring LC, Buckley A, Daynes RA. Presence of epidermal-derived thymocyte activating factor/interleukin 1 in normal human stratum corneum. J Clin Invest 1985; 76:1585.

74. Sauder DN, Katz SI. Immune modulation by epidermal cell products: possible role of ETAF in inflammatory and neoplastic skin diseases. J Am Acad Dermatol 1982; 7:651.

75. DiGiovine F, Duff G. Interleukin 1: the first interleukin. Immunol Today 1990;11:13.

76. Cork M, Duff G. Interleukin 1. In: Luger TA, Schwarz T, eds. Epidermal growth factors and cytokines. New York: Marcel Dekker Inc, 1994:19.

77. Nozaki S, Feliciani C, Sauder DN. Keratinocyte cytokines. Adv Dermatol 1992; 7:83.

78. Luger T, Schwarz T, eds. Epidermal growth factors and cytokines. New York: Marcel Dekker Inc, 1994.

79. Luger TA, Kock A, Danner M, et al. Production of distinct cytokines by epidermal cells. Br J Dermatol 1985; 113:145.

80. Kupper T, Horowitz M, Birchall N, et al. Hematopoietic, lymphopoietic and proinflammatory cytokines produced by human and murine keratinocytes. Ann NY Acad Sci 1988; 548:262.

81. Oxholm A, Oxholm P, Staberg B, Bendtzen K. Immunohistological detection of interleukin I-like molecules and tumor necrosis factor in human epidermis before and after UVB-irradiation in vivo. Br J Dermatol 1988; 118:369.

82. Baggiolini M, Dahinden CA. CC chemokines in allergic inflammation. Immunol Today 1994; 15:127.

82a. Konig A, Krenn V, Toksoy A, et al. Mig, GRO alpha and RANTES messenger RNA expression in the lining layer, infiltrates, and different leukocyte populations of synovial tissue from patients with rheumatoid arthritis, psoriatic arthritis, and osteoarthritis. Virchows Arch 2000; 436:449.

83. Hartschuh W, Weihe E, Reinecke M. Peptidergic (neurotensin, VIP, substance P) nerve fibres in the skin: immunohistochemical evidence of an involvement of neuropeptides in nociception, pruritus and inflammation. Br J Dermatol 1983; 109:14.

84. O'Shaughnessy DJ, McGregor GP, Ghatei MA, et al. Distribution of bombesin, somatostatin, substance-P and vasoactive intestinal polypeptide in feline and porcine skin. Life Sci 1983; 32:2827.

85. Hosoi J, Murphy GF, Egan CL, et al. Regulation of Langerhans cell function by nerves containing calcitonin gene-regulated peptide. Nature 1993; 363:159.

86. Foreman JC, Jordan CC, Oehme P, Renner H. Structure-activity relationships for some substance P-related peptides that cause wheal and flare reactions in human skin. J Physiol (Lond) 1983; 335:449.

87. Heinz-Erian P, Dey RD, Flux M, Said SI. Deficient vasoactive intestinal peptide innervation in the sweat glands of cystic fibrosis patients. Science 1985; 229:1407.

88. Winkelmann RK. Total plasma kininogen in psoriasis and atopic dermatitis. Acta Derm Venereol (Stockh) 1984; 64:261.

89. Toki N, Yamura T. Kinin-forming enzyme in human skin: the purification and characterization of a kinin-forming enzyme. J Invest Dermatol 1979; 73:297.

90. Hartschuh W, Weihe E, Yanaihara N, Reinecke M. Immunohistochemical localization of vasoactive intestinal polypeptide (VIP) in Merkel cells of various mammals: evidence for a neuromodulator function of the Merkel cell. J Invest Dermatol 1983; 81:361.

91. Hartschuh W, Reinecke M, Weihe E, Yanaihara N. VIP-immuno-reactivity in the skin of various mammals: immunohistochemical, radioimmunological and experimental evidence for a dual localization in cutaneous nerves and Merkel cells. Peptides 1984; 5:239.

92. Gu L, Polak JM, Tapia FJ, et al. Neuron-specific enolase in the Merkel cells of mammalian skin. Am J Pathol 1981; 104:63.

93. Gould VE, Moll R, Moll I, et al. Biology of disease: neuroendocrine (Merkel) cells of the skin: hyperplasias, dysplasias and neoplasms. Lab Invest 1985; 52:334.

94. Wick MR, Scheithauer BW. Primary neuroendocrine carcinoma of the skin. In: Wick M, ed. Pathology of unusual malignant cutaneous tumors. New York: Marcel Dekker Inc, 1985:107.

95. Pittelkow MR, Coffey RJ, Moses H. Transforming growth factor type β and other growth factors. In: Goldsmith L, ed. Physiology, biochemistry and molecular biology of skin. Oxford: Oxford University Press, 1991:351.

96. King LE, Stoscheck CM, Gates RE, Nanney LB. Epidermal growth factor and transforming growth factor α. In: Goldsmith L, ed. Physiology, biochemistry and molecular biology of skin. Oxford: Oxford University Press, 1991:329.

97. Pittelkow MR. Growth factors in cutaneous biology and disease. Adv Dermatol 1992; 7:55.

98. Coffey R Jr, Derynck R, Wilcox J, et al. Production and auto-induction of transforming growth factor-α human keratinocytes. Nature 1987; 328:817.

99. Pittelkow MR, Cook PW, Shipley GD, et al. Autonomous growth of human keratinocytes requires epidermal growth factor receptor occupancy. Cell Growth Differ 1993; 4:513.
100. Cook PW, Pittelkow MR, Keeble WN, et al. Amphiregulin mRNA is elevated in psoriatic epidermis and gastrointestinal carcinomas. Cancer Res 1992; 52:3224.
101. Hubner G, Alzheimer C, Werner S. Activin: a novel player in tissue repair processes. Histol Histopathol 1999; 14:295.
102. Longley BJ Jr, Morganroth GS, Tyrrell L, et al. Altered metabolism of mast-cell growth factor (*c-kit* ligand) in cutaneous mastocytosis. N Engl J Med 1993; 328:1302.

# CHAPTER 186

# THE ENDOCRINE ADIPOCYTE

REXFORD S. AHIMA AND JEFFREY S. FLIER

Mammals have evolved complex mechanisms to maintain a constant supply of energy for vital cellular functions during food deprivation. A major feature of this adaptation is the ability to store excess calories as triglycerides in adipose tissue. The breakdown of triglycerides is regulated by nutrient, neural, and hormonal factors, and results in the release of free fatty acids (FFAs), which are oxidized by a variety of tissues (e.g., muscle, liver, and kidney). Oxidation of FFAs also produces ketone bodies that can be utilized by the brain and other organs during fasting. Contrary to the prevailing view that adipocytes are specialized cells for the storage of fat, there is increasing evidence that adipocytes secrete into the bloodstream various factors with diverse systemic effects. The endocrine role of adipose tissue is best illustrated by the recently discovered hormone leptin.[1,2] Total leptin deficiency or leptin receptor abnormalities result in hyperphagia, hypothermia, diabetes, morbid obesity, and several neuroendocrine abnormalities—notably hypothalamic hypogonadism, impaired growth hormone (GH) and impaired thyrotropin secretion (TSH), and hypercorticism.[1,3,4] As is discussed later, leptin has been implicated in other roles, including regulation of neuroendocrine and immune function and development.[2,5]

Among the factors secreted by adipose tissue are steroids, components of the renin-angiotensin system (RAS), complement factors (i.e., adipsin, acylation-stimulating protein [ASP]), proinflammatory cytokines (tumor necrosis factor-α [TNF-α], and interleukin-6 [IL-6]), plasminogen activator inhibitor-1 (PAI-1), transforming growth factor-β (TGF-β), and tissue factor. While most of these products affect adipocytes and neighboring organs, they are also present in significant amounts in the circulation and are capable of regulating distant organs (Fig. 186-1). It has been suggested that alterations in the levels of adipocyte-derived hormones may mediate some of the metabolic, cardiovascular, and other complications associated with obesity (see Chaps. 125 and 126). In this chapter the authors review the current understanding of hormones and other products secreted by adipocytes, and their roles in normal physiologic regulation and disease.

## LEPTIN

Interest in the endocrine function of adipose tissue has increased extraordinarily following the discovery of leptin.[1,2] Leptin is a 167-amino-acid protein (relative mass of 16 kDa) with a helical structure that is similar to that of the cytokines, and is highly con-

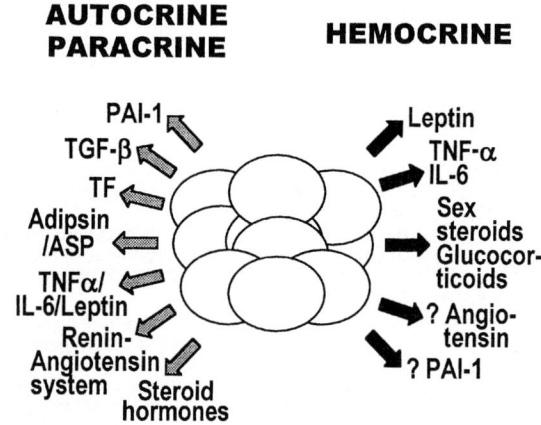

**FIGURE 186-1.** Adipose tissue synthesizes and secretes various hemocrine, paracrine, and autocrine factors. Sex steroids and glucocorticoid metabolism are regulated by aromatase and 17β-hydroxysteroid oxidoreductase, and 11β-hydroxysteroid dehydrogenase, respectively. (*PAI-1*, plasminogen activator inhibitor type 1; *TF*, tissue factor; *TGF-β*, transforming growth factor-β; *ASP*, acylation-stimulating protein; *TNF-α*, tumor necrosis factor α; *IL-6*, interleukin-6.)

served among mammalian species. It was named for its ability to decrease body weight and adiposity when injected into mice (Greek root *leptos* meaning thin).[6] Leptin is encoded by the *ob* gene and is expressed predominantly by adipocytes, although low levels have been detected in the placenta, skeletal muscle, and gastric and mammary epithelia under certain conditions.[2] Leptin appears to be secreted by the constitutive pathway, circulates as free and bound hormone, and is cleared mainly by the kidneys. Adipose tissue and plasma leptin concentrations are proportional to the amount of energy stored as fat, and obese individuals express higher levels of leptin than do lean individuals.[2,5] In addition, leptin levels are dependent on the state of energy balance, such that fasting results in a decrease in leptin while overfeeding increases leptin within hours in rodents and days in humans. The effects of nutrition on leptin are mediated in part by insulin. Insulin stimulates leptin synthesis in cultured adipocytes, and when infused in vivo. In contrast, leptin decreases in response to the fall in insulin with fasting and as a result of insulin deficiency in streptozocin-induced diabetes.

Leptin is regulated by other factors.[2,5] For example, leptin levels are higher in females than in age- and weight-matched males, and the sex difference is partly attributable to inhibition of leptin by androgens. Moreover, leptin production is higher in subcutaneous adipose tissue, which is more abundant in women. Leptin is increased in response to glucocorticoids, acute infection, and cytokines (TNF-α, interleukin-1 [IL-1], leukemia inhibitory factor). In contrast, cold exposure, β-adrenergic agonists, GH, thyroid hormone, smoking, and thiazolidinediones have been reported to decrease leptin. Some of these factors are likely to affect leptin synthesis directly, as regulatory elements for various nuclear transcription factors have been located in the *ob* gene promoter. Others affect leptin by actions to reduce adipose mass.

Leptin increases at night in humans (beginning of light cycle in rodents) and reaches a nadir in the morning (onset of dark cycle in rodents). The diurnal changes in leptin are reciprocal to glucocorticoids, and entrained by the timing of feeding.[7,8] An ultradian leptin rhythm has also been described in humans.[7] As with basal leptin secretion, the pulse amplitude of leptin is higher in females than in males. The factors responsible for pulsatile leptin secretion are yet to be determined, and may involve

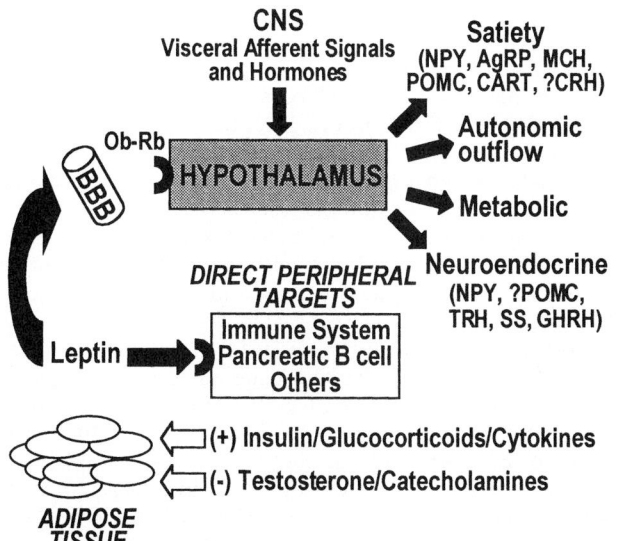

**FIGURE 186-2.** Regulation of leptin expression and sites of leptin action. Leptin levels increase with adiposity, and in response to insulin and glucocorticoids. Conversely, leptin decreases with fasting and in response to testosterone and catecholamines. Leptin is transported to neuronal targets in the hypothalamus, and regulates appetite, autonomic outflow, metabolism, and neuroendocrine function. The effects of leptin on satiety are likely to be mediated by a balance between *orexigenic peptides* (e.g., NPY, AgRP, and MCH) and *anorexigenic peptides* (e.g., POMC-precursor of α-MSH, CART, and possibly CRH) (see Chap. 125). Regulation of the neuroendocrine axis by leptin is thought to be mediated by NPY, POMC, TRH, and GHRH. Leptin also exerts direct effects on the immune system and pancreatic B cells. (*CNS,* central nervous system; *BBB,* blood–brain barrier; *Ob-Rb,* long-form leptin receptor; *NPY,* neuropeptide Y; *AgRP,* agouti-related peptide; *MCH,* melanin-concentrating hormone; *POMC,* proopiomelanocortin; *CART,* cocaine-and amphetamine-regulated transcript; *CRH,* corticotropin-releasing hormone; *TRH,* thyrotropin-releasing hormone; *GHRH,* growth hormone–releasing hormone; *SS,* somatostatin.)

an interaction between neural and humoral signals. Diurnal and ultradian leptin rhythms are positively correlated with female sex hormones, and may play a role in the pathogenesis of exercise-induced amenorrhea.[8]

At the time of its discovery, leptin was thought to represent the long-sought-after adipostatic factor. Based on parabiosis experiments more than two decades ago, it was predicted that body weight and adiposity were maintained at steady levels over long periods by a circulating satiety factor.[1,2] A rise in leptin with increasing adipose mass has been proposed to decrease body weight adiposity via negative feedback regulation.[1,2] This view of leptin as an antiobesity hormone was supported by the observation that peripheral, and more potently intracerebroventricular leptin injection, reduces the body weight of adipose mass through inhibition of food intake and increased energy expenditure.[2,6]

The effects of leptin on energy balance are mediated mainly by the hypothalamus and other brain regions (Fig. 186-2) (see Chap. 125). Consistent with this view, a saturable transport system for leptin has been demonstrated in the rodent brain.[9] The long leptin-receptor isoform (Ob-Rb), which mediates JAK-Stat (Janus kinase–signal transducer and activator of transcription) activation, is highly expressed in the hypothalamus, and has been colocalized with neuropeptide targets of leptin (e.g., neuropeptide Y [NPY], agouti-related peptide [AgRP], and proopiomelanocortin [POMC]).[2] Inhibition of appetite in response to leptin is thought to be mediated by decreased hypothalamic NPY levels and a rise in anorexigenic peptides (e.g., POMC [precursor of α-melanocyte–stimulating hormone, or α-MSH, in the brain], corticotropin-releasing hormone [CRH], and cocaine- and amphetamine-regulated peptide [CART]).[2,5] In contrast, short leptin-receptor isoforms that lack the intracellular protein motifs required for activation of the JAK-Stat signal-transduction pathway have a more widespread tissue distribution (e.g., choroid plexus, brain microvessels, kidneys, lungs, and liver) and may serve a transport role.

The notion that leptin functions primarily as an antiobesity hormone has to be reconciled with the inability of rising leptin levels to prevent common (diet-induced) obesity in humans and other mammals.[5] Obesity resulting from leptin deficiency or leptin-receptor abnormalities is extremely rare.[3,4] Rather, *most obesities are characterized by increased adipocyte leptin content and high circulating leptin levels.* It has been suggested that the apparent lack of response to elevated leptin levels represents a state of *leptin resistance.*[2,5] The mechanisms underlying leptin resistance may include abnormalities of leptin secretion, defective leptin transport into the brain, and/or reduced hypothalamic leptin signaling. A member of the suppressors of cytokine signaling family, SOCS-3, has been suggested as a mediator of leptin resistance in the brain.[10] It is also possible that leptin resistance is mediated in part by glucocorticoids and as yet undetermined factors.

The dominant physiologic role of leptin in energy homeostasis is likely to be *a signal for the metabolic and neuroendocrine adaptation to fasting.*[5,11] The fall in leptin, as energy stores in adipose tissue decline with fasting, results in a decrease in the levels of thyroid, growth, and reproductive hormones, and activation of the hypothalamic–pituitary–adrenal (HPA) axis (see Fig. 186-2). Leptin also mediates the reduction in cytokines produced by $T_H1$ cells and impairment of T-lymphocyte proliferation during fasting[12] (see Fig. 186-2). The neuroendocrine and metabolic adaptation to fasting is likely to be mediated by one or more of the neuropeptide targets of leptin (e.g., NPY, POMC, thyrotropin-releasing hormone [TRH], growth hormone–releasing hormone [GHRH], and somatostatin). Leptin's role in immune modulation is likely to be direct, as Ob-Rb is expressed by T lymphocytes.

Leptin regulates endocrine function apart from its role in energy balance.[5] For example, leptin restores pubertal maturation in *ob/ob* mice, and is capable of accelerating the timing of puberty in wild-type mice.[5,13,14] Leptin decreases glucocorticoid production by adrenal cortical cells in vitro, and when injected into rats, can blunt the activation of the HPA axis during restraint stress. Leptin is also capable of directly regulating CRH secretion by hypothalamic explants. Leptin regulates insulin production by pancreatic B cells and steroid secretion by ovarian granulosa cells, and affects the secretion of a variety of hormones by the pituitary gland. These endocrine targets express the long leptin receptor (albeit at low levels), so these effects of leptin are likely to be mediated directly. Leptin has been suggested as a mediator of the metabolic and cardiovascular complications of obesity.[15] A rise in leptin levels to levels as high as those observed in obesity leads to inhibition of glucose-stimulated insulin secretion, increased sympathetic nerve output in the splanchnic bed, and stimulation of diuresis. Leptin levels are positively correlated with blood pressure and have been associated with increased risk of cerebrovascular accidents.

A role of leptin during development is suggested by leptin synthesis by the placenta, and widespread tissue distribution of leptin and leptin receptors in murine fetuses. A rise in leptin has been observed in prepubertal boys and postnatal mice.[16,17] Leptin increases out of proportion to adipose mass during the prepubertal period and is postulated to influence gonadal maturation.[16] Leptin deficiency results in reduced brain weight, structural neuronal abnormalities, and defective expression of several neuronal and glial proteins in *ob/ob* and *db/db* mice.[18]

Chronic leptin treatment restores brain weight and some neuronal proteins in *ob/ob* mice, implying that it plays an important role in the postnatal development of the central nervous system.[18] Leptin also regulates the maturation of the hematopoietic system and stimulates angiogenesis.[19]

## PROINFLAMMATORY CYTOKINES

TNF-α and IL-6 have been implicated in fuel homeostasis, thermogenesis, and neuroendocrine regulation. Levels of both cytokines are stimulated by lipopolysaccharide, and they are thought to mediate weight loss, hypoglycemia, and lipolysis during sepsis (see Chap. 227).[20] The cellular actions of TNF-α are mediated by two receptors, p55 and p75.[21] TNF-α receptors are expressed on the cell surface in most tissues and are also present in the circulation.[21,22] It has been suggested that soluble TNF-α receptors inhibit TNF-α activity by competing with cell-surface receptors.[21] On the other hand, soluble TNF-α receptors stabilize TNF-α at low concentrations, and could potentiate TNF-α activity.[22] IL-6 binds to a receptor complex comprised of an 80-kDa ligand-binding glycoprotein and a 130-kDa signal-transduction glycoprotein (gp130).[23] A soluble IL-6 receptor is derived from proteolytic cleavage of the membrane-bound receptor and is likely to enhance IL-6 activity by forming a complex with IL-6 that then interacts with gp130 on the cell surface.[24] A soluble form of gp130 has been described, and is thought to antagonize IL-6 activity.[25]

TNF-α and IL-6 are produced in significant quantities by adipocytes and are involved in body weight regulation.[26,27] As with leptin, TNF-α and IL-6 levels increase with adiposity. TNF-α expression is also dependent on energy balance, as evidenced by increased expression in response to a high-fat diet and decreased expression with fasting. TNF-α and IL-6 affect insulin action, glucose homeostasis, and lipid metabolism. TNF-α has been proposed to increase insulin resistance by reducing insulin-receptor signaling and glucose transporter 4 (GLUT4) expression. Both TNF-α and IL-6 decrease insulin-stimulated glucose uptake by skeletal muscle. Moreover, TNF-α inhibits lipoprotein lipase activity while increasing hormone-sensitive lipase activity. The net effect of these actions is to increase lipolysis and decrease lipid accumulation; this may constitute a mechanism by which a rise in TNF-α levels can limit the tendency toward obesity. The precise role of increased adipocyte TNF-α in the insulin resistance of obesity in obese rodents and humans is controversial. Although targeted disruption of TNF-α has been reported to decrease body weight in lean mice, it does not prevent obesity in response to a high-fat diet or gold thioglucose treatment.[28] Furthermore, TNF-α deficiency resulted in a decrease in glucose and insulin, but did not restore insulin sensitivity in obese mice.[28] In contrast, another study has described an increase in insulin sensitivity in TNF-α-deficient mice on a high-fat diet, as well as in *ob/ob* mice lacking TNF-α.[29] In the same study, mutations of p55 and p75 TNF-α receptors were reported to improve insulin sensitivity in *ob/ob* mice.[29] These results are at odds with the apparent failure of targeted mutagenesis of p55 and p75 TNF-α receptors to affect glucose and insulin levels and insulin sensitivity in wild-type and *db/db* mice, as was reported in another study.[30]

Treatment with TNF-α and IL-6 decreases food intake and alters thermogenesis and neuroendocrine function.[31–33] For example, IL-6 administration activates the HPA axis, and suppresses the production of thyroid and reproductive hormones. However, it is not known whether TNF-α and IL-6 produced by adipose tissue have similar effects on the central nervous system and hormone regulation under normal physiologic conditions.

## STEROID HORMONES

Adipose tissue does not synthesize steroid hormones de novo. Rather, adipocytes and stromal cells *metabolize* sex steroids and glucocorticoids.[34] Furthermore, receptors for sex steroids and glucocorticoids are present in adipose tissue.[34] Adipose stromal cells express two enzymes involved in sex steroid metabolism. 17β-Hydroxysteroid oxidoreductase converts androstenedione (produced by the adrenal gland) to testosterone, and also metabolizes estrone to estradiol. Cytochrome P450-dependent aromatase is expressed by adipose tissue and converts androgens to estrogens. It has been suggested that local production of sex steroids influences regional adipocyte tissue development. Increased production of female sex steroids from androgen precursors is thought to result in a female-pattern fat distribution in obese males. In contrast, increased androgen production has been associated with central obesity in females.[35,36] The link between central obesity and insulin resistance, type 2 diabetes, dyslipidemia, and cardiovascular risk is well known.[37] Alterations in the relative concentrations of sex steroids by adipose tissue conversion may also lead to reproductive dysfunction and increase the risk of hormone-dependent cancers.

Glucocorticoids are important determinants of adiposity, as evidenced by hypercorticism in most rodent obese models and increased adipose mass in Cushing syndrome. Glucocorticoid action is regulated in part by the enzyme 11β-hydroxysteroid dehydrogenase (11βHSD), which catalyzes the interconversion of hormonally active cortisol to inactive cortisone. Two isoforms, 11βHSD-1 and 11βHSD-2, have been described.[38] 11βHSD-2 has a high affinity for cortisol (nM range), and inactivates cortisol in classic mineralocorticoid target tissues such as the kidney. 11βHSD-2 mutations are responsible for the syndrome of apparent mineralocorticoid excess, which is characterized by sodium retention, hypertension, and hypokalemia. 11βHSD-1 is expressed in adipose stromal cells and a variety of tissues, including liver, lung, kidney, and brain, and has a lower affinity for cortisol (mM range). It has a predominant oxoreductase activity (i.e., conversion of cortisone to cortisol) in adipose tissue and is increased in omental adipose stromal cells.[39] Expression of 11βHSD-1 in omentum is increased further by insulin and cortisol.[39] Results of in vivo studies suggest that alteration of the cortisol/cortisone ratio by 11βHSD-1 could influence the response of human subcutaneous abdominal adipose tissue to glucocorticoids.[40] Cortisol stimulates aromatase activity, and could potentially alter sex steroid conversion by adipose tissue. Increased production of cortisol as a result of increased 11βHSD activity in visceral adipose tissue has been proposed as an important regulator of fat distribution, and may mediate the well-known metabolic derangements associated with obesity.[36,37]

## RENIN-ANGIOTENSIN SYSTEM

Angiotensin II is a major regulator of salt and water balance and blood pressure (see Chap. 79). Angiotensinogen, the precursor protein, is produced mainly by the liver and is cleaved by renin into the decapeptide angiotensin I. Angiotensin I is subsequently converted to the octapeptide angiotensin II by angiotensin-converting enzyme (ACE). In the classic pathway, renin activity is localized mainly to the kidneys, while conversion of angiotensin I to angiotensin II by ACE occurs in the lungs.[41] Components of the RAS, which have also been identified in various tissues, may regulate tissue growth and development.[41] Angiotensinogen, renin, nonrenin-angiotensin enzymes (chymase, cathepsins D and G, and tonin), ACE, and angiotensin II receptors are expressed in adipose tissue,[42] consistent with involvement of tissue RAS in adipocyte function. In support of this view, angiotensin II stimulates prostacyclin synthesis, leading to adipocyte differentiation and lipogenesis.[43] Adipocyte angiotensinogen mRNA, and protein levels are decreased by fasting and increased in response to refeeding in rats.[44] Angiotensinogen production in epididymal fat is increased in *ob/ob* mice as compared with lean littermates.[44] These findings raise the possibility that the adipocyte RAS is involved in the pathogenesis of obesity. Abnormalities of the RAS are thought to mediate the cardiorenal complications of obesity; however, it is not known to what extent angiotensin production by adipocytes contributes to this process.

## PLASMINOGEN ACTIVATOR INHIBITOR-1

A link between increased visceral adiposity and cardiovascular risk has been established.[37] Obesity increases cardiovascular morbidity and mortality, in part through an increase in the incidence of thrombotic diseases (e.g., myocardial infarction, venous thrombosis, and pulmonary embolism). The expression of proteins involved in the coagulation and fibrinolytic pathways is altered in obesity, and is thought to contribute to the pathogenesis of cardiovascular disease.[45] PAI-1 inhibits the action of tissue plasminogen activator, a key enzyme involved in fibrinolysis. Therefore, it is likely that an increase in PAI-1 expression would increase the risk of thromboembolic disease. Consistent with this view, plasma PAI-1 levels have been shown to be elevated in survivors of myocardial infarction.[45] The major site of PAI-1 production is the liver. However, PAI-1 is also synthesized by adipose tissue in humans and rodents, and induced in 3T3-L1 adipocytes following differentiation into adipocytes.[46–48] Adipose tissue and plasma PAI-1 levels increase with obesity.[48] Furthermore, plasma PAI-1 levels increase in proportion to visceral (but not subcutaneous) fat area in obese humans.[48] These findings raise the possibility that a rise in PAI-1 levels as a result of increased production by visceral adipose tissue may serve as the link between adiposity and increased risk of thromboembolic disease in obesity.

## COMPLEMENT FACTORS

Various components of the alternate complement pathway are expressed by adipose tissue. The first of these gene products to be identified (*adipsin*) was cloned from a differentiated adipocyte cell line and shown to be identical to complement D.[29] Adipsin is synthesized and secreted by adipocytes. Studies in obese rodent models (*ob/ob*, *db/db*, neonatal monosodium glutamate–lesioned mice, and cafeteria-fed rats) have demonstrated a marked deficiency in adipsin expression.[49,50] The decrease in adipsin levels in obese rodents is mediated in part by glucocorticoids and insulin. The role of adipsin in human obesity is not known. Unlike what occurs in obese rodents, weight gain in humans is not associated with a decrease in adipsin.[51] Rather, plasma adipsin levels are elevated in obese individuals and are increased by feeding. Conversely, adipsin levels are decreased as a result of fasting, cachexia, and lipoatrophy.[51]

Adipsin could play a role in the pathogenesis of obesity by participating in the synthesis of acylation stimulating protein (ASP, C3adesArg).[52] ASP is highly expressed by mature adipocytes and is produced by the cleavage of C3a by carboxypeptidase. The formation of C3a complex from C3 requires factors B and D (adipsin). ASP facilitates the esterification and storage of fatty acids, through stimulation of diacylglycerol acyl transferase and glucose trans-

porters. Consistent with its role in lipogenesis, ASP is secreted in response to meals and facilitates the storage of triglycerides.

## REFERENCES

1. Zhang Y, Proenca R, Maffei M, et al. Positional cloning of the mouse obese gene and its human homologue. Nature 1994; 372:425.
2. Friedman JM, Halaas JL. Leptin and the regulation of body weight in mammals. Nature 1998; 395:763.
3. Montague CT, Farooqui S, Whitehead JP, et al. Congenital leptin deficiency is associated with severe early onset obesity in humans. Nature 1997; 387:903.
4. Clement K, Vaisse C, Lahlous N, et al. A mutation in the human leptin receptor gene causes obesity and pituitary dysfunction. Nature 1998; 392:398.
5. Flier JS. Clinical review 94: what's in a name? In search of leptin's physiologic role. J Clin Endocrinol Metab 1998; 83:1407.
6. Halaas J, Gajiwala K, Maffei M, et al. Weight-reducing effects of the plasma protein encoded by the obese gene. Science 1995; 269:543.
7. Licinio J, Mantzoros C, Negrao AB, et al. Human leptin levels are pulsatile and inversely related to pituitary-adrenal function. Nat Med 1997; 3:575.
8. Laughlin GA, Yen SS. Hypoleptinemia in women athletes: absence of a diurnal rhythm with amenorrhea. J Clin Endocrinol Metab 1997; 82:318.
9. Banks WA, Kastin AJ, Huang W, et al. Leptin enters the brain by a saturable system independent of insulin. Peptides 1996; 17:305.
10. Bjorbaek C, Elmquist JK, Franz JD, et al. Identification of SOCS-3 as a potential mediator of central leptin resistance. Mol Cell 1998; 1:619.
11. Ahima RS, Prabakaran D, Mantzoros C, et al. Role of leptin in the neuroendocrine response to fasting. Nature 1996; 382:250.
12. Lord GM, Matarese G, Howard JK, et al. Leptin modulates the T-cell immune response and reverses starvation-induced immunosuppression. Nature 1998; 294:897.
13. Chehab F, Lim M, Lu R. Correction of the sterility defect in homozygous obese female mice by treatment with the human recombinant leptin. Nat Genet 1996; 12:318.
14. Chehab FF, Mounzih K, Lu R, Lim ME. Early onset of reproductive function in normal female mice treated with leptin. Science 1997; 275:88.
15. Haynes WG, Sivitz WJ, Morgan DA, et al. Sympathetic and cardiorenal actions of leptin. Hypertension 1997; 30:619.
16. Mantzoros C, Flier JS, Rogol AD. A longitudinal assessment of hormonal and physical alterations during normal puberty in boys. V. Rising leptin levels may signal the onset of puberty. J Clin Endocrinol Metab 1997; 82:1066.
17. Devaskar SU, Ollesch C, Rajakumar RA, Rajakumar PA. Developmental changes in obese gene expression and circulating leptin peptide concentrations. Biochem Biophys Res Commun 1997; 238:44.
18. Ahima RS, Bjorbaek C, Osei SY, Flier JS. Regulation of neuronal and glial proteins by leptin: implications for brain development. Endocrinology 1999; 140:2755.
19. Sierra-Honigmann MR, Nath AK, Murakami C, et al. Biologic action of leptin as an angiogenic factor. Science 1998; 281:1683.
20. Grunfeld C, Feingold KR. Regulation of lipid metabolism by cytokines during host defense. Nutrition 1996; 12:S24.
21. Van-Zee KJ, Kohno T, Fischer E, et al. Tumor necrosis factor soluble receptors circulate during experimental and clinical inflammation and can protect against excessive tumor necrosis alpha in vitro and in vivo. Proc Natl Acad Sci U S A 1992; 89:4845.
22. Aderka D, Engelmann H, Maor Y, et al. Stabilization of the bioactivity of tumor necrosis factor by its soluble receptors. J Exp Med 1992; 175:323.
23. Kishimoto T, Hibi M, Murakami M, et al. The molecular biology of interleukin 6 and its receptor. Ciba Found Symp 1992; 167:5.
24. Gerhatz C, Dittrich E, Stoyan T, et al. Biosynthesis and half-life of the interleukin-6 receptor and its signal transducer gp 130. Eur J Biochem 1994; 223:265.
25. Yasukawa K, Fatatsugi K, Saito T, et al. Association of recombinant soluble IL-6 signal transducer, gp 130, with a complex of IL 6 and soluble IL-6 receptor, and establishment of an ELISA for soluble gp 130. Immunol Lett 1992; 31:123.
26. Stouhard JM, Romijn JA, Van-der-Poll T, et al. Endocrinologic and metabolic effects of interleukin-6 in humans. Am J Physiol 1990; 268:E813.
27. Hotamisligil GS, Arner P, Caro JF, et al. Increased adipose expression of human tumor necrosis factor and insulin resistance. J Clin Invest 1995; 95:2409.
28. Ventre T, Doebber T, Wu M, et al. Targeted disruption of the mouse tumor necrosis factor-α gene: metabolic consequences in obese and non-obese mice. Diabetes 1997; 46:1526.
29. Uysal KT, Wiesbrock MW, Marino MW, Hotamisligil GS. Protection from obesity-induced insulin resistance in mice lacking TNF-α function. Nature 1997; 389:610.
30. Schreyer SA, Chua SC, LeBoeuf RC. Obesity and diabetes in TNF-α receptor-deficient mice. J Clin Invest 1998; 102:402.
31. Tsigos C, Papanicolaou DA, Defensor R, et al. Dose effects of recombinant human interleukin-6 on pituitary hormone secretion and energy expenditure. Neuroimmunology 1997; 66:54.

32. Rivier C, Vale W. Cytokines act within the brain to inhibit luteinizing hormone secretion and ovulation in the rat. Endocrinology 1990; 127:849.

33. Kennedy JA, Wellby ML, Zotti R. Effect of interleukin-1 beta, tumor necrosis factor-alpha and interleukin-6 on the control of thyrotropin secretion. Life Sci 1995; 57:487.

34. Siiteri PK. Adipose tissue as a source of hormones. Am J Clin Nutr 1987; 45(Suppl 1):277.

35. Svedsen OL, Hassager C, Christiansen C. Relationships and independence of body composition, sex hormones, fat distribution and other cardiovascular risk factors in overweight postmenopausal women. Int J Obes 1993; 17:459.

36. Bjorntorp P. The regulation of adipose tissue distribution in humans. Int J Obes 1996; 20:291.

37. Larsson B, Svardsudd K, Welin L, et al. Abdominal adipose tissue distribution, obesity, and risk of cardiovascular disease and death: 13 year follow up of participants in the study of men born in 1913. Br Med J 1984; 288:1401.

38. Stewart PM. Cortisol, hypertension and obesity: the role of 11 beta hydroxysteroid dehydrogenase. J R Coll Physicians Lond 1998; 32:154.

39. Bujalska IJ, Kumar S, Stewart PM. Does central obesity reflect "Cushing's disease of the omentum"? Lancet 1997; 349:1210.

40. Katz JR, Mohamed-Ali V, Wood PJ, et al. An in vivo study of the cortisol-cortisone shuttle in subcutaneous abdominal adipose tissue. Clin Endocrinol (Oxf) 1999; 50:63.

41. Morgan L, Pipkin FB, Kalsheker N. Angiotensinogen: molecular biology, biochemistry and physiology. Int J Biochem Cell Biol 1996; 28:1211.

42. Karlsson C, Lindell K, Ottosson M, et al. Human adipose tissue expresses angiotensinogen and enzymes required for its conversion to angiotensin II. J Clin Endocrinol Metab 1998; 83:3925.

43. Darimont C, Vassaux G, Ailhaud G. Differentiation of preadipose cells: paracrine role of prostacyclin upon stimulation of adipose cells by angiotensin II. Endocrinology 1994; 135:2030.

44. Frederich RC, Kahn BB, Peach MJ, Flier JS. Tissue-specific nutritional regulation of angiotensinogen in adipose tissue. Hypertension 1992; 19:339.

45. Hamsten A, Wiman B, Faire UD, Blomback M. Increased plasma levels of rapid inhibitor of tissue plasminogen activator in young survivors of myocardial infarction. N Engl J Med 1985; 313:1557.

46. Morange PE, Aubert J, Peiretti F, et al. Glucocorticoids and insulin promote plasminogen activator inhibitor production by human adipose tissue. Diabetes 1999; 48:890.

47. Sakamoto T, Woodcock-Mitchell J, Marutsuka K, et al. TNF-alpha and insulin, alone and synergistically, induce plasminogen activator inhibitor-1 expression in adipocytes. Am J Physiol 1999; 276:C1391.

48. Shimomura I, Funahashi T, Takahashi M, et al. Enhanced expression of PAI-1 in visceral fat: possible contributor to vascular disease in obesity. Nat Med 1996; 2:800.

49. Flier JS, Lowell B, Napolitano A, et al. Adipsin: regulation and dysregulation in obesity and other metabolic states. Recent Prog Horm Res 1989; 45:567.

50. Flier JS, Cook KS, Usher P, Spiegelman BM. Severely impaired adipsin expression in genetic and acquired obesity. Science 1987; 237:405.

51. Napolitano A, Lowell BB, Damm D, et al. Concentrations of adipsin in blood and rates of adipsin secretion by adipose tissue in humans with normal, elevated and diminished adipose tissue mass. Int J Obes Relat Metab Disord 1994; 18:213.

52. Sniderman AD, Cianflone K. The adipsin-ASP pathway and regulation of adipocyte function. Ann Med 1994; 26:388.

# HERITABLE ABNORMALITIES OF ENDOCRINOLOGY AND METABOLISM

KENNETH L. BECKER, EDITOR

# CHAPTER 187

# INHERITANCE PATTERNS OF ENDOCRINOLOGIC AND METABOLIC DISORDERS

R. NEIL SCHIMKE

Most diseases of the endocrine system have a partial genetic component. In some, like the Turner and Klinefelter syndromes, a primary chromosome abnormality is clearly causative. In others, as exemplified by Graves disease and insulin-dependent diabetes mellitus, a genetic contribution is certain, but the precise molecular mechanism is unclear. The powerful new genetic techniques using restriction enzymes and cloned probes undoubtedly will answer the many questions still remaining about gene action in endocrine disease.

## MENDELIAN INHERITANCE

Mendelian or single-factor inheritance is subdivided on the basis of whether the gene is located on an *autosome* or on the X *chromosome.* If the mutant allele expresses itself in a single dose, the individual is said to be heterozygous for a *dominant* trait. If both alleles on homologous autosomes must be abnormal before the level of clinical detectability is reached, the condition is said to be *recessive.* A special situation exists for X-linked *recessive* disorders, because the hemizygous male bearing a gene for a recessive trait will show the condition, but an affected female ordinarily will be homozygous.

The elucidation of mendelian inheritance requires *pedigree analysis* and usually some knowledge of the trait. Most of the simply inherited disorders are assumed to arise because of *point mutations* (i.e., a change in a single base pair that generates a protein with one amino acid different from the normal). Whether such an alteration induces a true abnormality depends on the type of amino-acid substitution and its location in the protein. Population studies have established that many genes are polymorphic and that polymorphism does not invariably equate with disease or disability. Moreover, more complex alterations in DNA also can follow simple inheritance patterns, including mutation to terminating or stop codons, frame-shift mutations, and so forth.

The gene itself is neither dominant nor recessive; rather, this attribute arises from the sensitivity of the method of detection. For example, heterozygous carriers of recessive conditions commonly can be detected biochemically, but rarely is there clinical evidence of the gene because *recessive disorders* tend to result from defects in *enzyme proteins.* Alternatively, *dominant conditions* are more likely to be present if a *structural protein* is altered or some *regulatory mechanism* has been altered.

## AUTOSOMAL DOMINANT INHERITANCE

With autosomal dominant inheritance, only one of the two allelic genes on homologous chromosomes is abnormal (Fig. 187-1). Because these alleles separate at meiosis, half of the offspring of an affected individual also will be affected. Such expectations rarely occur except in very large families or unless family data are pooled. Thus, each child of a proband with a dominant trait has a 50% chance of being affected, and because

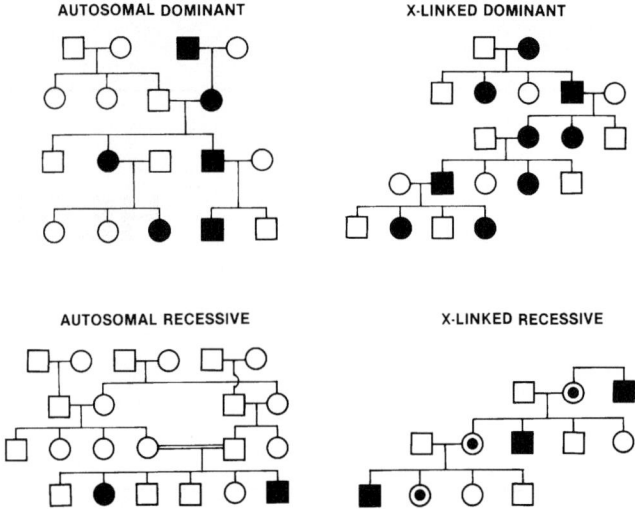

**FIGURE 187-1.** Idealized pedigrees. *Squares* are male, *circles* are female, and affected individuals are designated in *black. Half-darkened circles,* see discussion in X-Linked Inheritance section.

the condition is autosomal, there is ordinarily no sex predilection. Some individuals, who by pedigree analysis must be gene carriers, that is, have both an affected parent and an affected child, show no evidence of the condition. In these individuals, the gene is said to be *nonpenetrant* or *incompletely penetrant,* the term implying an all-or-none phenomenon. However, penetrance is relative, depending on the nature of the mutation and the ability to detect its presence. A gene deemed nonpenetrant simply on the basis of the family history may become penetrant when the unaffected members are examined by an experienced clinician. Penetrance is usually quoted as a percentage, for example, 90%, or as a proportion of 1, for example, 0. 9. This figure implies that 90% or 0.9 of gene carriers show evidence of the condition in some way. Estimations of penetrance are determined by the study of a number of families affected with the trait in question, not on a single family, no matter how large. As an example of reduced penetrance, consider family studies of multiple endocrine neoplasia syndrome type 1 (MEN1; see Chap. 188). The germline defect resides in a tumor-suppressor gene on chromosome 11. This lesion predisposes the heterozygote to endocrine tumors in the pituitary, parathyroid, and pancreas. However, to develop tumors in these respective endocrine organs, a somatic alteration in the normal allele must also occur (loss of heterozygosity). Hence, if 10% of gene carriers, as determined by direct molecular analysis, did not develop tumors in any of these endocrine glands during their lifetime, the MEN1 gene would be said to be only 90% penetrant. In this circumstance, the degree of penetrance of the gene obviously depends on the presence of the second event.

Another facet of dominant traits is that they tend to vary considerably in clinical expression, even within the same family. The reason for this variation is unknown but may depend on the efficiency of the opposite normal allele or on other modifying genes located elsewhere in the genome. Occasionally, a dominant trait appears in the absence of an affected antecedent. If nonpaternity can be excluded, such an occurrence represents a *new mutation.* Generally, the more lethal the disease, the more likely it is to result from a new mutation. In this setting, it is common to find that one or both parents are, on the average, older than the contemporary childbearing population.

The molecular events responsible for dominant expression of a single mutated gene are numerous, but some of the more common include haploinsufficiency with loss or diminution of overall function, mutations that cause overexpression or gain of function, and so-called dominant negative mutations in which the mutated gene product interferes in some way with the operation of the normal allele. As examples, individuals heterozygous for inactivating mutations in the low-density lipoprotein (LDL) receptor have familial hypercholesterolemia (see Chap. 163). Patients with germline activating mutations in the thyroid-stimulating hormone (TSH) and luteinizing hormone (LH) receptor have familial hyperthyroidism and precocious puberty, respectively.[1,2] In one dominantly inherited form of isolated growth hormone deficiency, a mutation in an exon-intron splice site led to the production of an abnormal molecule that effectively inactivated the product of the normal allele by a dominant negative effect.[3]

## AUTOSOMAL RECESSIVE INHERITANCE

The characteristic pedigree pattern with this form of inheritance is of affected sibs with unaffected parents (see Fig. 187-1). Occasionally, if the gene frequency is high enough, collateral relatives may be affected. The chances of heterozygous parents having a child with an autosomal recessive condition is 25%, but most families tend to be small, and a single case within a family is common. Clinical variability or *expressivity* tends to be less both within and between families than with autosomal dominant disorders. The rarer the condition, the more often one encounters *consanguinity* in the pedigree. Alternatively, if inbreeding is discovered on evaluation of the family history of a sporadic case of a condition, autosomal recessive inheritance becomes more likely. Some interfamilial variability may be due to the fact that affected individuals are compound heterozygotes; that is, each parent has contributed a different mutant allele. In other instances, phenotypic differences between families may be due to homozygosity for mutations at different sites within the gene. Rarely, a recessive trait may be uncovered in an otherwise heterozygous individual by a chromosome deletion or translocation in which the normal allele has been lost or its function interfered with by the chromosomal event.

Recessive traits tend to be enzyme deficiency states in which the homozygote has no or little enzyme activity. Half-normal enzyme activity characterizes the heterozygous parent, but this partial deficiency rarely causes any clinical signs or symptoms under ordinary circumstances. However, heterozygotes for some of the inborn errors of thyroxine ($T_4$) biosynthesis, for example, possibly could present with goiter and compensated hypothyroidism if they normally ingest a diet that is iodine deficient or rich in natural goitrogens.

Not all recessive disorders are enzymopathies. For example, homozygosity for a mutation in a transcription factor Pit-1 leads to defective lineage delineation of pituitary precursor cells such that affected individuals have congenital pituitary dwarfism with deficient production of thyroid stimulating hormone (TSH), growth hormone (GH), and prolactin.[4]

## X-LINKED INHERITANCE

Both dominant and recessive forms of X-linked inheritance are known, although the former is less common. With X-linked dominance (see Fig. 187-1), both males and females show the trait, but females are usually less severely affected because of the random inactivation that occurs with one of the X chromosomes in every female cell, the so-called *Lyon phenomenon*. This inactivation takes place early in gestation, and all the daughter cells of the original cell will have the same X chromosome inactivated, whether it is maternal or paternal in origin. Thus, a female with an X-linked dominant trait could be affected as severely as a hemizygous male or, at the opposite end of the spectrum, show no signs of the condition. The female phenotype usually is somewhere in the middle.

A good example of X-linked dominant inheritance is vitamin D–resistant rickets, in which affected females may show all of the classic features of rickets or be affected only on the basis of a low serum phosphate level. It is now known that the entire X chromosome is not inactivated, because genes on the terminal part of the short arm as well as on the long arm do remain active. Both X chromosomes are necessary for oogenesis, as evidenced by the gonadal findings in the Turner syndrome. *X-linked dominant* pedigrees may resemble autosomal dominant inheritance, the critical difference being the absence of male-to-male transmission in the former type. Usually an extensive kindred shows twice as many females affected as males, because affected men transmit the condition to all daughters and none of their sons, but affected women have a 50% chance of passing the condition to children of either sex.

With *X-linked recessive* inheritance (see Fig. 187-1), men typically are the only affected sex, although it is not uncommon to find partial expression of the trait in heterozygous female carriers, as expected under the Lyon hypothesis. Female carriers have a 50% chance of transmitting the condition to their sons, and the heterozygous state to their daughters, most of whom will be clinically unaffected. Other ways in which a female could be affected with an X-linked recessive trait would be if she were homozygotous or had the simultaneous presence of a 45,X karyotype. Even X-linked recessive traits in males exhibit genetic heterogeneity. For example, mutations of the X-linked androgen-receptor gene may give rise to an external genital phenotype that is totally female in appearance, is ambiguous, or is essentially male.[5] Further, another variant form of mild androgen insensitivity is due to a unique expansion of a polymorphic polyglutamine tract (CAGn) in exon 1. These individuals may show only mild gynecomastia as a limited expression of androgen insensitivity, but more significantly develop progressive spinal muscular atrophy (Kennedy disease).[6] How this alteration in the androgen receptor relates to the neuromuscular disease remains to be explained.

## MULTIFACTORIAL INHERITANCE

Multifactorial inheritance implies that multiple genes participate in the pathogenesis and that additional environmental elements play a role in modifying the threshold of expression. The more common endocrine diseases probably best fit this model, with the recurrence risk in a family being comparatively low. It has been estimated that for any given multifactorial trait, the chance of recurrence in a family is roughly the square root of the incidence at birth. Thus, for a condition such as congenital thyroid dysgenesis, which occurs in ~1 in 4000 births, the possibility of another affected child would be on the order of 1% to 2%. If more than one member of the nuclear family is affected, the recurrence risk increases, a situation quite dissimilar to mendelian inheritance, in which the risk remains the same in subsequent births no matter how many are affected. The risk also is increased for second-degree relatives of an index case, but to a considerably lesser extent. The more individuals in a family who are affected, the greater the genetic liability. The variation in expression of a multifactorial trait probably relates to natural polymorphisms that are present at virtually every gene locus. This normal variation also must modify the phenotypic threshold. Precisely what role the environmental influences have on phenotypic expression varies from trait to trait; they remain essentially undefined.

## CHROMOSOMAL INHERITANCE

Chromosomal inheritance is somewhat of a misnomer, because all genetic traits are inherited by means of the chromosomes. Nevertheless, there exist disorders caused by excesses or deficiencies of entire chromosomes or parts of chromosomes, and these often originate a characteristic phenotype (e.g., 45,X Turner syndrome or 47,XXY Klinefelter syndrome). These conditions arise by meiotic nondisjunction or by anaphase lag. In general, whole chromosome aberrations have low heritability. If the chromosomes become rearranged, as with breakage and translocation or by inversions, the meiotic process is more significantly disturbed. Aberrancy becomes both more frequent and potentially transmissible. Hence, the reproductive fitness of carriers of balanced reciprocal translocations may be reduced, and they may have a history of recurrent abortion, malformed infants, or even decreased fertility. More extended chromosome banding techniques supplemented by fluorescence in situ hybridization (FISH) have allowed the detection of small rearrangements and have facilitated diagnosis (see Chap. 90). These same techniques have helped explain certain traits that are uncommonly familial, but in which the individuals in question have a characteristic phenotype. Examples include some patients with the third/fourth branchial arch syndrome (DiGeorge syndrome), who have a visible or molecular deletion of the short arm of chromosome 22; the deletion comprises a number of genes that are important for the development of these embryologic structures, including the parathyroid glands.[7] If reproductive fitness is not impaired, such small deletions, if they arise spontaneously and not by imbalanced segregation from a translocation carrier, could be transmitted like a single gene autosomal dominant trait.

## MOSAICISM

In genetic parlance, mosaicism means the presence of two or more cell lines in the same individual. Mosaicism is by definition a postzygotic event. It may be chromosomal, due to nondisjunction, translocation, deletion, inversion, and so forth occurring at some unspecified time after fertilization or it may be due to a single gene mutation with preservation of both the normal and mutated cell lines. Clinicians are generally familiar with both of these types of mosaicism as they pertain to cancer. Probably the best-known example of a postzygotic chromosome alteration resulting in malignancy is the Philadelphia chromosome. This is due to a chromosomal rearrangement in the myeloid cell line that results from translocation of the c-*abl* protooncogene on chromosome 9 to the breakpoint cluster region (*bcr*) on chromosome 22, thereby facilitating the development of chronic myelogenous leukemia. Loss of function mutations in p53, a tumor-suppressor gene, is commonly seen as one of a series of somatic events in a host of malignancies.

Nonmalignant mosaicism can also result in phenotypic alterations. For example, postzygotic loss of an X chromosome in an XY individual may give rise to a phenotypic spectrum ranging from typical Turner syndrome to that of a normal male. Clearly, the phenotype will depend on the timing of the event and the ultimate fate of the progeny cells. Mosaicism for a mutation in the TSH-receptor gene with clonal expansion can result in a toxic thyroid adenoma.[8] A more general propensity for somatic mutation in the endocrine system is seen in the McCune-Albright syndrome wherein activating mutations in the G-protein intracellular signaling pathway may cause synchronous or metachronous production of acromegaly, thyrotoxicosis, and primary adrenal Cushing syndrome as well as precious puberty in a single individual.[9]

*Gonadal mosaicism* is a special circumstance in which two cell populations, one carrying a chromosome rearrangement or single gene alteration, the other being normal, coexist only (or are only demonstrable) in the gonads. Gonadal mosaicism is usually only revealed when otherwise normal parents have successive children with a specific trisomy, that is, familial Down syndrome, or multiple progeny with a known autosomal dominant disorder. The overall risk for disease recurrence in such families is unknown, but is likely small for most disorders, although it probably varies from trait to trait. For example, in the perinatal lethal form of osteogenesis imperfecta the requisite collagen mutation may be present in 5% to 8% of gametes.[10]

## MITOCHONDRIAL INHERITANCE

Mitochondria also contain DNA (mtDNA). The human mitochondrial genome is a 16,569-base-pair, circular, double-stranded DNA that contains ribosomal RNA and transfer RNA genes as well as certain structural genes, the latter coding for various enzymatic components of the electron transport chain. The remaining elements of this system are encoded by nuclear DNA and the derived polypeptides are incorporated into each mitochondrion. There are numerous copies of the mitochondrial chromosome per mitochondrion and multiple mitochondria per cell. The mtDNA replicates within the mitochondrion and each of these organelles divides by simple fission during cell division. Mutations occur in mtDNA such that the progeny of cells with mtDNA mutations may contain normal mtDNA (homoplasmy) or a mixture of normal and mutated mtDNA (heteroplasmy). The unique feature of mtDNA mutations is maternal inheritance, because only the ovum contributes mitochondria to the zygote. Because of heteroplasmy, there may be considerable variability in the phenotype of affected offspring in the same family.

Since mitochondria play a pivotal role in oxidative phosphorylation, mtDNA mutations, which commonly involve deletions as well as point mutations, tend to involve tissues with high energy requirements (e.g., brain, eye, and cardiac and skeletal muscle). At least two mitochondrial diseases, the Kearns-Sayre syndrome (myopathy, ophthalmoplegia, retinitis pigmentosa, heart block, diabetes) and a diabetes-deafness syndrome, illustrate that the pancreatic B cell also depends heavily on mitochondrial metabolism.[11,12]

## GENETIC HETEROGENEITY

Many heritable disorders, once thought to be single gene entities, are now known to have more than one cause; hence, they are heterogeneous. An obvious example would be the same condition with more than one mode of inheritance. Various abnormalities in $T_4$ biogenesis all present with euthyroid or hypothyroid goiter, but are due to different gene defects inherited in different ways (see Chap. 47). This is an example of *locus heterogeneity* in which different genes at different chromosomal sites (loci) are responsible for the same or a very similar phenotype. Even if the mode of inheritance is the same in different families, the demonstration of a different abnormal protein, as in the various enzymatic defects leading to the common phenotype of virilizing adrenal hyperplasia, establishes heterogeneity.

A somewhat different phenotype occasioned by different mutations within the same gene is termed *allele heterogeneity*. Thus, as previously mentioned, mild, moderate, and severe degrees of genital ambiguity are due to different molecular lesions in the androgen-receptor gene. The endocrine literature is replete with examples of this phenomenon, although precisely how these different mutations produce the altered phenotype is less well understood.

# GENETIC LINKAGE AND DISEASE ASSOCIATION

Linkage means that two genetic loci are within measurable physical proximity to one another on the same chromosome. Most, if not all, loci or sites potentially can be occupied by any number of different alleles. Therefore, it is the loci that are linked and not any two specific alleles. The usual technique used for *mapping genes* involves extended family studies seeking a linkage relationship between a given, simply inherited trait and various markers, such as blood groups or serum protein polymorphisms. The use of mouse-human hybrid cell lines, restriction endonuclease analysis, and other molecular techniques has facilitated mapping of the human genome.

Association is a statistical phenomenon. The well-known association of various human leukocyte antigen (HLA) alleles, particularly at the HLA-B and -D loci, with a number of autoimmune endocrine diseases is a good illustration. The current thinking is that the major histocompatibility region on chromosome 6 contains genes that predispose to organ-specific autoimmunity. Thus, the HLA alleles serve as markers for these immune response genes whose precise nature or existence remains unknown. The autoimmune endocrine diseases probably depend for their pathogenesis on a number of these predisposing genes, not all of which are located on chromosome 6, in concert with an environmental trigger (see Chaps. 194 and 197).

Some genes show both linkage and association. For example, the gene for the 21-hydroxylase deficiency form of congenital adrenal hyperplasia (see Chap. 77) is linked to the HLA-B locus. The deficiency state also is associated more commonly with HLA-B47 than would be expected by chance. A later-onset variant of 21-hydroxylase deficiency shows the same linkage phenomenon with the B locus, but it is associated with B14. The reasons for these associations are not clear.

# GENOMIC IMPRINTING

Genomic imprinting refers to differential genetic expression at a chromosomal or single gene level, depending on whether the genetic material in question was derived from the mother or father of the affected individual.[13] Imprinting is an exception to Mendelism. It has been known for some time that inheritance of the entire chromosome complement from a single parent results in lethality in utero. For example, it appears that paternal genes are important for the placenta and membranes; that is, a paternal diploid complement gives rise to a poorly formed embryo with well-developed extraembryonic tissues or a molar pregnancy, whereas the maternal haploid set is critical for the embryo itself, since a solely maternal chromosome set results in an embryo or teratoma with little membranous tissue. The inactivation of genes or genetic regions on the X chromosome in females is a classic type of imprinting. It is now known, however, that autosomal genes can be imprinted as exemplified by the molecular findings in the Prader-Willi and Angelman syndromes, respectively.[14] In the former disorder, loss of a paternal gene or genes on chromosome 15 gives rise to the characteristic phenotype, while a similar loss of the same genetic material from maternal chromosome 15 yields the latter disorder, which is quite distinct. As another example, familial glomus tumors (paragangliomas) only occur in a gene carrier if the transmitting parent is the father.[15] Why imprinted genes are necessary in humans, and indeed in mammals in general, is not known but probably has to do with the need for flexibility in gene control during crucial periods in growth and development.

# UNIPARENTAL DISOMY

The phenomenon of uniparental disomy, wherein a given individual has two copies of a single chromosome from one parent, could be loosely considered a special form of imprinting. In humans, uniparental disomy is caused primarily by nondisjunction in meiosis followed by trisomy or monosomy "rescue." If the two chromosomes in question are identical (isodisomic), it is assumed that mitotic nondisjunction of a monosomic conceptus occurred, whereas if the two parental chromosomes are not identical (heterodisomy), early chromosome loss in a trisomic embryo most likely took place. Uniparental inheritance of the aforementioned Prader-Willi and Angelman syndromes has been established, as has uniparental inheritance of cystic fibrosis, an autosomal recessive disease.[16]

# ANTICIPATION

*Anticipation* refers to progressively earlier age of onset of a dominantly inherited disease with each succeeding generation. For many years, anticipation was considered to be an ascertainment bias, with earlier detection being related to closer, earlier observation, looking for subtle signs of the disease in question. Molecular studies of a number of neurodegenerative diseases have now established the phenomenon as being real. For example, many genes contain repeated trinucleotide sequences that exhibit what might be considered a restrained polymorphism; that is, there is an upper and lower limit of triplet repeats in the general population that are allowable and do not produce disease. Once the upper threshold is exceeded the capacity for disease exists apparently by causing alteration in the respective protein product. Huntington chorea is the prototype in which inappropriate expansion of a CAG repeat sequence leads to progressively longer polyglutamine tracts in the protein huntingtin. Accumulation of the altered proteins in select cells of the central nervous system appears to promote neuronal apoptosis and progressive symptomatology.

Germline expansion of these triplet repeats (meiotic instability) has been seen in a number of disorders. Since there is a rough correlation between the size of the expansion and age of onset of disease, generational expansion accounts for anticipation. In some trinucleotide repeat disorders, such as myotonic dystrophy, the liability for progressive expansion, and hence, earlier onset of more severe disease is more marked when the mother is the affected parent.[17] In Huntington disease the opposite is true; that is, the father is the affected parent when the disease becomes clinically manifest within the first decade of life. The factors that promote these expansions and influence the sex predilection remain unknown.

Myotonic dystrophy features, in addition to muscle disease, male hypogonadism and diabetes in some patients. It has been suggested that postzygotic or somatic expansion of the relevant trinucleotide repeat (mitotic instability) could account for both the intra- and interfamilial variability of the nonmuscular effects of this pleiotropic gene.[18]

No pure example of triplet repeat disease has been seen in the endocrine system, although, as previously mentioned, expansion of a trinucleotide repeat in the androgen-receptor gene produces spinal muscular atrophy in addition to variable degrees of androgen insensitivity. However, this particular molecular lesion does not appear to exhibit anticipation.

# REFERENCES

1. Duprez L, Parma J, Van Sande J, et al. Germline mutations in the thyrotropin receptor gene cause non autoimmune autosomal dominant hyperthyroidism. Nature Genet 1994; 7:396.

2. Shenker A, Lane L, Kosugi S, et al. A constitutively activating mutation of the luteinizing hormone receptor in familial male precocious puberty. Nature 1993; 365:652.

3. Procter AM, Phillips JA III, Cooper DN. Molecular genetics of growth hormone deficiency. Hum Genet 1998; 103:255.

4. Pernasetti F, Milner RDG, Al Ashwal AAZ, et al. Pro 239 Ser: a novel recessive mutation of the Pit-1 gene in seven Middle Eastern children with growth hormone, prolactin and thyrotropin deficiency. J Clin Endocrinol Metab 1998; 83:2079.

5. Tsukada T, Inove M, Tachibana S, et al. An androgen receptor mutation causing androgen resistance in undervirilized male syndrome. J Clin Endocrinol Metab 1994; 79:1202.

6. Fischbeck KH. Kennedy disease. J Inherit Metab Dis 1997; 20:152.

7. Ryan AK, Goodship JA, Wilson DI, et al. Spectrum of clinical features associated with interstitial chromosome 22q11 deletions in a European collaborative study. J Med Genet 1997; 34:798.

8. Parma J, Duprez L, Van Sande J, et al. Somatic mutations in the thyrotropin receptor gene cause hyperfunctioning thyroid adenomas. Nature 1993; 365:649.

9. Weinstein LS, Shenker A, Gejman PV, et al. Activating mutations of the stimulatory G protein in the McCune-Albright syndrome. N Engl J Med 1991; 325:1688.

10. Byers PH, Tsipouras P, Bonadio JF, et al. Perinatal lethal osteogenesis imperfecta (OI type II): a biochemically heterogeneous disorder usually due to new mutations in the genes for type I collagen. Am J Hum Genet 1988; 42:237.

11. Moraes CT, De Mauro S, Zeviani M, et al. Mitochondrial DNA deletions in progressive external ophthalmoplegia and Kearns-Sayre syndrome. N Engl J Med 1989; 320:1293.

12. Velho G, Byrne MM, Clement K, et al. Clinical phenotypes, insulin secretion, and insulin sensitivity in kindreds with maternally inherited diabetes and deafness due to mitochondrial RNA Leu (UUR) gene mutation. Diabetes 1996; 45:478.

13. Hall JG. Genomic imprinting: review and relevance to human disease. Am J Hum Genet 1990; 46:857.

14. Smeets DFCM, Hamel BCJ, Nelen MR, et al. Prader-Willi syndrome and Angelman syndrome in cousins from a family with a translocation between chromosomes 6 and 15. N Engl J Med 1992; 326:807.

15. Milunsky J, De Stephano AL, Huang X-L, et al. Familial paragangliomas: linkage to chromosome 11q 23 and clinical implications. Am J Med Genet 1997; 72:66.

16. Ledbetter DH, Engel E. Uniparental disomy in humans: development of an imprinting map and its implications for prenatal diagnosis. Hum Mol Genet 1995; 4:1757.

17. Tsilfidis C, MacKenzie AE, Mettler G, et al. Correlation between CTG trinucleotide repeat length and frequency of severe congenital myotonic dystrophy. Nature Genet 1992; 1:192.

18. Richards RI, Sutherland GR. Heritable unstable DNA sequences. Nature Genet 1992; 1:7.

# CHAPTER 188

# MULTIPLE ENDOCRINE NEOPLASIA

GLEN W. SIZEMORE

## DEFINITION

Two distinct sets of multiple endocrine tumor associations have been recognized and well characterized. A classification system for these rare tumor associations was first proposed by Steiner and associates[1] and has been modified by the author and others (Table 188-1).

*Multiple endocrine neoplasia type 1* (MEN1) describes two or more of the major combinations of pituitary, pancreatic neuroendocrine, and parathyroid tumors, as well as other, less frequent tumors. Perhaps the first description of MEN1 should be attributed to Erdheim, who noted that patients with acromegaly had additional tumors of the pancreas and parathyroid glands.[2] The term *multiple endocrine adenomas* had been applied by Underdahl et al.[3] to 22 cases with tumors involving at least two of these glands.

**TABLE 188-1.**
**Multiple Endocrine Neoplasia: Organ Involvement**

**TYPE 1**
Pituitary
Pancreatic islet cell or enteropancreatic neuroendocrine
Parathyroid disease
Associated: carcinoid (bronchus, duodenum, thymus), thyroid, adenocortical, lipoma, facial angiofibromas, skin collagenomas

**TYPE 2**
*Type 2A*
Medullary thyroid carcinoma
Adrenomedullary disease–pheochromocytoma
Parathyroid disease
Normal phenotype
Associated: cutaneous lichen amyloidosis, Hirschsprung disease

*Type 2B*
Medullary thyroid carcinoma
Adrenomedullary disease–pheochromocytoma
Parathyroid disease is rare
Ganglioneuroma phenotype

**FAMILIAL MEDULLARY THYROID CARCINOMA (FMTC)**
Medullary thyroid carcinoma only

---

Wermer[4] reported multiple endocrine tumors in two consecutive generations of the same family, and he proposed a genetic origin. The genetic, pathologic, and clinical characteristics of patients with this syndrome have been summarized in many papers.[5-10]

*Multiple endocrine neoplasia type 2* (MEN2) describes the major combination of thyroid (medullary thyroid carcinoma [MTC]), adrenomedullary, and parathyroid tumors. Sipple[11] reported the autopsy findings in a patient with bilateral pheochromocytomas; bilateral carcinoma of the thyroid gland, which subsequently was shown to be MTC; and nodular enlargement of the one parathyroid gland that was identified. Numerous pathologic and clinical reports of similar cases followed.[12-18]

There are three variants of MEN2. The term *MEN2A* describes the condition in which affected patients have a normal physical appearance. The term *MEN2B* describes an unusual phenotype including eye and oral (mucosal, tongue) and labial ganglioneuromas, a marfanoid habitus, skeletal abnormalities, prominent corneal nerves, and general (not absolute) lack of parathyroid disease.[19] Familial medullary thyroid carcinoma (FMTC) describes affected members of families having heritable MTC only. Most probably, the term *MEN3* should be reserved for different sets of two or more heritable endocrine tumors, such as the syndrome of pheochromocytomas and islet cell tumor summarized by Carney et al.[20] In addition, there have been nonfamilial endocrine tumor associations such as papillary thyroid carcinoma and parathyroid adenoma; aldosterone-producing adrenocortical adenoma and parathyroid adenoma; and pituitary tumor, pheochromocytoma, and islet cell tumor.[21]

The *heritable* MEN syndromes share important characteristics, which contrast with those of *sporadic* endocrine tumors (e.g., genetic origin, precursor hyperplasias, malignant biologic behavior, multiplicity of involvement, and a clinical spectrum ranging from early occult hyperplasia to later symptomatic clinical tumors). Both MEN syndromes may be inherited with an autosomal dominant pattern of transmission. In MEN1, the genetic abnormality was mapped initially to chromosome 11 by linkage analysis.[22] Flanking DNA markers had suggested an 11q13 locus for the gene, and this was rapidly confirmed[23-25]; shortly thereafter, 32 different MEN1 germline mutations were found in 47 of 50 index cases studied at the National Institutes of Health.[26] In MEN2, the gene initially was assigned to chromosome 10 by linkage.[27,28] In MEN2A or FMTC, the most common abnormal genes on chro-

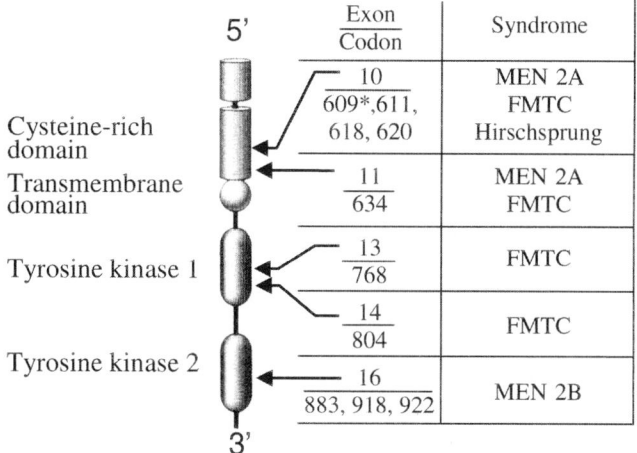

**FIGURE 188-1.** Diagrammatic representation of the most common sites of medullary thyroid carcinoma (*MTC*) and multiple endocrine neoplasia type 2 (*MEN2*) disease–causing mutations in the RET protooncogene on chromosome 10, including tabulation of the syndromes caused. (*FMTC,* familial medullary thyroid carcinoma.) (Adapted from Eng C. The RET protooncogene in multiple endocrine neoplasia type 2 and Hirschsprung's disease. N Engl J Med 1996;33f:943.)

mosome 10 are among the seven missense mutations of the RET protooncogene extracellular and transmembrane domains[29–31] (Fig. 188-1). In MEN2B, there are three missense mutations within the catalytic core of the RET tyrosine kinase domain.[32,33] Many infrequently occurring mutations are known (see Table 188-4), and new unusual ones are being found, including two de novo changes in one patient[33a] and a germline 9-base pair duplication in RET exon 8.[33b] In these syndromes, women and men are equally affected and there is variable penetrance of each major tumor component—both within and among affected families.

It has been suggested that the MTC and pheochromocytoma in MEN2 fit a "two-hit" mutational model.[34] The first event is a germinal mutation that makes cells susceptible to malignant transformation (C-cell and adrenomedullary hyperplasia). The second event is a somatic mutation that transforms a mutant cell into a tumor cell, with the tumors—MTC and pheochromocytoma—being multiple and presenting early. In sporadic neoplasms, both mutations occur in somatic cells; the tumors lack the precursor hyperplasias, are solitary, and present at later ages.

The term *neoplasia,* as opposed to the former term *adenomatosis,* emphasizes the malignant biologic behavior of some major components in these syndromes. In MEN1, pituitary carcinoma rarely occurs; however, 30% of the pancreatic neuroendocrine tumors are malignant. In MEN2, MTC always is malignant, as are ~10% of the pheochromocytomas.

*Multiplicity* is a hallmark. Not only are multiple endocrine glands involved, but also within these glands, the lesions are multicentric. Pituitary hyperplasia, as well as multiple pituitary adenomas, can occur. Seventy percent and 90% of gastrin-secreting and insulin-secreting pancreatic tumors, respectively, are multicentric, compared with 40% and 10%, respectively, of sporadic tumors. When adequate tissue has been examined, the MTC and adrenomedullary disease are always bilateral and multicentric. Rates of multiple gland parathyroid disease (generally hyperplasia) have ranged from 53% to 81% in MEN1 to as high as 100% in MEN2.

Glands in both syndromes, but particularly in MEN2, show convincing evidence of a pathologic spectrum ranging from initial hyperplasia to subsequent tumor.[35–37] The clinical spectrum is comparable; younger affected family members are asymptomatic, and disease generally does not manifest clinically until the second or later decades. Fortunately, family members who

**TABLE 188-2.**

**Multiple Endocrine Neoplasia Type 1: Tumor in 130 Patients at the National Institutes of Health**

| Tumor | Patients, No. (%) |
|---|---|
| *Parathyroid* | 129 (99) |
| *Enteropancreatic neuroendocrine tumor* | 86 (66) |
|   Gastrinoma | 61 (47) |
|   Insulinoma | 15 (12) |
|   Nonfunctioning tumor | 5 (4) |
|   Other* | 5 (4) |
| *Pituitary tumor* | 61 (47) |
|   Prolactinoma | 34 (26) |
|   Nonfunctioning tumor | 14 (11) |
|   Corticotropinoma | 9 (7) |
|   Somatotropinoma | 4 (3) |
| *Tumor in organ related to MEN* | |
|   Carcinoid | 21 (16) |
|   Bronchial | 11 (8) |
|   Gastric | 9 (7) |
|   Thymic | 1 (1) |
| *Adrenocortical tumor* | 21 (16) |
|   Nonfunctioning | 14 (11) |
|   Functioning | 7 (5) |
| *Thyroid tumor* | 16 (12) |
|   Follicular adenoma | 10 (8) |
|   Papillary carcinoma | 6 (5) |

*Glucagonoma, somatostinoma, and VIPoma.
(Adapted from Marx S, Spiegel AM, Skarulis M, et al. Multiple endocrine neoplasia type 1: clinical and genetic topics. Ann Intern Med 1998; 129:284.)

have inherited MEN usually can be recognized by identification of their DNA mutation, measurement of specific hormones indicating tumor, or recognition of biochemical or clinical changes related to tumor presence. Screening should be done for detection of disease early in the pathologic spectrum, so that early therapy may prevent unnecessary complications such as metastatic tumor, serious ulcer disease, fatal hypoglycemia, renal lithiasis, osteoporosis, or cardiovascular calamities.

## MULTIPLE ENDOCRINE NEOPLASIA TYPE 1

The incidence of principal organ involvement in patients with MEN1 has been reported in several publications.[5,8,26,38] The distribution in one series is outlined in Table 188-2. Differences in penetrance may reflect the type of study and the ages of the patients. MEN1 becomes manifest after the first decade, with symptoms developing in most patients in the third (women) and fourth (men) decades. The presenting features in 52 patients were ulcer disease in 40%, hypoglycemia in 31%, parathyroid disease in 15%, diarrhea in 6%, and pituitary disease in 6%.[15]

### PANCREATIC DISEASE

Enteropancreatic neuroendocrine tumors are present in 42% to 100% of patients with MEN1. Approximately 60% of these lesions are non–B-cell and 30% are B-cell tumors. Most secrete one hormone and produce a distinct clinical syndrome; a few secrete multiple substances and have a mixed presentation. Substances produced by these tumors include gastrin, insulin, glucagon, pancreatic polypeptide,[39] somatostatin,[26] vasoactive intestinal peptide,[40,41] serotonin, corticotropin, and calcitonin. Some tumors are nonfunctional even though they immunostain for multiple hormones. Thirty percent of the pancreatic tumors are malignant, but they often are indolent and cause death only through hormone secretion.

## GASTRIN-SECRETING TUMORS

Gastrinoma is the most common functioning enteropancreatic tumor. The clinical syndrome associated with excess gastrin secretion by non–B-cell tumors—the Zollinger-Ellison syndrome (ZES)[42]—does not differ between MEN1 and sporadic cases (see Chap. 220). Peptic ulcer occurs in 51% of cases and watery diarrhea in 13%.[5] As many as 65% of the ulcers are multifocal and often occur in atypical locations. Along with ulcer pain and esophagitis, patients often have complications such as multiple hemorrhages, pyloric obstruction, or perforation.

The diagnostic hallmarks of ZES are increased secretion of gastrin and gastric acid. One review summarizes the current evaluation and therapy.[43] A basal hourly acid output above 15 mEq is found in 68% to 97% of patients with ZES who have not had previous acid-reducing operations; this test excludes 88% to 96% of patients with ordinary duodenal ulcers. Gastrin values above 1000 pg/mL in patients with increased gastric acid secretion are diagnostic of ZES. However, many patients with ZES repeatedly have gastrin values that are only marginally elevated, so provocative tests are used to distinguish these patients from others with high gastric acid and high gastrin values—such as patients with retained gastric antrum, gastric outlet obstruction, renal failure, or antral G-cell hyperfunction-hyperplasia. The more sensitive and favored provocative test is an intravenous bolus of 2 U secretin (Kabi) per kilogram of body weight followed by sequential measurements of serum gastrin. An increase of gastrin by 200 pg/mL is regarded as diagnostic of ZES, with no false-positive responses and only occasional false-negative ones.[10,44]

Therapy for all varieties of gastrinoma still is evolving, is controversial, and is not uniformly satisfactory.[42,43,45,46] After surgical excision of their tumors, only 5% to 35% of patients are free from disease, tumor multiplicity, and frequent metastasis. Based on the experience in 14 cases, it was suggested that patients with MEN1 be excluded from abdominal surgery or be assigned a lower surgical priority because they had a greater chance for survival than did patients without MEN.[45] They also had a greater frequency of multicentricity—none of the nine patients who underwent surgery was cured (in four, the exploration was negative), and all had acceptable responses to medical therapy. Surgery is done only after various procedures have been done to localize tumor, such as angiography, computed tomography (CT), magnetic resonance imaging (MRI), transhepatic venous gastrin sampling, various isotopic liver-spleen scans, and upper gastrointestinal endoscopic ultrasonography.[47,48] Medical therapy is used initially in most patients. Presently, the National Institutes of Health (NIH) group suggests annual abdominal screens of unoperated gastrinoma patients with somatostatin-receptor scintigraphy[49] and CT or MRI. When tumors enlarge to greater than 3.0 cm, they are resected. The operation generally performed is a distal pancreatectomy with removal of tumor from other sites, particularly the microgastrinomas of the duodenum and peripancreatic lymph nodes. Medical therapy is used again in those whose symptoms persist after operation. Histamine$_2$-receptor antagonists, such as cimetidine (average dosage, 2.0–2.4 g per day), ranitidine (average dosage, 300–600 mg per day in divided doses), or famotidine, are used to reduce the predose gastric acid secretion to no more than 10 mEq per hour. Anticholinergic agents such as isopropamide are used to augment and prolong the effects of the histamine antagonist. These therapies adequately reduce gastric acid secretion in ~90% of all patients with ZES. However, many patients require progressive increases in the dosage of the histamine antagonist.

Omeprazole, a proton-pump inhibitor, which reduces the hydrogen, potassium adenosine triphosphatase, the enzyme responsible for gastric acid secretion, is used (average divided dosage, 60–120 mg per day).[50] Failure to respond to medical therapy mandates total gastrectomy. Even though long-term survival occurs in some patients because of slow tumor growth, the natural history of gastrinoma, with or without metastases, often is one of death from intractable ulcer disease, metastases, or surgical complications. In malignant gastrinoma, single or combination chemotherapeutic agents may be used: streptozocin, 5-fluorouracil, doxorubicin, dimethyltriazenoimidazol-carboximide, or octreotide acetate.[51] (see Chaps. 169 and 220).

## INSULIN-SECRETING AND MISCELLANEOUS TUMORS

Twelve percent to 30% of pancreatic tumors secrete insulin, and 10% secrete a mixture of gastrin and insulin. Both types may manifest clinically as hypoglycemia (i.e., headache, personality disturbance, dizziness, confusion, weakness, transient neurologic disturbances, convulsions, unconsciousness, coma, and death). The diagnosis of insulinoma is based on documentation of simultaneous fasting hypoglycemia of less than 45 mg/dL and an inappropriately high plasma insulin concentration of >10 μU/mL. Typical means used to accomplish this are either a 72-hour fast with sequential measurements of plasma glucose, insulin, and C-peptide or similiar measurements before and during induced hypoglycemia[52,53] (see Chap. 158). Insulinomas may often be localized by sequential measurement of hepatic vein insulin gradients after calcium infusion into pancreatic arteries.[54]

The initial therapy for insulinoma should be a distal pancreatectomy that removes ~85% of the gland.[55,56] This procedure is favored for three reasons. First, multicentric insulin-secreting tissue is present in 92% to 100% of patients with MEN1[55,57] compared with only 10% in those with sporadic tumors. Second, 5% to 15% of the tumors are malignant.[5,6] Finally, complications of pancreatic endocrine and exocrine insufficiency are greatly reduced compared with the frequency after total pancreatectomy (see Chap. 160). If hypoglycemia persists after surgery, diazoxide may be used; if metastatic disease is present, streptozocin, dacarbazine, or a somatostatin analog[58] may be used.

A glucagon-secreting tumor (see Chap. 220) without the necrolysis syndrome has been documented in a euglycemic woman with MEN1,[59] and hyperglucagonemia has been reported in five of six patients with MEN1.[60] Nonfunctioning A-cell adenomas also have been observed. Many reports of functioning glucagonomas are poorly documented, and in most suspected cases, cortisol or growth hormone excess or diabetes after pancreatectomy explains the hyperglycemia. Increased vasoactive intestinal peptide levels have been demonstrated, and one of the patients in the original Verner and Morrison[40] series who had watery diarrhea and hypokalemia (see Chaps. 182 and 220) had MEN1.

## PITUITARY DISEASE

The incidence of pituitary disease in MEN1 ranges from 47% (clinical) to 94% (autopsy).[5,8] There is a spectrum, ranging from hyperplasia through adenoma to cancer. In a large study, the tumor types and their frequencies were as follows: chromophobe, 44% (one cancer); eosinophilic, 35%; basophilic, 9%; mixed, 11%; and miscellaneous, 5%.[5] Manifestations of pituitary tumor accounted for only 4% of the presenting complaints in patients in that review, but may be as high as 32%. Tumor mass effects may produce headache, visual field abnormality, and monotropic or general hypopituitarism (see Chaps. 11, 17, and 19). The secretion of hormones by the tumor produces clinically identifiable endocrine manifestations: Prolactin causes galactorrhea-amenorrhea,[61,62] growth hormone causes acromegaly, and adrenocorticotropic hormone (ACTH) causes Cushing disease. Nonfunctioning pituitary tumors are in the minority. Presumably, many of the hyperplasias result from ectopic secretion of hypothalamic-releasing hormones by the pancreas or other primary syndrome tumors.[63]

The diagnosis and treatment of pituitary disease in MEN1 are similar to those of sporadic disease (see Chap. 17). The disease is confirmed by finding high or inappropriately low blood concentrations of prolactin, growth hormone, ACTH, or gonadotropins associated with an abnormality identified by gadolinium-enhanced MRI. Patients with prolactin-secreting microadenomas (see Chap. 13) may be treated with cabergoline, bromocriptine or pergolide unless subsequent mass effects dictate pituitary adenectomy. Macroadenomas, whether they secrete prolactin, growth hormone, ACTH, or nothing, require hypophysectomy, often followed by radiotherapy and medical therapy—such as octreotide for acromegaly. Larger or invasive tumors may require several treatment modalities. Endocrine deficiency states secondary to the tumor or its treatment necessitate replacement therapy.

## PARATHYROID DISEASE

Parathyroid disease is the most highly penetrant as well as earliest presenting manifestation of MEN1, affecting 87% to 99% of patients. In many families, this component is detected first, with the discovery of MEN1 occurring subsequently. This chronology may occur because the parathyroid disease matures earlier than other components; because screening serum calcium determinations may be used more frequently than other markers; and because kindred members may be incompletely studied. There is universal agreement that parathyroid hyperplasia, diffuse or asymmetric, is the rule in MEN1. Older patients may have superimposed adenomatous change. The parathyroid hyperplasia may be caused by a growth factor found in the plasma of patients with MEN1 that is highly mitogenic for bovine parathyroid cells.[64]

Although involvement of the parathyroid gland is the most frequent component, symptoms of hyperparathyroidism occur in only 9% to 30% of patients with MEN1.[5,6] The symptoms, signs, and complications of hyperparathyroidism are not significantly different from those in sporadic, familial, or MEN2–associated hyperparathyroidism (see Chap. 58). The diagnosis of parathyroid disease is established by finding increased concentrations of serum calcium and parathyroid hormone. Not all patients with familial hypercalcemia have MEN1. The differential diagnosis also includes other diseases inherited in an autosomal dominant pattern: familial hyperparathyroidism, MEN2A, and familial hypercalcemic hypocalciuria. The last disorder is suggested by an absence of clinical signs, normal concentrations of parathyroid hormone, onset of hypercalcemia in the first decade, hypermagnesemia, and a low urinary calcium/creatinine clearance ratio.[60] Because localization scans do not uniformly image all involved glands, they are not recommended.

The indications for parathyroidectomy in patients with MEN1 are similar to those in patients with sporadic disease: bone disease (low bone mineral density, increased bone alkaline phosphatase, radiographic evidence of periosteal resorption or osteitis fibrosa cystica fracture), renal disease (increasing creatinine, active metabolic stone disease, nephrocalcinosis), a serum calcium value of 11.0 mg/dL or higher, or other complications suspected to be secondary to the hypercalcemia (e.g., cardiac arrhythmias, depressive symptoms, fatigue). A lesser indication might be detection of hypercalcemia at an early age, which would create a longer period at risk for the development of complications. Operation to restore normal serum calcium and thus reduce gastrin and gastric acid secretion has also been advo-

cated. The surgical procedure of choice for all patients with MEN1 is subtotal parathyroidectomy with preservation of 30 to 50 mg parathyroid tissue or total parathyroidectomy with autotransplantation of some removed tissue. In patients with hyperplasia for whom an operation is performed, 93% are cured initially, but 23% also have permanent parathyroprivic hypoparathyroidism,[65] and about half of those who have initially successful operations develop recurrence in the long term. Because of the high rate of hypoparathyroidism, autotransplantation and cryopreservation of parathyroid tissue are recommended (see Chap. 62). In those who become permanently hypoparathyroid, human parathyroid hormone 1-34 treatment should be helpful.[65a]

## ASSOCIATED DISEASES

Carcinoid tumors may occur in the bronchus, gastroduodenum, and thymus of 5% to 9% of patients with MEN1.[66] They may be locally invasive, multifocal, and occasionally metastatic. Clinical symptoms are rare,[26] although occasional affected patients have a high urinary content of 5-hydroxyindoleacetic acid. Twelve to 18% of patients have thyroid disease, such as follicular adenoma, nodular hyperplasia, colloid goiter, diffuse enlargement with thyrotoxicosis, Hashimoto disease, or malignancy.[5,26] This does not represent an increased prevalence compared with the general population. Adrenocortical disease, including adenoma, diffuse hyperplasia, nodular hyperplasia, and, rarely, cancer, occurs in 10% to 38% of patients.[67] In one report, hypertension was associated with hyperaldosteronism.[5] Most of the adrenal abnormalities are nonfunctional and a few may be a reflection of pituitary or paraneoplastic ACTH secretion. Multiple subcutaneous, pleural, and retroperitoneal lipomas occur in 13% to 38% of patients.[68] The NIH group has noted that 88% of their patients have facial angiofibromas and 72% have skin collagenomas.

## SCREENING FOR MULTIPLE ENDOCRINE NEOPLASIA TYPE 1

Primary relatives of index cases with MEN1 and patients having certain diseases should be screened for MEN1. These diseases include ZES, insulinoma, or multiple gland hyperparathyroidism not associated with other known familial disease. MEN1 has been found in 26% to 33% of patients with ZES,[43,45] 4% to 10% of patients with insulinoma,[55] 14% of families with familial hyperparathyroidism, and 16% of patients with parathyroid hyperplasia.[60]

Before adulthood, major morbidity is rare and cancer related to MEN1 has not been reported; therefore, screening beginning at age 18 seems appropriate.[26] A positive family history is helpful; however, a negative family history does not rule out this entity. The screening history and physical examination should emphasize symptoms and signs of hypercalcemia, peptic ulcer disease, hypoglycemia, galactorrhea-amenorrhea, acromegaly, Cushing syndrome, visual changes, and hypopituitarism. In patients without evidence of disease, it is sufficient to measure serum calcium, gastrin, and prolactin.[69] The author is content to repeat core studies at intervals of 5 years in asymptomatic persons at risk. In such screening programs, asymptomatic hypercalcemia is the most frequently described abnormality. Routine screening with pancreatic polypeptide, growth hormone, cortisol, and MRI of the pituitary gland is inadvisable because of the low yield.

Commercial testing for the MEN1 germline mutation is not available at this writing. When it is, identification of the specific mutation in an index case should be done first. This will allow selective search by the laboratory for only 1 of the 32 currently known mutations; this should reduce cost. Identification of carrier status will focus subsequent core screening measurements on the affected and excuse the unaffected. This will provide a

**TABLE 188-3.**
**Multiple Endocrine Neoplasia Type 2A: Combinations of Thyroid, Adrenal, and Parathyroid Disease**

| Study | No. of Patients | MTC | MTC Only | MTC, PARA | MTC, PHEO | MTC, PARA, PHEO |
|---|---|---|---|---|---|---|
| | | | *Percentage Having* | | | |
| Sizemore et al., 1977[17] | 66 | 100 | 59 | 21 | 12 | 8 |
| Saad et al., 1984[71] | 31 | 100 | 42 | 10 | 35 | 13 |
| Wells et al., 1985[72]* | 122 | 100 | 47 | 20 | 18 | 15 |
| Total | 219 | 100 | 50 | 19 | 19 | 12 |

MTC, medullary thyroid carcinoma; PARA, parathyroid disease; PHEO, pheochromocytoma.
*Wells and colleagues, personal communication.

sense of relief and reduce laboratory test expenses for the unaffected.[70] For the 6% of MEN1–affected families who have no detected mutation as of yet, routine testing at selected intervals must go on. In MEN1 carriers, the author measures core serum calcium, prolactin, gastrin, growth hormone, and cortisol at intervals of 2 years. After an initially negative pituitary MRI scan, this test is repeated for clinical suspicion or at 5-year intervals.

## MULTIPLE ENDOCRINE NEOPLASIA TYPE 2

MEN2 has three subsets (see Table 188-1). Patients with MEN2A have a normal phenotype and commonly have parathyroid disease. Patients with MEN2B have the ganglioneuroma phenotype and only rarely have parathyroid disease. Patients with FMTC have MTC only. The incidence of principal organ involvement in patients with MEN2A has been reported in several publications and is summarized in Table 188-3. Precursor stages exist for all organ components: C-cell hyperplasia precedes MTC (Fig. 188-2); diffuse nonnodular adrenomedullary hyperplasia precedes pheochromocytoma, and occult, normocalcemic parathyroid hyperplasia is observed.[29–31] Generally, asynchronous clinical manifestations lead to detection, often beginning with the third decade. MTC is found in all patients for two reasons: its clinical presentation occurs earlier; and measurement of calcitonin, a tumor marker for MTC, provides an exquisitely sensitive means for the early detection of occult disease in family members at high risk. Both MTC and pheochromocytoma may cause death secondary to metastatic spread, and pheochromocytoma may cause hypertension- or hypotension-associated death. Occasional patients with MEN2A or FMTC may have cutaneous lichen amyloidosis, as well as Hirschsprung disease.[73–75]

### MULTIPLE ENDOCRINE NEOPLASIA TYPE 2B

The main features of the MEN2B syndrome are clearly established.[76–80] Hypotheses about the development of this phenotype, and the relationship of this "sympathoenteric lineage" to the RET mutation have been presented.[81] A marfanoid habitus is recognized by excessive limb length, loose-jointedness, scoliosis, and anterior chest deformities. However, these patients do not have the ectopia lentis and cardiovascular abnormalities of Marfan syndrome (see Chap. 189). The diffuse ganglioneuromatosis may present as yellow or white nodular or diffuse thickening of the tarsal plates of the eyes, associated with thickened corneal nerve fibers; pink, yellow, or translucent hemispherical nodules studding the tip and anterior third of the tongue; elon-

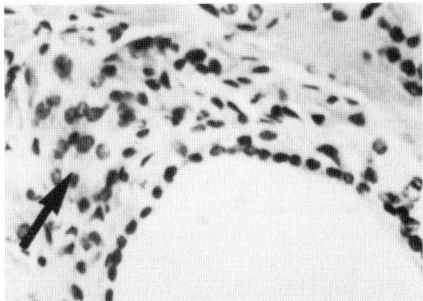
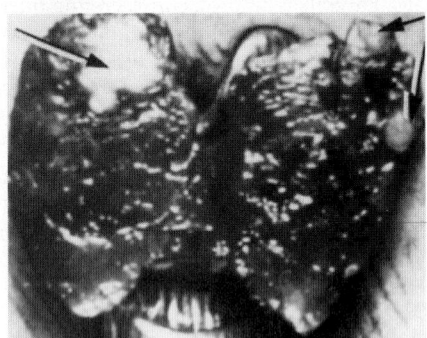
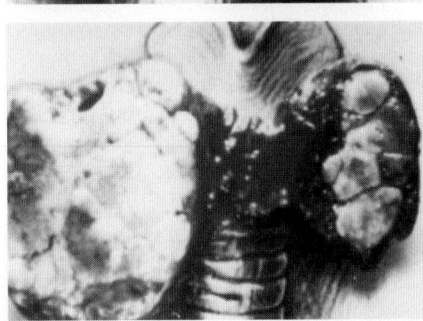

**FIGURE 188-2.** The spectrum of C-cell disease in a family with MEN2A. *Upper panel,* Microscopic example of the multicentric C-cell hyperplasia (*arrow*) found above the thyroid follicle in a 12-year-old girl. *Middle panel,* Surgical specimen showing 1.5-cm medullary thyroid carcinoma (*MTC; arrow*) in the right upper lobe and smaller lesions (*arrows*) in the left upper lobe of the girl's mother, age 29 years. *Lower panel,* Surgical specimen showing large masses of MTC in both lobes of the mother's 38-year-old brother. Larynx and trachea have been sketched.

gated projections posterior to each orolabial commissure; and nodules within the lips, causing them to appear everted, patulous, and lumpy (Fig. 188-3). These neural tumors are called *ganglioneuromas* rather than neuromas; they contain ganglion cells and tortuous nerve trunks with internal structural disarray. Functionally, alimentary ganglioneuromatosis produces gastrointestinal symptoms (constipation, diarrhea, dysphagia) and signs (megacolon, diverticulosis). The neuromuscular abnormalities range from localized (particularly to the peroneal muscles) to diffuse muscle weakness and may also be associated with sensory abnormalities.[78]

### MEDULLARY THYROID CARCINOMA

MTC originates from parafollicular, or C cells (so called because of their synthesis, storage, and secretion of calcitonin). The tumor has a solid, nonfollicular histologic pattern with amyloid in the stroma and a high incidence of lymph node metastases. In patients with MEN2, the MTC is located predominantly in the upper and middle thirds of the lateral thyroid lobes and, in contrast to sporadic MTC, is bilateral, multicentric, and almost universally associated with C-cell hyperplasia.

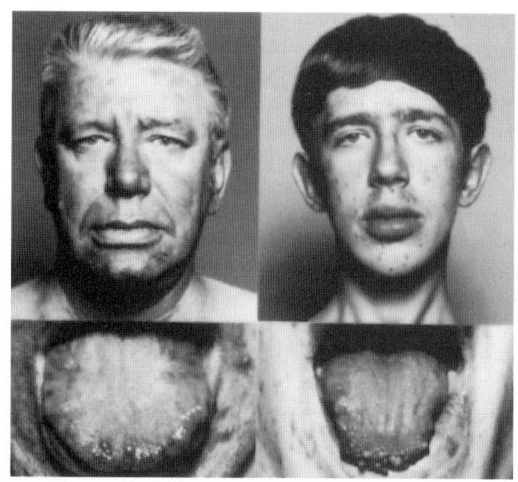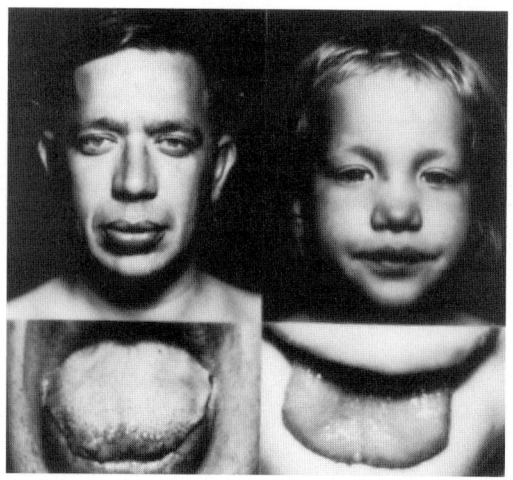

**FIGURE 188-3.** Abnormal facies, thickened lips, and ganglioneuromas of tongue in four affected members of a family with multiple endocrine neoplasia type 2B (*MEN2B*). *Left to right,* Grandfather, two sons, and 2-year-old granddaughter. (From Sizemore GW, Heath H III, Carney JA. Multiple endocrine neoplasia type 2. Clin Endocrinol Metab 1980; 9:299.)

## CLINICAL MANIFESTATIONS

One-third of all cases of MTC in patients with MEN2 present as a thyroid nodule, goiter, or mass, or as cervical lymphadenopathy, in the third to sixth decades. Less common clinical presentations include recognition because of an associated process, such as hyperparathyroidism, pheochromocytoma, or the ganglioneuroma phenotype in MEN2B. Rarely, there is an associated hereditary form of cutaneous lichen amyloidosis or Hirschsprung disease. Paraneoplastic syndromes occur: Cushing syndrome secondary to secretion of ACTH by the MTC; diarrhea, which is presumed to be caused by calcitonin-induced gastrointestinal secretion of water and electrolytes in persons with a large tumor volume; spontaneous or alcohol-induced flushing presumed to be caused by tumor secretion of other humoral substances—probably the vasodilating calcitonin gene–related peptide.[65–67] The remaining cases of MTC in patients with MEN2 are detected at earlier stages and ages through the screening of asymptomatic relatives at high risk.

## CALCITONIN TESTING

MTC secretes calcitonin, a biologic marker that is uniquely useful for detection and follow-up of MTC.[14,74] The measurement of this hormone is widely available and cost effective, making it applicable to large numbers of patients. It is a highly sensitive discriminator that detects, quantitatively, a difference between those with and those without MTC; when sensitive assays are used properly, there are few false-negative or false-positive responses. Several caveats apply to the use of calcitonin measurement in these patients. Clinicians are advised to ensure that referral laboratories have sufficiently standardized test information in normal persons so that the test they plan to use will allow detection of the majority of MTC-affected patients at a reasonable age. Hypercalcitonemia is not specific for MTC; for reviews of this subject, see Chapters 40 and 53. Stimulation testing should not be done in patients with unequivocally high calcitonin values, because rapid increases in the concentration of calcitonin or, probably, calcitonin gene–related peptide, have occasionally caused vasodilatation and shock in such patients.

Most patients with sporadic MTC have high basal concentrations of calcitonin.[17] However, 27% of patients with familial MTC—young patients with minimal tumor—have basal concentrations within the normal range, and repeated basal measurements alone are not helpful.[83] To identify C-cell hyperplasia or precursor forms of MTC, provocative tests of calcitonin secretion are needed to increase the marker's sensitivity. Tests using infusions of calcium, pentagastrin, or both appear to be best. Pentagastrin stimulation is particularly useful.[83,84] In this method, a bolus intravenous injection of 0.5 μg/kg is given over 5 seconds in 3.0 to 5.0 mL of 0.9% sodium chloride, and blood samples are taken at 0, 1.5 to 2.0, and 5 minutes for measurement of immunoreactive calcitonin. This test, when used with a well-standardized calcitonin assay, is a sensitive means of detecting and following MTC. The author's experience indicates that pentagastrin testing uniformly detects familial MTC before thyroidectomy in the 27% of patients who have normal basal calcitonin concentrations as well as the 15% who have false-negative responses to calcium infusion. In 20 years, the author has had only two initial false-negative results (which converted to positive at older ages) and two false-positive results. Others have obtained comparable results with a combined calcium-pentagastrin test.[85] In the latter procedure, a 1-minute injection of calcium, 2 mg/kg per minute, is followed by an injection of pentagastrin, 0.5 μg/kg in 5 seconds, with blood sampling during 15 minutes. At this time, pentagastrin is unavailable in the United States—a marketing decision. Although it remains available in Europe, many clinicians in the United States will have to use infusions of calcium as outlined in referral laboratory catalogs for stimulation testing.[86,87]

## SCREENING FOR MEDULLARY THYROID CARCINOMA MULTIPLE ENDOCRINE NEOPLASIA TYPE 2 KINDREDS

Genetic analysis of RET protooncogene mutations has been a major advance toward the goal of early detection of affected patients with presymptomatic and premetastatic MTC. Detection of the mutations causing MTC in patients within kindreds having MEN2 or FMTC allows gene carrier status to be established at birth in the majority of affected members in kindreds having risk, and should allow the same in persons who are at risk because of associated diseases. An international consortium that studied the mutations in 477 families in which two or more members had MTC has reported excellent results.[88] MEN2A mutations were correctly identified in 98% of affected families, MEN2B mutations were identified in 95% of affected families, and FMTC mutations were identified in 88% of affected families. The consortium also found that between 2% and 12% of these MTC-affected families, respectively, were not detected by genetic analysis. Perhaps other mutations will be found that explain the present false-negative percentage. This group and others have not yet reported false-positive results. The study also demonstrated a relationship between specific RET protooncogene mutations and the various MTC phenotypes (Table 188-4).

Initially, it was expected that all patients with MEN2 and a RET mutation would have medullary carcinoma or its precursor and that calcitonin testing would detect all. That is not the case. In MEN2, the clinical penetrance of the gene is not complete by age 70, and the prevalence of MTC detected by calcitonin testing through

**TABLE 188-4.**
**Mutations of the RET "Protooncogene" Associated with Multiple Endocrine Neoplasia (MEN) Type 2 and Familial Medullary Thyroid Carcinoma (FMTC)**

| Affected Codon | Amino Acid Change Normal>Mutant | Nucleotide Change Normal>Mutant | Syndrome | % of MEN2 Mutations |
|---|---|---|---|---|
| 532 | Glu Glu Cys | GAGGAGTGT | FMTC | <1 |
| 609 | Cys>Arg | TGC>CGC | MEN2A | <1 |
| | Cys>Gly | TGC>GGC | FMTC | |
| | Cys>Tyr | TGC>TAC | MEN2A | |
| | | | Hirsch-sprung | |
| 611 | Cys>Tyr | TGC>TAC | MEN2 | 2–3 |
| | Cys>Trp | TGC>TGG | FMTC | |
| | Cys>Phe | TGC>TTC | | |
| | Cys>Arg | TGC>CGC | | |
| | Cys>Gly | TGC>GGC | | |
| | Cys>Ser | TGC>AGC | | |
| 618 | Cys>Ser | TGC>AGC | MEN2A | 3–5 |
| | Cys>Gly | TGC>GGC | FMTC | |
| | Cys>Arg | TGC>CGC | | |
| | Cys>Phe | TGC>TTC | | |
| | Cys>Ser | TGC>TCC | | |
| | Cys>Tyr | TGC>TAC | | |
| 620 | Cys>Arg | TGC>CGC | MEN2A | 6–8 |
| | Cys>Tyr | TGC>TAC | FMTC | |
| | Cys>Phe | TGC>TTC | | |
| | Cys>Ser | TGC>TCC | | |
| | Cys>Gly | TGC>GGC | | |
| | Cys>Ser | TGC>AGC | | |
| | Cys>Trp | TGC>TGG | | |
| 630 | Cys>Tyr | TGC>TAC | MEN2A | |
| | Cys>Ser | TGC>TCC | FMTC | |
| | Cys>Phe | TGC>TTT | | |
| 634 | Cys>Ser | TGC>AGC | MEN2A | 80–90 |
| | Cys>Gly | TGC>GGC | | |
| | Cys>Arg | TGC>CGC | | |
| | Cys>Tyr | TGC>TAC | | |
| | Cys>Phe | TGC>TTC | | |
| | Cys>Ser | TGC>TCC | | |
| | Cys>Trp | TGC>TGG | | |
| 634,635 | Cys Arg>Trp Gly | TGC CGC>TGG GGC | MEN2A | |
| 635 | Thr Ser Cys Ala insertion | ACG AGC TGT GCC | MEN2A | <1 |
| 637 | Cys Arg Thr insertion | TGC CGC ACG | MEN2A | <1 |
| 768 | Glu>Asp | GAG>GAC | FMTC | 0–1 |
| 790 | Leu>Phe | TTG>TTC | MEN2A | <1 |
| | Leu>Phe | TTG>TTT | FMTC | |
| 791 | Tyr>Phe | TAT>TTT | FMTC | 0–1 |
| 804 | Val>Leu | GTG>TTG | MEN2A | <1 |
| | Val>Met | GTG>ATG | FMTC | |
| 883 | Ala>Phe | GCT>TTT | MEN2B | <1 |
| 891 | Ser>Ala | TCG>GCG | FMTC | <1 |
| 918 | Met>Thr | ATG>ACG | MEN2B | 3–5 |
| 922 | Ser>Tyr | TCC>TAC | MEN2B | <1 |

(Adapted from Gagel RF, Cote GJ. Pathogenesis of medullary thyroid cancer. In Fagin J, ed. Thyroid cancer. Kluwer Academic Publishers, 1998:85.)

age 31 is 93%.[89] These delayed expressions may be explained by slow growth of MTC in some patients, insensitive calcitonin assays, or, more probably, unknown epigenetic factors that translate the genetic message into a functional MTC. An analogy should help.

Although it is known that persons who have the BRCA 1 or 2 mutations have higher than normal risk for breast carcinoma, all persons with these mutations do not develop breast cancer within a few years of birth. The expression is delayed by unknown factors. Affected persons are advised to have long-term clinical follow-up and repeated mammograms. Gene mutations measure one thing, and stimulation tests or mammograms measure another. Therefore, direct comparisons seem somewhat futile. However, when done, the comparisons between RET and biochemical testing have favored RET, so mutation analysis is generally considered to be superior for detecting risk of MEN2. In a study comparing RET to calcitonin, it was found that 4 of 91 (4.3%) patients with MEN2A had false-negative calcitonin results (that is, they were RET-positive and calcitonin-negative); similarly, it was found that 5 of 51 (9.8%) patients with FMTC had false-negative calcitonin results; all of the "calcitonin-missed" patients were young—younger than 23 years.[90] Similar results were reported in a second study: 8 of 74 (11%) patients with MEN2, who were mutation-positive and had MTC, had false-negative calcitonin studies; all of these individuals were in the youngest or fifth generation of the 4 five-generation families that were studied.[91] These two studies also found false-positive pentagastrin results in 8% and 9% of mutation-negative MEN2 patients, respectively. In the second study, all of these were thought to have a nonprogressive C-cell hyperplasia, which probably represents a new entity not related to MEN2.[92]

The author's screening procedure follows: Each new case having MTC is screened for a RET mutation; these tests are now widely available. A positive result prompts screening for the mutation in all primary relatives. Those family members who are positive should have cervical exploration; those who are negative need no further evaluation unless indicated clinically at a later point. An initial negative result in the index case screened should be reassuring to family members, because it indicates a 98% chance that the tested patient and his family will not have MEN2. However, because 2% or 12% of index cases with MEN2 or FMTC, respectively, may be mutation-negative, the author advises primary relatives of mutation-negative index cases to be screened once with stimulated calcitonin tests. This reduces the risk of missing a truly affected patient to ~1%. If a mutation-negative, calcitonin-positive family is confirmed to have MTC, screening of the initially negative family members is performed again at ~1 year. If the patient is an adult and found to be negative, screening stops. If the patient is a child, screening continues at yearly intervals through age 18 years. When a mutation is found within a known affected family, confirmation of C-cell disease with pentagastrin testing probably is not necessary. However, a mutation in one person with a known associated disease (e.g., pheochromocytoma), who has no other MEN-affected family members, would cause the author to test with pentagastrin before recommending thyroidectomy. Patients who are mutation-positive–calcitonin-negative are uncommon. They should be provided with information about the inaccuracies of testing, genetic polymorphism, and other issues before undergoing thyroidectomy. At-risk patients who are mutation-negative and calcitonin-positive have been found to have an unusual form of C-cell hyperplasia.[92] In the familial setting, the C-cell disease is really preinvasive carcinoma or a carcinoma in situ. Outside the setting of MEN, one often finds C-cell hyperplasia in normal persons (who may have hypercalcitonemia), in older persons, and in those with hyperparathyroidism and high levels of gastrin.[92–94] In the author's experience, 19% of patients presumed to have sporadic disease were index cases to familial MTC,[6] and 4% to 8% of patients with presumed sporadic pheochromocytoma have MTC.[11,95] The author would not routinely screen persons with hyperparathyroidism or a solitary nodule for MTC using calcitonin measurements because his previous limited trials were unrewarding. Nonetheless, some reports[96,97] have suggested that such measurements will identify previously unsuspected cases of MTC. The author is concerned, however, that if widely applied using different immunoassays, some of which are insufficiently characterized or specific, there may be an unacceptably high rate of false positives similar to that in a case report of a patient with Hashimoto thyroiditis.[98] As the majority of MTC cases are sporadic, analysis for RET mutations will not be cost effective. Until further studies provide solutions to the nodule problem, the author will continue to use stimulated calcitonin tests only when the nodule workup has no suggestion of Hashimoto disease and the fine-needle aspiration results are quite atypical, unusual or strongly suggestive of MTC. Perhaps the use of RNA extracted from fine-needle aspiration biopsies as suggested by Takano, et al. will be helpful.[98a] Finally, thyroid scintiscan should not be used as a screening device because of low sensitivity.[99]

## TREATMENT

Patients with MTC should have total thyroidectomy at an early age after the exclusion, surgical excision, or medical treatment of any adrenomedullary disease.[100] Total thyroidectomy is recommended for several reasons: In MEN2, the tumor is bilateral; 19% of presumed sporadic cases are actually MEN2; and the report of a high calcitonin concentration after incomplete thyroidectomy mandates secondary surgery. In the hands of a skilled surgical team, the incidence of vocal cord paralysis and hypoparathyroidism should be low. The operation should include central lymph node clearance and ipsilateral functional or modified neck dissection for tumors >2.0 cm or if palpable adenopathy is present. The lymph nodes in the central compartment of the neck should be dissected at the time of primary total thyroidectomy, because metastasis frequently occurs in this region.[100] Lymph nodes in the lateral compartments of the neck should be sampled and, if tumor is found, lymphadenectomy should be done. If either the jugular vein or the sternocleidomastoid muscle is involved with tumor, resection is indicated. Whether to perform a modified neck dissection or a radical neck dissection is imperfectly known[100–102]; a retrospective, randomized trial of this question is needed. After surgery, all patients should receive replacement with levothyroxine and be evaluated with calcitonin stimulation tests. Those patients who have undetectable or normal immunoreactive calcitonin concentrations after surgery may be followed up with annual clinical review and provocative testing at intervals of 2 to 5 years. The author continues to recommend that children have thyroidectomy by age 5 for multiple reasons. Formed MTC has been found in children aged 6, 12, and 48 months. Metastatic MTC was found at age 5.5 years during primary surgery in a MEN2B patient who died with metastases at age 9.[103] An unreported MEN2A patient had metastases at age 6 years. There is no biochemical means to predict when metastasis will occur. When experienced endocrine surgeons perform the operation, recurrent nerve paralysis, permanent hypoparathyroidism, and anesthesia difficulties are reported to be negligible, and there is no study documenting increased complications in patients operated on at these young ages.[104–106] Pediatric endocrinologists have little difficulty managing thyroid hormone replacement in children. Clinicians are cautioned that avoidable delays in resection allow metastatic MTC, which causes significant morbidity and mortality.

A continuously developing picture suggests that the biologic virulence of MTC differs according to its associations, with most to least aggressive behavior as follows: MEN2B, sporadic disease, and MEN2A.[18,71,72,107] In one large group of patients, death from MTC has occurred in 50% of those with MEN2B, 31% of those with sporadic disease, and 9.7% of those with MEN2A.[72] In other large studies, 60% of patients with MEN2B have died of MTC, whereas the 10-year survival rate is 55% for sporadic cases and 95% for patients with MEN2A.[71,108] Multivariate analysis of these data suggests a 7.7-fold greater risk of dying of sporadic disease than of MEN2A–associated MTC. Factors having a negative effect on survival have been summarized: They include incomplete primary operation,

male sex, older age, large primary tumor size, extrathyroidal invasion, nodal metastasis, distant metastasis, high plasma CT, high carcinoembryonic antigen (CEA), negative tumor staining for amyloid, and the MEN2B phenotype.[109] In the author's continuing experience, no MEN2A patient who has had total thyroidectomy during the first decade of life has had detectable residual tumor. By contrast, the incidence of persistence progresses from 31% in those undergoing operation in the second decade to 67% in those operated on in the seventh decade.[17] Similarly, others have reported a 24% versus 1.5% mortality for patients with MEN2A in whom MTC was discovered when the tumor was symptomatic, compared with those in whom it was detected earlier through screening.[110] Furthermore, 19 of 22 patients identified by prospective screening were free of detectable disease after thyroidectomy.[111]

## POSTOPERATIVE FOLLOW-UP

After operation for MTC, a stimulated-calcitonin test is done as soon as patients have stable, normal serum calcium concentrations. If the calcitonin result is negative, repeat testing is advised in 1 year and then should continue at 2- to 5-year intervals. If the initial result is positive, repeat testing is done for confirmation. Because calcitonin is more sensitive and specific than other tumor markers for MTC, generally the author does not use markers such as CEA in the follow-up of patients. Patients who have high or steadily increasing CEA, particularly values that are relatively high compared to calcitonin, have advancing metastatic disease and a very poor prognosis.

What should be advised for patients who have occult MTC after primary operation (e.g., those with high immunoreactive calcitonin concentrations and, by the usual techniques, no overt disease)? Vigorous attempts should be made to eradicate persistent tumor in those having tumors with known biologic virulence such as MEN2B or sporadic MTC or those with some of the poor prognostic factors above. Three additional techniques may help determine which patients may have a poor prognosis. The first is immunostaining of primary tumors; patients with calcitonin-poor tumors have poor survivorship compared to those with calcitonin-rich tumors.[112] The second is measurement of the DNA content of tumors; tumors in nonsurviving patients with MTC have higher DNA contents than those in surviving patients.[113] The third is calculation of the doubling time of the calcitonin concentration; rapid doubling times have been reported in patients who have tumors that recur clinically within 5 years or that are associated with a reduced 3-year survival rate.[114] Because the long-term survival data clearly indicate that the natural history of MTC in MEN2A is biologically less aggressive, more conservative approaches are appropriate, unless the clinical course becomes virulent. In most patients with MEN2A who have occult disease and modestly elevated but relatively unchanging calcitonin concentrations during sequential follow-up, present data suggest that vigorous attempts to localize, to reoperate, or otherwise to eradicate tumor tissue are of little benefit.

The sites of MTC metastasis, in order of decreasing frequency, are cervical lymph nodes, lung, mediastinum, liver, bone, adrenal, heart, and pleura. Many techniques are available for the localization of metastases; their usefulness is summarized in Table 188-5.[115,116] Chest roentgenograms may show diffuse interstitial lung infiltrates, particularly in the middle and lower lobes. CT of the lungs, mediastinum, and liver may be helpful. Isotope scans may document bone metastasis, but are of little value in liver metastasis. Hepatic angiograms demonstrate vascular-pattern metastases of MTC more reliably than do isotope scans or CT. If these methods do not identify the sites of metastases, selective venous catheterization, with blood samples taken (with or without provocation) for calcitonin, locate more than half of persistent tumors. Reoperation surgery is recommended for multiple reasons: (a) when a combination of

**TABLE 188-5.**
**Medullary Thyroid Carcinoma: Localization of Metastases**

Thyrocervical ultrasound

Computed tomography

  Very good for chest disease

[111]Indium-octreotide

  Concentrates in >80% of metastases

  Poor visualization of <1.0 cm or liver metastases

  May visualize pheochromocytoma

[99m]Technetium (Tc)(V)-dimercaptosuccinic acid (DMSA)

  Concentrates in ~50% of metastases

[123 or 131]Iodine-metaiodobenzylguanidine (MIBG)

  Concentrates in ~40% of metastases

  Excellent for localizing pheochromocytoma

[99m]Tc(V)-sestamibi

  Limited studies; visualizes some metastases

[201]Thallium

  Limited studies

Radiolabeled anticarcinoembryonic antigen antibodies

  Limited studies

Angiography

  Good for liver metastases

Laparoscopic visualization

  Good for liver metastases

Selective venous catheterization with calcitonin measurement

  Excellent for liver disease

  Helpful for localizing disease to cervical area

  Difficult because of collateral circulation

localization studies suggests local rather than disseminated metastasis allowing a curative intent, (b) when vital structures need to be protected from tumor invasion, and (c) if debulking will reduce secondary side effects (such as medullary diarrhea).

Initial reoperation experience was disappointing; there were no cures, some complications, and occasional operative mortality. Recent experience with extensive microdissection operations done with curative intent has been better. Up to 38% of selected patients become calcitonin-negative after surgery with acceptable morbidity and no mortality.[117–119] It is hoped that these results will not deteriorate or will improve with increased experience and longer follow-up. Other therapies are less successful. Single-agent or combined chemotherapy has not cured patients and generally has not produced greater than a 33% partial response rate. Adjunctive radiotherapy, such as [131]iodine after thyroidectomy, does not improve survival rates or decrease the recurrence of MTC; therefore, it should not be used.[120] A doubled survival rate at 20 years has been shown in patients who receive radiation (either prophylactically or for extensive disease) compared with those who do not.[121] One group has documented eradication of microscopic disease and 30% (complete) to 45% (partial) remission rates of gross residual MTC by external radiation.[122] Another study showed that patients treated with external radiation after operation had survival rates similar to those of patients who underwent operation only, despite having more advanced disease.[123] The author has had radiated patients with similar long-term remissions. Thus, in patients with persistent, aggressive MTC, external radiotherapy seems reasonable (see also Chap. 40).

## ADRENOMEDULLARY DISEASE— PHEOCHROMOCYTOMA

The reported prevalence of adrenomedullary disease has ranged from 12% in a young population to 42% in a study of multiple, mature kindreds followed up for a longer period; the

penetrance in individual kindreds has ranged from 6% to 100%.[124] The pathologic spectrum extends from diffuse medullary hyperplasia to large, multilobular pheochromocytomas that occasionally involve accessory adrenal glands. MEN2 adrenal disease is uniformly bilateral and multicentric in an anatomic sense. Clinically, however, synchronously developed large adrenal masses are unusual; it is more common to encounter a larger tumor on one side and an impalpable hyperplasia or minimal tumor on the other. In an early personal series, tumors were malignant in 24% of cases.[36] However, the number of malignancies has been low——~10 cases. Symptomatic pheochromocytoma may dominate clinically in some families, but that is unusual.[125] The clinical syndrome in MEN2 is different from that in sporadic pheochromocytoma because one is looking for low-volume chromaffin-cell disease at earlier stages. Sustained hypertension is unusual. Patients may report anxiety, palpitations, and tachycardia early; headache, pallor, and perspiration are later symptoms. In a study of 17 patients, 8 were asymptomatic and 9 were symptomatic (paroxysms in 6, headache in 2, and dizziness in 1). Nine patients were normotensive, 7 were hypertensive, and 1 was hypotensive.[36] Episodic rather than sustained hypertension was the rule, and there was no increased incidence of orthostasis. Six of the patients (35%) died because of adrenomedullary disease (cerebral hemorrhage, hypotension, and metastasis in 2 cases each). Deaths resulting from this syndrome component should decrease with earlier case finding and improved physician awareness. Special problems remain in ensuring compliance with screening and in pheochromocytoma occurring during pregnancy, which may be fatal.[126]

The diagnosis of adrenomedullary disease is made by finding a high content of urinary epinephrine or a high urinary epinephrine/norepinephrine ratio.[127] Basal, supine plasma epinephrine also is used. Measurements of the urinary content of dopamine, metanephrine, and vanillylmandelic acid may be helpful, but are not as sensitive as the measurement of fractionated catecholamines. In normotensive patients who have normal urinary catecholamine and metabolite levels, results of stimulation tests with glucagon and histamine occasionally are useful.

CT and MRI do not detect adrenomedullary hyperplasia but do localize pheochromocytomas as small as 0.5 cm. [123]I- or [131]I-metaiodobenzylguanidine has been used to detect adrenomedullary disease in patients with MEN2.[128–130] In patients having normal or equivocal CT scan results, this radiolabeled scan has demonstrated a spectrum of adrenomedullary disease ranging from hyperplasia to bilateral pheochromocytomas (Fig. 188-4).

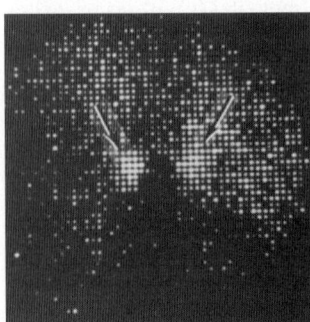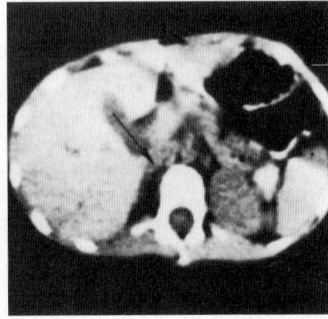

**FIGURE 188-4.** Posterior [131]iodine-metaiodobenzylguanidine (*MIBG*) scintiscan done at 48 hours (*left*) and abdominal computed tomographic (*CT*) scan (*right*) in a 14-year-old patient with multiple endocrine neoplasia type 2B (*MEN2B*). The scintiscan shows symmetric adrenal images (*arrows*). The CT scan shows normal right (*arrow*) and left (not shown) adrenal glands. Each adrenal gland weighed 6 g and contained macroscopic and microscopic hyperplasia. (From Valk TW, Frager MS, Gross MD, et al. Spectrum of pheochromocytoma in multiple endocrine neoplasia: a scintigraphic portrayal using [131]I metaiodobenzyl-guanidine. Ann Intern Med 1981; 94:762.)

All of these techniques for the detection of adrenomedullary disease have limitations in their sensitivity and specificity. However, they can be helpful when used for confirmation, rather than diagnosis, of adrenal disease.

When the diagnosis of adrenomedullary disease is established, appropriate α- and β-adrenergic blockade and glucocorticoid preparation should be commenced. Bilateral total adrenalectomy should be performed, which should include exploration of all paraganglionic areas, removal of extraadrenal paragangliomas, and examination of the liver for metastasis (i.e., pheochromocytoma or MTC). The author's recommendation for initial bilateral adrenalectomy is controversial but based on several observations.[131] First, there is a high likelihood of bilateral involvement; in the Mayo Clinic experience, the grossly uninvolved adrenal gland always was pathologically abnormal. Second, there is mortality associated with adrenomedullary disease, attributable both to the incidence of malignant pheochromocytoma and to the tumor's endocrine function. It is unknown at what tumor stage or size hyperfunction will cause hypertensive crisis or metastasis will occur. Third, a review of the clinical results in 72 patients indicates that 88% required total adrenalectomy, and that 55% of the 20 patients who had undergone initial unilateral adrenalectomy required completion of total adrenalectomy for clinical reasons within a mean period of 4.8 years.[131] The presence of an adrenal gland that is likely to be diseased requires sequential monitoring, resulting in more exposure to radiation and greater expense. Although patients with adrenal insufficiency require glucocorticoid and mineralocorticoid replacement and medical follow-up, the adrenalectomized state has not constituted an undue hazard (see also Chaps. 86, 87, and 89). Other groups think that only demonstrably enlarged or abnormal adrenal glands should be removed. They argue that initial unilateral adrenalectomy ameliorates the need for glucocorticoid and mineralocorticoid replacement for at least 5 to 8 years in some patients, and emphasize that death may occur due to adrenal insufficiency. The decision for unilateral or bilateral adrenalectomy is complex and should be considered on an individual basis after assessment of and discussion with each patient.

## PARATHYROID DISEASE

Clinical or anatomic evidence of parathyroid disease has been present in 29% to 64% of patients with MEN2A.[1,16,17,124] In the patients with parathyroid disease summarized in the cited publications, parathyroid hyperplasia was present in 84% and parathyroid adenoma in 16%. By contrast, overt parathyroid disease is distinctly uncommon in patients with MEN2B, although some have subtle microscopic abnormalities.

Patients with MEN2A seldom have symptoms of hypercalcemia. In patients who have clinical disease (recurrent nephrolithiasis, asymptomatic renal calculi, nephrocalcinosis, and chronic renal failure), there is no difference from sporadic hyperparathyroidism. The diagnosis is established for the clinical disease by finding simultaneous high serum calcium and immunoreactive parathyroid hormone concentrations. Patients with MEN2A also may have occult normocalcemic parathyroid hyperplasia. These normocalcemic patients have normal basal immunoreactive parathyroid hormone concentrations, yet, at cervical exploration, hyperplasia of one or more parathyroid glands is confirmed.[37] This occult disease may be predicted by finding failed suppression of parathyroid hormone during calcium infusion.

The indications for parathyroidectomy and the type of operation recommended are similar for patients with MEN2A and MEN1.[132] However, because the parathyroid disease more commonly is occult in MEN2A, and because the operation increases the incidence of hypoparathyroidism, the author recommends a conservative approach to parathyroidectomy in MEN2A:

### TABLE 188-6.
### Miscellaneous Diseases in Which Neoplasia of the Endocrine Glands May Occur

**GARDNER SYNDROME[133–135]**

Triad of familial polyposis coli, osteomas (e.g., bone, skull, mandible), and soft tissue tumors (e.g., epidermoid tumors of skin). The colonic polyps undergo malignant transformation. Hepatoblastomas may occur in childhood. Autosomal dominant inheritance; mutation of the adenomatous polyposis coli (APC) gene on chromosome 5q.

*Associated Endocrine Lesions*

Thyroid adenoma; thyroid carcinoma (usually papillary; often multicentric and bilateral; long-term prognosis following surgery is good).

Adrenal adenoma or carcinoma.

**PEUTZ-JEGHERS SYNDROME[136,137]**

Multiple lentigines (freckles) of skin (often the lips, eyelids, fingers, genitalia), and of the oral mucosa. Multiple benign hamartomatous polyps of the small intestine, and sometimes the stomach and colon (may cause bleeding, obstruction, intussusception). Adenocarcinomas of the bowel and pancreas may be associated. Breast tumors and tumors of uterine cervix are common. Autosomal dominant inheritance; mutation of the STK11/LKB1 gene on chromosome 19p, and perhaps another locus on 19q.

*Associated Endocrine Lesions*

Thyroid carcinoma (papillary carcinoma has been reported).

Ovarian cysts and tumors (sex cord tumors with annular tubules; Sertoli-cell tumors; may secrete estrogen, causing premature isosexual development).

Sertoli-cell tumor of testis (large cell; calcifying; may secrete estrogen and cause gynecomastia).

**CARNEY COMPLEX[138–142]**

Lentigines and blue nevi of skin, especially on the trunk and extremities. Myxoma of the heart (benign, usually involving left atrium) and myxomas of the skin. Breast lesions (myxoid fibromas and ductal adenomas; multiple; benign). Schwannomas (spinal roots, upper gastrointestinal tract, skin, and bones). Often, the schwannomas are psammomatous and melanotic; they may be benign, or metastatic and fatal. Autosomal dominant inheritance; genetic locus on chromosome 2p or 17q.

*Associated Endocrine Lesions*

Pituitary hyperplasia or tumor; may cause acromegaly.

Thyroid adenomas; 10% are malignant (usually follicular).

Primary pigmented nodular adrenocortical disease (nodules contain lipofuscin; often cause Cushing syndrome).

Pheochromocytoma (may be adrenal or extraadrenal).

Ovarian tumors.

Sertoli-cell tumor of testis (large cell; calcifying; may secrete estrogen).

Grossly enlarged glands should be removed, and the remaining glands should be marked to facilitate removal if there is future recurrence, or all glands should be removed with a portion of one being autotransplanted (see Chap. 62).

## OTHER MULTIPLE ENDOCRINE NEOPLASIA DISEASES

There are several other diseases in which neoplasia of the endocrine glands may be present, although among the persons afflicted with the syndrome, the associated neoplasms usually are less common than the neoplasms associated with the previously discussed multiple endocrine neoplasia entities. These other diseases include Gardner syndrome, Peutz-Jeghers syndrome, and Carney complex. The clinical characteristics of these diseases are listed in Table 188-6.

## REFERENCES

1. Steiner AL, Goodman AD, Powers SR. Study of a kindred with pheochromocytoma, medullary thyroid carcinoma, hyperparathyroidism and Cushing's disease: multiple endocrine neoplasia, type 2. Medicine (Baltimore) 1968; 47:371.

2. Erdheim J. Zur normalen und pathologischen Histologie der glandula Thyroidea, Parathyroidea und Hypophysis. Beitr Pathol Anat 1903; 33:1.

3. Underdahl LO, Woolner LB, Black BM. Multiple endocrine adenomas: report of eight cases in which parathyroids, pituitary and pancreatic islets were involved. J Clin Endocrinol Metab 1953; 13:20.

4. Wermer P. Genetic aspects of adenomatosis of endocrine glands. Am J Med 1954; 16:363.

5. Ballard HS, Frame B, Hartsock RJ. Familial multiple endocrine adenomapeptic ulcer complex. Medicine (Baltimore) 1964; 43:481.

6. Eberle F, Grun R. Multiple endocrine neoplasia, type I (MEN I). Ergeb Inn Med Kinderheilkd 1981; 46:76.

7. Yamagachi K, Kameya T, Abe K. Multiple endocrine neoplasia type 1. Clin Endocrinol Metab 1980; 9:261.

8. Majewski JT, Wilson SD. The MEN-I syndrome: an all or none phenomenon? Surgery 1979; 86:475.

9. Harrison TS, Thompson NW. Multiple endocrine adenomatosis-I and II. Curr Probl Surg 1975; 28.

10. Deveney CW, Deveney KS, Way LW. The Zollinger-Ellison syndrome: 23 years later. Ann Surg 1978; 188:384.

11. Sipple JH. The association of pheochromocytoma with carcinoma of the thyroid gland. Am J Med 1961; 31:163.

12. Cushman P Jr. Familial endocrine tumors: report of two unrelated kindred affected with pheochromocytomas, one also with multiple thyroid carcinomas. Am J Med 1962; 32:352.

13. Manning PC Jr, Molnar GD, Black BM, et al. Pheochromocytoma, hyperparathyroidism and thyroid carcinoma occurring coincidentally: report of a case. N Engl J Med 1963; 268:68.

14. Cance WG, Wells SA Jr. Multiple endocrine neoplasia type IIa. Curr Probl Surg 1985; 22:7.

15. Melvin KEW, Miller HH, Tashjian AH Jr. Early diagnosis of medullary carcinoma of the thyroid gland by means of calcitonin assay. N Engl J Med 1971; 285:1115.

16. Keiser HR, Beaven MA, Doppman J, Wells S Jr. Sipple's syndrome: medullary thyroid carcinoma, pheochromocytoma, and parathyroid disease. Ann Intern Med 1973; 78:561.

17. Sizemore GW, Carney JA, Heath H III. Epidemiology of medullary carcinoma of the thyroid gland: a 5-year experience (1971–1976). Surg Clin North Am 1977; 57:633.

18. Sizemore GW, Heath H III, Carney JA. Multiple endocrine neoplasia type 2. Clin Endocrinol Metab 1980; 9:299.

19. Chong GC, Beahrs OH, Sizemore GW, Woolner LB. Medullary carcinoma of the thyroid gland. Cancer 1975; 35:695.

20. Carney JA, Go VLW, Gordon H, et al. Familial pheochromocytoma and islet cell tumor of the pancreas. Am J Med 1980; 68:515.

21. Binkovitz LA, Johnson CD, Stephens DH. Islet cell tumors in von Hippel-Lindau disease: increased prevalence and relationship to the multiple endocrine neoplasias. AJR Am J Roentgenol 1990; 155:501.

22. Larsson C, Skogseid B, Oberg K, et al. Multiple endocrine neoplasia type 1 gene maps to chromosome 11 and is lost in insulinoma. Nature 1988; 332:85.

23. Chandrasekharappa SC, Guru SC, Manickam P, et al. Positional cloning of the gene for multiple endocrine neoplasia type 1. Science 1997; 279:404.

24. Agarwal SK, Kester MB, Debelenko LV, et al. Germline mutations of the MEN 1 gene in familial multiple endocrine neoplasia type 1 and related states. Hum Mol Genet 1997; 7:1169.

25. Lemmens I, Van de Ven WJ, Kas K, et al. Identification of the multiple endocrine neoplasia type 1 (MEN1) gene. The European Consortium on MEN1. Hum Mol Genet 1997; 7:1177.

26. Marx S, Spiegel AM, Skarulis M, et al. Multiple endocrine neoplasia type 1: clinical and genetic topics. Ann Intern Med 1998; 129:484.

27. Mathew CGP, Chin KS, Esaton DF, et al. A linked genetic marker for multiple endocrine neoplasia type 2A on chromosome 10. Nature 1987; 328:527.

28. Simpson NE, Kidd KK, Goodfellow PJ, et al. Assignment of multiple endocrine neoplasia type 2A to chromosome 10 by linkage. Nature 1987; 328:528.

29. Donis-Keller H, Dou S, Chi D, et al. Mutations in the RET proto-oncogene are associated with MEN2A and FWTC. Hum Mol Genet 1993; 2:851.

30. Mulligan LM, Kwok JBJ, Healey CS, et al. Germ-line mutations of the RET proto-oncogene in multiple endocrine neoplasia type 2A. Nature 1993; 363:456.

31. Mulligan LM, Eng C, Healey CS, et al. Specific mutations of the RET proto-oncogene are related to disease phenotype in MEN 2A and FMTC. Nat Genet 1994; 6:70.

32. Hofstra RM, Landavater RM, Ceccherini I, et al. A mutation in the RET proto-oncogene associated with multiple endocrine neoplasia type 2B and sporadic medullary thyroid carcinoma. Nature 1994; 367:375.

33. Eng C, Smith DP, Mulligan LM, et al. Point mutation within the tyrosine kinase domain of the RET proto-oncogene in multiple endocrine neoplasia type 2B and related sporadic tumours. Hum Mol Genet 1994; 3:237.

33a. Tessitore A, Simsi AA, Pasquali D, et al. A novel case of multiple endocrine neoplasia type 2A associated with two de novo mutations of the RET protooncogene. J Clin Endocrinol Metab 1999; 84:3522.

33b. Pigny P, Bauters C, Wemeau J-L, et al. A novel 9-base pair duplication in RET exon 8 in familial medullary thyroid carcinoma. J Clin Endocrinol Metab 1999; 84:1700.

34. Knudson AG Jr, Strong LC. Mutation and cancer: neuroblastomas and pheochromocytoma. Am J Hum Genet 1972; 24:514.

35. Wolfe HJ, Melvin KEW, Cervi-Skinner SJ, et al. C-cell hyperplasia preceding medullary thyroid carcinoma. N Engl J Med 1973; 289:437.

36. Carney JA, Sizemore GW, Sheps SG. Adrenal medullary disease in multiple endocrine neoplasia, type 2: pheochromocytoma and its precursors. Am J Clin Pathol 1976; 66:279.

37. Heath H III, Sizemore GW, Carney JA. Preoperative diagnosis of occult parathyroid hyperplasia by calcium infusion in patients with multiple endocrine neoplasia, type 2a. J Clin Endocrinol Metab 1976; 43:428.

38. Snyder N, Scurry M, Hughes W. Hypergastrinemia in familial multiple endocrine adenomatosis. Ann Intern Med 1974; 80:321.

39. Friesen SR, Kimmel JR, Tomita T. Pancreatic polypeptide as screening marker for pancreatic polypeptide apudomas in multiple endocrinopathies. Am J Surg 1980; 139:61.

40. Verner JV, Morrison AB. Islet cell tumor and a syndrome of refractory watery diarrhea and hypokalemia. Am J Med 1958; 25:374.

41. Brown CH, Crile G Jr. Pancreatic adenoma with intractable diarrhea, hypokalemia, and hypercalcemia. JAMA 1964; 190:142.

42. Zollinger RM, Ellison EC, O'Dorisio TM, Sparks J. Thirty years' experience with gastrinoma. World J Surg 1984; 8:427.

43. Jensen RT, Gardner JD, Raufman JP, et al. Zollinger-Ellison syndrome: current concepts and management. Ann Intern Med 1983; 98:59.

44. McGruigan JE, Wolfe MM. Secretin injection test in the diagnosis of gastrinoma. Gastroenterology 1980; 79:1324.

45. Malagelada J-R, Edis AJ, Adson MA, et al. Medical and surgical options in the management of patients with gastrinoma. Gastroenterology 1983; 84:1524.

46. Fishbeyn VA, Norton JA, Benya RV, et al. Assessment and prediction of long-term cure in patients with the Zollinger-Ellison syndrome: the best approach. Ann Intern Med 1993; 119:199.

47. Thompson NW, Vinik AI, Eckhauser FE. Microgastrinomas of the duodenum: a cause of failed operations for the Zollinger-Ellison syndrome. Ann Surg 1989; 209:396.

48. Rosch T, Lightdale CJ, Botet JF, et al. Localization of pancreatic endocrine tumors by endoscopic ultrasonography. N Engl J Med 1992; 326:1721.

49. Gibril F, Reynolds JC, Doppman JL, et al. Somatostatin receptor scintigraphy: its sensitivity compared with that of other imaging methods in detecting primary and metastatic gastrinomas. A prospective study. Ann Intern Med 1996; 125:26.

50. Bonfils S, Mignon M. Management of Zollinger-Ellison syndrome with gastric antisecretory drugs. Scand J Gastroenterol 1988; 23(Suppl 146):111.

51. Ellison EC, O'Dorisio TM, Woltering EA, et al. Suppression of gastrin and gastric acid secretion in the Zollinger-Ellison syndrome by long-acting somatostatin (SMS 201–995). Scand J Gastroenterol 1986; 21(Suppl 119):206.

52. Service FJ. Clinical presentation and laboratory evaluation on hypoglycemic disorders in adults. In: Service FJ, ed. Hypoglycemic disorders. Boston: GK Hall, 1983:73.

53. Service FJ, Horwitz DL, Rubenstein AH, et al. C-peptide suppression test for insulinoma. J Lab Clin Med 1977; 90:180.

54. Ram Z, Shawker TH, Bradford, MH, et al. Intraoperative ultrasound-directed resection of pituitary tumors. J Neurosurg 1995; 83:225.

55. Rasbach DA, van Heerden JA, Telander RL, et al. Surgical management of hyperinsulinism in the multiple endocrine neoplasia, type 1 syndrome. Arch Surg 1985; 120:584.

56. Demeure MJ, Klonoff DC, Karam JH, et al. Insulinomas associated with multiple endocrine neoplasia type 1: the need for a different surgical approach. Surgery 1991; 110:998.

57. Thompson NW, Lloyd RV, Nishiyama RH, et al. MEN1 pancreas: a histological and immunohistochemical study. World J Surg 1984; 8:561.

58. Osei K, O'Dorisio TM. The effects of a potent somatostatin analogue (SMS201-995) on serum glucose and gastro-entero-pancreatic hormones in a malignant insulinoma patient. Ann Intern Med 1985; 103:223.

59. Croughs RJM, Hulsmans HAM, Israel DE, et al. Glucagonoma as part of the polyglandular adenoma syndrome. Am J Med 1972; 52:690.

60. Marx SJ, Spiegel AM, Brown EM, Aurbach GD. Family studies in patients with primary parathyroid hyperplasia. Am J Med 1977; 62:698.

61. Levine JH, Sagel J, Rosebrock G, et al. Prolactin-secreting adenoma as part of the multiple endocrine neoplasia type 1 (MEN 1) syndrome. Cancer 1979; 43:2492.

62. Veldhuis JD, Green JE III, Kovacs E. Prolactin-secreting pituitary adenomas: association with multiple endocrine neoplasia, type I. Am J Med 1979; 67:830.

63. Ramsay JA, Kovacs K, Asa SL. Reversible sellar enlargement due to growth hormone-releasing hormone production by pancreatic endocrine tumors in an acromegalic patient with multiple endocrine neoplasia type 1 syndrome. Cancer 1988; 62:445.

64. Brandl ML, Zimering MB, Marx SJ, et al. Multiple endocrine neoplasia type 1: role of a circulating growth factor in parathyroid cell hyperplasia. In: Kleerekoper M, Krane SM, eds. Clinical disorders of bone and mineral metabolism. New York: Mary Ann Liebert, 1988:323.

65. van Heerden JA, Kent RB, Sizemore GW, et al. Primary hyperparathyroidism in patients with multiple endocrine neoplasia syndromes. Arch Surg 1983; 118:533.

65a. Wimer KK, Yanouski JA, Cutler GB Jr. Synthetic human parathyroid hormone 1–34 or calcitriol and calcium in the treatment of hypoparathyroidism. JAMA 1996; 276:631.

66. Williams ED, Celestin LR. The association of bronchial carcinoid and pluriglandular adenomatosis. Thorax 1962; 17:120.

67. Skogseld B, Larsson C, Lindgren P-G, et al. Clinical and genetic features of adrenocortical lesions in multiple endocrine neoplasia type 1. J Clin Endocrinol Metab 1992; 75:76.

68. Marshall AHE, Sloper JC. Pluriglandular adenomatosis of the pituitary, parathyroid and pancreatic islet cells associated with lipomatosis. J Pathol Bacteriol 1954; 68:225.

69. Marx SJ. Multiple endocrine neoplasia type 1. In: Vogelstein B, Kinzler KW, eds. The genetic basis of human cancer. New York: McGraw-Hill, 1998:489.

70. Wilson SD. Wermer's syndrome: multiple endocrine adenopathy, type I. In: Friesen SR, Bolinger RE, eds. Surgical endocrinology: clinical syndromes. Philadelphia: JB Lippincott Co, 1978:265.

71. Saad MF, Ordonez NG, Rashid RK, et al. Medullary carcinoma of the thyroid: a study of the clinical features and prognostic factors in 161 patients. Medicine (Baltimore) 1984; 63:319.

72. Wells SA Jr, Dilley WG, Farndon JA, et al. Early diagnosis and treatment of medullary thyroid carcinoma. Arch Intern Med 1985; 145:1248.

73. Nunziata V, Giannattasio R, Di Giovanni G, et al. Hereditary localized pruritus in affected members of a kindred with multiple endocrine neoplasia type 2A (Sipple's syndrome). Clin Endocrinol (Oxf) 1989; 30:57.

74. Gagel RF, Levy ML, Donovan DT. Multiple endocrine neoplasia type 2a associated with cutaneous lichen amyloidosis. Ann Intern Med 1989; 111:802.

75. Verdy M, Weber AM, Roy CC, et al. Hirschsprung's disease in a family with multiple endocrine neoplasia type 2. J Pediatr Gastroenterol Nutr 1982; 1:603.

76. Wagenmann A. Multiple Neurome des Auges und der Zunge. Zusammenkunft Dtsch Ophthalmol Ges 1922; 43:282.

77. Carney JA, Sizemore GW, Hayles AB. Multiple endocrine neoplasia, type 2b. Pathobiol Ann 1978; 8:105.

78. Dyck PJ, Carney JA, Sizemore GW, et al. Multiple endocrine neoplasia, type 2b: phenotype recognition; neurologic features and their pathologic basis. Ann Neurol 1979; 6:302.

79. Sizemore GW, Carney JA, Gharib H, Capen CC. Multiple endocrine neoplasia, type 2B: eighteen-year follow-up of a four-generation family. Henry Ford Hosp Med J 1992; 40:236.

80. Khairi MRA, Dexter RN, Dubzynski NJ, Johnston CC Jr. Mucosal neuroma, phytochromocytoma and medullary thyroid carcinoma: multiple endocrine neoplasia, type 3. Medicine 1975; 54:89.

81. Durbec PL, Larsson-Blomberg LB, Schuchgardt A, et al. Common origin and developmental dependence on C-RET of subsets of enteric and sympathetic neuroblasts. Development 1996; 122:349.

82. Melvin KEW, Miller HH, Tashjian AH Jr. Early diagnosis of medullary carcinoma of the thyroid gland by means of calcitonin assay. N Engl J Med 1971; 285:1115.

83. Sizemore GW. Medullary carcinoma of the thyroid gland and the multiple endocrine neoplasia type 2 syndrome. In: Spittel JA Jr, ed. Clinical medicine, vol 8. Philadelphia: Harper & Row, 1982:1.

84. Hennessy JF, Gray TK, Cooper CW, Ontjes DA. Stimulation of thyrocalcitonin secretion by pentagastrin and calcium in two patients with medullary carcinoma of the thyroid. J Clin Endocrinol Metab 1973; 36:200.

85. Wells SA Jr, Dilley WG, Farndon JA, et al. Early diagnosis and treatment of medullary thyroid carcinoma. Arch Intern Med 1985; 145:1248.

86. McLean GW, Rabin D, Moore L, et al. Evaluation of provocative tests in suspected medullary carcinoma of the thyroid: heterogeneity of calcitonin responses to calcium and pentagastrin. Metabolism 1984; 33:790.

87. Gharib H, Kao PC, Heath H III. Determination of silica-purified plasma calcitonin for the detection and management of medullary thyroid carcinoma: comparison of two provocative tests. Mayo Clin Proc 1987; 62:373.

88. Eng C, Clayton D, Schuffenecker I, et al. The relationship between specific RET proto-oncogene mutations and disease phenotype in multiple endocrine neoplasia type 2. JAMA 1996; 276:1575.

89. Easton DF, Ponder MA, Cummings T, et al. The clinical and screening age-at-onset distribution for the MEN 2 syndrome. Am J Hum Genet 1989; 44:208.

90. Heshmati HM, Gharib H, Khosla S, et al. Genetic testing in medullary thyroid carcinoma syndromes: mutation types and clinical significance. Mayo Clin Proc 1997; 72:430.

91. Lips CJM, Landsvater RM, Hoppener WM, et al. Clinical screening as compared with DNA analysis in families with multiple endocrine neoplasia type 2A. N Engl J Med 1994; 331:828.

92. LiVolsi VA. C cell hyperplasia/neoplasia. (Editorial). J Clin Endocrinol Metab 1997; 82:39.

93. Guyetant S, Rousselet M-C, Durigon M, et al. Sex-related C cell hyperplasia in the normal human thyroid: a quantitative autopsy study. J Clin Endocrinol Metab 1997; 82:42.

94. Biddinger PW, Brennan MF, Rosen PP. Symptomatic C cell hyperplasia associated with chronic lymphocytic thyroiditis. Am J Surg Pathol 1991; 15:599.

95. Neumann HPH, Berger DP, Sigmund G, et al. Pheochromocytomas, multiple endocrine neoplasia type 2, and von Hippel-Lindau disease. N Engl J Med 1993; 329:1531.

96. Pacini F, Fontanelli M, Fugazzola L, et al. Routine measurement of serum calcitonin in nodular thyroid disease allows the preoperative diagnosis of unsuspected sporadic medullary carcinoma. J Clin Endocrinol Metab 1994; 78:826.

97. Dunn J. When is a thyroid nodule a sporadic medullary carcinoma? (Editorial). J Clin Endocrinol Metab 1994; 78:624.

98. Uwaifo G, Remaley AT, Reynolds JC, et al. False hypercalcitoninemia in a patient with solitary thyroid nodule: should plasma calcitonin (CT) be used as a screening test for all thyroid nodules? Abstract 2454. The Endocrine Society 82nd Annual Meeting, Toronto, Canada: June 21–24, 2000.

98a. Takano T, Miyauchi A, Matsuzuka F, et al. Preoperative diagnosis of medullary thyroid carcinoma by RT-PCR using RNA extracted from leftover cells within a needle used for fine-needle aspiration biopsy. J Clin Endocrinol Metab 1999; 84:951.

99. Anderson RJ, Sizemore GW, Wahner HW, Carney JA. Thyroid scintigram in familial medullary carcinoma of the thyroid gland. Clin Nucl Med 1978; 3:147.

100. Russell CF, van Heerden JA, Sizemore GW, et al. The surgical management of medullary thyroid carcinoma. Ann Surg 1983; 197:42.

101. Miller HH, Melvin KEW, Gibson Tashjian AH Jr. Surgical approach to early familial medullary carcinoma of the thyroid gland. Am J Surg 1972; 123:438.

102. Brumsen C, Harm RH, Goslings BM, van de Velde CJH. Should patients with medullary thyroid carcinoma undergo extensive lymph node (re)operation to improve long-term survival? Henry Ford Hosp Med J 1992; 40:271.

103. Bartlett RC, Myall RW, Mandelstam P. A neuropolyendocrine system. Mucosal neuromas, pheochromocytoma and medullary thyroid carcinoma. Oral Surg Oral Med Oral Pathol 1971; 31:206.

104. Leape LL, Miller HH, Graze K, et al. Total thyroidectomy for occult familial medullary carcinoma of the thyroid in children. J Pediatr Surg 1976; 11:831.

105. Telander RL, Zimmerman D, Sizemore GW, et al. Medullary carcinoma in children: results of early detection and surgery. Arch Surg 1989; 124:841.

106. Decker RA, Toyama WM, O'Neal LW, et al. Evaluation of children with multiple endocrine neoplasia type IIb following thyroidectomy. J Pediatr Surg 1990; 25:939.

107. Raue F, Kotzerke J, Reinwein D, et al, and the German Medullary Thyroid Carcinoma Study Group. Prognostic factors in medullary thyroid carcinoma: evaluation of 741 patients from the German medullary thyroid carcinoma register. Clin Invest 1993; 71:7.

108. Gharib H, McConahey WM, Tiegs RD, et al. Medullary thyroid carcinoma: clinicopathologic features and long-term follow-up of 65 patients treated during 1946 through 1970. Mayo Clin Proc 1992; 67:934.

109. Heshmati HM, Gharib H, Sizemore GW. Advances and controversies in the diagnosis and management of medullary thyroid carcinoma. Am J Med 1997; 103:60.

110. Telenius-Berg M, Berg B, Hamberger B, et al. Impact of screening on prognosis in the multiple endocrine type 2 syndromes: natural history and treatment results in 105 patients. Henry Ford Hosp Med J 1984; 32:225.

111. Gagel RF, Tashjian AH Jr, Cummings T, et al. The clinical outcome of prospective screening for multiple endocrine neoplasia type 2a: an 18-year experience. N Engl J Med 1988; 318:478.

112. Saad MF, Ordonez NG, Guido JJ, Samaan NA. The prognostic value of calcitonin immunostaining in medullary carcinoma of the thyroid. J Clin Endocrinol Metab 1984; 59:850.

113. Bäckdahl M, Tallroth E, Auer G, et al. Prognostic value of nuclear DNA content in medullary thyroid carcinoma. World J Surg 1985; 9:980.

114. Miyauchi A, Onishi T, Morimoto S, et al. Relation of doubling time of plasma calcitonin levels to prognosis and recurrence of medullary carcinoma. Ann Surg 1984; 199:461.

115. Miyauchi A, Endo K, Ohta H, et al. $^{99m}$Tc(V)-dimercaptosuccinic acid scintigraphy for medullary thyroid carcinoma. World J Surg 1986; 10:640.

116. Clarke SEM, Lazarus CR, Wraight P, et al. Pentavalent [$^{99m}$Tc]DMSA, [$^{131}$I]MIGB, and [$^{99m}$Tc]MDP: an evaluation of three imaging techniques in patients with medullary carcinoma of the thyroid. J Nucl Med 1988; 29:33.

117. Tisell L-E, Hansson G, Jansson S, Salander H. Reoperation in the treatment of asymptomatic metastasizing medullary thyroid carcinoma. Surgery 1986; 99:60.

118. Moley JF, Dilley W, DeBenedetti MK. Improved results of cervical reoperation for medullary thyroid carcinoma. Ann Surg 1997; 225:734.

119. Buhr HJ, Kallinowski F, Raue F, et al. Microsurgical neck dissection for occult metastasizing medullary thyroid carcinoma; three year results. Cancer 1993; 72:3685.

120. Saad MF, Guido JJ, Samaan NA. Radioactive iodine in the treatment of medullary carcinoma of the thyroid. J Clin Endocrinol Metab 1983; 57:124.

121. Tubiana M. External radiotherapy and radioactive iodine in the treatment of thyroid cancer. World J Surg 1981; 5:75.

122. Simpson WJ, Palmer JA, Rosen IB, Mustard RA. Management of medullary carcinoma of the thyroid. Am J Surg 1982; 144:420.

123. Rougier P, Parmentier C, Laplanche A, Calmettes C. Medullary thyroid carcinoma: prognostic factors and treatment. Int J Radiat Oncol Biol Phys 1983; 9:161.

124. Howe JR, Norton JA, Wells SA Jr. Prevalence of pheochromocytoma and hyperparathyroidism in multiple endocrine neoplasia type 2A: results of long-term follow-up. Surgery 1993; 114:1070.

125. Lips CJM, Veer J, Struyvenberg A, et al. Bilateral occurrence of pheochromocytoma in patients with the multiple endocrine neoplasia syndrome type 2a (Sipple's syndrome). Am J Med 1981; 70:1051.

126. Moraca-Kvapilova L, Op de Coul AA, Merkus JM. Cerebral haemorrhage in a pregnant woman with a multiple endocrine neoplasia syndrome (type 2A or Sipple's syndrome). Eur J Obstet Gynecol Reprod Biol 1985; 20:257.

127. Gagel RS, Melvin KEW, Tashjian AH Jr, et al. Natural history of the familial medullary thyroid carcinoma-pheochromocytoma syndrome and the identification of the preneoplastic stages by screening studies: a 5-year report. Trans Assoc Am Physicians 1975; 88:177.

128. Sisson JC, Shapiro B, Bierwaltes WH. Scintigraphy with I-131 MIBG as an aid to the treatment of pheochromocytomas in patients with the multiple endocrine neoplasia type 2 syndromes. Henry Ford Hosp Med J 1984; 32:254.

129. Valk TW, Frager MS, Gross MD, et al. Spectrum of pheochromocytoma in multiple endocrine neoplasia: a scintigraphic portrayal using $^{131}$I metaiodobenzyl-guanidine. Ann Intern Med 1981; 94:762.

130. Sasaki Y, Klubo A, Kusakabe A, et al. The assessment of clinical usefulness of $^{131}$I-MIBG scintigraphy for localization of tumors of sympathetic and adrenomedullary origin—a report of multicenter phase III clinical trials. Kaku Igaku 1992; 9:1083.

131. van Heerden JA, Sizemore GW, Carney JA, et al. Surgical management of the adrenal glands in the multiple endocrine neoplasia 2 syndrome. World J Surg 1984; 8:612.

132. O'Riordain DS, O'Brien T, Grant CS, et al. Surgical management of primary hyperparathyroidism in multiple endocrine neoplasia types 1 and 2. Surgery 1993; 114:1037.

133. Traill Z, Tuson J, Woodham C. Adrenal carcinoma in a patient with Gardner's syndrome: imaging findings. AJR Am J Roentgenol 1995; 165:1460.

134. Hizawa K, Iida M, Hoyagi K, et al. Thyroid neoplasia and familial adenomatous polyposis/Gardner syndrome. J Gastroenterol 1997; 32:196.

135. Perrier ND, van Heerden JA, Goellner JR, et al. Thyroid cancer in patients with familial adenomatous polyposis. World J Surg 1998; 22:738.

136. Zung A, Shoham Z, Open M, et al. Sertoli cell tumor causing precocious puberty in a girl with Peutz-Jeghers syndrome. Gynecol Oncol 1998; 70:421.

137. Hertl MC, Wiebel J, Schafer H, et al. Feminizing Sertoli cell tumors associated with Peutz-Jeghers syndrome: an increasingly recognized cause of prepubertal gynecomastia. Plast Reconstr Surg 1998; 102:1151.

138. Stratakis CA, Kirschner LS, Taymans SE, et al. Carney complex, Peutz-Jeghers syndrome, Cowden disease, and Bannayan-Zonana syndrome share cutaneous and endocrine manifestations, but not genetic loci. J Clin Endocrinol Metab 1998; 83:2972.

139. Stratakis CA, Sarlis N, Kirschner LS, et al. Paradoxical response to dexamethasone in the diagnosis of primary pigmented nodular adrenocortical disease. Ann Intern Med 1999; 131:585.

140. Casey M, Mah C, Merliss AD, et al. Identification of a novel genetic locus for familial cardiac myxomas and Carney complex. Circulation 1998; 98:2560.

141. Kirschner LS, Taymans SE, Stratakis CA. Characterization of the adrenal gland pathology of Carney complex, and molecular genetics of the disease. Endocr Res 1998; 24:863.

142. Stratakis CA, Kirschner LS, Carney JA. Carney complex: diagnosis and management of the complex of spotty skin pigmentation, myxomas, endocrine overactivity, and schwannomas. Am J Med Genet 1998; 80:183.

# CHAPTER 189

# HERITABLE DISORDERS OF COLLAGEN AND FIBRILLIN

PETER H. BYERS

Collagens are ubiquitously distributed, are present in large amounts, and have important structural and functional properties, so that disorders of their structure and biosynthesis often have generalized phenotypic effects and may be fatal. Fibrillins, although less abundant, also are ubiquitously distributed; consequently, mutations in the genes that encode them may also be generalized in their effects. This chapter discusses the collagen and fibrillin families of proteins, the genes that code for them, the intracellular and extracellular processing of the proteins, and the mutations in the collagen and fibrillin genes and in the genes for the processing enzymes that lead to identifiable inherited disorders of connective tissue. More than 19 collagen types, encoded by more than 30 genes, and two fibrillins have been identified. Mutations in several of these genes have been characterized. They give rise to characteristic phenotypes, depending on the gene in which they occur and the nature and location of the mutation. Table 189-1 lists the collagen genes and their disorders. Because physicians seek information about named disorders and disease processes, this chapter is organized around those named heritable disorders of connective tissue in which molecular defects have been identified.[1–8]

## WHAT IS COLLAGEN, WHERE IS IT MADE, AND WHAT DOES IT DO?

The collagens are a family of more than 19 proteins, encoded by more than 30 genes, which have a similar core amino-acid sequence, contain three chains, form triple-helical structures, and contain the two characteristic amino acids, hydroxyproline and hydroxylysine (see Table 189-1). Some collagen molecules,

such as type I collagen, are heteropolymers, containing more than one type of chain, whereas others, such as types II and III, are homopolymers and contain three identical chains. Each collagen contains a long region, stretching from 600 to more than 1000 amino acids, characterized by the repeating Gly-X-Y unit, in which X and Y often are proline and hydroxyproline, respectively. In some collagens (the fibrillar collagens), this triplet domain is uninterrupted, but in most, several regions are found in which glycine is not in the third position. Each collagen has a characteristic tissue distribution, and mutations that affect the structure of one chain lead to phenotypes that reflect that distribution. For example, mutations in the chains of type I collagen frequently affect the skin, vessels, and bone; those in type II collagen alter the structure of cartilage; those in type III collagen affect skin, vessels, and bowel; and those in type VII collagen alter dermal-epidermal adhesion. Collagens play many roles in tissues, depending partly on the nature of the protein. For example, type I collagen provides tensile strength in skin, tendons, and fascia; is the chief structural component of many organ capsules; and, as the principal component of the cornea, facilitates light transmission. Type IV collagen, which is the primary component of basement membranes, separates epithelial cell layers from mesenchymal cells, an important function during tissue development.

Genes for most of the collagens have been characterized, and the chromosomal locations have been determined. The prototype genes—those for the chains of type I collagen, the most abundant collagen in the vertebrate body—provide models for gene structure, from which considerable divergence is seen. The *COL1A1* (α1[I]) and *COL1A2* (α2[I]) genes encode proteins that contain just over 1400 amino-acid residues. Although this would require ~5000 nucleotides of coding sequence, the coding sequences are interrupted by more than 50 intervening sequences, so that the *COL1A1* gene is 18 kilo–base pairs (kbp) in length, whereas the *COL1A2* gene is 38 kbp. The organization of the coding domains in each is similar: The long triple-helical domain of the protein (1014 amino acids in each) is coded for by 45 different coding regions (exons) interrupted by intervening or noncoding sequences (introns). A remarkable conservation of the intron-exon structure is found among several collagens, although the intron size and sequences differ widely from gene to gene. For example, almost the entire triple helical domain of the type X collagen gene (*COL10A1*) is contained in a single exon. In contrast, the *COL7A1* gene contains more than 100 exons, yet is contained within only 30 kbp of the genome.

The genes for the collagens are transcribed in the nucleus to form full-length transcripts from which the intervening sequences are removed to produce a mature mRNA molecule. Transcriptional efficiency may be controlled partly by various hormonal agents, including glucocorticoids, parathyroid hormone, and others, which may act in both a tissue- and collagen-specific manner. Along with transcriptional regulation, mechanisms are found that regulate collagen production at the level of translation of collagen mRNA, the rate of chain assembly to form molecules, and the rate of intracellular degradation of collagen molecules.

The mature mRNA is transported to the cytoplasm and translated on membrane-bound ribosomes of the rough endoplasmic reticulum (ER) (Fig. 189-1). The nascent polypeptide chain (a preproα chain) is directed to the lumen of the rough ER by the presence of signal sequences at the amino terminus. During translation and passage through the membrane, most of the prolyl residues in the Y position are hydroxylated by the enzyme prolyl 4-hydroxylase; a small number of prolyl residues in the X position are hydroxylated by a different hydroxylase; many Y-position lysyl residues are hydroxylated by lysyl hydroxylase; some of the hydroxylysyl residues are glycosylated, to

**TABLE 189-1.**
**Collagen Genes, Their Locations, and the Disorders That Result from Their Mutations**

| Collagen Type | Gene | Chromosomal Location | Protein | Disorders |
|---|---|---|---|---|
| I | COL1A1 | 17q21.31-q22.05 | proα1(I) | Osteogenesis imperfecta |
| | | | | Ehlers-Danlos syndrome type VIIA |
| | COL1A2 | 7q22.1 | proα2(I) | Osteogenesis imperfecta |
| | | | | Ehlers-Danlos syndrome type VIIB |
| | | | | Ehlers-Danlos syndrome type II |
| II | COL2A1 | 12q13.11-q13.2 | proα1(II) | Stickler syndrome type I |
| | | | | Wagner syndrome type II |
| | | | | Spondyloepiphyseal dysplasia congenita |
| | | | | Kniest dysplasia |
| | | | | Hypochondrogenesis |
| | | | | Achondrogenesis type II |
| | | | | Spondylo-metaphyseal-epiphyseal dysplasia (SMED), Strudwick type |
| III | COL3A1 | 2q31 | proα1(III) | Ehlers-Danlos syndrome type IV |
| | | | | Ehlers-Danlos syndrome type III (?) |
| IV | COL4A1 | 13q34 | proα1(IV) | |
| | COL4A2 | 13q34 | proα2(IV) | |
| | COL4A3 | 2q36-q37 | proα3(IV) | Alport syndrome, recessive |
| | COL4A4 | 2q36-q37 | proα4(IV) | Alport syndrome, recessive |
| | COL4A5 | Xq22 | proα5(IV) | Alport syndrome, X-linked |
| | COL4A6 | Xq22 | proα6(IV) | Alport syndrome, X-linked leiomyomatosis |
| V | COL5A1 | 9q34.2-q34.3 | proα1(V) | Ehlers-Danlos syndrome type I |
| | | | | Ehlers-Danlos syndrome type II |
| | COL5A2 | 2q31 | proα2(V) | Ehlers-Danlos syndrome type I |
| | COL5A3 | Not mapped | proα3(V) | |
| VI | COL6A1 | 21q22.3 | proα1(VI) | Bethlem myopathy |
| | COL6A2 | 21q22.3 | proα2(VI) | Bethlem myopathy |
| | COL6A3 | 2q37 | proα3(VI) | Bethlem myopathy |
| VII | COL7A1 | 3p21.3 | proα1(VII) | Epidermolysis bullosa, recessive dystrophic |
| | | | | Epidermolysis bullosa, dominant dystrophic |
| | | | | Epidermolysis bullosa, pretibial |
| VIII | COL8A1 | 3q12-q13.1 | proα1(VIII) | |
| | COL8A2 | 1p34.4-p32.3 | proα2(VIII) | |
| IX | COL9A1 | 6q13 | proα1(IX) | Multiple epiphyseal dysplasia |
| | COL9A2 | 1p33-p32.2 | proα2(IX) | Multiple epiphyseal dysplasia type II |
| | COL9A3 | 20q13.3 | proα3(IX) | Multiple epiphyseal dysplasia type III |
| X | COL10A1 | 6q21-q22.3 | proα1(X) | Metaphyseal chondrodysplasia, Schmid type |
| | | | | Spondylometaphyseal dysplasia, Japanese type |
| XI | COL11A1 | 1p21 | proα1(XI) | Stickler syndrome type III |
| | | | | Marshall syndrome |
| | COL11A2 | 6p21.3 | proα2(XI) | Stickler syndrome type II |
| | | | | Otospondylomegaepiphyseal dysplasia (OSMED) |
| | | | | Weissenbacher-Zweymuller syndrome |
| XII | COL12A1 | 6 | proα1(XII) | |
| XIII | COL13A1 | 10q22 | proα1(XIII) | |
| XIV | COL14A1 | 8q23 | proα1(XIV) | |
| XV | COL15A1 | 9q21-q22 | proα1(XV) | |
| XVI | COL16A1 | 1p34 | proα1(XVI) | |
| XVII | COL17A1 | 10q24.3 | proα1(XVII) | Epidermolysis bullosa, generalized atrophic benign |
| XVIII | COL18A1 | 21q22.3 | proα1(XVIII) | |
| XIX | COL19A1 | 6q12-q14 | proα1(XIX) | |

form glucosyl-galactosyl-hydroxylysine or the monosaccharide galactosyl-hydroxylysine; and one or more N-linked oligosaccharides are added to the precursor-specific polypeptides of most proα chains. The extent of lysyl hydroxylation differs widely among collagen types. In types I and III collagen, ~15% of the residues are hydroxylated; in type II collagen, ~50% are hydroxylated; and in type IV collagen, almost all of the lysyl residues in the Y position are hydroxylated.

Prolyl hydroxylation is a vital step in the formation of a stable collagen molecule, because its extent determines the melting point of the triple helix of the molecule: In the absence of any prolyl hydroxylation, the melting point of type I procollagen is ~27°C, whereas with complete hydroxylation, it is 42°C. The function of lysyl hydroxylation is less clear, although it appears to be important in the formation of stable intermolecular cross-links between collagen molecules in the extracellular matrix.

The completed proα chains of type I collagen are ~1400 amino acids in length (Fig. 189-2). Each chain has a propeptide-specific amino-terminal extension, which contains a globular domain and a collagen-like sequence; an amino-terminal telopeptide domain, which contains a peptidase cleavage site; a long central triple-helical domain, which is the Gly-X-Y triplet

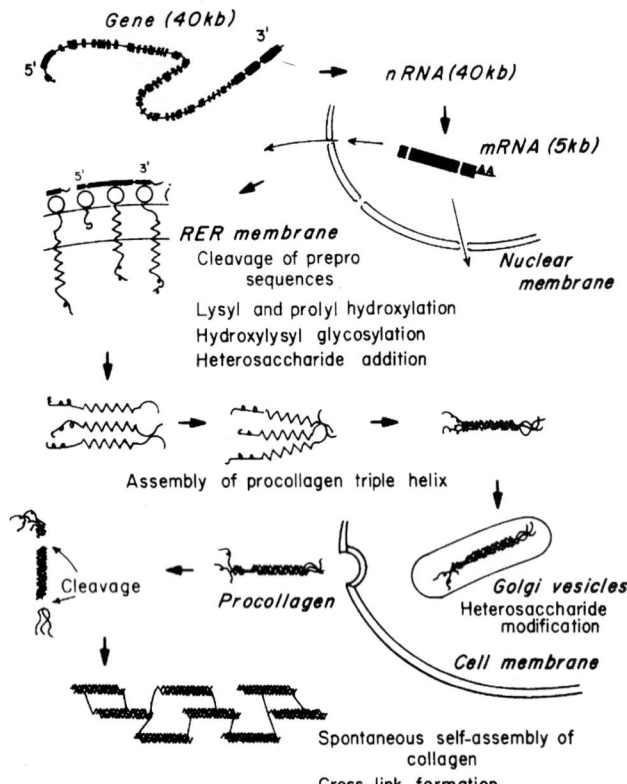

**FIGURE 189-1.** Schematic representation of the biosynthetic pathway of type I procollagen. The reactions depicted here can be generalized to all collagens. (*nRNA*, nuclear RNA; *mRNA*, messenger RNA; *RER*, rough endoplasmic reticulum.) (Modified from Byers PH, Barsh GS, Holbrook KA. Molecular pathology in inherited disorders of collagen metabolism. Hum Pathol 1982; 13:89.)

portion; a carboxyl-terminal telopeptide domain, which contains another peptidase cleavage site; and a carboxy-terminal extension of ~250 amino-acid residues, which contains a domain that governs chain selection during molecular assembly. The completed chains of type I procollagen are discharged into the lumen of the rough ER; the three chains of the molecule are assembled, stabilized by interchain disulfide bonds; and the triple helix is propagated toward the amino-terminal end of the molecule. The propagation of the triple-helical structure depends on the presence of glycine in every third position, and the structure is stabilized by hydrogen bonds that form between glycyl and hydroxyprolyl residues. The procollagen molecule is transported to the Golgi apparatus, where the N-linked oligosaccharide is converted to a high-mannose structure, and the mature molecule then is secreted into the extracellular space. After secretion, the amino-terminal and carboxy-terminal propeptide extensions are cleaved, each by a specific protease, and the resultant collagen molecule then aggregates with other molecules to form collagen fibrils.

The extent of processing differs among collagen types. The fibril structure is stabilized by the formation of intermolecular cross-links. These cross-links are formed after the oxidative deamination of lysyl residues in the amino-terminal and carboxyl-terminal telopeptide domains. These active aldehydes spontaneously condense with adjacent lysyl or hydroxylysyl residues and ultimately, in many molecules, go on to form stable cross-links derived from three lysyl or modified lysyl residues.

Although collagens form highly stable structures, a constant turnover occurs, which is mediated through extracellular matrix metalloproteinases, including collagenases—enzymes capable of hydrolyzing intact collagen molecules. The stability of a tissue is a fine balance between the biosynthetic activities and degradation of the connective tissue macromolecules. In some heritable disorders of collagen biosynthesis, this balance is lost.

## OSTEOGENESIS IMPERFECTA

Osteogenesis imperfecta (OI) is a group of inherited generalized connective tissue disorders of which the principal manifestation is bone fragility[9–11] (see Chap. 63). On the basis of the clinical findings, the mode of inheritance, and the radiologic picture, several types of OI have been described (Table 189-2). Determining which type of OI a patient has is important, because the natural history and recurrence risks in subsequent offspring differ. The discrimination of the different types of OI depends on the age of initial presentation, the family history, the presence or absence of bone deformity, and the radiographic appearance of the bones. Biochemical testing can be used to confirm the clinical impressions. Most of the forms of OI studied so far have resulted from mutations in the genes for the chains of type I collagen.[11] Because these molecules are synthesized by dermal fibroblasts in culture, biopsy of a small piece of skin (a 2-mm circle usually is sufficient), culture of dermal fibroblasts, and evaluation of collagen biosynthesis and structure constitute one test to determine the type of OI in a given patient; an alternative is the determination of the sequences of both type I collagen genes. The phenotypic differences reflect the nature and location of the mutation in the type I collagen genes. The following classification is most commonly used but, for a condition that varies almost continuously from lethal to mild, any attempt to create categories faces difficulty, and many people do not fit into the molds.

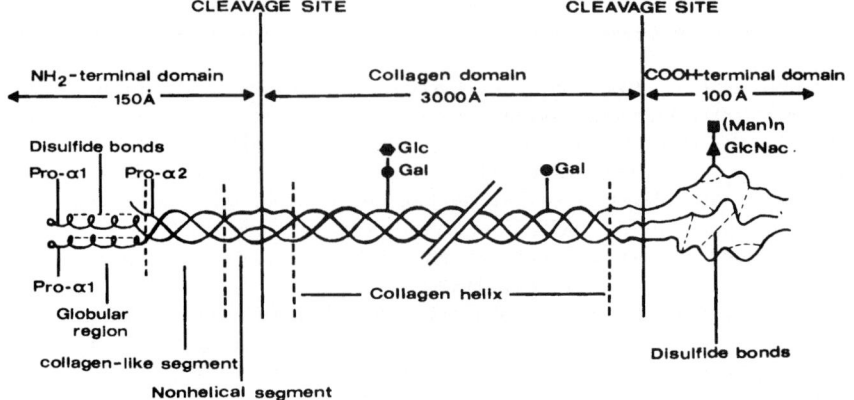

**FIGURE 189-2.** Schematic representation of type I procollagen, indicating different domains of the molecule. (Redrawn from Prockop DJ, Kivirikko KI, Tuderman L, Guzman NA. The biosynthesis of collagen and its disorders [first of two parts]. N Engl J Med 1979; 301:13.)

**TABLE 189-2.**

Classification, Clinical Characteristics, Mode of Inheritance, Biochemical Findings, and Ultrastructural Findings in Three Heritable Categories of Collagen Disorders

| Type | Clinical Features | Inheritance | Biochemical Findings | Ultrastructural Findings |
|---|---|---|---|---|
| **OSTEOGENESIS IMPERFECTA** | | | | |
| I Dominant with blue sclerae | | | | |
|   IA | Bone fragility, blue sclerae, hearing impairment. Postnatal onset of fractures, no dentinogenesis imperfecta, normal stature. | AD | Defective α1(I) gene expression | |
|   IB | Same as A, except accompanied by dentinogenesis imperfecta. | AD | Alterations in triple helix of type I collagen | |
| II Perinatal lethal | Intrauterine growth retardation, rhizomelic limb shortening and bowing. Death in the perinatal period. Dark blue sclerae. Minimal calvarial mineralization, broad "concertina" femurs, continuous beading of ribs, platyspondyly. | AD | Alterations in triple helix of type I collagen | |
| | | AR | Small deletion from α2(1) on background of nonfunctional α2(1) | |
| III Progressive deforming | Short stature, triangular facies, joint laxity. Radiographs at birth show decreased calvarial mineralization, thin ribs, thin long bones. Subsequently, cystic ends of long bones, many fractures, and bowing may occur. | AD | Alterations in triple helix of type I collagen. | |
| | | AR | Homozygous deletion of short region near carboxy-terminal end of α2(I) | |
| IV Dominant with normal sclerae, mild deformity | | | | |
|   IVA | Bone fragility, normal sclerae, no dentinogenesis imperfecta; variable short stature. | AD | Alterations in triple helix of type I collagen | |
|   IVB | Same as A, with dentinogenesis imperfecta. | | | |
| **MARFANOID SYNDROMES** | | | | |
| Marfan syndrome | Tall, thin, arachnodactyly, pectus deformities, scoliosis, joint laxity. Myopia, lens dislocation. Mitral valve prolapse, mitral insufficiency, aortic root dilatation, aortic insufficiency, aortic dissection. Onset of cardiovascular problems by third decade. | AD | Mutations in fibrillin 1 (chromosome 15) | |
| Contractural arachnodactyly | Contractures, arachnodactyly, ear deformities. No lens dislocation, cardiovascular findings generally are mild. | AD | Mutations in fibrillin 2 (chromosome 5) | |
| Marfanoid hypermobility | Similar to I, but with extreme joint hypermobility and later onset of cardiovascular problems. | AD | Not known | |
| Homocystinuria | Marfanoid habitus with arachnodactyly and pectus deformities, scoliosis unusual. Mild joint contractures, lens dislocation. Arterial thrombosis common. Mild to moderate mental retardation. | AR | Cystathionine β-synthases deficiency | |
| Mitral valve prolapse | Mitral prolapse, mild skeletal findings, including asthenic habitus, mild scoliosis and pectus deformities. | AD | Not known | |
| Isolated ectopia lentis | Ectopia lentis. Subtle skeletal findings but no aortic dilatation. | AD | Mutations in fibrillin 1 | |
| **EHLERS-DANLOS SYNDROME** | | | | |
| I Gravis | Soft, velvety skin; marked skin hyperextensibility, fragility, and easy bruisability; "cigarette paper" scars; large and small joint hypermobility; frequent venous varicosities; hernias. Prematurity. | AD | Abnormalities in type V collagen | Large collagen fibrils, many irregular in shape |
| II Mitis | Soft skin, moderate skin hyperextensibility and easy bruisability, moderate joint hypermobility; varicose veins and hernias are less common than in EDS I. Prematurity is rare. | AD | Abnormalities in type V collagen | Large collagen fibrils, many irregular in shape |
| III Benign familial hypermobility | Skin is soft but otherwise minimally affected; joint mobility is markedly increased and affects large and small joints; dislocation is common. | AD | Not known | Large collagen fibrils, many irregular in shape |
| IV Ecchymotic or arterial | Skin is thin or translucent or both; veins are readily visible over the trunk, arms, legs, and abdomen. Repeated ecchymosis with minimal trauma. Skin is not hyperextensible, and joints (except the small joints in the hands) usually are of normal mobility. Bowel rupture (usually affecting the colon) and arterial rupture are frequent and often lead to death; uterine rupture during pregnancy. | AD | Decreased or absent secretion of type III collagen; structurally abnormal type III collagen | Thin dermis, small fibers, often engorged cells in dermis, fibrils of variable size |
| V X-linked | Similar to EDS II; bruising may be more extensive. | XR | Not known | |
| VI Ocular | Soft, velvety, hyperextensible skin; hypermobile joints; scoliosis scarring less severe than in EDS I; some patients have ocular fragility and keratoconus. | AR | Lysyl hydroxylase deficiency | Small collagen bundles; fibrils normal or similar to those in EDS I |
| VII Arthrochalasis multiplex congenita | Soft skin, scars near normal. Marked joint hyperextensibility, congenital hip dislocation. | AD | Amino-acid substitution near the NH₂-terminal cleavage site of proα2(I) or proα1(I) | Irregular fibrils |
| | | AR | NH₂-terminal protease deficiency | Ribbon-like fibrils |
| VIII Periodontal | Marked skin fragility with abnormal, atrophic, pigmented scars; minimal skin extensibility; moderate joint laxity. Asthenic habitus, generalized periodontitis. | AD | Not known | Not known |
| IX | Soft, somewhat extensible skin; bladder diverticula; bladder rupture; rhizomelic shortening of arms with limitation of supination, occipital horns, broad clavicles. | XR | Abnormal copper utilization with multiple enzymopathy | Variable fibril diameter |
| X Fibronectin platelet defect | Soft, mildly hyperextensible skin; mild joint hypermobility; easy bruising. | AR | Fibronectin defect | Fibrils similar to EDS II |

*AD*, autosomal dominant; *AR*, autosomal recessive; *EDS*, Ehlers-Danlos syndrome; *NH₂-*, amino; *XR*, X-linked recessive.

## OSTEOGENESIS IMPERFECTA TYPE I

OI type I is inherited in an autosomal dominant manner. Typically, affected individuals have blue sclerae and normal stature. They rarely have dentinogenesis imperfecta and may experience from a few to more than 50 fractures (usually of the long bones) before puberty. The fracture frequency usually decreases about the time of puberty, suggesting that some hormonal change improves bone strength. The fractures heal without deformity. The frequency of this form of OI has been estimated at ~1 in 15,000, but because of the relatively mild presentation, it may go unidentified and thus may be more frequent.

The diagnosis of OI type I usually is suspected on the basis of a dominant family history, the observation of blue sclerae in the patient, and bone fractures. It is confirmed by measuring the production of type I procollagen by dermal fibroblasts in culture. Ordinarily, ~85% of the collagen synthesized by these cells is type I procollagen, and most of the remainder is type III procollagen. Cells from patients with OI type I synthesize approximately half the normal amount of type I procollagen but a normal amount of other proteins.

The decrease in type I procollagen production is caused by decreased synthesis of proα(I) chains that results from a decrease in the steady-state levels of cytoplasmic *COL1A1* mRNA.[12–14] Many different mutations in the *COL1A1* gene can cause the same phenotype. Most are premature chain terminations that result from point mutations, frame shift mutations,[15–17] or splice-site mutations that lead to frame shifts. Premature termination codons dramatically destabilize the mRNA that results from the mutant allele, so little is apparent in the cell.

No adequate treatment exists for OI type I that decreases the frequency of bone fracture or increases bone density. Agents that increase the production of type I collagen have therapeutic potential, but none has been effective in controlled tests. Treatment with bisphosphonates that decrease bone resorption is now being studied. The prenatal identification of affected fetuses can be accomplished by molecular diagnosis through either mutation detection or linkage.

## OSTEOGENESIS IMPERFECTA TYPE II

The perinatal lethal form of OI, OI type II, affects ~1 in 40,000 infants and is the most severe form of bone disease.[10,11,18] Affected infants have remarkably crumpled bones, a paucity of calvarial mineralization, and small thoracic cavities (Fig. 189-3). Death usually results from respiratory failure and frequently occurs during the first few hours after birth. More than 75% of these infants die during the first month, and none is known to have survived longer than a year. With the increasing use of early gestational ultrasonography, the disorder is being detected in a significant number of affected infants during the second trimester of pregnancy.

Although OI type II was originally thought to be an autosomal recessive disorder,[10,18] biochemical and molecular genetic studies indicate that in most infants this disorder is the result of new dominant mutations.[19] Rarely, these mutations are large insertions or deletions (of as many as 3.5 kbp) in either the *COL1A1* or *COL1A2* gene. Usually they are single nucleotide changes that cause substitutions for glycyl residues within the triple-helical domain in either of the chains.[11,20–28] These mutations decrease the thermal stability of the molecules into which the abnormal chains are incorporated, decrease the efficiency of secretion of those molecules, and decrease the amount of normal procollagen secreted.

This form of OI must be differentiated from some of the other lethal skeletal dysplasias and from hypophosphatasia. An experienced pediatric radiologist can help with this distinction, and the diagnosis can be confirmed by examination of the collagens synthesized by cultured fibroblastic cells.

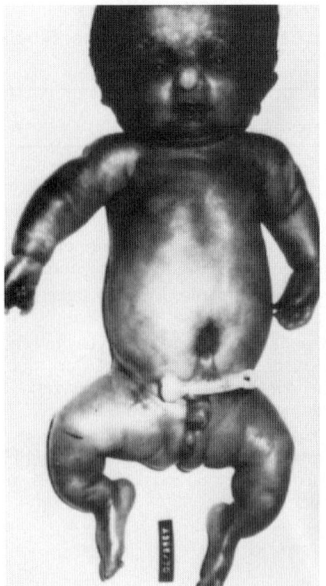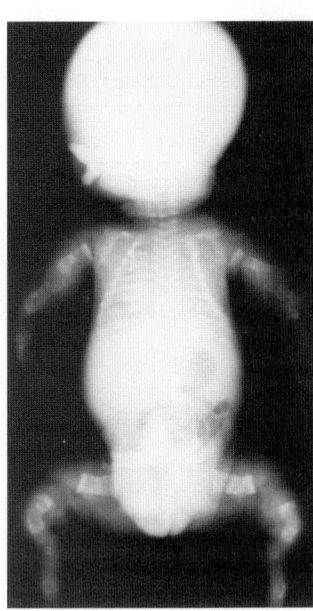

**FIGURE 189-3.** Osteogenesis imperfecta (*OI*) type II, the perinatal lethal form. *Left,* Infant who died in newborn period. Notice the beaked nose, the short, deformed limbs, and the position of legs. *Right,* Radiograph of infant with OI type II. Virtually no mineralization of calvarial bones is seen, the ribs are irregular, the bones of the limbs are all foreshortened, and the femurs appear telescoped. (From Hollister DW, Byers PH, Holbrook KA. Genetic disorders of collagen metabolism. Adv Hum Genet 1982; 12:1.)

Although OI type II usually results from a new dominant mutation, the observed recurrence risk is 2% to 6%. In almost all families, recurrence results from parental mosaicism for the mutation.[29] An autosomal recessive form also may exist but is rare.

Supportive care is appropriate, because no therapy alters the prognosis for these infants. Prenatal diagnosis should be offered in subsequent pregnancies in families to which an infant with OI type II has been born. Ultrasonographic examination of the fetus between 15 and 18 weeks of gestation reliably identifies the affected fetus. Prenatal diagnosis also can be performed by examination of the collagens synthesized by cells grown from chorionic villus biopsy specimens and by direct DNA analysis if the mutation is known.

## OSTEOGENESIS IMPERFECTA TYPE III

The progressive deforming variety of OI, OI type III, usually is recognized at birth because of slightly shorter stature and deformities resulting from in utero fractures (Fig. 189-4). Rare autosomal recessive and, more commonly, autosomal dominant forms of this type of OI are found.[30] Radiologically, the calvarium is undermineralized, the ribs are thin, the long bones are thin with evidence of fracture, and the skeleton is osteopenic. If no fractures are present at birth, they usually occur during the first year of life, when deformity becomes apparent. Angulation deformities of the tibias and the femurs reduce the efficiency of weight-bearing and increase the likelihood of fracture.

Treatment is directed toward providing a more functional anatomy, and in this group of children placement of intramedullary rods in long bones appears to improve the prognosis and may facilitate walking. For some children, bone fragility makes independent ambulation difficult in all but the most restricted circumstances, and motorized wheelchairs provide the most mobility. The growth of these children is limited, and adult height between 1 and 1.5 meters is common. Because of the bone fragility and ligamentous laxity, many of these children develop significant kyphoscoliosis and eventually experience pulmo-

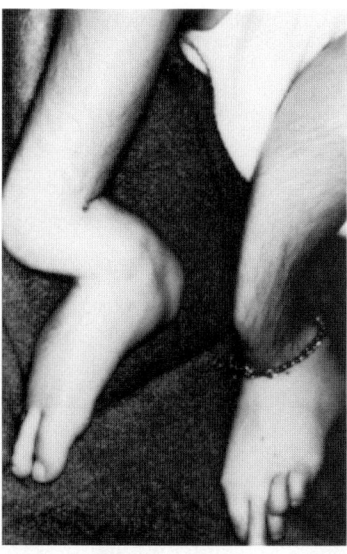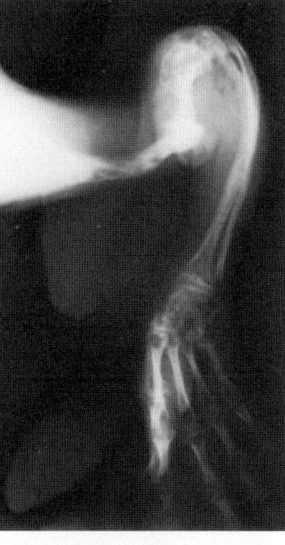

**FIGURE 189-4.** Osteogenesis imperfecta (*OI*) type III, the progressive deforming variety. *Left*, Marked bowing of lower legs in young man. *Right*, Radiograph of upper extremity in the same person. (From Hollister DW, Byers PH, Holbrook KA. Genetic disorders of collagen metabolism. Adv Hum Genet 1982; 12:1.)

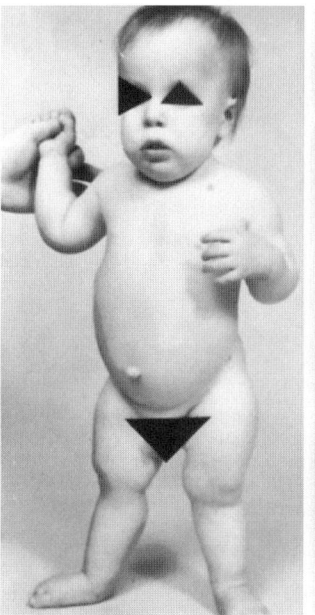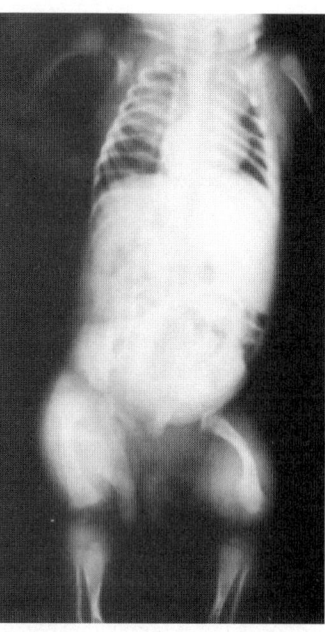

**FIGURE 189-5.** Osteogenesis imperfecta type IV. *Left*, A 13-month-old boy. *Right*, Radiograph showing short bowed femurs and deformities of his humeral and tibial bones. (From Wenstrup RJ, Hunter AGW, Byers PH. Osteogenesis imperfecta type IV: evidence of abnormal triple helical structure of type I collagen. Hum Genet 1986; 74:47.)

nary insufficiency. Sclerae often are pale blue at birth and become nearly normal by puberty. Dentinogenesis imperfecta is common, but hearing loss is rare. No medical therapy reliably decreases fracture frequency or increases growth and bone density. Observational studies of bisphosphonate use have suggested that they may increase bone density and perhaps reduce fracture risk, but more extensive study is required.

Although autosomal recessive[31,32] and autosomal dominant forms of OI type III have been identified, most affected individuals have dominant mutations in the type I collagen genes. Prenatal diagnosis is available by ultrasonography and by analysis of chorionic villus biopsy cells for abnormal proteins or the known mutations.

## OSTEOGENESIS IMPERFECTA TYPE IV

OI type IV is characterized by normal or grayish sclerae, mild to moderate deformity with some short stature, and autosomal dominant inheritance (Fig. 189-5). Some individuals have dentinogenesis imperfecta, but hearing loss seems rare. Infants often have mild shortness of stature and femoral bowing at birth, but in some, the diagnosis is delayed until the first fracture. As with the other forms of OI, fracture frequency decreases at the time of puberty but may increase at older ages, especially in women. Because of the deformities, some individuals benefit from insertion of rods during childhood, but medical therapies do not appear to modify the relatively mild natural history of this form of OI. Again, bisphosphonate treatment is being studied.

Linkage studies indicate that in some families, this phenotype results from mutations in the α2(I) gene.[33] Biochemical studies of type I collagen synthesized by cells from these patients confirm the linkage data and suggest that small deletions or single amino-acid substitutions for glycyl residues in the triple helical domains of the α1(I) and α2(I) chain cause this phenotype.[11,34]

## EHLERS-DANLOS SYNDROME

The Ehlers-Danlos syndrome (EDS) is a heterogeneous group of generalized connective tissue disorders in which the principal manifestations are skin fragility, skin hyperextensibility, and

joint hypermobility[4,35–38] (see Table 189-2). Genetic and biochemical studies had expanded the known types of EDS, but another classification has reduced some types into single categories.[39] EDS types I and II are known as the *classic form*; EDS type III is known as the *hypermobile form*; EDS type IV is termed the *vascular* or *ecchymotic form*; EDS type VI is known as the *ocular-scoliotic form*; and EDS type VII has been divided into the *arthrochalasis form* and *dermatosparaxis*. EDS type IX has been removed from the classification and renamed the *occipital horn syndrome*, a disorder that results from mutations in the *Menkes syndrome gene*, *ATP7A*. Distinguishing the different types is important, because in some forms (e.g., EDS type IV and EDS type VI) complications of arterial rupture may ensue, whereas for most of the other types life expectancy usually is normal and complications are modest. Some of the literature has not differentiated the types clearly, and, often, the complications inherent in EDS type IV are cited as characteristic of the syndrome as a whole.

## MILD TO MODERATE FORMS OF EHLERS-DANLOS SYNDROME

Several types of EDS, including types I, II, III, V, VIII, and X, have mild to moderate phenotypes and are rarely associated with lethal complications. The clinical findings in EDS types I and II may be dramatic, with markedly soft, velvety, hyperextensible skin; impressive joint hypermobility; easy bruising; and thin, atrophic, "cigarette-paper" scars (Fig. 189-6). In both forms, varicose veins are common, and in EDS type I, affected infants may be delivered prematurely. Although tissues are more friable than normal, most surgical procedures are tolerated well. Both of these conditions are inherited in an autosomal dominant fashion, and relatively little variation is found within families. Dermal collagen fibrils have a bizarre organization when viewed by electron microscopy.[36] Linkage to the *COL5A1*[40,41] and *COL5A2* genes has been identified, and mutations[42–45] in both genes have been observed in some families or individuals with EDS types I and II. A significant proportion of people with EDS type I or II probably have null mutations in the *COL5A1* gene.

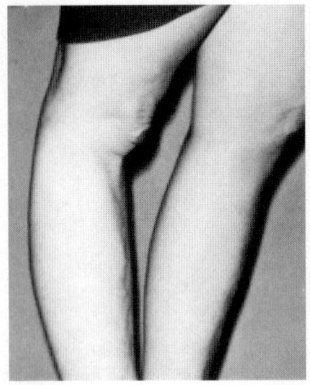 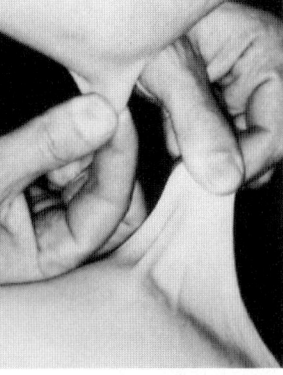

**FIGURE 189-6.** Ehlers-Danlos syndrome type I. *Left*, Genu recurvatum in a patient. Notice abnormal scars on both knees. *Right*, Marked skin hyperextensibility at elbow of a patient (*bottom*). A control is shown at the top. (From Hollister DW, Byers PH, Holbrook KA. Genetic disorders of collagen metabolism. Adv Hum Genet 1982; 12:1.)

In EDS type III, benign familial hypermobility, findings are limited to marked joint hypermobility. Although the skin often is soft, it is not hyperextensible, and scars are not abnormal. The principal complications are recurrent dislocation and early-onset degenerative joint disease. The condition is inherited in an autosomal dominant manner and probably is common in the general population. No biochemical defects have been identified.

EDS type V is distinguished from EDS type II by the X-linked recessive inheritance pattern. It appears to be rare. No biochemical defects have been identified,[37] and its existence has been disputed.[38]

EDS type VIII is inherited in an autosomal dominant manner. It is characterized by bruising; soft, hyperextensible skin; hypermobile joints; and periodontal disease. Loss of teeth by the early 20s is common.[46] No biochemical defects have been identified.

EDS type X is inherited in an autosomal recessive fashion. Only one family has been identified to date.[47] Joint hypermobility is mild; the chief finding is easy bruising. The disorder appears to result from an alteration in fibronectin that interferes with normal platelet aggregation.

## EHLERS-DANLOS SYNDROME TYPE IV

EDS type IV, the ecchymotic, arterial, or Sack-Barabas variety, is the most severe form of EDS and results from mutations in the *COL3A1* gene.[48–50] The disorder is inherited in an autosomal dominant fashion, but many of the patients are the only affected members of their families. Affected individuals have thin, translucent skin through which the venous pattern over the trunk, abdomen, and extremities is visible; minimal joint hypermobility, which may be limited to the small joints of the hands and feet; and marked bruising (Fig. 189-7). Often, the skin over the face has a parchment-like appearance, and the nose frequently is thin and beaked. Individuals with EDS type IV are at risk for arterial rupture, spontaneous rupture of the colon, and rupture of the gravid uterus.[38] Recurrent abdominal pain without significant other findings is common and may result from mural hemorrhage in the small bowel. The location of arterial hemorrhage determines the presenting symptoms in some patients (stroke, abdominal bleeding, limb compartment syndrome), whereas bowel rupture is the first complication seen in others.

The life span of individuals with EDS type IV is shortened, although survival into the seventh decade can be seen.[50] Causes of death include exsanguination from large-artery rupture, sepsis from bowel rupture, and shock from uterine rupture.

The complications of pregnancy, along with vascular rupture and uterine rupture, include tearing of the vaginal tissues during delivery. The risk of life-threatening or lethal complications during

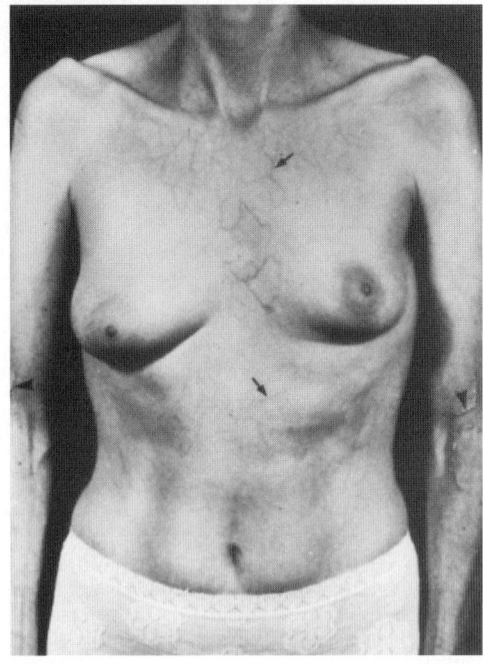

**FIGURE 189-7.** Ehlers-Danlos syndrome (*EDS*) type IV. This 26-year-old woman has a readily visible venous pattern over her trunk and abdomen (*arrows*). Linear markings in antecubital spaces (*arrowheads*) represent areas of elastosis perforans serpiginosa, a common accompaniment to EDS type IV. (From Byers PH, Holbrook KA, McGillivray B, et al. Clinical and ultrastructural heterogeneity of type IV Ehlers-Danlos syndrome. Hum Genet 1979; 47:141.)

pregnancy ranges from 8% to 15%.[51] Each affected woman should be aware of these potential risks. Furthermore, because of the autosomal dominant nature of inheritance in most families, the risk of having an affected infant is 50% for each pregnancy. Prenatal diagnosis by linkage analysis (using polymorphic restriction sites in the genes for type III collagen) is useful in some families,[45] and analysis of the type III collagen synthesized and secreted by cells from chorionic villus biopsy specimens may help in others.

EDS type IV results from abnormalities in the structure or expression of the genes for type III collagen.[49] No significant clinical variation appears to exist among families with different classes of mutations (e.g., point mutations that alter glycine residues, exon-skipping mutations, or large deletions).

The suspected diagnosis can be confirmed by examining the biosynthesis of type III procollagen by cultured dermal fibroblasts. Because of the nature of complications and the risks during surgery in this disorder, confirmation of the diagnosis is essential.

No medical treatment is available that increases the production of normal type III collagen.

## EHLERS-DANLOS SYNDROME TYPE VI

EDS type VI, the first true, heritable disorder of collagen metabolism to be described, is an autosomal recessive disorder that results from decreased activity of the enzyme lysyl hydroxylase because of mutations in the lysyl hydroxylase gene.[52–55] Some variation is found in the clinical phenotype, but a marfanoid habitus; soft, hyperextensible skin; joint hypermobility; scoliosis; and ocular fragility are the principal clinical features. Because many of the individuals identified have been children, the natural history of the disorder is not yet well understood. At least one patient appears to have died because of arterial rupture in later life.

The diagnosis is established most readily by the measurement of pyridinoline cross-links in urine.[56,57] These reflect the hydroxylation status of lysyl residues in collagen degradation products.

The lysyl hydroxylase gene responsible for hydroxylation of helical lysyl residues has been cloned (*PLOD1*), and several mutations have been identified, the most common of which is a duplication of exons 9–16.[58] Collagen fibrils in skin have a bizarre branching organization, similar to that seen in EDS type I.

Prenatal diagnosis has been attempted by the measurement of enzyme activity in amniotic fluid cells and has correctly predicted an unaffected but heterozygous infant[55]; molecular diagnosis would be more specific.

Although no specific therapy has been demonstrated, the use of pharmacologic doses of ascorbic acid, a cofactor for lysyl hydroxylase, has been advocated, and an increase in urinary excretion of hydroxylysine has followed ingestion of this vitamin.[54]

## EHLERS-DANLOS SYNDROME TYPE VII

EDS type VII is divided into two distinct phenotypes: *arthrochalasis multiplex congenita* (EDS types VIIA and VIIB) and *dermatosparaxis* (EDS type VIIC). EDS types VIIA and VIIB are characterized by marked joint hypermobility, multiple joint dislocations, and congenital hip dislocation. Initially, this disorder was thought to result from abnormalities in the enzyme that cleaves the amino-terminal propeptide extension from type I procollagen,[59] but restudy of some of the original patients and detailed study of the collagens synthesized by cells from several new patients have demonstrated that the mutations affect the cleavage of the $NH_2$-terminal propeptide of the substrate proα1(I) and proα2(I) chains.[60–62] No effective therapy, other than surgical repair of dislocation, is known.

Six children with defects in the procollagen N-protease have now been identified. They have very fragile skin, bruise easily, and have blue sclerae and very marked joint laxity.[63–65] Electron micrographs of their skin reveal very bizarre collagen fibrils. Mutations in the N-proteinase gene have been identified in all affected children.[65]

# DISORDERS RELATED TO OTHER COLLAGEN GENES

## CHONDRODYSPLASIAS

More than 150 varieties of chondrodysplasia, disorders of bone growth and structure, have been identified.[66–70] Within this relatively large group, only a few (some forms of achondrogenesis, spondyloepiphyseal dysplasia [SED], Stickler syndrome, and Kniest syndrome) result from mutations in the *COL2A1* gene that encodes the chains of type II collagen. These conditions share abnormalities of the articular cartilage and of the vitreous humor of the eye. These tissues contain collagen types II and XI; type XI collagen contains three chains, one encoded by the *COL2A1* gene, one by the *COL11A1* gene, and one by the *COL11A2* gene. This is a minor molecule in collagen. Mutations in the *COL11A1* gene cause a Stickler phenotype or a Stickler-Marshall picture, whereas those in the *COL11A2* gene cause a Stickler phenotype without ocular findings. Forms of metaphyseal dysplasia result from mutations in the type IX collagen genes. Mutations in the type X collagen gene result in the Schmid-type metaphyseal dysplasia. Other forms of chondrodysplasia result from mutations in other supporting matrix genes of cartilage.

## DISORDERS OF TYPE II, TYPE IX, TYPE X, AND TYPE XI COLLAGEN GENES

### STICKLER SYNDROME

Stickler syndrome, hereditary arthro-ophthalmodystrophy, is an autosomal dominant disorder characterized by early degenera-tive joint disease in the presence of a mild skeletal epiphyseal dysplasia, and vitreal degeneration with moderate to severe myopia and retinal detachment in some individuals.[71] Linkage studies in families with Stickler syndrome indicate genetic heterogeneity.[72] In most families with Stickler syndrome, mutations in the *COL2A1* gene have been identified that result in stop codons.[49] Heterogeneity has been found, and mutations in the *COL11A1* and *COL11A2* genes have been characterized. Although both cause the skeletal abnormalities, those in the *COL11A2* gene usually are not accompanied by ocular findings, because the *COL5A2* gene product, proα2(V), substitutes for proα2(XI) in the vitreous.

### SPONDYLOEPIPHYSEAL DYSPLASIA

SEDs are a group of chondrodysplasias in which the radiologic features include abnormal epiphyses, flattened vertebral bodies, and ocular involvement that ranges from myopia to vitreoretinal degeneration. A range of clinical expression is found, from mild short stature to very severe short stature, pulmonary compromise, and death in infancy. Analysis of type II collagen in articular cartilage from individuals with different forms of SED have demonstrated alterations in the amount and electrophoretic mobilities of the α1(II) chains in those tissues, compatible with mutations in the *COL2A1* gene.[49,73] Analysis of the *COL2A1* genes from several individuals with different forms of SED have identified mutations that include partial duplication of exon 48 with the resultant addition of 15 amino acids (duplication of residues 970–984 of the triple helix),[74] deletion of exon 48 from one allele,[75] substitution of the glycine at position 997 in the triple helix by serine,[76] a splice junction mutation that results in skipping the sequences of exon 20,[77] and, surprisingly, a substitution of cysteine for arginine at position 75 in the triple helical domain.[78]

### ACHONDROGENESIS/HYPOCHONDROGENESIS

The most severe end of the spectrum of chondrodysplasias in which evidence is found of involvement of the *COL2A1* gene is the achondrogenesis/hypochondrogenesis group. Infants with achondrogenesis have severe short-limbed dwarfism and die in the immediate perinatal period or in utero. Electron microscopic studies of cartilage from infants or fetuses with achondrogenesis/hypochondrogenesis have demonstrated marked dilation of the rough ER with electron-dense material and a paucity of fibrils in the extracellular matrix.[79] Several point mutations in the *COL2A1* gene have been identified in this disorder, resulting in substitution for glycine residues.[49] Too few mutations in the *COL2A1* gene have been identified to permit systematic genotype/phenotype analysis.

### MULTIPLE EPIPHYSEAL DYSPLASIA

Multiple epiphyseal dysplasia is characterized by autosomal dominant inheritance and short stature of varying severity with primary involvement of the epiphyses outside the spine. This family of disorders has been linked to mutations in genes of the type IX collagen family, and mutations have been identified in the *COL9A2* gene[80] and *COL9A3* gene.[81]

### METAPHYSEAL CHONDRODYSPLASIA OF SCHMID

The Schmid type of metaphyseal dysplasia is characterized by dominant inheritance, and bowing of the extremities.[82] Mild to moderate short stature is apparent in childhood. A variety of mutations in the *COL10A1* gene have been identified, most of which interfere with chain association.[83–86]

## ALPORT SYNDROME

Alport syndrome is characterized by progressive hereditary nephritis and sensorineural deafness that in some families is associated with ocular abnormalities, particularly lenticonus and macular changes.[87] The condition is inherited in an X-linked manner, with males likely to develop both hearing loss and renal dysfunction earlier than females in the same family. The renal basement membrane shows a characteristic array of findings that includes splitting and thinning of the glomerular basement membrane. Linkage studies showed the Alport gene[88–90] to be located at Xq13; shortly thereafter, a type IV collagen gene was identified that mapped to the same location.[90] In all families with X-linked nephritides, with or without significant deafness, the disorder has been linked to the *COL4A5* gene locus.

The mutational spectrum in the *COL4A5* gene is similar to that seen in other collagen genes. It has included multiexon deletions, point mutations within the triple-helical domain that substitute for glycine residues, and mutations within the non-collagenous carboxy-propeptide domain.[91]

Extensive deletions involving the 5' end of the *COL4A5* gene and a segment of the adjacent *COL4A6* gene can result in a form of Alport syndrome in which the renal disease is accompanied by diffuse esophageal leiomyomatosis.[92]

## DYSTROPHIC FORMS OF EPIDERMOLYSIS BULLOSA: DEFECTS IN TYPE VII COLLAGEN

Epidermolysis bullosa (EB) is a highly heterogeneous group of disorders in which blistering of the skin is the common unifying theme. Blistering occurs within the epidermis (simplex forms of EB), at the dermal-epidermal junction (junctional forms of EB), or within the dermis below the basement membrane (dystrophic forms of EB).[93]

### DYSTROPHIC FORMS OF EPIDERMOLYSIS BULLOSA

Dominantly inherited forms of dystrophic EB may be generalized in their distribution (blistering occurs early and is generalized; a later involvement of the limbs is seen, and scars forming while healing occurs), or may be more localized over the extremities with a preference for sites of trauma. Generally, this is most severe during the first 5 years of life.[94] Morphologic studies of the skin have indicated abnormalities in the structure or amount of anchoring fibrils or both. These structures course from the basement membrane zone into the upper portion of the papillary dermis and appear to be involved in maintaining dermal-epidermal integrity.[95] Anchoring fibrils consist largely, if not exclusively, of type VII collagen.[96] With the identification of polymorphic sites within the *COL7A1* gene in some families with abnormal anchoring fibrils, the disorder has been shown to be linked to the *COL7A1* gene. Many mutations have been identified.[97,98]

### RECESSIVE DYSTROPHIC FORMS OF EPIDERMOLYSIS BULLOSA

The severe recessive dystrophic forms of EB are characterized by generalized blistering in the newborn period, often present at birth, with scarring and progressive syndactyly from scars of the digital skin, mucosal involvement that leads to esophageal strictures, and consequent dysphagia. Protein and fluid loss through areas of chronic erosion may lead to infection and malnutrition. Survival is limited both by infection and by the consequences of involvement of the gastrointestinal tract. Early ultrastructural studies revealed abnormalities at the dermal-epidermal junction; subsequent analysis demonstrated that this is because of an absence or markedly diminished number of anchoring fibrils.[99]

Studies with antibodies known to react with type VII collagen have shown that staining at the epidermal-dermal junction is markedly diminished.[100] In some individuals, accumulation of type VII collagen within the basal epidermal cells reinforces the idea that the type VII collagen gene is the primary gene in which mutations produce the severe recessive dystrophic phenotype.[101] Studies of 25 families with more than one child with recessive dystrophic forms of EB have failed to demonstrate a single instance in which the siblings do not share the same *COL7A1* genotype, a finding consistent with the view that recessive inheritance of mutations in the *COL7A1* gene is the cause of the condition.[102] Many mutations have now been identified in the *COL7A1* gene.[99]

## MARFANOID SYNDROMES AND FIBRILLINOPATHIES

The term *fibrillinopathy*, however awkward, has emerged as a means to identify those disorders that result from mutations in the fibrillin genes. Two fibrillin genes, *FBN1* on chromosome 15 and *FBN2* on chromosome 5, have been identified and characterized.[103] These genes encode two distinct proteins that form part of the microfibrillar network in skin, vessels, and most other tissues. *Fibrillin 1* (the product of the *FBN1* gene) makes up the large part of the microfibrils that form the zonular fibrils of the lens—one of the clues that led to the identification of this gene as the host of mutations that result in Marfan syndrome.[104] The microfibrils are thought (in some tissues) to provide the scaffold on which elastin is deposited to form elastic fibers, although clearly in many regions they are devoid of associated elastin. *Fibrillin 2* appears early in vessel formation and is replaced later in development by fibrillin 1.[105]

The marfanoid syndromes are a *heterogeneous* group of connective tissue disorders, most of which are inherited in an autosomal dominant fashion, and are characterized by abnormalities of the cardiovascular system, the skeleton, and, often, the eyes.[106,107] These conditions include Marfan syndrome, contractural arachnodactyly, mitral valve prolapse syndrome, isolated ectopia lentis, and homocystinuria (see Table 183-2). Only the last is inherited in an autosomal recessive fashion.

### MARFAN SYNDROME

The classic variety of Marfan syndrome is inherited in an autosomal dominant fashion, although 15% to 20% of affected individuals represent new mutations.[107] Most affected individuals are tall and have long arms and legs, arachnodactyly, high arched palate, pectus deformities, and scoliosis; approximately half of the patients have lens dislocation.[108] Virtually all individuals develop mitral valve prolapse by puberty, and most are at risk to develop aortic dilatation, aortic insufficiency, and, ultimately, aortic dissection.[109,110] Cardiac complications, including both congestive heart failure resulting from valvular dysfunction and aortic dissection, usually are the chief causes of death in this disorder.

When the patient is first seen, a careful family history should be taken to determine which other family members are at risk. Height, upper and lower segment, and blood pressure in both arms should be measured, a slit-lamp examination of the dilated pupils should be performed, and an echocardiogram should be taken. All affected individuals should be followed at 1- to 2-year intervals. The echocardiogram should be repeated every other year before puberty and yearly in adult life. Yearly eye examinations should be performed to exclude glaucoma and assess lens status.

The most significant complication of Marfan syndrome is aortic dissection, which can lead to early death. Other complications include progressive scoliosis (which usually occurs during the pubertal growth spurt), excessive height, dural ectasia, and joint hypermobility. With the use of prophylactic aortic surgery to treat aortic dilatation before dissection,[110] life span is probably increasing, and a new range of age-related complications may appear. Treatment for the progressive scoliosis may include bracing and insertion of rods, especially if the thoracic space is compromised. Treatment of prepubertal children with androgens (for males) or estrogens (for females) to hasten epiphyseal closure can change projected growth patterns substantially.

Several lines of evidence have converged to demonstrate that the FBN1 gene harbors mutations that cause Marfan syndrome. Immunofluorescence studies of cells and tissue from people with Marfan syndrome indicated a lack of fibrillin in skin and cultured cells.[111] Linkage analysis with random markers identified a region on chromosome 15 that was linked.[112] Analysis of fibrillin synthesis by cells cultured from affected individuals confirmed abnormalities in synthesis and secretion.[113] Finally, the complementary DNA was cloned, linkage was established,[114] and mutations were identified.[103] More than 100 mutations have now been identified.[115]

The principal controversy in the care of patients with Marfan syndrome concerns the treatment of the cardiovascular complications. Most untreated individuals with this disease die from aortic and mitral insufficiency or, more commonly, aortic dissection.[106] Aneurysm formation usually precedes dissection or rupture. During the last several years, surgical technique and prosthetic materials have improved to the point that many medical centers recommend replacement of the ascending aorta and aortic valve by the time the aortic root reaches double the mean value (55–60 mm).[110] Still controversial is the question of whether medical therapy has a place in the treatment of aortic dilatation. The proposal has been made that all individuals with Marfan syndrome be treated with β-adrenergic blockers to decrease cardiac contractility. The results of a single therapeutic trial have been reported. These findings[116] indicate that some individuals with Marfan syndrome may benefit from treatment with β-blockers. Regardless, management of the nondilated aorta in patients with Marfan syndrome often involves treatment with β-blockers.

## CONGENITAL ARACHNODACTYLY

Congenital contractural arachnodactyly is characterized by joint contracture, rather than joint laxity, and a characteristic crumpled upper ear. Neither lens dislocation nor aortic dilatation is a feature of this condition. Linkage of the phenotype to polymorphic variants in the FBN2 gene on chromosome 5 was demonstrated when the gene was first identified,[114] and several mutations have now been identified. Interestingly, they appear to cluster in the central region of the gene,[117] and the phenotypes of mutations in other regions have not been convincingly demonstrated.

## MITRAL VALVE PROLAPSE SYNDROME

Mitral valve prolapse syndrome is inherited in an autosomal dominant manner with variable expression. Women appear to manifest the valvular findings more frequently than men. Affected individuals have mitral prolapse and frequently have subtle skeletal findings that suggest that they may have Marfan syndrome. They do not appear to be at risk for aortic valvular or aortic root complications, however, and they do not have lens dislocation. Concern about the family often is raised and, in some cases, the diagnosis of Marfan syndrome is mistakenly made.

## ISOLATED ECTOPIA LENTIS

Many of the features of Marfan syndrome, like mitral valve prolapse, may appear as isolated features. A rare example of this is isolated ectopia lentis, a dominantly inherited disorder in which aortic root dilatation and other features of Marfan syndrome are missing or exceedingly mild. The disorder results from mutations in FBN1.[118]

## REFERENCES

1. Piez KA, Reddi AH, eds. Extracellular matrix biochemistry. New York: Elsevier, 1984.
2. Prockop DJ, Kivirikko KI. Heritable diseases of collagen. N Engl J Med 1984; 311:376.
3. Hollister DW, Byers PH, Holbrook KA. Genetic disorders of collagen metabolism. Adv Hum Genet 1982; 12:1.
4. McKusick VA. Heritable disorders of connective tissue, 4th ed. St. Louis: CV Mosby, 1972.
5. Beighton P. McKusick's heritable disorders of connective tissue, 5th ed. St. Louis: CV Mosby, 1993.
6. Royce PM, Steinmann B. Connective tissue and its heritable disorders: molecular, genetic, and medical aspects. New York: Wiley-Liss, 1993.
7. Cheah KSE. Collagen genes and inherited connective tissue disease. Biochem J 1985; 229:287.
8. Byers PH. Disorders of collagen biosynthesis and structure. In: Scriver CR, Beaudet AL, Sly WS, Valle D, eds. The metabolic basis of inherited disease, 7th ed. New York: McGraw-Hill, 1995: 4029.
9. Smith R, Francis MJO, Houghton GF. Brittle bone disease: osteogenesis imperfecta. London: Butterworth, 1983.
10. Sillence DO, Senn A, Danks DM. Genetic heterogeneity of osteogenesis imperfecta. J Med Genet 1979; 16:101.
11. Dalgleish R. Mutations in type I and type III collagen genes. In: Humphries SE, Malcolm S, eds. From genotype to phenotype. Oxford: Bios Scientific Publishers, 1994:49.
12. Barsh GS, David KE. Type I osteogenesis imperfecta: a nonfunctional allele for proα1(I) chains of type I procollagen. Proc Natl Acad Sci U S A 1982; 79:3838.
13. Rowe DW, Shapiro JR, Poirier M, Schlesinger S. Diminished type I collagen synthesis and reduced α 1(I) collagen messenger RNA in cultured fibroblasts from patients with dominantly inherited (type I) osteogenesis imperfecta. J Clin Invest 1985; 76:604.
14. Sykes B, Ogilvie D, Wordsworth P, et al. Osteogenesis imperfecta is linked to both type I collagen structural genes. Lancet 1986; 2:69.
15. Willing MC, Cohn DH, Byers PH. Frameshift mutation near the 3' end of the COL1A1 gene of type I collagen predicts an elongated proα1(I) chain and results in osteogenesis imperfecta type I. J Clin Invest 1990; 85:282.
16. Willing MC, Purchno CJ, Atkinson M, Byers PH. Osteogenesis imperfecta type I is commonly due to a COL1A1 null allele of type I collagen. Am J Hum Genet 1992; 51:508.
17. Willing MC, Deschenes SP, Scott DA, et al. Osteogenesis imperfecta type I: molecular heterogeneity for COL1A1 null alleles of type I collagen. Am J Hum Genet 1994; 55:638.
18. Sillence DO, Barlow KK, Barber AP, et al. Osteogenesis imperfecta type II: delineation of the phenotype with reference to genetic heterogeneity. Am J Med Genet 1984; 17:407.
19. Byers PH, Tsipouras P, Bonadio JF, et al. Perinatal lethal osteogenesis imperfecta (OI type II): a biochemically heterogeneous disorder usually due to new mutation in the genes for type I collagen. Am J Hum Genet 1988; 42:237.
20. Barsh GS, Byers PH. Reduced secretion of structurally abnormal type I procollagen in a form of osteogenesis imperfecta. Proc Natl Acad Sci U S A 1981; 78:5142.
21. Williams CJ, Prockop DJ. Synthesis and processing of a type I procollagen containing shortened proα1 chains by fibroblasts from a patient with osteogenesis imperfecta. J Biol Chem 1983; 258:5915.
22. Chu M-L, Williams CJ, Pepe G, et al. Internal deletion in a collagen gene in a perinatal lethal form of osteogenesis imperfecta. Nature 1983; 304:78.
23. Chu M-L, Gargiulo V, Williams CJ, Ramirez F. Multiexon deletion in an osteogenesis imperfecta variant with increased type III collagen mRNA. J Biol Chem 1985; 260:691.
24. Barsh GS, Roush C, Bonadio J, et al. Intron-mediated recombination may cause a deletion in an α1 type I collagen chain in a lethal form of osteogenesis imperfecta. Proc Natl Acad Sci U S A 1985; 82:2870.
25. DeWet WJ, Pihlajaniemi T, Myers J, et al. Synthesis of a shortened proα2(I) chain and decreased synthesis of proα2(I) chains in a proband with osteogenesis imperfecta. J Biol Chem 1983; 258:7721.
26. Bonadio J, Byers PH. Subtle structural alterations in the chains of type I procollagen produce osteogenesis imperfecta type II. Nature 1985; 316:363.
27. Steinmann B, Rao VH, Bruckner P, et al. Cysteine in the triple-helical domain of one allelic product of the α1(I) gene of type I collagen produces a lethal form of osteogenesis imperfecta. J Biol Chem 1984; 259:11129.

28. Cohn DH, Byers PH, Steinmann B, Gelinas RE. Lethal osteogenesis imperfecta resulting from a single nucleotide change in one human pro α1(I) collagen allele. Proc Natl Acad Sci U S A 1986; 83:6045.

29. Cohn DH, Starman BJ, Blumberg B, Byers PH. Recurrence of lethal osteogenesis imperfecta due to parental mosaicism for a dominant mutation in a human type I collagen gene (COL1A1). Am J Hum Genet 1990; 46:591.

30. Sillence DO, Barlow KK, Cole WG, et al. Osteogenesis imperfecta type III: delineation of the phenotype with reference to genetic heterogeneity. Am J Med Genet 1986; 23:821.

31. Deak SB, Nicholls A, Pope FM, Prockop DJ. The molecular defect in a nonlethal variant of osteogenesis imperfecta: synthesis of proα2(I) chains which are not incorporated into trimers of type I procollagen. J Biol Chem 1983; 258:15192.

32. Pihlajaniemi T, Dickson LA, Pope FM, et al. Osteogenesis imperfecta: cloning of a pro-α2(I) collagen gene with a frameshift mutation. J Biol Chem 1984; 259:12941.

33. Tsipouras P, Myers JC, Ramirez F, Prockop DJ. Restriction fragment length polymorphism associated with the proα2(I) gene of human type I procollagen: application to a family with an autosomal dominant form of osteogenesis imperfecta. J Clin Invest 1983; 72:1261.

34. Wenstrup RJ, Cohn DH, Cohen Y, Byers PH. Arginine for glycine substitution in the triple helical domain of the products of one a2(I) collagen allele (COL1A2) produces the osteogenesis imperfecta type IV phenotype. J Biol Chem 1988; 263:7734.

35. Beighton P. The Ehlers-Danlos syndrome. London: William Heinemann, 1970.

36. Vogel A, Holbrook KA, Steinmann B, et al. Abnormal collagen fibril structure in the gravis form (type I) of the Ehlers-Danlos syndrome. Lab Invest 1979; 40:201.

37. Beighton P, Curtis D. X-linked Ehlers-Danlos syndrome type V: the next generation. Clin Genet 1985; 27:472.

38. Steinmann B, Royce PM, Superti-Furga A. The Ehlers-Danlos syndrome. In: Royce PM, Steinmann B, eds. Connective tissue and its heritable disorders: molecular, genetic, and medical aspects. New York: Wiley-Liss, 1993.

39. Beighton P, DePaepe A, Steinmann B, et al. Ehlers-Danlos syndrome: revisited nosology. Am J Med Genet 1998; 77:31.

40. Loughlin J, Irven C, Hardwick LJ, et al. Linkage of the gene that encodes the alpha 1 chain of type V collagen (COL5A1) to type II Ehlers-Danlos syndrome (EDS II). Hum Mol Genet 1995; 4:1649.

41. Burrows NP, Nicholls AC, Yates JR, et al. The gene encoding collagen alpha1(V) (COL5A1) is linked to mixed Ehlers-Danlos syndrome type I/II. J Invest Dermatol 1996; 106:1273.

42. Toriello HV, Glover TW, Takahara K, et al. A translocation interrupts the COL5A1 gene in a patient with Ehlers-Danlos syndrome and hypomelanosis of Ito. Nat Genet 1996; 13:361.

43. Burrows NP, Nicholls AC, Richards AJ, et al. A point mutation in an intronic branch site results in aberrant splicing of COL5A1 and in Ehlers-Danlos syndrome type II in two British families. Am J Hum Genet 1998; 63:390.

44. Nicholls AC, Oliver JE, McCarron S, et al. An exon skipping mutation of a type V collagen gene (COL5A1) in Ehlers-Danlos syndrome. J Med Genet 1996; 33:940.

45. Richards AJ, Martin S, Nicholls AC, et al. A single base mutation in COL5A2 causes Ehlers-Danlos syndrome type II. J Med Genet 1998; 35:846.

46. Stewart RD, Hollister DW, Rimoin DL. A new variant of the Ehlers-Danlos syndrome: an autosomal dominant disorder of fragile skin, abnormal scarring, and generalized periodontitis. Birth Defects 1977; 13(3B):85.

47. Arneson MA, Hammerschmidt DE, Furcht LT, King RA. A new form of Ehlers-Danlos syndrome: fibronectin corrects defective platelet function. JAMA 1980; 244:144.

48. Pope FM, Martin GR, Lichtenstein JR, et al. Patients with Ehlers-Danlos syndrome type IV lack type III collagen. Proc Natl Acad Sci U S A 1975; 72:1314.

49. Kuivaniemi H, Tromp G, Prockop DJ. Mutations in fibrillar collagens (types I, II, III, and XI), fibril-associated collagen (type IX), and network-forming collagen (type X) cause a spectrum of diseases of bone, cartilage, and blood vessels. Hum Mutat 1997; 9:300.

50. Pepin M, Schwarze V, Superti-Furga A, Byers PH. Clinical and genetic features of Ehlers-Danlos syndrome type IV, the vascular type. N Engl J Med 2000; 342:673.

51. Rudd NL, Nimrod C, Holbrook KA, Byers PH. Pregnancy complications in type IV Ehlers-Danlos syndrome. Lancet 1983; 1:50.

52. Pinnell SR, Krane SM, Kenzora JE, Glimcher MJ. A heritable disorder of connective tissue: hydroxylysine-deficient collagen disease. N Engl J Med 1972; 266:1013.

53. Steinmann B, Gitzelmann R, Vogel A, et al. Ehlers-Danlos syndrome in two siblings with deficient lysyl hydroxylase activity in cultured skin fibroblasts but only mild hydroxylysine deficient skin. Helv Paediatr Acta 1975; 30:255.

54. Elsas LJ, Miller RL, Pinnell SR. Inherited human collagen lysyl hydroxylase deficiency: ascorbic acid response. Pediatrics 1978; 92:378.

55. Dembure PP, Priest JH, Snoddy SC, Elsas LJ. Genotyping and prenatal assessment of collagen lysyl hydroxylase deficiency in a family with Ehlers-Danlos syndrome, type VI. Am J Hum Genet 1984; 36:783.

56. Pasquali M, Dembure PP, Still MJ, Elsas LJ. Urinary pyridinium cross-links: a noninvasive diagnostic test for Ehlers-Danlos syndrome type VI. N Engl J Med 1994; 331:132.

57. Steinmann B, Eyre DR, Shao P. Urinary pyridinoline cross-links in Ehlers-Danlos syndrome type VI. Am J Hum Genet 1995; 57:1505.

58. Heikkinen J, Toppinen T, Yeowell H, et al. Duplication of seven exons in the lysyl hydroxylase gene is associated with longer forms of a repetitive sequence within the gene and is a common cause for the type VI variant of Ehlers-Danlos syndrome. Am J Hum Genet 1997; 60:48.

59. Lichtenstein JR, Martin GR, Kohn L, et al. Defect in conversion of procollagen to collagen in a form of Ehlers-Danlos syndrome. Science 1973; 182:298.

60. Steinmann B, Tuderman L, Peltonen L, et al. Evidence for structural mutation of procollagen type I in a patient with the Ehlers-Danlos syndrome type VII. J Biol Chem 1980; 255:8887.

61. Cole WG, Chan D, Chambers GW, et al. Deletion of 24 amino acids from the proα1(I) chain of type I procollagen in a patient with the Ehlers-Danlos syndrome type VII. J Biol Chem 1986; 261:5496.

62. Byers PH, Duvic M, Atkinson M, et al. Ehlers-Danlos syndrome type VIIA and VIIB result from splice junction mutations or genomic deletions that involve exon 6 in the COL1A1 and COL1A2 genes of type I collagen. Am J Med Genet 1997; 72:94.

63. Smith LT, Wertelecki W, Milstone LM, et al. Human dermatosparaxis: a form of Ehlers-Danlos syndrome that results from failure to remove the amino-terminal propeptide of type I procollagen. Am J Hum Genet 1992; 51:235.

64. Nusgens BV, Verellen-Dumoulin C, Hermanns-Le T, et al. Evidence for a relationship between Ehlers-Danlos type VII C in humans and bovine dermatosparaxis. Nat Genet 1992; 1:214.

65. Colige A, Sieron AL, Li S-W, et al. Human Ehlers-Danlos type VII C and bovine dermatosparaxis are caused by mutations in the procollagen I N-proteinase gene. Am J Hum Genet 1999; 65:308.

66. Spranger JW, Langer LO, Wiedemann HR. Bone dysplasias: an atlas of constitutional disorders of skeletal development. Philadelphia: WB Saunders, 1974.

67. Rimoin DL. The chondrodystrophies. Adv Hum Genet 1975; 5:1.

68. Sillence DO, Horton WA, Rimoin DL. Morphologic studies in the skeletal dysplasia. Am J Pathol 1979; 96:813.

69. Spranger J. Radiologic nosology of bone dysplasias. Am J Med Genet 1990; 34:96.

70. Horton WA, Hecht JT. The chondrodysplasias. In: Royce PM, Steinmann B, eds. Connective tissue and its heritable disorders: molecular, genetic, and medical aspects. New York: Wiley-Liss, 1993:641.

71. Stickler GB, Belau PG, Farrell FJ, et al. Hereditary progressive arthroophthalmopathy. Proc Staff Meet Mayo Clin 1965; 40:433.

72. Snead MP, Yates JR. Clinical and molecular genetics of Stickler syndrome. J Med Genet 1999; 36:353.

73. Murray L, Bautista J, James PL, Rimoin DL. Type II collagen defects in the chondrodysplasias: I. Spondyloepiphyseal dysplasias. Am J Hum Genet 1989; 45:5.

74. Tiller GE, Rimoin DL, Murray LW, Cohn DH. Tandem duplication within a type II collagen gene (COL2A1) exon in an individual with spondyloepiphyseal dysplasia. Proc Natl Acad Sci U S A 1990; 87:3889.

75. Lee B, Vissing H, Ramirez F, et al. Identification of the molecular defect in a family with spondyloepiphyseal dysplasia. Science 1989; 244:978.

76. Chan D, Cole WG. Low basal transcription of genes for tissue-specific collagen by fibroblasts and lymphoblastoid cells: application to the characterization of a glycine 997 to serine substitution in α1(II) collagen chains of a patient with spondyloepiphyseal dysplasia. J Biol Chem 1991; 266:12487.

77. Tiller GE, Weis MA, Eyre DR, et al. An RNA splicing mutation (G+5IVS20) in the gene for type II collagen (COL2A1 produces spondyloepiphyseal dysplasia congenita (SEDC). Am J Hum Genet 1992; 51:A37. Abstract 136.

78. Reginato AJ, Passano GM, Neumann G, et al. Familial spondyloepiphyseal dysplasia tarda, brachydactyly, and precocious osteoarthritis associated with an arginine 75→cysteine mutation in the procollagen type II gene in a kindred of Chiloe Islanders. I. Clinical, radiographic, and pathologic findings. Arthritis Rheum 1994; 37:1078.

79. Godfrey M, Keene DR, Blank E, et al. Type II achondrogenesis-hypochondrogenesis: morphologic and immunohistopathologic studies. Am J Hum Genet 1988; 43:894.

80. Holden P, Canty EG, Mortier GR, et al. Identification of novel pro-α2(IX) collagen gene mutations in two families with distinctive oligo-epiphyseal forms of multiple epiphyseal dysplasia. Am J Hum Genet 1999; 65:31.

81. Paassilta P, Lohiniva J, Annunen S, et al. COL9A3: a third locus for multiple epiphyseal dysplasia. Am J Hum Genet 1999; 64:1036.

82. Lachman RS, Rimoin DL, Spranger J. Metaphyseal chondrodysplasia, Schmid type. Clinical and radiographic delineation with a review of the literature. Pediatr Radiol 1988; 18:93.

83. Warman ML, Abbott M, Apte SS, et al. A type X collagen mutation causes Schmid metaphyseal chondrodysplasia. Nat Genet 1993; 5:79.

84. McIntosh I, Abbott MH, Warman ML, et al. Additional mutations of type X collagen confirm COL10A1 as the Schmid metaphyseal chondrodysplasia locus. Hum Mol Genet 1994; 3:303.

85. Wallis GA, Rash B, Sykes B, et al. Mutations within the gene encoding the α1(X) chain of type X collagen (COL10A1) cause metaphyseal chondrodysplasia type Schmid but not several other forms of metaphyseal chondrodysplasia. J Med Genet 1996; 33:450.

86. Wallis GA, Rash B, Sweetman WA, et al. Amino acid substitution of conserved residue in the carboxyl-terminal domain of the α1(X) chain of type X

collagen occurs in two unrelated families with metaphyseal chondrodysplasia type Schmid. Am J Hum Genet 1994; 54:169.

87. Atkin CL, Gregory MC, Border WA. Alport syndrome. In: Schrier RW, Gotschalk CW, eds. Disease of the kidney, 4th ed. Boston: Little, Brown and Company, 1988:617.

88. Atkin CL, Hasstedt SJ, Menlove L, et al. Mapping of Alport syndrome gene to the long arm of the X chromosome. Am J Hum Genet 1988; 42:249.

89. Brunner H, Schroder C, Van Bennekom C, et al. Localization of the gene for X-linked Alport's syndrome. Kidney Int 1988; 34:507.

90. Flinter FA, Abbs S, Bobrow M. Localization of the gene for classic Alport syndrome. Genomics 1989; 4:335.

91. Martin P, Heiskari N, Zhou J, et al. High mutation detection rate in the COL4A5 collagen gene in suspected Alport syndrome using PCR and direct DNA sequencing. J Am Soc Nephrol 1998; 9:2291.

92. Antignac C, Zhou J, Sanak M, et al. Alport syndrome and diffuse leiomyomatosis: deletions in the 5' end of the COL4A5 collagen gene. Kidney Int 1992; 42(5):1178.

93. Fine J-D, Bauer EA, Briggaman RA, et al. Revised clinical and laboratory criteria for subtypes in inherited epidermolysis bullosa: a consensus report by the subcommittee on diagnosis and classification of the National Epidermolysis Bullosa Registry. J Am Acad Dermatol 1991; 24:119.

94. Bruckner-Tuderman L. Epidermolysis bullosa. In: Royce PM, Steinmann B, eds. Connective tissue and its heritable disorders: molecular, genetic, and medical aspects. New York: Wiley-Liss, 1993:507.

95. Palade G, Farquhar M. A special fibril of the dermis. J Cell Biol 1965; 27:215.

96. Keene DR, Sakai Y, Lunstrum GP, et al. Type VII collagen forms an extended network of anchoring fibrils. J Cell Biol 1987; 104:611.

97. Ryynanen M, Ryynanen J, Sollberg S, et al. Genetic linkage of type VII collagen (COL7A1) to dominant dystrophic epidermolysis bullosa in families with abnormal anchoring fibrils. J Clin Invest 1992; 89:974.

98. Pulkkinen L, Uitto J. Mutation analysis and molecular genetics of epidermolysis bullosa. Matrix Biol 1999; 18:29.

99. Tidman MJ, Eady RAJ. Evaluation of anchoring fibrils and other components of the dermal-epidermal junction in dystrophic epidermolysis bullosa by a quantitative technique. J Invest Dermatol 1985; 84:374.

100. Heagerty AHM, Kennedy AR, Leigh IM, et al. Identification of an epidermal basement membrane defect in recessive forms of dystrophic epidermolysis bullosa by LH7:2 monoclonal antibody: use in diagnosis. Br J Dermatol 1986; 115:125.

101. Smith LT, Sybert VP. Intra-epidermal retention of type VII collagen in a patient with recessive dystrophic epidermolysis bullosa. J Invest Dermatol 1990; 94:261.

102. Hovnanian A, Duquesnoy P, Blanchet-Bardon C, et al. Genetic linkage of recessive dystrophic epidermolysis bullosa to the type VII collagen gene. J Clin Invest 1992; 90:1032.

103. Dietz HC, Cutting GR, Pyeritz RE, et al. Marfan syndrome caused by a recurrent de novo missense mutation in the fibrillin gene. Nature 1991; 352:337.

104. Sakai LY, Keene DR, Engvall E. Fibrillin, a new 350-kDa glycoprotein, is a component of extracellular microfibrils. J Cell Biol 1986; 103:2499.

105. Zhang H, Hu W, Ramirez F. Developmental expression of fibrillin genes suggests heterogeneity of extracellular microfibrils. N Engl J Med 1999; 340(17):1307.

106. Pyeritz RE, McKusick VA. The Marfan syndrome: diagnosis and management. N Engl J Med 1979; 300:772.

107. De Paepe A, Devereux RB, Dietz HC, et al. Revised diagnostic criteria for the Marfan syndrome. Am J Med Genet 1996; 62:417.

108. Maumenee IH. The eye in the Marfan syndrome. Trans Am Ophthalmol Soc 1981; 79:684.

109. Pyeritz RE, Wappel MA. Mitral valve dysfunction in the Marfan syndrome. Am J Med 1983; 74:797.

110. Gott VL, Greene PS, Alejo DE, et al. Replacement of the aortic root in patients with Marfan's syndrome. N Engl J Med 1999; 340:1307.

111. Godfrey M, Menashe V, Weleber RG, et al. Cosegregation of elastin-associated microfibrillar abnormalities with the Marfan phenotype in families. Am J Hum Genet 1990; 46:652.

112. Kainulainen K, Pulkkinen L, Savolainen A, et al. Location on chromosome 15 of the gene defect causing Marfan syndrome. N Engl J Med 1990; 323:935.

113. Milewicz DM, Pyeritz RE, Crawford ES, Byers PH. Marfan syndrome: defective synthesis, secretion, and extracellular matrix formation of fibrillin by cultured dermal fibroblasts. J Clin Invest 1992; 89:79.

114. Lee B, Godfrey M, Vitale E, et al. Linkage of Marfan syndrome and a phenotypically related disorder to two different fibrillin genes. Nature 1991; 352(6333):330.

115. Collod-Beroud G, Beroud C, Ades L, et al. Marfan Database (third edition): new mutations and new routines for the software. Nucleic Acids Res 1998; 26:229.

116. Shores J, Berger KR, Murphy EA, Pyeritz RE. Progression of aortic dilatation and the benefit of long-term beta-adrenergic blockade in Marfan's syndrome. N Engl J Med 1994; 330:1335.

117. Park ES, Putnam EA, Chitayat D, et al. Clustering of FBN2 mutations in patients with congenital contractural arachnodactyly indicates an important role of the domains encoded by exons 24 through 34 during human development. Am J Med Genet 1998; 78:350.

118. Hayward C, Brock DJ. Fibrillin-1 mutations in Marfan syndrome and other type-1 fibrillinopathies. Hum Mutat 1997; 10:415.

# CHAPTER 190

# HERITABLE DISEASES OF LYSOSOMAL STORAGE

WARREN E. COHEN

## SPECTRUM OF LYSOSOMAL STORAGE DISEASES

At least 30, and possibly as many as 50, disorders of metabolism exist that cause the abnormal accumulation of metabolites in cell lysosomes. Although individually these disorders are rare, collectively they constitute a frequent cause of chronic illness and debilitation in childhood. The clinical manifestations of these disorders are diverse but they share a common pathogenesis, an insight into which requires a basic understanding of normal lysosomal function.

Lysosomes are organelles surrounded by a single membrane within which are packaged enzymes that normally degrade exogenous substances and the products of endogenous metabolism, and thus serve as the "waste disposal" system of the cell. Through this system of lysosomal enzymes, complex carbohydrates, lipids, and proteins are degraded sequentially. The enzymes of this system initially are synthesized in the endoplasmic reticulum. Multiple short oligosaccharide chains are then attached to them. They are further modified in the Golgi apparatus and eventually are packaged into lysosomes of various types, depending on the cell type and the particular metabolic pathway in which they will function.

Lysosomal storage disorders arise when a genetic defect causes deficient production or function of one or more of the lysosomal enzymes, with consequent abnormal accumulation of metabolites within the lysosome. The accumulation of these metabolites distends the lysosome and produces effects that are toxic to cell constituents. This disrupts normal cell function and eventually causes cell death. The clinical manifestations of any particular storage disorder are a consequence of the *specific enzyme or enzymes affected, the metabolic pathway in which they are involved, the alteration of cell function associated with abnormal lysosomal storage, and the particular tissues in which the affected enzymes normally function*. All lysosomal storage diseases are *progressive* because the process of lysosomal storage is continuous. Because many lysosomal enzymes participate in the metabolism of neural tissues, the *central and peripheral nervous systems* are affected in several of the lysosomal storage diseases, and this is manifest either by progressive psychomotor retardation or by any of various progressive neurologic signs and symptoms. The *diverse and multisystemic clinical manifestations* observed in these disorders demonstrate that normal lysosomal enzyme function is crucial to the health of many human tissues.

No simple clinical approach exists to the classification of this clinically diverse group of disorders. Thus, lysosomal storage disorders usually are classified not by their clinical manifestations, but rather according to the *nature of the macromolecule that is abnormally catabolized and consequently accumulates within the lysosome*. The *sphingolipidoses* are associated with the accumulation of complex lipids, the basic structure of which is sphingosine, a long-chain amino alcohol. The *mucopolysaccharidoses* (MPSs) are associated with the accumulation of complex protein-sugar macromolecules known as mucopolysaccharides or glycosaminoglycans. The *oligosaccharidoses* or *mucolipidoses* are associated with storage of complex glycoproteins. Within each of these biochemical categories is a diverse group of disorders, some with classically recognizable clinical and laboratory features and many with variant forms that are atypical in their clinical and biochemical findings[1-5] (Table 190-1). Increasingly, molecular genetic techniques are demonstrating the heterogeneity of lysosomal storage diseases. Many of the specific disorders that traditionally have been described by their clinical and biochemical features are now recognized to represent more than one genetic disorder. Some of this heterogeneity is explained by the fact that the same clinical and biochemical abnormality might result from the abnormal functioning of two or more different gene loci, but much of it may be due to different mechanisms of genetic mutation that result in varying degrees of dysfunction in a specific gene.[6]

# GANGLIOSIDOSES

## GM₁ GANGLIOSIDOSES

The GM₁ gangliosidoses are characterized by a deficiency of *GM₁ ganglioside β-galactosidase*, with the consequent accumulation of both GM₁ ganglioside and a keratan sulfate–like mucopolysaccharide.[7-10] Two classic clinical syndromes exist.

### INFANTILE GM₁ GANGLIOSIDOSIS

In infantile GM₁ gangliosidosis, symptoms usually are noted shortly after birth. Psychomotor retardation associated with hypotonia, poor suckling, lethargy, and hypoactivity are observed early. Weight gain is poor, and characteristic dysmorphic features appear early: frontal bossing, coarsened facial features, long philtrum, gingival hyperplasia, macroglossia, and, frequently, edema of the face and extremities. Visceral storage causes hepatosplenomegaly. Radiographs reveal characteristic changes in the spine and long bones. Over the first several months, the progressive psychomotor retardation becomes

more apparent, and the initial hypotonia gives way to spasticity with hyperreflexia and tonic spasms. A zone of retinal degeneration surrounding the normally red macula produces a macular cherry-red spot in approximately one-half of patients, but this may not be evident until after the age of 6 months. Slight corneal clouding may be present. Progression of the disorder renders the child deaf and blind, with decerebrate rigidity usually present by the age of 12 months; death usually occurs at approximately the age of 2 years.

### LATE INFANTILE GM₁ GANGLIOSIDOSIS

In late infantile GM₁ gangliosidosis, the symptoms do not manifest until the age of 1 to 2 years, when gait disturbance, ataxia, incoordination, and regression of language skills appear. As the disorder progresses, spasticity develops, and seizures frequently occur. These may become a difficult management problem. Unlike in the infantile form, the corneas are clear, no hepatosplenomegaly is present, and no significant bone changes are found on radiography. Abnormalities of cerebral cortex, white matter, and deep nuclei on magnetic resonance imaging have been reported.[11] Death usually occurs between the ages of 3 and 10 years, generally during an episode of pneumonia.

Several atypical variants of GM₁ gangliosidosis also have been described, including several with onset in later childhood.

## GM₂ GANGLIOSIDOSES

The GM₂ gangliosidoses are a group of disorders characterized by the inherited deficiency of the lysosomal enzyme *hexosaminidase*. The deficiency leads to an accumulation of GM₂ ganglioside, other glycosphingolipids, and various other metabolites.[10,12-16] The biochemical genetics of hexosaminidase function are complex because the activity of this enzyme involves at least two subunits, three isoenzymes, three gene loci, and at least one activator protein.[13] More than 20 forms of hexosaminidase deficiency are known.

**TABLE 190-1.**
**Clinical Aspects of Lysosomal Storage Disorders**

| Disease or Syndrome | Deficient Enzyme | Material Stored | Onset | Primary Organ Involvement | Comments |
|---|---|---|---|---|---|
| **GANGLIOSIDOSES** | | | | | |
| **Infantile GM₁** | β-galactosidase | GM₁ ganglioside | 6 mo–2 yr | CNS, liver, spleen, skeleton | PPMR, seizures, hepatosplenomegaly, cherry-red spot, spasticity, coarse facies, blindness, deafness |
| **Late infantile GM₁** | β-galactosidase | GM₁ ganglioside | 1–2 yr | CNS | PPMR, ataxia, incoordination, spasticity |
| **Tay-Sachs** | Hexosaminidase A | GM₂ ganglioside, other metabolites | 4–6 mo | CNS | PPMR, doll-like facies, macrocephaly, cherry-red spot, spasticity, blindness, seizures |
| **Sandhoff** | Hexosaminidase A or B | GM₂ ganglioside, other metabolites | 4–6 mo | CNS | PPMR, doll-like facies, macrocephaly, cherry-red spot, spasticity, blindness, seizures, mild hepatosplenomegaly |
| **GM₂ variants** | Hexosaminidase A, B, or both | GM₂ ganglioside, other metabolites | Varies | CNS, some PNS | Juvenile and adult onset; varied clinical presentations, including spinocerebellar degeneration, upper and lower motor neuron disease |
| **SPHINGOLIPIDOSES** | | | | | |
| **Gaucher type 1** | Glucocerebrosidase | Glucocerebroside | Varies | Spleen, liver, skeleton | Splenomegaly prominent, hepatomegaly, anemia, bone pain, characteristic radiographic bone changes, normal neurologic function |
| **Gaucher type 2** | Glucocerebrosidase | Glucocerebroside | 3–6 mo | CNS, spleen, liver, skeleton | Hepatosplenomegaly, PPMR, spasticity, cranial nerve dysfunction, seizures |
| **Gaucher type 3** | Glucocerebrosidase | Glucocerebroside | 6 mo–4 yr | CNS, spleen, liver, skeleton | Same as type 1, additionally with slowly progressive PPMR, ataxia, spasticity, seizures, oculomotor apraxia |
| **Niemann-Pick type A** | Sphingomyelinase | Sphingomyelin | 6 mo | CNS, liver, spleen | Failure to thrive, hepatosplenomegaly, PPMR, spasticity, cherry-red spot (50%), foam cells |
| **Niemann-Pick type B** | Sphingomyelinase | Sphingomyelin | | Liver, spleen, lungs | Hepatosplenomegaly, foam cells, normal neurologic function |

(continued)

**TABLE 190-1.**
**Clinical Aspects of Lysosomal Storage Disorders  (Continued)**

| Disease or Syndrome | Deficient Enzyme | Material Stored | Onset | Primary Organ Involvement | Comments |
|---|---|---|---|---|---|
| Niemann-Pick type C | ? | ? | 1–4 yr | CNS, liver, spleen | PPMR, hepatosplenomegaly, spasticity, ataxia, seizures, foam cells |
| Krabbe | Galactocerebrosidase | Galactocerebroside, psychosine | 0–6 mo | CNS, PNS | CNS and PNS demyelination, PPMR, irritability, spasticity, seizures, optic atrophy, blindness |
| Krabbe, atypical | Galactocerebrosidase | Galactocerebroside, psychosine | Varies | CNS, PNS | Variable clinical presentations, with PPMR, optic atrophy, spasticity, some with spinocerebellar degeneration |
| Metachromatic leukodystrophy | Arylsulfatase A | Cerebroside sulfate | 12–18 mo | CNS, PNS | CNS and PNS demyelination, PPMR, gait difficulty, spasticity mixed with signs of peripheral neuropathy |
| Metachromatic leukodystrophy, juvenile variant | Arylsulfatase A | Cerebroside sulfate | 3–16 yr | CNS, PNS | Behavioral difficulty, PPMR, gait difficulty, incontinence |
| Metachromatic leukodystrophy, adult variant | Arylsulfatase A | Cerebroside sulfate | 15+ yr | CNS, PNS | Emotional disturbance, PPMR, spasticity |
| Multiple sulfatase deficiency | Several sulfatases | Sulfate-containing glycolipids, MPS, and steroids | 1–2 yr | CNS, liver, spleen, skeleton | Coarse facies, dysostosis multiplex, hepatosplenomegaly, PPMR |
| Fabry | $\alpha$-Galactosidase A | Ceramide trihexoside | 4–5 yr | Skin, PNS, kidney, eye, cardiac vasculature, cerebral vasculature | Painful acrodysesthesias, angiokeratomas, corneal dystrophy, MI, CVA, hypertension, renal failure |
| **MUCOPOLYSACCHARIDOSES** | | | | | |
| Hurler (MPS IH) | $\alpha$-L-iduronidase | Dermatan sulfate, heparan sulfate | 1–2 yr | CNS, skeleton, liver, heart | PPMR, coarse facies, dysostosis multiplex, corneal clouding, deafness, heart failure, hepatosplenomegaly |
| Scheie (MPS IS) | $\alpha$-L-iduronidase | Dermatan sulfate, heparan sulfate | 2–7 yr | Eye, skeleton, heart | Corneal clouding, coarse facies, dysostosis multiplex, aortic valve disease, normal intellect |
| Hurler-Scheie (MPS IH/IS) | $\alpha$-L-iduronidase | Dermatan sulfate, heparan sulfate | 1–2 yr | Eye, skeleton, heart | Clinical features intermediate between those of MPS IH and MPS IS |
| Hunter (MPS II) | Iduronate sulfatase | Dermatan sulfate, heparan sulfate | 2–5 yr | CNS, skeleton, liver, heart | PPMR, coarse facies, dysostosis multiplex, nodular skin lesions, heart disease, hepatosplenomegaly |
| Sanfilippo (MPS III, types A, B, C, D) | Heparan N-sulfatase N-acetyl-$\alpha$-D-glucosaminidase<br><br>Acetyl coenzyme A: $\alpha$-glucosaminide-N-acetyl transferase<br><br>N-acetyl-$\alpha$-D-glucosaminide-6-sulfatase | Heparan sulfate | 2–3 yr | CNS, skeleton | PPMR, mild dysostosis multiplex, behavioral abnormalities, seizures |
| Morquio (MPS IV, types A, B) | Galactosamine-6-sulfate sulfatase $\beta$-galactosidase | Keratan sulfate | 1–2 yr | Skeleton | Characteristic skeletal changes, coarse facies, deafness, dental enamel hypoplasia, joint laxity, odontoid hypoplasia |
| Maroteaux-Lamy (MPS VI) | Arylsulfatase B | Dermatan sulfate | 2–3 yr | Skeleton | Coarse facies, dysostosis multiplex, corneal clouding |
| **MUCOLIPIDOSES** | | | | | |
| Sialidosis type I | $\alpha$-Neuraminidase | Sialyloligosaccharides | 8–25 yr | CNS, PNS, eye | Seizures, myoclonus, visual impairment, cherry-red spot, peripheral neuropathy |
| Sialidosis type II | $\alpha$-Neuraminidase | Sialyloligosaccharides | Varies | CNS, eye, skin | PPMR, coarse facies, dysostosis multiplex, visual impairment, cherry-red spot, angiokeratomas |
| Mannosidosis | Mannosidase | Oligosaccharides | 0–4 yr | CNS, eye, skeleton | PPMR, coarse facies, dysostosis multiplex, lenticular or corneal opacity, hepatosplenomegaly |
| Fucosidosis types I, II | Fucosidase | Oligosaccharides, sphingolipids | 0–2 yr | CNS, skeleton, liver, spleen | PPMR, coarse facies, dysostosis multiplex, hepatosplenomegaly, angiokeratomas |
| Aspartylglycosaminuria | Aspartyl-glycosaminidase | Glycoasparagines | 1–5 yr | CNS, eye | PPMR, coarse facies, sagging skin, lens opacities |
| I-cell (ML II) | N-acetylglucosamine-1-P-transferase | | 0–6 mo | CNS, skeleton, heart | PPMR, coarse facies, dysostosis multiplex, heart failure |
| Pseudo-Hurler polydystrophy (ML III) | N-acetylglucosamine-1-P-transferase | | 4–5 yr | Skeleton, eye | Coarse facies, dysostosis multiplex, corneal clouding |
| Mucolipidosis IV (ML IV) | | Gangliosides, glycosaminoglycans | 0–1 yr | CNS, eye | PPMR, corneal clouding |

*CNS,* central nervous system; *PPMR,* progressive psychomotor retardation; *PNS,* peripheral nervous system; *MI,* myocardial infarction; *CVA,* cerebrovascular accident; *MPS,* mucopolysaccharidosis; *ML,* mucolipidosis.

### TAY-SACHS DISEASE

Previously, the most common form of hexosaminidase deficiency was Tay-Sachs disease, a disorder that has become uncommon because of a widespread carrier detection program targeted at a well-defined population at risk for the disorder. Approximately 1 in 30 Jews of Eastern European (Ashkenazi) heritage are carriers of the autosomal recessive trait. Affected children with this disorder are deficient in *hexosaminidase A* and *hexosaminidase S*. They appear healthy during the first 4 to 6 months of life, after which signs of psychomotor deterioration appear. The earliest signs usually are hypotonia and inability to sit, followed by more obvious signs of regression of motor skills. An abnormal motor response to stimulation by sound and sometimes by light is characteristic of the disorder, appearing as an exaggerated infantile startle response. As the disorder progresses, weakness increases, and spasticity and hyperreflexia develop. A macular cherry-red spot is seen in 90% of cases, and by 12 to 18 months, severe visual impairment is present, with eventual blindness. During the second year, the intraneural accumulation of storage material leads to marked enlargement of the brain, reflected by markedly accelerated growth of the head circumference. Seizures occur; they may be generalized, minor motor, or myoclonic in character. By the age of 3 years, the child usually appears debilitated, with decerebrate rigidity, dementia, marked macrocephaly, blindness, and seizures. Most affected children die between the ages of 3 and 5 years; a few have survived longer.

### SANDHOFF DISEASE

Children with Sandhoff disease are deficient in *hexosaminidase A* and *hexosaminidase B*. The clinical picture is almost identical to that of infantile Tay-Sachs disease, but many children with Sandhoff disease also manifest moderate hepatosplenomegaly—a sign absent in Tay-Sachs disease. This disorder is rarer than Tay-Sachs disease and has no ethnic predilection.

### OTHER VARIETIES

Other variants of Tay-Sachs disease include disorders with onset in infancy, childhood, and adulthood.[14] Patients have been described with various symptom complexes, including a juvenile-onset disorder with manifestations similar to infantile Tay-Sachs, with blindness, seizures, and progressive psychomotor retardation. Molecular studies have demonstrated that the gene responsible for the juvenile disorder is allelic to the gene responsible for infantile Tay-Sachs disease.[15] Other such disorders include a disorder appearing as spinocerebellar degeneration, a disorder with a clinical picture resembling that of isolated lower motor neuron disease (similar to Kugelberg-Welander disease), and a disorder with signs of both upper and lower motor neuron dysfunction that resembles amyotrophic lateral sclerosis. Some individuals with hexosaminidase deficiency have no symptoms. Because of the wide variation of clinical manifestations in these disorders, a reasonable approach is to consider the possibility of hexosaminidase deficiency in virtually any individual with an unexplained degenerative neurologic disorder.

# SPHINGOLIPIDOSES

## GAUCHER DISEASE

Gaucher disease is a group of sphingolipidoses characterized by a deficiency of *glucocerebrosidase* with the consequent accumulation of glucocerebroside in body tissues.[17,18] The disorder is multisystemic and affects tissue macrophages of the reticuloendothelial system, primarily in the spleen, liver, bone, and lung. Macrophages in these tissues become laden with lipid, giving them a characteristic light-microscopic appearance ("Gaucher cells").

### TYPE 1 GAUCHER DISEASE

Type 1 Gaucher disease is by far the most common of the lysosomal storage disorders. Previously it was designated the "adult" form of Gaucher disease, but the onset of symptoms may be in childhood or adulthood, and many patients have no symptoms. Splenomegaly is the usual initial symptom; it may be associated with various degrees of anemia, thrombocytopenia, and leukopenia. Hepatomegaly usually is not as prominent and may appear later in the disease course. Any hepatic dysfunction usually is mild. Skeletal involvement produces various bone complications. Many patients experience episodes of severe bone pain similar to the crises of sickle cell disease. These episodes may be associated with fever and local swelling, erythema, and tenderness, and may be mistaken for osteomyelitis. Nonspecific chronic, mild joint pain is a common complaint. Other bone complications include a propensity to develop multiple fractures, vertebral collapse, and aseptic necrosis of the femoral head. Radiographs reveal osteopenia, cortical thinning, endosteal scalloping, cyst-like cavities, and characteristic Erlenmeyer-flask deformities of the distal femurs. Pulmonary complications are much less common and result from interstitial pulmonary infiltration. In those few patients who manifest severe liver dysfunction, associated pulmonary complications with intrapulmonary shunting occur. Patients with type 1 Gaucher disease exhibit no clinical signs of neurologic dysfunction. The clinical course of type 1 Gaucher disease is extremely variable. Most patients are affected only mildly; they may lead normal, productive lives, with minimal to mild disability and with normal longevity. Others may be severely debilitated, and death may occur in childhood. An increased incidence of multiple myeloma, leukemia, and Hodgkin disease is found among individuals with this disorder. Intravenous enzyme replacement therapy, using a modified form of the deficient enzyme that has been engineered to maximize cellular uptake, has been successful in treating the hematopoietic, hepatic, and skeletal abnormalities associated with type 1 Gaucher disease.[19]

### TYPE 2 GAUCHER DISEASE

Type 2 Gaucher disease has a characteristic clinical course. It was previously designated the "infantile" form of the disorder, and the age of onset usually is between 3 and 6 months. Hepatosplenomegaly is noted initially, followed by signs of neurologic dysfunction. The classic clinical triad of symptoms consists of trismus, strabismus, and head retroflexion. Spastic quadriparesis progresses rapidly, with associated hyperreflexia, cranial nerve dysfunction, and dysphagia. Seizures may occur but are not a common complication. As the disorder progresses, the child becomes hypotonic, lethargic, and apathetic. Most children die by the age of 1 year, and virtually none survive beyond the age of 2 years.

### TYPE 3 GAUCHER DISEASE

Type 3 Gaucher disease has characteristics intermediate between those of types 1 and 2, but the clinical presentation can be variable. Systemic complications are similar to those of type 1 Gaucher disease but in general may be more severe. Neurologic complications are of later onset and progress more slowly. They include ataxia, incoordination, myoclonus, seizures, a characteristic oculomotor apraxia (supranuclear eye movement disorder), and slowly progressive dementia.

### NIEMANN-PICK DISEASE

Niemann-Pick disease is a group of disorders characterized by the abnormal accumulation of sphingomyelin.[20–22] In two of the forms of the disorder, a deficiency of the lysosomal enzyme *sphingomyelinase* is found. In other variant forms, the nature of the biochemical abnormality is unclear.

### TYPE A NIEMANN-PICK DISEASE

Types A and B Niemann-Pick disease are associated with deficient sphingomyelinase activity. Type A disease is characterized by hepatosplenomegaly, which usually develops by the age of 6 months. It frequently is associated with failure to thrive. The enlargement of the liver precedes and is more prominent than enlargement of the spleen. Progressive neurologic deterioration ensues, with a loss of motor and cognitive skills, axial hypotonia coexistent with spasticity of the extremities, dysphagia, and blindness. A cherry-red macular spot is seen in approximately one-half the cases. As the disorder progresses, the child becomes increasingly cachectic, rigid, and opisthotonic. Foam cells (vacuolated histiocytes) are found in the bone marrow, peripheral blood, and other tissues, and are of diagnostic importance. Death usually occurs by the age of 3 years and frequently ensues after fulminant hepatic failure.

### OTHER TYPES OF NIEMANN-PICK DISEASE

In type B Niemann-Pick disease, hepatosplenomegaly becomes apparent in infancy or childhood. The nervous system is not involved, and no neurologic symptoms are present.

Other clinical forms that have been categorized as variants of Niemann-Pick disease are poorly understood. *Type C* is characterized by onset of mild hepatosplenomegaly in infancy or childhood associated with slowly progressive ataxia, dementia, and seizures. The disorder can be associated with childhood narcolepsy.[23] Foam cells are found in bone and liver biopsy specimens. Most affected patients die by the age of 20 years. A similar disorder, which is limited geographically to a coastal area in western Nova Scotia, has been designated *type D* disease. A few reported patients with visceral storage and foam cells have been designated as having *type E* Niemann-Pick disease. The biochemical defect in type C is caused by defective intracellular transport of exogenous cholesterol, resulting in the accumulation of unesterified cholesterol in the lysosome.[24]

### KRABBE DISEASE

Krabbe disease, or globoid cell leukodystrophy, is characterized by a deficiency of *galactocerebroside β-galactosidase*, which causes extensive demyelination of the central and peripheral nervous systems.[25–27] Neurologic symptoms usually are apparent by the age of 6 months, and some patients have symptoms at birth. In the classic disorder, the initial symptoms include hyperirritability and inexplicable crying, with episodes of tonic stiffening. Progressive development of spasticity is seen, and seizures frequently occur. Hyperreflexia, optic atrophy, opisthotonic posturing, and an arrest of head growth are noted, and deafness may occur. Tendon reflexes are diminished early in the course secondary to the peripheral neuropathy; later, the reflexes become hyperreactive. Nerve conduction velocities are delayed, and the cerebrospinal fluid protein level is elevated. No signs of visceral storage are seen. Late in the course, the child appears decerebrate, blind, and unresponsive to stimuli. Most affected children die by the age of 1 year, and virtually all die by the age of 2 years.

Several atypical clinical presentations have been reported, including later-onset forms featuring dementia, spasticity, and optic atrophy, as well as a late-onset disorder with spinocerebellar degeneration.

## METACHROMATIC LEUKODYSTROPHY

Metachromatic leukodystrophy is another disorder of myelin metabolism. It is caused by a deficiency of the lysosomal enzyme *arylsulfatase A* and is associated with the accumulation of cerebroside sulfate.[28–31] This disorder probably is the most common of the inherited leukodystrophies, which include disorders of lysosomal metabolism, disorders of peroxisomal metabolism, and disorders of uncertain etiology. In the classic disorder, affected children usually appear normal until the age of 12 to 18 months, at which time difficulty of gait becomes apparent. The initial signs and symptoms may differ depending on the balance of the effects of pyramidal tract dysfunction and of peripheral neuropathy. Some children have flaccid paraparesis and hyporeflexia, others have spasticity and hyporeflexia, and the remainder have spasticity and hyperreflexia. The onset of spastic weakness may be abrupt and asymmetric. As the disorder progresses, spastic quadriparesis and dementia ensue, and dysarthria and dysphagia are frequent problems. Visual impairment may occur, and various ophthalmologic findings may be present. Approximately one-third of patients have optic atrophy. Some individuals have a characteristic grayish discoloration of the macula, whereas others have a macular cherry-red spot. At the end stages of the disease, the child appears decerebrate, often with sensory-induced tonic spasms, pseudobulbar signs, and unresponsiveness. Death ensues after a course of several years. Bone marrow transplantation appears to slow the progression of the disease, but often the risks of the procedure outweigh the potential benefits by the time the diagnosis is made.

Several variant forms of metachromatic leukodystrophy have been described on clinical and biochemical grounds. In juvenile metachromatic leukodystrophy, symptoms appear between the ages of 3 and 16 years. In this disorder, school-age children frequently have behavioral abnormalities followed by incontinence and gait difficulty. The disorder progresses rapidly and renders the children debilitated, with spastic paraparesis, dementia, pseudobulbar signs, and tonic spasms. Most of these children die during the teenage years. In adult metachromatic leukodystrophy, progressive neurologic dysfunction often is heralded by behavioral and emotional abnormalities that frequently are mistaken for psychiatric illness. This form of the disease also is relentlessly progressive, ending in death after a variable period of neurologic deterioration.

Two biochemical variants of metachromatic leukodystrophy are important to note. In the rare disorder of multiple sulfatase deficiency, nine lysosomal sulfatases, including *arylsulfatase A*, are deficient. The clinical manifestations include features of late infantile metachromatic leukodystrophy and also of the mucopolysaccharide disorders, with coarse facial features, skeletal abnormalities, and hepatosplenomegaly. Finally, in a few patients with clinical and histopathologic features of metachromatic leukodystrophy, no deficiency of arylsulfatase A can be demonstrated. These patients lack an activator protein, saposin B, which is required for that enzyme to function.

## FABRY DISEASE

Fabry disease is a rare disorder characterized by a deficiency of α-*galactocerebrosidase A*, with the consequent accumulation of ceramide trihexoside in tissues.[32–34] This multisystemic disorder is transmitted as an X-linked recessive trait, but symptoms frequently occur in carrier females. A characteristic initial symptom is peculiar painful acrodysesthesias. Patients complain of severe pain of the hands and feet, often triggered during febrile illnesses or by exercise or exposure to heat. The pain can be debilitating and, because of its peculiar nature, often is attributed to a psychiatric disorder. The pain frequently responds to therapy with phenytoin sodium (Dilantin) or carbamazepine (Tegretol). Other clinical findings include angiokeratomas and a characteristic corneal dystrophy that is evident on slit-lamp examination. Vascular changes in the conjunctiva and retina also occur. The more serious complications of the disorder include angina and myocardial infarction, and progressive renal failure. Hemodialysis and renal transplantation have become lifesaving procedures for affected individuals. Neurologic complications do not arise secondary to intraneuronal storage, as seen in other lysosomal disorders, but rather due to cerebrovascular disease, which causes recurrent strokes. Death usually ensues at approximately the age of 40 years in affected males, but longer survival has been reported.

## MUCOPOLYSACCHARIDOSES

The MPSs are a heterogeneous group of disorders characterized by a deficiency of the enzymes involved in the catabolism of complex carbohydrate polymers called *glycosaminoglycans*.[35–43] These substances occur in large amounts in connective tissue of cartilage, bone, blood vessels, heart valves, skin, tendons, and cornea, and in lesser amounts in liver and brain. Thus, in storage disorders in which glycosaminoglycans accumulate, various multisystemic manifestations occur.

### HURLER SYNDROME

Hurler syndrome (MPS IH), the prototype of the MPS disorders, is characterized by a deficiency of α-L-*iduronidase*, which leads to the accumulation of dermatan sulfate and heparan sulfate. It is the most severe and most rapidly progressive of this group of disorders, usually resulting in death by the age of 10 years. After an initial period of normal development in infancy, affected children begin to display signs of progressive dementia, with the loss of previously acquired cognitive skills. Characteristic physical features develop with time and include coarse facies, macroscaphocephaly, sagittal sutural ridging, corneal clouding, prominent abdomen, hepatosplenomegaly, umbilical hernias, and thickened skin (Fig. 190-1). Skeletal involvement produces a characteristic

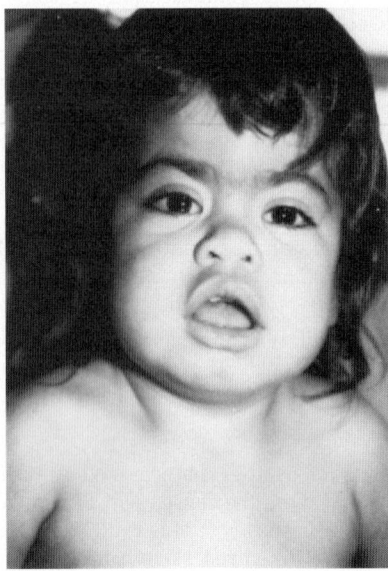

**FIGURE 190-1.** Hurler syndrome (mucopolysaccharidosis I) in a 17-month-old girl, who shows typical coarsening of facial features characteristic of several of the disorders of mucopolysaccharide metabolism. Although the classic "gargoyle" facial appearance often depicted in photographs of individuals with Hurler syndrome is usually more striking, this child's features are typical for a toddler with the disorder.

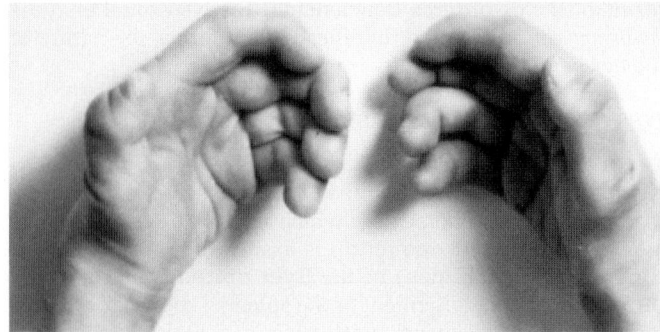

**FIGURE 190-2.** Claw-hand deformity of woman with Scheie syndrome (mucopolysaccharidosis IS). This progressive hand deformity is typical of that seen in several of the mucopolysaccharidoses and is extremely disabling.

clinical and radiographic picture that has been termed *dysostosis multiplex*. Clinical features of dysostosis include short stature, lumbar lordosis, thoracolumbar gibbus deformity, and joint stiffness, with claw-hand deformity (Fig. 190-2) and flexion contractures at the hips. Radiographic findings include hypoplastic vertebrae at the gibbus deformity with a broad-hook appearance, flaring of the iliac wings of the pelvis, coxa valga deformities, oar-shaped widened ribs, an absence of diaphyseal constriction of metacarpals, and widened shafts of the long bones. Neurologic complications include progressive dementia, seizures, spasticity, entrapment neuropathies (especially carpal tunnel syndrome), arachnoid cysts, sensorineural deafness, optic atrophy, and retinitis pigmentosa. The deposition of storage material in the meninges overlying the cerebral hemispheres frequently causes hydrocephalus, and a similar deposition in the meninges around the cervical spine causes the syndrome of pachymeningitis cervicalis circumscripta, with resultant spinal cord compression or nerve root involvement.

### SCHEIE SYNDROME

Scheie syndrome (MPS IS) is associated with the same enzyme deficiency as that in Hurler syndrome (α-L-iduronidase). MPS IS probably represents a different mutation at the same structural enzyme locus. Affected individuals have short stature, with coarse facies and signs of dysostosis multiplex. Visual impairment occurs because of severe corneal clouding, retinal pigmentary degeneration, and glaucoma. Cardiac involvement causes aortic stenosis, aortic regurgitation, or both. Neurologic complications include entrapment neuropathies, sensorineural deafness, and pachymeningitis cervicalis circumscripta. Intelligence is unaffected.

A variant of the α-iduronidase deficiency states is the *Hurler-Scheie syndrome (MPS IH/IS)*. Children with this disorder have clinical manifestations intermediate between those of the Hurler and Scheie syndromes.

### HUNTER SYNDROME

Hunter syndrome is associated with deficiency of the lysosomal enzyme *iduronidate sulfatase*, with accumulation of dermatan sulfate and heparan sulfate in body tissues. A broad range of severity is seen among children with this disorder, and affected individuals are loosely categorized as having either the "severe" or the "mild" form of the disorder. Features are similar to those seen in Hurler syndrome but generally are less severe, and survival is longer. Clinical features include dementia that usually is milder and less rapidly progressive than in Hurler syndrome, short stature, a characteristic pebbled appearance of the skin, coarse facies, hepatosplenomegaly, umbilical hernias, and dysostosis multiplex.

## SANFILIPPO SYNDROME

Sanfilippo syndrome (MPS III) is a clinically homogeneous group of disorders that are caused by four distinct deficiency states involving the following enzymes: *heparan-sulfate sulfatase* (type A); *N-acetyl-α-D-glucosaminidase* (type B); *N-acetyl-CoA acetyltransferase* (type C); and *N-acetylglucosamine-6-sulfate sulfatase* (type D).

The clinical course begins with a variable period of normal psychomotor development (usually 18 to 24 months) followed by a slowing, and then a plateau, of developmental progress. Normal development may be preserved for as long as 5 to 9 years. After the plateau of developmental progress is reached, a rapid mental deterioration ensues, usually with an onset between the ages of 3 and 5 years. Mental deterioration often is heralded by behavioral difficulties and sleep abnormalities and is rapidly progressive, with a rapid loss of language abilities. Physical signs, which usually are not striking, may include mild coarsening of the features, coarse hair, hirsutism, and macrocephaly. Mild dwarfing of stature and some radiographic signs of dysostosis multiplex are present. Seizures occur commonly.

## MORQUIO SYNDROME

Morquio syndrome (MPS IV) consists of two similar disorders characterized by a deficiency of *galactosamine-6-sulfate sulfatase* (type A) or *β-galactosidase* (type B). These disorders are manifest almost exclusively in the skeleton and through the secondary effects of these skeletal changes on the spinal cord. Intelligence usually is normal. Marked dwarfing of stature occurs, mild corneal clouding is present, and progressive deafness is almost invariable.

The skeleton is affected in a characteristic manner. Restricted joint movement and claw-hand deformities do not occur; several joints (especially the wrists) are excessively loose secondary to ligamentous laxity. The odontoid process is characteristically absent or markedly hypoplastic, and this, combined with laxity and redundancy of the paraspinal ligaments, causes cervical myelopathy secondary to atlantoaxial subluxation. This serious complication can be prevented by cervical spine fusion, which should be considered in all patients with the disorder.

## MAROTEAUX-LAMY SYNDROME

Maroteaux-Lamy syndrome (MPS VI) is characterized by a deficiency of *arylsulfatase B* and manifests clinically, in the severe or classic form, with coarse facial features, corneal clouding, short stature, and dysostosis multiplex with claw-hand deformity (Fig. 190-3). The course may be complicated by heart valve involvement, atlantoaxial subluxation, or hydrocephalus. Mental retardation is not associated with this disorder except as a complication of untreated hydrocephalus. Several patients have been reported with only mild features of the disorder.

## OTHER MUCOPOLYSACCHARIDOSES

Two other MPSs, *Sly syndrome (MPS VII)* and *DiFerrante syndrome (MPS VIII)*, are so rare that they are of no practical clinical importance.

## OLIGOSACCHARIDOSES (MUCOLIPIDOSES)

### SIALIDOSIS

Sialidosis constitutes a rare group of disorders associated with a deficiency of *N-acetylneuraminidase (sialidase)*, with the excretion of oligosaccharides containing sialic acid in the urine. The clinical

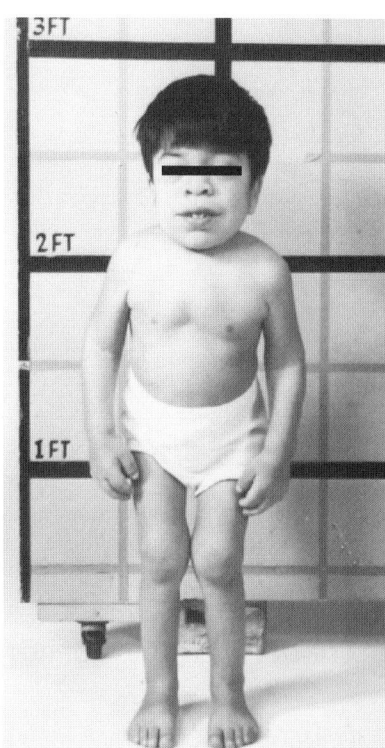

**FIGURE 190-3.** Eight-year-old boy with Maroteaux-Lamy syndrome (mucopolysaccharidosis VI). Note the coarsened facial features, extremely short stature, and claw-hand deformities. Mental retardation is not a feature of this disorder.

manifestations are variable,[44,45] and two classic syndromes have been delineated. In sialidosis type I, also known as the *cherry-red spot/myoclonus syndrome*, symptoms begin in adolescence, with progressive impairment of vision, a macular cherry-red spot, and severe myoclonus.[46] In sialidosis type II, symptoms begin in early or late childhood, with coarsened features suggestive of Hurler syndrome, dysostosis multiplex, hepatomegaly, and intellectual impairment.

### MANNOSIDOSIS

Mannosidosis is a rare disorder associated with a deficiency of *α-mannosidase*, with the excretion of oligosaccharides containing mannose in the urine.[45,47] The clinical features include mental retardation, coarsened facial features, dysostosis multiplex, hepatosplenomegaly, deafness, and recurrent infections.

### FUCOSIDOSIS

Fucosidosis is a heterogeneous group of rare disorders associated with a deficiency of *α-fucosidase*.[45,47] In fucosidosis type I, symptoms begin in infancy, with progressive psychomotor retardation, coarse facial features, hepatosplenomegaly, dysostosis multiplex, and seizures. In fucosidosis type II, the onset is in late childhood or adolescence, with progressive dementia, coarsened features, dysostosis multiplex, and skin changes; angiokeratomas similar to those seen in Fabry disease are present (Fig. 190-4).

### ASPARTYLGLYCOSAMINURIA

Aspartylglycosaminuria is a rare disorder associated with a deficiency of *N-aspartyl-β-glucosaminidase*.[45] The clinical features include mental retardation, behavioral difficulties, coarse facies, thickened and sagging skin, crystalline lens opacities, and a

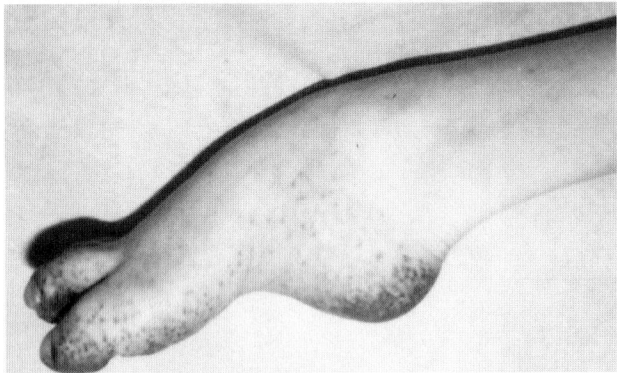

**FIGURE 190-4.** Typical angiokeratoma skin lesions in a boy with fucosidosis. The lesions are similar to those seen in Fabry disease.

slow course, with survival well into adulthood. The gene is common among the people of Finland, where this otherwise extremely rare disorder represents the third most common genetic cause of mental retardation.[48]

## CARBOHYDRATE-DEFICIENT GLYCOPROTEIN SYNDROME

Carbohydrate-deficient glycoprotein syndrome is a rare (though probably underdiagnosed) disorder for which the exact biochemical and molecular defects are not yet known. Clinical features include progressive psychomotor retardation, lipocutaneous abnormalities, liver dysfunction, retinal degeneration, episodic stupor or stroke-like events, and cerebellar hypoplasia.[49]

## I-CELL DISEASE (MUCOLIPIDOSIS II)

I-cell disease is associated with a deficiency of *N-acetylglucosamine 1-phosphotransferase*, an enzyme normally involved in the phosphorylation of mannose to newly synthesized lysosomal enzymes.[47,49,51–53] The result is that several lysosomal enzymes are deficient functionally because they have not undergone normal posttranslational modification. The incompletely modified enzymes are secreted rather than incorporated into lysosomes, and this causes a state of deficiency of multiple lysosomal enzymes. Symptoms arise during the first year of life, and the infant shows coarse features, dysostosis multiplex, joint contractures, gingival hyperplasia, and progressive psychomotor retardation (Fig. 190-5). Death usually occurs by the age of 5 years. The disorder is named for the characteristic inclusions seen on phase-contrast microscopy of cultured fibroblasts (inclusion cells).

## PSEUDO–HURLER POLYDYSTROPHY (MUCOLIPIDOSIS III)

The biochemical abnormality in pseudo-Hurler polydystrophy (mucolipidosis III) is similar to that in I-cell disease, but the clinical findings are different.[52] Affected individuals develop joint stiffness by the age of 4 to 5 years, with dysostosis multiplex, coarsened facial features, corneal clouding, and aortic or mitral valve disease. Intelligence may be normal or mildly impaired.

## MUCOLIPIDOSIS IV

The precise nature of the biochemical abnormality in mucolipidosis IV is unclear.[54] Affected children have corneal clouding and progressive psychomotor retardation. The diagnosis can be

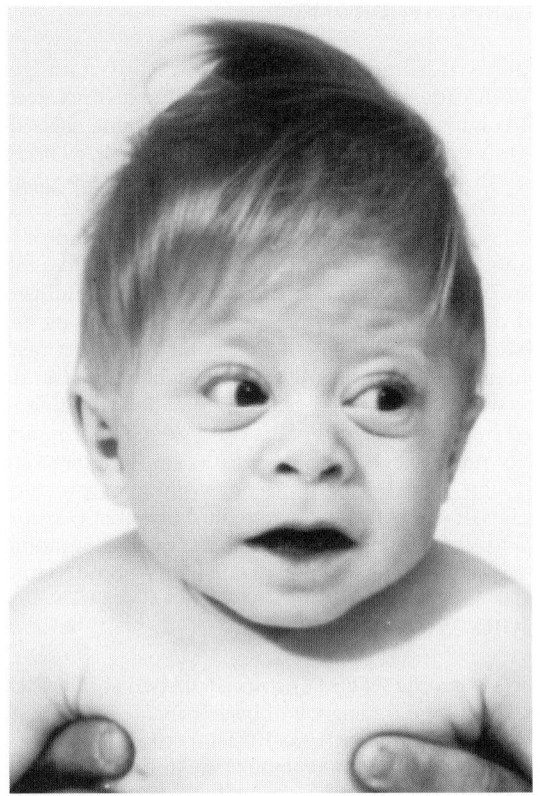

**FIGURE 190-5.** Eleven-month-old girl with I-cell disease (mucolipidosis II). Note the periorbital fullness and coarsened facial features, which, unlike those seen in the mucopolysaccharidoses, are evident during early infancy.

made by identification of the characteristic cytoplasmic inclusions in biopsy samples of the conjunctiva or the skin and also in histiocytes of aspirated bone marrow.

## DIAGNOSTIC CONSIDERATIONS

There is no simple, practical approach to the diagnostic evaluation of children in whom disorders of lysosomal metabolism are suspected. The laboratory evaluation of lysosomal enzyme function is tedious, expensive, and not widely available.[55] Therefore, a rational approach to these disorders involves the judicious use of diagnostic tests.[5] The tests frequently used in the diagnosis of lysosomal storage disorders are *skeletal radiography* (dysostosis multiplex), *nerve conduction velocity testing* (peripheral neuropathy), *ophthalmologic evaluation* (corneal clouding, macular changes), *neuropsychological testing* (psychomotor retardation), *urine mucopolysaccharide measurement*[56] (screening examination for several of the MPS disorders), *urine oligosaccharide measurement* (screening examination for several of the mucolipidoses), *electron microscopy of biopsy samples* (of skin, conjunctiva, rectal mucosa, liver), and *specific enzyme assays* (of leukocytes or skin fibroblasts).

The diagnostic evaluation must begin with a careful history and physical examination by an examiner experienced with these disorders. Using the historical and physical findings, a differential diagnosis usually can be attained based on the major features of the disorder, including the age of onset of symptoms and the cardinal clinical features (Table 190-2). Frequently, and especially in children with progressive neurologic deterioration, nonlysosomal disorders also must be considered in the differential diagnosis. Screening tests then can be used to narrow the scope of diagnostic possibilities (e.g., urine screening tests for muco-

**TABLE 190-2.**
**Diagnostic Considerations According to Symptom Complex**

**SEIZURES**
GM$_1$ gangliosidosis (infantile, late infantile)
Tay-Sachs disease
Sandhoff disease
Juvenile GM$_2$ gangliosidosis
Gaucher disease (types 2, 3)
Hurler syndrome
Hunter syndrome
Sanfilippo syndrome

**HEPATOSPLENOMEGALY**
GM$_1$ gangliosidosis (infantile)
Gaucher disease (types 1, 2, 3)
Sandhoff disease
Niemann-Pick disease (types A, B, C, D)
Hurler syndrome
Hunter syndrome
Mannosidosis
Fucosidosis

**COARSE FEATURES**
GM$_1$ gangliosidosis
Hurler syndrome
Hurler-Scheie syndrome
Hunter syndrome
Sanfilippo syndrome
Morquio syndrome
Sialidosis type II
Mannosidosis
Fucosidosis
Aspartylglycosaminuria
I-cell disease

**PROGRESSIVE PSYCHOMO-TOR RETARDATION**
GM$_1$ gangliosidosis (infantile, late infantile)
Tay-Sachs disease, Sandhoff disease, Gaucher disease (types 2, 3)
Niemann-Pick disease (types A, C, D)
Krabbe disease, metachromatic leukodystrophy, multiple sulfatase deficiency
Hurler, Hunter, Sanfilippo syndromes
Sialidosis type II
Mannosidosis, fucosidosis, aspartylglycosaminuria
I-cell disease, mucolipidosis IV

**PERIPHERAL NEUROPATHY**
Some GM$_2$ gangliosidosis variants
Krabbe disease
Metachromatic leukodystrophy
Fabry disease
Sialidosis type I

**ENTRAPMENT NEUROPATHIES**
Hurler disease
Hunter disease
Scheie disease
Pseudo–Hurler polydystrophy

**CHERRY-RED MACULAR SPOTS**
GM$_1$ gangliosidosis (infantile)
Tay-Sachs disease
Sandhoff disease
Niemann-Pick type A
Sialidosis (types I, II)
Metachromatic leukodystrophy
Multiple sulfatase deficiency

**DYSOSTOSIS MULTIPLEX**
GM$_1$ gangliosidosis (infantile)
Multiple sulfatase deficiency
Hurler disease
Hunter disease
Hurler-Scheie syndrome
Sanfilippo syndrome
Maroteaux-Lamy disease
Sialidosis type II
Fucosidosis (types I, II)
Mannosidosis
I-cell disease
Pseudo–Hurler polydystrophy

**MACROCEPHALY**
Tay-Sachs disease
Sandhoff disease
Hurler disease
Hunter disease

**EXAGGERATED STARTLE RESPONSE**
Tay-Sachs disease
Sandhoff disease
Juvenile GM$_2$ gangliosidosis
GM$_1$ gangliosidosis (infantile, late infantile)

**BLINDNESS**
GM$_1$ gangliosidosis (infantile, late infantile)
Tay-Sachs disease
Sandhoff disease
Juvenile GM$_2$ gangliosidosis
Sialidosis

**DEAFNESS**
GM$_1$ gangliosidosis (infantile)
Tay-Sachs disease
Hurler disease
Hurler-Scheie syndrome
Hunter disease
Morquio disease

**CORNEAL CLOUDING**
GM$_1$ gangliosidosis (infantile)
Hurler disease
Scheie disease
Hurler-Scheie disease
Morquio disease
Maroteaux-Lamy disease
Mannosidosis
Pseudo–Hurler polydystrophy
Mucolipidosis IV

---

polysaccharide excretion), and other procedures, such as a thorough ophthalmologic examination and radiographic evaluation, may be indicated. A particularly useful screening test is electron microscopic examination of biopsy material from skin, conjunctiva, or rectal mucosa for evidence of intralysosomal storage.

A definitive diagnosis rests on the laboratory demonstration of deficient activity of the specific lysosomal enzyme. This type of study should be performed only in qualified laboratories, where experience and careful controls enhance the validity of the findings. The diagnostician always must keep in mind that patients with these disorders often have unique clinical and biochemical findings. Finally, the use of molecular genetic analysis is becoming increasingly available to identify specific genetic mutations in many of the lysosomal disorders, and this can be a useful clinical tool, particularly when specific mutations correlate with clinical symptoms.

## MANAGEMENT ISSUES

A common misconception is that patients with "incurable" disorders such as the lysosomal storage disorders require no therapy. These patients present management problems that are among the most challenging in all of medical practice. Providing the parents of these affected children with the appropriate guidance, prognostic information, and emotional support to help them through what frequently is a lengthy and difficult struggle is a tremendous undertaking. Issues that are crucial to the care of patients with these disorders include control and management of seizures, feeding difficulties and nutritional disorders, hydrocephalus, joint contractures, pneumonia, urinary tract infections, hematologic abnormalities, orthopedic complications, spinal cord compression, peripheral nerve entrapment, chronic pain, visual and auditory impairment, sleep apnea, cardiovascular disease, cerebrovascular disease, renal failure, and hepatic failure, just to cite a few. The accomplishment of effective enzyme-replacement therapy for Gaucher disease is encouraging and may be a model for the future development of similar therapeutic interventions for the other lysosomal disorders.[57,58] The greatest challenge in the development of such interventions is how to deliver replacement enzyme across the blood–brain barrier to the cells of the brain, where most of the deleterious effects of enzyme deficiency occur. Bone marrow transplantation remains an alternative mode of therapy for many of these disorders, but the morbidity and mortality associated with this procedure make patient selection and timing difficult.[59] Ultimately, the ideal mode of therapy for lysosomal storage disease will come with the advent of successful human gene transplantation.[60]

### GENETIC ISSUES

The genetic aspects of the lysosomal storage disorders are extremely complex. The molecular defects are being elucidated by molecular genetic technology, which promises potentially curative approaches. With the exceptions of Hunter disease and Fabry disease (which are X-linked recessive), all of these disorders are *heritable autosomal recessive* conditions, and many have a characteristic ethnic predilection.[61] Clinically, these facts have several important implications. First, accurate diagnosis is crucial for accurate *genetic counseling*, which usually entails informing the parents of affected children that their risk for recurrence of the disorder is 25% with each subsequent pregnancy (see Chap. 187). Second, *prenatal diagnosis* is available for almost all of these disorders,[62] usually by specific enzyme assay of cultured amniocytes from amniocentesis or from chorionic villus biopsy specimens (Table 190-3). Third, *detection of the heterozygous carrier state* is possible for some of the disorders, usually by the demonstration of specific enzyme activity intermediate between the normal and the affected homozygote ranges. This often is useful for family members at risk for these disorders to determine who should undergo prenatal diagnostic studies, and has been used for mass screening programs for populations at risk, such as screening of the Ashkenazi Jewish population for Tay-Sachs disease. Finally, the new molecular genetic technology soon should allow the transplantation of normal genes into affected individuals.

**TABLE 190-3.**
**Genetic Aspects of Lysosomal Storage Disorders**

| Disease or Syndrome | Inheritance* | Ethnic Predilection | Recurrence Risk for Parents of Affected Child (%) | Prenatal Diagnosis Established |
|---|---|---|---|---|
| GM$_1$ gangliosidosis | AR | | 25 | Yes |
| Tay-Sachs | AR | Ashkenazi Jews | 25 | Yes |
| Sandhoff | AR | | 25 | Yes |
| Gaucher type 1 | AR | Ashkenazi Jews | 25 | Yes |
| Gaucher type 2 | AR | | 25 | Yes |
| Gaucher type 3 | AR | Norbottnian Swedes | 25 | Yes |
| Niemann-Pick type A | AR | Ashkenazi Jews | 25 | Yes |
| Niemann-Pick type B | AR | | 25 | Yes |
| Niemann-Pick type C | AR | | 25 | Yes |
| Niemann-Pick type D | AR | Western Nova Scotians | 25 | No |
| Krabbe | AR | | 25 | Yes |
| Metachromatic leukodystrophy | AR | Habbanite Jews (late infantile form) | 25 | Yes |
| Multiple sulfatase deficiency | AR | | 25 | Yes |
| Fabry | XR | | 50 (males affected) 50 (females carriers) | Yes |
| Hurler | AR | | 25 | Yes |
| Scheie | AR | | 25 | Yes |
| Hurler-Scheie | AR | | 25 | Yes |
| Hunter | XR | (?) Jews | 50 (males affected) 50 (females carriers) | Yes |
| Sanfilippo | AR | Prevalence of subtypes varies geographically | 25 | Yes (types A, B) |
| Morquio | AR | | 25 | Yes |
| Maroteaux-Lamy | AR | | 25 | Yes |
| Sialidosis type I | AR | (?) Italians | 25 | Yes |
| Sialidosis type II | AR | (?) Japanese | 25 | Yes |
| Mannosidosis | AR | | 25 | Yes |
| Fucosidosis | AR | Calabrians (Italy) | 25 | Yes |
| Aspartylglycosaminuria | AR | | 25 | Yes |
| I-cell disease | AR | | 25 | Yes |
| Pseudo–Hurler polydystrophy | AR | | 25 | No |
| Mucolipidosis IV | AR | Ashkenazi Jews | 25 | Yes |

*AR*, autosomal recessive; *XR*, X-linked recessive.

# REFERENCES

1. Rosenberg RN, Prusiner SB, DiMauro S, et al., eds. The molecular and genetic basis of neurological disease. Boston: Butterworth-Heinemann, 1993.
2. Adams R, Lyon G, Kolodny EH. Neurology of inherited metabolic diseases of children. New York: McGraw-Hill, 1996.
3. Scriver CR, Beaudet AL, Sly WS, Valle D, eds. The metabolic and molecular bases of inherited disease. New York: McGraw-Hill, 1995.
4. Kolodny EH, Cable WL. Inborn errors of metabolism. Ann Neurol 1982; 11:221.
5. Lowden JA. Approaches to the diagnosis and management of infants and children with lysosomal storage disease. In: Kaback MM, ed. Genetic issues in pediatric and obstetric practice. Chicago: Year Book Medical Publishers, 1981:267.
6. Beaudet AL, Scriver CR, Sly WS, et al. Genetics, biochemistry, and molecular basis of variant human phenotypes. In: Scriver CR, Beaudet AL, Sly WS, Valle D, eds. The metabolic and molecular bases of inherited disease. New York: McGraw-Hill, 1995.
7. Suzuki K. Gangliosides and disease: a review. Adv Exp Med Biol 1984; 174:407.
8. O'Brien JS, Ho MW, Veath ML, et al. Juvenile GM1-gangliosidosis: clinical, pathological, chemical, and enzymatic studies. Clin Genet 1972; 3:411.
9. Okada S, O'Brien JS. Generalized gangliosidosis: beta galactosidase deficiency. Science 1968; 160:1002.
10. Suzuki Y, Sakuraba H, Oshima A. β-Galactosidase deficiency: GM1 gangliosidosis and Morquio B disease. In: Scriver CR, Beaudet AL, Sly WS, Valle D, eds. The metabolic and molecular bases of inherited disease. New York: McGraw-Hill, 1995.
11. Chen CY. Neuroimaging findings in late infantile GM1 gangliosidosis. Am J Neuroradiol 1998; 19(9):1628.
12. Gravel RA, Clarke JTR, Kaback MM, et al. In: Scriver CR, Beaudet AL, Sly WS, Valle D, eds. The metabolic and molecular bases of inherited disease. New York: McGraw-Hill, 1995.
13. Sandhoff K, Kolter T. Biochemistry of glycosphingolipid degradation. Clin Chim Acta 1997; 266:51.
14. Johnson WG. The clinical spectrum of hexosaminidase deficiency states. Neurology 1981; 31:1453.
15. Petroulakis E, Cao Z, Clarke JTR, et al. W474C amino acid substitution affects early processing of the alpha-subunit of beta-hexosaminidase A and is associated with subacute G(M2) gangliosidosis. Hum Mutat 1998; 11:432.
16. Johnson WG, Wigger HJ, Karp HR, et al. Juvenile spinal muscular atrophy: a new hexosaminidase deficiency phenotype. Ann Neurol 1982; 11:11.
17. Winkelman MD, Banker BQ, Victor M, Moser HW. Non-infantile Gaucher's disease: a clinicopathologic study. Neurology 1983; 33:994.
18. Beutler E, Grabowski GA. Gaucher disease. In: Scriver CR, Beaudet AL, Sly WS, Valle D, eds. The metabolic and molecular bases of inherited disease. New York: McGraw-Hill, 1995.
19. Barton NW, Brady RO, Dambrosia JM, et al. Replacement therapy for inherited enzyme deficiency—macrophage-targeted glucocerebrosidase for Gaucher's disease. N Engl J Med 1991; 324:1464.
20. Crocker AC, Farber S. Niemann-Pick disease: a review of eighteen patients. Medicine (Baltimore) 1958; 37:1.
21. Yan-Go FL, Yanagihara T, Pierre RV, Goldstein NP. A progressive neurologic disorder with supranuclear vertical gaze paresis and distinctive bone marrow cells. Mayo Clin Proc 1984; 59:404.
22. Schuchman EH, Desnick RJ. Niemann-Pick disease types A and B: acid sphingomyelinase deficiencies. In: Scriver CR, Beaudet AL, Sly WS, Valle D, eds. The metabolic and molecular bases of inherited disease. New York: McGraw-Hill, 1995.
23. Challamel MJ, Mazzola ME, Nevsimalova S, et al. Narcolepsy in children. Sleep 1994; 17:17.
24. Pentchev PG, Vanier MT, Suzuki K, Patternson MC. Niemann-Pick disease type C: a cellular cholesterol lipidosis. In: Scriver CR, Beaudet AL, Sly WS, Valle D, eds. The metabolic and molecular bases of inherited disease. New York: McGraw-Hill, 1995.
25. Farrell DF, Swedberg K. Clinical and biochemical heterogeneity of globoid cell leukodystrophy. Ann Neurol 1981; 10:364.
26. Suzuki Y, Suzuki K. Krabbe's globoid cell leukodystrophy: deficiency of galactocerebrosidase in serum, leukocytes, and fibroblasts. Science 1971; 171:73.

27. Suzuki K, Suzuki Y. Galactosylceramide lipidosis: globoid cell leukodystrophy (Krabbe's disease). In: Scriver CR, Beaudet AL, Sly WS, Valle D, eds. The metabolic and molecular bases of inherited disease. New York: McGraw-Hill, 1995.

28. Kihara H. Genetic heterogeneity in metachromatic leukodystrophy. Am J Hum Genet 1982; 34:171.

29. Farooqui AA, Horrocks LA. Biochemical aspects of globoid and metachromatic leukodystrophies. Neurochem Pathol 1984; 2:189.

30. Hahn AF, Gordon BA, Hinton GG, Gilbert JJ. A variant form of metachromatic leukodystrophy without arylsulfatase deficiency. Ann Neurol 1982; 12:33.

31. Kolodny EH. Metachromatic leukodystrophy and multiple sulfatase deficiency: sulfatide lipidosis. In: Scriver CR, Beaudet AL, Sly WS, Valle D, eds. The metabolic and molecular bases of inherited disease. New York: McGraw-Hill, 1995.

32. Desnick RJ, Ioannou YA, Eng CM. α-Galactosidase A deficiency: Fabry disease. In: Scriver CR, Beaudet AL, Sly WS, Valle D, eds. The metabolic and molecular bases of inherited disease. New York: McGraw-Hill, 1995.

33. Menkes DL. Images in neurology: the cutaneous stigmata of Fabry disease: an X-linked phakomatosis associated with central and peripheral nervous system dysfunction. Arch Neurol 1999; 56(4):487.

34. Donati D, Novario R, Gastaldi L. Natural history and treatment of uremia secondary to Fabry's disease: an European experience. Nephron 1987; 46:353.

35. Dorfman A, Matalon R. The mucopolysaccharidoses: a review. Proc Natl Acad Sci U S A 1976; 73:630.

36. Kelly TE. The mucopolysaccharidoses and mucolipidoses. Clin Orthop 1976; 114:116.

37. McKusick VA, Pyeritz RE. Genetic heterogeneity and allelic variation in the mucopolysaccharidoses. Johns Hopkins Med J 1980; 146:71.

38. Neufeld EF. The biochemical basis of mucopolysaccharidoses and mucolipidoses. Prog Med Genet 1974; 10:81.

39. Neufeld EF, Muenzer J. The mucopolysaccharidoses. In: Scriver CR, Beaudet AL, Sly WS, Valle D, eds. The metabolic and molecular bases of inherited disease. New York: McGraw-Hill, 1995.

40. Van Schrojenstein-de Valk HM, van der Kamp JJ. Follow-up on seven adult patients with mild Sanfilippo B-disease. Prenat Diagn 1987; 7:603.

41. Wraith JE, Danks DM, Rogers JG. Mild Sanfilippo syndrome: a further cause of hyperactivity and behavioral disturbance. Med J Aust 1987; 147:450.

42. Colville GA. Sleep problems in children with Sanfilippo syndrome. Dev Med Child Neurol 1996; 38(6):538.

43. Sataloff RT, Schiebel BR, Spiegel JR. Morquio's syndrome. Am J Otol 1987; 8:443.

44. O'Brien JS, Warner TG. Sialidosis: delineation of subtypes by neuraminidase assay. Clin Genet 1980; 17:35.

45. Thomas GH, Beaudet AL. Disorders of glycoprotein degradation: In: Scriver CR, Beaudet AL, Sly WS, Valle D, eds. The metabolic and molecular bases of inherited disease. New York: McGraw-Hill, 1995.

46. Rapin I, Goldfischer S, Katzman R, et al. The cherry-red-spot–myoclonus syndrome. Ann Neurol 1978; 3:234.

47. Warner TG, O'Brien JS. Genetic defects in glycoprotein metabolism. Annu Rev Genet 1983; 17:395.

48. Mononen T, Mononen I, Matilainen R, Airaksinen E. High prevalence of aspartylglycosaminuria among school-age children in eastern Finland. Hum Genet 1991; 87:266.

49. Jaeken J, Hagberg B, Stromme P. Clinical presentation and natural course of the carbohydrate-deficient glycoprotein syndrome. Acta Paediatr Scand Suppl 1991; 375:6.

50. Whelan DT, Chang PL, Cockshott PW. Mucolipidosis II: the clinical, radiological and biochemical features in three cases. Clin Genet 1983; 24:90.

51. Leroy LG, Spranger JW, Feingold M, et al. I-cell disease: a clinical picture. J Pediatr 1971; 79:360.

52. Kornfeld S, Sly WS. I-cell disease and pseudo-Hurler polydystrophy: disorders of lysosomal enzyme phosphorylation and localization. In: Scriver CR, Beaudet AL, Sly WS, Valle D, eds. The metabolic and molecular bases of inherited disease. New York: McGraw-Hill, 1995.

53. Ben-Yoseph Y, Mitchell DA, Nadler HL. First trimester prenatal evaluation for I-cell disease by N-acetyl-glucosamine 1-phosphotransferase assay. Clin Genet 1988; 33:38.

54. Crandall BF, Phillipart M, Brown WJ, Bluestone DA. Mucolipidosis IV. Am J Med Genet 1982; 12:301.

55. Takahashi Y, Orii T. Diagnosis of subtypes of GM1 gangliosidosis in vitro and in vivo—using urinary oligosaccharides as substrates. Clin Chim Acta 1989; 179:219.

56. Whitley CB, Ridnour MD, Draper KA, et al. Diagnostic test for mucopolysaccharidosis. I. Direct method for quantifying excessive urinary glycosaminoglycan excretion. Clin Chem 1989; 35:374.

57. Brady RO, Barton NW. Enzyme replacement therapy for type 1 Gaucher disease. In: Desnick, ed. Treatment of genetic disease. New York: Churchill Livingstone, 1991:153.

58. Barton NW, Brady RO, Dambrosia JM, et al. Replacement therapy for inherited enzyme deficiency—macrophage-targeted glucocerebrosidase for Gaucher's disease. N Engl J Med 1991; 324:1464.

59. Barranger JA. Marrow transplantation in genetic disease. N Engl J Med 1984; 311:1629.

60. Hoogerbrugge PM, Valerio D. Bone marrow transplantation and gene therapy for lysosomal storage diseases. Bone Marrow Transplant 1998; 21 (Suppl 2):S34.

61. Zlotogora J, Zeigler M, Bach G. Selection in favor of lysosomal storage disorders? Am J Hum Genet 1988; 42:271.

62. D'Alton ME, Deherney AH. Prenatal diagnosis. N Engl J Med 1993; 328:114.

# CHAPTER 191

# HERITABLE DISEASES OF AMINO-ACID METABOLISM

HARVEY J. STERN AND JAMES D. FINKELSTEIN

The disorders of amino-acid metabolism are the most classic of the inherited metabolic disorders and have provided great insight into the pathogenesis, biochemistry, and treatment of human genetic disease. Sir Archibald Garrod, at the turn of the century, studied patients and families with alkaptonuria, cystinuria, pentosuria, and albinism.[1] From his studies of these amino-acid disorders, Garrod developed the conceptual framework for what he called "inborn errors of metabolism." Based on these observations, the one gene–one enzyme concept was proposed in the 1940s,[2] and shortly thereafter, the first enzyme defect in humans was described (methemoglobinemia). In 1949 Pauling and coworkers[3] demonstrated that mutations produced an alteration in the primary amino-acid sequence of a protein. This represented the beginning of the molecular age of human genetic research, which has evolved into the powerful and sophisticated methodologies of molecular biology and DNA-based diagnosis of human genetic diseases. With these discoveries has come an increasing appreciation of the molecular heterogeneity of these disorders, and the way in which various alterations of the amino-acid sequence of enzymatic or nonenzymatic proteins lead to major differences in the biochemical and clinical expression of disease in the patient.[4]

The elucidation and understanding of amino-acid disorders have paralleled the development of new laboratory methodologies to study the amino-acid composition of complex biologic fluids. Paper chromatography of urine followed by ninhydrin staining was the first technique to be widely used in the identification of patients with abnormal patterns of amino-acid excretion. Early column chromatography methods coupled to quantitative photometric ninhydrin analysis have been replaced by automated ion-exchange chromatography with computer-assisted data acquisition and calculation of results. Commercially available amino-acid analyzers can perform a complete physiologic analysis of plasma, urine, or cerebrospinal fluid in <3 hours. This is critical for rapid diagnosis of patients suspected of having amino-acid disorders, as well as for monitoring the effects of dietary or other therapies on amino-acid concentrations in patients with these diseases. Even more rapid techniques for the determination of amino- and organic-acid concentrations in biologic fluids have been developed using computer-assisted tandem mass spectrometry. These methods can analyze for multiple analytes in a matter of minutes and can be adapted for automated metabolic screening of newborns from blood spots using electrospray introduction of samples.[5]

The pathogenesis of genetic disorders of amino-acid metabolism can be grouped into *enzyme defects*, *defects in membrane transport*, and a *miscellaneous* class that would include the *storage diseases*. This classification is clearly a convenient artifact based on some functional attribute of the abnormal protein. Understanding of these complex biologic interrelationships has been aided by the development of more sensitive analytical techniques such as gas chromatography/mass spectrometry, by which the concentration of metabolic intermediates can be determined in patients suspected of having biochemical disorders. The structures of the amino acids are shown in Chapter 124, Figure 124-2. The endocrinologist must be aware of the existence of these disorders of amino-acid metabolism. With improved medical treatment of these patients, many are now able to reach adulthood, and they possibly face previously unappreciated medical complications. This is especially true of women during pregnancy and childbirth. In addition, asymptomatic carriers of metabolic disorders may indeed be susceptible to increased medical morbidity because of their heterozygous state. Because almost 1% of the population are carriers of an abnormal allele that has a homozygote frequency of 1 in 50,000, the consequences of metabolic disorders can no longer be considered to be limited to the "rare" patient.

## ENZYME DEFECTS

### GENERAL CONSIDERATIONS

The enzymatic defects constitute the largest and most diverse group of genetic disorders of amino-acid metabolism. Two considerations are relevant. First, multiple different genetic abnormalities may impair the same enzyme. Second, the resultant chemical abnormalities may involve metabolites distant from the affected enzyme.

The apparent deficiency of a specific enzyme may derive from either a defective rate of synthesis (*regulatory gene defect*) or from the synthesis of an abnormal protein (*structural gene defect*). The latter seems to be more frequent, and because the defect may occur at any one of a number of amino-acid positions, multiple abnormal alleles may impair the same enzyme protein. Often, the protein has some residual function, and the persistence of some enzyme activity is frequent, even in the homozygotic state. Along with these defects in apoenzyme synthesis, enzymatic activity can be compromised by defects in the synthesis of either coenzymes or cosubstrates. The methyltetrahydrofolate homocysteine methyltransferase reaction provides one example. Abnormalities of cosubstrate formation (methylene tetrahydrofolate reductase deficiency) and of coenzyme formation (impaired cobalamin metabolism), as well as defective synthesis of the apoenzyme, cause homocystinuria with hypomethioninemia.[6]

### CLINICAL SEQUELAE

The metabolic consequences, and therefore the clinical sequelae, of an enzyme defect are defined by (a) the location of the block, (b) the degree of impairment, and (c) the interrelations of the affected pathway. Figure 191-1 illustrates a hypothetical biochemical pathway and the potential effects of a deficiency in the enzyme that catalyzes the conversion of metabolite B to metabolite C. The concentration of B increases, as does that of A, if either the conversion of A to B is reversible or any of the metabolites distal to the block is a necessary and positive effector of that conversion. Conversely, the concentration of A may fall if any of the distal metabolites is a negative or feedback inhibitor of the A→B conversion. The concentrations of C, D, and E decline unless sustained by dietary intake or by an alternative means for synthesis.

Enzymatic sequences other than the primary pathway may be affected. For example, the accumulation of B may activate or enhance the alternative pathway, which leads to the synthesis of R, S, and T. The linked pathway M——→N→O is impaired if substrate C (or D and E) is a necessary cosubstrate in the conversion of M to N. Consequently, the concentration of M may increase, whereas that of N (and of other distal metabolites) may decrease. Finally, the primary defect may affect an apparently unrelated pathway if any of its component enzymes is affected by the change in the concentration of any of the metabolites in the primary, alternate, or linked sequences.

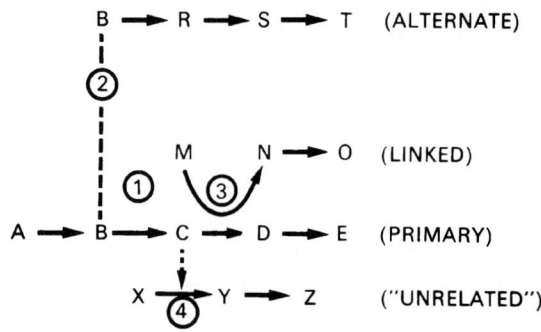

**FIGURE 191-1.** Hypothetical metabolic pathway. Letters represent the metabolites of the primary (*A–E*), linked (*M–O*), alternate (*B–T*), and "unrelated" (*X–Z*) sequences. Impairment of reaction 1 results in accumulation of B and activation of the alternative pathway. Linked pathway is limited by availability of C, which is shown as cosubstrate for reaction 3. The unrelated pathway is affected if C is an effector, either positive or negative, of reaction 4.

The clinical manifestations of many genetic disorders derive from these alterations in the concentrations of metabolites. Three types of abnormalities are common. Deficiencies may occur distal to the metabolic block or in linked pathways deprived of an essential cosubstrate. Conversely, potentially toxic increases in the concentrations of metabolites behind the impaired reaction may lead to the observed pathologic process. The third class of chemical abnormality, the appearance of abnormal metabolites, may be considered a variant of the second form, because the accumulation of normal metabolites activates an alternate enzymatic sequence. All three classes of abnormalities occur in most of the disorders, and the determination of which contributes most to the clinical syndrome is a prime consideration in the formulation of therapy.

### THERAPEUTIC STRATEGIES

The restoration of normal enzyme activity, which would provide optimal treatment, rarely is possible, although gene replacement may provide that capacity in the future. Current therapeutic strategies include restricted consumption of nutrients whose metabolites may accumulate, dietary supplementation with nutrients no longer synthesized in adequate amounts, and enhancement of residual enzymatic activity by the provision of increased concentrations of cofactors. The vitamin-responsive defects typify the last situation.[7]

### SPECIFIC DISORDERS

Table 191-1 summarizes the genetic disorders of amino-acid metabolism attributable to enzyme defects and their clinical expression.

#### HYPERPHENYLALANINEMIA

The phenylalanine hydroxylase reaction is the site of the metabolic impairment in all five variants of hyperphenylalaninemia. Types I, II, and III result from quantitative or qualitative defects in the synthesis of the apoenzyme. Failure to synthesize or maintain adequate concentrations of the cofactor tetrahydrobiopterin causes type IV (dihydropteridine reductase deficiency) and type V (dihydrobiopterin synthase deficiency). All five defects yield the same chemical abnormalities: an increase in the concentration of phenylalanine in the blood to >120 μmol/L and the urinary excretion of metabolites of this amino acid.

**TABLE 191-1.**
Genetic Disorders of Amino-Acid Metabolism Attributable to Enzyme Defects

| Disorder | Defect | Diagnosis | Clinical Expression |
|---|---|---|---|
| **AROMATIC AMINO ACIDS** | | | |
| Hyperphenylalaninemia | Phenylalanine hydroxylase | | |
|  Type I (phenylketonuria) | | Phenylalanine (B), phenylalanine metabolites (U) | Mental retardation, eczema |
|  Type II | | Same | Milder form of type I |
|  Type III | | Same | Transient |
|  Dihydropteridine reductase | | Same | Abnormal CNS development, seizures |
|  Dihydrobiopterin synthase | | Same | Same |
| **Tyrosinemia, type I** | Fumarylacetoacetate and maleylacetoacetate hydrolases | Tyrosine (B, U), methionine (B, U), succinylacetone (U), aminoaciduria (generalized) | Cirrhosis, hepatoma, Fanconi syndrome, porphyria |
| **Tyrosinemia, type II** | Tyrosine aminotransferase | Tyrosine (B, U), phenolic acids (U) | Mental retardation (?), corneal ulcers, keratoses (palms & soles) |
| **Alkaptonuria** | Homogentisic acid oxidase | Homogentisic acid (U) | Ochronosis (ears, sclerae), arthritis, cardiac valve stenosis |
| **Albinism** | | | |
|  Oculocutaneous | Tyrosinase | | Albinism involving hair, ocular defects with loss of binocular vision |
|  | Multiple forms | | As above; several involve hematologic functions |
|  Ocular | Multiple forms | | Ocular defects |
| **Histidinemia** | Histidase | Histidine (B, U), imidazoles (U) | Mental retardation (?), speech defects (?)/benign (?) |
| **SULFUR AMINO ACIDS** | | | |
| **Hypermethioninemia** | Methionine adenosyltransferase | Methionine (B, U), methionine sulfoxide (B, U) | Benign |
| **Homocystinuria** | Cystathionine synthase | Homocystine (B, U), methionine (B, U), decreased cysteine (B) | Thromboembolism, osteoporosis, mental retardation, ectopia lentis |
|  | Cobalamin metabolism | Homocystine (B, U), methylmalonic acid (B, U), cystathionine (U) | Retarded development, megaloblastic anemia, thromboembolism (?) |
|  | Methylenetetrahydrofolate reductase | Homocystine (B, U), cystathionine (U) | Thromboembolism, CNS dysfunction, mental retardation |
| **Cystathioninuria** | Cystathionase | Cystathionine (B, U), N-acetylcystathionine (B, U) | Benign |
| **Sulfocysteinuria** | Sulfite oxidase | Sulfocysteine (U) | Ectopia lentis, CNS dysfunction |
| **GLUTATHIONE METABOLISM** | | | |
| **Pyroglutamic aciduria** | Glutathione synthase (generalized) | 5-Oxoproline (B, U) | Acidosis, hemolytic anemia, CNS dysfunction |
| **Glutathione synthase deficiency** | Glutathione synthase (erythrocyte) | | Hemolytic anemia |
| **γ-Glutamylcysteine synthase deficiency** | Glutamate-cysteine ligase | Aminoaciduria (generalized), decreased glutathione (B) | Hemolytic anemia, spinocerebellar degeneration, neuromyopathy |
| **Glutathionuria** | γ-Glutamyltranspeptidase | Glutathione (B, U), cystine (B, U) | Mental retardation |
| **DIBASIC AMINO ACIDS AND UREA CYCLE** | | | |
| **Gyrate atrophy of choroid and retina** | Ornithine transaminase | Ornithine (B, U) | Retinal dysfunction with myopia, night blindness, tunnel vision; cataracts |
| **Hyperornithinemia with hyperammonemia** | Mitochondrial uptake of ornithine (?) | Ornithine (B), ammonia (B), homocitrulline (U) | Protein intolerance |
| **Hyperlysinemia** | | | |
|  Periodic | Lysine dehydrogenase | Lysine (B), ammonia (B) | Protein intolerance |
|  Persistent | Lysine ketoglutarate reductase | Lysine (B, U) | Mental retardation (?) |
| **Hyperammonemias** | Acetylglutamate synthetase | Ammonia (B) | Rare disorder |
|  | Carbamoyl phosphate synthase | Ammonia (B), aminoaciduria (generalized) | Protein intolerance |
|  | Ornithine carbamoyltransferase | Ammonia (B), orotic acid (U), decreased citrulline (B) | Protein intolerance, mental retardation |
| **Citrullinemia** | Argininosuccinate synthase | Ammonia (B), orotic acid (U), citrulline (B) | CNS dysfunction, hepatic steatosis |
| **Argininosuccinic aciduria** | Argininosuccinate lyase | Ammonia (B), argininosuccinate (B, U) | Psychomotor retardation, trichorrhexis |
| **Hyperargininemia** | Arginase | Ammonia (B), arginine (B, U), orotic acid (U), dibasic aminoaciduria, cystinuria | Spastic paraplegia |

(continued)

**TABLE 191-1.**
**Genetic Disorders of Amino-Acid Metabolism Attributable to Enzyme Defects (Continued)**

| Disorder | Defect | Diagnosis | Clinical Expression |
|---|---|---|---|
| **BRANCHED-CHAIN AMINO ACIDS** | | | |
| Hypervalinemia | Valine transaminase (?) | Valine (B, U) | One reported case |
| Hyperleucine-isoleucinemia | Leucine–isoleucine transaminase | Leucine (B), isoleucine (B), proline (B) | Only two sibs with associated hyperprolinemia |
| **Branched-chain ketoaciduria (maple syrup urine disease)** | Branched-chain 2-ketoacid decarboxylase (5 variants) | Leucine (B, U), isoleucine (B, U), valine (B, U), branched-chain ketoacids (B, U) | Ketoacidosis, neuromuscular retardation, hypoglycemia |
| **Isovaleric acidemia** | Isovaleryl-CoA dehydrogenase | Isovalerylglycine (U), isovaleric acid (B), hydroxyisovaleric acid (U) | Ketoacidosis, coma, leukopenia, thrombocytopenia |
| **Glutaric aciduria (type II)** | Electron transport flavoprotein (ETF) or ETF:ubiquinone oxidoreductase | Isobutyric acid (U), isovaleric acid (U), 2-methylbutyric acid (U), 2-hydroxyglutaric acid (U) | Nonketotic hypoglycemic acidosis |
| **3-Methylcrotonyl-CoA carboxylase deficiency** | 3-Methylcrotonyl carboxylase | 3-Hydroxyisovalerate (U), 3-methylcrotonylglycine (U) | Two cases resembling Werdnig-Hoffmann syndrome; one with metabolic acidosis |
| **3-Hydroxy-3-methyl-glutaryl-CoA carboxylase deficiency** | Hydroxymethylglutaryl-CoA carboxylase | Hydroxymethylglutarate (U), 3-methylglutarate (U), 3-methylglutaconate (U), 3-hydroxyisovalerate (U) | Hypoglycemia, ketoacidosis |
| **3-Ketothiolase deficiency** | 3-Ketothiolase | 2-Methyl-3-hydroxybutyrate (U), 2-methylacetoacetate (U), butanone (U) | Ketoacidosis |
| **OTHER NEUTRAL AMINO ACIDS** | | | |
| Hypersarcosinemia | Sarcosine dehydrogenase | Sarcosine (B, U) | Benign (?) |
| Nonketotic hyperglycinemia | Glycine cleavage complex | Glycine (B, U, CSF) | Mental retardation, seizures |
| Hyper-β-alaninemia | β-Alanine transaminase | β-Alanine (B, U), β-aminobutyrate (B, U), β-aminoisobutyrate (B, U), taurine (U) | One reported case |
| **Hypercarnosinuria** | Carnosinase (serum) | Carnosine (U) | Seizures with retardation (?) |
| Homocarnosinosis | Homocarnosinase (brain) | Homocarnosine (CSF) | CNS dysfunction |
| **ORGANIC ACIDEMIAS** | | | |
| **Propionic acidemias** | Propionyl-CoA carboxylase (2 variants) | Glycine (B, U), propionate (B, U), ammonia (B), methylcitrate (U), propionylglycine (U), 3-hydroxypropionate (U), tiglic acid (U) | Ketoacidosis, mental retardation |
| | Multiple carboxylases (defective biotin metabolism) | As above, plus β-methylcrotonylglycine (U), tiglyglycine (U), 3-hydroxyisovalerate (U) | Ketoacidosis, alopecia, eczematoid dermatitis |
| **Methylmalonic acidemias** | Methylmalonyl-CoA mutase | Methylmalonic acid (B, U), glycine (B, U), ammonia (B) | Ketoacidosis, hypoglycemia, hyperammonemia, pancytopenia |
| | Defective apoenzyme (2 variants) | Other metabolites as seen in propionic acidemia | |
| | Deficient coenzyme synthesis (2 variants) | | |
| **Methylmalonic acidemia with homocystinemia** | See sulfur amino-acid defects | | |
| **IMINO ACIDS** | | | |
| Hyperprolinemia | Proline oxidase | Proline (B, U), glycine (U), hydroxyproline (U) | Benign |
| | Pyrroline-5-carboxylate dehydrogenase | Above, plus pyrroline-5-carboxylate (U) | Benign |
| **Hyperhydroxyprolinemia** | Hydroxyproline oxidase | Hydroxyproline (B, U) | Benign |
| Hyperimidodipeptiduria | Prolidase | Imidodipeptides (U) | Mental retardation, dermatitis, infections, splenomegaly |

*B*, blood; *U*, urine; *CNS*, central nervous system; *CoA*, coenzyme A; *CSF*, cerebrospinal fluid.

The enzymatic impairment appears to be most complete in type I, which is classic phenylketonuria (PKU).[8,9] This disorder occurs in ~1 of every 10,000 births, and 2% of the population may be asymptomatic carriers. The dietary restriction of phenylalanine during the neonatal period is essential to prevent mental retardation in affected infants. The success of this therapy mandates the screening of all newborn infants, but testing can be useful only after the initiation of protein intake, for only then does the defect become manifest. The dietary restriction should be continued as long as possible, although maintenance of a protein-restricted diet becomes more difficult as the child enters adolescence. A prudent course is to maintain strict control through the first decade and then to periodically monitor the blood phenylalanine concentration as dietary intake is increased with the introduction of new foods. Note should be made, however, that multiple studies have shown a decline in school performance for older patients with PKU who go off a restricted diet.

The successful management of children with PKU has led to a new problem: the management of pregnancies of phenylketonuric women. During pregnancy, phenylalanine restriction is nec-

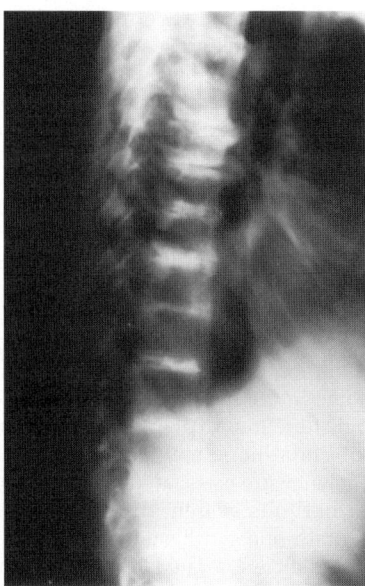

**FIGURE 191-2.** Alkaptonuria. Degeneration of intervertebral discs of lumbar spine is apparent; the joint spaces are narrowed, and the discs are calcified. Osteophyte formation is only moderate, and intervertebral ligaments are not calcified.

essary to prevent mental retardation, congenital heart disease, and other birth defects in the offspring.[10]

## TYROSINEMIA

Two defects cause the accumulation of tyrosine. A primary abnormality in tyrosine aminotransferase occurs in tyrosinemia type II (Richner-Hanhart syndrome). The clinical features include corneal ulcers, palmar and plantar keratoses, and possibly mental retardation, and are thought to derive from the intracellular crystallization of the amino acid. The primary defect in tyrosinemia type I (tyrosinosis) is a deficiency of fumarylacetoacetate hydrolase (type Ia) or maleylacetoacetate hydrolase (type Ib). Succinylacetone, a metabolite that accumulates, inhibits both tyrosine aminotransferase and porphobilinogen synthase. Moreover, succinylacetone impairs renal tubular function and methionine metabolism, resulting in a clinical syndrome that includes tyrosinemia, hypermethioninemia, liver cirrhosis, porphyria, and renal Fanconi syndrome. Primary hepatocellular carcinoma frequently occurs in survivors. Dietary restriction of tyrosine and phenylalanine, which is effective in type II tyrosinemia,[11] may not be sufficient therapy for tyrosinosis. Treatment with an inhibitor of 4-hydroxyphenylpyruvate dioxygenase (which leads to decreased production of succinylacetone) offers promising results.[12] Liver transplantation can be curative if performed before the development of hepatocellular carcinoma.

## ALKAPTONURIA

Although alkaptonuria is extremely rare, it is the disorder that led Garrod in 1902 to conceptualize the inborn errors of metabolism. The primary defect, deficiency of homogentisic acid oxidase, leads to the accumulation of that substrate and its derivatives in connective tissue. The resultant blue discoloration and arthritis characterize the condition, which is called ochronosis.[13] Intervertebral disc calcification is typical (Fig. 191-2). The oxidation of excreted homogentisic acid may cause a black discoloration of the urine, which is intensified by either exposure to air or alkalinization. No effective therapy for ochronosis is known. The gene for homogentisate 1,2-dioxygenase has been cloned and is located on human chromosome band 3q21-q23[12] This raises the possibility of using gene therapy in the future to replace this missing enzymatic function.[14]

## ALBINISM

The group of genetic diseases making up albinism includes the ten or more variants of oculocutaneous albinism (OCA) as well as the several forms of ocular albinism. The common characteristic is a derangement in melanin metabolism that leads to abnormal pigmentation of the eyes (in ocular albinism), or of the eyes, skin, and hair (in OCA). Although previously the classification of various forms of oculocutaneous albinism had been based on clinical findings, information regarding the fundamental molecular defects in the production and transport of melanin is now beginning to emerge.[15] The aggregate frequency of occurrence for this group of disorders approximates 1 in 10,000 among blacks and 1 in 20,000 among whites.

The absence of retinal pigmentation causes loss of acuity as well as nystagmus and photophobia. Most individuals with albinism lack binocular vision secondary to a failure of development of the normal decussation pattern of the optic nerve. In affected individuals, the fibers from the temporal retina cross at the optic chiasm instead of continuing on the same side as the eye of origin.

The variants of OCA differ in the degree of hypopigmentation of the hair and skin. Some of the syndromes have additional, unique abnormalities. The Hermansky-Pudlak form of OCA includes a mild coagulopathy secondary to platelet abnormalities,[16] the accumulation of storage material in the reticuloendothelial system and gastrointestinal mucosa, and the development of restrictive lung disease. In Chédiak-Higashi syndrome, another variant of OCA, leukocytes contain giant peroxidase-positive granules that seem to impair chemotaxis. This finding may explain the extreme vulnerability of these patients to severe, often lethal, infections as well as the subsequent development of lymphoreticular neoplasms.

## HOMOCYSTINURIAS

Homocysteine is a sulfhydryl amino acid formed by the demethylation of methionine. It is metabolized by either remethylation to methionine (with betaine or methyltetrahydrofolate as the methyl donor) or by the irreversible synthesis of cystathionine (transsulfuration).[17] Impairment of either pathway leads to the accumulation of homocysteine in tissues and blood, together with excretion of the amino acid in the urine.[18] Normal plasma contains homocysteine (the free thiol) and its disulfide derivatives—homocystine, homocysteine-cysteine mixed disulfide, and protein-homocysteine mixed disulfide. The latter is the predominant form.[19] The sum of all forms is termed *tHcy*, and the upper limit of normal ranges from 12 to 15 µmol/L—depending on the methodology and the laboratory. In addition to homocysteine accumulation, a defect in cystathionine-β-synthase (classic homocystinuria) is associated with the augmented resynthesis of methionine. Conversely, the impairment of methyltetrahydrofolate-homocysteine methyltransferase results in decreased levels of methionine and variable increases in the concentration of cystathionine. These differences, which are apparent on amino acid analysis of plasma, allow for the discrimination between the two classes of homocystinuria.[18]

The classic clinical expression of cystathionine synthase deficiency includes a marfanoid habitus (dolichostenomelia with pectus deformities), subluxation of the ocular lenses, osteoporosis, and thromboembolic episodes that often involve the major vessels.[18] Mental retardation is variable but may be constant within a pedigree. Response to therapy defines at least two major variants of this disorder. Large doses of pyridoxine normalize the amino acid concentrations and prevent the medical complications in approximately one-half of patients. The remaining patients are treated by dietary manipulations that reduce the accumulation of homocysteine. The program consists of methionine restriction and cyst(e)ine supplementation. Folic acid and betaine, the methyl donors for the two homocysteine methyltransferases, often are provided to augment homocysteine methylation. Both the success of these therapies and the fact that the untreated disease may become symptomatic after childhood make cystathionine synthase deficiency a clinical concern for adult medicine.[18,20]

Failure of homocysteine methylation results from impairment of the methyltetrahydrofolate-homocysteine methyltransferase reaction. This reaction is vulnerable to several genetic defects. Usually, the disorder derives from a defect in the synthesis of the cosubstrate, methyltetrahydrofolate,[21] or the coenzyme, methylcobalamin.[22] Patients with severe methylenetetrahydrofolate reductase deficiency may have vascular pathology and a variable spectrum of neuropsychiatric dysfunction. The clinical chemical findings in patients with defects in cobalamin absorption or metabolism are more complex, because the synthesis of adenosylcobalamin also may be limited. Thus, methylmalonic aciduria may accompany the homocystinuria. Furthermore, megaloblastic anemia with pancytopenia may occur in some patients. The aim of therapy in the remethylation defects is to reduce the concentration of homocysteine while increasing that of methionine. Some patients with deranged cobalamin metabolism respond to large doses of vitamin $B_{12}$; however, the effectiveness of folic acid in methylenetetrahydrofolate reductase deficiency is unproved. Betaine appears helpful in both conditions.

Due to the clinical observation that patients with classical homocystinuria (with plasma tHcy >100 µmol/L) have early onset thrombovascular disease, clinical studies were initiated to evaluate the clinical consequences of "hyperhomocysteinemia"—a more moderate elevation in plasma homocysteine concentration (usually in the range of 15–30 µmol/L). Although many reports identify increased plasma tHcy as an independent risk factor for vascular disease, the issue of causality remains unresolved.[23a,b] Until that relationship is clarified, there can be no consensus regarding the routine laboratory determination of plasma tHcy.[24a] Likewise, there is no agreement concerning the value of increasing folate intake, either by food fortification or dietary supplementation, in order to prevent thrombovascular disease, although such treatment does decrease plasma tHcy in most subjects. Lastly, the identification of the causes of hyperhomocysteinemia remains incomplete. Nutritional deficiencies, particularly of folate and cobalamin, are the basis for a large number of cases. The search for genetic factors has been less rewarding. Heterozygosity for cystathionine synthase deficiency does not appear to be a significant etiology. In contrast, homozygosity for an abnormal allele of methylenetetrahydrofolate reductase results in a thermolabile enzyme form that has increased vulnerability to folate deficiency.

### OTHER DISORDERS OF SULFUR AMINO ACID METABOLISM

Both cystathioninuria and hypermethioninemia may be benign metabolic defects.[18] The former derives from a deficiency in cystathionase. The accumulated cystathionine appears to be without toxicity, and the only consequence may be impairment in the conversion of methionine to cysteine. Dietary supplements of the latter amino acid may be appropriate, particularly during the neonatal period. Cystathioninuria is one of the pyridoxine-responsive defects, and treatment with this vitamin often reverses the biochemical abnormalities.

Hypermethioninemia results from a deficiency in the high-$K_m$ isoenzyme of methionine adenosyltransferase (MAT I/III), the enzyme that catalyzes the synthesis of S-adenosylmethionine (AdoMet) from methionine. Because the affected isoenzyme occurs primarily in the liver, the synthesis of AdoMet in other tissues should be unimpaired. However, the capacity for the catabolism of excessive quantities of methionine is limited. The absence of significant pathologic sequelae despite the accumulation of methionine suggests that methionine toxicity requires AdoMet synthesis. Several animal studies support this hypothesis. However, a report of CNS demyelination in a limited number of patients requires explanation.[24b]

### DISORDERS OF GLUTATHIONE METABOLISM

Glutathione, the tripeptide γ-glutamyl-cysteinyl-glycine, is the principal intracellular thiol and appears to be essential for the maintenance of other sulfhydryl compounds. This compound participates in the detoxification of peroxides and other chemical agents, and studies indicate another role for glutathione and γ-glutamylcysteine in the membrane transport of amino acids. These physiologic functions explain the clinical consequences of the disorders of glutathione metabolism.[25] Defects that cause glutathione deficiency are associated with erythrocyte hemolysis and central nervous system dysfunction. These defects include both glutathione synthase deficiency and γ-glutamylcysteine synthase deficiency. The latter, which impairs the synthesis of both transport glutamyl peptides, leads to a generalized aminoaciduria. The 5-oxoproline (pyroglutamic acid) excretion in glutathione synthase deficiency results from an overproduction of 5-oxoproline resulting from the failure of feedback inhibition. The effect of the accumulation of glutathione is uncertain; possibly the mental retardation reported in patients with γ-glutamyltranspeptidase deficiency is attributable to an ascertainment bias.

### DISORDERS OF THE UREA CYCLE

The function of the urea cycle is to dispose of waste nitrogen and synthesize arginine. The early diagnosis of the diseases resulting from disordered urea synthesis is essential to prevent the potentially irreversible changes in the central nervous system that can result from recurrent or chronic hyperammonemia. Patients may present in the neonatal period with lethargy, poor feeding, respiratory alkalosis, and vomiting, and rapidly progress to hyperammonemic coma, which is often fatal. Survivors are usually left with significant cognitive and motor deficits. In other cases, depending on the degree of enzyme deficiency and nitrogen load, clinical symptoms may not develop until adulthood. Women who carry the X-linked disorder ornithine transcarbamoylase deficiency may develop significant hyperammonemia during periods of metabolic stress, including childbirth. The differential diagnosis of urea cycle disorders includes transient hyperammonemia of the newborn, a relatively benign, transient, neonatal hyperammonemia; and the other inherited disorders listed in Table 191-1. Treatment by protein restriction may cause a deficiency of essential amino acids. Thus, a controlled diet containing the ketoacid analogs of the essential amino acids is preferable. Encouraging results have been reported for treatment with benzoic acid, sodium phenylbutyrate, or sodium phenylacetate.[26] Benzoate is conjugated with glycine to form hippurate, which is excreted by the kidney, and phenylacetate combines with glutamine. This process removes excess amino groups and reduces the hyperammonemia. Hemodialysis is usually required in the acutely ill newborn. Prenatal diagnosis of urea cycle disorders is now performed by DNA analysis of the affected enzyme. Biochemical analysis is not possible because urea cycle enzymes are not expressed in amniocytes or chorionic villous tissue.

### DISORDERS OF BRANCHED-CHAIN AMINO-ACID METABOLISM

The three neutral branched-chain amino acids—leucine, isoleucine, and valine—share a common pathway for initial catabolism. The sequence is transamination, oxidative decarboxylation of the ketoacid derivative, and dehydrogenation of the resultant acyl-coenzyme A (CoA) metabolites. As shown in Table 191-1, the reported biochemical defects in these pathways may be specific to one of the branched-chain amino acids or common to all three (maple syrup urine disease). Ketoacidosis and hypoglycemia are characteristic of several of these diseases. Only defects in the transaminases and ketoacid decarboxylases cause the accumulation of the corresponding amino acids. This is not true of the more distal enzymatic lesions of branched-chain amino-acid metabolism (i.e., isovaleric acidemia). The diagnosis of these disorders is made by organic-acid analysis of the urine using gas chromatography/mass spectrometry rather than amino-acid analyses. Treatment involves consumption of diets deficient in branched-chain amino acids.

## SHORT-CHAIN ORGANIC ACIDEMIAS

Propionyl-CoA is part of the final pathway common to the catabolism of multiple amino acids, sterols, and odd-chain fatty acids. The propionyl-CoA is carboxylated to form D-methylmalonyl-CoA, which, after racemization, is converted to succinyl-CoA. Recurrent metabolic acidosis, pancytopenia, growth failure, and mental retardation occur in patients with disorders of this pathway.

Defects in either the synthesis of the apoenzyme or the metabolism of the biotin cofactor may impair propionyl-CoA carboxylase and produce propionic acidemia. In multiple carboxylase deficiency, the biotin cofactor deficiency is shared by other mitochondrial carboxylases, and abnormalities of pyruvate and of methylcrotonyl metabolism are apparent. Similarly, the defect in methylmalonyl-CoA mutase in methylmalonic acidemia may be secondary to faulty synthesis of either the apoenzyme or the cobalamin coenzyme. If the cobalamin defect involves the synthesis of both adenosylcobalamin, the coenzyme for methylmalonyl-CoA mutase, and methylcobalamin, homocystinuria accompanies the methylmalonic aciduria.

# TRANSPORT DEFECTS

Transport enzymatic defects result in an "overflow" type of aminoaciduria. The increased concentration of the amino acid in the glomerular filtrate exceeds the capacity for tubular reabsorption, resulting in aminoaciduria. Moreover, the urine may contain other amino acids that share and compete for the same tubular transport mechanism. In contrast, syndromes also are found that derive from primary defects in epithelial transport. Although multiple organs may be affected, impairment of renal and small intestine absorption are the most relevant to the clinician. The characteristic biochemical abnormality is an aminoaciduria in the presence of a normal concentration of the substrate in the blood. Intestinal malabsorption of the same substrate may occur. Because epithelial transport systems may be specific for one amino acid or common to a defined group of amino acids, the disorders may involve one or more compounds. Of the disorders listed in Table 191-2, only methionine malabsorption and tryptophan malabsorption are limited to the gastrointestinal tract; each of the others involves the kidney and has variants with intestinal involvement.

The nature and the magnitude of the defect determine the clinical consequences. Intestinal malabsorption may lead to nutrient deficiency, as in the pellagra seen in Hartnup disease. Alternatively, metabolism of the nonabsorbed substrate by the intestinal flora may generate absorbable toxins. The aminoaciduria is rarely sufficient to cause plasma deficiency. In cystinuria, however, the urinary concentration of cystine may exceed the

**TABLE 191-2.**
**Genetic Disorders of Specific Amino-Acid Transport Mechanisms**

| Disorder | Amino Acids | Clinical Expression |
|---|---|---|
| CYSTINURIA | Cystine | Nephrolithiasis |
| | Ornithine | |
| | Arginine | |
| | Lysine | |
| HARTNUP DISEASE | Neutral (mono-amino–mono-carboxylic) | Dermatitis |
| | | Neuropsychiatric symptoms |
| | | Cerebellar ataxia |
| HYPERDIBASICAMINO-ACIDURIA | Ornithine | Protein intolerance |
| | Arginine | Mental retardation |
| | Lysine | Hepatosplenomegaly |
| | Citrulline | Cataracts |
| | | Skeletal defects |
| DICARBOXYLICAMI-NOACIDURIA | Aspartate | Hypoglycemia (inconstant) |
| | Glutamate | |
| FAMILIAL IMINOGLYCI-NURIA | Proline | Benign |
| | Hydroxyproline | |
| | Glycine | |
| METHIONINE MALAB-SORPTION | Methionine | Mental retardation |
| TRYPTOPHAN MALAB-SORPTION (BLUE DIAPER SYNDROME) | Tryptophan | Hypercalcemia |

solubility of the amino acid, and nephrolithiasis is the consequence (see Chap. 69).

Cystinuria is a relatively common defect with an estimated incidence of 1 in 7000 live births. Three variants can be defined on the basis of the degree of intestinal involvement (limited in type III) and the presence of detectable aminoaciduria in obligate heterozygotes (absent in type I). Nephrolithiasis is the only significant pathology and often appears in the second or third decade of life. Because the intestinal absorption of cysteine and cysteine-containing peptides is not impaired, dietary restriction is not effective. Therapy relies on increasing both the volume and the alkalinity of the urine.[27] Penicillamine, a thiol that forms more soluble disulfides with cysteine, may be tried in refractory cases. However, this drug can cause hepatic and renal dysfunction. Tiopronin, another thiol compound, appears to be less toxic.[28]

# STORAGE DISEASES

Cystinosis is the only known storage disorder of amino-acid metabolism.[29] The estimated incidence of this autosomal recessive disease approximates 1 in 200,000 live births. The fundamental defect is a failure of the transport of cystine out of the lysosomes. Consequently, cystine accumulates in these organelles and impairs the function of multiple tissues.

Nephropathic cystinosis is the most common and is the classic form of the disease. During the first decade of life, affected children show a marked retardation of growth without intellectual impairment. This effect may derive from the severe and progressive impairment of renal function. The initial abnormality is the failure of the tubular reabsorption of multiple solutes (glucose, amino acids, phosphate), together with both renal tubular acidosis and nephrogenic diabetes insipidus. Cystinosis is the most common identifiable cause of this Fanconi syndrome in children. Subsequently, glomerular damage begins to dominate the clinical picture, and renal failure usually is present by the

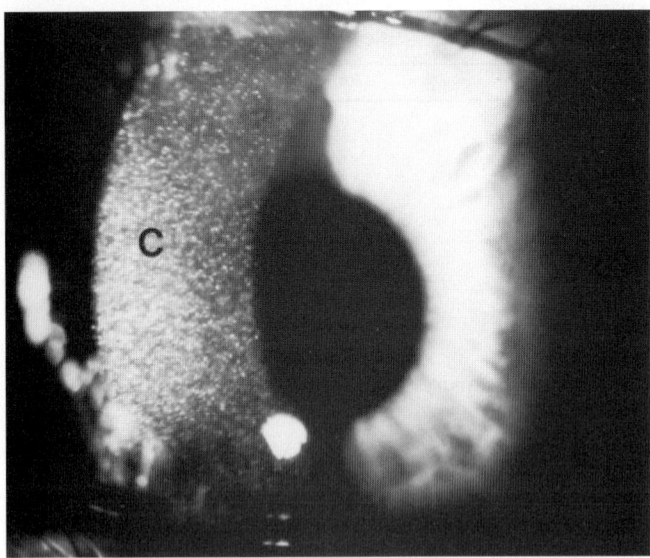

**FIGURE 191-3.** Cystinosis. Slit-lamp examination demonstrates extensive crystal deposits in the cornea (C).

end of the first decade, mandating transplantation or long-term dialysis to maintain life. The grafted kidney remains unaffected. Prolongation of life by renal transplantation has unmasked the more slowly occurring involvement of other organs. Cystine crystals in the cornea, conjunctivae, and irides (Fig. 191-3) are associated with severe photophobia and other ophthalmic symptoms. Hypothyroidism also is common. Hepatomegaly and splenomegaly occur in almost half of the patients.

Two other variants of cystinosis are both rare. A late-onset or adolescent form becomes apparent at a later age but then follows the same course.[30] Benign (adult) cystinosis spares the kidney, although cystine crystals occur in the cornea, conjunctivae, and bone marrow.

In the past, therapy for cystinosis had consisted of the meticulous management of the consequences of the progressive renal dysfunction. The finding that exogenous cysteamine mobilizes intralysosomal cystine, however, has provided the basis for more specific therapy. Unfortunately, this treatment does not restore lost functions; therefore, cysteamine therapy may be of maximal value in the prevention of the progression of cystinosis. Thus, early diagnosis remains essential. Specific evaluations of the younger siblings of known patients and of children with renal Fanconi syndrome are mandatory. Plasma cystine levels are normal; the increased urinary cystine excretion is part of a generalized aminoaciduria. Conversely, both excessive leukocyte cystine and corneal cystine crystals (observed by slit-lamp evaluation) are pathognomonic. Chorionic villus sampling allows prenatal detection; however, the advisability of maternal cysteamine therapy remains unclear.

Linkage analysis in families with cystinosis has localized the gene to the short arm of chromosome 17. Based on this information, a gene (*CTNS*) was identified of which the product (cystinosin) has the properties of a membrane transport protein. Mutation analysis of 108 nephropathic cystinosis patients found that 44% were homozygous for a 65-kb deletion of the cystinosis gene.[31,31a]

## DIAGNOSIS OF INHERITED DISORDERS OF AMINO-ACID METABOLISM

Many patients with inherited disorders of amino-acid metabolism are identified by newborn metabolic screening procedures, which are performed on blood spots obtained at the birth hospital. Currently, only a few states repeat the screen again at 2 to 3 weeks of age. The infant must have consumed a protein meal, and preferably at least two to three feedings, before the sample is obtained to ensure that elevated concentrations of amino acids will be detected. The trend of early discharge from the birth hospital, often within 24 hours of delivery, has led to the misdiagnosis of some affected newborns. For this reason, in cases of early hospital discharge, the recommendation is that newborn metabolic screening be repeated at the first pediatric visit to ensure identification of infants with amino-acid disorders. Most state newborn screening programs focus on diseases that have an initial asymptomatic period and for which an effective treatment exists to prevent irreversible pathology. PKU is the prototype disorder for which newborn screening was instituted, although most states also screen for tyrosinemia, maple syrup urine disease, biotinidase deficiency, and homocystinuria. A sibling of a patient with a known aminoacidopathy, in addition to undergoing newborn screening, should be evaluated by quantitative plasma amino-acid analysis as soon as protein-containing feedings are instituted.

In addition to identification by newborn screening programs, many patients with inborn errors of amino-acid metabolism are diagnosed when the astute clinician suspects a biochemical disorder. Pediatricians are most frequently involved, because they see the young patient with unexplained ketoacidosis, failure to thrive, formula intolerance, or developmental delay. Because of the organ-specific conditions associated with many of these disorders (Table 191-3), however, diagnosis by other physicians is not uncommon. The ophthalmologist may be the first to evaluate a patient with homocystinuria or gyrate atrophy of the choroid and retina, whereas the dermatologist may see the patient with alkaptonuria, albinism, or Hartnup disorder. Hematologists must be aware of the metabolic syndromes associated with severe anemia, pancytopenia, and other hematologic abnormalities. The nephrologist must consider cystinuria in young patients with nephrolithiasis, and unexplained thromboembolism or premature arteriosclerosis should alert the cardiologist to the possibility of homocystinuria. The endocrinologist, in particular, must be at least superficially familiar with these models of disordered metabolism, as well as their clinical manifestations.

Prenatal diagnosis is now possible for many disorders of amino-acid metabolism. Amniotic fluid may be directly analyzed for abnormal metabolites; alternatively, fetal tissue obtained by amniocentesis (at 15–17 weeks' gestation) or by chorionic villus sampling (at 10–12 weeks' gestation) can be used as source material for enzyme assays. The limited tissue distribution of many of the enzymes often restricts the applicability of enzymatic diagnosis. For example, phenylalanine hydroxylase (which is deficient in PKU) is not expressed in amniocytes or chorionic villus cells and is present only in liver. In some cases, diagnosis by fetal tissue sampling is theoretically possible but is associated with a significant risk of fetal loss. Many of these difficulties in prenatal testing are being overcome by the use of DNA-based diagnosis, because all cells with a nucleus share the same genetic characteristics. Another experimental approach involves obtaining and analyzing nucleated fetal red blood cells present in the maternal circulation.

Laboratory services used to diagnose and monitor patients with inborn errors of amino-acid metabolism are available through many commercial laboratories and in academic medical centers. The development of dedicated amino-acid analyzers allows rapid and accurate determination of amino-acid concentrations of biologic fluids. Although many laboratories still use paper chromatography of urine samples as a screening procedure, the speed and accuracy of quantitative plasma amino-acid analysis makes it the procedure of choice, and such analysis is

**TABLE 191-3.**
**Organ-Specific Involvement in Inherited Disorders of Amino-Acid Metabolism**

| Organ or Organ System | Disease or Condition | Amino-Acid Disorder |
|---|---|---|
| **EYES** | Ectopia lentis | Cystathionine synthase deficiency |
| | | Sulfocysteinuria |
| | | Gyrate atrophy |
| | Cataracts | Dibasicaminoaciduria |
| | Corneal crystals, photophobia | Cystinosis |
| | Corneal ulcers | Tyrosinemia type II |
| | Retinal degeneration | Gyrate atrophy |
| | Nystagmus, photophobia, no binocular vision | Albinism (all forms) |
| **SKIN AND HAIR** | Eczema | Phenylalaninemia type I |
| | Depigmentation | Oculocutaneous albinism |
| | Hypopigmentation | Phenylalaninemia |
| | | Cystinosis |
| | Palmar keratoses | Tyrosinemia type II |
| | Trichorrhexis nodosa | Argininosuccinic aciduria |
| | Alopecia with erythroderma | Multiple carboxylase deficiency |
| | Chronic dermatitis and leg ulcers | Hyperimidodipeptiduria |
| | Blue coloration of cartilage, tendons | Alkaptonuria |
| | Pellagra-like rash | Hartnup disease |
| **MUSCULO-SKELETAL** | Osteoporosis | Cystathionine synthase deficiency |
| | | Dibasicaminoaciduria |
| | Hyperextensible joints | Hyperimidodipeptiduria |
| | | Dibasicaminoaciduria |
| | Dolichostenomelia | Cystathionine synthase deficiency |
| | Arthritis | Alkaptonuria (ochronosis) |
| **CARDIOVAS-CULAR** | Thromboembolism | Cystathionine synthase deficiency |
| | | Methylenetetrahydrofolate reductase deficiency |
| | Aortic stenosis | Alkaptonuria |
| **LUNG** | Restrictive defect | Hermansky-Pudlak albinism |
| **GASTRO-INTESTINAL** | Colitis | Hermansky-Pudlak albinism |
| | Cirrhosis and hepatoma | Tyrosinemia type I |
| | Hepatomegaly (mild steatoses and dysfunction) | Urea cycle defects |
| | | Cystinosis |
| **KIDNEY** | Nephrolithiasis | Cystinuria |
| | Fanconi syndrome | Cystinosis |
| | | Tyrosinemia type I |
| | Aminoaciduria (generalized) | Carbamoyl phosphate synthase deficiency |
| | | Glutamylcysteine synthase deficiency |
| **BLOOD** | Hemolysis | Glutathione synthase deficiency |
| | | Glutamylcysteine synthase deficiency |
| | Megaloblastic anemia | Homocystinuria secondary to deranged cobalamin metabolism |
| | Pancytopenia | Methylmalonic acidurias |
| | Platelet defects | Hermansky-Pudlak albinism |
| | | Isovaleric acidemia |
| | Leukocyte defects | Chédiak-Higashi albinism |
| | | Isovaleric acidemia |
| | Porphyria | Tyrosinemia type I |

**TABLE 191-4.**
**Urine Screening Tests for Amino-Acid Disorders**

| Disorder | Result or Substance Detected |
|---|---|
| **FERRIC CHLORIDE TEST\*** | |
| Phenylketonuria | Blue-green |
| Tyrosinemia | Transient blue-green |
| Maple syrup urine disease | Blue, yellow, green |
| Hyperalaninemia | Yellow |
| Methionine malabsorption | Purple |
| Alkaptonuria | Dark brown |
| Histidinemia | Blue-green |
| **REDUCING SUBSTANCES (BENEDICT'S TEST)** | |
| Alkaptonuria | Homogentisic acid |
| Tyrosinemia | p-Hydroxyphenylpyruvate |
| **2,4-DINITROPHENYLHYDRAZINE TEST†** | |
| Yellow or red precipitate with ketoacids | |
| **CYANIDE-NITROPRUSSIDE TEST‡** | |
| Homocystinuria | Homocystine |
| | Homocysteine–cysteine mixed disulfide |
| Cystinuria | Cystine |
| Glutathionuria | Glutathione |

*Add $FeCl_3 \cdot 6 H_2O$ solution (10% w/v in 0.25 N HCl) dropwise to 1 mL of fresh urine. Any change in color from that of the ferric chloride solution constitutes a positive test.
†Mix with equal volume of 2,4-dinitrophenylhydrazine solution (0.5 g/dL in 2 N HCl).
‡Mix sodium cyanide solution (5% w/v in water) with equal volume of urine. Add 3–4 drops of fresh solution of a few crystals of sodium nitroprusside in water. Deep magenta color is positive; weak pink-orange is negative.

certainly indicated in any patient for whom there is a high suspicion of an aminoacidopathy. To avoid false-positive elevations due to the ingestion of protein, blood specimens should be obtained after a 12-hour fast in adults or after at least a 4- to 6-hour fast in young children. Quantitative amino-acid analysis of urine can also be performed, but the results are much more difficult to interpret than are those from plasma, owing to the much wider variation of normal urine amino-acid concentrations. Analysis of the cerebrospinal fluid glycine concentration is particularly useful in the diagnosis of nonketotic hyperglycinemia.

The urine metabolic screen (metabolic urinalysis) consists of a series of rapid screening tests that often provide the first clue to the presence of a metabolic disorder (Table 191-4). The ferric chloride test is the best known of these and is useful in the diagnosis of PKU, tyrosinemia, histidinemia, and alkaptonuria. Several drugs (phenothiazines, salicylates), as well as the presence of conjugated bilirubin, produce a positive result with the ferric chloride reagent. The 2,4-dinitrophenylhydrazine test detects 2-oxoacids and is useful in the diagnosis of maple syrup urine disease. Nitrosonaphthol reacts with tyrosine and its metabolites (tyrosinemia), and cyanide-nitroprusside detects sulfur amino acids (cystinuria, homocystinuria).

Many amino-acid disorders also produce disturbances in organic-acid excretion, because an early step in the catabolism of many amino acids is the removal of the amino group, which produces the corresponding organic acid. Analysis of urine organic-acid excretion by gas chromatography/mass spectrometry is an extremely sensitive and powerful tool that is widely available and, when used with plasma amino-acid analysis and urine metabolic screening, provides a comprehensive evaluation of the patient suspected of having an inborn error of metabolism. In some cases, the diagnosis of an amino-acid disorder can be confirmed by specific enzyme analysis in leukocytes, fibroblasts, or liver biopsy tissue. The limited tissue distribution and instability of some enzymes, however, and the accuracy of plasma amino-acid analysis in most cases make enzyme-based diagnosis unnecessary. New tests based on DNA technology may overcome the obstacles to enzyme-based analysis.

Identification of persons with amino-acid disorders by a finding of abnormalities in routine laboratory studies such as a chemistry panel is uncommon. Diagnosis, therefore, requires suspicion on the part of the clinician as well as the expertise of special laboratories that have experience in performing these complex studies. Clear communication between the referring physician and laboratory director is essential to ensure that appropriate studies are performed. This avoids a "shotgun" approach to metabolic evaluation, which, because of the labor-intensive nature of these studies, could result in a high expense for unnecessary testing. Referral to a regional clinic for metabolic disease (often located at academic medical centers) is recommended for patients with unusual or complex disorders.

## REFERENCES

1. Garrod AE. Croonian Lecture I: inborn errors of metabolism. Lancet 1908; 2:1.
2. Beadle GW. Genetic control of biochemical reactions. Harvey Lect 1945; 40:179.
3. Pauling L, Itano HA, Singer SJ, Wells IC. Sickle cell anemia: a molecular disease. Science 1949; 11:543.
4. Scriver CR, Beaudet AL, Sly WS, Valle D, eds. The metabolic basis of inherited disease, 7th ed. New York: McGraw-Hill, 1995.
5. Rashed MS, Ozand PT, Bucknall MP, Little D. Diagnosis of inborn errors of metabolism from blood spots by acylcarnitine and amino acid profiling using automated electrospray tandem mass spectrometry. Pediatr Res 1995; 38:324.
6. Finkelstein JD. Methionine metabolism in mammals: the biochemical basis of homocystinuria. Metabolism 1974; 23:387.
7. Scriver CR. Vitamin responsive inborn errors of metabolism. Metabolism 1973; 22:1319.
8. Scriver CR, Kaufman S, Eisensmith JL, Woo SL. The hyperphenylalaninemias. In: Scriver CR, Beaudet AL, Sly WS, Valle D, eds. The metabolic basis of inherited disease, 7th ed. New York: McGraw-Hill, 1995:1015.
9. Svensson E, Isellius L, Hagenfeldt L. Severity of mutation in the phenylalanine hydroxylase gene influences phenylalanine metabolism in phenylketonuria and hyperphenylalaninemia heterozygotes. J Inherit Metab Dis 1994; 17:215.
10. Lenke RR, Levy HL. Maternal phenylketonuria and hyperphenylalaninemia. N Engl J Med 1980; 303:1202.
11. Sammartino A, Carbella R, Cecio A, et al. The effect of diet on the ophthalmologic, clinical and biochemical aspects of Richner-Hanhart syndrome: a morphological ultrastructural study of the cornea and the conjunctiva. Int Ophthalmol 1987; 10:203.
12. Lindstedt S, Holme E, Lock EA, et al. Treatment of hereditary tyrosinaemia type I by inhibition of 4-hydroxyphenylpyruvate dioxygenase. Lancet 1992; 340:813.
13. Gaines JJ Jr. The pathology of alkaptonuric ochronosis. Hum Pathol 1989; 20:40.
14. Fernandez-Canon JM, Granadino B, Beltran-Valero de Bernabe D, et al. The molecular basis of alkaptonuria. Nat Genet 1996; 14:19.
15. Oetting WS, King RA. Molecular basis of albinism: mutations and polymorphisms of pigmentation genes associated with albinism. Hum Mutat 1999; 13:99.
16. Witkop CJ, Kromwiede M, Sedano H, White JG. Reliability of absent platelet dense bodies as a diagnostic criterion for Hermansky-Pudlak syndrome. Am J Hematol 1987; 26:305.
17. Finkelstein JD. Pathways and regulation of homocysteine metabolism in mammals. Semin Thromb Hemost 2000; 26:219.
18. Mudd SH, Levy HL, Skovby F. Disorders of transsulfuration. In: Scriver CR, Beaudet AL, Sly WS, Valle D, eds. The metabolic and molecular bases of inherited disease. New York: McGraw-Hill, 1995:1279.
19. Mudd SH, Finkelstein JD, Refsum H, et al. Homocysteine and its disulfide derivatives. A suggested consensus nomenclature. Arterioscler Throm Vasc Biol 2000; 20:1704.
20. Yap S, Naughten ER, Wilcken B, et al. Vascular complications of severe hyperhomocysteinemia in patients with homocystinuria due to cystathionine beta-synthase deficiency: effects of homocysteine-lowering therapy. Semin Thromb Hemost 2000; 26:335.
21. Rosenblatt DS. Inherited disorders of folate transport and metabolism. In: Scriver CR, Beaudet AL, Sly WS, Valle D, eds. The metabolic and molecular bases of inherited disease. New York: McGraw-Hill, 1995:3111.
22. Fenton WA, Rosenberg LE. Inherited disorders of cobalamin transport and metabolism. In: Scriver CR, Beaudet AL, Sly WS, Valle D, eds. The metabolic and molecular bases of inherited disease. New York: McGraw-Hill, 1995:3129.
23a. Refsum H, Ueland PM, Nygard O, Vollset SE. Homocysteine and cardiovascular disease. Annu Rev Medicine 1998; 49:31.
23b. Brattstrom L, Wilcken DEL. Homocysteine and cardiovascular disease: cause or effect. Am J Clin Nutr 2000; 72:315.
24a. Malinow MR, Bostom AG, Krauss RM. Homocyst(e)ine, diet and cardiovascular diseases. A statement for healthcare professionals from the Nutrition Committee, American Heart Association. Circulation 1999; 99:178.
24b. Chamberlin ME, Ubagai T, Mudd SH, et al. Demyelination of the brain is associated with methionine adenosyltransferase I/III deficiency. J Clin Invest 1996; 98:1021.
25. Meister A, Anderson ME. Glutathione. Annu Rev Biochem 1983; 52:711.
26. Brusilow SA, Horwich AL. Urea cycle enzymes. In: Scriver CR, Beaudet AL, Sly WS, Valle D, eds. The metabolic basis of inherited disease, 7th ed. New York: McGraw-Hill, 1995:1187.
27. Scriver CR. Cystinuria. N Engl J Med 1986; 315:1155.
28. Tiopronin for cystinuria. Med Lett Drugs Ther 1989; 31(Jan 27):7.
29. Gahl WA, Renlund M, Thoene JG. Lysosomal transport disorders: cystinosis and sialic acid storage disorders. In: Scriver CR, Beaudet AL, Sly WS, Valle D, eds. The metabolic basis of inherited disease, 6th ed. New York: McGraw-Hill, 1989:2619.
30. Gahl WA, Schneider JA, Aula PP. Lysosomal transport disorders: cystinosis and sialic acid storage disorders. In: Seriver CR, Beaudet AL, Sly WS, Valle D, eds. The metabolic and molecular basis of inherited disease. 7th edition. McGraw Hill, NY: 1995, 3763.
31. Shotelersuk V, Larson D, Anikster Y, et al. CTNS mutations in an American-based population of cystinosis patients. Am J Hum Genet 1998; 63:1352.
31a. Touchman JW, Anikster Y, Dietrich NL, et al. The genomic region encompassing the nephropathic cystinosis gene (CTNS). Genome Res 2000; 10:165.

# CHAPTER 192

# HERITABLE DISEASES OF PURINE METABOLISM

EDWARD W. HOLMES AND DAVID J. NASHEL

## GENERAL CONSIDERATIONS

Disorders of purine metabolism, which may be inherited or acquired, affect many organ systems, and clinical symptoms differ depending on the disorder and the particular organ systems affected. This chapter focuses on inherited defects, but, where appropriate, acquired defects also are cited for comparison. For some disorders, such as gout, it is difficult to separate inherited abnormalities completely from environmental influences, and the interplay between genetics and environment must be considered.

### SIGNS AND SYMPTOMS

*Arthritis* secondary to the deposition of monosodium urate crystals in synovial fluid is a prominent clinical manifestation of several inherited defects: hypoxanthine-guanine phosphoribosyltransferase (HPRT) deficiency, phosphoribosylpyrophosphate synthetase (PRPPS) overactivity, and glucose-6-phosphatase deficiency. *Nephrolithiasis* secondary to uric acid crystal formation in renal collecting structures also is a clinical feature of disorders such as HPRT deficiency and PRPPS overactivity, where uric acid is overproduced and excreted in the urine. Two other inherited defects, xanthine oxidase (XO) deficiency and adenine phosphoribosyltransferase (APRT) deficiency, lead to excessive excretion of the relatively insoluble purine bases xanthine and 2,8-dihydroxyadenine, respectively. Renal colic also develops in patients having these enzyme defects. *Neurologic symptoms*, including spasticity, choreoathetosis, mental retardation, and self-mutilation, ensue from high-grade deficiency of HPRT (Lesch-Nyhan syndrome), and autism may result from adenylosuccinate (S-AMP) lyase deficiency. *Immunodeficiency states* resulting from combined T- and B-cell defects or isolated T-cell defects are consequences of deficiencies of adenosine deaminase (ADA) and purine nucleoside phosphorylase (PNP), respectively. Patients with these enzyme deficiencies are subject to recurrent infections from an early age. *Metabolic myopathy symptoms*, including easy fatigability, muscle cramps, and myalgias, result from a deficiency of adenylate deaminase.

In most of these disorders, the enzyme defect is manifest in all tissues, and selective involvement of organ systems relates to

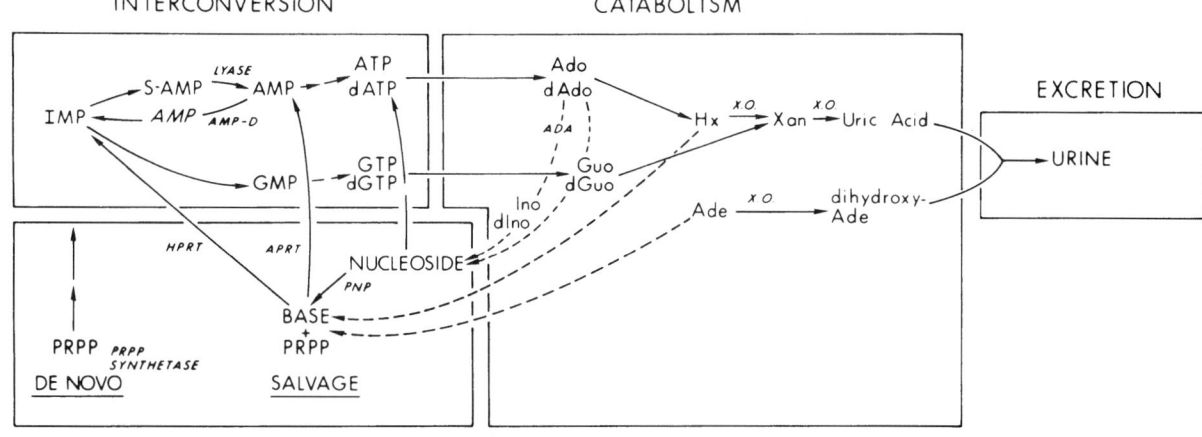

INTERCONVERSION                    CATABOLISM

FIGURE 192-1. Disorders of purine metabolism. Defects are broken down into derangements in purine synthesis, interconversion, catabolism, and excretion. (*PRPP*, phosphoribosylpyrophosphate; *IMP*, inosine monophosphate; *AMP*, adenosine monophosphate; *S-AMP*, succinyl-AMP; *GMP*, guanosine monophosphate; *Ado* and *dAdo*, adenosine and deoxyadenosine, respectively; *Guo* and *dGuo*, guanosine and deoxyguanosine, respectively; *Ino* and *dIno*, inosine and deoxyinosine, respectively; *Hx*, hypoxanthine; *Xan*, xanthine; *Ade*, adenine; *HPRT*, hypoxanthine-guanine phosphoribosyltransferase; *APRT*, adenine phosphoribosyltransferase; *PNP*, purine nucleoside phosphorylase; *lyase*, adenylosuccinate lyase; *AMP-D*, AMP deaminase; *ADA*, adenosine deaminase; *XO*, xanthine oxidase; *GTP*, guanosine triphosphate; *dGTP*, deoxyguanosine triphosphate; *ATP*, adenosine triphosphate; *dATP*, deoxyadenosine triphosphate.)

the accumulation of metabolic precursors or end products of purine metabolism in particular organs. However, in at least one condition, adenylate deaminase deficiency, the enzyme deficiency is localized to a specific tissue, skeletal muscle.

## CLASSIFICATION

Disorders of purine metabolism have been organized into categories of defects in *purine synthesis, catabolism, interconversion,* or *excretion.* Inspection of Figure 192-1 reveals numerous interconnections between the various components of the purine pathway. It follows that a primary defect in one component, such as purine synthesis, may lead to secondary changes in other components, such as purine catabolism and excretion. The clinical presentation is then influenced by the combined derangements in purine metabolism. For example, a person with a primary defect in purine synthesis develops hyperuricemia because of increased purine nucleotide production, with subsequent catabolism to uric acid. Hyperuricosuria is the result of increased uric acid production and excretion. Thus, gouty arthritis, a consequence of hyperuricemia, and renal calculi, a consequence of hyperuricosuria, reflect the secondary changes more than the primary derangement in purine metabolism. For other disorders, clinical manifestations may arise from a secondary effect on an entirely different metabolic system, such as a derangement in energy metabolism or DNA synthesis. Where known, interrelations between defects in purine metabolism and other pathways are pointed out; and to the extent possible, these derangements in metabolism are related to the symptoms and signs patients exhibit.

## DISORDERS OF PURINE SYNTHESIS

### CONSEQUENCES OF PURINE OVERPRODUCTION

Excessive rates of purine synthesis lead to excessive rates of uric acid production because urate is normally the end product of purine metabolism in humans.[1,2] Other mammals, except some species of New World apes, are able to oxidize urate to allantoin and other degradation products that are more soluble than urate

and uric acid. It is this poor solubility of urate and uric acid that leads to clinical problems in patients who overproduce purines.

The precipitation of urate, predominantly as the sodium salt, in cartilage, synovial membranes, and synovial fluid is responsible for initiating an inflammatory response leading to the acute attacks of arthritis that are characteristic of gout (Fig. 192-2). The arthritis typically is monoarticular in the early stages of gout but later may become polyarticular. Any joint lined with synovium may be affected, but distal joints are affected more often, and joints of the lower extremities are affected more often than joints of the upper extremities. After an acute attack of gouty arthritis, symptoms usually resolve completely, and the patient enters an *intercritical period* in which there are no symptoms. This symptom-free interval may last for years.[1,2]

Urate salt deposition is not limited to joints and periarticular structures, but also occurs in soft tissues throughout the body. These deposits, which usually are not inflammatory, are referred

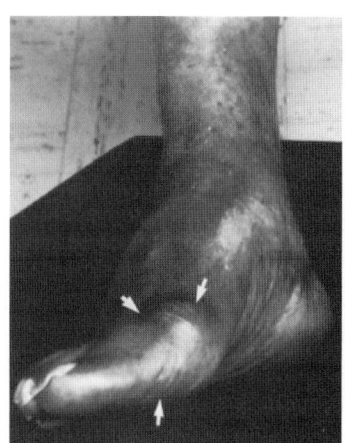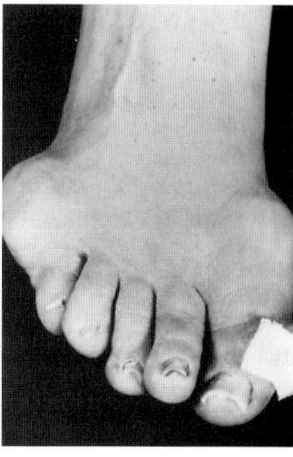

A,B

FIGURE 192-2. **A,** Acute attack of podagra (involvement of the big toe). Note the swollen area (*arrows*) and the shiny skin, which was warm to the touch. **B,** Chronic tophaceous gout affecting the first and fifth metatarsophalangeal joints. The bandage covers a draining tophaceous area. Initially, the patient had had recurrent attacks of pain of the metatarsophalangeal joint of the great toe (podagra).

to as *tophi*[3] (see Fig. 192-2). Subcutaneous tophi may ulcerate and drain urate crystals and, rarely, become secondarily infected. Tophi in the interstitium of the kidney may lead to fibrosis and mild renal insufficiency, a condition referred to as *urate nephropathy.*

Urate salts are unlikely to precipitate from extracellular fluids unless their concentration exceeds the solubility limit. For sodium urate, the predominant urate salt in body fluids, the solubility limit is ~7 mg/dL in serum. The distinction between a normal and an elevated serum urate concentration is somewhat arbitrary, because the statistical definition of hyperuricemia depends on the method by which urate is quantitated, the ethnic background of the population used to determine the statistical limits, and the environment in which the test population lives. For example, enzymatic methods for determining serum urate give results that are ~1 mg/dL lower than the colorimetric methods used in many automated clinical laboratories. The statistical definition of a normal urate concentration is confounded by the nonnormal distribution of urate concentrations in most populations, by differences in urate concentration among different ethnic groups, and by the effects of diet and other environmental factors on urate metabolism. In the authors' opinion, the most reasonable definition of hyperuricemia is that value at which urate concentration exceeds its solubility limit in body fluids, possibly leading to urate deposition and clinical symptoms. As mentioned earlier, when the urate concentration is >7 mg/dL, as determined by the enzymatic method, serum is supersaturated, and the patient is at risk for urate precipitation. If serum urate is determined by a colorimetric method that yields a higher value, the serum concentration that is saturating for urate may be 1 mg/dL higher. This chemical definition of hyperuricemia provides a uniform benchmark for monitoring patients of diverse ethnic backgrounds in different environmental situations. Its clinical utility is borne out by its widespread use.

Uric acid is much less soluble than its salt, but the pK of this acid (5.75) precludes its formation anywhere in the body except the urine. Patients who overproduce purines overexcrete uric acid in the urine; consequently, they are predisposed to the formation of uric acid calculi. Stone formation is exacerbated in patients who excrete a persistently acid urine, thereby favoring the formation of uric acid over that of urate. Patients who excrete low urine volumes, thereby increasing the concentration of uric acid, also are predisposed to stone formation. Rarely, uric acid excretion reaches extraordinary levels in patients with inherited defects in purine synthesis or in those with malignancies where accelerated cell turnover and nucleic acid catabolism lead to large increases in uric acid excretion. In these unusual situations, uric acid crystallizes in the collecting tubules, leading to acute renal failure. The latter condition is referred to as *acute uric acid nephropathy* to distinguish it from the urate nephropathy described earlier.[4]

*Hyperuricosuria,* or excessive uric acid excretion, is more difficult to define than hyperuricemia, because it depends on many factors, one of the most important being the purine content of the diet. On a purine-free diet, urate excretion normally is <600 mg per day.[1,2] The upper limit of "normal" on unrestricted diets is not well established, but most investigators believe that excretion in excess of 800 to 1000 mg uric acid per day is indicative of excessive uric acid production.

## CONTROL OF PURINE SYNTHESIS

Many conditions, some inherited, most acquired, influence purine synthesis and uric acid production. Table 192-1 provides a list of some of these conditions. Increased purine synthesis may arise from an enzyme defect causing a primary increase in

**TABLE 192-1.**
**Causes of Hyperuricemia in Humans**

---

**INCREASED PURINE BIOSYNTHESIS OR URATE PRODUCTION**
*Inherited enzymatic defects*
    Hypoxanthine-guanine phosphoribosyltransferase deficiency
    Phosphoribosylpyrophosphate synthetase overactivity
    Glucose-6-phosphatase deficiency
*Clinical disorders leading to purine overproduction*
    Myeloproliferative disorders
    Lymphoproliferative disorders
    Polycythemia vera
    Malignant diseases
    Hemolytic disorders
    Psoriasis
    Obesity
    Myocardial infarction
*Drugs or dietary habits*
    Ethanol
    Diet rich in purines
    Pancreatic extract
    Fructose
    Ethylamino-1,3,4-thiadiazole
    4-Amino-5-imidazole carboxamide riboside
    Vitamin $B_{12}$ (patients with pernicious anemia)
    Cytotoxic drugs
**DECREASED RENAL CLEARANCE OF URATE**
*Clinical disorders*
    Chronic renal failure
    Lead nephropathy
    Polycystic kidney disease
    Hypertension
    Dehydration
    Salt restriction
    Starvation
    Diabetic ketoacidosis
    Lactic acidosis
    Obesity
    Hyperparathyroidism
    Hypothyroidism
    Diabetes insipidus
    Sarcoidosis
    Toxemia of pregnancy
    Bartter syndrome
    Chronic beryllium disease
    Down syndrome
*Drugs or dietary habits*
    Ethanol
    Diuretics
    Low doses of salicylates
    Cyclosporine
    Ethambutol
    Pyrazinamide
    Laxative abuse (alkalosis)
    Levodopa
    Methoxyflurane

---

purine synthesis or may be a secondary response to increased purine catabolism.[5] Because of the exquisite control mechanisms that regulate purine synthesis, it can be difficult to tell whether purine production is being "pushed" by a primary increase in the rate of synthesis or "pulled" by a primary increase in purine catabolism. Work in many systems, including humans, has shown that the activity of the first enzyme unique to the pathway of purine biosynthesis, amidophospho-

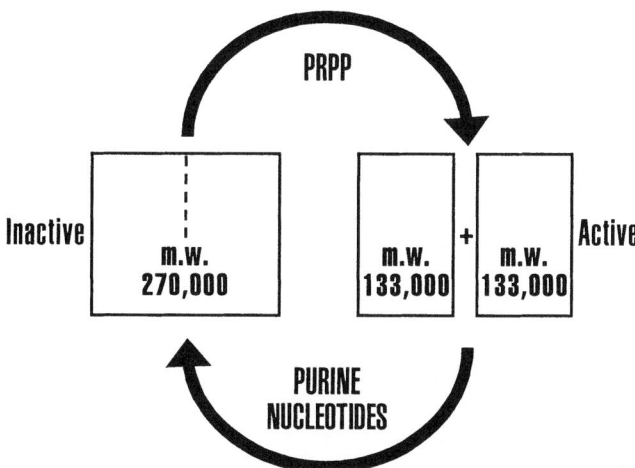

**FIGURE 192-3.** Role of phosphoribosylpyrophosphate (*PRPP*) and purine nucleotides in control of purine biosynthesis. Amidophosphoribosyltransferase, the enzyme that catalyzes the first and rate-limiting reaction in purine biosynthesis, assumes either an inactive (270,000 daltons) or active (133,000 daltons) conformation in the cell. The relative distribution between the active and inactive conformation is controlled by the relative concentrations of PRPP and purine nucleotides. (*m.w.*, molecular weight.)

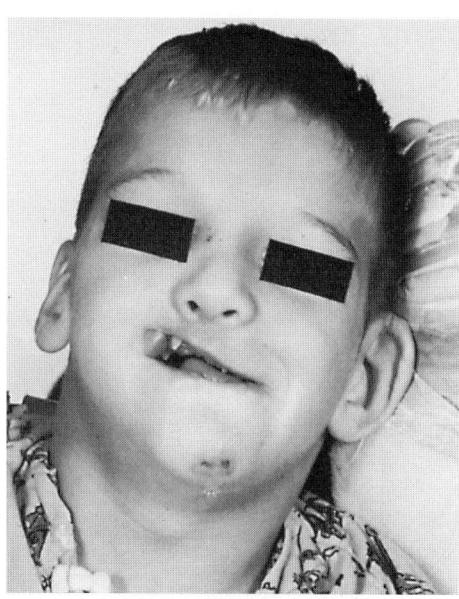

**FIGURE 192-4.** Lesch-Nyhan syndrome. Self-destructive behavior has resulted in injury to chin and bridge of nose and destruction of upper and lower lips.

ribosyltransferase, is controlled by the availability of its substrate, PRPP, and by the end products of the pathway, purine ribonucleotides (Fig. 192-3). The activity of the enzyme that catalyzes the rate-limiting step in the de novo pathway of purine synthesis is increased when the PRPP concentration in the cell rises, whereas the activity decreases when the concentration of purine nucleotide increases. Thus, there is a reciprocal relation between PRPP and purine nucleotide concentrations—increases in the former increase purine synthesis, as do decreases in the latter.

## PHOSPHORIBOSYLPYROPHOSPHATE SYNTHETASE OVERACTIVITY

PRPPS catalyzes a reaction in which the pyrophosphate group from adenosine triphosphate (ATP) is added to ribose-5-phosphate, creating an "activated" form of ribose-5-phosphate that participates in all reactions leading to purine, pyrimidine, and pyridine nucleotide synthesis. Overactivity of this enzyme is inherited as an autosomal dominant trait. The enzyme exists in an aggregate of two subunits encoded by genes on the X chromosome and two associating subunits encoded by genes on chromosome 17.[6] The principal clinical consequences of overactivity of PRPPS are hyperuricemia with gouty arthritis and tophi, as well as hyperuricosuria (often >1 g per day) with uric acid nephrolithiasis. The activity of this enzyme, which can be documented by assay of erythrocyte lysates, is increased in patients with primary gout and is not suppressed by allopurinol therapy.[7] A number of different types of enzymatic defects, including $K_m$ mutants and feedback-resistant mutants, account for overactivity of this enzyme, and all share the property of increasing the intracellular levels of PRPP. This increase in PRPP concentration activates the first enzyme in the de novo pathway of purine synthesis (see Fig. 192-3), with an increase in purine nucleotide formation. Subsequent catabolism of the purine nucleotides increases uric acid formation and excretion (see Fig. 192-1). Increased PRPP synthetase activity is a good example of a primary defect in purine synthesis "pushing" the catabolic and excretory components of the pathway.

## HYPOXANTHINE-GUANINE PHOSPHORIBOSYLTRANSFERASE DEFICIENCY

HPRT, another enzyme encoded by a gene on the X chromosome, catalyzes a significant reaction in the salvage pathway in which the purine bases, hypoxanthine and guanine, are phosphoribosylated to form purine nucleotides (see Fig. 192-1). This is one of the best studied of the human enzymatic deficiencies, including comprehensive metabolic studies in patients, biochemical analyses of cultured cells, and documentation of amino-acid changes in the HPRT protein and base substitutions in the HPRT gene.[8]

Two clinical syndromes are associated with this enzyme defect, which is inherited as an X-linked recessive disorder. *High-grade deficiencies* (<0.01% residual activity) cause the *Lesch-Nyhan syndrome*,[9] characterized by self-mutilation, choreoathetosis, mental retardation, and uric acid overproduction with gout and renal calculi (Figs. 192-4 and 192-5). Uric acid excretion reaches extraordinary levels, often exceeding 1 g per day in small children. The cause of the neurologic symptoms is not known but may be related to defects in neurotransmitter formation[9a] or in purine nucleotide synthesis in regions of the brain that have a limited capacity for de novo purine synthesis. The basal ganglia appear to be particularly susceptible to involvement.[9b] *Less severe or "partial" deficiencies* (>0.1% residual activity) of HPRT are associated with early (teenage)-onset gout and uric acid crystal formation (infancy), and, occasionally, acute renal insufficiency.[10] Neurologic symptoms either are absent or mild. Rarely, mothers of HPRT-deficient male children exhibit mild degrees of purine overproduction and late-onset gout, indicating that this disorder can be inherited as an incomplete X-linked dominant trait in unusual situations.

HPRT deficiency can be diagnosed readily by assay of erythrocyte lysates. A deficiency of this enzyme has two important consequences for purine synthesis: First, PRPP accumulates because it is not used in this salvage reaction, and second, purine nucleotide formation through salvage mechanisms is reduced (see Fig. 192-1). Consequently, there is increased activity of the first enzyme in the de novo pathway of purine synthesis (see Fig. 192-3). (HPRT deficiency is also discussed in the section Disorders of Purine Salvage.)

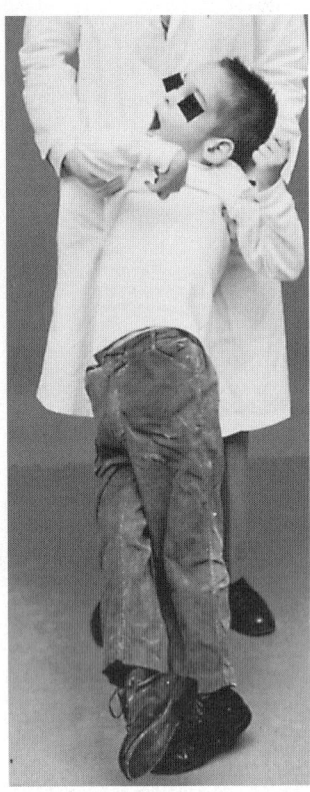

**FIGURE 192-5.** Lesch-Nyhan syndrome. Choreoathetosis of upper extremities and scissoring of lower extremities are typical of the spasticity observed in this disorder.

## MANAGEMENT OF PURINE OVERPRODUCTION

The treatment of purine overproduction states in patients with a primary derangement in purine synthesis, as in PRPP synthetase overactivity or HPRT deficiency, or in patients with a secondary increase in purine synthesis due to a primary defect in purine catabolism, is aimed at reducing uric acid formation. This is accomplished through the use of allopurinol, a drug that inhibits XO activity (Fig. 192-6; see Fig. 192-1). In the setting of Lesch-Nyhan syndrome, the use of allopurinol results in increased con-

centrations of hypoxanthine and xanthine in the urine. As a consequence, there is heightened risk of xanthine calculi formation. Sonography has been successfully used to detect these xanthine-containing calculi.[11] In patients with normal HPRT activity, the accumulation of hypoxanthine as a result of XO inhibition leads to increased purine base salvage and decreased de novo purine synthesis. This effect reduces the total amount of purine (hypoxanthine, xanthine, and uric acid) produced each day. XO inhibition also is beneficial because it replaces uric acid as the end product of purine metabolism with the more soluble purine base, hypoxanthine. The latter effect reduces urate and uric acid concentrations in serum and urine, respectively, thereby decreasing crystal formation in all patients with gout, even those with HPRT deficiency. In patients with normal HPRT activity, there is the added effect of decreased purine production. Although there still is no satisfactory treatment for the neurologic symptoms associated with HPRT deficiency, the production of a mouse model for Lesch-Nyhan syndrome[12] and the prospect of germline gene modification[13] raise the potential for somatic gene therapy and possibly even future treatment and prevention of this devastating disorder.

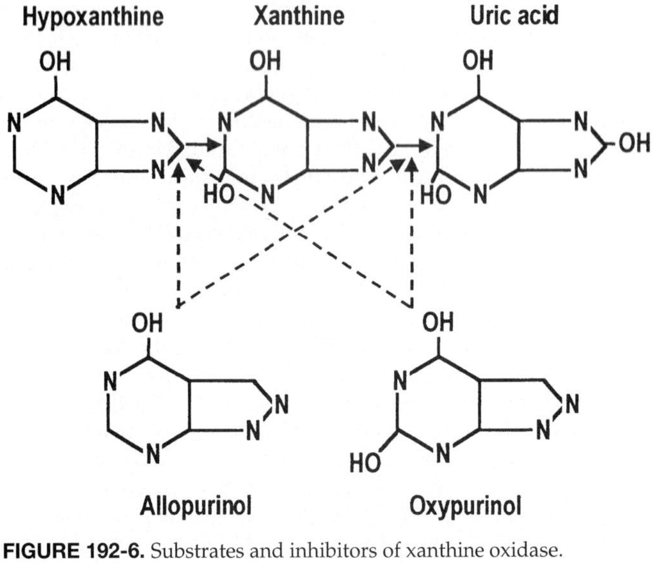

## DISORDERS OF PURINE SALVAGE

### HYPOXANTHINE-GUANINE PHOSPHORIBOSYLTRANSFERASE DEFICIENCY

HPRT deficiency is a disorder of *both purine base salvage and purine synthesis*. Failure to reuse hypoxanthine (and guanine) contributes to the excessive rate of uric acid production observed in patients with this enzyme defect. In normal persons, a large portion of the hypoxanthine produced each day through purine nucleotide catabolism is salvaged by the HPRT reaction. Loss of this salvage mechanism contributes to the excess production of uric acid characteristic of this disorder. Several mutations have been described.[13a]

### ADENINE PHOSPHORIBOSYL TRANSFERASE DEFICIENCY

Reutilization of the purine base, adenine, is catalyzed by APRT (see Fig. 192-1). This enzyme is the product of a gene different from that for HPRT. The salvage of adenine is quantitatively much less significant than that of hypoxanthine because human cells have a limited capacity to produce adenine. Thus, APRT deficiency has no discernible effect on purine nucleotide synthesis, and patients with this enzyme defect do not exhibit increased rates of purine synthesis and uric acid production. When adenine is not phosphoribosylated by APRT, this purine base becomes available for oxidation by XO (see Fig. 192-1). The affinity of APRT for adenine is considerably greater than that of XO, and in normal individuals, essentially all of the adenine is metabolized through the salvage pathway.

Symptoms in patients with APRT deficiency are the consequence of failure to "scavenge" or reuse the small amount of adenine produced or ingested each day.[14] Oxidation of adenine to 2,8-dihydroxyadenine leads to the formation of an extremely insoluble purine base, and crystals of 2,8-dihydroxyadenine form in the urine, causing renal calculi.[15] Complete deficiency of APRT is inherited as an autosomal recessive trait and can be diagnosed readily by assay of erythrocyte lysates. Recurrent radiolucent renal calculi may form in children and young adults with this enzyme defect. Renal insufficiency has developed in some patients. Occasionally, the stones have been misdiagnosed as uric acid calculi because of the similar physical properties of 2,8-dihydroxyadenine and uric acid. The treatment of this disor-

**Hypoxanthine**   **Xanthine**   **Uric acid**

**Allopurinol**   **Oxypurinol**

**FIGURE 192-6.** Substrates and inhibitors of xanthine oxidase.

der depends on early recognition of the type of stone being formed and institution of appropriate dietary (low purine) and drug therapy (allopurinol to inhibit XO). Partial deficiency of APRT appears to be a common genetic polymorphism. Generally it is of no clinical significance but has been associated with urolithiasis.[15]

Using gene-targeting, a mouse model of APRT deficiency has been generated. The kidney disease that ensues resembles that seen in humans and offers new avenues of research into this disorder.[16]

## DISORDERS OF PURINE CATABOLISM

Disorders in one portion of the purine pathway frequently lead to secondary changes in other parts of this pathway, as well as producing derangements in other metabolic pathways. This is best illustrated by the group of disorders categorized as defects in purine catabolism. Inherited defects in other pathways may alter purine catabolism, secondarily, and the resultant derangements in purine metabolism contribute to the symptoms observed in these patients.

### ADENOSINE DEAMINASE DEFICIENCY

Adenosine deaminase deaminates both adenosine and deoxyadenosine to form inosine and deoxyinosine, respectively (see Fig. 192-1). Deficiency of this enzyme activity, which is inherited as an autosomal recessive disorder, leads to profound lymphopenia.[17] Patients having this enzyme defect have reduced numbers of T and B cells, decreased immunoglobulin levels, and diminution in cellular and humoral immune responses. ADA deficiency accounts for a significant number of patients with severe combined immunodeficiency (SCID). These patients experience recurrent infections, and without therapy, they often die within the first few years of life. More recently, ADA deficiency has been recognized as a cause of lymphopenia and immunodeficiency in adults.[18]

ADA deficiency can be diagnosed by assay of any easily obtained tissue, such as erythrocytes. The deficiency leads to the accumulation of both adenosine and deoxyadenosine. The buildup of these naturally occurring purine nucleosides, particularly deoxyadenosine, may alter lymphocyte growth and function through derangements in purine, nucleic acid, or transmethylation reactions. The accumulation of deoxy-ATP may inhibit ribonucleotide reductase, leading to a decrease in DNA synthesis and lymphocyte replication. An accumulation of S-adenosylhomocysteine may inhibit transmethylation reactions. It is unclear why a generalized deficiency of ADA has such profound effects on lymphocytes while most other organs function normally, but the susceptibility of lymphocytes to ADA deficiency may be explained partly by other features of purine metabolism in lymphocytes that lead to the accumulation of deoxy-ATP or other purine intermediates in these cells.

The removal of deoxyadenosine and adenosine by replacement of ADA activity through red blood cell transfusion or bone marrow transplantation has restored immune function in some of these patients. Several SCID patients have been treated with injections of polyethylene glycol-modified bovine ADA, resulting in significant clinical improvement.[19] The successful cloning of the gene responsible for ADA deficiency has opened new avenues of therapeutic intervention for this disorder. In one of the first uses of gene transfer therapy, patients with SCID have been given infusions of genetically corrected T cells, resulting in improved immune status.[20]

## PURINE NUCLEOSIDE PHOSPHORYLASE DEFICIENCY

Purine PNP catalyzes the reaction in which inosine, deoxyinosine, guanosine, and deoxyguanosine undergo phosphorolysis to purine bases (see Fig. 192-1). PNP deficiency is characterized by recurrent infections with nonbacterial organisms, reflecting the primary defect in cellular immunity.[21] Laboratory tests reveal lymphopenia and a diminished number of T cells. Although there are normal numbers of B cells, their function may be significantly impaired. A confirmation of the diagnosis is obtained by the assay of erythrocyte lysates or other cell extracts.

The deficiency of PNP, which is inherited as an autosomal recessive trait, leads to the accumulation of several purine nucleosides, the most important of which is deoxyguanosine. Thus, deoxyguanosine triphosphate concentrations become elevated in T lymphocytes, leading to the inhibition of ribonucleotide reductase, a reduction in DNA synthesis, and the death of T cells. The prognosis in PNP deficiency usually is better than in ADA deficiency; the replacement of PNP activity by bone marrow transplantation or red blood cell infusion has been less successful.

### XANTHINE OXIDASE DEFICIENCY

XO catalyzes the last reactions in the purine catabolic pathway, that is, oxidation of hypoxanthine to xanthine and of xanthine to uric acid (see Fig. 192-1). This disorder is suspected in individuals with persistently low (<2 mg/dL) serum and urinary uric acid values.[22] The enzymatic confirmation requires liver or intestinal biopsy. The deficiency of this enzyme, which is inherited as an autosomal recessive trait, leads to an accumulation of hypoxanthine and xanthine. Increased urinary excretion of xanthine, which is quite insoluble, is responsible for the development of calculi in one-third of patients with XO deficiency. Fewer than 10% of these patients develop myopathic symptoms associated with deposition of xanthine and hypoxanthine crystals in skeletal muscle. More than 50% of individuals with this enzyme deficiency never report symptoms.

The deficiency of XO also has been associated with a deficiency of sulfite oxidase, another molybdenum-containing enzyme. In newborn infants with combined XO and sulfite oxidase deficiencies, neurologic symptoms, including tonic-clonic seizures, nystagmus, enophthalmos, and ocular lens dislocation, develop because of the sulfite oxidase deficiency.

Isolated XO deficiency may require no therapy if the patient is asymptomatic. Medical management of calculi with fluid and alkali is of some benefit; occasionally, surgical intervention is required. In children with combined XO and sulfite oxidase deficiency, neurologic symptoms have been refractory to therapy.

The hallmark of xanthinuria is hypouricemia (<2 mg/dL), a biochemical curiosity of no clinical consequence in its own right. However, hypouricemia may be a clue to underlying medical disorders or to the ingestion of a number of different types of drugs. Disorders and drug ingestions associated with hypouricemia are listed in Table 192-2. (See discussion of hypouricemia, later.)

### GLUCOSE-6-PHOSPHATASE DEFICIENCY

Glucose-6-phosphatase deficiency is not a primary disorder of purine metabolism, but is mentioned here because a secondary effect of this enzyme deficiency is accelerated purine nucleotide catabolism and a rebound increase in purine synthesis.[23] When patients with glucose-6-phosphatase deficiency fast, the accumulation of glucose-6-phosphate depletes the intracellular inorganic phosphate pools in the liver. This, in turn, leads to accelerated

**TABLE 192-2.**
**Potential Causes of Hypouricemia**

**DECREASED PRODUCTION**
*Congenital xanthine oxidase deficiency*
  Liver disease
  Allopurinol administration
  Low phosphoribosylpyrophosphate synthetase activity
  Purine nucleoside phosphorylase deficiency
**INCREASED EXCRETION**
*Disorders*
  "Isolated" defect in renal transport of uric acid (inherited)
  "Generalized" defect in renal tubular transport (Fanconi syndrome)
  Neoplastic diseases (multiple myeloma, bronchogenic carcinoma, others)
  Liver disease
  Wilson disease
  Cystinosis
  Heavy metal poisoning
  Galactosemia
  Hereditary fructose intolerance
  Pernicious anemia
  Acute intermittent porphyria
*Drugs and other chemicals*
  Acetohexamide
  Azauridine
  Benzbromarone
  Benziodarone
  Calcium ipodate
  Chlorporthixene
  Cinchophen
  Citrate
  Dicumarol
  Diflumidone
  Estrogens
  Ethyl biscoumacetate
  Ethyl *p*-chlorophenoxyisobutyric acid
  Glyceryl guaiacolate
  Glycine
  Glycopyrrolate
  Halofenate
  Iodopyracet
  Iopanoic acid
  Meglumine iodipamide
  *p*-Nitrophenylbutazone
  Orotic acid
  Outdated tetracyclines
  Phenindione
  Phenolsulfonphthalein
  Phenylbutazone
  Probenecid
  Salicylates (high doses)
  Sodium diatrizoate
  Sulfaethidole
  Sulfinpyrazone
  W 2354
  Zoxazolamine

hydrolysis of adenosine monophosphate (AMP) and guanosine monophosphate. Because of fasting, or after glucagon administration, there is an abrupt increase in uric acid formation. In response to the decrease in purine nucleotide pools, the feedback inhibition of de novo synthesis is diminished (see Fig. 192-3). The net effect of accelerated nucleotide catabolism is a rebound increase in purine production, and these patients go through cycles of increased catabolism followed by increased purine syn-

thesis. Hyperuricemia may be striking in glucose-6-phosphatase deficiency, and gouty arthritis is a prominent manifestation of this disorder, beginning in the late teens and early adulthood.

The cycle of accelerated purine nucleotide catabolism followed by increased purine synthesis is common to several acquired disorders of purine metabolism as well (see Table 192-1). This response has been studied extensively in patients who are given large doses of fructose,[24] and it may well account for the increase in purine synthesis observed in patients who ingest modest amounts of ethanol.[25] The latter association is particularly important clinically because of the strong link between alcohol ingestion and the development of hyperuricemia and gout. Ethanol produces hyperuricemia through another mechanism as well, lactic acidosis and decreased renal clearance of urate.[5]

## DISORDERS OF PURINE NUCLEOTIDE INTERCONVERSION

The two major classes of purine nucleotides—the adenylate compounds (ATP, adenosine diphosphate, and AMP) and the guanylate compounds (guanosine triphosphate, diphosphate, and monophosphate)—share a common nucleotide intermediate, inosine monophosphate, and interconversion between these two classes of purine nucleotides proceeds by way of this intermediate (see Fig. 192-1). Two inherited defects in this interconversion pathway have been recognized.

### ADENOSINE MONOPHOSPHATE DEAMINASE DEFICIENCY

AMP deaminase catalyzes the deamination of AMP to inosine monophosphate (see Fig. 192-1). Deficiency of the skeletal muscle isozyme of AMP deaminase, inherited as an autosomal recessive trait, leads to a selective loss of this enzyme activity in skeletal muscle.[26] Patients who are deficient in AMP deaminase activity exhibit a mild metabolic myopathy characterized by easy fatigability, myalgias, and muscle cramps with exercise. This disorder is suspected when patients are tested by ischemic exercise and fail to produce $NH_3$ while releasing normal amounts of lactate into the venous blood. The diagnosis is confirmed by enzyme assay of skeletal muscle biopsy specimens. The basis of the exercise-related symptoms in these patients is thought to be a disruption of the purine nucleotide cycle, a series of reactions especially active in skeletal muscle and important for maximal energy production during vigorous exercise. Because the deficiency is manifest only in skeletal muscle, this is the only organ that is affected by this enzyme deficiency. No effective therapy is available. Reassurance that this disorder is mild and usually nonprogressive, along with counseling regarding physical activity, is helpful to the patient in adjusting to the limitations imposed by this enzyme defect.

An isolated deficiency of AMP deaminase in erythrocytes has been reported. These individuals appear to be healthy and have no evidence of hemolysis.[27]

### ADENYLOSUCCINATE LYASE DEFICIENCY

Adenylosuccinate lyase cleaves S-AMP to AMP and fumarate (see Fig. 192-1). The deficiency of this enzyme, which presumably is inherited as an autosomal recessive trait, leads to variable reductions in S-AMP lyase activity in different tissues.[28] All of the symptoms resulting from this enzyme defect may not have been recognized as yet, and there is no clear-cut pathogenesis for the associated symptoms. The most striking clinical abnormality noted thus far is autism, suggesting that this enzyme defect has a particularly deleterious effect on the function of certain neurons. Skeletal muscle abnormalities also have been noted in some patients. Patients with this enzyme defect have a limited ability to synthesize adenine nucleotides, and excrete excessive amounts of succinyladenosine, a catabolic product of S-AMP, which is the basis of a urine test for this disorder.[29] The diagnosis may be confirmed by assay of cell lysates or biopsy specimens. No specific therapy is available thus far.

## DISORDERS OF URIC ACID EXCRETION

Reduced renal clearance of uric acid is a significant contributing factor, if not the primary cause, of hyperuricemia in many patients with gout.[1,2] Decreased urate clearance may occur in isolation, or it may be associated with increased uric acid production, as in obesity and ethanol consumption. Reduced renal urate clearance may be an inherited abnormality, associated with other medical disorders, or a result of drug or food ingestion (see Table 192-1). Clinical manifestations of decreased urate clearance include hyperuricemia, which may be asymptomatic, gouty arthritis, and tophi. The renal clearance of urate depends on glomerular filtration, urate secretion, and urate reabsorption. Other than conditions in which there is a clear reduction in glomerular filtration, such as renal insufficiency, the pathogenesis of decreased urate clearance is not known, because there is no reliable way to distinguish between abnormalities in urate secretion and reabsorption. Uricosuric agents (e.g., probenecid) are effective in restoring urate clearance to normal levels in most patients with glomerular filtration rates >60 mL per minute. However, treatment is reserved for those hyperuricemic patients with documented crystal deposition. Patients with gout in whom the glomerular filtration rate is <60 mL per minute are unlikely to respond to uricosuric drugs; therefore, allopurinol is the drug of choice.

## HYPOURICEMIA

Hypouricemia, arbitrarily defined as a serum urate concentration of <2 mg/dL, is detected in ~1% of hospitalized patients (see Table 192-2). The commonly held belief that uric acid has no physiologic usefulness has been called into question.[30] Nevertheless, hypouricemia on a nonrenal basis has not been shown to cause clinical problems. The principal importance of recognizing hypouricemia is the association of this laboratory abnormality with ingestion of certain types of drugs and acquired or inherited disorders that affect urate metabolism.[31] Renal hypouricemia is a genetic disease due to an isolated defect in tubular transport of urate.[32] Acute renal insufficiency and urolithiasis have been reported in this condition. In diabetics, a low serum uric acid level may relate to both renal tubular abnormalities and hyperuricosuria.[33]

## REFERENCES

1. Kelley WN. Gout and related disorders. In: Kelley WN, Harris ED Jr, Ruddy S, Sledge CB, eds. Textbook of rheumatology, 2nd ed. Philadelphia: WB Saunders, 1985:1397.
2. Holmes EW. Clinical gout and the pathogenesis of hyperuricemia. In: McCarty DJ, ed. Arthritis and allied conditions, 10th ed. Philadelphia: Lea & Febiger, 1985:1455.
3. Palmer DG, Highton J, Hessian PA. Development of the gout tophus. Am J Clin Pathol 1989; 91:190.
4. Holmes EW, Kelley WN. The renal pathophysiology of gout. In: Kurtzman NA, Martinez-Maldonado M, eds. Pathophysiology of the kidney. Springfield, IL: Charles C Thomas Publisher, 1977:696.
5. Palella TD, Fox IH. Hyperuricemia and gout. In: Scriver C, Beaudet AL, Sly WS, Valle DL, eds. The metabolic basis of inherited disease, 6th ed. New York: McGraw-Hill, 1989:965.
6. Katashima R, Iwahana H, Fujimura M, et al. Molecular cloning of a human cDNA for the 41-kDa phosphoribosylpyrophosphate synthetase-associated protein. Biochim Biophys Acta 1998; 1396:245.
7. Braven J, Hardwell TR, Hickling P, Whittaker M. Effect of treatment on erythrocyte phosphoribosyl pyrophosphate synthetase and glutathione reductase activity in patients with primary gout. Ann Rheum Dis 1986; 45:941.
8. Stout JT, Caskey CT. Hypoxanthine-guanine phosphoribosyltransferase deficiency, Lesch Nyhan syndrome and gouty arthritis. In: Scriver C, Beaudet AL, Sly WS, Valle DL, eds. The metabolic basis of inherited disease, 6th ed. New York: McGraw-Hill, 1989:1007.
9. Nyhan W. The recognition of Lesch-Nyhan syndrome as an inborn error of purine metabolism. J Inherit Metab Dis 1997; 20:171.
9a. Nyhan WL. Dopamine function in Lesch-Nyhan disease. Environ Health Perspect 2000; 108(Suppl 3):409.
9b. Visser JE, Bar PR, Jinnah HA. Lesch-Nyhan disease and the basal ganglia. Brain Res Brain Res Rev 2000; 32:449.
10. Hikita M, Hosoya T, Ichida K, et al. Partial deficiency of hypoxanthine-guanine phosphoribosyltransferase manifesting as acute renal damage. Intern Med 1998; 37:945.
11. Morino M, Shiigai N, Kusuyama H, Okada K. Extracorporeal shock wave lithotripsy and xanthine calculi in Lesch-Nyhan syndrome. Pediatr Radiol 1992; 22:304.
12. Wu CL, Melton DW. Production of a model for Lesch-Nyhan syndrome in hypoxanthine phosphoribosyltransferase-deficient mice. Nat Genet 1993; 3:235.
13. Wivel NA, Walters L. Germ-line gene modification and disease prevention: some medical and ethical perspectives. Science 1993; 262:533.
13a. Torres RJ, Mateos FA, Molano J, et al. Molecular basis of hypoxanthine-guanine phosphoribosyl transferase deficiency in thirteen Spanish families. Hum Mutat 2000; 15:383.
14. Simmonds HA, Van Acker KL, Sahofa AS. Adenine phosphoribosyltransferase deficiency. In: Scriver C, Beaudet AL, Sly WS, Valle DL, eds. The metabolic basis of inherited disease, 6th ed. New York: McGraw-Hill, 1989:1029.
15. Inagaki K, Muraoka A, Suehiro I, et al. Partial adenine phosphoribosyltransferase deficiency detected by ureterolithiasis. Intern Med 1998; 37:69.
16. Stockelman M, Lorenz J, Smith F, et al. Chronic renal failure in a mouse model of human adenine phosphoribosyltransferase deficiency. Am J Physiol 1998; 275:F154.
17. Kredich N, Hershfield MS. Immunodeficiency diseases caused by adenosine deaminase deficiency and purine nucleoside phosphorylase deficiency. In: Scriver C, Beaudet AL, Sly WS, Valle DL, eds. The metabolic basis of inherited disease, 6th ed. New York: McGraw-Hill, 1989:1045.
18. Ozsahin H, Arrendondo-Vega F, Santisteban I, et al. Adenosine deaminase deficiency in adults. Blood 1997; 89:2849.
19. Hershfield MS, Chaffee S, Sorensen RU. Enzyme replacement therapy with polyethylene glycol–adenosine deaminase in adenosine deaminase deficiency: overview and case reports of three patients, including two now receiving gene therapy. Pediatr Res 1993; 33(Suppl):S42.
20. Blaese RM. Development of gene therapy for immunodeficiency: adenosine deaminase deficiency. Pediatr Res 1993; 33(Suppl):S49.
21. Markert ML, Hershfield MS, Schiff RI, Buckley RH. Adenosine deaminase and purine nucleoside phosphorylase deficiencies: evaluation of therapeutic interventions in eight patients. J Clin Immunol 1987; 7:389.
22. Holmes EW, Wyngaarden JB. Hereditary xanthinuria. In: Scriver C, Beaudet AL, Sly WS, Valle DL, eds. The metabolic basis of inherited disease, 6th ed. New York: McGraw-Hill, 1989:1085.
23. Howell RR, Williams JC. The glycogen storage diseases. In: Stanbury JB, Wyngaarden JB, Fredrickson DS, et al., eds. The metabolic basis of inherited disease, 5th ed. New York: McGraw-Hill, 1983:141.
24. Ravio KO, Becker MA, Meyer LJ, et al. Stimulation of human purine synthesis de novo by fructose administration. Metabolism 1975; 24:861.
25. Faller J, Fox IH. Ethanol induced hyperuricemia: evidence for increased urate production by activation of adenine nucleotide turnover. N Engl J Med 1982; 307:598.
26. Sabina RL, Swain JL, Holmes EW. Myoadenylate deaminase deficiency. In: Scriver C, Beaudet AL, Sly WS, Valle DL, eds. The metabolic basis of inherited disease, 6th ed. New York: McGraw-Hill, 1989:1077.
27. Ogasawara N, Goto H, Yamada Y, et al. Complete deficiency of AMP deaminase in human erythrocytes. Biochem Biophys Res Commun 1984; 122:1344.
28. Jaeken J, Wadman SK, Duran M, et al. Adenylosuccinase deficiency: an inborn error of purine nucleotide synthesis. Eur J Pediatr 1988; 148:126.
29. Maddocks J, Reed T. Urine test for adenylosuccinase deficiency in autistic children. Lancet 1989; 1:158.
30. Becker BF. Towards the physiological function of uric acid. Free Radic Biol Med 1993; 14:615.
31. Wyngaarden JB, Kelley WN. Gout and hyperuricemia. New York: Grune & Stratton, 1976:395.
32. Hisatome I, Tanaka Y, Tsuboi M. Excess urate excretion correlates with severely acidic urine in patients with renal hypouricemia. Intern Med 1998; 37:726.
33. Shichiri M, Iwamoto H, Shiigai T. Diabetic renal hypouricemia. Arch Intern Med 1988; 147:225.

# PART XII

# IMMUNOLOGIC BASIS OF ENDOCRINE DISORDERS

LEONARD WARTOFSKY, EDITOR

# CHAPTER 193

# THE ENDOCRINE THYMUS

ALLAN L. GOLDSTEIN AND NICHOLAS R. S. HALL

The thymus gland generates humoral substances that can regulate a number of physiologic processes and stimulate directly the release of pituitary hormones or hypothalamic neurotransmitters and growth factors such as nerve growth factors.[1] Some of these humoral messengers, such as *thymosin $\alpha_1$ (T$\alpha_1$)*, are produced primarily in the thymus, whereas others (e.g., thymosin $\beta_4$ [T$\beta_4$], an actin-sequestering peptide) are more ubiquitous in nature and are found in highest concentrations not in the thymus, but rather in blood platelets, neutrophils, macrophages, and a wide variety of other cell types.[2] The physiologic systems that these products may regulate include body temperature, slow-wave sleep, and the release of proopiomelanocortin hormones and other pituitary peptides that are an integral part of the reproductive axis[3] as well as being involved in immune functions, wound healing, and angiogenesis (Table 193-1).

## STRUCTURE AND DEVELOPMENT OF THE THYMUS

The two lobes of the thymus gland are joined by connective tissue that forms a thin capsule. The thymus is located beneath the sternum of most mammals and consists of lobules that can be subdivided histologically.[4,5] The outer cortex contains lymphocytes undergoing mitosis at a high rate. These cells subsequently migrate from the cortex to the inner medullary region, where they undergo further differentiation. This differentiation can be influenced by humoral factors such as the thymosin peptides. Within the medulla are the thymic (Hassall) corpuscles that consist of layers of epithelial cells. These may constitute a source of thymosin or other immunomodulatory substances that can influence T-cell differentiation.

From the medulla, ~5% to 10% of mature T cells migrate out of the thymus gland to peripheral tissues, where they interact with antigens. A larger proportion of immature T cells undergo steroid-induced apoptosis and die within the thymus. The thymus gland performs a vital role, especially during the neonatal period, when the immune capabilities of the host are maturing. Neonatal thymectomy causes "wasting syndrome," which in certain strains of mice is characterized by marked lymphopenia and death. It also perturbs neuroendocrine functions, such as the reproductive axis. Similar consequences are associated with the congenital absence or hypoplasia of the thymus. This has been observed in both athymic or "nude" mice and in patients who have the DiGeorge syndrome (abnormal development of third and fourth pharyngeal pouches, with aplasia or hypoplasia of thymus and parathyroid glands). Immunologic function is impaired by the loss of T cells that regulate B cells and by the loss of effector T cells that normally play a direct role in host defense throughout life.

The comparatively high incidence of autoimmune and neoplastic disease associated with aging may be additional evidence for the crucial role that the thymus gland plays in host defense throughout life. Atrophy of the thymus gland occurs concomitantly with the increased incidence of these diseases. At birth, the human thymus gland weighs 10 to 15 g and then gradually develops until it attains 30 to 40 g at puberty. It then involutes as the individual ages.[6] The decline in weight involves both the medullary and cortical regions of the gland. Thymus

weight sometimes is expressed as a proportion of total body weight. When represented in this manner, the decline in weight appears to begin at a much earlier age.

## THE THYMUS AS AN ENDOCRINE GLAND

The thymus has an important endocrine function and can influence other hormonal systems. At the turn of the nineteenth century, this organ was implicated in regulating glucocorticoid release from the adrenal glands.[7] It also was considered a reproductive tissue after investigators found that some gonadal disorders could be successfully treated by the administration of thymic extracts.[8] However, until the discovery of the role of this gland as the "master gland" of the immune system in the early 1960s and the isolation of the thymosins, little was known about the chemical nature of the thymic products responsible for modulating the adrenal and reproductive hormonal circuits. Several of the bioactive thymosin peptides have been isolated and chemically characterized[9] (Table 193-2).

Two types of thymosin preparations have been evaluated using various bioassay systems. One is a partially purified product of bovine thymus called *thymosin fraction 5* (TF5). It consists of a mixture of peptides, some of which normally may be part of larger precursor molecules. This is true of T$\alpha_1$, a 28-amino-acid peptide that is contained within the NH$_2$-terminus of the 113-amino-acid peptide, prothymosin $\alpha$. Other peptides, such as T$\beta_4$, are present in higher concentrations in other tissues.[10] T$\beta_4$, which is an actin-sequestering peptide and a potent angiogenic factor, has been shown (both in vitro and in vivo) to accelerate wound healing.[10,11]

## THYMIC INFLUENCES ON THE PITUITARY-GONADAL AXIS

A number of investigators have evaluated the effects of different thymic extracts on the pituitary-gonadal axis. Early studies suffered because the preparations used were contaminated with impurities or were prepared in a manner that precluded draw-

**TABLE 193-1.**
**Immunotransmitters Produced by Immune System Cells That Are Biologically Active in the Central Nervous System**

| Immunotransmitter | Biologic Activity | Reference |
|---|---|---|
| Thymosin $\beta_4$ | Stimulates LHRH release from superfused hypothalamic tissue; regulates actin polymerization; stimulates angiogenesis and wound healing | 10,11,14 |
| Thymosin $\alpha_1$ | Stimulates pituitary-adrenal axis in vivo | 12 |
| Thymosin F5 | Stimulates pituitary-adrenal axis in vitro and in vivo; stimulates LHRH release from superfused hypothalamic tissue; stimulates prolactin and growth hormone in vitro | 14,21–23,26, 28,58–60 |
| Cytokines | Can stimulate pituitary-adrenal axis in vivo; decreases brain levels of norepinephrine; stimulates glial cells | 24,29,55 |
| | Stimulates thermoregulatory centers; stimulates slow-wave sleep | |
| C3a | Modulates feeding behavior | 56 |
| ACTH | A neural and pituitary peptide that also is produced by lymphocytes | 27 |
| $\beta$-Endorphin | A neural and pituitary peptide that also is produced by lymphocytes | 27 |
| Interferon-$\alpha$ | Induces lethargy and depression | 57 |

*ACTH*, corticotropin; *F5*, fraction 5; *LHRH*, luteinizing hormone–releasing hormone.

TABLE 193-2.
**Properties of Select Biologically Active Peptides Isolated from the Thymus**

| Name of Preparation | Chemical Properties | Biologic Effects |
|---|---|---|
| Thymosin $\alpha_1$ | Peptide of 28 residues, MW 3108, pI 4.2 | Enhances MIF, IFN, IL-2, and lympho-toxin production; modulates TdT activity; stimulates viral, fungal, and tumor immunity; increases IL-2–receptor expression; amplifies T-cell immunity in humans; angiogenic and wound healing properties; effective as a monotherapy or in combination with IFN in hepatitis B and C; prolongs survival in patients with lung cancer, hepatocellular carcinoma, and melanoma; increases efficacy of influenza and hepatitis vaccines in humans. |
| Prothy-mosin $\alpha$ | 113 amino acids, T$\alpha_1$ at NH$_2$-terminal position, MW 13,500 | Similar bioactivity to T$\alpha_1$ in protecting mice against opportunistic infection with *Candida albicans*; immunostimulatory in vitro. |
| Thymosin $\alpha_7$ | Acidic peptide, MW 2000, pI 3.5 | In vitro enhancement of suppressor T cells; expression of Lyt-1, -2, -3–positive cells. |
| Thymosin $\beta_4$ | Peptide of 43 residues, MW 4963, pI 5.1, sequence determined | Induces TdT in vivo and in vitro in bone marrow cells from normal and athymic mice; in vivo induction of TdT in thymocytes of immunosuppressed mice; stimulates release of LHRH; enhances thymocyte allogeneic MLR; induces TdT; suppresses allogeneic and syngeneic human MLR responses; actin-sequestering, promotes wound healing and angiogenesis. |

*MW*, molecular weight; *pI*, negative log of the isoelectric point; *IFN*, interferon; *IL-2*, interleukin-2; *MIF*, migration inhibition factor; *LHRH*, luteinizing hormone–releasing hormone; *MLR*, mixed leukocyte or lymphocyte reaction; *TdT*, terminal deoxynucleotidyl transferase.

ing conclusions about the chemical nature of the bioactive substance. More purified preparations have become available, and component peptides have been purified to homogeneity.

Working with the partially purified TF5 and other thymic factors, investigators had postulated that a product of the thymus gland acted at the level of the central nervous system (CNS)–pituitary axis to stimulate the release of reproductive hormones. This conclusion was based on experiments[12] in which animals that underwent hypophysectomy and thymectomy were used.

Several hormones were measured in laboratory rats that had undergone thymectomy within 24 hours of birth. Blood levels of two of these hormones, testosterone and luteinizing hormone (LH), were elevated at 30 days of age and then decreased at 60 days. The administration of TF5 reduced the extent of these changes and also restored the testes' weight loss that was observed after thymectomy. It was concluded that the site of action of certain of these effects was at the level of the brain or pituitary, because they failed to occur in animals that had undergone hypophysectomy.

A thymus-derived ubiquitous peptide that can modulate the reproductive axis is T$\beta_4$. Evidence that T$\beta_4$ can act on the hypothalamic–pituitary–gonadal axis included a series of studies in which various thymosin peptides were injected directly into the cerebroventricular system of chronically cannulated mice. This study[13] revealed that T$\beta_4$ but not T$\alpha_1$, which was used as a control peptide, was able to stimulate a significant release of LH.

Direct evidence that T$\beta_4$ is active at the level of the hypothalamus was provided by an in vitro superfusion model.[14] Rat hypothalamic and pituitary tissues were superfused with thy-mosin preparations, and LH was measured in the effluent. No change occurred in the amount of LH released when pituitary tissue alone was superfused, but when it was superfused in sequence with slices of medial basal hypothalamus, a significant release of LH was observed. It subsequently was found that luteinizing hormone–releasing hormone (LHRH) was stimulated by T$\beta_4$. These data generated with in vitro model systems confirmed the observation that T$\beta_4$ can stimulate the release of an important gonadotropin. Nonetheless, other thymosin peptides also may function in this capacity. For example, a series of T$\beta_4$ isoforms from the hypothalamus have been isolated, and their effects in modulating other hypothalamic and pituitary responses have been demonstrated.[15]

## THYMIC INFLUENCES ON PROLACTIN AND GROWTH HORMONE

Like LH, prolactin and growth hormone release are also stimulated by a component of TF5. The active peptide (termed *MB-35*) has sequence homology to a fragment of a nonhistone chromosomal protein.[16] When MB-35 is incubated with a prolactin and growth hormone–secreting pituitary cell line (GH3), both hormones are released.[16]

If thymosin peptides are proven to play a physiologic role in the modulation of reproductive and trophic hormone release, it may represent yet another mechanism by which the immune system can be regulated. Gonadal steroids, prolactin, and growth hormone alter various immune system measures. These range from the stimulation of macrophages by estrogen to potentiation of lymphocyte activity by prolactin and growth hormone.[17–20]

## THYMIC INFLUENCES ON THE HYPOTHALAMIC–PITUITARY–ADRENAL AXIS

Another hormonal system that may be regulated by products of the immune system is the hypothalamic–pituitary–adrenal axis. TF5 and a component of lymphokine-containing supernatant fluids each ultimately stimulate steroidogenesis, but apparently by different mechanisms. A component of TF5 stimulates glucocorticoid release in many species, including monkeys, rats, mice, and rabbits.[21–23] Moreover, supernatant fluids from stimulated lymphocytes are steroidogenic in rodents and humans.[24]

### PITUITARY EFFECTS

Evidence that the site of action is the pituitary gland includes a study[21] in which prepubertal monkeys were injected with a number of thymosin preparations before pituitary hormone release was measured. The administration of TF5 was followed by a time- and dose-dependent release of cortisol, adrenocorticotropic hormone (ACTH), and β-endorphin. The highest levels of ACTH preceded the peak in cortisol, suggesting that the corticosteroid release followed the ACTH release. The kinetics of β-endorphin release were similar to those of ACTH. When another group of monkeys underwent thymectomy, a significant reduction in circulating levels of ACTH and cortisol was noticed. TF5 also is steroidogenic in mice and rats, although only when basal levels of glucocorticoids are within a normal range. Stress-induced elevations are not affected.[22] A direct effect of T$\alpha_1$ on the concentration of pituitary hormones in plasma following third-ventricle injection in rats has been reported[25]; there is a significant decrease in plasma thyroid-stimulating hormone (TSH), ACTH, and prolactin.

Using in vitro models, it was confirmed that a site of action of TF5-induced steroidogenesis is the anterior pituitary gland.[26] First, TF5 and several purified component peptides were incubated with isolated adrenal fasciculata cells.[27] There was no effect on either corticosterone or cyclic AMP release. It was thought that thymosin might act synergistically with a suboptimal dose of ACTH, but when this combination was tested, no increase occurred in corticosterone release over the amount released by ACTH alone. Next, anterior pituitary cells either were superfused or maintained as primary cultures in the presence of TF5.[26] Although no evidence existed for TF5-stimulated ACTH release using the superfusion model, TF5 did stimulate ACTH release from cultured pituitary cell monolayers. This stimulative effect was dose dependent, with significant release of ACTH occurring with 125 µg/mL or more of TF5. An ACTH- and β-endorphin–secreting pituitary cell line (AtT20) also is responsive to TF5, releasing significant quantities of β-endorphin into the media after exposure to increasing concentrations of TF5.[28]

### CENTRAL NERVOUS SYSTEM–HYPOTHALAMIC EFFECTS

Although a component of TF5 can act directly at the level of the pituitary gland to stimulate the release of ACTH, lymphokine-containing supernatant fluids obtained from stimulated lymphocytes may have a CNS site of action. Hypothalamic levels of norepinephrine are significantly reduced in rats injected with this lymphokine preparation.[29] Because norepinephrine inhibits acetylcholine-induced corticotropin-releasing hormone secretions, it is hypothesized that the bioactive component works by way of a disinhibition mechanism.

## IMMUNE SYSTEM–NEUROENDOCRINE INTERRELATIONSHIPS

The steroidogenesis that occurs after exposure to immune system products may be part of a long feedback loop that ultimately serves to down-regulate the immune response.[30,30a] This hypothesis is based on several ideas. During an immune response, a rise in corticosterone coincides with the peak of antibody production.[29] Furthermore, relatively immature lymphocytes, especially those of the T-cell lineage, are most susceptible to corticosteroid-induced suppression because of the high density of glucocorticoid receptors (see Chap. 195). Thus, it would be this latter population of cells not sensitized by an immunogen that would be suppressed by the higher corticosteroid levels. Cells with high affinity for the immunogen would have differentiated into effector cells, thereby losing their corticosteroid sensitivity. This feedback loop presumably evolved for the purpose of fine-tuning the immune response, preventing the clonal expansion of lymphocytes with only moderate or weak affinity for the immunogen.

A second immunogen was injected at the time that antibodies to the first were at peak levels.[30] The antibody response to the second antigen was diminished, but only when the adrenal glands were present. Thus, the phenomenon of antigenic competition appears to arise partly from glucocorticoid release. This model system is not unique to the immune system. Within the context of sensory physiology, the inhibition of adjacent sensory nerves by the one that was stimulated has been well documented. Neurophysiologists describe this as "lateral inhibition." The difference is that in the nervous system the inhibitory signal is transmitted a distance of only a few angstroms across the synaptic cleft. In the immune system, the distance is several orders of magnitude greater and is facilitated by movements of thymic hormones via the blood from the thymus to the pituitary gland.

Precisely how the other hormones, the release of which also can be stimulated by thymosin peptides, accommodate this scenario is under investigation. Some of these hormones, such as ACTH and β-endorphin, are also produced by lymphocytes.[31] However, because all of the pituitary hormones that are stimulated by immune system products ultimately can modulate the course of

immunogenesis, it is likely that neuroendocrine circuits both regulate and are regulated by the endocrine immune system.[31a]

## ROLE OF ENDOCRINE THYMUS DURING ONTOGENY

A growing body of evidence[32,33] suggests that neonatal exposure to thymic peptides and cytokines (see Chaps. 173 and 174) can profoundly influence the physiology of the developing organism. Induction of endogenous cytokines after viral exposure is also able to influence the CNS and endocrine circuits of rodents. Exposure of newborn rats to Newcastle disease virus resulted in a significant reduction in testes and ovarian weight at 4 months of age.[33] Adrenal gland weight was significantly reduced in the female rats exposed to virus, but not in the males. Similarly, female rats infected with cytomegalovirus as newborns manifested an attenuated corticosterone response to a novel environment as adults. These changes may well be because of activation of the hypothalamic–pituitary–adrenal axis during a critical period of development when this neuroendocrine circuit would normally be quiescent. For example, 10-day-old rat pups have elevated ACTH and corticosterone levels during acute cytomegalovirus infection. This increase is both time and dose dependent and occurs during a developmental period when this circuit is less responsive to activation. It is unclear whether the results are because of a viral antigen acting directly within the brain, or whether they are subsequent to the production of immune system cytokines being secreted by virally sensitized cells. Evidence[34] strongly suggests that interleukin (IL)-1 is at least contributing to the activation of the hypothalamic–pituitary–adrenal axis. This cytokine, like cytomegalovirus, is able to stimulate ACTH and corticosterone release in a time- and dose-dependent manner that is similar to the pattern observed after exposure to the virus.

Viral- and cytokine-induced changes in brain processes during early development may influence the progression of certain forms of psychiatric illness. Historically, the word *thymus* is derived from the Greek word *thymos*, or mind. In view of the evidence linking thymosin peptides and cytokines with neurochemical events, it may be no coincidence that the word *athymia* is used to describe dementia as well as the absence of the thymus gland. Depression, schizophrenia, anxiety, and hyperactivity all have been linked with viral activation of the immune system, especially when viral exposure occurs during fetal development.[35] The potential mechanisms whereby the behavioral abnormalities might occur include focal damage to subcortical brain regions by the virus, cross-reacting antibodies, or the production of neuroactive cytokines. In light of the evidence that thymic products and cytokines can act in the brain, and that viral exposure is linked with psychiatric illness, further studies to determine a causal link between immune system activation and behavioral abnormalities are warranted.

### HOMEOSTATIC REGULATION OF THYMOCYTE DEVELOPMENT BY THYMOSIN $\alpha_1$

Glucocorticoid hormones can induce apoptosis in immature developing thymocytes. $T\alpha_1$ is a dose- and time-dependent antagonist of dexamethasone (DEX) and anti-CD3–induced DNA fragmentation of murine thymocytes in vitro.[36] Further studies of the mechanism of $T\alpha_1$ action have identified a $T\alpha_1$-sensitive thymocyte population[37] (Fig. 193-1). The authors have examined some of the molecular events associated with the $T\alpha_1$ antiapoptotic activity. Phenotypic analysis of the subpopulations of thymocytes, based on CD4 and CD8 expression, have revealed that $T\alpha_1$ exerts its effect on CD4+ CD8+ immature thy-

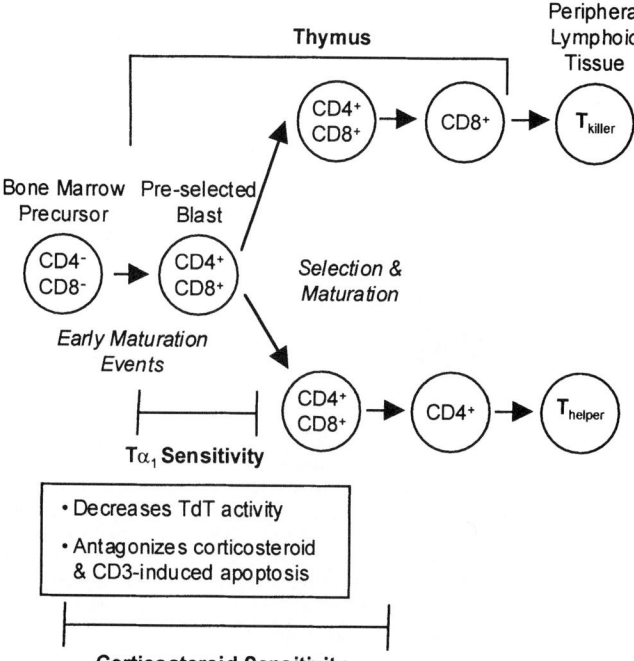

**FIGURE 193-1.** Proposed model for site of action of thymosin $\alpha_1$ ($T\alpha_1$) in thymocyte development. In the thymus, $T\alpha_1$ exerts its influence on the development of a population of immature CD4$^+$ CD8$^+$ T cells. $T\alpha_1$ antagonizes corticosteroid and anti-CD3–induced apoptosis, suggesting an influence on the preselection stages of cells destined to become T cells. (*TdT*, terminal deoxynucleotidyl transferase.)

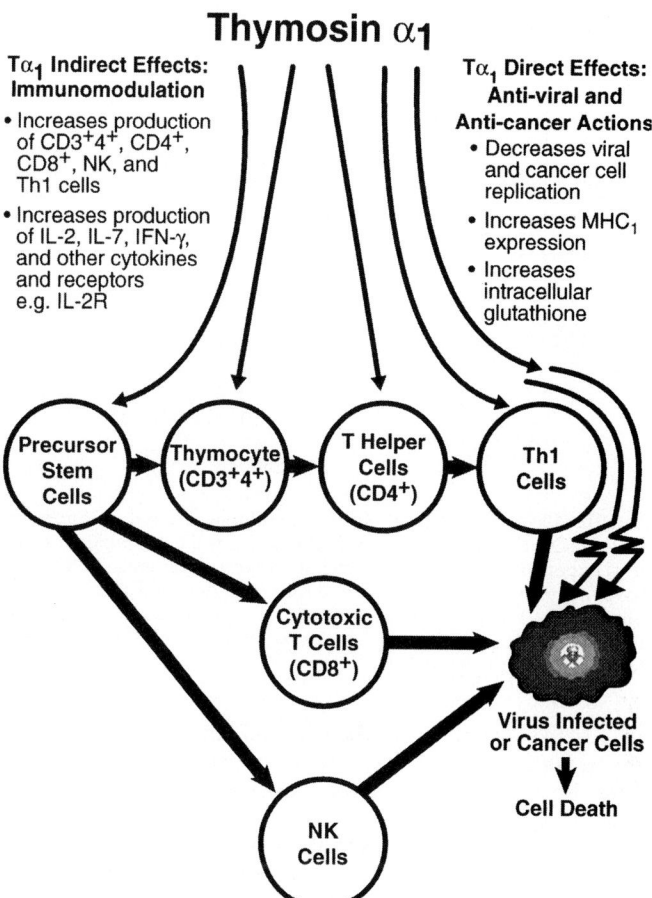

**FIGURE 193-2.** Mechanism of action of thymosin $\alpha_1$ ($T\alpha_1$): antiviral and anticancer properties. $T\alpha_1$ acts at the level of the immune system to modulate helper (*CD4$^+$*) T-cell responses and $T_H1$ cytokine responses and to stimulate natural killer (*NK*) and cytotoxic (*CD8$^+$*) T cells to kill virus-infected or cancer cells. $T\alpha_1$ also has direct effects on cancer or viral infected cells that lead to inhibition of cell growth or viral replication. (*IL*, interleukin; *IFN*, interferon; *MHC*, major histocompatibility complex.)

mocytes. $T\alpha_1$ treatment of thymocytes delays the production of free radicals, and the subsequent consumption of glutathione that is observed during both DEX and anti-CD3–induced apoptosis. These data suggest that $T\alpha_1$ exerts an influence on the development of a population of immature T cells in the thymus by affecting the sensitivity of thymocytes to apoptosis during the preselection stages of thymic development. The studies also suggest that the mechanism of $T\alpha_1$ action involves the induction of both cyclic adenosine monophosphate (cAMP)– and protein kinase C (PKC)–dependent second-messenger pathways.[37]

# THERAPEUTIC APPLICATIONS OF THE THYMOSINS

Thymosins have a broad spectrum of potential clinical applications in the treatment and diagnosis of diseases associated with deficiencies or imbalances of the immune system. Initial clinical trials were carried out with TF5. This preparation has been replaced by a synthetic $T\alpha_1$ peptide that is responsible for the major immunomodulatory activities in TF5. The mechanism of action of $T\alpha_1$ appears to be as an immunomodulator. $T\alpha_1$ can also act directly on virally infected or cancer cells to inhibit replication (Fig. 193-2).

## CANCER

Many cancers are associated with significant deficiencies in cellular immunity. In addition, standard treatments for cancer (i.e., surgery, radiotherapy, and chemotherapy) usually depress cellular immunity. In animal studies, TF5 and $T\alpha_1$ restore immunity and resistance to progressive tumor growth and reverse or ameliorate the immunosuppressive effects of chemotherapy or radiotherapy.[37a] Combinations of $T\alpha_1$ with interferon or IL-2 appear to be more effective than either agent alone.[38]

In a phase II trial, $T\alpha_1$ increased the disease-free interval, particularly in patients with nonbulky tumors, and prolonged survival in patients with non–small cell cancer of the lung as an adjunct to conventional radiotherapy.[39] A phase III trial conducted by the cooperative Radiation Therapy Oncology Groups confirmed this finding, in patients with nonbulky squamous cell non–small cell lung cancer.[40]

In patients with metastatic melanoma, $T\alpha_1$ increased the T-cell levels, natural killer (NK) activity, and survival obtainable with regimens of dacarbazine in combination with interferon or IL-2.[41] In 24 patients with hepatocellular carcinoma, the addition of $T\alpha_1$ increased the survival obtained with treatment by transcatheter arterial chemoembolization (TACE).[42] The survival advantage with $T\alpha_1$, which was significant at 18 months, was maintained to the most recent follow-up at 3 years (Fig. 193-3).

## AUTOIMMUNE DISEASES

Thymic peptides may be particularly useful in the treatment and control of autoimmune diseases. These diseases are distinguished by an abnormally overresponsive immune system, one that attacks not only harmful organisms and malignant cells but also the body's normal tissues. A frequent finding in many of these diseases is a deficiency of suppressor T cells. In preclinical studies, thymosins restored immune balance and increased the level of suppressor T cells. Studies with TF5 and $T\alpha_1$ in animals

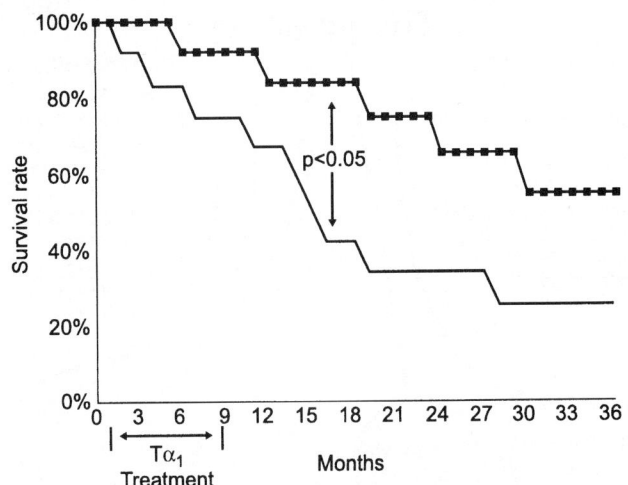

**FIGURE 193-3.** A combination of transcatheter arterial chemoembolization (*TACE*) and thymosin $\alpha_1$ (*T$\alpha_1$*) increases the probability of survival of patients with metastatic melanoma versus patients treated with TACE alone at 18 months ($p$ <.05). (From Stefanini GS, Faschi FG, Castelli E, et al. α1-Thymosin and transcatheter arterial chemoembolization in hepatocellular carcinoma patients: a preliminary experience. Hepatogastroenterology 1998; 45:209.)

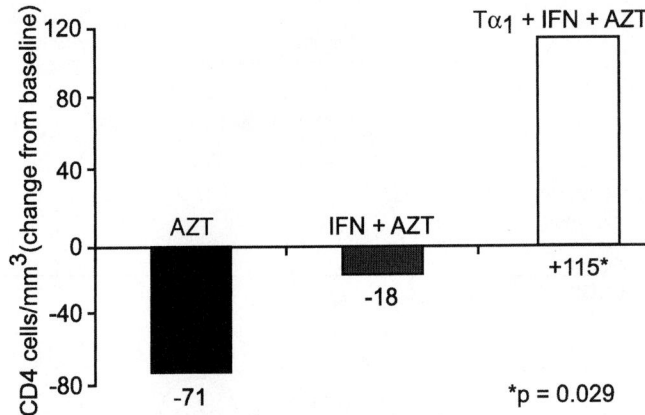

**FIGURE 193-4.** Thymosin $\alpha_1$ (*T$\alpha_1$*) in combination with interferon (*IFN*) and zidovudine (*AZT*) increases CD4 T-cell numbers in patients with human immunodeficiency virus. The figure shows the median change in CD4 cells/mm$^3$ at the end of 12 months of treatment relative to baseline for patients with baseline CD4 ≤350 mm$^3$. The three treatment groups were T$\alpha_1$ plus IFN-α plus AZT, IFN-α plus AZT, and AZT. (After Garaci E, Rocchi G, Perroni L, et al. Combination treatment with zidovudine, thymosin $\alpha_1$, and interferon-α in human immunodeficiency virus infection. Int J Clin Lab Res 1994; 24:23.)

suggest that juvenile-onset diabetes and other similar endocrine abnormalities have autoimmune components, and patients with those diseases may be candidates for experimental clinical studies with thymic hormones.

In pilot clinical studies, TF5 has relieved symptoms in rheumatoid arthritis, systemic lupus erythematosus, and Sjögren syndrome.[43]

## IMMUNODEFICIENCY DISEASES

Thymosins modulate immune activity and may be used to restore depressed immune systems. Most of the congenital immune deficiencies are T-cell dependent; that is, the defective immune activity is due to a partial or complete absence of mature T cells, resulting from a deficiency of thymic hormone production. (Also see ref. 43a.)

Overall, the response to therapy of patients with primary immunodeficiency diseases has been variable. A subgroup of patients with DiGeorge syndrome and some patients with combined immunodeficiency disorders appear to respond to TF5; however, the interpretation of their clinical status is often difficult. Randomized trials are difficult because of the rarity of the diseases. A patient with DiGeorge syndrome responded favorably to treatment with synthetic T$\alpha_1$.[44] Using a human thymus/bone marrow coculture, a clear effect of T$\alpha_1$ was demonstrated in enhancing CD34-positive T cells and in producing IL-7, a cytokine critical in the maturation of thymocytes.[45]

## INFECTIOUS DISEASES

Thymosins have been effective in improving immune responses and in arresting the progression of many viral, bacterial, and fungal infections in mice. In preclinical and clinical studies, thymosins and thymosin-like agents have increased T-cell numbers and functions and activated other antiviral lymphokines and macrophage cell populations. Preliminary results suggest that thymic hormones may be clinically effective in human viral diseases, such as viral hepatitis and influenza, and in the treatment of some bacterial, mycobacterial, and fungal diseases.

Many of these infections develop in patients with immunodeficiencies from other diseases and processes, particularly cancer patients during chemotherapy, patients with severe burns or massive trauma, patients with organ transplants, and patients with acquired immunodeficiency syndrome (AIDS; see Chap. 214).

A number of clinical trials have evaluated the efficacy of T$\alpha_1$ as an adjuvant in enhancing the efficacy of the hepatitis and influenza vaccines in patients treated with kidney dialysis.[46,47]

## HUMAN IMMUNODEFICIENCY VIRUS

In the United States and Italy, in vivo and in vitro studies suggest that thymosin may be useful in treating AIDS, particularly in combination with antivirals (see Chap. 214). A pilot study[48] in human immunodeficiency virus (HIV)–positive patients with helper/suppressor ratios of <1.2 showed that 60 mg of TF5 daily for 10 weeks was effective in significantly increasing functional immune responses; however, other surrogate markers were not changed. The successful use of T$\alpha_1$ in combination with other biologic response modifiers in several animal and human cancer models has permitted a novel potential use of T$\alpha_1$ to emerge in the treatment of AIDS. In multicenter studies,[49] a combination of T$\alpha_1$ and zidovudine (AZT) with interferon-$\alpha_1$ (IFN-α) was found to improve and maintain CD4 counts and to reduce HIV viral titers—as measured by polymerase chain reaction—in patients with AIDS (Fig. 193-4).

## HEPATITIS B AND C

The most clear-cut clinical indications for T$\alpha_1$ are in patients with chronic hepatitis B and hepatitis C. In a 12-patient placebo-controlled pilot study, T$\alpha_1$ significantly improved remission rates in advanced chronic hepatitis B.[50] These initial results stimulated further trials in the United States, China, the Philippines, and Italy. In a metaanalysis of the results of placebo-controlled trials that enrolled 223 patients, T$\alpha_1$ yielded significantly greater remission rates than placebo-treated or control patients.[51] In additional trials in hepatitis B, the combination of T$\alpha_1$ and interferon induced greater remission rates than did T$\alpha_1$ or interferon alone.[52]

Among 103 patients with hepatitis C in whom the remission rates with interferon alone were significantly greater than in placebo controls, the remission rates in patients treated with T$\alpha_1$ in combination with interferon were greater than those obtained with interferon alone[53] (Fig. 193-5).

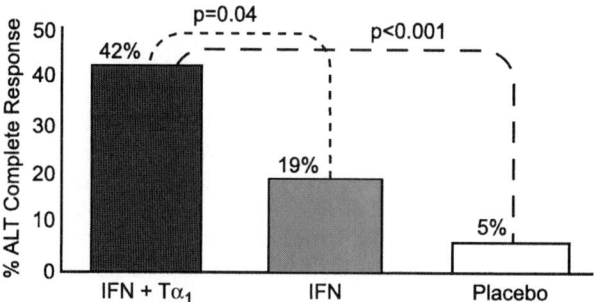

**FIGURE 193-5.** Thymosin $\alpha_1$ ($T\alpha_1$) improves the response of interferon (*IFN*) in patients with hepatitis C. This figure shows the complete biochemical response (*ALT*) at the completion of the 6 months of treatment. Patients were treated with either $T\alpha_1$ plus IFN-$\alpha_{2b}$, or IFN-$\alpha_{2b}$, or placebo for 6 months (n = 107 evaluable). (After Sherman KE, Sjögren M, Creager RL, et al. Combination therapy with thymosin α1 and interferon for the treatment of chronic hepatitis C infection: a randomized, placebo-controlled double-blind trial. Hepatology 1998; 27[4]:1128.)

## AGING

The discovery of a thymus and brain relationship may help in elucidating human aging. A predominant theory is that aging is partly related to the inability of the brain to produce and control certain hormones. Research in this area indicates that thymic hormones may be among the critical factors regulating brain hormonal activity, and thus may be a factor in the senescence of the immune system and other endocrine systems. The decline in thymic hormones and T-cell immunity corresponds with an increase in diseases of aging (see Chap. 199).

These studies suggest that it may be possible to improve immunologic responses in the elderly by manipulating the blood levels of thymic hormones.

In a 70-patient pilot trial and a 330-patient confirmatory trial in geriatric patients, $T\alpha_1$ significantly increased the antibody titers obtained with influenza vaccine.[54] The effect of $T\alpha_1$ was age-related, with the increases in antibody titers and decreases in pulmonary infections being confirmed in subjects 80 years of age or older.

There are a growing number of clinical studies and preclinical experiments with $T\alpha_1$ that point to an important role for this thymic peptide as an effective clinical medicinal in a variety of diseases.

## REFERENCES

1. Hall NR, McGillis JP, Spangelo BL, et al. Thymic hormone effects on the brain and neuroendocrine circuits. In: Guillemin R, Cohn M, Melnechuk T, eds. Neural modulation of immunity. New York: Raven Press, 1985:179.
2. Goldstein AL, Low TLK, Thurman GB, et al. Current status of thymosin and other hormones of the thymus gland. Recent Prog Horm Res 1981; 37:369.
3. Hall NR, McGillis JP, Spangelo BL, Goldstein AL. Evidence that thymosins and other biological response modifiers can function as immunotransmitters. J Immunol 1985; 135:806.
4. Di Marino V, Argeme MT, Brunet C, et al. Macroscopic study of the adult thymus. Surg Radiol Anat 1987; 9:51.
5. Wirt DP, Grogan TM, Nagle RB, et al. A comprehensive immunotopographic map of human thymus. J Histochem Cytochem 1988; 36:1.
6. Henry L, Anderson G. Epithelial-cell architecture during involution of the human thymus. J Pathol 1987; 152:149.
7. Sajous CEM. The thymus gland and the adrenals. In: Galoyan A, ed. The internal secretions and the principles of medicine. Philadelphia: FA Davis Co, 1903:171.
8. Anderson CT. The relationship between the thymus and reproduction. Physiol Rev 1932; 12:1.
9. Spangelo BL, Hall NR, Goldstein AL. Biology and chemistry of thymosin peptides: modulators of immunity and neuroendocrine circuits. Ann N Y Acad Sci 1987; 496:196.
10. Safer D, Elzinga M, Nachmias VT. Thymosin $\beta_4$ and Fx, an actin-sequestering peptide, are indistinguishable. J Biol Chem 1991; 266:4029.
11. Malinda KM, Goldstein AL, Kleinman HK. Thymosin $\beta_4$ stimulates directional migration of human umbilical vein endothelial cells. FASEB J 1997; 11:474.
12. Deschaux P, Massengo B, Fontanges R. Endocrine interaction of the thymus

with the hypophysis, adrenals and testes: effects of two thymic extracts. Thymus 1979; 1:95.
13. Hall NR, McGillis JP, Spangelo BL, et al. Evidence for a neuroendocrine-thymus axis mediated by thymic polypeptides. In: Serrou B, Rosenfeld C, Daniels JC, Saunders JP, eds. Current concepts in human immunology and cancer immunomodulation. New York: Elsevier–North Holland, 1982:653.
14. Rebar RW, Miyake A, Low TLK, Goldstein AL. Thymosin stimulates secretion of LH-releasing factor. Science 1981; 214:669.
15. Galoyan A. In: Biochemistry of Novel Cardioactive hormones and immunomodulators of the functional system neurosecretory hypothalamus-endocrine heart. Moscow: NAUKA Publishers, 1997:145.
16. Badamchiam M, Wang SS, Spangelo BL, et al. Chemical and biological characterization of MB-35: a thymic derived peptide that stimulates the release of growth hormone and prolactin from rat anterior pituitary cells. Prog Neuroendocrinimmunol 1990;3:258.
17. Hall NR, Spangelo BL, Farah JM Jr, et al. Immunotransmitters: a new class of neuroactive peptides produced by the lymphoid system that modulate both immune and neuroendocrine circuits. In: Oppenheim JJ, Jacobs DM, eds. Leukocytes and host defense. New York: Alan R. Liss, 1986:187.
18. Hall NR, Goldstein AL. Endocrine regulation of host immunity: the role of steroids and thymosins. In: Fenichel RL, Chirigos MA, eds. Immunomodulating agents: properties and mechanisms. New York: Marcel Dekker Inc, 1984:533.
19. Spangelo BL, Hall NR, Goldstein AL. Evidence that prolactin is an immunomodulatory hormone. In: MacLeod RM, Torner MO, Scapagnini U, eds. Prolactin: basic and clinical correlates. Padova, Italy: Liviana Press, 1985:343.
20. Spangelo BL, Hall NR, Ross PC, Goldstein AL. Stimulation of in vivo antibody production and concanavalin-A–induced mouse spleen cell mitogenesis by prolactin. Immunopharmacology 1987; 14:11.
21. Healy DL, Hodgen GD, Schulte HM, et al. The thymus-adrenal connection: thymosin has corticotropin-releasing activity in primates. Science 1983; 222:1353.
22. McGillis JP, Hall NR, Vahouny GV, Goldstein AL. Thymosin fraction 5 causes increased serum corticosterone in rodents in vivo. J Immunol 1985; 134:3952.
23. Sivas A, Uysal M, Oz H. The hyperglycemic effect of thymosin F5, a thymic hormone. Horm Metab Res 1982; 14:330.
24. Dumonde DC, Pulley MS, Hamblin AS, et al. Short-term and long-term administration of lymphoblastoid cell line lymphokine (LCL-LK) to patients with advanced cancers. In: Goldstein AL, Chirigos MA, eds. Lymphokines and thymic hormones: their potential utilization in cancer therapeutics. New York: Raven Press, 1982:301.
25. Milenkovic L, McCann SM. Effects of thymosin $\alpha_1$ on pituitary hormone release. Neuroendocrinology 1992, 55:14.
26. McGillis JP, Hall NR, Goldstein AL. Thymosin fraction 5 stimulates in vitro secretion of ACTH from cultured rat pituitaries. Life Sci 1988; 42:2259.
27. Vahouny GV, Kyeyune-Nyombi E, McGillis JP, et al. Thymosin peptides and lymphokines do not directly stimulate adrenal corticosteroid production in vitro. J Immunol 1983; 130:791.
28. Farah JM Jr, Hall NR, Bishop JF, et al. Thymosin fraction 5 stimulates secretion of immunoreactive beta-endorphin in mouse corticotropic tumor cells. J Neurosci Res 1987; 18:140.
29. Besedovsky HO, del Rey A, Sorkin E, et al. The immune response evokes changes in brain noradrenergic neurons. Science 1983; 221:564.
30. Besedovsky HO, Sorkin E. Network of immune-neuroendocrine interactions. Clin Exp Immunol 1977; 20:323.
30a. Savino W, Dardenne M. Neuroendocrine control of thymus physiology. Endocr Rev 2000; 21:412.
31. Johnson HM, Smith EM, Torres BA, Blalock JE. Regulation of the in vitro antibody response by neuroendocrine hormones. Proc Natl Acad Sci U S A 1982; 79:4171.
31a. Kavelaars A, Kuis W, Knpak L, et al. Disturbed neuroendocrine-immune interactions in chronic fatigue syndrome. J Clin Endocrinol Metab 2000; 85:692.
32. O'Grady MP, Hall NR. Interactions between the developing immune and neuroendocrine systems. In: Shair HN, Barr GA, Hofer MA, eds. Developmental psychobiology: new methods and changing concepts. New York: Oxford University Press, 1991:223.
33. O'Grady MP, Hall NR. Long term effects of neuroendocrine-immune interactions during early development. In: Ader R, Felten D, Cohen N, eds. Psychoneuroimmunology. New York: Academic Press, 1991:1067.
34. O'Grady MP, Hall NRS, Menzies RA. Interleukin-1B stimulates adrenocorticotropin and corticosterone release in 10 day old rat pups. Psychoneuroendocrinology 1993; 18:241.
35. Hall NRS, O'Grady MP, Menzies RA. Cytokines and the central nervous system: links with mental disorders. In: Kvetnansky R, McCarty R, Axelrod J, eds. Stress: neuroendocrine and molecular approaches, vol 2. New York: Gordon and Breach, 1992:585.
36. Osheroff, P. The effect of thymosin on glucocosticoid receptors in lymphoid cells. Cell Immunol 1981; 60:378.
37. Baumann CA, Badamchian M, Goldstein AL. Thymosin $\alpha_1$ antagonizes dexamethasone and CD3 induced apoptosis of CD4 and CD8 and thymocytes through the activation of cAMP and protein kinase C dependent second messenger pathways. Mech Aging Dev 1997; 94:85.
37a. Moody TW, Leyton J, Farah Z, et al. Thymosin $\alpha_1$, is chemopreventive for lung adenoma formation in A/J mice. Cancer Letters 2000; 155:121.
38. Lopez M. Biochemotherapy with thymosin $\alpha_1$, interleukin 2 and dacarbazine in patients with metastatic melanoma: clinical and immunological effect. Ann Oncol 1994; 5:741.
39. Schulof RS, Lloyd MJ, Cleary PA, et al. A randomized trial to evaluate the immunorestorative properties of synthetic thymosin $\alpha_1$ in patients with lung cancer. J Biol Resp Mod 1985; 4:147.

40. Chretien P. In: Maurer MR, Goldstein AL, eds. Thymic peptides in preclinical and clinical medicine. Munich: Zuckschwerdt Verlaq, 1997:152.

41. Favalli C. Combination therapy in malignant melanoma. In: Third International Symposium on Combination Therapies, Houston, TX: Institute for Advanced Studies in Immunology and Aging, 1997.

42. Stefanini GS, Faschi FG, Castelli E, et al. α1-Thymosin and transcatheter arterial chemoembolization in hepatocellular carcinoma patients: a preliminary experience. Hepatogastroenterology 1998; 45:209.

43. Lavastida MT, Goldstein AL, Daniels JC. Thymosin administration in autoimmune disorders. Thymus 1981; 2:287.

43a. Hatzakis A, Touloumi G, Karanicolas R, et al. Effect of recent thymic emigrants on progression of HIV-1 disease. Lancet 2000; 355:599.

44. Gupta S, Aggarwal S, Hguyen T. Accelerated spontaneous programmed cell death in lymphocytes in DiGeorge syndrome. J Allergy Clin Immunol 1997; 99(S3):11.

45. Knutsen AP, Freeman JJ, Mueller KR, et al. Thymosin α1 stimulates maturation of CD34 and stem cells into CD3+4+ in an in vitro thymic epithelial organ co-culture model. Int J Immunopharmacol 1999; 21:15.

46. Shen S, Corteza QB, Josselson J. Effects of thymosin alpha 1 on peripheral T-cell & hepatovax-B vaccination in previously non-responsive hemodialysis patients. Hepatology 1987; 7:1120A.

47. Shen S, Corteza QB, Josselson J. Age dependent enhancement of influenza vaccine responses by thymosin in chronic hemodialysis patients. In: Goldstein AL, ed. Biomedical advances in aging. New York: Plenum Press, 1990:523.

48. Schulof RS, Simon GL, Sztein MB, et al. Phase I/II trial of thymosin fraction 5 and thymosin α1 in HTLV-III-seropositive subjects. J Biol Resp Mod 1986; 5:429.

49. Garaci E, Rocchi G, Perroni L, et al. Combination treatment with zidovudine, thymosin α1, and interferon-α in human immunodeficiency virus infection. Int J Clin Lab Res 1994; 24:23.

50. Mutchnick MG, Appleman HD, Chung HT, et al. Thymosin treatment of chronic hepatitis B: a placebo controlled trial. Hepatology 1991; 14:409.

51. Niedzwiecki D, et al. The efficacy of thymosin α1 in chronic hepatitis B; a metaanalysis 1997. Data provided by SciClone Pharmaceuticals, Inc, San Mateo, CA.

52. Rasi G, Mutchnick MG, Di Virgilio D, et al. Combination low-dose lymphoblastoid interferon and thymosin α1 therapy in the treatment of chronic hepatitis B. J Viral Hepatitis 1996; 3:191.

53. Sherman KE, Sjogren M, Creager RL, et al. Combination therapy with thymosin α1 and interferon for the treatment of chronic hepatitis C infection: a randomized, placebo-controlled double-blind trial. Hepatology 1998; 27(4):1128.

54. McConnell L, Gravenstein S, Roecker E, et al. Augmentation of influenza antibody levels and reduction in attack rates in elderly subjects by thymosin α1. The Gerontologist 1989; 29:188A.

55. Krueger J, Dinarello C, Wolff M, et al. Sleep-promoting effects of endogenous pyrogen (interleukin-1). Am J Physiol 1984; 246:R994.

56. Schupf N, Williams CA, Hugh TE, Cox J. Psychopharmacological activity of anaphylatoxin C3a in rat hypothalamus. J Neuroimmunol 1983; 5:305.

57. Abrams PG, McClamrock E, Foon KA. Evening administration of alpha-interferon. N Engl J Med 1985; 312:443.

58. Spangelo BL, Hall NR, Dunn AS, Goldstein AL. Thymosin fraction 5 stimulates the release of prolactin from cultured GH3 cells. Life Sci 1987; 40:283.

59. Hall NRS, O'Grady M, Goldstein AL, Farah JM. Regulation of pituitary hormones by thymosins and other immune system products. In: Reif AE, Schlesinger M, eds. Cell surface antigen Thy-1, immunology, neurology and therapeutic applications. New York and Basel: Marcel Dekker Inc, 1989:469.

60. Farah JM, Bishop JF, Michel J, et al. Immune modulation of the hypothalamic-pituitary-adrenal axis: cellular effects of thymosin on clonal corticotropes. In: Breznitz S, Zinder O, eds. Molecular biology of stress. New York: Alan R. Liss, 1989:107.

# CHAPTER 194

# IMMUNOGENETICS, THE HUMAN LEUKOCYTE ANTIGEN SYSTEM, AND ENDOCRINE DISEASE

JAMES R. BAKER, JR.

Immunogenetics and the study of the human leukocyte antigen (HLA) system have made spectacular progress since "leukoagglutinating" antibodies (against the then unknown HLA) were discovered almost 50 years ago. Although the original interest in

HLA arose from its relation to histocompatibility (tissue typing and matching) in organ transplantation, it now is apparent that the HLA system is involved in the initiation and propagation of all immune activities.[1,2] This fact, and the known associations of certain subgroups of HLA with specific immunologic disorders, suggest that immunogenetics may be involved either directly or indirectly in the generation of autoimmunity and autoimmune endocrine disease. It is this involvement that now requires that the physician treating endocrine disorders understand the basis of immunogenetics.

## THE MAJOR HISTOCOMPATIBILITY COMPLEX IN HUMANS: STRUCTURE AND FUNCTION

The HLAs are structurally complex proteins with the remarkable property of being unique for each individual. The novel nature of each HLA is even more extraordinary because most of each antigen's structure is the same in all individuals. This is similar to antibody structure, in which most of the protein has a common structure, but the antigen-combining site is unique. In both cases, the common part of the molecule has a function (such as antigen presentation or immune clearance), whereas the unique determinants provide the specificity for this function.

The genes that code for the genetically restricted elements of the immune system are located in a cluster on the short arm of chromosome number 6, designated the major histocompatibility complex (MHC; Fig. 194-1). The MHC is divided into seven loci, based on physical location and the type of proteins they encode. The genes coding for class I HLA are located in the A, B, and C loci, and the antigens encoded by these loci are called HLA-A, -B, and -C, respectively. They encode variations of a 44-kDa immunoglobulin-like glycoprotein that is anchored to the cell through a transmembrane domain. This protein is noncovalently associated with a small, 12-kDa protein on the surface of the cell to form the functional molecule. The complex functions by presenting 8 to 12 amino-acid peptides to CD8 T cells in a manner that directs cytotoxic attack (Fig. 194-2). Class I antigens are essential to immune defenses against viruses and neoplasms, in which intracellular antigens must be targeted, and against infected or neoplastic cells. Class II HLA loci (also called the *HLA-D region products*) display at least three sets of antigens, designated DR, DQ, and DP. These genes are located in a separate locus that pro-

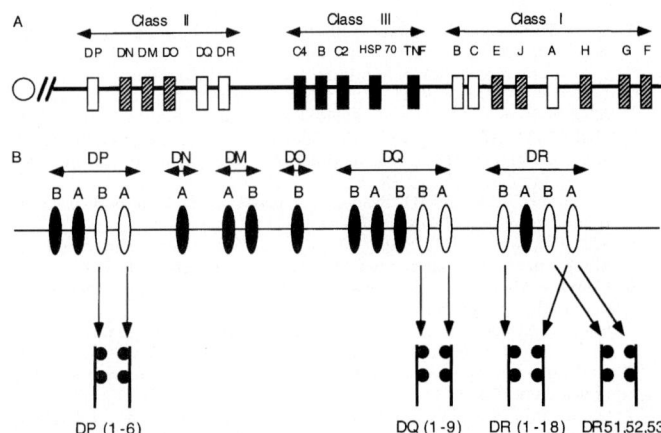

**FIGURE 194-1. A,** The major histocompatibility complex (*MHC*) gene loci on the short arm of chromosome number 6. MHC genes are *open boxes,* pseudogenes are *striped boxes,* and non–human leukocyte antigen genes are *black boxes.* **B,** Close-up of class II locus. Genes are *open ovals;* pseudogenes are *closed ovals.*

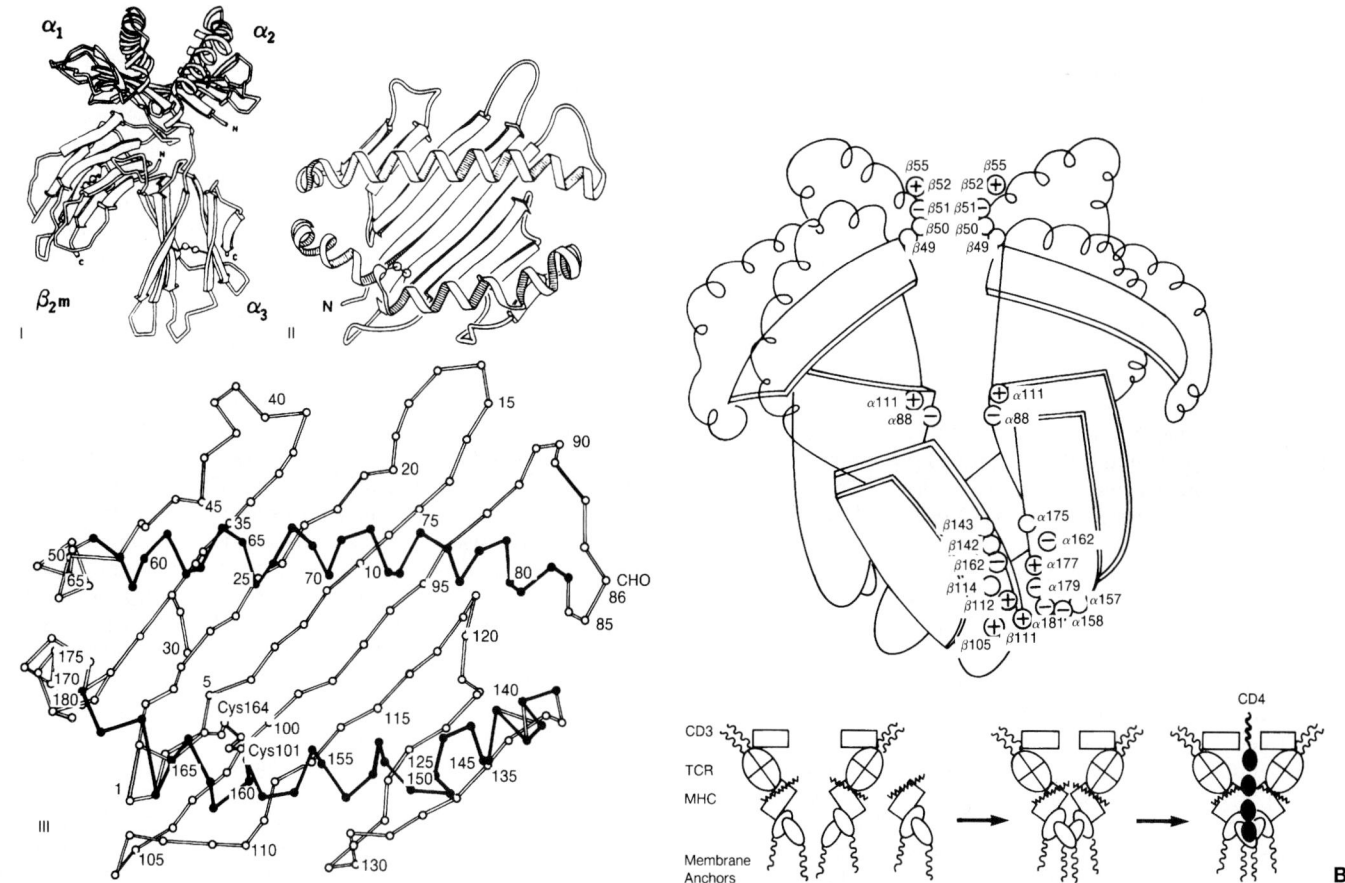

**FIGURE 194-2. A,** Three different views of the structure of the HLA class I antigen. The $\alpha_1$ and $\alpha_2$ domains form the peptide-binding groove, with an α-helix forming each side and a β-pleated sheet forming the floor. The amino-acid residues located at the sides of the peptide groove are the ones most likely to be involved in allotypic variations in structure of the antigens. (Adapted from Bjorkman PJ, Saper MA, Samraoui B, et al. Structures of the human histocompatibility antigen HLA-A2. Nature 1987; 329:506.) **B,** The structure of the HLA class II antigen. Note that, although the general structure (peptide-binding groove, etc.) is similar, both protein chains are transmembrane. In addition, the antigens form dimers. As is shown in the *lower panel*, forming dimers may be important in the interaction between class II antigens and T-cell antigen-receptor CD4 molecules, as well as in T-cell activation. (*MHC*, major histocompatibility complex; *TCR*, T-cell receptor.) (Adapted from Brown JH, Jardetzky TS, Gorge JC, et al. Three-dimensional structure of human class II histocompatibility antigen HLA-DR1. Nature 1993; 364:33.)

duces protein dimers more complicated than the class I antigens (see Fig. 194-1). The different types of class II antigens all are produced by two sets of genes that code transmembrane α and β chains, which have about the same molecular mass (34,000 and 28,000 Da, respectively). Both these chains are glycosylated and have complex structures. It is thought that the class II antigens have allotypic differences in three ways: in the proteins forming their two chains, in the carbohydrates on their chains, and in the conformation of the whole molecule attributable to the way in which the two chains interact. Because of this, the class II antigens display complex and diverse antigenicity. Remarkably, each class II locus codes for its protein in a different manner (see Fig. 194-1B). Class II antigens present foreign peptides to CD4 cells of the immune system. They are located primarily on antigen-presenting cells (e.g., macrophages, dendritic cells), and are essential in initiating both cellular and antibody immune responses. These antigens appear to accommodate peptides of more variable sizes and associate as dimers of two α- and β-chain complexes. This may be important for signaling through the T-cell antigen receptor.

Class III antigens are coded by genes in the C locus and include the complement proteins C2, C4, and properdin. There

also are polymorphisms of some of these genes; however, they number only two to four allotypes.

Class I and class II antigens from all loci have multiple allotypic (individual) forms, which are identified with a number after the locus name, such as HLA-B8. These assignments were initially made from antigen definitions developed using heterologous antisera (obtained mainly from multiparous women sensitized to HLA). The genes for the HLA also have been sequenced, and the sequence variations defining the allotypes are now known. These sequences are readily available in some excellent reviews.[3-5] There is marked allotypic heterogeneity in the HLA. Because each haplotype (set of chromosomes) has at least six loci (three class I and three class II) coding for six specific antigens, and because each individual has two haplotypes (one from each parent; 12 loci in all), it is highly unlikely that any two unrelated individuals would have the same HLAs (or the same "tissue type," as it is called in transplantation). Thus, it becomes clear how HLA is helpful in determining paternity, while being an effective barrier to organ transplantation. However, the phylogenetic basis for this variation is more important. The allotype differences in the MHC antigens ensure that individuals recognize antigens differently. This prevents the human species from being destroyed by an infectious agent that no one can recognize and respond to immunologically.

Recent advances in the understanding of the immune response have shown it to be regulated by the HLA system in both its initiating and terminal events. An understanding of this regulation can be gained by examining the types of cells that express the different classes of HLA. The class II antigens regulate the generation of the immune response and, under normal conditions, are expressed only on cells that present antigens to T cells, including dendritic cells, macrophages, and reticuloendothelial cells. Antigen is processed into peptides, which are then presented on the cell membrane by the HLA class II molecules. This combination of antigen and class II molecule then can be recognized by a T cell through its antigen receptor; however, this recognition can take place only if the two cells share the same class II molecules. In effect, this limits the earliest events in the generation of immune response to cells designed to present antigen and to antigens that appear foreign to the individual.[1,6] This restriction is important, because the population of T cells activated by antigen-presenting cells is then expanded and stimulated by *lymphokines* (such as interleukins-1 and -2; see Chap. 195), which are nonspecific. Thus, it is the initial, HLA-restricted antigen presentation that gives economy and specificity to the immune response.

B lymphocytes express both class I and class II antigens on their surfaces, and these antigens regulate antibody production. Antibody production usually requires the interaction of B cells and T cells, and this interaction probably takes place through class I and II antigen recognition on the surfaces of B cells.

The class I antigens, located on all the nucleated cells of the body, direct the targeting action of cytotoxic T cells. These T cells are important in the removal of virally infected cells and cancer cells, and attack only target cells that express the same class I HLA antigens. The ability to discriminate between self and foreign antigens is a result of the maturation of T cells in the thymus. Thus, the terminal event of the immune response shows a restriction to self much like the event at its initiation.

This regulatory network functions differently in organ transplantation, because allografts can elicit an immune response from the recipient without sharing any HLA. The reason for this is being clarified, and it appears that the "foreign" HLA of the donor organ is recognized as if it were self HLA in combination with foreign antigen.[7,8] Thus, allogenic differences in class II antigens can cause helper T-cell proliferation, and class I antigens from different individuals can serve as targets for cytotoxic T cells.

## INVOLVEMENT OF HLA IN THE DEVELOPMENT OF AUTOIMMUNITY

Because of the important role HLA plays in governing the immune response, it has long been suspected that the dysregulation of the immune system that permits autoimmunity might be related to faulty HLA presentation and restriction. There are several theories on the mechanisms underlying HLA-associated autoimmunity, which involve the class II antigens. These theories are based on the role of class II antigens in the generation of immune responses and on the statistical association between certain of these antigens and autoimmune diseases.

Of the many theories on the mechanisms whereby HLA serves in the development of autoimmunity, the one with the strongest support involves the presentation of antigenic peptides to T cells. T cells recognize foreign antigens in association with HLAs (see Fig. 194-2). Differences in the amino acids that form the walls of the peptide groove can result in great differences in the binding affinity of self-peptides, and in the confor-

mation of the peptide–MHC complex. T-cell antigen-receptor $\alpha$ and $\beta$ chains interact with the allotypic variable portions of the MHC antigens to recognize the combination of peptide and MHC molecule. This suggests either that certain HLA allotypes make self-antigens look foreign when the two are combined or that these allotypes generate a strong enough immune response to self-antigens to overcome T-cell suppression. This proposition has been generalized to suggest that there may be unique allotypes of class II antigens that can initiate strong immune responses to specific autoantigens.[8] There is indirect support for this view, because HLA-DR3 and other class II antigens have been associated with an increased risk for several autoimmune disorders. The most interesting example of how certain MHC allotypes might influence the development of autoimmune endocrine disease involves type 1 diabetes. It now appears that certain polymorphisms in the DQ$\beta$ gene code for allelic proteins that may relate to the presentation of autoantigenic peptides. This may help in the development of insulitis, with the resulting destruction of islet cells. These alleles result in only an eight-fold to ten-fold increase in the risk of disease development, however, so other factors, including environmental triggers, also are likely to be important. Final confirmation of these findings awaits the identification of the autoantigen peptides bound by these MHC antigens to evaluate how the polymorphisms alter presentation. This could lead to peptide-based therapies that block the development of autoimmune disease by preventing the binding of antigenic peptides to the MHC.

The other theory has to do with the expression of HLA class II determinants on the surfaces of cells that are not normally involved in immune processes. Because class II determinants usually are present only on the surfaces of reticuloendothelial and B cells, the ability to present antigens is restricted to these cell types. However, under certain circumstances, such as the influence of inflammatory hormones like interferon-$\gamma$ or tumor necrosis factor $\alpha$ (TNF-$\alpha$), almost any cell in the body will express class II antigens. When these antigens are expressed on endocrine cells, it is postulated that they can present the cells' own surface proteins as foreign antigens and so induce an autoimmune response. In this way, the expression of class II HLAs on the surface of thyroid cells might allow the presentation of thyroglobulin and microsomal antigens. This theory is supported by the findings that class II antigens are expressed on the surface of thyrocytes in patients with Graves disease and on pancreatic islet cells in patients with diabetes,[9] but there is no evidence that this phenomenon alone is sufficient to initiate autoimmunity. It is possible, however, that combined with unique allotypes of costimulating molecules, such as CTLA-4, T-cell activation is adequate to support or at least perpetuate autoimmunity.[10]

## HLA AND ENDOCRINE DISEASES

HLA has been related to autoimmune endocrine disease in two ways[6–15] (see Chap. 197). The first is through "disease associations," the finding that patients with a particular HLA are at significantly increased risk for the development of a particular disease. There are HLA associations for several endocrine diseases: subacute thyroiditis—B35, idiopathic Addison disease—DR3, Graves disease—DR3, myasthenia gravis—DR3, insulin-dependent (type 1) diabetes—DR3 or DR4, postpartum thyroiditis—DR3 or DR4, and Hashimoto thyroiditis—DR5. The definition of a disease association implies an etiologic connection between the antigen and the disease. This probably is not the case for most of the associations found with endocrine diseases, because many persons who do not have the associated HLA nevertheless develop the disease. It is likely that the associated antigens actually are "linked" (closely associated) to the true disease-associated antigen. Thus, those HLAs that are believed to be disease-associated actually may be markers for uncharacterized gene products that are responsible for disease susceptibility.[16]

Most HLA–disease associations (see earlier) are controversial. The cause for this controversy probably is the aforementioned fact that these associations actually are linkages that are not consistent in different population groups. For example, the initial observation that HLA-B8 was associated with Graves disease was actually an association with HLA-DR3, which is tightly linked to HLA-B8. The HLA-B8 association would not have been made in a genetic group in which HLA-B8 was not linked to HLA-DR3. The higher resolution of DNA genotyping of the class II genes has furthered and confirmed many of the Graves disease–MHC associations. The association with DR3 has been confirmed and may be explained in part by DQα501, which is in linkage disequilibrium with DR3.[17,18] Of interest, even the genotypic associations are not consistent across different racial and ethnic groups, bringing into question their role in the pathogenesis of this disorder.

The second HLA–disease relation is the haplotype linkage of HLA to disease found in family studies of inherited disorders. This relation does not imply an etiologic basis but simply links a disease gene with an HLA haplotype. This involves a comparison of haplotypes with the pattern of disease inheritance to detect affected individuals and carriers. The classic example of this type of linkage relates to 21-hydroxylase deficiency. The gene for this enzyme is located within the MHC (see Fig. 194-1) and, thus, is fortuitously tied to the HLA genes. Tissue typing of families with 21-hydroxylase deficiency reveals the affected haplotype, so that carriers of the disease and affected fetuses can be detected.

Although linkages already have provided clinically useful information, the clinical utility of HLA–disease associations is minimal. A clinical use has been suggested for the association of HLA-DR3 with Graves disease, because patients who have this antigen appear more likely to relapse after medical therapy.[19,20] This finding has been questioned, however, and relapses in Graves disease seem to have multiple causes.[20] It does appear that HLA associations may predict severity of illness in some patients with type 1 diabetes mellitus,[21,22] especially in certain racial groups.[23] The examination of DQ β-chain gene polymorphisms seems to offer a better basis for clinically relevant associations.[21,24,25] Other non-MHC genes also appear to be important in the genetic predisposition for these disorders.[26] Animal models of Graves disease that are dependent on antigen presentation by particular class II antigens may also provide insights into significant linkages.[27,28]

## REFERENCES

1. Pervis B. Internalization of lymphocyte membrane components. Immunol Today 1985; 6:45.
2. Bell JI, Todd JA, McDevitt HO. The molecular basis of HLA-disease association. In: Harris H, Hirschhorn K, eds. Advances in human genetics, vol 18. New York: Plenum Press, 1989:1.
3. Bodmer JG, Marsh SG, Albert ED, et al. Nomenclature for factors of the HLA system. Hum Immunol 1992; 34:4.
4. Marsh SG, Bodmer JG. HLA class II nucleotide sequences. Hum Immunol 1992; 35:1.
5. Browning MJ, Krausa P, Rowan A, et al. Tissue typing the HLA-A locus from genomic DNA by sequence-specific PCR: comparison of HLA genotype and surface expression on colorectal tumor cell lines. Proc Natl Acad Sci U S A 1993; 90:2842.
6. Burman KD, Baker JR Jr. Immune mechanisms in Graves disease. Endocr Rev 1985; 6:183.
7. Parham P. A repulsive view of MHC restriction. Immunol Today 1984; 5:89.
8. Todd JA. The role of MHC class II genes in susceptibility to insulin-dependent diabetes mellitus. Curr Top Microbiol Immunol 1990; 164:17.
9. Bottazzo GR, Pujol-Borrell R, Hanafusa T, Feldmann M. The role of aberrant HLA-DR expression and antigen presentation in the induction of endocrine autoimmunity. Lancet 1983; 2:1115.
10. Nistico L, Buzzetti R, Pritchard LE, et al. The CTLA-4 gene region of chromosome 2q33 is linked to, and associated with, type 1 diabetes. Belgian Diabetes Registry. Hum Mol Genet 1996; 5:1075.
11. Farid NR, Bear JC. The human major histocompatibility complex and endocrine disease. Endocr Rev 1981; 2:50.
12. Bjorkman PJ, Saper MA, Samraoui B, et al. Structure of the human class I histocompatibility antigen, HLA-A2. Nature 1987; 329:506.
13. Brown JH, Jardetzky TS, Gorga JC, et al. Three-dimensional structure of the human class II histocompatibility antigen HLA-DR1. Nature 1993; 364:33.
14. Gambelunghe G, Falorni A, Ghaderi M, et al. Microsatellite polymorphism of the NIHC class 1 chain-related (MIC-A and MIC-B) genes marks the risk for autoimmune Addison's disease. J Clin Endocrinol Metab 1999; 84:3701.
15. Gough SC. The genetics of Graves' disease. Endocrinol Metab Clin North Am 2000; 29:255.
16. Batchelor JR, McMichael AJ. Progress in understanding HLA and disease associations. Br Med Bull 1987; 43:156.
17. Hu R, Beck C, Chang YB, DeGroot LJ. HLA class II genes in Graves disease. Autoimmunity 1992; 12:103.
18. Yanagawa T, Mangklabruks A, Chang YB, et al. Human histocompatibility leukocyte antigen-DQA1 *0501 allele associated with genetic susceptibility to Graves disease in a Caucasian population. J Clin Endocrinol Metab 1993; 76:1569.
19. McGregor AM, Rees-Smith B, Hall R, et al. Prediction of relapse in hyperthyroid Graves disease. Lancet 1980; 1:1101.
20. Allannic H, Fauchet R, Lorcy Y, et al. A prospective study of the relationship between relapse of hyperthyroid Graves disease after antithyroid drugs and HLA haplotype. J Clin Endocrinol Metab 1982; 57:719.
21. Todd JA, Bell JI, McDevitt HO. HLA-DQ beta gene contributes to susceptibility and resistance to insulin-dependent diabetes mellitus. Nature 1987; 329:599.
22. Owerbach D, Gum S, Gabby KH. Primary associations of HLA-DQw8 with type I diabetes in DR4 patients. Diabetes 1989; 38:942.
23. Todd JA, Reed PW, Prins JB, et al. Dissection of the pathophysiology of type 1 diabetes by genetic analysis. Autoimmunity 1993; 15(Suppl):16.
24. Gregersen PK. HLA class II polymorphism: implications for genetic susceptibility to autoimmune disease. Lab Invest 1989; 239:1026.
25. Chuang LM, Wu HP, Chang CC, et al. HLA DRB1/DQA1/DQB1 haplotype determines thyroid autoimmunity in patients with insulin-dependent diabetes mellitus. Clin Endocrinol (Oxf) 1996; 45:631.
26. Merriman TR, Todd JA. Genetics of insulin-dependent diabetes; non-major histocompatibility genes. Horm Metab Res 1996; 28:289.
27. Shimojo N, Kohno Y, Yamaguchi K, et al. Induction of Graves-like disease in mice by immunization with fibroblasts transfected with the thyrotropin receptor and a class II molecule. Proc Natl Acad Sci U S A 1996; 93 (20):11074.
28. Kikuoka S, Shimojo N, Yamaguchi KI, et al. The formation of thyrotropin receptor (TSHR) antibodies in a Graves' animal model requires the N-terminal segment of the TSHR extracellular domain. Endocrinology 1998; 139(4):1891.

# CHAPTER 195

# T CELLS IN ENDOCRINE DISEASE

ANTHONY PETER WEETMAN

It has been traditional to categorize immune responses as *humoral* and *cell-mediated*, but the T cell plays a central role in both and, as discussed later, the relative importance of each is determined by the balance among subpopulations of T cells (Table 195-1). Autoimmunity is a major cause of endocrine disease, and T cells appear to be essential to its pathogenesis, directly through their effector functions and indirectly through their stimulation of B cells to produce autoantibodies. The initiation of the autoimmune response by *T-cell receptor* (TCR) recognition of the bimolecular complex formed from antigenic peptide and the major histocompatibility complex (MHC) molecule has been considered in Chapter 194. This section briefly reviews the control and diversity of autoreactive T cells, and then reviews the involvement of T cells in experimental and human endocrinopathies.

**TABLE 195-1.**
**Lexicon of Terms Used in Immunology**

| | |
|---|---|
| Anergy | A process of tolerance in which the T or B cell does not respond to an antigen, despite not being deleted. May be reversed under some circumstances. |
| Antibody | A protein secreted by B cells in response to a specific antigen to which the antibody binds. |
| Antigen | Any molecule, self or foreign, to which the immune system responds. |
| Antigen presentation | The first stage in a T-cell response to an antigen, in which the T cell is activated by an antigenic fragment plus MHC molecule, presented by an antigen-presenting cell (e.g., macrophage, dendritic cell). |
| Antiidiotypes | Antibodies that react with variable region antigenic determinants (idiotypes) on other antibodies; this interaction forms a network and may control the immune response. The term is often extended to T-cell receptor interactions. |
| Autoimmunity | The reaction of the immune system against self. Not all autoimmune responses result in autoimmune *disease*, which is a pathologic consequence of some autoimmune reactions. |
| B cell | Lymphocytes expressing surface immunoglobulin. Terminal differentiation produces antibody-secreting plasma cells. B cells can present antigen. |
| CD | Cluster of differentiation; cell-surface molecules defining the phenotype of a particular cell population (e.g., CD3 is a molecule expressed by T cells). |
| Central tolerance | Tolerance induced in the thymus. |
| Class I MHC molecule | Surface molecules encoded by the MHC class I region, which typically present endogenous antigen to CD8$^+$ T cells; important in T cell–mediated killing of target cells (e.g., after viral infection). |
| Class II MHC molecule | Surface molecules encoded by the MHC class II region that typically present exogenous antigen to CD4$^+$ T cells; important in the stimulation of $T_H$ subsets (e.g., helper cells for antibody production). |
| Clonal deletion | The induction of tolerance by the elimination of (self-reactive) T or B cells. T-cell deletion usually occurs within the thymus. |
| Complement | A series of proteins that mediate bacterial clearance, inflammation, and cell damage by membrane insertion. |
| Costimulation | The requirement for a second signal (e.g., B7), in addition to antigenic peptide plus class II molecule, in antigen presentation to a T cell. |
| Cytokine | Soluble factors released by many cell types, including those of the immune system. |
| Cytotoxicity | Killing of target cells by antibodies (through complement) or by cell-mediated events (T cells, NK cells). Cytotoxic T cells usually are CD8$^+$. |
| Dendritic cells | Potent, widespread antigen-presenting cells; unlike macrophages, they are poorly phagocytic and do not express immunoglobulin (Fc) or complement receptors. |
| Determinant spreading | The phenomenon of T cell–mediated responses occurring to increasing numbers of often cryptic epitopes on a molecule, after an initially restricted response to a critical epitope. |
| Effector cells | Immune cells carrying out a pathologic function (e.g., effector T cells killing a virally infected target cell). |
| Epitope | An antigenic determinant. T-cell epitopes are short peptides that bind to MHC class I or II molecules and are recognized by the T-cell receptor. B-cell epitopes usually are conformational (three-dimensional) structures on an antigen to which an antibody binds. |
| Germinal center | Complex structures made up of actively proliferating cells in lymphoid follicles. |
| Helper cell | A functional definition of the CD4$^+$ T-cell subpopulation that provides help for antibody synthesis and differentiation of other T cells. Often divided by the pattern of cytokine secretion into $T_H$1 and $T_H$2 cells. |
| Idiotypes | Unique determinants in the variable region of antibodies. The term also often is applied to unique determinants in the T-cell–receptor variable region. |
| Immune complex | Antigen bound to antibody, often together with complement components. |
| Immunoglobulin | The same as antibody. Each immunoglobulin has a basic structure of two identical heavy chains and two identical light chains. There are five classes of immunoglobulins: IgM, IgG, IgA, IgE, and IgD. Most pathologic antibodies are IgG. |
| Interferon | A group of cytokines with diverse functions that are broadly antiviral. Interferon-γ has several important immunologic effects. |
| Interleukin | Originally thought to be a group of diverse cytokines released only by cells of the immune system, but now (in some cases) known to have more diverse origins. |
| Lymphoid organs | The cells of the lymphoid system develop in primary lymphoid organs (thymus, liver, bone marrow) and migrate to the second lymphoid organs (spleen, lymph nodes, mucosa-associated lymphoid tissue). |
| Macrophages | Widespread phagocytic cells that can present antigen. |
| Major histocompatibility complex (MHC) | A large group of genes encoding proteins involved in immune recognition and signaling. The MHC in humans is termed HLA and lies on chromosome 6. |
| Memory cells | A functional definition of T or B cells that have encountered antigen during a primary immune response and, therefore, can respond promptly after a second encounter with the antigen. |
| Monoclonal | Cells or products derived from a single differentiated parent cell. |
| Naive cells | Lymphocytes that have not previously encountered a specific antigen. |
| Natural killer (NK) cells | Non-B, non-T lymphocytes that can kill a wide variety of target cells (e.g., tumor cells). |
| Peripheral tolerance | Tolerance induced outside the thymus, including at sites of autoimmune disease. |
| Polyclonal | Cells or products derived from many differentiated parent cells; a polyclonal immune response involves T or B cells expressing many different receptors or antibodies. |
| Primary response | The first encounter between the immune system and an antigen. Primary antibody responses are slower and weaker than secondary responses. |
| Secondary response | The response that occurs after rechallenge of the immune system with an antigen. |
| Self-tolerance | The mechanisms whereby the immune system fails to respond against self-antigens; failure of self-tolerance may result in autoimmunity. |
| Subclasses of antibodies | Classes of immunoglobulins can be divided into subclasses or isotypes with different functional properties (e.g., IgG$_4$ fails to fix complement, unlike IgG$_1$, IgG$_2$, and IgG$_3$). |
| Suppressor T cells | A functional definition of a group of T cells that can inhibit immune responses. Several mechanisms may explain suppression, and such T cells are likely to be heterogeneous. |
| T cells | Lymphocytes that develop in the thymus and express CD3 and T-cell receptors. There are many functional and phenotypic subpopulations. |
| T-cell receptor | The structure on T cells responsible for antigen recognition (in the context of an appropriate MHC molecule). Most T cells have a receptor comprised of α and β chains; a small population has a receptor made of γ and δ chains. |
| $T_H$ subsets | $T_H$1 cells mediate delayed-type hypersensitivity reactions and release cytokines such as interleukin-2, interferon-γ, and lymphotoxin. $T_H$2 cells provide help for B cells in antibody formation and release cytokines such as interleukin-4, interleukin-5, and interleukin-6. |
| Thymus | The primary lymphoid organ in the mediastinum in which T cells mature. Some T cells are positively selected, but self-reactive T cells are tolerized by deletion or anergy. |
| Tolerance | The mechanisms by which the immune systems fail to respond against an antigen. Tolerance to non–self-antigens can be induced experimentally. |
| Tumor necrosis factor (TNF) | TNF-α is made primarily by macrophages and TNF-β (lymphotoxin) by T cells. These cytokines may kill tumor cells but also have important effects on the immune system. |
| Variable (V) regions | The portions of the immunoglobulin heavy and light chains that show amino-acid sequence variation; this determines their antigen-binding specificity. The T-cell receptor chains also have variable regions that again are critical in antigen recognition. |

# T-CELL TOLERANCE

The key role of the immune system is to recognize and provide defense against foreign antigens, while at the same time avoiding harmful self-reactivity.[1,1a] A hierarchy of mechanisms prevents autoimmune disease. The most effective is the removal of all self-reactive T cells during ontogeny. This is known as *clonal deletion*, and it occurs in the thymus, as clearly demonstrated in animal models.[1,2] The mechanism for T-cell deletion is via *programmed cell death* or *apoptosis* and can occur in the thymic cortex at an early stage in development, when T cells are CD4+ CD8+, or later in the medulla, when cells are CD4+ CD8− or CD4− CD8+. Whether a particular T cell is deleted depends on the affinity of its specific TCR for the self-peptide–MHC complexes, which are presented to it. Because blood-borne self-proteins have only limited access to the thymic cortex, T-cell deletion at this site is probably limited to autoantigens produced by the cortical epithelial cells themselves. However, in the thymic medulla it is the dendritic cells that acquire a more generalized selection of autoantigens from the circulation and present these to potentially autoreactive T cells; those T cells with the highest affinity are deleted.[3] Autoreactive, mature T cells can also be deleted in the periphery at a later stage, either because they fail to be stimulated appropriately or because repeated antigenic stimulation leads to apoptosis, this being triggered by the interaction between Fas on the T cell and Fas ligand (FasL) on antigen-presenting cells.[4]

However, clonal deletion is imperfect, even in transgenic animals expressing abundant, selected self-antigens, and it is difficult to envisage the presentation of all possible autoantigens from endocrine and other tissues taking place within the developing thymus—assuming that they could be captured from the periphery. Clonal anergy is a second-line defense against autoreactive T cells escaping deletion,[2,5] and results from abortive antigen presentation in the absence of an appropriate costimulator (Fig. 195-1). The most clearly established costimulatory pathway (or second signal) involves the interaction of B7-1 (CD80) and B7-2 (CD86), found on dendritic cells, activated B cells, and macrophages (i.e., classic antigen-presenting cells) with their receptors, CD28 and CTLA-4, found on T cells.[6]

Engagement of CD28 by B7 delivers an activating signal, and prevents apoptosis, whereas CTLA-4 transduces a signal that inhibits interleukin-2 (IL-2) transcription and halts T-cell cycle progression, although the biochemical basis for this is unknown. When nonclassic antigen-presenting cells, such as thyroid cells, express MHC class II molecules in pathologic settings, they do not express B7, and T-cell interaction with presented self-antigen can lead to anergy or even deletion.[7] Thus, either the absence of costimulation, or the signal provided by CTLA-4, may induce anergy and self-tolerance. There are other molecules that have costimulatory function, including CD40 expressed on antigen-presenting cells, and CD40 ligand (CD154) on T cells. Interaction of these molecules leads both to direct costimulation of the T cell and to induction of expression of B7 and probably other costimulatory molecules. Provision of IL-2 can reverse anergy in certain settings, and this may provide an explanation for the induction of some types of autoimmune disease. The homeostasis mechanism that is employed in self-tolerance depends on a number of factors (Fig. 195-2).

A form of apparent tolerance is *clonal ignorance* in which T cells fail to respond to a particular autoantigen or epitope because this is not presented in a context in which the T cell can recognize it; in this state the T cell has not been actively blocked by anergy-inducing mechanisms. Therefore, it is possible that, under appropriate conditions, T-cell activation will occur. One such situation would be during an infection in which costimulatory signals become up-regulated, or previously hidden ("cryp-

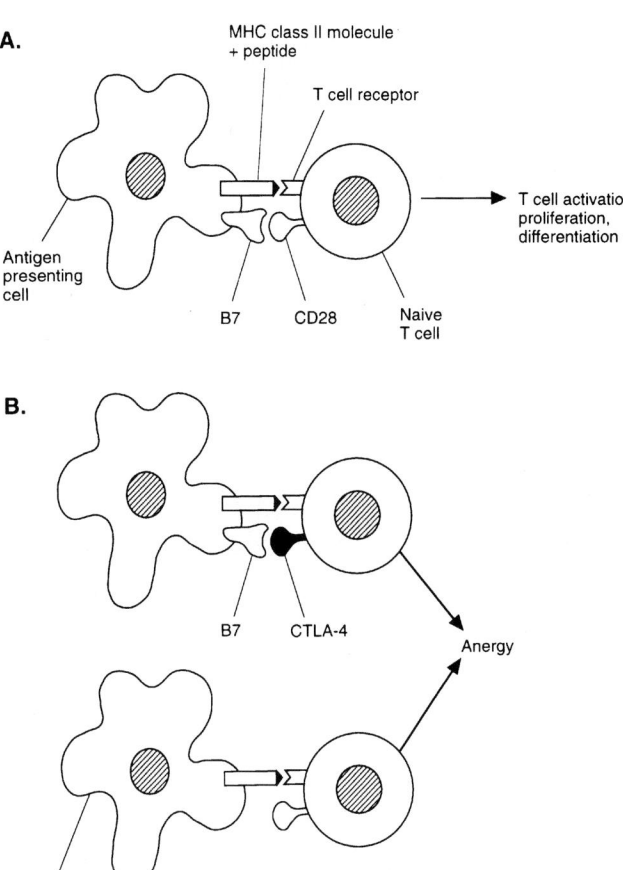

**FIGURE 195-1.** **A,** Mechanisms for anergy induction. The normal pathway for antigen presentation is shown. **B,** Failure to provide an appropriate costimulatory signal by B7 results in anergy. It should be noted that nonclassic antigen-presenting cells such as thyroid cells only express major histocompatibility complex (*MHC*) class II molecules when induced by interferon-γ under pathologic circumstances.

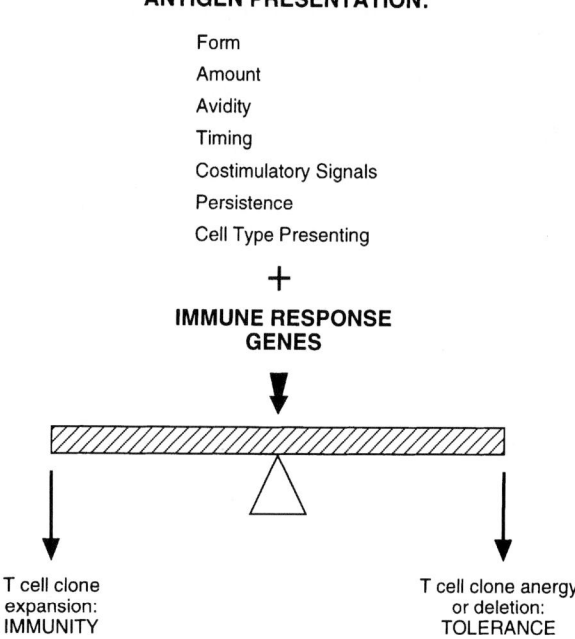

**FIGURE 195-2.** Factors in the balance between T-cell immunity and tolerance.

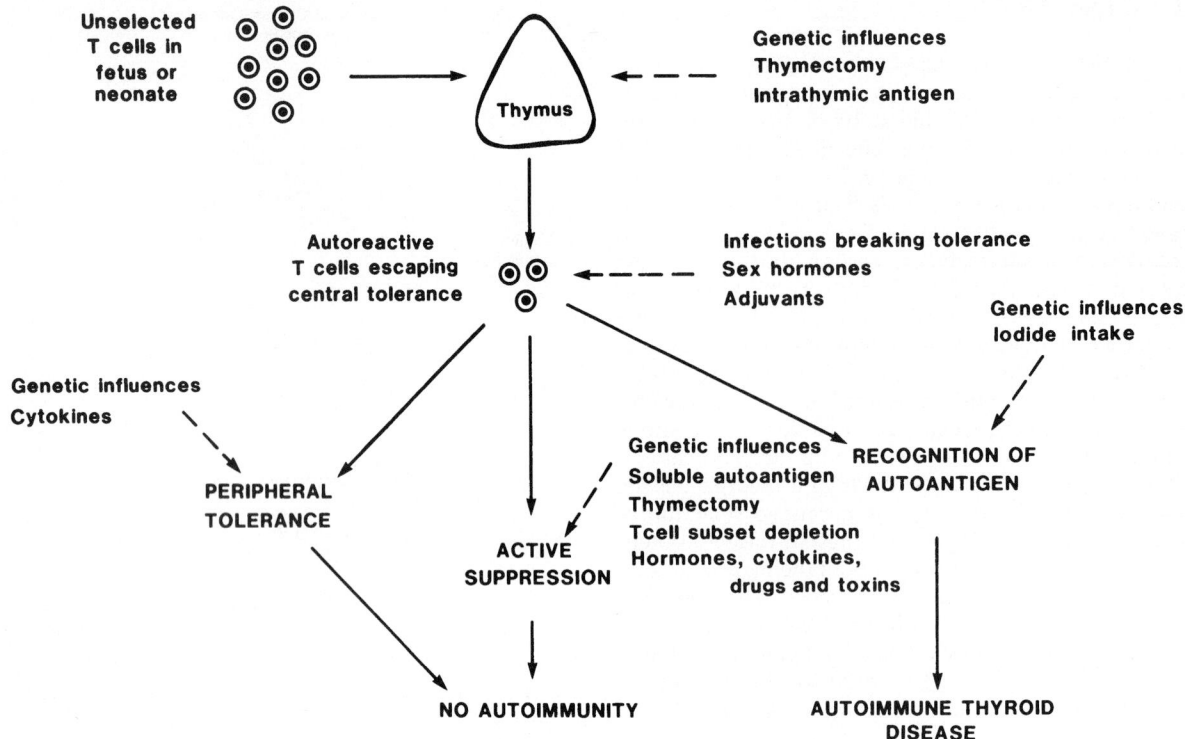

**FIGURE 195-3.** Influence of endogenous and exogenous factors on the balance of autoreactive T cells in experimental autoimmune thyroiditis. The likely sites at which manipulations of the immune system act are shown as broken lines. (From Weetman AP, McGregor AM. Autoimmune thyroid disease—further developments in our understanding. Endocr Rev 1994; 15:798.)

tic") epitopes become exposed.[8,8a] Autoreactive, cytotoxic CD8+ T cells may be less prone to deletion or anergy than CD4+ cells (because of differing antigen-presentation requirements), but remain harmless to the animal provided the autoantigen-specific CD4+ T cells are tolerized, because these are essential for helping to generate specific cytotoxic T-cell responses. Again, autoimmunity could result from a bypass of this control.

Finally, untolerized, self-reactive T cells can be actively controlled by suppressor mechanisms, for which there is strong evidence despite controversy over the mechanisms by which suppression is achieved.[9] This controversy has resulted in part from attempts to equate T-cell phenotypes with function, and from artifacts arising in vitro when testing for suppression. The effect of suppressor cells may be mediated by interaction between TCRs, by the suppressor TCR (antiidiotype) recognizing the TCR (idiotype) on a helper T cell, and by the cytokines released (see later). There also is evidence for the release of antigen-specific suppressor factors, possibly related to fragments of the TCR. As with deletion and anergy, suppression can be faulty and, thus, give rise to autoimmunity. The factors known to influence these protective mechanisms, using autoimmune thyroid disease as an example, are shown in Figure 195-3.

## T-CELL DIVERSITY

T cells can be characterized by their expression of diverse surface molecules. Of particular importance is the TCR responsible for antigen recognition. The TCR for most T cells is composed of an α and a β chain, but a minor population uses a γδ heterodimeric TCR. The role of these cells in autoimmunity is unclear, although they may be important in microbial defense. Restricted use of α

β TCRs by autoreactive T cells has been suggested in animal models such as experimental autoimmune encephalomyelitis (which parallels multiple sclerosis), in which the autoantigen is preferentially recognized by a TCR containing the Vα2 or Vα4 and Vβ8.2 sequences. Other Vα or Vβ sequences are not required for disease induction and there is homology between the encephalitogenic TCRs in mice and rats, although the MHC molecules and peptide epitopes recognized by the receptor differ. Based on these observations, new approaches to immunotherapy via the TCR are being developed.[10]

The search for similar TCR restriction in other autoimmune diseases, prompted by the potential for immunoregulatory treatment, has failed to show such clear restriction. It remains possible that TCR restriction is present during the earliest phase of disease, but T-cell recruitment then occurs as new autoantigenic epitopes are displayed ("determinant spreading"), leading to a diverse repertoire by the time the clinical condition is evident.[11] Selective inhibition of autoimmune disorders in humans by manipulating the TCR or antigenic peptide, therefore, seems unlikely at present.

The functional diversity of T cells depends on their cytokine secretion.[12] Cell-mediated and humoral immune responses are regulated by the $T_H0$, $T_H1$, and $T_H2$ subsets of CD4+ helper cells that make distinctive groups of cytokines (Table 195-2). TCR affinity and ligand density are critical factors in the selection of the CD4+ T-cell cytokine profile.[13] These subsets are particularly well defined in mice, but also can be identified in humans, although IL-2 and interleukin-10 (IL-10) secretion are features of both $T_H1$ and $T_H2$ human cells. Moreover, the $T_H1$ and $T_H2$ subpopulations are extremes, with many CD4+ cells making an intermediate array of cytokines, whereas cytotoxic CD8+ T cells secrete a more restricted cytokine profile, including interferon-γ (IFN-γ).

**TABLE 195-2.**
**Characteristics of Murine CD4+ T-Cell Subsets**

| | $T_H0$ | $T_H1$ | $T_H2$ |
|---|---|---|---|
| FUNCTION | | | |
| Delayed-type hypersensitivity | ? | ++ | – |
| B-cell help | ± | + | ++ |
| Eosinophil/mast cell production | ? | – | ++ |
| CYTOKINE RELEASE | | | |
| Interleukin-2 | + | ++ | – |
| Interleukin-3 | ++ | ++ | ++ |
| Interleukin-4 | – | – | ++ |
| Interleukin-5 | – | – | ++ |
| Interleukin-6 | – | – | ++ |
| Interleukin-10 | – | – | ++ |
| Interferon-γ | ++ | ++ | – |
| Tumor necrosis factor | ? | ++ | + |
| Lymphotoxin | ? | ++ | – |

Besides mediating their separate effector functions, the cytokines released by $T_H1$ and $T_H2$ produce reciprocal inhibition. IFN-γ antagonizes interleukin-4 (IL-4)–mediated B-cell stimulation, whereas IL-4 and IL-10 suppress the effect of IFN-γ and reduce delayed-type hypersensitivity. Such activities may be an explanation for some types of T-cell–mediated suppression and the activity of other cytokines, such as IL-2; transforming growth factor-β1 may also contribute to suppressor phenomena. Altering the balance in experimental models, by supplying exogenous cytokines or inhibiting endogenous release, can have a dramatic impact. For example, enhancing IL-4 production may be useful in suppressing harmful, $T_H1$-dependent tissue injury in some autoimmune conditions, provided the resulting stimulation of autoantibody production has no adverse sequelae.

## T-CELL EFFECTOR FUNCTIONS

As indicated earlier, cytokines are responsible for the T-cell help that is required for B cells to proliferate and differentiate into antibody-producing plasma cells. The appropriate, antigen-specific B cell is stimulated by the cognate interaction between it and the antigen-specific T cell, which is mediated by TCR recognition of MHC class II plus antigen on the B cell, and ensures the localized delivery of cytokines. B cells can take up specific antigen through surface antibodies, resulting in amplification of the immune response through this form of antigen presentation.

Cytotoxicity is produced primarily by CD8+ T cells, recognizing endogenous antigen presented by MHC class I molecules on the target cell surface. However, CD4+ cytotoxic cells do exist, although they are restricted by MHC class II molecules; these could play a role in autoimmune diseases, in which the injured tissue expresses class II molecules after local IFN-γ release. Cytotoxic T cells may use several mechanisms to kill cells: release of lymphotoxin and the membrane pore-forming protein, perforin, and interaction between FasL on the T cell and Fas on the target, leading to apoptosis in the latter.[14] Once cell killing has occurred, complement activation may follow and exacerbate injury without the need for antibodies. Finally, T cells may have indirect effects through cytokine release, including the activation of natural killer (NK) cells and macrophages, which in turn are cytotoxic, and the action of cytokines on the target cells themselves (i.e., inducing adhesion molecule and MHC class II expression) is important in enhancing tissue injury.

## T CELLS IN EXPERIMENTAL ENDOCRINE AUTOIMMUNITY

Clear evidence for the central role of T cells in autoimmune endocrine disease is provided by experiments on spontaneous and induced endocrinopathies in animals[15] (Table 195-3). Experimental autoimmune orchitis also can be induced by similar manipulation to oophoritis, but the human equivalent of this is unclear. Most information about the role of T cells has come from models of thyroiditis and type 1 diabetes mellitus, which, therefore, are considered in detail.

### EXPERIMENTAL AUTOIMMUNE THYROIDITIS

Thyroid infiltration by CD4+ and CD8+ T cells is an early feature of experimental autoimmune thyroiditis (EAT) and is independent of the production of thyroid antibodies. That autoreactive T

**TABLE 195-3.**
**Summary of the Main Animal Models of Autoimmune Endocrine Disease**

| Model | Putative Human Counterpart | Comments |
|---|---|---|
| Immunization-induced (mouse, rat, guinea pig, monkey) | Hashimoto thyroiditis<br>Addison disease<br>Autoimmune oophoritis<br>Autoimmune hypophysitis | Relies on injection of autoantigen with adjuvant: strain-dependent, transient, and transferred by T cells. |
| Thymectomy-induced (mouse, rat) | Hashimoto thyroiditis<br>Type 1 diabetes mellitus<br>Autoimmune oophoritis | May be combined with sublethal irradiation: strain-dependent and transferred by T cells. Cyclosporine A and reconstitution of T cell–depleted animals with T-cell subpopulations may induce similar diseases. |
| Spontaneous (chicken, mouse, rat) | Hashimoto thyroiditis<br>Type 1 diabetes mellitus | The Obese strain chicken develops thyroiditis, and NOD mouse and BB rat develop thyroiditis and diabetes. All are T cell–dependent. |
| Virus-induced (mouse, hamster) | Type 1 diabetes mellitus<br>Polyendocrine autoimmunity | Strain- and virus-dependent; autoimmune response may not be confined to endocrine system. |
| Transgenic mouse | Type 1 diabetes mellitus | Useful in delineating role of major histocompatibility complex (MHC) expression and cytokines in insulitis and diabetes. |
| Severe combined immunodeficiency mouse | Graves disease<br>Hashimoto thyroiditis | Immunodeficient mice allow long-term in vitro study of transplanted human tissues; animals do not develop disease. |
| Immunization with transfected fibroblasts | Graves disease | Uses fibroblasts transfected with MHC class II and thyroid-stimulating hormone receptor (TSH-R). |
| cDNA immunization | Graves disease | Allows production of TSH-R monoclonal antibodies. |

cells can escape tolerance is demonstrated clearly by the induction of EAT in genetically predisposed (good responder) mice after immunization with thyroglobulin (TG); in other strains, an adjuvant is required, in addition to TG, for EAT induction. This presumably enhances immunogenicity in a way that overcomes the more active suppression of these autoreactive T cells in poor responder strain mice. It is known that the tolerance state of the animal is dependent on the circulating TG level, with an exogenous or endogenous increase strengthening self-tolerance and protecting against EAT.[15a] This effect is mediated by CD4+ cells, which may in turn recruit CD8+ T cells to participate in active suppression of disease. The CD8+ population also is important for disease expression in this form of EAT, killing thyroid cells in vitro in a TG- and MHC-restricted fashion.[16]

A more chronic form of thyroiditis can be produced by T-cell manipulation in certain strains of mice and rats. Thymectomy, with or without irradiation or depletion of T cells by other means, induces disease in otherwise healthy animals, providing additional evidence that untolerized, self-reactive T cells exist normally, but are kept under active suppression.[15] Neonatal thymectomy may induce disease because T cells due to be depleted during early life are maintained, whereas thymectomy alone at a later stage (3 weeks old) in rats does not result in EAT because most such T cells have been tolerized. However, the addition of sublethal irradiation to the protocol may sufficiently impair the active suppression of the few remaining untolerized T cells for disease to result.

Spontaneous thyroiditis in the Obese strain chicken also depends on the presence of T cells: thymectomy prevents the disease when it is done at an early stage, but exacerbates it when it is done later, presumably because there is some, albeit imperfect, regulation of autoreactive T cells in these animals. It is important to emphasize that, although EAT often is regarded as a model for Hashimoto thyroiditis, most forms are reversible, thyroid destruction rarely is prominent, and overt hypothyroidism is not seen (except in the Obese strain chicken). This may be because the autoimmune response is directed against TG, which may more readily induce tolerance than the other key thyroid autoantigens, thyroid peroxidase (TPO) and thyroid-stimulating hormone receptor (TSH-R). Autoimmunity to these proteins has not yet been demonstrated in a homologous animal model.

### EXPERIMENTAL AUTOIMMUNE DIABETES MELLITUS

The demarcation between lymphocytic infiltration and destruction of a target organ, exemplified by EAT, also is found with experimental autoimmune diabetes mellitus, in which insulitis and diabetes may be independent. This is shown best using transgenic mice. In experiments designed to test whether MHC class II expression on endocrine cells could induce these to present self-antigen to T cells and lead to diabetes, transgenic mice were created whose B cells expressed a unique class II molecule under the influence of an insulin promotor. Such animals did not develop insulitis, and the T cells were tolerized rather than stimulated by the transgene class II molecule.[17] This is an example of peripheral tolerance, discussed earlier, in which failure to deliver a necessary costimulatory signal by the B cell has rendered the T cells anergic. Since this important finding, a wide variety of transgenic diabetes models have been developed which demonstrate the multiple checkpoints that normally exist to prevent autoimmune responses against the pancreatic B cells.[18]

Diabetes in the nonobese diabetic (NOD) mouse and BB rat, however, has close similarity to the human counterpart; both strains also develop thyroiditis. Insulitis appears ~4 weeks after birth in NOD mice, predominantly due to infiltration by CD4+ T cells, and many of these are activated, as judged by expression of IL-2 receptors.[19] Insulin-reactive T-cell clones can be isolated from NOD mice, and these show considerable restriction of Vα

but not Vβ TCR sequences.[20] However, this restriction does not appear to be the case for the T-cell response against other autoantigens involved in this model of diabetes. Of these autoantigens, 65-kDa glutamic acid decarboxylase (GAD-65) has received the most attention, and GAD-65–responsive T cells can be isolated from the spleens of young NOD mice before the emergence of other B-cell antigen responses. Furthermore, tolerance to GAD can be induced (by giving GAD intravenously, nasally, or intrathymically) in young NOD mice, and this prevents insulitis and diabetes; such tolerance may arise in part by biasing the T-cell response from a predominantly $T_H1$ destructive process to a $T_H2$ protective one.[21] Finally, a CD4+ T-cell line specific for a GAD peptide can transfer diabetes to NOD/SCID mice,[22] demonstrating directly the importance of GAD to this model, although not precluding the influence of other B-cell autoantigens.

It also is noteworthy that islet cells are class II–negative in NOD mice, and that islet cell–specific CD4+ T cells from these animals (as well as from strains that are not prone to diabetes) cannot be stimulated in vitro by islet cells alone, requiring, in addition, the presence of professional antigen-presenting cells.[17] For the response to GAD, B cells are crucial antigen-presenting cells, as B cell–deficient NOD mice fail to respond to this autoantigen.[23]

These features suggest that islet cell–reactive T cells commonly are present in diabetic and nondiabetic mice, and seem unlikely to undergo peripheral tolerance in the NOD model. Diabetes could result from infiltration of the islets by dendritic cells and macrophages, in response to a viral infection, and this reaction may be controlled by a variety of non-MHC genes, including those controlling cytokine responses. Coxsackie virus, frequently implicated in the pathogenesis of diabetes, can cause diabetes by initiating "bystander" damage; that is, local inflammation and islet cell destruction secondary to viral infection result in restimulation of resting autoreactive T cells.[24]

CD4+ T cells from diabetic NOD mice can transfer disease, but the CD4+ population in NOD mice that is not diabetic contains suppressor cells that inhibit the development of diabetes. Depending on the timing of disease, this may partly be due to the action of CTLA-4–mediated signals[25]; modulation of the balance between $T_H1$ and $T_H2$ cells is another possible explanation. The full diabetogenic capacity of CD4+ T cells requires the presence of CD8+ T cells, which depend on CD4+ inducer cells for their development. Again, timing is critical, with CD8+ T cells having adverse effects predominantly early (and possibly very late) in disease.[26] Islet cell destruction by MHC-restricted CD8+ T cells has been demonstrated in vitro; this may be mediated by perforin, Fas/FasL, and/or cytokines plus nitric oxide generation, so that cytotoxic T cell–mediated mechanisms are likely to be of major importance in this model.[26a]

Analogous findings have been made in the BB rat: CD4+ T cells infiltrate the islets early in the course of disease, diabetes can be transferred by activated T cells, and nondiabetic BB rats possess T cells that can inhibit the development of diabetes. BB rats have pronounced peripheral lymphopenia, resulting from a thymic abnormality, with reduced numbers of CD4+ cells and a virtual absence of CD8+ T cells. However, the remaining CD8+ T cells appear to be important in mediating disease, because diabetes cannot be transferred in their absence.[27]

## THE ROLE OF T CELLS IN HUMAN ENDOCRINOPATHIES

### AUTOIMMUNE HYPOTHYROIDISM

Thyroid infiltration by CD4+ and CD8+ T cells is an obvious feature of Hashimoto thyroiditis and, to a lesser extent, primary myxedema, and many of these cells are activated, as judged by the expression of class II molecules and IL-2 receptor. A broad range of cytokines is produced by the infiltrating T cells, including IL-2, IL-4, IL-6, IL-10, IFN-γ, and tumor necrosis factor (TNF), with no distinct pattern in CD4+ clones suggestive of the $T_H1$ and $T_H2$ subsets.[28] TCR V gene usage is generally unrestricted, but there is a limited restriction in the CD8+ population, the nature of which is unclear.[29]

Circulating T cells may show a reduction in the CD8+ population and an increase in activated T cells, but these features are common to many autoimmune disorders and their significance to the localized autoimmune response is unclear. However, it is this population that is readily accessible for in vitro study. Sensitization of these T cells to TG and TPO has been demonstrated in several assays; responses are generally weak, suggesting active suppression or a low frequency of untolerized antigen-specific T cells. Reliable assessment of suppressor activity in vitro is difficult, but some evidence suggests that there may be a relative defect in thyroid-specific T-suppressor cells in both autoimmune hypothyroidism and Graves disease.[30] How these exert their activities is unknown, and it remains possible that the defects seen are secondary rather than primary.

The identification of T-cell epitopes on TG and TPO has begun. In EAT, a likely major TG epitope consists of sequences flanking the hormonogenic site, and the iodine content of the thyroxine residue in this peptide influences its stimulatory capacity.[31] It is unknown whether the homologous sequence is an epitope in humans. The response of T cells to TPO is heterogeneous, with several peptides being recognized by different patients. These results are compatible with the polyclonality of the intrathyroidal T cells at the time clinical disease is apparent.

Expansion of infiltrating T cells in Hashimoto thyroiditis with IL-2 in vitro leads to nonspecific cytotoxic activity through the generation of lymphokine-activated killer cells; the role that these may play in vivo remains unknown. Cytotoxic T cells almost certainly kill thyroid cells in autoimmune hypothyroidism, via perforin, cytokines, and Fas-mediated apoptosis. The relative importance of these mechanisms is unclear. In addition, thyroid cells appear to express FasL as well as Fas in Hashimoto thyroiditis (expression being induced by cytokines); this could lead to an autocrine interaction and suicidal apoptosis, but the exact role remains to be established.[32] Thyroid follicular cells express the adhesion molecule ICAM-1 after stimulation with T-cell–derived cytokines in autoimmune thyroiditis, and this increases the ability of thyroid cells to bind cytotoxic T cells, with a subsequent increase in killing. Such cytokines also affect thyroid cell expression of MHC class I and II molecules, and membrane regulators of complement activation such as CD55 and CD59. In addition, they may impair the response of thyroid cells to TSH, thus contributing to the clinical disorder.

## GRAVES DISEASE

Although the proximal cause of Graves disease is the production of TSH-R–stimulating antibodies, it is almost certain that their production requires T-cell help.[32a] CD4+ and CD8+ T-cell infiltration is prominent in the thyroids of patients with Graves disease, although it is diminished after antithyroid drug treatment. Initial reports suggested that there was restricted TCR Vα gene usage in these organs, but this has not been confirmed by studies of TCR gene rearrangements, and even the IL-2 receptor–expressing population, believed to be activated in vitro, shows no Vα restriction when amplified TCR cDNA is examined.[33]

Convincing T-cell responses to intact TSH-R have not been demonstrated and, like TPO (to which these patients' T cells also respond), there appears to be heterogeneous recognition of TSH-R epitopes between patients.[34] Part of the difficulty in establishing T-cell lines and clones that recognize thyroid antigens in these

patients may arise from peripheral tolerance induction by the class II+ thyroid cells that appear in Graves disease and Hashimoto thyroiditis. Despite the original suggestion that this may confer antigen-presenting capacity on the thyroid cells, the T-cell responses seen are generally weak and could be the result of contaminating professional antigen-presenting cells. Moreover, thyroid cells do not express the costimulator B7, which appears to be essential in stimulating some CD4+ T cells, and can induce tolerance in certain T cells (representing a naive phenotype) in vitro.[7]

During the early phase of Graves disease, destructive mechanisms are usually absent, although several years after successful treatment with antithyroid drugs, hypothyroidism may supervene.

## THYROID-ASSOCIATED OPHTHALMOPATHY

Extraocular muscles are infiltrated by activated T cells in thyroid-associated ophthalmopathy (Fig. 195-4), and these release cytokines such as IFN-γ and TNF, which can stimulate glycosaminoglycan synthesis by the fibroblasts.[35] This in turn leads to edema, and the muscle swelling produces the clinical features of the disorder. Muscle cell destruction is not a prominent pathologic component; therefore, cytotoxic T cells do not appear to be involved. Orbital fibroblasts are recognized by T cells, making them a likely target of the autoimmune response.[36] Inconsistent eye muscle antibody responses are observed in patients with thyroid-associated ophthalmopathy, suggesting that this disease may be amenable to treatment by manipulating cytokines so that a $T_H2$-type response is promoted, but the absence of an animal model makes this difficult to assess. The autoantigen recognized by the infiltrating T cells probably is cross-reactive with a thyroid antigen, explaining the close association between thyroid and eye disease. Its identity is unknown; one possible candidate is the TSH-R or a fragment of it.

## TYPE 1 DIABETES MELLITUS

Insulitis is found in most patients with type 1 diabetes mellitus, and in rare cases in which characterization has been possible, these are a mixture of CD4+ and CD8+ T cells, together with NK and B cells.[37] As in autoimmune thyroid disease, activated T cells are increased in the circulation at the time of diagnosis, and recent progress has been made in identifying their reactivities. T-cell proliferation in response to fetal pig proislets can be

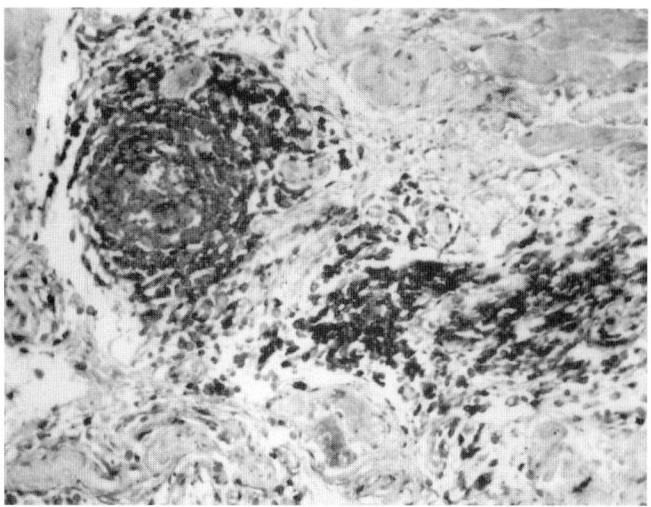

**FIGURE 195-4.** Lymphocytic infiltrate in the extraocular muscle in thyroid-associated ophthalmopathy. The section has been stained with the monoclonal antibody UCHL1 against CD45R0, showing that most lymphocytes are activated and memory T cells. (Original magnification ×400)

**TABLE 195-4.**
**Evidence for T-Cell Involvement in Autoimmune Endocrinopathies**

| Condition | T-Cell Infiltration of Target Organ | Functional Studies | Comments |
|---|---|---|---|
| Addison disease | Lymphocytic infiltration, but not well characterized | Circulating T cells stimulated by adrenal autoantigens | Activated T cells increased in circulation |
| Autoimmune oophoritis | Predominantly CD4+ T cells | Few reports with equivocal results | Activated T cells increased in circulation |
| Lymphocytic hypophysitis | CD4+ and CD8+ T cells | Not done | T-cell infiltration of infundibulum and posterior pituitary has been described in some cases of diabetes insipidus |
| Polyendocrine autoimmunity syndrome type I | Parathyroids not assessed | Not done with autoantigens | Generalized defects in T-cell function have been demonstrated, possibly responsible for candidiasis |

detected in ~70% of persons with preclinical diabetes (first-degree relatives of patients with diabetes who have islet cell antibodies), as well as in patients with overt diabetes.[38] Most attention has focused on GAD, which is a major target for autoantibodies in diabetes. This exists in 65- and 67-kDa forms, encoded by two separate genes, and T-cell reactivity to both has been detected in patients with preclinical and overt diabetes.[39,40] Two naturally processed epitopes of GAD have been identified that bind to human leukocyte antigen (HLA)-DRB1*0401, a susceptibility allele for diabetes.[38] This could lead to novel immunotherapy with modified peptides. Of considerable interest, persons with preclinical diabetes can be grouped into those with strong T-cell reactivity to GAD and those with high GAD antibody levels; few patients display both responses.[41] This suggests a dichotomy based on $T_H1$ and $T_H2$ responses that may be of prognostic and therapeutic importance. Furthermore, it has been shown that a bias toward a $T_H1$ T-cell response predisposes genetically at-risk individuals to develop diabetes, whereas an ongoing $T_H2$ response is protective.[42] However, this dichotomy is not universally accepted, and more work is required.[43]

The mechanisms involved in pancreatic B-cell destruction are unknown. The cytokines interleukin-1 (IL-1), IL-6, TNF, and IFN-$\gamma$ all have effects on B cells in vitro, ranging from ultrastructural changes to cell killing, and the specificity of these cytokines for the B cells within an islet could result from localized release and innate or acquired heightened sensitivity to their action. ICAM-1 expression is induced by IFN-$\gamma$ and TNF on all islet cells, which could increase B-cell killing by specific cytotoxic T cells. Fas/FasL-mediated apoptosis is also believed to play an important role in destruction.[4] Class II expression is induced on all islet cells by IFN-$\gamma$ and TNF, but the ability of human B cells to present antigen (in either a stimulating or a tolerizing form) is unclear.

## OTHER ENDOCRINOPATHIES

Evidence for the involvement of T cells in other autoimmune endocrine diseases is summarized in Table 195-4. These conditions have not received the same attention as thyroid disease and diabetes, but the clinical association between the various autoimmune endocrinopathies suggests a similar pathogenesis, and T cells are likely to play a central role in these disorders.

## REFERENCES

1. Mondino A, Khoruts A, Jenkins MK. The anatomy of T-cell activation and tolerance. Proc Natl Acad Sci U S A 1996; 93:2245.
1a. Romagnani S. T cell subsets (Th1 versus Th2). Ann Allergy Asthma Immunol 2000; 85:9.
2. Van Parijs L, Abbas AK. Homeostasis and self-tolerance in the immune system: turning lymphocytes off. Science 1998; 280:243.
3. Banchereau J, Steinman RM. Dendritic cells and the control of immunity. Nature 1998; 392:245.
4. Sakata K, Sakata A, Kong L, et al. Role of Fas/FasL interaction in physiology and pathology: the good and the bad. Clin Immunol Immunopathol 1998; 87:1.
5. Schwartz RH. Models of T cell anergy: is there a common molecular mechanism? J Exp Med 1996; 184:1.
6. Reiser H, Stadecker MJ. Costimulatory B7 molecules in the pathogenesis of infectious and autoimmune diseases. N Engl J Med 1996; 335:1369.
7. Marelli-Berg FM, Weetman AP, Frasca L, et al. Antigen presentation by epithelial cells induces anergic immunoregulatory CD45R0+ T cells and deletion of CD45RA+ T cells. J Immunol 1997; 159:5853.
8. Barnaba V, Sinigaglia F. Molecular mimicry and T cell-mediated autoimmune disease. J Exp Med 1997; 185:1529.
8a. Drakesmith H, Chain B, Beverley P. How can dendritic cells cause autoimmune disease? Immunol Today 2000; 21:214.
9. Bloom BR, Salgame P, Diamond B. Revisiting and revising suppressor T cells. Immunol Today 1992; 12:131.
10. Vandenbark AA, Chou YK, Whitham R, et al. Treatment of multiple sclerosis and T-cell receptor peptides: results of a double-blind pilot trial. Nature Med 1996; 2:1109.
11. Lehmann PV, Sercarz EE, Forsthuber T, et al. Determinant spreading and the dynamics of the autoimmune T-cell repertoire. Immunol Today 1993; 14:203.
12. Mosmann TR, Sad S. The expanding universe of T-cell subsets: Th1, Th2 and more. Immunol Today 1996; 17:138.
13. Murray JS. How the MHC selects Th1/Th2 immunity. Immunol Today 1998; 19:157.
14. Epstein FH. Lymphocyte-mediated cytolysis and disease. N Engl J Med 1996; 335:1651.
15. Weetman AP, McGregor AM. Autoimmune thyroid disease—further developments in our understanding. Endocr Rev 1994; 15:788.
15a. Seddon B, Mason D. Peripheral autoantigen induces regulatory T cells that prevent autoimmunity. J Exp Med 1999; 189:877.
16. Wan Q, McCormick DJ, David CS, et al. Thyroglobulin peptides of specific primary hormonogenic sites can generate cytotoxic T cells and serve as target autoantigens in experimental autoimmune thyroiditis. Clin Immunol Immunopathol 1998; 86:110.
17. Lo D, Burkly LC, Widera G, et al. Diabetes and tolerance in transgenic mice expressing class II MHC molecules in pancreatic beta cells. Cell 1988; 53:159.
18. André I, Gonzalez A, Wang B, et al. Checkpoints in the progression of autoimmune disease: lessons from diabetes models. Proc Natl Acad Sci U S A 1996; 93:2260.
19. Signore A, Pozzilli P, Gale EAM, et al. The natural history of lymphocyte subsets infiltrating the pancreas of NOD mice. Diabetologia 1989; 32:282.
20. Simone E, Daniel D, Schloot N, et al. T cell receptor restriction of diabetogenic autoimmune NOD T cells. Proc Natl Acad Sci U S A 1997; 94:2518.
21. Tian J, Clare-Salzler M, Herschenfeld A, et al. Modulating autoimmune responses to GAD inhibits disease progression and prolongs islet graft survival in diabetes-prone mice. Nature Med 1996; 2:1348.
22. Zekzer D, Wong FS, Ayalon O, et al. GAD-reactive CD4+ Th1 cells induce diabetes in NOD/SCID mice. J Clin Invest 1998; 101:68.
23. Falcone M, Lee J, Patstone G, et al. Lymphocytes are crucial antigen-presenting cells in the pathogenic autoimmune response to GAD65 antigen in non-obese diabetic mice. J Immunol 1998; 161:1163.
24. Horwitz MS, Bradley LM, Harbertson J, et al. Diabetes induced by Coxsackie virus: initiation by bystander damage and not molecular mimicry. Nature Med 1998; 4:781.
25. Lühder F, Höglund P, Allison JP, et al. Cytotoxic T lymphocyte-associated antigen 4 (CTLA-4) regulates the unfolding of autoimmune diabetes. J Exp Med 1998; 187:427.
26. Wang B, Gonzalez A, Genoist C, et al. The role of CD8+ T cells in the initiation of insulin-dependent diabetes mellitus. Eur J Immunol 1996; 26:1762.
26a. Graser RT, DiLorenzo TP, Wang F, et al. Identification of a CD8 T cell that can independently mediate autoimmune diabetes development in the complete absence of CD4 T cell helper functions. J Immunol 2000; 164:3913.
27. Edouard P, Hiserodt JC, Plamondon C, Poussier P. CD8+ T-cells are required for adoptive transfer of the BB rat diabetic syndrome. Diabetes 1993; 42:390.
28. Ajjan RA, Watson PF, McIntosh RS, et al. Intrathyroidal cytokine gene expression in Hashimoto's thyroiditis. Clin Exp Immunol 1996; 105:523.
29. McIntosh RS, Watson PF, Weetman AP. Analysis of the T cell receptor V$\alpha$ repertoire in Hashimoto's thyroiditis: evidence for the restricted accumulation of CD8+ T cells in the absence of CD4+ T cell restriction. J Clin Endocrinol Metab 1997; 82:1140.
30. Volpé R. Suppressor T lymphocyte dysfunction is important in the pathogenesis of autoimmune thyroid disease: a perspective. Thyroid 1993; 3:345.
31. Carayanniotis G, Rao VP. Searching for pathogenic epitopes in thyroglobulin: parameters and caveats. Immunol Today 1997; 18:83.

32. Arscott PL, Baker JR Jr. Apoptosis and thyroiditis. Clin Immunol Immunopathol 1998; 87:207.

32a. Sekine T, Kato R, Kato T, et al. Accumulation of identical T cell clones in the right and left lobes of the thyroid gland in patients with Graves' disease: analysis of T cell clonotype in vivo. Endocr J 2000; 47:127.

33. McIntosh R, Tandon N, Pickerill AP, et al. IL-2 receptor-positive intrathyroidal lymphocytes in Graves' disease: analysis of Vα transcript microheterogeneity. J Immunol 1993; 151:3884.

34. Fisfalen ME, Palmer EM, Van Seventer GA, et al. Thyroglobulin-receptor and thyroid peroxidase-specific T cell clones and their cytokine profile in autoimmune thyroid disease. J Clin Endocrinol Metab 1997; 82:3655.

35. Heufelder AE. Involvement of the orbital fibroblast and TSH receptor in the pathogenesis of Graves' ophthalmopathy. Thyroid 1995; 5:331.

36. Grubeck-Loebenstein B, Trieb K, Sztankay A, et al. Retrobulbar T cells from patients with Graves' ophthalmopathy are CD8+ and specifically recognize autologous fibroblasts. J Clin Invest 1994; 93:2738.

37. Foulis AK, Liddle CN, Farquharson MA, et al. The histopathology of the pancreas in type I (insulin-dependent) diabetes mellitus: a 25 year review of deaths in patients under 20 years of age in the United Kingdom. Diabetologia 1986; 29:267.

38. Harrison LC, Chu XC, DeAizpurua HJ, et al. Islet-reactive T cells are a marker of preclinical insulin-diabetes. J Clin Invest 1992; 89:1161.

39. Atkinson MA, Kaufman DL, Campbell L, et al. Response of peripheral-blood mononuclear cells to glutamate decarboxylase in insulin-dependent diabetes. Lancet 1992; 339:458.

40. Wicker LS, Chen S-L, Nepom GT, et al. Naturally processed T cell epitopes from human glutamic acid decarboxylase identified using mice transgenic for the type 1 diabetes-associated human MHC class II allele, DRB1*0401. J Clin Invest 1996; 98:2597.

41. Harrison LC, Honeyman MC, DeAizpurua HJ, et al. Inverse relation between humoral and cellular immunity to glutamic acid decarboxylase in subjects at risk of insulin-dependent diabetes. Lancet 1993; 341:1365.

42. Wilson SB, Kent SC, Patton KT, et al. Extreme Th1 bias of invariant Vα24JαQT cells in type 1 diabetes. Nature 1998; 391:177.

43. Almawi WY, Tamim H, Azar ST. T helper type 1 and 2 cytokines mediate the onset and progression of type 1 (insulin-dependent) diabetes. J Clin Endocrinol Metab 1999; 84:1497.

# CHAPTER 196

# B CELLS AND AUTOANTIBODIES IN ENDOCRINE DISEASE

ALAN M. MCGREGOR

The normal immune response involves the trapping, processing, presentation, and recognition of foreign antigen by accessory cells and T and B lymphocytes, and the subsequent generation of an immune response directed against the antigen that, in the case of B cells, is a humoral response, with the generation of antibodies directed against determinants on the target antigen (Table 196-1). These processes occur primarily within lymphoid tissue in which well-organized distributions of these cells ensure the ability to generate an appropriate immune response. Additionally, the cells involved in the immune response migrate not only through the lymphoid tissues but also throughout the body. This recirculation of lymphoid cells ensures that there is enhanced uptake and presentation of antigen to the appropriate sets of antigen-specific cells, and disseminates the immune response throughout the body.

## B-CELL DEVELOPMENT AND LOCALIZATION

In the embryo, B-lymphocyte generation occurs predominantly in sites of general hematopoiesis,[1] with the liver—an early site—followed in the later embryo and the adult by the bone marrow. The initial production of B cells from stem cells in these primary lymphoid organs occurs independently of antigen stimulation, unlike the process in secondary lymphoid organs.[2] The secondary lymphoid organs, which include the spleen, lymph nodes, and mucosal lymphoid tissues, are the major sites of the immune response in which lymphocyte activation and proliferation occur in response to exposure to foreign antigen. In contrast to T cells that undergo early thymic selection with the removal of newly formed T cells, which have specificity for self-antigens,[3] the selection of B cells with receptors, which have a high affinity for foreign antigen, takes place later during the immune response and involves the somatic mutation of immunoglobulin genes.[4]

Detailed organization of the tissues of the secondary lymphoid organs is critical for the initiation and regulation of antigen-driven proliferation and differentiation of lymphocytes, and for ensuring both easy access of the cells of the immune system to foreign antigen and the free movement of lymphocytes both within these lymphoid tissues and between them and the periphery. A number of key regions in these tissues are identified. A peripheral T-cell zone contains interdigitating (dendritic, accessory) cells and B cells, both of which express human leukocyte antigen (HLA) class II molecules and have the ability to internalize, process, and present peptides derived from foreign antigens in conjunction with major histocompatibility complex (MHC) class II molecules on their cell surfaces to the T cells in this zone. The B cell–rich follicles have a core consisting of a dense network of follicular dendritic cells that have the capacity to take up antigen and retain it for prolonged periods of time. B cells proliferate in these follicles and in doing so form germinal centers, which are the main sites for the affinity maturation of the antibody response.[5] Marginal zone B-cell areas are recognized as containing B cells, which, unlike the B cells in the germinal centers of follicles, are memory, and virgin B cells, which are larger, do not recirculate, and express little surface IgD immunoglobulin. The role of these B cells (which have a life span of 4–6 weeks if they are not activated by antigen) is to transport antigen, to ensure a rapid antibody response on sec-

**TABLE 196-1.**
**Characteristics of Human Immunoglobulins**

|  | IgG | IgA | IgM | IgD | IgE |
|---|---|---|---|---|---|
| Usual molecular form | Monomer | Mono/dimer | Pentamer | Monomer | Monomer |
| Subclasses | + | + | − | − | − |
| Molecular weight | 150,000 | 160–385,000 | 950,000 | 175,000 | 190,000 |
| Carbohydrate content (%) | 3 | 7 | 10 | 9 | 13 |
| Adult serum level (mg/dL) | 1250 ± 300 | 210 ± 50 | 125 ± 50 | 4 | 0.3 |
| Percentage of total serum Ig | 75–85 | 7–15 | 5–10 | 0.05 | 0.003 |
| Half-life (d) | 23 | 5.8 | 5.1 | 2.8 | 2.5 |

ondary exposure to antigen, and to respond directly to polysaccharide antigens. Although secondary lymphoid organs are significant sites of antibody production, this process tends to occur in regions away from the sites at which B cells are first activated by antigen. Immunocompetent T cells play a crucial role in the process of B-cell maturation in these secondary lymphoid tissues, with interaction between cell-surface receptors of T and B cells and cytokines providing important signals in the maturation process.

## B-LYMPHOCYTE DIFFERENTIATION

B-lymphocyte differentiation[5] can be divided into an antigen-independent stage, in which B lymphocytes are produced from stem cells in the bone marrow, and an antigen-driven proliferation and differentiation to both antibody-secreting plasma cells and memory B cells.[6] The earliest cell unequivocally committed to becoming a B lymphocyte is the pre-B lymphocyte, which expresses cytoplasmic μ immunoglobulin heavy (H) chains. Maturation of these pre-B cells leads to the expression of cytoplasmic light (L) chains and, thereafter, of membrane immunoglobulin. This is initially of the IgM class but is followed shortly by IgD expression, with these two membrane immunoglobulin classes sharing the same L-chain and H-chain variable regions so that they have the same specificity for antigen. These newly formed IgM+, IgD+ small B lymphocytes are the major B-cell population, and at this point in their life are mature and antigen responsive and also express on their cell surfaces a number of other molecules, including MHC class II determinants. The membrane immunoglobulins of the primary small B lymphocyte act as antigen receptors, thus allowing antigen to select the B cells committed to making immunoglobulin directed against the antigen.[7] From limiting dilution experiments, the frequency of antigen-responsive B cells is ~$10^{-4}$.

The process of lymphocyte activation, in which the small B lymphocytes proliferate and differentiate into antibody-secreting cells in response to antigen, occurs through a number of mechanisms.[8] For some antigens the process is T-cell independent and these responses typically lack memory and show only limited switching from IgM to other immunoglobulin classes. The optimum antibody response to protein antigens requires the participation of helper T lymphocytes, which must also be antigen specific. In this setting, T cells induce B-cell activation after T-cell recognition of antigen on the B-cell surface. For this process to be effective, however, primary helper T cells must first be primed; this process relies on the presentation of antigen by interdigitating dendritic cells to a primary helper T cell, with activation of the latter then allowing it to provide T-cell help for the generation of a B-cell antibody response. After B-cell activation, there is a decline in membrane immunoglobulin expression but a marked increase in MHC class I and class II molecule expression. Additionally, a number of activation antigens and the interleukin-2 receptor appear on the cell surface. In response to the primary encounter with antigen, recruited B cells may proliferate and differentiate into antibody-secreting cells or into small, longer life span memory cells. IgM+, IgD+ B cells make up >90% of the peripheral recirculating pool and are considered naive B cells. These cells can be differentiated from memory cells by the failure to demonstrate in them the characteristics of memory B cells, that is, clonal expansion and somatic mutation.[9] Unlike naive cells, memory B cells are IgG+, IgA+, or IgE+ cells. As part of the process of clonal expansion, differentiation, and immunoglobulin class switching that occurs after activation of B cells, the pathway along which the resulting centrocytes travel depends on the signals delivered, with signaling by CD40

directing these cells along the pathway of small, resting memory B cells; however, signaling by either interleukin-2 or soluble CD23 plus interleukin-1α results in the generation of plasmablasts and mature antibody-secreting plasma cells.[6] The increase in antibody affinity during the course of a response depends first on the selection of high-affinity H- and L-chain variable region combinations and second on the process of somatic hypermutation of V genes. Protein antigens, which require T-cell help to make optimal antibody responses, require contact-dependent helper signals from T cells to B cells, and lymphokines secreted by T cells, which are involved in B-cell maturation.[10] Interleukin-4 has a role in activating resting B cells, whereas interleukin-1 and -5 function to induce or maintain proliferation of activated B cells and interleukin-6 is involved in the late differentiation events that lead to the process of high-rate immunoglobulin secretion.

### CD5+ B CELLS

Conventional CD5− (B2) cells produce monoreactive, high-affinity, specific antibodies, primarily of the IgG class, in response to an antigen. This contrasts with the polyreactivity of natural antibodies that are predominantly of the IgM class of immunoglobulin. These antibodies occur independently of any known specific immunization, are of low affinity, are often directed against a variety of self-antigens, and are synthesized by CD5+ (B1) cells.[11] Whether these two cell populations share a common lineage remains controversial. Although the assumption has always been that most natural polyreactive antibodies generated by CD5+ cells do not arise from an antigen-driven process in which somatic mutations in V genes occur, evidence suggests that this may not be the case and that some polyreactive antibodies are, indeed, encoded in somatically mutated V genes. The assumption that natural polyreactive antibodies directed against self-determinants were unlikely to have any relevance to autoimmune disease processes is, likewise, being questioned with the demonstration that CD5+ B cells may, indeed, be capable of generating somatically mutated high-affinity autoantibodies similar to those detected in autoimmune states.

## IMMUNOGLOBULINS

Immunoglobulins are proteins that express antibody activity and represent the humoral arm of the immune response (Table 196-2; see Table 196-1). The humoral immune response has the capacity to recognize up to $10^7$ different antigenic molecules. To achieve this, enormous structural heterogeneity is required. A second important function of antibody molecules is the induction of a variety of effector functions, including activation of the complement cascade, macrophage phagocytosis, and extracellular killing mechanisms. Through these mechanisms, foreign antigens recognized by antibodies, and to which the antibodies

**TABLE 196-2.**
**Human Immunoglobulin G Subclass Characteristics**

|  | IgG$_1$ | IgG$_2$ | IgG$_3$ | IgG$_4$ |
|---|---|---|---|---|
| Secondary antibody response | + | + | + | + |
| Serum concentration (% of total IgG) | 60–65 | 20–25 | 5–10 | 3–6 |
| Complement fixation | ++ | + | +++ | − |
| Placental transport | + | + | + | + |
| Fc-receptor binding | +++ | − | +++ | ++ |
| Antibody response to polysaccharides | ++ | +++ | + | + |

are bound, are eliminated. Immunoglobulin structures are based on a four-chain subunit with two H chains and two L chains. Each chain has a variable part that is responsible for antibody diversity and a constant part that is responsible for the various effector functions. Interchain disulfide bonds link the chains and intrachain disulfide bonds provide internal stability. Based on structural differences in the constant parts of the H chains, the immunoglobulins can be divided into five classes (IgG, IgM, IgA, IgD, and IgE), four IgG subclasses (IgG$_1$, IgG$_2$, IgG$_3$, and IgG$_4$; see Table 196-2), and two IgA subclasses (IgA$_1$ and IgA$_2$). There are two types of L chains ($\kappa$ and $\lambda$) and all immunoglobulin molecules are of either the $\kappa$ or $\lambda$ type. The immunoglobulins are glycoproteins, with up to 10% of their content being carbohydrate. Some of the immunoglobulin molecules, particularly secretory IgA and IgM, have the ability to form high-molecular-weight polymers of the monomeric four-chain unit structure. Because any given plasma cell can only synthesize and express one type of H chain and one type of L chain, antibodies that are produced by an expanding clone of cells will consist of exactly the same H and L chains. Immunoglobulins make up ~20% of the total plasma proteins, with IgG being present at the highest concentration in serum at ~10 to 12 mg/mL. Enzyme digestion of immunoglobulin molecules creates well-defined and functionally active fragments. At physiologic pH, papain splits the IgG molecule into two identical Fab fragments—which are regions of the molecule involved in antigen binding—and a third fragment, the so-called Fc (crystallizable) fragment, which does not bind antigen but expresses many of the bioeffector properties of the IgG molecule previously described.

The constant (C) regions are generated from genes that encode for nine immunoglobulin H-chain classes and subclasses, and one $\kappa$ and four $\lambda$ L chains. The V-region polypeptide of the H chain is encoded for by three gene segments (V, D, J), and in the case of L chains, by only V and J gene segments.[12] Amino-acid variation occurs throughout the V gene but particularly in the hypervariable regions or complementarity-determining regions (CDRs). These are the parts of the molecule that are directly involved in antigen binding. Three CDRs from a single H chain and one CDR from an L chain come together to form a pocket into which the antigenic determinant fits. The remaining amino acids of the variable region are called the *framework region*, which constitutes ~75% of the total V region. These framework regions ensure the stability of the CDRs. There are six variable human H-chain gene families, seven variable V$\lambda$ L-chain families, and six variable V$\kappa$ L-chain families. Within each family, the number of genes varies considerably. A given variable gene (V, D, or J) can be associated with any of the H-chain C-region genes. Similarly, the constant $\kappa$ gene can use all of the different variable $\kappa$ genes, and the constant $\lambda$ gene can use all of the different variable $\lambda$-chain genes. The genes encoding the three different V regions (VH, V$\kappa$, and V$\lambda$) have different chromosomal locations (Table 196-3). The ability of H-chain C genes to use any V-D-J gene segments is crucial to the normal functioning of the humoral immune response in permitting H-chain V regions to be switched directly from one type of H chain to another, thus allowing maturation of the immune response, somatic mutation, and the selection of antibodies with the highest-affinity constants.

**TABLE 196-3.**
**Human Immunoglobulin Gene Chromosome Localization**

| Gene | Chromosome |
|---|---|
| Heavy chain | 14q32.3 |
| $\kappa$ Light chain | 2p12 |
| $\lambda$ Light chain | 22q11 |

## IMMUNOGLOBULIN GENE VARIABILITY

To recognize a huge variety of antigenic determinants, variability is required in the parts of the immunoglobulin molecule that both recognize and bind to antigen.[8] A number of mechanisms exist that allow the achievement of this goal. Gene rearrangement, in which chromosomal DNA is rearranged, takes place in the generation of mature immunoglobulin genes.[13] The two forms of gene rearrangement recognized are (a) V-D-J joining,[14] which is common to all immunoglobulin genes, and (b) immunoglobulin H-class switching, which is restricted to the immunoglobulin H-chain genes. The recombination activating genes (RAG-1 and RAG-2) activate the V-D-J recombinase that mediates V-D, D-J, and V-J joining. In the case of the immunoglobulin H-class switch, there is a switch from the expression of V$_H$DJ$_H$ joined to the C$\mu$ constant region to join with one of the other C$_H$ genes. This switch recombination process results in gene deletion of all the DNA between the recombining sequences. In addition to the variability afforded by inherited germline V$_H$ genes, as previously described, there is the potential for diversity, with the V-region repertoire being enhanced by somatic processes. Undoubtedly, there is an ability for somatic mutation to occur within V segments; this occurs particularly within the CDRs.[15]

## SELF-TOLERANCE AND ITS BREAKDOWN

Crucial to the normal immune response is the ability to discriminate between self- and non–self-determinants to prevent the possibility of immunologic attack on self and the development of autoimmune disease.[16] In the process of discriminating self from non-self, self-recognition is crucial for the induction of tolerance to autoantigens. Failure of appropriate self-recognition and, thus, the failure to delete self-reactive cells, both centrally (thymus, bone marrow) and in the periphery, during the ontogeny of the immune response result in autoimmune disease. Tolerance of lymphocytes results either from their deletion or the induction in them of a state of unresponsiveness (anergy). In the specific case of B-cell tolerance, B cells specific for membrane-bound antigen, which are present at high concentrations in the bone marrow or in the periphery, are clonally deleted.[17] Additionally, either in the bone marrow or in the periphery, B cells may be rendered anergic in response to soluble monovalent antigens. The absence of T-cell help also may induce a similar blockade in immunoglobulin secretion. Data from animal models suggest that an intrinsic defect in B cells in the absence of T cells may lead to the development of autoimmune disease. No data are available to determine whether differences exist between CD5$^+$ and CD5$^-$ cells in terms of their susceptibility to tolerance or autoreactivity. In the development of autoimmune disease, failure to delete or render autoreactive cells anergic is likely to be a major contributor to the process. Considerable evidence has accumulated to establish the existence of regulatory T cells that can down-regulate immune responses to self-antigens.[18] These CD4$^+$ regulatory T cells seem to require the cytokines transforming growth factor-$\beta$ (TGF-$\beta$) and interleukin-10 (IL-10) for the induction of immune suppression. Impairment of this function may be an important contributor to the induction of autoimmunity.

## AUTOIMMUNE DISEASE

Diseases that are autoimmune in origin are likely to be multifactorial in their etiology, with a number of genetic, constitutional, and environmental factors contributing to their development.

These diseases are loosely classified into organ-specific and non–organ-specific diseases, with the autoimmune endocrine diseases being entirely within the class of organ-specific diseases. The organ-specific autoimmune endocrine diseases may occur in isolation in individuals or may present alone or in combination in the affected individual, in the patient's family, or both. A number of criteria have been used to establish a disease as being autoimmune in origin; among these the demonstration of autoantibodies directed against target organ autoantigenic determinants in an endocrine gland is seen as being crucially important. The relatively easier ability to detect autoantibody activity, as opposed to cell-mediated autoreactivity, has, for too long, led to an uncritical assumption that the detection of antibodies is a likely reflection of a pathogenic role. With the recognition of the crucial role of cell-mediated destructive mechanisms in the autoimmune process and the characterization of the spectrum of autoantibody activities ranging from polyclonal low-affinity natural autoantibodies to highly specific, high-affinity monoclonal autoantibodies, there is clearly a need for careful reevaluation of the role of autoantibodies in the pathogenesis of the organ-specific autoimmune endocrine diseases.

The development of the $T_H1/T_H2$ paradigm for the cytokine secretion and function of CD4+ T cells is providing new insights into the underlying mechanisms leading to autoimmunity. Characterization of polymorphisms of genes for cytokines and their receptors is facilitating the identification of susceptibility loci for autoimmunity. The ability of environmental agents (infectious organisms) to alter cytokine profiles and induce autoimmunity is well recognized. With respect to the generation of an autoimmune response, it is likely that the pathogenic effector mechanism of autoantibody-mediated autoimmunity is related to a $T_H2$ response.

## AUTOANTIBODIES

While autoantibodies characterize many autoimmune diseases, their contribution to the pathogenic process has remained controversial; as markers both of likely disease development and of established disease as well as of disease severity, their role is not in doubt. However, as agents capable of causing disease, there is definite evidence in only very few autoimmune diseases. B cells that make pathologic autoantibodies should have been previously deleted or tolerized. Autoantibodies that are pathogenic are likely to have undergone isotype switching to IgG with the IgG subclass, which is controlled by CD4+ T-cell–secreted cytokines, determining the role of the autoantibody. Somatic mutation and secondary rearrangement (*receptor editing*) of V genes influence the antibody specificity for the determinants on the autoantigen against which it is directed. It is likely, therefore, that triggering antigenic epitopes recognized by antibodies will differ from the epitopes recognized once the disease is established.

To establish that an autoantibody has a pathogenetic role in a disease process, a number of criteria need to be met.[19,20] The autoantibody level in the circulation should correlate with the disease activity, the antigen against which it is directed should be characterized, and the antigen should be identifiable in the target organ, against which the antibody is assumed to be directed. Transfer of the antibody across the placenta with induction of autoimmune disease in the offspring of affected mothers, with the disease being transient and lasting as long as the antibodies are present in the neonatal circulation, is extremely strong evidence of the likely pathogenetic role of antibody. The improvement of disease by removal of autoantibody is again an important criterion of the likely pathogenetic role of the antibody. Additionally, evidence should accrue of the mechanism by which the antibody causes autoimmune damage, and

this should be demonstrable in the target organ. Where autoantigen is available, immunization in an animal model should induce antibodies similar to the human autoantibody, and lesions in the experimental animals induced by the autoantibody should be similar to those in the human setting. The location of likely target autoantigens is critically important in influencing the likely pathogenetic role of autoantibodies directed against these antigens. Where autoantibodies are directed against cell-surface targets, such as hormone receptors, little doubt exists regarding their pathogenetic role. If an autoantibody directed against an intracellular target is to be pathogenetic, then evidence must clearly show that the target autoantigen is released from the cell or exposed on the cell surface so that access to autoantibody occurs.[21]

## GRAVES DISEASE

The assumption, for many years, that Graves disease was due to autoantibodies that bind to the thyrotropin (thyroid-stimulating hormone; TSH) receptor on human thyroid follicular cells and that, through their interaction with the receptor, they stimulate thyroid hyperfunction by means of the adenylate cyclase system, has been proved beyond doubt with the successful cloning of the human TSH receptor[22] (see Chaps. 15, 42, and 197). Studies with the recombinant human receptor, expressed in Chinese hamster ovary cells, have demonstrated clear evidence of binding of antibodies from patients with Graves disease to the receptor and subsequent activation of the adenylate cyclase system in the Chinese hamster ovary cells. That these TSH-receptor antibodies cause Graves disease is not in doubt.[23] With the development of sensitive and specific assay systems for the measurement of TSH-receptor antibody activity, it is clear that these antibodies are specific for Graves disease and that the antibody level correlates with disease activity, with high levels of antibody being recorded during the phase of hyperthyroidism and with the antibody activity disappearing in most patients once the disease is controlled. Importantly, too, in women with high levels of antibody activity in the third trimester of pregnancy, antibodies that cross the placenta are capable of inducing transient neonatal hyperthyroidism in the offspring (see Chap. 47). The neonatal hyperthyroid syndrome lasts as long as the levels of maternal TSH-receptor antibody activity are high enough in the fetal circulation.

## LYMPHOCYTIC THYROIDITIS

Patients with lymphocytic thyroiditis can be divided on the basis of thyroid size into (a) those showing evidence of thyroid enlargement (goiter), who are defined as having Hashimoto thyroiditis, and (b) a subgroup of patients who demonstrate thyroid atrophy and are defined as having atrophic thyroiditis or primary myxedema (see Chap. 46). In both groups of patients, autoantibodies directed against thyroglobulin and the enzyme thyroid peroxidase (TPO) are detectable, with most patients having antibodies against TPO.[24] High levels of antibody to TPO of increased affinity and primarily of the IgG class predominate. These autoantibodies are directed against a spectrum of autoantigenic determinants; thus, they are not truly monoclonal in origin. It is unlikely that antibodies directed against thyroglobulin are of any pathogenetic significance, at least in humans. In contrast, antibodies directed against TPO may have an important role in thyroid destruction, because in addition to evidence that they bind to thyrocytes in vivo, there is clear evidence of the ability to kill thyrocytes in vitro in the presence of complement. Evidence as to whether these antibodies may directly interfere with TPO enzymatic activity remains controversial. In women with postpartum thyroid dysfunction, in whom high levels of antibody activity directed against TPO can be detected, these antibodies cross the placenta but show no evidence of interference with thyroid function in the neonate. The molecular cloning of TPO and attempts to establish animal models of autoimmune thyroid disease based on immunization with the antigen have contributed little to clarifying the potential role of autoantibodies directed against this thyroid target autoantigen in the pathogenesis of lymphocytic thyroiditis.

Within the subgroup of patients with primary myxedema, more convincing evidence of a likely role for pathogenetic autoantibodies has been demonstrated. In ~30% of patients with this condition, bioassay systems based on the ability of immunoglobulin from these patients to inhibit TSH-stimulated cyclic adenosine monophosphate (AMP) production by cultured human thyroid cells has demonstrated, beyond doubt, the existence of TSH-receptor blocking antibodies and their role in the development of thyroid failure in this group of patients.[23] Infants have been characterized in whom the transplacental passage of such antibody activity from the maternal circulation has resulted in transient neonatal hypothyroidism in the infant for as long as the antibody level was of a significantly high titer. Therefore, the concept has emerged of a spectrum of antibody activities directed against the TSH receptor; indeed, patients have been described in whom both blocking and stimulating activities have been detected and the level and affinity of the particular type of TSH-receptor autoantibody have determined, at any one time, whether the individual is hyperthyroid or hypothyroid. Despite the clear demonstration in a subgroup of patients, with primary myxedema, of TSH-receptor blocking antibody activity being responsible for the induction of their hypothyroidism, it is more likely in the majority of patients with lymphocytic thyroiditis that cell-mediated effector mechanisms leading to thyroid cell destruction have a more important role in the pathogenesis of this group of diseases.

## TYPE 1 DIABETES MELLITUS

In type 1 diabetes mellitus, the ability to detect, by indirect immunofluorescence, the presence of cytoplasmic islet cell antibodies has provided important serologic evidence of the likely role of autoimmunity in the development of type 1 diabetes[25] (see Chap. 136). Although these antibodies have provided a useful predictive marker for the increased risk of the development of type 1 diabetes, particularly in first-degree relatives of patients with the disease, the target autoantigen has remained poorly characterized. The description of a 64-kDa antigen and antibodies directed against this target has been followed by the identification of the antigen as the enzyme glutamic acid decarboxylase (GAD).[24a] GAD exists in at least two different isoforms with molecular masses of 65 kDa (GAD-65) and 67 kDa (GAD-67), respectively. Antibodies to GAD-67, however, are rare in patients with type 1 diabetes and in prediabetic individuals. In the nonobese diabetic (NOD) mouse model of type 1 diabetes, the expression of GAD-65 in islet B cells is required for the development of diabetes.[26] Other islet-specific autoantibodies directed against autoantigens including insulin and IA-2 (a tyrosine phosphatase) exist in the circulation of patients with type 1 diabetes. Continuing characterization of the autoantigenic targets in the pancreatic islet B cells will clarify the underlying autoimmune pathogenesis of type 1 diabetes; but all of the evidence available, particularly in animal models, indicates that T-cell–mediated destruction is the crucial process in the disease's development. Antibodies are more likely to be markers of prediction of disease development rather than causative agents.

## ADDISON DISEASE AND PRIMARY OVARIAN FAILURE

Autoimmune adrenocortical failure, traditionally called *idiopathic Addison disease*, can occur in isolation or as part of the autoimmune polyglandular syndromes, types I and II (see Chaps. 59, 76, and 197). In all three forms, the adrenal cortex is a target and autoantibodies reacting with steroid-producing cells in this site have been described. In patients with the type I polyglandular syndrome, antibodies have been detected that are directed against the cytochrome P450 enzyme, steroid 17α-hydroxylase, and against $P450_{scc}$. Both are enzymes specific to all steroid-producing cells but, in addition, they have antibodies directed against the adrenal-specific enzyme $P450_{c21}$ hydroxylase ($P450_{c21}$).[27] This contrasts with patients having the type II polyglandular syndrome or having isolated Addison disease, whose sera react almost exclusively with the $P450_{c21}$ enzyme.[28] In women with premature or primary ovarian failure, antibodies to the $P450_{scc}$ enzyme are also present.[29] Antibody activity is, therefore, clearly detectable in individuals with evidence of either adrenal or ovarian failure, but no data exist to demonstrate that these antibodies have any pathogenetic significance.

## REFERENCES

1. Uchida N, Fleming WH, Alpern EJ, Weissman IL. Heterogeneity of hematopoietic stem cells. Curr Opin Immunol 1993; 5:177.
2. Du Pasquier L. Phylogeny of B cell development. Curr Opin Immunol 1993; 5:185.
3. Von Boehmer H. Thymic selection: a matter of life and death. Immunol Today 1992; 13:454.
4. Burrows PD, Cooper MD. B cell development in man. Curr Opin Immunol 1993; 5:201.
5. Rolink A, Melchers F. Generation and regeneration of cells of the B lymphocyte lineage. Curr Opin Immunol 1993; 5:207.
6. Gray D. Immunological memory. Annu Rev Immunol 1993; 11:49.
7. Reth M. B cell antigen receptors. Curr Opin Immunol 1994; 6:3.
8. Berek C, Ziegner M. The maturation of the immune response. Immunol Today 1993; 14:400.
9. Berek C. Somatic mutation and memory. Curr Opin Immunol 1993; 5:218.
10. Clark AW, Ledbetter JA. How B and T cells talk to each other. Nature 1994; 367:425.
11. Kasaian MT, Casali O. Autoimmunity prone B-1 (CD5 B) cells, natural antibodies and self-recognition. Autoimmunity 1993; 15:315.
12. Alt FW, Honjo T, Rabbitts TH (eds). The immunoglobulin genes. New York: Academic Press, 1989.
13. Chen J, Alt FW. Gene rearrangement and B cell development. Curr Opin Immunol 1993; 5:194.
14. Schatz DG, Oettinger MA, Schlissel MS. V(D)J recombination: molecular biology and regulation. Annu Rev Immunol 1992; 10:359.
15. Berek C, Milstein C. Mutational drift and repertoire shift in the maturation of the immune response. Immunol Rev 1987; 96:23.
16. Nemazee D. Promotion and prevention of autoimmunity by B lymphocytes. Curr Opin Immunol 1993; 5:866.
17. Rolink A, Melchers F. Molecular and cellular origins of B lymphocyte diversity. Cell 1991; 66:1081.
18. Mason D, Powrie F. Control of immune pathology by regulatory T cells. Curr Opin Immunol 1998; 10:649.
19. Naparstek Y, Plotz PH. The role of autoantibodies in autoimmune disease. Annu Rev Immunol 1993; 11:79.
20. Diamond B, Katz JB, Paul E, et al. The role of somatic mutation in the pathogenic anti-DNA response. Annu Rev Immunol 1992; 10:731.
21. Banga JP, McGregor AM. Enzymes as targets for autoantibodies in human autoimmune disease: relevance to pathogenesis. Autoimmunity 1991; 9:177.
22. Misrahi M, Loosfelt H, Gross B, et al. Characterisation of the thyroid-stimulating hormone receptor. Curr Opin Endocrinol Diabetes 1994; 1:175.
23. Rapoport B, Chazenbalk GD, Jaume JC, McLachlan SM. The thyrotropin (TSH) releasing hormone receptor: interaction with TSH and autoantibodies. Endocr Rev 1998; 19:673.
24. Banga JP. Development in our understanding of the structure of thyroid peroxidase and the relevance of these findings to autoimmunity. Curr Opin Endocrinol Diabetes 1998; 5:275.
24a. Lohmann T, Hana M, Leslie RD, et al. Immune reactivity to glutamic acid decarboxylase 65 in stiffman syndrome and type 1 diabetes mellitus. Lancet 2000; 356:31.
25. Verge CF, Eisenbarth GS. Predicting and preventing insulin-independent diabetes mellitus. Curr Opin Endocrinol Diabetes 1994; 1:221.
26. Yoon J-W, Yoon C-S, Lim H-W, et al. Control of autoimmune diabetes in NOD mice by GAD expression or suppression in B (beta) cells. Science 1999; 284:1183.

27. Betterle C, Greggio NA, Volpato M. Autoimmune polyglandular syndrome type I. J Clin Endocrinol Metab 1998; 83:1049.

28. Betterle C, Volpato M, Pedini B, et al. Adrenal cortex autoantibodies and steroid producing cell autoantibodies in patients with Addison's disease. J Clin Endocrinol Metab 1999; 84:618.

29. Hoek A, Schoemaker J, Drexhage HA. Premature ovarian failure and ovarian autoimmunity. Endocr Rev 1997; 18:107.

# CHAPTER 197

# THE IMMUNE SYSTEM AND ITS ROLE IN ENDOCRINE FUNCTION

ROBERT VOLPÉ

This chapter discusses the immunologic aspects of the autoimmune endocrinopathies, particularly autoimmune thyroid disease (AITD) and insulin-dependent diabetes mellitus (type 1). General factors involved in these disorders are described first, followed by a consideration of the specific entities.

## GENETIC AND ENVIRONMENTAL FACTORS

The disturbances in immunoregulation that lead to organ-specific endocrine diseases are partly genetic and partly environmental.[1-3] Autoimmune endocrine diseases and those nonendocrine autoimmune disorders with which they are associated (Table 197-1) tend to aggregate in families, and more than one of these disorders may occur concomitantly within the same patient or his or her family. The modes of inheritance of these diseases do not follow simple genetic rules, and environmental factors such as stress, infection, trauma, drugs, nutrition, smoking, and aging may distort the penetrance and expressivity of these conditions by acting on the immune system.[4] The finding that the autoimmune endocrinopathies occur preferentially in individuals who have inherited certain major histocompatibility complex (MHC) gene markers (in humans, termed the *human leukocyte antigen [HLA] system*) definitely establishes the genetic influences in these disorders.[5,6] There tends to be a strong female preponderance in most of these autoimmune diseases, which

may be related partially to the influences of one gene on another[7] and partially to hormonal factors.[8]

## DISORDERED IMMUNE REGULATION IN AUTOIMMUNE ENDOCRINOPATHIES

Details of the immune system that relate to autoimmune endocrine diseases are described in Chapters 193 through 196, and only those elements that are necessary for an understanding of the entities themselves are presented in this chapter. The role of MHC in relation to these maladies is explained in Chapter 194, although Table 197-2 depicts the HLA associations that have been observed in these conditions.[9] The HLA system (which is essential for antigen processing and presentation) is important in the pathogenesis of the autoimmune disorders; while the HLA genes may not constitute the disease susceptibility genes, they nonetheless are crucial to the development of autoimmune diseases and possibly to their amplification.[5,6] It is now clear that other genes, not yet entirely characterized, also contribute to the etiology of these conditions[10] (see Chap. 194). The development of these diseases (including the disturbance in target cell function) depends on a complex interplay between the antigen, or antigens, on the target cells; the antigen-presenting cells (APC); the CD4 helper/inducer T lymphocytes; T-effector lymphocytes; the CD8 suppressor (regulatory)/cytotoxic T lymphocytes; B lymphocytes; antibodies; and various cytokines. In turn, these elements stimulate the target cell to express molecules of various types, such as intercellular adhesion molecule-1, heat shock proteins, class I and class II antigens, and other autoantigens, which further modify the immune response. Controversy still abounds about the nature of the autoimmune process, the role of the antigen and of antigen presentation, and the involvement of microorganisms in these mechanisms.[11,12]

Theoretical considerations that might account for the development of an organ-specific autoimmune process would be (a) an antigenic stimulus (however initiated, and including molecular mimicry) that would precipitate and even maintain the disorder—involving antigens originating from microorganisms with homology to target cell autoantigens, or with actual infections of the target cells; (b) a precipitating antigenic stimulus, but coupled with an underlying immune abnormality;

**TABLE 197-1.**
**Autoimmune Endocrinopathies and Some of the Nonendocrine Organ-Specific Autoimmune Disorders That May Be Associated**

| Endocrinopathies | Nonendocrine Diseases |
|---|---|
| Graves (Basedow, Parry disease) | Pernicious anemia |
| Hashimoto thyroiditis | Vitiligo |
| Idiopathic Addison disease | Myasthenia gravis |
| Insulinopenic diabetes mellitus | Sjögren syndrome |
| Autoimmune oophoritis and orchitis | Rheumatoid arthritis |
| Autoimmune hypoparathyroidism | Idiopathic thrombocytopenic purpura |
| Autoimmune hypophysitis | Chronic active hepatitis |
| Some cases of infertility caused by antisperm antibodies | Primary biliary cirrhosis |
| | Celiac disease |

(From Volpé R. Autoimmunity in endocrine disease. New York: Marcel Dekker Inc, 1985.)

**TABLE 197-2.**
**Associations between Human Leukocyte Antigen and Autoimmune Endocrinopathies and Some Related Disorders**

| Condition | HLA | Frequency (%) Patients | Frequency (%) Controls | Relative Risk |
|---|---|---|---|---|
| Idiopathic Addison disease | D/DR3 | 69 | 26.3 | 6.3 |
| Graves disease | D/DR3 | 56 | 26.3 | 3.7 |
| Insulin-dependent diabetes | D/DR3 | 56 | 28.2 | 3.3 |
| | D/DR4 | 75 | 32.2 | 6.4 |
| | D/DR2 | 10 | 30.5 | 0.2 |
| Myasthenia gravis | D/DR3 | 50 | 28.2 | 2.5 |
| Sjögren syndrome | D/DR3 | 78 | 26.3 | 9.7 |
| Atrophic thyroiditis* | DR3 | 64 | 23.8 | 5.7 |
| Goitrous thyroiditis* | DR5 | 53 | 26.3 | 3.1 |
| Pernicious anemia | Dw5 | 25 | 5.8 | 5.4 |
| Subacute thyroiditis | Bw35 | 70 | 14.6 | 13.7 |

*The relative risk indicates how many times more frequently the disease develops in individuals carrying the HLA antigen in question as compared with the frequency of the disease in individuals lacking the antigen. The data refer exclusively to white individuals.

(Reproduced from Svejgaard A, Platz P, Ryder LR. HLA and endocrine disease. In: Volpé R, ed. Autoimmunity in endocrine disease. New York: Marcel Dekker Inc, 1985:93.)

(c) the availability of costimulators; (d) abnormal antigen-specific induction of subsets of T lymphocytes because of an abnormal HLA-related gene or genes resulting in an operational disorder within the T lymphocytes; (e) mutation of appropriate T or B lymphocytes to form an abnormal clone or clones of lymphocytes interactive with a particular target organ (these would be autonomous and not subject to normal immunoregulation); and (f) a specific inherent defect in immunoregulation, probably due to somewhat reduced specific antigenic induction of regulatory (suppressor) T lymphocytes by virtue of a disorder in presentation of the specific antigen; this likely would be due to an abnormality or abnormalities of an HLA-related gene or genes. In the latter hypothesis, all that would be additionally necessary to precipitate the particular disease would be (a) the presence of the antigen without any need for it to be abnormal in quality or quantity, (b) availability of the antigen by means of an APC (e.g., the macrophage), (c) the presence of costimulators, (d) the appearance or availability of target cell–directed clones of helper T lymphocytes and B lymphocytes, and (e) perturbation of the immune system by such factors as stress, trauma, infection, drugs, smoking, and aging, which would be superimposed on the partial antigen-specific abnormality. The evidence favoring the latter hypothesis is increasingly compelling and is presented in this chapter.[13–15]

## DISORDERED SUPPRESSOR (REGULATORY) T LYMPHOCYTES

Although clonal deletion of autoreactive T lymphocytes in the thymus plays an important role in the development of tolerance to self-antigens, many autoreactive T lymphocytes reach the periphery where they remain unresponsive to the self-antigen. Both "anergy" and active suppression have been postulated to fulfill this role.[16] Anergic T lymphocytes can certainly be identified in the periphery, but this does not account for the observation that adoptive transfer of T lymphocytes from mice tolerant to a given antigen reduces the immune response to that same antigen in syngeneic recipients.[17] The best explanation for this result is that some T lymphocytes can suppress immune responses.

The previous skepticism regarding the nature or even existence of suppressor (regulatory) T lymphocytes has largely been laid to rest.[14,15] There is increasing evidence for a role for these cells in preventing autoimmune disease, and for a deficiency of these same cells in causing these disorders.[1,18] One theory approaches the problem of the control of self-reactivity from the perspective of a balance between the $T_H1$ and $T_H2$ pathways ($T_H1$ cells secrete interleukin-2 [IL-2] and interferon-$\gamma$, while $T_H2$ cells secrete IL-4, IL-5, and IL-10).[18] Cytokines act as chemical mediators that have widespread effects on immunocytes and other target cells (see Chaps. 173 and 228). According to this theory, failure of a target organ is caused by predominantly $T_H1$-mediated pathways, in which the target cells are destroyed by interferon-$\gamma$–activated scavenger macrophages. The $T_H1$-$T_H2$ balance theory emphasizes the reciprocal relationship between the $T_H1$ and $T_H2$ pathways, and suggests that if the $T_H1$ pathway is diverted into the $T_H2$ pathway the $T_H1$-mediated autoimmune reactivity is dampened. Thus, tolerance to self is not restored; rather, the harmful reaction to self is diverted to a less harmful reaction. Nonetheless, the hypothesis that protection from autoimmune destruction can be achieved by a $T_H1$ to $T_H2$ switch is, unfortunately, too simplistic. In many autoimmune conditions, both $T_H1$ and $T_H2$ cells exist.[16] It is now evident that there are regulatory T-lymphocyte populations other than those from $T_H2$ cells.[18] Antigen-specific suppressor T lymphocytes, which produce T-suppressor factor (TSF),[16] have been demonstrated. TSF is an antigen-specific glycosylation-inhibiting factor (GIF) that con-

tains a 55-kDa peptide, which has both a GIF determinant and a T-cell receptor (TCR) $\alpha$ determinant, and exhibits GIF bioactivity.

There has been no definitive evidence that a target cell abnormality or target cell injury or infection is necessary to induce these conditions,[13] although this notion has certainly had its advocates.[11,12] Moreover, the popular notion that molecular mimicry (i.e., homologies between microorganismal antigens and autoantigens) might play a role, while certainly a popular notion,[11] has not been established, and there is evidence against that hypothesis.[13] The author believes that no abnormalities, injuries, or infections of the target cell are required for the development of these diseases.[13] All that is required is that the normal target cell antigen or antigens be available to the T lymphocytes through APCs. The immunoregulatory disturbance is then sufficient to produce the disorder by virtue of the (partial) genetic abnormality of specific antigen induction of suppressor (regulatory) T lymphocytes, plus environmental factors (mentioned earlier), interacting with the immune system. Many membrane antigens circulate in solubilized form (e.g., the thyroid-stimulating hormone [TSH] receptor) and are thus available to the immune system.[19] Indeed, normal peripheral tolerance is maintained by low levels of autoantigen which activate suppressor (regulatory) T cells.[14] It would follow that genetic defects of specific antigen presentation (presumably of MHC and related genes) result in the specific autoantigen failing to activate the regulatory cells. This may prove to be the fundamental basis of organ-specific autoimmune disease.

## AUTOIMMUNE THYROID DISEASE

AITDs include Graves disease (GD) and Hashimoto thyroiditis (HT), as well as variants of the latter.[1,2,20–22] The clinical expression of these entities may be markedly different; yet there are genetic and pathogenic elements that are similar, if not identical, in both. Indeed, some investigators consider that these two conditions comprise opposite ends of a spectrum of the same disorder.[1,2] There are, however, elements that differ between these conditions and even between the variants of thyroiditis.

GD (see Chaps. 42 and 43) may be defined here as hyperthyroidism caused by the stimulation of the TSH receptor by an antibody (thyroid-stimulating antibody [TSAb]), and an appropriate new designation would be *autoimmune thyrotoxicosis*.

Autoimmune thyroiditis was first described by Hashimoto,[23] who reported four patients with goiter in whom the thyroid histologic appearance manifested diffuse lymphocytic infiltration, atrophy of parenchymal cells, fibrosis, and an eosinophilic change in some parenchymal cells (Askanazy or Hürthle cells). In the "chronic fibrous" variant, fibrosis predominates and lymphocytic infiltration is less evident. In lymphocytic thyroiditis of childhood and adolescence, fibrosis, Askanazy cells, and germinal centers are less obvious than in the adult form, and thyroid antibodies tend to be lower in titer, or even absent. Postpartum thyroiditis occurs a few months after delivery as a transient form of autoimmune thyroiditis; although it generally clears (almost) completely, it may later culminate in a chronic form. In "idiopathic myxedema" the gland is atrophied, rather than hypertrophied. There is also an atrophic asymptomatic form, which is occult, and often discovered only at autopsy. Those persons with no clinical features, but with circulating thyroid antibodies, can also be shown to have occult autoimmune thyroiditis; some of these may be shown to be in a state of "compensated hypothyroidism."[2] Although there may be subtle genetic and pathologic differences between these variants, the pathogenesis at least is similar; the term *autoimmune thyroiditis* is acceptable as a generic term for this group (see Chaps. 45 and 46).

**TABLE 197-3.**
**Immune Stigmata Associated with Graves Disease and Hashimoto Thyroiditis**

| Stigmata | Graves Disease | Hashimoto Thyroiditis |
|---|---|---|
| Lymphocytic infiltration in thyroid | Frequently present | Almost invariable |
| Immunoglobulins in thyroid stroma | Yes | Yes |
| Type of infiltrating lymphocytes | B and T | B and T, mostly $T_H 1$ |
| Immune complexes in circulation | Common | Common |
| Thymic enlargement | Common | Common |
| Lymphadenopathy and splenomegaly | Infrequent | — |
| Relative lymphocytosis | Common | — |
| Hypergammaglobulinemia | — | Common |
| Benefit from corticosteroid therapy | Yes | Yes |
| Thyroid-stimulating antibody | Almost all | Infrequent |
| Exophthalmos | Common | Occasional |
| Evidence of cell-mediated immunity | Yes | Yes |
| Regulatory cell defect | Yes | Yes |
| Other autoimmune diseases in patients | Yes (see Table 197-1) | Yes (see Table 197-1) |
| Thyroid antibodies in relatives | 50% | 50% |
| Thyroid and other autoimmune diseases in relatives | Common | Common |
| HLA relationships | Yes (see text) | Yes (see text) |
| Animal models | Experimental models | Spontaneous, experimental |

(From Volpé R, ed. Autoimmunity in endocrine disease. New York: Marcel Dekker Inc, 1985:112.)

HT may have increased in frequency in the last generation, perhaps owing to increased iodine intake over this time. (One possible mechanism for this observation is the increased immunogenicity of highly iodinated thyroglobulin, although the role for this in human AITD remains unclear.[24,25]) Approximately 3% of the population have some functional deficiency of the thyroid secondary to HT (much higher in women >50 years of age),[26] whereas up to 40% of elderly women have some degree of thyroidal lymphocytic infiltration, usually not recognized clinically.[2] The condition is probably slowly progressive in all, but only reaches overt hypothyroidism in a small percentage at the top of the disease "pyramid."[27] Approximately two-thirds of goiters in euthyroid adolescents are due to lymphocytic thyroiditis. GD is also common, occurring in ~1% of the population.[2]

In both GD and HT, there are several aspects that suggest the participation of an autoimmune process (Table 197-3). The overlap between GD and HT has long been recognized. Indeed, GD and HT frequently aggregate in the same families. There are several reports of identical twins, one with GD and the other with HT. In fact, both GD and HT can cohabit the same thyroid gland; the clinical expression will depend on which condition predominates.[2] As there remain several genetic, immunologic, laboratory, and clinical elements that differ between these maladies, they should be considered separate (albeit closely related) entities.

## HUMORAL IMMUNITY IN AUTOIMMUNE THYROID DISEASE

The initial observations included thyroid autoantibodies in the serum of patients with HT,[28] the induction of experimental thyroiditis in rabbits,[29] and the presence of an abnormal thyroid stimulator in the serum of some patients with GD, capable of stimulating the guinea pig thyroid gland.[30] This was termed *long-acting thyroid stimulator* (LATS) and proved to be an immunoglobulin G (IgG). It is now termed *TSAb*.[20]

The various antibodies that may be detected in AITD and their possible functions are documented in Table 197-4 and Figure 197-1. These are largely produced by intrathyroidal B lymphocytes, although help is required from T helper cells. TSAb has received the most attention because it acts to stimulate thyroid cells, resulting in hyperthyroidism; it is an antibody directed against epitope(s) on the extracellular domain of the TSH receptor and is an agonist of TSH; however, it stimulates

**TABLE 197-4.**
**Antigen-Antibody Systems Involved in Humoral Responses of Thyroid Autoimmune Disease**

| Antigen | Antibody (Function) | Antibody Detection |
|---|---|---|
| Thyroglobulin | Thyroglobulin antibody (no clear function) | Precipitin technique; tanned red cell hemagglutination; immunofluorescence on fixed thyroid sections; competitive binding radioimmunoassay; coprecipitation with $^{125}$I-thyroglobulin; microenzyme-linked immunoassay (enzyme-linked immunosorbent assay [ELISA]); plaque-forming assay |
| Thyroperoxidase | Thyroperoxidase (microsomal) antibody (cytotoxic in conjunction with lymphocytes) | Complement fixation; immunofluorescence on unfixed thyroid sections; cytotoxicity test on cultured thyroid cells; competitive binding radioimmunoassay; tanned red cell hemagglutination; micro-ELISA |
| Second colloid component | Colloid antigen-2 ($CA_2$) antibody (no clear function) | Immunofluorescence on fixed thyroid sections |
| Cell-surface antigens | Membrane antibodies (cytotoxic with lymphocytes) | Immunofluorescence on viable thyroid cells; hemadsorption; binding assays |
| Thyroxine and triiodothyronine | Thyroid hormone antibodies (bind and prevent hormone action) | Antigen-binding capacity |
| Antigen not defined | Growth-stimulating and growth-inhibiting antibodies (may induce or inhibit thyroid growth) | Effects on DNA content per thyroid cell nucleus or glucose-6-phosphate dehydrogenase (G6PD) activity per cell |
| Thyroid-stimulating hormone (TSH) receptor–related antigen | TSH-receptor antibodies (may stimulate thyroid cells, inhibit TSH effect, or do both or neither) | Stimulatory assays: Current terms employed for stimulatory assays include human thyroid stimulator, human thyroid-stimulating immunoglobulin (TSI), thyroid-stimulating antibody (TSAb) Long-acting thyroid stimulator (LATS) bioassay; colloid droplet formation in human thyroid slices; stimulation of human thyroid adenylate cyclase in vitro; cytochemical assay Binding assays: LATS protector assay; inhibition of $^{125}$I-thyrotropin binding to human thyroid membranes (thyrotropin displacement activity [TDA], TSH-binding–inhibitory immunoglobulin [TBII]); fat cell membrane radioligand assays; fat cell ELISA Inhibitory assays: thyrotropin-stimulating–blocking antibody (TSBAb) |

(From Volpé R, ed. Autoimmunity in endocrine disease. New York: Marcel Dekker Inc, 1985:127.)

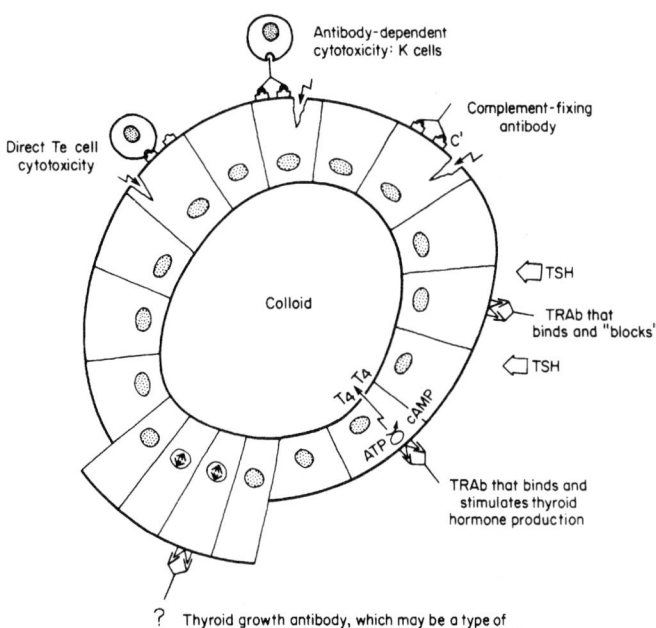

? Thyroid growth antibody, which may be a type of
TRAb that binds and stimulates follicular cell growth

**FIGURE 197-1.** Composite diagram of a thyroid follicle, showing possible immune effector mechanisms in autoimmune thyroid disease. Cytotoxic mechanisms include direct cytotoxicity by sensitized effector (*Te*) cells, antibody-dependent cytotoxicity by killer (*K*) cells armed with thyroid autoantibody, and cell lysis by complement-fixing thyroid autoantibody. The various types of thyrotropin receptor (*TSH-R*) antibodies (*TRAb*) have different mechanisms of action. One type binds to the TSH-R and blocks thyroid-stimulating hormone (*TSH*) from binding to or stimulating the receptor. Another type—thyroid-stimulating antibody (*TSAb*)—binds to and stimulates the TSH receptor, causing excess thyroid hormone production. Thyroid growth-promoting and -inhibiting antibodies remain controversial. ($T_4$, thyroxine; *ATP*, adenosine triphosphate; *cAMP*, cyclic adenosine monophosphate.) (Reproduced from Strakosch CR, Wenzel BE, Row VV, Volpé R. Immunology of autoimmune thyroid diseases. N Engl J Med 1982; 307:1499.)

the thyrocyte for several hours (compared to the short duration of stimulation by TSH).[2]

The original *LATS* assay was an in vivo guinea pig and, later, mouse assay.[31] Many other assays for the *TSH-receptor (TSH-R) antibodies* found in GD have now been described.[2] Since some of these antibodies are not stimulatory, the term *TSAb* should be used to refer only to those antibodies that cause increased cyclic adenosine monophosphate (cAMP) in thyroid cells. The radioligand assay that measures binding of IgG to the TSH receptor (by inhibition of binding of labeled TSH) is generally referred to as *thyrotropin-binding–inhibitory immunoglobulin* (TBII). In patients with GD specifically, there is a close correlation between TBII and TSAb, which may be useful in the diagnosis of that condition.[2] However, while TSAb is a TSH-R antibody demonstrable by the TBII assay, some IgGs that are positive in the TBII assay will not stimulate the thyroid cells, and some even inhibit TSH activity in vivo and in vitro (*thyroid-stimulating–blocking antibody, TSBAb*), and, thus, are capable of causing or contributing to hypothyroidism.[2] This most typically is associated with atrophic thyroiditis.[2] TSBAb has also been associated with transient neonatal hypothyroidism, due to passive placental transfer to the fetus.[2] While, presently, only functional assays (i.e., stimulation vs. inhibition) differentiate between the two antibodies, evidence suggests that they bind to different epitopes on the TSH receptor.[32]

By use of assays that measure the generation of cAMP in the human or in Fischer rat thyroid line-5 thyrocytes, several laboratories have demonstrated TSAb in the sera of ~95% of patients

with untreated GD.[2] TSAb in pregnant GD patients may rise in the first trimester, but tends to decline in the third trimester, and may sometimes temporarily disappear. However, in some cases, while it may have become reduced from very high levels, it may remain markedly elevated throughout pregnancy. In such instances, there is a very real possibility of fetal and neonatal hyperthyroidism, which can be a very serious illness. Since this is due to placental passive transfer of the antibody, it gradually declines over several weeks in the newborn; thus, treatment is necessary for only this length of time.[2] Following delivery, maternal TSAb may rebound to higher levels once again, sometimes leading to postpartum GD. TSAb tends to decline in many patients with long-term antithyroid drug therapy; while this, along with regression of the goiter, might suggest that the patient is in remission, sometimes the latter is very short-lived, and the disease recurs.[2] The continued presence of TSAb is associated with a high relapse rate, following discontinuance of medication.[2] TSAb will become further elevated after iodine-131 ($^{131}$I) therapy for several months as a result of the radiation-induced release of thyroid antigens, including TSH-R, and will then decline.[2] In all of these circumstances, TBII results will in general parallel those of TSAb, aside from the exceptions noted. TSAb may also transiently appear with liberation of membrane antigens in subacute or silent thyroiditis,[13] or due to molecular mimicry following acute yersiniosis[33]; in the latter patients, however, there was no evidence of thyroid dysfunction.[33] Thus, the presence of TSAb does not invariably signify a diagnosis of GD.

Other thyroid antibodies that are useful clinically are the thyroglobulin and thyroperoxidase (microsomal) antibodies. A high titer of thyroglobulin antibody, a non–complement-fixing antibody, is found in ~55% of patients with HT and 25% of patients with GD. It occurs less often in patients with thyroid carcinomas, and other (nonthyroidal) autoimmune diseases. Thyroperoxidase antibodies (TPO Ab; complement fixing) are found much more commonly in AITD than in thyroglobulin Ab, and have a much closer relationship with thyroid dysfunction and abnormal histology.[1,2] They are observed in ~95% of patients with HT, 90% of those with "idiopathic myxedema," and 80% of patients with GD; 72% of patients positive for TPO Ab manifest some degree of thyroid dysfunction (at least a state of compensated hypothyroidism, with high TSH values; patients with such antibodies in a state of compensated hypothyroidism will go on to overt hypothyroidism at the rate of 5–10% per year).[2] In terms of case-finding and cost reductions, performance of thyroglobulin Ab is hardly necessary; one study has shown that TPO Ab was the only positive test in 64% of all patients with positive tests, while thyroglobulin Ab was the only positive test in 1%.[34] The widespread practice of performing both tests increases the costs without an offsetting diagnostic gain.[34] Even low titers of TPO Ab correlate with thyroid lymphocytic infiltration.[2] High titers are highly suggestive of AITD, and very high titers are virtually diagnostic of AITD; nevertheless, a minority of patients with these disorders have only low titers or no detectable thyroid antibodies. The expression of recombinant TPO by the baculovirus system has allowed screening by an enzyme-linked immunosorbent assay (ELISA) for screening for AITD.[35] Low titers of TPO Ab are also observed in some cases of papillary thyroid carcinoma, nontoxic goiter, and subacute thyroiditis, as well as in many patients with no clinical evidence of thyroid disease.[2] When such antibodies are detected in women before or in early pregnancy, they tend to predict the later development of postpartum thyroiditis; moreover, these antibodies transiently increase in parallel with the functional abnormalities that occur with postpartum thyroiditis.[2] Thyroid antibodies in HT with elevated TSH values will generally decline with suppressive therapy of TSH by thyroxine ($T_4$).[2] They also often decline in patients with GD treated with antithyroid drug therapy.[2]

Antibodies to the thyroid hormones themselves are of clinical importance only when the thyroid gland is incapable of responding to excess TSH. In such instances, antibodies to $T_4$ and triiodothyronine ($T_3$) will reduce the free moiety; the addition of exogenous thyroid hormone may not yield the expected clinical improvement until the hormone-binding sites on the antibody are saturated. Moreover, in the presence of these antibodies, determination of thyroid hormone concentrations may misleadingly appear very high or low (depending on the assay system used) and conflict with the clinical presentation.[1,2] Antinuclear antibodies are also found in AITD, as are antibodies to cell membranes and to a colloid component other than thyroglobulin. Whether there are thyroid growth-promoting, or growth-inhibiting, antibodies separate from TSH-R antibodies remains controversial.[2]

Autoantibodies to a few other organs, such as gastric antigens, islet cell antigens, and others, are found more commonly in patients with AITD by virtue of the inheritance of more than one disease susceptibility gene situated in close proximity on chromosome 6. Antibodies against certain bacteria, such as *Yersinia enterocolitica*, are encountered commonly in AITD. This appears to arise from an artifact of homology between thyroid and bacterial antigens, and does *not* signify the presence or relevance of actual bacterial infection.[2,13]

## THE T LYMPHOCYTES IN AUTOIMMUNE THYROID DISEASE

Most intrathyroidal T lymphocytes are "primed" or activated cells, and in HT are $T_H1$-type cells; $T_H2$ cells are seldom found.[36] The proportion of intrathyroidal CD8+ clones versus CD4+ clones is greater than in the periphery. Studies in GD thyroids have had variable results. "Homing" of autologous lymphocytes to the thyroid has been demonstrated in AITD.[37] Restricted heterogeneity of TCR Vbβ gene expression in both GD and HT has been reported.[38]

Studies of antigen-specific regulatory T-lymphocyte function have yielded results of interest.[2,20,39] First, the idea that there could be an antigen-specific disorder in regulatory T lymphocytes seems more rational than that of a generalized disturbance in regulatory T-lymphocyte function, since the latter would result in multiple clinical disorders of immunoregulation, making it discordant with genetic observations in which AITD appears much more frequently in families in whom the propositus also has AITD (rather than other autoimmune disorders). There are several studies indicating the presence of an organ-specific defect in regulatory T lymphocytes in AITD, in which the observation does not relate to the thyroid function of the patient (i.e., whether the patient is hyperthyroid, euthyroid, or hypothyroid).[14,20,39–54] These studies have taken the form of measuring the impact of these cells specifically on antibodies directed against the target cell, or of reducing the sensitization of (helper) T cells against their specific antigen(s), without having a generalized effect as previously described. (Of course, under some conditions [e.g., hyperthyroidism] both effects may coexist.) Thyroid-specific antigens will not sufficiently activate CD8+ CD11b+ T lymphocytes ("pure" suppressor cells) from patients who have AITD, as well as irrelevant antigen, whereas in normal persons, CD8+CD11b+ T lymphocytes respond equally well to both relevant and irrelevant antigen.[53] Moreover, TSH-R will not activate CD8 T cells from patients with GD as well as control CD8 cells (from normal persons, and patients with HT, nontoxic goiter, and type 1 diabetes). Conversely, glutamic acid decarboxylase (GAD-65), the putative antigen of the pancreatic B cells, will not activate CD8 cells in patients with type 1 diabetes as well as CD8 cells from patients with GD

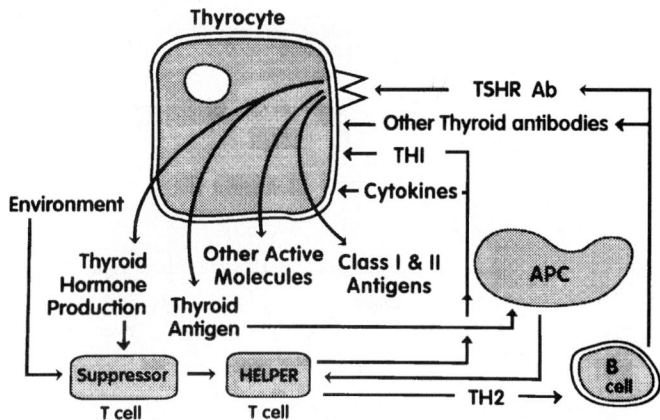

**FIGURE 197-2.** Hypothesis for the pathogenesis of autoimmune thyroid disease. The fundamental defect may relate to reduced activation by specific antigen (*Ag*; by means of an abnormality of specific antigen presentation by histocompatibility genes) of regulatory (suppressor) T lymphocytes (*Ts*). Precipitating environmental factors (e.g., stress, infection, trauma, drugs, smoking, and aging) may cause a reduction in nonspecific Ts function, thus adding to the antigen-specific Ts dysfunction. The result is to reduce suppression of thyroid-directed helper T lymphocytes ($T_H$ [$T_H1$ and $T_H2$]), allowing them to become activated in the presence of antigen-presenting cells (*APCs*; e.g., monocytes) and the thyroid antigens (which must "drive" the process, activating the helper T lymphocytes). Helper T lymphocytes may then act directly on the thyrocyte through production of cytokines, which are essential at every stage of the process, or may cooperate with cytotoxic cells to produce thyroid damage. The activated helper T lymphocytes will produce interferon-γ (*IFN-γ*) at close proximity to the thyrocytes, causing the latter to express class II antigens, which may initially promote anergy, but may later allow the thyrocyte to present antigen. Helper T lymphocytes will also "help" specific B lymphocytes to produce thyroid autoantibodies, which may add to the pathologic process. Certainly, thyroid-stimulating hormone (*TSH*) receptor autoantibodies play a major role in causing either thyroid stimulation (thyroid-stimulating antibody in Graves disease) or thyroid inhibition. Thyroid-stimulating antibody or TSH will enhance IFN-γ–induced thyrocyte HLA–DR expression and also increase thyroid antigen presentation, thus further stimulating helper T lymphocytes. Excess thyroid hormone further reduces nonspecific suppressor T-lymphocyte function and numbers, thus allowing further helper T-lymphocyte activation. These secondary processes thus tend to self-perpetuate the disease. (Reproduced from Volpé R. Immunology of autoimmune thyroid disease. In Volpé R, ed. The autoimmune endocrinopathies. Contemporary Endocrinology Series. Totowa, NJ: Humana Press, 1999:217.)

or HT and normal persons.[54] In animal models of AITD, there is also increasing evidence for a role for regulatory T lymphocytes in many studies.[14] The antigen-specific regulatory cell defect, which is partial or relative,[50–54] may be due to an abnormality of specific antigen presentation, resulting in reduced specific regulatory cell activation (Fig. 197-2). Whether antigen can be presented directly from thyroid follicular cells that lack some costimulators, or require professional APCs, has not been definitively settled.[20]

## THE ROLE OF THE ANTIGEN

There is no evidence for an alteration in the thyroid antigen.[2,13] AITD appears to be primarily a disorder of immunoregulation, with the organ dysfunction resulting from an antigen-specific attack mounted by inadequately suppressed lymphocytes directed toward these specific cellular targets. Certainly, the antigen must be available and presented to the T lymphocytes for this assault to occur. This requires expression of HLA-DR antigens on the APC[55]; this includes not only macrophages and dendritic cells, but thyroid cells can also express class I and class II antigens, although this may not be sufficient to present antigen directly[2,20]; however, it is now evident that thyrocyte HLA-DR expression is a secondary event, and that macrophages, lymphocytes, and the production of interferon-γ are all necessary for the thyroid cells to express HLA-DR after the initiation of the immune assault.[13] It has been suggested that the thyroid cell might be damaged by some external stimulus, then express HLA-DR as a consequence, and, thus, precipitate AITD,[12] but this notion does not withstand close scrutiny.[13] Rather, the evidence is consistent with the idea that the thyroid cell is initially normal, and expresses HLA-DR (as well as heat shock protein-72 and intercellular adhesion molecule-1, further amplifying the immune disorder[56]) as *consequences* of the immune disturbance. The notion that the primary event might be infective[11,12] is entirely speculative; the author has argued that the thyroid cell is a passive captive to immunologic events in AITD[13] and has postulated that the condition results from a disorder in immunoregulation, with environmental factors precipitating the disease by virtue of nonspecific effects on the immune system,[4] adding to the genetically induced specific partial defect.

## GENETIC CONTROL OF THE IMMUNE RESPONSE[5,6,10]

In mice, genes that map in the region that corresponds to the HLA-D locus in humans are responsible for controlling the response of T lymphocytes to a given antigen. In humans, GD is associated with HLA-DR3 (whites), while goitrous HT is associated with HLA-DR5, and atrophic thyroiditis with HLA-DR3. However, persons bearing HLA-DR3 have only a moderate increase of relative risk (three-fold); thus, this clearly does not represent the "disease susceptibility gene." The frequency of subjects positive for HLA-DQAl*0501 is significantly increased among white GD patients, markedly increasing the relative risk.[57] Patients with an autoimmune response to the TSH receptor (involving either stimulating or blocking antibodies) are genetically different in terms of HLA from patients whose thyroid autoimmune response does not involve TSH-R antibodies.[58] Nonetheless, other genes are undoubtedly involved in the pathogenesis of these disorders, but these are not well defined, and their role is not understood.[10,58]

## NATURE OF THE REMISSION OF GRAVES DISEASE

More than one form of clinical remission occurs in GD.[2] Surgical or [131]I destruction of sufficient tissue may prevent recurrence. Conversely, continuous immunologic thyroid destruction may bring about clinical remission, or even hypothyroidism. The latter may also result from a change in the nature of a TSH-R antibody from a stimulating to a blocking antibody.[2] Another important form of remission is one in which all immunologic stigmata of the disease disappear, including thyroid antibodies, TSAb, and evidence of sensitization of T lymphocytes.[59]

This form of remission may occur only in patients with a less severe defect in immunoregulation; in such patients, hyperthyroidism is initiated by some environmental insult acting on the immune system, converting an occult specific regulatory T-lymphocyte defect to an overt one. This is reversible when that circumstance is overcome. The restoration of an euthyroid state by whatever means (antithyroid drugs, [131]I, or surgery) should further relieve the situation because the effects of hyperthyroidism on the immune system would be reversed under these circumstances. Moreover, rest, the passage of time, the clearing of infection, the use of sedation, and other nonspecific measures each will serve to allow the partially defective immunoregulatory system to be restored to its previous functional capacity.[2,20]

Those persons with a presumed severe defect would not be expected to enter an immunologic remission, no matter how long their antithyroid drugs were continued. Only those remissions associated with spontaneous or iatrogenic thyroid destruction would occur in this group.

## IMPLICATIONS FOR THERAPY FOR GRAVES DISEASE

The understanding of the immune nature of GD has led to few changes in its management. Since patients with very large goiters rarely achieve immunologic remission, some selection for long-term antithyroid drug therapy can be made. It has been claimed that the antithyroid drugs are, themselves, immunosuppressive.[60,61] It is difficult, however, to reconcile this proposal with the fact that many patients continue to manifest immunologic activity throughout the course of treatment, no matter what dosage of antithyroid drug is used, and no matter how well the hyperthyroidism is controlled. It is also difficult to comprehend, because of the short duration of action of the drugs, how a long-term remission after cessation of therapy would persist. Moreover, the normalization of thyroid function is attended by normalization of the suppressor/helper T-lymphocyte ratio.[2] Thus, it seems more likely that the action of the antithyroid drugs on thyroid cells, normalizing all thyroid cell functions and restoring euthyroidism, is more decisive in bringing about remission than any direct immunosuppressive effect.[62] Indeed, evidence indicates that antithyroid drugs bring about remissions by a direct effect on thyrocytes, reducing thyrocyte-immunocyte signaling.[63,64]

The use of [131]I therapy de novo also is associated with immunologic perturbations, namely, a transient rise in TSAb and other thyroid autoantibodies, followed by an ultimate decline.[2] This may be due to the liberation of thyroid antigens, stimulating the already disturbed immune system.

Finally, subtotal thyroidectomy is often associated with a decline in TSAb activity, perhaps because most of the offending thyroid-committed lymphocytes are removed with the gland.[2] Recurrences after surgery would have to be associated with (a) sufficient remaining thyroid parenchyma to respond to TSAb and (b) sufficient remaining thyroid-committed lymphocytes to mount the immune attack.

The ophthalmopathy of GD is not discussed in these pages at length, since its pathophysiology is poorly understood, and there are no immune assays that are considered of general credence for use in diagnosis and management (see Chap. 43). However, the consensus is that the target cell is the retroorbital fibroblast, and the TSH-R is the chief candidate for an antigen that would cross-react with that cell.[1]

# THE IMMUNOLOGY OF TYPE 1 DIABETES

## GENETICS

It is evident that type 1 diabetes tends to aggregate in certain families and, thus, is genetically induced (see Chap. 136). The concordance rate in identical twins is ~50%; the disparity of the age at onset in the concordant twins suggests that the disease seems to occur at random in those predisposed to develop the disease.[1,2,65–67] This implies that there is, first, a genetic factor and, second, a nongenetic factor. This has prompted the search for environmental factors in the development of this disease, such as viruses, drugs, nutritional factors, and so forth. The most compelling evidence that this disease in humans could be caused by a virus was the finding of a Coxsackie virus B4, isolated from a child who had died with diabetic ketoacidosis and overwhelming viral infection.[68] However, a pathologic examination of the islets of Langerhans of this child demonstrated evidence of previous chronic B-cell damage that had preceded the acute viral infection.[69] (See also ref. 69a.)

Although there are experimental models that indicate that viruses may induce diabetes mellitus in vulnerable animals by infecting the islets, the evidence in humans is not compelling.[1,2,65–67] It is of considerable interest, however, that ~20% of children with congenital rubella will develop diabetes mellitus in later life.[65–67,70] This diabetes is somewhat atypical, in that it is often non–insulin dependent, although it usually does occur in patients who are HLA-DR3 and/or DR4 positive, many of whom express islet cell antibodies. In these cases, the diabetes does not occur at the time of the infection, but years later, and the same children have a high incidence of thyroid autoantibodies. It is likely that this is not because of viral-induced target cell damage, but is due to an effect of viruses on the immune system in genetically predisposed individuals. Another putative environmental factor may be a bovine albumin peptide found in cow's milk that cross-reacts with islet cell antigen, and has been proposed as a precipitating factor in inducing type 1 diabetes in susceptible individuals.[71] This hypothesis has been refuted.[72]

The genetic predisposition relates to genes in the region of the HLA-DR alleles residing on chromosome 6. Type 1 diabetes is associated with the HLA alleles DR3 and DR4.[5,6,73,74] Approximately 95% of persons with type 1 diabetes are positive for these alleles, as opposed to 40% of normal persons. Moreover, when siblings are identical for the HLA genes, the risk of diabetes is increased 90-fold, whereas a sibling having only one of the HLA loci in common with the diabetic sibling possesses a 37-fold increased risk.[73,74] On the other hand, an HLA-nonidentical sibling has a risk for this disease similar to that of the general population. As with AITD, however, the presence of these genes does not ensure the development of type 1 diabetes, because 40% of the population have these same genes and only a small proportion of them develop diabetes, unless they happen to be members of families in whom diabetes is already present. Moreover, there are patients with this disease who have neither DR3 nor DR4 alleles. Thus, it is believed that the diabetogenic genes reside close to these genes in linkage disequilibrium with them. In most whites with type 1 diabetes, HLA-DQ^beta sequences tend to share the common

characteristic of not encoding aspartic acid at the 57-amino-acid position of the HLA-DQ^beta peptide chain.[73] However, the HLA-DQ 3.2 (DQ^beta 1*0302) gene has been found to be the most prevalent susceptibility gene in white patients with this illness,[74] with a relative risk of 8. It, thus, is a susceptibility gene, but not sufficient by itself to precipitate the disease. Other genetic and environmental factors are required to add to this susceptibility, conspiring to induce type 1 diabetes. Patients with this illness often manifest autoantibodies to other organs, with an increased incidence of certain other organ-specific autoimmune diseases, most commonly AITD; these are generally related to HLA-DR3 alleles.

## IMMUNE PHENOMENA

In most patients with type 1 diabetes, the appearance of islet cell antibodies precedes overt diabetes, sometimes by many years, and occult changes in glucose metabolism may precede the overt expression of this condition.[65-67] Various anti-islet cell antibodies (ICA) have been described, with various methods of detection[75,76] (Table 197-5). Several groups have reported that up to 80% of patients have these antibodies at or before the onset of the disease.[77,78] Indeed, the presence of ICA combined with a decrease in the first phase of insulin secretion (<25 µu/mL) is predictive of the development of type 1 diabetes within 12 months, with a 95% probability.[79] However, some relatives who have developed such antibodies have not progressed to overt diabetes.[80] Nevertheless, of relatives with a single positive ICA test, 50% will develop this disease within 10 years.[81,82] The predictive value for health of negative ICA results is ~99%.[82] Strongly positive and persistent ICA (>40 JDF u) is the best predictor of forthcoming type 1 diabetes, particularly when combined with decreased insulin secretion.[83–86] The predictive value of ICA for development of type 1 diabetes within 10 years in first-degree relatives of patients with this illness increases from 40% at low levels of ICA to 100% at high levels, whereas the sensitivity is 88% at low levels and 31% at high levels.[85] Thus, the risk of this disease in relatives of propositi increases with the titer of ICA, is greater in multiplex families, and is increased in those <10 years of age with positive ICA.[86] It may also be noted that positive ICA values correlate with the rapid loss of C-peptide

**TABLE 197-5.**
**Major Islet Cell Antigens**

| Antigen | Localization | Autoantibody Assay | Significance |
|---|---|---|---|
| ICA antigen (?glycolipid) | All islet cells | Indirect immunofluorescence on frozen sections of human pancreas | ICA is the original immune marker of recent-onset and preclinical type 1 diabetes, but the chemical nature of the antigen remains an enigma. |
| Insulin | B cells | Immunoprecipitation of $^{125}$I-labeled insulin | Insulin autoantibodies in >50% of subjects with late preclinical and recent-onset type 1 diabetes; predominantly younger children in whom they denote a faster rate of B-cell destruction. |
| 65 kDa/GAD | B cells ?All islet cells (GAD also in neurons, testis, ovary) | Immunoprecipitation and ELISA | Positive in up to 80% of subjects with preclinical type 1 diabetes. |
| 37-kDa/40-kDa tryptic fragments of 64 kDa (not GAD) | B cells | Immunoprecipitation | Autoantibodies in up to 30% of preclinical and recent-onset type 1 diabetes subjects. |
|  | ?All islet cells |  | True prevalence and specificity unknown. |
| 38 kDa (protein partially purified from insulin secretory granule membrane) | Neuroendocrine secretory cell granule | Immunoprecipitation and immunoblotting | Target of T-lymphocyte lines generated from peripheral blood of subjects with recent-onset type 1 diabetes. |
| 52 kDa (carboxypeptidase H) | Neuroendocrine secretory cell granule | Screening of neonatal rat islet cDNA expression library with serum | Autoantibodies in 5 of 20 preclinical and 0 of 14 control subjects. True prevalence and disease specificity unknown. |

*cDNA*, complementary DNA; *ELISA*, enzyme-linked immunosorbent assay; *GAD*, glutamic acid decarboxylase; *ICA*, islet cell antigen.
(From Harrison LC. Islet cell antigens in insulin-dependent diabetes: Pandora's box revisited. Immunol Today 1992; 13:348.)

secretory capacity in newly diagnosed type 1 diabetes patients.[87] Conversely, not all patients who develop overt diabetes are positive for these antibodies.[88,89] The islet cell antibodies may be markers of ongoing B-cell destruction, but it is unlikely that they are pathogenic themselves. It is more likely that cytotoxic T lymphocytes, in conjunction with macrophages, induce the B-cell damage directly, with mediation by cytokines produced locally by the immunocytes.[90]

Although the responsible antigen has not been determined, a number of candidate autoantigens have been identified[75,76] (see Table 197-5), with GAD-65 as the leading contender.[91] This is an enzyme that catalyzes the conversion of glutamic acid to γ-aminobutyric acid (GABA), the major inhibitory neurotransmitter in the central nervous system.[76] The response of diabetic T lymphocytes to GAD-65 directly reflects the risk of progression of clinical type 1 diabetes.[92] However, it is not clear that antibodies to GAD have the same predictive value, since an inverse correlation of T-cell responses to GAD and antibodies to GAD have been shown.[76,92] In the acute, active phase of type 1 diabetes, there is an increase in activated T lymphocytes expressing the HLA-DR (Ia) antigen.[65-67,93] Indeed, there is evidence of aberrant expression of HLA-DR antigens on the cell surface of some B cells in this illness[93]; there is increasing evidence that HLA-DR expression on target cells is secondary to the immune assault itself, and, thus, is an intermediate step, rather than a primary precipitant.[13] The in vitro migration of lymphocytes from type 1 diabetic patients is inhibited by preparations of mammalian, including human, islets.[44,94] In studies with lymphocytes from such patients, there is evidence of lymphocyte-mediated cytotoxicity against an insulinoma cell line, and of inhibition of insulin release by isolated mouse islets.[95]

## EVIDENCE FOR AN ORGAN-SPECIFIC DEFECT IN IMMUNOSUPPRESSION

In the thymus and spleen of prediabetic nonobese diabetic (NOD) mice, there are CD4 immunoregulatory T cells that prevent diabetes onset in cotransfer experiments.[94] These suppressor cells are wiped out by thymectomy performed at 3 weeks of age and by administration of cyclophosphamide.[62] These regulatory T cells are presumably of the $T_H2$ type.

Studies on nonspecific and specific suppressor cell function in animal models and human type 1 diabetes have been performed.[46,94-99] Antigen-specific suppressor cell function was evaluated by suppressor cell activation with guinea pig islet cell homogenate, and measurement of cell proliferation rates demonstrated that specific suppressor cell activity was lower than that in the control population.[97]

T lymphocytes from patients with type 1 diabetes have been mixed with T lymphocytes from patients with GD in the migration inhibition factor (MIF) test,[46] to observe the response to human thyroid antigen, on the one hand, and to human islet cell antigen, on the other. Lymphocytes from the diabetic patients alone produced MIF in response to islet cell antigen, but this was abrogated when T lymphocytes from GD patients (positive alone in the MIF system against thyroid antigen but negative against islet cell antigen) were added. Thus, the Graves lymphocytes acted as "normal" T lymphocytes in inhibiting the diabetic lymphocytic response to islet cell antigen. Indeed, T lymphocytes from normal persons, but not those from other diabetic patients, also abrogate MIF production when added to the original diabetic T lymphocytes in response to the islet cell antigen. This would support the view that there is an organ-specific defect in suppressor T lymphocyte function in type 1 diabetic patients that is separate from that of GD.[46] Mention has been made in the section on AITD (see earlier) that there is reduced activation of diabetic suppressor T lymphocytes by GAD-65 (the

putative B-cell antigen), which is specific for this condition; these cells respond to irrelevant antigen normally.[54] Other investigators have shown that the cytotoxic effect on isolated rat islets of lymphocytes from newly diagnosed type 1 diabetics could be abolished by the addition of lymphocytes from healthy persons, but not by lymphocytes from other diabetic patients.[98] This also accords with the hypothesis of an organ-specific suppressor T-cell defect in type 1 diabetes.

In animal models of type 1 diabetes, there is also convincing evidence for a similar abnormality of suppressor T-cell function.[99] Such an abnormality may prove to be fundamental to the pathogenesis of the disease.

## GENERALIZED SUPPRESSOR T-LYMPHOCYTE FUNCTION

Some reports have indicated that there is a reduction in generalized suppressor T-lymphocyte function or numbers in the early phases of diabetes mellitus, but this appears to normalize as the disease stabilizes.[65-67] This may be analogous to the similar situation seen in severe hyperthyroidism. Conceivably, such generalized reductions in suppressor T-lymphocyte function or numbers may arise from some preceding stress or may be secondary to the stress of the metabolic disease itself. Stress may prove to be an important factor because it may be additive and superimposed on the organ-specific defect and, thereby, may act as a precipitant or a perpetuating factor, later subsiding as the environmental and metabolic disturbances abate. There is no convincing evidence for a target cell abnormality that precedes the disease. Similar to the thyroid cell in AITD, the B cells may be passive captives to immune events. The combination of an antigen-specific reduction in activation of suppressor T cells, plus the addition of any generalized disturbance in nonspecific suppressor T-cell function or numbers (resulting from variable environmental factors, such as stress, infection, trauma, and the like), could act additively to precipitate the disease. Thus, there is no need to invoke an antigenic disturbance in this theory. This would be in accord with the observation on transplanted pancreatic segments from three normal monozygotic twins (>15 years discordant) to their diabetic twinmates.[100] No immunosuppressive therapy was provided because the recipients were monozygotic twins. At first the diabetic state cleared, but within 4 months, lymphocytic infiltration appeared in the grafts, with B-cell destruction. Thus, without any apparent antigenic stimulation other than the presence of the normal islets, the immune system still was abnormal and capable of reestablishing the disease.

## IMMUNOTHERAPY

Interestingly, a fourth twin in the foregoing study, who also had been transplanted with a pancreatic segment, was treated prophylactically with azathioprine after the transplantation, and the diabetic state did not recur.[99] This raises the issue of immunotherapy in the treatment of type 1 diabetes, before total destruction of the B cells has occurred. Because B-cell destruction does proceed at a subclinical level for years before the onset of overt diabetes, it clearly would be of importance to predict which person is going to develop diabetes and to commence therapy before B-cell destruction is complete. This may soon be possible with new means of detecting antibodies or T-lymphocyte response to islet cell antigens, such as GAD-65.[92] It is well known that cyclosporine, an immunosuppressive agent, when given to newly diagnosed diabetic patients, will suppress the diabetic process, despite the considerable B-cell loss that has already occurred.[101] Azathioprine has also proved similarly useful.[102,103] Indeed, insulin administration itself, given before the development of frank type 1 diabetes, might prevent or delay the onset by "resting" the B cells and reducing the presentation of their antigens.[102,104] Immunotherapy with other models (e.g., T-cell vaccination,[105,106] and oral vaccination with myelin basic protein[107]) is being investigated. Vaccination with GAD-65 to susceptible, but not yet diabetic, mice has prevented the development of type 1 diabetes.[108,109] This is an exciting development in the quest for a means to prevent this very serious malady.

## INSULIN RESISTANCE DUE TO INSULIN-RECEPTOR ANTIBODIES

Brief mention should be made of this rare entity, which is not genetically related to type 1 diabetes or the other organ-specific endocrinopathies. It is termed *type B insulin resistance* and may be associated with profound hyperglycemia and acanthosis nigricans, although occasionally hypoglycemia may be noted when the insulin-receptor antibodies manifest an agonist, rather than antagonist, effect on insulin action.[110] However, insulin-receptor antibodies may be seen in occasional type 1 diabetic patients.[111]

# AUTOIMMUNE DISEASES OF ADRENALS, GONADS, PARATHYROIDS, AND PITUITARY

## ADDISON DISEASE

The original description by Addison[112] of 11 examples of this disorder included cases now recognized as idiopathic (now known to be autoimmune) adrenal atrophy, as well as tuberculosis of the adrenal gland and metastatic carcinoma. Although tuberculosis once accounted for most patients with Addison disease (see Chap. 213), autoimmune adrenalitis has become the most common form of this condition in Western countries.

There is ample evidence supporting an autoimmune basis for this disease.[1,2,18,113] The evidence derives from the histology of the disorder, the finding of autoantibodies against the adrenal cortex in many patients with this condition, the association with other organ-specific autoimmune disease, study of HLA antigens, genetic studies, and experimental observations.[1,2,18,113,113a]

In the human disease, both adrenal glands are found to be very small, and difficult to locate at autopsy. The capsule is generally thickened and the cortex is usually completely destroyed. The remaining adrenocortical cells may be single or in small clusters. A mononuclear cell infiltration is invariable, with lymphocytes, plasma cells, macrophages, and, occasionally, germinal centers. The few remaining parenchymal cells are surrounded by the heaviest infiltration of lymphocytes, and a variable amount of fibrosis is evident.[1,2,18,113]

### HUMORAL IMMUNITY

Antiadrenal antibodies are detectable in approximately two-thirds of patients with autoimmune Addison disease.[1,2,18,113] The means of detection have included the complement fixation test and immunofluorescence, but with identification of the actual antigens (21-hydroxylase in the adult disease and 17-hydroxylase in the type I childhood Addison disease),[18,113] Western blotting has been utilized. The adrenal antibodies tend to be more common in those patients with a short duration of disease, and in those who develop the disorder at an early age. The titers of adrenal antibodies are much lower than for thyroid or gastric antibodies in patients with AITD or pernicious anemia, respectively, but they may persist for many years after ade-

quate medical therapy. Such antibodies are found very rarely in the control population and are also quite rare in first-degree relatives of patients with Addison disease (providing that these relatives do not have idiopathic hypoparathyroidism). In "idiopathic" hypoparathyroidism, adrenal antibodies occur in 25% to 30% of patients.

In patients with Addison disease who have antiadrenal antibodies, there also may be antibodies that react with ovary, testis, and steroid-producing cells in the placenta. This cross-reacting antibody may be associated with primary ovarian failure. Although these are IgG antibodies and, therefore, can cross the placenta, there is no evidence that they cause damage to the fetal adrenal glands.

In patients with autoimmune Addison disease, there is a high prevalence of antibodies to other organ antigens, including not only steroid-producing cells, but also parathyroid, thyroid, islet cell antigens, or gastric antigens. There is also a higher prevalence of other overt organ-specific autoimmune diseases associated with these same antibodies (Table 197-6). Thus, in patients with autoimmune adrenal disease, careful consideration should be given to the probability that there will be other organ-specific autoimmune diseases, either in an overt or occult (serologic) form.

### GENETIC STUDIES

Autoimmune Addison disease tends to be familial. It generally is considered to be an autosomal recessive characteristic, although the inheritance has not been completely settled. There is an increased incidence of HLA-B8 and DR3 in whites, similar to that seen with GD. This is true, however, only with patients who do not have generalized candidiasis and hypoparathyroidism.

### OVARIAN FAILURE

Approximately 25% of women with autoimmune Addison disease have premature menopause or amenorrhea.[1,2,113] Most of these have circulating antibodies against steroid-secreting cells. Such antibodies are almost never detected in patients with amenorrhea that is not associated with Addison disease. The question

**TABLE 197-6.**

**Associated Organ-Specific Autoimmune Diseases in Patients with Autoimmune Adrenalitis (Addison Disease)**

| Associated Disorders | Middlesex Hospital Series | | Edinburgh Series | |
|---|---|---|---|---|
| | *No.* | *%* | *No.* | *%* |
| Primary ovarian failure | 25 | 8 | 51 | 18 |
| Thyroid disease | (56) | (19) | (46) | (16) |
| Primary thyrotoxicosis | 20 | 7 | 21 | 7 |
| Primary myxedema | 33 | 11 | 20 | 7 |
| Goitrous autoimmune thyroiditis | 3 | 1 | 5 | 2 |
| Insulin-dependent diabetes mellitus | 45 | 15 | 27 | 9 |
| Idiopathic parathyroid deficiency | 12 | 4 | 16 | 5.5 |
| Pernicious anemia | 7 | 2 | 12 | 4 |
| Positive prolactin-cell antibodies (?subclinical hypophysitis) | (12) | (4) | * | * |
| Number of patients affected | 118† | 40 | 106 | 37 |
| Total number of patients | 294 | | 289 | |

*Not tested.
†Discrepancy in numbers due to polyendocrine cases.
(From Doniach D, Bottazzo GF. Polyendocrine immune disease. In: Franklin EC, ed. Clinical immunology update. New York: Elsevier–North Holland, 1981:96; and Irvine WJ. Polyendocrine immune disease. In: Besser GM, ed. Advanced medicine, vol 13. Tunbridge Wells, England: Pittman, 1977:115.)

arises whether autoimmune gonadal failure is a closely associated, but separate, organ-specific autoimmune disease, or whether it results from cross-reactive antigens shared by gonads and adrenals. Certainly, some steroid cell antibodies are cross-reactive between adrenal, gonadal, and placental antigens. This would also explain the finding of antiovarian antibodies in some males with autoimmune adrenal failure. Sensitized T lymphocytes may be similarly cross-reactive.[1,2] In some instances, however, premature menopause, which is only occasionally of proven autoimmune etiology, may not be related to Addison disease.

Histologic features of the ovaries of patients with amenorrhea associated with autoimmune Addison disease will show lymphocytic infiltration and fibrous tissue, similar to that seen in AITD. Autoimmune testicular failure associated with Addison disease is uncommon; it generally is associated with polyendocrine autoimmune failure related to candidiasis and hypoparathyroidism.

## HYPOPARATHYROIDISM

Autoimmune hypoparathyroidism occurs mostly in children and adolescents, and is often associated with mucocutaneous candidiasis (type I polyendocrine autoimmune disease). Thus, it frequently is associated with Addison disease and other organ-specific autoimmune (see Chaps. 60 and 70) diseases.[1]

The pathologic picture is characterized by lymphocytic infiltration and atrophy. Antiparathyroid antibodies and evidence for cell-mediated immunity have been demonstrated.[1]

## HYPOPHYSITIS

There are an increasing number of cases of autoimmune hypophysitis being reported, all in women between the third and eighth decade.[2,114] In many of these patients, the diagnosis was made at autopsy. A conspicuous feature of this condition has been its association with pregnancy and the postpartum state. In many of the reported cases, the disease was detected after delivery, with the longest interval after gestation being 14 months. Possibly, cases that have been diagnosed as postpartum Sheehan syndrome may instead be examples of postpartum autoimmune pituitary disease, developing insidiously during and after pregnancy. Another prominent feature of autoimmune lymphocytic hypophysitis has been its association with other organ-specific autoimmune disorders, such as HT, adrenalitis, and pernicious anemia (see Chaps. 11 and 17).

## AUTOIMMUNE POLYENDOCRINE DISEASE

Theoretically, any patient with one expressed autoimmune endocrine disease showing serologic reactivity with another organ should be considered as potentially belonging to the polyendocrinopathies.[115,115a] Although many of these target organs are indeed endocrine glands, other nonendocrine organ-specific autoimmune diseases that are associated in increased frequency include pernicious anemia, myasthenia gravis, Sjögren disease, vitiligo, alopecia areata, chronic active hepatitis, idiopathic thrombocytopenic purpura, and rheumatoid arthritis.[116-119] Those patients with overt autoimmune diseases of these organs would belong to the categories depicted in Table 197-7.[115]

Of the categories listed in Table 197-7, only categories II and III are associated with definite HLA genes.[115] Category I, which seems to be the most severe form of autoimmune polyglandular endocrine failure, does not have any particular HLA type and generally occurs in children. Indeed, the inheritance has now been assigned to chromosome 21q22.3 (i.e., not part of the HLA system).[120] Possibly, in this condition, the putative suppressor T-

**TABLE 197-7.**
**Classification of Polyendocrine Autoimmune Disease**

I. Candidiasis, hypoparathyroidism, Addison disease (2 or 3 present)

II. Addison disease and thyroid autoimmune disease and/or type 1 diabetes mellitus

III. **a.** Thyroid autoimmune disease and type 1 diabetes mellitus

   **b.** Thyroid autoimmune disease and pernicious anemia

   **c.** Thyroid autoimmune disease and vitiligo and/or alopecia and/or other organ-specific autoimmune diseases not falling into the above categories

(From Neufeld M, Blizzard RM. Polyglandular autoimmune disease. In: Pinchera A, ed. Autoimmune aspects of endocrine disorders. New York: Academic Press, 1980:357.)

lymphocyte defect is more severe and more nonspecific than that seen in the other entities.

There are various other, rarer, polyendocrine autoimmune syndromes, such as central diabetes insipidus, autoimmune enteropathy, autoimmunity to gut hormone-secreting cells, and autoimmunity directed against specific prolactin cells in the anterior pituitary.[115]

The observation that all of the disorders listed in Table 197-1 have a close association with one another and often are associated with specific HLA genes suggests a very similar pathogenesis for all these autoimmune entities. It may well be that each disease has separate genes, and each a separate organ-specific defect in immunoregulation. Probably, the defect is an organ-specific abnormality in regulatory T-lymphocyte function, which is specific for each disease. The fact that some persons develop two or more diseases may relate to the inheritance of more than one closely related gene, or sets of genes. Nonetheless, much remains to be learned before these disorders are fully understood.[117,119]

## REFERENCES

1. Volpé R. The autoimmune endocrinopathies. Contemporary Endocrinology Series. Totowa, NJ: Humana Press, 1999:1.
2. Volpé R. Autoimmune diseases of the endocrine system. Boca Raton, FL: CRC Press, 1990:1.
3. Davies TF. Autoimmune endocrine disease. New York: John Wiley and Sons, 1983:1.
4. Plotnikoff N, Murgo A, Faith R, Wybran J. Stress and immunity. Boca Raton, FL: CRC Press, 1991:1.
5. Nepom GT, Erlich H. MHC class II molecules and autoimmunity. Ann Rev Immunol 1990; 90:493.
6. Nagataki S, Yamashita S, Tamai H. Immunogenetics of autoimmune endocrine disease. In: Volpé R, ed. Autoimmune diseases of the endocrine system. Boca Raton, FL: CRC Press, 1990:51.
7. Wachtel SS, Koo GC, Boyce EA. Evolutionary conservation of HY male antigen. Nature 1975; 254:270.
8. Kovacs W, Olsen N. Sex and autoimmune disease. In: Volpé R, ed. The autoimmune endocrinopathies. Contemporary Endocrinology Series. Totowa, NJ: Humana Press, 1999:183.
9. Svejgaard A, Platz P, Ryder LR. HLA and endocrine disease. In: Volpé R, ed. Autoimmunity in endocrine disease. New York: Marcel Dekker Inc, 1985:93.
10. Tomer Y, Steinberg D, Davies TF. Immunogenetics of autoimmune endocrine disease. In: Volpé R, ed. The autoimmune endocrinopathies. Contemporary Endocrinology Series. Totowa, NJ: Humana Press, 1999:57.
11. Tomer Y, Davies TF. Infection, thyroid disease and autoimmunity. Endocr Rev 1993; 14:107.
12. Martin A, Davies TF. T cells in human autoimmune thyroid disease: emerging data show lack of need to invoke suppressor T cell problems. Thyroid 1992; 2:247.
13. Volpé R. A perspective on human autoimmune thyroid disease: is there an abnormality of the target cell which predisposes to the disorder? Autoimmunity 1992; 12:3.
14. Volpé R. Suppressor T lymphocyte dysfunction is important in the pathogenesis of autoimmune thyroid disease. Thyroid 1993; 3:345.
15. Volpé R. Immunoregulation in autoimmune thyroid disease. Thyroid 1994; 4:157.
16. Iwatani Y. Normal mechanisms for tolerance. In: Volpé R, ed. The autoimmune endocrinopathies. Contemporary Endocrinology Series. Totowa, NJ: Humana Press, 1999:1.
17. Ishimura H, Kuchroo V, Abramson-Leeman S, Dorf ME. Comparison between helper and suppressor cell induction. Immunol Rev 1988; 106:93.

18. Drexhage HA. Autoimmune adrenocortical failure. In: Volpé R, ed. The autoimmune endocrinopathies. Contemporary Endocrinology Series. Totowa, NJ: Humana Press, 1999:309.

19. Murakami M, Miyashita K, Monden T, et al. Evidence that a soluble form of TSH receptor is present in the peripheral blood of patients with Graves' disease. In: Nagataki S, Mori T, Torizuka K, eds. 80 Years of Hashimoto disease. Amsterdam: Elsevier, 1993:683.

20. Volpé R. Immunology of autoimmune thyroid disease. In: Volpé R, ed. The autoimmune endocrinopathies. Contemporary Endocrinology Series. Totowa, NJ: Humana Press, 1999:217.

21. Weetman AP, McGregor AM. Autoimmune thyroid disease: further developments in our understanding. Endocr Rev 1994; 15:788.

22. Burman KD, Baker JR. Immune mechanisms in Graves' disease. Endocr Rev 1985; 6:183.

23. Hashimoto H. Zue Kenntnis der lymphomatosen Veranderung der Schilddruse (Struma lymphomatosa). Arch Klin Chir 1912; 97:219.

24. McGregor AM, Weetman AP, Ratanachaiyavong S, et al. Iodine: an influence on the development of autoimmune thyroid disease? In: Hall R, Kobberling J, eds. Thyroid disorders associated with iodine deficiency and excess. New York: Raven Press, 1985:209.

25. Sundick RS, Bagchi N, Brown TR. Mechanisms by which iodine induces autoimmunity. In: Drexhage HA, de Vijlder JJM, Wiersinga WM, eds. The thyroid gland, environment and autoimmunity. Amsterdam: Elsevier Science, 1990:13.

26. Helfand M, Redfern CC. Screening for thyroid disease: an update. Ann Intern Med 1998; 129:144.

27. Dayan CM. The natural history of autoimmune thyroiditis: how normal is autoimmunity? Proc R Coll Physicians Edinb 1996; 26:419.

28. Roitt IM, Doniach D, Campbell RN, Hudson RV. Autoantibodies in Hashimoto's disease (lymphadenoid goitre). Lancet 1956; 2:820.

29. Rose NR, Witebsky E. Studies on organ specificity: V. Changes in the thyroid glands of rabbits following active immunization with rabbit thyroid extracts. J Immunol 1956; 76:417.

30. Adams DD, Purves HD. Abnormal responses in the assay of thyrotrophin. Univ Otago Med School Proc 1956; 34:11.

31. McKenzie JM. Humoral factors in the pathogenesis of Graves' disease. Physiol Rev 1968; 48:252.

32. Nagayama Y, Wadsworth HL, Russo D, et al. Binding domains of stimulatory and inhibitory thyrotropin (TSH) receptor autoantibodies determined with chimeric TSH-lutropin/chorionic gonadotropic receptors. J Clin Invest 1991; 88:336.

33. Wolf M, Misaki T, Bech K, et al. Immunoglobulins of patients recovering from *Yersinia enterocolitica* infections exhibit Graves'-like activity in human thyroid membranes. Thyroid 1991; 1:315.

34. Nordyke RA, Gilbert FI, Miyamoto LA, Fleury KA. The superiority of antimicrosomal over antithyroglobulin antibodies for detecting Hashimoto's thyroiditis. Arch Intern Med 1993; 153:862.

35. Haubruck H, Mauch L, Cook NJ, et al. Expression of recombinant thyroid peroxidase by the bacillovirus system and its use in ELISA screening for diagnosis of autoimmune thyroid disease. Autoimmunity 1993; 15:275.

36. Bagnasco M, Pesce G. Autoimmune thyroid disease: immunological model and clinical problem. Fundam Clin Immunol 1996; 4:7.

37. Resetkova E, Nishikawa M, Mukuta T, et al. Homing of $^{51}$Cr-labelled human peripheral lymphocytes to Graves' disease tissue xenografted into SCID mice. Thyroid 1995; 5:293.

38. Davies TF, Concepcion ES, Ben-Nun A, et al. T cell receptor V gene use in AITD: direct assessment by thyroid aspiration. J Clin Endocrinol Metab 1993; 76:660.

39. Volpé R, Row VV. Role of antigen-specific suppressor T lymphocytes in the pathogenesis of autoimmune thyroid disease. In: Walfish PG, Wall JR, Volpé R, eds. Autoimmunity and the thyroid. Orlando, FL: Academic Press, 1985:79.

40. Gerstein H, Rastogi B, Iwatani Y, et al. The decrease in nonspecific suppressor T lymphocytes in female hyperthyroid patients is secondary to the hyperthyroidism. Clin Invest Med 1987; 10:337.

41. Grubeck-Loebenstein B, Derfler K, Kassal H, et al. Immunological features of non-immunogenic hyperthyroidism. J Clin Endocrinol Metab 1984; 60:150.

42. Okita N, Row VV, Volpé R. Suppressor T lymphocyte deficiency in Graves' disease and Hashimoto's thyroiditis. J Clin Endocrinol Metab 1981; 52:528.

43. Topliss DJ, Okita N, Lewis M, et al. Allosuppressor T lymphocytes abolish migration inhibition factor production in autoimmune thyroid disease: evidence from radiosensitivity experiments. Clin Endocrinol 1981; 15:335.

44. Topliss DJ, How J, Lewis M, et al. Evidence for cell-mediated immunity and specific suppressor T lymphocyte dysfunction in Graves' disease and diabetes mellitus. J Clin Endocrinol Metab 1983; 57:700.

45. Vento S, Hegarty JE, Bottazzo GF, et al. Antigen-specific suppressor cell function in autoimmune chronic active hepatitis. Lancet 1984; 1:1200.

46. Vento S, O'Brien CJ, Cundy T, et al. Cellular immunity and specific defects of T-cell suppression in patients with autoimmune thyroid disorders. In: Pinchera A, Ingbar SH, McKenzie JM, Fenzi GF, eds. Thyroid autoimmunity. New York: Plenum Press, 1987:304.

47. Noma T, Yata J, Shishiba Y, Inatsuki B. In vitro detection of antithyroglobulin antibody forming cells from the lymphocytes of chronic thyroiditis patients and analysis of their regulation. Clin Exp Immunol 1982; 49:465.

48. Mori H, Hamada N, DeGroot LJ. Studies in thyroglobulin-specific suppressor T cell function in autoimmune thyroid disease. J Clin Endocrinol Metab 1985; 61:306.

49. Tao TW, Gatenby PA, Leu SL, et al. Helper and suppressor activities of lymphocyte subsets on antithyroglobulin production in vitro. J Clin Endocrinol Metab 1985; 61:520.

50. Benveniste P, Row VV, Volpé R. Studies of the immunoregulation of thyroid autoantibody production in man. Clin Exp Immunol 1985; 61:274.

51. Iitaka M, Aquayo J, Iwatani Y, et al. Studies of the effect of suppressor T lymphocytes on the induction of antithyroid microsomal antibody-secreting cells in autoimmune thyroid disease. J Clin Endocrinol Metab 1988; 66:708.

52. Iitaka M, Aquayo J, Iwatani Y, et al. In vitro induction of antithyroid microsomal antibody secreting cells in peripheral blood mononuclear cells from normal subjects. J Clin Endocrinol Metab 1988; 69:749.

53. Yoshikawa N, Morita T, Resetkova E, et al. Reduced antigen-specific activation of suppressor T lymphocytes in autoimmune thyroid disease. J Endocrinol Invest 1993; 16:609.

54. Mukuta T, Yoshikawa N, Resetkova E, et al. Activation of T cell subsets by synthetic TSH receptor peptides and recombinant glutamate decarboxylase in autoimmune thyroid disease and insulin-dependent diabetes mellitus. J Clin Endocrinol Metab 1995; 80:1264.

55. Weetman AP, Volkman DJ, Burman KD, et al. The in vitro regulation of human thyrocyte HLA-DR antigen expression. J Clin Endocrinol Metab 1985; 61:817.

56. Arreaza G, Yoshikawa N, Resetkova E, et al. Expression of intercellular adhesion molecule-1 on human thyroid cells before and after xenografting in nude and severe combined immunodeficient mice. J Clin Endocrinol Metab 1995; 80:3224.

57. Yanagawa T, Mangklabruks A, Chang YB, et al. Human histocompatibility leukocyte antigen-DQA1*0501 allele associated with genetic susceptibility to Graves' disease in a Caucasian population. J Clin Endocrinol Metab 1993; 76:1569.

58. McLachlan S. The genetic basis of autoimmune thyroid disease: time to focus on chromosomal loci other than the major histocompatibility complex (HLA in man). J Clin Endocrinol Metab 1993; 77:605A.

59. How J, Topliss DJ, Strakosch C, et al. T lymphocyte sensitization and suppressor T lymphocyte defect in patients long after treatment for Graves' disease. Clin Endocrinol 1983; 18:61.

60. Weetman AP, McGregor AM, Hall R. Evidence for an effect of antithyroid drugs on the natural history of Graves' disease. Clin Endocrinol 1984; 21:163.

61. Ratanachaiyawong S, McGregor AM. Immunosuppressive effects of antithyroid drugs. Clin Endocrinol Metab 1985; 14:449.

62. Volpé R. Evidence that the immunosuppressive effects of antithyroid drugs are mediated through actions on the thyroid cell: a review. Thyroid 1994; 4:217.

63. Totterman TH, Karlsson FA, Bengtsson M, Mendel-Hartvig I. Induction of circulating activated suppressor-like T cells by methimazole therapy for Graves' disease. N Engl J Med 1987; 316:15.

64. Volpé R. Immunoregulation in autoimmune thyroid disease. N Engl J Med 1987; 316:44.

65. Eisenbarth GS. Autoimmune β cell insufficiency-diabetes mellitus type I. Triangle 1984; 23:111.

66. Rossini AA, Mordes JP, Like AA. Immunology of insulin dependent diabetes mellitus. Annu Rev Immunol 1985; 3:289.

67. Bach JF. Autoimmunity and type I diabetes. Trends Endocr Metab 1997; 8:71.

68. Yoon JW, Austin M, Onodera T, Notkins AL. Virus induced diabetes mellitus: isolation of a virus from the pancreas of a child with diabetic ketoacidosis. N Engl J Med 1979; 300:1173.

69. Gepts W. The pathology of the pancreas in human diabetes. In: Andreani A, DiMario U, Federlin KF, Heding LG, eds. Immunology and diabetes. London: Kimpton, 1984: 21.

69a. Varela-Calvino R, Sojarbi G, Arif S, Peakman M. T-cell reactivity to the P2C nonstructural protein of a diabetogenic strain of Coxsakie virus B4. Virology 2000; 274:56.

70. Menser MA, Forrest JM, Bransby JM. Rubella infection and diabetes mellitus. Lancet 1987; 1:57.

71. Karjalainen J, Martin JM, Knip M, et al. A bovine albumin peptide as a possible trigger of insulin dependent diabetes mellitus. N Engl J Med 1992; 327:302.

72. Atkinson MA, Bowman MA, Kao KJ, et al. Lack of immune responsiveness to bovine serum albumin in insulin-dependent diabetes. N Engl J Med 1993; 329:1853.

73. Todd JA, Bell JI, McDevitt HO. HLA-DQ$^{beta}$ gene contributes to susceptibility and resistance to insulin dependent diabetes mellitus. Nature 1987; 329:599.

74. Nepom GT. Immunogenetics and IDDM. Diab Rev 1993; 1:93.

75. Atkinson MA, MacLaren NK. Islet cell autoantigens in insulin dependent diabetes mellitus. J Clin Invest 1993; 92:1608.

76. Harrison LC. Islet cell antigens in insulin-dependent diabetes: Pandora's box revisited. Immunol Today 1992; 13:348.

77. Chase HP, Voss MA, Butler-Simon N, et al. Diagnosis of pre-type I diabetes. J Pediatr 1987; 111:807.

78. Ziegler AG, Ziegler R, Vardi P, et al. Life table analysis of progression to diabetes of anti-insulin autoantibody-positive relatives of individuals with type I diabetes. Diabetes 1989; 38:1320.

79. Dean BM, McNally JM, Bonifacio E, et al. Comparison of insulin autoantibodies in diabetes-related and healthy populations by precise displacement ELISA. Diabetes 1989; 38:12751.

80. Sachs JA, Cudworth AG, Jaraquemade D, et al. Type I diabetes and the HLA-D locus. Diabetologia 1980; 18:41.

81. Schatz DA, Winter WE, Maclaren NK. Immunology of diabetes mellitus. In: Volpé R, ed. Autoimmune diseases of the endocrine system. Boca Raton, FL: CRC Press, 1990:241.

82. Tarn AC, Thomas JN, Dean BM, et al. Predicting insulin dependent diabetes. Lancet 1988; 1:845.

83. McCulloch DK, Klaff LJ, Kahn SE, et al. Non-progression of subclinical beta cell dysfunction among first degree relatives of IDDM patients. Five year follow-up of the Seattle family study. Diabetes 1990; 39:549.

84. Bonifacio E, Bingley P, Shattock M, et al. Quantification of islet cell antibodies and prediction of insulin dependent diabetes. Lancet 1990; 335:147.

85. Riley WJ, Maclaren NK, Krischer J, et al. A prospective study of the development of diabetes in relatives of patients with insulin dependent diabetes. N Engl J Med 1990; 323:1167.

86. Peig M, Gomis R, Ercilla G, et al. Correlation between residual β cell function and islet cell antibodies in newly diagnosed type I diabetes: follow-up study. Diabetes 1989; 38:1396.

87. Spencer KM, Tarn A, Dean BM, et al. Fluctuating islet cell autoimmunity in unaffected relatives of patients with insulin dependent diabetes. Lancet 1984; 1:764.

88. Lernmark A, Baekkescov S. Islet cell antibodies—theoretical and practical implications. Diabetologia 1981; 24:431.

89. Brogren CH, Lernmark A. Islet cell antibodies in diabetes. J Clin Endocrinol Metab 1982; 11:409.

90. Nerup J, Mandrup-Poulsen T, Molvig J. The HLA-IDDM association: implications for the etiology and pathogenesis of IDDM. Diabetes Metab Rev 1987; 3:779.

91. Baekkeskov S, Aanstoot HJ, Fu Q, et al. The glutamate decarboxylase and 38 KD autoantigens in type I diabetes: aspects of structure and epitope recognition. Autoimmunity 1993; 15:24.

92. Harrison LC, Honeyman MC, DeAizpurua HJ, et al. Inverse relation between humoral and cellular immunity to glutamic acid decarboxylase in subjects at risk of insulin dependent diabetes. Lancet 1993; 341:1365.

93. Bottazzo GF, Dean BM, McNally JM, et al. In situ characterization of autoimmune phenomena and expression of HLA molecules in the pancreas in diabetic insulitis. N Engl J Med 1985; 313:353.

94. Nerup J, Andersen OO, Bendixen G, et al. Anti-pancreatic cellular hypersensitivity in diabetes mellitus. Diabetes 1971; 20:424.

95. Boitard C, Debray-Sachs M, Pouplard A, et al. Lymphocytes from diabetics suppress insulin release in vitro. Diabetologia 1981; 21:41.

96. Boitard C, Yasunami R, Dardenne M, Bach JF. T cell mediated inhibition of the transfer of autoimmune diabetes in NOD mice. J Exp Med 1989; 169:1669.

97. Fairchild RS, Kyner JL, Abdou NI. Suppressor cell dysfunction in insulin dependent diabetes. Diabetes 1980; 29:52A.

98. Lohmann D, Krug J, Lampeter EF, et al. Defect of suppressor cell activity and cell mediated anti-beta cell cytotoxicity in type I diabetes mellitus. Diabetologia 1986;29:421.

99. Boitard C, Timsit J, Larger E, et al. Pathogenesis of IDDM: immune regulation and induction of immune tolerance in the NOD mouse. Autoimmunity 1993; 15(Suppl):12.

100. Sutherland DER, Sibley R, Xu XZ, et al. Twin to twin pancreas transplantation reversal and re-enactment of the pathogenesis of type I diabetes. Trans Assoc Am Physicians 1984; 97:80.

101. Stiller CR, Dupre J. Immune interventional studies in type I diabetes mellitus: summary of the London (Canada) and Canadian-European experience. In: Eisenbarth GS, ed. Immunotherapy of diabetes and selected autoimmune diseases. Boca Raton, FL: CRC Press, 1989:73.

102. Harrison LC, Colman PG, Dean B, et al. Increase in remission rate in newly diagnosed type I diabetic subjects treated with azathioprine. Diabetes 1985; 34:1306.

103. Silverstein J, Maclaren N, Riley W, et al. Immunosuppression with azathioprine and prednisone in recent onset insulin dependent diabetes mellitus. N Engl J Med 1988; 319:599.

104. Muir A, Luchetta R, Song HY, et al. Insulin immunization protects NOD mice from diabetes. Autoimmunity 1993; 15:58A.

105. Boitard C. The differentiation of the immune system towards anti-islet autoimmunity: clinical prospects. Diabetologia 1992; 35:1101.

106. Formby B, Shao T. T cell vaccination against autoimmune diabetes in nonobese diabetic mice. Ann Clin Lab Sci 1993; 23:137.

107. Weiner HL. Treatment of autoimmune disease by oral tolerance to autoantigens. Autoimmunity 1993; 15:6.

108. Kaufman DL, Clare-Saizier M, Tian J, et al. Spontaneous loss of T-cell tolerance to glutamic acid decarboxylase in murine insulin-dependent diabetes. Nature 1993; 366:69.

109. Tisch R, Yang XD, Singer S, et al. Immune response to glutamic acid decarboxylase correlates with insulitis in non-obese diabetic mice. Nature 1993; 366:72.

110. Bloise W, Wajchenberg BL, Moncada VY, et al. Atypical antiinsulin receptor antibodies in a patient with type B insulin resistance and scleroderma. J Clin Endocrinol Metab 1989; 68:227.

111. Maron R, Elias D, Dejong BM, et al. Autoantibodies to the insulin receptor in juvenile onset insulin dependent diabetes. Nature 1983; 303:817.

112. Addison T. On the constitutional and local effects of disease of the suprarenal glands. In: Wilks S, Daldy T, eds. A collection of the published writings of the late Thomas Addison, M.D., physician to Guy's Hospital. London: New Sydenham Society, 1868:209.

113. Muir A, Schatz DH, MacLaren NK. Autoimmune Addison's disease. Springer Semin Immunopathol 1993; 14:275.

113a. de Carmo Silva R, Kater SA, Laureti S, et al. Autoantibodies against recombinant human steroidogenic enzymes 21-hydroxylase, side-chain cleavage and 17α-hydroxylase in Addison's disease and autoimmune polyendocrine syndrome Type III. Europ J Endocrinol 2000; 142:187.

114. Josse R. Autoimmune hypophysitis. In: Volpé R, ed. Autoimmune diseases of the endocrine system. Boca Raton, FL: CRC Press, 1990:331.

115. Bottazzo GF, Doniach D. Polyendocrine autoimmunity: an extended concept. In: Volpé R, ed. Autoimmunity and endocrine disease. New York: Marcel Dekker Inc, 1985:375.

115a. Ekwall O, Hedstrand H, Haavik J, et al. Pteridin-dependent hydroxylases as autoantigens in autoimmune polyendocrine syndrome type 1. J Clin Endocrinol Metab 2000; 85:2944.

116. Green ST, Ng JP, Chan-Lam D. Insulin dependent diabetes mellitus, myasthenia gravis, pernicious anemia, autoimmune thyroiditis and autoimmune adrenalitis in a single patient. Scott Med J 1988; 33:213.

117. Neufeld M, Blizzard RM. Polyglandular autoimmune disease. In: Pinchero A, ed. Autoimmune aspects of endocrine disorders. New York: Academic Press, 1980:357.

118. Irvine WJ. Autoimmunity in endocrine disease. In: Besser GM, ed. Advanced medicine, vol 13. Tunbridge Wells, England: Pittman, 1977;115.

119. Eisenbarth G, Maes M. Autoimmune polyendocrine syndromes. In: Volpé R, ed. The autoimmune endocrinopathies. Contemporary Endocrinology Series. Totowa, NJ: Humana Press, 1999:349.

120. Aaltonen J, Bjorses P, Sandkuijl L, et al. An autosomal locus causing autoimmune disease: autosomal polyglandular disease type I assigned to chromosome 21. Nat Genet 1994; 8:83.

# PART XIII

# ENDOCRINE AND METABOLIC DYSFUNCTION IN THE GROWING CHILD AND IN THE AGED

WELLINGTON HUNG, EDITOR

# CHAPTER 198

# SHORT STATURE AND SLOW GROWTH IN THE YOUNG

THOMAS ACETO, JR., DAVID P. DEMPSHER,
LUIGI GARIBALDI, SUSAN E. MYERS,
NANCI BOBROW, AND COLLEEN WEBER

## NORMAL LINEAR GROWTH, POSTNATAL

After birth, many infants shift from a growth rate that is determined by maternal factors to one that is increasingly related to the infant's own genetic background, as reflected by midparental size. Thus, for approximately two-thirds of normal infants, the linear growth rate shifts percentiles during the first 18 months of life. The number of infants shifting upward in growth rate and the number shifting downward are approximately equal. Normal full-term infants who are relatively small at birth but whose genetic background dictates a larger size accelerate toward the new growth rate soon after birth and achieve a new channel of growth by an average age of 13 months (Fig. 198-1).

Those infants who decelerate in their linear growth do so during the second to sixth months and achieve a new, lower growth channel by an average age of 13 months (Fig. 198-2). By the age of 18 months to 2 years, the shifts in growth rate usually cease, and growth proceeds along the same percentile.

## INTRAUTERINE GROWTH RESTRICTION/PREMATURITY

### INTRAUTERINE GROWTH RESTRICTION

Intrauterine growth restriction occurs in association with environmental, maternal, placental, and fetal factors.[1,1a] Whether different types of intrauterine growth restriction exist or whether the condition should be diagnosed solely on the basis of birth weight that is low for gestational age is unclear.[2,3] *Neonates with body weights of <10th percentile* are considered to have intrauterine growth restriction.

Two types of intrauterine growth restriction have been identified: *symmetric* and *asymmetric*. At birth, children with the symmetric type (type I) have the *same degree* of growth restriction in body weight, crown-heel length, and head circumference. Furthermore, postnatal growth is sluggish. Children with the asymmetric type (type II), which probably results from malnutrition,

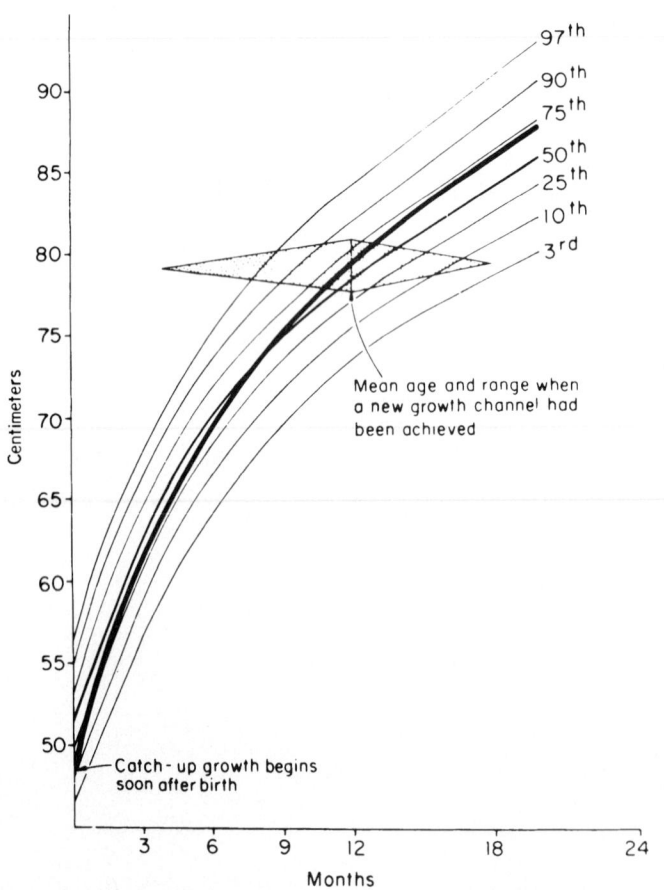

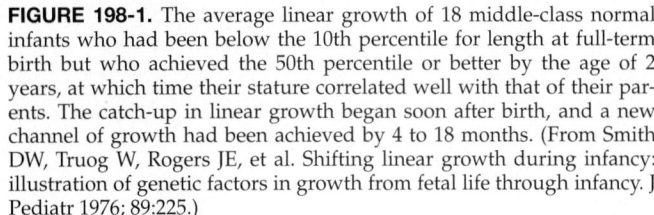

**FIGURE 198-1.** The average linear growth of 18 middle-class normal infants who had been below the 10th percentile for length at full-term birth but who achieved the 50th percentile or better by the age of 2 years, at which time their stature correlated well with that of their parents. The catch-up in linear growth began soon after birth, and a new channel of growth had been achieved by 4 to 18 months. (From Smith DW, Truog W, Rogers JE, et al. Shifting linear growth during infancy: illustration of genetic factors in growth from fetal life through infancy. J Pediatr 1976; 89:225.)

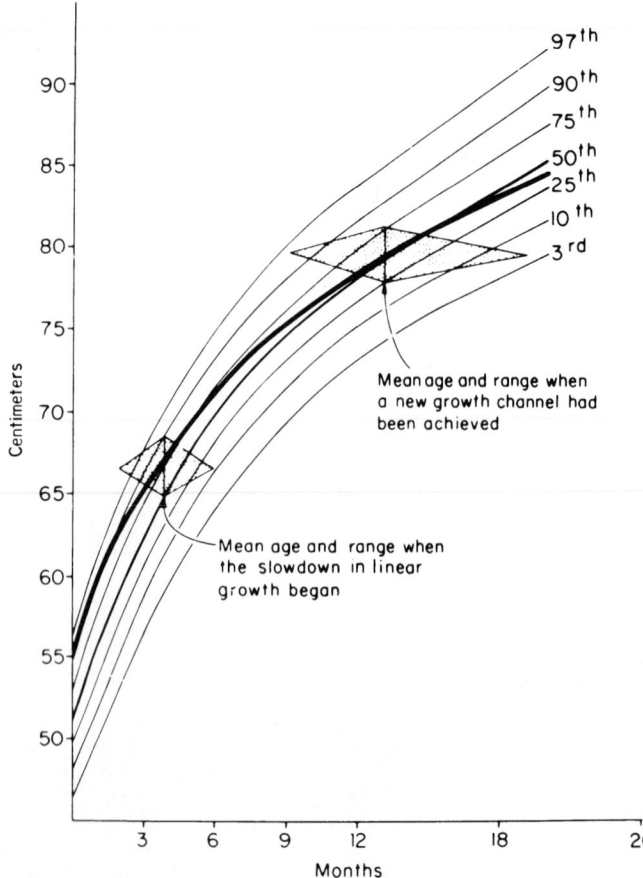

**FIGURE 198-2.** The average linear growth of 23 normal middle-class infants who had been at or above the 90th percentile for linear growth at full-term birth but who fell to the 50th percentile or less by 2 years of age, at which time their stature correlated well with that of their parents. The deceleration of linear growth did not begin until 2 to 7 months of age, and a new channel was achieved by 8 to 19 months. (From Smith DW, Truog W, Rogers JE, et al. Shifting linear growth during infancy: illustration of genetic factors in growth from fetal life through infancy. J Pediatr 1976; 89:225.)

have small skeletal dimensions for their gestational age as well as significant reductions in soft-tissue mass. These children tend to have more severe growth retardation.

Clinically, fetuses with intrauterine growth restriction are identifiable by ultrasonography. Therapies under investigation for fetal growth retardation include nutritional supplementation, oxygen therapy, and aspirin administration.[3]

Parents may not report to the physician that a short child has had intrauterine growth restriction. Important in the evaluation of such a child is a *review of past measurements*. An abnormally short child who is accelerating in growth probably does not require further laboratory evaluation. A child whose growth remains slow, however, should undergo additional testing.

## PREMATURITY

Infants *born before 37 weeks' gestation* are considered premature. Through the efforts of neonatologists, premature infants of extremely low birth weight (<1000 g) now survive. Although larger, healthy premature infants achieve normal length by 18 months of age, those with extremely low birth weight may not "catch up" until 8 years of age.[4–6] Some prematurely born children have intracranial damage and resultant growth hormone (GH) deficiency.

## THERAPY

In a study of 105 children who had intrauterine growth failure and remained small (3 standard deviations [SD] below the mean at a median chronologic age of 8.7 years), the mean height scores for chronologic age after 1, 2, and 3 years of GH treatment were –2.5 SD, –2.1 SD, and –1.9 SD, respectively. However, the effects of treatment on final adult height are not known.

## CHANGING GROWTH PATTERNS IN RECENT HISTORY

In industrialized nations, children now grow more rapidly during the first decade than did their ancestors in the nineteenth century. Peak height velocity in boys occurred at 14 years in the mid-twentieth century compared with 19 years in the nineteenth century. Boys achieved their final adult height at an average age of 19 years in 1960 compared with 23 years in 1850. The duration of growth was shorter in the mid-twentieth century, but final average adult heights had changed only moderately: from 168.5 cm to 176.5 cm (Fig. 198-3).

## POSTNATAL SOMATIC GROWTH IN INFANTS WITH ATYPICAL FETAL GROWTH PATTERNS[7]

Patterns of postnatal physical growth were studied in 61 full-term newborns with either normal or atypical somatic growth, based on *Rohrer's ponderal index* (weight in grams × 100 ÷ body length in centimeters).[7] Statistically significant and marked differences in postnatal growth were noted between short infants and infants with low ponderal indices.[7] The slow postnatal growth of the short infants appeared to be a continuation of their fetal growth pattern. On the other hand, infants born with low ponderal indices accelerated their weight gains and reversed the malnourished state in which they were born. These findings suggest the existence of two distinct types of fetal growth retardation. During the second year of life, these short-for-dates newborns continued to be abnormally short.

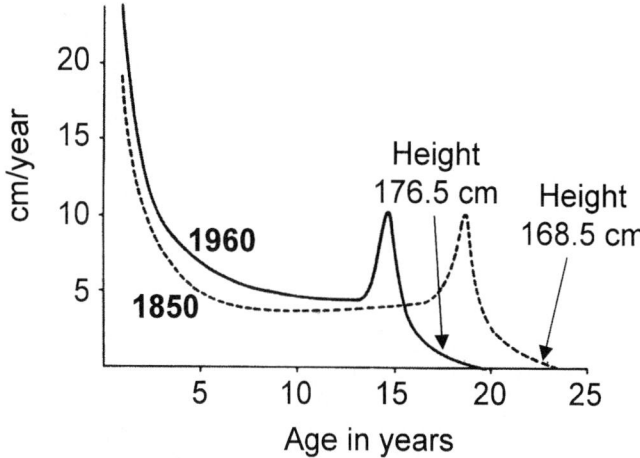

**FIGURE 198-3.** Accelerated maturation in 1960 in Netherland boys, who had a greater growth velocity and an earlier pubertal peak growth velocity and final height attainment than did those in 1850. Note that the predominant divergence in rate of growth is during childhood, and the peak growth velocity of puberty is of the same magnitude. (From Oppers VM. [academic thesis]. University of Amsterdam; 1963.)

## NORMAL SEXUAL MATURATION

More than 17,000 girls were examined by 225 clinicians in pediatric practices. At age 3 years, 3% of black and Puerto Rican girls and 1% of white girls showed breast tissue and/or pubic hair development, with proportions increasing to 27.2% (black and Puerto Rican) and 6.7% (white) at 7 years of age. At age 8, 48.3% of black and Puerto Rican girls and 14.7% of white girls had begun sexual development. At every age for each characteristic, black girls were more advanced than white girls. The mean ages of onset of breast development for black and white girls were 8.87 years (SD, 1.93) and 9.96 years (SD, 1.82), respectively; and for pubic hair development, 8.87 years (SD, 2.00) and 10.51 years (SD, 1.67), respectively. Menarche occurred at 12.16 years (SD, 1.21) in black girls and 12.88 years (SD, 1.20) in white girls.[8]

Boys mature more slowly than girls, and their rate of growth and maturation is less predictable. The onset of puberty is heralded by thinning and lengthening of the scrotum and enlargement of the testes at the age of 10 to 13.5 years. Linear growth accelerates, with a peak average yearly growth velocity of 9.5 cm (7–12 cm). The external genitalia usually are at Tanner stage IV (testicular volume 12 mL) at that time. Most linear growth has been achieved by the age of 18 years, with an average of 1 cm in additional growth taking place between the ages of 18 and 21 years.[9,10]

## PRECOCIOUS PUBERTY

### IDIOPATHIC PRECOCIOUS PUBERTY

Unusually early sexual maturation in girls presents a challenge to parents, physicians, and patients.[10a] Few long-term data are available on the spectrum of early sexual maturation. A small number of girls with *transient* (unsustained) central precocious puberty have been described. Thus, not all young girls with early puberty warrant therapy with gonadotropin-releasing hormone (GnRH) agonists. However, data on the natural history of either unsustained or slowly progressing early puberty in young girls are scant. The authors of a study involving 20 girls (with clinical features of central precocious puberty but without biochemical evidence of persistent pituitary hypothalamic–pituitary–ovarian axis activation) who were monitored without GnRH agonist treatment state that even patients with clinical characteristics of complete isosexual precocity may not warrant therapeutic intervention.[9] Girls with a *luteinizing hormone (LH) predominant response to exogenous GnRH* are probably good candidates for therapy, depending on age and adult height potential. The clinician should monitor patients with a *follicle-stimulating hormone (FSH) predominant response* and less marked bone age advancement for at least 6 months to insure that the early development is progressing before the initiation of therapy.

Effective drugs are available for children with idiopathic precocious puberty. Secondary sexual characteristics in females can spontaneously progress and regress.[8] An effective GnRH analog, administered monthly, has been developed for the treatment of patients (usually girls) with progressive precocious puberty.

For girls who develop secondary sexual characteristics at an unusually early age (e.g., 5 years), the recommendation is that the family and physician monitor the characteristics regularly over the next 6 months. If secondary sexual characteristics remain stable, no therapy is indicated. If acceleration occurs during the first 6 to 12 months, however, monthly injections of GnRH are indicated until the patient reaches age 10 to 12.[8,9]

## PRECOCIOUS PUBERTY IN GIRLS: ORGANIC VERSUS IDIOPATHIC

Formerly, precocious puberty in girls was particularly problematic from the standpoint of therapy (both medicinal and psychological). Also, few studies compared therapeutic results in cases with organic as opposed to idiopathic causation. Long-term observations of two groups of patients (one group with a hypothalamic hamartoma [n = 18] and a second group with idiopathic precocious puberty [n = 32]) have been reported. Those with idiopathic causation had been treated with deslorelin or histrelin for 3 to 10 years and were observed annually after discontinuation of treatment. No differences were seen in chronologic age or bone age between the patients with hypothalamic hamartoma and patients with idiopathic precocious puberty at the end of treatment or during GnRH-analog therapy.

Whereas mean peak LH levels in response to GnRH were higher in girls with hypothalamic hamartoma than in those with idiopathic precocious puberty both before treatment (165.5 vs. 97.5 mU/L) and at the end of therapy (6.8 vs. 3.9 mU/L), this difference did not persist at the posttherapy time points. Levels of LH, FSH, and estradiol declined into the pubertal range by 1 year posttherapy in both hypothalamic hamartoma and idiopathic cases.[11] (See Chap. 92 for a more extensive discussion of precocious puberty in both sexes and its causes.)

## INTERPRETATION OF CLINICAL INFORMATION

### HISTORY

Past height and weight measurements indicate the duration of the growth problem. Prolonged short stature dating to early childhood suggests a congenital disorder, whereas recent slowing of growth indicates an acquired problem. Patients whose growth and weight gain have accelerated with a change in caregivers may have been deprived in the past, and now thrive in the better environment.

Congenital GH deficiency (GHD) is associated with an increased incidence of excessive bleeding during pregnancy or complications during labor and delivery. An infant who is short for gestational age (i.e., has intrauterine growth failure) may continue to be significantly smaller than his or her peers.[1] Irradiation of the head can damage GH secretion; irradiation of the bones can inhibit subsequent growth of those particular bones. Glucocorticoids given in pharmacologic doses attenuate growth, but neurostimulant medications at standard dosages (<60 mg per day of methylphenidate) probably do not.

Teenagers with delayed puberty almost always have a close relative who has experienced a similar phenomenon. Mothers should determine the age at which close relatives experienced menarche and fathers should ask male relatives at what age they achieved adult height.

Children's heights correlate with those of their relatives, especially their biologic parents. When an abnormally short parent (3 SD or further below the mean) has an abnormally short child, the presence of a congenital disease resulting in abnormal genetic short stature (e.g., congenital GHD, a bone dysplasia, or congenital GH insensitivity) is suggested. Recurrent abdominal pain, diarrhea, and perianal fistula suggest Crohn disease. Because teenagers often feel uncomfortable discussing bowel habits, they should be approached diplomatically.

### USEFUL CLINICAL INFORMATION

In the initial evaluation of a patient with short stature or slow growth, the clinician must obtain a significant amount of clinical information. Parents, grandparents, caregivers, school personnel, referring physicians, and patients themselves can contribute. Table 198-1 summarizes the information that is especially helpful.

Most children with abnormal short stature or slowing of growth eat less than their peers. A recent marked decrease in appetite (food intake) is compatible with acquired problems such as chronic granulomatous disease, anorexia nervosa, or hypothalamic pituitary tumor. A hearty appetite suggests that the short patient has a malabsorption syndrome.

Polyuria and polydipsia (drinking water during the night) are associated with antidiuretic hormone deficiency, diabetes insipidus, or renal insufficiency. Decrease in visual acuity or visual fields, headaches, and recurrent vomiting suggest a space-occupying intracranial lesion.

The progression of sexual maturation at a normal age suggests normal gonadotropin secretion and normal gonads. This is found in patients with intrauterine dwarfism, skeletal dysplasia, or normal genetic short stature; in occasional patients with acquired GHD; and in some patients with drug-induced dwarfism. Puberty is delayed but normal in patients with familial delayed puberty and in some patients with drug-induced dwarfism. Incomplete or prolonged development of secondary sexual characteristics, or a combination of these, is found in most teenagers with congenital or acquired GHD, Turner syndrome, acquired hypothyroidism, mild Crohn disease, and Cushing disease or syndrome, and in those who engage in overly zealous exercise (e.g., 6 hours of gymnastics daily). Sexual infantilism (i.e., infantile testes in boys and absence of breast buds or labial hair in girls after 13 to 14 years of age) is found in many patients with acquired GHD.

Children, like adults, vary in their level of physical energy and in their sleep requirements. Abundant physical energy and an average or decreased sleep requirement are signs of relatively good health and can be seen in patients with familial delayed puberty, Turner syndrome, intrauterine growth failure, skeletal dysplasia, and normal genetic short stature, and in some patients with glucocorticoid-induced growth problems. Children who sleep during the day, rather than at night, may be

## TABLE 198-1.
### Helpful Information in the Initial Evaluation of Patients with Short Stature or Slowing of Growth

| History | Physical Examination |
|---|---|
| **PRESENT ILLNESS**<br>Past heights and weights: from well-baby visits or school nurses<br>**PAST MEDICAL HISTORY**<br>Complications during pregnancy, labor, delivery<br>Weight and gestational age at birth<br>Edema of hands and feet at birth<br>Irradiation<br>Medications: neurostimulants, glucocorticoids<br>Developmental history, including school performance<br>**FAMILY HISTORY**<br>Age of puberty and adult heights for parents, siblings, grandparents, uncles, aunts, and first cousins<br>**SYSTEM REVIEW**<br>Recurrent abdominal pain and diarrhea<br>Amount of food intake<br>Polyuria and polydipsia (awakening from sleep to drink)<br>Changes in vision, headaches, recurrent vomiting, and seizures<br>Progress of sexual maturation<br>Energy level, sleep pattern, and amount of exercise<br>**SOCIAL HISTORY**<br>Person who is raising the child<br>Source of income<br>Mental health of parents or caregiver<br>Occupation of parents or caregiver<br>Major problems of parents or caregiver | **GENERAL**<br>Interaction between parents and patient: eye contact, cuddling, gentle or rough handling, respect for patient's modesty<br>Indications of parental alcoholism (smell of alcohol)<br>Apparent age versus chronologic age<br>Alertness or apathy<br>Pudginess or scrawniness<br>Accurate height and weight<br>**BODY PROPORTIONS**<br>Upper/lower ratio<br>Comparison of arm span to length/height<br>**SKIN**<br>Unusual number of nevi<br>Dryness of elbows, knees<br>**MUSCULATURE** (in boys)<br>**HEAD:** Size in relation to height<br>**NECK:** Webbing, palpable thyroid<br>**FACIES:** Dysmorphic<br>**DENTITION:** Presence of permanent teeth; appropriate for age<br>**VOICE:** Timbre<br>**GENITALIA:** Stage of maturation<br>**HANDS:** Width of nails<br>**FEET:** Lymphedema<br>**ANUS:** Fistula |

emotionally deprived. GHD, hypothyroidism, and chronic inflammatory disease of the bowel have been associated with less abundant energy.

Infants and toddlers who feel well generally appear cheerful, whereas those with uncomfortable underlying diseases tend to be irritable. Recurrent early morning irritability that is relieved by eating breakfast occurs in patients with hypoglycemia caused by GHD and/or adrenocorticotropic hormone (ACTH) deficiency. An unusually placid and consistently cheerful teenage girl with short stature and delayed sexual maturation may have Turner syndrome (see Chaps. 90 and 92).

The social history can provide important clues to the environment in which the patient lives. A discordant environment (e.g., extreme marital problems, abusive or alcoholic parents or caregivers) is found in families of infants, toddlers, and children with slow growth resulting from deprivation.

## PHYSICAL EXAMINATION

Parents who hold infants and toddlers at a distance from their trunks and handle them roughly may not have bonded to them and may be depriving them.

Short children who look their chronologic age usually do not have familial delayed puberty, GHD, Turner syndrome, deprivation syndrome, Crohn disease, or hypothyroidism, but may have intrauterine growth failure, skeletal dysplasia, normal genetic short stature, or a drug-induced disorder.

Short infants who are extremely thin usually suffer from malnutrition. Children with "potbellies" and wasted buttocks may

be emotionally deprived as well. Short, pudgy children with pebbly fat over the abdomen may have GHD.

Disproportionate short stature occurs with many skeletal dysplasias and in patients whose spines have been damaged by irradiation or glucocorticoid therapy.

The overall demeanor can be alert or apathetic. Children who are not growing normally and who look apathetic may be emotionally and/or calorie deprived.

By the middle of the first decade, normal boys have visible and firm muscles. Good musculature is found in boys with normal genetic short stature, familial delayed puberty, skeletal dysplasia, intrauterine growth failure, or dysmorphic syndromes. It is not found in those with GHD, deprivation, chronic inflammatory disease of the bowel, or Cushing disease.

Short girls with many nevi may have Turner syndrome. Rough dryness, like sandpaper, over the elbows and knees suggests acquired primary hypothyroidism (see Chap. 47).

Often, the head of a child with short stature is somewhat smaller than average for chronologic age. A head that is larger than expected for chronologic age suggests the presence of a skeletal dysplasia. Webbing of the skin of the neck (from the mastoid bone to the acromial process) is found in some patients with Turner syndrome.

Delay in the eruption of permanent teeth is compatible with familial delayed puberty, congenital GHD, deprivation, acquired GHD, mild Crohn disease, Cushing disease, and some drug-induced disorders. Permanent teeth (see Chap. 217) erupt at a normal age with intrauterine growth failure, bone dysplasias, and normal genetic short stature.

Most boys and girls with congenital GHD have small-timbred voices.

Normal facies are seen in familial delayed puberty, intrauterine growth failure, normal genetic short stature, and acquired GHD, whereas abnormal facies are seen in congenital GHD or GH insensitivity, Turner syndrome, skeletal dysplasia, deprivation, acquired hypothyroidism, and Cushing disease (both spontaneous and iatrogenic).

Usually narrow nails occur in most girls with Turner syndrome. Lymphedema of one or both feet in a short girl is highly suggestive of this syndrome (see Chap. 92).

## DEFINITIONS

The following definitions are useful:

*Short stature, abnormal:* height at least 4 SD below the mean
*Short stature, possibly abnormal:* height 2 to 4 SD below the mean
*Normal short stature:* height 1 to 2 SD below the mean
*Slow growth, abnormal:* cessation of growth; relative decrease in height or length by >25 percentiles or by >1 SD in a child older than 18 months
*Slow growth, possibly abnormal:* <3.5 cm per year growth in height from 6 years of age to puberty

## CLASSIFICATION

Abnormal short stature or slow growth with good general health can arise from various disorders. Optimum therapy depends on accurate diagnosis.

Children with growth disorders are classified into two types: those in whom persistent short stature is the dominant feature, and those in whom slowing of growth, with or without short stature, is the major problem. Common causes of short stature are congenital and include familial delayed puberty, GHD, Turner syndrome, intrauterine growth failure, skeletal dysplasia, and normal genetic short stature. Common causes of slow

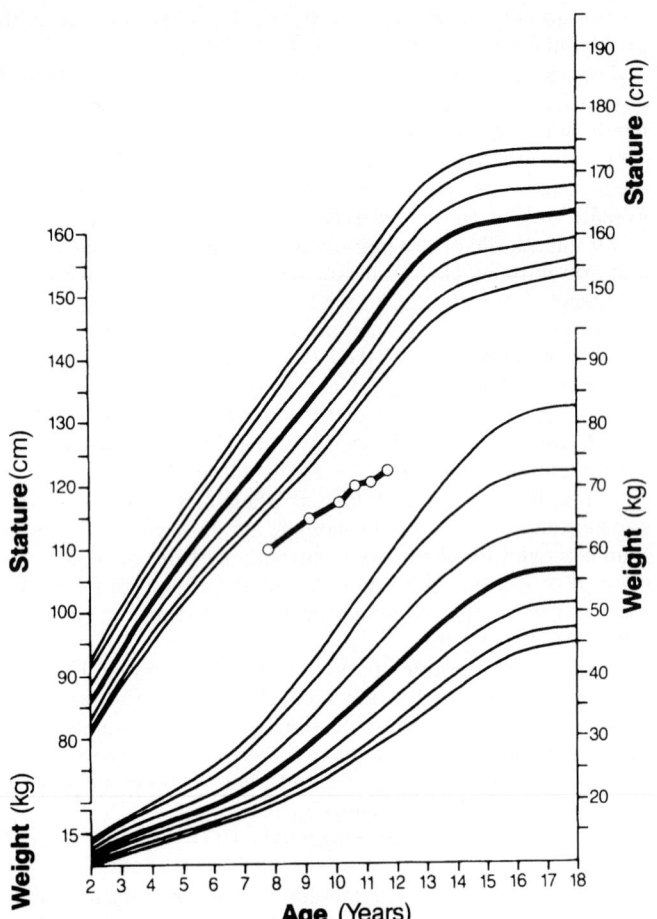

**FIGURE 198-4.** Growth curve of a typical girl with long-standing short stature, probably a congenital disorder.

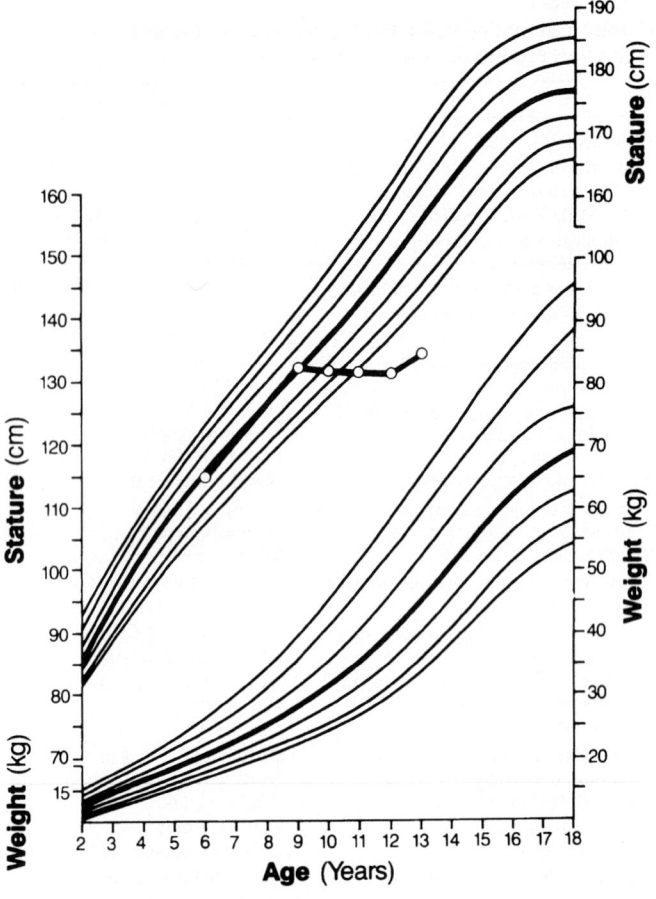

**FIGURE 198-5.** Growth curve of a typical boy who had grown normally, stopped growing, and then responded to growth hormone therapy.

growth are acquired and include deprivation, acquired GHD/ GH insensitivity, hypothyroidism, mild Crohn disease, and Cushing disease (spontaneous and glucocorticoid induced). Typical growth curves for the two types of growth problems are shown in Figures. 198-4 and 198-5.

# SHORT STATURE WITH OR WITHOUT SLOWING OF GROWTH

## FAMILIAL DELAYED PUBERTY

Associated with sexual maturation is a spurt in growth. The peak height velocity occurs at 14.1 ± 0.9 years in boys and at 12.2 ± 0.8 years in girls (mean ± SD).[12] Children who mature somewhat later than average are shorter than most of their peers throughout their teenage years. Almost always, a close relative has experienced a late but normal puberty. Because children with familial delayed puberty continue to grow for a longer period than usual, they achieve normal adult height. Anecdotal experience leads the authors to believe that, as adults, these men and women continue to look younger than their peers and are psychologically normal.

### PRESENTING MANIFESTATIONS

During the first decade of life, patients with familial delayed puberty, who usually are boys, have modest short stature (e.g., heights consistently 1 to 2 SD below the mean). During the second decade, they complain of absent puberty and an even

greater height discrepancy compared with their peers (2–3 SD below the mean). Patients vary in expressing their concern about their youthful appearance and sexual immaturity. Results of the system review are negative. The musculature is good and, except for delayed or absent sexual maturation, results of the physical examination are normal. This condition is much more common in boys than in girls, occurring in a ratio of ~10:1.

### CONFIRMATION OF THE DIAGNOSIS

The diagnosis of familial delayed puberty is suggested by a family history of late puberty. Ultimately, the diagnosis is confirmed when progressive sexual maturation and a pubertal growth spurt are observed. The bone age is delayed but usually is within normal limits.

Laboratory tests can be performed to detect rising serum testosterone levels, elevated serum LH levels during sleep, or elevated LH levels in response to stimulation with GnRH. In the experience of the authors, however, such tests are no more sensitive than a careful physical examination for the initial signs of puberty (lengthening of the scrotum and growth of the testes in boys, or breast budding and growth of pubic hair in girls).

In 45 sexually infantile boys aged 10.0 to 15.3 years, plasma testosterone levels were measured at 8:00 p.m. and again the next morning at 8:00 a.m.[13] Of those boys who had significant overnight elevations in testosterone, 58% achieved testicular volumes of 4 mL or more after 12 months and 89% after 21 months. Of those boys who had morning testosterone concentrations of ≥0.7 nmol/L (20 ng/dL), 77% entered puberty within 12 months and 100% did so within 15 months.

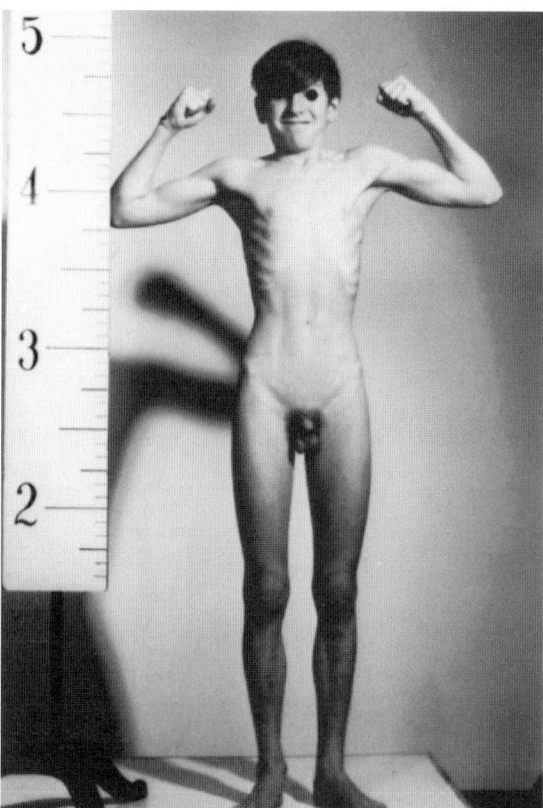

**FIGURE 198-6.** Eighteen-year-old boy with proportionate short stature, good musculature, recent appearance of secondary sexual characteristics, Tanner stage III genitalia, and a bone age of 14 years. His father completed sexual maturation and achieved full height at 21 years of age. Diagnosis: familial delayed puberty.

Boys in whom the initial signs of puberty have not developed by the age of 13.5 to 14 years and girls in whom they have not developed by the age of 13 to 13.5 years probably do not have familial delayed puberty, and require study for other causes of short stature or sexual immaturity (e.g., hypopituitarism, Turner syndrome, acquired hypothyroidism, hyperprolactinemia, or overzealous exercise).

### THERAPY AND PROGNOSIS

Because familial delayed puberty is a variation of the normal condition, supportive rather than hormonal therapy is needed. The natural history of the condition should be explained to patients and their parents: the children will continue to grow, but for a longer time than usual, and ultimately will achieve normal adult height. They will mature sexually, but at later age than usual. On return visits, the authors demonstrate to these patients that they have grown, gained weight, and acquired secondary sexual characteristics (Fig. 198-6). Many patients benefit from talking to a relative who has had a similar growth pattern, looking at old class pictures of that relative, and sharing humorous or trying experiences.

Occasionally, a boy is so upset by the delayed puberty that a short course of therapy is suggested with testosterone enanthate, 50 to 100 mg given intramuscularly once a month for 6 months and perhaps again the second year.[12] This results in some growth of the genitalia, an increase in muscle mass, and an increase in height, without undue acceleration of skeletal maturation. Used judiciously, such hormonal therapy does not seem to compromise the final adult height.[12]

Oxandrolone, 1.25 or 2.5 mg per day for 3 to 12 months, was administered to 40 boys with familial delayed puberty when the

volume of the testes was 4 mL and resulted in sustained growth acceleration.[13] (Ordinarily, boys experience acceleration in growth when the testes reach a volume of 10 mL.)

Although young women with familial delayed puberty or their parents rarely ask for female sex hormone therapy, ethinyl estradiol, 5 μg orally daily for 3 weeks out of 4 for 3 to 6 months, accelerates growth and, at least in some patients, initiates breast development.

These patients should avoid body contact sports, except with teammates of comparable weights. Girls should wear stylish clothes appropriate for their age.

Among 42 individuals with previously diagnosed constitutional delay of growth and puberty, both boys and girls achieved normal heights (~1 SD below the mean and 5 cm below target heights), based on midparental heights.[13] The discrepancy has been ascribed to a selection bias: the shortest children were referred for pediatric endocrinology consultation.[14] The 40 boys treated with an androgen grew to mean adult heights slightly greater than the predicted heights.[13]

Adult men with histories of constitutionally delayed puberty have decreased radial and spinal bone mineral density and may be at increased risk for osteoporotic fractures in old age.[15]

## CONGENITAL GROWTH HORMONE DEFICIENCY

The anterior pituitary gland secretes GH; the hypothalamus secretes GH-releasing hormone (GHRH) and somatostatin or GH release–inhibiting hormone. With the use of recombinant DNA probes, genes have been located on the long arm of chromosome 17 for GH, on chromosome 20 for GHRH, and on chromosome 3 for somatostatin.[16]

GH is essential for extrauterine growth. Congenital GHD varies from mild to marked in severity and results from disorders of the pituitary or hypothalamus. The underlying disorder can be heritable: X-linked recessive, autosomal dominant, or autosomal recessive. Congenital GHD can be associated with craniofacial midline defects (e.g., cleft lip or palate, single maxillary central incisor, or septo-optic dysplasia); it can arise from anatomic defects in the pituitary or from difficulties in pregnancy (e.g., early vaginal bleeding); or it can occur consequent to breech or forceps delivery and difficulties in the neonatal period (e.g., prematurity). Often, however, the origin of the deficiency is unknown (Fig. 198-7).

Other deficiencies of hypothalamic-pituitary hormones can be present. Thus, the natural history is variable and not fully delineated. Some patients with severe hypopituitarism probably die in the newborn period, whereas those who merely lack normal amounts of GH have pathologic short stature as adults. Adults with hypopituitarism develop atherosclerotic changes and die at a relatively early age.[17]

### PRESENTING MANIFESTATIONS

Most patients with GH and gonadotropin deficiency have short stature early in life and extreme short stature as well as sexual infantilism during the second decade. In the experience of the authors, children with isolated GHD come to the attention of physicians relatively late and with only moderately severe short stature. Other family members (e.g., parents or siblings) may be abnormally short. Some parents report that their short children lack physical strength and energy, and that permanent teeth erupt later than usual. Those who have both ACTH and GH deficiencies may have had symptoms of hypoglycemia (e.g., seizures, somnolence, irritability) during the newborn period and intermittently during the first decade of life. Neonatal hyperbilirubinemia can be associated with congenital GHD. Small external genitalia (penile length of <2.5 cm) can be one of the

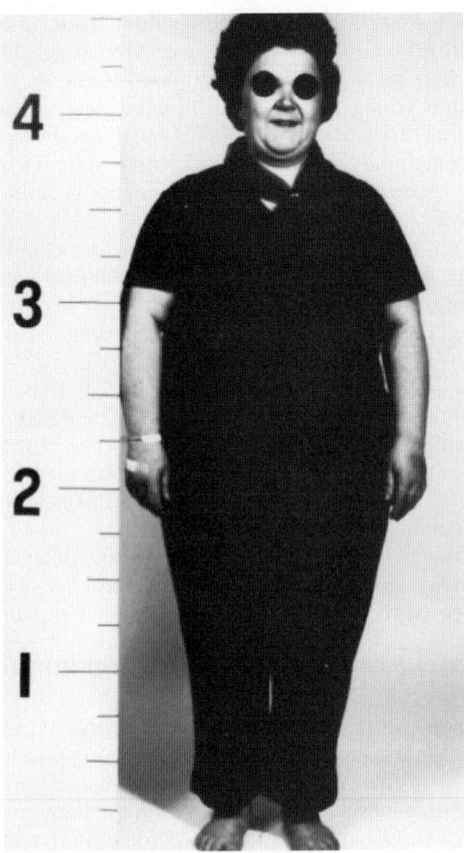

**FIGURE 198-7.** Adult with abnormal but proportionate short stature, obesity, and growth hormone deficiency. She is the mother of the boy in Figure 198-8.

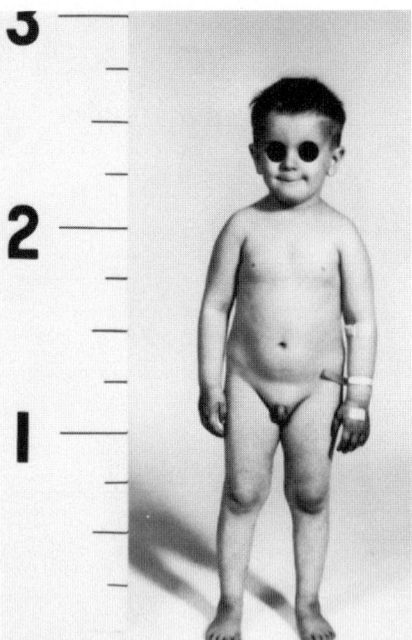

**FIGURE 198-8.** Seven-year-old boy with proportionate, but abnormal, short stature and low levels of growth hormone. Note youthful appearance, pudgy anterior thoracic and anterior abdominal walls, small normal external genitalia, and mottling of skin of lower extremities. He is the son of the woman in Figure 198-7.

presenting manifestations in male neonates and reflects GHD, gonadotropin deficiency, or both.

Septo-optic dysplasia is a defect of neuronal migration characterized by some or all of the following: absence of the septum pellucidum, optic nerve hypoplasia, hypopituitarism, diabetes insipidus, and mental retardation. Newborns with septo-optic dysplasia can have searching nystagmus secondary to blindness, as well as symptomatic hypoglycemia.

On physical examination, these patients have an unusually youthful appearance, small-timbred voice, and pudgy torso with dimpled abdominal fat. Boys can have an absence of good muscle development and small but normal external genitalia. Sexual infantilism can be present in both boys and girls (Fig. 198-8). Children with septo-optic dysplasia often have small optic globes, small optic nerve heads on funduscopic examination, normal or impaired vision, and normal or impaired intellect.

The authors evaluate proportional but unusually short children with bone age radiographs and measurements of serum insulin-like growth factor-I (IGF-I) and insulin-like growth factor–binding protein-3 (IGFBP-3) concentrations. In patients with GHD, bone ages usually are >2 SD below the mean and IGF-I concentrations are below the normal range for both chronologic and bone age. The serum IGF-I concentrations of normal children and those of children with hypopituitarism overlap, however, particularly during the first 5 years of life. Thus a low IGF-I concentration is a sensitive but nonspecific indicator of GHD in this age group. Measurement of the serum concentration of IGFBP-3 is a more specific test for GHD in young children.[18]

### LABORATORY DIAGNOSIS OF GROWTH HORMONE DEFICIENCY

**Diagnostic Difficulties.**   The diagnosis of GHD has been based on the presence of short stature, reduced growth rate, and bone age delay in the child who is unable to mount a GH secretory response to physiologic or pharmacologic stimuli.[19] Originally, an impaired GH secretory response was inferred from the patient's inability to tolerate an intravenous dose of insulin.[20] The tolerance test was refined by the polyclonal radioimmunoassay (RIA) for GH, which involved the direct measurement of GH in response to insulin-induced hypoglycemia, as well as other stimuli.[21] This also raised *the problem of defining the normal range of serum GH*, particularly when nonphysiologic stimuli are used.

Furthermore, a subgroup of children had been identified who had features of GHD and normal GH responses to pharmacologic stimulation, but decreased spontaneous secretion of GH in serial blood samples collected every 20 minutes for 24 hours. These children had short stature, delayed bone age, and low serum IGF-I concentrations, and their subnormal growth velocity was reported to have more than doubled after 1 year of GH therapy. This condition was called *GH neurosecretory dysfunction*. In these patients, GH secretion (expressed as mean GH concentration, peak frequency and amplitude, and area under the curve) was lower than in a normal control group, but higher than in children with classic GHD (Figs. 198-9, 198-10).[22,23]

In another study, integrated overnight GH secretory profiles were determined by pooling blood samples obtained through an indwelling catheter at 20-minute intervals from 8:00 p.m. to 8:00 a.m. on two consecutive nights in the hospital. The subjects had heights of <3rd percentile for age, height velocities of <25th percentile for age, or both. The investigators used the Hybritech immunoradiometric assay. Measurements of maximum stimulated GH concentrations correctly categorized 80% of children who had maximum nocturnal GH concentrations above or below 4 ng/mL. The remaining 20% of children had stimulated concentrations above this level. These investigators believe that it is common for stimulated GH concentrations to underestimate spontaneous GH secretion, and that the measurement of spontaneous GH secretion on a single night is more reliable for identifying children with low endogenous GH secretion than is the use of GH stimulation testing alone.[22,23]

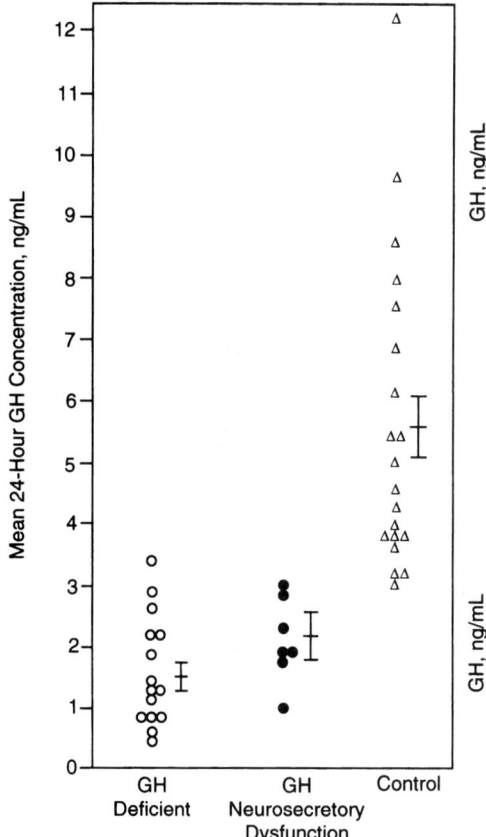

**FIGURE 198-9.** Mean 24-hour growth hormone (*GH*) concentrations in three patient groups (GH deficient, GH neurosecretory dysfunction, and control). The bar represents mean ± standard error of the mean. (From Spiliotis BE, August GP, Hung W, et al. Growth hormone neurosecretory dysfunction: a treatable cause of short stature. JAMA 1984; 251:2223.)

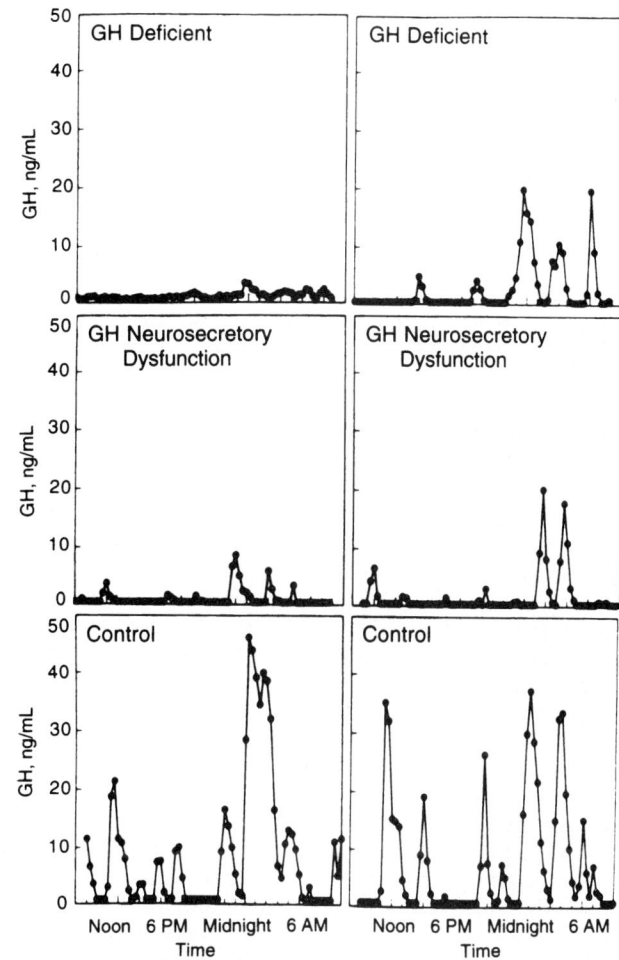

**FIGURE 198-10.** Representative 24-hour growth hormone (*GH*) secretory patterns in GH-deficient children, children with GH neurosecretory dysfunction, and control subjects. The GH-deficient children and those with GH neurosecretory dysfunction are in pubertal stage I. The control subject in the lower left panel is Tanner stage I and the control subject in the lower right panel is Tanner stage IV. (From Spiliotis BE, August GP, Hung W, et al. Growth hormone neurosecretory dysfunction: a treatable cause of short stature. JAMA 1984; 251:2251.)

The topic of GH neurosecretory dysfunction remains controversial.[24,25] The debate is fueled by the variability of GH secretion from day to day, both during sleep[26] and in response to stimulation tests[27]; by the limited use of electroencephalographic monitoring to document sufficient slow-wave sleep in most studies of spontaneous GH secretion; and by the absence of an ideal test of GH secretion. The positive short-term response to GH therapy described in patients with GH neurosecretory deficiency no longer is considered diagnostic of GHD, and the final heights of children with low spontaneous GH secretion who receive GH therapy are only minimally increased above those of untreated patients.[28,29]

During the 1960s and 1970s, serum GH levels were measured in children who had slept in the hospital, remained in bed in the morning, fasted, and had blood samples collected before, during, and after the administration of a stimulating agent.[30] Because of current insurance regulations, however, blood for GH measurements often must be obtained in ambulatory patients, under nonbasal conditions. The stimulated serum GH levels of normal ambulatory children are unknown.

Peak and integrated GH concentrations vary in normal children according to age: they are extremely high in the newborn period[31] and somewhat elevated during puberty. In 44 integrated studies involving nine prepubertal normal boys over a 1- to 3-year period, the mean 24-hour integrated concentrations of GH for individual profiles ranged from 1.1 to 7.0 ng/mL, with an intersubject coefficient of variation of 46%. Values for repeated studies performed on the same individual varied less, however, with a coefficient of variation of 26%. The physiologic

release of GH is regulated over time within characteristic, individually determined limits that vary predictably, but reciprocally, with body mass index (BMI).[32]

When the first polyclonal RIAs came into use, a consensus existed that a GH concentration of >5 ng/mL excluded GHD. This cutoff value subsequently rose to 7 ng/mL[25] and then to 10 ng/mL; however, data were inadequate to justify a cutoff point.[33] Moreover, 10% to 30% of normal children will "fail" a GH provocative test, and serial tests in the same child give variable results.[25] Eventually, a standard evaluation for GHD included two provocative tests, but the problem of defining a normal response remained. Because GH is secreted episodically, stimuli such as sleep, exercise, administration of hormones (insulin and glucagon), and administration of drugs (clonidine, L-dopa, arginine hydrochloride) were needed to elicit the secretory response. Administering drugs and hormones is easier in clinical practice, but it raises doubts about the relevance of such measurements to normal physiology.

GH provocative testing has come under further criticism because measurements diverge widely, depending on the immunoassay used.[34,35] Much of this variability can occur in the ranges of 5 to 15 ng/mL, directly affecting the diagnosis of GHD.

Some of the variability between assays can be explained by the complexity of the family of GH proteins present in the circulation. The main product of the normal GH gene is called *22 kDa GH* (see Chap. 12). A second product, the 20 kDa GH variant, results from alternative posttranscriptional messenger RNA splicing. Both 22 kDa GH and 20 kDa GH can be deamidated and acylated, and both can circulate as homo- or heterooligomers. Both are bound variably by at least two proteins in serum. One protein (growth hormone–binding protein, GHBP) binds with high affinity and relatively low capacity, whereas the other binds with lower affinity. Although 22 kDa GH is the major bioactive form in serum, only ~20% of immunoreactive GH is in this form. Another 20% binds to high-affinity GHBP to form a 90-kDa complex, and another 30% forms homo- or heterooligomers ("big GH," or "big-big GH"). Because the metabolic clearances of these forms vary, their relative proportions in serum change in temporal relation to secretory bursts from the pituitary. Thus, the above proportions represent only approximations, based on what is measured ~15 minutes after secretion.[36]

Polyclonal RIAs measure higher proportions of variants and oligomers. Many of the newer immunoradiometric and immunochemiluminometric assays using monoclonal antibodies to specific portions of the GH molecule measure secretory pulses of ~50% the magnitude of those detected by polyclonal RIAs.[34,37] Differences in basal GH concentrations are even more dramatic, probably because free 22 kDa GH is more rapidly metabolized and thus contributes less to the measured immunoactivity between secretory pulses.[37]

**Possible Responses to the Diagnostic Difficulties.** Clinicians have responded to the above difficulties and discrepancies in GH measurements in a variety of ways. One is to abandon or deemphasize the GH immunoassay and instead measure serologic markers of GH secretion (e.g., *IGF-I* and *IGFBP-3*).[38] These change little throughout the day and, in a sense, represent a biologic integration of GH secretory activity.[39] IGF-I also mediates many of the anabolic effects of GH. IGF-I assays are themselves technically difficult, largely because of interference from IGFBPs. Also, the normal range in the young child overlaps considerably with levels in the patient with hypopituitarism. GH secretion and IGF-I also diverge in chronic malnutrition. These problems may be less important with measurement of IGFBP-3. Given the difficulties, risks, and expense of GH provocative testing, assay of these two markers may prove to be a reasonable alternative to GH measurement; at the very least, they expand the knowledge of the GH-IGF axis.

A second response is to base GH therapy on auxologic criteria. In Australia, GH therapy has been started when height is <1 percentile for age and growth rate is <25 percentile for skeletal age.[40] Although GH provocative testing is retained for diagnostic purposes, patients with GHD and Turner syndrome comprised only half of the 3100 children treated. The empirical GH therapeutic trial also addressed the related controversy that some short, non–GH deficient children grow better, at least temporarily, on exogenous GH.

A third approach is to continue the search for standardized highly sensitive, biologically meaningful measurements of GH. In one promising approach, a monoclonal antibody and high-affinity GHBP are used in a "sandwich" assay to detect serum GH with the two exposed binding sites *necessary for in vivo GH activation of the GH receptor.*[41] High-sensitivity immunochemiluminometric assays are only now defining normal levels of GH in the basal state, in the aged, and in obese adults.[37]

As a practical matter, clinicians will continue to use the classic definitions of GHD not only to determine likely responsiveness to therapy but also to identify underlying pathologic causes for short stature (e.g., intracranial lesions). GH measurements can also identify the rare patient with a nonfunctioning GH gene. Thus, although the clinical indications for GH therapy expand, the diagnosis of GHD, determined with the help of IGF and IGFBP assays, continues to be a useful one. For those with organic disease, magnetic resonance imaging (MRI) has facilitated the diagnosis of pituitary disease based on a congenital anomaly of the hypothalamus-pituitary or a space-occupying lesion in the area. Nevertheless, scores of children receive human GH (hGH) because of short stature but do not necessarily have well-substantiated GHD. The usual subcutaneous dosage is 0.3 mg/kg per week in seven equal daily doses.

## ACQUIRED GROWTH HORMONE DEFICIENCY

Acquired abnormalities of the hypothalamic-pituitary area that inhibit GH synthesis or secretion produce a marked slowing or cessation of growth. Examples of such abnormalities include craniopharyngioma, histiocytosis X, severe trauma to the head, preventive cranial irradiation for acute lymphoblastic leukemia, and therapeutic irradiation with more than 20 to 40 Gy (2000–4000 rad) for neoplasms of the brain, face, head, or neck.

### PRESENTING MANIFESTATIONS

In addition to the growth problem, patients have a variety of complaints, including pituitary tumor with diabetes insipidus, visual problems, or increased intracranial pressure; and histiocytosis X with greasy, scaly scalp lesions (Fig. 198-11), chronically draining ears, and hepatosplenomegaly.[42] Patients who have received high-dose cranial irradiation are at risk for inappropriately early (precocious) puberty of central nervous system (CNS) origin, girls more commonly than boys.[43,44]

### CONFIRMATION OF THE DIAGNOSIS

As with congenital idiopathic GHD, acquired GHD is documented by serum GH determinations obtained during two stimulation studies, performed while the patient is euthyroid. Eventually, the bone age in acquired GHD is retarded. In some patients with prior cranial irradiation, only a neurosecretory disorder of GH secretion occurs.[45]

### THERAPY AND PROGNOSIS

The details of optimum therapy have not been determined for these tumors but include transsphenoidal excision and irradia-

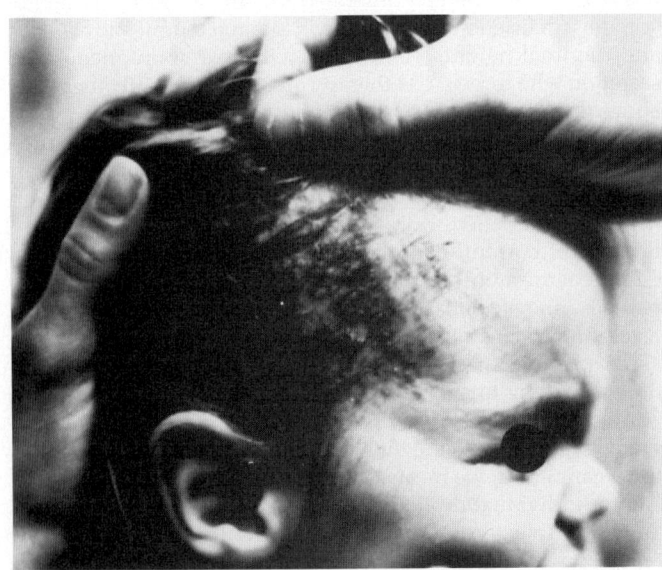

**FIGURE 198-11.** Chronic scaly, greasy scalp lesion of histiocytosis X.

tion. For histiocytosis X, most pediatric oncologists recommend the use of glucocorticoids and antimetabolites. Replacement hormonal therapy must include GH as well as any other hormones that are deficient. For patients with precocious puberty, therapy with a long-acting GnRH analog can be considered.

With a few exceptions, the prognosis for survival and growth has improved. Final adult heights are known for 30 patients with craniopharyngiomas who were treated with pituitary hGH. Most achieved a final height above the 3rd percentile, but none above the 50th percentile. Because these patients usually receive GH therapy before growth retardation is severe, the prognosis for achieving a normal adult height is better than that for patients with congenital GHD. Because of the localized invasive nature of some of the tumors, vision can be permanently impaired, and the life span shortened. Parents often ask whether therapy with hGH will exacerbate the neoplasia. Two studies suggest that hGH therapy itself does not increase the likelihood of tumor recurrence.[46,47]

## DIAGNOSTIC IMAGING IN GROWTH HORMONE DEFICIENCIES

With the use of MRI, almost 450 children with hypopituitarism and 46 healthy short children have been evaluated for pituitary abnormalities.[48,49] In a study of 101 consecutive patients with congenital idiopathic GHD, 59 had ectopia of the posterior pituitary or an interrupted pituitary stalk and 42 had a normal posterior pituitary. The pituitary volume was extremely small in the patients with ectopia and in those with normal glands that had severely narrowed stalks; the mean volume was significantly lower in these patients than in healthy short children. The investigators hypothesized defective induction of the mesobasal structure of the brain in the early embryo. The incidence of empty sella was 9% among patients with isolated GHD and 35% among those with multiple pituitary hormone deficiencies.

Prepubertal children with GHD have decreased bone density of the lumbar spine.[50]

Although short-term therapy with biosynthetic GH has produced no significant side effects, the safety of long-term therapy is unknown. Experience with other hormone therapies has shown that adverse effects can take years to emerge (e.g., administration of diethylstilbestrol to women pregnant with female fetuses led to subsequent malignancy of the external genitalia of the offspring). Thus, a cautious approach to hGH therapy is used. Meanwhile, the following guidelines are suggested:

1. Do *not* use for normal genetic short stature.
2. Consider for abnormal short stature of indeterminate cause for 1 year.
3. Validate the efficacy of treatment by obtaining careful height measurements during the 6 months before and the first year during therapy.
4. Continue therapy only if successful.

## THERAPY AND PROGNOSIS OF GROWTH HORMONE DEFICIENCIES

From the late 1950s until the mid-1980s, many clinicians investigated the response to treatment with human pituitary-derived GH. The Food and Drug Administration (FDA) withdrew this substance, however, because of the possibility of contamination with the Creutzfeldt-Jakob agent, which has caused the deaths of 12 patients treated with pituitary-derived hGH produced in the United States.[51] Because the incubation period can be as long as 35 years, patients who received hGH for the first time in 1985 may still be at risk for Creutzfeldt-Jakob disease in the early twenty-first century.

For infants and children with GHD, biosynthetic hGH is the drug of choice. It is commercially available in two forms, methionyl hGH (met-hGH, somatrem) and the natural sequence hGH (somatropin), both of which are equally effective in promoting linear growth. The current annual cost of biosynthetic GH for a 20-kg patient treated with 0.3 mg/kg per week is approximately $15,000.

In GH-deficient patients with abnormal short stature, the goal is to achieve normal stature during the first 3 to 4 years of GH therapy. Ideally, these children should grow at a rate of 1.5 times the mean growth rate for the bone age; for example, an 8-year-old boy with a bone age of 4 years should grow at a rate of $1.5 \times 7$ cm per year, or 10.5 cm per year.

Younger, smaller patients often respond well to smaller and less frequent doses, such as 0.15 mg/kg per week given in three separate injections on Monday, Wednesday, and Friday.[52,53] For those who achieve an optimum growth rate over a period of 6 months, the same dose per kilogram of body weight is continued at the same frequency. For those who grow significantly less, the frequency is increased to daily injections and, if necessary, the dosage is increased to 0.3 mg/kg per week or even 0.45 mg/kg per week. Older, larger patients should begin at 0.3 mg/kg per week. For those with hypoglycemia, daily injections are mandatory during the first decade. Once normal height has been achieved, the authors aim for a mean growth rate for bone age and offer "vacations" from treatment (e.g., for camping trips). European and a few American pediatric endocrinologists have treated patients with higher doses of GH (0.6 mg/kg per week). The intranasal administration of hGH results in a plasma peak similar to the physiologic and endogenous peak.[54] Figures 198-12, 198-13, and 198-14 illustrate excellent responses to growth hormone therapy in children with short stature of different causes.

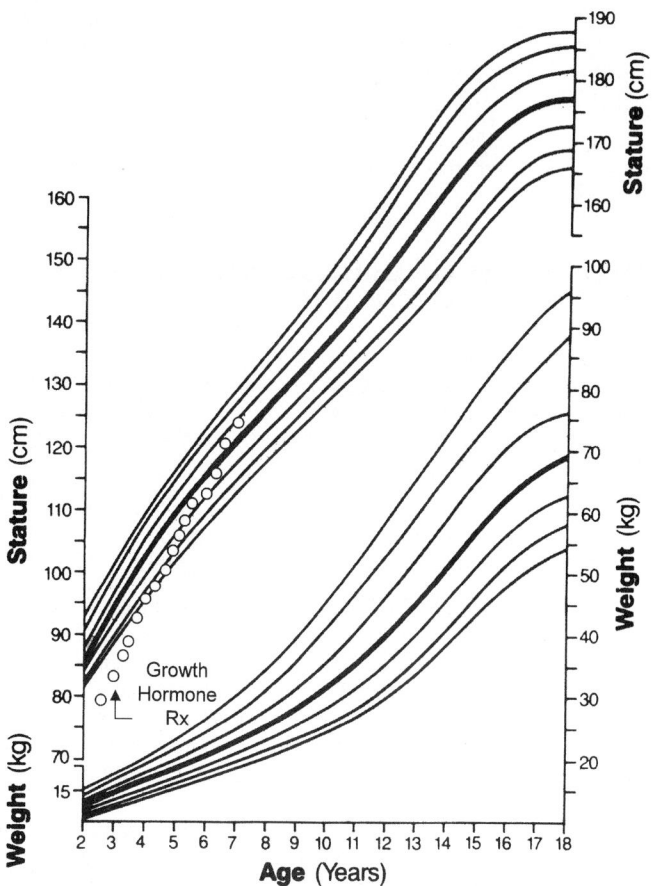

**FIGURE 198-12.** Growth curve of a boy with idiopathic hypopituitarism after commencement of growth hormone therapy.

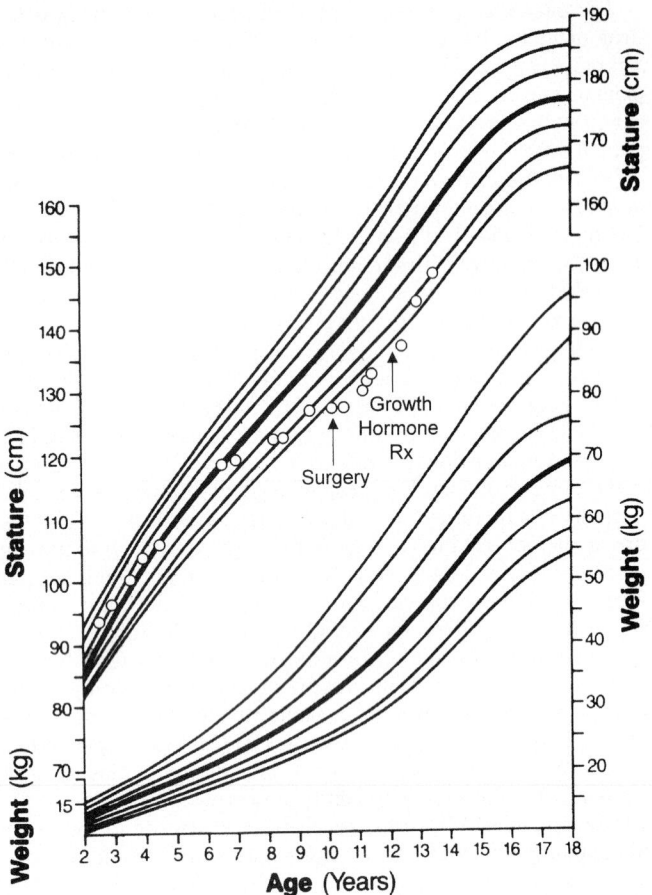

**FIGURE 198-13.** Growth curve of a 13-year-old boy with a history of craniopharyngioma removed 3 years previously. Growth hormone therapy was started at age 12.

Significant systemic levels of GH can be achieved in vivo by gene transfer into muscle cells, using either viral or DNA vectors.[55,56]

## TREATMENT OF GLUCOCORTICOID-INDUCED GROWTH SUPPRESSION

Growth failure commonly occurs in children treated with glucocorticoids because of blunting of GH release, of IGF-I bioactivity, and of collagen synthesis. Theoretically these effects could be reversed with GH therapy. In one study,[57] children meeting the following criteria were identified:

1. Treated with glucocorticoids and GH for >12 months
2. Known type and dosage of glucocorticoids
3. Height measurements taken for >12 months

Glucose, insulin, IGF-I, IGFBP-3, type I procollagen, osteocalcin, and glycosylated hemoglobin levels were monitored in a subset of 83 patients. Stimulated endogenous GH levels were <10 μg/L in 51% and <7 μg/L in 37%. The mean glucocorticoid dosage (expressed as prednisone equivalents) was 0.5 mg/kg per day. Initial evaluation revealed extreme short stature (mean height SD score of –3.7 cm), delayed skeletal maturation (mean delay of 3.1 cm per year), and slowed growth rates (mean of 3.0 cm per year). After 12 months of GH therapy (mean dosage of 0.29 mg/kg per week), the mean growth rate increased to 6.3 cm per year. The prednisone equivalent dosage and growth response to GH therapy were negatively correlated. Plasma concentrations of IGF-I, IGFBP-3, procollagen, osteocalcin, and gly-

cosylated hemoglobin increased with GH therapy, whereas glucose and insulin levels did not change. The results of GH therapy were as follows: (a) the growth-suppressing effects of glucocorticoids were counterbalanced, with a mean response that was double that of the baseline growth rate; (b) the responsiveness to GH was negatively correlated with the glucocorticoid dosage; and (c) the glycosylated hemoglobin levels increased slightly, but glucose and insulin levels were not altered.[57]

## INDICATIONS FOR GROWTH HORMONE TREATMENT IN PATIENTS WITHOUT GROWTH HORMONE DEFICIENCY

Although many GH-sufficient children who are abnormally short respond temporarily to therapy with GH, data are insufficient to indicate which of these children should be treated. Extensive research shows that children with Turner syndrome, renal insufficiency, glucocorticoid-induced dwarfism, and Prader-Willi syndrome experience accelerated growth. Less intensively studied children who also respond to GH treatment include those with intrauterine growth failure, Down syndrome, hypophosphatemic rickets, and meningomyelocele. The decision to treat with GH must be made by each patient's physician and family.[58-62]

The medical process influencing access to GH therapy for short stature in childhood has been examined by comparing coverage policies of U.S. insurers with treatment recommendations of U.S. physicians. Independent national representative surveys were mailed to insurers (private, Blue Cross/Blue Shield, health maintenance organizations [HMOs], programs for children with special health care needs, and Medicaid programs [n = 113]), primary care physicians (n = 1504), and pediatric endocrinologists (n = 534), with response rates of 75%, 60%, and 81%, respectively. Each survey included identical case scenarios. Primary care physicians were asked their decisions about referrals to pediatric endocrinologists. Endocrinologists were asked coverage decisions for GH therapy.

Insurance coverage decisions for GH in specific case scenarios were compared with recommendations of primary care physicians and pediatric endocrinologists. Physician recommendations and insurance coverage decisions differed strikingly. For example, although 96% of pediatric endocrinologists recommended GH therapy for children with Turner syndrome, insurer policies covered GH therapy for only 52% of these children. Overall, referral and treatment decisions by physicians resulted in recommendations for GH therapy in 78% of children with GHD, Turner syndrome, or renal failure; of those recommended for treatment, 28% were denied coverage by insurers. Similarly, GH therapy would be recommended by physicians for only 9% of children with idiopathic short stature, but insurers would not cover GH for the majority of these children. Furthermore, the data indicated considerable variation among insurers regarding coverage policies for GH.[63]

Final adult heights were reported for 15 normally short patients who were treated with GH for 4 to 10 years. The mean final heights did not differ from the mean pretreatment predicted adult heights.[28] For long-term results of GH therapy in girls with Turner syndrome, see later.

In a multicenter 5-year study of 121 patients treated with GH at 0.3 mg/kg per week for idiopathic short stature, IGF-I levels rose to a mean of 283 μg/L, within the normal range for age. Thyroxine, cholesterol, and triglyceride levels, blood chemistries, and blood pressure did not change significantly. Mean baseline and 2-hour postprandial blood glucose levels were unchanged, and fasting and postprandial insulin levels rose from low-normal levels to normal. The mean hemoglobin glycohemoglobin remained normal, and no metabolic side effects

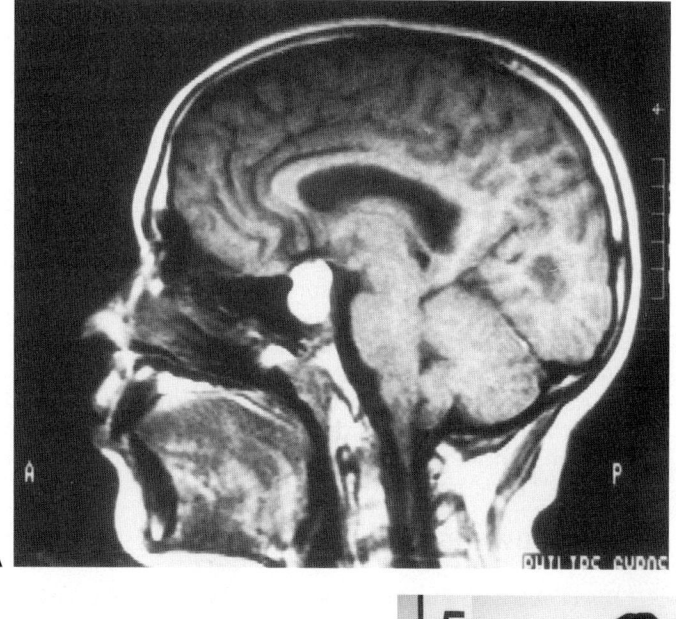

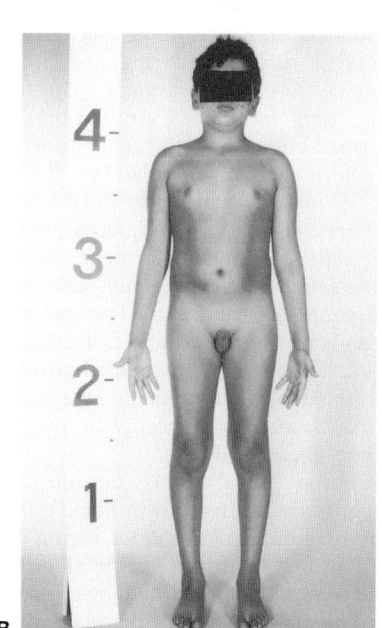

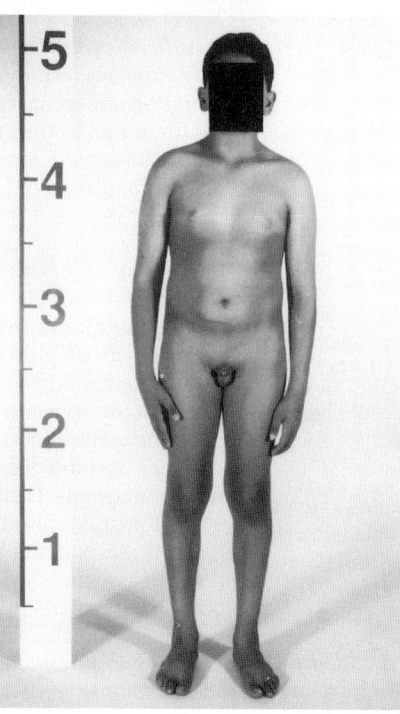

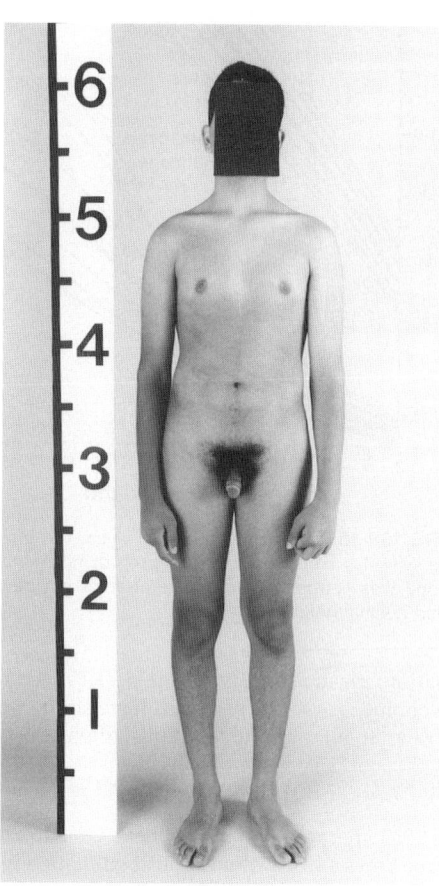

**FIGURE 198-14. A,** Large arachnoid cyst in a 14-year-old boy with hypopituitarism. **B,** He is short and sexually immature. The lesion was surgically removed. Growth hormone therapy was commenced, and, the following year, testosterone enanthate injections were commenced. **C,** Appearance at age 16. **D,** Appearance at age 17.

were seen. Although GH treatment in this group appears to be safe, continued surveillance is necessary.[64]

### TURNER SYNDROME

Turner syndrome is associated most commonly with a missing X chromosome (45,X) (see Chaps. 90 and 92). In the newborn period, the infant girl often has redundant skin at the nape of the neck and puffiness of the dorsum of the hands and feet. As the patient grows, the redundant skin may regress or it may progress and become more obvious. Usually the lymphedema of the hands and feet gradually wanes during the first decade of life. Among 594 Turner syndrome patients (age 1 month to 24 years) who were evaluated for congenital heart disease, the karyotype distribution was 45,X (54%), 45,X/46,XX mosaicism (13%), and

X-structural abnormalities (3.2%). A correlation was found between type of congenital heart defect and karyotype. The greatest prevalence of partial anomalous pulmonary venous drainage and aortic coarctation occurred in patients with the 45,X karyotype, whereas bicuspid aortic valve and aortic valve disease were more common in patients with X-structural abnormalities. The patients with severe dysmorphic signs showed a significantly higher relative risk of cardiac malformations.[65]

Patients with Turner syndrome respond to treatment with biosynthetic GH, although the linear growth is less than might be expected (Fig. 198-15). As a group, these girls are cheerful, reasonable students except for having more difficulty with mathematics and geography than is common. Because most lack ovarian endocrine tissue, female sex hormones are prescribed at an appropriate age and height. Because of a tendency for keloid

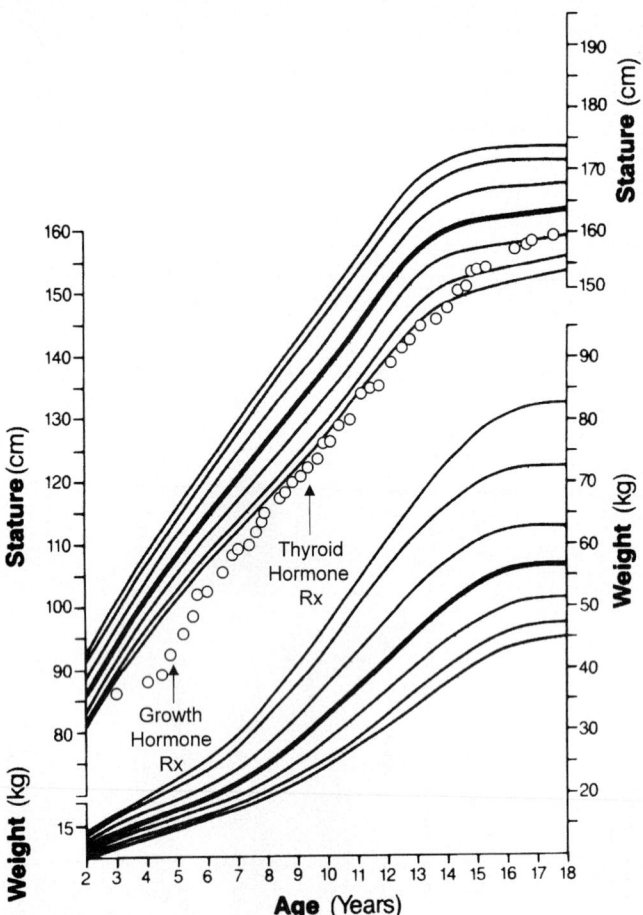

**FIGURE 198-15.** Growth curve of a 17-year-old girl with Turner syndrome. She has responded well to growth hormone therapy. Thyroid hormone was commenced later, because of hypothyroidism. She has attained normal height.

formation, plastic surgery on the neck is recommended only if the webbing is severe. These girls have strong maternal instincts, are drawn to infants, and, as adults, often adopt children.

### THERAPY AND PROGNOSIS

Since 1983, therapy with biosynthetic GH, initiated at 0.125 mg/kg three times a week, alone or in combination with oxandrolone, has been under study in 70 girls with Turner syndrome.[65] Thirty patients have completed treatment. Their mean height is 151.9 cm, which is greater than their originally projected mean adult height of 143.8 cm. At age 15 years, the authors initiate therapy with biosynthetic GH 0.3 to 0.375 mg/kg per week, in seven equal daily doses given subcutaneously. Some patients do not desire treatment, particularly those who have short stature within the normal range (often the offspring of relatively tall parents).

For complete feminization, most of these girls require replacement therapy with an estrogen and progesterone. Therapy is begun with 5 to 10 µg of ethinyl estradiol or 0.3 to 0.6 mg of conjugated estrogen given daily for 3 to 6 months. Thereafter, the estrogen is given on days 1 to 23 of each calendar month and medroxyprogesterone acetate, 2.5 to 5.0 mg, is given on days 10 to 23. Later, these patients can choose in vitro fertilization or adoption. (See also Ref. 65a.)

### PRADER-WILLI SYNDROME

Prader-Willi syndrome is a genetic, multistage disease of which the cardinal features are infantile hypotonia, obesity, short stat-

ure, typical facies, acromelia, hypogonadism, and intellectual impairment with aberrant behavior. Hypothalamic dysfunction has been hypothesized to underlie many of these features. Seventy percent of individuals have a paternally derived deletion of the long arm of chromosome 15, whereas the majority of the others have maternal disomy of chromosome 15.[66]

Individuals with Prader-Willi syndrome exhibit a gradual deceleration of linear growth, with short stature observed in most by 12 years. The mean adult height is 154 cm for men and 149 cm for women. Partial GHD appears to play a major role in the growth failure. Deficient spontaneous secretion and blunted responses to a variety of provocative stimuli have been demonstrated, even in children without marked obesity. IGF-I values are typically in the low-normal range.[67]

A randomized, controlled study of GH therapy in children with the Prader-Willi syndrome demonstrated a rapid linear growth and an improvement in body composition after 1 year.[68,68a] Long-term studies are under way.

### RENAL DWARFISM

The FDA has approved the use of GH for growth failure in renal insufficiency before transplantation. Several investigators are studying the response of patients with transplanted kidneys. Long-term (5-year) treatment with biosynthetic GH has been evaluated in 53 prepubertal short children with chronic renal failure who were receiving conservative treatment, or dialysis, or who had received renal transplantation.[69] Annual oral glucose tolerance tests (performed before and after renal transplantation) were compared with those of 12 age-matched children treated with biosynthetic GH for idiopathic short stature.

At the start of GH treatment, fasting levels of glucose, insulin, glycohemoglobin, triglycerides, and cholesterol, and insulin responses to oral glucose tolerance testing were significantly higher in all patient groups than in controls. Fasting and 2-hour postprandial glucose concentrations were correlated inversely with the glomerular filtration rate in all patients and correlated positively with age and the dosage of methylprednisolone in patients with renal transplants. Fasting insulin levels were positively correlated with glomerular filtration rate, age, and BMI.

In these patients with chronic renal failure, GH treatment was not associated with changes in fasting or stimulated glucose concentrations in any treatment group. In contrast, serum insulin levels increased during the first treatment year in all groups, resulting in a more marked elevation of integrated insulin levels in transplant and dialysis patients than in conservatively treated patients and control subjects. Hyperinsulinemia persisted in all treatment groups for up to 5 years of follow-up. Age, renal function, and weight were the major independent predictors of the insulin response to oral glucose tolerance testing in children with chronic renal failure. Long-term biosynthetic GH treatment does not affect oral glucose tolerance test results but aggravates the preexisting hyperinsulinemia in children with end-stage renal disease. In concert with the dyslipidemia of uremia, the GH-promoted hyperinsulinemia may contribute to the long-term risk for premature atherosclerosis in patients with childhood-onset chronic renal failure.[69]

### COMPLICATIONS OF GROWTH HORMONE THERAPY

Although some patients develop serum antibodies to GH during biosynthetic GH therapy, these antibodies do not produce immune complex disease and rarely inhibit growth. They do interfere with serum GH measurements. If antibodies develop, they usually do so within 3 to 6 months, and their appearance can be transient, especially in patients with low levels of binding. The methionyl GH is more likely to result in the formation of antibodies than is the native sequence.

A few patients with GHD have developed leukemia before, during, or after therapy with either pituitary-derived or biosynthetic GH. At risk are those who have undergone irradiation for brain tumors with or without GH therapy. In the United States, the incidence of leukemia is no higher in nonirradiated patients than in the general population.[70] A few patients have developed pseudotumor cerebri, which abated when GH treatment was discontinued.[71] Complications rarely occur from biosynthetic GH therapy; if acromegaloid facial features are noted, GH is discontinued for a few weeks and treatment is resumed at a lower dosage. Usually the undesirable facial features disappear.

Children with GHD who have gonadotropin sufficiency may need special attention. Because they are being treated with GH, puberty can begin at an inappropriately short height; thus, the final adult height can be compromised. The efficacy of GnRH analogs in retarding the onset of puberty in these patients is being evaluated. Preliminary data suggest that such combined therapy may be helpful in girls with central sexual precocity and severely compromised growth potential; it slows their sexual and skeletal maturation and may allow them to achieve a normal adult height.[72]

## GROWTH HORMONE INSENSITIVITY (LARON SYNDROME)

Patients with Laron syndrome have hypoglycemia and other clinical and laboratory signs of GHD but abnormally high concentrations of immunoreactive serum GH and decreased concentrations of IGF-I.[73] Since the original description, >200 such patients, mostly of Mediterranean or Indian descent, have been described.[74] Patients with Laron dwarfism have *GH insensitivity* due to a GH receptor deficiency. Therapy with IGF-I, 80 to 120 µg/kg twice daily, accelerated the growth of patients with Laron syndrome to 6.0 to 12 cm per year.[75,75a]

## RETESTING YOUNG ADULTS WITH CHILDHOOD-ONSET GROWTH HORMONE DEFICIENCY

Oral clonidine was used for a GH provocative test in 108 adult patients who had previously been treated with GH during childhood.[76] Basal IGF-I and IGFBP-3 levels and peak GH responses were compared to those of healthy adult controls. Seventy-nine patients had peak GH values of <7.5 µg/L (34 with isolated GHD), whereas 29 patients had a normal GH response (28 with previous isolated GHD). Thus, 45% of patients treated with GH during childhood because of isolated GHD had a normal GH response when retested in adulthood. Multiple regression analyses revealed that peak GH values were dependent on the degree of hypopituitarism, the BMI, and the duration of disease. IGF-I levels were below –2 SD in 60 of 79 GH-deficient patients and above –2 SD in 21 of 29 patients with a normal GH response. IGF-I and IGFBP-3 were significantly associated with GH response, whereas the BMI was significantly associated with IGFBP-3 but not with IGF-I.

Both IGF-I and IGFBP-3 serum concentrations are valuable diagnostic parameters in the evaluation of GHD in adults with childhood-onset disease. Reconfirming GHD is unnecessary in young adults who have two or more other pituitary hormone deficiencies.

The clinical relevance of the unfavorable lipid profile of patients with adult GHD and its improvement with biosynthetic GH treatment is apparent from a large retrospective epidemiologic study in Sweden. The overall mortality in 333 patients with hypopituitarism was found to be almost two-fold higher than in an age- and sex-matched normal population, despite adequate thyroid, adrenal, and sex hormone replacement. The increase in overall mortality was due largely to an increase in cardiovascular deaths (probably related to the GHD). However, long-term observations are needed to verify this hypothesis.[77]

Monitoring during the years of GH therapy should include measurement of fasting serum glucose and thyroxine levels and, in the second decade, observation for the appearance of secondary sexual characteristics. If gonadotropins are not secreted by age 14 to 15, administration of estrogen/progesterone to girls and testosterone enanthate to boys for a year is recommended. After 18 months, the patients should be reevaluated for the presence of FSH and LH, and treated accordingly.

When the patient has achieved a height satisfactory to him or her, GH treatment is discontinued and the patient is retested for GHD. If GH levels have not risen to normal, smaller regular doses of GH are recommended.

## GROWTH HORMONE DEFICIENCY IN ADULTS

Several benefits that GH replacement brings to some adults are now well documented.[78]

### YOUNG ADULTS WITH GROWTH HORMONE DEFICIENCY

The American College of Endocrinology recognizes the following benefits of GH therapy in GH-deficient adults: increase in bone density, increase in lean tissue, decrease in adipose tissue, bolstering of cardiac contractility, improvement in mood and motivation, increase in exercise capacity, and probably modulation of lipoprotein metabolism.

Acquired GHD in adult men is not associated with significant alterations in cognitive function as assessed by standardized tests, and long-term low-dose GH replacement therapy does not result in significant beneficial effects on cognitive function or quality of life.[79]

Evidence does suggest that GH-deficient adults are susceptible to development of premature cardiovascular disease.

### TREATMENT OF GROWTH HORMONE–DEFICIENT ADULTS

In young adults newly diagnosed with GHD, the starting dosage should be very low (0.1–0.4 mg subcutaneously per day), and the dosage should be gradually increased on the basis of clinical and biochemical responses assessed at monthly intervals. A maintenance dosage rarely exceeds 1.0 mg per day in patients >35 years of age, particularly in obese patients. GH should be administered daily. The best biochemical marker is IGF-I. Initially IGF-I should be measured monthly and later, semiannually.[80]

## GROWTH HORMONE FOR THE AGED

### GROWTH HORMONES AND COGNITIVE FUNCTIONING

The GH–IGF-I axis may be associated with cognitive functioning. Twenty-five healthy older men (65–76 years) with well-preserved functional ability participated in a study that used neuropsychological tests of general knowledge, vocabulary, basic visual perception, reading ability, visuoconstructive ability, perceptual-motor speed, mental tracking, and verbal long-term memory.[81] Performance on the last four tests declines with aging, whereas performance on the first four tests do not. The mean IGF-I level was 122 ng/mL (range 50–220 ng/mL). Subjects with higher IGF-I levels performed better on these tests. IGF-I may play a role in the age-related reduction of certain cognitive functions, specifically the speed of information processing.

## REVERSAL OF EARLY ATHEROSCLEROTIC CHANGES

Patients with hypopituitarism experience increased mortality from vascular disease. In these patients, early markers of atherosclerosis (i.e., increased carotid artery intima and media thickness and reduced distensibility) are more prevalent. As GH replacement can reverse some risk factors of atherosclerosis, the effect of GH treatment on morphologic and functional changes in the carotid and brachial arteries of GH-deficient adults has been studied.[82] GH-deficient men with hypopituitarism were treated with biosynthetic human GH (0.018 U/kg of body weight per day) for 18 months; the intima media thickness of the common carotid artery and the carotid bifurcation, and the flow-mediated endothelium-dependent dilatation of the brachial artery were measured by B-mode ultrasonography before and during therapy. The values were compared with those found for age-matched controls. Serum concentrations of lipoprotein(a), IGF-I, and IGFBP-3 were also measured. Before treatment, the intima media thickness of the common carotid artery and carotid bifurcation was significantly greater in GH-deficient men than in controls. GH treatment normalized the intima media thickness of the common carotid artery by 6 months and of the carotid bifurcation by 3 months.

GH treatment of hypopituitary GH-deficient men reverses early morphologic and functional atherosclerotic changes in major arteries and, if maintained, may reduce vascular morbidity and mortality. GH seems to act via IGF-I, which is known to have important effects on endothelial cell function.[82]

## CONGENITAL HYPOTHYROIDISM

The effects of congenital hypothyroidism have almost disappeared since the inception of the systematic screening of newborns. Nonetheless, *mothers with unrecognized hypothyroidism during pregnancy* can give birth to infants who are irreversibly brain damaged.[83] Thus, women planning a pregnancy should be screened for hypothyroidism.

Newborns with congenital hypothyroidism, as identified and confirmed in state screening laboratories, require lifelong thyroxine therapy. The dosage should be sufficient to keep the blood thyroxine and thyroid-stimulating hormone (TSH) concentrations normal for age. Normal levels in the newborn vary with duration of gestation and postgestational age (see *Handbook of Endocrine Sciences*, expected values and SI unit conversion tables, 4301 Lost Hills Road, Calabasas Hills, California 91301). If the initial results are abnormal, therapy should be started as soon as a second blood sample is drawn for blood thyroxine and TSH. In the interim, 8 to 14 μg/kg per day of oral thyroxine is prescribed. Then, if the results are completely normal, thyroxine can be discontinued. (Because of the seriousness of this problem, the authors use a laboratory that has established its own normal values.)

An elevated TSH level and normal thyroxine level suggest a lingual thyroid. This should be confirmed after 2 to 3 years of treatment. At this time, thyroxine can be temporarily discontinued, radioactive iodide administered, and the tongue scanned for a lingual thyroid.

In children who had documented congenital hypothyroidism, an attempt was made to assess the relationship between compliance to therapy and school achievement and cognitive test scores when the children were older.[83] At age 14, patients were studied at home via a battery of psychometric and school achievement tests. Also, blood was drawn for hormonal assays without forewarning. TSH and total thyroxine concentrations were measured. At 14 years, 16 of the 36 children with congenital hypothyroidism had poorly controlled hypothyroidism (TSH >15 mU/L). These 16 children also had thyroxine concentrations of <6.6 μg/dL. A second examination of the same children at 15 or 16 years of age disclosed significant improvements in hormonal levels without changes in thyroxine dosage. This suggested that the children were becoming more compliant. The improved hormonal concentrations at ages 15 to 16 years were accompanied by significant improvements in cognitive test results: the mean intelligence quotient (IQ) increased from 106 to 112 ($p = .002$). Patients with greater improvements in hormonal values had significantly greater improvements in their IQs.[83]

Earlier work had shown that the administration of oral thyroxine, 1.1 mg per square meter, once per week, resulted in normal blood triiodothyronine in a small series of patients. Thus, for noncompliant parents or patients, this once-weekly approach may be tried.[84]

## ACQUIRED PRIMARY HYPOTHYROIDISM

Normal levels of thyroid hormone are essential for optimal linear growth during extrauterine life; hence, inadequate levels retard growth.[85] Autoimmune chronic lymphocytic thyroiditis causes most of the acquired hypothyroidism seen in children and teenagers.[85a] Girls are at greater risk, as are patients with Down syndrome, Turner syndrome, Klinefelter syndrome, or type 1 diabetes. Occasionally, hypothyroidism is associated with a failure of ectopically placed thyroid tissue.

### PRESENTING MANIFESTATIONS

In addition to abnormally slow growth, most patients have only minimal complaints, such as decreased physical activity, increased need for sleep, and mild constipation. They usually perform well in school. Occasionally, pallor and rough, dry skin are marked. In patients with myxedema, the thyroid often cannot be visualized or palpated. Sexual maturation generally is delayed but can be precocious in cases of severe hypothyroidism. Postmenarchal girls have amenorrhea and, rarely, galactorrhea.

### ESTABLISHMENT OF THE DIAGNOSIS

Primary hypothyroidism is associated with a low serum thyroxine concentration and an elevated TSH. Delayed bone age, elevated serum prolactin (PRL) and creatine phosphokinase (CPK) levels, anemia (normocytic or macrocytic), and, on occasion, an enlarged sella (caused by hyperplasia or adenomatous transformations of the pituitary thyrotropes) also can be found. The presence of antithyroid antibodies (thyroglobulin, microsomal, or thyroid peroxidase), usually in low titers, suggests chronic lymphocytic thyroiditis. Compared with adults, children and teenagers with chronic thyroiditis have relatively low antithyroid antibody levels, often <1:64. The laboratory should be asked to provide the exact titer.

The authors often are asked to rule out hypothyroidism in children with exogenous obesity. Usually, this can be accomplished by physical examination. Patients with exogenous obesity have normal growth or tall stature, rosy cheeks, and soft, warm skin. These physical findings are incompatible with hypothyroidism.

### THERAPY AND PROGNOSIS

The authors treat patients who have hypothyroidism with L-thyroxine, 3.5 ± 0.3 μg/kg per day (100 μg/m² per day). For those who prefer, L-thyroxine can be administered once a week at a dosage of 1.1 mg/m².[86] The dosage should be regulated so that patients are clinically euthyroid and have normal serum thyroxine and TSH levels.

The prognosis for growth and good health is excellent (Figs. 198-16 and 198-17). With replacement therapy, some children

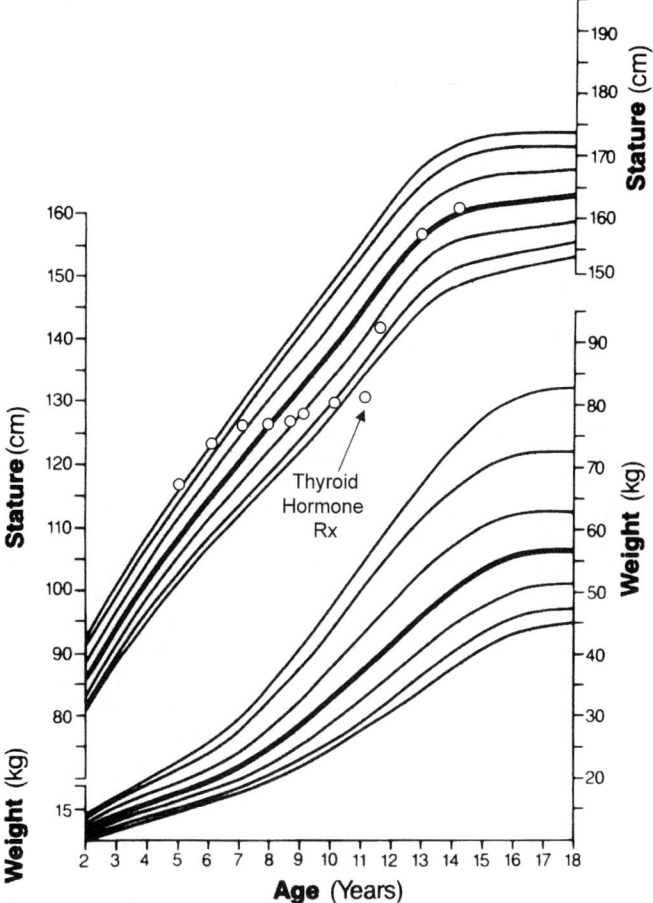

**FIGURE 198-16.** Growth curve of a 14-year-old girl with acquired primary hypothyroidism. Initially, this girl had nearly ceased growing after the age of 6. She responded dramatically to thyroid hormone therapy.

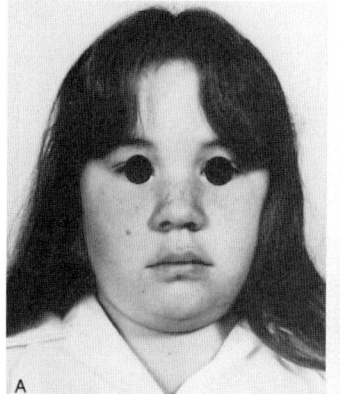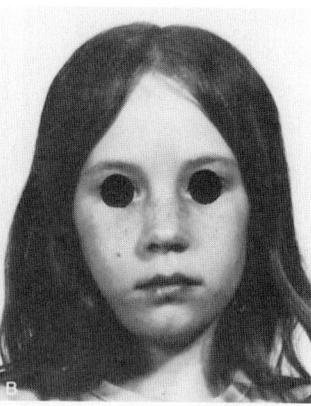

**FIGURE 198-17. A,** Hypothyroid 14-year-old girl with slowing of growth during previous 4 years, scant secondary sexual characteristics, and little physical energy. **B,** After 6 months of therapy with thyroxine.

experience a temporary deterioration in school performance, difficulty in interpersonal relationships (particularly with parents), and loss of scalp hair. Thyroid hormone replacement causes the enlarged ectopic thyroid tissue to disappear, the enlarged pituitary to shrink, and the anemia, precocious puberty, elevated PRL, and elevated CPK to resolve. If the bone age is unduly advanced, the sexual precocity may not resolve. Rarely, pseudotumor cerebri develops, but this abates with a reduction in the dosage of thyroxine. During therapy with physiologic dosages of L-thyroxine, acceleration in bone maturation without a proportional spurt in growth has been observed. Hence, patients may be shorter than expected as adults. For such individuals, the smallest dosage possible should be used to maintain a euthyroid state, both clinically and biochemically. Girls continue to grow after menarche, with a mean velocity of 4.1 cm per year.[87]

### MATERNAL HYPOTHYROIDISM AND CHILD DEVELOPMENT

The suggestion was made over three decades ago that mild maternal hypothyroidism alone was associated with lower IQs in the offspring.[88] Subsequently, TSH measurements in sera obtained at 17 weeks and stored for 8 years were used to screen 25,000 mothers for hypothyroidism.[89] The study groups were 48 untreated women with subclinical hypothyroidism, 14 hypothyroid women who had been treated before and during pregnancy, and 124 matched control women. When the children were 8 years of age, the results of neuropsychologic tests and the incidence of significant school problems for the children of the three

groups of mothers were compared. Outcomes for children of untreated hypothyroid women were significantly worse than for the children of control or treated hypothyroid mothers.

The risk of mental retardation in children of untreated subclinically hypothyroid mothers was ten times that in children with sporadic congenital hypothyroidism before neonatal screening was initiated. Very early screening and treatment of pregnant women could probably prevent this brain damage. The relative contributions of maternal and fetal deficiencies to the CNS developmental problems have not been established. Seven women with hypothyroidism had received a diagnosis and begun treatment before pregnancy. All their five surviving infants were considered to be mentally normal. Seven women who were first suspected of being hypothyroid during pregnancy had the diagnosis verified by thyroid function testing. Four of their five surviving infants were considered to be mentally retarded.

Thus, screening pregnant women for thyroid status and treating those with low thyroid function may prevent mental retardation in the infant.[89]

## SKELETAL DYSPLASIAS AND OTHER SYNDROMES

Skeletal dysplasias are associated with innate disorders of the cartilage and bone, probably metabolic in origin, so that the bones grow abnormally in length, shape, or both.[90–93] Although most of the skeletal dysplasias are transmitted as autosomal dominant traits, a few are autosomal recessive. The basic reasons for the anomalies are unknown. Final adult height varies with the underlying bone dysplasia from 61 to 152 cm (2 to 5 feet). Severe bone dysplasias can be associated with impaired hearing, weakness of the legs, and cardiopulmonary insufficiency.

The reader is referred to an international classification of the several dozen skeletal dysplasias.[90] Most of the patients have disproportionately short stature: the extremities usually are more affected than the trunk, or one portion of the extremities is more affected than the other. The diagnosis generally can be made from careful examination of a radiographic skeletal survey.[94] Bone age determinations are not reliable in these disorders.

### ACHONDROPLASIA

#### PRESENTING MANIFESTATIONS

Achondroplasia is the most common skeletal dysplasia, with a frequency of 1 in 26,000. The inheritance is autosomal dominant. Eighty percent of cases are spontaneous mutations.[95] Progres-

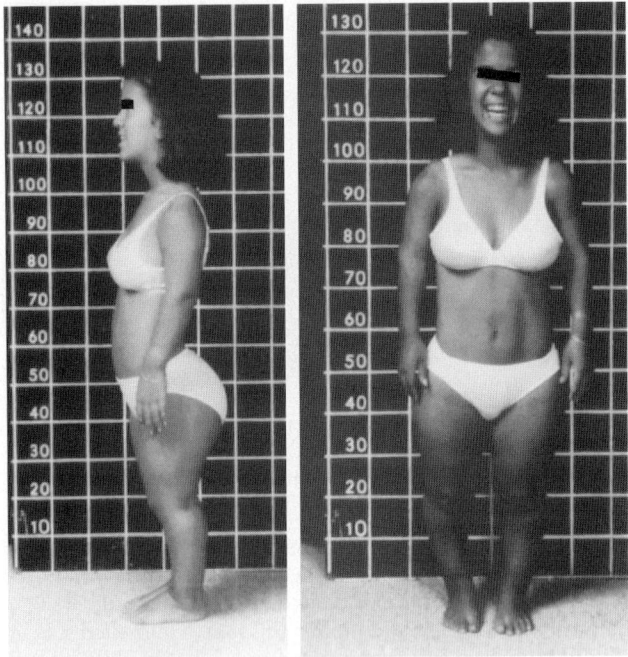

**FIGURE 198-18.** Young adult with achondroplasia. Note the relatively large head, short limbs, and exaggerated lumbar lordosis. (From Rimoin DL, et al. Growth Genet Horm 1991; 7[3]:5.)

sive deceleration of the growth rate begins in infancy. The mean adult height is 131 cm (51.5 in.) in men and 124 cm (49 in.) in women. The proximal limb shortening is readily apparent; the head is large, with a low nasal bridge and a prominent forehead. The usual lumbar lordosis is markedly exaggerated (Figs. 198-18 and 198-19). Because of hypotonia and the large head, motor development is slower than usual, but intellectual function is normal. In ~50% of adults, spinal cord or root compression

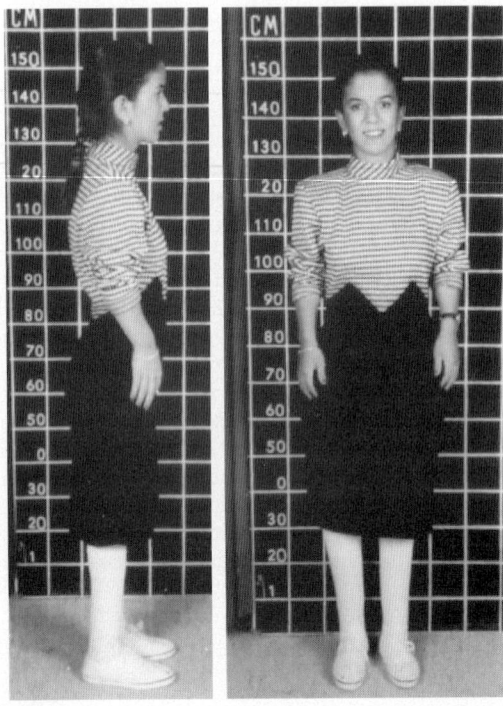

**FIGURE 198-19.** Same young adult as in Figure 198-18 after undergoing leg lengthening for achondroplasia. The final height was 61.5 in. (156.2 cm). (From Rimoin DL, et al. Growth Genet Horm 1991; 7[3]:5.)

occurs as a consequence of kyphosis, spinal stenosis, or an intravertebral disk lesion.

### ESTABLISHMENT OF THE DIAGNOSIS

The diagnosis of achondroplasia is clinical. Radiographs reveal a large calvarium; short ribs with anterior cupping; small, cube-shaped vertebral bodies; anterior "beaking" of the first or second lumbar vertebra, or both; small iliac wings with narrow greater sciatic notches; and short, broad tubular bones.

### THERAPY AND PROGNOSIS

Because the hydrocephalus arrests, shunt procedures rarely are necessary. For severely bowed legs, osteotomies are indicated. Short eustachian tubes can lead to frequent middle ear infections, and antibiotic therapy and tympanic tubes may be indicated. For weakness of the lower extremities, orthopedic surgery can be helpful. These infants usually are delivered by cesarean section.

Percutaneous limb-lengthening procedures can elongate the femur and tibia by up to 15 cm each.[96] These techniques are feasible in achondroplasia because of the excessive soft tissue and the tortuous nerves and blood vessels. Centers offering this surgery have widely varying age requirements, from 6 years and older to 14 years and older. The most common reasons for seeking surgery are poor body image and functional disability. One report describes a 94% satisfaction rate in 35 patients 2 to 5 years after surgery.[97] The efficacy of long-term GH therapy is being assessed; however, concern exists about worsening the narrowing of the foramen magnum and the spinal canal.

## HYPOCHONDROPLASIA

Hypochondroplasia is a condition with widely variable severity transmitted as an autosomal dominant trait. Short stature is obvious by 3 years of age.[98] The final adult height varies from 117 to 153 cm (46 to 60 in.) (Fig. 198-20).

### PRESENTING MANIFESTATIONS

These patients usually seek help in late childhood or adolescence for minimally disproportionate short stature with relatively short limbs, stubby hands and feet, and limitation of elbow extension and supination (Fig. 198-21).

### ESTABLISHMENT OF THE DIAGNOSIS

Especially helpful are radiographs that show mild V-shaped metaphyseal indentation and flaring, prominent bony sites of muscle attachment, bowing of the lower limbs, short femoral necks, a bony spinal canal narrowing caudally, and hypoplasia of the iliac bones with small greater sciatic notches.

### THERAPY AND PROGNOSIS

The efficacy of GH therapy is being assessed. Pregnant women with this disorder may require cesarean section.

## MULTIPLE EPIPHYSEAL DYSPLASIA SYNDROME

The multiple epiphyseal dysplasia syndrome is associated with a moderately short adult stature of 145 to 170 cm (57–67 in.), mottled epiphyses, and early osteoarthritis. It is inherited as an autosomal dominant trait with wide variability in expression.

### PRESENTING MANIFESTATIONS

Moderately short stature and waddling gait are evident by 2 to 10 years of age. Patients complain of pain and stiffness in the

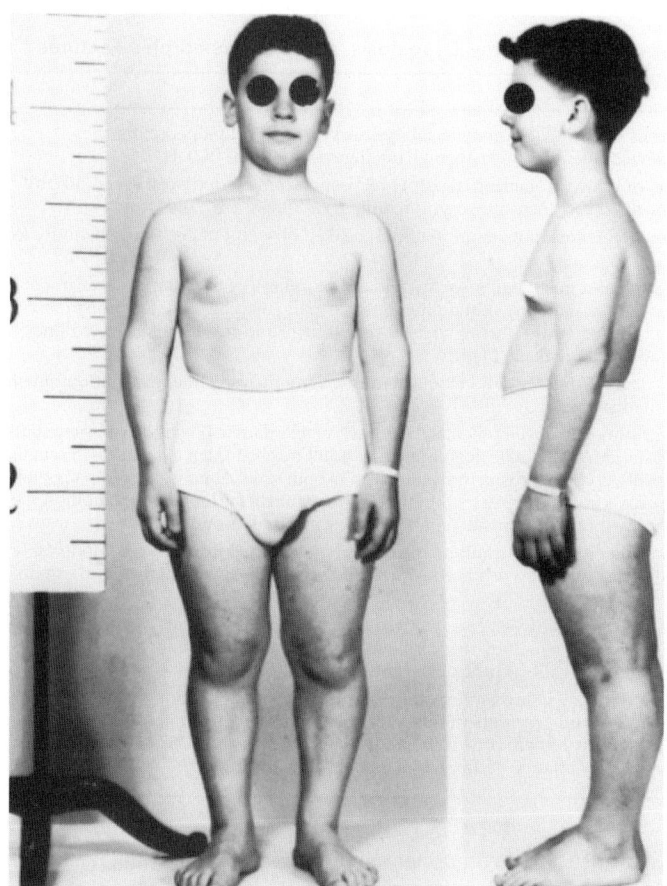

**FIGURE 198-20.** Nineteen-year-old boy with hypochondroplasia and abnormal short stature, but with normal proportions.

joints, especially the hips, as early as 5 years but usually not until the fourth decade.

### DIAGNOSIS AND THERAPY

On radiography, the epiphyses are late in ossifying and are small, irregular, and mottled; eventually, osteoarthritis occurs (Fig. 198-22). A short femoral neck, mild metaphyseal flare, and short metacarpals and phalanges are seen. No definitive therapy is available.

## OTHER SYNDROMES

Syndromes that feature proportionately short stature in the absence of chromosomal trisomy, dysostosis, or major dysmorphic features are listed in Table 198-2.

### NORMAL OR ABNORMAL GENETIC SHORT STATURE

Abnormal genetic short stature occurs when a child and a parent have heights of 4 SD or more below the mean.

Normal genetic short stature occurs when a child is short because the parents are normally short (i.e., within 2 SD of the mean).

### PRESENTING COMPLAINTS

These patients, often boys from middle- or upper-class families, seek help because they are somewhat smaller than their peers. The results of the physical examination, including signs of sexual maturation, are normal.

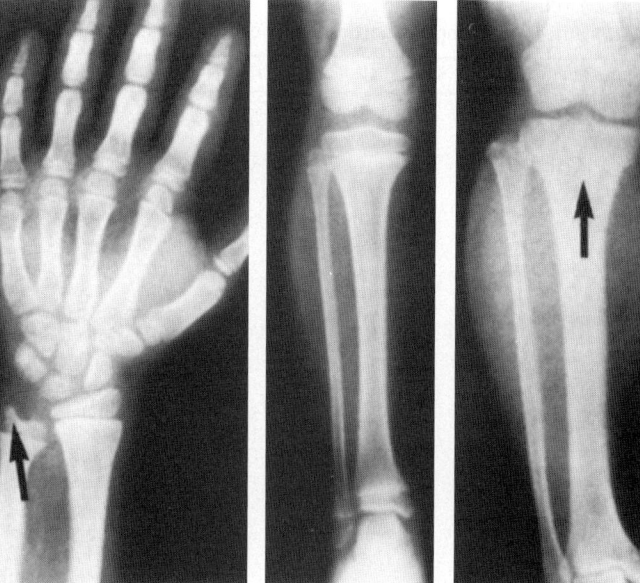

**FIGURE 198-21.** Hypochondroplasia. *Left,* radiograph of 10-year-old with slight ulnar shortening and metaphyseal flaring, with bulbous radial enlargement and elongation of the styloid process (*arrow*). *Middle,* radiograph of 7-year-old with elongation of the distal fibula and slight squaring off of the proximal tibial epiphysis. *Right,* radiograph of adult with more marked squaring of the proximal tibial epiphysis (*arrow*), with sharp flare of the metaphysis and elongation of the distal fibula with varus deformity of the ankle mortise. (From Beals RK. Hypochondroplasia: a report of five kindreds. J Bone Joint Surg 1969; 51:728.)

### ESTABLISHMENT OF THE DIAGNOSIS

The diagnosis is clinical. The height of both parents is measured and the data are plotted on the growth curve at 18 years of age. The parents' heights and the patient's height in terms of standard deviations are comparable. For example, if the patient's height is 2 SD below the mean, the height of one or both parents

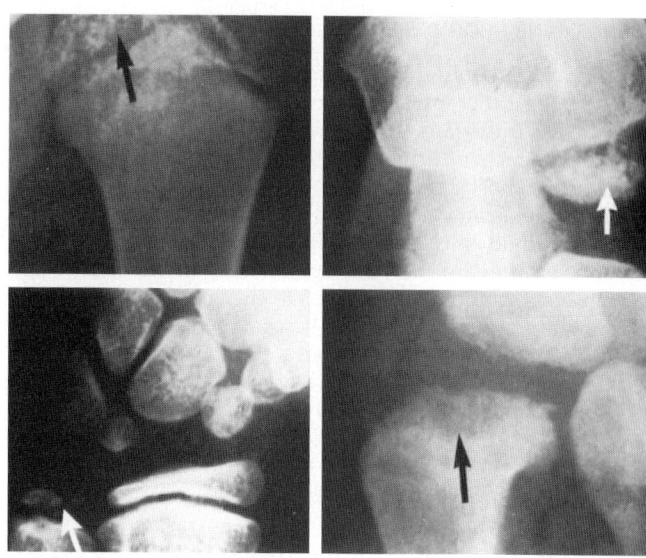

**FIGURE 198-22.** Multiple epiphyseal dysplasia syndrome. Late and irregular mineralization of epiphyses (*arrows*), which may be small or aberrant in shape, or both. (From Jones KL. Osteochondrodysplasias. Skeletal dysplasias and other disorders. In: Jones KL, ed. Smith's recognizable patterns of human malformation, 4th ed. Philadelphia: WB Saunders, 1988:331.)

**TABLE 198-2.**
**Syndromes Featuring Proportionate Short Stature in the Absence of Chromosomal Trisomy, Dysostosis, or Major Dysmorphic Features**

| Syndrome | Genetics | Clinical Features |
|---|---|---|
| FETAL ALCOHOL[74,75] | Environmental | Prenatal and postnatal growth deficiency of variable degree; facial dysmorphism (short palpebral fissures, smooth philtrum, microcephaly); developmental delay; average intelligence quotient (IQ): 60–70 |
| AARSKOG[76,77] | X-linked semi-dominant | Moderate short stature; hypertelorism, downward slanting of palpebral fissures, anteverted nostrils, broad philtrum; brachydactyly; inguinal hernias; "shawl" scrotum, cryptorchidism |
| COCKAYNE[78] | Autosomal recessive | Short stature; retinopathy; deafness; mental retardation; enophthalmos; beaked nose; cataracts; skin sensitivity to ultraviolet light |
| FANCONI PAN-CYTOPENIA[77,79] | Autosomal recessive | Mild to moderate short stature of prenatal and postnatal onset; hypoplasia or aplasia of the thumb; strabismus, microcephaly; mental retardation in 20% of patients; skin pigmentation; small genitalia/cryptorchidism in males; progressive bone marrow failure, generally starting at 5–10 years of age and resulting in severe pancytopenia and death; increased chromosomal breakage in vitro |
| LAURENCE-MOON-BIEDL[77,80] | Autosomal recessive | Moderately short stature; obesity; polydactylia and/or syndactylia; retinitis pigmentosa; mental retardation; small genitalia in males, variable hypogonadism |
| PRADER-WILLI[77,81–83] | Sporadic | Severe hypotonia and poor feeding in early infancy, developmental delay; mental retardation; progressive obesity starting in the first few years of life; short stature of moderate degree (average adult height 147 cm in females, 155 cm in males); small hands and feet; small penis, cryptorchidism, hypogonadism in both sexes; almond-shaped palpebral fissures, narrow biparietal diameter; occasionally, diabetes mellitus (type 2); deletion of the long arm of chromosome 15 is detected in >60% of cases, and virtually all the remaining patients have maternal disomy of 15q |
| RUSSELL-SILVER[77,84] | Sporadic | Short stature of prenatal onset (intrauterine growth retardation) and continuing postnatally; mildly to moderately short stature in childhood; triangular face with down-turned corners of the mouth, asymmetry of the extremities; clinodactyly of the fifth finger |
| ULLRICH-NOONAN[77,85] | Sporadic or autosomal dominant | Moderately short stature; epicanthal folds, ptosis, low-set ears, webbed neck; shield chest; mental retardation; pulmonic stenosis, septal defects; small penis, cryptorchidism, occasional hypogonadism; occasional lymphedema of the dorsum of hands and feet; improperly called Turner-like syndrome |
| WILLIAMS[77,86] | Sporadic | Prenatal and postnatal growth deficiency; mildly to moderately short stature in childhood; short palpebral fissures, depressed nasal bridge, anteverted nares, prominent lips with open mouth; mental retardation (average IQ: 50–60) with friendly personality; supravalvular aortic stenosis or other congenital heart disease or arterial anomaly; occasional hypercalcemia in early infancy ("idiopathic hypercalcemia of infancy") |

also should be ~2 SD below the mean (i.e., 152 cm [60 in] for the mother and 164 cm [64.5 in] for the father). Further evaluation is unnecessary; bone age is within normal limits. If the patient's height in standard deviations is significantly less than that of his parents (e.g., 4 SD below the mean), normal genetic short stature is not the cause and further evaluation is indicated. If the patient's height *and* a parent's height are >2 SD below the mean, both may have abnormal short stature and should be studied for a genetically controlled disease such as congenital GHD or skeletal dysplasia (e.g., hypochondroplasia, multiple epiphyseal dysplasia syndrome).

### THERAPY AND PROGNOSIS

No therapy is available for normal genetic short stature. Whether drug therapy for these normal children will ever be indicated is uncertain, given the difficulty of evaluating the long-term effects of drugs such as GH in healthy youngsters with normal short stature.

Most parents are reassured by the knowledge that their normally short child is healthy and will grow to adulthood like themselves as a normally short and functional individual. Affected teenage boys should be encouraged to engage in sports that they enjoy and that are safe (wrestling, baseball, swimming, tennis, ice skating, sailing) and to avoid sports that pose a potential risk (tackle football). They should be reassured that normally short girls are delighted to date normally short young men. Those parents, usually fathers, who find the diagnosis difficult to accept should be reassured repeatedly. Therapy for abnormal genetic short stature depends on the underlying disease.

## SLOW GROWTH WITH OR WITHOUT SHORT STATURE

### DEPRIVATION SYNDROME

Deprivation, caloric or emotional, slows weight gain and, eventually, linear growth. The type I deprivation syndrome has more

of a nutritional component and the type II syndrome has more of a psychosocial component.[98,99]

Type I deprivation syndrome is seen in infants and young children. For various reasons, these patients have not received enough food or, in some cases, enough attention. The parent or caregiver may be disorganized, inadequately trained, misguided, overwhelmed, or disturbed. This condition also has been described in the second decade of life.[100] Type II deprivation syndrome, the childhood variety, affects children older than 3 years and, occasionally, teenagers. Parents or caregivers, who frequently are alcoholics, abuse these children emotionally. Although the disorder occurs more often in the lower socioeconomic classes, the authors have documented the deprivation syndrome in the upper classes. Boys are affected most commonly.[101] At the initial evaluation, hypopituitarism, including GHD, often is present. Without intervention, the prognosis for normal growth and development is guarded to dismal for patients with both types of deprivation syndrome.

### PRESENTING MANIFESTATIONS

Infants with type I deprivation syndrome have slowing of growth, a scrawny appearance, and a relatively alert demeanor, although some look dejected. Kwashiorkor (see Chap. 127) rarely occurs in the United States. Eight patients, aged 14 to 27 months, were found to have consumed excessive amounts of fruit juice with resultant failure to thrive (abnormally low weight)[102]; however, these patients recovered after nutritional intervention. Sixteen extensively studied patients with nutritional dwarfing (aged 10 to 16 years) were found to have inappropriate eating habits and subnormal weight gain (accompanied by a proportionate decline in growth velocity), but no signs of emaciation. Parents reported that these children became satiated early during the course of a meal.[100]

Children with type II deprivation syndrome, those with "psychosocial dwarfism," generally are withdrawn, grow extremely slowly, and have delayed sexual maturation. Most have an appropriate weight for their height, and some resemble patients with celiac dwarfism, with protuberant abdomens and wasted buttocks. Eventually, a history emerges of polydipsia, polyphagia, stealing of food, eating from garbage cans, and drinking from toilet bowls. Developmentally, patients in both groups perform suboptimally.

### ESTABLISHMENT OF THE DIAGNOSIS

The gold standard for establishing the diagnosis of deprivation syndrome is the observation of accelerated weight gain in infants, and accelerated growth as well as weight gain in older children, when patients have new caretakers (e.g., hospitals or foster homes). Feeding should be increased gradually to the recommended number of kilocalories per kilogram of the ideal body weight for the patient's age. In infants, definitive weight gain occurs in ~2 weeks; in older children, acceleration of growth and weight gain can take several months. Laboratory studies are of little help in establishing the diagnosis. The bone age is retarded, particularly in patients with psychosocial dwarfism.

Infants whose linear growth rates are slowing (e.g., dropping from the 50th to the 20th percentile from the ages of 6 to 12 months, respectively) present diagnostic difficulties. Such infants may be perfectly normal and may simply be experiencing a shift from an intrauterine growth rate influenced by maternal factors to an extrauterine growth rate dictated by their own genetic backgrounds (i.e., midparental height). These normal infants establish their permanent normal growth rate (e.g., along the 20th percentile) by the age of 18 to 24 months.

### THERAPY AND PROGNOSIS

When the caretaker is disturbed, a new caretaker must be located. For some parents of malnourished infants, education in feeding is helpful. If a biologic parent is a psychologically disturbed caretaker, psychotherapy is essential. If the parent refuses psychotherapy or the infant does not improve rapidly, the physician must use every means necessary to place the child in a new permanent home.

With intervention, the long-term overall prognosis for children with type I deprivation syndrome is generally good. For children with type II deprivation syndrome, the long-term prognosis for growth and sexual maturation is favorable, and intellectual ability improves to some extent (Fig. 198-23). However, both intellectual function and emotional development are likely to be permanently compromised.[103]

### ATYPICAL CROHN DISEASE[104]

Crohn disease, a chronic inflammatory disease of the bowel of unknown etiology but with a strong genetic component, often interferes with growth and sexual maturation, probably as a result of chronic undernutrition, and secondarily, of low serum concentrations of IGF-I.[105] Several factors contribute to the nutritional problems, including increased nutrient losses and malabsorption.

### PRESENTING MANIFESTATIONS

Growth failure can herald Crohn disease. The weight often is more compromised than the height, and puberty is delayed but the patient looks well. Perianal fistulas are common. On questioning, patients may describe intermittent attacks of abdominal pain and diarrhea.

### CONFIRMATION OF THE DIAGNOSIS

Barium contrast radiographs of the small and large bowels often are characterized by an irregular mucosa or a cobblestone-like

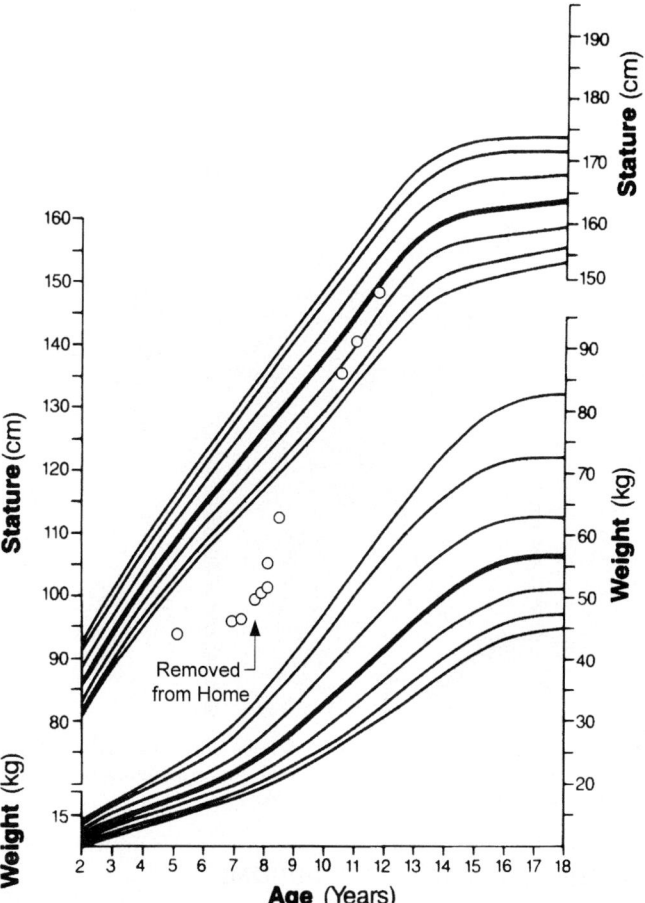

**FIGURE 198-23.** Growth curve of a girl with deprivation syndrome. Her growth as a young child was severely stunted, during which time she was being severely mistreated. She was removed from her home and responded remarkably to kindness and attention.

pattern, a thickened bowel, and the presence of enteric fistulas. The segmental distribution of the lesions frequently is diagnostic. Biopsy samples of the rectal mucosa obtained by colonoscopy show typical granulomas. The erythrocyte sedimentation rate usually is elevated, the bone age is retarded, and the hemoglobin and serum albumin levels occasionally are depressed.

### THERAPY AND PROGNOSIS

Control of the disease and provision of adequate nutrition are the prerequisites for growth, but an optimal method of accomplishing these goals has not been identified. Growth may accelerate with initial daily glucocorticoid therapy followed by alternate-day therapy in cases of stable disease.

Calories have been administered by central or peripheral intravenous hyperalimentation, elemental diets, and specialized formulas.[106] When the underlying disease is controlled, good nutrition alone, regardless of the method used to deliver it, stimulates growth. When disease activity cannot be stabilized and growth cannot be achieved with medical and nutritional support, surgical intervention should be considered. For growth to occur, resection must be performed before late puberty, all actively diseased bowel must be resected, and a prolonged disease-free postoperative period must be achieved. Ongoing nutritional therapy may augment the accelerated growth rate.[107]

The effects of various treatment plans on growth rate and final adult height require evaluation in large cooperative studies.

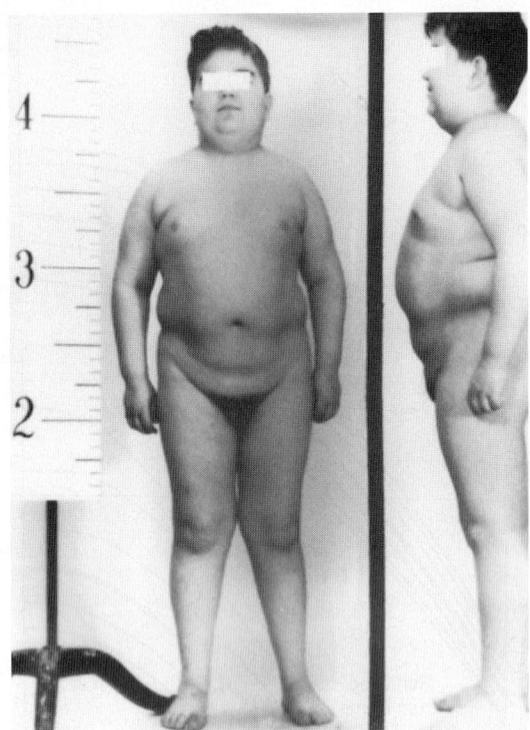

**FIGURE 198-24.** Seventeen-year-old boy with Cushing syndrome caused by bilateral adrenal hyperplasia. Note moon facies, buffalo hump, and obesity, especially of the trunk.

## CUSHING DISEASE OR SYNDROME

Patients with Cushing syndrome secrete excess cortisol and other adrenocortical hormones, usually continuously but sometimes periodically.[108] The underlying disease can be caused by an ACTH-secreting microadenoma of the pituitary (basophilic or mixed basophilic chromophobic, with a resultant bilateral adrenal hyperplasia) or by an adrenal tumor. Rarely, it is caused by a tumor secreting corticotropin-releasing hormone (CRH) or by an ectopic ACTH-producing tumor.[109] The natural history of Cushing disease (adrenal hyperplasia) is unknown, but rare cases of spontaneous remission have been reported.[110,111] Because many of the adrenal tumors are malignant, the mortality rate is high (see Chaps. 75 and 83). After the age of 7 years, the most common underlying problem is an ACTH-producing pituitary adenoma.[112,113]

### PRESENTING MANIFESTATIONS

Although Cushing disease is rare in the young, infants as well as teenagers can be affected. Usually, help is sought for the increasingly abnormal appearance—moon facies, obesity (especially of the trunk and face), purplish striae, hypertension, acne, emotional lability, and virilization (Fig. 198-24). A review of growth data invariably reveals a pathologically slow growth rate over months or years. The slowing of growth occasionally precedes the abnormal appearance by several months or years.

### CONFIRMATION OF THE DIAGNOSIS

The diagnosis of Cushing disease depends on the demonstration of pathologically elevated cortisol secretion—that is, elevated urinary free cortisol levels that cannot be suppressed with low doses of dexamethasone (see Chap. 77). The response to administration of larger doses of dexamethasone helps to localize the lesion. Suppression with high doses of dexamethasone

suggests the presence of adrenocortical hyperplasia caused by an abnormality of the hypothalamic-pituitary area, whereas failure to suppress is strongly suggestive of an adrenocortical tumor. Hypochloremic hypokalemic metabolic alkalosis can be present, and—in those cases caused by pituitary adenomas—late evening serum ACTH levels may be elevated. In a study of a short boy with periodic Cushing syndrome, the CRH test was found to be helpful. ACTH and cortisol concentrations were undetectable both in the basal state and after stimulation with CRH. As expected, the patient had bilateral micronodular adrenal hyperplasia at surgery.

In searching for a pituitary lesion, radiographs of the sella turcica, computed tomography of the pituitary area, MRI, petrosal sinus sampling, and, eventually, direct transsphenoidal visualization of the pituitary are helpful. For demonstrating the presence of an adrenal tumor, a radiograph of the abdomen can be useful to look for calcification of certain areas indicative of such a tumor. To reveal the tumor itself, ultrasonography, computed tomography, MRI, and radioactive iodocholesterol uptake can be used (see Chap. 88). In almost 300 patients, when plasma was sampled from the inferior petrosal sinuses with the conjunctive use of CRH, patients with Cushing disease could be distinguished from those with ectopic ACTH secretion.[114]

### THERAPY AND PROGNOSIS

Transsphenoidal microsurgery is the treatment of choice for patients with adrenal hyperplasia from a demonstrated pituitary tumor[115] (see Chap. 23). Results are excellent when the tumor is visualized and removed at surgery. Many of these patients become permanently glucocorticoid deficient. The former approach, bilateral adrenalectomy, rarely is indicated. Long-term remission has been reported with pituitary irradiation (see Chap. 22). Ketoconazole can facilitate regression of the stigmata of Cushing disease.[116]

Surgical excision is the treatment of choice for demonstrable adrenal tumors (see Chap. 89). Well-localized adenomas have a good prognosis. However, microscopic examination does not always distinguish benign from malignant lesions. The results of chemotherapy for malignant tumors are disappointing.

After successful therapy, the signs and symptoms of Cushing syndrome disappear, and many children grow in an accelerated fashion. As a group, they achieve a reasonable adult height.[112]

## IATROGENIC EFFECTS ON GROWTH

### STIMULANT MEDICATION

Certain neurostimulant drugs, especially methylphenidate but also pemoline and methamphetamine, can inhibit weight gain and growth before puberty but probably not after puberty. Desipramine does not inhibit the linear growth of children.[117–120]

### PRESENTING MANIFESTATIONS

Patients with attention deficit disorders who have been treated with neurostimulant drugs can have moderate slowing of growth and weight gain or even weight loss. Generally, these patients have received "high-normal" dosages (e.g., >1 mg/kg per day) of methylphenidate hydrochloride for many months. Anorexia is common and dose dependent, but abates with continued therapy. The results of physical examination usually are normal.

### ESTABLISHMENT OF THE DIAGNOSIS

The diagnosis is clinical and can be confirmed only when linear growth accelerates after cessation of the medication. Discontinuance of therapy during summer vacations seems to result in accelerated growth, but catch-up is incomplete. If linear growth does not increase during a drug "holiday," patients should be evaluated for other causes of slow growth.

### THERAPY AND PROGNOSIS

A controlled study involving 124 preadolescent boys with attention deficit/hyperactivity disorder (ADHD) has been reported.[120] Small but significant differences in height were found between children with and without ADHD. The height deficits were evident in early, but not late, adolescence, however, and were not related to the use of psychotropic medications. These data suggest that ADHD may be associated with temporary deficits in height gain through midadolescence that frequently normalize by late adolescence. This effect appears to be mediated by ADHD and not by its treatment. Thus, treatment with hGH is not indicated for this disorder.[120]

No definitive therapy is available, except for discontinuing drug therapy, decreasing a large dosage, or substituting desipramine. Thus, judicious prescribing of these drugs is important. During withdrawal, some children become temporarily hyperactive or depressed.

## PSYCHOSOCIAL MANAGEMENT OF SHORT STATURE

Current research builds on two decades of interest in psychosocial adjustment, personality and behavior factors, cognitive development, and school achievement, plus success in adulthood of children with diagnoses of GHD, constitutional delay of growth,[121-126] and Turner syndrome.[127-130] Interest is increasing in the effect of GH therapy on the cognitive and behavioral functioning of short children, regardless of whether they demonstrate GHD.[121,131-134] Societal bias toward tall stature from childhood through adulthood, even into the workplace, presents a challenge to the short individual in aspects of self-esteem, achievement, and acceptance. Therefore, their medical therapy is only one dimension of the care necessary to meet the multifaceted and variable needs of this population.

The overall goal for short children is to enable them to become financially self-supporting adults who hold jobs commensurate with their intellectual and educational ability, who function independently in their social environment, and who are satisfied with their lives. To maximize the possibility of success, physicians must interact with their patients in age-appropriate ways, being especially sensitive to the physical environment, to the use of language, and to the power and influence of the therapeutic relationship. The multidisciplinary team approach, including psychological intervention, skilled and compassionate nursing, and educational and vocational counseling, is most efficacious. Achieving realistic treatment expectations is essential.

In their interactions with short children, adults tend to infantilize, to overprotect, and to lower behavioral expectations. Some children respond by acting in a manner appropriate for their "height age" rather than their chronologic age. Short children may show a tendency to withdraw from their peer group and to continue this social isolation through adolescence and into adulthood. Boys, especially those with delayed onset or absence of puberty, may avoid interaction with male peers and form nonromantic liaisons with girls or younger children. Further social isolation, including rejection of dating and heterosexual interaction, and poor school achievement are additional risks. Accompanying these withdrawal syndromes are lack of assertiveness and ambition, anxiety, low self-esteem, and

dependency. GH therapy may add to the sense of well-being and overall health, thus leading to better psychological adjustment.[131,134] Children of all ages must be allowed assertively and politely to correct an adult who mistakes their age or remarks about their height in a derogatory manner. The support of the entire family, including siblings and parents, plays a crucial role in helping them to be emotionally expressive, competent, self-reliant, and independent.

Listening to parents, assessing their emotional capacity, and empowering and teaching them to meet the stresses of raising a child with a diagnosis of short stature are essential. Special issues relate to the language specific to the diagnosis of short stature. Sensitize parents to avoid the many "short"-related pejoratives in our language, such as calling someone "short-sighted" or referring to being "short-changed." Gender inequality creates a greater burden for males, because short females may be viewed as "cute" or "petite." Teaching parents to help their children to respond to teasing by bullies can be invaluable to the child who is not spontaneous in rebuffing a put-down with snappy repartee. Advise parents to encourage the development of hobbies, skills, and special talents that can help foster the high self-esteem that will cause peers to look up to their child. Specific suggestions include playing a musical instrument, singing, developing computer proficiency, debating, and engaging in arts and crafts such as painting, drawing, handicrafts, and sewing.

Children must wear age-appropriate clothing, and teens should be allowed to feel that peer group fashion trends are permitted. Creating a physical environment at home that fosters self-sufficiency and inclusion in family routines, including chores, should be stressed. Specific suggestions include making stepstools available, relaxing rules about climbing on counters, rearranging usual kitchen configurations, providing light switch pull cords, and lowering closet rods. Whether it be blocks added to bike pedals or devices to make driving accessible to the teen, these aids are necessary to foster a sense of self-worth and peer group inclusion. Celebrations of the ritual rites of passage, developmental milestones, and birthdays, particularly entrance into the teenage years, are pivotal times to enhance self-esteem.

Because short children tend to be at a physical disadvantage in body contact sports, encourage more personally self-competitive sports such as bettering one's own track record, rock climbing, tennis, golf, fishing, swimming, diving, skiing, martial arts, gymnastics, and wrestling in appropriate weight classes. Encourage individual problem solving; however, if, for example, the teen is self-conscious about changing clothes or showering in front of peers, altering of rigid school rules that may be changed only by the intervention of a parent or physician can save pain and humiliation. Allowing the individual to make his or her own choices and decisions fosters a sense of self-reliance.

Parents must be encouraged to be advocates for their short children at school, working closely with school personnel to preempt problems. Transition years when children move from elementary to middle and to high school may be times of increased stress when they have to redefine themselves in the hierarchy of their peer group. Special attention may be needed to insure that school achievement remains at the level of intellectual capacity. Relocating to a new community may increase stress and challenge academic and social adjustment.

As a group, short children have normal intellectual function. A few patients with GHD caused by tumors or by cranial irradiation may experience varying degrees of intellectual impairment. Some girls with Turner syndrome are at greater risk for visuospatial perception deficits that cause difficulties with directional sense and map and graph reading, as well as some inability to use a computer mouse. Learning environments should maximize the child's skills while removing distractions, anxiety, or overload. Remediation education should be instituted if specific math deficits are diagnosed. Vocational planning should be consistent with each individual's pattern of strengths and weaknesses.

The best means for part-time employment for teens and permanent employment for young adults may be through a friend or a nonjudgmental person who has had experience with people of short stature. Networks of such employers should be cultivated as a resource for this patient population. Role models in the community make ideal individuals to open doors and smooth the way for the short individual.

The formal support groups that have been established—such as Human Growth Foundation (www.hgfound.org), Magic Foundation for Children's Growth (www.magicfoundation.org) and Little People of America (www.lpaonline.org)—are important conduits for peer group interaction as well as information and family networking. The groups are an effective advocate-lobbying group in the health care and political arenas.

# REFERENCES

1. Cowett RM, Stern L. The intrauterine growth retarded infant: etiology, prenatal diagnosis, neonatal management, and long-term follow-up. In: Lifshitz F, ed. Pediatric endocrinology. New York: Marcel Dekker, 1985:109.
1a. Kramer MS, Seguin L, Lydon J, Galet L. Socio-economic disparities in pregnancy outcome: why do the poor fare so poorly? Paediatr Perinat Epidemiol 2000; 14:194.
2. Miller HC. Intrauterine growth retardation: past, present and future. Growth Genet Horm 1992; 8(3):5.
3. Warshaw JB. Intrauterine growth restriction revisited. Growth Genet Horm 1992; 8(1):5.
4. Cruise MO. A longitudinal study of the growth of low birth weight infants. I. Velocity and distance growth, birth to 3 years. Pediatrics 1973; 51:620.
5. Kitchen WH, Doyle LW, Ford GW. Very low birthweight and growth in infants with atypical fetal growth patterns. Am J Dis Child 1977; 131:1078.
6. Ross G, Lipper EG, Auld PAM. Growth achievement of very low birth weight premature children at school age. J Pediatr 1990; 117:307.
7. Holmes GE, Miller HC, Khatab H, et al. Postnatal somatic growth in infants with atypical fetal growth patterns. Am J Dis Child 1977; 131:1078.
8. Herman-Giddens ME, Slora EJ, Wasserman RC, et al. Secondary sexual characteristics and menses in young girls seen in office practice: a study from the pediatric research in office settings network. Pediatrics 1997; 99:505.
9. Palmert MR, Malvin HV, Boepple PA. Unsustained or slowly progressive puberty in young girls: initial presentation and long-term follow-up of 20 untreated patients. J Clin Endocrinol Metab 1999; 84:415.
10. Klein KO. Precocious puberty: who has it? Who should be treated? J Clin Endocrinol Metab 1999; 84:411.
10a. Lebrethon MC, Bourguignon JP. Management of central isosexual precocity: diagnosis, treatment, outcome. Curr Opin Pediatr 2000; 12:394.
11. Feuillam PP, Jones JV, Barnes K, et al. Reproductive axis after discontinuation of gonadotropin-releasing hormone analog. Treatment of girls with precocious puberty. Long-term follow-up comparing girls with hypothalamic hamartoma to those with idiopathic precocious puberty. J Clin Endocrinol Metab 1999; 84:44.
12. Butler GE, Sellar RE, Walker RF, et al. Oral testosterone undecaenoate in the management of delayed puberty in boys: pharmacokinetics and effects on sexual maturation and growth. J Clin Endocrinol Metab 1992; 75:37.
13. Wing-yee T, Boyukgelwiz A, Hindmarsh PC, et al. Long-term outcome of oxandrolone treatment in boys with constitutional delay of growth and puberty. J Pediatr 1990; 117:588.
14. LaFranchi S, Hanna CE, Mandel SH. Constitutional delay of growth: expected versus final adult height. Pediatrics 1991; 87:82.
15. Finkelstein JS, Neer RM, Biller BMK, et al. Osteopenia in men with a history of delayed puberty. N Engl J Med 1992; 326:600.
16. Wallis M. The molecular bases of growth hormone deficiency. Mol Aspects Med 1988; 10:429.
17. De Boer H, Blok G-J, Van der Veen E. Clinical aspects of growth hormone deficiency in adults. Endocr Rev 1995; 16:63.
18. Blum WF, Albertsson-Wikland K, Rosberg S, Rauke MB. Serum levels of IGF-I and IGFBP-3 reflect spontaneous growth hormone secretion. J Clin Endocrinol Metab 1993; 76:1612.
19. Frasier SD. A review of growth hormone stimulation tests in children. Pediatrics 1974; 53:929.
20. Lawson W. The diagnosis and treatment of endocrine disorders in childhood and adolescence. Springfield, IL: Charles C Thomas, 1950.
21. American Academy of Pediatrics Committee on Drugs and Committee on Bioethics. Considerations related to the use of recombinant human growth hormone in children. Pediatrics 1997; 99:122.
22. Spillotis BE, August GP, Hung W, et al. Growth hormone neurosecretory dysfunction: a treatable cause of short stature. JAMA 1984; 251:2223.
23. Daughaday WH. Recognition of growth hormone secretory disorders. (Editorial). JAMA 1984; 251:2251.
24. Moore WV, Donaldson DL, Hollowell JG, et al. Growth hormone secretory profiles: variation on consecutive nights. J Pediatr 1989; 115:51.
25. Frasier SD. A review of growth hormone stimulation tests in children. Pediatrics 1974; 53:929.
26. Rose SR, Ross JL, Uriarte M, et al. The advantage of measuring stimulated as compared with spontaneous growth hormone levels in the diagnosis of growth hormone deficiency. N Engl J Med 1988; 319:201.
27. Donaldson DL, Pan F, Hollowell JG, et al. Reliability of stimulated and spontaneous growth hormone (GH) levels for identifying the child with low GH secretion. J Clin Endocrinol Metab 1991; 72:647.
28. Loche S, Cambiaso P, Setzu S, et al. Final height after growth hormone therapy in non-growth-hormone-deficient children with short stature. J Pediatr 1994; 125:196.
29. Zadik Z, Mira U, Landau H. Final height after growth hormone therapy in peripubertal boys with a subnormal integrated concentration of growth hormone. Horm Res 1992; 37:150.
30. Frohman LA, Aceto T Jr, MacGillivray MH. Studies of growth hormone secretion in children: normal hypopituitary and constitutionally delayed. J Clin Endocrinol Metab 1967; 27:1409.
31. Cornblath M, Parker ML, Reisner SH, et al. Secretion and metabolism of growth hormone in premature and full term infants. J Clin Endocrinol Metab 1965; 25:209.
32. Martha PM Jr, Gorman KM, Blizzard RM, et al. Endogenous growth hormone secretion and clearance rates in normal boys, as determined by deconvolution analysis: relationship to age, pubertal status, and body mass. J Clin Endocrinol Metab 1992; 74:336.
33. Celniker AC, Chen AB, Wert RM Jr, Sherman BM. Variability in the quantity of circulating growth hormone using commercial immunoassays. J Clin Endocrinol Metab 1989; 68:469.
34. Granada ML, Sanmarti A, Lucas A, et al. Assay-dependent results of immunoassayable spontaneous 25-h growth hormone secretion in short children. Acta Paediatr Scand Suppl 1990; 370:63.
35. Baumann G. Growth hormone heterogeneity: genes, isohormones, variants, and binding proteins. Endocr Rev 1991; 12:424.
36. Chatelain P, Bouillat B, Cohen R, et al. Assay of growth hormone levels in human plasma using commercial kits: analysis of some factors influencing the results. Acta Paediatr Scand Suppl 1990; 370:56.
37. Rosenfeld RG, Albertsson-Wikland K, Cassorla F, et al. Diagnostic controversy: the diagnosis of childhood growth hormone deficiency revisited. J Clin Endocrinol Metab 1995; 80:1532.
38. Rosenfeld RG, Gargosky SE. Assays for insulin-like growth factors and their binding proteins: practicalities and pitfalls. J Pediatr 1996; 128:S52.
39. Werther GA. Growth hormone measurements versus auxologic treatment decisions: the Australian experience. J Pediatr 1996; 128:S47.
40. Strasburger CJ, Wu Z, Pflaum CD, Dressendorfer RA. Immunofunctional assay of human growth hormone in serum: a possible consensus for hGH measurement. J Clin Endocrinol Metab 1996; 81:2613.
41. L'Hermite-Balerjaux M, Copinschi G, Cauter EV. Growth hormone assays early to latest test generations compared. Clin Chem 1996; 42:1978.
42. Kaplan SA. Growth and growth hormone: disorders of the anterior pituitary. In: Kaplan SA, ed. Clinical pediatric and adolescent endocrinology, Philadelphia: WB Saunders, 1982:20.
43. Burstein S. Growth disorders after cranial irradiation in childhood. J Clin Endocrinol Metab 1994; 78:1280.
44. Ogilvy-Stuart AL, Clayton PE, Shalet SM. Cranial irradiation and early puberty. J Clin Endocrinol Metab 1994; 78:1282.
45. Blatt J, Bercu BB, Gillin JC, et al. Reduced pulsatile growth hormone secretion in children after therapy for acute lymphoblastic leukemia. J Pediatr 1984; 104:182.
46. Aceto T Jr, Frasier SD, Hayles AB, et al. Collaborative study of the effects of human growth hormone deficiency. I. First year of therapy. J Clin Endocrinol Metab 1972; 35:483.
47. Arslanian SA, Becker DJ, Lee PA, et al. Growth hormone therapy and tumor recurrence findings in children with brain neoplasms and hypopituitarism. Am J Dis Child 1985; 139:347.
48. Truilizi F, Scotti G, Di Natale B, et al. Evidence of a congenital midline brain anomaly in pituitary dwarfs: a magnetic resonance imaging study in 101 patients. Pediatrics 1994; 93:409.
49. Cacciari E, Zucchini S, Ambrosetto P, et al. Empty sella in children and adolescents with possible hypothalamic-pituitary disorders. J Clin Endocrinol Metab 1994; 78:767.
50. Baroncelli GI, Bertelloni S, Ceccarelli C, Saggese G. Measurement of volumetric bone mineral density accurately determines degree of lumbar undermineralization in children with growth hormone deficiency. J Clin Endocrinol Metab 1998; 83:3150.
51. Frasier SD, Foley TP Jr. Creutzfeldt-Jakob disease in recipients of pituitary hormones. J Clin Endocrinol Metab 1994; 78:1277.
52. Aceto T Jr, Sotos J, Garibaldi L, et al. Response to increasing doses of growth hormone (GH) in classic GH deficiency. Pediatr Res 1992; 31:71A.
53. Blethen SL, Compton P, Lippe B, et al. Factors predicting the response to

growth hormone (GH) therapy in prepubertal children with GH deficiency. J Clin Endocrinol Metab 1993; 76:574.

54. Hedin L, Olsson B, Diczfalusy M, et al. Intranasal administration of human growth hormone (hGH) in combination with membrane permeation enhancer in patients with GH deficiency: a pharmacokinetic study. J Clin Endocrinol Metab 1993; 76:962.

55. Dhawan J, Pan LC, Pavlath GK, et al. Systemic delivery of human growth hormone by injection of genetically engineered myoblasts. Science 1991; 254:1509.

56. Barr E, Leiden JM. Systemic delivery of recombinant proteins by genetically modified myoblasts. Science 1991; 254:1507.

57. Allen DB, Julius R, Breen TJ, Attie KM. Treatment of glucocorticoid-induced growth suppression with growth hormone. J Clin Endocrinol Metab 1998; 83:2824.

58. Hopwood NJ, Hintz RL, Gertner JM, et al. Growth response of children with non-growth-hormone deficiency and marked short stature during three years of growth hormone therapy. J Pediatr 1993; 123:215.

59. Allen DB, Frasier SD, Foley TP Jr, Pescowitz OH. Growth hormone for children with Down syndrome. (Editorial). J Pediatr 1993; 123:742.

60. Wilson DM, Lee PD, Morris AH, et al. Growth hormone therapy in hypophosphatemic rickets. Am J Dis Child 1991; 145:1165.

61. Rotenstein D, Reigel DH, Flom LL. Growth hormone accelerates growth of short children with neural tube defects. J Pediatr 1989; 115:417.

62. Angulo M, Castro-Magana C, Uy J. Pituitary evaluation and growth hormone treatment in Prader-Willi syndrome. J Pediatr Endocrinol 1991; 4:167.

63. Finkelstein BS, Silvers JB, Marrero U, et al. Insurance coverage, physician recommendations, and access to emerging treatments. Growth hormone therapy for childhood short stature. JAMA 1998; 279(9):663.

64. Saenger PH, Attie KM, DiMartino-Nardi J, et al. Metabolic consequences of 5-year growth hormone (GH) therapy in children treated with GH for idiopathic short stature. Genentech Collaborative Study Group. J Clin Endocrinol Metab 1998; 83:3115.

65. Rosenfeld RG, Frane J, Attie KM. Six-year results of a randomized prospective trial of human growth hormone and oxandrolone in Turner syndrome. J Pediatr 1992; 121:49.

65a. Chernausek SD, Attie KM, Cara JF, et al. Growth hormone therapy of Turner syndrome: the impact of age of estrogen replacement on final height. J Clin Endocrinol Metab 2000; 85:2439.

66. Holm VA, Cassidy SB, Butler MG, et al. Prader-Willi syndrome: consensus diagnostic criteria. Pediatrics 1993; 91:398.

67. Angulo M, Castro-Magana M, Mazur B, et al. Growth hormone secretion and effects of growth hormone therapy on growth velocity and weight gain in children with Prader-Willi syndrome. J Pediatr Endocrinol Metab 1996; 3:393.

68. Ritzen ME, Lindgren AC, Hagenäs L, Blichfeldt S, et al. Growth hormone treatment of children with Prader-Willi syndrome affects linear growth and body composition favourably. Acta Paediatr 1998; 87:28.

68a. Myers SE, Carrel AL, Whitman BY, Allen DB. Sustained benefit after 2 years of growth hormone upon body composition, fat utilization, physical agility, and growth in Prader-Willi syndrome. J Pediatr 2000; 137:42.

69. Haffner D, Schaefer F, Nissel R, et al. Effect of growth hormone treatment on the adult height of children with chronic renal failure. N Engl J Med 2000; 343:923.

70. Hintz RL. Untoward events in patients treated with growth hormone in the USA. Horm Res 1992; 38(Suppl 1):44.

71. Blethen SL. Pseudotumor cerebri: the national cooperative growth study. Contribution proceedings. 1993:14.

72. Kohn B, Julius JR, Blethen SL. Combined use of growth hormone and gonadotropin-releasing hormone analogues: the national cooperative growth hormone study experience. German Study Group for Growth Hormone Treatment in Chronic Renal Failure. Pediatrics 1999; 104:1014.

73. Laron Z, Pertzeland A, Mannheimer S. Genetic pituitary dwarfism with high serum concentrations of growth hormone: a new inborn error of metabolism? J Med Sci 1966; 2:152.

74. Rosenfeld RG, Rosenbloom AI, Guevara-Aguirre J. Growth hormone (GH) insensitivity due to primary GH receptor deficiency. Endocr Rev 1994; 15:369.

75. Clemmons DR, Underwood LE. Uses of human insulin-like growth factor-I in clinical conditions. J Clin Endocrinol Metab 1994; 79:4.

75a. Laron Z. The essential role of IGF-I: Lessons from the long-term study and treatment of children and adults with Laron syndrome. J Clin Endocrinol Metab 1999; 84:4397.

76. Juul A, Kastrup KW, Pedersen SA, et al. Growth hormone (GH) provocative retesting of 108 young adults with childhood-onset GH deficiency and the diagnostic value of insulin-like growth factor I (IGF-I) and IGF-binding protein-3. J Clin Endocrinol Metab 1997; 82:1195.

77. Rosen T, Bengtsson BA. Premature mortality due to cardiovascular disease in hypopituitarism. Lancet 1990; 336:285.

78. Sönksen PH, Weissberger AJ. Growth hormone deficiency in adults. Growth Genet Horm 1998; 14:41.

79. Baum HB, Katznelson L, Sherman JC, et al. Effects of physiological growth hormone (GH) therapy on cognition and quality of life in patients with adult-onset GH deficiency. J Clin Endocrinol Metab 1998; 83:3184.

80. Zimmerman D, Saenger PH, Gharib H. AACE clinical practice for growth hormone use in adults. Endocr Pract 1998; 4:165.

81. Aleman A, Verharr HJJ, DeHaan EHF, et al. Insulin-like growth factor-I and cognitive function in healthy older men. J Clin Endocrinol Metab 1999; 84:471.

82. Pfeiffer M, Verhorner R, Zizek B, et al. Growth hormone treatment reverses early atherosclerotic changes in GH-deficient adults. J Clin Endocrinol Metab 1999; 84:453.

83. Klein RZ, Arnold MB, Bigos ST, et al. Correlation of cognitive test scores and adequacy of treatment in adolescents with congenital hypothyroidism. J Pediatr 1994; 124:383.

84. Sekadde CB, Slaunwhite WR, Aceto T Jr. Rapid radioimmunoassay of triiodothyronine in clinical radioassay procedures: a compendium. In: Besch PK, ed. American Association of Clinical Chemists, 1975:292.

85. Jones KL. Achondroplasia syndrome. In: Jones KL, ed. Smith's recognizable patterns of human malformation, 5th ed. Philadelphia: WB Saunders, 1997:298.

85a. Hunter I, Greene SA, MacDonald TM, Morris AD. Prevalence and aetiology of hypothyroidism in the young. Arch Dis Child 2000; 83:207.

86. Sekadde CB, Slaunwhite WR Jr, Aceto T Jr, Murray K. Administration of thyroxine once a week. J Clin Endocrinol Metab 1975; 39:759.

87. Pantsiotou S, Stanhope R, Uruena M, et al. Growth prognosis and growth after menarche in primary hypothyroidism. Arch Dis Child 1991; 66:838.

88. Man EB, Jones WS. Thyroid function in human pregnancy, V. Am J Obstet Gynecol 1969; 104:898.

89. Haddow JE, Klein RZ, Mitchell ML, et al. Maternal thyroid deficiency during pregnancy and subsequent neuropsychological development of the child. N Engl J Med 1999; 341:549.

90. Beighton P, Giedion ZA, Gorlin R, et al. International classification of osteochondrodysplasias. Am J Med Genet 1992; 44:223.

91. Hall BD. Approach to skeletal dysplasia. Pediatr Clin North Am 1992; 39:279.

92. Shapiro F. Epiphyseal disorders. N Engl J Med 1987; 317:1702.

93. Jones KL. Osteochondrodysplasias. In: Jones KL, ed. Smith's recognizable patterns of human malformation, 5th ed. Philadelphia: WB Saunders, 1997.

94. Taybi H, Lachman RS. Radiology of syndromes, metabolic disorders, and skeletal dysplasias, 3rd ed. Chicago: Year Book, 1990:671.

95. Saleh M, Burton M. Leg lengthening: patient selection and management in achondroplasia. Orthop Clin North Am 1991; 22:589.

96. Lavini F, Renzi-Brivio L, de Bastianai G. Psychologic, vascular, and physiologic aspects of lower limb lengthening in achondroplastics. Clin Orthop 1990; 250:138.

97. Jones KL. Hypochondroplasia syndrome. In: Jones KL, ed. Smith's recognizable patterns of human malformation, 5th ed. Philadelphia: WB Saunders, 1997:304.

98. Powell GF, Brasel JA, Blizzard RM. Emotional deprivation and growth retardation simulating idiopathic hypopituitarism. I. Clinical evaluation of the syndrome. N Engl J Med 1967; 276:1271.

99. Powell GF, Brasel JA, Raiti S, et al. Emotional deprivation and growth retardation simulating idiopathic hypopituitarism. II. Endocrine evaluation of the syndrome. N Engl J Med 1967; 276:1279.

100. Sandberg DE, Smith MM, Fornari V, et al. Nutritional dwarfing: is it a consequence of disturbed psychosocial functioning? Pediatrics 1991; 88:926.

101. Rudolf MCJ, Hochberg Z. Annotation. Are boys more vulnerable to psychosocial growth retardation? Dev Med Child Neurol 1990; 32:1022.

102. Smith MM, Lifshitz F. Excess fruit juice consumption as a contributing factor in nonorganic failure to thrive. Pediatrics 1994; 93:438.

103. Money J, Annecillo C, Kelly JF. Growth of intelligence: failure and catch-up associated respectively with abuse and rescue in the syndrome of abuse dwarfism. Psychoneuroendocrinology 1983; 8:309.

104. Rosenthal SR, Snyder JD, Hendricks KM, Walker WA. Growth failure and inflammatory bowel disease. Approach to treatment of a complicated adolescent problem. Pediatrics 1983; 72:481.

105. Kirschner BS. Growth and development in chronic inflammatory bowel disease. Acta Paediatr Scand Suppl 1990; 366:98.

106. Polk DB, Hattner JAT, Kerner JA Jr. Improved growth and disease activity after intermittent administration of a defined formula diet in children with Crohn's disease. J Parenter Enteral Nutr 1992; 16:499.

107. Lipson AB, Savage MO, Davies PSW, et al. Acceleration of linear growth following intestinal resection for Crohn's disease. Eur J Pediatr 1990; 149:687.

108. Muguruza MTG, Chrousos GP. Periodic Cushing syndrome in a short boy: usefulness of the ovine corticotropin releasing hormone test. J Pediatr 1989; 115:270.

109. Preeyasombat C, Sikikulchayanonta V, Mahaclok Elert-Wattana P, et al. Cushing's syndrome caused by Ewing's sarcoma secreting corticotropin releasing factor-like peptide. Am J Dis Child 1992; 146:1103.

110. Putnam TI, Aceto T Jr, Abbassi V, Kenny FM. Cushing's disease with a spontaneous remission. Pediatrics 1972; 50:477.

111. Kammer H, Barton M. Spontaneous remission of Cushing's disease: a case report and review of the literature. Am J Med 1979; 67:519.

112. McArthur RG, Cloutier MD, Hayles AB, Sprague RF. Cushing's disease in children: findings in 13 cases. Mayo Clin Proc 1972; 47:318.

113. Thomas CG, Smith AT, Griffith JM, Askin FB. Hyperadrenalism in childhood and adolescence. Ann Surg 1984; 199:538.

114. Oldfield EG, Doppman JL, Nieman LK, et al. Petrosal sinus sampling with and without corticotropin-releasing hormone for the differential diagnosis of Cushing's syndrome. N Engl J Med 1991; 325:897.

115. Tyrell JB, Brooks RM, Fitzgerald PA, et al. Cushing's disease: selective transsphenoidal resection of pituitary microadenomas. N Engl J Med 1978; 298:753.

116. Sonino N, Boscaro M, Merola G, Mantero F. Prolonged treatment of Cushing disease by ketoconazole. J Clin Endocrinol Metab 1985; 61:718.

117. Roche AF, Lipman RS, Overall JE, Hung W. The effects of stimulant medication on the growth of hyperkinetic children. Pediatrics 1979; 63:847.

118. Dickinson LC, Lee J, Ringdahl IC, et al. Impaired growth in hyperkinetic children receiving pemoline. J Pediatr 1979; 94:538.
119. Vincent J, Varley CK, Leger P. Effects of methylphenidate on early adolescent growth. Am J Psychiatry 1990; 147:501.
120. Spencer T, Biederman J, Wilens T. Growth deficits in children with attention deficit hyperactivity disorder. Pediatrics 1998; 102:501.
121. Sandberg D. Short stature in middle childhood: a survey of psychosocial functioning in a clinic-referred sample. In: Stabler B, Underwood L, eds. Growth, stature, and adaptation. Chapel Hill, NC: University of North Carolina Press, 1994:19.
122. Stabler B, Underwood L, eds. Growth, stature, and adaptation. Chapel Hill, NC: University of North Carolina Press, 1994.
123. Zimet G. Psychosocial functioning of adults who were short as children. In: Stabler B, Underwood L, eds. Growth, stature, and adaptation. Chapel Hill, NC: University of North Carolina Press, 1994:73.
124. Sartorio A, Conti A, Molinari E, et al. Growth, growth hormone and cognitive functions. Horm Res 1996; 45:23.
125. Stabler B, Clopper RR, Siegel PT, et al. Links between growth hormone deficiency, adaptation and social phobia. Horm Res 1996; 45:30.
126. Burman P, Deijen JB. Quality of life and cognitive function in patients with pituitary insufficiency. Psychother Psychosom 1998; 67:154.
127. Lagrou K, Xhouret-Heinrichs D, Heinrichs C, et al. Age-related perception of stature, acceptance of therapy, and psychosocial functioning in human growth hormone-treated girls with Turner's syndrome. J Clin Endocrinol Metab 1998; 83:1494.
128. McCauley E. Self-concept and behavioral profiles in Turner Syndrome. In: Stabler B, Underwood L, eds. Growth, stature, and adaptation. Chapel Hill, NC: University of North Carolina Press, 1994:181.
129. Skuse D. Psychosocial functioning in the Turner Syndrome: a national survey. In: Stabler B, Underwood L, eds. Growth, stature, and adaptation. Chapel Hill, NC: University of North Carolina Press, 1994:151.
130. Rovet J. School outcome in Turner Syndrome. In: Stabler B, Underwood L, eds. Growth, stature, and adaptation. Chapel Hill, NC: University of North Carolina Press, 1994:165.
131. Cuttler L, Silvers JB, Singh J, et al. Short stature and growth hormone therapy. A national study of physician recommendation patterns. JAMA 1996; 276:531.
132. Hintz RL. Growth hormone treatment of idiopathic short stature. Horm Res 1996; 46:208.
133. Rao JK, Julius JR, Breen TJ, Blethen SL. Response to growth hormone in attention deficit hyperactivity disorder: effects of methylphenidate and pemoline therapy. Pediatrics 1998; 102(Suppl):497.
134. Stabler B, Siegel PT, Clopper RR, et al. Behavior change after growth hormone treatment of children with short stature. J Pediatr 1998; 133:366.

# CHAPTER 199

# ENDOCRINOLOGY AND AGING

DAVID A. GRUENEWALD AND ALVIN M. MATSUMOTO

The number of elderly people is growing faster than the population at large. The number of Americans older than age 65 years is expected to increase from 35 million in 2000 to 78 million in 2050. Furthermore, the number of the "oldest old," those older than age 85, is expected to increase from 4 million in 2000 to almost 18 million in 2050.[1]

Thus, the latter, most frail group of elderly people with the greatest burden of age-associated diseases is the group that is growing the most rapidly.[1a] Because endocrine diseases such as osteoporosis, type 2 diabetes mellitus, and hypothyroidism are extremely common in older people, adult endocrinologists will see an increasing proportion of elderly patients in their practices in the future.

With aging, changes occur in many parameters of endocrine function, such as decreases in growth hormone (GH) and gonadal steroid levels, and increases in cholesterol levels and adiposity. Many of these changes predispose to morbidity and mortality in later life; for example, ovarian failure affects bone mass and fracture risk. The effects of other age-related alterations (e.g., declin-

ing GH and testosterone levels) are of uncertain significance. Furthermore, the clinical presentation, diagnosis, treatment, and prognosis of certain endocrine diseases are altered with aging, greatly increasing the clinical challenges of evaluation and management in elderly patients. In turn, endocrine diseases in geriatric patients often have profound effects on functional status and quality of life, and these issues are often much more important to patients than the underlying diseases per se. Ultimately, the primary goal of medical management in elderly people is not to eliminate disease, but rather to help the older person achieve the highest possible level of functioning and quality of life.

## PRINCIPLES OF GERIATRIC ENDOCRINOLOGY

### IMPAIRED HOMEOSTASIS

Aging is characterized by a decline in functional reserve of major body organs, leading to impaired ability to restore equilibrium after environmental stresses. This age-related impairment of homeostatic regulation is evident in many endocrine functions but may become clinically evident only during acute or significant long-term stress. For example, fasting blood glucose levels exhibit very little change with normal aging, but after challenge with a glucose load, glucose levels increase more in healthy elderly people than in young adults. The function of endocrine systems may be maintained through homeostatic mechanisms and/or changes in hormone metabolism that offset the loss of function. For example, pituitary luteinizing hormone (LH) secretion and serum LH levels are increased in many elderly men and testosterone metabolism is decreased, thus compensating for a reduction in testicular testosterone secretion. In some cases, however, these changes are insufficient to maintain normal function with aging even under basal conditions. One example is aldosterone production, which declines disproportionately to its clearance rate with aging, a situation that leads to age-related decreases in basal plasma aldosterone levels.

Several principles of geriatric endocrinology illustrate the complexity and challenge of evaluating frail older patients with endocrine disease. These include the atypical presentations of illness; the presence of multiple coexisting medical problems; the large number of symptoms, signs, and abnormal laboratory findings often present in individual elderly patients; underreporting of symptoms; and problems in the cognitive, psychiatric, social, economic, and functional domains. Failure to appreciate these challenges and to appropriately assess older patients with these issues in mind may result in missed or incorrect diagnoses, inappropriate treatments, and poor functional outcomes.

### NONSPECIFIC AND ATYPICAL PRESENTATION

Endocrinopathies commonly present in elderly people with nonspecific, muted, or atypical symptoms and signs. For example, hypothyroidism and hyperthyroidism may present similarly in older adults with nonspecific symptoms, including weight loss, fatigue, weakness, constipation, and depression. The presentation of endocrine disease in geriatric patients may also be atypical compared with that in younger patients (e.g., apathy, depression, and psychomotor retardation may be associated with hyperthyroidism, and marked hyperglycemia and hyperosmolarity without ketoacidosis may be present in elderly patients with type 2 diabetes). In some patients, regardless of the cause of the illness, its manifestations may occur in the most compromised body system. Thus, in an older patient with underlying gait and balance abnormalities, falling may be the primary symptom of diseases as diverse as pneumonia, myocardial infarction, uncontrolled diabetes mellitus, or hypothyroidism. Illnesses may present in the guise of other disabling geriatric syndromes such as delirium, urinary incontinence, and dementia. Endocrine disorders may produce or be associated with any or all of these syndromes, so endocrinologists must have a basic understanding of these disorders. Several excellent reviews of these geriatric syndromes are available.[2–4]

## DIFFICULTIES IN LABORATORY EVALUATION

In addition to the atypical or nonspecific presentations of endocrine disease described earlier, with aging, it is increasingly common for illnesses such as hypothyroidism to present without any symptoms. The presence of disease may be appreciated only on routine laboratory screening, as in the case of asymptomatic hypercalcemia secondary to hyperparathyroidism. Furthermore, the presence of multiple medical problems and the use of multiple medications may confound the evaluation of older patients. For example, decreased serum thyroxine ($T_4$) and triiodothyronine ($T_3$) levels and alterations in the levels of serum thyroid-stimulating hormone may occur in elderly patients who are systemically ill or are taking certain medications (e.g., glucocorticoids, dopamine) but are euthyroid (euthyroid sick syndromes), giving a misleading impression of an endocrine abnormality.

The evaluation of the older patient is further complicated by the fact that normal ranges for endocrine laboratory tests are usually established in healthy young subjects and may not reflect normal values in healthy elderly people. Moreover, normative data for older populations are often confounded by the inclusion of subjects with age-associated diseases. Finally, most studies of aging and endocrine function in humans are cross-sectional rather than longitudinal and, therefore, may not accurately predict age-related changes within a given individual. Indeed, variability among individuals is a hallmark of aging.

## GERIATRIC ASSESSMENT AND TREATMENT

The onset of functional decline may be an important, and sometimes the only, clue to the development of an acute illness or exacerbation of a chronic disease in geriatric patients. Accordingly, a structured geriatric assessment should be a part of the clinical evaluation, especially in frail elderly patients. Functional assessment can detect impairments in physical function, cognition, emotional status, sensory capabilities, and activities of daily living that are not detected by standard clinical examinations,[5] and these impairments are often much more important to patients than the underlying diseases that give rise to them. Such an assessment can also help to determine the response to treatment and to predict the patient's ultimate degree of disability. A useful approach to general outpatient screening of older patients for functional disability has been suggested.[6] Patients with evidence of functional impairment on screening examination may benefit from a comprehensive functional assessment by an interdisciplinary care team. However, comprehensive evaluation is time consuming and expensive; therefore, it should be targeted to the most appropriate patients: frail or ill elderly people with a real or anticipated functional decline (including patients on the verge of requiring institutionalization), those with inadequate primary medical care, and those with poor economic and social support systems.[7]

Treatment decisions involving geriatric patients with endocrine disease must consider age-associated factors such as alterations in clearance rate and target-organ effects, coexisting

medical illnesses, and the medications taken by the patient. Older patients consume a disproportionate share of medications compared with the population at large. Moreover, drug toxicities are more frequent and severe in the elderly than in young patients receiving the same drug regimen.[3] Dysfunction in multiple organ systems together with cognitive and visual impairment further predispose older patients to adverse drug effects. As a result, older people are at high risk for the development of medication side effects and drug interactions secondary to polypharmacy. To minimize these risks, dosage levels for hormone replacement and medications must be adjusted for changes in clearance rate with aging, and patients should receive the lowest dosage of medication needed to achieve the therapeutic effect. New medications should be initiated using low doses and increased very gradually as needed. Finally, the medication regimen should be reviewed periodically, and medications no longer needed should be discontinued.

## HYPOTHALAMUS AND PITUITARY GLAND

### HYPOTHALAMUS

Studies directly assessing the effects of aging on parameters of hypothalamic neuroendocrine function in humans have not been performed. Some of these effects, however, can be inferred by assessing age-related alterations in circadian and ultradian rhythms (e.g., pulsatile release) of pituitary hormones and by determining pituitary hormonal responsiveness to administration of hypothalamic releasing hormones or to agents that either block end-organ feedback (e.g., clomiphene and metyrapone) or stimulate hypothalamic-pituitary hormonal secretion (e.g., stimulation of antidiuretic hormone [ADH] secretion by hypertonic saline administration or stimulation of GH secretion by insulin-induced hypoglycemia).

Age-related blunting of the circadian rhythm of LH pulse frequency has been observed in healthy elderly men, suggesting altered regulation of the gonadotropin-releasing hormone (GnRH) pulse generator with aging.[8] Furthermore, LH pulse frequency is relatively decreased despite reduced testosterone levels in some healthy elderly men as compared with young men, implying decreased GnRH pulse frequency in these older men.[9] Interestingly, despite this impairment in baseline LH pulse frequency with aging, fasting decreases LH pulse frequency in healthy young men but not in older men, indicating altered reproductive axis regulation in response to a fasting stress.[10] Finally, administration of naloxone, an opioid antagonist, does not increase LH pulse frequency in healthy older men as it does in young men, suggesting altered hypothalamic opioid regulation of LH secretion.[11] In contrast to the findings for the reproductive axis, adrenocorticotropic hormone (ACTH) pulse frequency, cortisol levels, and ACTH response to corticotropin-releasing hormone (CRH) stimulation are unchanged in healthy elderly compared with young men, suggesting that hypothalamic regulation of pituitary/adrenocortical function may be relatively unimpaired by aging.[12]

Hypothalamic-pituitary feedback sensitivity to some end-organ hormones is altered with aging. For example, most studies have found increased feedback sensitivity to testosterone with aging,[13,14] whereas glucocorticoid feedback sensitivity is decreased with aging.[15]

### POSTERIOR PITUITARY: ANTIDIURETIC HORMONE

The bulk of evidence suggests an increase in basal ADH levels with aging.[16] Furthermore, aging is associated with an increased

ADH responsiveness to osmotic stimuli such as hypertonic saline infusion, and pharmacologic inhibition of ADH secretion (e.g., with ethanol infusion) is impaired in elderly subjects compared with young adults.[17] Taken together with the age-associated decline in glomerular filtration rate, the increased prevalence of conditions such as congestive heart failure and hypothyroidism, and the use of sulfonylurea or diuretic medication, these changes in ADH secretion predispose elderly people to the development of hyponatremia by impairing free water clearance.

Elderly people are also at increased risk for dehydration and hypernatremia. Although ADH secretory capacity is unimpaired with aging, the renal response to ADH is blunted, possibly due to chronic exposure to elevated levels, resulting in decreased maximal urinary concentrating capacity.[16] Furthermore, baroreceptor responsiveness to ADH declines with aging, such that release in response to hypotension or hypovolemia is decreased and the risk of volume depletion is higher. Other factors predisposing older adults to water depletion include the impairment in thirst responses to dehydration[18] and the common occurrence of states that limit access to free water (e.g., altered mental status, immobility, and surgery).

## ANTERIOR PITUITARY

### GROWTH HORMONE

The GH axis undergoes significant alterations in many healthy elderly people (see Chap. 12). In adult men, GH secretion declines progressively after age 40, and by age 70 to 80 approximately half of all men have *no* significant GH secretion over a 24-hour period. Levels of plasma somatomedin C (insulin-like growth factor-I [IGF-I]) show a corresponding decline, such that by age 70 to 80, ~40% of subjects exhibit plasma IGF-I levels similar to those found in GH-deficient children (see Chaps. 12 and 173). These low IGF-I levels in octogenarians correlate with an absence of significant nocturnal GH pulses.[19] Circulating levels of IGF-binding protein-3 (IGFBP-3) also decrease with aging, but whether this affects the bioactivity of IGF-I in older adults is unclear.[20]

Based on animal studies, this dramatic decrease in GH secretion with aging is thought to be due primarily to decreased hypothalamic secretion of GH-releasing hormone (GHRH) and increased hypothalamic somatostatin production, rather than to an age-related decrease in pituitary GHRH responsiveness.[19,21] Furthermore, the ability of exogenous IGF-I to suppress serum GH levels decreases with advancing age in humans, suggesting that declining GH secretion with aging is not due to increased sensitivity to IGF-I negative feedback.[22] In line with these observations, normal GH and IGF-I levels can be achieved in GH-deficient elderly subjects with GHRH administration.[19] Of note, the magnitude of the increase in pulsatile GH secretion induced by fasting was found to be similar in elderly and young adult human subjects, although the absolute levels of GH secretion of older subjects were ~50% lower in both fed and fasted conditions.[23] These findings suggest that age-related hyposomatotropism may be partially reversible by lifestyle modifications such as changes in diet or exercise.

The GH response to various secretagogues (e.g., insulin, arginine, and L-dopa) and to GHRH is normal or reduced with aging. As with the thyrotropin-releasing hormone (TRH) stimulation test, a normal GH response may be useful in verifying intact pituitary (somatotrope) function. The insulin-tolerance test is considered the definitive test to diagnose GH deficiency in adults,[24] but in elderly people this test is associated with *increased risk* due to the high prevalence of ischemic heart disease in this population. The arginine-stimulation test[25] and the combined administration of arginine and GHRH[24] have been proposed as alternative methods for the assessment of GH secretion in older patients.

Many age-associated changes in body composition, such as increased adiposity and decreased muscle and bone mass, are similar to those associated with GH deficiency in younger patients.[21,26] This observation has led to the hypothesis that decreased GH secretion with aging contributes to alterations in body composition (including diminished muscle and bone mass) and increased frailty in older adults, and to the suggestion that GH supplementation might be clinically useful in preventing or reversing these age-related changes. As noted earlier, compared with young adults, many healthy older adults are deficient in GH and IGF-I, and frail elderly people living in nursing homes have even lower IGF-I levels than healthy elderly subjects.[27] Whether young adult or age-adjusted reference ranges are the most appropriate standards to use for older adults is unclear, however, and definitive criteria for clinically significant GH deficiency in elderly people have not been established.

Short-term GH replacement in older men with low plasma IGF-I levels was found to increase lean body mass by 9% and reduce fat mass by 14%.[28] These beneficial effects were sustained in a similar study over 1 year of follow-up and regressed partially after cessation of treatment, results which suggest that hyposomatotropism contributes to age-related alterations in body composition.[29] "Physiologic" replacement in elderly people, however, may require a lower dosage than in young adults.[30] Side effects such as carpal tunnel syndrome and gynecomastia were common in older subjects with plasma IGF-I levels exceeding 1.0 U/mL during treatment,[19] even though normal IGF-I levels in young adults may be as high as 1.5 U/mL. Moreover, whether GH supplementation can achieve meaningful improvements in functional status or quality of life in elderly people is unclear. In healthy older men with low IGF-I levels but intact functional capacity, GH replacement increased lean body mass and reduced adiposity but did not yield any discernible improvement in functional capacity.[31] GH supplementation, however, possibly could improve functioning in frail GH- and IGF-I–deficient elderly people with preexisting functional deficits.

Other abnormalities of GH secretion, including GH deficiency in adults with hypothalamic-pituitary disease, are covered in Chapter 12.

### PROLACTIN

No clinically significant changes in basal prolactin levels occur with aging. The amplitude of nocturnal pulsatile prolactin secretion, however, is lower in elderly than in young men; this may be due to age-related alterations in dopaminergic regulation of prolactin secretion.[32] Furthermore, several medications commonly used by elderly patients, including phenothiazines, metoclopramide, and cimetidine, inhibit dopamine secretion and sometimes cause elevated prolactin levels. Hypothyroidism increases hypothalamic TRH release, which in turn stimulates prolactin secretion. When hyperprolactinemia does occur, its clinical manifestations are usually subtle and often unrecognized. Prolactin excess has antigonadotropic effects; therefore, hyperprolactinemia causes secondary hypogonadism and may contribute to sexual dysfunction and bone loss. Less common manifestations of hyperprolactinemia in older people include gynecomastia and, rarely, galactorrhea.

### ADRENOCORTICOTROPIC HORMONE

No significant age-related changes occur in basal ACTH and cortisol levels, or in cortisol responses to exogenous ACTH stimulation. However, evidence obtained using stimuli such as metyrapone, insulin-induced hypoglycemia, or ovine CRH, with and without vasopressin, indicates that cortisol and ACTH responses to stimuli at or above the level of the anterior pituitary are increased or prolonged with aging.[33,34] Furthermore, the sensitivity of the hypothalamic–pituitary–adrenal (HPA) axis to glucocorticoid negative feedback is decreased with aging (see discussion of adrenal cortex physiology later).

### THYROID-STIMULATING HORMONE

Conflicting data have been reported on the effect of aging on thyroid-stimulating hormone (TSH) levels. Some studies have found unchanged or slightly increased TSH levels in normal elderly people, with elevated TSH occurring more commonly in females. However, TSH was found to decrease with aging in healthy subjects who were carefully selected to exclude subclinical primary hypothyroidism.[35,36] In fact, primary hypothyroidism is very common in older adults, with 3% of older men and 7% of elderly women having TSH levels >10 µU/mL.[37] In other cases, TSH levels were suppressed by concurrent glucocorticoid use, and by fasting and stress, which were associated with severe nonthyroidal illnesses. Thyroid responsiveness to TSH administration is preserved with normal aging, but the TSH response to TRH is diminished or even absent in healthy elderly people, particularly in men. Therefore, an abnormal TRH-stimulation test cannot be used to support a diagnosis of hyperthyroidism in elderly people. A normal TSH response to TRH may be useful in ruling out hyperthyroidism, but this test is rarely needed with the widespread availability of highly sensitive TSH assays. Finally, in young adults, TSH secretion exhibits a circadian variation, with the highest levels of TSH released during the night. This nocturnal TSH peak is blunted with aging, however, suggesting hypothalamic dysfunction.[38]

### GONADOTROPINS

In the early perimenopausal phase of the menopausal transition, the number of ovarian follicles gradually declines, leading to a reduction in inhibin-B production.[39] The decrease in negative feedback at the pituitary due to reduced inhibin-B levels is thought to be the primary stimulus leading to an increase of the serum follicle-stimulating hormone (FSH) levels that sustain inhibin-A and estradiol production until late in the menopausal transition.[39] Ultimately, inhibin A and estradiol levels decline and FSH levels increase substantially, marking the progression to late perimenopausal status—although LH levels do not increase during this period. After menopause, FSH levels are increased to a greater extent than are LH levels, although by 15 years postmenopause, LH levels fall to below premenopausal levels. Postmenopausal women exhibit an exaggerated gonadotropin response to GnRH, due to loss of negative feedback from ovarian hormones. Furthermore, older postmenopausal women exhibit lower basal 24-hour mean LH levels and greater suppression of LH and FSH secretion by estradiol than younger women with premature ovarian failure, suggesting hypothalamic-pituitary alterations in aging women.[40]

Aging men exhibit higher basal LH and FSH levels than younger men, but gonadotropin levels often remain within the normal range. Testosterone levels are decreased in many healthy older men with elevated gonadotropin levels, implying primary testicular failure. Furthermore, decreased LH pulse frequency (an indicator of hypothalamic GnRH pulse generator activity) is evident in some healthy elderly men despite reduced testosterone levels.[10,41] Evidence of altered pituitary function is also seen with aging, with slightly impaired LH responses to GnRH administration in elderly men compared with young men.[42] Decreased testosterone levels together with inappropriately normal (i.e., not elevated) gonadotropin levels

is a common finding in both healthy and systemically ill elderly men, suggesting secondary hypogonadism. Additional clinical and hormonal evidence of pituitary dysfunction is needed in these cases to justify imaging studies to rule out pituitary tumors.

## PITUITARY ADENOMAS AND THE EMPTY SELLA SYNDROME

The incidence of pituitary tumors is not markedly altered with aging.[43] Autopsy studies reveal that pituitary "incidentalomas" are common, occurring in 13% to 27% of subjects.[44] Most functioning adenomas are microscopic prolactin-producing tumors (see Chap. 13). In contrast, nonfunctioning adenomas are the most common type of pituitary tumors diagnosed during life in older adults, comprising 61% to 73% of cases.[44] Many of these apparently nonfunctioning adenomas, however, actually produce quantities of gonadotropins (especially FSH) or the α subunit of these glycoprotein hormones. Nonsecreting tumors and tumors that secrete LH, FSH, or α subunit are usually large at the time they are diagnosed, because few or no symptoms of hormonal hypersecretion occur. These tumors typically present with a mass effect, including visual field abnormalities and headaches, as incidental findings on imaging studies, or with manifestations of panhypopituitarism. Vision changes are the most common presentation of pituitary adenoma in elderly patients,[45] and for pituitary tumors to present with symptoms of hormonal overproduction (e.g., acromegaly or Cushing disease) is uncommon.

As in younger adults, management of large pituitary tumors usually involves transsphenoidal decompression and debulking, along with assessment of anterior pituitary hormone function and replacement of hormone deficiencies. Prolactinomas are managed medically with dopamine agonists, such as bromocriptine, pergolide, or cabergoline. Both transsphenoidal pituitary surgery and radiotherapy appear to be effective and relatively well tolerated by older patients who are appropriate candidates. The clinician may find it appropriate, however, to manage elderly patients with normal endocrine status and no visual field defects who are asymptomatic or at high surgical risk with only serial magnetic resonance imaging (MRI) and visual field assessment.[44]

Panhypopituitarism is difficult to diagnose in older patients because the symptoms are nonspecific and are difficult to distinguish from other common age-related symptoms. Among the presentations of hypopituitarism reported in case series of elderly patients are postural hypotension, recurrent falls, hyponatremia, weakness, weight loss, immobility, drowsiness and confusion, and urinary incontinence.[44] Elderly patients with panhypopituitarism require replacement of thyroid hormone and cortisol; the indications for replacement of estrogen, testosterone, and GH in these patients have not been as clearly established.[44]

With the widespread use of brain-imaging techniques such as computerized tomography (CT) and MRI, both pituitary masses and the empty sella syndrome are being identified with greater frequency. An MRI study of healthy young and elderly subjects reported that pituitary height and volume tends to decrease with aging, and empty sella was observed in 19% of elderly subjects but in none of the young subjects. No relationship was seen between pituitary volume and anterior pituitary hormone levels,[46] however, confirming other reports that *clinically apparent pituitary dysfunction is uncommon in empty sella syndrome*.[47] This study also found that the posterior pituitary bright signal on T1-weighted MRI, which is thought to reflect stored ADH-neurophysin complex, was not detected in 29% of healthy elderly subjects, whereas it was detected in all young adult subjects.[46] None of the subjects had clinical manifestations of diabetes insipidus, but plasma osmolarity and ADH levels were higher in the elderly subjects. Thus, the *absence of the posterior pituitary bright signal on T1-weighted MRI appears to reflect a physiologic depletion of ADH neurosecretory granules rather than a pathologic occurrence.* Based on the foregoing, the functional significance of an incidental finding of empty sella or altered posterior pituitary bright signal on MRI in apparently healthy elderly patients is unclear. In such patients, conservative management is appropriate, although visual field testing, and measurement of serum anterior pituitary hormone levels in patients with empty sella, are indicated to rule out subclinical pituitary dysfunction and suprasellar involvement.

## PINEAL GLAND AND MELATONIN

Interest is increasing in age-related alterations in the secretion of melatonin, a hormone involved in the organization of circadian and seasonal biorhythms that is produced by the pineal gland (see Chap. 10). Melatonin production is inhibited by light exposure, resulting in a robust circadian variation (levels high at night and low during the day) that is controlled by pacemaker neurons in the suprachiasmatic nucleus of the hypothalamus.[48] Melatonin has sedative effects, suggesting a role in sleep production, but its precise physiologic role has not been fully determined. Melatonin production is minimal in young infants but increases markedly after 3 months of age, reaching maximal nighttime levels by the age of 1 to 3 years. After early childhood, melatonin secretion gradually decreases, with a progressive decline continuing into old age.[49] The significance of this age-related decline in melatonin secretion is unclear, but proposals have been made in the lay press that age-related melatonin "deficiency" is related to a wide variety of age-associated conditions, including immune system deficiencies, cancer, and the aging process itself.[50] Based on such publicity, and the ready availability of melatonin supplements in the United States without a prescription, these supplements are enjoying wide use. The physiologic and pharmacologic effects of melatonin have *not* been thoroughly studied, however, and the long-term risks and benefits of melatonin-replacement therapy remain to be determined.

## THYROID GLANDS

### PHYSIOLOGY

The changes in thyroid physiology occurring with normal aging are summarized in Table 199-1. A reduction with aging in $T_4$ secretion by the thyroid is balanced by a decrease in $T_4$ clearance rate; therefore, serum $T_4$ levels do not change significantly with normal aging. Levels of the binding proteins thyroid-binding globulin (TBG) and thyroid-binding prealbumin (TBPA) are not markedly affected by aging; hence, no significant change occurs in total $T_4$ and $T_3$ resin uptake ($T_3RU$). $T_3$ levels are normal in healthy elderly people until extreme old age, when $T_3$ declines slightly,[35,51] but in the setting of nonthyroidal illness, extrathyroidal conversion of $T_4$ to $T_3$ by 5' deiodinase is often impaired, resulting in decreases in circulating $T_3$ levels.[52] Low serum total $T_3$ (*low $T_3$ syndrome*) is the most common thyroid function test abnormality in nonthyroidal illness and occurs in ~70% of hospitalized patients.[36,53] Serum reverse $T_3$ ($rT_3$) levels are increased in some elderly people, but this is associated with decreased food intake[52] or nonthyroidal illness[53] rather than aging per se,

**TABLE 199-1.**
**Alterations in Thyroid Physiology and Hormones with Aging**

$T_4$ production ↓
$T_4$ clearance ↓
$T_4$ to $T_3$ conversion ↓
$T_3$ clearance ↓
Serum total and free $T_4$ ↔
Serum total and free $T_3$ ↔/↓
Serum TSH ↔/↓
Radioactive iodine uptake ↓
Thyroid responsiveness to TSH ↔
TSH responsiveness to TRH ↓
TSH sensitivity to thyroid hormone feedback ↓

↓, decreased; ↔, unchanged; $T_4$, thyroxine; $T_3$, triiodothyronine; *TSH*, thyroid-stimulating hormone (thyrotropin); *TRH*, thyrotropin-releasing hormone.

and is due to a reduction in the metabolic clearance rate of $rT_3$ due to impaired 5' deiodinase activity. The effects of aging on TSH levels was discussed previously.

### LABORATORY DIAGNOSIS OF THYROID DISEASE IN OLDER PATIENTS

Muted, atypical, and often asymptomatic presentation of thyroid disease is the rule rather than the exception in elderly people, as discussed later. Accordingly, *laboratory screening* is the most reliable means to identify hypothyroidism and hyperthyroidism in the geriatric population. Office-based screening of women older than age 50 with a sensitive TSH test has been recommended to detect unsuspected hypothyroidism and hyperthyroidism, as the prevalence of overt thyroid dysfunction is 1.4% in this group.[54] Furthermore, the yield of the TSH test for hypo- and hyperthyroidism is sufficiently high to warrant testing elderly people of either sex who present for medical care—especially those with a recent decline in ability to perform activities of daily living or cognitive deterioration—and at the time of admission to the hospital, psychiatric unit, or nursing home. In addition, the possibility of altered thyroid status should be considered any time an elderly patient's clinical status deteriorates without a clear explanation.

In the nursing home population, routine screening and/or yearly monitoring of TSH levels have been recommended by some clinicians because of the high frequency of abnormalities in this group[55–57]; other physicians advocate an individualized approach to laboratory testing based on current health and functional status, and the wishes of the patient or surrogate decision maker regarding testing and treatment.[58]

### DIAGNOSIS OF HYPERTHYROIDISM

Highly sensitive TSH assays are adequate to screen for hyperthyroidism in relatively healthy elderly outpatients. The diagnosis should be confirmed using the free $T_4$ test, however, because systemic illnesses, malnutrition, and some medications commonly used by older patients (glucocorticoids, dopamine agonists, phenytoin) may suppress TSH levels.[59] Furthermore, many euthyroid patients with multinodular goiters have low TSH and normal $T_4$ levels, suggesting subclinical hyperthyroidism. *Most asymptomatic elderly patients with low serum TSH levels are euthyroid*; the majority of these patients have isolated suppression of TSH with normal $T_4$ and $T_3$ levels and normal TSH on repeat testing 4 to 6 weeks later.[59,60]

Additional testing is needed to confirm the diagnosis of hyperthyroidism in some older patients. "$T_3$ toxicosis" is more common with aging, especially in patients with toxic thyroid nodules. Patients with this disorder may exhibit a normal free $T_4$ or free $T_4$ index. In such cases, determination of free or total $T_3$ level is needed to diagnose hyperthyroidism. In contrast to thyrotoxicosis in young patients, an elevated $T_3$ level is specific but not sensitive for hyperthyroidism in an elderly patient. $T_3$ levels are elevated in only half of elderly hyperthyroid patients, compared with 87% of younger patients.[60] This is probably due to decreased $T_4$ to $T_3$ conversion secondary to normal aging and nonthyroidal disease in older people.

As in younger patients, the high $T_4$ syndrome (*euthyroid hyperthyroxinemia*) may also cause diagnostic confusion. Common causes of the high $T_4$ syndrome in elderly patients include acute psychiatric illness, use of some drugs, or other conditions associated with an acute reduction in $T_4$ to $T_3$ conversion (acute fasting, use of β-adrenergic blocking agents or glucocorticoids), and states associated with increased TBG (estrogen or opiate use, hepatitis). Patients with high $T_4$ syndrome have normal TSH levels and elevated total $T_4$ levels, often with elevated TBG concentrations (e.g., in liver diseases such as chronic hepatitis). Free $T_4$ levels may be elevated as well (e.g., in the setting of acute psychiatric illness). Abnormalities in thyroid function testing often resolve with treatment of the underlying condition or discontinuation of the responsible medication.

As noted earlier, the TRH-stimulation test is generally not helpful in diagnosing hyperthyroidism in older people, because the increase in TSH levels after TRH administration is often blunted or absent even in healthy elderly persons. A finding of an increase of >3 μU/mL in TSH over baseline levels after TRH administration, however, excludes hyperthyroidism at any age. Thyroid scanning and measurement of radioactive iodine uptake (RAIU) are sometimes helpful in confirming the diagnosis of hyperthyroidism and in defining the type of hyperthyroidism.

## DIAGNOSIS OF HYPOTHYROIDISM

In diagnosing hypothyroidism, the serum TSH level is the most sensitive indicator of primary hypothyroidism in elderly as in younger adults. Although an elevated TSH level alone usually indicates primary hypothyroidism, *TSH levels may be increased transiently during the recovery phase of an acute illness*. Primary hypothyroidism should, therefore, be confirmed by the finding of a reduced free $T_4$ index or level in association with an elevated TSH level, or a persistently elevated TSH level at a more distant time from the illness.

Some elderly patients with serious nonthyroidal illnesses have a decreased serum free $T_4$ index without elevation in serum TSH levels (*low $T_4$ syndrome*). In this syndrome, levels of thyroid hormone–binding proteins are decreased, and with severe illness, $T_4$ binding to TBG is decreased due to the presence of a $T_4$-binding inhibitor. Serum free $T_4$ levels are usually normal, and levels of $rT_3$ are usually elevated. These patients do not appear to benefit from thyroid hormone replacement. However, two other clinical situations may present with decreased serum free $T_4$ and free $T_4$ index and relatively normal TSH levels. Elderly patients with primary hypothyroidism may have suppressed TSH levels from fasting, acute illnesses such as head trauma, and use of medications (dopamine, phenytoin, glucocorticoids). TSH levels are not usually suppressed into the normal range in these patients, however. The other clinical situation is secondary hypothyroidism, which is uncommon in the elderly as in younger adults. Unlike in the low $T_4$ syndrome, in secondary hypothyroidism $rT_3$ levels are typically decreased, and panhypopituitarism is usually present. If secondary hypothyroidism is suggested by an inappropriately normal to low TSH level together with a low free $T_4$, measure-

ment of serum testosterone and gonadotropin levels and/or an ACTH-stimulation test may be useful.

## HYPERTHYROIDISM

Hyperthyroidism (see Chap. 42) is common in elderly people. Fifteen percent of patients with thyrotoxicosis are older than age 60, and estimates of the prevalence of hyperthyroidism in this population range from 0.5% to 3%.[36] Graves disease is the most common cause of hyperthyroidism in elderly people in the United States; however, toxic multinodular goiter and toxic adenomas are more common in older than in young adults. Many elderly patients with multinodular goiter have subclinical hyperthyroidism, with undetectable levels of TSH, free $T_4$ and $T_3$ levels within the normal range, and normal basal RAIU that cannot be fully suppressed with exogenous thyroid hormone.

As noted earlier, atypical disease presentations are common in geriatric patients with hyperthyroidism (Table 199-2). As with hypothyroidism, the presentation of thyrotoxicosis in elderly patients is often vague, atypical, or nonspecific, with symptoms often occurring in the most impaired organ system. Classic findings such as goiter, nervousness, ophthalmopathy, hyperactive reflexes, increased sweating, tremor, and heat intolerance are much less common in elderly than in younger patients with hyperthyroidism, whereas tachycardia, muscle atrophy, anorexia, and atrial fibrillation (often without a rapid ventricular

**TABLE 199-2.**
**Clinical Manifestations of Hyperthyroidism in the Elderly**

*Cardiovascular/pulmonary*
  Atrial fibrillation*
  Angina exacerbation*
  Dyspnea and other congestive heart failure symptoms*
  Palpitations
  Hypertension
  Tachycardia[†]
*Gastrointestinal*
  Constipation*
  Anorexia*
  Frequent bowel movements
  Polyphagia[†]
*Neuropsychiatric*
  Apathy*
  Depression
  Tremor[†]
  Nervousness[†]
  Hyperactive reflexes[†]
*Metabolic*
  Weight loss
  Heat intolerance[†]
  Hyperhidrosis[†]
  Polydipsia[†]
*Musculoskeletal*
  Osteoporosis
  Weakness
  Proximal muscle weakness
*Thyroid*
  Goiter[†]
*Ophthalmologic*
  Proptosis
  Lid lag[†]

*More common in elderly than in young adults.
[†]Less common in elderly than in young adults.

response) are more common manifestations.[36,60,61] Hyperthyroidism is present in 13% to 30% of elderly patients with atrial fibrillation, and estimates are that a low TSH concentration confers a three-fold increase in the risk of developing atrial fibrillation within a decade after the TSH abnormality is detected.[62] Furthermore, thyrotoxicosis in older patients may present with congestive heart failure. Unlike the situation with younger people, constipation is a *more* common presenting complaint than frequent bowel movements. Constitutional symptoms such as weight loss, weakness, nausea, and anorexia may be prominent; this may prompt clinicians to order unnecessary and extensive evaluations to rule out gastrointestinal malignancies. Other individuals present with *apathetic hyperthyroidism*, a common clinical manifestation in older patients but rarely if ever present in younger individuals. These patients demonstrate an absence of signs and symptoms of adrenergic hyperstimulation (e.g., tremor or hyperkinesis), a blunted affect or depression, and confusion or slowed mentation. Finally, hyperthyroidism increases the risk of developing osteoporosis and should be ruled out in those who present with decreased bone density. Not all studies, however, have found a relationship between low TSH levels and bone loss.[63,64]

Although the issue is somewhat controversial,[54,65] evidence exists that treatment of subclinical hyperthyroidism may be justified in elderly people, because of the increased risk of osteoporosis and cardiovascular complications.[36,65] An accurate assessment of thyroid function is essential, however, before initiating such treatment. For now, data from randomized, controlled trials of treatment for subclinical hyperthyroidism are not available to clarify the risks and benefits of this practice.

Administration of radioactive iodine (RAI) is the treatment of choice for thyrotoxicosis in most older patients. Patients with toxic multinodular goiter may require large or repeated doses of RAI. Treatment with antithyroid drugs such as propylthiouracil or methimazole is useful before RAI administration, both for symptom control and to reduce the likelihood of release of stored thyroid hormone and exacerbation of thyrotoxicosis from radiation thyroiditis. These drugs should be discontinued 1 week before RAI administration to optimize RAI uptake. In frail patients, an antithyroid drug can be resumed 3 to 5 days after RAI and continued for 1 to several months depending on the response to RAI. If not contraindicated, β-blockers can be given before and maintained after RAI for relief of symptoms such as tachycardia, tremor, and restlessness.

After RAI treatment, $T_4$ levels must be carefully followed for the emergence of hypothyroidism, or persistent or recurrent hyperthyroidism requiring retreatment. Moreover, the clearance rate of other medications may decrease after RAI treatment of the thyroid, such that drug levels may increase and dosage may need to be adjusted.

## HYPOTHYROIDISM

Hypothyroidism (see Chap. 45) is very common in the geriatric population. The reported prevalence of hypothyroidism in healthy elderly adults varies considerably depending on the population studied, with prevalence estimates of overt hypothyroidism ranging from 0.5% to 5% and of subclinical hypothyroidism, from 5% to 20% of adults older than age 60 years.[36] Most hypothyroidism in older adults is due to chronic autoimmune thyroiditis, as in younger patients.

The diagnosis of hypothyroidism is often overlooked in elderly people for several reasons. First, hypothyroidism usually has an insidious onset and a slow rate of progression. Second, physicians often fail to recognize typical clinical features of

hypothyroidism that in older people are similar to "normal" age-related changes (e.g., dry skin, poor skin turgor, weakness, slowed mentation, constipation) or to manifestations of coexisting disease (e.g., anemia, congestive heart failure, diabetes). Finally, as in hyperthyroidism, atypical or uncommon clinical findings may be the dominant or sole presenting manifestations of hypothyroidism in elderly patients (Table 199-3). In large studies of older patients with overt hypothyroidism, the diagnosis of hypothyroidism was recognized on clinical examination in <20% of cases.[66,67] These observations highlight the importance of laboratory screening in the diagnosis of hypothyroidism in elderly patients. Furthermore, the clinician should have a high index of suspicion for hypothyroidism when an elderly person's clinical status deteriorates.

Older patients with mild hypothyroidism may rapidly become severely hypothyroid in the setting of serious nonthyroidal illness. Many of the signs and symptoms of hypothyroidism improve or resolve with treatment, including deafness, ataxia, vertigo, hypoventilation, and myopathy. Although hypothyroidism is not a common cause of reversible dementia, and demented hypothyroid patients rarely regain normal cognition with thyroid replacement, cognitive function, overall func-

**TABLE 199-3.**
**Clinical Manifestations of Hypothyroidism in the Elderly**

*Cardiovascular*
  Bradycardia
  Congestive heart failure
  Pericardial effusion
  Hypertension
*Hematologic*
  Normocytic or macrocytic anemia (mild)
*Neuropsychiatric*
  Confusion
  Depression
  Irritability
  Dementia
  Paranoia
  Psychosis (myxedema madness)
  Myxedema coma
  Ataxia
  Cerebellar dysfunction
  Deafness
  Vertigo
  Peripheral neuropathy
*Metabolic*
  Weight loss
  Hypercholesterolemia
  Hypertriglyceridemia
*Musculoskeletal*
  Myopathy with weakness, easy fatigability
  Arthritis
  Carpal tunnel syndrome
*Electrolytic*
  Hyponatremia
*Laboratory findings*
  Elevated CPK, SGOT, and LDH levels
*Other*
  Pleural effusion
  Ascites
  Increased sensitivity to sedative drugs
  Decreased ventilatory drive

*CPK*, creatine phosphokinase; *SGOT*, serum glutamic-oxaloacetic transaminase; *LDH*, lactate dehydrogenase.

tional status, strength, and mood may improve with restoration of the euthyroid state.

Clinicians often encounter clinically euthyroid patients with elevated TSH levels but with free $T_4$ levels within the normal range. This picture of subclinical hypothyroidism is estimated to occur in 15% of people older than age 65 and is several times more common in women than in men. Overt hypothyroidism has been reported to occur in one-third of elderly subjects with elevated TSH levels within 4 years.[68] Older age, an initial TSH level of >20 µU/mL, and high titers of thyroid antimicrosomal antibodies are associated with an increased likelihood of eventual thyroid failure.[54]

Treatment with L-thyroxine may be beneficial for some elderly patients with subclinical hypothyroidism, with improvements in myocardial contractility and psychometric testing. The results of randomized trials of treatment for subclinical hypothyroidism have been mixed, however.[54] In those who are not started on L-thyroxine, the TSH level can be followed and thyroid replacement initiated if TSH levels progressively increase. Alternatively, L-thyroxine can be initiated at low dosages and carefully titrated to achieve normal serum TSH levels. Some physicians advise starting L-thyroxine treatment in all patients with serum TSH levels of ≥10 mU/L, as well as in those with both a borderline elevated TSH of between 5 and 10 mU/L and an abnormal elevation of thyroid antimicrosomal antibodies.[36]

Potential adverse effects such as exacerbation of myocardial ischemia and the patient's ability to comply with treatment should also be taken into consideration, however. Replacement should be with L-thyroxine in a reliable preparation of accurate dosage and predictable bioavailability. Thyroid hormone requirements decrease with age, due to a reduction in clearance rate; replacement dosages average 110 µg per day in elderly patients compared with 130 µg per day in younger patients.[60] With advancing age or declining nutritional status, a reduction in $T_4$ dosage may be necessary over time.

In most older patients, the initial replacement dosage is 25 µg per day, increasing by 25 µg every 4 weeks until serum TSH levels have normalized. In those with known cardiac disease, treatment is usually begun even more gradually, at an initial dosage of 12.5 to 25 µg per day, with increments every 4 weeks as tolerated. However, severely hypothyroid patients may require initial replacement doses of 50 to 100 µg orally, or up to 400 µg intravenously for myxedema stupor and coma, even with evidence of concomitant cardiac disease. In these markedly hypothyroid patients, the clinician is advised to test for the possibility of coexistent adrenal insufficiency and to protect against precipitation of adrenal crisis during thyroid replacement by giving stress dosages of glucocorticoid replacement (e.g., 200 mg hydrocortisone) before $T_4$ administration.

Although restoring the euthyroid state without exacerbating angina is not always possible, treatment of hypothyroidism should *not* be withheld based on the fear of an adverse effect of thyroid replacement. Treatment of patients with coexisting ischemic cardiac disease is individualized to reduce or eliminate symptoms of hypothyroidism without inducing intolerable anginal symptoms. Obtaining a baseline level of creatine phosphokinase (CPK), which can be elevated in some cases of hypothyroidism, in case the patient develops ischemic cardiac symptoms during initiation of treatment, may be useful.

Other areas of concern during thyroid-replacement therapy in older people include effects on dosages of other medications and avoidance of thyroid overreplacement. As hypothyroidism is corrected, the clearance rate of other medications may be affected, such that adjustments in dosage are required. Excessive $T_4$ replacement should be avoided, because it may result in decreased bone density and exacerbation of underlying heart disease, especially in high-risk osteopenic or cardiac patients. Finally, in patients with secondary hypothyroidism due to pituitary or hypothalamic disease, serum TSH levels cannot be used either to diagnose or to monitor thyroid hormone replacement as in those with primary hypothyroidism. Normalization of total or free $T_4$ levels should be the goal in these patients.

## NODULAR THYROID DISEASE AND THYROID CANCER

With aging, the thyroid gland becomes increasingly nodular, and the incidence of multinodular goiter increases. Estimates are that 90% of women older than age 70 and 60% of men older than age 80 have thyroid nodules, most of which are nonpalpable.[36]

Older patients with multinodular goiter are susceptible to iodine-induced thyrotoxicosis (e.g., after radiocontrast or amiodarone administration). Multinodular goiters frequently have functionally autonomous areas, and attempts to suppress the growth of these goiters with thyroid hormone may lead to iatrogenic hyperthyroidism. In elderly patients with nontoxic nodular goiter, surgical management is usually reserved for those with significant compressive symptoms, for those for whom suspicion of malignancy is high, or occasionally for patients with cosmetic concerns.

After age 50, the frequency of clinically evident solitary thyroid nodules decreases. However, even well-differentiated papillary and follicular carcinomas are more aggressive and are associated with increased mortality in elderly patients, so a careful evaluation is indicated when any new solitary nodule is noted or when the size of an existing nodule increases. Other clinical manifestations suggesting thyroid carcinoma include dysphagia, hoarseness, pain, adherence of the thyroid to adjacent structures, cervical lymphadenopathy, and a hard consistency of the thyroid. The incidence of both anaplastic thyroid carcinoma and thyroid lymphoma is higher in elderly than in younger adults.[36]

## DISORDERS OF PARATHYROID GLANDS AND CALCIUM METABOLISM

### AGING AND REGULATION OF SERUM CALCIUM

With aging, calcium homeostasis is preserved at the expense of elevated parathyroid hormone (PTH) levels and consequent reduction in bone mass. PTH protects against hypocalcemia by stimulating renal 1,25-dihydroxyvitamin D [1,25(OH)$_2$D] production, promoting calcium conservation by the kidney, and increasing bone resorption. With aging, however, PTH is less effective in stimulating 1,25(OH)$_2$D production, apparently due to decreased renal 1α-hydroxylase activity. The resulting decrease in 1,25(OH)$_2$D levels, together with impaired intestinal responsiveness to 1,25(OH)$_2$D action, in turn contribute to a decrease in intestinal absorption of dietary calcium that is evident by age 50 to 60 years.[69] Furthermore, decreased calcium absorption is exacerbated in some elderly individuals by decreased gastric acid secretion and lactase deficiency, which may result in avoidance of dairy products. In turn, a mild decrease in serum calcium levels and a reduction in renal clearance of PTH lead to a 30% increase in serum PTH levels between ages 30 and 80.[70] Serum calcium levels are normalized by the increased PTH levels, but bone resorption is increased relative to bone formation, resulting in loss of bone mass and increased fracture risk. Ultimately, these pathophysiologic changes result in type II osteoporosis and an increased risk of fractures in many elderly adults (see later).

## VITAMIN D DEFICIENCY

Dietary calcium intake is grossly inadequate in most older individuals.[71] As a consequence of age-related renal PTH resistance and intestinal 1,25(OH)$_2$D resistance, elderly people are unable to substantially increase intestinal absorption of calcium in response to a low-calcium diet and are, therefore, more dependent than young adults on adequate dietary calcium ingestion.[72,73] Age-related abnormalities in PTH secretion and bone turnover are not inevitable, however. Older women treated with 2400 mg per day of calcium for 3 years reversed these alterations,[74] and even 1000 mg per day significantly lowers PTH levels.[75] Furthermore, vitamin D deficiency commonly coexists with calcium deficiency in the elderly. In one study of elderly subjects performed in the United States, hypovitaminosis D was found in 38% of nursing home residents and 54% of homebound people residing in the community.[76] Vitamin D deficiency appears to be equally common in medical inpatients in the United States, occurring in 57% of unselected patients on a general medical ward, including substantial numbers of patients without apparent risk factors for vitamin D deficiency and those with vitamin D intakes above the recommended daily amount.[77] Vitamin D supplementation in postmenopausal women decreases PTH levels and bone turnover, and increases bone mineral density at the femoral neck.[78] Combined calcium and vitamin D supplementation reduces fracture rates in elderly women.[79] Based on these and other data, the current consensus is that an elemental calcium intake of at least 1000 to 1500 mg per day (and possibly more in some) is desirable in older adults, and adequate vitamin D intake (400 to 800 IU per day) must also be ensured.[80] The optimal amount of calcium needed to preserve bone mineral density in older women, however, is still unknown.

## PAGET DISEASE OF BONE

Paget disease of bone (see Chap. 65) rarely occurs before the age of 35 years. Its prevalence increases with aging, and it affects 2% to 5% of individuals >50 years of age, although significant geographic variation is found.[81] Commonly affected sites include the pelvis, spine, femur, and skull. Most people with Paget disease are asymptomatic, and the disorder is usually identified incidentally when radiographs are obtained for an unrelated indication, or an otherwise unexplained elevation in serum alkaline phosphatase is noted. In symptomatic patients, pain is the most common presenting symptom, usually localized to the affected bones. In one-third of cases, however, the pain is due to secondary osteoarthritic changes, often in the hips, knees, and vertebrae. Bony deformities occur in ~15% of patients at the time of diagnosis, usually involving the long bones of the lower extremities and often presenting as a bowing of the affected extremity. With involvement of the skull, compression of the eighth cranial nerve may result in sensorineural hearing loss. In patients with Paget disease of the hip joint, the results of total hip arthroplasty are comparable to those of hip arthroplasties performed in patients unaffected by Paget disease.[82] The bisphosphonates are the current treatment of choice and are effective in suppressing the accelerated bone turnover and bone remodeling that is characteristic of this disease.

# OSTEOPOROSIS

Osteoporosis is a major cause of morbidity and mortality in older people. Estimates are that 1.5 million fractures annually are a direct result of osteoporosis. By the age of 90 years, ~32% of women and 17% of men have fractured a hip.[83] Patients who fracture a hip are at a 10% to 20% increased risk of mortality over the following year[84] and have increased morbidity, including institutionalization and impairment in mobility and functional status.

Two clinical syndromes of osteoporosis have been proposed on epidemiologic and biochemical grounds.[85] Type I (*"postmenopausal"*) osteoporosis is thought to occur in women typically between 51 and 75 years old and is characterized by an accelerated rate of bone loss, mainly in trabecular bone, with distal radius and vertebral fractures. The loss of the direct restraining effects of estrogen on bone-cell function is thought to be the most important mediator of this accelerated bone loss, leading to increased sensitivity of bone to PTH and increased calcium release from bone.[86] PTH levels are slightly decreased at steady state in these patients. Type II (*"senile"*) osteoporosis is characterized by a late, slow phase of bone loss occurring in both men and women older than 70 years. This condition is associated with progressive secondary hyperparathyroidism and loss of both trabecular and cortical bone with vertebral and hip fractures. The proposal was originally made that type II osteoporosis is due primarily to decreased serum 1,25(OH)$_2$D levels and calcium malabsorption, resulting in a secondary increase in PTH levels and bone resorption. Subsequently, however, the proposal has been put forward that both the secondary hyperparathyroidism and the decreased bone formation characterizing this slow phase of bone loss are manifestations of underlying estrogen deficiency in *both* elderly men and elderly women, with loss of estrogen action resulting in net calcium wasting and in an increase in the level of dietary calcium intake required to maintain bone homeostasis.[86] Aging men have decreased circulating levels of both bioavailable estrogen and testosterone. Bioavailable estrogen levels appear to be a better correlate of bone mass than testosterone levels, supporting the hypothesis that estrogen deficiency is an important cause of bone loss in elderly men.[86]

As in younger patients, secondary causes of osteoporosis, osteomalacia, and primary hyperparathyroidism must be considered in the assessment of elderly osteopenic patients (Table 199-4). Osteomalacia due to vitamin D deficiency is relatively

**TABLE 199-4.**
**Causes of Osteopenia**

**OSTEOPOROSIS**
*Primary*
  Type I
  Type II
*Secondary*
  Excessive alcohol intake
  Smoking
  Glucocorticoid excess
  Anticonvulsant use (associated with both osteoporosis and osteomalacia)
  Hyperthyroidism
  Hyperprolactinemia
  Hypogonadism in men
  Malignancy, especially multiple myeloma
  Long-term heparin use
  Immobilization
  Rheumatoid arthritis
  Malnutrition
  Chronic liver disease (biliary cirrhosis)
**OSTEOMALACIA**
  Vitamin D deficiency
  Hypophosphatemia
  Miscellaneous (e.g., renal tubular acidosis)
**PRIMARY HYPERPARATHYROIDISM**

common in elderly people, particularly in those with a history of gastrectomy, chronic renal failure, malabsorption, or anticonvulsant use. Screening for osteomalacia is warranted in frail elderly people, including measurement of serum calcium and phosphate levels, which are decreased in vitamin D deficiency, and alkaline phosphatase level, which is increased. Findings of decreased 24-hour urinary calcium and serum 25-hydroxyvitamin D levels and increased PTH levels help to confirm the diagnosis.

## MANAGEMENT OF OSTEOPOROSIS

The management of osteoporosis and osteomalacia is discussed in detail in Chapters 64 and 63, respectively. The following points should be emphasized in the care of frail older patients with osteoporosis.

First, older people at risk for falling should be identified. Important risk factors for falls in elderly adults include cognitive impairment, abnormalities of gait and balance, use of multiple medications, use of psychoactive medications, nocturia, disabilities of the lower extremities, and environmental factors such as household clutter. Second, a performance-oriented assessment of gait and balance should be undertaken. Direct observation of gait and balance is probably more useful than the standard neuromuscular examination in identifying patients with increased fall risk and treatable mobility problems.[87–89] Assessment should include gait parameters (such as initiation of gait, step height, step length, step symmetry, path deviation, and trunk stability) and balance parameters (including ability to rise from a chair, immediate and sustained standing balance [with eyes open and closed], stability after sternal nudge, turning balance, and stability while looking upward or bending down). Management of patients at risk for falling may include treatment of underlying conditions contributing to falls (e.g., Parkinson disease, postural hypotension, foot disorders); minimization of medications increasing the risk of falling; gait retraining and strengthening; provision of assistive devices (e.g., a cane or walker); and environmental alterations (e.g., elimination of obstacles and clutter, provision of proper lighting and handrails).[88] Secondary causes of osteoporosis, such as alcoholism, glucocorticoid excess, hypogonadism in men, hyperthyroidism, and multiple myeloma, should be sought and treated.

For prophylaxis and for treatment of established osteoporosis, most women (and men) should ingest at least 1 to 1.5 g of elemental calcium per day beginning in the perimenopausal period, unless a contraindication such as a history of nephrolithiasis or hypercalciuria is present. Calcium carbonate is an inexpensive formulation that is acceptable for most patients, although calcium citrate is better absorbed by patients with achlorhydria. This should be accompanied by a daily multivitamin containing 400 to 800 IU of vitamin D. Intake of >1000 IU per day may cause increased bone resorption, although if biochemical evidence of osteomalacia is found, higher doses of vitamin D may be needed. Also, exercise is important.[89a]

Aside from calcium and vitamin D supplementation, estrogen-replacement therapy has been considered by some to be the treatment of first choice for established postmenopausal osteoporosis, based on long-term experience, well-documented effectiveness in preventing bone loss, and the potential for other benefits aside from its effects on bone. However, *relatively few data are available on the effects of estrogen use on rates of fracture* (especially hip fracture) in postmenopausal women.[90] Estrogens act primarily to prevent bone resorption, but the ability to *restore* lost bone mass may be minimal. Furthermore, evidence exists that the beneficial effects of estrogen replacement are more marked in women who begin treatment within five years after

menopause.[90] Therefore, maximum benefit from estrogen therapy is obtained by beginning use as soon as possible after menopause. Estrogens also play an important role in the treatment of type II osteoporosis,[91] however, and other studies have reported similar benefits from estrogen use on bone density, both in women older than age 70 and in younger women.[83] The optimal duration of estrogen use has not been established, but because cessation of estrogen treatment leads to resumption of bone loss, continuing treatment until age 65 to 70 or longer in those without contraindications to their use may be reasonable. Alternatively, the suggestion has been made that starting estrogen use at age 65 may provide almost as much protection against osteoporotic fractures as starting at menopause, and may reduce the risks of long-term estrogen therapy (see Chaps. 100 and 223 for discussions of the risks).[92,93] The selection of estrogen replacement regimens for elderly women is discussed later in the Menopause section.

The bisphosphonates alendronate and etidronate have been demonstrated to decrease the fracture rate in women with postmenopausal osteoporosis and are effective alternatives to estrogen therapy, especially for women who are concerned about the potential adverse effects of estrogens. Continuous high-dose etidronate may lead to impaired bone mineralization; therefore, etidronate must be given intermittently at a lower dosage (e.g., 400 mg per day for 2 weeks every 3 months).[94] An additive benefit of combined intermittent etidronate and cyclical estrogen and progesterone replacement on hip and spine bone mineral density was demonstrated over a 4-year period in postmenopausal women with established osteoporosis.[95] Low-dose alendronate (5 mg per day) prevents bone loss in postmenopausal women without established osteoporosis.[96,97] This approach is appropriate for those women who are at high risk for future fractures and who are unable or unwilling to take estrogen.[98] The efficacy and safety of other bisphosphonates (e.g., risedronate) in the prevention and treatment of osteoporosis are currently under investigation.

Calcitonin may be less effective in the prevention of bone loss in osteoporotic patients than estrogens or bisphosphonates, and its long-term efficacy in fracture prevention has not been as well documented. Raloxifene, a selective estrogen-receptor modulator, has been shown to increase bone density in postmenopausal women,[99] although to a smaller extent than estrogen replacement, and data regarding reduction in fractures are limited.[100] Although raloxifene does not appear to stimulate the endometrium in these women, it does decrease total and low-density lipoprotein (LDL) cholesterol levels. Unlike estrogens, however, raloxifene does not increase high-density lipoprotein (HDL) levels, and raloxifene is associated with an increased incidence of hot flushes, leg cramps, and thromboembolic events. Furthermore, no long-term data are available to assess the effects of raloxifene on the incidence of coronary heart disease (CHD) events, cognitive function, or the incidence of breast, ovarian, and uterine cancers.[100] At present, recommendation of other potential osteoporosis treatments such as fluoride, androgenic steroids, and parathyroid hormone injections is premature until studies are available that document improvements in osteoporotic fracture rates without significant adverse effects.

## HYPERCALCEMIA

### PRIMARY HYPERPARATHYROIDISM

Primary hyperparathyroidism occurs most commonly in adults between 45 and 60 years of age, although it may develop at any age. The condition occurs more often in women than in men by a ratio of nearly 3:1. The annual incidence of the disease is ~1 per 1000.[101] The diagnosis is often suspected based on a finding of elevated serum calcium levels on routine laboratory testing; indeed, asymptomatic hyperparathyroidism is by far the most common presentation.[102] Compared with younger patients, however, elderly people with primary hyperparathyroidism more often present with neuropsychiatric and neuromuscular symptoms, and with osteoporosis associated with fractures.[103] Other common complaints in older patients include altered mental status, fatigue, depression, weakness, personality change, memory loss, anorexia, and constipation.

The approach to the diagnosis and treatment of elderly patients with primary hyperparathyroidism is similar to that of younger patients (see Chap. 58).[102] Serum calcium level is high and phosphate level is often low to low normal, whereas alkaline phosphatase level is often high normal or mildly increased. Assays for intact PTH are the diagnostic tests of choice, and the presence of primary hyperparathyroidism is established by a high-normal or elevated PTH level in the setting of hypercalcemia. (Nonparathyroid causes of hypercalcemia are associated with undetectable or clearly decreased PTH levels. The most common cause of hypercalcemia in hospitalized patients is a malignancy producing a PTH-related protein [PTHrP] that can be measured in reference laboratories.) The skeletal effects of primary hyperparathyroidism are selective, with a reduction in cortical bone but relative protection against cancellous bone loss. Accordingly, bone densitometry is an important part of the evaluation of these patients, and measurements at the forearm and hip are the best indicators of cortical bone density (the latter is the most important site because of its significance as a risk factor for hip fracture).

Surgery is the only definitive treatment and is indicated in surgical candidates with markedly elevated serum calcium levels (>12 mg/dL), overt manifestations of primary hyperparathyroidism (e.g., nephrolithiasis), marked hypercalciuria, and markedly reduced cortical bone density. For the patients who are managed conservatively, checking serum calcium levels every 6 months and monitoring 24-hour urine calcium excretion, creatinine clearance, and bone densitometry annually is appropriate. These patients should be instructed to avoid thiazide diuretics and to avoid dehydration, but avoidance of dairy products is unnecessary. Most patients followed expectantly remain stable over time. Medical therapy for hyperparathyroidism may include administration of estrogens in women, oral phosphate in patients with low serum phosphate levels, and bisphosphonates.

### HYPERCALCEMIA OF MALIGNANCY

In most patients with malignancy-related hypercalcemia, an obvious neoplasm is evident on examination and routine diagnostic evaluation. Diagnostic possibilities include humoral hypercalcemia of malignancy, in which a PTHrP is produced by a cancer, usually of squamous cell type (e.g., lung, head, and neck), that occurs commonly in the elderly. In addition, multiple myeloma and some lymphatic tumors secrete osteoclast-activating factors, many of which are cytokines (e.g., lymphotoxin, interleukin-1, tumor necrosis factor). Treatment of hypercalcemia of malignancy includes volume repletion followed by immediate forced diuresis with saline infusion and furosemide. Parenteral bisphosphonates (e.g., pamidronate), calcitonin, or mithramycin should also be given, and the underlying malignancy should be treated if possible. Glucocorticoid therapy is reserved primarily for myeloma and lymphatic tumors. In elderly patients with advanced malignancies, short life expectancy, and poor functional status, not treating the hypercalcemia

may be appropriate and may provide a more comfortable mode of exit for these terminally ill patients.

## ADRENAL CORTEX

### PHYSIOLOGY

Decreased cortisol production is offset by decreased cortisol clearance, resulting in unchanged basal serum cortisol levels with aging. Urinary free cortisol levels are the same in elderly persons as in young adult subjects.[104] Stimulation of cortisol secretion by exogenous ACTH is unaltered with aging.[105] Furthermore, cortisol and ACTH responses to metyrapone, insulin-induced hypoglycemia, ovine CRH, and perioperative stress are normal or slightly prolonged in elderly subjects,[106,107] indicating an intact HPA axis responsiveness to stimulation with aging. In addition, ACTH pulse frequency is similar in healthy young and healthy elderly men, suggesting that baseline hypothalamic regulation of glucocorticoid function is intact with aging.[12] Clear evidence now exists, however, that feedback sensitivity to glucocorticoids decreases with aging.[15,108] Although the clinical implications of this decreased responsiveness to glucocorticoid feedback inhibition are uncertain, some have hypothesized that decreased negative feedback results in prolonged glucocorticoid exposure; this, in turn, damages hippocampal neurons regulating glucocorticoid secretion, leading to additional glucocorticoid hypersecretion and further damage to mechanisms regulating glucocorticoid feedback inhibition.[34,109] This process may be involved in mediating a "glucocorticoid cascade" of neurodegeneration in Alzheimer disease and, to a lesser extent, in the normal aging brain.[110] Thus, although the issue is still controversial, age-related glucocorticoid dysregulation may be a potentially modifiable risk factor for Alzheimer disease.

### LABORATORY DIAGNOSIS OF ADRENOCORTICAL DISEASE IN OLDER PATIENTS

Adrenal hyperfunction and hypofunction are less common in elderly than in middle-aged adults. However, manifestations that are associated with either adrenal hyperfunction (e.g., hypertension, obesity, and diabetes mellitus) or adrenal insufficiency (e.g., orthostatic hypotension and weight loss) occur more commonly in older than in young adults. Therefore, adrenal disease must be considered in the evaluation of elderly patients with these manifestations, and patients with suggestive findings on physical examination or laboratory screening should undergo further assessment. In addition, benign adrenal masses are common incidental findings observed during imaging procedures of the abdomen. Benign adenomas usually range in size from 1 to 6 cm and weigh 10 to 20 g, whereas malignant tumors generally weigh >100 g.[106,111] Incidentally detected adrenal masses of <3 cm in size probably do not need further evaluation or follow-up, and masses 3 to 6 cm in size may be followed with serial imaging studies. Hormone-secreting adrenal tumors and masses of >6 cm should probably be removed in patients who are appropriate candidates for surgery, although the natural history of incidentally discovered adrenal lesions in the elderly is unknown.

Several factors may interfere with testing of HPA axis function in the elderly. First, the excretion of steroids commonly measured in urine is decreased with renal impairment, and measurements are unreliable if the creatinine clearance is <50 mL per minute. This degree of renal insufficiency is common in elderly people. Nonetheless, serum creatinine levels may be relatively normal in these individuals due to an age-related decrease in muscle mass and creatinine production.[112] Second, cortisol clearance may be decreased in severely malnourished patients, resulting in falsely elevated cortisol levels. Third, the acute cortisol response to stress may be higher and more prolonged in elderly than in young adults; therefore, nonemergent testing of adrenal function should be deferred for at least 48 hours after major physiologic stresses such as trauma, surgery, and acute severe medical illnesses. Finally, agents such as phenytoin and phenobarbital induce liver metabolism of cortisol and other corticosteroids, and thereby may result in false-positive results on a dexamethasone-suppression test (i.e., failure of cortisol suppression) or decreased urinary 17-hydroxycorticosteroid levels (which are sometimes used as indices of cortisol secretion).

The results of provocative testing of HPA axis function, including cortisol responses to ACTH stimulation to rule out adrenal insufficiency, are unchanged with normal aging. However, some modifications in the approach to provocative testing may be required in elderly people. For example, measurement of the cortisol response to insulin-induced hypoglycemia is a reliable method to determine the presence of primary or secondary adrenal insufficiency, but this test is not usually used in frail older patients due to the *significant risks associated with severe hypoglycemia*. The standard metyrapone test may be used to confirm suspected adrenal insufficiency in those with a normal response to ACTH stimulation. This test, however, is often poorly tolerated by older patients, who may develop dizziness, nausea, and vomiting after receiving the drug. Intravenous infusions of metyrapone may be safer and better tolerated in elderly people.[106]

## HYPERADRENOCORTICISM

Hyperadrenocorticism is covered in detail in Chapter 75. Cushing disease appears most commonly in persons between 20 and 40 years of age, whereas the paraneoplastic ACTH syndrome is more common in elderly individuals, and often occurs in men older than age 50 with obvious neoplasms such as small cell lung cancer. Patients with the paraneoplastic ACTH syndrome typically present with cachexia (rather than a cushingoid appearance), hypokalemia, metabolic alkalosis, hyperglycemia, and hypertension. The most common cause of Cushing syndrome in elderly adults, however, as in other age groups, is the exogenous administration of glucocorticoids. Undesirable effects of glucocorticoid treatment are similar in elderly and in younger patients, but major adverse effects on function may occur in older people, including effects on the central nervous system (decreased cognition, confusion, depression, emotional lability, euphoria, psychosis), bone (osteoporosis, increased fracture risk), muscle (proximal wasting and weakness, decreased ambulation and transfers), skin (fragility), and glucose homeostasis (hyperglycemia).

When glucocorticoids must be used in the elderly patient, the minimum necessary dosage should be used for the shortest possible time. In addition, undesirable side effects of glucocorticoid administration should be mitigated by initiating bone-loss prevention measures as soon as corticosteroids are prescribed.[113] Baseline bone density should be determined before initiating long-term corticosteroid therapy and after 6 to 12 months of therapy. Treatments such as bisphosphonate or calcitonin may be considered for prevention of bone loss, but in any case should be initiated in patients who lose >5% of bone mass compared to baseline. Calcium supplementation with 1500 mg per day of elemental calcium, together with vitamin D, 800 IU per day, should be ensured to minimize bone loss caused by a corticosteroid-

induced decrease in intestinal calcium absorption and an increase in urinary calcium losses.

The exogenous administration of corticosteroids induces suppression of gonadotropins and sex steroids; therefore, sex hormone–replacement therapy should be considered unless contraindicated. For postmenopausal women, appropriate hormone-replacement regimens are the same as for women not receiving corticosteroids. Men with low testosterone levels should also be given hormone replacement, either with testosterone enanthate or testosterone cypionate, 100 to 200 mg intramuscularly every 2 weeks, or with daily transdermal application of a testosterone patch. The bisphosphonate alendronate (5 or 10 mg per day) or etidronate (administered cyclically, 400 mg per day for 14 days every 3 months) are effective in the primary and secondary prevention of bone loss in patients receiving glucocorticoid therapy.[114–116] Whether bisphosphonate treatment reduces fracture risk in patients with established corticosteroid-related osteoporosis is not yet clear, however. Calcitonin is also effective in the prevention and treatment of glucocorticoid-induced bone loss.[113,117] The restriction of dietary sodium and the administration of thiazide diuretics are useful to decrease corticosteroid-induced hypercalciuria, although the effects of these interventions on bone density have not been fully investigated.

## HYPOADRENOCORTICISM

Hypoadrenocorticism is covered in detail in Chapter 76. As in younger adults, iatrogenic adrenal failure secondary to long-term glucocorticoid administration is the most common cause of hypoadrenocorticism in elderly people. Only very uncommonly does autoimmune adrenocortical insufficiency present initially in an elderly patient. Some nonautoimmune causes of adrenal insufficiency occur more commonly in older adults, however, including tuberculosis, adrenal hemorrhage in patients taking anticoagulants, and metastatic involvement of the adrenals.[106] Some elderly patients with chronic adrenal insufficiency (e.g., secondary to hypopituitarism) present with nonspecific symptoms of "failure to thrive"—such as weight loss, anorexia, weakness, and decreased functional status. Moreover, one-third of older patients with adrenal insufficiency do not have hyperkalemia at initial presentation. Of note, compared with adrenal insufficiency in younger adults, adrenal insufficiency in the elderly has historically been more often fatal and more commonly diagnosed only at autopsy.[118] Therefore, a high index of suspicion is required to detect this treatable, life-threatening problem in many older patients.

Recovery of HPA axis responsiveness after cessation of glucocorticoid therapy is variable and in some individuals may not be complete even after several months. A number of factors may put older adults at higher risk to develop iatrogenic adrenal insufficiency. Elderly people who are on complicated medication regimens or who are cognitively impaired may become confused about their medications or forget to take them. High medication costs or medication-related side effects may cause older patients to discontinue their medicines abruptly without consulting their physicians. In addition, as noted earlier, the clinical manifestations of adrenocortical insufficiency are often nonspecific. When adrenocortical insufficiency due to cessation of long-term glucocorticoid therapy is suspected in an older person, an appropriate course is to perform the ACTH-stimulation test and institute therapy. As with younger adults, older people with persistent adrenocortical insufficiency should be given glucocorticoid replacement and coverage for major surgery and other stressful events until HPA axis function has recovered.

## ALDOSTERONE AND RENIN

Aldosterone secretion and clearance rates decrease with aging. In contrast to cortisol levels, however, basal plasma aldosterone levels are not maintained at normal levels in elderly subjects but decline by ~30% in healthy octogenarians compared with younger adults.[119] In response to dietary sodium restriction, aldosterone secretion increases three-fold in the young but only two-fold in older adults. These changes in aldosterone secretion with aging are thought to be due to corresponding reductions in plasma renin activity, which is decreased in the basal state and in response to sodium restriction or upright posture.[120] Furthermore, conversion of inactive to active renin is thought to be impaired with aging.[121] Age-related increases in atrial natriuretic hormone (ANH) secretion also contribute to the age-related decrease in aldosterone secretion by directly inhibiting aldosterone release and by inhibiting renal renin secretion, plasma renin activity, and angiotensin II levels. In addition, renal responsiveness to ANH is increased with aging, suggesting that ANH is an important contributor to age-related renal sodium losses.[16]

Declining aldosterone levels with aging predispose older people to renal salt wasting. Several other factors place elderly people at higher risk for volume depletion and dehydration, including decreased thirst sensation, increased ANH levels and renal ANH sensitivity, decreased renal ADH responsiveness, and possibly decreased renal-tubular responsiveness to aldosterone.[16] In addition, age-related hypoaldosteronism is characterized by a decreased aldosterone response to hyperkalemia, which may contribute to an increased susceptibility to hyperkalemia if other potassium regulatory systems fail.[122] Accordingly, elderly patients with hyporeninemic hypoaldosteronism are at higher risk of becoming hyperkalemic during treatment with potassium-sparing diuretics, β-blocking agents, or nonsteroidal antiinflammatory drugs. Older diabetic patients with renal insufficiency are particularly susceptible to this complication.

## ADRENAL ANDROGENS

Adrenal androgen secretion declines progressively beginning in the third decade, with plasma levels of the principal adrenal androgen, dehydroepiandrosterone (DHEA), declining to just 10% to 20% of young adult levels by the eighth and ninth decades.[123,124] This age-related decrease in DHEA levels is due to a reduction in adrenal DHEA secretion rather than to an increase in DHEA metabolism. Furthermore, the DHEA response to adrenal stimulation by ACTH is markedly decreased in older people. However, levels of DHEA and its sulfate, DHEAS, exhibit marked interindividual variability at all ages.

Epidemiologic data suggest that DHEA levels may play an important role in the deterioration of a variety of physiologic functions with aging. For example, low DHEA levels have been reported in states of poor health (e.g., after surgery or accidents) or in the setting of immunologic dysregulation (e.g., active rheumatoid arthritis or acquired immunodeficiency syndrome).[125] Other studies have reported positive correlations between plasma DHEA levels and vigor and longevity, and inverse correlations with cancers and cardiovascular disease.[126,127] Furthermore, high-functioning community-dwelling elderly subjects have higher levels of DHEAS than low-functioning subjects,[128] such that DHEAS levels are linked to functional status.

As a result of these associations, considerable interest has been generated in the potential therapeutic effects of DHEA administration in older adults. Data from randomized controlled trials in which DHEA was administered in dosages of 50 to 100 mg per day over a 6- to 12-month period have shown sub-jective improvements in physical and psychological well-being, increased serum IGF-I levels and, at higher dosages, increased lean body mass and muscle strength at the knee.[129] Levels of circulating lipids, glucose, and insulin as well as bone density were comparable in treated and placebo groups. Concerns remain, however, regarding the potential for androgenization in women, gynecomastia in men, possible adverse effects on lipoprotein metabolism at supraphysiologic doses, and potential hepatotoxicity.[130,131] Furthermore, DHEA is metabolizable to estrogens and to androgens, including testosterone and dihydrotestosterone,[125,129] and its effects on the risk of breast cancer in women and of prostate cancer in men have not been determined. Thus, although these data are potentially promising, the long-term safety and efficacy of DHEA treatment have *not* been established.

## CATECHOLAMINES

Norepinephrine (NE) is the principal neurotransmitter released by sympathetic postganglionic neurons. After release, most NE is taken up again into the axon terminals, whereas only a small fraction is released into the circulation.

Substantial evidence indicates that sympathetic nervous system (SNS) activity is increased with aging in humans. Basal plasma NE levels, and the NE secretory response to various stimuli such as upright posture and exercise, are increased with aging.[132,133] In contrast, circulating epinephrine levels and epinephrine responses to various stimuli exhibit little change with aging. Although sympathetic tone is increased with aging, physiologic responsiveness to both α- and β-adrenergic receptor–mediated stimulation appears to decrease with aging.[134] Decreased catecholamine responsiveness is thought to be due to changes at both the receptor and the postreceptor level.

The clinical effects of this age-related increase in sympathetic tone may include the development of hypertension. A number of studies have reported a correlation between hypertension and increased plasma NE levels in elderly people.[135] Body fat content is independently associated with both aging and plasma NE levels, however, suggesting that obesity may contribute to hypertension by increasing sympathetic tone, independent of the effects of aging per se.

Certain diseases commonly associated with aging may give rise to autonomic insufficiency with orthostatic hypotension, including Parkinson disease, multiple system atrophy, and diabetes mellitus. Moreover, certain drugs that interfere with SNS function may also cause orthostatic hypotension; these include antihypertensive agents such as clonidine and α-methyldopa and psychoactive drugs such as phenothiazines and tricyclic antidepressants. Other factors such as volume depletion, prolonged bed rest, and venous insufficiency may also cause or exacerbate postural hypotension. The management of orthostatic hypotension includes the treatment of hypovolemia, discontinuation of medications that may exacerbate postural hypotension, and instructing the patient to sit with legs dangling for several minutes before getting out of bed, to elevate the head of the bed at night, and to use elastic support stockings and an abdominal binder to promote venous return. Useful medications include caffeine, fludrocortisone to expand plasma volume, and midodrine, a sympathomimetic amine.

Postprandial hypotension is a common disorder involving SNS dysfunction in elderly people. It possibly results from inadequate SNS compensation for pooling of blood in the splanchnic vessels after a meal, impaired baroreceptor reflex function, impaired peripheral vasocontriction, release of vasoactive gastrointestinal peptides, and/or inadequate postprandial increases in cardiac output.[136] This condition is especially common in elderly hypertensive patients. Postprandial hypotension may be an important cause of syncope in elderly patients and should be considered in the evaluation of older people with unexplained syncope.[137] The management of this condition should include the avoidance of dehydration, discontinuation of unnecessary drugs that could exacerbate postprandial hypotension, consumption of frequent small meals, avoidance of alcohol, and avoidance of strenuous exercise within 2 hours after meals. Caffeine use has not been shown to be helpful in this condition.

# FEMALE REPRODUCTIVE AND ENDOCRINE FUNCTION: MENOPAUSE

The mean age for menopause in women, 51 years, has not changed significantly over the last century. Because life expectancy for women has increased markedly over the same period, however, most women can expect to spend more than one-third of their lives in the postmenopausal state. Accordingly, clinicians caring for perimenopausal and postmenopausal women must work closely with them to consider the potential impact of menopausal changes on future health and functional status.

Failure of ovarian end-organ function occurs by the fifth or sixth decade, with cessation of ovarian follicular development, estradiol secretion, and menstruation, and unresponsiveness to gonadotropin stimulation. Premenopausally, estradiol ($E_2$) and estrone ($E_1$) are secreted by maturing ovarian follicles and are produced by aromatization of ovarian and adrenal androgenic precursors in peripheral tissues. An elevation in serum FSH levels heralds the onset of menopause and is the most sensitive clinically available indicator of cessation of ovarian follicle development.[138] As noted in the discussion of gonadotropins earlier, levels of inhibin B appear to decline slightly before FSH levels increase,[39] but an inhibin-B assay is not yet clinically available. After menopause, circulating $E_2$ and $E_1$ are derived almost entirely from aromatization of adrenal androstenedione, and $E_1$ levels are higher than those of $E_2$. FSH levels increase to a greater extent than LH levels. Obese postmenopausal women exhibit increased production of adrenal androgenic precursors and increased peripheral aromatization of androgens to estrogens, especially to $E_1$, which is associated with a decreased risk of osteoporosis.

The manifestations of estrogen deficiency experienced by menopausal women are listed in Table 199-5. Vasomotor symptoms occur in three out of four women during the perimenopausal period[139] and may be associated with other symptoms such as palpitations, faintness, fatigue, and vertigo. These symptoms, along with atrophy of the sexual tissues, are relieved by estrogen replacement. Clonidine, methyldopa, or medroxyprogesterone may occasionally be effective for treating hot flushes in women who are unable to take estrogens.

As discussed earlier, long-term treatment with estrogens in postmenopausal women may prevent or delay the occurrence of osteoporosis and fractures. Furthermore, the incidence of coronary artery disease rises sharply in postmenopausal women, and some evidence from observational studies has suggested that estrogen replacement in postmenopausal women decreases the risk of cardiovascular disease by up to 50% compared with those not receiving estrogens.[83,140] This apparent cardioprotective effect of estrogens has been attributed to favorable effects on lipid metabolism, including decreased serum LDL and increased HDL cholesterol levels, and to other effects of estrogens on clotting mechanisms, glucose regulation, blood vessels, and myocardial tissue.[141] Cardiac catheterization studies have reported that women receiving estrogen replacement develop less severe coronary atherosclerosis, and that the greatest benefit of estrogens on

**TABLE 199-5.**
**Manifestations of Estrogen Deficiency in Menopausal Women**

*Primarily in the menopausal period*
  Vasomotor instability—"hot flushes"
    Spreading sensation of heat
    Palpitations
    Diaphoresis
    Sleep disturbances
  Irregular menstrual bleeding and eventual cessation of menses
  Neuropsychiatric symptoms probably related to low estrogen state
    Decreased concentration
    Irritability
    Anxiety
    Depressed mood
    Decreased libido (probably related to low testosterone levels)
  Alterations in lipid metabolism
    Increased LDL cholesterol
    Slight decline in HDL cholesterol
*Primarily postmenopausal*
  Urogenital atrophy
    Vulvar pruritus
    Dyspareunia
    Urinary complaints, including dysuria and stress incontinence
    Increased risk of pelvic prolapse due to loss of supporting structures
  Osteoporosis
  Increased risk of cardiovascular disease
  (?) Cognitive dysfunction
    Possible decreased short-term memory
    Possible increased risk of Alzheimer disease

*LDL,* low-density lipoprotein; *HDL,* high-density lipoprotein.

coronary disease is realized by women with more severe atherosclerosis at the time of the initial catheterization.[142,143]

The cardiovascular benefits of estrogen-replacement therapy have been called into question, however, by the results of the Heart and Estrogen/Progestin Replacement Study (HERS)—a randomized, placebo-controlled trial of hormone replacement for secondary prevention of CHD in postmenopausal women—which found *no* reduction in the rate of coronary events over a period of >4 years, with a tendency toward a higher coronary event rate in the treatment group in the first year and fewer events in years 4 and 5.[144] Furthermore, thromboembolic events were increased within the first year of therapy. Based on these data, *insufficient evidence* exists at this time to support the initiation of hormone-replacement therapy specifically to prevent coronary events in women with established CHD. Estrogen replacement possibly may be beneficial in the primary prevention of coronary events; however, data from randomized, controlled trials addressing this issue will not be available until the results of studies such as the Women's Health Initiative and the Women's International Study of Long Duration Oestrogen after Menopause (WISDOM) are completed.[145] Furthermore, given the trend toward a cardiovascular benefit after several years of treatment in the HERS study, continuing therapy for this indication in women who are already receiving replacement may be appropriate. Nevertheless, even long-term therapy may be associated with some risks. One large prospective observational study reported that overall mortality was reduced by 37% in women currently taking hormone replacement, but the magnitude of this apparent benefit decreased to 20% in those receiving therapy for >10 years.[146]

Some, but not all, evidence suggests that estrogen use may improve cognitive function in postmenopausal women with

**TABLE 199-6.**
**Contraindications to Postmenopausal Hormone Replacement**

*Contraindications*
    Known or suspected estrogen-dependent neoplasm
        Breast carcinoma
        Endometrial carcinoma
        Melanoma
    Vaginal bleeding of unknown origin
    Active liver disease or impairment in liver function
    Active or recent thrombophlebitis or thromboembolic disease
*Relative contraindications*
    History of endometrial hyperplasia
    Hypertension associated with estrogen use
    Uterine fibroids
    Active pancreatitis
    Familial hypertriglyceridemia
    Migraine headaches
    Endometriosis
    Gallbladder disease

Alzheimer disease (AD). Retrospective studies have found an inverse correlation between the dosage and duration of estrogen-replacement therapy and the incidence of AD,[147,148] and estrogen administration in small open trials appeared to improve cognition and mood in women with AD.[149,150] Moreover, some aspects of cognitive function were found to improve with transdermal estrogen replacement in a small double-blind, placebo-controlled trial of postmenopausal women with AD.[151] Larger prospective studies are needed, however, to document any alleged therapeutic role for estrogens in the treatment of AD.

Established risks associated with estrogen replacement include a nearly six-fold increase in the incidence of endometrial cancer in those receiving unopposed estrogen therapy. Coadministration of a progestin protects against this complication, however. The lifetime risk of developing breast cancer appears to be 10% to 30% higher in postmenopausal women receiving estrogen-replacement therapy for >10 years, and this risk must be weighed against the potential benefits of hormone replacement.[141] Hypercoagulability is a potential side effect of estrogen therapy. Estrogen use may also predispose to cholelithiasis and hypertriglyceridemia. Table 199-6 summarizes the contraindications to estrogen-replacement therapy.

In summary, further clarification of the risks and benefits of postmenopausal hormone-replacement therapy must await the completion of additional prospective, randomized, controlled trials such as the Women's Health Initiative. For the time being, the beneficial effects on bone density and urogenital atrophy, and—in the immediate postmenopausal period—the amelioration of vasomotor symptoms such as hot flushes, are the primary indications for hormone-replacement therapy in some postmenopausal women.

An estrogen-progestin combination is appropriate for women with an intact uterus to decrease the risk of endometrial cancer, although inclusion of a progestin may partially attenuate some of the favorable effects of estrogens on lipids, and the effects of progestins on cardiovascular risk are uncertain. Estrogens should be used alone in women who have had a hysterectomy. Many older women may prefer continuous rather than cyclic hormone administration, because objectionable resumption of menses often occurs with cyclic therapy. An appropriate continuous combined hormonal regimen for many of these women is 0.625 mg daily of an oral conjugated estrogen, together with 2.5 mg daily of medroxyprogesterone acetate. Potential disadvantages to this approach include the possibility of irregular bleeding and the relative lack of information on the effects of continuous progesterone on reduction in endometrial cancer risk and serum lipid levels. Furthermore, some women may experience weight gain and depression with daily progesterone administration. Patients should be informed that spotting often occurs during the first few months on this regimen, but that most women become amenorrheic after a year of treatment. For women who find a cyclic regimen suitable, 0.625 mg of conjugated estrogen may be used daily, with addition of a 10- to 14-day course of medroxyprogesterone acetate, 5 to 10 mg daily, every 3 or 4 months to induce withdrawal bleeding. This approach has the disadvantage of a greater likelihood of inducing menses, but menses will occur at a predictable time, and more is known about the effects of cyclic hormone regimens on uterine cancer risk and lipids. With either approach, very gradual introduction of conjugated estrogen may reduce unpleasant symptoms such as breast swelling, beginning with 0.3 mg every other day, advancing to 0.3 mg per day after 1 month and 0.625 mg per day the following month. Alternatives to conjugated estrogens include oral, transdermal, and vaginal estradiol preparations.

Alternatives to estrogen replacement are available for women who are unable or unwilling to take estrogens—specifically, the selective estrogen-receptor modulators such as raloxifene. As noted earlier, raloxifene has beneficial effects on bone mass and serum lipid levels. The increase in bone mass, however, may be less with raloxifene than with estrogen therapy, and although the reduction in total and LDL cholesterol levels is similar with estrogens and raloxifene, the latter does not increase HDL cholesterol levels.[100]

The effects of selective estrogen-receptor modulators on cardiovascular mortality and mortality due to all causes are unknown. In contrast to estrogens, raloxifene commonly produces hot flushes and is, therefore, not indicated for the treatment of vasomotor symptoms of menopause. Raloxifene has estrogen-antagonist effects on breast and uterine tissues, and does not cause endometrial hyperplasia. Tamoxifen, another estrogen antagonist, reduces the risk of invasive breast cancer in women who are at increased risk for breast cancer or who have a history of breast carcinoma in situ.[152] If raloxifene is shown to have similar effects, it may be particularly useful in women with risk factors for breast cancer or a history of the disease.

# MALE REPRODUCTIVE AND ENDOCRINE FUNCTION

## HORMONAL CHANGES

The age-related changes in reproductive function in men are less dramatic than those that occur in aging women. In aging men, reproductive changes occur gradually, exhibit considerable variation among individuals, and usually do not result in severe hypogonadism. A modest degree of primary testicular failure is evident in many healthy elderly men, as evidenced by decreases in daily sperm production, diminished total and free testosterone levels, and reduced testosterone responses to exogenous gonadotropin administration, together with increased serum gonadotropin levels.[42,153] Some medical illnesses and malnutrition may further impair testicular function, as can some medications (Table 199-7).[153a] In more frail older men, testicular failure is extremely common. For example, among male nursing home residents, 45% of individuals have been reported to exhibit testosterone levels within the hypogonadal range.[154] Some men,

**TABLE 199-7.**
**Medications Associated with Decreased Serum Testosterone Levels and Hypogonadism**

Opiates
Ethanol
Cytotoxic drugs
Cimetidine
Ketoconazole
Glucocorticoids
Phenytoin
Spironolactone

however, maintain serum testosterone levels within the normal range even after age 80.[42,153] In addition to primary testicular failure, subtle age-related changes occur in hypothalamic-pituitary control of testicular function, including decreased gonadotropin responsiveness to exogenous GnRH administration[42] and decreased LH pulse frequency in some healthy aging men.[41] Furthermore, many healthy older men have inappropriately normal gonadotropin levels (i.e., not elevated above the normal range) in the presence of low testosterone levels, suggesting secondary testicular failure.

A small number of aging men exhibit more obvious testicular failure, with total testosterone levels clearly below the lower limits of the normal range and clear manifestations of androgen deficiency (e.g., decreased libido and potency, osteoporosis, gynecomastia, and hot flushes). In the absence of contraindications, androgen replacement is indicated for these older men, as for young men. More often, however, the clinician is faced with an older patient with slightly decreased serum testosterone levels (e.g., 2.5 to 3.0 ng/mL) and nonspecific symptoms that may include impotence, loss of libido, muscle weakness, or osteopenia, and whether these men should be treated is unclear. In young hypogonadal men, androgens are important for the maintenance of normal bone and muscle mass, sexual drive, and erectile function.[42] The hypothesis has been raised that age-related androgen deficiency may contribute to declining muscle and bone mass and other concomitants of aging, but few randomized, controlled studies have been performed to determine whether androgen supplementation in older men is beneficial and whether the benefits outweigh the risks. Two reports involving a small number of older hypogonadal men found that testosterone administration for 3 months increased lean body mass, reduced biochemical indices of bone turnover, and increased libido, without adverse effects on lipid metabolism or symptoms of prostatism.[155,156] Another study of testosterone replacement over 12 months in older men with low testosterone levels found increases in grip strength but failed to demonstrate changes in body composition.[157] Several of the subjects were withdrawn from treatment, however, due to elevations in hematocrit. Finally, visceral fat mass and fasting blood glucose levels declined in middle-aged men receiving testosterone.[158] Although some placebo-controlled studies have shown improvements in some measures of strength with testosterone therapy, no data are yet available to show whether testosterone improves functional performance or quality of life in elderly men.[159] At the moment, larger and longer term studies are needed to determine the risks and benefits of androgen-replacement therapy before this approach can be recommended for aging men with slightly reduced testosterone levels.

Androgen-replacement therapy is discussed in detail in Chapter 119.

## SEXUAL ACTIVITY AND ERECTILE DYSFUNCTION

In general, sexual activity and libido decline with aging, although some healthy elderly men exhibit stable or increased sexual desire with aging.[160,161] Important determinants of sexual behavior in elderly men include perceived health status and the level of sexual activity during the younger years.

Kinsey estimated the prevalence of impotence to be 55% by the age of 75 years.[162] In contrast to the earlier view that most impotence is psychogenic, erectile dysfunction is now thought to have an organic basis in the large majority of cases. Furthermore, the prevalence of organic causes increases with advancing age.[163] Important contributors to impotence in older men include arterial and venous abnormalities, neuropathies, use of medications, and coexisting medical illnesses. The most common cause of erectile dysfunction in older men is vascular disease, with half of all men older than age 50 exhibiting evidence of impaired penile blood flow. Venous insufficiency (failure to occlude venous outflow) may occur due to leakage, arteriovenous malformations, or increased shunting between the corpora cavernosa and the glans. Although overt hypogonadism is present in <10% of elderly men with sexual dysfunction, hormonal alterations have been estimated to play a role in ~50% of cases.[163,164] In addition to androgen deficiency, endocrine disorders that may contribute to impotence include hypothyroidism and hyperthyroidism, hyperprolactinemia due to either medications or pituitary adenomas, Cushing syndrome, diabetes mellitus, and diseases involving the hypothalamus or pituitary (e.g., tumors).

The approach to diagnostic testing and management of erectile dysfunction in elderly patients is similar to that in younger men and is discussed in Chapter 117.

## OBESITY

Estimates are that, in the United States, 26% of white men and 37% of white women between the ages of 65 and 76 years are overweight.[165] Body weight generally increases with aging in young and middle-aged adults but begins to decline in the sixth and seventh decades.[166,167] Moreover, body composition is altered, with increasing total body adiposity and declining lean body mass (primarily muscle mass).[166,168] Mortality rates are increased at either extreme of body weight, with the lowest mortality at intermediate weights. The *body mass index* (BMI, a measure of weight standardized for height) associated with the lowest mortality increases progressively with aging, although a broad range of body weights appears to be acceptable. In men, however, the lowest mortality is observed in those of below-average weight, as long as the low weight is not caused by or associated with a disease.[169]

With advancing age, a progressive trend is seen toward the development of abdominal adiposity.[167] This central or upper body distribution of fat is associated with an increased prevalence and incidence of disorders such as hypertension, coronary artery disease, diabetes mellitus, and stroke, whereas lower body adiposity is relatively benign.[167]

Although population studies suggest that people with a BMI markedly above the mean have an increased mortality risk, weight reduction per se in obese older patients has not been shown to reduce morbidity and mortality. Furthermore, data from epidemiologic studies suggest that weight loss is associated with functional decline in some obese older patients.[170] However, weight loss in obese middle-aged and older men that was achieved over a 9-month period through modest reductions in energy intake was reported to improve coronary artery disease risk factors, including blood pressure, lipid profiles, and the glucose levels.[171] These findings suggest that weight control achieved through dietary modifications and appropriate exercise may be a useful primary preventive strategy to reduce the risk of coronary disease in middle-aged and older adults. Widespread implementation of this strategy will be a formidable challenge, however, and whether these benefits can be maintained for longer periods is unclear. Therefore, weight reduction should be considered primarily in obese individuals with other conditions that may benefit from weight loss, including those with type 2 diabetes mellitus, hypertension, degenerative joint disease of the lower extremities, and low back pain.[172]

Strategies for weight reduction in obese elderly people include dietary modification, with mild to moderate calorie restriction, an increase in complex carbohydrates, and a decrease in fat to <30% of total calories with a daily multivitamin supplement. An increase in dietary fiber may be appropriate in some individuals; meals with increased fiber take longer to ingest because of the increased need for chewing, and the larger size of food boluses leads to a greater feeling of satiety.[173] A decrease in dietary fat may promote mild weight loss even without calorie restriction, whereas patients may tend to regain the weight lost through calorie restriction alone. The patient's spouse should be included in these efforts, especially if the spouse cooks the meals. A graded aerobic exercise program is also advisable. Many older people find walking to be a suitable activity, and mall-walking programs are available for seniors in many communities. The risks and benefits of pharmacologic treatment of obesity with anorectic drugs such as adrenergic-receptor agonists or serotonergic agonists such as dexfenfluramine have not been determined in the elderly population, and these agents cannot be recommended at this time.[174]

## CARBOHYDRATE METABOLISM AND DIABETES MELLITUS

### EPIDEMIOLOGY

Fasting blood glucose levels increase minimally during normal aging, by ~1 mg/dL per decade.[175] The prevalence rate of diabetes mellitus increases markedly with aging, however, from <2% in American adults aged 20 to 39 years to 17.5% in women older than 75 years and 21.1% in men older than 75 years.[176] These figures were derived from the Third National Health and Nutrition Examination Survey, which used a fasting glucose level of ≥126 mg/dL (7.0 mmol/L) as the diagnostic criterion for diabetes (see discussion later). Nearly all elderly diabetic patients have type 2 diabetes, although with improvements in the care of younger adults with type 1 diabetes, an increasing number of these patients will survive to old age.

Unlike fasting glucose levels, which change little with aging, glucose tolerance declines progressively, with increases in plasma glucose levels of 9 to 10 mg/dL per decade after oral glucose challenge.[175] These age-related changes in glucose tolerance are reflected in a slight increase in glycosylated hemoglobin levels with aging.[51]

### PATHOGENESIS

The pathogenesis of age-related glucose intolerance is multifactorial, and involves alterations in insulin secretion as well as target-organ resistance to insulin action. Insulin-receptor number and binding are unaltered with aging, suggesting that insulin resistance is due to a postreceptor defect. Other factors contributing to age-related glucose intolerance and insulin resistance include obesity, abdominal adiposity, decreasing lean

body mass, a diet low in carbohydrates and high in fat, medication use, decreasing physical activity, and hypertension.[51] Glucose intolerance may not be inevitable with aging, however; at least some healthy nonobese older people show unaltered insulin sensitivity and B-cell function with aging.[177] Furthermore, a high-carbohydrate diet can improve glucose tolerance,[178] and physical training can improve insulin sensitivity.[179] In a study of exercise in very healthy elderly subjects, however, exercise-induced improvement in insulin sensitivity was counterbalanced by a reduction in insulin secretion, which resulted in no net change in glucose tolerance.[180]

Among those with impaired glucose tolerance, approximately one-third develop overt type 2 diabetes mellitus within 5 years. The progression to frank diabetes is thought to be determined by a combination of genetic predisposition (e.g., family history of diabetes or, in some cases, Native American, Hispanic, or black racial origin) and environmental factors such as sedentary lifestyle and obesity that contribute to insulin resistance. Many of those with both a genetic predilection to develop diabetes and permissive environmental factors develop insulin resistance with a compensatory hyperinsulinemia, but diabetes does not develop as long as insulin production is sufficient to overcome the insulin resistance. Obesity is associated with an increased risk of developing type 2 diabetes, especially in those exceeding 130% of ideal body weight and those with primarily abdominal adiposity. A multicenter study, the Diabetes Prevention Program, is currently under way to determine whether interventions such as dietary modification and exercise can delay or prevent the development of overt diabetes mellitus in high-risk individuals such as those with impaired glucose tolerance.

### CLINICAL PRESENTATION AND COMPLICATIONS OF DIABETES IN OLDER PATIENTS

Diabetes tends to present atypically in the elderly, often without classic symptoms such as polyuria and polydipsia (Table 199-8). The renal glucose threshold increases with advancing age; therefore, polyuria and polydipsia may not occur even with blood glucose levels well over 200 mg/dL (11.1 mmol/L). Common nonspecific presenting symptoms in older patients include weight loss, fatigue, weakness, cognitive impairment, urinary incontinence, or urinary tract infections. Diabetes may be completely asymptomatic in elderly people, however, and the diagnosis may be made only as a result of routine plasma glucose measurement. In fact, asymptomatic hyperglycemia may have been present for years before the diagnosis is appreciated. Furthermore, older patients may present initially with chronic complications of diabetes, such as nephropathy, peripheral neuropathy, cataracts, or symptoms of macrovascular disease, including myocardial infarction and stroke. Older patients not previously suspected of having diabetes may even present for the first time with an acute diabetic complication such as a hyperosmolar nonketotic state.

Older people with impaired glucose tolerance have an increased risk of macrovascular complications such as stroke and coronary artery disease, even in the absence of overt diabetes. This may be due to the hyperinsulinemia associated with glucose intolerance, which is independently associated with the risk of coronary artery disease. However, whether or not treatment of impaired glucose tolerance without diabetes in elderly people reduces the rate of macrovascular complications is unclear.

Older diabetic patients often have many complications of their disease. Manifestations of macrovascular disease, including amputation, myocardial infarction, and stroke, occur more commonly in elderly diabetic patients than in those without dia-

**TABLE 199-8.**
**Clinical Symptoms and Signs of Diabetes Mellitus in Older Patients**

*Constitutional*
  Fatigue
  Unexplained weight loss
*Eyes*
  Cataracts
  Background or proliferative retinopathy
*Nervous system*
  Pain
  Paresthesias
  Hypoesthesias
  Autonomic neuropathies
    Diarrhea
    Impotence
    Postural hypotension
    Overflow incontinence
  Cranial nerve palsies
  Muscle weakness
  Diabetic neuropathic cachexia and amyotrophy
  Coma (hyperosmolar nonketotic coma)
  Cognitive impairment
*Cardiovascular*
  Angina
  Silent ischemia
  Myocardial infarction
  Transient ischemic attack
  Stroke
  Diabetic foot ulcers
  Gangrene
*Genitourinary*
  Proteinuria
  Chronic renal failure
  Urinary incontinence
*Metabolic*
  Obesity
  Hyperlipidemia
  Osteoporosis
*Skin*
  Pruritus vulvae
  Intertrigo
  Bacterial infections
  Slow wound healing
*Infections*
  Urinary tract infections
  Reactivation of tuberculosis
  Oral thrush
  Vulvovaginitis, balanitis

betes.[181,182] Silent myocardial ischemia is more common in elderly diabetic patients, and diabetic patients tend to suffer more severe complications of myocardial infarction than nondiabetic individuals.

Microvascular complications are also extremely common in elderly diabetic patients. In the Framingham study, 19% of diabetic patients between 55 and 84 years of age had retinopathy, with an increasing prevalence and incidence with advancing age.[183] Both the degree of glycemic control and age itself are independent predictors of retinopathy in older diabetic patients,[184] and glycemic control is important in preventing the progression of retinopathy in this population.[185] End-stage renal disease is twice as common in elderly diabetic patients than in those of the same age without diabetes,[182] and the prevalence of diabetic nephropathy increases with age and the duration of

diabetes.[186] Older diabetic individuals are at significant risk for developing hyperkalemia secondary to hyporeninemic hypoaldosteronism. In these patients, hyperkalemia is commonly precipitated by addition of nonsteroidal antiinflammatory drugs, angiotensin-converting enzyme inhibitors, or β-blocking agents.

Older patients with diabetes are more likely to develop neuropathy within a decade of initial diagnosis than are younger patients. Certain diabetic neuropathic syndromes are seen almost exclusively in elderly patients, including diabetic amyotrophy, a progressive wasting of the pelvic girdle and thigh muscles that usually resolves spontaneously; and *diabetic neuropathic cachexia*, a self-limited disorder associated with anorexia, painful peripheral neuropathy, profound weight loss, and depression. The latter syndrome may mislead the clinician to perform an extensive evaluation to rule out malignancy.

Elderly diabetic patients are at higher risk than those without diabetes for the development of cataracts and glaucoma. In elderly patients whose cataracts cause significant visual impairment, cataract surgery may result in functional improvement. Poor glycemic control is associated with defects in cognitive functioning in elderly patients with type 2 diabetes, including learning and memory retrieval.[187] Therefore, the possibility of cognitive impairment should be considered in all elderly diabetic patients. Those with memory impairment may benefit from special counseling and use of memory aids, such as medication calendars and Medisets.

Hypoglycemia is the most common acute complication of diabetes in older patients. Many of the factors that complicate overall management of older diabetic individuals also contribute to an increased risk of hypoglycemia in these patients (Table 199-9). Furthermore, when hypoglycemia does occur, its presence may be unrecognized in the elderly and persist longer than in young patients because of decreased counterregulatory hormonal responses (*hypoglycemic unawareness*). Hypoglycemia may cause or contribute to myocardial ischemia and infarctions, strokes, cognitive impairment, and death in older patients who are already at increased risk for these problems.

## DIAGNOSTIC CRITERIA

The diagnosis of diabetes is easily made in older individuals presenting with an unequivocal elevation of plasma glucose and clinical symptoms and signs consistent with diabetes. Making the diagnosis is more difficult, however, when signs and symptoms are subtle, and plasma glucose is not as markedly elevated.

Based on the foregoing, it follows that screening is necessary to detect asymptomatic diabetes in elderly people. The best

**TABLE 199-9.**
**Factors Affecting Management of Hyperglycemia in Older Diabetic Patients**

Hypoglycemic unawareness
Coexisting acute and chronic medical illnesses
Cognitive impairment
Coexisting psychiatric illnesses
Polypharmacy
Use of medications affecting glucose homeostasis or food intake
Visual impairment
Decreased manual dexterity
Limited dietary preferences
Difficulties in obtaining, preparing, and ingesting food
Inadequate social support
Poverty
Difficulty obtaining medical care

available screening test is the fasting plasma glucose level, and the diagnosis of diabetes is established by documenting a *fasting blood glucose level of ≥126 mg/dL (7.0 mmol/L) on at least two occasions.* Fasting glucose levels of <110 mg/dL (6.1 mmol/L) are considered normal based on the American Diabetes Association diagnostic criteria, whereas intermediate values have been defined as impaired fasting glucose.[188] Previously, the recommended threshold for diagnosing diabetes was a fasting glucose level of ≥140 mg/dL (7.8 mmol/L). The rationale for the new, more stringent criterion was based on a consensus that the threshold of 140 mg/dL failed to identify a significant number of people at risk for the development of diabetes-related complications.[182] The new criterion is *not adjusted for age,* because a fasting glucose level of >126 mg/dL is thought to be an equally potent predictor of complications in elderly people and in younger adults. Furthermore, estimates are that one-third of elderly patients with diabetes remained undiagnosed using the threshold of 140 mg/dL.[182]

Diabetes screening in asymptomatic, undiagnosed adults is recommended every 3 years for all individuals older than age 45, or more often in those who are obese, have a first-degree relative with diabetes, are members of a high-risk ethnic population (e.g., black, Hispanic, or Native American), are hypertensive, have low HDL cholesterol and/or high triglyceride levels, or have a history of impaired glucose tolerance or impaired fasting glucose levels.[189] However, reductions in disease-specific outcomes as a result of screening asymptomatic elderly people for diabetes have not yet been demonstrated.[190] Furthermore, routine screening and yearly monitoring of fasting glucose levels have been recommended for nursing home residents.[57] This may be appropriate in some nursing home residents, but the physician must consider whether the patient or surrogate decision maker desires testing and treatment, whether the results would affect treatment decisions, and whether treatment would improve functional status and quality of life.

## MANAGEMENT

### GLYCEMIC CONTROL

Increasing evidence indicates that, as in type 1 diabetes, the *degree of hyperglycemia is a major determinant of morbidity in type 2 diabetes.* The Diabetes Control and Complications Trial (DCCT) reported a reduction in microvascular and neurologic complication rates in young individuals with type 1 diabetes who were treated with intensive insulin therapy,[191] raising the question of whether intensive intervention might similarly benefit patients with type 2 diabetes. The Wisconsin Epidemiologic Study of Diabetic Retinopathy found a relationship between the degree of hyperglycemia and the incidence and progression of microvascular and macrovascular complications in individuals with both type 1 and type 2 diabetes, but did not indicate whether intervention would be equally beneficial in the two disorders.[192,193] A small intervention trial of intensive insulin therapy versus conventional insulin therapy in patients with type 2 diabetes, however, demonstrated significant reductions in the development or progression of diabetic retinopathy, nephropathy, and neuropathy, as well as of macrovascular events in the intensively treated group.[194] Furthermore, the United Kingdom Prospective Diabetes Study of middle-aged type 2 diabetic patients reported that, over a 10-year period, intensive treatment with either oral hypoglycemic agents or insulin significantly reduced diabetes-related complications, especially microvascular events, although intensively treated patients experienced more hypoglycemic episodes.[195] These findings indicate that, in both type 1 and type 2 diabetes, optimizing glucose control is important in minimizing morbidity from this disease.

The management of diabetes in older patients must be individualized. Despite the foregoing observations, *tight* glycemic control is *not* an appropriate goal in many older patients with diabetes. As demonstrated in the DCCT and other trials, tight control involves an increased risk of hypoglycemia, even in young patients who are closely monitored. In elderly diabetic patients, this risk may be further increased by patients' tendency to err by up to 20% in their dosing of insulin.[196] Moreover, a variety of other coexisting medical, social, cognitive, economic, and functional problems may increase the risk of hypoglycemia or make accurate blood glucose monitoring difficult in frail older patients (see Table 199-9). Taken together, these problems often make efforts at rigorous glycemic control either unsafe or technically not feasible.

A major goal in all patients is to treat hyperglycemia to relieve symptoms while avoiding hypoglycemia. In many elderly diabetic patients, controlling glucose levels more rigorously in an attempt to minimize long-term complications such as macrovascular and microvascular disease is also appropriate, but the potential for benefit must be balanced with the risks of hypoglycemia and any practical constraints on more aggressive glucose control. The degree of glycemic control and other treatment goals should be agreeable to the patient, the physician, and the home caregivers assisting with diabetes care. A team approach is ideal for the care of older diabetic patients with complex medical, social, and functional issues. Available resources will determine the exact composition of the team, but one team member should be identified as a diabetes educator in charge of assessment, education, and follow-up.[197] Careful attention should be given to other risk factors for cardiovascular disease, such as systolic and diastolic hypertension, smoking, and hyperlipidemia; good foot care is essential.

The modalities available for the treatment of diabetes in elderly patients include diet, exercise, and the use of oral hypoglycemic agents and/or insulin, as in younger patients. Treatment of type 2 diabetes in older patients often begins with a trial of dietary therapy. No single approach can be uniformly recommended, however, as the following considerations demonstrate.

### DIET AND EXERCISE

The effects of dietary intervention in older diabetics have not been well studied, and in practice, marked changes in dietary habits may be difficult to achieve. Dietary alterations may adversely affect the patient's quality of life, and this must be considered along with the potential benefits of treatment. In contrast to younger patients with type 2 diabetes, many frail elderly diabetic patients are not overweight. In these patients, adequate nutrition and even weight gain are advisable. In older diabetic patients who are >20% above their ideal body weight, the goal of dietary therapy is long-term moderate weight reduction (not >5% to 10% reduction in body weight). Appropriate dietary prescriptions for these patients might include restriction of dietary fat to 25% to 30% of total calories, and moderate total calorie restriction (250 to 500 kcal per day reduction). In contrast, most patients who undertake a very low calorie diet eventually regain weight lost initially.[198]

The diet prescription should be simple and easy for the patient to understand, and should take the patient's food preferences and habits into consideration. Functional limitations affecting the elderly person's ability to eat, shop for food, and prepare meals should be assessed. Family members and others involved in meal preparation should be instructed in dietary recommendations and should be involved in helping the patient to comply. As with younger patients with type 2 diabetes, an intensive team approach to dietary therapy, together with regular exercise as indicated (see later) and active family involvement, is most likely to be successful.

Few data are available to indicate whether the benefits of regular exercise observed in younger patients with type 2 diabetes occur in older patients. Exercise training in some older type 2 diabetic patients may achieve modest improvements in glucose tolerance, although these benefits appear to be transitory if exercise is discontinued.[199] Exercise alone has not been shown to markedly improve glucose levels in patients with diabetes, but it may have significant benefits on cardiovascular function, hypertension, and lipid levels. Accordingly, recommending an exercise program for many older diabetic patients, with specific precautions, seems reasonable. Diabetic patients are at increased risk for silent myocardial ischemia, and those with proliferative retinopathy are susceptible to retinal detachments and vitreous hemorrhage; therefore, an exercise treadmill test and a careful retinal examination are advisable before an exercise program is initiated. Exercise should be aerobic and should be undertaken gradually under close supervision. Proper foot care, adequate glucose control before initiation of an exercise program, and avoidance of hypoglycemia are also essential.

## USE OF ORAL HYPOGLYCEMIC AGENTS

Oral agents are usually the next step in the treatment of type 2 diabetes that is not well controlled by diet and exercise, as in younger patients. Oral agents are particularly useful in treating obese or normal-weight elderly patients with visual problems, arthritis, or memory deficits, in whom insulin administration may be problematic. Sulfonylureas are traditionally the oral agents of first choice, although data from a long-term randomized, controlled trial of glucose-lowering agents in patients with type 2 diabetes suggested that metformin may be superior to other available agents in decreasing the incidence of diabetes-related complications in obese patients.[200] Advantages of using the sulfonylureas in older diabetic patients include their efficacy in lowering glucose levels, the simplicity of dosing regimens, long experience with these agents, and their relative safety. Underweight older diabetic patients often do not respond to sulfonylureas because they are relatively insulin deficient. Some elderly people are very sensitive to the hypoglycemic effects of these medications, however. Therefore, treatment of patients with mild to moderate hyperglycemia should begin with very low dosages (e.g., glipizide, 2.5–5.0 mg, or glyburide, 1.25–2.5 mg, each morning), with small incremental increases every 1 to 2 weeks if needed. Elderly diabetic patients with more marked hyperglycemia in the range of 300 to 400 mg/dL are unlikely to be adequately controlled with sulfonylurea therapy and may be better managed with insulin therapy.

Elderly people are at higher risk than younger patients for prolonged hypoglycemia due to the use of oral sulfonylureas.[201] Chlorpropamide is not recommended for use in the elderly due to its very long half-life, which may increase the risk of prolonged hypoglycemia. In addition, chlorpropamide also may cause hyponatremia due to inappropriate ADH secretion. Second-generation sulfonylureas (glipizide, glyburide) are preferable because they are nonionically bound to albumin in the circulation. As a result, these agents are not displaced from albumin by other anionic drugs such as warfarin and salicylates, and drug interactions are less likely to occur. Either of these agents is acceptable for initial use in most older patients with type 2 diabetes, and the reported incidence of hypoglycemia is similar in patients taking glyburide and in those taking glipizide.[202] In general, oral hypoglycemic agents should not be prescribed for patients with severe renal or hepatic failure, which may lead to drug accumulation and toxicity.

Several nonsulfonylurea oral hypoglycemic agents are now available. Metformin, a biguanide, is thought to act primarily by suppressing hepatic glucose production. In a 10-year, randomized, controlled trial comparing metformin treatment with sulfonylurea and insulin therapy in obese middle-aged patients with type 2 diabetes, metformin-treated subjects experienced fewer diabetes-related complications and lower overall mortality, as well as less weight gain and fewer hypoglycemic episodes, than did the other treatment groups.[200] Gastrointestinal discomfort is relatively common with metformin, although the appetite reduction and mild weight loss associated with its use may be potentially beneficial in some obese elderly patients. Severe lactic acidosis has been reported with metformin; therefore, the drug should be avoided in patients at risk for decreased tissue perfusion, for example, those with acute illnesses or congestive heart failure. Hepatic and renal insufficiency are other contraindications to its use.

Other available oral hypoglycemic agents include acarbose, an α-glucosidase inhibitor, and troglitazone, a thiazolidinedione. Acarbose inhibits the breakdown of ingested carbohydrates in the gastrointestinal tract, thus preventing their absorption. Diarrhea is a common side effect and potentially may be therapeutic in older people with constipation. Little information is available, however, regarding the tolerability and effectiveness of this agent in the older diabetic patient. Troglitazone, now off the market, acts by increasing insulin sensitivity. It had generally been well tolerated in clinical trials that had included older patients, but its disadvantages included its expense and the occurrence of severe hepatotoxicity and death in rare instances.[182] Monitoring of liver enzymes is mandatory for patients receiving drugs in this class, and they should not be used in patients with coexisting liver disease. Repaglinide is a nonsulfonylurea insulin secretagogue developed for the management of type 2 diabetes; available data suggest that the risk of hypoglycemic episodes may be lower with repaglinide than with sulfonylurea drugs such as glyburide.[203] However, its role in the treatment of elderly patients with type 2 diabetes has not been determined.

## INSULIN USE

Insulin is indicated for older insulinopenic patients and for patients with type 2 diabetes whose blood glucose cannot be adequately controlled with diet, exercise, and oral hypoglycemic agents. In these patients, the best approach is to begin with a low insulin dosage and to increase slowly as needed, while ensuring that the patient is never hypoglycemic. As with younger patients receiving insulin, prerequisites for safe insulin therapy include accurate home blood glucose monitoring and record keeping, and a stable pattern of food intake and activity throughout the day. In older patients who are unable to adjust their food intake regimen, the insulin regimen may have to be adjusted instead. Patients with visual or manual dexterity problems may require devices such as syringe magnifiers or dose gauges to help draw up the correct amount of insulin, or syringes with premeasured insulin doses.[204]

Lispro insulin, an insulin analog that more closely mimics the action of endogenous postprandial insulin release than regular insulin, may be useful in the management of diabetes in some elderly patients (see Chap. 143). Lispro insulin has a rapid onset of action and a short duration of action, and should be given within 15 minutes of meal consumption. It may be especially useful in elderly patients with erratic food intake patterns, because it can also be given immediately after a meal. Lispro insulin is also useful in older diabetic patients with impaired renal function, who are at increased risk of hypoglycemia due to the prolonged duration of action of regular insulin.[204]

In frail elderly patients with complex medical, cognitive, social, or functional problems (see Table 199-9), the insulin regimen should be kept as simple as possible to reduce medication errors and to improve compliance. Many elderly patients requiring insulin can be adequately managed with a single daily dose of intermediate-acting insulin in the morning. The *dawn phenomenon* is markedly reduced or absent in normal elderly people,[205] so for many elderly diabetic patients, giving a single dose in the evening may be inappropriate and could induce prolonged and unrecognized early morning hypoglycemia.

## LIPID LEVELS

In parallel with body weight, average total plasma cholesterol levels increase during early adulthood but level off beyond approximately age 50 in men and age 60 in women. In senescence, cholesterol and triglyceride levels may decline together with body weight, although all of these remain stable in some healthy elderly people. One longitudinal study reported declining HDL and LDL cholesterol levels with aging in healthy older men and women,[206] although women continue to have higher HDL levels, on average, than men of the same age.

HDL cholesterol levels are inversely associated with risk of coronary artery disease in older adults of both sexes,[207,208] whereas a high LDL level appears to be an important risk factor for coronary disease in older women.[209] Unlike in middle-aged adults, however, elevated total cholesterol levels do not strongly predict coronary events in elderly people, causing considerable controversy regarding the benefits of cholesterol screening in the older population. The presence of comorbidity or debilitation and their association with low cholesterol levels appear to account for this reduction in predictive capacity of cholesterol levels for coronary events in older people.[210] Extremes of cholesterol levels are associated with an increased mortality risk, with the lowest mortality risk in those with intermediate cholesterol levels.[211] These findings are consistent with the notion that a low cholesterol level in an older person may be a marker for frailty or serious underlying illnesses. Indeed, low total cholesterol levels are associated with early demise in nursing home residents and hospitalized patients.[212] On the other hand, long-standing or lifelong hypocholesterolemia is associated with a lower risk of cardiovascular disease.[213] Taken together, these observations suggest that judicious use of cholesterol screening may be indicated in more robust older adults.

Lowering of elevated cholesterol levels in middle-aged adults has been shown to reduce morbidity and mortality from CHD in randomized, controlled trials, not only in those with established atherosclerotic disease[214] but also in hypercholesterolemic men without a history of myocardial infarction.[215] Furthermore, lipid-lowering therapy decreased the number of coronary events in middle-aged subjects without hypercholesterolemia,[216] and reduced the coronary event rate in middle-aged subjects with average total cholesterol levels who did not have clinically evident CHD.[217] Taken together, these data indicate an important role for cholesterol screening and lowering in both primary and secondary prevention of CHD events in middle-aged patients.

No trials have been performed in an exclusively elderly population to determine whether cholesterol reduction decreases the occurrence of CHD in these patients. Secondary prevention trials (e.g., Scandinavian Simvastatin Survival Study [4S] and Cholesterol and Recurrent Events [CARE] trials), however, have shown benefits of cholesterol lowering in reducing CHD mortality in the subgroup of older subjects up to 75 years of age.[218,219] Moreover, in a trial of the use of a statin drug for primary prevention of CHD, the subset of older subjects up to 73 years old benefited from a reduction in CHD event rates.[217] Data are not yet available to indicate whether the benefits of cholesterol lowering in primary and secondary CHD prevention apply equally to people older than age 75. Many physicians have been reluctant to treat hypercholesterolemia aggressively in older patients because of concerns about efficacy, cost, side effects, decreasing strength of total cholesterol levels as a relative risk factor for CHD with aging, and the possibility of minimal benefit in patients with limited longevity. Because of the markedly increased prevalence of CHD with aging, however, the attributable risk, or amount of coronary artery disease risk due to hypercholesterolemia, is greater in the elderly population as a whole. Furthermore, lipid-lowering agents are effective in reducing lipid levels in the elderly, and no evidence is found to indicate that such therapy is less effective in preventing CHD-related morbidity and mortality in the elderly. In addition, angiographic studies in younger adults have shown regression of coronary artery plaques with lipid-lowering therapy, indicating the potential to alter the natural history of the atherosclerotic lesion.[220] Finally, stratification of data by age of subject in both primary and secondary prevention trials shows significant reduction in CHD events in both older and middle-aged adults.[215,216,218] Studies of the cost effectiveness of the use of statin drugs to lower cholesterol in those with and without preexisting CHD have yielded varying estimates of the cost of such treatment per year of life saved, but in general their cost effectiveness is greatest in patients with the highest risk of CHD.[221,222] Treatment of all patients without regard to CHD risk would be prohibitively expensive.

Based on these potential benefits, aggressive management of hypercholesterolemia may be appropriate in selected elderly patients, but the decision to treat should be made after carefully weighing individual factors, including overall health, patient motivation, the impact of atherosclerotic disease on quality of life, and the potential risks and benefits of therapy. Given the decreasing association between cholesterol levels and CHD with advancing age, whether or not lipid-lowering agents are helpful for primary prevention of CHD in the elderly is unclear. Lipid-lowering strategies for secondary prevention may be beneficial in patients with established atherosclerotic disease and a good life expectancy, whereas extremely old patients and those with marked functional limitations due to comorbid illnesses such as congestive heart failure, dementia, malignancies, and chronic renal or lung disease are unlikely to derive much benefit from lipid-lowering therapy. In all elderly patients, regardless of whether they are hypercholesterolemic, modification of other CHD risk factors including hypertension, smoking, and diabetes mellitus is the highest therapeutic priority, because treatment of these conditions has clearly been shown to benefit the elderly.[223]

According to the National Cholesterol Education Program guidelines, the approach to treatment initiation and the goals of treatment are similar in elderly and younger adults, and are based on both LDL cholesterol levels and CHD risk status.[214] As for young adults, older patients with one or more risk factors besides age (smoking, family history of CHD, diabetes, hypertension, HDL level of <35 mg/dL), who are good candidates for cholesterol-lowering therapy, should receive dietary intervention for LDL levels of ≥130 mg/dL, and drug treatment for LDL levels of ≥160 mg/dL. The presence of CHD, however, lowers these treatment initiation levels to ≥100 and ≥130 mg/dL, respectively.[214] Although these treatment guidelines have suggested a goal of <130 mg/dL for LDL levels in older patients with CHD risk factors and ≤100 mg/dL for those with established CHD,[214] increasing evidence suggests that HDL cholesterol levels should also be included in risk factor assessments, even in people without CHD.[217]

All of the cholesterol-lowering drugs have potential for significant toxicity in older patients and should be used in the lowest effective dosage. Bile salt resins may cause constipation and bloating, and can interfere with the absorption of many medications, including warfarin, digoxin, L-thyroxine, and antibiotics. Nicotinic acid use has a high incidence of side effects in older patients, including flushing of the skin, worsening of diabetes mellitus, elevation of liver function tests, and dry mouth and eyes. Gastrointestinal side effects and flushing can be minimized by initiating the drug at low dosages (e.g., 100 mg per day) and giving it only with meals. In general, the statin drugs (3-hydroxy-3-methylglutaryl coenzyme A [HMG CoA] reductase inhibitors) are better tolerated by older patients than the other cholesterol-lowering agents. Side effects are dose related and include gastrointestinal upset, elevation of liver function tests, and a severe myopathy syndrome that occurs more often with concomitant use of other lipid-lowering agents (gemfibrozil, nicotinic acid) or other drugs (e.g., erythromycin, cyclosporine).

# REFERENCES

1. Schneider EL. Aging in the third millennium. Science 1999; 283:796.
1a. Evans JG. Aging and medicine. 21st century review. J Intern Med 2000; 247:159.
2. Hazzard WR, Blass JP, Ettinger WH Jr, et al., eds. Principles of geriatric medicine and gerontology, 4th ed. New York: McGraw-Hill, 1999.
3. Minaker KL. What diabetologists should know about elderly patients. Diabetes Care 1990; 13(Suppl 2):34.
4. Kane RL, Ouslander JG, Abrass IB. Essentials of clinical geriatrics, 4th ed. New York: McGraw-Hill, 1999.
5. Fleming KC, Evans JM, Weber DC, Chutka DS. Practical functional assessment of elderly persons: a primary-care approach. Mayo Clin Proc 1995; 70:890.
6. Lachs MS, Feinstein AR, Cooney LM Jr, et al. A simple procedure for general screening for functional disability in elderly patients. Ann Intern Med 1990; 112:699.
7. Rubenstein LZ. Geriatric assessment: an overview of its impacts. Clin Geriatr Med 1987; 3:1.
8. Tenover JS, Matsumoto AM, Clifton DK, Bremner WJ. Age-related alterations in the circadian rhythms of pulsatile luteinizing hormone and testosterone secretion in healthy men. J Gerontol Biol Sci 1988; 43:M163.
9. Tenover JS, Matsumoto AM, Plymate SR, Bremner WJ. The effects of aging in normal men on bioavailable testosterone and luteinizing hormone secretion: response to clomiphene citrate. J Clin Endocrinol Metab 1987; 65:1118.
10. Bergendahl M, Aloi JA, Iranmanesh A, et al. Fasting suppresses pulsatile luteinizing hormone (LH) secretion and enhances orderliness of LH release in young but not older men. J Clin Endocrinol Metab 1998; 83:1967.
11. Vermeulen A, Deslypere JP, Kaufman JM. Influence of antiopioids on luteinizing hormone pulsatility in aging men. J Clin Endocrinol Metab 1989; 68:68.
12. Waltman C, Blackman MR, Chrousos GP, et al. Spontaneous and glucocorticoid-inhibited adrenocorticotropic hormone and cortisol secretion are similar in healthy young and old men. J Clin Endocrinol Metab 1991; 73:495.
13. Winters SJ, Sherins RJ, Troen P. The gonadotropin-suppressive activity of androgen is increased in elderly men. Metabolism 1984; 33:1052.
14. Winters SJ, Atkinson L. Serum LH concentrations in hypogonadal men during transdermal testosterone replacement through scrotal skin: further evidence that aging enhances testosterone negative feedback. Clin Endocrinol 1997; 47:317.
15. Wilkinson CW, Peskind ER, Raskind MA. Decreased hypothalamic-pituitary-adrenal axis sensitivity to cortisol feedback inhibition in human aging. Neuroendocrinology 1997; 65:79.
16. Miller M. Fluid and electrolyte homeostasis in the elderly: physiological changes of aging and clinical consequences. Baillières Clin Endocrinol Metab 1997; 11:367.
17. Helderman JH, Vestal RE, Rowe JW, et al. The response of arginine vasopressin to intravenous ethanol and hypertonic saline in man: the impact of aging. J Gerontol 1978; 33:39.
18. Phillips PA, Rolls BJ, Ledingham JG, et al. Reduced thirst after water deprivation in healthy elderly men. N Engl J Med 1984; 311:753.
19. Shetty KR, Duthie EHJ. Anterior pituitary function and growth hormone use in the elderly. Endocrinol Metab Clin North Am 1995; 24:213.
20. Martin FC, Yeo A-L, Sonksen PH. Growth hormone secretion in the elderly: aging and the somatopause. Baillières Clin Endocrinol Metab 1997; 11:223.
21. Corpas E, Harman SM, Blackman MR. Human growth hormone and human aging. Endocr Rev 1993; 14:20.
22. Chapman IM, Hartman ML, Pezzoli SS, et al. Effect of aging on the sensitivity of growth hormone secretion to insulin-like growth factor-I negative feedback. J Clin Endocrinol Metab 1997; 82:2996.
23. Hartman ML, Pezzoli SS, Hellman PJ, et al. Pulsatile growth hormone secretion in older persons is enhanced by fasting without relationship to sleep stages. J Clin Endocrinol Metab 1996; 81:2694.
24. Growth Hormone Research Society. Consensus guidelines for the diagnosis and treatment of adults with growth hormone deficiency: summary statement of the Growth Hormone Research Society workshop on adult growth hormone deficiency. J Clin Endocrinol Metab 1998; 83:379.
25. Toogood AA, Jones J, O'Neill PA, et al. The diagnosis of severe growth hormone deficiency in elderly patients with hypothalamic-pituitary disease. Clin Endocrinol 1998; 48:569.
26. Rudman D, Rao UMP. The hypothalamic-growth hormone-somatomedin C axis: the effect of aging. In: Morley JE, Korenman SG, eds. Endocrinology and metabolism in the elderly. Cambridge, MA: Blackwell Scientific Publications, 1992:35.
27. Rudman D, Shetty KR. Unanswered questions concerning the treatment of hyposomatotropism and hypogonadism in elderly men. J Am Geriatr Soc 1994; 42:522.
28. Rudman D, Feller AG, Nagraj HS, et al. Effects of human growth hormone in men over 60 years old. N Engl J Med 1990; 323:1.
29. Borst SE, Millard WJ, Lowenthal DT. Growth hormone, exercise, and aging: the future of therapy for the frail elderly. J Am Geriatr Soc 1994; 42:528.
30. Toogood AA, O'Neill PA, Shalet SM. Beyond the somatopause: growth hormone deficiency in adults over the age of 60 years. J Clin Endocrinol Metab 1996; 81:460.
31. Papadakis MA, Grady D, Black D, et al. Growth hormone replacement in healthy older men improves body composition but not functional ability. Ann Intern Med 1996; 124:708.
32. Greenspan SL, Klibanski A, Rowe JW, Elahi D. Age alters pulsatile prolactin release: influence of dopaminergic inhibition. Am J Physiol 1990; 258:E799.
33. Raskind MA, Peskind ER, Wilkinson CW. Hypothalamic-pituitary-adrenal axis regulation and human aging. Ann N Y Acad Sci 1994; 746:327.
34. Seeman TE, Robbins RJ. Aging and hypothalamic-pituitary-adrenal response to challenge in humans. Endocr Rev 1994; 15:233.
35. Mariotti S, Barbesino G, Caturegli P, et al. Complex alteration of thyroid function in healthy centenarians. J Clin Endocrinol Metab 1993; 77:1130.
36. Mariotti S, Franceschi C, Cossarizza A, Pinchera A. The aging thyroid. Endocr Rev 1995; 16:686.
37. Kunitake JM, Pekary AE, Hershman JM. Aging and the hypothalamic-pituitary-thyroid axis. In: Morley JE, Korenman SG, eds. Endocrinology and metabolism in the elderly. Cambridge, MA: Blackwell Scientific Publications, 1992:92.
38. Monzani F, Del Guerra P, Caraccio N, et al. Age-related modifications in the regulation of the hypothalamic-pituitary-thyroid axis. Horm Res 1992; 46:107.
39. Burger HG, Cahir N, Robertson DM, et al. Serum inhibins A and B fall differentially as FSH rises in perimenopausal women. Clin Endocrinol 1998; 48:809.
40. Santoro N, Banwell T, Tortoriello D, et al. Effects of aging and gonadal failure on the hypothalamic-pituitary axis in women. Am J Obstet Gynecol 1998; 178:732.
41. Deslypere JP, Kaufman JM, Vermeulen T, et al. Influence of age on pulsatile luteinizing hormone release and responsiveness of the gonadotrophs to sex hormone feedback in men. J Clin Endocrinol Metab 1987; 64:68.
42. Tenover JS. Male hormonal changes with aging. In: Morley JE, Korenman SG, eds. Endocrinology and metabolism in the elderly. Cambridge, MA: Blackwell Scientific Publications, 1992:243.
43. Sano T, Kovacs KT, Scheithauer BW, Young WFJ. Aging and the human pituitary gland. Mayo Clin Proc 1993; 68:971.
44. Turner HE, Wass JAH. Pituitary tumors in the elderly. Baillières Clin Endocrinol Metab 1997; 11:407.
45. Cohen DL, Bevan JS, Adams CBT. The presentation and management of pituitary tumours in the elderly. Age Ageing 1989; 18:247.
46. Terano T, Seya A, Tamura Y, et al. Characteristics of the pituitary gland in elderly subjects from magnetic resonance images: relationship to pituitary hormone secretion. Clin Endocrinol (Oxf) 1996; 45:273.
47. Brismar K, Efendic S. Pituitary function in the empty sella syndrome. Neuroendocrinology 1981; 32:70.
48. Brzezinski A. Melatonin in humans. N Engl J Med 1997; 336:186.
49. Penev PD, Zee PC. Melatonin: a clinical perspective. Ann Neurol 1997; 42:545.
50. Pierpaoli W, Regelson W, Colman C. The melatonin miracle: nature's age-reversing, disease-fighting, sex-enhancing hormone. New York: Simon & Schuster, 1995.
51. Hornick TR, Kowal J. Clinical epidemiology of endocrine disorders in the elderly. Endocrinol Metab Clin North Am 1997; 26:145.
52. Goichet B, Schlienger JL, Grunenberger F, et al. Thyroid hormone status and nutrient intake in the free living elderly. Eur J Endocrinol 1994; 130:244.
53. Chopra IJ. Euthyroid sick syndrome: is it a misnomer? J Clin Endocrinol Metab 1997; 82:329.
54. Helfand M, Redfern CC. Screening for thyroid disease: an update. Ann Intern Med 1998; 129:144.
55. Drinka PJ, Nolten WE. Prevalence of previously undiagnosed hypothyroidism in residents of a midwestern nursing home. South Med J 1990; 83:1259.
56. Joseph C, Lyles Y. Routine laboratory assessment of nursing home patients. J Am Geriatr Soc 1992; 40:98.
57. Ouslander JG, Osterweil D. Physician evaluation and management of nursing home residents. Ann Intern Med 1994; 121:584.
58. Evans JM, Chutka DS, Fleming KC, et al. Medical care of nursing home residents. Mayo Clin Proc 1995; 70:694.

59. Sawin CT, Geller A, Kaplan MM, et al. Low serum thyrotropin in older persons without hyperthyroidism. Arch Intern Med 1991; 151:165.

60. Mokshagundam S, Barzel US. Thyroid disease in the elderly. J Am Geriatr Soc 1993; 41:1361.

61. Trivalle C, Doucet J, Chassagne P, et al. Differences in the signs and symptoms of hyperthyroidism in older and younger patients. J Am Geriatr Soc 1996; 44:50.

62. Sawin CT, Geller A, Wolf PA, et al. Low serum thyrotropin concentrations as a risk factor for atrial fibrillation in older persons. N Engl J Med 1994; 331:1249.

63. Woeber KA. Subclinical thyroid dysfunction. Arch Intern Med 1997; 157:1065.

64. Bauer DC, Nevitt MC, Ettinger B, Stone K. Low thyrotropin levels are not associated with bone loss in older women: a prospective study. J Clin Endocrinol Metab 1997; 82:2931.

65. Cooper DS. Subclinical thyroid disease: a clinician's perspective. Ann Intern Med 1998; 129:135.

66. Sawin CT, Bigos ST, Land S, Bacharach P. The aging thyroid. Relationship between elevated serum thyrotropin level and thyroid antibodies in elderly patients. Am J Med 1985; 79:591.

67. Griffin JE. Review: hypothyroidism in the elderly. Am J Med Sci 1990; 299:334.

68. Rosenthal MJ, Hunt WC, Garry PJ, Goodwin JS. Thyroid failure in the elderly. Microsomal antibodies as discriminant for therapy. JAMA 1987; 258:209.

69. Mooradian AD. Mechanisms of age-related endocrine alterations, Part I. Drugs Aging 1993; 3:81.

70. Quesada JM, Coopmans W, Ruiz B, et al. Influence of vitamin D on parathyroid function in the elderly. J Clin Endocrinol Metab 1992; 75:494.

71. Heaney RP. Calcium, parathyroid function, bone, and aging. (Editorial). J Clin Endocrinol Metab 1996; 81:1697.

72. Ireland P, Fordtran JS. Effect of dietary calcium and age on jejunal calcium absorption in humans studied by intestinal perfusion. J Clin Invest 1973; 52:2672.

73. Armbrecht HJ. Calcium, vitamin D, and aging. In: Morley JE, Korenman SG, eds. Endocrinology and metabolism in the elderly. Cambridge, MA: Blackwell Scientific Publications, 1992:170.

74. McKane WR, Khosla S, Egan KS, et al. Role of calcium intake in modulating age-related increases in parathyroid function and bone resorption. J Clin Endocrinol Metab 1996; 81:1699.

75. Kochersberger G, Bales C, Lobaugh B, Lyles KW. Calcium supplementation lowers serum parathyroid hormone levels in elderly subjects. J Gerontol Med Sci 1990; 45:M159.

76. Gloth FMI, Gundberg CM, Hollis BW, et al. Vitamin D deficiency in homebound elderly persons. JAMA 1995; 274:1683.

77. Thomas MK, Lloyd-Jones DM, Thadhani RI, et al. Hypovitaminosis D in medical inpatients. N Engl J Med 1998; 338:777.

78. Ooms ME, Roos JC, Bezemer PD, et al. Prevention of bone loss by vitamin D supplementation in elderly women: a randomized double-blind trial. J Clin Endocrinol Metab 1995; 80:1052.

79. Chapuy MC, Arlot ME, Duboeuf F, et al. Vitamin D$_3$ and calcium to prevent hip fractures in the elderly woman. N Engl J Med 1992; 327:1637.

80. National Institutes of Health Consensus Conference. Optimal calcium intake. JAMA 1994; 272:1942.

81. Papapoulos SE. Paget's disease of bone: clinical, pathogenetic and therapeutic aspects. Baillières Clin Endocrinol Metab 1997; 11:117.

82. Ludkowski P, Wilson-McDonald J. Total arthroplasty in Paget's disease of the hip. A clinical review and review of the literature. Clin Orthop 1990; 255:160.

83. Ott SM. Osteoporosis and osteomalacia. In: Hazzard WR, Blass JP, Ettinger WH Jr, et al., eds. Principles of geriatric medicine and gerontology, 4th ed. New York: McGraw-Hill, 1999:1057.

84. Cooney LM. Hip fractures. In: Hazzard WR, Blass JP, Ettinger WH Jr et al., eds. Principles of geriatric medicine and gerontology, 4th ed. New York: McGraw-Hill, 1999:1547.

85. Riggs BL, Melton LJ III. Involutional osteoporosis. N Engl J Med 1986; 314:1676.

86. Riggs BL, Khosla S, Melton LJ III. A unitary model for involutional osteoporosis: estrogen deficiency causes both type I and type II osteoporosis in postmenopausal women and contributes to bone loss in aging men. J Bone Miner Res 1998; 13:763.

87. Tinetti ME. Performance-oriented assessment of mobility problems in elderly patients. J Am Geriatr Soc 1986; 34:119.

88. Kane RL, Ouslander JG, Abrass IB. Instability and falls. In: Kane RL, Ouslander JG, Abrass IB, eds. Essentials of clinical geriatrics, 4th ed. New York: McGraw-Hill, 1999:231.

89. Tinetti ME, Ginter SF. Identifying mobility dysfunctions in elderly patients: standard neuromuscular examination or direct assessment? JAMA 1988; 259:1190.

89a. Nguyen TV, Center JR, Eisman JA. Osteoporosis in elderly men and women: effects of dietary calcium, physical activity, and body mass index. J Bone Mineral Res 2000; 15:322.

90. Eastell R. Treatment of postmenopausal osteoporosis. N Engl J Med 1998; 338:736.

91. Lufkin EG, Wahner HW, O'Fallon WM, et al. Treatment of postmenopausal osteoporosis by transdermal estrogen administration. Ann Intern Med 1992; 117:1.

92. Ettinger B, Grady D. Maximizing the benefit of estrogen therapy for prevention of osteoporosis. Menopause 1994; 1:19.

93. Prelevic GM, Jacobs HS. Menopause and post-menopause. Baillières Clin Endocrinol Metab 1997; 11:311.

94. Watts NB, Harris ST, Genant HK, et al. Intermittent cyclic etidronate treatment of postmenopausal osteoporosis. N Engl J Med 1990; 323:73.

95. Wimalawansa SJ. A four-year randomized controlled trial of hormone replacement and bisphosphonate, alone or in combination, in women with postmenopausal osteoporosis. Am J Med 1998; 104:219.

96. Hosking D, Chilvers CED, Christiansen C, et al. Prevention of bone loss with alendronate in postmenopausal women under 60 years of age. N Engl J Med 1998; 338:485.

97. McClung M, Clemmesen B, Daifotis A, et al. Alendronate prevents postmenopausal bone loss in women without osteoporosis. Ann Intern Med 1998; 128:253.

98. Heaney RP. Bone mass, bone loss, and osteoporosis prophylaxis. (Editorial). Ann Intern Med 1998; 128:313.

99. Delmas PD, Bjarnason NH, Mitlak BH, et al. Effects of raloxifene on bone mineral density, serum cholesterol concentrations, and uterine endometrium in postmenopausal women. N Engl J Med 1997; 337:1641.

100. Khovidhunkit W, Shoback D. Clinical effects of raloxifene hydrochloride in women. Ann Intern Med 1999; 130:431.

101. Lyles KW. Hyperparathyroidism and Paget's disease of bone. In: Hazzard WR, Blass JP, Ettinger WH Jr, et al., eds. Principles of geriatric medicine and gerontology, 4th ed. New York: McGraw-Hill, 1999:1085.

102. Silverberg SJ, Bilezikian JP. Evaluation and management of primary hyperparathyroidism. J Clin Endocrinol Metab 1996; 81:2036.

103. Brickman AS. Primary hyperparathyroidism in the elderly. In: Morley JE, Korenman SG, eds. Endocrinology and metabolism in the elderly. Cambridge, MA: Blackwell Scientific Publications, 1992:215.

104. Barton RN, Horan MA, Weijers JWM, et al. Cortisol production rate and the urinary excretion of 17-hydroxycorticosteroids, free cortisol, and 6-beta-hydroxycortisol in healthy elderly men and women. J Gerontol Med Sci 1993; 48:M213.

105. Friedman M, Green MF, Sharland DG. Assessment of hypothalamic-pituitary-adrenal function in the geriatric age group. J Gerontol 1969; 24:292.

106. Tsagarakis S, Grossman A. The hypothalamic-pituitary-adrenal axis in senescence. In: Morley JE, Korenman SG, eds. Endocrinology and metabolism in the elderly. Cambridge, MA: Blackwell Scientific Publications, 1992:70.

107. Pavlov EP, Harman SM, Chrousos GP, et al. Responses of plasma adrenocorticotrophin, cortisol, and dehydroepiandrosterone to ovine corticotrophin-releasing hormone in healthy aging men. J Clin Endocrinol Metab 1986; 62:767.

108. Blichert-Toft M. Secretion of corticotrophin and somatotrophin by the senescent adenohypophysis in man. Acta Endocrinol (Copenh) 1975; 195(Suppl):11.

109. Stein-Behrens BA, Sapolsky RM. Stress, glucocorticoids and aging. Aging Clin Exp Res 1992; 4:197.

110. Sapolsky RM, Krey LC, McEwen BS. The neuroendocrinology of stress and aging: the glucocorticoid cascade hypothesis. Endocr Rev 1986; 7:284.

111. Gross MD, Shapiro B, Bouffard JA, et al. Distinguishing benign from malignant euadrenal masses. Ann Intern Med 1988; 109:613.

112. Beck LH. Aging changes in renal function. In: Hazzard WR, Blass JP, Ettinger WH Jr, et al., eds. Principles of geriatric medicine and gerontology, 4th ed. New York: McGraw-Hill, 1999:767.

113. Recommendations for the prevention and treatment of glucocorticoid-induced osteoporosis. American College of Rheumatology Task Force on Osteoporosis Guidelines. Arthritis Rheum 1996; 39:1791.

114. Adachi JD, Bensen WG, Brown J, et al. Intermittent etidronate therapy to prevent corticosteroid-induced osteoporosis. N Engl J Med 1997; 337:382.

115. Roux C, Oriente P, Laan R, et al. Randomized trial of effect of cyclical etidronate in the prevention of corticosteroid-induced bone loss. J Clin Endocrinol Metab 1998; 83:1128.

116. Saag KG, Emkey R, Schnitzer TJ, et al. Alendronate for the prevention and treatment of glucocorticoid-induced osteoporosis. N Engl J Med 1998; 339:292.

117. Montemurro L, Schiraldi G, Fraioli P, et al. Prevention of corticosteroid-induced osteoporosis with salmon calcitonin in sarcoid patients. Calcif Tissue Int 1991; 49:71.

118. Mason AS, Meade TW, Lee JA, Morris JN. Epidemiological and clinical picture of Addison's disease. Lancet 1968; 2:7571.

119. Flood C, Gherondache C, Pincus G, et al. The metabolism and secretion of aldosterone in elderly subjects. J Clin Invest 1967; 46:961.

120. Meneilly GS, Greenspan SL, Rowe JW, Minaker KL. Endocrine systems. In: Rowe JW, Besdine RW, eds. Geriatric medicine, 2nd ed. Boston: Little, Brown and Company, 1988:402.

121. Tsunoda K, Abe K, Goto T, et al. Effect of age on the renin-angiotensin-aldosterone system in normal subjects: simultaneous measurement of active and inactive renin, renin substrate and aldosterone in plasma. J Clin Endocrinol Metab 1986; 62:384.

122. Mulkerrin E, Epstein FH, Clark BA. Aldosterone responses to hyperkalemia in healthy elderly humans. J Am Soc Nephrol 1995; 6:1459.

123. Birkenhager-Gillesse EG, Derksen J, Lagaay AM. Dehydroepiandrosterone sulphate (DHEAS) in the oldest old, aged 85 and over. Ann N Y Acad Sci 1994; 719:543.

124. Orentreich N, Brind JL, Vogelman JH, et al. Long-term longitudinal measurements of plasma dehydroepiandrosterone sulfate in normal men. J Clin Endocrinol Metab 1992; 75:1002.

125. Baulieu E-E. Dehydroepiandrosterone (DHEA): a fountain of youth? (Editorial). J Clin Endocrinol Metab 1996; 81:3147.

126. Barrett-Connor E, Khaw KT, Yen SSC. A prospective study of dehydroepiandrosterone sulfate, mortality, and cardiovascular disease. N Engl J Med 1986; 315:1519.

127. Barrett-Connor E, Edelstein S. A prospective study of dehydroepiandrosterone sulfate and cognitive function in an older population: the Rancho Bernardo study. J Am Geriatr Soc 1994; 42:520.

128. Berkman LF, Seeman TE, Albert M, et al. High, usual and impaired functioning in community-dwelling older men and women: findings from the MacArthur Foundation research network on successful aging. J Clin Epidemiol 1993; 46:1129.

129. Yen SSC, Morales AJ, Khorram O. Replacement of DHEA in aging men and women: potential remedial effects. Ann N Y Acad Sci 1995; 774:128.

130. Milewich L, Catalina F, Bennett M. Pleotropic effects of dietary DHEA. Ann N Y Acad Sci 1995; 774:149.

131. Casson PR, Carson SA, Buster JE. Replacement dehydroepiandrosterone in the elderly: rationale and prospects for the future. Endocrinologist 1998; 8:187.

132. Veith RC, Featherstone JA, Linares OA, Halter JB. Age differences in plasma norepinephrine kinetics in humans. J Gerontol 1986; 41:319.

133. Sowers JR, Rubenstein LZ, Stern N. Plasma norepinephrine responses to posture and isometric exercise increase with age in the absence of obesity. J Gerontol 1983; 38:315.

134. Supiano MA, Halter JB. The aging sympathetic nervous system. In: Morley JE, Korenman SG, eds. Endocrinology and metabolism in the elderly. Cambridge, MA: Blackwell Scientific Publications, 1992:465.

135. Mooradian AD, Morley JE, Korenman SG. Endocrinology in aging. Dis Mon 1988; 34:398.

136. Jansen RW, Lipsitz LA. Postprandial hypotension: epidemiology, pathophysiology, and clinical management. Ann Intern Med 1995; 122:286.

137. Jansen RW, Connelly CM, Kelley-Gagnon MM, et al. Postprandial hypotension in elderly patients with unexplained syncope. Arch Intern Med 1995; 155:945.

138. Urban RJ. Neuroendocrinology of aging in the male and female. Endocrinol Metab Clin North Am 1992; 21:921.

139. Kronenberg F. Hot flashes: epidemiology and physiology. Ann N Y Acad Sci 1990; 592:52.

140. Noblett KL, Ostergard DR. Gynecologic disorders. In: Hazzard WR, Blass JP, Ettinger WH Jr, et al., eds. Principles of geriatric medicine and gerontology, 4th ed. New York: McGraw-Hill, 1999:797.

141. Pearce KF. Health care issues of older women. In: Hazzard WR, Blass JP, Ettinger WH Jr, et al., eds. Principles of geriatric medicine and gerontology, 4th ed. New York: McGraw-Hill, 1999:345.

142. Sullivan JM, Vander Zwaag R, Hughes JP, et al. Estrogen replacement and coronary artery disease: effect on survival in postmenopausal women. Arch Intern Med 1990; 150:2557.

143. Gruchow HW, Anderson AJ, Barboriak JJ, Sobocinski KA. Postmenopausal use of estrogen and occlusion of the coronary arteries. Am Heart J 1988; 115:954.

144. Hulley S, Grady D, Bush T, et al. Randomized trial of estrogen plus progestin for secondary prevention of coronary heart disease in postmenopausal women. JAMA 1998; 280:605.

145. Wren BG. Megatrials of hormonal replacement therapy. Drugs Aging 1998; 12:343.

146. Grodstein F, Stampfer MJ, Colditz GA, et al. Postmenopausal hormone therapy and mortality. N Engl J Med 1997; 336:1769.

147. Paganini-Hill A, Henderson VW. Estrogen deficiency increases the risk of Alzheimer's disease in women. Am J Epidemiol 1994; 140:256.

148. Henderson V, Paganini-Hill A, Emanuel C, et al. Estrogen replacement therapy in older women. Comparisons between Alzheimer's disease cases and nondemented control subjects. Arch Neurol 1994; 51:896.

149. Fillit H, Weinreb H, Cholst I, et al. Observations in a preliminary open trial of estradiol therapy for senile dementia-Alzheimer's type. Psychoneuroendocrinology 1986; 11:337.

150. Honjo H, Ogino Y, Naitoh K, et al. In vivo effects by estrone sulfate on the central nervous system—senile dementia (Alzheimer's type). J Steroid Biochem 1989; 34:521.

151. Asthana S, Craft S, Baker LD, et al. Cognitive and neuroendocrine response to transdermal estrogen in postmenopausal women with Alzheimer's disease: results of a placebo-controlled, double-blind, pilot study. Psychoneuroendocrinology 1999; 24(6):657.

152. Fisher B, Costantino JP, Wickerham DL, et al. Tamoxifen for prevention of breast cancer: report of the National Surgical Adjuvant Breast and Bowel Project P-1 Study. J Natl Cancer Inst 1998; 90:1371.

153. Swerdloff RS, Wang C. Androgen deficiency and aging in men. West J Med 1993; 159:579.

153a. Longcope C, Feldman HA, McKinlay JB, Araujo AB. Diet and sex hormone–binding globulin. J Clin Endocrinol Metab 2000; 85:293.

154. Rudman D, Mattson DE, Nagraj HS, et al. Plasma testosterone in nursing home men. J Clin Epidemiol 1988; 41:231.

155. Tenover JS. Effects of testosterone supplementation in the aging male. J Clin Endocrinol Metab 1992; 75:1092.

156. Morley JE, Perry HM III, Kaiser FE, et al. Effects of testosterone replacement therapy in old hypogonadal males: a preliminary study. J Am Geriatr Soc 1993; 41:149.

157. Sih R, Morley JE, Kaiser FE, et al. Testosterone replacement in older hypogonadal men: a 12-month randomized controlled trial. J Clin Endocrinol Metab 1997; 82:1661.

158. Marin P, Holmang S, Jonsson L, et al. The effects of testosterone treatment on body composition and metabolism in middle-aged obese men. Int J Obes Relat Metab Disord 1992; 16:991.

159. Bhasin S, Bagatell CJ, Bremner WJ, et al. Issues in testosterone replacement in older men. J Clin Endocrinol Metab 1998; 83:3435.

160. Pfeiffer E, Verwoerdt A, Wang HS. Sexual behavior in aged men and women. Arch Gen Psychiatry 1968; 19:753.

161. Schiavi RC, Schreiner-Engel P, Mandeli J, et al. Healthy aging and male sexual function. Am J Psychiatr 1990; 147:766.

162. Kinsey AC, Pomeroy WD, Martin CE. Sexual behavior in the human male. Philadelphia: WB Saunders, 1948.

163. Kaiser FE. Impotence in the elderly. In: Morley JE, Korenman SG, eds. Endocrinology and metabolism in the elderly. Cambridge, MA: Blackwell Scientific Publications, 1992:262.

164. Morley JE. Impotence. Am J Med 1986; 80:897.

165. Van Itallie TB. Health implications of overweight and obesity in the United States. Ann Intern Med 1985; 103:983.

166. Forbes GB, Reina JC. Adult lean body mass declines with age: some longitudinal observations. Metabolism 1970; 19:653.

167. Shimokata H, Tobin JD, Muller DC, et al. Studies in the distribution of body fat: I. Effects of age, sex, and obesity. J Gerontol Med Sci 1989; 44:M66.

168. Novak LP. Aging, total body potassium, fat-free mass, and cell mass in males and females between ages 18 and 85 years. J Gerontol 1972; 27:438.

169. Lee I, Manson JE, Hennekens CH, Paffenbarger RS Jr. Body weight and mortality: a 27-year follow-up of middle-aged men. JAMA 1993; 270:2823.

170. Launer LJ, Harris T, Rumpel C, Madans J. Body mass index, weight change, and risk of mobility disability in middle-aged and older women: the epidemiologic follow-up study of NHANES I. JAMA 1994; 271:1093.

171. Katzel LI, Bleecker ER, Colman EG, et al. Effects of weight loss vs aerobic exercise training on risk factors for coronary disease in healthy, obese, middle-aged and older men: a randomized controlled trial. JAMA 1995; 274:1915.

172. Harris T. Weight and age: paradoxes and conundrums. In: Hazzard WR, Blass JP, Ettinger WH Jr, et al., eds. Principles of geriatric medicine and gerontology, 4th ed. New York: McGraw-Hill, 1999:967.

173. Ortega RM, Andres P. Is obesity worth treating in the elderly? Drugs Aging 1998; 12:97.

174. Dvorak R, Starling RD, Calles-Escandon J, et al. Drug therapy for obesity in the elderly. Drugs Aging 1997; 11:338.

175. Shimokata H, Muller DC, Fleg JL, et al. Age as independent determinant of glucose tolerance. Diabetes 1991; 40:44.

176. Harris MI, Flegal KM, Cowie CC, et al. Prevalence of diabetes, impaired fasting glucose, and impaired glucose tolerance in U.S. adults. The Third National Health and Nutrition Examination Survey, 1988-1994. Diabetes Care 1998; 21:518.

177. Pacini G, Valerio A, Beccaro F, et al. Insulin sensitivity and beta-cell responsivity are not decreased in elderly subjects with normal OGTT. J Am Geriatr Soc 1988; 36:317.

178. Chen M, Halter JB, Porte DJ. The role of dietary carbohydrate in the decreased glucose tolerance of the elderly. J Am Geriatr Soc 1987; 35:417.

179. Tonino RP. Effect of physical training on the insulin resistance of aging. Am J Physiol 1989; 256:E352.

180. Kahn SE, Larson VG, Beard JC, et al. Effect of exercise on insulin action, glucose tolerance and insulin secretion in aging. Am J Physiol 1990; 258:E937.

181. Nathan DM, Singer DE, Godine JE, Perlmuter LC. Non-insulin-dependent diabetes in older patients. Complications and risk factors. Am J Med 1986; 81:837.

182. Halter JB. Diabetes mellitus. In: Hazzard WR, Blass JP, Ettinger WH Jr, et al., eds. Principles of geriatric medicine and gerontology, 4th ed. New York: McGraw-Hill, 1999:991.

183. Podgor MJ, Leske MC, Ederer F. Incidence estimates for lens changes, macular changes, open-angle glaucoma and diabetic retinopathy. Am J Epidemiol 1983; 118:206.

184. Naliboff BD, Rosenthal M. Effects of age on complications in adult onset diabetes. J Am Geriatr Soc 1989; 37:838.

185. Morisaki N, Watanabe S, Kobayashi J, et al. Diabetic control and progression of retinopathy in elderly patients: five-year follow-up study. J Am Geriatr Soc 1994; 42:142.

186. Scheen AJ. Non-insulin-dependent diabetes mellitus in the elderly. Baillières Clin Endocrinol Metab 1997; 11:389.

187. Gradman TJ, Laws A, Thompson LW, Reaven GM. Verbal learning and/or memory improves with glycemic control in older subjects with non-insulin-dependent diabetes mellitus. J Am Geriatr Soc 1993; 41:1305.

188. American Diabetes Association. Clinical practice recommendation 1998. Diabetes Care 1998; 21(Suppl 1):S1.

189. The Expert Committee on the Diagnosis and Classification of Diabetes Mellitus. Report of the Expert Committee on the Diagnosis and Classification of Diabetes Mellitus. Diabetes Care 1997; 20:1183.

190. Scheitel SM, Fleming KC, Chutka DS, Evans JM. Symposium on geriatrics, Part IX: geriatrics health maintenance. Mayo Clin Proc 1996; 71:289.

191. Diabetes Control and Complications Trial Research Group. The effect of intensive treatment of diabetes on the development and progression of long-term complications in insulin-dependent diabetes mellitus. N Engl J Med 1993; 329:977.

192. Skyler JS. Diabetic complications: the importance of glucose control. Endocrinol Metab Clin North Am 1996; 25:243.

193. Klein R. Hyperglycemia and microvascular and macrovascular disease in diabetes. Diabetes Care 1995; 18:258.

194. Ohkubo Y, Kishikawa H, Araki E, et al. Intensive insulin therapy prevents the progression of diabetic microvascular complications in Japanese patients with non-insulin-dependent diabetes mellitus: a randomized prospective 6-year study. Diabetes Res Clin Pract 1995; 28:103.

195. United Kingdom Prospective Diabetes Study Group. Intensive blood-glucose control with sulphonylureas or insulin compared with conventional treatment and risk of complications in patients with type 2 diabetes (UKPDS 33). Lancet 1998; 352:837.

196. Kesson CM, Bailie GR. Do diabetic patients inject accurate doses of insulin? Diabetes Care 1981; 4:333.

197. Funnell MM. Role of the diabetes educator for older adults. Diabetes Care 1990; 13(Suppl 2):60.

198. Franz MJ, Horton ES Sr, Bantle JP, et al. Nutrition principles for the management of diabetes and related complications. Diabetes Care 1994; 17:490.

199. Schwartz RS, Buchner DM. Exercise in the elderly: physiologic and functional effects. In: Hazzard WR, Blass JP, Ettinger WH Jr, et al., eds. Principles of geriatric medicine and gerontology, 4th ed. New York: McGraw-Hill, 1999:143.

200. UK Prospective Diabetes Study Group. Effect of intensive blood-glucose control with metformin on complications in overweight patients with type 2 diabetes (UKPDS 34). Lancet 1998; 352:854.

201. Asplund K, Wiholm BF, Lithner F. Glibenclamide-associated hypoglycemia: a report of 57 cases. Diabetologia 1983; 24:412.

202. Feldman JM. Review of glyburide after one year on the market. Am J Med 1985; 79(Suppl 3B):102.

203. Balfour JA, Faulds D. Repaglinide. Drugs Aging 1998; 13:173.

204. Benbarka MM, Prescott PT, Aoki TT. Practical guidelines on the use of insulin lispro in elderly diabetic patients. Drugs Aging 1998; 12:103.

205. Meneilly GS, Elahi D, Minaker KL, Rowe JW. The dawn phenomenon does not occur in normal elderly subjects. J Clin Endocrinol Metab 1986; 63:292.

206. Garry PJ, Hunt WC, Koehler KM, et al. Longitudinal study of dietary intakes and plasma lipids in healthy elderly men and women. Am J Clin Nutr 1992; 55:682.

207. Castelli WP, Garrison RJ, Wilson PW, et al. Incidence of coronary heart disease and lipoprotein cholesterol levels. The Framingham Study. JAMA 1986; 256:2835.

208. Corti M-C, Guralnik JM, Salive ME, et al. HDL cholesterol predicts coronary heart disease mortality in older persons. JAMA 1995; 274:539.

209. Zimetbaum P, Frishman WH, Ooi WL, et al. Plasma lipids and lipoproteins and the incidence of cardiovascular disease in the very elderly. Arterioscler Thromb 1992; 12:416.

210. Corti M-C, Guralnik JM, Salive ME, et al. Clarifying the direct relation between total cholesterol levels and death from coronary heart disease in older persons. Ann Intern Med 1997; 126:753.

211. Jacobs D, Blackburn H, Higgins M, et al. Report of the conference on low blood cholesterol: mortality associations. Circulation 1992; 86:1046.

212. Rudman D, Mattson DE, Nagraj HS, et al. Antecedents of death in the men of a Veterans Administration nursing home. J Am Geriatr Soc 1987; 35:496.

213. Hazzard WR. Dyslipoproteinemia. In: Morley JE, Korenman SG, eds. Endocrinology and metabolism in the elderly. Cambridge, MA: Blackwell Scientific Publications, 1992:406.

214. National Cholesterol Education Program Expert Panel. Summary of the second report of the National Cholesterol Education Program (NCEP) Expert Panel on Detection, Evaluation, and Treatment of High Blood Cholesterol in Adults (Adult Treatment Panel II). JAMA 1993; 269:3015.

215. Shepherd J, Cobbe SM, Ford I, et al. Prevention of coronary heart disease with pravastatin in men with hypercholesterolemia. N Engl J Med 1995; 333:1301.

216. Sacks FM, Pfeffer MA, Moye LA, et al. The effect of pravastatin on coronary events after myocardial infarction in patients with average cholesterol levels. N Engl J Med 1996; 335:1001.

217. Downs J, Clearfield M, Weis S, et al. Primary prevention of acute coronary events with lovastatin in men and women with average cholesterol levels: results of AFCAPS/TexCAPS. Air Force/Texas Coronary Atherosclerosis Prevention Study. JAMA 1998; 279:1615.

218. The Scandinavian Simvastatin Survival Study Group. Randomised trial of cholesterol lowering in 4444 patients with coronary heart disease: the Scandinavian Simvastatin Survival Study (4S). Lancet 1994; 344:1383.

219. Lewis SJ, Moye LA, Sacks FM, et al. Effect of pravastatin on cardiovascular events in older patients with myocardial infarction and cholesterol levels in the average range: results of the Cholesterol and Recurrent Events (CARE) trial. Ann Intern Med 1998; 129:681.

220. Blankenhorn DH, Azen SP, Kramsch DM, et al. Coronary angiographic changes with lovastatin therapy: the monitored atherosclerosis regression study (MARS). Ann Intern Med 1993; 119:969.

221. Johannesson M, Jonsson B, Kjekshus J, et al. Cost effectiveness of simvastatin treatment to lower cholesterol levels in patients with coronary heart disease. N Engl J Med 1997; 336:332.

222. Pharoah PD, Hollingworth W. Cost effectiveness of lowering cholesterol concentration with statins in patients with and without pre-existing coronary heart disease: life table method applied to health authority population. BMJ 1996; 312:1443.

223. Denke MA, Grundy SM. Hypercholesterolemia in elderly persons: resolving the treatment dilemma. Ann Intern Med 1990; 112:780.

# PART XIV

# INTERRELATIONSHIPS BETWEEN HORMONES AND THE BODY

KENNETH L. BECKER, EDITOR

# CHAPTER 200

# CEREBRAL EFFECTS OF ENDOCRINE DISEASE

HOYLE LEIGH

Hormones affect all organs of the body, and the brain is no exception (see Chap. 176). For example, even in utero, testosterone determines the formation of the "male brain," characterized by an absence of hypothalamic gonadotropic cyclicity; this early hormonal influence is associated with long-term behavioral effects. As many chapters of this textbook demonstrate, normal cerebral development and function are dependent on a normal hormonal milieu. Not surprisingly, many endocrine abnormalities can cause effects on the brain that are manifested by disorders in behavior, mood, and cognitive functions—symptoms that usually are attributed to psychiatric disorders.[1,2] In a study of 658 consecutively evaluated outpatients who had psychiatric syndromes, 9.1% had a medical disorder that explained their psychiatric complaints, and 46% had a previously undiagnosed medical illness.[3,4] In this study, 21 patients had an endocrine disorder; their average age was 37 years.

In a parallel study of 100 psychiatric inpatients, endocrine disorders were found in 17% of the 80 patients who had diagnosed physical illnesses. The endocrine dysfunction was responsible for more than one-third of all medical disorders that caused the psychiatric symptoms. Most patients were unaware that their psychiatric difficulties were because of medical illness, and their physicians had difficulty distinguishing the physical disorders that were associated with the psychiatric syndromes from "purely" psychiatric disorders given the psychiatric symptoms alone. Clearly, endocrine dysfunction must be ruled out before the diagnosis of a "functional" disorder is made in any patient who manifests psychiatric symptomatology.

*Cerebral cortical dysfunction* usually is manifested by *cognitive difficulties* (i.e., disturbances with orientation, memory, abstraction, and judgment). *Limbic system dysfunction* is manifested by problems with emotions (e.g., depression, mania, anxiety, and anhedonia [absence of pleasure from otherwise pleasurable acts]), as well as difficulties with instinctual behaviors such as appetite, sex, and aggression. Endocrine diseases often cause effects in many parts of the brain, so that one commonly sees complex psychiatric syndromes, such as *psychosis* (which includes disturbances of thought processes—a cortical function—as well as disturbances in emotions, such as flat affect or anxiety) and *depressive syndrome* (which includes depressive affect as well as anhedonia, suicidal ideations, and "vegetative" changes such as loss of appetite and sleep disturbance). *Anxiety* is one of the most common presenting symptoms of an endocrine dysfunction; endocrinopathy accounts for 25% of anxiety disorders in which a specific medical cause is found.[5] Table 200-1 lists descriptions of psychiatric syndromes.

## HYPOTHALAMIC DISORDERS

Lesions of the hypothalamus may cause bulimia (see Chap. 128), hypersomnia, anorexia, or impotence (see Chaps. 8 and 9). The associated autonomic dysfunction may mimic or actually produce an anxiety attack. Hypothalamic disorders often cause cerebral effects indirectly through their effects on the pituitary gland (see Chaps. 17 and 18). Drowsiness, confusion, irritability, hyperphagia, and depression are common psychiatric symptoms of hypothalamic disorders.[6]

**TABLE 200-1.**
**Psychiatric Syndromes Commonly Seen in Endocrinopathies**

**Organic brain syndrome:** Cerebral state characterized by global cognitive impairment because of a physical cause (e.g., delirium and dementia).

**Delirium:** Clouded state of consciousness having acute onset and fluctuating course. There is shifting, and difficulty in focusing and in sustaining attention. Perceptual disturbances such as illusions, hallucinations (especially visual and tactile types), and misinterpretations are common. Sleep–wakefulness cycle is often disturbed, leading to hypervigilance and difficulty in falling asleep. The patient exhibits somnolence or agitation, or alternates between the two states of motor activity. Key features of delirium are memory impairment (especially recent memory) and disorientation to time, place, and, infrequently, person. Confusion may be more severe in the evening.

**Dementia:** Loss of previously acquired intellectual abilities to the extent of social or occupational impairment. Persistent personality changes may accompany the disturbances in memory, abstract thinking, and other higher cortical functions. Level of consciousness does not fluctuate in dementia.

**Psychosis:** Syndrome characterized by disturbances in thought content and process, and by perceptual aberrations. Delusions, ideas of reference, and paranoid ideation are common. Thought processes may be incoherent, leading to looseness of association, poverty of content, and bizarre use of language. Hallucinations and illusions—especially visual, olfactory, or gustatory—are common in psychoses caused by endocrinopathies. Although the sensorium is usually clear in *functional* psychoses such as schizophrenia, features of delirium or dementia often coexist in endocrinopathic psychoses.

**Depression:** In a psychiatric context, denotes a syndrome characterized by affective, cognitive, and neurovegetative symptoms and signs. Whereas dysphoria is characteristic of depression, apathy and anhedonia are not infrequent. Feelings of hopelessness and helplessness, and suicidal thoughts, are common. There often is a decreased ability to concentrate and indecisiveness (pseudodementia of depression). Neurovegetative symptoms include insomnia (particularly, early morning awakening), hypersomnia, appetite changes (decrease or increase), and loss of libido. Psychomotor retardation or agitation may occur.

**The manic syndrome:** A state of elated, expansive, or irritable mood, with marked distractibility and flight of ideas. Self-esteem is often inflated, and patients involve themselves in activities with a high potential for self-harm without consideration of consequences. Hyperactivity, pressured speech, and a decreased need for sleep are common.

**Anxiety:** A common cerebral effect of endocrine disorders. The features include motor tension, inability to relax, autonomic hyperactivity with sweating, tachycardia, cold moist hands, dry mouth, lightheadedness, paresthesias, and often gastrointestinal or genitourinary complaints. Endocrine disorders account for approximately one-fourth of anxiety disorders in which a specific medical diagnosis is found.

## THE PITUITARY GLAND

In acromegaly, drowsiness, lethargy, and diminished libido have been reported. Personality change—decreased initiative, lack of spontaneity, and mood changes—may be prominent.

In hypopituitarism, there is typically a slow onset of a combination dementia-delirium, which sometimes is present up to 2 years before coming to medical attention.[7] The mental symptoms—commonly, confusion, disorientation, and drowsiness—may be the dominant features. Lethargy, anergy (asthenia), and depression may ensue. Psychosis and paranoid symptoms also may occur. There may be a personality change with brief episodes of irritability, argumentativeness, and a lack of initiative. When the onset of the hypopituitarism is rapid, however, the symptoms may be dramatic: lethargy rapidly progressing to stupor. In reversing the organic brain syndrome of hypopituitarism, both thyroid and corticosteroid replacement therapy are necessary.[8]

## THE THYROID GLAND

The mechanism whereby thyroid dysfunction affects the central nervous system (CNS) is probably related to changes in CNS receptor sensitivity to neurotransmitters and to changes of cellular metabolism. In hyperthyroidism, there may be an increase in the sensitivity of receptors to catecholamines, a decrease in the monoamine oxidase activity levels, and an increase in norepinephrine turnover rates. In hypothyroidism, there is depressed oxygen and glucose utilization by the CNS, decreased cerebral blood flow, and increased cerebrovascular resistance. Neurotransmitter receptors are also desensitized to the effects of catecholamines.

## HYPERTHYROIDISM

Some degree of thyrotoxic encephalopathy has been observed in 20% to 40% of cases of hyperthyroidism, but severe cognitive disorders are uncommon, except in the elderly. Decreased ability to concentrate and deficits in recent memory are common symptoms of the organic brain syndrome in hyperthyroidism. Also, in some patients antithyroid drugs may contribute to an organic brain syndrome.

Hyperthyroidism probably exacerbates preexisting thought disorder and prepsychotic personality traits. Symptoms of frank psychosis may occur in up to one-fifth of hyperthyroid patients.[8a,8b] The symptoms may be schizophreniform, with prominent paranoid symptoms, or they may manifest as manic psychoses with grandiose delusions, agitation, and irritability. Visual and auditory hallucinations may occur. Marked delirious states may signal impending thyroid storm in up to 5% of patients with this severe condition.[9]

Depression, along with anxiety and psychomotor agitation or retardation, may be the first symptoms of hyperthyroidism.[10] Chronic fatigue is an early symptom. Severe depression may precede the obvious clinical onset of thyrotoxicosis; it is one of the most outstanding psychiatric features of the illness and may continue after thyrotoxicosis subsides. In some elderly patients, particularly those with long-lasting thyroid illness, the depressive syndrome may be characterized by apathy and lethargy (*apathetic hyperthyroidism*),[11,12] accompanied by weight loss and tachycardia, with or without the presence of high-output congestive heart failure.[9,13] Antidepressant therapy usually is ineffective. The syndrome resolves with appropriate treatment of the thyrotoxicosis.

Anxiety, along with hyperactivity, nervousness, and motor tension with tremor, is observed in nearly half of hyperthyroid patients. Emotional lability and overreactivity are hallmarks of early hyperthyroidism. Diminished hearing, paresthesias, weakness, and at times bizarre neurologic symptoms may seem hysterical. Marital problems are common. Criminal behavior has been reported. Panic attacks and agoraphobia may occur.[14]

Most psychiatric symptoms of thyrotoxicosis are reversible with appropriate treatment of the underlying disease, but the manic or depressive syndrome may persist for considerable periods after a euthyroid state has been established.

## HYPOTHYROIDISM

Nearly every known type of psychiatric syndrome occurs in hypothyroidism. Psychiatric symptoms often precede a physically recognizable myxedematous state. Organic brain syndrome occurs in approximately one-third of these patients, impaired cognition occurs in more than 90%, and impaired recent memory is common. Delirium is unusual except in very rapid-onset cases (e.g., postthyroidectomy or antithyroid drug-induced hypothyroidism). A slow-onset dementia of long duration that has various degrees of reversibility is typical.[15–18] In elderly patients with concomitant cerebrovascular disorder, psychotic organic brain syndrome is common. There appears to be no consistent relationship between the severity of the physical symptoms and the severity of the psychiatric disorder.

Permanent intellectual and morphologic deficits occur if cretinism is not treated within the first year of life. In juvenile hypothyroidism, the mental disorder may appear 1 to 2 years after obvious somatic signs arise. Older children and adults show impaired recent memory; labored, slow mentation; and poor concentration. The "witzelsucht" or facetious humor of frontal lobe disorders also can be seen. There may be slowing and decreased amplitude on electroencephalography, and seizures may be present in severe cases.

Psychosis has been reported in more than 40% of hypothyroid patients. The psychosis is often rapid in onset, but it may be insidious in some patients. There are no specific symptoms for myxedema psychosis; however, depression, paranoid delusions, and vivid hallucinations are common. Thyroid replacement usually helps and leads to reversal of the symptoms within several weeks. The duration of hypothyroidism does not seem to be correlated with the response to treatment. Older patients seem to respond more rapidly to treatment. The psychosis may be irreversible if treatment is delayed.

Depression appears to be a concomitant of all grades of hypothyroidism, from the subclinical to the overt. It is marked in nearly half of myxedema patients. The incidence may be greater for those who have a first-degree relative who has a history of depression; suicidal and paranoid ideations often accompany this depression. The patients appear to be lethargic and have diminished mental effort and sexual interest. Patients may eventually become indifferent to their delayed cognitive processes. Typically, the depression does not respond to antidepressant medication and may also be resistant to thyroid replacement, requiring electroconvulsive therapy.[18] On the other hand, patients who have had depression for years may respond within a few days after the initiation of replacement therapy. No significant correlation between the severity of depression and the severity of myxedema has been observed.

In one study, nearly 10% of 100 patients with depression or anergia with unremarkable physical, neurologic, and routine laboratory evaluations were found to be hypothyroid.[19] "Postpartum blues" may be associated with decreased thyroid function.[20] In a study of mood disorder patients, there was an inverse relationship between serum thyroid-stimulating hormone (TSH) levels and global and regional cerebral blood flow and glucose metabolism.[21]

Mania may be the presentation of "myxedema madness," but the less dramatic and more common hypomanic symptoms include excitement, agitation, hostility, and hyperactivity. Thyroid hormone–induced mania is a distinct entity observed during the initial treatment of hypothyroid patients.[22] Nearly all of the affected patients have psychiatric symptoms at the time that medication is commenced. One-half of the patients have a past or family history of psychiatric disorder. More than 90% of the patients are women and have been hypothyroid for at least 6 months. The thyroid hormone therapy usually is excessive for a beginning dosage (see Chap. 45). In these cases, mania begins 4 to 7 days after medication is started, and lasts 1 to 2 weeks, resolving without sequelae, although the patient is at significant personal risk while manic. The syndrome consists of psychomotor agitation, persecutory delusions, elation, and irritability. Increased catecholamine activity and an abrupt increase in receptor sensitivity, both precipitated by too-rapid thyroid replacement, seem to play a role in this syndrome. Time-limited antipsychotic drug therapy with continuing medical treatment is usually effective.[23]

Anxiety and uncontrollable excitability may mark the presentation of some patients with myxedema. The anxiety is not related to the severity of myxedema, and it may persist even after thyroid replacement. There may be a personality change with chronic invalidism.

Often, no recovery is expected if the mental illness has a duration >2 years; the highest recovery rate (80%) from this condition is in those older than 50 years of age who have organic brain syndromes caused by the hypothyroidism. Once thyroid hormone therapy is commenced, the recovery from the mental disturbances of hypothyroidism often lags behind the restoration of normal metabolism, but occasionally mental improvement may precede major somatic changes.

## THE PARATHYROID GLAND AND DISORDERS OF CALCIUM METABOLISM

Parathyroid disorders affect the CNS by causing aberrations in calcium, phosphorus, and magnesium metabolism. Calcium enhances both the release and depletion of norepinephrine and dopamine β-hydroxylase.

### HYPERPARATHYROIDISM AND HYPERCALCEMIA

Confusion and delirious states may dominate the clinical picture in hyperparathyroidism.[24–27] The incidence of organic brain syndrome is 5% to 10%. The serum calcium level is closely correlated with the severity of psychiatric symptoms. Serum calcium levels of 12 to 16 mg/dL usually are associated with personality changes and affective disturbances. Acute organic brain syndromes with altered levels of consciousness, paranoid ideation, and hallucinations often occur at levels of 16 to 19 mg/dL. Somnolence and coma supervene at levels higher than 19 mg/dL.

The hypomagnesemia that occasionally is associated with hypercalcemia (see Chap. 68) also may play a role in the mental disturbances of some patients. These disorders include disorientation, confusion, and hallucinations. Also, reversible dementia may occur in the hypercalcemia of lithium-associated hyperparathyroidism.

Psychosis occurs in 5% to 20% of patients with hyperparathyroidism, largely depending on the level of serum calcium. The preponderant symptoms are hallucinations and delusions. Psychosis may appear abruptly while plasma calcium levels rise rapidly, necessitating rapid medical or surgical intervention. In such cases, paranoid states may begin to clear within 48 hours after the resection of a parathyroid adenoma.

Depression occurs in 5% to 20% of patients and may be associated with headaches. Usually, calcium levels are in the 12- to 16-mg/dL range, and fatigue with anergia develops first, at times insidiously, over years or decades. Anxiety and irritability are seen in up to one-third of the patients. Personality changes include fatigue, weakness, and anorexia.

The postoperative reversal[28] of many of the cerebral symptoms associated with hyperparathyroidism does not seem to be related to the duration of the illness, the severity of mental symptoms, or the patient's age. The depression of hyperparathyroidism usually reverses promptly after resection of the adenoma.

### HYPOPARATHYROIDISM

More than 40% of patients with hypoparathyroidism have an organic brain syndrome that may occur in the absence of tetany or seizures. Usually, this occurs within the first 3 to 4 months of the illness and tends not to recur with relapses. Sometimes, the psychiatric disturbances are the first and only manifestations of the disease observed—carpopedal spasm and convulsions may occur later.[8] A syndrome resembling delirium tremens may occur; typically, it resolves without sequelae when normal calcium levels are maintained.

Intellectual impairment is common in both hypoparathyroidism and pseudohypoparathyroidism. In pseudo-pseudohypopara-

thyroidism, intellectual impairment is seen in almost all of the patients who have psychiatric manifestations. Psychosis occurs in nearly 20% of patients with surgical hypoparathyroidism and less frequently in patients with idiopathic hypoparathyroidism.[29] Periodic psychosis associated with pseudo-pseudohypoparathyroidism has been reported.[30]

Depression is a common feature of patients with hypoparathyroidism as well as hyperparathyroidism. Feelings of guilt are described only rarely in depressed hypoparathyroid patients. Interestingly, the presence of guilt has been a clue to the hyperparathyroid etiology of an affective disorder. Well-defined mood swings have been reported in cases of surgical hypoparathyroidism. Anxiety and irritability are common.[31] Personality changes, such as obsessions, phobias, tics, social withdrawal, and irritability, may be prominent.[32]

Intellectual impairment improves with treatment of the hypocalcemia in most patients with surgical and idiopathic hypoparathyroidism and in one-third of patients with pseudohypoparathyroidism.

## THE ADRENAL CORTEX

The CNS effects of disorders of the adrenal cortex are related to the effects of corticosteroids, and perhaps also to the effects of changes of the levels of adrenocorticotropic hormone (ACTH) and corticotropin-releasing hormone. The concomitant abnormalities in glucose metabolism, electrolytes, and blood pressure also may play a role. Current evidence indicates that hypercortisolemia, often associated with stress, is toxic to certain cortical areas, including the hippocampus, and may contribute to various forms of psychopathology, including posttraumatic stress disorder, depression, and dementia.[33–35]

### CUSHING SYNDROME

Cushing syndrome is probably the endocrinopathy having the highest frequency of mental changes. Cerebral symptoms are more common in endogenous Cushing syndrome than in exogenous corticosteroid administration. Psychiatric symptoms predate the physical stigmata in 50% of the cases of Cushing syndrome. The greatest percentage of all mental changes in Cushing syndrome occurs in the bilateral adrenocortical hyperplasia secondary to a pituitary tumor (i.e., Cushing disease).[8]

Organic brain syndrome occurs in approximately one-third of patients with Cushing syndrome or with exogenous hypercortisolism, and can mimic the impaired concentration, delirium, and dementia of any organic, toxic, or metabolic disorder.[8b]

Psychosis occurs in 5% to 20% of patients with Cushing syndrome. Often, it is clinically indistinguishable from schizophrenia; the onset may be rapid, and it may occur early or late in the course of the illness; it is not related to the emotional reaction to the physical changes of the disorder. Paranoid states are more likely to occur in patients with the highest serum cortisol levels, but often these states do not seem to be related to predisposing personality factors.

Psychotic episodes occur in a similar percentage of patients who are receiving pharmacologic doses of corticosteroids.[8] Psychosis is twice as likely to occur during the first week of treatment. There is no characteristic pattern in corticosteroid-induced psychosis. The pattern ranges from schizophreniform, to affective, to delirium/dementia. The psychosis usually responds to chlorpromazine, or the equivalent, and spontaneous recovery occurs 2 weeks to 7 months after discontinuation of corticosteroids.[36] Occasionally, the psychosis may occur only after the corticosteroids are discontinued.

Depression occurs in more than half of the patients with Cushing syndrome. Some may attempt suicide. Suicidal ideation may first develop when physical signs and symptoms begin to resolve. Depression often antedates the physical findings. The depression in Cushing patients is often volatile, with rapid shifts in mood. Sadness and crying may occur without any depressing thought content. The duration of each depressive episode may last 1 to 2 days. Patients with high levels of both serum cortisol and ACTH generally have more serious depressive symptoms. Approximately 10% of patients who receive exogenous corticosteroids develop depression.[37]

Corticosteroid-induced euphoria, often with increased appetite and libido, occurs in at least 20% to 40% of patients receiving these medications, but it has been observed in fewer than 5% of those with endogenous Cushing syndrome.[8] In Cushing syndrome, loud rapid speech, increased energy, elation with hyperactivity, and rapid thoughts may be seen early in the disease process; later, this may lead to agitation, depression, or psychosis, as the disease progresses.

Acute episodes of anxiety occur in up to one-third of the patients with Cushing syndrome, and a milder degree of anxiety is common in patients receiving corticosteroids. Perceptual disorders occur in more than 10% of patients with Cushing syndrome, and these may be misinterpreted as hysterical in origin.

The treatment of Cushing syndrome (see Chap. 75) often induces a psychological improvement paralleling the resolution of physical signs. Corticosteroid-induced psychosis, however, may persist for some time, even after discontinuation of the drug.

### ADDISON DISEASE

Psychiatric symptoms are present in almost all cases of severe Addison disease (see Chap. 76). Memory impairment occurs in 75% of patients, and more severe organic brain syndrome in 5% to 20%. A profound perceptual impairment may occur, with a decreased threshold to tactile, auditory, gustatory, and olfactory stimuli, accompanied by impaired recognition and interpretation of sensory stimuli.[13]

Psychosis occurs in one-fourth of the cases and may include the symptoms of seclusiveness, negativism, poor judgment, agitation, hallucinations, delusions, and bizarre and catatonic posturing.

Approximately one-third of addisonian patients show depression, manifested by apathy or sad affect, fatigue, poverty of thought, and lack of initiative. Depression may antedate the physical signs. A subjective return of interest and energy occurs within days of corticosteroid replacement in Addison disease. However, the psychosis may persist for months after adequate replacement therapy. Also, acute mania can occur when a chronically hypoadrenal patient is administered corticosteroids for the first time.

### ADRENAL MEDULLA

Pheochromocytoma is often associated with an anxiety syndrome and sensations of impending doom.

### THE SEX HORMONES

Many forms of hypothalamic–pituitary–gonadal dysfunction may produce loss of libido and potentially reversible impotence. In hypogonadal men, androgen therapy may produce the side effects of insomnia, pressured thought, and irritability (see Chap. 115).

Seventy to 90% of women of childbearing age are considered to have some degree of the premenstrual tension syndrome, consisting of various emotional symptoms—emotional lability, irritability, depression, anxiety, crying spells, and fatigue[38] (see Chap. 99). Changes in appetite and craving for sweets may occur. However, fewer than one-third of these women are reported to change their daily routine because of the symptoms. The symptoms usually begin soon after ovulation and increase gradually, reaching a maximum ~5 days before menstruation. They dissipate rapidly once menstruation begins, and a peak of well-being often occurs during the mid- and late-follicular phase. Specific serotonin reuptake inhibitors seem to be effective in treating premenstrual tension syndrome.[39,40] "Postpartum blues," which occurs 1 to 2 weeks postpartum, may be due to withdrawal of endogenous progesterone or decreased thyroid hormone levels.[20,41]

In some women, anxiety, fatigue, emotional lability, depression, insomnia, tension, and difficulty in concentration are associated with the menopause (see Chap. 100). The degree of symptomatology seems to be related to the rate of withdrawal of the hormones (the most severe symptoms being associated with surgical menopause).

## HYPOGLYCEMIA, DIABETES, AND PANCREATIC DISORDERS

Anxiety occurs in 20% to 40% of patients with hypoglycemia. Behavioral disturbances associated with hypoglycemia can be quantified.[42] The perceptual disturbances associated with hypoglycemia together with fainting, confusion, and paresthesias may mimic hysteria. On the other hand, early symptoms of diabetes (e.g., blurred vision, polydipsia, polyuria, anorexia) also may mimic hysteria.

Many patients with hypoglycemia manifest an organic brain syndrome. However, cognitive function appears to be spared during mild reductions of plasma glucose and is dissociated from the adrenergic activation.[43] Mild delirium may occur at plasma glucose levels below 30 mg/dL and coma may occur at levels below 10 mg/dL (see Chap. 158). The rate of fall in plasma glucose is more important than the absolute level; therefore, a precipitous decrease to a normal level in a severe diabetic may cause delirium. On the other hand, high plasma glucose levels may cause a hyperosmolar encephalopathy. Both the clinical deterioration and the posttherapy improvement in the psychiatric symptoms of patients with hypoglycemia tend to lag behind the metabolic and electroencephalographic changes.[43a] Psychomotor retardation, depersonalization, and altered states of consciousness, which may mimic psychosis, are common in hypoglycemia. Chronic hypoglycemia of any etiology may present with depression.[44] Also, chronic hypoglycemia may mimic schizophrenia. In diabetics, varying degrees of intellectual deterioration may occur because of the multiple episodes of insulin-induced hypoglycemia and because of cerebral atherosclerosis.[45] Diabetes mellitus is a risk factor for dementia in later life.[46,47]

Interestingly, more than 50% of patients with pancreatitis have symptoms of psychosis, such as hallucinations (more commonly visual than auditory), which are not dependent on alcohol history.[48]

Inexplicably, depression and anxiety may be the presenting symptoms in patients with carcinoma of the pancreas and may predate physical signs and symptoms by 6 months to several years. At least 10% of pancreatic cancer patients have an associated psychiatric disorder of significant proportion; depression, anxiety, insomnia, and a feeling of impending doom are typically noticed. The sensorium is clear and, initially, a mild weight loss and complaints of pain are seen to variable extents. The depression is mild to moderate, without delusional content; feelings of guilt, worthlessness, or suicide are remarkably absent. The depression is usually resistant to antidepressant drugs. It is not known whether the cerebral symptomatology associated with carcinoma of the pancreas is humorally mediated.

## REFERENCES

1. Reus VI. Behavioral disturbances associated with endocrine disorders. Annu Rev Med 1986; 37:205.
2. Fava GA. Affective disorders and endocrine disease: new insights from psychosomatic studies. Psychosomatics 1994; 35:341.
3. Hall RCW, Popkin MK, DeVaul RA, et al. Physical illness presenting as psychiatric disease. Arch Gen Psychiatry 1978; 35:1315.
4. Hall RCW, Gardner ER, Stickney SK, et al. Physical illness manifesting as psychiatric disease: II. Analysis of a state hospital inpatient population. Arch Gen Psychiatry 1980; 37:989.
5. Hall RCW, Beresford TP, Gardner ER, Popkin MK. The medical care of psychiatric patients. Hosp Community Psychiatry 1982; 33:25.
6. Martin JB, Riskind PN. Neurologic manifestations of hypothalamic disease. Prog Brain Res 1992; 93:31.
7. Lipowski ZJ. Delirium: acute brain failure in man. Springfield, IL: Charles C Thomas Publisher, 1980.
8. Leigh H, Kramer SI. The psychiatric manifestations of endocrine disease. Adv Intern Med 1984; 29:413.
8a. Brownlie BE, Rae AM, Walshe JW, Wells JE. Psychoses associated with thyrotoxicosis–thyrotoxic psychosis: a report of 18 cases, with statistical analysis of incidence. Eur J Endocrinol 2000; 142:438.
8b. Forget H, Lacroix A, Somma M, Cohen H. Cognitive decline in patients with Cushing's syndrome. J Int Neuropsychol Soc 2000; 6:20.
9. Ettigi PG, Brown GM. Brain disorders associated with endocrine dysfunction. Psychiatr Clin North Am 1978; 1:117.
10. Trzepacz PT, McCue M, Klein I, et al. A psychiatric and neuropsychological study of patients with untreated Graves' disease. Gen Hosp Psychiatry 1988; 10:49.
11. Mintzer MJ. Hypothyroidism and hyperthyroidism in the elderly. J Fla Med Assoc 1992; 79:231.
12. Palacios A, Cohen MA, Cobbs R. Apathetic hyperthyroidism in middle age. Int J Psychiatry Med 1991; 21:393.
13. Devaris DP, Mehlman I. Psychiatric presentations of endocrine and metabolic disorders. Primary Care 1979; 6:245.
14. Orenstein H, Peskind A, Raskind MA. Thyroid disorders in female psychiatric patients with panic disorder or agoraphobia. Am J Psychiatry 1988; 145:1428.
15. Logotheis J. Psychiatric behavior as the initial indicator of adult myxedema. J Nerv Ment Dis 1963; 136:561.
16. Dugbaartey AT. Neurocognitive aspects of hypothyroidism. Arch Intern Med 1998; 13:1413.
17. Smith CL, Granger CV. Hypothyroidism producing reversible dementia: a challenge for medical rehabilitation. Am J Phys Med Rehabil 1992; 71:28.
18. Pitts FN, Guze SB. Psychiatric disorders and myxedema. Am J Psychiatry 1961; 118:142.
19. Gold MS, Pottash AC, Mueller EA III, Erxtein I. Grades of thyroid failure in 100 depressed and anergic psychiatric inpatients. Am J Psychiatry 1981; 138:253.
20. Ijuin T, Douchi T, Yamamoto S, et al. The relationship between maternity blues and thyroid dysfunction. J Obstet Gynecol Res 1998; 1:49.
21. Marangell LB, Ketter TA, George MS, et al. Inverse relationship of peripheral thyrotropin-stimulating hormone levels to brain activity in mood disorders. Am J Psychiatry 1997; 2:224
22. Josephson AM, McKenzie TB. Thyroid-induced mania in hypothyroid patients. Br J Psychiatry 1980; 137:222.
23. Irwin R, Ellis PM, Delahunt J. Psychosis following acute alteration of thyroid status. Aust N Z J Psychiatry 1997; 5:762.
24. Gatewood JW, Organ CH, Mead BT. Mental changes associated with hyperparathyroidism. Am J Psychiatry 1975; 132:129.
25. Agras S, Oliveau DC. Primary hyperparathyroidism and psychosis. Can Med Assoc J 1964; 91:1366.
26. Sier HC, Hartnell J, Morley JE, et al. Primary hyperparathyroidism and delirium in the elderly. J Am Geriatr Soc 1988; 36:157.
27. Solomon BL, Schaaf M, Smallridge RC. Psychologic symptoms before and after parathyroid surgery. Am J Med 1994; 96:101.
28. Joborn C, Hetta J, Lind L, et al. Self-rated psychiatric symptoms in patients operated on because of primary hyperparathyroidism and in patients with long-standing mild hypercalcemia. Surgery 1989; 105:72.
29. Pollard AJ, Prendergast M, al-Hammouri F, et al. Different subtypes of pseudohypoparathyroidism in the same family with an unusual psychiatric presentation of the index case. Arch Dis Child 1994; 70:99.
30. Furukawa T. Periodic psychosis associated with pseudo-pseudohypoparathyroidism. J Nerv Ment Dis 1991; 179:637.
31. Lawlor BA. Hypocalcemia, hypoparathyroidism, and organic anxiety syndrome. J Clin Psychiatry 1988; 49:317.
32. Peterson P. Psychiatric disorders in primary hyperparathyroidism. J Clin Endocrinol Metab 1968; 28:1491.
33. Kiraly SJ, Ancill RJ, Dimitrova G. The relationship of endogenous cortisol to psychiatric disorder: a review. Can J Psychiatry 1997; 42:415.
34. Holsboer F, Grasser A, Friess E. et al. Steroid effects on central neurons and implications for psychiatric and neurological disorders. Ann N Y Acad Sci 1994; 746:345.
35. Bremer JD, Randall P, Scott TM, et al. MRI-based measurement of hippocampal volume in patients with combat-related posttraumatic stress disorder. Am J Psychiatry 1995; 152:973.
36. Hall RCW, Popkin MK, Stickney SK, Gardner ER. Presentation of steroid psychoses. J Nerv Ment Dis 1979; 167:229.
37. Naber D, Sand P, Heigl B. Psychopathological and neuropsychological effects of 8-days' corticosteroid treatment. A prospective study. Psychoneuroendocrinology 1996; 21:25.
38. Wilson CA, Keye WR Jr. A survey of adolescent dysmenorrhea and premenstrual symptom frequency. J Adolesc Health 1989; 10:317.
39. Steiner M. Premenstrual dysphoric disorder. An update. Gen Hosp Psychiatry 1996; 18:244.
40. Eriksson E, Hedberg MA, Andersch B, et al. The serotonin reuptake inhibitor paroxetin is superior to the noradrenaline reuptake inhibitor maprotiline in the treatment of premenstrual syndrome. Neuropsychopharmacology 1995; 12:167.
41. Harris B, Lovett L, Newcombe RG, et al. Maternity blues and major endocrine changes: Cardiff Puerperal Mood and Hormone Study II. Br Med J 1944; 308:949.
42. Cox DI, Irvine A, Gonder-Frederick L, et al. Fear of hypoglycemia: quantification, validation, and utilization. Diabetes Care 1987; 10:617.
43. Ipp E, Forster B. Sparing of cognitive function in mild hypoglycemia: dissociation from the neuroendocrine response. J Clin Endocrinol Metab 1987; 65:806.
43a. Strachan MW, Deary IJ, Ewing FM, Frier BM. Recovery of cognitive function and mood after severe hypoglycemia in adults with insulin-treated diabetes. Diabetes Care 2000; 23:305.
44. Roy M, Collier B, Roy A. Excess of depressive symptoms and life events among diabetics. Comprehens Psychiatr 1994; 35:129.
45. Rovet JF, Ehrlich RM, Hoppe M. Specific intellectual deficits in children with early onset diabetes mellitus. Child Dev 1988; 59:226.
46. Stolk RP, Breteler MM, Ott A, et al. Insulin and cognitive function in an elderly population: the Rotterdam Study. Diabetes Care 1997; 5:792.
47. Leibson CL, Rocca WA, Hanson VA, et al. Risk of dementia among persons with diabetes mellitus: a population-based cohort study. Am J Epidemiol 1997; 4:301.
48. Schuster MM, Iber FL. Psychosis and pancreatitis. Arch Intern Med 1965; 116:228.

# CHAPTER 201

# PSYCHIATRIC-HORMONAL INTERRELATIONSHIPS

MITCHEL A. KLING, MARIANNE HATLE, RAMESH K. THAPAR, AND PHILIP W. GOLD

Extensive neuroendocrine research suggests an intimate linkage between neurohormonal functional activity and major components of the symptom complexes of illnesses such as major depression and anorexia nervosa. For instance, several aspects of the syndromes of mood and eating disorders suggest hypothalamic dysfunction. Thus, patients with depression often manifest disturbances in appetite, reproductive function (e.g., decreased libido and menstrual irregularities), sleep, cortisol secretion, and circadian periodicity. Anorexia nervosa is characterized not only by profound alterations in eating behavior, but also by marked changes in hypothalamic–pituitary–adrenal (HPA) regulation and gonadotropin secretion. The mechanism of these abnormalities in psychiatric populations is being explored. In addition, interest in neuroendocrine systems reflects the fact that the monoaminergic neurotransmitters, long thought to play a dominant role in major psychiatric illness, also modulate the synthesis and release of a number of hypothalamic peptides and pituitary hormones. Thus, examination of pituitary hormones in plasma can shed light on the functional activity of central biogenic amine systems. Moreover, the hypothalamic hormones are widely distributed throughout the brain, exert specific receptor-mediated bioactivity, and influence the functional activity of brain neurotransmitter systems (see Chap. 176). Several hypothalamic hormones also seem to coordinate complex behaviors and physiologic processes relevant to adaptation and the maintenance of internal homeostasis.

## MOOD DISORDERS

The major categories of mood disorders include *major depressive disorder* and *bipolar disorders*. Considerable clinical overlap is found in the depressive syndromes of these two conditions, but bipolar disorders differ in that they are also characterized by episodes of *mania* (in *bipolar I disorder*) or *hypomania* (in *bipolar II disorder*).

*Major depressive disorder* is defined as the occurrence of one or more episodes of the major depressive syndrome.[1] Although based exclusively on clinical criteria, the diagnosis of major depression leads to valid predictions concerning heritability, clinical manifestations, natural history, and response to treatment. In addition to the psychological pain of the disorder that is perhaps the cruelest symptom, patients with mood disorders also manifest symptoms suggestive of abnormalities in hypothalamic loci (controlling appetite, sexual function, circadian rhythms, and anterior pituitary function). Major depressive episodes tend to be recurrent, whether occurring as part of major depressive disorder (also known as *unipolar depression*) or as part of a bipolar disorder, and may increase in frequency and/or severity with advancing age. Major depressive episodes may also be superimposed on a more chronic, indolent depressive process (*dysthymia*) or associated with certain personality disorders, resulting in double depressions, or they may occur in other psychiatric disorders (e.g., schizophrenia, panic disorder, or substance use disorders) or in a number of medical conditions (e.g., thyroid or adrenal disease, hypercalcemia, heart disease, or cancer). In the latter cases, the diagnosis of an *organic mood syndrome* may be made, but the clinical picture and treatment implications are similar.

Data from numerous adoption and twin studies strongly suggest that vulnerability to mood disorders is heritable; however, nongenetic factors are involved in their phenotypic expression, as concordance rates in monozygotic twins are generally <100%. Most current evidence favors the existence of multiple susceptibility genes, each of relatively small effect.[2] Putative linkage markers for bipolar illness have been identified on chromosomes 18 and 21,[3,4] and others are under active investigation,[5] although specific susceptibility gene loci have yet to be defined. One factor hampering the search for such markers is a lack of specific biologic abnormalities in depressive illness, which would make phenotype definition more reliable. The diagnosis is currently made by carefully validated clinical criteria based on the evaluation of psychologic and physiologic symptoms. The standard diagnostic criteria in the United States are those of the *Diagnostic and Statistical Manual of Mental Disorders, Fourth Edition*,[1] which incorporates clinical signs of physiologic disturbances as well as affective and cognitive symptoms.

Clinical observations strongly suggest that the principal pathophysiologic alterations in the major depressive syndrome reflect changes in neuroendocrine regulation. Thus, major depressive illness is characterized by either anorexia or hyperphagia, decreased libido and menstrual irregularities, sleep disturbances, an apparent phase advance of rapid eye movement (REM) sleep and body temperature rhythms, and a diurnal variation in mood. Moreover, the finding of sustained hypercortisolism in patients with major depression[6] represents one of the best-validated and most extensively studied somatic abnormalities in biologic psychiatry. Other neuroendocrine abnormalities observed in depressed patients include alterations in hypotha-

lamic–pituitary–thyroid (HPT)[7] and growth hormone (GH) regulation. In addition, alterations in central neuropeptide systems have increasingly been implicated in the pathophysiology of mood disorders and may represent new targets for treatment of these disorders.

## SPECIFIC NEUROENDOCRINE ALTERATIONS IN PATIENTS WITH MAJOR DEPRESSIVE ILLNESS

### HYPOTHALAMIC–PITUITARY–ADRENAL AXIS

The existence of significant hypercortisolism in patients with major depression, particularly the *classic* or *melancholic subtype* of this disorder, has been demonstrated by a number of independent measures, including estimation of cortisol production rate, serial sampling of the diurnal cortisol secretory pattern, urinary free cortisol excretion, and escape of plasma cortisol levels from dexamethasone suppression.[6] Mechanistic studies suggest that the hypercortisolism reflects a defect at or above the level of the hypothalamus that results in the hypersecretion of corticotropin-releasing hormone (CRH). Thus, depressed patients manifest elevated plasma cortisol levels in association with an attenuated response of plasma adrenocorticotropic hormone (ACTH) to the administration of exogenous CRH.[8] This finding suggests a normal response of the pituitary corticotrope cell to cortisol negative feedback in depression and, thus, a suprapituitary locus of hypercortisolism. These attenuated ACTH responses to CRH in major depression contrast with those observed in patients with Cushing disease; in the latter, these responses are augmented despite profound hypercortisolism,[8] indicating a loss of cortisol negative-feedback sensitivity at the pituitary. Moreover, depressed patients demonstrate increased adrenocortical responsiveness to ACTH, as assessed either directly after ACTH infusions[9] or indirectly from the relative responses of ACTH and cortisol to CRH infusion.[8] This increased adrenocortical responsiveness to ACTH is consistent with the idea that depressive episodes (which tend to last weeks to months) are associated with the development of adrenal hyperplasia because of sustained hyperstimulation. This explains the typically "normal" basal plasma ACTH levels seen in depression, because smaller amounts of ACTH are required to generate the same cortisol response from hyperplastic than from normoplastic adrenal glands.

Direct measurements of CRH have been made in patients with depressive illness. Because CRH levels in peripheral blood are low and may reflect secretion from peripheral sites as well as any putative hypothalamic release,[10] most studies have focused on measuring CRH levels in the cerebrospinal fluid (CSF) (Fig. 201-1). These studies have suggested that CSF CRH levels are either frankly elevated or are inappropriately elevated for the degree of hypercortisolism manifested by these patients.[11] CSF CRH levels tend to decrease after successful treatment with electroconvulsive therapy[12] and antidepressants such as fluoxetine hydrochloride (Prozac).[13]

The putative hypersecretion of CRH in melancholic depression is of considerable interest in the light of data that the intracerebroventricular administration of CRH to experimental animals induces a series of complex physiologic and behavioral changes classically associated with stress (and depression).[14] These include not only hypercortisolism but also activation of the sympathetic nervous system, increased behavioral arousal, decreased sleep, decreased feeding, hypothalamic hypogonadism with decreased sexual behavior, and context-dependent changes in motor activity.

The idea that hypersecretion of CRH in several brain areas could account for a number of the cardinal symptoms of melancholic depression has led to increased interest in the develop-

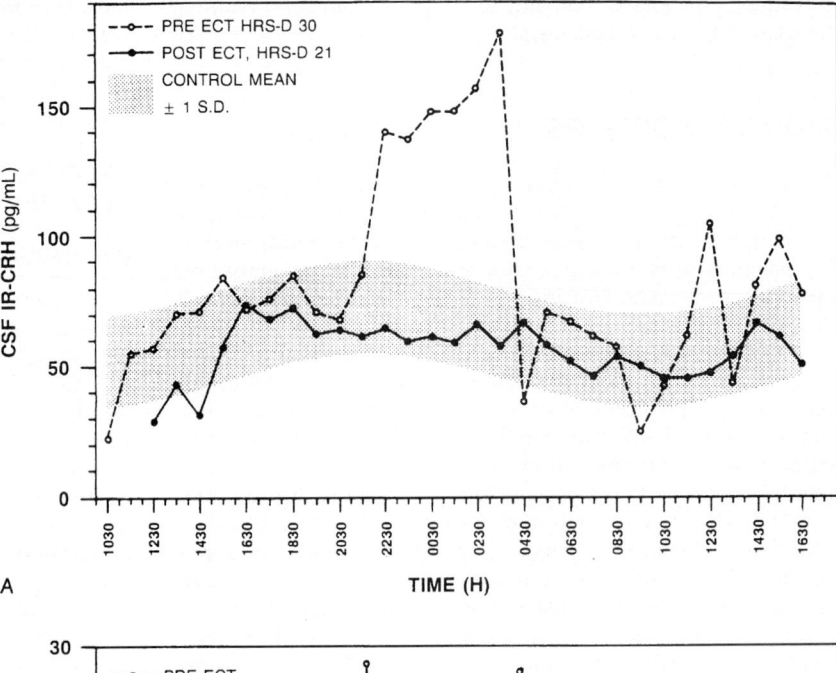

A

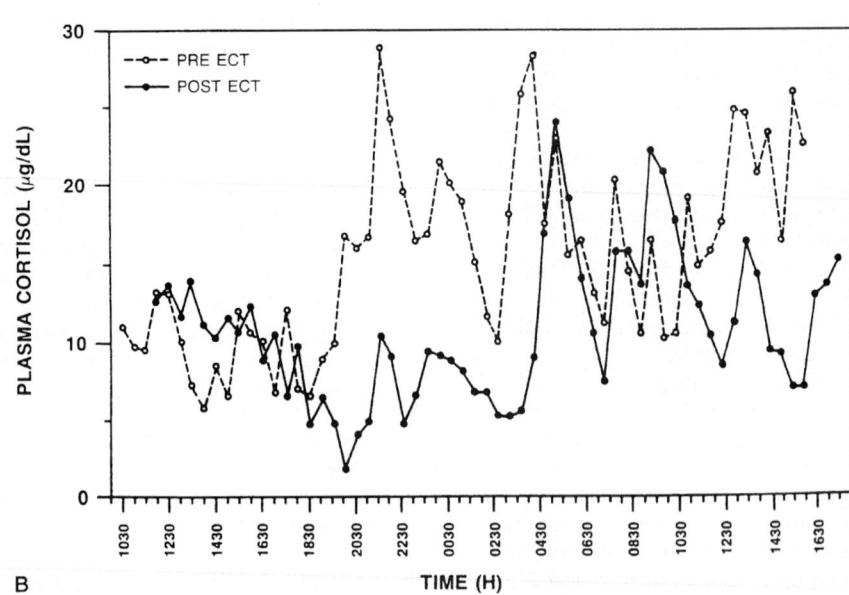

B

**FIGURE 201-1.** Effect of electroconvulsive treatment (*ECT*) on the pattern of cerebrospinal fluid (*CSF*) immunoreactive corticotropin-releasing hormone (*IR-CRH*) measured by serial sampling over 30 hours (**A**) and plasma cortisol measured every 30 minutes during study (**B**) in a 28-year-old white woman with melancholic depression. The patient was medication-free for both pretreatment and posttreatment studies. The shaded area in **A** represents the mean ± 1 standard deviation (*S.D.*) of sinusoidal fit for diurnal rhythm of CSF IR-CRH in six healthy volunteers. Before ECT, the increased CSF IR-CRH values in the early morning hours are superimposed on an apparently normal diurnal rhythm and are associated with, and slightly lag, the increased plasma cortisol values during late evening and early morning hours. After ECT, no such elevations in the early morning CSF IR-CRH levels are observed, whereas the plasma cortisol pattern reverts toward normal. (*HRS-D*, number of hourly samplings.) (From Kling MA, Geracioti TD, Licinio J, et al. Effects of electroconvulsive therapy on the CRH-ACTH-cortisol system in melancholic depression: preliminary findings. Psychopharmacol Bull 1994; 30:489. Data for healthy subjects are from Kling MA, Geracioti TD, De Bellis MD, et al. A significant diurnal rhythm of CSF immunoreactive corticotropin-releasing hormone in healthy volunteers: physiologic implications. J Clin Endocrinol Metab 1994; 79:233.)

ment of CRH antagonists as potential treatments for this disorder. Because peptide CRH antagonists are impractical for clinical use due to poor oral bioavailability and limited penetration of the blood–brain barrier, several pharmaceutical companies have been developing small-molecule-CRH antagonists with the desired characteristics for administration to patients. Preliminary studies with such agents in experimental animals indicate inhibitory effects on stress-related behaviors similar to those seen with peptide CRH antagonists.[15]

Some investigators have reported decreased CSF CRH levels in depressed patients.[16] These differences may reflect the existence of distinct syndromes of depression. Thus, although patients with classic melancholic depression show evidence of CRH hypersecretion, those with more "atypical" symptoms of fatigue, hyperphagia, hypersomnia, and mood reactivity have a pathologic decrease in CRH secretion.[17] Indeed, depression in patients with Cushing disease, who show markedly reduced CSF CRH levels,[18] tends to be associated with atypical features.[19] The existence of such pathophysiologic distinctions is an area of active investigation, not only because of the potential for identifying biologic markers that may be useful in diagnosis and in

genetic studies, but also because optimal treatment of atypical depressions may differ from that of melancholic depression.

## HYPOTHALAMIC–PITUITARY–GONADAL AXIS

The observation of a female preponderance in the prevalence of unipolar depression[20] stimulated interest in the potential role of gonadal dysfunction in the pathophysiology of this disorder. Indeed, early studies showed alterations in luteinizing hormone (LH) secretion in postmenopausal women with depression.[21] Moreover, major depression is frequently associated with loss of libido and, in some women, with menstrual disturbances, including secondary amenorrhea. Luteinizing hormone–releasing hormone (LHRH) secretion is believed to be under the tonic inhibitory control of β-endorphin secreted by the arcuate nucleus of the hypothalamus.[22] The injection of CRH into the arcuate nucleus appears to stimulate β-endorphin secretion from these neurons,[23] providing a possible mechanism for the inhibition of reproductive function associated with intracerebroventricular administration of this peptide. Moreover, glucocorticoids inhibit reproductive function at the hypothalamic, pituitary, and adrenal levels.[24] Hence, the pituitary-adrenal activation associated with depression can potentially act at multiple levels to inhibit both behavioral and physiologic aspects of reproductive function.

Epidemiologic studies indicate that the female preponderance in major depressive disorder appears to be confined to the reproductively active period,[25] when monthly cycling of estrogen and progesterone levels is occurring. Although social factors may influence the frequency with which men and women report depressive symptoms and may account in part for differences in the prevalence of depression in socioeconomic subgroups, research on the effects of estrogens on the central nervous system (CNS)[26] provides a possible neurobiologic basis for the age dependence of the male-female difference in the prevalence of major depression. Thus, several authors have suggested that periodic or sustained decreases in estrogen availability to the brain may deprive the organism of the normally neuroprotective effects of estrogens when continuously available at sufficient levels.[27–30] Although this hypothesis remains to be fully tested, controlled studies suggest that continuous administration of estrogens may have a beneficial effect in women with postpartum[31] or perimenopausal depression.[32,33]

### HYPOTHALAMIC–PIUITARY–THYROID AXIS

A number of disturbances in the regulation of thyroid function occur in depression.[34] Among these are a blunted response of thyrotropin (thyroid-stimulating hormone, TSH) to exogenous thyroid-releasing hormone (TRH) administration and an attenuation of the normal nocturnal rise of plasma TSH levels. Although basal plasma thyroxine ($T_4$) levels tend to be normal in depression, however, controversy exists about whether the abnormalities mentioned earlier represent a primary CNS disturbance that causes the hypersecretion of TRH (i.e., a form of tertiary hyperthyroidism) or whether thyrotrope responsiveness to TRH is impaired either by some nonspecific pituitary dysfunction or by increased secretion of some factor inhibitory to thyrotrope function. Exogenous thyroid hormones in physiologic doses (usually given as 25–50 μg of triiodothyronine [$T_3$] per day) can augment responses to antidepressants.[35] Based on the finding that most $T_3$ in brain derives from uptake and intracellular deiodination of $T_4$, rather than from direct $T_3$, the argument has been made that $T_3$ in this setting acts to reduce exposure of the CNS to thyroid hormone, thus correcting a putative tertiary hyperthyroidism in melancholic depression.[7] Alternatively, some have proposed that these doses correct a putative underlying alteration of β-adrenoceptor function in depression.[36]

Glucocorticoids have a number of effects on thyroid function, including a tendency to attenuate the responsivity of the thyrotrope to TRH. Moreover, Cushing syndrome is associated with a pattern of thyroid dysfunction similar to that observed in depression, including an attenuation of the nocturnal TSH rise, as well as a shift in thyroid hormone metabolism that causes decreased peripheral conversion of $T_4$ to $T_3$. Both of these findings are manifestations of the euthyroid sick state, a phenomenon that occurs in depression.[7] However, the precise relationship, if any, between HPA dysfunction and these thyroid alterations, and their clinical significance, remains to be fully elucidated (see Chap. 36).

An additional consideration is that mild hypothyroidism and/or antithyroid peroxidase antibodies may be found in individuals with both major depressive disorder and bipolar disorder,[37] and primary hypothyroidism is well known to occur in some patients given lithium for their mood disorder. Most clinicians use $T_4$ rather than $T_3$ in this setting. Identification and correction of mild hypothyroidism and/or subclinical autoimmune thyroiditis is important, not only because of the adverse health risks of these conditions[38] but also because subtle thyroid dysfunction may impair responsiveness to antidepressants.[36]

### GROWTH HORMONE

A number of studies suggest that alterations in GH regulation occur in depression. The GH responses to insulin-induced hypoglycemia, amphetamine, L-dopa, and clonidine are attenuated. However, the regulation of GH secretion involves the influences of multiple neurotransmitters (e.g., norepinephrine, dopamine, serotonin, γ-aminobutyric acid, and acetylcholine) that modulate the secretion of GH-releasing hormone (GHRH) and the release-inhibiting hormone, somatostatin (see Chap. 12). Moreover, GH secretion is subject to negative-feedback control by insulin-like growth factor-I (IGF-I), which had not been fully characterized when many of the earlier challenge studies were conducted. Thus, interpretation of the results of these studies is difficult.

The mean 24-hour plasma GH levels are increased in major depression, mostly because of an increased daytime or non–sleep-related secretion that more than counterbalances a decrease in sleep-dependent secretion.[39] These results are consistent with the notion that GH secretion tends to be increased in depression. Data suggest that this putative hypersecretion of GH in depression derives, as does the hypercortisolism in this disorder, from a suprapituitary disturbance. Thus, depressed patients show attenuated responses of GH to GHRH in association with increased basal IGF-I levels[35,36]; this finding provides further evidence for increased GH functional activity and intact somatotrope feedback responsiveness. Because glucocorticoids are known to interfere with IGF-I actions at the receptor level, however, the elevated GH and IGF-I levels could represent a compensatory response to a relative GH and IGF-I resistance syndrome.

### DECREASED BONE MINERAL DENSITY

Studies indicate that women with major depressive disorder have reduced bone mineral density.[40] The mechanism for this has not been established, but it appears to be associated with decreases both in bone resorption and in bone formation.[40] Nutritional factors, decreased activity levels, hypercortisolism, and hypoestrogenemia due to menstrual disturbances all may play a role, although levels of calcium, vitamin D, and parathyroid hormone (PTH) do not appear to be abnormal. Although this relationship is controversial,[40a] this finding might have important clinical implications, as it may place patients with major depression at increased risk for osteoporosis and fractures. Whether early treatment of depression helps to prevent or to reduce the severity of osteopenia and whether men with major depression are subject to the same risk is unknown, but these data suggest that bone density assessment and treatment should be considered in women with recurrent major depressive episodes.

### CENTRAL NEUROPEPTIDE SYSTEMS

A number of central neuropeptide systems have been examined in patients with major depressive disorder. Some of this work has involved measurement of neuropeptide levels in the cerebrospinal fluid. Data reviewed above provide the rationale for exploring the potential utility of nonpeptide CRH antagonists in mood and anxiety disorders,[15] which is an active area of drug development. In addition, neuropeptides such as somatostatin[41] have been examined.

Data have emerged suggesting that increased functional activity of the neuropeptide substance P may play a role in depressive and anxiety disorders.[42] Based on these data, nonpeptide substance P antagonists (which had already been in development for treatment of pain disorders, albeit with disappointing results) have been used in the treatment of major depressive disorder and have shown efficacy in preliminary studies.[42] Further studies are needed to determine whether these agents are safe and effective for treating depression and how they compare to existing agents.

## EATING DISORDERS

The major categories of eating disorders for which neuroendocrine data are available include *anorexia nervosa, bulimia nervosa,*[42a] and certain forms of obesity. Some related conditions, such as *binge eating disorder*[43] and *night eating syndrome,*[44] are currently being studied. This section focuses on neuroendocrine findings in anorexia nervosa and bulimia nervosa.

*Anorexia nervosa* is a syndrome characterized by decreased food intake and increased motor activity in the obsessive pursuit of thinness (see also Chap. 128). A related condition, *bulimia nervosa,* is characterized by episodic food binges and purging, and may either coexist with anorexia or occur as a separate entity without weight loss. These syndromes occur predominantly in young women, with an age of onset near the time of puberty. Anorexia nervosa carries one of the highest mortality rates of any psychiatric disorder, with estimates ranging from 5% to as high as 20%.[45]

Neuroendocrine abnormalities are among the cardinal manifestations of anorexia nervosa. The best described of these include hypercortisolism,[46] hypothalamic hypogonadism, alterations in the secretion of plasma and CSF vasopressin,[47] and decreased metabolic indices, including reduced thyroid function. Current areas of research include the adipocyte-derived hormone leptin[48] and the relationship between GH and IGF-I with respect to bone metabolism.[49] Some of these changes have also been observed in patients with bulimia. However, the study of disease mechanisms in these illnesses tends to be complicated by the often severe weight loss and/or changes in metabolic rate that accompany the disordered eating behavior. Thus, determining which alterations are primary and which are secondary to starvation or to repeated binging and purging is often difficult. Specific methodologic strategies for dealing with these potential confounding influences have included conducting studies in anorexic patients before and after refeeding (using behavioral programs in a controlled environment) and conducting studies in bulimic patients both while they are allowed to actively binge and purge and while after enforced abstinence from these behaviors. Examples of such studies are cited in the following sections.

### SPECIFIC NEUROENDOCRINE ABNORMALITIES IN PATIENTS WITH EATING DISORDERS

#### HYPOTHALAMIC–PITUITARY–ADRENAL AXIS

The underweight phase of anorexia nervosa is associated with profound hypercortisolism.[46,49a] Plasma and urinary free cortisol levels overlap with those seen in Cushing disease and often exceed those seen in all but the most severe depressions. In distinction to Cushing syndrome, however, the diurnal rhythm of plasma cortisol levels is preserved, although attenuated. This pattern is similar to that observed during starvation.[50] Pituitary-adrenal responses to CRH are qualitatively similar to those observed in depression and further suggest a CNS source of hypercortisolism. Thus, ACTH responses to CRH are attenuated in underweight anorexics in the face of elevated basal plasma cortisol levels (Fig. 201-2); this finding is compatible with normal corticotrope responsiveness to cortisol negative-feedback

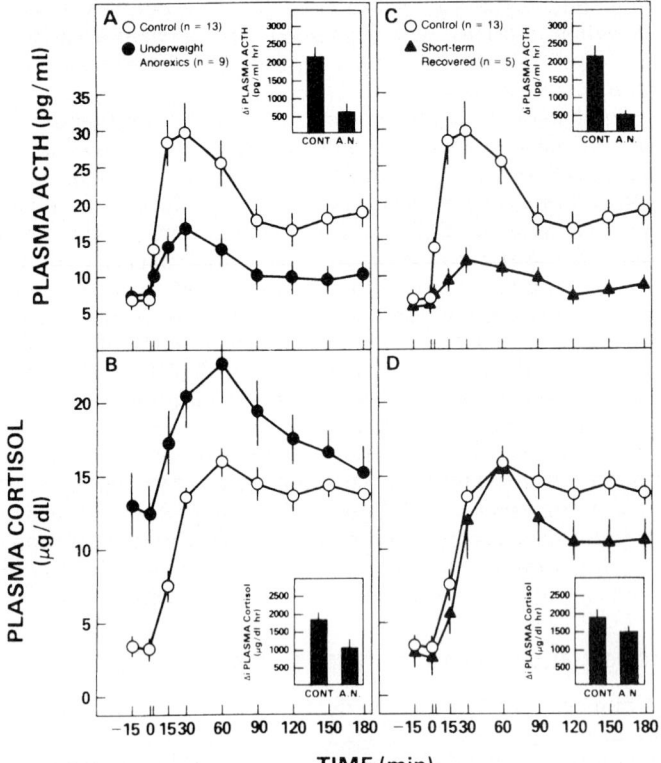

**FIGURE 201-2.** Response of plasma adrenocorticotropic hormone (*ACTH*) and cortisol to corticotropin-releasing hormone in control subjects and patients with anorexia nervosa while chronically underweight (**A** and **B**) and while in short-term recovery (**C** and **D**). (In the *Insets: Δi,* net integrated change [±1 standard error of the mean] in ACTH or cortisol; *CONT,* value in controls; *A.N.,* value in patients.) (From Gold PW, Gwirtsman H, Augerinos PC, et al. Abnormal hypothalamic-pituitary-adrenal function in anorexia nervosa: pathophysiologic mechanisms in underweight and weight-corrected patients. N Engl J Med 1986; 314:1335.)

and suggests that the hypercortisolism derives from an abnormality at or above the hypothalamus, which causes the hypersecretion of CRH.[51] A relatively greater response of cortisol than of ACTH after CRH administration suggests that a degree of adrenal hyperresponsiveness to ACTH has developed during the course of this illness. Finally, as in depression, basal plasma ACTH levels are not significantly different from normal (see Fig. 201-2), indicating that, to maintain the degree of hypercortisolism observed in these patients, the development of adrenal hyperresponsiveness causes a lower ACTH requirement than that of persons with normal adrenal responsiveness.

With short-term (3–4 week) recovery of normal or near-normal weight, plasma and urinary free cortisol levels return to normal,[51] suggesting resolution of the central defect that generates the hypercortisolism in the underweight phase. ACTH responses to CRH remain attenuated, however (see Fig. 201-2). Cortisol responses to CRH remain robust in relation to the ACTH responses in these patients, suggesting persistence of the apparent adrenal hyperresponsiveness to ACTH observed during the underweight phase. In patients studied after longer periods of weight recovery (>6 months), both ACTH and cortisol responses to CRH were normal, indicating that these abnormalities are not inherent pathophysiologic features of the illness but are related to the weight loss and its immediate aftermath. Similar findings have been obtained after administration of the glucocorticoid receptor antagonist RU-486,[52] further suggesting that the increased cortisol output in underweight patients is not purely due to glucocorticoid resistance.

Further supporting the hypothesis that hypercortisolism reflects hyperstimulation of the pituitary-adrenal axis by CRH are data that CSF CRH levels are significantly elevated in underweight anorexics.[53] Although CSF CRH levels partially normalized after the short-term correction of weight loss, they correlated positively with depression ratings at this time.[53] This finding reflected the fact that some patients remained both depressed and hypercortisolemic after correction of the weight loss, a situation associated with persistence of higher levels of CRH in the CSF. CSF levels of CRH seemed fully normalized in patients studied after ≥6 months of weight recovery.

Patients with bulimia tend to show more subtle evidence of disturbed pituitary-adrenal function than do underweight patients with anorexia nervosa. Normal-weight patients with bulimia (studied at >80% of average body weight) show a higher rate of nonsuppression of plasma cortisol in response to 1-mg overnight dexamethasone administration than do control subjects, but this rate is considerably less than that seen in underweight anorexic patients. Evidence of increased ACTH and cortisol secretion has been shown in normal-weight bulimic patients in association with attenuated ACTH and cortisol responses to CRH administration,[54] although some researchers have found normal ACTH and cortisol responses to CRH.[51] Further studies are required to clarify these apparent discrepancies.

## NEUROHYPOPHYSIAL HORMONES

Patients with anorexia nervosa demonstrate a number of abnormalities in the regulation of arginine vasopressin (AVP) secretion.[47] In particular, the underweight phase of the illness is associated with gross defects in the response of plasma AVP to osmotic stimuli such as hypertonic saline infusion. Hence, anorexic patients manifest either low basal levels of AVP that show a quantitatively subnormal response to increasing plasma sodium concentration, or a near-total disruption of the normal linear relationship between plasma AVP and sodium levels (Fig. 201-3). Such a defect in osmotically mediated vasopressin secretion previously has been described only in patients who manifest a CNS tumor that damages the osmostat, which is thought to reside in the anterior hypothalamus, but spares vasopressin neurosecretory neurons. Both patterns of the abnormal secretion of vasopressin in anorexia nervosa are slow to correct after refeeding and may take many months to normalize.

In most anorexic patients who showed disruption of osmotically mediated vasopressin secretion, a concomitant defect was found in the secretion of vasopressin into the CSF. The most consistent abnormality was a reversal of the normal plasma/CSF vasopressin ratio, which is usually less than unity.[47] These findings may be indicative of some degree of enhancement of central vasopressin secretion that may impair the responsiveness of the osmoreceptor and produce a dysregulation of peripheral vaso-

pressin secretion. Pathophysiologically, the data showing increased centrally directed AVP secretion in anorexia nervosa are intriguing in the light of data in animals demonstrating that AVP administration is associated with *delayed extinction* of (i.e., prolonged memories for) aversively learned behaviors.

Oxytocin, the levels of which decrease in underweight patients with anorexia and normalize after weight restoration, disrupts memory consolidation. The hypothesis has been put forward that the combination of increased central AVP and decreased oxytocin may help to account for the anorexic patient's exaggerated fear of the potential aversive consequences of food intake (i.e., weight gain) and to contribute to the preferential retention of these cognitive distortions as well as to inhibit the ability to incorporate new learning that would challenge these distortions.

Patients with bulimia have an attenuated response of plasma AVP to hypertonic saline infusion. The linear relationship between plasma AVP and plasma sodium is usually maintained,[55] although some investigators have found degrees of dysregulation similar to those seen in anorexic patients.[56] Patients with bulimia also have attenuated responses of AVP to insulin-induced hypoglycemia and metoclopramide administration.[7] CSF levels of AVP are slightly but significantly elevated, compared with those of healthy individuals.[57]

## HYPOTHALAMIC–PITUITARY–GONADAL AXIS

Menstrual disturbances are such an integral component of the clinical picture of anorexia nervosa that loss of menses has been incorporated into the diagnostic criteria for this illness.[1] Although the development of substantial weight loss is almost universally associated with secondary amenorrhea in patients with anorexia nervosa, loss or irregularity of menses may precede the onset of weight loss or other symptoms in up to 50% of cases.[58]

Several studies have shown decreased gonadotropin secretion in anorexia nervosa,[59–61] causing low and noncycling plasma estradiol levels. Pituitary LH and follicle-stimulating hormone (FSH) responses to LHRH generally are normal,[59] suggesting that the gonadotropin deficiency results from a loss of endogenous LHRH. A negative correlation between the degree of weight loss and the magnitude of LH and FSH responses[59] suggests that it is severe inanition that leads to hypothalamic hypogonadism in these patients.

As with depression, the abnormalities in hypothalamic–pituitary–gonadal (HPG) function may be partly secondary to hypercortisolism: increased CRH secretion may inhibit hypothalamic LHRH secretion,[23] and the resulting excess secretion of glucocorticoids may restrain gonadal function at the hypothalamic, pituitary, and gonadal levels.[24] Moreover, because sustained exercise can be associated with evidence of chronic hypercortisolism,[62] the increased physical activity that is characteristic of anorexia nervosa may indirectly contribute to the

**FIGURE 201-3.** Relationship between plasma arginine vasopressin (*pAVP*) and plasma sodium during intravenous hypertonic saline infusion in a control subject (**A**) contrasted with that in a recently recovered patient with anorexia nervosa (**B**). The shaded areas represent the range of all simultaneous plasma vasopressin and sodium values obtained during hypertonic saline infusion in 48 healthy adults. Notice that even though most of the arginine vasopressin values obtained during the infusion fall within the normal range, the pattern is qualitatively abnormal (i.e., it lacks the significant correlation between plasma vasopressin and plasma sodium that is invariably seen in controls). (*NS*, not significant; *L.D.*, limit of detectability of the assay [0.5 pg/mL].) (From Gold PW, Kaye W, Robertson GL, Ebert M. Abnormalities in plasma and cerebrospinal fluid arginine vasopressin in patients with anorexia nervosa. N Engl J Med 1983; 308:1117.)

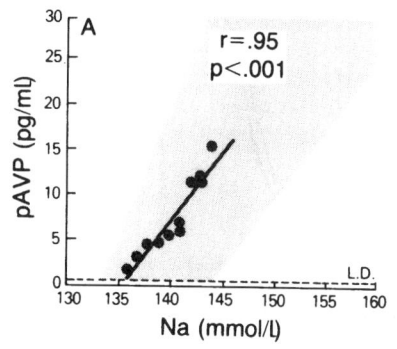
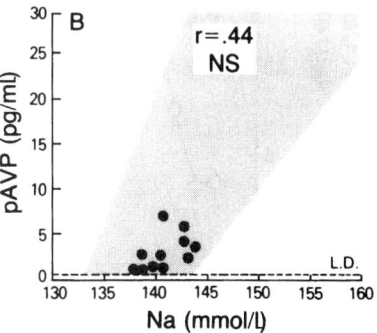

gonadal system dysfunction through effects on HPA function and may help to account for the onset of menstrual irregularities as an early manifestation of the illness.

## SYSTEMS INVOLVED IN THE REGULATION OF METABOLIC RATE

### HYPOTHALAMIC–PITUITARY–THYROID AXIS AND SYMPATHETIC SYSTEM

Basal thyroid hormone levels in anorexia nervosa tend to reflect a euthyroid sick pattern, with normal to low-normal serum $T_4$ levels, normal free $T_4$ levels, and decreased serum $T_3$ levels.[59–61] Increased reverse $T_3$ levels, a frequent concomitant of this syndrome, also have been reported. As in other clinical settings, these findings are thought to reflect decreased peripheral conversion of $T_4$ to $T_3$, with a relative increase in $T_4$ availability for inner-ring deiodination. The TSH responses to TRH are quantitatively normal but may be delayed, resembling the pattern seen in extreme starvation.[61]

Decreased plasma and urinary norepinephrine levels have also been observed in anorexic patients,[63] suggesting decreased sympathetic outflow. The reduced circulating levels of $T_3$ and catecholamines may help to account for the decreased resting metabolic rate and bradycardia that have been reported in anorexic patients and may represent an adaptive physiologic response to caloric restriction aimed at conserving skeletal muscle mass. Thus, fasting results in a rapid decrease in the peripheral conversion of $T_4$ to $T_3$ that is restored by carbohydrate loading. Similarly, food intake is associated with sympathetic activation (the thermic effect of food). Again, the presence of significant hypercortisolism would also be expected to contribute to the observed disturbances in thyroid function in underweight anorexic patients. The decreases in both thyroid and sympathetic function could represent an integrated metabolic adaptation to caloric restriction, as these two systems exert cooperative effects on thermogenesis and energy metabolism.[64] Refeeding leads to normalization of serum norepinephrine levels. $T_3$ levels also increase, but persistently low $T_3$ levels have been reported even after weight recovery in anorexic patients.[65]

Although many studies have shown reduced *resting metabolic rate (RMR)* in patients with anorexia nervosa, some have postulated that this finding is based on a prediction formula or regression equations that may overestimate the predicted RMR. Thus, RMR per kilogram of lean body mass in patients with anorexia nervosa, either while underweight or during early refeeding, was not significantly different from that of healthy volunteers.[65] RMR increased significantly after 2 weeks of refeeding, however, supporting the clinical observation that anorexic patients require high caloric intake to gain weight during this phase of treatment. Serum levels of norepinephrine and thyroid hormones do not appear to be correlated with RMR, although careful measurements of norepinephrine kinetics and metabolism have not been conducted in patients with anorexia nervosa.

Patients with bulimia show decreased thyroid and sympathetic indices and metabolic rates, particularly after prolonged abstinence from binging and purging.[66,67] These data are compatible with the idea that decreased energy requirements for weight maintenance may be a risk factor for eating disorders, although whether this is a preexisting condition or is secondary to abnormal food intake patterns has not been established.

### HYPOTHALAMIC–PITUITARY–SOMATOTROPIC FUNCTION: RELATION TO BONE METABOLISM

Patients with anorexia nervosa generally exhibit hypersecretion of GH, which is coupled with low levels of IGF-I; this suggests a peripheral GH resistance.[68,69] This state is thought to be caused by a deficiency of metabolic fuels (e.g., amino acids and glu-

cose), which in turn impairs the peripheral sensitivity to GH at the receptor and postreceptor level.[70] The hypothesis has been raised that the low IGF-I may play a role in the significant osteoporosis that is seen in >50% of patients by causing a reduction in bone matrix deposition. The osteoporosis is thought to be multifactorial, with hypogonadism, elevated cortisol levels, poor nutrition with inadequate intake of calcium and vitamin D, and excess physical activity contributing to the clinical picture.

Hypoestrogenemia may be a major contributing factor in the development of bone loss. The degree of spinal osteopenia seen in patients with anorexia nervosa, however, is greater than that seen in other states of comparable hypoestrogenemia (i.e., hyperprolactinemia and hypothalamic amenorrhea). Studies have failed to show a significant reversal or prevention of bone loss by estrogen/progesterone supplementation combined with calcium supplementation[71]; this contrasts with their marked efficacy in the treatment of postmenopausal women.

Although an inadequate intake of calcium and vitamin D can lead to osteopenia, calcium intake and vitamin D levels do not correlate with bone density in anorexia nervosa,[72] and calcium supplementation has failed to lead to increased bone density in this patient group.[71]

Prolonged undernutrition is likely a major factor in the development of bone loss. Bone density correlates with body composition indices such as body mass index (BMI) and fat mass in women with anorexia nervosa. IGF-I is a nutritionally regulated hormone with potent effects on bone formation. The IGF-I levels, which are reduced and correlate with bone loss in anorexia, increase with weight gain.[49,73] IGF-I may be important for bone formation[49] and may be useful in the treatment of osteoporosis in anorexic patients.

Plasma levels of the adrenal androgen dehydroepiandrosterone (DHEA), which can also be converted to estrogen, decrease in patients with anorexia nervosa.[74] These patients may have decreased adrenal 17–20 lyase activity, contributing to increased cortisol and decreased DHEA production.[75,76] As estrogens tend to inhibit bone resorption whereas androgens promote bone formation,[77] this would indicate that low DHEA levels may play a role in the development of osteoporosis in this patient group. Indeed, one study[74] indicates that DHEA treatment decreases N-terminal cross-linked telopeptide of type I collagen (a marker of bone resorption), while increasing osteocalcin (a marker of bone formation).

## LEPTIN

Leptin is a protein product of the *ob* gene in mice (see Chap. 186). It is produced by adipose tissue and appears to convey information regarding the bodily adipose tissue mass to neural systems in the hypothalamus that are involved in the regulation of food intake (see Chaps. 125, 126, and 186). The leptin level is positively correlated with the percentage of body fat in both obese individuals and those of normal body weight. Serum leptin levels are low in patients with anorexia nervosa[48] (in apparent relationship to BMI). This correlation becomes uncoupled at extremely low BMIs, however, indicating a possible threshold effect. Although one study[78] showed that short-term refeeding (3 days) of anorexic patients who had very low BMIs did not increase leptin levels, more long-term nutritional rehabilitation and weight gain leads to increased serum leptin. Higher leptin levels have been found in weight-recovering patients than in comparable controls.[48] These findings suggest that factors in addition to body fat mass have a role in regulating the serum leptin level. Indeed, insulin, cytokines, and possibly GH and corticosteroids may stimulate the release of leptin independently of body fat.[79–84] The relatively higher level of leptin seen in patients with anorexia nervosa has been hypothesized to contribute to the difficulties these patients have with weight restoration and maintenance. Leptin appears to affect several neuroendocrine mechanisms, and animal studies have shown that, during starvation, leptin plays a role in activating the HPG and thyroidal axes (while depressing the HPA axis).[85] (See also ref. 84a.) Some have proposed that the decreased leptin levels observed in anorexic patients may be responsible for the amenorrhea observed in these patients. Indeed, all weight-recovered anorexic patients with normal menstrual cycles have leptin levels above a certain threshold.[86] However, leptin levels are no different in weight-recovered amenorrheic and eumenorrheic patients. This indicates that leptin is a necessary, but not a sufficient, factor for the resumption of menses in patients with anorexia nervosa.[87]

## CENTRAL NEUROPEPTIDE SYSTEMS

Appreciation of the richness and complexity of the CNS regulation of food intake has increased profoundly. Much of this regulation takes place within the hypothalamus; the arcuate nucleus, ventromedial nucleus, lateral hypothalamic area, and paraventricular nucleus play major roles. Multiple neuropeptide systems appear to have a part in food intake regulation; these include proopiomelanocortin (POMC), neuropeptide Y (NPY), galanin, CRH, cholecystokinin, and more newly described peptides (e.g., orexin/hypocretin). Many of these neuropeptides have been found both in the brain and in the gut. Alterations in some of these neuropeptide systems have been described in patients with anorexia nervosa.[88]

Altered endogenous opioid activity may play a role in the disturbed feeding behavior seen in anorexia nervosa. Animal studies indicate that opioid agonists increase and opioid antagonists decrease food intake.[89] Underweight anorectics are reported to have lower CSF β-endorphin levels than healthy volunteers, whereas long-term weight-restored patients have normal CSF β-endorphin levels. Therefore, reduced β-endorphin activity may play a role in the refusal of food observed in anorectics.

NPY is one of the most potent stimulants of feeding behavior seen in the CNS. NPY, which is found in the hypothalamus, stimulates feeding behavior when injected intracerebroventricularly in animals. Studies of persons with anorexia nervosa indicate that underweight anorexic patients have significantly higher levels of CSF NPY than do controls and that this level normalizes after long-term weight restoration.[88] Possibly, this elevation represents a homeostatic mechanism to stimulate feeding, which, however, is ineffective within this patient group because of down-regulation of NPY receptors. NPY may play a role in the amenorrhea seen in anorexic patients by reducing LH, as NPY is involved in regulating the release of LHRH into the hypophysial circulation[90] (see Chap. 125).

Although these substances are technically difficult to study directly in human subjects, further research on the roles of these and other substances in food-intake-regulation is likely to have important implications for the pathophysiology of eating disorders and may identify new targets for pharmacologic treatment of these disorders.

## REFERENCES

1. American Psychiatric Association. Diagnostic and statistical manual of mental disorders, 4th ed. Washington: American Psychiatric Press, 1994.
2. Gershon ES, Badner JA, Goldin LR, et al. Closing in on genes for manic depressive illness and schizophrenia. Neuropsychopharmacology 1998; 18(4):233.
3. DePaulo JJ, McMahon FJ. Recent developments in the genetics of bipolar disorder. Cold Spring Harb Symp Quant Biol 1996; 61(783):783.
4. Berrettini W. Progress and pitfalls: bipolar molecular linkage studies. J Affect Disord 1999; 50(2–3):287.
5. Baron M. Genetic linkage and bipolar affective disorder: progress and pitfalls. Mol Psychiatry 1997; 2(3):200.
6. Stokes PE, Sikes CR. The hypothalamic-pituitary-adrenocortical axis in major depression. Neurol Clin 1988; 6(1):1.
7. Joffe RT, Levitt AJ. The thyroid and depression. In: Joffe RT, Levitt AJ, eds.

8. Gold PW, Loriaux DL, Roy A, et al. Responses to corticotropin-releasing hormone in the hypercortisolism of depression and Cushing's disease: pathophysiologic and diagnostic implications. N Engl J Med 1986; 314:1329.
9. Amsterdam JD, Winokur A, Abelman E, et al. Cosyntropin (ACTH 1–24) stimulation test in depressed patients and healthy subjects. Am J Psychiatry 1983; 140(907):907.
10. Orth DN. Corticotropin-releasing hormone in humans. Endocr Rev 1992; 13:164.
11. Mitchell AJ. The role of corticotropin releasing factor in depressive illness: a critical review. Neurosci Biobehav Rev 1998; 22(5):635.
12. Nemeroff CB, Bissette G, Akil H, Fink M. Neuropeptide concentrations in the cerebrospinal fluid of depressed patients treated with electroconvulsive therapy. Corticotrophin-releasing factor, beta-endorphin and somatostatin. Br J Psychiatry 1991; 158(59):59.
13. De Bellis MD, Gold PW, Geracioti TD Jr, et al. Association of fluoxetine treatment with reductions in CSF concentrations of corticotropin-releasing hormone and arginine vasopressin in patients with major depression. Am J Psychiatry 1993; 150(4):656.
14. Heinrichs SC, Menzaghi F, Pich EM, et al. The role of CRF in behavioral aspects of stress. Ann N Y Acad Sci 1995; 771:92.
15. Deak T, Nguyen KT, Ehrlich AL, et al. The impact of the nonpeptide corticotropin-releasing hormone antagonist antalarmin on behavioral and endocrine responses to stress. Endocrinology 1999; 140(1):79.
16. Geracioti TD, Orth DN, Ekhator NN, et al. Serial cerebrospinal fluid corticotropin-releasing hormone concentrations in healthy and depressed humans. J Clin Endocrinol Metab 1992; 74:1325.
17. Gold PW. The endocrinology of melancholic and atypical depression: relation to neurocircuitry and somatic consequences. Proc Assoc Am Physicians 1999; 111(1):22.
18. Kling MA, Roy A, Doran AR, et al. Cerebrospinal fluid immunoreactive corticotropin-releasing hormone and adrenocorticotropin secretion in Cushing's disease and major depression: potential clinical implications. J Clin Endocrinol Metab 1991; 72(2):260.
19. Dorn LD, Burgess ES, Dubbert B, et al. Psychopathology in patients with endogenous Cushing's syndrome: "atypical" or melancholic features. Clin Endocrinol (Oxf) 1995; 43(4):433.
20. Weissman MM, Klerman GL. Sex differences and the epidemiology of depression. Arch Gen Psychiatry 1977; 3:98.
21. Altman N, Sachar EJ, Gruen PH, et al. Reduced plasma LH concentration in postmenopausal depressed women. Psychosom Med 1975; 37:274.
22. Rivest S, Rivier C. The role of corticotropin-releasing factor and interleukin-1 in the regulation of neurons controlling reproductive function. Endocr Rev 1995; 16:177.
23. Sirinathsinghji DJS, Rees LH, Rivier J, Vale W. Corticotropin-releasing factor is a potent inhibitor of sexual receptivity in the female rat. Nature 1983; 305:232.
24. Chrousos GP, Torpy DJ, Gold PW. Interactions between the hypothalamic-pituitary-adrenal axis and the female reproductive system: clinical implications (NIH Conference). Ann Intern Med 1998; 129:229.
25. Bebbington PE, Dunn G, Jenkins R, et al. The influence of age and sex on the prevalence of depressive conditions: report from the National Survey of Psychiatric Morbidity. Psychol Med 1998; 28:9.
26. McEwen BS. Clinical Review 108: the molecular and neuroanatomical basis for estrogen effects on the central nervous system. J Clin Endocrinol Metab 1999; 84(6):1790.
27. Arpels JC. The female brain hypoestrogenic continuum from the premenstrual syndrome to menopause. J Reprod Med 1996; 41:633.
28. Fink G, Sumner BE, Rosie R, et al. Estrogen control of central neurotransmission: effect on mood, mental state, and memory. Cell Mol Neurobiol 1996; 16:325.
29. Seeman MV. Psychopathology in women and men: focus on female hormones. Am J Psychiatry 1997; 154:1641.
30. Archer JS. Relationship between estrogen, serotonin, and depression. Menopause 1999; 6:71.
31. Gregoire AJP, Kumar R, Everitt B, et al. Transdermal oestrogen for treatment of severe post-natal depression. Lancet 1996; 347:930.
32. Rubinow DR, Schmidt PJ, Roca CA. Estrogen-serotonin interactions: implications for affective regulation. Biol Psychiatry 1998; 44:839.
33. Joffe H, Cohen LS. Estrogen, serotonin, and mood disturbance: where is the therapeutic bridge? Biol Psychiatry 1998; 44:798.
34. Esposito S, Prange AJ, Golden RN. The thyroid axis and mood disorders: overview and future prospects. Psychopharmacol Bull 1997; 33(2):205.
35. Joffe RT. The use of thyroid supplements to augment antidepressant medication. J Clin Psychiatry 1998; 5(26):26.
36. Whybrow PC, Prange AJ. A hypothesis of thyroid-catecholamine receptor interaction: its relevance to affective illness. Arch Gen Psychiatry 1981; 38:106.
37. Haggerty JJ, Silva SG, Marquardt M, et al. Prevalence of antithyroid antibodies in mood disorders. Depress Anxiety 1997; 5(2):91.
38. Woeber KA. Subclinical thyroid dysfunction. Arch Intern Med 1997; 157(10):1065.
39. Mendlewicz J, Linkowski P, Kerkhofs M, et al. Diurnal hypersecretion of growth hormone in depression. J Clin Endocrinol Metab 1985; 60:505.
40. Michelson D, Stratakis C, Hill L, et al. Bone mineral density in women with depression. N Engl J Med 1996; 335(16):1176.
40a. Reginster JY, Deroisy R, Paul I, et al. Depressive vulnerability is not an independent risk factor for osteoporosis in postmenopausal women. Maturitas 1999; 33:133.
41. Kling MA, Rubinow DR, Doran AR, et al. Cerebrospinal fluid immunoreactive somatostatin concentrations in patients with Cushing's disease and

major depression: relationship to indices of corticotropin-releasing hormone and cortisol secretion. Neuroendocrinology 1993; 57(1):79.

42. Kramer MS, Cutler N, Feighner J, et al. Distinct mechanism for antidepressant activity by blockade of central substance P receptors. Science 1998; 281(5383):1640.

42a. Cotrufo P, Monteleone P, d'Istria M, et al. Aggressive behavioral characteristics and endogenous hormones in women with bulimia nervosa. Neuropsychobiology 2000; 42:58.

43. Yanovski SZ. Biological correlates of binge eating. Addict Behav 1995; 20(6):705.

44. Birketvedt GS, Florholmen J, Sundsfjord J, et al. Behavioral and neuroendocrine characteristics of the night-eating syndrome. JAMA 1999; 282:657.

45. Neumarker KJ. Mortality and sudden death in anorexia nervosa. Int J Eat Disord 1997; 21(3):205.

46. Licinio J, Wong ML, Gold PW. The hypothalamic-pituitary-adrenal axis in anorexia nervosa. Psychiatry Res 1996; 62(1):75.

47. Gold PW, Kaye W, Robertson GL, Ebert M. Abnormalities in plasma and cerebrospinal fluid arginine vasopressin in patients with anorexia nervosa. N Engl J Med 1983; 308:1117.

48. Eckert ED, Pomeroy C, Raymond N, et al. Leptin in anorexia nervosa. J Clin Endocrinol Metab 1998; 83(3):791.

49. Grinspoon S, Baum H, Lee K, et al. Effects of short term rhIGF-I administration on bone turnover in osteopenic women with anorexia nervosa. J Clin Endocrinol Metab 1996; 81:3864.

49a. Seed JA, Dixon RA, McCluskey SE, Yang AH. Basal activity of the hypothalamic–pituitary–adrenal axis and cognitive function in anorexia nervosa. Eur Arch Psychiatry Clin Neurosci 2000; 250:11.

50. Doerr P, Fichter M, Pirke KM, Lund R. Relationship between weight gain and hypothalamic pituitary adrenal function in patients with anorexia nervosa. J Steroid Biochem 1980; 13:529.

51. Gold PW, Gwirtsman H, Avgerinos PC, et al. Abnormal hypothalamic-pituitary-adrenal function in anorexia nervosa. Pathophysiologic mechanisms in underweight and weight-corrected patients. N Engl J Med 1986; 314(21):1335.

52. Kling MA, Demitrack MA, Whitfield HJJ, et al. Effects of the glucocorticoid antagonist RU 486 on pituitary-adrenal function in patients with anorexia nervosa and healthy volunteers: enhancement of plasma ACTH and cortisol secretion in underweight patients. Neuroendocrinology 1993; 57(6):1082.

53. Kaye WH, Gwirtsman H, George DT, et al. Elevated cerebrospinal fluid levels of immunoreactive corticotropin releasing hormone in anorexia nervosa: relationship to state of nutrition, adrenal function, and intensity of depression. J Clin Endocrinol Metab 1987; 64:203.

54. Mortola JF, Rasmussen DD, Yen SS. Alterations of the adrenocorticotropin-cortisol axis in normal weight bulimic women: evidence for a central mechanism. J Clin Endocrinol Metab 1989; 68(3):517.

55. Demitrack MA, Kalogeras KT, Altemus M, et al. Plasma and cerebrospinal fluid measures of arginine vasopressin secretion in patients with bulimia nervosa and in healthy subjects. J Clin Endocrinol Metab 1992; 74:1277.

56. Nishita JK, Ellinwood EHJ, Rockwell WJK, et al. Abnormalities in the response of plasma arginine vasopressin during hypertonic saline infusion in patients with eating disorders. Biol Psychiatry 1989; 26:73.

57. Chiodera P, Volpi R, Marchesi C, et al. Reduction in the arginine vasopressin responses to metoclopramide and insulin-induced hypoglycemia in normal weight bulimic women. Neuroendocrinology 1993; 57:907.

58. Morimoto Y, Oishi T, Hanasaki N, et al. Interactions among amenorrhea, serum gonadotropins and body weight in anorexia nervosa. Endocrinol Jpn 1980; 27:191.

59. Warren MP, Vande Wiele RL. Clinical and metabolic features of anorexia nervosa. Am J Obstet Gynecol 1973; 117:435.

60. Garfinkel RE, Brown GM, Stancer HC, Moldofsky H. Hypothalamic-pituitary function in anorexia nervosa. Arch Gen Psychiatry 1975; 32:739.

61. Vigersky RA, Loriaux DL, Anderson AE, Lipsett MB. Anorexia nervosa: behavioral and hypothalamic aspects. Clin Endocrinol Metab 1976; 5:517.

62. Luger A, Deuster PA, Kyle SB, et al. Acute hypothalamic-pituitary-adrenal responses to the stress of treadmill exercise: physiologic adaptations to physical training. N Engl J Med 1987; 316(21):1309.

63. Kaye WH, Jimerson DC, Lake CR, Ebert MH. Altered norepinephrine metabolism following long-term weight recovery in patients with anorexia nervosa. Psychiatry Res 1985; 14:333.

64. Landsberg L, Young JB. Endocrine changes in anorexia nervosa; an interpretation based on the metabolic adaptation to caloric restriction. In: Brown GM, Relchlin KS, eds. Neuroendocrinology and psychiatric disorder. New York: Raven Press, 1984:349.

65. Obarzanek E, Lesem M, Jimerson D. Resting metabolic rate of anorexia nervosa patients during weight gain. Am J Clin Nutr 1994; 60:666.

66. Altemus M, Hetherington MM, Flood M, et al. Decrease in resting metabolic rate during abstinence from bulimic behavior. Am J Psychiatry 1991; 148:1071.

67. Obarzanek E, Lesem MD, Goldstein DS, Jimerson DC. Reduced resting metabolic rate in patients with bulimia nervosa. Arch Gen Psychiatry 1991; 48:456.

68. Gianotti L, Broglio F, Aimaretti G, et al. Low IGF-I levels are often uncoupled with elevated GH levels in catabolic conditions. J Endocrinol 1998; 21:115.

69. Gianotti L, Rolla M, Arvat E, et al. Effect of somatostatin infusion on the somatotrope responsiveness to growth hormone-releasing hormone in patients with anorexia nervosa. Biol Psychiatry 1999; 45:334.

70. Thissen J, Keteslegers JM, Underwood LE. Nutritional regulation of the insulin like growth factors. Endocr Rev 1994; 15:80.

71. Klibanski A, Biller BM, Schoenfeld DA, et al. The effects of estrogen administration on trabecular bone loss in young women with anorexia nervosa. J Clin Endocrinol Metab 1995; 80(3):898.

72. Carmichael KA, Carmichael DH. Bone metabolism and osteopenia in eating disorders. Medicine 1995; 74:254.

73. Counts DR, Gwirtsman H, Carlsson LMS, et al. The effects of anorexia nervosa and refeeding on growth-hormone-binding protein, the IGFs and the IGF binding proteins. J Clin Endocrinol Metab 1992; 75:762.

74. Gordon CM, Grace E, Jean ES, et al. Changes in bone turnover markers and menstrual function after short-term oral DHEA in young women with anorexia nervosa. J Bone Miner Res 1999; 14(1):136.

75. Devesa J, Perez-Fernandez R, Bokser L, et al. Adrenal androgen secretion and dopaminergic activity in anorexia nervosa. Horm Metab Res 1987; 20:57.

76. Zumoff B, Walsh BT, Katz JL, et al. Subnormal plasma DHEA to cortisol ratio in anorexia nervosa: a second hormonal parameter of ontogenic regression. J Clin Endocrinol Metab 1983; 56:668.

77. Raisz LG, Wiita B, Artis A, et al. Comparison of the effects of estrogen alone and estrogen plus androgen on biochemical markers of bone formation and resorption in postmenopausal women. J Clin Endocrinol Metab 1996; 81:37.

78. Balligand JL, Brichard SM, Brichard V, et al. Hypoleptinemia in patients with anorexia nervosa: loss of circadian rhythm and unresponsiveness to short-term refeeding. Eur J Endocrinol 1998; 138(4):415.

79. Carro E, Senaris R, Considine RV, et al. Regulation of in vivo growth hormone secretion by leptin. Endocrinology 1997; 138:2203.

80. Bereis K, Vosmeer SUK. Effects of glucocorticoids and of growth hormone on serum leptin. Eur J Endocrinol 1996; 135:663.

81. Sarraf P, Frederich RC, Turner EM, et al. Multiple cytokines and acute inflammation raise mouse leptin levels: potential role in inflammatory anorexia. J Exp Med 1997; 185:171.

82. Grunfeld C, Zhao C, Fuller J, et al. Endotoxin and cytokines induce expression of leptin, the ob gene product, in hamsters. A role for leptin in the anorexia of infection. J Clin Invest 1996; 97:2152.

83. Malmstrom R, Taskinen MR, Daronen SLY-JH. Insulin increases plasma leptin concentrations in normal subjects and patients with NIDDM. Diabetologia 1996; 39:993.

84. Boden G, Chen X, Mazzoli MIR. The effect of fasting on serum leptin in normal human subjects. J Clin Endocrinol Metab 1996; 81:3419.

84a. Monteleone PD; Lieto A, Tortorella A, et al. Circulating Peptin in patients with anorexia nervosa, bulimia nervosa or binge-eating disorder: relationship to body weight, eating patterns, psychopathology and endocrine changes. Psychiatry Res 2000; 94:121.

85. Ahima R, Pkabakaran D, Mantzoros C, et al. Role of leptin in the neuroendocrine response to fasting. Nature 1996; 382:250.

86. Kopp W, Blum WF, Von PS, et al. Low leptin levels predict amenorrhea in underweight and eating disordered females. Mol Psychiatry 1997; 2(4):335.

87. Audi L, Mantzoros CS, Vidal PA, et al. Leptin in relation to resumption of menses in women with anorexia nervosa. Mol Psychiatry 1998; 3(6):544.

88. Kaye WH. Neuropeptide abnormalities in anorexia nervosa. Psychiatry Res 1996; 62(1):65.

89. Morley JE, Levine AS, Yim GK, Lowry MT. Opioid modulation of appetite. Neurosci Biobehav Rev 1983; 7:281.

90. Kalra SP, Allen LG, Clark JT, et al. Neuropeptide Y—an integrator of reproductive and appetitive functions. In: Moody TW, ed. Neural and endocrine peptides and behavior. New York: Plenum Press, 1986:353.

# C H A P T E R  2 0 2

# RESPIRATION AND ENDOCRINOLOGY

PRASHANT K. ROHATGI AND KENNETH L. BECKER

Hormones play a vital role in normal fetal lung maturation and also influence postnatal pulmonary structure and function. Therefore, it is not surprising that endocrine disease can exert profound effects on the respiratory system.

## INFLUENCE OF HORMONES ON FETAL LUNG MATURATION AND THE SURFACTANT SYSTEM

Pulmonary development is a continuous process that begins in the early embryo and continues for several years during postnatal life. A critical stage in prenatal lung development is the alveolar stage, beginning at 26 to 28 weeks, which is associated with the formation of rudimentary alveoli, the maturation of the sur-

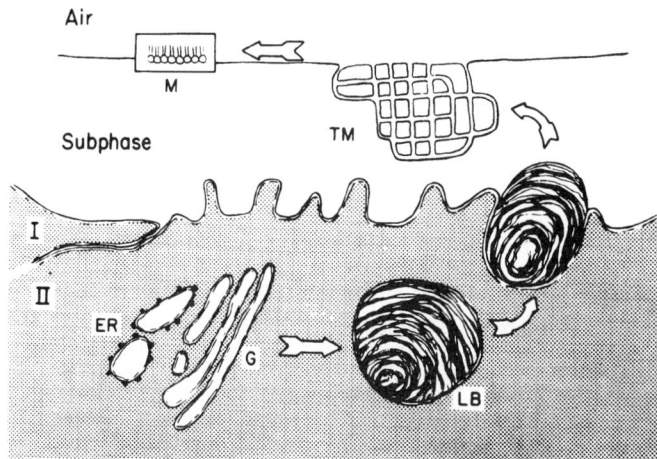

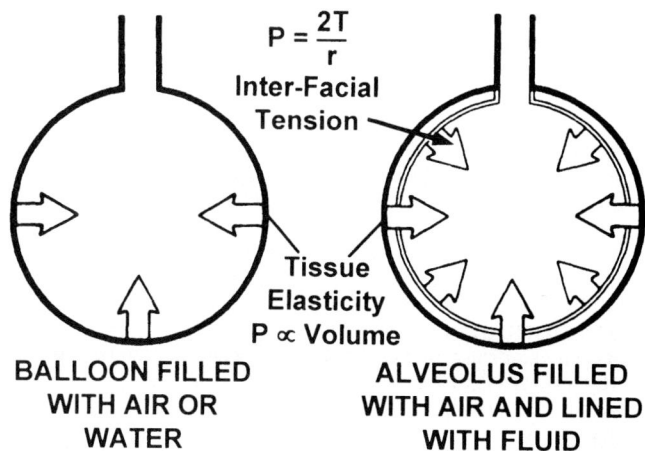

$$P = \frac{2T}{r}$$

Inter-Facial
Tension

Tissue
Elasticity
P ∝ Volume

**BALLOON FILLED WITH AIR OR WATER**

**ALVEOLUS FILLED WITH AIR AND LINED WITH FLUID**

**FIGURE 202-1.** Diagram of the formation and secretion of pulmonary surfactant by the type II epithelial cells (granular pneumocytes). After the migration of the lamellar bodies to the apex of the cell, they are extruded by exocytosis into the alveolar subphase and expand into tubular myelin (*TM*) figures. At the air-liquid interface, the figures spread into a monolayer (*M*). (*ER*, endoplasmic reticulum; *G*, Golgi apparatus; *LB*, lamellar bodies in which surfactant is stored.) (From Goerke J. Lung surfactant. Biochim Biophys Acta 1974; 344:241.)

**FIGURE 202-2.** The concept of interfacial tension and the physiologic role of surfactant: A rubber balloon filled with water or air (*left*) tends to empty because of the retractile pressure that is generated by the elasticity of the rubber. Similarly, in the lungs (*right*), the alveoli also generate retractile pressure because of tissue elasticity; this pressure is roughly proportional to the lung volume and is maximal at total lung capacity (i.e., the lung volume at maximal inspiration). Another dominant component of the total retractile pressure in the alveolus is that generated by surface tension due to (or because of) the air-liquid interface. Surface tension is a physical phenomenon inherent at interfaces between two dissimilar phases (in alveoli, it is the air-liquid interface), which generates a surface force that reduces the surface area (and consequently the volume) of the air-liquid interface. The retractile pressure caused by surface tension can be estimated from the Laplace relation $P = 2T/r$ ($P$ is pressure, $T$ is surface tension, and $r$ is alveolar radius). It is obvious from the relationship of T and r that the retractile pressure from surface tension increases with the decrease in the size of the alveoli and would be maximal toward the end of expiration. Thus, the transpulmonary pressure required to counterbalance the retractile force of tissue elasticity would be the least toward the end of expiration; however, the transpulmonary pressure required to counteract the surface tension and prevent the alveoli from total collapse during expiration would be highest during end-expiration. The pulmonary surfactant, which lines the alveoli and becomes more concentrated in the air-liquid interface during expiration, progressively reduces this interfacial tension during expiration and, thereby, decreases the levels of transpulmonary pressures required to prevent alveolar collapse. Furthermore, surfactant reduces the work of breathing and also prevents alveolar edema.

factant system (type II pneumocytes and their product surfactant), and the preparation of the liquid-filled lungs for their eventual extrauterine function of gas exchange.[1]

A close relationship exists between fetal viability and the maturation of the surfactant system.[2] Pulmonary surfactant (Figs. 202-1 and 202-2), which lines the alveolar spaces and small airways, is a complex mixture of lung proteins (10%) and lipids (90%), with dipalmitoylphosphatidylcholine (lecithin) being the major surface-active phospholipid component.

Apoproteins consist of four distinct lung-specific surfactant-associated proteins, SP-A, SP-B, SP-C, and SP-D. SP-A and SP-D are hydrophilic glycoproteins that contain a collagenous amino-terminal domain and a noncollagenous lectin-like carboxy-terminal domain. SP-B and SP-C are hydrophobic proteins. The genes for these proteins are expressed only in type II alveolar epithelial cells of the lungs and perhaps in certain bronchiolar epithelial cells that share the same embryonic lineage. Not only are these genes located on different chromosomes, but they respond differently to hormonal influences, suggesting that they are independently regulated. These proteins mediate the transformation of lamellar bodies into tubular myelin, accelerate the rate of adsorption and spreading of the phospholipids into a monolayer, help in phospholipid recycling and metabolism by facilitating the uptake of phospholipids by type II pneumocytes, and enhance pulmonary defense by modulating phagocytosis, bacterial killing, and chemotaxis of alveolar macrophages.[3,4]

The major function of surfactant is to reduce the surface tension that otherwise would be generated by the presence of the fluid-gas interface within the alveoli and small airways, thereby protecting alveoli from collapsing, reducing the work of breathing, and preventing alveolar edema. Neonates who lack a mature, "complete" surfactant system, or who have a deficiency of a specific component, develop neonatal respiratory distress syndrome (NRDS). The normal maturation of type II pneumocytes, and the synthesis and secretion of surfactant, is influenced by several hormones[5] (Table 202-1).

## GLUCOCORTICOIDS

The important physiologic role that glucocorticoids play in the regulation of the fetal surfactant system is suggested by the fol-

lowing observations in humans: (a) a surge in cortisol levels in amniotic fluid before the maturation of the surfactant system as evidenced by a rise in the lecithin/sphingomyelin (L/S) ratio in the amniotic fluid, (b) an inverse relationship between cortisol levels in cord blood and NRDS, and (c) the demonstration that the antepartum administration of glucocorticoids accelerates maturation of the surfactant system with a decrease in the incidence of NRDS in high-risk pregnancies.[5a] In animal studies, the antepartum administration of exogenous glucocorticoids is associated with binding of the hormone to its receptors in the cytosol and nucleus of type II pneumocytes, slowing of cytodifferentiation of type II pneumocytes into type I pneumocytes, ultrastructural evidence of maturation of type II pneumocytes with abundant lamellar inclusion bodies, and enhanced choline phosphate cytidyltransferase (CPCT) activity in the lung with an increase in choline incorporation into phosphatidylcholine. Moreover, there is a several-fold increase in surfactant phospholipid in bronchoalveolar lavage fluid and in the lungs, a significant increase in the L/S ratio in amniotic fluid, physiologic evidence of greater pulmonary distensibility and deflation stability, and an enhanced survival of the prematurely delivered fetus. In lung explant studies, glucocorticoids induce increases in SP-B and SP-C proteins and their messenger RNAs (mRNAs), whereas a variable response is observed in SP-A, depending on

**TABLE 202-1.**
The Influence of Hormones on Fetal Lung Maturation and Surfactant Synthesis

| | Glucocorticoids | Thyroid Hormone | Estrogen | Prolactin | Insulin* |
|---|---|---|---|---|---|
| RECEPTORS PRESENT IN THE LUNG | Yes | Yes | No | Yes | Yes |
| INDUCES MORPHOLOGIC CHANGES ASSOCIATED WITH MATURATION OF TYPE II PNEUMOCYTES | Yes | Yes | Yes | Yes | No |
| INDUCES CHANGES IN LUNG MECHANICS ASSOCIATED WITH REDUCED GAS-FLUID INTERFACIAL TENSION | Yes | Yes | — | — | No |
| CONCENTRATION OF LUNG AND AMNIOTIC FLUID SURFACE-ACTIVE PHOSPHOLIPIDS | Increase | Increase | Increase | Increase | Normal or reduced |
| PHOSPHOLIPID SYNTHESIS IN LUNG | Increase | Increase | Increase | Increase | Decrease |
| INDUCTION OF CPCT WITH INCORPORATION OF CHOLINE IN PHOSPHATIDYLCHOLINE | Yes | Yes | Yes | No | Inhibits |
| CONCENTRATION OF SURFACTANT | | | | | |
| PROTEIN A | Increase/decrease | Decrease | — | — | Decrease |
| PROTEIN B | Increase | Decrease | — | — | Decrease |
| PROTEIN C | Increase | Decrease | — | — | No effect |
| CONCENTRATION OF SURFACTANT | | | | | |
| PROTEIN A mRNA | Increase/decrease | No effect | Increase | — | Decrease |
| PROTEIN B mRNA | Increase | No effect | Increase | — | Decrease |
| PROTEIN C mRNA | Increase | No effect | Decrease | — | No effect |
| IMPROVES SURVIVAL | Yes | Yes | — | — | Yes? |

CPCT, choline phosphate cytidyltransferase; mRNA, messenger RNA.
*Based on studies of fetuses of diabetic mothers, it is difficult to separate the effects of insulin per se from the effects of changes in glucose levels.

the dose and duration of glucocorticoid administration. In vivo studies have demonstrated an increase in SP-A protein and mRNA, an increase in SP-B mRNA, and a decrease in SP-C mRNA.

## THYROID HORMONES

Thyroid hormones influence the maturation of the fetal lung and regulate surfactant synthesis. Low levels of thyroid hormones in cord blood have been found in neonates who develop NRDS. Interestingly, the intraamniotic injection of thyroxine to high-risk pregnant women whose infants were to be delivered prematurely induced changes in amniotic fluid typical for the mature fetal lung; perhaps more significantly, none of the premature babies developed NRDS. Type II pneumocytes have nuclear receptors for triiodothyronine. Hypothyroidism is associated with smaller type II pneumocytes, smaller and fewer lamellar bodies, and decreased synthesis of surfactant. After the administration of thyroid hormones, these morphologic changes reverse: There is increased choline incorporation into phosphatidylcholine subsequent to increased CPCT activity, increased fatty acid synthesis because of increased activity of fatty acid synthetase and acetyl coenzyme A carboxylase, augmented protein synthesis, improved lung mechanics, and increased recovery of surfactant from lung. Thyroid hormones do not enhance any of the surfactant proteins. In fact, they decrease SP-A and SP-B mRNA.

## ESTROGEN

In humans, a surge in blood estrogen levels precedes the increase in the L/S ratio in the amniotic fluid, and plasma estrogen levels are decreased in infants with NRDS. In addition, the administration of estrogen to pregnant women increases the L/S ratio in amniotic fluid. In animal studies, the administration of estrogen to mothers produces the following effects in the fetus: accelerated morphologic maturation of the lung, increased choline incorporation into phosphatidylcholine by stimulating the activity of CPCT, and an increased amount of surface-active

phospholipids recovered by lung lavage. These effects are mediated by estrogen-binding macromolecules in the cytosol of lung cells and not by classic estrogen receptors, which are lacking in the lung. Estrogen increases SP-A and SP-B mRNA, and decreases SP-C mRNA.

## PROLACTIN

The circumstantial evidence for a role of prolactin in the maturation of the surfactant system of humans includes the presence of receptors for prolactin in fetal lungs, the surge in prolactin levels in fetal blood that precedes and parallels the increase in the L/S ratio in amniotic fluid, and the presence of low cord blood prolactin levels in infants with NRDS. The role of this hormone in surfactant production also is supported by animal studies that have shown an increase in total phospholipids, phosphatidylcholine, and lecithin in lung tissue extracts of animals treated with prolactin, and a reduction in lung lavage phospholipids when animals were treated with bromocriptine, an inhibitor of prolactin secretion.

## INSULIN

The incidence of NRDS is increased six-fold in infants of mothers with diabetes because of a delay in the maturation of the lung and its surfactant system. Insulin receptors are present in fetal lung. Glucose freely crosses the placenta from mother to fetus and induces the fetal pancreas to produce more insulin. There is conflicting evidence concerning whether hyperinsulinemia or hyperglycemia is responsible for these adverse effects on the lung. In animals, fetal lung maturation has been studied by inducing diabetes in pregnant mothers with alloxan or streptozocin. These studies revealed morphologic evidence of delayed maturation, such as poorly developed alveoli, less well-differentiated epithelium, and intracellular accumulation of lamellar bodies in type II pneumocytes. Moreover, there was less retention of air on deflation, suggesting a propensity for alveolar collapse; reduced surface activity in lung lavage in association with diminished recovery of lecithin; decreased activity of CPCT; and diminished synthesis of lecithin, phosphatidylcholine, and phosphatidyl glycerol. Some of these findings may be due to an antagonism by insulin of the normal effects of cortisol on the enzymes of surfactant synthesis. Insulin decreases SP-A and SP-B proteins and their mRNAs, and has no effect on SP-C protein or its mRNA. Adequate glucose control of maternal diabetes appears to reduce the risk of fetal pulmonary immaturity.[6]

## OTHER HORMONES

Thyrotropin and corticotropin accelerate maturation of the surfactant system, presumably by increasing fetal thyroid hormones and glucocorticoids.[7] Interestingly, corticotropin also may act independently of its corticotropic effect. The administration of phospholipids extracted from the hypothalamus accelerates the maturation of the surfactant system, and this effect is not the result of increased availability of substrate for surfactant synthesis. Epidermal growth factor also may play a role in lung maturation.[8] In addition, decreased concentrations of mammalian bombesin have been found in the lungs of infants with NRDS.

## INFLUENCE OF DISORDERS OF THE ENDOCRINE SYSTEM ON THE RESPIRATORY SYSTEM

### HYPOTHALAMUS

Hypothalamic disorders can influence the respiratory tract by influencing the autonomic nervous system, by affecting the respiratory drive, or by producing hypopituitarism. The hypothalamus influences the cyclic changes in nasal resistance to airflow by affecting the sympathetic tone that controls blood flow, thereby modifying the turgidity of the mucosa and the humidification of inspired air. Patients with Kallmann syndrome, who have hypothalamic atrophy, lack cyclic changes in nasal resistance.[9] The hypothalamus also regulates the diurnal variation of bronchomotor tone by influencing the vagal tone; however, abnormalities of bronchomotor tone have not been evaluated in hypothalamic disorders. Intense hypothalamic stimulation following an acute intracranial pathology associated with increased intracranial pressure has been implicated in the pathogenesis of life-threatening neurogenic pulmonary edema.[10] In humans, hypothalamic dysfunction, initially suspected because of hyperphagia in patients with hypopituitarism, has been associated with central hypoventilation, depressed ventilatory response to inspired carbon dioxide, and hypoventilation during exercise.[11] Abnormal breathing patterns, including sleep apnea, have been described in Prader-Willi and Kleine-Levin syndromes associated with hypothalamic dysfunction.[12] Interestingly, corticotropin-releasing hormone is a respiratory stimulant in humans.[13]

### PITUITARY GLAND

Of the hormones produced by the pituitary gland, only growth hormone is known to have significant effects on the respiratory system. The effects of diminished as well as excessive secretion of growth hormone on the respiratory system depend on the age at which the disorder begins. This hormone influences growth and development maximally during childhood, to a limited extent in adulthood, and minimally, if at all, during fetal development.

### GROWTH HORMONE DEFICIENCY

Newborns with hypopituitarism are of normal length and weight and have normally developed lungs. Retardation in linear growth is apparent within the first few years of life and is associated with

a proportionate decrease in the size of the thorax and lungs, but there is no clinically recognizable respiratory impairment or changes in arterial blood gases. Although unproven, it is believed that these lungs would demonstrate fewer and smaller alveoli, as well as smaller bronchi and bronchioles.

In acquired causes of hypopituitarism, the growth is normal until somatotropic deficiency develops. A child who acquires growth hormone deficiency during adolescence will have poorly developed paranasal sinuses and smaller lungs.[14] The lungs would be expected to show small alveoli that are normal in number, because alveolar multiplication in humans is complete by preadolescence, and any further increase in lung volumes results primarily from increased size of the alveoli.

Patients with adult-onset hypopituitarism, who are being treated with replacement of thyroid, adrenal, and sex hormones, but not with growth hormone, have no clinically recognizable respiratory symptoms. However, pulmonary function studies demonstrate reduced static lung volumes, with disproportionate reductions in functional residual capacity and residual volume as well as increased lung elastic recoil, but normal respiratory muscle strength, flow rates, and gas exchange. Recurrent nasal polyps have been noted in Sheehan syndrome.[15] Although pituitary adenylate cyclase–activating peptide 38 is a potent endogenously produced dilator of human airways, its pathophysiologic effects are unknown.[15a]

### GROWTH HORMONE EXCESS

Persons with acromegaly die prematurely, and deaths attributed to respiratory disease are three times more frequent. This probably is related to adverse functional consequences of structural changes in the upper and lower respiratory tract, as described in Table 202-2.[16] On physical examination, the overgrowth of the ribs and the enlarged vertebral bodies may produce striking thoracic deformity (Fig. 202-3).

**Pulmonary Function Changes.** Persons with acromegaly have large lungs.[17] There is a significant correlation between the duration of acromegaly and lung size as measured by total lung capacity. The increase in total lung capacity with normal diffusing capacity seen in humans with acromegaly has been attributed to increase in size and perhaps to increase in number of alveoli.[18]

**Upper Airways Obstruction.** Persons with acromegaly have intrathoracic and extrathoracic airways obstruction. They are especially predisposed to upper airway obstruction because of (a) encroachment of the lumen of the upper airways by generalized thickening of the mucosa, (b) macroglossia (Fig. 202-4), and (c) narrowing of the opening between the vocal cords.[19] The last problem may result from hypertrophy of the vocal cords or from fixation of the vocal cords by any of the following mechanisms: enlargement of arytenoid cartilages with impaired mobility of cricoarytenoid joints; paralysis of the recurrent laryngeal nerve because of demyelination or stretching by overgrown laryngeal cartilaginous structures, or by an enlarged thyroid gland, which can occur in acromegaly; and myopathic changes in laryngeal muscles. The spectrum of obstruction ranges from physiologic evidence of upper airway obstruction without clinical manifestations, to chronic upper airway obstruction with hoarseness and dyspnea on exertion, to the development of acute upper airway obstruction with stridor during the induction of anesthesia, on extubation, or after acute viral upper respiratory tract infections (this may require emergency tracheotomy).

**Sleep Apnea.** Sleep apnea, primarily the obstructive form, has been recognized in patients with acromegaly and may be responsible for daytime somnolence, noisy snoring, and life-threatening arrhythmias during sleep.[20,21,21a] During these obstructive apneic episodes, there is no airflow at the entrance to the upper airways, in spite of persistent thoracic and abdominal

**TABLE 202-2.**
**Effect of Some Endocrine and Metabolic Disorders on the Respiratory System**

**GROWTH HORMONE DYSFUNCTION**

*Acromegaly*

**Structural changes**

Lower respiratory tract and thoracic cage

Thickening of clavicles and ribs because of periosteal bone growth

Clavicles and ribs lengthen because of endochondral proliferation, resulting in enlargement of the thoracic cavity

Thoracic kyphosis because of enlargement of vertebral bodies, narrowing of intervertebral disk spaces anteriorly, and limitation of anteflexion

Enlargement of lungs; this is more common in males, probably because of modulating effect of sex hormones

Narrowing of small airways

Lung ossification: pneumopathia osteoplastica racemosa

Upper respiratory tract

Excessive pneumatization of paranasal sinuses

Macroglossia with prognathism

Excessive deposition of connective tissue resulting in thickening, hypertrophy, and congestion of mucosa lining the upper airways

Narrowing of the opening between vocal cords

**Functional changes**

Total lung capacity, vital capacity, and other static lung volumes are greater than predicted for age, sex, and height

Increase in anatomic dead space proportional to increase in the size of the lungs

No evidence of intrathoracic large airway obstruction

Significant incidence of small airway narrowing

Evidence of extrathoracic airway obstruction

Normal diffusing capacity, but reduced transfer coefficient

Normal elastic recoil

Normal specific lung compliance

Normal or reduced inspiratory and expiratory muscle strength

**THYROID DYSFUNCTION**

*Hyperthyroidism*

Alterations in pulmonary function because of combination of myopathy, increase in basal metabolic rate, and increase in hypercapnic ventilatory drive

Exertional dyspnea and impaired cardiopulmonary exercise capacity

Worsening of coexistent asthma

*Hypothyroidism*

Alterations in pulmonary function caused by a combination of myopathy, diaphragmatic dysfunction, obesity, anemia, and cardiac dysfunction

Alveolar hypoventilation and $CO_2$ narcosis

Obstructive sleep apnea syndrome, disordered sleep architecture

Hoarseness caused by infiltration of vocal cords by myxomatous tissue

Nodular pulmonary parenchymal opacities caused by localized edema or myxomatous infiltration of lung

Pleural effusion

Amelioration of coexistent asthma

Leftward shift of oxygen-hemoglobin dissociation with worsening of tissue hypoxia

Pulmonary edema

**ABNORMALITIES OF CALCIUM AND PHOSPHATE METABOLISM**

*Hyperparathyroidism*

Metastatic pulmonary calcification

Subperiosteal resorption of distal ends of clavicle

Postparathyroidectomy improvement in pulmonary function, especially in asthmatics, is due to correction of metabolic acidosis and/or myopathy

*Hypoparathyroidism*

Tetany with laryngeal spasm

Increase in bronchomotor tone from spontaneous electrical activity in autonomic ganglia

*Hyperphosphatemia*

Has no respiratory consequences

*Hypophosphatemia*

Acute respiratory failure caused by respiratory muscle weakness

Adversely affects tissue oxygenation by (a) producing hemolytic anemia and (b) shifting oxygen-hemoglobin dissociation to left because of decreased synthesis of 2,3-diphosphatidylglycerol

*Rickets*

Rachitic rosary caused by bulge in the costochondral junction

Harrison groove caused by indentation of ribs at points of diaphragmatic insertion

Deformity of rib cage may lead to alveolar hypoventilation and respiratory failure

*Osteomalacia*

Pseudofractures in ribs and scapula

Kyphosis caused by biconcavity and loss of height of thoracic vertebrae

---

respiratory movement, suggesting occlusion of the upper airways. The fact that these apneic episodes occur only during sleep indicates that the occlusion is not related solely to anatomic narrowing of the airways, but also to superimposed abnormalities in upper airway function, which cause the oropharyngeal airway to collapse and occlude the airway. The collapse of the oropharynx is related to the interaction of at least three physiologic factors, all of which are operative in acromegaly: (a) Narrowing of the oropharyngeal lumen occurs caused by hyperplasia of soft tissues; (b) changes in the oronasopharynx take place, producing an increase in upstream airflow resistance, thereby leading to the development of greater subatmospheric pressure in the airways during inspiration; and (c) most importantly, during sleep, the inadequate increase in the tone of the upper airway muscles during inspiration results in their inability to prevent collapse of the upper airways during inspiration. Nasopharyngeal endoscopy performed during episodes of obstructive apnea has demonstrated collapse of the posterior and lateral hypopharyngeal walls during inspiration, before any posterior movement of the tongue.[22] The sleep apnea episodes may be responsive to treatment with bromocriptine and octreotide.[23,24] Polysomnographic studies in patients with acromegaly have found central sleep apnea to occur in ~50% of cases. The mechanism for altered respiratory control during sleep is not clear, but may be related to interaction of depressed levels of somatostatin, which is known to be involved in the control of breathing, and elevated levels of insulin-like growth factor-I.[25,26] In this regard, octreotide therapy has been reported to be useful.[27]

## THYROID GLAND (SEE TABLE 202-2)

### HYPERTHYROIDISM

**Pulmonary Function Changes.** Alterations in pulmonary function in persons with hyperthyroidism stem from the development of myopathy affecting respiratory muscles, including the diaphragm; increased central respiratory drive; and increased metabolism.[28] Total lung capacity and functional residual capacity usually are normal. However, vital capacity and maximum breathing capacity are reduced, primarily because of diminished muscle strength. Lung compliance is slightly decreased. Airway resistance is unaffected.

In persons with hyperthyroidism, basal oxygen consumption and the absolute oxygen consumption at each level of work are

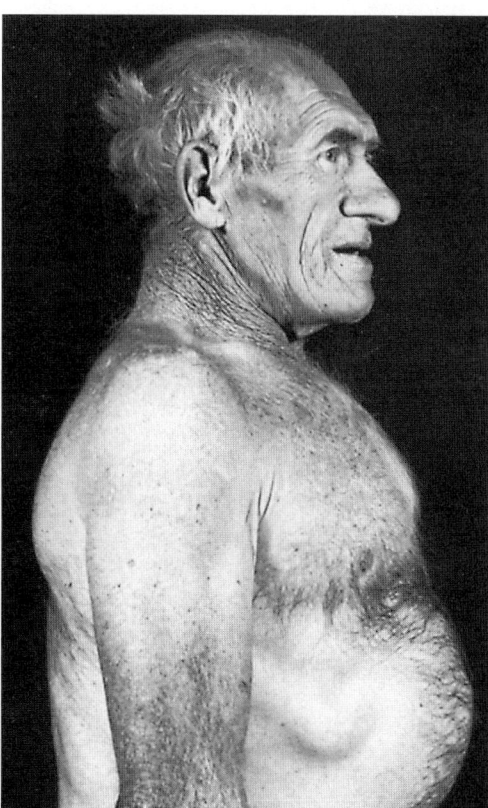

**FIGURE 202-3.** Kyphotic, deformed chest in a 65-year-old man with acromegaly. Note the increased anteroposterior diameter of the barrel-shaped thorax related to the transverse position of the thickened and lengthened ribs.

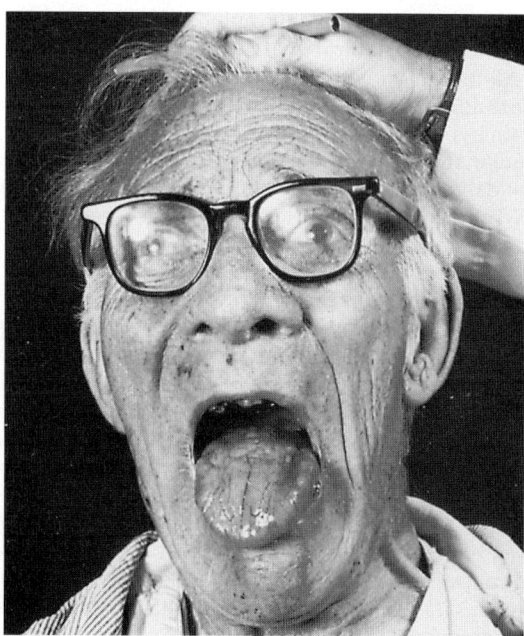

**FIGURE 202-4.** Macroglossia in a 70-year-old man with acromegaly. Note also the cranial nerve palsy, involving the extraocular muscles, that was due to the enlarging pituitary tumor. Other causes of macroglossia include hypothyroidism, amyloidosis, the Beckwith-Wiedemann syndrome, Down syndrome, Hurler syndrome (mucopolysaccharidosis I), hemangioma, lymphangioma, and plexiform neurofibromatosis.

increased, although the increment in oxygen consumption per unit increase in workload is comparable to that in normal persons. This requires an augmentation of ventilation. Because of muscle weakness and decreased lung compliance, this augmentation is achieved by increasing the frequency of breathing, rather than the tidal volume, and leads to increased dead-space ventilation, a disproportionate increase in minute ventilation, and dyspnea. Central respiratory drive in response to hypercapnia and hypoxia is increased, and, again, this disproportionate increase in minute ventilation is achieved predominantly by augmenting the frequency of breathing.[29,30]

**Bronchial Asthma.** The increase in bronchial reactivity and the worsening of coexistent asthma with the onset of hyperthyroidism are well established, although the mechanism remains unclear.[31] Hypotheses explaining the biochemical link between asthma and hyperthyroidism have centered around altered metabolism of catecholamines, corticosteroids, or arachidonic acid derivatives.[32] Although plasma catecholamine levels are low in hyperthyroidism, this is an unlikely explanation because the intracellular levels of cyclic adenosine monophosphate are higher than normal, and the tissue responsiveness to catecholamines is increased; both of these should cause improvement of bronchial asthma. In asthmatic patients with hyperthyroidism, there is an increased requirement for corticosteroids. However, serum cortisol is normal in hyperthyroidism despite increased endogenous catabolism, because of increased production. A finding, of uncertain significance, is that there is a shift in the metabolism of hydrocortisone toward its inactive 11-ketone metabolites. Hyperthyroidism is associated with an increase in cellular membrane phospholipids, the major source for arachidonic acid, and with an increase in the phospholipase activity that triggers the release of arachidonic acid from membrane phospholipids. Once freed, the

arachidonic acid is metabolized by one of the two membrane-bound enzymatic pathways (see Chap. 172). The lipoxygenase pathway leads to production of leukotrienes, the mediators of immunologically mediated asthma. The cyclooxygenase pathway leads to production of endoperoxides and prostaglandins that can produce bronchoconstriction. Furthermore, in hyperthyroidism, the activity of prostaglandin 15-hydroxydehydrogenase, which inactivates prostaglandins, is reduced. It is postulated that with the onset of hyperthyroidism, the accumulation of leukotrienes and prostaglandins in the lung, along with enhanced sensitivity of persons with asthma to these products, leads to a worsening of the asthma.

**Pulmonary Hypertension.** Primary pulmonary hypertension has been described with hyperthyroidism associated with Graves disease in neonates and adults, and multinodular toxic goiter.[33,34] Reversal of pulmonary hypertension with establishment of the euthyroid state suggests that this is due to an increase in pulmonary vascular reactivity; however, an autoimmune pathogenetic mechanism also has been suggested.

### HYPOTHYROIDISM

**Pulmonary Function Changes.** The primary effects of hypothyroidism on the respiratory system should be differentiated from secondary effects of obesity and cardiac dysfunction, which frequently accompany hypothyroidism. Hypothyroidism is associated with dysfunction of the diaphragm and other muscles of respiration.[35] Hypothyroid patients without obesity or cardiac dysfunction have normal lung volumes, airway conductance, and arterial blood gas values. However, maximum breathing capacity often is reduced as a consequence of muscle weakness, and pulmonary diffusing capacity can be reduced as a result of anemia. In hypothyroid, obese patients, the total lung capacity, vital capacity, maximum breathing capacity, and peak expiratory flow rate are reduced because of the combination of the obesity and muscle weakness. In severe hypothyroidism, the reduction of diffusing capacity is more than just a result of anemia, because it is not corrected by blood transfusion, suggesting the presence of structural changes within the alveolar membrane. All the abnormalities of pulmonary function correct with thyroxine administration. Bronchial reactivity increases in persons with hypothyroidism who do not have asthma.[36]

**Alveolar Hypoventilation.** Hypoxic and hypercapnic ventilatory drives are depressed in hypothyroidism. In severe hypothyroidism, a combination of depressed ventilatory drive and respiratory muscle weakness may produce alveolar hypoventilation and $CO_2$ narcosis, which may be lethal.[37,38] It responds to thyroid-replacement therapy.

**Sleep Apnea Syndrome.** The recognition that symptoms of excessive daytime somnolence, apathy, and lethargy are shared by patients with hypothyroidism and those with sleep apnea syndrome led to polysomnographic studies in patients with hypothyroidism.[39,40] Disturbances of sleep architecture and the presence of sleep apnea, predominantly obstructive sleep apnea, were found to be frequent, even when the patients were not obese. The frequency of apnea decreases with thyroxine therapy, even if there is no change in body weight.[41]

Multiple factors contribute to the pathogenesis of obstructive sleep apnea. They include narrowing of the upper airway orifice caused by myxomatous tissue infiltration of the tongue and pharyngeal structures; hypertrophy and hypotonia of the genioglossus caused by abnormalities of intrinsic contractile properties of the muscle; a preferential decrease in phasic inspiratory neural output to the upper airway musculature, including the genioglossus, as compared with the intercostal and diaphragmatic muscles; and a decrease in inspiratory effort. These findings suggest that the genioglossus and other pharyngeal muscles are unable to oppose the tendency for pharyngeal closure during inspiration when the pressure in the oropharynx is subatmospheric.

**Pleural Effusion.** Most pleural effusions result from heart disease, pericardial effusion, or ascites related to hypothyroidism. The mechanism responsible for these effusions is not well understood, but probably is related to alterations in pleural capillary permeability or extravasation of hygroscopic mucoproteins into the cavity. These effusions may be small or massive, unilateral or bilateral, and borderline between exudates and transudates, and they often exhibit little evidence of inflammation. Initially, neutrophils and, subsequently, lymphocytes are predominant in these effusions.[42]

**Pulmonary Edema.** The development of pulmonary edema secondary to upper airways obstruction related to deposition of myxomatous tissue in the larynx has been described in a patient with hypothyroidism.[43] In this respect, it is known that thyroid hormone upregulates alveolar epithelial fluid clearance.[43a]

## DISORDERS OF CALCIUM AND BONE METABOLISM (SEE TABLE 202-2)

### HYPERPARATHYROIDISM AND OTHER HYPERCALCEMIC DISORDERS

Hypercalcemia of diverse causes, when associated with renal insufficiency and consequent hyperphosphatemia, leads to the deposition of calcium salts within the alveolar septa. Acute deposition can lead to diffuse alveolar damage and adult respiratory distress syndrome,[44] whereas gradual deposition causes interstitial thickening and fibrosis and a restrictive pattern on pulmonary function testing. On the chest radiograph, an interstitial process may be seen that is commonly misinterpreted as pulmonary edema or idiopathic pulmonary fibrosis because the microdeposits of calcium usually are not apparent on radiographs.[45] Radionuclides used for bone imaging may localize in the lungs, and may suggest the diagnosis of metastatic pulmonary calcification before any radiographic changes can be recognized. Metastatic

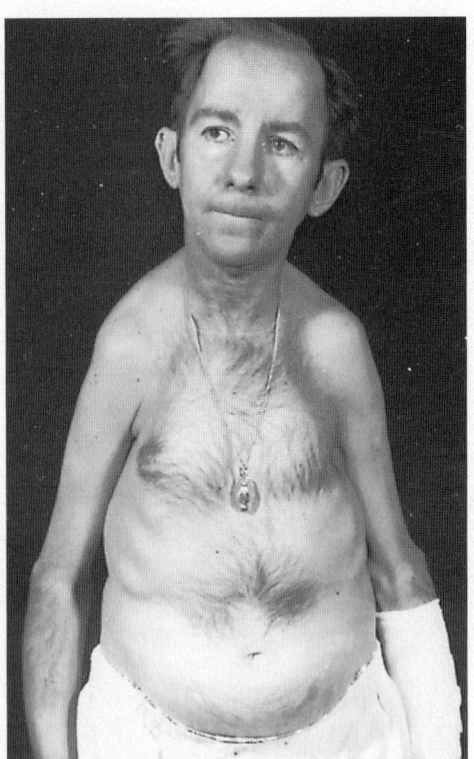

**FIGURE 202-5.** Forty-year-old man with long-lasting primary hyperparathyroidism that culminated in azotemia and osteodystrophy. Note the closeness of the ribs to the pelvis, and the effect of marked resorptive deformation of the clavicles.

pulmonary calcification may revert with normalization of the hypercalcemia.[46] Severe chest deformity may occur in primary hyperparathyroidism, particularly if azotemia supervenes (Fig. 202-5). An association between hypercalcemia and apnea in infants has been reported.[47]

### HYPOPARATHYROIDISM AND OTHER HYPOCALCEMIC DISORDERS

Hypocalcemia can affect the respiratory system by inducing spontaneous electrical activity (a) in the motor and sensory nerves, which produces tetanic laryngeal spasm, in which the vocal cords are fixed in the midline and cause stridor, crowing respiration, and sometimes asphyxiation,[48] and (b) in the autonomic ganglia, which may increase bronchomotor tone and lead to wheezing.[49]

### HYPERPHOSPHATEMIA AND HYPOPHOSPHATEMIA

Hyperphosphatemia has no respiratory consequences. Conversely, severe hypophosphatemia, with serum levels less than 1 mg/dL, produces generalized muscle weakness, including respiratory muscles, and can lead to acute respiratory failure.[50]

### RICKETS, OSTEOMALACIA, AND OSTEOPOROSIS

Rickets, osteomalacia, and osteoporosis are associated with defective mineralization of bones, which can affect the thorax. Their manifestations are listed in Table 202-2 (Fig. 202-6).

## ADRENAL CORTEX

### HYPERCORTISOLISM

Chronic excess secretion of cortisol, as in Cushing syndrome or from exogenous corticosteroid therapy, influences the respiratory system because of (a) a demineralization of bones with col-

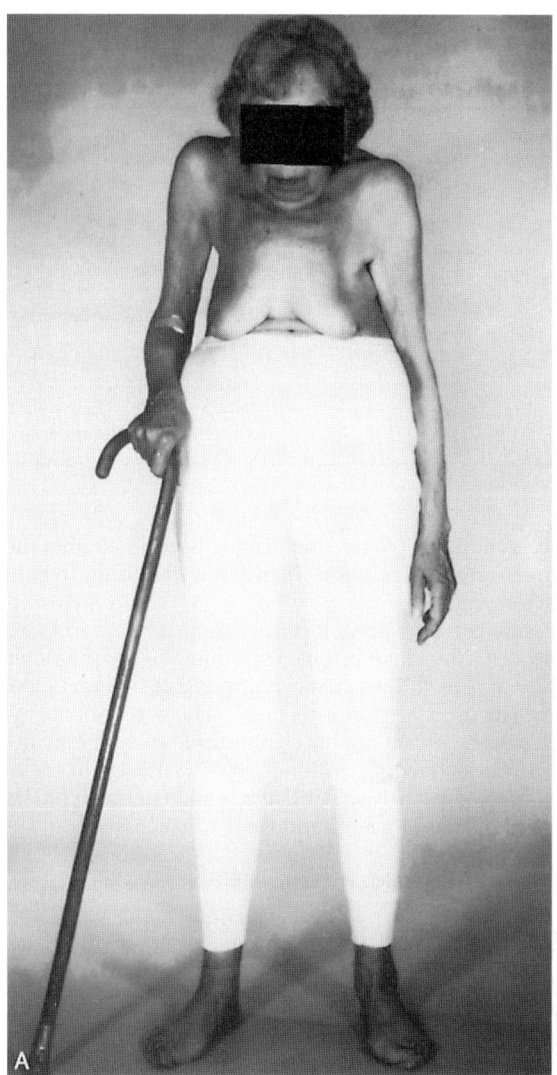
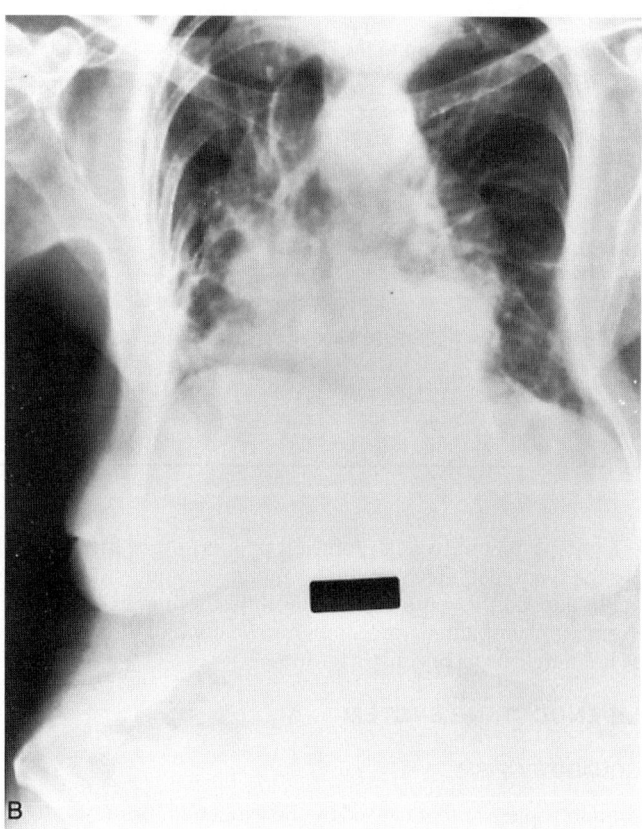

**FIGURE 202-6. A,** Osteoporotic 75-year-old woman with severe chest deformity and kyphosis. **B,** The chest radiograph demonstrates the markedly diminished intrathoracic volume. Note the inward curvature of the midportions of the lower ribs.

lapse of vertebral bodies; (b) a redistribution of subcutaneous fat causing truncal obesity, increased supraclavicular fat pads, and buffalo hump; (c) a modulation of allergic reactions with striking remissions of bronchial asthma and allergic rhinitis; and (d) an impairment of host defense ability to localize infections. As a result, patients with hypercortisolism may develop miliary tuberculosis, invasive pulmonary aspergillosis, pulmonary cryptococcosis, or *Pneumocystis carinii* pneumonia. Moreover, deposition of fat in the paracardiac areas and upper mediastinum in patients with hypercortisolism can be mistaken on a chest radiograph for lymphoma or a mediastinal disease process. Polysomnographic studies performed in patients with hypercortisolism, which is associated with the obesity and disordered sleeping pattern described earlier as a part of the depressive syndrome, also have demonstrated abnormal sleep architecture and obstructive sleep apnea.[51] Respiratory depression resulting in chronic respiratory failure has been reported in a patient with severe metabolic alkalosis associated with Cushing syndrome,[52] and exogenous corticosteroid therapy in patients with chronic obstructive pulmonary disease or asthma has been shown to contribute to respiratory muscle weakness.[53]

## HYPOCORTISOLISM

Increased production of reaginic antibody and increased sensitivity to bronchial anaphylactic reactions occur in adrenalectomized animals. In humans, atopic manifestations, such as bronchial asthma or allergic rhinitis, may be an uncommon presenting sign of Addison disease.[54,55]

## ADRENAL MEDULLA PHEOCHROMOCYTOMA

**Functional Hyperventilation Syndrome.** Catecholamine excess in pheochromocytoma can produce anxiety, tremulousness, changes in sleep patterns, paresthesias, and hyperventilation. These symptoms have led to a mistaken diagnosis of a functional hyperventilation syndrome.[56]

**Pulmonary Edema.** Epinephrine- and norepinephrine-induced pulmonary edema is a well-known phenomenon in experimental studies in animals. In humans, pulmonary edema has been reported with pheochromocytoma. This is thought to be due to left ventricular dysfunction, to postcapillary venoconstriction, or to the toxic effects of catecholamines on pulmonary capillary endothelial cells.[57] The development of pulmonary edema that follows the administration of β-adrenergic blockers without the concomitant administration of an α-adrenergic blocker results from the combination of vasoconstriction, mediated by unopposed α-adrenergic stimulation, and myocardial depression caused by interruption of β-adrenergic drive.[58]

**Amelioration of Bronchial Asthma.** Disappearance of bronchial asthma with the development of noradrenaline-secreting pheochromocytoma and its recurrence after the removal of the tumor have been described.[59] Excess circulating norepinephrine produces bronchodilation because airways have sparse, if any, α-

TABLE 202-3.
**Phenotypic Features Pertaining to the Respiratory System in Sex Chromosomal and Related Disorders Associated with Hypogonadism**

| | Ovarian Dysgenesis Syndrome | Ullrich-Noonan Syndrome | Klinefelter Syndrome |
|---|---|---|---|
| CHROMOSOMAL ABNOR-MALITIES | X monosomy<br>45X<br>Mosaic (45X/46XX), etc. | None<br>XX<br>XY | 47XXY<br>Mosaic (XY/XXY), etc. |
| PHENOTYPIC FEATURES PER-TAINING TO OR INFLUENC-ING RESPIRATORY SYSTEM | High arched palate<br>Micrognathia<br>Bifid uvula<br>Pectus excavatum<br>Shield chest<br>Pulmonary valvular stenosis | All features of Turner syndrome<br>Pulmonary valvular stenosis<br>Pulmonary lymphangiectasia producing interstitial markings and chylothorax | Eunuchoid habitus<br>Kyphosis<br>Pectus excavatum<br>Cleft palate<br>Bilateral aplasia mandibular rami and condyle<br>Increased frequency of restrictive defect rather than obstructive as had been suggested by earlier studies<br>Recurrent phlebothrombosis |

adrenergic receptors, but have a profusion of β receptors; therefore, only the β-agonist effects of the hormone become evident clinically. In addition, norepinephrine inhibits cholinergic discharge from parasympathetic preganglionic fibers and, thereby, reduces cholinergic bronchoconstrictor tone.

## FEMALE ENDOCRINE SYSTEM

### HYPERGONADOTROPISM

Hypergonadotropism, either caused by the exogenous administration of human menopausal gonadotropins for treating infertility or caused endogenously by a hydatidiform mole or chorioepithelioma, can lead to the formation of large theca lutein cysts and the ovarian hyperstimulation syndrome.[60] It is postulated that a metabolite elaborated from these overstimulated ovaries increases the permeability of the peritoneum, and possibly the pleura, and can lead to the development of massive ascites and pleural effusions with hypovolemia.

### HYPOGONADOTROPIC HYPOGONADISM

The prepubertal development of hypogonadotropic hypogonadism is associated with eunuchoid skeletal features. This causes a smaller thorax in proportion to height; hence, all the predicted lung volumes are overestimated because they are based on height, as well as age and sex. Thus, restrictive lung disease may be diagnosed mistakenly in these patients.

### ESTROGEN EFFECTS

No known respiratory abnormalities are associated with endogenous excess or deficiency of estrogen. However, the exogenous administration of estrogens in contraceptives is associated with an increased frequency of hay fever and a hypercoagulable state, manifested as pulmonary thromboembolism.

### PROGESTERONE

Hyperventilation during pregnancy results from the mechanical effects of the gravid uterus on the position and configuration of the diaphragm, increased metabolic demands, and the stimulatory effects of progesterone. That progesterone has stimulatory effects on respiration is suggested by the hyperventilation observed during the luteal phase of the menstrual cycle and the lack of this cyclic hyperventilation in postmenopausal women, and also by the stimulation of respiration in men with the administration of progesterone. Progesterone enhances the respiratory response to hypoxia and hypercapnia.[61] Thus, progesterone has been used therapeutically in treating the sleep apnea syndrome. When this drug is used in combination with estrogen, it reduces sleep-disordered breathing in postmenopausal women.[62]

Premenstrual exacerbation of asthma is believed to be caused by a cyclic decrease in progesterone and, perhaps, estrogen before menses.[63] These exacerbations can be prevented by the administration of progesterone.[64] The mechanism by which progesterone produces this effect is unknown. It may be related to a decrease in contractility of smooth muscle in the airways, regulation of microvascular leakage and edema in the bronchial mucosa, or the drug's immunosuppressive effects.

### MEIG SYNDROME AND PSEUDO-MEIG SYNDROME

Meig syndrome is characterized by the presence of ascites and hydrothorax in association with fibroma of the ovary, and their spontaneous resolution with removal of the tumor.[65] When observed with other ovarian neoplasms, the same phenomenon is termed pseudo-Meig syndrome. It is thought that fluid transudes from the ovarian lesion into the peritoneal cavity, from which it is transported to the thorax through transdiaphragmatic lymphatic channels. The fluid is a transudate, but it can be exudative, hemorrhagic, or rich in amylase if the tumor contains a high concentration of this enzyme and is undergoing hemorrhagic necrosis.

### OVARIAN DYSGENESIS SYNDROME AND ULLRICH-NOONAN SYNDROME

See Table 202-3 for a summary of phenotypic features relating to the respiratory system in patients with X-chromosome abnormalities and those with Ullrich-Noonan syndrome.

## MALE ENDOCRINE SYSTEM

### DISORDERS OF SEMINIFEROUS TUBULES

Testicular tubular disease has no effect on the respiratory tract, except when the same disease affects both of the organ systems, as in Kartagener syndrome.[66] This condition results from lack of dynein arms in the outer microtubules of the cilia and flagella. This ultrastructural defect reduces the motility of (a) embryonal cells, predisposing to the development of situs inversus; (b) spermatozoa, causing infertility; and (c) mucociliary transport in the paranasal sinuses and airways, leading to sinusitis and bronchiectasis.

### TESTOSTERONE EFFECT

A relationship between testosterone and respiratory disturbances during sleep is suggested by the higher frequency of obstructive sleep apnea in men than in premenopausal women, the higher frequency of disordered breathing during sleep in postmenopausal women compared with premenopausal women, the report of the development of central sleep apnea and blunted ventilatory response to $CO_2$ in a patient with hypogonadotropic hypogonadism after the administration of testosterone, and the report of the development of obstructive sleep apnea after therapy with testosterone in patients with a history of snoring.[67,68] Development of obstructive sleep apnea was related to an increase in supraglottic airway resistance resulting from hormonally induced hypertrophy of the soft tissues of the oronasopharynx. Furthermore, men with the sleep apnea syndrome often are impotent and have low concentrations of free and total testosterone that may be related to decreased steroidogenic activity of luteinizing hormone.[69]

### HYPOGONADAL DISORDERS

The prepubertal development of hypogonadotropic hypogonadism leads to testosterone deficiency and the somatic features of eunuchoidism. Kallmann syndrome is a familial hypogonadotropic hypogonadism associated with features of eunuchoidism, anosmia, or hyposmia caused by agenesis of the olfactory bulbs and tracts, midline defects such as cleft lip and cleft palate, and hypoplasia of the first rib.[70] Other hypogonadal disorders such as Klinefelter syndrome (Fig. 202-7)[71,72] and the Ullrich-Noonan syndrome[73] associated with thoracopulmonary abnormalities are detailed in Table 202-3. Although they do not have hypogonadism, eunuchoid-appearing patients with the inborn disease of collagen metabolism, Marfan syndrome, commonly have chest deformities as well as cystic lung disease.

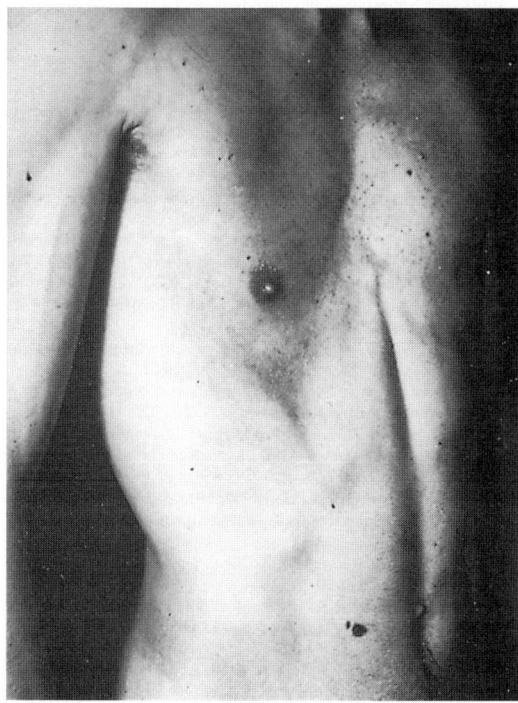

**FIGURE 202-7.** A chest deformity in a 25-year-old man with XXY Klinefelter disease. This patient also had a "straight-back syndrome" (loss of the normal mild thoracic kyphosis), which resulted in a reduced anteroposterior diameter of the chest and a markedly diminished total lung capacity. There was a loud systolic murmur heard best at the base of the heart.

## DIABETES MELLITUS

Diabetes mellitus is associated with widespread hormonal, metabolic, microvascular, and neuropathic abnormalities, leading to dysfunction of many organ systems, including the respiratory system.[74]

### PULMONARY INFECTIONS

Infection may be an immense problem in poorly controlled diabetes mellitus because of impaired chemotaxis, phagocytosis, and intracellular killing by granulocytes and mononuclear phagocytes. The diminished killing activity by alveolar macrophages is related to a depressed respiratory burst and a diminished superoxide anion production, probably because of decreased availability of NADPH (reduced form of nicotinamide adenine dinucleotide phosphate).[75] Poorly controlled diabetes predisposes to mycobacterial and fungal pulmonary infections, which also tend to be rapidly progressive. The increased susceptibility of patients with diabetes to zygomycosis (mucormycosis) may be related to an impaired ability of the alveolar macrophages to inhibit the germination of spores of this fungus.[76]

### ALTERATIONS IN PULMONARY MECHANICS

Abnormal pulmonary function has been found in 60% of a cross section of patients with diabetes. In some of these patients, the abnormalities are related to the obesity, congestive heart failure, and muscle weakness that are common in diabetes; in other patients, abnormal pulmonary function is noted in the absence of such confounding variables. The most consistent abnormalities are reduced lung volumes in young patients with insulin-dependent diabetes, reduced pulmonary elastic recoil and dynamic compliance in both young and adult patients with diabetes, and impaired diffusion.[77,78] Reduced lung volumes result from arthropathy affecting costovertebral joints,[79] or from nonenzymatic, glycosylation-induced alterations and the accumulation of connective tissue, including collagen, in the lungs. Impaired pulmonary diffusion is related to pulmonary microangiopathy that is characterized by thickening of epithelial and capillary basement membranes in the alveolar walls.[80] Impaired lung epithelial permeability has been documented using aerosol scintigraphy.[81]

### SUDDEN DEATH

Unexplained cardiorespiratory arrests in patients with diabetes and autonomic neuropathy may result from abnormal ventilatory responses to hypoxia, either because of reduced sensitivity of the central chemoreceptors or, more likely, because of neuropathy involving the vagus and glossopharyngeal nerves, which transmit afferent impulses from the carotid body and aortic arch chemoreceptors to the respiratory center. Studies evaluating the control of respiration in patients with diabetes have provided conflicting findings, with some investigators showing abnormal ventilatory responses to exercise, hypoxia, or hypercarbia, and others finding normal function.[82]

### SLEEP APNEA SYNDROME

Like patients with primary autonomic neuropathy (Shy-Drager syndrome), patients with diabetes who have autonomic neuropathy may have an increased prevalence of sleep-related breathing disorders that may be the basis for the unexplained cardiorespiratory deaths.[83,84] Although earlier studies in elderly patients with diabetic autonomic neuropathy had suggested a higher prevalence of hypopnea and sleep apnea, subsequent studies in younger diabetic patients, with and without autonomic neuropathy, have failed to confirm these findings.

## ADULT RESPIRATORY DISTRESS SYNDROME

Noncardiogenic pulmonary edema occurs during the treatment of diabetic ketoacidosis.[85] It may result from thickening of the basal lamina of alveolar capillaries, rendering them more permeable, especially during acidosis. Other factors that are implicated are development of cerebral edema causing neurogenic pulmonary edema or a decrease in the pressure gradient between the serum colloid oncotic pressure and the pulmonary capillary wedge pressure, leading to accumulation of fluid in the lungs.

## ALVEOLAR HYPOVENTILATION

Severe muscular weakness, leading to alveolar hypoventilation, has been reported when severe hypophosphatemia or hypokalemia develops during the treatment of diabetic ketoacidosis. This can be prevented and treated by repletion of phosphate or potassium.[86]

## BRONCHIAL ASTHMA

Asthma and diabetes rarely occur in the same patient; however, the development of hypoglycemia caused by either exogenous or endogenous insulin excess has been implicated in the exacerbation of bronchospasm in patients with asthma. The mechanism for this apparent exclusion between the two diseases is not understood but probably is related to genetic factors; to alterations in both insulin release and its hypoglycemic effect in atopic patients with asthma; to effects on the metabolism of cyclic nucleotides, which mediate smooth muscle contraction and relaxation in patients with diabetes; and to the effect of diabetic neuropathy on bronchomotor tone. Patients with diabetes who have autonomic neuropathy have reduced bronchial reactivity because of depression of cholinergic bronchomotor tone.[87,88]

## MISCELLANEOUS

Transient vocal cord paralysis,[89] apparently due to neuropathy, and persistent transudative pleural effusions related to left ventricular dysfunction and possibly other unknown factors, have been reported in patients with long-standing diabetes mellitus.[90] Massive pulmonary thromboembolism may develop secondary to the dehydration that occurs in diabetic ketoacidosis.[91]

# REFERENCES

1. Thurlbeck WM. Postnatal growth and development of the lung. Am Rev Respir Dis 1975; 111:803.
2. Farrell PM, Avery ME. Hyaline membrane disease. Am Rev Respir Dis 1975; 111:657.
3. Ballard PL. Hormonal regulation of pulmonary surfactant. Endocr Rev 1989; 10:165.
4. Floros J, Kala P. Surfactant proteins: molecular genetics of neonatal pulmonary diseases. Ann Rev Physiol 1998; 60:365.
5. Rooney SA. The surfactant system and lung phospholipid biochemistry. Am Rev Respir Dis 1985; 131:439.
5a. Spencer C, Heales K. Antenatal corticosteroids to prevent neonatal respiratory distress syndrome. BMJ 2000; 320:325.
6. Piper JM, Langer O. Does maternal diabetes delay pulmonary maturity? Am J Obstet Gynecol 1993; 168:783.
7. Morales WJ, O'Brien WF, Angel JL, et al. Fetal lung maturation: the combined use of corticosteroids and thyrotropin-releasing hormone. Obstet Gynecol 1989; 73:111.
8. Miettinen PJ, Warburton D, Bu D, et al. Impaired lung branching morphogenesis in the absence of functional EGF receptor. Dev Biol 1997; 186:224.
9. Galioto G, Mevio E, Galioto P, et al. Modifications of the nasal cycle in patients with hypothalamic disorders. Kallmann's syndrome. Ann Otol Rhinol Laryngol 1991; 100:559.
10. Brambrink AM, Dick WF. Neurogenic pulmonary edema. Pathogenesis, clinical picture and therapy. Anaesthesist 1997; 46:953.
11. Moskowitz MA, Fisher JN, Simpser MD, Strieder DJ. Periodic apnea, exercise hypoventilation and hypothalamic dysfunction. Ann Intern Med 1976; 84:171.
12. Sforza E, Krieger J, Geisert J, et al. Sleep and breathing abnormalities in a case of Prader-Willi syndrome. Acta Paediatr Scand 1991; 80:80.
13. Nink M, Salomon E, Coutinho M, et al. Corticotropin-releasing hormone (CRH) is a respiratory stimulant in humans: a comparative study of human and ovine CRH. Life Sci 1994; 54:1793.
14. Jain BP, Brody JS, Fisher AB. The small lung of hypopituitarism. Am Rev Respir Dis 1975; 108:49.
15. Hampal S, Bingham B, Desai P, et al. Recurrent simple nasal polyps associated with Sheehan's syndrome. J Otolaryngol 1992; 21:368.
15a. Kinhult J, Andersson JA, Uddman R, et al. Pituitary adenylate cyclase-activating peptide 38, a potent endogenously produced dilator of human airways. Eur Respir J 2000; 15:243.
16. Harrison BDW, Millhouse KA, Harrington M, Nabarro JDN. Lung function in acromegaly. Q J Med 1978; 47:517.
17. Brody JS, Fisher AB, Gocmen A, Dubois AB. Acromegalic pneumomegaly: lung growth in the adult. J Clin Invest 1970; 49:1051.
18. Donnelly PM, Grunstein RR, Peat JK, et al. Large lungs and growth hormone: an increased alveolar number? Eur Respir J 1995; 8:938.
19. Iandelli I, Gorini M, Duranti R, et al. Respiratory muscle function and control of breathing in patients with acromegaly. Eur Respir J 1997; 10:977.
20. Murrant NJ, Gatland DJ. Respiratory problems in acromegaly. J Laryngol Otol 1990; 104:52.
21. Mazon BJ, West P, Maclean JP, Kryger HG. Sleep apnea in acromegaly. Am J Med 1980; 69:615.
21a. Saeki N, Isono S, Nishino T, et al. Sleep disordered breathing in acromegalics—relation of hormonal levels and quantitative sleep study by means of bedside oximeter. Endocr J 1999; 46:585.
22. Cadieux RJ, Kales A, Senten RJ, et al. Endoscopic findings in sleep apnea associated with acromegaly. J Clin Endocrinol Metab 1982; 55:18.
23. Zlemer DC, Dunlap DB. Case report: relief of sleep apnea in acromegaly by bromocriptine. Am J Med Sci 1988; 295:49.
24. Buyse B, Michiels E, Bouillon R, et al. Relief of sleep apnoea after treatment of acromegaly: report of three cases and review of the literature. Eur Respir J 1997; 10:1401.
25. Grunstein RR, Ho KY, Sullivan CE. Sleep apnea in acromegaly. Ann Intern Med 1991; 115:527.
26. Grunstein RR, Ho KY, Berthon-Jones M, et al. Central sleep apnea is associated with increased ventilatory response to carbon dioxide and hypersecretion of growth hormone in patients with acromegaly. Am J Respir Crit Care Med 1994; 150:496.
27. Leibowitz G, Shapiro MS, Salameh M, Glaser B. Improvement of sleep apnea due to acromegaly during short-term treatment with octreotide. J Intern Med 1994; 236:231.
28. McElvaney GN, Wilcox PG, Fairbarn MS, et al. Respiratory muscle weakness and dyspnea in thyrotoxic patients. Am Rev Respir Dis 1990; 141:1221.
29. Massey DG, Becklace MR, McKenzie JM, Bates DV. Circulatory and ventilatory response to exercise in thyrotoxicosis. N Engl J Med 1967; 276:1104.
30. Kahaly G, Hellerman J, Mohr-Kahaly S, Treese N. Impaired cardiopulmonary exercise capacity in patients with hyperthyroidism. Chest 1996; 109:57.
31. Cockroft DW, Silverberg JDH, Dosman JA. Decrease in non-specific bronchial reactivity in an asthmatic following treatment of hyperthyroidism. Ann Allergy 1978; 41:160.
32. Hoult JRS, Moore P. Thyroid disease, asthma, and prostaglandin. Br Med J 1978; 1:366.
33. Thurnheer R, Jenni R, Russi EW, et al. Hyperthyroidism and pulmonary hypertension. J Intern Med 1997; 242:185.
34. O'Donovan D, McMahon C, Costigan C. Reversible pulmonary hypertension in neonatal Graves disease. Ir Med J 1997; 90:147.
35. Martinez FJ, Gomez MB, Celli BR. Hypothyroidism: a reversible cause of diaphragmatic dysfunction. Chest 1989; 96:1059.
36. Wieshammer S, Keck FS, Schauffelen AC, et al. Effects of hypothyroidism on bronchial reactivity in non-asthmatic subjects. Thorax 1990; 45:947.
37. Ladenson PW, Goldenheim PD, Ridgway EC. Prediction and reversal of blunted ventilatory responsiveness in patients with hypothyroidism. Am J Med 1988; 84:877.
38. Zwillich CW, Pierson DJ, Hofeldt FD, et al. Ventilatory control in myxedema and hypothyroidism. N Engl J Med 1975; 292:662.
39. Skatrud J, Iber C, Ewart R, et al. Disordered breathing during sleep in hypothyroidism. Am Rev Respir Dis 1981; 124:325.
40. Kapur VK, Koepsell TD, deMaine J, et al. Association of hypothyroidism and obstructive sleep apnea. Am J Respir Crit Care Med 1998; 158:1379.
41. Rajgopal KR, Abbrecht PH, Derderian SS, et al. Obstructive sleep apnea in hypothyroidism. Ann Intern Med 1984; 101:491.
42. Gottehrer A, Roa J, Stanford GG. Hypothyroidism and pleural effusions. Chest 1990; 98:1130.
43. Lopez A, Lorente JA, Jerez V, et al. Sleep apnea, hypothyroidism and pulmonary edema. Chest 1990; 97:763.
43a. Folkesson HG, Marlin A, Wang Y, et al. Dexamethasone and thyroid hormone pretreatment upregulate alveolar epithelial fluid clearance in adult rat. J Appl Physiol 2000; 88:416.
44. Khafif RA, Delima C, Silverberg A, et al. Acute hyperparathyroidism with systemic calcinosis. Arch Intern Med 1989; 149:681.
45. Hartman TE, Muller NL, Primack SL, et al. Metastatic pulmonary calcification in patients with hypercalcemia: findings on chest radiographs and CT scans. AJR Am J Roentgenol 1994; 162:799.
46. Weber CK, Friedrich JM, Merkle E, et al. Reversible metastatic pulmonary calcification in a patient with multiple myeloma. Ann Hematol 1996; 72:329.
47. Kooh S, Binet A. Hypercalcemia in infants presenting with apnea. Can Med Assoc J 1990; 143:509.

48. Williams GT, Brown M. Laryngospasm in hypoparathyroidism. J Laryngol Otol 1974; 88:369.
49. Aberg H, Johansson H, Werner I. Hyperparathyroidism and asthma. Lancet 1972; 2:381.
50. Newman JH, Neff TA, Ziporin P. Acute respiratory failure associated with hypophosphatemia. N Engl J Med 1977; 296:1101.
51. Shipley JE, Schteingart DE, Tandon R, et al. Sleep architecture and sleep apnea in patients with Cushing's disease. Sleep 1992; 15:514.
52. Tanaka M, Yano T, Ichikawa Y, et al. A case of Cushing's syndrome associated with chronic respiratory failure due to metabolic alkalosis. Intern Med 1992; 31:385.
53. Decramer M, Laquet LM, Fagard R, Ragiers P. Corticosteroids contribute to muscle weakness in chronic airflow obstruction. Am J Respir Crit Care Med 1994; 150:11.
54. Green M, Lim KH. Bronchial asthma with Addison's disease. Lancet 1971; 1:1159.
55. Saraclar Y, Turktas I, Adalioglu G, Tuncer A. Bronchial asthma with Addison's disease. Respiration 1993; 60:241.
56. Magarian GJ. Hyperventilation syndromes: infrequently recognized common expressions of anxiety and stress. Medicine (Baltimore) 1982; 61:219.
57. Fahmy N, Assaad M, Bathija P, Whittier FC. Postoperative acute pulmonary edema: a rare presentation of pheochromocytoma. Clin Nephrol 1997; 48:122.
58. Wark JD, Larkins RG. Pulmonary edema after propranolol therapy in two cases of phaeochromocytoma. Br Med J 1978; 1:1395.
59. Harvey JN, Dean HG, Lee MR. Recurrence of asthma following removal of a noradrenaline-secreting phaeochromocytoma. Postgrad Med J 1984; 60:364.
60. Shapiro AG, Thomas T, Epstein M. Management of hyperstimulation syndrome. Fertil Steril 1977; 28:238.
61. Bayliss DA, Millhorn DE. Central neural mechanisms of progesterone action. Application to the respiratory system. J Appl Physiol 1992; 73:393.
62. Pickett CK, Regensteiner JG, Woodard WD, et al. Progestin and estrogen reduce sleep-disordered breathing in post menopausal women. J Appl Physiol 1989; 66:1656.
63. Chandler MH, Schuldheisz S, Phillips BA, Muse KN. Premenstrual asthma: effect of estrogen on symptoms, pulmonary function, and beta 2 receptors. Pharmacotherapy 1997; 17: 224.
64. Beynon HLC, Garbett ND, Barnes PJ. Severe premenstrual exacerbations of asthma. Effect of intramuscular progesterone. Lancet 1988; 1:370.
65. Lemming R. Meigs syndrome and pathogenesis of pleurisy and polyserositis. Acta Med Scand 1960; 168:197.
66. Afzelius BA. A human syndrome caused by immotile cilia. Science 1976; 193:317.
67. Sandblom RE, Matsumoto AM, Schoene RB, et al. Obstructive sleep apnea syndrome induced by testosterone administration. N Engl J Med 1983; 308:508.
68. Johnson MW, Anch AM, Remmers JE. Induction of the obstructive sleep apnea syndrome in a woman by exogenous androgen administration. Am Rev Respir Dis 1984; 129:1023.
69. Grunstein RR. Metabolic aspects of sleep apnea. Sleep 1996; 19:S218.
70. Santen RJ, Paulsen A. Hypogonadotropic eunuchoidism: clinical study of the mode of inheritance. J Clin Endocrinol 1973; 36:47.
71. Gluck MC, Becker KL, Katz S. Pulmonary function of hypogonadal men before and after testosterone. Am Rev Respir Dis 1966; 94:676.
72. Morales P, Furest I, Marco V, et al. Pathogenesis of the lung in restrictive defects of Klinefelters syndrome. Chest 1992; 102:1550.
73. Baltaxe HA, Lee JG, Ehlers KH, Engle MA. Pulmonary lymphangiectasia demonstrated by lymphangiography in two patients with Noonan's syndrome. Radiology 1975; 115:149.
74. Strojek K, Ziora D, Sroczynski JW, et al. Pulmonary complications of type I (insulin dependent) diabetic patients. Diabetologia 1992; 35:1173.
75. Mohsenin V, Latifpour J. Respiratory burst in alveolar macrophages of diabetic rats. J Appl Physiol 1990; 68:2384.
76. Waldorf AR, Ruderman N, Diamond RD. Specific susceptibility to mucormycosis in murine diabetes and bronchoalveolar macrophage defense against *Rhizopus*. J Clin Invest 1984; 74:150.
77. Sandler M. Is the lung a "target organ" in diabetes mellitus. Arch Intern Med 1990; 150:1385.
78. Ljubic S, Metelko Z, Car N, et al. Reduction of diffusion capacity for carbon monoxide in diabetic patients. Chest 1998; 114:1033.
79. Schnapf BM, Banks RA, Silverstein JH, et al. Pulmonary function in insulin-dependent diabetes mellitus with limited joint mobility. Am Rev Respir Dis 1984; 130:930.
80. Vracko RD, Thorning D, Huang TW. Basal lamina of alveolar epithelium and capillaries. Quantitative changes with aging and in diabetes mellitus. Am Rev Respir Dis 1979; 120:973.
81. Caner B, Ugur O, Byraktar M, et al. Impaired lung epithelial permeability in diabetics detected by technetium-99m-DTPA aerosol scintigraphy. J Nucl Med 1994; 35:204.
82. Tantucci C, Scionti L, Bottini P, et al. Influence of autonomic neuropathy of different severities on the hypercapnic drive to breathing in diabetic patients. Chest 1997; 112:145.
83. Catterall JR, Calverley PMA, Ewing DJ, et al. Breathing, sleep, and diabetic autonomic neuropathy. Diabetes 1984; 33:1025.
84. Strohl KP. Diabetes and sleep apnea. Sleep 1996; 19:S225.
85. Hillerdal G, Wibell L. Adult respiratory distress syndrome and diabetes. Acta Med Scand 1982; 211:221.
86. Tillman CR. Hypokalemic hypoventilation complicating severe diabetic ketoacidosis. South Med J 1980; 73:231.
87. Villa MP, Cacciari E, Bernardi F, et al. Bronchial reactivity in diabetic patients. Relationship of duration of diabetes and degree of glycemic control. Am J Dis Child 1988; 142:726.
88. Santos e Fonesca CM, Manco JC, Gallo J, et al. Cholinergic bronchomotor tone and airway caliber in insulin-dependent diabetes mellitus. Chest 1992; 101:1038.
89. Kabadi UM. Unilateral vocal cord palsy in diabetic patient. Postgrad Med 1988; 84:53.
90. Chertow BS, Kadzielowa R, Burger AJ. Benign pleural effusions in long-standing diabetes mellitus. Chest 1991; 99:1108.
91. Quigley RL, Curran RD, Stagl RD, Alexander JC Jr. Management of massive pulmonary thromboembolism complicating diabetic ketoacidosis. Ann Thorac Surg 1994; 57:1322.

# CHAPTER 203

# THE CARDIOVASCULAR SYSTEM AND ENDOCRINE DISEASE

ELLEN W. SEELY AND GORDON H. WILLIAMS

Since the reports of Robert Graves and Thomas Addison in the mid-nineteenth century, deranged hormonal secretions have been known to alter substantially the function of the cardiovascular system. However, the magnitude of the interaction has begun to be appreciated only since the advent of precise measurement techniques for circulating hormone concentrations.[1] In fact, the heart has been added to the list of endocrine organs, with the evidence that it produces a circulating hormone (atrial natriuretic hormone; see Chap. 178).

## ACROMEGALY

The cardiac manifestations of acromegaly include enlargement of the heart, hypertension, premature coronary artery disease, cardiac arrhythmias, and congestive heart failure.[2] Indeed, a specific *acromegalic cardiomyopathy* has been suggested to account for patients with congestive heart failure[3] and cardiac arrhythmia in whom predisposing factors cannot be demonstrated.

### CARDIOMEGALY

After the fifth decade, nearly all patients with active acromegaly have cardiomegaly. In some, the dysfunction is so great that the ejection fraction is reduced. Because the enlargement of the heart is greater than the generalized organomegaly that is usually observed with this disease, the cause is probably more than the generalized effect of growth hormone on protein synthesis. Other contributing factors may include hypertension and atherosclerosis, both of which occur with increased frequency in acromegaly, and a cardiomyopathy. Focal cardiac interstitial fibrosis and a myocarditis also have occurred in most cases.[2] Because these patients may also have small vessel disease of the myocardium, diabetes, and hypertension, it is probable that a combination of factors contributes to the cardiac hypertrophy observed in acromegalics.[3a] Importantly, even short-term acromegaly affects the heart.[3b]

### HYPERTENSION

Hypertension is probably the most common cardiovascular manifestation, occurring in 15% to 50% of acromegalic patients.[4]

The frequency varies according to whether office or ambulatory blood pressures are assessed. Hypertensive acromegalics tend to be older and to have had their acromegaly longer than non-hypertensive patients. The underlying functional abnormality remains uncertain, but growth hormone, abnormal aldosterone secretion, and a pressor substance in the urine of acromegalics have been considered.

Several studies have suggested that the elevated growth hormone may be responsible for the hypertension: Pituitary irradiation and hypophysectomy reduce arterial pressure in hypertensive acromegalics; also, the administration of growth hormone can produce sodium retention and extracellular fluid volume expansion in normal persons.

An abnormality in the secretion of aldosterone may produce volume expansion and, secondarily, hypertension. Early studies suggested that aldosterone secretion is increased in many patients with acromegaly. However, more recent studies suggest that this is uncommon.[5] What frequently does occur is a change in the responsiveness of the adrenal gland and the peripheral vasculature to angiotensin II (AII). Thus, with sodium restriction, the aldosterone response to AII is decreased, whereas the vascular response is increased, compared with that of normal persons (see Chap. 79). These abnormalities are present in both hypertensive and normotensive acromegalics, although, perhaps, at a greater frequency in the hypertensives.[6] Whether this is related to the pathogenesis of the elevated arterial pressure or is a reflection of the expanded extracellular fluid volume is unclear.

## ATHEROSCLEROSIS

Because of growth hormone's major effect on carbohydrate and lipid metabolism, it is not surprising that premature atherosclerosis occurs in patients with acromegaly. It is uncertain, however, how frequently this tendency toward atherosclerosis occurs. One report[2] suggests that only 10% of acromegalics have major coronary artery disease.

## ACROMEGALIC CARDIOMYOPATHY

Several lines of evidence suggest that not all heart disease in acromegalics can be attributed to the increased prevalence of atherosclerosis and hypertension, leading some investigators to propose a specific acromegalic cardiomyopathy.[7–10] The evidence includes the following: (a) Ten percent to 20% of acromegalics have overt congestive heart failure and, in perhaps 25% of these, there is no known predisposing factor. (b) Approximately half of all patients with acromegaly, including patients without hypertension, have echocardiographic evidence of left ventricular hypertrophy (LVH),[7,8,10] the degree of which correlates reasonably well with the level of growth hormone. (c) Most patients with acromegaly who do not have hypertension or atherosclerosis have some clinical evidence of cardiac dysfunction, manifested by a shortening of the left ventricular (LV) ejection time and prolongation of the preejection period. (d) Nearly 50% of acromegalics have electrocardiographic abnormalities,[2] of which hypertension or atherosclerosis may account for 10% to 20%, but the remaining 30% remain unexplained. (e) Histologic studies of the heart show cellular hypertrophy, patchy fibrosis, and myofibrillar degeneration.[2] (f) Sudden death has been associated with inflammatory and degenerative changes in the sinoatrial and perinodal nerve plexus, as well as degeneration of the atrioventricular node.[5] (g) Finally, the acromegalic heart has a higher collagen content per gram of tissue than the normal myocardium. Thus, the evidence generally supports the hypothesis that there is a specific acromegalic cardiomyopathy. The presence of this cardiomyopathy, in turn, provides an explanation for the increased frequency of cardiac dysrhythmia and the difficulty in treating congestive heart failure with conventional therapy.

## TREATMENT OF CARDIOVASCULAR DISEASES IN ACROMEGALY

Acromegalics with cardiovascular abnormalities usually respond to conventional therapy for hypertension, heart failure, or arrhythmias. Those with hypertension, however, are more responsive to volume-depleting maneuvers (i.e., diuretics and sodium restriction) than the average person with essential hypertension. Also, acromegalics with congestive heart failure, without evidence of underlying hypertensive heart disease, often appear particularly resistant to conventional therapy. Absence of a clinical response in such patients suggests that vigorous efforts are needed to lower growth hormone levels (see Chap. 12). The use of somatostatin analogs is effective in reversing cardiac abnormalities in parallel with the fall in growth hormone.[10,11]

## GROWTH HORMONE'S EFFECT ON THE HEART

Increasing evidence suggests that while growth hormone excess (acromegaly) has profound adverse effects on the heart, growth hormone deficiency also is deleterious. Growth hormone replacement in deficient individuals improves cardiac performance. Furthermore, since growth hormone increases cardiac muscle mass, it may be useful in treating individuals with idiopathic dilated cardiomyopathy by reducing the size of the LV chamber size.[12]

# DISEASES OF THE THYROID

The relationship between thyroid and cardiac function is probably the most widely known interaction of an endocrine organ with the heart. These effects often are separated into two classes: (a) those that are indirect and appear to be mediated by the sympathetic nervous system, and (b) those that are directly mediated by thyroid hormone.[13]

## THE SYMPATHETIC NERVOUS SYSTEM AND THYROID DYSFUNCTION

Various theories have been proposed to explain altered sympathetic nervous system function in hyperthyroidism and hypothyroidism. Thyroid hormone has been suggested as a cause of an altered interrelationship between the sympathetic nervous system and the heart by increasing the activity of the sympathetic nervous system and by increasing the sensitivity of cardiac tissue to an unchanged level of sympathetic nervous system activity.

However, investigations seeking to show an increased activity of the sympathetic nervous system in hyperthyroidism have been conflicting and inconclusive. Studies of catecholamine levels in hyperthyroidism and hypothyroidism have shown that plasma and urinary levels of norepinephrine, epinephrine, and dopamine β-hydroxylase are low or normal in hyperthyroidism and normal or elevated in hypothyroidism.[14] Therefore, the direction of alteration of catecholamine levels does not appear to account for the clinical manifestations in these two conditions. Despite these conflicting data, it has been observed that β-adrenergic blockers, such as propranolol, improve or even eliminate many of the cardiac manifestations of hyperthyroidism. This observation, plus the fact that the clinical manifestations of hyperthyroidism parallel those of catecholamine excess, have led to the proposal that thyroid hormone enhances the sensitivity of cardiac tissue to catecholamines.

It has been clearly documented that the enhancement of catecholamine responsiveness induced by thyroid hormone results from an alteration in the activity of the β-adrenergic receptor–adenylate cyclase system.[15] Exogenous triiodothyronine ($T_3$) or thyroxine ($T_4$) increases the number of β-adrenergic receptors. Moreover, an increase in β-adrenergic receptor affinity has been demonstrated in the presence of thyroid hormone.

The observation that after β-adrenergic blockade dogs that are hyperthyroid have higher heart rates and greater myocardial contractility than when they were euthyroid supports the theory that thyroid hormone has an independent direct effect on the heart apart from that modulated by the sympathetic nervous system.[16] Additional support for this theory comes from experiments showing that chick embryonic heart cells increase their rate of beating with the addition of thyroid hormone. There is an augmentation of myocardial contractility of the right ventricular papillary muscle from hyperthyroid cats, manifested by an upward shift of the myocardial force velocity curve, increased velocity of myocardial fiber shortening, a decreased time to peak ejection during isometric contraction, and an augmentation of peak tension. Pretreatment of these hyperthyroid cats with reserpine to deplete catecholamines did not alter the effects of hyperthyroidism.

The direct effect of thyroid hormone on the heart appears to be mediated by changes in the level of messenger RNA (mRNA) for specific proteins.[13] As in other tissues, thyroid hormone increases the activity of the sodium pump in cardiac cells. In hypothyroid rats administered $T_3$, the activity of $Na^+$, $K^+$–adenosine triphosphatase (ATPase) and potassium-dependent $p$-nitrophenyl phosphatase in the heart increases by more than 50%.[17] Thyroid hormone also increases the synthesis of myosin, as well as increasing its contractile properties by increasing the more mobile myosin isoenzymes.[18] In thyrotoxicosis, there is an increased synthesis of a myosin isoenzyme with fast ATPase activity. This additional myosin ATPase may contribute to the increased cardiac contractility of the hyperthyroid heart, but it is unlikely to be the primary causative factor, because the administration of exogenous thyroid hormone increases contractility before an alteration of myosin ATPase activity occurs. Thus, an increasing body of evidence suggests that thyroid hormone also has extranuclear nonadrenergic-mediated effects. A specific effect on the activity of $Ca^{2+}$-ATPases has been proposed.[19]

## HYPERTHYROIDISM

### PHYSICAL FINDINGS

Many of the prominent clinical manifestations of hyperthyroidism are those of the cardiovascular system, such as tachycardia, palpitations, and systolic hypertension (see Chap. 42). Diastolic hypertension also may be seen, but it is not as typical as systolic hypertension. Additional cardiac findings on physical examination include a hyperactive precordium, a loud first heart sound, an accentuated pulmonic component to the second heart sound, and a third heart sound; the Means-Lerman scratch, a systolic scratch thought to result from the rubbing together of the pericardial and pleural surfaces by a hyperdynamic heart, may be heard at the second left intercostal space during expiration. A systolic flow murmur, representative of the hyperdynamic state, may be heard along the left sternal border. Moreover, a murmur of mitral valve prolapse, a click alone, or a click and a murmur may be heard. There appears to be an increased prevalence of mitral valve prolapse in patients with hyperthyroidism. A series[20] of 40 patients with active or previous hyperthyroidism had a 43% prevalence of mitral valve prolapse on echocardiogram compared with 18% of controls.

### HEMODYNAMIC EFFECTS

Patients with hyperthyroidism may have angina pectoris and congestive heart failure. Initially, it was thought that congestive heart failure occurred only in patients with underlying heart disease. However, in infants with neonatal hyperthyroidism (see Chap. 47) congestive heart failure has been seen without underlying cardiac disease. Also, congestive heart failure may be induced in experimental animals made hyperthyroid. Therefore, although congestive heart failure is a more common clinical manifestation in patients with underlying heart disease, hyperthyroidism may overstress even a normal heart.

Hemodynamic changes in hyperthyroidism include an increase in cardiac and stroke volume, mean systolic ejection rate, and coronary blood flow. The systolic ejection and/or ejection periods decrease, the pulse pressure widens, and systemic venous resistance decreases. The increase in cardiac output is greater than that expected by the increase in total body oxygen consumption; hence, it appears to be directly mediated by thyroid hormone effect on the heart independent of the effect of the thyroid hormone on general tissue metabolism.

### ELECTROCARDIOGRAPHIC FINDINGS

Electrocardiographic changes are nonspecific in hyperthyroidism. Approximately 40% of these patients have sinus tachycardia.[21] Also, atrial fibrillation occurs in ~15%. Intraatrial conduction disturbances may occur and be manifested by notching of the P wave in ~15% or by a prolonged PR interval in ~5% of these patients. Second- and third-degree heart block have also been observed, as well as intraventricular conductance defects, most commonly a right bundle branch block.

### THERAPY

The most effective treatment for cardiac dysfunction in hyperthyroidism is treatment of the hyperthyroidism itself. Often, no further therapy is required. In patients with angina pectoris, ~15% have resolution of symptoms when they become euthyroid.[22] A retrospective study of 163 patients with hyperthyroidism and atrial fibrillation reported that most revert to normal once they become euthyroid.

The most commonly used treatment of the cardiac manifestations of hyperthyroidism is a β-adrenergic blocking drug. These drugs can decrease heart rate in patients with sinus tachycardia and slow the rate of atrial fibrillation. In some patients with congestive heart failure caused by a hyperdynamic state, β-adrenergic blockade may even improve the congestive heart failure, although it must be administered cautiously and under close supervision. When congestive heart failure is severe, cardiac glycosides can be used. Patients with hyperthyroidism require higher doses of these drugs because of an increased volume distribution and because the hyperthyroidism decreases the enhancement of myocardial contractility produced by digitalis.

Atrial fibrillation reverts to normal sinus rhythm in most patients who become euthyroid. However, in patients who do not revert spontaneously, chemical or electrical cardioversion is indicated. Guidelines for the timing of cardioversion are based on the observations that 75% of hyperthyroid patients revert within 3 weeks of becoming euthyroid, and no spontaneous reversion occurs when the patients remain in atrial fibrillation more than 4 months after being rendered euthyroid.[23] Therefore, if a patient remains in atrial fibrillation for 16 weeks after achievement of the euthyroid state, cardioversion should be attempted.

A series[24] of 262 patients with hyperthyroidism and atrial fibrillation, reviewed in an 18-year retrospective study, showed a 10% incidence of arterial embolization. Patients with atrial fibrillation and mitral stenosis have a rate of embolization of 5% per year. Therefore, anticoagulation therapy should be used in patients with atrial fibrillation and hyperthyroidism unless there is a contraindication. Anticoagulation must be attempted cautiously, and with smaller doses than usual. The half-life of the clotting factors is shortened in hyperthyroidism; therefore, smaller-than-usual doses of warfarin derivatives can achieve adequate levels of anticoagulation. Finally, ipodate, used as a contrast agent for cholecystography, is beneficial in treating hyperthyroidism and its cardiac manifestations.[25]

## HYPOTHYROIDISM

### CLINICAL MANIFESTATION

The cardiac manifestations of hypothyroidism include cardiac enlargement with cardiac dilatation, sinus bradycardia, hypotension, distant heart sounds, edema, and evidence of congestive heart failure with ascites or orthopnea and paroxysmal nocturnal dyspnea. These full-blown clinical manifestations are seen infrequently, because hypothyroidism often is diagnosed at an earlier stage of the disease. Nevertheless, patients with hypothyroidism often complain of exertional dyspnea and, on physical examination, may have evidence of pleural effusions.

### HEMODYNAMIC EFFECTS

The hemodynamic manifestations of hypothyroidism include a decrease in cardiac output, stroke volume, and blood and plasma volumes. Similar to the delay in the relaxation phase of skeletal muscle that is seen in hypothyroidism, there is also a prolongation of the isovolumetric relaxation time of the heart on echocardiography, which returns to normal with thyroid replacement.[26] Contrary to the findings in hyperthyroidism, an increase in the preejection period and an increase in the ratio of preejection period to LV ejection time are observed. In severe hypothyroidism, there is increased capillary permeability leading to peripheral edema, with approximately one-third of all patients with myxedema developing pericardial effusions, increased interstitial edema, and pleural effusions seen on chest x-ray films. Thus, determining if these patients have congestive heart failure is often difficult. Invasive hemodynamic monitoring can differentiate these two conditions, because cardiac output rises with exercise in patients with hypothyroidism, whereas this rise does not occur if left heart failure is also present. Therefore, in most patients with hypothyroidism, although depressed myocardial contractility may be present, cardiac function remains sufficient to sustain the workload placed on the heart, because this workload itself is reduced.

### HYPERTENSION

Patients with hypothyroidism have a higher incidence of hypertension than the normal population.[27] In one series of 477 patients with hypothyroidism, 14.8% had hypertension (defined as a systolic/diastolic blood pressure above 160/95 mm Hg), as opposed to only 5.5% of 308 euthyroid patients who were age- and sex-matched. A significant correlation was observed between diastolic blood pressure and serum levels of $T_3$ or $T_4$. Of 14 patients who received thyroid replacement, 13 had normalization of their blood pressure.[27]

Because of changes in lipid metabolism observed in patients with hypothyroidism, the possibility of an increased risk of atherosclerosis has been raised. In hypothyroidism, there is elevation of cholesterol and triglycerides, and an impairment of free fatty acid mobilization, all of which are associated with prema-

ture coronary artery disease. Experimentally, atherosclerosis develops more readily in cholesterol-fed hypothyroid animals, compared with euthyroid animals. Moreover, patients with hypothyroidism have about twice the frequency of coronary atherosclerosis as do age- and sex-matched controls.

### ELECTROCARDIOGRAPHIC FINDINGS

The most common electrocardiographic finding in patients with hypothyroidism is sinus bradycardia. Also, there may be a low P-wave amplitude and prolongation of the QT interval.[28] There also is an increased duration of the QRS interval. The prolongation of the QRS and QT intervals may predispose to reentrant rhythms and may be an explanation for the increased incidence of ventricular arrhythmias occurring in patients with hypothyroidism. Furthermore, in patients with pericardial effusions, the electrocardiogram may show decreased voltage.

### ENZYME ABNORMALITIES

Laboratory abnormalities in patients with hypothyroidism may include an elevated creatine phosphokinase (CPK) concentration. This elevation may complicate the evaluation of patients with hypothyroidism and chest pain. The CPK level may be elevated in the absence of myocardial damage and, when levels are high, the MB band may be positive.[29]

### THERAPY

As with hyperthyroidism and cardiac dysfunction, the primary mode of treatment of cardiac dysfunction in the hypothyroid patient is correction of the thyroid abnormality itself (see Chap. 45). In patients who are hypothyroid and elderly, the thyroid hormone should be replaced cautiously because of the possibility of unmasking underlying organic heart disease. Depending on the clinical situation, an adequate starting dose of levothyroxine (L-thyroxine) is often 0.025 mg per day with an increase of 0.025 mg approximately every 2 weeks, with frequent monitoring of the patient's cardiovascular status. Serum thyroid-stimulating hormone (TSH) levels should be followed closely to determine when adequate replacement has been achieved. With the replacement of thyroid hormone, cardiovascular responses are rapid. In one series,[30] where full replacement of thyroid hormone was achieved, improvement in the preejection period and in the preejection period/LV ejection time ratio was seen within 1 week of treatment. Moreover, CPK levels and serum cholesterol levels normalized within 1 week of therapy.

In patients with true congestive heart failure, treatment is difficult because the heart's responsiveness to the cardiac glycosides is reduced substantially. The presence of ventricular arrhythmias should not be considered a contraindication for thyroid hormone replacement because these arrhythmias more often improve, rather than exacerbate, when thyroid hormone is given. Whether to treat patients with angina and hypothyroidism with thyroid hormone is uncertain because the angina may be exacerbated by hormone administration. However, there is also an increased risk during coronary artery bypass surgery in these patients if they are severely hypothyroid at the time of surgery. In most cases, at least partial thyroid hormone replacement is indicated, at which time, if angina persists, the patient may undergo coronary revascularization. After surgery, full thyroid replacement can be safely achieved.[31]

### AMIODARONE AND THYROID FUNCTION

The increasing use of amiodarone over the past 15 years for cardiac arrhythmia has substantially increased the number of cardiology patients with thyroid problems ranging from hypo- to hyperthyroidism. The most classic thyroid function test (TFT) findings in patients on amiodarone are upper range of normal $T_4$, low range of normal $T_3$, and a transient increase in TSH on initiation of treatment, with a subsequent fall to the low normal range.[32,33] These changes result in the clinical manifestations of hypo- or hyperthyroidism in 2% to 24% of patients.[32] Hypothyroidism is a more frequent manifestation in areas of adequate iodine intake such as the United States, whereas hyperthyroidism is more common in areas of low iodine intake such as Italy.

The mechanisms of amiodarone-induced thyroid dysfunction remain unclear. Several possibilities that have been proposed include (a) disturbance in iodine autoregulation, (b) induction of thyroid autoimmunity, and (c) direct thyroid cytotoxicity.

### PATIENT EVALUATION AND DIAGNOSIS

Because of the frequency of abnormalities in TFTs in patients on amiodarone and the potential impact of these abnormalities on cardiac function, routine testing is recommended. A suggested algorithim for management of patients receiving amiodarone is depicted in Figure 203-1.[32] Clinical indications for TFTs include classic manifestations of hyper- and hypothyroidism as well as deterioration of the underlying cardiac disorder. It is unusual for hypothyroidism to present after the first $1\frac{1}{2}$ years of treatment, whereas hyperthyroidism may present at any time. Diagnosis is made by the combination of corresponding clinical manifestations and an elevated or suppressed TSH.

### TREATMENT OF AMIODARONE-INDUCED THYROID DYSFUNCTION

Treatment is difficult because of the long half-life of amiodarone and the necessity of continuing treatment for some patients. When hypothyroidism occurs, L-thyroxine can be used. However, the treatment of hyperthyroidism is more complicated. If the drug is stopped, hyperthyroidism may take more than 6 months to resolve. During this period or in those patients who continue amiodarone therapy, medical treatment options include the use of corticosteroids, propylthiouracil (PTU), and perchlorate. In some cases, near-total thyroidectomy is the best option to allow continuation of amiodarone treatment. Radioiodine thyroid ablation is usually not successful due to the high total body and thyroid iodine load and resultant low thyroid iodine uptake.

# PARATHYROID DISEASES

The effect of parathyroid disease on the heart has been thought to be primarily due to hypercalcemia or hypocalcemia. However, it has been documented that parathyroid hormone (PTH) has a direct effect on the heart.[34] When PTH is added to isolated heart cells, there is an increase in chronotropy and inotropy.[35] The direct effect of PTH on the heart is probably mediated by the binding of PTH to receptors, which increases entry of calcium into the myocardial cell. In rat heart cells, PTH causes early cell death; therefore, the direct effects of PTH in hyperparathyroidism may be harmful.[35]

PTH has a mixed effect on blood pressure and vascular reactivity. Intact PTH levels are closely related to blood pressure, particularly in elderly subjects.[36] Subacute infusions of physiologic doses of PTH in humans modestly increase blood pressure.[37] In contrast, some osteogenic fragments of PTH are hypotensive.[38]

### HYPERPARATHYROIDISM

In patients with chronic hypercalcemia, there may be deposition of calcium in the heart valve, coronary arteries, myocardial

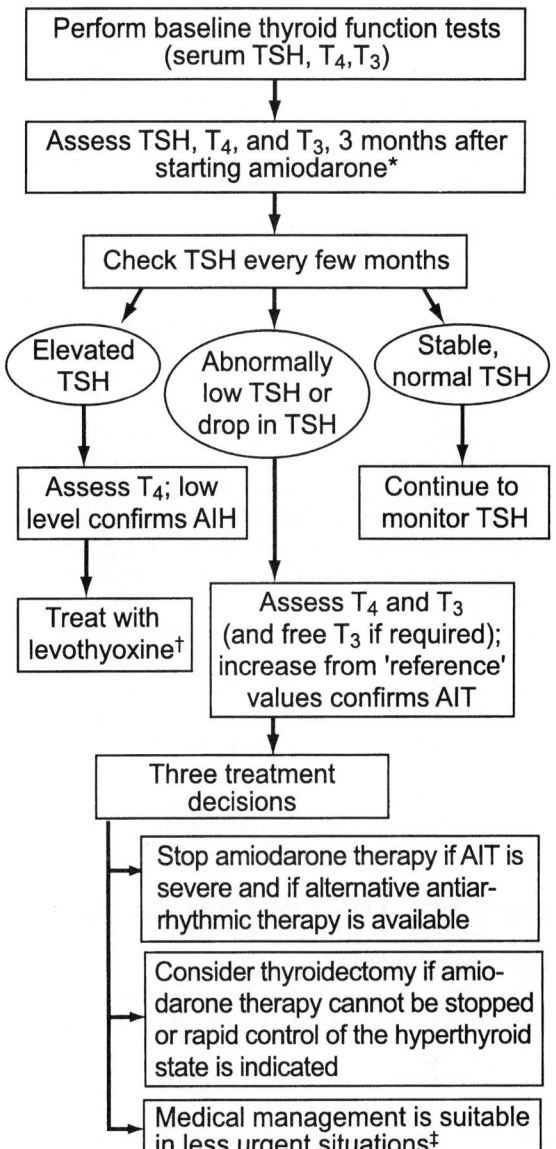

**FIGURE 203-1.** An algorithm for following thyroid function in patients on amiodarone. *Test should be performed as a baseline reference for future test results. †Goal is to increase serum thyroxine ($T_4$) to high normal or slightly above. (Do not attempt to normalize serum thyroid-stimulating hormone [*TSH*].) ‡Thionamides plus potassium perchlorate or prednisone for a short period of time might be helpful. β-Blockers can be added. ($T_3$, triiodothyronine; *AIH*, amiodarone-induced hypothyroidism; *AIT*, amiodarone-induced hyperthyroidism.) (From Harjari KJ, Licata AA. Effects of amiodarone on thyroid function. Ann Intern Med 1997; 126:63.)

fibers, and fibrous skeleton of the heart.[39] In hypercalcemic patients, the action potential plateau of cardiac fibers is shortened, thus decreasing the action potential duration that is reflected in the electrocardiographic finding of a shortened QT interval.[28] Arrhythmias may occur.[40,40a]

Patients with hyperparathyroidism and hypercalcemia have a higher prevalence of hypertension than normocalcemic matched controls. There are various mechanisms that have been proposed to account for the higher prevalence of hypertension. Whether PTH, itself, contributes to the pathogenesis of hypertension is unclear.[41] A hypertensive parathyroid-like factor has been proposed as the etiologic factor,[42] and it correlates with blood pressure in salt-sensitive essential hypertensive subjects.[43] Hypercalcemia may cause hypertension by inducing renal failure from nephrocalcinosis. In addition, there is increased myocardial contractility, peripheral resistance, and vascular sensitivity to vasoconstrictor agents, such as AII and norepinephrine. The most likely cause of the hypertension in patients with hyperparathyroidism is an elevation of peripheral resistance. A significant number of patients have resolution of the hypertension after surgical cure of their hyperparathyroidism.[44]

## HYPOPARATHYROIDISM

The effects on cardiac muscle of hypocalcemia due to hypoparathyroidism are opposite those of hypercalcemia; there is action potential prolongation that may prolong the QT interval.[28] Hypocalcemia also may have detrimental effects on cardiac function. In some patients with congestive heart failure and hypocalcemia, the heart failure did not respond to conventional therapy until the serum calcium concentration was normalized. Although experimentally a decrease in serum calcium concentration reduces cardiac contractility, heart failure is rarely seen in patients with hypocalcemia; therefore, it usually is the patient with an already compromised myocardial function who is susceptible to its effects. Besides the direct effects of the hypocalcemia on myocardial contractility, there is some evidence for a decrease in sodium excretion with hypocalcemia, which could be an additive factor in the development of congestive heart failure. Although most patients who develop myocardial dysfunction with hypocalcemia are patients with underlying cardiac disease, there have been several case reports of patients with no underlying cardiac disease who developed decreased myocardial function secondary to hypocalcemia resulting from hypoparathyroidism.[45]

## DISEASES OF THE ADRENAL GLAND

### CUSHING SYNDROME

Before the development of effective treatment for their disease, accelerated atherosclerosis was common in patients with Cushing syndrome; early death from either myocardial infarction, congestive heart failure, or stroke was the usual course. Although hypertension may partly contribute to the atherosclerosis, the accelerated atherosclerosis most likely is secondary to the lipid-mobilizing effects of cortisol. Excess cortisol production leads to hyperlipidemia and hypercholesterolemia, both of which may promote the development of atherosclerosis.

The pathophysiology of the hypertension in Cushing syndrome is uncertain. Initially, it was thought to be secondary to volume expansion because of cortisol's mineralocorticoid properties. However, studies[46] have been unable to support this hypothesis, except when the glucocorticoid levels exceed the capacity of the renal 11β-hydroxysteroid dehydrogenase. Other hypotheses include glucocorticoid potentiation of vascular smooth muscle response to the glucocorticoid itself[47] or to vasoconstrictor agents,[48] perhaps by suppressing nitric oxide production.[49] Glucocorticoids can also increase renin substrate.[50] With an increase in renin substrate, the elevated blood pressure would be secondary to the increased generation of AII. Finally, it has been proposed that glucocorticoids specifically increase renal vascular resistance, resulting in increased sodium retention.[51] Thus, it is likely that the pathophysiology of the hypertension is multifactorial, with volume expansion, increased production of AII, and increased sensitivity of the vascular smooth muscle to glucocorticoids and vasoactive agents all having a role.

In addition to efforts directed at lowering cortisol production, treatment of the cardiovascular manifestations of Cushing syndrome are aimed primarily at correcting the hypokalemia, if present, and lowering the blood pressure. Because these patients already have a tendency to lose potassium, treating the hypertension with potassium-losing diuretics must be done cautiously. Several studies have suggested that the hypertension may be more specifically treated with agents that block the release or action of renin (e.g., β-adrenergic blockers and converting enzyme inhibitors).[50] Because of their tendency toward hypokalemia, patients with Cushing syndrome should be treated cautiously with cardiac glycosides (see Chap. 75).

## HYPERALDOSTERONISM

Traditionally, aldosterone's effect on the cardiovascular system has been viewed as nonspecific and secondary to its effect on arterial pressure and potassium balance[52] (see Chap. 80). Thus, T- or U-wave abnormalities on the electrocardiogram, and premature ventricular contractions, as well as other arrhythmias caused by the hypokalemia, often are observed.[28] Evidence for LV hypertrophy, either on an electrocardiogram or on a chest x-ray film, also is common, particularly with long-standing primary aldosteronism. However, data suggest a much larger role for aldosterone in inducing cardiovascular injury.[53]

While LVH is common in primary aldosteronism, the LVH is greater than what would be expected for the degree of hypertension when compared to other secondary or primary forms of hypertension.[54,55] Arterial compliance is also inversely correlated to the level of aldosterone in subjects with hypertension.[56] These data suggest that aldosterone may have a direct effect on collagen formation—a hypothesis strongly supported by experimental data.[57] Aldosterone increases cardiac fibrosis independent of an AII effect in experimental animals.[58] Experimental studies also suggest that aldosterone induces strokes and renal disease,[59] which also occur with an increased frequency in the human hypertension that is associated with increased aldosterone production.[60] Finally, blockade of mineralocorticoid receptors by agents such as spironolactone or epleranone (not available in the United States) inhibits the development of fibrosis and/or reverses it.[61,62]

## ADRENAL INSUFFICIENCY

The most common cardiovascular finding in adrenal insufficiency (see Chap. 76) is arterial hypotension. In severe cases, the pressure has been in the range of 80/50 mm Hg, with a substantial postural fall. Heart size and the peripheral pulse also may be decreased. Most patients with chronic adrenal insufficiency have an abnormal electrocardiogram, with low or inverted T waves, sinus bradycardia, and prolongation of the $QT_c$ interval.[30] Twenty percent of these patients have conduction defects, with first-degree heart block being the most common. Paradoxically, changes secondary to hyperkalemia are not common, even though the serum potassium levels may be elevated. Interestingly, most of the cardiographic abnormalities do not respond to mineralocorticoid replacement, but do respond to glucocorticoid therapy.

## PHEOCHROMOCYTOMA

The major cardiovascular manifestation of pheochromocytoma is hypertension. Episodic discharge of catecholamines, reduction in plasma volume, and impaired sympathetic reflexes all contribute to the lability of blood pressure in these patients. Although some studies indicate that an absolute reduction in plasma volume exists only in a few cases, a number of observations strongly support the hypothesis that chronic volume depletion, to some extent, is present in most untreated patients with pheochromocytoma. For example, severe hypotension occurs with α-adrenergic blockade or removal of the tumor and is correctable by volume expansion. Impaired peripheral vascular reflexes are suggested by (a) orthostatic hypotension, (b) an increase in heart rate accompanied by decreased stroke volume, and (c) inadequate adjustment in peripheral vascular resistance.

In 75% of patients with pheochromocytoma, the electrocardiogram is abnormal.[28] The most common abnormalities include LVH, T-wave inversion, sinus tachycardia, and other alterations in rhythm such as supraventricular ectopic beats or paroxysmal supraventricular tachycardia. Depending on the level of blood pressure, changes are observed that are suggestive of myocardial damage, including transient ST segment elevation, diffuse T-wave inversions, and ST segment depressions. Because not all of the electrocardiographic changes can be attributed to hypertension or myocardial ischemia, a specific catecholamine-induced myocarditis has been proposed.[63] In one study, 50% of patients who died from pheochromocytoma had myocarditis, usually accompanied by LV failure and pulmonary edema.[63] Pathologically, the myocarditis consisted of focal necrosis with infiltration of inflammatory cells, contraction band necrosis, perivascular inflammation, and fibrosis.[63] Although there is evidence of atherosclerosis of the coronary arteries, medial thickening is the most common characteristic. Rats exposed to high levels of norepinephrine show similar changes in their coronary arteries.

# GONADAL HORMONES AND THE HEART

The effect of sex steroids on cardiovascular disease (CVD) has been investigated extensively, although there is still much debate over their role. The hypothesis that estrogens are protective against the development of atherosclerotic CVD is based on two observations. First, middle-aged men are at a higher risk for developing CVD than age-matched women. Second, this difference between men and women equalizes when postmenopausal women are compared with men of the same age. The mechanism whereby estrogens exert their protective effect is unclear and may involve effects on lipids, endothelial-dependent vasodilation, and blood pressure.

## POSTMENOPAUSAL HORMONE REPLACEMENT

Lower total cholesterol and higher high-density lipoprotein (HDL) cholesterol levels are seen in premenopausal women and postmenopausal women on estrogen. In the Postmenopausal Estrogen/Progestin Intervention (PEPI) study[64] of 875 women, higher HDL levels were seen in those taking unopposed estrogen (conjugated equine estrogen [CEE] 0.625 mg). However, the concomitant use of medroxyprogesterone, commonly used in clinical practice, tended to negate this benefit, while micronized progesterone did not.

An improvement in endothelial-dependent vasodilation has also been reported with unopposed estrogen therapy. This effect may be blunted or negated when medroxyprogesterone is added, but is maintained with the addition of natural progesterone.[65]

Although early oral contraceptives, containing higher doses of estrogens and varying progestins, were reported to cause hypertension, the doses of estrogen currently used for hormone-replacement therapy (HRT) have not been associated with hypertension. CEE appears to have a neutral effect on blood pressure, whereas estradiol may actually lower blood pressure.[66] Since estradiol is the primary estrogen of the premenopausal state, this may explain why hypertension is less common in pre- than in postmenopausal women. The rise in blood pressure following menopause may be one of the several contributors to the increase in CVD. The potential benefit of estradiol for HRT in this regard has not been evaluated.

Although epidemiologic studies had suggested a benefit to women using HRT on CVD, the Heart and Estrogen/Progestin Replacement Study (HERS)[67] did not. In a study of 2673 postmenopausal women with already established coronary heart disease, the use of CEE, 0.625 mg per day, and medroxyprogesterone, 2.5 mg per day, led to no improvement in future cardiac events. Indeed, in the first year of study, there was an increase in venous thromboembolism in the treatment group. Whether a benefit would have been seen in a primary prevention study remains to be seen, and should be answered by the Women's Health Initiative, scheduled for completion in 2006. Perhaps, if CEE does not give the CVD benefit of the premenopausal state, other estrogens (e.g., estradiol) might, and further studies of the impact of different estrogens on CVD will need to be carried out. Furthermore, the selective estrogen-receptor modulators will need to be evaluated in this regard.

## ORAL CONTRACEPTIVES

The use of oral contraceptive agents in the premenopausal woman has been associated with an increased risk of cardiovascular morbidity and mortality (see Chaps. 104 and 105). A three- to four-fold increase in incidence of deep venous thrombosis (DVT) has been reported.[68] This risk appears to be limited to women with other cardiovascular risk factors, such as smoking and hypertension. There also is a higher incidence of myocardial infarctions. These also may represent a thrombotic process, because in most myocardial infarctions a thrombosis forms on a preexisting substrate of a narrowing, which is secondary to atherosclerosis. This theory is supported by autopsy studies in women who have died from myocardial infarction while using oral contraceptives. They usually have thrombosis as a cause of their myocardial infarction.[69] As with DVT, women without underlying CVD do not appear to have increased risk. Changes in intrinsic coagulability induced by the oral contraceptives may account for the increased risk of thrombosis. Women with factor V Leiden mutations have a five- to ten-fold increased risk of thromboembolism.

In many women taking oral contraceptives, there is an elevation of blood pressure. The rise in blood pressure that develops in these patients is ascribed to the estrogen component, which increases the production of renin substrate by the liver. Although there is a small increase in blood pressure in many patients taking oral contraceptives, most do not develop clinical hypertension, suggesting that there are counterregulatory mechanisms that are brought into play in most women to compensate for the increase in renin substrate. It also has been theorized that women who develop clinical hypertension are those who are predisposed (e.g., family history of hypertension, renal disease).

# REFERENCES

1. Klee GG. Biochemical thyroid function testing. Mayo Clin Proc 1994; 69:469.
2. Ezzat S, Forster MJ, Berchtold P, et al. Acromegaly. Clinical and biochemical features in 500 patients. Medicine 1994; 73:233.
3. Aono J, Nobuoka S, Nagashima J, et al. Heart failure in three patients with acromegaly: echocardiographic assessment. Intern Med 1998; 37:599.
3a. Colao A, Baldelli R, Marzullo P, et al. Systemic hypertension and impaired glucose tolerance are independently correlated to the severity of the acromegalic cardiomyopathy. J Clin Endocrinol Metab 2000; 85:193.
3b. Fazio S, Cittadini A, Biondi B, et al. Cardiovascular effects of short-term growth hormone hypersecretion. Clin Endocrinol Metab 2000; 85:179.
4. Minniti G, Moroni C, Jaffrain-Rea ML, et al. Prevalence of hypertension in acromegalic patients: clinical measurement versus 24-hour ambulatory blood pressure monitoring. Clin Endocrinol 1998; 48:149.

5. Strauch G, Valloton MB, Touitou Y. The renin-angiotensin-aldosterone system in normotensive and hypertensive patients with acromegaly. N Engl J Med 1972; 287:795.

6. Moore TJ, Thein-Wai W, Dluhy RG, et al. Abnormal adrenal and vascular responses to angiotensin II and an angiotensin antagonist in acromegaly. J Clin Endocrinol Metab 1980; 51:215.

7. Lopez-Velasco R, Escobar-Morreale HF, Vega B, et al. Cardiac involvement in acromegaly: specific myocardiopathy or consequence of systemic hypertension? J Clin Endocrinol Metab 1997; 82:1047.

8. Fazio S, Cittadini A, Cuocolo A, et al. Impaired cardiac performance is a distinct feature of umcomplicated acromegaly. J Clin Endocrinol Metab 1994; 79:441.

9. Ozbey N, Oncul A, Bugra Z, et al. Acromegalic cardiomyopathy: evaluation of the left ventricular diastolic function in the subclinical stage. J Endocrinol Invest 1997; 20:305.

10. Baldelli R, Ferretti E, Jaffrain-Rea ML, et al. Cardiac effects of slow-release lanreotide, a slow-release somatostatin analog, in acromegalic patients. J Clin Endocrinol Metab 1999; 84:527.

11. Nishiki M, Murakami Y, Sohmiya M, et al. Histopathological improvement of acromegalic cardiomyopathy by intermittent subcutaneous infusion of octreotide. Endocrinol J 1997; 44:655.

12. Lombardi G, Colao A, Ferone D, et al. Effect of growth hormone on cardiac function. Horm Res 1997; 48:38.

13. Polikar R, Burger AG, Scherrer U, Nicod P. The thyroid and the heart. Circulation 1993; 87:1435.

14. Nishizawa Y, Hamada N, Fujii S, et al. Serum dopamine-beta-hydroxylase activity in thyroid disorders. J Clin Endocrinol Metab 1974; 39:599.

15. Hammond HK, White FC, Buxton ILO, et al. Increased myocardial beta receptors and adrenergic responses in hyperthyroid pigs. Am J Physiol 1987; 252:H283.

16. Rutherford JP, Vatner SF, Braunwald E. Adrenergic control of myocardial contractility in conscious hyperthyroid dogs. Am J Physiol 1980; 237:590.

17. Philipson KD, Edelman IS. Thyroid hormone control of Na$^+$/K$^+$-ATPase and K$^+$ dependent phosphatase in rat heart. Am J Physiol 1977; 232:C196.

18. Chizzonite RA, Everett AW, Clark WA, et al. Isolation and characterization of two molecular variants of myosin heavy chain from rabbit ventricle. Change in their content during normal growth and after treatment with thyroid hormone. J Biol Chem 1982; 257:2056.

19. Davis PJ, Davis FB. Acute cellular actions of thyroid hormone and myocardial function. Ann Thorac Surg 1993; 56(Suppl 1):S16.

20. Channick BJ, Adlin EV, Marks AD, et al. Hyperthyroidism and mitral valve prolapse. N Engl J Med 1981; 305:497.

21. Olshaasen K, Bischoff S, Kahaly G, et al. Cardiac arrhythmias and heart rate in hyperthyroidism. Am J Cardiol 1989; 63:930.

22. Sandler G, Wilson GM. The nature and prognosis of heart disease in thyrotoxicosis. A review of 150 patients treated with $^{131}$I. Q J Med 1959; 28:347.

23. Nakazawa HK, Sakurai K, Hamada N, et al. Management of atrial fibrillation in the post-thyrotoxic state. Am J Med 1982; 72:903.

24. Staffurth JS, Gibberd MC, Fui ST. Arterial embolism in thyrotoxicosis with atrial fibrillation. Br Med J 1977; 2:688.

25. Chopra IJ, Huang T-S, Hurd RE, Solomon DH. A study of cardiac effects of thyroid hormones: evidence for amelioration of the effects of thyroxine by sodium ipodate. Endocrinology 1984; 114:2039.

26. Shenoy MM, Goldman JM. Hypothyroid cardiomyopathy: echocardiographic documentation of reversibility. Am J Med Sci 1987; 294:1.

27. Saito I, Ito K, Saruta T. Hypothyroidism as a cause of hypertension. Hypertension 1983; 5:112.

28. Surawicz B, Manigiardi ML. Electrocardiogram in endocrine and metabolic disorders. In: Rios JC, ed. Clinical electrocardiographic correlation. Philadelphia: FA Davis Co, 1977:243.

29. Goldman J, Matz R, Mortimer R, Freeman R. High elevation of creatine phosphokinase in hypothyroidism. An isoenzyme analysis. JAMA 1977; 283:325.

30. Ladenson PW, Goldenheim PD, Cooper DS, et al. Early peripheral responses to intravenous L-thyroxine in primary hypothyroidism. Am J Med 1982; 73:467.

31. Drucker DJ, Burrow GN. Cardiovascular surgery in the hypothyroid patient. Arch Intern Med 1985; 145:1585.

32. Harjari KJ, Licata AA. Effects of amiodarone on thyroid function. Ann Intern Med 1997; 126:63.

33. Newman CM, Price A, Davies DW, et al. Amiodarone and the thyroid: a practical guide to the management of thyroid dysfunction induced by amiodarone therapy. Heart 1998; 79:121.

34. Stefenelli T, Mayr H, Berler-Klein J, et al. Primary hyperparathyroidism: incident of cardiac abnormalities and partial reversibility after successful parathyroidectomy. Am J Med 1993; 95:197.

35. Bogin E, Massry SG, Harary I. Effect of parathyroid hormone on rat heart cells. J Clin Invest 1981; 67:1215.

36. Morfis L, Smerdely P, Howes LG. Relationship between serum parathyroid hormone levels in the elderly and 24-h ambulatory blood pressures. J Hypertens 1997; 15:1271.

37. Fliser D, Franek E, Fode P, et al. Subacute infusion of physiological doses of parathyroid hormone raises blood pressure in humans. Nephrol Dial Transplant 1997; 12:933.

38. Whitfield JF, Morley P, Ross V, et al. The hypotensive actions of osteogenic and non-osteogenic parathyroid hormone fragments. Calcif Tissue Int 1997; 60:302.

39. Roberts WC, Waller BF. Effect of chronic hypercalcemia on the heart: an analysis of 18 necropsy patients. Am J Med 1981; 71:371.

40. Carpenter C, May ME. Case report: cardiotoxic calcemia. Am J Med Sci 1994; 307:43.

40a. Chang CJ, Chen SA, Tai CT, et al. Ventricular tachycardia in a patient with primary hyperparathyroidism. Pacing Clin Electro Physiol 2000; 23:534.

41. Hulter HN, Melby JC, Peterson JC, Cooke CR. Chronic continuous PTH infusion results in hypertension in normal subjects. J Clin Hypertens 1986; 2:360.

42. Pang PK, Benishin CG, Lewanczuk RZ. Parathyroid hypertensive factor: a circulating factor in animal and human hypertension. Am J Hypertens 1991; 4:472.

43. Resnick LM. Calciotropic hormones in salt-sensitive essential hypertension: 1,25-dihydroxyvitamin D and parathyroid hypertensive factor. J Hypertens 1994; 12(Suppl):S3.

44. Resnick LM. Calcium, parathyroid disease, and hypertension. Cardiovasc Rev Rep 1982; 3:1341.

45. Suzuki T, Ikeda U, Fujikawa H, et al. Hypocalcemic heart failure: a reversible form of heart muscle disease. Clin Cardiol 1998; 21:227.

46. Williamson PM, Kelly JJ, Whitworth JA. Dose-response relationships and mineralocorticoid activity in cortisol-induced hypertension in humans. J Hypertens 1996; 14(Suppl):S37.

47. Walker BR, Best R, Shackleton CH, et al. Increased vasoconstrictor sensitivity to glucocorticoids in essential hypertension. Hypertension 1996; 27:190.

48. Kalsner S. Mechanism of hydrocortisone potentiation of response to epinephrine and norepinephrine in rabbit aorta. Circ Res 1969; 24:383.

49. Kelly JJ, Mangos G, Williamson PM, Whitworth JA. Cortisol and hypertension. Clin Exp Pharmacol Physiol 1998; 25(Suppl):S51.

50. Krakoff L, Nicolis G, Amsel B. Pathogenesis of hypertension in Cushing's syndrome. Am J Med 1975; 58:216.

51. Gordon RD. Mineralocorticoid hypertension. Lancet 1994; 344:240.

52. Whitworth JA, Kelly JJ, Brown MA, et al. Glucocorticoids and hypertension in man. Clin Exp Hypertens 1997; 19:871.

53. Pessina AC, Sacchetto A, Rossi GP. Left ventricular anatomy and function in primary aldosteronism and renovascular hypertension. Adv Exp Med Biol 1997; 432:63.

54. Rossi GP, Sacchetto A, Pavan E, et al. Remodeling of the left ventricle in primary aldosteronism due to Conn's adenoma. Circulation 1997; 95:1471.

55. Shigematsu Y, Hamada M, Okayama H, et al. Left ventricular hypertrophy precedes other target-organ damage in primary aldosteronism. Hypertension 1997; 29:723.

56. Blacher J, Amah G, Girerd X, et al. Association between increased plasma levels of aldosterone and decreased systemic arterial compliance in subjects with essential hypertension. Am J Hypertens 1997; 10:1326.

57. Funck RC, Wilke A, Rupp H, Brilla CG. Regulation and role of myocardial collagen matrix remodeling in hypertensive heart disease. Adv Exp Med Biol 1997; 432:35.

58. Sun Y, Ramires FJ, Weber KT. Fibrosis of atria and great vessels in response to angiotensin II or aldosterone infusion. Cardiovasc Res 1997; 35:138.

59. Funder JW, Krozowski Z, Myles K, et al. Mineralocorticoid receptors, salt and hypertension. Recent Prog Horm Res 1997; 52:247.

60. Litchfield WR, Anderson BF, Weiss RJ, et al. Intracranial aneurysm and hemorrhagic stroke in glucocorticoid remediable aldosteronism. Hypertension 1998; 31:445.

61. Benetos A, Lacolley P, Safar ME. Prevention of aortic fibrosis by spironolactone in spontaneously hypertensive rats. Arterioscler Thromb Vasc Biol 1997; 17:1152.

62. Stier CT Jr, Chander PN, Zuckerman A, Rocha A. Vascular protective effect of a selective aldosterone receptor antagonist in stroke-prone spontaneously hypertensive rats. Am J Cardiol 2000; in press.

63. McManus BM, Fleury TA, Roberts WC. Fatal catecholamine crisis in pheochromocytoma: curable form of cardiac arrest. Am Heart J 1981; 102:930.

64. Writing Group for PEPI Trial. Effects of estrogen or estrogen/progestin regimens on heart disease risk factors in postmenopausal women: the postmenopausal estrogen/progestin interventions (PEPI) trial. JAMA 1995; 273:199.

65. Gerhard M, Walsh BW, Tawakol A, et al. Estradiol therapy combined with progesterone and endothelium-dependent vasodilation in postmenopausal women. Circulation 1998; 98:1158.

66. Seely EW, Walsh BW, Gerhard MD, Williams GH. Estradiol with or without progesterone and ambulatory blood pressure in postmenopausal women. Hypertension 1999; 33:1190.

67. Hulley S, Grady D, Bush T, et al. Randomized trial of estrogen plus progestin for secondary prevention of coronary heart disease in postmenopausal women. Heart and Estrogen/Progestin Replacement Study (HERS) Research Group. JAMA 1998; 280:605.

68. Mosca L, Manson JE, Sutherland SE, et al. Cardiovascular disease in women. A statement for healthcare professionals from the American Heart Association. Circulation 1997; 96:2468.

69. Psaty BM, Heckbert SR, Atkins D, et al. A review of the association of estrogens and progestins with cardiovascular disease in postmenopausal women. Arch Intern Med 1993; 153:1421.

# CHAPTER 204

# GASTROINTESTINAL MANIFESTATIONS OF ENDOCRINE DISEASE

ALLAN G. HALLINE

## HORMONES AND GASTROINTESTINAL FUNCTION

Gastrointestinal function involves a complex process of food transport, digestion, and absorption, secretion, and excretion. The normal function of the alimentary tract depends on a coordinated interaction of many different hormones and neuroendocrine substances; consequently, disorders of the endocrine system may have a profound effect on the gut. The gastrointestinal manifestations of endocrine disease are discussed here. The gastrointestinal symptomatology associated with diabetes is discussed in Chapter 149.

Moreover, various hormones and other chemical messengers that are synthesized within the gut serve to coordinate such important activities as gastric emptying, intestinal motility, biliary and pancreatic secretion, and mucosal absorption and secretion. Known collectively as the diffuse neuroendocrine system of the gut (see Chap. 175), these chemical messengers include peptides, prostaglandins, leukotrienes, serotonin, and histamine working in concert with the autonomic nervous system. The distinction between hormonal and neurologic influences becomes even more blurred with the localization of several of these gastrointestinal peptides (e.g., cholecystokinin) both within mucosal endocrine cells and the nerves of the gut (see Chap. 182). Other messengers such as vasoactive intestinal peptide (VIP) are located primarily in nerves and function as neurotransmitters, but they are released into local tissues or the bloodstream and also may serve a paracrine or hemocrine function.

## HORMONE-SECRETING TUMORS OF THE GUT

Certain hormone-secreting tumors of the gut are associated with profound gastrointestinal manifestations and may be part of, or even the presenting manifestation of, the multiple endocrine neoplasia (MEN) syndromes (see Chap. 188). The gut-related hormone-producing tumors (gastrinoma, vasoactive intestinal peptide–producing carcinoma [VIPoma], somatostatinoma, glucagonoma, carcinoid) and their clinical manifestations are discussed in Chapters 220 and 221. The Zollinger-Ellison (ZE) syndrome results from excessive neoplastic gastrin production, capable of inducing acid hypersecretion and severe ulceration of the duodenum and jejunum. This ulceration is often refractory to antacid or histamine $H_2$-receptor blocker therapy and may require high-dose proton-pump inhibitors such as omeprazole. One-third of ZE patients have diarrhea, which may be due to excessive gastric acid production, mucosal damage of the small bowel, and increased pancreatic and small bowel secretions. Inactivation of pancreatic lipase by the low pH in the intestinal lumen or precipitation of bile salts may cause steatorrhea. Moreover, the rugal folds of the stomach may become thickened because of the trophic influences of gastrin on the mucosa. VIP is a known secretagogue that may affect the small bowel. An excess production of this hormone, the so-called VIPoma, may produce watery diar-

rhea, hypokalemia, and achlorhydria (WDHA syndrome).[1] Other tumors producing glucagon, somatostatin, or serotonin also lead to well-characterized syndromes that may include effects on the gut. Tumor production of other chemical messengers, such as neurotensin, mammalian bombesin, and substance P, has not been associated with distinct clinical manifestations.

## IMPACT OF ENDOCRINE DISEASE ON THE GUT

### HYPOTHALAMUS-PITUITARY CONDITIONS

Diseases of the hypothalamus and pituitary gland usually are not associated with significant gastrointestinal complaints, except in relation to their effects on other hormones that likewise may alter digestive tract functions. The role of hypothalamic disease in disruption of human gastrointestinal physiology has yet to be clearly defined[2] (see Chap. 9). Normal pituitary function is required to maintain gastric acid secretion, perhaps related to the production of growth hormone. An increased frequency of colonic adenomatous polyps has been reported in patients with acromegaly[3] although others have found no increased prevalence of colonic polyps or other gastrointestinal neoplasms. Generally, in patients with diseases of the hypothalamus and pituitary gland, neurologic and other systemic manifestations are more significant than are gastrointestinal symptoms.

### THYROID DISORDERS

Abnormal gastrointestinal function frequently is encountered in patients with thyroid disorders and may be the initial or sole manifestation of either the hyperthyroid or hypothyroid state. This may result either from a direct mechanical effect of an enlarged thyroid gland or through the effects of increased or decreased thyroid hormone on the gut. In addition, disease affecting both the thyroid gland and the gut is well documented. For example, many reports have demonstrated concomitant thyroid conditions and gastrointestinal dysfunction,[4] including thyroid abnormalities in patients with Sjögren syndrome, pernicious anemia, gluten-sensitive enteropathy, nonspecific inflammatory bowel disease, primary biliary cirrhosis, and chronic active hepatitis—disorders commonly demonstrating immunologic features (see Chaps. 42 and 197).

#### GOITER AND COMPRESSION SYNDROMES

Esophageal compression from thyroid enlargement is common, and dysphagia may be seen in up to 30% of cases referred for thyroidectomy.[5,6] Dysphagia and symptoms of esophageal dysfunction occasionally may also be secondary to altered esophageal motility; in severe myxedema, megaesophagus rarely may be present. Patients with thyrotoxicosis also may develop dysphagia and evidence of altered esophageal motility.[7] In patients with large goiters, superior vena cava compression may lead to formation of "downhill" esophageal varices in up to 12%.[8] Rarely, upper gastrointestinal hemorrhage from esophageal varices may be the initial presentation of a substernal goiter.[9]

#### HYPERTHYROIDISM

Hyperthyroidism (see Chap. 42) commonly presents with increased appetite, weight loss, and more frequent bowel movements. Less often, thyrotoxic patients complain of watery stools and may even have steatorrhea; rarely, constipation is seen.[10] In elderly patients or in those with severe thyrotoxicosis, anorexia, nausea, and vomiting are sometimes seen and may contribute to weight loss.[11–13] Rarely, abdominal pain and functional duodenal obstruction have been reported.[14,15] The abdominal pain may be either chronic or acute in nature, at times simulating a "surgical" abdomen. Although the cause of this pain is unclear, it generally resolves promptly with correction of the hyperthyroid state. In the rare reported cases of functional duodenal obstruction, a history of significant weight loss is common and features similar to superior mesenteric artery syndrome are found.[14,15] When vomiting is significant, nasogastric suction may be required and treatment with rectal instillation of propylthiouracil has been successful.[15] Correction of hyperthyroidism results in gradual resolution of the obstruction. The degree of weight loss in hyperthyroidism is variable, but after successful treatment most patients return to their premorbid weight. Additional factors contributing to weight loss include increased metabolic rate and a decreased absorption of nutrients from the gut.

## HYPOTHYROIDISM

Hypothyroidism (see Chap. 45) may present with weight gain, diminished appetite, and clinical manifestations of altered intestinal motility, such as constipation, bloating, and flatulence. Usually, the weight gain is mild and is due to fluid retention that is associated with mucopolysaccharide deposition in various tissues and also occasionally to the presence of ascites (Fig. 204-1). However, weight loss and/or diarrhea may occur in hypothyroidism.[16] Intestinal hypomotility and pseudoobstruction are well described in hypothyroidism and may lead to unnecessary surgery.[17] Occasionally, intestinal atony may progress to massive bowel distention and result in perforation.[17]

In hypothyroidism abdominal pain may also occur. In myxedema, ~10% of patients insidiously develop nonspecific abdominal discomfort. When accompanied by bowel distention and elevated serum carcinoembryonic antigen levels (frequently seen in this disorder), the clinical picture may mimic colonic malignancy.

## PHYSIOLOGIC/LABORATORY STUDIES

Thyroid dysfunction can affect motility throughout the gastrointestinal tract.[18–20] In hyperthyroidism, oral-cecal transit

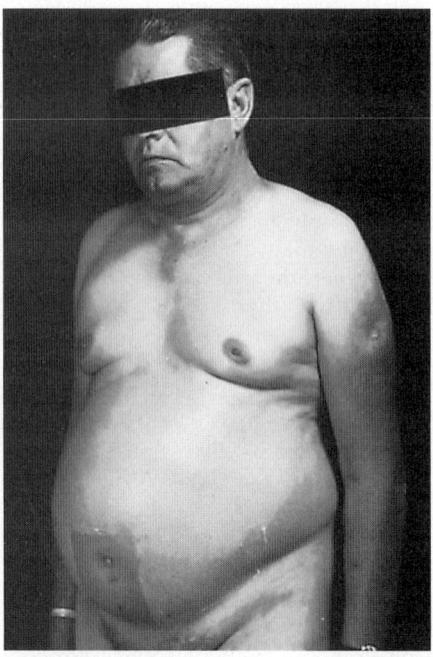

**FIGURE 204-1.** A 52-year-old hypothyroid man with ascites. Bilateral pleural effusions also were present.

time, evaluated by hydrogen breath tests, may be accelerated.[21] In hypothyroidism, gastric emptying is prolonged[18] and delayed small bowel and colonic transit has been documented, occasionally presenting as paralytic ileus or even as megacolon.[22] The frequency of intestinal slow-wave electrical activity, a cyclical depolarization of smooth muscle and an important determinant of motility, is increased in hyperthyroidism and decreased in hypothyroidism.[23]

Decreased salivary secretion has been described in both hyperthyroidism and hypothyroidism and may be secondary to coexisting Sjögren syndrome. Although decreased gastric acid secretion has been reported in many studies of both hyperthyroid and hypothyroid patients, a great deal of controversy remains, and these findings have not been confirmed.[19,24] In some cases, diminished acid production may be due to underlying pernicious anemia.[12]

Thyroid diseases also have been associated with mild abnormalities in intestinal absorption. For example, steatorrhea is described in more than 25% of hyperthyroid patients and appears to be due to the ingestion of large quantities of fat, as well as to rapid intestinal transit and reduced contact time with the small bowel mucosa.[13] Although abnormalities in pancreatic and biliary secretion may be detected in hyperthyroidism, they probably are not responsible for fat malabsorption. Thyrotoxic patients tend to have decreased calcium absorption from the jejunum and a resultant negative calcium balance. This defect may be due to increased mobilization of bone calcium, decreased parathyroid hormone (PTH) activity, and lowered plasma 1,25-dihydroxyvitamin D levels; yet, other mechanisms may be involved.[25] There appears to be no relationship between this decreased calcium absorption and the presence or absence of steatorrhea.

Elevated glucose tolerance curves are found in thyrotoxic patients, and flattened curves may be observed for hypothyroid patients. However, these findings may be accounted for by abnormal gastrointestinal transit, altered activity of the sympathetic nervous system, and changes in other carbohydrate-regulating hormones. D-Xylose absorption is normal in most instances of hyperthyroidism or hypothyroidism, further suggesting the absorptive integrity of the small bowel.[12] Yet, increased incidences of lactose intolerance, gluten-sensitive enteropathy, and nonspecific inflammatory bowel disease are found in association with either of these thyroid disorders.

Various histologic abnormalities of the gastrointestinal tract may be observed in patients with thyroid disorders, but no consistent abnormality has been confirmed. For example, there appears to be an increased frequency of atrophic gastritis in both hyperthyroidism and hypothyroidism, with an infiltration of lymphocytes and plasma cells occurring throughout the mucosa and submucosa of the entire gastrointestinal tract.[22,26] Furthermore, myxedematous infiltrations of the bowel wall occur in hypothyroidism, especially in the duodenum and colon.[2] However, these types of changes are not found universally, and their significance is uncertain.

Ascites is seen in <5% of myxedematous patients; the etiology remains unclear. Characteristically, the ascitic fluid has a high protein content (>2.5 g/dL) and a high serum-ascites albumin gradient (>1.1 g/dL).[27] It is often accompanied by pleural and pericardial effusions, and generally responds well to hormonal replacement (see Fig. 204-1).

## MEDULLARY THYROID CANCER AND MULTIPLE ENDOCRINE NEOPLASIA TYPE 2B SYNDROME

Up to 30% of patients with medullary thyroid carcinoma present with secretory diarrhea that is occasionally severe enough to cause dehydration and electrolyte abnormalities[28] (see Chap. 40).

Sometimes, it resolves on resection of the tumor but usually it occurs in patients with widely metastatic disease. The microscopic appearance of the small bowel is generally normal, and the etiology probably relates to altered secretory or absorptive function of the small intestinal mucosa. Others[29] have demonstrated that rapid colonic transport and a concomitant decrease in absorption may be more important in the pathogenesis of diarrhea. Calcitonin probably plays a central role in the production of this diarrhea; indeed, the infusion of this hormone into normal patients has been shown to lead to decreased intestinal absorption of water and electrolytes.[30] There is, however, poor correlation between the presence of diarrhea and the level of calcitonin; therefore, other humoral substances may be active. Besides calcitonin, medullary carcinoma of the thyroid may produce several humoral substances, such as VIP, prostaglandins, serotonin, kallikrein, and gastrin, all of which may have an effect on small bowel secretion or motility. Treatment with somatostatin analogs and interferon-$\alpha_{2b}$ may be effective in controlling diarrhea and flushing, since results with chemotherapy have been disappointing.[31]

Medullary thyroid carcinoma is associated with mucosal and submucosal ganglioneuromatosis of the bowel in patients with the MEN2B syndrome (see Chap. 188), which may alter motility throughout the gut. More than 90% of patients with MEN2B have gastrointestinal complaints.[32] Symptoms of colonic dysmotility are often the earliest manifestation of this inherited disorder and may present within the first few months of life. Constipation is the most frequent complaint but diarrhea is also seen. Radiographic studies often demonstrate proximal colonic dilatation and rectosigmoid narrowing similar to that observed in Hirschsprung disease.[32] Colonic diverticulosis is also common and, rarely, patients may present with a perforated diverticulum. In the esophagus, motility disorders may occasionally be seen, and dysphagia has been described.

## PARATHYROID GLAND DISORDERS

### HYPERPARATHYROIDISM

Symptomatic primary hyperparathyroidism (see Chap. 58) most commonly presents with renal or skeletal disease, but gastrointestinal manifestations may be seen in up to 35% of the patients. The reported frequency of abdominal symptoms varies according to the patient population and selection bias, the degree of hypercalcemia, and the duration of illness. With the advent of multichannel serum autoanalyzers, up to 50% of patients with hyperparathyroidism are being diagnosed on the basis of asymptomatic hypercalcemia.[33]

The most dramatic presentation of gastroenterologic manifestations occurs in the syndrome of so-called acute hyperparathyroidism, when the serum calcium level often exceeds 17 mg/dL. Such patients often present with severe abdominal pain, nausea, vomiting, lethargy, dehydration, and altered mental status that may progress to coma and seizures. In many of these cases, digestive tract symptoms predominate and peptic ulceration or pancreatitis is common.[34] Acute hyperparathyroidism can be life threatening and emergency parathyroidectomy may become necessary.

Primary hyperparathyroidism also is associated with frequent gastrointestinal symptoms that include anorexia, weight loss, nausea, vomiting, abdominal pain, and constipation.[34a] Although early studies described an increased incidence of peptic ulceration in hyperparathyroidism, this association has been disputed.[35] Any true association between these disorders is most often the result of a concurrent gastrinoma as part of the MEN1 syndrome. In patients with MEN1 and coexisting ZE syndrome and hyperparathyroidism, resection of the parathyroids alone has resulted in a significant reduction in serum gastrin levels,

acid secretion, and requirement for anti-ulcer medications,[36] lending further support to the association between hyperparathyroidism and peptic ulceration.

Hyperparathyroidism may be associated with acute or chronic pancreatitis in 3% to 7% of cases.[37] Elevated levels of both calcium and PTH have been implicated in the pathophysiology of this disease.[37a] Several examples of pancreatitis secondary to hypercalcemia from other causes, including administration of calcium chloride, vitamin D intoxication, and malignancy-associated hypercalcemia, have been reported.[37,38] PTH may also have direct toxic effects on the pancreas; however, none of these mechanisms has been unequivocally demonstrated in human subjects.

In acute pancreatitis, hypocalcemia has been attributed to the formation of calcium–fatty acid soaps in areas of fat necrosis, and also, a recognized abnormality of calcium homeostasis characterized by an impaired mobilization of calcium from bone and inadequate PTH release. Clinically, severe pancreatitis presenting with normal calcium levels, when ordinarily some degree of hypocalcemia is expected, should raise the suspicion of hyperparathyroidism.

Constipation may be seen in 30% of chronically hyperparathyroid patients and may relate to decreased smooth muscle tone or abnormal autonomic function of the gut. Moreover, hypercalcemia can lead to increased renal loss of free water, and to severe dehydration—a predisposing factor to constipation.

An association between hyperparathyroidism and esophageal dysfunction has been suggested, with symptoms of reflux reported in up to 60% of patients.[39] Esophageal manometry demonstrated reduced lower esophageal sphincter pressure, which normalized in most of these patients after parathyroidectomy. Although calcium infusion reduces lower esophageal sphincter tone in normal subjects, this result is unconfirmed; therefore, its mechanism and significance remain uncertain.

The prevalence of gallstone disease may be as high as 25% to 35% among patients with hyperparathyroidism, but a relationship between the two entities is controversial.

Carcinoid tumors, especially of the foregut, occur in association with both the MEN1 and MEN2 syndromes.[40] Thus, hyperparathyroidism should be considered in patients with carcinoids.[41]

### HYPOPARATHYROIDISM

Hypoparathyroidism (see Chap. 60) most commonly presents with neurologic and cardiac disease related to hypocalcemia; gastrointestinal symptoms are uncommon and a review[42] failed to mention any symptoms referable to the digestive tract. Yet, an association between idiopathic hypoparathyroidism and pernicious anemia has been recognized (see Chap. 197). In one study,[43] 9% of patients with idiopathic hypoparathyroidism had a diagnosis of pernicious anemia, and a slightly higher percentage had circulating antibodies against parietal cells. Gastric acid secretion ceases with serum calcium levels below 7.0 mg/dL, and the restoration of normal acid output follows correction of the hypocalcemia. The clinical significance of this finding is uncertain.

Several cases of idiopathic hypoparathyroidism in association with diarrhea and malabsorption have been reported. Usually, the small bowel architecture is normal, and the cause of the bowel dysfunction remains unclear. Correction of hypocalcemia generally improves the diarrhea.[44] However, one case report described a loss of small bowel villous architecture suggestive of celiac sprue; the patient responded to a gluten-free diet and not to correction of the hypoparathyroid state.[45]

## ADRENAL GLAND DISORDERS

Many studies suggest that normal human gastric acid secretion depends on an adequate production of adrenal corticosteroids, and diseases both of the adrenal cortex and medulla frequently may be associated with gastrointestinal symptoms and dysfunction. Evidence for this comes from the documentation of achlorhydria in up to 50% of patients with Addison disease (see Chap. 76) as well as the frequent finding of gastric atrophy in these cases.[46] Repletion with corticosteroids restores normal gastric acid secretion in many of these patients, but contrary data also exist.[46] The most common form of adrenal insufficiency seen today, idiopathic adrenal gland atrophy, often is presumed to be due to autoimmune mechanisms, and immune-mediated disease of the stomach is also a possibility in this clinical entity. For example, an increased incidence of pernicious anemia occurs in patients with idiopathic adrenal insufficiency, and up to 30% of the latter may have circulating antibodies reactive against parietal cells or intrinsic factor.[47] Clearly, the precise role of normal adrenal function in the maintenance of gastric secretion requires continued study.

### ADRENAL INSUFFICIENCY

Both acute and chronic adrenal insufficiency often are associated with gastrointestinal symptoms. Anorexia and weight loss are early manifestations in most cases and may progress to nausea and intractable vomiting.[48] Abdominal pain occurs in one-third of patients, although often mild and of a nonspecific character. In advanced cases, the abdominal pain occasionally may be severe and accompanied by tenderness and rigidity that simulate an acute "surgical" abdomen.[48] The etiology of these manifestations is unknown, but may be due, in part, to delayed gastric emptying[49] or altered intestinal motility,[50] and usually symptoms are relieved with correction of the hormone deficiencies. Nonetheless, adrenal insufficiency may be precipitated by the stress of intraabdominal sepsis and, thus, the clinical picture of an acute abdomen must be carefully assessed in these patients.

Diarrhea and steatorrhea have been described in a few cases of adrenal insufficiency.[51] The loss of fecal fat, electrolytes, and other nutrients may contribute to weight loss and hypotension and generally is corrected upon supplementation with corticosteroids.

### CUSHING SYNDROME

Cushing syndrome (see Chap. 75) is not associated with significant gastrointestinal disturbances, despite reports of increased serum gastrin levels[52] and excessive gastric acid secretion in this condition; for example, the incidence of peptic ulceration is not increased.[53] In normal human volunteers, chronic corticosteroid administration can increase both basal and stimulated gastric acid output[46]; long-term corticosteroid or adrenocorticotropic hormone (ACTH) administration also increases basal serum gastrin levels and the serum gastrin response to an ingested meal.[54] Although there are some who believe that exogenously administered corticosteroids play no role in the development of peptic ulcer disease,[55] others suggest that the incidence of ulcers actually may be slightly increased.[56]

### PHEOCHROMOCYTOMA

Gastrointestinal manifestations generally are not a predominant part of the clinical presentation of pheochromocytoma (see Chap. 86). However, one study revealed a high incidence of nausea and vomiting (50%), weight loss (40%), and abdominal pain (35%).[57] Several cases of adynamic ileus associated with pheochromocytoma have been reported, and constipation has been described in up to 8% of patients.[57] This may be due to high circulating levels of epinephrine and norepinephrine, both of which have an inhibitory effect on the smooth muscle of the gastrointestinal tract.[58] In fact, most cases have been associated with large adrenal tumors with the potential to release massive amounts of catecholamines

and cause decreased alimentary motility. Spasm of the intestinal vasculature may lead to ischemia of the gut and, thus, cases with bowel infarction[59] and gastrointestinal bleeding have been described.[58] Diarrhea and steatorrhea occasionally occur, with resolution of symptoms after resection of the pheochromocytoma. Although this may result from ischemic damage to the intestinal mucosa, occasionally diarrhea may be due to secretion by the tumor of other hormones, including VIP, somatostatin, calcitonin, or gastrin.[60,60a] Rare reports of hyperamylasemia and abdominal pain mimicking pancreatitis have been described in pheochromocytoma; however, there have been no documented cases of pancreatitis, and the amylase has been shown to arise from nonpancreatic sources.[61]

### SEX HORMONE–RELATED CONDITIONS

Various gastrointestinal symptoms caused by increased levels of female sex hormones have been suggested, based on observations made during pregnancy and in patients receiving hormonal therapy or taking oral contraceptives. Heartburn is a frequent complaint in up to 50% of pregnant women, occurring most often during the third trimester.[62] During pregnancy, there is a progressive fall in lower esophageal sphincter pressure and a decrease in esophageal peristalsis that returns to normal after delivery.[63] This appears to be due to raised levels of progesterone, a known smooth muscle relaxant, but other hormones including estrogen also may be important. Studies in normal women taking oral contraceptives have shown a reversible decrease in lower esophageal sphincter pressure when they are given a combination of the progestational agent, dimethisterone, and ethinyl estradiol in physiologic doses.[64]

A great deal of controversy exists over the effect of pregnancy on preexisting inflammatory bowel disease; however, most authors agree that pregnancy does not influence the severity or the frequency of exacerbation of Crohn disease or ulcerative colitis.[65]

The increased incidence of reversible ischemic colitis in young women using oral contraceptives, although rare, is well recognized.[66] Symptoms include abdominal pain, nausea, vomiting, and hematochezia. In mild cases, mucosal ulceration, erythema, or friability, often limited to the left colon, may be seen at colonoscopy. Usually, these findings resolve upon stopping the oral contraceptive; rarely, they may progress to mesenteric thrombosis and bowel infarction. This may be caused by an acquired resistance to activated protein C.[67]

Estrogens are a rare cause of pancreatitis, but when this does occur, it is often seen in patients with underlying lipid disorders.[68] In such cases, severe hypertriglyceridemia in response to estrogen administration may develop with levels often exceeding 1000 to 2000 mg/dL.[68] Pancreatitis during pregnancy has been related to the presence of gallstones in up to 90% of cases.[69] In a small percentage of cases, pancreatitis may be secondary to gestational hypertriglyceridemia.[70] Small intestinal transit is slowed during the second and third trimesters of pregnancy,[71] but the clinical significance of this is unclear.

Vomiting during pregnancy is common, and severe hyperemesis gravidarum may lead to dehydration and electrolyte and acid-base disturbances. Several hormones have been implicated, including human chorionic gonadotropin, estrogen, progesterone, thyroxine, and others; however, studies remain inconclusive.[72] Gastric slow-wave activity, a determinant of stomach emptying, has been shown to be frequently disrupted during pregnancy.[73] These effects have been duplicated in nonpregnant women with administration of progesterone alone, or with progesterone and estradiol at levels comparable to those found during pregnancy.[73]

# REFERENCES

1. O'Dorisio TM, Mekhjian HS, Gaginella TS. Medical therapy of VIPomas. Endocrinol Metab Clin North Am 1989; 18:545.
2. Grijalva CV, Novin D. The role of the hypothalamus and dorsal vagal complex in gastrointestinal function and pathophysiology. Ann N Y Acad Sci 1990; 597:207.
3. Ladas SD, Thalassinos NC, Ioannides G, Raptis SA. Does acromegaly really predispose to an increased prevalence of gastrointestinal tumors? Clin Endocrinol 1994; 41:597.
4. Counsell CE, Taha A, Ruddell WSJ. Coeliac disease and autoimmune thyroid disease. Gut 1994; 35:844.
5. Anders HJ. Compression syndromes caused by substernal goitres. Postgrad Med J 1998; 74:327.
6. Newman E, Shaha AR. Substernal goiter. J Surg Oncol 1995; 60:207.
7. Branski D, Levy J, Globus M, et al. Dysphagia as a primary manifestation of hyperthyroidism. J Clin Gastroenterol 1984; 6:437.
8. Schmidt KJ, Lindner H, Bungartz A, et al. Mechanical and functional complications in endemic struma. Munch Med Wochenschr 1976; 118:7.
9. Glanz S, Koser MW, Dallemand S, Gordon DH. Upper esophageal varices: report of three cases and review of the literature. Am J Gastroenterol 1982; 77:194.
10. Middleton WRJ. Thyroid hormones and the gut. Gut 1971; 12:172.
11. Scarf M. Gastrointestinal manifestations of hyperthyroidism: an analysis of 80 cases of hyperthyroidism with a report of 4 cases masked by digestive symptoms. J Lab Clin Med 1936; 21:1253.
12. Miller LJ, Gorman CA, Go VLW. Gut-thyroid interrelationships. Gastroenterology 1978; 75:901.
13. Thomas FB, Caldwell JH, Greenberger NJ. Steatorrhea in thyrotoxicosis: relation to hypermotility and excessive dietary fat. Ann Intern Med 1973; 78:669.
14. McClenathan JH, Wood BP. Hyperthyroidism as a cause of superior mesenteric artery syndrome. Am J Dis Child 1988; 142:685.
15. Cansler CL, Latham JA, Browne PM, et al. Duodenal obstruction in thyroid storm. South Med J 1997; 90:1143.
16. Stagias JG, Marignani P. Diarrhea, constipation, and hypothyroidism. J Clin Gastroenterol 1994; 18:347.
17. Bergeron E, Mitchell A, Heyen F, Dube S. Acute colonic surgery and unrecognized hypothyroidism: a warning. Dis Colon Rectum 1997; 40:859.
18. Kahraman H, Kaya N, Demircali A, et al. Gastric emptying time in patients with primary hypothyroidism. Eur J Gastroenterol Hepatol 1997; 9:901.
19. Dubois A, Goldman JM. Gastric secretion and emptying in hypothyroidism. Dig Dis Sci 1984; 29:407.
20. Wegener M, Wedmann B, Langhoff T, et al. Effect of hyperthyroidism on the transit of a caloric solid-liquid meal through the stomach, the small intestine, and the colon in man. J Clin Endocrinol Metab 1992; 75:745.
21. Papa A, Cammarota G, Tursi A, et al. Effects of propylthiouracil on intestinal transit time and symptoms in hyperthyroid patients. Hepatogastroenterology 1997; 44:426.
22. Duret RL, Bastenie PA. Intestinal disorders in hypothyroidism: clinical and manometric study. Dig Dis Sci 1971; 16:723.
23. Christensen J, Schedl HP, Clifton JA. The basic electrical rhythm of the duodenum in normal human subjects and in patients with thyroid disease. J Clin Invest 1964; 43:1659.
24. Miller LJ, Owyang C, Malagelada JR, et al. Gastric, pancreatic, and biliary responses to meals in hyperthyroidism. Gut 1980; 21:695.
25. Peerenboom H, Keck E, Kruskemper HL, Strohmeyer G. The defect of intestinal calcium transport in hyperthyroidism and its response to therapy. J Clin Endocrinol Metab 1984; 59:936.
26. Hellesen C, Friis T, Larsen E, Pock-Steen OC. Small intestinal histology, radiology and absorption in hyperthyroidism. Scand J Gastroenterol 1969; 4:169.
27. de Castro F, Bonacini M, Walden JM, Schubert TT. Myxedema ascites: report of two cases and review of the literature. J Clin Gastroenterol 1991; 13:411.
28. Hanna FW, Ardill JE, Johnston CF, et al. Regulatory peptides and other neuroendocrine markers in medullary carcinoma of the thyroid. J Endocrinol 1997; 152:275.
29. Rambaud JC, Jian R, Fluorie B, et al. Pathophysiological study of diarrhea in a patient with medullary thyroid carcinoma: evidence against a secretory mechanism and for the role of shortened colonic transit time. Gut 1988; 29:537.
30. Gray TK, Bieberdorf FA, Fordtran JS. Thyrocalcitonin and jejunal absorption of calcium, water, and electrolytes in normal subjects. J Clin Invest 1973; 52:3084.
31. Lupoli G, Cascone E, Arlotta F, et al. Treatment of advanced medullary thyroid carcinoma with a combination of recombinant interferon alpha-2b and octreotide. Cancer 1996; 78:1114.
32. O'Riordain DS, O'Brien T, Crotty TB, et al. Multiple endocrine neoplasia type 2B: more than an endocrine disorder. Surgery 1995; 118:936.
33. St. Goar WT. Gastrointestinal symptoms as a clue to the diagnosis of primary hyperparathyroidism: a review of 45 cases. Ann Intern Med 1957; 46:102.
34. Anglem TJ. Acute hyperparathyroidism: a surgical emergency. Surg Clin North Am 1966; 46:727.
34a. Lumachi F, Zucchetta A, Angelini F, et al. Tumors of the parathyroid glands. J Exp Clin Cancer Res 2000; 19:7.
35. Akerstrom G. Non-familial primary hyperparathyroidism. Semin Surg Oncol 1997; 13:104.
36. Norton JA, Cornelius MJ, Doppman JL, et al. Effect of parathyroidectomy in patients with hyperparathyroidism, Zollinger-Ellison syndrome, and multiple endocrine neoplasia type I: a prospective study. Surgery 1987; 102:958.
37. Carnaille B, Oudar C, Pattou F, et al. Pancreatitis and primary hyperparathyroidism: forty cases. Aust N Z J Surg 1998; 68:117.
37a. Mjaland O, Normann E. Severe pancreatitis after parathyroidectomy. Scand J Gastroenterol 2000; 35:446.
38. Fernandez del Castillo C, Harringer W, Warshaw A, et al. Risk factor for pancreatic injury after cardiopulmonary bypass. N Engl J Med 1991; 325:382.
39. Mowschenson PM, Rosenberg S, Pallotta J, Silen W. Effect of hyperparathyroidism and hypercalcemia on lower esophageal sphincter pressure. Am J Surg 1982; 143:36.
40. Duh QY, Hybarger CP, Geist R, et al. Carcinoids associated with multiple endocrine neoplasia syndromes. Am J Surg 1987; 154:142.
41. Rode J, Dhillon AP, Cotton PB, et al. Carcinoid tumour of the stomach and primary hyperparathyroidism: a new association. J Clin Pathol 1987; 40:546.
42. Breslau NA, Pak NYC. Hypoparathyroidism. Metabolism 1979; 28:1261.
43. Blizzard RM, Chee D, Davis W. The incidence of parathyroid and other antibodies in the sera of patients with idiopathic hypoparathyroidism. Clin Exp Immunol 1966; 1:119.
44. Peracchi M, Bardella MT, Conte D. Late-onset idiopathic hypoparathyroidism as a cause of diarrhoea. Eur J Gastroenterol Hepatol 1998; 10:163.
45. Matsueda K, Rosenberg IH. Malabsorption with idiopathic hypoparathyroidism responding to treatment for coincident celiac sprue. Dig Dis Sci 1982; 27:269.
46. Cushman P Jr. Glucocorticoids and the gastrointestinal tract: current status. Gut 1970; 11:534.
47. Irvine WJ, Barnes EW. Adrenocortical insufficiency. Clin Endocrinol Metab 1972; 1:549.
48. Sorkin SZ. Addison's disease. Medicine 1949; 28:371.
49. Valenzuela G, Davis T, McGroaty D, et al. Primary adrenal insufficiency: a new cause of reversible gastric stasis. Am J Gastroenterol 1990; 85:1626.
50. Phillips JD, Stelzner M, Zeng H, et al. Alterations in gastrointestinal motility during postoperative acute steroid withdrawal. Am J Surg 1991; 162:251.
51. Tobin MV, Aldridge SA, Morris AI, et al. Gastrointestinal manifestations of Addison's disease. Am J Gastroenterol 1989; 84:1302.
52. Lopez-Guzman A, Salvador J, Frutos R, et al. Hypergastrinaemia in Cushing's syndrome: pituitary origin or glucocorticoid-induced? Clin Endocrinol 1996; 44:335.
53. Kyle J, Logan JS, Neill DW, Welbourn RB. Influence of the adrenal cortex on gastric secretion in man. Lancet 1956; 1:664.
54. Seino S, Seino Y, Matsukura S, et al. Effect of glucocorticoids on gastrin secretion in man. Gut 1978; 19:10.
55. Conn HO, Blitzer BL. Nonassociation of adrenocorticosteroid therapy and peptic ulcer. N Engl J Med 1976; 294:473.
56. Messer J, Reitman D, Sacks HS, et al. Association of adrenocorticosteroid therapy and peptic ulcer disease. N Engl J Med 1983; 309:21.
57. Hume DM. Pheochromocytoma in the adult and in the child. Am J Surg 1960; 99:458.
58. Turner CE. Gastrointestinal pseudo-obstruction due to pheochromocytoma. Am J Gastroenterol 1983; 78:214.
59. Salehi A, Legome EL, Eichorn K, Jacobs RS. Pheochromocytoma and bowel ischemia. J Emerg Med 1997; 15:35.
60. Interlandi JW, Hundley RF, Kasselberg AG, et al. Hypercortisolism, diarrhea with steatorrhea, and massive proteinuria due to pheochromocytoma. South Med J 1985; 78:879.
60a. Van Eeckhart P, Shungu H, Descamps FX, et al. Acute watery diarrhea as the initial presenting feature of a pheochromocytoma in an 84-year-old female patient. Horm Res 1999; 52:101.
61. Perrier NA, van Heerden JA, Wilson DJ, Warner MA. Malignant pheochromocytoma masquerading as acute pancreatitis—a rare but potentially lethal occurrence. Mayo Clin Proc 1994; 69:366.
62. Van Thiel DH, Gavaler JS, Joshi SN, et al. Heartburn of pregnancy. Gastroenterology 1977; 72:666.
63. Singer AJ, Brandt LJ. Pathophysiology of the gastrointestinal tract during pregnancy. Am J Gastroenterol 1991; 86:1695.
64. Van Thiel DH, Gavaler JS, Stremple J. Lower esophageal sphincter pressure in women using sequential oral contraceptives. Gastroenterology 1976; 71:232.
65. Hanan IM, Kirsner JB. Inflammatory bowel disease in the pregnant woman. Clin Perinatol 1985; 12:669.
66. Deana DG, Dean PJ. Reversible ischemic colitis in young women. Association with oral contraceptive use. Am J Surg Pathol 1995; 19:454.
67. Mann DE, Kessel ER, Mullins DL, Lottenberg R. Ischemic colitis and acquired resistance to activated protein C in a woman using oral contraceptives. Am J Gastroenterol 1998; 93:1960.
68. Glueck CJ, Lang J, Hamer T, Tracey T. Severe hypertriglyceridemia and pancreatitis when estrogen replacement therapy is given to hypertriglyceridemic women. J Lab Clin Med 1994; 123:59.
69. McKay AJ, O'Neill J, Imrie CW. Pancreatitis, pregnancy and gallstones. Br J Obstet Gynaecol 1980; 87:47.
70. Roberts IM. Hyperlipidemic gestational pancreatitis. Gastroenterology 1993; 104:1560.
71. Lawson M, Kern F, Everson GT. Gastrointestinal transit time in human pregnancy: prolongation in the second and third trimesters followed by postpartum normalization. Gastroenterology 1985; 89:996.
72. Broussard CN, Richter JE. Nausea and vomiting of pregnancy. Gastroenterol Clin North Am 1998; 27:123.
73. Walsh JW, Hasler WL, Nugent CE, Owyang C. Progesterone and estrogen are potential mediators of gastric slow-wave dysrhythmias in nausea of pregnancy. Am J Physiol 1996; 270:G506.

## CHAPTER 205

# THE LIVER AND ENDOCRINE FUNCTION

NICOLA DE MARIA, ALESSANDRA COLANTONI, AND DAVID H. VAN THIEL

The liver is a hormone-responsive organ. Not only are numerous hepatic metabolic functions regulated by hormones, but the liver also is a principal site for hormone metabolism and clearance. In general, whereas the receptors for peptide hormones (e.g., insulin, glucagon, thyroid-stimulating hormone [TSH], adrenocorticotropic hormone [ACTH], and many small peptides [e.g., hypothalamic releasing factors]) are located on the surface of hepatocytes, the receptors for lipophilic hormones (e.g., steroid hormones) are located in either the cytosol or nucleus. Receptors for small neurotransmitters or signal transmitters present a mixed pattern: acetylcholine, $\alpha$-adrenergic neurotransmitter, and $\beta$-adrenergic agents are located on the cell surface. In contrast, the receptors for thyroid hormone are located within the cell, on mitochondria, and in the nucleus.

The response of liver cells to a hormone is dependent on the concentration of the hormone in extracellular fluid, the affinity of the hormone for its receptor, and the number of receptors present on or in the cell. At low hormonal concentrations, only those receptors with a high affinity are activated. With supraphysiologic amounts of hormone, nonclassic receptors can become activated and produce unusual biologic responses.

## GROWTH HORMONE

The growth-promoting actions of growth hormone (GH) are mediated by somatomedins (insulin-like growth factors) that are produced in the liver, as well as elsewhere, in response to GH stimulation (see Chap. 12). GH interacts with both "somatogenic" and "lactogenic" receptors located on the surface of hepatocytes.[1] The number of somatogenic receptors on liver cells is equal in men and women. In contrast, lactogenic receptors are present only in liver cells of women.[2,3] Prolactin (PRL) (see Chap. 13), unlike GH, binds only to the lactogenic receptors on liver cells. The number of these receptors is controlled by the levels of GH and PRL, and each of the two receptor classes is regulated independently.

### EFFECT OF GROWTH HORMONE ON THE LIVER

GH regulation of hepatic production of insulin-like growth factor-I (IGF-I) is mediated largely by somatogenic receptors (see Chap. 12).[4-6] GH stimulates hepatic protein synthesis and induces hepatic enzymes that regulate the flow of substrates into a number of metabolic pathways.[7-12] Moreover, GH is thought to be the factor that determines the sexually dimorphic pattern of hepatic drug metabolism.[13] The complex influences of GH on hepatic carbohydrate and lipid metabolism include both insulin-like and insulin antagonistic effects.

Hepatic somatomedin production is regulated predominantly by GH[14,15]; however, whether somatomedins are synthesized de novo or only released from storage sites remains unresolved. Subsequent to in vitro GH stimulation, protein synthesis inhibitors block IGF-I production, suggesting de novo synthesis rather than a simple release of stored IGF-I.[16] Malnutrition, a potent depressor of somatomedin, can block the effect

of GH. Thus, somatomedin concentrations are reduced in response to protein/calorie malnutrition or fasting and are not increased in response to administration of exogenous GH in these conditions.[17] The precise mechanisms by which nutritional factors modulate somatomedin production and release are unclear.

### EFFECT OF LIVER DISEASE ON GROWTH HORMONE HOMEOSTASIS

Because the liver is the major site of GH degradation, hepatocyte injury is associated with a reduction in GH clearance, and serum GH levels are increased in patients with chronic liver diseases. Thus, serum GH levels also correlate with the severity of the liver disease.[18,19] In cirrhotic patients, a wide variety of unusual physiologic stimuli (e.g., thyrotropin-releasing hormone [TRH] and oral glucose) enhance pituitary secretion of GH. In contrast, somatomedin concentrations are reduced in chronic liver diseases, correlating with the severity of the liver disease as manifested by a variety of biochemical indices (e.g., levels of serum albumin, alkaline phosphatase, and bilirubin).[20]

## THYROID HORMONES

The liver is the principal site for extrathyroidal thyroid hormone metabolism.[21] The liver is also responsible for sulfation, glucuronidation, and other phase II reactions of thyroid hormones. Thyroid hormone circulates bound to three different proteins that are synthesized in the liver: thyroxine ($T_4$)–binding globulin (TBG), $T_4$-binding prealbumin (TBPA), and albumin. These proteins determine the free $T_4$ ($FT_4$) level in plasma.

### EFFECT OF ACUTE LIVER DISEASE ON THYROID HORMONE HOMEOSTASIS

Patients with acute hepatitis have elevated serum levels of $T_4$ without clinical signs of hyperthyroidism.[22-25] The increase is caused by reduced clearance of thyroid hormone secreted by the thyroid gland and increased TBG concentrations occurring as part of the acute-phase response.[24] Both conditions resolve with clinical recovery. The increase in TBG concentration observed in acute hepatic injury may in part be due to an increased release from injured hepatocytes. A correlation is found between the changes observed in serum TBG levels and the aspartate aminotransferase levels that reflect the degree of hepatic injury.[23] The rise in serum $T_4$ levels coincides with the rise in serum TBG levels, and the continued euthyroid state of the patient is reflected by a lowered triiodothyronine ($T_3$) resin uptake and a normal $FT_4$ index. If a mistaken diagnosis of hyperthyroidism is entertained, a normal TSH response to TRH stimulation should exclude this possibility. In acute hepatitis, serum $T_3$ levels are highly variable. The increased reverse $T_3$ ($rT_3$) levels normalize with recovery,[23] and serum TSH concentrations generally are normal.[23]

The hepatic conversion of $T_4$ to $T_3$ is reduced in cases of acute liver injury.[26] The $rT_3$ levels are generally increased, however, whereas both total and free $T_3$ ($FT_3$) levels are reduced in acute hepatic failure.[27-29] Reduced levels of circulating $T_4$, $T_3$, and TBG are found in some cases of massive hepatic necrosis and in cases of fulminant hepatic failure.[27-29] The $T_3/T_4$ ratio has been proposed as an index of the severity of liver disease and as a prognostic factor in patients with fulminant hepatic failure and those with advanced liver disease awaiting liver transplantation.[29,30] Overall, the serum TSH level is usually normal in patients with acute hepatitis (TSH is considered to be the single best measure of thyroid hormone status in individuals with liver disease).[31]

## EFFECT OF CHRONIC LIVER DISEASE ON THYROID HORMONE HOMEOSTASIS

Alterations in thyroid hormone levels may occur with a variety of nonthyroidal illnesses, including liver diseases. Generally, these conditions are characterized by a decreased formation of $T_3$ from $T_4$ and an increase in serum levels of $rT_3$.[32–36] These changes occur as a consequence of a reduction in 5-monodeiodinase activity, which has the dual effect of decreasing $T_3$ production and consequently the clearance of $rT_3$.

Cirrhosis and other chronic liver diseases are associated with several important changes in the indices of thyroid hormone metabolism. Several patterns of thyroid hormone levels are recognized in individuals with various chronic liver diseases. An increase in serum total $T_4$ ($TT_4$) level, due to an increase in the serum level of TBG, occurs commonly in individuals with primary biliary cirrhosis and autoimmune chronic active hepatitis.[24] The $T_3$ resin uptake is reduced and the $FT_4$ index is normal. $T_3$ resin-binding ratios are ~50% higher in patients with chronic liver disease and primary biliary cirrhosis than in control subjects.[37] Many chronic parenchymal liver diseases, and also primary biliary cirrhosis, involve autoimmune phenomena, and coexistent autoimmune Hashimoto thyroiditis is found in 18% to 22% of such patients. The HLA antigens A1, B8, and DR3 are often found in subjects with HT and primary biliary cirrhosis, primary sclerosing cholangitis, and autoimmune chronic active hepatitis.

One of the consistent findings in chronic liver disease is a reduction in the serum $T_3$ level; lowest levels occur in end-stage cirrhosis. This finding is attributed to a reduced extrathyroidal and particularly hepatic conversion of $T_4$ to $T_3$ (resulting from reduced hepatic 5-monodeiodinase).[38–42] The percentage of $T_4$ that is converted to $T_3$ is reduced from 35.7% to 15.6% in cirrhotic patients.[43,44] Besides the low serum $T_3$, $rT_3$ levels are typically increased in chronic liver disease, possibly due to a reduced clearance because of the reduced 5-monodeiodinase activity. Serum levels of $rT_3$ have been used as a prognostic indicator for survival among patients waiting for orthotopic liver transplantation and those recovering from an episode of alcoholic hepatitis.[45–48] The circulating inhibitors of extrathyroidal conversion of $T_4$ to $T_3$, which are found in patients with liver cirrhosis,[49,50] also act as thyroid hormone–binding inhibitors; they are incompletely characterized. (Free fatty acids [FFAs] have been proposed as likely candidates for this activity.)

Patients with severe chronic liver disease, as well as those with other critical illnesses, often have reduced serum $TT_4$ and $T_3$ levels. The circulating $TT_4$ concentration is more severely reduced than is the $FT_4$, which usually is normal.[51] Mixed patterns have been described in patients with very advanced liver cirrhosis, in which $TT_3$ and $TT_4$ levels, as well as $FT_3$ and $FT_4$ levels, can be either increased or reduced. The absence of a consistent pattern in these individuals reflects the complexity of the metabolic alterations that occur in patients with end-stage liver disease.

Despite all the changes occurring in thyroid hormone levels in cirrhotic individuals, little or no change in the serum level of TSH occurs in the absence of overt thyroid disease. Basal levels are either normal or slightly increased.[52–55] Moreover, the TSH response to TRH is either normal or slightly exaggerated. These findings indicate an intact hypothalamic-pituitary axis regulation of thyroid function. Nevertheless, both the elevated serum level of cortisol seen in severely ill cirrhotic patients and their overall poor nutritional state may inhibit the thyrotrope response to low $T_3$ levels.[56,57] Thus, how the euthyroid state is maintained in patients with advanced liver disease and other critical illness in the face of markedly reduced $T_3$ concentrations is not entirely clear. The major tissue effects of $T_3$ are mediated via $T_3$ nuclear receptor proteins encoded by c-*erb*A genes (see Chap. 33). Two classes of $T_3$ receptors are found in humans (i.e., c-*erb*A–α and c-*erb*A–β).[58] The levels of c-*erb*A-α and c-*erb*A–β messenger RNA in monocytes and liver tissue are increased in cirrhotic patients.[59] This finding suggests an increased rate of $T_3$ receptor synthesis despite the presence of a reduced serum $T_3$ level. As a result, an euthyroid state is achieved in target tissues where $T_3$ receptors are expressed.

## HEPATIC ASPECTS OF DRUG-INDUCED ALTERATIONS OF THYROID HORMONES

Several drugs inhibit the enzymatic monodeiodination of $T_4$ to $T_3$, potentially causing hyperthyroxinemia. Most important for hepatologists are glucocorticoids, propranolol, and certain iodinated contrast reagents used in hepatobiliary scanning and other imaging procedures. Two distinct monodeiodinase enzymes are found within microsomes: the *type I* enzyme is present both in the liver and in the kidney; the *type II* is found solely in the pituitary gland. The drugs that have been reported to cause hyperthyroxinemia by inhibiting these enzymes can be divided into two categories—*drugs that inhibit only the type I enzyme alone and drugs that inhibit both enzymes.*

Drugs inhibiting only type I 5-deiodinase activity include high-dose propylthiouracil, dexamethasone, and propranolol.[60–62] Interestingly, propranolol is the only β-adrenergic blocker that inhibits the conversion of $T_4$ to $T_3$. The second group of drugs that inhibit both type I and type II enzymes includes amiodarone and the radiographic contrast agents iopanoic acid and ipodate, which are used for cholangiography.[63] All of these drugs contain iodine and have a structure that resembles that of thyroxine. The observed changes in thyroid function studies that occur after the use of these drugs include an increased serum $T_4$ and a decreased serum $T_3$ secondary to impaired peripheral conversion and clearance, a rise in serum $rT_3$, and a rise in serum TSH secondary to impaired $T_4$ conversion to $T_3$. Cholecystographic agents also elevate $T_4$ levels by inhibiting the hepatic uptake and binding of $T_4$.[63] Failure of a patient treated with amiodarone to develop hyperthyroxinemia should suggest the presence of hypothyroidism.[64,65] Finally, the clinical onset of Hashimoto thyroiditis after interferon-α therapy in patients with chronic viral hepatitis has been observed. Most such patients have low titers of antithyroid antibodies before starting interferon therapy.[66] Conversely, the safety of interferon treatment in patients with evidence of immune dysfunction, including the presence of antithyroid autoantibodies, has been confirmed.[67,68]

## THE LIVER IN THYROID GLAND DISEASE

### HYPERTHYROIDISM

Abnormal liver function tests may occur in 15% to 76% of individuals with hyperthyroidism.[65–68] The abnormalities observed include mild increases in serum glutamic-oxaloacetic transaminase (SGOT, AST), bilirubin, and, most commonly, alkaline phosphatase.[69] Alkaline phosphatase elevations can originate from liver or bone or both. The hepatic abnormalities seen in hyperthyroidism steadily improve slowly over many months as the patient returns to a euthyroid state.

Although elevated serum bilirubin occurs in hyperthyroidism, clinical jaundice develops infrequently. The pathogenesis of the hepatic dysfunction leading to jaundice is unclear, but it may be due to tissue hypoxia. Importantly, excess thyroid hormone increases the oxygen requirements for mitochondrial metabolism.[70] Moreover, hyperthyroidism affects both overall bile production and the amount of bile acids present in bile. These thyroid hormone–induced changes in the bile acid production and pool size may contribute to the pruritus occasionally associated with hyperthyroidism.[71]

### HYPOTHYROIDISM

No consistent or specific abnormalities of hepatic function are found in patients with hypothyroidism. Serum levels of SGOT may be abnormal in as many as 50% of these patients, however, suggesting coexistent hepatocellular disease. When the source of the transaminase elevation is investigated, however, concomitant increases in serum creatine kinase (MM isoenzyme) and aldolase levels usually indicate a skeletal muscle site of origin. In myxedema, release of these enzymes from muscle is increased and plasma clearance is decreased.

## HYPOTHALAMIC–PITUITARY–GONADAL AXIS

The normal function of the hypothalamic–pituitary–gonadal (HPG) axis is frequently disturbed by liver disease (see Chap. 16). Advanced cirrhosis in men is associated with phenotypic feminization, suggesting an alteration in plasma sex hormone levels. The findings of feminization are more pronounced in alcoholic individuals, because of their associated gonadal damage. The serum estrogen/androgen ratio of cirrhotic patients is usually increased; plasma testosterone and dehydroepiandrosterone sulfate (DHEAS) levels are reduced; and estradiol levels range from normal to moderately elevated.[72,73] Because estrogens can act as tumor promoters or at least as hepatocyte proliferation stimuli, estrogens may play a cocarcinogenic role in the development of hepatocellular carcinoma (HCC) in men with cirrhosis.[74,75] In hemochromatosis, the abnormal accumulation of iron in the hypothalamus, pituitary, and gonads can impair normal hormonal function (see Chaps. 116 and 131). In some patients, gonadotropin levels may be low despite advanced gonadal failure, indicating hypothalamic-pituitary involvement.[76–81] Thus, sexual dysfunction secondary to hypogonadotropic hypogonadism is a common complication of end-stage idiopathic hemochromatosis that can occur in the absence of clinically evident liver disease. Iron-mediated hepatic damage can play a contributory role late in the natural history of the disease. Hemochromatosis patients with cirrhosis have lower serum free testosterone and estradiol concentrations than do patients without cirrhosis.[82]

Historically, the description and characterization of sex hormone receptors have been limited to target tissues (e.g., ovary, testes, uterus, and prostate), sites where the levels of these somewhat labile proteins are maximal. Classic estrogen receptors (ERs), however, are present in both male and female liver.[83–88] These high-affinity ERs bind estradiol and various other estrogenic compounds (e.g., phytoestrogens, antiestrogens, and xenobiotics like chlorophenothane [DDT]).[83,87–91] Male liver contains ~25% of the ERs in female liver.[83] Androgens repress and castration increases the male ERs. Similarly, estrogen treatment of men increases hepatic ER activity. In women, the liver contains ~25% as many cytosolic ERs as does the uterus; hepatic ER activity differs from that of classic steroid-receptive tissues. Much higher doses of estrogen are required to translocate the ERs of the liver to the nucleus of the cell. Presumably, this occurs because the cytosolic metabolism of estrogen by the liver limits the availability of the steroid for its receptor.[92] Moreover, because of this metabolism within the liver cytosol, hepatic ERs are exposed to many different estrogenic metabolites and xenobiotics not found in classic ER-containing tissues.

The hepatic ER in humans has high affinity and low capacity; it is specific for both steroidal and nonsteroidal estrogens.[93]

**TABLE 205-1.**
**Sexual Dimorphism in Hepatic Processes**

| Elevated in Men | Elevated in Women |
|---|---|
| **MICROSOMAL OXIDATIVE ENZYMES** | **MICROSOMAL REDUCTIVE ENZYMES** |
| Estrogen 2-hydroxylase | Steroid 5α-reductase |
| 6α-Hydroxylase | |
| 16α-Hydroxylase | |
| Hexobarbital hydroxylase | |
| Benzo(α)pyrene hydroxylase | |
| **ENZYMES** | **ENZYMES** |
| Ethylmorphine demethylase | Bile acid sulfotransferase |
| Lidocaine N-demethylase | 15α-Hydroxylase (steroid sulfates) |
| Imipramine N-demethylase | Histidase |
| Imipramine N-oxidase | |
| Aminopyrine demethylase | |
| **RECEPTORS** | **RECEPTORS** |
| Androgen receptor | Estrogen receptor |
| | Prolactin receptor |
| | Low-density lipoprotein (LDL) receptor |
| **PROTEINS** | |
| β2-Microglobulin | |
| Male-specific estrogen binder (MEB) | |
| **SERUM PROTEINS** | **SERUM PROTEINS** |
| α1- Antitrypsin | Ceruloplasmin |
| | Sex steroid–binding globulin |
| | Transcortin |
| | Thyroxine-binding globulin |

Besides the cytosolic ER, human liver also contains ERs in the nuclear fraction,[94] suggesting that they are functional.

## SEXUAL DIMORPHISM OF HEPATIC FUNCTION

Men and women differ markedly in their ability to metabolize different classes of xenobiotics.[95–99] Generally, men have a higher hepatic content of microsomal oxidative enzymes, and women have a greater capacity for reductive activity (Table 205-1). Androgens appear to be the major steroids that determine the "masculine" pattern of hepatic metabolic function. In fact, most of the metabolic functions that are elevated in men require *androgen imprinting* (a brief surge of testicular androgen synthesis early in life) to achieve and maintain adult levels of masculine activities. The imprinting process occurs at the level of the hypothalamus or pituitary. Whether a direct effect of imprinting on the liver also occurs is unclear. Some imprinted functions require the constant presence of androgen after puberty for expression, whereas others retain partial activity even after castration. Certain enzymes (e.g., 5α-reductase; see Chap. 114) are low in livers of adult males but high in livers of women, presumably because of a "feminizing factor."

The pituitary plays an important role in the development of the sexually dimorphic male and female patterns of hepatic steroid- and drug-metabolizing enzyme systems. Developmentally, male and female rats have similar male-like hepatic enzyme patterns until ~30 days of age. Subsequently, in females, the hypothalamus secretes a "feminizing factor" (apparently GH) that induces the female pattern of hepatic steroid metabolism.[96,97]

A sexual difference is seen in the pattern of GH release.[100] The male pattern of GH secretion is programmed by the action of neonatal androgens at the level of the hypothalamus, as are those for luteinizing hormone (LH) and follicle-stimulating hormone (FSH). Moreover, feminization of hepatic steroid metabolism occurs in hypothalamectomized (HPX) male rats given GH (twice daily), ACTH, and $T_4$. Continuous administration of GH, mimicking the female pattern of GH secretion, feminizes hepatic steroid metabolism in normal and HPX males and "refeminizes" HPX and ovariectomized females.[101,102] Similarly, if male rats are castrated or treated with estrogen, a change to the female pattern of GH secretion is observed, concomitant with a change to the feminine pattern of hepatic steroid metabolism.[102,103] Collectively, these data suggest that female hepatic function, evidenced by higher hepatic PRL receptor levels, arises from continuous GH receptor occupancy, and that the male pattern originates as a result of a pulsatile pattern of GH receptor occupancy.

## ESTROGENS AND THE LIVER

Estrogen administration increases the synthesis of sex steroid–binding globulin, TBG, transcortin, ceruloplasmin, and other secretory proteins.[104–108] Estrogen also increases the number of hepatocyte low-density lipoprotein (LDL) receptors, thereby increasing hepatic uptake of LDL cholesterol from the blood.[109] Moreover, ovariectomized female rats given estrogen display an increase in very-low-density lipoprotein (VLDL) triglycerides, but not in cholesterol, compared with controls.

Estrogens promote the development of hepatic neoplasms associated with increased hepatocyte regenerative activity.[110] For example, estrogens promote diethylnitrosamine-induced liver tumors, and changes are found in the content and the distribution of ERs in the livers of patients with oral contraceptive–associated focal nodular hyperplasia and hepatic adenomas. This indicates a possible association between estrogen and its receptor, and the processes of hepatocyte proliferation and neoplasia.

The hepatocyte ER content increases sharply after partial hepatectomy, both in the cytosol and in the nuclear fraction. Simultaneously, the hepatic AR content declines in both the cytosol and the nucleus. The plasma estradiol levels increase, whereas testosterone levels decrease.[111,112] These changes do not occur after abdominal surgery without hepatic resection. Moreover, both in vitro and in vivo, tamoxifen, an antiestrogen, inhibits the proliferative response of liver cells.[113] These data strongly suggest that estradiol contributes to the hepatic regenerative process, and a feminization of the liver appears to be essential during the proliferative response of the liver to an injury.[114,115]

No alterations in the affinity of the ERs for estrogen occur with regeneration. The redistribution of the ERs from the cytosol to the nucleus occurs at the same time as the stimulation of DNA synthesis and reaches a maximum at 48 hours (the time at which the highest mitotic index occurs). Thus, the active translocation of the ERs into the nucleus correlates with several other markers of hepatocyte regeneration, including important biochemical functions (e.g., DNA polymerase activity, protein synthesis, and deoxythymidine kinase activity).

The effect of ER translocation after partial hepatectomy may be related to an increase in serum estradiol or to an increase in hepatic intracellular estradiol, resulting from a decrease in the estrogen-metabolizing capacity of the liver remnant. The fact that estrogen administration to nonhepatectomized rats causes a translocation of ERs to the nucleus, as well as increased liver weight and DNA synthesis, supports this view.

### ESTROGEN-INDUCED LIVER DISEASE

Numerous examples of liver-estrogen interactions have been associated with human liver disease. Women exposed to oral contraceptive steroids are at increased risk for hepatic neoplasms, jaundice, cholestatic hepatitis, gallstones, and hepatic vein thrombosis (*Budd-Chiari syndrome*). Pregnant women, who are exposed to gestational levels of both estrogenic and proges-

tational hormones, develop liver abnormalities (e.g., fatty liver of pregnancy, intrahepatic cholestasis of pregnancy, and gallstones).[116] The liver responds to estrogen exposure and also plays a major role in the metabolism of sex steroid hormones, converting them to less potent compounds. Many of these metabolites can alter the rate of metabolism and excretion of other hormones and drugs, further influencing the interaction between these compounds and the hepatocyte. For example, catechol estrogens, although weak, are noncompetitive inhibitors of the demethylation of mestranol, a 17α-ethinyl estrogen found in many oral contraceptive steroids. A reduction in their catabolism could expose the hepatocyte to higher levels of a potential hepatotoxin for long periods and thereby increase the likelihood of an untoward estrogen-hepatocyte interaction.

## ANDROGENS AND THE LIVER

Androgenic hormones exert powerful effects on the liver, whether directly or indirectly through their influence on the hypothalamus and pituitary. The presence of a hepatic androgen receptor (AR) is receiving increasing attention, especially with respect to its relationship with HCC. The AR content is higher in tumoral tissue than in nontumoral portions of the liver,[117] perhaps explaining the higher worldwide incidence of HCC in men than in women. This finding also supports the use of antihormonal therapy for the treatment of HCC, particularly in patients who express high AR levels.[118]

### ANDROGEN-INDUCED LIVER DISEASE

The use of androgenic anabolic steroids is associated with a significant risk of liver disease. The most common manifestation is a mild hepatic dysfunction without jaundice that resolves without sequelae on discontinuation of the drug. In contrast, androgen-induced cholestasis can be severe and may take weeks or months to resolve. The cholestasis is caused by a direct hepatotoxic effect of the drug, related to the alkyl group on the steroid nucleus at the $C_{17}$ position. Androgens also interfere with the excretion of conjugated bilirubin into the canaliculus. Other problems that occur with androgen treatment include peliosis hepatis and hepatic neoplasia. Some of the reported cases of HCC associated with androgen use have been disputed on pathologic grounds, however; some of them actually appear to be hepatic adenomas. Because many of the patients treated with anabolic steroids also have Fanconi anemia (which is associated with malignancy), independent of androgen exposure, the HCC occurring in androgen-treated patients may be a component of the underlying Fanconi syndrome rather than a consequence of the administered androgen.

## SEX HORMONE ALTERATIONS IN CIRRHOTIC SUBJECTS

Gynecomastia, impotence, loss of libido, and changes in body hair distribution are typical signs and symptoms in male patients with cirrhosis. The disturbances observed in the HPG axis in patients with liver disease vary, depending on the cause of the liver disease. Hypogonadism and feminization are common among individuals with chronic alcoholic liver disease. Hypogonadism alone is common in advanced hemochromatosis, whereas in patients with non–alcohol-related cirrhosis and in those without iron overload, such signs are much less prevalent and, when present, are much less severe.[119–121] Limited data are available concerning the alterations of the HPG axis in individuals with advanced non–alcohol-related liver disease. The levels of circulating testosterone and dehydroepiandrosterone are slightly decreased in nonalcoholic cirrhotic patients, whereas estradiol concentrations are usually normal. These abnormalities depend on the severity of liver disease and are more pronounced in individuals with higher Child-Pugh scores.[119,122] Gynecomastia and impotence occur in cirrhotic men and are enhanced by the frequent long-term use of the diuretic drug spironolactone (which is a competitive antagonist of aldosterone at mineralocorticoid receptors and can also bind to testosterone receptors). Spironolactone reduces testosterone levels and slightly increases estradiol levels.[123]

Among women with non–alcohol-related liver cirrhosis, amenorrhea occurs in up to 50% of cases. Irregular bleeding, oligomenorrhea, or metrorrhagia occurs in those with chronic liver disease without cirrhosis. As a consequence, conception and pregnancy are uncommon in women with advanced chronic liver disease. Many cirrhotic women manifest a state of hypogonadotropic hypogonadism that can be related to both malnutrition and an impaired intermediate metabolism.[124,125] In other cases, the plasma levels of both estradiol and testosterone are increased, in part due to a portosystemic recirculation of weak androgens with subsequent peripheral conversion to estrogens in fat as well as in other tissues. In cases of advanced liver disease complicated by the presence of hepatic encephalopathy, the central release of neuromediators (i.e., dopamine and norepinephrine) is altered, influencing the pulsatile release of gonadotropin-releasing factors from the hypothalamus. This may adversely affect neuroendocrine gonadal interrelationships. Decreased central levels of dopamine may contribute to the well-known hyperprolactinemia of cirrhotic patients, further compromising the release of gonadotropins.[124]

## GLUCOSE HOMEOSTASIS AND THE LIVER

The liver occupies a unique position in protein, carbohydrate, and lipid homeostasis. After feeding, the liver actively takes up glucose and uses it for fuel or stores it as glycogen. During fasting, the liver synthesizes glucose from amino acids. Because of these two opposing functions of storage and synthesis, the liver maintains a relatively stable plasma glucose concentration in the fasting and the fed state.

With the ingestion of a meal, a large bolus of glucose is delivered to the liver via the portal vein. The fact that the peripheral glucose concentration rises only slightly (50% above baseline) after a meal implies that the liver is the principal site of glucose uptake after a meal. With fasting or hypoglycemia, hepatic glycogen and peripheral proteins are broken down and made available to the liver as glucose precursor, so that the crucial energy needs of the body can be maintained.

The tight homeostatic control of peripheral glucose levels is maintained by hepatic glucose uptake in response to increases in portal venous glucose. This process does not appear to be insulin dependent, but results from the enzyme kinetics of the initial step in glucose handling by the hepatocyte. Specifically, by facilitated diffusion, glucose is taken up by the liver, and within the range of glucose concentrations experienced by the liver, this mechanism is saturated. Once glucose enters the hepatocyte, it is rapidly phosphorylated to glucose-6-phosphate (G6P) by glucokinase.

Although hepatic glucokinase is in relative excess compared with its substrate concentration, the amount of this enzyme within the liver is under the control of glucose and insulin. In the fasting state, or with acute insulin deficiency, the level of hepatic glucokinase declines. Conversely, during the fed state, the intrahepatic level of the enzyme increases, as does the glucose level.[126] Once glucose has been phosphorylated, it can be stored as glycogen or broken down to acetyl coenzyme A and further converted to an amino acid, fatty acid, or energy. In the fed state, glycogen synthesis predominates.

Insulin also appears to have an important effect on hepatic glucose production. Low doses of insulin inhibit glycogen breakdown, and high doses inhibit glucose synthesis from amino-acid precursors. Thus, low doses of insulin lead to hepatic glycogen accumulation by inhibiting its breakdown. At higher levels of insulin, both glycogenolysis and gluconeogenesis are inhibited. The net result is a smaller increase in the hepatic venous glucose concentration than would be expected, with storage of most of the ingested glucose as glycogen.

In the face of high splanchnic glucose concentrations, insulin stimulates a net hepatic glucose uptake.[127,128] Neither the ratio of insulin to glucagon nor the absolute amount of glucagon appears to be important in this process. This difference between portal venous and systemic insulin levels suggests that the liver is the major site of glucose regulation and is the main site of insulin degradation. This occurs because of binding of insulin to specific insulin receptors on the hepatocyte surface, followed by internalization of the receptor and its bound hormone, with the subsequent breakdown of the bound insulin by cytosolic proteases. The receptor is then recycled to the cell surface. Thus, the amount of insulin degraded by the liver is determined by the amount bound to hepatocyte receptors, which, in turn, depends on a variety of stimuli that control insulin receptor number, affinity, or both.

## GLUCOSE HOMEOSTASIS IN ACUTE LIVER FAILURE

Whereas glucose intolerance and insulin resistance are common features in acute hepatitis, hypoglycemia is a frequent complication of massive hepatic necrosis.[129–132] In acute hepatic failure, hypoglycemia can be symptomatic, persistent, and severe. Its prevention is based on a close monitoring of blood glucose levels as well as on the intravenous administration of high glucose loads. Also, because insulin and glucagon promote hepatic regeneration, their administration may have a beneficial effect in the treatment of acute liver failure.[133] The ability of the liver to produce glucose (as a result of glycogenolysis as well as gluconeogenesis) is reduced to a critical level in subjects with acute liver failure.[134] In addition, a state of hyperinsulinemia occurs, as a result of the loss of the normal metabolism of insulin by the liver. This situation is aggravated further by the portosystemic shunting of blood because of liver necrosis.[135]

## CONGENITAL DEFECTS OF HEPATIC GLUCONEOGENESIS

A deficiency of the enzyme fructose-1,6-diphosphatase occurs in humans.[136] Individuals with this deficiency are chronically ill, with metabolic acidosis and hepatomegaly, and manifest potentially lethal episodes of hypoglycemia that often are precipitated by infection or other metabolic stresses. The glycogenolytic system in these patients is intact; glucagon administration causes a hyperglycemic response if performed in the postprandial period. After a prolonged fast, however, no response occurs. This enzyme deficiency can be established by liver biopsy with subsequent assay of the activity of the enzyme fructose-1,6-diphosphatase.

Children with an absolute deficiency of the enzyme *phosphoenolpyruvate carboxykinase* manifest lactic acidosis and hypoglycemia associated with disturbances in pyruvate oxidation and organic acidemia (see Chap. 161).[137]

## HYPOGLYCEMIA DUE TO LIVER DISEASE

Hypoglycemia commonly occurs in Reye syndrome because of mitochondrial injury and the development of transient deficiencies of the mitochondrial enzymes pyruvate carboxylase and pyruvate dehydrogenase. The acquired deficiencies markedly limit the ability of the liver to convert gluconeogenic precursors, such as alanine and pyruvate, into glucose.

A similar form of hypoglycemia can occur in women with acute fatty liver of pregnancy. Hepatotoxin-induced liver disease, particularly that produced by mitochondrial toxins (e.g., phosphorus, chloroform, carbon tetrachloride, propylene glycol, and halothane) is frequently associated with hypoglycemia for similar reasons. These agents reduce gluconeogenesis because of transient hepatic injury or lethal hepatic necrosis, which is associated with a loss of pyruvate decarboxylase and pyruvate dehydrogenase activities within the liver.

Not unexpectedly, hypoglycemia can occur with massive hepatic necrosis due to any agent, virus, or drug, if the injury is severe enough or if hepatic infarction occurs.[138,139] Fortunately, the hepatic reserve for gluconeogenesis is substantial, and 85% to 95% of the liver must be dysfunctional before clinically important hypoglycemia occurs. When this does occur, the resulting hypoglycemia can be severe and usually exceeds that which can be explained by a reduction in gluconeogenesis alone. It seems to be compounded further by a loss of hepatic mechanisms for insulin degradation and glycogenolysis. Thus, the combination of insulin excess, inadequate gluconeogenesis, and inadequate glycogenolysis, all occurring together, produce the hypoglycemia. Because of the considerable hepatic reserve for gluconeogenesis, no consistent, direct association is found between hypoglycemia and any common hepatic injury or any laboratory parameter of hepatic function.

HCC is occasionally associated with the development of hypoglycemia, which occurs because of tumor production of massive amounts of insulin-like growth factors (see Chap. 219).

## GLUCOSE AND LIPID METABOLISM IN CIRRHOSIS

The liver disposes of the glucose load after meals and clears the portal venous blood of most of its insulin and glucagon. Much of the glucose cleared by the liver after a meal is stored within that organ as hepatic glycogen or is converted to triglycerides. High portal venous levels of insulin, low portal venous levels of glucagon, and an intact liver are required for these events to occur at normal rates.[52,140,141]

Several abnormalities of glucose metabolism occur in individuals with cirrhosis.[52,142–145] In end-stage liver disease, fasting hypoglycemia occurs as a result of impaired glycogen synthesis, impaired gluconeogenesis, and poor nutrition. Moreover, hypoglycemia indicates a very poor short-term prognosis. Normally, after an overnight fast, 70% to 80% of the glucose available in plasma is derived from hepatic glycogen. This decreases to 30% to 40% in cirrhotic patients, who have both a reduced hepatic glycogen content and liver cell dysfunction.[52,142–146]

The prevalence of overt glucose intolerance in cirrhotic patients varies greatly (54–92%).[147–150] Up to 40% of cirrhotic patients are diabetic.[147] The pathogenic mechanisms responsible for the glucose intolerance in cirrhotic individuals are incompletely understood, although a combination of impaired insulin secretion rate and reduced insulin sensitivity may be responsible. An elevated postprandial circulating insulin level and hyperglycemia are consistent features of advanced cirrhosis and strongly suggest peripheral insulin resistance. An increased rate of insulin secretion in response to intravenous hyperglycemic stimuli occurs in cirrhotic patients with impaired glucose tolerance and mild diabetes. The insulin response to an oral glucose load, however, appears to be blunted and is not significantly greater than that of control subjects until ≥90 minutes after the ingestion of a glucose load. An impaired glucose tolerance in

response to an oral glucose load has been reported in up to 80% of cirrhotic patients.[149] Moreover, an abnormal intravenous glucose intolerance (defined as a 2-hour serum glucose level of >7.8 mmol/L after 25 g intravenous glucose) was found in 19% of cirrhotic patients. The augmented insulin response to an intravenous glucose load supports the concept of an impaired pancreatic B-cell response to hyperglycemia. The late insulin response to an oral glucose load suggests that some intestinal factor(s) might be responsible for the changes in insulin secretion.[151]

Unlike insulin, C peptide is not degraded by the liver. In cirrhotic patients, increases in both C peptide and insulin levels have been reported during fasting and often in response to an oral glucose load. However, the C peptide/insulin ratio, an index of hepatic insulin uptake, is lower in cirrhotic patients than in controls. This finding suggests that cirrhotic individuals have a reduced hepatic uptake and degradation of insulin.[152–154] Clearly, the presence of hepatocyte dysfunction and both intrahepatic and extrahepatic portal systemic shunts in cirrhotic patients would be expected to contribute to the reduced hepatic insulin uptake and clearance of insulin. In healthy subjects, the insulin uptake by liver is ~50% of the insulin load. In patients with alcoholic liver cirrhosis, uptake has been estimated to be only 13%.[155] However, another study evaluating insulin and glucagon catabolism by hepatic tissue obtained from cirrhotic patients and controls failed to show a significantly reduced degradation of these two hormones.[156] Glucagon-like peptide-1 reverses the insulin secretion defects in liver cirrhosis.[156a]

Impaired negative feedback inhibition by circulating insulin levels in cirrhotic patients is yet another possible explanation for the hyperinsulinemia and insulin hypersecretion seen in cirrhosis. In normal subjects, C-peptide secretion is suppressed by as much as 50% after 30 minutes of a euglycemic hyperinsulinemic infusion.[157] In contrast, in cirrhotic patients insulin suppression is not achieved even after 120 minutes of a euglycemic hyperinsulinemic infusion. This finding suggests an insensitivity of B cells to suppression by insulin in cirrhotic patients.[158]

Non–insulin-dependent diabetes mellitus (type 2) is more common than insulin-dependent diabetes (type 1) in cirrhotic patients. Type 2 cirrhotic patients appear to have one or more insulin-receptor defects that contribute to their insulin resistance. This reduced sensitivity of cells to insulin may occur at either the insulin-receptor or postreceptor level. Moreover, an additional defect in glucose transport mechanisms may be present. Insulin binding to monocytes and adipocytes is reduced in cirrhotic subjects according to the severity of their glucose intolerance.[159,160] Presently, the evidence that altered insulin-receptor binding contributes to the insulin resistance seen in cirrhosis is inconclusive. The data supporting the possibility of a postbinding defect are much more convincing.[161,162] Examination of the transmembrane transport of labeled glucose in isolated adipocytes or skeletal muscle obtained from cirrhotic patients demonstrates a significant reduction in insulin-induced glucose uptake. Reduced levels of G6P are observed, whereas the activity of the phosphorylative chain is normal. Thus, insulin resistance in cirrhotic patients is characterized by reduced intracellular availability of G6P caused by a defect in glucose transport. Cirrhotic patients also may manifest a "glucose resistance," that is, a reduced tissue uptake of glucose that occurs independent of insulin. The insulin resistance in cirrhotic patients can be explained in part by the presence of circulating factors that antagonize insulin effects peripherally. Among the putative insulin antagonists present in the plasma of cirrhotic patients are the counterregulatory hormones (i.e., GH, glucagon, cortisol, and catecholamines). The malnutrition common to advanced cirrhosis also alters glucose homeostasis by reducing the intracellular availability of various cofactors for enzymes involved in overall glucose metabolism. The hyperglucagonemia that occurs in cirrhotic subjects[163–166] leads to a glucose overproduction, which contributes to the observed glucose intolerance. The data available for cirrhotic patients with impaired glucose tolerance fail to demonstrate a relationship between the degree of glucose intolerance and the level of hyperglucagonemia. Despite the hyperglucagonemia, hepatic glucose production is lower in cirrhotic patients than in normal individuals. This reflects both reduced hepatocyte function and reduced access of individual liver cells to glucose in portal venous blood. The possibility exists that, because of the portal systemic shunts within and around the liver in cirrhotic individuals, the diminished hepatocyte mass of cirrhotic patients actually experiences a reduced glucagon stimulus.

No relationship between the elevated cortisol levels and glucose intolerance has been reported in cirrhotic patients.[166] Thus, increased levels of adrenal counterregulatory hormones are unlikely to be related to their insulin resistance.

High plasma FFA levels have also been proposed as possible insulin antagonists in cirrhotic individuals. More important, basal FFA levels correlate with the degree of glucose intolerance observed.[166] In type 2 diabetes, elevated circulating FFA levels impair glucose utilization, especially in muscle tissue, thereby reducing the effect of insulin. A reduction in plasma FFA through the use of nicotinic acid is effective in ameliorating the glucose intolerance in individuals with type 2 diabetes without cirrhosis; however, it has little effect on the whole body insulin sensitivity seen in cirrhotic patients.

A malabsorption of lipids frequently occurs in patients with liver disease, not only in those with cholestasis but also in those with parenchymal liver disease. Moreover, lipid synthesis and transfer rates are impaired in cirrhotic patients. They have both impaired FFA synthesis and impaired VLDL production. In cirrhosis, plasma triglycerides are elevated and are carried by LDL rather than VLDL. In advanced liver disease, however, both plasma triglycerides and VLDL levels are reduced.

Of interest, diabetes-induced chronic vascular complications, such as diabetic retinopathy, are less frequent when diabetes is associated with chronic liver disease. Cirrhosis is a hypotensive condition, and the lower prevalence of hypertension in such patients may explain this observed reduction in vascular complications.[167]

# DIABETES MELLITUS AND THE LIVER

Diabetes mellitus comprises a group of heterogeneous disorders that are characterized by hyperglycemia and, in the more severe cases, ketosis and protein wasting. Diabetes is associated with an increased risk of certain associated diseases, including those involving the liver: *glycogenosis* (50% of those with type 1 diabetes), *fatty liver* (50% of those with type 2 diabetes), *steatonecrosis* (10–20% of those with type 2 diabetes), and *cirrhosis of the micronodular variety* (16% of those with type 2 diabetes).

## LIPID METABOLISM IN DIABETES MELLITUS

Hypercholesterolemia occurs in those with poorly controlled diabetes and improves with insulin therapy. Early studies demonstrated an increase in total body cholesterol synthesis in those with poorly controlled diabetes, which decreases with the initiation of better insulin therapy. In one study,[168] however, total body cholesterol synthesis increased in some diabetic patients after initiation of insulin therapy.

Animal data[169,170] demonstrate a decreased hepatic cholesterol synthesis in uncontrolled diabetes. This is difficult to explain in the face of an increased total body cholesterol synthesis, because normally the liver contributes more than half of the total cholesterol synthesis.[171] This may occur because intestinal

cholesterol synthesis markedly increases in experimentally induced diabetes. Cholesterol formed in the intestine is carried by chylomicrons to the liver, where it contributes to the regulation of hepatic cholesterol synthesis by negative feedback.[172]

A specific sequence of events has been suggested in experimentally induced diabetes. The observed increase in total body cholesterol synthesis is predominantly due to an increased intestinal cholesterol synthesis, which is partially offset by a diminished hepatic cholesterol synthesis. The institution of insulin therapy reestablishes a more normal rate of intestinal cholesterol synthesis and decreases the amount of cholesterol delivered to the liver from the intestine. This removes the suppression of hepatic cholesterol formation, accounting for the observed increase in hepatic cholesterol synthesis that accompanies the initiation of insulin therapy.

The liver is an important site of cholesterol synthesis and lipoprotein uptake and metabolism. Altered lipoprotein metabolism may contribute to the hypercholesterolemia observed in diabetic patients. Two defects in lipoprotein metabolism have been identified in diabetic individuals: an increased hepatic VLDL output and a decreased hepatic VLDL uptake. Because 20% of the VLDL particle is made up of cholesterol, the cholesterol concentration in plasma must increase as VLDL levels increase. The cholesterol carried in LDL, a particle that has a significant positive correlation with the development of atherosclerosis, is elevated in patients with type 1 diabetes mellitus. In humans, the LDL particle is formed almost exclusively from the hydrolysis of VLDL. LDL particles are cleared from the plasma by an LDL receptor–mediated mechanism. Quantitatively, however, the liver is thought to be the most important site of LDL cholesterol uptake (see Chap. 162).

## PROTEIN METABOLISM IN DIABETES MELLITUS

The liver uses endogenous and peripherally supplied amino acids and is exposed to high levels of portal venous amino acids absorbed from the intestinal tract after feeding. Fifty percent of the amino acids metabolized by the liver is derived from hepatic protein degradation.[173] The other half is derived from extrahepatic sources, either peripheral tissue sites or dietary sources. In the fed state, most amino acids delivered to the liver are derived from dietary proteins (90 g). Moreover, 50 g of amino acids are derived from exfoliated cell proteins that have been digested and absorbed by the intestine, 16 g are derived from secreted gastrointestinal enzymes, and 1 to 2 g are generated by exuded plasma proteins. In the fasting state, the total amount of amino acids that influx through the portal vein to the liver is reduced to approximately one-sixth of that found in the fed state and is derived almost exclusively from exfoliated intestinal cell protein. The liver adapts to this reduction in amino acids from the portal vein by metabolizing endogenous amino acids to supply its needs.

Hepatic protein synthesis is under hormonal control. This is true for proteins retained within the hepatocyte and for those manufactured in the liver and secreted into the systemic circulation. Adequate levels of insulin and glucagon are also necessary for the intrinsic hepatic protein synthesis that is observed during hepatic regeneration after injury. Both hormones appear to stimulate hepatic DNA synthesis, protein synthesis, and subsequent cell division. Secretory protein synthesis by the liver is modulated by fasting and by protein ingestion. Albumin synthesis promptly decreases with fasting. This reduction in albumin synthesis is associated with a decreased hepatic RNA concentration, a decreased hepatic protein concentration, and a reduced state of aggregation of the endoplasmic reticulum–bound polysomes. The free polysomes, however, do not appear to be affected significantly by fasting. These changes are quickly reversed with feeding or after amino-acid delivery to the liver.

Fasting affects the hepatic level of endoplasmic reticulum–bound polysomes, which are considered important in secretory protein synthesis, without affecting the hepatic levels of free polysomes, which are thought to be responsible for endogenous protein synthesis.

A basal insulin level is necessary to maintain the state of aggregation of the endoplasmic reticulum–bound polysomes for secretory protein synthesis. In insulin-deficient animals, a loss of rough endoplasmic reticulum occurs, together with a proliferation of smooth endoplasmic reticulum, a reduced amino-acid incorporation into protein, and a decreased amount of rough endoplasmic reticulum–bound ribosomes existing as polyribosomes. The relative sparing of the smooth endoplasmic reticulum suggests that patients with diabetes mellitus predominantly have a defect in secretory protein synthesis, although they maintain their synthesis of essential intracellular proteins.

## BILIARY LIPID SECRETION IN DIABETES MELLITUS

The influence of diabetes mellitus on biliary lipid secretion is seen most often in those with type 2 diabetes, who tend to be overweight and to secrete a lithogenic bile. When the duodenal bile obtained from patients with maturity-onset diabetes is compared with that of obesity-matched controls, however, the bile from both groups is similarly supersaturated.[174,175] This suggests that *obesity, rather than diabetes*, is the etiologic factor responsible for gallstones, which are common in patients with obesity and type 2 diabetes. Interestingly, nonobese Pima Indians with type 2 diabetes also secrete a supersaturated bile. (This phenomenon tends to occur in this group even when diabetes is not present. Nonobese, non-Indian patients with significant fasting hyperglycemia, who do not develop ketoacidosis, have an increase in bile acid and hepatic cholesterol synthesis without an increase in bile acid pool size or cholesterol saturation.) Therefore, in patients with type 2 diabetes, the secretion of a lithogenic bile appears to be related more to obesity than to a genetic predisposition associated with the diabetes.

The bile acid production and secretion rates in type 1 diabetes have not been investigated as carefully as those in type 2 diabetes. In a study[176] of 12 patients with type 1 diabetes who were not overweight, no increase in biliary cholesterol saturation was found. Moreover, the total biliary lipid concentration was found to be lower in the diabetic group than in the control group.

### EFFECT OF INSULIN THERAPY

Interestingly, insulin therapy changes the biliary saturation index. A lack of diabetic control is associated with increased bile salt synthesis and pool size, and insulin therapy decreases the bile salt secretion rate and reduces the bile acid pool size. This yields a net increase in the cholesterol saturation of bile. With experimentally induced diabetes, a decrease in hepatic cholesterol synthesis can be reversed with the institution of insulin therapy.

In humans, cholesterol synthesis appears to be an important determinant of biliary cholesterol secretion. Biliary cholesterol secretion is higher in those with uncontrolled and insulin-treated diabetes than in controls. A decrease in the bile acid pool size, associated with an increased secretion of biliary cholesterol, causes the formation of a supersaturated bile, a necessary prerequisite for gallstone formation. Therefore, by decreasing bile salt secretion and increasing biliary cholesterol secretion, insulin therapy can actually increase the risk for gallstone formation.

### CHOLELITHIASIS AND DIABETES

Many normal individuals secrete a supersaturated bile. Thus, the mere presence of a lithogenic bile does not completely explain the increased frequency of gallstones in diabetic individuals. The diabetic patient has another risk factor for gallstone formation not present in the normal population: decreased gallbladder contractility.[177,178] This decreased contractility results in incomplete emptying of the gallbladder, which promotes cholesterol nucleation; the result is stone formation and growth, particularly if the bile is supersaturated.

Data indicate that surgical intervention for gallstone disease in patients with diabetes and cholelithiasis is associated with a higher mortality rate than that seen in the normal population. In diabetic patients, emergency gallbladder surgery has been associated with a 10% to 20% mortality rate, compared with 1% to 4% in nondiabetic persons. These data prompted the suggestion that screening of patients with diabetes to identify silent gallstones should be considered, so that elective surgical intervention could be instituted before acute cholecystitis occurs. The available data,[179] however, suggest that the increased surgical risk observed in diabetic patients is primarily related to the coexistence of vascular and renal disease. In the diabetic patient without confounding vascular or renal disease, surgical intervention for acute cholecystitis is not associated with a mortality greater than that observed for the general population. Currently, whether elective surgery for silent gallstones in the subpopulation of diabetic patients with vascular or renal disease actually decreases the mortality rate from cholelithiasis is unclear.

## LIVER DISEASES ASSOCIATED WITH DIABETES

Various hepatic disorders are associated with diabetes mellitus. Moreover, several hepatic histopathologic lesions are observed with increased frequency in diabetic populations.

### GLYCOGEN DEPOSITION

The most common lesion seen in diabetes mellitus is an increase in liver glycogen, found both at autopsy and in biopsy material. The incidence rate of increased hepatic glycogen is as high as 80%. Increased glycogen deposits are observed especially in patients with brittle diabetes who are prone to hypoglycemia. Also, insulin therapy in these patients increases hepatic glycogen deposition further. Together, these findings suggest that an intermittent excess in insulin levels associated with exogenous insulin therapy causes the glycogen deposition and the associated hypoglycemia. The increased liver glycogen and the accompanying hepatomegaly can be quickly reversed if appropriate insulin therapy is instituted.

### FATTY LIVER

Fatty liver is defined as a hepatic accumulation of lipid, usually in the form of triglyceride, that exceeds 5% of the liver weight. An increase in lipolysosomes occurs in diabetic patients with fatty liver and apparently correlates with the level of increased serum cholesterol. Hypercholesterolemia may be an important contributing factor to the pathogenesis of the fatty liver associated with diabetes.

The prevalence of fatty liver in diabetic patients varies considerably, but biopsy studies reveal that ~50% of diabetic patients have excess fat in their livers. In several series of patients with fatty liver, diabetes was the cause in 4% to 46%. This wide range can be explained by the rate at which concurrent obesity is seen in those with type 2 diabetes. Because obesity appears to be a major cause of fatty liver, and because the incidence of fatty liver in patients with diabetes mellitus without concurrent obesity is unknown, isolating diabetes as the specific cause of the fatty liver in diabetic patients is extremely

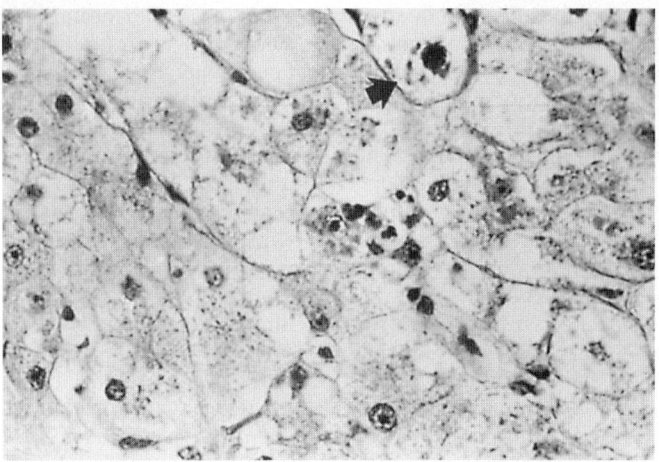

**FIGURE 205-1.** Photomicrograph of a fatty liver in a diabetic patient showing ballooned fat-filled hepatocytes and a Mallory lesion (*arrow*). ×400

difficult. Nevertheless, the presence of a fatty liver in diabetic patients correlates directly with age, inversely with the severity of the carbohydrate abnormality, and directly with the duration of the diabetes. However, it does not correlate with the degree of diabetic control.[180,181]

Rarely do patients with type 1 diabetes develop fatty liver. In contrast, in the type 2 diabetic population, fatty liver is found in >50% of patients. In this population, insulin insensitivity, rather than the degree of glucose intolerance, predicts the occurrence of fatty liver. Although patients with fatty livers often present with hepatomegaly, this finding is not invariably present. In diabetes, no abnormality of liver enzymes reliably predicts excess hepatic fat. Histologically, the fat appears as both large and small droplets within the hepatic cytosol (Fig. 205-1). With intensive fatty infiltration, the cytoplasmic fat coalesces into large droplets that displace the nucleus eccentrically. Presumably, in severe cases this can cause hepatocyte injury and death. In areas of severe fatty infiltration, an increase in connective tissue is occasionally seen. Inflammation, as manifested by the presence of polymorphonuclear cells, is typically absent.[182] Because of the poor correlation between the various laboratory tests for hepatic injury and function and the presence or absence of fat in liver cells, liver biopsy appears to be the only reliable way to make a reliable diagnosis of a fatty liver in diabetic and nondiabetic patients. Computed tomographic scanning has been somewhat helpful, whereas ultrasonographic techniques cannot distinguish fat from fibrosis.

The pathophysiologic mechanisms responsible for the development of a diabetic fatty liver are not understood completely. In diabetes mellitus, FFAs released from adipocytes are taken up by the liver in a concentration-dependent manner. The fate of these FFAs is either oxidation to ketone bodies, or esterification to phospholipids and triglycerides with subsequent excretion as part of VLDL particles. Fatty liver occurs when the rate of hepatic triglyceride synthesis exceeds the rate of hepatic secretion of VLDL. This can result from different mechanisms: (a) increased hepatic FFA concentrations derived from hepatic synthesis; (b) excess dietary intake or peripheral lipolysis; (c) decreased oxidation of fatty acids to ketone bodies; and (d) decreased output of triglycerides in VLDL particles. Which mechanism accounts for the development of fatty liver in any patient depends on the type of diabetes and the degree of diabetic control achieved.

Fatty liver seen in type 1 diabetes occurs only when diabetic control is inadequate. In the presence of reduced serum insulin levels, a marked increase in hepatic FFA concentrations occurs that stimulate ketone body production and hepatic triglyceride synthesis. Glucagon also inhibits triglyceride secretion as VLDL, but does not inhibit triglyceride synthesis. These data suggest that the fatty liver seen in those with poorly controlled type 1 diabetes is due to an increased influx of FFAs and impaired VLDL secretion of triglycerides.

In type 2 diabetes, the imbalance between hepatic triglyceride synthesis and VLDL secretion occurs for different reasons. Hepatic FFA concentrations are increased because of a greater intake of dietary fat and carbohydrate that contributes to elevated plasma FFA concentrations. Triglyceride synthesis is stimulated because of the increased hepatic FFA content from both endogenous and exogenous sources. Because no evidence exists to suggest that triglyceride secretion is impaired in type 2 diabetes, the intracellular lipid accumulation presumably occurs because the rate of triglyceride synthesis exceeds the liver's capacity to secrete newly formed triglyceride as VLDL.

The clinical significance of fatty liver in patients with diabetes mellitus is debatable. Generally, fatty liver is not believed to progress to more severe disease. In pancreatectomized dogs, however, the progression of fatty liver to fibrosis and cirrhosis has been documented. Similarly, serial liver biopsies in diabetic patients with fatty liver have demonstrated progression to cirrhosis. Also, fatty steatosis, pericentral fibrosis, and intracellular hyaline occurred in the livers of a small series of women with poorly controlled diabetes.[170] Steatonecrosis is seen more commonly in alcoholic individuals, in whom the presence of this histologic lesion is associated with a polymorphonuclear leukocytic inflammation not seen in diabetic patients. Despite the prevailing opinion that the fatty liver of diabetes does not lead to cirrhosis, many researchers report an increased prevalence of cirrhosis in diabetic patients. Approximately a four-fold increased incidence of cirrhosis occurs in diabetic patients.

### HEPATIC TOXICITY OF ORAL HYPOGLYCEMIC AGENTS

The treatment of diabetes with oral hypoglycemic agents (see Chap. 142) also appears to increase the risk for liver disease. The most commonly used group of oral hypoglycemics are the sulfonylurea agents (e.g., chlorpropamide, tolazamide, tolbutamide, acetohexamide, glyburide, and glipizide). These agents produce jaundice, although the frequency of reported hepatotoxic reactions varies with the particular agent used. The reported incidence of toxicity is greatest with chlorpropamide and has been reported at 0.5% to 1%.[183] Hepatic sulfonylurea toxicity usually consists of a cholestatic reaction, although hepatocellular injury or a mixed picture can be seen. Rarely, oral hypoglycemic agents are implicated as a cause of granulomatous liver disease.[184] Hepatocellular necrosis appears to be most common with acetohexamide.

## BONE AND CALCIUM METABOLISM

Both osteoporosis and osteomalacia occur in patients with longstanding liver disease. Defects in GH-binding protein and IGF concentrations contribute to the pathogenesis of these disorders in cirrhotic individuals.

Because of the hypoalbuminemia of many cirrhotic patients, the total calcium concentration often is low. Ionized calcium levels, however, are normal. Poor nutrition and alcohol-induced defects in the intestinal absorption of calcium are factors other than hypoalbuminemia that may contribute to the hypocalcemia.

In cirrhotic patients, parathyroid hormone (PTH) levels usually are normal. Nonetheless, PTH metabolism is altered. In patients with primary biliary cirrhosis, increased levels of the C-terminal PTH peptide, a proteolytic product of intact PTH, are found.[185] The biologic significance of increased levels of this 70-84 PTH product is unclear.

The liver also plays an important role in vitamin D metabolism. Most patients with liver disease have normal 1,25-hydroxyvitamin $D_3$ (1,25-OHD$_3$) and 25-hydroxyvitamin $D_3$ (25-OHD$_3$) levels, and only the few with very severe liver failure have reduced 25-OHD$_3$ levels. The exception to this rule is primary biliary cirrhosis, in which the incidence of 25-OHD$_3$ deficiency is high.

Among the mechanisms that explain the finding of reduced serum 25-OHD$_3$ concentrations in patients with cirrhosis is the reduced activity of 25-hydroxylase in the liver with an impaired conversion of vitamin $D_3$ to 25-OHD$_3$. Synthesis of vitamin D–binding protein by the liver is reduced.[186,187] Other factors that also may contribute to vitamin D deficiency in end-stage cirrhosis include decreased sun exposure, poor nutrition, intestinal malabsorption of vitamin D, and a disturbed enterohepatic circulation of the vitamin.

Osteoporosis is the most common bone disease seen in individuals with advanced liver disease (occurring in 21–39%).[188–190] Long-term immobility, poor nutrition, and a reduced muscle mass are features commonly noted in individuals with cirrhosis. Each of these factors can augment the development of osteoporosis. In addition, in primary biliary cirrhosis the proliferation of osteoblasts may be inhibited by increased levels of conjugated bilirubin.[191] Thus, prolonged hyperbilirubinemia may be an important factor in the pathogenesis of accelerated bone loss in patients with cholestatic liver disease.

In cirrhotic patients, histomorphometric evidence suggests that bone formation is reduced (low turnover), whereas bone resorption rates are normal.[186,188,192] A low osteocalcin level is a good marker of bone formation, and urinary pyridinium cross-link compounds reflect bone resorption rates. Both help to confirm the presence of a low bone turnover in the osteoporosis of cirrhotic patients.

## ALCOHOLIC LIVER DISEASE

### EFFECT OF ALCOHOL ON THE HYPOTHALAMIC–PITUITARY–GONADAL AXIS

#### ALCOHOLIC MEN

**Hypogonadism.**  Most alcohol-abusing male patients, particularly those with cirrhosis, present with signs of hypogonadism (e.g., loss of secondary male sex characteristics, testicular atrophy, and infertility)[193–199] (Fig. 205-2).

A reduction in circulating testosterone levels is the most common finding in alcoholic men with clinical manifestations of hypogonadism.[193,199] The toxic effect of alcohol rather than the presence of alcohol-induced cirrhosis may be responsible for the androgen deficiency of male alcoholics.[200–204] In fact, in experimental models, the reduction in circulating testosterone follows chronic alcohol feeding,[204a] even in the absence of liver injury. Several factors influence the impairment of testosterone biosynthesis caused by alcohol. Not only are ethanol and its metabolite, acetaldehyde, directly toxic to Leydig cells,[205,206] but a disruption of the hypothalamic–pituitary–gonadal axis also occurs as a consequence of alcohol abuse. A central defect at the level of the pituitary and/or hypothalamus that is associated with chronic alcohol intake contributes to the hypogonadism of alcoholic men.[193,207,208] Chronic alcohol exposure decreases circulating LH levels, and the response of LH to LH-releasing hormone (LHRH) is reduced in alcoholics.[209,210]

Hyperprolactinemia is often found in male alcoholics, particularly those with cirrhosis. Elevated PRL levels may participate in the pathogenesis of hypogonadism by inhibiting gonadotro-

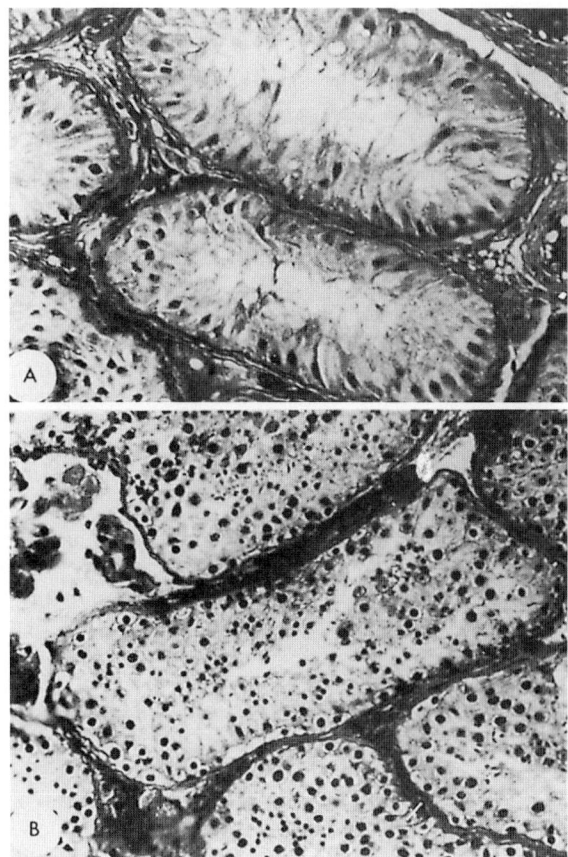

**FIGURE 205-2.** Photomicrographs of the testes obtained from (**A**) an alcoholic man with testicular atrophy and (**B**) a healthy control. ×400

pin secretion, thereby further decreasing sex hormone synthesis as well as germ cell production and maturation.[195,211]

Although, in the absence of liver disease, alcohol enhances the hepatic metabolism of testosterone, in the presence of cirrhosis, ethanol increases testosterone binding to the plasma androgen carrier sex hormone–binding globulin; this reduces the metabolic clearance rate of the hormone.[194]

**Feminization.**  Alcoholic men often manifest clinical gynecomastia, alterations in body fat distribution, and a female escutcheon. In addition, hyperestrogenization occurs in chronic alcoholic men.[212] Although alcohol abuse can cause hypogonadism even in the absence of liver disease, cirrhosis, acting in concert with alcohol, produces feminization. Alcoholic men with chronic liver disease have elevated circulating estradiol and estrone levels.[213] These are produced from weak androgens of adrenal gland origin.[209] In alcoholic men, although normal or slightly increased concentrations of estradiol are commonly found, levels of estrone are increased by the aromatization of androstenedione.[202] Both alcohol and acetaldehyde stimulate the adrenal cortex to increase the secretion of weak adrenal androgens that serve as estrogen precursors. Moreover, ethanol also increases the activity of aromatase, which converts androgens to estrogens. Normally, weak androgens are biotransformed by the liver and excreted in the urine; however, in liver disease, these hormones escape hepatic clearance and are shunted via venous collaterals to sites in the body where they undergo aromatization.[203]

The metabolic clearance rate for estradiol is normal in alcoholic subjects, even in the presence of advanced cirrhosis. On the other hand, in subjects with alcoholic cirrhosis, the reduced albumin may result in a relatively high level of free estrogen in the blood. Compounding this problem is the reduction in hepatic estrogen-binding proteins, which enables more estrogen receptors to produce an estrogenic effect.

### ALCOHOLIC WOMEN

**Hypogonadism.**    Alcohol abuse results in profound changes in the hormonal status, physical appearance, and reproductive performance of women. In women, chronic alcohol abuse may be associated with severe hypogonadism, as manifested by the loss of secondary sexual characteristics, amenorrhea, and early menopause, because the secretion of estrogens and gonadotropin is reduced. A reduction in estradiol and progesterone levels as well as ovulatory failure characterize the ovarian failure seen in alcoholic women. The ovulatory failure leads directly to infertility and to the absence of corpora lutea and the midcycle LH surge.[214–218]

Both increased PRL and decreased LH levels correlate with the severity of alcoholic liver disease as expressed by the Child-Pugh score. Such findings suggest that hormone levels may have a prognostic value in assessing the severity of liver disease.

**Endocrine Effect of Alcohol in Postmenopausal Women.** Normal postmenopausal women who drink moderately (one drink per day or less) have higher estradiol levels than do women who do not drink. Whether alcohol or estrogenic phytoestrogens (principal nutrients of plant origin in alcoholic beverages) are responsible for this effect is unclear. (Phytoestrogens interact with estrogen receptor–binding proteins and experimentally produce an estrogenic response that is dose dependent.[219])

In cirrhotic alcoholic postmenopausal women, estradiol levels are higher and testosterone levels are lower than in controls. The conversion of androgens to estrogens is enhanced by alcohol abuse in alcoholic cirrhotic postmenopausal women as it is in men. As a consequence of the increased levels of estrogen, the production and secretion of pituitary gonadotropins is reduced. Despite the increase in estrogen levels in alcoholic cirrhotic women, they appear to be defeminized, with a marked loss of secondary sex characteristics.[220,221]

### EFFECT OF ALCOHOL ON THYROID FUNCTION

Alcohol abuse has powerful effects on the hypothalamic–pituitary–thyroidal (HPT) axis and the thyroid gland. The severity of concomitant alcohol-induced liver disease is an important determinant of the severity of HPT axis disruption. Multiple thyroid function abnormalities may occur. Chronic alcoholism is associated with a marked decrease in thyroid volume[222] and thyroid stromal fibrosis.[223] However, no relationship between thyroid volume and fibrosis and any index of thyroid function has been reported.

Acute alcohol administration reduces $T_3$ levels both in alcoholic persons and in normal subjects by reducing hepatic deiodination of $T_4$ to $T_3$, due to an alcohol-induced hepatocellular injury.[224–226] A reduction in the circulating levels of $T_4$ and, to a greater extent, $T_3$ occurs in alcoholic subjects with liver disease.[227–231] Despite these alterations in the profiles of thyroid hormones, alcoholic patients remain clinically euthyroid.[228,232] TSH levels are usually within the normal range.[228,233–236]

The most consistent finding in alcoholic individuals is blunting of the TSH response to TRH, suggesting that a defect in the hypothalamic-pituitary axis occurs as a consequence of alcohol abuse.[237–240] In vitro, at physiologic doses, alcohol exposure modifies the number of TSH-binding sites on thyroid gland cell membranes as well as the thyroid response to TSH.[241] This may represent a self-correcting effort involving the HPT axis.

### EFFECT OF ALCOHOL ON GROWTH HORMONE AND PROLACTIN

In alcoholic persons, the increase in estrogen levels and the impaired synthetic ability of the liver due to the toxic effect of alcohol each contribute to a dysregulation of GH production and release (see Chap. 12). Chronic alcoholic subjects with cirrhosis have increased circulating levels of GH. A hypothalamic defect in neuroregulation of GH may exist in alcoholic patients with cirrhosis, as TRH abnormally stimulates the secretion of GH in alcoholic individuals with or without alcohol-induced liver disease, but not in normal volunteers.[242,243]

A single dose of ethanol does not affect PRL levels[244]; however, circulating PRL levels are increased in alcoholic individuals, particularly those with cirrhosis.[245] An increased abundance of PRL-secreting cells are found in the pituitaries of alcoholic cirrhotic patients.[246]

PRL secretion is regulated primarily through inhibitory mechanisms (see Chap. 13). Dopamine is the most important PRL-inhibiting factor.[247] In cirrhotic patients, dopaminergic drugs fail to suppress PRL and GH secretion, suggesting a dysregulation in dopaminergic systems, particularly in those patients with hepatic encephalopathy.[248] This abnormal GH and PRL secretion most likely occurs because of portal hypertension and portosystemic shunting of adrenergic monoamines and other substances that affect dopaminergic neuroreactivity at the level of the hypothalamus.[249,250] Hypersecretion of PRL has been implicated as one of the factors that mediate the ethanol-induced hypogonadism in male alcoholics. In experimental models, acute alcohol administration stimulates PRL secretion from the pituitary gland in a dose-dependent manner. Moreover, ethanol has a direct stimulatory effect on PRL secretion by the adenohypophysis.[251]

TRH stimulates the secretion of GH and PRL in individuals with alcohol-induced liver disease,[252–254] an effect not seen in normal subjects. The hypothesis has been raised that a dysregulation of TRH secretion in cirrhotic patients also contributes to the abnormalities of GH and PRL secretion, which are noted particularly in alcoholic cirrhotic patients.[236]

### EFFECT OF ALCOHOL ON BONE AND CALCIUM METABOLISM

The effect of alcohol on bone metabolism is multifactorial. Normal osteoblast function depends on an adequate state of nutrition and an intact endocrine system. The effect of alcohol on bone metabolism is a consequence of both direct toxicity and an indirect action through an impairment of the individual's hormonal and nutritional status. Hypophosphatemia is yet another factor that contributes to the osteodystrophy seen in chronic alcoholics.[255,256]

Alcoholic patients often present with a notable reduction in bone mass,[256a] of trabecular bone in particular, associated with increased bone fragility compared with age-matched controls.[257–261] Alcohol is thought to be responsible for the imbalance between bone formation and resorption. It decreases bone formation by reducing the number of osteoblasts.[262,263] Circulating levels of osteocalcin, a marker of osteoblast function, are reduced in chronic alcoholism.[264]

Liver disease, a condition that often accompanies chronic alcohol abuse, may itself be associated with disrupted bone metabolism (*hepatic osteodystrophy*). Osteoporosis occurs predominantly in hypogonadic individuals; reduced sex hormone concentrations may lead to a decreased activity of osteoblasts.[264] GH stimulates the proliferation of the osteoblasts and controls bone remodeling by modulating the production of IGF-I and IGF-II. Chronic alcohol abuse causes a reduction in both GH and IGF-I levels.[265]

Histomorphometric evidence of bone resorption is observed after moderate to heavy chronic alcohol intake. Osteoclasts are more abundant in bone biopsies obtained from alcoholic persons than in those from nonalcoholic individuals.[266] Moreover, alcohol seems to directly stimulate osteoclast activity in vitro.[267]

In alcoholic individuals with cirrhosis, both malabsorption of calcium and vitamin D deficiency contribute to a chronic hypocalcemia. Ethanol ingestion interferes with intestinal calcium absorption by reducing the duodenal transport of the calcium ion.[268,269] Moreover, alcohol ingestion is followed by an increased urinary excretion of both calcium and magnesium.[270,271]

The alterations in calcium homeostasis observed in alcoholic patients may be partly due to an alcohol-induced primary alteration of magnesium homeostasis, as magnesium is the principal regulator of PTH secretion and PTH action at peripheral tissue sites.[272-274] Chronic alcoholic individuals have PTH levels that are either elevated or at the upper level of the normal range.

## LIVER TRANSPLANTATION AND ENDOCRINE FUNCTION

Orthotopic liver transplantation (OLTx) is the treatment of choice for end-stage liver disease. Although OLTx is effective in correcting liver function in a short period of time, a complete correction of the various metabolic and hormonal imbalances associated with advanced liver disease is usually delayed. The immunosuppressive therapy required after transplantation to prevent graft rejection contributes largely to this phenomenon. In the first few months after OLTx, the high doses of corticosteroids and of tacrolimus or cyclosporine that are required are responsible for maintaining insulin resistance, impaired insulin secretion, and a hyperlipidemia consisting of hypertriglyceridemia and hypercholesterolemia. Both plasma glucagon and plasma insulin levels are higher than normal for several months after successful OLTx, presumably as a consequence of an overproduction of both hormones by the pancreas. Within 2 years posttransplantation, insulin and glucose metabolism normalizes. Protein metabolism remains altered, however, as several amino-acid transport systems in the hepatocyte are normally under neural control, and the transplanted liver is denervated. This, combined with the use of corticosteroids and cyclosporine or tacrolimus, probably accounts for the abnormality in substrate handling noted in individuals with liver transplants.

The cirrhosis-induced alteration of sex steroid homeostasis is significantly corrected after OLTx. Testosterone and gonadotropin levels usually return to normal within 6 months. A residual gonadal failure that may persist in patients with chronic alcoholism is associated with increased levels of FSH and LH. This residual hypergonadotropic hypogonadism is a consequence of an irreversible alcohol-induced gonadal injury. Finally, both cyclosporine and prednisone tend to reduce serum testosterone levels in men.

Usually, women achieve normal menstrual function and fertility after successful OLTx. A return of menses can occur as soon as 2 months post-OLTx. Pregnancy has been reported to occur as early as 3 weeks after OLTx. Pregnant transplant recipients require the same doses of immunosuppressive agents as their nonpregnant peers. Successful pregnancy has been reported, with no adverse fetal consequences of the administration of standard doses of immunosuppressive agents throughout the pregnancy. Maternal and perinatal outcomes are generally favorable. Pregnancies in transplant recipients require careful monitoring, however, because of an increased risk of preterm delivery, of preeclampsia, and of perineal infection in women who have undergone OLTx before their pregnancies.

## REFERENCES

1. Ranke MB, Stanley CA, Tenore A, et al. Characterization of somatogenic and lactogenic binding sites in isolated hepatocytes. Endocrinology 1976; 99:1033.
2. Postel-Vinay M-C, Cohen-Tanugi E, Charrier J. Growth hormone receptors in rat liver membranes: effects of fasting and refeeding, and correlation with plasma somatomedin activity. Mol Cell Endocrinol 1982; 28:657.
3. Delahaye-Zerras MC, Mertami H, Martini JF, et al. Expression of the growth hormone receptor gene in human digestive tissue. J Clin Endocrinol Metab 1994; 78:1473.
4. Bala RM, Bohnet HG, Carter JN, Friesen HG. Effect of ovine prolactin on serum somatomedin bioactivity in hypophysectomized female rats. Can J Physiol Pharmacol 1978; 56:984.
5. Francis MJO, Hill DJ. Prolactin-stimulated production of somatomedin by rat liver. Nature 1975; 255:167.
6. Holder AT, Wallis M. Actions of growth hormone, prolactin and thyroxine on serum somatomedin-like activity and growth in hypopituitary dwarf mice. J Endocrinol 1977; 74:223.
7. Cheek DB, Graystone JE. The action of insulin, growth hormone and epinephrine on cell growth in the liver, muscle, and brain of the hypophysectomized rat. Pediatr Res 1969; 3:77.
8. Wong BS, Chenoweth ME, Dunn A. Possible growth hormone control of liver glutamine synthetase activity in rats. Endocrinology 1980; 106:268.
9. Gebhardt R, Mecke D. The role of growth hormone, dexamethasone and triiodothyronine in the regulation of glutamine synthetase in primary cultures of rat hepatocytes. Eur J Biochem 1979; 100:519.
10. Korner A, Hogan BLM. The effect of growth hormone on inducible liver enzymes. In: Pecile A, Muller EE, eds. Growth and growth hormone. Amsterdam: Excerpta Medica, 1971:98.
11. Paleckar AG, Collipp PJ, Maddaiah VI. Growth hormone and rat liver mitochondria: effects on urea cycle enzymes. Biochem Biophys Res Commun 1981; 100:1604.
12. Raina A, Holtta E. The effect of growth hormone on the synthesis and accumulation of polyamines in mammalian tissues. In: Pecile A, Muller EE, eds. Growth and growth hormone. Amsterdam: Excerpta Medica 1972:143.
13. Gustafsson JA, Mode A, Norstedt G, et al. The hypothalamo-pituitary-liver axis: a new hormonal system in control of hepatic steroid and drug metabolism. In: Litwack G, ed. Biochemical actions of hormones, vol 7. New York: Academic Press, 1980:47.
14. D'Ercole AJ, Stiles AD, Underwood LE. Tissue concentrations of somatomedin C: further evidence for multiple sites of synthesis and paracrine or autocrine mechanisms of action. Proc Natl Acad Sci U S A 1984; 81:935.
15. Vassilopoulou-Sellin R, Phillips LE. Extraction of somatomedin activity from rat liver. Endocrinology 1982; 110:582.
16. Mayer PW, Schalch DS. Somatomedin synthesis by a subclone of Buffalo rat liver cells: characterization and evidence for immediate secretion of de novo synthesized hormone. Endocrinology 1983; 113:588.
17. Merimee TJ, Zapf J, Froesch ER. Insulin-like growth factors in the fed and fasted states. J Clin Endocrinol Metab 1982; 55:999.
18. Ilan Y, Oren R, Tur-Kaspa R. Elevated growth hormone levels in patients with non-alcoholic chronic liver disease. J Gastroenterol Hepatol 1993; 8:448.
19. Moller S, Gronbaek M, Main K, et al. Urinary growth hormone (U-GH) excretion and serum insulin-like growth factor 1 (IGF-1) in patients with alcoholic cirrhosis. J Hepatol 1993; 17:315.
20. Wu A, Grant DB, Hambley J, Levi AJ. Reduced serum somatomedin activity in patients with chronic liver disease. Clin Sci Mol Med 1974; 47:359.
21. Hepner GW, Chopra IJ. Serum thyroid hormone levels in patients with liver disease. Arch Intern Med 1979; 139:1117.
22. Vannotti A, Beraud T. Functional relationships between the liver, the thyroxine binding protein of serum, and the thyroid. J Clin Endocrinol Metab 1959; 19:466.
23. Gardner DF, Carithers RL, Utiger RD. Thyroid function tests in patients with acute and resolved hepatitis B virus infection. Ann Intern Med 1982; 96:450.
24. Schlusser GC, Schaffner F, Korn F. Increased serum thyroid hormone binding and decreased free hormone in chronic active liver disease. N Engl J Med 1978; 299:510.
25. Ross DS, Daniels GH, Dienstag JL, Ridgway EC. Elevated thyroxine levels due to increased thyroxine binding globulin in acute hepatitis. Am J Med 1983; 74:564.
26. Hepner GW, Chopra IJ. Serum thyroid hormone levels in patients with liver disease. Arch Intern Med 1979; 139:1117.
27. Pagliacci MC, Pelicci G, Francisci D, et al. Thyroid function tests in acute viral hepatitis: relative reduction in serum thyroxine levels due to $T_4$-TBG binding inhibitors in patients with severe liver cell necrosis. J Endocrinol Invest 1989; 12:149.
28. Van Thiel DH, Stone BG, Schade RR. The liver and its effect on endocrine function in health and diseases. In: Schiff L, Schiff ER, eds. Diseases of the liver. Philadelphia: JB Lippincott, 1987:129.
29. Kano T, Kojima T, Takahashi T, Muto Y. Serum thyroid hormone levels in patients with fulminant hepatitis: usefulness of $rT_3$ and the $rT_3/T_3$ ratio as prognostic indices. Gastroenterol Jpn 1987; 22(3):344.
30. Itoh S, Yamaha Y, Oda T, Kawagoe K. Serum thyroid hormone, triiodothyronine, thyroxine, and triiodothyronine/thyroxine ratio in patients with fulminant, acute, and chronic hepatitis. Am J Gastroenterol 1986; 81:444.

31. Faber J, Kirkegaard C, Rasmussen B, et al. Pituitary thyroid axis in critical illness. J Clin Endocrinol Metab 1987; 65:315.

32. Schimmel M, Utiger RD. Thyroidal and peripheral production of thyroid hormones: review of recent findings and their clinical implications. Ann Intern Med 1977; 878:760.

33. Chopra IJ, Hershman JM, Pardridge WM, Nicoloff JT. Thyroid function in nonthyroidal illness. Ann Intern Med 1983; 98:946.

34. Wartofsky L, Burman KD. Alterations in thyroid function in patients with systemic illness: the "euthyroid sick syndrome." Endocr Rev 1982; 3:164.

35. Kaptein EM, Grieb DA, Spencer CA, et al. Thyroxine metabolism in the low thyroxine state of critical nonthyroidal illnesses. J Clin Endocrinol Metab 1981; 53:764.

36. Baumgarten A, Rommelspacher H, Otto M, et al. Hypothalamic-pituitary-thyroid (HPT) axis in chronic alcoholism. I. HPT axis in chronic alcoholics during withdrawal and after three weeks of abstinence. Alcoholism 1994; 18:284.

37. Schussler GC, Schaffner F, Hurley J, Shapiro J. Thyroid function in primary biliary cirrhosis. Clin Res 1979; 27:259A.

38. Mendel CM, Cavalieri RR, Weisiger RA. Uptake of thyroxine by the perfused rat liver: implications for the free hormone hypothesis. Am J Physiol 1988; 255:E110.

39. Elta GH, Sepersky RA, Goldberg MJ, et al. Increased incidence of hypothyroidism in primary biliary cirrhosis. Dig Dis Sci 1982; 28:971.

40. Chopra IJ, Solomon DH, Chopra U, et al. Alterations in circulating thyroid hormones and thyrotropin in hepatic cirrhosis: evidence for euthyroidism despite subnormal serum triiodothyronine. J Clin Endocrinol Metab 1974; 39:501.

41. Itoh S, Matsuo S, Oda T, et al. Triiodothyronine level and triiodothyronine/thyroxine ratio in chronic hepatitis patients treated with prednisolone-withdrawal. Dig Dis Sci 1990; 35:1110.

42. Green JRB, Snitcher ES, Mowat NAG, et al. Thyroid function and thyroid regulation in euthyroid men with chronic liver disease. Clin Endocrinol (Oxf) 1977; 7:453.

43. Nomura S, Pittman CS, Chambers JB, et al. Reduced peripheral conversion of thyroxine to triiodothyronine in patients with hepatic cirrhosis. J Clin Invest 1975; 56:643.

44. Inada M, Sterling M. Thyroxine turnover and transport in Laënnec's cirrhosis of the liver. J Clin Invest 1967; 46:1275.

45. Van Thiel DH, Gavaler JS, Tarter RE, et al. Pituitary and thyroid hormone levels before and after orthotopic hepatic transplantation and their responses to thyrotropin-releasing hormone. J Clin Endocrinol Metab 1985; 60:569.

46. Israel Y, Walfish PB, Orrego H, et al. Thyroid hormones in alcoholic liver disease: effect of treatment with 6-N-propylthiouracil. Gastroenterology 1979; 76:116.

47. Walfish PG, Orrego H, Israel Y, et al. Serum triiodothyronine and other clinical and laboratory indices of alcoholic liver disease. Ann Intern Med 1979; 91:13.

48. Orrego H, Kalant H, Israel Y, et al. Effect of short-term therapy with propylthiouracil in patients with alcoholic liver disease. Gastroenterology 1979; 76:105.

49. Chopra IJ, Hung TS, Beredo A, et al. Serum thyroid hormone binding inhibitor in non-thyroidal illnesses. Metabolism 1986; 35:152.

50. Suzuki Y, Nanno M, Gemma R, Yoshimi T. Plasma free fatty acids: inhibitor of extrathyroidal conversion of $T_4$ to $T_3$ and thyroid hormone binding inhibitor in patients with various nonthyroidal illnesses. Endocrinol Jpn 1992; 39:445.

51. Woeber K, Maddux B. Thyroid hormone binding in nonthyroid illness. Metabolism 1981; 30:412.

52. Van Thiel DH. The liver and the endocrine system. In: Arias IM, Jakoby WB, Popper H, et al., eds. The liver: biology and pathobiology. New York: Raven Press, 1988:1007.

53. Van Thiel DH, Tarter R, Gavaler JS, et al. Thyroid and pituitary hormone responses to TRH in advanced nonalcoholic liver disease. J Endocrinol Invest 1986; 9:479.

54. Van Thiel DH, Gavaler JS, Tarter R, et al. Pituitary and thyroid hormone levels before and after orthotopic hepatic transplantation and their responses to thyrotropin-releasing hormone. J Clin Endocrinol Metab 1985; 60:569.

55. Van Thiel DH, Udani M, Schade RR, et al. Prognostic value of thyroid hormone levels in patients evaluated for liver transplantation. Hepatology 1985; 5:862.

56. Wilber JF, Utiger RD. The effect of glucocorticoids on thyrotropin secretion. J Clin Invest 1969; 48:2096.

57. Borst GC, Osburne RC, O'Brian JT, et al. Fasting decreases thyrotropin responsiveness to thyrotropin-releasing hormone: a potential cause of misinterpretation of thyroid function tests in the critically ill. J Clin Endocrinol Metab 1983; 57:380.

58. Sap J, Munoz A, Damm K, et al. The c-erb-A protein is a high-affinity receptor for thyroid hormone. Nature 1986; 324:635.

59. Williams GR, Franklyn JA, Neuberger JM, Sheppard MC. Thyroid hormone receptor expression in the "sick euthyroid" syndrome. Lancet 1989; 2:1477.

60. Silva JE, Larsen PR. Contributions of plasma triiodothyronine and local thyroxine monodeiodination to triiodothyronine to nuclear triiodothyronine receptor saturation in pituitary, liver and kidney of hypothyroid rats. J Clin Invest 1978; 61:1247.

61. Chopra IJ, Williams DE, Orgiazzi J, Solomon DH. Opposite effects of dexamethasone on serum concentrations of 3,3,5-triiodothyronine ($T_3$). J Clin Endocrinol Metab 1975; 41:911.

62. Cooper DS, Daniels GH, Ladenson PW, Ridgeway EC. Hyperthyroxinemia in patients treated with high-dose propranolol. Am J Med 1982; 73:867.

63. Felicetta JV, Green WL, Melp WB. Inhibition of hepatic binding of thyroxine by cholecystographic agents. J Clin Invest 1980; 65:1032.

64. Martino E, Safran M, Aghini-Lombardi F, et al. Environmental iodine intake and thyroid dysfunction during chronic amiodarone therapy. Ann Intern Med 1984; 101:28.

65. Amico JA, Richardson V, Alpert B, Klein I. Clinical and chemical assessment of thyroid function during therapy with amiodarone. Arch Intern Med 1984; 144:487.

66. Taniguchi Y, Murakami T, Nakanishi K, et al. Two cases of hypothyroidism associated with alpha-interferon therapy. Intern Med 1992; 31:373.

67. Fattovich G, Betterle C, Brollo L, et al. Autoantibodies during alpha-interferon therapy for chronic hepatitis B. J Med Virol 1991; 34:132.

68. Barreca T, Picciotto A, Franceschini R, et al. Long-term therapy with recombinant interferon alpha 2b in patients with chronic hepatitis C: effects on thyroid function and autoantibodies. J Biol Regul Homeost Agents 1993; 7:58.

69. Thompson P, Stru O. Abnormalities of liver function tests in thyrotoxicosis. Mil Med 1978; 143:548.

70. Goglia F, Liverini G, Lanni A, Barletta A. Mitochondrial DNA, RNA and protein synthesis in normal, hypothyroid and mildly hyperthyroid rat liver during cold exposure. Mol Cell Endocrinol 1988; 55:141.

71. Pauletzki J, Stellare F, Paumgartner GH. Bile acid metabolism in human hyperthyroidism. Hepatology 1989; 9:852.

72. Demelia L, Solinas A, Poma R, et al. Hypothalamo-pituitary-adrenal function in liver cirrhosis of viral etiology. Ann Ital Med Int 1991; 6:203.

73. Maruyama Y, Adachi Y, Aoki N, et al. Mechanism of feminization in male patients with non-alcoholic liver cirrhosis: role of sex hormone-binding globulin. Gastroenterol Jpn 1991; 26:435.

74. Farinati F, De Maria N, Fornasiero A, et al. Unresectable hepatocellular carcinoma: prospective controlled trial with the anti-estrogen drug tamoxifen in patients with unresectable hepatocellular carcinoma. Dig Dis Sci 1992; 37:659.

75. Frezza EE, Gerunda GE, Farinati F, et al. Sex hormones and trace elements in rat CCL4-induced cirrhosis and hepatocellular carcinoma. Eur J Cancer Prev 1993; 2:357.

76. Walton C, Kelly WF, Laing I, Bulock OE. Endocrine abnormalities in idiopathic haemochromatosis. Q J Med 1983; 52:99.

77. McNeil LW, McKee LC Jr, Lorber D, Robin D. The endocrine manifestations of hemochromatosis. Am J Med Sci 1983; 285:7.

78. Charbonnel B, Chupin M, LeGrand A, Guillon J. Pituitary function in idiopathic haemochromatosis. Acta Endocrinol (Copenh) 1981; 98:178.

79. Bezwoda WR, Bothwell TH, Vanderwalt LA, et al. An investigation into gonadal dysfunction in patients with idiopathic haemochromatosis. Clin Endocrinol (Oxf) 1977; 6:377.

80. Burrows GH, Barrea A. Copper stimulates the release of luteinizing hormone releasing hormone from isolated hypothalamic granulae. Endocrinology 1982; 115:1456.

81. Barrea A, Cho G. Evidence that copper-amino acid complexes are potent stimulators of the release of luteinizing hormone releasing hormone from isolated hypothalamic granulae. Endocrinology 1984; 115:936.

82. Piperno A, Rivolta MR, D'Alba R, et al. Preclinical hypogonadism in genetic hemochromatosis in the early stage of the disease: evidence of hypothalamic dysfunction. J Endocrinol Invest 1992; 15:423.

83. Eagon PK, Fisher SE, Imhoff AF, et al. Estrogen binding proteins in male rat livers: influences of hormonal changes. Arch Biochem Biophys 1980; 201:486.

84. Eagon PK, Zdunek JR, Van Thiel DH, et al. Alcohol-induced changes in hepatic estrogen binding proteins. Arch Biochem Biophys 1981; 211:48.

85. Aten RF, Dickson RB, Eisenbeld AJ. Estrogen receptor in adult male rat liver. Endocrinology 1978; 103:1629.

86. Powell-Jones W, Thompson C, Nayfeh SN, Lucier GW. Sex differences in estrogen binding by cytosolic and nuclear components of rat liver. J Steroid Biochem 1980; 13:219.

87. Norstedt G, Wrange O, Gustafsson JA. Multihormonal regulation of the estrogen receptor in rat liver. Endocrinology 1981; 108:1190.

88. Porter LE, Elm M, Van Thiel DH, Eagon PK. Hepatic estrogen receptor in human liver disease. Gastroenterology 1987; 92:735.

89. Powell-Jones W, Raeford S, Lucier GW. Binding properties of zearalenone myocotoxins to hepatic estrogen receptors. Mol Pharmacol 1981; 20:35.

90. Kneifel R, Katzenellenbogen BS. Comparative effects of estrogen and anti-estrogen on plasma renin substrate levels and hepatic estrogen receptors in rats. Endocrinology 1981; 108:545.

91. Kupfer D, Bulger WH. Estrogenic properties of DDT and its analogs. In: McLaughlin JA, ed. Estrogens in the environment. New York: Elsevier/North Holland, 1980:239.

92. Dickson RB, Eisenfeld AJ. 17-ethinylestradiol is more potent than estradiol in receptor interactions with isolated hepatic parenchymal cells. Endocrinology 1981; 108:1551.

93. Porter LE, Elm MS, Van Thiel DH, et al. Characterization and quantitation of human hepatic estrogen receptor. Gastroenterology 1983; 84:704.

94. Porter LE, Elm MS, Van Thiel DH, Eagon PK. Estrogen receptor in human liver nuclei. Hepatology 1984; 4:1085.

95. Colby HD. Regulation of hepatic drug and steroid metabolism by androgens and estrogens. In: Thomas JA, Singal RL, eds. Advances in sex hormone research. Baltimore: Urban and Schwartzenberg, 1980:346.

96. Bardin CW, Catteral JS. Testosterone: a major determinant of extragenital sexual dimorphism. Science 1981; 211:1285.

97. Gustafsson JA, Mode A, Norstedt G, et al. The hypothalamo-pituitary-liver axis: a new hormonal system in control of hepatic steroid and drug metabolism. Biochem Action Horm 1980; 7:47.

98. Gustafsson JA, Mode A, Norstedt G, et al. Sex steroid induced changes in hepatic enzymes. Annu Rev Physiol 1983; 45:51.

99. Roy AK, Chatterjee B. Sexual dimorphism in the liver. Annu Rev Physiol 1983; 45:37.

100. Eden S. Age- and sex-related differences in episodic growth hormone secretion in the rat. Endocrinology 1979; 105:555.

101. Mode A, Norstedt G, Simic B, et al. Continuous infusion of growth hormone feminizes hepatic steroid metabolism in the rat. Endocrinology 1981; 108:2103.

102. Mode A, Gustafsson JA, Jansson JD, et al. Association between plasma levels of growth hormone and sex differentiation of hepatic steroid metabolism in the rat. Endocrinology 1982; 111:1692.

103. Norstedt G, Palmiter R. Secretory rhythm of growth hormone regulates sexual differentiation of mouse liver. Cell 1984; 36:805.

104. Van Thiel DH, Gavaler JS. Sex steroids and the liver. In: Francavilla A, Panella C, DiLeo A, Van Thiel DH, eds. Liver and hormones. New York: Raven Press, 1987; 43:183.

105. Gilnoer D, McGuire RA, Gershengorn MC, et al. Effects of estrogen on thyrotropin-binding globulin metabolism in rhesus monkeys. Endocrinology 1977; 100:9.

106. Gilnoer DM, Gershengorn MC, DuBois A, Robbins J. Stimulation of thyroxine binding globulin synthesis by isolated rhesus monkey hepatocytes after in vitro β-estradiol administration. Endocrinology 1977; 100:807.

107. Moore DE, Kawagoe S, Davajan V, et al. An in vivo system in man for quantitation of estrogenicity: II. Pharmacologic in binding capacity of serum corticosteroid-binding globulin induced by conjugated estrogens, menstranol, and ethinyl estradiol. Am J Obstet Gynecol 1978; 130:482.

108. Song CS, Kappas A. Hormones and hepatic function. In: Schiff L, ed. Diseases of the liver, 4th ed. Philadelphia: JB Lippincott, 1975:163.

109. Windler EET, Kovaner PT, Chao Y-S, et al. The estradiol-stimulated lipoprotein receptor of rat liver: a binding site that mediates the uptake of rat lipoproteins containing apoproteins B and E. J Biol Chem 1980; 255:10.

110. Porter LE, Van Thiel DH, Eagon PK. Estrogens and progestins as tumor inducers. Semin Liver Dis 1987; 7:24.

111. Francavilla A, Gavaler JS, Makowka L, et al. Estradiol and testosterone levels in patients undergoing partial hepatectomy: a possible signal for hepatic regeneration? Dig Dis Sci 1989; 34:818.

112. Francavilla A, Eagon PK, Di Leo A, et al. Sex hormone-related functions in regenerating male rat liver. Gastroenterology 1986; 91:1263.

113. Francavilla A, Polimeno L, Di Leo A, et al. The effect of estrogen and tamoxifen in hepatocyte proliferation in vivo and in vitro. Hepatology 1989; 9:614.

114. Francavilla A, Di Leo A, Eagon PK, et al. Regenerating rat liver: correlation between estrogen receptor localization and deoxyribonucleic acid synthesis. Gastroenterology 1984; 86:552.

115. Fisher B, Gunduz M, Saffer EA, Zheng S. Relation of estrogen and its receptors to rat liver growth and regeneration. Cancer Res 1984; 44:2410.

116. Van Thiel DH, Gavaler JS. Pregnancy-associated sex steroids and their effects on the liver. Semin Liver Dis 1987; 7:1.

117. Eagon PK, Francavilla A, Di Leo A, et al. Quantitation of estrogen and androgen receptors in hepatocellular carcinoma and adjacent normal human liver. Dig Dis Sci 1991; 36:1303.

118. Eagon PK, Willett SM, Seguitti ML, et al. Androgen-responsive functions of male rat liver. Gastroenterology 1987; 93:1162.

119. Van Thiel DH, Gavaler JS, Spero JA, et al. Patterns of hypothalamic-pituitary-gonadal dysfunction in men with liver disease due to differing etiologies. Hepatology 1981; 1:39.

120. Van Thiel DH, Gavaler JS, Rosenblum E, Eagon PK. Effects of ethanol on endocrine cells: testicular effects. Ann N Y Acad Sci 1987; 492:287.

121. Van Thiel DH, Gavaler JS. Hypothalamic-pituitary-gonadal function in liver disease with particular attention to the endocrine effects of chronic alcohol abuse. Prog Liver Dis 1986; 8:273.

122. Bannister P, Oakes J, Sheridan P, Losowsky MS. Sex hormone changes in chronic liver disease: a matched study of alcoholic versus non-alcoholic liver disease. Q J Med 1987; 63:305.

123. Rose LI, Underwood RH, Newmark SR, et al. Pathophysiology of spironolactone-induced gynecomastia. Ann Intern Med 1977; 87:398.

124. Van Thiel DH, Gavaler JS, Schade RR. Liver disease and the hypothalamic pituitary gonadal axis. Semin Liver Dis 1985; 5:35.

125. Cundy TF, Butler J, Pope RM, et al. Amenorrhoea in women with non-alcoholic chronic liver disease. Gut 1991; 32:202.

126. Weinhouse S. Regulation of glucokinase in liver. In: Horecker BL, Stadtman ER, eds. Current topics in cellular regulation. New York: Academic Press, 1976:1.

127. Felig P, Wahren J. Influence of endogenous insulin secretion on splanchnic glucose and amino acid metabolism in man. J Clin Invest 1971; 50:1702.

128. Cherrington AD, Steiner KE. The effects of insulin on carbohydrate metabolism in vivo. J Clin Endocrinol Metab 1982; 11:307.

129. Chupin M, Charbonnel B, Le Bodic L, et al. Glucose tolerance in viral hepatitis. A study of twenty patients during the acute phase and after recovery. Diabetes 1978; 27:661.

130. Kaneko K, Arai M, Funatomi H, et al. Changes in immunoreactive insulin, C-peptide immunoreactivity, and immunoreactive glucagon in acute viral hepatitis. J Gastroenterol 1995; 30:624.

131. Sullivan SN, Chase RA, Christofides ND, et al. The gut hormone profile of fulminant hepatic failure. Am J Gastroenterol 1981; 76:338.

132. Samson RI, Trey C, Timme AH, Saunders SJ. Fulminating hepatitis with recurrent hypoglycemia and hemorrhage. Gastroenterology 1967; 53:291.

133. Bucher ML, Swaffield MN. Regulation of hepatic regeneration in rats by synergistic action of insulin and glucagon. Proc Natl Acad Sci U S A 1975; 72:1157.

134. Arky RA. Hypoglycemia associated with liver disease and ethanol. Endocrinol Metab Clin North Am 1989; 18:75.

135. Van Thiel DH. The liver and the endocrine system. In: Arias IM, Jakoby WB, Popper H, et al., eds. The liver: biology and pathobiology. New York: Raven Press, 1988:1007.

136. Tauton OD, Greene HC. Fructose-1,6-diphosphatase deficiency, hypoglycemia and a response to folate therapy in a mother and a daughter. Biochem Med 1978; 19:260.

137. Hommes FA, Bendienik E. Two cases of phosphoenolpyruvate carboxykinase deficiency. Acta Pediatr Scand 1976; 65:233.

138. Freinkel N, Cohn AK. Alcoholic hypoglycemia: a prototype of the hypoglycemias induced by fasting in diabetes. In: Ostram J, ed. New York: Elsevier, 1969:873.

139. Felig P, Brown WV, Levine RA, Klatskin G. Glucose homeostasis in viral liver disease. N Engl J Med 1979; 283:1436.

140. Jaspan JB, Huen AH, Morley CG, et al. The role of the liver in glucagon metabolism. J Clin Invest 1977; 60:421.

141. Shroyer LA, Varandani PT. Purification and characterization of rat liver cytosol neutral thiol peptidase that degrades glucagon, insulin and isolated insulin A and B chains. Arch Biochem Biophys 1985; 236:205.

142. Collins JR, Crofford OB. Glucose intolerance and insulin resistance in patients with liver disease. Arch Intern Med 1969; 124:142.

143. Kingston ME, Ashraf AM, Atiyeh M, Donnelly RJ. Diabetes mellitus in chronic active hepatitis and cirrhosis. Gastroenterology 1984; 87:688.

144. Conn HO, Schreiber W, Elkington SG. Cirrhosis and diabetes: association of impaired glucose intolerance with portal-systemic shunting in Laënnec's cirrhosis. Dig Dis Sci 1971; 16:227.

145. Johnston DG, Alberti KGMM, Faber OK, Binder C. Hyperinsulinism of hepatic cirrhosis: diminished degradation or hypersecretion. Lancet 1977; I:10.

146. Romijn JA, Endert E, Sauerwein HP. Glucose and fat metabolism during short-term starvation in cirrhosis. Gastroenterology 1991; 100:731.

147. Collins JR, Crofford OB. Glucose intolerance and insulin resistance in patients with liver disease. Arch Intern Med 1969; 124:142.

148. Kingston ME, Ali MA, Atiyeh M, Donnelly RJ. Diabetes mellitus in chronic active hepatitis and cirrhosis. Gastroenterology 1984; 87:688.

149. Conn HO, Schreiber W, Elkington SG. Cirrhosis and diabetes. II. Association of impaired glucose tolerance with portal-systemic shunting in Laënnec's cirrhosis. Am J Dig Dis 1971; 16:227.

150. Johnson DG, Alberti KG, Faber OK, Binder C. Hyperinsulinism of hepatic cirrhosis: diminished degradation or hypersecretion? Lancet 1977; 1:10.

151. Kruszynska YT, Home PD, McIntyre N. Relationship between insulin sensitivity, insulin secretion and glucose tolerance in cirrhosis. Hepatology 1991; 14:103.

152. Kasperska-Czyzykowa T, Heding LG, Czyzyk A. Serum levels of true insulin, C-peptide and proinsulin in peripheral blood of patients with cirrhosis. Diabetologia 1983; 25:506.

153. Ballmann M, Hartmann H, Deacon CF, et al. Hypersecretion of proinsulin does not explain the hyperinsulinaemia of patients with liver cirrhosis. Clin Endocrinol (Oxf) 1986; 25:351.

154. Proietto J, Dudley FJ, Aitken P, Alford FP. Hyperinsulinaemia and insulin resistance of cirrhosis: the importance of insulin hypersecretion. Clin Endocrinol (Oxf) 1984; 21:657.

155. Nygren A, Adner N, Sundblad L, Wiechel KL. Insulin uptake by the human alcoholic cirrhotic liver. Metabolism 1985; 34:48.

156. Antoniello S, La Rocca S, Cavalcanti E, et al. Insulin and glucagon degradation in liver are not affected by hepatic cirrhosis. Clin Chim Acta 1989; 183:343.

156a. Siegel EG, Seidenstüker A, Gallwitz B, et al. Insulin secretion defects in liver cirrhosis can be reversed by glucagon-like peptide-1. J Endocrinol 2000; 164:13.

157. Cavallo-Perin P, Bruno A, Nuccio P, et al. Feedback inhibition of insulin secretion is altered in cirrhosis. J Clin Endocrinol Metab 1986; 63:1023.

158. Petrides AS, Schulze-Berge D, Vogt C, et al. Glucose resistance contributes to diabetes mellitus in cirrhosis. Hepatology 1993; 18:284.

159. Taylor R, Heine RJ, Collins J, et al. Insulin action in cirrhosis. Hepatology 1985; 5:64.

160. Cavallo-Perin P, Cassader M, Bozzo C, et al. Mechanism of insulin resistance in human liver cirrhosis. Evidence of a combined receptor and postreceptor defect. J Clin Invest 1985; 75:1659.

161. Blei AT, Robbins DC, Drobny E, et al. Insulin resistance and insulin receptors in hepatic cirrhosis. Gastroenterology 1982; 83:1191.

162. Harewood MS, Proietto J, Dudley F, Alford FP. Insulin action and cirrhosis: insulin binding and lipogenesis in isolated adipocytes. Metabolism 1982; 31:1241.

163. Greco AV, Crucitti F, Ghirlanda G, et al. Insulin and glucagon concentrations in portal and peripheral veins in patients with hepatic cirrhosis. Diabetologia 1979; 17:23.

164. Petrides AS, Vogt C, Schulze-Berge D, et al. Pathogenesis of glucose intolerance and diabetes mellitus in cirrhosis. Hepatology 1994; 19:616.

165. Sherwin RS, Fisher M, Bessoff J, et al. Hyperglucagonemia in cirrhosis: altered secretion and sensitivity to glucagon. Gastroenterology 1978; 74:1224.

166. Riggio O, Merli M, Cangiano C, et al. Glucose intolerance in liver cirrhosis. Metabolism 1982; 31:627.

167. Vidal J, Ferrer JP, Esmatjes E, et al. Diabetes mellitus in patients with liver cirrhosis. Diabetes Res Clin Pract 1994; 25:19.

168. Frier BM, Saudek CD. Cholesterol metabolism in diabetes: the effect of insulin on the kinetics of plasma squalene. J Clin Endocrinol Metab 1979; 49:824.

169. Nakayama H, Nakagawa S. Influence of streptozotocin diabetes on intestinal 3-OH-3-methylglutaryl coenzyme A reductase activity in the rat. Diabetes 1977; 26:439.

170. Goodman MW, Michels LD, Keane WF. Intestinal and hepatic cholesterol synthesis in the alloxan diabetic rat. Proc Soc Exp Biol Med 1982; 170:286.

171. Turley SD, Dietschy JM. Cholesterol metabolism and excretion. In: Arias IM, Jakoby WB, Popper H, et al., eds. The liver: biology and pathobiology. New York: Raven Press, 1982:467.

172. Turley SD, Dietschy JM. Regulation of biliary cholesterol output in the rat: dissociation from the rate of hepatic cholesterol synthesis, the size of the hepatic cholesteryl ester pool, and the hepatic uptake of chylomicron cholesterol. J Lipid Res 1979; 20:923.

173. Tavill AS. Protein metabolism and the liver. In: Wright R, Alberti KGMM, Karan S, Millward-Sadler GH, eds. Liver and biliary disease. London: WB Saunders, 1979:83.

174. Meinders AE, Van Berge Henegouwen GP, Willekens FLA, et al. Biliary lipid and bile acid composition in insulin-dependent diabetes mellitus. Arguments for increased intestinal bacterial bile acid degradation. Dig Dis Sci 1981; 26:402.

175. John DW, Miller LL. Regulation of net biosynthesis of serum albumin and acute phase plasma proteins. J Biol Chem 1969; 244:6134.

176. Key PH, Bonorris GG, Coyne MJ, et al. Hepatic cholesterol synthesis: a determinant of cholesterol secretion in gallstone patients. Gastroenterology 1977; 72:1182.

177. Sarva RP, Shreiner DP, Van Thiel DH, Yingvorapant N. Gallbladder function: methods for measuring filling and emptying. J Nucl Med 1985; 26:140.

178. Evans DF, Cussler EL. Physiochemical considerations in gallstone pathogenesis. Hosp Pract 1974; 9:133.

179. Schneider HL, Hornback KD, Kniaz JL, Efrusy ME. Chlorpropamide hepatotoxicity: report of a case and review of the literature. Am J Gastroenterol 1984; 79:721.

180. Smals AG, Kloppenborg PW. Alcohol-induced Cushingoid syndrome. (Letter). Lancet 1977; 1:1369.

181. Cheah JS, Tan BY. Diabetes among different races in similar environment. In: Waldhausl WK, ed. Diabetes. Amsterdam: Excerpta Medica, 1979:326.

182. Hano T. Pathohistological study on the liver cirrhosis in diabetes mellitus. Kobe J Med Sci 1968; 14:87.

183. Bloodworth JMB, Hamwi GJ. Histopathologic lesions associated with sulfonylurea administration. Diabetes 1959; 10:90.

184. Goldstein MJ, Rothenberg AJ. Jaundice in a patient receiving acetohexamide. N Engl J Med 1966; 275:97.

185. Rittinghaus EF, Juppner H, Burdelski M, Hesch RD. Selective determination of C-terminal (70-84) hPTH: elevated concentrations in cholestatic liver disease. Acta Endocrinol 1986; 111:62.

186. Bouillon R, Auwerx J, Dekeyser L, et al. Serum vitamin D metabolites and their binding proteins in patients with liver cirrhosis. J Clin Endocrinol Metab 1984; 59:86.

187. Imawari M, Akanuma Y, Itakura H, et al. The effects of diseases of the liver on serum 25-OH vitamin D and on the serum binding protein for vitamin D and its metabolites. J Lab Clin Med 1979; 93:171.

188. Diamond T, Stiel D, Mason R, et al. Serum vitamin D metabolites are not responsible for low turnover osteoporosis in chronic liver disease. J Clin Endocrinol Metab 1989; 69:1234.

189. Diamond TH, Stiel D, Lunzer M, et al. Hepatic osteodystrophy: static and dynamic bone histomorphometry and serum bone Gla-protein in 80 patients with chronic liver disease. Gastroenterology 1989; 96:213.

190. Crippin JS, Jorgensen RA, Dickson ER, Lindor KD. Hepatic osteodystrophy in primary biliary cirrhosis. Effects of medical treatment. Am J Gastroenterol 1994; 89:47.

191. Janes C, Dickson ER, Bonde S, Riggs BL. Bilirubin inhibits proliferation in cultured normal human osteoblast-like cells: a possible mechanism for bone loss in primary biliary cirrhosis. (Abstract). Gastroenterology 1992; 102:A827.

192. Eastell R, Dickson ER, Hodgson SF, et al. Rates of vertebral bone loss before and after liver transplantation in women with primary biliary cirrhosis. Hepatology 1991; 14:296.

193. Van Thiel DH, Lester R, Sherins RJ. Hypogonadism in alcoholic liver disease: evidence for a double defect. Gastroenterology 1974; 67:1188.

194. Gordon GG, Olivo J, Rafii F, Southern AL. Conversion of androgens to estrogens in cirrhosis of the liver. J Clin Endocrinol Metab 1975; 40:1018.

195. Van Thiel DH, Gavaler JS, Lester R, Goodman MD. Alcohol induced testicular atrophy: an experimental model for hypogonadism occurring in chronic alcoholic men. Gastroenterology 1975; 69:326.

196. Van Thiel DH, Loriaux DL. Evidence for adrenal origin of plasma estrogens in alcoholic men. Metabolism 1979; 28:536.

197. Valimaki M, Salaspuro M, Harkonen M, Ylikahri R. Liver damage and sex hormones in chronic male alcoholics. Clin Endocrinol (Oxford) 1982; 17:469.

198. Longcope C, Pratt JH, Schneider S, Fineberg E. Estrogen and androgen dynamics in liver disease. J Endocr Invest 1984; 7:629.

199. Bannister P, Oakes J, Sheridan P, Losowsky MS. Sex hormone changes in liver disease. Q J Med 1987; 63:305.

200. Badr FM, Bartke A. Effect of ethyl alcohol on plasma testosterone levels in mice. Steroids 1974; 23:921.

201. Badr FM, Bartke A, Daiyerio S, Bugler W. Suppression of testosterone production by ethyl alcohol: possible mode of action. Steroids 1977; 30:647.

202. Gavaler JS, Van Thiel DH, Lester RR. Ethanol, a gonadal toxin in the mature rat of both sexes: similarities and differences. Alcohol Clin Exp Res 1980; 4:271.

203. Van Thiel DH, Gavaler JS, Eagon PK, et al. Alcohol and sex function. Pharmacol Biochem Behav 1980; 13:125.

204. Van Thiel DH, Gavaler JS, Rosenblum E, Tarter RE. Ethanol, its metabolism and hepatotoxicity as well as its gonadal effects: effects of sex. Pharmacol Ther 1989; 41:27.

204a. Tadic SD, Elms MS, Subbotin VM, Eagon PK. Hypogonadism precedes feminization in chronic alcohol-fed male rats. Hepatology 2000; 37:1135.

205. Cobb CF, Ennis MF, Van Thiel DH, et al. Acethaldehyde and ethanol as direct testicular toxins. Surg Forum 1978; 29:641.

206. Cobb CF, Van Thiel DH, Gavaler JS, Lester R. Effects of ethanol and acetaldehyde on the rat adrenal. Metabolism 1981; 30:537.

207. Van Thiel DH, Lester R, Vaitukaitis J. Evidence for a defect in pituitary secretion of luteinizing hormone in chronic alcoholic men. J Clin Endocrinol Metab 1978; 47:499.

208. Van Thiel DH, Gavaler JS. Endocrine effects of chronic alcohol abuse. Hypothalamic-pituitary-gonadal axis. In: Tarter RE, Van Thiel DH, eds. Alcohol and the brain. New York: Plenum Publishing, 1985:69.

209. Smanik EJ, Barkoukis H, Mullen KD, McCullogh AJ. The liver and its effect on endocrine function in health and disease. In: Shiff L, Shiff E, eds. Diseases of the liver. Philadelphia: JB Lippincott, 1993:1373.

210. Gavaler JS, Van Thiel DH. Endocrine consequences of alcohol abuse. In: Nemeroff CB, Loosen PT, eds. Handbook of psychoneuroendocrinology. New York: Guilford Press, 1987.

211. Carter JN, Tyson JE, Tolis G, et al. Prolactin-secreting tumors and hypogonadism in 22 men. N Engl J Med 1978; 299:847.

212. Van Thiel DH. Ethanol: its adverse effects upon the hypothalamic-pituitary-gonadal axis. J Lab Clin Med 1983; 101:21.

213. Olivo J, Gordon GG, Rafii F. Estrogen metabolism in hyperthyroidism and cirrhosis of the liver. Steroids 1975; 26:47.

214. Ryback RS. Chronic alcohol consumption and menstruation. JAMA 1977; 238:2143.

215. Jones-Saumty DJ, Fabian MS, Parsons OA. Medical status and cognitive functioning in alcoholic women. Alcohol Clin Exp Res 1981; 5:372.

216. James VH. The endocrine status of postmenopausal cirrhotic women. In: Langer M, Chiandussi L, Chopra IJ, Martini L, eds. The endocrine and the liver. New York: Academic Press, 1983:57.

217. Valimaki M, Pelkonen R, Salaspuro M, et al. Sex hormones in amenorreic women with alcoholic liver disease. J Clin Endocrinol Metab 1984; 59:133.

218. Becker U. The influence of ethanol and liver disease on sex hormones and hepatic oestrogen receptors in women. Dan Med Bull 1993; 40:447.

219. Gavaler JS, Van Thiel DH. The association between moderate alcoholic beverage consumption and serum levels of estradiol and testosterone levels in postmenopausal women: relationship to the literature. Alcohol Clin Exp Res 1992; 16:87.

220. Gavaler JS, Deal SR, Van Thiel DH, et al. Alcohol and estrogen levels in postmenopausal women: the spectrum of effect. Alcohol Clin Exp Res 1993; 17:786.

221. Gavaler JS. Alcohol effects on hormone levels in normal postmenopausal women and postmenopausal women with alcohol-induced cirrhosis. Recent Dev Alcohol 1995; 12:199.

222. Hegedus L. Decreased thyroid gland volume in alcoholic cirrhosis of the liver. J Clin Endocrinol Metab 1984; 55:930.

223. Hegedus L, Rasmussen N, Ravn V, et al. Independent effects of liver disease and chronic alcoholism on thyroid function and size: the possibility of a toxic effect of alcohol on the thyroid gland. Metabolism 1988; 37:229.

224. Green JRB, Strichter EJ, Mowat AG. Thyroid function and thyroid regulation in euthyroid men with chronic liver disease. Evidence of multiple abnormalities. Clin Endocrinol 1977; 7:453.

225. Yadav HS, Chandhurij BN, Mukherjee SK. Effect of ethyl alcohol on thyroidal iodine trapping and renal clearance of 131-I label in rats. Indian J Med Res 1978; 58:1421.

226. Van Thiel DH, Lester R. The effect of chronic alcohol abuse on sexual function. Clin Endocrinol Metab 1979; 8:499.

227. Israel Y, Walfish PG, Orrego H. Thyroid hormones in alcoholic liver disease. Effect of treatment with 6-N-propylthiouracil. Gastroenterology 1979; 76:116.

228. Chopra IJ, Solomon DH, Chopra U, et al. Alterations in circulating thyroid hormones and thyrotropin in hepatic cirrhosis: evidence for euthyroidism despite subnormal serum triiodothyronine. J Clin Endocrinol Metabol 1974; 39:501.

229. Orrego H, Kalant H, Israel Y. Effect of short-term therapy with propylthiouracil in patients with alcoholic liver disease. Gastroenterology 1979; 76:105.

230. Israel Y, Videla L, MacDonald A, Bernstein J. Metabolic alterations produced in the liver by chronic ethanol administration. Comparison between effects produced by ethanol and by thyroid hormones. Biochem J 1973; 134:523.

231. Nomura S, Pittman CS, Chamber JB. Reduced peripheral conversion of thyroxine to triiodothyronine in patients with hepatic cirrhosis. J Clin Invest 1975; 56:643.

232. Szilagi A. Thyroid hormones and alcoholic liver disease. J Clin Gastroenterol 1987; 9:189.

233. Knudsen M, Christensen H, Berlid D, et al. Hypothalamic-pituitary and thyroid function in chronic alcoholics with neurological complications. Alcohol Clin Exp Res 1990; 14:363.

234. Agner T, Hegen C, Andersen BN, Hegedus L. Pituitary-thyroid function and thyrotropin, prolactin, and growth hormone responses to TRH in patients with chronic alcoholism. Acta Med Scand 1986; 220:57.

235. Hasselbach HC, Bech K, Eskildsen PC. Serum prolactin and thyrotropin responses to thyrotropin-releasing hormone in men with alcoholic cirrhosis. Acta Med Scand 1981; 209:37.

236. Van Thiel DH, Gavaler JS, Sanghvi A. Lack of dissociation of prolactin responses to thyrotropin releasing hormone and metoclopramide in chronic alcoholic men. J Endocrinol Invest 1982; 5:281.

237. Loosen PT, Prange AJ. Alcohol and anterior pituitary secretion. Lancet 1977; 2:985.

238. Casacchia M, Rossi A, Stratta S. Thyrotropin-releasing hormone test in recently abstinent alcoholics. Psychiatr Res 1985; 16:249.

239. Dackis CA, Bailey J, Pottash ALC, et al. Specificity of the DST and the TRH test for major depression in alcoholics. Am J Psychiatry 1984; 141:680.

240. Garbutt JC, Mayo JP, Gillette GM, et al. Dose-response studies with thyrotropin-releasing hormone (TRH) in abstinent male alcoholics: evidence for selective thyrotroph dysfunction? J Stud Alcohol 1991; 52:275.

241. Clark OH, Gerend PL. Effect of ethyl alcohol on the TSH-receptor-cyclase system in thyroid and non-thyroid tissues. World J Surg 1986; 10:787.

242. Van Thiel DH, Gavaler JS, Wight WI, Abuid J. Thyrotropin releasing hormone (TRH) induced growth hormone (hGH) responses in cirrhotic men. Gastroenterology 1978; 75:66.

243. Franz AG. Prolactin. N Engl J Med 1978; 298:201.

244. Torro G, Kolodny RC, Jacobs LS. Failure of alcohol to alter pituitary and target organ hormone levels. Clin Res 1973; 21:505.

245. Van Thiel DH, McClain CJ, Elson MK, McMillin MJ. Hyperprolactinemia and thyrotropin releasing factor (TRH) responses in men with alcoholic liver disease. Alcoholism 1978; 2:344.

246. Jung Y, Russfield AB. Prolactin cells in the hypophysis of cirrhotic patients. Arch Pathol 1972; 94:265.

247. Weiner RI, Ganong WF. Role of brain monoamines and histamine in regulation of anterior pituitary secretion. Physiol Rev 1978; 58:905.

248. Borzio M, Calderara R, Ferrari C, et al. Growth hormone and prolactin secretion in liver cirrhosis: evidence for dopaminergic dysfunction. Acta Endocrinol 1981; 97:441.

249. Assad SN, Cunningham GR, Samaan NA. Abnormal growth hormone dynamics in chronic liver disease do not depend on severe parenchymal disease. Metabolism 1990; 39:349.

250. Bauer AGC, Wilson JHP, Lamberts SWJ, Blom W. Hyperprolactinemia in hepatic encephalopathy: the effect of the infusion of an amino-acid mixture with excess branched chain amino acids. Hepatogastroenterology 1983; 30:174.

251. Sato F, Nakamura K, Taguchi M, et al. Studies on the site of ethanol action in inducing prolactin release in male rats. Metab Clin Exp 1996; 45:1330.

252. Zanoboni A, Zanoboni-Muciaccia W. Gynaecomastia in alcoholic cirrhosis. Lancet 1975; 2:876.

253. Zanoboni A, Zanoboni-Muciaccia W. Elevated basal growth hormone levels and growth hormone response to TRH in alcoholic patients with cirrhosis. J Clin Endocrinol Metab 1977; 45:576.

254. Panerai AE, Salerno F, Mannesci M, et al. Growth hormone and prolactin response of thyrotropin-releasing hormone in patients with severe liver disease. J Clin Endocrinol Metab 1977; 45:134.

255. Stein JZ, Smith WO, Ginn HE. Hypophosphatemia in acute alcoholism. Am J Med Sci 1966; 252:78.

256. Knockel JP. The pathophysiology and clinical characteristics of severe hypophosphatemia. Arch Intern Med 1977; 137:203.

256a. Legroux-Gerot I, Blanckaert F, Solau-Gervais E, et al. Cases of osteoporosis in males. A review of 160 cases. Rev Rhum Engl Ed 1999; 66:404.

257. Nilsson BE. Conditions contributing to fracture of the femoral neck. Acta Clin Scand 1970; 136:383.

258. Baran DT, Teitelbaum SL, Bergfeld MA, et al. Effect of alcohol ingestion on bone and mineral metabolism in rats. Am J Physiol 1980; 238:E507.

259. Bikle DD, Genant HK, Cann C, et al. Bone disease in alcohol abuse. Ann Intern Med 1985; 103:42.

260. Kristensson H, Lunden A, Nilsson BE. Fracture incidence and diagnostic roentgen in alcoholics. Acta Orthop Scand 1995; 51:205.

261. Spencer H, Rubio N, Rubio E, et al. Chronic alcoholism. Frequently overlooked cause of osteoporosis in men. Am J Med 1986; 80:393.

262. Schnitzler CM, Solomon L. Bone changes after alcohol abuse. S Afr Med J 1984; 66:730.

263. Crilly RG, Anderson C, Hogan D, et al. Bone hystomorphometry, bone mass and related parameters in alcoholic males. Calcif Tissue Int 1988; 43:269.

264. Purohit V. Alcohol and osteoporosis. Introduction to the symposium. Alcohol Clin Exp Res 1997; 21:383.

265. Soszynski PA, Forhman LA. Inhibitory effects of ethanol on the growth hormone (GH)-releasing hormone–GH–insulin like growth factor-I axis in the rat. Endocrinology 1992; 131:2603.

266. Johnell O, Nilsson BE, Wiklund PE. Bone morphometry in alcoholics. Clin Orthop 1982; 165:253.

267. Cheung RCY, Gray C, Boyde A, Jones SJ. Effects of ethanol on bone cells in vitro resulting in increased resorption. Bone 1995; 16:143.

268. Krawitt EL. Effect of acute alcohol administration on duodenal calcium transport. Proc Soc Exp Biol Med 1974; 146:406.

269. Krawitt EL. Effect of ethanol ingestion on duodenal calcium transport. J Lab Clin Med 1975; 85:665.

270. Kalbfleisch JM, Lindenman RD, Ginn HE, Smith NO. Effects of ethanol administration on urinary excretion of magnesium and other electrolytes in alcoholic and normal subjects. J Clin Invest 1963; 42:1471.

271. Jones JE, Shane SR, Jacob WH, Flink EB. Magnesium balance studies in chronic alcoholism. Ann N Y Acad Sci 1969; 162:934.

272. Martin HE, McCuskey C, Tupikoua N. Electrolyte disturbance in acute alcoholism. Am J Clin Nutr 1959; 7:191.

273. Fankushen D, Roskin D, Dimich A, Wallack S. The significance of hypomagnesemia in alcoholic patients. Am J Med 1964; 37:802.

274. Rasmussen H. Parathyroid hormone calcitonin and the calciferols. In: Williams RH, ed. Textbook of endocrinology, 5th ed. Philadelphia: WB Saunders, 1974:686.

# CHAPTER 206

# EFFECTS OF NONRENAL HORMONES ON THE NORMAL KIDNEY

PAUL L. KIMMEL, ANTONIO RIVERA, AND PARVEZ KHATRI

## PATHWAYS OF HORMONAL ACTION ON THE KIDNEYS

Generally, there are four pathways by which renal function may be modified by hormones:

1. Changes in *systemic hemodynamics,* which may induce secondary changes in renal function
2. Changes in *glomerular hemodynamics,* such as afferent or efferent arteriolar tone
3. Changes in the *glomerular ultrafiltration coefficient*
4. Changes in the *tubular handling of solutes and water*

Many hormones profoundly affect normal renal function: mineralocorticoids, glucocorticoids, antidiuretic hormone (ADH), parathyroid hormone (PTH), calcitonin, insulin, glucagon, estrogen, progesterone, thyroid hormones, prolactin, catecholamines, growth hormone, and atrial natriuretic hormone (Table 206-1). Hormones regulate both active and passive transport processes in part through activation of channels, stimulating the synthesis of new channels, promoting redistribution of channels, or modulating the extent of active transport of various solutes at the level of the tubules. Such responses mediate the ability of the kidneys to respond to varying internal and external environmental stresses. These influences and responses are considered in this chapter.

## MINERALOCORTICOIDS

Mineralocorticoid receptors[1] are present in the cortical and medullary collecting and late distal convoluted tubules[2] (Fig. 206-1). These receptors are nonspecific, because they equivalently bind both mineralocorticoids and glucocorticoids.[3] However, glucocorticoids such as cortisol and corticosterone do not stimulate mineralocorticoid receptors in vivo because they are metabolized into inactive 11-keto congeners by the action of a specificity-conferring enzyme system, 11β-hydroxysteroid dehydrogenase (11-HSD).[4] Aldosterone is protected from inactivation by dehydrogenation. 11-HSD activity is inhibited by licorice, potentially increasing mineralocorticoid-mediated cellular responses.[5]

**TABLE 206-1.**
**Kidney Responses to Nonrenal Hormones***

| Hormone | Glomerular Filtration Rate | Renal Blood Flow | Urinary Sodium Excretion | Urinary Potassium Excretion | Urinary Calcium Excretion |
|---|---|---|---|---|---|
| Mineralocorticoids | NC | NC | ↓ | ↑ | NC or ↑ |
| Glucocorticoids | ↑ | ↑ | ± | ↑ | ↑ |
| Antidiuretic hormone | NC | NC | NC or ↑ | ?↑ | NC or ↑ |
| Parathyroid hormone | NC or ↓ | NC or ↑ | ↑ | ↑ | ↓ |
| Calcitonin | NC | NC | ↑ | ↑ | ↑ |
| Insulin | NC | NC | ↓ | ↓ | ↑ |
| Glucagon | ↑ | ↑ | ↑ | ↑ | ↑ |
| Estrogen | NC | NC | ↓ | NC | ↓ |
| Progesterone | ↑ | ↑ | ↑ | ± | — |
| Thyroid hormone | ↑ | ↑ | NC or ↑ | NC | ↑ |
| Prolactin | NC or ↑ | NC or ↑ | ↓ | ↓ | ↑ |
| α-Adrenergic agonists | ↓ | ↓ | ↓ | — | ?↑ |
| β-Adrenergic agonists | NC | ↑ | NC or ↑ | ?↓ | — |
| Growth hormone | NC or ↑ | ± | ↓ | ↓ | ↑ |
| Atrial natriuretic hormone | ↑ | NC | ↑ | ↑ | ?↑ |

*NC*, no change; ↓, decrease; ±, variable; ?, questionable; ↑, increase.
*This table summarizes the effects of several nonrenal hormones in intact, in vivo systems, representing studies in several species using physiologic and pharmacologic hormone dosages, various protocols, different study designs, and controls. Where data are available, results in humans are given.

Another area of current interest involves the interaction of aldosterone with membrane receptors that mediate physiologic changes through nongenomic mechanisms.[6]

Aldosterone mediates increased sodium reabsorption in distal nephron segments, which is characterized by increased luminal (apical) membrane sodium conductance, increased de novo synthesis of basolateral sodium-potassium adenosine triphosphatase (ATPase) and citrate synthase, and greater luminal electronegativity of the late distal convoluted, connecting, and collecting tubules.[7–10] After mineralocorticoid treatment, there is an increase in the basolateral membrane surface area of the principal cells of the connecting and collecting tubules. The cortical collecting duct is the main site affected.[11]

The gene encoding the *epithelial sodium channel* (ENaC), a multimeric protein composed of several subunits,[12] has been cloned. This channel is expressed in the distal convoluted tubule, the cortical collecting tubule, and the collecting duct.[12] Aldosterone induces activation of sodium channels within 1.5 to 3.0 hours as an early response, and synthesis of sodium channels over 6 to 24 hours as a late response. Aldosterone may also mediate changes in the subcellular localization of the channels.[13]

Mineralocorticoids do not directly affect glomerular filtration rate or renal blood flow.[14] The short-term administration of mineralocorticoids causes a decrease in urinary sodium excretion. During prolonged treatment with mineralocorticoids, urinary sodium excretion increases to normal levels. This phenomenon is known as *mineralocorticoid escape*. The immediate effect probably is mediated by changes in tubular sodium handling. The long-term effect likely reflects the balance of systemic and tubular influences on sodium excretion. This sodium retention, which is mediated by tubular mechanisms, causes progressive extracellular fluid volume expansion and usually an increase in systemic blood pressure. The volume expansion and increased renal arterial pressure cause inhibition of proximal tubular fluid reabsorption, resulting in increased urinary sodium excretion, opposing the distal tubular effects of the hormone[15,16] (see Table 206-1).

Aldosterone is necessary for the maintenance of maximum potassium excretion by the kidney, especially in the case of adaptation to a high-potassium diet (see Chap. 79). Aldosterone increases renal potassium excretion by increasing distal tubular Na⁺/K⁺-ATPase activity, by increasing its synthesis, and by targeting and insertion of new Na⁺/K⁺-ATPase units into the basolateral membrane.[17] Such changes mediate an increased renal tubular intracellular potassium concentration. Aldosterone increases basolateral potassium permeability as well as luminal cell membrane potassium conductance. Mineralocorticoids increase potassium secretion by the principal cells. A low-conductance potassium channel mediates potassium secretion across the apical membrane of principal cells in the cortical collecting tubule.[17] Aldosterone also enhances apical principal-cell potassium-channel density.[17] Increased potassium excretion results as a consequence of the increased negative transepithelial voltage potential difference, which varies directly with ambient mineralocorticoid levels. The net result of mineralocorticoid action is that urinary potassium excretion increases as the circulating potassium concentration falls. In the case of the physiologic response of mineralocorticoid synthesis to volume depletion, marked changes in potassium balance are limited since the urinary flow rate decreases. In instances of diuretic-induced volume depletion, the increased urinary flow rate in patients with secondary mineralocorticoid stimulation may be associated with marked increases in urinary potassium excretion and with the development of hypokalemia and a negative potassium balance.

The time courses of functional responses in the nephron segments are different for sodium and potassium transport.[17] It is unclear to what extent short-term changes in plasma aldosterone concentration alter renal potassium handling.[18]

The administration of mineralocorticoids to normal and mineralocorticoid-deficient persons increases urinary acidification by two mechanisms: increased hydrogen ion excretion and enhanced ammonia production.[19,20] Aldosterone increases hydrogen ion secretion by type A intercalated cells in the collecting duct via two mechanisms: direct stimulation of the proton pump (hydrogen-translocating ATPase), and, indirectly, by stimulating sodium influx, which creates a lumen-negative potential difference.[19] Studies in isolated collecting tubules demonstrate acute, non–sodium-dependent, in vitro influences on bicarbonate transport after mineralocorticoid treatment. Although bicarbonate reabsorption is stimulated by mineralocorticoids in the medullary collecting duct, an opposite effect occurs in the cortical collecting duct. Systemic acid-base balance may be a more important modulator of bicarbonate handling by the cortical collecting tubule than are mineralocorticoids.[21]

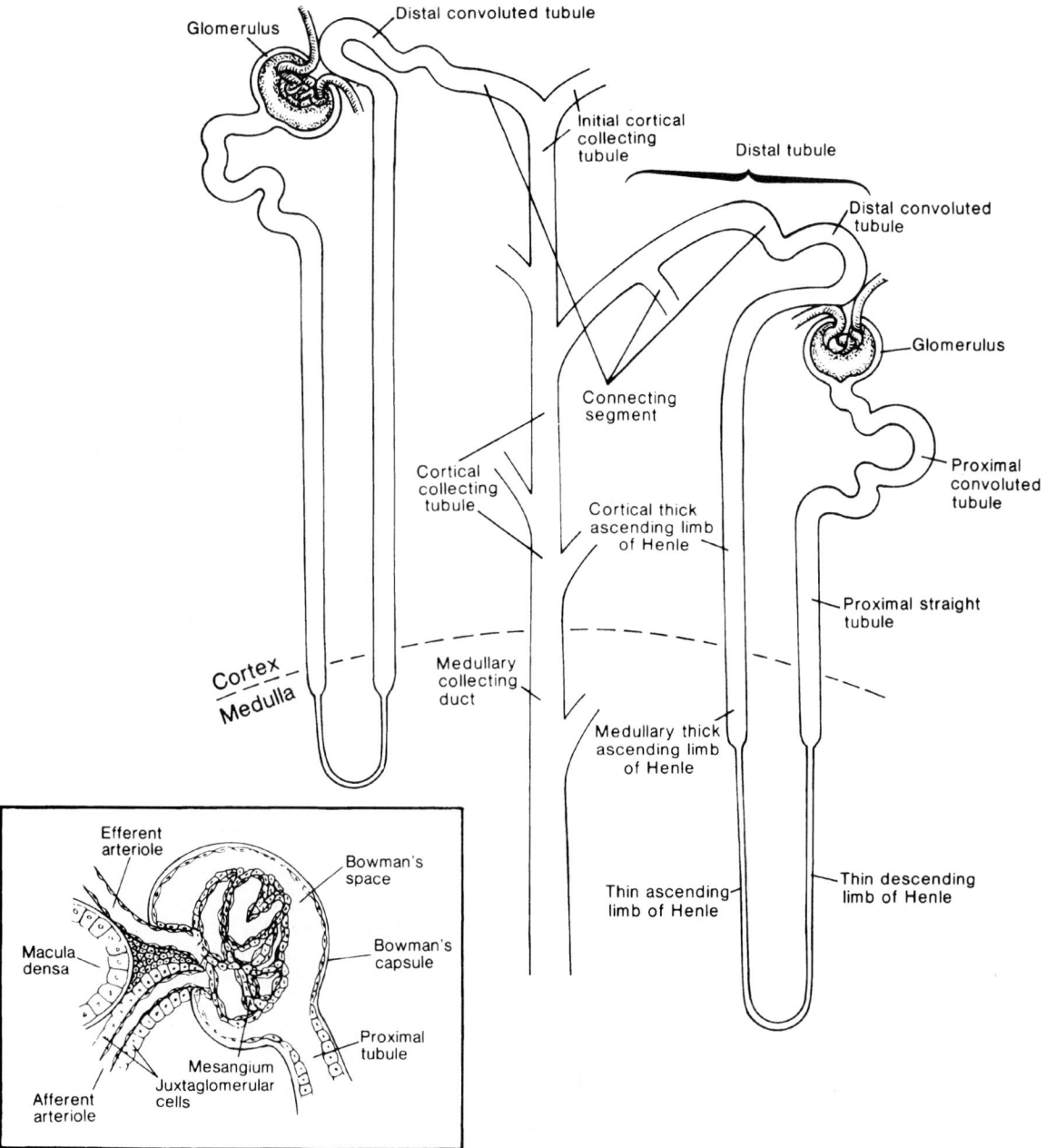

**FIGURE 206-1.** This figure provides a schema of the anatomy of the glomerulus and the various tubular segments that comprise the nephron, the functional unit of the kidney. The glomerulus is a capillary network, lined by endothelial cells, supported by a central region of mesangial cells and matrix material, within the Bowman capsule. An afferent arteriole enters each glomerulus at its hilum and subsequently divides into lobules, which form the glomerular tuft. The capillaries rejoin to form the efferent arteriole, which exits the glomerulus at the vascular pole. The proximal tubule originates from the urinary pole of the Bowman capsule and is composed of a convoluted and a straight section. The loop of Henle is composed of a thin segment, with descending and ascending portions, and a thick segment, with medullary and cortical portions. The distal convoluted tubule is variably composed of bright, granular, and light segments. The region of transition between the distal convoluted tubule and the collecting duct is the connecting segment, which is composed of a mixture of cells, including distal convoluted tubule, and connecting, intercalated, and principal cells. The collecting duct extends from the connecting segment in the cortex to the papillary tip and is divided into the cortical collecting tubule and the outer and inner medullary collecting ducts. The segments of the collecting duct are composed of varying proportions of principal and intercalated cells. The cellular composition and length of the individual nephron segments may vary with the species and the anatomic location of the glomerulus.

# GLUCOCORTICOIDS

Dexamethasone receptors have been identified in the proximal tubule and cortical collecting tubule, with a modest distribution in other nephron segments. The distribution of corticosterone receptors resembles that of mineralocorticoid receptors, although some also are located in the proximal tubule and thick ascending limb of Henle.[2] Glucocorticoid hormones activate both glucocorticoid and mineralocorticoid receptors located in the cytoplasm. In cells expressing 11-HSD (such as renal epithelia), glucocorticoids are metabolized and inactivated before they stimulate mineralocorticoid receptors.[4] When glucocorticoid or mineralocorticoid receptors are activated, they enter the nucleus and enhance transcription.[4]

Although exogenous glucocorticoids stimulate renal $Na^+$/$K^+$-ATPase, this does not occur with physiologic doses. Glucocorticoids do not affect citrate synthase production or the basolateral membrane area.

The direct effects of glucocorticoids on the kidney are difficult to evaluate, because glucocorticoid deficiency in humans is associated with alterations in cardiac output and changes in systemic hemodynamics. Moreover, animals that have undergone adrenalectomy or humans who have Addison disease have concurrent deficiencies in mineralocorticoid and catecholamine production. Glucocorticoids increase renal blood flow and glomerular filtration rate, without affecting glomerular or capillary pressure or permeability—essentially a vasodilatory effect.[22] Cortisone infusion decreases sodium excretion without affecting the excretion of chloride. Glucocorticoids may increase renal potassium excretion. The onset of the kaliuresis is more rapid and of shorter duration than that induced by mineralocorticoids, and it is relatively independent of dietary factors such as sodium and potassium intake. Because a direct, immediate action of glucocorticoids is not observed in the distal nephron, these effects on electrolyte excretion may be the result of changes in luminal flow and renal hemodynamics. It is possible that glucocorticoids modulate the level of sensitivity of the distal nephron to other factors that regulate ion transport.[18]

Although glucocorticoids stimulate renal gluconeogenesis and ammoniagenesis, and may affect luminal sodium and hydrogen ion exchange in the proximal tubule, a net effect on hydrogen ion secretion has been difficult to document.[2,23]

Acidosis increases adrenal secretion of glucocorticoids, which in turn increase proximal tubule apical membrane $Na^+$/$H^+$-antiporter activity in vivo; in vitro glucocorticoids enhance both the ability of acidosis to increase levels of cellular $Na^+$/$H^+$-exchanger 3 protein (likely through increasing synthesis) and the acidosis-induced trafficking of this protein to the apical membrane.[24] In this manner, glucocorticoids facilitate the renal response to systemic acidemia by facilitiating net hydrogen ion excretion.

In humans, the deficiency of glucocorticoids is associated with a renal diluting defect. The mechanism is controversial. Although in vitro data suggest that glucocorticoids directly influence distal tubular permeability to water, the impaired water excretory ability may result from concurrent alterations in glomerular filtration rate, plasma volume, ADH release, or distal tubular fluid delivery.[14]

Rapid administration of glucocorticoids does not change urinary calcium or magnesium excretion, although variable changes in urinary phosphate excretion have been reported. However, the long-term administration of glucocorticoids is associated with hypercalciuria and hypermagnesuria. The mechanism may be secondary to bone dissolution or an increase in plasma volume.[25]

## ANTIDIURETIC HORMONE

The action of ADH (arginine vasopressin [AVP]) is mediated through its binding to specific receptors.[26] $V_1$ receptors are found in the vascular smooth muscle and liver. $V_3$ receptors (also known as $V_{1b}$ receptors) are present in the neurons of the adenohypophysis and may play a role in mediating AVP-induced corticotropin secretion.[26] $V_2$ receptors are found in renal epithelial cells. Although the presence of the $V_2$ receptor in

endothelial cells has been inferred from pharmacologic studies, expression of its messenger RNA (mRNA) and protein has not yet been documented. ADH receptors have been localized in cells of the late distal convoluted tubules, the connecting tubule, the cortical collecting and medullary collecting ducts, and the glomerulus.[27,28] ADH-sensitive adenylate cyclase is found in isolated rabbit glomeruli, and contractile responses have been induced by ADH in cultured rat mesangial cells.[29] This may explain the mechanism whereby ADH decreases the glomerular ultrafiltration coefficient in rats, although the single nephron glomerular filtration rate remains unchanged.[30]

$V_2$-receptor transcripts are heavily expressed in cells of the renal connecting tubule and of the cortical, outer medullary, and inner medullary collecting ducts. Although the $V_2$ receptor is expressed in thick ascending limbs of the loops of Henle of the rat, its presence in this segment of the human nephron is currently debated. $V_2$ receptors on the basolateral membrane of the principal cells of the collecting ducts are activated by AVP binding. $V_2$ receptors are coupled to an adenylate cyclase stimulatory G protein (Gs). Binding of AVP to $V_2$ receptors on renal epithelial cells results in increased synthesis of cyclic adenosine monophosphate (cAMP), in activation of protein kinase A (PKA), and in increased synthesis of water channels (aquaporins [AQP]) and their cAMP-mediated incorporation into the luminal surface of these cells.[31,31a] At the collecting duct cell membranes, wide variations in permeability are achieved by differential regulation of the synthesis, trafficking, insertion, and removal of different types of aquaporins.[31]

At least five AQPs have been identified. AQP-1, AQP-2, AQP-3, and AQP-4 are found in the kidneys. AQP-1, or channel-forming integral membrane protein (CHIP), a 28-kDa protein, was the first molecular water channel identified. AQP-1 is expressed in mammalian red cells, renal proximal tubules, thin descending limbs, and other water-permeable epithelia. AQP-1 mediates isosmotic volume reabsorption in the proximal tubule and facilitates the function of the countercurrent multiplier in the loop of Henle. AQP-1 is localized in both apical and basolateral plasma membranes, where it may function both as an entry and as an exit route for transepithelial water transport. In contrast to AQP-2, limited amounts of AQP-1 are localized in membranes of vesicles or vacuoles. Tubule segments that are not water permeable (such as the thin and thick ascending limbs of the loop of Henle) do not express AQPs.

AQP-2 is the vasopressin-regulated water channel in renal collecting ducts. It is found from the connecting tubule, through the cortical collecting duct, and through the entire inner medullary collecting duct. ADH-induced PKA-mediated phosphorylation of the carboxy terminus of AQP-2 results in insertion and fusion of vesicles containing AQP-2 into the apical membrane, causing increased water permeability. AQP-2 is diffusely distributed in the cytoplasm in states of hydration. In contrast, apical localization of AQP-2 is intensified in dehydration or after vasopressin administration. These observations are thought to represent the insertion of preformed water channels by exocytosis into the apical plasma membrane from intracellular vesicles (the "shuttle hypothesis"). After the ADH-induced insertion of intracellular vesicles containing water channels into the apical membrane,[32] the tubular reabsorption of water is facilitated in the face of a renal osmotic gradient, decreasing free water excretion and producing relatively concentrated urine. In the absence of ADH, the water channels are transported into the cell for further processing or for subsequent reinsertion into the apical membrane[29,32] (see Chap. 25).

There are at least three ways in which AVP regulates the action of AQP-2: AVP regulates synthesis, controls trafficking from cytoplasm to the membrane, and regulates the balance between exocytosis and endocytosis of the water channels. Moreover, studies have provided evidence for the existence of vasopressin "escape," a selective down-regulation of AQP-2 expression, decreased cAMP signaling, and decreased activity of intracellular mediators—a process that occurs in states of AVP excess.[33,34] (See also ref. 34a.)

AQP-3 and AQP-4 are expressed in the basolateral membrane of cortical and medullary collecting-duct cells. AQP-3 is the water channel in basolateral membranes of renal medullary collecting ducts, and AQP-4 plays a critical role in the inner medullary collecting duct. Basolateral AQP-3 and AQP-4 mediate the exit of cell water, ultimately into the extracellular fluid.[31,35]

Genetic abnormalities in the regulation of synthesis of functional V$_2$ receptors and AQP-2 are associated with *nephrogenic diabetes insipidus*.[36] Calcium binding to the luminal calcium receptor of the inner medullary collecting duct cells causes endocytosis and down-regulation of AQP-2, reducing water permeability.[31,37] This may be one mechanism whereby hypercalcemia mediates decreased renal concentrating ability. A similar down-regulation has been noted in rats treated with lithium, and subjected to dietary potassium deprivation, perhaps explaining the concentration defect noted in patients with severe, prolonged hypokalemia.[38]

Increased sodium and potassium excretion are associated with the administration of ADH, but these effects are variable and may be species-specific. In humans, it is unclear whether such changes represent alterations in systemic hemodynamics secondary to mild volume expansion or a direct tubular influence of the hormone on electrolyte transport. ADH may stimulate sodium reabsorption in the loop of Henle, but may diminish it in the cortical collecting tubule.[39,40] Other studies demonstrate that the activity of ENaCs in cortical collecting-duct principal cells is regulated by ADH. ADH-induced increases in intracellular levels of cAMP result in insertion of channels into the plasma membrane and increased sodium reabsorption. The ADH effect is greater in the presence of aldosterone, but it is detectable even when the levels of circulating aldosterone are very low.[12]

Discrepancies in findings between different studies may have resulted from species differences, from variations in cell types studied, or from dietary conditions or technical approaches. ADH stimulates potassium secretion in the distal convoluted tubule, but has little effect on potassium transport in the cortical collecting tubule.[40,41] Patients with the syndrome of inappropriate ADH secretion may have hypercalciuria (see Chap. 27). Although the hypercalciuria has been attributed to volume expansion and increased sodium excretion, an in vitro study suggests that the hormone directly inhibits both calcium and phosphate reabsorption by the cortical collecting tubule.[42]

AVP also increases urea permeability in the inner medullary collecting duct. The gene encoding a renal urea transporter, UT-2 (UT-A2), was cloned in 1993.[43] Subsequently, several urea transporters have been identified in different tissues and species, some of which are vasopressin-responsive.[44] AVP stimulates the expression of an inner medullary collecting-duct urea transporter (UT-1, UT-A1)[45] and urea transport—which results in enhanced medullary tonicity (a phenomenon known as *"urea trapping"*)—thereby increasing the efficiency of the renal concentrating mechanism, especially in volume-depleted or dehydrated subjects. The physiologic roles and responses of this system in humans remain to be fully elucidated.

## PARATHYROID HORMONE

The PTH receptor (a member of the G protein–linked 7-membrane-spanning–receptor family) has been cloned in animals and humans,[46-48] and exhibits homology with the calcitonin receptor.[46] PTH receptors are found in the glomerulus, proximal tubule, medullary and cortical thick ascending limb of Henle, and early distal convoluted tubule.[27] Molecular biology studies of microdissected nephron segments demonstrate the presence of mRNAs coding for the parathyroid hormone/parathyroid hormone–related protein (PTH/PTHrP) receptor and an extracellular, G protein–coupled Ca$^{2+}$-sensing receptor (RaKCaR) in the glomeruli, proximal tubules, thick ascending limbs, distal convoluted tubules, and collecting ducts of rats and mice.[49,50] The reason for the differences noted in the distribution of receptor mRNA seen in these two studies is unclear.

The action of PTH probably is mediated primarily through cAMP (see Chap. 51). Renal PTH receptors are down-regulated when exposed to PTH. Binding of PTH to its receptor stimulates intracellular signaling by both cAMP and inositol-(1,4,5)-triphosphate (IP$_3$)/diacylglycerol (DAG) pathways.[51] After PTH binds to its receptor, Gs couples to adenylate cyclase and stimulates production of cAMP, which in turn activates PKA, while Gq couples to phospholipase C (PLC) to form IP$_3$ and DAG from phosphatidylinositol-(4,5)-biphosphate (PIP$_2$). IP$_3$ releases calcium from intracellular stores, and DAG stimulates protein kinase C (PKC) activity, ultimately mediating effects at the cell membrane.[52]

In thyroparathyroidectomized animals, PTH infusion diminishes whole kidney and single nephron glomerular filtration rates, most likely by reducing the glomerular ultrafiltration coefficient. Although volume depletion is a factor, PTH may partially mediate the decreased glomerular filtration rate seen in hypercalcemic patients with hyperparathyroidism. The physiologic role of PTH in modulating the glomerular filtration rate in humans is unclear.[53]

In clearance studies in humans, PTH infusion increases renal excretion of phosphate, sodium, potassium, and bicarbonate, and reduces the excretion of calcium and magnesium. The hormone inhibits the reabsorption of fluid, sodium, chloride, calcium, and phosphate in the proximal tubule of the dog and rat. High levels of PTH stimulate calcium and magnesium reabsorption in the thick ascending limb of Henle in the absence of substantial changes in sodium and chloride transport.[54-56] Microperfusion studies confirm that PTH stimulates calcium reabsorption in the distal convoluted tubule. Granular tubular epithelial cells are specifically involved. PTH stimulation of calcium uptake in the distal convoluted and connecting tubules occurs via apical calcium entry, most likely through the insertion of voltage-operated, dihydropyridine-sensitive calcium channels into the membrane. Stimulation of basolateral sodium/calcium exchanger and/or calcium/ATPase may also play a role in enhancing calcium reabsorption in these nephron segments.[55]

The hallmark of PTH action on the kidney is phosphaturia.[57] PTH stimulates gluconeogenesis and nonspecifically inhibits phosphate reabsorption, in the proximal straight tubule, via cAMP/PKA and IP$_3$/PKC pathways.[58] PTH decreases brush border membrane (BBM) sodium/phosphate cotransport and reduces the content of type II sodium/phosphate cotransporter protein.[59,60] Likewise, parathyroidectomy causes an increase in cotransporter protein levels.[60] Most of the effect of PTH on phosphate balance occurs in the distal nephron. PTH inhibits phosphate reabsorption in the late segments of the distal convoluted tubule.[58]

Renal 1α-hydroxylase activity is increased by PTH, thus enhancing the production of 1,25-dihydroxyvitamin D [1,25(OH)$_2$D] from 25-hydroxyvitamin D in the proximal convoluted tubule by a cAMP-mediated process.[61] Findings suggest that in addition to the proximal convoluted tubule, the murine distal convoluted tubule expresses a PTH-responsive 25-hydroxyvitamin D$_3$–24-hydroxylase, but the effects are mediated by different mechanisms.[62]

The role of PTH in modifying acid-base balance in humans is unclear. The immediate effect of the hormone is an inhibition of proximal tubular bicarbonate reabsorption. Although metabolic acidosis occurs with acute PTH infusion and in patients with hyperparathyroidism, the steady-state and long-term, direct renal effect of the hormone [in the absence of hypercalcemia and an increase of circulating 1,25(OH)$_2$D] appears to be an increase in renal bicarbonate reabsorption or distal tubular hydrogen ion secretion, causing metabolic alkalosis. PTH also indirectly stimulates distal tubular hydrogen ion secretion and titratable acid excretion by increasing phosphate delivery to the distal nephron.[63] The overall systemic effect may be modulated by time or by calcium and vitamin D homeostasis.[64]

## CALCITONIN

Calcitonin membrane receptors have been identified in renal cortical and medullary tissue.[65] Calcitonin-receptor mRNA is present in the cortical and medullary thick ascending limbs and the cortical collecting duct.[66] The calcitonin receptor is a G protein–coupled receptor with seven-membrane-spanning regions, coupled by Gs to adenylate cyclase. The PTH and calcitonin receptors are family members that have similar amino-acid sequences, although their ligands do not. Calcitonin-sensitive adenylate cyclase activity is found primarily in the thick ascending limb of Henle, distal convoluted tubule, and collecting tubule in humans.[67]

Calcitonin infusion causes natriuresis and kaliuresis in humans, but does not affect the glomerular filtration rate. High-dose infusion causes phosphaturia in humans, although the contribution of circulating PTH cannot be excluded. Calcitonin increases phosphate excretion in thyroparathyroidectomized animals and in humans with hypoparathyroidism, suggesting a direct renal effect. The increase in urinary magnesium excretion has been variable. Although calcitonin infusion in humans increases urinary calcium excretion, these findings are controversial and may depend on dosage or the species of the hormone. A direct renal effect on calcium handling is difficult to dissociate completely from its skeletal effects,[58] but studies suggest that calcitonin has a direct effect on distal convoluted tubule cells, leading to an increase in calcium reabsorption, which is mediated by calcium channels.[68] In the absence of ADH, calcitonin may play a role in the urinary-concentrating mechanism by stimulating adenylate cyclase pools, which are similar to those activated by ADH. In the absence of ADH, calcitonin causes an increase in calcium, magnesium, potassium, sodium, and chloride reabsorption by the loop of Henle.[39] Calcitonin stimulates 1α-hydroxylase activity in the proximal straight tubule through cAMP-independent mechanisms, although this effect may be species-specific.[61]

## INSULIN

Insulin binding occurs in the glomerulus, proximal tubule, distal convoluted tubule, and medullary ascending limb of Henle.[69] These sites, however, may be involved in insulin metabolism rather than mediation of tubular responses.[70] The functional significance of glomerular insulin receptors is unknown, because the administration of insulin to healthy humans does not affect the glomerular filtration rate.[71–73] The influence of insulin on tubular function is more significant. The binding of insulin to its receptor on the basolateral membrane of the proximal tubule cell initiates the phosphorylation of a receptor subunit. This activated subunit mediates the subsequent phosphorylation of intracellular protein substrates, which, in turn, mediate the hormone's physiologic effect.

Studies in animals and humans demonstrate that the administration of insulin decreases urinary sodium excretion in the absence of changes in plasma glucose, renal blood flow, or glomerular filtration rate.[71] In humans, insulin administration sufficient to achieve circulating levels between 41 and 90 μU/mL reduced sodium excretion in a dose-dependent manner, suggesting a distal nephron site of action.[72] This effect seems to be a direct one and has been documented in isolated perfused kidneys without changes in renal hemodynamics. Animal studies suggest that the response is dependent on ADH, but independent of the angiotensin and prostaglandin systems.[71]

Although sodium and hydrogen ion exchange may be increased, insulin decreases gluconeogenesis and sodium reabsorption by the proximal tubule.[74] Physiologic doses of insulin stimulate electrogenic sodium transport in experimental models of the cortical collecting duct[75] by mechanisms independent of transcription or protein synthesis. Aldosterone and insulin act independently to stimulate apical sodium entry into A6 epithelial cells by increasing the sodium channel density.[76] Insulin induces an increase in apical cell membrane sodium permeability, by increasing the number of activated sodium channels and the length of time they remain open.[77] The principal site of insulin action affecting urinary sodium excretion probably is the thick ascending limb of Henle or more distal segments of the nephron.[78] An insulin-responsive glucose transporter (GLUT4) is expressed at low levels in the kidney, primarily in the renal vasculature and in glomerular epithelial and mesangial cells.[79]

Insulin administration may decrease urinary potassium excretion, but the site and mechanism of action are obscure. An important factor may be the hormone's influence on extrarenal potassium disposition. The administration of insulin causes potassium uptake by the intracellular fluid, decreasing the plasma potassium concentration and the total potassium load presented for glomerular filtration and renal excretion. On the other hand, insulin decreases potassium secretion by the isolated perfused kidney without changing renal hemodynamics. This suggests a direct tubular effect of the hormone on potassium transport or an indirect diminution in renal potassium secretion secondary to the concurrent reduction in sodium excretion.[78]

The potential interactions in patients between hormonal effects on circulating ion levels and tubular functional changes are delineated in a clinical study of insulin administration during water diuresis, in which lithium, glucose, and/or sodium or potassium chloride were administered.[73] Potassium chloride infusion, to an extent that prevented the development of hypokalemia, but not sodium chloride repletion, abrogated the typical insulin-induced responses of urinary sodium and potassium excretion. Although the extent to which changes in potassium metabolism mediate insulin-induced renal tubular effects remains controversial, these results suggest that at least some of the findings in older clearance studies may have been affected by insulin-induced changes in circulating potassium levels, and that in vivo studies must be carefully designed and controlled to account for the multiple physiologic changes that occur in patients during hormone administration or dysregulation.

Insulin administration increases urinary calcium excretion, presumably acting at the proximal tubule, although a distal tubular effect is possible in humans. Urinary phosphate excretion decreases after insulin administration, as a result of increases in proximal tubular reabsorption.[78] Infusion of insulin in normal humans decreases both the renal clearance and fractional excretion of uric acid, perhaps as a result of the decreased sodium excretion.[80]

## GLUCAGON

Glucagon-induced adenylate cyclase activation has been documented in the thick ascending limb of Henle, distal convoluted tubule, cortical collecting tubule, and medullary collecting duct.[81] The glucagon receptors of the rat and human[82] have been cloned. The glucagon receptor, which is expressed in the kidney,[83-85] is a seven-transmembrane domain receptor with a conserved G protein–binding site and an amino-terminus domain that is involved in ligand binding.[85]

Glucagon infusion in supraphysiologic doses increases renal blood flow and glomerular filtration rate, associated with natriuresis, calciuria, and phosphaturia. Changes in electrolyte excretion depend on changes in renal hemodynamics, rather than direct tubular effects. No significant alterations in electrolyte transport have been documented in in vitro, isolated systems.[78] The effect of physiologic changes in the level of circulating glucagon on renal function is unclear.[86] In the absence of ADH, glucagon increases calcium, magnesium, and potassium reabsorption by the thick ascending limb of Henle.[87] Different cell types or pools of cAMP may be activated by each hormone.

## ESTROGEN

Estrogen receptors have been identified in rat renal tissue.[14,88,89] Estrogen receptors have been detected in renal tissue by direct methods, and their presence has been inferred as a result of responses after exposure to tamoxifen, a competitive inhibitor of estrogen.[90] The $\alpha$, but not the $\beta$, subtype estrogen receptor has been identified in the kidney.[90,91]

Interest has been directed toward understanding the effects of sex hormones in renal physiology since the progression of many renal diseases is slower in males than in females both in humans and in animal models.[92] $17\beta$-Estradiol increases growth of proximal tubular cells in culture, with a peak effect at $10^{-9}$ to $10^{-10}$ mol/L, but higher doses are inhibitory.[90] It increases the proliferation of mesangial cells at 10- to 100-nmol/L concentrations, but suppresses their proliferation at 10-$\mu$mol/L concentrations.[93] Moreover, it markedly suppresses mesangial-cell collagen synthesis at 1- and 10-$\mu$mol/L concentrations.[93] These effects may be mediated by antagonizing the actions of transforming growth factor-$\beta$.[94] Estrogen replacement therapy increases inducible nitric oxide synthase in the renal medulla of oophorectomized rats.[95]

Few data exist on the effects of estrogen on glomerular filtration rate and renal electrolyte handling.[96,97] Although the administration of estrogen to humans in physiologic doses has no influence on renal blood flow, glomerular filtration rate,[98] urine flow, or the tubular handling of glucose, estradiol administration causes sodium retention. The mechanism is unknown, but stimulation of the renin–angiotensin–aldosterone system or secondary systemic vasodilatation has been suggested to explain the diminution in sodium excretion.[99] Long-term estrogen administration decreases renal calcium excretion and phosphate reabsorption.[25] This may be the result of skeletal effects, rather than a direct renal effect.

## PROGESTERONE

Although definitive evidence of a progesterone receptor in the human kidney remains inconclusive, pharmacologic effects of this hormone may be manifested through interactions with other pathways. Progesterone binds to mineralocorticoid and glucocorticoid receptors and may act partly by competitively inhibiting aldosterone. Two isoforms of the progesterone receptor (hPR-A and hPR-B) have been identified.[100] The A form inhibits glucocorticoid, androgen, and mineralocorticoid receptor-mediated gene transcription. Progesterone at concentrations of $10^{-9}$ to $10^{-10}$ mol/L inhibited growth of rabbit proximal tubular cells in culture.[90]

Pharmacologic doses of progesterone have displaced aldosterone from binding sites in the toad bladder and have blunted its physiologic effects, but physiologic doses have had little influence on this system. Increased renal blood flow and glomerular filtration rate occur after the administration of pharmacologic doses of progesterone. Progesterone causes natriuresis and has been implicated in the blunting of mineralocorticoid-induced kaliuresis.[99,101]

## THYROID HORMONES

Hyperthyroidism has been associated with an increase in renal blood flow and glomerular filtration rate, and hypothyroidism has been associated with a diminution of these functions. These alterations have proved to be reversible after patients become euthyroid. Thyroxine supplementation in humans causes small increases in both glomerular filtration rate and renal blood flow. These changes may reflect effects on systemic hemodynamics. The maximum tubular reabsorption of glucose is increased in hyperthyroidism. Thyroid hormone supplementation enhances free water excretion, consistent with a renal concentrating defect. Both urinary diluting and, to a lesser extent, concentrating abilities are impaired in hypothyroidism. The mechanism is controversial: glucocorticoid deficiency, alterations in plasma volume and renal sodium reabsorption, increased ADH secretion, and decreased glomerular filtration rate and distal tubular fluid delivery have been implicated.

Hyperthyroidism has been associated with increased urinary calcium and magnesium excretion, and with tubular reabsorption of phosphate. These changes may be secondary to changes in ionized calcium or PTH levels, rather than to direct renal effects.[40] Thyroid hormones do, however, have a direct effect on phosphate transport in renal cells.[102] Renal phosphate reabsorption in proximal tubular BBM vesicles was increased in a dose-dependent manner in animals treated with triiodothyronine ($T_3$), while it was diminished in vesicles from hypothyroid rats.[103] The membrane findings occurred concurrently with consonant changes in levels of the sodium-phosphate transporter protein, and expression of the NPT-2 gene. These findings suggest a role for thyroid hormone in long-term regulation of phosphate homeostasis.

Animal studies have suggested a sodium reabsorptive defect in hyperthyroidism; however, the physiologic significance of this in humans is uncertain. Hypothyroidism may be associated with impaired renal tubular acidification. The mechanisms may involve abnormalities in sodium transport, carbonic anhydrase, or glutaminase activity.[104] Thyroid hormone also modulates $Na^+/K^+$-ATPase activity in the kidney.[61]

## PROLACTIN

Prolactin infusion results in an unchanged or slightly elevated glomerular filtration rate. Data on the effects of this hormone in humans remain scanty, but studies suggest decreases in urinary excretion of water, sodium, and potassium, and increases in urinary excretion of calcium.[105] Animal studies suggest direct effects on the renal tubular handling of sodium, potassium, water, and calcium.[101,106,107]

# CATECHOLAMINES

The direct effects of catecholamines on renal function have been difficult to ascertain. Endogenous catecholamines with different levels of α- and β-agonism affect systemic determinants of renal function, such as blood pressure, peripheral resistance, renal blood flow, and cardiac output. Adrenergic infusion also may modify the secretion of other hormones, such as ADH, renin, and prostaglandin E$_2$, which, in turn, affect renal function. Dopamine, and α- and β-adrenergic receptors, have been isolated from renal tissue.[108] β-Adrenergic receptors have been localized in glomeruli, the ascending limb of Henle, the distal convoluted tubule, and the collecting tubule.[109] Isoproterenol stimulates adenylate cyclase activity in the connecting and cortical collecting tubules.[81]

α-Adrenergic agents cause renal vasoconstriction, resulting in a dose-dependent decrease in glomerular filtration rate and renal blood flow, and an increase in the *filtration fraction* (i.e., glomerular filtration rate divided by renal plasma flow). β-Adrenergic agents have little effect on renal hemodynamics. The glomerular filtration rate tends to remain constant, in association with an increased renal plasma flow, resulting in a decreased filtration fraction.[108] Although norepinephrine receptors have been localized in the glomerulus, infusion of the hormone does not necessarily directly change the single nephron glomerular filtration rate, despite preferential vasoconstriction of the afferent arteriole.[110] Dopamine infusion at relatively low doses may specifically increase the glomerular filtration rate and urinary sodium excretion, most likely by changing renal hemodynamics.[103] Catecholamine infusions tend to decrease urinary sodium excretion, probably primarily as a result of an α-effect, perhaps mediated largely by changes in renal hemodynamics. In the isolated perfused kidney, this effect is blocked by propranolol, suggesting primarily a β-effect, but α$_2$-agonists also may decrease sodium excretion in this system.[111] Catecholamine infusions increase urinary calcium excretion in animals, an effect probably mediated by α-agonists. The mechanism may be unrelated to changes in renal sodium handling.[25]

Norepinephrine infusion increases free water excretion in humans and animals, in the absence of changes in the glomerular filtration rate, which is primarily an α-effect. β-Agonists usually cause antidiuresis, although this effect may be a result of ADH release (i.e., extrarenal).[108] β-Agonists do not affect the osmotic permeability of the cortical collecting tubule.[112]

The α$_2$-agonists specifically interfere with ADH-induced increases in osmotic permeability, presumably by interfering with the generation of cAMP.[113] The α$_2$-agonists inhibit cAMP formation by PTH in the proximal convoluted tubule and by ADH in the cortical collecting tubule, but not in the thick ascending limb of Henle.[114] α$_2$-Agonists inhibit AVP-stimulated water and urea permeability in the rat inner medullary collecting duct.[44] The α$_2$-agonists may antagonize the renal effects of other hormones that activate adenylate cyclase. α$_2$-Agonists stimulate Na$^+$/K$^+$-ATPase activity through PKC-mediated pathways, involving an increase in intracellular levels of IP$_3$ and DAG.[115]

In the proximal tubule, both α- and β-agonists stimulate fluid reabsorption.[61] In the late proximal tubule, α- and β-agonists have little effect, but dopamine decreases fluid reabsorption by non–cAMP-mediated events.[116] In the cortical collecting tubule, β-agonists decrease potassium secretion and increase chloride reabsorption, but have little effect on sodium reabsorption.[41,112]

# GROWTH HORMONE

Although growth hormone receptors have been identified in isolated proximal tubular basolateral membranes,[117] most of the renal effects of growth hormone appear to be mediated by its ability to stimulate the synthesis of insulin-like growth factors (IGFs), especially IGF-I.

Data concerning the role of growth hormone in renal function in normal humans are scanty and contradictory.[104,118–121] The rapid infusion of growth hormone has little influence on glomerular filtration rate, and renal plasma flow remains unchanged or decreases.[122] Animal studies have not suggested an acute effect of the hormone on glomerular filtration rate, renal blood flow, or the clearance of sodium, calcium, or phosphate.[123] Studies in patients with acromegaly (see Chap. 12) and in normal persons during the sustained administration of growth hormone suggest increased glomerular filtration rate, renal blood flow, and calcium and magnesium excretion.[104,118] The infusion of growth hormone in normal humans produces a delayed increase in glomerular filtration rate and renal plasma flow that correlates in time with increased levels of circulating IGF-I.[124] These findings explain the previous contradiction between the lack of change in glomerular filtration rate and renal plasma flow during short-term infusions with growth hormone, and the increments in glomerular filtration rate and renal plasma flow found in patients with acromegaly and normal humans during sustained administration of growth hormone. It is difficult to separate the direct renal effects on electrolyte transport from the systemic anabolic effects of the hormone.

Administration of growth hormone to subjects with ammonium chloride–induced acidosis increased urinary pH and net renal acid excretion, by increasing renal ammoniagenesis concurrently with increased sodium retention.[121]

Growth hormone enhances the reabsorption of phosphate in the proximal tubule.[118,125] This effect may be mediated by IGF-I.[117] The direct action of growth hormone to stimulate gluconeogenesis in the proximal tubule is not mediated by IGFs.[126] An effect of growth hormone to increase renal calcitriol synthesis may also be mediated by IGF-I.[127]

# ATRIAL NATRIURETIC HORMONE

Since the initial description of atrial natriuretic factor,[128] other similar peptides, secreted not only by the atria but also by the ventricles, brain, and kidneys, have been characterized.[129] This group of peptides rapidly and reversibly induces marked diuresis, natriuresis, kaliuresis, and reduction in blood pressure and extracellular volume[130–132] (see Chap. 178). Receptors for atrial natriuretic peptide (ANP) have been identified in the glomerulus and the inner medullary collecting duct.[129] ANPs increase renal plasma flow and glomerular filtration rate. The latter is mediated by a decrease in the afferent and an increase in the efferent arteriolar resistance, although an increase in the glomerular capillary ultrafiltration coefficient is involved in the response in dehydrated animals.[133] Simultaneous decreases in blood pressure and increases in glomerular filtration rate (in the absence of sustained changes in renal plasma flow or renal vascular resistance) cause a marked increase in filtration fraction, and make it difficult to evaluate the direct tubular effects of the peptides in vivo. ANPs interfere with the renin–angiotensin–aldosterone system by decreasing the secretion of renin and aldosterone. Moreover, ANPs may antagonize the actions of such vasoconstrictors as angiotensin II, norepinephrine, and ADH.[134] However, the action of ANPs may be offset in situations in which enhanced stimulation of the renin–angiotensin–aldosterone axis or the sympathetic nervous system occurs. Restoration of the natriuretic effects of ANPs may be seen in these settings after denervation or the administration of captopril.[133] The mechanism of action of ANPs is unclear, although preferential vasoconstriction of the efferent arteriole, an increase in the glomerular ultrafiltration coefficient, a direct effect on tubular sodium and water transport, and redistribution of renal blood flow all are possible factors mediating the integrated response.[135–137] ANP exerts inhibitory effects on NaCl reabsorption in the cortical collecting duct, and on sodium, chloride, and water reabsorption in the medullary collecting ducts.[138–142,142a] ANPs inhibit the tubular reabsorption of calcium, phosphorus, and magnesium, and also interfere with water reabsorption mediated by ADH.[143–146] The natriuretic effect probably is a combination of the increased glomerular filtration rate and changes in sodium reabsorption in the medullary collecting duct. These two mechanisms can be dissociated.[133] Increased circulating levels of ANP may partially mediate aldosterone escape.[15] Better understanding of the role of ANPs in sodium and fluid homeostasis may be achieved when specific antagonists become available for investigational use.

# REFERENCES

1. White PC. Disorders of aldosterone biosynthesis and action. N Engl J Med 1994; 331:250.
2. Marver D. Evidence of corticosteroid action along the nephron. Am J Physiol 1984; 246:F111.
3. Funder J. Corticosteroid receptors and renal 11β-hydroxysteroid dehydrogenase activity. Semin Nephrol 1990; 10:311.
4. Funder J. Mineralocorticoids, glucocorticoids, receptors and response elements. Science 1993; 259:1132.
5. Whorwood CB, Sheppard MC, Stewart PM. Licorice inhibits 11-beta-hydroxysteroid dehydrogenase messenger ribonucleic acid levels and potentiates glucocorticoid hormone action. Endocrinology 1993; 132:2287.
6. Wehling M. Specific, nongenomic actions of steroid hormones. Annu Rev Physiol 1997; 59:365.
7. Gary H. Regulation of Na+ permeability by aldosterone. Semin Nephrol 1992; 12:24.
8. Palmer LG, Frindt G. Regulation of apical membrane Na+ and K+ channels in rat renal collecting tubules by aldosterone. Semin Nephrol 1992; 12:37.
9. O'Neil RG. Aldosterone regulation of Na+ and K+ transport in cortical collecting duct. Semin Nephrol 1990; 10:365.
10. Marver D. Regulation of Na+/K+-ATPase by aldosterone. Semin Nephrol 1992; 12:56.
11. Kokko JP. Primary acquired hypoaldosteronism. Kidney Int 1985; 27:690.
12. Fyfe GK, Quinn A, Canessa CM. Structure and function of the Mec-ENaC family of ion channels. Semin Nephrol 1998; 18:138.
13. Garty H, Palmer LG. Epithelial sodium channels: function, structure and regulation. Physiol Rev 1997; 77:359.
14. Fanestil DD, Chun PS. Steroid hormones and the kidney. Annu Rev Physiol 1981; 43:637.
15. Haas JA, Knox FG. Mechanisms for escape from the salt-retaining effects of mineralocorticoids: role of deep nephrons. Semin Nephrol 1990; 10:380.
16. Stein JH. Hormones and the kidney. Hosp Pract (Off Ed) 1979; 14:91.
17. Giebisch G. Renal potassium transport: mechanisms and regulation. Am J Physiol 1998; 274:F817.
18. Field MJ, Giebisch GJ. Hormonal control of renal potassium excretion. Kidney Int 1985; 27:379.
19. Stone DK, Crider BP, Xie X-S. Aldosterone and urinary acidification. Semin Nephrol 1990; 10:375.
20. Perez GO, Oster JR. Acid-base pathophysiology in endocrine diseases. Mineral Electrolyte Metab 1985; 11:192.
21. Garcia-Austt J, Good D, Burg M, Knepper M. Deoxycorticosterone-stimulated bicarbonate secretion in rabbit cortical collecting ducts. Am J Physiol 1985; 249:F205.
22. Ichikawa I, Kon V. Hormonal regulation of glomerular filtration. Annu Rev Med 1985; 36:515.
23. Welbourne TC, Givens G, Joshi S. Renal ammoniagenic response to chronic acid loading: role of glucocorticoids. Am J Physiol 1988; 254:F134.
24. Ambuhl PM, Yang X, Peng Y, et al. Glucocorticoids enhance acid activation of the Na/H exchanger 3 (NHE3). J Clin Invest 1999; 103:429.
25. Sutton RAL, Dirks JH. Calcium and magnesium: renal handling and disorders of metabolism. In: Brenner BM, Rector FC, eds. The kidney. Philadelphia: WB Saunders, 1986:551.
26. Carmichael MC, Kumar R. Molecular biology of vasopressin receptors. Semin Nephrol 1994; 14:341.
27. Chabardes D, Gagnan-Brunette M, Imbert-Teboul M, et al. Adenylate cyclase responsiveness to hormones in various portions of the human nephron. J Clin Invest 1980; 65:439.
28. Abramow M, Beauwens R, Cogan E. Cellular events in vasopressin action. Kidney Int 1987; 32(Suppl 21):S56.
29. Handler JS, Orloff J. Antidiuretic hormone. Annu Rev Physiol 1981; 43:611.
30. Ichikawa I, Brenner BM. Evidence for glomerular actions of ADH and dibutyryl cyclic AMP in the rat. Am J Physiol 1977; 233:F102.
31. Zeidel ML. Recent advances in water transport. Semin Nephrol 1998; 18:167.
31a. Klussmann E, Maric K, Rosenthal W. The mechanisms of aquaporin control in the renal collecting duct. Rev Physiol Biochem Pharmacol 2000; 141:33.
32. Verkman AS. Mechanisms and regulation of water permeability in renal epithelia. Am J Physiol 1989; 257:C837.
33. Knepper MA. Molecular physiology of urinary concentrating mechanism: regulation of aquaporin water channels by vasopressin. Am J Physiol 1997; 272:F3.
34. Nielsen S, Fror J, Knepper MA. Renal aquaporins: key roles in water balance and water balance disorders. Curr Opin Nephrol Hypertens 1998; 7:509.
34a. Gustaffson CE, Katsura T, McKee M, et al. Recycling of AQP2 occurs through a temperature- and bafilomycin-sensitive trans-Golgi-associated compartment. Am J Physiol Renal Physiol 2000; 278:F317.
35. Frokiaer J, Marples D, Knepper MA, Nielsen S. Pathophysiology of aquaporin-2 in water balance disorders. Am J Med Sci 1998; 316:291.
36. Scheinman SJ, Guay-Woodford LM, Thakker RV, Warnock DG. Genetic disorders of renal electrolyte transport. N Engl J Med 1999; 340:1177.
37. Earm JH, Christensen BM, Frokiaer J, et al. Decreased aquaporin-2 expression and apical plasma membrane delivery in kidney collecting ducts of polyuric hypercalcemic rats. J Am Soc Nephrol 1998; 9:2181.
38. Marples D, Frokiaer J, Dorup J, et al. Hypokalemia-induced downregulation of aquaporin-2 water channel expression in rat kidney medulla and cortex. J Clin Invest 1996; 97:1960.
39. Elalouf JM, Roinel N, DeRouffignac C. ADH-like effects of calcitonin on electrolyte transport by Henles loop of rat kidney. Am J Physiol 1984; 246:F213.
40. Holt WF, Lechene C. ADH-PGE2 interactions in cortical collecting tubule. I. Depression of sodium transport. Am J Physiol 1981; 241:F452.
41. Kimmel PL, Goldfarb S. Effects of isoproterenol on potassium secretion by the cortical collecting tubule. Am J Physiol 1984; 246:F804.
42. Holt WF, Lechene C. ADH-PGE2 interactions in cortical collecting tubule. II. Inhibition of Ca and P reabsorption. Am J Physiol 1981; 241:F461.
43. You G, Smith CP, Kanai Y, et al. Cloning and characterization of the vasopressin-regulated urea transporter. Nature 1993; 365:844.
44. Sands JM. Regulation of renal urea transporters. J Am Soc Nephrol 1999; 10:635.
45. Terris J, Ecelbarger CA, Sands JM, Knepper MA. Long-term regulation of renal urea transporter protein expression in rat. J Am Soc Nephrol 1998; 9:729.
46. Juppner H, Abou-Samra AB, Freeman M, et al. A G protein-linked receptor for parathyroid hormone and parathyroid-hormone related peptide. Science 1991; 254:1024.
47. Bringhurst FR, Juppner H, Guo J, et al. Cloned, stably expressed parathyroid hormone/PTH related peptide receptors activate multiple messenger signals and biological responses in LLC-PK1 kidney cells. Endocrinology 1993; 132:2090.
48. Schneider H, Feyen JH, Seuwen K, Movva NR. Cloning and functional expression of a human parathyroid hormone receptor. Eur J Pharmacol 1993; 246:149.
49. Riccardi D, Lee WS, Lee K, et al. Localization of the extracellular Ca(2+)-sensing receptor and PTH/PTHrP receptor in rat kidney. Am J Physiol 1996; 271:F951.
50. Yang WT, Hassan S, Hyang YG, et al. Expression of PTHrP, PTH/PTHrP receptor and Ca²⁺-sensing receptor mRNAs along the rat nephron. Am J Physiol 1997; 272:F751.
51. Massry SG, Smogorzewski M. The mechanisms responsible for the PTH-induced rise in cytosolic calcium in various cells are not uniform. Mineral Electrolyte Metab 1995; 21:13.
52. Friedman PA, Coutermarsh BA, Kennedy SM, Gesek FA. Parathyroid hormone stimulation of calcium transport is mediated by dual signaling mechanisms involving protein kinase A and protein kinase C. Endocrinology 1996; 137:13.
53. Ichikawa I, Humes HD, Dousa TP, Brenner BM. Influence of parathyroid hormone on glomerular ultrafiltration in the rat. Am J Physiol 1978; 234:F393.
54. Friedman PA. Basal and hormone-activated calcium absorption in mouse renal thick ascending limbs. Am J Physiol 1988; 254:F62.
55. Friedman PA, Gesek F. Cellular calcium transport in renal epithelia: measurements, mechanisms and regulation. Physiol Rev 1995; 75:429.
56. Lau K, Bourdeau JE. Parathyroid hormone action in calcium transport in the distal nephron. Curr Opin Nephrol Hypertens 1995; 4:55.
57. Friedlander G. Autocrine/paracrine control of renal phosphate transport. Kidney Int 1998; 53:S65:S18.
58. Agus ZS, Wasserstein A, Goldfarb S. PTH, calcitonin, cyclic nucleotides and the kidney. Annu Rev Physiol 1981; 43:583.
59. Murer H, Lotscher M, Kaissling B, et al. Renal brush border membrane Na/Pi-cotransport: molecular aspects in PTH-dependent and dietary regulation. Kidney Int 1996; 49:1769.
60. Kempson SA, Lotscher M, Kaissling B, et al. Parathyroid hormone action on phosphate transporter mRNA and protein in rat renal proximal tubules. Am J Physiol 1995; 268:F784.
61. Kurokawa K. Cellular mechanisms and sites of hormone action in the kidney. In: Seldin DW, Giebisch G, eds. The kidney. New York: Raven Press, 1985:739.
62. Yang W, Friedman PA, Kumar R, et al. Expression of 25(OH)D₃ 24-hydroxylase in distal nephron: coordinate regulation by 1,25(OH)₂D₃ and cAMP or PTH. Am J Physiol 1999; 276:E793.
63. Stim JA, Bernardo AA, Arruda JA. The role of PTH and vitamin D in acid excretion and extrarenal buffer mobilization. Mineral Electrolyte Metab 1994; 20:60.
64. Hulter HN. Effects and interrelationships of PTH, Ca²⁺, vitamin D, and Pᵢ in acid-base homeostasis. Am J Physiol 1985; 248:F739.

65. Sexton PM, Adam WR, Mosely JM, et al. Localization and characterization of renal calcitonin receptors by in vitro autoradiography. Kidney Int 1987; 32:862.

66. Firsov D, Bellanger AC, Marsy S, Elaouf JM. Quantitative RT-PCR analysis of calcitonin mRNAs in the rat nephron. Am J Physiol 1995; 269:F702.

67. Morel F. Sites of hormone action in the mammalian nephron. Am J Physiol 1981; 240:F159.

68. Friedman PA, Gesek FA. Hormone-responsive $Ca^{2+}$ entry in distal convoluted tubules. J Am Soc Nephrol 1994; 4:1396.

69. Nakamura R, Emmanuel DS, Katz AI. Insulin binding sites in various segments of the rabbit nephron. J Clin Invest 1983; 72:388.

70. Nakamura R, Hayashi M, Emmanuel DS, Katz AI. Sites of insulin and glucagon metabolism in the rabbit nephron. Am J Physiol 1986; 250:F144.

71. Gupta AK, Clark RV, Kirchner KA. Effects of insulin on renal sodium excretion. Hypertension 1992; 19SI:I78.

72. Stenvinkel P, Bolinder J, Alvestrand A. Effects of insulin on renal hemodynamics and the proximal and distal tubular sodium handling in healthy subjects. Diabetologia 1992; 35:1042.

73. Friedberg CE, van Buren M, Bijlsma JA, Koomans HA. Insulin increases sodium reabsorption in diluting segment in humans: evidence for indirect mediation through hypokalemia. Kidney Int 1991; 40:251.

74. Hammerman M. Interaction of insulin with the renal proximal tubular cell. Am J Physiol 1985; 249:F1.

75. Rodriguez-Commes J, Isales C, Kalghati L, et al. Mechanism of insulin-stimulated electrogenic sodium transport. Kidney Int 1994; 46:666.

76. Blazer-Yost BL, Liu X, Helman SI. Hormonal regulation of EnaC: insulin and aldosterone. Am J Physiol 1998; 274:C1373.

77. Marunaka Y, Hagiwara N, Tohda H. Insulin activates single amiloride-blockable $Na^+$ channels in a distal nephron cell line (A6). Am J Physiol 1992; 263:F392.

78. Smith D, DeFronzo RA. Insulin, glucagon and thyroid hormone. In: Dunn MJ, ed. Renal endocrinology. Baltimore: Williams & Wilkins, 1983:367.

79. Brosius FC III, Briggs JP, Marcus RG, et al. Insulin-responsive glucose transporter expression in renal microvessels and glomeruli. Kidney Int 1992; 42:1086.

80. Quinones-Galvan A, Natali A, Baldi S, et al. Effect of insulin on uric acid excretion in humans. Am J Physiol 1995; 268:E1.

81. Morel F, Imbert-Teboul M, Chabardes D. Distribution of hormone-dependent adenylate cyclase in the nephron and its physiological significance. Annu Rev Physiol 1981; 43:569.

82. MacNeil DJ, Occi JL, Hey PJ, et al. Cloning and expression of a human glucagon receptor. Biochem Biophys Res Commun 1994; 198:328.

83. Dunphy JL, Taylor RG, Fuller PJ. Tissue distribution of rat glucagon receptor and GLP-1 receptor gene expression. Mol Cell Endocrinol 1998; 141:179.

84. Hansen LH, Abrahamsen N, Nishimura E. Glucagon receptor mRNA distribution in rat tissues. Peptides 1995; 16:1163.

85. Burcelin R, Katz EB, Charron MJ. Molecular and cellular aspects of the glucagon receptor. Diabetes Metab 1996; 22:373.

86. Premen AJ, Hall JE, Smith MJ Jr. Postprandial regulation of renal hemodynamics: role of pancreatic glucagon. Am J Physiol 1985; 248:F656.

87. Bailly C, Roinel N, Amiel C. PTH-like glucagon stimulation of Ca and Mg reabsorption in Henles loop of the rat. Am J Physiol 1984; 246:F205.

88. Hagenfeldt Y, Eriksson HA. The estrogen receptor in the rat kidney. Ontogeny, properties and effects of gonadectomy on its concentration. J Steroid Biochem 1988; 31:49.

89. Davidoof M, Caffier H, Schiebler T. Steroid hormone binding receptors in the rat kidney. Histochemistry 1980; 69:39.

90. Han HJ, Jung JC, Taub M. Response of primary rabbit kidney proximal tubule cells to estrogens. J Cell Physiol 1999; 178:35.

91. Kuiper GG, Carlsson B, Grandien K, et al. Comparison of the ligand binding specificity and transcript tissue distribution of estrogen receptors alpha and beta. Endocrinology 1997; 138:863.

92. Silbiger SR, Neugarten J. The impact of gender on the progression of chronic renal disease. Am J Kidney Dis 1995; 25:515.

93. Kwan G, Neugarten J, Sherman M, et al. Effects of sex hormones on mesangial cell proliferation and collagen synthesis. Kidney Int 1996; 50:1173.

94. Lei J, Sibiger S, Ziyadeh F, Neugarten J. Serum-stimulated alpha I type IV collagen gene transcription is mediated by TGF-β and inhibited by estradiol. Am J Physiol 1998; 24:F252.

95. Neugarten J, Ding Q, Friedman A, et al. Sex hormones and renal nitric oxide synthesis. J Am Soc Nephrol 1997; 8:1240.

96. Preedy JRK, Aitken EH. The effects of estrogen on water and electrolyte metabolism. J Clin Invest 1956; 35:423.

97. Johnson JA, Davis JO, Baumber S, Schineider EG. Effects of estrogen and progesterone on electrolytic balances in normal dogs. Am J Physiol 1970; 219:1691.

98. Dignam WS, Voskian J, Assali NS. Effects of estrogens on renal hemodynamics and excretion of electrolytes in human subjects. J Clin Endocrinol 1956; 16:1032.

99. Ferris TF, Francisco LL. Estrogen, progesterone and the kidney. In: Dunn MJ, ed. Renal endocrinology. Baltimore: Williams & Wilkins, 1983:462.

100. Vegeto E, Shahbaz MM, Wen DX, et al. Human progesterone receptor A form is a cell- and promoter-specific repressor of human progesterone receptor B function. Mol Endocrinol 1993; 7:1241.

101. Elkarib AO, Garland HO, Green R. Acute and chronic effects of progesterone and prolactin on renal function in the rat. J Physiol 1983; 337:389.

102. Beers KW, Dousa P. Thyroid hormone stimulates the $Na^+$-$PO_4$ symporter but not the $Na^+$-$SO_4$ in renal brush border. Am J Physiol 1993; 265:F2323.

103. Alcalde AI, Sarasa M, Raldua D, et al. Role of thyroid hormone in regulation of renal phosphate transport in young and aged rats. Endocrinology 1999; 140:1544.

104. Katz AI, Lindheimer MD. Actions of hormones on the kidney. Annu Rev Physiol 1977; 39:97.

105. Berl T, Better OS. Renal effects of prolactin, estrogen, and progesterone. In: Brenner BM, Stein JH, eds. Hormonal function and the kidney, contemporary issues in nephrology, vol 4. New York: Churchill Livingstone, 1979:194.

106. Stier CT Jr, Cowden EA, Friesen HG, Allison MEM. Prolactin and the rat kidney: a clearance and micropuncture study. Endocrinology 1984; 115:362.

107. Costanzo LS, Adler RA. Chronic prolactin excess causes hypercalciuria: a direct renal effect. Kidney Int 1986; 29:157.

108. Shrier RW. Effects of adrenergic nervous system and catecholamines on systemic and renal hemodynamics, sodium and water excretion and renin secretion. Kidney Int 1974; 6:291.

109. Munzel PA, Healy DP, Insel PA. Autoradiographic localization of β-adrenergic receptors in rat kidney slices using [125I]-iodocyanopindolol. Am J Physiol 1984; 246:F240.

110. Dworkin LD, Ichikawa I, Brenner BM. Hormonal modulation of glomerular function. Am J Physiol 1983; 244:F95.

111. Besarab A, Silva P, Landsberg L, Epstein F. Effects of catecholamines on tubular function in the isolated perfused rat kidney. Am J Physiol 1977; 233:F39.

112. Iino Y, Troy JL, Brenner BM. Effects of catecholamines on electrolyte transport in cortical collecting tubules. J Membr Biol 1981; 61:67.

113. Krothapalli RK, Duffy BW, Senekjian HO, Suki WN. Modulation of the hydroosmotic effect of vasopressin on the rabbit cortical collecting tubule by adrenergic agents. J Clin Invest 1983; 72:287.

114. Umemura S, Marver D, Smyth D, Pettinger W. $α_2$-Adrenoceptors and cellular cAMP levels in single nephron segments from the rat. Am J Physiol 1985; 249:F28.

115. Gesek FA. Alpha 2 adrenergic receptors activate phospholipase C in renal epithelial cells. Mol Pharmacol 1996; 50:407.

116. DiBona GF. Catecholamines and neuroadrenergic control of renal function. In: Dunn MJ, ed. Renal endocrinology. Baltimore: Williams & Wilkins, 1983:323.

117. Hammerman MR. The growth hormone-insulin-like growth factor axis in kidney. Am J Physiol 1989; 257:F503.

118. Feld S, Hirschberg R. Growth hormone, the insulin-like growth factor system, and the kidney. Endocr Rev 1996; 17:423.

119. Hirschberg R, Adler S. Insulin-like growth factor system and the kidney: physiology, pathophysiology, and therapeutic implications. Am J Kidney Dis 1998; 31:901.

120. Hammerman MR, Miller SB. Effects of growth hormone and the insulin-like growth factor on renal growth and function. J Pediatr 1997; 131:S17.

121. Sicuro A, Mahlbacher K, Hulter HN, Krapf R. Effects of growth hormone and systemic acid-base homeostasis in humans. Am J Physiol 1998; 24:F650.

122. Parving HH, Noer I, Mogensen CE, Svendsen PA. Kidney function in normal man during short-term growth hormone infusion. Acta Endocrinol (Copenh) 1978; 89:796.

123. Westby GR, Goldfarb S, Goldberg M, Agus ZS. Acute effects of bovine growth hormone on renal calcium and phosphate excretion. Metabolism 1977; 26:525.

124. Hirschberg R, Rabb H, Bergamo R, Kopple JD. The delayed effect of growth hormone on renal function in humans. Kidney Int 1989; 35:865.

125. Hammerman MR, Karl IE, Hruska KA. Regulation of canine renal vesicle Pi transport by growth hormone and parathyroid hormone. Biochim Biophys Acta 1980; 603:322.

126. Rogers SA, Hammerman MR. Growth hormone directly stimulates gluconeogenesis in canine renal proximal tubule. Am J Physiol 1989; 257:E751.

127. Wei S, Tanaka H, Seino Y. Local action of exogenous growth hormone and insulin-like growth factor-I on dihydroxyvitamin D production in LLC-PK1 cells. Eur J Endocrinol 1998; 139:454.

128. de Bold AJ, Borenstein HB, Veress AT, Sonnenberg H. A rapid and potent natriuretic response to intravenous injection of atrial myocardial extracts in rats. Life Sci 1981; 28:89.

129. Gunning ME, Brenner BM. Natriuretic peptides and the kidney: current concepts. Kidney Int 1992; 42(Suppl 38):S-127.

130. Espiner EA. Physiology of natriuretic peptides. J Intern Med 1994; 235:527.

131. Beland B, Tuchelt H, Bahr V, Oelkers W. The role of atrial natriuretic factor (alpha-human ANF-[99-126]) in the hormonal and renal adaptation to sodium deficiency. J Clin Endocrinol Metab 1994; 79:183.

132. Nicholls MG. The natriuretic peptide hormones. (Editorial and historical review). J Intern Med 1994; 235:507.

133. Awazu M, Ichikawa I. Biological significance of atrial natriuretic peptide in the kidney. Nephron 1993; 63:1.

134. Laragh JH. Atrial natriuretic hormone, the renin-aldosterone axis, and blood pressure-electrolyte homeostasis. N Engl J Med 1985; 313:1330.

135. Maack T, Camargo MJD, Kleinert HD, et al. Atrial natriuretic factor: structure and functional properties. Kidney Int 1985; 27:607.

136. Goetz KL. Physiology and pathophysiology of atrial peptides. Am J Physiol 1988; 254:E1.

137. Zeidel ML, Brenner BM. Action of atrial natriuretic peptides on the kidney. Semin Nephrol 1987; 7:91.

138. Butlen D, Mistaoui M, Morel F. Atrial natriuretic peptide receptors along the rat and rabbit nephrons: [125I] rat atrial natriuretic peptide binding in micro-

dissected glomeruli and segments of the rat and rabbit nephrons. Pflugers Arch 1987; 408:366.

139. Nonoguchi H, Sands JM, Knepper MA. ANF inhibits NaCl and fluid absorption in cortical collecting duct of rat kidney. Am J Physiol 1989; 256:F179.

140. Sonnenberg H, Honrath V, Chong CK, Wilson DR. Atrial natriuretic factor inhibits sodium transport in medullary collecting duct. Am J Physiol 1986; 250:F963.

141. Van de Stolpe A, Jamison RL. Micropuncture study of the effect of ANP on the papillary collecting duct in the rat. Am J Physiol 1988; 254:F477.

142. Ziedel ML. Medullary collecting duct sodium transport. Am J Physiol 1993; 295:F159.

142a. Holtback U, Kruse MS, Brismar H, Aperia A. Intrarenal dopamine coordinates the effect of antinatriuretic and natriuretic factors. Acta Physiol Scand 2000; 168:215.

143. Ortola FV, Ballermann BJ, Brenner BM. Endogenous ANP augments fractional excretion of Pi, Ca and Na in rats with reduced renal mass. Am J Physiol 1988; 255:F1091.

144. Dunn BR, Ichikawa I, Pfeffer JM, et al. Renal and systemic hemodynamic effects of synthetic atrial natriuretic peptide in the anesthetized rat. Circ Res 1986; 59:237.

145. Pollock DM, Arendshorst WJ. Effects of atrial natriuretic factor on renal hemodynamics in the rat. Am J Physiol 1986; 251:F795.

146. Dillingham MA, Anderson RJ. Inhibition of vasopressin action by atrial natriuretic factor. Science 1986; 231:1572.

---

# CHAPTER 207

# RENAL METABOLISM OF HORMONES

RALPH RABKIN AND MICHAEL J. HAUSMANN

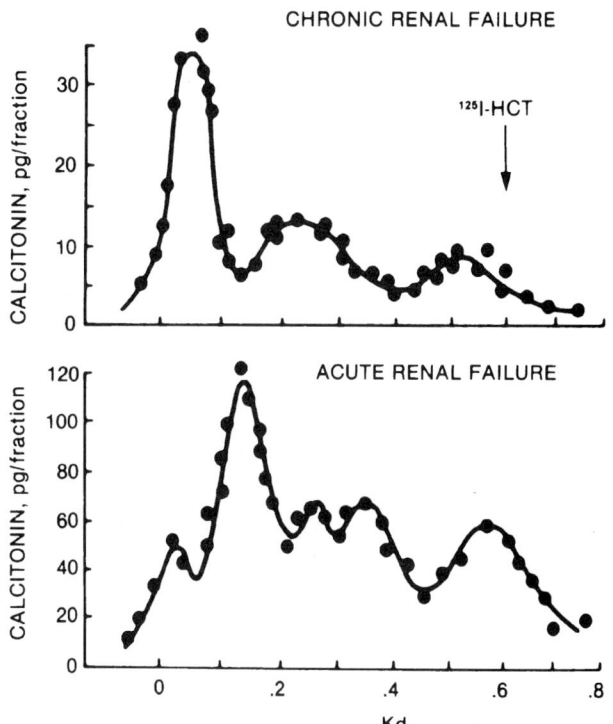

**FIGURE 207-1.** Gel filtration patterns of plasma from two patients with renal failure and elevated immunoreactive calcitonin levels. Samples of 2 mL were applied to a Bio Gel P-10 (1.5 × 100 cm) column, and 1-mL fractions were eluted with 0.2 M phosphate, pH = 7.4. *Arrow* indicates elution position of labeled monomer. Heterogeneity of molecular species is evident. ($^{125}$I-HCT, iodine-125 human calcitonin.) (From Lee JC, Parthmore JG, Deftos LJ. Immunochemical heterogeneity of calcitonin in renal failure. J Clin Endocrinol Metab 1977; 45:528.)

Three patterns of interaction occur among the kidney and hormones. The kidney may be the site of action, of production, or of degradation of hormones. The last interaction is the one discussed in this chapter. For peptide hormones, the kidney is a key site of metabolism and, together with the liver, accounts for most of their destruction.[1–6] A few hormones, however, including growth hormone (GH), calcitonin, and C peptide, are handled primarily by the kidney. The kidney plays a minor role in the metabolism of steroid hormones; these hormones circulate bound to large proteins and are not readily available for glomerular filtration. Hence, relatively small amounts are filtered, degraded by the kidney, or excreted in the urine.

The importance of the kidney in hormone metabolism becomes apparent in renal failure. Under these circumstances, the metabolic clearance rate (MCR) of hormones metabolized by the kidney is prolonged, and this may play a role in the pathogenesis of some of the endocrine manifestations associated with uremia. The situation may be compounded by uremic depression of extrarenal sites of hormone degradation and also by changes in hormone secretion. Prohormones and hormone metabolites may accumulate. Because commonly used hormone assays frequently do not distinguish between the bioactive and inactive forms of hormone, this potential pitfall must be considered when interpreting measured hormone levels in renal failure (Fig. 207-1). The following discussion regarding the physiology of hormone metabolism refers to data obtained in humans whenever possible.

## METABOLISM OF PEPTIDE HORMONES

The kidney extracts 16% to 45% of the various peptide hormones in the renal circulation. Occasionally, if the hormone is sensitive to enzymes in glomeruli and vascular endothelial cells (e.g., bradykinin, atrial natriuretic hormone), extraction may be as

high as 90%.[4] Depending on the contribution of extrarenal sites, the kidney may account for 30% to 80% of the total metabolism of a hormone (Table 207-1). An important feature of the renal removal process is that, unlike in the liver, saturation of uptake is difficult to achieve.[1] This largely reflects the dominant role of glomerular filtration in clearing hormones. Consequently, the kidney extracts peptide hormones from a constant volume of plasma per unit time, and the proportion of plasma hormone removed by the kidney remains constant through a broad range of plasma hormone concentrations. Thus, this system tends to maintain plasma hormone concentrations at basal levels. After a secretory stimulus and rise in plasma hormone concentration, the absolute amount of hormone removed increases proportionately; with return to the unstimulated state, the amount of hormone removed falls. This is not a true feedback regulatory mechanism, however. In severe renal failure, this system fails because renal blood flow is reduced, thereby decreasing delivery of hormone to the kidney. In addition, the kidney loses its ability to extract the hormone (Fig. 207-2).

Peptide hormones are removed from the renal circulation by two major pathways: *glomerular filtration* and *extraction from the postglomerular peritubular circulation* (Fig. 207-3).

### REMOVAL OF PEPTIDE HORMONES BY GLOMERULAR FILTRATION

Glomerular filtration serves as the predominant removal route for bioactive and inactive forms of peptide hormones.[3] Factors such as the size, conformation, and charge of the molecule affect the filtration rate. Thus, polymerization or protein binding, as occurs with insulin-like growth factor I (IGF-I), reduces filtra-

**TABLE 207-1.**
Contribution of the Kidney to the Metabolism of Polypeptide and Glycoprotein Hormones

| Hormone | Molecular Weight | MCR (mL/min/70 kg* or 1.73 m²†) | Renal Contribution to MCR (%) | Urinary Clearance (% GFR) | References |
|---|---|---|---|---|---|
| **POLYPEPTIDE HORMONES** | | | | | |
| Growth hormone | 21,500 | 210* | 65–70 | <1 | 12 |
| Parathyroid hormone | | | | | |
| 1-84 | 9500 | 1512* | 31‡ | 2 | 19 |
| 1-34 | | | 45‡ | | |
| COOH terminal | | | Major | | |
| Insulin | 6000 | 721§ | 33 | <1 | 10 |
| Proinsulin | 9000 | | 55‡ | | |
| C peptide | 3000 | | 69‡ | | |
| Calcitonin | 3400 | 154*§ | 64 | 4 | 2 |
| Glucagon | 3500 | 966* | 30 | 2 | 1 |
| Vasopressin | 1080 | 490† | 66 | 6 | 6, 18 |
| **GLYCOPROTEIN HORMONES** | | | | | |
| FSH | 30,000 | | 78‡ | 1.3‡ | 39 |
| LH | 30,000 | 43† | 94‡ | 1.0‡ | 39 |
| Erythropoietin | 34,000 | 17*§ | 32‡ | 0.3‡ | 40 |

*MCR*, metabolic clearance rate; *GFR*, glomerular filtration rate; *FSH*, follicle-stimulating hormone; *LH*, luteinizing hormone.
*Published results reported as mL/min/kg, here corrected to 70 kg for comparison.
†Published results reported as mL/min/m², here corrected to 1.73 m² for comparison.
‡Studies in animals.
§Calculated after intravenous administration of 10 IU/kg rEPO (human recombinant erythropoietin); erythropoietin; clearance decreases with increasing administered dose.

tion. Large polypeptide hormones (e.g., GH) are filtered slowly, at ~70% the rate of freely filtered molecules, and small peptides (e.g., angiotensin) probably pass through the glomerular filtration barrier without hindrance. The local destruction of hormone by the glomerulus is trivial for complex peptides such as parathyroid hormone (PTH). For less complex hormones such as angiotensin, bradykinin, and calcitonin, however, local destruction may account for a minor, but significant, portion of their metabolism.[5]

Specific receptors for many peptide hormones have been described in the glomerulus. The importance of these receptors is related to their roles in mediating the glomerular actions of their respective hormones. Accordingly, peptide hormones such as angiotensin, atrial natriuretic hormone, IGF-I, PTH, and vasopressin appear to modulate the glomerular filtration rate, and

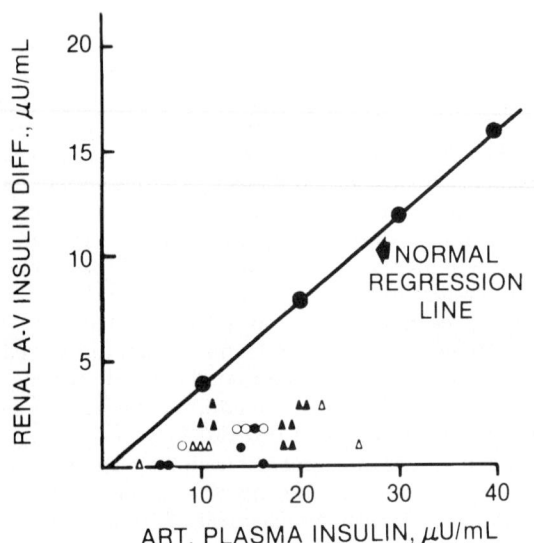

**FIGURE 207-2.** Relationship between plasma arterial (*ART.*) insulin concentration and renal arteriovenous (*A-V*) insulin difference in patients with advanced chronic renal failure. Under these circumstances, the kidney loses its ability to extract insulin. The regression line represents the relationship obtained in normal kidneys. The *closed circles* and *triangles* represent results for two diabetic patients, and the *open symbols* those for two nondiabetic subjects. (From Rabkin R, Simon NM, Steiner S, Colwell JA. Effect of renal disease on renal uptake and excretion of insulin in man. N Engl J Med 1970; 282:182.)

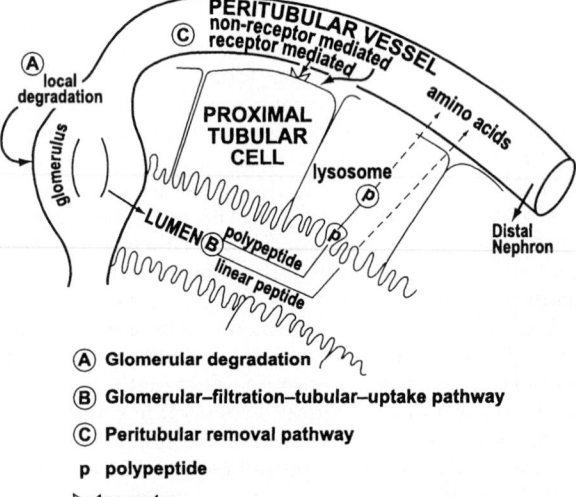

**FIGURE 207-3.** Pathways of peptide hormone degradation. A, Local degradation by the glomerulus represents a minor pathway for small hormones, such as angiotensin, bradykinin, and possibly calcitonin. B, Glomerular filtration and tubular reabsorption is the major pathway for all peptide hormones. Small linear peptides are hydrolyzed by the luminal membrane, but complex peptides require internalization before degradation. C, Peritubular removal occurs by receptor-mediated and non–receptor-mediated mechanisms. Receptor binding initiates hormone action, but its relationship to degradation is unknown. Degradation may be membrane associated or may require internalization. Peritubular removal probably occurs along the length of the nephron. (Modified from Rabkin R, Glaser T, Petersen J. Renal peptide hormone metabolism. Kidney 1983; 16:25.)

hormones such as insulin have important metabolic effects on the glomerulus (see Chap. 206).

After passage through the glomerular filtration barrier, peptide hormones enter the proximal tubular lumen, where, depending on their structure, they are *hydrolyzed on contact with the luminal membrane* or are *internalized by the tubular cell* (see Fig. 207-3). Both of these processes are highly efficient, because only a small percentage of the filtered load is excreted in the urine. Although the percentage excreted tends to be constant over physiologic plasma hormone levels, it rises in some instances. For example, at physiologic plasma levels, urinary arginine vasopressin (AVP) excretion represents 6% of the filtered load, but at higher levels, it reaches 24%.[6] This must be considered when measurements of urinary peptide hormone excretion are used as an indirect measure of endogenous hormone secretion. An even greater pitfall in the use of urine excretion rates is the fact that tubular dysfunction is associated with impaired tubular uptake of filtered peptide hormones.[1]

The biologic importance of proximal tubular destruction is that it serves as a means of conserving the constituent amino acids and of deactivating hormones such as angiotensin, atrial natriuretic hormone, and bradykinin, which may act from the luminal aspect of the tubules. This may prevent the unregulated action of filtered hormones on more distal nephron segments. Small linear peptides (e.g., angiotensin and bradykinin) are hydrolyzed within the proximal tubules by the peptidase-rich brush border membrane of the proximal tubule, and the metabolic products, predominantly amino acids, then are reabsorbed.[7]

As is the case for filtered proteins such as albumin, large, complex hormones (e.g., insulin, PTH, and GH) undergo relatively little or no brush border membrane hydrolysis. Internalization by the proximal tubular cell is a prerequisite for the degradation of these hormones.[1,3,8] Internalization occurs by endocytosis in the proximal renal tubule. This process is initiated by binding of the filtered hormone to the endocytic plasma membrane receptor megalin, originally named gp330.[8,9] To a much lesser extent endocytosis may be initiated by a charge-related interaction. In selected instances, as occurs with insulin, the hormone also may bind to specific sites in the brush border membrane.[10] The bound hormone is transported by endocytosis into the proximal tubular cell interior and delivered to the lysosomes. Although some degradation may occur in endosomes, most occurs in lysosomes. The released amino acids then are returned to the peritubular circulation. No evidence exists for significant transtubular transport of intact hormone. A small amount of internalized hormone, however, may be transported back to the cell surface in recycling endosomes to be released into the extracellular compartment, and certain hormones such as IGF-I are also transported to the nucleus.[11]

Although two major systems exist for degrading filtered peptide hormones—hydrolysis by brush border membranes and hydrolysis after internalization—these systems are not mutually exclusive and some overlap may occur. Degradation of some peptide hormones of intermediate complexity may involve both pathways, depending on their resistance to luminal hydrolysis. For example, luteinizing hormone–releasing hormone, a linear peptide with a C-terminal amide and an N-terminal pyroglutamyl residue, is incompletely degraded by the brush border membrane. Resultant peptide fragments and free amino acids, and perhaps some intact hormone, are absorbed, with further hydrolysis occurring within the cell. The liberated amino acids and some small peptide fragments then are released into the interstitial compartment. Calcitonin may be another hormone handled by both pathways.

## REMOVAL OF PEPTIDE HORMONES FROM THE POSTGLOMERULAR PERITUBULAR CIRCULATION

The kidney also removes peptide hormones from the postglomerular peritubular circulation, which is followed by binding of hormone to specific receptors in the basolateral membrane and by degradation.[1] Hormones such as insulin, PTH, calcitonin, vasopressin, and angiotensin are delivered to their receptors and initiate their actions through the peritubular route. The contribution of this pathway to the catabolism of each hormone varies. For example, estimates are that peritubular removal may account for ~40% of the total insulin extracted by the human kidney, but peritubular removal of GH is minimal.[1,12] For complex peptide hormones such as insulin, peritubular removal involves receptor-mediated endocytosis with intracellular degradation. For smaller, less complex peptide hormones, it is unclear whether receptor binding is a prerequisite for peritubular hormone degradation, whether degradation is membrane associated, and whether degradation follows internalization. Unlike the luminal aspect of the proximal tubular cell, the antiluminal aspect has a poorly developed endocytotic system. Significantly, degradation of hormone may not necessarily be complete; peritubular PTH and insulin catabolism is associated with the release of large fragments of unknown bioactivity along with the formation of products of complete degradation.[3,10]

## METABOLISM OF THE MAJOR PEPTIDE HORMONES

### GROWTH HORMONE

The kidney is the predominant site of GH metabolism. In rats, the kidneys account for 65% to 70% of the total MCR[1]; in humans, the kidneys are estimated to account for 25% to 53% of the total MCR.[12] The human data indicate that, when plasma GH levels are elevated, saturation of the extrarenal clearance pathways occurs, resulting in a greater contribution of the kidneys to the MCR. Renal clearance is achieved primarily by the glomerular filtration and proximal tubule degradative route; peritubular removal does occur, but it is a minor process. Some restriction of GH through the glomerular filtration barrier occurs, and indirect estimations suggest that the rate of GH filtration is 70% that of water. Restriction is partly the result of the complexing of GH to GH-binding proteins (GHBPs).[13] The principal GHBP in humans is derived from proteolytic cleavage of the full-length GH receptor and is identical to the extracellular domain of the receptor. Serum GHBP levels are, therefore, believed to reflect GH-receptor number and usually are low in advanced renal failure. Indeed GH resistance in uremia may be caused partly by a fall in receptor number.[13,14] Microperfusion and autoradiographic studies suggest that the filtered hormone is absorbed in the proximal tubule. This absorptive process is highly efficient, because <1% of filtered GH is excreted in the urine.[12] In renal failure, plasma GH levels often are elevated, the half-life of GH is prolonged by ~50%, and fractional urinary excretion is increased. The total GH MCR is depressed in renal failure because of loss of the renal metabolic pathway and depressed extrarenal clearance.[12] This accounts for the normal or elevated GH levels seen in patients with renal failure even though GH secretion is generally depressed (see Chap. 12).

### PROLACTIN

Prolactin (PRL) is structurally similar to GH and is handled by the kidney in a similar manner. The glomerular filtration and tubular degradative route accounts for most of the hormone removed, and little intact PRL appears in the urine. In normal persons, ~16% of circulating hormone is extracted during a single passage through the kidney. This value is smaller than the filtration fraction (i.e., the fraction of plasma water circulating through the glomerulus that is actually filtered) and indicates restricted PRL filtration. The true contribution of the kidney to the total metabolism of PRL in humans has not been established, but it is likely to be large, because renal failure is associated with a 33% reduction in the MCR.[1] In rats, the renal catabolism is responsible for 67% of the metabolism of PRL (see Chap. 13).[15]

## ARGININE VASOPRESSIN

The key sites of AVP removal are the splanchnic viscera (especially the liver) and the kidneys, with the latter accounting for ~67% of the total MCR.[6] During pregnancy, however, the MCR is increased as much as four-fold because of catabolism by the placenta and placentally derived vasopressinase.[16] AVP is a small cyclic peptide of 1080 Da. It is cleared from the renal circulation mainly by glomerular filtration (see Chap. 25). Filtered AVP is removed from the proximal tubular lumen by brush border membrane hydrolysis and by endocytosis, and only 6% of the filtered load is excreted in the urine at physiologic plasma AVP levels.[6,17] When plasma levels are elevated by infusions of AVP, the amount excreted in the urine rises markedly.[6,18] This may represent altered tubular uptake or tubular secretion of the hormone. Postglomerular peritubular removal also occurs and delivers the hormone to specific (V2) receptors that have been identified in the tubular basolateral membranes. Receptors are present in glomerular mesangial cells, and binding to these receptors initiates mesangial cell contraction and may modulate the glomerular filtration rate.

## PARATHYROID HORMONE

Parathyroid hormone (molecular mass, 9500 Da) is an 84-amino-acid single-chain peptide hormone. Its bioactivity is limited to the amino-terminal portion containing residues 1 through 34 (see Chap. 51). Tissue degradation causes the formation of the inactive COOH-terminal fragment (residues 53–84), the active amino-terminal fragment, and constituent amino acids. In normal persons, both the intact hormone and the COOH-terminal fragment are readily detectable in plasma. In patients with renal failure, the amino-terminal fragment may be detected. The two major fragments of PTH catabolism are cleaved from intact PTH (1–84) in the liver and, to a lesser extent, in the kidney and parathyroid glands. In vitro studies indicate that PTH degradation is calcium sensitive, but effects vary according to the organ. High calcium concentrations depress renal and hepatic degradation, but degradation by the parathyroid gland is stimulated.[19] The liver and the kidney are the principal sites of PTH metabolism; they are responsible for 61% and 31%, respectively, of the peripheral metabolism of intact PTH.[20] Although the liver removes intact hormone, cleaves it in the Kupffer cell, and then releases the COOH- and amino-terminal fragments, it is unable to extract these fragments from the circulation. The kidney, on the other hand, readily removes not only intact hormone but all circulating fragments. The amino-terminal fragment also is taken up by bone. The kidney clears PTH and its metabolites by glomerular filtration, followed by proximal tubular absorption and degradation. Glomerular degradation is negligible despite the presence of PTH receptors. The intact hormone and the amino-terminal fragment are removed from the postglomerular peritubular circulation (Fig. 207-4). This is followed by binding to PTH-specific receptors in the basolateral membrane of the

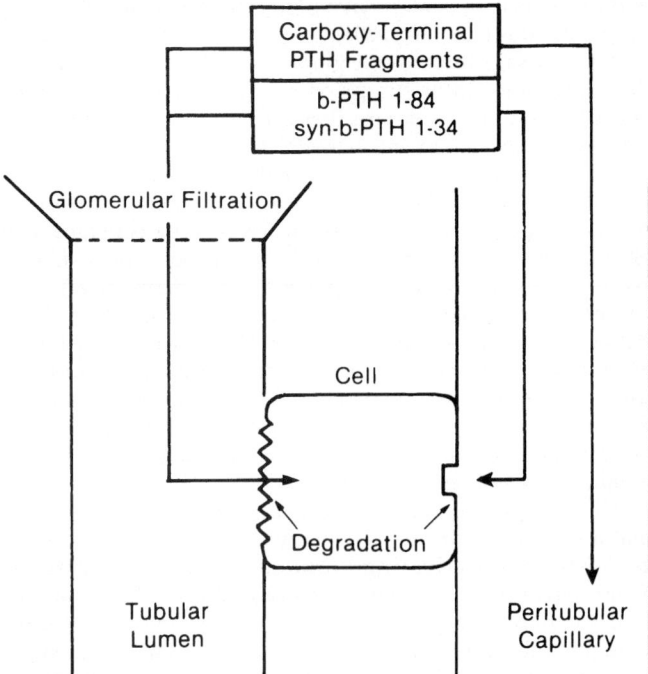

**FIGURE 207-4.** Pathways of renal clearance of parathyroid hormone (*PTH*) and its metabolites. Intact PTH and amino-terminal fragments are removed by filtration and by peritubular pathways. Filtration is the sole means of COOH-terminal fragment removal. (From Slatopolsky E, Martin K, Hruska K. Parathyroid hormone metabolism and its potential as a uremic toxin. Am J Physiol 1980; 239:F1.)

tubules, activation of the adenylate cyclase system, and degradation of the hormone. The COOH- and amino-terminal fragments are released into the renal circulation. Although the site of production of these fragments is uncertain, they probably are derived from intact hormone removed from the peritubular circulation.[19] Cathepsin D, isolated from bovine kidney lysosomes, cleaves intact PTH into complementary 1–34 and 35–84, or 1–37 and 38–84 fragments.[21] The 1–37 fragment is transitory, undergoing rapid hydrolysis to 1–34. Whether renal lysosomes are the source of the circulating fragments is questionable, however, because hydrolysis of peptides in these structures usually is complete.

## CALCITONIN

The major site of calcitonin metabolism is the kidney, which accounts for 67% of the total MCR of radiolabeled calcitonin.[22] Approximately 17% of the hormone in the renal circulation is extracted during a single passage through the kidney. Although it is difficult to detect in humans, a significant peritubular process for the removal of calcitonin has been observed in the isolated, perfused rat kidney. Calcitonin-specific (C1) receptors are present in renal basolateral membranes, and hormone binding is followed by activation of adenylate cyclase. This promotes an increase in distal nephron calcium and magnesium reabsorption.[1] Calcitonin-binding sites are present in tubular brush border membrane. Because these are not associated with adenylate cyclase activity, they may play a role in internalizing the hormone. Calcitonin receptors are also present in the juxtaglomerular apparatus and may be responsible for mediating the increase in plasma renin that follows calcitonin administration.[23] Major subcellular sites capable of calcitonin degradation include the brush border membrane, lysosomes, and cytosol.[22] The minor degrading activity associated with cortical basolateral membranes is located at a site distinct from the receptor. The glomeruli also may participate in calcitonin degradation (see Chap. 53).

## INSULIN

Endogenous insulin (molecular mass, 6000 Da) secreted by the pancreas enters the portal circulation, and during its first passage through the liver, 40% to 50% is extracted (see Chap. 134). Proinsulin also undergoes significant hepatic extraction, but the extraction of C peptide is negligible. On reaching the systemic circulation, insulin is removed by several tissues, including kidney, muscle, liver, and fat. The renal contribution to the systemic clearance of insulin, proinsulin, and C peptide averages 30%, 50%, and 70%, respectively.[10] In renal failure, the insulin MCR is prolonged because of loss of renal clearance and depressed extrarenal clearance. Furthermore, the relationship between insulin and C peptide is lost because of the greater contribution of the kidney to C-peptide metabolism.

Insulin and its related peptides are extracted from the renal circulation mainly by glomerular filtration. The filtered insulin is absorbed in the proximal tubule, and <1% appears in the urine. Besides filtration, a large amount is extracted from the peritubular circulation; in humans, this accounts for 40% of the total renal clearance. Insulin removed by this pathway undergoes partial and complete degradation.[1,24,25] The partially modified insulin molecule is similar in size to insulin but lacks immunoreactivity; whether this material retains bioactivity is unknown. Insulin-specific binding sites are present in isolated brush border and contraluminal membranes, suggesting that tubular uptake is partially receptor mediated.[10] The contraluminal receptors are not confined to the proximal tubule but are distributed throughout the nephron. Binding to the contraluminal, but not the brush border membrane, receptors is followed by phosphorylation of receptors. Thus, contraluminal receptors participate in hormone action, and brush border receptors probably serve a role in the absorption of filtered insulin. This is explained by the finding that megalin is the major brush border endocytotic receptor for insulin.[9] Insulin-degrading activity is present throughout the length of the nephron but is maximal in the proximal tubule, which is the predominant site of filtered insulin absorption[26] (Fig. 207-5). Subcellular sites of proximal tubular insulin-degrading activity have been identified and include lysosomes, endosomes, mitochondria, and cytosol,[27] although for all these sites to participate in the degradative process is improbable. Most likely, after the hormone undergoes endocytosis, it is transported in endosomes to the lysosomes. En route, degradation begins in endosomes, but most insulin is degraded after delivery to lysosomes.[24] A small portion of intact insulin and large insulin degradation products escape lysosomal delivery and recycle to the cell surface with the endosomes.[28] Brush border membranes and, to a lesser extent, contraluminal membranes exhibit some insulin-degrading activity. Although cultured glomerular endothelial cells degrade insulin, whether significant glomerular insulin degradation occurs in vivo is unclear.

## INSULIN-LIKE GROWTH FACTORS

The metabolism of the IGFs is more complex than that of insulin. More than 90% of the circulating IGF-I and IGF-II is complexed to high-affinity IGF-binding proteins (IGFBPs), of which IGFBP-3 is by far the most abundant. IGF-I (molecular mass, ~7500 Da), together with IGFBP-3 and an acid-labile subunit, form a 150-kDa complex from which IGF-I is released after proteolytic digestion. Because of the size of this complex, most circulating IGF-I is restricted from crossing the glomerular filtration barrier. Free IGF-I and IGF-I bound to low-molecular-weight binding

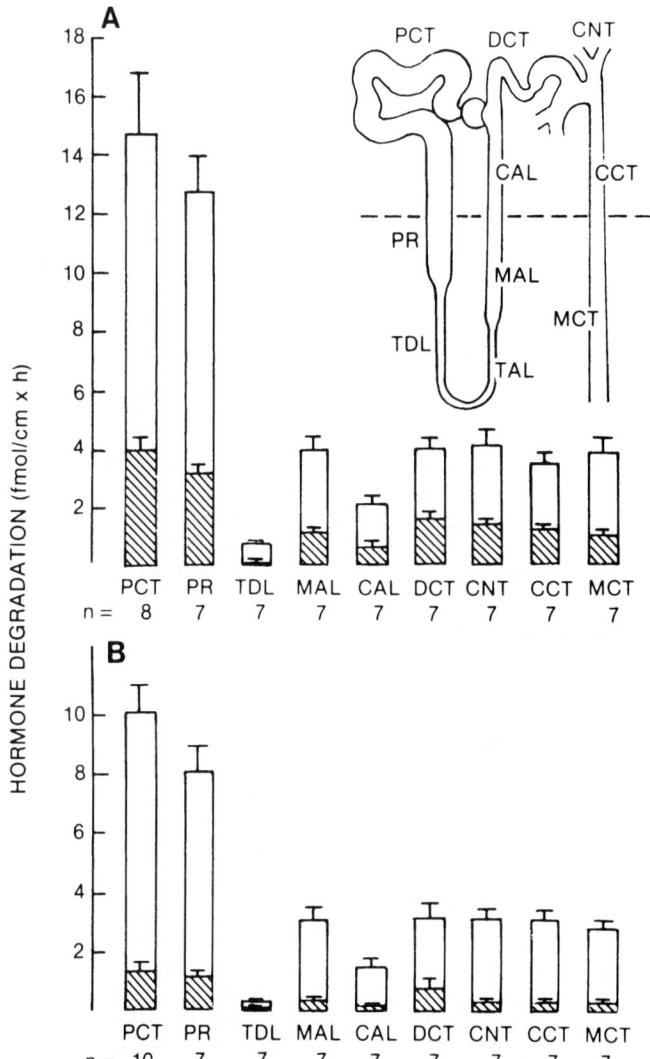

**FIGURE 207-5.** Glucagon (**A**) and insulin (**B**) degradation by isolated nephron segments. Degrading activity is maximal in the proximal tubule but is present throughout the nephron. (*PCT*, proximal convoluted tubule; *DCT*, distal convoluted tubule; *CNT*, connecting tubule; *CAL*, cortical ascending limb; *CCT*, cortical collecting tubule; *PR*, pars recta; *MAL*, medullary ascending limb; *TDL*, thin descending limb; *MCT*, medullary collecting tubule; *TAL*, thin ascending limb.) (From Nakamura R, Hayashi M, Emmanouel DS, Katz AI. Sites of insulin and glucagon degradation in the rabbit nephron. Am J Physiol 1986; 250:F144.)

proteins, especially IGFBP-1, are more readily filtered at the glomerulus. The IGF-I that does enter the tubular lumen is taken up by non–receptor-mediated endocytosis and transported to lysosomes, where degradation occurs; IGF-I and IGFBP-3 may also be transported into the nucleus.[11] Compared to insulin degradation, IGF-I degradation is slow. Uptake also may occur from the interstitial fluid and likely is mediated by basolateral tubular cell receptor–mediated endocytosis.[29] Only small amounts of IGF-I are measurable in urine. Animal studies suggest that the kidney is a major site of localization of injected IGF-I and IGF-II.[30] As the MCR of IGF-I is unaltered in humans with advanced renal failure, however, the human kidney is probably not a major site of clearance.[31] Plasma levels of IGFBP, especially IGFBP-1 and IGFBP-2, are elevated in chronic renal failure.[14] This restricts the extracellular volume into which IGF-I distributes, reducing its bioavailability and may partly explain the uremic resistance to IGF-I.[32]

## GLUCAGON

Glucagon is present in the circulation in several molecular forms. In normal persons, the bioactive 3500-Da species is predominant. This active form of glucagon is removed largely by the liver and kidneys, with these organs accounting for 30% and 24% of the total MCR, respectively.[1] Renal removal is predominantly by glomerular filtration, which is followed by degradation along the brush border membrane of the proximal tubules. The urinary loss of hormone is minimal. Glucagon is removed by the peritubular route, but this represents a minor pathway. Glucagon-degrading activity is maximal in the proximal tubules but also is present in distal nephron segments (see Fig. 207-5).[26] At a subcellular level, cytosol, lysosomes, and plasma membranes possess degrading activity. Brush border membranes are more active than are basolateral membranes.[33] The significance of the intracellular degrading activity is unclear, because most glucagon degradation probably occurs on the cell surface. In the rat, glucagon-specific receptors are lacking along the proximal tubules but occur along the thick ascending limb of Henle and the cortical tubules. These are sites of glucagon-sensitive adenylate cyclase (see Chap. 134).

## ATRIAL NATRIURETIC HORMONE

Atrial natriuretic peptide (ANP) is a 28-amino-acid peptide with powerful natriuretic and diuretic actions and is part of a larger family of peptides with similar action that also includes *brain natriuretic peptide* (BNP), *C-type natriuretic peptide* (CNP), and *urodilatin* or *renal natriuretic peptide* (RNP) (see Chap. 178). The kidneys contribute ~20% to the total MCR of ANP, and the renal extraction of ANP is 35% to 50%.[34,35] Renal clearance of ANP is by both the glomerular filtration pathway and a unique route that does not use glomerular filtration or the usual peritubular removal mechanisms but instead involves clearance by specific *clearance receptors* (C receptors). Binding to these receptors initiates endocytosis and delivery of the ligand to lysosomes, where it is degraded. The C receptors, unlike the other two ANP receptors, are not coupled to guanylate cyclase and do not mediate the natriuretic and hemodynamic actions of the natriuretic peptides. C receptors account for >95% of the ANP receptors in kidney cortex and have been found in mesangial and endothelial cells.[36] Overall, C receptors are quantitatively more important than glomerular filtration for the renal removal of ANP.

Filtered ANP is catabolized by renal tubular cells. Degradation is initiated at the luminal membrane by endopeptidase 24.11. This ectoenzyme inactivates ANP by opening its ring structure. Although all portions of the nephron possess ANP-degrading activity, the proximal tubular brush border is the renal site containing the most substantial endopeptidase 24.11 activity. When inhibitors of endopeptidase 24.11 are administered, filtered ANP is protected from luminal degradation and increased amounts of ANP immunoreactivity can be measured in urine.[37] Such endopeptidase inhibition enhances both natriuresis and the urinary excretion of cyclic guanosine monophosphate,[38] possibly by inhibiting proximal ANP degradation and, thus, allowing filtered ANP to exert its action at tubular sites usually protected by luminal hormone catabolism. As endopeptidase 24.11 inhibitors are not specific, however, their renal effects may also be mediated by inhibition of the degradation of other bioactive peptides such as bradykinin. ANP probably is not catabolized at the basolateral membrane of the proximal tubule, because this site contains little degrading activity.

## GLYCOPROTEIN HORMONES

The renal metabolism of the glycoprotein hormones—thyrotropin, follicle-stimulating hormone (FSH), luteinizing hormone (LH), human chorionic gonadotropin, and erythropoietin—has been less well studied than that of other peptide hormones. Nevertheless, the kidney is an important site of clearance of these hormones and their metabolites. The exact contribution of the kidney to the total MCR varies among hormones and may be determined partly by differences in molecular structure and charge. The renal metabolism of glycoprotein hormones is distinguished from nonglycosylated peptide hormone metabolism by several characteristics. The renal clearance of glycoprotein hormones is relatively slow (see Table 207-1). This arises largely from restricted glomerular filtration, probably due to the large size (>25,000 Da) and complex structure of glycoproteins. Furthermore, the absence of glycoprotein hormone–specific receptors excludes receptor-mediated removal.

The glycoprotein hormones have a relatively high urinary excretion rate (see Table 207-1). For example, the urinary excretion of FSH averages 43% of the total FSH renal clearance, but the urinary excretion of nonglycosylated hormones is less than 1% to 2% of the filtered load.[1] This indicates that the tubular absorption of filtered glycoproteins is less efficient. Despite the low renal clearance rate of glycoprotein hormones, the renal contribution to the total body MCR of glycoprotein hormones is relatively large. This reflects the slower total MCR of glycoprotein hormones.

In humans, urinary excretion accounts for ~5% and 25% of the total MCR of LH and human chorionic gonadotropin, respectively. This does not take into account the contribution of intrarenal degradation. In more detailed studies in the rat (see Table 207-1), the indirect estimates of the renal contribution to the MCR of LH, FSH, and erythropoietin averaged 94%, 78%, and 23%, respectively (see Chap. 16).[39,40]

## THYROID HORMONES

The thyroid hormones are released from the thyroid gland as the iodinated amino acids, thyroxine (3,5,3',5'-tetraiodothyronine; $T_4$) and, to a minor extent, 3,5,3'-triiodothyronine ($T_3$) (see Chap. 30). Like steroid hormones, they are transported in the plasma almost entirely in association with binding proteins. The metabolically active unbound $T_4$ and $T_3$ constitute 0.03% and 0.3% of total hormone, respectively. Most of the circulating $T_3$ is derived from the peripheral conversion of $T_4$. Other peripheral conversion products include the inactive 3,3',5'-triiodothyronine and 3,3'-diiodothyronine. The liver and kidneys are the major sites of conversion. The enzyme involved in this process, iodothyronine 5'-deiodinase, has been identified in microsomes.[41,42]

Both $T_4$ and $T_3$ are metabolized by the kidney and other organs through deamination and decarboxylation to form tetraiodothyroacetic acid and triiodothyroacetic acid. Approximately half of daily thyroid iodothyronine production is disposed of as urinary thyronine or as the acetic acid analog of thyronine.[43] Both of these products are completely deiodinated. More than half of infused $T_4$, however, is excreted in the urine as diiodometabolites. Because thyroid hormones are largely protein bound, the fraction extracted and excreted by the kidney is small; arteriovenous concentration differences are not detectable. The unbound $T_4$ and $T_3$, however, are freely filtered and excreted in the urine. During fasting, both mean $T_4$ and $T_3$ urinary excretion is decreased.[43a] Based on urine excretion rates, estimates are that ~65% of the filtered $T_4$ is reabsorbed by the tubules. Conversely, $T_3$ is added to the urine; this additional $T_3$ is derived from the intrarenal conversion of $T_4$. The kidney also contributes to the excretion of the glucuronide and sulfate conjugates that arise from liver metabolism.[44] In addition, significant peritubular removal of $T_4$ occurs; the $T_4$ is then converted to $T_3$ by 5'-deiodinase located on the cytoplasmic face of the proximal tubular basolateral membrane.[45,46] Renal disease is accompanied by alterations in thyroid hormone metabolism (see Chap. 209).[47]

## STEROID HORMONES

The major role of the kidney in steroid hormone metabolism is the elimination of metabolites. Metabolic processing of active hormone also occurs in the kidney, but this is a minor process. Conversely, the liver is the central site of steroid hormone inactivation and a minor site of elimination. These organ differences may be explained partly by the binding of circulating steroid hormones to albumin and certain globulins with a high affinity for specific steroids. Depending on the steroid, as much as 98% may be protein bound. Protein binding effectively restricts glomerular filtration. In contrast, metabolites circulate in free form and are readily eliminated by the kidney. The kidney filters circulating intact hormone that is not plasma protein bound, and also may remove intact hormone from the postglomerular peritubular circulation. Lipid-soluble steroids enter the tubular cell, where they interact with cytoplasmic receptors and undergo metabolic transformations.

## GLUCOCORTICOIDS

As with other steroids, the key role of the kidney in glucocorticoid metabolism is the excretion of metabolic products from extrarenal conversion. The liver is the major site of inactivation, accounting for 90% of the metabolism. The injection of radiolabeled cortisol is followed by the excretion of 90% of the radioactivity over 3 days. Less than 1% of the excreted radioactivity is associated with intact cortisol. In humans and several other species, cortisol is the most abundant corticosteroid synthesized by the adrenals, but in rabbits and rodents, the major product is corticosterone. In humans, 90% to 95% of the circulating cortisol is bound to the corticosteroid-binding globulin transcortin, or to albumin (see Chap. 72). The unbound form is freely filtered, and the lipid-soluble hormone is readily absorbed by the renal tubules, especially in the distal nephron. Altogether, between 60% and 90% of the filtered cortisol may be absorbed, and urinary excretion is low. Besides being filtered by the glomeruli, corticosterone may be extracted from the postglomerular peritubular circulation in the rat.[48] Although the kidney serves mainly as a site of elimination of hepatic metabolites, it also is the most important site of the conversion of cortisol to inactive cortisone.[49] This is significant because mineralocorticoid receptors bind cortisol and aldosterone with equal affinity, and circulating plasma cortisol levels are 500 times greater than plasma aldosterone levels. Thus, inactivation of cortisol is essential for aldosterone to mediate its specific regulatory actions. Abnormalities in conversion can result in pronounced clinical manifestations.

Normally, cortisol is converted to cortisone by 11β-hydroxysteroid dehydrogenase (11β-OHSD) expressed in two forms, 11β-OHSD1 and 11β-OHSD2.[49,50] The isoenzyme 11β-OHSD1 is located in proximal tubular cells and, by inactivating filtered glucocorticoids, limits the exposure of tubular cells to glucocorticoids. Low activity of this enzyme has been implicated in the development of renal cysts in cpk mice with hereditary cystic disease.[51] The isoenzyme 11β-OHSD2 is located in the distal nephron in aldosterone-sensitive collecting duct cells and allows aldosterone to act independently of glucocorticoids in the kidney.[52] When this enzyme is congenitally absent (syndrome of apparent mineralocorticoid excess[53]) or inactivated (as with glycyrrhetinic acid, a component of licorice), cortisol acts on renal mineralocorticoid receptors to stimulate potassium secretion, sodium avidity, and hypertension. Unidentified endogenous inhibitors of 11β-OHSD, which have been isolated from urine, are known as *glycyrrhetinic acid–like factors* or GALF.[54] Evidence also exists for the renal conversion of cortisol to 6β-hydroxycortisol by the enzyme 6β-hydroxylase. When enhanced, this pathway also may be responsible for the generation of hypertension.[55–57] Finally, the renal conversion of cortisol to 20-dehydrocorticosterone, which can inhibit AVP-stimulated water transport in toad bladder, has been reported.

## ALDOSTERONE

The major role of the kidney in aldosterone metabolism is the excretion of metabolites, which is achieved by glomerular filtration and tubular secretion. In humans, the kidney is one of the major extrahepatic sites for aldosterone metabolism.[58,59] Aldosterone circulates less firmly bound to plasma protein than do glucocorticoids; hence, it is cleared more rapidly from the plasma than are glucocorticoids, and the renal extraction is more prominent. The kidney extracts 10% of the hormone passing through it, but the liver extracts 92%. Free aldosterone is readily filtered at the glomerulus, and between 80% and 95% is absorbed by the proximal and distal nephron. The absorption is passive and is modulated by sodium and water movement. Aldosterone also is removed from the peritubular circulation. Thirty minutes after intravenous injection of [³H]-aldosterone in rats, 40% and 2.4% of the dose is present in the liver and kidney, respectively. Most of the radioactivity is present in the cytosol. The metabolic transformation of the hormone is rapid, and many metabolites formed locally and in the liver are found in the kidney.

Hepatic and renal aldosterone metabolism is sex dependent and affected by salt intake. Both the nature and the amount of kidney metabolites produced vary according to gender and the dietary sodium ingested. Most of the products of aldosterone metabolism in the kidney are polar-neutral hydroxylated compounds (nonconjugated) and nonpolar-reduced compounds. Moreover, sulfates and carboxylic acid metabolites also are formed. Studies in animals suggest that the nonpolar, ring A–reduced metabolites may be important in modulating or mediating the action of aldosterone.[58] Several of the reduced metabolites of aldosterone, although less active than the parent hormone, appear to possess some bioactivity. Whatever their role in the action of the hormone, the ultimate fate of the metabolites is excretion into the urine or entry into the circulation.

## REFERENCES

1. Rabkin R, Dahl DC. Renal uptake and disposal of proteins and peptides. In: Raub TJ, Audus KL, eds. Pharmaceutical biotechnology, vol. 5. Biological barriers to protein delivery. New York: Plenum Press, 1993:299.
2. Ardaillou R, Paillard F. Metabolism of polypeptide hormones by the kidney. Adv Nephrol Necker Hosp 1980; 9:247.
3. Maack T, Johnson V, Kau ST, et al. Renal filtration, transport, and metabolism of low-molecular-weight proteins: a review. Kidney Int 1979; 16(3):251.
4. Nasjlette A, Colessa-Chorerio J, McGiff JC. Disappearance of bradykinin in the renal circulation of dogs. Effects of kininase inhibition. Circ Res 1975; 37:59.
5. Thaiss F, Wolf G, Assad N, et al. Angiotensinase A gene expression and enzyme activity in isolated glomeruli of diabetic rats. Diabetologia 1996; 39(3):275.
6. Pruszczynski W, Caillens H, Drieu L, et al. Renal excretion of antidiuretic hormone in healthy subjects and patients with renal failure. Clin Sci 1984; 67:307.
7. Carone FA, Peterson DR. Hydrolysis and transport of small peptides by the proximal tubule. Am J Physiol 1980; 238:F151.
8. Christensen EI, Birn H, Verroust P, Moestrup S. Membrane receptors for endocytosis in the renal proximal tubule. Int Rev Cytol 1998; 180:237.
9. Orlando RA, Rader K, Authier F, et al. Megalin is an endocytic receptor for insulin. J Am Soc Nephrol 1998; 9(10):1759.
10. Rabkin R, Yagil C, Frank B. Basolateral and apical binding, internalization, and degradation of insulin by cultured kidney epithelial cells. Am J Physiol 1989; 257:E895.
11. Li W, Fawcett J, Widmer HR, et al. Nuclear transport of insulin-like growth factor-I and insulin-like growth factor binding protein-3 in opossum kidney cells. Endocrinology 1997; 138(4):1763.
12. Haffner D, Schaefer F, Girard J, et al. Metabolic clearance of recombinant human growth hormone in health and chronic renal failure. J Clin Invest 1994; 93:1163.
13. Baumann G. Growth hormone binding protein and free growth hormone in chronic renal failure. Pediatr Nephrol 1996; 10(3):328.

14. Tonshoff B, Blum WF, Mehls O. Derangements of the somatotropic hormone axis in chronic renal failure. Kidney Int Suppl 1997; 58:S106.

15. Emmanouel DS, Fong VS, Katz AI. Prolactin metabolism in the rat: role of the kidney in degradation of the hormone. Am J Physiol 1981; 249:F437.

16. Davison JM, Sheills EA, Philips PR, et al. Metabolic clearance of vasopressin and an analogue resistant to vasopressinase in human pregnancy. Am J Physiol 1993; 264:F348.

17. Claybaugh JR, Uyehara CF. Metabolism of neurohypophysial hormones. Ann N Y Acad Sci 1993; 689:250.

18. Moses AM, Steciak E. Urinary and metabolic clearances of arginine vasopressin in normal subjects. Am J Physiol 1986; 251:R365.

19. Hruska KA, Martin K, Mennes P, et al. Degradation of parathyroid hormone and fragment production by the isolated perfused dog kidney. J Clin Invest 1977; 60:501.

20. Hruska KA, Korkor A, Martin K, Slatopolsky E. Peripheral metabolism of intact parathyroid hormone. J Clin Invest 1981; 67:885.

21. Yamaguchi T, Fukase M, Nishikawa M, et al. Parathyroid hormone degradation by chymotrypsin-like endopeptidase in the opossum kidney cell. Endocrinology 1988; 123(6):2812.

22. Simmons RE, Hjelle JT, Mahoney C, et al. Renal metabolism of calcitonin. Am J Physiol 1988; 254:F593.

23. Chai SY, Christopoulos G, Cooper ME, Sexton PM. Characterization of binding sites for amylin, calcitonin, and CGRP in primate kidney. Am J Physiol 1998; 274(1 Pt 2):F51.

24. Duckworth WC, Bennett RG, Hamel FG. Insulin degradation: progress and potential. Endocr Rev 1998; 19(5):608.

25. Duckworth WC, Hamel FG, Liepnieks J, et al. Insulin degradation products from perfused rat kidney. Am J Physiol 1989; 256:E208.

26. Nakamura R, Hayashi M, Emmanouel DS, Katz AI. Sites of insulin and glucagon degradation in the rabbit nephron. Am J Physiol 1986; 250:F144.

27. Fawcett J, Rabkin R. Sequential processing of insulin by cultured kidney cells. Endocrinology 1995; 136:39.

28. Dahl DC, Tsao T, Duckworth WC, et al. Retroendocytosis of insulin in a cultured kidney epithelial cell line. Am J Physiol 1989; 257:C190.

29. Flyvbjerg A, Nielsen S, Sheikh I, et al. Luminal and basolateral uptake and receptor binding of IGF-I in rabbit renal proximal tubules. Am J Physiol 1993; 265:F624.

30. Ballard FJ, Knowles SE, Walton PE, et al. Plasma clearance and tissue distribution of labelled insulin-like growth factor-I (IGF-I), IGF-II and des(1–3)IGF-1 in rats. J Endocrinol 1991; 128:197.

31. Rabkin R, Fervenza FC, Maidment H, et al. Pharmacokinetics of insulin-like growth factor-1 in advanced chronic renal failure. Kidney Int 1996; 49(4):1134.

32. Hirschberg R, Adler S. Insulin-like growth factor system and the kidney: physiology, pathophysiology, and therapeutic implications. Am J Kidney Dis 1998; 31(6):901.

33. Talor Z, Emmanouel DS, Katz AI. Glucagon degradation by luminal and basolateral rabbit tubular membranes. Am J Physiol 1983; 244:F297.

34. Vierhapper H, Gasic S, Nowotny P, Waldhausl W. Renal disposal of human atrial natriuretic peptide in man. Metabolism 1990; 39:341.

35. Ruskoaho H. Atrial natriuretic peptide: synthesis, release, and metabolism. Pharmacol Rev 1992; 44(4):479.

36. Zhao J, Ardaillou N, Lu CY, et al. Characterization of C-type natriuretic peptide receptors in human mesangial cells. Kidney Int 1994; 46(3):717.

37. Walter M, Unwin R, Nortier J, Deschodt-Lanckman M. Enhancing endogenous effects of natriuretic peptides: inhibitors of neutral endopeptidase (EC.3.4.24.11) and phosphodiesterase. Curr Opin Nephrol Hypertens 1997; 6(5):468.

38. Lipkin GW, Dawnay AB, Harwood SM, et al. Enhanced natriuretic response to neutral endopeptidase inhibition in patients with moderate chronic renal failure. Kidney Int 1997; 52(3):792.

39. Emmanouel DS, Stavroyoulos T, Katz AI. Role of the kidney in metabolism of gonadotrophs in rats. Am J Physiol 1984; 247:E786.

40. Emmanouel DS, Goldwasser E, Katz AI. Metabolism of pure human erythropoietin in the rat. Am J Physiol 1984; 247:F168.

41. Goswami A, Rosenberg IN. Iodothyronine 5'-deiodinase in rat kidney microsomes. J Clin Invest 1984; 74:2097.

42. Morreale de Escobar G, Calvo R, Escobar del Ray F, Obregon MJ. Thyroid hormones in tissue from fetal and adult rats. Endocrinology 1994; 134:2410.

43. Chopra IJ, Boado RJ, Geffner DL, Solomon DH. A radioimmunoassay for measurement of thyronine and its acetic acid analog in urine. J Clin Endocrinol Metab 1988; 67:480.

43a. Rolleman EJ, Hennemann G, van Toor H, et al. Changes in renal tri-iodothyronine and thyroxine handling during fasting. Europ J Endocrinol 2000; 142:125.

44. Santini F, Hurd RE, Lee B, Chopra IJ. Sex related differences in iodothyronine metabolism in the rat: evidence for differential regulation among various tissues. Metabolism 1994; 43:793.

45. Lee WS, Berry MJ, Hediger MA, Larsen PR. The type I iodothyronine 5'-deiodinase messenger ribonucleic acid is localized to the S3 segment of the rat kidney proximal tubule. Endocrinology 1993; 132(5):2136.

46. Leonard JL, Ekenbarger DM, Frank SJ, et al. Localization of type I iodothyronine 5'-deiodinase to the basolateral plasma membrane in renal cortical epithelial cells. J Biol Chem 1991; 266(17):11262.

47. Kaptein EM. Thyroid hormone metabolism and thyroid diseases in chronic renal failure. Endocr Rev 1996; 17(1):45.

48. Hierholzer K, Schoneshofer M, Siebe H, et al. Corticosteroid metabolism in isolated rat kidney in vitro. I. Formation of lipid soluble metabolites from corticosterone (B) in renal tissue from male rats. Pflugers Arch 1984; 400(4):363.

49. Whitworth JA, Stewart PM, Burt D, et al. The kidney is the major site of cortisone production in man. Clin Endocrinol (Oxf) 1989; 31:355.

50. Funder JW, Pearce PT, Smith R, Smith AI. Mineralocorticoid action: target tissue specificity is enzyme, not receptor, mediated. Science 1988; 242(4878):583.

51. Aziz N, Maxwell MM, Brenner BM. Coordinate regulation of 11 beta-HSD and Ke 6 genes in cpk mouse: implications for steroid metabolic defect in PKD. Am J Physiol 1994; 267(5 Pt 2):F791.

52. Escher G, Frey BM, Frey FJ. 11 beta-hydroxysteroid dehydrogenase—why is it important for the nephrologist? (Editorial). Nephrol Dial Transplant 1995; 10(9):1506.

53. White PC, Mune T, Agarwal AK. 11 β-Hydroxysteroid dehydrogenase and the syndrome of apparent mineralocorticoid excess. Endocr Rev 1997; 18(1):135.

54. Lo YH, Sheff MF, Latif SA, et al. Kidney 11 β-HSD2 is inhibited by glycyrrhetinic acid-like factors in human urine. Hypertension 1997; 29(1 Pt 2):500.

55. Clore J, Schoolwerth A, Watlington CO. When is cortisol a mineralocorticoid? Kidney Int 1992; 42:1297.

56. Morris DJ, Latif SA, Rokaw MD, et al. A second enzyme protecting mineralocorticoid receptors from glucocorticoid occupancy. Am J Physiol 1998; 274(5 Pt 1):C1245.

57. Ghosh SS, Basu AK, Ghosh S, et al. Renal and hepatic family 3A cytochromes P450 (CYP3A) in spontaneously hypertensive rats. Biochem Pharmacol 1995; 50(1):49.

58. Morris DJ, Brem AS. Metabolic derivatives of aldosterone. Am J Physiol 1987; 252:F365.

59. Egfjord M. Corticosteroid metabolism in isolated perfused rat liver and kidney. Experimental studies with emphasis on aldosterone. Acta Physiol Scand Suppl 1995; 627:1.

## CHAPTER 208

# EFFECTS OF ENDOCRINE DISEASE ON THE KIDNEY

ELLIE KELEPOURIS AND ZALMAN S. AGUS

Endocrine disorders may affect the kidney in various ways. Hormone excess or deficiency states can directly alter tubular transport. Moreover, changes can be produced indirectly by alterations in the circulation, which modify renal hemodynamics and sodium transport. Many of the effects produced are not manifest clinically, but a few can be life threatening; some effects are diagnostically useful.

## PITUITARY DISEASE

Several aspects of renal function are regulated directly by the anterior and posterior pituitary gland through the secretion of various hormones, the most important of which is vasopressin (see Chaps. 23, 25, and 27). Two disorders of the anterior pituitary produce changes in renal function: acromegaly and hypopituitarism.

### ACROMEGALY

As part of the generalized visceromegaly, the kidneys of patients with acromegaly are hypertrophied and sometimes achieve a remarkably large size. The glomeruli are enlarged, and all tubular dimensions are increased. The glomerular filtration rate (GFR) and renal blood flow (RBF) are elevated 20% to 50% above normal.[1,2] Reversible prostatic enlargement is also common, even in men with hypogonadism.[3]

Generally, patients with acromegaly manifest a retention of water and electrolytes and an expanded plasma volume, which is appropriate for the degree of tissue growth and the consequent tissue perfusion requirements. The mechanisms by which this response occurs are unclear, but it is not the result of direct effects of growth hormone on renal sodium reabsorption.

Hypertension occurs in 30% to 50% of patients with acromegaly. Although hypervolemia contributes to the increased blood pressure, the role of the renin–angiotensin–aldosterone system is unclear. Serum renin and aldosterone levels are normal in acromegaly. These normal values in the face of hypervolemia probably reflect a physiologic resetting at a higher circulating blood volume. Rarely, aldosterone-producing adenomas have been described in conjunction with acromegaly, and they contribute to the blood pressure increase.

The electrolyte abnormality seen most frequently in acromegaly is hyperphosphatemia (~70% of patients). Serum phosphate often is elevated to levels of 5 to 6 mg/dL and has been used as a crude marker for the activity of the disease. The hyperphosphatemia reflects an increase in tubular phosphate reabsorption, which is independent of GFR and parathyroid hormone (PTH). The long-term, but not the short-term, administration of growth hormone increases tubular phosphate reabsorption; therefore, this effect may be mediated by a direct effect of insulin-like growth factor-I.[4]

Hypercalciuria also is seen in acromegaly and may present with or without nephrocalcinosis. The serum calcium level usually is normal but is mildly elevated in 15% of patients. Hypercalcemia occurs in some patients due to an increase in the endogenous production of calcitriol[5] but usually reflects coexisting primary hyperparathyroidism as part of multiple endocrine neoplasia syndrome, type 1 (see Chap. 188).

## HYPOPITUITARISM

A defect in water excretion occurs in almost all patients with panhypopituitarism. The incidence of hyponatremia (usually mild) may be ~50%. Associated hypothyroidism or hyperprolactinemia may alter the renal handling of water, but the renal defect in these patients results primarily from glucocorticoid deficiency.[1,6] On occasion, the hyponatremia may be severe and may be the presenting symptom in hypopituitarism.[7,8] It is thought to be due to inappropriate secretion of antidiuretic hormone (ADH) that is caused by cortisol (not aldosterone) deficiency.[6] The short-term parenteral administration of glucocorticoids is associated with the prompt restoration of normal diluting ability and a water diuresis in a dose-response fashion. The relationship between the plasma vasopressin level and plasma osmolality is also restored to normal. This observation can be used as a diagnostic maneuver in patients with unexplained hyponatremia. Although reduced GFR and increased permeability of the collecting duct in glucocorticoid deficiency contribute to the defect in water excretion, inappropriate secretion of ADH plays a major role (see Chap. 27). The rapid correction with hydrocortisone suggests that glucocorticoids modulate ADH secretion in response to changes in plasma osmolality. The hypersecretion of ADH and its lack of suppression by hypoosmolality may represent the loss of a normal feedback inhibition by cortisol. ADH is cosecreted with corticotropin-releasing hormone (CRH) from the hypothalamic paraventricular nuclei. With cortisol deficiency, an increase is seen in vasopressin messenger RNA as well as CRH and vasopressin immunoreactivity in these neurons.[9]

## THYROID DISORDERS

### HYPERTHYROIDISM

Although, in hyperthyroidism, alterations occur in renal hemodynamics and in the renal handling of water and electrolytes,

hyperthyroidism seldom produces clinical manifestations of renal dysfunction.[10–14] The RBF and GFR are increased because of renal vasodilation. The serum sodium concentration usually is normal, although studies demonstrate a mild impairment in maximal urinary concentration.[15] The washout of renal medullary hypertonicity by increased blood flow may be the cause of this concentrating defect. Mild polyuria may occur in some patients, usually when hyperthyroidism is complicated by hypercalcemia or hyperglycemia. In patients with thyrotoxicosis, severe dehydration and hypernatremia may develop, mainly because of excessive water loss from the skin and lungs, and inadequate water intake. Mild proteinuria is common.[16]

Although serum potassium generally is normal in hyperthyroidism, total body potassium often is decreased concomitantly with the loss of lean body mass. With control of the hyperthyroid state, body weight and total body potassium levels normalize. In a distinct group of thyrotoxic patients, periodic muscular paralysis in conjunction with episodic hypokalemia can occur. Hyperthyroid Asian men are at particular risk (estimated at 15–20%) of developing the disease.[17] The muscle function is improved with establishment of a euthyroid state and the administration of a β-adrenergic blocker. Use of β-blockers minimizes both the number and the severity of attacks, and often limits the fall in the plasma potassium concentration.[18]

The mechanism by which hyperthyroidism can produce hypokalemic periodic paralysis is not well understood. Thyroid hormone increases $Na^+$–$K^+$–adenosine triphosphatase (ATPase) activity (potassium is driven into cells), and thyrotoxic patients with periodic paralysis have higher $Na^+$–$K^+$–ATPase activity than those without paralytic episodes.[19] Excess thyroid hormone may predispose to paralytic episodes by increasing the susceptibility to the hypokalemic action of epinephrine or insulin.[18]

Hyperthyroidism often is associated with disorders of divalent ion homeostasis. Hypercalcemia may occur due to the direct effect of thyroid hormone on bone resorption, although osteoporosis seldom is encountered.[20] Total serum calcium is elevated in 10% to 20% of cases, and ionized serum calcium is increased in approximately half.[21–23] Usually, symptoms are minimal or absent because of the mild elevation, but with a greater increase, thirst and polyuria may occur. The hypercalcemia resolves after successful return to the euthyroid state and also can be controlled with β-adrenergic blocking drugs. If hypercalcemia does not resolve, the rare possibility of coexisting primary hyperparathyroidism should be considered. PTH levels should be measured, because thyrotoxicosis is associated with an increased incidence of parathyroid adenomas. Hypercalciuria is commonly seen in hyperthyroidism because of the increased filtered load of calcium resulting from increased GFR and the mobilization of bone calcium, and also from the suppression of PTH secretion caused by the increased serum calcium. Occasionally, the hypercalcemia and hypercalciuria are complicated by nephrocalcinosis and the development of nephrolithiasis.[16] Rarely, patients with nephrocalcinosis may manifest an overt, distal, renal tubular acidosis, but this also has been reported in patients without nephrocalcinosis. The autoimmune nature of thyroid disease may underlie an immunologic renal injury manifested as an acidification defect. Elevation of the serum phosphate concentration is common in hyperthyroidism, as a result of an increased tubular reabsorption of phosphate secondary to decreased PTH secretion and a direct effect of thyroid hormone, which increases proximal tubular phosphate reabsorption.[10] Hyperthyroidism also has been associated with mild hypomagnesemia caused by enhanced urinary excretion of magnesium resulting from the effects of the hypercalcemia or hypercalciuria, which inhibit magnesium transport in the loop of Henle.[24]

## HYPOTHYROIDISM

The kidney may undergo various structural and functional abnormalities in adult hypothyroidism. Anatomically, the most striking finding is the marked thickening of the glomerular and tubular basement membranes. Substances rich in mucopolysaccharides deposit in both these structures, as well as in renal blood vessels and the glomerular mesangium and renal interstitium. Cellular changes include vacuolization and periodic acid–Schiff–positive inclusion droplets. These changes are reversible after thyroid function is normalized. Mild proteinuria often is present, but the development of nephrotic syndrome is rare. An autoimmune glomerulonephritis associated with Hashimoto thyroiditis has been implicated in the development of nephrotic syndrome.

In myxedema, RBF and GFR are consistently depressed 25% to 40% below normal values.[25] These hemodynamic alterations reflect the hypodynamic state of the circulation and the renal vasoconstriction. The depressed cardiac output and, perhaps, the renal structural changes contribute to the fall in RBF and GFR.

Tubular reabsorptive and secretory processes generally are decreased and reverse rapidly with the achievement of an euthyroid state. In hypothyroidism, the most significant manifestation of changes in renal function is mild hyponatremia in 20% of patients, which results from an impairment in renal diluting capacity leading to water retention. Thyroid function should be evaluated in any patient with an otherwise unexplained reduction in the plasma sodium concentration. Severe hyponatremia may occur with myxedema coma. The major factor contributing to the water retention appears to be the lack of suppression of ADH secretion.[26] Measurements of circulating ADH levels have demonstrated elevated titers of the hormone that are not suppressed by water loading. Although a decrease in circulating blood volume may play a role, thyroid hormone deficiency probably causes impairment of the ability to respond to hypoosmolality similar to that which is observed in states of glucocorticoid deficiency.[26] ADH secretion may be regulated at a lower serum osmolality, causing a "reset-osmostat" condition.[27] Decreased delivery of tubular fluid to the distal diluting segments also has been implicated as a factor contributing to the diluting defect. This is caused by the hemodynamic alterations produced by a decreased cardiac output, which lead to a decrease in RBF and GFR, and to enhanced proximal tubular sodium and water reabsorption. Sodium chloride reabsorption in the diluting segments also may be diminished. In states of combined diabetes insipidus and hypothyroidism, the effect of thyroid deficiency in reducing free water clearance actually may be beneficial. In this situation, treatment with thyroid hormone may uncover a massive increase in urinary water losses. Regardless of the mechanism of the hyponatremia, normal water balance and correction can be rapidly achieved by the administration of thyroid hormone.

Myxedema is characterized by changes in the distribution of salt and water in the various body compartments. Thus, although total body sodium usually is increased, circulating blood volume often is low. This may be related partly to the binding of sodium to interstitial mucopolysaccharides. Total exchangeable potassium is either normal or decreased, but serum potassium is normal. The renal tubular transport of sodium and potassium generally is normal, although mild defects have been described in some instances. Usually, the kidney adequately regulates the renal excretion of sodium and potassium over a wide range of dietary intake. Similarly, acid-base regulation generally is intact in hypothyroidism. Hyperuricemia in adult men and postmenopausal women with myxedema often is caused by a renal impairment in uric acid excretion (i.e., decreased renal tubular secretion of urate).

Abnormalities in divalent ion metabolism in adult hypothyroidism often are mild and do not manifest as significant clinical problems. A generalized decrease in bone turnover is a common feature, associated with the decreased urinary and fecal excretion of calcium and phosphorus. Serum levels of calcium and phosphate are normal, but a loss of the circadian rhythm for serum and urinary phosphate has been reported, and modest hypermagnesemia frequently is encountered.[24]

# PARATHYROID DISORDERS

## PRIMARY HYPERPARATHYROIDISM

The renal effects of hyperparathyroidism are related principally to the degree and duration of hypercalcemia and the rate of onset of the elevation in the serum calcium concentration. Other features of hyperparathyroidism may play a role in the disturbances of water and electrolyte metabolism. These include renal phosphate wasting, stimulation of the renal production of 1,25-dihydroxyvitamin $D_3$ (by hypophosphatemia and PTH), and direct effects of high levels of circulating PTH.[28] Renal manifestations of primary hyperparathyroidism include decreased GFR, impaired urinary concentrating ability, reduced proximal phosphate reabsorption with consequent phosphaturia, hypercalciuria, nephrolithiasis, nephrocalcinosis, obstructive uropathy, distal renal tubular acidosis, hyperchloremic acidosis, hypertension, and normal or increased urinary excretion of magnesium.

Hypercalciuria is a characteristic feature of primary hyperparathyroidism. The elevated serum calcium seen in this disorder significantly increases the fractional excretion of calcium in the urine. The hypercalciuria is a major factor contributing to the development of renal calculi and nephrocalcinosis in primary hyperparathyroidism. In older series of patients with hyperparathyroidism, the incidence of stone disease exceeded 50%, but the early diagnosis and treatment of asymptomatic cases of hyperparathyroidism have led to a much lower incidence of renal calculi (20%).[29,30] In addition to calcium oxalate kidney stones, patients with primary hyperparathyroidism commonly have calcium phosphate stones because of the tendency of these patients to have an alkaline urine and the moderate enhancement of phosphate excretion that is present. Nephrocalcinosis, or renal parenchymal calcification, may be present; it is most commonly medullary but may be seen in the cortical areas of the kidney as well (Fig. 208-1). Nephrocalcinosis and nephrolithia-

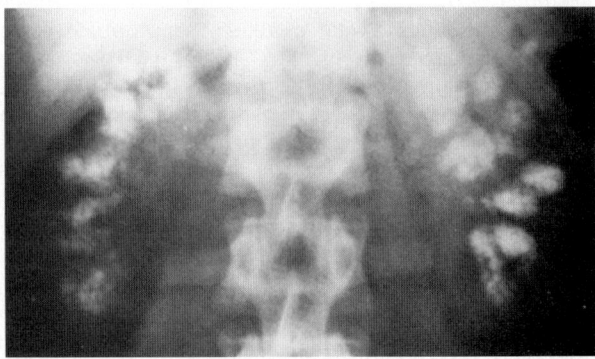

**FIGURE 208-1.** Radiographic appearance of bilateral medullary nephrocalcinosis in a patient with primary hyperparathyroidism. Deposits of calcium phosphate are localized primarily in the medulla (probably beginning in collecting ducts and spreading to periductal tissue). This may also occur in patients with renal tubular acidosis, chronic urinary tract infection, and idiopathic hypercalciuria.

sis are not necessarily associated. When detected on ordinary radiographic films, nephrocalcinosis usually is advanced and reflects severe renal parenchymal involvement. Earlier forms of the disease, not detected by conventional radiography, can be diagnosed by ultrasonography or computed tomography.[31]

Renal insufficiency may occur in hyperparathyroidism and is related to the degree and duration of hypercalcemia. Mild hypercalcemia alone is only rarely associated with renal insufficiency. In a series of patients with asymptomatic hyperparathyroidism and mild hypercalcemia (<11 mg/dL), normal renal function was maintained over a 30-month period of observation.[26] Acute and severe elevations of serum calcium (12–15 mg/dL) may lead to a reversible fall in GFR, mediated by direct renal vasoconstriction and natriuresis-induced volume contraction. Long-standing hypercalcemia and hypercalciuria lead to the development of chronic hypercalcemic nephropathy, which may be irreversible despite surgical cure of the hyperparathyroidism. This nephropathy has the clinical features of an interstitial nephritis, with polyuria, salt wasting, and hypertension. Hypertension, infection, stone disease, and obstruction all contribute to further loss of renal function. In the late stages of the disease, when renal insufficiency is severe, serum calcium may normalize; this is in contrast to the hypocalcemia that characterizes other conditions with the same magnitude of renal impairment. Some patients with long-standing azotemia have a normal or slightly increased serum calcium level. When the patient has no history of prior primary hyperparathyroidism, the occurrence of marked secondary hyperparathyroidism in states of chronic renal insufficiency could make the distinction between this entity and the chronic hypercalcemic nephropathy of primary hyperparathyroidism extremely difficult.

A defect in urinary concentrating ability is the most common renal functional abnormality seen with hypercalcemia.[28] The urinary osmolality is reduced, but the urine is rarely hypotonic. In some series, the incidence of symptomatic polyuria and polydipsia approaches 20%. This defect in urinary concentration is most likely the result of increased renal medullary blood flow contributing to a reduction of medullary hypertonicity and to decreased solute transport out of the loop of Henle.[32] Whether hypercalcemia interferes with the hydroosmotic response to ADH in the collecting tubule remains controversial.[28]

Renal tubular transport disorders are common in primary hyperparathyroidism. Reduced proximal tubular reabsorption of phosphate is a hallmark of this disease, and aminoaciduria can be demonstrated in 33% of patients. Serum magnesium is variable. PTH stimulates and hypercalcemia inhibits magnesium reabsorption in the loop of Henle. Thus, patients with hyperparathyroidism can have increased, normal, or decreased levels of serum magnesium.[33]

PTH and hypercalcemia exert demonstrable, but often not clinically apparent, effects on acid-base balance. PTH excess leads to bone resorption, associated with the dissolution of bone and release of buffers. Hypercalcemia of any cause may directly enhance the tubular reabsorption of bicarbonate and the excretion of increased amounts of net acid in the urine. High levels of PTH, however, tend to decrease tubular bicarbonate reabsorption, which may counteract the effect of hypercalcemia. The net effect on acid-base balance is a composite of opposing forces. The manifestation of marked hyperchloremic acidosis in primary hyperparathyroidism actually is uncommon and may reflect either very high levels of PTH or coexisting renal insufficiency.[34] Hypercalcemia also causes distal renal tubular acidosis.[35] Such a defect may lead to hypokalemia and hypocitraturia, which can contribute to renal calculi formation. Hyperparathyroidism also is associated with impaired renal urate excretion, and hyperuricemia and clinical gout may occur in these patients.

## HYPOPARATHYROIDISM

The absence or deficiency of PTH causes hypocalcemia, hyperphosphatemia, renal magnesium wasting, and glycosuria because of decreased insulin release. In this disorder, the reduction in the filtered load of calcium during hypocalcemia causes hypocalciuria. Because PTH directly stimulates renal calcium reabsorption, urinary calcium excretion, when factored for the filtered load, is higher than expected for the prevailing degree of hypocalcemia in hypoparathyroidism. This becomes an important issue when therapy for hypocalcemia is instituted.[24] When serum calcium is restored toward normal with vitamin D administration, frank hypercalciuria may occur. This can be complicated by renal calculi formation. For this reason, the goal of therapy is to raise the serum calcium level only to 8.5 to 9.0 mg/dL. Alternatively, thiazides can be used in combination with vitamin D to lower urine calcium excretion and permit a higher serum calcium level (see Chap. 60).

# DISORDERS OF THE ADRENAL CORTEX

## HYPERALDOSTERONISM

Primary aldosteronism resulting from an adrenal adenoma or, less commonly, from bilateral hyperplasia of the adrenal zona glomerulosa is characterized by sodium retention without edema, urinary potassium wasting, and excess urinary acid excretion causing a hypokalemic metabolic alkalosis.[1,36]

The clinical features of primary hyperaldosteronism are in part determined by the renal actions of aldosterone. The primary effect is to increase the number of open sodium channels in the luminal membrane of the principal cells in the cortical collecting tubule, leading to increased sodium reabsorption. The ensuing loss of cationic sodium makes the lumen electronegative, thereby creating an electrical gradient that favors the secretion of cellular potassium into the lumen through potassium channels in the luminal membrane. Clinically, these abnormalities are expressed as mild or moderate hypertension, muscle weakness that occasionally progresses to intermittent paralysis, paresthesias, and the signs and symptoms of tetany related to the hypokalemic alkalosis (see Chap. 80).

Aldosterone excess normally does not produce unremitting sodium retention.[1,37] This phenomenon is better appreciated by examining the effects of administering exogenous aldosterone to a normal person receiving a constant intake of sodium and potassium. Initially, urinary sodium excretion falls, urinary potassium excretion rises, and a modest expansion of the extracellular fluid (ECF) volume occurs. After 3 to 5 days, urinary sodium excretion begins to rise and approaches dietary intake, whereas potassium excretion remains at an elevated level. The renal adjustment that allows the experimental subject to return to sodium balance, albeit at the expense of a modest, sustained rise in ECF volume, is called *mineralocorticoid escape*. This response is induced by the volume expansion, because escape typically occurs in humans after a weight gain of ~3 kg. Tachyphylaxis to the cellular effects of aldosterone is not responsible for this phenomenon. Two factors appear to be important in the escape: increased secretion of atrial natriuretic peptide (ANP) induced by the hypervolemia[38] and pressure natriuresis.[39,40] The latter refers to the phenomenon in which increasing renal perfusion pressure (due, in this setting, to systemic hypertension) enhances sodium excretion.[40] How this occurs is not clear, but elevated renal interstitial pressure may indirectly diminish sodium reabsorption in the medullary segments.[41]

Studies of experimental animals have confirmed the role of both of these factors in aldosterone escape. Increased ANP release from the atria precedes the natriuresis, whereas blocking the action of ANP markedly attenuates the initial natriuresis and delays completion of the escape phenomenon.[38] The result is a reduction in tubular sodium reabsorption, possibly due to the effect of a circulating natriuretic hormone that inhibits transport at a distal site in the terminal nephron. Importantly, mineralocorticoid escape is restricted to sodium transport and does not include a reduction in urinary potassium excretion, so that potassium depletion proceeds unremittingly. Severe sodium restriction may limit the amount of potassium secreted in the collecting duct, a process largely dependent on the distal delivery of solute and on the tubular flow rate. Distal solute and water delivery are markedly reduced with sodium restriction, and the tubular flow rate becomes critically low, limiting the amount of potassium secretion despite high circulating levels of aldosterone.

Occasional patients with primary hyperaldosteronism due to an adrenal adenoma or hyperplasia are not hypokalemic at presentation for reasons that are not well understood.[42,43] The frequency with which this occurs is uncertain and has been addressed in rare hereditary disorders such as glucocorticoid-suppressible hyperaldosteronism (in which normal levels of ACTH are responsible for excess release of aldosterone) and Liddle syndrome (in which a primary, nonmineralocorticoid-mediated increase in sodium channel activity in the collecting tubules is present).[44,45] In both of these disorders, affected patients have hypertension, but their plasma potassium concentrations are normal.

The long-term administration of exogenous mineralocorticoids increases urinary excretion of calcium and magnesium as part of the renal response to volume expansion.[1] Serum calcium remains normal, however, possibly because of secondary stimulation of PTH secretion. Serum magnesium often is mildly depressed due to urinary magnesium wasting secondary to inhibition of sodium and magnesium transport in the loop of Henle.

The persistent mild volume expansion resets the osmostat, regulating ADH release and thirst upward. As a result, mild hypernatremia (144–147 mEq/L) often is seen in these patients.

Severe potassium depletion and hypokalemia can lead to a form of vasopressin-resistant (nephrogenic) diabetes insipidus. Polydipsia and polyuria develop, leading to excessive renal water losses and mild hypernatremia. The metabolic alkalosis that develops in primary aldosteronism can be worsened by the degree of hypokalemia. Although aldosterone directly stimulates hydrogen ion secretion in the cortical and medullary collecting ducts, severe hypokalemia also may contribute directly to the renal maintenance of metabolic alkalosis.

## HYPOALDOSTERONISM

Isolated hypoaldosteronism is a syndrome encompassing a heterogeneous group of conditions that share some common clinical findings, most notably hyperkalemia (Table 208-1) (see Chap. 79). Although hypoaldosteronism is most often related to hyporeninemia, factors other than low renin levels may be responsible for its development.[46,47] All patients with isolated hypoaldosteronism manifest a subnormal increase in the serum aldosterone level after a challenge with volume contraction. Although the baseline serum aldosterone level often is low, the occasional finding of a normal value represents an inappropriate response in the presence of an elevated serum potassium level, which, alone, normally should have a direct stimulatory effect on aldosterone secretion.

**TABLE 208-1.**
**Isolated Hypoaldosteronism Syndromes**

**HYPORENINEMIC HYPOALDOSTERONISM**
  Renal-tubulointerstitial disease (e.g., lead nephropathy)
  Diabetes mellitus
  Nephrosclerosis
  Drugs (e.g., nonsteroidal antiinflammatory agents, cyclosporine)
**HYPOALDOSTERONISM WITHOUT HYPORENINISM**
  Selective enzyme defects in aldosterone synthesis
  Long-term heparin therapy
  Angiotensin-converting enzyme inhibitors
  Human immunodeficiency virus infection
**MINERALOCORTICOID RESISTANCE**
  Pseudohypoaldosteronism
  Salt-losing nephropathies
  Obstructive uropathy
  Renal transplantation
  Sickle cell disease
  Systemic lupus erythematosus

The clinical presentation of isolated hypoaldosteronism is typical. Most patients are older and usually are asymptomatic. Almost 50% have diabetes mellitus or mild or moderate renal insufficiency. Asymptomatic hyperkalemia, not exceeding 6.5 mEq/L, occurs in 75% of these patients, and only a few have muscle weakness or cardiac bradyarrhythmias related to hyperkalemia. A common finding (50%) is hyperchloremic metabolic acidosis. Despite aldosterone deficiency, renal salt wasting is rare. Often, these patients manifest salt retention associated with congestive heart failure, edema, and hypertension. If dietary sodium restriction is imposed for the treatment of edema, however, negative sodium balance, intravascular volume depletion, and hypotension ensue. Under these conditions, hyperkalemia and hyperchloremic acidosis are markedly exaggerated. This most likely relates to the impaired delivery of solute to the distal nephron sites involved in potassium and hydrogen ion secretion. Thus, hospitalized patients seem to have more difficulty with hyperkalemia than do outpatients, who are less likely to adhere to rigid salt restriction.

The syndrome of hyporeninemic hypoaldosteronism has been described in patients with nephrotic syndrome secondary to membranous nephropathy. These patients are normotensive, usually have normal renal function and low plasma aldosterone with submaximal response to upright posture, and have episodes of sodium retention.

An unusual component of the impaired hydrogen ion secretion in hypoaldosteronism is the preserved ability to maximally acidify the urine (pH <5.3) during acid loading, unlike in other forms of distal renal tubular acidosis. The acidosis usually is mild and appears to be due primarily to decreased urinary ammonium excretion as well as a direct inhibitory effect of aldosterone deficiency on acid excretion. Chronic hyperkalemia produces inhibition of ammonium absorption in the medullary thick ascending limb of the loop of Henle. This, in turn, may lead to reduced ammonium secretion into the collecting duct and reduced urinary excretion.[48]

Hyperkalemia with mild renal impairment does not necessarily imply aldosterone deficiency but may represent tubular unresponsiveness. Other conditions associated with partial or complete renal tubular unresponsiveness to aldosterone include obstructive uropathy, renal transplantation, systemic lupus erythematosus, sickle cell disease, and acquired adult forms of pseudohypoaldosteronism (see Table 208-1).[46] Furthermore, various drugs can cause derangements in the renin-aldosterone system, leading to hyperkalemia. These include heparin, angiotensin-converting enzyme inhibitors, β-adrenergic blocking agents, and nonsteroidal antiinflammatory agents.

Low plasma sodium and elevated plasma potassium and renin in association with salt wasting and failure to thrive have been described in neonates with congenital hypoaldosteronism and corticosterone methyloxidase deficiency. The salt wasting is attributed to an enzymatic defect in the terminal aldosterone biosynthesis. This terminal defect is due to a homozygous deletion of codon 173 of the *CYP11B2* gene that encodes aldosterone synthase.[49]

Therapy for isolated hypoaldosteronism usually is not necessary unless symptomatic or severe hyperkalemia is present. The prudent approach is to eliminate any source of increased potassium intake; avoid drugs that predispose to hyperkalemia, including potassium-sparing diuretics; avoid marked salt restriction or volume contraction; and attempt to control the diabetes. Specific therapeutic interventions may be required in some conditions. Although treatment with fludrocortisone acetate (0.1 mg per day) corrects the mineralocorticoid deficiency, higher doses (up to 1 mg per day) often are required to overcome renal tubular resistance resulting from concomitant renal disease. Administration of mineralocorticoids in supraphysiologic doses can exacerbate hypertension or precipitate edema and congestive heart failure. In such conditions, the addition of a diuretic (e.g., furosemide or thiazides) is required.

## CUSHING SYNDROME

Although glucocorticoid hormones have only slight mineralocorticoid activity, when present in sufficiently large amounts in Cushing syndrome, they produce significant electrolyte abnormalities. These include increased sodium reabsorption and potassium and hydrogen ion secretion, which cause volume expansion, hypertension, and hypokalemic alkalosis.[37] Moreover, the catabolic effects of glucocorticoids cause loss of cellular potassium, which contributes to total body potassium depletion. The hypokalemia can accentuate the proximal muscle weakness and wasting induced by the catabolic effects of excess glucocorticoid on skeletal muscle. The electrolyte abnormalities are more pronounced in patients with particular forms of Cushing syndrome, such as in those with ACTH-producing carcinomas or those with adrenocortical carcinomas in which extremely high levels of glucocorticoids exert excessive mineralocorticoid activity. Patients with ACTH production by extrapituitary tumors often have severe muscle weakness as a result of the marked hypokalemia that is present.

The bone-demineralizing effects of glucocorticoid excess commonly lead to hypercalciuria, and nephrocalcinosis and renal calcium stones occasionally may be encountered.

Some patients with Cushing syndrome may manifest moderate diastolic hypertension secondary to the activation of renal tubular type 1 (mineralocorticoid) receptors by cortisol excess. They usually have severe hypercortisolism due to ectopic ACTH secretion.[50] The severely high serum cortisol levels overwhelm the kidney's ability to convert cortisol to cortisone. This results in activation of renal mineralocorticoid receptors and concurrent hypokalemia. This form of hypertension can be effectively treated with spironolactone to block mineralocorticoid activity.

## PRIMARY ADRENOCORTICAL INSUFFICIENCY

Adrenocortical hormone deficiency is characteristically associated with electrolyte and renal function abnormalities. In mild states of insufficiency, the condition may be chronic and may be tolerated reasonably well if adequate sodium intake is provided.

Mineralocorticoid deficiency causes urinary sodium wasting and diminished urinary excretion of potassium and hydrogen ion, and it is expressed clinically as ECF volume contraction, hyperkalemia, and metabolic acidosis. Glucocorticoid deficiency leads to a reduction in RBF and GFR, and these effects, coupled with the prevailing hypovolemia, can cause variable degrees of renal insufficiency. In stressful conditions, blood pressure may fall, cardiac output may diminish further, and severe renal insufficiency may develop. The hypotension is due primarily to volume depletion resulting from aldosterone deficiency. Serum concentrations of endothelin-1 (a vasoconstrictive peptide) and of adrenomedullin (a vasodilator peptide) are reported to be increased, but their contribution to the hypotension of primary adrenal insufficiency remains unknown.[51,52]

Hyponatremia resulting from an impairment in renal water excretion is present in 85% to 90% of patients with adrenocortical insufficiency. The impaired water excretion is attributable to a deficiency of both mineralocorticoid and glucocorticoid hormones. Glucocorticoid deficiency results in impaired renal diluting capacity and in an impairment of the systemic hemodynamics that normally provide a nonosmotic stimulus for ADH release. However, a more important mechanism in the hypersecretion of ADH, which is seen in cortisol deficiency, may be that ADH is an ACTH secretagogue, and ADH secretion is stimulated by CRH from the paraventricular nuclei in the hypothalamus. Cortisol exerts a negative feedback on CRH secretion and thereby on ADH secretion; this inhibitory effect is removed with adrenal insufficiency. Whether the effect of cortisol on ADH release is direct or is mediated by changes in the secretion of CRH is not known. Mineralocorticoid deficiency produces ECF volume contraction, which stimulates ADH secretion via the carotid sinus baroreceptors and decreases delivery of glomerular filtrate out of the proximal tubule to distal diluting segments. Although glucocorticoid replacement can lead to improved urinary dilution and partial correction of hyponatremia, in contrast to the situation in hypopituitarism, the full restoration of diluting capacity requires expansion of ECF volume by high salt intake and mineralocorticoid replacement. Glucocorticoid replacement also improves renal handling of acid loads.

These patients often have hyperkalemia (65%), which seldom is higher than 7 mEq/L; hyponatremia (90%), which rarely is below 120 mEq/L; hyperchloremic metabolic acidosis with a serum bicarbonate level usually between 15 and 20 mEq/L; and mild elevations in blood urea nitrogen and serum creatinine.

Hypercalcemia is seen in 6% of patients with adrenocortical insufficiency, and it appears to be more common in the autoimmune variety of the disease. Although the precise cause of the elevated serum calcium is unknown, the hemoconcentration associated with this disorder may increase the nonionic component of calcium. In addition, cortisol deficiency may lead to an increased sensitivity to vitamin D, and the subsequent increased intestinal calcium absorption, in conjunction with hypocalciuria caused by the volume contraction, may account for the unusual case with significant hypercalcemia. Hypocalcemia is rare in Addison disease and may be related to coexistent autoimmune disease with hypoparathyroidism.

## REFERENCES

1. Agus ZS, Goldfarb S. Renal function in adrenal and pituitary disease. In: Suki WN, Eknoyan G, eds. The kidney in systemic disease. New York: John Wiley and Sons, 1981:455.
2. Hoogenburg K, ter Wee PNI, Lieverse AG, et al. Insulin-like growth factor 1 and altered hemodynamics in growth hormone deficiency, acromegaly, and type 1 diabetes mellitus. Transplant Proc 1994; 26:505.
3. Coloa A, Marzullo P, Ferone D, et al. Prostatic hyperplasia: an unknown feature of acromegaly. J Clin Endocrinol Metab 1998; 83:775.

4. Quigley R, Baum M. Effects of growth hormone and insulin-like growth factor I on rabbit proximal convoluted tubule transport. J Clin Invest 1991; 88:368.

5. Eskildsen PC, Lund B, Sorensen OH, et al. Acromegaly and vitamin D metabolism: effect of bromocriptine. J Clin Endocrinol Metab 1979; 49:484.

6. Agus ZS, Goldberg M. Role of antidiuretic hormone in the abnormal water diuresis of anterior hypopituitarism in man. J Clin Invest 1971; 50:1478.

7. Oelkers W. Hyponatremia and inappropriate secretion of vasopressin in patients with hypopituitarism. N Engl J Med 1989; 321:492.

8. Lam KS, Kung AW, Young RT. Post irradiation hypopituitarism presenting as severe hyponatremia. Am J Med 1992; 92:219.

9. Wolfson B, Manning RW, Davis LG, et al. Co-localization of corticotropin releasing factor and vasopressin mRNA in neurones after adrenalectomy. Nature 1985; 315:59.

10. Smith D, DeFronzo RA. Insulin, glucagon and thyroid hormone. In: Dunn MJ, ed. Renal endocrinology. Baltimore: Williams & Wilkins, 1983:367.

11. Vaamonde CA, Michael UF. The kidney in thyroid dysfunction. In: Suki WN, Eknoyan G, eds. The kidney in systemic disease. New York: John Wiley and Sons, 1981:361.

12. Bradley SE, Stephan E, Coelho JB, Reville P. The thyroid and the kidney. Kidney Int 1974; 6:346.

13. Katz AI, Emmanouel DS, Lindheimer MD. Thyroid hormone and the kidney. Nephron 1975; 15:223.

14. Capasso G, DeSanto NG, Kinne R. Thyroid hormones and renal transport: cellular and biochemical aspects. Kidney Int 1987; 32:443.

15. Cutler RE, Glatte H, Dowling JT. Effect of hyperthyroidism on the renal concentrating mechanism in humans. J Clin Endocrinol Metab 1967; 27:453.

16. Ford HC, Lim WC, Chisnall WN, Pearce JM. Renal function and electrolyte levels in hyperthyroidism: urinary protein excretion and the plasma concentrations of urea, creatinine, uric acid, hydrogen ion and electrolytes. Clin Endocrinol (Oxf) 1989; 30:293.

17. Ko GT, Chow CC, Yeung VT, et al. Thyrotoxic periodic paralysis in a Chinese population. Q J Med 1996; 89:463.

18. Ober KP. Thyrotoxic periodic paralysis in the United States. Report of seven cases and review of the literature. Medicine 1992; 71:109.

19. Chan A, Shinde R, Cockram CS, et al. In vivo and in vitro sodium pump activity in subjects with thyrotoxic periodic paralysis. Br Med J 1991; 303:1096.

20. Adams PH, Jowsey J, Kelly PJ, et al. Effects of hyperthyroidism on bone and mineral metabolism in man. Q J Med 1967; 36:1.

21. Baxter JD, Bondy PK. Hypercalcemia of thyrotoxicosis. Ann Intern Med 1966; 65:42.

22. Frizel D, Malleson A, Marks V. Plasma levels of calcium and magnesium in thyroid disease. Lancet 1967; 1:1360.

23. Epstein FH, Freedman LR, Levitin H. Hypercalcemia, nephrocalcinosis and reversible renal insufficiency associated with hyperthyroidism. N Engl J Med 1958; 258:782.

24. Jones JE, Desper PC, Shane SR, Flink EB. Magnesium metabolism in hyperthyroidism and hypothyroidism. J Clin Invest 1966; 45:891.

25. DeRubertis FR Jr, Bloom ME, Mintz DH, et al. Impaired water excretion in myxedema. Am J Med 1971; 51:41.

26. Skowsky WR, Kikuchi TA. The role of vasopressin in the impaired water excretion of myxedema. Am J Med 1978; 64:613.

27. Discala VA, Kinney MJ. Effects of myxedema on the renal diluting and concentrating mechanism. Am J Med 1971; 50:325.

28. Kurkokawa K. Calcium-regulating hormones and the kidney. Kidney Int 1987; 32:760.

29. Mallette LE, Bilezikian JP, Heath DA. Primary hyperparathyroidism: clinical and biochemical features. Medicine (Baltimore) 1974; 53:127.

30. Purnell DC, Scholz DA, Smith LH, et al. Treatment of primary hyperparathyroidism. Am J Med 1974; 56:800.

31. Manz F, Jaschke W, Van Kaich G. Nephrocalcinosis in radiographs, computed tomography, sonography, and histology. Pediatr Radiol 1980; 9:19.

32. Goldfarb S, Agus ZS. On the mechanism of the polyuria of hypercalcemia. Am J Nephrol 1984; 4:69.

33. King RG, Stanbury SW. Magnesium metabolism in primary hyperparathyroidism. Clin Sci 1970; 39:281.

34. Coe FL. Magnitude of metabolic acidosis in primary hyperparathyroidism. Arch Intern Med 1974; 134:262.

35. Ferris R, Kashgarian M, Levitin H, et al. Renal tubular acidosis and renal potassium wasting acquired as a result of hypercalcemic nephropathy. N Engl J Med 1961; 265:924.

36. White PC. Disorders of aldosterone biosynthesis and action. N Engl J Med 1994; 331:250.

37. Higgins JT Jr, Mulrow PJ. Fluid and electrolyte disorders of endocrine diseases. In: Maxwell MH, Kleeman CR, eds. Clinical disorders of fluid and electrolyte metabolism. New York: McGraw-Hill, 1980:1291.

38. Yokota N, Bruneau BG, Kuroski de Bold AJ. Atrial natriuretic factor contributes to mineralocorticoid escape phenomenon. Evidence for a guanylate cyclase-medicated pathway. J Clin Invest 1994; 94:1938.

39. Hall JE, Granger JP, Smith MJ Jr, Premen AJ. Role of renal hemodynamics and arterial pressure in aldosterone "escape." Hypertension 1984; 6(2 Pt 2):I183.

40. Guyton AC. Blood pressure control—special role of the kidneys and body fluids. Science 1991; 252:1813.

41. Kinoshita Y, Knox FG. Role of prostaglandins in proximal tubular sodium reabsorption: response to elevated renal interstitial hydrostatic pressure. Circ Res 1989; 64:1013.

42. Bravo EL, Tarazi RC, Dustan HP, et al. The changing clinical spectrum of primary aldosteronism. Am J Med 1983; 74:641.

43. Gordon RD. Mineralocorticoid hypertension. Lancet 1994; 344:240.

44. Litchfield WR, Coolidge C, Silva P, et al. Impaired potassium-stimulated aldosterone production: a possible explanation for normokalemic glucocorticoid-remediable aldosteronism. J Clin Endocrinol Metab 1997; 82:1507.

45. Botero-Velez M, Curtis JJ, Warnock DG. Brief report: Liddle's syndrome revisited: a disorder of sodium reabsorption in the distal tubule. N Engl J Med 1994; 330:178.

46. DeFronzo RA. Hyperkalemia and hyporeninemic hypoaldosteronism. Kidney Int 1980; 17:118.

47. Smith JD, Bia MJ, DeFronzo RA. Clinical disorders of potassium metabolism. In: Arieff AI, DeFronzo RA, eds. Fluid electrolyte and acid-base disorders. New York: Churchill Livingstone, 1985:413.

48. DuBose TD Jr, Good DW. Chronic hyperkalemia impairs ammonia transport and accumulation in the inner medulla of the rat. J Clin Invest 1992; 90:1443.

49. Peter M, Nikischin W, Heinz-Eriau P, et al. Homozygous deletion of arginine-173 in the CYP11B2 gene in a girl with congenital hypoaldosteronism. Corticosterone methyloxidase deficiency type II. Horm Res 1998; 50:222.

50. Ulick S, Wang JZ, Blumenfeld JD, Pickering TA. Cortisol inactivation overload: a mechanism of mineralocorticoid hypertension in the ectopic adrenocorticotropin syndrome. J Clin Endocrinol Metab 1992; 74:963.

51. Letizia C, Centanni M, Scuro L, et al. High levels of endothelin-1 in untreated Addison's disease. Eur J Endocrinol 1996; 135:696.

52. Letizia C, Cerci S, Centanni M, et al. Circulating levels of adrenomedullin in patients with Addison's disease before and after corticosteroid treatment. Clin Endocrinol 1998; 48:145.

# CHAPTER 209

# ENDOCRINE DYSFUNCTION DUE TO RENAL DISEASE

ARSHAG D. MOORADIAN

The kidney has a central role in producing and metabolizing various hormones.[1,2] It synthesizes and secretes erythropoietin, 1,25-dihydroxycholecalciferol [$1,25(OH)_2D_3$], and renin (see Chaps. 54, 79, 183, and 212). Moreover, the kidney contributes to the metabolic clearance rates of insulin, glucagon, prolactin, parathyroid hormone (PTH), calcitonin, growth hormone (GH), and possibly leptin. In renal failure, the accumulation of bioinactive peptides with antigenic properties similar to those of the natural hormones causes an overestimation of the serum hormonal levels measured by radioimmunoassay.[2-4] Furthermore, the altered metabolic milieu in chronic renal failure (CRF) significantly influences the secretory rate of hormones and the sensitivity of target tissues to the hormonal effects. Table 209-1 summarizes many of the pathogenetic mechanisms of endocrine

**TABLE 209-1.**

**Pathogenetic Mechanisms of Endocrine Dysfunction in Chronic Renal Failure**

**INCREASED CIRCULATING HORMONE LEVELS**

Increased secretion (e.g., parathyroid hormone [PTH], aldosterone?)

Accumulation of immunoassayable hormone fractions that may lack bioactivity (e.g., glucagon, PTH, calcitonin, prolactin)

**DECREASED CIRCULATING HORMONE LEVELS**

Decreased secretion by diseased kidney (e.g., erythropoietin, renin, 1,25-dihydroxyvitamin $D_3$)

Decreased secretion by other endocrine glands (e.g., testosterone, estrogen, progesterone)

**DECREASED SENSITIVITY TO HORMONES**

Altered target tissue response (e.g., to insulin, glucagon, 1,25-dihydroxyvitamin $D_3$, erythropoietin, and PTH)

dysfunction in patients with CRF. The institution of dialysis or of kidney transplantation early in the course of renal failure may reverse many of these abnormalities, although dialysis may independently contribute to some hormonal derangements, such as menorrhagia, increased fecal thyroxine ($T_4$) excretion, or heparin-induced transient elevations of free $T_4$ levels.[1,5,6] Long-term erythropoietin therapy induces a significant decrease in GH, prolactin, follicle-stimulating hormone (FSH), and luteinizing hormone (LH) but does not change calcium-related hormones [PTH, calcitonin, $1,25(OH)_2D_3$].[7]

## ABNORMALITIES OF GROWTH HORMONE SECRETION

At least 50% of patients with uremia have elevated fasting GH levels and often exhibit a paradoxic rise in GH during the glucose-tolerance test.[1,6] Although the metabolic clearance rate of GH may be reduced in CRF, the elevated serum GH levels appear to result primarily from derangements in the central regulation of GH secretion. The GH response to insulin-induced hypoglycemia or levodopa (L-dopa) is exaggerated; thyrotropin-releasing hormone (TRH) administration causes an inappropriate GH secretory response, which is analogous to the response seen in patients with abnormal central GH regulation, such as patients with liver cirrhosis, anorexia nervosa, or acromegaly.[1,2]

Whether the elevated serum GH level occurring in azotemia contributes significantly to the glucose intolerance that may be seen in this condition is uncertain. Many children with chronic renal insufficiency and severe growth retardation have normal 24-hour GH secretion and normal or increased serum immunoreactive insulin-like growth factor-I (IGF-I) and -II (IGF-II) concentrations.[8] The cause of the growth retardation in children with uremia, despite normal or elevated GH levels, is multifactorial. Protein-calorie malnutrition, chronic acidosis, repeated infections, and decreased bioactive IGF-I are contributing factors.[9] The overall somatomedin activity on bioassay is decreased in renal failure, probably because of circulating inhibitors of low molecular weight. Dialysis increases somatomedin bioactivity, but there is little change in somatomedin levels on radioassay. Alterations in IGF-binding proteins (IGFBP) are also found in children with acute or chronic renal failure.[10] These changes include an increased serum IGFBP-2 and reduced serum IGFBP-3, along with increased urinary IGFBP-1 and absent urinary IGFBP-3.[10] In adults with CRF the immunoreactive fragments of IGFBP-3 are increased without a change in IGFBP-3 protease activity.[11] The metabolic clearance rate of exogenously administered IGF-I is not altered in CRF.[11]

## THYROID DYSFUNCTION

Structural changes in the thyroid gland occur in patients with CRF. The prevalence of goiter in patients with uremia may be as high as 58%. Its occurrence varies in different studies that have been reported from different geographic areas with different prevalence rates of endemic goiter.[1] However, the serum of patients on hemodialysis contains thyroid cell proliferation-inhibiting activity.[12] The clinical implications of this observation are not clear. The serum $T_4$ level is either normal or decreased, particularly in patients receiving long-term dialysis. The total serum triiodothyronine ($T_3$) level usually is decreased, whereas the $T_3$ resin uptake is either normal or increased. The incidence of abnormalities in thyroid function test results increases with the duration of hemodialysis. Unlike other chronic nonthyroidal illnesses, the total serum reverse $T_3$ ($rT_3$) level in patients with

uremia is not elevated, although the free $rT_3$ levels are increased (see Chaps. 30 and 36).

The underlying mechanisms of these alterations include decreased $T_4$ binding to serum proteins, poor peripheral conversion of $T_4$ to $T_3$, and impaired pituitary and thyroidal function.[13,14] A furan fatty acid and indoxyl sulfate in uremic sera inhibit hepatocyte transport and subsequent deiodination of $T_4$.[15] These substances may contribute to the low serum $T_3$ concentrations in patients with uremia. The plasma $T_4$-binding globulin concentrations usually are normal. The radioactive iodine uptake by the thyroid in patients with uremia is low when measured at 2 or 6 hours because of the dilution of the radioactive iodine by the high plasma levels of inorganic iodides. Conversely, the radioactive iodine uptake at 24 hours may be increased.[1,13] Iodine organification, as measured by the perchlorate discharge test, appears to be normal, but the salivary/plasma ratio of iodine-131 (a measure of iodine trapping) is increased.[13] The thyroid response to exogenous thyroid-stimulating hormone (TSH) is normal or decreased,[14] and the pituitary TSH response to exogenous TRH might be elevated or suppressed in some patients.[1,16] The thyroid function test results normalize after renal transplantation, with the exception of patients with subnormal TSH responses to TRH.[16] Presumably, this latter abnormality results from the suppression of TSH secretion by glucocorticoid therapy.

The physiologic significance of low thyroid hormone levels in renal failure is unclear. Clinically, it is difficult to exclude mild hypothyroidism in patients with uremia, who often have dry skin, lethargy, cold intolerance, and abnormal thyroid function test results. An elevated TSH level is the most useful index of hypothyroidism, necessitating thyroid-replacement therapy. Otherwise, the changes in thyroid hormone levels in patients with uremia are considered to be a physiologic adaptation to the disease state and do not require thyroid hormone replacement.

## PARATHYROID HORMONE AND RENAL OSTEODYSTROPHY

The most common metabolic bone disease occurring in patients with CRF is a mixture of osteitis fibrosa and osteomalacia; osteoporosis and osteosclerosis occur less frequently[1,2,2a] (see Chap. 61). The renal osteodystrophy is caused by the interplay of complex metabolic, nutritional, and cellular abnormalities that occur in uremia. Secondary hyperparathyroidism, chronic acidosis, vitamin D resistance secondary to decreased $1\alpha$-hydroxylation of 25-hydroxyvitamin D, and altered target organ sensitivity are the major causes of renal osteodystrophy.[17] Secondary hyperparathyroidism is an adaptive response to the progressive decline in the renal capacity to excrete phosphate.

Skeletal resistance to the action of PTH, impaired intestinal calcium absorption, and, possibly, reduced binding of $1,25(OH)_2D_3$ in the parathyroid glands contribute to the hypocalcemia and secondary hyperparathyroidism of patients with uremia.[17,18,18a] Occasionally, the parathyroid gland becomes autonomous with or without the development of adenomas (i.e., tertiary hyperparathyroidism). The high levels of COOH-terminal immunoreactive PTH should be interpreted with caution, because ~80% of serum PTH results from decreased renal and extrarenal clearance of PTH.[19] Moreover, aluminum toxicity can be confused with hyperparathyroidism when hypercalcemia occurs with a normal or modestly elevated PTH level along with radiologic evidence of osteitis fibrosa[20] (see Chaps. 61 and 131). It appears that the level of intact PTH (measured by sequential amino-terminal immunoextraction and PTH midregion radioimmunoassay), expressed as the percentage of total serum PTH midregion immunoreactivity, may distinguish between primary hyperparathyroidism and CRF.[21]

The role of calcitonin in renal osteodystrophy is controversial. Circulating levels of calcitonin in CRF are elevated and correlate directly with the phosphate/total calcium ratio[22] (see Chap. 53). It is not certain whether the elevated levels of red blood cell and white blood cell calmodulin (a ubiquitous, intracellular, calcium-binding protein) in patients receiving regular hemodialysis are related to the disturbances in calcium metabolism.[23] The judicious use of vitamin D compounds and phosphate binders, along with dietary measures and the correction of acidosis, are the mainstays of therapy for renal osteodystrophy. It appears that $1,25(OH)_2D_3$ or $1\alpha$-hydroxyvitamin $D_3$ supplementation normalizes the serum calcium level and suppresses secondary hyperparathyroidism, but may not heal the osteomalacia.[24] The therapeutic role of noncalcemic analogs of vitamin D, such as 22-oxacalcitriol, in the treatment of secondary hyperparathyroidism remains to be established.[25]

## ABNORMAL ADRENAL HORMONE METABOLISM

In patients with CRF, the excretion of urinary 17-hydroxycorticosteroids is diminished, increasing basal plasma levels of conjugated 17-hydroxycorticosteroids. However, the basal plasma cortisol levels usually are normal, although elevated levels of total and free plasma cortisol have been encountered occasionally.[1,2] The basal morning levels of adrenocorticotropic hormone (ACTH) are normal or slightly elevated. The cortisol secretory response to exogenous ACTH stimulation also is normal or elevated. The setpoint in the negative-feedback control of the hypothalamic–pituitary–adrenal system appears to be elevated; hence, the overnight dexamethasone suppression test or the classic 2-day dexamethasone suppression test may yield false-positive results.[26,27] If the duration of dexamethasone administration is prolonged, normal suppression of plasma cortisol may be achieved.[28] Subnormal responses to insulin-induced hypoglycemia and the single-dose metyrapone test (30 mg/kg) have been reported, but the cortisol response to major stress, such as surgery, is preserved. Although hemodialysis does not seem to remove much of the circulating cortisol, the metabolic clearance rate of cortisol is increased by 30% during dialysis.

It is not clear whether the increased corticotropin-releasing hormone-binding protein in uremia affects pituitary-adrenal axis physiology.[29]

The changes in aldosterone secretion in patients with uremia are controversial.[1,2] The plasma aldosterone level is normal in regularly dialyzed patients, but the response to posture and ACTH stimulation can be blunted. Conversely, elevated aldosterone levels with normal responses to various stimuli are found in patients with uremia who are not receiving regular dialysis. The metabolic clearance rate of aldosterone seems to be normal, because it is the liver that is responsible for the peripheral degradation of aldosterone. In the nephrotic syndrome, there is a reduced 11β-hydroxysteroid dehydrogenase activity, which may contribute to the exaggerated sodium retention in those patients.[29a]

Mild or moderate renal insufficiency occasionally is associated with impaired renin production and secretion, with consequent hypoaldosteronism. Diabetes mellitus and other diseases affecting the tubules and the interstitium of the kidney are the leading causes of the syndrome of hyporeninemic hypoaldosteronism, which is characterized by hyperkalemic, hyperchloremic metabolic acidosis out of proportion to the degree of renal insufficiency (see Chap. 81).

The plasma catecholamine levels usually are elevated in patients with CRF. However, low plasma epinephrine levels have been reported.[30] The loss of diurnal variation of the blood pressure in CRF with blunting of the nighttime decrease in blood pressure has been correlated with increased serum levels of vasoactive hormones such as angiotensin II, arginine vasopressin, and endothelin.[31]

## HYPOPHYSIAL-GONADAL DYSFUNCTION

### WOMEN

Infertility and amenorrhea without menopausal flushing occur frequently in women with uremia.[5,6] The lack of menopausal flushing is probably the result of an altered hypothalamic vasomotor center. The menses typically are irregular after dialysis is begun. Menstruation may remain scant, or menorrhagia may occur, which may require hysterectomy. Sexual dysfunction (e.g., loss of libido or orgasm) is common in women with uremia and appears to worsen after the initiation of dialysis. The hormonal derangements in premenopausal women with uremia include elevated serum prolactin levels, normal FSH levels, and mildly elevated LH levels, along with an increased LH/FSH ratio and low or low-normal serum estradiol, estrone, progesterone, and testosterone levels. Elevated circulating testosterone levels have been reported.[5,6] In women with uremia who have primary gonadal failure, the elevation of serum FSH and LH levels usually is similar to that observed in menopausal women without uremia. The normal pulsatile release of gonadotropin is lost in uremia, but the response to gonadotropin-releasing hormone and clomiphene appears to be normal, although the LH response to gonadotropin-releasing hormone may be prolonged and slow to return to the baseline. Exogenous estrogens, however, fail to induce LH release. Moreover, the cyclic release of LH, which is associated with positive estradiol feedback, is impaired; the negative estradiol feedback and the tonic gonadotropin secretion seem to be intact.[5,6] The hyperprolactinemia observed in women with uremia may contribute to gonadal dysfunction. The modest discrepancy between the prolactin levels on immunoassay and bioassay in patients with uremia indicates that the circulating prolactin is mostly bioactive.[3] Bromocriptine treatment may induce regular menstruation. Renal transplantation normalizes most of the hormonal levels of uremia, but normal menstruation is not always restored.

### MEN

Decreased libido, potency, and testicular size, with azoospermia and gynecomastia, are common manifestations of deranged hypophysial-gonadal function in men with uremia.[5,6] Men on hemodialysis or peritoneal dialysis more often have sexual desire disorder, sexual aversion disorder, and inhibited male orgasm compared to men with kidney transplants or rheumatoid arthritis.[32] Sexual dysfunction in these men is largely due to loss of sexual interest.[32]

The modest increase in circulating gonadotropin levels in the presence of profoundly decreased testosterone levels in some patients implies a defect of the hypothalamic-pituitary unit along with primary testicular failure. The serum concentration of sex hormone–binding globulin is normal, and the binding of testosterone to sex hormone–binding globulin is either normal or increased; hence, the low circulating testosterone levels cannot be attributed to alterations in binding of testosterone to plasma proteins. The testosterone response to the short-term administration of human chorionic gonadotropin is subnormal, but human chorionic gonadotropin treatment over months can yield normal testosterone levels, suggesting that the testicles have retained substantial reserve capacity. The gonadotropin response to gonadotropin-releasing hormone can be normal, blunted, or, more characteristically, exaggerated, and prolonged responses also have been reported. Thus, gonadal failure in men with uremia is secondary to two defects, one at the gonadal level and the other at the hypothalamic-pituitary level.

The suppression of hyperprolactinemia by bromocriptine may restore sexual function in some men. In patients with uremia who have zinc deficiency, sexual potency may be improved by treatment with pharmacologic doses of this trace metal[33] (see Chap. 131). Regular dialysis may improve libido and potency in some men, but more commonly, progressive deterioration of gonadal function occurs during long-term dialysis. Renal transplantation reverses gonadal dysfunction in many patients, but in some, hypogonadism may worsen. The deterioration is thought to be related to the effects of immunosuppressive agents on testicular function and of exogenous corticosteroids on LH release. In patients with low serum testosterone levels, therapy with a long-acting preparation of this hormone may be attempted. If medical therapy fails, some patients benefit from the surgical insertion of a penile prosthesis.

Delayed pubertal maturation in children can occur with CRF. In prepubertal boys with uremia, the serum LH and testosterone levels are normal, but the FSH level is elevated, suggesting that damage to the germinal epithelium may occur before the advent of spermatogenesis; Leydig cell function appears to be intact.[34]

## CARBOHYDRATE METABOLISM

*Uremic pseudodiabetes* refers to the state of carbohydrate intolerance in a nondiabetic patient in whom CRF develops.[35] It is attributed to decreased target tissue sensitivity to insulin, circulating insulin antagonists, and defective insulin release. Conversely, patients with diabetes who have CRF often have decreased daily insulin requirements because of decreased caloric intake and impaired renal and extrarenal (skeletal muscle) clearance of insulin. Spontaneous hypoglycemia has been reported in patients with CRF,[36] and has been attributed to inadequate glycogenolysis and substrate limitation of gluconeogenesis (see Chap. 158). Abnormalities of insulin receptor binding capacity and defects in postreceptor processes or cellular metabolism, such as impaired phosphorylation of glucose, may explain the impaired peripheral tissue responsiveness to insulin.[37]

The presence of circulating insulin antagonists in CRF has been suspected in pseudodiabetes because hemodialysis can correct glucose intolerance in patients with uremia. The nature of this antagonism is unknown. The plasma nonesterified fatty acid or elevated GH levels do not seem to play a significant role. Even more dubious is the role of hyperglucagonemia, because hemodialysis improves glucose intolerance despite persistently elevated glucagon levels. These results should be interpreted with caution because the measured total immunoreactive glucagon is a composite of three heterogeneous molecules with different molecular weights and bioactivities[4] (see Chap. 134). Alterations in the serum concentrations of potassium, calcium, and magnesium may contribute to the impaired insulin secretion found in patients with uremia. The high intracellular calcium content of pancreatic islets is associated with impaired cellular glucose metabolism and impaired glucose-induced insulin release. This defect is attributed to the secondary hyperparathyroidism of CRF.[38] Although glucose intolerance is common, fasting hyperglycemia usually indicates the development of frank diabetes mellitus.

Insulin is the treatment of choice for patients with uremia who have diabetes mellitus. Sulfonylurea agents can produce prolonged hypoglycemia in patients with renal failure and should not be used when creatinine levels are above 2 mg/dL. Metformin is contraindicated in renal failure because of the danger of lactic acidosis. Acarbose, an $\alpha$-glucosidase inhibitor, may

be used in those with predominantly postprandial hyperglycemia. However, this agent has not been adequately studied in subjects with renal failure. Home blood glucose monitoring is essential. Tests for urinary glucose are unreliable because of the altered renal tubular threshold of glucose with progressive deterioration of renal function. The glycosylated hemoglobin levels measured by affinity chromatography may underestimate the degree of glycemia in patients with uremia because of reduced red blood cell survival time. Alternatively, the glycemia is overestimated when glycosylated hemoglobin is measured by cation exchange chromatography, in which carbamylated hemoglobin interferes with the measurements.

## LIPID METABOLISM

Hypertriglyceridemia with elevated levels of very low-density lipoprotein occurs in at least 50% of patients with CRF, but elevated levels of cholesterol and low-density lipoprotein are found infrequently.[1,39] The serum levels of high-density lipoprotein (HDL) usually are low. The fasting plasma free fatty acid levels generally are normal, but plasma glycerol levels are increased. Whether this represents enhanced lipolysis is unclear. After heparin administration, plasma lipolytic activity and lipoprotein lipase activity of adipose tissue are impaired in patients with CRF. Long-term dialysis or the use of anabolic steroids to treat the anemia of CRF will aggravate the hypertriglyceridemia. The incidence of hypertriglyceridemia is not reduced by decreasing the dialysate glucose concentration. However, an intensified dialysis program may increase plasma lipolytic activity and lower the serum triglyceride level. Decreased plasma clearance of triglycerides and enhanced hepatic triglyceride synthesis secondary to hyperinsulinemia may explain the hypertriglyceridemia of renal failure. The serum lipid abnormalities may contribute to the pathogenesis of the accelerated atherosclerosis associated with uremia.

In the nephrotic syndrome, total cholesterol and triglyceride levels commonly are elevated, the $HDL_3$ level may be increased, and the $HDL_2$ level is decreased. The level of lipoprotein(a) may be elevated.[40]

## HORMONES INVOLVED IN WATER METABOLISM

The basal plasma concentration of antidiuretic hormone in patients with uremia usually is elevated above control levels, but the response to dialysis is inconsistent.[30,31] Atrial natriuretic hormone (ANH) appears to be elevated in the plasma of volume-overloaded children with CRF[41] and in patients with obstructive uropathy.[42] The significance of this finding is not clear (see Chap. 178). In contrast to the increased level of ANH, the plasma levels of a homologous peptide, the brain natriuretic peptide, are not increased in patients on dialysis.[43]

## GASTROINTESTINAL HORMONES

Hypergastrinemia caused by reduced renal clearance of gastrin is a common occurrence in patients with acute and chronic renal failure.[44] Whether the elevated plasma gastrin levels contribute to the high incidence of peptic ulcer disease in patients with uremia is unknown. In some patients with azotemia, achlorhydria associated with atrophic gastritis may contribute to the hypergastrinemia. Long-term erythropoietin therapy induces a significant decrease in plasma gastrin, glucagon, and pancreatic polypeptide levels.[7]

The clinical significance of decreased renal clearance of the other gut hormones, such as cholecystokinin, secretin, and gastric inhibitory peptide, is uncertain.[2]

## LEPTIN

Leptin is a peptide hormone produced by adipocytes and is implicated in regulating the adipose tissue mass through its central effects on feeding behavior and energy expenditure. It is also an important modulator of the neuroendocrine system (see Chaps. 126 and 186). In CRF, plasma leptin is higher than expected for body mass index.[45] It is possible that hyperleptinemia could contribute to the anorexia and poor nutritional status, as well as to some of the neuroendocrine changes found in subjects with renal failure.[45]

## REFERENCES

1. Mooradian AD, Morley JE. Endocrine dysfunction in chronic renal failure. Arch Intern Med 1984; 144:351.
2. Emmanouel DS, Lindheimer MD, Katz AI. Pathogenesis of endocrine abnormalities in uremia. Endocr Rev 1980; 1:28.
2a. Ritz E, Schomig M, Bommer J. Osteodystrophy in the millenium. Kidney Int Suppl 1999; 73:S94.
3. Mooradian AD, Morley JE, Korchik WP, et al. Comparison between bioactivity and immunoreactivity of serum prolactin in uraemia. Clin Endocrinol (Oxf) 1985; 22:241.
4. Kuku SF, Jaspan JB, Emmanouel DS, et al. Heterogeneity of plasma glucagon. Circulating components in normal subjects and patients with chronic renal failure. J Clin Invest 1976; 58:742.
5. Morley JE, Melmed S. Gonadal dysfunction in systemic disorders. Metabolism 1979; 28:1051.
6. Handelsman DJ. Hypothalamic-pituitary gonadal dysfunction in renal failure, dialysis and renal transplantation. Endocr Rev 1985; 6:151.
7. Kokot F, Wiecek A, Schmidt-Gayk H, et al. Function of endocrine organs in hemodialyzed patients on long-term erythropoietin. Artif Organs 1995; 19:428.
8. Hokken-Koelega AC, Hackeng WHL, Stijnen T, et al. Twenty-four-hour plasma growth hormone (GH) profiles, urinary GH excretion, and plasma insulin like growth factor-I and II levels in prepubertal children with chronic renal insufficiency and severe growth retardation. J Clin Endocrinol Metab 1990; 71:688.
9. Phillips LS, Unterman TG. Somatomedin activity in disorders of nutrition and metabolism. Clin Endocrinol Metab 1984; 13:145.
10. Powell DR, Durham SK, Brewer ED, et al. Effects of chronic renal failure and growth hormone on serum levels of insulin-like growth factor–binding protein 4 (IGFBP-4) and IGFBP-5 in children. J Clin Endocrinol Metab 1999; 84:596.
11. Rabkin R, Fervenza FC, Maidment H, et al. Pharmacokinetics of insulin-like growth factor-1 in advanced chronic renal failure. Kidney Int 1996; 49:1134.
12. Nishikawa M, Yoshikawa N, Yoshimura M, et al. Thyroid cell proliferation-inhibiting activity in serum of patients with chronic renal failure on hemodialysis. Endocr J 1996; 43:441.
13. Mooradian AD, Morley JE, Korchik WP, et al. Iodine trapping and organification in patients with chronic renal failure. Eur J Nucl Med 1983; 8:495.
14. Hardy MJ, Ragbeer SS, Nascimento L. Pituitary-thyroid function in chronic renal failure assessed by a highly sensitive thyrotropin assay. J Clin Endocrinol Metab 1988; 66:233.
15. Lim C-F, Bernard BF, DeJong M, et al. A furan fatty acid and indoxyl sulfate are the putative inhibitors of thyroxine hepatocyte transport in uremia. J Clin Endocrinol Metab 1993; 76:318.
16. Lim VS, Fang VS, Katz AI, Refetoff S. Thyroid dysfunction in chronic renal failure: a study of the pituitary thyroid axis and peripheral turnover kinetics of thyroxine and triiodothyronine. J Clin Invest 1977; 60:522.
17. Ritz E, Stefanski A. Endocrine disturbances of calcium metabolism in uremia: renal causes and systemic consequences. Kidney Int 1996; 49:1765.
18. Korkor AB. Reduced binding of [³H]1,25-dihydroxyvitamin D₃ in the parathyroid glands of patients with renal failure. N Engl J Med 1987; 316:1573.
18a. Block GA, Port FK. Re-evaluation of risks associated with hyperphosphatemia and hyperparathyroidism in dialysis patients: recommendations for a change in management. Am J Kidn Dis 2000; 35:1226.
19. Freitag J, Martin KJ, Hruska KA, et al. Impaired parathyroid hormone metabolism in patients with chronic renal failure. N Engl J Med 1978; 298:29.
20. Sherrard DJ, Ott SM, Andress DL. Pseudohyperparathyroidism syndrome associated with aluminum intoxication in patients with renal failure. Am J Med 1985; 79:127.
21. Lindall AW, Elting J, Ells J, Roos BA. Estimation of biologically active intact parathyroid hormone in normal and hyperparathyroid sera by sequential N-terminal immunoextraction and mid region radioimmunoassay. J Clin Endocrinol Metab 1983; 57:1007.
22. Silva OL, Becker KL, Shalhoub RJ, et al. Calcitonin levels in chronic renal disease. Nephron 1977; 19:12.
23. Mooradian AD, Morley JE, Levine AS, et al. The effects of chronic renal failure and hemodialysis on human red and white cell calmodulin levels. J Clin Endocrinol Metab 1984; 58:1010.
24. Bordier PH, Zingraff J, Gueris J, et al. The effect of 1-[OH]D₃ and 1,25-[OH]₂D₃ on the bone in patients with renal osteodystrophy. Am J Med 1978; 64:101.
25. Slatopolsky E, Berkoben M, Kelber J, et al. Effects of calcitriol and non-calcemic vitamin D analogs on secondary hyperparathyroidism. Kidney Int 1992; 42(Suppl 38):S43.
26. Wallace EZ, Rosman P, Toshav N, et al. Pituitary adrenocortical function in chronic renal failure: studies of episodic secretion of cortisol and dexamethasone suppressibility. J Clin Endocrinol Metab 1980; 50:46.
27. Rosman PM, Farag A, Peckham R, et al. Pituitary-adrenocortical function in chronic renal failure: blunted suppression and early escape of plasma cortisol levels after intravenous dexamethasone. J Clin Endocrinol Metab 1982; 54:528.
28. Workman RJ, Vaughn WK, Stone WJ. Dexamethasone suppression testing in chronic renal failure: pharmacokinetics of dexamethasone and demonstration of a normal hypothalamic-pituitary-adrenal axis. J Clin Endocrinol Metab 1986; 63:741.
29. Trainer PJ, Woods RJ, Korbonits M, et al. The pathophysiology of circulating corticotropin-releasing hormone-binding protein levels in the human. J Clin Endocrinol Metab 1998; 83:1611.
29a. Vogt B, Dick B, N'gankam V, Frey FJ, Frey BM. Reduced 11β-hydroxysteroid dehydrogenase activity in patients with the nephrotic syndrome. J Clin Endocrinol Metab 1999; 84:811.
30. Rauh W, Hund E, Sohl G, et al. Vasoactive hormones in children with chronic renal failure. Kidney Int 1983; 24:S27.
31. Jensen LW, Pedersen EB. Nocturnal blood pressure and relation to vasoactive hormones and renal function in hypertension and chronic renal failure. Blood Pressure 1997; 6:332.
32. Toorians AW, Janssen E, Laa E, et al. Chronic renal failure and sexual functioning: clinical status versus objectivity assessed sexual response. Nephrol Dialysis Transplant 1997; 12:2654.
33. Mahajan SK, Abbasi AA, Prasad AS, et al. Effect of oral zinc therapy on gonadal function in hemodialysis patients: a double-blind study. Ann Intern Med 1982; 97:357.
34. Ferraris J, Saenger P, Levine L, et al. Delayed puberty in males with chronic renal failure. Kidney Int 1980; 18:344.
35. De Fronzo RA, Andres R, Edgar P, Walker WJ. Carbohydrate metabolism in uremia. A review. Medicine (Baltimore) 1973; 52:469.
36. Arem R. Hypoglycemia associated with renal failure. Endocrinol Metab Clin North Am 1989; 18:103.
37. Smith D, De Fronzo RA. Insulin resistance in uremia mediated by postbinding defects. Kidney Int 1982; 22:54.
38. Fadda GZ, Hajjar S, Perna AF, et al. On the mechanism of impaired insulin secretion in chronic renal failure. J Clin Invest 1991; 87:255.
39. Avram MM, Goldwasser P, Burrell DE, et al. The uremic dyslipidemia: a cross-sectional and longitudinal study. Am J Kidney Dis 1992; 20:324.
40. Wheeler DC, Bernard DB. Lipid abnormalities in the nephrotic syndrome: causes, consequences, and treatment. Am J Kidney Dis 1994; 23:331.
41. Rascher W, Tulassey T, Lang RE. Atrial natriuretic peptide in plasma of volume-overloaded children with chronic renal failure. Lancet 1985; 2:303.
42. Gulmi FA, Moopan UM, Chou S, Kim H. Atrial natriuretic peptide in patients with obstructive uropathy. J Urol 1989; 142:268.
43. Akiba T, Tachibana K, Togashi K, et al. Plasma human brain natriuretic peptide in chronic renal failure. Clin Neph 1995; 44(Suppl 1):S61.
44. Korman MG, LaVer MC, Hansky J. Hypergastrinemia in chronic renal failure. Br Med J 1972; 1:209.
45. Howard JK, Lord GM, Clutterbuck EJ, et al. Plasma immunoreactive leptin concentration in end-stage renal disease. Clin Sci 1997; 93:119.

## CHAPTER 210

# NEUROMUSCULAR MANIFESTATIONS OF ENDOCRINE DISEASE

ROBERT B. LAYZER AND GARY M. ABRAMS

A broad range of neuromuscular symptoms are found in patients with endocrine and metabolic disease.[1] The most useful diagnostic approach is to place the patient's problem in a general category of neuromuscular symptoms and, by clinical and laboratory assessment, determine the *anatomic localization of the disorder within the motor unit* (Table 210-1). The most important localizing laboratory tests are the measurements of *serum enzyme*

**TABLE 210-1.**
**Survey of Neuromuscular Syndromes**

| Principal Symptom | Motor Unit Location | Neuromuscular Disorder | Endocrine or Metabolic Disease |
|---|---|---|---|
| ACUTE GENERAL-IZED WEAKNESS | Muscle | Reversible hypokalemic paraly-sis, myosin depletion | Hyperthyroidism, hyperaldosteronism, anorexia/bulimia, high-dose corticosteroid therapy |
| | | Rhabdomyolysis | Acute hypophosphatemia, hyperaldosteronism, high-dose corticosteroid therapy |
| | Neuromuscular junction | Acute myasthenic paralysis | Hypermagnesemia |
| | Peripheral nerve | Acute areflexic paralysis | Acute hypophosphatemia, hypoadrenalism |
| SUBACUTE AND CHRONIC GENER-ALIZED WEAKNESS | Muscle | Atrophic myopathy | Acromegaly, hyperthyroidism, hypothyroidism, osteomala-cia, chronic hypophosphatemia, hyperparathyroidism, Cushing disease/corticosteroid therapy |
| | | Necrotic myopathy | Hyperaldosteronism, anorexia/bulimia |
| | Neuromuscular junction | Myasthenia gravis | Hyperthyroidism, hypothyroidism |
| | Peripheral nerve | Polyneuropathy | Hyperthyroidism, hypothyroidism, adrenal myeloneuropa-thy, kwashiorkor/marasmus, GI surgery for obesity, diabe-tes mellitus, hypoglycemia |
| | | Carpal tunnel syndrome | Acromegaly, hypothyroidism, diabetes mellitus |
| MUSCLE SPASMS AND STIFFNESS | Muscle | Slow contraction and relaxation | Hypothyroidism |
| | | Myoedema | Hypothyroidism |
| | Peripheral nerve | Tetany | Hypocalcemia, hypomagnesemia, hypoparathyroidism, hyperaldosteronism, anorexia/bulimia |
| | Central nervous system | Ordinary cramps | Hypothyroidism |
| | | Painful reflex spasms | Hypoadrenalism |

*GI*, gastrointestinal.

*levels* reflecting muscle injury, especially creatine kinase (CK), and *electrodiagnostic tests* such as *electromyography* (EMG) and *tests of nerve conduction and neuromuscular transmission.*[2] *Muscle biopsy* (with routine and histochemical analysis) is used mainly in the pathologic classification of subacute and chronic myopa-thies; it adds little or nothing to the diagnosis of other neuro-muscular problems.

## PITUITARY DISORDERS

### ACROMEGALY

Patients with long-standing acromegaly often complain of diminished endurance, and ~40% have an overt myopathy, with mild proximal muscle weakness and atrophy.[3] Serum CK levels usually are normal, but EMG shows myopathic changes without irritable features. Muscle biopsy samples often show atrophy of type II muscle fibers and hypertrophy of type I fibers.[4] The weakness improves slowly after effective surgical treatment (see Chap. 12).

The carpal tunnel syndrome occurs in ~50% of patients with acromegaly, and subclinical nerve conduction abnormalities are found in 80% of asymptomatic cases.[5] Hand pain and paresthe-sias usually are bilateral and are associated with typical alter-ations of motor and sensory conduction in the median nerves at the wrists. After effective treatment of the pituitary tumor, the hand symptoms usually resolve within 6 weeks, although objec-tive signs improve much more slowly.[3] Other compression neu-ropathies may occur as a result of bone and soft tissue hypertrophy, and nerve roots sometimes are compressed in the vertebral foramina.

### NELSON SYNDROME

Although muscle weakness is uncommon in Nelson syndrome, in one study, myopathic and irritable EMG abnormalities were noted in each of five patients.[6] Serum CK levels were normal,

and muscle biopsies showed only a subsarcolemmal accumula-tion of lipid droplets within muscle fibers.

## THYROID DISORDERS

### HYPERTHYROIDISM

#### THYROTOXIC MYOPATHY

Thyrotoxic myopathy occurs in 60% to 80% of patients with hyperthyroidism. Painless muscle weakness and atrophy develop gradually, predominantly in the shoulder girdles and upper arms (Fig. 210-1); in the lower extremities, proximal weakness may be restricted to the hip flexors.[7] The reflexes often are brisk, and a few patients have prominent fasciculations (muscle twitches). EMG shows myopathic abnormalities in the proximal muscles, and these changes also are present in many patients who do not have overt weakness.[8] Serum CK activity is always normal, reflecting the paucity of muscle fiber damage seen in the muscle biopsy. The main pathologic finding is a non-selective atrophy of muscle fibers, which do not have the angu-lar conformation associated with denervation atrophy.

#### THYROTOXIC BULBAR MYOPATHY

Dysphagia occurs in ~16% of patients with thyrotoxic myopa-thy. Rarely, dysphagia is severe enough to cause aspiration of foods and liquids, and these patients are said to have thyrotoxic bulbar myopathy.[9] The pharyngeal weakness develops over a few weeks or months and may be accompanied by dysphonia, regurgitation of liquids through the nose, hoarseness, and weak-ness of the face, tongue, or eyes. Even respiratory weakness may occur. Although myasthenia gravis can produce similar symp-toms, these patients do not have pharmacologic, electrophysio-logic, or immunologic evidence of myasthenia.

All of the symptoms of thyrotoxic myopathy, including bul-bar weakness, resolve completely when the patients become euthyroid. Muscle power recovers in ~2 months, except in

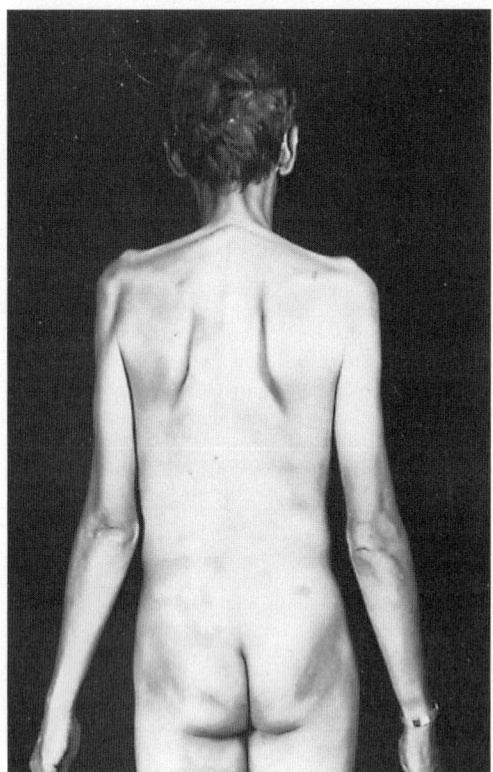

**FIGURE 210-1.** Thyrotoxic myopathy. The patient shows severe wasting of the shoulder girdle muscles, which are preferentially affected in this condition.

severe cases; muscle bulk is restored a little more slowly. Surprisingly, both bulbar weakness and limb weakness often improve during treatment with propranolol, even before antithyroid treatment is begun (see Chap. 42).

### MYASTHENIA GRAVIS

Myasthenia gravis occurs in <0.1% of patients with hyperthyroidism, but ~5% of patients with myasthenia develop hyperthyroidism or have a history of hyperthyroidism. In 25% of the latter cases, the two conditions appear simultaneously.[7] Like Graves disease, myasthenia gravis is an autoimmune disease associated with haplotypes HLA-B8 and HLA-D3 (see Chap. 194). Because propranolol has weak neuromuscular blocking properties, it should be used cautiously in patients with hyperthyroidism who have myasthenia. Treatment of the hyperthyroidism does not induce a remission of the symptoms of myasthenia.

### OTHER NEUROMUSCULAR FINDINGS

Approximately 12% of patients with hyperthyroidism have prominent fasciculations. Rarely, these patients manifest continuous, undulating fasciculations known as *myokymia*, which may involve the face, tongue, limbs, and trunk. Because fasciculations are caused by spontaneous discharges of motor nerves, these patients probably have a motor neuron disorder. A few patients even have pyramidal tract signs, producing a clinical picture easily mistaken for amyotrophic lateral sclerosis. The motor neuron signs all resolve after treatment of the hyperthyroidism. Rare reports are found of polyneuropathy in hyperthyroidism, with areflexia and weakness of the lower extremities (Basedow paraplegia).[10] Motor nerve conduction velocity usually is normal, suggesting that the neuropathy results from a disturbance of axonal function.

### HYPOKALEMIC PERIODIC PARALYSIS

The most distinctive complication of hyperthyroidism is hypokalemic periodic paralysis. This disorder is rare in Western countries, but among persons of Japanese or Chinese ancestry, periodic paralysis occurs in 8% to 34% of men with thyrotoxicosis and in 0.2% of women with thyrotoxicosis. It is linked to certain HLA antigens.[11,12] The signs of thyrotoxicosis may be extremely subtle in these highly susceptible patients. Native Americans and Filipinos also have an increased susceptibility. Approximately 90% of the patients are men, and the neuromuscular symptoms, like those of uncomplicated thyrotoxicosis, usually begin after the age of 20.

Generally, the disorder is clinically indistinguishable from familial hypokalemic periodic paralysis (Table 210-2). Weakness appears first in the proximal leg muscles and trunk, and becomes generalized over the course of several hours, sometimes affecting the respiratory and bulbar muscles. Fortunately, respiratory insufficiency is much rarer in the thyrotoxic than in the hereditary cases. Severe attacks occur during sleep and last as long as 12 hours, after which strength gradually returns, with the distal muscles recovering first. In the milder, daytime attacks, weakness may be confined to the legs; walking seems to hasten recovery, and strength returns in an hour or two. During an attack, the paralyzed muscles are flaccid and nontender. The

**TABLE 210-2.**
**Comparison of Hereditary and Acquired Forms of Hypokalemic Periodic Paralysis**

| History and Test Results | Hereditary | Thyrotoxic | Potassium Deficiency |
|---|---|---|---|
| AGE AT ONSET | Childhood or adolescence | After age 20 yr | Any age |
| FAMILY HISTORY | Usually positive | Negative | Negative |
| ATTACKS PRECIPITATED BY: | | | |
| CARBOHYDRATES | Yes | Yes | Yes |
| INSULIN | Yes | Yes | Yes |
| SALT | Yes | Yes | Yes |
| EPINEPHRINE | Yes | Yes | Yes |
| SLEEP | Yes | Yes | Yes |
| REST AFTER EXERCISE | Yes | Yes | Yes |
| SERUM POTASSIUM: | | | |
| DURING ATTACK | Low | Low | Low |
| BETWEEN ATTACKS | Normal | Normal | Low |
| METABOLIC ALKALOSIS OR ACIDOSIS | Absent | Absent | Often present |
| SERUM CREATINE KINASE ACTIVITY | Normal | Normal | Often increased |

tendon reflexes are diminished in proportion to the degree of weakness, and sensation is normal.

The serum potassium level is normal between attacks, falls as the attack develops, and returns to normal as strength recovers. These changes occur because large amounts of extracellular potassium move into muscle cells during an attack and move back into the blood during recovery. During a mild episode, however, the serum potassium level may not fall below the normal range. No other electrolyte abnormalities are seen. The serum CK activity remains normal, and EMG shows myopathic abnormalities in weak muscles.

Recovery from an acute attack can be hastened by the oral or intravenous administration of 80 to 100 mEq of potassium chloride over a period of 4 to 6 hours. Propranolol, in a dose of 40 mg four times daily, helps to prevent further attacks, and the attacks cease entirely within a few weeks after patients become euthyroid.[13]

The mechanism of thyrotoxic periodic paralysis is unknown.[14] In both the hereditary and acquired types, the paralyzed muscle fibers are depolarized and inexcitable, implying either an increased sodium permeability or a decreased potassium permeability of the plasma membrane. The large shift of potassium into muscle during the inception of an attack implies an active transport of this ion against a huge concentration gradient, requiring participation of the sodium-potassium pump. Insulin and β-adrenergic drugs, both of which can provoke attacks of paralysis, stimulate the sodium-potassium adenosine triphosphatase of muscle. Molecular studies have implicated a mutation in the gene coding for a voltage-sensitive calcium channel as the cause of familial hypokalemic periodic paralysis. Future research doubtless will focus on the effect of thyrotoxicosis on this membrane function.[15]

## HYPOTHYROIDISM

Neuromuscular symptoms are found in at least half of all patients with hypothyroidism, but they usually are not severe or disabling. The most frequent complaints relate to a physiologic disorder of muscle contraction, characterized by slowness of both contraction and relaxation. Contraction is slow because of a reduction in myosin adenosine triphosphatase activity, and relaxation is delayed because of the slow reaccumulation of calcium by the sarcoplasmic reticulum. These abnormalities produce muscle aches, a tendency for muscles to become stiff during exercise, and a consequent slowness of movement, symptoms often suggesting a rheumatic disorder. The well-known phenomenon of "hung-up" stretch reflexes has the same basis.

*Myoedema* is a small lump rising on the surface of a muscle when it is struck with a percussion hammer (Fig. 210-2). This electrically silent contraction is caused by a local release of calcium from the sarcoplasmic reticulum.[16] In patients with hypothyroidism, the mounding may persist for 30 to 60 seconds because of the slow reaccumulation of calcium within muscle fibers. (Myoedema also occurs in patients with cachexia, including those who have apathetic thyrotoxicosis.) Spontaneous muscle cramps also are common in hypothyroidism; like ordinary cramps, these are of neural origin and are not related to the disorder of muscle relaxation (Fig. 210-3A).

Muscle enlargement occurs in 19% of children with hypothyroidism, sometimes giving a remarkable "muscle-bound" appearance known as the *Kocher-Debré-Sémélaigne syndrome*[17] (Fig. 210-4). Less often, muscle enlargement is seen in adult patients who complain of muscle stiffness and pain, suggesting that work hypertrophy, related to prolonged muscle contraction, may be the cause.

Although the serum CK activity is increased in 90% of patients with hypothyroidism (probably because the enzyme is

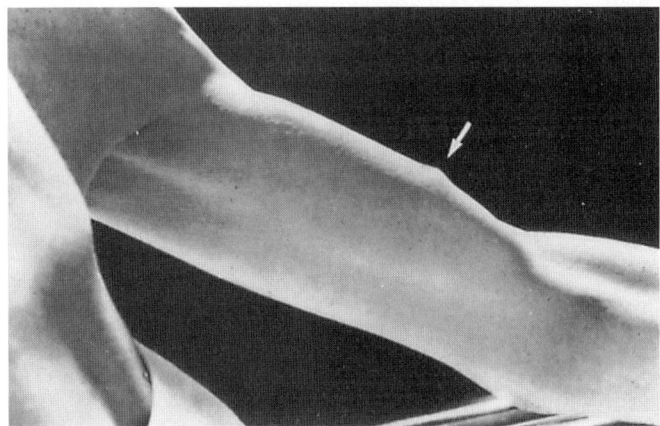

**FIGURE 210-2.** Myoedema in a patient with hypothyroidism. A small mound (*arrow*) is visible on the surface of the biceps muscle, which has just been struck by a percussion hammer. (From Salick AI, Colachis SC, Pearson CM. Myxedema myopathy: clinical, electrodiagnostic, and pathological findings in advanced case. Arch Phys Med Rehabil 1968; 49:230.)

cleared extremely slowly from the plasma), hypothyroid myopathy develops in only 25%.[18] Mild, proximal weakness appears slowly over many months, often accompanied by muscle pain, slowness, and stiffness. The affected muscles may be either enlarged or atrophied. Myopathic EMG changes are common, even in patients who are not weak. Fibrillations and other irritable features are seen occasionally.[19] Muscle biopsies show type II muscle fiber atrophy and a reduced proportion of type II muscle fibers, which contain increased numbers of central nuclei. With thyroid replacement, the muscle symptoms resolve in a few months. In rare cases, the myopathy can take a fulminating course, resulting in rhabdomyolysis and myoglobinuria.[20]

Carpal tunnel syndrome occurs in 15% to 30% of patients with hypothyroidism, usually causing bilateral hand symptoms. Among unselected patients with carpal tunnel syndrome, as many as 10% may have hypothyroidism. Surgery usually is not necessary, because the symptoms generally resolve with thyroid treatment. Minor signs of polyneuropathy, consisting of distal sensory impairment in the legs and absent ankle jerks, occur in ~10% of patients with hypothyroidism. Only a few cases of a moderately severe motor and sen-

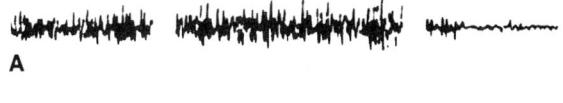

**A**

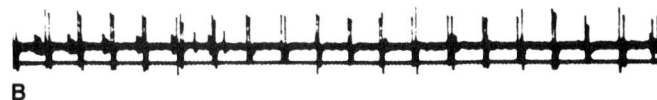

**B**

**FIGURE 210-3.** Electromyographic recordings of muscle spasms. **A,** Ordinary muscle cramps involve profuse, high-frequency discharges of motor unit potentials, waxing and waning in intensity. The abnormal muscle activity probably is triggered by spontaneous discharges arising in motor nerve terminals. **B,** In tetany, there is a rhythmic discharge of groups of two or more motor unit potentials, at a frequency of 5 to 15 Hz. The muscle discharges result from spontaneous activity arising in the proximal portions of peripheral nerves. (**A,** From Norris FH Jr, Gasteiger EL, Chatfield PO. An electromyographic study of induced and spontaneous muscle cramps. Electroencephalogr Clin Neurophysiol 1957; 9:139. **B,** From Kugelberg E. Activation of human nerves by ischemia. Trousseau's phenomenon in tetany. Arch Neurol Psychiatry 1948; 60:140.)

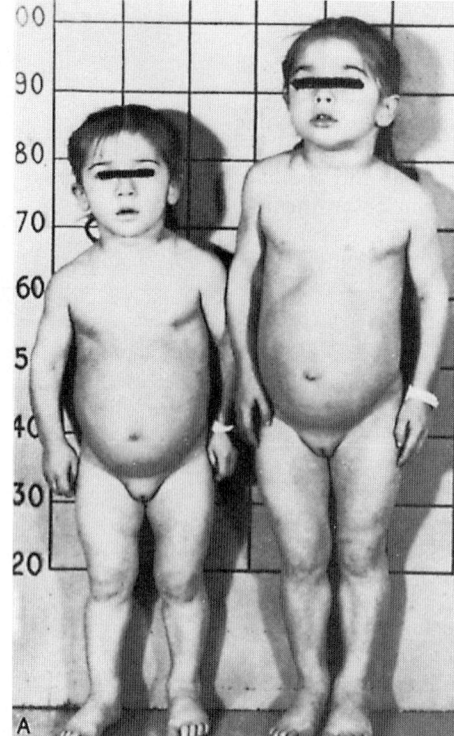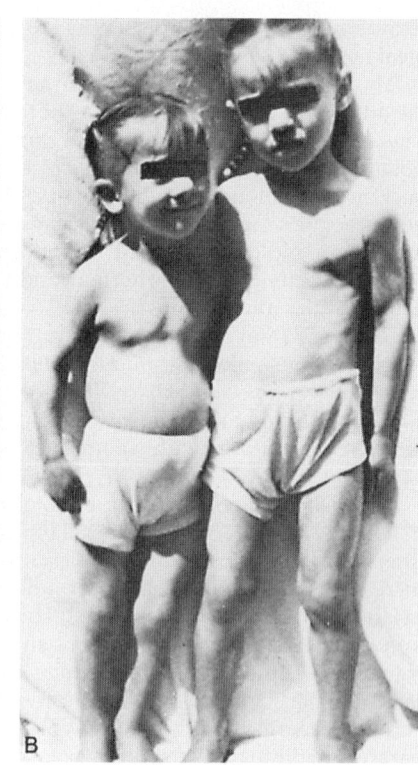

FIGURE 210-4. **A**, Muscle enlargement in two hypothyroid children (5 and 8 years of age) with Kocher-Debré-Sémélaigne syndrome. The athletic appearance is thought to result from work hypertrophy of muscle. The serum lactic dehydrogenase and glutamic-oxaloacetic transaminase levels were increased in both children, and the serum creatine phosphokinase level was increased in one. Electromyography and muscle biopsy were unremarkable. **B**, After thyroid hormone therapy, the musculature has normalized in appearance. (From Cross HE, Hollander CS, Rimain DL, McCusick VA. Familial agoitrous cretinism accompanied by muscular hypertrophy. Pediatrics 1968; 41:413.)

sory polyneuropathy have been reported; in these cases, motor nerve conduction velocity is reduced to a mild or moderate degree, and nerve biopsies reveal axonal degeneration.[21] Clinical recovery may be slow and incomplete because of the axonal damage. The spinal fluid protein concentration usually is increased in hypothyroidism, regardless of whether neuropathy is present.

As many as 6% of patients with *myasthenia gravis* have hypothyroidism, and autopsy studies show Hashimoto thyroiditis in 12% to 19% of patients with myasthenia.

## DISORDERS OF CALCIUM, PHOSPHORUS, AND MAGNESIUM METABOLISM

### HYPERCALCEMIA

Patients with hypercalcemia often complain of muscle weakness and fatigue, yet no firsthand descriptions exist of rapidly reversible muscle weakness in hypercalcemic states, and it is doubtful that hypercalcemia leads to a motor unit disorder. A few cases of pyramidal tract weakness have been reported, however. Hyperparathyroidism may be associated with a subacute or chronic myopathy.

### HYPOCALCEMIA

Hypocalcemia leads to *tetany*, which is characterized by spontaneous activity of the central and peripheral nervous systems (see Chap. 60). The cerebral form consists of epileptic seizures, and the peripheral form involves paresthesias and muscle spasms, reflecting repetitive discharges of sensory and motor nerves. The longer nerves tend to be activated first, and sensory nerves begin to discharge before motor nerves. An attack of tetany begins with paresthesias in the mouth, fingers, and toes, and proceeds to muscle twitching and spasms in the hands and feet. In severe cases, the spasms may spread to produce opisthotonus and laryngeal stridor.

Latent hypocalcemic tetany can be activated by hyperventilation, because alkalosis lowers the neural excitation threshold, and ionic hypocalcemia is present. Tetany also can be precipitated by the administration of potassium to patients with combined hypokalemia and hypocalcemia.[22] Nerve ischemia also activates latent tetany. This is the basis of the *Trousseau test*, in which a pneumatic cuff is placed around the upper arm and inflated above systolic pressure. In a person with latent tetany, paresthesias and tonic spasm of the intrinsic hand muscles appear within 3 minutes, producing the characteristic hand posture known as *main d'accoucheur* (Fig. 210-5). The Trousseau test is highly sensitive and specific for tetany. Tests of mechanical irritability of nerves (Chvostek and Schultze signs) are nonspecific and unreliable.[23] EMG recordings from the muscles undergoing tetanic spasm (see Fig. 210-3*B*) show a characteristic picture of groups of two or three motor unit potentials discharg-

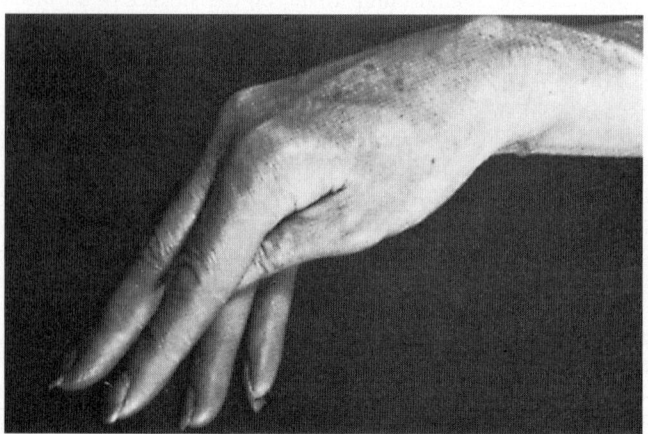

FIGURE 210-5. Tetany. This hand posture (main d'accoucheur) is caused by tonic spasm of the intrinsic hand muscles. (From Spillane JD. An atlas of clinical neurology, 3rd ed. London: Oxford University Press, 1982:295.)

ing rhythmically at a rate of 5 to 15 Hz.[24] The same EMG pattern occurs in tetany caused by alkalosis or hypomagnesemia.

## HYPERMAGNESEMIA

Magnesium, a nervous system depressant, blocks neuromuscular transmission by antagonizing the calcium-dependent release of acetylcholine from motor nerve terminals. A mild elevation of serum magnesium levels (3–5 mEq/L) paralyzes smooth muscle and autonomic nerves, causing dry mouth, flushed skin, hypotension, nausea, and vomiting. Levels above 5 mEq/L, and especially above 9 to 10 mEq/L, cause acute myasthenic paralysis, which includes respiratory and cranial muscles. Disturbances of cardiac conduction may occur if the magnesium level exceeds 10 mEq/L. Cerebral depression does not seem to occur in otherwise normal persons as long as respiration is adequate.[25] Clinical hypermagnesemia usually is caused by the use of magnesium-containing cathartics or antacids, especially in elderly persons or those with renal insufficiency.[26] The intravenous administration of 10 mL of 10% calcium gluconate reverses the paralysis temporarily, until the magnesium level can be lowered by hemodialysis or similar treatment (see Chap. 68).

## HYPOMAGNESEMIA

The main neuromuscular manifestations of magnesium deficiency are tetany and weakness. Magnesium and calcium, which act antagonistically at the neuromuscular junction, have synergistic actions in the excitability of peripheral nerves and brain. The tetany of magnesium deficiency has prominent cerebral features, such as tremor, myoclonus, seizures, and depression, as well as peripheral effects.[27] Carpopedal spasm occurs in hypomagnesemia, but in nearly every case, hypocalcemia (or at least a low ionized calcium concentration) also is present.[28] In practice, however, calcium is not an effective therapy for the tetany of magnesium deficiency, which responds only to magnesium replacement.

Muscle weakness and hyporeflexia occur in some patients, but whether these signs are related directly to magnesium deficiency or are caused by a secondary deficiency of potassium or phosphorus is unclear.

## HYPOPHOSPHATEMIA

Acute hypophosphatemia is encountered in malnourished patients who are given high-calorie feedings deficient in phosphorus. When serum phosphate levels fall below 1.0 mg/dL, disturbances of the central and peripheral nervous system may emerge. The central nervous system symptoms include confusion, coma, involuntary movements, and convulsions; peripheral symptoms consist of numbness and tingling of the face and distal extremities, multiple cranial nerve palsies, areflexic paralysis of the limbs, and acute respiratory failure.[29,30] Hypophosphatemia presumably produces neurologic symptoms by interfering with neuronal energy metabolism. Both the central and peripheral manifestations improve within a few hours when phosphorus is administered, although full recovery may take as long as 2 weeks.

The acute areflexic paralysis presumably is caused by a polyneuropathy. Acute hypophosphatemia also may be associated with *rhabdomyolysis* and *myoglobinuria*, especially during the hospital treatment of malnourished alcoholic patients and patients in diabetic coma. However, severe potassium deficiency may be a contributing factor in such cases. Subclinical muscle injury is common; a transient elevation of serum CK levels has been found in 36% of patients with acute hypophosphatemia.[31]

Chronic phosphorus deficiency may cause an osteomalacic myopathy, as described later.

## OSTEOMALACIA

An atrophic myopathy occurs frequently in vitamin D deficiency, whether of nutritional origin or secondary to malabsorption or vitamin D resistance (see Chap. 63).[32] These patients present a distinctive picture of osteomalacia, bone pain, and slowly progressive, proximal muscle weakness and atrophy that is more severe in the lower extremities. The EMG shows myopathic changes without irritability, the serum CK activity usually is normal, and muscle biopsy shows type II fiber atrophy. The mechanism of this myopathy is entirely unknown. Treatment with vitamin D restores muscle function over a period of many months, but large doses are required in patients with secondary vitamin D deficiency.

A similar myopathy occasionally occurs in patients with chronic renal failure who have uremic osteodystrophy.[33] In patients who are not undergoing dialysis, this complication may be related to impaired renal production of the active metabolite 1,25-dihydroxyvitamin $D_3$, but in patients undergoing long-term hemodialysis, aluminum intoxication may be an important factor (see Chaps. 61 and 131), and vitamin D therapy often is ineffective.[34] Exercise training substantially improves the work capacity of patients receiving hemodialysis.[35]

Chronic phosphorus depletion also causes osteomalacia and an atrophic myopathy.[32] Some cases are caused by inadequate phosphorus intake or overuse of phosphorus-binding antacids, but others are caused by renal phosphaturia (see Chap. 67). When renal hypophosphatemic osteomalacia is associated with a mesenchymal bone tumor, surgical removal of the tumor cures both the myopathy and the metabolic bone disease.[36]

## HYPERPARATHYROIDISM

Muscle weakness is uncommon in hyperparathyroidism, although many patients complain of weakness and fatigability.[36a] When weakness does occur, the hyperparathyroidism is likely to be of the secondary type (associated with osteomalacia), and the clinical picture is the same as in osteomalacic myopathy.[37] Interestingly, muscle strength is increased after surgery for primary hyperparathyroidism.[38]

## HYPOPARATHYROIDISM

Patients with parathyroid deficiency often experience hypocalcemic tetany. In addition, laboratory signs of a myopathy may be present, with moderate elevation of serum levels of CK and other enzymes, and scattered degeneration of muscle fibers on biopsy. Overt muscle weakness is uncommon, however.[39]

# ADRENAL DISORDERS

## HYPERALDOSTERONISM

The neuromuscular complications of hyperaldosteronism (see Chap. 80) result from chronic potassium depletion, which causes muscle weakness, and from the associated metabolic alkalosis, which induces tetany. Muscle weakness occurs in 73% of patients, and symptomatic tetany occurs in 20%.[40] Identical complications can result from the chronic ingestion of licorice (glycyrrhizic acid).

### ACUTE HYPOKALEMIC PARALYSIS

Three distinct syndromes of muscle weakness have been observed in patients with chronic potassium deficiency. Acute hypokalemic paralysis is clinically similar to the familial and

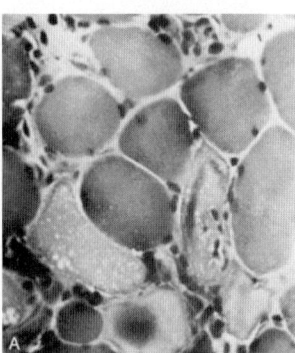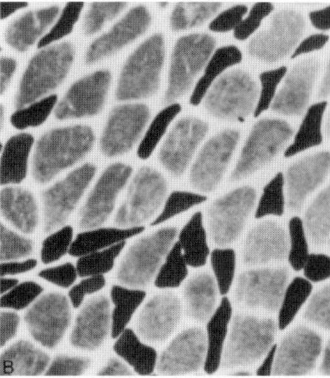

**FIGURE 210-6.** Muscle histopathology in hyperadrenal states. **A,** In hyperaldosteronism, potassium deficiency causes a subacute necrotizing myopathy, with vacuolar degeneration of scattered muscle fibers, some of which are undergoing phagocytosis. (Hematoxylin and eosin.) **B,** Corticosteroid myopathy causes selective atrophy of type II muscle fibers, which appear dark with this myosin adenosine triphosphatase stain. There is no structural damage in this atrophic myopathy. (**A,** From Atsumi T, Ishikawa S, Miyatake T, Yoshida M. Myopathy and primary aldosteronism: electronmicroscopic study. Neurology 1979; 29:1348. **B,** From Dubowitz V, Brooke MH. Muscle biopsy: a modern approach. Philadelphia: WB Saunders, 1978:79.)

thyrotoxic forms of periodic paralysis (see Table 210-2), except that respiratory paralysis is more common in potassium deficiency. The serum potassium level falls at the time of paralysis, as large amounts of extracellular potassium move into muscle. The administration of potassium restores muscle strength in a few hours. Between attacks of paralysis, the serum potassium level usually remains low, and alkalosis may be present. Serum electrolyte levels are normal between attacks of familial or thyrotoxic periodic paralysis.

### MYOPATHY

In other patients with chronic hypokalemia, a subacute or chronic myopathy develops, with gradually progressive weakness of the trunk and proximal limb muscles. The serum CK activity is moderately elevated and, on EMG, myopathic changes often are accompanied by fibrillations and other irritable features. Muscle biopsy shows scattered necrosis and vacuolar degeneration of muscle fibers (Fig. 210-6A), as well as regenerating muscle fibers.[41]

### RHABDOMYOLYSIS AND MYOGLOBINURIA

Rarely, muscle necrosis pursues a fulminating course, resulting in generalized rhabdomyolysis and myoglobinuria. The mechanism of muscle necrosis in chronic potassium deficiency is poorly understood; it may be related to a disturbance of muscle energy metabolism, perhaps at a mitochondrial level.

### CUSHING SYNDROME

Muscle wasting is a regular consequence of chronic exposure to glucocorticoid hormones, but overt muscle weakness is less common. Approximately 50% of patients with Cushing disease have muscle weakness (see Chap. 75). Weakness develops less often in patients receiving corticosteroid therapy, depending on the dose and duration of treatment.[42] At a dose of 15 mg of prednisone per day, corticosteroid myopathy develops in a few patients after many months; with massive corticosteroid doses, myopathy can appear in a few weeks.

Corticosteroid myopathy, whether endogenous or exogenous, is characterized by weakness and atrophy of the hip and thigh muscles, and, later, of muscles of the trunk (especially the anterior neck) and proximal upper extremities. Little or no pain is present. The affected muscles are flabby but not tender.[43] The serum CK activity is normal, and EMG shows only myopathic changes or, in early cases, no abnormality at all. Muscle biopsy shows muscle fiber atrophy, predominantly affecting type II fibers (see Fig. 210-6B). This pathologic change, which also is found in corticosteroid-treated patients who are not weak, suggests disuse atrophy, as if the affected muscle fibers were electrically inexcitable; however, the evidence for this is disputed.[44] Depending on the severity of the myopathy, the weakness resolves in a few weeks or months when corticosteroid therapy is withdrawn. Lowering the dose also may be sufficient, but knowing in advance what dose is safe is difficult. Less commonly, a severe, rapidly progressive myopathy, sometimes involving the respiratory muscles, has been seen in critically ill patients receiving high-dose steroid therapy after organ transplantation or during treatment for severe pulmonary disorders or sepsis. They usually have received neuromuscular blocking drugs. Serum CK levels may be normal or markedly elevated. Muscle biopsy in some cases shows a peculiar dissolution of the myosin thick filaments. The myopathy resolves gradually when steroid therapy is withdrawn.[45]

### ADRENAL INSUFFICIENCY

Subjective weakness and easy fatigue are leading symptoms of Addison disease, but objective weakness probably is uncommon. Spontaneous pain in the limbs or trunk was emphasized in early descriptions more than in recent accounts. However, a few patients with primary or secondary hypoadrenalism have come to medical attention because of bizarre, extremely painful muscle spasms and rigidity, mainly involving the trunk and lower extremities. The spasms are triggered by touching or manipulating the limbs, and thus resemble the reflex spasms of tetanus or of the stiff-man syndrome.[46–48] Some patients develop flexion contractures of the lower extremities. Glucocorticoid therapy relieves these symptoms, but mineralocorticoid therapy is ineffective (see Chap. 76).

### ACUTE AREFLEXIC PARALYSIS

The chronic hyperkalemia of adrenal insufficiency occasionally brings on an attack of acute areflexic paralysis, which may include respiratory, facial, or bulbar weakness. Clinically, this syndrome resembles an acute polyneuropathy, because reflexes are depressed or absent, and distal paresthesias and numbness usually are present.[49] An identical picture occurs in hyperkalemia resulting from chronic renal failure or from treatment with spironolactone or triamterene. Serum potassium levels during the attack usually are between 7.5 and 11.5 mEq/L; prompt treatment is required to prevent fatal cardiac arrhythmia. Depending on the circumstances, the intravenous administration of hydrocortisone, isotonic saline, sodium bicarbonate, glucose, and insulin should restore muscle power in a few hours, although reflexes and sensation may not return to normal for several days.

### ADRENOLEUKODYSTROPHY

A peripheral neuropathy may accompany progressive adrenal failure in patients with adrenoleukodystrophy, an X-linked recessive disorder of lipid metabolism. Testicular dysfunction is also common.[50] The neuropathy has been noted mainly in patients with the spinal form (adrenomyeloneuropathy), in whom progressive spastic paraplegia develops in the second or third decade of life.[51]

# GONADAL DISORDERS

A relative muscle hypertrophy occurs in both boys and girls with premature sexual development (see Chap. 92).

In male hypogonadism, the muscular development usually is diminished. This is particularly marked in men with prepubertal gonadal deficiency. Androgen replacement increases muscle mass in such cases, and preliminary studies suggest that androgen therapy may have a similar effect in normal elderly men.[52]

Gynecomastia and a variable degree of hypogonadism are among the clinical features of an X-linked type of hereditary spinal muscular atrophy known as *bulbospinal neuronopathy*. The disease has been traced to mutations within the androgen-receptor gene, consisting of enlargement of an unstable trinucleotide repeat.[53] Hypogonadism often occurs in myotonic muscular dystrophy.[53a]

# DISORDERS OF FUEL METABOLISM

## STARVATION

Prolonged starvation leads to the marked loss of fat and muscle tissue, a condition known as *cachexia*. A similar phenomenon occurs when catabolic processes are accelerated by infection, burns, trauma, or cancer. Despite their emaciated appearance, adult patients usually have normal muscle power as judged by standard clinical tests, and EMG shows no abnormality. Maximum muscle strength and exercise capacity are reduced in proportion to the reduction of muscle mass.[54] In the wasting syndrome of acquired immunodeficiency syndrome (AIDS), testosterone administration increases muscle mass and general well-being, but not functional exercise capacity.[55] In contrast, severely malnourished infants and children often exhibit generalized or proximal muscle weakness, hypotonia, and hyporeflexia, and electrodiagnostic tests reveal an axonal type of sensorimotor polyneuropathy.[56] These abnormalities are reversed with improved nutrition.

## OBESITY

The treatment of morbid obesity by gastrointestinal surgery, such as gastric partitioning or jejunoileal bypass, may cause a severe sensorimotor polyneuropathy, with electrophysiologic signs of axonal degeneration.

Thiamine deficiency has been implicated in the pathogenesis of this disorder.[57] Beriberi is still reported occasionally in otherwise healthy young Japanese men who engage in strenuous physical activity while consuming a carbohydrate-rich diet poor in thiamine.[58] The typical clinical picture includes a distal sensorimotor axonal polyneuropathy, pain and tenderness in the calf muscles, elevated serum CK levels, and edema of the face and ankles. Thiamine replacement leads to slow recovery.

Obesity is associated with carpal tunnel syndrome. The pathophysiologic mechanism is not clear.[59]

## ANOREXIA NERVOSA AND BULIMIA

The main neuromuscular complication of anorexia nervosa and bulimia is a subacute or chronic myopathy caused by chronic potassium depletion, which results from various combinations of starvation, self-induced vomiting, and concealed abuse of diuretics and laxatives.[60,61] The hypokalemic myopathy, similar to that caused by hyperaldosteronism, may be accompanied by alkalotic tetany, and hypovolemia may cause lassitude and orthostatic hypotension (see Chap. 128). Rarely, malnutrition alone, without vomiting or purging, causes an overt myopathy with respiratory muscle weakness, in the absence of electrolyte derangement.[62]

# DIABETES MELLITUS

The various forms of diabetic neuropathy are discussed in Chapter 148. A different complication, acute infarction of thigh muscles, has been reported in a few patients.[63] In this disorder, deep pain, swelling, and tenderness appear suddenly in one thigh. The condition resolves in a few weeks but is followed in a few months by a similar process in the other thigh. Most affected patients are women in the third and fourth decades of life. This rare condition requires a period of bed rest, with immobilization of the affected limb, to prevent hemorrhage in the damaged muscle.

# HYPOGLYCEMIA

Hypoglycemia influences muscle metabolism.[64] Patients with an insulinoma (see Chap. 158) may develop distal muscle weakness and atrophy, which often are worse in the upper extremities.[65] In 67% of patients, distal sensory symptoms also are present, and some have objective sensory deficits. The neuropathic symptoms may begin either abruptly or gradually, and usually are preceded by one or more episodes of hypoglycemic confusion or coma. Electrodiagnostic tests and autopsy studies suggest that the primary pathology is in the motor neurons of the spinal cord and in the dorsal root ganglia. After removal of the pancreatic tumor, motor and sensory function may show partial recovery, but most patients are left with some permanent deficits.

# REFERENCES

1. Layzer RB. Neuromuscular manifestations of systemic disease. Philadelphia: FA Davis Co, 1985.
2. Aminoff MJ. Electromyography in clinical practice, 3rd ed. New York: Churchill Livingstone, 1998.
3. Pickett JBE, Layzer RB, Levin SR, et al. Neuromuscular complications of acromegaly. Neurology 1975; 25:638.
4. Mastaglia FL. Pathological changes in skeletal muscle in acromegaly. Acta Neuropathol (Berl) 1973; 24:273.
5. Kameyama S, Tanaka R, Hasegawa A, et al. Subclinical carpal tunnel syndrome in acromegaly. Neurol Med Chir (Tokyo) 1993; 33:547.
6. Prineas J, Hall R, Barwick DD, Watson AJ. Myopathy associated with pigmentation following adrenalectomy for Cushing's syndrome. Q J Med 1968; 37:63.
7. Ramsay ID. Thyroid disease and muscle dysfunction. Chicago: Year Book Medical Publishers, 1974.
8. Puvanendran K, Cheah JS, Naganathan N, Wong PK. Thyrotoxic myopathy. A clinical and quantitative analytic electromyographic study. J Neurol Sci 1979; 42:441.
9. Kammer GM, Hamilton CR. Acute bulbar muscle dysfunction and hyperthyroidism. A study of four cases and review of the literature. Am J Med 1974; 56:464.
10. Feibel JH, Campa JF. Thyrotoxic neuropathy (Basedow's paraplegia). J Neurol Neurosurg Psychiatry 1976; 39:491.
11. McFadzean AJS, Yeung R. Periodic paralysis complicating thyrotoxicosis in Chinese. BMJ 1967; 1:451.
12. Tamai H, Tanaka K, Komaki G, et al. HLA and thyrotoxic periodic paralysis in Japanese patients. J Clin Endocrinol Metab 1987; 64:1075.
13. Yeung RTT, Tse TF. Thyrotoxic periodic paralysis. Effect of propranolol. Am J Med 1974; 57:584.
14. Layzer RB. Medical progress: periodic paralysis and the Na-K pump. Ann Neurol 1982; 6:547.
15. Ptacek LJ, Griggs RC, Tawil R, et al. Dihydropyridine receptor mutations cause hypokalemic periodic paralysis. Cell 1994; 77:863.
16. Mizusawa H, Takagi A, Sugita H, Toyokura Y. Mounding phenomenon. An experimental study in vitro. Neurology 1983; 33:90.
17. Najjar SS. Muscular hypertrophy in hypothyroid children: the Kocher-Debré-Sémélaigne syndrome. J Pediatr 1974; 85:236.
18. Karlsberg RP, Roberts R. Effect of altered thyroid function on plasma creatine kinase clearance in the dog. Am J Physiol 1978; 235:E614.
19. Rao SN, Katiyar BC, Nair KRP, Misra S. Neuromuscular status in hypothyroidism. Acta Neurol Scand 1980; 61:167.
20. Sekine N, Yamamoto M, Michikawa M, et al. Rhabdomyolysis and acute renal failure in a patient with hypothyroidism. Intern Med 1993; 32:269.
21. Pollard JD, McLeod JG, Angel Honnibal TG, Verheijden MA. Hypothyroid polyneuropathy. Clinical, electrophysiological and nerve biopsy findings in two cases. J Neurol Sci 1982; 53:461.
22. Navarro J, Oster JR, Gkonos PJ, et al. Tetany induced on separate occasions by administration of potassium and magnesium in a patient with hungry-bone syndrome. Miner Electrolyte Metab 1991; 17:340.

23. Schaff M, Payne CA. Diphenylhydantoin and phenobarbital in overt and latent tetany. N Engl J Med 1966; 274:1228.
24. Kugelberg E. Activation of human nerves by ischemia. Trousseau's phenomenon in tetany. Arch Neurol Psychiatry 1948; 60:140.
25. Somjen G, Hilmy M, Stephen CR. Failure to anesthetize human subjects by intravenous administration of magnesium sulfate. J Pharmacol Exp Ther 1966; 154:652.
26. Clark BA, Brown RS. Unsuspected morbid hypermagnesemia in elderly patients. Am J Nephrol 1992; 12:336.
27. Abbott LG, Rude RK. Clinical manifestations of magnesium deficiency. Miner Electrolyte Metab 1993; 19:314.
28. Zimmet P, Breidahl HD, Nayler WG. Plasma ionized calcium in hypomagnesemia. BMJ 1968; 1:622.
29. Furlan AJ, Hanson M, Cooperman A, Farmer RG. Acute areflexic paralysis. Association with hyperalimentation and hypophosphatemia. Arch Neurol 1975; 32:706.
30. Finck GA, Mai C, Gregor M. Passagere polyneuropathie mit Hirnnervenbeteiligung durch Hypophosphatämie. Nervenarzt 1979; 50:778.
31. Singhal PC, Kumar A, Desroches L, et al. Prevalence and predictors of rhabdomyolysis in patients with hypophosphatemia. Am J Med 1992; 92:458.
32. Schott GD, Wills MR. Muscle weakness in osteomalacia. Lancet 1976; 1:626.
33. Floyd M, Ayyar DR, Barwick DD, et al. Myopathy in chronic renal failure. QJM 1974; 53:509.
34. Ward MK, Feest TG, Ellis HA, et al. Osteomalacic dialysis osteodystrophy: evidence for a water-borne aetiological agent, probably aluminium. Lancet 1978; 1:841.
35. Moore GE, Parsons DB, Stray-Gundersen J, et al. Uremic myopathy limits aerobic capacity in hemodialysis patients. Am J Kidney Dis 1993; 22:277.
36. Pollack JA, Schiller AL, Crawford JD. Rickets and myopathy cured by removal of nonossifying fibroma of bone. Pediatrics 1973; 52:364.
36a. Deutch SR, Jonsen MB, Christiansen PM, et al. Muscular performance and fatigue in primary hyperparathyroidism. World J Surg 2000; 24:102.
37. Smith R, Stern G. Muscular weakness in osteomalacia and hyperparathyroidism. J Neurol Sci 1969; 8:511.
38. Chou FF, Sheen-Chen SM, Leong CP. Neuromuscular recovery after parathyroidectomy in primary hyperparathyroidism. Surgery 1995; 117:18.
39. Shane E, McClane KA, Olarte MR, Bilezikian JP. Hypoparathyroidism and elevated serum enzymes. Neurology 1980; 30:192.
40. Conn JW. Aldosteronism in man. Some clinical and climatological aspects. Part II. JAMA 1963; 183:871.
41. Atsumi T, Ishikawa S, Miyatake T, Yoshida M. Myopathy and primary aldosteronism: electronmicroscopic study. Neurology 1979; 29:1348.
42. Ross EJ, Linch DC. Cushing's syndrome killing disease: discriminatory value of signs and symptoms aiding early diagnosis. Lancet 1982; 2:646.
43. Afifi AK, Bergman RA, Harvey JC. Steroid myopathy. Clinical, histologic and cytologic observations. Johns Hopkins Med J 1968; 123:158.
44. Ruff RL, Stühmer W, Almers W. Effect of glucocorticoid treatment on the excitability of rat skeletal muscle. Pflugers Arch 1982; 395:132.
45. Lacomis D, Giuliani MJ, Van Cott A, Kramer DJ. Acute myopathy of intensive care: clinical, electromyographic and pathological aspects. Ann Neurol 1996; 40:645.
46. Castaigne P, Laplane D, Mauvais-Jarvis P, et al. Contractures des membres inférieurs au cours dun panhypopituitarisme. Ann Med Interne (Paris) 1975; 126:591.
47. George TM, Burke JM, Sobotka PA, et al. Resolution of stiff-man syndrome with cortisol replacement in a patient with deficiencies of ACTH, growth hormone, and prolactin. N Engl J Med 1984; 310:1511.
48. Lorish TR, Thorsteinsson G, Howard FM Jr. Stiff-man syndrome updated. Mayo Clin Proc 1989; 64:629.
49. Van Dellen RG, Purnell DC. Hyperkalemic paralysis in Addison's disease. Mayo Clin Proc 1969; 44:904.
50. Brenneman W, Kohler W, Zierz S, Klingmuller D. Testicular dysfunction in adrenomyeloneuropathy. Eur J Endocrinol 1997; 137:34.
51. Del Mastro RG, Bundey S, Kilpatrick MW. Adrenoleucodystrophy: a molecular genetic study in five families. J Med Genet 1990; 27:670.
52. Swerdloff RS, Wang C. Androgen deficiency and aging in men. West J Med 1993; 159:579.
53. La Spada AR, Wilson EM, Lubahn DB, et al. Androgen receptor gene mutations in X-linked spinal and bulbar muscular atrophy. Nature 1991; 352:77.
53a. Marchini C, Lonigro R, Verriello L, et al. Correlations between individual clinical manifestations and CTG repeat amplification in myotonic dystrophy. Clin Genet 2000; 57:74.
54. Lands L, Pavilanis A, Charge TD, Coates AL. Cardiopulmonary response to exercise in anorexia nervosa. Pediatr Pulmonol 1992; 13:101.
55. Grinspoon S, Corcoran C, Askari H, et al. Effects of androgen stimulation in men with AIDS-wasting syndrome. A double-blind, placebo-controlled trial. Ann Intern Med 1998; 128:18.
56. Chopra JS, Sharma A. Protein energy malnutrition and the nervous system. J Neurol Sci 1992; 110:8.
57. Maryniak O. Severe peripheral neuropathy following gastric bypass surgery for morbid obesity. Can Med Assoc J 1984; 131:119.
58. Yabuki S, Nakaya K, Sugimura T, et al. Juvenile polyneuropathy due to vitamin B$_1$ deficiency—clinical observations and pathogenetic analysis of 24 cases. Folia Psychiatr Neurol Jpn 1976; 30:517.
59. Stallings SP, Kasdan ML, Soergel TM, Corwin HM. A case-control study of obesity as a risk factor for carpal tunnel syndrome in a population of 600 patients presenting for independent medical examination. J Hand Surg 1997; 22:211.
60. Wolff HP, Vecsei P, Krück F, et al. Psychiatric disturbance leading to potassium depletion, sodium depletion, raised plasma-renin concentration, and secondary hyperaldosteronism. Lancet 1968; 1:257.
61. Mcloughlin DM, Wassif WS, Morton J, et al. Metabolic abnormalities associated with skeletal myopathy in severe anorexia nervosa. Nutrition 2000; 16:192.
62. Ryan CF, Whittaker JS, Road JD. Ventilatory dysfunction in severe anorexia nervosa. Chest 1992; 102:1286.
63. Barohn RJ, Kissel JT. Case-of-the-month: painful thigh mass in a young woman: diabetic muscle infarction. Muscle Nerve 1992; 15:850.
64. Winder WW, Carling JM, Duan C, et al. Muscle fructose-2, 6-bisphosphate and glucose-1-6-bisphosphate during insulin-induced hypoglycemia. J Appl Physiol 1994; 76:853.
65. Tintore M, Montalban J, Cervere C, et al. Peripheral neuropathy in association with insulinoma: clinical features and neuropathy of a new case. J Neurol Neurosurg Psychiatr 1994; 57:1009.

# CHAPTER 211

# RHEUMATIC MANIFESTATIONS OF ENDOCRINE DISEASE

DAVID J. NASHEL

Many of the earliest descriptions of endocrine dysfunction highlight symptomatology referable to the joints and periarticular structures. That perturbations of the endocrine system often are manifested by rheumatic complaints is not surprising. The principal elements of connective tissue are cells (e.g., fibroblasts, chondrocytes) and ground substance, which consists of fibers (collagen, reticulin, and elastin) and large proteoglycan molecules. Hormones play a substantial role in the growth of these cells, as well as in the synthesis and degradation of the macromolecules. Consequently, through the action of various hormones, endocrine glands directly affect the structure and function of the musculoskeletal system.[1]

## PITUITARY AND HYPOTHALAMIC DISORDERS

### ACROMEGALIC ARTHROPATHY

Joint and spine disorders are common in patients with acromegaly.[1a] The changes of acromegalic arthropathy stem from the effects of chronic elevation of growth hormone and insulin-like growth factor-I on cartilage and bone metabolism.[2] Initially, an accelerated and often nonuniform growth of chondrocytes occurs, resulting in an uneven thickening of the articular cartilage and fissuring of the surface layer. In addition, hypertrophy of the articular cartilage causes crepitation and a characteristic radiographic change of widened joint space. Synovial thickening frequently leads to pain and swelling about the joints. Eventually, ulcerations of the cartilage develop that, along with joint hypermobility, cause a process similar to degenerative joint disease. This severe degenerative process may dominate the clinical picture. Treatment of the underlying disease with octreotide has been associated with improvement in joint pain.[3] With the use of ultrasonography, a decrease in cartilage thickness after octreotide therapy has been demonstrated.[4,4a] In more severely affected large joints such as hips or knees, total joint arthroplasty may be required.

In the spine, thickening of the intervertebral disk causes the radiographic finding of an increased disk space. Marked osteophyte formation can occur, which explains the frequent complaints of backache. Yet, despite the bony overgrowth that occurs in the lumbar and thoracic vertebrae, spinal mobility often is maintained, perhaps because of increased laxity of the paraspinal ligaments.[1a]

# ACROMEGALIC NEUROMUSCULAR DISEASE

## CARPAL TUNNEL SYNDROME

Carpal tunnel syndrome is a common accompaniment of acromegaly. More than one-third of all patients with acromegaly have median nerve compression, and it frequently is bilateral.[5] The compression may stem from synovial edema and hyperplasia of tendons. Even in asymptomatic patients, median nerve conduction velocities are frequently abnormal.[6] Unlike acromegalic arthropathy, this syndrome is often rapidly abolished by treatment of the pituitary overactivity.

## MYOPATHY

Acromegaly is frequently accompanied by myopathy. This myopathic process is characterized by proximal muscle weakness, atrophy and, at times, myalgia.[7] Creatine kinase is variably elevated, and muscle biopsy demonstrates predominantly type II fiber atrophy.[8] In some cases the myopathy improves slowly after hypophysectomy.

## EXOGENOUS GROWTH HORMONE ABUSE

The use of synthetic growth hormone by athletes in an attempt to alter body composition and improve performance, although banned by regulatory committees, is an increasingly common problem in the sports environment. Clinicians need to be aware of the potential for these individuals to develop acromegalic complications similar to those noted above.

## HYPOTHALAMIC DISORDERS

Hypothalamic hypopituitarism may infrequently cause rheumatic complaints.[9] Conversely, this condition may result from injury to the hypothalamus and pituitary in the setting of temporal arteritis. Interestingly, the syndrome of inappropriate antidiuretic hormone secretion occurs in patients with polyarteritis nodosa and temporal arteritis.[10]

# THYROID DISEASE

## HYPOTHYROIDISM

Patients with hypothyroidism may have various rheumatic symptoms, ranging from generalized aching of joints and muscles to paresthesias of the fingers and acute arthritis. Thyroid studies should be considered in any patient who presents with such findings, especially elderly individuals, in whom unrecognized thyroid dysfunction is common.

### MYXEDEMA ARTHROPATHY

Swelling, pain, and stiffness of the large joints is a frequent accompaniment of myxedema.[11] The radiographic findings are nonspecific and may include joint space narrowing, osteolytic lesions, loose bodies, and chondrocalcinosis. The synovial fluid is characterized by a normal cell count, but often a striking increase in viscosity is seen.[12]

Typically, the patients are unresponsive to treatment with antiinflammatory drugs, but recover when given thyroid replacement.

### MYOPATHY AND FIBROMYALGIA SYNDROME (FIBROSITIS)

Muscle symptoms are common in untreated hypothyroidism.[13] Patients with hypothyroid myopathy usually have proximal

muscle weakness and often complain of myalgias or cramps. Because serum creatine kinase activity is often increased, sometimes markedly, the picture may simulate that of polymyositis.[14] Several cases of exercise-induced rhabdomyolysis in the setting of hypothyroidism have also been reported.[15] After thyroid-replacement therapy, the muscle and laboratory abnormalities resolve. Hypothyroidism should be considered in any case in which unexplained creatine kinase elevation occurs.

Because muscle stiffness is a common symptom in the hypothyroid patient, the disease may first be diagnosed as polymyalgia rheumatica, especially in the elderly. Other patients with subclinical hypothyroidism may have a fibromyalgia (fibrositis)-like picture,[16] characterized by the presence of widespread pain and stiffness, local tender points in some patients, and normal laboratory study results. The symptoms may be alleviated with the use of thyroid hormone–replacement therapy.

### CARPAL TUNNEL SYNDROME

Carpal tunnel syndrome is found in as many as 10% of patients with hypothyroidism, and it may be the presenting symptom. Compression of the median nerve probably arises from deposition of mucopolysaccharide in the carpal tunnel and from thickening of flexor tendon sheaths. Median nerve conduction abnormalities are common in untreated patients.[17] Surgical treatment usually can be avoided, because thyroid-replacement therapy often relieves the problem.

### GOUT AND HYPERURICEMIA

Hyperuricemia may result from impaired renal excretion of uric acid caused by diminished thyroid hormone. A significant increase in hypothyroidism was observed in patients with crystal-proven gouty arthritis: up to 40% in women and 15% in men.[18]

## HYPERTHYROIDISM

### THYROID ACROPACHY

Thyroid acropachy, an unusual manifestation of Graves disease, occurs in 0.1% to 1% of patients.[19] This syndrome consists of clubbing of the fingers, soft-tissue swelling of the hands and feet, and periosteal new bone formation (see Chap. 42). Exophthalmos and circumscribed (pretibial) myxedema are associated with thyroid acropachy so often that they are thought to be an integral part of the syndrome. A long interval may occur between the onset of hyperthyroidism and the development of acropachy. When it appears after therapy, it has been alleged to occur predominantly in those patients who are treated by thyroidectomy or radioactive iodine, as opposed to antithyroid drugs. A mild synovitis may be noted, and patients complain of stiffness in the affected extremities.

On radiographic examination, the periosteal bone reaction most commonly involves the diaphysial region of the metacarpal and metatarsal bones. This new bone formation has an irregular and lacy appearance. Thyroid acropachy must be differentiated from other conditions in which periosteal bone formation may be a prominent feature, such as hypertrophic pulmonary osteoarthropathy and pachydermoperiostosis (see Chap. 218).

### CARPAL TUNNEL SYNDROME

Several reports have been published of carpal tunnel syndrome occurring in the setting of Graves disease.[20] In a prospective study, carpal tunnel syndrome was found in 5% of patients at the time of diagnosis. The neurologic symptoms resolved with control of the endocrinopathy.[21]

## GIANT CELL ARTERITIS

Several studies have linked autoimmune thyroid disease (most often Graves disease) to the development of giant cell arteritis. In one study, 8.5% of patients with giant cell arteritis had a history of thyrotoxicosis.[22] Alternatively, in an investigation of patients with autoimmune thyroid disease, 2.8% of patients were found to have either polymyalgia rheumatica or giant cell arteritis.[23] Thus, particular attention should be given to the possible presence of arteritis in elderly women who have thyroid disease.

## DRUG-INDUCED RHEUMATISM

Rheumatic symptoms develop in some patients receiving thyroxine replacement for thyroid disease.[24] The clinical complaints include morning stiffness, weakness, and shoulder girdle pain, a constellation often seen in polymyalgia rheumatica. Antithyroid medications also have been associated with musculoskeletal symptoms. In this setting, patients may have severe arthralgias without swelling, often necessitating the use of antiinflammatory drugs for pain relief. These symptoms regress with time.

## HASHIMOTO THYROIDITIS

### CONNECTIVE TISSUE DISEASE

Lymphocytic (Hashimoto) thyroiditis may be associated with various connective tissue diseases, including rheumatoid arthritis, systemic lupus erythematosus (SLE), scleroderma, and Sjögren syndrome.[25] Moreover, patients with Hashimoto thyroiditis have an unusual syndrome of chest wall discomfort, notable for pain in the thoracic and shoulder girdle areas.[26] Patients complain of a dull, aching pain that is unrelated to respiration but may improve with changes in position. The extensive laboratory and radiographic evaluations that may be triggered by this symptom usually are unrevealing.

### SERONEGATIVE ARTHRITIS

Some patients who have seronegative (rheumatoid factor–negative) polyarthritis ultimately are found to have Hashimoto thyroiditis. The arthritis, which involves the hands and feet, is characterized by swelling, tenderness, and joint effusions. It differs from the arthritis associated with myxedema in that it is more inflammatory and does not improve with thyroid replacement.

## PARATHYROID DISEASE

### HYPERPARATHYROIDISM

Rheumatic symptoms develop in approximately half of all patients with primary hyperparathyroidism.[27] Myalgias are the most common complaint, and a mistaken diagnosis of polymyalgia rheumatica may be entertained when, in elderly patients, the complaints are limited to the shoulder girdle.

### HYPERPARATHYROID ARTHROPATHY

Patients with hyperparathyroidism often have articular symptoms involving the knees, wrists, shoulders, and hands. Because the presenting complaint of these patients may be polyarthritis, the condition initially may be misdiagnosed as rheumatoid arthritis. Joint lesions are postulated to result from a direct effect of parathyroid hormone on collagen, causing ligamentous laxity and joint instability.

A distinctive erosive arthritis also may occur, commonly involving the metacarpophalangeal and radiocarpal joints.[28] The erosions are not inflammatory and result from resorption and collapse of subchondral bone, with subsequent changes in the overlying cartilage. Unlike in rheumatoid arthritis, erosions are predominantly on the ulnar aspect of the joints, the joint space is not narrowed significantly, and the proximal interphalangeal joints are affected less often. A traumatic type of synovitis may ensue, followed by a secondary type of degenerative joint disease.[29]

Also noted is an unusual shoulder arthropathy consisting of intraarticular and periarticular erosions of the head of the humerus.[30] No calcium deposits are seen in the shoulder joints, and patients are asymptomatic. A similar arthropathy occurs in patients receiving long-term hemodialysis in whom secondary hyperparathyroidism develops.

Scintigraphy of joints with $^{99m}$technetium pyrophosphate appears to be more sensitive than standard radiography for revealing bone disease associated with hyperparathyroidism and for observing changes in joints after parathyroidectomy.

### CALCIUM PYROPHOSPHATE DIHYDRATE DEPOSITION DISEASE

In patients with hyperparathyroidism, chondrocalcinosis (articular cartilage calcification), the radiographic marker for calcium pyrophosphate dihydrate crystal deposition disease, is a relatively common finding, with a reported prevalence of 18% to 37%.[31] Interestingly, higher serum levels of parathyroid hormone and calcium, as well as larger size of the parathyroid gland, correlate with the development of chondrocalcinosis. Moreover, when many patients with chondrocalcinosis are examined, a higher than expected prevalence of both hypoparathyroidism and hyperparathyroidism is found, especially in more elderly patients.[32]

By 70 years of age, approximately half of all patients with hyperparathyroidism have radiographic evidence of cartilage calcifications. Such cartilage calcifications may be the only radiographic evidence for the diagnosis of hyperparathyroidism, because osteitis fibrosa cystica develops in less than half of these patients. These calcifications are most common in the wrists and knees (Fig. 211-1), and they take on a linear or punctate appearance much like that noted in primary chondrocalcinosis.

Most patients with chondrocalcinosis associated with hyperparathyroidism have hypercalcemia. However, normocalcemic hyperparathormonemia is found in some patients with primary

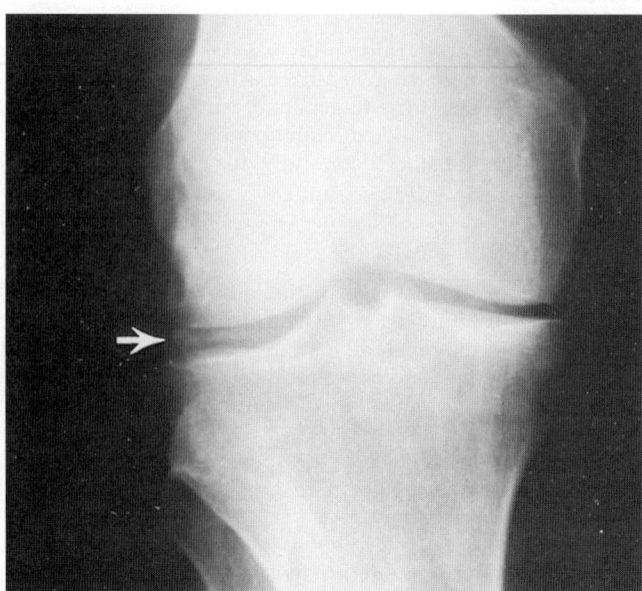

**FIGURE 211-1.** Chondrocalcinosis involving the fibrocartilage of the knee (*arrow*).

chondrocalcinosis. Chondrocalcinosis usually is absent in patients with secondary hyperparathyroidism, except in the setting of azotemic osteodystrophy and associated hypercalcemia.

### PYROPHOSPHATE ARTHROPATHY (PSEUDOGOUT) AND GOUT

Pseudogout occurs in patients with hyperparathyroidism and is found after the removal of parathyroid adenomas.[32a] Rapid shifts in calcium, as may occur after parathyroidectomy, may induce shedding of calcium pyrophosphate crystals into the joint, initiating synovitis. Just as a decrease in the serum calcium level may precipitate pseudogout, it also may cause acute calcific periarthritis.

Both hyperuricemia and gouty arthritis are reported in patients with hyperparathyroidism. Gout or hyperuricemia also may follow parathyroidectomy.[33]

### HYPOPARATHYROIDISM

Soft-tissue calcification involving the paraspinal region, as well as the shoulders and hips, is found in patients with idiopathic hypoparathyroidism. Calcifications of muscles and tendons, and paraspinal calcifications indistinguishable from diffuse idiopathic skeletal hyperostosis may occur.[34] Soft-tissue calcification also is a well-recognized complication of pseudohypoparathyroidism.

## CORTICOSTEROID-RELATED DISEASE

### HYPERCORTISOLISM: ASEPTIC NECROSIS

Aseptic (avascular) necrosis of bone may result from endogenous or exogenous hypercortisolism. Rarely, aseptic necrosis has been associated with functioning adrenal tumors and with Cushing disease.[35]

Approximately half of all patients with aseptic necrosis have received, or are receiving, corticosteroid therapy. Patients given corticosteroids after renal transplantation and for the treatment of SLE are particularly vulnerable.[36] Although the total dosage and duration of therapy are crucial factors in the etiology of aseptic necrosis, the administration of high dosages of corticosteroids for even a few weeks or months may be a more important predisposing factor.

The joints most frequently involved in aseptic necrosis are the hips, knees, and shoulders. Radiographic abnormalities may not become apparent for months to years after clinical symptoms begin. The earliest changes consist of subchondral radiolucencies, followed by the appearance of areas of sclerosis and osteoporosis. Later, changes in the bony contour and, finally, collapse and fragmentation of the bone may occur (Fig. 211-2).

For treatment purposes, recognizing the bone lesion in its earliest stages is important. If the presence of aseptic necrosis is strongly suspected, radionuclide bone scanning or magnetic resonance imaging are more likely to reveal the pathologic process in the initial stage than is radiography.

The treatment of avascular necrosis is controversial. If it is feasible, consideration should be given to discontinuing the use of or decreasing the dosage of any concurrent corticosteroid therapy. When disease of the femoral head is recognized in an early phase, some investigators advocate a core decompression procedure.[37] With more advanced disease, surgical joint replacement often is necessary.

### HYPOCORTISOLISM

Some patients who have been treated with corticosteroids for extended periods develop rheumatic symptoms when the dos-

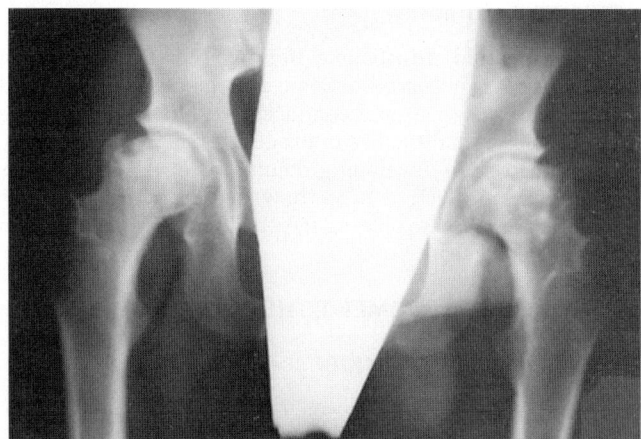

**FIGURE 211-2.** Aseptic (avascular) necrosis in a patient who had received long-term treatment with corticosteroids. Advanced disease is present involving both femoral heads, with flattening and collapse of the articular surfaces.

age is tapered or abruptly discontinued. This has been termed the *steroid withdrawal syndrome*.[38] Often, these symptoms cannot be correlated with suppression of hypothalamic–pituitary–adrenal function.

Myalgias and periarticular discomfort have been reported in the setting of adrenal insufficiency.[39] Some of these patients have radiologically identifiable tendon calcifications.[40]

## SEX HORMONES

The sex hormones have important immunoregulatory effects.[41] Generally, androgens suppress immunoreactivity, whereas estrogens augment this process. Alterations in hormone levels, as well as therapy with these agents, may induce or alter the course of certain autoimmune disorders.

### ORAL CONTRACEPTIVES

#### SYSTEMIC LUPUS ERYTHEMATOSUS

Estrogens appear to play an important role in the pathogenesis of SLE. The female predominance in the disease, the observation of abnormal estrogen metabolism in lupus patients, and studies in murine models of SLE all support this concept. Some women taking oral contraceptives show positive results on tests for antinuclear antibodies (see Chaps. 104 and 105), whereas some develop Raynaud phenomenon, arthralgias, or overt arthritis.[42] Usually, the symptoms resolve when use of the drug is discontinued. Sometimes, however, the clinical and laboratory findings persist and a syndrome indistinguishable from SLE ensues. Then, the use of oral contraceptives may have unmasked subclinical SLE.

Whether oral contraceptive use exacerbates preexistent SLE is a matter of some dispute. Some clinicians believe that they are safe to use if the underlying disease is inactive.[43] Others avoid using these drugs in the belief that they often cause a flare in disease activity. Some patients with underlying renal disease are reported to have serious worsening of their kidney lesions and to develop deep venous thrombosis in the presence of high levels of antiphospholipid antibodies.[44] The potential for oral contraceptives to induce an increase in disease activity appears to be associated with the estrogen content, even when they are used in low dosages.[45] Alternatively, progesterone preparations do not have this effect and are preferred in patients with SLE for whom other contraceptive methods are not feasible.

### RHEUMATOID ARTHRITIS

Just as rheumatoid arthritis may improve during pregnancy, a salutary effect is observed in some patients with rheumatoid arthritis who are given oral contraceptives. In addition, some evidence is seen that the use of exogenous sex hormones may decrease the risk of developing rheumatoid arthritis.[46] Rather than having a protective effect, however, oral contraceptives may modify the disease process, thereby preventing progression to more severe disease.[47]

## HORMONE-REPLACEMENT THERAPY

### SYSTEMIC LUPUS ERYTHEMATOSUS

With the increasing use of postmenopausal estrogen hormone-replacement therapy (HRT), concerns have arisen as to whether this therapy increases the risk for development of SLE or whether it might exacerbate existing disease. One study has shown that, although short-term estrogen exposure was not associated with increased risk, use of estrogen for 2 or more years significantly increased the chances of developing SLE.[48] The risk was somewhat diminished when estrogen was used in combination with progestins.

The effect of HRT in patients with existing lupus disease has been examined in follow-up studies of 1 and 3 years' duration respectively.[49,50] In neither study was the risk of disease flare increased during the observation period.

### RHEUMATOID ARTHRITIS

Osteoporosis is a significant complication of rheumatoid disease and its treatment with corticosteroids. Although HRT has not been shown to significantly alter rheumatoid arthritis disease activity, it does improve bone density and contributes to a patient's sense of well-being.[51] Measurement of markers of bone metabolism reveal that HRT reduces bone resorption even in patients receiving corticosteroids.[52]

## DIABETES MELLITUS

Several rheumatic syndromes occur in patients with both insulin-dependent (type 1) and non–insulin-dependent (type 2) diabetes mellitus.[53] Because the course of these syndromes usually is insidious, their presence may not be appreciated nor their relationship to diabetes recognized. These musculoskeletal disorders fall into two general categories: those involving the periarticular structures and those affecting the joints and juxta-articular bone.

### PERIARTICULAR DISEASE

#### ADHESIVE CAPSULITIS

Periarthritis, adhesive capsulitis, and frozen shoulder are names given to a process in which the joint capsule is thickened, causing painful and diminished motion of the shoulder. This condition often is associated with calcific tendinitis and has been found in 10% of patients with type 1 and 22% of patients with type 2 diabetes.[54] For most patients, recovery of motion occurs within 6 months, and those that fail to respond to conservative management may benefit from arthroscopic release.[55]

#### REFLEX SYMPATHETIC DYSTROPHY

The appellation *reflex sympathetic dystrophy* is used interchangeably with such terms as shoulder-hand syndrome, Sudeck atrophy, algodystrophy, and posttraumatic osteoporosis (see Chap. 64). The reflex sympathetic dystrophy syndrome is characterized by pain or burning in the extremity and signs of vasomotor dysfunction. This dystrophic process may develop in patients with diabetes who are taking insulin or oral hypoglycemic agents, and even in patients with mild cases of diabetes who are receiving no treatment.[56]

Characteristically, swelling and pain occur on motion of the joints, often leading to serious disability if not treated aggressively. The radiographic appearance is one of patchy osteoporosis. Several forms of treatment, including corticosteroid therapy, calcitonin therapy, and sympathectomy, have been used, with varying degrees of success. Physiotherapy with early mobilization is particularly important.[57]

### DIABETIC HAND

In diabetes, the hand often is a mirror of the diffuse metabolic disturbances occurring throughout the body. Many of the rheumatic hand syndromes that complicate the diabetic process can be traced to the underlying pathologic changes in microvasculature, connective tissue, and peripheral nerves that exist in this disease.

#### LIMITED JOINT MOBILITY (CHEIROARTHROPATHY)

Only in the last decade has the syndrome of limited joint mobility (LJM) gained widespread recognition.[58] This disorder typically involves the joints of the hands. The fourth and fifth fingers are affected initially by limitation of motion, but, mostly, the process is painless. This disorder is found most commonly in young patients with type 1 diabetes, with as many as 42% of individuals affected. A simple screening test for LJM is to ask the patient to place both hands together as if in prayer. Normally, the palmar surfaces of the fingers can be approximated, but in LJM, a perceptible gap is apparent (Fig. 211-3).

The LJM syndrome also occurs in adults with type 1 and type 2 diabetes.[59] As many as 45% of adults with type 2 diabetes have evidence of LJM. Furthermore, the decreased mobility is not restricted to the hand; it often affects other joints of the upper extremity and foot, and may lead to significant functional deficits. Interestingly, women with LJM and type 1 diabetes have been reported to have a high prevalence of fibrous breast masses.[60]

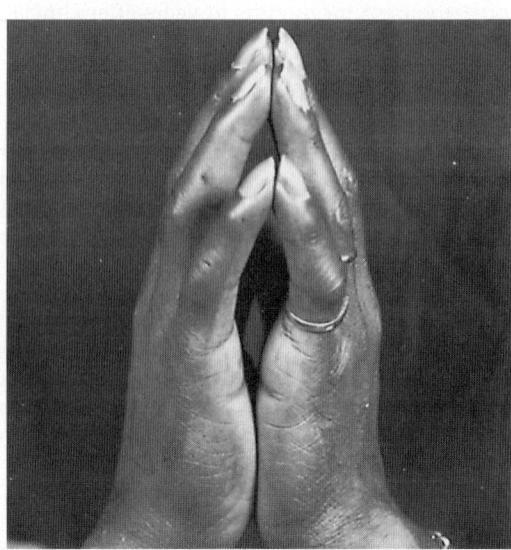

**FIGURE 211-3.** Limited joint mobility of the hands (cheiroarthropathy) in a patient with type 1 diabetes.

## PSEUDOSCLERODERMA

Many patients with more severe LJM syndrome have scleroderma-like skin changes.[61] The skin has a tight, waxy appearance, primarily on the dorsal aspect of the hands. Histologic examination shows dermal fibrosis (increased collagen) and a reduction in the number of skin appendages. In children and adolescents it is said to be the earliest complication of diabetes that is apparent on clinical examination. Digital sclerosis also may occur in adults with type 2 diabetes.

## FLEXOR TENOSYNOVITIS

Tenosynovitis of the flexor tendon of the finger is noted in both type 1 and type 2 diabetes.[62] The tendon sheaths often are thickened because of an accumulation of fibrous tissue, with resultant pain and crepitation along with reduced motion of the affected fingers. When perceptible nodules are found on the palmar aspect of the metacarpophalangeal joints, palpation usually is painful. Often, swelling of the fingers, a diminished grasp, and worsening of the symptoms on repeated use of the hand occur. It is not unusual for flexor tenosynovitis to occur in conjunction with carpal tunnel syndrome, and it may be a factor in the development of LJM.[63]

## DUPUYTREN CONTRACTURE

Dupuytren contracture, a nodular thickening of the palmar fascia, is a frequent accompaniment of diabetes and is reported in as many as 14% of those with type 1 and type 2 diabetes.[64] Conversely, diabetes mellitus has been diagnosed in as many as 37% of patients who have Dupuytren contracture.[65] It generally is a painless process and is seen more often in women and the elderly. The patient usually has tethering of the skin of the palm or fingers, as well as nodules and digital contractures. Some of these findings are easily confused with other hand complications of diabetes, such as tenosynovitis and LJM, with which it is associated.[66] Thus, the reported incidence of this disease may not be correct.

In patients with diabetes, Dupuytren disease seems to be milder than the contracture that is familial or associated with alcoholism. Another differential feature is the more common involvement of the third finger and the tendency for the fifth digit to be spared. In those cases in which significant functional disability occurs, fasciotomy or fasciectomy may be a useful procedure.

## CARPAL TUNNEL SYNDROME

Of the diseases associated with carpal tunnel syndrome, diabetes is one of the most common. Carpal tunnel syndrome affects up to 35% of diabetic patients.[67] Typically, patients complain of numbness or tingling in the distribution of the median nerve. The symptoms often are worse at night and may awaken patients from sleep. Confirmatory tests include the Tinel sign (paresthesia elicited by tapping over the volar aspect of the wrist) and the Phalen sign (symptoms when the wrist is held in extreme flexion). In most cases, nerve conduction studies reveal a delayed transmission of impulses through the carpal tunnel.

If the median nerve entrapment is severe, substantial muscle atrophy and loss of hand function may result. Local measures such as corticosteroid injection and splinting of the wrist may be helpful in alleviating compression of the nerve. If symptoms persist, surgical incision of the transverse carpal ligament may be required. For some patients with diabetes, abnormal results on median nerve conduction studies may represent intrinsic neuropathy rather than extrinsic compression[68]; in such patients, surgery is contraindicated. More complete electrodiagnostic studies will reveal abnormalities in ulnar nerve impulse transmission as well.

## TREATMENT OF THE DIABETIC HAND

Although therapy for diabetic hand complaints often is unsatisfactory, several novel approaches to this complex disorder have been developed. Several of the secondary complications of diabetes, including dysfunction of certain connective tissues (tendons and ligaments),[69] have been linked to excessive accumulations of sorbitol. Studies of certain aldose reductase inhibitors have been undertaken to determine whether these complications can be ameliorated. One inhibitor, sorbinil, has been found to be useful in treating LJM syndrome.[70] Tolrestat, another aldose reductase inhibitor, has shown promise in patients with carpal tunnel syndrome,[71] but it is too early to tell whether it will attenuate connective tissue complications. Another interesting approach to LJM has been the attempt to improve diabetes control. Several patients given insulin infusion pumps have shown a decrease in skin thickness when measured at various body sites.[72]

Corticosteroid injection is effective in treating diabetic tenosynovitis and may benefit associated LJM.[63] Tenolysis also has been successful in improving function and reducing pain caused by tenosynovitis.

## JOINT DISEASE

### NEUROARTHROPATHY (CHARCOT JOINT)

As a result of sensory neuropathy, a destructive arthropathy (Charcot joint) affecting the lower extremities develops in some patients with diabetes.[73] Rarely, it may present as an initial manifestation of diabetes. Both trauma and diminished pain perception appear to play major roles in the development of this arthropathy. The most common sites of involvement are the tarsal, tarsometatarsal, metatarsophalangeal, and ankle joints. Although callosities and plantar ulcerations often are noted in the region of the metatarsophalangeal joints, swelling and signs of inflammation are seen more frequently with ankle involvement. Radiologically identifiable changes include disruption of the joint surface, bony fragmentation, and dislocation (Fig. 211-4).

A Charcot joint may be difficult to differentiate by radiography from osteomyelitis, which also commonly affects the diabetic foot. Magnetic resonance imaging and indium-111–labeled white blood cell (WBC) scintigraphy are useful in differentiating between these conditions.[74]

In the active phase of the arthropathy, the mainstay of treatment is avoidance of weight-bearing. The site and type of involvement may dictate more specific therapy such as internal fixation or arthrodesis.[75]

## OTHER RHEUMATIC DISEASES ASSOCIATED WITH DIABETES

Isolated reports have been published of an association between type 1 diabetes and rheumatoid arthritis, and an increased prevalence of type 1 diabetes in close relatives of patients with rheumatoid arthritis. These findings may relate to certain histocompatibility antigens known to be common to both disorders. A study of hospitalized rheumatoid patients, however, found no unusual concurrence of diabetes.

Several autoimmune phenomena have been described in patients with type 2 diabetes (see Chap. 146). Many patients have high titers of antinuclear antibodies, and some fulfill the criteria for SLE. Furthermore, glomerular disease typical of lupus nephritis may develop in some cases.

Hyperuricemia and gouty arthritis are often noted in the diabetic population. This relationship is particularly evident in patients with the insulin-resistance syndrome (syndrome X) (see Chap. 145).

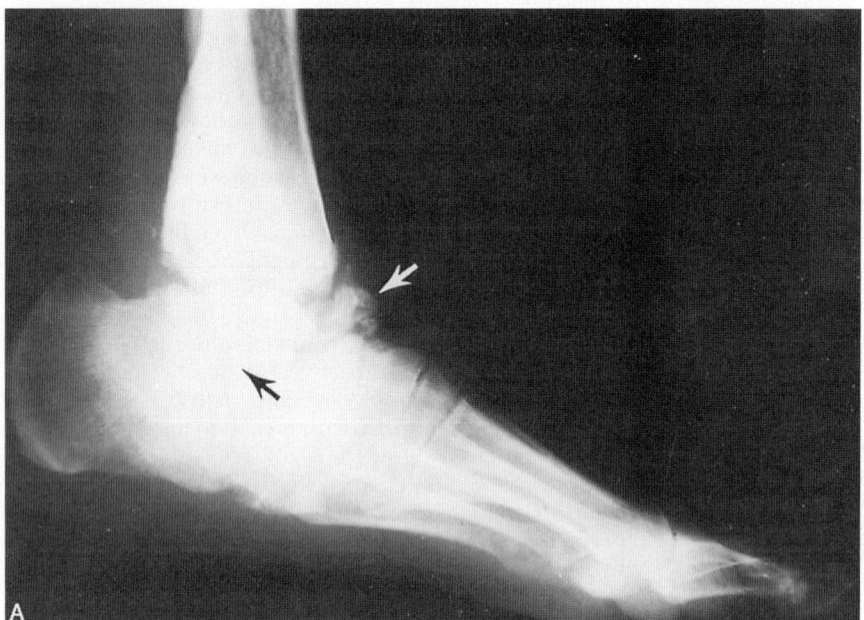
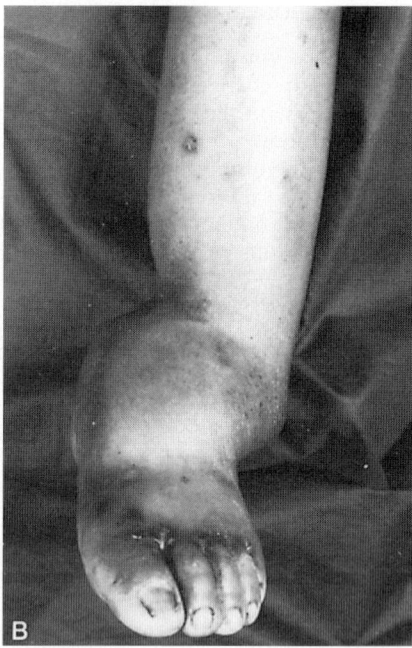

**FIGURE 211-4. A,** Neuroarthropathy (Charcot joint) in diabetes mellitus. Fragmentation of bone, osteophytosis (*white arrow*), and disruption of subtalar and talonavicular articulations (*black arrow*) are apparent. **B,** Another patient with diabetic neuroarthropathy leading to loss of the plantar arch and severe deformity of the foot, which subsequently required amputation. (**A,** From Nashel DJ. A diabetic with persistent ankle swelling. Drug Therapy 1983; 13:87.)

## MISCELLANEOUS ENDOCRINE DISORDERS

Hyperuricemia has been noted in several patients with congenital vasopressin-resistant (nephrogenic) diabetes insipidus. Some patients also have had attacks of acute gouty arthritis. Although the cause of the increased serum urate is unclear, certain data suggest that it results from a renal tubular defect.

## REFERENCES

1. Liote F, Orcel P. Osteoarticular disorders of endocrine origin. Baillieres Best Pract Res Clin Rheumatol 2000; 14:251.
1a. Podgorski M, Robinson B, Weissberger A, et al. Articular manifestations of acromegaly. Aust N Z J Med 1988; 18:28.
2. Lieberman SA, Bjorkengren AG, Hoffman AR. Rheumatologic and skeletal changes in acromegaly. Endocrinol Metab Clin North Am 1992; 21:615.
3. Newman CB, Melmed S, George A, et al. Octreotide as primary therapy for acromegaly. J Clin Endocrinol Metab 1998; 83:3034.
4. Colao A, Marzullo P, Vallone G, et al. Reversibility of joint thickening in acromegalic patients: an ultrasonography study. J Clin Endocrinol Metab 1998; 83:2121.
4a. Colao A, Marzullo P, Vallone G, et al. Ultrasonographic evidence of joint thickening reversibility in acromegalic patients treated with lanreotide for 12 months. Clin Endocrinol 1999; 51:611.
5. O'Duffy JD, Randall RV, MacCarty CS. Median neuropathy (carpal tunnel syndrome) in acromegaly. Ann Intern Med 1973; 78:379.
6. Kameyama S, Tanaka R, Hasegawa A, et al. Subclinical carpal tunnel syndrome in acromegaly. Neurol Med Chir (Tokyo) 1993; 33:547.
7. Pickett JB, Layzer RB, Levin SR, et al. Neuromuscular complications of acromegaly. Neurology 1975; 25:638.
8. Khaleeli AA, Levy RD, Edwards RH, et al. The neuromuscular features of acromegaly: a clinical and pathological study. J Neurol Neurosurg Psychiatry 1984; 47:1009.
9. Yunus M, Masi AT, Allen JP. Hypothalamic hypopituitarism presenting with rheumatologic symptoms. Arthritis Rheum 1981; 24:632.
10. Luzar MJ, Whisler RL, Hunder GG. Syndrome of inappropriate antidiuretic hormone secretion in association with temporal arteritis. J Rheumatol 1982; 9:957.
11. Bland JH, Frymoyer JW. Rheumatic syndromes of myxedema. N Engl J Med 1970; 282:1171.
12. Dorwart BB, Schumacher HR. Joint effusions, chondrocalcinosis and other rheumatic manifestations in hypothyroidism. Am J Med 1975; 59:780.
13. Khaleeli AA, Griffith DG, Edwards RH. The clinical presentation of hypothyroid myopathy and its relationship to abnormalities in structure and function of skeletal muscle. Clin Endocrinol (Oxf) 1983; 19:365.
14. Ciompi ML, Zuccotti M, Bazzichi L, Puccetti L. Polymyositis-like syndrome in hypothyroidism: report of two cases. Thyroidology 1994; 6:33.
15. Sekine N, Yamamoto M, Michikawa M, et al. Rhabdomyolysis and acute renal failure in a patient with hypothyroidism. Intern Med 1993; 32:269.
16. Wilke WS, Sheeler LR, Makarowski WS. Hypothyroidism with presenting symptoms of fibrositis. J Rheumatol 1981; 8:626.
17. Cruz MW, Tendrich M, Vaisman M, Novis SA. Electroneuromyography and neuromuscular findings in 16 primary hypothyroidism patients. Arq Neuropsiquiatr 1996; 54:12.
18. Erickson AR, Enzenauer RJ, Nordstrom DM, Merenich JA. The prevalence of hypothyroidism in gout. Am J Med 1994; 97:231.
19. Moule B, Grant MC, Boyle IT, May H. Thyroid acropachy. Clin Radiol 1970; 21:329.
20. Beard L, Kumar A, Estep HL. Bilateral carpal tunnel syndrome caused by Graves' disease. Arch Intern Med 1985; 145:345.
21. Roquer J, Cano JF. Carpal tunnel syndrome and hyperthyroidism. A prospective study. Acta Neurol Scand 1993; 88:149.
22. Thomas RD, Crift DN. Thyrotoxicosis and giant-cell arteritis. BMJ 1974; 2:408.
23. Dent RG, Edwards OM. Autoimmune thyroid disease and the polymyalgia rheumatica-giant cell arteritis syndrome. Clin Endocrinol (Oxf) 1978; 9:215.
24. Delamere JP, Scott DL, Felix-Davies DD. Thyroid dysfunction and rheumatic diseases. J R Soc Med 1982; 75:102.
25. Gaches F, Delaire L, Nadalon S, et al. Frequency of autoimmune diseases in 218 patients with autoimmune thyroid pathologies. Rev Med Interne 1998; 19:173.
26. Becker KL, Ferguson RH, McConahey WM. The connective tissue diseases and symptoms associated with Hashimoto's thyroiditis. N Engl J Med 1963; 268:277.
27. Helliwell M. Rheumatic symptoms in primary hyperparathyroidism. Postgrad Med J 1983; 59:236.
28. Resnick DL. Erosive arthritis of the hand and wrist in hyperparathyroidism. Radiology 1974; 110:263.
29. Bywaters EGL, Dixon ASJ, Scott JT. Joint lesions of hyperparathyroidism. Ann Rheum Dis 1963; 22:171.
30. Nussbaum AJ, Doppman JL. Shoulder arthropathy in primary hyperparathyroidism. Skeletal Radiol 1982; 9:98.
31. Yashiro T, Okamoto T, Tanaka R, et al. Prevalence of chondrocalcinosis in patients with primary hyperparathyroidism in Japan. Endocrinol Jpn 1991; 38:457.
32. Alexander GM, Dieppe PA, Doherty M, Scott DGI. Pyrophosphate arthropathy: a study of metabolic associations and laboratory data. Ann Rheum Dis 1982; 41:377.
32a. Caramaschi P, Biasi D, Carletto A, et al. Calcium pyrophosphate dihydrate crystal deposition disease and primary hyperparathyroidism associated with rheumatoid arthritis: description of 3 cases. Clin Exp Rheumatol 2000; 18:110.
33. Kiss ZS, Neale FC, Posen S, Reed CS. Acute arthritis and hyperuricemia following parathyroidectomy. Arch Intern Med 1967; 119:279.
34. Lambert RG, Becker EJ. Diffuse skeletal hyperostosis in idiopathic hypoparathyroidism. Clin Radiol 1989; 40:212.

35. Sharon P, Kaplinsky N, Leiba S, Frankl O. Aseptic necrosis of head of femur: presenting manifestation in Cushing's disease. J Rheumatol 1977; 4:73.

36. Mok CC, Lau CS, Wong RW. Risk factors for avascular bone necrosis in systemic lupus erythematosus. Br J Rheumatol 1998; 37:895.

37. Powell ET, Lanzer WL, Mankey MG. Core decompression for early osteonecrosis of the hip in high risk patients. Clin Orthop 1997; 335:181.

38. Dixon RB, Christy NP. On the various forms of corticosteroid withdrawal syndrome. Am J Med 1980; 68:224.

39. Calabrese LH, White CS. Musculoskeletal manifestations of Addison's disease. Arthritis Rheum 1979; 22(5):558.

40. Benhamou CL, Halimi D, Luton JP, et al. Manifestations osteoarticulaires au cours des insuffisances surrenales. Rev Rhum Mal Osteoartic 1984; 51:69.

41. Talal N. Sex steroid hormones and systemic lupus erythematosus. Arthritis Rheum 1981; 24:1054.

42. Bole GG Jr, Friedlaender MH, Smith CK. Rheumatic symptoms and serological abnormalities induced by oral contraceptives. Lancet 1969; 1:323.

43. Buyon JP. Oral contraceptives in women with systemic lupus erythematosus. Ann Med Interne (Paris) 1996; 147:259.

44. Julkunen HA. Oral contraceptives in systemic lupus erythematosus; side-effects and influence on the activity of SLE. Scand J Rheumatol 1991; 20:427.

45. Jungers P, Dougados M, Pelissier C, et al. Influence of oral contraceptive therapy on the activity of systemic lupus erythematosus. Arthritis Rheum 1982; 25:618.

46. Hazes JM, van Zeben D. Oral contraception and its possible protection against rheumatoid arthritis. Ann Rheum Dis 1991; 50:72.

47. Spector TD, Hochberg MC. The protective effect of the oral contraceptive pill on rheumatoid arthritis: an overview of the analytic epidemiological studies using meta-analysis. J Clin Epidemiol 1990; 43:1221.

48. Meier CR, Sturkenboom MC, Cohen AS, Jick H. Postmenopausal estrogen replacement therapy and the risk of developing systemic lupus erythematosus or discoid lupus. J Rheumatol 1998; 25:1515.

49. Kreidstein S, Urowitz MB, Gladman DD, Gough J. Hormone replacement therapy in systemic lupus erythematosus. J Rheumatol 1997; 24:2149.

50. Mok CC, Lau CS, Ho CT, et al. Safety of hormonal replacement therapy in post-menopausal patients with systemic lupus erythematosus. Scand J Rheumatol 1998; 27:342.

51. MacDonald AG, Murphy EA, Capell HA, et al. Effects of hormone replacement therapy in rheumatoid arthritis: a double blind placebo-controlled study. Ann Rheum Dis 1994; 53:54.

52. Hall GM, Spector TD, Delmas PD. Markers of bone metabolism in post-menopausal women with rheumatoid arthritis. Effects of corticosteroids and hormone replacement therapy. Arthritis Rheum 1995; 38:902.

53. Rosenbloom AL, Silverstein JH. Connective tissue and joint disease in diabetes mellitus. Endocrinol Metab Clin North Am 1996; 25:473.

54. Arkkila PE, Kantola IM, Viikari JS, Ronnemaa T. Shoulder capsulitis in type I and II diabetic patients: association with diabetic complications and related diseases. Ann Rheum Dis 1996; 55:907.

55. Ogilvie-Harris DJ, Myerthall S. The diabetic frozen shoulder: arthroscopic release. Arthroscopy 1997; 13:1.

56. Lequesne M, Dang N, Bensasson M, Mery C. Increased association of diabetes mellitus with capsulitis of the shoulder and shoulder-hand syndrome. Scand J Rheumatol 1977; 6:53.

57. Gordon N. Reflex sympathetic dystrophy. Brain Dev 1996; 18:257.

58. Rosenbloom AL. Limitation of finger joint mobility in diabetes mellitus. J Diabetes Complications 1989; 3:77.

59. Fitzcharles MA, Duby S, Waddell RW. Limitation of joint mobility (cheiroarthropathy) in adult noninsulin-dependent diabetic patients. Ann Rheum Dis 1984; 43:251.

60. Soler NG, Khardori R. Fibrous disease of the breast, thyroiditis, and cheiroarthropathy in type I diabetes mellitus. Lancet 1984; 1:193.

61. Seibold JR. Digital sclerosis in children with insulin-dependent diabetes mellitus. Arthritis Rheum 1982; 25:1357.

62. Gamstedt A, Holm-Glad J, Ohlson CG, Sundstrom M. Hand abnormalities are strongly associated with the duration of diabetes mellitus. J Intern Med 1993; 234:189.

63. Sibbitt WL Jr, Eaton RP. Corticosteroid responsive tenosynovitis is a common pathway for limited joint mobility in the diabetic hand. J Rheumatol 1997; 24:931.

64. Arkkila PE, Kantola IM, Viikari JS. Dupuytren's disease: association with chronic diabetic complications. J Rheumatol 1997; 24:153.

65. Machtey I. Dupuytren's contracture and diabetes. J Rheumatol 1988; 15:879.

66. Pal B, Griffiths ID, Anderson J, Dick WC. Association of limited joint mobility with Dupuytren's contracture in diabetes mellitus. J Rheumatol 1987; 14:582.

67. Renard E, Jacques D, Chammas M, et al. Increased prevalence of soft tissue hand lesions in type 1 and type 2 diabetes mellitus: various entities and associated significance. Diabetes Metab 1994; 20:513.

68. Valensi P, Giroux C, Seeboth-Ghalayini B, Attali JR. Diabetic peripheral neuropathy: effects of age, duration of diabetes, glycemic control, and vascular factors. J Diabetes Complications 1997; 11:27.

69. Eaton RP. The collagen hydration hypothesis: a new paradigm for the secondary complications of diabetes mellitus. J Chronic Dis 1986; 39:763.

70. Eaton RP, Sibbitt WL Jr, Shah VO, et al. A commentary on 10 years of aldose reductase inhibition for limited joint mobility in diabetes. J Diabetes Complications 1998; 12:34.

71. Monge L, De Mattei M, Dani F, et al. Effect of treatment with an aldose-reductase inhibitor on symptomatic carpal tunnel syndrome in type 2 diabetes. Diabet Med 1995; 12:1097.

72. Lieberman LS, Rosenbloom AL, Riley WJ, Silverstein JH. Reduced skin thickness with pump administration of insulin. N Engl J Med 1980; 303:940.

73. Sinha S, Munichoodappa CS, Kozak GP. Neuro-arthropathy (Charcot joints) in diabetes mellitus. Medicine (Baltimore) 1972; 51:191.

74. Lipman BT, Collier BD, Carrera GF, et al. Detection of osteomyelitis in the neuropathic foot: nuclear medicine, MRI and conventional radiography. Clin Nucl Med 1998; 23:77.

75. Simon SR, Tejwani SG, Wilson DL, et al. Arthrodysis as an early alternative to nonoperative management of Charcot arthropathy of the diabetic foot. J Bone Joint Surg Am 2000; 82-A:939.

# CHAPTER 212

# HEMATOLOGIC ENDOCRINOLOGY

HARVEY S. LUKSENBURG, STUART L. GOLDBERG, AND CRAIG M. KESSLER

The primary functions of the blood are to provide tissue oxygenation and immune defense, and to maintain hemostasis. To accomplish these tasks, the bone marrow must produce $10^{11}$ mature cells per day in a tightly controlled fashion. Hematopoietic regulatory proteins, known as *cytokines*, aid in this control through endocrine, paracrine, and autocrine mechanisms. Recent advances in the understanding of this process have had clinical impact in the fields of transplantation, gene therapy, and supportive care. This chapter provides a brief overview of hematopoiesis, hematopoietic regulatory factors, and the effect of classic endocrine disorders on the blood system. Cytokines are discussed extensively from an overall endocrine viewpoint in Chapter 173 and from an immunologic viewpoint in Chapters 193 to 197.

## THE STEM CELL HYPOTHESIS

The stem cell model of hematopoiesis proposes that blood elements are derived from the progeny of a few primitive ancestral cells. These undifferentiated "stem cells" possess the capacity for self-renewal and the ability to differentiate into all the elements necessary to sustain hematologic function (Fig. 212-1). This hierarchical concept has been supported by studies in a lethally irradiated mouse model in which multilineage hematopoietic cell colonies of clonal origin form in the spleen after donor marrow infusions. Suspensions from these splenic colonies (called *colony-forming units–spleen [CFU-S]*) can successfully serve as the source of stem cells in second transplants.[1] Subsequent in vivo transplantation experiments and in vitro colony analyses have characterized a candidate human stem cell with self-renewal and differentiation properties. Subset surface marker examination indicates that the human stem cell resides in the CD34+, Thy-1+, Rho123lo, c-kit R+, DR−, CD45 RO+, and Lin− population.[2] Final isolation, purification, and expansion of the true human stem cell holds great potential for gene therapy and marrow transplantation.

## REGULATION OF HEMATOPOIESIS

Current theories on hematopoiesis hold that most human stem cells are in a resting G0 phase. As the stem cell enters an active cycle, asymmetric quantal division occurs, allowing one daughter cell to remain a pluripotent stem cell. The other daughter cell, however, begins a differentiation process during which each subsequent division leads to progressive lineage restriction and

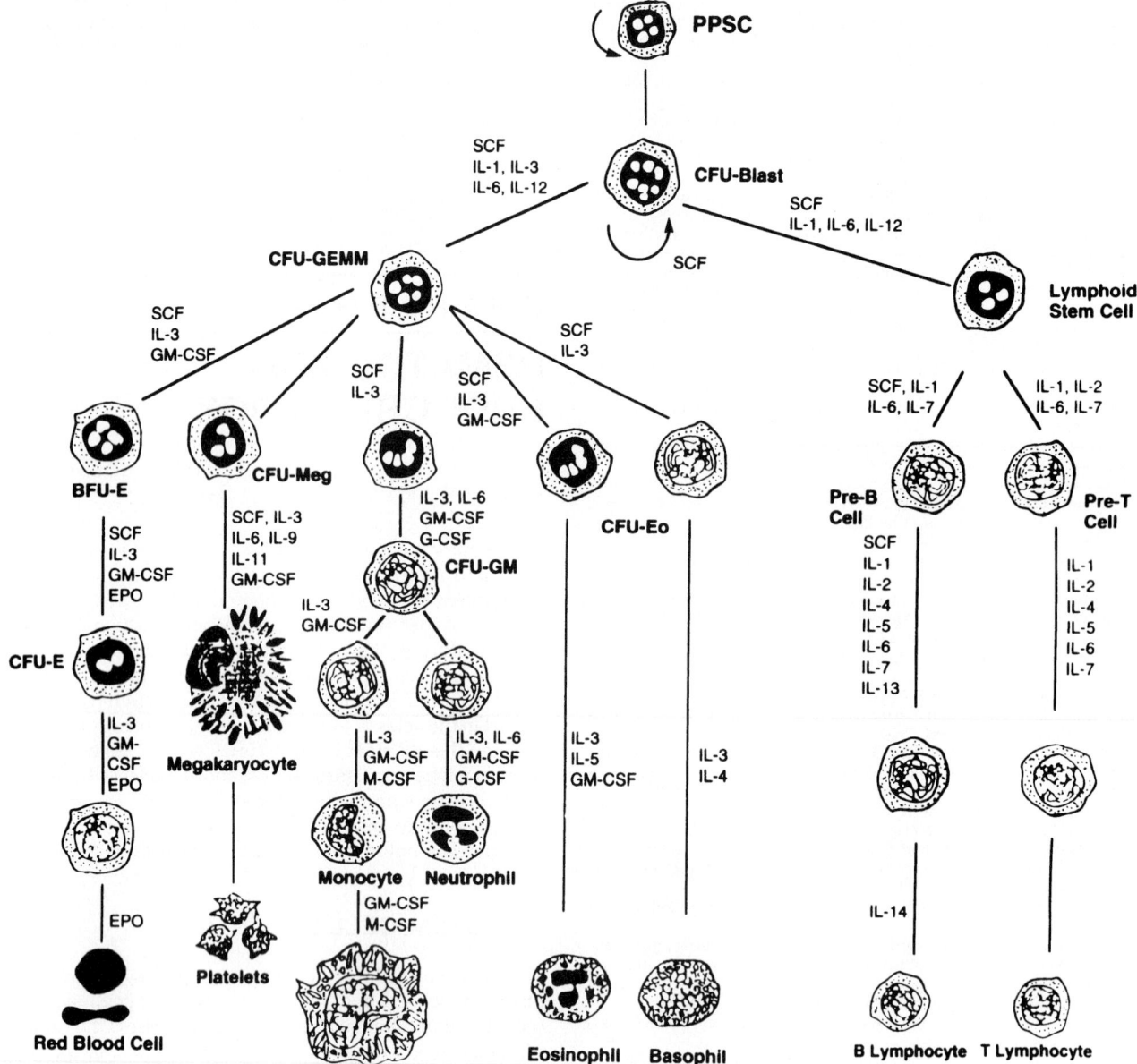

**FIGURE 212-1.** Stem cell model of hematopoiesis. A single pluripotential stem cell (*PPSC*) has the capacity for self-renewal and the ability to differentiate into all the hematopoietic lineages. Multiple regulatory proteins facilitate this differentiation. (*BFU*, burst-forming unit; *CFU*, colony-forming unit; *CSF*, colony stimulating factor; *E*, erythroid; *Eo*, eosinophil; *EPO*, erythropoietin; *G*, granulocyte; *GM*, granulocyte macrophage; *IL*, interleukin; *M*, monocyte/macrophage; *MEG*, megakaryocyte; *PPSC*, pluripotential stem cell; *SCF*, stem cell factor; *IL*, interleukin.)

the acquisition of surface receptors for regulatory proteins. The initial path of differentiation (i.e., whether it becomes a red blood cell, white blood cell, or platelet) seems to be a random event. Regulatory cytokines perform permissive rather than obligatory roles in differentiation. As shown in Figure 212-1, there is significant redundancy in hematopoietic control. Many cytokines exert multiple effects, stimulatory and inhibitory, on multiple target cells of both early and late stages of differentiation. The reliance on combinations of regulatory proteins rather than on a single protein allows broader enhancement of cell production and cellular responses, and augmentation of differentiation commitment in responding cells.[3] More than 50 regulatory proteins have been identified (Table 212-1). The complexity and redundancy of this system provide the flexibility and immediate adaptability necessary to respond to constantly changing environmental and physiologic stresses.

## CLINICAL USE OF HEMATOPOIETIC GROWTH FACTORS

Several hematopoietic growth factors have been purified, cloned, and commercially developed for clinical use. These hematologic hormones have found applications in the supportive care of patients with various blood diseases.[4–6]

### ERYTHROPOIETIN

Erythropoietin is the primary regulator of erythrocyte (red blood cell) production.[7] Although erythropoietin has actions on both primitive (burst-forming unit) and committed (colony-forming unit) erythroid progenitor cells, it is unlike most hematologic regulators in that it has no effect on the terminal differentiated cell. Mature red blood cells lack erythropoietin receptors, are enucle-

## TABLE 212-1.
### Hematopoietic Growth Factors, Interleukins, and Cytokines*

Angiogenin
Epidermal growth factor (EGF)
**Erythropoietin (EPO)**
Fibroblast growth factor, acidic
Fibroblast growth factor, basic
Fibroblast growth factor-3
Fibroblast growth factor-4
Fibroblast growth factor-5
Fibroblast growth factor-6
Fibroblast growth factor-7
**Granulocyte colony stimulating factor (G-CSF)**
**Granulocyte/macrophage colony stimulating factor (GM-CSF)**
Heparin-binding EGF-like growth factor
Hepatocyte growth factor
Interferon-$\alpha$/$\beta$
Interferon-$\gamma$
**Insulin-like growth factor-I**
**Insulin-like growth factor-II**
**Interleukin-1$\alpha$**
**Interleukin-1$\beta$**
Interleukin-1 receptor antagonist
Interleukin-2
**Interleukin-3**
**Interleukin-4**
**Interleukin-5**
**Interleukin-6**
Interleukin-7
Interleukin-8
**Interleukin-9**
Interleukin-10
**Interleukin-11**
Interleukin-12
Interleukin-13
Interleukin-14
IP-10 (interferon-$\gamma$–induced protein 10)
**Leukemia inhibitory factor (LIF)**
Low molecular weight B-cell growth factor
**Macrophage colony-stimulating growth factor (M-CSF)**
Monocyte chemotactic protein-1
Macrophage inflammatory protein-1$\alpha$
Macrophage inflammatory protein-1$\beta$
Melanoma growth-stimulating activity
Nerve growth factor
Oncostatin M
Platelet-derived endothelial cell growth factor
Platelet-derived growth factor
Regulated upon activation, normal T expressed, and presumably secreted
  (RANTES)
**Stem cell factor**
Transforming growth factor-$\alpha$
Transforming growth factor-$\beta$
Tumor necrosis factor $\alpha$
Tumor necrosis factor $\beta$
Vascular endothelial growth factor

*Many cytokines have multiple functions, including both growth-regulatory and immunologic activity. This table represents a simplification of the most important action. Primary growth regulator cytokines appear in **boldface**.
(Courtesy of R & D Systems, Inc, Minneapolis, MN.)

etin synthesis in adults occurs in the kidney by interstitial cells adjacent to the proximal convoluted tubules; the remaining 10% is produced in the liver. The rate of renal synthesis parallels the need for oxygen-carrying capacity, mediated in part through prostaglandin E release during hypoxia. A physiologic feedback control mechanism is hypothesized to exist. The site of the renal oxygen "sensor" remains unknown, but probably consists of a heme-related protein because exposure to carbon monoxide effectively blocks erythropoietin production. Patients with chronic renal insufficiency typically have low erythropoietin production and low serum concentrations, leading to the development of normocytic, normochromic anemia. In diseases of target organ failure, such as aplastic anemia, the feedback control mechanism results in markedly increased levels of erythropoietin production. In iron-deficiency anemia (a target organ disease), an inverse linear relationship exists between hemoglobin and erythropoietin levels in the serum. Anemia is commonly found in patients with both solid and hematologic malignancies and may be a major cause of fatigue. The anemia of malignancies (and inflammatory states) is characterized by an inappropriately low level of erythropoietin for a given hematocrit (as compared to anemia due to iron deficiency). This decreased responsiveness to erythropoietin in the anemias of inflammation and malignancy may be modulated by interleukin-1, tumor necrosis factor, and other cytokines. For example, in patients with anemia due to inflammatory bowel disease, an inverse correlation was found between the level of hemoglobin and the ability of monocytes to secrete interleukin-1$\beta$. While most of the patients responded to exogenous erythropoietin, the patients with the highest monocytic secretion of interleukin-1$\beta$ had no response.[8] Nevertheless, in most patients with the anemias of inflammation, malignancy, or acquired immunodeficiency syndrome (AIDS), administration of pharmacologic amounts of erythropoietin can lead to an increase in the hematocrit.[9]

The gene for erythropoietin, coded on the long arm of chromosome 7, was cloned in 1985. A recombinant form of erythropoietin, produced in Chinese hamster ovary cells, is available for clinical use. This glycosylated product has a molecular mass of 29,900 daltons. Clearance of erythropoietin is increased with multiple exposures through a non-antibody–mediated mechanism. The peak serum level with subcutaneous dosing occurs at 12 to 24 hours and the half-life is 20 hours.

In patients with chronic renal insufficiency who are undergoing renal dialysis, the administration of recombinant erythropoietin, 50 U/kg subcutaneously three times per week, leads to increased hematocrit levels, reduced transfusion requirements, and improved quality-of-life parameters.[10] Failure to respond to therapy may indicate coexisting iron or nutritional deficiencies, aluminum toxicity, secondary hyperparathyroidism (see later), or an underlying primary hematologic or inflammatory disorder. Erythropoietin, 150 U/kg given subcutaneously three times per week, has also been effective in reducing the need for transfusional support among patients with cancer who are receiving repetitive chemotherapy.[11,12] Patients with human immunodeficiency virus (HIV) infection who are anemic may benefit from erythropoietin, at a dosage of 150 U/kg three times per week. The decline in the use of azidothymidine (AZT), which can be associated with severe anemia, has also led to decreased transfusion requirements in these patients. A serum erythropoietin level of <500 mU/mL can be used to identify HIV-infected patients who are likely to respond.[13]

## GRANULOCYTE COLONY STIMULATING FACTOR

A decrease in the number of functioning neutrophils represents the most important risk factor for the development of infection in patients with cancer who are receiving myelotoxic chemo-

ate, and do not divide. Erythropoietin also has minor effects on megakaryopoiesis (platelet production), although the clinical relevance of these effects is probably insignificant.

Erythropoietin acts as a true hormone and is produced at a site distant from its target organ. Ninety percent of erythropoi-

therapy and in individuals with congenital neutropenias such as chronic granulomatous disease and cyclic neutropenia. As the neutrophil count declines, the risk of infection increases. Absolute neutrophil counts of <500 cells/mm³ are associated with more than 70% of bacterial septic episodes and with 90% of disseminated fungal infections among patients with cancer.[14]

Granulocyte colony stimulating factor (G-CSF) plays a major role in the regulatory control of both the production and the function of neutrophils.[15] Coded by a gene on the long arm of chromosome 17, G-CSF is produced by a variety of cells, including neutrophils, endothelial cells, fibroblasts, and cells of the bone marrow stroma. In contrast to the other major neutrophil cytokine, granulocyte/macrophage colony stimulating factor (GM-CSF), G-CSF is not elaborated by T-cell lymphocytes. G-CSF accelerates the maturation and marrow transit time of neutrophils by stimulating the colony-forming unit–granulocyte and the pre–colony-forming unit pool. This results in a rapid increase in the peripheral neutrophil count. G-CSF also acts to enhance neutrophil migration by working as a weak chemoattractant. Vascular endothelial cells proliferate and migrate under stimulation from G-CSF. Increases in serum levels of G-CSF are noted in patients with elevated neutrophil counts during active infection. Thus, G-CSF may act in a true hormonal fashion during stress conditions.

## GRANULOCYTE/MACROPHAGE COLONY STIMULATING FACTOR

GM-CSF exerts stimulatory effects on both the early and late stages of the hematopoietic differentiation cascade.[16] This results in increased numbers of neutrophils, monocytes, and eosinophils. GM-CSF also has numerous effects on mature cells, including stimulation of neutrophil expression of cellular adhesion molecules, locomotion, responsiveness to chemotactic and biosynthetic factors, augmentation of the respiratory burst, and release of other cytokines, all of which contribute to an increase in the ability of neutrophils to control infection. Macrophage and eosinophil activity against infection are similarly increased.

GM-CSF is produced by activated T-cell and B-cell lymphocytes, endothelial cells, mast cells, fibroblasts, macrophages, mesothelial cells, and osteoblasts. Unlike G-CSF, GM-CSF cannot be detected in the serum during physiologic states, suggesting that GM-CSF acts primarily in a paracrine fashion. The gene for GM-CSF is located on the long arm of chromosome 5 in a region containing several hematopoietic and immunologic regulator genes. Deletion of this region may lead to myelodysplasia (the 5q minus syndrome).

## CLINICAL USES OF GRANULOCYTE COLONY STIMULATING FACTOR AND GRANULOCYTE/ MACROPHAGE COLONY STIMULATING FACTOR

Given the importance of neutropenia as an infectious risk factor after chemotherapy, it is not surprising that recombinant G-CSF and GM-CSF have become essential components in the supportive care of some patients with cancer, especially those patients who receive highly myelosuppressive chemotherapy regimes. Most studies have not shown a benefit for these drugs in decreasing the period of severe neutropenia (an absolute neutrophil count of ≤500 cells/mm³) in chemotherapy regimes that result in neutropenia of short duration (less than a week).[17] The use of G-CSF in acute myelogenous leukemia, with the goal of reducing the incidence of severe infection, has shown only modest reductions in days with fever, days with severe neutropenia, and length of hospitalization.[18] However, no adverse effects of G-CSF have been seen, such as stimulation of leukemic growth.

In patients undergoing bone marrow transplantation, both GM-CSF and G-CSF can shorten the period of neutropenia and, thus, lead to a reduction in infections in patients who have undergone either autologous or allogeneic bone marrow transplantation.[19,20] The technique of peripheral stem cell transplantation utilizes G-CSF as an effective agent in mobilizing CD34+ hematopoietic stem cells from their usual location in the bone marrow, into the peripheral blood, where they can then be collected. These stem cells are then reinfused after patients have received myeloablative chemotherapy.[21,22]

There has been a resurgence of interest in granulocyte transfusions, as an adjunct in the therapy of infections that occur in patients with prolonged neutropenia due to the chemotherapy of acute leukemia. This increased interest has been due to the feasibility of collecting large amounts of functional neutrophils from normal donors who have been "primed" with G-CSF (and often with corticosteroids). The administration of G-CSF results in much higher circulating granulocyte counts in the peripheral circulation. The donors then undergo leukopheresis, and the product is then infused into the neutropenic recipients. A number of clinical trials are currently in progress assessing the efficacy of this therapy.[23,24]

Patients with HIV are prone to develop neutropenia. The common causes are drug-induced (nonchemotherapy), secondary to HIV effects on the bone marrow or to chemotherapy for non-Hodgkin lymphoma. G-CSF is well tolerated and effective in stimulating neutrophil recovery in these situations. GM-CSF has been shown to be associated with an increased replication of HIV-1.[25] However, clinical studies have not demonstrated either accelerated disease progression or an increase in p24 levels in patients treated with GM-CSF.[26] Treatment with G-CSF, 5 μg/kg given intravenously or subcutaneously, is usually well tolerated. Bone pain, occurring at the time of neutrophilic recovery, is the most common adverse effect, and may be severe enough to warrant narcotic analgesia.[27]

## THROMBOPOIETIN (TPO)

Since the 1950s, investigators have appreciated that plasma, urine, and serum from animals and humans contained bioactivity that regulated the production of platelets from megakaryocytes. The search for a lineage-specific growth factor for platelet production became more intensive during the last several years, when it became clear that the cytokines that are known to have some effect on megakaryocyte production (e.g., the interleukins, IL-3, IL-6, and IL-11) did not seem to fully possess the properties of thrombopoietin.

The cloning of TPO is the result of a remarkable chain of basic research investigations. In 1986, a murine retrovirus isolate, the myeloproliferative leukemia virus (MPLV), was reported to provoke an acute hematologic disorder in mice that resembled a myeloproliferative syndrome, in which all three cell lineages were dramatically increased.[28] Cultures of the bone marrows of these cells formed terminally differentiated erythroid, myeloid, and megakaryocytic colonies without the addition of any exogenous interleukins, colony stimulating factors, erythropoietin, or any conditioned medium. This led to characterization of a transforming gene carried by the retrovirus, v-*mpl*. Analysis of the amino-acid sequence of the v-*mpl* protein revealed striking similarity to eight cloned hematopoietic cytokine receptors (IL-2-Rβ chain, IL-3R, IL-4R, GCSFR, GMCSFR, etc.), the so-called *hematopoietin receptor superfamily.*[29] The v-*mpl* coded for a cytokine receptor that had not yet been characterized—it was termed an "orphan" receptor. Further work showed that the human counterpart of v-*mpl*, c-*mpl*, was expressed in megakaryocytes, strongly suggesting that it was the receptor for a ligand that regulated megakaryocytic growth. The c-*mpl* ligand has been cloned; it has properties that had been predicted as being consistent with TPO.[30,31]

The gene for TPO maps to the long arm of chromosome 3. It is a polypeptide of 355 amino acids. There are currently two products available for clinical trials: recombinant human TPO, which consists of the entire polypeptide, and a truncated protein that contains only the part that binds to the receptor, and has polyethylene glycol (PEG) added (PEG-conjugated human megakaryocyte growth and development factor).

To date, the clinical trials have been conducted in patients receiving chemotherapy that is known to cause thrombocytopenia in a significant proportion of patients. These initial trials have demonstrated that patients who receive this growth factor have less severe suppression of their platelet counts and require shorter time periods before their platelet counts reach normal levels.[32–34]

IL-11 is a cytokine that functions as a maturation factor for megakaryocytes; it has been shown to decrease the extent of chemotherapy-induced thrombocytopenia seen in patients being treated for malignancies. IL-11 is currently the only cytokine approved by the Food and Drug Administration for stimulation of platelet production.[35]

Other growth factors, which have been found to have platelet stimulatory effects, include stem cell factor (c-*kit* ligand), the ligand for a receptor found on early hematopoietic cells. Stem cell factor is more effective when used in concert with other growth factors. PIXY321 is an engineered fusion growth factor consisting of IL-3 and GM-CSF. In vitro activities have indicated that PIXY321 would have superior multilineage hematopoietic stimulatory effects as compared to the use of IL-3 and GM-CSF combined. However, phase I trials in breast cancer and non-Hodgkin lymphoma failed to demonstrate any advantage as compared to G-CSF and were also associated with a greater incidence of adverse effects.[36,37]

# HEMATOLOGIC EFFECTS OF ENDOCRINE DISORDERS

Dysfunction of classic endocrine organs frequently results in alteration of the hematologic system.[38,39] In most disorders, the complex interplay between traditional hormones and hematopoietic cytokines is incompletely understood. However, correction of the underlying endocrine disorder usually leads to improvement in hematologic status.

## DISORDERS OF THE PITUITARY GLAND

Hypopituitarism is commonly complicated by a normochromic, normocytic anemia and bone marrow findings of severe erythroid hypoplasia.[40] It is hypothesized that the anemia is related to a deficiency of anterior lobe hormones because the surgical removal, in rats, of the posterior and intermediate lobes does not cause changes in erythropoiesis.[41] Because the clinical findings of the anemia are similar to those observed in patients who have undergone thyroidectomy or in patients with myxedema, deficiencies of thyroid-stimulating hormone may be the primary cause. However, hormonal replacement studies have not produced conclusive results to confirm this hypothesis. Several other pituitary hormones, including adrenocorticotropin, gonadotropin, and growth hormones (GH), which have modulating effects on red blood cell production, may play important additional roles.[42] Leukopenia has also been noted in patients with pituitary dysfunction. It is unknown which of the pituitary hormones (or combinations) is responsible.

Although many hormones secreted by the pituitary may have secondary effects on hematopoiesis through their actions on target organs, only GH has been implicated as a direct regulator of hematopoiesis.[43] It appears that most of the effects on erythropoiesis through GH are mediated by insulin-like growth factor-I (IGF-I).[44] While receptors for both GH and IGF-I are found on erythroid precursors, in vitro studies have demonstrated that physiologic concentrations of IGF-I are required to stimulate erythroid colony growth, whereas supraphysiologic concentrations of GH are required to achieve the same effect.[38,45] In erythroid cell cultures, erythropoietin is the major growth factor required for proliferation and maturation. However, IGF-I is required for late cell maturation. Without IGF-I, late erythroid cells in culture have a markedly defective morphology.[46] GH also acts on early erythroid cells to assist in the transition from $\gamma$-chain to $\beta$-chain hemoglobin synthesis.[47] In adults with GH deficiency, mild increases in the hemoglobin are seen after 120 weeks of therapy with human recombinant GH.[48] GH also plays a role in white blood cell production through a process mediated by IGF-I.

One clinical entity where IGF-I seems to play a more important role is polycythemia vera (PV). In 1974, it was found that bone marrow erythroid cells from patients with PV could proliferate in vitro without a requirement for erythropoietin, which is necessary for normal erythropoiesis.[49] However, it was later demonstrated that PV erythropoietic precursors were hypersensitive to IGF-I.[50] The levels of the major binding protein for IGF-I, IGFBP-3, were more than four-fold higher in patients with PV than either in controls or in patients with secondary erythrocytosis. When erythroid precursor cells from PV were incubated with IGF-I in the presence of IGFBP-3, the degree of hypersensitivity was pronounced, with stimulation of growth seen at IGF-I concentrations of $10^{-14}$ mol/L.[51] A patient with both acromegaly and PV normalized his hematocrit after removal of a GH-secreting pituitary adenoma.[52]

Vasopressin and its synthetic analog desmopressin (DDAVP, 1-desamino-8-D-arginine-vasopressin) cause a rapid rise in factor VIII and von Willebrand factor levels through posttranslational mechanisms, possibly by the release of von Willebrand factor from intracellular storage sites in endothelial cells. Desmopressin is a strong agonist of the vasopressor $V_2$ receptors, which also mediate water resorption in the renal collecting ducts. Therapeutically, this effect has been used in the treatment of patients with *type I von Willebrand disease* (who have decreased amounts of normally functioning von Willebrand factor). The hormone is variably effective in *type IIA* von Willebrand disease and may be contraindicated in the *type IIB* variant. DDAVP is currently the treatment of choice for the temporary correction of bleeding or as prophylaxis for surgical procedures in patients with type I von Willebrand disease of mild and moderate severity. It is also useful in selected patients with mild hemophilia A and in patients with both acquired and hereditary qualitative disorders of platelet dysfunction.[53,54] Desmopressin can be administered through either the intravenous or intranasal route.

## THYROID HORMONE EFFECTS

Abnormalities of the hematologic system are common in patients with thyroid diseases. Thyroid hormones are primary regulators of the basal metabolic rate and, therefore, are linked to tissue oxygen consumption. Tissue hypoxia leads, by erythropoietin-driven renal mechanisms, to increases in erythropoiesis, iron turnover, and red blood cell mass. Thyroid hormones also cause a favorable shift in the oxygen saturation curve, by increasing erythrocyte 2,3-diphosphoglycerate, which favors unloading of oxygen to tissues.[55] Further stimulation of erythro-

**TABLE 212-2.**
**Red Cell Effects of Thyroid Disease**

**HYPOTHYROIDISM**

| | |
|---|---|
| Anemia | Common (up to one-third). Often a physiologic response to a decrease in oxygen requirement resulting in a decrease in erythropoietin and a decrease in erythropoiesis. Concurrent fall in plasma volume masks degree of red blood cell mass reduction. Bone marrow hypoplasia. Nutritional defects may play a role. |
| Microcytic anemia | Seen in up to 15%. Frequently secondary to concurrent iron deficiency (caused by decreased iron absorption from hypochlorhydria, or excessive blood loss caused by platelet/coagulation abnormalities or menorrhagia). |
| Normochromic anemia | Typical of the physiologic anemia of hypothyroidism. |
| Macrocytic anemia | Most common deficiency morphologic abnormality (more than one-third of cases). May reflect vitamin $B_{12}$ deficiency (associated with pernicious anemia or hypochlorhydria) or folic acid deficiency. |

**HYPERTHYROIDISM**

| | |
|---|---|
| Erythrocytosis | Physiologic increase in red blood cell mass is virtually never apparent because of the concurrent increase in plasma volume. |
| Anemia | Less common than in hypothyroidism (10–20%). |
| Microcytic anemia | Most common morphology (approximately one-third of cases), even in the absence of anemia. Iron deficiency is usually not the cause. Corrects with treatment of the thyroid. |
| Normochromic anemia | Occasionally seen. May be caused by defective iron utilization. |
| Macrocytic anemia | Most often associated with vitamin $B_{12}$ or folic acid deficiency, both of which occur because of increased metabolism. Increased frequency of pernicious anemia. |

(Modified from Ansell JE. The blood in thyrotoxicosis, and the blood in hypothyroidism. In: Braverman LE, Utiger RD, eds. The thyroid: a fundamental and clinical text. Philadelphia: JB Lippincott Co, 1991:785.)

poiesis through noncaloric, nonerythropoietin mechanisms has been proposed. In hypophysectomized rats, thyroxine ($T_4$) causes increased erythropoiesis despite polycythemia, an effect independent of the degree of oxygen consumption.[56] L-$T_4$, D-$T_4$, L-triiodothyronine ($T_3$), and reverse $T_3$ are also able to stimulate erythropoiesis in vitro in erythropoietin-primed colonies.[57] The effect of $T_4$ is mediated through β-adrenergic receptors on the erythroid cell membrane and nucleus, and can be inhibited by the β-adrenergic blocker propranolol.[58] Additional effects of thyroid hormones on red blood cell production include a decrease in osmotic fragility, an increase in glucose-6-phosphate dehydrogenase activity, and an increase in hemoglobin δ-chain synthesis and, thus, on hemoglobin $A_2$ concentration.[59]

The clinical effects of thyroid disorders on red blood cell production are shown in Table 212-2. Although thyroid hormones stimulate red blood cell production, an expansion in plasma volume in thyrotoxicosis prevents the clinical expression of thyroid hormone–induced polycythemia. By contrast, anemia occurs in 8% to 20% of patients with hyperthyroidism and is frequently secondary to coexisting disorders such as pernicious anemia (PA)[60] (Fig. 212-2). Approximately one-third of patients with thyrotoxicosis have antibodies to gastric parietal cells. Conversely, half of all patients with PA have antibodies to the thyroid.[61] Overall, PA occurs in 1% to 3% of patients with Graves disease, and Graves disease occurs in 8% of American patients with PA.

Hypothyroidism is frequently accompanied by anemia[62] (see Table 212-2). Although macrocytosis is observed most commonly, normochromic and microcytic anemias also may be seen. Microcytic anemia also may be secondary to iron deficiency from the menorrhagia of hypothyroidism. PA is also common; gastric antibodies are noted in 27% of patients with hypothy-

roidism and intrinsic factor antibodies are observed in 6%.[63] Overall, 7% to 12% of patients with hypothyroidism have clinical PA and an additional 10% have latent PA[64] (see Chap. 45).

Thyroid hormones have relatively few effects on white blood cell production. Mild increases in lymphocytes, especially T lymphocytes, and generalized lymphadenopathy have been noted rarely in hyperthyroidism. Half of all individuals with hyperthyroidism have asymptomatic enlargement of the spleen.[65] Granulocyte production appears not to be affected.

Iatrogenic granulocytopenia due to antithyroid medications can be a life-threatening condition. Approximately 0.5% to 1.0% of patients receiving methimazole, carbimazole, or propylthiouracil develop agranulocytosis.[66] In most drug-induced cases, mild neutropenia usually resolves within 7 days of discontinuing use of the medication (see Chap. 42). In a group of Japanese patients with Graves disease, a strong correlation was seen between the risk of methimazole-induced agranulocytosis and the human leukocyte antigen (HLA) class II allele DRB1*08032, suggesting a role for T lymphocyte–mediated autoimmunity in this syndrome.[67]

Thyrotoxicosis occasionally has been associated with thrombocytopenia.[68] Although originally thought to be immune-mediated, splenic sequestration of platelets (in enlarged spleens) may play a role. The autoimmune thrombocytopenia of Graves disease may respond to treatment with antithyroid medications alone.[69] Patients with normal platelet counts may have easy bruising due to qualitative platelet abnormalities from increased platelet-associated immunoglobulins. Of course, easy bruising may also be due to thrombocytopenia. Coagulation abnormalities in hyperthyroidism include increased levels of factor VIII coagulant activity, elevated levels of von Willebrand factor, and prolongation of euglobulin lysis.[70]

In hypothyroidism, qualitative as opposed to quantitative platelet abnormalities predominate. Prolongation of the bleeding time and an increased response to aspirin challenges are observed.[71] A subset of patients with hypothyroidism will present with clinical evidence of von Willebrand disease (i.e., with mucosal bleeding or menorrhagia). In these patients the typical laboratory manifestations of *type I von Willebrand disease* are seen (low factor VIII, low ristocetin cofactor activity, and low von Willebrand factor antigen levels). These levels will normalize with thyroid-replacement therapy.[72,73] In contradistinction to pathologic thyroid excess states, hypothyroidism may be associated with depressed factor VIII levels and increased fibrinolysis, with accelerated euglobulin lysis times.

## PARATHYROID GLAND AND ABNORMALITIES OF CALCIUM METABOLISM

Abnormalities of calcium metabolism, including those caused by parathyroid disease, are associated with a variety of hematologic changes. A normochromic, normocytic anemia complicates the clinical course of ~20% of patients with primary hyperparathyroidism; a similar anemia is frequently noted in the secondary hyperparathyroidism of chronic renal insufficiency.[74,75] Parathyroidectomy may result in improvement of the anemia in both settings. These changes have led to the hypothesis that parathyroid hormone (PTH) is the uremic "toxin" responsible for the anemia associated with chronic renal failure.[75a] Supporting this view is the finding that PTH can suppress normal erythropoiesis in vitro.[76] However, the reversal of the anemia of renal failure with the administration of erythropoietin has challenged the central role of PTH.

While erythropoietin administration to patients with renal failure results in correction of the anemia of renal disease in the majority of patients, ~20% to 25% require higher than usual

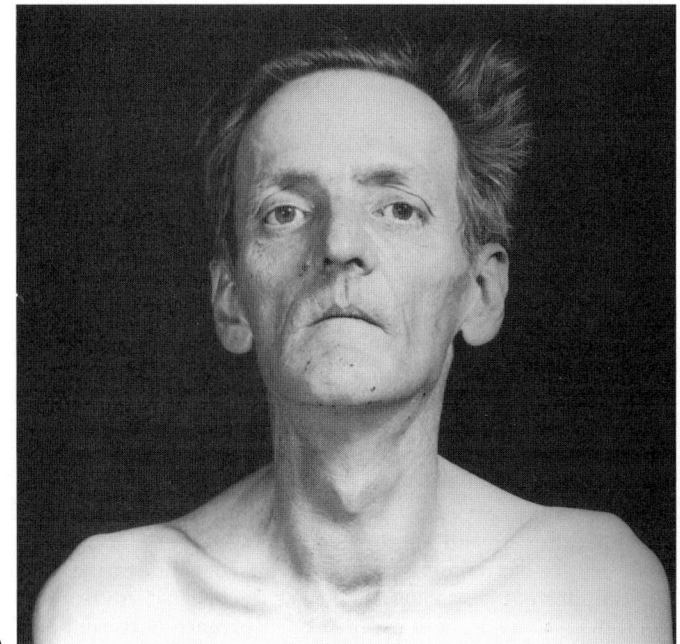
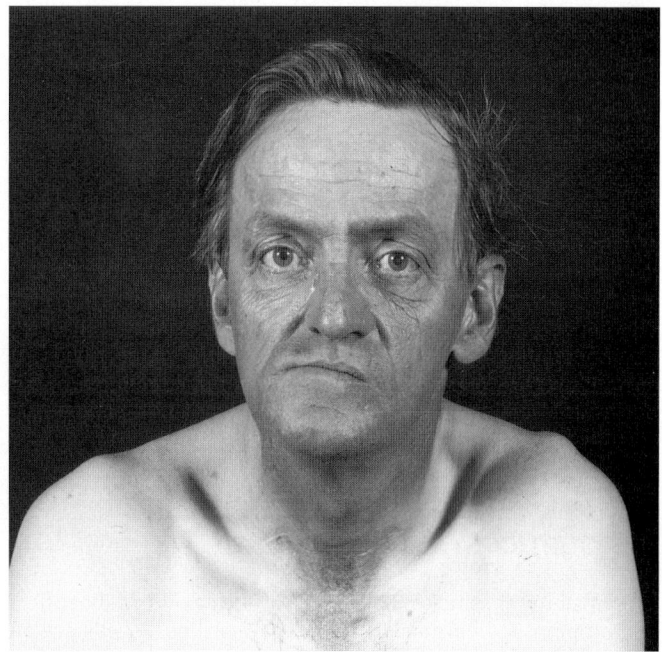
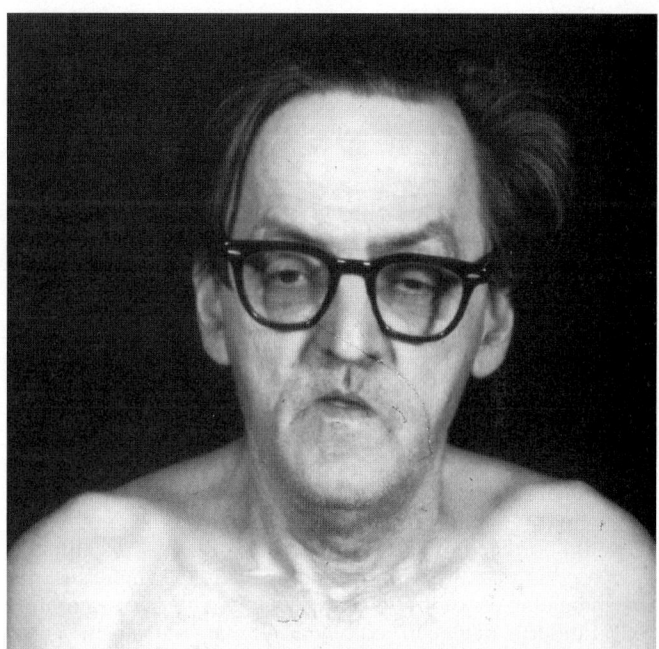

**FIGURE 212-2. A,** A 56-year-old man with Graves disease. He had lost considerable weight, and was pale because of an anemia that was normochromic and normocytic. **B,** Five months after subtotal thyroidectomy (he had refused radioiodine treatment), his anemia had resolved. **C,** Two years later, the patient complained of severe weakness and symptoms of peripheral neuropathy. Again, he was pale. A macrocytic anemia was present, and pernicious anemia was diagnosed. He responded to vitamin $B_{12}$ therapy.

dosages of the drug (>100 U/kg 3 times per week). In a study of serum PTH levels and bone histomorphometry in patients with both normal and excessive erythropoietin requirements, the highest erythropoietin requirements were found in those with the highest serum PTH levels, the greatest evidence of osteoclastic changes on bone biopsy, and the presence of bone marrow fibrosis. These findings suggest that excessive serum PTH levels may interfere with erythropoiesis by inducing marrow fibrosis.[77] Patients with erythropoietin resistance due to secondary hyperparathyroidism may respond to parathyroidectomy with lowering of erythropoietin requirements by 30% to 50%.[78] Intravenous calcitriol also was effective in reducing erythropoietin requirements and increasing the hematocrit in 19 of 28 patients.[79]

Although patients with defects in the receptor for $1,25(OH)_2D_3$ typically have no clinical abnormalities of hematopoiesis, hypoproliferative anemia and impairment of phagocy-

tosis have been noted in children with rickets.[80] Direct effects of vitamin D on the hematopoietic system include inhibition of the release of cytokines (GM-CSF, IL-2, and interferon-γ), stimulation of macrophage-related enzymes and activity, and promotion of macrophage and myeloid leukemia cell differentiation.

## PANCREATIC DYSFUNCTION

Patients with diabetes mellitus occasionally may have a hypoproliferative anemia. This anemia is most often due to chronic renal disease or chronic infection. There is a small group of patients with normal renal function who have an anemia due to low serum erythropoietin levels.[80,81,81a] Acute acidosis, such as in ketoacidosis, also may lead to hemolysis. The finding of anemia in patients with diabetes is paradoxic because several factors in diabetes should lead to erythrocytosis. In vitro, insulin has a stimulatory effect on the growth of red blood cell precursors, but it is not known whether this has any clinical significance in patients with diabetes.[82] Glycosylation of hemoglobin A to hemoglobin $A_{1c}$ results in impaired binding of 2,3-diphosphoglycerate and an increase in hemoglobin oxygen affinity.[83] In addition, ketoacidosis leads to decreased levels of 2,3-diphosphoglycerate that further impair oxygen delivery to tissue.[84] These changes in oxygen delivery should result in an increase in erythropoietin production and, eventually, erythrocytosis; however, clinically this is not observed.

Impaired granulocyte function has also been noted in patients with poorly controlled diabetes.[85,86] These alterations may result in the increased susceptibility to bacterial infections commonly seen in patients with diabetes. Other immunologic abnormalities include abnormal leukocyte migration, elevated spontaneous secretion of immunoglobulins, and abnormal levels of circulating T lymphocytes.[87] Hyperinsulinemia, associated with impaired glucose tolerance, enhances the potential for acute thrombosis.[87a]

## ABNORMALITIES OF ADRENAL FUNCTION AND CORTICOSTEROID HORMONES

Corticosteroid hormones have a multitude of actions that affect hematopoiesis. Pharmacologic doses of corticosteroids are an important part of the treatment of immune-mediated cytopenias. Corticosteroid hormones reduce antibody-mediated red blood cell and platelet destruction by reducing immunoglobulin synthesis and decreasing immunoglobulin binding to target cells and macrophages. They also increase the rate of red blood cell and platelet production directly. An increase in the total white blood cell count, initially caused by the release of granulocytes from the marrow reserve and subsequently sustained by the true stimulation of granulocyte production, is also observed during corticosteroid therapy. Simultaneously, a reduction in the total lymphocyte count occurs, which may be a desired effect in patients with hematologic lymphoproliferative malignancies or autoimmune diseases. Diagnostically, a rise in the total granulocyte count after an infusion of corticosteroids, epinephrine, or both has been used to document the ability of patients with granulocytopenia to respond to stress or infectious challenges, and can differentiate between benign neutropenia and states of decreased myeloid reserve.[88]

Adrenal insufficiency, such as that observed in Addison disease or in laboratory animals undergoing adrenalectomy, results in a mild normochromic anemia. Because the plasma volume is decreased in patients with hypoadrenalism, the slight declines in hemoglobin concentration and hematocrit may not accurately reflect the true degree of red blood cell mass decrement. These effects can be corrected with adrenal hormone replacement. Hypoadrenalism also may result in leukopenia, eosinophilia, and a relative lymphocytosis.

Conversely, hyperadrenalism, occurring in Cushing syndrome and congenital adrenal hyperplasia, may result in polycythemia.[89] Patients with primary hyperaldosteronism, Bartter syndrome, and pheochromocytoma also may exhibit polycythemia. In these diseases, erythropoietin levels often are elevated. Surgical removal of the tumor and appropriate medical therapy result in normalization of the erythropoietin level and correction of the polycythemia.

## GONADAL DYSFUNCTION

Gonadal hormones play an important role in hematopoiesis, as evidenced by the 1- to 2-g difference in hemoglobin concentrations between adult men and women. Hemoglobin concentrations increase in both sexes between the ages of 2 and 14 years. However, between the ages of 14 and 20 years, hemoglobin levels increase in men and decrease in women.[90] Testosterone metabolites function as stimulants of red cell production through at least two different mechanisms: direct stimulation of erythroid precursors and increasing erythropoietin production.[91] The 5α-metabolites augment the release of erythropoietin from the kidney, whereas the 5β-metabolites recruit inactive erythroid stem cells into an erythropoietin-responsive phase.[92] Attempts to stimulate hematopoiesis in patients with bone marrow failure syndromes and myelodysplastic syndromes using exogenous androgens are only rarely successful and are frequently complicated by virilizing side effects, hepatotoxicity, and fluid retention. Testicular hypogonadism (e.g., Klinefelter syndrome [XXY]) is associated with a mild anemia that is corrected during testosterone therapy.

Androgens have been used to treat disorders of the coagulation system. Idiopathic thrombocytopenic purpura (ITP), is a chronic autoimmune disorder that is due to autoantibodies directed against platelet glycoproteins. The major clinical manifestation is thrombocytopenia, which can be mild and asymptomatic or severe and life-threatening. Like other autoimmune diseases, ITP has a predilection for women of childbearing ages. The initial treatment usually consists of corticosteroids; however, many patients will experience recurrence of thrombocytopenia when steroids are tapered. The definitive therapeutic procedure is splenectomy; by removing the spleen, the major site of platelet destruction is eliminated. In addition, the spleen is a major source of autoantibody production; ~60% of patients who undergo splenectomy will have a satisfactory increase in their platelet count. Patients who relapse after splenectomy may continue to respond to steroid therapy, but in an effort to avoid the complications of chronic steroid therapy, a number of drug regimes have been assessed. One of the drugs that has been used in patients who relapse postsplenectomy is danazol, which is an impeded androgen. A review of a number of small series in which danazol has been used has shown that 24% of patients will respond with normal platelet counts, while 16% will have platelet counts of >50,000/μL for varying durations. Therapeutic responses to danazol may require at least 3 to 6 months of therapy. Some patients have had unmaintained remissions after 1 year of therapy.[93] Danazol has also been found to be effective in autoimmune hemolytic anemia.[94]

Antithrombin III deficiency and protein C deficiency are two hereditary conditions in which decreased levels of the respective proteins lead to an increased risk for venous thrombotic disease. The anabolic steroids, stanozolol and danazol, increase the levels of antithrombin III and protein C in some patients.[95,96]

In contrast, estrogens suppress erythropoiesis and granulopoiesis by inducing changes in the hematopoietic microenvironment of the bone marrow.[97] In laboratory animals, large doses of estrogens cause an estrous-associated aplastic anemia, blunted responses to erythropoietin, and decreased numbers of colony-forming units–spleen. The effect of estrogens on hemostasis is more complex. Whether estrogens cause direct suppression of thrombopoiesis and platelet counts in humans is unknown. However, the incidence of ITP is significantly elevated in women compared to men.

Estrogens, whether administered in the form of oral contraceptives or as postmenopausal hormone replacement, are associated with an increased risk for venous thromboembolism. Two large epidemiologic studies have implicated older formulations of oral contraceptives as a risk factor for thromboembolic disease.[98,99] While the amount of estrogens has been decreased since the 1960s, the most recent oral contraceptives, which contain <50 μg ethinyl estradiol, are *still associated* with an increased risk of thromboembolic disease. For individuals who take oral contraceptives, the relative risks for nonfatal thrombotic events is 3.8, and for fatal thrombotic events, 2.1. The third-generation oral contraceptives contain the progestins desogestral or gestodene. Oral contraceptives that contain either of these compounds are associated with much *higher risks* of venous thromboembolism than the second-generation oral contraceptives that contain levonorgestrel as the progestin.[100]

A subgroup that is at a particularly high risk of venous thromboembolic disease while on estrogen contraceptives are women who have the *factor V Leiden gene*. This mutation, which is present in ~5% of whites of northern European descent, is a known risk factor for venous thrombosis in both sexes. However, the combination of heterozygosity for factor V Leiden adds a multiplicative increase to the already increased risk associated with oral contraceptive use and yields a 30-fold increase in the risk of thrombosis.[101] The risk for patients with homozygous factor V Leiden who take oral contraceptives is *several hundred-fold*.[102]

Postmenopausal hormonal therapy with estrogens is also associated with an increased risk of venous thromboembolism. There have been five observational studies, which have shown an increased risk of thrombosis that is two to four times as high as in women who do not take estrogens.[103]

The slight hypercoagulable state induced by estrogen therapy has been used clinically to shorten the bleeding time of patients with uremia.[104] Estrogens also stimulate increased production of von Willebrand factor protein by endothelial cells and increase factor VIII levels by unclear mechanisms.

Inhibin, a glycoprotein produced by Sertoli cells in men and granulosa cells in women, causes inhibition of erythropoiesis. Activin A, a glycoprotein homodimer composed of two β units of inhibin, conversely causes stimulation of erythropoiesis. It is believed that the β subunits of these glycoproteins cause the effect indirectly through the release of cytokines.[105]

## HEMATOLOGIC ASPECTS OF PREGNANCY

The many alterations of hormonal status that occur during pregnancy induce numerous changes in hematologic and hemostatic function.[106] During pregnancy, the total red blood cell mass expands by ~20% to 30%. However, a simultaneous increase in plasma volume (40%–60%) results in the hydremia of pregnancy. Thus, a fall in the hematocrit to ~30% to 32% and decreased hemoglobin to ~10 g/dL are common. The expanded blood pool compensates for the increased metabolic and perfusion needs of the fetus. The cause of the increased red blood cell mass is unknown, although stimulation of erythropoietin secretion by placental lactogen has been noted in the mouse model.[107]

A true anemia occurring during pregnancy is most frequently the result of a deficiency of iron, folate, or both.[107a] During pregnancy, ~1000 mg of iron is required by the developing fetus. Iron is preferentially transferred across the placenta even if the mother is deficient. Folate deficiency also may occur because of a similar increase in the need for this essential cofactor by the fetus. Although folate deficiency traditionally results in a macrocytic anemia, concomitant iron deficiency (a microcytic anemia) and changes in blood plasma volume frequently mask the ability of automated size determinations to distinguish the cause or the mixed character of the anemia.

An elevation of the white blood cell count, with an outpouring of early forms, Doehle bodies, and increased cytoplasmic granulation, may occur during pregnancy and probably results from increased glucocorticoid production during the pregnant state. In an uncomplicated pregnancy, platelet counts tend to decrease slightly within the normal range as the pregnancy approaches term.[108] Thrombocytopenia in the expectant mother represents an abnormal state and requires investigation. The incidence of immune-mediated thrombocytopenic purpura is

slightly elevated during pregnancy. Management of this disorder remains controversial. Corticosteroid therapy is typically recommended as a first maneuver (in nondiabetic, normotensive women), with intravenous γ-immunoglobulins reserved for corticosteroid-refractory or steroid-intolerant patients. Because the fetus is also a candidate for the development of thrombocytopenia as a result of transplacental transfer of antiplatelet immunoglobulin G (IgG), sampling of fetal scalp venous blood during labor or periumbilical vein sampling before labor has been used by some to indicate the need for operative delivery.

Preeclampsia and eclampsia are associated with abnormal platelet-endothelium interactions. Platelet consumption is considered a major component of this hypertensive disorder. A decrease in antithrombin III levels and an elevation of dimers of fibrin split products may be observed. Thrombocytopenia and a hemolytic anemia are components of the HELLP syndrome (hemolysis with elevated liver enzymes and low platelets) that also may present as hypertension, edema, and proteinuria. Thrombotic thrombocytopenic purpura, a disease consisting of thrombocytopenia, microangiopathic hemolytic anemia, fever, renal insufficiency, and neurologic dysfunction, is a life-threatening complication that requires emergency diagnosis and therapy, typically with plasmapheresis.

Disseminated intravascular coagulation (DIC) represents the most frequent cause of life-threatening bleeding during pregnancy. DIC caused by the unrecognized slow release of the products of conception into the systemic circulation during fetal death in utero has become a rare occurrence because of improvement in diagnostic ultrasound techniques. However, DIC that accompanies abruptio placentae and amniotic fluid embolism remains a life-threatening disease. DIC may complicate hypertonic saline and urea-induced abortions. These complications usually disappear shortly after the uterus is evacuated, although temporary use of heparin to control DIC may be required while preparing for definitive surgery.

A hypercoagulable state with progressive increases in the concentration of clotting factors and a decrease in fibrinolytic capacity occurs during normal pregnancy.[109] This change in the hemostatic state probably serves to prevent postpartum hemorrhage. However, the hypercoagulable state together with venostasis caused by direct compression of the inferior vena cava by the enlarged uterus and the relaxation of the musculature of the venous vessels, which also increase stasis, result in a markedly increased risk of lower-extremity deep venous thrombosis. If deep venous thrombosis develops during pregnancy, or if the pregnant woman is considered to be at high risk because of previous episodes of deep venous thrombosis or pulmonary embolus, subcutaneous dose-adjusted heparin therapy is the treatment of choice. Warfarin is not recommended in the first trimester because of fetal wastage and frequent teratogenicity. There is controversy about the use of warfarin at any time during pregnancy.

## NUTRITIONAL DEFICIENCIES AND ANOREXIA NERVOSA

Iron deficiency, resulting from decreased intake or excessive blood loss, leads to impairment of hemoglobin synthesis with a resultant microcytic anemia. A diagnosis of iron-deficiency anemia requires a search for an underlying cause, although replacement therapy can be initiated concurrently. Deficiencies of folic acid or vitamin $B_{12}$ lead to megaloblastic changes, which are the result of impaired DNA synthesis. Clinically, these vitamin deficiencies may result in megaloblastic anemia, giant band leukocytes, and dysplasia of platelets.

Severe restriction of calorie intake, such as that which occurs during fad diets, starvation, or anorexia nervosa, may be accompanied by many endocrine and hematologic abnormalities. During severe protein starvation, anemia may occur as a result of a relative increase in plasma volume and a concurrent decrease in red blood cell production. Patients with anorexia nervosa and bulimia may have pancytopenia.[110] The bone marrow in these patients becomes infiltrated with an interstitial ground substance (amorphous eosinophilic material) in a process known as gelatinous transformation. Necrosis of marrow cells also may occur. An anemia characterized by irregularly shaped red blood cells (acanthocytes) and a decrease in the white blood cell count may be noted. Although decreased circulating levels of immunoglobulins and components of the complement cascade may develop, patients are not at increased risk of infection and T-cell lymphocyte function typically remains normal. Severe thrombocytopenia with clinical evidence of bleeding may occur in as many as 10% of patients. Deficiencies of vitamin K–dependent coagulation factors can be noted.

# REFERENCES

1. Till JE, McCulloch EA. Direct measurement of the radiation sensitivity of normal mouse bone marrow cells. Radiat Res 1961; 14:213.
2. Baum CM, Uchida N, Peault B, Weissman IL. Isolation and characterization of hematopoietic progenitor and stem cells. In: Forman SJ, Blume KG, Thomas ED, eds. Bone marrow transplantation. Cambridge, MA: Blackwell Science, 1994:53.
3. Metcalf D. Hematopoietic regulators: redundancy or subtlety? Blood 1993; 82:3515.
4. Gabrilove JL, Golde DW. Hematopoietic growth factors. In: DeVita VT Jr, Hellman S, Rosenberg SA, eds. Cancer: principles & practice of oncology. Philadelphia: JB Lippincott Co, 1993:2275.
5. Robinson BE, Quesenberry PJ. Hematopoietic growth factors: overview and clinical applications (Pts I, II, III). Am J Med Sci 1990; 300:163.
6. Mazanet R, Griffin JD. Hematopoietic growth factors. In: Armitage JO, Antman KH, eds. High-dose cancer therapy: pharmacology, hematopoietins, stem cells. Baltimore: Williams & Wilkins, 1992:289.
7. Krantz SB. Erythropoietin. Blood 1991; 77:419.
8. Schreiber S, Howaldt S, Schnoor MS, et al. Recombinant erythropoietin for the treatment of anemia in inflammatory bowel disease. N Engl J Med 1996; 334:619.
9. Spivak JL. Recombinant erythropoietin and the anemia of cancer. Blood 1994; 84:997.
10. Eschbach J, Kelly M, Haley R, et al. Treatment of the anemia of progressive renal failure with recombinant human erythropoietin. N Engl J Med 1989; 321:158.
11. Jilani SM, Glaspy JA. Impact of epoetin alfa in chemotherapy-associated anemia. Semin Oncol 1998; 25:571.
12. Thatcher N. Management of chemotherapy-induced anemia in solid tumors. Semin Oncol 1998; 25(Suppl 7):23.
13. Henry DH. Experience with epoetin alfa and acquired immunodeficiency syndrome anemia. Semin Oncol 1998; 25(Suppl 7):64.
14. Bodey GP, Buckley M, Sathe YS, et al. Quantitative relationships between circulating leukocytes and infection in patients with acute leukemia. Ann Intern Med 1966; 64:328.
15. Metcalf K, Begley CJ, Johnson GR, et al. Biologic properties in vitro of a recombinant granulocyte-macrophage colony-stimulating factor. Blood 1986; 67:37.
16. Sieff CA, Emerson SG, Donahue RE, et al. Human recombinant granulocyte-macrophage colony stimulating factor: a multilineage hematopoietin. Science 1985; 230:1171.
17. American Society of Clinical Oncology. Update of recommendations for the use of hematopoietic colony-stimulating factors: evidence-based clinical practice guidelines. J Clin Oncol 1996; 14:1957.
18. Heil G, Hoelzer D, Sanz MA, et al. A randomized, double-blind, placebo-controlled, phase III study of filgrastim in remission induction and consolidation therapy for adults with de novo acute myeloid leukemia. Blood 1997; 90:4710.
19. Nemunaitis J, Rosenfeld CS, Ash R, et al. Phase III randomized, double-blind placebo-controlled trial of rhGM-CSF following allogeneic bone marrow transplantation. Bone Marrow Transplant 1995; 15:949.
20. Klumpp TR, Mangan KF, Goldberg SL, et al. Granulocyte colony-stimulating factor accelerates neutrophil engraftment following peripheral-blood stem-cell transplantation: a prospective, randomized trial. J Clin Oncol 1995; 13:1323.
21. Bensinger WI, Weaver CH, Appelbaum FR, et al. Transplantation of allogeneic peripheral blood stem cells mobilized by recombinant human granulocyte colony-stimulating factor. Blood 1995; 85:1655.
22. Schmitz N, Linch DC, Dreger P, et al. Randomised trial of filgrastim-mobilised peripheral blood progenitor cell transplantation versus autologous bone-marrow transplantation in lymphoma patients. Lancet 1996; 347:353.
23. Caspar CB, Seger RA, Burger J, et al. Effective stimulation of donors for granulocyte transfusions with recombinant methionyl granulocyte colony-stimulating factor. Blood 1993; 81:2866.
24. Bensinger WI, Price TH, Dale DC, et al. The effects of daily recombinant human granulocyte colony-stimulating factor administration on normal granulocyte donors undergoing leukapheresis. Blood 1993; 81:1883.
25. Kitano K, Abboud CN, Ryan DH, et al. Macrophage-active colony stimulating factors enhance human immunodeficiency virus type 1 infection in bone marrow stem cells. Blood 1991; 77:1699.
26. Levine JD, Allan JD, Tessitore JH, et al. Recombinant human granulocyte-macrophage colony-stimulating factor ameliorates zidovudine-induced neutropenia in patients with acquired immunodeficiency syndrome (AIDS)-related complex. Blood 1992; 78:3148.
27. Scadden DT. Hematologic disorders and growth factor support in HIV infection. Hematol Oncol Clin North Am 1996; 10:1149.
28. Wendling F, Varlet P, Charon M, Tambourin P. MPLV: a retrovirus complex inducing an acute myeloproliferative leukemia disorder in mice. Virology 1986; 149:242.
29. Vigon I, Mornon JP, Cocault L, et al. Molecular cloning and characterization of MPL, the human homolog of the v-mpl oncogene: identification of a member of the hematopoietic growth factor receptor superfamily. Proc Natl Acad Sci U S A 1992; 89:5640.
30. de Sauvage F, Hass PE, Spencer SD, et al. Stimulation of megakaryocytopoiesis and thrombopoiesis by the c-mpl ligand. Nature 1994; 369:533.
31. Kaushansky K, Lok S, Holly RD, et al. Promotion of megakaryocyte progenitor expansion and differentiation by the c-mpl ligand thrombopoietin. Nature 1994; 369:568.
32. Fanucchi M, Glaspy J, Crawford J, et al. Effects of polyethylene glycol-conjugated recombinant human megakaryocyte growth and development factor on platelet counts after chemotherapy for lung cancer. N Engl J Med 1997; 336:404.
33. Basser RL, Rasko JE, Clarke K, et al. Randomized, blinded, placebo-controlled phase I trial of pegylated recombinant human megakaryocyte growth and development factor with filgrastim after dose-intensive chemotherapy in patients with advanced cancer. Blood 1997; 89:3118.
34. Vadhan-Raj S. Recombinant human thrombopoietin: clinical experience and in vivo biology. Semin Hematol 1998; 35:261.
35. Maslak P, Nimer S. The efficacy of IL-3, SCF, IL-6, and IL-11 in treating thrombocytopenia. Semin Hematol 1998; 35:253.
36. O'Shaughnessy J, Tolcher A, Risenberg D, et al. Prospective, randomized trial of 5-fluorouracil, leucovorin, doxorubicin and cyclophosphamide chemotherapy in combination with the interleukin-3/granulocyte-macrophage colony-stimulating factor fusion protein (PIXY321) versus GM-CSF in patients with advanced breast cancer. Blood 1996; 87:205.
37. Vose J, Pandite L, Beveridge R, et al. Phase III study comparing PIXY 321 and GM-CSF following autologous bone marrow transplantation in patients with non-Hodgkin's lymphoma. Blood 1995; 86(Suppl 1):972a.
38. Dainiak N. Hematologic manifestations of endocrine disorders. In: Hoffman R, Benz EJ Jr, Shattil SJ, et al, eds. Hematology: basic principles and practice. New York: Churchill Livingstone, 1991:1747.
39. Erslev AJ. Anemia of endocrine disorders. In: Williams WJ, Beutler E, Erslev AJ, Lichtman MA, eds. Hematology. New York: McGraw-Hill, 1990:444.
40. Daughaday WH, Williams RH, Daland GA. The effect of endocrinopathies on the blood. Blood 1948; 3:342.
41. Van Dyke DC, Garcia JF, Simpson ME, et al. Maintenance of circulating red cell volume in rats after removal of the posterior and intermediate lobes of the pituitary. Blood 1952; 7:1017.
42. Ferrari E, Ascari E, Bossoto PA, Barosi G. Sheehan's syndrome with complete bone marrow aplasia: long-term results of substitution therapy with hormones. Br J Haematol 1976; 33:575.
43. Golde DW, Bersch N, Li CH. Growth hormones: species-specific stimulation of erythropoiesis in vitro. Science 1976; 196:1112.
44. Merchav S, Tatarsky I, Hochberg Z. Enhancement of erythropoiesis in vitro by human growth hormone is mediated by insulin-like growth factor I. Br J Haematol 1988; 70:267.
45. Claustres M, Chatelain P, Sultan C. Insulin-like growth factor I stimulates human erythroid colony formation in vitro. J Clin Endocrinol Metab 1987; 65:78.
46. Muta K, Krantz SB, Bondurant MC, et al. Distinct roles of erythropoietin, insulin-like growth factor I, and stem cell factor in the development of erythroid progenitor cells. J Clin Invest 1994; 94:34.
47. Hoffman R, Dainiak N, Coupal E, et al. Hormonal influences on globin chain synthesis of fetal cord BFU-E in vitro. In: Stamatoyannopoulos G, Nienhuis AW, eds. Cellular and molecular regulation in hemoglobin switching. Orlando, FL: Grune & Stratton, 1979:389.
48. Ten Have SM, van der Lely AJ, Lamberts SW. Increase in haemoglobin concentration in growth hormone deficient adults during human recombinant growth hormone replacement therapy. Clin Endocrinol (Oxf) 1997; 47:565.
49. Prchal JF, Axelrad AA. Bone marrow responses in polycythemia vera. N Engl J Med 1974; 290:1382.
50. Correa P, Eskinazi D, Axelrod A. Circulating erythoid progenitors in polycythemia vera are hypersensitive to insulin-like growth factor 1 in vitro: studies in an improved serum-free medium. Blood 1994; 83:99.
51. Mirza A, Ezzat S, Axelrad A. Insulin-like growth factor binding protein-1 is elevated in patients with polycythemia vera and stimulates erythroid burst formation in vitro. Blood 1997; 89:1862.
52. Grellier P, Chanson P, Casadevall N, et al. Remission of polycythemia vera after surgical cure of acromegaly. Ann Intern Med 1996; 124:495.
53. Lethagen S. Desmopressin (DDAVP) and hemostasis. Ann Hematol 1994; 69:173.
54. Mannucci PM. Desmopressin (DDAVP) in the treatment of bleeding disorders: the first 20 years. Blood 1997; 90:2515.
55. Synder LM, Reddy WJ. Thyroid hormone control of erythrocyte 2,3-diphosphoglyceric acid concentrations. Science 1970; 169:879.
56. Meineke HA, Crafts RC. Evidence for a non-caloriogenic effect of thyroxin on erythropoiesis as judged by radioiron utilization. Proc Soc Exp Biol Med 1964; 117:520.

57. Golde DW, Bersch N, Chopra IJ, Cline MJ. Thyroid hormones stimulate erythropoiesis in vitro. Br J Haematol 1977; 37:173.
58. Boussios T, McIntyre WR, Gordon AS, Bertles JF. Receptors specific for thyroid hormones in nuclei of mammalian erythroid cells: involvement in erythroid cell proliferation. Br J Haematol 1982; 51:99.
59. Kuhn JM, Riew M, Rochette J, et al. Influence of thyroid status on hemoglobin A2 expression. J Clin Endocrinol Metab 1983; 57:344.
60. Reddy J, Brownlie BEW, Heaton DC, et al. The peripheral blood picture in thyrotoxicosis. NZ Med J 1981; 93:143.
61. Doniach D, Roitt IM, Taylor KB. Autoimmune phenomena in pernicious anemia. Br Med J 1963; 1:1374.
62. Ansell JE. The blood in hypothyroidism. In: Braverman LE, Utiger RD, eds. The thyroid: a fundamental and clinical text. Philadelphia: JB Lippincott Co, 1991:1022.
63. Ardeman S, Chanarin I, Krafchik B, Singer W. Addisonian pernicious anemia and intrinsic factor antibodies in thyroid disorders. Q J Med 1966; 35:421.
64. Tudhope GR, Wilson GM. Deficiency of vitamin B12 in hypothyroidism. Lancet 1962; 1:703.
65. Metcalfe-Gibson C, Keddie N. Spleen size and previous tonsillectomy in autoimmune disease of the thyroid. Lancet 1978; 1:944.
66. Wall JR, Fang SL, Kuroki T, et al. In vitro immunoreactivity to propylthiouracil, methimazole, and carbimazole in patients with Graves' disease: a possible cause of antithyroid drug-induced agranulocytosis. J Clin Endocrinol Metab 1984; 58:868.
67. Tamai H, Sudo T, Kimura A, et al. Association between the DRB1*08032 histocompatibility antigen and methimazole-induced agranulocytosis in Japanese patients with Graves disease. Ann Intern Med 1996; 124:490.
68. Herman J, Resnitzky P, Fink A. Association between thyrotoxicosis and thrombocytopenia. Isr J Med Sci 1978; 14:469.
69. Hofbauer LC, Spitzweg C, Schmauss S, et al. Graves disease associated with autoimmune thrombocytopenic purpura. Arch Intern Med 1997; 157:1033.
70. Farid NR, Griffiths BL, Collins JR, et al. Blood coagulation and fibrinolysis in thyroid disease. Thromb Haemost 1976; 35:415.
71. Edson JR, Fecher DR, Doe RP. Low platelet adhesiveness and other hemostatic abnormalities in hypothyroidism. Ann Intern Med 1975; 82:342.
72. Dalton RG, Dewar MS, Savidge GF, et al. Hypothyroidism as a cause of acquired von Willebrands disease. Lancet 1987; 1:1007.
73. Myrup B, Bregengard C, Faber J. Primary hemostasis in thyroid disease. J Intern Med 1995; 238:59.
74. Boxer H, Ellman L, Geller R, et al. Anemia in primary hyperparathyroidism. Arch Intern Med 1977; 13:588.
75. Zingraff J, Drueke T, Marie T, et al. Anemia and secondary hyperparathyroidism. Arch Intern Med 1978; 138:1650.
75a. Gallieni M, Corsi C, Brancaccio D. Hyperparathyroidism and anemia in renal failure. Am J Nephrol 2000; 20:89.
76. Meyets D, Bogin A, Dukes P, et al. Effect of parathyroid hormone on erythropoiesis. J Clin Invest 1981; 67:1263.
77. Rao DS, Shih MS, Mohini R. Effect of serum parathyroid hormone and bone marrow fibrosis on the response to erythropoietin in uremia. N Engl J Med 1993; 328:171.
78. Goicoechea M, Gomez-Campdera F, Polo JR, et al. Secondary hyperparathyroidism as cause of resistance to treatment with erythropoietin: effect of parathyroidectomy. Clin Nephrol 1996; 45:420.
79. Goicoechea M, Vazques MI, Ruiz MA, et al. Intravenous calcitriol improves anaemia and reduces the need for erythropoietin in haemodialysis patients. Nephron 1998: 78:23a.
80. Reichel H, Koeffler HP, Norman AW. The role of vitamin D endocrine system in health and disease. N Engl J Med 1989; 320:980.
81. Kojima K, Totsuka Y. Anemia due to reduced serum erythropoietin concentration in non-uremic diabetic patients. Diabetes Res Clin Pract 1995; 27:229.
81a. Cotroneo P, Maria Ricerca B, Todaro L, et al. Blunted erythropoietin response to anemia in patients with type 1 diabetes. Diabetes Metab Res Rev 2000; 16:172.
82. Kallab AM, Dabaghian G, Terjanian T. Anemia secondary to low erythropoietin in a patient with normal renal function. Mt Sinai J Med 1997; 64:406.
83. Bersch N, Groopman JE, Golde DW. Natural history and biosynthetic insulin stimulate the growth of human erythroid progenitors in vitro. J Clin Endocrinol Metab 1978; 55:1209.
84. Bunn HF, Briehl RW. The interaction of 2,3-2 diphosphoglycerate with various human hemoglobins. J Clin Invest 1970; 49:1008.
85. Ditzel J, Standl E. The problem of tissue oxygenation in diabetes mellitus. Acta Med Scand (Suppl) 1975; 578:59.
86. Molan CM, Beaty HN, Bagdade JD. Further characterization of the impaired bactericidal function of granulocytes in patients with poorly controlled diabetes. Diabetes 1978; 27:889.
87. Horita M, Suzuki H, Onodera T, et al. Abnormalities of immunoregulatory T-cell subsets in patients with insulin-dependent diabetes mellitus. J Immunol 1982; 129:1426.
87a. Meigs JB, Mittleman MA, Nathan DM, et al. Hyperinsulinemia, hyperglycemia, and impaired hemostasis. The Framingham Offspring Study. JAMA 2000; 283:221.
88. Dale DC, Fanci AS, DuPont G IV, Wolff SM. Comparison of agents producing a neutrophilic leukocytosis in man: hydrocortisone, prednisone, endotoxin, and etiocholanone. J Clin Invest 1975; 56:808.
89. Plotz CM, Knowlton AI, Regan C. The natural history of Cushing's syndrome. Am J Med 1952; 13:579.
90. Hawkins WW, Speck E, Keonard VG. Variations of a hemoglobin level with age and sex. Blood 1954; 9:999.
91. Besa EC. Hematologic effects of androgens revisited: an alternative therapy in various hematologic conditions. Semin Hematol 1994; 31:134.
92. Gorshein D, Hait WN, Besa EC, et al. Rapid stem cell differentiation induced by 19-nortestosterone decanoate. Br J Haematol 1974; 26:215.
93. McMillan R. Therapy for adults with refractory chronic immune thrombocytopenic purpura. Ann Intern Med 1997; 126:307.
94. Ahn YS, Harrington WJ, Mylvaganam R, et al. Danazol therapy for autoimmune hemolytic anemia. Ann Intern Med 1989; 107:177.
95. Winter JH, Fenech A, Bennett B, et al. Prophylactic antithrombotic therapy with stanazolol in individuals with familial antithrombin III deficiency. Br J Haematol 1984; 57:527.
96. Gonzalez R, Albeca I, Sala N, et al. Protein C deficiency response to danazol and DDAVP. Thromb Haemost 1985; 53:320.
97. Crandall TL, Joyce RA, Boggs DR. Estrogens and hematopoiesis: characterization and studies on the mechanism of neutropenia. J Lab Clin Med 1980; 95:857.
98. Vessey MP, Mann JI. Female sex hormones and thrombosis. Epidemiological aspects. Br Med Bull 1978; 34:157.
99. Bottiger LE, Boman G, Eklund G, Westerholm B. Oral contraceptives and thromboembolic disease: effects of lowering estrogen content. Lancet 1980; 1:1097.
100. Helmerhorst FM, Bloemenkamp KW, Rosendaal FR, et al. Oral contraceptives and thrombotic disease: risk of venous thromboembolism. Haemost Thromb 1997; 78;327.
101. Vandenbroucke JP, Koster T, Briet E, et al. Increased risk of venous thrombosis in oral contraceptive users who are carriers of factor V Leiden mutation. Lancet 1994; 344:1453.
102. Dahlback B. Resistance to activated protein C as risk factor for thrombosis: molecular mechanisms, laboratory investigation and clinical management. Semin Hematol 1997; 34:217.
103. Grady D, Saway G. Postmenopausal hormone therapy increases risk of deep vein thrombosis and pulmonary embolism. Am J Med 1998; 105:41.
104. Livio M, Mannucci PM, Vigano G, et al. Conjugated estrogens for the management of bleeding associated with renal failure. N Engl J Med 1986; 315:731.
105. Broxmeyer HE, Lu L, Cooper S, et al. Selective and indirect modulation of human amultipotential and erythroid hematopoietic progenitor cell proliferation by recombinant human activin and inhibin. Proc Natl Acad Sci U S A 1988; 85:9052.
106. Duffy TP. Hematologic aspects of pregnancy. In: Hoffman R, Benz EJ Jr, Shattil SJ, et al, eds. Hematology: basic principles and practice. New York: Churchill Livingstone, 1991:1707.
107. Jepson JH, Lowenstein L. The effect of testosterone, adrenal steroids, and prolactin on erythropoiesis. Acta Haematol 1970; 38:292.
107a. Allen LH. Anemia and iron deficiency: effects on pregnancy outcome. Am J Clin Nutr 2000; 71[5 Suppl]:1280S.
108. Sill PR, Lind T, Walker W. Platelet values during normal pregnancy. Br J Obstet Gynaecol 1985; 92:48.
109. Burns MM. Emerging concepts in the diagnosis and management of venous thromboembolism during pregnancy. J Thromb Thrombolysis 2000; 10:59.
110. Waren WP, Van de Wicke RI. Clinical and metabolic features of anorexia nervosa. Am J Obstet Gynecol 1973; 117:435.

# CHAPTER 213

# INFECTIOUS DISEASES AND ENDOCRINOLOGY

CARMELITA U. TUAZON AND STEPHEN A. MIGUELES

## INFECTIOUS DISEASES CAUSING HORMONAL OR METABOLIC DISORDERS

The clinician must be aware of the many *infectious diseases that can cause hormonal and metabolic disorders*. Similarly, there are a surprising number of *hormonal disorders that may be associated with or predispose to certain infectious diseases*.

In addition, drugs such as the corticosteroids may have adverse, as well as beneficial, effects in the occurrence or treatment of infectious diseases. Finally, there are several antimicrobials that can exert endocrine effects.

### HYPOTHALAMIC-PITUITARY INFECTIONS

Infections involving the hypothalamic-pituitary systems are rare, but can cause important clinical manifestations, such as diabetes insipidus, impairment of temperature regulation, and anterior pituitary hypofunction (see Chaps. 9 and 11). A wide variety of etiologies have been implicated, including bacterial, mycobacterial, fungal, parasitic, and viral infections.

Hypothalamic-pituitary bacterial infections occur as rare complications of an adjacent bacterial meningitis or as a focal abscess formation. Such involvement has been reported with pneumococcal, streptococcal, listerial, or tuberculous meningitis. Pituitary abscesses can be classified as primary (occurring within a previously healthy gland) or secondary (occurring within and sharing radiologic characteristics with an existing lesion). Approximately 33% of pituitary abscesses are secondary, arising within preexisting pituitary lesions (e.g., adenomas, craniopharyngioma, and Rathke cleft cyst).[1,2] Even in the absence of a tumor or other mass lesion, hypothalamic-pituitary abscesses may occur as a complication after sphenoid sinusitis or cavernous thrombophlebitis. Infectious isolates of the pituitary abscess or of the adjacent foci have included *Staphylococcus aureus*, *Staphylococcus epidermidis*, *Streptococcus pneumoniae*, *Streptococcus pyogenes*, *Escherichia coli*, *Salmonella typhi*, *Neisseria* species, *Citrobacter diversus*, diphtheroids, *Actinomyces*, *Mycobacterium tuberculosis*, and syphilis.[3,4]

Children in developing countries have a predilection for tuberculous meningitis. Hypopituitarism can occur after this condition, with growth hormone and gonadotropin deficiency being the most common abnormalities. Clinicians should be aware of the possibility of growth hormone deficiency in children with tuberculous meningitis because they may benefit from hormone-replacement therapy.[5]

Shock resulting from infection also may cause pituitary necrosis of sudden onset, similar to the Sheehan syndrome, which is associated with peripartum hemorrhage (see Chaps. 11 and 17). A case of partial hypopituitarism has been reported after septic peritonitis with shock, complicating a perforated appendix.[6] Toxic shock syndrome has been reported subsequent to hypophysectomy by the transsphenoidal route. In this setting, removal of the nasal tampon is a lifesaving procedure.[7]

Hypothalamic-pituitary infection may be difficult to diagnose. Signs of pituitary insufficiency may not occur until >50% of the gland is destroyed. Some reported cases have been discovered only at autopsy.[3] The clinical presentation may vary, but usually is related to the symptoms of a mass lesion (i.e., headache and vision disturbance). The endocrine dysfunction may manifest as amenorrhea, polydipsia, polyuria, or panhypopituitarism.

Radiologic findings of a pituitary abscess reveal changes consistent with an expanding mass in the sella turcica. The pressure of an expanding mass may lead to erosion of the walls of the sella turcica, with depression of the floor into the sphenoid sinus and upward rotation and osteoporosis of the anterior and posterior clinoids.[8–10] With computed tomographic (CT) scans and magnetic resonance imaging (MRI), suprasellar extension may be seen. Although these techniques are useful in defining the anatomic location and characteristics of an abscess of the hypothalamic-pituitary region, it may be difficult to distinguish such an abscess from tumor.[9,10] Even before the development of MRI, it had been suggested that the presence of diabetes insipidus (DI) could help to differentiate pituitary abscess from an adenoma. DI occurs in only 10% of patients with adenomas as compared to almost half of patients with an abscess.[2]

Treatment of a pituitary abscess usually consists of the administration of antibiotics combined with surgical drainage, using the transsphenoidal approach with drainage into the sphenoid sinus.

Fungal infections of the pituitary caused by *Histoplasma capsulatum*, *Coccidioides immitis*, *Blastomyces dermatitidis*, *Sporothrix schenckii*, *Candida* species, and *Aspergillus* species have been described. They usually are associated with disseminated diseases and immunosuppression.

Parasitic infections of the pituitary are extremely rare. Pituitary involvement has been described in patients with disseminated toxoplasmosis. An intrasellar hydatid cyst also has been reported. Amebic brain abscess and malaria have been associated with pituitary necrosis. African trypanosomiasis (SS) is an anthropozoonosis transmitted by the tsetse fly. Infection with *Trypanosoma brucei* in humans is associated with adynamia, lethargy, anorexia, and more specifically, amenorrhea/infertility in women and loss of libido/impotence in men. Evidence suggests that experimental infection with *T. brucei* species causes polyglandular endocrine failure by local inflammation of the pituitary, thyroid, adrenal, and gonadal glands. In a study of Ugandan patients with untreated SS, there was a high prevalence of hypogonadism (85%), hypothyroidism (50%), and adrenal insufficiency (27%). Pituitary function tests suggested an unusual, combined central (hypothalamic/pituitary) and peripheral defect in hormone secretion. The presence of hypopituitarism correlated with high cytokine concentrations (i.e., tumor necrosis factor-α [TNF-α], interleukin-6 [IL-6]), and direct parasitic infiltration of the endocrine glands, is involved in the pathogenesis of SS-associated endocrine dysfunction.[11]

Viral infections may alter hypothalamic-pituitary function or cause actual necrosis of the gland. All of the herpesviruses, as well as influenza, measles, mumps, poliomyelitis, Coxsackie B, rabies, St. Louis encephalitis, rubella, and epidemic hemorrhagic fever, have been implicated.[3]

## THE THYROID

### INFECTIONS OF THE THYROID

Infections of the thyroid gland are uncommon. Clinically, they may be divided into two categories: *acute suppurative thyroiditis*, usually caused by bacterial, fungal, mycobacterial, or parasitic infections, and *subacute thyroiditis*, more commonly attributed to a viral etiology[12] (see Chap. 46).

Of 224 reported cases of acute suppurative thyroiditis, 68% were bacterial, 9% were mycobacterial, 5% were parasitic, and 3% were the result of syphilitic gummatous infections.[13]

Acute bacterial thyroiditis may occur in patients of any age; it is more common in women and in persons with preexisting thyroid disease. The thyroid infection often is preceded by infection elsewhere in the body, usually the upper respiratory tract, throat, or head and neck. Clinical manifestations include anterior neck pain, tenderness, and dysphagia; the area may be warm and erythematous. Unilateral vocal cord paralysis has been reported as a complication of acute suppurative thyroiditis.[14] Often, there is fever and concurrent pharyngitis. Other than the leukocytosis (frequently more than 10,000 cells, usually neutrophilia), laboratory data, including thyroid function tests, usually are normal. The most frequent bacterial isolates include *S. aureus*, *S. pyogenes*, *S. pneumoniae*, and *Enterobacter* species.[12,13] Other bacteria—*Actinomyces*, *Salmonella*, *Klebsiella pneumoniae*, and *Brucella*—have been isolated.[15] In rare circumstances, some multisystemic infections (e.g., Lyme disease) can be superimposed on severe primary hypothyroidism such that if the thyroidal symptoms are sufficiently advanced and pronounced, the nonspecific symptoms of *Borrelia* infections are easily overlooked.[16] Fine-needle aspiration, with or without ultrasonographic guidance, may aid in the diagnosis.[17] The treatment of acute bacterial thyroiditis consists of rest, local heat, and appropriate antibiotics. If an abscess occurs as a complication, surgical drainage should be performed (Fig. 213-1).

A role for *Yersinia enterocolitica* has been proposed in patients with Graves disease, nontoxic goiter, and other thyroid disorders on the basis of the presence of antibodies in their sera. In the United States and Israel, where serotype 0:3 is not commonly

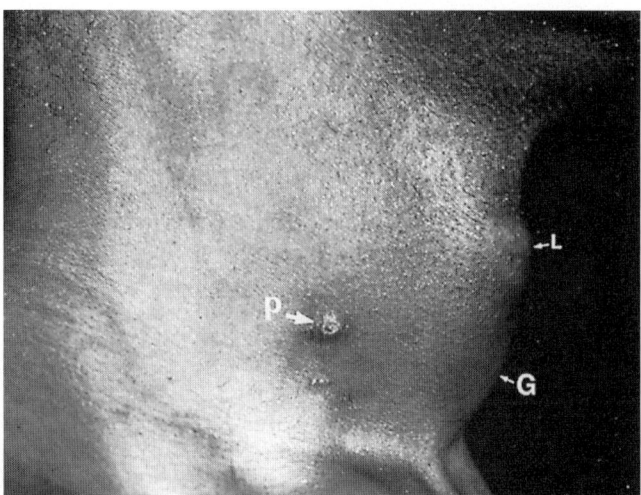

**FIGURE 213-1.** A 25-year-old man with thyroid abscess caused by bacterial infection after attempted intravenous heroin injection. At first, it was thought that he had subacute granulomatous thyroiditis. Usually, immediate incision and drainage are necessary for this life-threatening condition. Note the initial pustule. (*G*, goiter; *L*, larynx; *P*, pustule.)

isolated, 0:3 antibody titers greater than 1:8 were reported in 52% of patients with thyroid disorders—a finding that suggests the occurrence of a cross-reaction rather than a causal relation in these patients. Cross-reactivity may occur at the level of the receptor for thyroid-stimulating hormone (TSH).[18]

*Helicobacter pylori*, a newly recognized pathogen, has a markedly increased prevalence in patients with autoimmune atrophic gastritis (87.5%). Anti–*H. pylori* immunoglobulin G (IgG) levels and results of breath tests are also higher in patients with Graves disease and Hashimoto thyroiditis. A positive linear regression has been found between the levels of microsomal autoantibodies and anti–*H. pylori* IgG in patients with atrophic thyroiditis. Such a relationship suggests that the *H. pylori* antigen may be involved in the development of autoimmune atrophic thyroiditis or that autoimmune function in atrophic thyroiditis may increase the likelihood of *H. pylori* infection.[19]

The incidence of tuberculosis (TB) of the thyroid gland is difficult to assess. Previous reports were based mainly on the presence of granulomas on tissue biopsy without cultures; such findings easily could represent sarcoidosis, syphilis, or granulomatous thyroiditis. In one review of bacteriologically proven TB of the thyroid, most cases were associated with coexistent disseminated infection. Compared with patients who had nontuberculous bacterial thyroiditis, fever, pain, and tenderness were less prominent and symptoms had been present longer.[13] Rarely, TB of the thyroid may present as an isolated area of thyroiditis in the form of a nodular lesion.[20] On rare occasions, atypical mycobacterium (e.g., *Mycobacterium avium intracellulare*) has been reported as a cause of suppurative thyroiditis.[21]

Of 31 reported cases of thyroiditis caused by fungi, *Aspergillus* infections were most common, accounting for >80% of cases, with *C. immitis*, *Candida* species, and *Allescheria boydii* implicated in the remaining 15% of cases.[13] Aspergillosis of the thyroid usually is a manifestation of disseminated disease and is seen in immunocompromised hosts. The diagnosis most often is made at autopsy. The pathogenesis probably is by hematogenous spread to the thyroid, with subsequent formation of focal abscesses, and with patchy hemorrhagic lesions from vascular invasion by the fungus. Therapy for disseminated infection usually consists of high doses of amphotericin B. Coccidioidomycosis of the thyroid is very rarely recognized antemortem.[22] Cases usually occur as part of a fatal disseminated infection. Treatment

may require surgery as well as antifungal therapy (e.g., fluconazole or amphotericin B).

The authors treated a patient with underlying sickle cell disease and sarcoidosis who was receiving low-dose corticosteroid therapy and had an abscess of the thyroid caused by *Cryptococcus neoformans*. The infection failed to clear with amphotericin B therapy but subsequently responded to fluconazole.

Parasitic infections of the thyroid are extremely rare. A few cases of thyroidal echinococcal infection have been reported, which usually present as a chronic, slow-growing mass, with signs and symptoms of compression. The initial diagnosis at the time of surgery generally is a nontoxic goiter. Cysticercosis of the thyroid also has been reported.[13] Severe hypothyroidism was reported in a patient with chronic intestinal giardiasis due to isolated levothyroxine malabsorption. Treatment with metronidazole resulted in complete elimination of the parasites and recovery of regular intestinal thyroid hormone absorption.[23]

Syphilitic gumma of the thyroid gland is extremely rare. This infection mimics a slow-growing tumor; the most common symptoms are those of local compression.[13]

Thyroiditis is a rare manifestation of disseminated disease with the protozoan *Pneumocystis carinii*. One patient, who was chemically euthyroid at the time of diagnosis, became hypothyroid during therapy and required the use of thyroid hormone replacement.[24]

Infectious agents have been implicated in the pathogenesis of autoimmune thyroid disease.[25] Classic autoimmune thyroid disease (i.e., Graves disease and Hashimoto thyroiditis) has been shown to be associated with a variety of infectious agents (e.g., *Y. enterocolitica* and retroviruses), while infection of the thyroid gland (e.g., subacute thyroiditis and congenital rubella) has been shown to be associated with autoimmune thyroid phenomena.[25]

Subacute thyroiditis is a remitting inflammatory disease of the thyroid gland that may be caused by a viral infection; mumps, measles, influenza, Coxsackie virus, St. Louis encephalitis, cytomegalovirus (CMV), and infectious mononucleosis all have been reported.[26,27] However, it has been difficult to culture virus or to demonstrate viral inclusion bodies. Therefore, in most cases, the actual role of viral agents in the etiology of thyroiditis is merely a supposition.

### EUTHYROID SICK SYNDROME

The euthyroid sick syndrome refers to an alteration of thyroid function that occurs in patients with various nonthyroid illnesses, such as chronic renal failure, liver disease, stress, drug use, starvation, surgery, fever, and infection (see Chap. 36). Of the infections involved, sepsis probably is implicated most commonly, but pyelonephritis, pulmonary infections, viral hepatitis, other viral infections, typhoid fever, brucellosis, and malaria also have been reported.[28–30]

The euthyroid sick syndrome has been estimated to occur in ~50% of all patients in the medical intensive care unit setting, many of whom have severe infections. The prognosis correlates with the level of serum thyroxine ($T_4$). Of a large number of patients studied with nonthyroid illness, 84% with a $T_4$ level <3 µg/dL died, whereas only 15% of those with a $T_4$ level >5 µg/dL died.[31] As patients recover, there may be a transient, slight rise in the serum TSH level.[3] Subsequently, when the serum triiodothyronine ($T_3$) level begins to rise, the TSH level normalizes.

Patients with the euthyroid sick syndrome are clinically euthyroid, but have a low serum $T_3$ level and a high reverse $T_3$ level. The serum total $T_4$ level may be low, high, or normal, and the TSH level often is normal. The depression of serum $T_3$ is thought to result from an impaired peripheral conversion of $T_4$ to $T_3$, which, in turn, may cause a relative increase of $T_4$ or an increased reverse T$_3$. A decreased total T$_4$ level may occur because of a reduction of thyroid-binding globulin in patients who are malnourished. Moreover, a thyroid hormone–binding inhibitor has been described that may interfere with thyroid-binding globulin binding of T$_4$, such that the total T$_4$ level is decreased but the free T$_4$ level remains normal.

Infection may cause the euthyroid sick syndrome; among those who already have the syndrome for other reasons, the incidence of complicating infection also is high. It has been suggested that thyroid hormone–binding inhibitor may be similar in structure to a phagocytosis inhibitor, and that small amounts of thyroid hormone–binding inhibitor can inhibit the phagocytosis of *E. coli* in some tissues.

## DISORDERS OF CALCIUM AND PHOSPHATE IN RELATION TO INFECTIOUS DISEASES

### HYPOCALCEMIA AND THE TOXIC SHOCK SYNDROME

Hypocalcemia is a common finding in patients with toxic shock syndrome. The hypocalcemia has been thought to result from concurrent hypoalbuminemia. The severity of the hypocalcemia often is correlated with the inflammatory response.[31a] However, studies have indicated that the hypocalcemia often occured in conjunction with elevated concentrations of serum immunoreactive calcitonin,[32] which now has been found to be due to increased procalcitonin and other calcitonin precursors (Chap. 53). Often, hypophosphatemia is present.[32a]

### HYPOCALCEMIA DURING SEPSIS AND OTHER INFECTIONS

A low ionized calcium level is common during bacterial sepsis and has been implicated as a prognostic factor. In a study of 60 critically ill patients with bacterial sepsis, 20% had ionic hypocalcemia.[33] A significant mortality was observed among patients with hypocalcemia (up to 50%), compared with patients who had normal calcium levels (29%). Interestingly, only patients with gram-negative sepsis had hypocalcemia. The two most common organisms isolated from blood cultures were *E. coli* and *Pseudomonas aeruginosa*. Serum calcium concentrations normalized in each of those patients with sepsis who survived. Hypocalcemia in the patients with sepsis resulted from an efflux of calcium from the vascular space that was not met by a concomitant influx. The cause of defective calcium influx appeared to be multifactorial and resulted from acquired parathyroid gland insufficiency, renal 1α-hydroxylase insufficiency, dietary vitamin D deficiency, and acquired tissue resistance to calciferol.

The role that calcium plays in sepsis is not clear. Patients with sepsis often have decreased plasma ionized calcium levels. It appears that calcium replacement would be beneficial for normal cardiovascular and cellular function. However, in experimental models of septic shock, in hypocalcemic animals, calcium replacement resulted in increased mortality.[34,35] Studies on animal models of sepsis demonstrated increased intracellular free calcium levels, which may contribute to cellular injury.[35] The administration of exogenous calcium may act to increase the intracellular flux of calcium, leading to detrimental effects on the cell. The mechanism for the increase in intracellular calcium during sepsis is not known. Mediators of septic shock such as bacterial endotoxin or tumor necrosis factor do not alter lymphocyte free intracellular calcium levels in vitro; however, incubation with lysophosphatidylcholine (an endogenous membrane lipid) significantly increases intracellular free calcium levels.[36] Additional animal studies, which investigated the blockade of calcium influx with calcium-channel blockers, led to improved survival.[37,38] Dantrolene, which is thought to reduce intracellular calcium by decreas-

ing calcium release from the sarcoplasmic reticulum, also may have beneficial effects on cellular function during sepsis.[39] The question of whether to replace calcium in patients with hypocalcemia remains unanswered. No human trials have been performed.

A temporary decrease in the serum calcium level also has been described in patients with hypoparathyroidism who are treated with cholecalciferol during febrile illness.[40]

### HYPERCALCEMIA IN GRANULOMATOUS AND VIRAL INFECTIONS

Hypercalcemia can be associated with chronic granulomatous processes and chronic infection. Increased production of dihydroxyvitamin D by activated macrophages has been shown to be the cause in most cases. Hypercalcemia occasionally occurs in patients with TB.[41] Often, normocalcemia is present at the time of hospital admission, and hypercalcemia develops after patients are in the hospital, are eating, and are taking multivitamins containing vitamin D. The increased serum calcium responds to a corticosteroid suppression test. Usually, serum calcium levels normalize spontaneously. Many of these patients have hyperglobulinemia. Their serum phosphate concentrations generally are normal. It has been postulated that the tuberculous lymph nodes of these patients contain the 1α-hydroxylase enzyme, which induces an increased production of 1,25-dihydroxyvitamin D$_3$, leading to the hypercalcemia.

Coccidioidomycosis and, occasionally, other fungal infections (i.e., histoplasmosis) are associated with hypercalcemia. Hypercalcemia was reported in a patient with *Nocardia asteroides* pericarditis correlated with the duration of infection. The hypercalcemia resolved after treatment of *N. asteroides* with sulfisoxazole.[42]

Adult T-cell leukemia (ATL) caused by human T-cell leukemia virus (HTLV)-I infection is associated with hypercalcemia in >66% of patients. A parathyroid hormone–related protein, which is implicated in the hypercalcemia of ATL, is transactivated by the HTLV-I and HTLV-II tax proteins.[43]

### HYPOPHOSPHATEMIA

Hypophosphatemia occurs in approximately one-third of all patients with *Legionella pneumophila* pneumonia. In one study, 10 of 18 patients had serum phosphate levels of <2.5 mg/dL; 5 patients had levels of <2.0 mg/dL. Hypophosphatemia tended to occur within the first 72 hours of illness and was not associated with common causes of phosphate depletion, such as starvation, respiratory alkalosis, or excessive carbohydrate intake.[44]

The toxic shock syndrome secondary to *S. aureus* infection also may be a cause of hypophosphatemia, perhaps because of increased calcitonin precursor levels (Chap. 53). In addition, it has been postulated that staphylococcal toxins may alter phosphate metabolism.[45]

Hypophosphatemia has been recognized in gram-negative sepsis and, rarely, in gram-positive sepsis. High levels of inflammatory cytokines and their receptors are correlated with sepsis and positive blood cultures.[46] Hypophosphatemia occurs in meningococcal infection in children and is an early indication of sepsis in critically ill newborns.[47]

Therapy consists of treating the underlying disorder and, in severe cases, providing phosphate replacement. Anticytokine strategies may reverse hypophosphatemia and other parameters of sepsis.

In patients with septic shock, severe hypophosphatemia may be considered as a superimposed cause of myocardial depression, inadequate peripheral vasodilatation, and acidosis. A rapid correction of hypophosphatemia may have beneficial effects both in myocardium and in the vascular system.[48]

## INFECTIONS OF THE PANCREAS

Infections of the pancreas are varied and can interfere with both endocrine and exocrine function. Pancreatic abscess frequently develops as a complication of pancreatitis. Bacterial etiologies usually are polymicrobial, with enteric organisms such as *E. coli* and *Enterobacter* species; gram-negative anaerobes are the most common. *S. aureus* and *Candida* species also have been reported in pancreatic abscess. Optimal therapy involves either percutaneous or surgical drainage of the abscess, in addition to the administration of appropriate antimicrobial agents. The mortality from an undrained abscess is extremely high. Therefore, the prognosis is greatly affected by the ability to drain the abscess adequately.[49]

*M. tuberculosis* infection presenting as pancreatitis or pancreatic abscess has been reported in patients.[50] Establishing the diagnosis of tuberculous abscess is important because the response to therapy generally is excellent.

Enteroviruses have been examined for their possible role in the etiology of insulin-dependent (type 1) diabetes mellitus for nearly 40 years, yet the evidence remains inconclusive.[51] The mechanism of acute cytolytic infection of B cells, which was proposed in earlier studies, appears to be incompatible with the long preclinical period of autoimmunity preceding type 1 diabetes.[51] Various factors contribute to the development of the disease, including the strain of the virus, the genetic predisposition of the host, and additional environmental factors that maintain the disease process. Human studies that show an association between Coxsackie virus infection and acute pancreatitis are further supported by the extensive data from mouse studies, which demonstrate that some serotypes (i.e., $B_4$, $B_3$) are trophic for the exocrine pancreas.[52]

The advent of pancreatic transplantation for end-stage type 1 diabetes has been associated with infectious complications including fungal and viral opportunistic pathogens associated with immunosuppression. There appears to be a significant incidence of intraabdominal infections related to the transplantation surgery. CMV pancreatitis is a rare complication after pancreatic transplantation and can result in allograft rejection.[53] Ganciclovir is efficacious in the treatment of invasive CMV in solid organ transplants.

## INFECTIONS OF THE ADRENAL GLANDS

Neonatal adrenal abscess is a rare finding, with only 15 cases reported. Two cases of adrenal abscess in adults have been reported with presentation of fever, flank pain, and leukocytosis.[54,55] Rarely, adrenal abscess can be a complication of an adrenal fine-needle biopsy.[56]

Although Waterhouse-Friedrichsen syndrome is the classic finding of bilateral adrenal hemorrhage associated with *Neisseria meningitidis*, it has been reported in patients with *Haemophilus influenzae*,[57] *S. pyogenes*,[58] and *S. pneumoniae*[59,60] infections. This syndrome should be considered in any patient with infection and evidence of adrenal insufficiency. Syphilitic gumma of the adrenal gland resulting in adrenal insufficiency has also been reported in a patient with meningovascular syphilis.[61]

Although infections, particularly tuberculosis (TB), have been implicated in Addison disease, the current leading cause is autoimmune destruction of the adrenal glands (see Chap. 76). Infections typically go undiagnosed because the extent of involvement of the gland in certain infections (e.g., North American blastomycosis) must approximate 95% before clinical symptomatology occurs. Even if overt hypoadrenalism occurs, patients may die before the diagnosis is considered, and the clinical indications of the disease may be masked by other organ damage from infection or by intercurrent disease states.[62]

Etiologic agents that have been implicated in Addison disease include fungi; *H. capsulatum* is the most common, confirmed in >80% of autopsied patients with subacute progressive disseminated histoplasmosis.[63] CT scans typically demonstrate bilateral enlargement with a low attenuation center of increased density at the gland perimeter.[64] Rarely, unilateral gland enlargement can be seen; therefore, clinicians should include *H. capsulatum* and other granulomatous diseases and tumors in the differential diagnosis of unilateral adrenal gland enlargement.[65] Cryptococcosis, sporotrichosis, coccidioidomycosis, and blastomycosis also have been reported. In the United States, mycobacterial infections of the adrenal gland, especially *M. tuberculosis*, which formerly was the most common cause, still occur, and probably rank fairly close to *H. capsulatum* in prevalence. It is estimated that 5% to 10% of patients with subacute progressive, disseminated histoplasmosis will develop adrenal insufficiency despite antifungal therapy.

In endemic areas, *H. capsulatum* causes Addison disease as commonly as do autoimmune disorders. In Venezuela and Brazil, South American blastomycosis is the leading cause of Addison disease.

In some patients with infections involving the adrenal glands, the clinical and laboratory evidence of the adrenal insufficiency may be the presenting manifestations. Depending on the endemicity of the area, the presence or absence of a positive tuberculin test result, and evidence of tuberculous or fungal infection elsewhere, once hypoadrenalism has been documented, empiric treatment with antituberculous agents or with antifungal therapy may be begun, along with appropriate corticosteroid therapy.

Several clinical findings may be useful in determining the cause of adrenal destruction in Addison disease: the duration of the illness, the increase in size of the adrenal glands on abdominal CT scanning, and the presence of adrenal calcification. The diagnosis of Addison disease, whether secondary to fungal infection or to TB, should be suggested if a calcified adrenal gland is visualized on routine radiographs of the abdomen. However, calcification of the adrenal glands may occur without adrenal insufficiency. TB of the adrenal glands (like histoplasmosis) may cause adrenal enlargement with or without calcification (observable on abdominal CT scan); however, granulomatous adrenal TB may cause Addison disease without either calcification or abnormal gland enlargement.[66]

Similarly, in patients with overt adrenal insufficiency, calcification detected by radiography or by CT images of the abdomen suggests TB or fungal infection and excludes idiopathic adrenal atrophy (Fig. 213-2). In one study, 9 of 17 patients (53%) with TB and Addison disease had calcification on abdominal imaging, whereas none of the 16 patients with idiopathic atrophy had evidence of adrenal calcification.[67] Other processes causing adrenal calcification include hemorrhage, metastatic melanoma, pheochromocytoma, and adrenal carcinoma.

The size of the adrenal glands varies with the cause of adrenal disease and with the duration of adrenal insufficiency. Those patients with relatively short illnesses caused by TB or fungi have enlarged adrenals, whereas those with a longer disease duration have small glands.[67]

The possibility of some improvement in adrenal function after treatment of the underlying systemic disease further justifies an effort to diagnose the cause of Addison disease. Thus, the finding of enlarged adrenal glands in a patient with Addison disease warrants serious consideration of an open adrenal biopsy.[67] Unless the glands have been completely destroyed, treatment may result in normalization of serum cortisol levels and an associated improvement of symptoms related to the adrenal insufficiency.

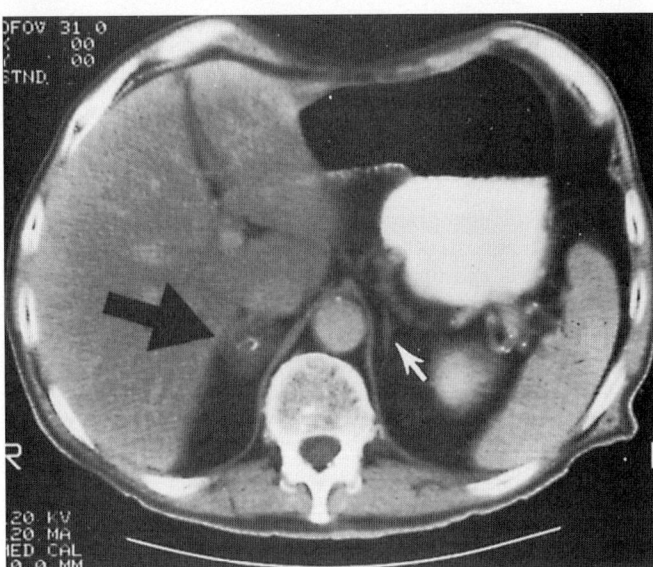

**FIGURE 213-2.** Abdominal computed tomographic scan of a 72-year-old man with adrenal tuberculosis. Note the enlarged right adrenal gland with calcification (*large arrow*). The contralateral adrenal (*small arrow*) is normal in size and shape.

## INFECTIONS OF THE GONADS

Infections of the testicles usually result from spread of disease from the epididymis or prostate. In younger heterosexual men, infections with *Neisseria gonorrhoeae* or *Chlamydia trachomatis* are most common, whereas in older men, *Enterobacter* or *Pseudomonas* species are the more frequent causes. Homosexual males of all age groups are more likely to have urogenital infections caused by enteric pathogens.[68] Salmonella infection has been reported in a preexisting hydrocele (as a cause of epididymoorchitis) and also in a preexisting ovarian cyst.[69] These infections are diagnosed easily, respond readily to antimicrobial therapy, and usually do not cause infertility.

Mumps virus is the most common viral cause of epididymoorchitis and occurs in 20% to 30% of postpubertal men with mumps infection. Two-thirds of cases of mumps orchitis occur during the first week of the illness, and another one-fourth arise during the second week. The gonadal involvement may precede the parotitis, or may occur as the only manifestation of mumps. The clinical presentation usually is high-grade fever, chills, headache, vomiting, and testicular pain. On physical examination, the testicle generally is warm, swollen, and tender, with accompanying erythema of the scrotum. Epididymitis is seen in 85% of the cases, and usually precedes the orchitis. The testis may be enlarged three to four times its normal size. Fifty percent of cases show some degree of atrophy when the testes are examined months to years later. The concern about sexual impotence and sterility secondary to mumps orchitis has been exaggerated. Men with unilateral orchitis need not worry about sterility, although they may suffer emotionally from the possible small testis.[70] Even those with bilateral involvement should be assured that impotence or sterility is uncommon. However, gynecomastia is common after either unilateral or bilateral orchitis (see Chap. 120). Testicular malignancy after atrophy of the testis caused by mumps orchitis has been reported. With mumps vaccination, such complications are observed less frequently. Limited experience with the use of interferon (IFN)-$\alpha_{2a}$ has achieved both clinical improvement and resolution of mumps infections without any after effects.[71] In the setting of postpuberty mumps, treatment with IFN may prevent testicular atrophy and the resulting infertility.

Other viruses that rarely may be associated with epididymoorchitis are the Epstein-Barr virus, echovirus 6, group B Coxsackie virus, and Coxsackie virus A9. Varicella-zoster virus has been reported to cause orchitis in children and also appears to result in a high incidence of testicular atrophy.[72] Parvovirus B19 DNA sequences have been demonstrated in the testicular tissue of 85% of patients with germ-cell tumors. It has been hypothesized that this virus plays a role in the development of testicular germ-cell tumors or stimulates the growth of these tumor cells.[73]

Tuberculous orchitis occurs in somewhat fewer than 5% of cases of miliary TB. In as many as 83% to 100% of cases, the testicles become infected by an ipsilateral tuberculous epididymis. Epididymal infection can occur by hematogenous seeding, lymphatic spread, or retrograde canalicular spread through the vas deferens. The epididymis and testes share the same blood supply. Involvement of the epididymis occurs more frequently and usually precedes orchitis. Hematogenous spread probably is less common than canalicular or lymphatic spread.

Male fertility decreases markedly in chronic genital TB.[74] Impotence seldom occurs, except occasionally as a psychogenic manifestation. However, abnormal semen analysis is common and includes decreased ejaculate volume, blockage of flow through the epididymal tubules and vas deferens, secondary testicular atrophy, decreased sperm count, and poor sperm motility.

The earliest symptoms in patients with tuberculous epididymitis are scrotal swelling in 74% to 91% and local epididymal pain in 12% to 43%. Urinary tract symptoms usually are absent in patients with epididymoorchitis. Physical examination may reveal a palpable, irregular, and nodular epididymis that later may increase in size. The epididymis becomes less indurated because of caseation necrosis and adheres to the scrotal skin. The scrotal skin loses its normal rugosity because of edema. Forty percent to 50% of patients with advanced disease may have scrotal fistulas with purulent discharge.

Nontuberculous mycobacteria, including *Mycobacterium kansasii*, *Mycobacterium fortuitum*, and *M. avium-intracellulare*, are rare causes of granulomatous epididymitis and prostatitis. Leprous testicular involvement leads to testicular atrophy and the secondary development of gynecomastia. Usually, patients have concomitant cutaneous and neurologic evidence of leprosy.

In 4% to 20% of cases of brucellosis, epididymoorchitis may occur. Syphilitic orchitis is unusual and, most commonly, is a manifestation of congenital infection. Syphilitic gummas may develop in the epididymis and cause anterior draining scrotal sinuses.

Fungal causes of orchitis usually are *B. dermatitidis* or *C. immitis*. Four percent to 22% of cases of disseminated blastomycosis present with genitourinary tract involvement.[75] Epididymoorchitis caused by *B. dermatitidis* is a chronic process with multiple recurrences that, in some patients, may be complicated by a draining scrotal sinus tract. Genital tract involvement with *C. immitis* is rare and need not result from renal infection in disseminated disease. *C. immitis* can be isolated from urine culture in at least 9% of patients with coccidioidomycosis.[76]

In early stages of filariasis, acute recurrent febrile episodes of orchitis and epididymitis can occur, with a clinical presentation of swelling and inflammation that may be difficult to differentiate from pyogenic and granulomatous infections.

Infection of the female gonads is not common. Tuboovarian abscess occurs as a result of ascending genital infection. The responsible bacterial flora are variable and can include *N. gonorrhoeae*, gram-negative enteric organisms, and anaerobes such as *Bacteroides fragilis*. *Chlamydia trachomatis* is a common cause of lower genital tract infections in women. Evidence suggests that *C. trachomatis* can persist in the female genital tract in an unculturable state. Immunoglobulin A (IgA) antibodies to two chlamydial antigens and heat shock protein have been detected in the follicular fluid of patients experiencing in vitro fertilization (IVF) failure, indicating that persistent upper genital tract chlamydial infection may contribute to IVF failure in some women.[77]

There have been numerous reports of actinomycotic infection of the ovary, which usually is associated with an intrauterine contraceptive device. The indolent course of this infection often leads to the inappropriate initial diagnosis of ovarian malignancy.[78] *Actinomyces* infection of the upper genital tract may be clinically inapparent. When *Actinomyces*-like organisms are detected on cervical cytologic smears, removal of an intrauterine device should be considered.[79]

Parasitic infection as a cause of infertility in women is rare. A parasitic infection presenting as a coincidental finding has been reported in one patient.[80] Moving microfilariae of *Mansonella perstans* were found in the aspirated follicular fluid of a patient undergoing IVF with embryo transfer because of tubal pathology caused by *C. trachomatis*.

## HYPOGLYCEMIA AS A MANIFESTATION OF SEPSIS

The association between hypoglycemia and infection first was described in pediatric patients with overwhelming meningococcemia and adrenal hemorrhage. In addition, symptomatic hypoglycemia has been reported in the setting of sepsis associated with extensive burns, viral hepatitis, varicella, pertussis, and fulminant pneumococcal infection, as well as in patients with *Clonorchis sinensis* infestation complicated by suppurative cholangitis. A description of nine patients with overwhelming sepsis complicated by hypoglycemia called attention to this finding as an important clue to the presence of the sepsis; the prognosis was poor.[81] The association of hypoglycemia and sepsis is more common in the setting of cirrhosis. In one study, asymptomatic hypoglycemia was demonstrated in 15 of 30 cirrhotic patients with septicemia.[82] In the 15 patients with hypoglycemia, severe circulatory failure was observed.

The exact mechanism of the hypoglycemia that may occur during sepsis is unknown. Experimentally, direct inhibition of gluconeogenesis and depletion of hepatic glycogen secondary to endotoxin have been suggested as possible mechanisms. Another metabolic factor that has been proposed is the shift to anaerobic metabolism that requires more energy when hypotension and diminished tissue perfusion occur as a result of sepsis. In neonates with bacteremia, increased peripheral utilization of glucose appears to be the primary mechanism for the hypoglycemia. In vitro studies have demonstrated that the utilization of glucose by bacteria is not responsible for the hypoglycemia in sepsis.

In studies of glucose metabolism in patients with severe malaria,[83] the basal plasma glucose utilization is increased ~50%. Prevention and treatment of early hypoglycemia should be based on adequate glucose replacement.

Other conditions in which impairment of glucose turnover has been reported include *Plasmodium falciparum* malaria and enteric fever.[84] Glucose turnover is 20% greater in malaria than in enteric fever. Such a finding may reflect increased noninsulin-mediated glucose uptake in *P. falciparum* malaria and/or impaired gluconeogenesis in enteric fever and may have implications for metabolic complications and the clinical management of these disorders.

## HORMONAL DISORDERS ASSOCIATED WITH OR PREDISPOSING TO INFECTIOUS DISEASES

### ENDOCRINOPATHY AND CANDIDIASIS

Chronic mucocutaneous candidiasis is a recurrent and persistent candidal infection of the skin, nails, and mucous membranes that often is resistant to prolonged, conventional therapy. This condition is not a single disease entity, but represents the final common pathway in patients with one or more immunologic abnormalities. Various associated defects of cell-mediated immunity have been described. The most common immune defect is the failure of T cells to respond to candidal antigen, which causes an anergic response to candidal skin testing.[85]

The spectrum of chronic mucocutaneous candidiasis may vary from mild oral thrush and nail infections to generalized involvement of the skin, scalp, and mucous membranes. Rarely, patients with the disease have developed severe invasive fungal infections, such as candidal and cryptococcal meningitis and disseminated histoplasmosis.[86]

The association of chronic mucocutaneous candidiasis with abnormalities of one or more endocrine disorders is known as the *candidiasis endocrinopathy syndrome*. Although the pathogenesis still is unclear, a genetic component with an autosomal recessive mode of inheritance has been suggested. Many of these patients have antibodies to various endocrine organs and other tissues, implicating an autoimmune disorder. Nonendocrine abnormalities, such as thymoma, myasthenia gravis, pernicious anemia, chronic hepatitis, psoriasis, and dental dysplasia, also have been described (also see Chaps. 60 and 197).

Because endocrinopathy may develop several years after the onset of symptoms of chronic mucocutaneous candidiasis, it is important to monitor laboratory parameters in these patients on a yearly basis (fasting plasma glucose, thyroid function tests, serum calcium, phosphate, electrolytes, cortisol) and to watch for signs and symptoms of endocrine abnormalities.[87] In patients with endocrinopathy in whom candidal infections develop, a negative skin test result to *Candida* antigen may suggest the diagnosis of chronic mucocutaneous candidiasis. The major immune defect associated with this condition is failure of T-cell lymphocytes to respond to stimulation with the antigen.

The skin manifestations of chronic mucocutaneous candidiasis are difficult to treat. It is important to consider *Candida* as an opportunistic infection that is a manifestation of an underlying immune deficiency. Diagnosis and treatment of the underlying disorder should be the priority. Attempts to modulate the immune system have been tried with transfer factor, levamisole, cimetidine, and thymic tissue transplants. The present treatment of choice for mucocutaneous *Candida* infections consists of long-term oral therapy (more than 6 months) with the new triazole agents, fluconazole or itraconazole.[88,89] Oral ketoconazole also has shown promising results, but this drug may inhibit gonadal and adrenal steroidogenesis.

### HYPOTHYROIDISM

Hypothyroidism has been associated with an increased susceptibility to bacterial infections. These patients may have weakened respiratory muscles, reduced respiratory drive, hypoxemia, and pleural effusions, all of which may predispose them to upper respiratory tract infections, empyema, and pneumonia (see Chap. 45). Pericardial effusions in patients with hypothyroidism have been complicated by bacterial pericarditis.[90]

Once infection has occurred, myxedema coma may develop in patients with hypothyroidism. In this state, intubation and the placement of multiple intravenous tubes and urinary catheters often predispose patients to aspiration pneumonia, catheter-related sepsis, and urinary tract infection. In such cases, the diagnosis of infection may be delayed because these patients can be afebrile and have a low white blood cell count.

Sepsis induces profound effects on the hypothalamic–pituitary–thyroid axis, with acute depression of $T_3$. The role of the thyroid hormone in sepsis is still unknown. In one study using thyroidectomized rats, the hyperdynamic phase of sepsis was abolished, and the mortality was increased.[91] $T_4$ replacement in the animals decreased mortality from sepsis. Experimental studies in sepsis-induced hypothyroid rats suggested that correction of the hypothyroid state with exogenous $T_3$ improved respiratory function.[92] These studies suggest that intact thyroid function may be important in the response of the body to infection.

One patient developed autoimmune hypothyroidism with antithyroid autoantibodies and seronegative rheumatoid-like arthritis after 7 months of IFN-α therapy for chronic active hepatitis C.[93] Hepatitis C virus (HCV) infection may play an adjuvant role in the triggering of immunomediated complications secondary to IFN-α therapy.[94]

## CUSHING SYNDROME

The excessive endogenous production of corticosteroids may predispose to the development of opportunistic infection in patients with Cushing syndrome (see Chap. 75).[94a] The many reports of *P. carinii* pneumonia, invasive aspergillosis, cryptococcosis, superficial cutaneous infections, and oral candidiasis in patients with Cushing syndrome emphasize the susceptibility of these patients to opportunistic infections.[95] In one brief report, 45% of patients with Cushing syndrome had superficial cutaneous and mucosal fungal infections, including tinea versicolor, onychomycosis, and oral candidiasis. Often, these were the initial clinical manifestations of endogenous hypercortisolism, frequently predating the diagnosis.[96]

Of interest is the observation that there is a direct correlation between the risk of infection and the degree of hypercortisolism.[97] Patients with Cushing disease are less prone to infection than are those with Cushing syndrome caused by paraneoplastic adrenocorticotropic hormone (ACTH) production or adrenal tumors. Interestingly, there is a correlation between the degree of hypercortisolism and the type of infection. *P. carinii* pneumonia tends to occur in patients with severe hypercortisolism, whereas cryptococcosis tends to occur in those with lesser degrees of hypercortisolism. Successful treatment of opportunistic infection often depends on lowering the plasma cortisol level to a physiologic range.

## HORMONE THERAPY AND INFECTIONS

### CORTICOSTEROIDS AND INCREASED SUSCEPTIBILITY TO INFECTIONS

Corticosteroids may enhance susceptibility to infection. These drugs may exert antiinflammatory effects; they decrease the availability of inflammatory cells, interfere with the functions of these cells when they reach the injured site, and suppress the noncellular components of the inflammatory response (see Chap. 78).

Overall, the incidence of spontaneous infections in patients receiving corticosteroid therapy is low. Infections are more common in patients receiving >20 to 40 mg prednisone, or its equivalent, daily. Patients who are receiving corticosteroids for collagen vascular diseases, such as systemic lupus erythematosus or rheumatoid arthritis, definitely have a higher incidence of bacterial infections. When these drugs are administered on an alternate-day regimen, infectious complications are less common.

Certain types of bacterial infections tend to occur more often in patients treated with corticosteroids. Of these, staphylococci, gram-negative organisms, *Listeria*, and TB are most common. The only bacterial infection that clearly is exacerbated by corticosteroid therapy is TB. Tuberculin-positive persons are at high risk for the development of TB, whereas in tuberculin-negative persons, TB rarely is documented. Isoniazid prophylaxis is indicated in patients who are tuberculin-positive and are receiving large doses of corticosteroids or other immunosuppressive agents.

Patients receiving corticosteroids appear to have an increased susceptibility to systemic fungal infections. One-third of all patients with candidal infections are receiving concurrent corticosteroid therapy. Cryptococcal infections also are more prevalent in corticosteroid-treated patients than in the general population. Systemic and pulmonary aspergillosis occur mostly in patients treated with corticosteroids or ACTH injections. Nocardial infections are fairly common among transplant recipients being treated with corticosteroids.

Some evidence suggests that varicella-zoster, herpes simplex, and CMV infections are enhanced by corticosteroid therapy. In addition, patients receiving corticosteroids are reported to have decreased resistance to malaria, amebiasis, and strongyloidiasis. Susceptibility to *P. carinii* pneumonia is enhanced markedly by corticosteroids.

## THERAPEUTIC USE OF CORTICOSTEROIDS IN INFECTIONS

Corticosteroids have been used in acute infections to reduce fever and decrease inflammation, edema, or symptoms of toxicity.[98] Table 213-1 summarizes some of the infectious diseases for which the use of corticosteroids appears to be of benefit.

Despite the use of antimicrobial therapy and sophisticated intensive care support, septic shock remains a serious life-threatening illness, with a high mortality. Corticosteroids have been used in the treatment of septic shock for several years. However, their efficacy remains controversial.

Corticosteroids exert multiple effects on the human body, which may explain the conflicting results concerning their value in septic shock. Theoretically, they inhibit the mobilization of

**TABLE 213-1.**

**Some Infectious Diseases in Which Corticosteroids May Be of Benefit**

| Disease | Comments |
|---|---|
| BACTERIAL MENINGITIS (*HAEMOPHILUS INFLUENZAE*) IN CHILDREN | Reduces cerebral edema, decreases incidence of complications (i.e., hearing loss, hydrocephalus) |
| BRAIN ABSCESS | Reduces cerebral edema, prevents cerebral herniation |
| CHRONIC OBSTRUCTIVE PULMONARY DISEASE, ASTHMA | Reduces inflammation |
| INFECTIOUS MONONUCLEOSIS | Reduces pharyngeal edema and enlarged tonsils; also used to treat associated thrombocytopenic purpura, hemolytic anemia, neurologic symptoms, pericarditis, myocarditis |
| OCULAR INFECTIONS, UVEITIS, CHORIORETINITIS SECONDARY TO TOXOPLASMOSIS, HISTOPLASMOSIS, OR LYME BORRELIOSIS | Reduces inflammation |
| *PNEUMOCYSTIS CARINII* PNEUMONIA | Reduces inflammation; improves gas exchange |
| PERTUSSIS | Reduces severity and duration of illness |
| RHEUMATIC FEVER | Reduces fever, toxicity, cardiac failure |
| TUBERCULOUS MENINGITIS | Reduces cerebral edema |
| TUBERCULOUS PERICARDITIS | Reduces fibrosis, scarring |
| TYPHOID FEVER | Reduces fever, toxicity, mortality |
| VIRAL HEPATITIS | Used in fulminant hepatitis or hepatitis B surface antigen (HbsAg)–negative patients with progressive disease; not useful in HbsAg-positive patients with chronic active hepatitis |

polymorphonuclear cells in the intravascular space, thereby preventing capillary leakage, which can lead to hypovolemia and hypoperfusion of vital organs. However, corticosteroids also suppress the immune system, such that patients may be unable to mount an adequate bactericidal response to infection.

The use of intravenous high-dose corticosteroids in septic shock has been controversial. In a randomized, prospective study of 54 patients, corticosteroids provided transient improvement in the sepsis-related shock syndrome only if they were administered within 4 hours of the onset of symptoms, but they did not improve the overall survival of patients with severe, late septic shock.[99] In a multicenter, placebo-controlled, double-blind, randomized trial of 382 patients, a higher mortality was noted in the corticosteroid-treated patients who had elevated serum creatinine levels.[100] An additional large multicenter trial has reported no benefit from corticosteroid treatment.[101]

Adrenal insufficiency may be a feature of septic shock patients who do not respond to conventional treatment. A standard 250-μg dose of ACTH is adequate for detecting adrenal insufficiency. Steroid supplementation appears to improve short-term survival when adrenal insufficiency occurs. The overall mortality is worse in patients with septic shock and adrenal insufficiency as compared to those with an adequate adrenal response.[102]

## CORTICOSTEROIDS IN OTHER INFECTIONS

Infectious agents induce inflammation as the body's response to wall off and eliminate the organism. Some inflammation probably is beneficial; however, an excess of swelling and edema associated with the inflammatory process can be detrimental. Glucocorticosteroids are potent antiinflammatory agents that can be used to decrease the inflammation associated with selected infectious processes. A consensus article from the Infectious Diseases Society of America outlines the guidelines for the use of systemic corticosteroids in infectious diseases.[103] Infections for which steroids are clearly indicated are few, and include *P. carinii* pneumonia, severe cases of typhoid fever, and tuberculous pericarditis. Other infections for which steroids probably are beneficial include bacterial meningitis in children and tuberculous meningitis. Corticosteroids do have a clear benefit for some of the complications of infectious processes, such as cerebral edema secondary to brain abscess or airway obstruction from Epstein-Barr virus. The judicious use of such drugs for these and other complications should be determined on an individual basis. Corticosteroids should not be used in cases of cerebral malaria, viral hepatitis, or gram-negative septic shock.

## HUMAN GROWTH HORMONE THERAPY AND CREUTZFELDT-JAKOB DISEASE

Creutzfeldt-Jakob disease (CJD), a form of transmissable spongiform encephalopathy (TSE), is a subacute degenerative infection of the central nervous system, which has a prolonged incubation period of several years and usually affects older adults. There were isolated reports of young adults who died of degenerative neurologic disease compatible with CJD.[104] All patients had been receiving long-term therapy with pituitary-derived human growth hormone for the treatment of hypopituitarism. It was postulated that one or more of the large pools of pituitary glands used to make the human growth hormone extract may have been infected with CJD, and purified human growth hormone was withdrawn from use. Biosynthesized growth hormone is now used instead (see Chaps. 12, 18, and 198).

In France, 51 of 968 children treated with human growth hormone lots produced between January 1984 and March 1985

developed CJD by the end of 1996. In an epidemiologic investigation of the risk of transmission of CJD, the risk for iatrogenic CJD in patients exposed to contaminated human growth hormone lots was estimated to be 0.06%.[105]

The iatrogenic cases have a genotype frequency similar to that of sporadic CJD. This suggests that there may be highly susceptible individuals and that sporadic CJD may have an environmental origin.[106] These data serve to emphasize the importance of homozygous codon 129 in determining the risk of incurring CJD after exposure to a TSE agent.[106] Pooled data from all identified and tested cases of iatrogenic CJD support the hypothesis that the prion protein (PrP) gene and homozygosity at codon 129 increase susceptibility to iatrogenic infections.

## MISCELLANEOUS ENDOCRINE EFFECTS OF ANTIMICROBIALS

Several adverse endocrine reactions and altered endocrine test results have been reported among patients receiving various antimicrobials. It is well known that cephalosporins can produce a false-positive test result for glycosuria when the reducing method is used. Patients with diabetes who are receiving oral hypoglycemic agents, such as tolbutamide and chlorpropamide, may experience hypoglycemic episodes if coexistent sulfonamide therapy is begun. Such interaction may be related to protein binding of the sulfonamides.

Rarely, trimethoprim-sulfamethoxazole (TMP-SMX) has been associated with the development of hypoglycemia in patients with renal failure.[107] Similar to sulfonylureas, sulfonamides are thought to cause hypoglycemia by increasing pancreatic secretion of insulin.

Because rifampin causes increased clearance of $T_4$, hypothyroidism may develop in patients with marginal pituitary or thyroid disease. The dose of $T_4$ may need to be increased in patients with hypothyroidism who already are receiving replacement therapy.[108]

Rifampin causes adrenal crisis in patients with Addison disease who are receiving adequate corticosteroid replacement therapy. This drug can induce liver enzymes that enhance corticosteroid metabolism. In patients with Addison disease, it has been recommended that treatment with rifampin be accompanied by doubling or tripling the dose of adrenal corticosteroids to maintain adequate replacement.[109]

A syndrome of nephrogenic diabetes insipidus has been reported with demeclocycline.[110]

Many antibiotics have adverse effects on spermatogenesis. DNA flow cytometry of testicular fluid has been used to evaluate testicular function quantitatively. Animal experiments suggest that TMP-SMX, nitrofurantoin, ofloxacin, and doxycyline significantly alter spermatogenesis. Ciprofloxacin, norfloxacin, and lomefloxacin have no apparent effect on spermatogenesis as measured by DNA flow cytometry.[111]

Pentamidine, an antiparasitic agent, is one of the diamidine compounds that were developed originally as hypoglycemic agents. Hypoglycemia may be responsible for the neurotoxicity that may occur during or soon after the initiation of therapy with pentamidine for *P. carinii* infection or African sleeping sickness. Interestingly, diabetes mellitus also has been reported with the use of pentamidine; the drug may have a direct toxic effect on the B cells of the pancreas.[112]

Ketoconazole, a drug generally used in fungal infections, was used in high doses (400 mg given orally every 8 hours) in nine patients with advanced prostate cancer (see Chap. 225). It was noted that this drug caused long-term suppression of androgen production and that the degree of suppression was proportional to the serum levels of the drug.[113] Decreased biosynthesis of corticosteroids also occurs.[114,115] In addition, ketoconazole has been implicated in the development of primary hypothyroidism in two relatives with chronic mucocutaneous candidiasis.[116] Other untoward effects include gynecomastia.

The new antifungal agents, fluconazole and itraconazole, have been evaluated in many large-scale trials and appear to have no effect on serum testosterone levels. Fluconazole has been reported to cause hypoglycemia by increasing the effects of oral hypoglycemic agents.

Potassium iodide solution used in the treatment of lymphocutaneous sporotrichosis has been associated with subclinical hypothyroidism.[117]

Aminoglycoside and amphotericin B therapy produces magnesium wasting, as well as other electrolyte abnormalities, and results in hypocalcemia.[118]

Vidarabine therapy for disseminated varicella-zoster infection has been implicated in one case of the syndrome of inappropriate antidiuretic hormone secretion.[119]

# REFERENCES

1. Jain KC, Varma A, Mahapatra AK. Pituitary abscess: a series of six cases. Br J Neurosurg 1997; 11:139.
2. Thomas N, Wittert GA, Scott G, Reilly PL. Infection of a Rathke's cleft cyst: a rare cause of pituitary abscess. Case illustration. J Neurosurg 1998; 89:682.
3. Berger SA, Edberg SC, David G. Infectious diseases of the sella turcica. Rev Infect Dis 1986; 8:747.
4. Shanley DJ, Holmes SM. *Salmonella typhi* abscess in a craniopharyngioma: CT and MRI. Neuroradiology 1994; 36:35.
5. Lam KS, Sham MMK, Tam SCF, et al. Hypopituitarism after tuberculous meningitis in childhood. Ann Intern Med 1993; 118:701.
6. Arafah BM, Salit IS. Partial hypopituitarism following septic peritonitis with shock. Arch Intern Med 1978; 138:1272.
7. Mohsenipour I, Deusch E, Twerdy K, Semenitz E. Toxic shock syndrome in transsphenoidal neurosurgery. Acta Neurol Chir 1994; 128:169.
8. Fong TC, Johns RD, Long M, Myles ST. CT of pituitary abscess. AJR Am J Roentgenol 1985; 144:1141.
9. Wolansky LJ, Gallagher JD, Heary RI, et al. MRI of pituitary abscess: two cases and review of the literature. Neuroradiology 1997; 39:499.
10. Sidhu PS, Kingdon CC, Strickland NH. Case report: CT scan appearances of a pituitary abscess. Clin Radiol 1994; 49:427.
11. Reincke M, Arlt W, Heppner C, et al. Neuroendocrine dysfunction in African trypanosomiasis. The role of cytokines. Ann N Y Acad Sci 1998; 840:809.
12. Hay ID. Thyroiditis: a clinical update. Mayo Clin Proc 1985; 60:836.
13. Berger SA, Zonszein J, Villamena P, Mittman N. Infectious diseases of the thyroid gland. Rev Infect Dis 1983; 74:2.
14. Boyd CM, Esclamado RM, Telian SA. Impaired vocal cord mobility in the setting of acute suppurative thyroiditis. Head Neck 1997; 19:235.
15. Azizi F, Katchoui A. Brucella infection of the thyroid gland. Thyroid 1996; 6:461.
16. Paparone PW. Hypothyroidism with concurrent Lyme disease. J Am Osteopath Assoc 1995; 95:435.
17. Clair MR, Mendelblait S, Baim RES, et al. Sonographic features of acute suppurative thyroiditis. J Clin Ultrasound 1983; 11:222.
18. Cover TL, Aber RC. *Yersinia enterocolitica*. N Engl J Med 1989; 321:16.
19. DeLuis DA, Valera C, deLa Calle H, et al. *Helicobacter pylori* infection is markedly increased in patients with autoimmune atrophic thyroiditis. J Clin Gastroenterol 1998; 26:259.
20. Barnes P, Weathersome R. Tuberculosis of the thyroid: two case reports. Br J Dis Chest 1979; 73:187.
21. Robillon JF, Sadoul JL, Guerin P, et al. *Mycobacterium avium intracellulare* suppurative thyroiditis in a patient with Hashimoto's thyroiditis. J Endocrinol Invest 1994; 17:133.
22. Smilack JD, Argueta R. Coccidioidal infection of the thyroid. Arch Intern Med 1998; 158:89.
23. Seppel T, Rose F, Schiaghecke R. Chronic intestinal giardiasis with isolated levothyroxine malabsorption as a reason for severe hypothyroidism—implications for localization of thyroid hormone absorption in the gut. Exp Clin Endocrinol Diabetes 1996; 104:180.
24. Drucker DJ, Bailey D, Rotstein L. Thyroiditis as the presenting manifestation of disseminated extrapulmonary *Pneumocystis carinii* infection. J Clin Endocrinol Metab 1990; 71:1663.
25. Tomer Y, Davies TF. Infection, thyroid disease and autoimmunity. Endocr Rev 1993; 14:107.
26. Pennel JS, Tomkin GH. Sub-acute thyroiditis and hepatitis in a case of infectious mononucleosis. Postgrad Med 1978; 54:351.
27. Frank TS, LiVolsi VA, Connor AM. Cytomegalovirus infection of the thyroid in immunocompromised adults. Yale J Biol Med 1987; 60:1.

28. Wartofsky L, Burman KD. Alterations in thyroid functions in patients with systemic illness: "the euthyroid sick syndrome." Endocr Rev 1982; 3:164.
29. Chopra IJ, Hershman JM, Pardridge WM, Nicoloff JT. Thyroid function in non-thyroidal illnesses. Ann Intern Med 1983; 98:946.
30. Post FA, Soule SG. Willcox PA, Levitt NS. The spectrum of endocrine dysfunction in active pulmonary tuberculosis. Clin Endocrinol (Oxf) 1994; 40:367.
31. Slag MF, Morley JE, Elsson MK, et al. Hypothyroxemia in critically ill patients as a predictor of high mortality. JAMA 1981; 245:43.
31a. Lind L, Carlstedt F, Rastad J, et al. Hypocalcemia and parathyroid hormone secretion in critically ill patients. Crit Care Med 2000; 28:93.
32. Müller B, Becker KL, Kränzlin M, et al. Disordered calcium homeostasis of sepsis: association with calcitonin precursors. Europ J Clin Invest 2001; in press.
32a. Miller DW, Slovis CM. Hypophosphatemia in the emergency department therapeutics. Am J Emerg Med 2000; 18:457.
33. Zaloga GP, Chernow B. The multifactorial basis for hypocalcemia during sepsis. Ann Intern Med 1987; 107:36.
34. Malcolm DS, Zaloga GP, Holaday JW. Calcium administration increases the mortality of endotoxic shock in rats. Crit Care Med 1989; 17:900.
35. Zaloga GP, Sager A, Prielipp R, et al. Calcium administration decreases survival and exacerbates endotoxemia during peritonitis. Chest 1990; 98:1355.
36. Zaloga OP, Washburn D, Black KW, Prielipp R. Human sepsis increases lymphocyte intracellular calcium. Crit Care Med 1993; 21:196.
37. Bosson S, Kuenzig M, Schwartz SI. Increased survival with calcium antagonists in antibiotic treated bacteremia. Circ Shock 1986; 16:69.
38. Lee HC, Lum BKB. Protective action of calcium entry blockers in endotoxin shock. Circ Shock 1986; 18:193.
39. Song SK, Karl IE, Ackerman JJH, Hotchkiss RS. Increased intracellular Ca$^{2+}$: a critical link in the pathophysiology of sepsis? Proc Natl Acad Sci U S A 1993; 90:3933.
40. Harkowitz ME, Rosen JF, Smith C. 1,25-Dihydroxy-vitamin D treated hypoparathyroidism: thirty-five patient years in ten children. J Clin Endocrinol Metab 1982; 55:727.
41. Shai F, Baker RK, Addrizzo JR, Wallach S. Hypercalcemia in mycobacterial infection. J Clin Endocrinol Metab 1972; 34:251.
42. Dockrell DH, Poland GA. Hypercalcemia in a patient with hypoparathyroidism and *Nocardia asteroides* infection: a novel observation. Mayo Clin Proc 1997; 72:157.
43. Prager D, Rosenblatt JD, Ejima E. Hypercalcemia, parathyroid hormone-related protein expression and human T-cell leukemia virus infection. Leuk Lymphoma 1994; 14:395.
44. Kirby BD, Snyder KM, Meyer RD, Finegold SM. Legionnaires' disease: clinical features of 24 cases. Ann Intern Med 1978; 89:297.
45. Chesney RW, Chesney PJ, David JP, Segar WE. Renal manifestations of staphylococcal toxic-shock syndrome. Am J Med 1981; 71:583.
46. Barak V, Schwartz A, Kalickman I, et al. Prevalence of hypophosphatemia in sepsis and infection: the role of cytokines. Am J Med 1998; 104:40.
47. Storm W. Identification of early sepsis by serial phosphate determination in critically ill newborns. Acta Paediatr Acad Sci Hung 1980; 21:253.
48. Bollaert PE, Levy B, Nace L, et al. Hemodynamic and metabolic effects of rapid correction of hypophosphatemia in patients with septic shock. Chest 1995; 107:1698.
49. Becker JM, Pemberton JH, Diamgno EP, et al. Prognostic factors in pancreatic abscess. Surgery 1984; 96:455.
50. Stambler JB, Klibaner MI. Tuberculous abscess of the pancreas. Gastroenterology 1982; 83:922.
51. Graves PM, Norris JM, Pallansch MA, et al. The role of enteroviral infections in the development of IDDM: limitations of current approaches. Diabetes 1997; 46:161.
52. Ramsingh AI. Coxsackieviruses and pancreatitis. Front Biosci 1997; 2:53.
53. Margreiter R, Schmid T, Dunser M, et al. Cytomegalovirus (CMV) pancreatitis: a rare complication after pancreas transplantation. Transplant Proc 1991; 23:1619.
54. Echaniz A, De Miguel J, Arnal A, Pedreira JD. *Escherichia coli* abscess as an adrenal mass. Ann Intern Med 1985; 103:481.
55. O'Brien WM, Copeland CJ, Klappenback RS, Lynch JH. Computed tomography of adrenal abscess. J Comput Assist Tomogr 1987; 11:550.
56. Masmiquel L, Hernandez-Pascual C, Simo R, Mesa J. Adrenal abscess as a complication of adrenal fine-needle biopsy. Am J Med 1993; 95:244.
57. McKinney WP, Agner RC. Waterhouse-Friderichsen syndrome caused by *Haemophilus influenzae* type b in an immunocompetent young adult. South Med J 1989; 82:1571.
58. Gertner M, Rodriquez L, Barnett SH, Shah K. Group A beta-hemolytic streptococcus and Waterhouse-Friderichsen syndrome. Pediatr Infect Dis J 1992; 11:595.
59. Ryan CA, Wenman W, Henningsen C, Tse S. Fatal childhood pneumococcal Waterhouse-Friderichsen syndrome. Pediatr Infect Dis J 1993; 12:250.
60. Bramley PN, Shah P, Williams DJ, Losowsky MS. Pneumococcal Waterhouse-Friderichsen syndrome despite a normal spleen. Postgrad Med 1989; 65:687.
61. Ilogu N, Daidone P, Stefan T, et al. Neurosyphilis and syphilitic gumma of the adrenal gland. Clin Infect Dis 1998; 26:224.
62. Chandler PT. Addison's disease secondary to North American blastomycosis. South Med J 1977; 70:863.
63. Goodwin RA Jr, Shapiro JL, Thurman GH, et al. Disseminated histoplasmosis. Clinical and pathologic correlations. Medicine 1980; 59:1.
64. Wilson DA, Muchmore HG, Tisdal RG, et al. Histoplasmosis of the adrenal glands studied by CT. Radiology 1984; 150:779.
65. Swartz MA, Scofield RH, Dickey WD, et al. Unilateral adrenal enlargement due to *Histoplasma capsulatum*. Clin Infect Dis 1996; 23:813.

66. Kelestimur F, Ozbaker O, Sagdam A. Acute adrenocortical failure due to tuberculosis. J Endocrinol Invest 1993; 16:281.

67. Vita JA, Silverberg SA, Goland RS, et al. Clinical clues to the cause of Addison's diseases. Am J Med 1985; 78:461.

68. Berger RE, Kessler D, Holmes KK. Etiology and manifestations of epididymitis in young men: correlations with sexual orientation. J Infect Dis 1987; 155:1341.

69. Lalitha MK, John R. Unusual manifestations of salmonellosis—a surgical problem. Q J Med 1996; 87:301.

70. Baum SG, Litman N. Mumps virus. In: Mandell G, ed. Principles and practice of infectious diseases II. New York: Churchill Livingstone 1995:1496.

71. Ruther U, Stilz S, Rohl E, et al. Successful interferon alpha 2 therapy for a patient with acute mumps orchitis. Eur Urol 1995; 27:174.

72. Turner RB. Orchitis as a complication of chickenpox. Pediatr Infect Dis J 1987; 6:489.

73. Gray A, Guillou L, Zufferey J, et al. Persistence of parvovirus B$_{19}$ DNA in testis of patients with testicular germ cell tumours. J Gen Virol 1998; 79:573.

74. Gorse GP, Belshe RB. Male genital tuberculosis: a review of the literature with instructive case reports. Rev Infect Dis 1985; 7:511.

75. Sarosi GA, Davies SF. Blastomycosis. Am Rev Respir Dis 1979; 120:911.

76. Drutz DJ, Catanzaro A. Coccidioidomycosis (Pt II). Am Rev Respir Dis 1978; 117:727.

77. Neuer A, Lam KN, Tiller FW, et al. Humoral immune response to membrane components of *Chlamydia trachomatis* and expression of human 60 kDa heat shock protein in follicular fluid of in vitro fertilization patients. Hum Reprod 1997; 12:925.

78. Hoffman MS, Roberts WS, Solomon P, et al. Advanced actinomycotic pelvic inflammatory disease simulating gynecologic malignancy. J Reprod Med 1991; 36:543.

79. Dehal SA, Kaplan MA, Brown R, et al. Clinically inapparent tuboovarian actinomycosis in a women with an IUD. A case report. J Reprod Med 1998; 43:595.

80. Govde AJ, Schats R, Van Berlo PJ, Clasesen FA. An unexpected guest in follicular fluid. Hum Reprod 1996; 11:531.

81. Miller SI, Wallace RJ, Musher DM, et al. Hypoglycemia as a manifestation of sepsis. Am J Med 1980; 68:649.

82. Nouel X, Bernuan J, Rueff B, Benhamou JP. Hypoglycemia: a common complication of septicemia in cirrhosis. Arch Intern Med 1981; 141:1477.

83. Binh TP, Davis TM, Johnston W, et al. Glucose metabolism in severe malaria: minimal model analysis of the intravenous glucose tolerance test incorporating a stable glucose level. Metabolism 1997; 46:1435.

84. Singh B, Choo KE, Ibrahim J, et al. Non-radioisotopic glucose turnover in children with falciparum malaria and enteric fever. Trans R Soc Trop Med Hyg 1998; 92:532.

85. Dwyer JM. Chronic mucocutaneous candidiasis. Annu Rev Med 1981; 32:491.

86. Kauffman CA, Shea MJ, Frame PT. Invasive fungal infections in patients with chronic mucocutaneous candidiasis. Arch Intern Med 1981; 141:1076.

87. Dolen J, Varma SK, South MA. Chronic mucocutaneous candidiasis endocrinopathies. Cutis 1981; 28:592.

88. Hay RJ. Overview of studies of fluconazole in oropharyngeal candidiasis. Rev Infect Dis 1990; 12(Suppl 3):S334.

89. Burke WA. Use of itraconazole in a patient with chronic mucocutaneous candidiasis. J Am Acad Dermatol 1989; 21:1309.

90. Lieber IH, Rensimer ER, Erickson CD. Campylobacter pericarditis in hypothyroidism. Am Heart J 1981; 102:462.

91. Moley JF, Ohkawa M, Chaudry IH. Hypothyroidism abolishes the hyperdynamic phase and increases susceptibility to sepsis. J Surg Res 1984; 36:265.

92. Dulchavsky SA, Kennedy PR, Geller ER, et al. T$_3$ preserves respiratory function in sepsis. J Trauma 1991; 31:753.

93. Pittau E, Bogliolo A, Tinti A, et al. Development of arthritis and hypothyroidism during alpha-interferon therapy for chronic hepatitis. J Clin Exp Rheumatol 1997; 15:415.

94. Vallisa D, Cavanna L, Berti R, et al. Autoimmune thyroid dysfunction in hematologic malignancies treated with alpha-interferon. Acta Haematol 1995; 93:31.

94a. Sarlis NJ, Chanock SJ, Nieman LK. Cortisolemic indices predict severe infections in Cushing syndrome due to ectopic production of adrenocorticotropin. J Clin Endocrinol Metab 2000; 85:42.

95. Bakker RC, Gallas PR, Romiju JA, Wiesinger WM. Cushing's syndrome complicated by multiple OI. J Endocrinol Invest 1998; 21:329.

96. Findling JW, Tyrell JB, Aron DC, et al. Fungal infections in Cushing's syndrome. Ann Intern Med 1981; 95:392.

97. Graham BS, Tucker WS. Opportunistic infections in endogenous Cushing's syndrome. Ann Intern Med 1984; 101:334.

98. Hoffman SL, Punjabi NH, Kumala S, et al. Reduction of mortality in chloramphenicol-treated severe typhoid fever by high dose dexamethasone. N Engl J Med 1984; 310:82.

99. Sprung CL, Caralis PV, Marcial EH, et al. The effects of high dose corticosteroids in patients with septic shock. N Engl J Med 1984; 311:1137.

100. Bone RC, Fisher CJ, Clemmer TP, et al. A controlled clinical trial of high-dose methylprednisolone in the treatment of severe sepsis and septic shock. N Engl J Med 1987; 317:653.

101. The Veterans Administration Systemic Sepsis Cooperative Study Group. Effect of high-dose glucocorticoid therapy on mortality in patients with clinical signs of systemic sepsis. N Engl J Med 1987; 317:659.

102. Soni A, Pepper GM, Wyrwrinski PM, et al. Adrenal insufficiency occurring during septic shock: incidence, outcome and relationship to peripheral cytokine levels. Am J Med 1995; 98:266.

103. McGowan JE, Chesney PJ, Crossley KB, LaForce NC. Guidelines for the use of systemic glucocorticosteroids in the management of selected infections. Clin Infect Dis 1992; 165:1.

104. Koch TK, Berk BO, DeArmand SJ, Gravina RF. Creutzfeldt-Jakob disease in a young adult with idiopathic hypopituitarism: possible relation to the administration of cadaveric human growth hormone. N Engl J Med 1985; 313:731.

105. Hurtland d'Aignaux J, Alperovitch A, Maccario J. A statistical model to identify the contaminated lots implicated in iatrogenic transmission of Creutzfeldt-Jakob disease among French human growth hormone recipients. Am J Epidemiol 1998; 146:597.

106. Deslys JP, Marco D, Dormont D. Similar genetic susceptibility in iatrogenic and sporadic Creutzfeldt-Jakob disease. J Gen Virol 1994; 75:23.

107. Lee AJ, Maddix DS. Trimethoprim-sulfamethoxazole induced hypoglycemia in a patient with acute renal failure. Ann Pharmacother 1997; 31:727.

108. Isley WL. Effect of rifampin therapy on thyroid function tests in a hypothyroid patient on replacement L-thyroxine. Ann Intern Med 1987; 107:517.

109. Kyriazopoulou V, Parapousi O, Vagenakis AG. Rifampicin-induced adrenal crisis in addisonian patients receiving corticosteroid replacement therapy. J Clin Endocrinol Metab 1984; 59:1204.

110. Roth H, Becker KL, Shalhoub RJ, Katz S. Nephrotoxicity of demethylchlortetracycline hydrochloride. Arch Intern Med 1967; 120:433.

111. Crotty KL, May R, Kulvicki A, et al. The effect of antimicrobial therapy on testicular aspirate flow cytometry. J Urol 1995; 153:835.

112. Pearson RD, Hewlett EL. Pentamidine for the treatment of *Pneumocystis carinii* pneumonia and other protozoal diseases. Ann Intern Med 1986; 103:782.

113. Heyns W, Drochmans A, VanderSchuerren E, Verhoeven G. Endocrine effects of high-dose ketoconazole therapy in advanced prostatic cancer. Acta Endocrinol (Copenh) 1985; 110:276.

114. Couch RM, Muller J, Perry YS, Winter JS. Kinetic analysis of inhibition of human adrenal steroidogenesis by ketoconazole. J Clin Endocrinol Metab 1987; 65:551.

115. Britton H, Shehab Z, Lightner E, et al. Adrenal response in children receiving high doses of ketoconazole for systemic coccidioidomycosis. J Pediatr 1988; 112:488.

116. Tanner AR. Hypothyroidism after treatment with ketoconazole. Br Med J 1987; 294:125.

117. Lesher JL Jr, Fitch MH, Dunlap DB. Subclinical hypothyroidism during potassium iodide therapy for lymphocutaneous sporotrichosis. Cutis 1994; 53:128.

118. Davis SV, Murray JA. Amphotericin B, aminoglycosides, and hypomagnesemic tetany. Br Med J 1986; 292:1395.

119. Semel JD, McNerney JJ Jr. SIADH during disseminated herpes varicella-zoster infections: relationship to vidarabine therapy. Am J Med Sci 1986; 291:115.

# CHAPTER 214

# ENDOCRINE DISORDERS IN HUMAN IMMUNODEFICIENCY VIRUS INFECTION

STEPHEN A. MIGUELES AND CARMELITA U. TUAZON

Endocrine dysfunction may arise during any stage of infection with the human immunodeficiency virus (HIV). Etiologies include direct viral-induced tissue damage, perturbations related to inflammatory mediators of the host response, parenchymal infiltration by opportunistic pathogens or neoplasms, adverse medication effects, and/or a nonspecific consequence of chronic illness. The spectrum of manifestations ranges from subclinical hypothalamic-pituitary dysregulation to states of overt glandular insufficiency. While the former does not typically require hormone replacement, the latter may be life-threatening if misdiagnosed or inadequately treated. The advent of highly active antiretroviral therapy (HAART) has enabled many HIV-infected patients to enjoy improved health and prolonged survival. However, the recent emergence of a host of endocrinologic/metabolic abnormalities in a subset of HAART recipients may negatively impact the quality of life and future well-being of these individuals. In this chapter, the

**TABLE 214-1.**
**Common Endocrine Disorders in Human Immunodeficiency Virus (HIV)–Infected Patients**

| Endocrine Gland | Endocrine Abnormality |
|---|---|
| HYPO-THALAMIC-PITUITARY | Nonspecific hypothalamic-pituitary dysfunction due to severe illness and/or direct effect of HIV |
| | Syndrome of inappropriate antidiuretic hormone (SIADH) secretion |
| | Growth failure in children |
| | GH resistance in the AIDS-wasting syndrome (AWS) |
| ADRENAL | Drug-induced adrenal dysfunction |
| | Adrenal insufficiency/glucocorticoid resistance |
| | CMV adrenalitis |
| | Reduced adrenal androgen levels |
| THYROID | Subclinical hypothyroidism |
| | Nonelevated $rT_3$, $\uparrow$TBG, $\downarrow$/normal $T_4$ and $T_3$ with complicated, advanced HIV infection |
| | *Pneumocystis carinii* thyroiditis |
| GONADS | Hypogonadotropic hypogonadism |
| | Hypogonadism→wasting |
| ENDOCRINE PANCREAS | Increased insulin sensitivity and clearance |
| | Drug-induced endocrine dysfunction manifested as hypoglycemia or hyperglycemia |
| | HAART→insulin resistance |
| PARATHYROID | Relative hypoparathyroidism |
| ELECTROLYTES | Hypotonic hyponatremia (most commonly hypo-volemic or euvolemic with $\uparrow$ADH) |
| | Hypokalemia (due to dehydration or an adverse medication effect) |
| | Drug-induced hypocalcemia |

$\uparrow$, increased; $\downarrow$, decreased; *GH*, growth hormone; *CMV*, cytomegalovirus; *$rT_3$*, reverse triiodothyronine; *TBG*, thyroid-binding globulin; *$T_4$*, thyroxine; *$T_3$*, triiodothyronine; *HAART*, highly active antiretroviral therapy; *ADH*, antidiuretic hormone.

authors review the more frequent endocrine disorders (Table 214-1) associated with HIV infection and provide a general approach to diagnosis and management.

## HYPOTHALAMIC-PITUITARY FUNCTION

Autopsy series have revealed that an array of pathologic processes can damage the hypothalamus and pituitary gland in patients with the acquired immunodeficiency syndrome (AIDS; see Chap. 11). The most frequent abnormalities are varying degrees of infarction and necrosis, occurring in 10% of cases. Infiltration by various pathogens, including cytomegalovirus (CMV), *Toxoplasma gondii*, *Pneumocystis carinii*, *Mycobacterium tuberculosis*, *Cryptococcus neoformans*, and *Aspergillus*, has also been documented in the setting of disseminated disease and/or diffuse central nervous system (CNS) infection. Malignant destruction is extremely rare, but peripheral adenohyphophyseal involvement by cerebral lymphoma has been reported.[1]

CNS toxoplasmosis and hypothalamic CMV infection have become manifest as frank panhypopituitarism in a few HIV-infected individuals, a rare occurrence in contrast to the frequent subtle alterations detected in hypothalamic-pituitary function.[2,3]

The growth hormone (GH)–insulin-like growth factor-I (IGF-I) axis has been evaluated in HIV-infected children experiencing growth failure. IGF-I levels are reduced in a subset of these children despite normal basal and stimulated GH concentrations in most instances.[4] Malnutrition cannot explain these findings in the majority of cases. In vitro resistance to the growth-promoting effects of GH, IGF-I, and insulin in symptomatic HIV-infected children with normal plasma IGF-I levels has been demonstrated.[5] Acquired GH resistance has also been implicated in the pathogenesis of HIV-related wasting in adult men.[6]

Posterior pituitary function may be impaired in HIV disease. The syndrome of inappropriate antidiuretic hormone (SIADH) secretion has been described in hospitalized HIV-infected patients (see Chap. 27); several of these had been diagnosed with *P. carinii* pneumonia (PCP) and were receiving trimethoprim-sulfamethoxazole. The latter can potentiate renal-salt wasting. SIADH has also been reported in HIV-infected patients with CNS disease and other pulmonary lesions and appears to be more prevalent in patients more seriously affected by AIDS.[7] Identification and treatment of underlying disease processes and fluid restriction in moderate cases remain cornerstones of therapy.

Patients with AIDS have been infrequently reported to have central (neurogenic) diabetes insipidus (DI) and intracranial infections—including herpetic meningoencephalitis, cerebral toxoplasmosis, and CMV encephalitis.[8] Nephrogenic DI has occurred in the setting of foscarnet administration for CMV retinitis.[9] Central DI can often be successfully managed with intranasal desmopressin acetate (DDAVP), while nephrogenic DI can be improved by use of amiloride, hydrochlorothiazide, and indomethacin.[10]

**Drugs (Table 214-2).** Reversible panhypopituitarism and elevated IGF-I levels have been associated with interferon-$\alpha$ therapy for HCV infection.[11] Likewise, SIADH has occurred in HIV-infected patients receiving vidarabine and pentamidine.

## THE HYPOTHALAMIC–PITUITARY–ADRENAL AXIS

The adrenal gland is the most adversely affected endocrine organ in autopsy series of patients with AIDS.[12] CMV-inclusion bodies have been identified in 40% to 88% of cases.[10] While frank hypoadrenalism has been reported in a few patients with CMV adrenalitis, tissue destruction is typically <70% and rarely exceeds the 90% considered necessary to produce functional impairment.[12] Infiltration by *C. neoformans*, *Histoplasma capsulatum*, *T. gondii*, Microsporidia, *Mycobacterium avium* complex, *M. tuberculosis*, Kaposi sarcoma, and non-Hodgkin lymphoma has also been demonstrated at postmortem examination. Adrenal insufficiency resulting from bilateral adrenal abscesses has been described in the setting of disseminated infection with *Nocardia asteroides*.[13] Other pathologic findings include hemorrhage, infarction, and cortical lipid depletion.[12]

The pathogenic significance of antiadrenal antibodies in patients with HIV infection remains to be determined. Secondary adrenal insufficiency has been attributed to direct invasion of the hypothalamic-pituitary region by HIV, opportunistic pathogens (*T. gondii*, CMV), Kaposi sarcoma, or lymphoma.

Clinically significant adrenal insufficiency occurs in ~5% to 10% of untreated patients with advanced HIV infection. While basal serum cortisol levels are typically normal in most HIV-infected persons, elevations have been observed during all stages of disease. In hypercortisolemic patients, serum ACTH concentrations lie above, below, or within the normal range.[14–16] Suppressed circadian secretion of ACTH in one study was attributed to noncorticotropin adrenal stimulation.[15] Elevated ACTH levels may arise from a hypothalamic activation that is directly induced by HIV viral proteins or is mediated by inflammatory cytokines. Additionally, a syndrome of glucocorticoid resistance has been described in some HIV-infected patients that is characterized by hypercortisolemia, increased serum levels of ACTH, impaired dexamethasone suppression, and clinical hypoadrenalism.[16] Mononuclear cells from these individuals

**TABLE 214-2.**
**Endocrinologic Side Effects of Medications Used in the Treatment of Human Immunodeficiency Virus Infection**

| Drugs | Indication/Use | Mechanism | Clinical Effect |
|---|---|---|---|
| **Amphotericin B** | Fungal infections | Renal insufficiency/type I RTA | Hypokalemia<br>Hypomagnesemia, hypocalcemia<br>Sodium abnormalities (less common) |
| **Anabolic steroids (nandrolone,\* oxandrolone)** | AIDS-related wasting | Anabolic steroids with less androgenic properties than testosterone | Lipid abnormalities<br>Impaired glucose tolerance |
| **Anticonvulsants (phenobarbital, phenytoin)** | Neoplastic or infectious CNS lesions | Inducers of hepatic cytochrome P450 enzymes→accelerated steroid hormone clearance | Hypothyroidism in patients with limited thyroid reserve or without replacement dosage adjustments<br>Adrenal insufficiency in patients with limited adrenal reserve or without replacement dosage adjustment |
| **Cyclophosphamide** | Lymphoma | Gonadal toxicity | Ovarian failure, amenorrhea<br>Testicular failure |
| **Didanosine (ddI)** | Antiretroviral agent (nucleoside analog) | Pancreatic toxicity | Pancreatitis<br>Hyperglycemia |
| **Foscarnet** | CMV disease (retinitis, encephalomyelitis, esophagitis, colitis) Resistant HSV disease | Nephrotoxicity/complexes with ionized calcium<br>Nephrogenic diabetes insipidus (DI) | Hypocalcemia, hypophosphatemia<br>Hypomagnesemia, hypokalemia (less common)<br>Hypernatremia |
| **Ganciclovir** | CMV disease (retinitis, encephalomyelitis, esophagitis, colitis) | Inhibition of testicular steroidogenesis (uncommon) | Hypogonadism (uncommon) |
| **Glucocorticoids** | *P. carinii* pneumonia, ITP, aphthous ulcers, CNS mass lesions, LIP, nephropathy, lymphoma | Counterregulatory hormones | Hyperglycemia/diabetes mellitus<br>Cushing syndrome |
| **Growth hormone** | AIDS-related wasting | ↑IGF-I levels, counterregulatory hormone | Hyperlipidemia<br>Hyperglycemia/diabetes mellitus |
| **Interferon-α** | Immunomodulator used in Kaposi sarcoma, HCV infection | Autoimmunity<br><br>Unknown | Hypothyroidism/hyperthyroidism<br>Diabetes mellitus<br>Reversible panhypopituitarism (uncommon)<br>↑IGF-I levels |
| **Interleukin-2** | Immunomodulator | Unknown | (?) Hypothyroidism |
| **Ketoconazole** | Fungal infections | Decreased adrenal and gonadal steroidogenesis<br><br>Reduced 1,25 dihydroxyvitamin D formation<br>Induction of hepatic cytochrome P450 enzymes | Adrenal insufficiency in patients with marginal adrenal reserve<br>Decreased testosterone levels/hypogonadism<br>Decreased total calcium levels<br>Hypothyroidism |
| **Megestrol acetate** | AIDS-related wasting | Intrinsic glucocorticoid-like activity→suppression of hypothalamic–pituitary–adrenal axis<br><br>Progestational activity→suppression of hypothalamic–pituitary–gonadal axis | Hyperglycemia/diabetes mellitus<br>Cushing syndrome (uncommon)<br>Adrenal insufficiency with abrupt discontinuation<br>Decreased testosterone levels/hypogonadism |
| **Opiates** | Analgesia | Inducer of hepatic cytochrome P450 enzymes→accelerated steroid hormone clearance<br><br>Unknown | Hypothyroidism in patients with limited thyroid reserve or without replacement dosage adjustments<br>Adrenal insufficiency in patients with limited adrenal reserve or without replacement dosage adjustment<br>Hypogonadotropic hypogonadism |
| **Protease inhibitors (saquinavir, ritonavir, indinavir, nelfinavir)** | Antiretroviral agents | Exact mechanism unknown/?inhibition of proteins involved with lipid metabolism | Abnormal fat redistribution/lipodystrophy<br>Insulin resistance/impaired glucose tolerance/diabetes mellitus<br>Hypertriglyceridemia<br>Hypercholesterolemia |
| **Pentamidine** | *P. carinii* pneumonia | Pancreatic toxicity<br><br>Nephrotoxicity/inhibition of distal tubular sodium transport/SIADH | Pancreatitis<br>Acute hypoglycemia<br>Chronic hyperglycemia/diabetes mellitus<br>Hyperkalemia<br>Hypocalcemia<br>Hyponatremia |
| **Rifampin/rifabutin** | *M. tuberculosis*<br>*M. avium complex* | Inducers of hepatic cytochrome P450 enzymes→accelerated steroid hormone clearance | Hypothyroidism in patients with limited thyroid reserve or without replacement dosage adjustments<br>Adrenal insufficiency in patients with limited adrenal reserve or without replacement dosage adjustment |
| **Testosterone** | Hypogonadism<br>AIDS-related wasting\* | Anabolic steroid with potent androgenic properties | Lipid abnormalities (↓HDL)<br>Glucose intolerance<br>Testicular atrophy |
| **Trimethoprim–sulfamethoxazole** | *P. carinii* pneumonia<br>Activity against *T. gondii*<br>Bacterial infections | Trimethoprim:<br>Distal tubular sodium channel inhibitor/SIADH<br>Sulfamethoxazole:<br>Interstitial nephritis<br>Pancreatic toxicity<br>Sulfonylurea-like stimulation of islet B cells | Hyperkalemia<br>Hyponatremia<br>Hyporeninemic hypoaldosteronism, hyponatremia, hyperkalemia<br>Pancreatitis<br>Hypoglycemia (uncommon) |

↑, increased; ↓, decreased; *RTA*, renal tubular acidosis; *AIDS*, acquired immunodeficiency syndrome; *CNS*, central nervous system; *CMV*, cytomegalovirus; *HSV*, herpes simplex virus; *P. carinii*, *Pneumocystis carinii*; *ITP*, idiopathic thrombocytopenic purpura; *LIP*, lymphocytic interstitial pneumonitis; *IGF-I*, insulin-like growth factor-I; *HCV*, hepatitis C virus; *SIADH*, syndrome of inappropriate antidiuretic hormone; *M.*, *Mycobacterium*; *HDL*, high-density lipoprotein; *T. gondii*, *Toxoplasma gondii*.
\*Not yet granted approval for this indication.

have increased numbers of glucocorticoid receptors, which have decreased affinity for hormone. Discrepant adrenocorticotropic hormone (ACTH) values among study subjects may also relate to varying degrees of stress and a prior history of opiate abuse. Heightened corticotropin-releasing hormone (CRH) secretion occurs with advanced HIV infection.[17]

ACTH-stimulation testing in HIV-infected individuals yields an adequate cortisol response in most patients. A profile consisting of normal or elevated basal serum cortisol levels and a marginal response to ACTH provocation is suggestive of diminished adrenal reserve. Furthermore, results of CRH-stimulation testing in some HIV-infected patients are compatible with blunted pituitary-adrenal responsiveness that may become more prevalent with advanced disease.[17]

Inflammatory cytokines are likely to be involved in the aberrations of the hypothalamic–pituitary–adrenal (HPA) axis, which occurs in HIV disease. Interleukin (IL)-1 and tumor necrosis factor-α (TNF-α), which are produced by macrophages in response to HIV infection, have been shown to stimulate adrenal cortisol secretion directly. Additionally, interactions between viral proteins and lymphocytes influence IL-6 production. Both IL-1 and IL-6 promote release of hypothalamic CRH and pituitary ACTH; serum concentrations of these cytokines correlate significantly with cortisol levels in HIV-infected patients. Glucocorticoids, in turn, are potent regulators of lymphocyte function and cytokine expression. Furthermore, receptors for CRH and ACTH have been identified on lymphocytes. These findings attest to the complexity of the neuroendocrine-immune interactions that appear to influence HIV infection.[18]

Clinically significant mineralocorticoid deficiency is rare in HIV-infected patients despite the tendency toward mild reductions in basal aldosterone levels. While normal increases of plasma aldosterone in response to provocative stimuli have been documented at various stages of infection,[14] an impaired response to ACTH stimulation is not necessarily predictive of the development of clinically significant hypoaldosteronism.[19]

Basal adrenal androgen levels are lower in most HIV-infected patients as compared to healthy controls and fail to rise in response to ACTH stimulation at all stages of HIV infection.[19] Dehydroepiandrosterone (DHEA) concentrations correlate with CD4+ cell counts and are independent predictors of disease progression in asymptomatic patients.[20] The strong inverse correlation between CD4+ cell counts and cortisol/DHEA ratios has aroused discussion regarding the likelihood that an elevated ratio prompts a transition in cytokine production that modulates progressive HIV infection.[21] The observation that products of the 17-deoxysteroid pathway are diminished despite normal or elevated cortisol levels in HIV-infected individuals (along with the aforementioned findings) may simply reflect a shift in adrenal steroid biosynthesis, which favors cortisol production as an adaptation to physiologic changes arising from progressive HIV infection.[14]

Hypoadrenalism should be considered in patients with advanced HIV disease, disseminated opportunistic infections, and/or a compatible clinical picture (e.g., unexplained nausea, abdominal pain, weight loss, fatigue, hyperpigmentation, orthostasis, hyponatremia, hyperkalemia, hypoglycemia, or metabolic acidosis). Stress doses of hydrocortisone (100 mg every 8 hours) should be administered to any patient with suspected adrenal crisis while awaiting diagnostic confirmation. A random morning cortisol concentration <10 μg/dL (280 nmol/L) is suggestive of adrenal insufficiency, whereas a value >20 μg/dL (540 nmol/L) virtually excludes it. ACTH (cosyntropin) provocation should be performed with basal hypocortisolemia or a high clinical suspicion of adrenal insufficiency. Definitions of normal values are the same as for seronegative patients. A

low or inappropriately normal ACTH level accompanying a reduced cortisol response is compatible with secondary adrenal insufficiency. Evaluation of the other hypothalamic-pituitary axes should be performed; elevated corticotropin levels are consistent with primary adrenal insufficiency. Individuals exhibiting an abnormal response to ACTH stimulation should receive maintenance glucocorticoid therapy (30 mg per day hydrocortisone) and dose escalation during acute stress. Fludrocortisone (0.1 mg per day) is usually indicated for patients with primary adrenal insufficiency. The approach to patients with high-normal basal cortisol levels and a marginal response to provocative testing is less straightforward. Given concern for worsening immunosuppression, the potential acceleration of wasting, and further inhibition of the HPA axis, sequential provocative testing may help to identify the appropriate timing of replacement therapy in such patients. However, brief courses of glucocorticoid therapy during acute stress should be considered.

Despite the mild hypercortisolemia reported in HIV-infected patients, Cushing syndrome is rare. Iatrogenic Cushing syndrome secondary to administration of megestrol acetate, a progestational appetite stimulant with intrinsic glucocorticoid-like activity, has been reported[22] (see Chap. 75).

Indications for glucocorticoid administration in HIV-infected patients include moderate to severe PCP (arterial $PO_2$ <70 mm Hg), idiopathic thrombocytopenic purpura, aphthous ulceration, cerebral edema resulting from CNS mass lesions, lymphoid interstitial pneumonitis, nephropathy, and palliation of disseminated *M. avium* complex. No difference in survival or in the risk of most AIDS-related complications (except esophageal candidiasis) was associated with a 21-day tapering course of adjunctive corticosteroids for the treatment of PCP in a large cohort study. However, concern for induction of worsening immunosuppression and exacerbation of HIV-related infections is appropriate with prolonged treatment courses.[23]

**Drugs (see Table 214-2).** The antifungal agent ketoconazole inhibits steroidogenesis and could induce adrenal insufficiency in patients with limited adrenal reserve.[19] Due to suppression of the HPA axis, megestrol acetate should be tapered when ceasing therapy, as abrupt discontinuation has resulted in adrenal insufficiency. Inducers of the cytochrome P450 enzymes such as rifampin, anticonvulsants, and opiates may precipitate hypoadrenalism in patients with marginal reserve due to accelerated hepatic steroid metabolism.

## THE HYPOTHALAMIC–PITUITARY–THYROIDAL AXIS

Infiltration of the thyroid gland by a number of opportunistic disease processes has been reported in HIV-infected patients, but clinically significant thyroid dysfunction only results from marked parenchymal destruction.

*P. carinii* thyroiditis represents the most common HIV-associated thyroid infection.[24] A painful, enlarging neck mass is a typical presentation. Disruption of glandular architecture leading to states of thyroid excess or deficiency has been reported. Antithyroid antibodies are usually negative and radionuclide scanning is of low yield. The diagnosis may be established with Gomori methenamine silver staining of a fine-needle aspirate. Treatment with systemic anti-*Pneumocystis* medications and supportive care has resulted in normalization of thyroid function. Aerosolized pentamidine, administered as prophylaxis for PCP, is a risk factor for extrapulmonary, including thyroidal, pneumocystosis.[24]

While CMV inclusions within the thyroid gland have been detected in autopsy series of AIDS patients, clinical evidence of antemortem thyroid dysfunction was lacking. Subclinical thyroid infection with *M. tuberculosis* and *M. avium* complex has also been reported in HIV-infected patients. A biochemical profile consistent with the euthyroid sick syndrome has resulted from thyroid infiltration with *C. neoformans* and *Aspergillus*. A large thyroid abscess caused by *Rhodococcus equi* has been described in an HIV-infected man with a pulmonary focus.[25]

Thyroid involvement by metastatic Kaposi sarcoma has been reported. In one case, hypothyroidism resulted from extensive glandular invasion in a patient presenting with neuropsychiatric deterioration.[26] HIV-associated lymphoma involving the thyroid gland has not been reported. Individuals with autoimmune thyroid disease and HIV-related immune dysfunction may be at an increased risk for primary thyroid lymphoma.

Overt hypothyroidism or hyperthyroidism does not occur at an increased frequency in patients with HIV disease as compared to patients with other nonthyroidal illnesses. While most individuals with early infection and stable body weight maintain normal thyroid function, a unique thyroid profile has been observed in some that may become more pronounced with disease progression.[27] Features include high serum total thyroxine ($T_4$) and thyroxine-binding globulin (TBG) levels, normal serum triiodothyronine ($T_3$) levels, and reduced reverse $T_3$ ($rT_3$) values. Inappropriately normal $T_3$ levels despite progressive HIV disease may reflect dysregulation of the hypothalamic–pituitary–thyroidal axis and may promote protein catabolism.[27]

A decline in serum thyroid hormone concentrations does occur during episodes of severe intercurrent infection and with the progressive debilitation seen in advanced disease. Contrasting with the usual pattern observed in nonthyroidal illness, low $rT_3$ levels have been demonstrated at all stages of HIV infection.[27] In one series, $rT_3$ levels and $rT_3/T_4$ ratios were low in HIV-infected outpatients but normal in those requiring hospitalization. The pathophysiologic significance of nonelevated $rT_3$ levels is unknown.

TBG levels rise with progressive stages of HIV infection in both adults and children. While concurrent acute hepatitis is responsible in some cases, the exact mechanism is unclear; this warrants consideration as one interprets total $T_3$ and $T_4$ measurements.

In HIV-infected patients, thyrotropin (thyroid-stimulating hormone; TSH) levels are high-normal when compared to seronegative controls (see Chap. 15). A highly significant correlation has been found between higher mean 24-hour TSH concentrations and a greater mean TSH-pulse amplitude in stable HIV-infected outpatients. Compared to normal controls, higher peak thyrotropin-releasing hormone (TRH)–stimulated TSH levels have also been described in these individuals. These alterations may represent a state of compensated primary hypothyroidism (induced by HIV infection), which differs from the thyroid dysfunction observed in non-HIV, nonthyroidal illnesses.[28]

Thyroid indices classic for the euthyroid sick syndrome are not uncommon in advanced, complicated HIV infection.[29] Those at particular risk include patients with wasting syndrome and severe AIDS-related infections and neoplasms.[30]

Inflammatory cytokines influence thyroid hormone metabolism. TNF-$\alpha$ infusion produces a "euthyroid sick" pattern in normal patients.[31] An increase in hepatic type I 5'-deiodinase activity and inhibition of the effects of TSH on the thyroid gland in TNF-$\alpha$–treated mice have been demonstrated.[32] The former phenomenon may contribute to the relatively elevated $T_3$ levels and depressed $rT_3$ concentrations observed in these animals. Similarly, when cultured human thyrocytes are exposed to IL-1, TNF-$\alpha$, and interferon-$\gamma$, they exhibit impaired iodine organification and de novo synthesis of thyroid hormones.[33]

As previously suggested, thyroid function tests may have predictive value in HIV-infected individuals. The low levels of $T_3$ and $T_4$ accompanying severe AIDS-related complications have been associated with increased mortality.[27,29] Nonsurviving hospitalized patients with PCP were more likely to have decreased $T_3$ levels. TBG levels have been shown to be inversely correlated with CD4+ counts in HIV-infected persons.[27] Furthermore, thyroid hormones may directly influence the progression of HIV disease. Clinical hypothyroidism has been implicated in delaying the onset of full-blown AIDS. Conversely, low levels of $T_3$ may enhance viral transcriptional activity by facilitating the interaction between the long terminal repeat (LTR) of HIV-1 and the thyroid hormone $T_3$ receptor $\alpha$.[34]

Although these alterations in hormone levels must be considered when interpreting laboratory values, primary thyroid disease can still be readily diagnosed on the basis of routine thyroid function testing (e.g., TSH, free $T_4$) in HIV-infected patients. Discrimination between secondary hypothyroidism and the sick euthyroid syndrome may pose a greater diagnostic challenge and require provocative testing and further pituitary evaluation. Radioactive thyroid scanning in the setting of hyperthyroidism and fine-needle aspiration biopsy of a thyroid nodule are recommended as with seronegative patients. After establishing a diagnosis of hypothyroidism, replacement $T_4$ therapy should be initiated with caution at low starting doses, as AIDS-related wasting may be exacerbated. Graves disease has been described in a small number of patients on a stable antiretroviral regimen that had been successfully treated with antithyroid drugs or ablative radioactive iodine.[35] Antimicrobial therapy and supportive care may suffice for patients with infectious thyroiditis (see Chap. 46).

**Drugs (see Table 214-2).** Rifampin, which may be used in the treatment of mycobacterial disease, and ketoconazole induce hepatic cytochrome P450 enzymes and accelerate thyroid hormone clearance. Patients already receiving thyroid-replacement therapy may require dosage escalation and patients with marginal reserve may develop clinically apparent hypothyroidism. Interferon-$\alpha$, used in the treatment of Kaposi sarcoma and hepatitis C infection, has been implicated in autoimmune thyroid disease manifesting as hyperthyroidism or hypothyroidism. Evidence has suggested that IL-2 may precipitate thyroid dysfunction.[36]

## THE HYPOTHALAMIC–PITUITARY–GONADAL AXIS

Postmortem examination of men dying from AIDS has revealed frequent histopathologic changes in the genital system. Common findings include testicular tubular hyalinization, decreased spermatogenesis, thickened basement membranes, peritubular fibrosis, Leydig cell hypoplasia, and epididymal obstruction.[37] As occurs in other endocrine glands, infiltration of the testes has been described in patients with disseminated CMV, *M. avium* complex, *M. tuberculosis*, *T. gondii*, and *H. capsulatum*.[37] *T. gondii* may cause clinical orchitis. Epididymal destruction by metastatic Kaposi sarcoma and testicular involvement by lymphoma have also been reported. HIV-related proteins have been demonstrated by various techniques in gonadal tissue and may directly induce pathologic changes.[38] Furthermore, the increased prevalence of sexually transmitted diseases among homosexual men appears to represent a risk factor of testicular pathology.[37] A review of ovarian histopathology in HIV-infected women has not been conducted.

Isolation of replication-competent virus from seminal cells of a few HIV-infected men despite long-term viral suppression with HAART and without detectable levels of viral RNA in the plasma or semen suggests that the genital tract is a sanctuary for HIV replication.[38]

Causes of subnormal testosterone levels in patients with HIV infection include pituitary or hypothalamic dysfunction, gonadotropin resistance, testicular failure due to neoplastic or infectious destruction, adverse medication effects, illicit drug use, or a nonspecific response to chronic illness.[39] In early infection, testosterone concentrations are either normal or increased.[15,29] In advanced disease, hypogonadism occurs at a greater frequency.[15,29] Indeed, symptomatic hypogonadism represents one of the most prevalent endocrine abnormalities in AIDS patients, occurring in 29% to 50% of untreated patients with full-blown AIDS.[29] Common complaints include decreased libido, impotence, fatigue, depression, loss of body hair, and muscle wasting. Reduced testosterone levels in AIDS patients correlate with a decline in lymphocyte counts.[15,29] The AIDS wasting syndrome (AWS) is associated with a significant reduction in testosterone concentrations as compared to HIV-infected patients without wasting and similar CD4+ counts.[40] In a majority of hypogonadal patients, serum gonadotropin levels are low or inappropriately normal, consistent with hypogonadotropic hypogonadism. Primary hypogonadism has been discovered in up to 25% of androgen-deficient patients.[40]

Abnormalities of the hypothalamic–pituitary–gonadal axis may contribute to gonadal dysfunction at any stage of HIV infection. Elevations of total and free testosterone, basal luteinizing hormone (LH), and gonadotropin-releasing hormone (GnRH)–stimulated LH in one series of HIV-infected patients suggest a relatively early alteration at the hypothalamic-pituitary level.[41] Disturbed testosterone circadian rhythmicity has been described and probably also reflects central dysregulation.[15] Prolactin concentrations are typically within the normal range in HIV-infected patients,[41] but modest elevations may have contributed to abnormal gonadal function in some individuals with wasting.[40] Secondary hypogonadism has been reported in patients with generalized and/or cerebral infection with CMV, *P. carinii*, and *T. gondii*.[2] As with other severe illnesses, hypogonadotropic hypogonadism may occur as a nonspecific consequence of chronic HIV disease related to cachexia, malnutrition, prolonged fever, and superimposed opportunistic infections.[29] Cytokines have once again been implicated.

Data regarding gonadal dysfunction in women with HIV infection are sparse. Similar patterns of menstruation between HIV-infected women and seronegative controls have been observed by some investigators, yet others have reported a higher frequency of amenorrhea among HIV-infected women with weight loss.[42,43] In one study, amenorrhea had an overall prevalence of 20%, with a higher rate (38%) observed in women with the AWS. Furthermore, a relationship between amenorrhea and decreased muscle mass was found to be independent of body weight or CD4+ count. Androgen levels (free testosterone and DHEA-S) were decreased significantly in women with wasting, and correlated with diminished muscle mass, suggesting an association between gonadal function and body composition in HIV-infected women. Gonadotropin levels were reduced, consistent with hypogonadotropic hypogonadism.

Several investigators have found normal serum sex hormone–binding globulin (SHBG) levels at all stages of HIV infection, whereas others have demonstrated serum concentrations significantly exceeding levels in normal controls.[40,44] The higher SHBG-association constant for testosterone, which has been noted in the sera of AIDS patients when compared to patients with earlier stages of disease, results in lower free testosterone levels.[44] A similar pattern has been observed in HIV-infected women, suggesting that the unbound fraction is a better index of androgen function.[43]

Androgen deficiency is easily diagnosed by obtaining morning blood for serum testosterone, prolactin, and follicle-stimulating hormone (FSH)/LH levels. As patients may have elevations of SHBG, free testosterone levels are more sensitive indicators of hypogonadism.

Hormone-replacement therapy is indicated in symptomatic male patients with reduced testosterone levels, including individuals with the AWS.[44a] Improvements in libido and sexual function, mood, appetite, and overall quality of life have been reported in HIV-infected patients receiving therapy. Testosterone supplementation in eugonadal HIV-infected patients with the wasting syndrome, in chemically hypogonadal patients without wasting or other obvious clinical manifestations of testosterone deficiency, and in HIV-infected women requires further investigation. Some patients who continue to report symptoms despite serum concentrations within the "normal range" do note improvements, with levels exceeding the upper limit of normal. In these individuals, free or bioavailable testosterone may be a better marker of androgen function.

Testosterone is available in injectable forms and as transdermal patches. A typical starting dose for the injectable, long-acting preparations is 200-mg intramuscular injections every 2 weeks (an average of 100 mg per week), but this may require adjustment to effect a clinical response. Transdermal systems are also available. They have the advantages of eliminating first-pass hepatic metabolism, maintaining the normal circadian variation, minimizing central feedback inhibition, and avoiding several of the complications associated with intramuscular delivery. Concerns include variations in absorption, a requirement to wear the patch 22 to 24 hours per day, the potential for skin irritation, maintenance of adhesion during exercise and in hot weather, and excessive cost.

**Drugs (see Table 214-2).** Similar to its effect on the adrenal glands, ketoconazole is also known to inhibit gonadal steroidogenesis, thereby causing reduced serum testosterone levels. Ganciclovir has been associated with inhibition of steroidogenesis. Megestrol acetate lowers serum testosterone levels through central feedback inhibition. This has been offered as an explanation for the greater fat accrual versus lean body mass seen with treatment. Opiate abuse may lead to hypogonadotropic hypogonadism.[10] Gonadal dysfunction has followed administration of cyclophosphamide for the treatment of AIDS-related lymphoma. Regimens including doxorubicin and dacarbazine have been associated with transient reductions in sperm counts.

## LIPID METABOLISM

Serum triglyceride levels increase with progressive HIV infection due to both decreased clearance and increased production of the very low-density lipoprotein (VLDL) fraction[45] (see Chaps. 162 and 163). A reduction in lipoprotein lipase activity has been demonstrated in AIDS patients. However, some investigators maintain that the most striking defect is the paradoxical increase in hepatic de novo lipogenesis (DNL), the synthesis of fat from carbohydrate precursors.[46] This effect appears to be more pronounced with disease progression. Elevated peripheral lipolysis may also contribute to this enhanced VLDL production.

These disturbances in lipid metabolism likely result from the influence of cytokines. Recombinant TNF-α, IL-1, and interferon-α have all been shown to lower lipoprotein lipase activity, to decrease the synthesis of fatty acids, and to increase lipolysis in cultured fat cells.[45] The predominant in vivo effect of TNF-α, IL-1, IL-6, and interferon-α on lipid metabolism is the stimulation of DNL without a significant decline in triglyceride clearance.[45]

Serum cholesterol, high-density lipoprotein (HDL), and low-density lipoprotein (LDL) levels are reduced in HIV-infected patients not receiving protease inhibitors (PIs).[45] These alterations are observed even in clinically stable patients without evidence of malabsorption, appear relatively early in HIV infection, and do not necessarily correlate with disease progression. Elevations have been reported in the LDL subclass LDL-B, as occur in other syndromes of hypertriglyceridemia and low HDL.[47] The mechanism underlying the hypocholesterolemia seen in HIV infection has not been defined but may relate to the same processes leading to an accumulation of the VLDL fraction.

Impressive hypertriglyceridemia and hypercholesterolemia have been demonstrated in recipients of PI-containing antiretroviral therapy.

## THE WASTING SYNDROME

Severe, progressive weight loss is a well-known complication of HIV infection and remains a major cause of morbidity and mortality. The AWS has been defined as >10% unintentional loss from baseline weight in the absence of identifiable opportunistic infections, malignancies, or illnesses—other than HIV infection itself. Recognition of this condition in an HIV-infected individual establishes the diagnosis of AIDS. Most patients with AIDS in industrialized nations have intermittent episodes of accelerated weight loss despite maintenance of a normal baseline weight. With disease progression, recovery from these periods is less complete, producing an overall loss of body cell mass and further debilitation.[30] Lean body cell mass refers to metabolically active, nonadipose tissue and appears to be a better predictor of mortality. While HAART has enhanced survival and has reversed weight loss for many patients, body composition abnormalities have continued to emerge. Three distinct, yet not mutually exclusive, patterns of wasting/weight loss exist in the current era of HAART: (a) a more chronic form as seen in simple starvation, (b) the altered nutrient partitioning and hypermetabolism characteristic of the classic wasting syndrome,[48] and (c) regional wasting with abnormal fat redistribution (reported in a subset of patients receiving antiretroviral therapy).

The dominant pattern of weight loss observed in some HIV-infected patients resembles simple starvation. The rate of weight loss is relatively slow, is generally associated with gastrointestinal dysfunction, is predominantly comprised of fat depletion, and may be accompanied by a compensatory reduction in the resting energy expenditure (REE).[48] Decreased serum triglyceride concentrations are not uncommon. Additionally, an appropriate accrual of lean body mass along with fat tissue results with refeeding. Important factors leading to reduced caloric intake include anorexia, taste alteration, oral and/or esophageal lesional pain (related to aphthous ulceration or infection by *Candida* species, herpes simplex virus [HSV], or CMV), nausea, vomiting, fatigue, and neuropsychiatric illness acting either alone or in combination. Medications used in the treatment of HIV disease may be contributory. Malabsorption due to gastrointestinal infection or neoplasia is not rare in patients with HIV disease and may significantly impair nutrient uptake.

Hypermetabolism, a state of increased energy expenditure, results from overwhelming infection or trauma and leads to weight loss. Lean-body-mass preservation may not be achieved despite increased caloric administration. In a subset of individuals with AIDS, a pattern of wasting with similar pathophysiologic features predominates.[30] Instead of the preferential depletion of fat tissue as occurs with nutrient deprivation, the metabolic derangements in these patients permit muscle protein catabolism and a state of negative nitrogen balance. Hypertriglyceridemia, an inappropriate elevation of REE,[30] and a poor lean-body-mass response to refeeding despite increases in fat stores are other characteristics. For these reasons, body fat content may not be a reli-

able marker of wasting in AIDS. Secondary infection is an important determinant of energy balance. It has been shown that the critical factor promoting accelerated weight loss in this setting is the failure to compensate adequately for decreased caloric intake (caused by anorexia) with a reduction in REE.[30]

Although the precise pathogenesis of the AWS has not been elucidated, the host response to infection is likely to occupy a central role. In patients with AIDS, there have been strong positive correlations both between serum triglycerides and circulating levels of interferon-$\alpha$ and between serum concentrations of this cytokine and progressive HIV infection.[45] Additionally, IL-6 concentrations are elevated in HIV-infected patients, rise with advanced disease, and clearly promote hypertriglyceridemia. Levels of TNF-$\alpha$ do not differ significantly between AIDS patients and control subjects; nonetheless, anorexia, hypermetabolism, increased protein turnover, and hypertriglyceridemia follow administration of recombinant TNF-$\alpha$ to normal human subjects.[30] While these relationships suggest causality, a definite link between these cytokines, the presence and severity of hypertriglyceridemia, and the AWS remains to be established.[30]

DNL is elevated in patients with the AWS. It has been suggested that this paradoxical anabolism of fat during ongoing muscle degradation may be a marker of an underlying metabolic abnormality that leads to poor nutrient partitioning.[46] Ingested calories are shunted into wasteful lipogenesis instead of being directed into lean body tissue. As mentioned previously, inflammatory cytokines have again been implicated. Futile cycling of substrates occurs in the AWS and may be involved pathogenically.

Endocrine abnormalities are likely to contribute to the multifactorial etiology of the AWS. Thyroid dysfunction may predispose to the AWS but a clear association is lacking. A correlation between hypogonadism and poor preservation of lean body mass has been well documented.[40,49] A loss of lean body mass and deterioration in exercise capacity were found to be highly correlated with reduced androgen levels in hypogonadal men with the AWS.[40] Testosterone-replacement therapy restored anabolic capacity in this group of patients.[50] Gender-specific body composition may provide additional support for a hormonal influence on the development of the AWS. Although androgen deficiency is also common in women with wasting (and may contribute to decreased muscle mass), women appear to experience a greater relative loss of fat than lean mass with progressive degrees of wasting in contrast to men.[43] In a pilot study of transdermal testosterone administration in women with the ASW, the lower dose (estimated delivery rates, 150 vs. 300 $\mu$g/day) was associated with augmented serum free testosterone levels and positive trends in weight and quality of life. The weight accrued was primarily composed of fat.[43a] GH resistance may be involved in the pathogenesis of HIV-related wasting.[6,50] Increased basal GH secretion and pulse frequency in association with reduced IGF-I concentrations among hypogonadal and eugonadal men with wasting has been described. Following testosterone administration, decreases in GH levels in hypogonadal patients were inversely related to the magnitude of change in lean body mass.[50] No differences in GH or IGF-I levels have been noted in women with advanced wasting compared to age-matched healthy controls; this may partially explain the disproportionate loss of fat mass compared to lean mass in women with the AWS.[43]

### TREATMENT OF THE WASTING SYNDROME

The initial approach to the HIV-infected patient with wasting is a nutritional evaluation to assess the adequacy of caloric intake and a rigorous search for treatable opportunistic infections. Potent antiretroviral therapy for those with uncontrolled HIV infection may also promote weight gain. Therapeutic interventions include those that enhance caloric intake (nutritional supplementation, appetite stimulants) or modify abnormal metabolic and/or endocrinologic processes (anabolic/hormonal therapy, cytokine inhibition).

Those individuals most likely to benefit from enteral support include patients with anorexia, patients with neuropsychiatric illness, or patients with a bypassable mechanical obstruction who retain intact absorptive capacity. Parenteral feeding has been used in individuals with severe bowel dysfunction. While quality of life may be enhanced in some patients, prolonged survival or improved immunologic parameters have not been documented.

Appetite stimulants, like dronabinol and the progestational agent megestrol acetate, can lead to increased caloric intake but have not been associated with significant increases in lean body mass.[51] Adverse effects may be considerable. Concerns with megestrol acetate include adrenal insufficiency following abrupt discontinuation and suppressed androgen function. The latter effect might account for limited lean-body-mass accrual with treatment. Appetite stimulants may be most beneficial as short-term therapy in patients with active secondary infections and/or during the early stages of wasting.

Men with AIDS-related wasting and documented androgen deficiency are likely to derive sustained benefit from testosterone replacement, with increases in lean body mass and improvements in quality of life.[50,50a] Testosterone supplementation in eugonadal HIV-infected patients with the AWS requires further investigation. While female patients might also benefit from replacement therapy, efficacy has not been established, and the optimal dosing strategy remains to be defined. Testosterone is available as short-acting injections (propionate), esterified long-acting injections (enanthate and cypionate), and patches. Concerns with the intramuscular preparations include lack of circadian variation in delivery, fluctuating clinical effects due to a peak supraphysiologic concentration that gradually wanes, painful administration, requirement for an office visit in some cases, and an infrequent allergy to the oil vehicle.

Chemical modification of testosterone has allowed the synthesis of agents with greater anabolic effects and minimal androgenic properties. In open-label studies, the oral agent oxandrolone and the injectable testosterone analog nandrolone decanoate have been shown to significantly increase weight and lean body mass.[50a] In a randomized, placebo-controlled trial, the combination of progressive resistance exercise occurring with a moderately supraphysiologic androgen regimen that included oxandrolone was associated with significantly greater increases in tissue accrual and strength than exercise with physiologic testosterone replacement alone in eugonadal HIV-infected men with weight loss.[52] The long-term efficacy of such treatment is unknown. Furthermore, use of anabolic steroids may be limited by cost, liver function abnormalities, hepatic tumors, glucose intolerance, and hyperlipidemia (see Table 214-2).

Recombinant human growth hormone (rhGH) was granted accelerated approval in 1996 for the treatment of AIDS-related wasting. Significant increases in weight, lean body mass, and treadmill work output were observed among treated patients in a prospective, randomized, double-blind, placebo-controlled study.[53] Considerations related to rhGH therapy include side effects (edema, arthralgias, myalgias, hyperglycemia, and carpal tunnel syndrome), lack of long-term follow-up, lack of a demonstrated survival benefit, unknown durability of response with discontinuation of treatment, and limited experience in women. Due to the prohibitive cost and aforementioned concerns, rhGH should be reserved for individuals with the AWS who have failed or are poor candidates for alternative therapies. The addition of insulin-like growth factor I provides no further advantage.[50a]

The role of cytokines as mediators of AWS has been addressed. A significant increase in lean body mass was demonstrated with thalidomide at dosages of 300 to 400 mg per day in patients with wasting.[54] Inhibition of TNF-α production by monocytes is the presumed mechanism. The toxicity profile of thalidomide precludes recommendation of this agent as first-line treatment for HIV-related wasting. Other cytokine inhibitors (cyproheptadine, ketotifen, fish oil, N-acetylcysteine) are being studied in clinical trials to determine efficacy and safety. Pentoxifylline has not been shown to be effective. These agents should be reserved for patients with wasting who have failed treatment with appetite stimulants and/or who are poor candidates for anabolic/hormonal therapies.

## ABNORMAL FAT REDISTRIBUTION SYNDROME(S)/PERIPHERAL LIPODYSTROPHY

PI-containing regimens are standard of care for HIV-infected patients due to improved clinical, immunologic, and virologic responses.[55] While the incidence of AIDS-related wasting has decreased in the current era of HAART, reports of body composition changes in a subset of treated individuals are accumulating. Various nomenclatures and the existence of several overlapping syndromes have been suggested. Some claim that "lipodystrophy" is a misnomer, as it has historically connoted an absolute loss of fat mass and does not account for the adipose accumulations observed at other sites in the same patient. Alternative descriptive terms that have been used are Crix belly, protease paunch, benign symmetric lipomatosis, and pseudo-Cushing syndrome[56] (see Chap. 75). The *HIV-associated fat redistribution* (HAFR) is described herein as a single clinical entity. The constellation of features includes subcutaneous fat wasting in the face, glutei, and extremities; increased central adiposity in the visceral, dorsocervical ("buffalo hump"), supraclavicular, and submandibular areas (Fig. 214-1); breast enlargement; hyperlipidemia; insulin resistance; and hyperglycemia[57,58] (Table 214-3; see Table 214-2). Estimated prevalence rates vary due to lack of a precise case definition but have ranged from 5% to 64% in various studies. Women and men seem to be affected equally, and the syndrome has been reported in children.

Measurements of body composition with dual energy x-ray absorptiometry (DEXA) or computed tomographic (CT) imaging have demonstrated comparable body weight and fat-free mass among patients receiving PIs, patients not receiving PIs, and healthy controls. However, a lower overall fat mass in each body region, except the central abdomen, has also been reported.[57,58] Quantification of visceral abdominal fat using CT scanning has revealed increased indices in patients (being treated with indinavir) who reported abdominal fullness, distention, and bloating. An intermediate amount of visceral fat was detected in asymptomatic indinavir recipients.[57]

While hyperlipidemia occurs in untreated HIV-infected patients and may be a direct effect of PIs, greater serum lipid elevations have been reported in individuals with HAFR versus PI-treated patients without the syndrome.[58] With enhanced survival attributed to HAART and clinical similarities between HAFR and syndrome X, there is growing concern for accelerated atherosclerosis and associated vascular complications induced by the metabolic derangements seen in many of these patients. Additionally, relatively high rates of infection with organisms such as chlamydia and CMV may incur additional risk.[59] Reports of a few HIV-infected patients with PI-associated hyperlipidemia experiencing premature coronary artery disease have already appeared in the literature.[60]

Although evidence supporting a relationship between use of PIs and the development of HAFR is compelling, causality has not been confirmed. Furthermore, the syndrome has been observed in untreated patients as well as in patients treated with protease-sparing regimens, suggesting that an alternative mechanism may also be operative.[61] In any event, a class-specific

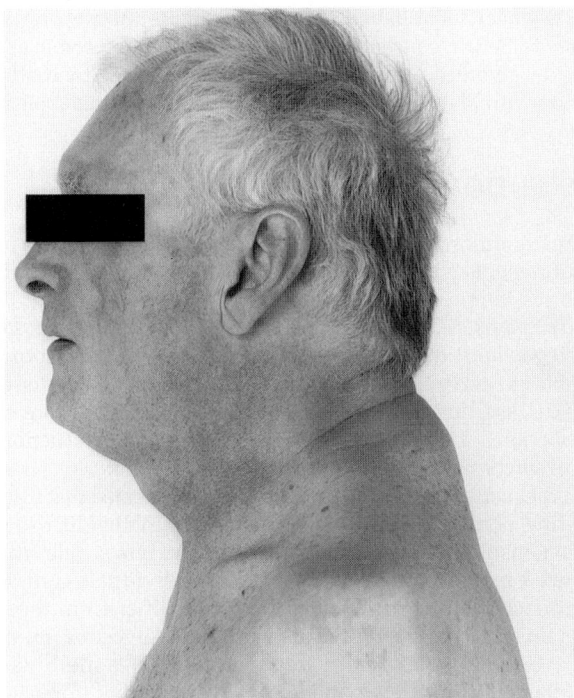

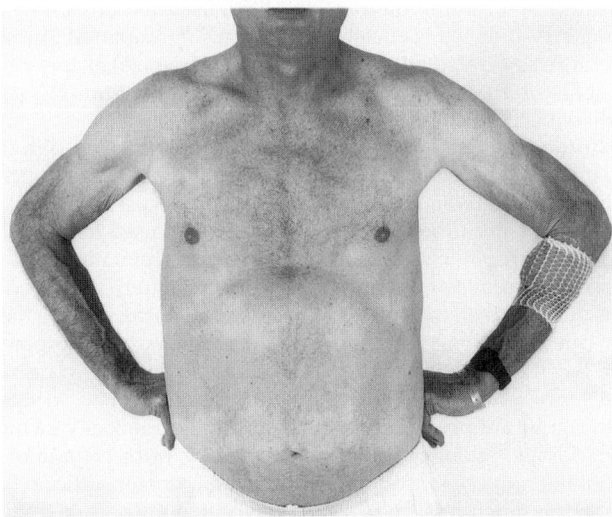

**FIGURE 214-1.** This 60-year-old man developed facial wasting, submandibular adiposity, a dorsocervical fat accumulation (*top panel*), peripheral fat wasting, and increased abdominal girth (*bottom panel*) 27 months after beginning indinavir-based highly active antiretroviral therapy.

**TABLE 214-3.**
**Features of Human Immunodeficiency Virus–Associated Fat Redistribution Syndrome(s)**

**PHYSICAL FINDINGS**
*Fat wasting*
  Face (preauricular, periorbital, and temporal fat loss; prominent nasolabial folds)
  Extremities (prominent vasculature; increased muscular appearance)
  Gluteal thinning
*Central adiposity*
  Increased abdominal girth
  Dorsocervical ("buffalo hump")
  Supraclavicular
  Submandibular
  Breast enlargement
**LABORATORY ABNORMALITIES**
  Hypercholesterolemia
    Elevated low-density lipoprotein (LDL) fraction
    Reduced high-density lipoprotein (HDL) fraction
  Hypertriglyceridemia
  Hyperinsulinemia
  Increased C-peptide levels
  Increased insulin-resistance scores (insulin-tolerance test and homeostasis model)
  Impaired glucose tolerance (oral glucose-tolerance test)
  Elevated fasting glucose

mechanism appears likely as the syndrome has been reported with use of all of the currently approved PIs (saquinavir, ritonavir, nelfinavir, and indinavir). Specific features may occur at variable frequencies with different agents. HAFR appears to be most pronounced in those receiving dual PI therapy with ritonavir-saquinavir.[58] Saquinavir seems to be the least diabetogenic.[62] The hyperlipidemia is more severe among individuals receiving a ritonavir-containing regimen.[58,63]

The median time to onset of the syndrome(s) of abnormal fat redistribution after initiating therapy was 10 months in one large study.[58] A significantly longer duration of treatment with PIs has been reported in patients who have developed HAFR than in individuals who have not.[58] The lipid abnormalities and hyperglycemia may occur earlier than the morphologic changes.

A specific mechanism whereby PIs could lead to abnormal fat redistribution has not been elucidated. Interference with the hepatic degradation of glucagon, insulin, and insulin-like

growth factor, which results in primary hyperinsulinemia and the eventual emergence of insulin resistance, has been hypothesized.[64] A more recently postulated mechanism involves binding of these antiretroviral agents with two proteins important in lipid metabolism—the low-density lipoprotein–receptor-related protein (LRP) and the cytoplasmic retinoic-acid–binding protein type 1 (CRABP-1).[65] They share ~60% homology with the catalytic region of HIV-1 protease. Proportional to individual drug potency and the degree of cytochrome P450 antagonism, hyperlipidemia and peripheral adipocyte apoptosis ensue, culminating in visceral adiposity and insulin resistance.[65] Based on in vitro data, insulin resistance due to selective inhibition of the intrinsic transport activity of the predominant glucose transporter GLUT4 by the PIs has also been suggested.[65a]

An alteration in glucocorticoid metabolism related to PI therapy or to HIV infection itself may be involved.[56,66] Modest elevations in serum cortisol levels are rare in patients with HAFR. However, a tissue-specific paracrine effect independent of hypercortisolemia might result from PI-induced inhibition of cytochrome P450 steroid metabolism or from heightened sensitivity of regional adipocytes to glucocorticoids as a direct effect of these medications. Alternatively, the HIV *vpr* gene product, which has been reported to stimulate the glucocorticoid receptor directly, may exert a localized effect on adipocyte cortisol metabolism that only becomes manifest with weight recovery during treatment.[67] As most patients with HAFR have responded favorably to HAART, marked changes in viral burden and improved immune function may be operative.[68]

Laboratory abnormalities in patients with HAFR include elevated levels of triglycerides, cholesterol, insulin, C peptide, and other markers of insulin resistance.[58] The incidence of hyperglycemia has been reported to be 0.7% to 6.5% in patients being treated with PIs.[62] Impaired glucose tolerance (as assessed by oral glucose-tolerance testing) appears to occur more frequently than hyperglycemia or overt diabetes mellitus.[62,68] Dexamethasone suppression testing typically yields normal results, excluding a diagnosis of Cushing syndrome (see Chap. 75). Systematic evaluation of the HPA axis showed that patients with HAFR had normal diurnal cortisol secretion, normal cortisol secretory dynamics following ovine CRH administration, normal levels of binding globulins, and normal glucocorticoid receptor and affinity.[68]

Establishing a diagnosis of HAFR is complicated by the lack of a precise case definition. On physical examination, particular attention should be directed to the face (preauricular, periorbital, and temporal fat pad loss; prominent nasolabial folds; accentuated zygomata), neck (submandibular, supraclavicular, and dorsocervical adiposity), extremities (prominent vasculature with increased muscular appearance), buttocks (thinning), and abdomen (increasing girth; see Table 214-3). A baseline weight should be obtained. Supporting laboratory data include elevations of serum triglycerides, total and LDL cholesterol, fasting blood glucose, insulin, and C-peptide levels. An abnormal oral glucose-tolerance test might assist in making a diagnosis and possibly predict future severity. It may be prudent to check glucose homeostasis and fasting lipids at regular intervals. No formal recommendations can be made regarding regional fat mass quantification with DEXA or CT imaging. The diagnosis is less certain in the setting of recent or ongoing treatment with glucocorticoids, megestrol acetate, anabolic steroids, or immunomodulators.

Data regarding therapy for the HIV-associated fat redistribution are sparse. Liposuction allowed one patient with a bulky dorsocervical fat pad to regain full neck mobility.[56] Another patient with elevated basal urine free cortisol levels experienced some reduction in the size of his dorsocervical fat accumulation with ketoconazole therapy.[56] Some patients have derived benefit from switching or eliminating PIs from the combination.[58,62] The lipid abnormalities and hyperglycemia appear more likely to improve with switching PIs than are other features of the syndrome. Causality needs to be verified before recommendations regarding a change in PIs can be generalized. Moreover, there remains the serious consequence of progressive HIV infection with discontinuation of a potent regimen. A hypogonadal patient experienced marked improvements in his appearance and restoration of insulin sensitivity within 4 months of initiating testosterone cypionate.[69] Androgen replacement carries the risk of exacerbating the lipid disorder. Recombinant human GH may ameliorate some of the morphologic abnormalities but may worsen the lipid profile or precipitate hyperglycemia.

Some preliminary data suggest that patients with PI-associated hyperlipidemia can be managed following National Cholesterol Education Program (NCEP) guidelines.[63] A fasting lipid profile at baseline and 3 to 6 months after initiating PI-containing therapy has been recommended in an attempt to identify individuals who may benefit from treatment. Given the increased risk of pancreatitis associated with severe hypertriglyceridemia, treatment should be strongly considered for serum triglyceride levels >1000 mg/dL. Significant reductions in total cholesterol and total triglycerides in patients treated with gemfibrozil, 600 mg twice a day, and/or atorvastatin (starting at 10 mg per day) have been noted.[63] Caution is advised when using a fibrate in combination with the statin drugs due to an increased risk of myositis. If treatment with a lipid-lowering agent becomes necessary, a statin that is not exclusively metabolized by the cytochrome P450 3A4 isoform (e.g., pravastatin or fluvastatin) may minimize the potential for drug interactions with the PIs. Modification of other reversible cardiac risk factors such as hypertension and tobacco use should be included in risk-reduction counseling.

The hyperglycemia observed in patients with HAFR is generally nonketotic and responsive to treatment with sulfonylureas or insulin. Most patients do not require discontinuation of PI-containing therapy. Given the strong likelihood that insulin resistance is pathophysiologic, metformin might prove to be efficacious. Preliminary data indicate that relatively low dosages of this agent relieve hyperinsulinemia in HIV-infected patients with fat redistribution and abnormal glucose homostasis.[69a] Guidelines

have not been established regarding glucose monitoring in PI recipients. Serum concentrations of the oral hypoglycemic agents glipizide, glyburide, or tolbutamide may be affected by coadministration with PIs by influencing cytochrome P-450 metabolism.

## THE ENDOCRINE PANCREAS

Pancreatic abnormalities have been identified at autopsy in up to 50% of patients with AIDS[70] (see Chap. 133). Nonspecific inflammation is the predominant finding. Infiltration by CMV, HSV, *M. tuberculosis*, *M. avium* complex, *C. neoformans*, *Aspergillus* species, *T. gondii*, *P. carinii*, *Cryptosporidium parvum*, Microsporidia, lymphoma, and Kaposi sarcoma usually occurs with disseminated disease, but rarely results in clinically significant endocrine dysfunction.[71] Hypoglycemia due to pancreatic destruction by Kaposi sarcoma has been reported[70] (see Chap. 158).

Studies conducted in the pre-HAART era revealed that insulin-requiring nonoxidative glucose disposal, hepatic glucose production, insulin clearance, and peripheral insulin sensitivity are enhanced in symptomatic HIV-infected individuals compared to seronegative controls.[72] These findings differ from those of sepsis, in which insulin resistance and hyperglycemia are common.[73] Spontaneous insulin-requiring diabetes mellitus has been diagnosed in a few patients without apparent opportunistic infection or autoimmunity and has raised the possibility of direct HIV-induced islet cell dysfunction.[70,70a] Impaired glucose tolerance associated with HAART and syndrome(s) of abnormal fat redistribution has received considerable attention. The presumed mechanism is insulin resistance.

**Drugs (see Table 214-2).** Several medications used in the treatment of HIV disease are toxic to the pancreas. Acute pancreatitis is the main clinical manifestation, but glucose homeostasis may also be perturbed. Pentamidine, an agent used in the treatment and prophylaxis of PCP, causes hypoglycemia in ~25% of recipients because of insulin release from acutely damaged B cells.[70] This adverse effect has appeared weeks after ceasing therapy due to the long tissue half-life.[74] In some patients, progressive B-cell destruction may ensue, ultimately leading to insulin deficiency and frank diabetes mellitus. Risk factors associated with significant pentamidine-induced B-cell cytotoxicity include high dosage, prolonged duration of therapy, prior pentamidine treatment, intravenous administration, and renal insufficiency.[70] Although much less frequent, dysglycemia has occurred with aerosolized pentamidine.[70] Serum glucose concentrations should be monitored during intravenous pentamidine therapy, and patients should be advised of the warning symptoms of hypoglycemia and diabetes. Symptomatic hypoglycemia should prompt glucose administration and discontinuation of the drug. Individuals experiencing hyperglycemia typically have reduced serum C-peptide concentrations and require insulin administration.

Stimulation of B-cell insulin secretion by the sulfonamide component of trimethoprim-sulfamethoxazole is the presumed mechanism for the rare association of this agent with hypoglycemia.[71] Interferon-α, megestrol acetate, and didanosine have been reported to result in hyperglycemia and frank diabetes in patients with AIDS.[70]

## ELECTROLYTE AND MINERAL METABOLISM

The same principles guiding the evaluation and treatment of electrolyte disorders in seronegative patients should be applied to HIV-infected individuals. Attempts should be made to identify and eliminate any precipitating factors with special attention directed to recently administered medications.

**Hyponatremia.** Hyponatremia is the most common electrolyte disturbance in HIV-infected patients, occurring in up to 50% of hospitalized patients and in ~20% of ambulatory patients.[7] Hypovolemic hyponatremia results from excessive cutaneous, renal, or gastrointestinal fluid losses. Renal-salt wasting has been associated with pentamidine and amphotericin B.[7] Excessive hypotonic solution administration should be avoided, as it may further dilute the serum sodium concentrations. As adrenocortical deficiency is causal in a minority of patients, exclusion of this entity should be considered, based on the associated findings (e.g., hyperkalemia, metabolic acidosis) and/or refractoriness to fluid replacement. Sulfonamide-induced interstitial nephritis producing hyporeninemic hypoaldosteronism has been described in recipients of trimethoprim-sulfamethoxazole. Furthermore, trimethoprim inhibits sodium channels in the distal nephron, mimicking the action of a potassium-sparing diuretic[75] (see Table 214-2). Euvolemic hyponatremia may be a manifestation of SIADH. Primary polydipsia in the setting of dementia has also been reported.

**Hypernatremia.** Hypernatremia results from dehydration when free water deficits exceed sodium wasting. Increased insensible losses associated with fever and impaired urinary concentrating capacity related to certain medications (e.g., amphotericin B) have been etiologic. Central (neurogenic) DI occurs rarely in HIV-infected patients with CNS disease[8] and nephrogenic DI has occurred with foscarnet administration for CMV retinitis[9] (see Table 214-2).

**Hypercalcemia.** Hypercalcemia is caused by neoplastic, infectious, or granulomatous processes in HIV-infected patients and results mostly from the extrarenal conversion of 25-hydroxyvitamin D to 1,25-dihydroxyvitamin D by 1α-hydroxylase occurring within immune cells[39] (see Chap. 59). Besides lymphoma, raised serum calcium levels have complicated infections with *C. neoformans*, disseminated CMV, *M. avium* complex, and *P. carinii* in HIV-infected individuals.[10,39] The hypercalcemia appearing in patients coinfected with human T-cell lymphotropic virus type 1, a retrovirus linked to T-cell leukemia and lymphoma, has been attributed to viral-induced production of IL-2 and/or parathyroid hormone (PTH)–related peptide.[39]

**Hypocalcemia.** As in seronegative individuals, hypocalcemia has been described in HIV-infected patients with sepsis, hypoalbuminemia, and impaired vitamin D metabolism due to renal insufficiency or malabsorption. Elevated circulating free fatty acids may reduce serum calcium levels by enhancement of calcium binding to albumin. Relative hypoparathyroidism determined by reductions of PTH at baseline and following ethylenediaminetetraacetic acid (EDTA)–induced hypocalcemia has been demonstrated in patients with AIDS. These findings correlated with the degree of hypocalcemia. Destructive infiltration by opportunistic pathogens (e.g., *P. carinii* or CMV) or direct invasion by HIV due to expression of CD4-like surface molecules on parenchymal cells could be pathogenic. Frank hypoparathyroidism in a patient presenting with muscle cramps, tetany, and undetectable serum PTH levels has also been described. The significance of modest reductions in serum calcium concentrations, which are associated with advanced HIV infection, increased circulating TNF-α levels, and reduced concentrations of 1,25-dihydroxyvitamin D in some patients, is unknown.[76]

Adverse medication effects account for a majority of cases of hypocalcemia in HIV-infected patients. While foscarnet complexes with ionized calcium in a dose-dependent manner, renal tubular damage may also be operative in some cases given the association with hypomagnesemia and hypokalemia.[77] Since total calcium levels may not be altered, the ionized fraction should be monitored during treatment in those who develop compatible symptoms. Pentamidine-induced hypocalcemia has been reported and may be profound if concurrently administered with foscarnet.[78] Ketoconazole can interfere with vitamin D metabolism and exacerbate hypocalcemia. Marked hypo-

magnesemia resulting from amphotericin B therapy potentiates hypocalcemia through inhibition of PTH release as well as induction of peripheral PTH resistance (see Table 214-2).

**Hyperkalemia.** HIV-related causes of hyperkalemia include primary adrenal insufficiency, hyporeninemic hypoaldosteronism, and adverse effect of medications.[39] Pentamidine induces hyperkalemia by interfering with distal sodium transport (see Table 214-2). Mechanisms responsible for raised serum potassium concentrations with trimethoprim-sulfamethoxazole therapy have been discussed.

**Hypokalemia.** Malnutrition, gastrointestinal fluid losses, foscarnet administration, and amphotericin B–related renal tubular acidosis have been associated with hypokalemia in HIV-infected patients.

## REFERENCES

1. Mosca L, Costanzi G, Antonacci C, et al. Hypophyseal pathology in AIDS. Histol Histopathol 1992; 7:291.
2. Milligan SA, Katz MS, Craven PC, et al. Toxoplasmosis presenting as panhypopituitarism in a patient with the acquired immune deficiency syndrome. Am J Med 1984; 77:760.
3. Sullivan WM, Kelley GG, O'Connor PG, et al. Hypopituitarism associated with a hypothalamic CMV infection in a patient with AIDS. (Letter). Am J Med 1992; 92:221.
4. Schwartz LJ, St. Louis Y, Wu R, et al. Endocrine function in children with human immunodeficiency virus infection. Am J Dis Child 1991; 145:330.
5. Geffner ME, Yeh DY, Landaw EM, et al. In vitro insulin-like growth factor-I, growth hormone, and insulin resistance occurs in symptomatic human immunodeficiency virus-1–infected children. Pediatr Res 1993; 34:66.
6. Frost RA, Fuhrer J, Steigbigel R, et al. Wasting in the acquired immune deficiency syndrome is associated with multiple defects in the serum insulin-like growth factor system. Clin Endocrinol (Oxf) 1996; 44:501.
7. Tang WW, Kaptein EM, Feinstein EI, Massry SG. Hyponatremia in hospitalized patients with the acquired immunodeficiency syndrome (AIDS) and the AIDS-related complex. Am J Med 1993; 94:169.
8. Keuneke C, Anders HJ, Schlondorff D. Adipsic hypernatremia in two patients with AIDS and cytomegalovirus encephalitis. Am J Kidney Dis 1999; 33:379.
9. Navarro JF, Quereda C, Gallego N, et al. Nephrogenic diabetes insipidus and renal tubular acidosis secondary to foscarnet therapy. Am J Kidney Dis 1996; 27:431.
10. Sellmeyer DE, Grunfeld C. Endocrine and metabolic disturbances in human immunodeficiency virus infection and the acquired immune deficiency syndrome. Endocr Rev 1996; 17:518.
11. Del Monte P, Bernasconi D, De Conca V, et al. Endocrine evaluation in patients treated with interferon-alpha for chronic hepatitis C. Horm Res 1995; 44:105.
12. Glasgow BJ, Steinsapir KD, Anders K, Layfield LJ. Adrenal pathology in the acquired immune deficiency syndrome. Am J Clin Pathol 1985; 84:594.
13. Arabi Y, Fairfax MR, Szuba MJ, et al. Adrenal insufficiency, recurrent bacteremia, and disseminated abscesses caused by *Nocardia asteroides* in a patient with acquired immunodeficiency syndrome. Diagn Microbiol Infect Dis 1996; 24:47.
14. Membreno L, Irony I, Dere W, et al. Adrenocortical function in acquired immunodeficiency syndrome. J Clin Endocrinol Metab 1987; 65:482.
15. Villette JM, Bourin P, Doinel C, et al. Circadian variations in plasma levels of hypophyseal, adrenocortical and testicular hormones in men infected with human immunodeficiency virus. J Clin Endocrinol Metab 1990; 70:572.
16. Norbiato G, Bevilacqua M, Vago T, et al. Cortisol resistance in acquired immunodeficiency syndrome. J Clin Endocrinol Metab 1992; 74:608.
17. Azar ST, Melby JC. Hypothalamic-pituitary-adrenal function in non-AIDS patients with advanced HIV infection. Am J Med Sci 1993; 305:321.
18. Chrousos GP. The hypothalamic-pituitary-adrenal axis and immune-mediated inflammation. N Engl J Med 1995; 332:1351.
19. Findling JW, Buggy BP, Gilson IH, et al. Longitudinal evaluation of adrenocortical function in patients infected with the human immunodeficiency virus. J Clin Endocrinol Metab 1994; 79:1091.
20. Mulder JW, Frissen PH, Krijnen P, et al. Dehydroepiandrosterone as predictor for progression to AIDS in asymptomatic human immunodeficiency virus-infected men. J Infect Dis 1992; 165:413.
21. Clerici M, Trabattoni D, Piconi S, et al. A possible role for the cortisol/anti-cortisols imbalance in the progression of human immunodeficiency virus. Psychoneuroendocrinology 1997; 22:S27.
22. Steer KA, Kurtz AB, Honour JW. Megestrol-induced Cushing's syndrome. Clin Endocrinol (Oxf) 1995; 42:91.
23. Gallant JE, Chaisson RE, Moore RD. The effect of adjunctive corticosteroids for the treatment of *Pneumocystis carinii* pneumonia on mortality and subsequent complications. Chest 1998; 114:1258.
24. Heufelder AE, Hofbauer LC. Human immunodeficiency virus infection and the thyroid gland. Eur J Endocrinol 1996; 134:669.
25. Martin-Davila P, Quereda C, Rodriguez H, et al. Thyroid abscess due to *Rhodococcus equi* in a patient infected with the human immunodeficiency virus. Eur J Clin Microbiol Infect Dis 1998; 17:55.

26. Mollison LC, Mijch A, McBride G, Dwyer B. Hypothyroidism due to destruction of the thyroid by Kaposi's sarcoma. Rev Infect Dis 1991; 13:826.

27. LoPresti JS, Fried JC, Spencer CA, Nicoloff JT. Unique alterations of thyroid hormone indices in the acquired immunodeficiency syndrome (AIDS). Ann Intern Med 1989; 110:970.

28. Hommes MJ, Romijn JA, Endert E, et al. Hypothyroid-like regulation of the pituitary-thyroid axis in stable human immunodeficiency virus infection. Metabolism 1993; 42:556.

29. Raffi F, Brisseau JM, Planchon B, et al. Endocrine function in 98 HIV-infected patients: a prospective study. AIDS 1991; 5:729.

30. Grunfeld C, Feingold KR. Metabolic disturbances and wasting in the acquired immunodeficiency syndrome. N Engl J Med 1992; 327:329.

31. van der Poll T, Romijn JA, Wiersinga WM, Sauerwein HP. Tumor necrosis factor: a putative mediator of the sick euthyroid syndrome in man. J Clin Endocrinol Metab 1990; 71:1567.

32. Ozawa M, Sato K, Han DC, et al. Effects of tumor necrosis factor-alpha/cachectin on thyroid hormone metabolism in mice. Endocrinology 1988; 123:1461.

33. Sato K, Satoh T, Shizume K, et al. Inhibition of $^{125}$I organification and thyroid hormone release by interleukin-1, tumor necrosis factor-alpha, and interferon-gamma in human thyrocytes in suspension culture. J Clin Endocrinol Metab 1990; 70:1735.

34. Rahman A, Esmaili A, Saatcioglu F. A unique thyroid hormone response element in the human immunodeficiency virus type 1 long terminal repeat that overlaps the Sp1 binding sites. J Biol Chem 1995; 270:31059.

35. Gilquin J, Viard JP, Jubault V, et al. Delayed occurrence of Graves' disease after immune restoration with HAART. Highly active antiretroviral therapy. Lancet 1998; 352:1907.

36. Sumida S, Miller K, Vogel S, et al. Hypothyroidism is associated with IL-2 therapy in a randomized controlled trial of IL-2 for the treatment of HIV infection. Abstracts of the 36th Annual Meeting of the Infectious Diseases Society of America, Denver, 1998.

37. De Paepe ME, Waxman M. Testicular atrophy in AIDS: a study of 57 autopsy cases. Hum Pathol 1989; 20:210.

38. Zhang H, Dornadula G, Beumont M, et al. Human immunodeficiency virus type 1 in the semen of men receiving highly active antiretroviral therapy. N Engl J Med 1998; 339:1803.

39. Hofbauer LC, Heufelder AE. Endocrine implications of human immunodeficiency virus infection. Medicine (Baltimore) 1996; 75:262.

40. Grinspoon S, Corcoran C, Lee K, et al. Loss of lean body and muscle mass correlates with androgen levels in hypogonadal men with acquired immunodeficiency syndrome and wasting. J Clin Endocrinol Metab 1996; 81:4051.

41. Merenich JA, McDermott MT, Asp AA, et al. Evidence of endocrine involvement early in the course of human immunodeficiency virus infection. J Clin Endocrinol Metab 1990; 70:566.

42. Ellerbrock TV, Wright TC, Bush TJ, et al. Characteristics of menstruation in women infected with human immunodeficiency virus. Obstet Gynecol 1996; 87:1030.

43. Grinspoon S, Corcoran C, Miller K, et al. Body composition and endocrine function in women with acquired immunodeficiency syndrome wasting. J Clin Endocrinol Metab 1997; 82:1332.

43a. Miller K, Corcoran C, Armstrong C, et al. Transdermal testosterone administration in women with acquired immunodeficiency syndrome wasting: a pilot study. J Clin Endocrinol Metab 1998; 83:2717.

44. Martin ME, Benassayag C, Amiel C, et al. Alterations in the concentrations and binding properties of sex steroid binding protein and corticosteroid-binding globulin in HIV+ patients. J Endocrinol Invest 1992; 15:597.

44a. Bhasin S, Storer TW, Javanbakht M, et al. Testosterone replacement and resistance exercise in HIV-infected men with weight loss and low testosterone levels. JAMA 2000; 283:763.

45. Grunfeld C, Pang M, Doerrler W, et al. Lipids, lipoproteins, triglyceride clearance, and cytokines in human immunodeficiency virus infection and the acquired immunodeficiency syndrome. J Clin Endocrinol Metab 1992; 74:1045.

46. Hellerstein MK, Grunfeld C, Wu K, et al. Increased de novo hepatic lipogenesis in human immunodeficiency virus infection. J Clin Endocrinol Metab 1993; 76:559.

47. Feingold KR, Krauss RM, Pang M, et al. The hypertriglyceridemia of acquired immunodeficiency syndrome is associated with an increased prevalence of low density lipoprotein subclass pattern B. J Clin Endocrinol Metab 1993; 76:1423.

48. Strawford A, Hellerstein M. The etiology of wasting in the human immunodeficiency virus and acquired immunodeficiency syndrome. Semin Oncol 1998; 25:76.

49. Dobs AS, Few WL 3rd, Blackman MR, et al. Serum hormones in men with human immunodeficiency virus-associated wasting. J Clin Endocrinol Metab 1996; 81:4108.

50. Grinspoon S, Corcoran C, Askari H, et al. Effects of androgen administration in men with the AIDS wasting syndrome. A randomized, double-blind, placebo-controlled trial. Ann Intern Med 1998; 129:18.

50a. Corcoran C, Grinspoon S. Treatments for wasting in patients with the acquired immunodeficiency syndrome. N Engl J Med 1999; 340:1740.

51. Oster MH, Enders SR, Samuels SJ, et al. Megestrol acetate in patients with AIDS and cachexia. Ann Intern Med 1994; 121:400.

52. Strawford A, Barbieri T, Van Loan M, et al. Resistance exercise and supraphysiologic androgen therapy in eugonadal men with HIV-related weight loss. A randomized controlled trial. JAMA 1999; 281(14):1282.

53. Schambelan M, Mulligan K, Grunfeld C, et al. Recombinant human growth hormone in patients with HIV-associated wasting. A randomized, placebo-controlled trial. Serostim Study Group. Ann Intern Med 1996; 125:873.

54. Reyes-Teran G, Sierra-Madero JG, Martinez del Cerro V, et al. Effects of thalidomide on HIV-associated wasting syndrome: a randomized, double-blind, placebo-controlled clinical trial. AIDS 1996; 10:1501.

55. Carpenter CC, Fischl MA, Hammer SM, et al. Antiretroviral therapy for HIV infection in 1997. Updated recommendations of the International AIDS Society-USA panel. JAMA 1997; 277:1962.

56. Miller KK, Daly PA, Sentochnik D, et al. Pseudo-Cushing's syndrome in human immunodeficiency virus-infected patients. Clin Infect Dis 1998; 27:68.

57. Miller KD, Jones E, Yanovski JA, et al. Visceral abdominal-fat accumulation associated with use of indinavir. Lancet 1998; 351:871.

58. Carr A, Samaras K, Burton S, et al. A syndrome of peripheral lipodystrophy, hyperlipidaemia and insulin resistance in patients receiving HIV protease inhibitors. AIDS 1998; 12:F51.

59. Danesh J, Collins R, Peto R. Chronic infections and coronary heart disease: is there a link? Lancet 1997; 350:430.

60. Henry K, Melroe H, Huebsch J, et al. Severe premature coronary artery disease with protease inhibitors. Lancet 1998; 351:1328.

61. Lo JC, Mulligan K, Tai VW, et al. "Buffalo hump" in men with HIV-1 infection. Lancet 1998; 351:867.

62. Walli R, Herfort O, Michl GM, et al. Treatment with protease inhibitors associated with peripheral insulin resistance and impaired oral glucose tolerance in HIV-1-infected patients. AIDS 1998; 12:F167.

63. Henry K, Melroe H, Huebesch J, et al. Atorvastatin and gemfibrozil for protease-inhibitor-related lipid abnormalities. (Letter). Lancet 1998; 352:1031.

64. Martinez E, Gatell J. Metabolic abnormalities and use of HIV-1 protease inhibitors. Lancet 1998; 352:821.

65. Carr A, Samaras K, Chisholm DJ, Cooper DA. Pathogenesis of HIV-1-protease inhibitor-associated peripheral lipodystrophy, hyperlipidaemia, and insulin resistance. Lancet 1998; 351:1881.

65a. Murata H, Hruz PW, Mueckler M. The mechanism of insulin resistance caused by HIV protein inhibitor therapy. J Biol Chem 2000; 275(27):20251.

66. Hirsch MS, Klibanski A. What price progress? Pseudo-Cushing's syndrome associated with antiretroviral therapy in patients with human immunodeficiency virus infection. Clin Infect Dis 1998; 27:73.

67. Kino T, Gragerov A, Kopp JB, et al. The HIV-1 virion-associated protein vpr is a coactivator of the human glucocorticoid receptor. J Exp Med 1999; 189:51.

68. Yanovski JA, Miller KD, Kino T, et al. Endocrine and metabolic evaluation of human immunodeficiency virus-infected patients with evidence of protease inhibitor-associated lipodystrophy. J Clin Endocrinol Metab 1999; 84:1925.

69. Saint-Marc T, Touraine JL. "Buffalo hump" in HIV-1 infection. (Letter). Lancet 1998; 352:319.

69a. Hadigan C, Corcoran C, Basgoz N, et al. Metformin in the treatment of HIV lipodystrophy syndrome: a randomized controlled trial. JAMA 2000; 284(4):472.

70. Brivet FG, Naveau SH, Lemaigre GF, Dormont J. Pancreatic lesions in HIV-infected patients. Baillieres Clin Endocrinol Metab 1994; 8:859.

70a. Hadigan C, Corcoran C, Stanley T, et al. Fasting hyperinsulinemia in human immunodeficiency virus-infected men: relationship to body composition, gonadal function, and protease inhibitor use. J Clin Endocrinol Metab 2000; 85:35.

71. Cappell MS, Hassan T. Pancreatic disease in AIDS—a review. J Clin Gastroenterol 1993; 17:254.

72. Hommes MJ, Romijn JA, Endert E, et al. Insulin sensitivity and insulin clearance in human immunodeficiency virus-infected men. Metabolism 1991; 40:651.

73. Grunfeld C, Feingold KR. The metabolic effects of tumor necrosis factor and other cytokines. Biotherapy 1991; 3:143.

74. Waskin H, Stehr-Green JK, Helmick CG, Sattler FR. Risk factors for hypoglycemia associated with pentamidine therapy for *Pneumocystis* pneumonia. JAMA 1988; 260:345.

75. Hsu I, Wordell CJ. Hyperkalemia and high-dose trimethoprim/sulfamethoxazole. Ann Pharmacother 1995; 29:427.

76. Haug CJ, Aukrust P, Haug E, et al. Severe deficiency of 1,25-dihydroxyvitamin D3 in human immunodeficiency virus infection: association with immunological hyperactivity and only minor changes in calcium homeostasis. J Clin Endocrinol Metab 1998; 83:3832.

77. Gearhart MO, Sorg TB. Foscarnet-induced severe hypomagnesemia and other electrolyte disorders. Ann Pharmacother 1993; 27:285.

78. Youle MS, Clarbour J, Gazzard B, Chanas A. Severe hypocalcaemia in AIDS patients treated with foscarnet and pentamidine. Lancet 1988; 1:1455.

# CHAPTER 215

# THE EYE IN ENDOCRINOLOGY

ROBERT A. OPPENHEIM AND WILLIAM D. MATHERS

The eye is frequently a window into the systemic conditions of the body. There is no better illustration of this than the interrelationship between the eye and the endocrine system. Many changes, subtle and gross, are manifested in the *eye* by normal fluctuations in hormones, exogenous hormones, endocrine disorders, and metabolic abnormalities.

## OCULAR EFFECTS OF NORMAL HORMONAL FLUCTUATION

### MENSTRUAL CYCLE

Studies of the serum levels of luteinizing hormone, follicle-stimulating hormone, estriol, progesterone, and testosterone throughout the menstrual cycle, combined with determinations of intraocular pressure, anterior chamber depth, corneal thickness, outflow facility, and tear production, established no statistically valid correlation between any of these physiologic measurements and the hormonal fluctuations.[1,2]

### PREGNANCY

Both physiologic and pathologic ocular changes occur during *pregnancy.* In addition, there are several preexisting ocular conditions that are either exacerbated or ameliorated by pregnancy.[3]

#### PHYSIOLOGIC OCULAR CHANGES DURING PREGNANCY

**Visual Acuity.** Blurred vision due to a *change in refraction* commonly occurs during pregnancy and usually resolves after delivery. The index of refraction of the cornea may change due to changes in corneal thickness.

**Lids.** *Chloasma,* the increased pigmentation of the cheeks that often occurs in pregnancy, can also involve the eyelids. It is caused by increased melanocyte stimulation and resolves after delivery.[4] *Ptosis,* or droopiness of the upper lid, is a well-documented complication of lumbar anesthesia during childbirth.[5] Ptosis associated with miosis and anhidrosis (i.e., *Horner syndrome*) has also been noted to occur with the use of lumbar anesthesia at the time of delivery.[6]

**Conjunctiva.** Conjunctival vessels undergo a progressively decreased flow of blood during pregnancy that is manifested by a decrease in the number of visible conjunctival capillaries.[7] Subconjunctival hemorrhages have also been observed during pregnancy and resolve with no sequelae.

**Cornea.** Corneal sensitivity decreases after the 31st week of pregnancy with a return to normal by 6 to 8 weeks postpartum.[8] A slight increase in corneal thickness, perhaps due to edema, also occurs and is a possible cause of new-onset contact lens intolerance during pregnancy.

**Intraocular Pressure.** A reduction in intraocular pressure usually occurs in pregnancy, probably as a result of an increase in outflow facility, which is especially evident during the last trimester.[9]

#### PATHOLOGIC OCULAR CHANGES DURING PREGNANCY

*Preeclamptic-eclamptic hypertensive retinopathy* can occur after the 20th week of pregnancy. Findings on fundus examination include narrowing of the arterioles, flame-shaped hemorrhages, cotton-wool spots, retinal edema, and disc swelling. There is a correlation between the severity of the retinopathy and the risk that the mother will have permanent renal damage,[10] as well as the risk that the fetus will die.[11] Ten percent of patients with eclampsia and 1% to 2% of patients with severe preeclampsia have *exudative retinal detachment,* which usually resolves within weeks after delivery.[12,13] Occasionally, residual retinal pigment epithelial (RPE) alterations may cause decreased visual acuity. Indocyanine green (ICG) angiography suggests that damage to the choroidal vasculature compromises the overlying RPE, leading to subretinal exudation.[14] Transient *cortical blindness*[15] and *acute ischemic optic neuropathy*[16] have also been associated with toxemia.

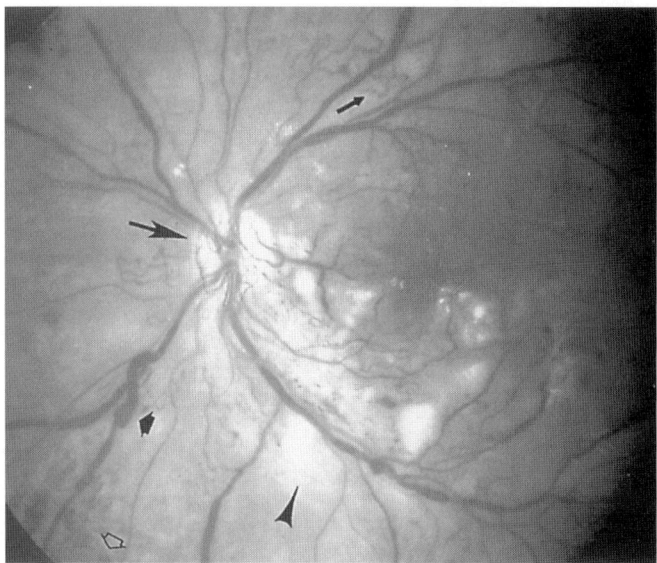

**FIGURE 215-1.** Fundus of a 26-year-old woman who had a 15-year history of juvenile-onset diabetes mellitus before pregnancy. Her proliferative diabetic retinopathy (*PDR*) quickly progressed during pregnancy. Typical changes of PDR seen here are neovascularization of the retina (*thin small arrow*), neovascularization of the optic disc (*large arrow*), cotton-wool spots (*arrowhead*), retinal hemorrhage (*arrow outline*), and irregular venous dilation (*short fat arrow*).

In *central serous choroidopathy* (CSC), dysfunction of the RPE allows serous fluid to leak under the retina, causing elevation of the macula. Subretinal exudates are seen in a high proportion of patients during pregnancy, as compared to the incidence of CSC in nonpregnant patients.[17] The condition usually resolves spontaneously after delivery.[18]

*Pseudotumor cerebri* (idiopathic intracranial hypertension) is a condition in which there is increased intracranial pressure with papilledema in the presence of normal results on head imaging scan and normal cerebrospinal fluid composition. Symptoms may include headache, visual obscurations, and visual field loss. It may be associated with pregnancy; however, nonpregnant pseudotumor cerebri patients are typically overweight women of childbearing age.[3,19]

#### EFFECTS OF PREGNANCY ON PREEXISTING OCULAR CONDITIONS

Two ocular conditions are known to improve with pregnancy: *glaucoma,* by virtue of decreased intraocular pressure (see earlier), and *intraocular inflammation.*[20] Both sarcoid uveitis and Vogt-Koyanagi-Harada syndrome have been noted to improve during pregnancy and to rebound after delivery.[20,21] It is postulated that this is due to the increased cortisol in the bloodstream during pregnancy and to the subsequent reduction that occurs after childbirth.

The possibility of exacerbation of *diabetic retinopathy* during pregnancy is an extremely important clinical issue. The presence of diabetic retinopathy before pregnancy and the degree of its severity determine the course of this condition during pregnancy. It is therefore recommended that women with diabetes undertake childbearing at a young age, before retinopathy has developed.[22] Of women with diabetes who do not have retinopathy before pregnancy, only ~10% develop mild retinopathy that usually regresses after delivery.[3] Background diabetic retinopathy tends to progress transiently during pregnancy.[23,24] These patients should undergo dilated fundus examination every trimester. The real concern is for women who have proliferative diabetic retinopathy before pregnancy. Approximately 50% of these patients experience vision-threatening progression of their retinopathy during pregnancy[3] (Fig. 215-1). Therefore, it is recommended that patients with proliferative retinopathy undergo panretinal photocoagulation before conceiving. Dilated fundus examination should be performed once a month during the pregnancy. Without close supervision and treatment, pregnancy in a woman with proliferative diabetic retinopathy can lead to irreparable loss of sight. Although the pathogenesis is unclear, one hypothesis suggests that there is an absence of autoregulation, which leads to increased retinal blood flow in the presence of a hyperdynamic circulation during pregnancy.[25]

*Graves disease*, which is common in young women, can be aggravated by pregnancy. It also may present during pregnancy. Because many of the symptoms of Graves disease, such as heat intolerance, tachycardia, and emotional fragility, are also seen in pregnancy, the ocular signs of exophthalmos and lagophthalmos may be important clues that a pregnant patient also has Graves disease.[3]

*Uveal melanomas* have been noted to grow during pregnancy.[26] Studies suggest that women with uveal melanoma are not at increased risk for metastases and that women with posterior uveal melanoma have a similar 5-year survival compared with nonpregnant women.[27,28]

Just as the normal pituitary is known to enlarge in pregnant women, so do *pituitary adenomas*.[3] Pituitary adenomas that previously caused no symptoms may do so for the first time during pregnancy. Affected women have headache, decreased visual acuity, and visual field disturbances such as bitemporal hemianopsia. The symptoms usually resolve after delivery with spontaneous regression of the tumor. Bromocriptine, which has been shown to produce regression of the tumor, appears not to be detrimental to the developing fetus. Pituitary adenoma enlargement during pregnancy also can be caused by pituitary apoplexy, which can threaten the mother's life. A woman with a known pituitary adenoma who develops a headache or a new visual field defect should undergo magnetic resonance imaging and, possibly, lumbar puncture to rule out subarachnoid hemorrhage from the tumor.

*Meningiomas*, which typically grow in a chronic and insidious manner, may demonstrate an accelerated course producing relatively acute vision loss during pregnancy. This accelerated growth pattern is probably hormone related. Many cases of meningioma have presented during pregnancy.[29]

## MENOPAUSE

In clinical practice, the most commonly recognized effect of menopause on the eye is the occurrence of dry eyes due to lacrimal insufficiency. This traditionally has been associated with the decrease in estrogen levels that occurs after menopause. However, treatment with exogenous estrogen does not modify this dryness. In addition, lacrimal insufficiency also occurs with increased frequency during pregnancy and the use of estrogen-containing birth control pills, when estrogen and prolactin levels are elevated. This has led some investigators to speculate that the hormonal mediator of the lacrimal gland is androgen, rather than estrogen.[30] Androgen levels are decreased during the high-estrogen states of pregnancy and oral contraceptive use. When ovarian function declines during menopause, both estrogens and androgens decrease. Studies also suggest that prolactin, in addition to androgens, is involved in regulating exocrine secretion of the lacrimal gland.[31]

## OCULAR EFFECTS OF EXOGENOUS HORMONES

### CORTICOSTEROIDS

Hormones have many effects on the eye when they are used as therapeutic agents for both eye disease and systemic diseases.

The most common hormonal preparations used in the treatment of eye diseases are *corticosteroids*, such as prednisolone, dexamethasone, fluorometholone, and rimexolone. Along with antibiotics, topical steroids and oral prednisone play a central role in the medical armamentarium of ophthalmologists. Their tremendous usefulness stems from both their antiinflammatory and immunosuppressive effects.

### ANTIINFLAMMATORY EFFECTS

Inflammation in the eye can cause scarring and opacification of ocular structures that can lead to loss of vision. Corticosteroids are frequently used to diminish inflammation after eye surgery such as cataract extraction, refractive surgery, and corneal transplantation. In addition, these agents are used to treat most forms of uveitis involving either the anterior or posterior segment. Although topical application is effective for anterior segment inflammation, uveitis involving structures posterior to the ciliary body requires periocular injection or systemic administration. Corticosteroids are also a mainstay of therapy for other forms of ocular inflammation, such as scleritis, optic neuritis, temporal arteritis, and cystoid macular edema.

### IMMUNOLOGIC SUPPRESSION

Topical and systemic corticosteroids are used to control harmful immunologic activity. They are essential after corneal transplant surgery to prevent and, when relevant, reverse rejection of the graft. Ocular infections, such as bacterial keratitis and endophthalmitis, are also treated with topical corticosteroids once the eye infection is believed to be sterile after the initiation of antibiotic treatment. Finally, there is a wide range of ocular immunologic conditions that resolve in response to corticosteroid treatment. One example is the type IV immune response that causes phlyctenular keratitis, an allergic response that involves the limbus and mimics a corneal ulcer. When herpes simplex antigens remain in the corneal stroma after the infection resolves, a protracted immunologic response, mediated by both T and B cells, can cause pain and clouding of the cornea. Corticosteroids are the only drugs used routinely to suppress this deleterious response.

### SIDE EFFECTS AND COMPLICATIONS

Topical and systemic corticosteroid therapy can be associated with multiple ocular complications. The risk is directly related to increased length of treatment, and all patients started on topical corticosteroid therapy must receive close follow-up to monitor for complications. The most common side effects are glaucoma and posterior subcapsular cataracts. Twenty-five percent of patients who receive topical corticosteroids have an increase in intraocular pressure. Some preparations, such as fluorometholone and rimexolone, are less likely to increase intraocular pressure. It is common for patients with systemic conditions such as sarcoidosis, rheumatoid arthritis, or lupus, who have been treated long-term with systemic corticosteroids, to have advanced cataracts necessitating extraction. Microbial infections can be tragically exacerbated by the use of corticosteroids. Bacterial and fungal keratitis can be made worse if topical corticosteroids are initiated prematurely. The use of topical corticosteroids in the presence of actively replicating herpes simplex virus in the corneal epithelium may cause rapid acceleration of the infection, as well as corneal perforation. Finally, topical steroids can accelerate corneal melts by increasing collagenase activity, although topical steroids may be helpful if there is associated corneal stromal infiltration. Systemic corticosteroid use or withdrawal may be associated with pseudotumor cerebri.

## OVARIAN STEROIDS

### HARMFUL EFFECTS OF ORAL CONTRACEPTIVES

*Oral contraceptives* have no known therapeutic benefits in the treatment of eye disease; however, they have been implicated in the pathogenesis of many types of eye disease.[32] Numerous case reports and studies have indicated that these drugs can affect nearly every part of the eye.[33] Oral contraceptive use has been associated with edema of the eyelids and conjunctiva, subconjunctival hemorrhage, conjunctivitis, and allergic reactions. Other studies have described vascular complications, such as central retinal vascular occlusions, retinal periphlebitis, and retinal hemorrhages.[34–36,36a] In addition, macular edema, central serous chorioretinopathy, and RPE disturbances have been reported.[37] Many cases of optic neuritis and retrobulbar neuritis have been associated with oral contraceptives. These agents are well-known causes of pseudotumor cerebri, which manifests itself as papilledema and can easily be confused with optic neuritis.

Finally, many subjective visual disturbances can be attributed to oral contraceptives.[38] Photophobia, glare, transient blurring of vision, difficulty in focusing, and other similar symptoms frequently occur in patients taking these agents. The role of oral contraceptive–induced migraine in these events remains obscure, but undoubtedly plays a part (see Chap. 105).

### NONSTEROIDAL ANTIESTROGENS

*Tamoxifen* is an antiestrogen that prevents estrogen stimulation of breast cancer cells. It is the treatment of choice in women with estrogen receptor–positive advanced breast cancer. Ocular complications include corneal opacities (cornea verticillata; Fig. 215-2), optic nerve toxicity, and retinopathy. Retinal abnormalities include bilateral macular edema and yellow-white dots in the paramacular and foveal areas. Most ocular changes are reversible after the withdrawal of tamoxifen.[39]

*Clomiphene* is a competitive antagonist of estrogen receptors that is used to stimulate ovulation in the treatment of female infertility. Ocular side effects include blurred vision and scintillating scotomas that are dose-related and reversible on discontinuation of the drug. Changes in retinal cell function have been reported. Visual abnormalities are considered a contraindication to continuing use of this medication.

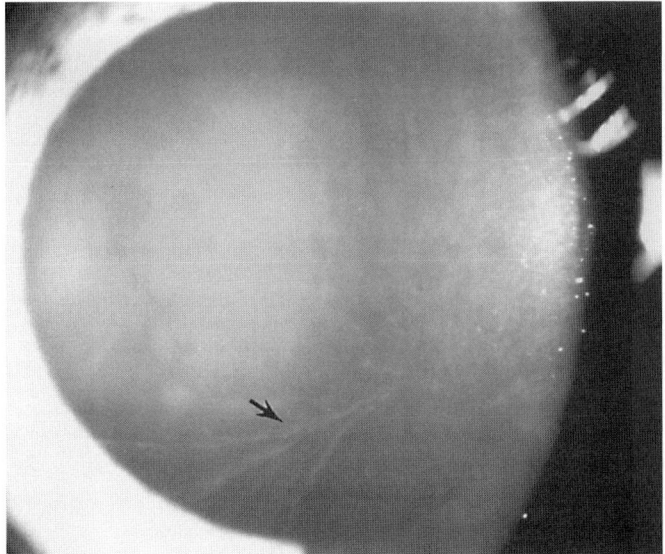

**FIGURE 215-2.** Whorl-like opacities (*arrow*) seen in the corneal epithelium as seen in patients with Fabry disease or with tamoxifen administration.

## OCULAR EFFECTS OF ENDOCRINE DISORDERS

Two common endocrine disorders have frequent and often severe involvement of the eyes: *diabetes mellitus* and *Graves disease*. So extensive is the eye involvement in these conditions that an entire chapter in this text is devoted to each of them (see Chaps. 43 and 151). Patients should be referred to an ophthalmologist at the time diabetes is diagnosed. The ophthalmologist will perform a baseline and thereafter yearly eye examination to monitor not only the development of diabetic retinopathy and macular edema, but also primary open-angle glaucoma (which occurs with increased frequency in patients with diabetes). Careful monitoring and timely treatment of these two conditions can reduce potential loss of vision. Diabetes can also contribute to the development of many other eye conditions, including cranial nerve abnormalities (such as isolated third, fourth, or sixth cranial nerve palsies) as well as acute disc edema and mucormycosis (a rare but life-threatening orbital infection). Finally, patients with diabetes are at increased risk for cataracts (posterior subcapsular cataracts) and often experience sudden shifts in refraction due to acute hyperglycemia.

Thyroid ophthalmopathy is clinically apparent in ~50% of patients with *Graves disease*.[40] Clinical signs range from asymptomatic exophthalmos to vision-threatening optic neuropathy. Intensive medical or surgical treatment is required in only ~4% of cases.[40] Most patients with Graves disease who have no readily apparent eye findings can be demonstrated to have more subtle eye changes when examined with orbital ultrasound or magnetic resonance imaging. Any patient with Graves disease who complains of eye discomfort or decreased vision should promptly undergo a complete eye examination.

With the exception of diabetes mellitus and Graves disease, all other endocrine disorders that involve the eyes are less common and, in most cases, less pervasive. However, all aspects of the eye and ocular adnexa can be affected by endocrine conditions. Knowledge of these associations and observation of these ocular findings can serve as important clues to what may be an otherwise diagnostically elusive condition. For example, the presence of a subluxated lens can confirm the diagnosis of *Marfan syndrome*, and a *Kayser-Fleischer* ring can help in the diagnosis of *Wilson disease*.

A description of ocular signs that are associated with endocrine conditions is provided here, beginning from the ocular adnexa and proceeding from the front to the back of the eye. The endocrine and metabolic disorders that are associated with each of these eye signs are summarized in Table 215-1. It should be noted that the differential diagnosis of these eye signs includes many ocular and systemic conditions that are not included here.

### ORBIT

Endocrine and metabolic conditions are often associated with changes in the location of the globe in relationship to the bony cavity that contains it. The most common cause of both unilateral and bilateral *exophthalmos*, or protrusion of the eye, is thyroid ophthalmopathy. *Hypothyroidism* and several other disorders are also associated with *enophthalmos*, or recession of the globe within the orbit. Changes in the distance between the two orbits can also be affected by endocrine conditions. *Hypertelorism* is increased separation between the bony orbits, and *hypotelorism* is decreased separation between the orbits.

Changes in the size and shape of the osteal bones and their cavities are also associated with systemic disease. Endocrine and metabolic conditions are associated with *deep-set eyes*, a prominent *supraorbital ridge*, and *hypertrophy of the orbital bones*. Additional associations are *osteolysis of the bony orbit, erosion of the lateral wall of the optic canal, and enlargement of the superior orbital fissure*.

**TABLE 215-1.**
**Ocular Conditions and Their Endocrine and Metabolic Associations**

**ORBIT**

*Exophthalmos*

Brown tumor of hyperparathyroidism

Cretinism (hypothyroidism)

Cushing syndrome

Graves disease

Hunter syndrome (MPS II-H)

Hurler syndrome (MPS I-H)

Hypophosphatasia (phosphoethanolaminuria)

Obesity

Pseudotumor cerebri

Scheie syndrome (MPS I-S)

Thyroid disorder

*Enophthalmos*

Cretinism (hypothyroidism)

Maple syrup urine disease (branched-chain ketoaciduria)

Morquio syndrome (MPS IV)

*Hypertelorism*

Cretinism (hypothyroidism)

Ehlers-Danlos syndrome

Hunter syndrome (MPS II-H)

Hurler syndrome (MPS I-H)

Infantile hypercalcemia with supravalvular aortic stenosis (Williams syndrome)

Maple syrup urine disease

Marfan syndrome

Morquio syndrome (MPS IV)

*Hypotelorism*

Maternal phenylketonuria fetal defects

Turner syndrome

*Deep-Set Eyes*

Lowe syndrome (oculocerebrorenal syndrome)

Marfan syndrome

*Prominent Supraorbital Ridge*

Hurler syndrome (MPS I-H)

Marfan syndrome

*Hypertrophy of Orbital Bones*

Acromegaly

*Osteolysis of Bony Orbit*

Hyperparathyroidism

*Erosion of Optic Canal (Lateral Wall)*

Craniopharyngioma

Pituitary tumor

*Enlargement of Superior Orbital Fissure*

Pituitary neoplasm

*Extraocular Muscle Enlargement on Computed Tomography (CT)*

Acromegaly

Graves disease

*Orbital Bruit (Bilateral)*

Hyperthyroidism

*Ptosis*

Abetalipoproteinemia

Addison disease

Corticosteroid ptosis (prolonged use of topical corticosteroids)

**LIDS**

*Ptosis*

Cretinism

Eclampsia and preeclampsia

Ehlers-Danlos syndrome

Graves disease

Hunter syndrome

Hurler syndrome (MPS I-H)

Hyperparathyroidism

Hyperthyroidism

Hypocalcemia

Hypoparathyroidism

Laurence-Moon-Biedl syndrome

Maple syrup urine disease

Morquio syndrome

Normal pregnancy

Obesity (floppy eyelid syndrome)

*Horner Syndrome*

Pituitary tumor

*Lid Retraction*

Graves disease

Dalrymple sign—widening of palpebral fissure

Stellwag sign—retraction of upper lid associated with infrequent or incomplete blinking

*Lid Lag*

Excess intake of thyroid hormone

Graves disease

*Ectropion*

Congenital ectropion

Lowe syndrome

*Facial Palsy*

Diabetes mellitus (Willis syndrome)

*Blepharospasm*

Addison disease

Hypocalcemia (in hypoparathyroidism)

*Infrequent Blinking*

Thyrotoxicosis (Stellwag sign)

Including exophthalmic ophthalmoplegia

*Lid Edema*

Angioneurotic edema caused by corticosteroids

Hyperthyroidism

Stasis, including premenstrual edema

*Mongoloid Obliquity*

Laurence-Moon-Biedl syndrome

Prader-Willi syndrome

*Epicanthus*

Abetalipoproteinemia

Ehlers-Danlos syndrome

Hurler syndrome

Infantile hypercalcemia

Laurence-Moon-Biedl syndrome

Lowe syndrome

Turner syndrome

*Hyperpigmentation*

Adrenocorticotropic hormone (ACTH) therapy

ACTH-secreting pituitary tumors

Addison disease

Estrogen therapy

Gaucher disease (cerebroside lipidosis)

Hemochromatosis

Melasma

Niemann-Pick disease (essential lipid histiocytosis)

Porphyria cutanea tarda

Pregnancy

Wilson disease

*Hypopigmentation*

Corticosteroids

Fanconi syndrome

Homocystinuria

Hyperthyroidism (Graves disease)

Hypopituitarism

Phenylketonuria

Vitiligo (in autoimmune adrenal or thyroid disease)

*Xanthelasma*

Diabetes mellitus

Hyperlipemia

*Thickened Eyelids*

Acromegaly

Congenital hypothyroidism

*Trichomegaly (Long Lashes)*

Isolated adrenal malfunction and ovarian atrophy

*Madarosis (Loss of Lashes)*

Ehlers-Danlos syndrome

Hyperthyroidism

Hypocalcemia

Hypoparathyroidism

Hypothyroidism

Pituitary insufficiency

Pituitary necrosis (Simmonds-Sheehan syndrome)

*Poliosis*

Albinism

Werner syndrome (progeria of adults)

*Coarse Eyebrows*

Congenital hypothyroidism (cretinism)

CPD syndrome (chorioretinopathy and pituitary dysfunction)

Hunter syndrome (MPS II)

Hurler syndrome (MPS I)

Sanfilippo syndrome (MPS III)

*Hertogh Sign (Loss of Outer Third of Eyebrow)*

Hypogonadism

Hypothyroidism

**LACRIMAL SYSTEM**

*Dry Eye*

Multiple mucosal neuromas

Pheochromocytoma

*Bloody Tears*

Vicarious menstruation with ectopic tissue

*Excessive Tears*

Morquio syndrome (MPS IV)

Thyrotoxicosis

**EXTRAOCULAR MUSCLES**

*Strabismus*

Arylsulfatase A deficiency syndrome

Diabetes mellitus

Ehlers-Danlos disease

Gangliosidosis

Infantile (GM$_1$)

Juvenile (GM$_2$)

Gaucher disease

Gout

Graves disease

Homocystinuria

Hurler disease (mucopolysaccharidosis type I)

Hutchinson syndrome (adrenal cortex neuroblastoma with orbital metastasis)

Hypocalcemia

Infantile hypercalcemia with supravalvular aortic stenosis (Williams syndrome)

Laurence-Moon-Biedl syndrome

Lowe syndrome

Marfan syndrome

Maple syrup urine disease

Prader-Willi syndrome (hypotonia-obesity syndrome)

Pseudohypoparathyroidism

Tay-Sachs disease (familial amaurotic idiocy)

*Cyclic Strabismus*

Graves disease

*Vertical Nystagmus*

Diabetes mellitus

*Nystagmus*

Abetalipoproteinemia

Chédiak-Higashi syndrome (anomalous leukocytic inclusions with constitutional stigmata)

Eclampsia and preeclampsia

Gangliosidosis (generalized gangliosidosis, infantile)

Hermansky-Pudlak syndrome (oculocutaneous albinism and hemorrhagic diathesis; MPS I-H)

Hurler syndrome

Hypervitaminosis D and other forms of hypercalcemia

Hypothyroidism (cretinism)

Laurence-Moon-Biedl syndrome (retinal pigmentosa–polydactyly–adiposogenital syndrome)

Lowe disease (oculocerebrorenal syndrome)

Marfan syndrome

Obesity (cerebral-ocular-skeletal anomalies syndrome)

Ocular albinism (Nettleship-Falls and Forsius-Eriksson types–X-linked)

Prader-Willi syndrome (hypotonia-obesity syndrome)

Pseudohypoparathyroidism

Tay-Sachs disease

Werner syndrome (progeria of adults)

Wilson disease (hepatolenticular degeneration)

*Pendular Nystagmus*

Albinism

Laurence-Moon-Biedl syndrome (retinal pigmentosa–polydactyly–adiposogenital syndrome)

*Periodic Alternating Nystagmus*

Diabetes mellitus

*Ocular Bobbing*

Encephalopathy of GM$_2$ gangliosidoses

(continued)

**TABLE 215-1.**
**Ocular Conditions and Their Endocrine and Metabolic Associations (Continued)**

*Paralysis of Third Cranial Nerve*
 Cavernous sinus syndrome
  Pituitary adenoma (lateral extension)
 Diabetes (usually pupil-sparing)
*Paralysis of Fourth Cranial Nerve*
 Intracranial
  Craniopharyngioma
  Diabetes
*Paralysis of Sixth Cranial Nerve*
 Cretinism
 Diabetes mellitus
 Gaucher disease (cerebroside lipidosis)
 Massive pituitary adenoma
*External Ophthalmoplegia*
 Abetalipoproteinemia
 Diabetes mellitus (Willis disease)
 Refsum syndrome (phytanic acid α-hydroxylase deficiency)
*Internuclear Ophthalmoplegia*
 Fabry disease (α-galactocere-brosidase deficiency)
*Painful Ophthalmoplegia*
 Diabetic ophthalmoplegia
*Double Elevator Palsy*
 Graves disease
*Transient Ophthalmoplegia*
 Wilson disease
*Poor Convergence*
 Graves disease (Möbius sign)
 Paralysis of third nerve (see earlier)
*Divergence Paralysis*
 Diabetes mellitus (vascular disease)
**CONJUNCTIVA**
*Congestion of Conjunctiva*
 Gout
 Hyperparathyroidism
 Hypoparathyroidism
 Hypothyroidism
*Chronic Mucopurulent Conjunctivitis*
 Gout
*Conjunctival Aneurysms, Varicosities, Tortuosities, and Telangiectasias*
 Diabetes
 Fabry disease (diffuse angiokeratosis)
*Conjunctival Xerosis*
 Sjögren syndrome (keratoconjunctivitis sicca), seen in association with autoimmune thyroid disease
 Vitamin A deficiency (seen in pregnancy)
*Subconjunctival Hemorrhage*
 Diabetes (due to fragility of vessel walls)
 Ehlers-Danlos syndrome
*Conjunctival Hyperpigmentation*
 Addison disease
**GLOBE**
*Microphthalmia*
 Colobomatous microphthalmia
  Laurence-Moon-Biedl syndrome
 Noncolobomatous microphthalmia
  Lowe syndrome
*Buphthalmos*
 Hurler syndrome
 Lowe syndrome

*Soft Globe*
 Diabetic coma
**SCLERA**
*Episcleritis*
 Addison disease
*Scleritis*
 Cretinism (hypothyroidism)
 Gout
 Porphyria cutanea tarda
*Staphyloma of Sclera*
 Ehlers-Danlos syndrome
 Hyperparathyroidism
 Marfan syndrome associated with myopia
 Porphyria cutanea tarda
*Blue Sclera*
 Ehler-Danlos syndrome
 Hallermann-Streiff syndrome (bird-faced dwarf )
 Hypophosphatasia (phosphoetha-nolaminuria)
 Lowe syndrome
 Marfan syndrome
 Osteogenesis imperfecta
 Phenylketonuria
 Pseudohypoparathyroidism
 Pseudoxanthoma elasticum
 Scleral thinning secondary to scleritis
 Werner syndrome (adult progeria)
*Dilated Episcleral Vessels*
 Endocrine exophthalmos of rapid development
*Scleral Rigidity*
 Decreased scleral rigidity
 Graves disease
 Increased scleral rigidity
 Diabetes mellitus
**CORNEA**
*Microcornea*
 Ehlers-Danlos syndrome
 Laurence-Moon-Biedl syndrome
 Marfan syndrome
*Megalocornea*
 Lowe syndrome
 Marfan syndrome
 Osteogenesis imperfecta
 Scheie syndrome (MPS I-S)
*Hyperplastic Corneal Nerves*
 Multiple endocrine neoplasia type 2B
*Increased Visibility of Corneal Nerves*
 Refsum syndrome
*Corneal Anesthesia*
 Diabetes mellitus
 Metachromatic leukodystrophy (arylsulfatase-A deficiency)
 Nephropathic cystinosis
*Band-Shaped Keratopathy*
 Gout
 Hypercalcemia
 Hyperparathyroidism
 Hypophosphatasia
 Paget disease
 Renal failure, associated with Fanconi syndrome (cystinosis)
*Sclerocornea*
 Hurler syndrome

*Corneal Opacity, Diffuse*
 Cystinosis
 Fabry disease
 $GM_1$ gangliosidosis type I deficiency
 Hurler syndrome
 Maroteaux-Lamy syndrome (MPS VI)
 Morquio syndrome
 Mucopolysaccharidosis
 Multiple sulfatase deficiency
 Pseudo-Hurler polydystrophy (mucolipidosis III)
 Scheie syndrome
 Sialidosis, Goldberg type
*Corneal Opacification in Infancy*
 Corneal lipidosis
 Lowe syndrome
 Mucolipidosis
  Generalized gangliosidosis ($GM_1$ gangliosidosis I and II)
  Lipomucopolysaccharidosis
  Pseudo-Hurler polydystrophy
 Mucopolysaccharidoses
  Hurler syndrome
  Maroteaux-Lamy syndrome
  Morquio syndrome
  Scheie syndrome
 Riley-Day syndrome
 Von Gierke disease
*Corneal Opacity, Localized*
 Fucosidosis
*Cornea Verticillata*
 Fabry disease
 Tamoxifen administration
*Corneal Crystals*
 Cystinosis syndrome
 Gout
 Hyperthyroidism
*Cornea Plana*
 Marfan syndrome
*Keratoconus*
 Apert syndrome (acrocephalosyndactylia)
 Ehlers-Danlos syndrome
 Laurence-Moon-Biedl syndrome
 Marfan syndrome
 Pseudoxanthoma elasticum
*Punctate Keratitis*
 CRST syndrome (Calcinosis, *Raynaud* phenomenon, *Sclero-dactyly, Telangiectasia*)
 Diabetes mellitus
 Graves disease
 Hypothyroidism
 Riley-Day syndrome
*Filamentary Keratitis*
 Diabetes mellitus
*Keratitis Sicca*
 Autoimmune thyroid disease
 Diabetes mellitus
*Anterior Corneal Mosaic*
 Endocrine exophthalmos
*Corneal Dermoids*
 Incontinentia pigmenti
*Pannus*
 Hypothyroidism

*Interstitial Keratitis*
 Incontinentia pigmenti
*Corneoscleral Keratitis*
 Gout
*Marginal Corneal Ulcers*
 Gout
*Pigmentation of Cornea*
 Metallic pigmentation
  Wilson disease (Kayser-Fleischer ring)
 Yellow discoloration
  Tangier disease
*Anterior Embryotoxon*
 Alport syndrome (hereditary nephritis-deafness syndrome)
 Familial hypercholesterolemia
*Staphyloma of Cornea*
 Occurs in advanced keratoconus (see earlier)
*Trigger Mechanisms for Recurrent Herpes Simplex Keratitis*
 Menses
*Corneal Disease Associated with Lenticular (Lens) Problems*
 Addison disease
 Apert syndrome
 Cataracts
 Corneal ulcers
 Ehlers-Danlos syndrome
 Hypoparathyroidism
 Keratic moniliasis
 Keratoconjunctivitis
 Lowe syndrome
 Marfan syndrome
 Mucolipidosis IV
 Pseudohypoparathyroidism
 Refsum syndrome
 Sanfilippo syndrome (MPS III)
 Scheie syndrome
 Werner syndrome
*Corneal Disease Associated with Retinal Problems*
 Apert syndrome
 Cystinosis
 Ehlers-Danlos syndrome
 Fabry disease
 Hunter syndrome
 Hurler-Scheie syndrome
 Hurler syndrome
 Hyperlipoproteinemia
 Hyperparathyroidism
 Idiopathic hypercalcemia
 Marfan syndrome
 Mucolipidosis IV
 Porphyria cutanea tarda
 Refsum syndrome
 Scheie syndrome
 Von Gierke disease (glycogen storage disease type I)
 Werner syndrome
**INTRAOCULAR PRESSURE**
*Hypotony*
 Diabetes mellitus
 Homocystinuria
 Morquio syndrome

(continued)

**TABLE 215-1.**
**Ocular Conditions and Their Endocrine and Metabolic Associations (Continued)**

*Glaucoma*
Acromegaly
Cretinism
Cushing syndrome
Diabetes mellitus
Ehlers-Danlos syndrome
Homocystinuria
Hunter syndrome
Hurler syndrome
Hyperthyroidism
Lowe syndrome
Marfan syndrome
Multiple endocrine neoplasia type 1
Scheie syndrome
Sulfite oxidase deficiency
*Elevated Intraocular Pressure in Upgaze*
Graves ophthalmopathy
*Glaucoma Associated with Shallow Anterior Chamber*
Cystinosis
*Conditions Simulating Congenital Glaucoma*
Cystinosis
Familial lipidosis
Glycogen storage disease type I
Hurler disease
Incontinentia pigmenti
Maroteaux-Lamy disease
Morquio syndrome
Riley-Day syndrome
Scheie disease
**ANTERIOR CHAMBER**
*Hyphema*
Diabetes mellitus
*Iris Processes*
Marfan syndrome
Mucopolysaccharidoses
**PUPIL**
*Mydriasis*
Lowe syndrome
*Fixated Pupil*
Diabetic ophthalmoplegia (usually spares pupillary fibers)
*Miosis*
Argyll Robertson pupil
Diabetes mellitus
Lowe syndrome
Marfan syndrome
Morquio syndrome
Refsum disease
Horner syndrome
*Afferent Pupillary Defect*
Diabetic retinopathy
**IRIS**
*Aniridia*
Homocystinuria syndrome
*Iris Coloboma*
Laurence-Moon-Biedl syndrome
Marfan syndrome
*Rubeosis Iridis*
Diabetes mellitus

*Heterochromia*
Incontinentia pigmenti
*Iris Atrophy*
Diabetes mellitus
Homocystinuria
Hurler syndrome
**LENS**
*Anterior Subcapsular Cataracts*
Addison disease
Albinism
Diabetes mellitus
Hypothyroidism
Tyrosinosis
Werner syndrome
Wilson disease
*Nuclear Cataracts*
Maple syrup urine disease
Von Gierke disease (glycogen storage disease type I)
*Lamellar Cataracts*
Galactokinase deficiency
Hypophosphatasia
Mannosidosis
Marfan syndrome
*Punctate Cataracts*
Cretinism
Galactokinase deficiency
Hypercalcemia
Lowe syndrome
Pseudohypoparathyroidism
*Posterior Subcapsular Cataract*
Abetalipoproteinemia
Diabetes mellitus
Fabry disease
Hypoparathyroidism
Incontinentia pigmenti
Laurence-Moon-Biedl syndrome
Refsum disease
Werner syndrome
*Iridescent Crystalline Deposits in Lens*
Cretinism
Hypocalcemia
*Posterior Lenticonus*
Lowe syndrome
*Microphakia or Spherophakia*
Homocystinuria
Hyperlysinemia
Lowe syndrome
Marfan syndrome
*Dislocated Lens*
Ehlers-Danlos syndrome
Homocystinuria
Hyperlysinemia
Marfan syndrome
Pseudoxanthoma elasticum
Sulfite oxidase deficiency
*Lenticular Disease Associated with Corneal Problems*
Diabetes mellitus
Fabry disease
Wilson disease
*Syndromes and Diseases Associated with Cataracts*
Abetalipoproteinemia
Addison syndrome

Albinism
Cretinism
Diabetes mellitus
Fabry disease
Galactokinase deficiency
Galactose-transferase deficiency
Hagberg-Santavuori syndrome (hereditary encephalopathy, microcephaly, optic atrophy)
Homocystinuria
Hypercalcemia
Hypoglycemia (in infants)
Hypoparathyroidism
Hypophosphatasia
Incontinentia pigmenti
Laurence-Moon-Biedl syndrome
Lowe syndrome
Mannosidosis
Maple syrup urine disease
Marfan syndrome
Morquio syndrome
Multiple sulfatase deficiency
Osteogenesis imperfecta congenita
Passow syndrome (congenital syringomyelia)
Prader-Willi syndrome (hypogenital dystrophy with diabetic tendency)
Refsum disease
Tyrosinosis
Wilson disease
Zellweger syndrome (cerebrohepatorenal syndrome)
*Spasm of Accommodation*
Diabetes mellitus
*Paresis of Accommodation*
After pregnancy
Diabetes mellitus
Lactation
**VITREOUS**
*Vitreous Hemorrhage*
Diabetes mellitus
**RETINA**
*Anatomic Classification of Macular Diseases*
Nerve fiber–ganglion cell layers
Goldberg disease (β-galactosidase deficiency)
Jansky-Bielschowsky disease (gangliosidosis GM$_2$ type III)
Mucolipidoses
Sphingolipidoses
Vogt-Spielmeyer disease (hereditary cerebroretinal degeneration, mental retardation)
Outer plexiform layer
Cystoid macular degeneration
Diabetes mellitus
Lipid deposits in macula secondary to vascular disease in retina
Diabetes mellitus
Bruch membrane
Angioid streaks
Acromegaly
Ehlers-Danlos syndrome
Pseudoxanthoma elasticum

*Cotton-wool spots*
Diabetic retinopathy
Toxemia retinopathy of pregnancy
*Dilated Retinal Veins and Retinal Hemorrhages*
Diabetes mellitus
Porphyria cutanea tarda
*Retinovitreal Hemorrhage in Young Adults*
Diabetes mellitus
Incontinentia pigmenti
*Macular Hemorrhage in Young Adults*
Angioid streaks
Diabetic retinopathy
*Hard Exudates*
Diabetes mellitus
*Macular Edema*
Diabetes mellitus
Fabry disease
Hunter syndrome
Hurler syndrome
*Parafoveal Telangiectasia*
Diabetes mellitus
*Aneurysmal Dilation of Retinal Vessels*
Diabetes mellitus
*Neovascularization of the Retina*
Diabetes mellitus
Ehlers-Danlos syndrome
*Generalized Arterial Narrowing*
Adrenal tumor hyperaldosteronism
Cushing disease
Hunter syndrome
Jansky-Bielschowsky disease (gangliosidosis GM$_2$ type III)
Pheochromocytoma
Sanfilippo syndrome
Tay-Sachs disease (amaurotic familial idiocy)
Toxemia of pregnancy
Zellweger syndrome (cerebrohepatorenal syndrome)
*Retinitis or Pseudoretinitis Pigmentosa*
Abetalipoproteinemia
Cystinosis
Haltia-Santavuori syndrome (neuronal ceroid lipofuscinosis)
Hunter syndrome (MPS II)
Hurler syndrome (MPS I)
Hypophosphatasia
Infantile phytanic acid storage disease
Kearns-Sayre syndrome (external ocular muscle myopathy, blepharoptosis, mental deficiency, heart block, and occasional hypothyroidism)
Laurence-Moon-Biedl syndrome
Mucolipidosis IV
Multiple sulfatase deficiency
Pseudohypoparathyroidism
Refsum disease
Sanfilippo syndrome (MPS III)
Scheie syndrome (MPS I-S)
Stock-Spielmeyer-Vogt syndrome

*(continued)*

**TABLE 215-1.**
**Ocular Conditions and Their Endocrine and Metabolic Associations** (Continued)

*Retinal "Sea Fans"*
Diabetes mellitus
Incontinentia pigmenti
*Retinal Vascular Tumors and Angi-
omatosis Retinal Syndromes*
Pheochromocytoma
*Retinal Vascular Tortuosity*
Fabry disease
Maroteaux-Lamy syndrome
(MPS type VI)
*Lipemia Retinalis*
Diabetes mellitus with hyper-
lipemia
Hypothyroidism, untreated
Idiopathic hypercalcemia
Primary hyperlipoproteinemia
Progressive lipodystrophy
Secondary hyperlipoproteinemia
*Central Retinal Vein Occlusion*
Diabetes mellitus
*Cholesterol Emboli of Retina*
Diabetes mellitus
*Retinal Artery Occlusion*
Fabry disease
Homocystinuria
*Cherry-Red Spot in Macula*
β-Galactosidase deficiency
Hurler syndrome
Lipomucopolysaccharidoses
Multiple sulfatase deficiency
Sphingolipidoses
Farber syndrome (congenital
soft tissue nodules, muscle
hypotonia, mental retar-
dation with ceramide dep-
osition)
Gangliosidosis GM type 2
Gaucher disease
Goldberg syndrome
Infantile metachromatic dys-
trophy
Niemann-Pick disease
Sandhoff disease (ganglioside
storage disorder)
Stock-Spielmeyer-Vogt syn-
drome
Tay-Sachs disease
*Macular Hypoplasia*
Albinism
*Bull's Eye Macular Lesion*
Ceroid lipofuscinosis
Stock-Spielmeyer-Vogt
syndrome
*Pigmentary Changes in Macula*
Abetalipoproteinemia
Vogt-Spielmeyer disease
Gangliosidosis GM$_2$ type 3
Hunter disease (MPS II)
Hurler syndrome (MPS I-H)
Refsum disease (phytanic acid
storage disease)
Sanfilippo syndrome (MPS III)
Scheie syndrome (MPS I-S)
Tangier disease

Tay-Sachs disease (gangliosidosis
GM$_2$ type I)
*White or Yellow Flat Macular Lesion
and Pigmentary Change*
Diffuse leukoencephalopathy
Gaucher disease
*Macular Pucker*
Diabetes mellitus
*Pigmented Fundus Lesions*
Abetalipoproteinemia
Incontinentia pigmenti
Laurence-Moon-Biedl syndrome
Lignac-Fanconi syndrome
Refsum disease
*Pale Fundus Lesions*
Generalized pallor
Albinism
Fabry disease
Gaucher disease
Hyperlipemia
Lipidoses
Congenital
Gangliosidosis GM$_2$ type III
Kufs disease (inherited pro-
gressive mental deterio-
ration with ceroid-
lipofuscin deposition
systemically)
Stock-Spielmeyer-Vogt syn-
drome
Tay-Sachs disease
Localized pale areas
Hypercholesterolemia
Incontinentia pigmenti
Laurence-Moon-Beidl syn-
drome
Lignac-Fanconi syndrome
Refsum syndrome
*Retinal Detachment*
Apert syndrome
Ehlers-Danlos syndrome
Homocystinuria
Incontinentia pigmenti
Marfan syndrome
Norrie syndrome (X-linked blind-
ness, deafness, and mental
retardation)
Toxemia of pregnancy
Warburg syndrome (recessive
hydrocephalus, cryptorchid-
ism, micropenis, and eye abnor-
malities)
*Peripheral Retinal Degeneration*
Cystinosis
*Crystalline Retinopathy*
Cystinosis
**CHOROID**
*Angioid Streaks*
Acromegaly
Diffuse lipomatoses
Ehlers-Danlos syndrome
Pseudoxanthoma elasticum
*Choroidal Neovascularization*
Angioid streaks
Osteogenesis imperfecta

*Ischemic Infarcts of Choroid
(Elschnig Spots)*
Toxemia of pregnancy
*Choroidal Ischemia*
Toxemia of pregnancy
*Choroidal Folds*
Graves disease
*Choroidal Hemorrhage*
Diabetes mellitus
Ehlers-Danlos syndrome
*Choroidal Detachment*
Diabetes mellitus
Toxemia of pregnancy
*Syndromes Associated with Uveitis*
Glaucoma
Homocystinuria
*Conditions Simulating Posterior
Uveitis in Children*
Cystinosis
**OPTIC NERVE**
*Papilledema*
Endocrine exophthalmos
Pseudotumor cerebri
Addison disease
Diabetes mellitus
Fabry disease
Hunter syndrome
Hyperparathyroidism
Hypocalcemia
Hypoparathyroidism
Idiopathic hypercalcemia
Maroteaux-Lamy syndrome
Menarche
Menses
Mucolipidosis III
Obesity
Oral contraceptives
Pregnancy
Pseudohypoparathyroidism
Systemic corticosteroids
*Optic Neuritis*
Diabetes mellitus
Hyperthyroidism
Hypoparathyroidism
Hypothyroidism
*Ischemic Optic Neuropathy*
Diabetes mellitus
*Optic Nerve Drusen*
Diabetes mellitus
Pituitary tumor
Pseudoxanthoma elasticum
*Optic Atrophy*
Abetalipoproteinemia
Albinism
Cretinism
Cushing syndrome
Diabetes mellitus
Galactosylceramide lipidosis
Gangliosidosis GM$_1$ type 2
Gangliosidosis GM$_2$ type 3
Homocystinuria
Hunter syndrome
Hurler syndrome
Hyperparathyroidism

Hypophosphatasia
Hypopituitarism
Infantile type neuronal ceroid
lipofuscinosis
Laurence-Moon-Biedl syndrome
Maple syrup urine disease
Maroteaux-Lamy disease
Metachromatic leukodystrophy
Morquio syndrome
Mucolipidosis IV
Niemann-Pick disease
Passow syndrome
Pituitary gigantism
Porphyria cutanea tarda
Refsum disease
Riley-Day syndrome
Sanfilippo disease
Stock-Spielmeyer-Vogt syn-
drome
Tay-Sachs disease
Von Gierke disease (glycogen
storage disease type I)
Zollinger-Ellison syndrome
*Optic Nerve Hypoplasia*
Albinism
Children of diabetic mothers
Osteogenesis imperfecta
Pituitary abnormalities
Diabetes insipidus
Growth retardation
Neonatal hypoglycemia
*Neovascularization of Optic Disc*
Incontinentia pigmenti achromi-
ans
**VISUAL DISTURBANCE**
*Acquired Myopia*
Albinism
Diabetes mellitus
Hypothyroidism
Toxemia of pregnancy
*Myopia*
Ehlers-Danlos syndrome
Homocystinuria
Laurence-Moon-Biedl syndrome
Marfan syndrome
Scheie syndrome
*Acquired Hyperopia*
Diabetes mellitus
*Cortical Blindness*
Galactosemia
Pompe disease (glycogen storage
disease type II)
Tay-Sachs disease
*Blindness in Childhood*
Laurence-Moon-Biedl syndrome
Marfan syndrome
Metachromatic leukodystrophy
Niemann-Pick disease
Sandhoff disease (ganglioside
storage disorder with GM$_2$
accumulation)
*Night Blindness*
Refsum syndrome
Retinitis pigmentosa

(Adapted from Roy FH, ed. Ocular differential diagnosis, 5th ed. Philadelphia: Lea & Febiger, 1993.)

Besides the globe, the orbit contains nerves, fat, blood vessels, and the extraocular muscles. Several endocrine conditions, such as thyroid ophthalmopathy and acromegaly, cause *enlargement of the extraocular muscles* that is seen on orbital imaging. Another orbital sign that requires a special test for detection is an *orbital bruit*. This is the audible flow of blood that can be heard with a stethoscope held over the orbit. It is associated with hyperthyroidism.

## LIDS

Endocrine and metabolic disorders associated with abnormalities of the eyelids are particularly common. In addition, of all ocular abnormalities, those of the lids are among the most easily detected by the internist because they are signs that can be noted on general inspection without the use of specialized ophthalmic equipment such as the slit lamp or indirect ophthalmoscope.

Many of the changes of the lids are only cosmetically important. More serious, mostly because they threaten the health of the underlying cornea, are abnormalities that change the relationship of the lids to the globe and abnormalities in a patient's blink. *Ptosis*, or droopiness of the upper lid, if severe, can impair a person's visual field. *Horner syndrome*, which is caused by paralysis of the sympathetic nerve supply, is manifested by a droopy eyelid and a pupil that is smaller than the pupil of the fellow eye. The disparity in pupil size is greater in dim illumination. One cause of Horner syndrome is a pituitary tumor. *Lid retraction* is present when the lower eyelid exposes sclera, or the white of the eye, beneath the inferior limbus or when the upper eyelid is at or above the superior limbus. The limbus is the sclerocorneal junction. In *lid lag*, the eyelids briefly lag behind when the patient looks down. Both lid retraction and lid lag are common signs in patients with Graves disease. In *ectropion*, the lid margin turns out from the globe.

Abnormalities in blinking that are related to endocrine conditions include facial palsy, *blepharospasm*, and infrequent blinking. In facial palsy, which can be caused by diabetes mellitus, the patient cannot close the lids on the involved side because of paralysis of the facial muscles supplied by the seventh cranial nerve. The inability to blink leads to corneal exposure and, if not treated, can cause serious corneal damage. Blepharospasm is involuntary twitching, blinking, or closure of the eyelids. It is associated with Addison disease (see Chap. 76) and hypoparathyroidism.

*Mongoloid obliquity* is the term used when the temporal corner of the eye is higher than the nasal corner. *Epicanthus* refers to a congenital fold of skin that overlies the inner canthus of the eye. It simulates the appearance of the eye turning in. Changes in the pigmentation of the lid skin have multiple endocrine associations and include both *hyperpigmentation* and *hypopigmentation*.

Growths on the lids include *xanthelasma* (or *xanthoma*), which are yellowish fatty deposits on the eyelid (Fig. 215-3). These are frequently seen in lipid disorders (see Chap. 163).

Alterations in the texture, amount, growth pattern, and color of the eyebrows and lashes are also manifestations of endocrine disorders. These include *trichomegaly* (long lashes), *madarosis* (loss of lashes), and *poliosis* (whitening of the lashes or brows). In some conditions, especially several of the mucopolysaccharidoses, *coarse eyebrows* are noted. The *Hertogh sign* refers to the lack of the outer third of the eyebrows and can occur in patients with hypothyroidism (Fig. 215-4).

## EXTRAOCULAR MUSCLES

The extraocular muscles are the muscles associated with movements of the globe. Thus, pathology involving these muscles or their nerve supply is manifested by abnormalities in eye movement, including involuntary movement, weakened movement, and paralysis.

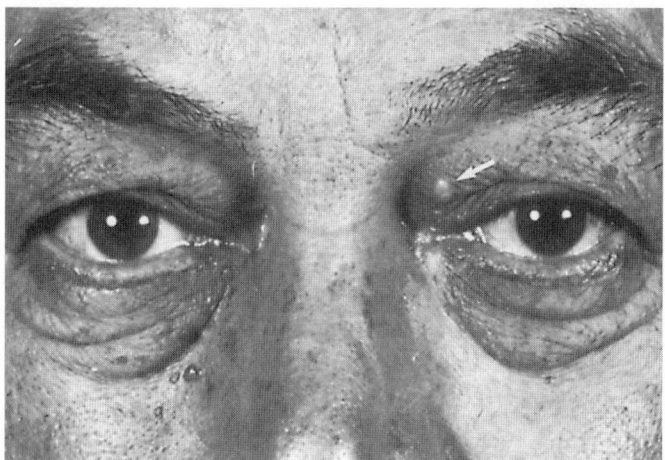

**FIGURE 215-3.** Palpebral xanthoma (xanthelasma) of the eyelid (*arrow*) in a patient with mild familial hypercholesterolemia.

*Strabismus* refers to misalignment or dissociation of the eyes (i.e., when the two eyes are not looking in the same direction). The most common examples of this are *esotropia* (the eye turned in) and *exotropia* (the eye turned out). *Cyclic strabismus* is a manifest strabismus that recurs regularly.

*Nystagmus* refers to involuntary repetitive oscillating movements of the eyes in the horizontal, vertical, or rotary directions. In *pendular nystagmus*, the oscillations are smooth and equal in velocity in both directions. In *periodic alternating nystagmus*, there are rhythmic jerk-type movements in one direction for 60 to 90 seconds and then in the reverse direction for 60 to 90 seconds.

*Ocular bobbing* is present when both eyes move together spontaneously by intermittently dropping downward a few millimeters and then returning to the straight-ahead position.

Several cranial nerves are devoted to innervating the extraocular muscles, and lesions anywhere along these nerves can have an effect on ocular movement. *Paralysis of the third cranial nerve* is manifested by (a) droopiness of the eyelid; (b) limitation of the ability to look up, down, and in; and (c) if the pupil is involved, a dilated, unreactive pupil (Fig. 215-5). *Paralysis of the fourth cranial nerve* causes superior oblique muscle palsy that results in limitation of the eye's ability to look down and in. *Paralysis of the sixth cranial nerve* causes a palsy of the lateral rectus muscle resulting in limitation of temporal gaze in that eye. Paralysis of any of these three nerves can be caused by diabetic neuropathy.

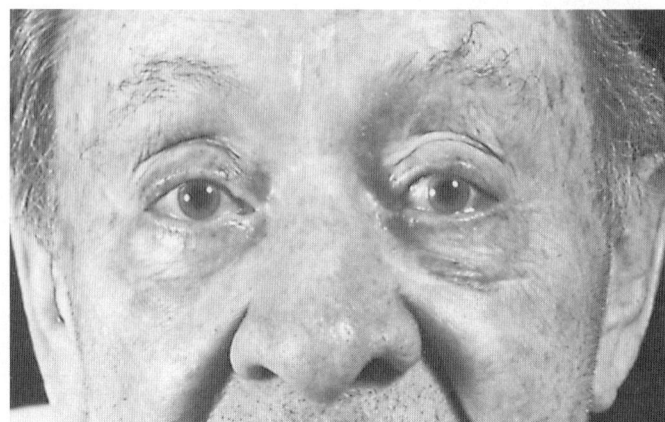

**FIGURE 215-4.** Loss of eyelashes and outer third of eyebrows in a patient with previously diagnosed hypothyroidism. With thyroid hormone therapy, the patient currently is euthyroid. The eyelashes did not return.

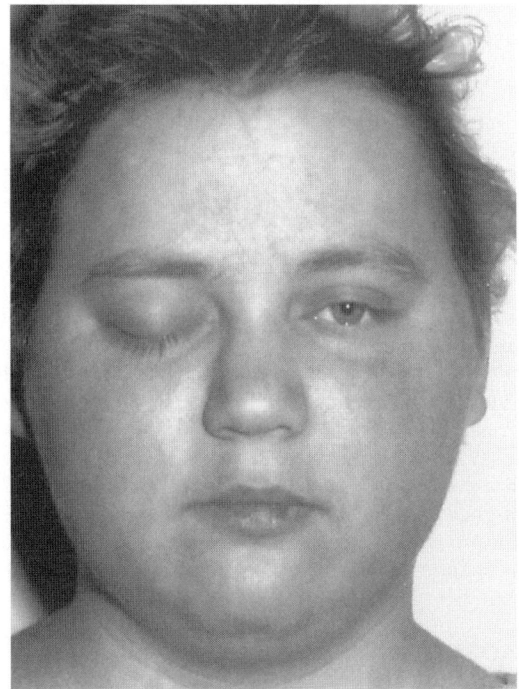

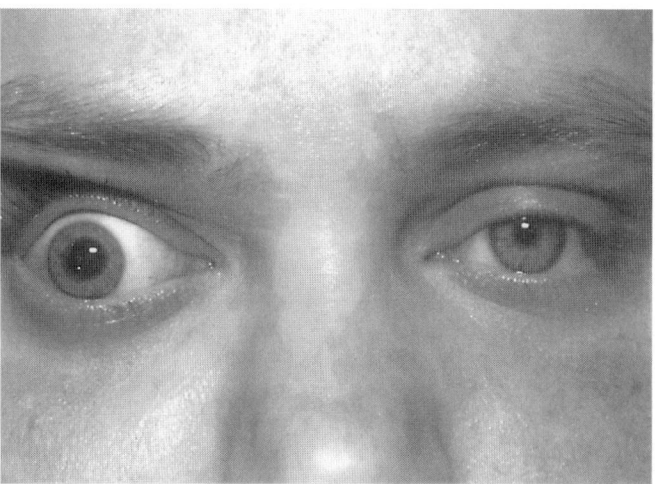

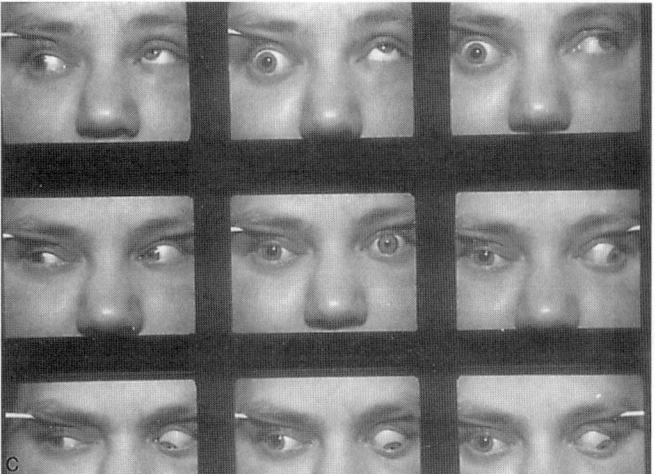

**FIGURE 215-5.** A 22-year-old woman with Cushing syndrome secondary to an adrenocorticotropic hormone–producing pituitary tumor. There is a third cranial nerve palsy on the right side due to tumor compression, as manifested by ptosis (**A**), a dilated pupil (**B**), and loss of the right eye's ability to look up, down, and medially (**C**). In the central picture (**C**), the patient is looking straight ahead. The remaining pictures are located in a position that corresponds to the direction of the patient's gaze. For example, in the upper left photograph, the patient is looking up and to the right. Note the inability of the right eye to look up.

*External ophthalmoplegia*, or generalized paralysis of the extraocular muscles, is manifested by a droopy eyelid and inability to move the eye. *Internuclear ophthalmoplegia* refers to a situation in which the ability to move one eye inward is decreased or lost, with concomitant nystagmus of the fellow eye when it tries to look outward.

*Double elevator palsy* is characterized by limitation of upward gaze in the involved eye and a turning downward of that eye when looking straight ahead.

*Poor convergence* refers to the inability to move the eyes inward to fixate on a close object. *Divergence paralysis* is an esodeviation, that is, a latent or manifest turning in of the eye that is greater at distance than at near.

### CONJUNCTIVA

The conjunctiva is the transparent, vascularized membrane that covers the inner surface of the eyelids and the globe adjacent to the cornea. *Congestion of the conjunctiva* refers to the injection of the conjunctival vessels, giving the appearance of a "red eye."

*Chronic mucopurulent conjunctivitis* refers to chronic hyperemia of the conjunctiva that is accompanied by a mucopurulent discharge.

### GLOBE

Congenital systemic conditions can affect the size of the globe. *Microphthalmos* refers to a small globe, whereas *buphthalmos* refers to a large globe.

### SCLERA

The sclera is the white, avascular supportive wall of the eye. The episclera is the vascularized connective tissue located between the sclera and the overlying conjunctiva.

*Episcleritis* is a sectoral, although sometimes diffuse, erythema of the eyes resulting from engorgement of the large vessels that can be seen beneath the conjunctiva. These vessels blanch with the application of topical epinephrine. Episcleritis is accompanied by ocular discomfort as opposed to severe pain, which occurs in scleritis.

*Scleritis,* or inflammation of the sclera, is manifested by engorgement of the large vessels beneath the conjunctiva that do not blanch with the application of topical phenylephrine.

A *staphyloma* of the sclera refers to a localized area of thinned sclera that bulges outward. In *blue sclera*, the sclera has a blue coloration.

### CORNEA

The cornea is one of the parts of the eye most commonly involved by systemic disease. Endocrine and metabolic abnormalities can affect the size, shape, and clarity of this normally transparent structure.

*Microcornea* refers to a cornea that is <10 mm in diameter, whereas *megalocornea* refers to a cornea that is >14 mm in diameter. The term *hyperplastic corneal nerves* refers to an overgrowth of corneal nerves ≤20 times the normal number.[41] *Band keratopathy* is a type of corneal opacification that consists largely of sub-

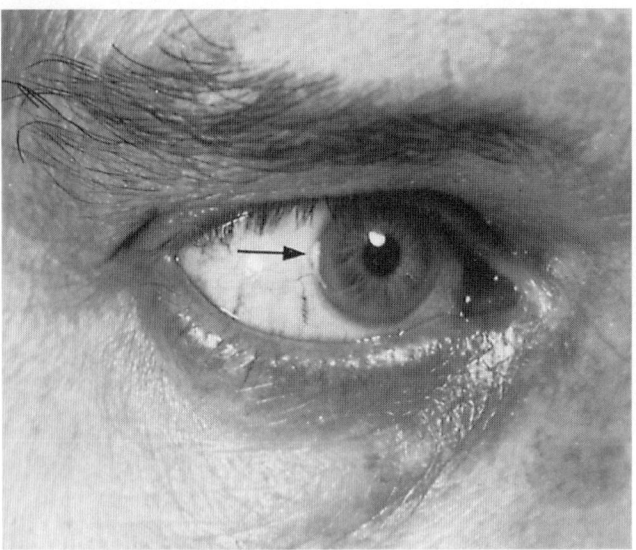

**FIGURE 215-6.** Patient with hyperparathyroidism and band keratopathy (*arrow*). Note the gray-white calcification that is interspersed with dark areas, which represents clear cornea.

epithelial calcium deposits. It extends as a horizontal band across the cornea in the area that is exposed between the eyelids (Fig. 215-6). Band keratopathy typically occurs with chronic ocular inflammation, but it can also be associated with systemic conditions that cause hypercalcemia. *Sclerocornea* is a cornea that, in its periphery or entirety, resembles the opaque connective tissue of sclera.

Many systemic conditions, including most mucopolysaccharidoses, cause *diffuse opacification of the cornea*, often starting in infancy. *Cornea verticillata* (see Fig. 215-2) is the whorl-like pattern of powdery opacities in the corneal epithelium that is seen in Fabry disease or with tamoxifen administration. *Corneal crystals* are punctate opacities seen in the cornea in cystinosis (Fig. 215-7).

In addition to its clarity, the shape of the cornea is an important factor in good visual acuity. In *cornea plana*, the corneal curvature is flatter than normal. *Keratoconus* is a noninflammatory

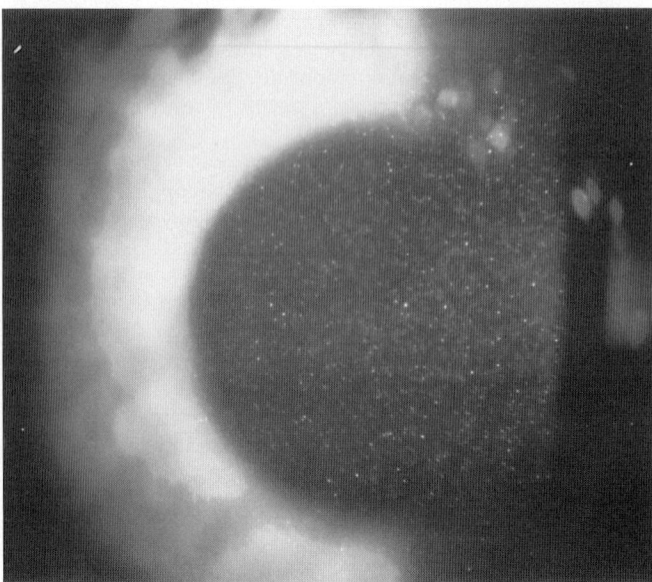

**FIGURE 215-7.** Corneal crystals in a patient with cystinosis.

thinning of the central or paracentral cornea, which results in a cone-shaped cornea.

The surface of the cornea can also be altered. In *punctate keratitis*, there is a speckled irregularity of the corneal epithelium that can be seen by applying a drop of fluorescein and observing the cornea with a blue light. In *filamentary keratitis*, threads of devitalized corneal epithelium are attached by one end to the corneal surface. Both of these conditions are seen in *keratitis sicca*, a dry eye that manifests secondary corneal changes. *Anterior corneal mosaic*[41] is a pattern of fluorescein pooling in the corneal epithelium that can be induced by exerting pressure on the eye, such as when the lids fit tightly over the globe in exophthalmos.

*Corneal dermoids* are congenital, yellowish, fatty tumors on the corneal limbus. *Pannus* is the superficial vascularization of the cornea.

Two systemically related conditions involving the corneal stroma are *interstitial keratitis*, or inflammation of the stroma, and *marginal corneal ulcers*. In an ulcer, there is a corneal defect in which there is a localized lack of epithelium with underlying stromal changes, such as thinning and infiltration of white blood cells.

## INTRAOCULAR PRESSURE

A certain range of normal intraocular pressure is necessary for the health of the eye. Intraocular pressure can be pathologically decreased (*hypotony*) or increased (*glaucoma*). In Cushing syndrome, ~25% of affected patients have increased intraocular pressure. This is the same percentage of the general population that responds with a rise in pressure when treated with exogenous corticosteroids.[41a] Because of the increased distensibility of the sclera in infancy, congenital glaucoma, in contrast to adult-onset glaucoma, causes the globe to be enlarged.

## ANTERIOR CHAMBER

The anterior chamber is usually filled with clear aqueous humor. Pathologic changes include *hyphema*, or blood in the anterior chamber, which can be caused by diabetes mellitus when an iris with neovascularization associated with diabetic retinopathy bleeds. Chronic angle-closure glaucoma results when *peripheral anterior synechiae*, areas of sheet-like scarring, seal the angle of the anterior chamber. *Iris processes* are fine ligaments that follow the normal curve of the anterior chamber angle.

## PUPIL

Endocrine and metabolic conditions can affect the pupil's size and response to light. *Mydriasis* is a dilated pupil, whereas *miosis* is a constricted pupil. A special example of miosis is an *Argyll Robertson pupil*, which is seen most commonly with neurosyphilis. Besides being miotic, these pupils have light-near dissociation: They do not react (constrict) in response to light, but their near response is intact. An eye with an *afferent pupillary defect* has loss of direct response to light: It dilates, as opposed to constricts, when a light is shined into it.

## IRIS

*Aniridia* is complete or partial absence of the iris. An *iris coloboma* is an iris defect resulting from failure of the fetal tissue to close in embryonic life. In *heterochromia*, the irises of the two eyes are different colors. *Rubeosis iridis* is neovascularization of the iris, notably present in severe diabetic retinopathy.

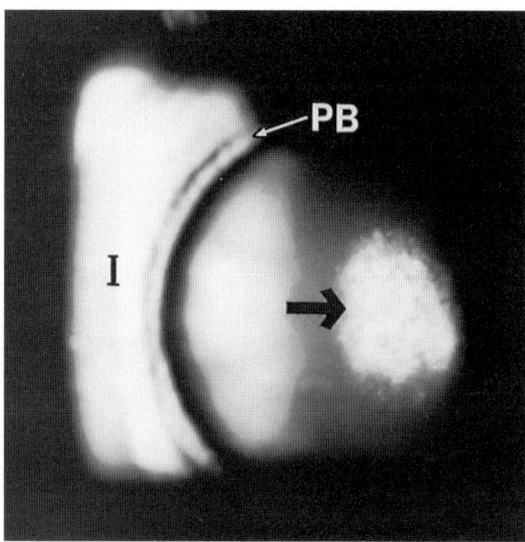

**FIGURE 215-8.** Posterior subcapsular cataract. Note the white opacification forming on the central posterior lens surface on the inside of the basement membrane capsule (*arrow*). (*I*, iris; *PB*, papillary border.) (Courtesy of William J. Shields, CRA.)

## LENS

The most common pathologic changes induced in the lens are decreased clarity, seen in *cataracts*, and changes in size or shape. Most types of cataracts vary in regard to the part of the lens that is opaque. *Posterior subcapsular cataracts* form as a white, dense layer on the inside of the posterior capsule of the lens (Fig. 215-8). This type of cataract is typical of that which is induced by trauma or corticosteroids. *Nuclear sclerosis* is associated with diffuse, yellow discoloration of the nucleus (the central part of the lens; Fig. 215-9). *Cortical cataracts* form white, linear, radiating spokes in the middle layers of the lens (Fig. 215-10). Left untreated, all progressive forms of cataract eventually develop the uniform, white appearance of a *mature cataract*.

Approximately 50% of patients with untreated hypoparathyroidism exhibit some degree of *cataract* formation.[42,43] At first, these cataracts may appear as bilateral, small, polychromatic deposits in the cortex that may be seen only with the slit lamp. When treated

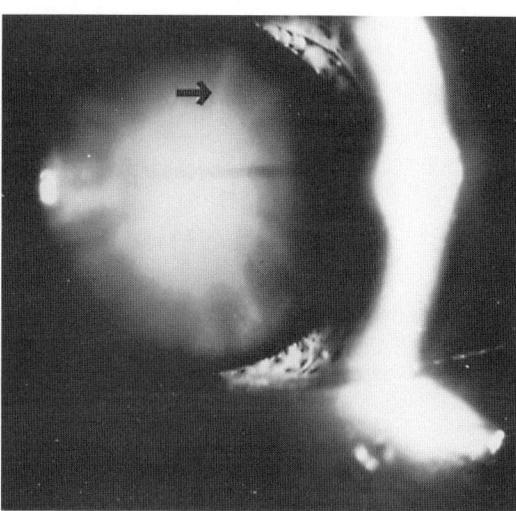

**FIGURE 215-10.** Cortical spoking cataract. Note the spokes of lens opacification (*arrow*) radiating from the center of the lens cortex. (Courtesy of William J. Shields, CRA.)

adequately, further cataract development is arrested; otherwise, the condition progresses, and dense, white cataracts form.

Cataracts are found in several syndromes characterized by hypogonadism and testicular failure,[44] such as myotonic dystrophy. In addition, patients with cretinism also develop visually significant focal cortical opacities. In infants, hypoglycemia may be associated with cataract formation, but this does not occur in adults.[45,46] Posterior subcapsular and cortical cataract formation commonly occurs in patients with diabetes mellitus. Although patients with Cushing syndrome are subjected to high levels of cortisol, they do not develop the posterior subcapsular cataracts that are seen with parenteral or topical administration of corticosteroids.

*Microphakia* is a small lens and *spherophakia* is a highly spherical lens. In *lenticonus*, there is a conical deformation of the lens surface. In *paresis of accommodation*, there is an inability to focus on near objects due to loss of ability to change the shape of the lens.

A *dislocated lens* is one that is displaced from its normal position. If it is only partially displaced, or subluxated, it can still be seen within the pupillary area (Fig. 215-11). In *Marfan syndrome*,

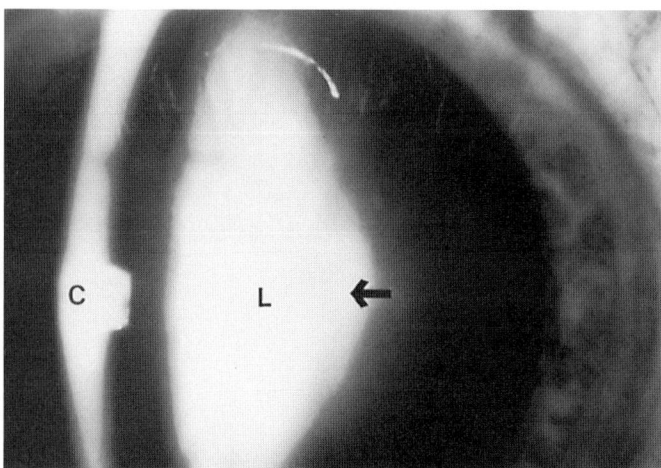

**FIGURE 215-9.** Nuclear sclerosis cataract. Note the increased density in the center of the lens (*arrow*), which clinically has a yellow coloration when viewed with a slit lamp. (*C*, cornea; *L*, lens.) (Courtesy of William J. Shields, CRA.)

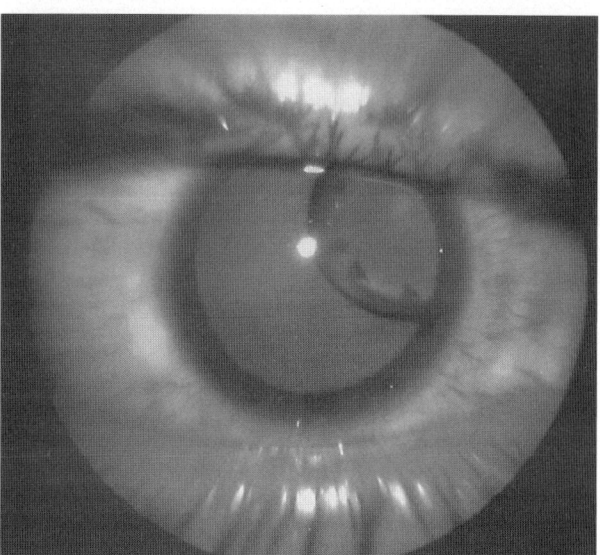

**FIGURE 215-11.** Subluxated lens as seen through a dilated pupil on slit lamp examination. The lens is displaced temporally and superiorly, as is often seen in Marfan syndrome.

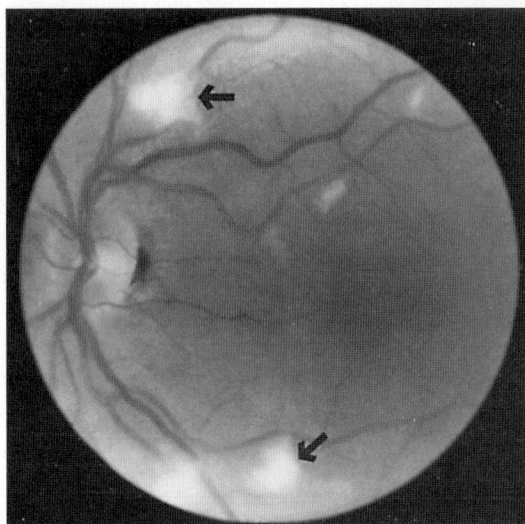

**FIGURE 215-12.** Cotton-wool spots on the retina. Infarcts of the nerve fiber layer have caused white opacification of the retina (*arrows*). (Courtesy of William J. Shields, CRA.)

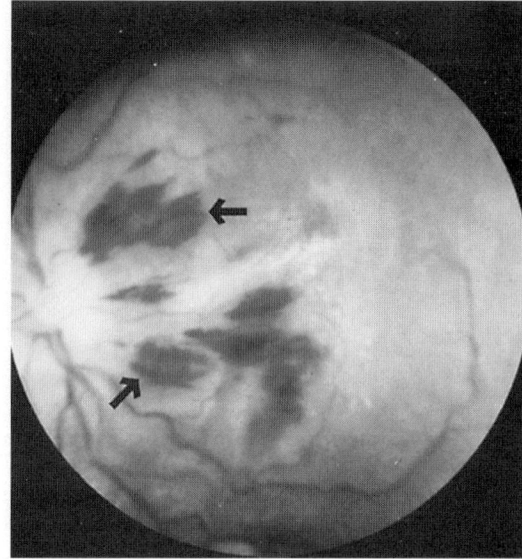

**FIGURE 215-13.** Flame hemorrhages. These red streaks of hemorrhage (*arrows*) are confined to the nerve fiber layer. (Courtesy of Peter Y. Evans, MD.)

the *lens* typically subluxates temporally and superiorly. In patients in whom Marfan syndrome is suspected, the presence of a subluxated lens can help confirm the diagnosis. In *homocystinuria*, the position of the subluxated *lens* is usually medial and inferior.

### RETINA/CHOROID

The most common endocrine disorder affecting the retina is diabetes mellitus (see Chap. 151). The retinal lesions frequently associated with diabetes include cotton-wool spots, retinal hemorrhages, hard exudates, and retinal edema. However, these lesions are also found in other endocrine abnormalities. *Cotton-wool spots*—soft, white infarcts of the nerve fiber layer—are seen in many conditions that cause focal retinal ischemia, including toxemia, hypertension, and collagen vascular disease (Fig. 215-12; see Fig. 215-1). *Retinal hemorrhages* lying on the surface of the retina are called preretinal hemorrhages, while those within the nerve fiber layer form flame-shaped hemorrhages (Fig. 215-13). In deeper layers of the retina, hemorrhages may appear as small, round dots. *Hard exudates* are yellowish deposits caused by partially absorbed serous fluid; they are seen in the deep retinal layers and often form a ring around areas of vascular incompetence and leakage. Any condition that leads to increased vascular permeability can cause the formation of hard exudates. Retinal or macular edema often accompanies hard exudates. Retinal ischemia can eventually lead to neovascularization, when tufts of small new vessels proliferate on the surface of the retina and grow into the vitreous cavity. These vessels are especially important to identify because they indicate severe disease and the need for laser photocoagulation therapy. Laser treatment destroys retinal and choroidal tissue and is used to treat neovascularization from any cause. The mechanism by which laser treatment causes retinal ischemia to improve is unknown.

Other vascular abnormalities are seen in diabetic retinopathy. *Parafoveal telangiectasias* are microvascular anomalies involving the capillary network around the fovea. *Retinal sea fans* are peripheral retinal neovascularizations in the shape of a fan.

Many of the pathologic changes that frequently are associated with diabetic retinopathy also may be seen in patients with pheochromocytoma, Cushing syndrome, or hypertensive retinopathy.[47,48] Cotton-wool spots, retinal hemorrhages, and edema are typical findings in severe hypertension. Irregular venous dilation (see Fig. 215-1), sclerosis of the arteries, and arteriovenous nicking also may be found (Fig. 215-14). Sclerotic arteries appear narrower than normal, because as the vessel walls thicken, the central core of blood becomes narrower and increasingly difficult to observe. The relatively mild hypertension that is associated with hyperaldosteronism is accompanied by minimal retinal changes. However, marked retinopathy can occur in rare instances.

Neovascularization is not usually associated with hypertensive retinopathy. However, affected patients often have optic nerve ischemia with disc edema, as well as a pattern of lipid deposition in the nerve fiber layer around the fovea that is called a *macular star* (Fig. 215-15). This results from hard exudates (lipid) that are deposited in a radial pattern around the fovea, where the nerve fiber layer has a radial configuration.

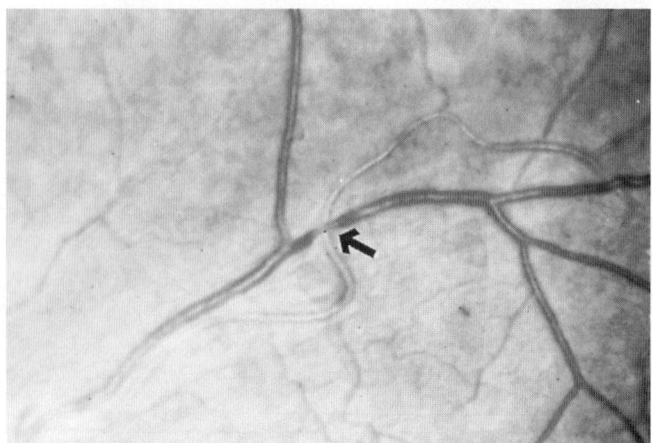

**FIGURE 215-14.** Arteriovenous nicking. Note the deformation and narrowing of the retinal vein as it crosses over a retinal artery (*arrow*). (Courtesy of Peter Y. Evans, MD.)

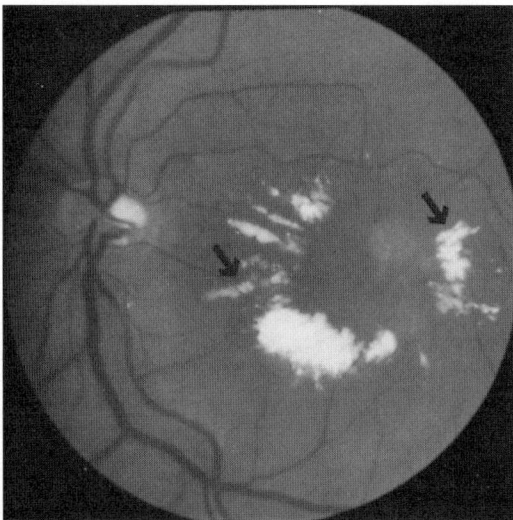

**FIGURE 215-15.** Macular star. Deposits of serum lipids are confined to the nerve fiber layer, which has a radiating configuration (*arrows*) around the macula. (Courtesy of Peter Y. Evans, MD.)

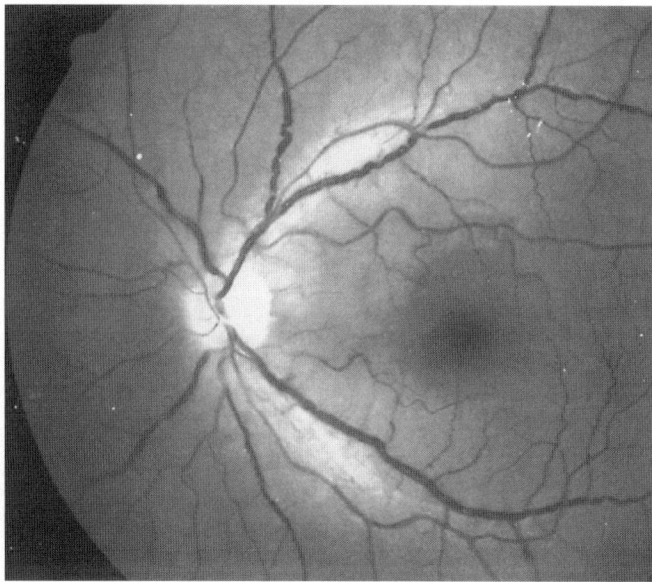

**FIGURE 215-17.** Corkscrew tortuosity of retinal vessels in a patient with Fabry disease. Compare with the normal retinal vessels in Figure 209-18*B*.

Endocrinologists also should be familiar with the appearance of *retinitis pigmentosa*,[49–51] the characteristic findings of which include clumps of pigment that form a bone-corpuscle pattern (pigmentary retinopathy) in the midperiphery of the retina (Fig. 215-16). The pigment comes from RPE cells, found deep in the retina, which migrate to the surface and collect along blood vessels. The optic disc is pale and waxy, and a decrease in the caliber of the blood vessels is evident. Certain syndromes, such as *Laurence-Moon-Biedl syndrome*,[52] are associated with retinitis pigmentosa combined with hypogonadism.[53] The "progressive external ophthalmoplegia plus" of *Kearns-Sayre syndrome* is associated with retinitis pigmentosa, heart block, and, in some patients, hypoparathyroidism.[54,55] Moreover, pseudohypoparathyroidism, and also hypophosphatasia, may coexist with retinitis pigmentosa.

Several other diseases of interest to the endocrinologist have retinal manifestations. A patient with angiomata of the retina may have the *von Hippel-Lindau syndrome*; if the patient also has hypertension, this may suggest a coexistent pheochromocytoma (see Chap. 86).

Numerous other vascular abnormalities of the retina are associated with endocrine diseases. Tortuosity of retinal vessels (Fig. 215-17) is seen in Fabry disease. In *lipemia retinalis*, there is a yellowish or white appearance to the retinal arterioles and venules. This condition is seen with hyperlipoproteinemia.

Retinal vascular occlusion can cause sudden, painless loss of vision. In *central retinal vein occlusion*, which is also associated with diabetes, massive retinal hemorrhages and dilated retinal vessels are seen on examination. *Cholesterol emboli* are seen as bright yellow plaques within a retinal arteriole. In *retinal artery occlusion*, there is diffuse whitening of the retina and a *cherry-red spot* in the center of the macula. This area remains red because its blood supply comes from the unaffected choroidal circulation. The etiology of this spot is different from that of the cherry-red spot associated with Tay-Sachs disease, which results from the deposition of storage material (sphingolipids) within the retina (Fig. 215-18).

Another macular condition is *macular hypoplasia*, which is incomplete development of the macula and is commonly seen in albinism. A *bull's-eye macular lesion* is a macula that has abnormal concentric rings around it. Multiple conditions are associated with *pigmentary changes in the macula*, including the mucopolysaccharidoses. In *macular pucker*, there are fine wrinkles around the macula caused by a preretinal membrane. A characteristic finding known as *angioid streaks* (because they resemble blood vessels) develops in patients with acromegaly. These streaks result from breaks in Bruch membrane, which lies underneath the retina (Fig. 215-19). Sometimes, neovascularization from the choroid penetrates these breaks, causing subretinal bleeding. Angioid streaks also occur in pseudoxanthoma elasticum, Paget disease, sickle cell anemia, and *Ehlers-Danlos syndrome*. *Ischemic infarcts of the choroid* appear as yellowish spots with central pigmentation. They are seen in toxemia of pregnancy.

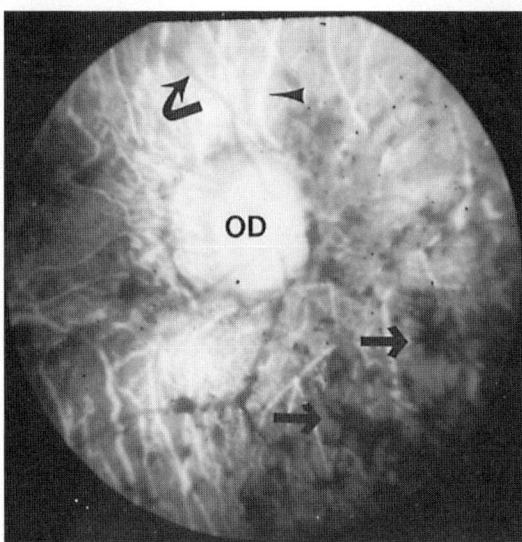

**FIGURE 215-16.** Pigment clumping in retinitis pigmentosa. Note that the pigment on the retinal surface (*straight arrows*) of the optic disc (*OD*) is pale, the waxy retinal vessels are narrowed (*curved arrow*), and the deeper choroidal vessels can readily be seen through the atrophic retina (*arrowhead*). (Courtesy of Peter Y. Evans, MD.)

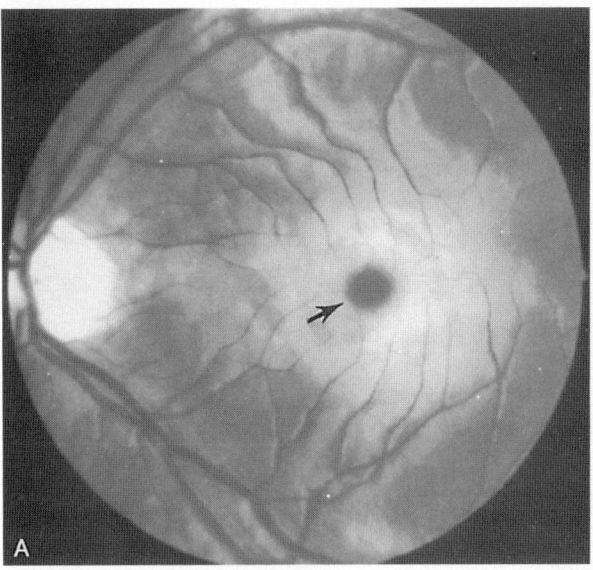 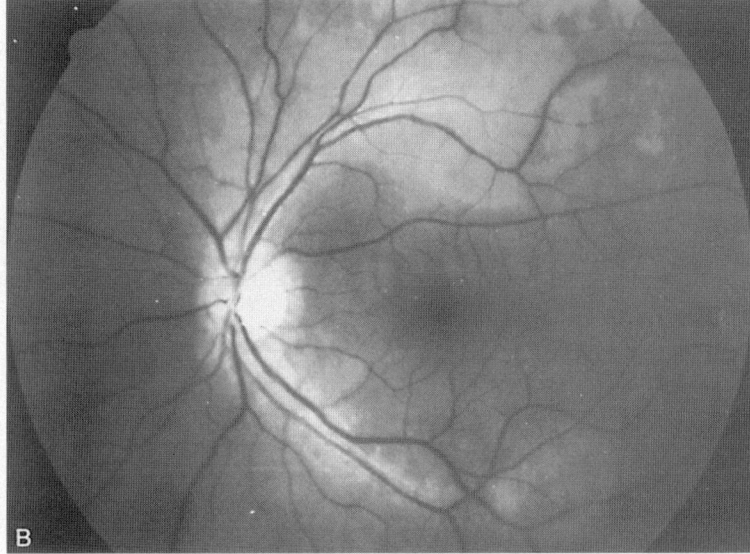

**FIGURE 215-18.** Cherry-red spot appearance (*arrow*) of macula in patient with Tay-Sachs disease (**A**). Compare to normal macula (**B**).

## OPTIC NERVE

The *optic nerve* is a relatively easy structure to observe using a direct ophthalmoscope and is preferably viewed through a dilated pupil. It should be examined for evidence of swelling, which produces elevation, and for atrophy. Although the direct ophthalmoscope does not provide a stereoscopic view, with experience, elevation of the optic disc is readily appreciated. Optic disc swelling results from the interruption of axonal transport. Blood vessels, particularly the small vessels lining the rim of the disc, appear to be engorged. Flame-shaped hemorrhages may also be found along the disc margin, which is obscured by the swollen axons.

The differential diagnosis of *optic disc edema* is extensive. Optic disc edema may be seen in endocrine conditions including diabetes, hyperthyroidism, pregnancy, Addison disease, hypoparathyroidism, and hyperparathyroidism.[56,57]

In *papilledema*, there is optic disc edema due to increased intracranial pressure. On examination, there is usually bilateral (often asymmetric) elevation of the optic discs with a diminished or absent central depression (Fig. 215-20). Spontaneous venous pulsations are absent. Note that these pulsations may be absent in 20% of normal patients.

*Pseudotumor cerebri* refers to papilledema associated with elevated cerebrospinal fluid pressure in the presence of a normal head imaging scan and normal cerebrospinal fluid composition.

*Optic neuritis* is usually unilateral and causes an acute impairment of vision. The inflammation is retrobulbar in two-thirds of cases with a normal-appearing optic disc initially. Greater than 60% of patients with optic neuritis will develop multiple sclerosis.

*Ischemic optic neuropathy* results from infarction of the optic nerve. It causes acute loss of vision. The optic disc is usually swollen, and flame-shaped hemorrhages are often present. Anterior ischemic optic neuropathy may be arteritic (related to giant cell

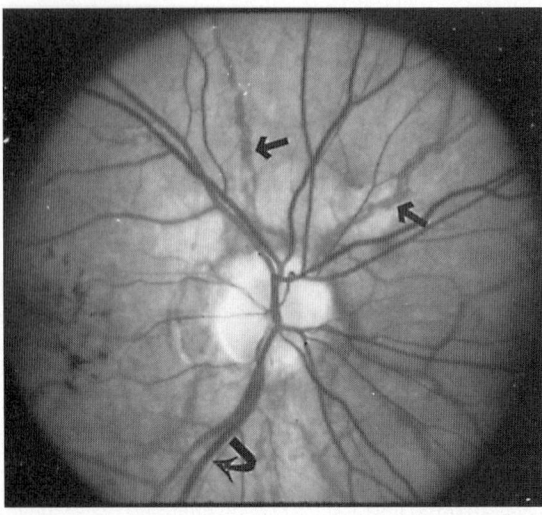 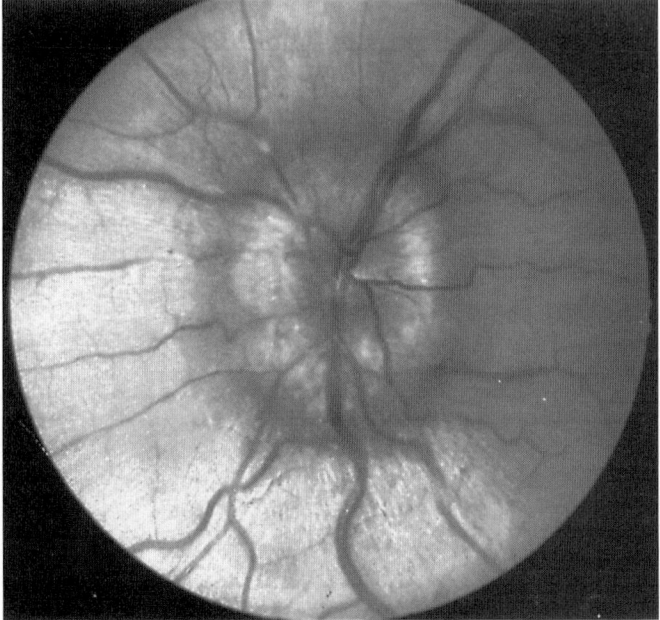

**FIGURE 215-19.** Angioid streaks. Breaks in the Bruch membrane (*straight arrows*) form cracks that resemble retinal vessels (*curved arrow*). (Courtesy of William J. Shields, CRA.)

**FIGURE 215-20.** Patient with papilledema; there is swelling of the optic disc as a result of increased intracranial pressure. Note the loss of the central cup.

arteritis) or nonarteritic. *Giant cell arteritis*, occurring predominantly in patients older than 55 years, should be suspected, especially if relevant symptoms are present. These symptoms include headache, scalp pain, weight loss, fever, malaise, temporal tenderness, jaw claudication, and polymyalgia rheumatica.

*Optic nerve drusen* are hyaline-like bodies within the optic nerve. If they are superficial, the drusen look like yellow globules clustered on the surface of the optic nerve head. If they are located deeper within the nerve head, they are not directly visible and are a cause of pseudopapilledema.

*Optic atrophy* is recognized by optic disc pallor, with associated changes in retinal vessels, that is accompanied by visual dysfunction. Pathologically, this is due to shrinkage of the optic nerve as a result of any process that causes degeneration of the axons in the anterior visual system. Many endocrine and metabolic abnormalities are associated with optic atrophy.

*Optic nerve hypoplasia* refers to an optic disc that is underdeveloped. The disc is usually pale and smaller than normal. It is one of the causes of decreased vision or blindness in newborn infants. Septooptic dysplasia, or de Morsier syndrome, is optic nerve hypoplasia associated with midline cerebral defects, such as absence of the septum pellucidum. Optic nerve hypoplasia is also associated with various pituitary abnormalities, including growth hormone deficiency, hypothyroidism, diabetes insipidus, and neonatal hypoglycemia.[58–60] It is standard practice for an ophthalmologist who is caring for an infant with optic nerve hypoplasia to obtain a magnetic resonance imaging study to rule out an absent septum pellucidum and to refer the patient for a pediatric endocrine evaluation. Approximately 10% of eyes from patients with bilateral optic nerve hypoplasia have vision of 20/60 or better.[61]

## OCULAR EFFECTS OF METABOLIC DISEASES

Many metabolic abnormalities are accompanied by significant ocular changes (Table 215-2). In some cases, changes noted in the

**TABLE 215-2.**
**Metabolic Disease Affecting the Eye**

| Disease or Disorder | Basic Defect/ Abnormality | Lids/Orbit/ Motility | Conjunctiva/Sclera/ Cornea | Iris/Lens/ Glaucoma | Retina | Optic Nerve |
|---|---|---|---|---|---|---|
| **AMINO ACID AND/OR ENZYMATIC ABNORMALITIES** | | | | | | |
| Albinism | Tyrosinase deficiency | Nystagmus; strabismus | | Iris transillumination | Pale fundus; foveal hypoplasia | |
| Alkaptonuria | Homogentisic acid oxidase deficiency | | Cornea pigmentation; brown scleral deposits (ochronosis) | | | |
| Cystinosis | Lysosomal storage disorder | | Conjunctival and corneal crystals | Iris crystals | Peripheral retinitis pigmentosa | |
| Familial dysautonomia (Riley-Day syndrome) | Dopamine-β-hydroxylase deficiency | Exotropia | Corneal ulcer; decreased corneal sensation; alacrima | | | |
| Homocystinuria | Cystathionine β-synthase deficiency | | | Ectopia lentis; myopia (often inferonasal); secondary glaucoma; cataracts; optic atrophy | Peripheral retinal degeneration | |
| Hyperlysinemia | Hydroxylysine kinase deficiency | | | Ectopia lentis; spherophakia | | |
| Hyperornithinemia | Ornithine transferase deficiency | | | Cataracts; myopia | Gyrate atrophy of the retina and choroid; night blindness | |
| Hypophosphatasia | Alkaline phosphatase deficiency | Proptosis | Band keratopathy | | | Papilledema |
| Lowe oculocerebrorenal syndrome | Unknown | | | Congenital cataract, glaucoma; miosis | Albinism | |
| Phenylketonuria (Folling disease) | Phenylalanine hydroxylase deficiency | | Photophobia | Cataracts | | |
| Hereditary xanthinuria-sulfite oxidase deficiency (combined deficiency) | Xanthine oxidase and sulfite oxidase deficiency | | | Ectopia lentis | | Optic atrophy |
| Tyrosinemia II | Tyrosine aminotransferase deficiency | | Conjunctival plaques Corneal ulcers (pseudo-dendrite appearance—i.e., linear branching); corneal vascularization | | | |
| **LIPOPROTEIN AND LIPID METABOLISM DISORDERS** | | | | | | |
| Abetalipoproteinemia (Bassen-Kornzweig syndrome) | β-Lipoprotein deficiency | Ptosis; ophthalmoplegia | | Cataracts | Atypical retinitis pigmentosa | |
| Hyperlipoproteinemia | | | | | | |
| Type I | Lipoprotein lipase deficiency | Eruptive xanthomas of lid; nystagmus | | | Lipemia retinalis; retinal hemorrhages; salmon-colored retina; retinal deposits | |

(continued)

**TABLE 215-2.**
**Metabolic Disease Affecting the Eye  (Continued)**

| Disease or Disorder | Basic Defect/ Abnormality | Lids/Orbit/ Motility | Conjunctiva/Sclera/ Cornea | Iris/Lens/ Glaucoma | Retina | Optic Nerve |
|---|---|---|---|---|---|---|
| Type II (hyperbetalipoproteinemia) | Abnormal function of the low-density lipoprotein (LDL) receptor | Xanthelasma | Corneal arcus; conjunctival xanthoma | | | |
| Type III (broad-beta disease) | Abnormal levels of triglycerides, cholesterol, and β-lipoproteins | Xanthelasma | Corneal arcus | | Lipemia retinalis | |
| Type IV (hyperprebetalipoproteinemia) | Increased triglycerides | Eruptive xanthomas | | | Lipemia retinalis | |
| Type V (hyperprebetalipoproteinemia and hyperchylomicronemia) | Fasting chylomicronemia and increased very-low-density lipoprotein (VLDL) | Eruptive xanthomas | Dry eye | | Lipemia retinalis; retinal and choroidal xanthomas | |
| Fish eye disease | Increased levels of triglycerides | | Corneal opacification | | | |
| Lecithin-cholesterol acyltransferase deficiency (LCAT disease) | Lecithin-cholesterol acyltransferase deficiency | | Corneal deposits; corneal arcus | | | |
| Refsum disease | Phytanic acid α-hydroxylase deficiency | | Thick, hazy corneal epithelium; higher visibility of corneal nerves | Cataracts; miosis | Pigmentary retinopathy; night blindness | |
| Tangier disease | High-density lipoprotein deficiency | | Corneal stromal opacities; corneal arcus | | | |
| Lipomucopolysaccharidosis (MLS I), or sialidosis | Sialidase deficiency | | Corneal opacities | | Cherry-red macula | |
| Mucolipidosis II (MLS II, or I-cell disease) | Deficiency of unknown acid adrolases | | Corneal opacities | Glaucoma; lens opacities | Cherry-red macula | |
| Mucolipidosis III (MLS III, or pseudo-Hurler polydystrophy) | Deficiency of unknown acid hydrolases | | Corneal opacities | | | |
| Mucolipidosis IV | Deficiency of unknown acid hydrolases | Puffy lids; convergent strabismus | Corneal clouding | | | |
| **LYSOSOMAL ENZYME DISORDERS** | | | | | | |
| Glucosylceramide lipidosis (Gaucher disease), types I, II, and III | Glucocerebrosidase deficiency | Oculomotor apraxia | | Brownish scleral discoloration | Cherry-red macula | |
| Angiokeratoma corporis diffusum (Fabry disease) | Ceramide trihexosidase deficiency | Periorbital edema; nystagmus | Corneal epithelial whorl-like deposits; tortuous conjunctival vessels (corneal verticillata) | Posterior spoke-like cataracts | Tortuous retinal vessels; retinal or macular edema | Papilledema; optic atrophy |
| Ceramidase deficiency (Farber lipogranulomatosis) | Lysosomal acid ceramidase deficiency | | Conjunctival granulomas; corneal opacities | Lens opacities | Gray retina; cherry-red spots | |
| Orthochromic leukodystrophy (Pelizaeus-Merzbacher) | Myelin metabolism defects | | | | | Optic atrophy |
| Gangliosidosis GM$_1$, type 1 (Landing disease) | Acid β-galactosidase A, B, C deficiency | | Corneal clouding | | Cherry-red spot retinal hemorrhages | |
| Gangliosidosis GM$_1$, type 2 (Derry disease or juvenile generalized gangliosidosis) | β-Galactosidase B and C deficiency | Nystagmus | | | Pigmentary retinopathy | Optic atrophy |
| Gangliosidosis GM$_2$, type 1 (Tay-Sachs disease) | N-acetylhexosaminadase A deficiency | | | | Cherry-red spot | Optic atrophy |
| Gangliosidosis GM$_2$, type 2 (Sandhoff disease) | N-acetylhexosaminadase A deficiency | | | | Cherry-red spot | Optic atrophy |
| Gangliosidosis GM$_2$, type 3 (juvenile Tay-Sachs or Batten disease) | Partial deficiency of hexosaminadase A | | | | Cherry-red spot | Optic atrophy |
| Fucosidosis | Lysosomal α-fucosidase deficiency | | Tortuous conjunctival vessels; diffuse corneal opacities | | Retinal vascular tortuosity | Optic atrophy; cortical blindness |
| Globoid cell leukodystrophy (Krabbe disease) | Galactosylceramide-β-galactosidase deficiency | | | | | |
| Lactosylceramidosis | Lactosylceramide galactosyl hydrolase deficiency | | | | Macular grayness or redness | Optic atrophy |
| Metachromatic leukodystrophy | Arylsulfatase A deficiency | Abnormal extraocular movements | Corneal clouding | Papillary abnormalities | Cherry-red spot | |

(continued)

**TABLE 215-2.**
Metabolic Disease Affecting the Eye  (Continued)

| Disease or Disorder | Basic Defect/ Abnormality | Lids/Orbit/ Motility | Conjunctiva/Sclera/ Cornea | Iris/Lens/ Glaucoma | Retina | Optic Nerve |
|---|---|---|---|---|---|---|
| Sphingomyelin lipidosis (Niemann-Pick disease) | Sphingomyelinase deficiency | Periorbital puffiness | Corneal clouding | Yellowish discoloration of lens | Cherry-red spot; macula | |
| Type A | Sphingomyelinase deficiency | | | | Cherry-red spot | |
| Type B | Sphingomyelinase deficiency | | | | Macular halo syndrome | |
| Type C | Esterification of cholesterol metabolically blocked | Paralysis of downgaze; progression to total supranuclear ophthalmoplegia | | | | |
| Type D | Unknown | No ocular manifestations | | | | |
| Type E | Unknown | | | | Possible cherry-red spot | |
| **MUCOPOLYSACCHARIDOSES** | | | | | | |
| Hurler syndrome (mucopolysaccharidosis I-H) | α-L-Iduronidase deficiency | | Early corneal clouding | | Pigmentary retinopathy | |
| Scheie disease (mucopolysaccharidosis I-S; formerly MPS-V) | α-L-Iduronidase deficiency | | Corneal clouding | | Pigmentary retinopathy | |
| Hurler-Scheie compound (mucopolysaccharidosis I-H/S) | α-L-Iduronidase deficiency | | Corneal clouding | | | |
| Hunter syndrome (mucopolysaccharidosis II) | Iduronate sulfate deficiency | | Late corneal clouding | | Pigmentary retinopathy | |
| Sanfilippo syndrome, type A (mucopolysaccharidosis II-A) | Heparan sulfatase deficiency | | | | Pigmentary retinopathy | |
| Sanfilippo syndrome, type B (mucopolysaccharidosis III-B) | N-acetyl-α-D-glucosaminidase deficiency | | | | Pigmentary retinopathy | |
| Morquio syndrome (mucopolysaccharidosis IV-A) | N-acetylgalactosamine-6-sulfatase deficiency | | Corneal clouding | | | |
| Maroteaux-Lamy syndrome (mucopolysaccharidosis VI) | Arysulfatase B deficiency | | Corneal clouding | | | |
| Sly disease (mucopolysaccharidosis VII) | β-Glucuronidase deficiency | | Corneal clouding | | | |
| Mucosulfatidosis | Multiple sulfatase deficiencies | | | | | Optic atrophy |
| **MISCELLANEOUS HERITABLE METABOLIC DEFECTS, DISORDERS** | | | | | | |
| Alström syndrome | Unknown | | | | Retinitis pigmentosa | |
| Laurence-Moon-Biedl syndrome | Unknown | | | | Retinitis pigmentosa | |
| Ullrich-Noonan syndrome (male Turner syndrome) | Unknown | Epicanthal folds; anti-Mongoloid slant of eyes | | | | |
| Werner syndrome | Unknown | | | Juvenile cataracts | | |
| **CONNECTIVE TISSUE DISORDERS** | | | | | | |
| Ehlers-Danlos syndrome, type VI | Lysyl hydroxylase deficiency | Redundant folds of eyelids; easily everted upper lid; strabismus | Microcornea; blue sclera; ocular fragility; keratoconus | Myopia | Retinal angioid streaks | |
| Marfan syndrome | Connective tissue defect | | | Ectopia lentis (superior and temporal dislocation); myopia | Spontaneous retinal detachment | |
| Osteogenesis imperfecta | Defects in type 1 collagen biosynthesis | | Blue sclera; keratoconus | | | |
| Pseudoxanthoma elasticum | Connective tissue defect | | | | Retinal angioid streaks; retinal hemorrhage | |
| **CARBOHYDRATE METABOLISM DISORDERS** | | | | | | |
| Galactosemia | Galactose-1-phosphate-uridyltransferase or galactokinase deficiency | | | Cataract soon after birth | | |
| Von Gierke disease | Glucose-6-phosphatase deficiency | | | | Multiple, bilateral, yellow, paramacular lesions | |

(continued)

**TABLE 215-2.**
**Metabolic Disease Affecting the Eye (Continued)**

| Disease or Disorder | Basic Defect/ Abnormality | Lids/Orbit/ Motility | Conjunctiva/Sclera/ Cornea | Iris/Lens/ Glaucoma | Retina | Optic Nerve |
|---|---|---|---|---|---|---|
| Mannosidosis | Lysosomal α-mannosi-dase deficiency | | | Posterior spoke-like cataracts | | |
| **METAL METABOLISM DISORDERS** | | | | | | |
| Hemochromatosis | Hemosiderin deposi-tion | Hyperpigmenta-tion of lid mar-gins | Increased melanin deposits in perilimbal bulbar conjunctiva (pathognomonic) | | | |
| Wilson disease (hepato-lenticular degenera-tion) | Copper deposition; diminished cerulo-plasmin | | Kayser-Fleischer ring (rusty brown ring at limbal cornea) | Sunflower cataract (radiating deposits on ante-rior lens capsule) | | |
| **PURINE METABOLISM DISORDERS** | | | | | | |
| Gout | Urate deposition | | Corneal cysts; band kerat-opathy; conjunctivitis; episcleritis; scleritis | | | |
| Xanthinuria | Xanthine oxidase defi-ciency | Enophthalmos; nystagmus | | Brushfield spots; lens dislocation | | |
| **PORPHYRIN DISORDERS** | | | | | | |
| Congenital erythropoietic porphyria | Overproduction of porphyrins (type I) | Ectropion; loss of lashes; bilateral exophthalmos; loss of eyebrows | Conjunctival scarring; decreased corneal sen-sitivity; corneal scar-ring; scleromalacia | | Retinal hemor-rhages; choriore-tinitis | Optic atro-phy |

eye are the first indication of the underlying metabolic abnor-mality, and may lead directly to the diagnosis. For example, con-genital cloudy corneas suggest the presence of one of the mucopolysaccharidoses, whereas lens dislocation suggests homocystinuria (see Chap. 191) or Marfan syndrome.

Examination of the fundus in patients with hyperlipidemias sometimes reveals arteries that appear creamy white instead of blood red, particularly in patients with hypertriglyceridemia (see Table 215-2 and Chap. 163). Mucolipidoses and glycogen storage diseases[62] manifest a cherry-red spot, indicating an abnormal deposition in the retina that spares the central fovea and creates the red-centered white appearance.

Many of these findings can be identified readily by an expe-rienced clinician without sophisticated instrumentation. Fre-quently, this responsibility falls to the physician who first examines the patient. Thus, it is essential that endocrinologists be skilled and diligent in the basic ocular examination.[63] When a particular finding or lesion has been identified or is suspected, a more detailed and complete ocular examination can be con-ducted by an ophthalmologist.

## EFFECTS OF BLINDNESS ON THE ENDOCRINE SYSTEM

The bulk of the interaction of endocrinology with ophthalmol-ogy consists of the effect of the endocrine system on the eyes. *Blindness* is a case in which an ocular condition can have an effect on the endocrine system.

The role of *light* in synchronizing the circadian rhythms of various hormones has been investigated by researchers studying blind subjects. No difference was found in the diurnal rhythms of follicle-stimulating hormone and testosterone in a study com-paring these rhythms in blind and sighted men. However, there was an apparent "phase shift" in circulating cortisol levels in the blind subjects, and the cortisol cycle appeared to be independent of the follicle-stimulating hormone and testosterone diurnal cycles.[64] Peak levels of serum cortisol in these individuals occurred between 8:00 a.m. and 4:00 p.m., whereas in sighted subjects, peak levels occurred at 8:00 a.m. and progressively declined between 8:00 a.m. and 4:00 p.m. (See also ref. 65.)

Blindness also appears to have effects on other hormonal lev-els and functions. Long-term testicular function was altered when 1-month-old rats were blinded.[66] Testosterone secretion in blinded rats was consistently lower than that in control animals. In humans, blindness was reported to be associated with decreased urinary excretion of 17-ketosteroids and gonadotro-pins, and this effect was more pronounced when blindness occurred before puberty. Pineal gland activity (see Chap. 10) appeared to mediate the decrease in gonadal function associated with blindness.

## REFERENCES

1. Feldman F, Bain J, Matuk A. Daily assessment of ocular and abnormal vari-ables throughout the menstrual cycle. Arch Ophthalmol 1978; 96:1835.
2. Leach NO, Wallis NE, Lothringer LL, Olson JA. Corneal hydration changes during the normal menstrual cycle. J Reprod Med 1971; 6:15.
3. Sunness J. The pregnant woman's eye. Surv Ophthalmol 1988; 32:219,228,231,233.
4. Pritchard JA, MacDonald PC, Grant NF. Williams obstetrics, 17th ed. Nor-walk, CT: Appleton-Century-Crofts, 1985:137.
5. Sanke RL. Blepharoptosis as a complication of pregnancy. Ann Ophthalmol 1984; 16:720.
6. Schachner SM, Reynolds AC. Horner's syndrome during lumbar epidural analysis for obstetrics. Obstet Gynecol 1982; 59(Suppl):315.
7. Landesman R. Retinal and conjunctival vascular changes in normal and tox-emic pregnancy. Bull NY Acad Med 1955; 31:376.
8. Millodot M. The influence of pregnancy on the sensitivity of the cornea. Ophthalmology 1977; 61:646.
9. Horven I, Gjonnaess H. Corneal indentation pulse and intraocular pressure in pregnancy. Arch Ophthalmol 1974; 91:92.
10. Dieckmann WJ. The toxemias of pregnancy, 2nd ed. St. Louis: Mosby, 1952:240.
11. Sadowsky A, Serr DM, Landau J. Retinal changes and fetal prognosis in the toxemias of pregnancy. Obstet Gynecol 1956; 8:426.
12. Fry WE. Extensive bilateral retinal detachment in eclampsia with complete reattachment. Arch Ophthalmol 1929; 1:609.
13. Hallum AV. Eye changes in hypertensive toxemia of pregnancy. JAMA 1936; 106:1649.
14. Valluri S, Adelberg DA, Curtis RS, Olk RJ. Diagnostic indocyanine green angiography in preeclampsia. Am J Ophthalmol 1996; 122:672.
15. Arvlkumaran S, Gibb DMF, Rauf M, et al. Transient blindness associated with pregnancy-induced hypertension. Br J Obstet Gynaecol 1988; 92:847.
16. Beck RW, Gamel JW, Willcourt RJ, et al. Acute ischemic optic neuropathy in severe preeclampsia. Am J Ophthalmol 1980; 90:342.
17. Sunness JS, Haller JA, Fine SL. Central serous chorioretinopathy and preg-nancy. Arch Ophthalmol 1993; 111:360.

18. Bedrossian R. Central serous retinopathy and pregnancy. (Letter). Am J Ophthalmol 1974; 78:152.

19. Digre KB, Varner MW, Corbett JJ. Pseudotumor cerebri and pregnancy. Neurology 1984; 34:721.

20. Maycock RL, Sullivan RD, Greening RR, Jones R. Sarcoidosis and pregnancy. JAMA 1957; 164:158.

21. Snyder DA, Tessler HH. Vogt-Koyanagi-Harada syndrome. Am J Ophthalmol 1980; 90:69.

22. Cassar J, Hamilton AM, Kohner EM. Diabetic retinopathy in pregnancy. Int Ophthalmol Clin 1978; 18:179.

23. Ohrt V. The influence of pregnancy on diabetic retinopathy with special regard to the reversible changes shown in 100 pregnancies. Acta Ophthalmol (Copenh) 1984; 62:603.

24. Moloney JBM, Drury MI. The effect of pregnancy on the natural course of diabetic retinopathy. Am J Ophthalmol 1982; 93:745.

25. Chen HC, Newsom RSB, Patel V, et al. Retinal blood flow changes during pregnancy in women with diabetes. Invest Ophthalmol Vis Sci 1994; 35:3199.

26. Seddon JM, MacLaughlin DT, Albert PM, et al. Uveal melanomas presenting during pregnancy and the investigation of estrogen receptors in melanomas. Br J Ophthalmol 1982; 66:695.

27. Egan KM, Walsh SM, Seddon JM, Gragoudas ES. An evaluation of the influence of reproductive factors on the risk of metastases from uveal melanoma. Ophthalmology 1993; 100:1160.

28. Shields CL, Shields JA, Eagle RC, et al. Uveal melanoma and pregnancy. Ophthalmology 1991; 98:1667.

29. Wan WL, Geller JL, Feldon SE, Sadun AA. Visual loss caused by rapidly progressive intracranial meningiomas during pregnancy. Ophthalmology 1990; 97:18.

30. Warren DW. Hormonal influences on the lacrimal gland. Int Ophthalmol Clin 1994; 34(1):19.

31. Mathers WD, Stovall D, Lane JA, et al. Menopause and tear function: the influence of prolactin and sex hormones on human tear production. Cornea 1998; 17:353.

32. Radnot M, Follman P. Ocular side-effects of oral contraceptives. Ann Clin Res 1972; 5:197.

33. Davidson SI. Reported adverse effects of oral contraceptives on the eye. Trans Ophthalmol Soc UK 1971; 91:561.

34. Stowe GC, Zakov ZN, Albert DM. Central retinal vascular occlusions associated with oral contraceptives. Am J Ophthalmol 1978; 86:798.

35. Svarc ED, Werner D. Isolated retinal hemorrhages associated with oral contraceptives. Am J Ophthalmol 1977; 84:50.

36. Rock T, Dinar Y, Romem M. Retinal periphlebitis after hormonal treatment. Ann Ophthalmol 1989; 21:75.

36a. Lake SR, Vernon SA. Emergency contraception and retinal vein thrombosis. Br J Ophthalmol 2000; 84:144.

37. Giovannini A, Consolani A. Contraceptive-induced unilateral retinopathy. Ophthalmologica 1979; 179:302.

38. Voke J. Colour vision and the pill. Nurs Times 1974; 70:139.

39. Gerner E. Ocular toxicity of tamoxifen. Ann Ophthalmol 1989; 21:420.

40. Netland PA, Dallon RL. Thyroid ophthalmopathy. In: Albert GM, Jakobiec FA, eds. Principles and practice of ophthalmology, vol 5. Philadelphia: WB Saunders, 1994:2937.

41. Roy FH. Ocular differential diagnosis, 5th ed. Philadelphia: Lea & Febiger, 1993:289,316.

41a. Tripathi RC, Parapuram SK, Tripathi BJ, et al. Corticosteroids and glaucoma risk. Drugs Aging 1999; 15:439.

42. Mahto RS. Ocular features of hypoparathyroidism. Br J Ophthalmol 1972; 56:546.

43. Blake J. Eye signs in idiopathic hypoparathyroidism. Trans Ophthalmol Soc U K 1976; 96:448.

44. Lundberg PO. Hereditary myopathy, oligophrenia, cataract, skeletal abnormalities and hypergonadotropic hypogonadism. Eur Neurol 1973; 10:261.

45. Chlack LT Jr. Mechanism of "hypoglycemic" cataract formation in the rat lens. I. The role of hexokinase instability. Invest Ophthalmol 1975; 14:746.

46. Merin S, Crawford JS. Hypoglycemia and infantile cataract. Arch Ophthalmol 1971; 86:495.

47. Saadat H, Bahrami Y. Blindness: a postoperative complication of pheochromocytoma. Virginia Med 1977; 104:38.

48. Hagler WS, Hyman BN, Waters WC. Von Hippel's angiomatosis retinae and pheochromocytoma. Trans Am Acad Ophthalmol Otolaryngol 1971; 75:1022.

49. Brown AC, Pollard ZF, Jarret H. Ocular and testicular abnormalities in alopecia areata. Arch Dermatol 1982; 118:546.

50. Chang RJ, Davidson BJ, Carlson HE, et al. Hypogonadotropic hypogonadism associated with retinitis pigmentosa in a female sibship: evidence for gonadotropin deficiency. J Clin Endocrinol Metab 1981; 53:1179.

51. Edwards JA, Sethi PK, Scoma AJ, et al. A new familial syndrome characterized by pigmentary retinopathy, hypogonadism, mental retardation, nerve deafness and glucose intolerance. Am J Med 1976; 60:23.

52. Rizzo JF, Berson EL, Lessell S. Retinal and neurologic findings in Laurence-Moon-Bardet-Biedl phenotype. Ophthalmology 1986; 93:1452.

53. Lee ES, Galle PC, McDonough PG. The Laurence-Moon-Bardet-Biedl syndrome. Case report and endocrinologic evaluation. J Reprod Med 1986; 31:353.

54. Brownlie BEW, Newton OAG, Singh SP. Ophthalmopathy associated with primary hypothyroidism. Acta Endocrinol (Copenh) 1975; 79:691.

55. Pellock JM, Behrens M, Lewis L, et al. Kearns Sayre syndrome and hypoparathyroidism. Ann Neurol 1978; 3:455.

56. Bajandas FJ, Smith JL. Optic neuritis in hypoparathyroidism. Neurology 1976; 26:451.

57. Murphy KJ. Papilloedema due to hyperparathyroidism. Br J Ophthalmol 1974; 58:694.

58. Costin G, Murphree AL. Hypothalamic-pituitary function in children with optic nerve hypoplasia. Am J Dis Child 1985; 139:249.

59. Hoyt WF, Koplan SL, Grumbach MM, et al. Septo-optic dysplasia and pituitary dwarfism. Lancet 1970; 1:893.

60. Sheridan SJ, Robb RM. Optic nerve hypoplasia and diabetes insipidus. J Pediatr Ophthalmol 1978; 15:82.

61. Siatkowski RM, Sanchez JC, Andrade R, Alvarez A. The clinical, neuroradiographic, and endocrinologic profile of patients with bilateral optic nerve hypoplasia. Ophthalmology 1997; 104:493.

62. Collins JE, Leonard JV. Hepatic glycogen storage disease. Br J Hosp Med 1987; 38:168.

63. Newell FW. Ophthalmology. Principles and concepts, 5th ed. St. Louis: Mosby, 1985:165.

64. Bodenheimer S, Winter JSD, Faiman C. Diurnal rhythms of serum gonadotropins, testosterone, estradiol and cortisol in blind men. J Clin Endocrinol Metab 1973; 37:472.

65. Lockley SW, Skene DJ, James K, et al. Melatonin administration can entrain the free-running circadian system of blind subjects. J Endocrinol 2000; 164:R1.

66. Kinson G, Liu CC. Long-term testicular responses to blinding in rats. Life Sci 1974; 14:2179.

---

# CHAPTER 216

# OTOLARYNGOLOGY AND ENDOCRINE DISEASE

STEPHEN G. HARNER

Endocrine diseases can manifest themselves in four ways that are of concern to the otolaryngologist. The first is when head and neck manifestations are a major component of the disease (e.g., the hearing loss that occurs in Pendred syndrome) (see Chap. 47). The second is when certain findings are commonly associated with the disease but are not invariably present (e.g., mixed hearing loss and Paget disease). Another situation of concern is when certain findings are occasionally present and are thought to be a part of the disease process or condition, but the relationship is unclear (e.g., facial palsy in pregnancy). Finally, some associations between clinical findings and endocrine disease have been accepted but may be no more than a chance relationship (e.g., Ménière syndrome and diabetes mellitus).

A thorough otolaryngologic workup includes history-taking; a specialized physical examination; tests such as audiometry, electronystagmography, posturography, and brainstem evoked response audiometry; appropriate imaging studies; fiberoptic examination; voice analysis; and biopsy. The features evaluated include hearing loss, voice change, nasal obstruction, neck masses, and dizziness. In this way, the cause of the disorder and the appropriate mode of therapy are determined.

## HYPOTHALAMUS

Several of the processes that cause altered hypothalamic activity appear to be associated with a vasomotor rhinitis. Moreover, some genetically induced syndromes affect the hypothalamus and have other associated otolaryngologic findings. Laurence-Moon-Biedl syndrome (a syndrome characterized by retinitis pigmentosa, polydactylism, mental defects, and hypogonadism) and Alström syndrome (an autosomal recessive disorder marked by hypogonadism, atypical retinitis pigmentosa, and diabetes mellitus) often are associated with obesity and sensori-

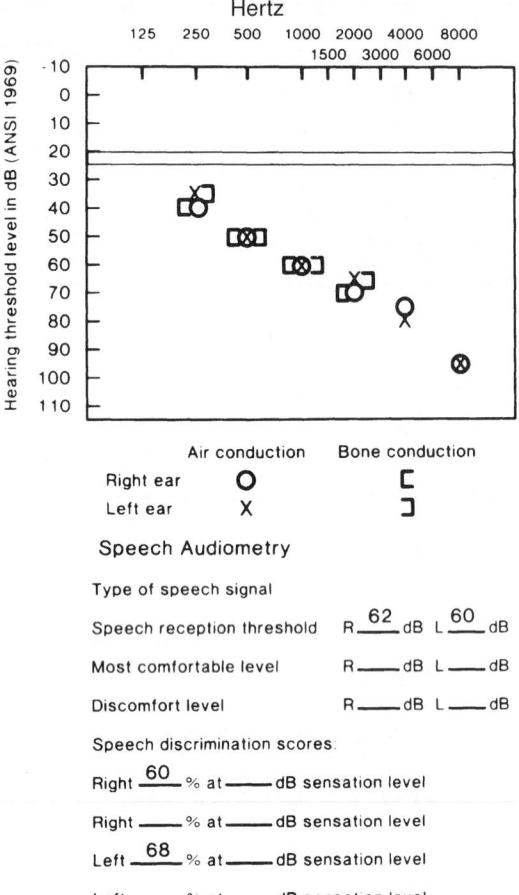

**FIGURE 216-1.** Typical sensorineural hearing loss, which is equal in both ears. The air and bone responses are identical. Notice that bone conduction cannot be tested at intensities of >70 dB. Speech reception threshold is the sound intensity at which the subject begins to hear words. Speech discrimination is the ability to understand a list of unrelated words. Sensorineural hearing loss is the most common type of loss. Treatment usually involves the use of hearing aids and aural rehabilitation. (*ANSI*, American National Standards Institute.)

neural hearing loss as well (Fig. 216-1). Deafness is associated with diabetes insipidus in the DIDMOAD syndrome[1] (*d*iabetes *i*nsipidus, *d*iabetes *m*ellitus, *o*ptic *a*trophy, and *d*eafness). In olfactory-genital dysplasia (Kallmann syndrome), anosmia is the primary feature (see Chap. 115).[1a] Craniopharyngiomas (see Chap. 11) are congenital cysts that arise in the basisphenoid and may erode into the pituitary and hypothalamus. This tumor usually appears as a cystic mass in the sphenoid and nasopharynx; it may be detected on the basis of clinical signs or on an imaging study of the sinuses. The treatment options include transoral and transnasal resections.

## PITUITARY GLAND

In acromegaly, the tongue is increased in size. Also, most affected patients have a change in voice that consists of decreased pitch and a huskier sound. Occasionally, the recurrent laryngeal nerve is stretched, which causes vocal cord paralysis. If the condition does not improve spontaneously, the voice change can be treated by thyroplasty.

A patient may develop diabetes insipidus as a result of trauma to the skull base secondary to an operation or a disease process that is otolaryngologic in origin. Large pituitary tumors can infiltrate the sinuses.

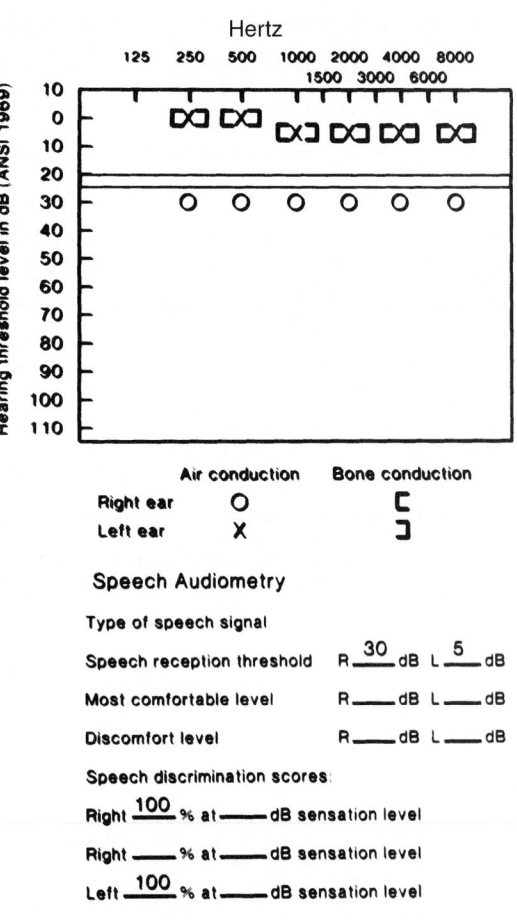

**FIGURE 216-2.** Audiogram demonstrates normal hearing in the left ear and conductive hearing loss in the right ear. Notice that the air conduction levels in the right ear are separated from the bone conduction markers. The speech reception threshold corresponds to the air conduction level. Speech discrimination scores are normal in both ears. This type of hearing loss usually is associated with some malfunction in the ossicular chain, tympanic membrane, or external ear canal. Surgical correction usually is possible. (*ANSI*, American National Standards Institute.)

The major interest of the otolaryngologist in pituitary disease has been patient management. The transseptal-transsphenoidal surgical approach is primarily a team procedure in which the rhinologist provides access for the neurosurgeon.[2,3] This type of cooperative effort has markedly improved the management and outcome of these patients (see Chap. 23).

## THYROID GLAND

With hyperthyroidism (thyrotoxicosis, Graves disease), a patient may have a goiter and Graves ophthalmopathy. Often, the otolaryngologist is involved in the surgical management of the ophthalmopathy. Transantral orbital decompression is the most widely used surgical procedure for this condition.[4] This procedure allows removal of the inferior and medial orbital walls to provide space for the excess tissue in the sinuses. No external incisions are necessary, and complications are minimal. Endoscopic decompression has been described and appears successful (see Chap. 43).[5]

A number of pertinent findings are associated with myxedema (hypothyroidism). A conductive hearing loss secondary to serous otitis media may be present (Fig. 216-2). Also, a sensorineural hearing loss may be present. The conductive loss usually resolves with treatment, but the sensorineural loss generally persists. Generalized mucosal edema produces nasal obstruction, thickened tongue, facial edema, hoarseness, and slowed speech. Although diagnosis is rarely a problem, if doubt arises, biopsy of the nasal mucosa can be performed and will reveal an increase in acid mucopolysaccharide content.

Carcinoma of the thyroid may present as a mass in the gland, a neck mass of unknown cause, or a cause of vocal cord paralysis. Vocal cord paralysis secondary to recurrent laryngeal nerve involvement or surgical trauma often responds to thyroplasty, arytenoidectomy, or other appropriate therapy.[6,7] When the tumor is under control, the customary practice is to wait 6 months before instituting therapy. If the prognosis is poor, however, and the patient is having trouble with aspiration or a weak voice, the therapy is performed immediately. Acute bacterial thyroiditis (see Chaps. 46 and 213) may be associated with a large neck mass, hoarseness, vocal cord paralysis, or a compromised airway. In such cases, tracheostomy or vocal cord injection with fat may be indicated.

An infant with congenital hypothyroidism (cretinism) usually presents with a severe sensorineural hearing loss (see Fig. 216-1), a broad flat nose, and a high-pitched cry[8] (see Chap. 47). Correction of the hypothyroidism improves the voice, but the hearing loss remains. In Pendred syndrome[9]—a rare congenital syndrome associated with bilateral sensorineural hearing loss and a euthyroid goiter—the hearing loss involves high-frequency sound primarily, is of varying severity, and is nonreversible. The goiter results from a defect in the organification of thyroid hormone. Thyroid function tests are normal, and the diagnosis is confirmed using a perchlorate washout test. No treatment is available, but genetic counseling may be appropriate.[10] Another nontreatable syndrome—Hollander syndrome—is characterized by progressive sensorineural hearing loss and euthyroid goiter.

## CALCIUM AND PHOSPHATE METABOLISM

Patients with hyperparathyroidism may have hearing loss, dysphagia, fasciculations of the tongue, tumors of the facial bones, and lesions of the oral mucosa. The hearing loss is sensorineural and nonreversible (see Fig. 216-1). The lesions seen in the facial bones are called brown tumors (osteitis fibrosa cystica). These lesions are benign, are most often located in the maxilla, and need not be excised unless they cause functional or cosmetic problems. The nodular lesion of the oral mucosa, called epulis, requires no therapy. Hyperparathyroidism is an important component of multiple endocrine neoplasia (MEN) (see Chap. 188). In MEN type 1, the findings may include those of hyperparathyroidism, pituitary tumor, and pancreatic tumor. In MEN type 2A, hyperparathyroidism, pheochromocytoma, and medullary thyroid carcinoma (occasionally presenting as a neck mass) are found. In MEN type 2B, the findings include medullary thyroid cancer, pheochromocytoma, and neuromas involving the mucosa lining the lips, oral cavity, nose, larynx, and eyes; hyperparathyroidism is rare. These neuromas are histologically benign, but their presence should alert the clinician to the possibility of a MEN syndrome. In any patient suspected of having MEN type 2A or 2B, the clinician must screen for pheochromocytoma preoperatively. If a secreting pheochromocytoma is present, anesthesia and surgery are exceedingly risky.[11]

Hypercalcemia that is unrelated to parathyroid malfunction may be seen with malignant lesions involving the head and neck region and with sarcoidosis (see Chap. 59). Careful head and neck examination should reveal any primary cancer. Sarcoidosis causes many characteristic findings in the head and neck region.[12,13] Granular lesions of the nasal mucosa, ulcers of the larynx, neck masses, and swelling of the salivary glands are commonly seen. Hypoparathyroidism with hypocalcemia pro-

duces nerve irritability, which causes laryngeal stridor, laryngospasm, and a positive Chvostek sign (see Chap. 60). Frequently, this hypoparathyroidism is a sequela of a surgical procedure in the neck. Severe hypocalcemia and hypomagnesemia can cause bilateral vocal cord paralysis.[14]

Hypophosphatasia, as well as hyperphosphatasia, has been reported to occur in infants found to have an associated hearing loss.[15]

## METABOLIC BONE DISEASE

Several metabolic diseases of bone produce significant otolaryngologic findings, one of which is Paget disease of the bone (see Chap. 65). This is a disease process that has truly protean manifestations that are revealed in middle and old age. Skull changes are relatively common, as is involvement of the temporal bone. Clinically, a significant number of these patients have hearing loss. Classically, this loss begins as a mixed hearing loss and then becomes purely sensorineural (Fig. 216-3). Moreover, these

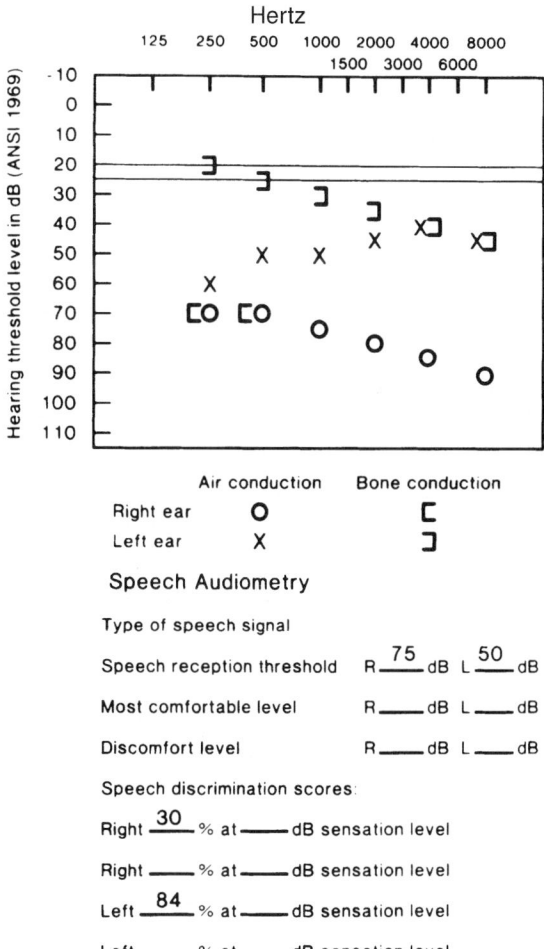

**FIGURE 216-3.** Audiogram reflects the type of hearing loss that is often seen with Paget disease of the bone. In the left ear, a mixed hearing loss is present: part of the loss is sensorineural and part is conductive. Notice the separation, in the low frequencies, between air conduction and bone conduction levels on the left side. The speech reception threshold corresponds to the air conduction level, but speech discrimination remains fairly good at this point. The hearing level in the right ear is fairly typical of end-stage Paget disease of the temporal bone. This is a fairly severe sensorineural hearing loss with poor speech discrimination. In such cases, the mixed hearing loss might occur relatively early in the course of the disease, whereas the sensorineural hearing loss might occur relatively late. (*ANSI*, American National Standards Institute.)

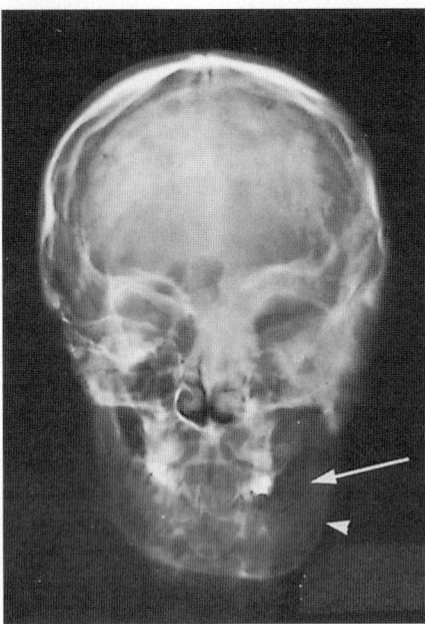

**FIGURE 216-4.** Radiograph showing fibrous dysplasia of the left maxilla. Severe cystic involvement (*arrow*), overall expansion of the bone, and extreme thinning of the cortex (*arrowhead*) are evident. Notice the asymmetry of the orbits, as well as the gross deformity of the left orbit.

patients can have tinnitus and vertigo, which seem to be related to the disease.[16] Calcitonin therapy may halt the progress of the involvement.[17]

Osteogenesis imperfecta is a genetically induced disease with varying levels of involvement[18] (see Chaps. 66, 70, and 189). Affected patients may have a conductive hearing loss secondary to involvement of the ossicular chain. Clinically and histologically, the condition is identical to otosclerosis. Surgical treatment and use of hearing aids may be necessary. At operation, if the incus is involved, performing a stapedectomy may not be possible.

In fibrous dysplasia (see Chap. 66), the maxilla is the bone most commonly involved in the head (Fig. 216-4). Mass lesions can form anywhere, leading to cosmetic and functional problems.[19,20] These lesions can be debulked or removed, but they have a tendency to recur. Malignant transformation is rare but is more likely if the patient has been irradiated.[21]

Osteopetrosis (Albers-Schönberg disease) may have otologic complications as well. The involvement varies greatly from patient to patient, but the temporal bone is commonly affected.[22] Temporal bone disease causes sensorineural and conductive hearing losses. Usually, these are not treatable except with a hearing aid. Moreover, facial paralysis may be seen; this tends to be recurrent, and decompression often is advised. Dental caries occurs frequently and is severe. This condition may cause osteomyelitis of the mandible, which is difficult to control.

## ADRENAL CORTEX

Patients with adrenal insufficiency (Addison disease) may present with sunken eyes, dry tongue, and hyperpigmentation of the skin and tongue (see Chap. 76). Endolymphatic hydrops (Ménière syndrome), dysosmia, and dysgeusia all have been reported to occur with adrenal insufficiency. Adrenocortical hyperactivity (Cushing disease) causes moon facies and prominent supraclavicular fat pads.

## PREGNANCY

The most common otolaryngologic abnormality related to pregnancy is a severe vasomotor rhinitis. This usually arises in the second or third trimester. No predisposing factors have been identified. Treatment with decongestants is of limited benefit. Another unusual finding is hoarseness, which arises from vascular engorgement of the true and false vocal cords. An extremely dry throat—*laryngitis sicca gravidarum*—occasionally is seen. All of these conditions resolve after delivery. Finally, the incidence of facial paralysis is three times greater in pregnant women than in nonpregnant women; the cause for this is unknown, and treatment usually is limited to careful observation.[23]

## DIABETES MELLITUS

Sensorineural hearing loss has been reported to appear earlier and is more severe in diabetic individuals than in the normal population. When diabetic patients are compared with a general population of the same age and sex, however, no difference in hearing levels is found.[24,25] Other conditions that have been thought to be more prevalent in diabetic persons are Ménière syndrome, facial nerve palsy (Bell palsy), and vocal cord paralysis, but none of these has been conclusively shown to be more common in these patients than in the population as a whole.

Infections are a great problem in diabetic individuals. Two infectious processes are unique and are reviewed in some detail. The first is *malignant (necrotizing) external otitis,* a disease that affects elderly diabetic patients.[26,27] It is a unilateral process that begins as a routine external otitis. Despite therapy, it evolves from a soft tissue infection into an osteomyelitis of the temporal bone and eventually involves the base of the skull. *Pseudomonas aeruginosa* is the major pathogen. The cardinal symptoms are severe otalgia and otorrhea. Granulation tissue is present at the anterior junction of the bony and the cartilaginous external auditory canal. The clinical appearance is deceptively mild, and the course of the disease is prolonged. Once the bone is involved, cranial nerve deficits develop. The facial nerve is the one most commonly affected, but cranial nerves VI through XII can be involved. If more than one cranial nerve is affected, the prognosis is poor. The treatment must be aggressive and multifaceted. Local treatment consists of placing an antibiotic-soaked wick in the ear canal. Systemic therapy uses an aminoglycoside and one of the synthetic penicillins. Prolonged therapy with a cephalosporin or fluoroquinolone may be effective.[28] Treatment must be continued for at least 4 weeks, and probably for 6 weeks. Surgical management is limited to debridement of the temporal bone, usually a radical mastoidectomy. Controlling the diabetes concurrently and monitoring renal function is imperative. Treatment must be continued until all clinical evidence of the disease disappears, the erythrocyte sedimentation rate normalizes, the gallium bone scan improves, and radiographic evidence of resolution is noted.[29] At one time, the mortality rate associated with this disease was 50%, but it is now around 10% (see Chap. 152).

The second infection of concern is *mucormycosis*. The two forms seen in the head and neck region are the rhino-orbital-cerebral form and the otic form.[30–33,33a] The nasal form presents with blindness, ophthalmoplegia, proptosis, facial swelling, palatal ulcer, or disorders of consciousness. Examination reveals brick red or black areas within the nasal cavity. Biopsy confirms the clinical impression of mucormycosis. The otic presentation usually is accompanied by otorrhea, followed by facial paralysis and then altered sensorium. Treatment must be prompt and aggressive. The diabetes must be controlled, because ketoacidosis and dehydration are invariably present at the onset of the disease. Systemic therapy is initiated with amphotericin B. Surgical debridement is more important in mucormycosis than in malignant otitis externa. Surgical management involves the removal of all necrotic tissue and the establishment of drainage from areas of infection. If the facial or optic nerve is involved, decompression is indicated. The mortality rate associated with this condition is 40%.

## HYPOGLYCEMIA

Reactive postprandial hypoglycemia[34] has been associated with Ménière syndrome, fluctuating hearing loss, and episodic vertigo.[35] Although some authors believe that hypoglycemia plays a major role in the evolution of these symptom complexes, the objective data are not impressive. The subjective nature of the symptoms and the tendency for remission to occur make scientific evaluation difficult.

## LIPID METABOLISM

Hyperlipidemia causes characteristic xanthomas of the face and may be associated with sensorineural hearing loss.[36] The view once was that patients with Ménière syndrome, fluctuating hearing loss, episodic imbalance, and premature hearing loss often had hyperlipidemia.[37] Most of those studies had flaws in their design, and hyperlipidemia probably is not a significant factor in these conditions. In abetalipoproteinemia, which is a rare recessive disorder, the presenting features include ataxia, acanthocytosis, and sensorineural hearing loss.[38]

## REFERENCES

1. Ito H, Takamoto T, Nitta M, et al. DIDMOAD (diabetes insipidus, diabetes mellitus, optic atrophy and deafness) syndrome associated with myocardial disease. Jpn Heart J 1988; 29:371.
1a. Jenkin A, Renner D, Hahn F, Larsen J. A case of primary amenorrhea, diabetes and anosmia. Gynecol Endocrinol 2000; 14:65.
2. Laws ER Jr, Thapar K. Surgical management of pituitary adenomas. Baillières Clin Endocrinol Metab 1995; 9:391.
3. Carrau RL, Jho HD, Ko Y. Transnasal-transsphenoidal endoscopic surgery of the pituitary gland. Laryngoscope 1996; 106:914.
4. Harner SG. Orbital decompression techniques. In: Gorman CA, Waller RR, Dyer JA, eds. The eye and orbit in thyroid disease. New York: Raven Press, 1984:221.
5. Metson R, Shore JW, Gliklich RE, Dallow RL. Endoscopic orbital decompression under local anesthesia. Otolaryngol Head Neck Surg 1995; 113:661.
6. Bauer CA, Valentino J, Hoffman HT. Long-term result of vocal cord augmentation with autogenous fat. Ann Otol Rhinol Laryngol 1995; 104:871.
7. Netterville JL, Aly A, Ossoff RH. Evaluation and treatment of complications of thyroid and parathyroid surgery. Otolaryngol Clin North Am 1990; 23:529.
8. Chaouki ML, Maoui R, Benmiloud M. Comparative study of neurological and myxoedematous cretinism associated with severe iodine deficiency. Clin Endocrinol (Oxf) 1988; 28:399.
9. Friis J, Johnsen T, Feldt-Rasmussen U, et al. Thyroid function in patients with Pendred's syndrome. J Endocrinol Invest 1988; 11:97.
10. Maisel RH, Brown DR, Ritter FN. Endocrinology. In: Paparella MM, Shumrick DA, eds. Otolaryngology, vol 1. Philadelphia: WB Saunders, 1980:779.
11. Werbel SS, Ober KP. Pheochromocytoma. Update on diagnosis, localization, and management. Med Clin North Am 1995; 79:131.
12. Krespi YP, Kuriloff DB, Aner M. Sarcoidosis of the sinonasal tract: a new staging system. Otolaryngol Head Neck Surg 1995; 112:221.
13. Benjamin B, Dalton C, Croxson G. Laryngoscopic diagnosis of laryngeal sarcoid. Ann Otol Rhinol Laryngol 1995; 104:529.
14. Lye WC, Leong SO. Bilateral vocal cord paralysis secondary to treatment of severe hypophosphatemia in a continuous ambulatory peritoneal dialysis patient. Am J Kidney Dis 1994; 23:127.
15. Schuknecht HF. Pathology of the ear. Cambridge, MA: Harvard University Press, 1974:172.
16. Harner SG, Rose DE, Facer GW. Paget's disease and hearing loss. Otolaryngology 1978; 86:869.
17. El Samma M, Linthicum FH Jr, House HP, House JW. Calcitonin as treatment for hearing loss in Paget's disease. Am J Otolaryngol 1986; 7:241.

18. Bergstrom L. Osteogenesis imperfecta: otologic and maxillofacial aspects. Laryngoscope 1977; 87(Suppl):1.
19. Feldman MD, Rao VM, Lowry LD, Kelly M. Fibrous dysplasia of the paranasal sinuses. Otolaryngol Head Neck Surg 1986; 95:222.
20. Megerian CA, Sofferman RA, McKenna MJ, et al. Fibrous dysplasia of the temporal bone: ten new cases demonstrating the spectrum of otologic sequelae. Am J Otol 1995; 16:408.
21. Sofferman RA. Cysts and bone dyscrasias of the paranasal sinuses. In: English GM, ed. Otolaryngology, vol 2. Philadelphia: Harper & Row, 1985:13.
22. Stocks RM, Wang WC, Thompson JW, et al. Malignant infantile osteopetrosis: otolaryngological complications and management. Arch Otolaryngol Head Neck Surg 1998; 124:689.
23. Hilsinger RL Jr, Adour KK. Idiopathic facial paralysis, pregnancy, and the menstrual cycle. Ann Otol Rhinol Laryngol 1975; 84:433.
24. Harner SG. Hearing in adult-onset diabetes mellitus. Otolaryngol Head Neck Surg 1981; 89:322.
25. Duck SW, Prazma J, Bennett PS, Pillsbury HC. Interaction between hypertension and diabetes mellitus in the pathogenesis of sensorineural hearing loss. Laryngoscope 1997; 107:1596.
26. Chandler JR. Malignant external otitis and osteomyelitis of the base of the skull. Am J Otol 1989; 10:108.
27. Slattery WH 3rd, Brackmann DE. Skull base osteomyelitis. Malignant external otitis. Otolaryngol Clin North Am 1996; 29:795.
28. Levenson MJ, Parisier SC, Dolitsky J, Bindra G. Ciprofloxacin: drug of choice in the treatment of malignant external otitis (MEO). Laryngoscope 1991; 101:821.
29. Grandis JR, Curtin HD, Yu VL. Necrotizing (malignant) external otitis: prospective comparison of CT and MR imaging in diagnosis and follow-up. Radiology 1995; 196:499.
30. Vessely MB, Zitsch RP 3rd, Estrem SA, Renner G. Atypical presentations of mucormycosis in the head and neck. Otolaryngol Head Neck Surg 1996; 115:573.
31. Sugar AM. Mucormycosis. (Review). Clin Infect Dis 1992; 1(Suppl 14):S126.
32. Harril WC, Stewart MG, Lee AG, Cernoch P. Chronic rhinocerebral mucormycosis. Laryngoscope 1996; 106:1292.
33. Gussen R, Canalis RF. Mucormycosis of the temporal bone. Ann Otol Rhinol Laryngol 1982; 91:27.
33a. Ferguson BJ. Mucormycosis of the nose and paranasal sinuses. Otolaryngol Clin North Am 2000; 33:349.
34. Betteridge DJ. Reactive hypoglycemia. BMJ 1987; 295:286.
35. de Vincentiis I, Ralli G. New pathogenetic and therapeutic aspects of Ménière's disease. Adv Otorhinolaryngol 1987; 37:97.
36. Pulec JL, Pulec MB, Mendoza I. Progressive sensorineural hearing loss, subjective tinnitus and vertigo caused by elevated blood lipids. Ear Nose Throat J 1997; 76:716.
37. Spencer JT Jr. Hyperlipoproteinemia and inner ear disease. Otolaryngol Clin North Am 1975; 8:483.
38. Liston S, Meyerhoff WH. Metabolic hearing loss. In: English GM, ed. Otolaryngology, vol 1. Philadelphia: Harper & Row, 1985:9.

# CHAPTER 217

# DENTAL ASPECTS OF ENDOCRINOLOGY

ROBERT S. REDMAN

Most of the major circulating hormones are important in the normal growth and development of the orofacial region, including the teeth, and most of them also participate in the maintenance of the health and integrity of these structures. Consequently, hormonal abnormalities commonly have dental and oral manifestations. Many of these oral signs and symptoms, and the endocrinopathies and other disorders with which they may be associated, are summarized in Tables 217-1 and 217-2.

## ONTOGENY OF THE OROFACIAL STRUCTURES

When one considers the potential for hormonal effects on the development of mature oral structures, two phenomena must be examined. First, with regard to tooth development, the various

**TABLE 217-1.**
**Dental and Orofacial Abnormalities That May Be Associated with Specific Metabolic or Endocrine Disorders**

| Dental or Oral Abnormality | Metabolic or Endocrine Disorders |
| --- | --- |
| **TEETH** | |
| Enamel hypoplasia, hypocalcification | Cretinism; juvenile myxedema; rickets; hypophophatasia; pseudohypophosphatasia; hypoparathyroidism, including APECS; pseudohypoparathyroidism; fluorosis |
| | *To be distinguished from:* amelogenesis imperfecta; results of local trauma or severe systemic illness in infancy or early childhood |
| Dental hypoplasia, hypocalcification | Cretinism; juvenile myxedema; rickets; familial hypophosphatemia; hypophosphatasia and pseudohypophosphatasia; hypoparathyroidism and APECS |
| | *To be distinguished from:* dentinogenesis imperfecta; results of trauma or illness in early childhood |
| Short roots, occluded pulp chambers | Cretinism; myxedema |
| | *To be distinguished from:* regional odontodysplasia |
| Short roots, enlarged pulp chambers | Pseudohypoparathyroidism |
| | *To be distinguished from:* dentinogenesis imperfecta; dentinal dysplasia |
| Dental defects leading to periapical infection | Vitamin D–resistant rickets (familial hypophosphatemia) |
| Delayed eruption | Cretinism; myxedema; hypopituitarism; rickets |
| Precocious eruption | Hyperthyroidism; congenital adrenal hyperplasia; precocious puberty |
| **BONES OF THE MAXILLA AND MANDIBLE** | |
| Hypocalcification (developmental) | Cretinism; juvenile myxedema; rickets; hypophosphatasia; pseudohypophosphatasia; familial hypophosphatemia |
| Hypocalcification (postdevelopmental) | Decreased estrogen (postmenopause); hyperparathyroidism; vitamin D deficiency; long-term inadequate dietary calcium or high dietary phosphate/calcium ratio |
| Loss of lamina dura | Hyperparathyroidism; vitamin D deficiency (osteomalacia and rickets); renal dialysis |
| Central (intraosseous) giant cell lesions | Hyperparathyroidism; renal dialysis |
| Underdevelopment; relative maxillary prognathism | Pituitary dwarfism; cretinism; juvenile myxedema |
| | *To be distinguished from:* Down syndrome |
| Postpubertal enlargement | Acromegaly (greater degree of enlargement in the mandible than in the maxilla) |
| | *To be distinguished from:* Paget disease of bone (in which the enlargement is usually greater in the maxilla) |
| **ORAL MUCOSA** | |
| Macroglossia (secondary to edema) | Hypothyroidism at any age |
| | *To be distinguished from:* cellulitis; lymphangioma; amyloidosis; relative or absolute hyperplasia (true macroglossia), as in Down syndrome and acromegaly |
| Amyloidosis ($\beta_2$-microglobulin) | Renal dialysis (ABM2 amyloidosis) |
| | *To be distinguished from:* all other types of amyloidosis |
| Glossodynia; metallic taste | Diabetes; decreased estrogen (postmenopause); also occurs in conjunction with pernicious or iron deficiency anemia and ingestion of bismuth and lead |
| Candidiasis | |
| Acute pseudomembranous type (tongue, buccal mucosa, gingiva) | Greater incidence in diabetic patients than in normal population |
| | If lesions are resistant to antifungal therapy, APECS, hyperadrenocorticism (including corticosteroid therapy) and hypoparathyroidism should be considered. Also occurs in immune deficiencies, both congenital and acquired (AIDS). |
| Chronic hyperplastic type (tongue, buccal mucosa, and especially the labial angular commissures) | Hypoparathyroidism, APECS; hyperadrenocorticism; also occurs in immune deficiencies, including AIDS |
| | *To be distinguished from:* Angular cheilosis associated with closed bite or nutritional deficiencies; premalignant dyskeratosis; carcinoma; also occurs in immune deficiencies, including AIDS |
| Atrophic type (especially focal on tongue and hard palate) | Greater prevalence in diabetic patients than in general population |
| | *To be distinguished from:* median rhomboid glossitis; benign migratory glossitis; glossitis secondary to anemia or vitamin B deficiency. also occurs in immune deficiencies, including AIDS |
| Patchy melanin pigmentation (buccal, labial, and gingival mucosa) | Hypoadrenocorticism |
| | *To be distinguished from:* amalgam tattoo; bismuth or lead deposits; pigmentations associated with African or Mediterranean ancestry; nevus; melanoma; Peutz-Jeghers syndrome |
| Aphthae; herpes labialis | Frequently associated with menses |
| Hyperplastic gingivitis; pyogenic granuloma | Increased female sex hormones, as occur in pregnancy, hypergonadism, use of oral contraceptives, or estrogen therapy; diabetes |
| | *To be distinguished from:* hyperplastic gingivitis due to vitamin C deficiency and medications such as phenytoin (Dilantin), cyclosporine, and nifedipine |
| Periodontitis that is progressive despite treatment | Poorly controlled diabetes; hyper- and hypothyroidism; hyperparathyroidism; hyperadrenocorticism; renal dialysis; also occurs in immune deficiencies |
| **SALIVARY GLANDS** | |
| Xerostomia | Diabetes |
| | *To be distinguished from:* postirradiation atrophy and fibrosis of salivary glands; Sjögren syndrome; and the effects of medications such as diuretics and antipsychotics |
| Bilateral, generalized enlargement, especially the parotid glands | Diabetes |
| | *To be distinguished from:* alcoholism; chronic undernutrition; Sjögren syndrome; iodine therapy (iodine mumps); bismuth ingestion; sarcoidosis |

*APECS,* autoimmune polyendocrinopathy candidiasis syndrome; *AIDS,* acquired immunodeficiency syndrome.

**TABLE 217-2.**
**Reported Effects of Various Endocrine Conditions on the Sense of Taste***

| Abnormality/Disorder | Effect |
|---|---|
| HYPOGONADOTROPIC HYPOGONADISM (KALLMANN SYNDROME) | Decreased sense of taste (largely attributable to loss of sense of smell); defects are irreversible. |
| HYPOTHYROIDISM | Distortion of taste (dysgeusia), as well as hyposmia; decreased taste acuity, especially to bitter stimuli. Defects are reversible with thyroid hormone therapy. |
| HYPERCALCEMIA | Bitter taste in mouth; reversible with normalization of serum calcium levels |
| PSEUDOHYPOPARATHYROIDISM | Impaired taste for sour and bitter (as well as impaired olfaction) |
| ADDISON DISEASE | Lowered threshold for the sensation of saltiness; reversible with corticosteroid therapy |
| GONADAL DYSGENESIS | Variable disorders of gustatory (as well as olfactory) functions |
| DIABETES MELLITUS | Blunted sensation for sweetness and generalized decreased taste acuity for saltiness and bitterness; metallic taste |

*Taste (gustation) is an extremely adaptive chemical sense. The thousands of taste buds are located mostly on the dorsal surface of the tongue but also are located on palatal, pharyngeal, and buccal mucosae. Taste buds consist of supporting cells and gustatory cells. The latter cells, which respond to dissolved substances, are supplied afferently by the facial nerve (anterior two-thirds of the tongue), glossopharyngeal nerve (posterior one-third of the tongue), and vagus nerve (throat); the impulses eventually arrive in the parietal cortex, where they are intermixed with sensations of touch, temperature, and smell.

stages of odontogenesis occur at different ages for each pair of teeth. The first *primary teeth* are initiated at ~6 weeks after conception, whereas the last *secondary teeth* (the third molars) finish root formation at ~20 years after birth.[1] Thus, significant deviations from the normal chronology of tooth eruption (Fig. 217-1) can be an important sign of endocrinopathy, as well as of metabolic or nutritional problems. Furthermore, any part of a tooth that has completely calcified undergoes no significant further developmental changes in shape or composition. Thus, the duration, as well as the severity, of hormonal changes determine which parts of which teeth are affected. Once the teeth have fully formed and erupted, they can be altered only by destructive processes, such as periodontitis and caries, and their capacity for repair is limited. Therefore, abnormalities of shape or mineralization that are restricted to certain teeth also may serve as a permanent record, indicating when and for how long an endocrinopathy has been a factor (Fig. 217-2). Second, the maxilla, mandible, and most of the facial bones grow by intramembranous ossification, except for epiphyseal plate-like growth in a rim of hyaline cartilage on the head of each mandibular condyle. This cartilage persists in the adult.[2] Thus, with appropriate hormonal stimulation, during adulthood, the facial bones and both jaws can enlarge by accretion, but the mandible also can elongate from the condyles.

## PITUITARY GLAND

Experiments in which the incisors continuously erupt have indicated the relative importance of the pituitary and several of its target endocrine gland hormones in the production of dental and alveolar bone abnormalities in hypopituitarism.[3] In hypophysectomized rats, the rate of eruption progressively slows, then ceases, and the incisors become reduced in size and misshapen. Amelogenesis, morphogenesis, and rate of eruption are largely restored by thyroxine administration, whereas dentino-

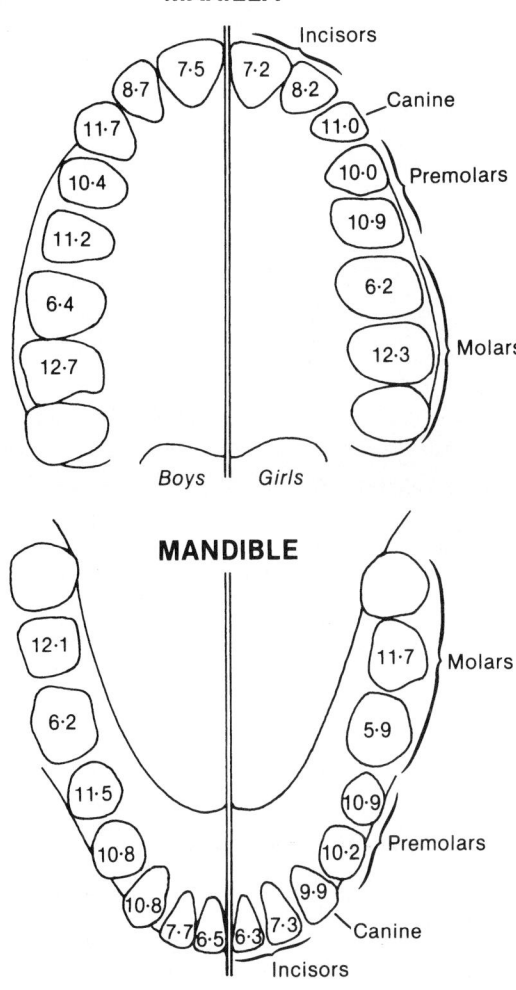

**FIGURE 217-1.** Chronology of eruption of the permanent, or secondary, teeth. Eruption time, as depicted in this diagram, is defined as the time when the tooth first pierces the gingiva and becomes visible in the oral cavity. The numbers within the teeth designate the mean eruption times in years and months; example, the maxillary central incisors (next to the midline) erupt at the age of 7 years, 5 months in boys, and 7 years, 2 months in girls. The third molars ("wisdom teeth") contain no numbers because their eruption times are extremely variable and are, therefore, of little use as a sign of metabolic or hormonal disturbance. Of the deciduous teeth (not shown), the mandibular incisors usually erupt first, beginning at ~6 months after birth, followed by the first molars, canines, and second molars. Notice that when the deciduous molars are shed, they are replaced by the permanent premolars. All of the deciduous teeth usually have erupted by the age of 2 years. Like the permanent teeth, the deciduous teeth tend to erupt earlier in girls than in boys. (Modified from Sinclair D. Human growth after birth. London: Oxford University Press, 1978:103.)

genesis and alveolar bone growth nearly normalize with growth hormone supplementation. Decreased levels of adrenocortical hormones also may participate in the abnormal morphogenesis of the incisors.

### HYPOPITUITARISM

In pituitary dwarfism (growth hormone deficiency), eruption of both primary and secondary dentitions is delayed, and shedding of the primary teeth is delayed.[3–6] The crowns of the teeth reportedly are smaller than normal, although some researchers have suggested that the crowns appear smaller only because

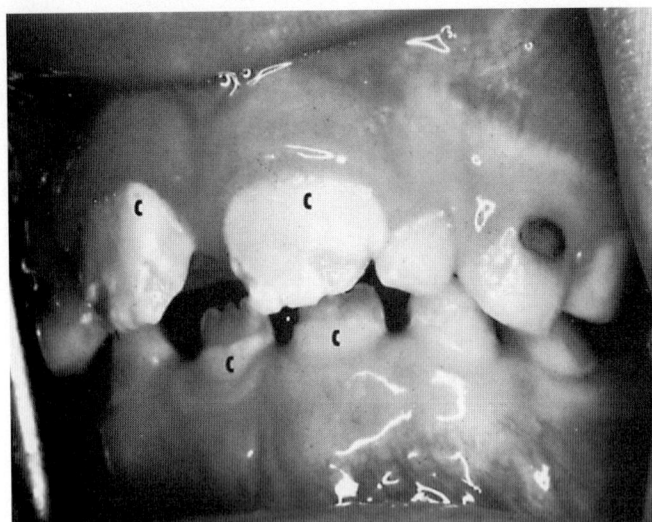

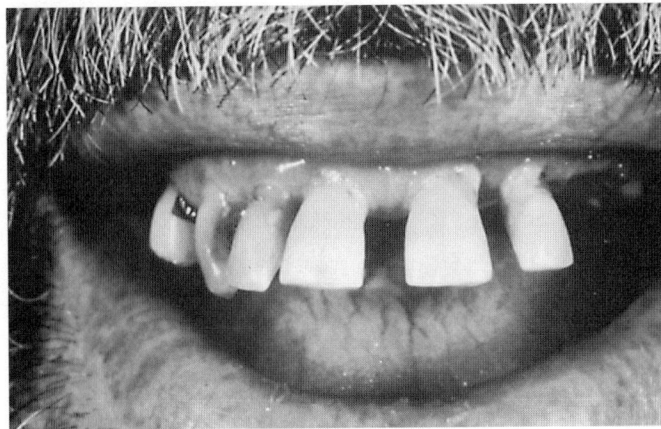

**FIGURE 217-3.** The maxillary anterior teeth of a 52-year-old man with acromegaly are pictured. Notice the wide spaces between the teeth, as well as their anterior inclination.

**FIGURE 217-2.** Severe hypoplasia of enamel and dentin. The parents of this 7-year-old girl were unsure of the nature of her illness in early childhood. The limitation of the dental defect to the incisal third of the secondary teeth, of which only the central incisors (c) have erupted, would be compatible with the onset of an endocrinopathy, such as hypothyroidism, shortly after birth and its subsequent diagnosis and appropriate treatment at 14 to 16 months of age. (Courtesy of Douglas J. Sanders, DDS.)

they are incompletely erupted.[3] Also, the roots of the teeth are noticeably stunted.[3–6] The overall growth of the jaws is retarded, with the maxilla being less affected than the mandible.[3] In this condition, the alveolar (tooth-supporting) regions of both jaws grow at a disproportionately reduced rate. Consequently, the dental arches are too small to accommodate all of the teeth, causing crowding and malocclusion.[3,5,6] Hypofunction of the salivary glands also may occur, leading to increased dental caries and periodontitis.[6]

Adult-onset panhypopituitarism has no specific effects on the teeth, but characteristic orofacial changes include thinning of the mucosa of the lips and an immobile facial expression.[3]

## HYPERPITUITARISM

Growth hormone excess that occurs before puberty (gigantism) causes progressive, symmetric enlargement of the jaws, tongue, and teeth,[3,6] and the eruption of the teeth is accelerated.[3] Orofacial features of acromegaly emerge when the hyperpituitarism continues past, or begins after, 8 to 10 years of age.[3–5] The jaws and facial bones enlarge disproportionately in relation to most of the bones of the skull because resumption of osseous growth is more vigorous in the intramembranous bones. Moreover, endochondral ossification resumes in the hyaline cartilage of the heads of the mandibular condyles, and the mandibular angles become flattened. This causes progressively more severe mandibular prognathism. The palatal arch is flattened, and panoramic dental radiographs may demonstrate enlarged maxillary sinuses. The periosteum of the jaws may become ossified at points of attachment of the muscles and tendons. The crowns of the teeth are not enlarged, but often excessive deposition of cementum on the roots (hypercementosis) occurs. The tongue may become so large that indentations form where it encroaches on the teeth. Partly from this pressure, and partly from the enlargement of the jaws, the teeth become spaced and outwardly tipped (Fig. 217-3). The nose and lips also are enlarged, adding to the general coarsening of the facial features (see Chap. 12).

Enlargement of the bones of the face and skull, and spacing and hypercementosis of the teeth can occur in osteitis deformans (Paget disease of bone).[3,4] In contrast to that associated with acromegaly, however, the enlargement in this disease is limited to the bones. The lips may become thinner because of stretching, and the maxilla tends to enlarge disproportionately to the mandible, producing an anterior open bite and a maxillary prognathism. Also, the jaws and skull bones are especially inclined to exhibit radiolucency (osteoclastic stage) and fuzzy (cotton-wool) radiodensity (osteoblastic stage).

## THYROID GLAND

The serum concentration of thyroid hormone is low in neonatal rats and mice but increases to adult levels between 2 and 3 weeks of age. When this rise is prevented by thyroidectomy, the weaning process, tooth eruption, and maturation of the salivary glands are all retarded but not prevented.[7–9] Rodent parathyroid glands are enclosed in the poles of the thyroid gland, and surgical removal of the thyroid eliminates both glands. Similar developmental retardation occurs when hypothyroidism is induced by propylthiouracil, however, and is prevented with timely replacement of thyroxine.[7] This indicates that the effects are attributable to the lack of thyroxine and not to any disturbance of parathyroid hormone. Furthermore, the administration of thyroxine to suckling mice and rats induces precocious development of salivary glands[8] as well as of the teeth.[3] Also, in mature rats and mice, deficiency of thyroxine causes up to 50% reductions in salivary flow and of gland stores of amylase, protease, and other salivary proteins.[9] These findings suggest that decreased salivary function, as well as the previously observed enamel hypocalcification, may contribute to the increased dental caries that occur in juvenile hypothyroidism.

Of note, the major salivary glands actively concentrate iodine from body fluids.[9] This does not complicate radioiodine uptake or scanning tests of the thyroid because of the relatively small amounts used, the lesser uptake by the salivary glands, and the anatomic separation of these organs and the thyroid gland. If radioiodine is used to destroy thyroid tissue in a patient with thyroid hyperplasia, adenoma, or carcinoma, however, the salivary glands also may be seriously damaged.[10,11] The resulting xerostomia may be permanent, and rampant caries and periodontal destruction follow unless long-term, specific dental care is instituted in a timely manner. Appropriate care includes scrupulous oral hygiene, frequent professional dental cleanings, use of saliva substitutes for oral moistness and comfort, and the daily topical application of a fluoride gel onto the teeth.

## HYPOTHYROIDISM

Cretinism is characterized by maxillary prognathism because the underdevelopment of the maxilla is less severe than that of the mandible.[3,6] Radiographic examination often reveals hypocalcification of the jaws, and sometimes abnormal development of the sinuses or nonunion of the mandibular symphysis is seen. The characteristic facies consists of a concave nasal bridge and flared alae nasi; stiff facial expression, thickened lips and enlarged tongue, owing to doughy, nonpitting edema; and a mouth held partly open because of the lack of room for the tongue inside the underdeveloped mandible.[3,6] The somewhat similar facies in Down syndrome arises from a disproportionately underdeveloped maxilla and a relative macroglossia that is not associated with edema.[3] In both juvenile myxedema and cretinism, development of the teeth is retarded, frequently with hypocalcification, enamel hypoplasia (see Fig. 217-2), persistence of large pulp chambers, and open apical foramina.[5] Eruption of both dentitions and shedding of the primary dentition are generally (but erratically) delayed.[3-6] This, and the underdevelopment of the jaws, causes a malocclusion that may be severe and also may be complicated by spreading and flaring of the teeth secondary to pressure from the enlarged tongue.

Hypothyroidism at any age seems to predispose affected patients to excessive dental caries, as well as to accelerated alveolar bone loss in both dentulous areas (periodontitis) and edentulous ridges (atrophy).[5,6] The increased caries and periodontitis are related to hyposalivation and to the drying effects of mouth breathing caused by the enlarged, protruding tongue.[6] Adults with myxedema also develop thickened lips and a swollen tongue (from edema). Pressure from the latter, in conjunction with an exacerbation of periodontitis, may cause spreading and splaying of the teeth.[3-5] Generally, the earlier that childhood hypothyroidism is treated, the greater is the success in preventing or reversing orofacial maldevelopment, except for the affected parts of dentin and enamel that have completed all phases of development.

Hypothyroid patients often are unable to tolerate prolonged dental procedures. Also, they usually have an exaggerated response to premedication with narcotics or barbiturates.[5]

## HYPERTHYROIDISM

In children, hyperthyroidism accelerates the development of the teeth and jaws, but maldevelopment is unusual.[3,5] Malocclusion results occasionally when shedding of primary teeth and eruption of secondary teeth are disproportionately precocious to jaw growth. Usually, the teeth are normal in terms of size, morphology, and calcification. Periodontitis may begin at an unusually early age, and both caries and periodontitis reportedly are exacerbated in hyperthyroidism at any age. In severe hyperthyroidism, rapid bone demineralization, manifested radiographically as osteoporosis of the jaws and loss of alveolar bone in both dentulous and edentulous areas.

People with hyperthyroidism are likely to be poor dental patients because they are unable to hold still for dental procedures and are likely to develop cardiac arrhythmias.[3,4,6] The anxiety, stress, and trauma associated with dental treatment thus may precipitate a medical emergency in the dental office. In particular, the use of epinephrine and other vasoconstrictors in local anesthetics is contraindicated.[6]

# CALCIUM AND PHOSPHORUS METABOLISM

Hypoplasia of enamel and dentin, marked chronologic deviations in eruption and exfoliation of teeth, loss of radiodensity of the jawbones (especially the lamina dura), and the presence of giant cell lesions in the jaws may alert the dentist to previously undiagnosed disorders of calcium and phosphorus metabolism. Abnormalities of mineral metabolism that produce oral signs and symptoms include disturbances of particular nutritional factors (calcium, fluoride, vitamin D) or hormones (parathyroid hormones, adrenal corticosteroids), and renal function.

## NUTRITIONAL FACTORS

Calcium deficiency may be an important factor in osteoporosis, which may accentuate alveolar bone loss in edentulous ridges.[3]

Fluoride deficiency has only one overt oral effect: a greatly increased susceptibility to dental caries. It also may contribute to osteoporosis when calcium intake is inadequate. Dental fluorosis, or mottled (hypoplastic) enamel, occurs with increasing frequency and severity when fluoride concentrations exceed 1.0 ppm in the drinking water if it is ingested while tooth development and calcification are in progress[3] (see Chap. 131). When the water supply contains <0.7 ppm fluoride, dietary fluoride supplements for infants (drops) and children (tablets) can significantly reduce subsequent caries. Vitamin D deficiency in children (rickets) causes hypocalcification of the dentin, enamel, and alveolar bone, and delays the eruption of both dentitions.[3] The hypocalcified dentin is characterized histologically by a wide predentin zone and excessive amounts of interglobular dentin. The crowns may be pitted, stained, or even deformed. In dental radiographs, the crown may have radiolucent spots or striations. In adults with vitamin D deficiency (osteomalacia), the maxilla and mandible are hypomineralized. Radiographic examination reveals prominent marrow spaces, thin cortices, fading or loss of trabeculae, and thinning or even loss of the lamina dura. The teeth are not affected and may seem unusually dense in contrast to the reduced mineral content of the bone.

The dentinal hypocalcification is more severe in vitamin D–resistant rickets (familial hypophosphatemia) than in ordinary rickets, and is associated with hypoplasia.[3] Frequently, clefts and tubular defects are seen near the pulp horns, and oral microorganisms often invade the pulp in the absence of caries. Consequently, multiple periapical infections and fistulas develop. The lamina dura may be reduced or absent, and the cementum may be hypoplastic.

Both hypophosphatasia and pseudohypophosphatasia cause premature exfoliation of the deciduous teeth, apparently because of a lack of cementogenesis. Occasionally, the teeth and alveolar bones are sufficiently hypocalcified to be demonstrably less radiodense, and the pulp chambers may be abnormally large.[3,5]

## PARATHYROID HORMONE

In hypoparathyroidism of infancy or early childhood, hypoplasia or even aplasia of the teeth may occur.[3] The hypoplasia affects both enamel and dentin, and often results in short, blunted roots, malformed teeth, delayed eruption, and impaction. When it occurs as part of the autoimmune polyendocrinopathy candidiasis syndrome (APECS), superficial mucocutaneous candidiasis frequently precedes any of the other signs or symptoms[3] (see Chaps. 60 and 197). Acute exacerbations of the oral mucosal lesions usually can be controlled with topical anti-

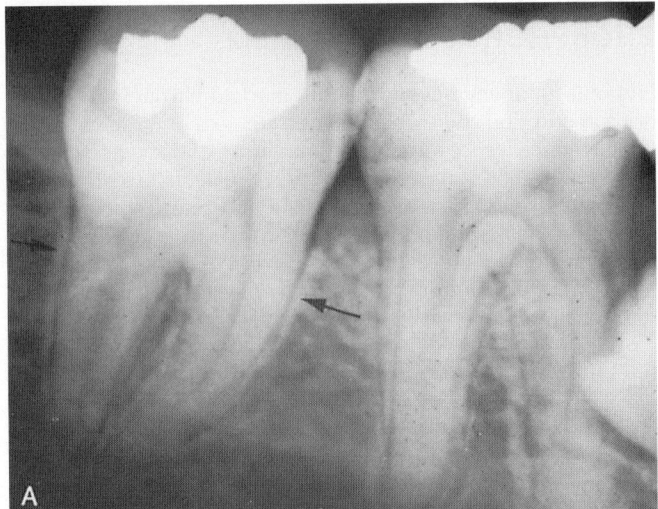

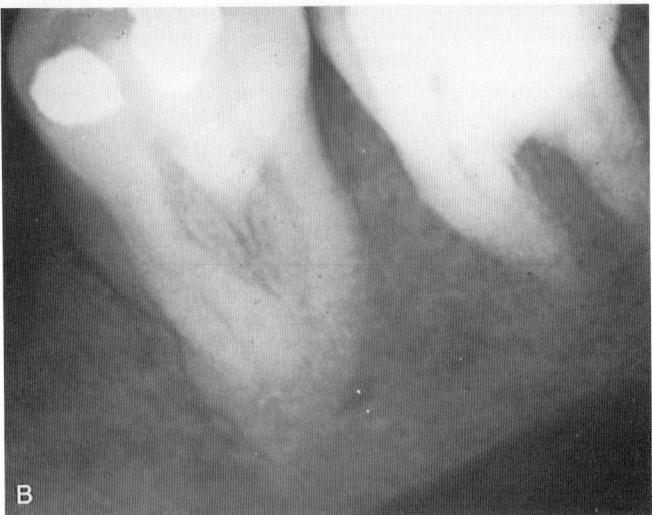

**FIGURE 217-4.** Periapical radiographs of mandibular molars. **A,** In a normal patient, the lamina dura (*arrow*) and the bony trabeculae are thick and dense. **B,** By contrast, the lamina dura is virtually absent and the trabeculae are thinner and much less radiodense in this patient with hyperparathyroidism. (Courtesy of John N. Trodahl, DDS.)

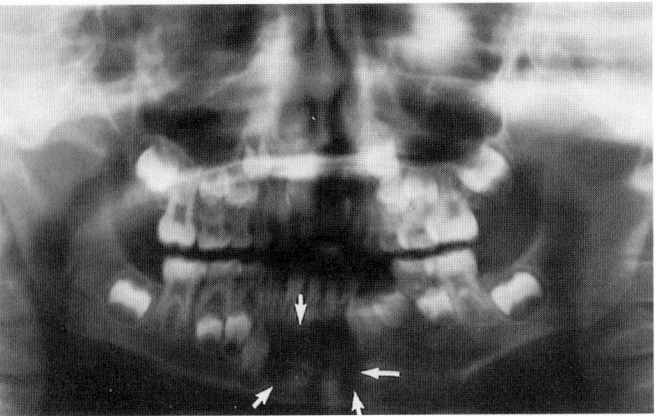

**FIGURE 217-5.** Radiograph of a central giant cell granuloma in the mandible of a 7-year-old girl. The circumscribed, multilocular, radiolucent region (*arrows*) initially appeared (when the child was 5 years old) as a small radiolucent area in the premolar region. No evidence of hyperparathyroidism was seen in this patient. (Courtesy of L. Stefan Levin, DDS.)

fungal agents, but the lesions are subject to recurrence when therapy is discontinued. Angular cheilosis, however, is nearly constant, and seldom completely regresses with antifungal therapy. Enamel hypoplasia occurs in many cases. Frequently, the enamel is affected before the onset of any of the endocrinologic disorders. This supports the notion that the syndrome may be caused by episodes of autoimmune destruction limited to certain organs. Tooth eruption and occlusion seem to be unaffected. Hypoparathyroidism occurring after puberty does not affect tooth development or eruption but may cause circumoral paresthesia and predispose to oral candidiasis.[6]

Pseudohypoparathyroidism is characterized by microdontia, occluded pulp chambers, short roots, hypoplastic enamel, osteodentin, and multiple impacted teeth.[3,4]

Hyperparathyroidism, whether primary or secondary, produces characteristic changes in dental radiographs.[3–6] The bones of the maxilla and mandible are generally less radiodense than normal, and often have a ground-glass appearance. Frequently, the lamina dura is greatly reduced or even lost (see Fig. 217-4). In time, discrete radiolucent areas appear and enlarge. These are osteoclastomas that are histologically identical to the giant cell granuloma (Fig. 217-5), a lesion

that occurs almost exclusively in the jaws. Thus, if a circumscribed lesion of the maxilla or mandible is diagnosed as a central (arising from within the bone) giant cell granuloma, the patient should be referred for investigation of possible hyperparathyroidism. The less uncommon peripheral (arising from or near the surface of the bone) giant cell granuloma apparently is not associated with hyperparathyroidism[12]; however, tests for hyperparathyroidism still would be prudent if more than a superficial cupping of the underlying bone is present, or if multiple lesions occur.

Dental treatment of the patient with parathyroid disease must involve a consultation between the dentist and the physician, because abnormal blood calcium levels can precipitate medical emergencies such as cardiac arrhythmias, bronchospasm, laryngospasm, and convulsions.[6]

## RENAL FUNCTION

Azotemic osteodystrophy may affect oral and facial bones via negative calcium balance (osteoporosis or osteomalacia) or secondary hyperparathyroidism (as described earlier), or both.[3] Patients with renal failure who are treated by dialysis or renal transplantation are prone to accelerated alveolar bone loss and, therefore, require recurrent dental treatment.[13]

A form of amyloidosis (AB2M) that is peculiar to long-term renal dialysis (10 years or more) results from a gradual accumulation of $\beta_2$-microglobulin in the blood and tissues (Fig. 217-6). The crystals have a pathognomonic ultrastructural appearance, resembling shocks of wheat, rather than the wind-scattered look of all other forms of amyloid. Although the principal site for significant deposits is the skeleton, typical lingual manifestations can occur.[14] The substitution of biocompatible for cellulosic membranes in the dialysis equipment slows the process and greatly reduces the incidence of the disorder. Nonetheless, periodic inspections of the oral soft tissues for signs of amyloidosis are indicated after 8 to 10 years of hemodialysis.

## ADRENAL GLANDS

Experiments in young rats and mice indicate that corticosteroids are much less important than growth hormone and thy-

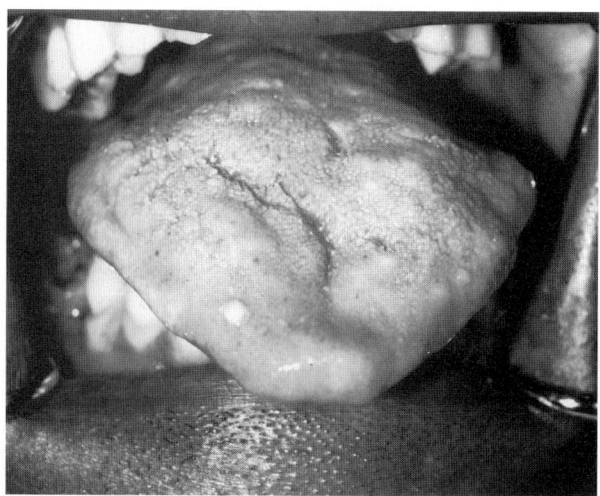 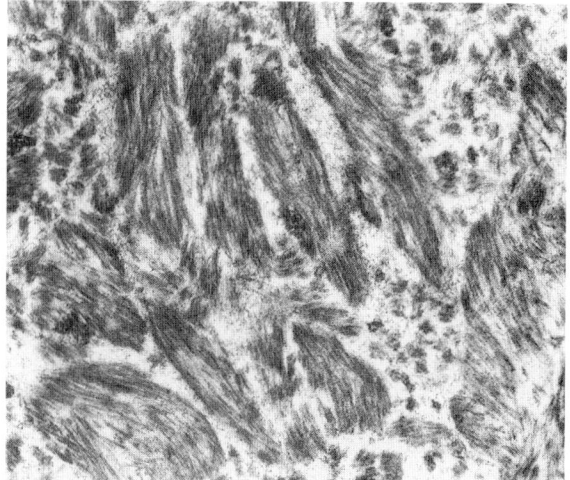

A        B

**FIGURE 217-6.** Lingual amyloidosis caused by inadequate removal of $\beta_2$-microglobulin from blood during long-term renal hemodialysis. **A,** The initial presentation as yellow nodules with foci of hypervascularity. The amyloid deposits in these lesions and in the thyroid gland were shown to be composed of accumulations of $\beta_2$-microglobulin by immunohistochemistry and electron microscopy. **B,** Electron micrograph demonstrating the pathognomonic stacking of the lingual amyloid crystals. × 21,600 (From Guccion JG, Redman RS, Winne CE: Hemodialysis-associated amyloidosis presenting as lingual nodules. Oral Surg 1989; 68:618.)

roxine in odontogenesis.[3] They are nearly as essential as thyroxine, however, in the maturation of the salivary glands that is associated with weaning. Glucocorticosteroids also affect the composition of saliva in mature rats[9] (see Thyroid). Administration of high doses of corticosteroids during pregnancy causes an increased incidence of cleft palate in mice and rabbits, but only in strains that are prone to the spontaneous development of this defect.[3] Therefore, the clinical significance of this observation is unclear.

## HYPOADRENOCORTICISM

The appearance of irregularly shaped, blotchy melanin patches on the oral mucosa is often an early sign of Addison disease[3–6] (see Chap. 76). The color varies from brown to blue-black, and characteristically affects the buccal mucosa near the commissures first, then spreads posteriorly. In time, the tongue and gingiva may be affected. Melanin pigmentation of the oral mucosa is common in persons from the Mediterranean region or those of African ancestry, but the involved areas tend to be evenly colored, and a correlation is seen between the inherent darkness of the person's skin and the extent and darkness of the oral pigmentation. The pigment usually affects the attached, but not the marginal, gingivae. The gingival pigmentation associated with heavy metal poisoning affects mostly the marginal gingivae; with lead poisoning, the deposits are gray, whereas with bismuth poisoning, they are blue-black.[3]

Other oral pigmented spots that must be considered include ephelides, pigmented macules, nevi, melanomas, amalgam tattoos (silver amalgam dust embedded in tissues during polishing and shaping of restorations), and the labial, lingual, and buccal mucosal spots associated with Peutz-Jeghers syndrome.

Dental procedures may precipitate an adrenal crisis in patients with Addison disease or in those who recently were receiving long-term, high-dose corticosteroid therapy.[3,4,6] The dentist should confer with the patient's physician regarding the need for antibiotic coverage, a preoperative boost in corticosteroid dosage, or hospitalization (see Chaps. 76 and 78).

## HYPERADRENOCORTICISM

Cushing syndrome, as well as exogenous corticosteroid therapy, can cause osteoporosis and an increased susceptibility to periodontitis and oral candidiasis.[3] The gingivae may be edematous and bleed easily.[6] In children, accelerated tooth development has been reported, but most cases have occurred in conjunction with the adrenogenital syndrome, in which increased androgen levels are common.[3,5]

The dentist should know whether a patient is receiving adrenocortical medication, because all but the lowest doses significantly interfere with healing and the patient's resistance to infection. Other considerations in the dental management of patients with hypoadrenocorticism include caution in the use of sedatives that can depress respiration, and, in cases of hyperadrenocorticism, care to provide adequate support of weakened vertebrae.[6] Similarly, patients requiring long-term treatment with corticosteroids should receive timely dental care, so that periodontal bone loss and serious oral infections may be avoided.

Hyperaldosteronism decreases both the flow rate and the sodium/potassium ratio in saliva. A failure of the sodium/potassium ratio to normalize after adrenal surgery indicates incomplete removal of the causative adenoma.[15]

## ADRENAL MEDULLA

Headaches occurring in conjunction with hypersecretion of catecholamines, such as with pheochromocytomas, may resemble the pain of temporomandibular joint dysfunction (TMD) and related conditions. Therefore, for patients with episodic pain symptoms of TMD that do not respond to conservative treatment, a prudent approach is to look for signs and symptoms of pheochromocytoma, for example, hypertension and excessive perspiration, during the pain episodes.[6]

Of the multiple endocrine neoplasia (MEN) syndromes, only MEN2B has significant oral manifestations. These include multiple nodular ganglioneuromas of the tongue and lips and a high-arched palate[6] (see Chap. 188).

Dentists caring for patients with any of the MEN syndromes or with sporadic pheochromocytoma should not use epinephrine in local anesthetics or gingival retraction cords.[6]

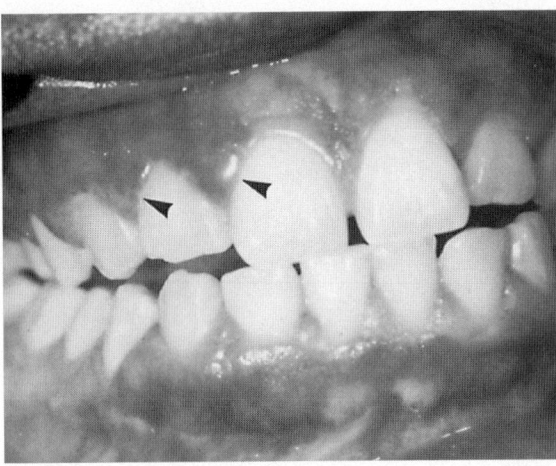

**FIGURE 217-7.** Hyperplastic marginal gingivitis (*arrowheads*) was evident in this 22-year-old woman who was 8 months pregnant at the time of this examination. Five weeks after delivery of her baby, the patient returned for dental treatment, at which time the gingivitis had completely regressed.

## SEX HORMONES

The granular ducts in the submandibular salivary glands of rats and mice differentiate after puberty. The number and size of the granules in these ducts, as well as the amount of proteases, epidermal growth factor, nerve growth factor, and a host of other enzymes and hormones they contain, all are greater in male than in female rodents.[16] Gonadectomy eliminates this sexual dimorphism, decreasing the volume of granular ducts less in the females than in the males. Consistent with these observations is the fact that, when testosterone is administered to female rodents or to gonadectomized rodents of either sex, a much greater degree of differentiation of the granular ducts is achieved than with any of the female hormones. These differences in hormonal responsiveness appear to be due to the greater number of androgen receptors in the glands, and to the fact that a much larger proportion of these receptors are occupied by testosterone, and thus activated, in male than in female rodents.[16] On the other hand, estrogen receptors are found in salivary glands of female rats, and the peroxidase activity in these glands is estrogen responsive.[17]

### WOMEN

Pregnancy frequently produces a florid marginal gingivitis (Fig. 217-7), from which a pyogenic granuloma ("pregnancy tumor") sometimes emerges.[3,4,6] The gingivitis and smaller pyogenic granulomas (those <1.0 cm in diameter) usually regress completely after parturition. Scrupulous oral hygiene tends to minimize these gingival lesions but does not prevent them entirely. Oral contraceptive use also seems to exacerbate gingivitis. Pregnancy and estrogen therapy also have been implicated in the development of both peripheral and central giant cell granulomas.[18] Excessive emesis with pregnancy can erode the enamel of teeth, particularly the lingual surfaces of the maxillary incisors. Some women tend to develop recurrent herpes labialis or oral mucosal aphthae in conjunction with menstruation.[3]

Postmenopausal oral changes can include osteoporosis involving the jaws and facial bones, mild to moderate atrophy of the oral epithelium, mild xerostomia, and glossodynia.[3,4] Possibly related to the last two changes is a significant drop in the flow rate, pH, and buffering effect of whole stimulated saliva in postmenopausal women, which is reversed with hormone-replacement therapy.[19]

### MEN

Testosterone and other androgens are primarily responsible for the generally larger size attained by males, and this size differential encompasses the jaws and orofacial bones. The greater bone mass causes greater general radiodensity on dental radiographs; thus, gender must be considered when evaluating bone density.

## PANCREAS: DIABETES MELLITUS

Experimentally induced diabetes in rats has significant effects on the salivary glands.[20] Growth and development are markedly retarded, with the granular ducts being most affected. In older rats, atrophy of the granular ducts and accumulation of lipid droplets in the acinar cells occur. Glandular stores of the salivary enzymes peroxidase and protease are greatly diminished.

Insulin and glucagon immunoreactivity is present in the parenchymal cells of both rat and human salivary glands. Although purified extracts are bioactive, salivary gland glucagon is not released by stimuli that effect pancreatic glucagon secretion.[21,22]

Diabetes mellitus adversely affects resistance to oral infection and, in turn, significant oral infection can adversely affect the management of diabetes. Therefore, dental care is an important adjunct to the management of diabetes in patients with natural teeth.[3,6,23] Oral signs and symptoms of diabetes mellitus include periodontitis, enlarged salivary glands, taste impairment (*hypogeusia*),[24] disturbances of taste (*dysgeusia*, especially the presence of a metallic taste), glossodynia, dry mouth, and increased susceptibility to oral candidiasis.

In some patients with poorly controlled diabetes, the salivary glands, especially the parotid glands, are enlarged (Fig. 217-8).

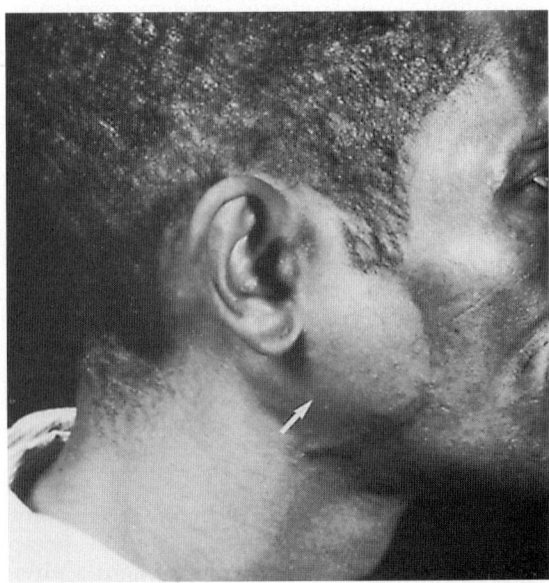

**FIGURE 217-8.** Parotid gland hypertrophy (*arrow*) in a 28-year-old patient with poorly controlled type 1 diabetes.

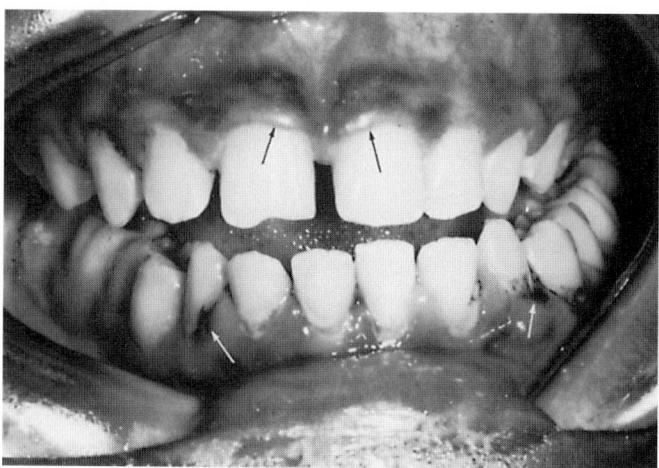

**FIGURE 217-9.** Severe marginal gingivitis and early periodontitis developed in a 38-year-old man 8 months after the onset of type 2 diabetes. Notice the shiny, swollen gingival margins (*black arrows*) and gingival bleeding (*white arrows*). The gingivae were much improved 2 weeks after dental prophylaxis and resumption of acceptable oral hygiene practices.

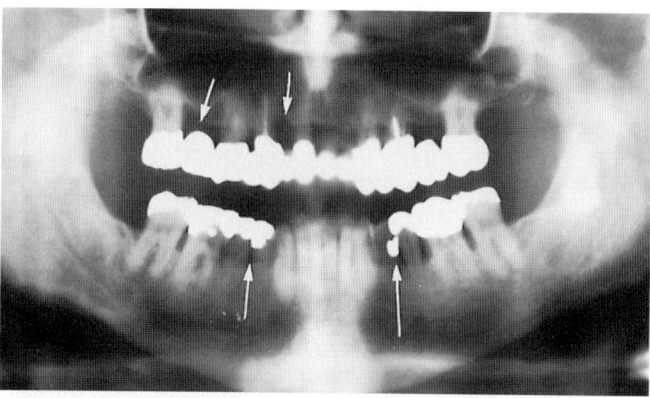

**FIGURE 217-11.** This panoramic dental radiograph shows advanced periodontal destruction and alveolar bone loss in a 64-year-old man. Onset of type 2 diabetes had occurred at the age of 60 years. In the intervening 3 years, three acute exacerbations had occurred, accompanied by abscess formation and mobility of teeth, when the patient had neglected his oral hygiene. With each episode, the patient's need for insulin increased significantly until dental treatment brought the oral infection under control. Notice that the crest of the alveolar bone (*arrows*) has receded to a line that is midway between the crowns and the root apices (tips) of the teeth. (Courtesy of Cullen C. Ward, DDS.)

The enlargement is bilateral, firm, smooth, and painless, and often persists after the diabetes is brought under control. Similarly enlarged salivary glands can occur in generalized undernutrition, chronic alcoholism, and Sjögren syndrome (see Table 217-1).

A slow but inexorably progressive periodontitis associated with a poor response to treatment occurs in some diabetic individuals even when their blood glucose is generally well controlled. When diabetes is poorly controlled, rapidly progressive periodontal destruction is a frequent occurrence (Figs. 217-9 through 217-11). Multiple and recurrent periodontal abscesses are characteristic of both situations. The substitution of blood glycated hemoglobin or of fructosamine for blood glucose as the indicator of diabetes control has clarified and strengthened the previously somewhat inconsistent correlation between such control and the severity of periodontal disease.[25]

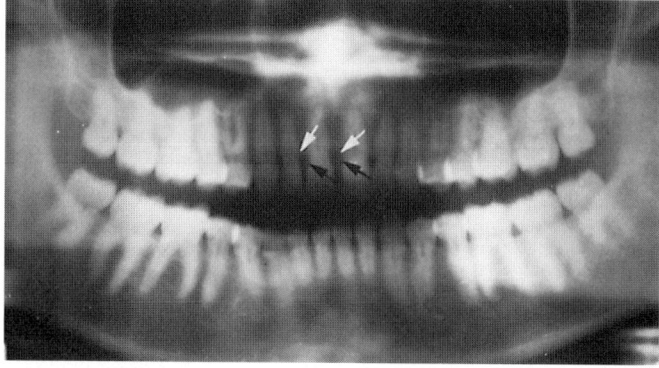

**FIGURE 217-10.** Panoramic dental radiograph of the patient depicted in Figure 217-8. Significant alveolar bone loss is evident among the maxillary incisors, where the crests of the interdental ridges (*white arrows*) were 2 to 3 mm below the lateral cementoenamel junctions (*black arrows*).

The xerostomia and altered taste that are seen in some diabetic patients are caused mostly by polyuria and resultant dehydration, but they also may be partially attributable to salivary gland dysfunction. These symptoms usually are relieved when the diabetes is controlled.

Oral candidiasis is more common among diabetic persons than among the general population because of reduced immunologic resistance, decreased salivary flow, and increased glucose in the oral fluids and tissues of the former.[23,26,27] The increased prevalence is independent of ABH(O) secretor status.[26] The best-known form of this disease is acute pseudomembranous candidiasis, or thrush, in which soft, creamy white plaques cover an erythematous mucosa (Fig. 217-12*A*). This form usually responds to topical antifungal therapy and recurs infrequently in diabetics whose disease is well controlled. Two similar, but apparently etiologically distinct, lesions affecting the dorsum of the tongue are more common among diabetic patients than among normal subjects.[28] One of these—median rhomboid glossitis (see Fig. 217-12*B*)—has a controversial etiology. Although it was once thought to be a developmental anomaly, many now believe it to be a form of chronic hyperplastic candidiasis. It seldom regresses completely or permanently with antifungal therapy, however, and, despite reports to the contrary, it does occur in infants and children. Therefore, the view that this condition is a developmental anomaly still has merit. The other lesion is a focal, atrophic variety of candidiasis. It sometimes occurs close to the same site as does median rhomboid glossitis but usually is more anterior and differs from the latter in the lack of hyperplasia except for the occasional appearance of a thin white plaque (see Figs. 217-12*C* and *D*).

Extensive and tenacious oral involvement with one or more of the forms of candidiasis (atrophic, pseudomembranous, or chronic hyperplastic) is likely to be a sign of a suppressed or defective immune system. For example, this type of involvement is common in patients with APECS[3] and acquired immunodeficiency syndrome (AIDS).[29]

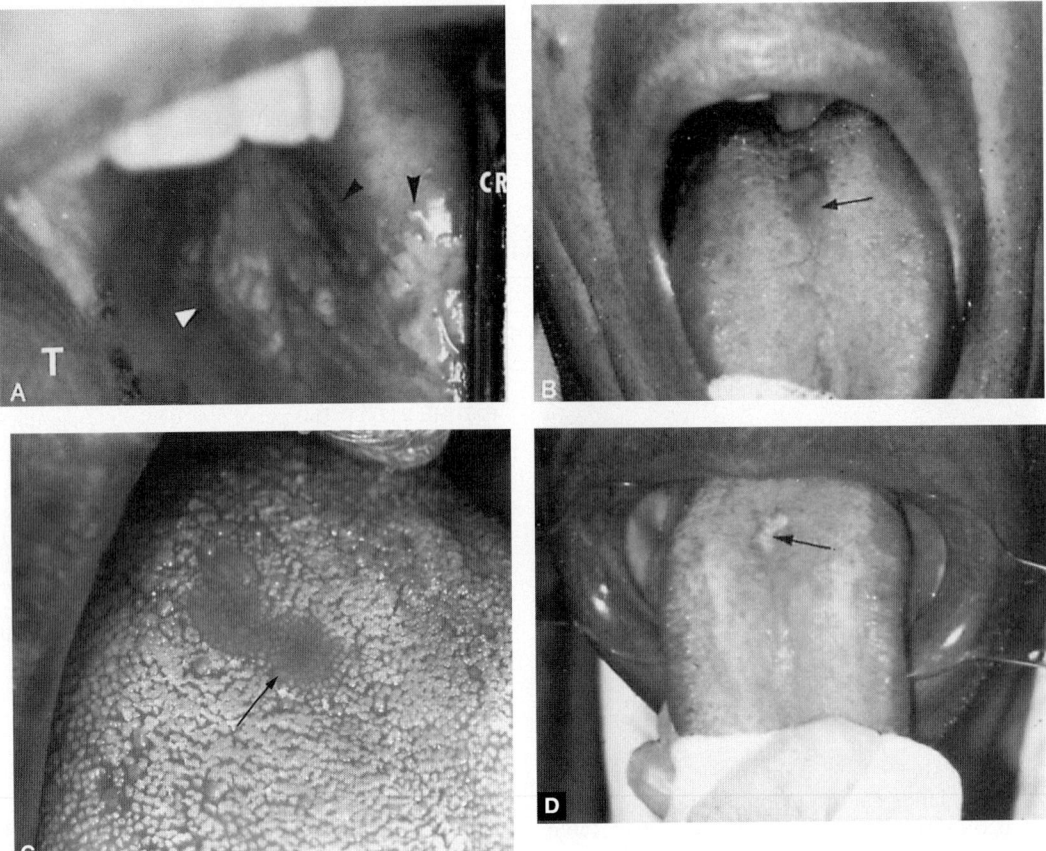

**FIGURE 217-12.** Three different types of oral candidiasis occurring in diabetic patients. **A,** Acute pseudomembranous oral candidiasis (thrush) in a 42-year-old woman. A lateral view of the retracted left buccal mucosa shows raised, curd-like plaque (*arrowheads*). Onset of the disease occurred 1 week after the patient began a 2-week course of penicillin for an upper respiratory tract infection. Nystatin oral suspension was prescribed, and the lesions healed within 3 days despite continuation of the penicillin. Nystatin was discontinued at the conclusion of the penicillin therapy, and the candidiasis did not recur. (*CR,* cheek retractor; *T,* tongue.) **B,** Median rhomboid glossitis (*arrow*) is evident as a lumpy bald patch on the dorsum of the tongue just anterior to the vallate papillae. The incidence of this benign, usually asymptomatic lesion is reported to be disproportionately high among diabetic patients, and many of the patients studied have been infected superficially with *Candida* organisms. **C,** Atrophic candidiasis presenting as a discrete erythematous patch with atrophic papillae. The lesion appeared on the right dorsum of the tongue of a 32-year-old man while his type 2 diabetes was poorly controlled. **D,** Focal, slightly hyperplastic candidiasis in a 64-year-old diabetic man who was a heavy cigarette smoker. In this case, both diabetes and smoking were considered to be etiologic factors. The thin, firm, white plaque on an erythematous base is a recurrent lesion. Although its location near the midline is somewhat anterior to where median rhomboid glossitis occurs, it is close enough to be confused with the latter. A previous patch in a more anterior and lateral location had been shown to be a result of infection with *Candida albicans* (confirmed by biopsy and culture), and a good response had been achieved after 2 weeks of treatment with nystatin troches dissolved in the mouth twice daily. This subsequent lesion also disappeared after 2 weeks of nystatin therapy.

# REFERENCES

1. Ten Cate AR. Tooth eruption. In: Bhaskar SN, ed. Orban's oral histology and embryology, 10th ed. St. Louis: CV Mosby, 1986:361.
2. Sharawy M, Bhussry BR, Suarez FR. Temporomandibular joint. In: Bhaskar SN, ed. Orban's oral histology and embryology, 10th ed. St. Louis: CV Mosby, 1986:395.
3. Shafer WG, Hine MK, Levy BM, Tomich CE. A textbook of oral pathology, 4th ed. Philadelphia: WB Saunders, 1983:56,616.
4. Snyder MB. Endocrine disease and dysfunction. In: Lynch MA, ed. Burket's oral medicine: diagnosis and treatment, 8th ed. Philadelphia: JB Lippincott, 1984:812.
5. Pindborg JJ. Pathology of the dental hard tissues. Copenhagen: Munksgaard, 1970:140,178.
6. Bricker SL, Langlais RP, Miller CS. Endocrine system. In: Bricker SL, Langlais RP, Miller CS, eds. Oral diagnosis, oral medicine, and treatment planning, 2nd ed. Philadelphia: Lea & Febiger, 1994:421.
7. Blake HH, Henning SJ. Effect of propylthiouracil dose on serum thyroxine, growth and weaning in young rats. Am J Physiol 1985; 248:R524.
8. Redman RS. Development of the salivary glands. In: Sreebny LM, ed. The salivary system. Boca Raton, FL: CRC Press, 1987:1.
9. Johnson DA. Regulation of salivary glands and their secretions by masticatory, nutritional, and hormonal factors. In: Sreebny LM, ed. The salivary system. Boca Raton, FL: CRC Press, 1987:135.
10. Wiesenfeld D, Webster G, Ferguson MM, et al. Salivary gland dysfunction following radioactive iodine therapy. Oral Surg 1983; 55:138.
11. Laupa MS, Toth BB, Keene HJ, Sellin RV. Effects of radioactive iodine therapy on salivary flow rates and oral *Streptococcus mutans* in patients with thyroid cancer. Oral Surg 1993; 75:312.
12. Smith BR, Fowler CB, Svane TJ. Primary hyperparathyroidism presenting as a peripheral giant cell granuloma. J Oral Maxillofac Surg 1988; 46:65.
13. Sowell SB. Dental care for patients with renal failure and renal transplants. J Am Dent Assoc 1982; 104:171.
14. Guccion JG, Redman RS, Winne CE. Hemodialysis-associated amyloidosis presenting as lingual nodules. Oral Surg 1989; 68:618.
15. Wotman S, Goodwin FJ, Mandel ID, Laragh JH. Changes in salivary electrolytes following treatment of primary aldosteronism. Arch Intern Med 1969; 124:477.
16. Gresik EW. The granular convoluted tubule (GCT) of rodent submandibular glands. Microsc Res Tech 1994; 27:1.
17. Laine M, Tenuovo J. Effects on peroxidase activity and specific binding of the hormone 17β-oestradiol and rat salivary glands. Arch Oral Biol 1983; 28:847.

18. Flaggert JJ III, Heldt LV, Gareis FJ. Recurrent giant cell granuloma occurring in the mandible of a patient on high dose estrogen therapy for the treatment of Soto's syndrome. J Oral Maxillofac Surg 1987; 45:1074.
19. Laine M, Leimola-Virtanen R. Effect of hormonal replacement therapy on salivary flow rate, buffer effect and pH in perimenopausal and postmenopausal women. Arch Oral Biol 1996; 41:91.
20. Anderson LC. Hormonal regulation of salivary glands, with particular reference to experimental diabetes. In: Garrett JR, Ekström J, Anderson LC, eds. Glandular mechanisms of salivary secretion. Basel: Karger, 1998:200
21. Bhathena SJ, Smith SS, Voyles NR, et al. Studies on submaxillary gland immunoreactive glucagon. Biochem Biophys Res Commun 1977; 74:1574.
22. Smith PH, Toms BB. Immunocytochemical localization of insulin- and glucagon-like peptides in rat salivary glands. J Histochem Cytochem 1986; 34:627.
23. Murrah VA. Diabetes mellitus and associated oral manifestations: a review. J Oral Pathol 1985; 14:271.
24. Le Floch J-P, Le Lievre G, Sadorn J, et al. Taste impairment and related factors in type 1 diabetes mellitus. Diabetes Care 1989; 12:173.
25. Unal T, Firatli E, Sivas A, Meric H, Hikmet O. Fructosamine as a possible monitoring parameter in non-insulin dependent diabetes patients with periodontal disease. J Periodontol 1993; 64:191.
26. Lamey P-J, Darwaza A, Fisher BM, et al. Secretor status, candidal carriage and candidal infection in patients with diabetes mellitus. J Oral Pathol 1988; 17:354.
27. Guggenheimer J, Moore PA, Rossie K, et al. Insulin-dependent diabetes mellitus and oral soft tissue pathologies: II. Prevalence and characteristics of Candida and Candidal lesions. Oral Surg Oral Med Oral Pathol Oral Radiol Endod 2000; 89:570.
28. Redman RS. Glossitis, median rhomboid type. In: Buyse ML, ed. Birth defects encyclopedia. Cambridge, MA: Blackwell Scientific Publications, 1990:417.
29. Pindborg JJ. Oral candidiasis in HIV infection. In: Robertson PB, Greenspan JS, eds. Perspectives on oral manifestations of AIDS. Littleton, MA: PSG Publishing, 1988:77.

# CHAPTER 218

# THE SKIN AND ENDOCRINE DISORDERS

JO-DAVID FINE, ADNAN NASIR, AND KENNETH L. BECKER

The endocrine system greatly influences the skin, both during the normal maturational and aging processes and in the course of several endocrine- or metabolism-related disease states.[1] In many cases, skin findings are the first disease indicators to be recognized by the astute clinician. In this chapter, the major cutaneous manifestations of several physiologic and disease states are emphasized. Detailed discussions of the extracutaneous and biochemical aspects of these conditions can be found elsewhere in this book.

## CUTANEOUS MANIFESTATIONS OF PHYSIOLOGIC ENDOCRINE STATES

### NEONATAL, PREPUBERTAL, AND POSTPUBERTAL PERIODS

Newborn human skin appears to contain most, if not all, of the well-characterized structural antigens, including epidermal cell surface antigens, keratins, basement membrane components, and collagens, that are present in adult skin. Despite this, some differences exist—most notably, the amount and distribution of terminal hair, the activity of glandular structures, and the pigmentation in some areas of the body. Many of these differences are regulated by the endocrine system. For example, terminal hair development in the axillary and pubic regions in both sexes, and in the bearded area in men, is absent until puberty, unless precocious puberty supervenes. Similarly, significant sebaceous and apocrine gland activity and their associated diseases,

including acne and hidradenitis suppurativa, as well as genital hyperpigmentation, usually are lacking in normal individuals until the onset of puberty. Seborrheic dermatitis, a common inflammatory condition of sebaceous glands characterized by mild erythema and scale, usually becomes clinically manifest at or after puberty. Seborrheic dermatitis occasionally is observed transiently in neonates, however (as are mild clitoral hypertrophy and vaginal discharge in the female neonate and gynecomastia in the male neonate), as a result of the presence of circulating maternal hormones within the infant. As discussed in Chapter 101, measurable aberrations in one or more hormones may be seen in some individuals with severe acne, and such patients may experience clinical improvement with administration of dexamethasone or androgen antagonists.

## PREGNANCY

During pregnancy, increased pigmentation develops in the genital and perianal regions, areolae, umbilicus, and linea nigra. Such hyperpigmentation subsides several months after the completion of pregnancy. Similarly, increased gingival tissue and inflammation, and an increase in the number or size of some skin tumors, including neurofibromas, nevi (moles), and skin tags (fibroma molluscum gravidarum), may occur.[2] At least in the case of nevi, this is most likely attributable to the effects of elevated estrogen levels on estrogen receptors present on nevus cell membranes. Another pigmentary disorder that is usually associated with pregnancy (or the use of oral contraceptives) is *melasma*, sometimes referred to as the "mask of pregnancy." This condition is characterized by the development of irregular, brownish discoloration, which at times becomes confluent, along the lateral aspects of the face, cheeks, forehead, and upper lip. In contrast to other pigmentary changes associated with pregnancy, however, melasma may persist for years afterward in some individuals and may become more pronounced with repeated sunlight exposure.

Other skin findings that may be associated with pregnancy include hyperhidrosis, hypertrichosis, urticaria, dermatographism, cutaneous flushing, other vascular changes, diffuse hair loss, and nail abnormalities. Vascular findings may include palmar erythema, telangiectases, spider angiomas, and pyogenic granulomas. Other skin diseases that may be exacerbated by pregnancy include acne, eczema, erythema multiforme, and malignant melanoma. In addition to these, several other specific skin conditions may arise during pregnancy, including herpes gestationis, pruritic urticarial papules and plaques of pregnancy (PUPPP), impetigo herpetiformis (a form of pustular psoriasis), pruritus gravidarum, papular dermatitis of pregnancy (of Spangler), and immune progesterone dermatitis of pregnancy.

Herpes gestationis (also called gestational pemphigoid) is a markedly pruritic vesiculobullous disorder that usually arises during the second or third trimester, waxes and wanes during the course of the pregnancy, flares at the time of delivery, and slowly diminishes in disease activity several weeks to months later.[3] Some patients experience disease recurrence, at times earlier or more severe, during successive pregnancies. In addition, affected individuals frequently experience flares during menses or after the initiation of treatment with oral contraceptives, findings that suggest a significant influence by the endocrine system in the perpetuation of disease activity. Despite this, however, no consistent aberrations in hormonal levels have been demonstrated in such patients. Because of the severity of symptoms and extent of disease, most patients require treatment throughout pregnancy with systemic corticosteroids or dapsone. Evidence to suggest that this disease is also immunologically mediated includes the demonstration of C3 and, less frequently, immunoglobulin G (IgG), which is bound, in vivo, to the basement membrane zone of lesional and perilesional skin. In addition, some patients' sera contain circulating IgG autoantibodies or a complement-fixing factor (herpes gestationis factor) capable of binding in vitro to the basement membrane zone of normal human skin. The target of these autoantibodies is bullous pemphigoid antigen-2, also known as *type XVII collagen*, a 180-kDa protein that is a normal structural component of the hemidesmosome and is one of two target antigens associated with bullous pemphigoid. These serum factors may be transmitted transplacentally to the infant, resulting in the transient development of similar eruptions in some newborn infants. Two other important aspects of this disease include an increased risk of morbidity and mortality (≤30%) in the fetus[4] and a markedly increased frequency of histocompatibility antigens HLA-DR3 and HLA-DR4 in affected mothers.[5]

By contrast, PUPPP is a markedly pruritic eruption that is seen in the latter portion of the third trimester and is characterized by the presence of variably sized red papules, urticarial plaques, and infrequent vesicles, often initially arising within the striae distensae.[6] Unlike with herpes gestationis, no fetal problems, immunologic abnormalities, or associations with HLA are seen in PUPPP.

Immune progesterone dermatitis of pregnancy is a rare disorder characterized by the appearance, during the first trimester, of a papulopustular eruption over the extremities, anterior thighs, and buttocks.[7] Affected patients have been reported to have numerous laboratory abnormalities, including peripheral eosinophilia, hypergammaglobulinemia, elevated serum histamine levels, elevated plasma β-estradiol levels, and slightly decreased urinary levels of 17-hydroxysteroids and 17-ketosteroids. Intradermal challenge with progesterone reportedly reproduces the disease histologically. Similarly, symptoms have been exacerbated and reduced in such patients after the introduction of progesterone- and estrogen-containing oral contraceptives, respectively.

Papular dermatitis of pregnancy (of Spangler) is a rare, severely pruritic eruption that can develop at any time during the course of pregnancy, clears rapidly after delivery, and may recur in future pregnancies.[8] As with herpes gestationis, a 30% incidence rate of fetal mortality (stillbirths, spontaneous abortions) has been reported in untreated cases. This eruption is characterized by the development of erythematous papules, crusts, excoriations, and postinflammatory hyperpigmentation. Associated endocrinologic abnormalities include elevated urinary levels of human chorionic gonadotropin, decreased plasma hydrocortisone levels with foreshortened half-life, and reduced or low-normal 24-hour urinary estrogen levels. Although diethylstilbestrol is no longer an acceptable mode of therapy, in the past affected patients were treated successfully with this agent. In addition, fetal loss appeared to be prevented by treatment with systemic corticosteroids.

Other conditions associated with pregnancy include impetigo herpetiformis, intrahepatic cholestasis of pregnancy, and occasionally diffuse nonscarring alopecia. Impetigo herpetiformis is not related to staphylococcal impetigo. It is instead a variant of severe, generalized pustular psoriasis, which occurs in the third trimester, is characterized by a high incidence of fetal and maternal mortality, and is associated with several endocrine abnormalities, including hypoparathyroidism and decreased urinary levels of pregnanediol, androsterone, and dehydroepiandrosterone. Intrahepatic cholestasis of pregnancy (pruritus gravidarum) occurs during the third trimester and may recur in subsequent pregnancies or after the initiation of oral contraceptive therapy. This disorder is characterized by laboratory and clinical findings that are consistent with cholestasis, including hyperbilirubinemia, jaundice, generalized pruritus, nausea, and vomiting.

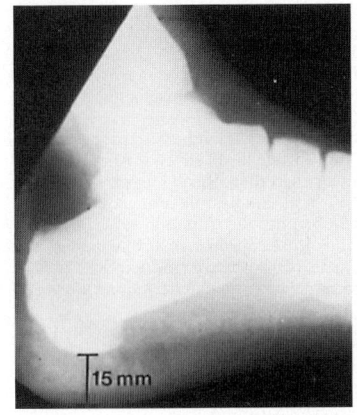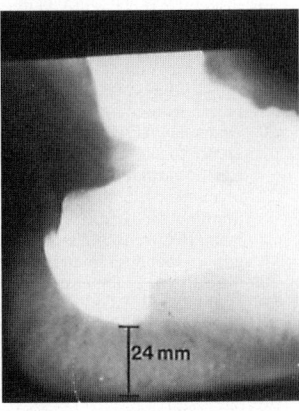

**FIGURE 218-1.** Radiograph of the foot of a patient with acromegaly (*right*) and a normal person (*left*). The heel pad distance is measured at the shortest distance between the calcaneus and plantar surface of the skin. In one study, most acromegalic patients had heel pad distance values of >20 mm (mean, 25.6 mm), whereas nearly all of the normal subjects had values of ≤20 mm.[36] Although this phenomenon is of pathophysiologic interest, a valid diagnosis is based on growth hormone studies.

Hair growth may increase during pregnancy. One explanation is that estrogen has been noted to prolong the anagen phase of the hair growth cycle. Postpartum hair loss can occur several weeks to months after delivery and may be related to reduced estrogen and progesterone levels.

## CUTANEOUS MANIFESTATIONS OF DISEASES OF SPECIFIC ENDOCRINE GLANDS

### PITUITARY GLAND

At least three disorders of hypersecretion by the anterior pituitary gland are associated with skin findings. In acromegaly (see Chap. 12), these include coarse, leathery, thickened skin with increased markings and deepened furrows (on the scalp this is referred to as cutis verticis gyrata because of its resemblance to the gyri of the cerebral cortex); hyperhidrosis; increased skin oiliness; hyperpigmentation; an increased amount and coarseness of body hair; increased numbers and sizes of skin tags (fibroma molluscum); thickening of the eyelids, nose, and lower lip; and acanthosis nigricans, which is characterized by hyperpigmentation and a velvet-like or increasingly papillomatous exaggeration of skin markings in usually symmetrical but localized regions (lateral neck, axillae, inguinal folds) (Figs. 218-1 and 218-2).

In Cushing disease, as well as in other conditions leading to the overproduction of adrenocorticotropic hormone (ACTH), generalized hyperpigmentation may develop as a result of the stimulation of epidermal melanocytes by this hormone and by related peptides of its precursor molecule. Pituitary microadenomas causing hyperprolactinemia may present with associated hirsutism.

Skin findings associated with panhypopituitarism include absent axillary and pubic hair, soft and finely textured skin (with fine facial wrinkling in some patients), and generalized pallor (including of the nipples) (Fig. 218-3). If hypogonadism is also present, a juvenile scalp hair pattern (i.e., lacking frontal recession) is observed.

### THYROID GLAND

In hyperthyroidism, the skin appears red, smooth, and warm, velvety, and moist to touch, the latter feature being attributable

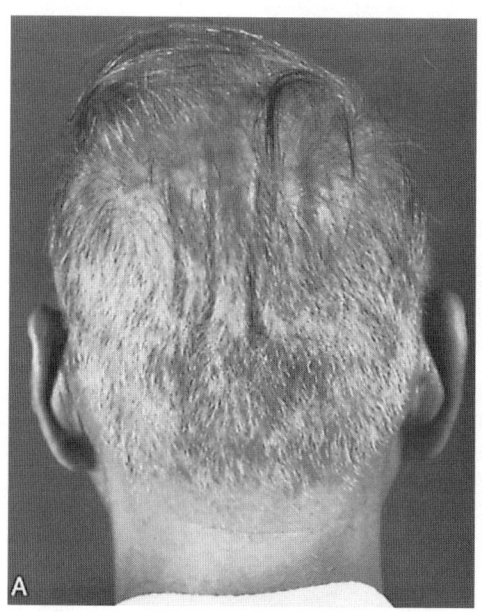

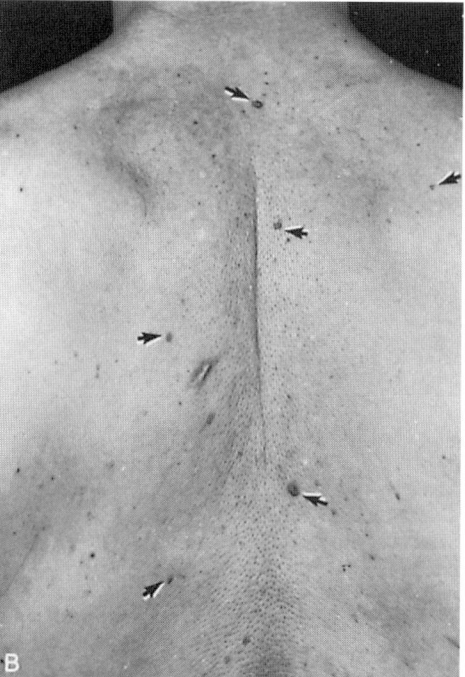

**FIGURE 218-2.** **A,** Cutis verticis gyrata in a man with acromegaly. The skin of the scalp has a corrugated appearance and forms elevated folds and intervening furrows that are not obliterated by traction. This condition may be familial (occurring mostly in men, and associated with increased facial creases), idiopathic, or secondary, as in acromegaly. **B,** Acrochordons (skin tags, fibroma molluscum) on the back of a man with acromegaly. These soft sessile or pedunculated lesions vary in size from 1 to 3 mm and, in whites, are flesh colored or brownish. They may appear on the neck, eyelids, upper chest, back, axillae, groin, or other folds of the body. They are characterized by a hyperplastic epidermis and a central connective tissue core. They are often seen in obesity and in association with acanthosis nigricans. The lesions may be removed by electrodesiccation, by cautery, or by scissors or a scalpel.

to generalized hyperhidrosis.[9] The face may be flushed and the palms may exhibit a marked redness (localized or diffuse), both of which are a reflection of cutaneous vasodilatation and increased blood flow. The scalp hair is finely textured, soft, and somewhat fragile. Other hair changes may include hirsutism, leukotrichia (Fig. 218-4), alopecia areata (a presumptive autoimmune disorder characterized by circular, well-circumscribed hair loss), and, at times, rather diffuse alopecia. Diffuse hyperpigmentation of the skin, similar to that seen in Addison disease, may occur in hyperthyroidism, although oral involvement is reportedly absent in the latter condition. The nails may become soft, shiny, and onycholytic (i.e., the nail separates from the dis-

tal nail bed [Fig. 218-5]), or concave, widened, irregular, and/or darkened. Other skin findings may include vitiligo (an autoimmune phenomenon manifested by discrete areas of depigmentation), urticaria, dermatographism, and generalized pruritus (Fig. 218-6; see Chap. 42).

By contrast, the skin in hypothyroidism (see Chap. 45) appears boggy but nonpitting, coarse, dry (the result of diminished eccrine and sebaceous gland activity), cool (owing to reduced core body temperature and cutaneous vasoconstriction), and pale. In more profound disease, nonpitting puffiness or edema may be observed in the face, eyelids, and hands. When the face is markedly affected, it may appear to be expressionless,

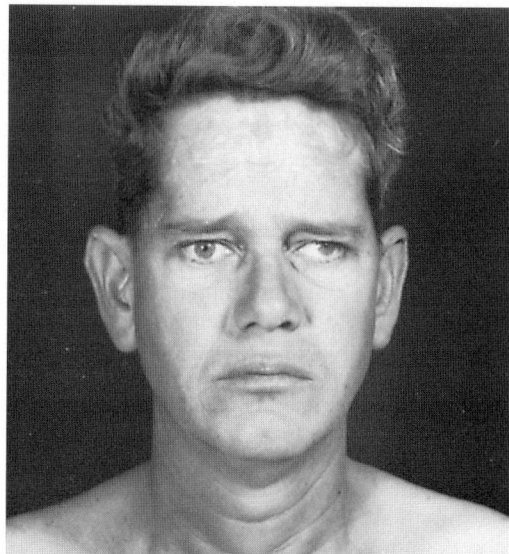

**FIGURE 218-3.** A 30-year-old man with panhypopituitarism subsequent to the surgical removal of a nonfunctioning pituitary tumor. The skin is soft and wrinkled. Marked pallor and an absence of facial hair are apparent. Notice the extraocular muscle palsy that is secondary to cranial nerve involvement by the lesion.

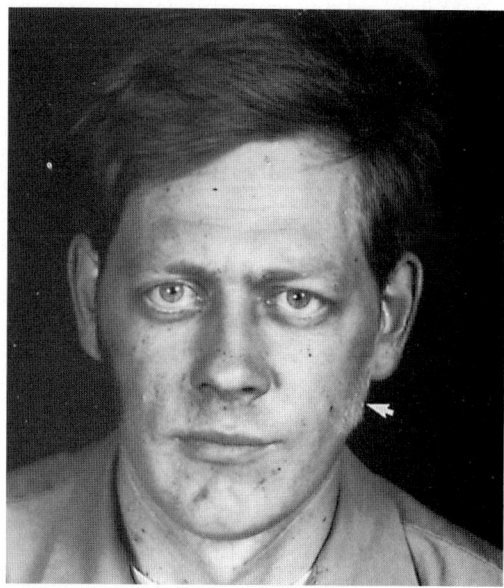

**FIGURE 218-4.** A young man, who is now euthyroid, shown several weeks after a course of radiation therapy for Graves disease. During this time, he developed leukotrichia of the left sideburn (*arrow*). Notice the slight residual exophthalmos on the right.

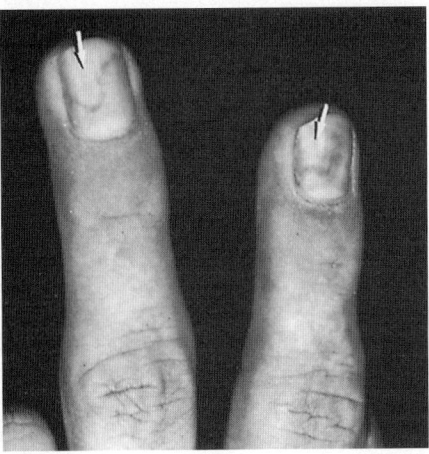

**FIGURE 218-5.** Onycholysis (Plummer sign) in a hyperthyroid man with Graves disease. Notice the separation of the nails from the nail beds (*arrows*).

owing to the loss of normal skin creases and markings. The tongue also may become markedly enlarged in myxedema. When hypopituitarism is also present, normally pigmented areas, such as the nipples, may become lightened. Some background yellowish discoloration may also be observed in hypothyroidism, reflecting carotene accumulation within the horny layer of the skin as a result of associated carotenemia. The hair appears dull, coarse, and brittle. In some patients, diffuse hair loss may occur, including over the scalp, the lateral thirds of the eyebrows (referred to as madarosis), the beard, and the genital regions. The nails are thin, striated, and brittle. In some patients, pruritus may be significant, possibly a reflection of extensive skin dryness and secondary inflammation. Localized or symmetrically distributed, matted telangiectases (the latter on the fingertips) and eruptive or tuberous xanthomas have also been observed in some patients with myxedema (Figs. 218-7 through 218-9).

In congenital hypothyroidism (cretinism), skin findings include thickened, dry, cool, yellowish skin; coarse scalp hair; and a mottled reticulate or livedo pattern on the extremities (see Chap. 47). Other findings may include enlargement of the

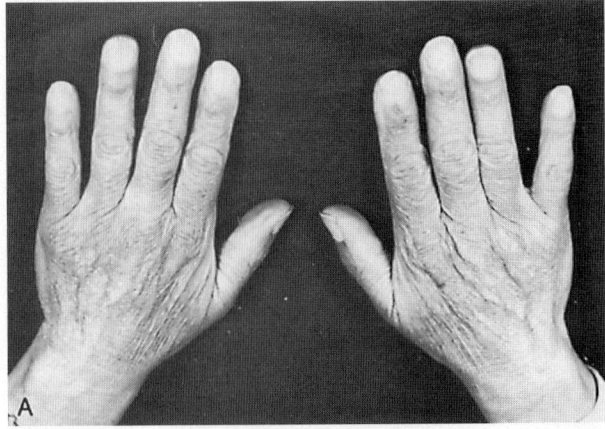

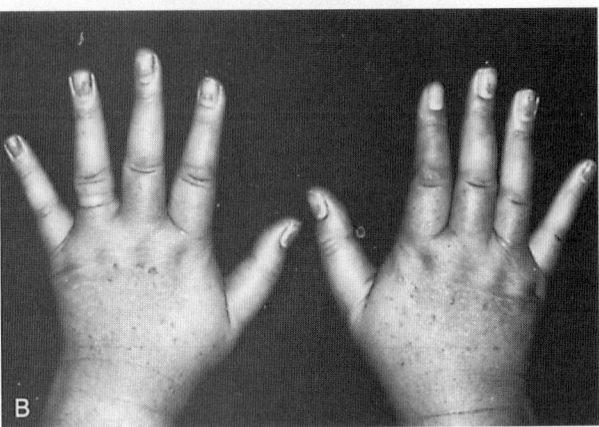

**FIGURE 218-7. A,** Severe dryness of the skin in a 45-year-old man with hypothyroidism secondary to Hashimoto thyroiditis. **B,** Nonpitting puffiness of the hands in a 22-year-old woman with hypothyroidism of 2 years' duration subsequent to radiation therapy for Graves disease.

tongue, protuberant lips, thickened and everted eyelids, a flattened nose, and confluence of the eyebrows. At puberty, pubic and axillary hair is either sparse or absent.

Pretibial myxedema is seen most commonly in patients with Graves disease, although it may occur less frequently in those who are euthyroid or hypothyroid. Pretibial myxedema most often develops symmetrically on the anterior lower extremities, although occasionally it is observed elsewhere (including the dorsal aspects of the hands, arms, face, and trunk). Rarely, it is localized to scar tissue.[9a] Typically, these lesions appear as skin-colored, yellowish, or somewhat violaceous plaques or nodules with a waxy texture, dilated follicular orifices ("peau d'orange"), and, at times, overlying hypertrichosis (see Chap. 42). Such lesions can be readily differentiated from necrobiosis lipoidica diabeticorum, because the latter have overlying telangiectatic vessels, tend to ulcerate centrally, and usually become atrophic rather than verrucous with time (see Chap. 153). With progression, areas of pretibial myxedema may become so thickened that they simulate the late acral skin changes of elephantiasis (elephantiasis verrucosa nostra). In some patients, the latter changes may actually produce distal deformative swelling. Occasionally, patients with pretibial myxedema also develop acquired keratoderma (excessive hyperkeratinization) of the palms, which rapidly improves with thyroxine therapy. Studies[10,11] in tissue culture suggest that patients with pretibial myxedema contain within their sera one or more heat-stable factors capable of inducing mucopolysaccharide biosynthesis by normal fibroblasts. In addition, this response appears to be site specific to the skin, because it occurs in fibroblasts from the

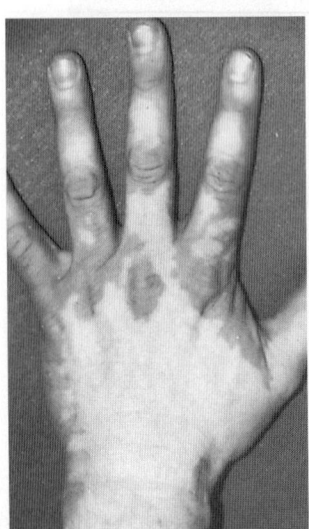 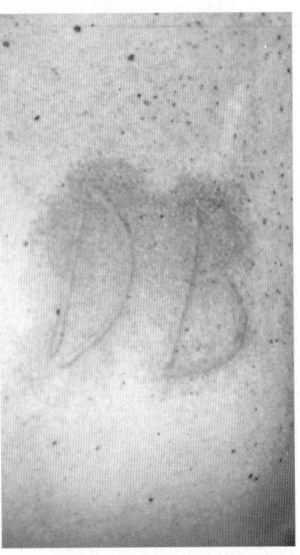

**A,B**

**FIGURE 218-6. A,** Progressive depigmentation, referred to as vitiligo, involving the hand. **B,** Dermatographism, a form of physical urticaria, on the trunk of an affected patient.

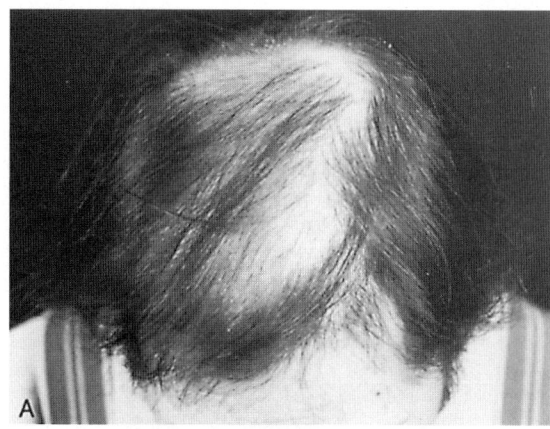

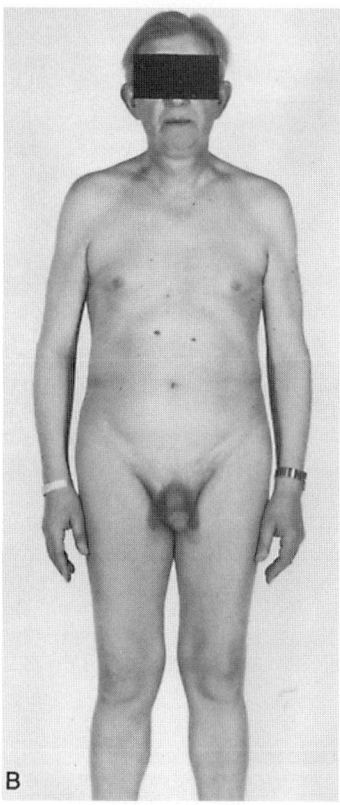

**FIGURE 218-8. A,** Severe alopecia in a 45-year-old man with hypothyroidism. **B,** Diffuse loss of body hair in a man with hypothyroidism.

pretibial areas of normal subjects and of patients with pretibial myxedema but not in fibroblasts from other regions of the body. Such findings correlate with the usually pretibial distribution of lesions, as well as the histologic and biochemical findings of increased mucin, hyaluronic acid, and dermatan sulfate within the affected dermis.

Thyroid acropathy is characterized by diaphyseal, periosteal proliferation of the distal long bones and phalanges, with overlying swelling of soft tissues. It is seen in some patients with pretibial myxedema and exophthalmic thyrotoxicosis (see Chap. 43).[11a]

Finally, the incidence of hyperthyroidism and hypothyroidism appears to be increased in patients with dermatitis herpetiformis. In a series of 305 patients with dermatitis herpetiformis followed for 10 years,[12] 4.3% had autoimmune thyroid disease, whereas only 1% developed vitiligo (the latter rate is not significantly different from that of the general population). Dermatitis herpetiformis is an intensely pruritic autoimmune vesiculobullous disorder that usually affects young adults and is characterized by the following: the occurrence of grouped, symmetrically distributed vesicles and crust (most often on the elbows, knees, buttocks, shoulders, and scalp); histologic, if not clinical, evidence of associated gluten-sensitive enteropathy; and immunoglobulin A (IgA) in vivo bound within the uppermost portion of the dermis.[13] Although the nature of the association between thyroid disease and dermatitis herpetiformis is poorly understood, it may simply reflect the increased prevalence of the HLA-B8 haplotype in patients with thyroid disorders and dermatitis herpetiformis.

Irradiation to the neck may produce hypothyroidism. As a correlate, the overlying skin may appear poikilodermatous or show other features of chronic radiodermatitis. In one series, for example, therapeutic neck irradiation was associated with characteristic skin changes in 57% of cases and hypothyroidism in 14%.[14]

## PARATHYROID GLANDS

The skin findings in hypoparathyroidism may include scaliness, dryness, and, in autoimmune hypoparathyroidism, altered pigmentation (hyperpigmentation or vitiligo).[15] Hair loss, which may either be mild or extensive, also may occur. The nails may be thin, brittle, and horizontally ridged. Associated skin disorders may include impetigo herpetiformis (see the previous discussion on the skin signs of pregnancy), candidiasis (Fig. 218-10), and exfoliative dermatitis. In contrast, calciphylaxis (described later) may be a manifestation of hyperparathyroidism.

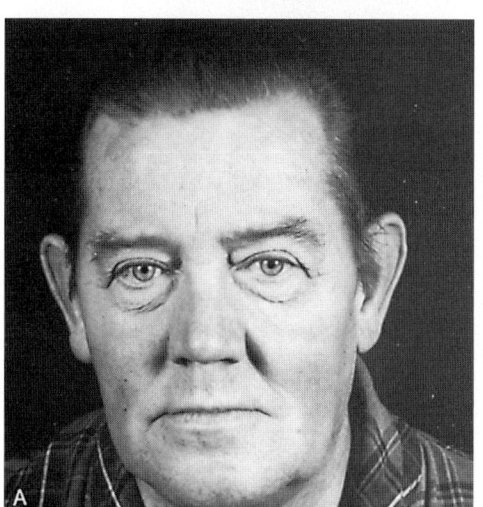

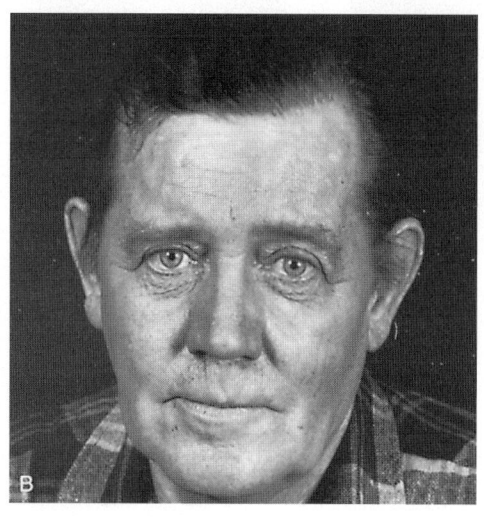

**FIGURE 218-9.** A 46-year-old man with hypothyroidism (**A**) before and (**B**) 6 months after treatment with thyroid hormone. Notice the more alert appearance, the darker skin, the increased sebaceous secretion, and the increased facial hair after therapy.

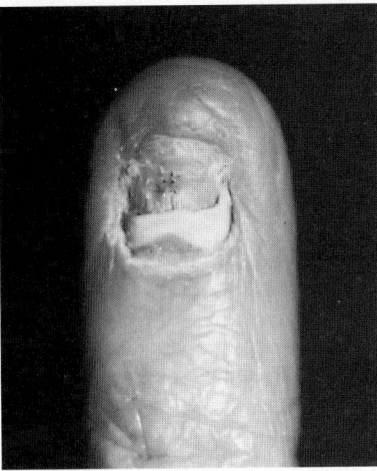

**FIGURE 218-10.** Brittleness, dystrophy, discoloration, and loss of the distal nail plate are evident in a patient with candidiasis of the nails.

## ADRENAL GLANDS

In Cushing syndrome (see Chap. 75), body fat tends to become centripetally distributed, leading to the characteristic appearance of exaggerated fat pads in the supraclavicular areas, posterior base of the neck (buffalo hump [Fig. 218-11A]), and cheeks (moon facies). The skin is somewhat atrophic as a result of the loss of dermal collagen and mucopolysaccharides, which, at least in part, contributes to its noticeably fine texture, the development of violaceous striae (on abdomen, thighs, arms), easy bruisability, plethoric-appearing facies, and prolonged wound healing. In addition, hirsutism and acne (see Fig. 218-11B) may develop, the latter of which may, at times, be severe. Primary pigmented nodular adrenocortical disease (Carney complex), an autosomal dominant disorder, is associated with familial multiple neoplasia (schwannomas and pituitary, adrenal, thyroid, heart, and eyelid tumors), multiple lentigines, blue nevi, myxomas, Cushing syndrome, and various other endocrine disor-

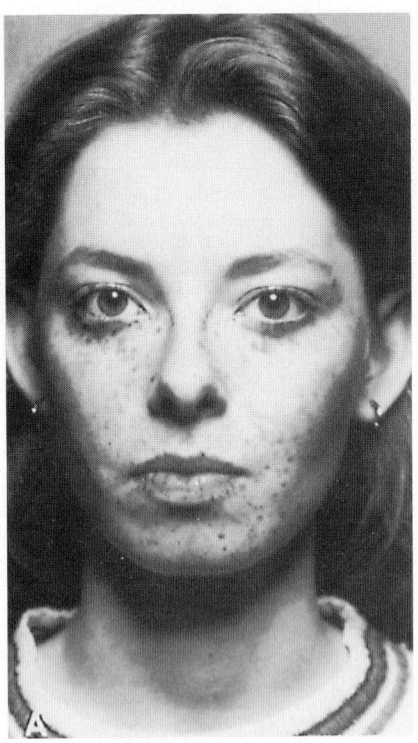

**FIGURE 218-12.** This young woman with multiple facial freckles has pigmented nodular adrenocortical disease (Carney complex). (From Carney JA, Gordon H, Carpenter PC, et al. The complex of myxomas, spotty pigmentation and endocrine overactivity. Medicine 1985; 64:270.)

ders (i.e., acromegaly from a growth hormone–producing adenoma)[16,16a] (Fig. 218-12).

In adrenal virilizing syndromes, female patients may exhibit multiple cutaneous findings. These may include hirsutism, marked male-pattern alopecia or baldness, thickening of the skin, male escutcheon, and acne (see Chap. 77).

In Addison disease (see Chap. 76), the major cutaneous finding is generalized hyperpigmentation of the skin and associated

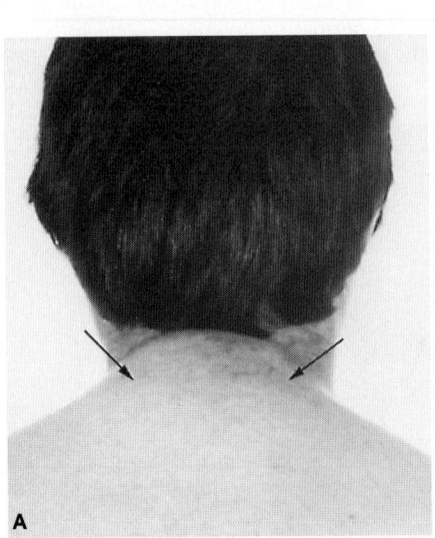

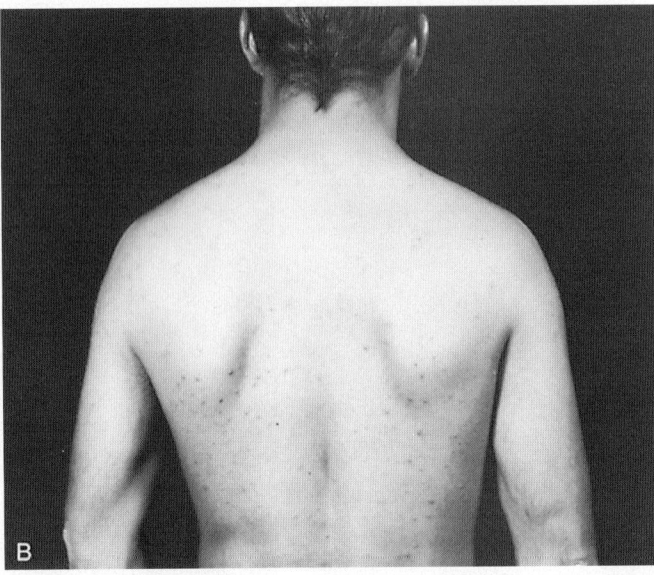

**FIGURE 218-11. A,** A 25-year-old woman with a cervicodorsal fat pad (buffalo hump) (*arrows*) associated with Cushing disease. Also notice the increased amount of fine hair over the woman's back. **B,** Acne of sudden onset on the back of a young man being treated with high doses of prednisone.

mucous membranes. This pigmentation, which is tan to bronze in color, is accentuated in exposed areas (i.e., the face), in flexural folds and creases (palms, knuckles, elbows), in sites of trauma (i.e., scars), and in skin regions that are normally pigmented (areolae, genitalia, some nevi, linea alba in pregnant women). In the oral cavity, the gums, buccal mucosa, and tongue all may be involved, and may appear blue-black in longstanding disease. Other mucosal surfaces, including the conjunctiva and vagina, also may become hyperpigmented. Similarly, hair becomes darker in color and nails may develop darkened longitudinal bands (see Chap. 14). In addition to hyperpigmentation, a subset of patients with Addison disease also develop areas of vitiligo.

## PANCREAS

The most common pancreatic disorder with skin manifestations is diabetes mellitus. Associated findings are discussed in detail in Chapter 153. Also, Chapter 163 discusses the skin manifestations of the hyperlipemias, some of which may be associated with disordered carbohydrate metabolism.

Glucagon-producing islet cell tumors of the pancreas are associated with a distinctive eruption—referred to as necrolytic migratory erythema—as well as systemic symptoms and findings that include weakness, weight loss, and diarrhea. Laboratory evaluation may reveal markedly elevated plasma glucagon levels, normocytic normochromic anemia, elevated sedimentation rate, hyperglycemia, hypocholesterolemia, and hypoaminoacidemia[17] (see Chap. 220).

Necrolytic migratory erythema is characterized by a symmetrical annular or arciform array of erythema, scale, papules, erosions, crusts, flaccid bullae, and postinflammatory hyperpigmentation. Typically, the advancing border may appear vesiculopustular, whereas the receding border is denuded. This eruption usually develops on the face, lower abdomen, groin, perineum, buttocks, thighs, and distal extremities. Given this morphology, only a limited differential diagnosis exists, including pemphigus, zinc deficiency (inherited [acrodermatitis enteropathica] or acquired), and extensive candidiasis.

Other findings associated with glucagonoma include glossitis, stomatitis, angular cheilitis, blepharitis, scalp alopecia, and thin and friable nails. Usually, necrolytic migratory erythema rapidly disappears after successful surgical removal of the glucagon-secreting tumor.

Several other diseases involving the pancreas, in addition to diabetes mellitus and glucagonoma, are associated with skin changes, including pancreatitis, adenocarcinoma of the pancreas, and hemochromatosis. In acute or fulminant pancreatitis, for example, suppurative panniculitis may develop. These lesions, which reflect saponification and necrosis of subcutaneous tissue secondary to the effects of elevated serum levels of lipolytic enzymes, are variably sized, painful nodules that are palpable deep within the skin and that characteristically drain, exuding an oily discharge to the skin surface. Identical lesions may also occur in the setting of pancreatic adenocarcinoma. Recurrent migratory superficial thrombophlebitis, usually seen on the upper extremities, is also a marker for internal malignant disease, including pancreatic adenocarcinoma. In hemochromatosis (a disorder of excessive iron absorption or parenteral iron loading), multiple organs may be involved, including the pancreas. Involvement of the latter may lead to the development of diabetes.[18] The cutaneous findings associated with hemochromatosis (see Chap. 131) include localized to generalized bronze or bluish gray discoloration, dryness, skin atrophy, hair loss (truncal, axillary, suprapubic), palmar erythema, and spider angiomas, of which the latter two features most likely reflect cirrhosis and its associated hyperestrogenic state. The bronze skin discoloration in hemochromatosis has been attributed to increased melanin content within the

epidermis, whereas the bluish hue is believed to be the result of iron deposition within sweat glands. This discoloration initially develops on exposed areas of the body and is most intense over the face, arms, genitalia, and body folds. A number of studies have linked a novel major histocompatibility complex class I–like gene called *HLA-H* with hemochromatosis. This gene has also been implicated in porphyria cutanea tarda.[19,20]

## MISCELLANEOUS CONDITIONS INVOLVING THE SKIN AND ENDOCRINE SYSTEM

### ACANTHOSIS NIGRICANS

As previously described, acanthosis nigricans is usually a localized process characterized by hyperpigmentation, papillomatous velvety hyperproliferation, and dermal glycosaminoglycan deposition of the skin.[21] For practical purposes, acanthosis nigricans can be thought of as arising primarily in three subsets of patients. In the first subset, a very mild clinical variant, sometimes referred to as "benign" acanthosis nigricans, develops along the sides of the neck, in the axillary vaults, and in the inguinal folds and perineal region. This form is associated with obesity and with onset at puberty or afterward (Fig. 218-13). This benign acanthosis nigricans, however, also has been reported in a number of other unrelated conditions, such as acromegaly, pituitary and hypothalamic tumors or lesions (sarcoidosis), Cushing disease, adrenal insufficiency, polycystic ovary syndrome, chondrodystrophy, Wilson disease, lupoid hepatitis, hepatic cirrhosis, Rud syndrome (lamellar ichthyosis, dwarfism, hypogonadism, mental retardation, and epilepsy), Bloom syndrome (photosensitivity, facial telangiectasia, short stature, and neoplasia), and drug use (diethylstilbestrol, corticosteroids, and nicotinic acid). The second group of patients with associated benign acanthosis nigricans, which is often extensive or generalized in distribution, are those with syndromes of insulin-resistant diabetes mellitus (see Chap. 146). In the third form of the disease, which is often referred to as "malignant" acanthosis nigricans, the eruption appears de novo, usually after the age of 50 to 55 years, and is associated with occult malignant diseases, the most common of which is adenocarcinoma of the stomach (see Chap. 219).

### MULTIPLE ENDOCRINE NEOPLASIA

The cutaneous manifestations that occur in patients with various types of multiple endocrine neoplasia (MEN) may reflect the particular organs involved (e.g., the parathyroid, pituitary, and pancreatic islet cells in MEN type 1 [MEN1]). In addition, patients with MEN1 develop multiple angiofibromas, collagenomas, epidermal inclusion cysts, leiomyomas, and lipomas.[22] Tumors in

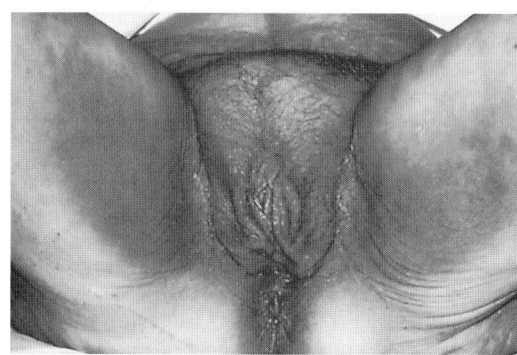

**FIGURE 218-13.** The vulva and medial thighs of this woman with acanthosis nigricans are hyperpigmented and have a velvet-like appearance (see Chap. 146).

patients with MEN1 show deletion of the *MEN1* gene, suggesting loss of heterozygosity.[23] In MEN2A, no specific skin markers are present, whereas in MEN2B (medullary carcinoma of the thyroid and pheochromocytoma), extensive neuromas may occur and may involve the mucous membranes. In addition, evidence of diffuse lentigos, café-au-lait spots, neuromas, or neurofibromas may be present (see Chap. 188).

## VITILIGO

Vitiligo, which was mentioned earlier, is a presumptive autoimmune condition characterized by the development of symmetrical depigmentation (either localized or generalized) of the skin. It usually occurs in the absence of endocrine disease; however, a subset of patients may develop vitiligo before, at the same time, or after the appearance of one or more endocrine conditions, including thyroid disease, Addison disease, diabetes mellitus, and hypoparathyroidism. For example, ~7% of patients with Graves disease, and 15% of those with Addison disease, have been reported to have vitiligo. Furthermore, vitiligo may be seen in some patients who are diagnosed as having autoimmune polyglandular failure syndrome, and various autoantibodies (including antibodies directed against thyroid, adrenal, and parietal cells) may be detectable in the sera of some patients with vitiligo, even in the absence of definable endocrinopathy (see Chap. 197).

## LIPODYSTROPHIES

Lipodystrophies are characterized by localized, partial, or generalized loss of subcutaneous tissue. Localized lipodystrophy (see Chaps. 143 and 153) occurs primarily at sites of insulin injection. Although it has been a problem in the past, lipodystrophy is seen less commonly in patients who are using the newer, more purified or synthetic insulin preparations. In partial (progressive cephalothoracic) lipodystrophy, which has a 20% incidence of associated diabetes mellitus, an initial loss of subcutaneous tissue in the facial area leads to marked coarsening of the facial features. With time, this process slowly progresses inferiorly. A generalized form of lipodystrophy (Lawrence-Seip syndrome), which is characterized by autosomal recessive transmission and onset at puberty, also may occur. This form is associated with insulin-resistant diabetes mellitus, hyperthyroidism, and acanthosis nigricans. Affected patients may also manifest cirrhosis, epilepsy, mental retardation, xanthomas, or osteoporosis (see Chap. 146).

## BUSCHKE SCLEREDEMA

Buschke scleredema is characterized by the sudden onset of diffuse symmetrical, nonpitting, woody induration of the skin. This usually develops first in the posterior and lateral aspects of the neck, but it may progress over a period of several weeks to months to include the upper trunk, back, and arms and, rarely, other areas of the body. The affected skin is usually flesh-colored. When the induration is pronounced, some areas may actually have a peau d'orange appearance (Fig. 218-14). The face, when affected, may become expressionless. Although this disorder usually affects only the skin, other tissues rarely may become involved, including the tongue, pharynx, conjunctiva, heart, and pleura. Diabetes mellitus is seen in many of these patients. Others may have multiple myeloma.[23a] The etiology of this condition is unknown. Both adults and children may be affected, and many experience a preceding infection, which is most often streptococcal in nature. Histochemical studies suggest increased collagen synthesis and, in some cases, increased deposition of acid mucopolysaccharides within the dermis. In most patients, this disorder spontaneously resolves within 6 to 24 months; however, in others, it may persist for years or indefinitely.

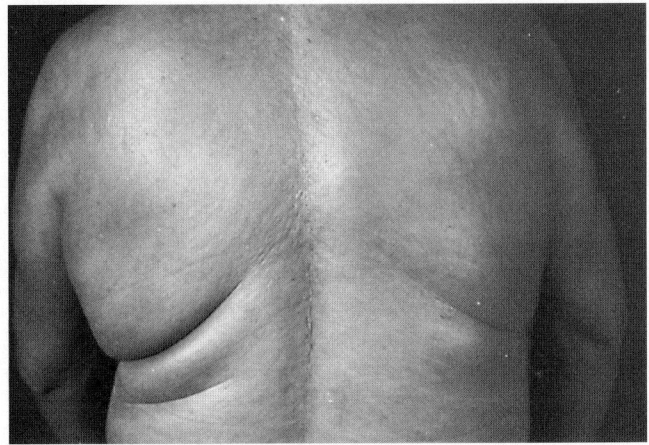

**FIGURE 218-14.** Buschke scleredema in a man with type 2 diabetes mellitus. Notice the thickened, infiltrated, peau d'orange appearance of the skin of the back.

## CUTANEOUS CALCIFICATION

Calcification may occur in localized or more generalized areas of skin and other organs as a result of (a) preceding tissue injury (dystrophic calcification), (b) markedly elevated calcium-phosphorus product (metastatic calcification), or (c) unknown causes (as in the case of calcinosis circumscripta or universalis). When present within the skin, asymptomatic papules or nodules are usually seen. In some situations, these lesions may break down, leading to drainage of chalky material. Among endocrine conditions associated with metastatic calcification to the skin, hyperparathyroidism and hypoparathyroidism must be considered in the differential diagnosis (Fig. 218-15). In one unique clinical disorder—calciphylaxis—painful ischemic ulcerations may develop on the fingers, legs, and thighs of patients with secondary or tertiary hyperparathyroidism who are undergoing maintenance hemodialysis or who have functioning renal homografts.[24,25] Although the mechanism for this phenomenon

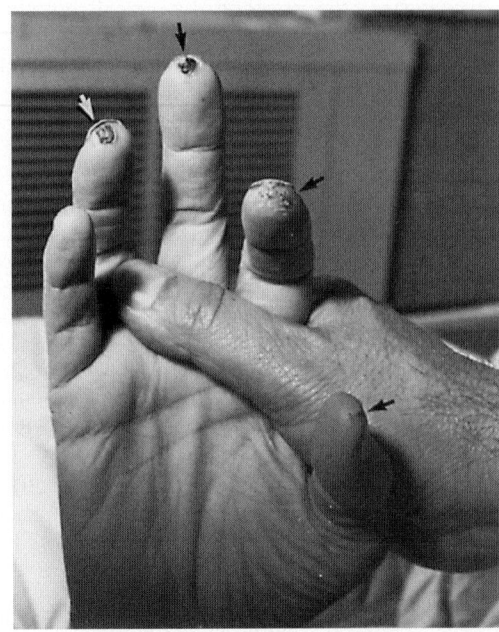

**FIGURE 218-15.** Severe calcinosis cutis in a patient who has hyperparathyroidism secondary to prolonged renal failure and who is on dialysis. Multiple ischemic ulcerations of the fingers are visible (*arrows*).

is still poorly understood, it appears in part to involve arterial insufficiency and ischemic necrosis in conjunction with medial calcification of dermal and subcutaneous arterioles and arteries. Although patients on long-term dialysis commonly develop metastatic calcification of various organs, the skin is involved only rarely.[26] Calciphylaxis is estimated to occur in 1% of patients with end-stage renal disease each year. Nonhealing lesions may become secondarily infected, leading to sepsis and death. Although lower extremities are typically involved, truncal or proximal lesions tend to be associated with a poorer prognosis. In some patients, parathyroidectomy may lead to dramatic healing of ulcers.[27] Some patients have subsequently developed tertiary hyperparathyroidism from increased mobilization of $Ca^{2+}/PO_4^{3-}$ stores in the viscera and lungs.[28]

## OTHER METABOLIC DISORDERS WITH CUTANEOUS MANIFESTATIONS

Albright syndrome (i.e., McCune-Albright syndrome) consists of the triad of localized hyperpigmentation, often unilateral lesions of fibrous dysplasia affecting the long bones of the extremities or pelvis, and precocious puberty. The characteristic skin lesion in this syndrome is a solitary, often large, brown macule with jagged borders that is located on the same side of the body as the underlying bony abnormalities. In addition, oral hyperpigmentation may be seen in some patients.

A separate entity, Albright hereditary osteodystrophy (AHO), is a disorder characterized by a unique body habitus (short stature, round facies, hand abnormalities [brachydactyly, short 4th and 5th metacarpals/tarsals, long index finger, depressed knuckles]), developmental delay, cataracts, cutaneous calcifications, radiographic abnormalities (thickened calvarium, basal ganglia calcifications), hypocalcemic tetany, elevated parathyroid hormone (PTH) and hyperphosphatemia.[29] Cutaneous findings in AHO include dermal and subcutaneous firm nodules. The overlying skin may be normal in appearance, pigmented, translucent, or opaque. A rim of erythema and slight tenderness may be present. Occasionally, firm calcifying erythematous plaques are noted. Lesions may be solitary or multiple and tend to occur around the joints of the extremities. Some lesions may progress to ulceration and extrusion of chalky material. Other associated endocrine findings include hyperprolactinemia, partial antidiuretic hormone resistance, and hyper- or hypothyroidism. Some patients may have diminished olfaction.[30] Approximately half of these patients have the type IA disorder, which is caused by a defective G protein that couples the PTH receptor to the cytoplasm. A temperature-sensitive type IA variant is found that is associated with precocious puberty in males. Type IB is associated with no electrolyte or PTH abnormalities (misnamed as pseudopseudohypoparathyroidism). Type II has an unknown underlying defect. Albright hereditary osteodystrophy is not to be confused with McCune-Albright syndrome. Ironically, both disorders were described as distinct entities by the same investigator and have subsequently been found to be caused by a defect in the same G protein.

Neurofibromatosis is an autosomal dominant disorder characterized by the development of usually widespread tumors (neurofibromas) on the skin, as well as in other organs, including the nervous system, eye, gastrointestinal tract, and bone.[31] Less than 1% of patients with neurofibromatosis develop a pheochromocytoma. A pathognomonic skin finding in neurofibromatosis is axillary freckling. Other characteristic skin lesions include café-au-lait spots (Fig. 218-16) (>75% of affected patients have six or more with a diameter of at least 1.5 cm), soft pedunculated or firmer nonpedunculated neurofibromas, and, rarely, large lobulated masses (plexiform neuromas) containing tumors arranged along peripheral nerves.[32]

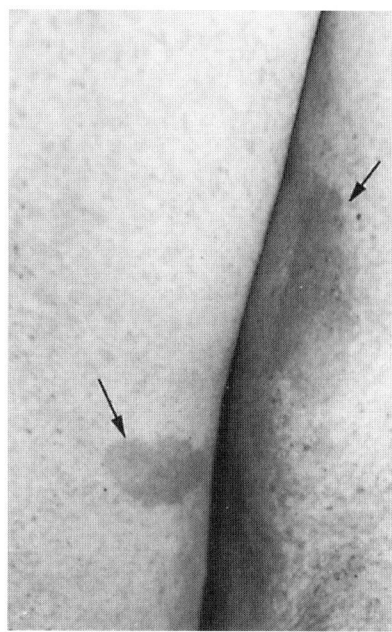

**FIGURE 218-16.** Discrete, hyperpigmented macules (*arrows*), referred to as café-au-lait spots, are visible on the backs of the legs of a patient with neurofibromatosis.

Werner syndrome[33] is an autosomal recessive condition that is associated with endocrine abnormalities, such as diabetes mellitus, hypogonadism, osteoporosis, metastatic subcutaneous calcifications, and impotence. The skin typically shows patches of scleroderma-like changes and marked, premature wrinkling (Fig. 218-17).

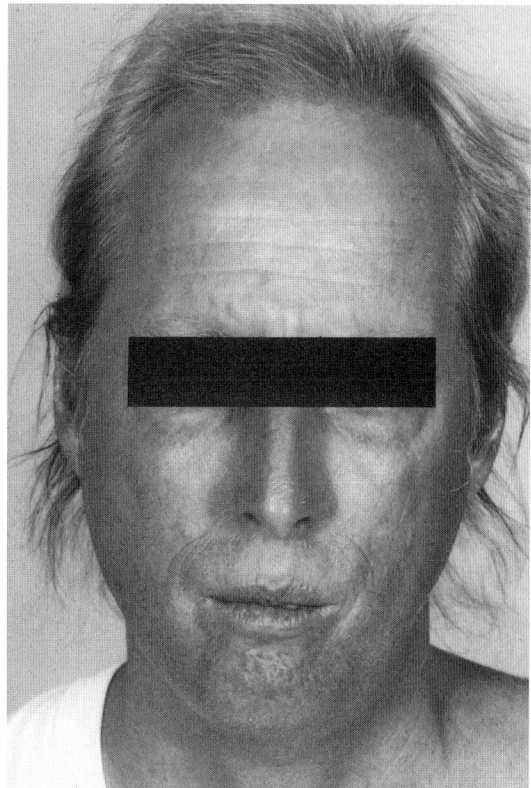

**FIGURE 218-17.** A 45-year-old man with Werner syndrome. Note the wrinkled, thin skin, graying and thinned hair, and overall aged appearance.

Many other metabolic disorders, both acquired and inherited, have prominent cutaneous manifestations. Although a detailed discussion of each of these conditions is beyond the scope of this chapter, salient features of several of these diseases are summarized in Table 218-1.[34–37]

**TABLE 218-1.**
**Selected Metabolic Disorders with Cutaneous Manifestations**

| Disease | Mode of Transmission | Metabolic Defect | Clinical Findings | |
|---|---|---|---|---|
| | | | *Skin* | *Extracutaneous* |
| **DISORDERS OF AMINO ACID METABOLISM**[*34–37] | | | | |
| PHENYLKETONURIA | AR | Phenylalanine hydroxylase deficiency (owing to defective dihydrobiopterin biosynthesis, or deficient dihydropteridine reductase in 10% of affected patients) | Fair complexion; blond or light hair; atopic eczema; sclerodermoid changes (in lower extremities); atrophoderma; linear scleroderma | Blue eyes; neurologic deterioration; skeletal changes (microcephaly, short stature, syndactyly, pes planus); pyloric stenosis |
| HOMOCYSTINURIA | AR | Cystathionine synthetase deficiency | Fair complexion; fine, light hair; malar blush; livedo reticularis | Ocular changes (e.g., glaucoma, dislocated lens, proptosis); neurologic abnormalities (seizures, mental retardation); skeletal disorders (disproportion, various deformities, vertebral osteoporosis, high arched palate); hepatomegaly; premature atherosclerosis (strokes, myocardial infarcts); thromboembolic phenomena |
| ALKAPTONURIA | AR | Homogentisic acid oxidase deficiency | Gray discoloration (eyelids, tarsal plate, pinna, hands, nasal tip, malar face, flexural areas) | Ocular discoloration (gray) (sclera, conjunctiva, cornea); spinal changes (e.g., lumbosacral spondylosis); severe degenerative arthritis; calculi (prostatic, renal); aortic valve murmurs |
| HARTNUP DISEASE | AR | Defective amino acid transport (renal, intestinal) | Photoeruption (pellagra-like); abnormal hair | Neurologic changes (ataxia, dementia, spasticity); short stature; diarrhea; glossitis, stomatitis |
| TYROSINEMIA (TYPE II; RICHNER-HANHART SYNDROME)[34] | ?AR | Absent tyrosine aminotransferase | Painful palmoplantar keratoses | Corneal ulcers and clouding; photophobia |
| **DISORDERS OF LIPID METABOLISM**[†] | | | | |
| FABRY DISEASE | XR | Galactosidase A deficiency | Angiokeratomas (diffuse; especially affecting the umbilicus, knees); telangiectases; turtle-back nails; defective sweating | Angiokeratomas (oral mucosa, tongue, conjunctiva); severe peripheral neuralgias; fever; distal arthropathy; corneal opacities; aneurysmal dilatations (conjunctival veins); renal failure; hypertension; atherosclerosis; pulmonary disease |
| REFSUM DISEASE | AR | Phytanic acid α-hydroxylase deficiency | Acquired ichthyosis | Ocular changes (night blindness, altered visual fields, retinitis pigmentosa, cataracts); impaired hearing; neurologic abnormalities (e.g., ataxia, polyneuropathy); renal disease; skeletal deformities |
| **DISORDERS OF METAL METABOLISM**[‡] | | | | |
| WILSON DISEASE | AR | Abnormal copper metabolism | Hyperpigmentation (legs); easy bruisability; azure lunulae (nails) | Pigmented corneal ring (Kayser-Fleischer ring); neurologic changes (cerebellar, pyramidal, pseudobulbar); psychiatric symptoms; hepatic disease (hepatitis, cirrhosis); hypersplenism; hemolytic anemia; skeletal changes; renal calculi, arthralgias; cardiac disease (rare) |
| MENKES SYNDROME | XR | Abnormal copper transport | Abnormal hair (pili torti) | Failure to thrive; hypothermia; recurrent infections (respiratory and gastrointestinal); neurologic abnormalities (retardation, seizures, spasticity); deafness; blindness |
| ACRODERMATITIS ENTEROPATHICA[36] | AR | Zinc deficiency | Symmetric erosions, crusts, vesicles; hyperkeratotic areas (periorificial, acral, perianal, intergluteal); nail dystrophy; alopecia | Failure to thrive; malabsorption; diarrhea; growth retardation; photophobia |

*AR*, autosomal recessive; *XR*, X-linked recessive.
[*]See Chap. 191.
[†]See Chap. 163.
[‡]See Chap. 131.

# PIGMENTARY ALTERATIONS AND THE ENDOCRINE SYSTEM

As previously discussed, many endocrine disorders are characterized by generalized or focal increased or decreased pigmentation of the skin. Techniques are available to quantify skin pigmentation.[38] For example, *hyperpigmentation* may occur with Addison disease, ACTH-producing tumors of the pituitary gland, paraneoplastic ACTH secretion, and POEMS syndrome (*p*eripheral neuropathy, *o*rganomegaly, *e*ndocrine dysfunction, *m*onoclonal gammopathy, and *s*kin pigmentation).[32,39] *Hypopigmentation* may accompany panhypopituitarism, hypogonadism (particularly in the male patient), and vitiligo (in polyglandular autoimmune deficiency).

# REFERENCES

1. Fine JD, Moschella SL. Diseases of nutrition and metabolism. In: Moschella SL, Hurley HJ, eds. Dermatology, 2nd ed. Philadelphia: WB Saunders, 1985:1422.
2. Costello MJ. Eruptions of pregnancy. N Y State J Med 1941; 41:849.
3. Katz SI, Hertz KC, Yaoita H. Immunopathology and characterization of the herpes gestationis factor. J Clin Invest 1976; 57:1434.
4. Lawley TJ, Stingl G, Katz SI. Fetal and maternal risk factors in herpes gestationis. Arch Dermatol 1978; 114:552.
5. Shornick JK, Stastny P, Gilliam JM. High frequency of histocompatibility antigens HLA-DR3 and DR4 in herpes gestationis. J Clin Invest 1981; 68:553.
6. Lawley TJ, Hertz KC, Wade TR, et al. Pruritic urticarial papules and plaques of pregnancy. JAMA 1979; 241:1696.
7. Bierman SM, Ackerman AB, Katz SI. Autoimmune progesterone dermatitis of pregnancy. Arch Dermatol 1973; 107:896.
8. Spangler AS, Emerson K Jr. Estrogen levels and estrogen therapy in papular dermatitis of pregnancy. Am J Obstet Gynecol 1971; 110:534.
9. Lang PC. Cutaneous manifestations of thyroid disease. Cutis 1978; 21:862.
9a. Pujol RM, Monmany J, Bague S, Alomar A. Graves' disease presenting as localized myxoedematous infiltration in a smallpox vaccination scar. Clin Exp Dermatol 2000; 25:132.
10. Cheung H, Nicoloff JT, Kamiel MB, et al. Stimulation of fibroblast biosynthetic activity by serum of patients with pretibial myxedema. J Invest Dermatol 1978; 71:12.
11. Jolliffe DS, Gaylarde PM, Brock AP, Sarkany I. Pretibial myxedema: stimulation of mucopolysaccharide production of fibroblasts by serum. Br J Dermatol 1979; 100:557.
11a. Suzuki H, Shimura H, Haraguchi K, et al. Exophthalmos, pretibial myxedema, osteoarthropathy syndrome associated with papillary fibroelastoma in the left ventricle. Thyroid 1999; 9:1257.
12. Reunala T, Collin P. Diseases associated with dermatitis herpetiformis. Br J Dermatol 1997; 136:315.
13. Zone JJ, Petersen MJ. Dermatitis herpetiformis. In: Thiers BH, Dobson RL, eds. Pathogenesis of skin disease. New York: Churchill Livingstone, 1986:159.
14. August M, Wang J, Plante D, Wang CC. Complications associated with therapeutic neck radiation. J Oral Maxillofac Surg 1996; 54:1409.
15. DePadova-Elder SM, Ditre CM, Kantor GR, et al. Candidiasis endocrinopathy syndrome. Arch Dermatol 1994; 130:19.
16. Carney JA, Gordon H, Carpenter PC, et al. The complex of myxomas, spotty pigmentation and endocrine overactivity. Medicine 1985; 64:270.
16a. Watson JC, Stratakis CA, Bryant-Greenwood PK, et al. Neurosurgical implications of Carney complex. J Neurosurg 2000; 92:413.
17. Kahan RS, Perez-Figaredo RA, Neimanis A. Necrolytic migratory erythema. Distinctive dermatosis of the glucagonoma syndrome. Arch Dermatol 1977; 113:792.
18. Bassett ML, Haliday JW, Powell LW. Hemochromatosis—newer concepts: diagnosis and management. Disease-a-Month Series 1980; 26:1.
19. Feder JN, Gnirke A, Thomas W, et al. A novel MHC class I-like gene is mutated in patients with hereditary hemochromatosis. Nat Genet 1996; 13:399.
20. Bonkovsky HL, Poh-Fitzpatrick M, Pimstone N, et al. Porphyria cutanea tarda, hepatitis C, and HFE gene mutations in North America. Hepatology 1998; 27:1661.
21. Matsuoka LY, Wortsman J, Gavin JR, Goldman J. Spectrum of endocrine abnormalities associated with acanthosis nigricans. Am J Med 1987; 83:719.
22. Darling TN, Skarulis MC, Steinberg SM, et al. Multiple facial angiofibromas and collagenomas in patients with multiple endocrine neoplasia type 1. Arch Derm 1997; 133:853.
23. Pack S, Turner ML, Zhuang Z, et al. Cutaneous tumors in patients with multiple endocrine neoplasia type 1 show allelic deletion of the MEN1 gene. J Invest Derm 1998; 110:438.
23a. Grudeva-Popuva J, Dobrev H. Biomechanical measurement of skin distensibility in scleredema of Buschke associated with multiple myeloma. Clin Exp Dermatol 2000; 25:247.
24. Gipstein RM, Coburn JW, Adams DA, et al. Calciphylaxis in man: a syndrome of tissue necrosis and vascular calcification in 11 patients with chronic renal failure. Arch Intern Med 1976; 136:1273.
25. Mehregan DA, Winkelmann RK. Cutaneous gangrene, vascular calcification, and hyperparathyroidism. Mayo Clin Proc 1989; 64:211.
26. De Graaf P, Ruiter DJ, Scheffer E, et al. Metastatic skin calcification: a rare phenomenon in dialysis patients. Dermatologica 1980; 161:28.
27. Angelis M, Wong LL, Myers SA, Wong LM. Calciphylaxis in patients on hemodialysis: a prevalence study. Surgery 1997; 122:1083.
28. Zouboulis CC, Blume-Peytavi U, Lennert T, et al. Fulminant metastatic calcinosis with cutaneous necrosis in a child with endstage renal disease and tertiary hyperparathyroidism. Br J Dermatol 1996; 135:617.
29. Van Dop C, Bourne HR. Pseudohypoparathyroidism. Annu Rev Med 1983; 34:259.
30. Doty RL. Olfactory dysfunction in type I pseudohypoparathyroidism: dissociation from Gsα protein deficiency. J Clin Endocrinol Metab 1997; 82:247.
31. Hofman KJ. Diffusion of information about neurofibromatosis type 1 DNA Testing. Am J Med Genet 1994; 49:299.
32. Martuza RL, Eldridge R. Neurofibromatosis 2. N Engl J Med 1988; 318:684.
33. Bauer EA, Uitto J, Tau ML, Holbrook KA. Werner's syndrome: evidence for preferential regional expression of a generalized mesenchymal cell defect. Arch Dermatol 1988; 124:90.
34. Goldsmith LA. Tyrosine-induced skin disease. Br J Dermatol 1978; 98:119.
35. Fine JD, Wise TG, Falchuk KH. Zinc in cutaneous disease and dermatologic therapeutics. In: Moschella SL, ed. Dermatology update: reviews for physicians. New York: Elsevier, 1982:299.
36. Steinbach HL, Russell W. Measurement of the heel pad as an aid to diagnosis of acromegaly. Radiology 1964; 82:418.
37. Case Records of the Massachusetts General Hospital. Case 10-1987. N Engl J Med 1987; 316:606.
38. Bech-Thomsen N, Angelo HR, Wulf HG. Arch Dermatol 1994; 130:464.
39. Schulz W, Domenico D, Nand S. POEMS syndrome associated with polycythemia vera. Cancer 1989; 63:1175.

# HORMONES AND CANCER

KENNETH L. BECKER, EDITOR

# CHAPTER 219

# PARANEOPLASTIC ENDOCRINE SYNDROMES

KENNETH L. BECKER AND OMEGA L. SILVA

## DEFINITION

In addition to being a local disorder of tissue growth and a source of potential metastases, cancers often have important systemic metabolic manifestations. These remote biologic effects sometimes can dominate the other clinical effects of the malignant process.[1,2] As discussed in other chapters of this text, many humoral manifestations are attributable to a neoplasm of a tissue that normally is the predominant site of production of a hormone (e.g., pituitary prolactinoma and galactorrhea; adrenal cortical adenoma and Cushing syndrome; thyroid adenoma and hyperthyroidism). However, if clinical manifestations are the result of hormones secreted by tumors emanating from tissues that normally do not secrete them into the blood at significant levels, they are termed *paraneoplastic endocrine syndromes.*

Despite the extraordinary cellular differentiation and organization seen in humans, most normal tissues retain the ability to secrete many hormones, albeit some more efficiently than others (see Chap. 175). This inherent secretory capacity is shared by the neoplasms derived from these tissues. A cancer often reflects the innate humoral characteristics and secretory potentials of its cell of origin. Thus, conceptually, the elaboration of a hormone by a neoplasm is not really "ectopic"; it is "eutopic," but quantitatively abnormal.

## PATHOGENESIS

Some tumors that produce paraneoplastic endocrine syndromes (e.g., small cell lung cancer,[3] carcinoid tumor, Merkel cell tumor) arise from the diffuse neuroendocrine system (see Chap. 175). Although the primordial tissues engendering such neoplastic lesions initially were thought to have a common embryonic origin, this theory is no longer tenable. The neuroendocrine cancers do not share common embryonic precursors. Also, many paraneoplastic syndromes originate from tumors that are not neuroendocrine.

In attempting to explain why a tumor produces hormones, investigators have stressed the fact that the DNA complement within each normal somatic cell is identical; that is, in each specific cell, some functions normally are repressed (e.g., a gene that codes for a certain hormone). Therefore, hormone-secreting cancers are viewed as exhibiting selective derepression of the genome, allowing synthesis of the hormone. Others attribute the hormonal elaboration by cancer to a failure of differentiation of undifferentiated, totipotential stem cells.

## CRITERIA

Certain traditional criteria have been proposed for accepting a group of symptoms and signs as a paraneoplastic endocrine syndrome[4] (Table 219-1). These idealized criteria have not been met for several bona fide paraneoplastic syndromes, however, and often are unnecessary for making the diagnosis.

**TABLE 219-1.**
**Criteria for Defining a Paraneoplastic Endocrine Syndrome***

Documentation, in a patient with a neoplasm, of the presence of a syndrome known to be caused by a certain hormone.

Measurement of increased levels of the hormone in the serum, the urine, or both. (Investigatively, comparison of the potency of the hormone by immunologic means [e.g., radioimmunoassay], by its receptor affinity [e.g., radioreceptor assay], and by its biologic effects [e.g., bioassay] may be informative.)

Determination of an arteriovenous gradient for the hormone indicating active secretion.

Demonstration of hormone concentrations in the neoplastic tissues that are greater than those found in the normal adjacent tissue. (Such studies can be performed quantitatively [e.g., radioimmunoassay or bioassay] or qualitatively [immunohistochemical methods].)

Demonstration in the tumor of messenger RNA coding for the hormone in question.

Demonstration that removal of the tumor (by surgery) or other antitumor effect (e.g., by chemotherapy) causes remission of the paraneoplastic syndrome.

Return of the hormonal syndrome with recurrence of the tumor.

*Not all these criteria must be met in any given patient before the clinical diagnosis of a paraneoplastic endocrine syndrome can be established.

## GENERAL PRINCIPLES

A common feature of most paraneoplastic endocrine syndromes is the elaboration of peptide hormones. De novo steroid synthesis by cancer usually requires adrenal, gonadal, or placental tissue, and de novo thyroid hormone synthesis requires thyroidal or teratomatous tissue (see Chap. 204).

Moreover, biogenic amines (i.e., histamine, serotonin) play significant roles in some paraneoplastic manifestations. Prostaglandin secretion also may be important (see Chap. 172).

When encountering most paraneoplastic endocrine syndromes, the physician already is conscious of the associated neoplasm. Nonetheless, sometimes the syndrome precedes the diagnosis of the tumor; indeed, marked endocrine effects may mask the tumor, averting attention to inappropriate therapeutic approaches. Although a paraneoplastic endocrine syndrome might constitute an interesting but relatively harmless occurrence (e.g., acanthosis nigricans, hypertrophic osteoarthropathy), it also might contribute directly to the patient's premature demise (e.g., hypercalcemia, syndrome of inappropriate antidiuresis [SIAD]).

Although tumors sometimes produce the same hormone as related normal cells, they often produce and secrete much greater quantities.[5] Moreover, such tumors frequently secrete other hormones that may be secreted by their normal cellular counterparts in minute amounts. The clinical effects of the polyhormonal potential of many of these tumors are unknown.

Generally, hormones secreted by cancers are not unique in chemical structure. Nonetheless, the distribution of the molecular forms of the secreted peptide frequently is abnormal. In particular, precursor forms with high molecular weight often predominate. This probably reflects a deficient or incomplete posttranslational modification; or it may signify an alternative means of secretion.[6] Because these precursors often have less or no bioactivity, a clinical syndrome may not occur, despite an extraordinarily high level of radioimmunoassayable hormone in the serum. Most tumors producing such peptides remain clinically silent.

Furthermore, the finding of high serum hormone levels emanating from a tissue other than a classic endocrine gland is not a specific indicator of neoplasia. Irritated, hyperplastic, or premalignant tissues or lesions also may secrete increased levels of peptide hormones (e.g., in chronic obstructive pulmonary disease, chronic bronchitis of smokers, regional ileitis, and ulcerative colitis).

Morphologically, in contrast to normal, anatomically discrete endocrine organs, hormone-secreting neoplasms often do not possess a highly structured and coordinated neural control.

Metabolically, the neoplastic cells in most paraneoplastic syndromes often do not respond to the usual physiologic control mechanisms that modulate normal hormone secretion (i.e., physiologic secretagogues, feedback suppression). Although exceptions exist, this relative autonomy may be of considerable diagnostic use.

Last, the hormonal secretion by cancer may serve as an important biomarker for its presence, its response to therapy, and its relapse.

# SPECIFIC PARANEOPLASTIC ENDOCRINE SYNDROMES

This chapter discusses the paraneoplastic endocrine syndromes of certain cancers, including those in which the humoral mediator is suspected but not yet identified. Brief mention also is made of possible humoral syndromes that arise as a result of the effect of neoplasia on noncancerous tissue. Hormone-secreting tumors of the pancreas and of the neuroendocrine cells of the gut (e.g., insulinoma, gastrinoma) are discussed elsewhere (see Chaps. 158 and 220). Although several humoral syndromes associated with other neuroendocrine tumors are mentioned, they also are discussed in other chapters.

## PARANEOPLASTIC GROWTH HORMONE–RELEASING HORMONE SYNDROME

Although far less common than hypothalamic-pituitary acromegaly, the syndrome of acromegaly that is secondary to the tumoral secretion of growth hormone–releasing hormone (GHRH) is a fascinating and instructive example of a paraneoplastic endocrine syndrome.[7,8] Normally, GHRH circulates at low or undetectable levels, although appreciable levels are found in the hypothalamic-hypophysial portal system. Some tumors secrete large amounts of GHRH, causing acromegaly. The secreted GHRH is the same as that in the human hypothalamus; both the 44- and 40-amino-acid hormones are found.[9]

Two lesions, in particular, may produce the syndrome: bronchial carcinoid and pancreatic islet cell tumor. In addition, GHRH is found in some carcinoid tumors involving the gastrointestinal tract and thymus, as well as in pheochromocytoma, medullary thyroid cancer, and small cell lung cancer. Although it is also in the blood of some patients with these tumors, however, it does not necessarily cause symptoms and signs of acromegaly.

Patients with the full-blown syndrome of paraneoplastic GHRH secretion have the classic appearance of acromegaly (see Chap. 12), but often it is of more rapid onset. The serum levels of GHRH frequently exceed 200 pg/mL. The high serum levels of the hormone cause hyperplasia of the pituitary somatotropes, with consequent hypersecretion of growth hormone. As in hypothalamic-pituitary acromegaly, serum growth hormone levels are not suppressed after the administration of oral glucose; however, in contrast to classic acromegaly, patients with the paraneoplastic GHRH syndrome may have a markedly increased serum growth hormone response to insulin-induced hypoglycemia.[10] Usually, the sella turcica is not enlarged, and examination by computed tomography or nuclear magnetic resonance imaging yields normal results. Occasionally, however, an enlarged sella is seen[11]; some cases apparently eventuate in pituitary tumors.

Pituitary surgery is not indicated in this syndrome. If feasible, the cancerous lesion should be removed. If surgery is successful, it should cause regression of the acromegalic syndrome. Medical treatment with bromocriptine often successfully suppresses the growth hormone level; the somatostatin analog octreotide acetate also has been useful in this regard.[12]

Paraneoplastic secretion of growth hormone is very rare. A case has been described in which acromegaly was apparently due to secretion of this hormone by a non-Hodgkin lymphoma.[12a]

## PARANEOPLASTIC CORTICOTROPIN-RELEASING HORMONE SYNDROME

Corticotropin-releasing hormone (CRH) has been found in bronchial carcinoid tumors and in small cell carcinoma of the lung. Rarely, high serum levels of this hormone stimulate the pituitary gland to produce excess adrenocorticotropic hormone (ACTH). In such cases, the increased ACTH levels cause bilateral adrenal hyperplasia, and the resultant hypercortisolism results in Cushing syndrome[13,14] (see Chap. 75).

## PARANEOPLASTIC ADRENOCORTICOTROPIC HORMONE SYNDROME

The paraneoplastic ACTH syndrome (or ectopic ACTH syndrome) is caused by the secretion of ACTH by a nonpituitary neoplasm, which results in bilateral adrenal hyperplasia and manifestations of Cushing syndrome. This condition is more common than Cushing disease. Two-thirds of the cases of paraneoplastic ACTH syndrome are attributable to bronchogenic cancer. The principal offender is small cell cancer of the lung; occasionally, pulmonary adenocarcinoma also has been implicated. Another common cause is the relatively benign bronchial carcinoid tumor.[15] Other, less frequent causes are thymic tumor (usually benign, and often of carcinoid histology), islet cell carcinoma of the pancreas,[16] medullary thyroid cancer, pheochromocytoma, and colon carcinoma.

Manifestations of the syndrome are influenced not only by the level of ACTH secretion but also by the bioactivity of the hormone. Many nonpituitary tumors that secrete ACTH typically remain biologically silent because of the secretion of bioinactive precursors of ACTH—big ACTH—that make up preproopiomelanocortin and its related products, including multiple immunologic forms of β-endorphin.[17] Simultaneous assays of receptor-active ACTH and immunoactive ACTH have confirmed the inactivity of many of the secreted hormones. Thus, although approximately one-third of patients with small cell cancer of the lung have increased serum ACTH levels by radioimmunoassay, only 1% to 2% have hypercortisolism.

Clinically, because of the close association with small cell lung cancer, the fact that many patients with the syndrome are men older than 40 years who abuse tobacco is not surprising. (This is in direct contrast to Cushing disease, which occurs in younger persons and has a strong female predilection.) The tumor type is important; in patients with slow-growing bronchial carcinoid often the disease onset is gradual and insidious, the duration of symptoms may span months to several years, and the classic cushingoid features (facial plethora, moon facies, easy bruising, hirsutism, truncal obesity, and atrophy of the extremities) develop over a prolonged period.[18] In such patients, the tumor may be occult and difficult to localize; however, computerized tomography often is helpful.[19,20]

Because of the increased secretion of ACTH and its precursor (proopiomelanocortin), the level of melanocyte-stimulating hormone (MSH) activity (α-MSH within the ACTH molecule, and β-MSH within the β-lipotropin molecule) increases (see Chap. 14). Consequently, these patients may manifest marked hyperpigmentation that is similar in appearance to that encountered in Addison disease (Fig. 219-1).

Patients with more aggressive malignant disease (e.g., small cell lung cancer [see Fig. 219-1], pancreatic adenocarcinoma) often do not have centripetal obesity. Commonly, the onset is acute, the symptoms have been present for several weeks at the

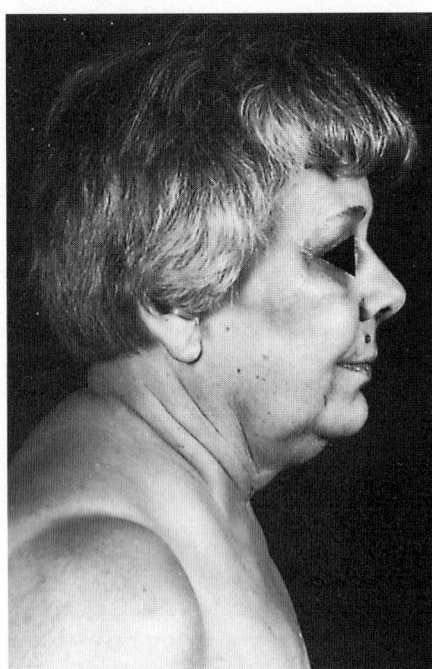

**FIGURE 219-1.** Patient with paraneoplastic adrenocorticotropic hormone syndrome secondary to small cell cancer of the lung. Note the darkening of the skin, the fullness of the cheeks and the supraclavicular fossae, and the cervicodorsal hump.

time of examination, and obvious, rapid weight loss occurs. Often, the serum ACTH level is even higher than that in patients with carcinoid tumor, and the resultant hyperpigmentation is more pronounced. Other manifestations may include edema, muscle weakness, hypertension, severe hypokalemic alkalosis, and hyperglycemia. A clear-cut parallelism between clinical findings, tumor type, and duration of the neoplasm is not always present, however.

Laboratory studies of patients with the paraneoplastic ACTH syndrome may reveal normal or decreased serum potassium levels. Hypokalemia occurs much more commonly in this syndrome than in either pituitary Cushing disease or Cushing syndrome secondary to adrenal adenoma. Any unprovoked hypokalemia (i.e., in a patient not taking diuretics or laxatives) merits further investigation. Metabolic alkalosis and hyperglycemia may be present. The demonstration of hypercortisolism is essential to the diagnosis. Commonly, the serum cortisol level is extremely high—higher than that seen in most patients with Cushing disease (although the serum cortisol elevation in patients with carcinoid tumor often is moderate). The normal diurnal cortisol rhythmicity (see Chap. 6) is abolished, and a large day-to-day variability in the serum cortisol level often is seen. Rarely, periodic hypersecretion may be encountered, with intervals of days to weeks of normal levels interspersed among periods marked by increased values. Increased levels of serum dehydroepiandrosterone sulfate and urinary 17-ketosteroids may help to distinguish between Cushing syndrome caused by paraneoplastic ACTH production and Cushing syndrome caused by unilateral adrenal adenoma, the latter of which is characterized by normal values.

Although exceptions exist, many patients with the paraneoplastic ACTH syndrome do not exhibit suppression of serum cortisol or urinary 17-hydroxycorticosteroid levels with daily administration of 8 mg of dexamethasone orally (2 mg every 6 hours for 2 days). Most patients with Cushing disease, however, do exhibit such suppression (see Chaps. 74 and 75). In contrast to the marked responsiveness of serum 11-deoxycortisol and

urinary 17-hydroxycorticosteroid levels to the administration of metyrapone that usually occurs in patients with Cushing disease, those with the paraneoplastic ACTH syndrome generally are unresponsive.

In the paraneoplastic ACTH syndrome, serum ACTH levels usually are high, and several other hormones, such as calcitonin, arginine vasopressin (AVP), somatostatin, or vasoactive intestinal peptide, may simultaneously be produced. (The β-MSH–secreting tumor does not constitute a clinical entity that is distinct from the paraneoplastic ACTH syndrome.) The injection of CRH may induce a further increase in serum ACTH levels in Cushing disease, but not in the paraneoplastic ACTH syndrome.[21]

Localization studies are essential to the workup of these patients. Chest radiography, sputum cytology, and bronchoscopy often facilitate the diagnosis of small cell lung cancer. Results of computed tomographic and magnetic resonance imaging studies of the pituitary are normal. Similar studies of the chest or abdomen may reveal the tumor, and imaging of the abdomen often demonstrates bilateral adrenal hyperplasia. (In one instance, a pheochromocytoma that secreted ACTH was diagnosed in a patient with bilateral enlarged adrenal glands, one of which also contained a focal mass.) Bilateral, simultaneous inferior petrosal sinus sampling of patients with paraneoplastic ACTH syndrome generally reveals no unilateral ACTH gradient and demonstrates ACTH levels that are less than those derived from venous catheterization samples of the tumor effluent (e.g., mediastinal veins). The simultaneous administration of CRH further increases the utility of the procedure.[22] Somatostatin-receptor scintigraphy may be used to demonstrate the location of the tumor-producing lesion.[23] Occasionally, percutaneous needle aspiration of tumor tissue, with assay of the intracellular ACTH, has confirmed the diagnosis.[24]

The ideal therapy for the paraneoplastic ACTH syndrome is extirpation of the neoplasm. If this is not feasible, some patients respond, albeit transiently, to chemotherapy. If the neoplasm cannot be treated successfully, adrenocortical hyperactivity can be mitigated with drugs, such as mitotane (o,p'-DDD), aminoglutethimide, metyrapone, or ketoconazole.[25] Such therapy may lead to prolonged control of the hypercortisolemia.[26] In addition, such drugs can be administered before surgery in patients whose primary neoplasms are resectable, but whose Cushing syndrome initially might make an operation too hazardous.

## PARANEOPLASTIC ARGININE VASOPRESSIN SYNDROME

SIAD is characterized by the excretion of a hypertonic urine despite an expanded extracellular volume. SIAD can arise from *central* mechanisms (acute or chronic disorders of the central nervous system, drugs), or from *peripheral* mechanisms, in which case the secretion of AVP by a neoplasm is a common offender.[27] This paraneoplastic AVP syndrome also has been termed *tumoral hyponatremia*[28] (see Chaps. 25 and 27).

AVP and oxytocin, as well as the carrier protein neurophysin, are found within such cancers, and cell cultures of the tumor also secrete the precursor peptide, propressophysin. In 80% of cases, the tumor causing SIAD is small cell cancer of the lung[29]; although it often is an incidental finding, as many as one-third of patients with this type of cancer have some degree of the syndrome. Other tumors that have been known to cause SIAD include those involving the pancreas, thymus, and breast. Occasionally, a cancerous lesion that does not directly secrete AVP can produce this syndrome through a central mechanism (e.g., metastases to the brain).

The symptoms and signs of SIAD are attributable to water intoxication and hyponatremia, and may range in severity from having no effect to being life-threatening. They may include nausea, weakness, and central nervous system effects, such as confusion or obtundation, all of which may be easily misconstrued as being caused by the malignant disease. The central nervous system effects may progress to convulsions and, sometimes, frank coma. Laboratory studies reveal hyponatremia (and consequent hypoosmolality: <270 mOsm/kg) and hypochloremia; serum potassium levels usually are normal. A concurrently voided specimen of urine shows inappropriate levels of sodium (or increased osmolality) in comparison with the serum hypoosmolality. The determination of serum AVP is not essential to the diagnosis; levels of the hormone need not appear to be inappropriately high.

Some patients with pulmonary disorders, such as acute pneumonitis or advanced tuberculosis, also may manifest SIAD, allegedly as a result of alterations in thoracic baroreceptor control mechanisms. However, the syndrome is more likely attributable to AVP secretion by stimulated or hyperplastic pulmonary neuroendocrine cells (see Chap 177).

The hyponatremia of tumor-associated SIAD must be distinguished from that occurring with solute depletion, as well as with other conditions, such as adrenal insufficiency, hypopituitarism, hypothyroidism, congestive heart failure, cirrhosis of the liver, and renal disease. The initial therapy is water restriction. In emergencies, intravenous saline with furosemide-induced diuresis is used. Various drugs (lithium, hydantoin sodium, demethylchlortetracycline) also have been used (see Chap. 177). Many patients with small cell cancer of the lung exhibit a striking remission after radiotherapy, combined chemotherapy, or both, in which case the SIAD ceases, only to return with recurrence of the neoplasm. In rare instances, however, patients with this cancer may be cured.

Some patients with hyponatremia and inappropriate sodium loss have paraneoplastic secretion of *atrial natriuretic hormone*. This may occur in patients with small cell cancer of the lung.[30,31]

## PARANEOPLASTIC HYPERCALCEMIA

The most common paraneoplastic endocrine syndrome is hypercalcemia. It also constitutes the most frequent form of hypercalcemia seen in hospitalized patients (see Chap. 59). Of all the paraneoplastic syndromes, hypercalcemia is the most life-threatening. Although the basic mechanism usually is excess bone resorption, increased tubular reabsorption of calcium also may be a factor.

The symptoms and signs of the hypercalcemia associated with malignant disease do not differ markedly from those seen in other forms of hypercalcemia. The confusion and weakness may be attributed erroneously to the spread of the cancer or to chemotherapy. With the exception of lymphoma, multiple myeloma, and breast cancer, the associated hypercalcemia usually occurs late in the course of the disease. Its history is short, the onset often is abrupt, erratic day-to-day variations in the level may occur, and it is often a harbinger of imminent death. Nephrocalcinosis or nephrolithiasis usually is not seen, and no subperiosteal bone resorption or bone cysts are present; only rarely does extraosseous metastatic calcification occur. Commonly, the hypercalcemia is precipitated by volume depletion, resulting in a decreased glomerular filtration rate with renal retention of calcium. The condition is worsened by immobilization.

Among solid tumors, the principal causes of the hypercalcemia associated with malignant disease are breast cancer (50% of all patients with metastatic mammary cancer have an episode of hypercalcemia); lung cancer; squamous cell cancer of the head, neck, esophagus, and cervix; and cancer of the kidney, ovary, and bladder. Of the lung cancers associated with hypercalcemia,

squamous cell carcinoma is the most common, adenocarcinoma occurs somewhat less frequently, large cell cancer is uncommon, and small cell carcinoma is rare. Of the hematologic malignant diseases causing hypercalcemia, multiple myeloma is the most common; among the leukemias, acute leukemia is the most common; and among the lymphomas, the histiocytic variety is particularly prone to cause the syndrome.

The humoral factors causing the paraneoplastic hypercalcemia of malignant disease are discussed in Chapter 59. Hardly ever do solid tumors produce parathyroid hormone (PTH).[32] Rather, solid tumors often secrete PTH-related protein (PTHrP), which binds to PTH receptors and induces bone resorption and phosphaturia.[33–35] Hematologic malignancy also can cause hypercalcemia via secretion of PTHrP.[36] Some homology is found between PTHrP and PTH in the amino-terminal region. However, PTHrP does not react with antisera to PTH. PTHrP is the principal tumor-derived factor causing the hypercalcemia of malignancy, but its expression by a cancer does not necessarily obligate the occurrence of hypercalcemia.[37]

PTHrP is expressed at low levels in normal tissues (see Chap. 52).[38] Its gene expression and secretion are regulated, in part, by peptide growth factors, such as transforming growth factor-β and epidermal growth factor.[39] Cellular transformation by the *ras* and *src* oncogenes has been shown to increase the gene expression markedly.[40] In patients with PTHrP-induced hypercalcemia, the serum calcium levels do not necessarily correlate with the serum hormonal levels. Nevertheless, the elevated serum levels of PTHrP, as well as the hypercalcemia, may return to normal after successful surgical removal of the tumor.[41] In addition to having a hypercalcemic effect, PTHrP likely stimulates the growth of some malignant cells in an autocrine fashion.[37,42]

Other humoral factors that are produced either by solid tumors or by hematologic neoplasms have been implicated in hypercalcemia, again because of their bone-resorbing effects. For example, multiple myeloma often produces osteoclast-activating factors, which are made up of one or several cytokines (e.g., interleukin-1β, lymphotoxin, interleukin-6) emanating directly from the neoplastic plasma cell.[43] Multiple myeloma also may produce tumor necrosis factor β, a cytokine that is normally secreted by monocytes and macrophages and that also causes bone resorption. Several other growth factors resorb bone and are secreted by various neoplasms in patients with associated hypercalcemia, including epidermal growth factor and transforming growth factor (see Chap. 50).

In some patients with lymphoma, the hypercalcemia may be due to increased 1α-hydroxylation of 25-hydroxyvitamin D [25(OH)D] by malignant histiocytes.[44] Normal activated T lymphocytes also can induce this transformation. Although prostaglandin E$_2$ is produced by some neoplasms, serum levels do not appear to be sufficiently high to enhance bone resorption to the extent of producing hypercalcemia; moreover, inhibitors of prostaglandin synthesis have no effect on most patients with neoplastic hypercalcemia.

Usually, the initial therapy for the hypercalcemia of malignant disease is intravenous physiologic saline; rehydration alone may dramatically reduce or even normalize the hypercalcemia. Other modes of therapy (plicamycin, calcitonin, phosphate, corticosteroids, gallium nitrate[45]) are discussed elsewhere (see Chaps. 53, 58, and 59). The most effective and least toxic therapy for the hypercalcemia associated with solid tumors, however, is intravenous pamidronate sodium.[46] Patients with the highest PTH-related protein levels tend to be somewhat more resistant to therapy and have the worst prognosis. Nevertheless, they usually respond to higher doses and increased frequency of pamidronate therapy. In the future, immunoneutralization of PTHrP could be a novel mode of treatment.[46a]

## PARANEOPLASTIC OSTEOMALACIA

Osteomalacia or rickets secondary to the secretion of a humoral substance by a tumor (paraneoplastic osteomalacia, oncogenous osteomalacia) is being diagnosed with surprising frequency (see Chap. 63). Affected patients have a deficiency of serum calcitriol, as well as renal phosphate wasting.[47,48] The syndrome has been reproduced by transplantation of tumor tissue into athymic nude mice. The mechanism appears to be twofold: an inhibition of 1α-hydroxylation, which prevents 25(OH)D from being metabolized to the more active l,25-dihydroxyvitamm D [l,25(OH)$_2$D], and an effect on the proximal nephron, which promotes phosphaturia. In this regard, tumor extracts from patients with this syndrome have been found to stimulate PTH-responsive renal adenylate cyclase.

Clinically, paraneoplastic osteomalacia most commonly occurs in young adults. The symptoms often are severe and include skeletal pain, muscle weakness and cramps, and, sometimes, fracture. The illness may confine the patient to the chair or bed. The symptoms of this syndrome may be present for months or years before being recognized.

The lesions producing paraneoplastic osteomalacia have been well described as "strange tumors in strange places."[49] Most of them are slow growing, benign, and extremely vascular mesenchymal tumors involving soft tissue or bone.[50,50a] Frequently, they are small (as small as 1 cm in diameter) and difficult to find, although they also may be large. Hemangiomatous lesions are encountered most often—specifically, cavernous hemangioma, hemangiopericytoma, angiofibroma, angiosarcoma, and others.[51] Other tissue diagnoses include soft-tissue myxoma, osteoblastoma, ossifying mesenchymal tumor, neurofibromatosis, schwannoma, and prostatic cancer. In many of these lesions, multinucleated giant cells, resembling osteoclasts, have been described. The unusual locations of these tumors have included the nasopharynx, the maxilla, and the palm of the hand (Fig. 219-2).

Paraneoplastic osteomalacia should be suspected in any patient with osteomalacia for which no obvious cause (e.g., malabsorption syndrome) or familial history is found. Most patients have hypophosphatemia; serum alkaline phosphatase levels usually are increased. Serum calcium levels are normal or only slightly decreased. Why the stimulation of PTH-responsive receptors is not accompanied by hypercalcemia is unknown; perhaps only renal receptors, and not those of bone, are stimulated. Serum 25(OH)D levels are normal; however, despite the presence of hypophosphatemia (which should stimulate 1α-hydroxylation), serum levels of l,25(OH)$_2$D are decreased. Serum PTH and calcitonin levels are normal. Even with hypophosphatemia, phosphaturia occurs, as demonstrated by a decreased tubular reabsorption of phosphate. The proximal renal tubular dysfunction may be accompanied by aminoaciduria and glucosuria (plasma glucose levels are normal). Histomorphologic analysis of a biopsy of nondecalcified iliac crest bone confirms the excess osteoid.

When it is found in association with osteoblastic metastases, prostate cancer, as well as breast cancer, also may cause osteomalacia (and sometimes hypocalcemia) because of the high calcium and vitamin D requirements of the rapidly forming new bone. These patients manifest hypophosphatemia, increased alkaline phosphatase levels, and, importantly, low serum 25(OH)D levels.[52] Another clinical entity that may be confused with paraneoplastic osteomalacia is found rarely in patients with multiple myeloma or chronic lymphatic leukemia. It is termed *light-chain nephropathy* and causes decreased tubular reabsorption of phosphate and hypophosphatemia, as well as aminoaciduria, glucosuria, and impaired renal acidification.[53] Presumably, vitamin D metabolism is normal.

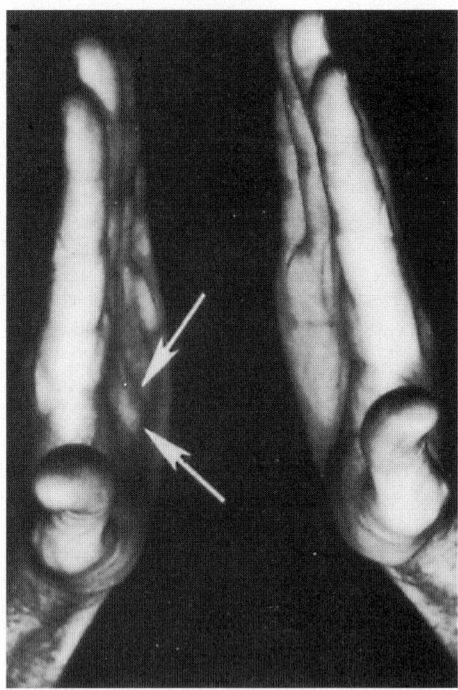

**FIGURE 219-2.** A nontender, firm nodule (*arrows*) measuring 2 × 3 cm is evident on the palm of this 34-year-old man with severe osteomalacia. Bone pain and muscle weakness disappeared after removal of the lesion, and previously undetectable serum levels of 1,25-dihydroxyvitamin D returned to normal. The lesion was a benign tumor composed of hyaline cartilage and osteoclast-like giant cells. (From Weiss D, Barr RS, Weidner N, et al. Oncogenic osteomalacia: strange tumors in strange places. Postgrad Med J 1985; 61:349.)

Therapy for paraneoplastic osteomalacia consists of extirpation of the tumor, which is followed by spontaneous cure of the bone abnormality. After operation, serum l,25(OH)$_2$D levels rapidly normalize. Even the partial removal of an offending tumor may be beneficial. If surgery cannot be performed, or if the causative neoplasm cannot be found, treatment includes large doses of 1,25(OH)$_2$D daily (up to 3 μg per day) plus oral phosphate. Often, the clinical response to this treatment is only partial. The patient's serum should be monitored, because hypercalcemia may occur if the bone lesions heal.

## PARANEOPLASTIC SECRETION OF HUMAN CHORIONIC GONADOTROPIN

Human chorionic gonadotropin (hCG) is a glycoprotein hormone of ~45,000 Da that is made up of two dissimilar, noncovalently joined subunits, each of which is encoded by different genes. The α subunit is identical to that in luteinizing hormone, follicle-stimulating hormone, and thyroid-stimulating hormone, whereas the β subunit differs and confers biologic specificity to the hormone (see Chaps. 15 and 16).

The principal source of serum hCG is the syncytiotrophoblast cell of the normal placenta (see Chaps. 108, 111, and 112). Moreover, hCG is widely distributed at low concentrations in many, perhaps all, normal tissues. Except in pregnancy, however, serum hCG levels are extremely low or undetectable.

Large amounts of hCG may be secreted from trophoblastic tumors, including gestational tumors (hydatidiform mole, choriocarcinoma), gonadal tumors with trophoblastic elements, and extragonadal nongestational choriocarcinoma (see Chaps. 111 and 112). Hormone production in these cases is not really paraneoplastic because the tumor involves tissue components that normally would be expected to produce considerable amounts of the hormone. However, nontrophoblastic tumors also may produce levels of hCG that are sufficiently high to cause clinical manifestations.

Interestingly, ovarian and testicular tumors (see Chaps. 102 and 122) commonly secrete hCG. Although areas suggestive of trophoblastic tissue may be found on histologic examination, this is not obligatory. For example, 25% of pure seminomas of the testis are associated with increased serum hCG levels. As mentioned earlier, extragonadal, nongestational, choriocarcinomatous-appearing lesions occur rarely. These lesions are usually midline in location (mediastinum, pineal gland, retroperitoneum, bladder), and are more prevalent in men[54] than in women. Rarely, they may be nonmidline (lung, kidney, colon). Whether such lesions are caused by incomplete or aberrant migration of primordial germ cells, metastases from occult (or regressed) lesions of the gonads or placenta, metaplastic differentiation of epithelial cells, or persistence of totipotential cells from early embryogenesis is unknown.

The nontrophoblastic tumors that may secrete large amounts of hCG include lung cancer (mostly large cell), gastrointestinal tumors (especially those involving the stomach and functioning islet cell lesions), breast cancer, melanoma, and hepatoblastoma. The serum gonadotropin levels are not suppressible with androgen or estrogen administration.[55]

The clinical manifestations of tumoral secretion of hCG depend on the level of the hormone and the age and sex of the patient. Most patients, particularly those with nontrophoblastic tumors, have no symptoms. Infants or children with the rare malignant hepatoblastoma may have precocious pseudopuberty.[56] Boys, in particular, are affected, perhaps because of the luteinizing hormone–like activity of hCG and its lack of follicle-stimulating hormone activity. The precocious puberty is isosexual, manifested by the early appearance of secondary sex characteristics, increased body hair, and an enlarged penis. Because of the absence of follicle-stimulating hormone, the testes usually exhibit interstitial cell hyperplasia without seminiferous tubule maturation or spermatogenesis, and they remain rather small in size. One-third of these hepatoblastomas are resectable, and the symptoms may remit. Similar cases may occur among patients with trophoblastic teratomas or pinealomas.

Women with high levels of serum hCG often have dysfunctional uterine bleeding, whereas affected men commonly have gynecomastia and, often, impotence. Whether the gynecomastia is the result of the stimulation of secretion of sex steroids from the testes or of the direct production of sex hormones by the tumor tissue is uncertain. Thyrotoxicosis can occur with high levels of serum hCG because of its thyroid-stimulating hormone–like effects[57]; this condition may be seen in some women with choriocarcinoma (see Chaps. 15, 42, and 112), but it also occurs, albeit rarely, in men with testicular cancer.

Care should be exercised in interpreting serum hCG levels because sensitive assays may detect hCG in normal persons, and slight increases may occur in patients with gastrointestinal inflammatory diseases, such as ulcerative colitis, regional ileitis, and, rarely, duodenal ulcer. In addition, some hCG radioimmunoassays cross-react with other glycoprotein hormones. Antisera raised to the isolated, purified β subunit of hCG (the β-subunit assay) also detect intact hCG but do not cross-react with luteinizing hormone. In addition, new, highly specific β-subunit assays are available.[58,59] Boys with precocious pseudopuberty secondary to hCG have serum testosterone levels that are inappropriately high for their age. Adult men and women have no consistent pattern of abnormality in terms of either serum androgen or estrogen levels. Some men with gynecomastia secondary to increased serum hCG may have a decreased androgen/estrogen ratio. Patients with hCG-induced thyrotoxicosis have abnormal results on several thyroid function tests.

## PARANEOPLASTIC HYPOGLYCEMIA

Occasionally, patients have hypoglycemia secondary to extrapancreatic tumors.[60] Usually, these are large neoplasms located within the thorax or abdomen; often, the abdominal lesions are behind the peritoneum. Many of these tumors, which most commonly are mesenchymal, fibrous neoplasms, are benign; others are sarcomas.

The cell types that have been encountered include fibroma, fibrosarcoma, mesothelioma, neurofibroma, neurofibrosarcoma, liposarcoma, rhabdomyosarcoma, spindle cell sarcoma, hemangiopericytoma, and leiomyosarcoma.[61] Lymphoma and lymphosarcoma also have been implicated. Other tumors have included malignant phyllodes tumor of the breast,[62] bronchial or ileal carcinoid, gastric and colon carcinoma, hypernephroma, adrenal carcinoma, and hepatoma. The last of these often occurs in men.

The mechanism of the hypoglycemia is uncertain. Because the tumors are large, they were thought to arise as a result of the utilization of glucose by the neoplastic tissue. However, this is not a valid conclusion. Nor do the tumors release insulin; in most studies, radioimmunoassayable serum insulin levels are diminished. In some reports, serum levels of nonsuppressible insulin-like protein, a high-molecular-weight substance whose action is not suppressed by insulin antibody, are increased.[63] Usually, serum growth hormone levels are suppressed. In other studies, increased levels of a labile material such as insulin-like growth factor (IGF) that is similar[64] or identical[65] to IGF-II have been found in serum.[66] In one study, this material was receptor active and presumably bound to insulin receptors, but by immunoassay was not recognized as IGF-II.[67] Acidic gel filtration of sera of patients with tumor-associated hypoglycemia demonstrated the presence of a large-molecular-weight IGF-II (big IGF-II), an incompletely processed IGF-II precursor. Levels normalized after removal of the tumor.[68] Still another mechanism was postulated on the basis of a case report in which a large increase in the number of insulin receptors was seen. This increase suggests an augmented utilization of glucose by normal body tissues resulting from an acquired, hormone-induced proliferation of receptors.[69]

Care should be taken not to confuse paraneoplastic hypoglycemia with the glycolysis that may occur in vitro in blood obtained from patients with hematologic malignant disease who have greatly increased leukocyte counts (e.g., those with acute or chronic myeloid leukemia).[70] In such patients, the freshly drawn blood is normoglycemic.

Clinically, patients with paraneoplastic hypoglycemia manifest symptoms when fasting; in severe cases, symptoms may occur spontaneously. Patients may have histories of sweating, hunger, headache, visual disturbances, or confusion. If the onset is gradual, behavioral problems may occur. Commonly, the ingestion of food brings relief. Patients with intractable disease may become comatose, however, despite the fact that they are not in a fasting state.

The treatment of paraneoplastic hypoglycemia involves surgery. Most patients do not survive unless the lesion is resectable, in which case the hypoglycemia may resolve—either permanently if the lesion is benign, or transiently if it is malignant. Before operation, continuous glucose infusion may be necessary. Diazoxide therapy is helpful only occasionally.

## PARANEOPLASTIC HYPERRENINISM

Occasionally, renin may be produced autonomously by a neoplasm (also called *tumoral hyperreninism* or *primary hyperreninism*). Because renin normally is produced by the kidney, the fact that this syndrome most commonly occurs in conjunction with renal neoplasms is not surprising. In patients with a benign renal cyst, renin excess probably is attributable to localized ischemia of the adjacent renal cortex. In rare cases, however, the excess may be caused by primary renin secretion by a juxtaglomerular tumor (also called *renal hemangiopericytoma*). These tumors usually are small, occur in children and young adults, and, on microscopic examination, resemble the normal juxtaglomerular apparatus.[71] In addition, young children with paraneoplastic hyperreninism may have a Wilms tumor (nephroblastoma). In adults, renal adenocarcinoma occasionally is implicated.

Extrarenal tumors also can cause hyperreninism.[72] Such lesions have included adenocarcinoma of the pancreas, adenocarcinoma and small cell carcinoma of the lung, adrenocortical adenoma,[73] ovarian cancer (especially the Sertoli cell type[74]), and a benign, tumor-like condition of the subcutaneous tissue termed *angiolymphoid hyperplasia with eosinophilia*.[75] In some of these tumors, most of the secreted renin is in the form of relatively inactive precursors. Normally, the hormone is biosynthesized as a preprorenin molecule and then is converted into prerenin, which subsequently is processed into a smaller, active renin. This posttranslational processing may be deficient in neoplasms.

Most patients with paraneoplastic hyperreninism have severe hypertension that is resistant to therapy, although occasionally, the hypertension may be mild. Usually, β-adrenergic blockade is unsuccessful, and captopril, an angiotensin-converting enzyme inhibitor, is only variably effective. Retinal hemorrhages may occur and, because of the secondary hyperaldosteronism, a persistent hypokalemia may be present. The plasma renin levels may be extremely high. Generally, procedures that increase renin in normal persons (i.e., salt restriction, diuresis, or both) do not further increase hormonal levels in patients with this syndrome because of a loss of the physiologic regulatory controls. Nevertheless, attempts to use saralasin, an angiotensin II antagonist, or other pharmacologic blockade agents as diagnostic tools have yielded inconsistent results. When hyperreninism has been caused by a renal lesion, venous catheterization studies have demonstrated lateralization of the hyperreninism, whereas an increased venous tumor/kidney renin ratio has been demonstrated in cases in which an extrarenal lesion has been involved. The hypertension and hypokalemia usually respond to chemotherapy or to extirpative surgery.

Paraneoplastic production of angiotensin I may also cause hypertension (e.g., from hepatocellular carcinoma).[76] In this syndrome, the serum level of angiotensin I is high, but that of renin is normal.

### PARANEOPLASTIC ERYTHROCYTOSIS

Erythrocytosis (polycythemia) may be caused by various benign or malignant tumors that contain and secrete erythropoietin. Not surprisingly, because erythropoietin is produced by the normal kidney, various renal lesions have been found to secrete this hormone (e.g., hypernephroma, which is responsible for 50% of such cases; renal cyst; Wilms tumor; and metanephric adenoma or adenofibroma[77]). However, extrarenal tumors also can produce the syndrome.

Three extrarenal tumors, in particular, seem to be involved more often than others: uterine fibroma, cerebellar hemangioblastoma, and hepatocellular carcinoma.[78,79] Cerebellar hemangioblastoma, a tumor that occurs predominantly in girls, may be associated with increased erythropoietin levels in the cerebrospinal fluid, as well as in the blood. The lesion, when transplanted to the athymic nude mouse, has caused erythrocytosis. One study of hepatocellular cancer in South African blacks revealed that, although 23% of the 65 patients had increased serum levels

of erythropoietin, only 1 patient had erythrocytosis. This finding suggests that either the secreted hormone often is inactive, or erythropoiesis is inhibited, a phenomenon that occurs in advanced cancer. Other tumors causing this syndrome include pheochromocytomas,[80] uterine myomas, and ovarian tumors.

Because of the hormonal stimulation that is involved in the proliferation and differentiation of erythrocyte progenitor cells, patients with paraneoplastic erythrocytosis have an increased red blood cell count, increased hemoglobin and hematocrit values, and an elevated red blood cell mass. No splenomegaly is seen as may occur in polycythemia vera. Erythropoietin is found within the tumor, either by immunostaining methods or by direct assay. Moreover, serum and urine erythropoietin levels, as measured by radioimmunoassay or bioassay, may be increased.

Erythropoietin levels also are increased in secondary erythrocytosis attributable to cyanotic heart disease or chronic obstructive pulmonary disease. In these patients, however, the cause is tissue hypoxia, and blood gas determinations demonstrate hypoxemia. In polycythemia vera, a primary bone marrow disorder, serum erythropoietin is either decreased or undetectable.

Remission of paraneoplastic erythrocytosis generally is effected by successful, complete excision of the tumor. Perioperative complications, such as hemorrhage and thromboembolism, may occur. Therefore, prophylactic phlebotomies have been advocated to reduce the red blood cell mass before surgery.

### COMBINED PARANEOPLASTIC ENDOCRINE SYNDROMES

Commonly, cancers that cause an endocrine syndrome as a result of the secretion of a specific hormone also are found to secrete other hormones, such as neurotensin, calcitonin, somatostatin, or vasoactive intestinal peptide. In most such cases, no clinical manifestations are evident. Occasionally, however, patients may manifest combined endocrine syndromes, as in the case of a small cell cancer of the lung that secretes ACTH and vasopressin, resulting in Cushing syndrome and inappropriate secretion of ADH, or an ACTH- and CRH-secreting bronchial carcinoid tumor that produces adrenal hyperplasia both directly and through pituitary stimulation.[81] Small cell cancer of the trachea has been reported to cause both Cushing syndrome due to ACTH secretion and paraneoplastic osteomalacia.[82] Reports have been published of a gastrin- and GHRH-secreting pancreatic islet cell tumor that has caused both the Zollinger-Ellison syndrome and acromegaly,[83] as well as a gastrin- and ACTH-secreting pancreatic islet cell tumor that has produced the Zollinger-Ellison syndrome and Cushing syndrome.[84] Often, primary liver cell carcinoma is associated with erythropoietin-induced polycythemia, as well as with hypercalcemia and hypoglycemia.[85]

### PARANEOPLASTIC SECRETION OF OTHER KNOWN PEPTIDE HORMONES WITH NO ASSOCIATED ENDOCRINE SYNDROME

*Calcitonin* is one of the most common hormones to be secreted by tumors. Hypercalcitonemia occurs not only in medullary thyroid carcinoma (see Chap. 40) but also in 10% to 30% of other malignant neoplasms. In these cases, preferential secretion of procalcitonin is seen. Particularly high values are seen in cases of small cell lung cancer and pulmonary carcinoid tumors (see Chap. 177). Clinically, the measurement of this hormone in blood or urine may be a biomarker for the progression of a tumor or its response to therapy.[86] No specific syndrome is known to be caused by hypercalcitonemia. Serum calcium levels and bone architecture remain normal.

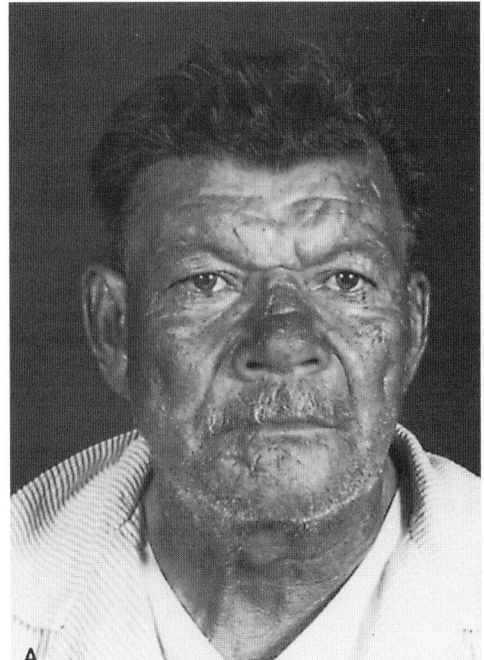

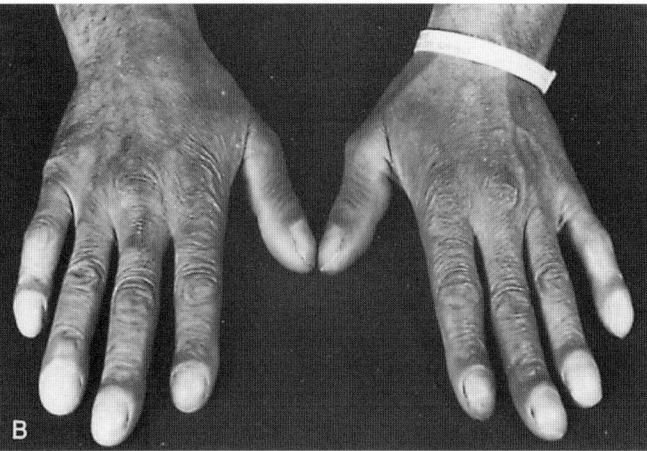

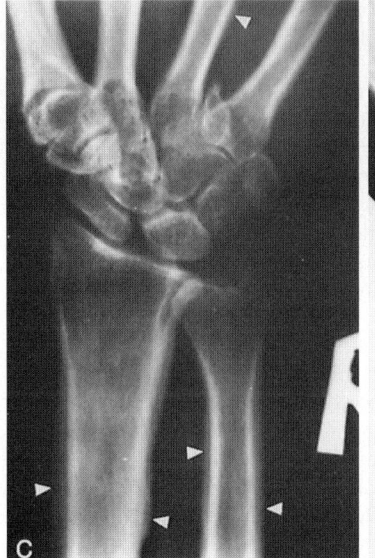

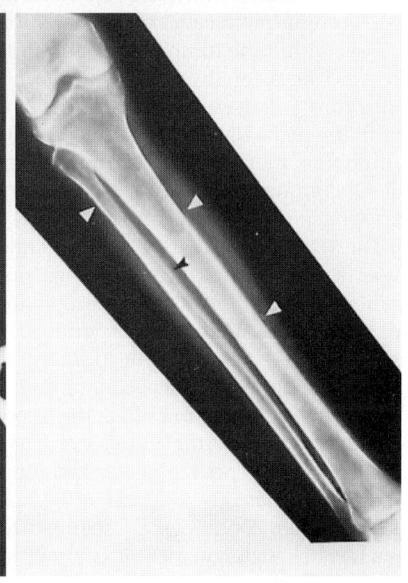

**FIGURE 219-3.** A patient with pachydermoperiostitis (thickened facies, hypertrophic osteoarthropathy, and underlying malignancy). The patient had epidermoid carcinoma of the lung. **A,** Note the coarsening of the facial features, including the prominent creases of the forehead, the deep nasolabial folds, and the broad nose. The skin is very oily. **B,** Marked clubbing of the digits is evident. **C,** Radiographs of a patient with this syndrome reveal periostitis of the long bones (*arrowheads*), especially the distal ends.

*Neurotensin, somatostatin,* and *cholecystokinin* also are commonly secreted by tumors without obvious clinical effects. Conceivably, these hormones may participate in the general systemic effects that often accompany malignant disease, such as fatigue, depression, nausea, anorexia, and weight loss.

Rare and insufficiently documented cases of the extrapituitary production of thyroid-stimulating hormone have been reported. However, most patients with hyperthyroidism secondary to associated nonpituitary, nonthyroidal malignant disease are thyrotoxic because of the thyroid-stimulating effects of high serum levels of hCG produced by trophoblastic tumors (see Chaps. 15 and 42).

*Human chorionic somatomammotropin,* also termed *human placental lactogen,* has been reported to have been produced by a large cell lung cancer in a patient who also had gynecomastia. However, subsequent documentation of a specific syndrome has not been forthcoming.

Alleged cases of lung cancer in which tumoral secretion of growth hormone was associated with hypertrophic pulmonary osteoarthropathy have been reported. However, the validity of this phenomenon remains uncertain.

Little evidence exists of a syndrome attributable to prolactin secretion by a tumor of nonpituitary origin. Although this hormone has been found in both the normal and cancerous uterine cervix, the patients with malignancy do not usually have hyperprolactinemia.[87]

## SUSPECTED PARANEOPLASTIC ENDOCRINE SYNDROMES

### HYPERTROPHIC OSTEOARTHROPATHY

Hypertrophic osteoarthropathy (Bamberger-Marie syndrome) is a progressive, bilaterally symmetric, periosteal reaction involving the bones of the fingers and toes. It commonly affects the distal long bones and joints as well. The thickened, clubbed-appearing digits have been referred to as *acropachy* (Fig. 219-3B). Often, the disease is associated with a malignant process.

Patients may note progressive disfigurement, or, if the onset is sudden, patients may be surprised when the examiner calls attention to the enlarged fingers. If present, the arthralgia of the fingers, wrists, knees, and ankles may be confused with rheumatoid arthritis. On physical examination, the digits have a widened transverse diameter. Obliteration of the normal angle between the distal phalanges and the nails adds to the drumstick appearance. The nails may be fluctuant to the touch and slightly mobile. In addition, the hands and feet may appear enlarged, and the wrists and ankles may be thickened. In such cases, periarticular swelling of the soft tissues, which are tender and slightly warm, may also occur. Occasionally, joint effusions may be palpated. A sample of the synovial fluid is "noninflammatory"; counts seldom are >500 leukocytes/mm$^3$.

Rarely, the facial skin may be thickened and seborrheic, with deep furrows, increased nasolabial folds, a corrugated brow, and a broad nose. These findings may impart an acromegalic appearance to the patient (see Fig 219-3*A*). On radiographic examination, evidence often is seen of periosteal new bone formation in the proximal phalanges. The metacarpals, the distal ends of the radius and ulna, the tibia and fibula, and the distal femur also may show involvement (see Fig. 219-3*C*). In severe cases, thick, multilayered, new bone formation is present with periosteal elevation and an underlying rarefaction of the outer portions of the original cortex, which imparts an "onionskin" appearance. Later, fusion of old and new bone may occur. A radionuclide bone scan usually reveals increased uptake of contrast material in the involved areas.

The underlying pathology in many patients with hypertrophic osteoarthropathy is malignant disease. Probably 90% of such cases are attributable to intrathoracic cancers, of which the predominant form is bronchogenic cancer. The most common cell type is epidermoid cancer (especially if pleural involvement or necrosis within the tumor is present), followed by adenocarcinoma, and, occasionally, large cell cancer. (Small cell cancer of the lung rarely causes this syndrome.[88]) Other intrathoracic lesions that may be implicated include mesothelioma, mediastinal lymphoma, metastatic cancer involving the lungs, and thymoma. Uncommon extrathoracic causes include carcinoma of the nasopharynx or gastrointestinal tract, and osteogenic sarcoma. The syndrome also may occur in childhood.[89,90]

Hypertrophic osteoarthropathy also may occur in chronic nonmalignant conditions, such as bronchiectasis, cyanotic congenital heart disease, subacute bacterial endocarditis, ulcerative colitis, or cirrhosis of the liver. In addition, endocrinologists may see this condition in patients with the hyperthyroidism associated with Graves disease but not in the hyperthyroidism accompanying toxic adenomatous goiter (see Chap. 42).

Another form of hypertrophic osteoarthropathy—*hereditary acropachy*—is not associated with cancer or with any of the previously mentioned benign conditions. Sometimes, this condition is inherited as a mendelian dominant trait; commonly, it begins in puberty. The term *pachydermoperiostosis*[91] should be reserved for the primary or idiopathic variety of hypertrophic osteoarthropathy (Fig. 219-4), whereas *pachydermoperiostitis* is the correct term for the secondary form, which is associated with a known, underlying condition.

Clinically, a severe case of hypertrophic osteoarthropathy may be mistaken for rheumatoid arthritis. Occasionally, the finding of hypertrophic osteoarthropathy may precede a clinical diagnosis of malignant disease, and hence may first call attention to the presence of the neoplasm. Rarely, a patient may not manifest any signs or symptoms indicating the presence of an underlying malignant lesion for several months. In many patients, the erythrocyte sedimentation rate is increased, probably reflecting the presence of a neoplasm. The serum alkaline phosphatase level may be normal or increased.

Most likely, hypertrophic osteoarthropathy is humorally mediated. Vascular endothelial growth factor may play a role.[91a] The mediastinum, and the pleura in particular, is rich in vagal innervation, and it has been postulated that an abnormal vagal afferent reflex, instituted by a thoracic lesion, can induce a local or central release of vasoactive or growth-promoting substances.

Aspirin and other nonsteroidal antiinflammatory agents may provide symptomatic relief if joint pain or joint effusions occur. Successful surgical extirpation or chemotherapy may reverse the joint swellings and may even induce partial remission of the bone changes.[92,93]

## ACANTHOSIS NIGRICANS

Acanthosis nigricans is an acquired, bilaterally symmetric, cutaneous lesion characterized by a piling up of the skin, which

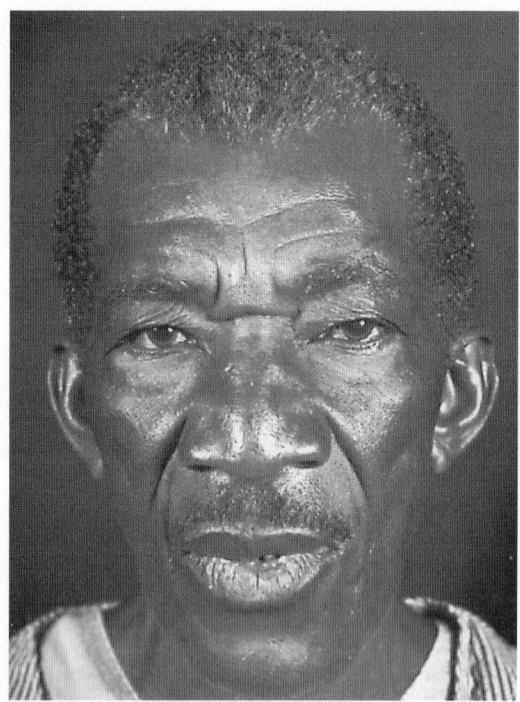

**FIGURE 219-4.** Patient with pachydermoperiostosis (thickened facies, hypertrophic osteoarthropathy, no associated malignancy). Affected patients have marked clubbing of the digits as well as radiographic evidence of periostitis of the long bones, especially the distal ends. This condition is inherited as a mendelian dominant trait.

assumes a brown to black coloration and a velvety consistency. Commonly, many local, tiny, pedunculated, papillomatous overgrowths (skin tags) also are present. Usually, the condition is nonpruritic.

The darkened, verrucous-appearing skin lesion occurs in flexural areas, such as the axillae, the back and sides of the neck, the antecubital fossae, beneath the folds of pendulous abdominal fat, behind the knees, between the thighs, and, sometimes, on the face (circumoral and nasolabial regions) (see Chap. 218). In these relatively moist regions, the piling up of the epidermis parallels the body creases in a striate fashion. The condition occurs in all races. Histologic examination reveals hyperkeratosis, a thickened stratum corneum, papillary hypertrophy, and an increase in the pigmented basal layers.

Traditionally, acanthosis nigricans has been classified as either benign or malignant. A common, but not universal, characteristic associated with the benign variety is a cellular resistance to insulin action (see Chap. 146).[94] In some manner, this metabolic defect, which does not always result in frank diabetes, induces an overgrowth of epidermal cells that may be hormonally mediated, perhaps involving blood-borne trophic factors. The more common benign form of acanthosis nigricans usually occurs in relatively young persons who are obese or who have obesity-related ovarian dysfunction (polycystic ovary syndrome) (see Chaps. 96 and 101). Other associated metabolic or endocrine conditions include congenital lipodystrophy, acromegaly, and Cushing disease. In nearly all cases, the coexistent skin lesions progress with time.

The malignant form of acanthosis nigricans, so named because of its association with internal tumors, may occur at any age but is most common among older persons.[95] Often, affected patients are not obese. The most common causative lesion is gastrointestinal adenocarcinoma (e.g., involving the stomach [in two-thirds of the cases], the gallbladder, or the rectum). Other causes include ovarian carcinoma and lymphoma. The neoplasm invariably is highly malignant and usually is inoperable because of the presence of metastases. Although acanthosis nigricans can precede any clinical manifestations of the underlying neoplasm,[95a] it generally coincides with detection of the tumor and worsens with the progress of the malignancy. Oral lesions may occur. Some believe that pruritic involvement of the palms and soles is a clue to the presence of underlying neoplasia. In cancer, transforming growth factor-α may be one of the humoral causes of acanthosis nicricans.[96] Occasionally, cases have been reported in which successful surgery or chemotherapeutic treatment of the neoplasm was associated with reversal of the skin lesion.[97]

## MISCELLANEOUS POSSIBLY PARANEOPLASTIC ENDOCRINE SYNDROMES

Several other syndromes that are associated with neoplasms may be humorally mediated. *Paraneoplastic eosinophilia,* described in association with large cell cancer of the lung, is characterized by marked eosinophilia and diffuse eosinophilic infiltration of nearly all tissues. Increased serum eosinophilic colony-stimulating factor and eosinophilic chemotactic factor have been detected.[98] The expression of adhesion molecules may also play a role.[98a] Lung cancer also may be associated with an absolute *neutrophilia* and, in some instances, *thrombocytosis.* In such cases, granulocyte/macrophage colony-stimulating factors may be secreted.[99–101] In some patients, the neutrophilia rapidly resolves after surgical removal of the primary lesion. *Acquired hypertrichosis lanuginosa* ("malignant down")[102] is found in patients with late-stage widespread cancer, commonly involving the gastrointestinal tract and occasionally involving other locations.[103] The face, neck, and trunk exhibit long, fine, silky, unpigmented hair (Fig 219-5). Conceivably, the condition may be due to the secretion of a growth factor.

The *sign of Leser-Trélat* (sudden onset of seborrheic keratoses in association with an internal malignant lesion) may be caused by the production of transforming growth factor-α by the neoplasm. Such a condition has been postulated in one patient with melanoma and also was associated with acanthosis nigricans and multiple acrochordons (skin tags).[104]

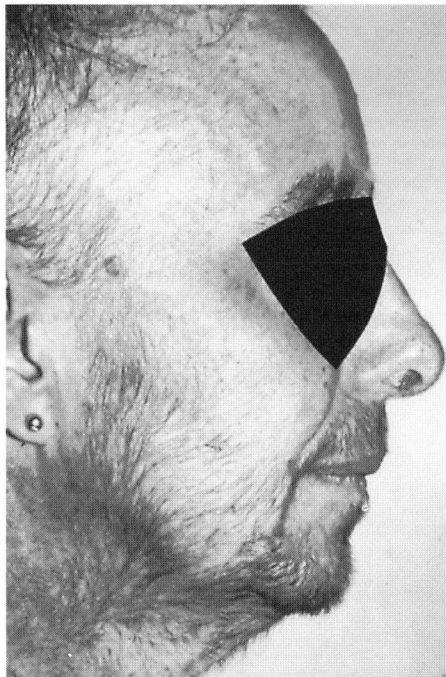

**FIGURE 219-5.** Woman with acquired hypertrichosis lanuginosa associated with metastatic sarcoma.

*The spontaneous regression of metastases after excision of the primary lesion* has been described in ~80 patients, mostly men, whose pulmonary metastases regressed after nephrectomy for renal cell carcinoma.[105] A similar phenomenon has been described in malignant melanoma. Conceivably, the removal of the primary lesion arrests the secretion of a growth factor that either had been stimulating or maintaining the viability of the metastases.

Several other syndromes associated with cancer have no evidence of humoral mediation but merit further endocrine investigation. The *Eaton-Lambert myasthenic syndrome,* characterized by proximal muscle weakness in association with small cell cancer of the lung, was formerly thought to be mediated by a hormone. It is caused by an autoantibody to the tumor that cross-reacts with determinants at the motor nerve terminal.[106] Similarly, the cerebellar degeneration associated with malignant disease may be attributable to autoantibodies.[107] Severe constipation occurring in several patients with ovarian carcinoid tumors has been attributed to secretion of peptide YY, a substance known to inhibit intestinal motility.[108] Malignant hemangioendotheliomas have been reported to secrete endothelin and to cause hypertension.[109]

## HORMONE-MEDIATED EFFECT OF NEOPLASIA ON THE BODY

Neoplasia frequently is associated with asthenia, negative nitrogen balance, and severe wasting. Sometimes, these symptoms occur even if the causative lesion is relatively small. Usually, the patient loses weight despite deliberate attempts to overeat. The hormone tumor necrosis factor α, which is produced by endotoxin-stimulated macrophages, inhibits lipoprotein lipase activity in adipocytes and induces a loss of triglycerides from this tissue[110]; it also causes an anemia.[111] The extent to which this substance, or other cytokines, might contribute to the cachexia of cancer, either by direct production from the neoplasm[112,113] or by other tissues that react to the malignant lesion,[114] is unknown. Tumor cells, as well as T lymphocytes, may produce humoral *tumor angiogenesis factors*[115] that stimulate new blood vessel growth, which, in turn, assists in the perpetuation and propagation of the malignant neoplasm.

Lastly, some tumor cells produce humoral factors that inhibit the growth of other cell lines of cancer (e.g., secretion of transforming growth factor-β by breast cancer cell lines after treatment with antiestrogens inhibits the growth of an estrogen receptor-negative human breast cancer cell line[116]).

## REFERENCES

1. De Bustros A, Baylin SB. Hormone production by tumors: biological and clinical aspects. Clin Endocrinol Metab 1985; 14:221.
2. Howlett TA, Rees LH. Ectopic hormones. In: Cohen MP, Foa PP, eds. Special topics in endocrinology and metabolism, vol 7. New York: Liss, 1985:1.
3. Becker KL, Gazdar AF. What can the biology of small cell cancer of the lung teach us about the endocrine lung? Biochem Pharmacol 1985; 34:155.
4. Lupulescu A. Cancer and ectopic hormones: clinical and biological aspects. In: Hormones and carcinogenesis. New York: Praeger Publishers, 1983:276.
5. LeRoith D, Roth J. Syndromes associated with inappropriate hormone synthesis by tumors: an evolutionary interpretation. Recent Results Cancer Res 1985; 99:209.
6. Gumbiner B, Kelly RB. Two distinct intracellular pathways transport secretory and membrane glycoproteins to the surface of pituitary tumor cells. Cell 1982; 28:51.
7. Losa M, von Werder K. Pathophysiology and clinical aspects of the ectopic GH-releasing hormone syndrome. Clin Endocrinol 1997; 47:123.
8. Shimon I, Melmed S. Growth hormone and growth hormone-releasing hormone producing tumors. Cancer Treat Res 1997; 89:1.
9. Frohman LA, Jansson J-O. Growth hormone-releasing hormone. Endocr Rev 1986; 7:223.
10. Boizel R, Halimi S, Labat F, et al. Acromegaly due to a growth hormone-releasing hormone-secreting bronchial carcinoid tumor. J Clin Endocrinol Metab 1987; 64:304.

11. Ezzat S, Asa SL, Stefaneanu L, et al. Somatotroph hyperplasia without pituitary adenoma associated with a long standing growth-hormone releasing hormone-producing bronchial carcinoma. J Clin Endocrinol Metab 1994; 78:555.

12. Barkan AL, Shenker Y, Grekin RJ, Vale WW. Acromegaly from ectopic growth hormone-releasing hormone secretion by a malignant carcinoid tumor. Successful treatment with long-acting somatostatin analogue SMS 201-995. Cancer 1988; 61:221.

12a. Beuschlein F, Strasburger CJ, Siegerstetter V, et al. Acromegaly caused by secretion of growth hormone by a non-Hodgkin's lymphoma. New Engl J Med 2000; 342:1871.

13. Carey RM, Varma SK, Drake CR Jr, et al. Ectopic secretion of corticotropin-releasing factor as a cause of Cushing's syndrome. A clinical morphologic, and biochemical study. N Engl J Med 1984; 311:13.

14. Zarate A, Kovacs K, Flores M, et al. ACTH and CRF-producing bronchial carcinoid associated with Cushing's syndrome. Clin Endocrinol (Oxf) 1986; 24:523.

15. Hofland J, Schneider AJ, Cuesta MA, Meijer S. Bronchopulmonary carcinoids associated with Cushing's syndrome—report of a case and an overview of the literature. Acta Oncol 1993; 32:571.

16. Jensen RT. Pancreatic endocrine tumors: recent advances. Ann Oncol 1999; 10(Suppl 4):170.

17. White A, Clark AJL. The cellular and molecular basis of the ectopic ACTH syndrome. Clin Endocrinol (Oxf) 1993; 39:131.

18. Cederna P, Eckhauser FE, Kealey GP. Cushing's syndrome secondary to bronchial carcinoid secretion of ACTH: a review. Am Surg 1993; 59:438.

19. Howlett TA, Drury PL, Perry L, et al. Diagnosis and management of ACTH-dependent Cushing's syndrome: comparison of the features in ectopic and pituitary ACTH production. Clin Endocrinol (Oxf) 1986; 24:699.

20. Horton KM, Fishman EK. Cushing syndrome due to a pulmonary carcinoid tumor: multimodality imaging and diagnosis. J Comput Assist Tomogr 1998; 22:804.

21. Chrousos GP, Schulte HM, Oldfield EH, et al. The corticotropin-releasing factor stimulation test: an aid in the evaluation of patients with Cushing's syndrome. N Engl J Med 1984; 310:622.

22. Cizza G, Chrousos GP. Adrenocorticotrophic hormone-dependent Cushing's syndrome. Cancer Treat Res 1997; 89:25.

23. Tremble JM, Buxton-Thomas M, Hopkins D, et al. Cushing's syndrome associated with a chemodectoma and a carcinoid tumour. Clin Endocrinol 2000; 52:789.

24. Doppman JL, Loughlin T, Miller DL, et al. Identification of ACTH-producing intrathoracic tumors by measuring ACTH levels in aspirated specimens. Radiology 1987; 163:501.

25. Shepherd FA, Hoffert B, Evans WK, et al. Ketoconazole. Use in the treatment of ectopic adrenocorticotropic hormone production and Cushing's syndrome in small cell lung cancer. Arch Intern Med 1985; 145:863.

26. Comi RJ, Gorden P. Long-term medical treatment of ectopic ACTH syndrome. South Med J 1998; 91:1014.

27. Robertson GL. Cancer and inappropriate antidiuresis. In: Ruddon RW, ed. Biological markers of neoplasia: basic and applied aspects. Amsterdam: Elsevier North Holland, 1978:277.

28. Verbalis JG. Tumoral hyponatremia. Arch Intern Med 1986; 146:1686.

29. Sorensen JB, Kristjansen PEG, Osterlind K, et al. Syndrome of inappropriate antidiuresis in small-cell lung cancer. Acta Med Scand 1987; 222:155.

30. Bliss DP Jr, Battey JF, Linnoila RI, et al. Expression of the atrial natriuretic factor gene in small cell lung cancer tumors and tumor cell lines. J Natl Cancer Inst 1990; 82:305.

31. Kamoi XX, Ebe T, Hasegawa A, et al. Hyponatremia in small cell lung cancer: mechanisms not involving inappropriate ADH secretion. Cancer 1987; 60:1089.

32. Rizzoli R, Pache J-C, Didierjean L, et al. A thymoma as a cause of true ectopic hyperparathyroidism. J Clin Endocrinol Metab 1994; 79:912.

33. Rankin W, Grill V, Martin TJ. Parathyroid hormone-related protein and hypercalcemia. Cancer 1997; 80(Suppl 8):1564.

34. Strewler GJ, Stern PH, Jacobs JW, et al. Parathyroid hormone-like protein from human renal carcinoma cells. J Clin Invest 1987; 80:1803.

35. Stewart AF, Elliot J, Burtis WJ, et al. Synthetic parathyroid hormone-like protein–(1–74): biochemical and physiological characterization. Endocrinology 1989; 124:642.

36. Firkin F, Schneider H, Grill V. Parathyroid hormone-related protein in hypercalcemia associated with hematological malignancy. Leuk Lymphoma 1998; 29:499.

37. Dunne FP, Rollason T, Ratcliffe WA, et al. Parathyroid hormone-related gene expression in invasive cervical tumors. Cancer 1994; 74:83.

38. Vasavada RC, Garcia-Ocana A, Massfelder T, et al. Parathyroid hormone-related protein in the pancreatic islet and the cardiovascular system. Recent Prog Horm Res 1998; 53:305.

39. Tait DL, McDonald PC, Casey ML. Parathyroid hormone-related protein expression in gynecic squamous carcinoma cells. Cancer 1994; 73:1515.

40. Li X, Drucker DJ. Parathyroid hormone-related peptide is a downstream target for ras and src activation. J Biol Chem 1994; 269:6263.

41. Ratcliffe WA, Bonden SJ, Dunne FP, et al. Expression and processing of parathyroid hormone-related protein in a pancreatic endocrine cell tumor associated with hypercalcemia. Clin Endocrinol (Oxf) 1994; 40:679.

42. Iwamura M, Abrahamsson PA, Foss KA, et al. Parathyroid hormone-related protein: a potential autocrine growth regulator in human prostate cancer cell lines. Urology 1994; 43:675.

43. Roodman GD. Mechanisms of bone lesions in multiple myeloma and lymphoma. Cancer 1997; 80 (Suppl 8):1557.

44. Mudde AH, Van den Berg H, Boshuis PG, et al. Ectopic production of 1,25 dihydroxyvitamin D by B-cell lymphoma as a cause of hypercalcemia. Cancer 1987; 59:1543.

45. Warrell RP Jr, Israel R, Frisone M, et al. Gallium nitrate for acute treatment of cancer-related hypercalcemia. Ann Intern Med 1988; 108:669.

46. Wimalawansa SJ. Significance of plasma PTH-rp in patients with hypercalcemia of malignancy treated with bisphosphonate. Cancer 1994; 73:2223.

46a. Ogata E. Parathyroid hormone–related protein as a potential target of therapy for cancer-associated morbidity. Cancer 2000; 88(12 Suppl):2909.

47. Ryan EA, Reiss E. Oncogenous osteomalacia. Review of the world literature of 42 cases and report of two new cases. Am J Med 1984; 77:501.

48. Shane E, Parisien M, Henderson JE, et al. Tumor-induced osteomalacia: clinical and basic studies. J Bone Miner Res 1997; 12:1502.

49. Weiss D, Barr RS, Weidner N, et al. Oncogenic osteomalacia: strange tumors in strange places. Postgrad Med J 1985; 61:349.

50. Nelson AE, Robinson BG, Mason RS. Oncogenic osteomalacia: is there a new phosphate regulating hormone? Clin Endocrinol 1997; 47:635.

50a. Reyes-Mugica M, Arnsmeier SL, Backeljaun PF, et al. Phosphaturic mesenchymal tumor-induced rickets. Pediatr Dev Pathol 2000; 3:61.

51. Baronofsky SI, Kalbhen CL, Demos TC, Sizemore GW. Oncogenic osteomalacia secondary to a hemangiopericytoma of the hip: case report. Can Assoc Radiol J 1999; 50:26.

52. Charhon SA, Chapux MC, Delvin EE, et al. Histomorphometric analysis of sclerotic bone metastases from prostatic carcinoma with special reference to osteomalacia. Cancer 1983; 51:918.

53. Rao DS, Parfitt AM, Villanueva AR, et al. Hypophosphatemic osteomalacia and adult Fanconi syndrome due to light-chain nephropathy. Am J Med 1987; 82:333.

54. Kathuria S, Jablokow VR. Primary choriocarcinoma of mediastinum with immunohistochemical study and review of the literature. J Surg Oncol 1987; 34:39.

55. Becker KL, Cottrell J, Moore CF, et al. Endocrine studies in a patient with a gonadotropin-secreting bronchogenic carcinoma. J Clin Endocrinol Metab 1968; 28:809.

56. Navarro C, Corretger JM, Sancho A, et al. Paraneoplastic precocious puberty. Report of a new case with hepatoblastoma and review of the literature. Cancer 1985; 56:1725.

57. Norman RJ, Green-Thompson RW, Jialal I, et al. Hyperthyroidism in gestational trophoblastic neoplasia. Clin Endocrinol (Oxf) 1981; 15:395.

58. Hay DL. Histological origins of discordant chorionic gonadotropin secretion in malignancy. J Clin Endocrinol Metab 1988; 66:557.

59. O'Connor JF, Schlatterer JP, Birken S, et al. Development of highly sensitive immunoassays to measure human chorionic gonadotropin, its β-subunit, and core fragment in the urine: application to malignancies. Cancer Res 1988; 48:1361.

60. Daughaday WH. Hypoglycemia in patients with non-islet cell tumors. Endocrinol Metab Clin North Am 1989; 18:91.

61. Touyz R, Plitt M, Rumbak M. Hypoglycemia associated with a lung mass. Chest 1986; 89:289.

62. Kataoka T, Haruta G, Goto T, et al. Malignant phyllodes tumor of the breast with hypoglycemia: report of a case. Jpn J Clin Oncol 1998; 28:276.

63. Li TC, Reed CE, Stubenbord WT Jr, et al. Surgical cure of hypoglycemia associated with cystosarcoma phyllodes and elevated nonsuppressible insulin-like protein. Am J Med 1983; 74:1080.

64. Ron D, Powers AC, Pandian MR, et al. Increased insulin-like growth factor II production and consequent suppression of growth hormone secretion: a dual mechanism for tumor-induced hypoglycemia. J Clin Endocrinol Metab 1989; 68.701.

65. Horiuchi T, Shinohara Y, Sakamoto Y, et al. Expression of insulin-like growth factor II by a gastric carcinoma associated with hypoglycemia. Virchows Arch 1994; 424:449.

66. Rose MG, Tallini G, Pollak J, Murren J. Malignant hypoglycemia associated with a large mesenchymal tumor: case report and review of the literature. Cancer J Sci Am 1999; 5:48.

67. Merimee TJ. Insulin-like growth factors in patients with non-islet cell tumors and hypoglycemia. Metabolism 1986; 35:360.

68. Zapf J. IGFs: function and clinical importance. Role of insulin-like growth factor (IGF) II and IGF binding proteins in extrapancreatic tumor hypoglycemia. J Intern Med 1993; 234:543.

69. Stuart CA, Price MJ, Peters EJ, et al. Insulin receptor proliferation: a mechanism for tumor-associated hypoglycemia. J Clin Endocrinol Metab 1986; 63:879.

70. Al Hilali MM, Majer RV, Penney O. Hypoglycemia in acute myelomonoblastic leukaemia: report of two cases and review of published work. BMJ 1984; 289:1443.

71. Pedrinelli R, Graziadei L, Taddei S, et al. A renin-secreting tumor. Nephron 1987; 46:380.

72. Morris BJ, Pinet F, Michel JB, et al. Renin secretion from malignant pulmonary metastatic tumour cells of vascular origin. Clin Exp Pharmacol Physiol 1987; 14:227.

73. Kawai M, Sahashi K, Yamase H, et al. Renin-producing adrenal tumor: report of a case. Surg Today 1998; 28:974.

74. Korzets A, Nouriel H, Steiner Z, et al. Resistant hypertension associated with a renin-producing ovarian Sertoli cell tumor. Am J Clin Pathol 1986; 85:242.

75. Fernandez LA, Olsen TG, Barwick KW, et al. Renin in angiolymphoid hyperplasia with eosinophilia. Arch Pathol Lab Med 1986; 110:1131.

76. Arai H, Saitoh S, Matsumoto T, et al. Hypertension as a paraneoplastic syndrome in hepatocellular carcinoma. J Gastroenterol 1999; 34:530.

77. Grignon DJ, Eble JN. Papillary and metanephric adenomas of the kidney. Semin Diagn Pathol 1998; 15:41.

78. Rosenlof K, Fyhrquist F, Gronhagen-Riska C. Erythropoietin and renin substrate in cerebellar hemangioblastoma. Acta Med Scand 1985; 218:481.

79. Okabe T, Urabe A, Kato T, et al. Production of erythropoietin-like activity by human renal and hepatic carcinomas in cell culture. Cancer 1985; 55:1918.

80. Shulkin BL, Shapiron B, Sisson JC. Pheochromocytoma, polycythemia, and venous thrombosis. Am J Med 1987; 83:773.

81. Schteingart DE, Lloyd RV, Akil H, et al. Cushing's syndrome secondary to ectopic corticotropin-releasing hormone-adrenocorticotropin secretion. J Clin Endocrinol Metab 1986; 63:770.

82. Van Heyningen C, Green AR, MacFarlane IA, Burrow CT. Oncogenic hypophosphatemia and ectopic corticotrophin secretion due to oat cell carcinoma of the trachea. J Clin Pathol 1994; 47:80.

83. Wilson DM, Ceda GP, Bostwick DG, et al. Acromegaly and Zollinger-Ellison syndrome secondary to an islet cell tumor. J Clin Endocrinol Metab 1984; 59:1002.

84. Maton PN, Gardner JD, Jensen RT. Cushing's syndrome in patients with the Zollinger-Ellison syndrome. N Engl J Med 1986; 315:1.

85. Teniola SO, Ogenleye IO. Paraneoplastic responses in primary liver cell carcinoma in Nigeria. Trop Geogr Med 1994; 46:20.

86. Silva OL, Broder LE, Doppman JL, et al. Calcitonin as a marker for bronchogenic cancer: a prospective study. Cancer 1979; 44:680.

87. Macfee MS, McQueen J, Strayer DE. Immunocytochemical localization of prolactin in carcinoma of the cervix. Gynecol Oncol 1987; 26:314.

88. Yacoub MH. Relation between the histology of bronchial carcinoma and hypertrophic pulmonary osteoarthropathy. Thorax 1965; 20:537.

89. Ilhan I, Kutluk T, Gogus S, et al. Hypertrophic pulmonary osteoarthropathy in a child with thymic carcinoma: an unusual presentation in childhood. Med Pediatr Oncol 1994; 23:140.

90. Roebuck DJ. Skeletal complications in pediatric oncology patients. Radiographics 1999; 19:873.

91. Rimoin DL. Pachydermoperiostosis (idiopathic clubbing and periostitis): genetic and physiologic considerations. N Engl J Med 1965; 272:923.

91a. Silveira LH, Martinez-Lavin M, Pineda C, et al. Vascular endothelial growth factor and hypertrophic osteoarthropathy. Clin Exp Rheumatol 2000; 18:57.

92. Evans WK. Reversal of hypertrophic osteoarthropathy after chemotherapy for bronchogenic carcinoma. J Rheumatol 1980; 7:93.

93. Nishi K, Matsamura M, Myou S, et al. Two cases of pulmonary hypertrophic osteoarthropathy associated with primary lung cancer, in which symptoms were rapidly improved by resection of the primary lesions. Nippon Kyobu Shikkan Gakkai Zasshi 1994; 32:271.

94. Stuart CA, Driscoll MS, Lundquist KF, et al. Acanthosis nigricans. J Basic Clin Physiol Pharmacol 1998; 9:407.

95. Curth HO, Hilberg AW, Machacek GF. The site of histology of the cancer associated with malignant acanthosis nigricans. Cancer 1962; 15:364.

95a. Yeh JS, Munn SE, Plunkett TA, et al. Coexistence of acanthosis nigricans and the sign of Leser-Trelat in a patient with gastric adenocarcinoma. J Am Acad Dermatol 2000; 42:357.

96. Koyama S, Ikeda K, Sato M, et al. Transforming growth factor-alpha (TGF-alpha)-producing gastric carcinoma with acanthosis nigricans. J Gastroenterol 1997; 32:71.

97. Pfeifer SL, Wilson RM, Gawkrodger DJ. Clearance of acanthosis nigricans associated with the HAIR-AN syndrome after partial pancreatectomy: an 11-year follow-up. Postgrad Med J 1999; 75:421.

98. Kodama T, Takada K, Kameya T, et al. Large cell carcinoma of the lung associated with marked eosinophilia. Cancer 1984; 54:2313.

98a. Ali S, Kaur J, Patel KD. Intercellular cell adhesion molecule-1, vascular cell adhesion molecule-1, and regulated on activation normal T cell expressed and secreted are expressed by human breast cancer cells and support eosinophil adhesion and activation. Am J Pathol 2000; 157:313.

99. Ascensao JL, Oken MM, Ewing SL, et al. Leukocytosis and large cell lung cancer. Cancer 1987; 60:903.

100. Adachi N, Yamaguchi K, Morikana T, et al. Constitutive production of multiple colony-stimulating factors in patients with lung cancer associated with neutrophilia. Br J Cancer 1994; 69:125.

101. Watanabe M, Ono K, Ozeki Y, et al. Production of granulocyte-macrophage colony-stimulating factor in a patient with metastatic chest wall large-cell carcinoma. Jpn J Clin Oncol 1998; 28:559.

102. Hovenden AL. Acquired hypertrichosis lanuginosa associated with malignancy. Arch Intern Med 1987; 147:2013.

103. Farina MC, Tarin N, Grilli R, et al. Acquired hypertrichosis lanugosa: case report and review of the literature. J Surg Oncol 1998; 68:199.

104. Nakano E, Sonoda T, Fujiaka H, et al. Spontaneous regression of pulmonary metastases after nephrectomy for renal cell carcinoma. Eur Urol 1984; 10:212.

105. Ellis DL, Kafka SP, Chow JC, et al. Melanoma, growth factors, acanthosis nigricans, the sign of Leser-Trélat, and multiple acrochordons. N Engl J Med 1987; 317:1582.

106. Roberts A, Perera S, Lang B, et al. Paraneoplastic myasthenic syndrome IgG inhibits 45 $Ca^{2+}$ flux in a human small cell carcinoma line. Nature 1985; 317:737.

107. Wang A-M, Leibowich S, Ridker PM, David WS. Paraneoplastic cerebellar degeneration in a patient with ovarian carcinoma. AJNR Am J Neuroradiol 1988; 9:216.

108. Motoyama T, Katayama Y, Watanabe H, et al. Functioning ovarian carcinoids induce severe constipation. Cancer 1992; 70:513.

109. Yokokawa K, Tahara H, Kohno M, et al. Hypertension associated with endothelin-secreting malignant hemangioendothelioma. Ann Intern Med 1991; 114:213.

110. Beutler B, Cerami A. Cachectin (tumor necrosis factor): a macrophage hormone governing cellular metabolism and inflammatory response. Endocr Rev 1988; 9:57.

111. Moldawer LL, Marano MA, Wei H, et al. Cachectin/tumor necrosis factor-α alters red blood cell kinetics and induces anemia in vivo. FASEB J 1989; 3:1637.

112. Balkwill F, Burke F, Talbot D, et al. Evidence for tumor necrosis factor/cachectin production in cancer. Lancet 1987; 1:1229.

113. Barber MD, Ross JA, Fearon KC. Disordered metabolic response with cancer and its management. World J Surg 2000; 24:681.

114. Ikemoto S, Sugimura K, Yoshida N, et al. TNF alpha, IL-1 beta and IL-6 production by peripheral blood monocytes in patients with renal cell carcinoma. Anticancer Res 2000; 20:317.

115. Hadar EJ, Ershler WB, Kreisle RA, et al. Lymphocyte-induced angiogenesis factor is produced by L3T4+ murine T lymphocytes, and its production declines with age. Cancer Immunol Immunother 1988; 26:31.

116. Knabbe C, Lippman ME, Wakefield LM, et al. Evidence that transforming growth factor-beta is a hormonally regulated negative growth factor in human breast cancer cells. Cell 1987; 48:417.

# CHAPTER 220

# ENDOCRINE TUMORS OF THE GASTROINTESTINAL TRACT

SHAHRAD TAHERI, KARIM MEERAN, AND STEPHEN BLOOM

Endocrine tumors of the gastrointestinal tract (*gastroenteropancreatic neuroendocrine tumors*) arise mostly in the pancreas (Fig. 220-1) and can be broadly subdivided into *functioning* and *nonfunctioning* tumors. Functioning tumors secrete peptides that can cause recognizable clinical syndromes. These tumors often are slow growing, and, usually, their clinical manifestations are entirely due to excess peptide hormone secretion. Because these tumors are slow growing, palliation is possible in metastatic disease by suppressing peptide release or by blocking the action of the peptide hormone. Nonfunctioning tumors have a worse prognosis and generally present with local pressure symptoms from the primary tumor and/or metastases, or with symptoms of malignancy such as anorexia and weight loss.

Although functioning tumors produce and tend to secrete predominantly a single major peptide, usually resulting in a defined clinical syndrome, these tumors frequently produce other peptides, either at the time of presentation or later in the progression of the tumor. The clinical picture may, therefore, change over time, particularly after therapeutic intervention

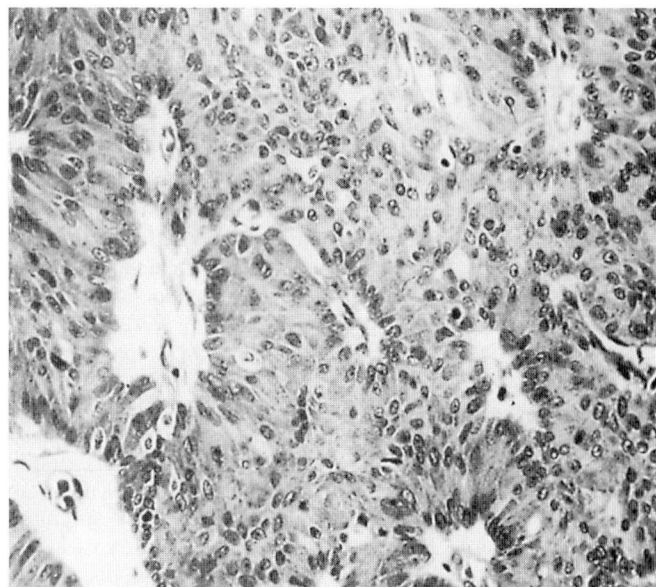

**FIGURE 220-1.** Hematoxylin and eosin stain of a pancreatic endocrine tumor. The lesion shows a solid growth pattern of regular cells with regular nuclei. Nucleoli can be seen in some cells, but mitotic figures are absent. (Bouin's fixation ×400)

such as tumor debulking, when the initial excess hormone may be superseded by a new principal hormone producing a different clinical picture. Because gastrointestinal endocrine tumors may be associated with the syndrome of multiple endocrine neoplasia type 1 (MEN1) (see Chap 188), which has features of parathyroid disease, pituitary tumor, and pancreatic tumor, the clinician must take a detailed family history at presentation, regularly investigate baseline pituitary function, and measure serum calcium in these patients. The aim of this chapter is to review the various gastrointestinal tumors and the major treatment modalities for these lesions, such as somatostatin analog therapy and hepatic tumor embolization.

## GASTRINOMA

In 1955, Zollinger and Ellison described a syndrome of intractable peptic ulcer disease and gastric acid hypersecretion that was secondary to a non–B cell pancreatic tumor.[1] Not until more than a decade later were these tumors found to secrete the hormone gastrin. Gastrin acts through CCK-A receptors on parietal cells of the stomach to stimulate acid secretion and also has a trophic role on the gastric mucosa.[2,3] Gastrin-producing tumors have an annual incidence of one per million. The mean age at the onset of symptoms is 50 years, and a male preponderance is seen. Up to one-third of gastrinomas are associated with MEN1, and up to one-half of MEN1 patients develop gastrinomas. Some sporadic cases are due to MEN1 gene mutations.[3a] The majority of gastrinomas arise in the *gastrinoma triangle*, an area containing the duodenum, the pancreatic head, and the hepatoduodenal ligament. Because gastrin is *not* normally detected in the *adult* pancreas but *is* present in the fetal pancreas, gastrin secreted by pancreatic gastrinomas represents *oncofetal expression of the gastrin gene* in these tumors. At presentation, up to 50% of patients with gastrinoma have metastases, mainly to the liver.

As with other gastrointestinal endocrine tumors, the diagnosis of gastrinoma, or Zollinger-Ellison syndrome, requires a high degree of clinical alertness. Although the peptic ulcer may be quite typical in behavior, the diagnosis certainly should be contemplated in patients with *unusual or complicated ulcer disease that is refractory to treatment which includes* Helicobacter pylori *eradication.*[4] *Gastric mucosal hypertrophy*, seen endoscopically or radiologically, should raise the suspicion of gastrinoma. In addition to symptoms of peptic ulcer disease, *esophagitis* and *diarrhea* are common manifestations. The increased acid secretion secondary to elevated gastrin levels neutralizes digestive enzymes and damages the intestinal mucosa; this may result in diarrhea. A diarrhea that persists in spite of fasting and that is relieved by drugs that inhibit acid secretion, such as $H^+$-$K^+$ adenosine triphosphatase (ATPase) inhibitors, should raise the possibility of a gastrinoma.

Once the diagnosis of gastrinoma is suspected, it must be confirmed by the demonstration of high levels of fasting serum gastrin in the face of high basal gastric acid secretion. Several other conditions can result in raised gastrin levels (Table 220-1), but most commonly acid antisecretory drug therapy is the cause. Therefore, in the diagnostic work-up of a suspected gastrinoma, acid antisecretory drugs, such as $H_2$ blockers and $H^+$-$K^+$ ATPase inhibitors, should be discontinued—for at least 72 hours in the case of $H_2$ blockers and for at least 14 days in the case of $H^+$-$K^+$ ATPase inhibitors. This may not be possible for a patient who is dependent on such medications for symptom control, and the *secretin provocative test* may then be used. Because hypercalcemia can raise gastrin levels, in patients with MEN1 syndrome, hyperparathyroidism needs to be excluded first before a diagnosis of gastrinoma is made.

In gastrinoma patients, basal acid output is usually >15 mEq/hour in patients without previous gastric surgery and is

**TABLE 220-1.**
**Causes of Elevated Plasma Gastrin Levels**

General: response to a meal, renal failure, hepatic failure, stress
Drugs: $H_2$ blockers, proton pump inhibitors
Pernicious anemia
*Helicobacter pylori* infection
Hypercalcemia
Intestinal resection
Inflammatory bowel disease
Antral remnant
Gastrinoma

>5 mEq/hour in patients with previous gastric surgery. The secretin provocative test is usually carried out in patients with borderline gastrin levels and equivocal acid-secretion results. In normal individuals, the administration of secretin *suppresses* gastrin secretion, but in gastrinoma patients a *paradoxical rise* in gastrin levels occurs in response to secretin. (The fasted patient is given 2 U/kg of secretin intravenously, and blood is collected for gastrin measurement at 2, 5, 10, and 20 minutes; in the presence of gastrinoma, gastrin levels increase by at least 50% from baseline.) Up to 87% of patients with gastrinoma demonstrate a positive response to secretin.

If the diagnosis of gastrinoma is confirmed biochemically, tumor localization is carried out to identify the small proportion of patients (9%) with localized disease, because these persons may benefit from curative surgery. Radiolabeled octreotide scanning provides the most useful information regarding the primary tumor and any metastases (see Chap. 169).[5,6] As with other neuroendocrine tumors, the detection of radiolabeled octreotide binding also identifies patients who may respond best to therapy with somatostatin analogs. Magnetic resonance imaging (MRI) provides information regarding hepatic metastases but is not helpful in localizing the primary tumor. Small tumors may be detected with endoscopic ultrasonography and/or selective arterial angiography in combination with computed tomographic (CT) scanning. On occasion, intraarterial secretin injection at the time of angiography may help localize the gastrinoma (see Chap. 159). Surgical exploration, often in conjunction with intraoperative ultrasonography, duodenal transillumination, and duodenotomy, may be necessary to localize any solitary tumor not detected by the above imaging techniques.

Fortunately, symptomatic control can be achieved, without many side effects, with acid antisecretory drugs (particularly $H^+$-$K^+$ ATPase inhibitors) at dosages titrated to the patient's response. The aim of therapy is to reduce gastric acid secretion to <10 mEq per hour (5 mEq per hour in patients with previous acid-reducing surgery) for the hour before the next dose of the drug.

Somatostatin analogs and gastric surgery may be necessary in a few patients. Once symptomatic control is achieved, persons with solitary tumors should undergo surgical removal of the lesion in an attempt at cure. If metastatic disease is present, symptoms can often be controlled well with $H^+$-$K^+$ ATPase inhibitors for many years. If symptoms become difficult to control, however, or if the tumor behaves more malignantly than expected, then use of somatostatin analogs, tumor debulking surgery, cytotoxic chemotherapy, interferon-$\alpha$ therapy, hepatic tumor embolization, and/or treatment with radiolabeled somatostatin analogs are available options.

Combination chemotherapy with streptozotocin and chlorozotocin or doxorubicin has been found to be useful in malignant gastrinoma. Each therapy results in tumor regression with a median duration of up to 18 months. Some gastrinoma patients benefit from hepatic tumor embolization as a means of reducing local pressure symptoms. Although interferon-α therapy can result in tumor regression in some patients, its side effects, such as severe influenza-like symptoms, are not well tolerated. Liver transplantation in association with removal of the primary tumor has been attempted in gastrinoma patients, but at present this approach is unlikely to be used routinely because tumor recurrence is common.

The 5-year survival of patients with liver metastases is only 20%, compared with 81% in those with no metastases. The effect of treatment in gastrinoma is evaluated by measurement of serial fasting gastrin levels and imaging techniques. Other gut hormones and calcium levels are also measured regularly. The serum calcium level is particularly useful because gastrinomas may secrete PTH-related protein (PTHrP), and also because patients with MEN1 syndrome may develop hyperparathyroidism. The management of nonmetastatic gastrinoma in patients with MEN1 has been difficult because of a lack of information regarding the natural history of the gastrinoma in these patients and because they may have multiple duodenal microgastrinomas.[7] These patients are also more prone to the development of gastric carcinoids than are patients with sporadic gastrinomas.

## VIPoma

Many types of tumors are associated with diarrhea, but in 1958, Verner and Morrison described two cases in which a pancreatic tumor appeared to be responsible.[8,9] These tumors were later found to secrete vasoactive intestinal peptide (VIP)[10] and other peptides derived from the same preprohormone as VIP (e.g., peptide histidine methionine [PHM]). VIPomas (see Chap. 182) have an annual incidence of 1 in 10 million. The mean age at presentation is 49 years, with a slight female preponderance. The majority of VIPomas arise from the pancreas (90%). Extrapancreatic VIPomas occur along the autonomic nervous system, in the retroperitoneum, lungs, jejunum, liver, and adrenal glands. Pancreatic VIPomas are usually solitary (1–7 cm diameter); 37% to 68% have metastasized at the time of diagnosis, usually to the liver and regional lymph nodes.

The clinical and biochemical features of the VIPoma syndrome provide a valuable insight into the physiologic actions of VIP and related peptides[11,12] (Table 220-2). Elevated circulating VIP results in *severe secretory diarrhea with massive fluid, chloride, bicarbonate, potassium, and magnesium losses from the small intestine. Hypochlorhydria*, which occurs in 73% of cases, is due to inhibition of gastric acid secretion via somatostatin release. Stool volumes can reach up to 20 L per day, despite fasting. Potassium losses may rise to >400 mEq per day. In the early stages, this is usually intermittent, but with progressive tumor growth, it becomes continuous and can be life-threatening. The stool is otherwise normal and does not contain mucus or blood. Steatorrhea is not a feature. The severe potassium loss can result in temporary quadriplegia and is frequently accompanied by a metabolic acidosis due to bicarbonate loss in the stool. The average duration of symptoms before diagnosis is ~3 years. Other features of the VIPoma syndrome are *hypercalcemia, glucose intolerance,* and *mild diabetes mellitus.* In up to 20% of patients, flushing of the head and trunk may occur in association with a *patchy erythematous rash.*

The diagnosis of VIPoma depends on the demonstration of *secretory diarrhea associated with elevated fasting plasma VIP levels* (usually >200 pg/mL). On the whole, a stool volume of <700 mL per day excludes the diagnosis of VIPoma, but one must bear in mind that the diarrhea may be intermittent. The plasma levels of PHM, pancreatic polypeptide, and neurotensin may also be elevated. Because VIPomas are large at presentation, they can be localized by ultrasonography, CT, and radiolabeled somatostatin-receptor scintigraphy. Up to 87% of VIPomas express somatostatin receptors. Rarely, small tumors are present that may require more invasive localization techniques such as arteriography.

Treatment of VIPoma patients requires supportive measures to restore fluid, potassium, and acid-base balance. Specific therapy involves the use of somatostatin analogs, which not only inhibit VIP secretion but also independently reduce intestinal secretions. Second-line agents include glucocorticoids, indomethacin, lithium carbonate, and phenothiazines. Surgical tumor debulking is also beneficial in symptom control. VIPomas are sensitive to cytotoxic chemotherapy; often good response is seen to combination therapy with streptozotocin and 5-fluorouracil. Treatment with monoclonal antibodies against VIP may prove to be beneficial in the future.

## GLUCAGONOMA

Glucagonomas are mostly of pancreatic origin (see Chap. 134) and secrete glucagon and other products of the preproglucagon gene (see Chap. 182). These tumors have an annual incidence of 1 in 20 million, so that they are one of the rarest of gut endocrine tumors.[13] The median age at presentation is 62 years, and a slight female preponderance is seen. The majority of glucagonomas are sporadic. Approximately 20% occur in association with the MEN1 syndrome. The nonspecific nature of the symptoms associated with glucagonoma can delay the diagnosis for up to 10 years. This may account for the fact that at the time of presentation >70% of the patients have metastatic disease (usually in the liver and regional lymph nodes).

The most characteristic feature of the glucagonoma syndrome is the presence of a *necrolytic migratory erythematous rash* (Fig. 220-2).[14] The rash usually starts in the groin and perineum and then gradually migrates to the distal extremities. Typically, the initial lesions are erythematous macules, which become raised and bullous. Then the lesions break down and heal, often leaving a residual area of hyperpigmentation. The rash is intensely painful and pruritic, and secondary bacterial and fungal infections are common. The underlying cause of the rash is unknown, but several factors such as direct action of glucagon on the skin, amino-acid and fatty acid deficiency, and zinc deficiency have been implicated

**TABLE 220-2.**
**Mechanisms of Vasoactive Intestinal Peptide (VIP) Syndrome**

| Sign/Symptom | Mechanism |
|---|---|
| Secretory diarrhea | VIP stimulation of intestinal chloride secretion via cyclic adenosine monophosphate |
| | VIP stimulation of pancreatic and hepatobiliary secretions |
| Hypokalemia | Passive losses in stool |
| | Secondary hyperaldosteronism |
| Hypomagnesemia | Losses in stool |
| Hypercalcemia | Acidosis |
| | Hyperparathyroidism |
| | Direct action of VIP on bone |
| Metabolic acidosis | Bicarbonate loss in stool |
| Hypochlorhydria/achlorhydria | VIP inhibition of gastric acid secretion |
| Hyperglycemia | Glycogenolytic effect of VIP on the liver |
| | Effect of prolonged hypokalemia on pancreatic B cells |
| | Hypercalcemia |
| Flushing | VIP action as peripheral vasodilator |

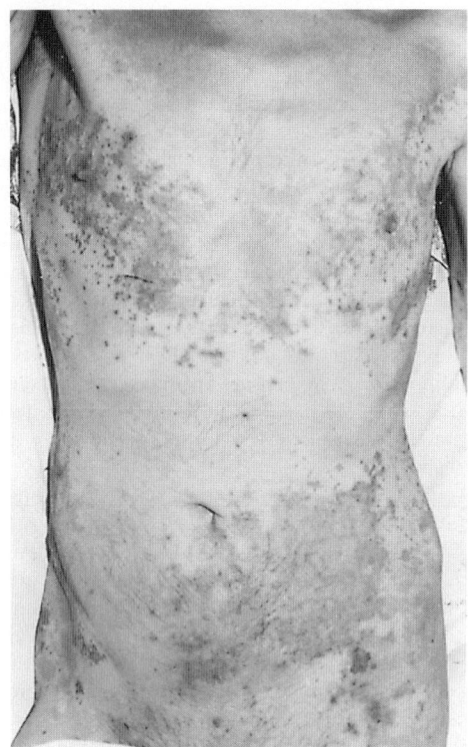

**FIGURE 220-2.** Truncal rash in a patient with a glucagonoma. (From Bloom SR, Polak JM. Glucagonoma syndrome. Am J Med 1987; 82[Suppl 5B]:25.)

in its etiology. The rash is commonly associated with mucosal involvement, which results in *stomatitis, cheilitis,* and *glossitis. Cachexia* is a common feature of glucagonoma and may mislead the physician into believing that a more aggressive tumor, such as pancreatic carcinoma, is responsible for the patient's symptoms. As glucagon opposes the effects of insulin on blood glucose homeostasis, *impaired glucose tolerance,* which usually results in *mild diabetes,* is also a manifestation of the glucagonoma syndrome. Other manifestations of glucagonoma include *normocytic normochromic anemia, dystrophy of the nails, diarrhea, a tendency to venous thrombosis and pulmonary embolism,* and *neuropsychiatric symptoms.* Paraneoplastic syndromes, such as optic atrophy, have also been reported in association with glucagonoma.

The diagnosis of glucagonoma depends greatly on clinical suspicion. Once the diagnosis is considered, measurement of a highly elevated plasma glucagon value after an overnight fast is confirmatory. Plasma glucagon levels may be increased in patients with prolonged fasting, renal and hepatic failure, diabetic ketoacidosis, or therapy with oral contraceptives or danazol, and in those with trauma, burns, sepsis, or Cushing syndrome. These conditions are easily distinguishable from glucagonoma, however, and rarely result in markedly raised glucagon levels. A rare condition associated with elevated glucagon levels is *familial hyperglucagonemia.*[15] Cosecretion of a second gut hormone is common, and one-fifth of glucagonoma patients also have elevated gastrin levels, which may cause acid hypersecretion. Elevated plasma insulin, pancreatic polypeptide, VIP, and urinary 5-hydroxyindoleacetic acid levels have all been observed with glucagonoma. Secretion of other cleavage products of preproglucagon by these tumors may result in gastrointestinal mucosal hypertrophy.

The majority of glucagonomas are large and metastatic at presentation. Tumor localization can be achieved with ultrasonography, CT, or visceral angiography (see Chap. 159). Somatostatin-receptor scintigraphy is most useful for determining the extent of metastatic disease.[15a] Endoscopic ultrasonography is sensitive in the detection of pancreatic primary tumors, but limited penetration reduces the detection of distant spread. Localized solitary tumors may require multiple techniques for localization.

Localized, solitary glucagonomas should be surgically excised to aim for a cure, whereas palliative measures are used for metastatic disease. The glucagonoma rash responds to oral and topical zinc, and somatostatin analogs. Longer acting somatostatin analogs and longer lasting preparations of octreotide are likely to be increasingly used.[16,17] With time, the tumor may become less responsive to such therapy, and increasing doses and/or surgery or induced embolization to reduce tumor bulk may be required. Control of cachexia is extremely difficult and may require dietary intervention such as consumption of a high-protein diet. Glucose intolerance may require insulin therapy. Aspirin has been advocated for prevention of thrombotic episodes, and anticoagulant therapy is used for patients with proven thrombosis. Psychiatric symptoms, such as psychosis or depression, require appropriate psychiatric assessment and treatment. The available palliative measures directed at the tumor and its metastases include surgical debulking of the tumor, hepatic tumor embolization, and cytotoxic chemotherapy. Glucagonomas are relatively insensitive to chemotherapeutic agents, but occasionally a patient may benefit from this treatment modality.

## SOMATOSTATINOMA

Somatostatinomas[18] are extremely rare tumors with an annual incidence of ~1 in 40 million. They occur mostly in the pancreas but can also arise in the duodenum. Duodenal somatostatinomas may be associated with neurofibromatosis type 1 (von Recklinghausen disease) and pheochromocytoma.[19] Duodenal somatostatinomas usually present early with obstructive symptoms and only rarely result in the tumor syndrome. Pancreatic tumors present late, with hepatic metastases, and often with the tumor syndrome characterized by the triad of *cholelithiasis, diabetes,* and *steatorrhea. Hypoglycemia* may occasionally occur and is likely to be caused by larger molecular forms of somatostatin.[20,21] Other features include *anemia, hypochlorhydria, postprandial fullness,* and *weight loss.* Occasionally, somatostatinomas may secrete adrenocorticotropic hormone (ACTH), resulting in Cushing syndrome. The diagnosis of somatostatinoma is confirmed by detection of highly elevated plasma somatostatin levels. Tumor localization uses the same techniques as described for other endocrine tumors of the gut. Treatment is mainly surgical. The palliative measures used are similar to those used for other gastrointestinal endocrine tumors.

### PPoma

Many types of pancreatic endocrine tumors also secrete pancreatic polypeptide (PP).[22–24] Elevated plasma PP levels can, therefore, be used as a marker of gastrointestinal endocrine tumors, particularly VIPomas (see Chap 182). Rare tumors produce only PP, but this does *not* result in any unique clinical or biochemical features. Histologically, the tumors are usually composed of mixed cell types, one of which can be immunocytochemically identified as producing PP.

### NEUROTENSINOMA

Neurotensin is a 13-amino-acid peptide released from N cells in the small intestine. Neurotensin immunoreactivity has also been detected in enteric neurons. The hormone is produced by a small number of pancreatic endocrine tumors, which usually also produce VIP.[25] When infused in humans, neurotensin causes increased watery secretions from the small intestine and frequent defecation.[26] Neurotensin may therefore *contribute* to the clinical features of the VIPoma syndrome. When neurotensin is the sole product of an endocrine tumor, however, *no* clinical features occur. (Presumably, escape occurs from long-continued elevations of plasma neurotensin.) Neurotensin is also detected in non-endocrine tumors in the gastrointestinal tract, suggesting that it may have growth regulatory functions in the pancreas and colon.

## ENTEROGLUCAGONOMA

In the intestinal mucosa, proglucagon-derived peptides are synthesized and released by L cells of the terminal ileum and colon.[27] Proglucagon undergoes tissue-specific posttranslational processing in the pancreas and intestine. In the pancreas, the end products of proglucagon processing are glucagon, glicentin-related pancreatic polypeptide (GRPP), and a large major fragment. In the intestine, the products are glucagon-like peptide-1 (GLP-1), glucagon-like peptide-2 (GLP-2), and glicentin (or enteroglucagon). Interest in these peptides as intestinal growth factors began with the observation that intestinal villous hypertrophy occurred in a patient with a tumor that was secreting proglucagon-derived peptides. Resection of the tumor resulted in the normalization of the previously increased blood levels of these peptides and regression of intestinal villous hypertrophy (see Chap. 160).[28] Further evidence was provided by the fact that, after small bowel resection, proglucagon messenger RNA expression was increased in the remnant intestine. Other studies have reported that overexpression of the glucagon gene or exogenously administered proglucagon-derived peptides in rodents are associated with bowel growth and regeneration.[29] Although initially the belief was that enteroglucagon was the growth factor released by the tumor described (hence, the name "enteroglucagonoma"), *GLP-2*, a 33-amino-acid peptide, appears to be the *mediator of epithelial cell proliferation* in the gut.[30]

## OTHER ENDOCRINE TUMORS OF THE GUT

Gastrointestinal endocrine tumors may secrete PTHrP, resulting in hypercalcemia. The *hypercalcemia* can be controlled by regular infusion of bisphosphonates, hepatic tumor embolization, and surgical debulking. Tumors have been described that secrete growth hormone–releasing hormone (GHRH), causing acromegaly, and ACTH, causing Cushing syndrome. These may occur either alone or in association with other gastrointestinal hormone tumor syndromes. Numerous other peptides have been detected either in the plasma or in tissue from endocrine tumors of the gut. These include neuropeptide Y (NPY), neuromedin-B, calcitonin gene–related peptide (CGRP), motilin, and bombesin, but these are not associated with specific clinical syndromes.

## TUMOR MARKERS

No generally useful tumor marker exists for gastrointestinal endocrine tumors. Some interest has been shown in the use of chromogranins and neuron-specific enolase (NSE) as markers. Histochemically, chromogranins and NSE have been used for some time in the immunocytochemical identification of neuroendocrine tumors.[31] In neuroendocrine tumors, a correlation is seen between tumor burden and circulating chromogranin A

levels; the highest levels of chromogranin A are seen in metastatic disease.[32] Small gastrinomas can result in high plasma chromogranin A levels, because gastrin causes hyperplasia of enterochromaffin-like cells that also secrete chromogranin A. Severe renal failure can result in elevated plasma chromogranin A levels comparable to levels seen with neuroendocrine tumors. Chromogranin A is most useful as a marker of nonfunctioning tumors. The peptide *GAWK*,[33] the product of chromogranin B, is also a useful marker for neuroendocrine tumors, as are secretoneurins.[33a] The role of the above tumor markers remains to be defined, but at present they are *not* routinely used in the diagnosis and follow-up of patients.

## SOMATOSTATIN THERAPY

Somatostatin analogs are commonly used in the treatment of gut endocrine tumors. Somatostatin has widespread inhibitory effects in the gastrointestinal tract.[34] It is used to reduce the secretion of peptides from endocrine tumors and also has antineoplastic actions.[35] Somatostatin has a half-life of <3 minutes (thus, the need to develop analogs with longer half-lives). The octapeptide octreotide, which was the first such analog introduced for clinical use (see Chap. 169),[36] usually is administered subcutaneously, three times a day, because its effects last from 6 to 8 hours. A slow-release depot form of octreotide (octreotide LAR [long-acting release]) is administered intramuscularly every 4 weeks. Lanreotide is another cyclic octapeptide and can be given subcutaneously, intravenously, or in a slow-release depot form (lanreotide LAR, administered once every 2 weeks). Five different types of somatostatin receptor (sst) have been cloned.[37] The somatostatin analogs in clinical use bind with high affinity to $sst_2$ and $sst_5$, but with ten-fold lower affinity to $sst_3$ and with little or no affinity to $sst_1$ and $sst_4$.[38] Novel radiolabeled somatostatin analogs are being investigated for the treatment of gastrointestinal endocrine tumors.[39]

Treatment with somatostatin analogs has several side effects, including nausea, abdominal cramps, flatulence, and malabsorption. Long-term treatment results in the formation of cholesterol gallstones and biliary sludge, which do not cause symptoms in the majority of patients. Tachyphylaxis to the actions of these analogs may occur, requiring the use of increasing doses and/or hepatic tumor embolization and surgery to reduce the tumor bulk.

## TUMOR EMBOLIZATION

Hepatic tumor embolization is an important palliative approach in the treatment of metastatic gastrointestinal endocrine tumors (Fig. 220-3). Hepatic metastases are particularly dependent on blood supply from the hepatic artery, whereas normal liver tissue receives the majority of its blood supply from the portal vein. Injection of inert microspheres into branches of the hepatic artery supplying the tumor results in tumor infarction and regression while leaving the proximal artery patent. This is superior to occlusion of the hepatic artery branches, which cannot be repeated. Tumor revascularization occurs, resulting in symptom recurrence after 6 months in up to half the cases.

The careful selection of patients for embolization is vital. Establishing that the portal vein is patent is important. If >50% of the liver parenchyma is replaced by tumor, embolization may precipitate fulminant hepatic failure. Other contraindications to tumor embolization include blood coagulation disorders, intercurrent infection, and end-stage disease. Embolization can result in the release of numerous vasoactive peptides from the tumor and,

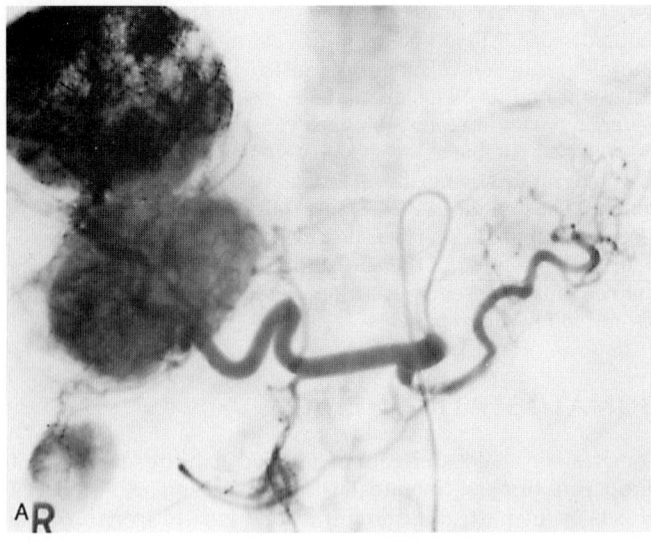

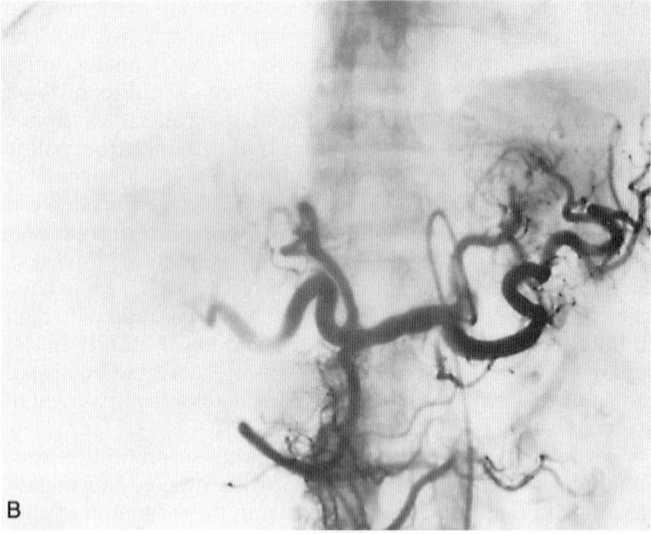

**FIGURE 220-3. A,** Hepatic arteriogram showing three large hepatic metastases in the right lobe. **B,** Hepatic arteriogram of the same patient after hepatic artery embolization, which completely occluded the arterial supply to the secondary tumors seen in **A.**

therefore, a hypotensive crisis. Patients are prepared for the procedure by prehydration. An octreotide infusion is used to block the effects of the peptides. Intravenous aprotinin and prophylactic broad-spectrum antibiotics are also administered to minimize the risks of the procedure. The procedure may result in fever, malaise, nausea, vomiting, abdominal pain, and paralytic ileus. Fever necessitates appropriate microbiologic investigations; in such cases, the development of a hepatic abscess should be excluded by abdominal ultrasonographic examination. Fortunately, complications of tumor embolization are rare in the hands of an experienced operator. Chemoembolization, using agents such as doxorubicin and iopamidol, has been advocated in the treatment of metastatic neuroendocrine tumors. Morbidity is reported to be less than for cytotoxic chemotherapy or for embolization alone.

## REFERENCES

1. Zollinger RM, Ellison EH. Primary peptic ulceration of the jejunum associated with islet cell tumors of the pancreas. Ann Surg 1955; 142:709.
2. Polak JM, Bloom SR. Review: The enterochromaffin-like cell, intragastric acidity and the trophic effects of plasma gastrin. Aliment Pharmacol Ther 1988; 2:291.
3. Walsh JH. Gastrin. In: Walsh JH, Dockray GJ, eds. Gut peptides. New York: Raven Press, 1994:75.
3a. Goebel SU, Heppner C, Burns AL, et al. Genotype/phenotype correlation of multiple endocrine neoplasia type 1 gene mutations in sporadic gastrinomas. J Clin Endocrinol Metab 2000; 85:116.
4. Jensen RT. Gastrointestinal endocrine tumours. Gastrinoma. Baillière's Clin Gastroenterol 1996; 10(4):673.
5. Modlin IM, Tang LH. Approaches to the diagnosis of gut neuroendocrine tumors: the last word (today). Gastroenterology 1997; 112:583.
6. Hammond PJ, Jackson JA, Bloom SR. Localization of pancreatic endocrine tumors. Clin Endocrinol 1994; 40:3.
7. Jensen RT. Management of the Zollinger-Ellison syndrome in patients with multiple endocrine neoplasia type 1. J Intern Med 1998; 243:477.
8. Verner JV, Morrison AB. Islet cell tumor and a syndrome of refractory diarrhea and hypokalemia. Am J Med 1958; 25:374.
9. Park SK, O'Dorisio MS, O'Dorisio TM. Gastrointestinal endocrine tumours. Vasoactive intestinal polypeptide-secreting tumours: biology and therapy. Baillières Clin Gastroenterol 1996; 10(4):673.
10. Bloom SR, Polak JM, Pearce AGE. Vasoactive intestinal peptide and watery-diarrhoea syndrome. Lancet 1973; 2:14.
11. Dockray G. Vasoactive intestinal polypeptide and related peptides. In: Walsh JH, Dockray GJ, eds. Gut peptides. New York: Raven Press, 1994:447.
12. O'Dorisio TM. VIP and watery diarrhea. In Bloom SR, ed. Gut hormones. Edinburgh: Churchill Livingstone, 1978:581.
13. Frankton S, Bloom SR. Gastrointestinal endocrine tumours. Glucagonomas. Baillières Clin Gastroenterol 1996; 10(4):673.
14. Bloom SR, Polak JM. Glucagonoma syndrome. Am J Med 1987; 82:25.
15. Boden G, Owen OE. Familial hyperglucagonemia: an autosomal dominant disorder. N Engl J Med 1977; 296:534.
15a. Johnson DS, Coel MN, Bornemann M. Current imaging and possible therapeutic management of glucagonoma tumors. Clin Nuclear Med 2000; 25:120.
16. Arnold R, Frank M. Gastrointestinal endocrine tumours. Gastrointestinal endocrine tumours: medical management. Baillières Clin Gastroenterol 1996; 10(4):737.
17. Trautman ME, Neuhaus C, Lenze H, et al. The role of somatostatin analogs in the treatment of endocrine gastrointestinal tumors. Horm Metab Res 1995; 27:24.
18. Kreijs GJ, Orci L, Conlon JM, et al. Somatostatinoma syndrome. N Engl J Med 1979; 301:285.
19. Griffiths DF, Williams GT, Williams ED. Duodenal carcinoid tumors, phaeochromocytoma and neurofibromatosis: islet cell tumor, phaeochromocytoma and the von Hippel-Lindau complex: two distinctive neuroendocrine syndromes. Q J Med 1987; 64:769.
20. Penman E, Lowry PJ, Wass JAH, et al. Molecular forms of somatostatin in normal subjects and patients with pancreatic somatostatinomas. Clin Endocrinol (Oxf) 1980; 12:611.
21. Bloom SR, Polak JM. Somatostatin. BMJ 1987; 295:288.
22. Vinik AI, Strodel WE, Eckhauser FE, et al. Somatostatinomas, PPomas, neurotensinomas. Semin Oncol 1987; 14:263.
23. Adrian TE, Lettenthal LO, Williams SJ, Bloom SR. Secretion of pancreatic polypeptide in patients with pancreatic endocrine tumors. N Engl J Med 1986; 315:287.
24. Polak JM, Bloom SR, Adrian TE, et al. Pancreatic polypeptide in insulinomas, gastrinomas, VIPomas and glucagonomas. Lancet 1976; 1:328.
25. Blackburn AM, Bryant MG, Adrian TE, Bloom SR. Pancreatic tumors producing neurotensin. J Clin Endocrinol Metab 1981; 52:820.
26. Calam J, Unwin R, Peart WS. Neurotensin stimulates defaecation. Lancet 1983; 1:737.
27. Holst JJ. Enteroglucagon. Ann Rev Physiol 1997; 59:257.
28. Bloom SR. An enteroglucagon tumor. Gut 1972; 13(7):520.
29. Drucker DJ, Erlich, P, Asa SL, et al. Induction of intestinal epithelial proliferation by glucagon-like peptide 2. Proc Natl Acad Sci U S A 1996; 93 (15):7911.
30. Hussain MA. A biological function for glucagon-like peptide 2. Eur J Endocr 1998; 139:265.
31. Bishop AE, Polak JM. Gastrointestinal endocrine tumours. Pathology. Baillières Clin Gastroenterol 1996; 10(4):555.
32. Nobels FRE, Kwekkeboom DJ, Bouillon R, et al. Chromogranin A: its clinical value as marker of neuroendocrine tumors. Eur J Clin Invest 1998; 28:431.
33. Sekiya K, Ghatei MA, Salahuddin MJ, et al. Production of GAWK (Chromogranin-B 420-493)-like immunoreactivity by endocrine tumors and its possible diagnostic value. J Clin Invest 1989; 83:1834.
33a. Ischia R, Gasser RW, Fischer-Collorie R, et al. Levels and molecular properties of secretoneurin-immunoreactivity in the serum and urine of control and neuroendocrine tumor patients. J Clin Endocrinol Metab 2000; 85:355.
34. Chiba T, Yamada T. Gut somatostatin. In: Walsh JH, Dockray GJ, eds. Gut Peptides. New York: Raven Press, 1994:123.
35. Pollack MN, Schally AV. Mechanisms of antineoplastic action of somatostatin analogs. Proc Soc Exp Biol Med 1998; 217:143.
36. Lamberts SWJ, Van der Lely A-J, De Herder WW, et al. Octreotide. N Engl J Med 1996; 334(4):246.
37. Patel YC, Greenwood MT, Panetta R, et al. The somatostatin receptor family. Life Sci 1995; 57(13):1249.
38. De Herder WW, Hofland LJ, Van der Lely AJ, Lamberts SW. Gastrointestinal endocrine tumours. Peptide receptors in gut endocrine tumors. Baillières Clin Gastroenterol 1996; 10(4):571.
39. Virgolini I. Mark Forster Award Lecture. Receptor nuclear medicine: vasointestinal peptide and somatostatin receptor scintigraphy for diagnosis and treatment of tumour patients. Eur J Clin Invest 1997; 27 (10):793.

# CHAPTER 221

# CARCINOID TUMOR AND THE CARCINOID SYNDROME

PAUL N. MATON

Carcinoids are found in 1% of autopsies, but clinical data suggest an incidence of 2 cases per 100,000 per year.[1] Although the incidence of subclinical gastric carcinoids has probably been underestimated,[2,3] most carcinoids remain localized and are not clinically significant. The major interest in these tumors relates to the few that produce 5-hydroxytryptamine and other substances and cause flushing, diarrhea, heart disease, and asthma—the carcinoid syndrome.[3,4]

## CELL OF ORIGIN

Carcinoids are neuroendocrine tumors that usually arise from enterochromaffin (EC) cells, which are found scattered throughout the body but occur principally in the submucosa of the intestine and main bronchi.[3,4] The EC cell population is heterogeneous, which may explain the variety of features associated with carcinoid tumors (Table 221-1). Some EC cells are argentaffinic, whereas others are argyrophilic (see Chap. 175). Furthermore, some EC cells contain peptides, such as substance P, enkephalins, or motilin.[3] Most gastric carcinoids arise not from EC cells but from enterochromaffin-like (ECL) cells, which may be important in the production of histamine.[2,5]

## PATHOLOGY

Carcinoid tumors are benign or of low-grade malignancy. Some authors, however, have included more aggressive "atypical" carcinoids and even highly malignant neuroendocrine carcinomas in accounts of carcinoids.[6] The relative distribution of carcinoid tumors, their propensity to metastasize, and their ability to cause the carcinoid syndrome are given in Table 221-2. One analysis of 8000 carcinoids[1] showed appendiceal carcinoids to be the most common. Overall, 75% of carcinoids occur in the gut, 24% in the lungs, and only 1% in other sites. Eighty percent of small intestinal carcinoids (which may be multiple) occur within 60 cm (2 ft) of the ileocecal valve, and 85% of bronchial carcinoids are in the main bronchi. The primary tumors tend to remain small and to extend outward, away from the lumen. They then spread to local lymph nodes. A marked fibrotic reaction may occur, which, with midgut carcinoids, may distort the gut and mesentery, and sometimes cause intestinal obstruction or vascular occlusion. Further spread occurs to the peritoneum or liver, and distant metastases may occur at almost any site; such distant lesions may include osteolytic and osteoblastic bone metastases.[3,7,8]

Most gastric ECL cell carcinoids are under the influence of gastrin. In patients with hypergastrinemia due to gastric atrophy (with or without pernicious anemia) or Zollinger-Ellison syndrome with multiple endocrine neoplasia type 1 (MEN1), a generalized hypertrophy of ECL cells is present that in some cases leads to the formation of multiple carcinoids.[2,5] The many small polyps (sometimes numbering in the hundreds) that are seen initially depend on gastrin but may become autonomous. Metastases to lymph nodes are rare[6] but are more common in sporadic (non–hypergastrinemia-associated) ECL cell carcinoids (see Table 221-2).

Carcinoids may contain and secrete various peptides and amines, and some carcinoids, particularly those of the foregut, can produce other clinical syndromes with or without the carcinoid syndrome. Carcinoids that secrete insulin, growth hormone, corticotropin, β-melanocyte–stimulating hormone, gastrin, calcitonin, substance P, growth hormone–releasing hormone, and bombesin-like peptides have been described.[3] Many carcinoids secrete chromogranin, a peptide common to many neuroendocrine tumors.[9]

Carcinoid tumors of the stomach can occur in MEN1. The MEN1 gene, a tumor suppressor gene, is on chromosome 11 (11q13). In MEN1 patients gastric carcinoids (like parathyroid and islet cell tumors) exhibit loss of heterozygosity at 11q13 with deletion of the wild-type allele.[10] This developmental mechanism is also true for lung carcinoids (and possibly for sporadic gut carcinoids,[10,11] but not for thymic carcinoids[12]), irrespective of MEN1.[13,14]

The carcinoid syndrome is much rarer than carcinoid tumors: the estimated incidence is approximately three cases per million population per year. The syndrome occurs only when vasoactive substances reach the systemic circulation; therefore, most gut carcinoids cause the syndrome only when hepatic metastases are present. Even then, the carcinoid syndrome occurs only in a few cases (see Table 221-2), and the histamine-type syndrome caused by gastric carcinoids has been described in less than ten cases (all carcinoids were sporadic ECL cell carcinoids). Ovarian and bronchial tumors, which drain directly into the systemic circulation, can cause the carcinoid syndrome without metastases; however, with bronchial carcinoids, metastases are usually present. Rarely, medullary carcinoma of the thyroid and small cell tumors of the lung cause the syndrome.

**TABLE 221-1.**
**Characteristics and Embryologic Derivation of Carcinoid Tumors**

| | Site of Tumor | | |
|---|---|---|---|
| | *Foregut* | *Midgut* | *Hindgut* |
| **HISTOLOGIC FEATURES** | Trabecular | Solid mass of cells | Mixed |
| **APPEARANCE OF CYTOPLASMIC GRANULES (ELECTRON MICROSCOPY)** | Variable density, 180 μm diameter | Uniformly dense, 230 μm diameter | Variable density, 190 μm diameter |
| **STAINING:** | | | |
| NSE | Positive | Positive | Positive |
| SILVER | Argyrophilic or negative | Argentaffin | Negative |
| **TUMOR PRODUCTS** | 5-HTP, peptides; histamine (gastric) | 5-HT | None |
| **METASTASES TO BONE AND SKIN** | Common | Unusual | Common |

*NSE*, neuron-specific enolase; *5-HTP*, 5-hydroxytryptophan; *5-HT*, 5-hydroxytryptamine.

**TABLE 221-2.**
**Ability of Carcinoid Tumors to Metastasize and Produce the Carcinoid Syndrome**

| | No. of Cases | | |
| --- | --- | --- | --- |
| | Total | With Metastases | With Carcinoid Syndrome |
| **FOREGUT** | | | |
| Esophagus | 2 | — | — |
| Stomach* | | | |
|   With gastric atrophy | 197 | 17 | — |
|   With ZES | 21 | 12 | — |
|   Sporadic† | 32 | 17 | 9 |
| Duodenum | 115 | 23 | 4 |
| Pancreas | 5 | 1 | 1 |
| Gallbladder | 18 | 6 | 1 |
| Bile duct | 5 | — | — |
| Ampulla | 7 | 1 | — |
| Larynx | 4 | 2 | — |
| Bronchus | >500‡ | >100‡ | 66 |
| Thymus | 74 | 19 | — |
| **MIDGUT** | | | |
| Jejunum | 56 | 20 | 91 |
| Ileum | 1013 | 355 | — |
| Meckel diverticulum | 44 | 8 | 6 |
| Appendix | 1687 | 34 | 6 |
| Colon | 89 | 53 | 5 |
| Liver | 4 | — | — |
| Ovary | 34 | 2 | 17 |
| Testis | 2 | — | 1 |
| Cervix | 33 | 8 | 1 |
| **HINDGUT** | | | |
| Rectum | 573 | 18 | 1 |

ZES, Zollinger-Ellison syndrome.
*From Rindi G, Luinetto O, Cornaggia M, et al. Three subtypes of gastric argyrophil carcinoid and the gastric neuroendocrine carcinoma: a clinical pathologic study. Gastroenterology 1993; 104:994.
†Not associated with hypergastrinemia.
‡Only approximate data are available.

## CLINICAL FEATURES

### CARCINOIDS WITHOUT SYSTEMIC FEATURES

Carcinoids without systemic features occur most commonly in the appendix and small intestine[1] (see Table 221-2) and usually are found incidentally at surgery.[3,4,7,8] Small intestinal carcinoids are usually symptomless but, occasionally, cause intestinal obstruction or vascular occlusion. Ileal tumors generally are not demonstrated by simple radiology; therefore, barium infusion studies or angiography is required.[15] Duodenal and gastric carcinoids most often are found incidentally at endoscopy. Colonic, rectal, and esophageal carcinoids also may be found incidentally or may cause obstruction.[16] Bronchial carcinoids may be discovered as a coin lesion on chest radiographs or may be seen at bronchoscopy. They also may present with cough, wheeze, hemoptysis, or segmental obstruction and infection. Mediastinal and ovarian carcinoids appear as masses.[17] Most carcinoids occur as an isolated disease, but associations are seen between foregut carcinoids and MEN1; between gastric carcinoids and hypergastrinemia, whether due to achlorhydria or to Zollinger-Ellison syndrome, especially as part of MEN1[18]; between ampullary carcinoids and von Recklinghausen disease[3]; and between renal carcinoids and horseshoe kidney.[19] The diagnosis of all carcinoids without systemic features depends on the histologic structure and staining.

## CARCINOID SYNDROME

The carcinoid syndrome[3,4,7,8] is characterized by flushing, diarrhea, and heart disease, although the relative importance of the symptoms varies in different patients, reflecting differences in tumor origin, bulk, tumor products, and length of history. The primary tumor may have been removed many years before the development of the syndrome, or it may never have become clinically evident. Most patients with the carcinoid syndrome, however, have an ileal tumor, with evident hepatic metastases at the time of presentation (see Table 221-2).

Carcinoid flushing is erythematous, and principally affects the upper part of the body. Some patients are unaware of the flushing, whereas others are distressed by it. Flushes may be brief or prolonged. They often are spontaneous, but they may be precipitated by alcohol, certain foods, abdominal palpation, or anxiety. Several patterns of flushing have been described,[7] but only two are clinically distinctive. Gastric carcinoids may produce a bright red, geographic flush, often precipitated by food consumption.[20] Bronchial carcinoids may cause severe prolonged flushes with salivation, lacrimation, sweating, facial edema, palpitations, diarrhea, and hypotension. After many months of flushing, a fixed, facial telangiectasia, edema, and cyanotic plethora may occur.

Diarrhea occurs in most cases, although it is less evident with gastric carcinoids. In some patients, diarrhea is related to episodes of flushing; in others, the two seem independent. Watery diarrhea is more frequent than malabsorption and is due to increased motility and possibly intestinal secretion, but intermittent intestinal obstruction, cholorrheic diarrhea after previous intestinal resection for tumor, or vascular insufficiency or lymphatic obstruction may occur in some patients. Abdominal pain may be due to these abnormalities or to necrosis of hepatic metastases.

Heart disease occurs in ~30% of patients. Insidious right heart failure often worsens during periods of flushing, and, in such cases, tricuspid regurgitation or stenosis is typical; less commonly, pulmonary stenosis may occur. The left side of the heart also may be involved, usually in association with bronchial carcinoids. The heart disease is caused by a unique form of fibrosis that involves the endocardium and valves.[21,21a] Fibrosis in other sites can cause constrictive pericarditis, retroperitoneal fibrosis, pleural thickening,[22] and Peyronie disease.

Wheezing occurs in 10% of patients and can be the presenting feature. A pellagra-like syndrome may occur, and confusional states have been described with foregut carcinoids. Rarely, patients experience arthralgia or a myopathy.[23]

## PATHOGENESIS OF THE CARCINOID SYNDROME

The flushing is poorly understood but may be due to the release of kinins in some patients.[24,25] Carcinoids contain kallikrein, an enzyme that, when released into the circulation spontaneously or stimulated by alcohol or catecholamines, acts on plasma kininogens to generate bradykinin[3,7] (see Chap. 170). In gastric carcinoids, the distinctive flush is mediated by histamine (see Chap. 181). The diarrhea is caused largely by 5-hydroxytryptamine (serotonin) through its effects on gut motility. The 5-hydroxytryptamine also contributes to the asthma and is probably implicated in the cardiac fibrosis. The diversion of tryptophan to the tumor for 5-hydroxytryptamine synthesis can lead to reduced protein synthesis, with hypoalbuminemia, and to nicotinic acid deficiency, with pellagra.[26]

The prostaglandins[27] and many gut peptides[28] probably are not mediators of the flushing or diarrhea in most patients. The role of other peptides such as substance P or other tachykinins (neurokinin A, neuropeptide K) has yet to be fully evaluated.[25]

# DIAGNOSIS OF THE CARCINOID SYNDROME

Once the carcinoid syndrome has been considered, confirmation of the diagnosis is often not difficult and rests on clinical features, measurement of the principal 5-hydroxytryptamine metabolite in urine (5-hydroxyindoleacetic acid [5-HIAA]) and, occasionally, the provocation of flushing with epinephrine.[3,4,7,8] In a patient who flushes, who has an enlarged liver, and in whom urinary 5-HIAA excretion is >30 mg per day (normal is <10 mg per day), the diagnosis is obvious. Diagnostic difficulties may arise in patients who flush for other reasons, in patients with carcinoid syndrome in whom the flushing is not apparent, or in patients with modestly elevated urinary 5-HIAA.[8a] The differential diagnosis of flushing includes menopausal flushing, reactions to alcohol and glutamate, side effects of drugs (such as chlorpropamide, calcium-channel blockers, and nicotinic acid), other tumors, chronic granulocytic leukemia, idiopathic flushing, and systemic mastocytosis[29,30] (see Chap. 181). None of these conditions increases urinary 5-HIAA, and in none does epinephrine provoke flushing as it does in the carcinoid syndrome. A positive response to epinephrine also may help to confirm the diagnosis of carcinoid syndrome in patients without apparent flushing. When urinary 5-HIAA is only modestly elevated, other causes must be excluded; excretion rates of up to 25 mg per day have been described in Whipple disease, celiac disease, tropical sprue, and pancreatic islet tumors other than carcinoids. Furthermore, the ingestion of 5-hydroxytryptamine-containing foods, such as pineapples, avocados, walnuts, or bananas, can increase 5-HIAA excretion, and more than 30 drugs are known to cause falsely high or low urinary 5-HIAA values.[31] If the clinician has any doubt about the diagnosis, urinary collections should be performed with the patient abstaining from all medications.

# PROGNOSIS

In the carcinoid tumor registry, the age-adjusted 5-year survival in patients with local disease was 99% for appendiceal tumors and >75% for tumors from all sites. In patients with distant metastases, the 5-year survival was 30% or less.[32] One analysis indicates an overall 5-year survival of 50%, with 45% of carcinoids having metastasized at the time of diagnosis.[1] In the largest reported series of patients with the carcinoid syndrome, the median survival from first flush was 3 years but survival ranged up to 17 years.[8] The median survival in patients with heart disease was 14 months, and in patients with a large tumor burden (5-HIAA level of >150 mg per day), it was 11 months.

# TREATMENT

## CONTROL OF THE TUMOR

Except in the case of gastric ECL cell carcinoids that are of low malignancy and can be observed for some years, surgery should be considered in all patients because the resection of local disease can result in cure of carcinoid tumors, and in cure of the carcinoid syndrome due to some bronchial and ovarian tumors.[33] Interestingly, the appropriate surgery for multiple gastric carcinoids in patients with gastric atrophy is not removal of the tumors, but removal of the gastric antrum, leading to normalization of plasma gastrin and tumor regression.[5] Resection of isolated hepatic metastases detected by computed tomographic scan or somatostatin analog scintigraphy[34–36] also may be markedly beneficial in selected cases[7,8]; however, in the presence of extensive metastases, partial hepatic resection is not warranted, nor is removal of the primary tumor unless it is causing local problems. Hepatic transplantation has been beneficial on occasion.[37] Chemotherapy for carcinoid tumors has been disappointing, with responses occurring in a minority and lasting only a mean of 7 months.[8] Single agents have produced responses in up to 30%, streptozocin being the most effective agent. Various combinations of streptozocin with 5-fluorouracil, cyclophosphamide, and doxorubicin have produced response rates of up to 35%.[8] Given the variation in tumor growth, questionable efficacy, and undoubted toxicity of chemotherapy, as well as the availability of other symptomatic therapy, chemotherapy should be reserved for advanced tumors that are actively growing. Administration of interferon-α, 3 to 6 million IU per day subcutaneously, reduces tumor size in ~15% of cases and stabilizes tumor size in another 30% to 40%.[8,38–41] Octreotide acetate, used mainly for its effect on symptoms (see later), reduces tumor bulk in ~5% and stabilizes tumor size in another 20%.[42–44] Radiotherapy is useful only for symptomatic therapy of bone and skin metastases.

Hepatic artery occlusion leads to selective necrosis of hepatic metastases. Surgical ligation of the hepatic artery has been used to necrose the hepatic tumor in the carcinoid syndrome,[8] but percutaneous arterial embolization is less traumatic, more selective, and can be repeated.[45–47] Embolization, alone or in combination with chemotherapy,[8,48] can produce a striking relief of symptoms and reduction in urinary 5-HIAA levels, even in patients with symptoms that are resistant to other modes of therapy. Complete remissions of up to 30 months have been reported. Second remissions may follow repeat embolizations, and survival may be prolonged.

## CONTROL OF SYMPTOMS

Many patients have considerable hepatic tumor, yet they remain well, apart from occasional flushing or diarrhea.[3,7] They should be advised to avoid precipitants of flushing and to supplement their diet with nicotinamide. Heart failure can be treated with diuretics, asthma with albuterol (salbutamol) (which does not precipitate flushing), and diarrhea with loperamide. If patients require further therapy, various other agents may be tried. For diarrhea, cyproheptadine, 4 to 8 mg every 6 hours, is the best oral agent.[49] In the rare patient with carcinoid syndrome due to a gastric carcinoid, a combination of diphenhydramine 50 mg every 6 hours, together with an $H_2$ antagonist (e.g., cimetidine 300 mg every 6 hours), has proved effective for flushes.[50] For most patients, however, the most effective agent for both diarrhea and flushes is the long-acting somatostatin analog octreotide acetate (100–500 μg every 8–12 hours or the long-acting formulation every 24 hours subcutaneously), which has produced responses in >80% of patients.[43,44,51] Another somatostatin analog, lanreotide, is also effective. Interferon-α, used principally for its effect on the tumor, reduces flushing and diarrhea in ~50% of patients[8,38–40] (see Chap. 169). If drugs fail to control symptoms, hepatic embolization should be considered. Progressive cardiac disease can be halted only by removal of the tumor and cure of the carcinoid syndrome, but the occasional, carefully selected patient may benefit from tricuspid valve replacement.[7,52]

Anesthetics, surgery, chemotherapy, and hepatic artery occlusion can precipitate extremely severe flushing with hypotension—a *carcinoid crisis.* The risk of developing such a crisis can be reduced by appropriate premedication, careful monitoring, the judicious use of anesthetic drugs and techniques, and avoidance of flush-provoking agents, such as catecholamines.[45,46,53] Should a crisis occur, hypotension should be treated with octreotide acetate 100 µg intravenously, which should be available whenever patients with the carcinoid syndrome undergo procedures.[54] If octreotide acetate is not available, intravenous methoxamine, 3 to 5 mg, can be used. Other pressor agents should be avoided.

# REFERENCES

1. Modlin IM, Sandor A. An analysis of 8305 cases of carcinoid tumors. Cancer 1997; 79:813.
2. Rindi G, Luinetto O, Cornaggia M, et al. Three subtypes of gastric argyrophil carcinoid and the gastric neuroendocrine carcinoma: a clinical pathologic study. Gastroenterology 1993; 104:994.
3. Maton PN, Hodgson HJF. Carcinoid tumours and the carcinoid syndrome. In: Bouchier IAD, Allan RN, Hodgson HJF, Keighly MRB, eds. Textbook of gastroenterology. London: Bailliere-Tindall, 1984:620.
4. Feldman JM, Zakin D, Dannenberg AJ. Carcinoid tumors and syndrome. Semin Oncol 1987; 14:237.
5. Maton PN, Dayal Y. Clinical implications of hypergastrinemia. In: Zakim DH, Dannenberg AJ, eds. Peptic ulcer disease and other acid-related disorders. New York: Academic Research Associates, 1991:213.
6. Bordi C, Falchetti A, Azzoni C, et al. Aggressive forms of gastric neuroendocrine tumors in multiple endocrine neoplasia type 1. Am J Surg Pathol 1997; 21:1075.
7. Grahame-Smith DG. The carcinoid syndrome. London: William Heinemann, 1972.
8. Moertel CG. An odyssey in the land of small tumors. J Clin Oncol 1987; 5:1503.
8a. Nuttall KL, Pingree SS. The incidence of elevations in urine 5-hydroxyindoleacetic acid. Ann Clin Lab Sci 1998; 28:167.
9. Nobels FR, Kwekkeboom DJ, Coopmans W. Chromogranin A as a serum marker for neuroendocrine neoplasia: comparison with neuron–specific enolase and the alpha-subunit of glycoprotein hormones. J Clin Endocrinol Metab 1997; 82:2622.
10. Debelenko LV, Emmert-Buck MR, Zhuang Z, et al. The multiple endocrine neoplasia type 1 gene locus is involved in the pathogenesis of type II gastric carcinoids. Gastroenterology 1997; 113:773.
11. Jakobovitz O, Nass D, De Marco L, et al. Carcinoid tumors frequently display genetic abnormalities involving chromosome 11. J Clin Endocrinol Metab 1996; 81:164.
12. Teh BT. Thymic carcinoids in multiple endocrine neoplasia type 1. J Intern Med 1998; 243:501.
13. Dong Q, Debelenko LV, Chandrasekharappa SC, et al. Loss of heterozygosity at 11q13: analysis of pituitary tumors, lung carcinoids, lipomas, and other uncommon tumors in subjects with familial multiple endocrine neoplasia type 1. J Clin Endocrinol Metab 1997; 82:1416.
14. Walch AK, Zitzelsberger HF, Aubele MM, et al. Typical and atypical carcinoid tumors of the lung are characterized by 11q deletions as detected by comparative genomic hybridization. Am J Pathol 1998; 153:1089.
15. Jeffree MA, Barter SJ, Hemingway AP, Nolan DJ. Primary carcinoid tumors of the ileum: the radiological appearances. Clin Radiol 1984; 35:451.
16. Spread C, Berkel H, Jewell L, et al. Colon carcinoid tumors: a population-based study. Dis Colon Rectum 1994;37:482.
17. Wang DY, Chang D-B, Kuo S-H, et al. Carcinoid tumors of the thymus. Thorax 1994; 49:357.
18. Hakanson R, Sundler F, eds. Mechanisms for the development of gastric carcinoids: proceedings of an international symposium. Digestion 1986; 35(Suppl 1):1.
19. Krishnan B, Truong LD, Saleh G, et al. Horseshoe kidney is associated with an increased relative risk of primary renal carcinoid tumor. J Urol 1997; 157:2059.
20. Roberts LJ, Marney SR, Oates JA. Blockade of the flush associated with metastatic gastric carcinoid by combined $H_1$ and $H_2$ receptor antagonists: evidence for an important role of $H_2$ receptors in human vasculature. N Engl J Med 1979; 300:236.
21. Wikowske MA, Hartman LC, Mullaney CJ, et al. Progressive carcinoid heart disease after resection of primary ovarian carcinoid. Cancer 1994; 73:1889.
21a. Sakai D, Mukakami M, Kasazoe K, Tsutsumi Y. Ileal carcinoid tumor complicating carcinoid heart disease and secondary retroperitoneal fibrosis. Pathol Int 2000; 50:404.
22. Moss SF, Lehner PJ, Gilbey SG, et al. Pleural involvement in the carcinoid syndrome. Q J Med 1993; 86:49.
23. Lederman RJ, Bukowski RM, Nickelson P. Carcinoid myopathy. Cleve Clin J Med 1987; 54:299.
24. Lucas KJ, Feldman JM. Flushing in the carcinoid syndrome and plasma kallikrein. Cancer 1986; 58:2290.
25. Grahame-Smith DG. What is the cause of the carcinoid flush? Gut 1987; 28:1413.
26. Swain CP, Tavill AS, Neale G. Studies of tryptophan and albumin metabolism in a patient with carcinoid syndrome, pellagra and hypoproteinemia. Gastroenterology 1976; 74:484.
27. Metz SA, McRae JR, Robertson PR. Prostaglandins as mediators of paraneoplastic syndromes: review and update. Metabolism 1981; 30:299.
28. Long RG, Peters JR, Bloom SR, et al. Somatostatin, gastrointestinal peptides and the carcinoid syndrome. Gut 1981; 22:549.
29. Wilkin JK. Flushing reactions: consequences and mechanisms. Ann Intern Med 1981; 95:468.
30. Aldrich LB, Moattari R, Vinik AI. Distinguishing features of idiopathic flushing and carcinoid syndrome. Arch Intern Med 1988; 148:2614.
31. Young DS, Pestaner LC, Gibberman V. Effects of drugs on clinical laboratory tests. Clin Chem 1975; 21:398D.
32. Godwin JD. Carcinoid tumors: an analysis of 2837 cases. Cancer 1975; 36:560.
33. Norton JA. Neuroendocrine tumors of the pancreas and duodenum. Curr Probl Surg 1994; 31:77.
34. Kwekkeboom DJ, Krenning EP, Bakker WH, et al. Somatostatin analog scintigraphy in carcinoid tumors. Eur J Nucl Med 1993; 20:283.
35. Kwekkeboom DJ, Krenning EP. Somatostatin receptor scintigraphy in patients with carcinoid tumors. World J Surg 1996; 20:157.
36. Kisker O, Weinel RJ, Geks J, et al. Value of somatostatin receptor scintigraphy for preoperative localization of carcinoids. World J Surg 1996; 20:162.
37. Le-Treut YP, Delpero JR, Dousset B, et al. Results of liver transplantation in the treatment of metastatic neuroendocrine tumors. A 31–case French multicentric report. Ann Surg 1997; 225:355.
38. Oberg K, Eriksson B. Role of interferons in the management of carcinoid tumors. Br J Hematol 1991; 79(Suppl 1):74.
39. Janson ET, Oberg K. Long-term management of the carcinoid syndrome: treatment with octreotide alone and in combination with alpha interferon. Acta Oncol 1993; 32:225.
40. Öberg K, Norheim I, Lind E, et al. Treatment of malignant carcinoid tumors with human leukocyte interferon. Cancer Treat Rep 1986; 70:1296.
41. Oberg K. Advances in chemotherapy and biotherapy of endocrine tumors. Curr Opin Oncol 1998; 10:58.
42. Arnold R, Benning R, Neuhaus C, et al. Gastroenteropancreatic endocrine tumors: effect of Sandostatin on tumor growth. The German Sandostatin Study Group. Metabolism 1992; 41(Suppl 2):116.
43. Kvols LK, Moertel CG, O'Connell MJ, et al. Treatment of the malignant carcinoid syndrome. N Engl J Med 1986; 315:663.
44. Gorden P, Comi RJ, Maton PN, Go VLW. Somatostatin and somatostatin analogue (SMS 201–995) in treatment of hormone-secreting tumors of the pituitary and gastrointestinal tract and non-neoplastic diseases of the gut. Ann Intern Med 1989; 110:35.
45. Maton PN, Camilleri M, Griffin G, et al. The role of hepatic arterial embolisation in the carcinoid syndrome. BMJ 1983; 287:932.
46. Martensson H, Norbin A, Bengmark S, et al. Embolisation of the liver in the management of metastatic carcinoid tumors. J Surg Oncol 1984; 27:152.
47. Ruszdiewski P, Malka D. Hepatic arterial chemoembolization in the management of advanced digestive endocrine tumors. Digestion 2000; 62(Suppl 1):79.
48. Drougas JG, Anthony LB, Blain TK, et al. Hepatic artery chemoembolization for management of patients with advanced metastatic carcinoid tumors. Am J Surg 1998; 175:408.
49. Moertel CG, Kvols LK, Rubin J. A study of cyproheptadine in the treatment of metastatic carcinoid tumor and the malignant carcinoid syndrome. Cancer 1991; 67:33.
50. Oates JA. The carcinoid syndrome. N Engl J Med 1986; 315:702.
51. Saslow SB, O'Brien MD, Camilleri M, et al. Octreotide inhibition of flushing and colonic motor dysfunction in carcinoid syndrome. Am J Gastroenterol 1997; 92:2250.
52. Codd JE, Prozda J, Merjavy J. Palliation of carcinoid heart disease. Arch Surg 1987; 122:1076.
53. Törnebrandt K, Nobin A, Ericsson M, Thompson D. Circulation, respiration and serotonin levels in carcinoid patients during neuroleptic anaesthesia. Anaesthesia 1983; 38:957.
54. Marsh HM, Martin JK Jr, Kvols LK, Moertel CG. Carcinoid crisis during anesthesia: successful treatment with somatostatin analogue. Anesthesiology 1987; 66:89.

# CHAPTER 222

# HORMONES AND CARCINOGENESIS: LABORATORY STUDIES

JONATHAN J. LI AND SARA ANTONIA LI

The resurgence and rapid growth of the field of hormonal carcinogenesis—the role of hormones in the etiology and growth of cancer—are due in large part to growing concerns regarding two of the most common human cancers, breast and prostate.[1–4] Although other hormone-associated cancers occur at lower fre-

**TABLE 222-1.**
**Animal Models in Hormonal Carcinogenesis**

| Hormone | Species | Organ Site | Incidence (%) | References |
|---|---|---|---|---|
| 17β-E$_2$, DES, E$_1$ | Hamster | Kidney | 90–100 | 7, 39, 43, 44 |
| EE | Hamster | Liver | 25–35 | 45 |
| EE + ANF | Hamster | Liver | 100 | 46 |
| 17β-E$_2$/DES + PRL | Mouse | Testis | 30–70 | 37, 38 |
| 17β-E$_2$, E$_1$, DES | Rat | Mammary gland | 70–100 | 9, 14, 16, 17 |
| 17β-E$_2$, DES | Mouse | Cervix/uterus | 20–60 | 28–29 |
| DES | Monkey | Uterus | 70 | 33 |
| DES, 17β-E$_2$ | Rat | Pituitary | 15–85 | 34–36 |
| MPA | Mouse | Mammary gland | 60 | 20 |
| 17β-E$_2$ + T/DES | Hamster | Ductus deferens | 100 | 31, 63 |
| 17β-E$_2$/DES + P | Rat | Mammary gland | 100 | 19 |
| 17β-E$_2$ + T/T | Rat | Prostate | 20–100 | 11, 47, 48 |

*17β-E$_2$*, 17β-estradiol; *DES*, diethylstilbestrol; *E$_1$*, estrone; *EE*, ethynylestradiol; *ANF*, α-naphthoflavone; *PRL*, prolactin; *MPA*, medroxyprogesterone acetate; *T*, testosterone; *P*, progesterone.

quencies, they are also of clinical importance; these include endometrial, ovarian, testicular, cervicovaginal, pituitary, thyroid, and sex hormone–related hepatic neoplasms.[5–7] That these cancers cannot be attributable to any specific exogenous physical, environmental, or dietary factor is becoming increasingly clear. Despite the long history of hormonal carcinogenesis research, the precise mechanism whereby hormones affect neoplastic transformation remains elusive. A better understanding of the effect of hormones, both ovarian/testicular and pituitary, on normal cellular processes of growth and differentiation is needed to ascertain more precisely their involvement in neoplastic development. Nevertheless, after intensive study,[8] some of the cellular and molecular alterations elicited by hormones during tumorigenesis are beginning to be revealed.

That hormones can induce neoplasms in experimental animals has been known for >60 years.[9] Moreover, with a few notable exceptions, for nearly every human neoplasm with a hormonal association, a corresponding animal tumor model can be induced by hormones alone. Of the various hormonal agents, sex hormones, particularly estrogens[9a] and to a lesser extent progesterone and prolactin (PRL) in women, and androgens in men, have been associated with tumor induction.

## GENERAL CONSIDERATIONS

Hormones can affect neoplastic processes by acting either as the sole etiologic agent or in conjunction with physical agents (i.e., ionizing radiation) or nonhormonal chemical carcinogens.[8] A number of general mechanisms exist whereby hormones may modify a target tissue during one or more phases of the events initiated by carcinogenic events, such as viral infection, chemical

exposure, or exposure to ionizing radiation. For example, hormones may be involved in (a) promotional or carcinogenic effects, (b) alterations of the host immune system, (c) activation of viruses, and (d) modification of hormone receptors or alteration of metabolic rates affecting carcinogen activation. The primary concern of this chapter, however, is *the induction of tumors, benign and malignant, by hormones, either endogenously produced or exogenously administered.* The concept that a given hormone acts specifically on individual target organs or tissues is somewhat misleading, because most organs or tissues are differentially sensitive to various hormones acting alone, or in concert with or opposition to, other hormones. The general characteristics of hormonal carcinogenesis are (a) tissue, strain, and species specificity; (b) long induction period; (c) sustained and prolonged hormone exposure; and (d) cellular proliferation. Sex hormones have been implicated in the induction and growth of a wide variety of experimental tumors as summarized in Table 222-1. A common characteristic during endocrine-induced tumorigenesis appears to be a prolonged and severe derangement in normal homeostasis and regulatory relationships as a result of chronic hormone exposure.

Although the minimum oncogenic dose for a given sex hormone to elicit a high incidence of tumors at any tissue site is not precisely known, clearly the conditions required to induce a high tumor yield do not require particularly high concentrations of hormones, either at the serum or tissue level (Table 222-2). For example, the serum level of 17β-estradiol (17β-E$_2$) in a female ACI rat in estrus is 75 to 80 pg/mL,[10] and the sustained oncogenic dose required to elicit a high incidence of mammary tumors is only twice estrous levels. Such levels approach those found during pregnancy in this species. In the male Syrian hamster, continuous administration of exogenous 17β-E$_2$ induces

**TABLE 222-2.**
**Sex Hormone Levels Required for Experimental Hormonal Carcinogenesis**

| Hormone | Species | Organ | Serum (ng/mL) | Tissue (pg/mg protein) | Reference |
|---|---|---|---|---|---|
| 17β-E$_2$ | Hamster | Kidney | 1.9–2.7 | 4.5–5.4 | 11 |
| 17β-E$_2$ | Rat | Mammary gland | 0.18–0.21 | ND | 10 |
| 17β-E$_2$ | Rat | Prostate | 0.045 | 0.10* | 12 |
| Testosterone | | | 2.3 | 0.90† | |

*17β-E$_2$*, 17β-estradiol; *ND*, not determined.
*pg/g tissue.
†ng/g tissue.

renal tumors, and the serum estrogen levels are approximately seven-fold higher than the mean estrous levels found in normal untreated females (see Table 222-2). The $17\beta$-$E_2$ levels in the male kidney are equal to or slightly lower than those found in the uterus during estrus, however, because this organ site has only modest ability to concentrate estrogens.[11] Similarly, even lower levels of estrogen and androgen are required to induce a high incidence of prostate carcinomas in the male Noble rat.[12]

## EXPERIMENTAL ANIMAL MODELS

Numerous murine and one primate species develop tumors in response to sex hormone exposure alone. Although some of these hormone-induced tumor models either may involve viral mediation or may arise in conjunction with the stimulation of other pertinent hormonal factors, most are considered to be the result of the direct carcinogenic action of the hormonal agents themselves. The induction of tumors by hormones characteristically occurs in hormone-dependent target tissues. The Syrian hamster kidney model is included in this group because it is essentially an estrogen-responsive target organ.[7,11]

### MAMMARY GLAND

More than 65 years ago, Lacassagne[9] first demonstrated that long-term estrone ($E_1$) administration induced a high frequency of mammary cancer in male mice. Subsequent studies showed that numerous other mouse strains were also susceptible to the carcinogenic action of estrogens at this tissue site.[13] Whereas, in the past, the suggestion was that estrogens were direct carcinogens, the belief now is that, in mice, sex hormones alone cannot effect a high incidence of mammary tumors in the absence of a mouse mammary tumor virus (MMTV) or chemical carcinogen exposure. The lack of an established viral association in rats, however, suggests that mammary tumor induction by female sex hormones in susceptible strains may result from direct hormonal action. High incidences (54–100%) of mammary tumors have been elicited with natural and synthetic estrogens, including $E_1$, $17\beta$-$E_2$, ethynylestradiol (EE), and diethylstilbestrol (DES), in both male and female Noble, Wistar, Long-Evans, and ACI rats after 5.0 to 10.0 months of continuous estrogen treatment (Fig. 222-1).[6,10,14] As in the mouse, genetic factors also clearly play a significant role in the induction of mammary tumors by estrogens in the rat. Despite the marked differences in incidence between the sexes in humans, the lack of a sex difference in the ability of estrogens to induce mammary tumors in the rat may actually be analogous to the situation seen in humans. For instance, the strongest risk factor for breast cancer in men is known to be Klinefelter syndrome, a condition resulting from inheritance of an extra X chromosome and characterized by testicular dysfunction and gynecomastia.[15] This finding clearly indicates that breast cancer in men develops under conditions favoring excessive endogenous estrogen levels. Pertinent distinctions can be made between mammary tumors in the rat induced by estrogen and by a chemical carcinogen (e.g., dimethylbenzanthracene [DMBA], N-nitrosomethylurea [NMU]). Estrogen-induced primary mammary neoplasms exhibit a modest but distinct frequency of metastases (~15%) to other tissue sites, including lymph nodes, liver, and lung,[16,17] whereas rat mammary tumors induced by chemical carcinogens do not exhibit any significant metastatic potential.[18] Approximately 85% of the mammary tumors originating in rats are estrogen dependent, similar to breast cancer in postmenopausal women, whereas most (~90%) of the mouse mammary tumors are estrogen independent.[18] Also, PRL plays a permissive, if not essen-

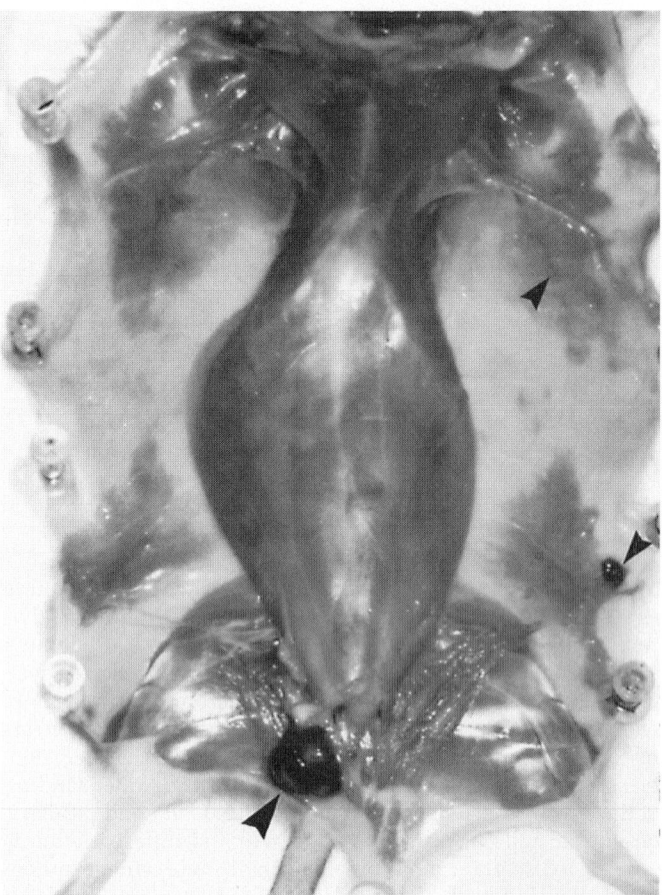

**FIGURE 222-1.** Mammary gland carcinomas (*arrowheads*) induced after continuous administration of $17\beta$-estradiol for 6 months to a female ACI rat. Hormone pellets (20-mg pellet containing 4 mg of $17\beta$-estradiol) were renewed every 4 months to maintain constant estrogen levels. Serum estradiol concentrations were 165 to 170 pg/mL throughout the treatment period.

tial, role in the induction of mammary tumors by estrogen in most rat strains.[14] Finally, combined estrogen and progesterone treatment has been shown to induce a higher incidence of mammary tumors in Wistar-WAG rats than estrogen exposure alone.[19] Of interest, however, medroxyprogesterone acetate (MPA, Provera) is capable of inducing mammary tumors in mice in the absence of added estrogen.[20]

The biosynthesis of the estrogens $E_1$ and $17\beta$-$E_2$ from their androgen precursors, androstenedione and testosterone, is catalyzed by aromatase, a microsomal cytochrome P450-dependent enzyme. In postmenopausal women with breast cancer, aromatase activity in the peripheral tissues is a major endogenous source of estrogen for tumor growth.[21,22] The dynamics of androgen and estrogen production and metabolism, particularly the percentage of peripheral aromatization in nonhuman primates (cynomolgus, rhesus, and baboons), closely resembles that in humans.[23] This is not found in murine species. Primate species have been used as models of human peripheral aromatization to test the therapeutic effects of steroidal and nonsteroidal aromatase inhibitors in vivo.[24]

### OVARY

Presently, an animal model for hormonally induced epithelial ovarian tumors does not exist. Nevertheless, granulosa cell tumors of the ovary develop in 25% to 50% of BALB/c mice when they are implanted with progesterone pellets.[25] In one study, 19-norprogesterone was more effective than progesterone in inducing these neoplasms. The contraceptive agents norethindrone and norethynodrel elicited a 52% incidence of ovarian tumor. Castrated rats with intrasplenic ovarian transplants that resulted in constant high levels of gonadotropins showed a high frequency of tumors in the transplanted ovaries.[26] The resulting ovarian tumors were thecal granulosa cell tumors, however, and were not of epithelial origin. In these rats, the long-term excess of gonadotropins is believed to be largely responsible for promoting ovarian tumor development.

## UTERUS

Despite the well-established association between estrogen and endometrial cancer in women,[4] an animal model of similar hormonally induced cancer at this site is lacking. Although endometrial tumors are produced with a high incidence in rabbits after estrogen treatment, these adenocarcinomas are preceded by cystic hyperplasia, which occurs spontaneously with high frequency (75%) in aging animals.[27] Endometrial carcinomas in the uterine horns have also been induced with either DES or 17β-E$_2$ in mice.[28] Uterine carcinomas were observed in 90% of mice receiving DES for 5 days neonatally.[29] The induction of these uterine tumors was age and dose dependent. In addition, these uterine tumors were estrogen dependent because they partially regressed after ovariectomy and, when transplanted into nude mice, required estrogen for continued growth. The involvement of a MMTV in mice uterine tumor development remains a possibility. Similarly, estrogen-dependent uterine tumors can be induced in hamsters when DES is administered to newborn animals.[30] Finally, a high incidence of uterine leiomyosarcomas has been induced in hamsters after combined estrogen and androgen treatment.[31] Interestingly, the addition of progesterone to this combined treatment inhibited the induction of these uterine smooth muscle cell tumors. Particularly relevant is the induction of uterine mesotheliomas in a nonhuman primate species (squirrel monkey) after prolonged treatment with either DES or estradiol benzoate.[32]

## CERVIX-VAGINA

Cervical or vaginal squamous cell carcinomas occur after prolonged estrogen administration in C3H, C57, and BC mouse strains.[33] Moreover, no spontaneous occurrence of such tumors has been reported. Generally, the belief is that these tumorigenic effects are produced by the direct carcinogenic action of estrogens. Also, prolonged testosterone administration causes cervical tumors in female hybrid mice.

## PITUITARY GLAND

Some strains of mice and rats are highly susceptible to the induction of pituitary tumors by estrogens, whereas other strains are largely resistant.[34,35] Males appear to be more susceptible to estrogen-induced pituitary tumors than females. Once pituitary tumors develop in mice, they do not regress after estrogen treatment ceases. Histologically, these tumors are described as chromophobe adenomas. The predominant secretion of these tumors is PRL, and growth-promoting properties as well as adrenocorticotropin-like effects have been reported. These pituitary tumors can be induced either by natural steroidal estrogens or by synthetic steroidal and stilbene estrogens. Intermediate-lobe pituitary adenomas also have been induced in rats and hamsters after prolonged estrogen treatment.[36] Present evidence indicates that these pituitary tumors are also induced by direct hormonal action.

## TESTES

The induction of testicular tumors in mice with estrogens has been studied extensively. Initially, malignant tumors of the interstitial cells were reported to develop in the A1 strain of mice receiving 17β-E$_2$.[37] Since then, similar testicular tumors have been induced with high incidence in other mouse strains, including BALB/c, A$_{Bi}$, and ACrg, but not in several other strains.[38] As a consequence of estrogen treatment of susceptible mice, alterations in androgen biosynthetic enzyme systems, transient induction of DNA synthesis, and a greater nuclear estrogen content in Leydig cells may contribute to their neoplastic transformation.[38] Apparently, the pituitary plays a permissive role in estrogen-induced testicular tumors, because hypophysectomy prevents the appearance of these tumors.

## KIDNEY

The most extensively studied experimental model in hormonal carcinogenesis is the estrogen-induced renal carcinoma of the Syrian hamster. Long-term exposure of either castrated or intact male hamsters (but not female hamsters) to either steroidal or stilbene estrogens results in essentially 100% incidence of multiple bilateral renal neoplasms.[39] Because the reproductive and urogenital tracts of the Syrian hamster arise from the same embryonic germinal ridge, the kidney of this species appears to have carried over genes that are expressed and responsive to estrogens. Complete chemoprevention of renal tumorigenesis can be effected by administering the estrogen concomitantly with androgen, progesterone, antiestrogens, or EE.[40,41] Evidence strongly indicates that the estrogen-induced renal tumor arises primarily from undifferentiated committed epithelial stem cells in the interstitium.[42] Not all estrogens are equally active in inducing these renal tumors.[43] With the exception of EE, which elicits only a 10% renal tumor incidence, potent estrogens (17β-E$_2$, DES, hexestrol, and 11β-methoxyethinylestradiol [Moxestrol]) exhibit high incidences of renal neoplasms compared with weak estrogens (estriol, 4-hydroxyestrone). Moreover, estrogens that possess low or negligible estrogenic activity (17α-E$_2$, β-dienestrol, 2-hydroxy-estradiol) do not induce kidney tumors. The lack of strong carcinogenic activity of EE in the hamster kidney, despite its known potent estrogenic activity, may be the result of a differential effect of EE on the proliferation of a subset of renal tubule cells, rather than on the stem cells residing in the interstitium.[41]

One of the most unusual features of the Syrian hamster kidney is its ability to behave as an estrogen-responsive and estrogen-dependent organ. Estrogen treatment elevates the level of estrogen receptors and induces progesterone receptors in the kidney. These effects are characteristic of estrogen action in target tissues. A comprehensive model for estrogen carcinogenicity in the hamster kidney is proposed (Fig. 222-2). Briefly, estrogens induce proliferation of preexisting estrogen-sensitive interstitial cells, as well as reparative proliferation secondary to cellular damage. The proliferation of the interstitial cells leads to aneuploidy and chromosomal instability, resulting in gene overexpression, amplification, and suppression (specifically, protooncogene, and suppressor gene expression) and eventually leads to tumor formation via a multistep process.[44]

## LIVER

A few hepatic tumors have been induced in mice, rats, and hamsters by various synthetic estrogens and progestins.[45] A 20% to 30% incidence of liver tumor has been reported in hamsters after long-term administration of EE. However, in the presence of

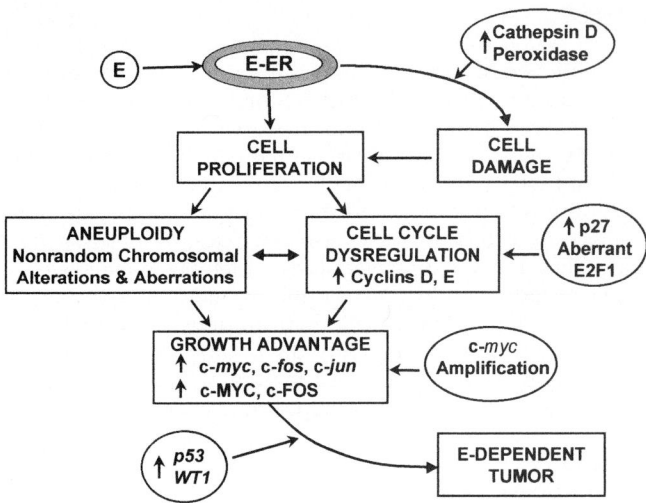

**FIGURE 222-2.** Multistep model for estrogen-induced carcinogenesis in the Syrian hamster kidney. (*E*, estrogen; *ER*, estrogen receptor; *E2F1*, transcription factor E2F1; *WT1*, suppressor gene Wilm tumor 1.)

0.3% α-naphthoflavone (ANF) in the diet, or in a 20-mg pellet form, EE administration induced an 80% to 100% incidence of hepatocellular carcinomas in castrated male hamsters.[46] Because ANF is not known to behave as a carcinogen or to possess substantial mutagenic activity, the belief is that it modifies the metabolism of synthetic estrogens, thus enhancing their carcinogenicity by increasing the amount of the parent hormone. A cocarcinogenic role for ANF cannot be ruled out, however, in the induction of these hamster liver tumors.[46]

## PROSTATE

Long-term exposure of either Noble or Lobund Wistar rats to testosterone results in prostatic carcinomas.[47] Tumor incidence was 50% when testosterone treatment was applied for 13 months and then $E_1$ was substituted for 6 months. Maximum tumor yields were obtained when testosterone plus $17\beta$-$E_2$ was given for 19 months, with the tumor incidence approaching 90%.[48] The resultant tumor nodules attained only microscopic proportions, however, somewhat limiting the usefulness of this model. Similar simultaneous exposure to testosterone plus $17\beta$-$E_2$ for 4 months resulted in consistent dysplastic lesions in the dorsolateral lobe of the prostate in Noble rats.[49] When testosterone was replaced by dihydrotestosterone, the active androgen in many species, prostatic tumors were not seen.[50] These data suggest that $17\beta$-$E_2$ may be involved in the etiology of these prostatic neoplasms, because testosterone is known to enhance proliferative activity at this organ site. Current evidence suggests that estrogen, acting on the androgen-supported prostate, induces cell proliferation through a receptor-mediated process.[51]

## DUCTUS DEFERENS AND SCENT GLAND

As with tumors in the Noble rat prostate model, other hormone-induced tumors also require the presence of two hormones, both estrogen and androgen. Examples are a leiomyosarcoma induced in the hamster ductus deferens[31] and an unknown type of epithelial tumor induced in the scent gland after long-term coadministration of these gonadal hormones.[52] Although, presently, the relationship between these hormones in inducing these tumors is not well understood, the scent gland tumor is a particularly interesting model system because androgen is

required for preneoplasia, and estrogen is required for full tumor development.[52]

## PERINATAL EFFECTS

Perinatal effects of estrogens have been studied extensively in the mouse.[53] When these animals receive prenatal and neonatal exposure to DES or $17\beta$-$E_2$, cervicovaginal adenosis and adenocarcinomas occur in females, and testicular lesions occur in the rete testis of the males. The mechanism for these transplacental and perinatal effects remains to be elucidated.

# HORMONES AS COCARCINOGENS OR PROMOTERS

Finally, hormones can act as cocarcinogens or promoters in conjunction with either physical carcinogens (e.g., ionizing radiation) or chemical carcinogens (DMBA, diethylnitrosamine [DEN], N-nitrosobutylurea [NBU]) at different organ sites. For example, either DES or EE plus x-ray treatments yields a high incidence of mammary tumors in female ACI rats, a rat strain that is relatively insensitive to radiation treatment alone.[54] These same hormones are capable of promoting mammary tumors in other rat strains exposed to DMBA and DEN/NBU.[55]

## IN VITRO CELL CULTURE MODELS

Hormonal effects on in vitro cell transformation and mutagenic assays have important implications regarding the role of these substances in oncogenic processes. Hormonal agents have yielded some negative results in numerous in vitro tests, including lack of gene mutations in the *Salmonella typhimurium* assay. Positive findings in other in vitro cell assay systems are significant, however, and strongly suggest the possibility that hormones may possess epigenotoxic characteristics that could affect in vivo malignant cell transformation.[56]

## SYRIAN HAMSTER EMBRYO CELL SYSTEM

One of the most intensively studied in vitro assays is the Syrian hamster embryo (SHE) cells in culture.[57] In this assay system, DES and some of its metabolites induce morphologic and neoplastic transformation of SHE cells. However, no detectable gene mutations at two genetic loci were found. In the presence of a rat postmitochondrial supernatant fraction, DES also induced unscheduled DNA synthesis.

## BALB/C 3T3 CELL SYSTEM

Another in vitro cell system that has been studied in considerable detail is the BALB/c 3T3 cell system.[58] In this system, $17\beta$-$E_2$, DES, and $E_1$ induce a statistically significant cell transformation frequency. The natural steroidal estrogens require three- to five-fold higher concentrations than DES to induce an equivalent transformation frequency.

## OTHER CELL SYSTEMS

In other systems studied,[59] DES induced gene mutations in mouse lymphoma cells in the presence of a rat liver postmitochondrial supernatant, and unscheduled DNA synthesis in HeLa cells in the presence of the same postmitochondrial supernatant fraction. Sister chromatid exchanges have been induced in human fibroblasts and lymphocytes in culture by DES but not by $17\beta$-$E_2$.

The major drawbacks of the cells used in most short-term systems include the fact that many are not primarily of epithelial origin, they are not considered target cells for sex hormones, and in many instances they are neoplastic.

## METABOLISM AND COVALENT BINDING STUDIES

Investigations in both animal models and short-term in vitro cell culture assays provide indirect evidence for the bioactivation of sex hormones as a pertinent aspect of hormone-induced tumor cell transformation. In this regard, estrogens have been more extensively studied. Based on numerous reports, no doubt exists that estrogens can form reactive species capable of covalent binding to cellular macromolecules.[60] Whether such reactive intermediates have any involvement in initiating oncogenesis in whole animal systems remains controversial, however, because of the high microsomal protein and hormone concentrations required to demonstrate their formation.[61]

## GROWTH FACTOR AND ONCOGENE INVOLVEMENT

An analysis of carcinogenesis, especially hormonal carcinogenesis, must include consideration of the possible role of growth factors and oncogenes in these processes.[62] This is especially pertinent because many growth factors produced by normal cells are involved, singly or in combination with other mitogens, in the proliferation of specific target cells, both normal and neoplastic. Growth factors such as insulin-like growth factors (IGF) and transforming growth factors (TGF) can be produced by target cells. Also, the likelihood is that transformed cells may both synthesize and respond to growth factors and, consequently, proliferate independently through autocrine secretion. Thus, growth factors, which are basically peptide hormones, may be involved in the regulation of growth of both normal and neoplastic endocrine tissues. In vitro studies with serum-free media have clearly shown the proliferative effects of epidermal growth factor (EGF) and TGF-α on endocrine target cells.

Oncogenes, including cellular protooncogenes, are thought to play an important role in carcinogenesis in animals and humans, perhaps through their proliferative functions. Oncogenes could participate in carcinogenesis in several ways. Some of them possibly may be coding for growth factors or their receptors. The *onc* gene of simian sarcoma virus (*sis*) is almost identical to a gene coding for a precursor of one polypeptide chain of platelet-derived growth factor (PDGF).[63] The expression of the c-*sis* protooncogene is known to be under androgenic control in a ductus deferens smooth muscle tumor cell line (DDTMF-2). Moreover, these cells synthesize and secrete a PDGF-like growth factor that is implicated in the autocrine regulation of $DDT_1MF-2$ cell proliferation.[64] In addition, studies of the amino-acid sequence of immunoaffinity-purified EGF receptor have shown that the v-*erb*-B oncogene of avian erythroblastosis virus may encode for a truncated receptor lacking the external ligand-binding domain for EGF. These findings provide direct evidence that oncogenes may contribute to malignant cell transformation by inappropriate production of growth factors or through expression of uncontrolled growth factor receptor functions, causing unregulated cell proliferation.

Although little is known about the expression of oncogenes by endocrine target cells, prolonged hormonal stimulation, a prerequisite for hormonal carcinogenesis, may cause inappropriate gene overexpression, amplification, and suppression. For estrogens, immediate estrogen response genes (e.g., c-*myc*, c-*fos*, c-*jun*) may be overexpressed.[7] Moreover, cell-cycle genes as well

as their regulatory genes (e.g., *p16*, *p21*, *p27*) may be deregulated and frequently overexpressed.

In conclusion, many chemical and physical agents are known to be involved in carcinogenesis in animals and humans. These agents have been classified into various categories, such as initiators, promoters, cocarcinogens, and others. Hormones probably possess one or more of these characteristics, depending on the experimental model system in question. A unique and fundamental feature of carcinogenesis resulting from hormonal imbalance is the consistent finding that transformation usually follows a discrete pathway from normal cell hyperplasia to hormone-responsive and hormone-dependent neoplasia to hormone-independent neoplasia (i.e., autonomous tumors). Both hormone-induced and chemical carcinogen–induced tumors require a long latent period. Unlike hormonally induced cancers, however, cancers that are induced by chemical carcinogens in endocrine glands or in their target tissues usually do not depend on hormones for their growth. An exception to this general rule is the chemical carcinogen–induced mammary cancer in rats. What the nature of hormonal involvement is and whether hormones have a direct or indirect influence in one or more parts of the sequence of events leading to carcinogenesis remain to be elucidated. However, hormone-mediated genomic instability may be a key element common to a number of different hormonally induced model systems at various organ sites.

## REFERENCES

1. Colditz GA, Stampfer MJ, Willett WC, et al. Prospective study of estrogen replacement therapy and risk of breast cancer in postmenopausal women. JAMA 1990; 264:2648.
2. Toniolo PG. Endogenous estrogens and breast cancer risk: the case for prospective cohort studies. Environ Health Perspect 1997; 105:587.
3. Ross RK, Bernstein L, Lobo RA, et al. 5-Alpha-reductase activity and risk of prostate cancer among Japanese and U.S. white and black males. Lancet 1992; 339:887.
4. Colditz GA, Hankinson SE, Hunter DJ, et al. The use of estrogens and progestins and the risk of breast cancer in postmenopausal women. N Engl J Med 1995; 332:1589.
5. Hertz R. An appraisal of the concepts of endocrine influence on etiology, pathogenesis, and control of abnormal and neoplastic growth. Cancer Res 1957; 17:423.
6. Nandi S. Role of hormones in mammary neoplasia. Cancer Res 1978; 38:4046.
7. Hou X, Li JJ, Chen WB, et al. Estrogen-induced protooncogene and suppressor gene expression in the hamster kidney: significance for estrogen carcinogenesis. Cancer Res 1996; 56:2616.
8. Li JJ, Li SA. The effect of hormones on tumor induction. I. Brief overview of the endocrine system. II. Hormonal carcinogenesis. III. Effect of hormones on carcinogenesis by non-hormonal chemical agents. In: Arcos JC, Argus MF, Woo WT, eds. Chemical induction of cancer. Boston: Birkhauser, 1996:397.
9. Lacassagne A. Apparition de cancers de la mamelle chez la souris male, soumise á des injections de folliculine. Compt Rend Acad Sci 1932; 195:630.
9a. Lippert TH, Seeger H, Mueck AO. The impact of endogenous estradiol metabolites on carcinogenesis. Steroids 2000; 65:357.
10. Shull JD, Spady TJ, Snyder M, et al. Ovary-intact, but not ovariectomized female ACI rats treated with 17β-estradiol rapidly develop mammary carcinomas. Carcinogenesis 1997; 18:1595.
11. Li SA, Xue Y, Xie Q, et al. Serum and tissue levels of estradiol during estrogen-induced renal tumorigenesis in the Syrian hamster. J Steroid Biochem Mol Biol 1994; 48:283.
12. Leav I, Ho S-M, Ofner P, et al. Biochemical alterations in sex hormone induced hyperplasia and dysplasia of the dorsolateral prostates of Noble rats. J Natl Cancer Inst 1988; 80:1045.
13. Rudali G, Coezy E, Frederic F, et al. Susceptibility of mice of different strains to the mammary carcinogenic action of natural and synthetic oestrogens. Prev Europ Etudes Clin Biol 1971; 16:425.
14. Blankenstein MA, Broerse JJ, van Zwieten MJ, et al. Prolactin concentration in plasma and susceptibility to mammary tumors in female rats from different strains treated chronically with estradiol 17β. Breast Cancer Res Treat 1984; 4:137.
15. Thomas DB, Jimenez LM, McTieman A, et al. Breast cancer in men: risk factors with hormonal implications. Am J Epidemiol 1992; 135:734.
16. Dunning WF, Curtis MR, Segaloff A. Strain differences in response to diethylstilbestrol and the induction of mammary gland and bladder cancer in the rat. Cancer Res 1947; 7:511
17. Cutts JH, Noble RL. Estrone-induced mammary tumors in the rat. I. Induction and behavior of tumors. Cancer Res 1964; 24:1116.

18. Nandi S, Yang J, Guzman R. Hormones and the cellular origin of mammary cancer: a unifying hypothesis. In: Li JJ, Li SA, Gustafsson JA, et al., eds. Hormonal carcinogenesis, vol II. New York: Springer-Verlag, 1996:11.

19. Hannouche N, Samperez S, Riviere MR, Jouan P. Estrogen and progesterone receptors in mammary tumors induced in rats by simultaneous administration of 17β-estradiol and progesterone. J Steroid Biochem 1982; 17:415.

20. Lanari C, Molinolo AA, Dosne Pasqualini C. Induction of mammary adenocarcinomas by medroxyprogesterone acetate in BALB/c female mice. Cancer Lett 1986; 33:215.

21. Varela, RM, Dao TL. Estrogen synthesis and estradiol binding by human mammary tumors. Cancer Res 1978; 38:2429.

22. Longcope C, Femino A, Johnston ON. Androgen and estrogen dynamics in the female baboon (Papio anubis). J Steroid Biochem 1988; 31:195.

23. Brodie AMH, Hammond JO, Ghosh M, et al. Effect of treatment with aromatase inhibitor 4-hydroxyandrostenedione on the nonhuman primate menstrual cycle. Cancer Res 1989; 49:4780.

24. Dukes M, Edwards PN, Large M, et al. The preclinical pharmacology of "Arimidex" (Anastrozole; ZD1033)—a potent, selective aromatase inhibitor. J Steroid Biochem Mol Biol 1996; 58:439.

25. Lipschutz A, Iglesias R, Pamosevick V, et al. Ovarian tumors and other ovarian changes induced in mice by two 19-nor contraceptives. Br J Cancer 1967; 21:153.

26. Biskind GR, Kordan B, Biskind MS. Ovary transplanted to spleen in rats: the effect of unilateral castration, pregnancy, and subsequent castration. Cancer Res 1950; 10:309.

27. Griffiths CT. Effects of progestins, estrogens, and castration on induced endometrial cancer in rabbits. Surg Forum 1963; 14:399.

28. Highman B, Greeman DL, Norvell MJ, et al. Neoplastic and preneoplastic lesions induced in female C3H mice by diets containing diethylstilbestrol or 17β-estradiol. J Environ Path Toxicol 1980; 4:81.

29. Newbold RR, Bulock BC, McLachlan JA. Uterine adenocarcinomas in mice following developmental treatment with estrogens: a model for hormonal carcinogenesis. Cancer Res 1991; 50:7677.

30. Leavitt WW, Evans RW, Hendry WJ III. Etiology of DES-induced uterine tumors in Syrian hamster. In: Leavitt WW, ed. Hormones and cancer. New York: Plenum Publishing, 1982:63.

31. Kirkman H, Algard FT. Characteristics of an androgen/estrogen-induced uterine smooth muscle cell tumor of the Syrian hamster. Cancer Res 1970; 30:794.

32. McClure HM, Graham CE. Malignant uterine mesotheliomas in squirrel monkeys following diethylstilbestrol administration. Lab Animal Sci 1973; 23:493.

33. Bischoff F. Carcinogenic effects of steroids. Adv Lipid Res 1969; 7:165.

34. Banerjee SK, Zoubine MH, Sarkar DK, et al. 2-Methoxy estradiol blocks estrogen-induced rat pituitary tumor growth and tumor angiogenesis: possible role of vascular endothelial growth factor. Anticancer Res 2000; 20:2641.

35. Nakagawa K, Ohara T, Tashiro K. Pituitary hormones and prolactin-releasing activity in rats with primary estrogen-induced pituitary tumors. Endocrinology 1980; 106:1033.

36. Koneff AA, Simpson ME, Evans HM. Effect of chronic administration of diethylstilbestrol on the pituitary and other endocrine organs of hamsters. Anat Rec 1946; 94:169.

37. Bonser GM, Robison JM. The effects of prolonged estrogen administration upon male mice of various strains: development of testicular tumors in the strong A strain. J Pathol Bacteriol 1940; 51:9.

38. Sato B, Spomer W, Huseby RA, Samuels LT. The testicular estrogen receptor system in two strains of mice differing in susceptibility to estrogen-induced Leydig cell tumors. Endocrinology 1979; 104:822.

39. Kirkman H. Estrogen-induced tumors of the kidney. III. Growth characteristics in the Syrian hamster. Natl Cancer Inst Monogr 1959; 1:1.

40. Li JJ, Cuthbertson TL, Li SA. Inhibition of estrogen carcinogenesis in the Syrian golden hamster kidney by antiestrogens. J Natl Cancer Inst 1980; 64:795.

41. Li JJ, Hou X, Bentel JM, et al. Prevention of estrogen carcinogenesis in the hamster kidney by ethynylestradiol: some unique properties of a synthetic estrogen. Carcinogenesis 1998; 19:471.

42. Oberley TD, Gonzalez A, Lauchner LJ, et al. Characterization of early lesions in estrogen-induced renal tumors in the Syrian hamster. Cancer Res 1991; 51:1922.

43. Li JJ, Li SA, Klicka JK, et al. Relative carcinogenic activity of various synthetic and natural estrogens in the hamster kidney. Cancer Res 1983; 43:5200.

44. Li SA, Hou X, Li JJ. Estrogen carcinogenesis: a sequential, epi-genotoxic multi-stage process. In: Li JJ, Li SA, Gustafsson JA, et al., eds. Hormonal carcinogenesis, vol II. New York: Springer-Verlag, 1996:200.

45. Li JJ, Kirkman H, Li SA. Synthetic estrogens and liver cancer: Risk analysis of animal and human data. In: Li JJ, Nandi S, Li SA, eds. Hormonal carcinogenesis, New York: Springer-Verlag, 1992:217.

46. Li JJ, Li SA. High incidence of hepatocellular carcinoma after synthetic estrogen administration in Syrian hamsters fed α-naphthoflavone: a new tumor model. J Natl Cancer Inst 1984; 73:543.

47. Drago JR. The induction of Nb rat prostatic carcinomas. Anticancer Res 1984; 4:255.

48. Ofner P, Bosland MC, Vena RL. Differential effects of diethylstilbestrol and estradiol-17β in combination with testosterone on rat prostate lobes. Toxicol Appl Pharmacol 1992; 112:300.

49. Bruchovsky N, Lesser B. Control of proliferative growth in androgen responsive organs and neoplasms. Adv Sex Horm Res 1976; 2:1.

50. Pollard M, Snyder DL, Lochert PH. Dihydrotestosterone does not induce prostate adenocarcinoma in L-W rats. Prostate 1987; 10:325.

51. Ho S-M, Yu M, Leav I, Viccione T. The conjoint action of androgens and estrogens in the induction of proliferative lesions in the rat prostate. In: Li JJ, Nandi S, Li SA, eds. Hormonal carcinogenesis. New York: Springer-Verlag, 1992:18.

52. Kirkman, H, Algard FT. Androgen-estrogen-induced tumors I. The flank organ (scent gland) chaetepithelioma of the Syrian hamster. Cancer Res 1964; 24:1569.

53. Bern HA, Talamantes FJ. Neonatal mouse models and their relation to disease in the human female. In: Herbst SL, Bern HA, eds. Developmental effects of diethylstilbestrol (DES) in pregnancy. New York: Thieme-Stratton, 1981:129.

54. Holtzman S, Stone JP, Shellabarger CJ. Synergism of estrogens and x-rays in mammary carcinogenesis in female ACI rats. J Natl Cancer Inst 1981; 67:455.

55. Russo IH, Russo J. Mammary gland neoplasia in long-term rodent studies. Environ Health Perspect 1996; 104:938.

56. Li JJ. Perspectives in hormonal carcinogenesis: animal models to human disease. In: Huff J, Boyd J, Barrett JC, eds. Cellular and molecular mechanisms in hormonal carcinogenesis: environmental influences. Philadelphia: Wiley-Liss 1996:447.

57. Tsutsui T, Degen GH, Schiffmann D, et al. Dependence on exogenous metabolic activation for induction of unscheduled DNA synthesis in Syrian hamster embryo cells by diethylstilbestrol and related compounds. Cancer Res 1984; 44:184.

58. Friedrich U, Thomale J, Nass G. Induction of malignant transformation by various chemicals in BALB/3T3 clone A31-1-1 cells and biological characterization of some transformants. Mutation Res 1985; 152:113.

59. Rao PN, Engelberg J. Structural specificity of estrogens in the induction of mitotic chromatid non-disjunction in HeLa cells. Exp Cell Res 1967; 48:71.

60. Tsibris JCM, McGuire PM. Microsomal activation and binding to nucleic acids and proteins. Biochem Biophys Res Commun 1977; 78:411.

61. Beleh MA, Lin YC, Brueggemeier RW. Estrogen metabolism in microsomal, cell, and tissue preparations from kidney and liver from Syrian hamster. J Steroid Biochem Mol Biol 1995; 52:479.

62. Schavorovsky OG, Rozados VR, Gervasoni SI, Matar P. Inhibition of ras oncogene: a novel approach to antineoplastic therapy. J Biomed Sci 2000; 7:292.

63. Waterfield MD. Oncogenes may encode a growth factor or part of the receptor for a growth factor. Br J Cancer 1984; 50:242.

64. Smith RG, Nag A, Syms AJ, Norris JS. Steroid regulation of receptor concentration and oncogene expression. J Steroid Biochem 1986; 24:51.

# CHAPTER 223

# SEX HORMONES AND HUMAN CARCINOGENESIS: EPIDEMIOLOGY

ROBERT N. HOOVER

Because of the central role that the hormonal milieu plays in various carcinogenic processes, clinical endocrinologists must be aware of malignancies to which their patients may be predisposed, either because of the nature of their illness or because of the nature of the hormonal therapy being instituted.

## CARCINOGENESIS AND ENDOGENOUS SEX HORMONE STATUS

Endogenous hormone status has long been thought to be an important factor in the etiology of a number of human malignancies. This belief has been based on animal carcinogenesis studies (see Chap. 222), the responsiveness of a number of tumors to hormonal manipulation (see Chaps. 224 and 225), the relationship of risk of certain tumors to a variety of reproductive and other factors thought to influence hormonal status, and the simple fact that some organs depend on hormonal status for their normal function.[1] Speculation about a causal role for hormones has focused on malignancies of the female breast and the reproductive tract. Some evidence for hormonal carcinogenesis has been observed for a variety of other tumors, however, including prostate, liver, testis, thyroid, and gallbladder cancers, and malignant melanoma. Despite these long-standing suspicions, little success has been achieved in identifying the specific hormonal factors that might be responsible for these tumors, with the possible exception of endometrial cancer.

## CARCINOGENESIS AND EXOGENOUS SEX HORMONE THERAPY

Within the last 50 years, a new element in the area of hormonal influences on cancer risks has been added, that of exogenous sex hormone exposure. Pharmacologic levels of estrogens, progestins, androgens, and pituitary trophic hormones, alone or in combination, have been administered to large segments of the population for various reasons. These large-scale "natural experiments" have provided more specific insights into the relationship between hormonal factors and several different malignancies.[2] Moreover, enthusiasm has grown for the widespread treatment of relatively healthy segments of the population (e.g., women receiving oral contraceptive agents or menopausal replacement therapy). Considerable interest has arisen in the use of estrogens for postmenopausal prevention of osteoporosis and osteoporotic fractures[3] (see Chaps. 64 and 100). Some evidence supports the long-suspected potential of menopausal estrogens to prevent clinical coronary heart disease.[4] In addition, within the general population, a substantial increase has been seen in the use of dietary supplements, many of which have significant hormonal activity (e.g., androstenedione, melatonin). Because of this enthusiasm on the part of physicians and the public, appropriate evaluations of the carcinogenic consequences of these exposures have become important to public health, as well as to understanding the biology of the tumors involved.

## ENDOMETRIAL CANCER

### ENDOGENOUS FACTORS IN ENDOMETRIAL CANCER

The cancer for which the evidence for both an endogenous and an exogenous hormonal cause is best established is endometrial cancer.

Various factors related to endogenous hormone production have been associated with endometrial cancer.[5] Medical conditions related to increased risk include functional (estrogen-secreting) ovarian tumors, the polycystic ovary syndrome, diabetes mellitus, and hypertension. Reproductive factors, including nulliparity and a late natural menopause, also have consistently been found to be related to increased risk. Some dietary factors also seem to influence risk. Obesity is a risk factor and a vegetarian diet is a possible protective factor.[6] Age, a determinant of levels of most endogenous hormones, also influences endometrial cancer risk in a unique manner. Endometrial cancer rates are extremely low in women younger than 45 years of age, rise precipitously among women in their late 40s and throughout their 50s (much more dramatically than for other tumors), and then decline in women approximately age 60 and older (Fig. 223-1).

### EXOGENOUS SEX HORMONES AND ENDOMETRIAL CANCER

Exposure to exogenous hormones also has been linked to endometrial cancer.[5]

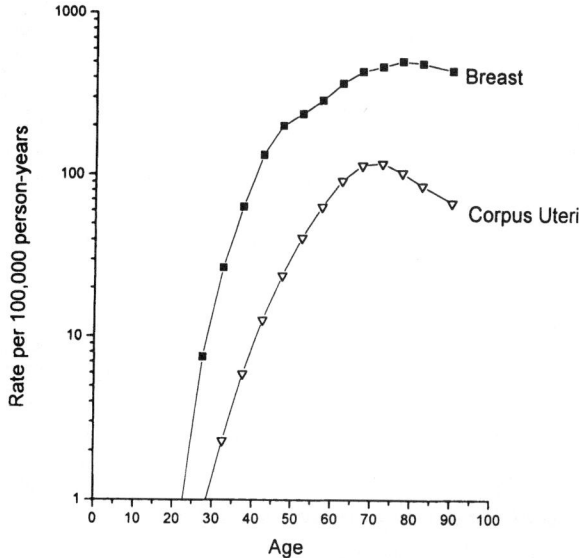

**FIGURE 223-1.** Age-specific incidence rates for breast and uterine corpus cancers among white women during 1986 through 1990. (Data from the Surveillance, Epidemiology and End Results Program.)

### ESTROGENS AND ENDOMETRIAL CANCER

Estrogen-replacement therapy of 2 years or longer for menopausal women is associated with an excess *relative risk* of endometrial cancer. Table 223-1 shows estimated relative risks (i.e., the risk of the disease among those exposed to estrogen therapy compared with the risk among those not exposed).[7–14] The relative risk among users compared with nonusers ranges from two-fold to eight-fold. It increases even further with long duration of use and with high average daily doses. Thus far, every type of estrogen that has been investigated has shown this relationship, including conjugated equine estrogens, ethinyl estradiol, and diethylstilbestrol (DES). The highest risk occurs among current users. The risk declines with each year after cessation of use, although apparently some residual excess risk is present even 10 years after cessation. The risk is highest for early-stage malignancies, but a two-fold to three-fold excess risk is seen for the advanced stages of disease as well.

### EFFECT OF ESTROGEN AND PROGESTERONE IN SEQUENCE

A profound trend has been seen away from unopposed estrogen treatment of menopausal symptoms and toward treatment with

**TABLE 223-1.**

**Relative Risks\* of Endometrial Cancer Associated with Menopausal Estrogen Use from Selected Case-Control Studies**

| Reference | Source of Controls | Overall RR | RR among Long-Term Users[†] |
|---|---|---|---|
| Ziel and Finkle[7] | Health plan | 7.6 | 13.9 |
| Mack et al.[8] | Retirement community | 5.6 | 8.8 |
| Gray[9] | Private practice | 3.1 | 11.6 |
| Pike et al.[10] | Community | 2.1 | 24.2 |
| Green et al.[11] | General population | 3.7 | 16.3 |
| Hulka et al.[12] | Gynecology patients | 1.8 | 4.1 |
| Shapiro et al.[13] | Hospital patients | 3.9 | 6.0 |
| Brinton et al.[14] | Community | 3.0 | 6.0 |

*RR*, relative risk.

\*Risk of cancer relative to a risk of 1.0 for women who never used menopausal estrogens.

[†]Definition of *long-term* varied from ≥5 to ≥15 years.

a sequence of an estrogen that is then combined with a progestin. Substantial evidence[15] indicates that such cyclic treatment reduces the frequency of hyperplasia and atypical hyperplasia associated with unopposed estrogen treatment. Although the epidemiologic data concerning endometrial cancer risk are still developing, certain patterns are emerging. The risk of endometrial cancer is lower among women using the combined regimen than among women using estrogen alone.[10,16] Evidence implies that, at least in the short term, the risk is related to the *number of days that a progestin is used with estrogen in a monthly cycle.* Those using the progestin for ≥10 days per month, including those using the combined regimen continuously, have a risk similar to that of women not using any hormone-replacement therapies. Those using progestins for <10 days per month have a risk that is substantially greater and may be close to that of women using estrogen alone. The risks associated with long-term use of these regimens are not yet clear.

### ORAL CONTRACEPTIVES AND ENDOMETRIAL CANCER

Oral contraceptives also have been studied extensively in relation to endometrial cancer, after the observations in the early 1970s that young women receiving sequential oral contraceptives (particularly dimethisterone and ethinyl estradiol [Oracon]) were developing endometrial cancer.[17] Subsequent investigations estimated that such women were at a two-fold to eight-fold excess risk of developing this tumor. On the other hand, nonsequential combination oral contraceptives clearly are related to decreased risks of endometrial cancer (Table 223-2). Relative risks of 0.4 to 0.5 have been observed, indicating a 50% to 60% protection associated with such use.[18–23] Some evidence also is seen of increased levels of protection with increased years of use. The effects of stopping use are unclear. Three studies[20,21,23] have noted that the protection was substantial among current users and subsided after cessation. These studies, however, disagreed on the duration of protection after stopping. In addition, most studies have observed profound interaction between other endometrial cancer risk factors and the associations with combination oral contraceptive use. Specifically, the protective effect is attenuated among the obese,[24] among long-term estrogen users,[23] and among the multiparous. Although the same interactions have not been found in all studies, these observations are consistent with a situation in which a number of these risk factors operate through common or highly correlated hormonal mechanisms.

### TAMOXIFEN AND ENDOMETRIAL CANCER

Case reports of endometrial cancers after tamoxifen treatment for breast cancer led to a series of case-control and cohort stud-

ies, as well as systematic reviews of the original clinical trials of tamoxifen treatment. A consistent *increased risk of two- to seven-fold among tamoxifen-treated subjects* was seen in these investigations, including a relative risk of 2.5 in a large clinical trial of tamoxifen therapy for breast cancer prevention in women without breast cancer.[25] This was viewed as entirely consistent with tamoxifen's organ-specific effects: acting as an estrogen agonist in the endometrium, while acting as a potent estrogen antagonist in the breast.

### MECHANISMS OF ACTION

A unified theory[26] of how these risk factors operate has been proposed (Fig. 223-2). Most known risk factors are associated with increased levels of circulating estrogens, particularly estrogens not bound to protein. Clearly also related are the age effects and the use of combination oral contraceptives, which probably modify the increased risk associated with estrogen level through the modulating effects of progestogens. Furthermore, although nulliparity, diabetes, hypertension, and race have not yet been included in this scheme, they possibly will be as our knowledge of basic endocrinology expands.

Few attempts have been made to actually test this theory. Specifically, only two reasonably sized epidemiologic investigations have assessed endogenous hormone levels, and only one of these attempted to determine if hormone levels actually explained questionnaire-based risk factors.[27] In this study, although elevated risks were seen with elevated estrogen levels, the risks were much lower than anticipated. In addition, the risks associated with the factor thought most likely to operate

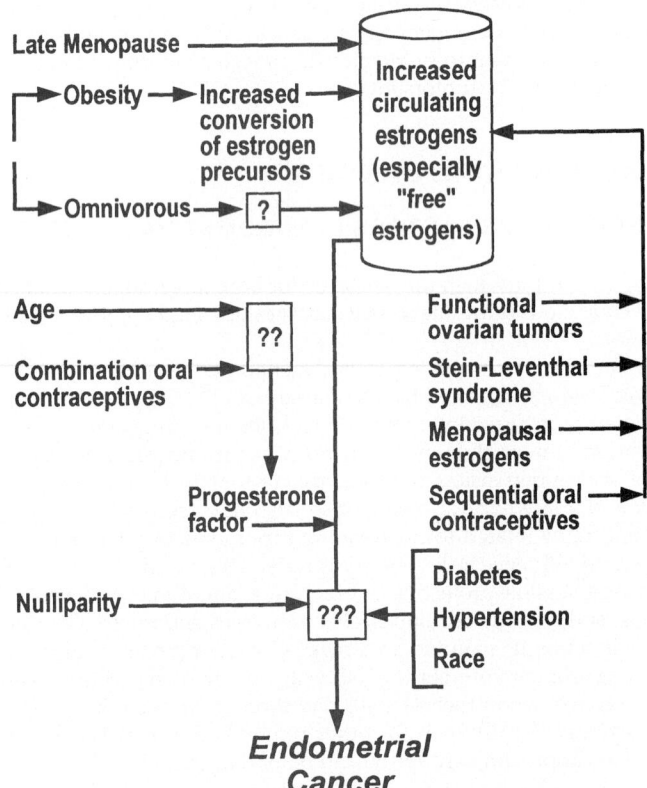

**FIGURE 223-2.** Risk factors for endometrial cancer and their possible modes of action. (From Brinton LA, Hoover RN. Epidemiology of gynecologic cancers. In: Hoskins WJ, Perez CA, Young RC, eds. Principles and practice of gynecologic oncology. Philadelphia: Lippincott–Raven Publishers, 1997:3.)

**TABLE 223-2.**
**Relative Risks\* of Endometrial Cancer Associated with Combination Oral Contraceptive Use from Five Case-Control Studies**

| Reference | Source of Controls | Overall RR | RR among Long-Term Users† |
|---|---|---|---|
| Weiss and Sayvetz[18] | General population | 0.5 | |
| Kaufman et al.[19] | Hospital patients | 0.5 | 0.3 |
| Hulka et al.[20] | Community | 0.4 | 0.3 |
| Stanford et al.[23] | Community | 0.4 | 0.2 |
| CDC[22] | General population | 0.5 | 0.6 |

*RR*, relative risk; *CDC*, Centers for Disease Control and Prevention.
\*Risk of cancer relative to a risk of 1.0 for women who never used oral contraceptives.
†Definition of *long-term* varied from ≥4 to ≥10 years.

through circulating estrogen levels—obesity—was unchanged when controlled for estrogen levels. Thus, although the model is attractive, additional work is needed to determine its place in the understanding of endometrial carcinogenesis. Even so, the model does suggest several promising lines of future clinical, epidemiologic, and laboratory research.

Perhaps most important to an understanding of carcinogenesis is the clarification of the precise mechanism by which circulating estrogens produce endometrial cancer. Several possibilities have been proposed: that estrogens are complete carcinogens themselves; that they promote initiated cells; or that they simply stimulate growth and, thereby, offer a greater opportunity for abnormal cells to arise or for carcinogens to act on vulnerable genetic material. The epidemiologic evidence strongly favors the argument that estrogens act at a relatively late stage in the process of carcinogenesis. If estrogens are promoters, however, no initiators of the process are readily apparent.

# BREAST CANCER

The hormonal etiology of breast cancer is well accepted, but no accepted unified model for the mechanism exists. Several hormonal hypotheses have been suggested, but extensive supporting data are lacking.

## ENDOGENOUS FACTORS IN BREAST CANCER

The importance of the ovary in breast cancer etiology is demonstrated by its relationship to a number of breast cancer risk factors.[28] Earlier age at menarche is associated with high risk of breast cancer. Similarly, later age at natural menopause also is associated with elevated risks. Surgical removal of the ovaries before natural menopause reduces risk of breast cancer, and the earlier the operation, the lower the risk. The shape of the age-incidence curve for this disease (see Fig. 223-1) has been interpreted as showing that the onset of ovarian activity early in life determines the slope of the curve, and that a reduction in this ovarian factor around the time of menopause is responsible for the change in the slope of the curve at ~50 years of age.

Other risk factors for breast cancer also have been established. *A history of breast cancer in a first-degree relative elevates a woman's risk of contracting breast cancer two-fold to five-fold.* Historical observations of a protection against breast cancer associated with an increase in parity were found to reflect the influence of the age at first birth. A woman who has her first child after the age of 30 years has approximately two-fold to three-fold the risk of breast cancer of a woman who had her first child when younger than 18 years of age. Nulliparous women have approximately the same risk as those women who had their first child at 30 years of age, whereas women who have a first birth after this age actually experience a greater risk than do nulliparous women. Investigations[29] have implied that increased parity may indeed diminish the risk of breast cancer, even when controlled for age at first birth. Benign breast disease, particularly that containing hyperplastic or dysplastic elements, places a woman at a two-fold to five-fold excess risk of subsequent breast cancer.[30] Body size also relates to breast cancer risk. Height or frame size is positively associated with risk. Obesity, or an increasing body mass index, is associated with an increased breast cancer risk among menopausal women, and a decreased breast cancer risk among premenopausal women.[31] Evidence implies that increased weight contributes as a risk factor only in the years immediately before diagnosis, suggesting that the mechanism involved operates very late in the process of breast carcinogenesis.[32]

## INFLUENCE OF DIET

Diet, particularly a diet high in caloric and/or fat intake, is strongly suspected of playing a role, because of worldwide differences in breast cancer rates. Asian populations have rates five-fold to six-fold lower than those seen in the United States and Western Europe. Migrants from Japan and China to the United States experience risks that rise toward the levels of whites over the course of two generations of residence within the United States. Whereas some direct support[33] for these dietary hypotheses has been proposed, a number of studies[34-37] have found no relationship, and the entire area remains controversial.

## HYPOTHESES FOR THE HORMONAL CAUSATION OF BREAST CANCER

A unifying hormonal hypothesis for breast cancer is frequently speculated to be possible, because even the nonovarian risk factors actually may operate through a hormonal mechanism. Perhaps the simplest of these models[38] is that breast cancer risk reflects total lifetime, or perhaps total early life, dose of estrogens. Related to this is the unopposed-estrogen hypothesis,[39] which also assumes that estrogens are the important risk factor but emphasizes the relative protective role of progesterone. Other hypotheses have suggested that, rather than total estrogens, specific individual estrogens and/or their metabolites may be the operative agents, in keeping with their differing carcinogenic or mitogenic potencies.[40,41] Another hypothesis[42] holds that the proportion of free versus protein-bound estrogen determines a woman's breast cancer and endometrial cancer risk. Speculation has also arisen that progesterone might actually be hazardous rather than protective because, contrary to its action on the endometrium, it seems to act as a mitogen within the breast ductal epithelium. Historically, androgens had been viewed as protective through their antiestrogenic action. Subsequently, however, laboratory and epidemiologic studies have suggested the opposite, perhaps due to the roles of androgens as precursors of estrogen synthesis.[43] Finally, pituitary hormones and prolactin in particular have been suggested as being primarily involved in breast carcinogenesis.[44,45]

Confirmation for these hypotheses has been sought by measuring levels of various hormones: first, in breast cancer patients and controls either at the time of diagnosis or at some time before; and second, in women with different levels of known risk factors, to determine whether the risk factors operate through specific hormones. In general, these studies have tended to find higher estrogen levels in women with breast cancer than in controls, at least among menopausal women. The level of difference has been highly variable, however, and often restricted to subgroups of women that also differ from study to study. Interestingly, subsequent studies have also noted elevations of several different adrenal androgens in women with breast cancer.[43] Studies of hormonal profiles related to various breast cancer risk factors have been few and have produced little in terms of consistent patterns. As a result, although they add to the evidence that estrogens are related to breast cancer risk, taken together, all of these laboratory-epidemiologic studies fail to rule out any of the proposed models of endogenous hormone effects as a partial explanation, and they also fail to support any one model as the unified explanation, perhaps because the women are being tested at ages other than those critical for breast cancer risk modification. Or, perhaps, the premise of a unifying hypothesis is incorrect.

Thus, although the evidence that breast cancer is a tumor of hormonal etiology is overwhelming, all of the specific endogenous hormones involved and their relative roles remain elusive.

**TABLE 223-3.**
**Relative Risk\* of Breast Cancer Associated with Hormone Replacement Therapy (HRT) by Duration of Use and Time Since Last Use**

| Last Use before Diagnosis | Duration of Use (Years) | | | | |
|---|---|---|---|---|---|
| | <1 | 1–4 | 5–9 | 10–14 | ≥15 |
| <5 years | 0.99 | 1.08 | 1.31[†] | 1.24[†] | 1.56[†] |
| ≥5 years | 1.12 | 1.12 | 0.90 | | |
| | | | | 0.95 | |

\*Relative to a risk of 1.00 for those who never used HRT.
[†]$p < .05$.
(Adapted from Collaborative Group on Hormonal Factors in Breast Cancer. Breast cancer and hormone replacement therapy: collaborative reanalysis of data from 51 epidemiological studies of 52,705 women with breast cancer and 108,411 women without breast cancer. Lancet 1997; 350:1047.)

**TABLE 223-4.**
**Relative Risk\* of Breast Cancer Associated with Oral Contraceptive Use by Duration of Use and Time Since Last Use**

| Last Use before Diagnosis | Duration of Use (Years) | | | |
|---|---|---|---|---|
| | <1 | 1–4 | 5–9 | ≥10 |
| Current | 1.18 | 1.27[†] | 1.21[†] | 1.29[†] |
| 1–4 years | 1.05 | 1.12 | 1.26[†] | 1.14[†] |
| 5–9 years | 1.05 | 1.05 | 1.13[†] | 1.14[†] |
| ≥10 years | 1.03 | 0.99 | 0.97 | 1.01 |

\*Relative to a risk of 1.00 for those who never used oral contraceptives.
[†]$p < .05$.
(Adapted from Collaborative Group on Hormonal Factors in Breast Cancer. Breast cancer and hormonal contraceptives: collaborative reanalysis of individual data on 53,297 women with breast cancer and 100,239 women without breast cancer from 54 epidemiological studies. Lancet 1996; 374:1713.)

## EXOGENOUS SEX HORMONES AND BREAST CANCER

Because of the pharmacologic levels of exposure, the impact of exogenous hormones should be more easily discerned than that of endogenous levels. Consistent findings have also been elusive, however, for hormone-replacement therapy (HRT) and oral contraceptive use.

### HORMONE-REPLACEMENT THERAPY AND BREAST CANCER

The widespread use of noncontraceptive estrogens seems to be an ideal natural experiment through which to evaluate some of the more prominent hormonal hypotheses about breast cancer etiology. The relationship has been controversial because of conflicting evidence. After two decades of small clinical studies suggesting that HRT was unrelated to, or even protective against, breast cancer, a retrospective cohort study[46] released in 1976 suggested a relatively small overall excess risk (30%) among conjugated estrogen users, which reflected a two-fold excess risk among long-term users. Since then, numerous studies of this issue have been conducted. Virtually none has found evidence of protection. *Most, but not all, have found some evidence of increased risk*, but the increases in relative risks were small; often showed inconsistencies with respect to issues of dose, duration, and recency of use; and frequently varied within subgroups of women defined by the presence or absence of various breast cancer risk factors. Although the increases in *relative risk* were relatively small, because of the frequency of use of HRT and the frequency of breast cancer, the *absolute risks and number of cases involved* could be of substantial public health consequence. This is the type of situation in which an ambitious effort to combine all of the available data into a pooled analysis would be particularly useful. Such an effort was published in 1997 (Table 223-3).[47] The combination of information from >50,000 patients with breast cancer and >100,000 control women from 51 epidemiologic investigations demonstrated a *stable and consistent pattern of risk.* HRT was associated with an increased breast cancer risk that was related both to recency and to duration of use. Specifically, risk was highest for current users and declined in proportion to the time since stopping use, so that no excess risk was noted for those who had stopped HRT 5 or more years before diagnosis. Among those using HRT within the 5 years before diagnosis, the excess relative risk rose with increasing duration of use to ~60% excess risk among those who had taken HRT for ≥15 years. When examined with respect to the presence or absence of other breast cancer risk factors, the patterns of risk associated with HRT were remarkably consistent except with regard to body mass: lean women had higher increases in relative risk associated with HRT than did heavier women. As with endometrial cancer, risks were

greater for less clinically advanced disease. Consistent with this, a study of a large series of cases from a prospective investigation found that, although breast cancer risk was elevated for HRT users, survival after breast cancer was better for those who were recent users at the time of diagnosis than for past users or those who had never used HRT.[48] This survival advantage did decrease with time after diagnosis, however, and eventually disappeared.

As for endometrial cancer, the issue of what impact the use of the combined estrogen and cyclic progestin regimen has on breast cancer has become a major research focus. The first studies[49,50] to evaluate this issue found that, in contrast to the pattern for endometrial cancer, the excess risk associated with estrogen replacement was not reduced in those also receiving cyclic progestins (Table 223-4). In fact, some indicated that the excess risk might actually be higher.[50a,50b,50c]

Noncontraceptive hormonal exposures other than the use of menopausal estrogen are relatively rare and generally have not been investigated. A notable exception is the study of the risk of breast cancer among women who took DES during a pregnancy to prevent a spontaneous abortion. Women participating in three clinical trials of DES use have been evaluated for long-term sequelae, and three follow-up studies of exposed women have also been reported.[51] Two of the three clinical trials showed evidence of excess breast cancer risk. Two of the cohort studies revealed overall excesses of ~50%. In the first systematic assessment of breast cancer risk among those exposed to DES in utero, no overall difference in risk was noted.[52] Although these results are comforting, because the average age of the group studied was only 38, more follow-up is necessary before final conclusions can be reached.

Although some controversy remains concerning causality, practically, the prudent course is to assume that high cumulative doses of noncontraceptive estrogens are related to a 50% to 80% excess breast cancer risk among current or recent users of these drugs, and risk-benefit decisions about drug use should be made on this assumption.

### ORAL CONTRACEPTIVES AND BREAST CANCER

The extensive use of oral contraceptives (see Chaps. 104 and 105) since they were licensed for use in the United States also seems to be a promising natural experiment, as well as an important public health issue. Overall, the results of studies of the effects of oral contraceptive use have been more consistent than those for menopausal estrogen use, although these findings are somewhat surprising. Because oral contraceptives so clearly alter the hormonal milieu, most investigators had predicted that oral contraception, particularly of long duration, would have a substantial impact on subsequent breast cancer risk. Whether this effect would be hazardous or beneficial was hotly debated. Most studies, however, have found essentially no overall relationship between the use of oral contraceptives and the risk of breast cancer.

The large number of studies of this issue and the large size of some of these studies have allowed assessments of risk according to different patterns of use and in multiple subgroups. Accordingly, a variety of questions were raised. The inconsistencies across studies prompted a large pooled analysis similar to that described above for HRT.[53] The considerable power resulting from the inclusion of >53,000 cases yielded consistent findings that were similar in many respects to those seen for HRT. *Breast cancer risk is increased in oral contraceptive users, but only among relatively recent users and to a lesser extent than for HRT.* Specifically, compared with those who had never used such contraceptives, the risks were 24% higher for current users, 16% higher for those who stopped use in the 5 years before diagnosis, and 7% higher for those who stopped 5 to 9 years earlier. These findings were remarkably consistent across various levels of other breast cancer risk factors. Also, as with the findings for HRT, these risks were more pronounced for less clinically advanced disease.

### TAMOXIFEN AND BREAST CANCER

An ancillary observation made during the conduct of clinical trials on the effect of tamoxifen treatment for breast cancer was the dramatic reduction in the risk of development of a new breast cancer in the contralateral breast in the tamoxifen-treated groups. This led to the development of several randomized clinical trials of tamoxifen as a preventive agent in women at high risk of breast cancer but without a prior history of the disease. The largest such trial found a 49% reduction in the incidence of breast cancer in the tamoxifen group, coming entirely from a 69% reduction in estrogen receptor–positive tumors.[25] Significant side effects occurred. In addition to the increase in risk of endometrial cancer noted above, the rates of stroke, pulmonary embolism, and deep-vein thrombosis also increased in the tamoxifen-treated group. The results of this trial have spurred enthusiasm for tests of the efficacy of related compounds that might carry a smaller risk of serious side effects.

### FUTURE IMPERATIVES

Clearly, the long-term consequences of oral contraceptive use on breast cancer risk will remain a research subject for many years. Only now are substantial numbers of women who used oral contraceptives for 5 or more years early in their reproductive lives entering the ages of high breast cancer risk. Thus, the final conclusion on long-term sequelae of oral contraceptive use must be postponed.

The current enthusiasm for cyclic estrogen-progestogen treatment of menopausal symptoms offers the opportunity to investigate an exposure of particular relevance to a number of the etiologic theories concerning the hormonal basis of breast cancer. Continued development of such studies seems to warrant a high priority, both on this basis and because of the sudden onset of treatment of a large population of healthy women with this currently understudied drug combination therapy.

In addition, because of the lack of practical opportunities to prevent breast cancer by altering known risk factors, enthusiasm has grown for the use of potentially chemopreventive drugs, most of which have a hormonal action. The tamoxifen experience continues, but other even more imaginative regimens have been suggested.[54] As for tamoxifen therapy, such treatments are likely to have unanticipated consequences, as well as, one hopes, the desired result. Thus, close study of such

treatment groups may provide unique insights into hormonal carcinogenesis in human populations.

## OVARIAN CANCER

Much less is known about risk factors for ovarian cancer than about risk factors for cancers of the endometrium and breast. Until the late 1970s, the issue was little studied, but several extensive epidemiologic investigations have been undertaken.

### ENDOGENOUS FACTORS IN OVARIAN CANCER

Only a few risk factors for ovarian cancer have been identified in these investigations, and they account for only a small proportion of the disease. However, the few factors consistently identified clearly imply a hormonal cause for this malignancy.[5] First of all, parity is protective, with the risk of the disease being highest among nulliparous women and declining by 70% among those with three or more live births. Independent of nulliparity, a three-fold to five-fold excess risk among women who have had medical consultation for infertility is consistently found. The consistent finding of a 30% to 40% reduced risk associated with a prior tubal ligation or hysterectomy has been hypothetically attributed to the compromised ovarian function resulting from reduced blood flow. Few other risk factors reflecting endogenous hormonal status have been identified for ovarian cancer, and none with any consistency among studies.

### HORMONE-REPLACEMENT THERAPY AND OVARIAN CANCER

HRT, primarily with estrogens, has been studied in various case-control and follow-up studies over the last 15 years. Most studies have found no consistent association between menopausal estrogen use and the risk of ovarian cancer. The overall relative risks in these studies have been close to 1.0 and yielded no evidence of higher risks for longer duration or higher dosages of estrogen. One investigation[55] found an increased risk of ovarian cancer among women who received both conjugated estrogens and DES for the treatment of menopausal symptoms. The number of cases in this study was limited, however, and the finding has not been confirmed.

### ORAL CONTRACEPTIVES AND OVARIAN CANCER

Oral contraceptive use, by contrast, appears to exert a *marked protective effect.* The effect seems to be related to duration, with those using oral contraceptives for >5 years having an ~50% to 70% reduced risk of the disease.[56]

The encouraging nature of this result has overshadowed some inconsistencies among individual studies. Whether these differences reflect chance biases in some studies, the influences of varying patterns of use between studies, or meaningful biologic interactions remains unclear. Critical comparisons of the existing studies and new data may enhance the understanding of ovarian carcinogenesis and clarify risk-benefit issues, particularly as demographic patterns of oral contraceptive use continue to change. In particular, the influence of cessation of use on risk for ovarian cancer merits more study.

### INFERTILITY TREATMENT

A history of drug therapy for infertility has been linked to increased ovarian cancer risk.[56,57] Generally, the lack of attempts to seek medical records to validate these reports and the difficulties in appropriately assessing the effect of a treatment (e.g., ovulation-stimulating drugs) for a condition (infertility) that is itself related to ovarian cancer risk has prevented a comprehensive interpretation of these reports. With the increasing number of therapeutic options for treatment of infertility, much more focus on better assessments should be a high priority.

## MECHANISMS

The increased risk associated with infertility coupled with the decreased risk associated with increased parity and the extended use of oral contraceptives, and the lack of an association with HRT implicate ovulation and perhaps gonadotropin stimulation of the ovary in its carcinogenesis. Decreased stimulation should reduce the risk, and those conditions associated with enhanced stimulation should elevate the risk. If this unifying hypothesis were supported by further evidence, it would have direct implications for the consequences of several trends in endocrine therapy and would emphasize the need for appropriate evaluation of the effects of ovulation-stimulating drugs.

## CANCER OF THE UTERINE CERVIX

### RISK FACTORS AND CERVICAL CANCER

Most findings from studies[58] of cervical cancer are consistent with primary involvement of a venereal agent. The two major factors that elevate a woman's risk of this malignancy are having a large number of different sexual partners and having first intercourse at an early age. In addition, among women with only one sexual partner, the more sexual partners her mate has had, the higher her risk of cervical cancer. Clinical, laboratory, and epidemiologic work have definitively implicated *papilloma viruses* as the key infectious factor in this disease.[59]

The strength of sexual, social, and specific infectious risk factors have tended to obscure other factors that might contribute to this disease. For example, cigarette smoking is a risk factor, even after control for sexual variables.[60] The presence of tobacco metabolites in cervical mucus provides a plausible biologic rationale for the role of tobacco.

### ORAL CONTRACEPTIVES AND CERVICAL CANCER

Potential hormonal risk factors for cervical cancer have not been systematically sought, but the cervix is a target organ for several of the sex hormones and, therefore, a likely candidate for the modification of tumor incidence by hormonal factors. Studies[61] linking increased risk to multiparity after appropriate control for sexual and viral risk factors support this notion. In addition, several case-control and follow-up studies *have linked oral contraceptive use to cervical neoplasia*.[62–65]

### IN UTERO DIETHYLSTILBESTROL EXPOSURE AND CERVICAL CANCER

A systematic follow-up of women who were exposed in utero to DES has revealed a higher incidence of cervical intraepithelial neoplasia among these women than among women unexposed to the drug.[66] The data are preliminary and need confirmation, but further support the belief that the uterine cervix is an endocrine target organ whose neoplastic potential may depend on hormonal influences.

## OTHER GYNECOLOGIC CANCERS AND EXOGENOUS SEX STEROIDS

The causal relationship between DES exposure in utero and the subsequent occurrence of *clear cell carcinomas of the vagina and cervix* is well established.[66a] This relationship was first observed in the early 1970s, and in the first directly observed estimate, the rate was reported as approximately one case per 1000 exposed female offspring.[52] An interesting feature of this malignancy is the incidence by age. The patients seem to be diagnosed primarily from preadolescence through 30 years of age. The slope of the attack rate curve is particularly steep from 11 through 20 years of age.[67] This implies that the onset of puberty is required for expression of the carcinogenic effect and may indicate a promotional role for endogenous hormones in completing the carcinogenic effect of DES.

Several studies have linked long-term use of oral contraceptives to increased risk of *trophoblastic disease* (see Chaps. 111 and 112), whereas others have suggested that such use may increase the risk of malignant sequelae after mole evacuation. Several other investigations[5] have failed to find these effects, however, so that this is an important area for future investigations designed to address these differences.

## MALE GENITAL CANCERS AND SEX STEROIDS

The roles of sex hormones in male genital cancers have not been well studied, but substantial reason exists to believe that hormonal factors do operate.

Because of its relative rarity, *testicular cancer* has not often been the subject of major analytic epidemiologic investigations (see Chap. 122). Studies of testicular cancer in relatively young men, and other studies of cryptorchidism (a major risk factor for this tumor), have implied that high levels of circulating estrogens (from either an endogenous or exogenous source) in a pregnant woman could place a male offspring exposed in utero at a high subsequent risk of these conditions.[68] These preliminary findings indicate the need for attention to hormonal risk factors for testicular cancer.

Although *prostate cancer* is a common malignancy among men in the United States, little is known with certainty about its etiology in humans. Many investigators hypothesize a hormonal influence based on the role of sex hormones in the development and maintenance of normal prostatic function, experimental evidence, the responsiveness of prostatic cancer to therapeutic hormonal manipulation, and limited clinical data. Some of the descriptive risk factors for this disease, including racial and ethnic variation, have also been speculated to operate through a hormonal mechanism. Prominent hormonal hypotheses[69–71] suggest an increased risk of prostatic cancer caused by increased levels of testosterone or dihydrotestosterone, increased levels of insulin-like growth factors, decreased levels of estrogen, increased levels of prolactin, differential activity of 5α-reductase, or some combination of these. Despite the frequency of the malignancy and the concerns over a hormonal etiology, few epidemiologic data exist to address these hypotheses. This lack of analytic studies stems partly from doubts that hormonal patterns in patients with prostatic cancer accurately reflect the premorbid patterns, and partly from the technical difficulties in assaying for the particular hormones of primary interest. Current enthusiasm for treatment of benign prostatic hypertrophy with finasteride, an inhibitor of 5α-reductase, should result in large groups of men with lowered levels of dihydrotestosterone and compensatory rises in testosterone; this may provide insights into the role of these hormones in prostate cancer etiology.

## LIVER CANCER AND SEX STEROIDS

Hormones have been linked to liver tumors in men and women. The androgenic-anabolic steroids and oral contraceptives have been implicated.

### ANDROGENIC-ANABOLIC STEROIDS AND LIVER CANCER

Androgenic-anabolic steroids in the form of oxymetholone or methyltestosterone derivatives were first linked to hepatocellular carcinoma by case reports[72] of patients undergoing long-term therapy for aplastic anemia. Patients with Fanconi anemia seemed to be at special risk, consistent with their heritable predisposition to acute leukemia and other cancers.[73] Liver tumors also have occurred when the steroids were used to treat conditions other than aplastic anemia, and some tumors have regressed on drug withdrawal. Although these findings are provocative, they are difficult to interpret because other risk factors for primary liver cancer, particularly the presence of hepatitis B virus, have not been evaluated in these studies, and these factors may be more common in these conditions. Resolution of these methodologic concerns was not important until the abuse of these androgenic drugs by body builders and other athletes became common (see Chap. 119).

### ORAL CONTRACEPTIVES AND BENIGN LIVER TUMORS

A number of clinical reports[74] describing the development of benign liver tumors in young women receiving oral contraceptives have appeared in the literature. These tumors were highly vascular and often presented as emergencies with abdominal hemorrhage and shock. Two analytic case-control studies[75,76] have linked these tumors to the use of oral contraceptives. The risk for users of 3 to 5 years was ~100 times that of nonusers, and the risk for users of 7 years or more was ~500 times that of nonusers. The risks also appear to be higher for users older than 30 years of age and for users of relatively high potency pills. Although the relative risk is high, the absolute risk is not large for this rare tumor. The risk of hepatocellular adenoma among women younger than 30 years of age may be no more than 3 in 100,000 contraceptive users per year. Over this age, the absolute risk probably is greater but has not been precisely estimated. A study concluded that these high relative risks are more likely related to the high-dose preparations used in the early years of oral contraception and that current dosage regimens are associated with substantially smaller increases in risk.[77]

### ORAL CONTRACEPTIVES AND LIVER CANCER

Because of the findings of these benign tumors and the role of the liver in metabolizing steroid hormones, much concern has been expressed over the potential for a relationship between oral contraceptive use and the risk of malignant liver tumors. Thus, the reports of a duration-related excess risk of this tumor with oral contraceptive use from six case-control investigations in the 1980s was further cause for substantial concern. The overall excesses were around 2.5-fold for women who had "ever used" oral contraceptives and more than nine-fold for long-term users.[78] All of these reports were from countries with low incidence rates of primary liver cancer and the number of cases in each study was limited, ranging from 12 to 26 patients. A study[79] in the United States

that included 76 women who died of this tumor has confirmed these excess risks. Two investigations[80,81] conducted in high-risk countries have not noted an excess risk with contraceptive use, but in each instance the numbers of long-term users were few.

## OTHER TUMORS

For some time, the speculation has been that endogenous hormones, particularly estrogens, might figure in the etiology of *malignant melanoma*. One follow-up study and one case-control study[82,83] conducted in the late 1970s implied that oral contraceptive users may be at 50% to 80% increased risk for this tumor. Partially because of the marked rise in incidence of malignant melanoma during the 1960s and 1970s, this finding caused considerable concern. Critical reviews noted the equally impressive rise in the incidence of skin melanoma among men and pointed out that the two positive studies had not obtained information on other possible risk factors that might be related to oral contraceptive use, particularly the duration of exposure to sunlight. Several investigations were launched to assess this issue. Although the results have been mixed, the level of concern has declined.

Also, in the late 1970s, reports were published of a number of clinical series of cases of pituitary adenoma among young women, a high proportion of whom had recently stopped using oral contraceptives. Subsequent investigations[84] have indicated that this association probably was not causal but reflected the increased use of computed tomography in detection of pituitary abnormalities among women with postcontraceptive menstrual disorders.

A number of other tumors have been suggested to be related to sex hormone levels because of a higher incidence among women than among men, a relationship to reproductive characteristics, or isolated observations of altered frequency among exogenous hormone users. In this category are cancers of the *gallbladder, thyroid, kidney, colon,* and *lung.* Most of the observations concerning cancers at these sites remain preliminary and speculative, but they clearly mark these tumors as candidates for more analytical assessments in the future.

## REFERENCES

1. International Agency for Research on Cancer. Evaluation of the carcinogenic risk of chemicals to man. In: Sex hormones, 2nd ed, vol 21. Lyon, France: IARC, 1979:11.
2. Bernstein L, Henderson BE. Exogenous hormones. In: Schottenfeld D, Fraumeni JF Jr, eds. Cancer epidemiology and prevention. New York: Oxford University Press, 1996:462
3. Johnson SR. Menopause and hormone replacement therapy. Med Clin North Am 1998; 82:297.
4. Barrett-Connor E, Grady D. Hormone replacement therapy, heart disease, and other considerations. Annu Rev Public Health 1998; 19:55.
5. Brinton LA, Hoover RN. Epidemiology of gynecologic cancers. In: Hoskins WJ, Perez CA, Young RC, eds. Principles and practice of gynecologic oncology. Philadelphia: Lippincott–Raven Publishers, 1997:3.
6. Armstrong BK. The role of diet in human carcinogenesis with special reference to endometrial cancer. In: Watson JD, Hiatt HH, Winsten JA, eds. Origins of human cancer. New York: Cold Spring Harbor Laboratory, 1977:557.
7. Ziel HK, Finkle WD. Increased risk of endometrial cancer among users of conjugated estrogens. N Engl J Med 1975; 293:1167.
8. Mack TM, Pike MC, Henderson BE, et al. Estrogens and endometrial cancer in a retirement community. N Engl J Med 1976; 294:1262.
9. Gray LA Sr, Christopherson WM, Hoover RN. Estrogens and endometrial carcinoma. Am J Obstet Gynecol 1977; 49:385.
10. Pike MC, Peters RK, Cozen W, et al. Estrogen-progestin replacement therapy and endometrial cancer. J Natl Cancer Inst 1997; 89:1110.
11. Green PK, Weiss NS, McKnight B, et al. Risk of endometrial cancer following cessation of hormone use. Cancer Causes Control 1996; 7:575.
12. Hulka BS, Fowler WC Jr, Kaufman DG, et al. Estrogen and endometrial cancer: cases and two control groups from North Carolina. Am J Obstet Gynecol 1980; 137:92.
13. Shapiro S, Kaufman DW, Slone D, et al. Recent and past use of conjugated estrogens in relation to adenocarcinoma of the endometrium. N Engl J Med 1980; 303:485.

14. Brinton LA, Hoover RN, et al. Estrogen replacement therapy and endometrial cancer risk: unresolved issues. Obstet Gynecol 1993; 81:265.
15. Whitehead MI, Townsend PT, Pryse-Davies J, et al. Effects of estrogen and progestins on the biochemistry and morphology of the postmenopausal endometrium. N Engl J Med 1981; 305:1599.
16. Persson I, Adami H-O, Bergkvist L, et al. Risk of endometrial cancer after treatment with estrogens alone or in conjunction with progestogens: results of a prospective study. BMJ 1989; 298:147.
17. Silverberg SG, Makowski EL. Endometrial carcinoma in young women taking oral contraceptive agents. Obstet Gynecol 1975; 46:503.
18. Weiss NS, Sayvetz TA. Incidence of endometrial cancer in relation to the use of oral contraceptives. N Engl J Med 1980; 302:551.
19. Kaufman DW, Shapiro S, Slone D, et al. Decreased risk of endometrial cancer among oral-contraceptives users. N Engl J Med 1980; 303:1045.
20. Hulka BS, Chambless LE, Kaufman DG, et al. Protection against endometrial carcinoma by combination-product oral contraceptives. JAMA 1982; 247:475.
21. Henderson BE, Casagrande JT, Pike MC, et al. The epidemiology of endometrial cancer in young women. Br J Cancer 1983; 47:749.
22. The Centers for Disease Control Cancer and Steroid Hormone Study. Oral contraceptive use and the risk of endometrial cancer. JAMA 1983; 249:1600.
23. Stanford JL, Brinton LA, Berman ML, et al. Oral contraceptives and endometrial cancer: do other risk factors modify the association? Int J Cancer 1993; 54:243.
24. Gangemi M, Meneghetti G, Dredebon O, et al. Obesity as a risk factor for endometrial cancer. Clin Exp Obstet Gynecol 1987; 14:119.
25. Fisher B, Costantino JP, Wickerham DL, et al. Tamoxifen for prevention of breast cancer: report of the National Surgical Adjuvant Breast and Bowel Project P-1 study. J Natl Cancer Inst 1998; 90:1371.
26. Hoover RN. Hormonal, infectious, and nutritional aspects of cancer of the female reproductive tract. In: Harris CC, ed. Biochemical and molecular epidemiology of cancer. New York: Alan R Liss, 1985:313.
27. Potischman N, Hoover RN, Brinton LA, et al. Case-control study of endogenous steroid hormones and endometrial cancer. J Natl Cancer Inst 1996; 88:1127.
28. Henderson BE, Pike MC, Ross RK. Breast cancer. In: Schottenfeld D, Fraumeni JF Jr, eds. Cancer epidemiology and prevention. New York: Oxford University Press, 1996:1022.
29. Tulinius H, Day NE, Johannesson G, et al. Reproductive factors and risk for breast cancer in Iceland. Int J Cancer 1978; 21:724.
30. Dupont WD, Page DL. Risk factors for breast cancer in women with proliferative breast disease. N Engl J Med 1985; 312:146.
31. Hunter DJ, Willett WC. Diet, body size, and breast cancer. Epidemiol Rev 1993; 15:110.
32. Ziegler RG, Hoover RN, Nomura AMY, et al. Relative weight, weight change, height, and breast cancer risk in Asian-American women. J Natl Cancer Inst 1996; 88:650.
33. Schatzkin A, Greenwald P, Byar DP, Clifford CK. The dietary fat–breast cancer hypothesis is alive. JAMA 1989; 261:3284.
34. Phillips RL, Garfinkel L, Kuzona JW, et al. Mortality among California Seventh-Day-Adventists for selected cancer sites. J Natl Cancer Inst 1980; 65:1097.
35. Kinlen LJ. Meat and fat consumption and cancer mortality: a study of strict religious orders in Britain. Lancet 1982; 1:946.
36. Jones DY, Schatzkin A, Green SB, et al. Dietary fat and breast cancer in the National Health and Nutrition Examination Survey I epidemiologic follow-up study. J Natl Cancer Inst 1987; 79:465
37. Holmes MD, Hunter DJ, Colditz GA, et al. Association of dietary intake of fat and fatty acids with risk of breast cancer. JAMA 1999; 281:914.
38. Key TA, Pike MC. The role of oestrogens and progestogens in the epidemiology and prevention of breast cancer. Eur J Cancer 1988; 24:29.
39. Sherman BM, Korenman SG. Inadequate corpus luteum function: a pathophysiological interpretation of human breast cancer epidemiology. Cancer 1974; 33:1306.
40. Cole P, MacMahon B. Oestrogen fractions during early reproductive life in the aetiology of breast cancer. Lancet 1969; 1:604.
41. Bradlow L, Telang NT, Osborn MP. Estrogen metabolites as bioreactive modulators of tumor initiators and promotors. Adv Exp Med Biol 1996; 387:285.
42. Reed MJ, Beranek PA, Cheng RW, et al. The distribution of oestradiol in plasma from postmenopausal women with or without breast cancer: relationships with metabolic clearance rates of oestradiol. Int J Cancer 1985; 35:457.
43. Dorgan JF, Longcope C, Stephenson HE Jr, et al. Serum sex hormone levels are related to breast cancer risk in postmenopausal women. Environ Health Perspect 1997; 105(Suppl 3):583.
44. Musey V, Collins DC, Musey PI, et al. Long-term effect of a first pregnancy on the secretion of prolactin. N Engl J Med 1987; 316:229.
45. Hankinson SE, Willett WC, Michand DS, et al. Plasma prolactin levels and subsequent risk of breast cancer in postmenopausal women. J Natl Cancer Inst 1999; 91:629.
46. Hoover RN, Gray LA, Cole P, MacMahon B. Menopausal estrogens and breast cancer. N Engl J Med 1976; 295:401.
47. Collaborative Group on Hormonal Factors in Breast Cancer. Breast cancer and hormone replacement therapy: collaborative reanalysis of data from 51 epidemiological studies of 52,705 women with breast cancer and 108,411 women without breast cancer. Lancet 1997; 350:1047.
48. Schairer C, Gail M, Byrne C, et al. Estrogen replacement therapy and breast cancer survival in a large screening study. J Natl Cancer Inst 1999; 91:264.
49. Bergkvist L, Adami H-O, Persson I, et al. The risk of breast cancer after estrogen and estrogen-progestin replacement. N Engl J Med 1989; 321:293.
50. Schairer C, Byrne C, Keyl PM, et al. Menopausal estrogen and estrogen-progestin replacement therapy and risk of breast cancer. Cancer Causes Control 1994; 5:491.
50a. Schairer C, Lubin J, Troisi R, et al. Menopausal estrogen and estrogen-progestin replacement therapy and breast cancer risk. JAMA 2000; 283:485.
50b. Willett WC, Colditz G, Stampfer M. Postmenopausal estrogens—opposed, unopposed, or none of the above. JAMA 2000; 283:534.
50c. Ross KK, Paganini-Hill A, Wan PC, Pike MC, et al. Effect of hormone replacement therapy on breast cancer risk: estrogen versus estrogen plus progestin. J Natl Cancer Inst 2000; 92:328.
51. DES Task Force. Report of the 1985 DES Task Force. Bethesda, MD: National Cancer Institute, 1985:1.
52. Hatch EE, Palmer JR, Titus-Ernstoff L, et al. Cancer risk in women exposed to diethylstilbestrol in utero. JAMA 1998; 280:630.
53. Collaborative Group on Hormonal Factors in Breast Cancer. Breast cancer and hormonal contraceptives: collaborative reanalysis of individual data on 53,297 women with breast cancer and 100,239 women without breast cancer from 54 epidemiological studies. Lancet 1996; 374:1713.
54. Spicer DV, Ursin G, Parisky YR, Pearace JG. Changes in mammographic densities induced by a hormonal contraceptive designed to reduce breast cancer risk. J Natl Cancer Inst 1994; 86:431.
55. Hoover R, Gray LA Sr, Fraumeni JF Jr. Stilbestrol (diethylstilbestrol) and the risk of ovarian cancer. Lancet 1977; 1:533.
56. Whittemore AS, Harris R, Itnyre J, et al. Characteristics relating to ovarian cancer risk: collaborative analysis of 12 U.S. case-control studies. Am J Epidemiol 1992; 136:1184.
57. Rossing MA, Daling JR, Weiss NS. Ovarian tumors in a cohort of infertile women. N Engl J Med 1994; 331:771.
58. Schiffman MH, Brinton LA, Devesa SS, Fraumeni JF Jr. Cervical cancer. In: Schottenfeld D, Fraumeni JF Jr, eds. Cancer epidemiology and prevention. New York: Oxford University Press, 1996:1090.
59. Schiffman MH, Bauer HM, Hoover RN, et al. Epidemiologic evidence showing that human papillomavirus infection causes most cervical intraepithelial neoplasia. J Natl Cancer Inst 1993; 85:958.
60. Brinton LA, Schairer C, Haenszel W, et al. Cigarette smoking and invasive cervical cancer. JAMA 1986; 255:3265.
61. Brinton LA, Reeves WC, Brenes MM, et al. Parity as a risk factor for cervical cancer. Am J Epidemiol 1989; 130:486.
62. World Health Organization Collaborative Study of Neoplasia and Steroid Contraceptives. Invasive cervical cancer and combined oral contraceptives. BMJ 1985; 290:961.
63. Brinton LA, Huggins GR, Lehman HF, et al. Long-term use of oral contraceptives and risk of invasive cervical cancer. Int J Cancer 1986; 38:339.
64. Bosch FX, Munoz N, DeSanjose S, et al. Risk factors for cervical cancer in Colombia and Spain. Int J Cancer 1992; 52:750.
65. Eluf-Neto J, Booth M, Munoz N. Human papillomavirus and invasive cervical cancer in Brazil. Br J Cancer 1994; 69:114.
66. Robboy SJ, Noller KL, O'Brien P, et al. Increased incidence of cervical and vaginal dysplasia in 3980 diethylstilbestrol-exposed young women. JAMA 1984; 252:2979.
66a. Herbst AL. Behavior of estrogen-associated female genital tract cancer and its relation to neoplasia following intrauterine exposure to diethylstilbestrol (DES). Gynecologic Oncology 2000; 76:147.
67. Herbst AL. Clear cell adenocarcinoma and the current status of DES-exposed females. Cancer 1981; 48:484.
68. Depue RH. Maternal and gestational factors affecting the risk of cryptorchidism and inguinal hernia. Int J Epidemiol 1984; 13:311.
69. Ross RK, Bernstein L, Lobo RA, et al. 5-Alpha-reductase activity and risk of prostate cancer among Japanese and U.S. white and black males. Lancet 1992; 339:887.
70. Ross RK, Schottenfeld D. Prostate cancer. In: Schottenfeld D, Fraumeni JF Jr, eds. Cancer epidemiology and prevention. New York: Oxford University Press, 1996:1180.
71. Chan JM, Stampfer MJ, Giovannucci E, et al. Plasma insulin-like growth factor-I and prostate cancer risk: a prospective study. Science 1998; 279:563.
72. Hoover R, Fraumeni JF Jr. Drug-induced cancer. Cancer 1981; 47:1071.
73. Okuyama S, Mishina H. Fanconi's anemia as nature's evolutionary experiment on carcinogenesis. Tohoku J Exp Med 1987; 153:87.
74. Baum JK, Holtz F, Bookstein JJ, Klein EW. Possible association between benign hepatomas and oral contraceptives. Lancet 1973; 2:926.
75. Edmondson HA, Henderson B, Benton B. Liver-cell adenomas associated with the use of oral contraceptives. N Engl J Med 1976; 294:470.
76. Rooks JB, Ory HW, Ishak KG, et al. Epidemiology of hepatocellular adenoma: the role of oral contraceptive use. JAMA 1979; 242:644.
77. Heinemann LA, Weimann A, Gerken G, et al. Modern oral contraceptive use and benign liver tumors: the German benign liver tumor case-control study. Eur J Contracept Reprod Health Care 1998; 3:194.
78. Prentice RL. Epidemiologic data on exogenous hormones and hepatocellular carcinoma and selected other cancers. Prev Med 1991; 20:38.
79. Hsing AW, Hoover RN, McLaughlin JK. Oral contraceptives and primary liver cancers among young women. Cancer Causes Control 1992; 3:43.
80. World Health Organization Collaborative Study of Neoplasia and Steroid Contraceptives. Combined oral contraceptives and liver cancer. Int J Cancer 1989; 43:254.
81. Kew MC, Song E, Mohammed A, Hodkinson J. Contraceptive steroids as a risk factor for hepatocellular carcinoma: a case/control study in South African black women. Hepatology 1990; 11:298.
82. Beral V, Ramcharan S, Faris R. Malignant melanoma and oral contraceptive use among women in California. Br J Cancer 1977; 36:804.
83. Holman CDJ, Armstrong BK, Heenan PJ. Cutaneous malignant melanoma in women: exogenous sex hormones and reproductive factors. Br J Cancer 1984; 50:673.
84. Pituitary Adenoma Study Group. Pituitary adenomas and oral contraceptives: a multicenter case-control study. Fertil Steril 1983; 39:752.

# CHAPTER 224

# ENDOCRINE TREATMENT OF BREAST CANCER

GABRIEL N. HORTOBAGYI

Breast cancer is the most common cancer in women in all the Western industrialized nations. In the United States, estimates are that 176,300 new cases of breast cancer are currently diagnosed, of which 1300 occur in men.[1] Worldwide, estimates were that close to 1 million new cases of breast cancer would be diagnosed in women in 1999. Epidemiologic studies have demonstrated major differences in the incidence of this disease in different countries, suggesting that genetic and environmental factors play an important role in its etiology.[2] The incidence of breast cancer has been increasing over the last three decades. Current projections indicate that one of every nine American women will develop this disease during her lifetime.

Estimates have been made that 43,300 women currently die of breast cancer in the United States, making this tumor the second most common cause of cancer death in women, exceeded only by lung cancer. Despite increasing incidence rates, death rates remained constant but have started to decrease since 1990.[3] The last several decades have witnessed substantial improvement in the understanding of the development and biology of this disease, and modern clinical trial methodology has led to improvements in early diagnosis and therapy.

## DIAGNOSIS, PATHOLOGY, AND STAGING

Most breast cancers diagnosed are in the form of a discrete mass. For this reason, regular physical examination of the breasts by primary physicians, as well as by men and women themselves, is an important diagnostic tool. Modern x-ray mammography, however, is the most sensitive diagnostic technique. It can detect tumor nodules as small as 3 to 5 mm (and, increasingly, even tumors at the noninvasive stage) by detecting microcalcifications or architectural distortions of the breast parenchyma. Used systematically in screening programs and combined with physical examination, x-ray mammography can detect most breast cancers in the earliest stages and can reduce the disease-specific death rate by 25% to 30%.[4]

Although multiple histologic types of breast cancer are found, *infiltrating ductal carcinoma*, not otherwise specified, is the most common (65%), followed by *infiltrating lobular carcinoma*. Several uncommon types also are seen that, together, represent <5% of breast malignancies.[5] The various subtypes of breast cancer have different biologic characteristics, including steroid-receptor content, cytokinetic properties, grade of differentiation, metastatic capability, and expression of growth factors and growth factor receptors. Stage by stage, the different histologic subtypes have varying prognoses after appropriate local or regional therapy.

The most widely accepted staging classification for breast cancer is the *Tumor/Node/Metastases (TNM) classification* proposed by the Union Internationale Contre le Cancer (UICC) and the American Joint Commission on Cancer.[6] With optimal therapy, estimates are that 10-year survival rates for patients with stages 0, I, II, III, and IV disease are 98%, 80%, 65%, 45%, and <5%, respectively. All patients with primary operable breast cancer (stage 0, I, or II) initially are treated surgically with either total mastectomy or wide excision with axillary dissection. For all patients with positive axillary lymph nodes and many without, primary treatment includes adjuvant systemic therapy and, in the case of partial mastectomy, radiotherapy.

## MECHANISM OF ACTION OF ENDOCRINE THERAPY

The influence of hormones in the etiology of breast cancer is described in Chapters 222 and 223. During the process of transformation, neoplasms derived from hormone-dependent tissues retain such hormonal dependency. Estimates are that 30% of breast carcinomas retain hormone dependence. Steroid hormone action is known to be mediated through specific receptors for estrogens, progesterone, androgens, and corticosteroids. Sixty percent to 80% of primary breast cancers contain high concentrations of *estrogen receptors*.[7] This percentage is substantially higher for male breast cancers. Although progression to metastatic and refractory disease is associated with a decrease in the percentage of receptor-positive tumors, most metastatic breast tumors still express steroid hormone receptors. A smaller proportion of breast cancers (45% to 60%) express *progesterone receptors,* and these usually are found in estrogen receptor–positive tumors. The presence of progesterone receptors is thought to represent an intact steroid hormonal pathway. *Androgen and corticosteroid receptors* are found in a smaller percentage of breast cancers, and their role in the cause and modulation of breast carcinoma is less well understood. Estrogens (and presumably other steroid hormones) stimulate the production of autocrine and paracrine growth factors by the tumor cells and surrounding stroma.[8] These growth factors, in turn, stimulate or inhibit the growth of the tumor and modulate its interactions with the stroma. Several excellent reviews have been published on this aspect of the pathophysiology of breast carcinoma.

Interference with any step of the hypothalamic–pituitary–gonadal–steroid receptor pathway can inhibit the growth and proliferation of hormone-dependent tumor cells and represents, in general terms, endocrine therapy.

### TYPES OF ENDOCRINE THERAPY

Endocrine interventions are frequently used for the treatment of primary and metastatic breast carcinoma in both men and women. Table 224-1 shows the various hormonal therapy options available. Endocrine therapy can be viewed as *interfering with the production of steroid hormones* (major ablative procedures, steroid synthesis inhibitors) or *interfering with hormonal action* (most "additive" therapies, including estrogens, selective estrogen-receptor modulators [SERMs] or antiestrogens, androgens, and progestins).

#### INTERFERENCE WITH STEROID HORMONE PRODUCTION

**Ovarian Ablation.** Ovarian ablation is the oldest form of endocrine therapy, first described in 1896. It remains an effective, although infrequently used, hormonal treatment for premenopausal women.[9] Ovarian ablation can be performed by surgical removal of the ovaries or by radiotherapy. The latter requires 2 to 3 months for maximal ablation of ovarian function, which is a disadvantage in the treatment of symptomatic patients. On the other hand, ovarian ablation by radiotherapy is noninvasive. Ovarian ablation produces major objective tumor regressions in one-third of unselected patients with metastatic breast cancer and in ~60% of those with tumors

**TABLE 224-1.**
**Hormonal Therapies for Metastatic Breast Cancer**

**INHIBITION OF ESTROGEN PRODUCTION**

*Ovarian ablation*
  Surgical oophorectomy
  Ovarian irradiation
*Inhibitors of pituitary function*
  LHRH analogs
    Leuprolide
    Buserelin
    Gonadorelin
    Goserelin*
*Aromatase inhibitors*
  Anastrozole*
  Letrozole
  Formestane (4-Hydroxyandrostenedione)
  Aminoglutethimide
  Exemestane
*Adrenal inhibitors*
  Aminoglutethimide*
  Trilostane
*Glucocorticoids*
  Prednisone*
  Dexamethasone
  Hydrocortisone
*Hormone withdrawal*
*Selective estrogen receptor modulators (antiestrogens)*
  Tamoxifen*
  Toremifene
  Raloxifene
  Trioxifene
  Droloxifene
  Keoxifene
  Zindoxifene
  ICI 164,384
  ICI 182,780
  Idoxifene
*Pharmacologic estrogen therapy*
  Ethinyl estradiol*
*Androgens*
  Fluoxymesterone*
  Testolactone
  Calusterone
*Progestins*
  Megestrol acetate*
  Medroxyprogesterone acetate

    *LHRH*, luteinizing hormone releasing hormone.
    *Most frequently used agent.

positive for estrogen receptors. The average duration of response is 1 year, although a few patients derive long-term benefits that last for several years. Over the short term, ovarian ablation is a safe, well-tolerated procedure. Acute side effects include hot flashes, alterations in mood, and other symptoms of estrogen deprivation. Long-term consequences include accelerated loss of bone mineral density and alterations in the blood lipid profile that indicate an increased risk of coronary artery disease.[10] Ovarian ablation has been largely displaced by the use of antiestrogens and gonadotropin-releasing hormone analogs.

In the United States, surgical ablation is preferred over radiotherapy. Since the appearance of antiestrogens, ovarian ablation has been used less commonly because its therapeutic effects are transient, whereas the estrogen deprivation it causes is permanent. Ovarian ablation is a cheap, safe, and effective procedure, however, and is a useful endocrine maneuver when questions exist about the possibility of close follow-up or of compliance with oral medication regimens.

**Surgical Adrenalectomy and Hypophysectomy.** Surgical adrenalectomy and hypophysectomy are of historical interest only, because these two major surgical ablative procedures are no longer performed for breast cancer therapy. Previously they had been used as second-line endocrine manipulations after ovarian ablation. They have been totally replaced by therapy with inhibitors of steroid synthesis and of aromatase. Their purpose was to eliminate adrenal steroidogenesis. After either procedure, lifetime mineralocorticoid and glucocorticoid replacement therapy was required. In addition, even in expert hands, both procedures were associated with a small, but definite, mortality rate.

**Medical Adrenalectomy.** Aminoglutethimide suppresses adrenal steroid synthesis by inhibiting the conversion of cholesterol to pregnenolone.[11] Administered at doses of 500 to 1000 mg per day orally, it also is a moderately effective aromatase inhibitor. Aminoglutethimide is effective in patients with absent or inactive ovaries. Because it also inhibits glucocorticoid synthesis, hydrocortisone replacement usually is administered to prevent the development of an adrenocorticotropic hormone override mechanism. Direct comparisons between aminoglutethimide therapy and surgical adrenalectomy have documented equivalence, at the very least, and even suggest a superiority for medical adrenalectomy.[12] Surgical adrenalectomy is associated with a small, but definite, mortality risk. Aminoglutethimide can be administered to any patient without risk of mortality.

The common side effects of aminoglutethimide therapy include nausea, somnolence, and a mucocutaneous rash (Table 224-2). Aminoglutethimide often was used as second- or third-line hormonal therapy before the advent of selective aromatase inhibitors for treatment of women after natural or iatrogenic menopause.

**Aromatase Inhibitors.** Aromatase is an enzyme complex consisting of a cytochrome P450 hemoprotein and a flavoprotein reduced nicotinamide-adenine dinucleotide phosphate (NADPH)–cytochrome P450 reductase.[12] It is needed for the 3-hydroxylation step in the conversion of androstenedione to estrone, and subsequently to estradiol at peripheral tissues. Aromatase is substantially concentrated in adipose and hepatic tissues. The enzyme has no effect on glucocorticoid, androgen, or mineralocorticoid production. Therefore, aromatase inhibition is applicable only to postmenopausal (or oophorectomized) women in whom estrogen production is predominantly from peripheral sources. Type 1 aromatase inhibitors are substrate analogs. With these agents, the enzyme binds covalently and irreversibly to the inhibitor. Type 2 inhibitors (such as aminoglutethimide) reversibly inhibit cytochrome P-450. Whereas suicide inhibitors are exclusively steroidal, competitive inhibitors need not be.

The first aromatase inhibitor discovered, aminoglutethimide, has a double mechanism of action: inhibition of the conversion of cholesterol to pregnenolone, and inhibition of androgens to estrogens by inhibition of aromatase. Because its aromatase-inhibiting activity is modest and it produces multiple side effects, it has been totally displaced by new aromatase inhibitors.[13]

TYPE 1 AROMATASE INHIBITORS. The earliest of the new inhibitors, *formestane* (or *4-hydroxyandrostenedione*), has no estrogenic properties and is rapidly metabolized by the liver.[14,15] By

TABLE 224-2.
Commonly Encountered Toxicity of Hormonal Therapies (Percentages)

| Toxic Effect/ Symptoms | SERMs | Progestins | Androgens | Aromatase Inhibitors | LHRH Analogs |
|---|---|---|---|---|---|
| Nausea | 10 | 11 | 18 | 10–16 | 5–19 |
| Vomiting | 10 | 5 | 11 | 10–12 | 5–19 |
| Anorexia | 1 | — | — | 7–9 | — |
| Diarrhea | — | — | — | 9 | 7 |
| Weight gain | 1 | 18 | 71 | 3–4 | — |
| Vaginal bleeding | 1 | 5–8 | — | 2–3 | 4–28 |
| Edema | 1 | 5–19 | 16 | 8–10 | 2 |
| Hypercalcemia | 4–3 | 5–10 | 10 | — | — |
| Hoarseness | — | — | 61 | — | — |
| Hirsutism | — | 1–5 | 52 | — | — |
| Baldness | <1 | Rare | 22 | — | — |
| Increased libido | — | — | 37 | — | — |
| Acne | — | <5 | 30 | — | — |
| Phlebitis | 1 | 2 | — | 0–3 | 1 |
| Hot flashes | 8 | 10 | — | 5–13 | 19–51 |
| Rash | 1–2 | 4 | — | 6–7 | 4 |
| Headache | 1–4 | Rare | — | 12–20 | 15 |
| Depression | 1–5 | 1 | — | — | — |
| Fatigue | 1–8 | Rare | — | 18 | — |
| Flare | 5–9 | — | 2–4 | — | 15 |
| Thrombocytopenia | 4–6 | Rare | — | — | — |
| Leukopenia | 1–6 | Rare | — | — | — |
| Amenorrhea | 25 | 37 | ? | — | 100 |
| Cushingoid facies | — | 1–12 | 2.8 | — | — |
| Hypertension | — | <1–3 | — | 3 | <1 |
| Muscle cramps | — | 3–16 | 1 | — | — |
| Perspiration | — | 5–17 | <1 | 2 | — |
| Dizziness | — | — | — | — | 9 |
| Ataxia | — | — | — | — | 25–75 |
| Endometrial cancer | 2.2* | <1 | — | — | — |

*SERMs*, selective estrogen-receptor modulators; *LHRH*, luteinizing hormone releasing hormone.

*Relative risk of developing toxicity after prolonged exposure, compared with patients not exposed to hormone.

(Modified from Hortobagyi GN, Dhingra K. Breast cancer. In: Mazzaferri EL, Samaan NA, eds. Endocrine tumors. Boston: Blackwell Scientific Publications, 1993:818.)

intramuscular administration, its half-life is 5 to 10 days. It has an excellent therapeutic index and requires no glucocorticoid replacement.

*Exemestane* is another type 1 steroidal inhibitor approved for this purpose. In clinical trials it was superior to megestrol acetate in second-line therapy. In addition, it shows no cross resistance with type II aromatase inhibitors.[15a]

The primary action of *trilostane* is aromatase inhibition, but it also inhibits the 3β-hydroxysteroid dehydrogenase. Its level of activity is similar to that of aminoglutethimide. However, this drug also causes nausea, vomiting, lethargy, and diarrhea, side effects that result in poorer tolerance than of 4-hydroxyandrostenedione.

TYPE 2 AROMATASE INHIBITORS. Two type 2 aromatase inhibitors are available: anastrozole and letrozole.[16,17] Both agents have excellent antitumor activity and an excellent tolerance profile, similar to that of the SERMs. Both anastrozole and letrozole have greater efficacy, in terms of higher response rates and longer survival, than does megestrol acetate.[18] In one randomized trial, letrozole showed similar superiority over aminoglutethimide. Based on these results, anastrozole and letrozole

have replaced the progestins and aminoglutethimide in the second-line treatment of metastatic breast cancer. Both agents are currently under evaluation for first-line treatment of metastatic breast cancer and are being compared with tamoxifen as adjuvant agents for treatment of primary breast cancer. *Fadrozole* demonstrated antitumor efficacy similar to that of established aromatase inhibitors or other hormonal agents.[19] It is well tolerated, although nausea, vomiting, anorexia, headache, rash, and other minor adverse effects have been reported. *Pyridoglutethimide* is an aminoglutethimide analog with encouraging preliminary results in early clinical trials. Neither of these latter two drugs will undergo additional development, however. The major advantage of the selective aromatase inhibitors over their predecessors is a better therapeutic index.

**Inhibitors of Pituitary Function.** *Luteinizing hormone-releasing hormone (LHRH) agonists (buserelin, goserelin, leuprolide)* produce long-lasting inhibition of luteinizing hormone and follicle-stimulating hormone release after a transient initial increase. Their action also could be described as pharmacologic ovarian ablation, because they inhibit ovarian estradiol release by ~90%.[20,21] In addition, some authors have hypothesized that LHRH analogs may have direct effects on breast cancer cells; however, this action remains speculative. LHRH analogs are primarily effective in premenopausal women. Ten percent or fewer of postmenopausal women respond to this therapy. LHRH analogs also are effective in male breast cancer.

## INTERFERENCE WITH HORMONAL ACTION

The endocrine therapies described in this section act not by inhibiting or preventing hormonal production or release but by interfering with the effects of hormones on the end organ (i.e., the breast cancer cell).

**Selective Estrogen-Receptor Modulators (Antiestrogens).** Antiestrogens initially were developed in the search for better contraceptives.[22] Although their efficacy as antifertility drugs was limited, they were found to cause regression of breast cancer cells. Tamoxifen is known to bind competitively to the estrogen receptor, but it also has multiple additional effects on the cancer cell.[23] It can lower the production of insulin-like growth factor-I and transforming growth factor-α; it blocks angiogenesis and induces the production of transforming growth factor-β, calmodulin, and protein kinase C. It also has been reported to increase natural killer cell activity. Tamoxifen has a multitude of actions, all of which affect breast cancer cells unfavorably. Clinical trials have demonstrated that tamoxifen, administered orally at 20 to 40 mg on a daily basis, produces tumor regression of established metastatic breast cancer in ~30% of unselected patients and in 50% to 60% of patients with estrogen receptor–positive tumors. The responses last 12 months, on average. In addition, another 20% to 30% of women have stable disease for periods that exceed 3 to 6 months and, in some cases, even longer. Because tamoxifen has excellent tolerance, it has become the front-line hormonal treatment of choice for untreated metastatic breast cancer. No apparent dose-response correlation exists for tamoxifen, and the drug has been administered safely for periods that exceed 5 years. In a small percentage of patients (<10%), an initial, short-lasting *tumor flare* may occur, starting within the first week or two of administration of this agent. This may be manifested as increased bone pain, development of hypercalcemia, and, occasionally, even a slight increase in tumor dimensions. Flare usually predicts response to therapy, and close follow-up with active symptomatic support is appropriate. If tumor flare symptoms appear late (>3 weeks after initiation of therapy), they represent progression of disease and should prompt the discontinuation of tamoxifen and a change in therapy.

Tamoxifen is a mixed estrogen agonist and antagonist. The tumor flare reaction probably is secondary to its agonist activity. Other agonist effects of tamoxifen include the preservation or enhancement of bone mineral density, a decrease in cholesterol level, and additional modifications of the serum lipid profile that may lead to a reduction in the risk of coronary artery disease. Tamoxifen also has been associated with endometrial hyperplasia, an increased frequency of ovarian cysts, and an apparent increased incidence of endometrial carcinomas.

Several new SERMs have been extensively tested. Toremifene is approved for the management of metastatic, estrogen receptor–positive breast cancer, whereas raloxifene was approved for the prevention of osteoporosis.[24,25] Both agents are under additional evaluation in comparison with tamoxifen in randomized clinical trials. Other SERMs (idoxifene, droloxifene, etc.) are under development. These agents, however, appear to be no more effective, nor less toxic, than tamoxifen.

Tamoxifen has been compared in randomized clinical trials to oophorectomy, adrenalectomy, and the use of megestrol acetate, aminoglutethimide, estrogens, and other hormonal agents in the treatment of breast cancer. In all trials, tamoxifen has had at least equivalent efficacy and less toxicity than the other hormonal treatments under study.[9]

**Estrogens.** Second to ovarian ablation, estrogens probably are the oldest form of hormonal therapy. Estrogens are thought to act through the estrogen-receptor mechanism, and their antitumor efficacy is similar to that described for tamoxifen. Common side effects include nausea, vomiting, fluid retention, increased risk of thrombotic phenomena, tumor flare, urinary incontinence, and vaginal bleeding. When compared with tamoxifen, estrogens were found to be more toxic and less well tolerated, but they are also less expensive than tamoxifen and several of the other modern hormonal therapies. They were used as the first modality of hormonal therapy for postmenopausal women for many years but were displaced by SERMs and aromatase inhibitors.

**Progestins.** The development of new synthetic progestational agents led to their evaluation for the treatment of breast cancer.[9,26] Numerous clinical trials demonstrated that these agents are effective in producing tumor regression in 20% to 40% of patients with metastases and, in general, are well tolerated. In the United States, the most commonly used progestational agent for this purpose is megestrol acetate, whereas in Europe and South America, it is medroxyprogesterone acetate. Other progestational agents are of historical interest only. Although responses to progestin therapy correlate with estrogen-receptor content, no evidence exists that progesterone-receptor content is a better predictor of response for this group of agents than for other hormonal treatments. Toxicity is clearly dose related. At high doses, substantial weight gain, fluid retention, and other toxicities become prominent. Some studies have suggested that higher doses of progestins are more effective in the treatment of breast cancer than are lower doses, but controversy is ongoing about this dose-response correlation. At low doses, the efficacy and tolerance of progestins appear to be similar to those of tamoxifen. Based on these studies, progestins were used as first-line or second-line therapy for metastatic breast cancer until they were rapidly displaced by selective aromatase inhibitors.

High-dose progestins also have been used for palliative treatment of patients with advanced cancer, in whom anorexia, weight loss, and a decreasing sense of well-being all can be reversed by the administration of these agents.

**Androgens.** Androgen therapy also is an effective approach to the endocrine treatment of breast cancer, but the virilizing effects make it intolerable to many women. Newer semisynthetic testosterone derivatives, such as fluoxymesterone and danazol, are better tolerated, with fewer virilizing effects. Nevertheless, with long-term therapy, all these agents can produce hirsutism, deepening of the voice, clitoral hypertrophy, male pattern alopecia, and increased libido. Like other hormonal agents, androgens also can cause tumor flare. Androgens are generally considered somewhat less effective than other additive hormonal therapies, such as antiestrogens and progestins.[26] Although this is not clearly established, the therapeutic index of the new antiestrogens, aromatase inhibitors, and LHRH analogs is clearly superior to that of androgens. Androgens, like estrogens, can be valuable therapeutic tools when cost is an important consideration, and especially when good tolerance can be established in an individual patient.

**Corticosteroids.** The antitumor efficacy of corticosteroids is poorly documented for metastatic breast cancer but is considered to be ~10%. In some trials, no antitumor activity has been documented. More importantly, the long-term administration of glucocorticoids is associated with potentially severe and intolerable side effects. Therefore, glucocorticoids are not recommended as antitumor agents for breast cancer.

Glucocorticoids, however, have a specific role in the management of well-defined complications of breast cancer. High-dose glucocorticoid therapy is administered for short periods to patients with central nervous system metastases and for spinal cord compression, and some experts also use it during the management of acute hypercalcemia of malignancy. Its antiemetic effects are also well known.

**Antiandrogens.** *Flutamide* and *cyproterone acetate* have been evaluated in a few clinical trials. Their efficacy against metastatic breast cancer appears limited. At this point, these agents have no role in the standard treatment of breast carcinoma.

**Antiprogestins.** *Mifepristone* (RU-486) has had limited evaluation in treatment of metastatic breast cancer. Although antitumor activity has been demonstrated, the drug also is accompanied by antiglucocorticoid activity, which limits its long-term administration. Newer antiprogestins with limited or no antiglucocorticoid effects are being developed.

**Hormone Withdrawal.** After the administration of estrogens, androgens, and antiestrogens, withdrawal of the hormonal agent on the appearance of progressive disease can induce an (additional) objective regression of tumor deposits.[9] The mechanism of this phenomenon is poorly understood, although laboratory experiments with tamoxifen have suggested that, after long-term suppression of breast cancer cell lines by this agent, some cells become dependent on (or stimulated by) continued exposure to tamoxifen.[27] If, at the time of tumor progression, tamoxifen is removed, a secondary inhibition of these tumor cells can be observed. The hormone withdrawal response has been poorly documented in the literature and is based mostly on retrospective reports that suggest a frequency of 10% to 20%; however, its occurrence is considered real by most experts. In at least one prospective trial of tamoxifen withdrawal, up to 40% of patients progressing on tamoxifen had a response or prolonged stability after antiestrogen withdrawal.[28] Importantly, a hormone withdrawal response is reported almost exclusively in patients with an intervening response to hormonal therapy. The occurrence of a hormone withdrawal response after clear hormonal therapy failure is negligible. For patients with indolent metastatic disease, especially those who have no symptoms at the time of secondary progression after an intervening response to additive hormonal therapy, a period of 2 or 3 months of observation to detect a hormone withdrawal response might be appropriate.

**Combination Hormonal Therapy.**    Many attempts have been made to combine hormonal therapies for breast cancer, based on the hypothesis that blocking different pathways of the hypothalamic–hypophysial–gonadal–breast cell pathway may produce a more complete hormonal blockade and, therefore, increase therapeutic efficacy. Although initial reports regarding the addition of corticosteroids to oophorectomy or tamoxifen suggested a higher response rate, these results could not be confirmed by larger prospective, randomized trials. Higher response rates have been reported when fluoxymesterone was added to tamoxifen. A few preliminary reports of prospective randomized trials strongly suggest that combinations of newer hormonal agents (LHRH analogs) with tamoxifen might be more effective than either agent alone.[29,30] The mature results of these trials are awaited with interest. Until then, no role exists for the routine use of combined hormonal therapy for the treatment of primary or metastatic breast cancer.

## COMBINED HORMONAL THERAPY AND CHEMOTHERAPY

Metastatic breast cancer is moderately sensitive to cytotoxic therapy. More than 40 individual agents have demonstrated therapeutic efficacy, producing 20% to 50% objective regression rates. Because hormonal therapy and cytotoxic therapy are thought to act by different mechanisms, and because the two modalities produce different patterns of toxicity, the hypothesis was raised that their combined use might result in enhanced therapeutic efficacy without increased toxicity. Numerous prospective randomized trials have been conducted using a combination of simultaneous chemotherapy and hormonal therapy.[31,32] In most cases, the hormonal agent was either ovarian ablation (or LHRH analogs) or tamoxifen, although several trials used progestins or androgens. Some of these trials showed increased response rates, and a few demonstrated a slight prolongation of response duration. None of them, however, demonstrated an increase in median survival or in long-term survival in patients with metastatic breast cancer. Based on these results, the *sequential* use of hormonal therapy and chemotherapy is considered the optimal way to provide palliative therapy to patients with metastatic breast cancer.

The consensus of the oncology community on this combination is clearly different in the adjuvant setting (see later).

## HORMONAL THERAPY FOR MALE BREAST CANCER

As noted earlier, breast cancer is more often hormone receptor–positive in men than in women. This also has been confirmed clinically by the more frequent observation of responses to hormonal therapy in men than in women.[33,34] Gonadal ablation (orchiectomy) has demonstrated efficacy against metastatic breast cancer and, until the appearance of tamoxifen and other SERMs, was the hormonal therapy of choice. Orchiectomy has been reported to produce overall response rates of 30% to 80% in men with metastatic breast cancer. The median duration of response after orchiectomy was 22 months in one collective series, which is almost twice as long as for women treated with ovarian ablation. Adrenalectomy also has been used in men with breast cancer, with a high response rate and response duration. As in women with breast cancer, however, adrenalectomy has been displaced by noninvasive hormonal manipulations.

Tamoxifen is the hormonal treatment of choice for male breast cancer. More than 50% of unselected patients with metastatic breast cancer respond, as do 80% of patients with estrogen receptor–positive tumors. The experience with other SERMs in male breast cancer is quite limited. Other hormonal agents with demonstrated efficacy against metastatic breast cancer in men are progestins, aminoglutethimide, estrogens, and antiandrogens. Anecdotal reports have shown antitumor activity of androgens and corticosteroids in men with breast cancer. However, these reports are based on only a few patients. Combined hormonal therapy has not been extensively evaluated in males.

## OPTIMAL SEQUENCING OF HORMONAL TREATMENTS

Patients with metastatic breast cancer often respond to more than one hormonal manipulation. Evidently, no complete cross-resistance exists between the various endocrine interventions in use today. Consequently, sequential hormonal manipulations have been successful in offering quality palliation for these patients.

Table 224-3 documents the recommended sequence of hormonal treatments. For *premenopausal* women, tamoxifen, toremifene, or ovarian ablation appears to be the treatment of choice. LHRH analogs can substitute for ovarian ablation. The selection between these two modalities depends on patient pref-

**TABLE 224-3.**
**Optimal Sequence of Hormonal Therapies**

| | Premenopausal | | | | Postmenopausal |
|---|---|---|---|---|---|
| **FIRST LINE** | **SERM** (or oophorectomy or LHRH analog) | → | If no response ↓↓↓↓ | ← | **SERM** (or aromatase inhibitor) ↓ |
| | If response ↓↓ | | | | If response ↓ |
| **SECOND LINE** | **LHRH analog** (or oophorectomy, or SERM) | → | If no response ↓↓↓↓ | ← | **Aromatase inhibitor** (or SERM or hormone withdrawal or megestrol acetate) ↓ |
| | If response ↓↓ | | | | |
| **THIRD LINE** | **Megestrol acetate** (or androgens) | → | If no response ↓↓↓↓ Chemotherapy | ← | **Megestrol acetate** (or androgens) |

*SERM*, selective estrogen-receptor modulator; *LHRH*, luteinizing hormone releasing hormone.

erence, cost, possibility of follow-up, and predicted compliance with treatment.

After an intervening response to tamoxifen, ovarian ablation can be an effective second-line therapy. Conversely, after an objective response to ovarian ablation, tamoxifen can be an effective second-line regimen. As an alternative, progestins can serve as second-line or third-line therapy or, after ovarian ablation, selective aromatase inhibitors also might serve this purpose. Androgens can be used as third-line or fourth-line treatment for premenopausal patients.

For *postmenopausal* patients, either antiestrogens (SERMs) or selective aromatase inhibitors are the hormonal therapy of choice. Either of these agents also can serve as effective second-line therapy after the other, whereas progestins are usually reserved for third-line hormonal treatment.

Formerly these hormonal manipulations were generally accepted to have equal efficacy. However, clinical trials demonstrate the therapeutic superiority of aromatase inhibitors over progestins and aminoglutethimide. Therefore, the selection of hormonal therapy or the sequence of administration of hormonal therapies is now based not only on the *toxicity profile* of the various treatments but also on a rational ranking by efficacy (see Table 224-2).

## SELECTION OF THERAPY FOR METASTATIC BREAST CANCER

Patients with newly developed metastatic breast cancer are evaluated to assess the probability of short-term catastrophic complications or severe symptoms (bone fractures, spinal cord compression, hepatic or pulmonary failure). This evaluation is based on the location and extent of metastatic lesions, the duration of the disease-free interval (the interval between initial diagnosis and first evidence of metastases), the number of years since menopause, the tumor's estrogen-receptor or progesterone-receptor status, and the patient's overall general condition. For patients at low risk for catastrophic complications, hormonal therapy is usually the treatment of choice and should be instituted (see Table 224-3).[35] If an initial response occurs to hormonal therapy, then sequential hormonal therapy should be administered until breast cancer becomes clearly hormone refractory. At that time, combination chemotherapy and comprehensive supportive care should be introduced.

For all other patients, combination chemotherapy is the initial treatment of choice. Although some of these patients might benefit from hormonal therapy, this usually is reserved for the time when the probability of response to chemotherapy declines, and hormonal therapy becomes a reasonable or equivalent choice.

## ADJUVANT HORMONAL THERAPY

Over the last 20 years, adjuvant systemic therapy has come to be considered an integral and necessary part of the comprehensive treatment of primary breast cancer. Based on individual prospective, randomized trials and on a metaanalysis of the world literature, three modalities of adjuvant systemic treatment have been shown to improve disease-free and overall survival rates at 5, 10, and 15 years after diagnosis: *adjuvant SERM (antiestrogen) therapy*,[36] adjuvant ovarian ablation,[37] and *adjuvant chemotherapy*.[38] The world overview included >220,000 women evaluated and treated in >405 clinical trials. An in-depth statistical analysis of these data indicated that adjuvant antiestrogen therapy reduced annual recurrence rates by ~26.4% and annual mortal-

ity rates by ~14.5%. A somewhat greater reduction was seen for node-positive breast cancer, and a more modest one for node-negative tumors. Additional analyses of the data showed no evidence of a dose-response rate with tamoxifen, but did suggest that the duration of administration of adjuvant tamoxifen was critical for optimal results and that the extent of benefit was directly proportional to the duration of administration of treatment. Indirect comparisons from the world overview and direct comparisons of shorter versus longer duration of therapy in prospective randomized clinical trials have demonstrated that administration of tamoxifen for 5 years resulted in a 43% reduction in odds of recurrence and a 23% reduction in odds of death. This would translate into a 15.2% absolute reduction in recurrences and a 10.9% absolute reduction in deaths for lymph node–positive patients.[36] The results with 5 years of tamoxifen therapy were similar for younger and older women, contrary to earlier observations with short-term use (1–2 years) of tamoxifen. In addition, in terms of both recurrence and mortality rates, the efficacy of adjuvant tamoxifen was directly proportional to the estrogen-receptor content of the tumor. Women with estrogen receptor–negative tumors fail to benefit from adjuvant tamoxifen therapy. Adjuvant tamoxifen also has been correlated with a 39% *decrease in the incidence of contralateral* breast cancers and with a 12% decrease in deaths not related to breast cancer, especially cardiovascular deaths. Although toremifene is under evaluation in clinical trials of adjuvant therapy, no information is yet available on its therapeutic index for this indication.

The proportional reduction in annual odds of recurrence after adjuvant polychemotherapy was 35% for women younger than age 50, and 20% for those aged 50 to 69 in one metaanalysis. The corresponding proportional reductions in odds of death were 27% and 11%, respectively.[38] The proportional reductions were similar for women with node-positive and node-negative tumors. The benefits from chemotherapy were independent of hormone-receptor status.

The third world overview provided evidence to support the hypothesis that adding chemotherapy to tamoxifen treatment, or tamoxifen treatment to chemotherapy, improved the therapeutic efficacy of adjuvant systemic treatments in women younger than 50 years. For women older than 50 years, the evidence in favor of combined tamoxifen and combination chemotherapy has been shown to be even stronger.[38] The increased benefit from combined chemotherapy and hormonal therapy applies to women with hormone receptor–positive tumors.

Adjuvant ovarian ablation has undergone limited evaluation. The data available show that this approach resulted in a substantial decrease in the odds of recurrence and death at 5, 10, and 15 years after diagnosis.[37] In relative terms, the benefit from ovarian ablation for premenopausal patients appeared similar to the benefit obtained with combination chemotherapy in the same group of patients. In the only direct comparison performed, however, patients with estrogen receptor–positive tumors had greater benefit from ovarian ablation than from CMF (cyclophosphamide, methotrexate, 5-fluorouracil) therapy, whereas the opposite results were observed in patients with estrogen receptor–negative tumors.[39] Table 224-4 outlines the current recommendations for selecting the appropriate adjuvant systemic therapy, based on the data obtained thus far.

## ADJUVANT SYSTEMIC THERAPY FOR MALE BREAST CANCER

No controlled trials have been conducted for male breast cancer because of the rarity of this malignancy. However, reports

## TABLE 224-4.
## Selection of Adjuvant Therapies for Patients with Primary Breast Cancer

| Patient Characteristics | Estrogen-Receptor Status | |
|---|---|---|
| | *Positive* | *Negative* |
| **Age younger than 50 years** | | |
| *NODE NEGA-TIVE* | | |
| <1 cm | No therapy or tamoxifen | No therapy or chemotherapy |
| ≥1 cm | Tamoxifen or ovarian ablation or chemotherapy + tamoxifen | Chemotherapy |
| *NODE POSI-TIVE* | Chemotherapy + tamoxifen | Chemotherapy |
| **Age older than 50 years** | | |
| *NODE NEGA-TIVE* | | |
| <1 cm | No therapy or tamoxifen | No therapy or chemotherapy |
| ≥1 cm | Tamoxifen or chemotherapy + tamoxifen | Chemotherapy |
| *NODE POSI-TIVE* | Chemotherapy + tamoxifen | Chemotherapy |

based on retrospective evaluation of patient groups treated with either adjuvant chemotherapy or adjuvant hormonal therapy have been published.[33] Comparison with historical controls suggested that adjuvant CMF therapy, adjuvant CAF or FAC (cyclophosphamide, Adriamycin [doxorubicin], 5-fluorouracil) therapy, and adjuvant tamoxifen therapy produced a distinct reduction in the odds of recurrence and death for men with breast cancer. No reports have been published concerning the efficacy of adjuvant orchiectomy or other hormonal manipulations in male breast cancer.

### CHEMOPREVENTION TRIALS

On the basis of the marked reduction in the incidence of second primary or contralateral breast cancers observed in patient groups who received adjuvant tamoxifen therapy,[36] and because of the extensive preclinical and epidemiologic evidence implicating estrogens in the etiology of breast cancer, several prospective clinical trials were initiated to determine whether administration of an antiestrogen (or SERM) can reduce the incidence of breast cancer in high-risk groups of women. The group from the Royal Marsden Hospital (London) conducted an 8-year feasibility trial with 2000 women randomized to tamoxifen or placebo. This trial demonstrated the overall feasibility of such a trial, as well as the good tolerance and virtual absence of life-threatening toxicities.[40] A somewhat larger trial involving average-risk women who had also undergone a hysterectomy was completed in Italy.[41] To date, no significant differences have been detected. The National Surgical Adjuvant Breast and Bowel Project (NSABP) reported the initial results of a randomized clinical trial in which >13,300 high-risk women received 5 years of treatment with either placebo or tamoxifen.[42] After a mean follow-up of 4 years, a 49% reduction was seen in the incidence of breast carcinomas in the tamoxifen group. This reduction was observed in all age groups and included both invasive and noninvasive breast cancers. Osteoporotic fractures were also reduced; in exchange, an increase was seen in the incidence of endometrial cancers and thromboembolic events. This seminal trial opened the doors for additional trials of chemopre-

vention and provided support for the first effective preventive intervention for breast cancer in high-risk women. Simultaneously, a large randomized trial of raloxifene therapy for women at high risk of osteoporosis showed a similar reduction in the incidence of breast cancer.[43] These data suggested that SERMs were effectively reducing the incidence of breast cancer. A second randomized NSABP trial comparing 5 years of tamoxifen therapy with administration of raloxifene (a SERM with antiestrogenic effects on the endometrium) has started patient accrual.

### CONCLUSION

The rapid expansion of our knowledge of the complex biology of breast cancer and the integration of hormonal effects, growth factors, signal transduction, and growth inhibition of complex feedback loops have led to the development of the first steps in biologic therapy and to the promise that systemic therapy for breast cancer will change substantially in the coming years. Because growth stimulatory and growth inhibitory factors appear to be partially under hormonal control, systemic treatments based on the modulation of growth factor activity are currently being tested. These developments may provide a better understanding of this complex disease and tools for its more effective treatment.

### REFERENCES

1. Landis SH, Murray T, Bolden S, Wingo PA. Cancer statistics, 1999. CA Cancer J Clin 1999; 49:8.
2. Miller AB. Breast cancer epidemiology, etiology, and prevention. In: Harris JR, Hellman S, Henderson IC, Kinne DW, eds. Breast diseases. Philadelphia: JB Lippincott, 1987:87.
3. Chu KC, Tarone RE, Kessler LG, et al. Recent trends in U.S. breast cancer incidence, survival, and mortality rates. J Natl Cancer Inst 1996; 88:1571.
4. Kerlikowske K, Grady D, Rubin SM, et al. Efficacy of screening mammography. A meta-analysis [see comments]. JAMA 1995; 273:149.
5. Fisher ER, Gregorio RM, Fisher B, et al. The pathology of invasive breast cancer. Cancer 1975; 36:1.
6. Fleming ID, Cooper JS, Henson DE, et al. AJCC cancer staging manual, 5th ed. Philadelphia: Lippincott–Raven Publishers, 1997.
7. Jordan VC. Studies on the estrogen receptor in breast cancer—20 years as a target for the treatment and prevention of cancer. Breast Cancer Res Treat 1995; 36:267.
8. Lippman ME, Dickson RB. Growth control of normal and malignant breast epithelium. In: Ragaz J, Simpson-Herren L, Lippman ME, Fisher B, eds. Effects of therapy on biology and kinetics of the residual tumor, part A: preclinical aspects. New York: Wiley-Liss, 1990:147.
9. Buzdar AU, Hortobagyi G. Update on endocrine therapy for breast cancer. (Review). Clin Cancer Res 1998; 4:527.
10. Oliver MF, Boyd GS. Effect of bilateral ovariectomy on coronary-artery disease and serum-lipid levels. Lancet 1959; ii:690.
11. Santen RJ, Worgul TJ, Lipton A, et al. Aminoglutethimide as treatment of postmenopausal women with advanced breast carcinoma. Ann Intern Med 1982; 96:94.
12. Harris AL. Could aminoglutethimide replace adrenalectomy? (Review). Breast Cancer Res Treat 1985; 6:201.
13. Ibrahim NK, Buzdar AU. Aromatase inhibitors: current status. (Review). Am J Clin Oncol 1995; 18:407.
14. Brodie AMH. Aromatase inhibitors in the treatment of breast cancer. J Steroid Biochem Mol Biol 1994; 49:281.
15. Dowsett M, Mehta A, King N, et al. An endocrine and pharmacokinetic study of four oral doses of formestane in postmenopausal breast cancer patients. Eur J Cancer 1992; 28:415.
15a. Kaufmann M, Bajetta E, Dirix LY, et al. Exemestane is superior to megestrol acetate after tamoxifen failure in postmenopausal women with advanced breast cancer: results of a phase III randomized double-blind trial. The Exemestane Study Group. J Clin Oncol 2000; 18:1399.
16. Hortobagyi GN, Buzdar AU. Anastrozole (Arimidex), a new aromatase inhibitor for advanced breast cancer: mechanism of action and role in management. (Review). Cancer Invest 1998; 16:385.
17. New aromatase inhibitors for breast cancer. (Review). Drug Ther Bull 1997; 35:55.
18. Buzdar AU, Jonat W, Howell A, et al. Anastrozole versus megestrol acetate in the treatment of postmenopausal women with advanced breast carci-

noma: results of a survival update based on a combined analysis of data from two mature phase III trials. Arimidex Study Group. Cancer 1998; 83:1142.

19. Raats JI, Falkson G, Falkson HC. A study of fadrozole, a new aromatase inhibitor, in postmenopausal women with advanced metastatic breast cancer. J Clin Oncol 1992; 10:111.

20. Taylor CW, Green S, Dalton WS, et al. Multicenter randomized clinical trial of goserelin versus surgical ovariectomy in premenopausal patients with receptor-positive metastatic breast cancer: an intergroup study. J Clin Oncol 1998; 16:994.

21. Nicholson RI, Walker KJ, Walker RF, et al. Review of the endocrine actions of luteinising hormone-releasing hormone analogues in premenopausal women with breast cancer. Horm Res 1989; 32(Suppl 1):198.

22. Lerner LJ, Jordan VC. Development of antiestrogens and their use in breast cancer: eighth Cain Memorial Award lecture. (Review). Cancer Res 1990; 50:4177.

23. MacGregor JI, Jordan VC. Basic guide to the mechanisms of antiestrogen action. [Review]. Pharmacological Reviews 1998; 50:151.

24. Buzdar AU, Hortobagyi GN. Tamoxifen and toremifene in breast cancer: comparison of safety and efficacy. (Review). J Clin Oncol 1998; 16:348.

25. Delmas PD, Bjarnason NH, Mitlak BH, et al. Effects of raloxifene on bone mineral density, serum cholesterol concentrations, and uterine endometrium in postmenopausal women [see comments]. N Engl J Med 1997; 337:1641.

26. Pritchard KI. Endocrine therapy for breast cancer. [Review] [53 refs]. Oncology (Huntington) 2000; 14:483.

27. Gottardis MM, Jordan VC. Development of tamoxifen-stimulated growth of mcf-7 tumors in athymic mice after long-term antiestrogen administration. Cancer Res 1988; 48:5183.

28. Taylor SG, Gelman RS, Falkson G, Cummings FJ. Combination chemotherapy compared to tamoxifen as initial therapy for stage IV breast cancer in elderly women. Ann Intern Med 1986; 104:455.

29. Klijn JG, Beex LV, Mauriac L, et al. Combined treatment with buserelin and tamoxifen in premenopausal metastatic breast cancer: a randomized study. J Natl Cancer Inst 2000; 92:903.

30. Buzzoni R, Biganzoli L, Bajetta E, et al. Combination goserelin and tamoxifen therapy in premenopausal advanced breast cancer: a multicentre study by the ITMO group. Italian Trials in Medical Oncology. Br J Cancer 1995; 71:1111.

31. Buzdar AU. Combined chemohormonal therapy for metastatic breast cancer. In: Kimura K, Yamada K, Carter SC, Griswold DP, eds. Cancer chemotherapy: challenges for the future. Amsterdam: Excerpta Medica, 1990:257.

32. Sheth SP, Allegra JC. What role for concurrent chemohormonal therapy in breast cancer? (Review). Oncology (Huntingt) 1987; 1:19.

33. Jaiyesimi IA, Buzdar AU, Sahin AA, Ross MA. Carcinoma of the male breast. Ann Intern Med 1992; 117:771.

34. Hecht JR, Winchester DJ. Male breast cancer. (Review). Am J Clin Pathol 1994; 102:S25.

35. Hortobagyi GN. Treatment of breast cancer. (Review). N Engl J Med 1998; 339:974.

36. Tamoxifen for early breast cancer: an overview of the randomised trials. Early Breast Cancer Trialists' Collaborative Group. Lancet 1998; 351:1451.

37. Ovarian ablation in early breast cancer: overview of the randomised trials. Early Breast Cancer Trialists' Collaborative Group [see comments]. Lancet 1996; 348:1189.

38. Polychemotherapy for early breast cancer: an overview of the randomised trials. Early Breast Cancer Trialists' Collaborative Group. Lancet 1998; 352:930.

39. Scottish Cancer Trials Breast Group and ICRF Breast Unit GH, London. Adjuvant ovarian ablation versus CMF chemotherapy in premenopausal women with pathological stage II breast carcinoma: the Scottish trial. Lancet 1993; 341:1293.

40. Powles T, Eeles R, Ashley S, et al. Interim analysis of the incidence of breast cancer in the Royal Marsden Hospital tamoxifen randomised chemoprevention trial [see comments]. Lancet 1998; 352:98.

41. Veronesi U, Maisonneuve P, Costa A, et al. Prevention of breast cancer with tamoxifen: preliminary findings from the Italian randomised trial among hysterectomised women. Italian Tamoxifen Prevention Study [see comments]. Lancet 1998; 352:93.

42. Fisher B, Costantino JP, Wickerham DL, et al. Tamoxifen for prevention of breast cancer: report of the National Surgical Adjuvant Breast and Bowel Project P-1 Study. J Natl Cancer Inst 1998; 90:1371.

43. Cummings SR, Eckert S, Krueger KA, et al. The effect of raloxifene on risk of breast cancer in postmenopausal women: results from the MORE randomized trial. Multiple Outcomes of Raloxifene Evaluation. JAMA 1999; 281:2189.

## CHAPTER 225

# ENDOCRINE ASPECTS OF PROSTATE CANCER

CHULSO MOON AND CHRISTOPHER J. LOGETHETIS

## PROSTATE CANCER

Prostate cancer is the most common type of hormone-dependent tumor in the United States and is present at autopsy in 30% of men older than 60 years of age.[1] Prostate cancer is now second only to lung cancer as a cause of cancer-related deaths in the United States, and predictions had estimated >317,000 new cases and 41,400 deaths due to prostate cancer.[1] Concepts about the endocrine dependence of prostate cancer result largely from the work of Dr. Charles Huggins, who postulated that endocrine-dependent tumors in general, and prostate cancer in particular, contain malignant cells that require hormones for cellular viability and proliferative capacity.[2] Thus, treatments designed to induce hormone deprivation would be expected to produce tumoricidal effects and the amelioration of clinical signs and symptoms, if not cure. He demonstrated dramatic regressions of prostate cancer in response to surgical orchiectomy or suppression of androgens with estrogens such as diethylstilbestrol (DES). These observations provided the rationale for endocrine therapy for a number of tumors. Although the hope for cure was not fulfilled, his conceptual approach led to a wide variety of studies, including tumor induction with hormones, receptors as mediators of hormone action, and the use of antihormones to block the mitotic effects of androgens on tumor growth.

### INCIDENCE

Prostate cancer is detected initially in one of three ways: (a) during investigation of suspicious signs and symptoms, (b) incidentally at the time of surgery for other reasons, and (c) at autopsy. The yearly incidence differs for each mode of detection. Prostate cancer is suspected in patients with symptoms of bone pain caused by metastases or with a firm nodule on routine prostate examination. This form of clinically evident prostate cancer is second only to that of the lung in frequency among men in the United States, and ~300,000 new cases are diagnosed yearly. Each year, ~40,000 men die of prostate cancer after its clinical presentation—a number that represents 10% of all male cancer deaths. The second type, occult prostate cancer, is found incidentally at the time of transurethral resection of the prostate, performed as treatment for presumed prostatic hypertrophy. Several thousand new cases are detected yearly in this manner. Only a small fraction of men die from this relatively benign form of prostate cancer. The third mode of detection, which involves the routine examination of the prostate at autopsy, uncovers prostate cancer in >30% of men older than 60 years of age. Autopsy-detected prostate cancer[3] is clinically insignificant because symptoms are rarely present before death. These cancers are localized and are never the cause of death of the patient.

The three modes of detection of prostate cancer emphasize its wide biologic spectrum of aggressivity. This fundamental concept has important clinical implications for the choice of appropriate therapy. Highly variable biologic behavior is not unique to prostate cancer; it is also a characteristic of the endocrine-dependent tumors of thyroid, breast, and endometrium. Thyroid and endometrial cancers, but not breast cancers, frequently are detected for the first time at autopsy.

## ETIOLOGY

The causes of prostate cancer remain unknown.[4] A higher than expected prevalence among relatives suggests genetic factors,[4a] but histocompatibility antigen typing has shown no confirmatory associations. The higher incidence and mortality for American blacks than for whites also raise the possibility of genetic interactions. Environmental factors or ascertainment bias also could explain this difference, however, and this possibility is suggested by the six-fold lower rate of prostate cancer in Nigerian blacks than in American blacks. Androgens have been considered as possible promoters or initiators of prostate cancer in men. Support for this hypothesis includes the following: eunuchs rarely develop prostate cancer; exogenous androgens or estrogens can induce prostate cancer in an animal model; and, in humans, most prostatic cancers are hormone dependent. However, no consistent abnormalities of androgen production, metabolism, or circulating levels or tissue sensitivity to testosterone have been observed in men with prostate cancer. Exposure to chemicals, dietary factors, or sexual transmission of an infecting agent remains an additional, albeit unproved, etiologic possibility. Protein translation products (i.e., p21 protein) of the c-*ras* oncogene have been detected in prostate cancer tissue. This is probably the result of secondary oncogene activation during the process of tumor evolution, rather than indication of a prior retrovirus infection.[5] A role for inactivation of tumor suppressor genes has also been proposed.[6]

## PATHOLOGY

The analysis of tissue sections provides a potential means of predicting the biologic behavior of prostate cancer. Many pathologic classification systems are available. Histologic criteria developed by Gleason[7] included the degree of glandular differentiation and structural architecture of a specimen viewed at low-power magnification. The Gleason score correlates with patient prognosis when groups of men are studied[8] (Fig. 225-1). The scoring methods developed later added the features of cellular anaplasia, the degree of nuclear roundness, and the appearance of nucleoli as additional criteria. Critiques of each method emphasize problems with the lack of scoring reproducibility among individual observers, the variability of grades within the same tumor, and the lack of predictive power for the individual patient as opposed to groups of patients. Hence, histologic grading scores generally have not been used as the basis for making therapeutic decisions, and no single grading system is universally accepted. Nonetheless, the clinician may wish to use the information gained from histologic assessment when determining the aggressiveness of the therapeutic strategy to be chosen for an individual patient.[9,10] Nuclear DNA ploidy has been proposed as an important and independent prognostic variable for patients with stage C and D1 disease.[11,12] Patients having tumors with DNA tetraploid or aneuploid patterns experienced tumor progression sooner and died earlier than patients with diploid tumors.[11,12]

The detection of an early premalignant lesion has been difficult, but one study has suggested that pS2 immunoreactivity could be useful for the diagnostic evaluation of early premalignant lesions in the setting of a negative tumor biopsy.[13] Prostate tissue obtained from patients without malignant disease consistently lacked pS2 protein expression. In contrast, nonneoplastic

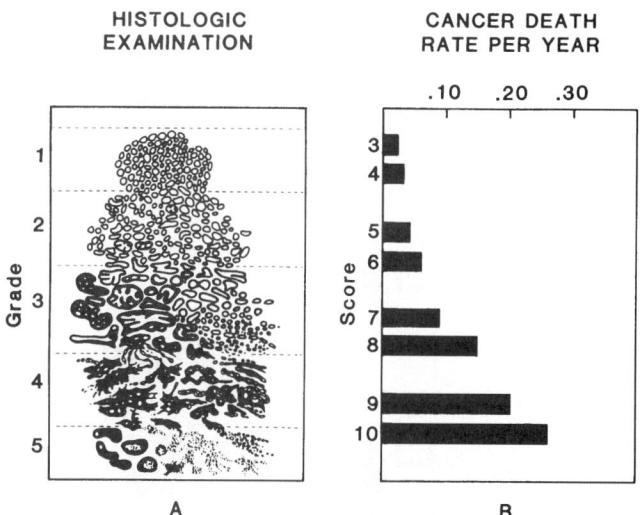

**FIGURE 225-1.** **A,** Histologic grading system of Gleason.[7] Tumors are graded 1 to 5 based on the degree of glandular differentiation and structural architecture. Tumors commonly contain more than one histologic grade. To take this characteristic into account, the grades are added together and become the Gleason histologic score. This provides the scaling effect of averaging, but without division by 2. In general, histologic grades 1 and 2 become histologic scores 3 and 4 as shown on panel **B**. **B,** Correlation of Gleason histologic score with cancer death rate per year. (Modified from Gleason DF. Histologic grading and clinical staging of carcinoma of the prostate. In: Tannenbaum M, ed. Urological pathology: the prostate. Philadelphia: Lea & Febiger, 1977:171.)

prostatic tissue from patients with locally advanced prostate cancer exhibited a variable degree of pS2 expression in the normal or hyperplastic gland and in intraepithelial hyperplasia adjacent to the cancerous lesion. Also, the expression of this pS2 was closely associated with neuroendocrine differentiation. From many ongoing studies, several other gene markers are expected to be found to facilitate the determination of the degree of tumor progression.

## CLINICAL STAGING

Clinical staging of prostate cancer provides the major means of determining prognosis and is widely used (Fig. 225-2). Treatment decisions depend heavily on this parameter.

Patients thought to have local disease after initial clinical assessment often have occult spread to lymph nodes or to distant sites at the time of surgical exploration for staging. Therefore, surgical staging is required when the results would influence treatment decisions. Initially, noninvasive studies, including skeletal survey, intravenous pyelogram, measurement of serum acid phosphatase levels and levels of more sensitive markers such as serum prostate-specific antigen[14] values, bone scans, and, when indicated, magnetic resonance imaging and sonograms[14a] are ordered. The finding of metastases or extensive local spread by these methods obviates the need for surgical staging. If these test results are negative, however, then surgical exploration of the lymph nodes usually is required. The yield of this procedure in detecting occult spread is 2% in stage A1, 23% in stage A2, 18% in stage B1, 35% in stage B2, and 46% in stage C.[15] Surgical staging is important particularly for patients with disease of clinical stages A2 and B who are being considered for curative surgical therapy and who would not be candidates for such treatment if positive nodes were detected at the time of surgical exploration.

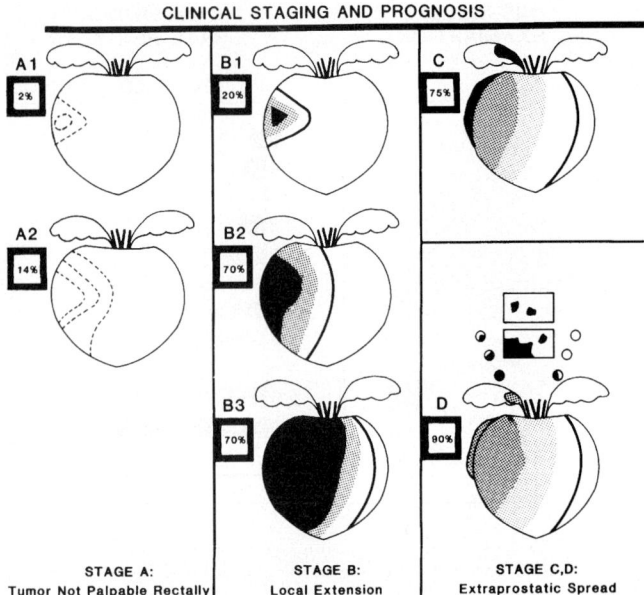

CLINICAL STAGING AND PROGNOSIS

A1 2%

A2 14%

B1 20%

B2 70%

B3 70%

C 75%

D 80%

STAGE A:
Tumor Not Palpable Rectally

STAGE B:
Local Extension

STAGE C,D:
Extraprostatic Spread

**FIGURE 225-2.** Clinical staging systems in general use. Stage A represents occult disease found at the time of transurethral resection of the prostate for the suspected clinical diagnosis of benign prostatic hypertrophy. Subsets A1 and A2 depend on the number of tissue chips found to contain cancer. Stage B disease is palpable clinically and is divided into subsets representing various degrees of involvement of the prostate. Stage C represents local extraprostatic metastasis contiguous to the gland, and Stage D, distant lymph node, bone, or other metastases. Approximate percentage of patients dead at 5 years is indicated by the *heavy squares* containing percentages drawn for each category. Prognostic data represent a compilation of information from varying time intervals. (Summarized from Catalona WJ, ed. Endocrine therapy. In: Prostate cancer. New York: Grune & Stratton, 1984:40.)

## TUMOR BIOLOGY

A stem cell model has been proposed for the organization of the prostatic epithelium. This model explains the growth and transformation of normal epithelium into cancer cells.[16] According to this model, the prostate has three basic layers: secretory luminal, basal, and endocrine paracrine cells. The proliferative compartment, which is located in the basal cell layer, usually is androgen independent but contains androgen-responsive target cells. During the malignant transformation, the proliferative zone is shifted to luminal cell types with formation of neoplastic basement membranes. These proliferative changes in prostate cancer are exclusively restricted to exocrine cell types, and the majority of exocrine cells are androgen dependent, whereas endocrine-differentiated cells lack the nuclear androgen receptor. A small stem cell population located in the basal cell layer is the source for all epithelial layers in the normal, hyperplastic, and neoplastic cells. This differentiating process (from basal cells to secretory luminal cells) via intermediate phenotypes is induced by circulating androgen and largely depends on the androgen-responsive target cells in the basal cell layers.

The biologic behavior of neuroendocrine lineage cells is quite different from that of exocrine lineage cells and usually is more aggressive. A study of a transgenic mouse model of metastatic prostate cancer has shown that the neuroendocrine cell lineage (from several cell types) is exquisitely sensitive to transformation.[17] The simian virus 40 T antigen was expressed in a subset of neuroendocrine cells in all lobes of mouse prostate. After 7 weeks, prostatic intraepithelial neoplasias developed and rapidly progressed to local invasion. After 6 months, these tumors

metastasized to lymph nodes, liver, lung, and bone; this tumor was not androgen dependent. Neuroendocrine differentiation was strongly associated with the progression of the disease in the presence of endocrine therapy.[18]

At the time of clinical diagnosis of this tumor, heterogeneous subpopulations of malignant cells with varying characteristics are present.[19,20] Some of the cells are absolutely hormone dependent and die when deprived of their androgen support. Others, the hormone-sensitive population, grow faster when stimulated with androgen but become quiescent and enter the $G_0$ (resting) stage of the cell cycle on androgen deprivation. Still other clones of cells (hormone independent) grow in the complete absence of androgenic stimulation.

The relative numbers of each of these three cell types determine whether the initial response of the patient to androgen deprivation consists of objective tumor regression, stabilization of disease, or continued progression. In general, when highly stringent criteria are applied, 40% of men with prostate cancer exhibit objectively measurable tumor regression and a further 40% experience disease stabilization when deprived of androgens.[21,22] At most, only 10% to 20% of tumors continue to grow after androgen deprivation and, thus, consist exclusively of hormone-independent cells.

The proportion of each cell type changes progressively in response to hormonal treatment. After initial hormonal deprivation, the subsets of cells that are absolutely hormone independent at the outset continue to grow and gradually repopulate the tumor. Hence, hormonal treatment does not cure patients, and therapy is nearly always followed, within months to years, by relapse. In all patients, the hormone-independent cells represent almost all of those within the tumor at the time of the patient's death.

The natural history of prostatic cancer cells entering $G_0$ during hormonal deprivation (i.e., the hormone-sensitive population) is less well known. The readministration of androgens after initial deprivation elicits marked increases in bone pain and objective tumor progression in nearly 80% of patients with prostate cancer.[23] This observation provides evidence for the persistence of hormone-sensitive cells in most patients. In some patients, these cells appear to regrow in the presence of much lower amounts of androgen. Objective responses to secondary hormonal therapy, such as hypophysectomy, adrenalectomy, antiandrogens, or medical adrenalectomy, probably occurs from a response of the substantial fraction of such cells that had begun to regrow.

## GENETICS

Several studies have provided insights regarding the relationships between tumor suppressor or transcriptional factors and the development, progression, or endocrine characteristics of prostate cancer.

The study of genetic changes with comparative hybridization techniques has shown that losses of several chromosomal sites (8p, 13q, 6q, 16q, 18q, 9q) are common changes in primary tumors, a finding which suggests that deletion-inactivation of putative tumor-suppressor genes at these sites is likely to contribute to the development of prostatic cancer.[24] Likewise, through the identification of homozygous deletions in malignant tissue, chromosome band 12p12-13 has been suggested as a potential location of a novel tumor-suppressor gene for advanced prostate cancer.[25] Although the gene has not yet been isolated, this study should facilitate the identification of genes involved in the progression of prostate adenocarcinoma. Also, p53 mutations are frequently associated with increased metastases. In one study, these mutations were found at approximately twice the frequency in metastatic prostate cancer as in unselected samples of primary prostatic cancer.[26]

Immunohistochemical staining for the expression of the *KAI1* gene (a metastatic suppressor gene for prostatic cancer) correlates with tumor characteristics.[27] In benign prostatic hyperplasia tissues, *KAI1* protein is uniformly expressed in the glandular cell membrane at cell-to-cell borders. This protein is similarly expressed in untreated prostate cancer, but the percentage of protein-positive cells correlates inversely with the Gleason pattern and clinical stage. Also, this protein was not expressed in either primary or metastatic cancer tissue from patients who died after relapse from endocrine therapy.

Presently, the molecular mechanism for the growth-promoting effects of androgens is not clearly understood, but one study has shown a close correlation between *pRB* gene expression (one of the transcriptional factors involved in the suppression of carcinogenesis) and androgen-receptor activity.[28] In this study, overexpression of the *pRB* gene increased androgen-receptor transcriptional activity; loss of *pRB* protein inhibited androgen-receptor functions. Also, the suggestion has been made that the loss of *pRB* activity during the progression of cancer may directly decrease the response to androgens. Likewise, a transcriptional factor, ETS2, is critical to the maintenance of the transformed state of human prostate cancer cell lines. When the action of this protein was blocked, the transformed properties were reduced.[29]

## HORMONE DEPENDENCE

Androgenic effects mediated through the action of dihydrotestosterone are responsible for stimulation of prostatic cancer growth. The exact nature of the stimulatory process is unknown, and it may reflect a secondary enhancement of androgen-dependent growth factors or direct proliferative effects of the androgens themselves. Nonetheless, dihydrotestosterone must first bind to nuclear receptors in prostate carcinoma tissue to initiate the events leading to tumor growth. Thus, therapies for prostate cancer are designed to lower the tissue levels of dihydrotestosterone or to antagonize its action at the receptor level.

Human prostate cancer also may be estrogen dependent. Estrogen receptors can be demonstrated in some human prostate cancers.[30] Objective responses, albeit in <10% of patients, occur during the administration of the antiestrogen tamoxifen.[31] Regressions in up to 15% of patients treated with DES, after surgical castration, have been reported, but they are incompletely substantiated.[32] In experimental systems, estrogens can affect the concentration of androgen receptors present. This information leaves open the possibility of direct estrogen effects on prostate cancer, but it does not suggest a major role for them.

Prolactin enhances androgen uptake into rat ventral prostate nuclei and potentiates the effects of exogenous androgen. However, inhibitors of prolactin secretion, such as bromocriptine, are ineffective in patients with prostate cancer. Hypophysectomy, although highly effective in relieving bone pain, may act through lowering of adrenal androgens rather than by a prolactin mechanism. Thus, the clinical importance of prolactin in prostate cancer remains doubtful. Insulin-like growth factors (IGFs) have also been postulated to play a role in prostate cancer growth. IGF-binding protein-2, the main IGF-binding protein produced by prostate epithelial cells, is elevated in the serum of prostate cancer patients.[33] Furthermore, the degree of elevation correlates with the prostate-specific antigen level and stage of the tumor.[33]

## SOURCES OF ANDROGENS

Dihydrotestosterone, the major active androgen, is primarily a peripheral conversion product of secreted testosterone (see Chap. 114). In adult men, 95% of the 7000 µg of testosterone produced is secreted by the testes. Testosterone is converted in peripheral tissues to dihydrotestosterone at a rate of 500 µg daily. A large fraction of the dihydrotestosterone present in benign and malignant prostatic tissue is produced locally in the prostate gland from testicular testosterone. Thus, the testis is, by far, the major source of androgen.[34]

The adrenal gland provides the remaining 5% of androgen produced in adult men. Approximately 200 µg of testosterone is secreted directly by the adrenal glands, and another 200 µg is derived from adrenal androstenedione, which is then converted peripherally to testosterone.[35] The 400 µg of testosterone originating from these two adrenal sources is then converted to ~25 µg of dihydrotestosterone daily. An additional pathway involves the peripheral conversion of dehydroepiandrosterone and its sulfate into dihydrotestosterone. Although the exact quantitative significance of this pathway is unknown, 2% of an injected dose of radiolabeled dehydroepiandrosterone can be found later in the prostate as dihydrotestosterone.[36,37]

## TUMOR MARKERS OF ANDROGEN DEPENDENCE

No specific hormonal or receptor measurements are available that allow the precise biochemical characterization of tumors as androgen dependent or independent. In contrast to the situation in breast cancer, the measurement of androgen receptors in prostate cancer has not been established as a practically useful method of predicting responses to endocrine therapy. The first androgen-receptor assays were nonspecific and detected the presence of testosterone-estrogen–binding globulin as well as progestin receptors in human prostatic cancer tissue.[38] Early reports correlating the presence of androgen receptor with response to endocrine therapy, thus, should be viewed with caution. Advances such as the development of specific radioactive tracers (i.e., R-1881) for use as ligands, the addition of triamcinolone to eliminate progestin-receptor binding, the use of sodium molybdate as a stabilizer, and the use of nuclei as a source of receptor enable the accurate measurement of the androgen receptor. Correlations of androgen receptor and clinical response by use of these methods are preliminary. In three studies,[38–40] androgen receptors were detected in prostatic cancer tissue in all patients, even in those not responding to endocrine therapy. These data suggest that the initial response to therapy cannot be predicted by androgen-receptor measurements, but they do appear to provide prognostic information. In patients with androgen-receptor–rich tumors (i.e., >500 fmol/mg DNA), responses to endocrine therapy often persisted for >1 year, whereas relapse occurred within 1 year in all patients with receptor-poor tumors (i.e., levels of <500 fmol/mg). In addition, the level of nuclear androgen receptor correlated with the duration of patient survival.

Potentially more predictive assays are being validated and correlated with clinical responses. One approach involves the measurement of the nuclear matrix fraction of androgen receptor and another the levels of nuclear dihydrotestosterone mass. However, the level of precision required to differentiate the 20% of patients who do not respond to endocrine therapy from the total pool of patients may not be achievable. Practically speaking, the acceptable approach is probably to treat all prostate cancer patients with hormonal therapy, because it is known that 80% will respond. Receptor measurements, then, are not critically important. In marked contrast, predictive receptor tests are essential in breast cancer patients, because only 30% respond to hormonal therapy, and receptor assays identify the 70% of women whose breast cancer is not hormone responsive (see Chap. 224).

# HORMONAL TREATMENT OF PROSTATE CANCER

## INITIATING TREATMENT

The decision on when to begin hormonal therapy is a major question in prostate cancer. Because cure with hormones is not possible, the two goals of treatment are to relieve the patient's symptoms and to increase the life expectancy. If treatment is advocated before symptoms develop, the therapy must improve the length of patient survival. Historically, controlled studies in the 1940s suggested survival benefit from endocrine therapy and, therefore, patients were treated at the time of initial diagnosis. However, the rigorously controlled series of Veterans Administration Cooperative Urological Research Group (VACURG) trials[41] during the 1960s indicated no survival benefit from early endocrine therapy. Since then, standard practice is to withhold hormonal therapy until metastatic (stage D) disease is present and patients are symptomatic.

Treatment of asymptomatic patients with stage D disease should be based on demonstration of a survival benefit. Reanalysis of the VACURG studies[42] has revealed that younger patients with high-grade tumors may experience prolongation of survival if given hormonal therapy at the time of diagnosis. A retrospective study[43] has also indicated that patients with stage D1 disease and diploid tumors experienced a survival benefit from radical prostatectomy and adjuvant hormonal therapy. Whereas these studies suggest a survival advantage from early hormonal therapy in some groups of asymptomatic patients with stage D disease, prospective trials are needed to substantiate these findings.

## CHOOSING ENDOCRINE THERAPY

### ORCHIECTOMY

Which endocrine therapy to use initially is also a major question (Fig. 225-3). In the VACURG study,[41,44] treatment with various dosages of estrogen was compared with orchiectomy and with the combination of orchiectomy plus estrogen therapy. The results show that orchiectomy is as effective in inducing tumor regression as is an optimal dosage of estrogen. In addition, orchiectomy is not associated with accelerated cardiovascular disease or with other indirect complications of therapy that can occur with estrogens. The operative risks, especially when local anesthesia is used, are minimal. Impotence occurs as frequently after castration (i.e., nearly always) as with other standard endocrine

therapies. Also, patient compliance and assurance that testicular androgens are completely suppressed are not considerations once an adequate orchiectomy has been performed.

### ESTROGEN THERAPY

Before the studies of the gonadotropin-releasing hormone (GnRH) superagonist analogs (GnRH-A), estrogen administration was the preferred form of "medical castration." The rationale is to inhibit release of luteinizing hormone (LH) by the pituitary and, thereby, lower plasma androgens to castrate levels. The VACURG studies[41] identified several problems with estrogen therapy and emphasized their critical dependence on the dosage administered. Excessive amounts of estrogen accelerate cardiovascular morbidity, whereas insufficient dosages do not completely suppress testosterone levels. Specifically, 5 mg of DES daily suppresses testosterone to the same extent as surgical orchiectomy and reduces deaths from prostate cancer. This dosage, however, accelerates cardiovascular deaths to the extent that the antitumor effect is offset. On the other hand, 0.2 mg of DES daily neither retards tumor growth nor accelerates cardiovascular disease. An intermediate dosage of 1 mg daily appeared to retard prostate cancer growth while causing no apparent excess in cardiovascular risk. Based on this observation, 1 mg of DES daily is a commonly recommended estrogen dosage (Table 225-1).

After the VACURG studies, however, additional clinical trials[45] indicated that administration of 1 mg of DES daily does not inhibit testosterone to the extent achieved by surgical castration. Testosterone levels may rise abruptly within 12 hours of omitting a single dose, a problem that often could occur in a poorly compliant patient. For this reason, many experts recommend a 3-mg daily dose. A limited study,[46] however, demonstrated increased cardiovascular toxicity at the 3-mg dose level. These data suggest that it may not be possible to completely suppress testicular androgens without enhancing the risk of cardiovascular death.

Estrogens other than DES have been used to treat prostate cancer, but they are less well studied. The synthetic estrogen chlorotrianisene (TACE) was found to produce no testosterone suppression. Incomplete dose-response characterizations are available for these alternative estrogens, a fact that precludes their use for prostate cancer.

Estrogen therapy is associated with other, less serious, side effects. Tender gynecomastia occurs commonly but can be prevented by prophylactic irradiation of the breasts. Fluid retention with edema occurs commonly, and the potential exists for

**FIGURE 225-3.** Diagrammatic representation of various forms of endocrine therapy currently used for prostatic cancer. Primary therapy is directed toward removal of testicular androgens and includes surgical castration or medical castration with estrogens (diethylstilbestrol, *DES*) or gonadotropin-releasing hormone superagonist analogs (*GnRH-As*). Ketoconazole is used experimentally to inhibit testicular androgen biosynthesis, and antiandrogens are used to block androgen action on the prostatic tumor tissue. Secondary therapy is directed toward blockade of adrenal androgen sources. Aminoglutethimide in combination with hydrocortisone produces a medical adrenalectomy to inhibit androgen biosynthesis, and antiandrogens are used to block androgen action. (*LH*, luteinizing hormone; *FSH*, follicle-stimulating hormone; *ACTH*, adrenocorticotropic hormone.) (From Santen RJ. The testis. In: Felig P, Baxter JD, Broadus AE, Frohman LA, eds. Endocrinology and metabolism. New York: McGraw-Hill, 1987:891.)

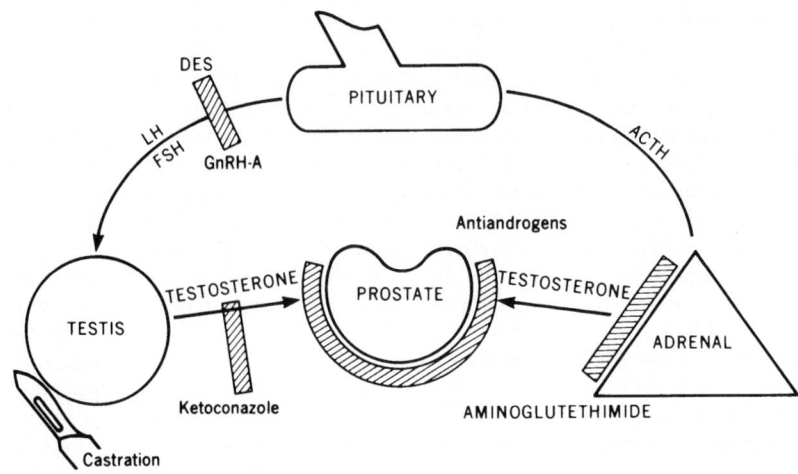

**TABLE 225-1.**
**Hormonal Therapy for Prostate Cancer**

| Modality | Drug | Recommended Dosage | Special Problems |
|---|---|---|---|
| **PRIMARY** | | | |
| Surgical orchiectomy | | | Unacceptable to many patients |
| Estrogens | DES* | 3 mg daily | Acceleration of cardiovascular disease |
| | DES | 1 mg daily | Lack of complete testicular androgen suppression |
| GnRH superagonist analogs | D-Leu-6-GnRH proethylamide | 7.5 mg IM once monthly | Requires once-monthly injection of biodegradable material |
| | Goserelin acetate | 3.6 mg IM once monthly | Requires once-monthly injection of biodegradable material |
| **SECONDARY** | | | |
| Medical adrenalectomy | Aminoglutethimide + hydro-cortisone | 250 mg, 2–4 times daily 20 mg, twice daily | Drug-related side effects |
| High-dose estrogen | DES diphosphate | 500–2000 mg IV | Requires intravenous administration daily for 5 days |
| Oral estrogens | DES | 3 mg daily | Efficacy questioned |
| Antiandrogen | Flutamide | 750 mg daily in divided doses | Methemoglobinemia |
| **UNAPPROVED IN UNITED STATES** | | | |
| Antiandrogen | Cyproterone acetate | 250 mg daily | Liver toxicity |
| Androgen synthesis inhibitor | Ketoconazole[†] | 1200 mg daily | Liver toxicity |

*DES*, diethylstilbestrol; *GnRH*, gonadotropin releasing hormone.
*The appropriate dosage of DES is not uniformly agreed on.
[†]Approved in the United States as an antifungal agent but not as an androgen synthesis inhibitor.

exacerbation of congestive heart failure. Nausea also may be a problem.

## THERAPY WITH GONADOTROPIN-RELEASING HORMONE SUPERAGONIST ANALOGS

Highly potent agonist analogs of GnRH, the GnRH-A, have been approved for use in prostate cancer. These compounds paradoxically inhibit LH secretion by the pituitary and, thereby, suppress testicular testosterone production.[47] Under normal physiologic circumstances, the pituitary is exposed to episodic pulses of GnRH released by the hypothalamus in response to signals from a "pulse generator." The amplitude and frequency of GnRH pulses control the amount of both LH and follicle-stimulating hormone (FSH) released. The exposure of the pituitary to constant, rather than episodic, GnRH renders the pituitary refractory to GnRH stimulation through receptor down-regulation and postreceptor inhibition. As a result, plasma levels of LH, FSH, and testosterone decline. The superagonist analogs of GnRH mimic the effects of constant GnRH infusions because of their prolonged duration of action and their high potency (i.e., 50 to 200 times greater than that of native GnRH) (see Chap. 16).

Clinically, the GnRH-A stimulate LH three-fold to four-fold and testosterone two-fold for 1 to 2 weeks on initiation of therapy.[48] Thereafter, LH is profoundly depressed, and the plasma testosterone level falls from ~500 ng/dL to castrate levels of 15 ng/dL. The rapidity of initial suppression depends on the dosage and accelerates with increasing amounts. No escape from inhibition occurs during ≤2 years of continuous therapy[49] (Fig. 225-4). The initial rise in testosterone causes a transient flare in 5% to 10% of patients that has occasionally resulted in spinal cord compression and death. This complication can be prevented by concomitant administration of antiandrogen therapy. The development of GnRH antagonists will also obviate the flare phenomenon because these compounds are devoid of agonistic activity.

During initial studies with the GnRH-As, divergent results for suppression of plasma LH levels by radioimmunoassay were reported. Variable findings ranged from elevated to marked suppression of gonadotropin levels. Highly sensitive LH bioassays,[48] however, uniformly detect profound LH suppression during GnRH-A therapy. The discrepancy between the levels of LH measured by radioimmunoassay and LH levels measured

by bioassay results partly from the continued secretion of the immunologically recognizable but bioinactive LH α subunit. In addition, physicochemical studies[50] suggest that the carbohydrate content of LH is altered during GnRH therapy. This change reduces the intrinsic bioactivity of LH and the biologic/immunologic activity ratios.

The rationale for using GnRH-A is to induce a medical castration selectively and without unwanted toxicity or side effects. Initial studies compared testosterone and dihydrotestosterone levels in patients treated with GnRH-A and with surgical orchiectomy and demonstrated an equivalent degree of androgen suppression. Hormonal effects with the GnRH-A were selective because no alterations of adrenal, thyroid, parathyroid, or pancreatic function were observed. Full biochemical batteries revealed no unexpected toxicity. Objective regressions occurred as frequently as would be expected with orchiectomy.

The clinical use of the GnRH analogs was then further validated by a direct comparison with estrogen therapy.[21] Patients with stage D disease were stratified to ensure clinical comparability and randomized to treatment with GnRH-A (leuprolide acetate [Lupron]) or DES, 3 mg per day. The percentage of patients with objective disease response and the duration of these effects did not differ for the two treatments (Fig. 225-5). Cardiovascular and other side effects appeared to be more pronounced with DES than with the GnRH-A. Although additional experience is required, that the GnRH-A will be shown to cause accelerated cardiovascular deaths is considered highly unlikely.

Initially, a major problem with GnRH-A therapy was the requirement for daily subcutaneous administration. Second- and third-generation formulations have been developed. Administration by nasal spray, a second-generation development, allows only 2% to 5% absorption of the drug; significantly higher levels of testosterone were measured during GnRH-A therapy administered by nasal spray (i.e., buserelin, 1.5 mg per day) than with therapy by the subcutaneous route.[51] The third-generation approach—use of a once-monthly biodegradable preparation—appears highly effective, well tolerated, and acceptable to patients. In one randomized study,[22] microcapsules of D-Trp-GnRH suppressed testosterone to an extent similar to that of orchiectomy. Clinical tumor regression and stabilization did not differ for the orchiectomy and GnRH-A treatment groups. No unexpected toxicity occurred with this

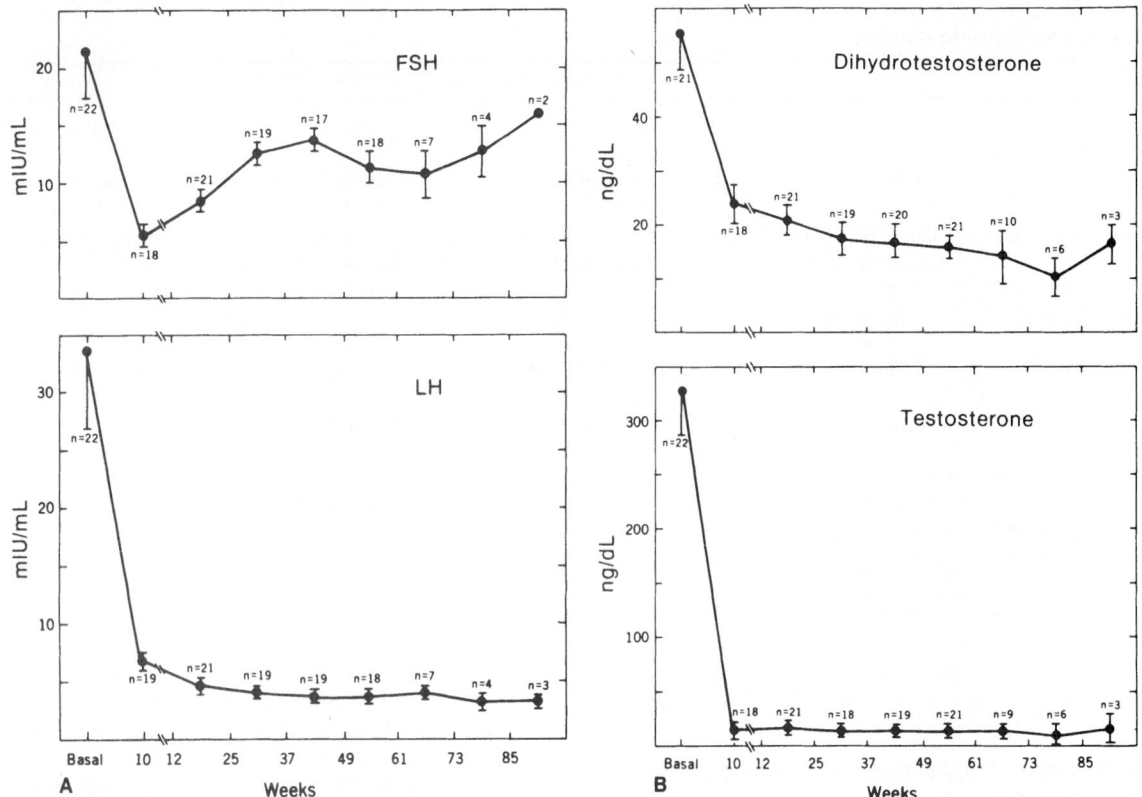

**FIGURE 225-4.** Levels of plasma luteinizing hormone (*LH*) and follicle-stimulating hormone (*FSH*) (**A**) and testosterone and dihydrotestosterone (**B**) in men with prostate cancer receiving a gonadotropin-releasing hormone superagonist analog for at least 1 year. The number (*n*) of men receiving therapy at each time point is indicated. (From Santen RJ, Demers LM, Max DT, et al. Long-term effects of administration of a gonadotropin-releasing hormone superagonist analog in men with prostatic carcinoma. J Clin Endocrinol Metab 1984; 58:397.)

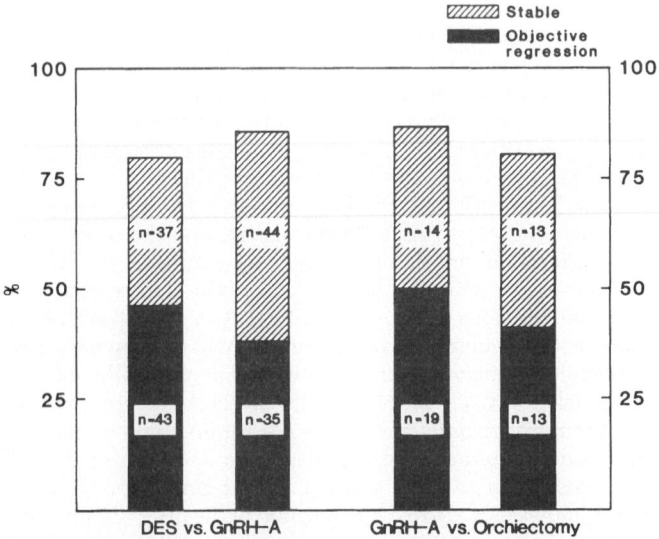

**FIGURE 225-5.** The responses produced by orchiectomy, 3 mg of diethylstilbestrol (*DES*) daily, and the gonadotropin-releasing hormone superagonist analog (*GnRH-A*) are equivalent. One randomized study compared 3 mg of DES with GnRH-A (*left*) and another compared GnRH-A with surgical orchiectomy (*right*). Duration of responses is also similar. (Data adapted from the Leuprolide Study Group. Leuprolide vs diethylstilbestrol for metastatic prostatic cancer. N Engl J Med 1984; 311:1281; and from Parmar H, Phillips RH, Lightman SL, et al. Randomized controlled study of orchidectomy vs. long-acting D-Trp-6-LHRH microcapsules in advanced prostatic cancer. Lancet 1985; 2:1201.)

form of drug administration. Another preparation, biodegradable goserelin acetate (Zoladex), has shown similar hormonal and clinical results in open trials.[52–54] A long-acting form of D-Leu-GnRH is approved for treatment of prostate cancer in the United States. This preparation (leuprolide acetate) requires only once-monthly injections.[55] Most investigators recommend continuing GnRH-A treatment on disease relapse (in conjunction with secondary therapy) because of the persistence of some androgen-sensitive cells despite escape from primary endocrine treatment.

### OTHER PRIMARY ENDOCRINE THERAPIES

Two additional strategies as primary therapy to reduce the effect of androgens on prostatic cancer tissue have been studied. One involves a reduction of androgen biosynthesis by the testes, and the other uses antiandrogens to inhibit the actions of male hormones on cancer cells.

**Ketoconazole.** Only one inhibitor of androgen biosynthesis, ketoconazole, is sufficiently potent to significantly reduce plasma testosterone and dihydrotestosterone levels in men. With other inhibitors of testicular steroidogenesis, such as aminoglutethimide, the initial decrease in testosterone induces a reflex rise in LH that can overcome the blockade. Ketoconazole initially was used as an antifungal agent, but it later was found to be an inhibitor of the $C_{17,20}$ lyase enzyme. This cytochrome P-450–mediated step catalyzes the conversion of 17α-hydroxyprogesterone to androstenedione, the immediate precursor of testosterone. Administration of 1200 mg of ketoconazole daily, an amount six times the dosage commonly used for antifungal therapy, continuously suppresses plasma testosterone values to levels approaching, but not reaching, those observed after castration. Preliminary reports[56] suggest a rate of objective disease regression similar to that occurring after orchiectomy. The lack of complete androgen suppression with ketoconazole, however, probably limits its clinical application.

Also, a potential drawback of ketoconazole therapy is the incidence of hepatotoxicity. Minor elevations of liver enzymes commonly occur, but serious reactions are observed in ~1 in 7000 patients. Fatalities from hepatic failure occurred before this effect was recognized, but prospective monitoring of hepatic enzymes should allow this drug to be given safely.

**Flutamide.** The use of antiandrogens for prostate cancer is analogous to the use of antiestrogens for breast cancer. Two agents have been extensively studied: flutamide, a nonsteroidal antiandrogen, and cyproterone acetate, a potent steroidal antiandrogen with major progestational activity (see Chap. 119). Both flutamide and cyproterone acetate bind to androgen receptors and block the cellular effects of circulating testosterone and dihydrotestosterone. Flutamide is nearly unique among hormonal antagonists in not possessing weak hormone agonist activity. Blockade of the androgen negative-feedback system results in reflex increments in serum LH, testosterone, and dihydrotestosterone levels. The peripheral effects of these reflex androgen increments, however, appear to be blocked nearly completely by flutamide. Available for clinical use in the United States and Canada, flutamide has induced disease regressions at the same rate, and for the same duration, as DES in a multicenter trial. Of interest in these early studies was the lower incidence of impotence reported by patients taking this agent than by those taking DES. Flutamide causes a minor degree of methemoglobinemia, a biochemical problem that has not, as yet, generally caused significant clinical signs or symptoms. Beyond this, flutamide generally is well tolerated and effective.[57] Unlike DES, it has caused no acceleration of cardiovascular disease and no thrombophlebitis.

**Cyproterone Acetate.** Cyproterone acetate is a potent antiandrogen that, in addition, exerts hormone agonist effects through the progestin receptor. The progestin effect not only prevents the reflex rise in LH expected from an antiandrogen but actually suppresses LH. Consequently, the action of cyproterone acetate is dual: it acts on the pituitary to suppress LH secretion and on tumor tissue to antagonize androgen actions. This agent clearly induces tumor regression in patients with prostate cancer, and it generally is well tolerated. Although it was originally thought to have considerable liver toxicity, this does not appear to be the case. This agent was used infrequently in the United States in the past, and its exact role remains to be defined.[58,59]

## PERSPECTIVES ON CHOICE OF THERAPY

Surgical orchiectomy appears preferable for the initial treatment of prostate cancer. The operation is relatively minor and can be performed under local anesthesia, if desired. Rapid and complete cessation of testicular androgen secretion ensues, and patient compliance after surgery is not a factor. Unwarranted cardiovascular or other toxic side effects are unknown. The incidence of impotence and loss of libido is the same as with other available therapies.

In actual practice, nearly half of patients in the United States prefer a form of medical castration for psychological or other reasons. The two available alternatives (i.e., Food and Drug Administration approved) include administration of DES and GnRH-A by subcutaneous injection. The greater safety of the GnRH-A agents favors their use over DES. Formerly, daily sub-

cutaneous injections were required if GnRH-A therapy was chosen. A large proportion of patients did not accept this approach because the alternative was oral medication in the form of DES. Medical castration with GnRH-A can be achieved with a once-a-month injection of biodegradable material. Commercially available preparations include leuprolide acetate and goserelin acetate. This treatment schedule is well tolerated by patients and should not be associated with cardiovascular complications. Cost is the limiting factor. Nonetheless, for the reasons discussed, the long-acting GnRH analogs are preferable to the use of estrogens when medical castration is the chosen therapy.

## MECHANISM OF HORMONE RESISTANCE

The progression of prostate cancer during endocrine therapy is a major clinical problem for which the molecular mechanisms are poorly understood. Overexpression of amplified genes was suggested as the main mechanism for the acquisition of resistance to anticancer agents in vitro. Amplification of the androgen-receptor gene also occurs in the setting of in vivo endocrine failure.[60] Comparative genomic hybridization has shown amplification of the Xq11-q13 region only in recurring tumors obtained from patients during androgen deprivation therapy and has not been found in tumor samples obtained from the same patients before therapy.

Presently, many different causative mechanisms are suggested for in vivo endocrine resistance.[61] Many involve the androgen-receptor gene and its complex downstream signaling pathways. These can be categorized as follows: (a) conversion of inactive adrenal precursor steroids into bioactive androgens, (b) androgen-receptor mutations, which produce an androgen-receptor protein with altered transactivational properties (e.g., activation by other steroids), (c) increased expression of androgen receptor as a result of gene amplification, (d) autoactivation of androgen-receptor protein by means of a protein kinase or various androgen-independent growth factors, (e) increased activation of downstream genes, (f) possible activation of several downstream genes by androgen-receptor signaling and other growth factor pathways, and possible sharing between androgen receptors and growth factors of downstream mechanisms for cell proliferation, and (g) possible blocking by antiapoptotic genes of the programmed cell death normally induced by androgen deprivation.

The resulting recurrent tumor growth may not be exclusively androgen independent, but rather a significant fraction of tumors may exist that are highly dependent and, perhaps, hypersensitized to the remaining androgens. The distinction between these two alternatives is important for developing more rational and effective therapies for advanced prostate cancer.

## SECONDARY ENDOCRINE TREATMENTS

The initial responses to hormonal treatment in prostate cancer patients persist for a median duration of 12 to 18 months. After relapse, several means of further reducing hormone secretion remain. Controversy exists, however, over the efficacy of any of the secondary maneuvers. The dispute rests on two issues: the degree of production of androgens or preandrogens by the adrenal glands, and the persistence of hormonally dependent cells in the tumor. Evidence for the existence of androgen-dependent subpopulations that persist after surgical orchiectomy comes from several observations. Objective responses to surgical adrenalectomy or hypophysectomy and to medical adrenalectomy with aminoglutethimide occur in 10% to 20% of castrate men with prostate cancer.[62,63] Early studies[23] of androgen administration to such patients, a maneuver analogous to DES administration to breast cancer patients, resulted in increased bone pain or objective disease progression in nearly three-fourths of the patients. This progression was mediated presumably by persisting androgen-dependent cells.

Additional factors have tempered enthusiasm for secondary endocrine therapy. Responses consist predominantly of the stabilization of disease or relief of bone pain; fewer men experience objective tumor regression. In contrast with the situation in breast cancer, receptor determinations have not been shown to identify the subset of patients who will respond objectively. The average duration of benefit is short, with a median of only 6 months. These factors, when weighed against the morbidity of surgical hypophysectomy or adrenalectomy, argue convincingly against the use of surgical ablation as a form of secondary therapy.

Nontoxic medical treatments to inhibit androgen biosynthesis or to antagonize androgen action, on the other hand, would be warranted, even if responses are short-lived. Several approaches have been evaluated. The combination of aminoglutethimide and hydrocortisone inhibits adrenal androgen production in castrate patients and is tolerated, although associated with troublesome side effects. Measurable disease regression occurred in 15% of 350 patients treated with this approach, and objective stabilization was seen in another 20%. A further 20% reported relief of bone pain even while their tumors were progressing.[63,64] These rates of response are similar to those observed from available chemotherapeutic regimens. On the other hand, side effects from aminoglutethimide and hydrocortisone were substantial and included a transient skin rash and dose-dependent lethargy, ataxia, and drowsiness. Coexisting renal disease often necessitates a reduction in aminoglutethimide dosage to reduce side effects. Some patients require mineralocorticoid replacement because of the inhibition of aldosterone secretion induced by blockade of the 18-hydroxylase step, another action of aminoglutethimide. Generally, these side effects are less than those produced by chemotherapy, the alternative modality selected for such patients.

Antiandrogen therapy provides another means of neutralizing the effects of adrenal androgens in castrate men with prostate cancer. Flutamide[57,65] and cyproterone acetate are also active in the same proportion of patients as is medical adrenalectomy.[58,62] Ketoconazole, an inhibitor of adrenal as well as testicular androgen biosynthesis, is modestly active and has been shown to induce remissions in 14% of patients with refractory disease.[66] Each of these agents could be considered for patients relapsing slowly after castration. Flutamide is preferable because of its favorable profile of side effects.

### DIETHYLSTILBESTROL AND DIETHYLSTILBESTROL DIPHOSPHATE

On relapse after castration, patients have been reported to respond to the administration of estrogens. Whether these responses reflect further androgen suppression in patients with a few residual Leydig cells or a direct estrogen effect is unknown. Approaches include the use of 3 mg of DES daily or intermittent intravenous administration of DES diphosphate (Stilphostrol), a soluble estrogen, in high doses.[67] The place of either of these treatments has not been precisely defined.

### ESTRAMUSTINE

Theoretically, a single molecule containing both an estrogen receptor–binding site and a cytotoxic region would allow concentration of drug at the site of estrogen receptors. Estramustine phosphate sodium (Emcyt), an estrogen/nitrogen mustard analog, was initially synthesized for this purpose.[68] Later data indicated that this compound bound with only weak affinity to the estrogen receptor but unexpectedly concentrated in malignant prostatic cancer tissue by binding to prostatic proteins. Although estramustine is active against prostatic cancer, its actions relate more to its chemotherapeutic potency than to the estrogen moiety. Its use should be considered in patients with prostate cancer who are candidates for chemotherapy.

## PERSPECTIVES ON CHOICE OF SECONDARY HORMONAL THERAPY

The major decision at the time of prostate cancer relapse after medical or surgical castration is whether to use hormonal therapy or chemotherapy. Patients with a rapid downhill course with widespread systemic metastases probably should receive chemotherapy. Conversely, a slower disease course allows time to observe a potential response to hormonal therapy. Even though only 10% to 20% of patients experience objective tumor regressions, the relief of bone pain in an additional 20% to 40% can be beneficial. Hormonal therapy does not preclude concomitant radiotherapy to focal symptomatic metastases. Flutamide would be the preferable agent, with ketoconazole and aminoglutethimide/hydrocortisone as additional choices. DES or DES diphosphate is also used in these patients, but the frequency of beneficial responses is poorly defined.

## CYTOTOXIC CHEMOTHERAPY

Although, during the last four decades, numerous clinical trials of single-agent or combination chemotherapy have failed to show any consistently effective chemotherapeutic agents, most clinicians agree that cytotoxic therapy might yield subjective and objective improvement. To date, however, all of the cytotoxic chemotherapy studies performed on patients who progressed despite hormonal therapy have been disappointing.[69] Such patients have shown objective or subjective response rates of <20% and no predictable improvement in pain, serum marker levels, or quality of life.

## NEWER EXPERIMENTAL APPROACHES

### COMPLETE ANDROGEN BLOCKADE

An important strategy for the endocrine treatment of prostate cancer is complete androgen blockade.[70] The rationale for this approach rests on three observations. First, the adrenal glands contribute 5% of the total androgen pool. Second, the concentrations of dihydrotestosterone in prostate cancer tissue of patients fall by only 50% to 80% after surgical orchiectomy, and after castration, dihydrotestosterone levels still are higher in that tissue than in nonandrogen target tissues. Third, in vitro systems demonstrate a log-dose response effect of androgens, which extends over a 3-log range from $10^{-10}$ to $10^{-8}$ mol/L. After surgical castration, plasma testosterone levels fall over only a 1.5-log range by 95% from $10^{-10}$ to $0.5 \times 10^{-9}$ mol/L (i.e., 300 ng/dL to 15 ng/dL). Therefore, surgical castration might diminish the bioeffects of androgen on tumor cells by only 75%, whereas 25% remains from adrenal sources. The ablation of adrenal as well as testicular androgens (i.e., complete androgen blockade) might then produce more efficacious results in patients.

On the basis of this rationale, the treatment is a combination of either orchiectomy or GnRH-A therapy to eliminate testicular androgens, and a nonsteroidal antiandrogen (either flutamide or anandron [RU-23908]) to block adrenal androgen action. This regimen of complete androgen blockade is used for patients with stage C and D disease. In an early nonrandomized study, 95% of men responded objectively and the median survival at 2 years was 95%. These results are superior to those historically reported with orchiectomy or GnRH therapy alone. Randomized studies suggest that the efficacy of complete androgen blockade may not be as optimistic as initially suggested. The Southwest Oncology Group (SWOG) conducted the largest study, in conjunction with the Eastern Cooperative Oncology Group (i.e., the Intergroup Study). The initial report[71] indicated that prolongation of disease-free survival with complete androgen blockade was only ~3 months. Three French studies[72] reported similar findings.

One of the observations from the Intergroup Study is that a subset of men with limited disease may benefit to a greater extent from complete androgen blockade than do unselected patients. Among the men in the overall study, a subset of ~15% (41 men in each arm) had stage D disease with metastases limited either to axial (but not appendicular) bone or to local lymph nodes. Survival in this subset of patients appears to be substantially prolonged by the combined use of a GnRH-A plus an antiandrogen than by GnRH-A alone. An update of the Intergroup Study[73] revealed that in the subset of patients with minimal disease and excellent performance status, the median duration of survival in the combined therapy group was 61 months compared with 41 months for patients treated with leuprolide plus placebo. Median survival of the entire group was 35.1 months in the leuprolide-flutamide arm compared with 29.3 months in the leuprolide-placebo arm.[73]

The concept of complete androgen blockade remains somewhat controversial. Although not all studies have confirmed the advantages of combination versus single-modality therapy,[74] the use of maximal androgen blockade is gaining use. One possible explanation for the positive results observed with complete androgen blockade is that the antiandrogen merely blocks early tumor flare induced by GnRH-A therapy and, thus, prolongs patient survival. This hypothesis, however, is not supported by the finding that addition of the antiandrogen nilutamide to surgical castration improved clinical outcome over castration alone, both in terms of response rate (46% vs. 20%, $p = .001$) and overall survival (24.3 vs. 18.9 months, $p = .048$).[75]

Two other regimens also have been used to produce complete androgen blockade. In one, GnRH-A treatment is combined with ketoconazole.[64] In another, megestrol acetate is combined with low dosages of DES.[37] The progestational effects of megestrol act synergistically with DES to suppress LH and FSH secretion. In addition, megestrol probably also inhibits testosterone biosynthesis directly at the testicular level and suppresses adrenal androgens through its glucocorticoid actions. Results on responses to both regimens are preliminary.[76]

Although the use of hormone-cytotoxic conjugates (e.g., estramustine phosphate sodium, an alkylating agent–estradiol hybrid) does not increase survival, clinical improvement occurs in 10% to 20% of patients. Ongoing clinical trials using these agents in combination with other chemotherapeutic agents should soon reveal the effectiveness of such combinations.[77,78]

## ANDROGEN STIMULATION PLUS CHEMOTHERAPY

Another experimental approach is based on the rationale that prostate tumor cells are relatively resistant to chemotherapy because of their inherently slow doubling time. In this concept, transient stimulation of tumor cells with androgen would enhance their sensitivity to chemotherapy. Application of this strategy in an animal model of hormone-dependent prostate can-

cer demonstrated enhanced tumor regression and animal survival when chemotherapy was preceded by a period of androgen depletion and transient androgen repletion.[79] The only randomized trial[80] testing this concept did not demonstrate objective benefit from androgen stimulation when final data analyses were complete, although preliminary reports[64] were encouraging. The prevention of undue toxicity from androgen stimulation required that all patients receive screening myelograms and intravenous pyelograms before treatment. Those with impending spinal cord or urethral compression were eliminated from the trial because of fear of an initial worsening of their disease. The study included only patients relapsing after initial castration. On the basis of these results, androgen priming should not be recommended in routine clinical practice. Its potential merit earlier in the disease course should be tested in controlled clinical trials.

## EARLY CYTOTOXIC THERAPY

The suggestion has been made that prostate cancer may be more responsive to cytotoxic therapy if therapy is given before endocrine therapy and at a time of smaller tumor burden. A study in which chemotherapy was given for D2 disease before any endocrine therapy showed that, although the response rates may have been higher (30%) than for patients treated later in the course of disease, these responses were short-lived.[81] A second approach to early cytotoxic therapy is the combined use of hormonal manipulation and chemotherapy in untreated D2 disease. In a trial of orchiectomy or DES (3 mg per day) plus a CA regimen consisting of cyclophosphamide (500 to 650 mg/m²) and doxorubicin (20 to 30 mg/m²) every 21 days for 1 year,[82] no survival benefit was detected for patients who received CA early over those who progressed after DES/orchiectomy and then received CA. Too few patients were in this trial, however, to optimally detect an increase in survival; therefore, this combination therapy should be recommended only to patients expected to do poorly with endocrine therapy.

The role of vitamin D analogs as an antiproliferative, prodifferentiating, and proapoptotic agent in prostate cancer merits further study.[83]

## NEWER AGENTS

The recognition that increased bone resorption occurs in the presence of osteoblastic metastasis provides the rationale for the use of inhibitors of bone resorption in prostate cancer. Evidence indicates that administration of the bisphosphonate pamidronate provides significant improvement in bone pain and patient mobility. The treatment also produced significant decreases in the indices of bone turnover and stabilization of worsening bone scans in some patients.[84] Further controlled studies of bisphosphonate therapy in metastatic prostate cancer are warranted to assess the full therapeutic potential of this form of treatment.

The antiparasitic agent suramin has been tested in patients with hormone-refractory prostate cancer. The rationale for its use derives from the broad-spectrum anti–growth factor action of the drug.[85] In phase I clinical trials, its use has decreased the level of prostate-specific antigen by >75% in 70% to 80% of cases and reduced tumor masses in many patients with advanced prostate cancer.[86,87] Toxicity can be severe, however; therefore, patients should be considered for suramin therapy only in the context of clinical trials.

Encouraging results have been obtained with combinations of estramustine and either vinblastine, etoposide, or paclitaxel. Preclinical data suggest that these combinations may exert their effects through inhibition of microtubule function.[86]

# REFERENCES

1. Parker SL, Tong T, Bolden S, et al. Cancer Statistics 1996. CA Cancer J Clin 1996; 46:5.
2. Welsch CW. Host factors affecting the growth of carcinogen-induced rat mammary carcinomas: a review and tribute to Charles Brenton Huggins. Cancer Res 1985; 45:3415.
3. Holund B. Latent prostatic cancer in consecutive autopsy series. Scand J Urol Nephrol 1980; 14:29.
4. Catalona WJ, ed. Epidemiology and etiology. In: Prostate cancer. New York: Grune & Stratton, 1984:1.
4a. Ozen M, Pathak S. Genetic alterations in human prostate cancer: a review of current literature. Anticancer Res 2000; 20:1905.
5. Viola MV, Fromowitz F, Oravez S, et al. Expression of ras oncogene p21 in prostate cancer. N Engl J Med 1986; 314:133.
6. Gao X, Honn KV, Grignon D, et al. Frequent loss of expression and loss of heterozygosity of the putative tumor suppressor gene DCC in prostate carcinomas. Cancer Res 1993; 53:2723.
7. Gleason DF. Histologic grading and clinical staging of carcinoma of the prostate. In: Tannenbaum M, ed. Urologic pathology: the prostate. Philadelphia: Lea & Febiger, 1977:171.
8. Gleason DF, Mellinger GT, Veterans Administration Cooperative Urological Research Group. Prediction of prognosis for prostatic adenocarcinoma by combined histological grading and clinical staging. J Urol 1974; 111:58.
9. Catalona WJ, ed. Pathology. In: Prostate cancer. New York: Grune & Stratton, 1984:15.
10. Diamond DA, Berry SJ, Umbricht C, et al. Computerized image analysis of nuclear shape as a prognostic factor for prostatic cancer. Prostate 1982; 3:321.
11. Nativ O, Winkler HZ, Raz Y, et al. Stage C prostatic adenocarcinoma: flow cytometric nuclear DNA ploidy analysis. Mayo Clin Proc 1989; 64:911.
12. Winkler HZ, Rainwater LM, Myers RP, et al. Stage D1 prostatic adenocarcinoma: significance of nuclear DNA ploidy patterns studied by flow cytometry. Mayo Clin Proc 1988; 63:103.
13 Bonkhoff H, Stein U, Welter C, et al. Differential expression of the pS2 protein in the human prostate and prostate cancer: association with malignant changes and neuroendocrine differentiation. Hum Pathol 1995; 26:824.
14. Carter HB. Current status of PSA in the management of prostate cancer. Adv Surg 1994; 27:81.
14a. Lavoipierre AM. Ultrasound of prostate and testicles. World J Surg 2000; 24:198.
15. Donohue RE, Mani JH, Whitesel JA, et al. Pelvic lymph node dissection: guide to patient management in clinically locally confined adenocarcinoma of prostate. Urology 1982; 20:559.
16. Bonkhoff H, Remberger K. Differential pathways and histologenetic aspects of normal and abnormal prostatic growth: a stem cell model. Prostate 1996; 28:98.
17. Garabedian EM, Hunphrey PA, Gordon JI. A transgenic mouse model of metastatic prostate cancer originating from neuroendocrine cells. Proc Natl Acad Sci U S A 1995; 26:15382.
18. Krijen JL, Bogdanowicz JF, Seldenrijk CA, et al. The prognostic value of neuroendocrine differentiation in adenocarcinoma of the prostate in relation to progression of disease after endocrine therapy. J Urol 1997; 158:171.
19. Isaacs JT, Coffey DS. Adaptation versus selection as the mechanism responsible for the relapse of prostatic cancer to androgen ablation therapy as studied in the Dunning R3327H adenocarcinoma. Cancer Res 1981; 41:5070.
20. Partin AW, Coffey DS. Benign and malignant prostatic neoplasms: human studies. Recent Prog Horm Res 1994; 49:293.
21. The Leuprolide Study Group. Leuprolide vs diethylstilbestrol for metastatic prostatic cancer. N Engl J Med 1984; 311:1281.
22. Parmar H, Phillips RH, Lightman SL, et al. Randomized controlled study of orchidectomy vs. long-acting D-Trp-6-LHRH microcapsules in advanced prostatic cancer. Lancet 1985; 2:1201.
23. Fowler JE Jr, Whitmore WF Jr. The response of metastatic adenocarcinoma of the prostate to exogenous testosterone. J Urol 1981; 126:372.
24. Visakorpi T, Kallioniemi AH, Syvanen AC, et al. Genetic changes in primary and recurrent prostate cancer by comparative genomic hybridization. Cancer Res 1995; 55:342.
25. Kibel AS, Schutte M, Kern SE, et al. Identification of 12p as a region of frequent deletion in advanced prostate cancer. Cancer Res 1998; 58:5652.
26. Meyers FJ, Gumerlocj PH, Chi SG, et al. Very frequent p53 mutations in metastatic prostate carcinoma and in matched primary tumors. Cancer 1998; 83:2534.
27. Ueda T, Ichikawa T, Tamaru J, et al. Expression of KA1 protein in benign prostatic hyperplasia and prostate cancer. Am J Pathol 1996; 149:1435.
28. Lu J, Danielsen M. Differential regulation of androgen and glucocorticoid receptors by retinoblastoma protein. J Biol Chem 1998; 273:31528.
29. Sementchenko VI, Schweinfest CW, Papas TS, et al. ETS2 function is required to maintain the transformed state of human prostate cancer cells. Oncogene 1998; 17:2883.
30. Wolf RM, Schneider SL, Pontes JE, et al. Estrogen and progestin receptors in human prostatic carcinoma. Cancer 1985; 55:2477.
31. Glick JH, Wein A, Padavic K, et al. Phase II trial of tamoxifen in metastatic carcinoma of the prostate. Cancer 1982; 49:1367.
32. Klugo RC, Farrah RN, Cerny JC. Bilateral orchiectomy for carcinoma of prostate: response to serum testosterone and clinical response to subsequent estrogen therapy. Urology 1981; 17:49.

33. Cohen P, Peehl DM, Stamey TA, et al. Elevated levels of insulin-like growth factor-binding protein-2 in the serum of prostate cancer patients. J Clin Endocrinol Metab 1993; 76:1031.
34. Santen RJ. The testis. In: Felig P, Baxter J, Broadus A, Frohman L, eds. Endocrinology and metabolism, 2nd ed. New York: McGraw-Hill, 1986:821.
35. Sanford EJ, Paulsen DF, Rohner TJ, et al. The effects of castration on adrenal testosterone secretion in men with prostatic carcinoma. J Urol 1977; 118:1019.
36. Harper ME, Pike A, Peeling WB, Griffiths K. Steroids of adrenal origin metabolized by human prostatic tissue both in vivo and in vitro. J Endocrinol 1984; 60:117.
37. Geller J. Rationale for blockade of adrenal as well as testicular androgens in the treatment of advanced prostate cancer. Semin Oncol 1985; 12(Suppl 1):28.
38. Connolly JG, Mobbs EG. Clinical applications and value of receptor levels in treatment of prostate cancer. Prostate 1984; 5:477.
39. Trachtenberg J, Walsh PC. Correlation of prostatic nuclear androgen-receptor content with duration of response and survival following hormonal therapy in advanced prostatic cancer. J Urol 1982; 127:466.
40. Ghanadian R, Auf G, Williams G, et al. Predicting the response of prostatic carcinoma to endocrine therapy. Lancet 1981; 2:1418.
41. Byar DP. The Veterans Administration Cooperative Urological Group's studies of cancer of the prostate. Cancer 1973; 32:1126.
42. Byar DP, Corle DK. Hormone therapy for prostate cancer: results of the Veterans Administration Cooperative Urological Research Group studies. In: National Cancer Institute Monographs, no 7. Washington: US Government Printing Office, 1988:165.
43. Zincke H, Bergstralh EJ, Larson-Keller JJ, et al. Stage D1 prostate cancer treated by radical prostatectomy and adjuvant hormonal treatment. Cancer 1992; 70(Suppl):311.
44. Catalona WJ, ed. Endocrine therapy. In: Prostate cancer. New York: Grune & Stratton, 1984:145.
45. Beck PH, McAninch JW, Goebel JL, Stutzman RE. Plasma testosterone in patients receiving diethylstilbestrol. Urology 1978; 11:157.
46. Glashan RW, Robertson MRG. Cardiovascular complications in the treatment of prostatic carcinoma. Br J Urol 1981; 53:624.
47. Santen RJ, Manni A, Harvey H. Gonadotropin releasing hormone (GnRH) analogs for the treatment of breast and prostatic carcinoma. Breast Cancer Res Treat 1986:129.
48. Warner B, Worgul TJ, Drago J, et al. Effects of very high-dose D-leucine-6-gonadotropin-releasing hormone proethylamide on the hypothalamic-pituitary testicular axis in patients with prostatic cancer. J Clin Invest 1983; 71:1842.
49. Santen RJ, Demers LM, Max DT, et al. Long-term effects of administration of a gonadotropin-releasing hormone superagonist analog in men with prostatic carcinoma. J Clin Endocrinol Metab 1984; 58:397.
50. Evans RM, Doelle GC, Lindner J, et al. A luteinizing hormone releasing hormone agonist decreases biologic activity and modifies chromatographic behavior of luteinizing hormone in man. J Clin Invest 1984; 73:262.
51. Santen RJ, English HF, Warner BA. GnRH superagonist treatment of prostate cancer: hormonal effects with and without an androgen biosynthesis inhibitor. In: Labrie F, Belanger A, DuPont A, eds. LHRH and its analogues: basic and clinical aspects. Amsterdam: Excerpta Medica, 1984:336.
52. Ahmed SR, Grant J, Shalet SM, et al. Preliminary report on use of depot formulation of LHRH analog, ICI 118630 (Zoladex) in patients with prostatic cancer. BMJ 1985; 289:185.
53. Debruyne FM, Denis L, Lunglmayer G, et al. Long-term therapy with a depot luteinizing hormone-releasing hormone analogue (Zoladex) in patients with advanced prostatic carcinoma. J Urol 1988; 140:775.
54. Ahmann FR, Citrin DL, deHaan HA, et al. Zoladex: a sustained-release, monthly luteinizing hormone-releasing analogue for the treatment of advanced prostate cancer. J Clin Oncol 1987; 5:912.
55. Kruger H, Mohring K, Dorsam J, Vecsei P. The slow release form of leuprolide (TAP 144 SR) in the treatment of prostatic carcinoma: a hormonal profile. In: Proceedings of International Symposium on Endocrine Therapy, Monaco, November 19–21, 1988. Abstract A16.
56. Denis L, Mahler D. Ketoconazole in the treatment of prostate cancer. In: International Symposium on Hormonal Manipulation of Cancer: peptides, growth factors and new antisteroidal agents, June 4–6, 1986.
57. Sogani PC, Whitmore WF Jr. Experience with flutamide in previously untreated patients with advanced prostatic cancer. J Urol 1979; 122:640.
58. Smith RB, Walsh PC, Goodwin WE. Cyproterone acetate in the treatment of advanced carcinoma of the prostate. J Urol 1973; 110:106.
59. Beurton D, Grall J, Davody P, Cukier J. Treatment of prostatic cancer with cyproterone acetate as monotherapy. Prog Clin Biol Res 1987; 243A:369.
60. Visakorpi T, Hyytinen E, Kovisto P, et al. In vivo amplification of androgen receptor gene and progression of human prostate cancer. Nat Genet 1995; 9:401.
61. Koivisto P, Kolmer M, Visakorpi T, et al. Androgen receptor gene and hormonal therapy failure of prostate cancer. Am J Pathol 1998; 152:1.
62. Brendler H. Adrenalectomy and hypophysectomy for prostatic cancer. Urology 1973; 2:99.
63. Worgul TJ, Santen RJ, Samojlik E, et al. Clinical and biochemical effect of aminoglutethimide in the treatment of advanced prostatic carcinoma. J Urol 1983; 129:51.
64. Santen RJ, English H, Rohner T, et al. Androgen depletion/repletion in combination with chemotherapy: strategy for secondary treatment of metastatic

prostatic cancer. In: Schroeder FH, Richards B, eds. EORTC Genitourinary Group monograph 2 (part A): Therapeutic principles in metastatic prostatic cancer. New York: Alan R Liss, 1985:359.

65. Sogani PC, Ray B, Whitmore WF Jr. Advanced prostatic carcinoma: fluta-mide therapy after conventional endocrine treatment. Urology 1975; 6:164.

66. Trump DL, Havlin KH, Messing EM, et al. High-dose ketoconazole in advanced hormone-refractory prostate cancer: endocrinologic and clinical effects. J Clin Oncol 1989; 7:1093.

67. Susan LP, Roth RB, Adkins WC. Regression of prostatic cancer metastasis by high doses of diethylstilbestrol diphosphate. Urology 1976; 7:598.

68. Benson RC, Wear JB, Gill GM. Treatment of Stage D hormone resistant car-cinoma of the prostate with estramustine phosphate. J Urol 1979; 121:452.

69. Eisenberger MA. Chemotherapy for prostate carcinoma. National Cancer Institute Monographs, no 7. Washington, DC: US Government Printing Office, 1988:151.

70. Klotz L. Hormone therapy for patients with prostate carcinoma. Cancer 2000; 88(12 Suppl):3009.

71. Crawford CD, Eisenberger MA, McLeod DG, et al. A controlled trial of leu-prolide with and without flutamide in prostatic carcinoma. N Engl J Med 1989; 321:419.

72. Brisset JM, Bertagna C, Fist J, et al. Total androgen blockade vs. orchiectomy in stage D prostate cancer. Monograph Series of European Organization, Research and Treatment, 1987:17.

73. Eisenberger M, Crawford Ed, McCleod D, et al. A comparison of leuprolide and flutamide vs. leuprolide alone in newly diagnosed stage D2 prostate cancer. (Abstract). Proc Am Soc Clin Oncol 1992; 11:201.

74. Denis L, Mettlin C. Conclusions. Cancer 1990; 66(Suppl):1086.

75. Beland G, Elhilai M, Fradet Y, et al. A controlled trial of castration with and without nilutamide in metastatic prostatic carcinoma. Cancer 1990; 60(Suppl):1074.

76. Crombie C, Raghaven D, Page J, et al. Phase II study of megestrol acetate for metastatic carcinoma of the prostate. Br J Urol 1987; 59:443.

77. Loeng SA, Beckley S, Brandy MF, et al. Comparison of estramustine phos-phate, methotrexate and *cis*-platinum in patients with advanced, hormone refractory prostate cancer. J Urol 1983; 129:1001.

78. Pienta KJ, Reidman B, Hussian M. Phase II evaluation of oral estramustine and oral etoposide in hormone-refractory adenocarcinomas of prostate. J Clin Oncol 1994; 12:2005.

79. English HF, Heitjan DF, Lancaster, et al. Beneficial effects of androgen-primed chemotherapy in the Dunning R3327 G model of prostatic cancer. Cancer Res 1991; 51:1760.

80. Manni A, Bartholomew M, Caplan R, et al. Androgen priming and chemo-therapy in advanced prostate cancer. Evaluation of determinants of clinical outcome. J Clin Oncol 1988; 6:1456.

81. Seifter EJ, Bunn PA, Cohen MH, et al. A trial of combination chemotherapy followed by hormonal therapy for previously untreated metastatic carci-noma of prostate. J Clin Oncol 1986; 4:1365.

82. Osborne CK, Blumenstein B, Crawford ED, et al. Combined versus sequen-tial chemo-endocrine therapy in advanced prostate cancer: final results of a randomized Southwest Oncology Group study. J Clin Oncol 1990; 8:1675.

83. Feldman D, Zhao X-Y, Krishan AV. Editorial mini-review: vitamin D and prostate cancer. Endocrinology 2000; 141:5.

84. Clarke NW, Holbrook IB, McClure J, et al. Osteoclast inhibition by pamidronate in metastatic prostate cancer: a preliminary study. Br J Cancer 1991; 63:420.

85. Small EJ, Meyer M, Marshall ME, et al. Suramin therapy for patients with symptomatic hormone-refractive prostate cancer. J Clin Oncol 2000; 18:1440.

86. Myers C, Cooper M, Stein C, et al. Suramin: a novel growth factor antago-nist with activity in hormone-refractory metastatic prostate cancer. J Clin Oncol 1992; 10:881.

87. Eisenberger MA, Reyno LM, Jodrell DI, et al. Suramin, an active drug for prostate cancer: interim observations in a Phase I trial. J Natl Cancer Inst 1993; 85:611.

# CHAPTER 226

# ENDOCRINE CONSEQUENCES OF CANCER THERAPY

DAIVA R. BAJORUNAS

Survival statistics for cancer have improved dramatically dur-ing the past three decades. Overall, with aggressive multimodal-ity therapy, nearly 60% of newly diagnosed cancer patients can expect to survive beyond 5 years after diagnosis. Clinical cancer research efforts, therefore, increasingly focus on longer-term medical, psychologic, and economic effects of such treatment.

Endocrine system dysfunction as a consequence of chemother-apy, radiotherapy, and immunotherapy for malignancies is recog-nized with increasing frequency.[1] Prominent among acute effects are disordered glucose and mineral metabolism, hyperlipidemia, and cytokine-induced autoimmune thyroiditis (Tables 226-1 and 226-2). Long-term adverse effects of chemotherapy and radiother-apy on hypothalamic-pituitary, thyroid, parathyroid, and gonadal function continue to be well described in the literature, and the multifactorial nature of osteopenia in cancer survivors is being defined. These late sequelae remain the most clinically rel-evant endocrine complications of cancer therapy; they have prompted vigorous efforts at early detection and treatment as well as a search for measures to reduce or prevent such morbidity.

## THERAPY-INDUCED HYPOTHALAMIC-PITUITARY GLAND DYSFUNCTION

Iatrogenic hypothalamic-pituitary dysfunction commonly occurs after cranial irradiation for leukemia and tumors of the head and neck region, or with total body irradiation (TBI) in bone marrow transplantation (BMT). In patients receiving incidental hypotha-lamic-pituitary axis (HPA) irradiation in doses of up to 70 Gy, the risk of endocrine deficiencies may exceed 90%.[2] Growth hormone (GH) secretion is the first to fail after cranial radiation, and, in chil-dren, GH deficiency and premature sexual development are the most common therapy-induced neuroendocrine problems.[2,3] In adults, hyperprolactinemia is commonly observed, and complete or partial gonadotropin deficiency, tertiary hypothyroidism, or decreased thyrotropin (thyroid-stimulating hormone, TSH) reserve occur progressively in descending order of frequency. Whereas clinically significant adrenal insufficiency is relatively uncommon, subtle abnormalities in adrenal function may be present in up to one-third of patients. More than one-half of irradiated patients have manifest dysfunction of multiple endocrine axes. Inexplica-bly, diabetes insipidus does not occur after external radiation, even in patients with therapy-induced panhypopituitarism.

The available data indicate that the hypothalamus is more commonly the site of damage than is the pituitary.[2] Hypotha-lamic blood flow is reduced after cranial irradiation,[4] and incon-gruent GH secretory dynamics (normal responses to provocative stimuli, subnormal spontaneous secretion) and dose-dependent alteration in circadian/ultradian GH rhythms and pulsatility[5] suggest neurosecretory or regulatory dysfunction. Anterior pitu-itary responses to testing with hypothalamic peptides are charac-teristic of pathologically documented hypothalamic disease, and satisfactory end-organ responses to long-term treatment with gonadotropin- or GH-releasing hormone (GnRH, GHRH) have been described.[6,7] Data[8] suggest that a hierarchy of sensitivity to radiation damage exists, with the most vulnerable being extrahy-pothalamic neurotransmitter control of GH.

Both the total dose of cranial radiation and the fraction sizes determine the frequency of neuroendocrine dysfunction. GH deficiency and precocious puberty have been noted after con-ventional fractionated HPA irradiation with doses of ≥18 Gy, and after total doses as low as 9 to 10 Gy when given in a single dose, as in TBI for BMT.[3] A significant inverse relationship is seen between the dose of radiation and the stimulated peak GH responsiveness. Hypothalamic-pituitary radiation doses of >24 Gy place patients at high risk of developing GH deficiency.[5,9] The central nervous system is more sensitive to radiation at an early age; for any given dose of irradiation, the incidence of GH deficiency is lower in adults than in children, and the very young child who receives craniospinal irradiation is most at risk of extreme short stature. In adults, hyperprolactinemia or defi-ciencies of gonadotropins, TSH, or adrenocorticotropic hor-mone (ACTH) are very uncommon at doses under 40 to 50 Gy.[3]

**TABLE 226-1.**
**Effects of Chemotherapy on Endocrine Function**

| Chemotherapeutic Agents | Endocrine Function |
|---|---|
| *HYPOTHALAMUS-PITUITARY* | |
| Busulfan; 6-mercaptopurine | Secondary adrenal insufficiency* |
| L-Asparaginase[†] | ↓ TSH release |
| Vincristine (animal data) | ↓ GH release |
| Cyclophosphamide; vincristine; vinblastine; melphalan; cisplatin | Inappropriate vasopressin secretion (SIADH) |
| *THYROID* | |
| L-Asparaginase | ↓ TBG levels |
| 5-Fluorouracil; mitotane | ↑ TBG levels |
| BVP (bleomycin, vinblastine, cisplatin) chemotherapy | ↓ Thyroid hormone clearance (? via ↓ deiodinase activity) |
| Vinblastine (animal data) | ↓ Thyroidal hormone secretion |
| [131]I-containing radiopharmaceuticals; aminoglutethimide; vincristine, carmustine (or lomustine), procarbazine; mechlorethamine, vinblastine, procarbazine*[†] | ↑ TSH; ↓ T$_3$ , T$_4$ |
| Cisplatin, vinblastine; busulfan, cyclophosphamide | ↑ TSH; normal T$_3$, T$_4$ |
| Dactinomycin | ↑ Radiosensitization |
| Multidrug chemotherapy | ↑ Calcitonin levels* |
| *PARATHYROID* | |
| Vinblastine, L-asparaginase (animal data); multidrug chemotherapy for acute leukemia and breast cancer* | ↓ PTH secretion |
| *PANCREAS* | |
| Vincristine; L-asparaginase; streptozocin; plicamycin; mitomycin C, 5-fluorouracil | ↓ Insulin secretion |
| Cyclophosphamide | Autoimmune diabetes |
| Dacarbazine, mitomycin, doxorubicin, cisplatin, GM-CSF[†] | ↑ Insulin secretion, ↓ insulin action |
| L-Asparaginase[†] | ↑ Glucagon secretion |
| *ADRENAL* | |
| 5-Fluorouracil; 5-fluorodeoxyuridine | ↓ In vitro steroidogenesis |
| Mitotane; aminoglutethimide | ↓ Cortisol, ± ↓ aldosterone |
| *RENAL* | |
| Cisplatin; multidrug chemotherapy for ALL, AML[†] | ↓ 1,25-dihydroxyvitamin D, ↓ Ca, ↓ Mg |
| Ifosfamide; streptozocin | Nephrogenic DI |
| *BONE* | |
| Chlorambucil | ↑ Bone mineral density* |
| Plicamycin; dactinomycin; cisplatin,* estramustine | ↓ Bone resorption |
| ATRA | ↑ Ca, ↑ bone resorption |
| Methotrexate; doxorubicin (animal data); multidrug chemotherapy for ALL;[†] cisplatin, doxorubicin, cyclophosphamide | Osteopenia |
| Dactinomycin | ↑ Radiosensitization |
| Ifosfamide | Rickets |
| *METABOLIC DISORDERS* | |
| Multidrug chemotherapy for leukemias, lymphomas and (rarely) solid tumors | Tumor lysis syndrome, with ↑ P, ↓ Ca, ↑ K, ↑ uric acid |
| Mitotane; isotretinoin; etretinate; L-asparaginase; tamoxifen; cisplatin*; 5-fluorouracil | ↑ Cholesterol |
| Isotretinoin; etretinate; acitretin; ATRA; L-asparaginase; tamoxifen; 5-fluorouracil (animal data) | ↑ Triglycerides |

↓, decreased; ↑, increased; *TSH,* thyroid-stimulating hormone; *GH,* growth hormone; *SIADH,* syndrome of inappropriate secretion of antidiuretic hormone; *TBG,* thyroxine-binding globulin; *T$_3$,* triiodothyronine; *T$_4$,* thyroxine; *PTH,* parathyroid hormone; *GM-CSF,* granulocyte-macrophage colony-stimulating factor; *ALL,* acute lymphoblastic leukemia; *AML,* acute myeloblastic leukemia; *DI,* diabetes insipidus; *ATRA,* all-*trans* retinoic acid.
*Requires further substantiation.
[†]Concomitant corticosteroid administration.

**TABLE 226-2.**
**Endocrine Effects of Immune Modulators in Cancer Therapy**

| Immune Modulators | Endocrine Effect |
|---|---|
| Interleukin-2 | Thyroid dysfunction, ± hyperthyroidism or hypothyroidism (± LAK), on an autoimmune basis in some; acute painless thyroiditis; autoimmune hyperglycemia, with insulin and/or islet cell autoantibodies (± LAK); dyslipidemia, with ↓ TC, ↓ HDL-C, ↓ LDL-C, ↑ remnant lipoproteins, ↑ TG (± interferon-α, isotretinoin); ↓ testosterone, nl LH, ↓ DHEA; ↑ cortisol, ↑ β-endorphin, ↓ melatonin |
| Interleukin-4 | ↓ Bone resorption, ↓ calcium (animal data) |
| Interleukin-6 | ↓ TSH, ↓ T$_3$, ↓ or nl T$_4$, ↑ rT$_3$ |
| Interferons | α, γ: Thyroid dysfunction, ± hyperthyroidism, or hypothyroidism, on an autoimmune basis in some; autoimmune diabetes; ↑ TG |
| | α: Insulin allergy; ↓ TC, ↓ HDL-C, ↓ LDL-C |
| | β: ↑ Cortisol, ↑ ACTH, ↑ prolactin, ↑ GH, ↑ urinary free cortisol |
| | γ: Hyperglycemia with insulin resistance; ↑ cortisol; ↑ ACTH, ↑ GH; ↓ osteoclast formation (animal data) |
| Tumor necrosis factor | ↑ Cortisol, ↑ ACTH; exacerbation of hypothyroidism; autoimmune thyroid dysfunction (with interleukin-2); ↓ HDL-C, ↑ TG; ↑ glucagon |
| Cyclosporine A | ↑ TC, ↑ LDL-C |

↓, decreased; ↑, increased; *LAK,* lymphokine-activated killer cells; *TC,* total cholesterol; *HDL-C,* high-density lipoprotein cholesterol; *LDL-C,* low-density lipoprotein cholesterol; *TG,* triglycerides; *nl,* normal; *LH,* luteinizing hormone; *DHEA,* dehydroepiandrosterone; *TSH,* thyroid-stimulating hormone; *T$_3$,* triiodothyronine; *T$_4$,* thyroxine; *rT$_3$,* reverse triiodothyronine; *ACTH,* adrenocorticotropic hormone; *GH,* growth hormone.

Slowed growth velocity that is inappropriate for a child's age and stage of puberty is a very common, but not universal, outcome of GH deficiency in this setting. Age at irradiation is correlated not only with final height, with the youngest at irradiation having the worst growth prognosis, but also with the age at onset of puberty.[10] The majority of subjects who experience premature sexual maturation also have GH deficiency, and early puberty contributes to their poor growth.[3,10] An inverse relationship exists between time since therapy and stimulated peak GH responsiveness[11] (Fig. 226-1). In contrast to findings in patients with isolated idiopathic GH deficiency, young adults with radiation-induced GH dysfunction rarely revert to normal GH status.[12]

Little direct evidence exists that cytotoxic drugs impair anterior pituitary function (see Table 226-1). Growth deceleration in children has been seen to occur during antileukemic multimodality therapy, however, with some degree of "catch-up" growth occurring after completion of chemotherapy.[13] Moreover, final height as well as growth velocity after craniospinal irradiation for brain tumors is more profoundly affected in children who have received adjuvant chemotherapy than in those receiving craniospinal irradiation alone, suggesting potentiation of radiation-induced growth failure by the chemotherapy.[10] Cancer patients receiving chemotherapy regimens that include short-term, high-dose courses of corticosteroids are at risk for the development of adrenal suppression, which does not necessarily correlate with either the corticosteroid dosage or the duration of therapy. Impaired release of other pituitary hormones in response to provocative stimulation also can occur in such patients and is not inconsistent with the well-known multiple effects of corticosteroids on hypothalamic-pituitary function.

## PREVENTION AND TREATMENT

Routine hypothalamic-pituitary shielding during cranial radiation, dose targets of ≤18 Gy, and, in patients undergoing BMT, fractionation of TBI are measures that can provide some degree

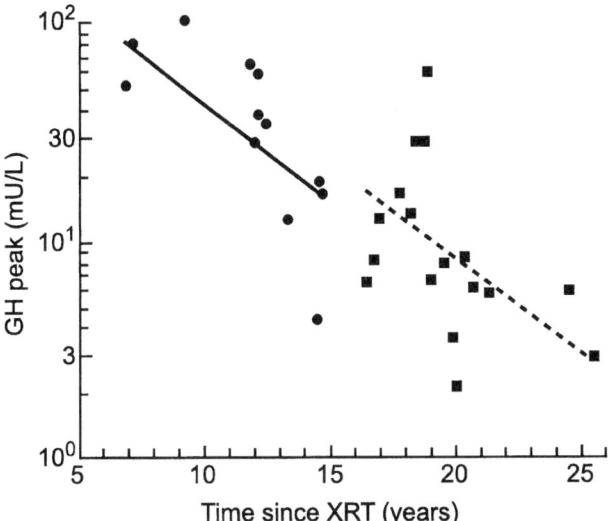

**FIGURE 226-1.** Relationship between the time since cranial irradiation (*XRT*) and the peak growth hormone (*GH*) response to an insulin-tolerance test in 32 adults who had received XRT in childhood as part of their treatment for acute lymphoblastic leukemia. The fitted lines are from the regression of log 10 of the peak GH response on time since therapy and dose group. *Solid circles* depict the subjects who received 18 Gy XRT; *solid squares* depict the subjects who received 24–25 Gy XRT. (Reprinted from Brennan BMD, Rahim A, Mackie EM, et al. Growth hormone status in adults treated for acute lymphoblastic leukaemia in childhood. Clin Endocrinol 1998; 48:777.)

of endocrine protection. Nevertheless, all patients who have received incidental hypothalamic-pituitary irradiation should undergo periodic evaluation for the integrity of the hypothalamic-pituitary target organ axes. In survivors of childhood leukemia, growth deceleration may occur after an interval of improved growth; therefore, all such patients should be followed until they have attained their final heights. As false-negative results may be common in children who have demonstrated slowed growth velocities after such irradiation, the wise course is to conduct pharmacologic testing for GH reserve with at least two agents, preferably including a carefully supervised insulin-induced hypoglycemic stimulus, which may provide a discriminatory advantage. A single plasma determination of insulin-like growth factor–binding protein-3 (IGFBP-3) is not a useful screening test for GH deficiency in this population. Pituitary size visualization with magnetic resonance imaging correlates with nocturnal GH secretion, but its utility in evaluating GH secretory capacity is unknown.[14]

In children with documented GH deficiency and growth retardation caused by HPA irradiation, GH replacement therapy should be initiated as promptly as is prudent—generally, in most institutions, after a 1-year disease-free interval. Although GH replacement can cause a gratifying increase in growth velocity, the final height, especially in children who have received craniospinal irradiation, is often significantly less than the midparental height. Concomitant therapy to suppress puberty should be considered in GH-deficient patients with early puberty who have a poor predicted final height. Traditionally, GH therapy in children has been discontinued when final height has been achieved. However, awareness is growing of adverse effects of adult GH deficiency. Altered body composition, physical performance, psychological well-being, and substrate metabolism, as well as an increased risk of cardiovascular disease and osteopenia, have been reported.[15] GH replacement corrects or improves many of these alterations, although longer-term effects have not been fully addressed. Although data from long-

term studies of children with both solid tumors and hematologic malignancies suggest that no increased risk of cancer recurrence is associated with GH therapy,[15] the safety of long-term GH replacement in an adult cancer population remains to be established. Replacement hormonal therapy should be instituted in patients shown to be hypothyroid, hypoadrenal, or hypogonadal. Infusion therapy with GnRH can induce ovulatory cycles in a small number of patients after cranial irradiation.[6] Overt clinical adrenal insufficiency after short-term, high-dose corticosteroid administration is rare, but patients so treated should undergo testing of adrenal reserve and are candidates for corticosteroid coverage if exposed to acute stress.

Although the highest incidence of endocrine complications after hypothalamic-pituitary irradiation occurs within the first 5 years after therapy, life-long surveillance in this population appears to be warranted.

## THERAPY-INDUCED THYROID GLAND DISEASE

### THYROID TUMORS

Abnormalities of thyroid morphology, including focal hyperplasia, single or multiple adenomas, chronic lymphocytic thyroiditis, colloid nodules, and fibrosis, are frequently found in patients exposed to radiation for nonmalignant conditions. Palpable thyroid lesions occur in 20% to 30% of an irradiated population, whereas a 1% to 5% prevalence of palpable nodular thyroid disease is found in the general population.[16] In patients who received head and neck irradiation for childhood cancer (thyroid dose, 22.5–40 Gy), thyroid sonography performed a decade later detects widespread abnormalities.[17] Nearly all patients have diffuse atrophy; half have discrete nodularity, with 39% developing new focal abnormalities at follow-up 6 to 18 months later.

The thyroid is one of the organs most sensitive to the neoplastic effects of radiation. Direct or incidental thyroid irradiation increases the risk of well-differentiated thyroid cancer, usually papillary, with an excess relative risk of 7.7 per Gy reported in a pooled analysis of seven studies in nearly 120,000 subjects.[18] In patients treated for childhood malignancies, the risk of secondary thyroid cancer is increased 15- to 53-fold.[19,20] Thyroid cancer risk increases with duration of follow-up. Although it appears to peak at 15 to 19 years after treatment, an excess risk is still apparent at 40 or more years after treatment.[18] At lower-dose exposures, the dose response is linear, even down to 0.10 Gy, with some indication of a leveling off at the high end of the radiation dose curve ($\geq$60 Gy).[18,20] The risk is highest after radiation at a young age (Fig. 226-2). A pattern of oncogene involvement that may be characteristic of radiation-induced thyroid cancers is suggested by detection of *p53* mutations (usually confined to anaplastic thyroid cancers) and a distinct pattern of *ret* oncogene rearrangements, a highly prevalent molecular alteration in thyroid tumors that developed in children after the Chernobyl reactor accident.[21,22] Data[23] suggest that a DNA repair defect is likely to be present in patients with radiation-associated thyroid tumor. The mortality does not seem to differ from that seen in nonirradiated thyroid cancer patients.[19]

Iodine-131 ($^{131}$I), used in the diagnosis and treatment of Graves disease and thyroid cancer for nearly 50 years, remains the most frequently used radioisotope for radioimmunotherapy in cancer patients. Previous epidemiologic studies of patients who had been treated with $^{131}$I failed to reveal an increased risk of thyroid cancer.[24] Although most of these patients were adults, children whose thyroid glands had received as much as 2 Gy of $^{131}$I irradiation also showed no increased risk of thyroid cancer.

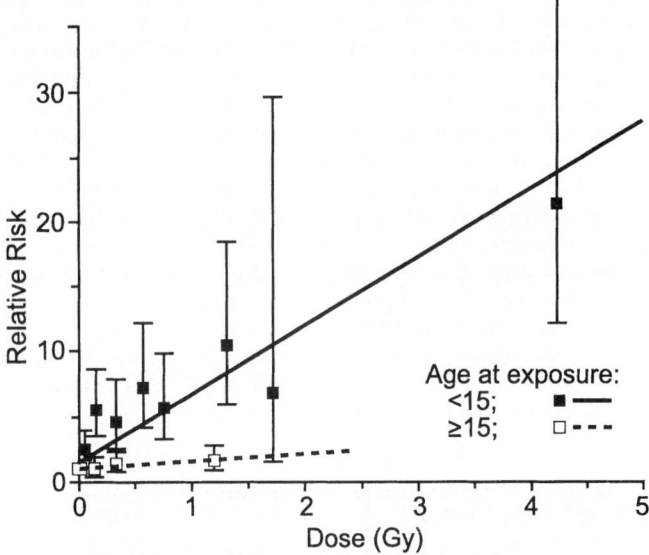

**FIGURE 226-2.** Relative risk of thyroid cancer after exposure to external radiation: a pooled analysis of seven studies.[18] (Reprinted from Ron E, Saftlas AF. Head and neck radiation carcinogenesis: epidemiologic evidence. Otolaryngol Head Neck Surg 1996; 115:403.)

These findings suggested that [131]I was less carcinogenic than acute exposure to x-rays. However, public interest in the late health effects of [131]I was rekindled by the 1986 Chernobyl nuclear reactor accident, which released very large amounts of [131]I and short-lived radioiodines into the atmosphere. In those exposed to thyroid doses of ≥0.1 to >10 Gy, after a short latency period, a markedly increased rate of childhood papillary thyroid cancer has now been reported, with a calculated excess relative risk of 22 to 90 per Gy.[24,25] A small but statistically significant increased risk in thyroid cancer mortality after [131]I treatment for adult hyperthyroidism has been reported after long-term follow-up (mean, 21 years).[26]

No excess risk of thyroid cancer has been described after exposure to alkylating agents or vinca alkaloid treatment, when radiation exposure is controlled for; however, a suggestion is seen of increased risk (relative risk, 39; 95% confidence interval, 1.6–947) in those receiving higher dose radiation (≥10 Gy) and dactinomycin than in those receiving radiation alone.[20]

## THYROID DYSFUNCTION

Primary hypothyroidism is the most common clinical consequence of irradiation of the thyroid in patients who have received therapeutic doses to the cervical area (30–70 Gy).[19] In patients with Hodgkin disease, one-half to two-thirds of those receiving incidental thyroidal irradiation can be expected to develop elevated TSH levels, with half frankly hypothyroid at presentation.[27] Most reports cite a 30% to 40% incidence of hypothyroidism in head and neck cancer patients. Almost twice as many have overt hypothyroidism as have subclinical hypothyroidism (an isolated TSH elevation with normal serum thyroxine and triiodothyronine), a pattern opposite to that seen in Hodgkin patients.[28]

The prevalence of thyroid dysfunction in patients with Hodgkin disease and other lymphomas appears somewhat increased compared with that in patients with carcinoma of the head and neck treated by radiotherapy alone, despite the fact that the latter group of patients generally receive higher doses of neck irradiation and frequently undergo hemithyroidectomy.

Information has been conflicting regarding the role of the iodine load associated with the use of radiographic contrast agents (especially the ethiodized oil used in lymphangiography) in predisposing such patients to radiation injury of the thyroid. More recently, a time-adjusted multivariate analysis of data for patients with Hodgkin disease, which accounted for other potentially important variables, found lymphangiography to be the only variable that significantly influenced the development of hypothyroidism.[29]

Other cancer populations at risk for primary thyroid dysfunction after cancer therapy are being identified. In children and adolescents treated for acute lymphoblastic leukemia with cranial or craniospinal irradiation, subtle primary hypothyroidism is relatively common, with significantly elevated mean nadir diurnal TSH and mean peak nocturnal TSH levels reported.[30] Among patients receiving single-fraction TBI for BMT in childhood, 73% develop overt (15%) or subclinical (58%) hypothyroidism within a mean follow-up period of 3.2 years; fractionating the irradiation results only in transiently elevated TSH levels in 25%.[31] Spinal axis irradiation for central nervous system malignancies results in hypothyroidism in 20% to 68% of children.[19]

Irradiation-induced hypothyroidism shows a dose dependency, with the prevalence and severity of thyroid dysfunction lower in patients receiving <30 Gy to the neck[27] (Fig. 226-3). In patients with head and neck cancer, hemithyroidectomy in the setting of thyroidal irradiation results in a three-fold to four-fold higher prevalence of thyroid dysfunction. Most investigators have not found age at irradiation to be a risk factor when the data are controlled for radiation doses. Whereas the actuarial risk for the development of hypothyroidism after incidental thyroidal irradiation increases most rapidly in the first 5 years after therapy, continued deterioration of thyroid function occurs (see Fig. 226-3). Recovery of euthyroid function, although reported, remains distinctly uncommon.

Graves hyperthyroidism, with or without infiltrative ophthalmopathy, has been reported to occur 3 weeks to 18 years

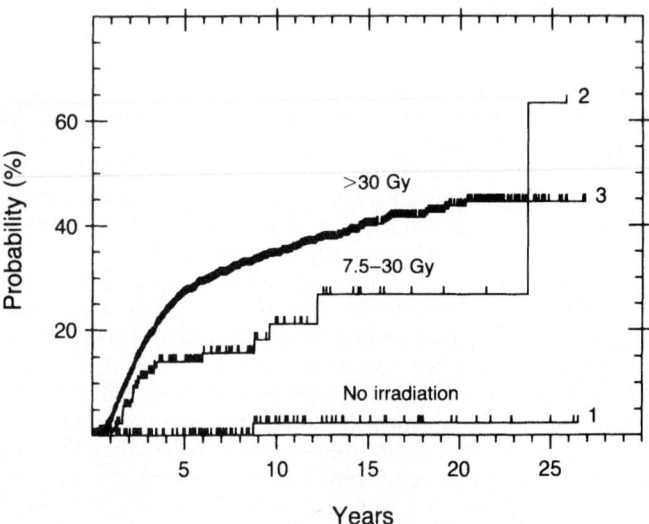

**FIGURE 226-3.** Actuarial risk of hypothyroidism in 1787 patients treated for Hodgkin disease from the time of initial therapy. *Curve 1* represents the risk for 110 patients who did not undergo irradiation of the thyroid; *curve 2*, the risk for 140 patients who received 7.5 to 30 Gy; and *curve 3*, the risk for 1537 patients who received >30 Gy. The differences between curves 1 and 2 (*p* = .0001), curves 2 and 3 (*p* = .0083), and curves 1 and 3 (*p* <.0001) were all significant by the Gehan test. (Reprinted from Hancock SL, Cox RS, McDougall IR. Thyroid diseases after treatment of Hodgkin's disease. N Engl J Med 1991; 325:599.)

after incidental thyroidal irradiation for nonthyroidal neoplastic disease, with a risk that is 7.2 to 20.4 times the expected risk.[27] One-third of the patients in whom Graves hyperthyroidism developed had been receiving thyroxine before its onset. The reason for development of autoimmunity is unknown, but irradiation-induced thyroidal damage possibly may cause a subsequent release of thyroid antigens, and a triggered immunologic reaction causes both the hyperthyroidism and the ophthalmopathy.[32] Silent thyroiditis (transient hyperthyroidism with a low radioiodine uptake) may also occur.[33]

Conflicting data continue to be reported on the role of chemotherapy in radiation-induced thyroid dysfunction. In patients with Hodgkin disease, one multivariate analysis found chemotherapy to be a more important factor in the development of hypothyroidism than an increasing dose of radiation,[27] whereas another, performed in a similar population, found no effect.[29] Information about the effect of chemotherapeutic agents alone on thyroid function is sparse (see Table 226-1). Elevated serum TSH levels have been reported to occur in 44% of patients with lymphoma after chemotherapy alone, a prevalence higher than expected that has not been confirmed. Cisplatin and vinblastine have been implicated in subtle thyroidal dysfunction, and subclinical hypothyroidism after a cyclophosphamide-busulfan pre-BMT regimen has been reported in isolated cases.

Thyroid dysfunction has been reported in 15% to 30% of patients with cancer who receive immunotherapy with interleukin-2 (IL-2) and interferon-α, with or without lymphokine-activated killer cells (see Table 226-2). In a prospective study[34] of such patients receiving IL-2 alone, 41% of initially euthyroid patients developed thyroid dysfunction, with 35% becoming hypothyroid. Although the hypothyroidism is mild and reversible in the majority, symptomatic hypothyroidism necessitated thyroid hormone replacement in 9%. Hyperthyroidism occurred in 7% of patients receiving high-dose IL-2. Elevated titers of antithyroglobulin and antimicrosomal antibodies have been reported in such patients.

## PREVENTION AND TREATMENT

Few measures are effective in preventing treatment-induced thyroid dysfunction. Excluding the thyroid from the fields of irradiation may risk cervical lymph node recurrence in lymphoma or head and neck cancer. The administration of thyroxine before irradiation does not prevent subsequent hypothyroidism. Moreover, no convincing evidence exists that long-term suppressive thyroid hormone therapy reduces either the incidence of benign thyroid nodularity or the incidence of subsequent cancer in patients with incidental thyroidal irradiation who lack either laboratory or clinical evidence of thyroid abnormalities.

Thyroid function testing should be performed routinely in all asymptomatic patients who have received incidental thyroidal irradiation, semiannually for the first 5 years, then annually. Patients with Hodgkin disease and radiation-induced pericarditis should always be evaluated for hypothyroidism because a causal association may exist between these two radiation-induced complications. Serum thyroglobulin determinations may identify patients who should be examined and followed more carefully for thyroid nodules and cancer. Thyroid sonography is more sensitive than physical examination and scanning, but as detected nodules are so prevalent, care in interpretation is advised.

In patients with documented overt hypothyroidism, thyroid hormone replacement should be initiated with thyroxine. Patients with radiation-induced subclinical hypothyroidism should also, in all likelihood, be treated. Such patients may manifest subtle abnormalities in myocardial contractility and may

also be at risk for hypercholesterolemia and accelerated atherosclerosis. Moreover, experimental evidence in animals suggests that an elevated TSH level in the presence of irradiation-damaged thyroid tissue is carcinogenic. Although conclusive evidence that this indeed occurs in the human is lacking, more palpable thyroidal abnormalities and all the thyroid cancers found in a large cohort of such patients occurred in patients not receiving thyroxine,[27] and a longer duration of a raised TSH is associated with focal sonographic abnormalities.[17] Although transient elevations in TSH levels can occur, a reasonable assumption is that, in most patients with subclinical hypothyroidism, progression to more overt dysfunction will occur.

In a substantial number of patients with palpable irradiation-induced thyroid nodules, no clinical suspicion of thyroid cancer, and benign cytology on thyroid needle aspiration, suppressive therapy with thyroid hormone has led to complete regression in the first year of therapy. If surgery is performed for benign thyroid nodules, a high recurrence rate is reported, which can be decreased by thyroid hormone therapy. The management of thyroid cancer in this population does not differ from management for malignancy not induced by radiation.

## RADIATION-INDUCED PARATHYROID DISEASE

Hyperparathyroidism has been found in 5% to 11% of irradiated patients. Rarely, this has been due to parathyroid carcinoma. In up to 30% of patients presenting with primary hyperparathyroidism, a history of prior low-dose external irradiation for benign disease can be elicited. This incidence of irradiation history is considerably higher than that seen in control patients. The latency period is protracted (mean, 30–47 years) and radiation doses are low (<7.5 Gy). Age at therapy is not a significant predictor. Data[35] suggest that a very high proportion of patients exposed to childhood radiation who subsequently manifest hyperparathyroidism also develop thyroid tumors (84%), including thyroid cancer (31%). Hyperparathyroidism has not been clearly identified to occur after cancer therapy, perhaps because of the associated high dose of irradiation.[36] Conversely, high-dose radiation may cause a hypoparathyroid tendency.[37]

## POSTTHERAPY GONADAL DYSFUNCTION

### OVARIAN DYSFUNCTION

Human ovaries acquire their lifetime quota of oocytes before birth; the number declines at a biexponential rate thereafter.[38] Although an upper limit for the dose of radiation that causes death in 50% of human oocytes has been estimated to be 4 Gy,[39] the clinical consequences of radiation-induced ovarian damage depend on the age of the patient and the status of her follicular development, as well as on the ability of the primordial oocytes to survive the damage. Although permanent menopause can be caused by a radiation exposure of ~6 Gy in women aged 40 years or older, the dose level with 50% probability of causing permanent sterility in young women is ~20 Gy over a 6-week period.[40] Radiation-induced ovarian damage is dose dependent: a 68% prevalence of persistent amenorrhea was detected in long-term survivors of childhood cancer when both ovaries were within abdominal radiotherapy fields (mean estimated ovarian tissue dose, ~32 Gy).[41] Damage to the ovary is increased if the radiation dosage is delivered in a smaller number of fractionated doses: 97% of 2068 women failed to menstruate again after two to four fractionated doses of 6.25 to 10.5 Gy (estimated ovarian dose,

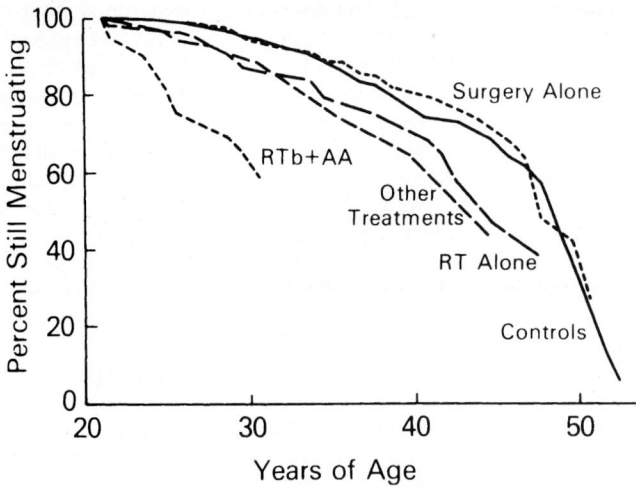

**FIGURE 226-4.** Proportion still menstruating among cancer survivors diagnosed between the ages of 13 and 19 years, grouped by the type of treatment received and compared with the proportion of controls still menstruating (Kaplan-Meier curves). Survivor and control cohorts only. (*RTb + AA*, radiotherapy below the diaphragm plus alkylating agents; *RT*, radiotherapy.) (Reprinted from Byrne J, Fears TR, Gail MH, et al. Early menopause in long-term survivors of cancer during adolescence. Am J Obstet Gynecol 1992; 166:788.)

3.6–7.2 Gy).[42] Radioiodine ablation therapy, which is performed after thyroidectomy for thyroid cancer, is followed by transient ovarian failure, particularly among older women. Commonly, a temporary amenorrhea occurs during the first year, which is associated with increased serum gonadotropins.[43]

Although data to the contrary are found, treatment with radiation fields that exclude the pelvis appears to confer little risk of permanent ovarian failure.[44] Transposition of the ovaries (oophoropexy) before irradiation, with a consequent reduction in the dose delivered to the shielded ovaries to a maximum of 6 Gy, reduces the incidence of amenorrhea by >50%.[45] Lateral rather than medial transposition of the ovaries is preferred if irradiation of the pelvic lymph nodes is planned, although this procedure may not be uniformly effective.[46]

Women receiving chemotherapy as well as subdiaphragmatic irradiation appear to be at an even higher risk of gonadal failure[47] (Fig. 226-4). That the toxicity is additive might be anticipated from the similar histologic appearance of ovaries exposed to either treatment modality alone: stromal fibrohyalinization, necrotic vasculitis, hemorrhage, absence of growing follicles, and reduction of the number of small primordial follicles have been documented. Even in children treated with combined-modality therapy, autopsy studies have shown extreme ovarian damage, with only 3% of the small follicle complement of the ovary surviving.[48] In all patients with hematologic malignancies, BMT after multiagent cytotoxic chemotherapy, with or without TBI, results in symptomatic ovarian failure, with amenorrhea and sonographically documented reduction in ovarian size associated with follicular depletion.[49] Ovarian recovery after TBI and BMT has been reported, however.[50] The actuarial chance of having a menstrual period at 10 years after BMT was 100% in girls who were premenarchal at therapy and 36% in those who were postmenarchal; in the latter group, the rate was 100% if the patient was younger than 18 years of age at transplant and 15% if she was older than 18 years.

At least 50% of women treated with combination chemotherapy containing alkylating agents or procarbazine, or both, become amenorrheic[51] (Table 226-3). Elevated serum gonadotropin levels and low plasma estradiol levels comparable with

**TABLE 226-3.**
**Drugs Causing Infertility**

| Definite | Probable |
|---|---|
| Chlorambucil | Doxorubicin |
| Cyclophosphamide | Vinblastine |
| L-Phenylalanine mustard | Cytosine arabinoside |
| Nitrogen mustard | Nitrosoureas |
| Busulfan | Etoposide (VP-16-213) |
| Procarbazine | Cisplatin |
| Thiotepa | Amsacrine (M-AMSA) |
| | Carmustine |
| | Lomustine |
| | Mitomycin C |
| | Dactinomycin |

| Unlikely/Rare | Unknown |
|---|---|
| Methotrexate | Interleukin-2 |
| 5-Fluorouracil | Interferon-α |
| 6-Mercaptopurine | Paclitaxel |
| Vincristine | |
| Azathioprine | |
| L-Asparaginase | |
| Bleomycin | |
| Carboplatin | |
| Dacarbazine | |

(Adapted from Gradishar WJ, Schilsky RL. Ovarian function following radiation and chemotherapy for cancer. Semin Oncol 1989; 16:425; and from Shahin MS, Puscheck E. Reproductive sequelae of cancer treatment. Obstet Gynecol Clin North Am 1998; 25;423.)

those seen in postmenopausal women confirm the presence of primary gonadal failure. Based on data from 3628 premenopausal women treated for breast cancer with adjuvant chemotherapy (regimens composed of cyclophosphamide, methotrexate, and fluorouracil given for at least 3 months), the incidence of chemotherapy-related amenorrhea is 68% (95% confidence interval, 66–70%).[52] The risk of ovarian dysfunction varies according to the chemotherapy regimen used (Table 226-4) and is strongly age dependent. In a follow-up of patients treated with nitrogen mustard, vincristine, procarbazine, and prednisone chemotherapy for Hodgkin disease, up to 90% of women

**TABLE 226-4.**
**Gonadal Toxicity of Combination Chemotherapy Regimens**

| Toxic | Less Toxic | Least Toxic |
|---|---|---|
| MVPP or MOPP | ABVD | VAPEC-B |
| ChlVPP/EVA | ChlVPP | VACOP-B |
| COPP | CHOP | MACOP-B |
| BEAM | | VEEP |
| COPP/ABVD | | |
| CMF | | |
| Bu/Cy | | |

*MVPP*, mechlorethamine, vinblastine, procarbazine, prednisolone; *MOPP*, mechlorethamine, vincristine, procarbazine, prednisone; *ChlVPP/EVA*, chlorambucil, vinblastine, procarbazine, prednisolone/etoposide, vincristine, doxorubicin; *COPP*, cyclophosphamide, vincristine, procarbazine, prednisone; *BEAM*, BiCNU (carmustine), etoposide, ara-C, melphalan; *COPP/ABVD*, cyclophosphamide, vincristine, procarbazine, prednisone/cyclophosphamide, vincristine, procarbazine, prednisone; *CMF*, cyclophosphamide, methotrexate, 5-fluorouracil; *BuCy*, busulfan, cyclophosphamide; *ABVD*, cyclophosphamide, vincristine, procarbazine, prednisone; *CHOP*, cyclophosphamide, doxorubicin, vincristine, prednisolone; *VAPEC-B*, vincristine, doxorubicin, prednisolone, etoposide, cyclophosphamide, bleomycin; *VACOP-B*, vinblastine, doxorubicin, prednisolone, vincristine, cyclophosphamide, bleomycin; *MACOP-B* (as VACOP-B except mustine in place of vinblastine); *VEEP*, vincristine, etoposide, epirubicin, prednisolone.

(Adapted from Howell S, Shalet S. Gonadal damage from chemotherapy and radiotherapy. Endocrinol Metab Clin North Am 1998; 27:927.)

older than 25 years at diagnosis developed amenorrhea, whereas 80% of those younger than 25 years at diagnosis continued to menstruate normally. The outlook for therapy of childhood malignancies remains more optimistic. Normal or early pubertal development and menarche have been reported in girls treated for acute lymphoblastic leukemia despite biochemical evidence of primary gonadal damage,[53] and 87% of girls treated for Hodgkin disease in childhood have normal menstrual function at a median follow-up of 9 years.[54]

The adverse impact of cancer and its therapy on sexual function is well described. Vaginal dryness, reduced sexual desire, reduced ability to have orgasm, and less enjoyment of sexual intercourse are the most frequently reported factors that affect the sexuality of patients with gynecologic malignancies, many of whom have been rendered menopausal by cancer therapy.[55] However, a high prevalence of global sexual dysfunction has been reported in younger women with breast cancer and those who are pre-BMT that is not clearly associated with ovarian failure. No long-term outcomes of sexual dysfunction obtained from longitudinal data have been reported, although an ongoing prospective multi-center trial assessing gonadal function, sexuality, and quality of life in women after breast cancer diagnosis should help address these important issues.

In women who remain fertile after chemotherapy, no evidence of an increase in birth defects during subsequent pregnancies is seen.[56,57] Uterine volume, musculature, and blood flow are irreversibly affected by high-dose irradiation in childhood; these abnormalities are not improved by physiologic sex steroid replacement.[58] In pregnancies after BMT that includes TBI, an increased risk of spontaneous abortion has been reported, and pregnancies in all women who receive marrow transplant are likely to be accompanied by preterm labor and delivery of offspring with low or very low birth weight.[59] In women receiving donated embryos, prior exposure to chemotherapy has been shown to lead to greater pregnancy wastage, possibly due to altered endometrial integrity.[60]

### PREVENTION AND TREATMENT

Transposition of the ovaries to allow better shielding during radiotherapy is of use in some women. Animal models suggest that suppression of the pituitary-gonadal axis may provide some protection against ovarian follicular depletion. Although preliminary data[61] from a study using a GnRH agonist during chemotherapy for lymphoma suggest that ovarian protection may be possible, most clinical trials in which oral contraceptives or GnRH antagonists are used to suppress ovarian function during chemotherapy have shown disappointing results. Cryopreservation of oocytes before cancer therapy is not a feasible option, given the technical challenges and the inherent time constraints. Cryopreservation of embryos is much more successful, but delay to cancer treatment also precludes its use. Cryopreserved ovarian tissue, however, has been shown to maintain postthaw follicular viability; such tissue, obtained from cancer patients before cancer therapy and reimplanted on the completion of treatment, may provide an avenue for the maintenance of endogenous ovarian function in women who would otherwise be rendered infertile.[62]

Currently, all women who have successfully completed cancer therapy should be followed at half-yearly or yearly intervals. If oligomenorrhea or secondary amenorrhea develops, determination of serum gonadotropin levels can help ascertain if it is a consequence of primary ovarian failure or is secondary to hypothalamic-pituitary dysfunction. In the latter patients, one should search carefully for nutritional, emotional, or stress-related factors; hypothyroidism; or hyperprolactinemia. In most patients, however, amenorrhea after cytotoxic therapy is due to primary

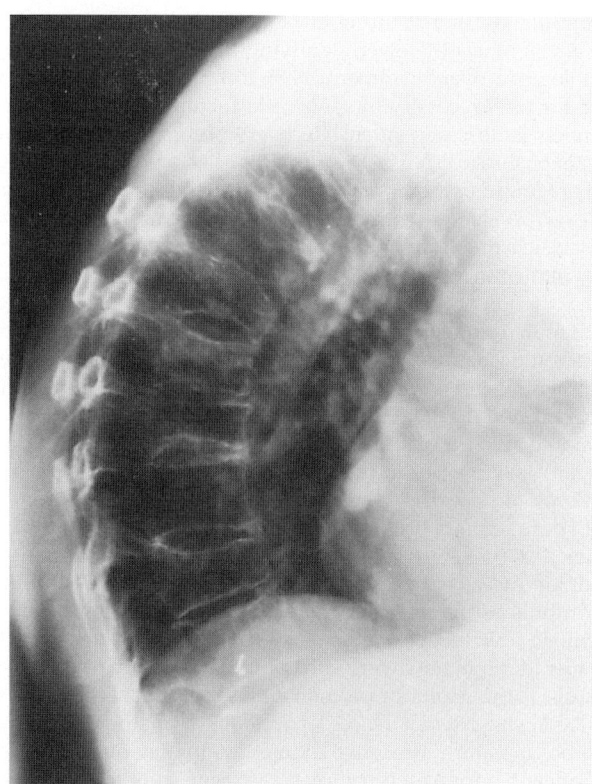

**FIGURE 226-5.** Radiographic appearance of osteoporosis in a patient with Hodgkin disease and therapy-induced premature menopause. Marked osteopenia is apparent on this radiograph of the thoracic spine of a 59-year-old woman who developed treatment-related premature menopause at age 43 after receiving radiation therapy for Hodgkin disease. She did not receive hormone-replacement therapy. Severe compression fractures are noted at T6, T8, and T10. A moderate compression fracture has developed in the T7 vertebral body in the past year.

gonadal failure, and no therapeutic options are available to reverse the induced ovarian damage or to speed recovery of the remaining ovarian follicles.

Serious and disturbing hot flashes, decreased libido, irritability, dyspareunia, and depression commonly occur in women rendered prematurely menopausal after cancer therapy, and decreased bone mineral density can occur in this population (Fig. 226-5) (see Chap. 100). Thus, in patients in whom gonadal failure has been confirmed and for whom no contraindication to hormone-replacement therapy (HRT) exists, treatment with estrogen and progesterone should be instituted promptly, preferably in a continuous sequential or continuous combined regimen, and parameters of bone mineralization should be monitored over time in this high-risk population. Use of selective estrogen-receptor modulators may be considered in postmenopausal women at high risk for osteoporosis who are not current candidates for HRT. The safety of estrogen use in menopausal survivors of breast cancer is being assessed by several large ongoing cooperative trials.

### TESTICULAR DYSFUNCTION

The testis is one of the most radiosensitive tissues, and very low doses of radiation cause significant impairment of function. The effect of graded doses of testicular irradiation (0.08–6 Gy) on spermatogenesis in healthy fertile men has been well documented.[63,63a] Spermatogonia are the most radiosensitive cell type; both morphologic and quantitative changes are observed at all dosage levels. At doses of 2 to 3 Gy, spermatocytes are unable to complete maturation division; at doses of 4 to 6 Gy, the resultant spermatozoa are significantly fewer, signifying covert spermatid damage. Histologic recovery commences at 6 to 7.5 months; however, the time for total recovery of sperm production and germinal cell numbers is dose dependent. Recovery occurs in 9 to 18 months after exposure to 0.2 to 1 Gy, 30 months after exposure to 2 to 3 Gy, and not until 5 or more years after exposure to 4 to 6 Gy. Although the exact level required is not known, a single radiation exposure must be in a much larger dose to produce permanent sterility, perhaps in the range of 10 to 20 Gy.

Irradiation of the testis during radiotherapy usually involves fractionated exposures; although it is unproved in humans, fractionation probably causes more stem cell killing than do single treatments. Men who are given abdominal irradiation (inverted Y, pelvic, and inguinal field) for Hodgkin disease receive a considerable amount of scatter irradiation to the testes. Total doses of 1.4 to 3 Gy can produce complete aspermia in most such men, and only one-fourth of these patients had oligospermia or normal sperm counts at the time of retrospective analysis.[64] Low doses (0.2–0.7 Gy) of scatter irradiation during treatment for Hodgkin disease can result in transient injury to the seminiferous tubule as manifested by elevations of follicle-stimulating hormone (FSH). Levels return to normal within 12 to 24 months after irradiation, however, with complete recovery of spermatogenesis. A threshold for permanent testicular damage of 1.2 Gy has been suggested.[65] Dose-dependent spermatogenic damage also occurs after radioactive iodine therapy for thyroid cancer; significant impairment of spermatogenesis is found in men receiving multiple doses totaling 100 or more mCi (equivalent to a testicular radiation dose of 0.5–1 Gy).[66] Below a dose of 12 Gy, testosterone levels tend to be normal, although luteinizing hormone levels may be raised; after a dose of 20 Gy, however, Leydig cell function is significantly impaired. A greater vulnerability to radiation-induced Leydig cell damage is noted in prepubertal boys than in adult males. Other reported complications of pelvic irradiation are the development of impotence and psychogenic sexual dysfunction.

The effect of cytotoxic agents on testicular germinal tissue is radiomimetic, and usually the germ cells are more selectively damaged (see Table 226-3). Testicular biopsy specimens show peritubular fibrosis, with or without hyalinosis, absent or scattered spermatogonia (Sertoli-cell-only or germinal aplasia), and well-preserved Leydig cells. Elevated serum FSH levels confirm germinal cell aplasia; however, decreased serum testosterone levels with elevated serum luteinizing hormone levels, gynecomastia, increased serum estradiol levels, and decreased libido and sexual performance have infrequently been observed. An analysis of 30 studies of male gonadal function after various chemotherapy regimens has shown testicular dysfunction to occur in 45%.[67] Although evidence of recovery of testicular function with time is found, testicular biopsy specimens have shown significant morphologic abnormalities as late as 62 months after treatment for Hodgkin disease. In ~90% of patients with up to 6 to 8 years of follow-up, persistent azoospermia has occurred when six or more cycles of combination chemotherapy containing alkylating agents and procarbazine were used as therapy. A consistent, dose-dependent, and reversible suppression of plasma testosterone levels has been observed during cancer therapy with the cytokine interleukin-2.[68]

Results are more encouraging for patients with various neoplasms treated with alternative (newer) chemotherapeutic regimens, such as has been reported for patients with acute lymphoblastic leukemia or testicular cancer[69] (see Tables 226-3 and 226-4). In lymphoma patients treated with the combination chemotherapy cyclophosphamide, doxorubicin, vincristine, and prednisone plus bleomycin, with or without radiotherapy,

gonadal recovery was noted by 7 years in two-thirds of the patients who were rendered aspermic during treatment. The pelvic radiotherapy dose and cumulative cyclophosphamide dose of >9.5 g/m$^2$ were independent significant determinants of recovery.[70] At one time, a prepubertal age in a patient undergoing chemotherapy was thought to be protective. Long-term studies, however, indicate a high incidence of germinal cell damage in boys treated before adulthood for Hodgkin disease.[71] In an assessment of fertility after chemotherapy for testicular germ cell cancers, the prechemotherapy sperm count had the strongest predictive value for recovery.[72] Several reports, however, have shown decreased potential fertility and testicular histologic abnormalities in pretherapy semen analysis specimens and testicular biopsy material in patients with malignant disease, especially those with Hodgkin disease and those with testicular carcinoma. These findings raise important questions about the impact of the underlying disease per se on the degree of infertility seen after therapy.

In addition to impairment of steroidogenesis and sperm production, chemotherapy-induced increased aneuploid frequency and an increase in chromosomal abnormalities have been demonstrated in patients treated for various malignancies.[73] Data concerning the outcome of pregnancies, however, have not shown any increase in genetically mediated birth defects, altered sex ratios, or birth weight effects in the offspring of cancer survivors,[69] possibly as a result of selection bias against genetically abnormal sperm.

### PREVENTION AND TREATMENT

In a murine model, the use of a GnRH analog has provided impressive testicular protection from histologically detectable cyclophosphamide-induced damage. These results indicate that inhibition of the pituitary-gonadal axis might reduce the rate of spermatogenesis and render the testis less susceptible to the effects of chemotherapy. However, subsequent clinical and experimental trials with such analogs, with or without testosterone, in patients undergoing cancer therapy have shown no beneficial effect. As animal data suggest that hormonal treatment may enhance the recovery of spermatogenesis from surviving stem cells rather than protect the cells from damage during cytotoxic or radiation insult, continuing suppressive therapy in patients for a fixed time after completion of irradiation or chemotherapy may prove more successful.[69]

Semen cryopreservation with artificial insemination has become standard practice and should be offered to all men before cytotoxic cancer therapy. Long-term experience with this practice has suggested that a prefreeze sperm motility of ≥15% predicts a postthaw motility of >10%.[74] Newer methods of assisted reproductive techniques, such as intracytoplasmic sperm injection, permit conception even in cases of severe oligo-asthenospermia; the success rate with this technique in cancer patients is ~20% per cycle.[75] A future consideration is stem cell autoimplantation after freeze storing before the start of sterilizing therapy, a technique demonstrated with donor stem cells in animals.[76] For men with uncommon therapy-related hypogonadism, treatment with transdermal or parenteral testosterone preparations, given in physiologic replacement doses, can result in improvement in mood, physical strength, libido, and potency.

## EFFECTS OF THERAPY ON BONE

Abnormal bone mineral density is an increasingly recognized long-term consequence of cancer therapy, described in both males and females, adults and children. Altered mineral metabolism has been noted in children with acute leukemia at diagnosis, probably secondary to the leukemic process, which becomes more prevalent with treatment.[77] Various metabolic abnormalities have been described in such patients (see Table 226-1). The most obvious contributor to the therapy-related skeletal morbidity seen in young leukemic patients is corticosteroid therapy; however, long-term untreated GH deficiency may also participate in the pathogenesis of this bone loss. Osteoporosis is common among patients undergoing marrow transplantation. Among the mechanisms invoked are the baseline disease, the use of immunosuppressive drugs, and, in women, estrogen deficiency. Hypogonadism in women is well established as a cause of osteoporosis, and after treatment for Hodgkin disease, young, prematurely menopausal women have been shown to have reductions in bone mass comparable to that seen in normal postmenopausal women several decades older but equally estrogen deficient.[78] In such patients, however, additional adverse effects of chemotherapy have been suggested.[78,79] The pretherapy lean body mass is the most important predictor of subsequent bone mineral loss in patients undergoing anticancer chemotherapy.

# REFERENCES

1. Yeung SJ, Chiu AC, Vassilopoulou-Sellin R, Gagel RF. The endocrine effects of nonhormonal antineoplastic therapy. Endocr Rev 1998; 19:144.
2. Constine LS, Woolf PD, Cann D, et al. Hypothalamic-pituitary dysfunction after radiation for brain tumors. N Engl J Med 1993; 328:87.
3. Sklar CA, Constine LS. Chronic neuroendocrinological sequelae of radiation therapy. Int J Radiat Oncol Biol Phys 1995; 31:1113.
4. Chieng PU, Huang TS, Chang CC, et al. Reduced hypothalamic blood flow after radiation treatment of nasopharyngeal cancer: SPECT studies in 34 patients. Am J Neuroradiol 1991; 12:661.
5. Blatt J, Lee P, Suttner J, Finegold D. Pulsatile growth hormone secretion in children with acute lymphoblastic leukemia after 1800 cGy cranial radiation. Int J Radiat Oncol Biol Phys 1988; 15:1001.
6. Hall JE, Martin KA, Whitney HA, et al. Potential for fertility with replacement of hypothalamic gonadotropin-releasing hormone in long term female survivors of cranial tumors. J Clin Endocrinol Metab 1994; 79:1166.
7. Ogilvy-Stuart AL, Stirling HF, Kelnar CJH, et al. Treatment of radiation-induced growth hormone deficiency with growth hormone-releasing hormone. Clin Endocrinol 1997; 46:571.
8. Jorgensen EV, Schwartz ID, Hvizdala E, et al. Neurotransmitter control of growth hormone secretion in children after cranial radiation therapy. J Pediatr Endocrinol 1993; 6:131.
9. Shalet SM, Crowne EC, Didi MA, et al. Irradiation-induced growth failure. Baillières Clin Endocrinol Metab 1992; 6:513.
10. Ogilvy-Stuart AL, Shalet SM. Growth and puberty after growth hormone treatment after irradiation for brain tumours. Arch Dis Child 1995; 73:141.
11. Brennan BMD, Rahim A, Mackie EM, et al. Growth hormone status in adults treated for acute lymphoblastic leukaemia in childhood. Clin Endocrinol 1998; 48:777.
12. Nicolson A, Toogood AA, Rahim A, Shalet SM. The prevalence of severe growth hormone deficiency in adults who received growth hormone replacement in childhood. Clin Endocrinol 1996; 44:311.
13. Schriock EA, Schell MJ, Carter M, et al. Abnormal growth patterns and adult short stature in 115 long-term survivors of childhood leukemia. J Clin Oncol 1991; 9:400.
14. Talvensaari KK, Lanning M, Paakko E, et al. Pituitary size assessed with magnetic resonance imaging as a measure of growth hormone secretion in long term survivors of childhood cancer. J Clin Endocrinol Metab 1994; 79:1122.
15. Carroll PV, Christ ER, Bengtsson BA, et al. Growth hormone deficiency in adulthood and the effects of growth hormone replacement: a review. J Clin Endocrinol Metab 1998; 83:382.
16. DeGroot LJ. Effects of irradiation on the thyroid gland. Endocrinol Metab Clin North Am 1993; 22:607.
17. Healy JC, Shafford EA, Reznek RH, et al. Sonographic abnormalities of the thyroid gland following radiotherapy in survivors of childhood Hodgkin's disease. Br J Radiol 1996; 69:617.
18. Ron E, Lubin JH, Shore RE, et al. Thyroid cancer after exposure to external radiation: a pooled analysis of seven studies. Radiat Res 1995; 141:259.
19. Hancock SL, McDougall IR, Constine LS. Thyroid abnormalities after therapeutic external radiation. Int J Radiat Oncol Biol Phys 1995; 31:1165.
20. Tucker MA, Morris Jones PH, Boice Jr JD, et al. Therapeutic radiation at a young age is linked to secondary thyroid cancer. Cancer Res 1991; 51:2885.
21. Fogelfeld L, Bauer TK, Schneider, et al. p53 Gene mutations in radiation-induced thyroid cancer. J Clin Endocrinol Metab 1996; 81:3039.
22. Nikiforov YE, Rowland JM, Bove KE, et al. Distinct pattern of ret oncogene rearrangements in morphological variants of radiation-induced and sporadic thyroid papillary carcinomas in children. Cancer Res 1997; 57:1690.
23. Leprat F, Alapetite C, Rosselli F, et al. Impaired DNA repair as assessed by the "Comet" assay in patients with thyroid tumors after a history of radiation therapy: a preliminary study. Int J Radiat Oncol Biol Phys 1998; 40:1019.
24. Becker DV, Robbins J, Beebe GW, et al. Childhood thyroid cancer following the Chernobyl accident. Endocrinol Metab Clin North Am 1996; 25:197.
25. Likhtarev I, Kairo I, Tronko ND, et al. Thyroid cancer risk to children calculated. Nature 1998; 392:31.
26. Ron E, Morin Doody M, Becker DV, et al. Cancer mortality following treatment for adult hyperthyroidism. JAMA 1998; 280:347.
27. Hancock SL, Cox RS, McDougall IR. Thyroid diseases after treatment of Hodgkin's disease. N Engl J Med 1991; 325:599.
28. Constine LS. What else don't we know about the late effects of radiation in patients treated for head and neck cancer? Int J Radiat Oncol Biol Phys 1995; 31:427.
29. Fein DA, Hanlon AL, Corn BW, et al. The influence of lymphangiography on the development of hypothyroidism in patients irradiated for Hodgkin's disease. Int J Radiat Oncol Biol Phys 1996; 36:13.
30. Pasqualini T, McCalla J, Berg S, et al. Subtle primary hypothyroidism in patients treated for acute lymphoblastic leukemia. Acta Endocrinol 1991; 124:375.
31. Thomas BC, Stanhope R, Plowman PN, Leiper AD. Endocrine function following single fraction and fractionated total body irradiation for bone marrow transplantation in childhood. Acta Endocrinol 1993; 128:508.
32. Wasnich RD, Grumet FC, Payne RO, Kriss JP. Graves' ophthalmopathy following external neck irradiation for nonthyroidal neoplastic disease. J Clin Endocrinol Metab 1973; 37:703.
33. Petersen M, Keeling CV, McDougall IR. Hyperthyroidism with low radioiodine uptake after head and neck irradiation for Hodgkin's disease. J Nucl Med 1989; 30:255.
34. Krouse RS, Royal RE, Heywood G, et al. Thyroid dysfunction in 281 patients with metastatic melanoma or renal carcinoma treated with interleukin-2 alone. J Immunother Emphasis Tumor Immunol 1995; 18:272.
35. Cohen J, Gierlowski TC, Schneider AB. A prospective study of hyperparathyroidism in individuals exposed to radiation in childhood. JAMA 1990; 264:581.
36. Redman JR, Bajorunas DR. Therapy-related thyroid and parathyroid dysfunction in patients with Hodgkin's disease. In: Lacher MJ, Redman JR, eds. Hodgkin's disease: the consequences of survival. Philadelphia: Lea & Febiger, 1989:222.
37. Glazebrook GA. Effect of decicurie doses of radioactive iodine 131 on parathyroid function. Am J Surg 1987; 154:368.
38. Faddy MJ, Gosden RG, Gougeon A, et al. Accelerated disappearance of ovarian follicles in mid-life: implications for forecasting menopause. Hum Reprod 1992; 7:1342.
39. Wallace WHB, Shalet SM, Hendry JH, et al. Ovarian failure following abdominal irradiation in childhood: the radiosensitivity of the human oocyte. Br J Radiol 1989; 62:995.
40. Lushbaugh CC, Ricks RC. Some cytokinetic and histopathologic considerations of irradiated male and female gonadal tissues. Front Radiat Ther Oncol 1972; 6:228.
41. Stillman RJ, Schinfeld JS, Schiff I, et al. Ovarian failure in long-term survivors of childhood malignancy. Am J Obstet Gynecol 1981; 139:62.
42. Doll R, Smith PG. The long-term effects of x-irradiation in patients treated for metropathia haemorrhagica. Br J Radiol 1968; 41:362.
43. Raymond JP, Izembart M, Marliac V, et al. Temporary ovarian failure in thyroid cancer patients after thyroid remnant ablation with radioactive iodine. J Clin Endocrinol Metab 1989; 69:186.
44. Madsen BL, Giudice L, Donaldson SS. Radiation-induced premature menopause: a misconception. Int J Radiat Oncol Biol Phys 1995; 32:1461.
45. Thomas PRM, Winstanly D, Peckham MJ, et al. Reproductive and endocrine function in patients with Hodgkin's disease: effects of oophoropexy and irradiation. Br J Cancer 1976; 33:226.
46. Hadar H, Loven D, Herskovitz P, et al. An evaluation of lateral and medial transposition of the ovaries out of radiation fields. Cancer 1994; 74:774.
47. Byrne J, Fears TR, Gail MH, et al. Early menopause in long-term survivors of cancer during adolescence. Am J Obstet Gynecol 1992; 166:788.
48. Himelstein-Braw R, Peters H, Faber M. Influence of irradiation and chemotherapy on the ovaries of children with abdominal tumours. Br J Cancer 1977; 36:269.
49. Chatterjee R, Mills W, Katz M, et al. Prospective study of pituitary-gonadal function to evaluate short-term effects of ablative chemotherapy or total body irradiation with autologous or allogenic marrow transplantation in post-menarcheal female patients. Bone Marrow Transplant 1994; 13:511.
50. Spinelli S, Chiodi S, Bacigalupo A, et al. Ovarian recovery after total body irradiation and allogeneic bone marrow transplantation: long-term follow up of 79 females. Bone Marrow Transplant 1994; 14:373.
51. Gradishar WJ, Schilsky RL. Ovarian function following radiation and chemotherapy for cancer. Semin Oncol 1989; 16:425.
52. Bines J, Oleske DM, Cobleigh MA. Ovarian function in premenopausal women treated with adjuvant chemotherapy for breast cancer. J Clin Oncol 1996; 14:1718.
53. Quigley C, Cowell C, Jimenez M, et al. Normal or early development of puberty despite gonadal damage in children treated for acute lymphoblastic leukemia. N Engl J Med 1989; 321:143.
54. Sy Ortin TT, Shostak CA, Donaldson SS. Gonadal status and reproductive function following treatment for Hodgkin's disease in childhood: The Stanford experience. Int J Radiat Oncol Biol Phys 1990; 19:873.

55. Lalos O, Lalos A. Urinary, climacteric and sexual symptoms one year after treatment of endometrial and cervical cancer. Eur J Gynaec Oncol 1996; 17:128.
56. Sorosky JI, Sood AK, Buekers TE. The use of chemotherapeutic agents during pregnancy. Obstet Gynecol Clin North Am 1997; 24:591.
57. Mensley ML, Reichman BS. Fertility and pregnancy after adjuvant chemotherapy for breast cancer. Crit Rev Oncol Hematol 1998; 28:121.
58. Critchley HO, Wallace WH, Shalet SM, et al. Abdominal irradiation in childhood: the potential for pregnancy. Br J Obstet Gynaecol 1992; 99:392.
59. Sanders JE, Hawley J, Levy W, et al. Pregnancies following high-dose cyclophosphamide with or without high-dose busulfan or total-body irradiation and bone marrow transplantation. Blood 1996; 87:3045.
60. Sauer MV, Paulson RJ, Ary BA, Lobo RA. Three hundred cycles of oocyte donation at the University of Southern California: assessing the effect of age and infertility diagnosis on pregnancy and implantation rates. J Assist Reprod Genet 1994; 11:92.
61. Blumenfeld Z, Avivi I, Linn S, et al. Prevention of irreversible chemotherapy-induced ovarian damage in young women with lymphoma by a gonadotrophin-releasing hormone agonist in parallel to chemotherapy. Hum Reprod 1996; 11:1620.
62. Donnez J, Bassil S. Indications for cryopreservation of ovarian tissue. Hum Reprod Update 1998; 4:248.
63. Rowley MJ, Leach DR, Warner GA, Heller CG. Effect of graded doses of ionizing radiation on the human testis. Radiat Res 1974; 59:665.
63a. Beumer TL, Roepers-Gajadien HL, Gademan IS, et al. Apoptosis regulation in the testis: involvement of Bcl-2 family members. Mol Reprod Dev 2000; 56:353.
64. Ogilvy-Stuart AL, Shalet SM. Effect of radiation on the human reproductive system. Environ Health Perspect 1993; 101(Suppl 2):109.
65. Centola GM, Keller JW, Henzler M, Rubin P. Effect of low-dose testicular irradiation on sperm count and fertility in patients with testicular seminoma. J Androl 1994; 15:608.
66. Handelsman DJ, Turtle JR. Testicular damage after radioactive iodine (I-131) therapy for thyroid cancer. Clin Endocrinol (Oxf) 1983; 18:465.
67. Rivkees SA, Crawford JD. The relationship of gonadal activity and chemotherapy-induced gonadal damage. JAMA 1988; 259:2123.
68. Meikle AW, Cardoso de Sousa JC, Ward JH, et al. Reduction of testosterone synthesis after high dose interleukin-2 therapy of metastatic cancer. J Clin Endocrinol Metab 1991; 73:931.
69. Howell S, Shalet S. Gonadal damage from chemotherapy and radiotherapy. Endocrinol Metab Clin North Am 1998; 27:927.
70. Pryzant RM, Meistrich ML, Wilson G, et al. Long-term reduction in sperm count after chemotherapy with and without radiation therapy for non-Hodgkin's lymphomas. J Clin Oncol 1993; 11:239.
71. Heikens J, Behrendt H, Adriaanse R, Berghout A. Irreversible gonadal damage in male survivors of pediatric Hodgkin's disease. Cancer 1996; 78:2020.
72. Lampe H, Horwich A, Norman A, et al. Fertility after chemotherapy for testicular germ cell cancers. J Clin Oncol 1997; 15:239.
73. Robbins WA. Cytogenetic damage measured in human sperm following cancer chemotherapy. Mutation Res 1996; 355:235.
74. Padron OF, Sharma RK, Thomas Jr AJ, Agarwal A. Effects of cancer on spermatozoa quality after cryopreservation: a 12-year experience. Fertil Steril 1997; 67:326.
75. Costabile RA, Spevak M. Cancer and male factor infertility. Oncology 1998; 12:557.
76. Brinster RL, Zimmermann JW. Spermatogenesis following male germ-cell transplantation. Proc Natl Acad Sci U S A 1994; 91:11298.
77. Halton JM, Atkinson SA, Fraher L, et al. Altered mineral metabolism and bone mass in children during treatment for acute lymphoblastic leukemia. J Bone Miner Res 1996; 11:1774.
78. Redman JR, Bajorunas DR, Wong G, et al. Bone mineralization in women following successful treatment of Hodgkin's disease. Am J Med 1988; 85:65.
79. Douchi T, Kosha S, Kan R, et al. Predictors of bone mineral loss in patients with ovarian cancer treated with anticancer agents. Obstet Gynecol 1997; 90:12.

# PART XVI

# ENDOCRINOLOGY OF CRITICAL ILLNESS

ERIC S. NYLÉN, EDITOR

# CHAPTER 227

# CRITICAL ILLNESS AND SYSTEMIC INFLAMMATION

GARY P. ZALOGA, BANKIM BHATT, AND PAUL MARIK

Endocrinology is predominantly the study of *homeostatic* systems; thus, the fact that endocrine perturbations occur as a consequence of critical illness has been recognized since the seminal works of Bernard, Cannon, Cuthbertson, Selye, and others is not surprising. The notion of a *general adaptation syndrome* has been further refined by placing it within the context of a complex of inflammatory, immune, and endocrine mediators. Importantly, the full expression of this response involves mutual and reciprocal interaction among these compartments. Central to understanding the organism's response and recovery from critical illness has been the unveiling of the role of inflammatory mediators and the embracing of the concept of systemic inflammation.

*Critical illness is an acute medical condition that is immediately or imminently life-threatening.* One or more organ systems deteriorate to such an extent that they can no longer support the independent functioning of the patient (e.g., cardiac failure, renal failure, respiratory failure). Common to many forms of critical illness are *activation of systemic inflammatory cascades* and *decreased perfusion of one or more organ systems*. Critical illness differs from *terminal illness* in that it is *potentially reversible*. Critically ill patients are usually managed in an *intensive care unit* where they receive temporary physiologic support concurrent with the management of their acute medical condition. Shock, trauma, burns, systemic infections, and organ ischemia are common examples of critical illnesses.

## IMMUNE SYSTEM AND INFLAMMATORY MEDIATORS

A primary function of the immune system is the *removal of foreign antigens* (e.g., invading organisms, malignant cells, and necrotic tissue), a role that is vital to the survival of the host. Cytokines are soluble proteins that activate and regulate T and B lymphocytes and mediate many of the manifestations of the inflammatory response. They are produced by a wide variety of hematopoietic and nonhematopoietic cells (see Chap. 173). Like hormones, they mediate communication between cells in the body by hemocrine, autocrine, and paracrine mechanisms. They also circulate in the blood, thereby producing systemic effects distant from their sites of synthesis via distinct and specific receptors. Although the view once was that endocrine glands did not synthesize or respond directly to cytokines, evidence now demonstrates that not only do they respond directly to cytokines but they also synthesize and secrete these mediators. *Cytokines* differ from classic hormones in their *redundancy*[1] (different cytokines have similar functions). In addition, cytokines are *pleiotropic* in that they are able to act on many different cell types.

The cytokines are conveniently divided into three groups: *immunoregulatory* cytokines that are involved in the activation, growth, and differentiation of lymphocytes, monocytes, and leukocytes (i.e., interleukin-2 [IL-2], interleukin-3 [IL-3], interleukin-4 [IL-4]); *proinflammatory* cytokines that are produced predominantly by mononuclear phagocytes in response to infectious agents (i.e., interleukin-1β [IL-1β], tumor necrosis factor-α [TNF-α], interleukin-6 [IL-6]); and *antiinflammatory* cytokines (i.e., IL-4, IL-6, interleukin-10 [IL-10], interleukin-13

[IL-13], and transforming growth factor-β [TGF-β]). Some cytokines (e.g., IL-4 and IL-6) have *overlapping* actions.

Although monocytes, macrophages, and CD4-$T_H$ (helper) cells are the most important sources of cytokines, they are also produced by many other cells, including glial cells, Kupffer cells, keratinocytes, bone marrow stromal cells, mast cells, eosinophils, fibroblasts, endothelial cells, gut mucosal cells, mesangial cells, and endocrine glands. Monocytes and macrophages are the principal sources of the proinflammatory cytokines. CD4-$T_H$ cells develop into two distinct subsets of cells, $T_H$1 and $T_H$2 cells.[2] $T_H$1 cells (T helper cell subtype 1) secrete IL-2, TNF, and interferon-γ (IFN-γ), and are the principal effectors of cell-mediated immunity against intracellular microbes. $T_H$2 cells (T helper cell subtype 2), on the other hand, secrete IL-4, IL-5, IL-10, and IL-13, which largely inhibit macrophage function.[2,3] A number of factors play a role in driving native CD4-$T_H$ cells toward $T_H$1 or $T_H$2 cells, including antigen-presenting cells, hormones, and cytokines.[2] Glucocorticoids enhance $T_H$2 activity and synergize with IL-4, whereas dehydroepiandrosterone and IFN-γ enhance $T_H$1 activity.[4,5]

Cytokine receptors are predominantly integral *plasma membrane glycoproteins* with *three distinct domains*: (a) a *recognition domain* protruding from the plasma membrane that confers specificity with regards to ligand binding; (b) a *hydrophobic region* spanning the plasma lipid bilayer; and (c) the *cytoplasmic domain*, located on the inner surface of the plasma membrane, which has intrinsic enzyme activity. All the cytokine receptors are associated with one or more members of the *Janus kinases*, which couple ligand binding to tyrosine phosphorylation of various known signaling proteins and transcription factors termed the *signal transducers* and *activators of transcription* (Stats).[6]

## SYSTEMIC INFLAMMATION

The idea that cytokines play pivotal roles in the pathogenesis of sepsis is based on several lines of evidence: (a) intravenous administration of cytokines (i.e., TNF-α, IL-1) induces a sepsis-like syndrome in animals and humans; (b) inhibition of the effects of some cytokines (i.e., TNF-α, IL-1) by administration of neutralizing antibodies, soluble cytokine receptors, or receptor antagonists attenuates sepsis in animals; (c) administration of antiinflammatory cytokines such as IL-10 mitigates severe sepsis in animals; and (d) plasma levels of cytokines (i.e., TNF-α, IL-1, IL-6, IL-8, and macrophage-migration inhibitory factor [MIF]) increase in models of sepsis as well as in human sepsis, and the levels generally reflect the severity of sepsis. Further evidence that cytokines are essential for the manifestations of sepsis is derived from knock-out models. TNF-deficient mice are resistant to the lethality of lipopolysaccharide (LPS).[7] Transgenic TNF-receptor (TNF-R55) knock-out mice do not display hemodynamic or systemic immune alterations to intravenous LPS.[8,9] Transgenic mice lacking the IL-1 converting enzyme are resistant to the effects of LPS.[10] Mice lacking IL-1 receptor antagonist (IL-1ra) are more susceptible than controls to lethal endotoxemia, and IL-1ra overproducers are protected from the lethal effects of endotoxemia.[11]

In patients with sepsis, TNF-α is the first proinflammatory cytokine released, followed by IL-1 and IL-6.[12,13] TNF-α and IL-1 (the most important proinflammatory cytokines) are closely related biologically, act synergistically, and are largely responsible for the clinical manifestations of sepsis.[12–18] IL-6 is not a proximal inflammatory cytokine; it does not cause shock in mice or primates.[19] Nuclear factor-κB (NF-κB), which plays a critical role in the transcriptional induction of proinflammatory mediators,[20,20a] is activated by endotoxin, viruses, oxidants, TNF-α, and platelet-activating factor (PAF).[21,22] In addition to activating a proinflammatory cytokine cascade, inflammatory stimuli acti-

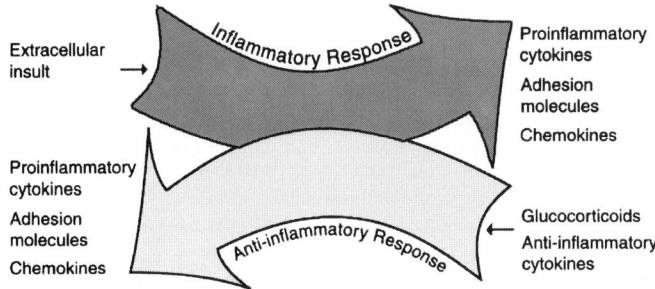

**FIGURE 227-1.** Balance of proinflammatory and antiinflammatory forces in systemic inflammation. (Modified from McKay LI, Cidlowski JA. Molecular control of immune/inflammatory responses: interactions between nuclear factor-kappa B and steroid signaling pathways. Endocr Rev 1999; 20:435.)

**TABLE 227-1.**
**Criteria for Systemic Inflammation (Systemic Inflammatory Response Syndrome)**

| Two or more of the following: | |
| --- | --- |
| Temperature | >38°C or <36°C |
| Heart rate | >90 beats/min |
| Respiratory rate | >20 breaths/min |
| White blood cell count | >12.0 × 10⁹/L, <4.0 × 10⁹/L, or >0.1 immature forms (bands) |

vate the production of specific cytokine-neutralizing molecules, which include cytokine receptors and cytokine-receptor antagonists. Circulating soluble cytokine receptors result from proteolytic cleavage of the extracellular binding domain of the receptors.[23] Soluble cytokine receptors from both of the TNF receptors (p75 and p55), the IL-1 receptor, and the IL-6 receptor have been identified. The release of surface receptors may down-regulate membrane cytokine receptor responsiveness, with circulating receptors acting as a buffer for the free cytokines in the circulation. Additional factors, such as suppressors of cytokine signaling, (i.e., SOCS 1–7), modulate the response via effects on Janus kinase (JAK)–Stat kinase activity.

After the release of IL-1 and TNF-α, antiinflammatory cytokines (i.e., IL-4, IL-10, IL-13, and TGF-β) are released into the circulation. The production of antiinflammatory cytokines is associated with a switch from T$_H$1 to T$_H$2 activation. The antiinflammatory cytokines suppress the expression of the genes for IL-1 and TNF-α and inhibit antigen presentation by monocytes as well as T- and B-lymphocyte function. IL-1ra is released into the circulation, and binds to and neutralizes IL-1. *The role of the antiinflammatory cytokines is to limit the inflammatory response* (Fig. 227-1). If the compensatory antiinflammatory response is excessive, it manifests clinically as anergy, immune depression, and an increased susceptibility to infection, known as the *compensatory antiinflammatory response syndrome (CARS)*.[24,25] In most healthy persons, the body is able to achieve a *balance between proinflammatory and antiinflammatory mediators*, and homeostasis is restored. In some persons, however, this *balance is upset*, which results in *systemic inflammatory response syndrome* (SIRS) (Table 227-1) and can progress to *multisystem organ dysfunction* (MODS).[24,25,25a] The systemic inflammatory response is seen in association with a large number of clinical conditions. Besides *infectious* insults that may produce SIRS (characterized by fever, tachycardia, tachypnea, and leukocytosis), *noninfectious* causes include pancreatitis, ischemia, trauma and tissue injury, hypovolemic shock, drugs, and immune-mediated injuries. Although a similar pathogenesis and pathophysiology are assumed to underlie the various clinical entities that comprise SIRS, the nature of the precipitating insult as well as other factors such as genetic polymorphism, sex, age, race, and nutritional status likely affect the production of inflammatory mediators and their interactions.

The properties and bioeffects of the relevant cytokines are summarized in Table 227-2.

## TUMOR NECROSIS FACTOR

TNF-α is produced by mononuclear cells, whereas TNF-β (lymphotoxin) is produced by T lymphocytes. TNF-α shares 28% amino-acid homology with TNF-β. Both cytokines bind to the same receptors, but their synthesis is differentially regulated. Active TNF-α consists of a trimer of three identical polypeptide chains with molecular masses of 17 kDa each. The 17-kDa subunits are released from a 26-kDa membrane-associated precursor protein by proteolytic cleavage. The enzyme that processes precursor TNF-α is a microsomal metalloprotease, TNF-α-converting enzyme (TACE).[26–28] Nitric oxide plays a regulatory role in the activation of metal-dependent proteases.[29] Synthetic inhibitors of metalloproteases prevent the processing of the TNF-α precursor with decreased production of TNF-α, as well as release of the 55-kDa and 75-kDa TNF receptors. They do not affect the release of other cytokines.[30–33]

Although many factors lead to the release of TNF-α, the most important and well studied is *endotoxin* (i.e., *LPS*). Endotoxin released from bacteria binds with a 60-kDa protein (LPS-binding protein or LBP), normally present in the blood. The LPS-LPB complex, in turn, binds to a 55-kDa cell-surface receptor on monocytes (the CD-14 molecule), activating the monocyte.[34,35] Teichoic acid and peptidoglycan from gram-positive bacteria activate monocytes and macrophages and induce the production of TNF-α by a CD-14–independent pathway.[36] Exposure of macrophages to endotoxin results in a three-fold increase in the transcriptional rate of the TNF-α gene, which is mediated through the induction of the transcription factor NF-κB, a heterodimeric protein that is normally found in the cytoplasm bound to its 37-kDa inhibitor (IκB) until a stimulatory signal is sensed at the cell surface. Several signal-transduction pathways may be involved in NF-κB activation, but all act by means of protein kinases that phosphorylate and degrade IκB.

The production of TNF-α is tightly controlled. Transcription of TNF-α genes is regulated by nuclear transcription factors (e.g., NF-κB) and suppressed by a variety of repressors. Furthermore, the messenger (mRNA) transcripts of TNF-α have short half-lives. Differences in the regulatory sequences of the TNF-α gene may influence the response to TNF-α after microbial challenge. In patients with severe sepsis, genomic polymorphism within the TNF-α locus is associated with TNF-α production and patient outcome.[37] Various agents are known to modulate the biosynthesis of TNF-α by macrophages (e.g., norepinephrine, PAF, granulocyte-macrophage colony-stimulating factor, C5a, engagement of CD11b/CD18, and nitric oxide may enhance the synthesis of TNF-α by macrophages). Agents that increase intracellular cyclic adenosine monophosphate (e.g., β-agonists, prostaglandin E$_2$, and phosphodiesterase inhibitors) decrease TNF-α mRNA in response to LPS.[38] Glucocorticoids decrease the production of the proinflammatory cytokines and mediators, probably by activating glucocorticoid receptors that bind to activated NF-κB and prevent gene transcription.[39] In addition, IL-4, IL-10, IL-13, and TGF-β decrease TNF-α synthesis. The activity of TNF-α in biologic fluids is controlled by a number of mechanisms. Proteinases released by activated neutrophils can inactivate TNF-α, and the increased circulating soluble TNF receptors (sTNF-R) in sepsis bind 90% of the free TNF-α. Although sTNF-Rs significantly attenuate TNF-α activity, this inhibition is unlikely to be sufficient to neutralize the toxic activities of TNF in sepsis, because even at the highest concentrations of sTNF-R, 10% of TNF-α is still active.

**TABLE 227-2.**
**Cytokine Actions**

| Cytokine | Source | Major Actions |
|---|---|---|
| **IMMUNOREGULATORY** | | |
| IL-2 | Activated T cells | T & B cell growth and differentiation; immunoglobulin secretion by B cells; NK cell growth and activity; production of IFN-$\gamma$ and TNF-$\beta$ |
| IL-4 | $T_H2$ cells | T & B cell growth and differentiation |
| IL-5 | T cells; mast cells, eosinophils | Differentiation of B cells and eosinophils; chemotaxis |
| IL-7 | Bone marrow stromal cells | Pre–B and pre–T cell growth and maturation |
| IL-11 | Bone marrow stromal cells | Megakaryocyte colony formation, myelopoiesis, erythropoiesis, lymphopoiesis |
| IFN-$\gamma$ | Activated T cells | Antiviral activity; activates monocytes, macrophages, neutrophils; NK cells; T-cell cytotoxicity |
| **PROINFLAMMATORY** | | |
| IL-1$\beta$ | Macrophages; T & B cells; endothelial cells | Activates T, B, NK cells, neutrophils; induces proinflammatory cytokines, coagulation, fibrinolysis; mediates acute-phase response; down-regulates IL-1ra; increases ACTH, endorphins, vasopressin, somatostatin release |
| TNF-$\alpha$ | Macrophages, activated T & B cells | See Table 227-3 |
| IL-6 | Many cells including macrophages, activated T & B cells, endothelial cells, smooth muscle cells, fibroblasts, mast cells, intestinal cells | Activates T & B cells; acute-phase proteins; activates phospholipase $A_2$ |
| IL-8 | Monocytes, macrophages, neutrophils, endothelial cells | Neutrophil and basophil chemotaxis; neutrophil activation |
| MCP-1, MCP-2, MCP-3 | Monocytes, macrophages, fibroblasts, B cells, endothelial cells | Chemotactic for monocytes; release of lysosomal enzymes and superoxide anion; stimulates eosinophils and basophils |
| MIP-1 | T & B cells | Chemotactic for monocytes; expression of $\beta$-1 integrins |
| RANTES | T cells, platelets, renal epithelium, mesangial cells | Chemotactic for monocytes, CD4 cells, eosinophils, basophils |
| **ANTIINFLAMMATORY** | | |
| IL-1ra | Monocytes, macrophages | Inhibits IL-1$\alpha$ and IL-1$\beta$ |
| IL-4 | $T_H2$ cells | Induces IL-1ra, IL-10; inhibits antigen presentation; inhibits production of IL-1, TNF, IL-8 |
| IL-6 | Many cells, including macrophages, activated T & B cells, endothelial cells, smooth muscle cells, mast cells | Decreases TNF production; induces IL-1ra and sTNF-R55 |
| IL-10 | Activated T & B cells | Inhibits IFN, IL-1, IL-6, and TNF production; induces IL-1ra |
| IL-13 | $T_H2$ cells | B cell growth and differentiation; promotes IL-1ra production; inhibits IL-1, IL-6, IL-8, IL-10, TNF, IFN-$\alpha$ production |

*IL,* interleukin; *NK,* natural killer; *TNF,* tumor necrosis factor; $T_H2$, helper T lymphocyte type 2; *IFN,* interferon; *ACTH,* adrenocorticotropic hormone; *MCP,* monocyte chemotactic protein; *MIP,* macrophage inflammatory protein; *RANTES,* regulation on activation, normal T-expressed and secreted; *IL-1ra;* interleukin-1 receptor antagonist.

TNF-$\alpha$ release into the circulation during endotoxemia occurs in a stereotypical pattern. Within minutes after intravenous endotoxin administration, a burst of TNF-$\alpha$ occurs that peaks in 90 to 120 minutes. TNF-$\alpha$ is then cleared quickly, with circulating levels becoming undetectable within 4 to 6 hours.[40,41] Repeat administration of endotoxin is followed by a markedly attenuated or absent secondary release of TNF-$\alpha$. TNF-$\alpha$ down-regulation occurs independent of IL-1, because IL-1 production is not attenuated after a second endotoxin dose.[42,43] The serum half-life of recombinant TNF-$\alpha$ is short (i.e., 20 to 40 minutes).[41,44,45] These data suggest that most patients with acute-onset sepsis have a peak TNF-$\alpha$ level very early in the course of the illness.

Two different TNF receptors (TNF-Rs), which have been cloned and characterized in most cells and tissues, have molecular masses of 55 kDa (TNF-R55) and 75 kDa (TNF-R75). Similar to other receptors, TNF-Rs have an extracellular domain, a single hydrophobic transmembrane region, and an intracellular domain. A TNF-$\alpha$ trimer has three binding sites for TNF-R, each located at the interface between two subunits. Thus, one TNF trimer molecule can cross-link up to three TNF-Rs. In vitro studies indicate that the cytotoxic and most inflammatory effects are triggered by TNF-R55, whereas the proliferative effects are triggered by TNF-R75.[46]

Circulating TNF-$\alpha$ is principally responsible for the release of its receptors into the circulation.[3,23,47–49] The levels of soluble TNF receptors may, thus, reflect the TNF-$\alpha$ levels.[50] Soluble TNF-R concentrations show a dose-dependent increase to peak concentrations within 2 hours; however, in contrast to TNF-$\alpha$ levels, TNF-R concentrations remain elevated for 48 hours. Furthermore, animals pretreated with antibody to TNF-$\alpha$ have reduced circulating levels of TNF-R.

TNF-$\alpha$ and IL-1 have many overlapping actions and synergisms. Binding of TNF-$\alpha$ and IL-1 to their cellular receptors induces activation and generation of a number of secondary messengers mediated by G proteins, adenylate cyclase, phospholipase $A_2$ and C, and oxygen free radicals. In addition, a number of genes are transcribed, including those for *intracellular adhesion molecule-1 (ICAM-1)* and *endothelial-leukocyte adhesion molecule (ELAM)*; the clotting and fibrinolytic proteins, tissue factor, urokinase-type plasminogen activator, and plasminogen activator inhibitor-1; the proinflammatory cytokines IL-4, IL-6, and IL-8; the antiinflammatory cytokines IL-4, IL-10, and IL-1RA; phospholipase $A_2$; inducible nitric oxide synthetase; and cyclooxygenase. The biologic and clinical effects of TNF-$\alpha$ are summarized in Tables 227-3 and 227-4.

### INTERLEUKIN-1$\beta$

Interleukin-1 shares many functional and biologic characteristics with TNF-$\alpha$. The IL-1 family of cytokines consists of three peptides, IL-1$\alpha$, IL-1$\beta$, and IL-1RA, that are encoded by three distinct genes. IL-1$\alpha$ and IL-1$\beta$ activate the same receptors and, therefore, have similar biologic properties. IL-1$\beta$, the predominant form of this mediator, is produced by activated mononu-

**TABLE 227-3.**
**Biologic Effects of Tumor Necrosis Factor α**

**ACTIVATES MANY CELLS INCLUDING:**
  Macrophages, lymphocytes, neutrophils, eosinophils
  Fibroblasts, osteoclasts, chondrocytes
  Endothelial cells, neural cells
**EXPRESSION OF ADHESION MOLECULES**
  ICAM-1, ELAM, VCAM-1
**ACTIVATES CYCLOOXYGENASE, PHOSPHOLIPASE A₂, NITRIC**
    **OXIDE SYNTHETASE**
  Production of PAF, PGE₂, PGI₂, NO
**ACTIVATES COMPLEMENT**
**CYTOKINES AND HEMATOPOIETIC FACTORS**
  Proinflammatory cytokines: IL-1, IL-6, IL-8, MCP-1
  Antiinflammatory cytokines: IL-4, IL-10, IL-1ra
  PDGF, IL-2
**COAGULATION SYSTEM**
  Activates contact system
  Increases urokinase-type plasminogen activator
  Increases plasminogen activator inhibitor
  Down-regulates thrombomodulin
**VASCULAR SYSTEM**
  Endothelin-1
**NEUTROPHILS**
  Expression of surface adhesion molecules, C3B receptors, L-selectin
  Superoxide production
  Phagocytosis, enzyme release

*ICAM-1,* intracellular adhesion molecule-1; *ELAM,* endothelial-leukocyte adhesion molecule; *PAF,* platelet-activating factor; *PGE₂,* prostaglandin E₂; *PGI₂,* prostaglandin I₂; *NO,* nitric oxide; *IL,* interleukin; *IL-1ra,* interleukin-1 receptor antagonist; *MCP,* monocyte chemotactic protein; *PDGF,* platelet-derived growth factor.

**TABLE 227-4.**
**Clinical Effects of Tumor Necrosis Factor α**

**INCREASED VASCULAR PERMEABILITY**
**MYOCARDIAL DEPRESSION**
**HYPOTENSION**
**COAGULATION**
**FIBRINOLYSIS**
**PULMONARY HYPERTENSION**
**MICROTHROMBI**
**CATABOLISM**

clear cells. The mature 17-kDa form is released from a 31-kDa precursor via proteolytic cleavage by a cysteine proteinase, the IL-1β–converting enzyme, or caspase-1.[51]

As with TNF, two IL-1 receptors have been isolated: IL1-RI and IL1-RII. IL1-RI is found on most cells of the body, whereas IL1-RII is restricted to B cells, neutrophils, and bone marrow cells. IL1-RI mediates signaling of cells by IL-1, whereas IL1-RII competes with IL1-RI for IL-1, acting as a *decoy receptor.* Under physiologic conditions, only a few hundred IL-1Rs are found per cell, but under inflammatory conditions receptor levels increase to 20,000 per cell. IL-1α and IL-1β mimic many of the bioactivities of TNF-α. Infusion of either form into humans causes fever, hemodynamic abnormalities, anorexia, malaise, arthralgia, headache, and neutrophilia (i.e., signs of sepsis). The activity of IL-1 in biologic fluids is regulated by the production and release of IL-1ra, which is a pure competitive antagonist of IL-1β.

### INTERLEUKIN-6

IL-6 is produced not only by immune cells but also by many nonimmune cells (e.g., osteoblasts, keratinocytes, and intestinal epithelial cells). It is involved in inflammation and the regulation of endocrine and metabolic function. It is secreted during stress of diverse origins, probably through β-adrenergic receptor mechanisms, and is a major mediator of the *stress-response.*[52]

IL-6 exerts its effects by binding to specific receptors (IL-6Rs) that are structurally related to receptors for IL-2, IL-3, IL-5, and IL-7. The IL-6R, which has a very short intracytoplasmic component, is associated with a second membrane protein (termed *gp130*) that is responsible for signal transduction. Evidence is found for IL-6 antagonists in vivo. Unlike TNF-α and IL-1, IL-6 does not cause the septic response when injected into animals or into transgenic mouse models.[53–59]

IL-6 stimulates growth of some cells and inhibits that of others. It is a growth and differentiation factor for T and B lymphocytes and is responsible for the stimulation of acute-phase proteins, fever, bone resorption, and thrombopoietic activity. Although once thought to be a proinflammatory cytokine, IL-6 also has antiinflammatory properties. IL-6 reduces TNF-α production and causes the induction of circulating IL-1ra and sTNF-R55.[60,61] It is a potent inhibitor of matrix metalloproteinases that are responsible for the release of active TNF-α.[62] IL-6 increases the liver production of acute-phase proteins, which are believed to attenuate the effects of proinflammatory mediators.[63] IL-6 also has proinflammatory effects and induces the expression of phospholipase A₂, which plays a central role in inflammation by producing potent lipid mediators (e.g., leukotrienes, prostaglandins, and PAF).[64,65]

A number of studies in diverse groups of patients with sepsis have demonstrated a strong association between IL-6 levels and outcome.[66–73] In addition, IL-6 levels appear to correlate with the severity of sepsis (see Chapter 228, Fig. 228-3). IL-6 levels in patients with sepsis may reflect effects of IL-1 and TNF-α.[74]

### INTERLEUKIN-8

A salient feature of acute and chronic inflammation is the infiltration of the affected tissues by polymorphonuclear and mononuclear cells. This *recruitment of inflammatory cells* is directed mainly by a number of structurally related cytokines, the *chemokines.* IL-8 precursor protein is synthesized as a single 99-amino-acid peptide chain. The 79-amino-acid mature form is proteolytically cleaved at the amino-terminus to yield various forms with slightly different biologic properties. The predominant form of IL-8 consists of 72 amino acids. Two different types of IL-8 receptors are found, IL-8Rα and IL-8Rβ, which are members of a superfamily of receptors coupled to guanine nucleotide–binding proteins. IL-8 is produced by a variety of cells, including monocytes, macrophages, neutrophils, and endothelial cells. TNF-α, IL-1, and endotoxin release IL-8, which has remarkable specificity for neutrophils and basophils. It has chemoattractant activity and is able to induce degranulation, to elicit a respiratory burst, and to activate arachidonate-5-lipoxygenase in neutrophils.

### INTERLEUKIN-10

IL-10 (a peptide of 160 amino acids and a molecular mass of 16.5 kDa), like IL-4 and IL-13, is produced by T_H2 cells. Its receptor has a molecular mass of 90 to 100 kDa and has structural homology with the IFN-γ receptor. IL-10 is a potent inhibitor of the synthesis and release of proinflammatory cytokines (i.e., TNF-α, IL-1, IL-6, IL-8), probably by inhibition of transcription of the genes for these cytokines.[75–77] IL-10 inhibits antigen-stimulated T-cell proliferation by decreasing the surface expression of major histocompatibility complex II molecules.[78] It also inhibits tissue factor expression and induction of procoagulant activity on monocytes.

### INTERLEUKIN-4 AND INTERLEUKIN-13

IL-4 and IL-13 are synthesized by $T_H2$ cells and macrophages, as well as certain CD8 T cells, mast cells, and B cells. IL-4 promotes differentiation of CD4-$T_H$ cells into $T_H2$ cells. IL-4 inhibits $T_H1$ cells and decreases antibody-dependent cell-mediated cytotoxicity. IL-13 decreases production of IL-1, IL-8, macrophage inflammatory peptide-1, and nitric oxide, and increases production of IL-1ra and IL-1RII.

## INFLAMMATORY MEDIATORS AND ENDOCRINE ACTION

*Neuroendocrine* changes are an important and essential component of the response to critical illness, as the immune and neuroendocrine systems share numerous regulatory factors. This *system of shared regulators* allows *one system to modulate functions of the other* (see Fig. 227-2). Most endocrine cells are affected by *cytokines*, and major alterations in hormonal balance accompany the acute-phase response. The *reciprocal interactions between the immune, endocrine, and nervous systems* are extremely complex. For example, in addition to cytokine receptors, *immune cells contain receptors for classic endocrine hormones* (e.g., corticosteroids, insulin, prolactin, growth hormone [GH], estradiol, testosterone, β-adrenergic agonists, acetylcholine, endorphins, enkephalins, substance P, somatostatin, and vasoactive intestinal peptide [VIP][1]). In addition, immune cells (i.e., leukocytes) *synthesize classic hormones* (e.g., adrenocorticotropic hormone [ACTH], β-endorphin, GH, prolactin, VIP, and substance P) (see Chap. 180). On the other hand, classic endocrine organs contain receptors for cytokines and other immune-derived products as well as for hormones. In particular, interleukin receptors (i.e., IL-6, IL-1) have been identified on pituitary, adrenal, thyroid, pancreas, testicular, and ovarian tissues. These tissues also synthesize various cytokines. Interestingly, stimulation of immune or neuroendocrine cells with specific cytokines or hormones *often alters responses* to other hormones or cytokines.

Evidence is increasing that cytokines contribute to the pathogenesis of immune-mediated target cell damage, leading to *functional insufficiency of various endocrine glands* (i.e., hypophysitis, thyroiditis, parathyroiditis, adrenalitis, insulitis) (see Chaps. 46, 60, 76, 137).

Cytokines affect endocrine glands at many different levels. In particular, they affect the release of hormones from the hypothalamus and the pituitary. They also act on the pituitary as paracrine and/or autocrine regulators, modulating hormone secretion and cell growth. The major cytokines that affect the hypothalamic-pituitary axis are IL-1, IL-2, IL-6, TNF, and IFN. The predominant effects of these cytokines are stimulation of the hypothalamic–pituitary–adrenal (HPA) axis (see Chap. 229), suppression of the hypothalamic–pituitary–gonadal (HPG) axis and hypothalamic–pituitary–thyroid (HPT) axis, and release of GH (see Chap. 230).

### HYPOTHALAMUS

Numerous cytokines are expressed in the central nervous system (CNS).[79] IL-1, IL-6, and TNF-α are synthesized in the hypothalamus[80] and alter anterior pituitary function via the portal circulation. In particular, IL-1 is abundantly expressed in the paraventricular nucleus, the arcuate nucleus, and the median eminence.[80] Although cytokines are produced in the brain, cir-

culating cytokines also enter the brain through the organum vasculosum (no blood–brain barrier) and alter hypothalamic function.

Immune stimulation (i.e., inflammation) increases the activity of the HPA axis, a phenomenon directly and indirectly mediated through cytokines.[81] Corticotropin-releasing hormone (CRH) and arginine vasopressin (AVP) are released by cytokines and play important roles in the release of ACTH. CRH and AVP release are also modulated by catecholamines, prostaglandins, and nitric oxide, mediators released by cytokines. In addition, endotoxemia and tissue inflammation up-regulate brain levels of TNF-α, IL-1β, and IL-6, providing additional mechanisms whereby inflammation stimulates the brain.

IL-1, IL-2, IL-6, IL-8, and TNF stimulate hypothalamic release of CRH.[82] These cytokines activate the HPA axis independently and in combination; their effects are synergistic.[83–88] They are effective when produced by the brain (paracrine) or from the circulation. In humans, IL-6 increases serum ACTH and cortisol levels beyond those achieved by CRH. This effect is mediated through the combined release of CRH and AVP from the hypothalamus.[89,90] In addition, IL-1 stimulates expression of proopiomelanocortin (POMC), the precursor for ACTH. IFN-γ has an inhibitory effect on the release of CRH,[80] and TGF selectively blocks acetylcholine-stimulated CRH release from the hypothalamus.[91] Immunoneutralization of CRH blocks cytokine stimulation of ACTH release and glucocorticoid secretion, suggesting that the major effects of cytokines on the HPA axis are through CRH.

IL-1 and TNF mediate their hypothalamic stimulatory effects via generation of second messengers (i.e., prostaglandins, norepinephrine, nitric oxide). The mechanism by which IL-2 activates the release of CRH is activation of IL-2 receptors on cholinergic interneurons near cell bodies of CRH neurons in the paraventricular nucleus.[92] The release of acetylcholine from these interneurons stimulates muscarinic-type receptors that, in turn, stimulate the release of CRH.[92] This release of CRH can be blocked by atropine.[92]

IL-1β, IL-2, IL-6, and IFN-α enhance the release of AVP in hypothalamic cells, whereas TGF-β selectively blocks acetylcholine release of AVP.[91] Cytokines also affect other hypothalamic hormones such as gonadotropin-releasing hormone (GnRH), growth hormone–releasing hormone (GHRH), and thyrotropin-releasing hormone (TRH). IL-1 indirectly inhibits the release of GnRH from the hypothalamus via CRH, AVP, norepinephrine, prostaglandins, excitatory amino acids, and endorphins.[93–97] IL-1 and TNF-α stimulate the release of somatostatin.[98–100] Both IL-1 and TNF inhibit the release of TRH, and IL-1 also stimulates the release of dopamine and somatostatin, which, in turn, strongly inhibit the synthesis of TRH.[93,94]

Somatostatin inhibits release of GH by the pituitary.[79] On the other hand, IL-6 enhances GH secretion, whereas IL-1 and TNF-α both stimulate and inhibit GH release. IL-1 is a weak stimulator of GHRH release from the hypothalamus. IFN-γ blocks GHRH-dependent release of GH. Although cytokines have inhibitory effects on hypothalamic signals for GH secretion, GH levels are elevated during inflammatory diseases, the acute-phase response, and experimental endotoxemia. Perhaps the IL-6 effects on the pituitary predominate.

### PITUITARY GLAND

The pituitary gland expresses cytokines and their receptors[101,102] (e.g., IL-6 is produced in anterior pituitary cells[1]). Interestingly, this production of IL-6 is induced by LPS, TNF, IL-1β, IFN-γ, and prostaglandin $E_2$ and is inhibited by glucocorticoids. IL-2 receptor transcripts and protein products are colocalized in ACTH-, prolactin-, and GH-producing cells. IL-2 and IL-6 are involved in the autocrine/paracrine regulation of normal and tumor anterior pituitary hormone–producing cell growth.[101] IL-1β has been localized to cytoplasmic granules in anterior pituitary cells and colocalizes with TSH. IL-1 regulates the growth of normal pituitary cells, whereas IL-1ra, which blocks this action, is expressed in pituitary adenomas (mainly GH and ACTH). In ACTH-producing cells, IL-1 enhances glucocorticoid feedback, stimulating glucocorticoid response-element transcriptional activity. Constitutive production of TNF-α mRNA also occurs in the pituitary.[1] Cytokines act as inter/autocellular factors that regulate not only the function but also the growth of anterior pituitary cells.[101]

In the pituitary, IL-1, IL-2, IL-6, TNF-α, and IFN-γ stimulate the release of ACTH.[80] IL-1 also stimulates the expression of the POMC gene,[100] the common precursor of ACTH, endorphins, and α-melanocyte–stimulating hormone.

In addition to ACTH, the cytokines affect other anterior pituitary hormones (e.g., luteinizing hormone [LH], follicle-stimulating hormone [FSH], GH, and TSH). IL-1 stimulates LH via IL-6, whereas it inhibits FSH release.[103,104] IL-6 causes increased release of GH from the pituitary, whereas IL-1 and TNF-α have divergent effects on GH secretion.[93,94,105,106] IFN-γ interferes with GHRH-dependent release of GH.[94] The release of TSH is enhanced directly by IL-1 and IL-6[103,107] and indirectly by IL-1.

The prolactin receptor is a member of a larger family, known as the *cytokine class 1 receptor superfamily*, which currently has > 20 different members. Prolactin receptors are widely distributed throughout the body and have diverse actions, including immune regulation.[108] Prolactin promotes antibody production and macrophage function. IL-1 stimulates dopamine release and inhibits VIP and TRH secretion in the hypothalamus, resulting in a pronounced inhibition of prolactin secretion. On the other hand, IL-1 stimulates the release of IL-6 from the folliculostellate cells of the anterior pituitary, thereby stimulating the release of prolactin from lactotropes.[109] IL-1, TNF-α, and IFN-γ have both stimulatory and inhibitory effects on TRH/VIP-stimulated prolactin secretion.[93,94,110–116] The net effect of cytokines is inhibition of prolactin secretion, which during the acute-phase response may help down-regulate the immune response to inflammation.

Hormones of the posterior pituitary are also affected by the cytokines. IL-1 stimulates the secretion of AVP via norepinephrine and angiotensin II.[94] IL-1 also stimulates the secretion of several neuropeptides that augment the release of oxytocin.[117]

## PANCREAS

Cytokines have multiple effects on carbohydrate, lipid, and protein metabolism. IL-1 enhances uptake of glucose by renal tubular cells,[118] adipose cells,[119] synoviocytes,[120] and fibroblasts.[121,122] The combination of IFN-γ and TNF-α increases uptake of glucose in fibroblasts.[122] In animals without endogenous insulin production, IL-1 causes a decrease in blood glucose by increasing the activity of hepatic 5-hydroxytryptamine.[123] In addition, IL-1 decreases lipid uptake from the intestine and into peripheral tissues.[124] It also stimulates proteolysis.[125] IFN-γ causes insulin resistance, increased insulin clearance, impaired glucose tolerance, and increased counterregulatory hormone responses.[126] TNF-α causes hyperglycemia and hypertriglyceridemia by increasing liver triglyceride production.[127] Long-term infusion of TNF-α causes insulin resistance,[128] whereas neutralization of TNF-α improves insulin resistance.[129,130]

Insulin secretion from the pancreas is directly and profoundly affected by cytokines.[131–133] At low concentrations of IL-1, glucose-stimulated insulin secretion is increased.[134] At higher concentrations of IL-1, glucose-stimulated insulin

secretion is inhibited.[135] These effects are associated with an increase or reduction in preproinsulin gene transcription/translation, protein biosynthesis, oxygen consumption, and oxidative metabolism. With prolonged IL-1 incubation, pancreatic B cells are destroyed via apoptosis.[136] The cytotoxic effects of IL-1 may contribute to the pathogenesis of autoimmune diabetes mellitus.

In vitro, low concentrations of IL-6 augment glucose-stimulated insulin release.[137] IL-6, TNF-α, and IFN-γ at high concentrations inhibit glucose-stimulated insulin release.[138,139] In combination with TNF-α, TNF-β, IFN-γ, and IL-1, IL-6 synergizes to inhibit the release of insulin and causes the destruction of pancreatic B cells.[140,141]

In general, low levels of cytokines stimulate insulin secretion, whereas high concentrations of proinflammatory cytokines inhibit insulin secretion. The elevated blood glucose concentrations seen in critically ill patients (i.e., *stress hyperglycemia*) result from a *combination of insulin resistance and impaired insulin secretion induced by proinflammatory cytokines*.

In addition to effects on insulin, interleukins alter the secretion of glucagon. IL-1 causes increased secretion of glucagon from islets.[142] Prolonged incubation of islets with IL-1 causes functional inhibition of glucagon secretion and A-cell toxicity.[135,136] Hyperglucagonemia seen in patients with inflammation and infection probably results partially from elevated levels of IL-1 and TNF-α. Glucagon assists with substrate mobilization during the acute-phase response.

## THYROID

IL-1 and TNF inhibit TRH release. IL-1 also stimulates release of somatostatin and dopamine, which serve to inhibit TRH synthesis.[143,144] In contrast, IL-1 and IL-6 stimulate TSH release by the pituitary.[143] However, IL-1, TNF, IL-6, and IFN-γ reduce expression of TSH receptors[143] and thus inhibit the thyroidal axis. The effect of these cytokines on TRH release predominates over the pituitary effects and is believed to contribute to low TSH concentrations during the acute-phase response. The predominant effects of cytokines on the HPT axis are inhibitory.[143,145–147] Release of cytokines from immune and nonimmune cells during illness and inflammatory states contributes to the euthyroid sick syndrome. In addition, thyrocyte-produced cytokines and cytokines produced by intrathyroidal immune cells (i.e., lymphocytes, monocytes) may modulate thyroid function, growth, and response to immune attack.

## ADRENAL GLAND

IL-1 immunoreactivity is found in noradrenergic chromaffin cells in the adrenal gland.[1] Adrenal production of IL-1α is decreased by systemic administration of cholinergic agonists. On the other hand, endotoxin increases production of adrenal IL-1α. Immunoreactive IL-1 is also present in cultured sympathetic ganglia. The release of IL-6, which is synthesized by adrenal zona glomerulosa cells, is stimulated by IL-1 (α and β), ACTH, endotoxin, prostaglandin E₂, and angiotensin. Fetal, but not adult, adrenal glands express TNF-α.

Cytokines activate the HPA axis[79,81] and increase glucocorticoid secretion. At the level of the adrenal cortex, IL-1, IL-2, IL-6, TNF-α, and IFN-α stimulate glucocorticoid secretion in isolated adrenal glands and hypophysectomized animals.[79] IL-6 production by the adrenal gland further contributes to glucocorticoid secretion.

Interestingly, IL-6 inhibits hepatic synthesis of corticosteroid-binding globulin, increasing free cortisol concentrations (and cortisol bioavailability). In addition to directly stimulating adrenal glucocorticoid secretion, TNF-α also inhibits the glucocorticoid response to ACTH via a nitric oxide–dependent mechanism.[79] TNF-β also inhibits glucocorticoid production. Prolonged overproduction of TNF may contribute to adrenal insufficiency in the chronically critically ill.

Glucocorticoids produced by the adrenal gland decrease CRH and ACTH release via a negative-feedback mechanism. They also decrease production of cytokines by mononuclear cells, down-regulating the immune system and decreasing the inflammatory response.

### GONADS

The testes and ovaries synthesize cytokines and contain receptors for cytokines.[1] These cytokines play important roles in the regulation of gonadal function and may play a role in inflammatory destruction of these glands.

IL-1 inhibits GnRH secretion from the hypothalamus.[79] On the other hand, IL-6 stimulates pituitary synthesis of LH. IL-1 can stimulate LH release via IL-6. IL-1 inhibits FSH release, whereas Sertoli cells produce IL-1 and express TNF receptors. TNF-α blocks gonadotropin-stimulated inhibin synthesis, decreasing negative feedback on FSH secretion. Leydig cells also make IL-1 and express TNF receptors. IL-1, IL-2, and TNF-α inhibit testosterone synthesis. Testosterone, in turn, inhibits IL-1 secretion from mononuclear cells. Overall, the effects of cytokines on the hypothalamic–pituitary–testosterone axis are complex but may contribute to *hypogonadotropic hypogonadism during illness.*

An intraovarian cytokine system of agonists, receptors, and antagonists also exists.[79] Theca cells express IL-1R, TNF-α, and TGF-β; granulosa cells express IL-1, IL-1R, IL-6, TNF-α, and TGF-β; and oocytes express TNF-α and TGF-β. IL-1 stimulates progesterone secretion from theca cells, whereas TNF-α has both stimulatory and inhibitory effects. Theca-cell androgen synthesis is inhibited by TNF-α. In granulosa cells, IL-1 and TNF-α interfere with sex hormone production; TNF-α inhibits estrogen synthesis, whereas IL-1, IL-6, and TNF-α inhibit progesterone synthesis. Sex steroids also inhibit cytokine production.[79] Estrogens inhibit IL-1, IL-6, and TNF-α production, and progesterone and androgens inhibit IL-1 synthesis by mononuclear cells. Overall, cytokines (especially IL-1) participate in follicle growth and maturation, luteal growth, and luteolysis. The inhibitory effects on gonadotropin-stimulated sex steroid production by cytokines may contribute to hypogonadotropic hypogonadism, anovulation, oligomenorrhea and amenorrhea, and infertility during inflammatory processes.

## SUMMARY

The *acute-phase response*, a *generalized host reaction to a variety of pathologic processes*, is characterized by *activation of the immune and neuroendocrine systems* (Fig. 227-2). Like classic hormones, cytokines have autocrine, paracrine, and hemocrine effects. Most endocrine cells produce cytokines, contain cytokine receptors, and are affected by cytokines. Cytokines are responsible for many of the neuroendocrine alterations that accompany the acute-phase response and systemic inflammation. These changes include increased levels of epinephrine, cortisol, aldosterone, insulin, glucagon, GH, prolactin, and AVP, and reduced levels of thyroid hormones and gonadal steroids. Not only do cytokines affect endocrine cells, but endocrine hormones affect immune-cell function and cytokine secretion. The result is *an integrated immunoendocrine network.* Improved understanding of the actions of cytokines on endocrine cells and the effects of endocrine hormones on immune cells may lead to new therapeutic approaches to both inflammatory and endocrine diseases.

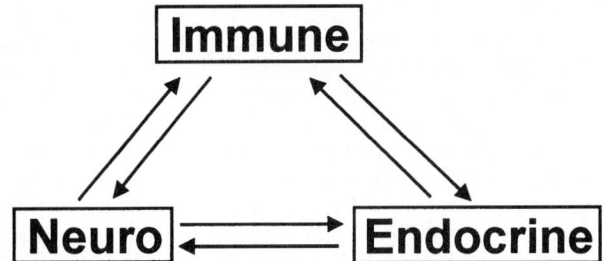

**FIGURE 227-2.** Reciprocal interactions of immune-neuro-endocrine systems in critical illness.

## REFERENCES

1. Besedovsky HO, Del Rey A. Immune-neuroendocrine interactions: facts and hypotheses. Endocr Rev 1996; 17:64.
2. Romagnani S. Biology of human TH1 and TH2 cells. J Clin Immunol 1995; 15:121.
3. Curfs JH, Meis JF, Hoogkamp-Korstanje JA. A primer on cytokines: sources, receptors, effects, and inducers. Clin Microbiol Rev 1997; 10:742.
4. Daynes RA, Meikle AW, Araneo BA. Locally active steroid hormones may facilitate compartmentalization of immunity by regulating the types of lymphokines produced by helper T cells. Res Immunol 1991; 142:40.
5. Rook GAW, Hernandez-Pando R, Lightman SL. Hormones, peripherally activated prohormones and regulation of the Th1/Th2 balance. Immunol Today 1994; 15:301.
6. Ihle JN. Cytokine receptor signaling. Nature 1995; 377:591.
7. Marino MW, Dunn A, Grail D, et al. Characterization of tumor necrosis factor-deficient mice. Proc Natl Acad Sci U S A 1997; 94:8093.
8. Peschon JJ, Torrance DS, Stocking KL, et al. TNF receptor-deficient mice reveal divergent roles for p55 and p75 in several models of inflammation. J Immunol 1998; 160:943.
9. Pfeffer K, Matsuyama T, Kundig T. Mice deficient for the 55-kd tumor necrosis factor receptor are resistant to endotoxic shock, yet succumb to *L. monocytogenes* infection. Cell 1993; 73:457.
10. Li P, Allen H, Banerjee S, et al. Mice deficient in IL-1β-converting enzyme are defective in production of mature IL-1β and resistant to endotoxic shock. Cell 1995; 80:401.
11. Hirsch E, Irikura VM, Paul SM, Hirsh D. Functions of interleukin 1 receptor antagonist in gene knockout and overproducing mice. Proc Natl Acad Sci U S A 1996; 93:11008.
12. Hack CE, Aarden LA, Thijs LG. Role of cytokines in sepsis. Adv Immunol 1997; 66:101.
13. Thijs LG, Hack CE. Time course of cytokine levels in sepsis. Intensive Care Med 1995; 21(Suppl 2):S258.
14. Okusawa S, Gelfand JA, Ikejima T. Interleukin 1 induces a shock like state in rabbits: synergism with tumor necrosis factor and the effect of cyclooxygenase inhibition. J Clin Invest 1988; 81:1162.
15. Fong Y, Tracey KJ, Moldawer LL, et al. Antibodies to cachectin/tumor necrosis factor reduce interleukin 1β and interleukin 6 appearance during lethal bacteremia. J Exp Med 1989; 170:1627.
16. Tracey KJ, Fong Y, Hesse DG, et al. Anti-cachectin/TNF monoclonal antibodies prevent septic shock during lethal bacteraemia. Nature 1987; 330:662.
17. Tracey KJ, Beutler B, Lowry SF, et al. Shock and tissue injury induced by recombinant human cachectin. Science 1986; 234:470.
18. Kumar A, Thota V, Dee L, et al. Tumor necrosis factor alpha and interleukin 1β are responsible for in vitro myocardial cell depression induced by human septic shock serum. J Exp Med 1996; 183:949.
19. Dinarello CA, Cannon JG, Mancilla J. Interleukin-6 as an endogenous pyrogen: induction of prostaglandin $E_2$ in brain but not peripheral blood mononuclear cells. Brain Res 1991; 562:199.
20. Barnes PJ, Karin M. Nuclear factor-κB—a pivotal transcription factor in chronic inflammatory diseases. N Engl J Med 1997; 336:1066.
20a. Paterson RL, Galley HF, Phillon TK, Webster NR. Increased nuclear factor kappa B activation in critically ill patients who die. Crit Care Med 2000; 28:1047.
21. Carter AB, Monick MM, Hunninghake GW. Lipopolysaccharide-induced NF-kappaB activation and cytokine release in human alveolar macrophages is PKC-independent and TK- and PC-PLC dependent. Am J Respir Cell Mol Biol 1998; 18:384.
22. Blackwell TS, Christman JW. The role of nuclear factor-kappa B in cytokine gene regulation. Am J Respir Cell Mol Biol 1997; 17:3.
23. Lantz M, Gullberg U, Nilsson E, Olsson I. Characterization in vitro of a human tumor necrosis factor-binding protein. A soluble form of a tumor necrosis factor receptor. J Clin Invest 1990; 86:1396.
24. Bone RC. Sir Isaac Newton, sepsis, SIRS and CARS. Crit Care Med 1996; 24:1125.

25. Bone RC, Grodzin CJ, Balk RA. Sepsis: a new hypothesis for pathogenesis of the disease process. Chest 1997; 112:235.

25a. Papathanassoglou ED, Moynihan TA, Ackerman MH. Does programmed cell death (apoptosis) play a role in the development of multiple organ dysfunction in critically ill patients? Crit Care Med 2000; 28:537.

26. Moss ML, Jin SL, Becherer JD, et al. Structural features and biochemical properties of TNF-alpha converting enzyme (TACE). J Neuroimmunol 1997; 72:127.

27. Moss ML, Jin SL, Milla ME, et al. Cloning of a disintegrin metalloproteinase that processes precursor tumour-necrosis factor-α. Nature 1997; 385:733.

28. Black RA, Rauch CT, Kozlosky CJ, et al. A metalloproteinase disintegrin that releases tumour-necrosis factor-alpha from cells. Nature 1997; 385:729.

29. Murrell GA, Jang D, Williams RJ. Nitric oxide activates metalloprotease enzymes in articular cartilage. Biochem Biophys Res Commun 1995; 206:15.

30. Solomon KA, Covington MB, DeCicco CP, Newton RC. The fate of pro-TNF-alpha following inhibition of metalloprotease-dependent processing to soluble TNF-alpha in human monocytes. J Immunol 1997; 159:4524.

31. Gallea-Robache S, Morand V, Millet S, et al. A metalloproteinase inhibitor blocks the shedding of soluble cytokine receptors and processing of transmembrane cytokine precursors in human monocytic cells. Cytokine 1997; 9:340.

32. Solorzano CC, Ksontini R, Pruitt JH, et al. A matrix metalloproteinase inhibitor prevents processing of tumor necrosis factor alpha (TNF alpha) and abrogates endotoxin-induced lethality. Shock 1997; 7:427.

33. Gearing AJ, Beckett P, Christodoulou M, et al. Matrix metalloproteinases and processing of pro-TNF-alpha. J Leukoc Biol 1995; 57:774.

34. Wright SD, Ramos RA, Tobias PS. CD 14, a receptor for complexes of LPS and LPS binding protein. Science 1990; 249:1431.

35. Gallay P, Barras C, Tobias PS, et al. Lipopolysaccharide (LPS)-binding protein in human serum determines the tumor necrosis factor response of monocytes to LPS. J Infect Dis 1994; 170:1319.

36. Heumann D, Barras C, Severin A, et al. Gram-positive cell walls stimulate synthesis of tumor necrosis factor alpha and interleukin-6 by human monocytes. Infect Immun 1994; 62:2715.

37. Stuber F, Petersen M, Bokelmann F, Schade U. A genomic polymorphism within the tumor necrosis factor locus influences plasma tumor necrosis factor-alpha concentrations and outcome of patients with severe sepsis [see comments]. Crit Care Med 1996; 24:381.

38. Trinchieri G. Regulation of tumor necrosis factor production by monocyte-macrophages and lymphocytes. Immunol Res 1991; 10:8.

39. Van der Poll T, Buller HR, ten Cate H, et al. Activation of coagulation after administration of tumor necrosis factor to normal subjects. N Engl J Med 1990; 322:1622.

40. Hesse DG, Tracey KJ, Fong Y, et al. Cytokine appearance in human endotoxemia and primate bacteremia. Surg Gynecol Obstet 1988; 166:147.

41. Beutler BA, Milsark IW, Cerami A. Cachectin/tumor necrosis factor: production, distribution, and metabolic fate in vivo. J Immunol 1985; 135:3972.

42. Zuckerman SH, Evans GF, Butler LD. Endotoxin tolerance: independent regulation of interleukin-1 and tumor necrosis factor expression. Infect Immun 1991; 59:2774.

43. Salkowski CA, Vogel SN. Lipopolysaccharide increases glucocorticoid receptor expression in murine macrophages. A possible mechanism for glucocorticoid-mediated suppression of endotoxicity. J Immunol 1992; 149:4041.

44. Waage A. Production and clearance of tumor necrosis factor in rats exposed to endotoxin and dexamethasone. Clin Immunol Immunopathol 1987; 45:348.

45. Palladino MAJ, Shalaby MR, Kramer SM, et al. Characterization of the antitumor activities of human tumor necrosis factor-alpha and the comparison with other cytokines: induction of tumor-specific immunity. J Immunol 1987; 138:4023.

46. Friers W. Tumor necrosis factor: characterization at the molecular, cellular and in vivo levels. FEBS Letters 1991; 285:199.

47. Lantz M, Malik S, Slevin ML, Olsson I. Infusion of tumor necrosis factor (TNF) causes an increase in circulating TNF-binding protein in humans. Cytokine 1990; 2:402.

48. Kern WV, Engel A, Kern P. Soluble tumor necrosis factor receptors in febrile neutropenic cancer patients. Infection 1995; 23:64.

49. Van Zee KJ, Kohno T, Fischer E, et al. Tumor necrosis factor soluble receptors circulate during experimental and clinical inflammation and can protect against excessive tumor necrosis factor alpha in vitro and in vivo. Proc Natl Acad Sci U S A 1992; 89:4845.

50. Redl H, Schlag G, Adolf GR, et al. Tumor necrosis factor (TNF)-dependent shedding of the p55 TNF receptor in a baboon model of bacteremia. Infect Immun 1995; 63:297.

51. Cerretti DP, Kozlosky CJ, Mosley B, et al. Molecular cloning of interleukin beta converting enzyme. Science 1992; 256:97.

52. Papanicolaou DA, Wilder RL, Manolagas SC, Chrousos GP. The pathophysiologic roles of interleukin-6 in human disease. Ann Intern Med 1998; 128:127.

53. Blackwell TS, Christman JW. Sepsis and cytokines: current status. Br J Anaesth 1996; 77:110.

54. Dinarello CA. Interleukin-1 and interleukin-1 antagonism. Blood 1991; 77:1627.

55. Wewers MD, Rinehart JJ, She Z-W. Tumor necrosis factor infusions in humans' prime neutrophils for hypochlorous acid production. Am J Physiol Lung Cell Mol Physiol 1990; 259:L276.

56. Pfeffer K, Matsuyama T, Kundig T. Mice deficient for the 55-kd tumor necrosis factor receptor are resistant to endotoxic shock, yet succumb to L. monocytogenes infection. Cell 1993; 73:457.

57. Smith JW, Urba WJ, Curti BD. The toxic and hematologic effects of interleukin-1 alpha administered in a phase I trial of patients with advanced hematologic malignancies. J Clin Oncol 1992; 10:1140.

58. Woodroofe C, Muller W, Ruther U. Long-term consequences of interleukin-6 overexpression in transgenic mice. DNA Cell Biol 1992; 11:587.

59. Preiser JC, Schmartz D, van der Linden P, et al. Interleukin-6 administration has no acute hemodynamic or hematologic effects in the dog. Cytokine 1991; 3:1.

60. Tilg H, Trehu E, Atkins MB, et al. Interleukin-6 (IL-6) as an anti-inflammatory cytokine: induction of circulating IL-1 receptor antagonist and soluble tumor necrosis factor receptor p55. Blood 1994; 83:113.

61. Mizuhara H, O'Neill E, Seki N, et al. T cell activation-associated hepatic injury: mediation by tumor necrosis factors and protection by interleukin 6. J Exp Med 1994; 179:1529.

62. Shingu M, Miyauchi S, Nagai Y, et al. The role of IL-4 and IL-6 in IL-1-dependent cartilage matrix degradation. Br J Rheumatol 1995; 34:101.

63. Alcorn JM, Fierer J, Chojkier M. The acute-phase response protects mice from D-galactosamine sensitization to endotoxin and tumor necrosis factor-alpha. Hepatology 1992; 15:122.

64. Crowl RM, Stoller TJ, Conroy RR, Stoner CR. Induction of phospholipase A$_2$ gene expression in human hepatoma cells by mediators of the acute phase response. J Biol Chem 1991; 266:2647.

65. Shrikant P, Weber E, Jilling T, Benveniste EN. Intercellular adhesion molecule-1 gene expression by glial cells. Differential mechanisms of inhibition by IL-10 and IL-6. J Immunol 1995; 155:1489.

66. Casey LC, Balk R, Bone RC. Plasma cytokine and endotoxin levels correlate with survival in patients with sepsis syndrome. Ann Intern Med 1993; 119:771.

67. Presterl E, Staudinger T, Pettermann M, et al. Cytokine profile and correlation to the APACHE III and MPM II scores in patients with sepsis. Am J Respir Crit Care Med 1997; 156:825.

68. Helfgott DC, Tatter SB, Santhanam RH, et al. Multiple forms of IFN-beta/IL-6 in serum and body fluids during acute bacterial infection. J Immunol 1989; 142:948.

69. Calandra T, Gerain J, Heumann D, et al. High circulating levels of interleukin-6 in patients with septic shock: evolution during sepsis, prognostic value and interplay with other cytokines. Am J Med 1991; 91:23.

70. Meduri GU, Headley S, Kohler G, et al. Persistent elevation of inflammatory cytokines predicts a poor outcome in ARDS. Plasma IL-1 beta and IL-6 levels are consistent and efficient predictors of outcome over time. Chest 1995; 107:1062.

71. Antonelli M, Raponi GM, Martino P, et al. High IL-6 serum levels are associated with septic shock and mortality in septic patients with severe leukopenia due to hematological malignancies. Scand J Infect Dis 1995; 27:381.

72. Damas P, Canivet J-L, De Groote D, et al. Sepsis and serum cytokine concentrations. Crit Care Med 1997; 25:405.

73. Damas P, Ledoux D, Nys M, et al. Cytokine serum level during severe sepsis in human IL-6 as a marker of severity. Ann Surg 1992; 215:356.

74. Dinarello CA. Proinflammatory and antiinflammatory cytokines as mediators in the pathogenesis of septic shock. Chest 1997; 112:321S.

75. Lalani I, Bhol K, Ahmed AR. Interleukin-10: biology role in inflammation and autoimmunity. Ann Allergy Asthma Immunol 1997; 79:469.

76. Berg DJ, Kuhn R, Rajewsky K, et al. Interleukin-10 is a central regulator of the response to LPS in murine models of endotoxic shock and the Shwartzman reaction but not endotoxin tolerance. J Clin Invest 1995; 96:2339.

77. Howard M, Muchamuel T, Andrade A, Menon S. Interleukin-10 protects mice from lethal endotoxemia. J Exp Med 1993; 177:1205.

78. de Waal Malefyt R, Haanen J, Spits H. IL-10 and viral IL-10 strongly reduced antigen specific T cell proliferation by diminishing the antigen presenting capacity of monocytes via down regulation of class major histocompatibility complex expression. J Exp Med 1991; 174:915.

79. Mandrup-Poulsen T, Nerup J, Reimers JI, et al. Cytokines and the endocrine system. I. The immunoendocrine network. Eur J Endocrinol 1995; 133:660.

80. Mandrup-Poulsen T, Nerup J, Reimers JI, et al. Cytokines and the endocrine system. I. The immunoendocrine network. Eur J Endocrinol 1995; 133:660.

81. Turnbull AV, Lee S, Rivier C. Mechanisms of hypothalamic-pituitary-adrenal axis stimulation by immune signals in the adult rat. Ann N Y Acad Sci 1998; 840:434.

82. Chrousos GP. The hypothalamic-pituitary-adrenal axis and immune-mediated inflammation. N Engl J Med 1995; 332:1351.

83. Imura H, Fukata J, Mori T. Cytokines and endocrine function: an interaction between the immune and neuroendocrine systems. Clin Endocrinol 1991; 35:107.

84. Bernardini R, Kamilaris TC, Calogero AE, et al. Interactions between tumor necrosis factor-α, hypothalamic corticotropin-releasing hormone and adrenocorticotropin secretion in the rat. Endocrinology 1990; 126:2876.

85. Sapolsky R, Rivier C, Yamamoto G, et al. Interleukin-1 stimulates the secretion of hypothalamic corticotropin-releasing factor. Science 1987; 238:522.

86. Naitoh Y, Fukata J, Tominaga T, et al. Interleukin-6 stimulates the secretion of adrenocorticotropic hormone in conscious, free-moving rats. Biochem Biophys Res Commun 1988; 155:1459.

87. Perlstein RS, Mougey EH, Jackson WE, Neta R. Interleukin-1 and interleukin-6 act synergistically to stimulate the release of adrenocorticotropic hormone in vivo. Lymphokine Cytokine Res 1991; 10:141.

88. Perlstein RS, Whitnall MH, Abrams JS, et al. Synergistic roles of interleukin-6, interleukin-1, and tumor necrosis factor in adrenocorticotropin response to bacterial lipopolysaccharide in vivo. Endocrinology 1993; 132:946.

89. Mastorakos G, Chrousos GP, Weber JS. Recombinant interleukin-6 activates the hypothalamic-pituitary-adrenal axis in humans. J Clin Endocrinol Metab 1993; 77:1690.

90. Mastorakos G, Weber JS, Magiakou MA, et al. Hypothalamic-pituitary-adrenal axis activation and stimulation of systemic vasopressin secretion by recombinant interleukin-6 in humans: potential implications for the syndrome of inappropriate vasopressin secretion. J Clin Endocrinol Metab 1994; 79:934.

91. Raber J, Sorg O, Horn TF, et al. Inflammatory cytokines: putative regulators of neuronal and neuro-endocrine function. Brain Res Brain Res Rev 1998; 26:320.

92. McCann SM, Lyson K, Karanth S, et al. Mechanism of action of cytokines to induce the pattern of pituitary hormone secretion in infection. Ann N Y Acad Sci 1995; 771:386.

93. Scarborough DE. Cytokine modulation of pituitary hormone secretion. Ann N Y Acad Sci 1990; 594:169.

94. Jones TH, Kennedy RL. Cytokines and hypothalamic-pituitary function. Cytokine 1993; 5:531.

95. Rivest S, Lee S, Attardi B, Rivier C. The chronic intracerebroventricular infusion of interleukin-1β alters the activity of the hypothalamic-pituitary-gonadal axis of cycling rats. I. Effect of LHRH and gonadotropin biosynthesis and secretion. Endocrinology 1993; 133:2424.

96. Bonavera JJ, Kalra SP, Kalra PS. Evidence that luteinizing hormone suppression in response to inhibitory neuropeptides β-endorphin, interleukin-1β, and neuropeptide K may involve excitatory amino acids. Endocrinology 1993; 133:178.

97. Rettori V, Gimeno MF, Karara A, et al. Interleukin 1α inhibits prostaglandin E₂ release to suppress pulsatile release of luteinizing hormone but not follicle-stimulating hormone. Proc Natl Acad Sci U S A 1991; 88:2763.

98. Scarborough DE. Somatostatin regulation by cytokines. Metabolism 1990; 39:108.

99. Scarborough DE, Lee SL, Dinarello CA, Reichlin S. Interleukin-1β stimulates somatostatin biosynthesis in primary cultures of fetal rat brain. Endocrinology 1989; 124:549.

100. Brown SL, Smith LR, Blalock JE. Interleukin 1 and interleukin 2 enhance proopiomelanocortin gene expression in pituitary cells. J Immunol 1987; 139:3181.

101. Arzt E, Paez Pereda M, Costas M, et al. Cytokine expression and molecular mechanisms of their auto/paracrine regulation of anterior pituitary function and growth. Ann N Y Acad Sci 1998; 840:525.

102. Arzt E, Stalla GK. Cytokines: autocrine and paracrine roles in the anterior pituitary. Neuroimmunomodulation 1996; 3:28.

103. Spangelo BL, Judd AM, Isakson PC, MacLeod RM. Interleukin-6 stimulates anterior pituitary hormone release in vitro. Endocrinology 1989; 125:575.

104. Murata T, Ying SY. Effects of interleukin-1 beta on secretion of follicle stimulating hormone (FSH) and luteinizing hormone (LH) by cultured rat anterior pituitary cells. Life Sci 1991; 49:447.

105. Walton PE, Cronin MJ. Tumor necrosis factor-α inhibits growth hormone secretion from cultured anterior pituitary cells. Endocrinology 1989; 125:925.

106. Nash AD, Brandon MR, Bello PA. Effects of tumor necrosis factor-alpha on growth hormone and interleukin 6 mRNA in ovine pituitary cells. Mol Cell Endocrinol 1992; 84:R31.

107. Bernton EW, Beach JE, Holaday JW, et al. Release of multiple hormones by a direct action of interleukin-1 on pituitary cells. Science 1987; 238:519.

108. Bole-Feysot C, Goffin V, Edery M, et al. Prolactin (PRL) and its receptor: actions, signal transduction pathways and phenotypes observed in PRL receptor knockout mice. Endocr Rev 1998; 19:225.

109. Yamaguchi M, Matsuzaki N, Hirota K, et al. Interleukin 6 possibly induced by interleukin 1β in the pituitary gland stimulates the release of gonadotropins and prolactin. Acta Endocrinol 1990; 122:201.

110. Schettini G, Florio T, Meucci O, et al. Interleukin-1-β modulation of prolactin secretion from rat anterior pituitary cells: involvement of adenylate cyclase activity and calcium mobilization. Endocrinology 1990; 126:435.

111. Schettini G, Landolfi E, Grimaldi M, et al. Interleukin 1 beta inhibition of TRH stimulated prolactin secretion and phosphoinositide metabolism. Biochem Biophys Res Commun 1989; 165:496.

112. Yamaguchi M, Koike K, Yoshimoto Y, et al. Effect of TNF-α on prolactin secretion from rat anterior pituitary and dopamine release from the hypothalamus: comparison with the effect of interleukin 1β. Endocrinol Jpn 1991; 38:357.

113. Koike K, Hirota K, Ohmichi M, et al. Tumor necrosis factor-α increases release of arachidonate and prolactin from rat anterior pituitary cells. Endocrinology 1991; 128:2791.

114. Walton PE, Cronin MJ. Tumor necrosis factor-α and interferon-γ reduce prolactin release in vitro. Am J Physiol 1990; 259:E672.

115. Koike K, Masumoto N, Kasahara K, et al. Tumor necrosis factor-α stimulates prolactin release from anterior pituitary cells: a possible involvement of intracellular calcium mobilization. Endocrinology 1991; 128:2785.

116. Yamaguchi M, Koike K, Matsuzaki N, et al. The interferon family stimulates the secretions of prolactin and interleukin-6 by the pituitary gland in vitro. J Endocrinol Invest 1991; 14:457.

117. Naito Y, Fukata J, Shindo K, et al. Effects of interleukins on plasma arginine vasopressin and oxytocin levels in conscious, freely moving rats. Biochem Biophys Res Commun 1991; 174:1189.

118. Kohan DE, Schreiner GF. Interleukin-1 modulation of renal epithelial glucose and amino acid transport. Am J Physiol 1988; 254:F879.

119. Garcia-Welsh A, Schneiderman JS, Baly DL. Interleukin-1 stimulates glucose transport in rat adipose cells. Evidence for receptor discrimination between IL-1β and IL-1α. FEBS Lett 1990; 269:421.

120. Hernvann A, Aussel C, Cynober L et al. IL-1β, a strong mediator for glucose uptake by rheumatoid and non-rheumatoid cultured human synoviocytes. FEBS Lett 1992; 303:77.

121. Bird TA, Davies A, Baldwin SA, Saklavala J. Interleukin 1 stimulates hexose transport in fibroblasts by increasing the expression of glucose transporters. J Biol Chem 1990; 265:13578.

122. Taylor DJ, Faragher EB, Evanson JM. Inflammatory cytokines stimulate glucose uptake and glycolysis but reduce glucose oxidation in human dermal fibroblasts in vitro. Circul Shock 1992; 37:105.

123. Endo Y, Suzuki R, Kumagai K. Interleukin 1-like factors can accumulate 5-hydroxytryptamine in the liver of mice and can induce hypoglycaemia. Biochem Biophys Acta 1985; 840:37.

124. Argiles JM, Lopez-Soriano F, Evans RD, Williamson DH. Interleukin-1 and lipid metabolism in the rat. Biochem J 1989; 259:673.

125. Zamir O, Hasselgren P-O, Von Allmen D, Fischer JE. In vivo administration of interleukin-1α induces muscle proteolysis in normal and adrenalectomized rats. Metabolism 1993; 42:204.

126. Koivisto VA, Pelkonen R, Cantell K. Effect of interferon on glucose tolerance and insulin sensitivity. Diabetes 1989; 38:641.

127. Feingold KR, Soued M, Staprans I, et al. Effect of tumor necrosis factor (TNF) on lipid metabolism in the diabetic rat. Evidence that inhibition of adipose tissue lipoprotein lipase activity is not required for TNF-induced hyperlipidemia. J Clin Invest 1989; 83:1116.

128. Lang CH, Dobrescu C, Bagby GJ. Tumor necrosis factor impairs insulin action on peripheral glucose disposal and hepatic glucose output. Endocrinology 1992; 130:43.

129. Hotamisligil GS, Shargill NS, Spiegelman BM. Adipose expression of tumor necrosis factor α: direct role in obesity-linked insulin resistance. Science 1993; 259:87.

130. Hofmann C, Lorenz K, Braithwaite SS, et al. Altered gene expression for tumor necrosis factor α and its receptors during drug and dietary modulation of insulin resistance. Endocrinology 1994; 134:264.

131. Mandrup-Poulsen T, Helquist D, Molvig J, et al. Cytokines as immune effector molecules in autoimmune endocrine disease with special reference to insulin-dependent diabetes mellitus. Autoimmunity 1989; 4:191.

132. Sandler S, Eizirik DL, Svensson C, et al. Biochemical and molecular actions of interleukin-1 on pancreatic β cells. Autoimmunity 1991; 10:241.

133. Purrello F, Buscema M. Effects of interleukin-1β on insulin secretion by pancreatic beta-cells. Diab Nutr Metab 1993; 6:295.

134. Palmer JP, Helquist S, Spinas GA, et al. Interaction of β-cell activity and IL-1 concentration and exposure time in isolated rat islets of Langerhans. Diabetes 1989; 38:1211.

135. Mandrup-Poulsen T, Bendtzen K, Nerup J, et al. Affinity-purified human interleukin 1 is cytotoxic to isolated islets of Langerhans. Diabetologia 1986; 39:63.

136. Mandrup-Poulsen T, Egeberg J, Nerup J, et al. Ultrastructural studies of time-course and cellular specificity of interleukin 1 mediated islet cytotoxicity. Acta Path Microbiol Immunol Scand 1987; 95:55.

137. Buschard K, Aaen K, Horn T, et al. Interleukin 6: a functional and structural in vitro modulator of beta cells from islets of Langerhans. Autoimmunity 1990; 5:185.

138. Southern C, Schultser D, Greene IC. Inhibition of insulin secretion from rat islets of Langerhans by interleukin-6. Biochem J 1990; 272:243.

139. Bendtzen K, Mandrup-Poulsen T, Nerup J, et al. Cytotoxicity of human p17 interleukin-1 for pancreatic islets of Langerhans. Science 1986; 232:1545.

140. Mandrup-Poulsen T, Bendtzen K, Dinarello CA, Nerup J. Human tumor necrosis factor potentiates human interleukin-1 mediated rat pancreatic beta-cell cytotoxicity. J Immunol 1987; 139:4077.

141. Rabinovitch A, Sumoski W, Rajotte RV, Warnock GL. Cytotoxic effects of cytokines on human pancreatic islet cells in monolayer culture. J Clin Endocrinol Metab 1990; 71:152.

142. Helqvist S, Zumsteg UW, Spinas GA, et al. Repetitive exposure of pancreatic islets to interleukin-1β. An in vitro model of pre-diabetes? Autoimmunity 1991; 10:311.

143. Mandrup-Poulsen T, Nerup J, Reimers JI, et al. Cytokines and the endocrine system. II. Roles in substrate metabolism, modulation of thyroidal and pancreatic endocrine cell functions and autoimmune endocrine diseases. Eur J Endocrinol 1996; 134:21.

144. Jones TH, Kennedy RL. Cytokines and hypothalamic-pituitary function. Cytokines 1993; 5:531.

145. Dubuis JM, Dayer JM, Siegrist-Kaiser CA, Burger AG. Human recombinant interleukin-1B decreases plasma thyroid hormone and thyroid stimulating hormone levels in rats. Endocrinology 1988; 123:2175.

146. Van der Poll T, Romijn JA, Wiersinga WM, Sauerwein HP. Tumor necrosis factor: a putative mediator of the sick-euthyroid syndrome in man. J Clin Endocrinol Metab 1990; 71:1567.

147. Bartalena L, Grasso L, Brogioni S, Martino E. Interleukin-6 effects on the pituitary-thyroid axis in the rat. Eur J Endocrinol 1994; 131:302.

# CHAPTER 228

# ENDOCRINE MARKERS AND MEDIATORS IN CRITICAL ILLNESS

ABDULLAH A. ALARIFI, GREET H. VAN DEN BERGHE, RICHARD H. SNIDER, JR., KENNETH L. BECKER, BEAT MÜLLER, AND ERIC S. NYLÉN

*Inflammation* is the response to an injury (e.g., infection, trauma, heat, cold, locally toxic chemicals, etc.). It is characterized by vasodilatation with increased blood flow, increased capillary permeability resulting in passage of macromolecules and fluid into the interstitial space, chemoattraction of hematopoietic cellular elements to the site of injury, stimulation of neutrophilic phagocytosis, and activation of monocytes. The inflammatory response is mediated by a multitude of humoral substances including several cytokines, which emanate from cells of the immune system as well as many other cells throughout the body. These have a particularly key role in stimulating, perpetuating, and/or modulating the inflammatory response. Some of the cytokines are *proinflammatory*, some are *antiinflammatory*, and some manifest *either* of these functions, depending on their local or systemic concentration, and the coexisting chemical or hormonal milieu.

*Stress* can be defined as any condition that threatens to disrupt the equilibrium of bodily functions (i.e., *homeostasis*). Stress is a somewhat broader and less specific term than inflammation and usually includes in its definition the response of the immune, neural, and endocrine systems to a concurrent perturbation or injury. Previously, the concept of stress had focused primarily on the hypothalamic–pituitary–adrenal (HPA) axis, the catecholamines, and glucose and insulin metabolism. The histopathologic changes, physiologic alterations, and hormonal and cytokine responses observed in many studies, however, have documented a substantial overlap between the concepts of "inflammation" and "stress."

The appellation *critical illness* is best applied to a *life-threatening condition that merits intensive medical and/or surgical intervention.* The patient with critical illness is always under stress and, not uncommonly, manifests some or all of the physiologic and biologic characteristics of inflammation.

Generally, different stressors evoke a multihormonal and selective response, the magnitude of which frequently correlates with the degree and type of stress. Although the endocrine changes during stress are well documented, their mechanisms, their extent, their timing, their duration, the prognostic value of these changes, and whether they are *adaptive* or *maladaptive* (i.e., harmful) are much less well understood. In the short term, stress-induced changes in endocrine function are generally adaptive: they promote optimal intravascular volume, perfusion pressure, and substrate availability. Nonetheless, if the stress is prolonged or if the homeostatic response is inadequate, the endocrine response can contribute to a worsened clinical status and, hence, to the potential need for therapeutic interventions (see Chaps. 230 and 232).

Much of our current understanding of the endocrine response to stress originated with Bernard's concept of the *"internal environment."* Cannon coined the term *homeostasis* to describe the complete bioresponse necessary to maintain a steady state and documented the role of the sympathoadrenal system. Selye described the enlargement of the adrenal cortex in response to diverse noxious agents (later termed the *general adaptation syndrome*); this shifted attention to the HPA axis. Later, the role of glucocorticoids in stress was redefined as *the modulation of other adaptive responses (especially those involving proinflammatory cytokines), thereby protecting the host from the effects of "overreaction."*[1] Further clarifying the endocrine response to stress has been the emerging recognition of the cytokines as pivotal mediators and the endocrine endothelium as an essential site of activation in critical illness (see Chap. 227). Also, the expression of heat-shock protein in stress tolerance at the cellular level, its involvement in mediating the immune response to stress, and its potential protective effect appear to provide another fundamental component. Finally, as discussed in Chapter 227, a hallmark of the stress response is a multidirectional immunoneuroendocrine interaction (see Chap 227, Fig 227-2).[2,3]

## GLUCOCORTICOIDS

The most accepted explanation for the increased requirement of circulatory glucocorticoids in response to stress is that, although they exert a permissive action during periods of no stress (allowing other hormones and factors to maintain homeostasis[4]), they exert a regulatory role during stress.[1] These regulatory effects are essential in preventing immunotoxicity.[1] The secretion of glucocorticoids is part of a closed, feedback-loop system that is ideal for providing physiologic levels at all times, while also allowing for an emergency override via the central nervous system (CNS) (see Chap. 229). This is the single most important stress-response system, without which survival is unlikely.[5]

Critical illness induces an increase in the serum cortisol concentration,[6] the extent of which is determined by the type and severity of stress. Elevated cortisol levels can block the HPA response to minor stress but do not alter the response to major stress. Generally, the HPA responds in a graded fashion to increasing stress.[7] In surgery, the degree of activation depends on the type and extent of surgery and anesthesia.[8] Reversal of general anesthesia is also a potent stimulator of adrenocorticotropic hormone (ACTH) secretion.[9] (Interruption of the neural connections from the operative site can block the rise in ACTH and cortisol.[10]) Typically, the serum cortisol increase is in response to corticotropin-releasing hormone (CRH) and ACTH stimulation. These increases are associated with loss of circadian rhythm, resistance to dexamethasone suppression, and hyperresponsiveness to CRH stimulation.[9] Both ACTH and CRH levels decrease to below presurgical levels by the first postoperative day. In contrast, elevations in ACTH and CRH due to sepsis may last for several days; the cortisol levels remain high, gradually returning to normal.[11] Suppressed ACTH levels indicate the restoration of normal feedback sensitivity, whereas high cortisol secretion, in the presence of low ACTH levels, indicates either an increased adrenal sensitivity to ACTH, cortisol resistance, or the presence of alternative pathway(s) for cortisol secretion (see Chaps. 229 and 232). Thus, clinical assessment of adrenal function based on the cortisol concentration can be misleading (see Chap. 232). Another change that occurs in critical illness is the shift of adrenal steroid production from mineralocorticoid and androgens to cortisol.[12]

Associations between the severity of injury and the degree of HPA activation have been reported.[13] For example, the Glasgow Coma Score is significantly correlated with cortisol concentrations in patients who have experienced both head and systemic injuries.[14] Furthermore, serum cortisol concentrations typically correlate inversely with critical illness outcome.[13,14]

Glucocorticoids stimulate gluconeogenesis in the liver, kidney, and skeletal muscle; inhibit glucose uptake; and facilitate the synthesis and release of catecholamines (see Chap. 73). They also inhibit the secretion and action of insulin and stimulate the secretion of glucagon, causing protein wasting and inhibition of protein synthesis in skeletal muscle. Thus, although the importance of glucocorticoids to survival is well recognized, just how these effects influence the adaptation to stress is less clear. The hypercortisolism elicited by critical illnesses can be interpreted as an attempt by the body to mute its own inflammatory cascade and thus protect itself against possible endogenous overreaction.[1] Moreover, the acute cortisol-induced metabolic effects provide immediately available energy and postpone anabolism. Nonetheless, the benefit of prolonged hypercortisolism is questionable, as it may lead to immune suppression, stress hyperglycemia, myopathy, a catabolic state, and impaired healing.

At the cellular level, glucocorticoids act via ligand binding to a superfamily of nuclear receptors (see Chap. 73). As transcriptional modifiers (regulators), they affect the expression of a variety of genes, thereby serving as an important antiinflammatory force that is counteracted by proinflammatory cytokines and transcriptional factors (e.g., nuclear factor-κB) (see Chap. 227, Fig. 227-1).[15] Despite a half-century of extensive research into the actions of glucocorticoids, their multifaceted actions have yet to be fully unraveled.[16]

## CATECHOLAMINES

The control center of the stress response is located in the cerebral cortex, limbic system, hypothalamus, and brainstem (see Chap. 229). Various noxious stressors cause increased activity of the sympathetic nervous system (SNS) and adrenal medulla. This results in secretion of epinephrine and norepinephrine from the adrenal medulla and norepinephrine from the sympathetic nerve terminals, respectively (norepinephrine comprises ~20% of adrenal medullary catecholamine secretion). Although most norepinephrine is taken up by presynaptic neurons, some "overflow" into the plasma occurs, serving as an indicator of sympathetic neuronal activity. Increasingly, this stress response appears to show specificity (i.e., the degree of the response and the ratio of epinephrine to norepinephrine secretion depend on the specific type of stress).

The catecholaminergic response, which is rapid and transient, can be attenuated by epidural analgesia.[17] The *severity* of the stressor determines the *degree* of the catecholamine response[18]; *however, the catecholamine concentration is not predictive of the final outcome in critically ill patients.*[19] With prolonged stress, marked compensatory changes occur in the adrenal medulla, including increased activity of the enzymes involved in catecholamine biosynthesis and elevated tissue concentrations of catecholamines. These changes in enzymatic activity are regulated to varying degrees by glucocorticoids, ACTH, and neuronal activity.[20]

The released catecholamines trigger metabolic and hemodynamic changes characteristic of the "flight or fight" response, which range from increased blood pressure to increased glycogenolysis.

Catecholamines have direct effects on the metabolism of lipids, proteins, and carbohydrates, and on regulatory hormones (e.g., insulin and glucagon).[21] They augment hepatic glucose output by stimulating both gluconeogenesis and glycogenolysis, increase lipolysis, inhibit insulin secretion, impair tissue sensitivity to insulin, and increase glucagon and growth hormone secretion.[21,22]

As with the HPA axis, multidirectional effects are also found between the SNS and cytokines. Infusion of tumor necrosis factor-α (TNF-α) or interleukin-1 (IL-1) causes a rapid and marked increase of catecholamines.[23] Norepinephrine inhibits lipopolysaccharide (LPS)-induced TNF-α and IL-6 release in human whole blood; this effect is blocked by β antagonism, suggesting that norepinephrine may modulate ongoing cytokine production in acute sepsis.[24]

## THYROID HORMONES

The changes in thyroid function during acute critical illness are well known[25] (see Chaps. 36 and 232). During a mild illness, triiodothyronine ($T_3$) production is rapidly decreased by inhibition of conversion of thyroxine ($T_4$) to $T_3$, with a reciprocal increase in reverse $T_3$ ($rT_3$; *low $T_3$ syndrome*). With an increase in severity of illness, $T_4$ decreases (*low $T_4$ syndrome*). The serum thyroid-stimulating hormone (thyrotropin, TSH) concentration also may be low or normal. The nocturnal rise in serum TSH concentrations may be blunted, but usually the serum TSH response to thyrotropin-releasing hormone (TRH) is normal.[26] Among patients in intensive care units (ICUs), up to 70% have low $T_3$ syndrome and 22% have low $T_4$ syndrome.[27] Transient elevations in serum TSH concentrations precede the eventual normalization of serum $T_4$ concentrations during recovery from the critical illness.[28] These changes occur within hours. Declines in $T_4$ and $T_3$ levels are apparent within a few hours of injury[29] and become maximal within 4 days.[30] Reverse $T_3$ peaks at 12 hours after injury and returns to normal by 2 weeks.[31]

The magnitude of thyroid function changes in patients with critical illness varies with the severity of the illness. The degree of $T_3$ suppression with concomitantly low TSH correlates positively with the severity and duration of disease, and correlates negatively with outcome.[32] Decreased $T_4$ concentration correlates with increased mortality; total $T_4$ levels of <3 μg/dL have been associated with a mortality rate of up to 84%.[27] Nonetheless, administration of $T_4$ to critically ill patients with low serum $T_4$ concentrations is not beneficial (see Chap. 232).[33]

Several mechanisms may contribute to these changes. The 5'-monodeiodination decreases when caloric intake is low and/or in the presence of any degree of illness. High serum cortisol concentrations, circulating inhibitors of deiodinase activity, drugs that inhibit 5'-monodeiodinase activity, and cytokines (e.g., TNF-α and IL-6) have all been implicated. The serum $T_4$ levels become low because of variable reductions in the serum concentrations of thyroid hormone–binding proteins or the presence of circulating substances that inhibit $T_4$ binding to the binding proteins.

## GROWTH HORMONE

Growth hormone (GH) is elevated in most stress states (and also exhibits a reduced oscillatory activity), whereas insulin-like growth factor-I (IGF-I), IGF-binding protein-3 (IGFBP-3), and IGF-II levels are decreased.[34] The response of IGF-I to exogenous recombinant human GH (rhGH) is also attenuated. The serum IGF-I (as well as IGF-I messenger RNA) decreases, probably due to the uncoupling of the GH–IGF-I axis by inhibitory cytokines and the modulation of IGFBP-1 and IGF-I by catabolic hormones, primarily glucagon.[35] Thus, acute critical illness appears to be characterized by a *GH-resistant state.*

Minimal pain or discomfort results in a variable GH response.[36] Major trauma and surgery cause significant increases in GH levels that last for several hours; levels return to normal by the first postoperative day in most individuals.[36,37] The GH response to surgery is blocked with spinal or epidural anesthesia.[38] GH levels are markedly elevated with acute, severe illness, such as trauma with shock or sepsis.[39] Although hypoglycemia is a potent stimulator of GH secretion,[40] this may be a specific effect of the fall in glucose and not a nonspecific "stress" effect. In most individuals, acute exercise results in GH release in proportion to the degree of exertion.[41] A poor response to GH-releasing hormone (GHRH) correlates with mortality after severe head injury.[42]

GH, acting via IGF-I, is an anabolic hormone. It promotes protein synthesis (increasing nitrogen retention), decreases protein catabolism (decreasing urea nitrogen), and enhances fat mobilization. All of these actions are of potential benefit during acute catabolic stress. Physiologic levels of GH enhance lipolysis and ketonemia, but these actions are not apparent in the presence of physiologic levels of insulin.[43] GH has antiinsulin-like effects that may be relevant in critical illness; these effects decrease glucose uptake into some tissues.[44]

## PROLACTIN

Prolactin (PRL) has long been known to be one of the pituitary hormones released by stress.[36] The stress-induced rise in PRL generally consists of a doubling or tripling, which lasts <1 hour. Hypoglycemia is also a well-known stimulator of PRL release (at least doubling baseline levels); the maximum rise occurs between 40 and 90 minutes. PRL levels, which increase within 15 to 20 minutes after seizure, have been used to differentiate between epilepsy and pseudoseizures.[45]

The PRL effect is to promote lactation; however, its significance during critical illness may be related to its reported immune modulation.[1] In this regard, the use of dopamine infusion, common in the ICU, impacts negatively on circulating PRL levels.[46]

## SEX STEROIDS

In critically ill patients, sex steroids and gonadotropins show a rapid fall, regardless of the type of insult.[47,48] Most commonly, acutely critically ill patients exhibit evidence of hypogonadotropic hypogonadism, associated with an attenuated luteinizing hormone (LH) pulse.[49] LH and follicle-stimulating hormone (FSH) levels actually are appropriately elevated in only 31% of critically ill postmenopausal women and are in the hypogonadotropic range in 25%.[50] Furthermore, these patients have a blunted response to gonadotropin-releasing hormone (GnRH) stimulation; the low levels persist until clinical recovery.[51] CRH and cortisol impair reproductive function both peripherally and centrally,[52] and a correlation is seen between the suppression of the reproductive axis and the score on Acute Physiology and Chronic Health Evaluation II (APACHE II).[53] On admission to the ICU, testosterone levels are low; they decrease further in nonsurvivors but increase in survivors (Fig. 228-1).[54] Interestingly, estradiol levels may be elevated in men and postmenopausal women with critical illness.

Dehydroepiandrosterone sulfate (DHEAS) is abundantly secreted by the adrenal cortex; it is under pituitary control, possibly involving ACTH. The concentration of DHEAS decreases gradually with advancing age and acutely in severe illness.[47] This steroid, which is thought to be bioinactive, is peripherally converted into active dehydroepiandrosterone (DHEA), which is a weak androgen but a potent modulator of the immune response.[2] Both DHEA and DHEAS concentrations are consistently lower in patients experiencing severe illnesses,[47,55] and the DHEA response to ACTH administration is blunted,[12] possibly due to the altered adrenal steroidogenesis in critical illness.

## ARGININE VASOPRESSIN

Blood levels of arginine vasopressin (AVP), which is secreted primarily in response to hypovolemia and hyperosmolarity, are increased in response to stress. Many other stimuli exist for AVP

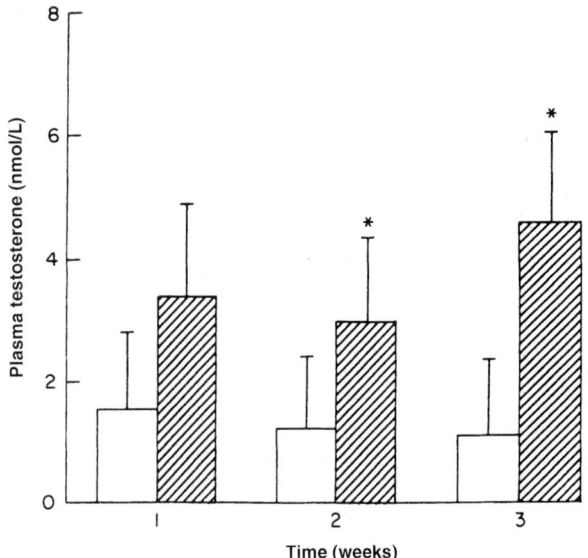

**FIGURE 228-1.** Mean testosterone levels of intensive care unit patients 3 weeks after admission (level in normal subjects, 12–40 nmol/L). *Unfilled bars* show values for survivors and *hatched bars* for nonsurvivors. *Asterisks* indicate a statistically significant difference between levels in survivors and nonsurvivors (p <.05). (From Dong Q, Hawker F, McWilliam D, et al. Circulating immunoreactive inhibin and testosterone levels in men with critical illness. Clin Endocrinol [Oxf] 1992; 36:399.)

release, however, including pain, nausea, head injury, epinephrine, cytokines (IL-1 and IL-6), and numerous drugs. AVP interacts with three receptors ($V_1$–$V_3$). Hypovolemia is the most potent stimulus for AVP secretion in the acute setting. Secreted AVP stimulates the renal $V_2$ receptor, resulting in the accumulation of cyclic adenosine monophosphate (cAMP). This induces antidiuresis. In contrast, stimulation of renal $V_1$ receptors results in the production of cyclic guanosine monophosphate and diuresis. AVP may be responsible for the hyponatremia frequently seen in postsurgical and critically ill patients. Apart from its known antidiuretic and vasopressor effects, AVP enhances ACTH release, potentiates CRH effects on ACTH secretion,[56] and increases glucose levels.[57]

The physiologic role of AVP in metabolism is uncertain. The hyperglycemic effect of AVP appears to be due both to increased glucagon secretion and to increased hepatic glucose production.

## RENIN AND ALDOSTERONE

In critical illness, hypotension and volume depletion activate the renin–angiotensin–aldosterone axis. In addition, hypersecretion of ACTH may produce secondary hyperaldosteronism, independent of volume status. Aldosterone increases within minutes of surgery and remains elevated for several days.[58] The magnitude and duration of the rise in aldosterone levels after injury are dependent on sodium intake. In some 20% of critically ill patients, renin and aldosterone production become dissociated, a condition termed *hyperreninemic hypoaldosteronism*. Because of increased renin levels, even "normal" aldosterone levels are inappropriate. This syndrome has been associated with an increased severity of the underlying disease and increased mortality.[59] It is also thought to be due to altered adrenal steroidogenesis.

## INSULIN AND GLUCAGON

In stress states, hyperglycemia is a strong stimulus for insulin release; however, the mildly elevated insulin level is inappropriate and probably reflects the dominant α-adrenergic inhibitory activity (i.e., a state of relative hypoinsulinism).[60] In heatstroke, trauma,[61] and burns,[62] the insulin levels are higher but are inappropriately low for the corresponding glucose levels.

Hyperglycemia inhibits glucagon secretion, whereas stress-associated increases in adrenergic stimulation, aminoacidemia, cortisol, and TNF-α augment glucagon release.[63] Glucagon levels are reported to be high in many stress situations (e.g., infections,[64] trauma,[61] hyperthermia,[65] hypoglycemia, burns, heatstroke, and myocardial infarction[66]). In the more severe cases, this vigorous response may be delayed up to 12 hours after trauma[67] and up to 1 to 3 days after burn injury.[68] The magnitude of glucagon increase in the survivors of heatstroke is proportional to the severity of illness (as judged from APACHE II score), an effect similar to that reported with burn size.[69] Although hyperglucagonemia has been postulated to be advantageous to survival in stress situations, this has never been demonstrated.[61] The issue deserves further scrutiny, because glucagon is a recognized antishock and inotropic hormone.[70]

## PARATHYROID HORMONE, VITAMIN D, AND MINERAL METABOLITES

Ionized hypocalcemia is common during critical illness,[71] particularly in patients with acute sepsis,[72] and is associated with increased mortality.[73] The multiple causes of hypocalcemia during critical illness relate to dietary vitamin D deficiency, failure to hydroxylate 25-hydroxyvitamin $D_3$, and cytokine effects. Because early studies failed to demonstrate increased serum parathyroid hormone (PTH) levels in critically ill patients, hypofunction of the parathyroid glands was postulated.[72,74–76] This view has been challenged by experimental data in acute pancreatitis,[77] however, and by clinical studies (using improved assays) that have demonstrated increases in serum PTH, which are related to the severity of disease and mortality.[78–82] In addition, the administration of parenteral parathyroid extract to hypocalcemic, critically ill patients increases levels of serum ionized calcium and urinary cAMP as in controls, indicating PTH-responsive target organs.[74,83] Thus, a suppression of parathyroid function or of hormone action cannot explain the ionized hypocalcemia found in critically ill patients. PTH secretion has been examined in patients with inflammation resulting from rheumatoid arthritis. The PTH response to lowering of calcium with EDTA is decreased from that of controls, implicating a suppressive effect of inflammation on the parathyroid glands.[84] IL-1 inhibits PTH secretion in bovine parathyroid cells in vitro[85] due to increased expression of the calcium-sensing receptor gene. Interestingly, PTH inhibits both B and T lymphocytes.[86,87]

Endotoxin administration in experimental sepsis decreases levels of circulating calcium; however, the cause is unclear in these animal models. Cytokines released during endotoxemia and infections (including calcitonin precursors)[88,88a] are implicated in the pathophysiology of the hypocalcemia. Furthermore, the extracellular hypocalcemia may be associated with intracellular hypercalcemia (see Chap. 232).

Cytokines play major roles in resorption (release of calcium) and formation of bone: TNF-α, IL-1, and IL-6 act synergistically to increase osteoclastic activity[89,90] and to stimulate bone calcium release. Both IL-6 and TNF-α correlate with markers of bone resorption in patients with hyperparathyroidism,[91,92] and IL-6 is thought to be a mediator of PTH, stimulating bone resorption.[93,94] TNF-α and IL-1 also down-regulate PTH receptors in osteoblasts,[95] decreasing their response to PTH and contributing to bone resorption. ICU care is associated with impaired nutrition and immobilization; this is of potential importance as a cause of clinical osteoporosis. Circulating alkaline phosphatase levels or cross-links in the urine as markers of bone resorption can be elevated, especially in prolonged critical illness.

The suggestion has been made that vitamin D modulates cytokine release. Administration of calcitriol to uremic patients increases IL-6 and IL-1 levels and reduces TNF-α levels, irrespective of PTH and calcium concentrations.[96]

Whether increased serum lactate levels influence ionized hypocalcemia in critically ill patients is controversial.[97,98] The prevalence and significance of hypomagnesemia or hypophosphatemia in critically ill patients are also unclear (see Chap. 232).

## METABOLIC MARKERS

The metabolic response to stress injury includes impaired carbohydrate metabolism, enhanced protein breakdown with a negative nitrogen balance, increased use of lipids as oxidative fuel, and increased energy expenditure.[99] The use of metabolic marker(s) to assess severity of illness is logical, because the response is the integration of multiple variables (i.e., hormones and other mediators) that may have synergistic or opposing effects on different tissues. The most commonly used markers are glucose and lactate.

Carbohydrate metabolism has been studied in various stress states.[100–103] In all of these cases, hepatic insulin resistance (i.e., increased hepatic glucose production) and peripheral insulin resistance (i.e., reduced glucose disposal) have been documented. Similar metabolic effects have been observed with combined infusion of catabolic hormones (i.e., cortisol, glucagon, and epinephrine) in normal subjects.[104] The combination of the increased hepatic glucose production with the decrease in glucose utilization results in *stress hyperglycemia*. The positive correlation between hyperglycemia and the severity of illness has been reported in association with surgery,[105] trauma,[106] the shock state,[107] stroke,[108] and myocardial infarction.[109] In myocardial infarction,[109,110] in stroke,[111] and in severe head injury,[112] the presence of hyperglycemia (in the nondiabetic patient) predicts a worse outcome. In patients experiencing cardiac arrest, higher blood glucose levels have been detected in those in whom resuscitation was delayed or prolonged.[113] Therefore, in at least some stress conditions, hyperglycemia may be a predictor of a poor outcome.

Hypoglycemia in nondiabetic patients is most frequently encountered in critical illness in the setting of acute adrenal, pituitary, renal, or hepatic failure, or severe sepsis. The hypoglycemia is most likely due to a substrate limitation of gluconeogenesis and inadequate glycogenolysis.[114] In addition, peripheral glucose uptake is enhanced in the hypermetabolic septic state.[115]

Serum IGFBP-1 also appears to predict outcome in prolonged critical illness. This small IGFBP produced in the liver is distinct from other IGFBPs in that it is acutely regulated by metabolic stimuli.[116] Insulin is inhibitory, whereas hepatic substrate deprivation and hypoxia are stimulatory, in the regulation of IGFBP-1.[117,117a] Moreover, an inverse correlation is seen between IGFBP-1 and IGF-I and the GH-dependent IGFBP-3 and acid-labile subunit (ALS) in critical illness, which is consistent with the inverse regulation of IGFBP-1 by GH.[118] The higher IGFBP-1 levels that have been observed in those who do not survive prolonged illness coincide with lower insulin concentrations, despite the fact that glucose levels are similar to those in survivors. (Because those who do not survive are thought to be more insulin resistant, even insulin secretion may be impaired in patients in the ICU for long periods.) In adverse metabolic conditions, the hepatocyte alters its production of IGFBPs, suppressing IGF-I and ALS while stimulating the production of IGFBP-1. This may occur via increased levels of hepatocyte cAMP and/or via changes in the

**TABLE 228-1.**
**Human Acute-Phase Proteins**

**PROTEINS WHOSE PLASMA CONCENTRATIONS INCREASE**

*Complement system*
  Factor B
  Cl inhibitor
  C4b-binding protein
  Mannose-binding lectin

*Coagulation and fibrinolytic system*
  Fibrinogen
  Plasminogen
  Tissue plasminogen activator
  Urokinase
  Protein S
  Vitronectin
  Plasminogen activator inhibitor-1

*Antiproteases*
  $\alpha_1$-Protease inhibitor
  $\alpha_1$-Antichymotrypsin
  Pancreatic secretory trypsin inhibitor
  Inter-$\alpha$-trypsin inhibitors

*Transport proteins*
  Ceruloplasmin
  Haptoglobin
  Hemopexin

*Participants in inflammatory responses*
  Secreted phospholipase $A_2$
  Lipopolysaccharide-binding protein
  Interleukin-1–receptor antagonist
  Granulocyte colony-stimulating factor

*Others*
  C-reactive protein
  Serum amyloid A
  $\alpha_1$-Acid glycoprotein
  Fibronectin
  Ferritin
  Angiotensinogen

**PROTEINS WHOSE PLASMA CONCENTRATIONS DECREASE**

  Albumin
  Transferrin
  Transthyretin
  $\alpha_2$-HS glycoprotein
  Alpha-fetoprotein
  Thyroxine-binding globulin
  Insulin-like growth factor I
  Factor XII

$\alpha_2$-HS, $\alpha_2$-Heremans Semid-glycoprotein.
(Adapted from Gabay C, Kushner I. Acute-phase proteins and other systemic responses to inflammation [published erratum in N Engl J Med 1999 340:1376]. N Engl J Med 1999; 340:448.)

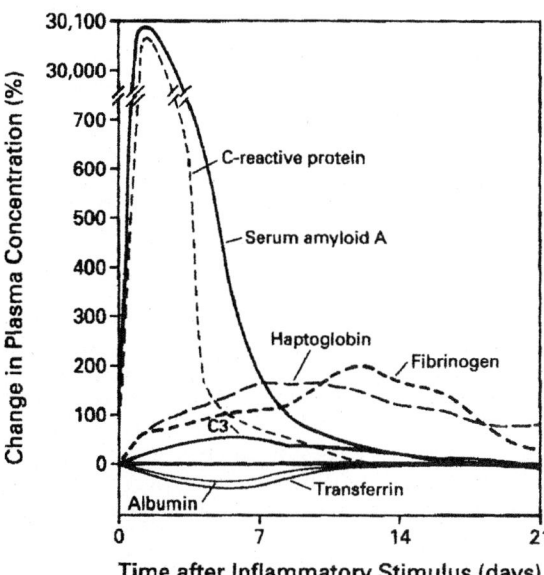

**FIGURE 228-2.** Secretion and time course of several acute-phase proteins after an inflammatory stimulus. (*C3*, complement 3.) (From Gabay C, Kushner I. Acute-phase proteins and other systemic responses to inflammation [published erratum in N Engl J Med 1999 340:1376]. N Engl J Med 1999; 340:448.)

patients, serial determinations of blood lactate levels are predictors of the development of multiple organ failure and death.[124] In this respect, the duration of lactic acidosis is important.[124,125]

The systemic response to inflammation includes changes in the concentrations of a variety of plasma proteins known as the *acute-phase proteins* (APPs; Table 228-1).[126] The concentration of some APPs (e.g., C-reactive protein) increases, whereas that of others (e.g., albumin, transferrin, and lipoproteins) decreases. These changes largely reflect hepatic production. Many of the endocrine mediators of critical illness, chief among them cytokines such as IL-6, mediate these changes. The magnitude of change varies depending on the individual protein under examination and the condition causing the changes (Fig. 228-2). The role of APPs such as C-reactive protein may involve modulation of the inflammatory response.[126]

## ENDOCRINE MEDIATORS

Many, if not most, of the clinical, metabolic, and humoral changes associated with critical illness stem from the unleashing of an uncontrolled inflammatory response. The recognition that critical illness leads to similar inflammatory responses, irrespective of the nature of the insult, has led to a better understanding of its pathogenesis. The characterization of the roles of causative mediators (e.g., cytokines and hormones; see Chap. 227) is important not only for prognostication and illness severity assessment, but also for the development of novel therapeutic approaches.

The identification of any single humoral factor or combination of factors as a mediator is a challenging task, and new mediators are continually being identified. The mediators can be local and/or general. They include leukocyte products, vascular products, local tissue factors, and products originating from diverse (parenchymal) sources. All of these products have been investigated, individually and in combination, in a variety of critical illnesses. In general, the magnitude of the rise in these mediators correlates with the severity of illness. Moreover, some of them have been found to be predictive of outcome.

pulsatility of GH.[119] Furthermore, IGFBP-1 expression is influenced by nitric oxide via its effects on oxygen sensing.[119a]

Lactate is the consequence of anaerobic metabolism, resulting from the relative tissue hypoxia or hypoperfusion; therefore, its measurement is used to assess the severity of the critical illness. Considerable evidence supports an inverse relationship between hyperlactatemia and survival. Several clinical studies have correlated blood lactate levels to the mortality rate in septic shock, as in other forms of circulatory shock.[120–122] Other studies have related blood lactate levels to the development of organ failure and mortality after severe trauma.[123] Furthermore, in septic shock

## LEUKOCYTE PRODUCTS

Several studies have demonstrated leukocyte activation with the release of mediators (sometimes toxic) in trauma and sepsis. Neutrophils are the fastest in responding to the inflammation. Activation of neutrophils occurs via endotoxins, complements, cytokines (IL-1, IL-8, and TNF-α), and other inflammatory mediators.[127,128] The level of elastase, a proteinase derived from activated neutrophils, is a convenient measure of their activation. In critically ill patients, significantly elevated elastase levels are predictive of multiple organ failure and are predictive of mortality in polytrauma.[127,129] The elevated elastase levels also correlate well with the severity of illness.[127,129]

The functions of leukocytes are altered after infection and injury (e.g., chemotaxis, adhesion, and phagocytosis).[130] Alteration in neutrophil function has been associated with adult respiratory distress syndrome (ARDS) and systemic inflammatory response syndrome (SIRS).[130,131] Neutrophils play a significant role in the tissue destruction associated with inflammation.[132]

## VASCULAR PRODUCTS

The endothelium is an active endocrine organ with hemocrine and paracrine properties. It is also an active transfer system between the blood, cellular, and fluid compartments.

**Nitric Oxide.** Endothelium-derived vasoactive factors include the endothelium-derived relaxing factor, nitric oxide (NO),[133] and the endothelins, which have potent vasoconstriction properties.[134] NO is rapidly produced from L-arginine by NO synthase, which occurs in three different isoforms (see Chap. 179). NO, a potent vasodilator, has been implicated in platelet and neutrophil inhibition, neurotransmission, and immune modulation.[135] NO also decreases endothelin levels. It has been reported to be high in cases of burn injury,[136] sepsis,[137] and heatstroke.[135] In heatstroke, the excessive NO production is proportional to the severity of illness.[135] The NO increase in critical illness is thought to be due to increased NO formation caused by the inducible form of NO synthase, which is under the influence of various proinflammatory cytokines. The serum NO level has been used as a predictor of postoperative morbidity.[138] NO excess is thought to be responsible, at least in part, for the hypotension seen in septic patients.[139]

**Endothelin-1.** Endothelin-1, a very potent vasoconstrictor produced by the action of endothelin-converting enzyme on big endothelin-1 (see Chap. 179), stimulates the production of endothelial NO. Endothelin is elevated in sepsis[140] and heatstroke.[141]

Under normal conditions, NO action plays a dominant role in the basal regulation of blood pressure, whereas endothelin has a minor influence. In several disease states, including critical illness, the levels of both endothelin-1 and NO are elevated, and the new balance of these opposing forces determines the outcome in a process that is still poorly understood.[142]

**Adhesion Molecules.** During the inflammatory response, up-regulated endothelial cell–surface receptors (known as "adhesion molecules") interact with circulatory leukocytes. This interaction mediates the participation of the leukocytes in the inflammatory response and their subsequent infiltration into damaged tissue. Endothelial activation/dysfunction is commonly identified as an important step in the progression of any critical illness that leads to multiple organ failure. Many different mediators and cytokines induce the expression of adhesion molecules. Soluble forms of these adhesion molecules have been found in sera of patients with various conditions.[143] Four families of adhesion molecules are found. The *immunoglobulin superfamily* (e.g., the vascular cell adhesion molecule [VCAM] and intercellular adhesion molecule [ICAM]), the *integrin family*, the *selectins*, and the *cadherins*.[143]

All adhesion molecules (ICAM, VCAM, and, most notably, E-selectin) increase in critical illness, and the concentration increases further with the onset of organ dysfunction and failure.[144] The plasma concentrations of these molecules are markedly higher in nonsurviving than in surviving critically ill patients.[145] The significance of this rise is unknown, but it probably reflects the severity of the endothelial dysfunction rather than a direct contribution to multiple organ failure.

**Complement.** The complement system is composed of a cascade of proteins that mediate inflammation and promote the phagocytosis of microorganisms. The system can be activated by antibody-antigen binding (classic pathway) or by multiple other substances (the alternative pathway). Endothelial damage can activate the system.[146]

Activation of the complement cascade has been documented in various critical illnesses, including trauma, sepsis, and burns.[131,147,148] In trauma, C3a/C3 increases with illness severity as evidenced by a positive correlation with APACHE II score. In addition, the level of C3a/C3 is significantly higher in nonsurvivors than in survivors.[127]

**Kinins.** Kinins arise from the action of enzymes (the kallikreins) on kininogens to liberate the kinins, bradykinin, and kallidin (see Chap. 170). The kinins are associated with vasodilation, vascular leakage, and the release of cytokines, eicosanoids, and NO during SIRS. The kinins, which are produced during the early phases of inflammation, have been assigned a mediator role in septic states.

**Coagulation Factors.** Inflammation promotes coagulation, including down-regulation of the anticoagulant protein C. Activated protein C interacts with protein S, which by inactivating factors Va and VIIIa dampens thrombin formation. Importantly, the degree to which protein C is decreased in sepsis is predictive of adverse outcome.[149] Studies in meningococcal sepsis, for example, suggest that replacement of protein C may be beneficial.[150]

## OXYGEN FREE RADICALS

Oxygen free radicals are formed from various sources, including catecholamine oxidation, neutrophils, and the xanthine-xanthine oxidase system.[151,152] Numerous studies have unequivocally demonstrated a role for various oxygen free radicals in the pathogenesis of sepsis and other critical illnesses.[153] Levels of antioxidant vitamins (oxygen free radical scavengers) are lower in septic patients with multiple organ failure than in septic patients without such failure.[154,155]

In various clinical trials and experimental models, the use of antioxidants has usually, but not always, improved outcome as measured by improved neutrophil function, reduced tissue injury, and improved survival.[156]

Oxygen free radicals contribute to the cellular toxicity associated with severe illness. This is manifested by increased membrane permeability, intracellular overload, capillary leak, and vascular tone alterations.[153]

## PRODUCTS FROM DIVERSE CELLULAR SOURCES

**Cytokines.** Cytokines are a ubiquitous group of peptide mediators produced by leukocytes, endothelial cells, epithelial cells, macrophages, and many other cells (see Chaps. 173, 174, and 227). Of particular importance with regard to the stress response and SIRS are proinflammatory cytokines, such as TNF-α, IL-1, and IL-6. These cytokines are elevated in infections,[157] trauma,[158] surgery,[159] and burns.[160] The circulating levels of these cytokines (e.g., TNF-α and IL-1) may not necessarily correlate with the severity of illness,[161,162] because circulating inhibitors exist, and cytokines often act via paracrine means. Unlike TNF-α and IL-1, IL-6 exhibits consistently high levels that correlate positively with illness severity (Fig. 228-3). Furthermore, higher levels predict worse outcome.[162] In patients with the sepsis syndrome, blood levels of IL-8 correlate positively with the levels of IL-6; however, the IL-8 rise is transient and levels decrease regardless of outcome.[163] Only in septic shock do IL-8 levels correlate with fatal outcome and multiple organ failure.[164]

The importance of the bioeffects of cytokines in mediating the stress response is illustrated by reports that administration of TNF-α to healthy individuals causes hemodynamic and metabolic changes similar to the abnormalities that occur in sepsis.[165] The metabolic and hemodynamic consequences of cytokines have been investigated in many animal models with similar results. TNF-α causes hyperglycemia and insulin resistance,[166,167] whereas IL-1 and IL-6 seem to have similar effects in blocking insulin signal transduction.[168]

**Eicosanoids.**    Arachidonic acid is released from the cell membrane after any significant traumatic or septic event. The metabolism of arachidonic acid results in production of prostaglandin via the cyclooxygenase pathway or of leukotrienes via the lipoxygenase pathway (see Chap. 172). Arachidonic acid metabolites are involved in both the early and the late responses to thermal injury.[169] The vasodilator prostaglandin $I_2$ ($PGI_2$) and the vasoconstrictor thromboxane $A_2$ ($TXA_2$) are elevated in the plasma of burn victims.[170] $TXA_2$ and/or $PGI_2$ may affect blood flow and distribution in sepsis.[170] In trauma patients, prostaglandin $E_2$ and leukotrienes are significantly elevated.[171] The use of cyclooxygenase inhibitors in critically ill patients has produced mixed results,[152,172] possibly because of marked effects not only on cyclooxygenase but also on the neutrophil accumulation at the site of inflammation.[173]

**Calcitonin Precursors.**    In critically ill patients (e.g., those with sepsis, burns, pneumonitis, heatstroke, multitrauma, etc.), levels of calcitonin precursors (CTpr), including procalcitonin (ProCT), typically are very markedly elevated (sometimes up to thousands of times) and correlate significantly with the outcome (Fig. 228-3).[174,175] In contrast, mature calcitonin remains in the normal range or is only slightly elevated.[174] Intravenous injection of endotoxin from *Escherichia coli* into normal humans[88] produces a prolonged decrease in the total serum calcium concentration that parallels the increase in CTpr (which peaks at 6–8 hours, maintains a plateau for 24 hours, and remains elevated for a prolonged period). Importantly, the hypocalcemia persists even after the normalization of TNF-α and IL-6 concentrations,[88] possibly suggesting a continued hypocalcemic effect of the persistently elevated CTpr. Other studies have uncovered a potential role of Ctpr as a toxic mediator: infusion of ProCT in experimental sepsis increases mortality, whereas infusion of ProCT-reactive antiserum enhances survival.[176] These studies suggest a novel, specific mechanism of host response to a microbial infection that challenges the current physiologic paradigm of the *CALC-I* gene (see Chap. 53). In the absence of infection, the transcription of the *CALC-I* gene is suppressed and largely restricted to a selective expression in the neuroendocrine cells found mainly in the thyroid and the lung. In these neuroendocrine cells, the mature, yet relatively inactive, hormone is processed and stored in secretory granules.[177] A microbial infection induces an ubiquitous, yet very specific, increase of *CALC-I* gene transcription and translation, and a release of CTpr into the circulation by virtually all tissues and cell types throughout the body.[178] Thus, the transcriptional regulation of the *CALC-I*

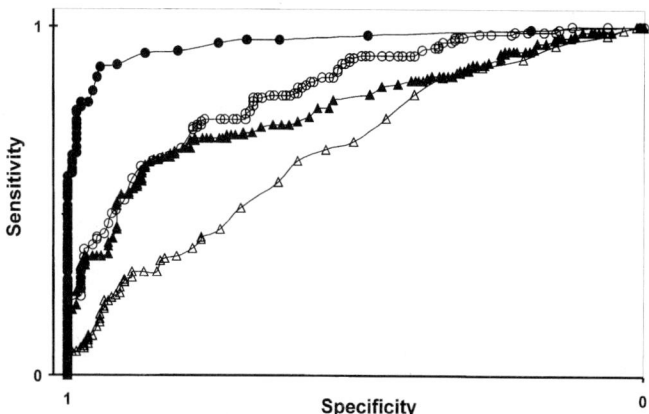

**FIGURE 228-3.** Sensitivity and specificity (i.e., receiver operating curve) of several markers for the severity of systemic inflammation in intensive care unit patients. Daily values of calcitonin precursors (*filled circles*), interleukin-6 (*closed triangles*), C-reactive protein (*open circles*), and lactate (*open triangles*) are shown for patients with the diagnoses of sepsis, severe sepsis, or septic shock. Near-optimal sensitivity and specificity is achieved by calcitonin precursor measurement, whereas lactate levels are equivalent to random correlation.

gene in sepsis appears to be stimulus related, rather than tissue specific. This increased transcription and translation is mediated by as yet unknown factors and might be induced either directly via microbial toxins or indirectly via a humoral or cell-mediated host response. The predominance of prohormonal CTpr indicates a constitutive pathway in cells lacking secretion granules and, hence, a bypassing of much of the enzymatic processing.[179,180] This dually regulated transcriptional activity of the *CALC-I* gene to yield either endocrine or cytokine-like products may be the prototype of a novel class of "hormokine" mediators.

**Cellular Stress Products: Heat Shock Proteins.**    Individual cells exposed to stress express genes encoding a group of proteins referred to as the *heat shock proteins (HSPs)*. (The original stimulus used was heat, hence the name.) Exposure to heavy metals, metabolic poisons, hypoxia, hypoglycemia, and various in vivo insults (e.g., ischemia/perfusion) also increase the expression of HSPs.[181] This response seems to be universally conserved in cells from all organisms studied. Most of these proteins are expressed constitutively at low levels in normal cells, where they function to facilitate many aspects of protein maturation and to interact as *"molecular chaperones."* The increase in stress protein expression occurring after a cellular exposure to insult confers added protection to the cell against future insults from unrelated stressors.[181,182] Of particular interest is the demonstration that the deliberate induction of the stress protein response by hyperthermia or the administration of sodium arsenite has a protective effect against subsequent experimental sepsis.[183,184] The clinical importance of the stress proteins is apparent in their response to infectious agents, toxins, vaccines, and cancer. Stress proteins are expressed locally in the intact animal in response to injury[185,186] and more diffusely in response to a generalized stress such as heat.[187] The homeostatic role of stress protein expression in response to surgical stress in animals and its modulation by stress hormones is currently being investigated.[188,189] The direct effects of HSPs on stress are still being sought experimentally,[190] specifically in relation to their protective effects against the toxicity and cell death that are mediated by the inflammatory reaction products.

TABLE 228-2.
**Additional Candidate Markers and Mediators of Critical Illness**

| Putative Marker/<br>Mediator | Changes | References |
|---|---|---|
| Adrenomedullin | ↑ | 191 |
| ANH | ↓ (mechanical ventilation with high PEEP)<br>or | 192 |
| | ↑ with MI | 193 |
| Endorphins | ↑ | 194 |
| Histamine | ↑ | 195, 196 |
| HMG-1 | ↑ | 197 |
| Kinin | ↑ | 198 |
| Leptin | ↑ | 199 |
| MIF | ↑ | 200 |
| NPY | ↑ | 201 |
| PAF | ↑ | 202, 203 |
| Serotonin | ↑ | 204 |
| VIP | ↑ | 205 |

*ANH*, atrial natriuretic hormone; *PEEP*, positive end-expiratory pressure; *MI*, myocardial infarction; *HMG-1*, high mobility group-1; *MIF*, macrophage migration inhibitory factor; *VIP*, vasoactive intestinal polypeptide; *NPY*, neural peptide Y; *PAF*, platelet-activating factor.

## ADDITIONAL CANDIDATE MARKERS AND MEDIATORS OF CRITICAL ILLNESS

Although many other hormones and humoral factors have been studied in relation to critical illness, no data are available regarding their roles as markers or mediators. The relationship between the changes in these hormones/factors and the severity or outcome of critical illnesses have yet to be established (Table 228-2).

## REFERENCES

1. Munck A, Guyre PM, Holbrook NJ. Physiological functions of glucocorticoids in stress and their relation to pharmacological actions. Endocr Rev 1984; 5:25.
2. Reichlin S. Neuroendocrine-immune interactions. N Engl J Med 1993; 329:1246.
3. Besedovsky HO, del Rey A. Immune-neuroendocrine circuits: integrative role of cytokines. Front Neuroendocrinol 1992; 13:61.
4. Ingle DJ. Permissibility of hormone action: a review. Acta Endocrinol (Copenh) 1954; 17:172.
5. Ganong WF. The stress response—a dynamic overview. Hosp Pract 1988; 23:155.
6. Hume DM, Bell CC, Bartter F. Direct measurement of adrenal secretion during operative trauma and convalescence. Surgery 1962; 52:174.
7. Chernow B, Alexander HR, Smallridge RC, et al. Hormonal responses to graded surgical stress. Arch Intern Med 1987; 147:1273.
8. Raff H, Norton AJ, Flemma RJ, Findling JW. Inhibition of the adrenocorticotropin response to surgery in humans: interaction between dexamethasone and fentanyl. J Clin Endocrinol Metab 1987; 65:295.
9. Udelsman R, Norton JA, Jelenich SE, et al. Responses of the hypothalamic-pituitary-adrenal and renin-angiotensin axes and the sympathetic system during controlled surgical and anesthetic stress. J Clin Endocrinol Metab 1987; 64:986.
10. Engquist A, Brandt MR, Fernandes A, Kehlet H. The blocking effect of epidural analgesia on the adrenocortical and hyperglycemic responses to surgery. Acta Anaesthesiol Scand 1977; 21:330.
11. Siegel RA, Grinspoon SK, Garvey GJ, Bilezikian JP. Sepsis and adrenal function. Trends Endocrinol Metab 1994; 5:324.
12. Parker LN, Levin ER, Lifrak ET. Evidence for adrenocortical adaptation to severe illness. J Clin Endocrinol Metab 1985; 60:947.
13. Span LF, Hermus AR, Bartelink AK, et al. Adrenocortical function: an indicator of severity of disease and survival in chronic critically ill patients. Intensive Care Med 1992; 18:93.
14. Woolf PD. Hormonal responses to trauma. Crit Care Med 1992; 20:216.
15. McKay LI, Cidlowski JA. Molecular control of immune/inflammatory responses: interactions between nuclear factor-kappa B and steroid receptor-signaling pathways. Endocr Rev 1999; 20:435.
16. Sapolsky RM, Romero LM, Munck AU. How do glucocorticoids influence stress responses? Integrating permissive, suppressive, stimulatory, and preparative actions. Endocr Rev 2000; 21:55.
17. Engquist A, Fog-Moller F, Christiansen C, et al. Influence of epidural analgesia on the catecholamine and cyclic AMP responses to surgery. Acta Anaesthesiol Scand 1980; 24:17.
18. Frayn KN, Little RA, Maycock PF, Stoner HB. The relationship of plasma catecholamines to acute metabolic and hormonal responses to injury in man. Circ Shock 1985; 16:229.
19. Wortsman J, Frank S, Cryer PE. Adrenomedullary response to maximal stress in humans. Am J Med 1984; 77:779.
20. Axelrod J, Reisine TD. Stress hormones: their interaction and regulation. Science 1984; 224:452.
21. Cryer PE. Physiology and pathophysiology of the human sympathoadrenal neuroendocrine system. N Engl J Med 1980; 303:436.
22. Deibert DC, DeFronzo RA. Epinephrine-induced insulin resistance in man. J Clin Invest 1980; 65:717.
23. Van der Poll T, Romijn JA, Endert E, et al. Tumor necrosis factor mimics the metabolic response to acute infection in healthy humans. Am J Physiol 1991; 261:E457.
24. Van der Poll T, Jansen J, Endert E, et al. Noradrenaline inhibits lipopolysaccharide-induced tumor necrosis factor and interleukin 6 production in human whole blood. Infect Immun 1994; 62:2046.
25. Wartofsky L, Burman KD. Alterations in thyroid function in patients with systemic illness: the "euthyroid sick syndrome." Endocr Rev 1982; 3:164.
26. Romijn JA, Wiersinga WM. Decreased nocturnal surge of thyrotropin in nonthyroidal illness. J Clin Endocrinol Metab 1990; 70:35.
27. Slag MF, Morley JE, Elson MK, et al. Hypothyroxinemia in critically ill patients as a predictor of high mortality. JAMA 1981; 245:43.
28. Hamblin PS, Dyer SA, Mohr VS, et al. Relationship between thyrotropin and thyroxine changes during recovery from severe hypothyroxinemia of critical illness. J Clin Endocrinol Metab 1986; 62:717.
29. Woolf PD, Lee LA, Hamill RW, McDonald JV. Thyroid test abnormalities in traumatic brain injury: correlation with neurologic impairment and sympathetic nervous system activation. Am J Med 1988; 84:201.
30. Ziegler MG, Morrissey EC, Marshall LF. Catecholamine and thyroid hormones in traumatic injury. Crit Care Med 1990; 18:253.
31. Phillips RH, Valente WA, Caplan ES, et al. Circulating thyroid hormone changes in acute trauma: prognostic implications for clinical outcome. J Trauma 1984; 24:116.
32. Rothwell PM, Lawler PG. Prediction of outcome in intensive care patients using endocrine parameters. Crit Care Med 1995; 23:78.
33. Brent GA, Hershman JM. Thyroxine therapy in patients with severe nonthyroidal illnesses and low serum thyroxine concentration. J Clin Endocrinol Metab 1986; 63:1.
34. Ross R, Miell J, Freeman E, et al. Critically ill patients have high basal growth hormone levels with attenuated oscillatory activity associated with low levels of insulin-like growth factor-I. Clin Endocrinol (Oxf) 1991; 35:47.
35. Nygren J, Sammann M, Malm M, et al. Distributed anabolic hormonal patterns in burned patients: the relation to glucagon. Clin Endocrinol (Oxf) 1995; 43:491.
36. Noel GL, Suh HK, Stone JG, Frantz AG. Human prolactin and growth hormone release during surgery and other conditions of stress. J Clin Endocrinol Metab 1972; 35:840.
37. Newsome HH, Rose JC. The response of human adrenocorticotrophic hormone and growth hormone to surgical stress. J Clin Endocrinol Metab 1971; 33:481.
38. Hagen C, Brandt MR, Kehlet H. Prolactin, LH, FSH, GH and cortisol response to surgery and the effect of epidural analgesia. Acta Endocrinologica 1980; 94:151.
39. Carey LC, Cloutier CT, Lowery BD. Growth hormone and adrenal cortical response to shock and trauma in the human. Ann Surg 1971; 174:451.
40. Fish HR, Chernow B, O'Brian JT. Endocrine and neurophysiologic responses of the pituitary to insulin-induced hypoglycemia: a review. Metabolism 1986; 35:763.
41. Lin T, Tucci JR. Provocative tests of growth-hormone release. A comparison of results with seven stimuli. Ann Intern Med 1974; 80:464.
42. Gottardis M, Nigitsch C, Schmutzhard E, et al. The secretion of human growth hormone stimulated by human growth hormone releasing factor following severe cranio-cerebral trauma. Intensive Care Med 1990; 16:163.
43. Gerich JE, Lorenzi M, Bier DM, et al. Effects of physiologic levels of glucagon and growth hormone on human carbohydrate and lipid metabolism. Studies involving administration of exogenous hormone during suppression of endogenous hormone secretion with somatostatin. J Clin Invest 1976; 57:875.
44. Davidson MB. Effect of growth hormone on carbohydrate and lipid metabolism. Endocr Rev 1987; 8:115.
45. Pritchard PB 3d, Wannamaker BB, Sagel J, Daniel CM. Serum prolactin and cortisol levels in evaluation of pseudoepileptic seizures. Ann Neurol 1985; 18:87.
46. Van den Berghe G, de Zegher F. Anterior pituitary function during critical illness and dopamine treatment. Crit Care Med 1996; 24:1580.
47. Lephart ED, Baxter CR, Parker CR Jr. Effect of burn trauma on adrenal and testicular steroid hormone production. J Clin Endocrinol Metab 1987; 64:842.
48. Woolf PD, Hamill RW, McDonald JV, et al. Transient hypogonadotropic hypogonadism caused by critical illness. J Clin Endocrinol Metab 1985; 60:444.

49. Van den Berghe G, de Zegher F, Lauwers P, Veldhuis JD. Luteinizing hormone secretion and hypoandrogenaemia in critically ill men: effect of dopamine. Clin Endocrinol (Oxf) 1994; 41:563.

50. Gebhart SS, Watts NB, Clark RV, et al. Reversible impairment of gonadotropin secretion in critical illness. Observations in postmenopausal women. Arch Intern Med 1989; 149:1637.

51. Dolecek R, Dvoracek C, Jezek M, et al. Very low serum testosterone levels and severe impairment of spermatogenesis in burned male patients. Correlations with basal levels and levels of FSH, LH and PRL after LHRH + TRH. Endocrinol Exp 1983; 17:33.

52. Rivier C, Rivest S. Effect of stress on the activity of the hypothalamic-pituitary-gonadal axis: peripheral and central mechanisms. Biol Reprod 1991; 45:523.

53. Spratt DI, Cox P, Orav J, et al. Reproductive axis suppression in acute illness is related to disease severity. J Clin Endocrinol Metab 1993; 76:1548.

54. Dong Q, Hawker F, McWilliam D, et al. Circulating immunoreactive inhibin and testosterone levels in men with critical illness. Clin Endocrinol (Oxf) 1992; 36:399.

55. Wade CE, Lindberg JS, Cockrell JL, et al. Upon-admission adrenal steroidogenesis is adapted to the degree of illness in intensive care unit patients. J Clin Endocrinol Metab 1988; 67:223.

56. Plotsky PM, Bruhn TO, Vale W. Central modulation of immunoreactive corticotropin-releasing factor secretion by arginine vasopressin. Endocrinology 1984; 115:1639.

57. Spruce BA, McCulloch AJ, Burd J, et al. The effect of vasopressin infusion on glucose metabolism in man. Clin Endocrinol (Oxf) 1985; 22:463.

58. Le Quesne LP, Cochrane JP, Fieldman NR. Fluid and electrolyte disturbances after trauma: the role of adrenocortical and pituitary hormones. Br Med Bull 1985; 41:212.

59. Rolih CA, Ober KP. The endocrine response to critical illness. Med Clin North Am 1995; 79:211.

60. Halter JB, Beard JC, Porte D Jr. Islet function and stress hyperglycemia: plasma glucose and epinephrine interaction. Am J Physiol 1984; 247:E47.

61. Lindsey A, Santeusanio F, Braaten J, et al. Pancreatic alpha-cell function in trauma. JAMA 1974; 227:757.

62. Jahoor F, Herndon DN, Wolfe RR. Role of insulin and glucagon in the response of glucose and alanine kinetics in burn-injured patients. J Clin Invest 1986; 78:807.

63. Rorsman P, Ashcroft FM, Berggren PO. Regulation of glucagon release from pancreatic A-cells. Biochem Pharmacol 1991; 41:1783.

64. Rocha DM, Santeusanio F, Faloona GR, Unger RH. Abnormal pancreatic alpha-cell function in bacterial infections. N Engl J Med 1973; 288:700.

65. Tatar P, Vigas M, Jurcovicova J, et al. Increased glucagon secretion during hyperthermia in a sauna. Eur J Appl Physiol 1986; 55:315.

66. Willerson JT, Hutcheson DR, Leshin SJ, et al. Serum glucagon and insulin levels and their relationship to blood glucose values in patients with acute myocardial infarction and acute coronary insufficiency. Am J Med 1974; 57:747.

67. Meguid MM, Brennan MF, Aoki TT, et al. Hormone-substrate interrelationships following trauma. Arch Surg 1974; 109:776.

68. Shuck JM, Eaton P, Shuck LW, et al. Dynamics of insulin and glucagon secretions in severely burned patients. J Trauma 1977; 17:706.

69. Vaughan GM, Becker RA, Unger RH, et al. Nonthyroidal control of metabolism after burn injury: possible role of glucagon. Metabolism 1985; 34:637.

70. Pollack CV Jr. Utility of glucagon in the emergency department. J Emerg Med 1993; 11:195.

71. Zaloga GP, Malcolm D, Chernow B, Holaday J. Endotoxin induced hypocalcemia results in defective calcium mobilization in rats. Circ Shock 1988; 24:143.

72. Taylor B, Sibbald WJ, Edmonds MW, et al. Ionized hypocalcemia in critically ill patients with sepsis. Can J Surg 1978; 21:429.

73. Desai TK, Carlson RW, Geheb MA. Prevalence and clinical implications of hypocalcemia in acutely ill patients in a medical intensive care setting. Am J Med 1988; 84:209.

74. Robertson GM Jr, Moore EW, Switz DM, et al. Inadequate parathyroid response in acute pancreatitis. N Engl J Med 1976; 294:512.

75. Weir GC, Lesser PB, Drop LJ, et al. The hypocalcemia of acute pancreatitis. Ann Intern Med 1975; 83:185.

76. Zaloga GP, Chernow B. The multifactorial basis for hypocalcemia during sepsis. Studies of the parathyroid hormone vitamin D axis. Ann Intern Med 1987; 107:36.

77. Izquierdo R, Bermes E Jr, Sandberg L, et al. Serum calcium metabolism in acute experimental pancreatitis. Surgery 1985; 98:1031.

78. Burchard KW, Gann DS, Colliton J, Forster J. Ionized calcium, parathormone, and mortality in critically ill surgical patients. Ann Surg 1990; 212:543.

79. Burchard KW, Simms HH, Robinson A, et al. Hypocalcemia during sepsis. Relationship to resuscitation and hemodynamics. Arch Surg 1992; 127:265.

80. McKay C, Beastall GH, Imrie CW, Baxter JN. Circulating intact parathyroid hormone levels in acute pancreatitis. Br J Surg 1994; 81:357.

81. Carlstedt F, Lind L, Rastad J, et al. Parathyroid hormone and ionized calcium levels are related to the severity of illness and survival in critically ill patients. Eur J Clin Invest 1998; 28:898.

82. Carlstedt F, Lind L, Wide L, et al. Serum levels of parathyroid hormone are related to the mortality and severity of illness in patients in the emergency department. Eur J Clin Invest 1997; 27:977.

83. Sibbald WJ, Sardesai V, Wilson RF. Hypocalcemia and nephrogenous cyclic AMP production in critically ill or injured patients. J Trauma 1977; 17:677.

84. Af Ekenstam E, Benson L, Hallgren R, et al. Impaired secretion of parathyroid hormone in patients with rheumatoid arthritis: relationship to inflammatory activity. Clin Endocrinol (Oxf) 1990; 32:323.

85. Nielsen P, Rasmussen A, Butters R, et al. Inhibition of PTH secretion by interleukin-1 beta in bovine parathyroid glands in vitro is associated with an up-regulation of the calcium-sensing receptor mRNA. Biochem Biophys Res Commun 1997; 238:880.

86. Jiang Y, Yoshida A, Ishioka C, et al. Parathyroid hormone inhibits immunoglobulin production without affecting cell growth in B cells. Clin Immunol Immunopathol 1992; 65:286.

87. Klinger M, Alexiewicz JM, Linker IM, et al. Effect of parathyroid hormone on human T cell activation. Kidney Int 1990; 37:1543.

88. Dandona P, Nix D, Wilson MF, et al. Procalcitonin increase after endotoxin injection in normal subjects. J Clin Endocrinol Metab 1994; 79:1605.

88a. Müller B, Becker KL, Känzlin M, et al. Disordered calcium homeostasis of sepsis and association with calcitonin precursors. Eur J Clin Invest 2000; 30:823.

89. Weryha G, Leclere J. Paracrine regulation of bone remodeling. Horm Res 1995; 43:69.

90. Skerry TM. The effects of the inflammatory response on bone growth. Eur J Clin Nutr 1994; 48:S190.

91. Grey A, Mitnick M, Shapses S, et al. Circulating levels of interleukin-6 and tumor necrosis factor-alpha are elevated in primary hyperparathyroidism and correlate with markers of bone resorption—a clinical research study. J Clin Endocrinol Metab 1996; 81:3450.

92. Silverberg S, Bilezikian J. Cytokines in primary hyperparathyroidism—factors that matter. J Clin Endocrinol Metab 1996; 81:3448.

93. Greenfield EM, Gornik SA, Horowitz MC, et al. Regulation of cytokine expression in osteoblasts by parathyroid hormone: rapid stimulation of interleukin-6 and leukemia inhibitory factor mRNA. J Bone Miner Res 1993; 8:1163.

94. Greenfield EM, Shaw SM, Gornik SA, Banks MA. Adenyl cyclase and interleukin-6 are downstream effectors of parathyroid hormone resulting in stimulation of bone resorption. J Clin Invest 1995; 96:1238.

95. Katz MS, Gutierrez GE, Mundy GR, et al. Tumor necrosis factor and interleukin-1 inhibit parathyroid hormone responsive adenylate cyclase in clonal osteoblast-like cells by down-regulating parathyroid hormone receptors. J Cell Physiol 1992; 153:206.

96. Riancho JA, Zarrabeitia MT, de Francisco AL, et al. Vitamin D therapy modulates cytokine secretion in patients with renal failure. Nephron 1993; 65:364.

97. Cooper DJ, Walley KR, Dodek PM, et al. Plasma ionized calcium and blood lactate concentrations are inversely associated in human lactic acidosis. Intensive Care Med 1992; 18:286.

98. Aduen J, Bernstein WK, Miller J, et al. Relationship between blood lactate concentrations and ionized calcium, glucose, and acid-base status in critically ill and noncritically ill patients. Crit Care Med 1995; 23:246.

99. Frayn KN. Hormonal control of metabolism in trauma and sepsis. Clin Endocrinol (Oxf) 1986; 24:577.

100. Black PR, Brooks DC, Bessey PQ, et al. Mechanisms of insulin resistance following injury. Ann Surg 1982; 196:420.

101. Wolfe RR, Durkot MJ, Allsop JR, et al. Glucose metabolism in severely burned patients. Metabolism 1979; 28:1031.

102. Clowes GH Jr, O'Donnell TF Jr, Ryan NT, Blackburn GL. Energy metabolism in sepsis: treatment based on different patterns in shock and high output stage. Ann Surg 1974; 179:684.

103. Brandi LS, Santoro D, Natali A, et al. Insulin resistance of stress: sites and mechanisms. Clin Sci 1993; 85:525.

104. Gore DC, O'Brien R, Reines HD. Derangements in peripheral glucose and oxygen utilization induced by catabolic hormones. Crit Care Med 1993; 21:1712.

105. Thorell A, Efendic S, Gutniak M, et al. Development of postoperative insulin resistance is associated with the magnitude of operation. Eur J Surg 1993; 159:593.

106. Stoner HB, Frayn KN, Barton RN, et al. The relationships between plasma substrates and hormones and the severity of injury in 277 recently injured patients. Clin Sci 1979; 56:563.

107. Carey LC, Lowery BD, Cloutier CT. Blood sugar and insulin response of humans in shock. Ann Surg 1970; 172:342.

108. Power MJ, Fullerton KJ, Stout RW. Blood glucose and prognosis of acute stroke. Age Ageing 1988; 17:164.

109. Oswald GA, Smith CC, Betteridge DJ, Yudkin JS. Determinants and importance of stress hyperglycaemia in non-diabetic patients with myocardial infarction. BMJ (Clin Res Ed) 1986; 293:917.

110. Lakhdar A, Stromberg P, McAlpine SG. Prognostic importance of hyperglycaemia induced by stress after acute myocardial infarction. BMJ (Clin Res Ed) 1984; 288:288.

111. Woo J, Lam CW, Kay R, et al. The influence of hyperglycemia and diabetes mellitus on immediate and 3-month morbidity and mortality after acute stroke. Arch Neurol 1990; 47:1174.

112. Young B, Ott L, Dempsey R, et al. Relationship between admission hyperglycemia and neurologic outcome of severely brain-injured patients. Ann Surg 1989; 210:466.

113. Longstreth WT Jr, Diehr P, Cobb LA, Pagliara AS. Neurologic outcome and blood glucose levels during out-of-hospital cardiopulmonary resuscitation. Neurology 1986; 36:1186.

114. Garber AJ, Bier DM, Cryer PE, et al. Hypoglycemia in compensated chronic renal insufficiency. Substrate limitation of gluconeogenesis. Diabetes 1974; 23:982.
115. Wolfe RR, Elahi D, Spitzer JJ. Glucose and lactate kinetics after endotoxin administration in dogs. Am J Physiol 1977; 232:E180.
116. Yeoh SI, Baxter RC. Metabolic regulation of the growth hormone independent insulin-like growth factor binding protein in human plasma. Acta Endocrinol 1988; 119:465.
117. Lewitt MS, Baxter RC. Inhibitors of glucose uptake stimulate the production of insulin-like growth factor binding protein-1 (IGFBP-1) by human fetal liver. 1990; 126:1527.
117a. Tazuke SI, Mazure N, Sugawara J, et al. Hypoxia stimulates insulin-like growth factor binding protein-1 (IGFBP-1) gene expression in HepG2 cells: a possible model for IGFB-1 expression in fatal hypoxia. Proc Natl Acad U S A 1998; 95:10188.
118. Norrelund H, Fisker S, Vahl N, et al. Evidence supporting a direct suppressive effect of growth hormone on serum IGFBP-1 levels, experimental studies in normal, obese and GH-deficient adults. Growth Horm IGF Res 1999; 9:52.
119. Van den Berghe G, Baxter RC, Weekers F, et al. A paradoxical gender dissociation within the growth hormone/insulin-like growth factor axis during protracted critical illness. J Clin Endocrinol Metab 2000; 85:183.
119a. Sugawara J, Suh D-S, Faessen GH, et al. Regulation of insulin-like growth factor-binding protein-1 by nitric oxide under hypoxic conditions. J Clin Endocrinol Metab 2000; 85:2714.
120. Rashkin MC, Bosken C, Baughman RP. Oxygen delivery in critically ill patients. Relationship to blood lactate and survival. Chest 1985; 87:580.
121. Vincent JL, Dufaye P, Berre J, et al. Serial lactate determinations during circulatory shock. Crit Care Med 1983; 11:449.
122. Weil MH, Afifi AA. Experimental and clinical studies on lactate and pyruvate as indicators of the severity of acute circulatory failure (shock). Circulation 1970; 41:989.
123. Roumen RM, Redl H, Schlag G, et al. Scoring systems and blood lactate concentrations in relation to the development of adult respiratory distress syndrome and multiple organ failure in severely traumatized patients. J Trauma 1993; 35:349.
124. Bakker J, Gris P, Coffernils M, et al. Serial blood lactate levels can predict the development of multiple organ failure following septic shock. Am J Surg 1996; 171:221.
125. Abramson D, Scalea TM, Hitchcock R, et al. Lactate clearance and survival following injury. J Trauma 1993; 35:584.
126. Gabay C, Kushner I. Acute-phase proteins and other systemic responses to inflammation [published erratum in N Engl J Med 1999 340:1376]. N Engl J Med 1999; 340:448.
127. Redl H, Schlag G, Bahrami S, et al. Experimental and clinical evidence of leukocyte activation in trauma and sepsis. Prog Clin Biol Res 1994; 388:221.
128. Cioffi WG, Burleson DG, Pruitt BA Jr. Leukocyte responses to injury. Arch Surg 1993; 128:1260.
129. Nuytinck JK, Goris JA, Redl H, Littleton M. Posttraumatic complications and inflammatory mediators. Arch Surg 1986; 121:886.
130. Rivkind AI, Siegel JH, Guadalupi P, Littleton M. Sequential patterns of eicosanoid, platelet, and neutrophil interactions in the evolution of the fulminant post-traumatic adult respiratory distress syndrome. Ann Surg 1989; 210:355.
131. Bengtsson A. Cascade system activation in shock. Acta Anaesthesiol Scand 1993; S98:7.
132. Weiss SJ. Tissue destruction by neutrophils. N Engl J Med 1989; 320:365.
133. Cobb JP, Cunnion RE, Danner RL. Nitric oxide as a target for therapy in septic shock. Crit Care Med 1993; 21:1261.
134. Levin ER. Endothelins. N Engl J Med 1995; 333:356.
135. Alzeer AH, Al-Arifi A, Warsy AS, et al. Nitric oxide production is enhanced in patients with heat stroke. Intensive Care Med 1999; 25:58.
136. Preiser JC, Reper P, Vlasselaer D, et al. Nitric oxide production is increased in patients after burn injury. J Trauma 1996; 40:368.
137. Kilbourn RG, Griffith OW. Overproduction of nitric oxide in cytokine-mediated and septic shock. J Natl Cancer Inst 1992; 84:827.
138. Van Dissel JT, Groeneveld PH, Maes B, et al. Nitric oxide: a predictor of morbidity in postoperative patients? Lancet 1994; 343:1579.
139. Kilbourn RG, Jubran A, Gross SS, et al. Reversal of endotoxin-mediated shock by NG-methyl-L-arginine, an inhibitor of nitric oxide synthesis. Biochem Biophys Res Commun 1990; 172:1132.
140. Weitzberg E, Lundberg JM, Rudehill A. Elevated plasma levels of endothelin in patients with sepsis syndrome. Circ Shock 1991; 33:222.
141. Bouchama A, Hammami MM, Haq A, et al. Evidence for endothelial cell activation/injury in heatstroke. Crit Care Med 1996; 24:1173.
142. Warner TD. Relationships between the endothelin and nitric oxide pathways. Clin Exp Pharmacol Physiol 1999; 26:247.
143. Frenette PS, Wagner DD. Adhesion molecules—Part 1. N Engl J Med 1996; 334:1526.
144. Cowley HC, Heney D, Gearing AJ, et al. Increased circulating adhesion molecule concentrations in patients with the systemic inflammatory response syndrome: a prospective cohort study. Crit Care Med 1994; 22:651.
145. Boldt J, Wollbruck M, Kuhn D, et al. Do plasma levels of circulating soluble adhesion molecules differ between surviving and nonsurviving critically ill patients? Chest 1995; 107:787.
146. Hansson GK, Lagerstedt E, Bengtsson A, Heideman M. IgG binding to cytoskeletal intermediate filaments activates the complement cascade. Exp Cell Res 1987; 170:338.
147. Davis CF, Moore FD Jr, Rodrick ML, et al. Neutrophil activation after burn injury: contributions of the classic complement pathway and of endotoxin. Surgery 1987; 102:477.
148. Heideman M, Hugli TE. Anaphylatoxin generation in multisystem organ failure. J Trauma 1984; 24:1038.
149. Esmon CT. Regulation of blood coagulation. Biochim Biophys Acta 2000; 1477:349.
150. Ettingshausen E, Veldmann A, Beeg T, et al. Replacement therapy with protein C concentrate in infants and adolescents with meningococcal sepsis and purpura fulminans. Semin Thromb Hemost 1999; 25:537.
151. Ikeda Y, Long DM. The molecular basis of brain injury and brain edema: the role of oxygen free radicals. Neurosurg 1990; 27:1.
152. Hebert JC, O'Reilly M, Bednar MM. Modifying the host response to injury. The future of trauma care. Surg Clin North Am 1995; 75:335.
153. Zimmerman JJ. Defining the role of oxyradicals in the pathogenesis of sepsis. Crit Care Med 1995; 23:616.
154. Borrelli E, Roux-Lombard P, Grau GE, et al. Plasma concentrations of cytokines, their soluble receptors, and antioxidant vitamins can predict the development of multiple organ failure in patients at risk. Crit Care Med 1996; 24:392.
155. Goode HF, Cowley HC, Walker BE, et al. Decreased antioxidant status and increased lipid peroxidation in patients with septic shock and secondary organ dysfunction. Crit Care Med 1995; 23:646.
156. Maderazo EG, Woronick CL, Hickingbotham N, et al. A randomized trial of replacement antioxidant vitamin therapy for neutrophil locomotory dysfunction in blunt trauma. J Trauma 1991; 31:1142.
157. Offner F, Philippe J, Vogelaers D, et al. Serum tumor necrosis factor levels in patients with infectious disease and septic shock. J Lab Clin Med 1990; 116:100.
158. Cinat M, Waxman K, Vaziri ND, et al. Soluble cytokine receptors and receptor antagonists are sequentially released after trauma. J Trauma 1995; 39:112.
159. Sakamoto K, Arakawa H, Mita S, et al. Elevation of circulating interleukin 6 after surgery: factors influencing the serum level. Cytokine 1994; 6:181.
160. Cannon JG, Friedberg JS, Gelfand JA, et al. Circulating interleukin-1 beta and tumor necrosis factor-alpha concentrations after burn injury in humans. Crit Care Med 1992; 20:1414.
161. Billiau A, Vandekerckhove F. Cytokines and their interactions with other inflammatory mediators in the pathogenesis of sepsis and septic shock. Eur J Clin Invest 1991; 21:559.
162. Barriere SL, Lowry SF. An overview of mortality risk prediction in sepsis. Crit Care Med 1995; 23:376.
163. Hack CE, Hart M, van Schijndel RJ, et al. Interleukin-8 in sepsis: relation to shock and inflammatory mediators. Infect Immun 1992; 60:2835.
164. Marty C, Misset B, Tamion F, et al. Circulating interleukin-8 concentrations in patients with multiple organ failure of septic and nonseptic origin. Crit Care Med 1994; 22:673.
165. Van der Poll T, Romijn JA, Endert E, et al. Tumor necrosis factor mimics the metabolic response to acute infection in healthy humans. Am J Physiol 1991; 261:E457.
166. Hotamisligil GS, Spiegelman BM. Tumor necrosis factor alpha: a key component of the obesity-diabetes link. Diabetes 1994; 43:1271.
167. Stephens JM, Pekala PH. Transcriptional repression of the GLUT4 and C/EBP genes in 3T3-L1 adipocytes by tumor necrosis factor-alpha. J Biol Chem 1991; 266:21839.
168. Hotamisligil GS, Murray DL, Choy LN, Spiegelman BM. Tumor necrosis factor alpha inhibits signaling from the insulin receptor. Proc Natl Acad Sci U S A 1994; 91:4854.
169. Jin LJ, LaLonde C, Demling RH. Lung dysfunction after thermal injury in relation to prostanoid and oxygen radical release. J Appl Physiol 1986; 61:103.
170. Youn YK, LaLonde C, Demling R. The role of mediators in the response to thermal injury. World J Surg 1992; 16:30.
171. Fauler J, Tsikas D, Holch M, et al. Enhanced urinary excretion of leukotriene E4 by patients with multiple trauma with or without adult respiratory distress syndrome. Clin Sci 1991; 80:497.
172. Rockwell WB, Ehrlich HP. Ibuprofen in acute-care therapy. Ann Surg 1990; 211:78.
173. Higgs GA, Eakins KE, Mugridge KG, et al. The effects of non-steroid antiinflammatory drugs on leukocyte migration in carrageenin-induced inflammation. Eur J Pharmacol 1980; 66:81.
174. Whang KT, Steinwald PM, White JC, et al. Serum calcitonin precursors in sepsis and systemic inflammation. J Clin Endocrinol Metab 1998; 83:3296.
175. Müller B, Becker KL, Schächinger H, et al. Calcitonin precursors are reliable markers of sepsis in a medical intensive care unit. Crit Care Med 2000 28(7):2445.
176. Nylen ES, Whang KT, Snider RH Jr, et al. Mortality is increased by procalcitonin and decreased by an antiserum reactive to procalcitonin in experimental sepsis [see comments]. Crit Care Med 1998; 26:1001.
177. Becker KL, Nylén ES, Cohen R, Snider RH. Calcitonin: structure, molecular biology, and actions. In: Bilezikien JP, Raisz LG, Rodan GA, eds. The principles of bone biology. San Diego, CA: Academic Press, 1996:471.
178. Müller B, Vath S, Becker K, et al. Calcitonin precursors (CTpr) emanate from several tissues throughout the body in sepsis. Intensive Care Med 1999; 25:S140.
179. Snider RH Jr, Nylen ES, Becker KL. Procalcitonin and its component peptides in systemic inflammation: immunochemical characterization. J Investig Med 1997; 45:552.
180. Burgess TL, Kelly RB. Constitutive and regulated secretion of proteins. Annu Rev Cell Biol 1987; 3:243.
181. Minowada G, Welch WJ. Clinical implications of the stress response. J Clin Invest 1995; 95:3.
182. Welch WJ. How cells respond to stress. Sci Am 1993; 268:56.
183. Ribeiro SP, Villar J, Downey GP, et al. Sodium arsenite induces heat shock protein-72 kilodalton expression in the lungs and protects rats against sepsis. Crit Care Med 1994; 22:922.

184. Villar J, Ribeiro SP, Mullen JB, et al. Induction of the heat shock response reduces mortality rate and organ damage in a sepsis-induced acute lung injury model. Crit Care Med 1994; 22:914.
185. Vass K, Welch WJ, Nowak TS Jr. Localization of 70-kDa stress protein induction in gerbil brain after ischemia. Acta Neuropathol (Berl) 1988; 77:128.
186. Gower DJ, Hollman C, Lee KS, Tytell M. Spinal cord injury and the stress protein response. J Neurosurg 1989; 70:605.
187. Blake MJ, Gershon D, Fargnoli J, Holbrook NJ. Discordant expression of heat shock protein mRNAs in tissues of heat-stressed rats. J Biol Chem 1990; 265:15275.
188. Udelsman R, Blake MJ, Stagg CA, et al. Vascular heat shock protein expression in response to stress. Endocrine and autonomic regulation of this age-dependent response. J Clin Invest 1993; 91:465.
189. Udelsman R, Blake MJ, Stagg CA, Holbrook NJ. Endocrine control of stress-induced heat shock protein 70 expression in vivo. Surgery 1994; 115:611.
190. Jacquier-Sarlin MR, Fuller K, Dinh-Xuan AT, et al. Protective effects of hsp70 in inflammation. Experientia 1994; 50:1031.
191. Ueda S, Nishio K, Minamino N, et al. Increased plasma levels of adreno-medullin in patients with systemic inflammatory response syndrome. Am J Resp Crit Care Med 1999; 160:132.
192. Frass M, Watschinger B, Traindl O, et al. Atrial natriuretic peptide release in response to different positive end-expiratory pressure levels. Crit Care Med 1993; 21:343.
193. Gutierrez-Marcos FM, Fernandez-Cruz A, Gutkowska J, et al. Atrial natriuretic peptide in patients with acute myocardial infarction without functional heart failure. Eur Heart J 1991; 12:503.
194. Pasi A, Moccetti T, Legler M, et al. Elevation of blood levels of beta-endorphin-like immunoreactivity in patients with shock. Res Commun Chem Pathol Pharmacol 1983; 42:509.
195. Ennis M, Sangmeister M, Neugebauer E, et al. Plasma histamine levels in polytraumatized patients. Agents Actions 1990; 30:271.
196. Neugebauer E, Lorenz W. Causality in circulatory shock: strategies for integrating mediators, mechanisms and therapies. Prog Clin Biol Res 1988; 264:295.
197. Wang H, Bloom O, Zhang M, et al. HMG-1 as a late mediator of endotoxin lethality in mice. Science 1999; 285:248.
198. O'Donnell TF Jr, Clowes GH Jr, Talamo RC, Colman RW. Kinin activation in the blood of patients with sepsis. Surg Gynecol Obstet 1976; 143:539.
199. Bornstein SR, Licinio J, Tauchnitz R, et al. Plasma leptin levels are increased in survivors of acute sepsis: associated loss of diurnal rhythm, in cortisol and leptin secretion. J Clin Endocrinol Metab 1998; 83:280.
200. Calandra T, Echtenacher B, Le Roy D, et al. Protection from septic shock by neutralization of macrophage migration inhibitory factor. Nature Med 2000; 6:164.
201. Watson JD, Sury MR, Corder R, et al. Plasma levels of neuropeptide tyrosine Y (NPY) are increased in human sepsis but are unchanged during canine endotoxin shock despite raised catecholamine concentrations. J Endocrinol 1988; 116:421.
202. Hosford D, Paubert-Braquet M, Braquet P. Platelet-activating factor and cytokine interactions in shock. Resuscitation 1989; 18:207.
203. Bussolino F, Porcellini MG, Varese L, et al. Intravascular release of platelet activating factor in children with sepsis. Thromb Res 1987; 48:619.
204. Sibbald W, Peters S, Lindsay RM. Serotonin and pulmonary hypertension in human septic ARDS. Crit Care Med 1980; 8:490.
205. Revhaug A, Lygren I, Jenssen TG, et al. Vasoactive intestinal peptide in sepsis and shock. Ann N Y Acad Sci 1988; 527:536.

# CHAPTER 229

# THE HYPOTHALAMIC–PITUITARY–ADRENAL AXIS IN STRESS AND CRITICAL ILLNESS

STEFAN R. BORNSTEIN AND GEORGE P. CHROUSOS

## DEFINITION OF STRESS AS A STATE OF THREATENED HOMEOSTASIS

*Stress* is the state of threatened homeostasis. Threatening stimuli or stressors activate an integrated adaptive response, the purpose of which is to *maintain homeostasis*. Dysregulation of this response in either direction, hypofunction or hyperfunction, may influence the course of a disease or may produce disease.

Indeed, neuroendocrine, neural, and immune responses during a stressful situation are involved in the pathophysiology of many common health problems in modern societies and influence the course and outcome of critical illness.

## CONCEPTS OF STRESS AND DISEASE

The term *strain* was first used in physics to mean the force of pressure applied on a material body. This was measured in units of weight per unit of surface area. The term *stress*, on the other hand, was used to express the *resistance* of this body to strain. At the beginning of the century, Walter Cannon extrapolated such concepts from the theory of elasticity and Hook's law described at the end of the 1700s to living organisms.

The concept of stress is applicable to the entire field of biology. Living matter responds to disturbing forces or *stressors* first by transient adaptation, and then by plastic, long-term, and, occasionally, permanent changes. The idea that the natural state is not static but dynamic was originally proposed by Chinese, Greek, and Roman philosophers. Heraclitus, for example, was among the first to suggest that all things are constantly undergoing dynamic changes. Empedocles based his theory of life on the dynamic opposition-alliance of life elements, with "harmony" or equilibrium a necessary condition for survival. Later, Hippocrates defined health as a balance of the elements of life and stated that disease was due to disharmony among these elements; thus he excluded the intervention of supernatural forces.[1,2]

These general ideas of harmony within living matter were later adopted by Greco-Roman philosophers and physicians. Epicurus and Antiphon applied the same concept in the idea of the harmony of behavior and recognized the importance of the mind in maintaining the balance or equilibrium of bodily functions. These concepts were well recognized through the ancient centuries. They were lost in the Middle Ages but flourished again during the Renaissance and were nicely enunciated in the work of the English physician Thomas Sydenham in the seventeenth century. In the mid-nineteenth century, Claude Bernard introduced his influential theory of the constant "milieu intérieur," which proposed the existence of a crucial dynamic internal physiologic and biochemical equilibrium. This led to the development of the cybernetic concept of feedback regulation of vital parameters. In the early twentieth century, Cannon first developed the theory of strain/stress and coined the term "homeostasis" to describe true coordinated physiologic processes maintaining the steady state of temperature, pH, and osmotic pressure of internal fluids. Cannon also introduced the role of the adrenomedullary system in maintaining homeostasis and proposed the concept of the "fight or flight" reaction.

Hans Selye further elucidated and popularized the concept of stress and the relationship between stress and disease. He proposed the existence of a *stress* or *general adaptation syndrome* as the coordinated multifaceted "nonspecific" response of the body to any threatening force. In addition, he introduced the idea that the amount and perceived "control" of stress was important and that stress might have both positive and negative behavioral and somatic sequelae depending on intensity, duration, quality, and perception of control.[1-4] With the advent of modern technologies, the stress response is no longer believed to be nonspecific. Rather, it is thought to be tailored to the *stressor* and gradually to lose specificity as the intensity of the *stressor* increases.

## HYPOTHALAMIC–PITUITARY–ADRENAL AXIS AND STRESS

The physiologic response to stress involves activation of stress regulatory centers in the central nervous system (CNS), with consequent stimulation of the hypothalamic–pituitary–adrenal (HPA) axis and the autonomic nervous system. The stress system influences other endocrine systems (i.e., those controlling gonadal, thyroidal, and growth functions) and exerts complex effects on the immune/inflammatory reaction. The principal CNS centers of the stress system are the corticotropin-releasing hormone (CRH)/arginine vasopressin (AVP) and locus ceruleus–norepinephrine neurons of the hypothalamus and brainstem, respectively, which regulate the HPA axis and the sympathetic nervous system. The end hormones of these systems, glucocorticoids and the catecholamines, act to maintain behavioral, cardiovascular, metabolic, and immune homeostasis during stress.[1,2,5–7,7a]

## CORTICOTROPIN-RELEASING HORMONE—CENTRAL INTEGRATOR OF THE STRESS RESPONSE

Ovine CRH, a 41-amino-acid peptide, was isolated and sequenced in 1981.[8] Human CRH, identified later, differs from ovine CRH by seven amino acids and is metabolized more rapidly than the ovine analog in humans. Both ovine and human CRH have been synthesized and used in clinical research and practice.[6–9] CRH has proven useful in the differential diagnosis of Cushing syndrome and adrenal insufficiency.[6–9]

Hypothalamic paraventricular nucleus (PVN) CRH-secreting neurons innervate and stimulate cell bodies of the locus ceruleus/noradrenergic centers of the arousal and sympathetic nervous systems in the brainstem. Therefore, CRH is a central coordinator of both the HPA axis and the arousal/sympathetic nervous system. CRH also elicits specific stress-related behaviors. Delivery of intracerebroventricular CRH to rats, mice, and nonhuman primates leads to a spectrum of behavioral and physical manifestations typical of those of acute stress and/or chronic, intense anxiety.[10] These include tachycardia, increased arterial pressure, reduced appetite and sexual activity, social withdrawal, and psychomotor retardation or agitation, depending on the context.[1,7]

CRH receptors are of at least two different types. They mediate all of the aforementioned effects and are widespread throughout the CNS. They are also present in the PVN and CRH/locus ceruleus/norepinephrine cell bodies and in limbic structures.[2] CRH neurons in the central nucleus of the amygdala may have unique roles. Evidence exists that they elicit a fear/anxiety reaction, possibly in response to mental associations. Free, active CRH availability at the receptor level is regulated by a specific CRH-binding protein (CRH-BP).[11]

## NEURAL CONTROL OF THE HYPOTHALAMIC–PITUITARY–ADRENAL AXIS

Studies of the neural control of the HPA axis are important for at least two reasons: first, through measurements of hormones, such as adrenocorticotropic hormone (ACTH) and cortisol, they provide information about brain function; and, second, they help elucidate the pathogenesis of several common behavioral, metabolic, and immune system disorders in which a large body of evidence shows concomitant brain–HPA axis dysfunction.[1,5,7]

The available animal and human studies with pharmacologic agents indicate a stimulatory role for brain noradrenergic, serotonergic, and cholinergic pathways on CRH release, an inhibitory role for γ-aminobutyric acid (GABA) pathways via the GABA (A) benzodiazepine receptor, and an inhibitory role for central opioidergic and substance P–ergic pathways. Neuropeptide Y (NPY), which is colocalized in adrenergic projections and is also secreted by NPY-containing neurons of the arcuate nucleus of the hypothalamus, stimulates CRH secretion.[5]

The noradrenergic neuronal axes and terminals arise primarily from the A1, A2, and A6 areas of the brainstem and the

adrenergic neuronal axes and terminals from the C1, C2, and C3 areas. The locus ceruleus and/or its vicinity has rich CRH fiber innervation and local application of CRH stimulates firing by the locus ceruleus. Thus, a reciprocal stimulatory relation between PVN CRH neurons and locus ceruleus/noradrenergic neurons exists that links the arousal/sympathetic nervous system (adrenomedullary and sympathoneural) and the HPA axis responses to stress.[1,4]

In addition, a direct neuroadrenocortical axis exists.[12–16] In isolated perfused porcine adrenal glands, adrenal cortisol can be released immediately through splanchnic nerve activation mediated by catecholamines and intraadrenal neuropeptides.[17–19] Therefore, in stress a complex central and peripheral interaction is found between the HPA axis and the autonomic nervous system.[1,5,12,20,21,21a]

## HYPOTHALAMIC–PITUITARY–ADRENAL AXIS INTERACTIONS WITH THE IMMUNE SYSTEM

Glucocorticoids have strong antiinflammatory and immunosuppressive effects and, thus, are used in the treatment of many inflammatory/autoimmune and allergic diseases. Glucocorticoids influence the trafficking of circulating leukocytes and inhibit many functions of lymphocytes and immune accessory cells. They suppress the activation of these cells by immune stimuli, repress the production of proinflammatory cytokines and other mediators of inflammation, and increase resistance of target tissues to certain cytokines[1,5,22–25] (see Chap. 227). Glucocorticoids preferentially suppress certain types of T lymphocytes, such as T helper 1 ($T_H$1) lymphocytes, as well as stimulate apoptosis of eosinophils and certain groups of T cells (Fig. 229-1). These effects depend on the alteration of the transcription rates of glucocorticoid-responsive genes and/or changes in the

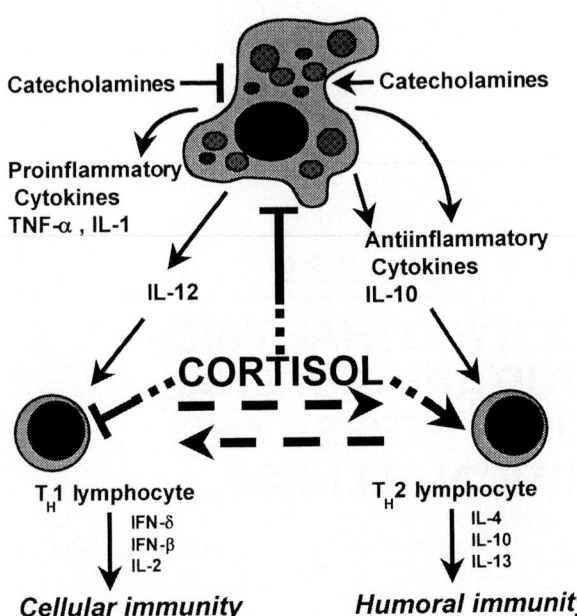

**FIGURE 229-1.** Cortisol regulates both cellular and humoral immunity. It inhibits monocyte/macrophage and helper T lymphocyte type 1 ($T_H$1) functions and suppresses proinflammatory cytokines. On the other hand, the production of antiinflammatory cytokines is enhanced. (*TNF-α*, tumor necrosis factor-α; *IL*, interleukin; $T_H$2, helper T lymphocyte type 2; *IFN*, interferon.) (Modified from Meduri GU, Chrousos GP. Duration of glucocorticoid treatment and outcome in sepsis: is the right drug used the wrong way? Chest 1998; 114:355.)

stability of the messenger RNA of several proteins that regulate inflammation.[25a] The effects of the glucocorticoids are receptor-mediated and may be direct through binding to glucocorticoid-response elements of DNA, or indirect through interaction with other transcription factors, such as activator protein-1 (AP-1) or nuclear factor-κB (NF-κB), which are involved in growth and inflammatory processes.[25]

Activation of the immune system leads to activation of the HPA axis. The links between the immune system and the HPA axis are the inflammatory cytokines, especially tumor necrosis factor α (TNF-α), interleukin-1 (IL-1), and interleukin-6 (IL-6)[22,26] (see Chaps. 173 and 227). At inflammatory sites, TNF-α is secreted first, then IL-1, followed by IL-6. TNF-α and IL-1 stimulate each other's secretion, whereas IL-6 inhibits secretion of both TNF-α and IL-1. CRH-neutralizing antisera and/or antagonists block the acute effects of each of the three inflammatory cytokines on the HPA axis.[5] An immune-HPA negative-feedback loop is closed by glucocorticoids, which repress the synthesis and secretion of these cytokines. Systemic IL-6 concentrations also increase during stress unrelated to inflammation, presumably stimulated by catecholamines acting through β2-adrenergic receptors. IL-6 has been shown to stimulate the HPA axis both at the level of the hypothalamus and pituitary gland and directly at the adrenal gland.[27–29]

Chronic activation of the HPA axis or inflammation results in reciprocally protective adaptations of the immune response and axis.

## ADRENAL GLANDS IN STRESS

The adrenal gland has an impressive capacity to adapt to various forms of acute and chronic stress. After central activation of the HPA axis, ACTH triggers a physiologic, molecular, and morphologic response of the adrenal cortex. This leads to glucocorticoid release, to up-regulation of steroidogenic cytochrome P450 messenger RNAs, and to conspicuous structural changes of the adrenal gland, characterized by both hypervascularization and cellular hypertrophy and hyperplasia. These morphologic changes are mirrored on the ultrastructural level: adrenocortical cells increase the number of their mitochondria and smooth endoplasmic reticulum to increase sites for steroidogenesis, whereas their inner membranes form a dense vesicular pattern.[30]

The adrenal gland, as the end organ of the human stress system, reacts with these morphologic changes in many clinical situations that involve severe or chronic stress. Severe subacute stress (i.e., major surgery) or lingering affective disorders, chronic infections, and chronic autoimmune diseases are frequently associated with overt adrenal alterations. In these states, dissociation between central activation of the HPA axis and the adrenal cortex may occur.[31] Thus, frequently, ACTH levels are low for the corresponding chronically elevated concentrations of glucocorticoids and the hypertrophy/hyperplasia of the adrenal gland. This dissociation suggests a long-term reset of the HPA axis maintained by central stimuli and/or the presence of extrapituitary mechanisms of adrenal regulation that can be both neural and immune.[12,31]

## STRESS SYSTEM DISORDERS

Alteration in the functioning of the stress system may be responsible for unexplained human disorders. Thus, major melancholic depression is associated with mild cortisol hypersecretion; the pituitaries[32] and adrenals[33] of depressed patients are enlarged. Likewise, the ACTH response to CRH is blunted, suggesting endogenous CRH hypersecretion and consequent CRH-receptor down-regulation.[5] Autopsy studies of depressed human subjects and individuals who have committed suicide have demonstrated adrenal hypertrophy/hyperplasia,[34] decreased CRH-binding sites in limbic areas,[35] and increased numbers of CRH and AVP neurons in the hypothalamic PVN. Evidence exists of chronic CRH hypersecretion in the posttraumatic stress disorder of the young, who are particularly vulnerable to anxiety and depression.[5] This suggests that central CRH hypersecretion is involved in the pathophysiology of melancholic depression and anxiety disorders. In addition, other disorders such as chronic active alcoholism, the metabolic syndrome, anorexia nervosa, and obsessive-compulsive disorder show an increased HPA activity.[7]

Central CRH hyposecretion has been hypothesized in atypical/seasonal depression, the chronic fatigue/fibromyalgia syndromes, and the postpartum period, as well as in subjects who have increased susceptibility to alcoholism.[5,7,36] Patients with the chronic fatigue and fibromyalgia syndromes have decreased urinary free cortisol excretion, perhaps owing to low central CRH secretion,[37,38] and patients with rheumatoid arthritis show decreased responsiveness of the HPA axis to inflammatory stimuli. Lewis rats, which have a hypoactive CRH neuron, are prone to alcohol addiction and autoimmune/inflammatory phenomena. Children of alcoholics, who are more vulnerable to alcoholism, also have an impaired HPA axis. This may lead to the conclusion that central CRH hyposecretion is a predisposing factor for autoimmune disorders and alcoholism in humans.[5]

In summary, dysregulation or altered regulation of the HPA axis is involved in the pathophysiology of many of the major human disorders, including psychiatric, metabolic, and autoimmune states (Table 229-1).

# HYPOTHALAMIC–PITUITARY–ADRENAL AXIS AND CRITICAL ILLNESS

The endocrine response to the stress of critical illness may influence its outcome. Two main questions need to be addressed:

**TABLE 229-1.**

**States Associated with Dysregulation or Altered Regulation of the Hypothalamic–Pituitary–Adrenal (HPA) Axis**

| Increased HPA Activity | Decreased HPA Activity | Disrupted HPA Activity |
| --- | --- | --- |
| Severe chronic disease | Atypical depression | Cushing syndrome |
| Melancholic depression | Seasonal depression | Glucocorticoid deficiency |
| Anorexia nervosa | Chronic fatigue syndrome | Glucocorticoid resistance |
| Obsessive-compulsive disorder | Fibromyalgia | |
| Panic disorder | Hypothyroidism | |
| Chronic excessive exercise | Adrenal suppression | |
| Malnutrition | Obesity ("hyperserotonergic" form) | |
| Diabetes mellitus | Nicotine withdrawal | |
| Hyperthyroidism | Vulnerability to inflammatory disease (Lewis rat) | |
| Central obesity | Rheumatoid arthritis | |
| Childhood sexual abuse | Premenstrual tension syndrome | |
| Pregnancy | Postpartum mood and inflammatory disorders | |
| | Vulnerability to alcoholism | |

(Modified from Chrousos GP, Gold PW. The concepts of stress and stress system disorders. Overview of physical and behavioral homeostasis. JAMA 1992; 267:1244.)

*(a) What is a normal homeostatic endocrine stress response to severe illness and what defines a clinically important deviation? (b) Should we intervene endocrinologically, why, and when?*

## ACTIVATION OF THE HYPOTHALAMIC–PITUITARY–ADRENAL AXIS IN CRITICAL ILLNESS

The fact that severe acute stress leads to a strong activation of the HPA axis is well established. After car accidents or during major surgery or sepsis, the human body can increase its glucocorticoid production by 5- to 10-fold. An adequate increase in glucocorticoid production is crucial for survival and is required by the organism to cope with the severe stress.[39] On the other hand, elevation of plasma levels of cortisol contributes to the hyperglycemia, leukocytosis, and hypercatabolism seen in most forms of critical illness. Likewise, high glucocorticoid levels suppress the immune system, as well as the reproductive, growth, and thyroid axes.[40] The first of these effects may be necessary to restrain the inflammatory response from overreacting, but it may also be responsible for the unrestrained progression of an infection.

The acute increase in cortisol levels is caused by activation of the PVN CRH and AVP neurons. The amplitude and synchronization of CRH and AVP pulses in the hypophyseal portal system are increased. In the presence of hypotension or volume depletion, recruitment of AVP from the magnocellular neurons secreted both into the hypophysial portal system via collateral neuroaxons and into the systemic circulation takes place.[5,41] Depending on the cause of the acute illness, other factors, such as angiotensin II, opioids, and other neuropeptides, regulate the activity of PVN CRH and AVP neurons and the effects of these neuropeptides on the pituitary corticotropes.[5] Peripheral infectious or inflammatory signals, such as endotoxin, inflammatory cytokines, and other mediators of inflammation, directly stimulate the hypothalamus, pituitary, and/or adrenal cortices[1,42,43,43a] (see Chap. 227). Acute interactions of the HPA axis with the adipostatic hormone leptin suggest a close link of the metabolic system with stress regulation in severe illness.[42,44,45] Finally, glucocorticoids influence the major regulatory systems that are involved in the maintenance of arterial blood pressure (Fig. 229-2).

Non–ACTH-mediated regulation of adrenocortical function plays a role in maintaining high glucocorticoid levels in critical illness.[31] The dissociation of plasma ACTH concentrations and cortisol secretion in critical illness could not be explained by the different kinetics of these hormones. Thus, suppression of ACTH secretion with dexamethasone did not prevent a rise in plasma cortisol in response to surgical stress, whereas it did so in response to the stress of exercise.[46,47] In postoperative patients, patients with bacterial sepsis, and patients with late-stage human immunodeficiency virus disease, persistently elevated cortisol levels were accompanied by low or normal plasma ACTH values.[31,48] Some patients in intensive care units have a markedly altered responsiveness of their pituitary corticotropes to suppression with dexamethasone and stimulation with CRH. In these patients, an altered pituitary glucocorticoid feedback and a hypersecretion of peptides with CRH- or ACTH-like activity may be involved in the regulation of the HPA axis.[49] High endothelin or β-endorphin levels exerting a positive drive on the adrenal cortex have also been implicated in the non–ACTH-mediated regulation of glucocorticoid release during critical illness. Furthermore, IL-6 has been demonstrated to stimulate adrenal cortisol secretion directly.[28,29,49a] Therefore, an extrapituitary-adrenocortical stress response may have been designed by nature as an ancillary regulatory mechanism to cope with these extreme situations[31] (Fig. 229-3).

Although in severe stress of limited duration (as in sepsis) the maintenance of high glucocorticoid production is beneficial and desirable, long-term activation of this extrapituitary-adrenocortical stress system may have devastating side effects due to the chronically elevated glucocorticoid levels, as described earlier. In addition, chronic hyperstimulation of the adrenal cortex in conjunction with overexpression or aberrant expression of receptors for neuropeptides, neurotransmitters, or cytokines may lead to adrenal tumor formation and possibly non–ACTH-mediated Cushing syndrome (see Chap. 75).[50,51] Therefore, understanding the mechanisms of HPA activation in the various forms of acute and chronic stress during critical illness will help in developing more specific and more efficient diagnostic and therapeutic strategies.

## CUSHING SYNDROME AND CRITICAL ILLNESS

Cushing syndrome with high plasma cortisol levels can cause severe immunosuppression; therefore, patients with hypercortisolemia are at risk for both bacterial and multiple opportunistic infections.[52,53] This is especially true for patients with paraneoplastic (ectopic) ACTH syndrome who present with very high cortisol levels (>2000 nmol/L) (see Chap. 219). Indeed, the risk of infection has been shown to increase with the amount of endogenous cortisol production.[53] Because the high levels of cortisol suppress the fever response and elevate white blood cell levels, these clinical signs are not reliable. Therefore, prompt antibiotic treatment must be initiated, and the clinician must remain vigilant for infectious complication in these immunosuppressed patients. Frequent pathogens in patients with paraneoplastic ACTH Cushing syndrome include *Pneumocystis carinii, Aspergillus, Nocardia, Cryptococcus, Candida,* herpes viruses, and also bacterial agents.[52–56] Some studies have even recommended prophylactic therapy for *P. carinii* in patients with Cushing syndrome when plasma cortisol levels are >2500 nmol/L.[56]

Patients with Cushing syndrome who are critically ill and who cannot take oral adrenolytic therapy (such as metyrapone or ketoconazole) may benefit from parenteral administration of etomidate.[57–63] Intravenous administration of etomidate reportedly has been used to control hypercortisolemia for over

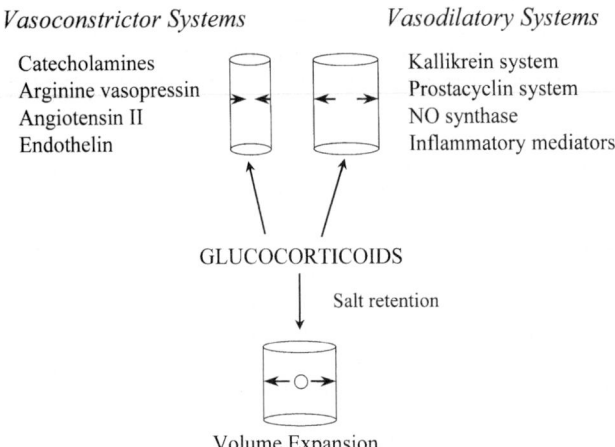

*Vasoconstrictor Systems*

Catecholamines
Arginine vasopressin
Angiotensin II
Endothelin

*Vasodilatory Systems*

Kallikrein system
Prostacyclin system
NO synthase
Inflammatory mediators

GLUCOCORTICOIDS

Salt retention

Volume Expansion

**FIGURE 229-2.** Effects of glucocorticoids on arterial blood pressure. Glucocorticoids potentiate the effects of vasoconstrictor systems and inhibit those of vasodilatory systems, but, through their mineralocorticoid properties, retain salt and increase blood volume. Tumor necrosis factor-α and interleukin-1, both of which are inhibited by glucocorticoids, represent major vasodilatory and permeability stimulants during the inflammatory stress of sepsis, septic shock, and adult respiratory distress syndrome. (*NO,* nitrous oxide.) (Modified from Meduri GU, Chrousos GP. Duration of glucocorticoid treatment and outcome in sepsis: is the right drug used the wrong way? Chest 1998; 114:355.)

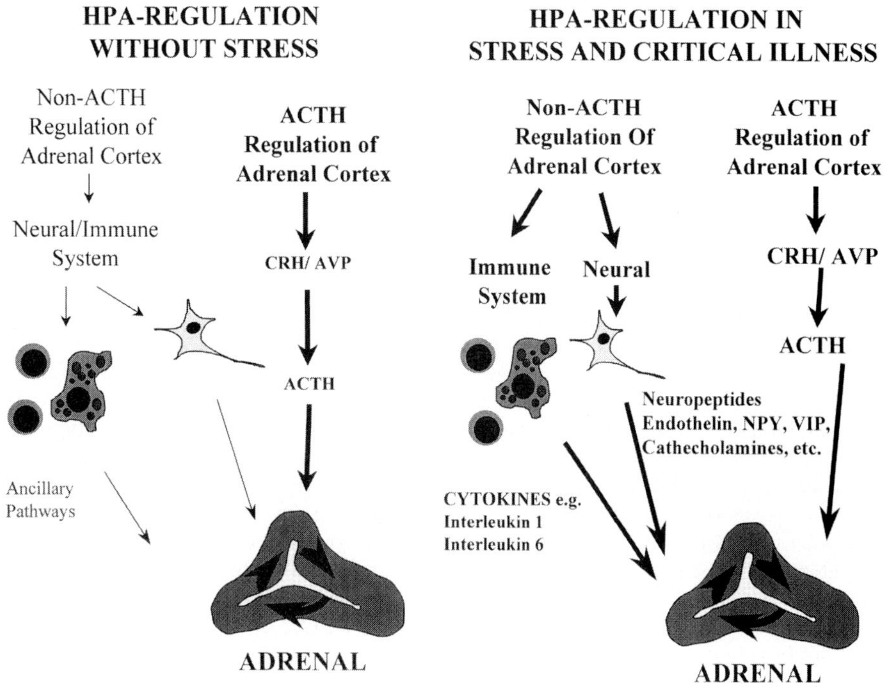

FIGURE 229-3. Adrenocorticotropic hormone (*ACTH*) is the main regulator of adrenocortical cortisol production. Under normal conditions, extrapituitary regulation of adrenocortical function is mediated by the immune system, and in adults the autonomic nervous system is less prominent (**A**). In severe stress and prolonged critical illness, however, non–ACTH-mediated mechanisms participate in the maintenance of high glucocorticoid levels (**B**). (*HPA*, hypothalamic–pituitary–adrenal; *CRH*, corticotropin-releasing hormone; *AVP*, arginine vasopressin; *NPY*, neuropeptide Y; *VIP*, vasoactive intestinal polypeptide.) (Modified from Bornstein SR, Chrousos GP. ACTH- and non-ACTH-mediated regulation of the adrenal cortex: neural and immune inputs. J Clin Endocrinol Metab 1999; 84:1729).

## DYSFUNCTION OF THE HYPOTHALAMIC–PITUITARY–ADRENAL AXIS IN CRITICAL ILLNESS

An abnormal hormonal response due to a defect in HPA functioning with primary or secondary adrenocortical insufficiency (see Chap. 76) can suddenly progress into an acute life-threatening condition that mimics critical illness of many different etiologies. Adrenal insufficiency is indeed an insidious disorder with rapid downhill progression and can be lethal if not diagnosed and treated in time.

In patients admitted to an intensive care unit who present with hypovolemic shock, hyperkalemia, hyponatremia, and hypoglycemia, the diagnosis of acute adrenal insufficiency must be considered. This diagnosis should also be suspected in any patient with a history of an underlying adrenal or pituitary disorder, in patients treated with suppressive doses of glucocorticoids (e.g., for rheumatoid arthritis, asthma, inflammatory bowel disease, etc.), or in patients with severe sepsis, acquired immunodeficiency syndrome (AIDS), disorders requiring anticoagulant therapy, or end-stage malignancies. In any case, if acute adrenal insufficiency is suspected, immediate replacement of glucocorticoids and fluids is essential for survival and should be initiated before the diagnosis can be confirmed through endocrine testing. Therefore, immediate therapeutic interventions include sampling blood for subsequent cortisol and ACTH measurement and simultaneously administering 2 mg per day of intravenous dexamethasone or 100 mg of hydrocortisone every 8 hours.[39] A heightened clinical awareness allows successful management of this critical condition. However, routine screening of adrenocortical function is not justified for this rare disorder.[64]

Although overt adrenocortical insufficiency is a rare medical emergency, occult hypoadrenalism has been reported more frequently. Transient and/or functional hypoadrenalism has been demonstrated in patients with multisystem critical illness[65] or surgical critical illness[66] and in patients with AIDS.[67] This relative hypoadrenalism may be much more frequent than is cur-

2 months in a patient with severe ectopic ACTH Cushing syndrome due to a pancreatic islet cell tumor who developed life-threatening peritonitis after perforation of the duodenum.[57]

rently recognized, because the cortisol response to the standard 250 µg cosyntropin test may be falsely normal.[65]

The mechanisms of an impaired or suboptimal adrenal response in some patients with critical illness remain to be elucidated. Both extra- and intraadrenal factors may be involved. In critically ill patients with acute sepsis, several peptides and cytokines that have been shown to suppress glucocorticoid production are elevated. Thus, atrial natriuretic hormone, leptin, and TNF, which have been demonstrated to inhibit adrenal cortisol production, are elevated in patients with severe illness[26,44,49,68,69] (see Chap. 227).

On the other hand, human adrenocortical cells of the inner zona fasciculata and zona reticularis express major histocompatibility complex (MHC) class II molecules and the apoptosis protein Fas (CD95) receptor.[70,71] Conceivably, therefore, in critical illness due to acute severe inflammation, lymphocytes passing through the adrenal cortex may trigger an MHC class II/CD 95–mediated cell death in the inner zone of the adrenal cortex, which contributes to the previously described impairment of adrenal androgen and, occasionally, cortisol secretion in prolonged sepsis.[72,73,73a]

Finally, in patients who maintain high glucocorticoid levels, resistance of tissues to circulating glucocorticoids may contribute to the septic shock syndrome. Cytokines, including IL-1, IL-6, interferon-α, and the combination of IL-2 and IL-4,[5] can cause glucocorticoid resistance in part by reducing glucocorticoid–receptor-binding affinity. This may involve interactions of cytokine-stimulated transcription factors AP-1 and NF-κB with the glucocorticoid receptor. Acquired tissue resistance to glucocorticoids may also contribute to the late stages of AIDS.[25,74] The elevation of glucocorticoid secretion in patients with sepsis and septic shock may not be up to the requirement of the inflammatory response due to tissue resistance. Therefore, exogenous administration of glucocorticoids at doses that are pharmacologic for normal persons may be necessary to achieve an adequate "replacement" in septic patients.[75]

High plasma cortisol levels, like a high Apache II score, seem to correlate with the severity of disease in critically ill patients. However, both high and low glucocorticoid levels have been associated with poor survival. Considering the diverse mechanisms of HPA axis regulation in these patients, the determination of single plasma cortisol levels may not provide an answer regarding prognosis of the patient or the potential benefit of glucocorticoid therapy. Transient hypoadrenalism may aggravate the adverse effects of severe inflammation. During sepsis, glucocorticoids ensure metabolic substrate availability, sustain the blood pressure, and restrain the immune system from producing host tissue damage. Although controlled clinical trials of the once-popular regimen of a short-term (24- to 48-hour) course of glucocorticoids suggested that such therapy was ineffective, other studies have identified critically ill patients with clinical features consistent with hypoadrenalism, such as hypotension, who exhibit relatively low "basal" plasma cortisol levels (<15 µg/dL) and who respond clinically to glucocorticoid therapy (see Chap. 232).

Most patients with sepsis have clearly elevated cortisol levels with normal ACTH levels and elevated levels of inflammatory cytokines (Fig. 229-4). In contrast to high-dose pharmacologic steroid therapy, modest supraphysiologic and prolonged administration of hydrocortisone or synthetic glucocorticoids may be beneficial in critical illness. Indeed, renewed interest is being shown in glucocorticoid therapy for patients with severe sepsis, septic shock, and adult respiratory distress syndrome (ARDS). Several double-blind, randomized trials of prolonged glucocorticoid treatment reported significant clinical improvement and a significantly decreased mortality.[75–77] Why do these studies report success, in contrast to earlier randomized, multicenter trials[78–80] that failed to find any benefits? Important differences exist in the new approach with regard to initiation of treatment, dosage of glucocorticoids, and duration of treatment. In contrast to previous trials, treatment was started *immediately* (2 mg/kg per day of methylprednisolone or equivalent), doses were 6 to 140 times *lower*, and glucocorticoids were administered over a *prolonged period of time* (5–32 days).[75,77] In fact, prolonged glucocorticoid treatment has been shown to be necessary to achieve an adequate and efficient suppression of the inflammatory cytokines that are major players in the aggressive and protracted host defense response in sepsis.[75]

In experimental acute lung injury, glucocorticoid treatment led to a decrease in edema and lung collagen formation.[81] When the glucocorticoids were discontinued, however, these positive effects were abrogated.[82] In clinical studies, premature discontinuation of prolonged glucocorticoid treatment in septic shock and in ARDS was shown to be associated with worsening of the disease due to a rebound of the inflammatory response. Thus, if treatment is stopped too early, not only are early treatment benefits lost but also the patients deteriorate; this provides a possible explanation for the discrepancies with previous studies.[75,82]

In addition to corticosteroid replacement, therapeutic intervention directed against other components of the HPA axis may turn out to be useful in the treatment of critically ill patients. CRH, the main regulator of the HPA axis, is expressed outside the central nervous system, and peripheral CRH secreted in inflammatory sites acts as a local proinflammatory modulator. In preclinical studies, novel CRH-receptor type I antagonists have been effective in suppressing the HPA axis and inflammation.[83,84,85]

In conclusion, the regulation and functioning of the HPA axis in critical illness is still far from understood. Although no argument exists about the need for glucocorticoid treatment for patients with a known defect in HPA function, further double-blind, controlled studies are required to define the correct treatment for patients with no obvious impairment of the HPA axis who, however, might benefit from moderate-dose, prolonged glucocorticoid therapy because of transient glucocorticoid resistance of target tissues, including the immune and cardiovascular systems.

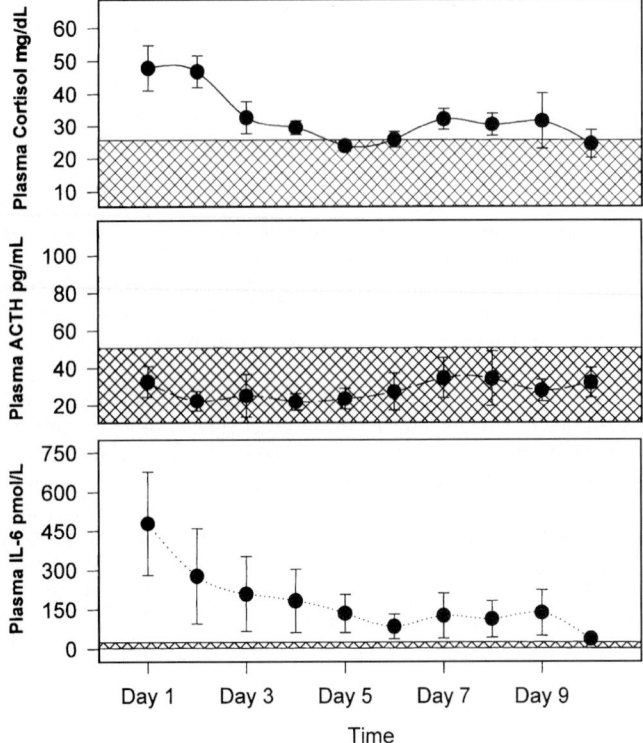

**FIGURE 229-4.** Time course of plasma cortisol, adrenocorticotropic hormone (*ACTH*), and interleukin-6 (*IL-6*) secretion in 12 critically ill patients in an intensive care unit. All patients fulfilled the clinical criteria for sepsis and all patients survived the critical disease. Both cortisol and IL-6 levels are high over a prolonged period of time (11 days), whereas ACTH levels remain in the normal range.

## REFERENCES

1. Chrousos GP. Stressors, stress, and neuroendocrine integration of the adaptive response: The 1997 Hans Selye Memorial Lecture. Ann N Y Acad Sci 1998; 851:311.
2. Bolis CL, Licinio J, ed. Stress and the nervous system. Geneva: World Health Organization, 1998. WHO/RPS/98.2.
3. Bornstein SR, Feindel W, Jouvet M, et al. Stress and adaptation: from Selye's concept to application of modern formulations. (Summary). Geneva: World Health Organization, 1998. WHO/RPS/98.3.
4. Goldstein DS. Stress response patterns. In: Goldstein DS, ed. Stress, catecholamines, and cardiovascular disease. New York: Oxford University Press; 1995:287.
5. Torpy DJ, Chrousos GP. General adaptation syndrome: an overview. In: Ober KP, ed. Contemporary endocrinology: endocrinology of critical disease. Totowa, NJ: Humana Press, 1997:1.
6. Orth DN. Corticotropin-releasing hormone in humans. Endocr Rev 1992; 13:164.
7. Chrousos GP, Gold PW. The concepts of stress and stress system disorders. Overview of physical and behavioral homeostasis. JAMA 1992; 267:1244.
7a. Sapolsky RM, Romero M, Munck AU. How do glucocorticoids influence stress responses? Integrating permissive, suppressive, stimulatory, and preparative actions. Endocr Rev 2000; 21:55.
8. Vale W, Spiess J, Rivier C, Rivier J. Characterization of a 41-residue ovine hypothalamic peptide that stimulates secretion of corticotropin and beta-endorphin. Science 1981; 213:1394.
9. Schurmeyer TH, Averginos PC, Gold PW, et al. Human corticotropin-releasing factor in man: pharmacokinetic properties and dose response of plasma adrenocorticotropin and cortisol secretion. J Clin Endocrinol Metab 1984; 59:1103.
10. Gold PW, Goodwin FK, Chrousos GP. Clinical and biochemical manifestations of depression. Relation to neurobiology of stress. N Engl J Med 1988; 319:348.
11. Zhao XJ, Hoheisel G, Schauer J, Bornstein SR. Corticotropin-releasing hormone-binding protein and its possible role in neuroendocrinological research. Horm Metab Res 1997; 29:373.
12. Ehrhart-Bornstein M, Hinson JP, Bornstein SR, et al. Intraadrenal interactions in the regulation of adrenocortical steroidogenesis. Endocr Rev 1998; 19:101.
13. Bornstein SR, Vaudry H. Paracrine and neuroendocrine regulation of the adrenal gland: basic and clinical aspects. Horm Metab Res 1998; 30:292.
14. Pignatelli D, Magalhaes MM, Magalhaes MC. Direct effects of stress on adrenocortical function. Horm Metab Res 1998; 30:464.
15. Engeland WC. Functional innervation of the adrenal cortex by the splanchnic nerve. Horm Metab Res 1998; 30:311.

16. McDonald TJ, Nathaniels PW. The involvement of innervation in the regulation of fetal adrenal steroidogenesis. Horm Metab Res 1998; 30:297.

17. Bornstein SR, Ehrhart-Bornstein M, Scherbaum WA, et al. Effects of splanchnic nerve stimulation on the adrenal cortex may be mediated by chromaffin cells in a paracrine manner. Endocrinology 1990; 127:900.

18. Bornstein SR, Ehrhart-Bornstein M. Ultrastructural evidence for a paracrine regulation of the rat adrenal cortex mediated by the local release of catecholamines from chromaffin cells. Endocrinology 1992; 131:3126.

19. Haidan A, Bornstein SR, Glasow A, et al. Basal steroidogenic activity of adrenocortical cells is increased tenfold by co-culture with chromaffin cells. Endocrinology 1998; 139:772.

20. Pacak K, Baffi JS, Kvetnansky R, et al. Stressor-specific activation of catecholaminergic systems: implications for stress-related hypothalamic-pituitary-adrenocortical responses. Adv Pharmacol 1998; 42:561.

21. Pacak K, Palkovits M, Yadid G, et al. Heterogeneous neurochemical responses to different stressors: a test of Selye's doctrine of nonspecificity. Am J Physiol 1998; 275:R1247.

21a. Merke DP, Chrousos GP, Eisenhofer G, et al. Adrenomedullary dysplasia and hypofunction in patients with congenital hyperplasia. N Engl J Med 2000 (in press).

22. Sternberg EM, Chrousos GP, Wilder RL, Gold PW. The stress response and the regulation of inflammatory disease: NIH combined clinical staff conference. Ann Intern Med 1992; 117:854.

23. Elenkov IJ, Papanicolaou DA, Wilder RL, Chrousos GP. Effects of glucocorticoids and catecholamines on human interleukin-12 and interleukin-10 production: implications for the effect of stress on immunity and the Th1/Th2 balance. Proc Am Assoc Physicians 1996; 108:374.

24. Mosmann TR, Sad S. The expanding universe of T-cell subsets: Th1, Th2 and more. Immunol Today 1996; 17:138.

25. Bamberger CM, Schulte HM, Chrousos GP. Molecular determinants of glucocorticoid receptor function and tissue sensitivity to glucocorticoids. Endocr Rev 1996; 17:245.

25a. Franchimont D, Galon J, Gardina M, et al. Inhibition of Th1 immune response by glucocorticoids: dexamethasone selectively inhibits IL-12 induced stat4 phosphorylation in T lymphocytes. J Immunol 2000; 15:1768.

26. Marx C, Ehrhart-Bornstein M, Scherbaum WA, Bornstein SR. Regulation of adrenocortical function by cytokines: relevance for immune-endocrine interaction. Horm Metab Res 1998; 30:416.

27. Papanicolaou DA, Wilder RL, Manolagas SC, Chrousos GP. The pathophysiologic roles of interleukin-6 in human disease. Ann Intern Med 1998; 128:127.

28. Päth G, Bornstein SR, Ehrhart-Bornstein M, Scherbaum WA. Interleukin-6 and the interleukin-6 receptor in the human adrenal gland: expression and effects on steroidogenesis. J Clin Endocrinol Metab 1997; 82:2343.

29. Päth G, Bornstein SR, Späth-Schwalbe E, Scherbaum WA. Direct effects of interleukin-6 on human adrenal cells. Endocr Res 1996; 22:867.

30. Bornstein SR, Ehrhart-Bornstein M, Güse-Behling H, Scherbaum WA. Structure and dynamics of adrenal mitochondria following stimulation with corticotropin releasing hormone (CRH). Anat Rec 1992; 234:255.

31. Bornstein SR, Chrousos GP. ACTH- and non-ACTH-mediated regulation of the adrenal cortex: neural and immune inputs. J Clin Endocrinol Metab 1999; 84:1729.

32. Krishnan KRR, Doraiswamy PM, Lurie SN, et al. Pituitary size in depression. J Clin Endocrinol Metab 1991; 73:256.

33. Amsterdam J, Marinelli D, Arger P, Winokur A. Assessment of adrenal gland volume by computed tomography in depressed patients and healthy volunteers: a pilot study. Psychiatry Res 1987; 21:189.

34. Willenberg HS, Bornstein SR, Dumser T, et al. Morphological changes in adrenals from victims of violent suicides in relation to altered apoptosis. Endocr Res 1998; 24:963.

35. Nemeroff CB, Owens MJ, Bissette G, et al. Reduced corticotropin releasing factor binding sites in the frontal cortex of suicide victims. Arch Gen Psychiatry 1988; 45:577.

36. Wand GS, Dobs AS. Alterations in the hypothalamic-pituitary-adrenal axis in actively drinking alcoholics. J Clin Endocrinol Metab 1991; 72:1290.

37. Demitrack MA, Dale JK, Straus SE, et al. Evidence of impaired activation of the hypothalamic-pituitary-adrenal axis in patients with chronic fatigue syndrome. J Clin Endocrinol Metab 1991; 73:1224.

38. Griep EN, Boerdma JW, de Kloet ER. Altered reactivity of the hypothalamic-pituitary-adrenal axis in the primary fibromyalgia syndrome. J Rheumatol 1993; 20:469.

39. Salem M, Guarino AH, Chernow B. Adrenal dysfunction in the intensive care unit. In: Shoemaker WC, Ayres SM, Grenvik A, Holbrook PR, ed. Textbook of critical care, 3rd ed. Philadelphia: WB Saunders, 1995.

40. Chrousos GP, Torpy DJ, Gold PW. Interaction between the hypothalamic-pituitary-adrenal axis and the female reproductive system: clinical implications. Ann Intern Med 1998; 129:229.

41. De Bold CR, Sheldon WR, DeCherney GS, et al. Arginine vasopressin potentiates adrenocorticotropin release induced by ovine corticotropin-releasing factor. J Clin Invest 1984; 73:533.

42. Bornstein SR, Preas HL, Chrousos GP, Suffredini AF. Circulating leptin levels during acute experimental endotoxinemia and anti-inflammatory therapy in humans. J Infect Dis 1998; 178:887.

43. Reincke M, Allolio B, Wurth G, Winkelmann W. The hypothalamic-pituitary-adrenal axis in critical illness: response to dexamethasone and corticotropin-releasing hormone. J Clin Endocrinol Metab 1993; 77:151.

43a. Bornstein SR. Cytokines and the adrenal cortex: basic research and clinical implications. Curr Opin Endocrinol Diabetes 2000; 7:128.

44. Bornstein SR, Licinio J, Tauchnitz R, et al. Plasma leptin levels are increased in survivors of acute sepsis: associated loss of diurnal rhythm, in cortisol and leptin secretion. J Clin Endocrinol Metab 1998; 83:280.

45. Bornstein SR. Is leptin a stress related peptide? Nature Med 1997; 3:937.

46. Naito Y, Fukata J, Tamai S, et al. Biphasic changes in hypothalamo-pituitary-adrenal function during the early recovery period after major abdominal surgery. J Clin Endocrinol Metab 1991; 73:111.

47. Calogero AE, Norton JA, Sheppard BC, et al. Pulsatile activation of the hypothalamic-pituitary-adrenal axis during major surgery. Metabolism 1992; 41:839.

48. Siegel LM, Grinspoon SK, Garvey GJ, Bilezikan JP. Sepsis and adrenal function. Trends Endocrinol Metab 1994; 5:324.

49. Vermes I, Beishuizen A, Hampsink RM, Haanen C. Dissociation of plasma adrenocorticotropin and cortisol levels in critically ill patients: possible role of endothelin and atrial natriuretic hormone. J Clin Endocrinol Metab 1995; 80:1238.

49a. Franchimont O, Bouma G, Galon J, et al. Adrenocortical activation in murine colitis. Gastroenterology 2000; 119 (in press).

50. Bornstein SR, Stratakis CA, Chrousos GP. Adrenocortical tumors: recent advances in basic concepts and clinical management. Ann Intern Med 1999; 130:759.

51. Willenberg HS, Stratakis CA, Marx C, et al. Aberrant interleukin-1 receptors in a cortisol-secreting adrenal adenoma causing Cushing's syndrome. N Engl J Med 1998; 339:27.

52. Graham BS, Tucker WS. Opportunistic infections in endogenous Cushing's syndrome. Ann Intern Med 1984; 101:334.

53. Sarlis NJ, Chanock SJ, Nieman LK. Cortisolemic indices predict severe infection in Cushing's syndrome due to ectopic production of adrenocorticotropin. J Clin Endocrinol Metab 2000; 85(1):42.

54. Kramer M, Corrado ML, Bacci V, et al. Pulmonary cryptococcosis and Cushing's syndrome. Arch Intern Med 1983; 143:2179.

55. Sieber SC, Dandurand R, Gelfman N, et al. Three opportunistic infections associated with the ectopic corticotropin syndrome. Arch Intern Med 1989; 149:2589.

56. Bakker RC, Gallas PRJ, Romijin JA, Wiersinga WM. Cushing's syndrome complicated by multiple opportunistic infections. J Endocrinol Invest 1998; 21:329.

57. Drake WM, Perry LA, Hinds CJ, et al. Emergency and prolonged use of intravenous etomidate to control hypercortisolemia in a patient with Cushing's syndrome and peritonitis. J Clin Endocrinol Metab 1998; 83:3542.

58. Verhelst A, Trainer PJ, Howlett TA, et al. Short- and long-term responses to metyrapone in the medical management of 91 patients with Cushing's syndrome. Clin Endocrinol (Oxf) 1991; 35:169.

59. Sonino N, Boscaro M, Paoletta A, et al. Ketoconazole treatment in Cushing's syndrome: experience in 34 patients. Clin Endocrinol (Oxf) 1991; 35:347.

60. Allolio B, Stuttmann R, Fischer H, et al. Long-term etomidate, and adrenocortical suppression. Lancet 1983; 2:626.

61. Lambert A, Mitchell R, Frost J, et al. Direct in vitro inhibition of adrenal steroidogenesis by etomidate. Lancet 1983; 2:1085.

62. Schulte HM, Benker G, Reinwein D, et al. Infusion of low dose etomidate: correction of hypercortisolemia in patients with Cushing's syndrome and dose-response relationship in normal subjects. J Clin Endocrinol Metab 1990; 70:1426.

63. Gartner R, Albrecht M, Muller OA. Effect of etomidate on hypercortisolism due to ectopic ACTH production. Lancet 1986; 1:275.

64. Span LF, Hermus AR, Bartelink AK, et al. Adrenocortical function: an indicator of severity of disease and survival in chronic critically ill patients. Intensive Care Med 1992; 18:93.

65. Baldwin WA, Allo M. Occult hypoadrenalism in critically ill patients. Arch Surg 1993; 128:673.

66. Mackenzie JS, Burrows L, Burchard KW. Transient hypoadrenalism during surgical critical illness. Arch Surg 1998; 133:489.

67. Stolarczyk R, Rubio SI, Smolyar D, et al. Twenty-four-hour urinary free cortisol in patients with acquired immunodeficiency syndrome. Metabolism 1998; 47:690.

68. Bornstein SR, Uhlmann K, Haidan A, et al. Evidence for a novel peripheral action of leptin as a metabolic signal to the adrenal gland. Leptin inhibits cortisol release directly. Diabetes 1997; 46:1235.

69. Glasow A, Haidan A, Hilbers U, et al. Expression of ob receptor in normal human adrenal and adrenal tumors: differential regulation of adrenocortical and adrenomedullary function by leptin. J Clin Endocrinol Metab 1998; 83:4459.

70. Khoury EL, Greenspan JS, Greenspan FS. Adrenocortical cells of the zona reticularis normally express HLA-DR antigenic determinants. Am J Pathol 1987; 127:580.

71. Marx C, Bornstein SR, Wolkersdörfer GW, et al. Relevance of major histocompatibility complex class II expression as a hallmark for the cellular differentiation in the human adrenal cortex. J Clin Endocrinol Metab 1997; 82:3136.

72. Wolkersdörfer GW, Bornstein SR. Tissue remodelling in the adrenal gland. Biochem Pharmacol 1998; 56:163.

73. Marx C, Wolkersdörfer GW, Bornstein SR. A new view on immune-adrenal interactions: role for Fas and Fas-ligand? Neuroimmunomodulation 1998; 5:5.

73a. Bornstein SR, Wolkersdörfer GW, Preas HL II, et al. Plasma dehydroepiandrosterone (DHEA) levels during acute experimental endotoxemia and antiinflammatory therapy in humans. Crit Care Med 2000; 28:2103.

74. Norbiato G, Bevilacqua M, Vago T, et al. Cortisol resistance in acquired immunodeficiency syndrome. J Clin Endocrinol Metab 1992; 74:608.

75. Meduri GU, Chrousos GP. Duration of glucocorticoid treatment and outcome in sepsis: is the right drug used the wrong way? Chest 1998; 114:355.

76. Bollaert PE, Charpentier C, Levy B, et al. Reversal of late septic shock with supraphysiological doses of hydrocortisone. Crit Care Med 1998; 26:645.

77. Meduri GU, Headley AS, Golden E, et al. Effect of prolonged methylprednisolone therapy in unresolving acute respiratory distress: a randomized controlled trial. JAMA 1998; 279:159.

78. Bone RC, Fisher CJ Jr, Clemmer TP, et al. Early methylprednisolone treatment for septic syndrome and the adult respiratory distress syndrome. Chest 1987; 92:1032.

79. Sprung CL, Caralis PV, Marcial EH, et al. The effects of high-dose corticosteroids in patients with septic shock. N Engl J Med 1984; 311:1137.

80. Bernard GR, Luce JM, Sprung CL, et al. High-dose corticosteroids in patients with the adult respiratory distress syndrome. N Engl J Med 1987; 317:1565.

81. Hesterberg TW, Last JA. Ozone-induced acute pulmonary fibrosis in rats—prevention of increased rates of collagen synthesis by methylprednisolone. Am Rev Respir Dis 1981; 123:47.

82. Kehrer JP, Klein-Szanto AJP, Sorensen EMB, et al. Enhanced acute lung damage following corticosteroid treatment. Am Rev Respir Dis 1984; 130:256.

83. Bornstein SR, Webster EL, Torpy DJ, et al. Chronic effects of a nonpeptide corticotropin-releasing hormone type I receptor antagonist on pituitary-adrenal function, body weight, and metabolic regulation. Endocrinology 1998; 139:1546.

84. Webster EL, Torpy DJ, Elenkov IJ, Chrousos GP. Corticotropin-releasing hormone and inflammation. Ann N Y Acad Sci 1998; 840:21.

85. Willenberg HS, Bornstein SR, Hiroi N, et al. Effects of a type 1 antagonist on human adrenal function. Mol Psych 2000; 5:137.

---

# CHAPTER 230

# NEUROENDOCRINE RESPONSE TO ACUTE VERSUS PROLONGED CRITICAL ILLNESS

GREET H. VAN DEN BERGHE

## METABOLIC AND IMMUNOLOGIC RESPONSE TO CRITICAL ILLNESS

Throughout evolution, the human species has been selected to survive disease and trauma by the development of defense mechanisms to allow humans to withstand insults—most of them accompanied by temporary starvation—without having to rely on external support. The defensive metabolic response has been described as consisting, first, of an early and brief "ebb phase," during which metabolism and tissue perfusion are jointly reduced and selectively directed toward vital organs such as the brain[1]; subsequently, a hypermetabolic "flow phase" ensues, with activated lipolysis, gluconeogenesis, and protein degradation providing the metabolic substrates for inflammation, for host defense and survival, and for the onset of the healing process.[1–3] If recovery does not follow and exogenous substrates are not provided by refeeding, the adaptive hypercatabolic defense mechanism will use all available vital protein, unequivocally leading to death. This constellation of acute catabolic changes is thought to be evoked at least partly by endocrine changes, which consistently have been viewed as adaptive and beneficial for survival. Endocrine responses include release of catecholamines and glucagon, peripherally regulated alterations in insulin release and sensitivity, activation of the hypothalamic–pituitary–adrenocortical axis (HPA), hypersecretion of prolactin (PRL) and growth hormone (GH) in the presence of low circulating levels of insulin-like growth factor-I (IGF-I), and inactivation of peripheral thyroid hormones and gonadal function[4–11] (see Chap. 228). To what extent some of these defense mechanisms may fail to respond or, alternatively, may hyperrespond and, as a consequence, be harmful, is still unclear. Because they have been continuously selected by the challenges of nature and time, however, little argument presently exists for medical interference with the adaptive endocrine changes that occur during the first hours to days after injury or onset of severe illness.

The development of intensive care unit (ICU) medicine over the past three decades has enabled humans to survive previously lethal conditions such as extensive burn injury, multiple trauma, sepsis, and shock. Although resuscitation is possible, advanced ICU medicine still cannot prevent the development of a chronic phase in which nutritional and vital organ function support, which is clearly beyond the capacity of the natural defense systems, is often required for weeks or months. In the pre-ICU era, patients experiencing these conditions died; therefore, nature is unlikely to have been able to select adequate coping mechanisms for this chronic phase of critical illness and for the ICU care conditions in which survival is made possible. The developments within acute medicine and ICU care have unmasked a particular *wasting syndrome* that was previously unknown: Despite feeding, protein continues to be lost from vital organs and tissues due to both activated degradation and suppressed synthesis, whereas reesterification (instead of oxidation) of free fatty acids allows fat to accumulate, not only in adipocytes but also in organs such as the liver and the pancreas.[12,13] This paradoxic metabolic condition is no longer accompanied by targeted inflammation but rather by an *immune paralysis* or an impaired capacity of the immune system to respond appropriately to an additional toxic or infectious challenge. This condition in itself may become problematic when it lasts for several weeks. Impaired capacity to synthesize protein underlies the inability to restore normal protein content and thereby hampers recovery of the dysfunctioning systems.[13] Muscle atrophy and weakness are some of the most overt functional consequences of protein wasting and provoke, among other problems, failure of the muscular ventilatory system, thus perpetuating the need for mechanical ventilation. Atrophy of the intestinal mucosa and disturbed motility of the gastrointestinal tract prolong the need for parenteral feeding. Fatty infiltration of the liver hampers its vital metabolic role. In addition, delayed tissue repair and immune dysfunction jeopardize the healing process. Hence, dependency on ICU care support is further prolonged.[14,15] The development of this wasting syndrome and ensuing ICU dependency appears to be primarily related not to the type of the initial disease or trauma, but rather to the *duration of the critical condition*.[13] In clinical practice, a limited number of patients on ICUs who have survived an acute life-threatening insult *continue to occupy high-dependency beds for a long time* because of the functional consequences of this particular catabolic state and require a considerable fraction of the resources for ICU care.[14,15] Many of these "long-stay" patients ultimately die from (infectious) complications, to which they are increasingly vulnerable.[14,15]

The anterior pituitary gland has long been known to play a crucial role in normal metabolic and immunologic homeostasis (see Chaps. 227 and 229). Data on pituitary function and its regulation during prolonged critical illness have been scarce, however, and data from models of the acute catabolic state (such as healthy starved volunteers or patients undergoing the perioperative phase of elective surgery, the admission phase of trauma, or acute infection) had been extrapolated—without validation—to this type of protracted catabolic state. The neuroendocrine changes in protracted critical illness are, in fact, quite different from those documented during the first hours or days after onset of a life-threatening disease or trauma.[16–19] This observation was only possible after elimination of important confounding factors such as concomitant medication (e.g., dopamine infusion, which has been shown to profoundly suppress anterior pituitary function).[6,7,16] The novel concept that acute and prolonged critical illness represent *different* neuroendocrine paradigms appears to clarify many of the apparent paradoxes currently found in the literature.

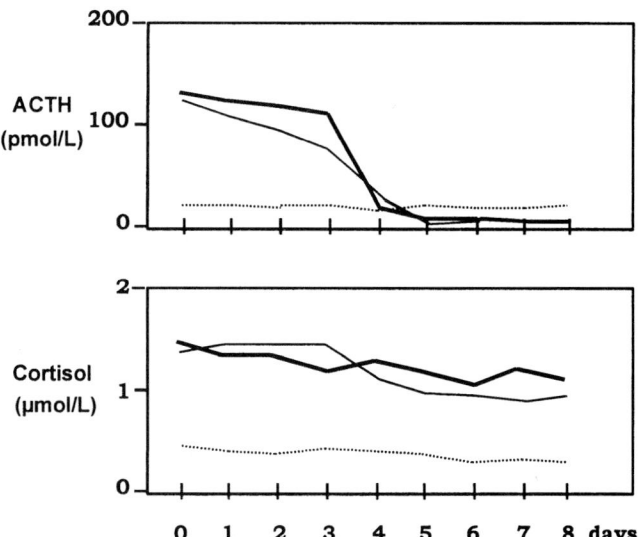

**FIGURE 230-1.** Pituitary-adrenocortical response to severe illness. Mean plasma concentrations of adrenocorticotropic hormone (*ACTH*) and cortisol in patients with sepsis (*thick line*) or multiple traumas (*thin line*) during 8 days after admission to the intensive care unit, in comparison with control subjects (*dotted line*). The initial phase is characterized by an activation of the hypothalamic–pituitary–adrenocortical axis, whereas the subsequent phase is associated with high cortisol and paradoxically low ACTH levels. (Adapted from Vermes I, Bieshuizen A, Hampsink RM, Haanen C. Dissociation of plasma adrenocorticotropin and cortisol levels in critically ill patients: possible role of endothelin and atrial natriuretic hormone. J Clin Endocrinol Metab 1995; 80:1238.)

This chapter makes clear that the acute phase is characterized mainly by an actively secreting anterior pituitary gland and a peripheral inactivation or inactivity of anabolic hormones, whereas *prolonged critical illness is marked by a uniformly reduced neuroendocrine stimulation*, independent of the patient's age, gender, body mass index, or type of underlying disease (Fig. 230-1). The question that arises from this concept is whether the neuroendocrine alterations present during prolonged critical illness should be considered as a *beneficial adaptation* or, rather, as a *neuroendocrine dysfunction*.

## BIPHASIC NEUROENDOCRINE RESPONSE TO CRITICAL ILLNESS

### ADRENOCORTICAL FUNCTION

The activity of the HPA axis displays a biphasic pattern during the course of critical illness.[20] By 1856, Brown-Séquard had noted that immediate postoperative survival depends on adrenal function (see Chap. 74).[21] The high serum cortisol concentrations present during the initial phase after surgery, trauma, or sepsis are associated with augmented adrenocorticotropic hormone (ACTH) release, which, in turn, is driven by corticotropin-releasing hormone (CRH), cytokines, and the noradrenergic system[4,22–24] (see Chaps. 227–229). Concomitantly, circulating levels of angiotensin II and aldosterone are elevated.[25] The acute cortisol-induced shifts in carbohydrate, fat, and protein metabolism selectively and instantly provide energy to vital organs, such as the brain, and postpone anabolism. Intravascular fluid retention and the enhanced inotropic and vasopressor response to catecholamines and angiotensin II, respectively, offer hemodynamic advantages in the "fight or flight" reflex. In addition, as

virtually all components of the immune response are inhibited by cortisol, the hypercortisolism elicited by acute disease or trauma can be interpreted as an attempt of the organism to mute its own inflammatory cascade, thus protecting itself against overresponses.[26] Therefore, available evidence is still compatible with the time-honored view that the hyperactive state of the HPA axis in acute illness is part of the "wisdom of the body."[27–29]

In prolonged critical illness, serum ACTH is low whereas cortisol concentrations usually remain elevated; this indicates that cortisol release in this phase may be driven by an alternative pathway, possibly involving endothelin[20] (see Chap. 229). Why ACTH levels are low in prolonged critical illness is unclear; a role for atrial natriuretic peptide[20] or substance P[23] has been suggested. In contrast to the situation with serum cortisol, circulating levels of adrenal androgens such as dehydroepiandrosterone sulfate (DHEAS), which has immunostimulatory effects on type 1 helper T cells ($T_H1$), are low during prolonged critical illness.[30–32] Moreover, despite increased plasma renin activity, paradoxically decreased concentrations of aldosterone are found in protracted critically ill patients.[33] This constellation suggests a *shift of pregnenolone metabolism away from both mineralocorticoid and adrenal androgen pathways toward the glucocorticoid pathway, orchestrated by a peripheral drive*. Also the latter mechanism may ultimately fail, as indicated by a substantially higher incidence of adrenal insufficiency in prolonged critical illness.[34] Hypercortisolism in the chronic phase of critical illness probably continues to exert its beneficial hemodynamic effects. The benefit for the host defense of a sustained hypercortisolism in the presence of low levels of DHEAS could be questioned, however, as prolonged imbalance between immunosuppressive and immunostimulatory hormones of adrenocortical origin may participate in the increased susceptibility to infectious complications. Other conceivable—although still unproven—drawbacks include impaired wound healing and myopathy, which are often observed during prolonged critical illness.

### SOMATOTROPIC AXIS

The acute-phase response of the somatotropic axis—as evoked by trauma, surgery, or acute infectious disease—has a characteristic presentation. First, circulating levels of GH are elevated[5] (Fig. 230-2). Normally, the serum profile of GH consists of peaks alternating with troughs in which levels are virtually undetectable (see Chap. 12). In acute illness, the total amount of GH released from the somatotropes appears to be increased, and interpulse concentrations of GH are relatively high.[6,7] Second, serum concentrations of IGF-I are low.[6,35,36] The concurrence of elevated GH levels and decreased IGF-I levels has been interpreted as resistance to GH that may be related to decreased GH-receptor expression.[36] Third, changes occur in the circulating IGF-binding proteins (IGFBPs), which regulate IGF-I plasma half-life and bioavailability.[37] The low serum concentrations of IGF-I are associated with low levels of IGFBP-3 and acid-labile subunit (ALS).[11,35,38] The synthesis of these three polypeptides is normally up-regulated by GH and, together, they form a 150-kDa ternary complex in the circulation.[37] In acute illness, increased IGFBP-3–protease activity has been reported, resulting in increased dissociation of IGF-I from the ternary complex and a shortening of the IGF-I plasma half-life.[11,35] IGFBP-1, which normally binds only a small amount of IGF-I compared with IGFBP-3, remains in the circulation, often in quite elevated concentrations.[38,39] As serum concentrations of free fatty acids and glucose are elevated by the acute stress response, and as nonfasting insulin levels are also increased, the possibility exists that the abundantly released GH still exerts direct lipolytic and insulin-antagonizing actions, whereas its indirect

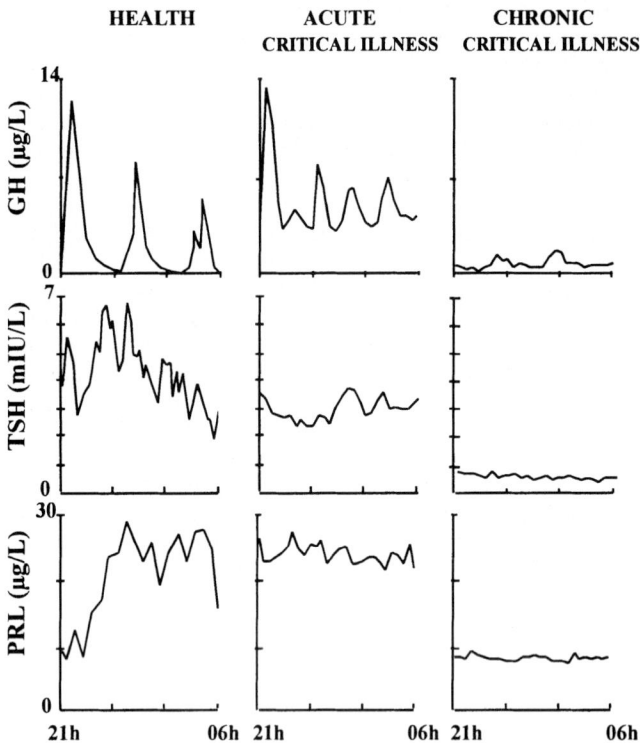

**HEALTH**   **ACUTE CRITICAL ILLNESS**   **CHRONIC CRITICAL ILLNESS**

**FIGURE 230-2.** Nocturnal serum concentration profiles of growth hormone (*GH*), thyroid-stimulating hormone (*TSH*), and prolactin (*PRL*), illustrating the differences between the initial phase and the chronic phase of critical illness in an intensive care setting. (Adapted from Van den Berghe G, de Zegher F, Bouillon R. Acute and chronic critical illness as different neuroendocrine paradigms. J Clin Endocrinol Metab 1998; 83:1827.)

somatotropic effects are attenuated. Inflammatory cytokines may be among the mediators of the aforementioned changes. Alternatively, because most conditions of acute stress are accompanied by starvation or at least a degree of protein malnutrition, nutritional factors may also be involved.[36,40–42] So, in the acute phase of life-threatening disease or trauma, presently *no* solid pathophysiologic basis exists for endocrine intervention. Accordingly, ongoing trials of exogenous GH administration are not expected to demonstrate major benefit in the acute phase of illness.

During prolonged critical illness, a *different* set of changes in the somatotropic axis has been documented. First, the pattern of GH secretion in this condition has been characterized as having a substantially reduced pulsatile fraction (Fig. 230-3) (especially in women)[42a], whereas the nonpulsatile or tonic fraction is still somewhat elevated and the number of pulses is rather high. This pattern results in mean serum GH concentrations that are within normal limits.[17] Moreover, GH is released in an erratic fashion, as indicated by a high calculated approximate entropy.[17,43] At least two hypothalamic regulatory factors, GH-releasing hormone (GHRH) and somatostatin (SRIH), are known to act in concert on the somatotropes to evoke pulsatile GH secretion. A complex interaction with several other neural and hormonal feedback networks results in the normal "volleyed burst-like" pattern, with intravolley peaks proposed to reflect GHRH bursts during nadirs of SRIH secretion. A family of GH-releasing peptides (GHRPs) has been developed that acts at the pituitary gland and the hypothalamus to release GH through activation of a specific receptor that is distinct from the GHRH receptor.[44] Although the exact mechanism of action of these peptides has not been conclusively elucidated, they seem to act in concert

with GHRH, perhaps in part as functional SRIH antagonists. An endogenous GHRP-like ligand and a hypothalamic *U-factor* (unknown factor) by which these GH-releasing peptides affect GH release are postulated but have not yet been identified. The hypothalamic and pituitary receptor for these peptides has been cloned.[45] The blunted and irregular GH secretory pattern observed in prolonged critical illness does not appear to be due to a limited pituitary capacity to synthesize GH, as the somatotropes release large amounts of GH on stimulation with GH secretagogues (Fig. 230-4).[46] The pronounced GH release in response to an intravenous bolus of GHRP, and even more so in response to the combination of GHRH and GHRP,[46] is remarkable, as it appears to overcome a number of normally inhibiting factors present in this condition, such as the nonfasting state; high circulating levels of glucose, insulin, and cortisol; low testosterone levels in males; and sometimes obesity. In prolonged critical illness, the GH response to a GHRH bolus does not appear to be as exaggerated as that to GHRP, suggesting that if a hypothalamic drive of the somatotropic axis is less available, this deficiency is more likely to include the endogenous GHRP-like ligand, rather than GHRH. A reduced inhibitory SRIH tone would be expected to enhance the responses both to GHRH and to GHRP, as well as spontaneous GH secretion. The continuous infusion of GHRP, in contrast to GHRH infusion, has also been documented to substantially increase pulsatile and basal GH secretion without altering the high GH burst frequency[17,19] (Fig. 230-5). Infusing GHRH together with GHRP synergistically increases GH secretion in this condition of prolonged stress.

Second, the reduced amount of GH that is released in pulses during prolonged critical illness appears to be *positively* correlated with low circulating levels of IGF-I (see Fig. 230-3), IGFBP-3, and ALS.[17,19] Indeed, when pulsatile GH secretion falls below a critical threshold during the chronic phase of illness, circulating IGF-I and ALS progressively decrease over time.[19] Low serum IGF-I and, even more so, low levels of ALS are markers of protein wasting in this condition.[11,47] These findings suggest that the neuroendocrine component of the somatotropic axis may participate in the pathogenesis of the wasting syndrome in prolonged critical illness. Infusion of GH secretagogues during this chronic phase of critical illness[17,19] allows the whole somatotropic axis to be reactivated, as evidenced by amplified pulsatile GH secretion followed by increases in the circulating levels of IGF-I, IGFBP-3, and ALS (see Fig. 230-5). Moreover, close correlations have been observed between total or pulsatile GH secretion, on the one hand, and markers of GH responsiveness—in particular, serum levels of IGF-I, ALS, and, to a lesser extent, IGFBP-3—on the other. The correlations documented between variables of GH secretion and indices of responsiveness to GH have exponential regression lines (see Fig. 230-5). This relationship indicates that circulating IGF-I, IGFBP-3, and particularly ALS further increase in proportion to GH secretion up to a certain point, beyond which further increases of GH secretion apparently have little or no additional effect. Of note, the latter point corresponds to a pulsatile GH secretion of ~200 μg/Lv (distribution volume) over ≤9 hours, a value that can be evoked by the infusion of GHRP alone. Together, these findings indicate the presence of considerable responsiveness to restored endogenous pulsatile GH secretion during prolonged critical illness; they thus further delineate its distinct pathophysiologic paradigm, as opposed to that of the acute phase, which is thought to be primarily a condition of GH resistance.[6]

The pathophysiologic basis for *failure to secrete stored GH during prolonged critical illness*, in contrast to starvation or acute illness, is not entirely clear.[17] ICU procedures such as continuous parenteral feeding are unlikely to be important determinants, as intravenous infusion of glucose and fat have been shown to suppress rather than stimulate the responses to GHRPs. Circulating

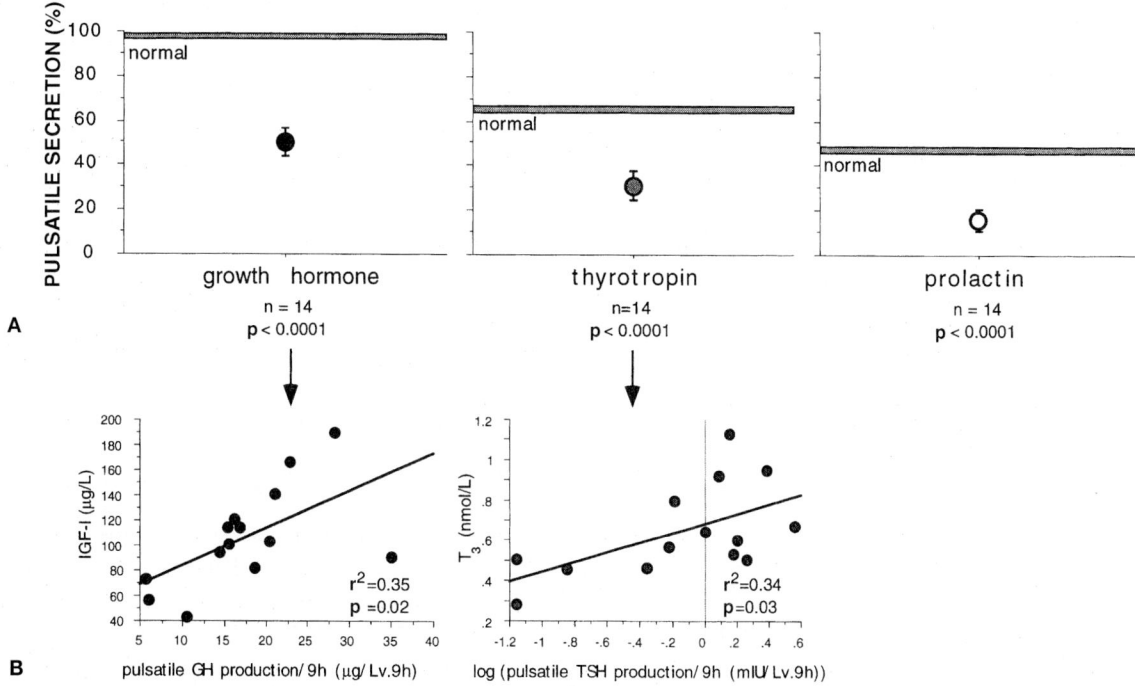

**FIGURE 230-3. A,** In patients with prolonged critical illness, in the presence of low-normal nocturnal serum concentrations (growth hormone [*GH*]: 1.5 ± 0.24 µg/L; thyroid-stimulating hormone [*TSH*]: 1.25 ± 0.42 mIU/L; prolactin [*PRL*]: 9.4 ± 0.9 µg/L), the fraction of hormone released in a pulsatile fashion was consistently reduced for all three hormones (GH: 51 ± 6% vs. normal mean 99%; TSH: 32 ± 6% vs. normal 65%; and PRL: 16 ± 3% vs. normal 48%). Time series were obtained between 9 p.m. and 6 a.m. (Values are mean ± standard error of the mean.) **B,** The reduced nocturnal pulsatile GH and TSH production, calculated with deconvolution analysis as the amount of hormone released in a pulsatile fashion per liter of distribution volume (*Lv*) over 9 hours, correlated positively with, respectively, low circulating insulin-like growth factor-I (*IGF-I*; 106 ± 11 µg/L) and low triiodothyronine (*T₃*; 0.64 ± 0.06 nmol/L). (Adapted from Van den Berghe G, de Zegher F, Veldhuis JD, et al. The somatotropic axis in critical illness: effect of continuous GHRH and GHRP-2 infusion. J Clin Endocrinol Metab 1997; 82:590; and from Van den Berghe G, de Zegher F, Veldhuis JD, et al. Thyrotropin and prolactin release in prolonged critical illness: dynamics of spontaneous secretion and effects of growth hormone secretagogues. Clin Endocrinol 1997; 47:599.)

substances released as a consequence of the inflammatory response to disease or trauma (e.g., tumor necrosis factor-α [TNF-α] and other interleukins) are also candidates to play a role in the pathogenesis of altered GH-secretory control. The circulating levels of these cytokines, however, are often low to undetectable in the chronic phase of critical illness. Alternatively, adaptive mechanisms within the central nervous system, possibly mediated by endogenous dopamine or serotonin, may modulate regulation of GH secretion during chronic stress. As the spontaneous GH secretion is suppressed, which is in contrast to the pronounced responses to GH secretagogues, an altered SRIH secretion alone is unlikely to explain the complete picture. The observed GH-releasing effect of GHRP infusion indicates at least some availability of endogenous GHRH to maintain the synthesis of GH during critical illness. Therefore, a lack of GHRP in combination with a reduced SRIH tone would provide a suitable explanation for the findings in prolonged critical illness.[17,19,46] Infusing GHRP in this condition could accordingly be interpreted as a hypothalamic replacement therapy. From a therapeutic perspective, this provides a pathophysiologic basis for exploring the safety and efficacy of GH-secretagogue administration as a strategy to counter the wasting syndrome and, consequently, to accelerate the process of recovery from prolonged critical illness.

In summary, the *acute* stress-regulated changes within the somatotropic axis appear to consist primarily of an *activated GH secretion and a peripheral shift toward its direct effects*, whereas the *chronic* phase is mainly characterized by a relative *hyposomatotro-*

*pism with a hypothalamic component.* When a *renewed acute phase,* such as an intercurrent infection or an urgent surgical intervention, complicates the chronic phase, *protease activity reappears in serum, and blood levels of IGFBP-3 and IGF-I drop.*[34] In other words, repetitive episodes of GH resistance may appear on a background of relative hyposomatotropism, thus forming mixed conditions that may be difficult to interpret and may explain some of the apparent paradoxes on this issue. Infusion of GH secretagogues precisely in the chronic phase of critical illness amplifies GH secretion, which is followed by a rise in the somatomedins. Supplying a hypothalamic releasing factor allows for feedback inhibition and for peripheral adjustment of metabolic pathways according to the needs determined by the disease. Thus, infusing GH secretagogues may be a safer strategy than the administration of human recombinant GH and/or IGF-I for reversing the wasting syndrome of prolonged critical illness.

### THYROID AXIS

Critical illness is characterized by multiple and complex alterations in the thyroid axis (see Chaps. 30–33).[9,48] Again, a dual presentation appears to exist: Mainly, changes occur in peripheral metabolism, binding, and receptor occupancy of thyroid hormones during acute illness and/or starvation, and a low activity state of primarily neuroendocrine origin occurs in prolonged critical illness (see Fig. 230-3). Mixed forms are again possible and may further complicate the difficult interpretation of thyroid function tests in this setting.

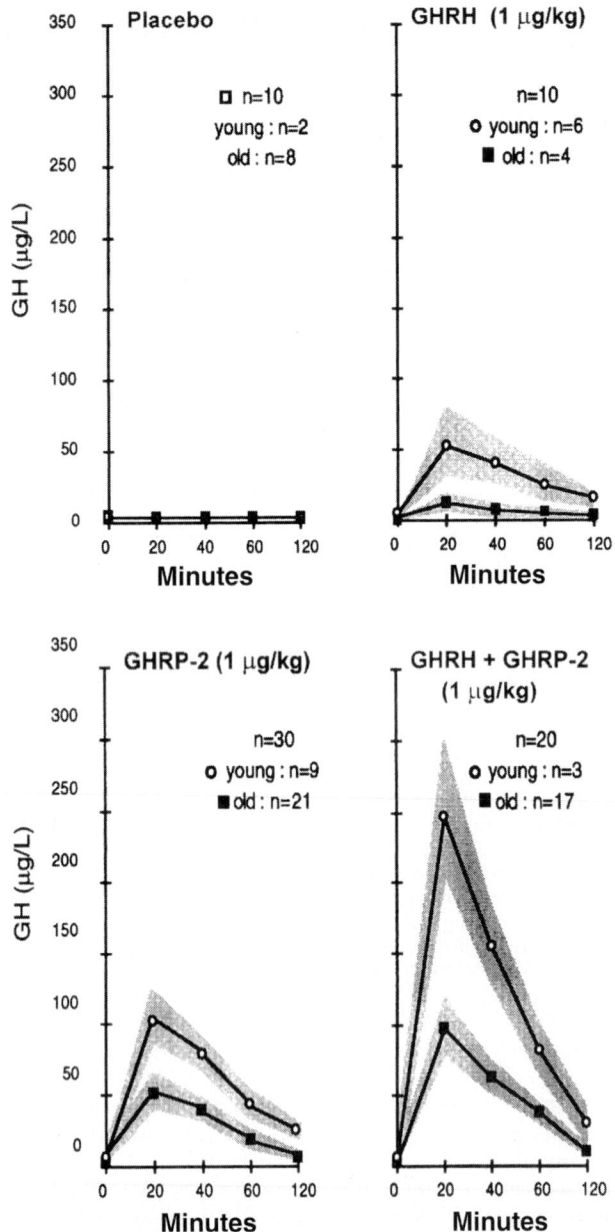

**FIGURE 230-4.** The somatotropes appear to readily release large amounts of growth hormone (*GH*) on stimulation with GH secretagogues. Shown are the serum peak GH responses to placebo, growth hormone–releasing hormone (*GHRH*; 1 µg/kg intravenously [*IV*]), GH-releasing peptide-2 (*GHRP-2*; 1 µg/kg IV), and GHRH plus GHRP-2 (1 + 1 µg/kg IV) obtained in 11 younger critically ill patients (age 28 ± 2.6 years, *open circles*) and 29 older critically ill patients (age 66 ± 2 years, *squares*). *Lines* interlink mean values; *shaded area* indicates mean ± standard error of the mean. (Reproduced from Van den Berghe G, de Zegher F, Bowers CY, et al. Pituitary responsiveness to growth hormone [GH] releasing hormone, GH-releasing peptide-2 and thyrotropin releasing hormone in critical illness. Clin Endocrinol 1996; 45:341.)

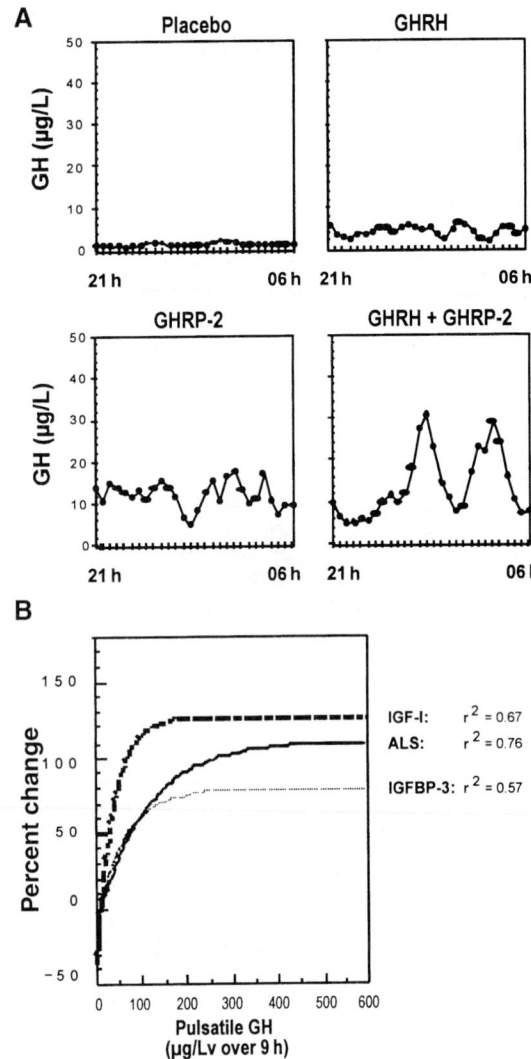

**FIGURE 230-5. A,** Nightly serum growth hormone (*GH*) profiles in the prolonged phase of illness, illustrating the effects of continuous infusion of placebo, growth hormone–releasing hormone (*GHRH*; 1 µg/kg per hour), GH-releasing peptide-2 (*GHRP-2*; 1 µg/kg per hour), or GHRH plus GHRP-2 (1 + 1 µg/kg per hour). Age range of the patients was 62 to 85 years; duration of illness was from 13 to 48 days. Infusions were started 12 hours before the beginning of the respective profiles. **B,** Exponential regression lines have been reported between pulsatile GH secretion and the changes in circulating insulin-like growth factor-I (*IGF-I*), acid-labile subunit (*ALS*), and insulin-like growth factor–binding protein-3 (*IGFBP-3*) obtained with 45-hour infusion of either placebo, GHRP-2, or GHRH plus GHRP-2. They indicate that the parameters of GH responsiveness increase in proportion to GH secretion up to a certain point, beyond which a further increase of GH secretion has apparently little or no additional effect. In the chronic, nonthriving phase of critical illness, GH sensitivity is clearly present; in contrast, the acute phase of illness is thought to be primarily a condition of GH resistance. (**A,** Adapted from Van den Berghe G, de Zegher F, Veldhuis JD, et al. The somatotropic axis in critical illness: effect of continuous GHRH and GHRP-2 infusion. J Clin Endocrinol Metab 1997; 82:590; and from Van den Berghe G, de Zegher F, Baxter RC, et al. On the neuroendocrinology of prolonged critical illness: effect of continuous thyrotropin-releasing hormone infusion and its combination with growth hormone-secretagogues. J Clin Endocrinol Metab 1998; 83:309. **B,** Adapted from Van den Berghe G, de Zegher F, Baxter RC, et al. On the neuroendocrinology of prolonged critical illness: effect of continuous thyrotropin-releasing hormone infusion and its combination with growth hormone-secretagogues. J Clin Endocrinol Metab 1998; 83:309.)

Acute illness or trauma induces alterations in thyroid function within hours. Although serum levels of thyrotropin (thyroid-stimulating hormone, TSH) usually remain normal, circulating triiodothyronine ($T_3$) levels drop rapidly (partly due to decreased conversion of thyroxine [$T_4$] to $T_3$ by 5'-deiodinase).[49] An increased turnover of thyroid hormones may also be involved.[50] The magnitude of the $T_3$ drop within 24 hours reflects the severity of illness.[51,52] Serum reverse $T_3$ (r$T_3$) levels increase, partly due to reduced r$T_3$ degradation.[48] In animal models, hepatic nuclear $T_3$ receptors appear to decrease in number and in occupancy.[53,54] The absence of a TSH elevation in the face of low $T_3$ feedback suggests that a degree of suppression or setpoint alteration also occurs at the hypothalamic-pituitary level.[55–57] Experimental data suggest that enhanced nuclear $T_3$-receptor occupancy within the thyrotropes as well as a reduced expression of the prothyrotropin (TRH) messenger RNA in the paraventricular nucleus could be involved.[56,57] The cytokines TNF-$\alpha$, IL-1, and IL-6 have been investigated as putative mediators of the acute low $T_3$ syndrome.[57–60] Although these cytokines are capable of mimicking the acute stress-induced alterations in thyroid status, cytokine antagonism in sick mice failed to restore normal thyroid function.[61] Endogenous thyroid hormone analogs resulting from alternative deamination and decarboxylation, such as triiodothyroacetic and tetraiodothyroacetic acid, may also participate in the pathogenesis of the low $T_3$ syndrome by blunting the TSH response to low thyroid hormone feedback and by competing with active thyroid hormone for binding to transport proteins.[62,63] Finally, low concentrations of binding proteins and inhibition of hormone binding, transport, and metabolism by elevated levels of free fatty acids and bilirubin have been proposed as factors contributing to the low $T_3$ syndrome at the tissue level.[64] Teleologically, the acute changes in the thyroid axis that occur during starvation have been interpreted as an attempt to reduce energy expenditure[65] and, thus, represent an appropriate response that does not warrant intervention. Whether this is also applicable to other acute stress conditions is conceivable but unproven.

Alterations in the thyroid axis during the prolonged phase of ICU–dependent critical illness appear to be different. Essentially, in the presence of mean nocturnal serum TSH concentrations at the low limit of the normal range, pulsatile TSH secretion is substantially diminished and *positively* related to low serum levels of $T_3$.[18,19] (see Fig. 230-3). The normally occurring nocturnal TSH surge was consistently found to be absent, independent of concomitant sleep.

The suggestion has been made that the low TSH levels of the low $T_3$ syndrome reflect an adaptive pituitary suppression in response to thyroid hormone levels that may be perceived as relatively high for the catabolic condition. According to this hypothesis, one would expect a negative or no correlation between circulating $T_3$ and pituitary TSH secretion. The finding of a positive correlation between reduced pulsatile TSH secretion and serum $T_3$ does not support this hypothesis. The alternative concept of a *true central hypothyroidism* is more plausible. The observation of a normal mean number of TSH bursts and the absence of the nightly TSH surge both support this concept. The exact mechanisms underlying *central hypothyroidism accompanying prolonged critical illness* are still unclear. As TRH is thought to determine the TSH setpoint for feedback inhibition by peripheral thyroid hormone levels, a secretory deficiency of hypothalamic TRH or decreased responsiveness to TRH may be involved. The observation that hypothalamic TRH gene expression is *positively* related to serum $T_3$ after death from prolonged critical illness[66] and the finding that an increase in serum TSH is a marker of the onset of recovery from severe illness[55] support the hypothesis of hypothalamic TRH deficiency. Endogenous dopamine could also play a role, because dopamine has been found to blunt TSH, PRL, and GH secretory patterns in a similar fashion during critical illness, and to decrease pituitary responsiveness to TRH.[16] Likewise, alterations in somatostatin or cortisol secretion could be involved.[67] Endogenous thyroid hormone analogs resulting from alternative deamination and decarboxylation, such as triiodothyroacetic acid and tetraiodothyroacetic acid, may also participate in a decreased pituitary responsiveness to TRH.[62,68,69] Finally, intrapituitary or circulating cytokines may modulate pituitary hormone release.[60,70] The normal TSH pulse frequency during critical illness suggests that the still unidentified pacemakers governing pulsatile hormone release by the thyrotropes are not altered. Uncertainty remains as to whether the low serum and tissue $T_3$ concentrations[71] are involved

in several problems specifically associated with prolonged critical illness, such as diminished cognitive status with lethargy[72]; somnolence or depression; ileus and gallbladder dysfunction; pleural and pericardial effusions; glucose intolerance and insulin resistance; hyponatremia; normocytic normochromic anemia; and deficient clearance of triglycerides.

The hypothesis of a low $T_3$ syndrome of neuroendocrine origin during prolonged critical illness has been further explored by investigating the effect of TRH administration.[19] The thyroid axis of patients in the ICU for long periods can indeed be reactivated by a continuous infusion of TRH, producing TSH secretion in addition to increases in circulating thyroid hormones (Fig. 230-6). Interestingly, coinfusion of TRH and GH-secretagogues has been

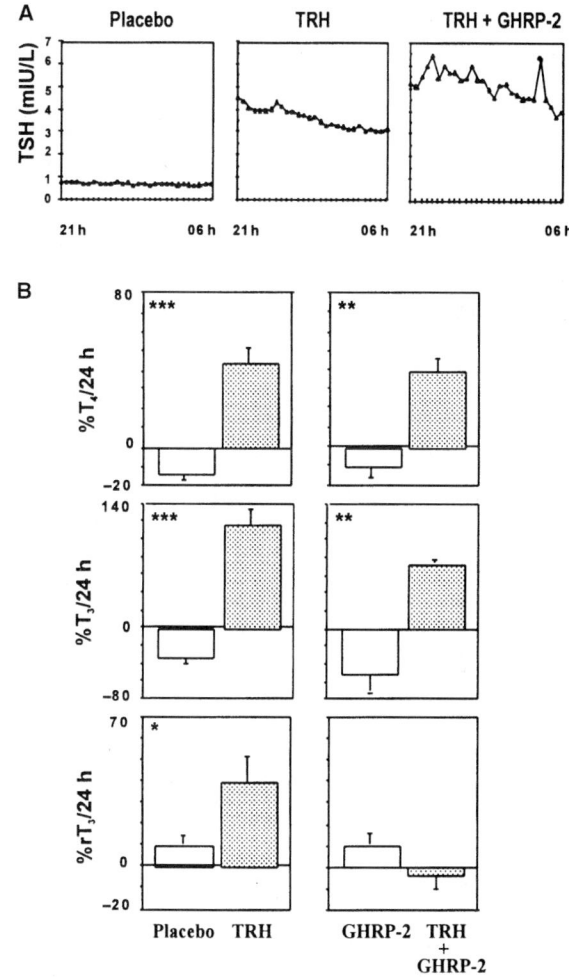

**FIGURE 230-6.** **A,** Nightly serum thyroid-stimulating hormone (*TSH*) profiles in the prolonged phase of illness (duration of illness, 15–18 days; patients' ages, 69–80 years), illustrating the effects of continuous infusion of placebo, thyrotropin-releasing hormone (*TRH*; 1 μg/kg per hour), and TRH plus growth hormone–releasing peptide-2 (*GHRP-2*; 1 + 1 μg/kg per hour). Although TRH elevated TSH secretion, the addition of GHRP-2 to the TRH infusion appeared necessary to increase its pulsatile fraction. **B,** Continuous administration of TRH (1 μg/kg per hour), infused alone or together with GHRP-2 (1 μg/kg per hour), induces a significant rise in serum thyroxine ($T_4$) and triiodothyronine ($T_3$) within 24 hours. The reverse $T_3$ ($rT_3$) level is increased after infusion of TRH alone (n = 8), but not if TRH is coinfused with GHRP-2 (n = 6). Studied patients were ill for 12 to 59 days; age range was 32 to 87 years. Data are presented as the mean ± standard error of the mean. *$p < .05$; **$p < .001$; ***$p < .0001$. (Adapted from Van den Berghe G, de Zegher F, Baxter RC, et al. On the neuroendocrinology of prolonged critical illness: effect of continuous thyrotropin-releasing hormone infusion and its combination with growth hormone-secretagogues. J Clin Endocrinol Metab 1998; 83:309.)

found to be necessary to increase the *pulsatile* fraction of TSH release. Moreover, continuous infusion of TRH alone results in a striking increase not only of serum $T_4$ and $T_3$ but also of circulating $rT_3$, indicating incomplete peripheral conversion of increased $T_4$ into $T_3$. When TRH was infused together with GHRP or with both GHRH and GHRP, circulating $rT_3$ was not altered. This finding suggests that the concomitant increase of GH secretion amplifies the efficacy of the peripheral conversion of increased $T_4$ into $T_3$, as has been defined in earlier independent studies of GH action (see Fig. 230-6). The effect of TRH infusion in critically ill patients seems to be self-limiting; once serum $T_3$ approaches the upper-normal range, the TSH response to TRH decreases (Fig. 230-7). Thus, TRH infusion does not appear to overcome the negative feedback exerted by thyroid hormones at the pituitary level, which serves as a safety mechanism preventing overstimulation of the thyroid gland. Consequently, the continuous infusion of TRH (as compared to $T_4$ or $T_3$ administration) theoretically appears to be a safer strategy for driving the thyrotropic axis in prolonged critical illness.[19] Moreover, TRH infusion in this condition allows for peripheral shifts in thyroid hormone metabolism to occur in response to the specific metabolic needs imposed by

intercurrent acute insults. This may reflect another safety aspect, which may explain why earlier therapeutic attempts using $T_4$ or $T_3$ administration have failed to demonstrate clinical benefit.[73,74]

## GONADAL AXIS

A variety of catabolic states are associated with low serum testosterone levels in men. These conditions include starvation,[75,76] the acute posttraumatic phase,[8,77] burn injury,[78,79] psychological and physical stress,[80,81] and prolonged critical illness.[82] *Acute injury* appears to lead primarily to an *immediate and direct gonadal suppression*. Indeed, low testosterone concentrations and increased levels of luteinizing hormone (LH) are evoked by the acute stress of surgery, in the presence of normal levels of follicle-stimulating hormone (FSH) and inhibin.[8,77,83] The mechanisms underlying the decreased Leydig cell responsiveness in humans remain largely unknown. A role for inflammatory cytokines (IL-1 and IL-2) is possible, as suggested by experimental studies.[84,85] Teleologically, it may be appropriate that androgen secretion is switched off in circumstances of acute stress.

When a severe stress condition is *prolonged, hypogonadotropic hypogonadism ensues.*[78,86] The decrease in gonadotropin secretion apparently occurs within a shorter time frame than the suppression of ACTH, GH, and TSH.[77] In men with long-term critical illness, mainly the pulsatile fraction of LH release appears to be attenuated.[82] A reversible reduction of LH and FSH secretion—and of serum estradiol concentrations—has also been observed in critically ill women and has been correlated with outcome.[86–88] Endogenous dopamine or opiates could be involved in the pathogenesis of hypogonadotropic hypogonadism, as iatrogenic factors such as exogenous dopamine and opioids may further diminish blunted LH secretion.[82,89] Animal data suggest that prolonged exposure of the brain to IL-1 could also play a role by suppressing LH-releasing hormone (LHRH) synthesis.[84]

The pioneering studies evaluating androgen treatment as an anabolic strategy for protein wasting induced by critical illness failed to demonstrate conclusive clinical benefit.[90] In view of the secretory characteristics of the other anterior pituitary hormones during prolonged critical illness, the therapeutic potential of androgens should perhaps be reappraised in a combined treatment regimen. In analogy with the strategy for reactivating the somatotropic and thyrotropic axes, the effects of pulsatile gonadotropin-releasing hormone (GnRH) administration, alone and in combination with GHRP and TRH, during the prolonged phase of critical illness are currently being explored.

## PROLACTIN

Serum PRL has long been known to rise in response to acute physical or psychological stress in humans,[5] a rise that may be mediated by cytokine or dopaminergic pathways.[91,92] Although PRL appears to have immunostimulatory properties in animal models and in humans,[92] whether the rise in serum PRL in response to acute illness or trauma contributes to the initially activated immune response remains unclear.

In prolonged critical illness, PRL is no longer elevated, and the secretory pattern is characterized by a reduction in the pulsatile fraction[18,19] (see Figs. 230-2 and 230-3). Whether the blunted secretory pattern of PRL secretion plays a role in the anergic immune dysfunction or in the increased susceptibility for infections characterizing the chronically ill is unknown.[15,93] Dopamine, which is often infused as an inotropic and vasoactive supportive agent in ICU-dependent patients, has been found to suppress PRL secretion (in addition to DHEAS secretion) without altering elevated serum cortisol levels.[31,69] It also has been shown to concomitantly aggravate both T-lymphocyte dysfunction and impaired neutrophil chemotaxis in this condition.[94]

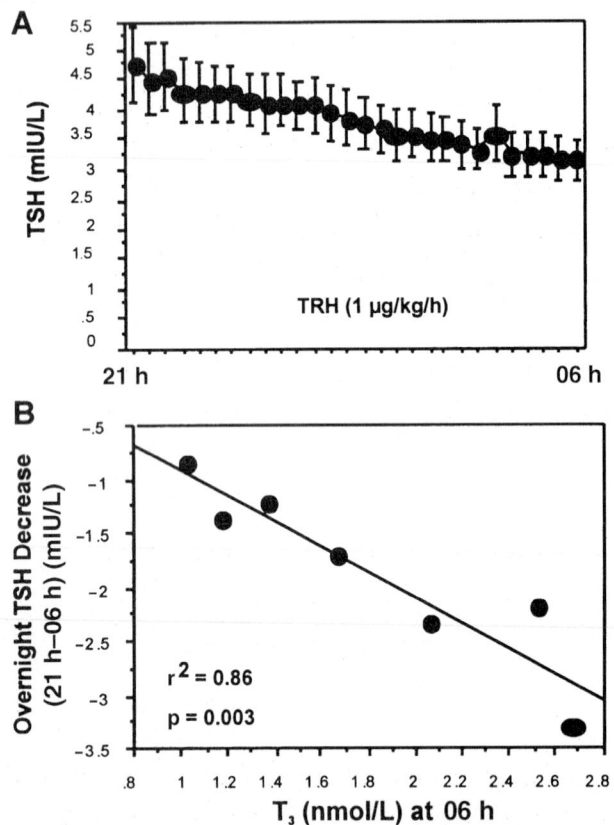

**FIGURE 230-7.** The effect of thyrotropin-releasing hormone (*TRH*) infusion in prolonged critically ill patients appears to be self-limiting. Once serum triiodothyronine (*$T_3$*) approaches the upper-normal range, the thyroid-stimulating hormone (*TSH*) response to TRH decreases, suggesting feedback inhibition. **A,** Serum TSH concentrations (mean ± standard error of the mean) between 9 p.m. and 6 a.m. during a TRH infusion (1 μg/kg per hour) that was started at 9 a.m. (n = 8). In all but one patient, the TSH concentration was significantly lower at 6 a.m. than at 9 p.m. **B,** The overnight TSH decrease (difference between 6 a.m. and 9 p.m. serum TSH concentrations) correlated with the serum $T_3$ concentration measured at the end of the TRH infusion (at 6 a.m.). (Reproduced from Van den Berghe G, de Zegher F, Veldhuis JD, et al. Thyrotropin and prolactin release in prolonged critical illness: dynamics of spontaneous secretion and effects of growth hormone secretagogues. Clin Endocrinol 1997; 47:599.)

# CONCLUSION

Acute and prolonged critical illness are *different* neuroendocrine paradigms and should, perhaps, be approached with different therapeutic strategies. The acute response to severe illness or trauma consists primarily of an actively secreting anterior pituitary gland and a peripheral inactivation or inactivity of anabolic target-organ hormones. These changes may contribute to the provision of metabolic substrates essential for survival, to postponement of energy- and substrate-consuming anabolism, and to the activation of the immune response, while the host is being protected against deleterious systemic effects of the latter. At present, *no* pathophysiologic basis exists for hormonal treatment in this acute phase. The development of modern ICU care led to survival from previously lethal conditions and unmasked newly recognized disorders such as the wasting syndrome. In the chronic phase of critical illness, a uniformly reduced pulsatile secretion of the different anterior pituitary hormones has been found to underlie impaired secretory activity of target tissues, a finding that was independent of the patient's age, gender, body mass index, or type of underlying disease. Cortisol secretion appears to be a notable exception and is usually maintained through a peripheral drive. An acute event complicating the chronic phase of illness, such as an intercurrent infection or a surgical intervention in a patient with a long stay in the ICU, may be accompanied by mixed acute/prolonged endocrine patterns, which are difficult to interpret and may account for some of the apparently conflicting data in the literature.[95] That the reduced neuroendocrine stimulation distinctly present in the chronic phase of illness has been selected for by evolution and should accordingly be considered as time honored and appropriate is unlikely. The hypothesis of a reduced neuroendocrine drive can be validated by studying the effects either of combined peripheral hormonal substitution or of hypophysiotropic-releasing peptide administration. Selected pituitary-dependent axes have been shown to be readily reactivated in the chronic phase of critical illness, with preserved pulsatility and peripheral responsiveness. Intervening at the hypothalamic-pituitary level may eventually appear to be a safer strategy than the administration of peripheral hormones, as the presence of active feedback inhibition and the allowance for alterations in the peripheral activity of these pathways protects from dose-related side effects at a time when determining what is a "normal" or "optimal" circulating level of peripheral hormones is difficult, if not impossible.

# REFERENCES

1. Cuthbertson DP. Observations on the disturbance of metabolism produced by injury to the limbs. QJM 1932; 25:233.
2. Kinney JM, Duke JH, Long CL, Gump FE. Tissue fuel and weight loss after injury. J Clin Pathol 1970; 23:65.
3. Cahill GF. Starvation in man. N Engl J Med 1970; 12:668.
4. Chrousos GP. The hypothalamic-pituitary adrenal axis and immune-mediated inflammation. N Engl J Med 1995; 332:1351.
5. Noel GL, Suh HK, Stone SJG, Frantz AE. Human prolactin and growth hormone release during surgery and other conditions of stress. J Clin Endocrinol Metab 1972; 35:840.
6. Ross R, Miell J, Freeman E, et al. Critically ill patients have high basal growth hormone levels with attenuated oscillatory activity associated with low levels of insulin-like growth factor-1. Clin Endocrinol 1991; 35:47.
7. Voerman HJ, Strack van Schijndel RJM, de Boer H, et al. Growth hormone: secretion and administration in catabolic adult patients, with emphasis on the critically ill patient. Neth J Med 1992; 41:229.
8. Wang C, Chan V, Yeung RTT. Effect of surgical stress on pituitary-testicular function. Clin Endocrinol 1978; 9:255.
9. Chopra IJ. Euthyroid sick syndrome: is it a misnomer? J Clin Endocrinol Metab 1997; 82:329.
10. Utiger RD. Decreased extrathyroidal triiodothyronine production in nonthyroidal illness: benefit or harm? Am J Med 1980; 69:807.
11. Baxter RC. Acquired growth hormone insensitivity and insulin-like growth factor bioavailability. Endocrinol Metab 1997; 4(Suppl B):65.
12. Streat SJ, Beddoe AH, Hill GL. Aggressive nutritional support does not prevent protein loss despite fat gain in septic intensive care patients. J Trauma 1987; 27:262.
13. Gamrin L, Essén P, Forsberg AM, et al. A descriptive study of skeletal muscle metabolism in critically ill patients: free amino acids, energy-rich phosphates, protein, nucleic acids, fat, water, and electrolytes. Crit Care Med 1996; 24:575.
14. Madoff RD, Sharpe SM, Fath JJ, et al. Prolonged surgical intensive care. A useful allocation of medical resources. Arch Surg 1985; 120:698.
15. Goins WA, Reynolds HN, Nyanjom D, Dunham CM. Outcome following prolonged intensive care unit stay in multiple trauma patients. Crit Care Med 1991; 19:339.
16. Van den Berghe G, de Zegher F. Anterior pituitary function during critical illness and dopamine treatment. Crit Care Med 1996; 24:1580.
17. Van den Berghe G, de Zegher F, Veldhuis JD, et al. The somatotropic axis in critical illness: effect of continuous GHRH and GHRP-2 infusion. J Clin Endocrinol Metab 1997; 82:590.
18. Van den Berghe G, de Zegher F, Veldhuis JD, et al. Thyrotropin and prolactin release in prolonged critical illness: dynamics of spontaneous secretion and effects of growth hormone secretagogues. Clin Endocrinol 1997; 47:599.
19. Van den Berghe G, de Zegher F, Baxter RC, et al. On the neuroendocrinology of prolonged critical illness: effect of continuous thyrotropin-releasing hormone infusion and its combination with growth hormone-secretagogues. J Clin Endocrinol Metab 1998; 83:309.
20. Vermes I, Bieshuizen A, Hampsink RM, Haanen C. Dissociation of plasma adrenocorticotropin and cortisol levels in critically ill patients: possible role of endothelin and atrial natriuretic hormone. J Clin Endocrinol Metab 1995; 80:1238.
21. Brown-Séquard CE. Recherches expérimentales sur la physiologie et la pathologie des capsules surrénales. C R Acad Sci Paris 1856; 43:422.
22. Rivier C, Vale W. Modulation of stress induced ACTH release by corticotropin-releasing factor, catecholamines and vasopressin. Nature 1983; 305:325.
23. Dallman MF. Stress update: adaptation of the hypothalamic-pituitary-adrenal axis to chronic stress. Trends Endocrinol Metab 1993; 4:62.
24. Harbuz MS, Rees RG, Eckland D, et al. Paradoxical responses of hypothalamic corticotropin-releasing factor (CRF) messenger ribonucleic acid (mRNA) and CRF peptide and adenohypophysial proopiomelanocortin mRNA during chronic inflammatory stress. Endocrinology 1992; 130:1394.
25. O'Leary E, Hubbard K, Tormey W, Cunningham AJ. Laparoscopic cholecystectomy: hemodynamic and neuroendocrine responses after pneumoperitoneum and changes in position. Br J Anaesth 1996; 76:640.
26. Munck A, Guyre P, Holbrook N. Physiological functions of glucocorticoids during stress and their relation to pharmacological actions. Endocr Rev 1984; 5:25.
27. Starling EH. The wisdom of the body. The Harveian Oration delivered to the Royal College of Physicians, London, 1923. London: H. K. Lewis, 1923.
28. Cannon WB. The wisdom of the body. New York: WW Norton, 1932.
29. Selye H. The physiology and pathology of exposure to stress. Montreal: Acta, 1950.
30. Suzuki T, Suzuki N, Daynes RA, Engleman EG. Dehydroepiandrosterone enhances IL2 production and cytotoxic effector function of human T-cells. Clin Immunol Immunopathol 1991; 61:202.
31. Parker LN, Levin ER, Lifrak ET. Evidence for adrenocortical adaptation to severe illness. J Clin Endocrinol Metab 1985; 60:947.
32. Van den Berghe G, de Zegher F, Schetz M, et al. Dehydroepiandrosterone sulphate in critical illness: effect of dopamine. Clin Endocrinol 1995; 43:457.
33. Zipser RD, Davenport MW, Martin KL, et al. Hyperreninemic hypoaldosteronism in the critically ill: a new entity. J Clin Endocrinol Metab 1981; 53:867.
34. Barquist E, Kirton O. Adrenal insufficiency in the surgical intensive care unit patient. J Trauma 1997; 42:27.
35. Timmins AC, Cotterill AM, Cwyfan Hughes SC, et al. Critical illness is associated with low circulating concentrations of insulin-like growth factors-I and -II, alterations in insulin-like growth factor binding proteins, and induction of an insulin-like growth factor binding protein 3 protease. Crit Care Med 1996; 24:1460.
36. Hermansson M, Wickelgren RB, Hammerqvist F, et al. Measurement of human growth hormone receptor messenger ribonucleic acid by a quantitative polymerase chain reaction-based assay: demonstration of reduced expression after elective surgery. J Clin Endocrinol Metab 1997; 82:421.
37. Baxter RC. Insulin-like growth factor binding proteins in the human circulation: a review. Horm Res 1994; 42:140.
38. Ghahary A, Fu S, Shen YJ, et al. Differential effects of thermal injury on circulating insulin-like growth factor binding proteins in burn patients. Mol Cell Biochem 1994; 135:171.
39. Ross RJM, Miell JP, Holly JMP, et al. Levels of GH-binding activity, IGFBP, insulin, blood glucose and cortisol in intensive care patients. Clin Endocrinol 1991; 35:361.
40. Hartman ML, Veldhuis JD, Johnson ML, et al. Augmented growth hormone secretory burst frequency and amplitude mediate enhanced GH secretion during a two day fast in normal men. J Clin Endocrinol Metab 1992; 74:757.
41. Thissen JP, Ketelslegers J-M, Underwood LE. Nutritional regulation of insulin-like growth factors. Endocr Rev 1994; 15:80.
42. Souba WW. Nutritional support. N Engl J Med 1997; 336:41.

42a. Van den Berghe GH, Baxter RC, Weekers F, et al. A paradoxical gender dissociation within the growth hormone/insulin-like growth factor/axis during protracted critical illness. J Clin Endocrinol Metab 2000; 85:183.

43. Pincus SM. Approximate entropy as a measure of system complexity. Proc Natl Acad Sci U S A 1991; 88:2297.

44. Bowers CY, Momany FA, Reynolds GA, Hong A. On the in vitro and in vivo activity of a new synthetic hexapeptide that acts on the pituitary to specifically release growth hormone. Endocrinology 1984; 114:1537.

45. Howard AD, Feighner SD, Cully DF, et al. A receptor in pituitary and hypothalamus that functions in growth hormone release. Science 1996; 273:974.

46. Van den Berghe G, de Zegher F, Bowers CY, et al. Pituitary responsiveness to growth hormone (GH) releasing hormone, GH-releasing peptide-2 and thyrotropin releasing hormone in critical illness. Clin Endocrinol 1996; 45:341.

47. Hawker FH, Steward PM, Baxter RC, et al. Relationship of somatomedin-C/insulin-like growth factor-I levels to conventional nutritional indices in critically ill patients. Crit Care Med 1987; 15:732.

48. Wartofsky L, Burman KD. Alterations in thyroid function in patients with systemic illness: the "euthyroid sick syndrome." Endocr Rev 1982; 3:164.

49. Chopra IJ, Huang TS, Beredo A, et al. Evidence for an inhibitor of extrathyroidal conversion of thyroxine to 3,5,3'-triiodothyronine in sera of patients with non-thyroidal illness. J Clin Endocrinol Metab 1985; 60:666.

50. Kaptein EM, Grieb DA, Spencer C, et al. Thyroxine metabolism in the low thyroxine state of critical non-thyroidal illnesses. J Clin Endocrinol Metab 1981; 53:764.

51. Schlienger JL, Sapin R, Capgras T, et al. Evaluation of thyroid function after myocardial infarction. Ann Endocrinol 1991; 52:283.

52. Rothwell PM, Lawler PG. Prediction of outcome in intensive care patients using endocrine parameters. Crit Care Med 1995; 23:78.

53. Carr FE, Seelig S, Mariash CN, et al. Starvation and hypothyroidism exert an overlapping influence on rat hepatic messenger RNA activity profiles. J Clin Invest 1983; 72:154.

54. Thompson P Jr, Burman KD, Lukes YG, et al. Uremia decreases nuclear 3,5,3'-triiodothyronine receptors in rats. Endocrinology 1980; 107:1081.

55. Bacci V, Schussler GC, Kaplan TC. The relationship between serum triiodothyronine and thyrotropin during systemic illness. J Clin Endocrinol Metab 1982; 54:1229.

56. St. Germain DL, Galton VA. Comparative study of pituitary-thyroid economy in fasting and hypothyroid rats. J Clin Invest 1985; 75:679.

57. Kakucska I, Romero LI, Clark BD, et al. Suppression of thyrotropin-releasing hormone gene expression by interleukin-1-beta in the rat: implications for nonthyroidal illness. Neuroendocrinology 1994; 59:129.

58. Van der Poll T, Romijn JA, Wiersinga WM, Sauerwein HP. Tumor necrosis factor: a putative mediator of the sick euthyroid syndrome in man. J Clin Endocrinol Metab 1990; 71:1567.

59. Stouthard JML, van der Poll T, Endert E, et al. Effects of acute and chronic interleukin-6 administration on the thyroid hormone metabolism in humans. J Clin Endocrinol Metab 1994; 79:1342.

60. Van der Poll T, van Zee K, Endert E, et al. Interleukin-1 receptor blockade does not affect endotoxin-induced changes in plasma thyroid hormone and thyrotropin concentration in man. J Clin Endocrinol Metab 1995; 80:1341.

61. Boelen A, Platvoet-ter Schiphorst MC, Bakker O, Wiersinga WM. The role of cytokines in the LPS-induced sick euthyroid syndrome in mice. J Endocrinol 1995; 146:475.

62. Carlin K, Carlin S. Possible etiology for euthyroid sick syndrome. Med Hypotheses 1993; 40:38.

63. Everts ME, Visser TJ, Moerings EP, et al. Uptake of triiodothyroacetic acid and its effect on thyrotropin secretion in cultured anterior pituitary cells. Endocrinology 1994; 135:2700.

64. Lim CF, Doctor R, Visser TJ, et al. Inhibition of thyroxine transport into cultured rat hepatocytes by serum of non-uremic critically ill patients: effects of bilirubin and non-esterified fatty acids. J Clin Endocrinol Metab 1993; 76:1165.

65. Gardner DF, Kaplan MM, Stanley CA, Utiger RD. Effect of triiodothyronine replacement on the metabolic and pituitary responses to starvation. N Engl J Med 1979; 300:579.

66. Fliers E, Guldenaar SEF, Wiersinga WM, Swaab DF. Decreased hypothalamic thyrotropin-releasing hormone gene expression in patients with nonthyroidal illness. J Clin Endocrinol Metab 1997; 82:4032.

67. Faglia G, Ferrari C, Beck-Peccoz P, et al. Reduced plasma thyrotropin response to thyrotropin releasing hormone after dexamethasone administration in normal humans. Horm Metab Res 1973; 5:289.

68. Van den Berghe G, de Zegher F, Lauwers P. Dopamine and the sick euthyroid syndrome in critical illness. Clin Endocrinol 1994; 41:731.

69. Van den Berghe G, de Zegher F, Vlasselaers F, et al. Thyrotropin releasing hormone in critical illness: from a dopamine-dependent test to a strategy for increasing low serum triiodothyronine, prolactin and growth hormone. Crit Care Med 1996; 24:590.

70. Damas P, Reuter A, Gysen P, et al. Tumor necrosis factor and interleukin-1 serum levels during severe sepsis in humans. Crit Care Med 1989; 17:975.

71. Arem R, Wiener GJ, Kaplan SG, et al. Reduced tissue thyroid hormone levels in fatal illness. Metabolism 1993; 42:1102.

72. Vaughan GM, Mason AD, McManus WF, Pruitt BA Jr. Alterations of mental status and thyroid hormones after thermal injury. J Clin Endocrinol Metab 1985; 60:1221.

73. Brent GA, Hershman JM. Thyroxine therapy in patients with severe nonthyroidal illnesses and low serum thyroxine concentrations. J Clin Endocrinol Metab 1986; 63:1.

74. Becker RA, Vaughan GM, Ziegler MG, et al. Hypermetabolic low triiodothyronine syndrome in burn injury. Crit Care Med 1982; 10:870.

75. Klibanski A, Beitens IZ, Badger TM, et al. Reproductive function during fasting in man. J Clin Endocrinol Metab 1981; 53:258.

76. Veldhuis JD, Iranmanesh A, Evans WS, et al. Amplitude suppression of the pulsatile mode of immunoradiometric LH release in fasting-induced hypoandrogenemia in normal men. J Clin Endocrinol Metab 1993; 76:587.

77. Wang C, Chan V, Tse TF, Yeung RT. Effect of acute myocardial infarction on pituitary testicular function. Clin Endocrinol 1978; 9:249.

78. Vogel AV, Peake GT, Rada RT. Pituitary-testicular axis dysfunction in burned men. J Clin Endocrinol Metab 1985; 60:658.

79. Lephart ED, Baxter CR, Parker CR Jr. Effect of burn trauma on adrenal and testicular steroid hormone production. J Clin Endocrinol Metab 1987; 64:842.

80. Kreutz LD, Rose RM, Jennings JR. Suppression of plasma testosterone levels and psychological stress: a longitudinal study of young men in officer candidate school. Arch Gen Psychiatry 1972; 26:479.

81. Aakvaag A, Bentdal O, Quigstad K, et al. Testosterone and testosterone binding globulin in young men during prolonged stress. Int J Androl 1978; 1:22.

82. Van den Berghe G, de Zegher F, Lauwers P, Veldhuis JD. Luteinizing hormone secretion and hypoandrogenemia in critically ill men: effect of dopamine. Clin Endocrinol 1994; 41:563.

83. Dong Q, Hawker F, McWilliam D, et al. Circulating immunoreactive inhibin and testosterone levels in patients with critical illness. Clin Endocrinol 1992; 36:399.

84. Rivier C, Vale W. In the rat, interleukin 1-a acts at the level of the brain and the gonads to interfere with gonadotropin and sex steroid secretion. Endocrinology 1989; 124:2105.

85. Guo H, Calkins JH, Sigel MM, Lin T. Interleukin-2 is a potent inhibitor of Leydig cell steroidogenesis. Endocrinology 1990; 127:1234.

86. Woolf PD, Hamill RW, McDonald JV, et al. Transient hypogonadotropic hypogonadism caused by critical illness. J Clin Endocrinol Metab 1985; 60:444.

87. Van Steenbergen W, Naert J, Lambrecht S, et al. Suppression of gonadotropin secretion in the hospitalized postmenopausal female as an effect of acute illness. Neuroendocrinology 1994, 60:165.

88. Spratt DI, Cox P, Orav J, et al. Reproductive axis suppression in acute illness is related to disease severity. J Clin Endocrinol Metab 1993; 76:1548.

89. Cicero TJ, Bell RD, Wiest WG, et al. Function of the male sex organs in heroin and methadone users. N Engl J Med 1975; 292:882.

90. Tweedle D, Walton C, Johnston IDA. The effect of an anabolic steroid on postoperative nitrogen balance. Br J Clin Pract 1972; 27:130.

91. Ben-Jonathan N. Dopamine: a prolactin-inhibiting hormone. Endocr Rev 1985; 6:564.

92. Reichlin S. Neuroendocrine-immune interactions. N Engl J Med 1993; 329:1246.

93. Meakins JL, Pietsch JB, Bubenick O, et al. Delayed hypersensitivity: indicator of acquired failure of host defenses in sepsis and trauma. Ann Surg 1977; 188:241.

94. Devins SS, Miller A, Herndon BL, et al. Effects of dopamine on T-lymphocyte proliferative responses and serum prolactin concentrations in critically ill patients. Crit Care Med 1992; 263:9682.

95. Van den Berghe GH. Increased mortality associated with growth hormone treatment in critically ill adults. N Engl J Med 2000; 342:135.

# CHAPTER 231

# FUEL METABOLISM AND NUTRIENT DELIVERY IN CRITICAL ILLNESS

THOMAS R. ZIEGLER

## HORMONAL RESPONSES AND FUEL METABOLISM IN CRITICAL ILLNESS

Critical illness after stresses such as major trauma, sepsis/infection, burns, or severe inflammation induces a complex hormonal milieu associated with classic alterations in amino acid, fat, and carbohydrate metabolism.[1-5] In comparison with healthy individuals, patients with severe illness exhibit major changes in endocrinologic functions, including activation of the hypothalamic–pituitary–adrenocortical (HPA) axis, increased secretion of counterregulatory hormones, release of cytokines from stimulated immune cells and other cell types, altered thyroid hormone metabolism, diminished secretion of gonadal steroids, decreased circulating levels of insulin-like growth factor-I (IGF-I) and its major carrier protein IGF-binding protein-3 (IGFBP-3), and peripheral tissue resistance to anabolic hormones (insulin, growth hormone [GH], and IGF-I) (see Chaps. 227–230). Stimulation of protein breakdown by cytokines and counterregulatory hormones and decreased secretion and/or tissue resistance to endogenous anabolic mediators are major contributors to the marked protein-catabolic response that is characteristic in critical illness.[6]

As outlined later, these hormonal alterations serve to increase availability of metabolic substrates and fuels (e.g., glucose, amino acids, free fatty acids) critical for organ function, wound healing, and host survival. Concomitantly, anabolic and reproductive functions are inhibited. The stimuli that induce the classic neuroendocrine responses to stress are common and frequently recurrent in intensive care unit (ICU) patients. These include hemorrhage and volume depletion, decreased oxygen availability, acidosis, fever, infection, inflammation, traumatic tissue damage, pain, and emotional stress.[1,2] If the inciting events are minor and limited in duration, restoration of metabolic and immune homeostasis occurs as the patient recovers. With severe or persistent stress, however, hormonally mediated events contribute to the patient's morbidity and prolong the convalescence (Fig. 231-1). For example, skeletal muscle atrophy and weakness due to peripheral amino-acid mobilization, infection associated with hyperglycemia, and tissue injury due to the effects of cytokines and cortisol may occur.[7,8]

## METABOLIC RESPONSE PATTERNS IN INTENSIVE CARE UNIT PATIENTS

Temporally distinct metabolic response patterns have been described after severe trauma or burn injury. The early *ebb phase* and the later *postresuscitation flow phase* are followed by the period of convalescence (Table 231-1). The effects of severe illness on fuel metabolism are largely mediated by the classic endocrine hormones, although the contribution of numerous cytokines is being increasingly elucidated.[1–4] Temporal responses have been better defined in patients experiencing traumatic injury than in patients with sepsis or other medical conditions, in whom the timing of the initiating stress may be uncertain. The ebb phase occurs during the first 24 to 36 hours after injury when fluid volume may be depleted, cardiac function is diminished, and tissue perfusion is reduced.[2] In trauma patients, this acute period is often characterized by a general reduction in metabolic rate and oxygen consumption and/or by reduced body temperature. Nitrogen loss is generally minor, whereas lipolytic and endogenous glucose production rates are increased to provide critical metabolic fuels (i.e., free fatty acids and glucose) to vital organs such as cardiac muscle and brain. Counterregulatory hormone concentrations are increased whereas insulin levels are generally reduced at this early time point.[1,2]

After resuscitation, the *hypermetabolic/catabolic flow phase* occurs. This period may last several weeks, depending on the nature, severity, and repetition of the inciting illness or injury and on the patient's response to medical or surgical therapy (see Table 231-1).[1,2] The flow phase is characterized by increased metabolic rate (i.e., energy expenditure and oxygen consumption), increased cardiac output, and frequently fever. Net erosion of lean body mass is typical. The whole body protein

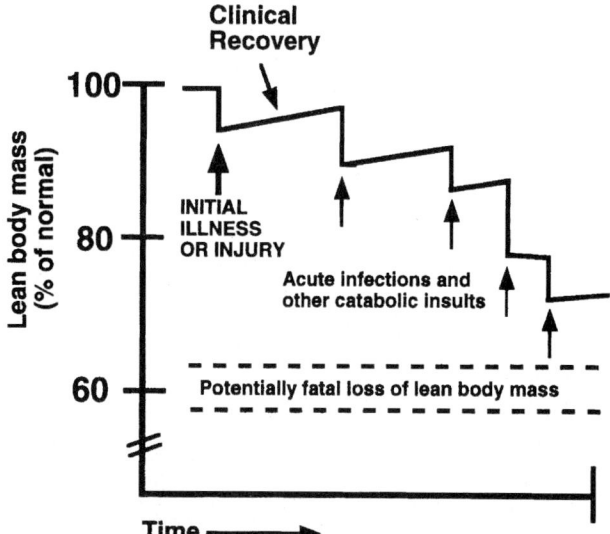

**FIGURE 231-1.** Net body protein breakdown and loss of lean body mass is typical in critical illness. This catabolic response is commonly manifested as a wasting of skeletal muscle (the major repository of body protein) over time, and a negative nitrogen balance (reflecting whole body nitrogen/protein losses). This figure illustrates the decline in lean body mass as a percentage of normal during the initial inciting illness or injury (*thick arrow*) and the slow accrual of lean tissue with clinical recovery and nutritional support. With repeated or prolonged catabolic insults (*thin arrows*), progressive loss of lean tissue occurs despite appropriate delivery of nutrients because of counterregulatory hormonal signals and decreased secretion and/or resistance to anabolic hormones.

synthetic rate is increased (primarily due to increased hepatic production of acute-phase proteins), but the rate of protein synthesis is exceeded by the rate of protein degradation. This leads to a negative nitrogen balance and erosion of skeletal muscle. Net protein catabolism is generally of greater magnitude earlier in the course of critical illness. Body nitrogen loss in ICU settings is directly related to the degree of catabolic stress.[9]

Mechanisms regulating erosion of body protein during illness remain incompletely understood but undoubtedly involve increased secretion of counterregulatory hormones working in concert with proinflammatory cytokines. In studies of healthy adults infused with combinations of glucagon, hydrocortisone, and epinephrine, additive effects of these hormones to increase the nitrogen loss, the insulin resistance, and the metabolic rate were observed.[2,3] Hormonal/cytokine signals interrelate with other mechanisms favoring net protein breakdown, such as malnutrition, metabolic acidosis, and muscle disuse (e.g., bed rest). The amino acids released from skeletal muscle (particularly glutamine and alanine, which comprise as much as 70% of total amino acids released) serve an important role as substrates for activated gluconeogenesis, whereas glutamine is a key metabolic fuel for the gut mucosa and immune cells.[10]

Marked changes in carbohydrate and lipid metabolism occur during the flow phase of critical illness (see Table 231-1). Increased rates of endogenous glucose production (especially by liver) and increased glucose uptake by tissues (especially the reticuloendothelial system, wounds, gut, and immune cells) are seen.[1] Elevated blood glucose and insulin levels are due to a combination of endogenous glucose production via glycogenolysis and gluconeogenesis combined with insulin resistance.[3] Insulin resistance in ICU patients is probably largely due to the effects of counterregulatory hormones (e.g., cortisol, norepinephrine, epinephrine, glucagon), in combination with

**TABLE 231-1.**
**Classic Metabolic Responses after Severe Injury***

| | Ebb Phase (Initial 24–36 Hours) | Flow Phase (Initial Weeks after Resuscitation) | Convalescence |
|---|---|---|---|
| Body temperature | Often reduced | Increased | Normalized |
| Cardiac output | Reduced | Increased | Normalized |
| Oxygen consumption | Reduced | Increased | Normalized |
| Body nitrogen loss | Reduced | Increased | Normalized |
| Endogenous glucose production (glycogenolysis, gluconeogenesis) | Increased | Increased | Normalized |
| Glucose uptake by tissues (especially spleen, liver, and immune cells) | Increased | Increased | Normalized |
| Lipolysis | Increased | Increased | Normalized |
| Plasma free fatty acids | Increased | Increased | Normalized |
| Plasma lactate | Normal | Increased | Normalized |
| Plasma glucose | Increased | Increased | Normalized |
| Plasma insulin | Reduced | Increased | Normalized |
| Counterregulatory hormones | Increased | Increased | Normalized |
| Insulin resistance | Yes | Yes | No |

*Responses vary as a function of the nature, timing and severity of illness, nutrient provision, drug administration, and other factors.

responses to local and circulating cytokines (especially interleukin-6 [IL-6] and tumor necrosis factor [TNF]).[4] In later or prolonged endotoxemia and septic shock, clinical observations and studies of animal models demonstrate that glycogenolysis and gluconeogenesis rates may actually decrease. Accelerated glucose uptake by macrophage-rich tissues may persist, however, and lead to *hypoglycemia* in some cases of severe illness (especially in hepatic failure) if exogenous glucose is not provided.[1] Underlying molecular events associated with tissue insulin resistance in septic and critically ill patients are beginning to be elucidated.[8] Activated lipolysis and increased plasma free fatty acid levels are characteristic of the flow phase of critical illness.[1,2] Along with providing endogenous glucose and amino acids as outlined earlier, this metabolic response also serves to provide fuel substrates critical for wound healing, tissue repair, synthesis of acute-phase proteins, and host defense.

The alterations in plasma hormones and fuel metabolism during catabolic illness are affected by numerous factors, including the nature and severity of the injury or illness, patient age, underlying nutritional status, administration of drug (e.g., corticosteroids, pressor agents), time course of catabolic stress, and efficacy of therapy.[1,2] In addition to changes in amino-acid, carbohydrate, and lipid metabolism, ICU patients manifest increased micronutrient losses in urine, especially of zinc and water-soluble vitamins.[10] During convalescence, the metabolic alterations of the flow phase are generally normalized, depending on the underlying illness and response to therapy[1,2] (see Table 231-1).

## CENTRAL AND PERIPHERAL HORMONAL RESPONSES IN CRITICAL ILLNESS

The central and peripheral hormonal responses observed in the first several days after the onset of major illness may be distinguished from changes characteristic of prolonged, chronic catabolic conditions (i.e., >10 days postinjury) (see Chap. 230).[4] In the acute period, the secretory activity of the anterior pituitary is generally augmented, with increased blood levels of adrenocorticotropic hormone (ACTH), prolactin, luteinizing hormone, and GH.[11] In contrast, plasma thyroid-stimulating hormone (TSH) levels are usually within normal limits; however, they may be decreased, possibly due to increased endogenous cortisol and dopamine release or their exogenous administration. In patients requiring prolonged care, the secretory activity of these anterior pituitary hormones is often suppressed, and plasma levels are reduced toward or below the normal range.[4,11] Exceptions to this pattern are blood TSH levels, which occasionally increase during recovery, and levels of arginine vasopressin (AVP), which are often elevated acutely and may remain so during prolonged critical illness.[12,13]

*Impaired anterior pituitary hormone secretion results in a proportionate decrease of the respective peripheral target organ hormones over time, except for cortisol, of which the circulating levels remain high despite decreased ACTH concentrations.[11]*

### HYPOTHALAMIC–PITUITARY–ADRENAL AXIS

In contrast to the general observation of increased plasma cortisol levels, adrenal *hypofunction* is not uncommon in some groups of septic and critically ill patients.[14] Subnormal plasma cortisol levels in response to standard stimulation tests, with or without blunted aldosterone responses, appear to predict increased morbidity and mortality in ICU patients.[14]

Glucocorticoids increase peripheral amino-acid efflux from skeletal muscle, facilitating gluconeogenesis by liver and kidney.[1,2] In adipose tissue, cortisol stimulates lipolysis and inhibits glucose uptake, resulting in elevated plasma free fatty acids, triglycerides and glycerol.[1,2] In contrast to the increase in cortisol synthesis and secretion, critical illness is associated with a dissociated, reduced production of the androgens dehydroepiandrosterone (DHEA) and DHEA sulfate (DHEAS) by the adrenal glands[11,15] (Table 231-2). Blood androstenedione concentrations have been reported to be decreased in burn patients, but they are elevated in critically ill nonburn patients.[15] DHEA and DHEAS concentrations are consistently decreased after severe illnesses or burns, and the DHEA response to ACTH administration is blunted.[15]

### THYROID AXIS

Within hours of acute illness or trauma, circulating levels of triiodothyronine ($T_3$) decline, due to inhibited peripheral conversion of thyroxine ($T_4$) to $T_3$ and/or increased turnover of thyroid hormones in the hypermetabolic phase of illness[4,16] (see Chaps. 228 and 232). Changes in thyroid hormone levels in ICU patients mirror the severity and duration of illness and correlate negatively with outcome variables.[7] Central hypothyroidism has been hypothesized to contribute to the catabolic state of prolonged critical illness, because normal concentrations of plasma and tissue $T_3$ are necessary for pro-

**TABLE 231-2.**

**Endocrine Responses in Acute versus Prolonged Critical Illness***

| | Acute (Initial 7–10 Days) | Prolonged (>10 Days) |
|---|---|---|
| Cortisol | ↑↑ | ↑ |
| Adrenal androgens | ↓ | ↓ |
| Aldosterone | ↑ | NL to ↓ |
| Glucagon | ↑↑ | ↑ |
| Insulin | NL to ↓ | ↑ |
| Catecholamines | ↑↑ | ↑ |
| Triiodothyronine (total) | ↓↓ | ↓ |
| Thyroxine (total) | NL to ↑ | NL to ↓ |
| IGF-I | ↓ | ↓ |
| IGFBP-3 | ↓ | ↓ |
| Testosterone | ↓ | ↓ |
| Cytokines (TNF, IL-1, IL-6) | ↑ | NL |

↑, increased blood levels; ↓, decreased blood levels; *NL*, generally normal blood levels; *IGF*, insulin-like growth factor; *IGFBP*, IGF-binding protein; *TNF*, tumor necrosis factor; *IL*, interleukin.

*Responses vary as a function of the nature, timing and severity of illness, underlying nutritional status, drug administration, and other factors. Alterations in growth hormone and thyroid-stimulating hormone pulse amplitude and/or pulse number also may occur.

tein synthesis, lipolysis, fuel utilization by muscle, and GH secretion.[1,2,17] Thyroid hormones may induce protein catabolism when levels are increased, however; thus, the low $T_3$ syndrome may be an adaptive response to conserve body protein, as in simple malnutrition.[1]

### PITUITARY-GONADAL AXIS

Serum testosterone levels in men decrease markedly in a number of catabolic states, including malnutrition and critical illness.[4,18] Acute injury results in Leydig cell suppression, as evidenced by low serum testosterone concentrations in association with elevated plasma luteinizing hormone (LH) concentrations but normal levels of follicle-stimulating hormone (FSH) and inhibin in plasma.[4,19] In women, prolonged critical illness is associated with a decrease in both FSH and LH levels.[20] In men, prolonged critical illness and hypoandrogenemia is associated with *low* LH concentrations.[4] Administration of dopamine and long-term administration of opioids result in additional suppression of gonadotrope function.[18] The magnitude of the decrease in plasma testosterone correlates with the severity of the insult in prolonged coma after trauma.[21] Recovery of gonadal function may take weeks, even months, after recovery from critical illness. Thus, prolonged hypogonadism, especially in men, may delay anabolism and clinical recovery.

### GROWTH HORMONE–INSULIN-LIKE GROWTH FACTOR AXIS

Malnutrition, exogenous and endogenous glucocorticoids, somatostatin, and drugs (e.g., dopamine) can attenuate pulsatile GH secretion and result in low concentrations of IGF-I. In critically ill patients the rise in GH concentrations coupled with low levels of IGF-I may serve to shift metabolic responses to those directly induced by GH, including lipolysis and insulin antagonism, and to concomitantly attenuate protein-sparing anabolic effects mediated by IGF-I.[5,6]

A summary of peripheral endocrine response patterns for major body hormones in acute versus prolonged critical illness is given in Table 231-2 (also see Chap. 230). The onset of clinical recovery is characterized by *restored sensitivity of the anterior pituitary to reduced feedback control.*[4,11,13]

# NUTRITIONAL SUPPORT IN CRITICAL ILLNESS

## GENERAL CONCEPTS

The primary focus of nutritional support in critically ill patients is to supply adequate energy, protein, and micronutrients (e.g., vitamins, minerals, electrolytes) to facilitate organ function, wound and tissue healing, and, thus, patient recovery. Protein is critical for organ structure and function, and a significant erosion of lean tissue is associated with a worsened clinical outcome, including diminished immune function, increased rates of infection, decreased wound healing, skeletal muscle dysfunction, and delayed convalescence.[9,10] This relationship is especially apparent in those with preexisting malnutrition before the onset of severe catabolic stress. Direct cause-and-effect relationships between nutritional status and patient outcomes are difficult to prove, however, because malnutrition reflects, in part, the severity or nature of the underlying illness.[22] Nonetheless, a reasonable assumption is that the provision of nutritional support in critically ill adult and pediatric patients is beneficial if feeding is not possible for 5 to 7 days.[23]

The goal of nutritional support is to maintain organ structure and function and to support body metabolism and protein synthesis. Thus, major objectives of nutritional and metabolic support in malnourished or catabolic patients are to detect and correct preexisting depletion of macro- and micronutrients, attenuate progressive protein wasting, optimize fluid and electrolyte status, and, thus, reduce morbidity related to malnutrition.[10,23] Parenteral and enteral nutritional support is *adjunctive* to primary therapies (e.g., fluid resuscitation, oxygen delivery, abscess drainage, and provision of antibiotics). Use of parenteral nutrition (PN) and tube feedings has become a standard of care in most ICUs throughout the world. Few objective data from properly designed, randomized, controlled studies are available to determine the true efficacy of, and the indications for, nutritional support in critical illness.[24] Nonetheless, several clear indications exist for the use of PN and tube feedings in critically ill patients (Table 231-3).

### NUTRITIONAL ASSESSMENT

Nutritional assessment in the hospital setting involves an integration of several factors, including medical/surgical history, type and severity of the acute underlying illness, physical examination findings, weight loss history, prior dietary intake pattern, evaluation of current organ function, and fluid status and

**TABLE 231-3.**

**Some Clinical Indications for Specialized Enteral or Parenteral Nutrition (PN) Support in Critically Ill Patients**

Food intake not possible for >5–7 days due to underlying illness

Severe catabolic stress (e.g., burns, trauma, sepsis)

Major gastrointestinal operations (PN)

Medical illness associated with prolonged gastrointestinal dysfunction (diarrhea, nausea/vomiting) and/or illness in which oral food intake is contraindicated:

Bone marrow transplantation

Inflammatory bowel disease

Pancreatitis

High-output enterocutaneous fistula

Ileus or bowel obstruction

Short bowel syndrome

Preexisting moderate to severe protein-energy malnutrition and inability to maintain adequate enteral feeding to promote anabolism (PN)

**TABLE 231-4.**
**Components of Comprehensive Nutritional Assessment in Hospitalized Patients**

**PHYSICAL EXAMINATION**
  Skeletal muscle and fat wasting
  Skin lesions suggestive of micronutrient deficiency
  Fluid status
**BODY WEIGHT PATTERN**
  Current body weight as percentage of ideal body weight
  Usual body weight
  Percentage weight loss over past several weeks and months
**DIETARY INTAKE PATTERN**
  Food intake pattern
  Previous intravenous or enteral nutritional support
  Use of nutritional supplements
**INTESTINAL TRACT FUNCTION**
  Gastrointestinal symptoms (nausea, emesis, diarrhea, steatorrhea)
  Delayed gastric emptying, gastroparesis, ileus, obstruction, intraabdominal infection, perforation, hemorrhage
**SELECTED SERUM OR PLASMA BIOCHEMICAL INDICES**
  Standard organ function indices (liver and renal function tests), blood glucose
  Electrolytes, including calcium, magnesium, and phosphorus
  Triglycerides
  Vitamins and mineral levels (e.g., serum zinc, vitamin C), if suggested by physical examination, by dietary history, or by underlying illness
  Serum proteins (e.g., albumin, prealbumin) are not helpful in the intensive care unit setting (values markedly influenced by degree of stress and by fluid status)

selected biochemical values (Table 231-4). Circulating concentrations of proteins (e.g., albumin, prealbumin, IGF-I, transferrin, and retinol-binding protein) generally are *not* useful as indices of the underlying nutritional status in ICU patients. Plasma levels of these proteins are markedly affected by nonnutritional factors (e.g., fluid status, decreased hepatic synthesis and increased metabolic clearance associated with inflammation or infection).[22,23] Because of the long turnover of albumin (18–21 days), levels in blood remain low despite adequate feeding.

The basic principle in considering PN therapy is that the patient must be unable to achieve adequate energy, protein, and micronutrient intake via the enteral route with oral food, liquid supplements, or tube feedings. Compared with PN, enteral feeding is much less expensive, maintains intestinal mucosal structure and function, is safer in terms of mechanical and metabolic complications, and is associated with reduced rates of nosocomial infections.[23,24] Thus, the *enteral route of feeding should be used whenever possible.*

## PROVISION OF ENERGY AND PROTEIN

Studies on nutrient utilization efficiency in severely catabolic patients suggest that lower amounts of total energy (calories) and protein should be administered than have been routinely given in the past.[22,23] Excessive dietary calories and protein loads (hyperalimentation) may induce metabolic complications, including carbon dioxide overproduction, azotemia, hyperglycemia, electrolyte alterations, and hepatic dysfunction.[24] Energy intake should be advanced slowly over several days after the initiation of specialized feeding to provide maintenance energy intake. Energy requirements may be estimated using standard equations (e.g., the *Harris-Benedict equation*) that incorporate the patient's age, sex, weight, and height to determine *basal energy expenditure (BEE):*

BEE for males (kcal/24 hours) = 66.5 + (13.8 × kg body weight) + (5.0 × height in cm) – (6.8 × age in years)

BEE for females (kcal/24 hours) = 655.1 + (9.6 × kg body weight) + (1.8 × height in cm) – (4.7 × age in years)

The BEE is then multiplied by factors to account for activity (1.2 to 1.3 times BEE, unless the patient is sedated), and occasionally for illness severity, to arrive at the energy prescription. The estimated maintenance energy requirement is ~1.3 times BEE.[23,24] In obese subjects (defined as >20% above ideal body weight), the *adjusted body weight* should be used in the calculation of energy and protein needs:

Adjusted body weight = (current weight – ideal body weight [from standard tables or equations] × 0.25) + ideal body weight

The estimated dry weight should be used to determine energy and protein needs (see later) in settings of peripheral or central edema due to fluid overload or the capillary leak syndrome.

Energy expenditure varies considerably from day to day in critically ill ICU patients. In light of the complications related to overfeeding outlined earlier, energy provision in the range of 25 to 30 kcal/kg per day is generally safe for most ICU patients and for stable patients without severe malnutrition.[23,24] In clinically stable non-ICU patients with severe malnutrition who require nutritional repletion, 35 to 40 kcal/kg per day may be provided, with careful monitoring of serum chemistries, as outlined later. Carbon dioxide overproduction, as evidenced by an indirect calorimetry-derived respiratory quotient of >1.0 (the ratio of carbon dioxide production to oxygen consumption) was not uncommon in the past, when ICU patients routinely received excessive energy doses. This complication is unusual, however, with current standards of nutritional care in ICU settings.

Dextrose in PN or tube feeds should be given at a dosage not to exceed 5 mg/kg per minute (~500 g per day for a 70-kg person).[23] Catabolic patients are unable to efficiently oxidize larger carbohydrate loads, which may induce hyperglycemia, hepatic steatosis, and/or excessive carbon dioxide production over time. Dextrose should provide 70% to 80% of nonprotein energy, unless the patient is hyperglycemic. In this case, the dextrose load should be reduced and/or regular insulin should be provided in parenteral feeding or as a separate insulin drip to maintain blood glucose between 100 and 150 mg/dL.[25]

Intravenous lipid emulsions are used to provide essential linoleic and linolenic fatty acids or as an energy source, and are generally infused over a 24-hour period in patients requiring PN. The maximal recommended rate of fat emulsion infusion is ~1.0 g/kg per day.[23] ICU patients generally clear intravenous fat emulsions well from plasma; however, large doses of fat emulsion have been associated with impaired reticuloendothelial function and possibly immune suppression. Serum triglycerides should be monitored serially to assess the clearance of the intravenous fat emulsion. The triglyceride levels should be maintained at <400 to 500 mg/dL to decrease the risk of pancreatitis or diminished pulmonary diffusion capacity in patients with severe chronic obstructive lung disease.[23]

Guidelines for protein administration are given in Table 231-5. Studies of ICU patients indicate that protein loads of >2.0 g/kg per day are not efficiently used for protein synthesis, and the excess may be oxidized, contributing to azotemia. In most catabolic patients requiring specialized feeding, a generally recommended protein dose is 1.5 g/kg per day in individuals with normal renal function.[9,23] The administered protein dosage should be adjusted downward as a function of the degree of azotemia and hyperbilirubinemia. This strategy takes into account the relative inability of ICU patients to efficiently use exogenous nutrients and the knowledge that most protein and lean tissue repletion occurs over a period of several weeks to months during convalescence. Adequate nonprotein energy is essential to allow amino acids to be effectively used for protein

**TABLE 231-5.**
Guidelines for Protein Administration in Hospitalized Patients

| Condition | Protein Intake Goal* (g/kg/day) |
|---|---|
| Malnourished, clinically stable | 1.5–2.0 |
| Mild to moderate catabolic stress | 1.2–1.5 |
| Critically ill | 1.2–1.5 |
| Encephalopathy | 0.6 |
| Hepatic failure | 0.6–1.0 |
| Renal failure, not dialyzed | 0.6–0.8 |
| Renal failure, dialyzed | 1.2 |

*Protein load is adjusted proportional to hepatic and renal function indices.

**TABLE 231-6.**
Guidelines for Electrolyte and Micronutrient Administration
in Parenteral Nutrient (PN) Solutions*

| Element | Peripheral PN | Central PN |
|---|---|---|
| Potassium (mEq/L) | 20–40 | 40–60 |
| Sodium (mEq/L) | 30–75 | 50–75 |
| Phosphorus (mmol/L) | 5–8 | 10–15 |
| Calcium (mEq/L) | 5 | 5 |
| Magnesium (mEq/L) | 5–8 | 15 |
| Multivitamins | Standard products available to admix | |
| Trace elements | Standard products available to admix | |
| Vitamin K (mg/day) | 1 | 1 |

*Electrolytes are adjusted as indicated to maintain serially measured serum levels within the normal range; the percentage of sodium and potassium salts as chloride is increased to correct metabolic alkalosis, and the percentage of salts as acetate is increased to correct metabolic acidosis.

synthesis. The nonprotein calorie/nitrogen ratio used in most centers ranges from 100:1 to 150:1 (nitrogen = protein/6.25). Highly catabolic patients are given protein loads at the lower end of this range, assuming near-normal renal and hepatic function.[9,23]

To diminish the risk of phlebitis, peripheral vein PN solutions provide low concentrations of dextrose (<7 %) and amino acids (<4%) with a large proportion of energy as fat (50% to 60% of total calories). Because fluid restriction precludes the use of large fluid volumes for intravenous feedings, peripheral vein PN is generally not indicated in ICU patients requiring intravenous feeding. Central venous administration of PN containing hypertonic dextrose, fat, and higher amino-acid concentrations allows maintenance energy and protein needs to be met with as little as 1 L of PN volume.

A large variety of tube-feeding products are available for clinical use. The specific product chosen depends on the clinical condition and underlying organ function.[26] Thus, liquid diet formulas designed for use in patients with renal failure contain low protein and electrolytes and are concentrated in calories (2 kcal/ mL) to allow minimal fluid intake. Formulas providing concentrated calories are also used in patients with fluid overload. More "elemental" tube-feeding products (i.e., containing peptides or free amino acids, simple sugars, and medium-chain triglycerides as opposed to intact protein, starches, and long-chain fats) are used in cases of gut mucosal inflammation or atrophy and in the short-gut syndrome. For most ICU patients, however, standard nonelemental enteral formulas delivered via nasogastric or postpyloric routes are very well tolerated.[23,26]

### MICRONUTRIENT ADMINISTRATION

A standard of care during specialized feeding is maintenance of normal blood levels of glucose, electrolytes, and, if measured, vitamins and minerals. Malnourished patients frequently exhibit whole body depletion of intracellular electrolytes, which, depending on the status of hydration, may or may not be reflected in abnormally low serum levels. Plasma levels of potassium, magnesium, and especially phosphorus may markedly decrease during rapid nutritional repletion due to an insulin-induced intracellular shift (*refeeding syndrome*).[23,24] In patients with normal renal function, the dosage of electrolytes required to maintain normal plasma levels is directly related to the dosage of administered dextrose. Table 231-6 shows typical dosage ranges for daily PN electrolyte concentrations in central venous PN formulas (which generally contain 15% to 25% dextrose) and peripheral vein PN solutions (which generally provide 5% dextrose).

Specific requirements for intravenous trace elements and vitamins in various catabolic states have not been rigorously defined, and therapy is directed at meeting the recommended dietary allowances (RDA) for micronutrients, with adjustments based on

intravenous delivery.[24] Zinc is an important nutrient for immune function, wound healing, protein synthesis, and gastrointestinal mucosal regeneration. Supplemental zinc (and possibly supplements of other trace elements such as selenium) may be indicated for patients with burns, large wounds, severe pancreatitis, and/ or significant gastrointestinal fluid losses. Approximately 12 mg of zinc are lost per liter of small bowel fluid, and the urinary excretion of zinc increases dramatically as a function of the degree of catabolic stress. Thus, with serum zinc levels and/or urinary excretion used as a guide to therapy, the administration of 5 to 10 mg per day of additional zinc intravenously (or 200 to 400 mg of zinc sulfate per day enterally) during catabolic illness reduces the risk of continued total body zinc depletion. Data also suggest that a depletion of thiamine is not uncommon in patients receiving long-term diuretic therapy.[24]

## BIOCHEMICAL MONITORING

Serial monitoring of plasma glucose, electrolytes, and triglycerides and assessment of renal, hepatic, and pulmonary function in ICU patients to determine the metabolic response is critical, especially during periods of clinical instability.[23] The nutrient mix is adjusted to maintain normal blood concentrations of standard substances and to minimize metabolic complications. When the patient's condition is extremely unstable, providing a lowered amount or even discontinuing specialized feeding may be necessary until organ function stabilizes. Few objective clinical data are available to guide the timing of nutrient administration in ICU patients who are unable to tolerate oral food. The current standard of care in most critical care units is to provide specialized PN (if the gut is not functional) or enteral tube feeding within 5 to 7 days after admission; in practice, however, nutritional support is often provided several days sooner.[23] The indications for, and utility of, specialized nutritional support in critical illness will be further defined after the completion of ongoing randomized controlled trials.[27]

## REFERENCES

1. Hasselgren P-O. Mediators, hormones, and control of metabolism: regulation of protein, carbohydrate and lipid metabolism during critical illness. In: Fischer JE, ed. Nutrition and metabolism in the surgical patient. Boston: Little, Brown and Company, 1996:57.
2. Bessey PQ. Metabolic response to trauma and infection. In: Fischer JE, ed. Nutrition and metabolism in the surgical patient. Boston: Little, Brown and Company, 1996:601.
3. Bessey PQ, Lowe KA. Early hormonal changes affect the catabolic response to trauma. Ann Surg 1993; 218:476.

4. Van den Berghe G, de Zegher F, Bouillon R. Clinical review 95: acute and prolonged critical illness as different neuroendocrine paradigms. J Clin Endocrinol Metab 1998; 83:1827.

5. Ferrando AA. Anabolic hormones in critically ill patients. Curr Opin Nutr Metab Care 1999; 2:171.

6. Frost RA, Lang CH. Growth factors in critical illness: regulation and therapeutic aspects. Curr Opin Nutr Metab Care 1998; 1:195.

7. Jarek MJ, Legare EJ, McDermott MT, et al. Endocrine profiles for outcome prediction from the intensive care unit. Crit Care Med 1993; 21:543.

8. Hasselgren P-O, Fischer JE. Counter-regulatory hormones and mechanisms in amino acid metabolism with special reference to the catabolic response in skeletal muscle. Curr Opin Nutr Metab Care 1999; 2:9.

9. Ziegler TR, Nattakom TV. Amino acid support in catabolic states. In: L Cynober, ed. Amino acid metabolism in health and nutritional diseases. Boca Raton, FL: CRC Press, 1995:399.

10. Ziegler TR, Leader LM, Jonas CR, Griffiths DP. Adjunctive therapies in specialized nutrition support. Nutrition 1997; 9(Suppl):64S.

11. Chrousos GP. The hypothalamic-pituitary-adrenal axis and immune-mediated inflammation. N Engl J Med 1995; 332:1351.

12. Reichlin S. Mechanisms of disease: neuroendocrine-immune interactions. N Engl J Med 1993; 329:1246.

13. Van den Berghe G, de Zegher F. Anterior pituitary function during critical illness and dopamine treatment. Crit Care Med 1996; 24:1580.

14. Briegel J, Schelling G, Haller M, et al. A comparison of the adrenocortical response during septic shock and after complete recovery. Intensive Care Med 1996; 22:894.

15. Parker LN, Levin ER, Lifrak ET. Evidence for adrenocortical adaptation to severe illness. J Clin Endocrinol Metab 1985; 60:947.

16. Brent GA, Hershman JM. Thyroxine therapy in patients with severe nonthyroidal illnesses and low serum thyroxine concentration. J Clin Endocrinol Metab 1986; 63:1.

17. Becker RA, Vaughan GM, Ziegler MG, et al. Hypermetabolic low triiodothyronine syndrome in burn injury. Crit Care Med 1982; 10:870.

18. Van den Berghe G, de Zegher F, Lauwers P, Veldhuis JD. Luteinizing hormone secretion and hypoandrogenemia in critically ill men: effect of dopamine. Clin Endocrinol 1994; 41:563.

19. Wang C, Chan V, Yeung RTT. Effect of surgical stress on pituitary-testicular function. Clin Endocrinol 1978; 9:255.

20. Van Steenbergen W, Naert J, Lambrecht S, et al. Suppression of gonadotropin secretion in the hospitalized postmenopausal female as an effect of acute illness. Neuroendocrinology 1994; 60:165.

21. Fleischer AS, Rudman DR, Payne NS, Tindall GT. Hypothalamic hypothyroidism and hypogonadism in prolonged traumatic coma. J Neurosurg 1978; 49:650.

22. Klein S, Kinney J, Jeejeebhoy K, et al. Nutrition support in clinical practice: review of published data and recommendations for future research directions. JPEN J Parenter Enteral Nutr 1997; 21:133.

23. ASPEN Board of Directors. Guidelines for the use of parenteral and enteral nutrition in adult and pediatric patients. JPEN J Parent Enteral Nutr 1993; 17:1SA.

24. Heyland DK, MacDonald S, Keefe L, Drover JW. Total parenteral nutrition in the critically ill patient: a meta-analysis. JAMA 1998; 280:2013.

25. Ziegler TR, Smith RJ. Parenteral nutrition in patients with diabetes mellitus. In: Rombeau JL, Caldwell MD, eds. Clinical nutrition: parenteral nutrition, vol 2. Philadelphia: WB Saunders, 1993:649.

26. Shikora SA, Ogawa AM. Enteral nutrition and the critically ill. Postgrad Med J 1996; 72:395.

27. Jonas CR, Pucket AB, Jones DP, et al. Plasma antioxidant status after high dose chemotherapy: a randomized trial of parenteral nutrition in bone marrow transplantation patients. Am J Clin Nutrition 2000; 72:181.

# CHAPTER 232

# ENDOCRINE THERAPEUTICS IN CRITICAL ILLNESS

ERIC NYLÉN, GARY P. ZALOGA, KENNETH L. BECKER,
KENNETH D. BURMAN, LEONARD WARTOFSKY,
BEAT MÜLLER, JON C. WHITE, AND ABDULLAH A. ALARIFI

The progressively aging population is subject to chronic debilitating illnesses. The care of critical illness in this population, as well as in the newborn and infant, has become an ever-increasing clinical and societal task. Furthermore, despite aggressive therapeutic management, the mortality associated with critical illness

in all age groups remains dismally high. The finding that the normal systemic response to illness may actually become maladaptive to the host in critical illness (see Chaps. 228, 229, and 230) has encouraged new and innovative strategies and an extensive reappraisal of current therapeutic practices. As suggested in this chapter, the use and levels of hormones and hormone-like substances have been, and continue to be, an important consideration in the treatment of critically ill patients.

## ADRENAL FUNCTION IN THE CRITICALLY ILL PATIENT: A DIAGNOSTIC UNCERTAINTY

A particularly important challenge in the treatment of critical illness is the *identification* of the very rare patient who has coexistent primary or secondary hypoadrenalism—lethal but treatable conditions for which replacement therapy is urgent. A number of reports of dramatic hemodynamic responses to the empirical administration of glucocorticoids to critically ill patients have suggested that adrenal deficiency may be somewhat more common than realized (e.g., it has been suggested that up to 30% of HIV patients are hypoadrenal). Nonetheless, nearly all studies have shown that most critically ill patients tend to have relatively *high* basal serum cortisol.[1-3] Some authors have hypothesized that those critically ill patients who *do not* have increased serum cortisol levels may have a "relative adrenal insufficiency" (also called "occult hypoadrenalism," "subclinical hypoadrenalism," or "unrecognized hypoadrenalism").[4,5] Some investigators have arbitrarily placed critically ill patients in this category if serum levels of cortisol are <20 μg/dL[4]; others use levels of <18 μg/dL.[6] A large number of septic patients who recover *without* cortisol therapy, however, have even lower levels. Moreover, in sepsis, a single serum cortisol value often is *invalid*, because of the wide variations that occur.[2,7] Furthermore, the serum cortisol level may not be indicative of concurrent tissue needs.

### RELATIVE ADRENAL INSUFFICIENCY

A review of the literature reveals as invalid the view that an alleged relative adrenal insufficiency (based solely on a finding of basal cortisol values in the upper range for healthy individuals) will impact harmfully on the outcome of a critical illness (e.g., sepsis). Indeed, most studies either show that serum cortisol levels have *no* correlation with outcome[2] or find that high basal cortisol values actually correlate with *increased* mortality.[7-9]

### FUNCTIONAL HYPOADRENALISM

Other investigators have advocated the use of the rapid intravenous adrenocorticotropic hormone (ACTH) test to evaluate adrenal function and to predict mortality. An insufficient response has been termed "functional hypoadrenalism" (also called "adrenocortical dysfunction," "transient hypoadrenalism," or "adrenal hyporesponsiveness").[2,10-12] ACTH has been administered at doses of 250 μg, 1 μg, or 1 μg followed in 1 hour by 250 μg.[13] The precise minimal level to be achieved or the increase in cortisol that is required for the response to be considered normal in the critically ill patient is controversial, and no consensus exists on the interpretation.[13,14] In addition, because the response to ACTH varies considerably, even if the levels seen in unstressed patients are attained, the finding can be falsely reassuring.[15] Moreover, even immediately before death, septic patients may continue to respond to ACTH. Thus, a lack of agreement is found as to whether any correlation exists between a low cortisol response to ACTH and mortality.

The difficulty in accepting these concepts of "relative adrenal insufficiency" or "functional hypoadrenalism" in critical illness (based on either baseline cortisol levels or the ACTH test) arises not only from the contradictory results, but also from the erroneous assumption that critically ill patients in general should have a "normally" responding hypothalamic–pituitary–adrenal (HPA) axis (see Chaps. 227 and 228).

**Relative Cortisol Resistance.** Studies of the HPA-immune interaction during stress[16] have suggested that a state of relative cortisol resistance (akin to the relative insulin resistance in critical illness) may be present. Thus, certain severe immune-mediated inflammatory states can cause glucocorticoid resistance in target tissues.[16] For example, in rheumatoid arthritis, the concentration of glucocorticoid receptors in circulating leukocytes is reduced.[17] Furthermore, glucocorticoid-resistant asthma is also associated with increased expression of glucocorticoid receptor-β (GR-β) in the peripheral blood and airway cells.[18,19] GR-β induces glucocorticoid insensitivity by antagonizing the transactivating activity of the classic GR type II. This GR-β expression is cytokine inducible.[18] Whether this GR-β expression is responsible for the cortisol resistance in the acquired immunodeficiency syndrome (AIDS),[20] however, or whether such a mechanism can be found in critical illness, is unknown. Nonetheless, proinflammatory cytokines do induce glucocorticoid insensitivity (see Chap. 229), and the beneficial effect of hydrocortisone in some patients with septic shock may not necessarily be related to adrenocortical insufficiency.[21]

**Alternative Adrenal Assessment.** Theoretically, the degree of relative cortisol resistance might be assessed by a bioresponse (or lack thereof) to glucocorticoids. One such assessment strategy might be to determine the extent to which high C-reactive protein (CRP) levels, found in patients with the systemic inflammatory response syndrome (SIRS), are reduced by a hydrocortisone infusion.[22] Potentially, such an approach might improve the selection of cases for the appropriate application of glucocorticoid therapy and provide an objective assessment of the effectiveness of therapy. Unless the cortisol level is extremely low, clearly a need exists to apply alternative or new techniques to the clinical assessment of adrenal function. The fact that glucocorticoid deficiency causes eosinophilia and hypotension (particularly when the hypotension is vasopressor resistant) can be put to good use in the assessment process. The suggestion has been made that such findings be used along with the cortisol concentration to improve evaluation in cases of suspected adrenal insufficiency.[23]

Presently, unless the serum cortisol levels are extremely low, to identify the rare patient with bona fide primary hypoadrenalism, the clinician must rely foremost on a detailed history (e.g., autoimmune status, history of tuberculosis or other infections such as meningococcemia, previous glucocorticoid usage [including megestrol acetate], exposure to adrenotoxic agents [ketoconazole, phenytoin, etomidate], and risk factors for adrenal hemorrhage), physical examination (e.g., hyperpigmentation, vitiligo, loss of pubic/axillary hair), and ancillary supportive information (e.g., levels of serum electrolytes, glucose). A reasonable course, for the occasional, selected, extremely ill patient without established hypoadrenal findings, might be the use of near-physiologic doses of cortisol, especially if the patient is already vasopressor dependent.

# GLUCOCORTICOIDS

## RATIONALE FOR USAGE

Shortly after its initial identification, purification, and structural elucidation, *endogenous* cortisol was found to exert marked effects in protecting against stress and combating inflammation. Certainly, the clinical benefits of *exogenous* use of cortisol, corti-

**TABLE 232-1.**

**Physiologic/Pharmacologic Effects of Glucocorticoids That May Reduce an Inflammatory Response***

Stabilize lysomal membranes and, hence, diminish the release of proteolytic enzymes.

Inhibit synthesis of prostaglandins and leukotrienes.

Counteract norepinephrine vasoconstriction.

Decrease the migration of leukocytes and macrophages to areas of injury.

Induce lymphopenia (e.g., apoptosis).

Induce eosinopenia and, hence, decrease enzyme release from their granules.

Blunt transcriptional and posttranscriptional production and release of proinflammatory cytokines (e.g., tumor necrosis factor).

Inhibit the formation of histamine.

Lower fever by diminishing interleukin-1β production.

Mobilize amino acids; augment their transport into liver and decrease their transport into extrahepatic tissues.

Mobilize fatty acids.

Decrease utilization of glucose by cells.

Increase gluconeogenesis.

Diminish antibody production by B lymphocytes.

Diminish capillary and venule pressure, thus favoring reabsorption of interstitial fluid.

Decrease oxygen free radicals.

*Many of these effects also play a role in combating stress.

sone, and their synthetic analogs in the treatment of the allergic inflammatory reactions of urticaria, asthma, and anaphylaxis, as well as in the autoimmune inflammation that is characteristic of illnesses such as rheumatoid arthritis, have been amply confirmed. Furthermore, many in vitro and in vivo experiments have demonstrated the multiple antiinflammatory and anti-stress effects of glucocorticoids (Table 232-1).

## SUPRAPHYSIOLOGIC GLUCOCORTICOID THERAPY

Is a supraphysiologic dose of exogenously administered glucocorticoid more beneficial to a critically ill patient than an adequate endogenous secretion of cortisol? This highly controversial question has been debated for a half century. Because of the marked increase of blood pressure in hypotensive addisonian patients in response to the administration of cortisol, evaluation of supraphysiologic glucocorticoid therapy in sepsis, an illness that is often marked by dramatic hypotension (commonly a preterminal event) had seemed logical. Furthermore, *adrenalectomized* animals fare poorly when subjected to infection or administered endotoxin or cytokines, and this phenomenon is reversible after the administration of glucocorticoids.

Some clinical studies have, indeed, supported the use of pharmacologic doses of glucocorticoids in septic and critically ill patients who have no apparent adrenal insufficiency.[21,22] Many of these studies, however, have involved too few patients for valid conclusions to be drawn. In this regard, two metaanalyses of the literature have been particularly informative. One of these found (by duplicate, independent review of 124 published articles) nine randomized, controlled trials in which high dosages of corticosteroids (e.g., 30 mg/kg prednisolone every 4–6 hours for 1–4 doses) had been administered to patients with sepsis and septic shock.[24] Corticosteroids were found to *increase mortality* in patients with overwhelming infection and had *no* beneficial effect in a subgroup with septic shock. Furthermore, a trend was seen toward increased mortality from secondary infections among those treated with corticosteroids, and gastrointestinal bleeding was slightly increased. Thus, this review found *no support for the use of sup-*

raphysiologic doses of corticosteroids and suggested that they may, indeed, be harmful. In another large study of nine reports involving 537 patients who were treated with high-dose glucocorticoids for sepsis and septic shock, no significant beneficial effect of therapy was found.[25] Except in one patient with outlying results, in whom a beneficial effect was noted, high-dose glucocorticoid administration was significantly harmful (odds ratio, 0.70; 95% confidence interval, 0.54–0.91, p = .008). The authors of this study concluded: "inhibition of inflammation can be dangerous, either by inducing immunosuppression and worsening infection and outcome, or by altering normal regulation of inflammation in such a way as to produce harm independent of infection, or by both mechanisms."

These results notwithstanding, in other studies, the use of moderate supraphysiologic doses of hydrocortisone (e.g., 200–300 mg) has resulted in an improvement in hemodynamic parameters, thereby leading to reversal of shock and allowing for vasopressor therapy cessation.[21,22] These studies, however, were too small to demonstrate statistical significance for organ failure or for death, although a positive trend was noted. These and other studies,[26] as well as an improved understanding of the corticosteroid-immune interaction, have rekindled interest in the use of glucocorticoids as therapeutic adjuvants (immune modulators).

Very little definitive advice can be offered concerning the use of glucocorticoids in critical illness in general, or in critically ill patients who meet either some of the aforementioned contradictory basal cortisol criteria for "relative adrenal insufficiency" or the contradictory ACTH-stimulation criteria for "functional hypoadrenalism." The potential dangers of such therapy (as demonstrated by metaanalysis) should be a cause for concern. Nonetheless, conceptually, our evolving understanding of the interconnected molecular actions of glucocorticoids vis-à-vis proinflammatory cytokines, as well as the nonadrenal actions of glucocorticoids with respect to catecholamines and adrenergic receptors, indicates that an appropriate use of these agents might, conceivably, be useful. For example, the administration of glucocorticoids in certain specific conditions (e.g., tuberculosis,[27] pediatric meningitis,[28] typhoid fever,[29] Pneumocystis carinii pneumonia in AIDS,[30] and acute spinal cord injury[31]) has been reported to be beneficial.[32] Possibly, resolution of issues such as the appropriate dosage and timing, intermittent versus continuous infusion, and the use of hydrocortisone versus synthetic agents may provide much-needed clinical information.

## CATECHOLAMINES

Shock is associated with an early and marked elevation in serum levels of catecholamines, resulting in enhanced vasoconstriction, increased inotropy, and chronotropy. Critical illness often necessitates pressor support (along with concurrent fluid resuscitation), for which a variety of catecholaminergic agents are used.[33] These agents have a wide variety of hemodynamic actions, which are exerted through multiple adrenergic receptors located in the myocardium and in the vascular and pulmonary smooth muscle (Table 232-2). The different adrenergic receptors, which have different specificities for agonists and different signaling properties, are located at differing sites. In general, $\alpha_1$-receptors mediate arterial vasoconstriction, and $\alpha_2$-receptors cause constriction of venous capacitance vessels and inhibit the release of norepinephrine. The $\beta_1$-receptors enhance myocardial contractility and performance, and $\beta_2$-receptors mediate bronchial and vascular smooth muscle relaxation. Dopamine 1 receptors ($DA_1$) increase perfusion to the kidney, splanchnic bed, and brain. Dopamine 2 receptors ($DA_2$) may cause vasodilation and inhibit norepinephrine release.

**TABLE 232-2.**
**Catecholaminergic Agents and Their Respective Receptor Affinities**

| Drug | $\alpha$ | $\beta_1$ | $\beta_2$ | $DA_1$ | $DA_2$ |
|---|---|---|---|---|---|
| Dobutamine | 1 | 3 | 1 | 0 | 0 |
| Dopexamine | 0 | 1 | 3 | 2 | 2 |
| Dopamine | 2 | 2 | 2 | 3 | 3 |
| Epinephrine | 3 | 3 | 2 | 0 | 0 |
| Isoproterenol | 0 | 3 | 3 | 0 | 0 |
| Norepinephrine | 3 | 1 | 0 | 0 | 0 |
| Phenylephrine | 3 | 0 | 0 | 0 | 0 |

$DA_1$ and $DA_2$ are the dopamine 1 and 2 receptors, respectively. Relative potency is indicated; 0 = no effect, 3 = most potent.

The infusion of low doses of dopamine (0.5–3 µg/kg/minute) causes mainly $DA_1$-receptor stimulation with possible vasodilation in renal, splanchnic, cerebral, and coronary vascular beds without associated changes in heart rate or blood pressure. Higher doses of dopamine (2–5 µg/kg/minute) stimulate $\beta_1$-receptors and inotropy, whereas yet higher doses (5 to 10 µg/kg/minute) result in $\alpha$ effects (albeit less potent than those achieved with norepinephrine). Dopamine is often the first-line agent to combat mild to moderate hypotension, oliguria, and circulatory depression, especially in the early phases of septic shock. This agent exerts a diuretic effect, increasing the renal tubular sodium excretion. Dopamine frequently is used in combination with other inotropic agents such as dobutamine.

Dopamine has multiple effects on anterior pituitary hormone secretion: It suppresses prolactin, luteinizing hormone (LH), growth hormone (GH), and thyroid-stimulating hormone (TSH), and decreases dehydroepiandrosterone sulfate (DHEAS) but not cortisol (see Chap. 230). Therefore, the use of dopamine may have aggravating influences on immunity and catabolism.

Dobutamine (2–12 µg/kg/minute) is a complex synthetic agent consisting of two stereoisomers having opposing actions. It has predominantly a $\beta_1$ action, however, with greater inotropic than chronotropic effects. It is commonly used in the presence of poor left ventricular function; it increases cardiac output and oxygen delivery in states of compromised tissue perfusion, avoiding the $\alpha$ effects of norepinephrine, epinephrine, or dopamine. Its vasodilatory action may enhance organ perfusion, provided that hypotension is avoided. Dobutamine, like dopamine, can decrease TSH levels.[34]

Dopexamine (0.9–5 µg/kg/minute) is a synthetic catecholamine with a strong $\beta_2$ action and weaker $\beta_1$ and $DA_1$ and $DA_2$ receptor actions. It has the combined properties of dopamine plus dobutamine infusion. It has no $\alpha$ actions. Dopexamine causes vasodilatation in the renal, splanchnic, coronary, skeletal, and pulmonary vascular beds, and enhances inotropic and chronotropic activity.

Norepinephrine (0.05–0.5 µg/kg/minute) is a potent pressor agent with predominant $\alpha$ effects. In addition to its $\beta_1$ actions, it exerts an increased inotropy and chronotropy. As it is the most potent vasoconstrictor agent available, total peripheral resistance (via $\alpha$ effects) occurs at higher doses. It may, however, cause vasoconstriction in mesenteric and coronary beds with resultant splanchnic and myocardial ischemia. Arterial blood pressure may increase, so that increased renal blood flow is induced. The norepinephrine dose should be gradually titrated. Low doses have $\beta_1$ effects and higher doses have $\alpha$ effects. Norepinephrine is often a second-line agent after the failure of therapy with dopamine or dobutamine. Dobutamine is the agent of choice in congestive heart failure, because its inotropic support is combined with mild vasodilation. On the other hand, norepinephrine is the agent of choice in most inflammatory conditions (associated with low systemic resistance) because its inotropic effects are combined with vasoconstriction.

*Epinephrine* is often used in anaphylactic shock, cardiac arrest, or cardiogenic shock. A dosage of <0.01 μg/kg per minute may decrease blood pressure via dilatation of vascular beds in skeletal muscle. A dosage of 0.02 to 0.1 μg/kg per minute exerts $\beta_1$ and $\alpha$ effects (with weak $\beta_2$ action) and increases heart rate, cardiac output, and stroke volume. Dosages of >0.2 μg/kg per minute increase total peripheral resistance via $\alpha$ vasoconstrictive predominance. Further dosage elevation (>0.3 μg/kg/minute) may cause decreased perfusion and gastric ulceration. The $\alpha$ response enhances coronary artery perfusion and is helpful during cardiopulmonary resuscitation. Epinephrine is associated with dysrhythmias, myocardial ischemia, lactic acidosis, hyperglycemia, increased free fatty acid levels, and hypokalemia.

Catecholamine action is highly dependent on the concentrations of adrenergic receptors, their respective affinities for different catecholamines, and reciprocal interactions. These variables often are significantly altered in critical illness. For example, a relative $\beta$-adrenergic hyporesponsiveness (i.e., desensitization) of the heart is frequently seen, and the interactions of the stereoisomers of dobutamine are unpredictable. Furthermore, glucocorticoids have potent modulatory influences on several aspects of catecholamine action, including up-regulation of $\beta$-receptors. The physician should, therefore, watch for unexpected responses. The future use of nitric oxide inhibitors may decrease the need for the use of catecholamines.[35]

# THYROID HORMONES

Serum thyroid hormone levels exhibit fairly consistent alterations in systemic nonthyroidal illness (NTI). Typically TSH and free thyroxine ($T_4$) are normal and total triiodothyronine ($T_3$) is decreased.[36–40] These findings are thought to represent a homeostatic mechanism by which the body decreases thyroid hormone action by diminishing the effects of the bioactive hormone, $T_3$. Despite the belief that these changes might be homeostatic, studies have been performed in which either $T_3$ or $T_4$ has been administered to patients to detect any potential benefits.[41–47] Because NTI occurs in many patients with systemic illness, and because the morbidity and mortality rate of such illness is high, determining whether thyroid hormone administration is beneficial or detrimental is important.

## THYROID HORMONE CHANGES IN NONTHYROIDAL ILLNESS

The most consistent finding in NTI is that serum total $T_3$ and free $T_3$ are decreased below the normal range, especially in cases in which the total $T_4$ concentration is also subnormal (see Chap. 36; Fig. 36-1). In general, the greater the severity of disease, the lower the serum $T_3$ levels. Typically, serum total $T_4$ levels are decreased in patients with more chronic and severe systemic illness; indeed, total $T_4$ levels of <4 μg/dL are associated with increased mortality. Studies have shown inconsistent results with regard to free $T_4$, depending on the analytical techniques used (i.e., equilibrium dialysis, direct measurement, or ultrafiltration; see Chap. 33). In most studies, patients with NTI have either normal or decreased serum free $T_4$.[48–50] Although the total $T_3$ may be decreased in patients with NTI, a relatively large number may have normal free $T_3$ levels.[51] The sera of NTI patients may contain substances (e.g., free fatty acids) that are capable of inhibiting the binding of $T_4$ and/or $T_3$ to serum-binding proteins.[52]

When a third-generation assay is used, serum TSH concentrations are usually found to be normal, although they may be slightly decreased. For TSH to be undetectable (i.e., <0.01 μU/mL) due to NTI alone is extremely unusual.[53] Various pharmacologic agents used in critical illness (e.g., dopamine and glucocorticoids) may decrease TSH levels significantly; thus, in some studies, excluding the effects of these drugs may be difficult.[54,55] An unresolved issue is whether the measured TSH is appropriately bioactive.[56]

## PERIPHERAL ACTIONS OF THYROID HORMONES

Although *serum levels* of thyroid hormones are important, the critical issues with respect to thyroid hormone action are *tissue concentrations* and *nuclear receptor occupancy.* These are difficult to determine in humans. Serum from NTI patients may inhibit $T_4$ entry into hepatocytes compared with normal serum[57]; the mechanism for this is unknown. In a pathologic study, the $T_3$ concentrations of tissue obtained from NTI patients were found to be 0.9 and 3.7 (nmol/kg wet weight) in liver and kidney, respectively, compared with 3.7 and 12.9 in control tissues ($p$ <.01).[58] The anterior pituitary $T_3$ content was 3.7 in NTI patients versus 6.8 in controls. The cerebral cortex and hypothalamus of NTI patients also had relatively lower tissue concentrations. Interestingly, the $T_3$ content of skeletal muscle and cardiac tissue $T_3$ appeared to be higher in NTI patients than in controls, although this difference was not statistically significant.

## ARE PATIENTS WITH NONTHYROIDAL ILLNESS EUTHYROID OR HYPOTHYROID?

Clinically, determining whether the patient with NTI is euthyroid is difficult, because many of the classic signs and symptoms that are commonly found in hypothyroidism may be observed. For example, patients in an intensive care unit (ICU) may manifest hypotension, dry skin, bradycardia, and hypothermia. Furthermore, as discussed earlier, whether the serum thyroid hormone and TSH levels obtained in the ICU setting accurately reflect tissue thyroid hormone status is unknown. Conceivably, a "normal" TSH level might be inappropriately low for the level of serum $T_4$ and free $T_4$, especially in relation to the hepatic and anterior pituitary concentrations of $T_3$. Although $T_3$ receptor occupancy has not been studied, anterior pituitary $T_3$ concentrations would seem to be critical; however, pituitary function is normal in NTI.[59] Alternatively, the hypothalamic TRH synthesis and concentration may be decreased in NTI and, as a result, the TSH and thyroid hormone secretion would be diminished.[37] This is supported by the finding of decreased TRH mRNA in the periventricular nucleus of a single subject who died with systemic illness and NTI.[60] A decreased hypothalamic TRH concentration in NTI could be related to cytokine changes (e.g., increased IL-6) (see Chap. 227) or to increased endogenous glucocorticoid secretion.[61]

Nevertheless, the TSH level probably does accurately reflect the amount of thyroid hormone available in the pituitary and probably also reflects the thyroid hormone concentrations of the tissues.

## TREATMENT OF NONTHYROIDAL ILLNESS

In several studies, patients with NTI have been treated with $T_3$ or $T_4$.[41–47] These studies are of limited applicability, however, because they generally have involved a small number of patients in diverse populations.

**Animal Studies.** In an experimental model of sepsis, both pulmonary elasticity and respiratory drive were improved by injection of 15 μg/kg $T_3$.[62] In another study, injection of $T_3$ (10 μg/100 g body weight) into rats with streptococcal pneumonia improved outcome.[63] Other animal studies indicate that $T_4$ administration is associated with less post–cardiac arrest and neurologic defects,[64] and that $T_3$ therapy may increase cardiac reperfusion and inotropy after heart transplantation.[65] No evidence of tissue hypothyroidism or altered urinary nitrogen excretion was found in rats treated with turpentine oil (a model of NTI),[66] and thyroid hormone administration was not associated with any proven benefit. On the other hand, $T_3$ administration to pigs with myocardial ischemia was associated with improved cardiac function.[67]

**Human Studies.** The best large-scale studies in humans have administered $T_3$ to patients who have undergone coronary artery bypass surgery (CABG).[42,43,45,67a] In one prospective, randomized clinical trial, 211 patients undergoing CABG were randomized to receive either an intravenous infusion of $T_3$ (0.8 μg/kg followed by 0.12 μg/kg per hour for 6 hours), dopamine (5 μg/kg/m²), or placebo.[43] Serum $T_3$ levels decreased in the dopamine and placebo groups but did not decrease in the $T_3$ treatment group. No significant differences were seen in hemodynamic variables or inotropic drug requirements among the groups (see Chap. 36; Fig. 36-6). A similar prospective, randomized study of CABG patients was performed in which one group received $T_3$ (0.8 μg/kg followed by 0.113 μg/kg per hour infusion for 6 hours).[42] The postoperative cardiac index was higher in the $T_3$-treated group (2.97 vs. 2.67 L/minute/m²) than in the placebo group, and systemic vascular resistance was lower (1073 vs. 1235 dyne·sec·cm⁻⁵). No differences were seen in the incidence of cardiac arrhythmias, mortality, or the requirement for medications. $T_3$ administration in these studies was not associated with significant improvement.[45]

The effect of $T_3$ administration on recovery rate and mortality in patients with burn injuries has also been evaluated.[44] A dose of 200 μg $T_3$ restored serum $T_3$ concentrations but did not affect mortality or the basal metabolic rate compared with placebo.

Patients with NTI and a serum $T_4$ level of <5 μg/dL were randomly assigned to a control regimen or $T_4$ treatment (1.5 μg/kg) for 14 days.[41] In the $T_4$-treated group, serum $T_4$ concentrations normalized on day 5. The control group had a significant rise in total $T_3$ on day 7, but this rise was delayed until day 10 in the treatment group. TSH was reduced in the treatment group. The mortality rate was equivalent in both groups (~75%), and the baseline $T_3$/$T_4$ ratios predicted outcome regardless of treatment group.

The possible adverse effects of $T_3$ administration on muscle protein catabolism during fasting has been studied in obese patients in fed and fasted states.[46] During the fasting stage, patients received 5 to 10 μg of $T_3$ every 4 hours orally to maintain a normal $T_3$ concentration ($T_3$ usually decreases during fasting). In this study, $T_3$ administration blunted the expected decrease in 3-methylhistidine excretion (reflecting muscle catabolism), results which suggested that the fasting-associated decrease in serum $T_3$ may be homeostatic in nature.

In summary, no compelling evidence exists to support the utility of $T_4$ or $T_3$ administration in NTI patients. Nevertheless, evidence accrued in one disease state may not be applicable to others. Moreover, knowing which end points, other than mortality, are relevant is difficult.

## CLINICAL APPROACH TO PATIENTS WITH NONTHYROIDAL ILLNESS

In the evaluation of possible thyroid dysfunction, the patient should be examined thoroughly, and the physician should look for evidence of previous thyroid surgery and signs suggestive of hypothyroidism (i.e., enlarged thyroid gland, dry skin, cardiac

arrhythmias, pericardial effusion, hypothermia, and/or delayed reflex return). Some of these signs may be extremely difficult to detect in the ICU patient, who typically has multiple medical problems, may have had a tracheotomy, and may be receiving medication for sedation. The physician should obtain as complete a history as possible from medical records and from the patient and/or relatives to ascertain whether the patient has had thyroid disease or has received surgery or radioactive iodine for an overactive thyroid and also whether a family history of disease is present. Of course, thyroid function tests and measurement of antibodies may be helpful.

Evaluating a patient who may have secondary hypothyroidism is particularly difficult. In this case, an assessment for papilledema, visual field alteration, and involvement of other pituitary hormones is important. Medications also need to be reviewed, with special emphasis on dopamine and glucocorticoids, both of which may suppress serum TSH concentrations.[36–40,54,55] Dilantin and phenobarbital[68] may also influence the hypothalamic–pituitary–thyroid axis, as do many other drugs (see Chap. 15), and to accurately assess the clinical and biochemical thyroid state of ICU patients who are receiving these agents is virtually impossible. Frequently, these patients may have had a computed tomography or magnetic resonance imaging of the head without attention to the pituitary gland, studies that may be helpful in delineating possible pathology.

**Normal Thyroid-Stimulating Hormone Level.** Excluding those patients receiving medications known to affect TSH, a normal TSH suggests that the patient is euthyroid and does not require L-thyroxine therapy. A normal free $T_4$ level would support this view. If the free $T_4$ level is <0.2 ng/dL (normal 0.8–1.8 ng/dL) in the presence of a normal TSH level, however, consideration of L-thyroxine therapy probably is warranted, because only a few euthyroid patients with systemic illness have such a low free $T_4$. Theoretically, administration of reverse $T_3$ might be useful. An elevated level suggests altered homeostatic $T_4$ conversion to reverse $T_3$ rather than to $T_3$; a decreased level suggests decreased production of $T_4$ and possibly hypothyroidism.[69] Nevertheless, only rarely is the reverse $T_3$ determination of value for treatment purposes.[70]

**Subnormal Thyroid-Stimulating Hormone Level.** In the circumstance of a normal or decreased free $T_4$ level and a subnormal (but detectable) TSH value, if the patient is not taking medications known to alter TSH values, the physician should ensure that the remainder of the pituitary gland function is normal and that no hypothalamic or pituitary involvement by a mass or infiltrative disease is present. If the TSH is *undetectable*, however, efforts should be made to rule out mass involvement of the pituitary gland.

**High Thyroid-Stimulating Hormone Level.** If the TSH level is >10 μU/mL, especially if the free $T_4$ is decreased and a reasonable clinical suspicion of hypothyroidism exists, the physician should recommend L-thyroxine therapy. Although several potential regimens are available for treatment with $T_4$ and/or $T_3$, L-thyroxine is preferable, usually in dosages of 50 to 100 μg per day (the dosage depends on the level of suspicion of hypothyroidism and the general medical and cardiac condition). If the TSH level is between 5 and 10 μU/mL (assuming the patient is not in recovery from systemic illness), repeating the laboratory determination several times over the next few days is reasonable; if the values are consistently elevated, the patient could be treated with L-thyroxine or simply followed very closely with frequent physical examinations and repeat thyroid function tests. Occasionally, a patient with hypothyroidism may not have an elevated TSH. For example, fasting decreases serum TSH concentrations in euthyroid healthy individuals,[71] and in certain circumstances of bona fide hypothyroidism, the TSH level may be lower than expected. (For example, the authors saw an extremely ill patient with metastatic cancer in the ICU who had a serum TSH of 10 to 20 μU/mL. Fortuitously, a serum sample obtained 1 week earlier when the patient had been relatively stable had revealed the TSH level to be 80 μU/mL. This patient was not receiving medications known to decrease serum TSH. Although this represents a single case, such a phenomenon is a cause for concern.) Certainly, the presence of a decreased serum free $T_4$ level in association with an elevated TSH level adds considerable support for a diagnosis of primary hypothyroidism.

**Undetectable Level of Thyroid-Stimulating Hormone.** Occasionally hyperthyroidism is suspected in a patient with NTI.[72,73] The serum TSH will be undetectable, the free $T_4$ will be high normal or elevated, and the free $T_3$ may be inappropriately normal or elevated. Determining which patients should be treated with antithyroid agents may be difficult, because clinical findings such as tachycardia may also be related to the underlying medical illness. Often, obtaining radioactive iodine uptake results is difficult. Treatment is usually with methimazole (e.g., 5–15 mg per day) or propylthiouracil (50–150 mg per day) with frequent monitoring of leukocytes and liver function test results. Several days to weeks is required for these antithyroid agents to have maximal inhibitory effect on thyroid hormone synthesis. Iodine or ipodate should be administered only in emergencies.

In conclusion, NTI is seen in multiple disorders that tend to yield similar thyroid function test results (i.e., normal free $T_4$ and TSH in conjunction with decreased total and/or free $T_3$). *Most of these patients should be considered to be euthyroid and should not be treated with thyroid hormones.* Patients with elevated TSH levels, especially in conjunction with decreased free $T_4$, should be considered for L-thyroxine treatment. The clinical context, including the medical history and physical examination, must be considered in the decision to treat any given patient. Differences in approach to patients with NTI will continue until further information regarding its etiology, pathophysiology, and response to treatment in different patient populations are better understood.

# GROWTH HORMONE AND INSULIN-LIKE GROWTH FACTOR-I

Critical illness has considerable impact on the GH/insulin-like growth factor-I (IGF-I) axis, leading to a *GH-resistant state* (see Chap. 228). Typically a marked increase in serum GH is seen, accompanied by a concomitant decrease in serum IGF-I, insulin-like growth factor–binding protein-3 (IGFBP-3), acid-labile subunit (ALS) levels, and IGF-I mRNA. In an attempt to abrogate the associated hypermetabolic response to critical illness, treatment with human recombinant growth hormone (rhGH) has been evaluated. In general, this hormone, in a wide dosage range (from 0.03 mg/kg/day to 10 mg/kg/day), is typically administered during the first days of admission and continued from a few days to as long as 4 weeks. Metabolic studies of protein kinetics in normal subjects have shown improvement in protein balance and increased free fatty acid and glycerol levels. Concurrently, serum IGF-I levels often are increased (similar results are found in subjects who are nutritionally deprived or malnourished).[74]

Despite the improved metabolic impact in normal and malnourished subjects, the efficacy of rhGH treatment of critically ill patients remains less certain. In burn cases, some reports suggest improved nitrogen balance, perhaps related to the dosage of this hormone. Children with burns who are treated with 0.2 mg/kg per day appear to have improved wound healing and a

decreased period of hospitalization.[75] Although malnourished patients with chronic obstructive pulmonary disease (COPD) appear to gain weight and have improved respiratory function, attempts to hasten the weaning of respiratory-dependent patients have not been successful. Several studies, involving both the critically ill and those with sepsis, also show an improvement in nitrogen balance that is linked to enhanced IGF-I levels; however, the eventual outcome is unaffected, although the depression of hand grip strength is minimized.[76] An adequate concurrent caloric supplementation is important for effective GH action (see Chap. 231).

Many of the anabolic actions of GH are mediated by IGF-I levels, which often are decreased in malnourished and/or critically ill patients. Studies using exogenously administered IGF-I, however, have had inconsistent results, perhaps related to the dose achieved. Increased survival has been reported in a phase II study of head injury patients.[77] An alternative approach, which avoids the risk of hyperglycemia from GH and hypoglycemia from IGF-I, uses a combination of GH and IGF-I. (This approach may also overcome the weak anabolic effects of IGF-I as well as the decrease in GH via negative feedback.) GH secretagogues and stable synthetic analogs have potent stimulatory effects on GH secretion via specific GH secretagogue receptors in the hypothalamus and the pituitary (see Chaps. 12 and 230). The infusion of GH-releasing peptide-2, but not of GH-releasing hormone (GHRH) or TRH, into patients with prolonged critical illness synchronized the temporal release of GH, TSH, and prolactin from the pituitary (see Chap. 230 and Fig. 230-4). An oral analog of the GH secretagogue peptide, GH-releasing peptide-6, improved the nitrogen balance in catabolic stress.[78]

Although the safety and efficacy of GH replacement appears to be confirmed for patients with *documented GH deficiency* (see Chap. 17), the benefits in *critically ill patients with GH resistance* are more controversial. Two large phase III, multicenter, prospective, double-blind, randomized, placebo-controlled studies were performed that included 532 patients who had undergone abdominal surgery, cardiac surgery, or multiple trauma, or who had acute respiratory failure; patients with type 1 diabetes, chronic renal failure, burns, organ transplants, acute central nervous system damage, liver dysfunction, or septic shock were excluded.[79] A mean dose of 0.1 mg/kg of body weight of rhGH (or placebo) was administered to patients from the fifth ICU day for up to 21 days. In the two parallel studies, the relative risk of death was 1.9 (95% confidence interval, 1.3–2.9) and 2.4 (95% confidence interval, 1.6–2.9). Multiple organ failure, septic shock, and uncontrolled infection were more prevalent in the GH-treated patients. In contrast, in other studies, administration of GH to victims of burns and trauma appeared to produce some benefit without excess death. A reappraisal of studies in which rhGH was given to pediatric burn victims or to adults with hypopituitarism did not reveal a similar safety issue.[80,81] The cause of this difference in outcome is unclear, but the timing of rhGH administration may be important. Experimentally, GH-primed animals experience a potentiation of the detrimental effects of endotoxin.[82] Timing in relation to the effects on pituitary function of a prolonged stay in the ICU (see Chap. 230) may be an additional factor to be considered.

In summary, certain metabolic parameters characteristic of this GH-resistant state (e.g., low IGF-I) can be ameliorated by the exogenous administration of rhGH and/or IGF-I. Clearly, more detailed information about timing, dosage, and possible immune enhancement must be obtained to establish both the safety and efficacy of such treatment. Therapeutic intervention with GH in *established* GH deficiency, however, appears to have a beneficial impact (see Chap. 12); although this application has not been studied specifically, these patients should be considered for rhGH replacement during critical illness. Critical illness and the associated GH-resistant state in the *absence* of GH deficiency provides a different challenge, however, and requires alternative approaches, as exemplified by the use of GH secretagogue peptides.

## ANABOLIC STEROIDS

Alternative anabolic strategies to GH and IGF-I use, such as androgen replacement, have received scant studies other than in AIDS.[83]

## POSTERIOR PITUITARY HORMONES

The posterior pituitary hormone arginine vasopressin (AVP) plays an essential role in cardiovascular regulation via stimuli mediated by hyperosmolality and hypovolemia (see Chap. 25). The $V_1$ AVP receptor signals vasoconstrictive responses, whereas the $V_2$ receptor impacts the movement of free water across the distal nephron via recruitment of aquaporin channels. Activation of AVP secretion also increases the release of ACTH. In general, the antidiuretic response to AVP occurs at concentrations much lower than those needed for pressor response.

Several AVP analogs are available with differing affinities for the $V_1$ and $V_2$ receptors. The infusion of AVP ($V_1$ and $V_2$ action) causes vasoconstriction in most vascular beds. The decreased splanchnic and portal blood flow has been used to control bleeding from esophageal varices as well as in other types of gastrointestinal bleeding (e.g., Mallory-Weiss tears, gastritis, diverticuli, and ulcers). Transcatheter intraarterial delivery of vasopressin (0.2 U/minute to 0.4 U/minute) results in capillary vasoconstriction and muscle wall contraction of the gastrointestinal tract. Vasopressin can also lead to myocardial infarction (MI), stroke, and bowel ischemia. In contrast to the negligible pressor effect of AVP in normal subjects, the pressor response to an infusion of AVP in vasodilatory septic shock is augmented, suggesting a hypersensitivity state.[84] AVP has also been used to control and prevent bleeding in patients with a variety of hemostatic disorders (e.g., hemophilia A, type 1 von Willebrand disease, cardiac surgery, uremia, and sickle cell crisis). In certain conditions (e.g., endstage congestive heart failure), a low-dose infusion (i.e., 1 IU/hour) of AVP can minimize the vasoconstrictive side effects, exerting instead a beneficial diuretic action.[85] Low-dose vasopressin restores diuresis both in patients with hepatorenal syndrome and in anuric patients with end-stage heart failure. Administration of vasopressin has been reported to enhance survival after cardiopulmonary resuscitation.[86]

Hyponatremia, as in the syndrome of inappropriate antidiuresis (see Chap. 27), is a common sequela of pain, nausea, hypoxia, and drugs. It is an important risk marker of mortality in hospitalized patients. In addition to the traditional approach of water restriction for patients with the syndrome of inappropriate secretion of antidiuretic hormone, novel analogs that act as selective $V_2$ receptor antagonists are available.[87,88] These analogs can enhance free water clearance, while maintaining effective arterial blood volume in edema, congestive heart failure, cirrhosis, and nephrosis.

## PANCREATIC HORMONES

**Insulin.** Administration of insulin is life-saving in diabetic ketoacidosis. The increased morbidity and mortality in diabetic patients who experience stroke, MI, or other insults underscore the importance of insulin therapy for hyperglycemia in these patients. In nondiabetic patients experiencing an MI, hyperglycemia on admission is a poor prognostic factor.[89] In a randomized trial, insulin-glucose infusion followed by subcutaneous insulin in diabetic patients with acute MI improved the long-term prognosis.[90] This benefit of strict glycemic control extended to patients who previously had poor metabolic control (as evidenced by high levels of hemoglobin $A_{1c}$ on admission).[91,92] In nondiabetic patients who develop stress hyperglycemia, insulin should be used to treat the moderate to severe hyperglycemia to prevent acute associated complications (e.g., hyperosmolar state, polyuria, volume depletion, and electrolyte disturbances). The benefit of control of milder stress hyperglycemia, however, has been less studied.

Hyperkalemia is a frequent occurrence in ICU patients and can be life-threatening. Insulin and glucose infusion is very useful in the acute treatment of this condition[93] but is less effective for critically ill patients owing to their relative insulin resistance.

In spite of the relative insulin resistance of critically ill patients, the use of insulin for its anabolic effect, in combination with total parenteral nutrition, has been advocated to counter the effect of catabolic hormones (i.e., to decrease protein catabolism and nitrogen loss).[93,94]

**Glucagon.** In addition to having well-known metabolic effects (see Chap. 182), glucagon, in pharmacologic doses, has cardiovascular (positive inotropic and chronotropic action), gastrointestinal, hepatobiliary, and urinary effects (smooth muscle relaxation). Intramuscular glucagon increases blood glucose faster than does oral glucose; the use of glucagon to treat hypoglycemia acutely is indicated when the patient cannot be given oral glucose or when intravenous access is not available. The prolonged use of glucagon in this setting is limited by the depletion of glycogen storage that commonly occurs in alcoholics, in malnourished patients, and in patients with liver or adrenal failure.[95]

The positive inotropic and chronotropic effect of glucagon is independent of catecholamine release or of adrenergic receptors. Because of these cardiac properties, it has been successfully used to treat cardiogenic shock and congestive heart failure, and to reverse bradycardia and hypotension due to β-blocker overdose.[96] Glucagon has also been useful in other shock states such as calcium-channel blocker overdose[97] and refractory anaphylactic shock.[98] In experimental models, glucagon was used with success in hypovolemic and septic shock,[96] and in ventricular standstill.[97]

To take advantage of glucagon's esophageal sphincter–relaxing properties, this agent has been used intravenously, either alone or in combination with other modalities (e.g., medical and interventional), to treat esophageal food impaction.[97]

Glucagon has also been used for its smooth muscle–relaxing properties, but with less success, in asthma, choledochoduodenal spasm, biliary colic, acute diverticulitis, renal colic, and intussusception.[97] The suppressive action of glucagon on pancreatic enzymes was the basis for an inconclusive trial in acute pancreatitis.[97]

**Somatostatin.** Somatostatin has multiple inhibitory effects on hormones. It decreases upper gastrointestinal motility and secretion, and diminishes pancreatic secretion (see Chaps. 169 and 182). This hormone inhibits the release of vasodilator hormones and indirectly causes splanchnic vasoconstriction; it decreases portal venous inflow, portal pressures, and azygous flow.

In addition to its known use in cases of acromegaly and other neuroendocrine tumors, somatostatin and one of its analogs (octreotide) have many useful applications in critical illness. They can, for example, control bleeding from esophageal varices. They are more effective than placebo or vasopressin and have fewer side effects than vasopressin.[99] They are as effective as sclerotherapy for the acute management of variceal bleeding[100]; in combination with sclerotherapy, they are more effective than sclerotherapy alone or band ligation alone.[101] Their use in upper gastrointestinal nonvariceal bleeding can be beneficial in some patients.[102] Neither natural somatostatin nor octreotide improves the course of acute pancreatitis. Octreotide use in pancreatic fistulas and pseudocysts markedly reduces fluid production.[103] This agent has been used to prevent and treat carcinoid crisis,[104] and also can possibly be of use in combination with insulin to normalize the abnormal glucose metabolism occurring in critical illness.[105] In persistent neonatal hyperinsulinemic hypoglycemia, octreotide treatment may obviate the need for surgery.[106]

Somatostatin also has significant immunomodulatory properties (e.g., suppression of tumor necrosis factor [TNF] levels).[107]

## MINERAL METABOLITES

Levels of the divalent cations—calcium, magnesium, and phosphorus—are frequently abnormal in critically ill patients. The role of manipulation of these cations in the treatment of the hypocalcemic, hypomagnesemic, and hypophosphatemic disorders that are encountered in critically ill patients is discussed in this section.

### HYPOCALCEMIA

Calcium circulates in the blood in bound, chelated, and ionized forms (see Chaps. 49 and 60). Critically ill patients frequently have low total serum calcium levels as a result of decreased concentrations of albumin and diminished albumin binding of calcium. Numerous formulae to correct the measured total serum calcium levels for alterations in the albumin level have proved to be unreliable.[108,109] Ionized calcium levels (the bioactive calcium fraction) are readily available on most blood gas analyzers. Blood for ionized calcium measurement should be obtained anaerobically just before analysis (using calcium heparin or a minimal heparin technique). The ionized calcium level should be determined for patients with suspected hypocalcemia (usually based on a low total serum calcium concentration). Many critically ill patients with low total serum calcium levels (even after correction for albumin) have normal ionized calcium concentrations. Some debate exists regarding the normal level of ionized calcium; the commonly cited normal range is 1.05 to 1.3 mmol/L.

The administration of calcium to critically ill patients is believed to be detrimental and to be associated with cell injury.[109–113] Intracellular calcium overload is a common mechanism for cell injury and death, especially when associated with tissue ischemia or systemic inflammation. Most individuals with ionized hypocalcemia are thought to have elevated free intracellular calcium concentrations.[110,114] Importantly, no study to date has shown calcium administration to be beneficial in critically ill patients with mild to moderate ionized hypocalcemia (i.e., 0.7–1.05 mmol/L). Some studies have shown that moderate degrees of ionized hypocalcemia are *protective* during various critical illnesses (e.g., shock, sepsis).[110,111] Calcium administration increases vascular tone and blood pressure in most critically ill patients, irrespective of their ionized calcium levels. Interestingly, calcium administration does not increase cardiac output or organ blood flow in most critically ill patients (unless severe ionized hypocalcemia is present). In fact, studies in both animals and humans indicate that calcium administration is associated with catecholamine resistance (perhaps as a result of intracellular calcium overload).[115–117] Thus, calcium should be administered only to critically ill patients with *severe ionized hypocalcemia* (<0.7 mmol/L), symptomatic hypocalcemia, or as an antagonist to hyperkalemia, hypermagnesemia, or calcium-channel blocker toxicity.

Ionized hypocalcemia, which is part of the acute-phase response, probably evolved to be protective during critical illness. Thus, overaggressive repletion may be detrimental to the patient. The decrease in circulating ionized calcium levels that is observed during critical illness results from a variety of causes, including hyperphosphatemia, hypermagnesemia, hypomagnesemia, deficiency of 1,25-dihydroxyvitamin D, acquired parathyroid hormone deficiency, tissue sequestration of calcium, and high levels of calcitonin precursors.[118] The underlying cause of ionized hypocalcemia (i.e., sepsis, hypomagnesemia) must be treated. Drugs that aggravate the hypocalcemia (i.e., loop diuretics, phosphate) should be discontinued, if possible. Magnesium and phosphorus levels should be measured in patients with ionized hypocalcemia, and these levels should be corrected if abnormal (see later). Administration of calcium to hyperphosphatemic patients can result in calcium phosphate precipitation, organ injury, and death. In addition, normalization of circulating calcium levels in the presence of severe alterations in magnesium is difficult. If clinically indicated, blood should be sent for analysis of intact parathyroid hormone and vitamin D levels. Symptomatic ionized hypocalcemia is rare in critically ill patients with levels of >0.7 mmol/L. *Thus, the recommendation is to treat only those patients with ionized calcium levels of <0.7 mmol/L or with symptoms thought to be related to the hypocalcemia.* Bolus intravenous administration of calcium is short-lived and associated with adverse effects (e.g., hypertension, vasoconstriction, and nausea/vomiting). The emergency management of ionized hypocalcemia should be accomplished by administering a small bolus of elemental calcium (50–100 mg over 5–10 minutes) followed by a continuous intravenous infusion of elemental calcium (0.5–1.0 mg/kg/hour). The choice of calcium salt is of little clinical importance. Because the elemental calcium content of calcium salts varies, however, the quantity of salt required to deliver specified amounts of elemental calcium differs. The response to calcium differs significantly among individuals and depends on renal function and the status of the parathyroid hormone–vitamin D axis. Thus, ionized calcium levels should be followed closely during therapy, and the rate of infusion should be adjusted to keep ionized calcium levels between 0.8 to 1.0 mmol/L. Patients also should have adequate intravascular volume during treatment to minimize toxic actions of calcium.

Calcium is irritating to veins and should be diluted before administration or administered into a central vein. Calcium chloride should not be injected intramuscularly; however, when intravenous access is not available, calcium gluceptate can be administered intramuscularly (but only in an emergency). Calcium salts should not be admixed with carbonates, phosphates, sulfates, or tartrates in parenteral solutions. Calcium should be given cautiously to patients receiving digitalis because calcium increases the toxic effects of this drug on the heart.

The response to calcium therapy is monitored by following blood ionized calcium levels, vital signs, clinical symptoms, and the electrocardiogram. Levels of magnesium, phosphorus, potassium, and creatinine should also be checked at periodic intervals (i.e., every 6–12 hours during initial therapy). Once ionized calcium is at the desired level and the patient is stable, the patient may be switched to enteral calcium. Most patients with persistent hypocalcemia require 2 to 4 g of elemental calcium per day in divided doses (i.e., every 6 hours). If enteral calcium alone is insufficient to maintain near normal ionized calcium levels, vitamin D should be added.

The adverse effects of calcium administration are similar to those of hypercalcemia (see Chap. 58). Hypercalciuria is common during long-term treatment and may result in development of renal calculi or nephrocalcinosis. Other common side effects include hypertension, flushing, and nausea or vomiting (see Chaps. 49 and 60).

## HYPOMAGNESEMIA

Hypomagnesemia is common in critically ill patients.[109] However, because magnesium circulates in the blood in ionized, chelated, and bound forms (similar to calcium) (see Chap. 68), many patients with hypomagnesemia have normal ionized magnesium levels. Ionized magnesium measurement (via ion-selective electrode) is available in some centers; however, the electrode is unstable, and the test is expensive. In addition, blood magnesium levels frequently do not reflect tissue magnesium status, and the physiologic actions of magnesium are such that increasing the levels within the normal or slightly elevated ranges is not harmful and may be protective (i.e., it may prevent arrhythmias, tissue ischemia, and organ injury). Thus, treating with magnesium is cheaper and physiologically more beneficial, provided severe hypermagnesemia can be excluded (based on a normal or low total serum magnesium level). Furthermore, hemodynamically stable patients with normal renal function who are not receiving magnesium supplements rarely if ever develop significant hypermagnesemia.

The treatment of hypomagnesemia consists of magnesium repletion and elimination of the cause of the hypomagnesemia. Most hypomagnesemic patients in the ICU develop magnesium depletion secondary to gastrointestinal or renal losses. If possible, use of drugs that increase magnesium loss in the urine (i.e., diuretics, aminoglycosides, amphotericin B, and cyclosporine B) or via the gastrointestinal tract (i.e., laxatives) should be halted. If these drugs cannot be stopped, repletion may need to be continued during and after drug therapy. Concomitant electrolyte disturbances may require treatment during the magnesium repletion. The most common electrolyte disturbances resulting from hypomagnesemia are hypokalemia and hypocalcemia.

The amount, route, and duration of magnesium repletion depend on the cause and severity of depletion. Mild hypomagnesemia (i.e., <1.4 mg/dL) can be treated with diet (or enteral feeding) alone. Moderate (1.0–1.4 mg/dL) and severe (<1.0 mg/dL) hypomagnesemia should be treated with enteral and/or parenteral magnesium supplementation. For severe or life-threatening hypomagnesemia, intravenous administration of magnesium sulfate (1–2 g, 8–16 mEq) over 5 to 10 minutes followed by 0.5 to 1.0 g per hour as an infusion is recommended. The dosage should be reduced for patients with renal insufficiency. Serum magnesium levels should be monitored every 4 to 6 hours during initial therapy. Levels of <3.5 mg/dL are safe. Serum potassium levels also should be monitored during magnesium therapy and should be maintained within the normal range. Once serum magnesium levels are normalized, stable patients may be switched to oral magnesium repletion. Magnesium supplementation should be continued for at least 3 to 5 days to allow for repletion of intracellular stores. Once magnesium repletion is achieved, patients should receive maintenance doses of magnesium (by enteral or parenteral routes) to avoid future depletion syndromes. Most adults with normal renal function require 0.4 mEq/kg per day orally or 0.1 to 0.2 mEq/kg per day intravenously plus replacement of any concomitant excess losses (i.e., in urine, gastrointestinal secretions). Bolus doses of magnesium are quickly excreted in the urine; therefore, repeated small doses or continuous infusion is preferred over large intermittent bolus doses. When given enterally, magnesium oxide is preferable. Magnesium-containing antacids are poorly absorbed from the gastrointestinal tract, and large doses of enteral magnesium can cause diarrhea. During magnesium treatment, serum levels of magnesium, potassium, calcium, and creatinine should be monitored; blood pressure, heart rate, and clinical status (i.e., deep tendon reflexes, neuromuscular strength, mental status, respiratory function) should be checked; and, occasionally, an electrocardiogram should be taken (especially if the patient has arrhythmias).

Controversy is found in the literature regarding the use of magnesium for the treatment of cardiac arrhythmias in patients with underlying ischemic cardiac disease. Nonetheless, most studies indicate that magnesium has antiarrhythmic, antiischemic, cytoprotective, and antiatherosclerotic properties. Most studies indicate that magnesium decreases arrhythmias in patients after MI[119–121] and coronary artery bypass surgery. Furthermore, some studies indicate an improvement in outcome after myocardial ischemia.[119–121] The authors believe that intravenous administration of magnesium for the treatment of arrhythmias in patients with myocardial ischemia and infarction is justified.

## HYPOPHOSPHATEMIA

Hypophosphatemia commonly becomes life-threatening at serum phosphorus levels of <1 mg/dL. Patients with such levels should receive aggressive phosphorus repletion.[109] Cell dysfunction is frequent when circulating phosphorus levels remain <2 mg/dL, and patients with these levels usually benefit from phosphorus supplementation. The therapy for hypophosphatemia includes discontinuance of agents that may be contributing to low phosphorus levels (i.e., phosphorus-binding antacids, diuretics, refeeding[122]), treatment of the underlying disease, and therapeutic phosphorus repletion.

When the phosphorus level is <1 mg/dL, phosphorus should be administered intravenously. It should be given cautiously because it may precipitate with calcium. If phosphorus depletion is recent (i.e., total body stores are only mildly depleted), 0.6 mg/kg per hour (0.02 mmol/kg/hour) should be administered; if phosphorus depletion is prolonged and multifactorial, 0.9 mg/kg per hour (0.03 mmol/kg/hour) should be given. Circulating phosphorus levels should be checked every 6 to 12 hours during initial therapy and further replacement adjusted accordingly. Hyperkalemia may occur if phosphorus is administered as the potassium salt. Phosphorus is cleared by the kidneys, and the rate of administration usually must be decreased in patients with renal insufficiency. Enteral phosphorus is best administered to patients once phosphorus levels are within the low-normal range; when intracellular depletion is severe, this usually takes 5 to 7 days. Once repleted, patients should receive maintenance doses of phosphorus to prevent further depletion (i.e., 1000–1200 mg/day in divided doses every 6 hours, plus replacement of any excess losses). The most common side effect of enteral phosphorus administration is diarrhea (see Chap. 67). During therapy, phosphorus, calcium, potassium, and creatinine levels should be monitored.

# MODULATORS OF IMMUNITY

The field of immunology began with the seminal work of Edward Jenner, who, in 1796, immunized patients with cowpox to protect them from the more deadly virus, smallpox. Subsequently, the initial paradigm was that each immunoglobulin was preprogrammed to protect the host against invasion by a specific foreign substance (an *antigen*). It was also learned that immunoglobulins retain memory of exposure to a specific antigen, allowing them to mount a more acute protective response to a second exposure to the same antigen. This initial scheme has expanded enormously over the last century into an entire branch of science involving transplantation, oncology, autoimmune disorders, allergy, trauma, inflammation, sepsis, and critical illness. Advances in genetics and molecular biology have further expanded these boundaries. In fact, so many cells, mediators, messengers, receptors, and so on, have been identified that precisely distinguishing the field of immunology from endocrinology has become impossible. Cytokines, which play a large role in inflammation and immunity (see Chaps. 173, 174, and 227), are signaling proteins secreted by effector cells, much like traditional hormones. Indeed, many of the mediators that play principal roles in the immune response act via autocrine, paracrine, juxtacrine, and hemocrine pathways (see Chap. 1). Other effectors (e.g., calcitonin precursors), which have been traditionally classified as hormones, act in the inflammatory cascade in a manner similar to cytokines. Importantly, modulation of circulating mediators of the inflammatory response during critical illness may have therapeutic implications.[123]

**Tumor Necrosis Factor-α.** Tumor necrosis factor-α (TNF-α) is a recognized principal proximal mediator of the inflammatory response (see Chap. 227). Serum levels of this cytokine typically increase shortly after a discrete inflammatory insult and return to baseline within hours. A series of animal and human clinical trials have evaluated the effects of blocking the actions of TNF-α in inflammatory disorders associated with high levels of this cytokine. Monoclonal antibodies,[124] chimeric, humanized monoclonal antibodies,[125] and an antibody fragment (MAK 195 F)[126] have all been used with variable success. Animal experiments using these immunotherapies appeared promising but were followed by disappointing clinical trials.[125–128] None of the three antibodies tested decreased the 28-day mortality in septic patients. Recombinant TNF receptor–immunoglobulin G fusion protein is soluble in plasma and has a 50-fold greater affinity for the TNF-α molecule than does the membrane-bound receptor. Human trials of two of these fusion-type receptors have had inconsistent results, with some doses causing increased mortality and others showing marginal benefits.[129,130]

Results from systemic attack on the TNF effector cell axis have been disappointing in sepsis and SIRS. On the other hand, trials of TNF down-regulation in chronic inflammatory conditions such as rheumatoid arthritis and ulcerative colitis have been more promising.[131] Alternative approaches that have been tried include use of TNF-α-converting enzyme (TACE), which converts inactive TNF-α to its active form,[131] and inhibitors of nuclear factor-κB.[132]

**Interleukin-1β.** Interleukin-1β (IL-1β) is the predominant form of IL-1 in humans and is one of the most potent of the proinflammatory cytokines (see Chaps. 173, 174, and 227). Like TNF-α, it is considered to be a principal proximal mediator/initiator of the inflammatory cascade. The margin between clinical benefit and unacceptable toxicity is narrow, however, and IL-1β has come to be regarded as a toxic agent.[133] It has a number of features that allow its effects to be carefully regulated. IL-1β is synthesized as an inactive precursor, proIL-1β, which must be converted into its bioactive form by IL-1β–converting enzyme (ICE).[134] A naturally occurring antagonist, IL-1 receptor antagonist (IL-1ra), is also found.[135] Although structurally similar to IL-1, it is inactive. It downregulates the response to IL-1 through competition for the IL-1 receptor. Two IL-1 receptors are found: types I and II. The type II receptor form does not appear to have signal transduction capability and may be a decoy to limit the amount of IL-1 available to the functioning type I receptors.[136] The most promising strategy for IL-1 down-regulation was thought to

be administration of IL-1ra. Produced by recombinant technology, IL-1ra effectively blocks expression of IL-1.[137] The results of several clinical trials, however, have not demonstrated a decrease in mortality for patients with lethal systemic inflammation associated with its use.[138] The two endogenous soluble IL-1 receptors also bind IL-1.[139] No clinically relevant effects of their use other than a mild antiinflammatory response has been demonstrated.[140]

**Interleukin-6.** IL-6 is a pleiotropic cytokine that is under hormonal regulation (see Chaps. 173, 174, and 227). Its primary function is the regulation of the hepatic acute-phase response[141] via a transmembrane receptor (gp130). In healthy individuals, IL-6 levels are almost undetectable, but levels become significantly higher in a variety of inflammatory conditions. Thus, IL-6 is believed to mediate some of the toxicity associated with these disorders. Efforts to block or modulate IL-6 include the use of neutralizing monoclonal antibodies in patients with hematologic malignancy and autoimmune disease (with only marginal effects).[142] A receptor antagonist is also being investigated. The principal clinical use of IL-6 is as a marker for the severity of illness.

**Interleukin-8.** IL-8 is another pleiotropic cytokine involved in tumor growth, immunoglobulin E production, and angiogenesis (see Chaps. 173, 174, and 227). It also plays a role in the inflammatory cascade, in which it acts as a factor for chemotaxis, including the migration of neutrophils into areas of tissue damage.[143] Its production is, in turn, induced by IL-1, TNF, endotoxin, and other proinflammatory mediators. Although IL-8 is considered harmful, this view is most likely an oversimplification. Presumably, chemotaxis of neutrophils to areas of injury is a protective phenomenon in some situations. Despite good arguments that IL-8 is an important cytokine for normal host defense, blocking of IL-8 in conditions in which neutrophil chemotaxis is no longer beneficial (e.g., adult respiratory distress syndrome [ARDS]) may be advantageous.

**Interleukin-10.** IL-10 functions as an antiinflammatory cytokine causing inhibition of proinflammatory cytokines such as IL-1β, TNF-α, IL-6, and IL-8 (see Chaps. 173, 174, and 227).[144] It is produced late in the course of the inflammatory response and is considered to serve a regulatory role by opposing the actions of proinflammatory mediators. Although early studies demonstrated that infusing IL-10 decreased mortality in an endotoxin injection model,[145] it did not successfully decrease morbidity or mortality in a more relevant model of sepsis.[146] Supplementation with supraphysiologic amounts does not seem to hold much promise.

**Platelet-Activating Factor.** Platelet-activating factor (PAF) is a bioactive biolipid that is produced by endothelial cells, neutrophils, and lymphocytes. It is implicated in the pathogenesis of inflammatory states and organ dysfunction, especially those associated with pancreatitis. In animal trials, PAF antibodies as well as naturally occurring PAF-receptor antagonists (PAFRa) have been administered to subjects with sepsis and other inflammatory conditions. Although the results of animal experiments were promising, the clinical trials have been disappointing. Administration of PAFRa to patients with suspected sepsis (due to gram-positive and gram-negative organisms) did not reduce the 28-day mortality.[147] A naturally occurring PAF acetylhydrolase (PAF-AH) also exists that degrades PAF and is part of the body's effort to regulate the inflammatory response. In animal studies, recombinant PAF-AH has had marked antiinflammatory effects.[148] Its use in pancreatitis is also being investigated.

**Nitric oxide.** Nitric oxide (NO) is a ubiquitous, low-molecular-weight, membrane-permeable gas, the production of which is under tight regulation and the effects of which are far-reaching (see Chaps. 179 and 228). NO is produced in multiple cells under the direction of NO synthase (NOS). It causes smooth muscle relaxation by activating soluble guanylate cyclase and increasing intracellular cyclic guanosine monophosphate.[149] The constitutive isoform of NOS is determined by calcium levels in neurons (nNOS) and endothelial cells (eNOS) and produces only small amounts of NO. The inducible form of NOS (iNOS) is stimulated by mediators of inflammation and leads to a larger and more sustained production of NO.[150] The results of increased NO include bacterial lysis, vasoplegia, and myocardial depression. One of the hallmarks of inflammation and sepsis is vasodilation leading to hypotension. The vasodilation is due, in large part, to the smooth muscle dilation caused by excessive levels of NO. Decreasing the levels of NO has been attempted in patients with systemic inflammation. At least four agents have been used for this purpose. N-nitro-L-arginine methyl ester (L-NAME) and N-monomethyl-L-arginine (L-NMMA) are NOS inhibitors that decrease levels of NO. Two other agents (e.g., diasporin–cross-linked hemoglobin and pyridoxilated hemoglobin polyethylene) scavenge NO after it is produced. Although studies of the use of these four agents have shown an increase in blood pressure with decreasing NO levels,[151–154] no consistent improvement in outcome has been seen. In fact, one study demonstrated an increase in mortality in endotoxemic subjects with decreasing NO.[152] This maladaptive effect of NO depletion has multiple causes. Because of its ubiquitous nature, NO is almost certainly involved in the maintenance of homeostasis when not secreted in supraphysiologic amounts. Indeed, selective blockade of iNOS and not the constitutive forms of NOS may increase survival.[154] Although vasoconstriction raises blood pressure, it may also decrease cardiac output and decrease blood flow to critical areas. In fact, supplemental NO has been given therapeutically to patients with pulmonary hypertension and ARDS, a frequent concomitant of systemic inflammation.[155] The combination of a systemic NOS inhibitor with inhalational NO has been tried.[156] Although NO is undoubtedly an important molecule, it has not yet proved to be a clinically useful target for therapeutic modulation.

**Other Mediators.**    Other mediators have been identified or targeted for immune modulation. Prominent among these are arachidonic acid metabolites (e.g., prostaglandins, leukotrienes, and cytochrome P450 products); the complement cascade; the kinin family (e.g., bradykinin and histamine); oxygen free radicals; phagocytic proteinases (e.g., elastase and cathepsin B); other cytokines; and calcitonin precursor peptides.

Levels of the calcitonin precursors increase markedly in response to severe inflammation, infection, and sepsis (see Chaps. 53 and 228) and have very long serum half-lives, making them promising markers and potential therapeutic targets, particularly in view of the salutary responses of some species of septic animals to immunoneutralization.[157,158] Protein C and its anticoagulant properties are suppressed by the inflammatory process; augmentation of serum levels shows some promise for improving outcome.[159]

## THERAPEUTIC CONSIDERATIONS

Therapeutic considerations based on interventions involving the complex array of mediators, receptors, naturally occurring antagonists, converting enzymes, and other elements have been reviewed.[160] Although most of these modalities have had some success in experimental studies, they have failed to consistently increase survival in clinical trials.[161] A number of reasons have been cited for these repeated failures.

The inflammatory response is a complicated cascade of events involving multiple mediators and multiple pathways. Blocking or diminishing one of these pathways may not be sufficient to affect the overall expression. (This has led to the suggestion that several of these agents be used together as an "antiinflammatory cocktail," so that multiple pathways are blocked simultaneously.)

Furthermore, the timing of therapeutic intervention has also been questioned. Timing is probably crucial, insofar as the transient elevations of some of these mediators *may already have occurred* and returned to baseline before intervention has been initiated. This is especially true for the most proximal proinflammatory mediators. In most clinical conditions, the inflammatory cascade has already been stimulated before the patient's illness has been recognized. To block these mediators once this recognition has occurred may be too little and/or too late. In support of this contention, some of these interventions have proved effective when instituted before an inflammatory stimulus but not after the inflammatory cascade has been activated.

Investigators have been using severity-of-illness scores (e.g., Acute Physiology and Chronic Health Evaluation [APACHE] scores) to select patients who may be helped by some of these interventions. The development of markers that have prognostic significance would be even more useful, however. If such a marker were also a mediator contributing to the severity of illness, it would constitute an ideal therapeutic target. Also, interventions directed toward "late mediators" such as calcitonin precursors and high mobility group-1 (see Chap. 228) are quite likely to prove more useful.

Better diagnostic tools and prognostic indicators would likely help to identify subsets of patients from among those with systemic inflammation. Each of these subsets might respond favorably to different treatment modalities, some of which may have already been developed. Thus, although no single magic bullet yet exists to treat all varieties of systemic inflammation, a whole arsenal of weapons undoubtedly will become available (and may already be available) to use against its many clinical presentations.

As knowledge of the pathophysiology of sepsis and other conditions associated with critical illness improves, and as further interventional strategies are evaluated, real progress will be achieved.

## REFERENCES

1. Lamberts SWJ, Bruining HA, De Jong FH. Corticosteroid therapy in severe illness. N Engl J Med 1997; 337:1285.
2. Schein RMH, Sprung CL, Marcial E, et al. Plasma cortisol levels in patients with septic shock. Crit Care Med 1990; 18:259.
3. Reincke M, Allolio B, Wurthe G, Winklemann W. The hypothalamic-pituitary-adrenal axis in critical illness: response to dexamethasone and corticotropin-releasing hormone. J Clin Endocrinol Metab 1993; 77:151.
4. Rivers E, Blake HC, Dereczyk B, et al. Adrenal dysfunction in hemodynamically unstable patients in the emergency department. Acad Emerg Med 1999; 6:626.
5. Baldwin WA, Allo M. Occult hypoadrenalism in critically ill patients. Arch Surg 1993; 128:673.
6. Martinez FJ, Lash RW. Endocrinologic and metabolic complications in the intensive care unit. Clin Chest Med 1999; 20:401.
7. Moran A, Chapman MJ, O'Fathartaigh MS, et al. Hypocortisolemia and adrenocortical responses and onset of septic shock. Intensive Care Med 1994; 20:489.
8. Span L, Hermus A, Bartelink A, et al. Adrenocortical function. An indication of severity of disease and survival in chronic critically ill patients. Intensive Care Med 1992; 18:93.
9. Sibbald WJ, Short A, Cohen MP, Wilson RF. Variation in adrenocortical responses during severe bacterial infections. Ann Surg 1977; 186:29.
10. Drucker D, Shandling M. Variable adrenocortical function in acute medical illness. Crit Care Med 1985; 13:477.
11. Mackenzie JS, Burrows L, Burchara KW. Transient hypoadrenalism during surgical critical illness. Arch Surg 1998; 133:199.

12. Soni A, Pepper GM, Wyrinski PM, et al. Adrenal insufficiency occurring during septic shock: incidence, outcome, and relationship to peripheral cytokine levels. Am J Med 1995; 98:266.

13. May ME, Carey RM. Rapid adrenocorticotropic hormone test in practice: retrospective review. Am J Med 1985; 79:679.

14. Masterson GR, Mostafa SM. Adrenocortical function in critical illness. Br J Anaesth 1998; 81:308.

15. Streeten DHP, Anderson GH, Bonaventura NM. The potential for serious consequences from misinterpreting normal responses to the rapid ACTH test. J Clin Endocrinol Metab 1996; 81:285.

16. Chrousos GP. The hypothalamic-pituitary-adrenal axis and immune-mediated inflammation. N Engl J Med 1995; 332:1351.

17. Schlaghecke R, Kornely E, Wollenhaupt J, et al. Glucocorticoid receptors in rheumatoid arthritis. Arthritis Rheum 1992; 35:740.

18. Leung DYM, Hamid Q, Vottero A, et al. Association of glucocorticoid insensitivity with increased expression of glucocorticoid receptor beta. J Exp Med 1997; 186:1567.

19. Hamid QA, Wenzel SE, Hauk PJ, et al. Increased glucocorticoid receptor beta in airway cells of glucocorticoid-insensitive asthma. Am J Resp Crit Care Med 1999; 159:1600.

20. Norbiato G, Bevilacqua M, Vago T, et al. Cortisol resistance in acquired immunodeficiency syndrome. J Clin Endocrinol Metab 1992; 74:608.

21. Bollaert PE, Charpentier C, Levy B, et al. Reversal of late septic shock with supraphysiologic doses of hydrocortisone. Crit Care Med 1998; 26:645.

22. Briegel J, Forst H, Haller M, et al. Stress doses of hydrocortisone reverse hyperdynamic septic shock: a prospective, randomized, double-blind, single-center study. Crit Care Med 1999; 27:723.

23. Beishuizen A, Vermes I, Hylkema BS, Haanen C. Relative eosinophilia and functional adrenal insufficiency in critically ill patients. Lancet 1999; 353:1675.

24. Cronin L, Cook DJ, Carlet J, et al. Corticosteroid treatment for sepsis: a critical appraisal and metaanalysis of the literature. Crit Care Med 1995; 23:1430.

25. Freeman BD, Eichacker PQ, Natanson C. The role of inflammation in sepsis and septic shock: a meta analysis of both clinical and preclinical trials of anti-inflammatory therapies. In: Gallin JI, Snyderman R, eds. Inflammation: basic principles and clinical correlates. Philadelphia: Lippincott Williams & Wilkins, 1999:Chap. 61, 965.

26. Schneider AJ, Voerman HJ. Abrupt hemodynamic improvement in late septic shock with physiological doses of glucocorticoids. Intensive Care Med 1991; 17:436.

27. Dooley DP, Carpenter JL, Rademacher S. Adjunctive corticosteroid therapy for tuberculosis: a critical reappraisal of the literature. Clin Infect Dis 1997; 25:872.

28. Lebel MH, Freij BJ, Syrogiannopoulos GA, et al. Dexamethasone therapy for bacterial meningitis. Results of two double-blind, placebo-controlled trials. N Engl J Med 1988; 319:964.

29. Hoffman SL, Punjabi NH, Kumala S, et al. Reduction of mortality in chloramphenicol-treated severe typhoid fever by high-dose dexamethasone. N Engl J Med 1984; 310:82.

30. Montaner JS, Lawson LM, Levitt N, et al. Corticosteroids prevent early deterioration in patients with moderately severe *Pneumocystis carinii* pneumonia and the acquired immunodeficiency syndrome (AIDS). Ann Intern Med 1990; 113:14.

31. Bracken MB, Shepard MJ, Collins WF, et al. A randomized, controlled trial of methylprednisolone or naloxone in the treatment of acute spinal-cord injury. Results of the Second National Acute Spinal Cord Injury Study. N Engl J Med 1990; 322:1405.

32. McGowan JE Jr, Chesney PJ, Crossley KB, LaForce FM. Guidelines for the use of systemic glucocorticosteroids in the management of selected infections. Working Group on Steroid Use, Antimicrobial Agents Committee, Infectious Diseases Society of America. J Infect Dis 1992; 165:1.

33. Mackenzie JS, Burrows L, Buchard KW. Treatment of hypoadrenalism during surgical critical illness. Arch Surg 1998; 133:199.

34. Kulka PJ, Tryba M. Inotropic support of the critically ill patient. A review of the agents. Drugs 1993; 45:654.

35. Stanford GG. Use of inotropic agents in critical illness. Surg Clin North Am 1991; 71:683.

36. Wartofsky L, Burman KD. Alterations in thyroid function in patients with systemic illness: the "euthyroid sick syndrome." Endocr Rev 1982; 3:164.

37. DeGroot LJ. Dangerous dogmas in medicine: the nonthyroidal illness syndrome. J Clin Endocrinol Metab 1999; 84:151.

38. McIver B, Gorman CA. Euthyroid sick syndrome: an overview. Thyroid 1997; 7:125.

39. Docter R, Krenning EP, de Jong M, Hennemann G. The sick euthyroid syndrome: changes in thyroid hormone serum parameters and hormone metabolism. Clin Endocrinol 1993; 39:499.

40. Wartofsky L, Burman KD, Ringel M. Trading one "dangerous dogma" for another? Thyroid hormone treatment of the "euthyroid sick syndrome." J Clin Endocrinol Metab 1999; 84:1759.

41. Brent GA, Hershman JM. Thyroxine therapy in patients with severe nonthyroidal illness and low serum thyroxine concentration. J Clin Endocrinol Metab 1986; 63:1.

42. Klemperer JD, Klein I, Gomez M, et al. Thyroid hormone treatment after coronary-artery bypass surgery. N Engl J Med 1995; 333:1522.

43. Bennett-Guerrero E, Jiminez JL, White WD, et al. Cardiovascular effects of intravenous triiodothyronine in patients undergoing coronary artery bypass graft surgery. JAMA 1996; 275:687.

44. Becker RA, Vaughan GM, Ziegler MG, et al. Hypermetabolic low triiodothyronine syndrome of burn injury. Crit Care Med 1982; 10:870.

45. Burman KD. Is triiodothyronine administration beneficial in patients undergoing coronary artery bypass surgery? JAMA 1996; 275:687.

46. Burman KD, Wartofsky L, Dinterman RE, et al. The effect of $T_3$ and reverse $T_3$ administration on muscle protein catabolism during fasting as measured by 3-methylhistidine excretion. Metabolism 1979; 28:805.

47. Dulchavsky SA, Ksenzeko SM, Saba AA, et al. Triiodothyronine ($T_3$) supplementation maintains surfactant biochemical integrity during sepsis. J Trauma 1995; 39:53.

48. Surks MI, Hupart KH, Pan C, Shapiro LE. Normal free thyroxine in critical nonthyroidal illnesses measured by ultrafiltration of undiluted serum and equilibrium dialysis. J Clin Endocrinol Metab 1988; 67:1031.

49. Melmed S, Geola FL, Reed AW, et al. A comparison of methods for assessing thyroid function in nonthyroidal illness. J Clin Endocrinol Metab 1982; 54:300.

50. Kaptein EM, MacIntyre SS, Weiner JM, et al. Free thyroxine estimates in nonthyroidal illness: comparison of eight methods. J Clin Endocrinol Metab 1981; 54:300.

51. Chopra IJ. Simultaneous measurement of free thyroxine and free 3,5,3'-triiodothyronine in undiluted serum by direct equilibrium dialysis/radioimmunoassay: evidence that free triiodothyronine and free thyroxine are normal in many patients with the low triiodothyronine syndrome. Thyroid 1998; 8:249.

52. Jaume JC, Mendel CM, Frost PH, et al. Extremely low doses of heparin release lipase activity into the plasma and can thereby cause artifactual elevations in the serum free thyroxine concentrations as measured by equilibrium dialysis. Thyroid 1996; 6:79.

53. Franklyn JA, Black EG, Betteridge J, Sheppard MC. Comparison of second and third generation methods for measurement of serum thyrotropin in patients with overt hyperthyroidism, patients receiving thyroxine therapy, and those with nonthyroidal illness. J Clin Endocrinol Metab 1994; 77:1368.

54. Van den Berghe G, de Zegher F, Lauwers P. Dopamine and the sick euthyroid syndrome in critical illness. Clin Endocrinol 1994; 41:731.

55. Samuels MH, McDaniel PA. Thyrotropin levels during hydrocortisone infusions that mimic fasting-induced cortisol elevations: a clinical research center study. J Clin Endocrinol Metab 1997; 82:3700.

56. Persani L, Borgato S, Romoli R, et al. Changes in the degree of sialylation of carbohydrate chains modify the biological properties of circulating thyrotropin isoforms in various physiological and pathological states. J Clin Endocrinol Metab 1998; 83:2386.

57. Sarne DH, Refetoff S. Measurement of thyroxine uptake from serum by cultured human hepatocytes as an index of thyroid status: reduced thyroxine uptake from serum of patients with nonthyroid illness. J Clin Endocrinol Metab 1985; 61:1046.

58. Arem R, Wiener GJ, Kaplan SG, et al. Reduced tissue thyroid hormone levels in fatal illness. Metabolism 1993; 42:1102.

59. Faber J, Kirkegaard C, Rasmussen B, et al. Pituitary-thyroid axis in critical illness. J Clin Endocrinol Metab 1987; 65:315.

60. Fliers E, Guldenaar SEF, Wiersinga WM, Swaab DF. Decreased hypothalamic thyrotropin-releasing hormone gene expression in patients with nonthyroidal illness. J Clin Endocrinol Metab 1997; 82:4032.

61. Papanicolau DA, Wilder RL, Manolagas SC, Chrousos GP. The pathophysiologic role of interleukin-6 in human disease. Ann Intern Med 1998; 128:127.

62. Dulchavsky SA, Kennedy PR, Geller ER, et al. $T_3$ preserves respiratory function in sepsis. J Trauma 1991; 31:753.

63. Little JS. Effect of thyroid hormone supplementation on survival after bacterial infection. Endocrinology 1985; 117:1431.

64. D'Alecy LG. Thyroid hormone in neural rescue. Thyroid 1997; 7:115.

65. Jeevandam V. Triiodothyronine: spectrum of use in heart transplantation. Thyroid 1997; 7:139.

66. Chopra IJ, Huang TS, Chen Y-S, Chu SH. Evidence against replacement doses of thyroid hormones in nonthyroidal illnesses: studies using turpentine oil injected rat. J Endocrinol Invest 10:559.

67. Hsu R-B, Huang T-S M, Chen Y-S, Chi S-H. Effect of triiodothyronine administration in experimental myocardial injury. J Endocrinol Invest 1995; 18:702.

67a. Bettendorf M, Schmidt KG, Grulich-Henn J, et al. Tri-iodothyronine in children after cardiac surgery: a double-blind, randomized, placebo-controlled study. Lancet 2000; 356:529.

68. Smith PJ, Surks MI. Multiple effects of 5,5'-diphenylhydantoin on the thyroid hormone system. Endocr Rev 1984; 5:514.

69. Zaloga GP, Chernow B, Smallridge RC, et al. A longitudinal evaluation of thyroid function in critically ill surgical patients. Ann Surg 1985; 201:456.

70. Burmeister LA. Reverse $T_3$ does not reliably differentiate hypothyroid sick syndrome from euthyroid sick syndrome. Thyroid 1995; 5:435.

71. Borst GC, Osburne RC, O'Brian JT, et al. Fasting decreases thyrotropin responsiveness to thyrotropin-releasing hormone: a potential cause of misinterpretation of thyroid function tests in the critically ill. J Clin Endocrinol Metab 1983; 57:380.

72. Ross DR. Subclinical thyrotoxicosis. In: Braverman LE, Utiger RD, eds. Werner and Ingbar's the thyroid, 7th ed. New York: Lippincott–Raven Publishers, 1995:1016.

73. Samuels MH. Subclinical thyroid disease in the elderly. Thyroid 1998; 8:803.

74. Manson JM, Smith RJ, Wilmore DW. Growth hormone stimulates protein synthesis during hypocaloric parenteral nutrition: role of hormonal-substrate environment. Ann Surg 1988; 208:136.

75. Herndon DN, Barrow RE, Kunkel KJ, et al. Effects of recombinant human growth hormone on donor-site healing in severely burned children. Ann Surg 1990; 212:424.

76. Jiang Z-M, He G-Z, Zhang S-Y, et al. Low dose growth hormone and hypocaloric nutrition attenuate the protein-catabolic response after major operation. Ann Surg 1989; 210:513.

77. Hatton J, Rapp RP, Kudsk KA, et al. Intravenous insulin-like growth factor-1 (IGF-1) in moderate-to-severe head injury. J Neurosurg 1997; 86:779.

78. Murphy MG, Plunkett LM, Gertz BJ, et al. MK-677, an orally active growth hormone secretagogue, reverses diet-induced catabolism. J Clin Endocrinol Metab 1998; 83:320.

79. Takala J, Ruokonen E, Webster NR, et al. Increased mortality with growth hormone treatment in critically ill patients. N Engl J Med 1999; 341:785.

80. Ramirez RJ, Wolf SE, Barrow RE, Herndon DN. Growth hormone in pediatric burns: a safe therapeutic approach. Ann Surg 1998; 228:439.

81. Bengtsson BA, Koppeschaar HPF, Abs R, et al. Growth hormone replacement therapy is not associated with any increase in mortality. J Clin Endocrinol Metab 1999; 84:4291.

82. Liao W, Rudling M, Angelin B. Growth hormone potentiates the in vivo biological activities of endotoxin in the rat. Eur J Clin Invest 1996; 26:254.

83. Chang DW, DeSanti L, Demling RH. Anticatabolic and anabolic strategies in critical illness. A review of current treatment modalities. Shock 1998; 10:155.

84. Landry DW, Levin HR, Gallant EM, et al. Vasopressin pressor hypersensitivity in vasodilatory septic shock. Crit Care Med 1997; 25:1279.

85. Eisenman A, Armali Z, Enat R, et al. Low-dose vasopressin restores diuresis both in patients with hepatorenal syndrome and in anuric patients with end-stage heart failure. J Intern Med 1999; 246:183.

86. Lindner KH, Dirks B, Strohmenger H-U, et al. Randomized comparison of epinephrine and vasopressin in patients with out-of-hospital ventricular fibrillation. Lancet 1997; 349:535.

87. Naito A, Ohtake Y, Hasegaw H, et al. Pharmacological profile of VP-343, a novel selective vasopressin $V_2$ antagonist. Biol Pharm Bull 2000; 23:182.

88. Chan WY, Wo NC, Stovey ST, et al. Discovery and design of novel and selective vasopressin and oxytocin agonists and antagonists: the role of bioassays. Exp Physiol 2000; 85:7S.

89. Mak KH, Mah PK, Tey BH, et al. Fasting blood sugar level: a determinant for in-hospital outcome in patients with first myocardial infarction and without glucose intolerance. Ann Acad Med Singapore 1993; 22:291.

90. Bellodi G, Manicardi V, Malavasi V, et al. Hyperglycemia and prognosis of acute myocardial infarction in patients without diabetes mellitus. Am J Cardiol 1989; 64:885.

91. Malmberg K, Ryden L, Efendic S, et al. Randomized trial of insulin-glucose infusion followed by subcutaneous insulin treatment in diabetic patients with acute myocardial infarction (DIGAMI study): effects on mortality at 1 year. J Am Coll Cardiol 1995; 26:57.

92. Malmberg K, Norhammar A, Wedel H, Ryden L. Glycometabolic state at admission: important risk marker of mortality in conventionally treated patients with diabetes mellitus and acute myocardial infarction: long-term results from the Diabetes and Insulin-Glucose Infusion in Acute Myocardial Infarction (DIGAMI) study. Circulation 1999; 99:2626.

93. Blumberg A, Weidmann P, Shaw S, Gnadinger M. Effect of various therapeutic approaches on plasma potassium and major regulating factors in terminal renal failure. Am J Med 1988; 85:507.

94. Cuthbertson DP. Alterations in metabolism following injury. Injury 1980; 11:175.

95. Wolfe RR. Substrate utilization/insulin resistance in sepsis/trauma. Baillières Clin Endocrinol Metab 1997; 11:645.

96. Hall-Boyer K, Zaloga GP, Chernow B. Glucagon: hormone or therapeutic agent? Crit Care Med 1984; 12:584.

97. Pollack CV Jr. Utility of glucagon in the emergency department. J Emerg Med 1993; 11:195.

98. Zaloga GP, DeLacey W, Holmboe E, Chernow B. Glucagon reversal of hypotension in a case of anaphylactoid shock. Ann Intern Med 1986; 105:65.

99. Imperiale T, Teran J, McCullough A. A meta-analysis of somatostatin versus vasopressin in the management of acute esophageal variceal hemorrhage. Gastroenterology 1995; 109:1289.

100. Sung J, Chung S, Lai C, et al. Octreotide infusion or emergency sclerotherapy for variceal haemorrhage. Lancet 1993; 342:637.

101. Besson, I, Ingrand P, Person B, et al. Sclerotherapy with or without octreotide for acute variceal bleeding. N Engl J Med 1995; 333:555.

102. Jenkins SA, Poulianos G, Coraggio F, Rotondano G. Somatostatin in the treatment of non-variceal upper gastrointestinal bleeding. Digestive Dis 1995; 310:1495.

103. Shulkes A, Wilson JS. Somatostatin in gastroenterology. BMJ 1994; 308:1381.

104. Warner R, Mani S, Profeta J, Grunstein E. Octreotide treatment of carcinoid hypertensive crisis. Mt Sinai J Med 1994; 61:349.

105. Arnold J, Campbell IT, Hipkin LJ, et al. Manipulation of substrate utilization with somatostatin in patients with secondary multiple organ dysfunction syndrome. Crit Care Med 1995; 23:71.

106. Glaser B, Hirsch HJ, Landau H. Persistent hyperinsulinemic hypoglycemia of infancy: long-term octreotide treatment without pancreatectomy. J Pediatr 1993; 123:644.

107. Karalis K, Mastorakos G, Chrousos G, Tolis G. Somatostatin analogues suppress the inflammatory reaction in vivo. J Clin Invest 1994; 93:2000.

108. Zaloga GP, Chernow B, Cook D, et al. Assessment of calcium homeostasis in the critically ill surgical patient. The diagnostic pitfalls of the McLean-Hastings nomogram. Ann Surg 1985; 202:587.

109. Zaloga GP, Roberts PR. Calcium, magnesium and phosphorus disorders. In Grenvik A, Ayres SM, Holbrook PR, Shoemaker WC, eds. Textbook of critical care, 4th ed. Philadelphia: WB Saunders, 2000:862.

110. Zaloga GP, Malcolm D. Calcium as a mediator in septic shock. In Neugebauer E, Holaday J, eds. Handbook of mediators in septic shock. Boca Raton, FL: CRC Press, 1993:475.

111. Malcolm DS, Zaloga GP, Holaday JW. Calcium administration increases the mortality of endotoxic shock in rats. Crit Care Med 1989; 17:900.

112. Zaloga GP, Sager A, Prielipp R, Word K. Low dose calcium administration increases mortality during septic peritonitis. Circ Shock 1992; 37:226.

113. Cheung JY, Bonventre JV, Malis CD, Leaf A. Calcium and ischemic injury. N Engl J Med 1986; 314:1670.

114. Zaloga GP, Washburn D, Black KW, Prielipp R. Human sepsis increases lymphocyte intracellular calcium. Crit Care Med 1993; 21:196.

115. Zaloga GP, Willey S, Malcolm D, et al. Hypercalcemia attenuates blood pressure response to epinephrine. J Pharmacol Exp Ther 1988; 247:949.

116. Zaloga GP, Strickland RA, Butterworth JF, et al. Calcium attenuates epinephrine's beta-adrenergic effects in postoperative heart surgery patients. Circulation 1990; 81:196.

117. Butterworth JF, Zaloga GP, Prielipp RC, et al. Calcium inhibits the cardiac stimulating properties of dobutamine but not amrinone. Chest 1992; 101:174.

118. Müller B, Becker KL, Schächinger H, et al. Calcitonin precursors are reliable markers of sepsis in a medical intensive care unit. Crit Care Med 2000; 28:977.

119. Teo KK, Yusuf S, Collins R, et al. Effects of intravenous magnesium in suspected acute myocardial infarction: an overview of randomized trials. BMJ 1991; 303:1499.

120. Lau J, Antman EM, Jimenez-Silva J, et al. Cumulative meta-analysis of therapeutic trials for myocardial infarction. N Engl J Med 1992; 327:248.

121. Woods KL, Fletcher S, Roffe C, et al. Intravenous magnesium sulphate in suspected acute myocardial infarction: results of the second Leicester Intravenous Magnesium Intervention Trial (LIMIT-2). Lancet 1992; 339:1553.

122. Marik PE, Bedigian MK. Refeeding hypophosphatemia in critically ill patients in an intensive care unit. Arch Surg 1996:1043.

123. Bohrer H, Nawroth PP. Nuclear factor κB—a new therapeutic approach? Intensive Care Med 1998; 24:1129.

124. Exley LR, Cohen J, Burman W. Monoclonal antibodies to TNF-α in severe septic shock. Lancet 1990; 335:1275.

125. Clark MA, Plank LD, Connolly AB, et al. Effect of a chimeric antibody to tumor necrosis factor-α on cytokine responses in patients with severe sepsis—a randomized, clinical trial. Crit Care Med 1998; 26:1650.

126. Reinhart K, Wiegand-Lohnert C, Grimminger F, et al. Assessment of the safety and efficacy of the anti-tumor necrosis factor monoclonal antibody-fragment, MAK195F, in patients with sepsis and septic shock: a multicenter, randomized, placebo-controlled, dose-ranging study. Crit Care Med 1996; 24:773.

127. Abraham E, Wunderink R, Silverman H, et al. Efficacy and safety of monoclonal antibody to human tumor necrosis factor alpha in patients with sepsis syndrome. JAMA 1995; 273:934.

128. Cohen J, Carlet J. INTERCEPT: an international multi-center, placebo-controlled trial of monoclonal antibody to human tumor necrosis factor-alpha in patients with sepsis. International Sepsis Trial Study Group. Crit Care Med 1996; 24:1431.

129. Abraham E, Glauser MP, Butler T, et al. p55 tumor necrosis factor receptor fusion protein in the treatment of patients with severe sepsis and septic shock. A randomized controlled multi-center trial. Ro 45-2081 Study Group. JAMA 1997; 277:1531.

130. Fisher CJJ, Agosti JM, Opal SM, et al. Treatment of septic shock with tumor necrosis factor receptor:Fc fusion protein. N Engl J Med 1996; 334:1697.

131. Ksontini R, MacKay SL, Moldawer LL. Revisiting the role of tumor necrosis factor alpha and the response to surgical injury and inflammation. Arch Surg 1998; 133:558.

132. Karin M. The NF-kappa B activation pathway: its regulation and role in inflammation and cell survival. Cancer J Sci Am 1998; 4:S92.

133. Dinarello CA. Interleukin-1. Cytokine Growth Factor Rev 1997; 8:253.

134. Dinarello CA. Interleukin-1 beta, interleukin-18, and the interleukin-1 beta converting enzyme. Ann N Y Acad Sci 1998; 856:1.

135. Dinarello CA, Thompson RC. Blocking IL-1: interleukin-1 receptor antagonist in vivo and in vitro. Immunol Today 1991; 12:440.

136. Pruitt JH, Copeland EM, Moldawer LL. Interleukin-1 antagonism in sepsis, systemic inflammatory response syndrome and septic shock. Shock 1995; 3:235.

137. Hannum CH, Wilcox CJ, Arend WP, et al. Interleukin-1 receptor antagonist activity of a human interleukin-1 inhibitor. Nature 1990; 343:336.

138. Fisher CJ, Dhainaut JF, Opal SM, et al. Recombinant human interleukin-1 receptor antagonist in the treatment of patients with sepsis syndrome: results from a randomized, double-blind, placebo-controlled trial. JAMA 1994; 271:1836.

139. Symons JA, Young PR, Duff GW. Soluble type II interleukin-1 (IL-1) receptor binds and blocks processing of IL-1 beta precursor and loses affinity for IL-1 receptor antagonist. Proc Natl Acad Sci U S A 1995; 92:1714.

140. Preas HL, Reda D, Tropea M, et al. Effects of recombinant soluble type I interleukin-1 receptor on human inflammatory responses to endotoxin. Blood 1996; 88:2465.

141. Sehgal PB, Greininger G, Tosato G. Regulation of the acute phase and immune responses: interleukin-6. Ann N Y Acad Sci 1989; 557:1.

142. Beck JT, Su-Ming H, Wijdenes J. Brief report: alleviation of systemic manifestations of Castleman's disease by monoclonal anti-interleukin-6 antibody. N Engl J Med 1994; 330:602.

143. Baggiolini M, Walz A, Kunkel SL. Neutrophil-activating peptide-1/interleukin-8, a novel cytokine that activates neutrophils. J Clin Invest 1989; 84:1045.

144. De Waal Malefyt R, Abrams J, Bennet B, et al. Interleukin 10 (IL-10) inhibits cytokine synthesis by human monocytes: an autoregulatory role of IL-10 produced by monocytes. J Exp Med 1991; 174:1209.

145. Gerard C, Bruyns C, Marchant A, et al. Interleukin 10 reduces the release of tumor necrosis factor and prevents lethality in experimental endotoxemia. J Exp Med 1993; 177:547.

146. Remick DG, Garg SJ, Newcomb DE, et al. Exogenous interleukin-10 fails to decrease the mortality or morbidity of sepsis. Crit Care Med 1998; 26:895.

147. Dhainaut JA, Tenaillon A, Hemmer M, et al. Confirmatory platelet-activating factor receptor antagonist trial in patients with severe Gram-negative bacterial sepsis: a phase III, randomized, double-blind, placebo-controlled, multicenter trial. Crit Care Med 1998; 26:1963.

148. Tjoelker LW, Wilder C, Eberhardt C, et al. Anti-inflammatory properties of a platelet activating factor acetylhydrolase. Nature 1995; 374:549.

149. Palmer RM, Ashton DS, Moncada S. Vascular endothelial cells synthesize nitric oxide from L-arginine. Nature 1988; 333:664.

150. Forstermann U, Schmidt HH, Pollock JS. Isoforms of nitric oxide synthetase: characterization and purification from different cells. Biochem Pharmacol 1991; 42:1849.

151. Freeman BD, Zeni F, Banks SM, et al. Response of the septic vasculature to prolonged vasopressor therapy with N-monomethyl-L-arginine and epinephrine in canines. Crit Care Med 1998; 26:877.

152. Cobb JP, Natanson C, Banks SM, et al. N-amino-L-arginine, an inhibitor of nitric oxide synthase, raises vascular resistance but increases mortality rates in awake canines challenged with endotoxin. J Exp Med 1992; 176:1175.

153. Reah G, Bodenham AR, Mallick A, et al. Initial evaluation of diasporin cross-linked hemoglobin (DCLHb) as a vasopressor in critically ill patients. Crit Care Med 1997; 25:1480.

154. Fisher SR, Bone HG, Powell WC, et al. Pyridoxalated hemoglobin polyoxyethylene conjugate does not restore hypoxic pulmonary vasoconstriction in ovine sepsis. Crit Care Med 1997; 25:1551.

155. Aranow JS, Zhuang J, Wang H, et al. A selective inhibitor of inducible nitric oxide synthase prolongs survival in a rat model of bacterial peritonitis: comparison with two nonselective strategies. Shock 1996; 5:116.

156. Roissant R, Falke KJ, Lopez F, et al. Inhaled nitric oxide for the adult respiratory distress syndrome. N Engl J Med 1993; 328:399.

157. Nylén ES, Whang KT, Snider RH, et al. Mortality is increased by procalcitonin and decreased by an antiserum reactive to procalcitonin in experimental sepsis. Crit Care Med 1998; 26:1001.

158. Wagner KA, Vath S, Nylén ES, et al. Immunoneutralization of elevated calcitonin precursors markedly attenuates the harmful physiologic response to sepsis. 40th Interscience Conference on Antimicrobial Agents and Chemotherapy. Toronto, Canada, 2000; 873:52.

159. Ettinghausen CE, Veldmann A, Beeg T, et al. Replacement therapy with protein C concentrate in infants and adolescents with meningococcal sepsis and purpura fulminans. Semin Thromb Hemost 1999; 25:537.

160. Wheeler AP, Bernard GR. Treating patients with severe sepsis. N Engl J Med 1999; 340:207.

161. Natanson C, Esposito CJ, Banks SM. The siren's song of confirmatory sepsis trials: selection bias and sampling error. Crit Care Med 1998; 26:1927.

# PART XVII

# ENDOCRINE AND METABOLIC EFFECTS OF TOXIC AGENTS

KENNETH L. BECKER, EDITOR

# CHAPTER 233

# ENDOCRINE-METABOLIC EFFECTS OF ALCOHOL

ROBERT H. NOTH AND ARTHUR L. M. SWISLOCKI

The adverse effects of alcohol on reproductive function have been recognized since biblical times. Shakespeare observed that "it [drink] provokes the desire, but it takes away the performance" (*Macbeth* II.iii.34). In modern times, the list of alcohol-related endocrine-metabolic disorders has greatly expanded. Because the prevalence of alcohol abuse is at least 5% in the U.S. population, these disorders are commonly encountered and mislead unwary clinicians. Although much has been learned about the endocrine-metabolic effects of alcohol, information is often incomplete or apparently conflicting.[1-4] In epidemiologic studies, alcohol dose is difficult to quantitate because of the variability in the alcohol content of alcoholic drinks (Table 233-1) and different patterns of drinking. Drinkers may not report intake accurately. In clinical studies, multiple variables can influence outcome, such as the dose, route, and time course of alcohol administration; age, gender, and nutritional state of subjects; type of alcoholic beverage; recent alcohol exposure; psychological stress; use of tobacco or other drugs; and coexisting other diseases. Comparisons between studies are thus difficult. The potential mechanisms of action of alcohol are also multiple. Ethanol acts directly on cell membranes and on intracellular metabolism but at the same time can have indirect effects mediated by, for example, the stress of acute intoxication or withdrawal, or nausea and vomiting. By-products of ethanol metabolism such as acetaldehyde and lactic acid produce toxic effects of their own. With prolonged abuse of alcohol, tissue damage becomes a factor. When residual effects of prior intake have resolved, and whether underlying genetic endocrine-metabolic differences exist between alcoholic individuals and the rest of the population, are difficult to know. Considering this complexity, the inconsistencies that are the hallmark of this literature are not surprising. Methodologic details are often critical for the correct interpretation of results.

## EFFECTS OF ALCOHOL ON THE PITUITARY GLAND

The diuretic effect of alcohol and its pituitary dependence are well known. Alcohol ingestion initially suppresses both plasma vaso-

pressin and thirst.[5-7] This results in a water diuresis, which produces increasing volume contraction and rising serum osmolality, even after correction for the contribution from serum alcohol (which is freely permeable). After several hours, plasma vasopressin returns to baseline, limiting any further diuresis and dehydration. In effect, the osmostat is transiently reset to a somewhat higher plasma osmolality. Other factors may be involved, however, because some investigators have failed to find a significant decrease in serum arginine vasopressin (AVP) accompanying the water diuresis during acute alcohol ingestion.[8] Severe alcohol intoxication in persons with chronic alcoholism, but not in nonalcoholic individuals, may have the opposite effect on vasopressin, resulting in elevated serum levels.[9] Regulation of vasopressin in patients with Korsakoff syndrome may be erratic, indicating a possible role of central nervous system damage in these individuals.[10] The degree of volume contraction, which in some studies measures almost a liter, may be sufficient to reduce atrial stretch and suppress atrial natriuretic peptide, as well as stimulate other volume-regulated hormones such as renin and catecholamines.[5] During withdrawal, vasopressin responsiveness is restored or even enhanced and antidiuresis results. Thirst returns and generally no specific therapy is required. During severe symptomatic withdrawal, however, a prolonged augmentation of serum vasopressin levels may occur in spite of reversal of hypertonicity, which may cause hyponatremia.[11] Hyponatremia may also occur in severe alcoholic liver disease because of nonosmotic stimuli to vasopressin secretion. Severe hyponatremia can also result from chronic alcohol intake linked with high fluid intake and low solute intake (*beer drinker's potomania*). Under these conditions, despite vasopressin suppression, the capacity of the kidney to eliminate an adequate amount of water may be exceeded because of limited solute availability. The evaluation and treatment of alcohol-related hyponatremia should be the same as for hyponatremia of any other cause (see Chap. 27).

Serum growth hormone increases during acute alcohol intoxication. In individuals with chronic alcoholism who have Korsakoff psychosis (thiamine deficiency, amnesia, imaginary reminiscences, diencephalic involvement), the serum growth hormone response to insulin hypoglycemia is blunted, although generally not absent.[12] Severe alcohol dependence is associated with diminished growth hormone release through dopaminergic mechanisms. Growth hormone release by other stimuli often remains normal in alcoholism. In addition to its effects on growth hormone, alcohol will increase IGFBP-1 and decrease IGF-1; the effects on growth are unknown.[12a]

Serum prolactin also tends to rise during acute alcohol intoxication and withdrawal, and also is increased in actively drinking alcoholic individuals.[12b] Basal levels are generally normal in abstinent alcoholic patients, but the response to dopaminergic and serotoninergic stimuli is blunted, at least in the short term.[13-15]

**TABLE 233-1.**
**Alcohol, Carbohydrate, and Calorie Content of Commonly Used Alcoholic Beverages**

| Type of Alcoholic Beverage | Usual Portion | | Ethyl Alcohol* (g) | CHO (g) | kcal |
| | *g* | *fl oz* | | | |
|---|---|---|---|---|---|
| DISTILLED SPIRITS: GIN, RUM, VODKA, WHISKEY† | 42 | 1.5 | 14 | 0.0 | 97 |
| WINES | 103 | 3.5 | 9–17 | 2.5–17.0 | 70–158 |
| BEER | 356 | 12 | 12.8 | 13.2 | 146 |
| BEER, LIGHT | 354 | 12 | 11.3 | 4.6 | 99 |
| COCKTAILS | 60–220 | 2–8 | 14–22 | 0.3–40.0 | 110–260 |

*CHO*, carbohydrate.
*Caloric content of ethyl alcohol is ~7 kcal/g.
†Data given for 80 proof liquor (40% alcohol by volume); one jigger = 42 g (1.5 fl oz).
(Adapted from Pennington JAT. Bowes and Church's food values of portions commonly used, 17th ed. Philadelphia: Lippincott–Raven Publishers, 1998:3–6, 315.)

# EFFECTS OF ALCOHOL ON THE THYROID GLAND

The thyroid-pituitary axis is relatively resistant to alcohol. Basal serum thyroid hormone levels and thyrotropin (thyroid-stimulating hormone) levels and their responses to thyrotropin-releasing hormone are unaltered by short-term alcohol administration.[16,17] Chronic alcoholism, however, even in the absence of clinical alcoholic liver disease, is often associated with one or more of the following abnormalities: a blunted thyrotropin response to thyrotropin-releasing hormone and lower levels of serum total thyroxine, triiodothyronine, thyroid-binding globulin, and free thyroxine.[18-21] No unifying hypothesis has emerged to explain these changes, and they tend to resolve after withdrawal. A difficult-to-prove hypothesis is that alcoholism is associated with a genetic abnormality in neuroregulation of pituitary hormones, including thyrotropin. Alcohol liver damage reduces conversion of thyroxine to triiodothyronine, significantly altering serum thyroid hormone values but not producing clinical hypothyroidism (see Chap. 36).

# EFFECTS OF ALCOHOL ON THE ADRENAL GLANDS

The term *pseudo-Cushing syndrome* has been applied to the Cushing-like features occurring in some alcoholic individuals. Although nearly the full spectrum of clinical and laboratory findings of true Cushing syndrome has been described, most cases are mild and incomplete and resolve spontaneously with abstinence.[1,22,23] Furthermore, clinical and laboratory findings may be dissociated, resulting in misdiagnosis if alcoholism is unrecognized.[24] No good data are available on the incidence of this syndrome, but it is uncommon. Nonsuppressibility of serum cortisol by low-dose dexamethasone as an isolated abnormality may occur in up to 20% of noncirrhotic alcoholic patients and generally resolves within 2 weeks of abstinence from alcohol.[25,26] In individuals with chronic alcoholism who have features of Cushing syndrome, adrenocorticotropic hormone (ACTH) levels may be normal or elevated. Increased urinary free cortisol has been reported. Occasionally, serum cortisol may be markedly elevated and nonsuppressible even on high-dose dexamethasone, mimicking the paraneoplastic ACTH syndrome.

Central activation of the hypothalamic–pituitary–adrenal (HPA) axis by chronic alcohol abuse is a key factor in pseudo-Cushing syndrome. In nonalcoholic volunteers, acute alcohol ingestion in amounts sufficient to raise blood alcohol above 100 mg/dL generally increases serum cortisol levels.[1,23] The timing of this increase is variable, however, and it may sometimes result more from nausea or withdrawal than from a direct effect of alcohol.[27] Lesser amounts of alcohol fail to increase serum cortisol[22,28] and blunt ACTH responsiveness to other stimuli, including corticotropin-releasing hormone (CRH), metyrapone, and hypoglycemia. During withdrawal and early abstinence in nondepressed chronic alcoholic patients, cerebrospinal fluid levels of CRH are increased.[29] Pituitary ACTH and β-endorphin responses to multiple stimuli, including CRH, hypoglycemia, naloxone, and heat stress, are blunted, whereas serum cortisol levels are normal to high.[30,31] In experimental animals, activation of the HPA axis by alcohol is dependent on intact CRH receptors on pituitary cells.[32] These findings, together with the existence of the pseudo-Cushing syndrome, including lack of suppressibility of cortisol by dexamethasone, support the hypothesis that clinically significant chronic stimulation of the HPA axis occurs during heavy habitual drinking. The clinical implications of this, including effects on the immune system,

reproductive system, intermediary metabolism, behavior, and bone metabolism, are considerable. The hypothesis has also been raised that abnormalities in this system are markers for susceptibility to alcoholism.[33]

# EFFECTS OF ALCOHOL ON THE GONADS

In chronic alcoholic men, both hypogonadism (testicular atrophy, impotence, loss of libido, decreased hair growth, reduced prostate size, and oligospermia) and feminization (gynecomastia, vascular spiders, and female fat distribution) are recognized.[34] In women, amenorrhea, and occasionally menorrhagia, are observed, along with a decrease in fertility. Animal studies document a hypothalamic site of action for alcohol, but human studies are inconclusive on this point. Alcoholic men do display a blunted luteinizing hormone (LH) and follicle-stimulating hormone (FSH) response to clomiphene, suggesting either pituitary or hypothalamic dysfunction. Studies with luteinizing hormone–releasing hormone (LHRH) generally have shown a normal LH response, but some investigators[1] argue that this is inappropriately low relative to the hypogonadal state. A transient blunting of the LH and FSH responses to LHRH has been observed in alcoholic men, with normalization after 5 weeks of abstinence.[35] Although alcoholic men demonstrate abnormal LH dynamics, the LH level increases during withdrawal and may remain elevated during abstinence. An elevated LH suggests testosterone biosynthetic defects.[36] Abstinence also results in normalization of the estradiol level. Postmenopausal women with alcohol-induced cirrhosis of the liver have higher estradiol levels and lower LH and FSH levels than do controls.[37] Although data in women are limited, most studies fail to show either hypothalamic or pituitary effects of alcohol on gonadotropin levels. The long-term administration of alcohol to female rats induces decreased ovarian size, absent corpora lutea, and changes typical of estrogen deficiency in the uteri and fallopian tubes. Specific ovarian effects of alcohol in women have not been well evaluated, although in cultured human granulosa cells alcohol has been shown to acutely inhibit the progesterone and estradiol responses to LH.[38] Hormonal and ultrasonographic data suggest that even heavy alcohol use results in only minor permanent effects on ovarian function, at least until development of cirrhosis.[39] In contrast, testicular effects of alcohol have been well documented.[40] Serum testosterone is reduced by both long-term and relatively short-term (days) administration of ethanol. Simultaneously elevated serum LH levels suggest a primary testicular effect. The short-term administration of alcohol decreases LH binding to testicular receptors, whereas long-term exposure decreases the number of these receptors. Alcohol also directly impedes testosterone synthesis by affecting several enzymes in the synthetic pathway. Furthermore, while ethanol is metabolized, it competes with retinol for alcohol dehydrogenase and decreases conversion of retinol to retinal (vitamin A), which is required for spermatogenesis. Interestingly, despite these effects, one study[41] failed to show a significant association between the level of alcohol consumption in men and fertility in couples attending an infertility clinic. On the other hand, autopsy studies have documented spermatogenic arrest in 52% of heavy drinkers (compared to 19% of controls); 10% of drinkers (0% of controls) had Sertoli-cell-only syndrome.[42]

The cause of feminization in chronic alcoholism is less clear. Despite testicular injury, the alcoholic individual with cirrhosis maintains a normal to slightly elevated estrogen level. Although this may relate partly to decreased hepatic clearance of estrogen, the predominant effect seems to be increased peripheral conversion of adrenally derived androgens into estrogens. Peripheral conversion from androstenedione to estradiol via aromatase is enhanced in patients with chronic alcoholism, at least during withdrawal.[36]

The optimal treatment of hypogonadism in the alcoholic patient is cessation of alcohol consumption, and anecdotal evidence exists that in the early stages the lesion is reversible. In nonalcoholic and alcoholic patients with cirrhosis, liver transplantation leads to improvement but not normalization of gonadal function.[43,44] In the event that the damage is irreversible, therapy with testosterone may be considered, but its safety and efficacy in this setting remain to be proved. Gynecomastia is a reported complication. A potential but unproved benefit, however, is improved preservation of bone, already damaged by the direct effects of alcohol. (See later and Chaps 116, 120, and 205.)

## ALCOHOL, BLOOD PRESSURE, AND ELECTROLYTES

Epidemiologic data clearly document a dose-dependent increase in both systolic and diastolic blood pressure with increasing alcohol consumption,[45] usually beginning with consumption of more than two to three drinks per day. Ingestion of more than six drinks per day increases the systolic blood pressure by ~10 mm Hg, with a lesser increase in diastolic pressure. In the Multiple Risk Factor Intervention Trial (MRFIT) study involving over 11,000 participants, alcohol intake correlated positively with blood pressure both at baseline and during treatment across all groups.[46] Withdrawal frequently results in substantial transient increases in blood pressure. Restriction of chronic heavy intake of alcohol lowers blood pressure.[47,48] During abstention, blood pressures are lower than during withdrawal, and ventricular function improves.[49] Acute alcohol loading has a variable effect, depending on factors such as dose and recent alcohol exposure.[50] At least one study, however, using 24-hour ambulatory blood pressure recording, showed an initial vasodepressor effect.[51] In young healthy abstinent social drinkers, mild acute intoxication potentiated the decrease of blood pressure to orthostatic stress.[51a] Left ventricular mass correlated positively and independently with alcohol intake in the Framingham study,[52] indirectly suggesting a significant net increase in average blood pressure while drinking. The blood pressure effect of alcohol may depend on an individual's apolipoprotein E phenotype.

The mechanisms of these cardiovascular effects probably are multiple. The sympathetic nervous system (SNS) is activated by acute intoxication, causing the pulse rate to increase, but vasoconstrictor effects may be opposed by a direct vasodilator effect of alcohol.[53,54] Increases in plasma and urine catecholamine levels during acute intoxication and withdrawal can mimic pheochromocytoma. The renin–angiotensin–aldosterone system is affected by multiple factors.[2,55] During acute alcohol ingestion, plasma renin activity generally rises,[27] but the plasma aldosterone response is variable. During withdrawal, both renin and aldosterone levels rise. The most likely stimulus for renin secretion is reduced plasma volume,[55] which results from suppression of vasopressin or gastrointestinal fluid losses; however, SNS stimulation and electrolyte changes probably have a role as well. The role of factors such as increased cortisol and vasopressin secretion and electrolyte changes, including intracellular magnesium, calcium, and potassium, is unclear.

Treatment of any form of hypertension in alcoholic individuals is compromised by the hypertensive effects of alcohol and by poor compliance with antihypertensive medication regimens. Also, the side effects of antihypertensive therapy are increased. Diuretics worsen the tendency toward both hypokalemia and hypomagnesemia in alcoholic patients; they must be used with caution and measures must be taken to minimize these effects. Combined use of clonidine and a nonselective β-adrenergic blocker is potentially catastrophic if both alcohol and medications

are stopped at the same time; marked hypertension may result from the concurrent activation of β-adrenergic vasoconstriction and lingering blockade of $\beta_2$-vasodilation. Adequate control of hypertension often is achieved only with cessation of drinking.

Hypokalemia and decreased total body potassium are common during withdrawal in people who chronically abuse alcohol. Hypokalemia can contribute to weakness, myopathy, and cardiac arrhythmias. Because acute alcohol intoxication does not directly cause renal potassium wasting, secondary factors, including secondary hyperaldosteronism, are responsible. Poor dietary intake and gastrointestinal losses can aggravate the situation. Transcellular shifts in potassium caused by increased plasma catecholamine levels and ethanol-induced changes in membrane $Na^+$–$K^+$–adenosine triphosphatase have been postulated. Therapy consists of potassium replacement and close monitoring of serum potassium concentrations. Full replacement can require days to weeks, depending on the total body deficit and ongoing potassium losses. Refractory hypokalemia may result from hypomagnesemia, which is frequently present and requires concurrent correction.[56]

## EFFECTS OF ALCOHOL ON MINERAL METABOLISM

Hypocalcemia is a common complication of chronic alcoholism. In nonhospitalized, otherwise healthy alcoholic persons, mean serum total calcium usually is 0.2 to 0.3 mg/dL lower than for control subjects. Data on serum-ionized calcium in uncomplicated alcoholism are limited. In advanced cirrhosis, hypocalcemia may occur in one-third of cases; however, it usually is explained by decreased protein-bound calcium. Tetany in these patients is rare. When severe hypocalcemia is encountered, secondary causes must be considered, including pancreatitis, rhabdomyolysis,[57] vitamin D deficiency, and, most commonly, hypomagnesemia (see Chap. 60).[58,59]

In experimental studies[60] in healthy *nonalcoholic* volunteers, ethanol ingestion caused significant renal tubular dysfunction, including substantial increases in urinary calcium and magnesium excretion.[61,62] Changes in serum total and ionized calcium are less consistent, but some studies[60–62] document a delayed 2% to 4% decline after the urinary losses. Sensitive assays demonstrate a transient decrease in serum parathyroid hormone (PTH), followed by a rebound to above baseline values.[61,62] These findings are supported by studies in patients with chronic alcoholism withdrawn from alcohol, who experience an increase in serum ionized calcium[60,63] coincident with a decrease in urinary calcium losses.[60] Reported PTH values in actively drinking alcoholic individuals are variable, probably dependent on the level of alcohol intake and other factors.[62,64–66] Relative to the low serum ionized calcium found in intoxicated alcoholic patients, however, even the normal level of PTH found in some studies is inappropriately low and suggests factors other than hypoparathyroidism as the primary cause of this hypocalcemia.[67] Although initial data[65,68] had indicated an increase of serum calcitonin with acute alcohol ingestion, this has not been corroborated.[61] Decreased serum levels of vitamin D metabolites in chronic alcoholic patients are reported,[64,66] but the cause and clinical significance of these observations is unclear. In the absence of signs of tetany, cardiac arrhythmias, or identifiable secondary causes, the patient with mild hypocalcemia of alcoholism should be evaluated and observed but not treated. In most cases, serum calcium normalizes without specific therapy other than alcohol withdrawal.

Hypomagnesemia (see Chap. 68) is common and clinically significant in the alcoholic patient. It is involved in the pathogenesis of alcohol withdrawal tremor, delirium, seizures, and cardiac arrhythmias.[2,69,70] Hypomagnesemia in the alcoholic individual can mimic hypoparathyroidism, including severe hypocalcemia and hyperphosphatemia, but causes both suppression of PTH secretion and resistance to PTH action. Acute alcohol ingestion induces urinary magnesium loss comparable with calcium loss.[61,62] When patients with chronic alcoholism abstain, serum magnesium rises.[60,63] Poor nutritional intake, malabsorption, secondary hyperaldosteronism, and diuretic therapy can contribute to further magnesium depletion. Although serum magnesium correlates poorly with intracellular magnesium, it is the only feasible clinical measurement. Magnesium therapy is usually indicated for serum concentrations of <1.8 mg/dL, but symptoms and complications possibly related to hypomagnesemia are often overlooked and need to be taken into account (see Chap. 68).[70]

Hypophosphatemia is also common in alcoholism and occurs in up to 30% of hospitalized alcoholic patients. Factors contributing to hypophosphatemia include renal loss,[60] poor intake, diarrhea, and the use of phosphate-binding antacids. Furthermore, glucose administration can produce a precipitous fall in serum phosphorus through transcellular shifts.[2] Close monitoring is required. The indications and approach to therapy are the same as for hypophosphatemia of any other cause (see Chap. 67).

Osteoporosis occurs with increased frequency in alcoholic individuals. Fractures are common in the alcoholic individual, but so is trauma. Bone mineral density measured by absorptiometry is generally decreased[71–73] although not all studies have demonstrated this.[63–66,68] Bone histomorphology shows evidence of a marked decrease in the rate of bone formation in actively drinking alcoholic patients,[64,71,72] an abnormality that is possibly reversible with cessation of drinking.[64] Markers of bone formation, including serum osteocalcin,[64–66,74,75] are correspondingly low. In some studies, bone formation has been decreased even in the absence of abnormalities in mineral metabolism.[71,72] Markers of bone resorption, including deoxypyridinium crosslinks, are normal or even increased, suggesting an imbalance between bone formation and resorption.[75,76] These findings together suggest that, in addition to its effect on the renal tubule, alcohol ingestion exerts a direct selective toxic effect on the osteoblast. Despite this rationale for bone loss in alcoholic patients, the evaluation of osteopenia in these patients should include a search for other causative factors, including osteomalacia associated with vitamin D deficiency and use of antiseizure medications (see Chap. 63). Treatment of osteoporosis in alcoholism is cessation of alcohol intake and use of dietary supplements, including calcium, magnesium, and vitamin D. Aseptic osteonecrosis of the femoral head is often associated with heavy alcohol intake but appears to be linked with bone marrow edema and dysfunction rather than a primary bone disease.[77]

# EFFECTS OF ALCOHOL ON FUEL METABOLISM

The effects of alcohol on carbohydrate metabolism in humans are complex, and plasma glucose levels may increase or decrease depending on conditions.[78] In lean Japanese men, for example, heavy alcohol consumption appears to be associated with an increased risk of type 2 diabetes, while in heavier men, moderate alcohol consumption may reduce this risk.[78a] In most studies, basal serum insulin levels are not altered by acute ethanol ingestion, but the preadministration of ethanol enhances the insulin response to glucose.[79] This may explain the frequent occurrence of hypoglycemic reactions after drinking gin and sweet tonic. Ethanol pretreatment also enhances the insulin response to arginine and tolbutamide. Light to moderate consumption of alcohol (10 to 30 g per day) is associated with increased insulin sensitivity.[80–82] The beneficial effect on insulin sensitivity of moderate alcohol use may account for the observed effect of alcohol on high-density lipoprotein (HDL) cholesterol.[83] On the other hand, acute alcohol administration blunts insulin-stimulated glucose uptake.[84] Insulin target

tissues are affected as well: chronic alcohol intake causes an increase in muscle glycogen concentration and a decrease in pyruvate kinase.[85] Alcohol abuse also affects hepatic intermediary metabolism: hepatic steatosis has been associated with hepatic insulin resistance and obesity in drinkers.[86] Withdrawal of alcohol in alcoholic persons is associated with reduced levels of circulating insulin, related to increased hepatic extraction.[87] Thus, although the effects of alcohol are complex, the overall impact favors an increase in blood sugar. Heavy drinking in nondiabetic persons is associated with slight increases in fructosamine,[88] and moderate drinking in patients with type 2 (non–insulin-dependent) diabetes mellitus is associated with increased glycohemoglobin.[89] This is countered by the observation that alcohol interferes with carbohydrate metabolism before and after anaerobic exercise and may reduce the availability of glucose under these conditions.[90]

Alcohol leads to increases or decreases in body weight,[91] depending on whether alcohol is substituted for other calories or taken in addition to them.[92] Some data suggest that in alcoholics, lipids may be a preferred energy source. On the other hand, other data suggest that the oxidation of alcohol produces acetate, which may inhibit lipolysis and lead to a preferential use of carbohydrate as an energy source. Although calorimetric data suggest that alcohol energy can be counted similarly to that of carbohydrate,[92] some propose that alcohol be regarded as a fat exchange, with one drink equivalent to two fat exchanges. This does not account for carbohydrate in beer or wine.[93] Part of alcohol's caloric impact can be explained by an "oxidative hierarchy," in which alcohol, carbohydrate, and protein elicit adjustments in their oxidation in response to intake, whereas fat does not; fat balance is therefore easily displaced, so that fat is stored and not oxidized.[94] Alcohol intake, like obesity, is positively correlated with blood leptin concentrations and may thus play a role in the regulation of energy homeostasis.[95] The primary route of alcohol detoxification is through oxidation; the dominant position of alcohol oxidation is explained by the absence of feedback control.[91] Despite the presumed increase of leptin, diets high in alcohol have no inhibitory effect on fat intake, with the consequence of higher daily energy intake and an increased risk of positive energy balance.[96] This effect on energy balance can be substantial. Ethanol provides 7 kcal/g and is very efficiently absorbed.[97] When alcohol intake is <5% of daily caloric intake, however, no net effect on body weight is seen.[98]

When ethanol is administered in the fed state, plasma glucose typically increases, probably because of glycogenolysis after ethanol-induced epinephrine release. After 18 to 24 hours' fasting in normal adults, however, glycogen stores become depleted and the inhibitory effect of ethanol on gluconeogenesis predominates.[99] The oxidation of ethanol increases the hepatic ratio of the reduced form of nicotinamide adenine dinucleotide (NADH) to the unreduced form (NAD$^+$), thereby opposing conversion of lactate to pyruvate and of glutamate to α-ketoglutarate, and inhibits gluconeogenesis (Fig. 233-1). Ethanol also inhibits gluco-

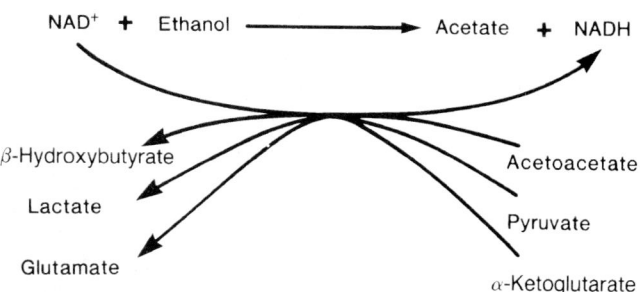

**FIGURE 233-1.** Effect of ethanol oxidation on key redox pairs involved in gluconeogenesis, ketosis, and lactate production. (*NAD$^+$*, nicotinamide adenine dinucleotide; *NADH*, reduced nicotinamide adenine dinucleotide.)

neogenesis from glycerol. Alanine production or release from skeletal muscle also may be depressed.[99] The summation of these effects makes severe hypoglycemia a real danger when alcohol is ingested in the fasting state. Failure to recognize this entity has caused many deaths, particularly in younger individuals, in whom altered mental status may erroneously be attributed to intoxication rather than to hypoglycemia. Clearly, the chronic alcohol abuser with significantly impaired liver function is at particular risk, because glycogen stores will be limited. Inhibition of gluconeogenesis may persist beyond the state of intoxication; therefore, fasting hypoglycemia can occur in the absence of detectable blood ethanol if liver glycogen has not been replenished (see Chaps. 158 and 205). The risk of hypoglycemia may be enhanced by $H_2$-receptor antagonists (drugs that may be heavily used in patients with alcohol-related gastric disturbances). This may result from particular effects of these drugs on glucose metabolism, including intensified alcohol oxidation resulting in suppressed hepatic gluconeogenesis, as well as a possible increase in the metabolism of sulfonylureas.[100]

Alcohol-associated ketoacidosis occurs typically in persons with chronic alcoholism, who, after a binge, develop nausea and vomiting and discontinue food and ethanol intake.[99,101] The anion-gap acidosis generally is mild, with serum bicarbonate values in the range of 10 to 15 mEq/L, levels somewhat lower than those resulting from fasting alone. Serum glucose is usually normal, but it may be low or, when in association with acute pancreatitis, it may be transiently mildly elevated. Qualitative testing results for ketones may be negative or borderline positive, but specific measurement of β-hydroxybutyrate shows a pronounced elevation. When starvation is combined with the stress of alcohol withdrawal, counterregulatory hormones—including catecholamines, cortisol, growth hormone, and glucagon—are released; serum insulin declines. The net result is the release of free fatty acids from fat depots and enhanced ketone formation by the liver. Because of the increased hepatic $NADH/NAD^+$ ratio, β-hydroxybutyrate production predominates. Because only acetoacetate and acetone are measured by the nitroprusside reaction (Acetest, Ketostix), ketosis may clinically be missed. The ketosis usually reverses promptly with administration of glucose and saline. Hyperglycemia occasionally may require insulin administration. Because the redox pair, lactate and pyruvate, also are affected by the metabolism of ethanol, ethanol can exacerbate lactic acidosis resulting from other causes, such as dehydration.[102] Given these profound and complex effects of alcohol on fuel metabolism, one should perhaps not be surprised that a form of non–insulin-dependent diabetes, distinct from type 2 diabetes mellitus, has been described in lean adults with no family history of diabetes but with long histories of alcohol abuse. This entity reflects both pancreatic destruction and peripheral insulin resistance. Metformin should be used cautiously, if at all, in these patients because of presumed hepatic dysfunction predisposing to lactic acidosis.[103]

Consumption of alcoholic beverages in moderation—for example, in amounts containing up to 1 oz of alcohol daily—probably does not affect glucose control in diabetics; therefore, the usual recommendation of total abstention seems inappropriate. Patients with type 2 diabetes, whether diet or medication controlled, have no increased risk of hypoglycemia when alcohol is consumed with a meal.[104,105] The effect of wine on glucose metabolism may be in part mediated by the tannin content (i.e., of red wine).[105a] However, the routine ingestion of alcoholic beverages contributes calories, from alcohol itself (7 kcal/g) and from carbohydrate, and may be a cause of obesity (see Table 233-1). Furthermore, diabetic patients taking either sulfonylurea drugs or insulin should be cautioned to eat regularly when drinking ethanol to avoid glycogen depletion and the risk of

hypoglycemia. Drinking, excluding food, and taking antidiabetic medication is a potentially fatal, yet not rare, scenario. As in those with alcoholic ketoacidosis, the ketotic diabetic patient who drinks also has an increased β-hydroxybutyrate/acetoacetate ratio, causing conventional measurements of ketones to underestimate the degree of ketosis. Lactic acidosis, a metabolic disturbance with an increased prevalence in diabetic individuals, is potentially exacerbated by excessive ethanol ingestion. This is of particular concern in those patients treated with metformin, in whom the risk of lactic acidosis, although small, is exacerbated by dehydration and liver disease. Heavy alcohol consumption may be associated with an increased incidence of proliferative and exudative retinopathy.[106] Finally, diabetics need to be vigilant in monitoring and managing their disease. Impairment of mentation may cause significant morbidity in these patients. Of note, the use of the thiazolidinediones alone is not associated with increased risk of hypoglycemia when alcohol is consumed in moderation.[107] The use of alcohol by diabetic patients may impact, and reflect, treatment compliance and quality of life.[108] Although alcohol may have cardioprotective effects on the lipid profile, fibrinolytic activity, and insulin resistance, its major problem in diabetic patients is the induction and masking of hypoglycemia, and it should therefore be consumed with meals. The risk of neuropathy and gastritis is also increased.

Typically, the hyperlipemic response to ethanol is modest, although extraordinary levels are occasionally seen.[109] Diabetic individuals, patients with pancreatitis, and those with type IV hyperlipidemia may show great increases in triglyceride levels after ethanol ingestion, as may an occasional person in the absence of any apparent underlying cause. A diagnosis of type IV hyperlipidemia may be incorrectly made in some otherwise normal individuals who exhibit hyperlipemia only after ethanol ingestion. The ethanol effect on hyperlipemia is both dose and duration dependent and bears some relationship to the presence of a fatty liver. In animals, increased production of triglyceride-rich very low-density-lipoproteins (VLDLs) and HDLs by the liver are the primary effects of continued ethanol ingestion, although increases in all classes are seen.[110] The mechanism is less clear in humans, although rapid increases in triglyceride and phospholipid in low-density lipoproteins, VLDL, and HDL occur.[111,112] The pattern is independent of the presence or absence of liver disease; however, severe liver parenchymal disease attenuates the hyperlipemic effect in humans.[113] Pancreatitis can be induced by hyperlipemia, but probably accounts for only a small proportion of these cases in chronic alcoholism. Although abstention is the cornerstone of the therapy for ethanol-induced hyperlipemia, an argument can be made for offering pharmacotherapy to any patient with fasting triglycerides in excess of 500 to 1000 mg/dL to prevent pancreatitis (see Chap. 164).

In epidemiologic studies, chronic heavy intake of alcohol is associated with increases in both overall mortality and cardiovascular mortality, but light to moderate intake (1 to 2 drinks per day) is consistently associated with decreased coronary heart disease.[114,115] The apparent protective effect may result at least in part from an increase in HDL, including $HDL_2$.[116,117] Low-dose alcohol consumption (1 beer per day) may increase serum apolipoprotein A-I, possibly also lowering cardiovascular risk.[116] In addition, alcohol may reduce atherogenic risk by suppressing smooth muscle proliferation.[118] Alcohol may also protect against cardiovascular disease by lowering fibrinogen, and thereby reducing a tendency toward thrombosis. This relationship is U-shaped, and is seen at both extremes of alcohol consumption, particularly in men. This effect may be more pronounced with wine and spirits than with beer and cider. Because of the paucity of long-term controlled clinical trials and the known substantial risks of alcohol intake, however, alcohol generally is not recommended as prophylaxis for cardiovascular disease.

# MISCELLANEOUS ENDOCRINE-METABOLIC EFFECTS OF ALCOHOL

The facial flushing that accompanies alcohol ingestion in 3% to 12% of whites and >50% of Asians is possibly related to acetaldehyde production.[119] Also, ethanol-induced facial flushing is an occasional complication of therapy of diabetes mellitus with chlorpropamide. Both prostaglandins and endogenous opioids have been postulated to mediate this response. Finally, ethanol ingestion induces a flushing attack in approximately one-third of patients with the carcinoid syndrome and has been used as a diagnostic test.

The association between chronic alcoholism and gout (see Chap. 192) has been recognized for centuries, but the underlying mechanism remains uncertain.[120] Ethanol-induced lacticacidemia can suppress the renal excretion of uric acid, but data dispute whether fractional renal excretion of urate is in fact decreased in alcoholic persons. Increased uric acid production may produce hyperuricemia,[121] but in addition, alcoholic individuals have gout attacks at a lower serum urate level than nonalcoholic individuals, and multiple factors likely are involved. Gout, hypertension, and chronic nephritis may occur together as a result of lead intoxication. Moonshine whiskey is a potential source of lead intoxication in these cases of "saturnine" gout. Skeletal muscle myopathy may be found in a majority of individuals with chronic alcoholism. Although not well correlated with levels of alcohol intake, the myopathy may be a result of reduced skeletal muscle protein synthesis.[122]

# REFERENCES

1. Noth RH, Walter RM Jr. The effects of alcohol on the endocrine system. Med Clin North Am 1984; 68:133.
2. Kaysen G, Noth RH. The effects of alcohol on blood pressure and electrolytes. Med Clin North Am 1984; 68:221.
3. Williams HE. Alcoholic hypoglycemia and ketoacidosis. Med Clin North Am 1984; 68:33.
4. Adler RA. Clinical review 33: clinically important effects of alcohol on endocrine function. J Clin Endocrinol Metab 1992; 74:957.
5. Leppäluoto J, Vuolteenaho O, Arjamaa O, Ruskoaho H. Plasma immunoreactive atrial natriuretic peptide and vasopressin after ethanol intake in man. Acta Physiol Scand 1992; 144:121.
6. Collins GB, Brosnihan B, Zuti RA, et al. Neuroendocrine, fluid balance, and thirst responses to alcohol in alcoholics. Alcohol Clin Exp Res 1992; 16:228.
7. Eisenhofer G, Johnson RH. Effects of ethanol ingestion on thirst and fluid consumption in humans. Am J Physiol 1983; 244:R568.
8. Taivainen H, Laitinen K, Tahtela R, et al. Role of plasma vasopressin in changes of water balance accompanying acute alcohol intoxication. Alcohol Clin Exp Res 1995; 19:759.
9. Hirschl MM, Derfler K, Bieglmayer C, et al. Hormonal derangements in patients with severe alcohol intoxication. Alcohol Clin Exp Res 1994; 18:761.
10. Emsley RA, Roberts MC, Taljaard C, et al. Vasopressin secretion and memory impairment in alcoholic Korsakoff's syndrome. Alcohol Alcohol 1995; 30:223.
11. Trabert W, Caspari D, Bernhard P, Biro G. Inappropriate vasopressin secretion in severe alcohol withdrawal. Acta Psychiatr Scand 1992; 85:376.
12. Eisenhofer G, Johnson RH, Lambie DG. Growth hormone, vasopressin, cortisol, and catecholamine responses to insulin hypoglycemia in alcoholics. Alcohol Clin Exp Res 1984; 8:33.
12a. Rojdmark S, Rydvald Y, Aquilonius A, et al. Insulin-like growth factor (IGF-I) and IGF-binding protein-I concentrations in serum of normal subjects after alcohol ingestion: evidence for decreased IGF-I bioavailability. Clin Endocrinol 2000; 52:313.
12b. Frias J, Rodriguez R, Torres JM, et al. Effects of acute alcohol intoxication on pituitary-gonadal axis hormones, pituitary-adrenal axis hormones, beta endorphin and prolactin in human adolescents of both sexes. Life Sci 2000; 67:1081.
13. Schmidt LG, Dettling M, Graef KJ, et al. Reduced dopaminergic function in alcoholics is related to severe dependence. Biol Psychiatry 1996; 39:193.
14. Coiro V, Vescovi PP. Alcoholism abolishes the growth hormone response to sumatriptan administration in man. Metabolism 1995; 44:1577.
15. Farren CK, Ziedonis D, Clare AW, et al. D-fenfluramine-induced prolactin responses in postwithdrawal alcoholics and controls. Alcohol Clin Exp Res 1995; 19:1578.
16. Van Thiel DH, Smith WI, Wright C, Abuid J. Elevated basal and abnormal thyrotropin-releasing hormone-induced thyroid-stimulating hormone secretion in chronic alcoholic men with liver disease. Alcohol Clin Exp Res 1979; 3:302.
17. Ylikahri RH, Huttenen MO, Harkonen M, et al. Acute effects of alcohol on anterior pituitary secretion of the tropic hormones. J Clin Endocrinol Metab 1978; 46:715.
18. Knudsen GM, Christensen H, Berild D, et al. Hypothalamic-pituitary and thyroid function in chronic alcoholics with neurological complications. Alcohol Clin Exp Res 1990; 14:363.
19. Hegedüs L, Rasmussen N, Ravn V. Independent effects of liver disease and chronic alcoholism on thyroid function and size: the possibility of a toxic effect of alcohol on the thyroid gland. Metabolism 1988; 37:229.
20. Pienaar WP, Roberts MC, Emsley RA, et al. The thyrotropin releasing hormone stimulation test in alcoholism. Alcohol Alcohol 1995; 30:661.
21. Garbutt JC, Mayo JP, Little KY, et al. Dose-response studies with thyrotropin-releasing hormone: evidence for differential pituitary responses in men with major depression, alcoholism, or no psychopathology. Alcohol Clin Exp Res 1996; 20:717.
22. Jeffcoate W. Alcohol-induced pseudo-Cushing's syndrome. Lancet 1993; 341:676.
23. Veldman RG, Meinders AE. On the mechanism of alcohol-induced pseudo-Cushing's syndrome. Endocr Rev 1996; 17:262.
24. Kapcala LP. Alcohol-induced pseudo-Cushing's syndrome mimicking Cushing's disease in a patient with an adrenal mass. Am J Med 1987; 82:849.
25. Willenbring ML, Morley JE, Niewoehner CB, et al. Adrenocortical hyperactivity in newly admitted alcoholics: prevalence, course and associated variables. Psychoneuroendocrinology 1984; 9:415.
26. Kirkman S, Nelson DH. Alcohol-induced pseudo-Cushing's disease: a study of prevalence with review of the literature. Metabolism 1988; 37:390.
27. Inder WJ, Joyce PR, Wells JE, et al. The acute effects of oral ethanol on the hypothalamic-pituitary-adrenal axis in normal human subjects. Clin Endocrinol 1995; 42:65.
28. Waltman C, Blevins LS Jr, Boyd G, Wand GS. The effects of mild ethanol intoxication on the hypothalamic-pituitary-adrenal axis in nonalcoholic men. J Clin Endocrinol Metab 1993; 77:518.
29. Adinoff B, Anton R, Limnoila M, et al. Neuropsychopharmacology 1996; 15:288.
30. Costa A, Bono G, Martignoni E, et al. An assessment of hypothalamo-pituitary-adrenal axis functioning in non-depressed, early abstinent alcoholics. Psychoneuroendology 1996; 21:263.
31. Inder WJ, Joyce PR, Ellis MJ, et al. The effects of alcoholism on the hypothalamic-pituitary-adrenal axis: interaction with endogenous opioid peptides. Clinical Endocrinology 1995; 43:283.
32. Rivier C. Alcohol stimulates ACTH secretion in the rat: mechanisms of action and interactions with other stimuli. Alcohol Clin Exp Res 1996; 20:240.
33. Gianoulakis C, Krishnan B, Thavundayil J. Enhanced sensitivity of pituitary β-endorphin to ethanol in subjects at high risk of alcoholism. Arch Gen Psychiatry 1996; 53:250.
34. Van Thiel DH, Gavaler JS. The adverse effects of ethanol upon hypothalamic pituitary gonadal function in males and females compared and contrasted. Alcoholism 1982; 6:179.
35. Iranmanish A, Veldhuis JD, Samojlik E, et al. Alterations in the pulsatile properties of gonadotropin secretion in alcoholic men. J Androl 1988; 9:207.
36. Heinz A, Rommelspacher H, Graf KJ, et al. Hypothalamic-pituitary-gonadal axis, prolactin, and cortisol in alcoholics during withdrawal and after three weeks of abstinence: comparison with healthy control subjects. Psychol Res 1995; 56:81.
37. Gavaler JS, Van Thiel DH. Hormonal status of postmenopausal women with alcohol-induced cirrhosis: further findings and a review of the literature. Hepatology 1992; 16:312.
38. Saxena S, Meehan D, Coney P, Wimalasena J. Ethanol has direct inhibitory effects on steroidogenesis in human granulosa cells: specific inhibition of LH action. Alcohol Clin Exp Res 1990; 14:522.
39. Valimaki MJ, Laitinen A, Tiitinen A, et al. Gonadal function and morphology in non-cirrhotic female alcoholics: a controlled study with hormone measurements and ultrasonography. Acta Obstet Gynecol Scand 1995; 74:462.
40. Bannister P, Lowosky MS. Ethanol and hypogonadism. Alcohol Alcohol 1987; 22:219.
41. Dunphy BC, Barratt CL, Cooke ID. Male alcohol consumption and fecundity in couples attending an infertility clinic. Andrologia 1991; 23:219.
42. Pajarinen JT, Karhunen PJ. Spermatogenic arrest and "Sertoli cell-only" syndrome—common alcohol-induced disorders of the human testis. Int J Androl 1994; 17:292.
43. Handelsman DJ, Strasser S, McDonald JA, et al. Hypothalamic-pituitary-testicular function in end-stage non-alcoholic liver disease before and after liver transplantation. Clin Endocrinol 1995; 43:331.
44. Guechot J, Chazouilleres O, Loria A, et al. Effect of liver transplantation on sex-hormone disorders in male patients with alcohol-induced or post-viral hepatitis advanced liver disease. J Hepatol 1994; 20:426.
45. Beilin LJ, Puddey IB. Alcohol and hypertension. Clin Exp Hypertens [A] 1992; 14:119.
46. Stamler J, Caggiula AW, Grandits GA. Relation of body mass and alcohol, nutrient, fiber, and caffeine intakes to blood pressure in the special intervention and usual care groups in the Multiple Risk Factor Intervention Trial. Am J Clin Nutr 1997; 65(Suppl):338S.
47. Puddey IB, Parker M, Beilin LJ, et al. Effects of alcohol and caloric restrictions on blood pressure and serum lipids in overweight men. Hypertension 1992; 20:533.
48. Hsieh S-T, Saito K, Miyajima T, et al. Effects of alcohol moderation on blood pressure and intracellular cations in mild essential hypertension. Am J Hypertension 1995; 8:696.
49. Rajzer M, Kawecka-Jaszcz K, Czarnecka D, et al. Blood pressure insulin resistance and left ventricular function in alcoholics. J Hypertension 1997; 15:1219.
50. Potter JF, Beevers DG. Factors determining the acute pressor response to alcohol. Clin Exp Hypertens [A] 1991; 13:13.

51. Kawano Y, Abe H, Kojima S, et al. Acute depressor effect of alcohol in patients with essential hypertension. Hypertension 1992; 20:219.

51a. Narkiewicz K, Cooley RL, Sommers VK. Alcohol potentiates orthostatic hypotension: implications for alcohol-related syncope. Circulation 2000; 101:398.

52. Manolio TA, Levy D, Garrison RJ. Relation of alcohol intake to left ventricular mass: the Framingham study. J Am Coll Cardiol 1991; 17:717.

53. Van de Borne P, Mark AL, Montano N, et al. Effects of alcohol on sympathetic activity, hemodynamics, and chemoreflex sensitivity. Hypertension 1997; 29:1278.

54. Iwase S, Matsukawa T, Ishihara S, et al. Effect of oral ethanol intake on muscle sympathetic nerve activity and cardiovascular functions in humans. J Auton Nerv Syst 1995; 54:206.

55. Nieminen MM. Renin-aldosterone axis in ethanol intoxication during sodium and fluid repletion versus depletion. Int J Clin Pharmacol Ther Toxicol 1983; 21:552.

56. Whang R. Magnesium deficiency: pathogenesis, prevalence and clinical implications. Am J Med 1987; 82(Suppl 3A):24.

57. Knochel JP. Serum calcium derangements in rhabdomyolysis. N Engl J Med 1985; 305:161.

58. Blachley JD, Knochel JP. Ethanol and minerals. Pharmacol Ther 1987; 33:435.

59. Zakhari S, Altura BM. Alcohol and magnesium. Symposium. Alcohol Clin Exp Res 1994; 18:1037.

60. De Marchi S, Cecchin E, Basile A, et al. Renal tubular dysfunction in chronic alcohol abuse: effects of abstinence. N Engl J Med 1993; 329:1927.

61. Laitinen K, Lamberg-Allardt C, Tunninen R, et al. Transient hypoparathyroidism during acute alcohol intoxication. N Engl J Med 1991; 324:721.

62. Laitinen K, Tühtelü R, Vülimüki M. The dose-dependency of alcohol-induced hypoparathyroidism, hypercalciuria, and hypermagnesuria. Bone Miner 1992; 19:75.

63. Laitinen K, Lamberg-Allardt C, Tunninen R, et al. Bone mineral density and abstention-induced changes in bone and mineral metabolism in noncirrhotic male alcoholics. Am J Med 1992; 93:642.

64. Lindholm J, Steiniche T, Rasmussen E, et al. Bone disorder in men with chronic alcoholism: a reversible disease? J Clin Endocrinol Metab 1991; 73:118.

65. Rico H. Alcohol and bone disease. Alcohol Alcohol 1990; 25:345.

66. Laitinen K, Vülimüki M. Alcohol and bone. Calcif Tissue Int 1991; 49(Suppl):S70.

67. Laitinen K, Tahtela R, Luomanmaki K, Valimaki MJ. Mechanisms of hypocalcemia and markers of bone turnover in alcohol-intoxicated drinkers. Bone Miner 1994; 24:171.

68. Williams GA, Bowser EN, Hargis GK, et al. Effect of alcohol on parathyroid hormone and calcitonin secretion in man. Proc Soc Exp Biol Med 1978; 159:187.

69. Flink EB. Magnesium deficiency in alcoholism. Alcohol Clin Exp Res 1986; 10:590.

70. Rivlin RS. Magnesium deficiency and alcohol intake: mechanisms, clinical significance and possible relation to cancer development (a review). J Am College Nutrition 1994; 13:416.

71. Bikle DD, Genant HK, Cann C, et al. Bone disease in alcohol abuse. Ann Intern Med 1985; 103:42.

72. Diamond T, Stiel D, Lanzer M, et al. Ethanol reduces bone formation and may cause osteoporosis. Am J Med 1989; 86:282.

73. Gonzalez-Calvin JL, Garcia-Sanchez A, Bellot V, et al. Mineral metabolism, osteoblastic function and bone mass in chronic alcoholism. Alcohol Alcohol 1993; 28:571.

74. Laitinen K, Kürkküinen M, Lalla M, et al. Is alcohol an osteoporosis-inducing agent for young and middle-aged women? Metabolism 1993; 42:875.

75. Nyquist F, Ljunghall S, Berglund M, Obrant K. Biochemical markers of bone metabolism after short and long time ethanol withdrawal in alcoholics. Bone 1996; 19:51.

76. Kline RF. Alcohol-induced bone disease: impact of ethanol on osteoblast proliferation. Alcohol Clin Exp Res 1997; 21:392.

77. Hernigou P, Beaujean F. Abnormalities in the bone marrow of the iliac crest in patients who have osteonecrosis secondary to corticosteroid therapy or alcohol abuse. J Bone Joint Surg 1997; 79-A:1047.

78. Lang CH, Molina PE, Skrepnick N, et al. Epinephrine-induced changes in hepatic glucose production after ethanol. Am J Physiol 1994; 266:E863.

78a. Tsumura K, Hayashi T, Suematsu C, et al. Daily alcohol consumption and the risk of type 2 diabetes in Japanese men. Diabetes Care 1999; 22:1432.

79. Metz R, Bergen S, Mako M. Potentiation of the plasma insulin response to glucose by prior administration of alcohol. Diabetes 1969; 18:517.

80. Facchini F, Chen Y-DI, Reaven GM. Light-to-moderate alcohol intake is associated with enhanced insulin sensitivity. Diabetes Care 1994; 17:115.

81. Kiechl S, Willeit J, Poewe, W, et al. Insulin sensitivity and regular alcohol consumption: large, prospective, cross sectional population study (Bruneck study). Br Med J (Clin Res Ed) 1996; 313:1040.

82. Lazarus R, Sparrow D, Weiss ST. Alcohol intake and insulin levels. The Normative Aging Study. Am J Epidemiol 1997; 145:909.

83. Van de Wiel A. Alcohol and insulin sensitivity. Neth J Med 1998; 52:91.

84. Spolarics Z, Bagby GJ, Pekala PH, et al. Acute alcohol administration attenuates insulin-mediated glucose use by skeletal muscle. Am J Physiol 1994; 267(6 Pt 1):E886.

85. Vernet M, Cadefau JA, Balague A, et al. Effect of chronic alcoholism on human muscle glycogen and glucose metabolism. Alcohol Clin Exp Res 1995; 19:1295.

86. Ikai E, Ishizaki M, Suzuki Y, et al. Association between hepatic steatosis, insulin resistance and hyperinsulinaemia as related to hypertension in alcohol consumers and obese people. J Hum Hypertension 1995; 9:101.

87. Piccardo MG, Pacini G, Nardi E, et al. Beta-cell response and insulin hepatic extraction in noncirrhotic alcoholic patients soon after withdrawal. Metabolism 1994; 43:367.

88. Kallner A, Blomquist L. Effect of heavy drinking and alcohol withdrawal on markers of carbohydrate metabolism. Alcohol Alcohol 1991; 26:425.

89. Ben G, Gnudi L, Maran A, et al. Effects of chronic alcohol intake on carbohydrate and lipid metabolism in subjects with type II (non-insulin-dependent) diabetes. Am J Med 1991; 90:70.

90. Heikkonen E, Ylikahri R, Roine R, et al. Effect of alcohol on exercise-induced changes in serum glucose and serum free fatty acids. Alcohol Clin Exp Res 1998; 22:437.

91. Sonko BJ, Prentice AM, Murgatroyd PR, et al. Effect of alcohol on postmeal fat storage. Am J Clin Nutr 1994; 59:619.

92. Murgatroyd Pr, Van De Ven ML, Goldberg CGR, Prentice AM. Alcohol and the regulation of energy balance: overnight effects on diet-induced thermogenesis and fuel storage. Br J Nutr 1996; 75:33.

93. Bell DS. Alcohol and the NIDDM patient. Diabetes Care 1996; 19:509.

94. Prentice AM. Manipulation of dietary fat and energy density and subsequent effects on substrate flux and food intake. Am J Clin Nutr 1998; 67(3 Suppl):535S.

95. Mantzoros CS, Liolios AD, Tritos NA, et al. Circulating insulin concentrations, smoking, and alcohol intake are important independent predictors of leptin in young healthy men. Obesity Res 1998; 6:179.

96. Tremblay A, Wouters E, Wenker M, et al. Alcohol and a high-fat diet: a combination favoring overfeeding. Am J Clin Nutr 1995; 62:639.

97. Addolorato G, Capristo E, Greco AV, et al. Energy expenditure, substrate oxidation, and body composition in subjects with chronic alcoholism: new findings from metabolic assessment. Alcohol Clin Exp Res 1997; 21:962.

98. Cordain L, Bryan ED, Melby CL, Smith MJ. Influence of moderate daily wine consumption on body weight regulation and metabolism in healthy free-living males. J Am Coll Nutr 1997; 16:134.

99. Lieber CS, Gordon GC, Southren AL. The effects of alcohol and alcoholic liver disease on the endocrine system and intermediary metabolism. In: Lieber CS, ed. Medical disorders of alcoholism, pathogenesis and treatment. Philadelphia: WB Saunders, 1982:65.

100. Czyzyk A, Lao B, Szutowski M, et al. Enhancement of alcohol-induced hypoglycaemia by H₂-receptor antagonists. Arzneimittelforschung 1997; 47:746.

101. Fulop M, Hoberman HD. Alcoholic ketoacidosis. Diabetes 1984; 24:785.

102. Kreisberg RA, Owen WC, Siegel AM. Hyperlacticacidemia in man: ethanol-phenformin synergism. J Clin Endocrinol Metab 1972; 34:29.

103. Greenhouse L, Lardinois CK. Alcohol-associated diabetes mellitus. A review of the impact of alcohol consumption on carbohydrate metabolism. Arch Fam Med 1996; 5:229.

104. Christiansen C, Thomsen C, Rasmussen O, et al. The acute impact of ethanol on glucose, insulin, triacylglycerol, and free fatty acid responses and insulin sensitivity in type 2 diabetes. Br J Nutr 1996; 76:669.

105. Christiansen C, Thomsen C, Rasmussen O, et al. Effect of alcohol on glucose, insulin, free fatty acid and triacylglycerol responses to a light meal in non-insulin-dependent diabetic subjects. Br J Nutr 1994; 71:449.

105a. Gin H, Rigalleau V, Caubet O, et al. Effects of red wine, tannic acid, or ethanol on glucose tolerance in non-insulin-dependent diabetic patients and on starch digestibility in vitro. Metabolism 1999; 48:1179.

106. Young RJ, McCulloch DK, Prescott RJ, Clarke BF. Alcohol: another risk factor for diabetic retinopathy. BMJ 1984; 288:1035.

107. Foot EA, Eastmond R. Good metabolic and safety profile of troglitazone alone and following alcohol in NIDDM subjects. Diabetes Res Clin Pract 1997; 38:41.

108. Cox WM, Blount JP, Crowe PA, Singh SP. Diabetic patients' alcohol use and quality of life: relationships with prescribed treatment compliance among older males. Alcohol Clin Exp Res 1996; 20:327.

109. Lieber CS. Ethanol and lipid disorders, including fatty liver, hyperlipemia, and atherosclerosis. In: Lieber CS, ed. Medical disorders of alcoholism: pathogenesis and treatment. Philadelphia: WB Saunders, 1982:141.

110. Baraona E, Savolainen M, Karsenty C, et al. Pathogenesis of alcoholic hypertriglyceridemia and hypercholesterolemia. Trans Assoc Am Physicians 1983; 96:306.

111. Taskinen M-R, Valimaki M, Nikkila EA, et al. Sequence of alcohol-induced initial changes in plasma lipoproteins (VLDL and HDL) and lipolytic enzymes in humans. Metabolism 1985; 34:112.

112. Frohlich JJ. Effects of alcohol on plasma lipoprotein metabolism. Clin Chim Acta 1996; 246:39.

113. Duhamel G, Nalpas B, Goldstein S, et al. Plasma lipoprotein and a lipoprotein profile in alcoholic patients with and without liver disease: on the relative roles of alcohol and liver injury. Hepatology 1984; 4:577.

114. Criqui MH. Alcohol and coronary heart disease: consistent relationship and public health implications. Clin Chim Acta 1996; 246:51.

115. Solomon CG, Hu FB, Stampfer MJ, et al. Moderate alcohol consumption and risk of coronary artery disease among women with type 2 diabetes mellitus. Circulation 2000; 102:494.

116. Moore RD, Smith CR, Kwiterovich PO, et al. Effect of low-dose alcohol use versus abstention on apolipoproteins A-1 and B. Am J Med 1988; 84:884.

117. Gaziano JM, Buring JE, Breslow JL, et al. Moderate alcohol intake, increased levels of high-density lipoprotein and its subfractions, and decreased risk of myocardial infarction. N Engl J Med 1993; 329:1829.

118. Locher R, Suter PM, Vetter W. Ethanol suppresses smooth muscle cell proliferation in the postprandial state: a new antiatherosclerotic mechanism of ethanol? Am J Clin Nutr 1998; 67:338.

119. Tsukamoto S, Muto T, Nagoya T, et al. Determinations of ethanol, acetaldehyde and acetate in blood and urine during alcohol oxidation in man. Alcohol Alcohol 1989; 24:101.

120. Vamvakas S, Teschner M, Bahner U, Heidland A. Alcohol abuse: potential role in electrolyte disturbances and kidney diseases. Clin Nephrol 1998; 49:205.

121. Faller J, Fox IH. Ethanol-induced hyperuricemia: evidence for increased urate production by activation of adenine nucleotide turnover. N Engl J Med 1982; 307:1598.
122. Preedy VR, Peters TJ. Alcohol and skeletal muscle disease. Alcohol Alcohol 1990; 25:177.

# CHAPTER 234

# METABOLIC EFFECTS OF TOBACCO, CANNABIS, AND COCAINE

OMEGA L. SILVA

The use of tobacco products is known to be associated with oral and lung cancer, heart disease, and chronic obstructive lung diseases. Although the influence of tobacco and marijuana on the endocrine and metabolic systems has not been emphasized in the general medical literature and textbooks, the research literature on this subject is abundant.

## ENDOCRINE EFFECTS OF TOBACCO

Smoke generated from the burning of tobacco is an exceedingly complex mixture of more than 4000 compounds. One of the principal components, nicotine, is a volatile, natural alkaloid named after Jean Nicot, the French ambassador to Portugal who introduced the tobacco leaf to France. The absorption of nicotine from inhaled tobacco smoke is nearly as rapid as from an intraarterial injection. Nicotine exerts many of its effects by binding to specific acetylcholine receptors on postganglionic cells within the autonomic ganglia and elsewhere. This plant alkaloid shares with acetylcholine a quaternary ammonium group and resembles acetylcholine in the spacing of its positive and negative charges. Nicotine is both a stimulant and a depressant, depending on timing and dosage. Pharmacologically, the *nicotinic cholinomimetic effect* on postsynaptic receptors is blocked by quaternary ammonium derivatives (i.e., hexamethonium, pentolinium, mecamylamine). Acetylcholine also may exert a *muscarinic cholinomimetic effect,* duplicated by pilocarpine or bethanechol and blocked by atropine.[1] That nicotine, a drug which mimics the actions of an endogenous neurotransmitter, produces many endocrine effects is not surprising. Smoking delivers 0.05 to 2.5 mg of nicotine per cigarette. The peak nicotine level in the blood of a smoker after 5 to 10 minutes of smoking is 35 ng/mL, and the peak of a snuff taker is 40 ng/mL.

## POSTERIOR PITUITARY HORMONES

Many smokers have noticed that smoking cigarettes can counteract the diuretic effect of alcohol. Acutely, nicotine stimulates the release of antidiuretic hormone (ADH).[2] In addition, ADH may exert a vasoconstrictive effect on the coronary arteries.[3] In long-term smokers, smoking a cigarette increases serum ADH and also decreases skin blood flow; both phenomena are blocked by a specific ADH antagonist.

## ANTERIOR PITUITARY HORMONES

Serum prolactin levels are significantly lower in both male and female infertile smokers who smoke >10 cigarettes per day. Cig-

arette smoking may increase dopamine excretion centrally, reducing serum prolactin levels.[4] If injected subcutaneously, nicotine reduces both serum prolactin and luteinizing hormone (LH) levels in animals. Male long-term smokers have increased serum follicle-stimulating hormone concentrations.

## THYROID GLAND

In Sweden, the frequency of goiter is higher among smokers (30%) than among nonsmokers (16%). A higher incidence of goiter in smokers (15%) than in nonsmokers (9%) also was found in a Danish study; in this study, serum thyroglobulin levels were higher and thyrotropin (thyroid-stimulating hormone) levels were lower in long-term smokers, but no difference was found in levels of serum thyroxine ($T_4$), triiodothyronine ($T_3$), and reverse $T_3$.[5]

Another study, which used plasma cotinine, thiocyanide, and blood carboxyhemoglobin levels to measure the degree of short-term cigarette smoking, found lower serum $T_3$ and $T_4$ levels but the same levels of thyrotropin in long-term smokers. These studies were done 30 to 60 minutes after cigarette smoking, which may reflect both immediate and long-term effects.[6]

Women with hypothyroidism who smoke have a greater degree of hypothyroidism and higher serum low-density lipoprotein than in nonsmoking hypothyroid women. These findings suggest an alteration of thyroid function as well as blunted thyroid hormone action.[7]

Graves ophthalmopathy is more common and severe among tobacco smokers. Interestingly, several constituents of tobacco smoke have known antithyroid properties. Smoking increases levels of plasma thiocyanate, which enters the thyroid by the same active transport system as iodide and competitively inhibits the uptake, activation, and organification of iodide by the follicular cell. Pyridine compounds in tobacco can inhibit the peripheral conversion of $T_4$ to $T_3$, as well as the activation, organification, and coupling pathways (i.e., the peroxidase-dependent reactions) in the follicular cell. These factors may promote goiter formation, a protective mechanism against development of hypothyroidism. Infants of smoking mothers have relative thyroidal hyperfunction at birth.[8]

Serum calcitonin levels increase acutely after cigarette smoking.[9] This appears to emanate from the lung, however, rather than the thyroid gland (see Chap. 177).

## CALCIUM AND BONE METABOLISM

Cigarette smoking is a risk factor for osteoporosis.[10] Also, smoking hinders bone healing after injuries or surgery.[11]

## ADRENAL GLANDS

Studies of the effect of cigarette smoking on the adrenal glands of humans have had discordant results. In one study, urinary levels of 17- and 11-hydroxycorticoids and catecholamines in smokers did not significantly differ from those in nonsmokers. Conversely, an investigation of the relationship between changes in plasma nicotine, adrenocorticotropic hormone (ACTH), and cortisol levels after smoking by men found significant rises of serum cortisol levels in 73% and of ACTH levels in 45% after a high-nicotine cigarette (2 mg) was smoked, but no changes after a low-nicotine cigarette (0.48 mg) was smoked. The serum ACTH increase occurred if nausea occurred.[12] Long-term smokers are particularly prone to the development of the acute hypercortisolemia of smoking.[13] In postmenopausal women, long-term smoking is associated with increased plasma levels of the adrenal androgens dehydroepiandrosterone sulfate and androstenedione.[14]

After a 12-hour abstinence from smoking, men with hypertension who were receiving no medication had a significant, immediate rise in plasma aldosterone, cortisol, ACTH, and catecholamine levels after smoking. A later rise in plasma renin activity occurred, which was associated with a transient, but significant, increase in blood pressure and pulse rate.[15]

Plasma norepinephrine and epinephrine levels have been determined in smokers before and after adrenergic blockade. Before blockade, they were increased, with an associated increase in pulse rate, blood pressure, and blood lactate/pyruvate ratio. These effects were blocked by the prior administration of phentolamine and propranolol.[16] These circulatory changes preceded plasma increases in catecholamine levels and, therefore, probably were mediated by a neurocrine effect of norepinephrine from adrenergic axon terminals. The effect of the release of catecholamines on coronary artery disease or on acute coronary events must be determined in humans; in animals, smoking and acute myocardial ischemia synergistically produce ventricular fibrillation. Furthermore, smoking decreases the level of high-density lipoprotein.

## GONADAL AND REPRODUCTIVE FUNCTION

Evidence suggests that women who smoke have an increased frequency of menstrual disorders and decreased fertility.[17] Women who smoke have earlier menopause.[18,18a] The percentage of postmenopausal women, standardized according to age, rises with the amount of smoking. For example, of those women aged 44 to 53 years who never smoked, only 35% were postmenopausal, compared with 49% of those who smoked more than one pack per day. Ex-smokers (who stopped at least 1 year earlier) and smokers consuming less than one-half pack per day had intermediate percentages of 36% and 43%, respectively. In another study, current smokers reached menopause an average of 1.7 years earlier than did nonsmokers. Two mechanisms have been proposed for the earlier menopause in smokers: nicotine may directly affect the interplay of hormones involved in the menopausal process, or the cigarette smoke may induce secretion of hepatic enzymes that affect the metabolism of estrogen.[19]

Partly associated with the earlier menopause and lower body weight seen in female smokers, postmenopausal osteoporosis shows a higher incidence in smokers. Male smokers have a higher incidence of osteoporosis as well.[20]

The Apgar scores of the offspring of women who smoke are lower at 1 and 5 minutes after birth and are inversely proportional to the amount of cigarettes smoked by the mother during pregnancy. Furthermore, the hemoglobin and hematocrit of the newborn are increased in proportion to the extent of maternal smoking.

Maternal tobacco smoking disturbs the endocrine states of the human fetus, resulting in increased serum levels of prolactin, growth hormone, and insulin-like growth factor-I.[21]

In one study of almost 7000 women, smokers had a stillbirth rate three times as high as that of nonsmokers. The neonatal death rate was equal in smokers and nonsmokers.[22] In most studies, little correlation is seen between maternal smoking and congenital malformations.

Mothers who smoke produce smaller infants.[23] Although all investigations are not in accord, one study found that serum levels of human placental lactogen were significantly lower in pregnant smokers than in nonsmokers. This relationship persisted throughout pregnancy.[24] A direct correlation is seen between the level of human placental lactogen and birth weight. Maternal serum chorionic gonadotropin and estradiol levels also are decreased in smokers.[25] Estriol excretion, an index of intrauterine fetal growth, does not differ in smoking and nonsmoking pregnant women. More data are required to determine the extent to which serum hormone levels during pregnancy may be correlated with smoking and lower-birth-weight infants. Reduced placental blood flow may be responsible for the decreased serum human placental lactogen and chorionic gona-

dotropin levels, as well as the low birth weight. In sheep, however, short-term smoking or nicotine administration has little effect on uterine blood flow. Nevertheless, babies born to mothers at higher altitudes, presumably with less available oxygen, have lower birth weights than do the babies of mothers at sea level. Some investigators, however, believe the low birth weights of these infants result from low maternal weight gain during pregnancy rather than from hormonal mediation.

In studies of infertile men, semen analyses have shown a significantly greater percentage of abnormal spermatozoa in the tobacco smokers.[26,27] Cigarette smoking is associated with lowered sperm density.[28] In one study, men who were smokers had significantly higher serum follicle-stimulating hormone levels and lower cortisol and testosterone levels, along with an increased percentage of abnormal spermatozoa. In dogs, long-term cigarette smoking increases the hepatic metabolism of testosterone.[29] Current cigarette smokers have higher endogenous serum estrogen levels than do nonsmokers.[30] Erectile dysfunction may occur.[31]

## DIABETES MELLITUS

Generally, persons with diabetes smoke fewer cigarettes than do persons without diabetes. Smoking is less common in older patients with diabetes than in younger ones. The largest group of ex-smokers among patients with diabetes are middle-aged females. Nevertheless, heavy users of cigarettes have an increased risk of type 2 diabetes.[31a]

The suggestion has been made that chronic hypoxia caused by carbon monoxide in smoke and an increased tendency for platelet aggregation might play a role in diabetic microangiopathy. A study was made of 181 patients with diabetic retinopathy to determine whether smoking influenced the incidence or severity of retinopathy.[32] Although the degree of control of diabetes was not ascertained, the incidence of retinopathy rose in smokers with increasing duration of diabetes, and the incidence of proliferative retinopathy rose with increase in tobacco consumption. No such association between proliferative retinopathy and duration of diabetes was found among nonsmokers. Other researchers have reported a relationship between diabetic retinopathy in men and smoking.[33] A large study of Oklahoma Native Americans with type 2 diabetes, however, found no relationship between smoking and retinopathy, and another study of a different ethnic group also found no association.[34,35]

In patients with type 1 diabetes, the frequency of diabetic nephropathy is significantly higher among cigarette smokers, and the condition progresses more rapidly.[36] Furthermore, a correlation between smoking and both nephropathy and retinopathy in men, but not in women, has been reported.

A consensus exists that smoking exacerbates the coronary and peripheral vascular disease of persons with and without diabetes. The influence of smoking on diabetic neuropathy has been insufficiently studied, although many reports of smoking-related neuropathic syndromes have appeared.

Cigarette smoking raises blood levels of endothelin-1. This hormone may play an important role in the development of atherosclerosis in smokers with or without diabetes.[37]

In patients with diabetes, cigarette smoking may affect insulin requirements. In one study of long-term smokers, subcutaneous insulin absorption was not influenced by the short-term effect of cigarettes. On the other hand, smokers with diabetes have been reported to have 15% to 20% higher insulin requirements than nonsmokers with diabetes, as well as 30% higher serum triglyceride concentrations. In another study, however, patients with type 1 diabetes had no change in insulin sensitivity.[38]

In smokers without diabetes, chain smoking increased the 40- and 60-minute serum glucose levels and decreased the 120-minute level of the oral glucose-tolerance test. Compared with nonsmokers without diabetes and with ex-smokers, chain smokers without diabetes had a lower glucose disappearance constant in the intravenous glucose-tolerance test.[39]

Thus, evidence suggests that cigarette smoking in patients with diabetes increases the incidence of retinopathy and nephropathy. Moreover, the possibility of increased insulin requirements and the higher incidence of coronary and peripheral vascular disease in smokers are ample reasons to insist that patients with diabetes not smoke and to provide programs and encouragement to help them to quit.[40]

## BODY WEIGHT AND CALORIC REGULATION

Many investigations have found that smokers tend to weigh less than nonsmokers and that weight gain occurs after cessation of smoking.[41] Oral satisfaction and keeping one's hands occupied are two often-quoted explanations. Cigarette smoking has been linked to a decreased sense of taste, which may be relieved by cessation of smoking. Moreover, one postulation is that some ex-smokers who gain weight have lost an acquired signal to terminate eating, which had been provided by the cigarette smoked after the meal.

Smokers eat less sugar and fewer fatty foods than do nonsmokers. Evidence is found, however, that smokers actually consume more calories than their heavier counterparts but may be more "energy efficient," storing energy in protein rather than fat. Pregnant women who smoke consume more food than do control patients who do not smoke, but gain less weight during pregnancy. Nicotine may modulate gastrointestinal peptides, such as cholecystokinin, involved in regulation of feeding.[42]

An unexplored subject is the effect, if any, of "passive" smoking (environmental cigarette smoke) on the endocrine system.[43,44]

## ENDOCRINE EFFECTS OF MARIJUANA

Cannabis (hashish, marijuana) is obtained from the flowering tops of hemp plants. It is a psychoactive substance that usually is smoked. Its principal psychoactive ingredient is L-Δ-9-tetrahydrocannabinol (THC). Despite its illegal status in the United States, it has become a widely used social drug. Its long-term use alters the activities of the endogenous cerebral opiate system and the catecholaminergic and histamine systems. Many of the endocrine and metabolic effects of marijuana are mediated by hypothalamic responses. In long-term users of this drug, a tolerance to some effects develops. Many of the changes appear to be reversible.

Marijuana affects gonadal function. Sporadic cases of gynecomastia have occurred, that are probably related to this substance.[45] Men who otherwise were healthy but who smoked marijuana on a long-term basis were reported to have lower plasma testosterone levels and sperm counts than did nonsmokers. Some studies in humans have shown a depression of plasma testosterone levels after marijuana smoking, which sometimes was associated with lower levels of plasma LH.[46,47]

Studies using male rats, mice, monkeys, pigeons, and toads have shown that cannabis extract (THC), usually given parenterally or inhaled, reduces the weight of the male reproductive glands (i.e., seminal vesicles, prostate, epididymis, and seminiferous tubules) and decreases sperm production.[48] Plasma levels of growth hormone are decreased after THC treatment. Some of these effects are mediated by the hypothalamic-pituitary axis. In the female animal, marijuana inhibits the secretion of LH and follicle-stimulating hormone, and decreases plasma levels of prolactin.

In rats, cannabis resin depresses radioactive iodine uptake in the thyroid gland. Body temperature was decreased in another study.

In animals, levels of adrenal cortical hormones increase after short-term cannabinoid administration; this effect is thought to be mediated through the hypothalamic-pituitary axis.[48] In men,

marijuana smoking caused an acute increase of serum cortisol levels.[49] Another study of the acute effects of marijuana smoking has shown no difference in serum cortisol levels after ACTH administration between normal men and those who smoked marijuana on a long-term basis.[50] Plasma catecholamine levels appear to decrease with administration of THC.[51]

THC crosses the placenta. Although teratogenic effects in humans have not been confirmed, growth retardation and delayed development have been observed in infants of mothers who smoked marijuana.[52,53]

## ENDOCRINE EFFECTS OF COCAINE

Cocaine is an alkaloid obtained from the leaves of coca plants (*Erythroxyloncoca*) an evergreen shrub that grows at relatively high altitudes. Cocaine exerts many endocrine effects. Some of the data appear contradictory because of the paucity of human studies and the differences between short- and long-term administration.

Magnetic resonance imaging studies of men who abuse opiates and cocaine reveal an increased pituitary volume.[54] More than one-third of cocaine-dependent patients have hyperprolactinemia.[55] In cocaine-dependent men, intravenous cocaine acutely increases serum ACTH levels. This is mediated via corticotropin-releasing hormone (CRH).[56] Human cocaine addicts, however, fail to exhibit the normal increase in prolactin, ACTH, β-endorphin, or cortisol after a hyperthermic stress.[57] In female monkeys in the early follicular stage, cocaine acutely increases LH levels and also enhances gonadotropin-releasing hormone–induced stimulation of LH secretion. It disrupts menstrual and ovarian cyclicity.[58,58a]

Clinically, humans who use cocaine extensively do not appear to have altered thyroid function. However, there is a blunted response of thyroid stimulating hormone to thyroid releasing hormone administration.[59] In laboratory animals, cocaine induces a central stimulation of the sympathoadrenal neural axis and may play a role in the pressor and tachycardic effects of the drug.[60]

Gonadal and reproductive function may be affected by cocaine. In rats, cocaine significantly reduces ovulation rates.[61] Long-term administration of cocaine to rats causes testicular lesions; this may be due to ischemia secondary to local vasoconstriction.[62] Human cocaine addicts have decreased sperm concentrations. In addition, human sperm may act as a vector to transport cocaine into the ovum, resulting in the abnormal development that occasionally occurs in the offspring of cocaine-exposed men.[63] Cocaine passes the placenta. Cocaine usage during pregnancy impairs transplacental amino-acid transport.[64] Maternal cocaine use may affect the endocrine homeostasis of the fetus and newborn.[65] In humans, the cortisol response of the newborn to stress is blunted.

The short-term administration of cocaine to pregnant ewes increases both maternal and fetal glucose and lactate levels.[66] Patients with diabetes who are undergoing dialysis and use cocaine have an increased rate and greater severity of infections (e.g., cellulitis, abscess, and sepsis).[67]

In addition to cocaine and marijuana, other street drugs (e.g., heroin, amphetamines, hallucinogens, volatile substances, phencyclidine [PCP]) merit ongoing study concerning possible endocrine and metabolic effects.

## REFERENCES

1. Day MD. Autonomic pharmacology. Experimental and clinical aspects. New York: Churchill Livingstone, 1979.
2. Seckl JR, Johnson M, Shakespear C, Lightman SL. Endogenous opioids inhibit oxytocin release during nicotine-stimulated secretion of vasopressin in man. Clin Endocrinol (Oxf) 1988; 28:509.
3. Waeber B, Schaller M, Nussberg J, et al. Skin blood flow reduction induced by cigarette smoking: role of vasopressin. Am J Physiol 1984; 247:H895.

4. Andersen AN, Semczuk M, Tabor A. Prolactin and pituitary-gonadal function in cigarette smoking infertile patients. Andrologia 1984; 16:391.

5. Christensen SB, Ericsson UB, Janzon L, et al. Influence of cigarette smoking on goiter formation, thyroglobin, and thyroid hormone levels in women. J Clin Endocrinol Metab 1984; 58:615.

6. Sepkovic DW, Haley NJ, Wynder EL. Thyroid activity in cigarette smokers. Arch Intern Med 1984; 144:501.

7. Müller B, Zulewski H, Huber P, et al. Impaired action of thyroid hormone associated with smoking in women with hypothyroidism. N Engl J Med 1995; 333:964.

8. Meberg A, Marstein S. Smoking during pregnancy—effects on the fetal thyroid function. Acta Paediatr Scand 1986; 75:762.

9. Tabassian AR, Nylén ES, Giran AE, et al. Evidence for cigarette smoke-induced calcitonin secretion from lungs of man and hamster. Life Sci 1988; 42:2323.

10. Thomas TN. Lifestyle risk factors for osteoporosis. Medsurg Nurs 1997; 6:275.

11. Haverstock BD, Mandracchia VJ. Cigarette smoking and bone healing: implications in foot and ankle surgery. J Foot Ankle Surg 1998; 37:69.

12. Cherek DR, Smith JE, Lanc JD, Branchi JT. Effect of cigarettes on saliva cortisol levels. Clin Pharmacol Ther 1982; 32:765.

13. Gossain VV, Sherma NK, Srivastava L, et al. Hormonal effects of smoking. II. Effects on plasma cortisol, growth hormone, and prolactin. Am J Med Sci 1986; 291:325.

14. Khaw K-T, Tazuke S, Barrett-Connor E. Cigarette smoking and levels of adrenal androgens in postmenopausal women. N Engl J Med 1988; 318:1705.

15. Baer L, Radichevich I. Cigarette smoking in hypertensive patients: blood pressure and endocrine responses. Am J Med 1985; 78:564.

16. Cryer PE, Haymond MW, Santiago JV, Shah SD. Norepinephrine and epinephrine release and adrenergic mediation of smoking associated hemodynamic and metabolic events. N Engl J Med 1976; 295:753.

17. Weisberg E. Smoking and reproductive health. Clin Reprod Fertil 1985; 3:175.

18. McKinlay SM, Bifano NL, McKinlay JB. Smoking and age at menopause in women. Ann Intern Med 1985; 103:350.

18a. Cooper GS, Sandler DP, Bohlig M. Active and passive smoking and the occurrence of natural menopause. Epidemiology 1999; 10:771.

19. Michnovicz JJ, Hershcopf RJ, Naganuma H, et al. Increased 2-hydroxylation of estradiol as a possible mechanism for the anti-estrogenic effect of cigarette smoking. N Engl J Med 1986; 315:1305.

20. Seeman E, Melton LJ III, O'Fallon WM, Riggs BL. Risk factors for spinal osteoporosis in men. Am J Med 1983; 75:977.

21. Beratis NG, Varvarigou A, Makri M, Vagenakis AG. Prolactin, growth hormone and insulin-like growth factor-I in newborn children of smoking mothers. Clin Endocrinol (Oxf) 1994; 40:179.

22. Schwartz D, Goujard J, Kaminski A, et al. Smoking and pregnancy. Results of a prospective study of 6989 women. Rev Eur Etud Clin Biol 1972; 18:867.

23. Kramer MS. Socioeconomic determinants of intrauterine growth retardation. Eur J Clin Nutr 1998; 52(Suppl 1):S29.

24. Boyce A, Schwartz D, Hubert C, et al. Smoking, human placental lactogen and birth weight. Br J Obstet Gynaecol 1975; 82:964.

25. Bernstein L, Pike MC, Lobo RA, et al. Cigarette smoking in pregnancy results in marked decrease in maternal hCG and oestradiol levels. Br J Obstet Gynaecol 1989; 96:92.

26. Evans HJ, Fletcher J, Torrance M, Hargreave TB. Sperm abnormalities and cigarette smoking. Lancet 1981; 1:627.

27. Shaarawy M, Mahmoud KZ. Endocrine profile and semen characteristics in male smokers. Fertil Steril 1982; 38:255.

28. Vine MF, Margolin BH, Morrison HI, Huka BS. Cigarette smoking and sperm density: a meta-analysis. Fertil Steril 1994; 61:35.

29. Mittler JC, Pogach L, Ertel NH. Effects of chronic smoking on testosterone metabolism in dogs. J Steroid Biochem 1983; 18:759.

30. Barrett-Connor E, Khaw KT. Cigarette smoking and increased endogenous estrogen levels in men. Am J Epidemiol 1987; 126:187.

31. Jeremy JY, Mikhailidis DP. Cigarette smoking and erectile dysfunction. J R Soc Health 1998; 118:151.

31a. Perrson PG, Carlsson S, Svanstrom L, et al. Cigarette smoking, oral moist snuff use and glucose intolerance. J Intern Med 2000; 248:103.

32. Paetkau ME. Diabetic retinopathy and smoking. Lancet 1978; 2:1098.

33. Walker JM, Cove DH, Beevers DG, et al. Cigarette smoking, blood pressure and the control of blood glucose in the development of diabetic retinopathy. Diabetes Res 1985; 2:183.

34. West KM, Stober JA. Smoking and diabetic retinopathy. Lancet 1978; 2:49.

35. Klein R, Klein BE, Davis MD. Is cigarette smoking associated with diabetic retinopathy? Am J Epidemiol 1983; 118:228.

36. Sauiski PT, Didurget U, Mühlauser I, et al. Smoking is associated with progression of diabetic nephropathy. Diabetes Care 1994; 17:126.

37. Haak T, Dungmann E, Raab C, Usadel KH. Preliminary report: elevated endothelin-1 levels after cigarette smoking. Metabolism 1994; 43:267.

38. Helve E, Yki-Jarvinen H, Koivisto VA. Smoking and insulin sensitivity in type I diabetic patients. Metabolism 1986; 35:874.

39. Janzon L, Berntorp K, Hanson M, et al. Glucose tolerance and smoking: a population study of oral and intravenous glucose tolerance tests in middle-aged men. Diabetologia 1983; 25:86.

40. Willett WC, Green A, Stampfer MF, et al. Relative and absolute excess risks of coronary heart disease among women who smoke cigarettes. N Engl J Med 1987; 317:1303.

41. Wack JT, Rodin J. Smoking and its effects on body weight and the systems of caloric regulation. Am J Clin Nutr 1982; 35:366.

42. Chowdhury P, Inoue K, Rayford PL. Effect of nicotine on basal and bombesin stimulated canine plasma levels of gastrin, cholecystokinin and pancreatic polypeptide. Peptides 1985; 6:127.

43. Byrd JC, Shapiro RS, Schiedermayer DL. Passive smoking: a review of medical and legal issues. Am J Public Health 1989; 79:209.

44. Cigarette smoking. Focus on the workplace. N Y State J Med 1989; 89:1.

45. Cates W Jr, Pope JN. Gynecomastia and cannabis smoking. A nonassociation among US Army soldiers. Am J Surg 1977; 134:613.

46. Barnett G, Chiang CW, Licko V. Effects of marijuana on testosterone in male subjects. J Theor Biol 1983; 104:685.

47. Kolodny RC, Lessin RC, Toro G, et al. Depression of plasma testosterone with acute marijuana administration. In: Brande MC, Szara J, eds. The pharmacology of marijuana. New York: Raven Press, 1976:217.

48. Mendelson JH, Mello NJ. Effects of marijuana on neuroendocrine hormones in human males and females. Natl Inst Drug Abuse Res Monogr Ser 1984; 44:97.

49. Cone EJ, Johnson RE, Moore JD, Roache JD. Acute effects of smoking marijuana on hormones, subjective effects and performance in male human subjects. Pharmacol Biochem Behav 1986; 24:1749.

50. Perez-Reyes M, Brine D, Wall ME. Clinical study of frequent marijuana use: adrenal cortisol reserve, metabolism of a contraceptive agent and development of tolerance. In: Dornbush RL, Freedman AM, Fink M, eds. Chronic cannabis use. New York: New York Academy of Sciences, 1976:173.

51. Harclerode J. Endocrine effects of marijuana in the male: preclinical studies. Natl Inst Drug Abuse Res Monogr Ser 1984; 44:46.

52. Smith CG, Asch RH. Acute, short-term, and chronic effects of marijuana on the female primate reproductive function. Natl Inst Drug Abuse Res Monogr Ser 1984; 44:82.

53. Hatch EE, Bracken MB. Effect of marijuana use in pregnancy on fetal growth. Am J Epidemiol 1986; 124:986.

54. Teoh SK, Mendelson JH, Woods BT, et al. Pituitary volume in men with concurrent heroin and cocaine dependence. J Clin Endocrinol Metab 1993; 76:1529.

55. Kranzler HR, Wallington DJ. Serum prolactin level, craving, and early discharge from treatment in cocaine-dependent patients. Am J Drug Alcohol Abuse 1992; 18:187.

56. Sarnyai Z. Neurobiology of stress and cocaine addiction. Studies on corticotropin-releasing factor in rats, monkeys, and humans. Ann N Y Acad Sci 1998; 851:371.

57. Vescovi PP, Coiro V, Volpi R, et al. Hyperthermia in sauna is unable to increase the plasma levels of ACTH/cortisol, beta-endorphin and prolactin in cocaine addicts. J Endocrinol Invest 1992; 15:671.

58. Mello NK, Mendelson JH, Kelly M, Bowen CA. The effects of cocaine on basal and human chorionic gonadotropin-stimulated ovarian steroid hormones in female rhesus monkeys. J Pharmacol Exp Ther 2000; 294:1137.

59. Vescovi PP, Pezzarossa A. Thyrotropin-releasing hormone-induced GH release after cocaine withdrawal in cocaine addicts. Neuropeptides 1999; 33:522.

60. Tella SR, Schindler CW, Goldberg SR. Cocaine: cardiovascular effects in relation to inhibition of peripheral neuronal monoamine uptake and central stimulation of the sympathoadrenal system. J Pharmacol Exp Ther 1993; 267:153.

61. Barroso-Moguel R, Mendez-Armenta M, Villeda-Hernandez J. Testicular lesions by chronic administration of cocaine in rats. J Appl Toxicol 1994; 14:37.

62. Li H, George VK, Crawford SC, Dhabuwala CB. Effect of cocaine on testicular blood flow in rats: evaluation by percutaneous injection of xenon-133. J Environ Pathol Toxicol Oncol 1999; 18:73.

63. Yazigi RA, Odem RR, Polakoski KL. Demonstration of specific binding of cocaine to human spermatozoa. JAMA 1991; 266:1956.

64. Pastrakuljic A, Derewlany I.O, Koren G. Maternal cocaine use and cigarette smoking in pregnancy in relation to amino acid transport and fetal growth. Placenta 1999; 20:499.

65. Chiriboga CA. Neurological correlates of fetal cocaine exposure. Ann N Y Acad Sci 1998; 846:109.

66. Owiny JR, Sadowsky D, Jones MT, et al. Effect of maternal cocaine administration on maternal and fetal glucose, lactate, and insulin in sheep. Obstet Gynecol 1991; 77:901.

67. D'Elia JA, Weinrauch LA, Paine DF, et al. Increased infection rate in diabetic dialysis patients exposed to cocaine. Am J Kidney Dis 1991; 18:349.

# CHAPTER 235

# ENVIRONMENTAL FACTORS AND TOXINS AND ENDOCRINE FUNCTION

LAURA S. WELCH

In the 1960s, the populations of various bird species in the United States began to decline. Thinning eggshells and decreased survival of the young were caused by the effects of the pesticide dichlorodiphenyltrichloroethane (DDT) on the endocrine and other body systems of the birds. This important discovery sparked increasing research on the effects of environmental toxins on both animal and human health.

Now, years later, although these observations have caused public and governmental concern, knowledge of the effects of environmental and industrial chemicals on the endocrine system of humans still is incomplete. A ban on, or restriction on use of, many persistent organic pollutants has resulted in a definite decrease in the body burden of these chemicals in humans and other animals. What level is "safe" and will not result in an endocrine-like effect is an area of active debate.[1,1a] Research is providing important information, but many of the effects of environmental substances on people are uncovered because astute clinicians remember to take occupational histories and to look for the causes of clusters of specific diseases. Only by the routine incorporation of occupational and environmental histories into clinical practice can physicians identify causal relationships.[2]

This chapter reviews the known and probable effects of environmental and occupational exposures on the endocrine system. Endocrine responses to physical or chemical agents and the role of the endocrine system in modulating toxic effects are described. Data from animal experiments are presented to elucidate the mechanism of human toxicity.[3,4] The importance of taking occupation into account in the treatment of endocrine disorders is discussed. The environmental agents alcohol, smoking, and drugs are discussed in Chapters 233, 234, and 239, respectively.

## HYPOTHALAMUS

Beryllium, a metal widely used in specialty alloys (Table 235-1), causes a syndrome with many of the manifestations of sarcoidosis. Berylliosis can present as an acute or subacute disease, which usually includes chest disease as a prominent manifestation. The differentiation of berylliosis from sarcoidosis depends on a history of beryllium exposure and either the documentation of a body burden of beryllium or the demonstration of activation of lymphocytes, obtained from blood or bronchial lavage, on exposure of the cells to the metal. Berylliosis may affect the hypothalamus in the same way as sarcoidosis (see Chap. 9): the granulomatous involvement of the hypothalamus can cause posterior or anterior pituitary dysfunction.

## PITUITARY GLAND

Lead exposure in a battery plant has caused decreased levels of serum thyroid-stimulating hormone (TSH), thus reducing serum thyroxine ($T_4$) concentrations. Response to thyrotropin-releasing hormone stimulation was flat or delayed, suggesting anterior pituitary involvement.[5,6] Moreover, subtle effects on the pituitary have been found in monkeys exposed to lead.[7] Removal of the patients from the lead exposure was followed by improvement after months to years, but the natural history of this dysfunction still is not clear. The patients studied had non-specific symptoms, such as fatigue, headache, muscle pains, and impotence, that may have resulted from the known central nervous system effects of lead.

Styrene causes a rise in serum prolactin and growth hormone levels in exposed workers; levels of prolactin increase as the exposure increases.[8] Styrene is a solvent used extensively in the manufacture of reinforced plastics, such as boat hulls or molded chairs. In humans, styrene and similar solvents cause dose-related effects on visual-motor, visual-perceptive, and memory functions. In rabbits, styrene depletes striatal and tuberoinfundibular levels of catecholamines, and a similar phenomenon probably occurs in humans. Prolactin is the hormone most likely to be affected by such involvement because it is regulated directly by dopaminergic feedback.

The effects of toxins on sexual function are discussed later; some of these effects may be due to effects on the pituitary as well.

## THYROID GLAND

Many chemicals affect human and animal thyroid function.[8a] Table 235-1 lists these chemicals and the jobs and industries in which workers may be exposed. Generally, most of the chemicals cause goiter or hypothyroidism. For some of the compounds, the mechanism of action is well understood.

In addition, many naturally occurring substances act as goiter-producing agents, and sporadic outbreaks of endemic goiter have been traced to them.[9] These compounds include thiouracil, thiocyanates, and thiourea. Plants in the cabbage family cause goiter in animals and have caused an outbreak in people drinking milk from cows feeding on these plants. The active ingredient in these plants is a thiocyanate that inhibits organic iodination in the thyroid (see Chaps. 30 and 38).

Many compounds affecting the thyroid are used in industry. Ethylene thiourea is used as an accelerator in the manufacture of rubber and as a chemical intermediate in the manufacture of pesticides, fungicides, dyes, and chemicals. It is in the same chemical class as propylthiouracil and has been used previously in the treatment of thyrotoxicosis. One study showed that men working as rubber mixers with significant exposure to ethylene thiourea dust had serum $T_4$ levels that were significantly lower than those of a control group, although all levels were within the normal range. One of the men had an increased serum TSH level.[10]

Halogenated aromatic hydrocarbon compounds affect thyroid function in humans and animals. Table 235-1 describes where these compounds are found in the environment. Figure 235-1 displays some of the most common chemicals in this group. Polybrominated biphenyls (PBBs) caused primary hypothyroidism in 11% of men working in a PBB production facility. The serum free $T_4$ level was decreased, and the serum TSH level was elevated. Thyroid antimicrosomal antibodies were present.[11] Although PBBs are no longer produced, they still are found in the environment. Polychlorinated biphenyls (PCBs) appear to mimic $T_4$ structurally.[12,13,13a]

The pesticide hexachlorobenzene (HCB) causes thyroid enlargement in humans. In the 1950s, an epidemic of HCB poisoning occurred in Turkey; 4000 persons were affected, and 400 died. Seed grain had been treated with HCB and, during a period of famine, local farmers used the seed for baking bread. A subset of these persons were studied again between 1977 and 1981. The major effect was the development of a syndrome of porphyria cutanea tarda and joint disease. Moreover, 40% had thyroid enlargement, which affected 60% of the women and 27% of the men in the subset. Two of these persons underwent thyroidectomy, and no malignant changes were noted.[14] Experimentally, feeding HCB to rats has been found to decrease $T_4$ levels.[15] This effect results from interference with plasma thyroid transport protein by the hydroxylated metabolites of HCB and from increased metabolism of $T_4$ induced by HCB.[16]

Several polychlorinated compounds, such as 2,3,7,8-tetrachlorodibenzo-*p*-dioxin (TCDD, or dioxin), PCBs, and PBBs, have similar biologic effects. This observation has led to the discovery of a specific receptor, called the *Ah receptor*, for these compounds.[17,18] The Ah receptor is similar in structure to steroid receptors, but the endogenous ligand remains unknown. Future work should determine the role of this receptor in the endocrine toxicity of these compounds. The administration of TCDD and PCBs to rats decreases serum $T_4$ concentrations.[18a] Histologically, hyperplasia and hypertrophy of thyroid follicular cells are

**TABLE 235-1.**
**Toxins Associated with Endocrine Dysfunction**

| Affected Function or Organ | Toxin | Job or Industry with Risk |
|---|---|---|
| **HYPOTHALAMUS** | Beryllium | Alloy manufacture, in particular alloys for the aircraft and aerospace industry; beryllium-copper in dental alloys |
| **PITUITARY GLAND** | Lead | Foundry work, other metal manufacture and use; paints and pigments, especially removal of old paint (e.g., ironworking, welding, house renovation) |
| | Styrene | Solvent used in manufacture of reinforced plastics (e.g., fiberglass, molded chairs, boats) |
| **THYROID GLAND** | Radiation | Medical and nuclear industries, therapeutic or diagnostic exposure |
| | *Brassica* plants | Food |
| | Thioureas | Chemical intermediates in synthesis of specialty chemicals |
| | Lead | See under pituitary gland |
| | Halogenated aromatics: | |
| | Hexachlorobenzene (HCB) | Formerly used as a pesticide (still used in other countries); waste product of chemical manufacture and a contaminant of pesticide manufacture |
| | Polybrominated biphenyls (PBBs) | Formerly used as flame retardants, widespread in the environment as a contaminant because of long-term chemical stability |
| | Polychlorinated biphenyls (PCBs) | Formerly used as oil in transformers, as a lubricating oil, for insulated wires, as plasticizers, and in other uses; now banned from new use; existing products still used |
| | 2,3,7,8-Tetrachloro-dibenzo-*p*-dioxin (TCDD, dioxin) | Contaminant of the manufacture of chlorophenols and other chlorinated aromatic compounds |
| **CALCIUM AND BONE METABOLISM** | Beryllium | See under hypothalamus |
| | Lead | See under pituitary gland |
| | Fluoride | Extraction of aluminum from cryolite (sodium aluminum fluoride); manufacture of fertilizer from rock; hydrofluoric acid in electrolyte reduction processes |
| | Aluminum | Processing of aluminum |
| | Radium | Previously used for fluorescent dials on watches; not used since 1960s |
| **ADRENAL GLANDS** | Glucocorticoids | Manufacture of glucocorticoids |
| | Paraquat | Hazard from herbicide ingestion |
| | Carbon tetrachloride | Solvent used in many industries |
| **FEMALE SEXUAL FUNCTIONING** | Estrogens | Manufacture of estrogens |
| | Polycyclic aromatic hydrocarbons | By-product of fossil fuel use; generated in significant amounts in producing coke from coal in iron and steel industry |
| | Halogenated aromatics | See under thyroid gland |
| | Dichlorodiphenyltrichloroethane (DDT) | Formerly used as a pesticide; still in the environment due to long-term chemical stability |
| | HCB | See under thyroid gland |
| **MALE SEXUAL FUNCTIONING** | Carbon disulfide | Solvent used in the production of viscous rayon and in the manufacture of optical glass and of pesticides |
| | Dibromochloropropane (DBCP) | Pesticide manufacture and use (banned in the United States) |
| | Ethylene glycol ethers | Solvent in widespread use |
| | Lead | See under pituitary gland |
| | Carbaryl | Pesticide manufacture and use |
| | Kepone | Pesticide manufacture and use |
| | Physical factors: | |
| | Heat | Many sources |
| | Radiation | See under thyroid gland |
| **SUSPECTED TESTICULAR TOXINS (BASED ON ANIMAL DATA)** | Arsenic | Used in many businesses and manufacturing processes |
| | Benzene | Solvent used in many processes |
| | 3,4-Benzopyrene | Chemical reagent |
| | Boron | Preservative; painting; other manufacturing |
| | Cadmium | Metals manufacture, batteries |
| | Chloroprene | Rubber manufacture |
| | Ethylene oxide | Fumigant and sterilizing agent in hospitals |
| | Ethylene dibromide | Fumigant |
| | Epichlorhydrin | Solvent |
| | Halothane | Anesthetic gas |
| | Methyl chloride | Chemical intermediate in various industrial processes |
| | Nitrous oxide | Anesthetic agent |
| | PBBs | See under thyroid gland |
| | Trichloroethylene | Solvent used in many industries |
| | Triethyleneamine | Used in various manufacturing processes |
| **DIABETES** | N-3-pyridylmethyl-N-*p*-nitrophenylurea (Vacor) | Pesticide |
| **HYPOGLYCEMIA** | Parathion | Insecticide |
| | Ackee fruit | Edible fruit |
| **LIPIDS** | TCDD | See under thyroid gland |
| | PCBs | See under thyroid gland |
| | Carbon disulfide | Solvent used in the production of viscous rayon and in the manufacture of optical glass and of pesticides |

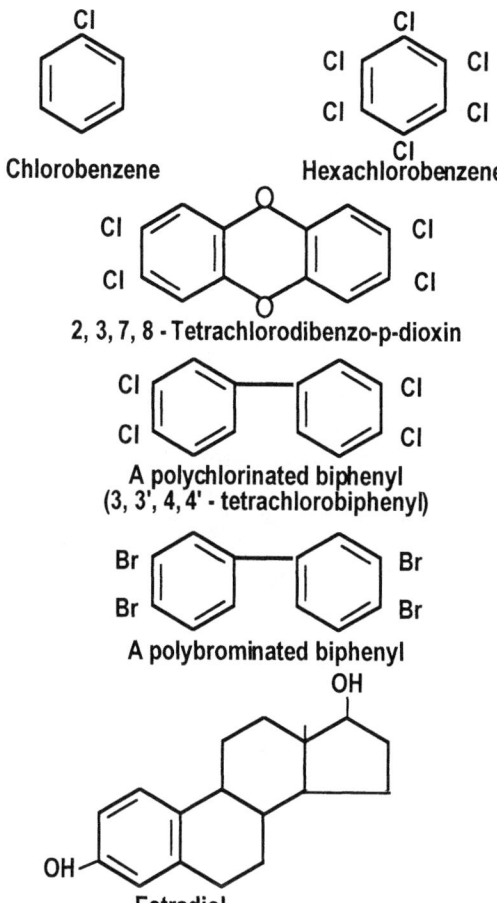

**FIGURE 235-1.** The chemical structures of several halogenated aromatic hydrocarbon compounds. Note the structural similarities among the group and the similarity to estradiol and diethylstilbestrol (see Fig. 235-2).

seen. These chemicals seem to impair the release of thyroid hormone. Studies of the effect of organochlorine compounds on birds demonstrate definite effects on thyroid function.[19] At low levels of exposure, DDT caused hyperthyroidism in pigeons; at higher levels, it caused hypothyroidism. Herring gulls from polluted areas of the Great Lakes had goiters and decreased serum triiodothyronine ($T_3$) and $T_4$ levels. Examination of the thyroid glands demonstrated a decreased colloid content, epithelial hyperplasia, and decreased follicular size. In addition, several bird species had abnormal incubating behavior, which was linked to abnormalities of both sex and thyroid hormones. No studies of the effects of DDT and TCDD on human thyroid function are available, but a reasonable suspicion is that exposure to a chlorinated aromatic compound may contribute to thyroid disease. An occupational history should concentrate on intense or prolonged exposure to any substances in this category.

A series of pesticides were administered to ewes, and chlorpyrifos, lindane, 2,4-D, and pentachlorophenol produced a marked decrease in $T_4$ levels.[20]

Physical agents also cause thyroid disease. Radiation causes thyroid cancer, both from gamma irradiation and from thyroid uptake of the radioactive iodine released in nuclear tests (see Chap. 40). The inhabitants of the Marshall Islands were exposed to radioactive fallout from test detonation of an atomic bomb in 1954. Subsequent studies showed a high incidence of thyroid neoplasms and hypothyroidism.[21,22] A risk may exist from lower levels of radioactive iodine exposure from above-ground testing and nuclear accidents, from radioiodine, and from occupational, therapeutic, or diagnostic exposure to radiation.[23,24]

## CALCIUM AND BONE METABOLISM

Beryllium and lead interact with calcium metabolism. Other metals, such as radium, aluminum, and fluoride, are stored in bone and can cause adverse health effects.

Berylliosis can mimic sarcoidosis and can be associated with hypercalcemia. Removal from beryllium exposure is an essential aspect of the treatment of this disease.[25]

Lead is widespread in the environment. It is used in gasoline additives, in metal alloys, and in paints and pigments (see Table 235-1). Lead accumulates in the body, and significant stores are present in bone. Although the mechanism is poorly understood, lead is handled in the body like the calcium ion, and some endocrine disorders that affect calcium balance may affect lead balance in lead-exposed patients. In addition, lead may be directly toxic to osteoblasts.[26] Hyperparathyroidism, immobilization, and treatment with corticosteroids may cause an elevation in the blood lead level and may precipitate symptoms of lead toxicity. Men working in lead industries develop an acute mononeuropathy from bed rest, perhaps from bone resorption.[27] Table 235-1 lists jobs with potential lead exposure.

Fluoride is stored in bone, and significant doses cause osteosclerosis as part of the syndrome of fluorosis. Table 235-1 lists potential sources of exposure in the occupational setting (see Chap. 131).

Ingested radium is deposited in bone. The use of radium salts in the 1920s and 1930s in luminescent paint for clocks and watches caused jaw necrosis, osteosarcoma, and aplastic anemia in the watch painters, who pointed their brushes by touching them to the tips of their tongues.[28] The use of radium for fluorescence ceased in the 1960s.

Aluminum also is deposited in bone if ingested and predominantly in the lungs if inhaled. Aluminum may cause a vitamin D–resistant osteomalacia (see Chaps. 61 and 131).

## ADRENAL GLANDS

Adrenocortical suppression has occurred in men working in the manufacture of potent synthetic glucocorticoids, even though they adhered to recommended safety precautions in the workplace. In one man, adrenal insufficiency resulted after the exposure suddenly stopped.[29]

Paraquat is a commonly used herbicide that has caused death after accidental or intentional ingestion. It causes pulmonary toxicity. A dozen fatal cases of diffuse bilateral adrenal necrosis have been reported in patients with paraquat poisoning; this may occur in only the most severe cases of poisoning.[30] These cases point to the importance of considering corticosteroid replacement therapy in patients with paraquat poisoning.

Many toxic substances are not harmful until metabolized. This metabolism occurs in the microsomal P450 enzyme system of the adrenals; these enzymes catalyze hydroxylation reactions for the production of adrenal glucocorticoids and mineralocorticoids. The system also acts rapidly on foreign compounds. For example, dichlorodiphenyldichloroethane (DDD) is an insecticide that induces a selective necrosis of the zonae fasciculata and reticularis of the adrenal cortex. Adrenal metabolism of DDD causes this toxicity. This discovery led to the development of the active isomer *o,p*'-DDD (mitotane), now used in the treatment of inoperable adrenal carcinoma. The insecticide is no longer used in the United States.

One review suggests that the adrenal cortex may be more vulnerable to chemically induced injury than are other endocrine tissues.[31] Local activation probably is involved in the adrenocortical necrosis seen with carbon tetrachloride. This agent is metabolized by microsomal monooxygenases in the liver to a highly reactive trichloromethyl radical.[32]

## SEXUAL AND ENDOCRINE FUNCTION IN WOMEN

Toxic exposures can cause two types of female sexual dysfunction. Exposure may interfere with endocrine functioning and, if the exposure occurs during pregnancy, the toxins may affect fetal development.

Much of the study of the effects of environmental exposures on female reproduction has focused on abnormal fetal growth and development or fetal loss. The direct toxic effects on the fetus are not discussed in this chapter, except for those affecting the developing fetal endocrine system.[33,34]

Exposures to toxins can affect the development of the fetal endocrine system, including the development of reproductive organs and their subsequent functioning. The administration of estrogens has a feminizing effect on male embryos and causes abnormal genitourinary development. Exposure of animals to polyaromatic hydrocarbons in utero causes the loss of ovarian follicles in the newborn; no studies of this effect in humans have been performed.[34]

Many environmental compounds (e.g., chlorinated aromatic hydrocarbons) have estrogen-like activity (see Table 235-1). For example, TCDD (dioxin) exposure has been reported to reduce serum levels of follicle-stimulating hormone, luteinizing hormone, and testosterone in men.[35] Assessment of the effect of these compounds is complicated, for a specific compound may be an estrogen agonist in one tissue and an antagonist in another. Exposure to these compounds in the environment usually is to a mixture of endocrine-active compounds, so predicting the effect is difficult.[36]

Estrogenic activity of many of these compounds is known to impair reproductive function in adults of either sex. For example, occupational exposure to estrogens in pharmaceutical manufacture caused irregular menses and infertility.[37] High-level exposures have been shown to affect wildlife populations. At this time, little direct evidence is found that exposures to ambient levels of estrogenic compounds affects reproductive health in humans. Some studies suggest that exposure to estrogenic compounds increases the risk of breast cancer,[38,39] but others do not.[40–42]

Milk production is mediated by hormones. Although toxic exposures have not been shown to interfere with the endocrine aspects of breast-feeding, significant concentrations of toxic chemicals may be excreted in breast milk.[43,44]

DDT, methoxychlor, and other DDT derivatives cause an increase in uterine weight and endometrial hyperplasia. DDT binds to estrogen receptors and induces estrogen-sensitive protein synthesis. Low-level exposure to TCDD caused a high incidence of endometriosis in rhesus monkeys[45]; other studies are investigating this effect in humans. Moreover, the injection of DDT into gull eggs caused feminization of the male embryos, similar to the effect of estradiol administration. The cyclodiene insecticides have similar estrogenic activity.[44]

Plants, especially legumes such as soya and clover, contain *phytoestrogens*. Structurally, these compounds are phenols rather than steroids; they have both weak estrogenic and antiestrogenic activity (Fig. 235-2). Resveratrol, a phytoestrogen in grapes, which is present in red wine, is a mixed agonist/antagonist for estrogen receptors alpha and beta.[45a] When herbivorous animals eat large amounts of plants containing these compounds, they may have prolonged periods of estrus. Diets high in clover have caused reproductive disorders, including infertility, in other animals.[46–48] Daidzein, a phytoestrogen precursor in soya, is metabolized to equol, a compound with weak estrogenic activity. Feed containing soya has caused uterotropic effects in rats, and a high-soya diet in men caused a 1000-fold

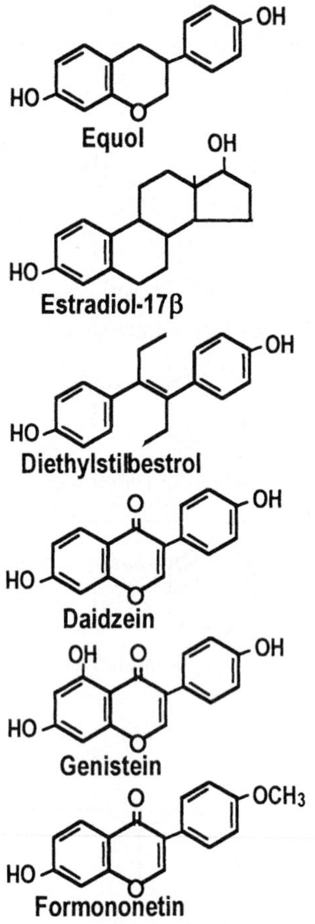

**FIGURE 235-2.** Chemical structures of equol, the phytoestrogen formed in the gastrointestinal tract of humans and animals; estradiol; the potent synthetic estrogen, diethylstilbestrol; and several phytoestrogens of plant origin. (From Sectell KDR, Doriello SD, Hulme P, et al. Nonsteroidal estrogens of dietary origins: possible roles in hormone dependent disease. Am J Clin Nutr 1984; 40:569.)

increase in the urinary excretion of equol.[49,50] Whether these phytoestrogens can cause similar effects in humans and animals is unknown. Potentially, high-soya diets could cause reproductive abnormalities in men and women, and the amount of phytoestrogens in the diet could affect rates of breast cancer or other estrogen-responsive diseases.

The toxic effects of HCB have included hirsutism.

## SEXUAL AND ENDOCRINE FUNCTION IN MEN

Gynecomastia may occur as a result of hepatic injury from carbon tetrachloride or other industrial toxins. In these conditions, hepatic inactivation of endogenous estrogens is diminished.[51] Gynecomastia also has been reported in workers engaged in the manufacture of stilbestrol.[52] Organochlorine insecticides, such as lindane, have estrogenic activity, and extensive exposure could cause gynecomastia.[53] Presumably, the ingestion of large amounts of phytoestrogens could cause gynecomastia.

The effects of environmental exposures on male fertility have been studied extensively in humans. At least half a dozen agents cause semen abnormalities, and others cause testicular toxicity in animals.[54] Much of the research followed the discovery that the pesticide dibromochloropropane caused an epidemic of infertility in workers involved in its manufacture; 13% of the exposed group had azoospermia, and another 30% had oligospermia (see Table 235-1). For the substances that have been investigated in humans, the mechanism in most cases is a direct toxic effect on the testes, rather than suppression of the hypothalamic-pituitary axis. In these studies, serum follicle-stimulating hormone levels are normal unless azoospermia results, at which time they rise. The mechanism of action of the ethylene glycol ethers has been studied extensively in animals; they directly affect the early pachytene spermatocyte.

Some animal experiments suggest that a toxic effect on testicular function is mediated by hypothalamic dysfunction. For example, methyl chloride suppresses the release of luteinizing hormone–releasing hormone, causing a decreased sperm count.[55] Evidence exists that lead may suppress pituitary function, causing testicular atrophy. However, testicular biopsies of azoospermic men exposed to lead have revealed fibrosis, suggesting a direct testicular effect as well.[56] Significant exposure to lead (blood levels of 23–98 μg/dL) were associated with abnormal sperm morphology and, to some degree, with sperm immotility.[57]

Toxins may act at many stages of sperm development, causing abnormal sperm count, motility, or morphology. The initial studies in men primarily looked at sperm count per cubic centimeter (density) and sperm count per ejaculate as end points. Motility and morphology traditionally have been assessed in a relatively subjective manner, and these measures were fairly insensitive for detection of subtle differences between groups in an epidemiologic study. In recent years, the use of videomicrography for assessing sperm motility and computer-generated scoring systems for evaluating sperm morphology have allowed objective measurement of semen production (see Chaps. 114 and 118).

## FUEL METABOLISM

### DIABETES MELLITUS

Environmental factors may play a role in the development of type 1 diabetes mellitus. An acute diabetes-like syndrome was reported from poisoning with an insecticide, N-3-pyridyl-methyl-N-p-nitrophenylurea (Vacor).[58] This chemical is structurally related to alloxan and streptozocin, which induce islet cell failure. Whether low doses of similar chemicals could contribute to the development of diabetes is unknown. A study in Taiwan suggests that long-term arsenic exposure may induce diabetes mellitus in humans.[59]

### HYPOGLYCEMIA

Severe hepatic deficiency caused by environmental toxins can produce hypoglycemia. Parathion, an insecticide, can lower blood glucose levels in animals and has caused hypoglycemia in at least one case of human exposure.[60]

The ingestion of the unripe fruit of the ackee tree (primarily eaten in Jamaica) causes a poisoning that includes severe hypoglycemia. The fruit contains two toxins, L-α-aminomethyl-enecyclopropylproprionic acid and its α-glutamyl conjugate, which inhibit transport of long-chain fatty acids into mitochondria, suppress oxidation, and inhibit gluconeogenesis.[61]

### LIPIDS

TCDD and related aromatic halogenated hydrocarbons induce changes in animal lipid metabolism, including fatty liver. Serum triglyceride and free fatty acid levels may be increased at low doses, and both serum total cholesterol and high-density lipoprotein cholesterol levels may be increased at higher doses.[62]

TCDD exposure leads to depletion of brown adipose tissues of rats. This causes a significant energy imbalance, with less efficient energy use and subsequent wasting. Wasting has not been reported in humans, although lipid metabolism may be impaired.

In humans exposed to PCBs, elevated serum triglyceride levels have been reported. The clinical significance is unknown, but this elevation may serve as a useful marker of exposure. Carbon disulfide, a solvent, causes elevation of serum cholesterol levels in exposed workers.[63] Some phytoestrogens increase resistance of low-density lipoprotein to oxidation.[64] Some have lipid-lowering effects.[65]

## OCCUPATIONAL FACTORS

The natural history of many of the chemically induced endocrine disorders discussed is obscure. As a general principle, removal from exposure to a toxin may cause regression of the disease, unless irreversible anatomic alterations have occurred. Removal from work must be prescribed with an understanding of the financial and legal implications.[25,33]

Some occupations entail risks to persons with coexistent endocrine disorders; these need to be considered in the treatment of the disease. The occupational factor most likely to have an effect is heat. Patients with diabetes insipidus, Addison disease, hypoaldosteronism, and diabetes mellitus require special education about fluid balance in job environments with significant risk for heat stress. These include bakeries; brick-firing and ceramics kilns; electrical utilities (especially boiler maintenance); food canneries; iron, nonferrous, and steel foundries; laundries; chemical, glass, and rubber plants; mines; outdoor locations in hot weather; restaurant kitchens; smelting facilities; and steam tunnels. Occupational exposure to cold also has endocrine effects. For example, one study has demonstrated an adaptive decrease in thyroid hormone–binding capacity with increases of free $T_4$ and $T_3$.[66]

That environmental and occupational agents can influence the endocrine system is now apparent. As our awareness of the omnipresent and often unsuspected toxins in our environment increases, and as our ability to detect subtle endocrine disorders improves, many additional and previously unsuspected relationships undoubtedly will appear.[25,67]

## REFERENCES

1. Crisp TM, Clegg ED, Cooper RI, et al. Environmental endocrine disruption: an effects assessment and analysis. Environ Health Perspect 1997; 1:11.
1a. Cooper RL, Kavlock RJ. Endocrine disruptors and reproductive development: a weight-of-evidence review. J Endocrinol 1997; 152:159.
2. Butterworth KR, Mangham BA. The application of clinical toxicology. Crit Rev Toxicol 1987; 18:81.
3. Clayton GD, Clayton FE. Patty's industrial hygiene. New York: John Wiley and Sons, 1981.
4. Doull J, Klaassen CD, Amdur MO, eds. Casarett and Doull's toxicology. New York: Macmillan, 1980.
5. Robins JM, Cullen MR, Conners BB. Depressed thyroid indexes associated with occupational exposure to inorganic lead. Arch Intern Med 1983; 143:220.
6. Gustafson A, Heder P, Schutz A, Skerfving S. Occupational lead exposure and pituitary function. Int Arch Occup Environ Health 1989; 61:277.
7. Foster WG, McMahon A, YoungLai EV, et al. Reproductive endocrine effects of chronic lead exposure in the male cynomolgus monkey. Reprod Toxicol 1993; 7:203.
8. Mutti A, Vescovi PP, Falzoi M, et al. Neuroendocrine effects of styrene on occupationally exposed workers. Scand J Work Environ Health 1984; 10:225.
8a. Brucker-Davis F. Effects of environmental synthetic chemicals on thyroid function. Thyroid 1998; 8:827.
9. Van Etten CH. Goitrogens. In: Liener IE, ed. Toxic constituents of plant foodstuffs. New York: Academic Press, 1969:103.
10. Smith DM. Ethylene thiourea: thyroid function in two groups of exposed workers. Br J Ind Med 1984; 41:362.

11. Bahn A, Mills J, Snyder P, et al. Hypothyroidism in workers exposed to polybrominated biphenyls. N Engl J Med 1980; 302:31.
12. McKinney JD, Waller CL. Polychlorinated biphenyls as hormonally active structural analogues. Environ Health Perspect 1994; 102:290.
13. Safe S. Toxicology, structure-function relationship, and human and environmental health impacts of polychlorinated biphenyls: progress and problems. Environ Health Perspect 1993; 100:259.
13a. Brouwer A, Longnecker MP, Birnbaum LS, et al. Characterization of potential endocrine-related health effects at low-dose levels of exposure to PCBs. Environ Health Perspect 1999; 107:639.
14. Peters HA, Gocmen A, Cripps DJ, et al. Epidemiology of hexachlorobenzene-induced porphyria in Turkey. Arch Neurol 1980; 39:744.
15. Van Raaij JAGM, Frijters CMG, Van den Berg KJ. Hexachlorobenzene induced hypothyroidism. Biochem Pharmacol 1993; 46:1385.
16. Den Besten C, Bennik MHJ, Bruggleman I, et al. The role of oxidative metabolism in hexachlorobenzene-induced porphyria and thyroid hormone homeostasis: a comparison with petachlorobenzene in a 13-week feeding study. Toxicol Appl Pharmacol 1993; 119:181.
17. Vanden Heuvel JP, Lucier G. Environmental toxicity of polychlorinated dibenzo-*p*-dioxins and polychlorinated dibenzofurans. Environ Health Perspect 1993; 100:189.
18. Whitlock JP. Genetic and molecular toxicity of 2,3,7,8-tetrachlorbenzo-*p*-dioxin action. Annu Rev Pharmacol Toxicol 1990; 30:251.
18a. Kohn MC. Effect of TCDD on thyroid hormone homeostasis in the rat. Drug Chem Toxicol 2000; 23:259.
19. Rattner BA. Endocrine responses to avian environmental pollutants. J Exp Zool 1984; 232:683.
20. Rawlings NC, Cook SJ, Waldbillig D. Effects of the pesticides carbofuran, chlorpyrifos, dimethoate, lindane, triallate, trifluralin, 2,4-D, and pentachlorophenol on the metabolic, endocrine and reproductive endocrine system in ewes. J Toxicol Environ Health 1998; 54:21.
21. Conrad RA, Paglia DE, Larsen PR. Review of medical findings in a Marshallese population 26 years after accidental exposure to radioactive fallout. Upton, NY: Brookhaven National Laboratory, 1980. Brookhaven National Laboratory report 51261.
22. Larsen PR, Conrad RA, Knudsen KD. Thyroid hypofunction after exposure to fallout from a hydrogen bomb explosion. JAMA 1982; 247:1571.
23. Reizenstein P. Carcinogenicity of radiation doses caused by the Chernobyl fallout in Sweden and prevention of possible tumors. Med Oncol Tumor Pharmacother 1987; 4:1.
24. Zeighami EA, Morris MD. Thyroid cancer risk in the population around the Nevada test site. Health Phys 1986; 50:19.
25. Rosenstock L, Cullen MR. Clinical occupational medicine. Philadelphia: WB Saunders, 1994.
26. Klein RF, Wiren KM. Regulation of osteoblastic gene expression by lead. Endocrinology 1993; 132:2531.
27. Cagin CR, Diloy-Puray M, Westerman MP. Bullets, lead poisoning and thyrotoxicosis. Ann Intern Med 1978; 89:509.
28. Hunter D. The diseases of occupations. London: English Universities Press, 1975:879.
29. Newton RW, Browning MC, Iqbal J, et al. Adrenocortical suppression in workers manufacturing synthetic glucocorticoids. BMJ 1978; 1:73.
30. Reif RM, Lewinsohn G. Paraquat myocarditis and adrenal cortical necrosis. J Forensic Sci 1983; 28:505.
31. Ribelin WE. Effects of drugs and chemicals upon the structure of the adrenal gland. Fundam Appl Toxicol 1984; 4:105.
32. Colby HD, Eacho PI. Chemically induced adrenal injury: role of metabolic activation. In: Thomas JA, ed. Endocrine toxicology. New York: Raven Press, 1985:35.
33. Welch LS. Decision making about reproductive hazards. Semin Occup Med 1986; 1:97.
34. Paul M. Clinical evaluation and management. In: Occupational and environmental reproductive hazards: a guide for clinicians. Baltimore: Williams & Wilkins, 1993:113.
35. Egeland GM, Sweeney MH, Fingerhut MA, et al. Total serum testosterone and gonadotropins in workers exposed to dioxin. Am J Epidemiol 1994; 139:272.
36. Safe S, Commor K, Rananoorthy K, et al. Human exposure to endocrine-active compounds: hazard assessment problems. Regul Toxicol Pharmacol 1997; 26:52.
37. Bulger WH, Kupfer D. Estrogenic activity of pesticides and other xenobiotics. In: Thomas JA, ed. Endocrine toxicology. New York: Raven Press, 1985.
38. Wolff MS, Toniolo PG, Lee EW, et al. Blood level of organochlorine residues and risk of breast cancer. J Natl Cancer Inst 1993; 85:648.
39. Dewailly E, Dodin S, Verreault R, et al. High organochlorine body burden in women with estrogen receptor positive breast cancer. J Natl Cancer Inst 1994; 86:232.
40. Van't Veer P, Lobbezoo IE, Martin-Moreno JM, et al. DDT (dicophane) and postmenopausal breast cancer in Europe: case-control study. BMJ 1997; 31:81.
41. Lopez-Carrillo L, Blair A, Lopez-Cervantes M, et al. Dichlorodiphenyl-trichloroethane serum levels and breast cancer risk: a case-control study from Mexico. Cancer Res 1997; 57:3728.
42. Hunter DJ, Hankinson SE, Laden F, et al. Plasma organochlorine levels and the risk of breast cancer. N Engl J Med 1997; 337:1253.
43. Wolff MS. Occupationally derived chemicals in breast milk. In: Mattison DR, ed. Reproductive toxicology, vol 117. New York: Alan Liss, 1983:259.
44. Kacew S. Adverse effects of drugs and chemicals in breast milk on the nursing infant. J Clin Pharmacol 1993; 33:213.
45. Rier HE, Martin DC, Bowman RE, et al. Endometriosis in Rhesus monkeys (*Macaca mulatta*) following chronic exposure to 2,3,7,8-tetrachlorbenzo-*p*-dioxin. Fundam Appl Toxicol 1993; 21:433.
45a. Bowers JL, Tyulmenkov VV, Jernigan SC, Klinge CM. Resveratrol acts as a mixed agonist/antagonist for estrogen receptors alpha and beta. Endocrinology 2000; 141:3657.
46. Bennetts HW, Underwood EJ, Shier FL. A specific breeding problem of sheep on subterranean clover pastures in Western Australia. Aust Vet J 1946; 22:2.
47. Kallela K, Heinonen H, Saloniemi H. Plant oestrogens; the cause of decreased fertility in cows. A case report. Nord Vet Med 1984; 36:124.
48. Lightfoot RJ, Croker KP, Neil HG. Failure of sperm transport in relation to ewe infertility following prolonged grazing on oestrogenic pasture. Aust J Agric Res 1967; 18:755.
49. Drane HM, Patterson DSP, Roberts BA, Saba N. The chance discovery of oestrogenic activity in laboratory rat cake. Food Chem Toxicol 1975; 13:491.
50. Sectell KDR, Doriello SD, Hulme P, et al. Nonsteroidal estrogens of dietary origin: possible roles in hormone dependent disease. Am J Clin Nutr 1984; 40:569.
51. Morrione T. Effects of estrogens on the testes in hepatic insufficiency. Arch Pathol 1944; 37:38.
52. Fitzsimmons M. Gynaecomastia in stilboestrol workers. Br J Ind Med 1944; 1:235.
53. Raizada RB, Pushpa M, Saxena I, et al. Weak estrogenic activity of lindane in rats. J Toxicol Environ Health 1980; 6:483.
54. Wyrobek AJ, Gordon LA, Bulchart JG. An evaluation of human sperm as indicators of chemically induced alterations of spermatogenic function: a report of the US Environmental Protection Agency Gene-Tox Program. Mutat Res 1983; 114:77.
55. Chapin RE, White RD, Morgan KT, Bus JS. Studies of lesions induced in the testis and epididymis of F-344 rats by inhaled methyl chloride. Toxicol Appl Pharmacol 1984; 76:328.
56. Cullen MR, Robins JM, Eskenazi B. Adult inorganic lead intoxication—presentation of 31 new cases and a review of recent advances in the literature. Medicine (Baltimore) 1983; 62:221.
57. Robins TG, Bornman MS, Ehrlich RI, et al. Semen quality and fertility of men employed in a South African lead acid battery plant. Am J Ind Med 1997; 32:369.
58. Pesticidal diabetes. (Editorial). BMJ 1979; 2:292.
59. Lai M-S, Hsueh Y-M, Chen C-J, et al. Ingested inorganic arsenic and prevalence of diabetes mellitus. Am J Epidemiol 1994; 139:484.
60. Hruban Z, Schulman S, Warner NE, et al. Hypoglycemia resulting from insecticide poisoning. JAMA 1969; 184:509.
61. Tanaka K, Kean EA, Johnson B. Jamaica vomiting sickness. Biochemical investigation of two cases. N Engl J Med 1976; 295:461.
62. Poland A, Knutson JC. 2,3,7,8-Tetrachlorodibenzo-*p*-dioxin and related halogenated aromatic hydrocarbons: examination of the mechanism of toxicity. Annu Rev Pharmacol Toxicol 1982; 22:517.
63. Lillis R. Carbon disulfide. In: Rom WN, ed. Environmental and occupational medicine. Boston: Little, Brown and Company, 1983:627.
64. Wiseman H, O'Reilly JD, Adlercreutz H, et al. Isoflavone phytoestrogens consumed in soy decrease F(2)-isoprostane concentrations and increase resistance of low-density lipoprotein to oxidation in humans. Am J Clin Nutr 2000; 72:395.
65. Lissin LW, Cooke JP. Phytoestrogens and cardiovascular health. J Am Coll Cardiol 2000; 35:1403.
66. Solter M, Brkic K, Petek M, et al. Thyroid hormone economy in response to extreme cold exposure in healthy factory workers. J Clin Endocrinol Metab 1989; 68:168.
67. Rom WN, ed. Environmental and occupational medicine. Boston: Little, Brown and Company, 1992:3.

# PART XVIII

# ENDOCRINE DRUGS
# AND VALUES

KENNETH L. BECKER, EDITOR

# CHAPTER 236

# COMPENDIUM OF ENDOCRINE-RELATED DRUGS

DOLLY MISRA, MICHELLE FISCHMANN MAGEE,
AND ERIC S. NYLÉN

There has been a great proliferation of preparations used in the clinical practice of endocrinology, and this will undoubtedly increase further with time. Any drug that is to be entered into the market in the United States goes through a rigorous certification procedure that may last for years, until it is "approved" for use in humans by the U.S. Food and Drug Administration (FDA). The manufacturer must first obtain an approved New Drug Application (NDA) from the FDA. A Notice of Claimed Investigational Exemption for a New Drug (IND) must then be accepted by the FDA. Subsequently, the drug is entered into phase I trials in normal subjects to identify "tolerable" dose ranges. In phase II trials, limited numbers of patients are treated with the drug to establish efficacy and doses. Finally, phase III involves more extensive clinical trials in patients. After a drug has been approved and is in clinical use, there is an ongoing process of postmarketing surveillance, whereby all reports of adverse effects, additional clinical experience, and other relevant data must be submitted by the manufacturer to the FDA.

Drugs are approved for use for specific indications. The FDA does not attempt to compel prescribers to adhere to officially labeled uses. Unlabeled uses are considered to be proper if based on "rational scientific theory, reliable medical opinion, or controlled clinical studies."

For all prescription drugs, FDA-approved labeling must be contained in the package insert or official label. This provides a summary of information about the "chemical and physical nature of the product, its pharmacology, the indications and contraindications, the means of administration, the appropriate dosage, side effects and adverse reactions, how the drug is supplied, and any other information pertinent to its safe and effective use." The *Physicians' Desk Reference* (PDR) is mainly a compilation of these official labels.

The use of any drug during pregnancy should be considered only if clearly needed. Before using a drug in a pregnant woman, one should consider its potential to cause harm to the fetus. The FDA has established five pregnancy categories for drugs. On the basis of the degree of documentation required concerning the validity of the relationship, these categories indicate the potential for a drug to cause birth defects and also the drug risk/benefit ratio in pregnancy.

This chapter is a practical listing of many drugs in current use in the clinical practice of endocrinology. The information in Table 236-2, which follows, provides specifics for each drug, including preparations available, indications for use, dose ranges and rates of administration, and other comments that the authors feel are germane to the agents' use. Where such specifics are discussed in detail in other parts of this textbook, the reader is referred to the relevant chapter. This table is intended as a useful lexicon of the available drugs and many of their proprietary (trade) names. Their use is not necessarily being recommended. The indications, dose, side effects, precautions, and usage in pregnancy are presented in an abbreviated form, and the following references should be checked for more complete details.

*The United States Pharmacopeia (USP DI), Drug Information for the Health Care Professional* 2000. Published by an alliance between the United States Pharmacopeial Convention and Micromedex, Inc. Contains specific pharmacological information on drugs, including formulae, formulations of preparations, and assays for identification. On-line access: www.micromedex.com/uspdi

*Drug Facts and Comparisons,* 2000. Facts and Comparisons Division of JB Lippincott Co, Philadelphia. A comprehensive drug information compendium whose core of information is derived from the most current FDA-approved package literature, updated monthly. On-line access: www.drugfacts.com

*Physicians' Desk Reference,* 2001. Medical Economics Inc, Oradell, New Jersey. Product overviews of selected drugs, usually based on official package circulars. On-line access: www.pdr.net

*Physicians' Desk Reference for Nonprescription Drugs,* 2001. Medical Economics Inc, Oradell, New Jersey. A guide to the contents of many nonprescription drugs.

*Drug Information,* 2000. Compiled by American Hospital Formulary Service and published by the American Society of Health-System Pharmacists, Inc, Bethesda. A detailed guide of drugs and their use.

*The Medical Letter.* Bi-weekly publication of evidence-based drug data. On-line access: www.medletter.com

**TABLE 236-1.**
**Index of General Categories of Drugs Found in Table 236-2**

**TABLE 236-2. Endocrine Related Drugs** (Approved Use, Unlabeled Use or Investigational)*

**DRUGS ARE LISTED BY CATEGORY OR ALPHABETICALLY. A LOCATION INDEX IS ON THE PRIOR PAGE.**
(See Indicated Chapters, References, *Physicians' Desk Reference*, and *Drug Facts and Comparisons* for More Complete Information)

## ABBREVIATIONS

| | | | | | | | | |
|---|---|---|---|---|---|---|---|---|
| ac | = | before meals (ante cibum) | h | = | hour(s) | qd | = | every day (quaque die) |
| ad lib | = | as required (ad libitum) | hs | = | bedtime | qid | = | four times daily (quarter in die) |
| amp(s) | = | ampule(s) | IC | = | intracutaneous | qod | = | every other day |
| aq | = | water (aqua) | IM | = | intramuscular | qoh | = | every other hour |
| bid | = | twice daily (bis in die) | IV | = | intravenous | RDA | = | recommended dietary |
| BMD | = | bone mineral density | kg | = | kilogram(s) | | | allowance |
| BMI | = | body mass index | LFT | = | liver function test | RNA | = | ribonucleic acid |
| Ca | = | cancer | m | = | meter(s) | Rx | = | therapy |
| cal | = | calorie | max | = | maximum | SC | = | subcutaneous |
| cap(s) | = | capsule(s) | mCi | = | milliCurie(s) | SL | = | sublingual |
| CBC | = | complete blood count | mEq | = | milliequivalent(s) | soln | = | solution(s) |
| CHF | = | congestive heart failure | mg | = | milligram(s) | stat | = | immediately (statin) |
| CNS | = | central nervous system | min | = | minute(s) | suspn | = | suspension(s) |
| concn | = | concentration(s) | mL | = | milliliter(s) | tab(s) | = | tablet(s) |
| d | = | day(s) | mm | = | millimeter(s) | tid | = | three times daily (ter in die) |
| dL | = | deciliter(s) | ng | = | nanogram(s) | $t^1/_2$ | = | half-life |
| DNA | = | deoxyribonucleic acid | pc | = | after meals (post cibum) | U | = | unit(s) |
| Dx | = | diagnosis | po | = | by mouth (per os) | USP | = | United States Pharmacopeia |
| equiv | = | equivalent | ppm | = | parts per million | vag | = | vaginal |
| g | = | gram(s) | prn | = | as needed (pro re nata) | wk | = | week(s) |
| GI | = | gastrointestinal | PSA | = | prostate specific antigen | µg | = | microgram |
| gr | = | grain(s) | q | = | each (quaque) | yr | = | year(s) |
| gtt(s) | = | drop(s) (gutta) | | | | | | |

| Drug | Trade Names and Preparations |
|---|---|

**ADRENAL STEROID INHIBITORS**

| **I. AMINOGLUTETHIMIDE** | Cytadren      250 mg/tab |
|---|---|

**INDICATIONS:** For control of cortisol secretion in selected patients with Cushing syndrome: (1) until definitive Rx can be performed; (2) if surgery and/or irradiation Rx fail to control cortisol secretion; (3) if definitive Rx is not feasible; (4) as palliative Rx for metastatic adrenal Ca or paraneoplastic ACTH-producing tumors [see Chaps. 21, 75 and 219]. Unlabeled uses: (1) Rx of advanced breast Ca postmenopause [see Chap. 224]; (2) Rx of metastatic prostate Ca [see Chap. 225].

- - - - - - -

**DOSE:** Initial dosage: 250 mg po q 6 h. May be increased by 250 mg/d q 1-2 wk to dosage of 2 g/d.

- - - - - - -

**ACTIONS AND SIDE EFFECTS:** Reversibly inhibits conversion of cholesterol to Δ-5-pregnenolone; reduces adrenal secretion of glucocorticoids, mineralocorticoids and sex steroids. May cause adrenal insufficiency, hypotension, hypothyroidism, drowsiness, skin rash, nausea, anorexia, fever, marrow suppression, masculinization in females, precocious puberty in males, LFT abnormalities. Give both gluco- and mineralocorticoid Rx if adrenal insufficiency occurs; do not replace with dexamethasone, since aminoglutethimide increases its rate of metabolism. May be teratogenic in humans and rats. Effects may be overcome in Cushing disease by increased ACTH secretion.

| **II. CYPROHEPTADINE HYDROCHLORIDE** | (tabs) | mg/tab | (syrup) | mg/5 mL |
|---|---|---|---|---|
| | Cyproheptadine HCl | 4 | Cyproheptadine HCl | 2 |
| | Periactin | 4 | Periactin | 2 |

**INDICATIONS:** (1) Investigationally to control ACTH secretion in Cushing disease or Nelson syndrome [see Chaps. 21 & 75]; (2) carcinoid syndrome for control of symptoms; (3) Rx of prostate Ca [see Chap. 225].

- - - - - - -

**DOSE:** Initial dosage: 4 mg po tid. May be increased over 2 wk to maximum of 32 mg/d, or 0.5 mg/kg, in 4-6 divided doses.

- - - - - - -

**ACTIONS AND SIDE EFFECTS:** Antihistamine, anticholinergic, and serotonin antagonist. May decrease pituitary ACTH secretion in adenomas. Side effects similar to those of other antihistamines. Use with caution in: narrow-angle glaucoma, asthma, urinary retention, cardiovascular disease, hypertension, gastric outlet obstruction.

| **III. IMIDAZOLES** | |
|---|---|
| **A. KETOCONAZOLE** | Nizoral      200 mg/scored tab |

**INDICATIONS:** Used investigationally in: (1) Cushing syndrome for palliative or preoperative Rx [see Chaps. 21 & 75]; (2) prostate Ca to decrease androgen production [see Chap. 225]; (3) testing of gonadotropin reserve in the male; (4) selected cases of precocious puberty; (5) the management of hirsutism and ovarian hyperandrogenism.

- - - - - - -

**DOSE:** Beneficial effects shown in Cushing syndrome at dosages of 200-1200 mg/d. Divided dosages up to 600 mg po/d for precocious puberty.

- - - - - - -

**ACTIONS AND SIDE EFFECTS:** An antifungal agent that is a potent inhibitor of gonadal and adrenal steroid synthesis. Inhibits: $C_{17-20}$ lyase, side-chain cleavage enzyme, 11ß-hydroxylase, 18-hydroxylase. Side effects include adrenal insufficiency, impotence, gynecomastia, oligospermia, gastrointestinal disturbances, hepatic toxicity, potentiation of anticoagulants and corticosteroids. Long-term safety in children not determined. Requires gastric acidity for dissolution; avoid concomitant antacids, anticholinergics and $H_2$ blockers, or delay administration by 2 h.

* The authors and editor appreciate the assistance of Roberta L. Brown, Pharm. D., in the verification of this table and other pertinent pharmaceutical information in this textbook.

| B. ETOMIDATE | Amidate | 2mg/mL injection |
|---|---|---|

**INDICATIONS:** Unlabeled emergency use in ectopic Cushing disease.

**DOSE:** 1.2-2.5 mg/h.

**ACTIONS AND SIDE EFFECTS:** Non-barbiturate hypnotic without analgesic activity. Used for induction of general anesthesia. May cause acute adrenal insufficiency.

| IV. METYRAPONE | Metopirone | 250 mg/cap |
|---|---|---|

**INDICATIONS:** (1) Dx of hypothalamic-pituitary ACTH function [see Chap. 241]; (2) control of cortisol secretion in Cushing syndrome [see Chaps. 21 and 75].

**DOSE:** (1) For Dx of hypothalamic-pituitary ACTH function [see Chap. 241]; (2) Cushing syndrome dosage is 250-500 mg po tid.

**ACTIONS AND SIDE EFFECTS:** Inhibits conversion of 11-deoxycortisol to cortisol by 11ß-hydroxylase. Side effects include abdominal discomfort, dizziness, headache, rash, and adrenal insufficiency. Erroneous Dx test results may occur if cyproheptadine or phenytoin is taken within 2-3 wk, or if on estrogen Rx.

| V. MITOTANE (o,p'-DDD) | Lysodren   500 mg/tab | |
|---|---|---|

**INDICATIONS:** (1) Palliative Rx of Ca of the adrenal cortex; (2) unlabeled: as adjunctive Rx in selected patients with Cushing disease [see Chaps. 21 and 75].

**DOSE:** Start with 2-6 g/d in 3 or 4 divided doses. Increase incrementally to 9-10 g/d. Dose is adjusted according to side effects and response. Maximum tolerated dosage varies from 2-16 g/d (usually 9-10 g). May need up to 3 months of maximum tolerated dose for response to occur. For unlabeled Rx in selected patients with Cushing disease: initially 500 mg po/d, up to a max of 6 g/d in 3-4 divided doses.

**ACTIONS AND SIDE EFFECTS:** Selectively toxic to adrenal cortical cells by an unknown mechanism. Temporarily inhibits or permanently destroys adrenal tissue depending on dose given. Side effects commonly include GI disturbances, CNS effects (lethargy, somnolence, dizziness, vertigo), dermatitis, cystitis, hematuria, flushing, hypertension and adrenal insufficiency. Behavioral and neurologic impairment may result from prolonged Rx.

| VI. TRILOSTANE | Modrastane | 30 & 60 mg/cap |
|---|---|---|

**INDICATIONS:** Temporary control of hypercortisolism in selected patients with Cushing syndrome [see Chaps. 21 and 75].

**DOSE:** Start with 30 mg po qid. May be increased q 3-4 d up to total dose of 360 mg. Dosages >480 mg/d are not recommended.

**ACTIONS AND SIDE EFFECTS:** Trilostane reversibly inhibits 3ß-hydroxysteroid dehydrogenase, causing decreased production of cortisol and aldosterone. Contraindicated in severe hepatic or renal disease. Side effects include abdominal discomfort or pain, diarrhea, oral or nasal burning, headache, myalgia, arthralgia and skin rash. May prevent maximal adrenal response in a stressed patient or when used in combination with other adrenal steroid inhibitors. May also cause orthostatic hypotension by its suppression of aldosterone production.

| Drug | Trade Names and Preparations |
|---|---|

**ADRENOCORTICOTROPIC HORMONE (ACTH)**

**INDICATIONS:** Assessment of adrenocortical function. Disorders that respond to glucocorticoid therapy also respond to ACTH if the adrenal cortex is intact [see Chap. 78].

| I. CORTICOTROPIN | Powder: | | Repository: | |
|---|---|---|---|---|
| | ACTH | 40 U/vial | ACTH-80 | 80 U/mL |
| | Acthar | 25 or 40 U/vial | H.P. Acthar Gel | 40 or 80 U/mL |
| | Corticotropin | 40 U/vial | | |

**INDICATIONS:** Limited use in testing adrenocortical function and disorders responsive to corticosteroids.

**DOSE:** Use as much as 80 U as a single injection for test of adrenal responsiveness.

**ACTIONS AND SIDE EFFECTS:** Prepared from animal pituitaries. Higher risk of allergic reactions than for the synthetic analog of ACTH, cosyntropin (below). May be used as a Rx agent. If used long-term, patients should be monitored for side effects of hypercortisolism. These preparations are all for IM or SC injection. "ACTH" and Acthar also may be given IV for Dx purposes. The others all are repository gels and are not for IV use.

| II. COSYNTROPIN | Cortrosyn | 250 µg per vial |
|---|---|---|

**INDICATIONS:** (1) The short ACTH stimulation test is used as a *screening* test of adrenocortical function in the assessment of hypothalamic-pituitary-adrenal function in patients treated with glucocorticoids. (2) The long ACTH stimulation test is performed in the evaluation of adrenal insufficiency when the response to the short test is abnormal. It helps to delineate whether the source is primary or central. It is the preferred preparation for Dx testing of adrenocortical function. Given IM or IV.

**DOSE:** 1 µg or 250 µg bolus push. See Chapters 74 and 241 for use in ACTH stimulation tests.

**ACTIONS AND SIDE EFFECTS:** A synthetic corticotropin analog of the first 24 amino acids of the corticotropin molecule, which possesses full bioactivity. Not used as a Rx agent [see Chaps. 78 and 241].

| Drug | Trade Names and Preparations |
|---|---|

**ANDROGENS**

### I. TESTOSTERONE
### A. TRANSDERMAL SYSTEM

| | | mg/d | | mg/d |
|---|---|---|---|---|
| Testoderm | 4 & 6 | Androderm | 2.5 & 5 |
| Testoderm TTS | 5 | AndroGel 1% | 50, 75 & 100 |
| Testoderm + adhesive | 6 | | |

**INDICATIONS:** Replacement therapy for conditions associated with a deficiency or lack of endogenous testosterone (i.e., congenital and acquired primary and hypogonadotropic hypogonadism).

**DOSE:** Testoderm should be applied to dry shaven scrotal skin every 22-24 h. Total testosterone measurement should be determined after 3-4 wk of Rx 2-4 h after application. Testoderm TTS may be applied to skin of arm, back, or upper buttocks every 24 h. Serum testosterone concentrations should be measured 2-4 h after application. Androderm may be applied to skin of back, abdomen, upper arms, or thighs at bedtime. Serum testosterone concentrations should be measured the morning after application. AndroGel 1% (i.e., 5G delivers 50 mg testosterone) is applied once daily to clean dry intact skin of shoulders, upper arms, or abdomen. Do not apply gel to genitals. Avoid showering or swimming for about 5-6 h. Check testosterone level after 14 days.

**SIDE EFFECTS:** See discussion below.

### B. TESTOSTERONE SUBCUTANEOUS IMPLANT

| | |
|---|---|
| Testopel | 75 mg pellets |

**INDICATIONS:** As for the transdermal system (see above).

**DOSE:** In androgen-deficient males, use 150-450 mg SC q 3-6 mo. Adjust dose as follows: implant two 75 mg pellets for each 25 mg testosterone propionate required weekly.

**SIDE EFFECTS:** See discussion below.

### II. TESTOSTERONE (In Aqueous Suspension)

| | | mg/mL | | mg/mL | | mg/mL |
|---|---|---|---|---|---|---|
| Testosterone (Aq) | 25, 50 & 100 | Testamone | 100 | | |
| Histerone 100 | 100 | Testandro | 100 | | |

### III. TESTOSTERONE DERIVATIVES
#### A. 17β-Hydroxyl Esterification

| | | | | | | |
|---|---|---|---|---|---|---|
| **1. NANDROLONE DECANOATE IN OIL** | Nandrolone decanoate D | 50, 100 & 200 | Androlone-D | 200 | Hybolin Decanoate | 50 & 100 |
| | | | Deca-Durabolin | 50, 100 & 200 | Neo-Durabolic | 50 & 200 |
| **2. NANDROLONE PHENPROPIONATE IN OIL** | Nandrolone phenpropionate | 25 & 50 | Durabolin | 25 & 50 | Nandrobolic | 25 |
| | | | Hybolin Improved | 50 | | |
| **3. TESTOSTERONE CYPIONATE IN OIL** | Testosterone cypionate | 100 & 200 | Depo-Testosterone | 100 & 200 | Duratest-100 | 100 |
| | depAndro 100 | 100 | Depotest 100 | 100 | Duratest-200 | 200 |
| | depAndro 200 | 200 | Depotest 200 | 200 | | |
| **4. TESTOSTERONE ENANTHATE IN OIL** | Testosterone enanthate | 100 & 200 | Andropository-200 | 200 | Durathate-200 | 200 |
| | Andro L.A. 200 | 200 | Delatestryl | 200 | Everone | 200 |
| **5. TESTOSTERONE PROPIONATE IN OIL** | Testosterone propionate | 100 | | | | |

#### B. 17α-Alkylation

| | | | | | | |
|---|---|---|---|---|---|---|
| | (tabs) | mg/tab | (tabs) | mg/tab | (tabs) | mg/tab |
| **1. FLUOXYMESTERONE** | Fluoxymesterone | 10 | Halotestin | 2, 5 & 10 | (All contain tartrazine) | |
| **2. METHYLTESTOSTERONE** | (tabs) | mg/tab | (buccal tabs) | mg/tab | (caps) | mg/tab |
| | Methyltestosterone | 10 & 25 | Methyltestosterone | 10 | Testred | 10 |
| | Android-10 | 10 | Oreton Methyl | 10 | Virilon | 10 |
| | Android-25 | 25 | | | | |
| | Oreton Methyl | 10 | | | | |
| **3. OXANDROLONE** | Oxandrin | 2.5 | | | | |
| **4. OXYMETHOLONE** | Anadrol-50 | 50 | | | | |
| **5. STANOZOLOL** | Winstrol | 2 | | | | |

**INDICATIONS:** See Chapter 119 for clinical uses and abuses of androgens. Also see Chapter 92, use in delayed puberty; Chapter 18, pediatric dose in pituitary hormonal deficiency; Chapter 17, replacement dose in adult hypopituitarism; Chapter 224, use in breast Ca. The aqueous testosterone preparations and 17ß-Hydroxyl esterification derivatives are for use by IM injections. 17ß-Hydroxyl derivatives are in oil and are long-acting. 17α-Alkylation derivatives are po preparations. Bioavailability of po 17α-Alkylation derivatives is lessened by passage through the hepatic circulation. Also, they have potential hepatotoxicities. The so-called anabolic steroids are related to testosterone; they have a high anabolic/low androgenic ratio, and have been prescribed for weight gain in underweight, recently ill patients; for osteoporosis; for reversal of nitrogen loss during corticosteroid Rx; for certain varieties of anemia; and for hereditary angioedema. These agents include nandrolone phenpropionate, nandrolone decanoate, oxandrolone, oxymetholone, and stanozolol.

**DOSE:** See Chapters in Indications.

**ACTIONS AND SIDE EFFECTS:** Side effects include virilization in the female, hepatotoxicity, prostatic hypertrophy, inhibition of spermatogenesis, gynecomastia, acne, baldness, hirsutism, polycythemia, sleep apnea, hyperlipidemia, edema, and/or hypercalcemia with malignancy or immobilization. Periodic evaluation of LFT, PSA, lipids, and CBC is recommended. Their use has been much abused [see Chap. 119]. Rule out pregnancy if considering use of any androgen in a woman.

| IV. DANAZOL | Danocrine | 50, 100 & 200 mg/cap |
|---|---|---|

**INDICATIONS:** (1) May be used to induce medical "pseudomenopause" in endometriosis; (2) fibrocystic disease of breast if severe pain and tenderness; (3) prophylactically in hereditary angioedema. Unlabeled uses: premenstrual syndrome [see Chap. 99], precocious puberty, gynecomastia, menorrhagia, idiopathic immune and lupus-associated thrombocytopenias, autoimmune hemolytic anemia.

------------------------------------------------------------------------------------------------------------------------

**DOSE:** Dosage must be individualized. In females, start only during menses or with negative pregnancy test. For mild endometriosis, initially use 200-400 mg/d in 2 divided doses. Severe cases may require up to 800 mg/d in 2 divided doses. Dosage is adjusted according to response [see Chap. 98]. Rx is continued for 3-6 mo; may extend to 9 mo. In fibrocystic breast disease, dosage is 100-400 mg/d in 2 divided doses. In hereditary angioedema, initial dosage is 200 mg bid to tid.

------------------------------------------------------------------------------------------------------------------------

**ACTIONS AND SIDE EFFECTS:** Synthetic androgen derivative of 17α-ethinyltestosterone. Side effects include: androgenization, hypoestrogenicity and hepatic dysfunction. Exclude Ca of the breast before Rx. Long-term experience limited. Androgenic effects may not reverse when drug is stopped [see Chap. 98].

| Drug | Trade Names and Preparations |
|---|---|

**ANTIANDROGENS**

| I. BICALUTAMIDE | Casodex | 50 mg tab |
|---|---|---|
| II. FLUTAMIDE | Eulexin | 125 mg cap |

**INDICATIONS:** Treatment in combination with GnRH analogs for stage $D_2$ prostate Ca [see Chap. 225]. The flutamide GnRH combination is also indicated in the treatment of stage $B_2$ to C prostate Ca in conjunction with radiation therapy. Unlabeled uses include hirsutism and prostatic hyperplasia.

------------------------------------------------------------------------------------------------------------------------

**DOSE:** Casodex 50 mg po qd. Eulexin 250 mg po tid q8h.

------------------------------------------------------------------------------------------------------------------------

**ACTIONS AND SIDE EFFECTS:** All agents are nonsteroidals with antiandrogenic properties. Contraindicated in pregnant women. Common side effects include hot flushes, diarrhea, gynecomastia, nausea, and impotence. Rarely causes reversible elevation in LFT and jaundice.

| III. NILUTAMIDE | Nilandron | 50 mg tab |
|---|---|---|

**INDICATIONS:** Treatment in combination with surgical castration for treatment of stage $D_2$ metatstatic prostatic Ca.

------------------------------------------------------------------------------------------------------------------------

**DOSE:** 300 mg po qd for 30 days, then 150 mg po qd.

------------------------------------------------------------------------------------------------------------------------

**ACTIONS AND SIDE EFFECTS:** As above. Impaired adaptation to darkness. Rarely, interstitial pneumonitis. Baseline chest x-ray should be obtained.

| IV. FINASTERIDE | Proscar | 5 mg/tab | Propecia | 1 mg/tab |
|---|---|---|---|---|

**INDICATIONS:** Proscar for benign prostatic hyperplasia. Propecia for androgenetic alopecia. Unlabeled use for adjuvant monotherapy following radical prostatectomy.

------------------------------------------------------------------------------------------------------------------------

**DOSE:** Proscar 5 mg po qd. May take 6-12 months to see response. Propecia 1 mg po qd. Generally takes 3 or more months to see benefit.

------------------------------------------------------------------------------------------------------------------------

**ACTIONS AND SIDE EFFECTS:** A competitive and specific inhibitor of type II 5α-reductase reducing conversion of testosterone to dihydrotestosterone. Contraindicated in women who are or may potentially be pregnant, and women should not handle crushed or broken tablets. PSA levels drop in patients with benign prostatic hyperplasia or prostate Ca, but does not indicate a beneficial effect.

| Drug | Trade Names and Preparations |
|---|---|

**ANTITHYROID DRUGS**

| I. Thionamide Derivatives | (tabs) | mg/tab |
|---|---|---|
| A. METHIMAZOLE | Tapazole | 5 & 10 |
| B. PROPYLTHIOURACIL | Propylthiouracil (PTU) | 50 |

**INDICATIONS:** Used in medical management of Graves disease or toxic nodular goiter [see Chap. 42]. Propylthiouracil may be preferred to methimazole in treatment of (1) severe hyperthyroidism including thyroid storm, because it blocks peripheral conversion of $T_4$ to $T_3$; (2) hyperthyroidism in pregnancy, because less placental transfer and no teratogenic effects reported. Dosage here should be adjusted to keep $T_4$ in upper-normal range; (3) lactation (only if patient insists, with scrupulous monitoring of infant's thyroid function. PTU crosses into breast milk less than methimazole). Frequently possible to maintain patients on once-daily dosing with methimazole.

------------------------------------------------------------------------------------------------------------------------

**DOSE:** See Chapters in Indications.

------------------------------------------------------------------------------------------------------------------------

**ACTIONS AND SIDE EFFECTS:** Use has been associated with aplasia cutis in the fetus, but the significance of this finding has been questioned. Agranulocytosis, skin rash, jaundice, abnormal LFT.

| II. Iodide-Containing Compounds | Soln: | |
|---|---|---|
| A. IODIDES | Potassium iodide | 1 g potassium iodide/mL |
| | Pima | 325 mg potassium/5 mL syrup |
| | SSKI | 1 g potassium iodide/mL |
| | Strong Iodine soln: | |
| | (Lugol's) | 5% iodine + 10% potassium iodide soln |
| | Tabs: | |
| | Thyro-Block | 130 mg potassium iodide tabs |
| | Injection: | |
| | Sodium Iodide | 10% sodium iodide for injection in 10 mL amps |

**INDICATIONS:** (1) Thyroid storm $\geq 1$ h after ß-adrenergic blocker and thionamide Rx instituted; (2) postradioactive iodine Rx to control hyperthyroidism, while awaiting the therapeutic radioactive effect. Iodide started about 5 d after radioactive iodine administration; (3) preparation of hyperthyroid patient for surgery: Iodide given for about 10 d before; (4) radiation exposure emergencies to block thyroidal uptake of iodine.

**DOSE:** In hyperthyroidism, dosage generally is 5 drops of soln po tid or 1 tab tid [see Chapter 42 for adult doses, Chapter 47 for pediatric doses]. In radiation exposure, the recommended dosages are: age <1 yr =1/2 tab or 3 drops po qd; >1 yr=1 tab or 6 drops po/d. In thyroid storm, the parenteral dosage of sodium iodide is 2 g/d.

**ACTIONS AND SIDE EFFECTS:** Considered "non-routine" agents in Rx of hyperthyroidism. See Chapters 37, 42 and 47 for specifics regarding uses, mechanisms of action and adverse reactions. Administration in multinodular goiter may lead to an increase in thyroid hormone levels and thyrotoxicosis. Thyro-Block tabs are available only to state and federal agencies. Caution: test for idiosyncrasy before giving iodide parenterally.

| B. Cholecystographic Dyes | | |
|---|---|---|
| 1. IOCETAMIC ACID | Cholebrine | 62% iodine as 750 mg tabs |
| 2. IOPANOIC ACID | Telepaque | 66.7% iodine as 500 mg tabs |
| 3. IPODATE SODIUM | Bilivist | 61.4% iodine as 500 mg caps |
| | Oragrafin Sodium | 61.4% iodine as 500 mg caps (contains tartrazine) |
| 4. IPODATE CALCIUM | Oragrafin Calcium | 61.7% iodine as 3 g/pack oral suspension |
| 5. TYROPANOATE SODIUM | Bilopaque | 57.4% iodine as 750 mg caps |

**INDICATIONS:** May be used for short-term early Rx of hyperthyroidism or as an adjunct to thionamides.

**DOSE:** 500-1000 mg po/d.

**ACTIONS AND SIDE EFFECTS:** Iopanoic acid may not be effective as long-term Rx in Graves disease; $T_3$ reduction may not be sustained.

| C. Radioactive Iodine | | |
|---|---|---|
| SODIUM $^{131}$I | Iodotope | 8-100 mCi/cap; 7.05 mCi/mL oral soln |
| | Sodium Iodide I$^{131}$ Therapeutic | 0.75-100 mCi; cap; 3.5-150 mCi/vial soln |

**INDICATIONS:** Sodium $^{131}$I is indicated for: (1) Hyperthyroidism [Graves, toxic solitary or multiple nodular goiter]; (2) papillary and follicular Ca of the thyroid.

**DOSE:** $^{131}$I dose calculated by gland size and radioactive iodine uptake [see Chap. 42]. Toxic multinodular goiter may be relatively resistant to its effects. The usual dose of $^{131}$I in thyroid Ca is 50 mCi to ablate the thyroid bed and 100-150 mCi as a Rx dose.

**ACTIONS AND SIDE EFFECTS:** Half-life of $^{131}$I is 8.06 d. ß-Radiation causes 90% of the local effect and $\gamma$, 10% [see Chaps. 40, 42 and 47].

| Drug | Trade Names and Preparations |
|---|---|

## AROMATASE INHIBITORS

| I. ANASTROZOLE | Arimidex | 1 mg/tab |
|---|---|---|

**INDICATIONS:** Treatment in advanced breast Ca and in postmenopausal women with disease progression following antiestrogen Rx.

**DOSE:** 1 mg po qd.

**ACTIONS AND SIDE EFFECTS:** A nonsteroidal competitive inhibitor of aromatase enzyme that prevents conversion of androgens to estrogens. Generally well-tolerated. May cause diarrhea, nausea, hot flashes, headache and edema.

| II. LETROZOLE | Femara | 2.5 mg tabs |
|---|---|---|

**INDICATIONS:** Same as anastrozole.

**DOSE:** 2.5 mg qd.

**SIDE EFFECTS:** Same as anastrozole.

| III. TESTOLACTONE | Teslac | 50 mg tabs |
|---|---|---|

**INDICATIONS:** Adjuvant Rx for palliative treatment of advanced or disseminated breast Ca in postmenopausal women, when hormonal Rx is indicated. May also be used in premenopausal women after ovarian function has been terminated. Unlabeled use in congenital adrenal hyperplasia and gynecomastia.

**DOSE:** 250 mg po qid.

**SIDE EFFECTS:** A synthetic antineoplastic agent that inhibits steroid aromatase activity. The inhibition may be noncompetitive and irreversible. Occasionally, rash, paresthesia, increased blood pressure, acne, edema, glossitis, anorexia, nausea, and vomiting.

| Drug | Trade Names and Preparations |
|---|---|

## BISPHOSPHONATES

| I. ALENDRONATE SODIUM | Fosamax | 5, 10 & 40 mg tabs |
|---|---|---|

**INDICATIONS:** (1) Prevention and treatment of osteoporosis, including the osteoporosis associated with glucocorticoids. (2) Symptomatic Paget disease of the bone.

**DOSE:** Prevention of osteoporosis: 5 mg tab po qd with 8 ounces of water at least 30 min before food, beverage, or other medications. Patients should avoid lying down for at least 30 min after ingestion. Treatment of osteoporosis (men and women): 10 mg tab po qd. Treatment of Paget disease of bone: 40 mg tab po qd for 6 months. Retreatment in patients with relapse may be considered after a 6-month drug-free period. Periodic alkaline phosphatase measurement is recommended. Adequate calcium and vitamin D should be ensured.

**ACTIONS AND SIDE EFFECTS:** Contraindicated in patients with hypocalcemia or hypersensitivity to any components. Not recommended for patients with creatinine clearance < 35 mL/min or patients with abnormalities of esophagus that delay emptying (e.g., stricture or achalasia).

| II. ETIDRONATE DISODIUM | Didronel 200 & 400 mg tabs    Didronel IV 300 mg/6 mL soln |
|---|---|

**INDICATIONS:** (1) Symptomatic Paget disease of bone [see Chap. 65]; (2) prevention and Rx of heterotopic ossifications following total hip replacement or spinal injury; (3) hypercalcemia of malignancy that persists after hydration [see Chap. 59]; (4) unlabeled use in postmenopausal osteoporosis. Maximum improvement seen within 6 mo. Some patients have been treated by IV for up to 7 successive d. Results in Rx of myositis ossificans are equivocal.

--------

**DOSE:** Initial Rx for symptomatic Paget disease of bone: 5-10 mg/kg/d po for no longer than 6 mo or 11-20 mg/kg/d not to exceed 3 mo. Retreatment may be started, if indicated, after 3 mo off drug. Eating should be avoided for 2 h before and after the daily dose is taken. Initial Rx for hypercalcemia of malignancy: 7.5 mg/kg/d in 250 mL normal saline IV over 2 h for 3 d. Tabs may be started the day after last infusion. The dosage then is 20 mg/kg/d for 30 d. If hypercalcemia recurs, retreatment may be started 7 d after last dose given. In osteoporosis, intermittent cyclical use of 400 mg/d usually is followed by calcium.

--------

**ACTIONS AND SIDE EFFECTS:** Safety of long-term continuous Rx not established. Reduced doses required if impaired renal function. Contraindicated if serum creatinine >5 mg/dL. Follow renal function in all patients. Side effects include nausea, diarrhea, vomiting, and inhibition of bone mineralization.

| III. PAMIDRONATE DISODIUM | Aredia 30, 60 & 90 mg powder for injection |
|---|---|

**INDICATIONS:** (1) Hypercalcemia of malignancy; (2) Paget disease; (3) unlabeled use is (a) postmenopausal osteoporosis, (b) symptomatic bone metastasis, (c) hyperparathyroidism, (d) glucocorticoid-induced bone loss, (e) reduce bone pain in metastatic prostate Ca, (f) immobilization-induced hypercalcemia.

--------

**DOSE:** 60-90 mg for moderate hypercalcemia. 90 mg in severe hypercalcemia. Give as a single dose IV over 24 h or alternatively 60 mg IV over 4 h. Consider retreatment after 7d to allow for initial response. Use same dose for the second treatment. Dilute to 30 mg/10 mL and add 1 L 0.45% or 0.9% NaCl or 5% dextrose.

--------

**ACTIONS AND SIDE EFFECTS:** Pamidronate, unlike etidronate, inhibits bone resorption without inhibiting bone formation and mineralization. Pamidronate Rx has resulted in decreased serum phosphate. Reversible nephropathy has been associated with IV bolus of pamidronate in animals. Hypocalcemia has been reported in 6-12% of patients receiving pamidronate Rx. Other side effects include fever and infusion site reaction.

| IV. RISEDRONATE SODIUM | Actonel 5 & 30 mg tabs |
|---|---|

**INDICATIONS:** (1) Paget disease of bone; (2) Prevention and Rx of bone loss in postmenopausal women; (3) Glucocorticoid-induced osteoporosis.

--------

**DOSE:** (1) Rx 30 mg po with 6-8 ounces water at least 30 min before first food or drink of the day and avoid lying down for 30 min after administration. Duration of treatment is 2 months. (2) 5 mg qd for osteoporosis.

--------

**ACTIONS AND SIDE EFFECTS:** Contraindicated in patients with hypocalcemia or hypersensitivity to any component. Not recommended in patients with creatinine clearance < 30 mL/min. Should be used with caution in patients with a history of upper GI disorders. Most commonly reported side effects were diarrhea, arthralgia, and nausea. No osteomalacia noted.

| V. TILUDRONATE SODIUM | Skelid 240 mg/tab |
|---|---|

**INDICATIONS:** Paget disease of bone.

--------

**DOSE:** Rx 480 mg po qd with 6-8 ounces plain water. Do not take within 2 h of food. Duration of Rx is 3 months.

| Drug | Trade Names and Preparations |
|---|---|

**CALCITONIN**

| I. CALCITONIN-SALMON | Calcimar 200 IU/mL soln in 2 mL vials   Miacalcin 200 IU/mL soln in 2 mL vials |
|---|---|
| | Osteocalcin 200 IU/mL soln in 2 mL vials   Salmonine 200 IU/mL soln in 2 mL vials |

**INDICATIONS:** (1) Symptomatic Paget disease [see Chaps. 53 and 65]; (2) hypercalcemia [see Chap. 53]; (3) osteoporosis [see Chaps. 53 and 64].

--------

**DOSE:** For dosage, see Chapters in Indications. For skin testing of salmon calcitonin, inject 0.1 mL of a 10 IU/mL soln IC on the inner aspect of the forearm. More than mild erythema or wheal at 15 min is a positive response.

--------

**ACTIONS AND SIDE EFFECTS:** Side effects of Rx include rash, nausea, vomiting, diarrhea, facial flushing. Systemic allergic reactions may occur. Skin testing should be done. Calcimar and Miacalcin are salmon calcitonin preparations. When they are administered over a prolonged period, antibodies may be formed that can interfere with its effects.

| II. CALCITONIN-SALMON | Miacalcin 200 IU/0.09 mL Nasal spray in 2 mL bottles |
|---|---|

**INDICATIONS:** Rx of postmenopausal osteoporosis. Mainly improves BMD of vertebrae. Analgesic activity may alleviate bone pain.

--------

**DOSE:** 200 IU (1 puff) qd intranasally, alternating nostrils daily. Adequate vitamin D and calcium should be ensured. Baseline and periodic nasal examinations are recommended.

--------

**ACTIONS AND SIDE EFFECTS:** Most commonly rhinitis, epistaxis, and sinusitis. No serious allergic reactions have been reported; however, skin testing should be considered for patients with suspected sensitivity to calcitonin.

| Drug | Trade Names and Preparations |
|---|---|

**CALCIUM**

| (% Calcium: mEq Ca$^{2+}$/g) | |
|---|---|

**INDICATIONS:** (1) Dietary supplement, when calcium intake from the diet may be inadequate; (2) calcium deficiency states including: hypoparathyroidism, rickets, osteomalacia, hypocalcemia of the newborn, osteoporosis; (3) magnesium intoxication [see Chap. 68]; (4) hyperkalemia with ECG changes; (5) acute Rx of load-dependent hyperphosphatemia [see Chap. 67]; (6) renal osteodystrophy [see Chap. 61].

**DOSE:** As a dietary supplement, give sufficient quantity to ensure a total calcium intake [diet plus supplement] of 1000 mg/d in adults and 1500 mg/d in pregnant and lactating women and postmenopausal women [see Chap. 64]. For calcium deficiency states, doses of calcium up to 1000-2500 mg po qd may be necessary. See Chapters 60, 63 and 64 for rationale for selecting a dose in various disorders. For magnesium intoxication, 500 mg calcium is given IV. Further doses should be given only if patient does not show signs of recovery. For hyperkalemia with ECG changes, see under calcium gluconate below. For renal osteodystrophy, 1500 mg of elemental calcium qd may be given.

**ACTIONS AND SIDE EFFECTS:** High-fiber diets may decrease calcium absorption. Patients taking calcium supplements should be warned of the symptoms of hypercalcemia, particularly if they also are taking vitamin D preparations. Intravenous calcium should not be used while on digoxin, if possible, as marked bradycardia may result.

**Note**: The calcium preparations below are listed by tablet size or suspension concentration, *followed by the number of mg of elemental calcium contained in each unit in parentheses.* (There also are numerous preparations containing combinations of calcium plus vitamin D, with or without phosphorus.)

| **I. CALCIUM ACETATE** (25 : 12.6) | (tabs) | mg (mg $Ca^{2+}$/tab) |
|---|---|---|
| | Calphron | 667 (169) |
| | PhosLo | 667 (169) |

**INDICATIONS:** Control of hyperphosphatemia in end-stage renal disease. Does not promote aluminum absorption. Calcium acetate taken with meals combines with dietary phosphate to form insoluble calcium phosphate that is excreted in the feces.

**DOSE:** Recommended dose is 2 tabs with each meal. May need 3-4 tabs per meal to lower phosphate to < 6 mg/dL, as long as hypercalcemia does not occur.

| **II. CALCIUM CARBONATE** ($CaCO_3$) (40 : 20) | (caps) | mg (mg $Ca^{2+}$/tab) | (tabs) | mg (mg $Ca^{2+}$/tab) | (tabs) | mg (mg $Ca^{2+}$/tab) |
|---|---|---|---|---|---|---|
| | Calci-Mix | 1250 (500) | Calci-Chew | | Os-Cal 500 | |
| | | | (chewable) | 1250 (500) | (also chewable) | 1250 (500) |
| | (powder) | | Calcium 600 | 1500 (600) | Oysco 500 | |
| | Calcarb-HD | 6500 (2400) | Caltrate 600 | 1500 (600) | (chewable) | 1250 (500) |
| | | | Caltrate Jr | | Oyst-Cal 500 | 1250 (500) |
| | (tabs) | | (chewable) | 750 (300) | Oystercal 500 | 1250 (500) |
| | Calcium | | Femcal | 250 (100) | Oyster Shell | |
| | Carbonate | 650 (260) | Florical caps or tabs | | calcium 500 | 1250 (500) |
| | | 1250 (500) | (+8.3 mg NaF) | 364 (145.6) | Tums 500 | |
| | Cal-plus | 1500 (600) | Gencalc 600 | 1500 (600) | (chewable) | 1250 (500) |
| | Calciday-667 | 667 (266.8) | Nephro-Calci | 1500 (600) | Viactiv | |
| | | | | | (chewable) | (500) |

**INDICATIONS:** Should be taken with meals to ensure optimum absorption. It provides an efficient form of oral calcium supplement.

**ACTIONS AND SIDE EFFECTS:** Oyster-shell preparations are impure, containing possible contaminants. Calcium carbonate and other calcium preparations often have many extraneous constituents (e.g., polyethylene glycol, polysorbate 80, paraben, povidone, edible gray ink, titanium dioxide, etc.), which usually do not appear on the label. The effects of such substances when taken for many years has not been determined. Rugby Labs makes a 10 gr [650 mg] tab which contains $CaCO_3$ [260 mg of elemental Ca], microcrystalline cellulose, and carmellose sodium. Viactiv comes in the following flavors: caramel, milk chocolate, mocha, and mochaccino.

| **III. CALCIUM CHLORIDE** ($CaCl_2$) (27.2 : 13.6) | Calcium chloride | 10 mL soln in amps, vials, & syringes that contain calcium: 1 g $CaCl_2$ (272 mg Ca) |
|---|---|---|

**INDICATIONS:** For IV use when urgent administration of calcium is required, i.e., in the setting of symptomatic hypocalcemia, ECG changes and/or cardiac dysfunction (see Chap. 232).

**DOSE:** The usual IV dose is about 500 mg. The rate at which it is given should not exceed 1 mL/min.

**ACTIONS AND SIDE EFFECTS:** This compound is very irritating and may cause severe necrosis and sloughing if extravasated. Hence, the use of calcium gluconate is preferable.

| **IV. CALCIUM CITRATE** (21 : 10.5) | (tabs) | mg (mg $Ca^{2+}$/tab) |
|---|---|---|
| | Citracal | 950 (200) |
| | Citracal Liquitab | 2375 (500) effervescent with aspartame |

**INDICATIONS:** Calcium citrate is more soluble, and its absorption is less dependent on gastric acidity than that of calcium carbonate. Calcium citrate may have the best absorption of all of the oral calcium preparations [see Chap. 64].

| **V. CALCIUM GLUBIONATE** (6.5 : 3.3) | (5 mL syrup) | mg/tsp (mg $Ca^{2+}$/tsp) |
|---|---|---|
| | Neo-Calglucon | 1800 (115) |

**INDICATIONS:** For oral calcium supplementation.

**ACTIONS AND SIDE EFFECTS:** Diarrhea.

| **VI. CALCIUM GLUCEPTATE** (8.2 : 4.1) | (5 mL) | mg/mL (mg $Ca^{2+}$/mL) |
|---|---|---|
| | Calcium gluceptate | 220 (18) |

**INDICATIONS:** For IV or IM administration of calcium.

**DOSE:** In adults, 5-20 mL IV or 2-5 mL IM into the gluteal region or lateral thigh.

**ACTIONS AND SIDE EFFECTS:** Generally is well tolerated but may cause mild local reactions following intramuscular injection.

| **VII. CALCIUM GLUCONATE** (9 : 4.5) | Intravenous: |
|---|---|
| | Calcium Gluconate 10% soln in amps and vials. 10 mL contains 1 g (90 mg $Ca^{2+}$) of calcium gluconate. |

| Oral: | mg/tab | (mg Ca$^{2+}$/tab) |
|---|---|---|
| Calcium gluconate | 500 | (45) |
| | 650 | (59) |
| | 975 | (88) |
| | 1000 | (90) |

**INDICATIONS:** (1) Acute hypocalcemic crisis with tetany, laryngospasm, or seizures; (2) severe hypocalcemia with symptoms, but without tetany; (3) hyperkalemia with ECG changes. (Calcium gluconate is the agent of choice for Rx of hypocalcemic crisis. Calcium gluconate also is available in tablet form, but is seldom used orally because of its low calcium content.)

---

**DOSE:** In adults in acute hypocalcemic crisis, 10-20 mL calcium gluconate may be given over 10 min IV. In children, the dosage is 2 mg/kg elemental calcium. In adults with severe hypocalcemia, a continuous IV infusion, containing 5-6 amps (10 mL of 10% soln/amp) of calcium gluconate/L of IV fluid, may be given at a rate of 100-125 mL/h. In hyperkalemia with ECG changes, 5-10 mL of a 10% soln of calcium gluconate is injected over 2 min IV. This dosage may be repeated in 5 min.

---

**ACTIONS AND SIDE EFFECTS:** Calcium gluconate does not cause venous irritation, but may cause skin necrosis if extravasated in infants. Serum calcium levels must be monitored closely when IV calcium is being given. Calcium antagonizes the cardiac and neuromuscular toxicities of hyperkalemia. In this setting, it should be given with the patient on an ECG monitor [see Chap. 60].

| VIII. CALCIUM LACTATE (13 : 6.5) | (tabs) | mg/tab | (mg Ca$^{2+}$/tab) |
|---|---|---|---|
| | Calcium lactate | 325 | (42) |
| | | 650 | (85) |

**INDICATIONS:** Oral supplementation. (It is readily absorbed. A large number of tablets are required for a therapeutic effect.)

| IX. CALCIUM PHOSPHATE A. TRICALCIUM PHOSPHATE (38.8 : 19.4) | (tabs) | mg/tab | (mg Ca$^{2+}$/tab) |
|---|---|---|---|
| | Posture | 1565 | (600) |

**INDICATIONS:** Oral calcium supplementation.

| Drug | Trade Names and Preparations |
|---|---|

## CLOMIPHENE CITRATE

| (scored tabs) | mg/tab | (scored tabs) | mg/tab | (scored tabs) | mg/tab |
|---|---|---|---|---|---|
| Clomiphene citrate | 50 | Clomid | 50 | Serophene | 50 |

**INDICATIONS:** Ovulatory failure in patients desiring pregnancy. Unlabeled use: has been tried in Rx of male infertility.

---

**DOSE:** See Chapter 97 for Rx protocol in ovulation induction. Unlabeled use: in male infertility, dosage is 25 mg/d for 25 d with 5 d off, or 100 mg/d on Mondays, Wednesdays and Fridays.

---

**ACTIONS AND SIDE EFFECTS:** Clomiphene citrate is a nonsteroidal, triphenylethylene derivative that is similar to tamoxifen. Its actions in the stimulation of ovulation probably result from binding to estrogen receptors as a mixed agonist/antagonist. Clomiphene citrate should not be used in patients with liver disease.

| Drug | Trade Names and Preparations |
|---|---|

## CORTICOTROPIN-RELEASING HORMONE (CRH)

| CORTICORELIN OVINE TRIFLUTATE | | |
|---|---|---|
| | Acthrel | 100 µg/vial |

**INDICATIONS:** The CRH stimulation test may be useful in (1) differential Dx of: (a) the forms of Cushing disease or syndrome; (b) adrenal insufficiency of primary, pituitary, or suprapituitary type; (c) Cushing syndrome and hypercortisolism of psychiatric origin; (2) Postoperative functional capacity of pituitary corticotropin in Cushing disease.

---

**DOSE:** Single IV dose of 1 µg/kg over 30 seconds (use of heparin soln to maintain IV cannula is not recommended).

---

**ACTIONS AND SIDE EFFECTS:** CRH is the hypothalamic releasing factor for ACTH. Human CRH is a 40 amino acid molecule. Human and ovine CRH differ by seven amino acids. Ovine CRH is about five times more potent, mainly because of its longer effect on ACTH and cortisol secretion. Side effects seen in patients receiving a 1 µg/kg dose of CRH include facial and upper body flushing and an increase in heart rate. Side effects are minimized by slow bolus [see Chaps. 74, 75 and 241].

| Drug | Trade Names and Preparations |
|---|---|

## DEMECLOCYCLINE HCL

| | Declomycin | 150 mg caps |
|---|---|---|
| | | 150 & 300 mg tabs |

**INDICATIONS:** Infections due to various microorganisms. Unlabeled use: syndrome of inappropriate secretion of antidiuretic hormone [SIADH].

---

**DOSE:** In adults, for SIADH, the dosage is 600-1200 mg/d in divided doses, or 13-15 mg/kg.

---

**ACTIONS AND SIDE EFFECTS:** Demeclocycline is a tetracycline derivative. It induces a nephrogenic form of diabetes insipidus. Follow renal function closely. May cause photosensitivity. Should not be used in children [see Chap. 27].

| Drug | Trade Names and Preparations |
|---|---|

## DOPAMINE AGONISTS

| I. BROMOCRIPTINE MESYLATE | Parlodel | 2.5 mg scored tabs & 5 mg caps |
|---|---|---|

**INDICATIONS:** (1) Amenorrhea/galactorrhea or infertility associated with hyperprolactinemia; (2) prolactin-secreting pituitary adenoma [see Chap. 21]; (3) acromegaly, particularly when associated with hyperprolactinemia.

------

**DOSE:** Rx may be initiated with 1.25 mg po at bedtime, with food. Dosage may be increased q few d to 1.25 mg bid or tid. Subsequent increases may be made by 2.5-5 mg increments. In prolactinoma, a good response generally is seen with dosages of 5-15 mg/d [see Chaps. 13 and 21]. In the suppression of lactation, the dosage is 2.5 mg/d to 2.5 mg tid for 14-21 d. In acromegaly, usual dosage is 20-30 mg/d. Maximum dosage should not exceed 100 mg/d.

------

**ACTIONS AND SIDE EFFECTS:** Bromocriptine mesylate is a semisynthetic ergot alkaloid that is a dopamine agonist. It inhibits prolactin secretion in humans and may inhibit growth hormone secretion in patients with acromegaly. Nausea, headaches, dizziness and Raynaud phenomenon.

| II. CABERGOLINE | Dostinex | 0.5 mg/scored tab |
|---|---|---|

**INDICATIONS:** Hyperprolactinemic disorders. May be used in patients intolerant or resistant to bromocriptine.

------

**DOSE:** Rx initiated with 0.25 mg po 1x/wk. Dose may be increased by 0.25 mg 2x/wk. Max dose 1 mg 2x/wk.

------

**ACTIONS AND SIDE EFFECTS:** Dopamine $D_2$ receptor agonist. Nausea, headaches, vomiting, dizziness, and hypotension.

| III. PERGOLIDE MESYLATE | Permax | 0.05, 0.25 & 1 mg tabs |
|---|---|---|

**INDICATIONS:** Adjunctive Rx in Parkinson disease. Unlabeled use in hyperprolactinemic states.

------

**DOSE:** 0.05 mg/d on first 2 days. Increase gradually by 0.1 or 0.15 mg q 3 days for 12 days. Increase by 0.25 mg/day q 3 days until optimal response is achieved. Administer tid.

------

**ACTIONS AND SIDE EFFECTS:** Dopamine receptor agonist at $D_1$ and $D_2$ receptors. It is 10-1000 times more potent than bromocriptine in lowering prolactin. Side effects include hypotension (to which tolerance often develops), hallucinosis (no tolerance observed), atrial premature contractions, and sinus tachycardia.

| Drug | Trade Names and Preparations |
|---|---|

## ERECTILE DYSFUNCTION DRUGS

| I. ALPROSTADIL | Caverjet | 6.15, 11.9, 23.2 & 46.4 µg powder (5, 10, 20 & 40 µg/mL solution, respectively) |
|---|---|---|
| | Edex | 6.225, 12.45, 24.9 & 49.8 µg (5, 10, 20 & 40 µg/mL, respectively) powder |
| | MUSE | 125, 250, 500, and 1000 µg pellets |

**INDICATIONS:** Erectile dysfunction due to neurogenic, vasculogenic, psychogenic, or mixed causes.

------

**DOSE:** Dose should be individually titrated by physician. Intracavernosal injection is performed dorso-laterally in the proximal third of the penis, alternating the side used. Start with 1.25-2.5 µg and adjust ≤ 3 times/wk. Intraurethral administration results in a response within 10 min with a duration of up to 1 h.

------

**ACTIONS AND SIDE EFFECTS:** Preparation is prostaglandin $E_1$. Priapism, penile fibrosis (< 3%), penile pain (37%), hypotension.

| II. SILDENAFIL CITRATE | Viagra | 25, 50 & 100 mg tabs |
|---|---|---|

**INDICATIONS:** Erectile dysfunction.

**DOSE:** Usually ~ 1h before sexual activity (can be taken 4 h to 30 min before sexual activity). The max dose is 100 mg once per day. Increased plasma levels are seen in those > 65, hepatic impairment, severe renal failure (creatinine clearance < 30 mL/min), and concomitant use of P4503A4 inhibitors (erythromycin, ketoconazole, itraconazole).

------

**ACTIONS AND SIDE EFFECTS:** Sildenafil is a selective competitive inhibitor of cyclic guanosine monophosphate-specific phosphodiesterase type 5. The etiology for erectile dysfunction should be established and treated accordingly. Concurrent or intermittent use of nitrates in any form is contraindicated due to potentiation of hypotension. Approximately 130 patients have died in the United States, mostly from cardiovascular events, including myocardial infarction. Most patients had preexisting cardiovascular risk factors. Transient, dose-related impairment of blue-green color discrimination may occur, and patients with diabetic retinopathy or retinitis pigmentosa should use the drug with caution.

| Drug | Trade Names and Preparations |
|---|---|

## ERYTHROPOIETIN

| EPOETIN ALFA | Epogen | 2000, 3000, 4000, 10,000 & 20,000 U/mL in 1 mL vials (also 2 mL for 10,000) |
|---|---|---|
| | Procrit | 2000, 3000, 4000, 10,000 & 20,000 U/mL in 1 mL vials (also 2 mL for 10,000) |

**INDICATIONS:** For anemia of chronic renal failure, zidovudine therapy and HIV, and non-myeloid malignancies. Unlabeled use: (1) procurement of autologous blood; (2) orthostatic hypotension; (3) pruritus associated with renal failure.

------

**DOSE:** Starting dosage: 50-100 U/kg IV or SC 3x/wk. Maintenance dosage should be individualized. When the hematocrit reaches 30-36%, the dosage should be decreased by approx 25 U/kg to avoid exceeding the target range. Iron status and iron supplementation should be evaluated.

------

**ACTIONS AND SIDE EFFECTS:** Epoetin alfa is a 165 amino acid glycoprotein which is biologically identical to erythropoietin. It is manufactured by recombinant DNA technology [see Chap. 212]. Hypertension and seizures may occur. Blood pressure should be monitored and controlled. Iron supplementation is recommended.

| Drug | Trade Names and Preparations |
|------|------------------------------|

## ESTROGENS

**INDICATIONS:** (1) Menopausal symptoms [Menop]; (2) hypogonadism [Repl]; (3) osteoporosis prevention [as for "Repl" below]; (4) dysfunctional uterine bleeding; (5) constituent in oral contraceptive pills; (6) breast Ca; (7) prostate Ca. (Generally, estrogens for contraception, osteoporosis prevention, menopausal symptoms, and as replacement Rx may be given cyclically [days 1-25] and in combination with a progestin [days 16-25 of the month]. See Chapter 64 for use of estrogens in prevention of osteoporosis, Chapter 224 for use in breast Ca, Chapter 225 for use in prostate Ca.

-------------------------------------------------------------------------------------------------------

**DOSE:** The estrogen dose is titrated in each patient for optimum relief of symptoms; the smallest possible dose that achieves these goals should be used.

-------------------------------------------------------------------------------------------------------

**SIDE EFFECTS:** *Estrogen side effects and contraindications to use must be considered before institution of Rx* [see Chaps. 100, 104 and 105]. Estrogens cannot be used in pregnancy, since there is an increased risk of vaginal and cervical Ca and vaginal adenosis in female offspring and anomalies of the genitourinary tract and abnormal semen quality in male offspring. May also cause an increased risk of congenital heart disease and limb reduction defects.

### I. CONJUGATED EQUINE ESTROGENS

Oral:
  Premarin — 0.3, 0.625, 0.9, 1.25 & 2.5 mg tabs

Parenteral:
  Premarin Intravenous — 25 mg/vial

**DOSE:** *Oral:* Menop 0.3-1.25 mg po/d. Repl 0.625-1.25 mg po/d. Dysfunctional uterine bleeding 2.5-5 mg/po in divided doses x 1 wk. Breast Ca 10 mg tid po x ≥ 3 mo. Prostate Ca 1.25-2.5 mg tid. *Intravenous:* Dysfunctional uterine bleeding 25 mg IV or IM.

### II. CONJUGATED SYNTHETIC ESTROGENS

Cenestin — 0.625 & 0.9 mg tab

**DOSE:** Menopause 0.625-1.25 mg po qd.

### III. STEROIDAL ESTROGENS
#### A. ESTRADIOL

Oral:
  Estrace — 0.5, 1 & 2 mg micronized tabs
  Estradiol — 0.5, 1 & 2 mg tabs

**DOSE:** *Oral:* Menop & Repl 0.5-2 mg po qd.

#### B. ESTRADIOL CYPIONATE IN OIL

Estradiol cypionate — 5 mg/mL in oil
Depo-Estradiol Cypionate — 5 mg/mL in oil
depGynogen — 5 mg/mL in oil
DepoGen — 5 mg/mL in oil

**DOSE:** Repl 1.5-2 mg IM/mo. Menop 1-5 mg IM q 3-4 wk.

#### C. ESTRADIOL VALERATE IN OIL

Estradiol valerate — 20 & 40 mg/mL in oil
Delestrogen — 10, 20 & 40 mg/mL in oil
Estra-L 40 — 40 mg/mL in oil
Gynogen L.A. 20 — 20 mg/mL in oil
Valergen 20 — 20 mg/mL in oil
Valergen 40 — 40 mg/mL in oil

**DOSE:** Menop 10-20 mg IM q 4-6 wk. Prostate Ca 30 mg IM q 1-2wk.

#### D. ESTRONE AQUEOUS SUSPENSION

Estrone Aqueous — 5 mg/mL aq suspn for IM injection only
Kestrone 5 — 5 mg/mL aq suspn for IM injection only

**DOSE:** Prostate Ca 2-4 mg IM 2-3x/wk. Menop & Repl 0.1-2 mg/wk in single or divided doses.

#### E. ESTROPIPATE (Piperazine Estrone Sulfate)

Estropipate — 0.625, 1.25, 2.5 & 5 mg tabs
Ogen — 0.625, 1.25, 2.5 mg tabs
Ortho-Est — 0.625 & 1.25 mg tabs

**DOSE:** Menop 0.625-5 mg po/d. Repl 1.25-7.5 mg po/d.

#### F. ESTERIFIED ESTROGENS

Estratab — 0.3, 0.625 & 2.5 mg tabs
Menest — 0.3, 0.625, 1.25 & 2.5 mg tabs

**DOSE:** As for conjugated estrogens.

#### G. ETHINYL ESTRADIOL

Estinyl — 0.02, 0.05, 0.5 mg tabs

**DOSE:** Menop 0.02-0.05 mg po/d. Dysfunctional uterine bleeding 0.05-0.1 mg po/d x 10 d. Breast Ca 1 mg tid. Prostate Ca 0.15-2 mg po/d..

#### H. MESTRANOL

Mestranol — (see below in Indications)

#### I. ESTRAMUSTINE PHOSPHATE SODIUM

Emcyt — 140 mg caps, contain 12.5 mg sodium

**DOSE:** Prostate Ca 280-420 mg po/d in 2-4 divided doses.

**INDICATIONS:** Premarin Intravenous is given IV or IM for Rx of abnormal uterine bleeding caused by hormonal imbalance. Estrace is micronized to prevent inactivation. The onset of action of estradiol cypionate and estradiol valerate is slow and erratic. Their duration of action is variable and may range from 3-4 d to 3-4 wk. Estropipate is piperazine estrone sulfate. Esterified estrogens are a combination of sodium salts of sulfated esters of estrogenic substances. Ethinyl estradiol is used in oral contraceptive pills. It undergoes an extensive first-pass metabolism; 5 µg of ethinyl estradiol may be equivalent to 0.625 mg of conjugated estrogens for menopausal replacement Rx. Mestranol is a constituent of certain oral contraceptive pills. Mestranol is the 3-methyl ether of ethinyl estradiol. It is demethylated in vivo to ethinyl estradiol. Estramustine phosphate sodium is nitrogen mustard linked to estradiol. It can produce a similar response to DES in the Rx of prostate Ca. Polyestradiol phosphate provides continuous levels of estradiol in inoperable prostate Ca. See Chapter 225 for general considerations regarding the Rx of prostate Ca.

### IV. TRANSDERMAL ESTROGENS
#### A. ESTROGEN (ESTRADIOL)

| | mg/24 h | | mg/24 h |
|---|---|---|---|
| Alora | 0.05, 0.075 & 0.1 | FemPatch | 0.025 |
| Climara | 0.05, 0.075 & 0.1 | Vivelle | 0.0375, 0.05, 0.075 & 0.1 |
| Esclim | 0.025, 0.0375, 0.05, 0.075 & 0.1 | Vivelle-Dot | 0.0375, 0.05, 0.075 & 0.1 |
| Estraderm | 0.05 & 0.1 | | |

**DOSE:** Apply to clean dry skin avoiding breasts and areas exposed to sunlight. Climara & Fempatch apply weekly. All others are applied twice a week. For menopausal symptoms initiate with the lowest dose necessary to control symptoms. Women without uterus can use continuously. Women with uterus should have combination progestin or use cyclically 3 wk on and 1 wk off. For prevention of postmenopausal bone loss initiate with 0.05 mg/d.

| **B. ESTROGEN/PROGESTERONE** | | mg/24 h (estradiol) | mg/24 h (norethindrone acetate) |
|---|---|---|---|
| | Combipatch | 0.05 | 0.14 |
| | | 0.05 | 0.25 |

**INDICATIONS:** For women with intact uterus for treatment of menopausal vascular symptoms and vulvar and vaginal atrophy.

**DOSE:** Apply to lower abdomen twice in a week. May be used continuously or in combination with estrogen only patch for 2 wk, combined patch for 2 wk.

| **V. VAGINAL ESTROGENS** | Cream: | | | | |
|---|---|---|---|---|---|
| | Estrace | 42.5 g (0.1 mg estradiol/g) | Estring | 2 mg estradiol in ring |
| | Ogen | 42.5 g (1.5 mg estropipate/g) | Vagifem | 25 μg tab |
| | Ortho Dienestrol | 78 g (0.1% dienestrol) | | (estradiol hemihydrate) |
| | Premarin | 42.5 g (0.625 conjugated estrogens/g) | | |

**INDICATIONS:** Atrophic vaginitis and Kraurosis vulvae.

**DOSE:** Use lowest dose that will control symptoms and disseminate as promptly as possible. Attempt to taper or discontinue at 3-6 month intervals. Estropipate and conjugated estrogens, 0.5-2 g/d should be administered cyclically (3 wk on & 1 wk off). Estradiol cream, 2-4 g/d and dienestrol, 1-2 applicators full, qd for 1-2 wk, then gradually reduce to half the dose for similar period. Maintenance dose of 1 g or 1 applicator full 1-3 x /wk. Estradiol ring is inserted into upper 1/3 of vaginal vault and should remain in place continuously for 3 months, after which time it should be removed and, if appropriate, replaced. Estradiol hemihydrate 1 tab vaginally once daily for 2 wk. Maintanance dose is 1 tab 2 x/wk.

| **VI. ESTROGEN & PROGESTE-RONE COMBINED** | Premphase | 0.625 mg conjugated estrogens d 1-14 | Prempro | 0.625 conjugated estrogen + |
|---|---|---|---|---|
| | | 0.625 conjugated estrogens + 5 mg | | 5 mg medroxyprogesterone |
| | | medroxyprogesterone acetate d 15-28 | | 0.625 conjugated estrogen + |
| | | | | 2.5 mg medroxyprogesterone |

**DOSE:** These products are dispensed in "EZ Dial" dispensers that organize the tablets into 28 d doses. Similar to oral contraceptives.

| **VII. ESTROGEN & ANDROGEN COMBINATIONS** | Oral: | |
|---|---|---|
| | Estratest H.S. | 0.625 mg esterified estrogen + 1.25 mg methyltestosterone |
| | Estratest | 1.25 mg esterified estrogen + 2.5 mg methyltestosterone |
| | Menogen H.S. | 0.625 mg esterified estrogens + 1.25 mg methyltestosterone |
| | Menogen | 1.25 mg esterified estrogens + 2.5 mg methyltestosterone |
| | Premarin with methyltestosterone | 0.625 mg conjugated equine estrogens + 5 mg methyltestosterone |
| | | 1.25 mg conjugated equine estrogens + 10 mg methyltestosterone |

**INDICATIONS:** Rx for severe vasomotor symptoms associated with menopause that are not responding to estrogen only. Do not use for depression or nervousness.

| **Drug** | **Trade Names and Preparations** | | | | | |
|---|---|---|---|---|---|---|
| **FLUORIDE** | | | | | | |
| | (tabs) | mg NaF/tab | (mg F/tab) | (tabs) | mg NaF/tab | (mg F/tab) |
| | Fluoride | 2.2 | (1) chewable tabs | Pharmaflur df | 2.2 | (1) |
| | | | and lozenges | Pharmaflur 1.1 | 1.1 | (0.5) |
| | Fluoride Loz | 2.2 | (1) tabs | Pharmaflur | 2.2 | (1) |
| | Fluoritab | 1.1 & 2.2 | (0.55 & 1) tabs | | | |
| | Flura | 2.2 | (1) tabs | | | |
| | Flura-Loz | 2.2 | (1) lozenges | (drops) | mg NaF/drop | (mg F/drop) |
| | Karidium | 2.2 | (1) lozenges | Fluoritab | 0.55 | (0.25) |
| | Luride | | | Flura-Drops | 0.55 | (0.25) |
| | Lozi-Tabs | 0.5, 1.1 & 2.2 | (0.25, 0.5 & 1) | Karidium | 0.275 | (0.125) |
| | | | chewable tabs | Luride | 1.1 | (0.5) |
| | Luride-SF | | | NaF | 0.275 | (0.125) |
| | Lozi-Tabs | 2.2 | (1) chewable tabs | Pediaflor | 1.1 | (0.5) |
| | NaF | 1.1 | (0.5) in regular & | Phos-Flur | 0.44 | (0.2) |
| | | 2.2 | (1) chewable tabs | | | |

**INDICATIONS:** Prevention of dental caries. Unlabeled use: Rx of established osteoporosis [see Chap. 64]. Sodium fluoride [NaF] increases trabecular bone mass and skeletal density. It is not clear if this leads to a reduction in fractures. In Rx of osteoporosis, calcium and vitamin D also should be given. Commercial products contain relatively small amounts of NaF; in osteoporosis, a large number of tabs must be taken daily. For dental use, many liquid preparations are available as po rinses.

**DOSE:** 1 mg/kg of NaF po/d for the Rx of established osteoporosis. Doses <50 mg/d may have fewer side effects.

**ACTIONS AND SIDE EFFECTS:** Do not use in renal insufficiency, since toxic levels may accumulate. Large doses may cause gastrointestinal symptoms, skeletal fluorosis (crippling skeletal fluorosis with bone fractures may be higher in areas with naturally high fluoride intake), and osteomalacia.

| Drug | Trade Names and Preparations |
|---|---|

## GLUCOCORTICOIDS

**INDICATIONS:** (1) Replacement Rx in adrenocortical deficiency states; (2) anti-inflammatory or immunosuppressive Rx; (3) other endocrine uses include congenital adrenal hyperplasia [see Chap. 77], granulomatous thyroiditis [see Chap. 46] and hypercalcemic states [see Chap. 59]. Unlabeled endocrine uses include Graves ophthalmopathy [start at 60 mg prednisone/d] and hirsutism [start dexamethasone at 0.5 mg/d]. (For a complete discussion of glucocorticoid Rx and relative potencies, see Chapter 78.)

--------------------------------------------------------------------------------

**DOSE:** Doses must be individualized. For replacement Rx, corticosteroids are given in physiologic doses. For anti-inflammatory or immunosuppressive Rx, corticosteroids are given in pharmacologic doses. Generally, the lowest possible dose that will provide the desired end result should be used to minimize adverse reactions.

--------------------------------------------------------------------------------

**ACTIONS AND SIDE EFFECTS:** Avoid Rx in fungal infection. Avoid live virus vaccines. Monitor for hypertension, hyperglycemia, infections, GI bleeding. Adrenal insufficiency may occur if doses omitted or stress is superimposed.

| | |
|---|---|
| **I. Betamethasone**<br>  **A. BETAMETHASONE** | Celestone      0.6 mg scored tabs; 0.6 mg/5 mL sorbitol-containing syrup in 120 mL (< 1% ethanol) |

**DOSE:** The replacement dosage is approx 0.6-0.75 mg/d po.

| | | |
|---|---|---|
| **B. BETAMETHASONE**<br>    **SODIUM PHOSPHATE** | Betamethasone sodium phosphate | 4 mg/mL in 5 mL vials |
| | Celestone phosphate | 4 mg/mL in 5 mL vials |
| | Cel-U-Jec | 4 mg/mL in 5 mL vials |
| | Selestoject | 4 mg/mL in 5 mL vials |

**DOSE:** Initial dosage may vary up to 9 mg/d for systemic (IV) and local uses.

| | | |
|---|---|---|
| **C. BETAMETHASONE**<br>    **SODIUM PHOSPHATE**<br>    **AND BETAMETHASONE**<br>    **ACETATE** | Celestone Soluspan | 3 mg betamethasone acetate plus 3 mg betamethasone sodium phosphate/mL in 5 mL vials. |

**DOSE:** Initial dosage is 0.5-9.0 mg/d. Not for IV use.

**INDICATIONS:** The biologic $t^1/_2$ of betamethasone is 36-54 h. May be used in the Rx of arthritis, bursitis, tenosynovitis and dermatologic conditions.

| | | |
|---|---|---|
| **II. CORTISONE** | Cortisone acetate | 5, 10 and 25 mg/white scored tab |
| | Cortone acetate | 25 mg/white scored tab; 50 mg/mL suspn for IM use |

**INDICATIONS:** (1) Replacement in chronic adrenal insufficiency; (2) congenital adrenal hyperplasia. (The biologic $t^1/_2$ of cortisone is 8-12 h. It is converted to cortisol readily.)

| | | |
|---|---|---|
| **III. Dexamethasone**<br>  **A. DEXAMETHASONE** | Dexamethasone | 0.25,0.5,0.75,1,1.5,2,4 & 6 mg tabs; 0.5 mg/5 mL elixir; 0.5 mg/5 mL po soln with sorbitol (no ethanol) |
| | Decadron | 0.5,0.75 & 4 mg tabs; 0.5 mg/5 mL elixir (5% ethanol) |
| | Dexameth | 0.5,0.75,1.5 & 4 mg tabs |
| | Dexamethasone<br>  Intensol | 0.5 mg/0.5 mL oral soln (30% ethanol) |
| | Dexone | 0.5,0.75,1.5 & 4 mg/tab |
| | Hexadrol | 1.5 & 4 mg/tab; 'Therapeutic Pack' containing six 1.5 mg & eight 0.75 mg tabs; 0.5 mg/5 mL elixir (5% ethanol) |

**INDICATIONS:** (1) Replacement or suppressive Rx; (2) dexamethasone suppression testing for the evaluation of Cushing syndrome [see Chaps. 74, 75, and 241]; (3) may be used to treat a patient in whom the Dx of adrenal insufficiency is strongly suspected while diagnostic ACTH stimulation testing is performed. In dosages up to 1-2 mg IV q 6 h, it will not interfere with assays for cortisol. (The biologic $t^1/_2$ of dexamethasone is 36-54 h.)

--------------------------------------------------------------------------------

**DOSE:** The replacement dosage of dexamethasone is approx 0.75-1 mg/d in the adult.

| | | | | |
|---|---|---|---|---|
| **B. DEXAMETHASONE**<br>    **ACETATE** | Dexamethasone acetate | Dalalone L.A. | Decaject-L.A. | Dexone LA |
| | Cortastat-LA | Decadron-L.A. | Dexasone-L.A. | Solurex LA |
| | (All the above products are available as a 8 mg/mL acetate suspn in 5 mL vials. Decadron-L.A. also is available in 1 mL vials.) | | | |
| | Dalalone D.P. | 16 mg/mL acetate suspn in 1 & 5 mL vials (not for intralesional use) | | |

**INDICATIONS:** For systemic, intralesional, intra-articular, or soft tissue uses. (Dexamethasone acetate is a long-acting preparation that is not for IV use.)

--------------------------------------------------------------------------------

**DOSE:** Not for IV use. 8-16 mg IM at 1-3 wk intervals for systemic use; 4-16 mg at 1-3 wk intervals for intra-articular or soft tissue use; 0.8-1.6 mg for intralesional use (except Dalalone D.P.).

| | | | | |
|---|---|---|---|---|
| **C. DEXAMETHASONE**<br>    **SODIUM PHOSPHATE** | Dexamethasone sodium phosphate | Decaject | | Dexone |
| | Cortastat | Dexacen-4 | | Hexadrol Phosphate |
| | Dalalone | Dexasone | | Solurex |
| | Decadron Phosphate | | | |
| | (All the above products are available as 4 mg/mL dexamethasome sodium phosphate soln for injection.) | | | |
| | Dexamethasone sodium phosphate | 10 mg/mL injection | | |
| | Hexadrol Phosphate | 10 & 20 mg/mL injection | | |
| | Decadron Phosphate | 24 mg/mL injection | | |

**INDICATIONS: (1)** May be used in Rx of cerebral edema and in the neurosurgical patient in the perioperative period in high doses. (2) May be used for intra-articular, intralesional, or soft tissue Rx. (Dexamethasone sodium phosphate also is available in 10 and 24 mg/mL soln [IV use only]; Hexadrol Phosphate in 10 and 20 mg/mL soln and disposable syringes; Decadron Phosphate in 24 mg/mL soln [IV use only].)

--------------------------------------------------------------------------------

**DOSE:** Dosage generally is 0.5-9 mg/d IV or IM. Daily dosages are about 1/3-1/2 of the po dose given q 12 h. An example of a regimen which may be used in the neurosurgical setting is 10 mg IV as an initial dose, followed by 4 mg IM q 6 h for several d. As soon as the patient's condition permits, switch to po dexamethasone, 1-3 mg q 8 h, and subsequently taper off over 5-7 d.

| D. DEXAMETHASONE SODIUM PHOSPHATE W/LIDOCAINE | Decadron W/Xylocaine | 4 mg dexamethasone sodium phosphate and 10 mg lidocaine HCl/mL soln in 5 mL vials |
|---|---|---|

**INDICATIONS:** Soft tissue injection, bursitis, tenosynovitis, intra-articular. (Prompt activity.)

----

**DOSE:** 0.1-0.75 mL depending on site to be injected.

| IV. Hydrocortisone (Cortisol) A. HYDROCORTISONE (Cortisol) | Hydrocortisone | 10 & 20 mg/tab |
|---|---|---|
| | Cortef | 5, 10 & 20 mg/white scored tab |
| | Hydrocortone | 10 & 20 mg/white scored tab |

**INDICATIONS:** Commonly used for replacement Rx in chronic adrenal insufficiency and for the Rx of congenital adrenal hyperplasia. Hydrocortisone is chemically identical to cortisol.

----

**DOSE:** Maintenance dosage of hydrocortisone in the adult is approx 20-30 mg po/d. In chronic adrenal insufficiency may be given as 20 mg in the am and 10 mg in the pm to simulate the normal adrenal secretory pattern. In congenital adrenal hyperplasia, the dose may be given as 10 mg in the am and 20 mg in the pm to provide maximal suppression of ACTH secretion. In children, the maintenance dosage is 25 $mg/m^2/d$ [also see Chap. 83]. The dosage of hydrocortisone IM injection usually is 1/3-1/2 the po dose q 12 h [see Chaps. 76 and 77].

| B. HYDROCORTISONE ACETATE | Hydrocortisone acetate | 25 & 50 mg/mL suspn |
|---|---|---|
| | Hydrocortone acetate | 25 & 50 mg/mL suspn |

**INDICATIONS:** Intralesional, intra-articular or soft tissue injection only. (Hydrocortisone acetate has a low solubility that provides a sustained duration of action.)

| C. HYDROCORTISONE SODIUM PHOSPHATE | Hydrocortone Phosphate | 50 mg/mL soln for injection in 2 & 10 mL vials; may be given IV, IM, or SC |
|---|---|---|
| D. HYDROCORTISONE SODIUM SUCCINATE | A-HydroCort | 100 & 250 mg/2 mL vial; 500 mg/4 mL vial; 1000 mg/8 mL vial (IV or IM) |
| | Solu-Cortef | 100 & 250 mg/2 mL vial; 500 mg/4 mL vial; 1000 mg/8 mL vial (IV or IM) |

**INDICATIONS:** Hydrocortisone sodium succinate is a water soluble salt that has a rapid onset of action. It is commonly the preparation of choice when stress doses of corticosteroids are to be administered IV or IM.

----

**DOSE:** The dosage for injection usually is 1/3-1/2 the po dose q 12 h. In acute adrenal insufficiency, dosages up to 100 mg may be given q 8 h IV or IM. In the perioperative period, 50 mg IV may be given on-call to the operating room, followed by 50 mg q 8 h for first 24 h after surgery. Tapering then is carried out as rapidly as possible, depending on the underlying disease process and the patient's general condition.

| V. Methylprednisolone A. METHYLPREDNISOLONE | Methylprednisolone | 4 & 16 mg/tab |
|---|---|---|
| | Medrol | 2, 4, 8, 16, 24 (with tartrazine) & 32 mg/scored tab |

**INDICATIONS:** The biologic $t^{1}/_{2}$ of methylprednisolone is 18-36 h. Medrol Dosepak, 4 mg tabs [containing 21 tabs], is available for a short, 6 d course of tapering dosage. Also available as a generic.

----

**DOSE:** The maintenance dosage of methylprednisolone is approx 4 mg po/d in the adult.

| B. METHYLPREDNISOLONE ACETATE | (suspn) | mg/mL | (suspn) | mg/mL | (suspn) | mg/mL |
|---|---|---|---|---|---|---|
| | Methylprednisolone acetate | 20, 40 & 80 | Depo-Medrol | 20, 40 & 80 | Duralone-80 | 80 |
| | | | Depoject | 40 & 80 | Medralone 40 | 40 |
| | Adlone | 40 & 80 | Depopred-40 | 40 | Medralone 80 | 80 |
| | depMedalone 40 | 40 | Depropred-80 | 80 | M-Prednisol-40 | 40 |
| | depMedalone 80 | 80 | Duralone-40 | 40 | M-Prednisol-80 | 80 |

**INDICATIONS:** For IM, intra-articular and intralesional injections. Not for IV use. May be used as weekly IM injections for prolonged effect. (The low solubility results in a sustained effect.)

| C. METHYLPREDNISOLONE SODIUM SUCCINATE | Methylprednisolone sodium succinate | 40, 125, 500 & 1000 mg vials for use by IV or IM injection |
|---|---|---|
| | A-methapred | 40, 125, 500 & 1000 mg vials for use by IV or IM injection |
| | Solu-Medrol | 40, 125, 500, 1000 & 2000 mg vials for use by IV or IM injection |

**INDICATIONS:** Methylprednisolone sodium succinate has a high solubility, which provides a rapid onset of action when given IV or IM.

----

**DOSE:** See Chapter 78 for considerations in dosing, including use in the perioperative period and in acute bronchospasm.

| VI. Prednisolone A. PREDNISOLONE | Prednisolone | 5 mg/tab & 15 mg/5 mL syrup | Delta-Cortef | 5 mg/tab | Prelone | 5 & 15 mg/5 mL syrup |
|---|---|---|---|---|---|---|

**INDICATIONS:** (1) Replacement Rx in secondary adrenal insufficiency or salt-retaining forms of congenital adrenal hyperplasia; (2) with a mineralocorticoid in replacement Rx for primary adrenal insufficiency or salt-wasting forms of congenital adrenal hyperplasia. Prednisolone is a Δ-1 analog of hydrocortisone. Its biologic $t^{1}/_{2}$ is 18-36 h.

----

**DOSE:** The maintenance dosage of prednisolone is approximately 5 mg/d in the adult.

| B. PREDNISOLONE ACETATE | (suspn) | mg/mL | (suspn) | mg/mL | (suspn) | mg/mL |
|---|---|---|---|---|---|---|
| | Prednisolone acetate | 25 & 50 | Key-Pred 50 | 50 | Predcor-50 | 50 |
| | Key-Pred 25 | 25 | Predalone 50 | 50 | | |

**INDICATIONS:** Intralesional, IM, intra-articular, or soft tissue injection only. Not for IV use.

| C. PREDNISOLONE SODIUM PHOSPHATE | Soln for injection: | mg/mL | Oral liquid: | mg/mL |
|---|---|---|---|---|
| | Hydeltrasol | 20 | Pediapred | 1 |
| | Key-Pred-SP | 20 | | (5 mg/tsp) |

**INDICATIONS:** Oral liquid is used in pediatrics for endocrine, anti-inflammatory, and antiallergic purposes. Injection is water soluble; rapid action and short duration. For intra-articular, intralesional, soft tissue injection, IM or IV use.

| D. PREDNISOLONE TEBUTATE | (suspn) | mg/mL | (suspn) | mg/mL |
|---|---|---|---|---|
| | Prednisolone tebutate | 20 | Prednisol TBA | 20 |

**INDICATIONS:** For intrabursal, intra-articular, or IM use. The combined acetate and sodium phosphate salts of prednisolone allow for a rapid onset and a prolonged activity.

## VII. PREDNISONE

| (tabs) | mg/tab | (tabs) | mg/tab | (oral soln) | mg/5 mL |
|--------|--------|--------|--------|-------------|---------|
| Prednisone | 1, 5, 10, 20 & 50 | Panasol-S | 1 | Liquid Pred (syrup) | 5 |
| Deltasone | 2.5, 5, 10, 20 & 50 | Prednicen-M | 5 | Prednisone Intensol | |
| Meticorten | 1 | Sterapred DS | 10 | Concentrate (30% ethanol) | 5 |
| Orasone | 1, 5, 10, 20 & 50 | | | | |

**INDICATIONS:** Indications for prednisone are the same as those for prednisolone. It also commonly is used in anti-inflammatory, or immunosuppressive Rx. Prednisone is a Δ-1 analog of cortisone. It is converted in the liver to prednisolone, the active compound. Conversion may be impaired in subjects with liver disease. The biologic $t^1/_2$ of prednisone is 18-36 h.

------------------------------------------------

**DOSE:** Maintenance dose of prednisone and of prednisolone is approx 5-7.5 mg/d in the adult.

## VIII. Triamcinolone
### A. TRIAMCINOLONE

| (tabs) | mg/tab | (tabs) | mg/tab | (syrup) | mg/5 mL |
|--------|--------|--------|--------|---------|---------|
| Triamcinolone | 4 | Atolone | 4 | Kenacort | 4 |
| Aristocort | 4 & 8 | Kenacort | 4 & 8 | (with tartrazine) | |

**INDICATIONS:** The biologic $t^1/_2$ of triamcinolone is 18-36 h.

------------------------------------------------

**DOSE:** Maintenance dosage in the adult is approximately 4 mg/d.

### B. TRIAMCINOLONE ACETONIDE

| (suspn) | mg/mL | (suspn) | mg/mL | (suspn) | mg/mL |
|---------|-------|---------|-------|---------|-------|
| Triamcinolone acetonide | 40 | Tac-3 | 3 | Triamonide 40 | 40 |
| Kenaject-40 | 40 | Tac-40 | 40 | Tri-Kort | 40 |
| Kenalog-10 | 10 | Triam-A | 40 | Trilog | 40 |
| Kenalog-40 | 40 | | | | |

**INDICATIONS:** Triamcinolone acetonide has an extended duration of action that may persist for several wk.

------------------------------------------------

**DOSE:** Triamcinolone acetonide is given by IM, intra-articular, intrasynovial, and intralesional routes only. Not for IV use.

### C. TRIAMCINOLONE DIACETATE

| (suspn) | mg/mL | (suspn) | mg/mL | (suspn) | mg/mL |
|---------|-------|---------|-------|---------|-------|
| Triamcinolone | 40 | Aristocort Forte | 40 | Triamolone 40 | 40 |
| Amcort | 40 | Clinacort | 40 | Trilone | 40 |
| Aristocort Intralesional | 25 | Triam Forte | 40 | Tristoject | 40 |

**INDICATIONS:** For IM, intralesional and intra-articular use. Not for IV use. (Prompt onset of action and longer duration of effect. IM dose has been given once weekly.)

### D. TRIAMCINOLONE HEXACETONIDE

| (suspn) | mg/mL | (suspn) | mg/mL | (suspn) | mg/mL |
|---------|-------|---------|-------|---------|-------|
| Aristospan Intralesional | 5 | Aristospan Intra-articular | 20 | | |

**INDICATIONS:** Triamcinolone hexacetonide has a prolonged duration of action.

------------------------------------------------

**DOSE:** Triamcinolone hexacetonide is given by the intra-articular and intralesional routes. Not for IV use.

---

| Drug | Trade Names and Preparations |
|------|------------------------------|

## GONADOTROPIN RELEASING HORMONE (GnRH)

| **I. GONADORELIN HCl** | Factrel | 100 & 500 µg/vial |
|------------------------|---------|-------------------|

**INDICATIONS:** (1) Evaluation of anterior pituitary gonadotropic functional capacity [see Chap. 241]; (2) assessment of residual anterior pituitary gonadotropic function in the presence of a pituitary tumor or lesion or following surgical or radiation Rx [see Chap. 241]. Unlabeled use: (1) induction of ovulation; (2) treatment of precocious puberty; (3) treatment of hypothalamic amenorrhea [see Chap. 97].

------------------------------------------------

**DOSE:** In induction of ovulation, GnRH is delivered in a pulsatile fashion, with pulse frequencies from 60-120 min, in doses from 10-25 µg/pulse if delivered SC by infusion pump or 1-5 µg/pulse if delivered IV [see Chap. 97]. For gonadotropin testing: 100 µg SC or IV.

------------------------------------------------

**ACTIONS AND SIDE EFFECTS:** Gonadorelin is a synthetic preparation of luteinizing hormone releasing hormone [LHRH]/gonadotropin releasing hormone [GnRH] which is identical in structure to the naturally occurring hormone. The GnRH stimulation test should not be performed in patients taking androgens, estrogens, progestins, or glucocorticoids because these drugs directly affect pituitary secretion of gonadotropins. Phenothiazines, dopamine antagonists, spironolactone, levodopa, and digoxin also should be avoided. Side effects of gonadorelin include: headache, nausea, lightheadedness, abdominal discomfort, and flushing.

| **II. GONADORELIN ACETATE** | Lutrepulse | 0.8 & 3.2 mg powder |
|-----------------------------|------------|---------------------|

**INDICATIONS:** Rx of primary hypothalamic amenorrhea.

------------------------------------------------

**DOSE:** Infusion 3-5 µg q 60-90 min via Lutrepulse pump.

------------------------------------------------

**ACTIONS AND SIDE EFFECTS:** Local effects at site of infusion and ovarian hyperstimulation.

---

| Drug | Trade Names and Preparations |
|------|------------------------------|

## GONADOTROPIN RELEASING HORMONE-AGONISTS (GnRH-A/LHRH-A)

| **I. GOSERELIN ACETATE** | Zoladex | 3.6 & 10.8 mg implant in preloaded syringes |
|--------------------------|---------|----------------------------------------------|

**INDICATIONS:** Palliative treatment of advanced carcinoma of the prostate and endometriosis.

------------------------------------------------

**DOSE:** 3.6 mg SC q 28 d for prostatic Ca. Rx for 6 mo in cases of endometriosis. Alternatively, 10.8 mg SC q 28 d for 3 mo.

------------------------------------------------

**ACTIONS AND SIDE EFFECTS:** Synthetic decapeptide analog of GnRH with similar action and precautions as other GnRH agonists. When used in Rx of prostate Ca, side effects include a flare of bone pain in the first 4-10 d, which may be attenuated by the prior and concomitant use of flutamide. May be dangerous in patients with spinal cord impingement by tumor. Side effects otherwise appear to be minor.

| II. HISTRELIN ACETATE | Supprelin | 120 µg/0.6 mL, 300 µg/0.6 mL & 600 µg/0.6 mL for injection |
|---|---|---|

**INDICATIONS:** Rx of central precocious puberty.

**DOSE:** 10 µg/kg SC qd.

**ACTIONS AND SIDE EFFECTS:** Hypersensitivity, vasodilation, and headaches.

| III. LEUPROLIDE ACETATE | Lupron | 5 mg/mL soln for injection in 2.8 mL multiple-dose vials |
|---|---|---|
| | Lupron Depot | 3.75 & 7.5 mg powder for injection in a single-dose vial |
| | Lupron Depot-Ped | 7.5, 11.25 & 15 mg powder in a single dose kit |

**INDICATIONS:** (1) Palliative Rx of symptomatic, metastatic prostate Ca [see Chap. 225]; (2) treatment of gonadotropin-dependent precocious puberty [see Chaps. 16, 21 and 92]; (3) endometriosis; and (4) central precocious puberty. Unlabeled uses: (1) breast, ovarian, endometrial Ca, leiomyoma uteri; (2) infertility; and (3) prostatic hyperplasia.

**DOSE:** Usually effective as a single qd SC injection. In the Rx of prostate Ca, Lupron is given in a dose of 1 mg SC qd. Lupron Depot is given IM in a dosage of 7.5 mg q mo.

**ACTIONS AND SIDE EFFECTS:** GnRH superagonists have a greater potency and longer duration of action than naturally occurring GnRH. Initial doses cause an increase in serum LH, FSH, estrogen, and androgen levels. Administration for >2-4 wk causes down-regulation of pituitary gonadotropin receptors and a fall in androgens in males to castrate levels and of estrogens in premenopausal females to postmenopausal levels. Side effects when used in Rx of prostate Ca include a flare of bone pain in the first 4-10 d, which may be attenuated by the prior and concomitant use of flutamide. May be dangerous in patients with spinal cord impingement by tumor. Side effects otherwise appear to be of a minor nature.

| IV. NAFARELIN ACETATE | Synarel | 2 mg/mL nasal soln (one spray = 200 µg) |
|---|---|---|

**INDICATIONS:** Rx of endometriosis and central precocious puberty.

**DOSE:** Dosage for endometriosis is 400 µg/d. Dosage for central precocious puberty is 1600 µg/d up to 1800 µg/d.

**ACTIONS AND SIDE EFFECTS:** Rhinitis and hypoestrogenemia.

| Drug | Trade Names and Preparations |
|---|---|

## GONADOTROPIN RELEASING HORMONE-ANTAGONIST

| GANIRELIX ACETATE | Antagon | 250 µg/5 mL prefilled syringe |
|---|---|---|

**INDICATIONS:** Inhibition of premature LH surges during controlled ovarian hyperstimulation.

**DOSE:** 0.25 mg daily SC.

**ACTIONS AND SIDE EFFECTS:** Synthetic decapeptide generated by amino acid substitution of native GnRH. Competitively blocks GnRH receptors. Pregnancy must be excluded. Should not be used in patients with hypersensitivity to GnRH.

| Drug | Trade Names and Preparations |
|---|---|

## GONADOTROPINS

| I. CHORIONIC GONADOTROPIN, HUMAN (hCG) | Chorionic gonadotropin | 5-10-20,000 U.S.P. units with 10 mL diluent, for IM use only |
|---|---|---|
| | A.P.L. | 5-10-20,000 U.S.P. units with 10 mL diluent, for IM use only |
| | Chorex-5 & 10 | 5-10,000 U.S.P. units with 10 & 25 mL diluent, for IM use only |
| | Choron 10 | 10,000 U.S.P. units with 10 mL diluent, for IM use only |
| | Gonic | 10,000 U.S.P. units with 10 mL diluent, for IM use only |
| | Pregnyl | 10,000 U.S.P. units with 10 mL diluent, for IM use only |
| | Profasi | 5-10,000 U.S.P. units with 10 mL diluent, for IM use only |

**INDICATIONS:** Rx of infertility: (1) In females: (a) in the induction of ovulation in combination with menotropins; (b) for Rx of luteal phase defect; (2) in males (a) in selected cases of hypogonadotropic hypogonadism; (b) prepubertal cryptorchidism not due to anatomical obstruction.

**DOSE:** See Chapter 97 for protocol for ovulation induction. One regimen for Rx of male hypogonadotropic infertility is 2000 IU of hCG IM 2-3 x/wk. After 18-24 mo, hMG may be added.

**ACTIONS AND SIDE EFFECTS:** hCG is a placental hormone extracted from the urine of pregnant women. Biologically, hCG mimics the action of LH. Headaches, irritability, gynecomastia, and precocious puberty.

| II. FOLLITROPINS | | |
|---|---|---|
| A. FOLLINOTROPIN ALPHA | Gonal-F | 75 & 150 IU |
| B. FOLLINOTROPIN BETA | Follistim | 75 IU |
| C. UROFOLLINOTROPIN | Fertinex | 75 & 150 IU/mL |

**INDICATIONS:** (1) Ovulation induction in anovulatory infertile women; (2) Follicle stimulation in ovulatory women undergoing "Assisted Reproductive Technologies."

**DOSE:** See protocol for ovulation induction.

**ACTIONS AND SIDE EFFECTS:** Urofollinotropin is highly purified FSH extracted from the urine of postmenopausal women. Follinotropin alfa and beta are human FSH preparations of recombinant DNA origin. Follinotropins stimulate ovarian follicular growth. Treatment with hCG may be needed in the absence of an endogenous LH surge. Ovarian hyperstimulation syndrome, multiple pregnancies, ovarian enlargement, thromboembolic events, and acute respiratory distress syndrome.

| III. MENOTROPINS (hMG) | Pergonal | 75 IU each of FSH and LH activity per 2 mL amp of hMG |
| | | 150 IU each of FSH and LH activity per 2 mL amp of hMG |

**INDICATIONS:** (1) Induction of ovulation in selected patients who do not respond to clomiphene, or do not produce endogenous gonadotropins; (2) with hCG in Rx of hypogonadotropic or idiopathic male infertility when no response to clomiphene.

-------------------------------------------------------------------------------------------------------------------------

**DOSE:** See Chapter 97 for protocol for ovulation induction using hMG-hCG. In male infertility, the dosage of hMG is 25-75 IU 3 x/wk with hCG injections 2 x/wk.

-------------------------------------------------------------------------------------------------------------------------

**ACTIONS AND SIDE EFFECTS:** hMG is a preparation of human menopausal gonadotropins extracted from the urine of postmenopausal women. Side effects include hyperstimulation syndrome and gynecomastia.

| Drug | Trade Names and Preparations |
|------|------------------------------|

## GROWTH HORMONE (GH)

| SOMATROPIN | Genotropin | 1.5, 5.8 & 13.8 mg/mL (5 & 12 mg cartridge may be used with pen). |
| | Humatrope | 5 mg (~ 13 IU) per vial |
| | Norditropin | 4 & 8 mg per vial (also available in cartridge for the Nordipen) |
| | Nutropin | 5 & 10 mg (~ 13 & 26 IU) per vial |
| | Nutropin AQ | 10 mg (~30 IU) |
| | Saizen | 5 mg per vial |
| | Serostim | 5,6 mg per vial |
| **SOMATREM** | Protropin | 5 & 10 mg (~ 13 & 26 IU) per vial |

**INDICATIONS:** (1) Rx of pediatric GH deficiency (GHD); (2) adult GHD; (3) pediatric chronic renal insufficiency; (4) Turner syndrome; (5) cachexia treatment of AIDS. Somatropin and somatrem are synthetic preparations of GH. Somatropin is identical to human pituitary GH, while somatrem has an additional methionine.

-------------------------------------------------------------------------------------------------------------------------

**DOSE:** General guidelines for indication #1 are 0.18-0.3 mg/kg total weekly dose divided into 3-7 injections/wk SC or IM. For indication #2, 0.375 mg/kg total weekly dose divided into 3-7 injections/wk SC or IM. For indication #3, 0.35 mg/kg total weekly dose divided into qd SC injections. (In hemodialysis, administer hs or 3-4 h post dialysis. With chronic cycling peritoneal dialysis give q morning. In chronic ambulatory dialysis, give q hs.) For indication #4, 0.002-0.006 mg/kg (Nutropin AQ only) SC qd. Starting dose is titrated q 6 wk to maximum of 0.0125 mg/kg/d. For indication #5, 0.1 mg/kg (Serostim only) SC hs.

-------------------------------------------------------------------------------------------------------------------------

**ACTIONS AND SIDE EFFECTS:** In children: injection site reactions, lipoatrophy, headache, hematuria, hypothyroidism, mild hyperglycemia. A small number of patients may develop antibodies to protein that may interfere with growth response. Relationship between leukemia and GH Rx is uncertain. Benign intracranial hypertension may occur soon after initiation of Rx. A dose reduction or discontinuation resolves signs and symptoms. Contraindicated with any evidence of neoplastic activity. Discontinue if any evidence of tumor growth. Do not use with fused epiphyses. Concomitant glucocorticoid Rx may inhibit the growth promoting effects of GH. Baseline and periodic thyroid function studies, fundoscopic exams, and bone age should be monitored. Patients should be observed for glucose intolerance. Use with caution in patients with diabetes. Patients with endocrine disorders have a higher incidence of slipped capital femoral epiphyses. Patients with chronic renal insufficiency should have baseline X-rays of the hip to monitor for renal osteodystrophy and avascular necrosis of the femoral head. Patients with Turner syndrome should be evaluated carefully for otitis media and other ear disorders while on GH Rx.
In adults: Patients with childhood GHD should be reevaluated before replacement with GH. Patients should be monitored with IGF-I levels q 6 wk while titrating dose. Side effects include edema, arthralgias, carpal tunnel syndrome, rarely malignant transformation of nevi, gynecomastia, and pancreatitis.

| Drug | Trade Names and Preparations |
|------|------------------------------|

## GROWTH HORMONE RELEASING HORMONE (GHRH)

| I. SERMORELIN ACETATE | Geref | 0.5 & 1 mg per vial | Geref Diagnostic | 50 µg per vial |

**INDICATIONS:** (1) Treatment of idiopathic GH deficiency (GHD) in children with growth failure; (2) Dx aid for GHD.

-------------------------------------------------------------------------------------------------------------------------

**DOSE:** For Dx GH testing: 1 µg/kg IV. For Rx, 30 µg/kg SC/d hs. All children should be prepubescent. Geref Dx test should be performed in all children. Those who do not achieve a peak GH level > 2 ng/mL should be excluded from receiving Geref Rx. Treatment response is best when initiated at a bone age ≤ 7.5 years for females and ≤ 8 years for males. Relative GH response to stimulation is not predictive of growth response. Height shoud be assessed at least q 6 months. Treatment should be discontinued when the epiphyses are fused. Patients who fail to respond should be reevaluated, and a change to Rx with GH should be considered. Baseline & periodic thyroid function and bone age should be monitored. Concomitant glucocorticoid Rx may inhibit growth promoting effects.

-------------------------------------------------------------------------------------------------------------------------

**ACTIONS AND SIDE EFFECTS:** Sermorelin is the acetate salt of an amidated synthetic 29 amino acid peptide (GHRH$_{1-29}$) that corresponds to the amino terminal segment of human GHRH, which is composed of 44 amino acids. It is the shortest fragment of GHRH known to possess full bioactivity. Brief local injection reactions, rarely headache and flushing, dysphagia, dizziness, hyperactivity, somnolence, and urticaria. Side effects with Dx use include flushing, injection site pain, redness and/or swelling, nausea, headache, vomiting, dysgeusia, pallor, and chest tightness.

| Drug | Trade Names and Preparations |
|------|------------------------------|

## HYPERGLYCEMIC AGENTS

| I. DIAZOXIDE | | |
| A. Oral Preparation | Proglycem | 50 mg/cap; 50 mg/mL oral suspn |

2159

**DOSE:** Dosage must be individualized. Adults and children: 3-8 mg/kg/d in 2-3 equal doses q 8-12 h. Infants and neonates: 8-15 mg/kg/d in 2-3 equal doses q 8-12 h.

| B. Parenteral Preparation | Hyperstat IV | 300 mg in 20 mL amp |
| | Diazoxide Injection | 15 mg/mL vial in 10 mL or 20 mL vials |

**DOSE:** Adults: 1-3 mg/kg (up to 150 mg) as a bolus into a peripheral vein. May be repeated at 5 to 15 min intervals.

**INDICATIONS:** (1) Hypoglycemia caused by hyperinsulinism; (2) hypertensive crisis. Oral preparations may be used for persistent hypoglycemia caused by hyperinsulinism in adults with islet cell neoplasia and in infants and children with leucine sensitivity, islet cell hyperplasia, nesidioblastosis, and islet cell neoplasms. Parenteral preparations may be used for the emergency lowering of blood pressure. Insulin or tolbutamide will reverse the hyperglycemic effects. When given po, onset of action is <1 h and duration of action is <8 h. Reduces blood pressure by causing relaxation of smooth muscle in arterioles. When given IV, a response is seen within 5 min. Duration of effect usually is <12 h. Not the agent of first choice for hypertensive crisis.

**DOSE:** Dosage must be individualized. Adults and children: 3-8 mg/kg/d in 2-3 equal doses q 8-12 h. Infants and neonates: 8-15 mg/kg/d in 2-3 equal doses q 8-12 h.

**ACTIONS AND SIDE EFFECTS:** Diazoxide is related to thiazide diuretics. Diazoxide raises blood glucose by inhibition of insulin release and by an extrapancreatic effect. May cause fluid retention by decreasing excretion of sodium and water. Other side effects include gastrointestinal disturbances; acute pancreatitis; thrombocytopenia; leukopenia; rise in serum uric acid, AST, alkaline phosphatase, and BUN levels; fall in creatinine clearance; nephrotic syndrome; hematuria; extrapyramidal signs; hirsutism; skin rashes; galactorrhea; and advance in bone age. Moreover, parenteral preparation also may cause severe hypotension and cerebral and myocardial ischemia. Blood glucose levels must be monitored closely during Rx to avoid hyperglycemia. Blood pressure must be monitored closely to avoid hypotension.

| II. GLUCAGON | Glucagon | Glucagon 'Emergency Kit' for Low Blood Sugar. |
| | | Glucagon Diagnostic Kit. |
| | | Lyophilized for injection in 1 mg vials with 1 mL of diluent. |

**INDICATIONS:** Emergency Rx of severe hypoglycemia. Diagnostic aid in radiologic examination of gastrointestinal tract when diminished intestinal motility would be advantageous. Unlabeled uses include Rx of (a) propranolol overdose, (b) cardiovascular emergencies, and (c) food impaction of the esophagus, and (d) Dx aid for insulinoma and pheochromocytoma [see Chap. 241], and for differentiation of type 1 and type 2 diabetes mellitus using C-peptide measurements. Glucagon will not raise glucose levels if glycogen stores are depleted. Once a patient who has been unconscious because of hypoglycemia has been aroused, food should be given by mouth to prevent recurrence.

**DOSE:** For hypoglycemia, 0.5-1.0 mg of glucagon SC, IM, or IV. Dosage may be repeated at 15-20 min intervals for 2 or 3 doses, if no response is obtained.

**ACTIONS AND SIDE EFFECTS:** Side effects include nausea, vomiting, and allergy.

| III. GLUCOSE | | |
| A. ORAL PREPARATIONS OF D-GLUCOSE | Glutose | 80 g bottle gel & 25 g tube (no dye) |
| | Insta-Glucose | 30.8 g tubes gel (cherry) |
| | Insulin Reaction | 25 g tubes gel (lime) |
| | B-D Glucose | 5 g chewable tabs |

**INDICATIONS:** Rx of hypoglycemia. (Glucose provides 4 Cal/g. It must be swallowed to be absorbed. Response should begin about 10 min after glucose ingestion. Glucose is not absorbed from the buccal cavity.)

**DOSE:** 10-20 g po. The dosage may be repeated in 10 min if necessary.

**ACTIONS AND SIDE EFFECTS:** Oral preparations should not be given to an unconscious patient, since this may lead to aspiration.

| B. PARENTERAL PREPARATIONS OF DEXTROSE IN WATER (D-%-W) | | mL | | mL |
|---|---|---|---|---|
| | D-2.5-W | 1000 | D-30-W | 500 & 1000 |
| | D-5-W | 10, 25, 50, 100, 150, 250, 500 & 1000 | D-40-W | 500 & 1000 |
| | D-10-W | 3, 250, 500 & 1000 | D-50-W | 50, 500, 1000 & 2000 |
| | D-20-W | 500 & 1000 | D-60-W | 500 & 1000 |
| | D-25-W | 10 | D-70-W | 70, 1000 & 2000 |

**INDICATIONS:** A constant infusion of a D-5-containing soln should be given to any patient who is being treated with an insulin drip or to any insulin-dependent diabetic who is not eating, to avoid hypoglycemia. Also may be used in Rx of hypoglycemia from other causes. Hypertonic dextrose solutions (D-10-W to D-70-W) most commonly are used in admixtures for total parenteral nutrition Rx (TPN). If hyperglycemia is induced during administration of these soln for TPN, insulin may be mixed into the soln directly. Hypertonic soln should be given into central veins to avoid irritation. Constant infusion of D-10-W may be used to maintain a euglycemic state in patients with prolonged episodes of hypoglycemia. D-50-W is used in the emergency Rx of insulin-induced hypoglycemia when the patient is too obtunded or confused to be treated po. In the adult, the usual dose for the treatment of insulin-induced hypoglycemia is one 50 mL amp of D-50-W IV. This may be repeated if no response is obtained. Once a patient who has been unconscious because of hypoglycemia has been aroused, food should be given by mouth to prevent recurrent hypoglycemia.

**DOSE:** Dosage and rate of administration of IV soln must be titrated to blood glucose levels in the individual patient.

**ACTIONS AND SIDE EFFECTS:** Local effects at site of injection with febrile response and phlebitis. The serum potassium level should be monitored while dextrose-containing IV soln is being administered, to avoid hypokalemia.

| IV. STREPTOZOCIN | Zanosar | 100 mg/mL in 1 g vials |

**INDICATIONS:** The management of metastatic islet cell tumors including insulin and noninsulin-secreting B cell and non-B cell neoplasms and malignant carcinoid tumors [see Chap. 220]. Streptozocin is a nitrosourea that is taken up by pancreatic islet cells. It is used as a chemotherapeutic agent in Rx of malignant islet cell tumors.

**DOSE:** 1-1.5 g/m$^2$/wk or 500 mg/m$^2$ IV qd for 5 d q 6 wk.

**ACTIONS AND SIDE EFFECTS:** Dose-related nephrotoxicity is the major side effect of streptozocin. Other side effects include nausea, vomiting, hepatotoxicity, fever, and eosinophilia.

| Drug | Trade Names and Preparations |
|---|---|

## INSULIN

**INDICATIONS:** (1) Type 1 diabetes mellitus; (2) type 2 diabetes mellitus that cannot be controlled by diet and exercise alone; (3) diabetes in pregnancy; (4) emergency Rx of hyperkalemia given with glucose. Purified pork or human insulins should be used preferentially in the following settings: (a) intermittent insulin Rx [e.g., gestational diabetes mellitus, perioperative management of hyperglycemia in noninsulin-requiring type 2 diabetics]; (b) immunologic insulin resistance; (c) lipodystrophy at injection sites; (5) they may also be used in any newly diagnosed diabetic or any patient in whom control is less than optimal with other preparations. Humalog, Humulin R and Velosulin BR insulins are used in insulin pumps.

---

**COMMENTS:** Insulin preparations generally are divided into four classes based on their action profiles following SC administration: rapid, short, intermediate, and long-acting [see Chap. 143]. Dose must be individualized. Onset, peak, and duration of activity vary considerably according to site and depth of injection and interindividual differences. All patients being treated with insulin should be warned of the signs and symptoms of hypoglycemia and hyperglycemia. All insulins come in 10 mL vials. Several insulins also come in cartridges for use in insulin pen delivery systems. NovoNordisk manufactures 1.5 & 3.0 mL cartridges containing Regular, NPH, or 70/30 U100 insulin. Lilly manufactures 1.5 mL cartridges containing Humalog, NPH, 70/30, or Humalog 75/25 U100 insulin. Pen delivery systems may offer increased portability and the ease of "dialing in" an insulin dose.

Insulin sources in the table following are abbreviated as follows: H = human; P = pork; B = beef; rDNA = recombinant DNA technology (y = yeast; b = bacteria); enz. m-p = enzymatically modified pork insulin.

---

**DOSE:** See Chapter 143.

---

**ACTIONS AND SIDE EFFECTS:** Hypoglycemia; hypokalemia (see Chap. 143). Follow $K^+$ closely when using IV insulin infusions. May cause systemic allergy (see Chap. 143), lipodystrophy, or lipohypertrophy.

---

| I. Rapid-Acting<br>**LISPRO** | Humalog | H rDNA analog (b) | | |
|---|---|---|---|---|

**COMMENTS:** Modified by reversal of amino acids at positions 28 & 29 of the insulin B-chain. (Aspart [B28] is another rapid acting H rDNA analog.)

---

| II. Short-Acting<br>**A. REGULAR**<br>**(Insulin Injection)** | Humulin-R<br>Regular Iletin II<br>Novolin R | H rDNA (b)<br>P<br>H rDNA (y) | Regular Purified Pork Insulin<br>Velosulin Human BR | P<br>H enz. m-p |
|---|---|---|---|---|

**DOSE:** See Chapter 143.

| **B. U-500** | Regular (Concentrated) Iletin II | H rDNA(b) | | |
|---|---|---|---|---|

**INDICATIONS:** For Rx in diabetics with marked insulin resistance for administration of large doses in a reasonable volume. Concentration is 500 units/mL.

---

**DOSE:** See Chapter 143.

---

| III. Intermediate-Acting<br>**A. LENTE**<br>**(Insulin Zinc Suspension)** | Humulin L<br>Lente Iletin I | H rDNA (b)<br>B & P | Novolin L<br>Lente Iletin II | H rDNA (y)<br>Purified P |
|---|---|---|---|---|
| **B. NPH**<br>**(Isophane Insulin Suspn)** | Humulin N<br>NPH Iletin II | H rDNA (b)<br>P | Novolin N | H rDNA (y) |

**DOSE:** See Chapter 143.

---

| IV. Mixtures of Short- and<br>Intermediate-Acting<br>**(Isophane Insulin Suspn and**<br>**Insulin Injection)** | Humulin 70/30<br>Humulin 50/50 | H rDNA (b)<br>H rDNA (b) | Humalog 75/25<br>Novolin 70/30 | H rDNA<br>H rDNA (y) |
|---|---|---|---|---|

**INDICATIONS:** Fixed ratio mixtures of 70% NPH & 30% Regular, 50% NPH & 50% Regular, or 75% lisproprotamine and 25% lispro. Useful in patients for whom the addition of short-acting insulin would be beneficial, and for whom mixing by the patient is not feasible or not desirable.

---

**DOSE:** See Chapter 143.

---

| V. Long-Acting<br>**ULTRALENTE**<br>**(Insulin Zinc Suspn, Extended)** | Humulin U Ultralente | H rDNA (b) | Glargine | H rDNA |
|---|---|---|---|---|
| **DOSE:** See Chapter 143. | | | | |

<br>

| Drug | Trade Names and Preparations |
|---|---|

## LIPID-LOWERING AGENTS

**INDICATIONS:** Consider drug Rx for (1) hypercholesterolemia, after maximal effort at diet Rx, if LDL >100 mg/dL with definite coronary heart disease [CHD] or Diabetes Mellitus, if LDL > 130 mg/dL without CHD but with two or more risk factors, or if LDL > 160 mg/dL without CHD and fewer than two risk factors; (2) hypertriglyceridemia after maximal effort at diet Rx, risk factor modification, and exercise if (a) triglycerides 250-500 mg/dL and LDL elevated, HDL depressed, or a positive family history of coronary artery disease or (b) triglycerides >500 mg/dL. Diet Rx is the cornerstone of hyperlipidemia Rx and must be continued concurrently with any drug Rx. Factors to which hyperlipidemia may be secondary (e.g., hypothyroidism, diabetes mellitus, alcohol consumption), must be treated with specific Rx. Lipid levels should be monitored at regular intervals. Oat bran, psyllium mucilloid, fish oil, and plant stanol and sterol esters have lipid-lowering effects. Although not now specifically recommended for Rx of hyperlipidemia, they may play an adjunctive role. For mechanisms of action of individual lipid-lowering agents see Chapter 164.

| I. Bile Acid Sequestrants | |
|---|---|

**INDICATIONS:** (1) Adjunctive Rx of elevated LDL cholesterol; (2) pruritus associated with biliary tree obstruction. Unlabeled use in diabetic diarrhea and hyperthyroidism. (Maximum possible lowering of LDL with these agents alone is about 20%.)

---

**DOSE:** All dosages cited are for adults. Other drugs should be taken 1 h before or 4 h after, to avoid their malabsorption.

**ACTIONS AND SIDE EFFECTS:** Contraindicated in the presence of total biliary tree obstruction or hypersensitivity [pruritus, urticaria] to bile acid sequestrants. Side effects include GI manifestations such as nausea and constipation, which usually decline over several months of Rx; interference with absorption of fat-soluble vitamins and various medications including digoxin, thyroxine, and anticoagulants [see Chap. 164]. Safety for use in pregnancy or during nursing has not been determined. Their use may lead to elevation in triglyceride levels.

| A. CHOLESTYRAMINE | | |
|---|---|---|
| | Questran | 4 g/9 g powder (sucrose) |
| | Cholestyramine | 4 g/5.5 g powder (aspartame) |
| | Prevalite | 4 g/5.5 g powder (aspartame) |
| | Questran Light | 4 g/5 g powder (sucrose, aspartame) |
| | LoCHOLEST | 4 g/9g powder (fructose, sorbitol, sucrose. Strawberry flavor) |
| | LoCHOLEST Light | 4 g/7.5g powder (aspartame, fructose, mannitol, sorbitol, 3.93 mg phenylalanine. Strawberry flavor) |

**DOSE:** Begin with 4 g bid. Titrate upward at 1 wk intervals to 12 g bid or 8 g tid. Mix dose well in 6 oz of preferred liquid, soup, pureed fruit, or jello, before taking. Do not take dry.

| B. COLESTIPOL | | |
|---|---|---|
| | Colestid | 300 & 500 g bottles; 5 g single dose packets,1 g tabs & granules, and 5 & 7 g powder |

**DOSE:** Begin with 5 g po bid. Titrate upward at 1 wk intervals to 15 g bid or 10 g tid. Mix as for cholestyramine above. Maximum dose is 16 g/d.

## II. Fibric Acid Derivatives

**INDICATIONS:** Type II, IV and V hyperlipidemias. These agents predominantly lower triglycerides and VLDL levels. They lower LDL cholesterol less predictably. Gemfibrozil increases HDL levels.

| A. CLOFIBRATE | Clofibrate | 500 mg caps | Atromid-S | 500 mg caps |
|---|---|---|---|---|

**INDICATIONS:** Rx of type III hyperlipidemia that does not respond to dietary Rx, and for diet-resistant types IV and V for which triglyceride values are higher than 750 mg/dL and there is risk of pancreatitis.

**DOSE:** 1 g po bid.

**ACTIONS AND SIDE EFFECTS:** Side effects of clofibrate include cholelithiasis, myositis, and enhanced action of warfarin. May be associated with excess mortality from gastrointestinal disease, including Ca [see Chap. 164]. May lead to elevations of serum AST and ALT, and proteinuria.

| B. FENOFIBRATE | Tricor | 67, 134 & 200 mg caps |
|---|---|---|

**INDICATIONS:** Types IV and V hyperlipidemia.

**DOSE:** Start 67 mg qd. Max dose is 201 mg with meals (67 mg tid).

**ACTIONS AND SIDE EFFECTS:** Cholelithiasis, myositis, decreased clearance in renal insufficiency.

| C. GEMFIBROZIL | Gemfibrozil | 600 mg caps | Lopid | 600 mg tabs |
|---|---|---|---|---|

**INDICATIONS:** Rx for hypertriglyceridemia in adults with serum triglyceride values higher than 750 mg/dL [types IV and V] who do not respond to dietary Rx and in whom there is risk of pancreatitis. Low HDL syndrome.

**DOSE:** 600 mg po bid ac.

**ACTIONS AND SIDE EFFECTS:** Side effects of gemfibrozil include gastrointestinal discomfort, elevation of serum LFT, hypokalemia, anemia, leukopenia, and enhanced action of warfarin.

## III. HMG-CoA REDUCTASE INHIBITOR

| | | |
|---|---|---|
| A. ATORVASTATIN | Lipitor | 10, 20 & 40 mg tabs (max 80 mg/d) |
| B. CERIVASTATIN | Baycol | 0.2, 0.3, 0.4 & 0.8 mg tabs (max 0.8 mg/d) |
| C. FLUVASTATIN | Lescol | 20 & 40 mg caps (max 80 mg/d) & 80 mg XL |
| D. LOVASTATIN | Mevacor | 10, 20 & 40 mg tabs (max 80 mg/d) |
| E. PRAVASTATIN | Pravachol | 10, 20 & 40 mg tabs (max 40 mg/d) |
| F. SIMVASTATIN | Zocor | 5, 10, 20, 40 & 80 mg tabs (max 80 mg/d) |

**INDICATIONS:** Highly effective in lowering total and LDL cholesterol as an adjuvant to diet (refer to cited references for specific uses in Rx of elevated triglycerides, atherosclerosis retardation, coronary events and myocardial infarction).

**DOSE:** See Chapters 163 and 164.

**ACTIONS AND SIDE EFFECTS:** Check LFT q 6-12 wk. Use with caution if liver disease history. May cause myalgia; discontinue if markedly elevated plasma CPK. Increased association with rhabdomyolysis in transplant recipients on cyclosporine, erythromycin, gemfibrozil, and niacin use. Side effects among these drugs are similar.

| IV. NEOMYCIN SULFATE | (tabs) | mg/tab | (5 mL oral soln) | mg |
|---|---|---|---|---|
| | Neomycin sulfate | 500 | Mycifradin Sulfate | 125 |
| | Neo-tabs | 500 | Neo-fradin | 125 |

**INDICATIONS:** Unlabeled use: Elevated LDL cholesterol in type IIa hyperlipidemia, only if there is prior failure to respond to conventional Rx and high risk of ischemic heart disease. Elevated Lp(a).

**DOSE:** Adult dosage for the unlabeled use (below): 0.5 g/d to a maximum of 2 g/d.

**ACTIONS AND SIDE EFFECTS:** Contraindicated in renal insufficiency because it may cause nephrotoxicity and ototoxicity.

| V. NICOTINIC ACID | | | | |
|---|---|---|---|---|
| | Nicotinic acid | 50, 100, 250 & 500 mg tabs | Niacor | 500 mg tabs |
| | Nicotinic acid | 250 & 500 mg timed-release tabs | Niaspan | 375, 500, 750 & 1000 mg tabs |
| | | | Nico-400 | 400 mg timed release caps |
| | Nicotinic acid | 125, 250, 400 & 500 mg caps | Nicobid | 125, 250 & 500 mg timed-release caps |
| | Nicotinic acid | 100 mg/mL injection | Nicolar | 500 mg tabs (contains tartrazine) |
| | Nia-Bid | 400 mg timed-release caps | Nicotinex | 50 mg/5 mL elixir |

|  | Niac | 300 mg timed-release caps | Slo-Niacin | 250, 500 & 750 mg timed release tabs |
|  | Niacels | 400 mg timed-release caps |  |  |

**INDICATIONS:** (1) Advocated as adjunctive Rx in diet nonresponders with elevated LDL cholesterol or triglycerides; (2) elevated triglycerides; (3) used in lower doses for Rx of niacin deficiency.

------------------------------------------------------------------------------------------------------------------------------------

**DOSE:** Begin with 100 mg po tid. Increase slowly up to 2 g tid, with or after meals. Niaspan is used qhs.

------------------------------------------------------------------------------------------------------------------------------------

**ACTIONS AND SIDE EFFECTS:** If flushing occurs, it may be alleviated by administration of one aspirin given 30 min before the scheduled dose. Nicotinic acid may exacerbate glucose intolerance, and the slow-release preparations are associated with increased risk of liver toxicity.

| Drug | Trade Names and Preparations | | | |
|------|------|------|------|------|

### LITHIUM

| I. LITHIUM CARBONATE | Lithium carbonate | 300 mg tabs; 150, 300 & 600 mg caps | Lithobid | 300 mg slow-release tabs |
|------|------|------|------|------|
|  | Eskalith | 300 mg caps & tabs | Lithonate | 300 mg caps |
|  | Eskalith CR | 450 mg controlled-release tabs | Lithotabs | 300 mg tabs |
|  | Lithane | 300 mg tabs and caps |  |  |
| **II. LITHIUM CITRATE** | Lithium Citrate | 8 mEq lithium (as citrate, equiv to 300 mg lithium carbonate)/5 mL syrup | | |

**INDICATIONS:** Manic episodes of bipolar disorder and maintenance Rx. Unlabeled uses: Rx of the syndrome of inappropriate secretion of antidiuretic hormone [SIADH] and of hyperthyroidism [see Chaps. 27 and 42].

------------------------------------------------------------------------------------------------------------------------------------

**DOSE:** For unlabeled use in SIADH (below), the dose is 600-1200 mg/d, in divided doses. For acute mania, about 600 mg po tid is used. Dosage must be individualized according to serum levels and clinical response.

------------------------------------------------------------------------------------------------------------------------------------

**ACTIONS AND SIDE EFFECTS:** Lithium in the Rx of SIADH may be associated with multiple side effects and inconsistent results. The drug may cause neurologic, cardiovascular, and other toxicities. It interferes with the action of vasopressin on the renal tubule. Lithium and sodium compete for reabsorption in the proximal renal tubule. Use may exacerbate hyponatremia. Serum levels must be followed closely to avoid toxicity, although side effects may occur at levels which are not very high. Hypothyroidism may occur with long-term Rx. Hyperthyroidism also has occurred.

| Drug | Trade Names and Preparations | |
|------|------|------|

### MAGNESIUM

| I. MAGNESIUM CHLORIDE (MgCL$_2$) | Magnesium chloride | Solutions: 20% (1.97 mEq/mL) in 50 mL vials |
|------|------|------|
|  | Slow-Mag | 64 mg tabs (approx 12% elemental Mg) |
| **II. MAGNESIUM GLUCONATE** | Almora | 500 mg tabs (approx 5.4% elemental Mg) |
|  | Mag | 500 mg tabs (approx 5.4% elemental Mg) & 54 mg/5 mL |
| **III. MAGNESIUM HYDROXIDE (Mg[OH]$_2$)** | Magnesium | 400 mg tabs |
|  | Milk of Magnesia | 325 mg tabs; 400 mg/5 mL |
|  | Concentrated Phillips Milk of Magnesia | 800 mg/5 mL (sorbitol, sugar. Strawberry, orange & vanilla creme flavors) |
| **IV. MAGNESIUM LACTATE** | Mag-Tab SR | 84 mg Mg, caplets, sustained release |
| **V. MAGNESIUM OXIDE (MgO)** | Mag-200 | 400 mg tabs |
|  | Mag-Ox 400 | 400 mg tabs |
|  | MaOx | 420 mg tabs (with tartrazine) |
|  | Uro-Mag | 140 mg caps (84.5 mg magnesium) |
| **VI. MAGNESIUM SULFATE (MgSO$_4$)** | Magnesium Sulfate | Solutions: 10% (0.8 mEq/mL) in 20 & 50 mL vials & 20 mL amps; 12.5% (1 mEq/mL) in 20 mL vials; 50% (4 mEq/mL) in 2, 10, 20 & 50 mL vials, 5 & 10 mL syringes, and 2 & 10 mL amps (~10% elemental Mg) |
|  | Epsom Salt | 40 mEq magnesium sulfate/5 g granules |
| **VII. MAGNESIUM AMINO ACIDS CHELATE** | Chelated Magnesium | 500 mg tabs (100 mg magnesium) |

**DOSE:** If using MgSO$_4$ for mild magnesium deficiency in adults, 1 g (8.1 mEq) (2 mL of 50% soln) is given IM q 6 h for 4 doses. For severe magnesium deficiency in adults with seizures or tetany, one may give up to 2 mEq/kg (0.5 mL of the 50% MgSO$_4$ soln) IM; or 5 g (40 mEq as the 50% MgSO$_4$ soln in 1 L D-5-W) IV over 3 h [also see Chap. 68].

------------------------------------------------------------------------------------------------------------------------------------

**INDICATIONS:** (1) Hypomagnesemia; (2) hyperalimentation; (3) control of hypertension, encephalitis, and convulsions associated with acute nephritis in children; (4) toxemia/eclampsia of pregnancy; (5) saline laxative. [1 g elemental Mg = 82.3 mEq or 41.2 mmol.] Mild depletion of magnesium may be corrected with po magnesium carbonate, chloride, gluconate, hydroxide, or oxide salts. Magnesium chloride has greater solubility and may be absorbed better than the other preparations. Moderate to severe depletion usually is treated by the administration of parenteral magnesium sulfate. Urine output should be maintained at 100 mL q 4 h and serum magnesium levels should be closely monitored during parenteral Rx.

------------------------------------------------------------------------------------------------------------------------------------

**DOSE:** For po magnesium supplementation in adults and older children, 5 mg magnesium/kg/d is given.

------------------------------------------------------------------------------------------------------------------------------------

**ACTIONS AND SIDE EFFECTS:** Excess oral magnesium salts cause diarrhea. Use with caution in patients with renal insufficiency. Magnesium toxicity is characterized by flushing, hypotension, paralysis, hypothermia, and cardiac and CNS depression [see Chap. 68].

| Drug | Trade Names and Preparations |
|---|---|
| **METYROSINE** | |
| | Demser          250 mg caps |

**INDICATIONS:** Pheochromocytoma, particularly in the preoperative preparation of patients for surgery. Also may be used if surgery is not possible or in cases of malignant pheochromocytoma. It is important to maintain adequate hydration during Rx [see Chap. 86].

**DOSE:** Starting dosage is 250 mg po q 6 h. May be increased by 250 to 500 mg/d to a maximum dose of 4 g/d in divided doses.

**ACTIONS AND SIDE EFFECTS:** Metyrosine, α-methyl-L-tyrosine, inhibits tyrosine hydroxylase, which is the enzyme that catalyzes the first, rate-limiting step in the synthesis of catecholamines. It is not recommended for use in children <12 yr. Side effects include sedation, extrapyramidal signs, crystalluria, diarrhea, eosinophilia and elevation of LFT levels. (Adequate hydration of 2 L/d should be ensured.)

| Drug | Trade Names and Preparations |
|---|---|
| **MINERALOCORTICOID** | |
| **FLUDROCORTISONE ACETATE** | Florinef Acetate          0.1 mg tabs |

**INDICATIONS:** Replacement of mineralocorticoid function in (1) adrenal insufficiency [see Chap. 76]; (2) salt-wasting forms of congenital adrenal hyperplasia [see Chap. 77]; (3) hypoaldosteronism [see Chap. 81]. Unlabeled use: the management of chronic orthostatic hypotension.

**DOSE:** In primary adrenal insufficiency, the starting dosage of fludrocortisone is 0.05-0.1 mg po/d. The maintenance dosage usually is 0.1 mg/d. Up to 0.2 mg/d may be required. In salt-losing congenital adrenal hyperplasia, the dosage is 0.1 to 0.2 mg po/d.

**ACTIONS AND SIDE EFFECTS:** Fludrocortisone acetate acts on the distal renal tubule to promote the reabsorption of sodium and to increase excretion of potassium and hydrogen ions. The dosage must be adjusted according to the clinical response and serum electrolyte levels. This drug is the only po mineralocorticoid available. It is a fluorinated derivative of cortisol. It has only minimal glucocorticoid activity and, if cortisol deficiency is present, it must be used in conjunction with a predominantly glucocorticoid drug. Desoxycorticosterone acetate [DOCA] and desoxycorticosterone pivalate are no longer available in the United States. Use of fludrocortisone acetate may produce fluid retention, hypertension, congestive heart failure, hypokalemia, and headaches. Fluid and electrolyte status must be monitored closely. Possesses glucocorticoid activity and can cause withdrawal symptoms.

| Drug | Trade Names and Preparations |
|---|---|
| **OBESITY MANAGEMENT DRUGS** | |
| **I. ORLISTAT** | Xenical          120 mg caps |

**INDICATIONS:** Management of obesity (BMI $\geq$ 30 kg/m$^2$ or $\geq$ 27 kg/m$^2$ with additional risk factors (e.g., diabetes, hypertension, dyslipidemia) when used in conjunction with dieting.

**DOSE:** 120 mg with each meal containing fat (during or up to 1 h after the meal). A daily vitamin containing fat-soluble vitamins 2 h before or after orlistat is recommended.

**ACTIONS AND SIDE EFFECTS:** Orlistat is a reversible lipase inhibitor which leads to undigested triglycerides. Mostly mild & transient GI side effects, including oily evacuation & spotting, flatus with discharge, increased defecation, and fecal incontinence.

| **II. SIBUTRAMINE** | Meridia          5, 10 & 15 mg caps |
|---|---|

**INDICATIONS:** Management of obesity (BMI $\geq$ 30 kg/m$^2$ or $\geq$ 27 kg/m$^2$ with additional risk factors (e.g., diabetes, hypertension, dyslipidemia) when used in conjunction with dieting.

**DOSE:** 10 mg/d with or without food. Max dose is 15 mg/d.

**ACTIONS AND SIDE EFFECTS:** Reuptake inhibitor of norepinephrine, serotonin, and dopamine via liver-generated primary and secondary metabolites. Contraindicated with concurrent use of monoamine oxidase inhibitors and agents associated with the "serotonin syndrome." Can increase systolic and diastolic blood pressure by a mean of 1-3 mm Hg and heart rate by 4-5 beats/min. Pulmonary hypertension has been associated with other agents that cause the release of serotonin.

| Drug | Trade Names and Preparations |
|---|---|
| **ORAL CONTRACEPTIVES** | **(see Chaps. 104 and 105)** |

| Drug | Trade Names and Preparations |
|---|---|
| **ORAL HYPOGLYCEMIC AGENTS** | |
| **I. INSULIN SECRETAGOGUES** **A. SUFONYLUREAS** "First-Generation Agents" | |
| **1. ACETOHEXAMIDE** | Acetohexamide     250 & 500 mg tabs     Dymelor     250 & 500 mg tabs |

**DOSE:** Acetohexamide: Begin Rx with 500 mg po/d, in 2 divided doses. Some give once daily Rx if total qd dose is 1 g or less. Maximum daily dose is 1500 mg.

| **2. CHLORPROPAMIDE** | Chlorpropamide | 100 & 250 mg tabs | Diabinese | 100 & 250 mg tabs |
|---|---|---|---|---|

**DOSE:** Chlorpropamide: Begin Rx with 250 mg po/d, except in the elderly, in whom the initial dosage should be 100-125 mg/d. The maximum effective dosage is 500 mg/d.

| **3. TOLAZAMIDE** | Tolazamide | 100, 250 & 500 mg tabs | Tolinase | 100, 250 & 500 mg tabs |
|---|---|---|---|---|

**DOSE:** Tolazamide: Begin Rx with 100 to 250 mg po/d. Maximum dosage is 1000 mg/d. If >500 mg/d is required, dose should be divided.

| **4. TOLBUTAMIDE** | Tolbutamide | 500 mg tabs | Orinase | 250 & 500 mg tabs |
|---|---|---|---|---|

**DOSE:** Tolbutamide: Begin Rx with 1-2 g po/d. Maximum dose is 3 g/d in 2 divided doses.

**"Second-Generation Agents"**

| **1. GLIPIZIDE** | Glucotrol | 5 & 10 mg scored tab | Glucotrol XL | 2.5, 5 & 10 mg scored tab |
|---|---|---|---|---|

**DOSE:** Glucotrol: Begin Rx with 5 mg po/d. If elderly or if liver disease, begin with 2.5 mg/d. Maximum dosage is 40 mg/d. Give bid if dose is >20 mg/d. Should be taken 30 min before meals, since food delays its absorption. Starting dose of Glucotrol XL is 5 mg qd; maximum dose is 20 mg qd not at meal times.

| **2. GLYBURIDE** | Glyburide | 1.25, 1.5, 2.5, 3, 4.5, 5, 6 mg scored tabs | | |
|---|---|---|---|---|
| **(Glibenclamide)** | DiaBeta | 1.25, 2.5 & 5 mg scored tabs | Micronase | 1.25, 2.5 & 5 mg scored tabs |
| | Glynase | 1.5, 3 & 6 mg scored tabs | Glucovance | 1.25/250, 2.5/500 & 5/500 tabs |

**DOSE:** Glyburide: Begin Rx with 2.5 to 5 mg po/d. If elderly, start with 1.25 or 1.5 mg. Give bid if dose is >10 mg/d. Should be taken with meals. Maximum dose is 20 mg/d for DiaBeta and Micronase and 12 mg/d for Glynase. (Glucovance contains glyburide and metformin. Starting dose is 1.25/250 mg qd or bid.)

| **3. GLIMEPIRIDE** | Amaryl | 1, 2 & 4 mg scored tabs. | | |
|---|---|---|---|---|

**DOSE:** Glimepiride: Begin Rx with 1-2 mg po/d. Impaired renal function, begin Rx with 1 mg po/d. Take with first meal of day. Usual dose range is 1-4 mg po/d. Maximum dose is 8 mg/d.

**INDICATIONS:** Type 2 diabetes mellitus, if diet and exercise Rx alone are not successful in achieving adequate serum glucose control. (The designations "first-" and "second-generation" for oral hypoglycemic agents are based on the time-course of their development rather than a clear-cut Rx advantage of the second group over the first. The second-generation agents are more potent on a mg/mg basis and the two groups differ in their lipophilic properties. If a patient is well-controlled on one agent, there usually is no reason to switch to another.)

---

**ACTIONS AND SIDE EFFECTS:** Adverse reactions to oral hypoglycemic agents include hypoglycemia, gastrointestinal disturbances, cholestatic jaundice, skin rashes, and hematologic dyscrasias. Patients should be told to notify physician if they have symptoms of hypoglycemia or hyperglycemia, or if they develop fever, sore throat, or unusual bruising or bleeding. See Chapter 142 for a full discussion of these agents. The duration of action of any one of these agents [see Chap. 142] should be taken into consideration when making a Rx decision regarding its use. The long $t_{1/2}$ of chlorpropamide gives it a prolonged hypoglycemic effect. Hypoglycemia may need to be aggressively treated, including hospitalization. In addition to IV dextrose, charcoal hemoperfusion shortened the $t_{1/2}$ of chlorpropamide in one patient with drug-induced hypoglycemia in association with renal failure. Rx with octreotide has also been reported to be useful in drug-induced hypoglycemia. Drugs that compete for protein-binding sites may potentiate hypoglycemic effects of first-generation agents. Acetohexamide is the only sulfonylurea with uricosuric properties. Difference in bioequivalence of generics for these agents may be a problem. Chlorpropamide may be used in Rx of nephrogenic diabetes insipidus in a dose of 125-250 mg/d. Tolazamide has a mild diuretic effect that may make it useful in patients with a tendency for fluid retention. Rx with sulfonylureas is contraindicated in the presence of known hypersensitivity to these agents, in type 1 diabetes mellitus, in pregnancy or lactation, and in the presence of significant liver or renal disease. Sulfonylureas, particularly chlorpropamide, may cause a disulfuram-like reaction when used in conjunction with alcohol. They may cause hyponatremia owing to potentiation of the effect of vasopressin on the kidney (particularly chlorpropamide). The toxicities associated with the use of tolbutamide, glyburide, glimepiride, and glipizide generally are low.

| **B. MEGLITINIDES** | | | | |
|---|---|---|---|---|
| **REPLAGINIDE** | Prandin | 0.5, 1 & 2 mg tabs | | |

**INDICATIONS:** Type 2 diabetes mellitus if diet & exercise Rx are not successful in achieving adequate serum glucose control. Approved indications for Rx are same as for monotherapy or in combination with metformin.

---

**DOSE:** Begin Rx with 0.5 mg if Rx naïve or $A_{1c}$ < 8; 1-2 mg if prior antihyperglycemic agent Rx or $A_{1c} \geq 8$. Take within 30 min prior to meal with 2-4 meals daily. Skip dose if meal to be missed. Add dose if meal added. May Rx smaller dose with bedtime snack. Max dose is 16 mg/d. Initial dose adjustment not necessary in renal insufficiency, increases should be made with care. Use with caution if impaired liver function as repaglinide & metabolites may accumulate.

---

**ACTIONS AND SIDE EFFECTS:** Hypoglycemia, upper respiratory tract infection, diarrhea, constipation, back or chest pain. In < 1% subjects in clinical trials, elevated LFT, thrombocytopenia, leukopenia, and anaphylactic reaction (one subject) have been reported. Hypoglycemic action may be potentiated by protein-bound drugs. Contraindicated for Rx of type 1 diabetes. Not recommended for use in pregnancy or lactation.

| **II. BIGUANIDES** | | | | |
|---|---|---|---|---|
| **METFORMIN** | Glucophage | 500, 850, & 1000 mg tabs | Glucovance | 1.25/250, 2.5/500 & 5/500 mg tabs |

**INDICATIONS:** Type 2 diabetes mellitus if diet & exercise Rx are not successful in achieving adequate serum glucose control. May be used in combination with an insulin secretagogue (sulfonylurea or repaglinide) or with insulin. Tends to lower LDL cholesterol, triglycerides and weight, so may be helpful in improving cardiovascular risk factor profile. Confirm normal renal function pre-Rx. Metformin use is CONTRAINDICATED in: renal insufficiency (serum creatinine $\geq 1.4$ mg/dL in females & $\geq 1.5$ mg/dL in males; if $\geq 80$ years old unless creatinine clearance is normal); CHF on pharmacologic Rx; liver disease; alcohol abuse; metabolic or diabetic ketoacidosis; presence of sepsis, hypotension, hypoxemia, or use of intravascular iodinated contrast agents. Metformin should be withheld from patients undergoing contrast studies from the time of the procedure until 48 hr afterwards and may be restarted when renal function is known to be normal. Use of metformin in pregnancy or lactation is not recommended.

---

**DOSE:** Begin Rx for monotherapy with 500 mg po bid or 850 mg po/d. If elderly or adding to insulin, Rx begins with 500 mg po/d. Give with meal. Titrate dose upward by 500 mg/wk or by 850 mg every 2 wk. Usual dose range 500-2,000 mg/d given bid or tid. Max dose is 2550 mg/d.

---

**ACTIONS AND SIDE EFFECTS:** Up to 30% incidence of mild GI side effects, including nausea, bloating, loose stools. Usually resolve after 2-3 weeks of ongoing Rx. If GI symptoms more pronounced (e.g., vomiting, diarrhea), use should be discontinued; may note metallic taste in mouth at start of Rx; up to 9% develop subnormal, asymptomatic vitamin $B_{12}$ levels; lactic acidosis is rare (0.03 cases/1,000 patient years; up to 50% of cases fatal). Occurrence of lactic acidosis associated with presence of renal insufficiency, CHF or Rx, and/or hypoxemia, dehydration, sepsis, and hypertension; therefore, AVOID USE of metformin in these clinical settings. Monitor hematology & renal function on ongoing basis in long-term Rx.

| III. ALPHA-GLUCOSIDASE INHIBITORS | | |
|---|---|---|
| A. ACARBOSE | Precose | 50 & 100 mg tabs scored |
| B. MIGLITOL | Glyset | 25, 50 & 100 mg tabs |

**INDICATIONS:** Type 2 diabetes mellitus if diet & exercise Rx are not successful in achieving adequate serum glucose control. May be used in combination with sulfonylurea. Alpha-glucosidase inhibitors lower postprandial blood glucose levels. Contraindicated in Rx for: ketoacidosis; chronic intestinal disease, including inflammatory bowel disease, malabsorption syndromes, or any disorder predisposing to intestinal obstruction. Not recommended for use in pregnancy, lactation, or if serum creatinine > 2 mg/dL.

------

**DOSE:** Begin Rx with 25 mg po tid. Increase at 4-8 wk intervals to max dose of 100 mg tid. Take with first bite of each main meal. In patients ≤ 60 kg, max dose of Precose is 50 mg tid.

------

**ACTIONS AND SIDE EFFECTS:** Flatulence, diarrhea, and abdominal pain. Rarely (19/500,000) mild LFT abnormalities with acarbose (predisposing factor ≤ 60 kg on 100 mg tid). Alpha-glucosidase inhibitors when used as monotherapy do not cause hypoglycemia. If hypoglycemia occurs when used in combination therapy with other classes of oral agents, glucose, not sucrose, must be used for treatment.

| IV. THIAZOLIDINEDIONES | | |
|---|---|---|
| A. ROSIGLITAZONE | Avandia | 2, 4 & 8 mg tabs |

**INDICATIONS:** Type 2 diabetes mellitus if diet & exercise Rx are not successful in achieving adequate serum glucose control. May be used as monotherapy or in combination with metformin or sulfonylureas. Use of Avandia is contraindicated if known hypersensitivity to the product or any of its components. It should not be used in pregnancy or lactation or for treatment of type 1 diabetes with ketoacidosis. Use with caution in CHF III & IV.

------

**DOSE:** Begin Rx with 4 mg po/d. May be increased to 8 mg po/d after 12 wk Rx. Max recommended dose is 8 mg po/d. May be given as once daily dose in AM or in divided doses bid. As thiazolidinediones induce nuclear protein synthesis through the PPAR-γ receptor, time to onset of action is 1-2 wk. No dose adjustment required in elderly, renal impairment, or hemodialysis. Can be taken with or without meals.

------

**ACTIONS AND SIDE EFFECTS:** In premenopausal, anovulatory patients with insulin resistance, Avandia Rx may result in resumption of ovulation. These patients may be at risk for pregnancy (Avandia has no clinically relevant effect on pharmacokinetics of oral contraceptives); anemia, edema (4.8%); and 2 cases to date of Avandia-induced hepatotoxicity. Because of adverse experience with hepatotoxicity with troglitazone (another thiazolidinedione), periodic LFTs in patients on Avandia Rx is recommended as follows: at baseline, if LFT normal, initiate Avandia Rx & test every 2 mo the first year and periodically thereafter. If LFT > 2.5x upper limit of normal at baseline or during Rx, should be evaluated to determine the cause. Rx under these circumstances should proceed only with caution & more frequent LFTs. Drug should be stopped if LFT ≥ 3x upper limit of normal.

| B. PIOGLITAZONE | Actos | 15, 30 & 45 mg tabs |
|---|---|---|

**INDICATIONS:** Monotherapy as an adjunct to diet and exercise in type 2 diabetes. Combination Rx with sulfonylureas, metformin, or insulin.

------

**DOSE:** Start 15 or 30 mg po/d without regard to meals; do not exceed 45 mg/d.

------

**ACTIONS AND SIDE EFFECTS:** Do not start if have baseline liver abnormalities or LFTs > 2.5x the upper limit of normal. LFT should be monitored as per Avandia guidelines.


| Drug | Trade Names and Preparations | | |
|---|---|---|---|
| **OXYTOCIN** | | | |
| | Oxytocin | 10 U/mL for injection | Syntocinon |
| | Pitocin | 10 U/mL for injection | |

| | | | |
|---|---|---|---|
| Syntocinon | 10 U/mL for injection |
| | 40 U/mL in nasal spray |

**INDICATIONS:** (1) Medical induction of labor; (2) to augment labor in selected patients with uterine dysfunction; (3) prevention of postpartum uterine atony or hemorrhage; (4) promotion of milk letdown in lactation.

------

**DOSE:** (1), (2) and (3) IV (drip) infusion: 1-2 mU/min; max 20 mU/min.

------

**ACTIONS AND SIDE EFFECTS:** Oxytocin is an octapeptide produced in the hypothalamus and stored in the posterior pituitary. It has uterine-stimulating, vasopressor, and antidiuretic properties, and stimulates the milk let-down reflex. All synthetic oxytocic products are potentially dangerous to mother and fetus and should be used only in a closely monitored setting. Monitor for overstimulation of the uterus, hypertension, water intoxication, and fetal distress.


| Drug | Trade Names and Preparations |
|---|---|
| **PARATHYROID HORMONE (TERIPARATIDE ACETATE)** | |
| | Parathar | 200 U hPTH powder in a 10 mL vial with a 10 mL vial of diluent |

**INDICATIONS:** Dx agent to assist in determining whether hypocalcemia may be due to hypoparathyroidism or pseudohypoparathyroidism. Teriparatide acetate is a synthetic form of human parathyroid hormone made up of the 1-34 fragment [NH$_2$-terminal region] of native PTH.

------

**DOSE:** For dosages, see Chapter 241.

------

**ACTIONS AND SIDE EFFECTS:** Subjects may note paresthesias, a metallic taste, pain at the injection site, nausea, cramps, urge to defecate, or diarrhea.

| Drug | Trade Names and Preparations |
|---|---|

**PHENOXYBENZAMINE**

| | |
|---|---|
| Dibenzyline | 10 mg caps |

**INDICATIONS:** Management of pheochromocytoma to control hypertension [see Chap. 86]. Unlabeled use in micturition disorders (neurogenic bladder, sphinctorial outlet obstruction, partial prostatic obstruction) in a dose of 5-60 mg/d.

------------------------------------------------------------------------

**DOSE:** In adults, initial dosage is 10 mg po bid. May be increased qod until the desired blood pressure response is achieved. Usual dose is 20-40 mg, bid or tid. Dosage must be individualized. For doses in children, see Chapter 87.

------------------------------------------------------------------------

**ACTIONS AND SIDE EFFECTS:** Phenoxybenzamine is an α-adrenergic receptor-blocking agent. If tachycardia develops during its use, a ß-adrenergic receptor-blocking agent may be added. Important to maintain adequate hydration during Rx. Side effects include postural hypotension, cardiac arrhythmias, miosis, and inhibition of ejaculation. Should be used with caution in patients with atherosclerosis or renal disease.

| Drug | Trade Names and Preparations |
|---|---|

**PHENTOLAMINE**

| | |
|---|---|
| Phentolamine mesylate    5 mg/2 mL vial     Regitine   5 mg/1 mL vial | |

**INDICATIONS:** Management of pheochromocytoma for the control of blood pressure in hypertensive crisis or in the perioperative period. Unlabeled use in the control of hypertensive crisis associated with withdrawal from clonidine or propranolol Rx or secondary to MAO inhibitor/sympathomimetic amine interactions. Also may be useful in controlling other effects of excessive epinephrine, such as respiratory depression and convulsions [see Chap. 86]. It also has been used in combination with papaverine and prostaglandin $E_1$ as an intracavernosal injection for impotence.

------------------------------------------------------------------------

**DOSE:** Phentolamine, 5 mg, in the adult, or 1 mg in the child, is given IV or IM 1-2 h preoperatively, or IV as needed for control of blood pressure. These doses may be repeated.

------------------------------------------------------------------------

**ACTIONS AND SIDE EFFECTS:** Phentolamine is an α-adrenergic receptor-blocking agent. It causes cardiac stimulation. It has a rapid onset and short duration of action. Maintain adequate hydration during Rx. Side effects include severe hypotension, tachycardia, cardiac arrhythmias, flushing, nausea, vomiting, and diarrhea. Should be used with extreme caution in patients with atherosclerosis because myocardial and cerebrovascular infarction have occurred following its use.

| Drug | Trade Names and Preparations |
|---|---|

**PHOSPHORUS**

| **I. Oral** | K-Phos Neutral | 250 mg phorphorus/tab | Neutra-Phos-K | 250 mg phosphorus powder |
|---|---|---|---|---|
| | Neutra-Phos | 250 mg phosphorus powder | Uro-KP-Neutral | 250 mg phosphorus/tab |
| **I. Intravenous** | Potassium phosphate | 224 mg monobasic & 236 mg dibasic potassium phosphate/mL (3 mmol phosphate & 4.4 mEq potassium/mL) in 5 & 15 mL vials and 50 mL bulk additive vials | | |
| | Sodium phosphate | 276 mg monobasic & 142 mg dibasic sodium phosphate/mL (3 mmol phosphate & 4 mEq sodium/mL) in 15 & 30 mL vials | | |

**INDICATIONS:** (1) Phosphate depletion; (2) dietary phosphorus supplementation, particularly if the diet is restricted or if needs are increased; (3) Rx of hypercalcemia in certain circumstances when serum phosphate levels are low [see Chaps. 58 and 59]; (4) hypophosphatemic rickets [see Chap. 63]; (5) X-linked hypophosphatemic rickets [see Chap. 70]; (6) adult hypophosphatasia [see Chap. 67]. (1 mmol of phosphorus = 31 mg.) K-Phos Neutral tabs have 1.1 mEq $K^+$ and 13 mEq $Na^+$ each. They contain dibasic sodium phosphate anhydrous, monobasic sodium phosphate, and monobasic potassium phosphate. Neutra-Phos has 7.1 mEq $K^+$ and 7.1 mEq $Na^+$/cap or 75 mL of po soln. It contains monobasic and dibasic sodium and potassium phosphates. Neutra-Phos-K contains 14.2 mEq $K^+$/cap or per 75 mL of po soln. It contains dibasic and monobasic potassium phosphate. Uro-KP-Neutral tabs contain 1.3 mEq $K^+$ and 10.8 mEq $Na^+$ each. They consist of disodium and dipotassium phosphate anhydrous and monobasic sodium anhydrous phosphate.

------------------------------------------------------------------------

**DOSE:** For phosphate depletion, 2.5 to 3.5 g of phosphate po/d in 4 equally divided doses. For hypercalcemia with low serum phosphate, 250 mg po qid. For hypophosphatemic rickets, 2-4 g po/d in divided doses. For X-linked hypophosphatemic rickets, 1-4 g po/d. For adult hypophosphatasia, 1.25-3 g po/d.

------------------------------------------------------------------------

**ACTIONS AND SIDE EFFECTS:** Phosphorus replacement products contain significant amounts of sodium or potassium and should be used with caution if a patient is on a sodium or potassium-restricted diet. Serum calcium, phosphate, and creatinine levels should be followed closely in any patient being treated, since renal failure may occur. Use is contraindicated in the presence of severely impaired renal function, hyperphosphatemia, Addison disease, or hyperkalemia. Should be used with caution in certain conditions including renal insufficiency, liver disease, dehydration, and congestive heart failure. Most commonly experienced side effects are gastrointestinal upset and diarrhea. IV phosphorus Rx should be used *only if absolutely* necessary in the rare patient with life-threatening hypophosphatemia who cannot be controlled using any other approach, and then with *extreme caution* because it may cause severe soft tissue calcification, renal cortical necrosis, and shock [see Chap. 59].

| Drug | Trade Names and Preparations |
|---|---|

**PROGESTINS**    (*Caution: progestins during pregnancy may be teratogenic. Rule out pregnancy before use.*)

| **I. DESOGESTREL** | |
|---|---|
| **DOSE:** Constituent with estrogen, of oral contraceptive pills. | |
| **II. ETHYNODIOL DIACETATE** | |
| **DOSE:** Constituent of oral contraceptive pills. | |

| | | | | | |
|---|---|---|---|---|---|
| **III. HYDROXYPROGESTERONE CAPROATE IN OIL** | Hydroxyprogesterone caproate | 125 & 250 mg/mL in oil | Hylutin | 125 & 250 mg/mL in oil | |

**DOSE:** For menstrual disorders, 125 to 250 mg IM.

---

**IV. LEVONORGESTREL**

**DOSE:** Constituent with estrogen, of oral contraceptive pills & Norplant.

---

**V. MEDROXYPROGESTERONE ACETATE**

| Oral: | | | |
|---|---|---|---|
| Medroxyprogesterone acetate | 2.5, 5 & 10 mg tabs | Cycrin | 2.5, 5 & 10 mg tabs |
| Amen | 10 mg tabs | Provera | 2.5, 5 & 10 mg tabs |
| Curretab | 10 mg tabs | | |
| Injection: | | | |
| Depo-Provera | 150 mg/mL aqueous suspn for IM injection | | |

**DOSE:** For amenorrhea and dysfunctional uterine bleeding, 5-10 mg po qd x 5-10 d. For endometriosis, 30 mg po/d. For replacement hormonal Rx, 5-10 mg po/d for each of the last 12 to 15 d of the mo in which estrogen is administered.

---

**VI. MEGESTROL ACETATE** — Megestrol acetate — 20 & 40 mg tabs — Megace — 20 & 40 mg tabs & 40 mg/mL suspn

**DOSE:** Palliative Rx: breast Ca, 40 mg po qid; endometrial Ca, 40 to 320 mg po/d in divided doses. In cachexia initial dose is 800 mg/d.

---

**VII. NORETHINDRONE**

| Micronor | 0.35 mg tabs |
|---|---|
| Norlutin | 5 mg tabs |
| NorQD | 0.35 mg tabs |

**DOSE:** For amenorrhea and dysfunctional uterine bleeding, 5-20 mg po/d days 5-25 of the menstrual cycle. For endometriosis, 10 mg po/d x 14 d, then increase dose by 5 mg increments every 2 wk to maximum dose of 30 mg/d. Also used in doses of 0.35-2 mg/pill as constituent of oral contraceptive pills.

---

**VIII. NORETHINDRONE ACETATE** — Aygestin — 5 mg tabs

**DOSE:** For replacement Rx, 2.5 mg po/d days 16-25 of the menstrual cycle. For amenorrhea and dysfunctional uterine bleeding, 2.5-10 mg po/d days 5-25. For endometriosis, 5 mg po/d x 14 d, then increase the dose by 2.5 mg increments q 2 wk to a maximum dose of 15 mg/d. Constituent of oral contraceptive pills in dosages of 1, 1.5 and 2.5 mg/pill.

---

**IX. NORGESTIMATE**

**DOSE:** Constituent with estrogen, of oral contraceptive pills.

---

**X. NORGESTREL** — Ovrette — 0.075 mg/tab

**DOSE:** Also available as a constituent, with estrogen, of oral contraceptive pills.

---

**XI. PROGESTERONE**
**A. Progesterone in Oil** — Progesterone in oil — 50 mg/mL
**B. Progesterone Powder** — Progesterone powder — 1, 10, 25, 100 & 1000 g (for prescription compounding)

**DOSE:** For Dx use in amenorrhea, 100 to 200 mg IM. For dysfunctional uterine bleeding and amenorrhea 5-10 mg qd x 6 days

**C. MICRONIZED PROGESTE-RONE** — Prometrium — 100 & 200 mg caps

**DOSE:** For secondary amenorrhea 400 mg po q hs x 10 d. For hormone replacement Rx, 200 mg po q hs x 12 d for every 28 d cycle. Synthesized from yam plant sources. Contraindicated in patients with peanut allergy.

**D. MICRONIZED PROGESTE-RONE GEL** — Crinone — 8% (90 mg) applicator

**DOSE:** For secondary amenorrhea, 8% gel dose intravaginally qd for up to 6 doses. Gel may also be used in Assisted Reproductive Technology.

---

**INDICATIONS:** (1) Ethynodiol diacetate used in po contraceptive pills; (2) hydroxyprogesterone caproate used for menstrual disorders; (3) medroxyprogesterone used for amenorrhea and dysfunctional uterine bleeding, endometriosis, and replacement hormonal Rx in combination with estrogens; (4) megestrol acetate used for palliative Rx of breast Ca and endometrial Ca; (5) norethindrone used for amenorrhea and dysfunctional uterine bleeding, endometriosis, and contraceptive pills; (6) norethindrone acetate used for replacement hormonal Rx in combination with estrogens, amenorrhea and dysfunctional uterine bleeding, endometriosis, and constituent of progestin only contraceptive pills; (7) norgestrel used as progestin-only contraceptive pill and constituent of contraceptive pills; (8) progesterone used for dysfunctional uterine bleeding and for Dx evaluation of amenorrhea. Progestins are used for wide variety of Dx and Rx purposes including contraception, dysfunctional uterine bleeding, amenorrhea, premenstrual syndrome, endometriosis, postmenopausal replacement Rx, palliative Rx of endometrial and breast Ca, suppression of postpartum lactation, chronic anovulatory syndrome and hypoventilation syndromes. Ethynodiol diacetate is converted to norethindrone in vivo. Duration of action of hydroxyprogesterone caproate is 9-17 d. Levonorgestrel has no first-pass effect. It has pronounced androgenic effects. Medroxyprogesterone acetate is commonly used in clinical practice in the evaluation of amenorrhea to induce endometrial sloughing, and in combination with estrogens for replacement Rx. In replacement Rx, doses of 2.5 or 5 mg medroxyprogesterone acetate/d may be given if progestin side effects are a problem. Duration of Rx with this agent as well as dose may be responsible for the endometrial protective effect of progestins. Depo-Provera is used as a contraceptive agent. The androgenic effects of norethindrone are minor to moderate. Norethindrone acetate is twice as potent as norethindrone. It has no androgenic effects. Norgestrel has pronounced androgenic effects. It also is used in the Progestasert intrauterine device. For use of progestins in oral contraception and menopause [see Chaps. 100, 104 and 105].

---

**ACTIONS AND SIDE EFFECTS:** Breakthrough bleeding, change in menstrual flow, amenorrhea, breast tenderness, masculinization, jaundice.

---

| Drug | Trade Names and Preparations |
|---|---|

**SERM (SELECTIVE ESTROGEN RECEPTOR MODULATORS)**

**I. RALOXIFENE HCL** — Evista — 60 mg tab

**INDICATIONS:** Prevention of osteoporosis in postmenopausal women. Improves hip, spine, and total body BMD. Inconsistent effects on forearm BMD. May improve lipid profiles ($\downarrow$ LDL, Lp[a], and fibrinogen).

---

**DOSE:** 60 mg po/d. Adequate vitamin D and calcium should be ensured. Cholestyramine should not be coadministered with raloxifene due to reduction in absorption. INR should be monitored in patients on warfarin Rx. (Recommended that Evista is discontinued at least 72 h prior to and during prolonged immobilization.)

---

**ACTIONS AND SIDE EFFECTS:** Has estrogen-like effects on bone and lipid metabolism; lacks effects on uterus and breast tissue. Contraindicated in women who may become pregnant, patients with history of thromboembolic events or known hypersensitivity to raloxifene or other constituents of the tablets. Most common side effects are hot flashes and leg cramps. Rarely, thromboembolic events.

| **II. TAMOXIFEN CITRATE** | Nolvadex | 10 & 20 mg tabs | Tamoxifen | 10 & 20 mg tabs |
|---|---|---|---|---|

**INDICATIONS:** (1) Adjunctive Rx in postmenopausal women with estrogen receptor-positive breast Ca; (2) also may be used in premenopausal breast Ca patients who are estrogen receptor-positive [see Chap. 224]; (3) advanced breast Ca in women and men. Unlabeled use in mastalgia [10 mg/d x 4 mo] and for decreasing the size and pain of gynecomastia.

---

**DOSE:** The usual dosage is 10 or 20 mg po bid.

---

**ACTIONS AND SIDE EFFECTS:** A nonsteroidal antiestrogenic agent. Side effects include nausea, vomiting, and hot flashes. Bone pain and hypercalcemia may follow initiation of Rx due to tumor flare. May have estrogen-like effect in utero, causing endometrial hyperplasia and/or Ca. Rarely, increases LFT.

| **III. TOREMIFENE CITRATE** | Fareston | 60 mg tabs |
|---|---|---|

**INDICATIONS:** Treatment in combination with surgical castration for treatment of stage $D_2$ metatstatic prostatic Ca.

---

**DOSE:** 60 mg po qd.

---

**ACTIONS AND SIDE EFFECTS:** Same as tamoxifen

| **Drug** | **Trade Names and Preparations** |
|---|---|

**SOMATOSTATIN ANALOG**

| **OCTREOTIDE ACETATE** | Sandostatin | 0.05, 0.10, 0.2, 0.50 & 1 mg in 1 mL amp |
|---|---|---|
| | | 200, 500 & 1000 µg in 5 mL multidose vials |
| | Sandostatin LAR | 10, 20 & 30 mg in 5 mL vials |

**INDICATIONS:** Rx of (a) acromegaly, (b) symptomatic metastatic carcinoid tumors, and (c) vasoactive intestinal peptide-secreting tumors (VIPomas; see Chap. 220). Also unlabeled use in a variety of neuroendocrine disorders [see Chap. 169].

---

**DOSE:** Rx is initiated with 50 µg SC bid to tid. The dosage then is increased q 2 wk according to the patient response and tolerance [see Chap. 169]. Sandostatin may also be given IV diluted. If patient responds well to sandostatin, sandostatin LAR may be used beginning with 20 mg IM intragluteally q 4 wk for 3 months. Dosage may be adjusted to 10-30 mg IM monthly based on response. Patients with carcinoids and VIPoma should be maintained on daily SC Sandostatin for at least 2 wk with initial LAR injection while adjusting therapeutically effective levels of LAR. Patients on dialysis generally require lower maintenance doses.

---

**ACTIONS AND SIDE EFFECTS:** Rx may be associated with cholelithiasis; it is recommended that patients on extended Rx be evaluated periodically by ultrasound of the gallbladder and bile ducts. Adverse reactions, which may be seen in 3-10% of patients, include nausea, injection site pain, diarrhea, abdominal pain/discomfort, loose stools, and vomiting.

| **Drug** | **Trade Names and Preparations** |
|---|---|

**SPIRONOLACTONE**

| | Spironolactone | 25 mg tabs | Aldactone | 25, 50 & 100 mg tabs |
|---|---|---|---|---|

**INDICATIONS:** (1) Primary aldosteronism [see Chap. 80]; (2) certain edematous conditions when some potassium retention is desired or other Rx fails, e.g., congestive heart failure, cirrhosis of the liver with ascites, nephrotic syndrome; (3) essential hypertension; (4) hypokalemia. Unlabeled use: hirsutism [see Chap. 101].

---

**DOSE:** For primary aldosteronism, 100-400 mg po/d in divided doses. For certain edematous conditions, the initial dosage is 100 mg/d in single or divided doses. The maintenance dosage is 25-200 mg/d. For essential hypertension, 50-100 mg/d in single or divided doses. For hypokalemia, 25-100 mg/d. For hirsutism, dosages of 50-200 mg/d have been used. Many hirsute patients require 200 mg/d.

---

**ACTIONS AND SIDE EFFECTS:** Spironolactone is an aldosterone antagonist. It binds competitively in the distal renal tubule and promotes sodium excretion and potassium retention. It also has antiandrogenic effects. Should not be used in a patient with significantly impaired renal function from any cause, or in any patient who is hyperkalemic. Must be evaluated periodically for the presence of hyperkalemia and/or hyponatremia. Has been shown in rats to produce dose-related adenomas of the thyroid and testis, malignant breast tumors, proliferative changes in the liver, and hepatocellular Ca. The drug and its metabolites may cross the placenta and into breast milk. They can cause feminization of the male rat fetus. Should *not* be used in pregnancy. Side effects also include abdominal cramps and diarrhea, lethargy, headaches, confusion, ataxia, impotence, gynecomastia, menstrual irregularities, postmenopausal bleeding, skin rashes, and fever.

| **Drug** | **Trade Names and Preparations** |
|---|---|

**THYROID HORMONE**

| **I. Natural Products** | Thyroid U.S.P. | 15, 30, 60, 120, 180 & 300 mg tabs |
|---|---|---|
| **DESICCATED THYROID** | Armour Thyroid | 15, 30, 60, 90, 120, 180, 240 & 300 mg tabs |
| **(THYROID U.S.P.)** | Thyrar | Bovine: 30, 60 & 120 mg tabs |
| | S-P-T | Pork thyroid in soybean oil: 60, 120, 180 & 300 mg caps |

| | Thyroid Strong | 50% stronger than thyroid U.S.P.: 30, 60 & 120 mg tabs; 30, 60, 120 & 180 mg sugar-coated tabs |
|---|---|---|

**DOSE:** Doses must be individualized with follow-up thyroid function tests to assess levels. The starting dose of desiccated thyroid is 15-30 mg po qd, depending on clinical setting. Maintenance dosages are 60-120 mg/d (1 grain = 60 mg).

| II. Synthetic Preparations<br>A. LEVOTHYROXINE SODIUM<br>(L-THYROXINE, T₄) | | (Note: doses are in *micrograms*) |
|---|---|---|
| | Levothyroxine sodium | 100 (white), 150 (blue), 200 (pink) & 300 (green) µg tabs and IV 200 & 500 µg/vial |
| | Levothroid | 25 (orange), 50 (white), 75 (gray), 88 (green), 100 (yellow), 112 (rose), 125 (purple) 137 (blue), 150 (blue), 175 (turquoise), 200 (pink) & 300 (green) µg tabs. Available as an IV preparation: 200 & 500 µg/vial |
| | Levoxyl | 25 (orange), 50 (white), 75 (purple), 88 (olive), 100 (yellow), 112 (rose), 125 (brown) 137 (aqua), 150 (blue), 175 (turquoise), 200 (pink) & 300 (green) µg scored tabs. |
| | Synthroid | 25 (orange), 50 (white), 75 (violet), 88 (olive), 100 (yellow), 112 (rose), 125 (brown), 150 (blue), 175 (lilac), 200 (pink) & 300 (green) µg scored tabs. Available as an IV preparation: 200 & 500 µg/vial |
| | Eltroxin | 50, 100, 150, 200 & 300 µg tabs |
| | Levo-T | 25, 50, 75, 100, 125, 150, 200 & 300 µg tabs |

**DOSE:** The initial and maintenance dosage of levothyroxine used depends on the age of the patient, the indication for its use, the severity of hypothyroidism, and the presence of concurrent medical conditions, such as coronary artery disease. A reasonable eventual maintenance dosage in adults is 1.7 µg/kg/d. Dosage must always be titrated to clinical response and thyroid function tests. Levothyroxine is administered IV in the Rx of myxedema coma.

| B. LIOTHYRONINE SODIUM<br>(T₃) | | (Note: doses are in *micrograms*) | | |
|---|---|---|---|---|
| | Liothyronine sodium | 25 µg tabs | Triostat | 10 µg/mL injection |
| | Cytomel | 5, 25 & 50 µg tabs | | |

**DOSE:** The usual dosage of T₃ in adults is 25-75 µg qd. (Some subdivide the dosage tid.)

| C. LIOTRIX (T₄ & T₃) | Thyrolar | Strengths: "¹/₄" (violet/wh.), "¹/₂" (peach/wh.), "1" (pink/wh.), "2" (green/wh.) & "3" (yellow/wh.) |
|---|---|---|

**INDICATIONS:** Thyroid preparations are used for (1) Rx of hypothyroidism and (2) TSH suppression.

*Natural thyroid products* are derived from beef or pork sources. Desiccated thyroid and thyroglobulin are thought by many to be obsolete. Their standardization is inexact and their shelf-lives are limited.

*Levothyroxine* is the synthetic sodium salt of the L isomer of T₄. Its t¹/₂ is about 1 wk. A steady-state serum level is reached after about 4 wk on a given dose. FDA standardization procedures recently have been improved. Bioequivalence may vary between brands, and it is suggested that they not be interchanged. See Chapters 45 and 199 for initiation guidelines for adults and Chapter 47 for pediatric doses. 0.1 mg of levothyroxine = approximately 1 gr thyroid USP.

*Liothyronine sodium* is the synthetic sodium salt of the L isomer of T₃. T₃ is rapidly metabolized and excreted. Its t¹/₂ is 1-2 d. Serum levels fluctuate widely. Postabsorptive T₃ peaks could be dangerous in the elderly and in subjects with coronary artery disease. Liothyronine is not recommended for routine thyroid hormone replacement Rx. T₃ is used (1) to prepare patients for scanning for presence of metastatic thyroid Ca in order to allow for a relatively short period between discontinuation of thyroid hormone Rx and scanning; (2) may be used in the performance of a T₃ suppression test, where it must be used with caution because it may precipitate angina pectoris or myocardial infarction; (3) myxedema coma [use injectable form q 4 hr at a rate of 65 µg/d. The initial dose ranges from 25 to 50 µg. In patients with known cardiovascular disease, start with 10 to 20 µg.

*Liotrix* is a mixture of synthetic T₄ and T₃ in a 4:1 ratio. Generally, there is no clinical advantage to its use over that of T₄ alone. All strengths of Euthroid, except "2," contain tartrazine. 60 mg of Liotrix = approximately 1 gr thyroid USP. The reference strength of Euthroid "1" = 60 µg T₄ + 15 µg T₃. This provides a so-called "thyroid equivalent" of 60 mg. Reference strength of Thyrolar "1" = 50 µg T₄ + 12.5 µg T₃. This provides a "thyroid equivalent" of 60 mg.

**ACTIONS AND SIDE EFFECTS:** Side effects of thyroid hormone Rx generally reflect hyperthyroidism secondary to overdosage. Rarely, hypersensitivity reactions may occur to vehicles in tablets.

| Drug | Trade Names and Preparations |
|---|---|

**THYROTROPIN (TSH)**

| THYROGEN | Thytropar | 1.1 mg vials & 10 mL diluent (10 IU of thyrotropic activity/vial) |
|---|---|---|

**INDICATIONS:** Adjunctive diagnostic tool for serum thyroglobulin testing with or without radioiodine imaging in the follow-up of patients with thyroid cancer [see Chap. 40].

**DOSE:** 0.9 mg IM q 24 h for 2 doses or q 72 h for 3 doses. Radioiodine administration should be given 23 h following the final thyrogen dose. Scanning is typically done 48 h after radioiodine administration and 72 h after final thyrogen dose.

**ACTIONS AND SIDE EFFECTS:** Purified recombinant form of human TSH produced by recombinant DNA technology. Side effects include nausea, weakness, dizziness, headache, and vomiting with overdosage.

| Drug | Trade Names and Preparations |
|---|---|

**THYROTROPIN RELEASING HORMONE (TRH, Protirelin)**

| | Thypinone | 500 µg/mL in 1 mL | Thyrel TRH | 500 µg/mL in 1 mL amps |
|---|---|---|---|---|
| | Relefact TRH | 500 µg/mL in 1 mL amps | | |

**INDICATIONS:** Dx agent in the assessment of (1) thyroid function; (2) pituitary or hypothalamic dysfunction; (3) adequacy of thyrotropin suppression in patients on thyroid hormone Rx [see Chap. 241].

**DOSE:** In the TRH stimulation test, protirelin is administered as a 500 µg bolus in adults. In children aged 6-16 years, 7 µg/kg, up to 500 µg.

**ACTIONS AND SIDE EFFECTS:** Protirelin is a synthetic tripeptide thyrotropin releasing hormone. It causes release of thyroid stimulating hormone and prolactin from the anterior pituitary. In acromegaly, about 2/3 of patients will have a paradoxical rise of growth hormone levels in response to protirelin. Side effects, usually minor, occur in about 50% of patients and include transient hypo- or hypertension, nausea, flushing, urge to urinate, abdominal discomfort, a metallic taste in the mouth, and headache. Occasionally a patient may experience chest or throat tightness. Rarely, seizures may occur in persons with predisposing central nervous system disease and amaurosis has occurred transiently in patients with pituitary tumors.

| Drug | Trade Names and Preparations |
|---|---|

### VASOPRESSIN DERIVATIVES

| **I. DESMOPRESSIN ACETATE** | DDAVP | 0.1 and 0.2 mg tabs |
|---|---|---|
| | DDAVP | nasal spray pump (Nasal soln of 0.1 mg/mL) |
| | DDAVP | rhinal tube delivery system (Nasal soln of 0.1 mg/mL) |
| | DDAVP | injection 4-15 μg/mL |
| | Stimate | 0.15 mg/mL nasal soln |

**DOSE:** In Rx of neurogenic diabetes insipidus, dose of DDAVP in adults is 0.5-1 mL/d (2-4 μg) IV or SC in 2 divided doses; 0.1-0.4 mL/d (10-40 mg) intranasally in 2-3 doses (100 μg = 100 IU AVP), or 0.05 mg po bid starting dose (0.1-1.2 mg/d). Enuresis: 2 puffs (0.2 mL; 20 μg) intranasally q hs (10-40 μg range); or 0.2 mg po q hs starting (0.2-0.6 mg range).

| **II. LYPRESSIN** | Diapid | 0.185 mg/mL in 8 mL bottles of nasal spray (1 spray = approx 2 posterior pituitary pressor U) |
|---|---|---|

**DOSE:** The usual dose for adults and children is 1 or 2 sprays into each nostril qid. An additional bedtime dose may be required to prevent nocturia.

| **III. VASOPRESSIN** | Vasopressin | 20 pressor U/mL in 0.5 or 1 mL amps for injection, IM or SC |
|---|---|---|
| | Pitressin Synthetic | 20 pressor U/mL in 0.5 or 1 mL amps for injection, IM or SC |

**DOSE:** Pitressin synthetic, 5-10 U, usually yields a full physiologic response in adults. In diabetes insipidus, the dosage is 5-10 U bid to tid IM or SC as needed, or intranasally on cotton pledgets, by spray or by dropper.

**INDICATIONS:** (1) Central diabetes insipidus (intranasal, oral, parenteral); (2) primary nocturnal enuresis (intranasal); (3) congenital bleeding disorders (intranasal or parenteral). Unlabeled uses include (1) management of bleeding esophageal varices; (2) congenital and acquired bleeding disorders.

----------------------------------

**ACTIONS AND SIDE EFFECTS:** These agents are derivatives of vasopressin, a posterior pituitary hormone. They have pressor and antidiuretic hormone activity. See Chapter 26 for their use in diabetes insipidus. Desmopressin acetate is 1-deamino-8-D-arginine vasopressin. It is a synthetic analog of arginine vasopressin. A single dose has an antidiuretic effect that lasts 8-20 h. By injection, its antidiuretic effect is about 10 times as potent as by the nasal route. DDAVP presently is the drug of choice in Rx of diabetes insipidus. Lypressin is 8-lysine vasopressin, which has antidiuretic activity and vasopressor effects. The peak of antidiuretic effect is 30-60 min. Its duration of action is 3-8 h. It is useful in patients who become unresponsive or have reactions to other preparations. May induce vasoconstriction if taken in excess. Pitressin is synthetic 8-arginine vasopressin. The duration of action of vasopressin is 2-8 h, and of vasopressin tannate is 24-96 h. Fluid and electrolyte status should be monitored closely to avoid fluid overload and hyponatremia. Use with caution in patients with atherosclerosis or hypertension. Side effects include hypersensitivity reactions, tremor, vertigo, abdominal cramps, bronchoconstriction, and anaphylaxis.

| Drug | Trade Names and Preparations |
|---|---|

### VITAMIN D

| **I. CALCIFEDIOL** (25[OH]D$_3$) | Calderol | 20 & 50 μg/cap |
|---|---|---|

**INDICATIONS:** (1) Renal osteodystrophy in the presence of hypocalcemia, hyperparathyroidism, osteomalacia, or proximal myopathy [see Chap. 61]; (2) hypoparathyroidism [see Chap. 60]; and (3) osteoporosis. (Calcifediol is 25-hydroxycholecalciferol or 25(OH)D$_3$. The time to optimal Rx effect is 2-4 wk. Serum calcium levels must be monitored closely and patients should be warned of the symptoms of hypercalcemia. For a discussion of individual agents, see Chapter 63.)

----------------------------------

**DOSE:** For renal osteodystrophy, 20 to 100 μg po/d. For hypoparathyroidism, 50-200 μg po/d. Some give Rx on alternate days.

| **II. CALCITRIOL** (1,25[OH]$_2$D$_3$) | Oral: | |
|---|---|---|
| | Rocaltrol | 0.25 & 0.5 μg/cap |
| | Injection: | |
| | Calcijex | 1 & 2 μg/mL for IV injection |

**INDICATIONS:** (1) Renal failure in the presence of hypocalcemia, osteodystrophy, tertiary hyperparathyroidism, osteomalacia, or proximal myopathy [see Chap. 61]; (2) hypoparathyroidism [see Chap. 60]; (3) pseudohypoparathyroidism; (4) osteomalacia; (5) tumor-induced osteomalacia; (6) X-linked hypophosphatemic rickets [see Chaps. 63 and 70]; (7) vitamin D-dependent rickets type I [see Chaps. 63 and 70]; and (8) vitamin D-dependent rickets type II [see Chap. 70]. Calcitriol is 1,25-dihydroxycholecalciferol [1,25(OH)$_2$D$_3$]. The time to optimal Rx effect for this preparation is 1-3 d. Because of its short time to onset and offset of action, calcitriol is the preparation of choice in Rx of hypocalcemia in pregnancy. It is commonly used in the Rx of renal osteodystrophy in the presence of the indications listed here. In the Rx of osteomalacia, if hypophosphatemia is present, phosphate also is added to the Rx regimen. In vitamin D-dependent rickets type II, parenteral calcium Rx may be necessary to heal the bone disease. Calcium levels should be checked at least twice weekly until the dose of calcitriol is established.

----------------------------------

**DOSE:** Starting po dosage is 0.25 μg/d. In dialysis patients, increase by 0.25 μg as needed at 4-8 wk intervals up to 1 μg/d. In hypoparathyroidism, increase at 2-4 wk intervals to 0.5-2 μg/d in adults; to 0.25-0.75 μg/d in children 1-5 yr. Other doses: 0.5-2 μg/d in X-linked hypophosphatemic rickets; 0.5-3 μg po/d in vit. D-dependent rickets type I. Also see Chapter 70; doses as high as 15-20 μg/d may be required in vitamin D-dependent rickets type II.

| **III. CHOLECALCIFEROL** (Vitamin D$_3$) | Delta-D | 400 IU tabs |
|---|---|---|
| | Vitamin D$_3$ | 1000 IU tabs |

**INDICATIONS:** (1) Dietary vitamin D supplementation and (2) Rx of vitamin D deficiency. (1 mg = 40,000 IU vitamin D activity.)

----------------------------------

**DOSE:** 400-1000 IU po/d.

| IV. DIHYDROTACHYSTEROL (DHT) | DHT | 0.125, 0.2 & 0.4 mg tabs; 0.2 mg/mL Intensol soln (20% ethanol); 0.2 mg/5 mL oral soln (4% ethanol) |
| | Hytakerol | 0.125 mg caps; 0.25 mg/mL in oil |

**INDICATIONS:** (1) Hypoparathyroidism and tetany [see Chap. 60]. Unlabeled use: Renal osteodystrophy in the presence of hypocalcemia, secondary hyperparathyroidism, osteomalacia, or proximal myopathy. DHT is a synthetic reduction product of tachysterol and is very similar to vitamin $D_3$. It is hydroxylated in the liver, but does not require renal activation. Its time to optimal Rx effect is 1-2 wk. It has only weak antirachitic activity [1/450 that of vitamin D]. 1 mg of DHT is equivalent to about 3 mg [120,000 IU] of vitamin $D_2$. Monitor serum calcium.

------------------------------------------------------------------------

**DOSE:** In renal osteodystrophy, DHT dose is 0.20-2.0 mg po/d. In hypoparathyroidism, maintenance dose is 0.2-1 mg po/d.

| V. ERGOCALCIFEROL (Vitamin $D_2$) | Drops: | |
| | Calciferol Drops | 8,000 IU/mL in 60 mL dropper |
| | Drisdol | 8,000 IU/mL in 60 mL dropper bottle |
| | Vitamin D Oral Drops | 8,000 IU/mL in 60 mL dropper bottle |
| | | |
| | Caps or Tabs: | |
| | Vitamin D | 50,000 IU/cap |
| | Calciferol | 50,000 IU/tab |
| | Drisdol | 50,000 IU/cap (with tartrazine) |
| | (Many over-the-counter small-dosage forms are available, e.g., 400, 800 & 1000 IU/cap or tab) | |
| | | |
| | Injection, IM: | |
| | Calciferol in oil | 500,000 IU/mL |

**INDICATIONS:** (1) Hypoparathyroidism [see Chap. 60]; (2) pseudohypoparathyroidism; (3) malabsorption of vitamin D; (4) vitamin D-resistant rickets; (5) vitamin D-deficient rickets [see Chap. 63]; and (6) vitamin D-dependent rickets type II [see Chaps. 63 and 70]. Ergocalciferol is vitamin $D_2$. 1.25 mg provides 50,000 IU of vitamin D activity. Its time to optimal Rx effect is 4-6 wk. This is the least expensive vitamin D preparation available. 400 IU/d of vitamin $D_2$ satisfies daily allowances for most age groups. Monitor serum calcium. Vitamin D-dependent rickets type II may respond to Rx with vitamin $D_2$. For malabsorption, ergocalciferol may be given IM.

------------------------------------------------------------------------

**DOSE:** In hypoparathyroidism in adults, dosage is 1.25-5 mg (50,000-200,000 IU) po/d [see Chap. 60]. In vit. D-resistant rickets: 12,000 to 500,000 IU/d po in adults; 1000-16,000 IU/d po in children. If compliance is a problem, 600,000 IU may be given po or IM for 1 dose [also see Chap. 70]. In vit. D-deficient rickets: 5,000-10,000 IU/d po until bone is healed. The dose then is reduced to 400 IU po/d.

| VI. PARICALCITOL (19-NOR-1α, 25-DIHYDROXY VITAMIN D) | | |
| | Zemplar | 5 µg/mL 1 & 2 mL vials |

**INDICATIONS:** Prevention and Rx of secondary hyperparathyroidism associated with chronic renal failure.

------------------------------------------------------------------------

**DOSE:** 0.04-0.1 µg/kg IV with dialysis no more frequently than qod. Adjust by 2-4 µg every 2-4 wk as needed.

------------------------------------------------------------------------

**ACTIONS AND SIDE EFFECTS:** Vitamin D products may cause hypercalcemia and the calcium-phosphate product should not exceed 70. Early symptoms include weakness, headache, somnolence, nausea, vomiting. Late symptoms include polyuria, polydipsia, irritability, generalized vascular calcification.

# CHAPTER 237

# REFERENCE VALUES IN ENDOCRINOLOGY

D. ROBERT DUFOUR

Laboratory tests are widely used by endocrinologists in the diagnosis and monitoring of disease. On receiving the results of such tests, the first thing physicians do is check to see whether the results are "normal" by comparing them with a list of values prepared by the laboratory, which commonly are referred to as "normal ranges." Textbooks often provide such lists. Although comparing a test result to a published standard may seem simple, many considerations may influence the interpretation. This chapter, instead of simply providing a list of normal values, discusses the factors that may affect the interpretation of test results as well as common situations that may change test results. Table 237-1, at the end of the chapter, lists common factors that may influence the results of each of these tests.

## REFERENCE RANGES: DO THEY MEAN "NORMAL"?

### DEFINITIONS OF NORMAL

Although one review documented seven possible meanings of the word *normal*, to most endocrinologists and their patients, normal is synonymous with *absence of disease*.[1] By corollary, *abnormal* indicates the presence of disease, which has caused a change from the normal, healthy state. A second common meaning of normal, which is derived from statistics, is often used by scientists: *a bell-shaped frequency distribution in which 95% of all results are within 2 standard deviations (SD) of the average value.* Although these two definitions do not necessarily describe the same thing, they frequently are used interchangeably in medicine, particularly in the interpretation of laboratory results.[2,3]

### REFERENCE VALUES

All clinical pathology laboratories publish a list of reference values. Until recently, these were called *tables of normal values*, with the laboratory using the term *normal* in the sense of the second definition given earlier. *Reference value* now is widely used to indicate that the value provides a reference, something to be used for comparison with a test result, rather than a declaration of values expected in normal, healthy persons.[4] This subtle but important difference is the source of much confusion among physicians seeking to interpret the results of laboratory tests. Less commonly, reference values may be established for disease, such as expected values of glycated hemoglobin in persons with varying degrees of glycemic control. Because the principles and assumptions used in establishing such reference values are similar, this latter type of reference range is not discussed further here.

### ESTABLISHMENT OF A REFERENCE RANGE

Reference ranges can be established in several ways. A sample of suitable size is needed to guarantee the statistical validity of results. Usually, 100 to 200 persons constitute a sample large enough to be valid but small enough to be workable. For many difficult or expensive procedures, published reference ranges may be based on results from fewer than 20 persons.

**Representative Sampling.**    The first assumption is that the sample is representative of the population that ultimately will be tested. Most volunteers are hospital employees, blood donors, or medical students. None of these groups is necessarily representative of the population that eventually will be examined.[5] This is especially a problem in inner city and charity hospitals, in which the usual volunteers are not likely to be from the same population as the patients. If the sample is not representative, the reference range may or may not be valid, but its validity cannot be tested.

**Absence of Disease.**    A second assumption is that no persons in the sample group have the diseases for which the testing is being done. This is important for disorders with a high prevalence of asymptomatic disease. An example is the current widespread effort to screen the U.S. population for risk factors for coronary artery disease. Autopsy studies show a high incidence of atherosclerosis in persons without symptoms.[6] Serum cholesterol is thought to be related to the development of atherosclerotic plaques.[7,8] To develop a reference range for serum cholesterol levels to separate persons without atherosclerosis from those with atherosclerosis, a sample of persons without atherosclerosis would have to be selected. This is not commonly done. Until the late 1980s, most laboratories used reference ranges derived from "normal" volunteers, many of whom actually had atherosclerosis. This led to extremely wide reference ranges in which virtually no one except those with familial hypercholesterolemia had abnormal results.[9] Currently, "reference" values for cholesterol are based on the risk of development of coronary artery disease, rather than the selection of "typical" values.[10] (Other common disorders that may affect laboratory tests are diabetes mellitus, hypertension, and alcohol abuse.)

**Conditions of Testing.**    Although the method used for obtaining samples is not commonly considered, differences in patient preparation and the technique used for venipuncture can affect test results.[11] Fasting increases bilirubin and uric acid levels, whereas glucose, triglycerides, and insulin levels increase after meals. A number of constituents show diurnal variation, including cortisol, osteocalcin, and urinary excretion of collagen fragments (N-telopeptide, deoxypyridinoline). If all volunteers are requested to come in after an overnight fast (a common instruction given by laboratories), then reference ranges will be valid only for comparing samples obtained under those conditions.[5] In most clinical settings, patients are seen at other times of the day for blood drawing, and they may have results outside the reference range solely for that reason.

In an elegant series of experiments, the effect of various forms of prevenipuncture position on test results was evaluated.[12] Drawing blood after the person stood and walked for 30 minutes before sitting down increased the apparent concentrations of proteins and protein-bound molecules (which affect many of the tests related to endocrine evaluation) by 3% to 5% over those obtained after the same person had been sitting for 30 minutes. If the person had been supine for 30 minutes before venipuncture, a 5% to 10% decrease was seen in the same constituents. Because the first condition describes the common procedure for obtaining blood from outpatients, and the second describes the usual method of obtaining blood from inpatients, different interpretations of results could easily be made. In virtually all laboratories, reference ranges are derived using samples obtained from ambulatory persons, so that some results are 8% to 15% higher than expected for supine inpatients.

### STATISTIC INTERPRETATION

**Mean and Standard Deviation.**    The typical approach in evaluating the data is to consider the central 95% of all values as the reference range. In most laboratories, this is determined by

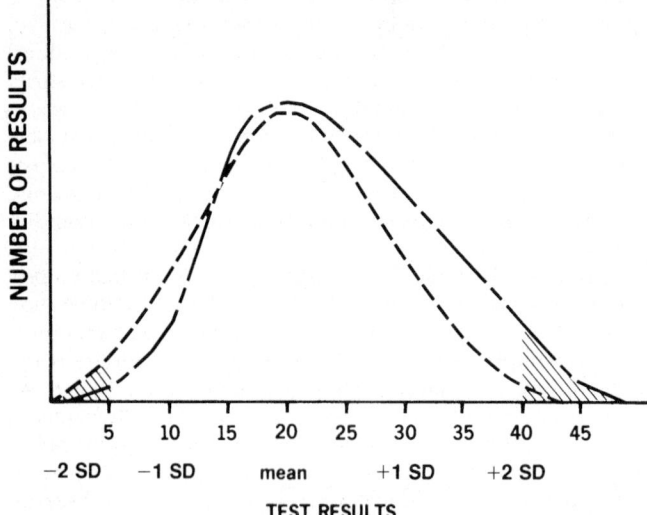

**FIGURE 237-1.** This skewed distribution of test results is typical of the pattern observed for many serum constituents. Using the mean ± 2 standard deviations (*SD*) as reference limits would falsely classify results between 0 and 5 as normal and results between 40 and 45 as abnormal.

calculating the mean and SD and defining the reference limits as the mean ± 2 SD. Several problems are associated with this seemingly simple statistical procedure. The assumption is that the data are graphically distributed in a bell-shaped fashion, that is, as the Gaussian or normal distribution. For many parameters, distribution of results is not symmetric but is skewed to one side or the other.[13] Often, the degree of skewing of the data is not enough to invalidate the assumption that values within 2 SD of the mean include 95% of all data points. Some statistical tests demonstrate whether the degree of skewing is too great for this assumption to be used.[14] Many laboratories neither inspect the data for skewing nor use these statistical tests to determine whether skewing is too great; they simply define the reference range as the mean ± 2 SD. Figure 237-1 illustrates the consequences of this approach. If values are skewed toward higher concentrations, >5% of the sample have results above the upper reference limit, and the converse is true for values skewed to lower concentrations. Even if valid sampling techniques are used, such statistical errors lead to incorrect reference limits. Evaluation of the sensitivity of several statistical techniques to differences in data distributions has shown that some are virtually unaffected by skewing of results.[15]

**Limitations of Gaussian Statistics.** An even more important problem is associated with this method of defining limits of a reference range: Gaussian statistics describe the distribution of repeated measurements of the same parameter.[16] For example, if 100 different scales were used to measure one person's weight, the chance would be 95% that the actual weight would lie within 2 SD of the average value for all weight measurements. When results obtained from populations are described, no valid statistical reason exists for selecting these limits as defining an expected range of normality. Once limits are set to include only the central 95% of all values as normal, then 5% of results from the sample are considered to be outside the reference limits, even though all persons in the sample originally were considered normal. Thus, if reference limits are used as a guide to what is normal in the medical sense, then 5% of results from the sample must indicate disease. This same condition holds true for each test performed. If each test assays an independent variable, and results for each test are distributed randomly in the population, then the likelihood that *n* tests are within the reference

range is $(0.95)^n$. The likelihood (*p*) that all independent test values are within the reference ranges (assuming that reference limits include 95% of all values) is as follows for different values of *n*: $n = 1, p = .95; n = 2, p = .90; n = 6, p = .74; n = 10, p = .60; n = 12, p = .54; n = 15, p = .46; n = 20, p = .36; n = 24, p = .29$. As *n* becomes larger and approaches the number of tests commonly included in screening profiles by many laboratories, most patients should have at least one result outside the reference limits solely because of the chance distribution of results.

Because of this statistical fact, results outside reference values are frequently produced, even for apparently healthy persons. The author has been using results of medical students' laboratory tests to illustrate this phenomenon to the students for several years. When samples were taken from 597 healthy medical students, and reference values were defined as within 2 SD of the average, only 65% of students had all "normal" test results; 27% had one "abnormal" test result; and 8% had more than one "abnormal" test result. When the central 95% of the distribution was used as the reference values (because several tests showed statistically significant skewness), the results were similar (64% had all "normal" results, 27% had one "abnormal" result, and 9% had two or more "abnormal" results), although in ~15% of students, the two methods disagreed on the number of "abnormal" results. Several publications have highlighted this statistical phenomenon and have used it to suggest that widespread screening programs are unlikely to be beneficial, because most "abnormal" results are probably the result of random statistical occurrences.[17,18] The statistical assumptions of independence become more complicated, however, because the results of many commonly measured tests change in parallel, rather than independently (i.e., sets of compounds such as serum electrolytes; calcium, phosphate, and magnesium; blood urea nitrogen and creatinine; and triiodothyronine [$T_3$], thyroxine [$T_4$], and thyroid-stimulating hormone [TSH]).

Another assumption limiting the use of reference values is that results are randomly distributed in the population, and that an individual is no more likely to have any one result than another. Many studies have shown that each individual maintains concentrations of many critical parameters within an extremely narrow range and, thus, results would not be randomly distributed in the population.[19–21] The ratio of average variation within an individual to the variation within a population has been termed the *index of individuality*. An index below 1.4 suggests that standard reference ranges will be insensitive markers of significant changes in the condition of a person. As an example, the range of cholesterol values seen in the medical students (central 95% of values) is from 126 to 252 mg/dL. In contrast, the average day-to-day variation in cholesterol level in a person in relation to his or her average blood cholesterol level is ~6% (1 SD). Thus, significant changes in serum cholesterol can occur without producing an "abnormal" result. Other common tests with small individual variation in results include calcium, alkaline phosphatase, and thyroid function tests.

## IMPLICATIONS OF A REFERENCE RANGE

The usefulness of reference ranges depends on the techniques used to establish them. Even if all of the influences have been considered, it does not follow that a result within the reference range indicates health or that a result outside the reference range indicates disease. Because the reference range is a descriptive statistic of the sample (and, if valid sampling techniques were used, of the population), then results outside the reference range indicate only that an individual is not from the same population. This could be due to disease, to population differences, or to physiologic variations in the individual. Similarly, a result within the reference range does not guarantee health, because some diseases may have a high enough prevalence in the population that the test cannot separate healthy and diseased individuals. These observations have led to several alternatives to reference ranges.

## MEDICAL DECISION LEVELS

Medical decision levels are cutoff points that reliably indicate disease or the need for additional action.[22] The limits for these values usually are wider than those for reference ranges, so that finding a result beyond these limits as a result of chance alone would be uncommon. Because they indicate the need for medical intervention, less reason exists to consider qualifying factors in interpreting results. Tables of medical decision levels are found in several articles, and one book gives medical decision levels for 137 tests.[23] Decision levels may prove useful for analytes that are commonly subject to minor, physiologic variations.

### SENSITIVITY AND SPECIFICITY

*Sensitivity* refers to the ability to detect disease, expressed as percentage of patients with disease having an abnormal test result. *Specificity* refers to the ability to exclude disease, expressed as percentage of persons without disease having a normal test result. One limitation of medical decision levels is that, although they are highly specific for disease, they tend to be less sensitive and are of less use in screening persons for early stages of a disease process that produces gradual changes in test results. Figure 237-2 shows the effect of changing the reference limits of a test to improve either sensitivity or specificity: Improving the sensitivity and specificity of a given test simultaneously is impossible. For most disease-test combinations, sensitivity and specificity are unknown.[24] In addition, the use of sensitivity and specificity has been criticized, because values usually are derived by applying the test to patients with known disease, which was confirmed by some other technique of equal or greater specificity and sensitivity. The original results for sensitivity and specificity are unlikely to remain valid when the same test is used for patients with fewer manifestations of disease.[25]

### RELATIVE OPERATING CHARACTERISTIC CURVES

*Relative operating characteristic (ROC)* curves are a graphic depiction of sensitivity and specificity over a continuous range of cutoff points or decision levels.[26] Typically, sensitivity is plotted in an ascending fashion on the Y-axis and specificity is plotted in a descending fashion on the X-axis. Such graphs are useful for selecting optimal decision points to use in diagnosing disease and for comparing the performance of diagnostic tests. The point closest to the upper left corner of the graph (perfect performance) correctly classifies the greatest percentage of patients. For comparison of two or more tests, the curve closer to the upper left corner performs better in clinical usage. Decision points can be selected to give high sensitivity or high specificity, depending on the use of the test. When medical decision levels are used, the specificity is increased to virtually 100%, meaning that all abnormal results indicate disease. Figure 237-3 illustrates a typical ROC curve for a diagnostic test. Several possible cutoff points are indicated, showing why medical decision levels have a lower sensitivity than other possible decision levels.

### INTERLABORATORY DIFFERENCES

Because laboratories use many different techniques for measuring most analytes, different cutoff values may be needed for different laboratories. Thus, some time will be required before enough universally applicable formulas are available for diagnosis of disease by laboratory tests alone.

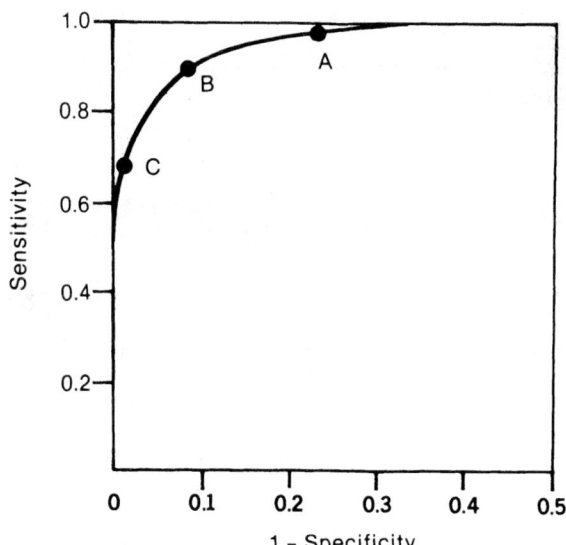

**FIGURE 237-3.** This relative operating characteristic curve illustrates the results obtained in several screening programs for primary hyperparathyroidism. *Point A* represents a serum calcium level of 10.0 mg/dL; all patients with primary hyperparathyroidism continuously have serum calcium levels above this value, but ~30% of normal persons have one or more values above this. *Point B* represents an upper reference limit of 10.5 mg/dL. Approximately 90% of serum calcium values from patients with primary hyperparathyroidism fall above this level; 5% to 8% of values from normal persons are above it, usually due to hemoconcentration. *Point C* is the medical decision level of 11.0 mg/dL recommended by Statland.[26] Only 70% of values from patients with primary hyperparathyroidism are above this level, but it reliably indicates an elevated serum calcium value of clinical significance.

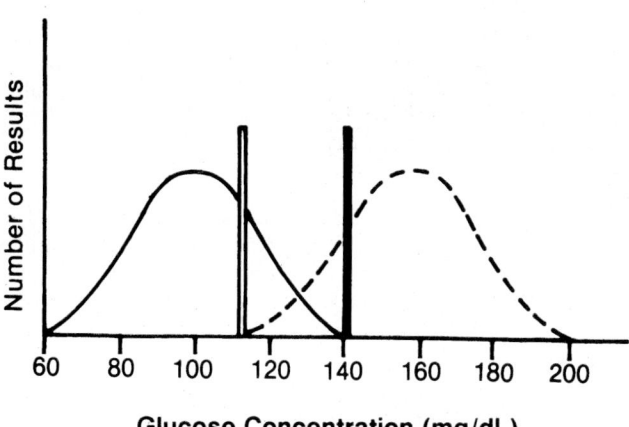

**Glucose Concentration (mg/dL)**

**FIGURE 237-2.** The distribution of fasting glucose levels in patients with normal glucose tolerance (*solid line*) and those with "diabetic" glucose tolerance (*dotted line*) illustrates the impossibility of improving both sensitivity and specificity simultaneously. Use of a fasting glucose level of 140 mg/dL (*solid bar*) to predict abnormal glucose tolerance excludes all persons with normal glucose tolerance (specificity 100%), but it misses 40% of those with abnormal glucose tolerance (sensitivity 60%). With use of a fasting glucose level of 115 mg/dL (*open bar*), sensitivity is improved to 100%, but specificity falls to 75%. With any value between these two points, specificity improves and sensitivity falls. Moving below 115 or above 140 mg/dL lowers specificity or sensitivity, respectively, without improving the other component.

## INDIVIDUAL REFERENCE RANGES

Another approach is the use of *individual reference ranges*.[4,27] The concentrations of many analytes are closely regulated in most individuals, so that the variation within a person is much smaller than the variation between persons.[19–21] With the feasibility of performing widespread population screening for different disease states and the common practice of doing "profiles" of laboratory tests as part of periodic physical examinations, a database exists for determining a person's typical concentrations of several analytes. If the results of laboratory tests are available on computers, this analysis is easier to perform. One way in which these ranges can be useful is in diagnosing myocardial infarction. In one common approach, standard reference ranges are used and serum isoenzyme determinations of creatine kinase are obtained only if the enzyme levels exceed the reference limit. In several studies, many patients with apparent myocardial infarction had extremely low baseline values for serum creatine kinase and showed acute rises in the level of this enzyme that did not exceed the upper reference limit.[28,29] Thus, comparing a patient's test results to his or her own values improves the sensitivity of creatine kinase measurements for diagnosing myocardial infarction.[30]

The use of individual reference ranges should better define the expected limits of normal physiologic changes and provide the ultimate in sensitivity for early detection of disease. As discussed earlier, intraindividual variation is generally much less than the variation seen in the population.[31] The major impediments are the extremely high cost of screening the population using every conceivable test and the enormous amount of data storage capacity required. Another possible problem is the lack of acceptable reference ranges for allowable changes in an individual. Although the studies cited provide approximate reference ranges for intraindividual variation, they are not all inclusive, and a wide difference is seen in the values given. Moreover, data suggest that intraindividual variation is greater in persons with certain disease processes.[32] A range that may detect early changes in healthy persons may be a false-positive indicator of impending complications in persons with disorders such as diabetes. Despite these problems, the use of individual reference ranges probably will increase.

## COMMON CAUSES OF "ABNORMAL" ENDOCRINE TEST RESULTS

Although reference ranges often are used to define "normal," results outside reference limits are commonly seen when no evidence of an underlying disease process is present. In this section, some frequent causes of variation in laboratory test results are described. A more complete listing is available in Table 237-1 at the end of this chapter.

### PHYSIOLOGIC INFLUENCES ON ENDOCRINE TEST RESULTS

The effects of normal physiologic changes in a patient are not often considered in interpreting laboratory findings, yet they are commonly the explanation for an unexpected test result.

#### DIET

Occasionally, dietary factors are responsible for unexpected changes, either due to the ingestion of food (e.g., transient alkalosis, intracellular shifts in phosphate, release of intestinal alkaline phosphatase into the circulation, elevated levels of hormones) or due to the chemical substances in food that cause physiologic changes (e.g., caffeine-induced catecholamine release).[33,34]

### DIURNAL AND PULSATILE RHYTHMS

Diurnal variation is a well-known phenomenon for cortisol and adrenocorticotropic hormone, but smaller degrees of diurnal variation also are found for other hormones, including prolactin, TSH, and testosterone.[35–37] Marked diurnal variation in serum iron concentrations is a common finding, and many hormones, such as gonadotropins, growth hormone, and prolactin, are released in a pulsatile fashion, such that interpreting a single test result is difficult.[38] Even for substances measured by common hematology and chemistry tests, a significant diurnal variation is seen.[38a] For measurement of most pituitary hormones, pooling several serum samples and assaying the pooled specimen provides a more accurate indication of average hormone concentration and pituitary function. For most other tests, consistently sampling in the early morning yields more reproducible results.

### PHYSICAL AND EMOTIONAL STRESS

Exercise leads to the release of catecholamines, prolactin, and muscle-specific enzymes into the circulation.[39] Even mild exercise can cause a marked increase in the frequency of menstrual irregularities,[39a] probably due to hormonal changes. Stress leads to catecholamine release; prolonged stress can cause marked changes in the concentrations of various blood lipids and hormones.[40–42] An entire section of this book (Part XVI) is devoted to the endocrine changes seen in acute illness.

### AGE

The values of many serum constituents change markedly in concentration during a person's lifetime. Although it is accepted that values may differ in children (see Chaps. 7, 18, 47, 70, 83, 87, 90–92, 157, 161, and 198), changes also occur at other times in life. For example, testosterone and renin decrease with increasing age in adults, and alkaline phosphatase and parathyroid hormone (PTH) levels continue to increase in persons older than 50 years. (Also see Chap. 199.)

### RACE

For many commonly measured parameters, values in persons of African ancestry are different from those in persons of European ancestry; differences in other races have not been evaluated as carefully. For example, blacks tend to have higher values for high-density lipoprotein cholesterol and PTH, but lower values for vitamin D metabolites and renin.

### SEX

Obvious differences are found between the sexes in levels of sex hormones and prolactin, but women and men often have different concentrations of many of the analytes commonly measured. Serum levels of free $T_4$ and copper are higher in women, but lower values for renin, aldosterone, and most blood lipids also are the rule.

### MENSTRUATION AND PREGNANCY

During the normal menstrual cycle, in addition to the obvious changes in levels of estrogens and progesterone, levels of vasopressin, prolactin, and PTH increase. The onset of menstruation causes a fall in serum sodium and phosphate levels, and a rise in renin and aldosterone concentrations. Pregnancy induces some unexpected changes: Levels of PTH, calcitonin, cortisol, and aldosterone increase, and fasting levels of glucose and glycohemoglobin (hemoglobin $A_{1c}$) fall. The effects of pregnancy may last long after the baby is delivered. Studies have shown lower levels of prolactin and dehydroepiandrosterone in women who have borne children than in those who have never been pregnant.

## HEIGHT AND WEIGHT

A person's height and weight are related to the concentrations of several substances. In children, a positive correlation is seen between height and serum alkaline phosphatase levels. Weight is much more closely associated with the concentrations of several parameters, especially in obese persons, who have higher serum concentrations of cortisol, insulin, and glucagon, but lower than normal levels of gonadotropins and sex hormone–binding globulin. Weight loss in obese persons causes changes, such as a fall in renin and aldosterone levels (see Chap. 126).

## ALTITUDE

Changes in the concentrations of many analytes are found in persons living at altitudes above 5000 ft. Although some of these changes are transient, occurring only during the process of acclimatization, others appear to persist. Persons living at these heights tend to have higher levels of erythropoietin and lower levels of renin, angiotensin II, and aldosterone.

## EFFECTS OF DRUGS ON ENDOCRINE TEST RESULTS

Drugs affect laboratory tests by two mechanisms.[43] The first is a direct pharmacologic effect of the drug, such as hypokalemia due to diuretic therapy. Although most endocrinologists are familiar with this particular effect, many unfamiliar drug effects occur. For example, anticonvulsants increase levels of alkaline phosphatase (and related enzymes such as γ-glutamyltransferase), prolactin, and vasopressin, but decrease total and free $T_4$ and 25-hydroxyvitamin D levels, as well as urinary excretion of corticosteroid metabolites.[44]

A second type of drug interference results from cross-reaction in the assay. Two common examples are the cross-reaction of phenothiazines with some assays for urinary metanephrine, and the cross-reaction of certain cephalosporins with many assays for creatinine.[45,46] Usually, information on the medications being taken by each patient tested is not given to the laboratory; even if this information were available, screening all test requests manually to detect possible drug-test interferences would be virtually impossible. With the increasing use of computers, however, it should be possible to construct a program to review the pharmacy record for each patient and search for drug interferences when abnormal results are encountered. Several comprehensive lists of drug effects on laboratory tests are available,[47,48] and a compendium of drug effects on endocrine laboratory tests is provided in Chapter 239.

## HEMOCONCENTRATION

Hemoconcentration causes an increase in proteins (e.g., albumin) and, consequently, in the level of protein-bound substances in the blood. The common causes of hemoconcentration are dehydration, postural differences, and the use of tourniquets during blood collection, but evaporation of serum after collection may produce the same effect. Ambulatory patients have a mild degree of relative hemoconcentration as a result of the shift of extracellular fluid from intravascular to extravascular locations, caused by the increased hydrostatic pressure in the upright position.[12] This causes an increase of 3% to 5% in the concentration of proteins and protein-bound substances (e.g., some hormones, lipids, and ions such as Mg, Ca, and Fe). A similar hemoconcentrating effect is produced by leaving on a tourniquet for as little as 40 seconds while drawing blood.[12] The suggested approach is to use a tourniquet only after a vein has been located and the skin has been prepared; longer use can cause 5% to 10% hemoconcentration. Fist clenching during blood collection, with a tourniquet applied, leads to leakage of muscle contents, especially potassium, which can increase by 1 to 1.5 mmol/L in as little as 1 minute.

The combined effects of posture and tourniquet use may cause a 10% to 20% increase in the apparent concentration of proteins. In one study, 15% of all persons evaluated for hypercalcemia eventually were found to have normal serum calcium levels; hypercalcemia was artifactual as a result of concentration of serum proteins.[49] In the author's laboratory, 5% to 10% of persons with "hypercalcemia" have serum albumin levels of >4.5 g/dL on initial study; usually, their calcium levels are within the reference range if their blood was collected (without prolonged use of a tourniquet) after they sat for 30 minutes. In one year, two patients were admitted for the evaluation of "hypercalcemia" that was found to be caused by hemoconcentration.

## CHANGES AFTER COLLECTION OF SPECIMENS

Difficulties occasionally arise from changes that occur in the test tube during or after specimen collection. Some of the more common specimen-related problems include hemolysis, which increases the apparent concentration of all abundant substances within cells, such as potassium, phosphate, magnesium, and enzymes; and delay in transport of the specimen to the laboratory, which allows utilization and exhaustion of glucose, after which the cells leak their intracellular contents.[50,51] Less commonly, extremely high white blood cell or platelet counts cause difficulties; the former increases the rate of glucose use, and the latter leads to the release of potassium during coagulation.[52,53] In rare instances, an interaction occurs between a substance in the collection tube and the patient's blood that causes artifactual abnormalities, such as an increase in potassium induced by heparin in patients with extremely high lymphocyte counts.[54] Renin levels increase with storage in ice water, as a result of the conversion of prorenin to renin.[55]

## CLERICAL AND ANALYTIC ERRORS

A final source of unexpected test results may be the laboratory itself if the results reported are not matched to the correct patient. Although all laboratories strive to minimize errors, such mistakes do occur. Clerical errors in specimen identification, which can occur at any time from collection to final reporting, are the single most common cause (25%) of erroneous results.[56] Less commonly, actual errors in performing the test cause incorrect results.

Explainable causes of abnormal laboratory test results always should be considered. These factors are likely if the result is only minimally outside the reference limits; if evidence exists of hemoconcentration, such as a serum albumin level above the reference limit; if patients are receiving multiple medications; or if results from the current specimen differ markedly from previous results for a patient who is clinically stable. In any of these circumstances, the best approach is to contact the laboratory and submit a new specimen. Many reference laboratories perform repeated testing at no charge or at a reduced rate to maintain good customer relationships and to document possible causes of unexpected results.

## USE OF LABORATORY TESTS IN DIAGNOSIS

Although the major purpose of this chapter is to familiarize the endocrinologist with the techniques used in laboratories that can influence the interpretation of laboratory tests, it would not be complete without a brief discussion of the uses of laboratory tests in endocrine diagnosis.

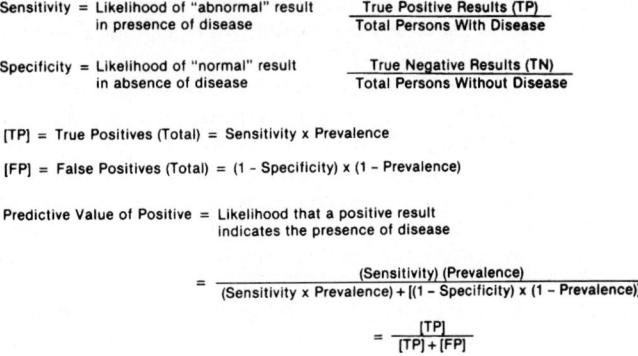

**FIGURE 237-4.** Bayes' theorem. The predictive value of a positive result answers the question: What is the likelihood that a positive result indicates the presence of disease? For any disease, increasing sensitivity or specificity of the tests used increases the predictive value. The major determinant of predictive value is disease prevalence. If the prevalence is low, then the true-positive results (*TP*) become small compared with false-positive results (*FP*), because TP = sensitivity × prevalence. The equation then reduces to TP/FP, or TP/[(1 – specificity) × (1 – prevalence)]. Because (1 – prevalence) is ~1, the predictive value is [sensitivity/([1 – specificity] × prevalence)] × prevalence.

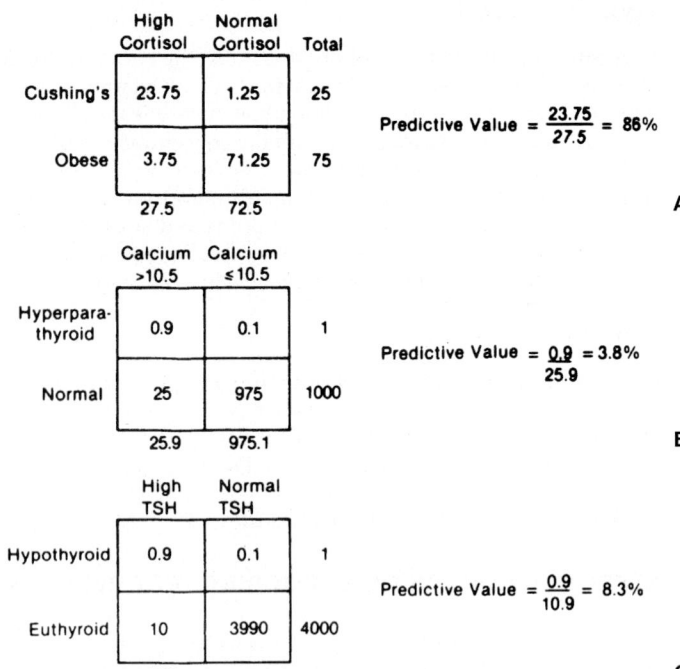

**FIGURE 237-5.** Examples of the use of Bayes' theorem. **A,** In obese patients with abdominal striae and centripetal obesity, the frequency of Cushing syndrome is ~25%. In testing 100 patients using urinary free cortisol levels, the sensitivity and specificity are each ~95%. The predictive value of elevated urinary free cortisol levels in this setting is 86%; thus, the certainty of diagnosis is increased from 25% to the higher figure by using this one test. **B,** In screening for primary hyperparathyroidism, ~90% of all serum calcium values in affected persons are above 10.5 mg/dL. Because this is the upper reference limit, 2.5% of normal persons have a serum calcium value above this figure by chance alone. In screening studies, the prevalence of hyperparathyroidism is ~1:1000. The likelihood that a serum calcium value above 10.5 mg/dL represents primary hyperparathyroidism, given only the result of the calcium test, is 3.5%. **C,** Neonatal hypothyroidism screening programs sometimes use measurements of thyroid-stimulating hormone (*TSH*) in cord blood for the initial test. Because ~10% of cases are due to hypothalamic-pituitary insufficiency, the sensitivity of such testing is 90%. The cutoff value is >3 standard deviations above the mean value for normal neonates; this excludes 99.75% of normal infants. Because the prevalence of hypothyroidism is ~1:4000 newborns, the predictive value of an elevated TSH level is ~8%, but most affected infants have an elevated TSH level. Thus, when 4000 infants are screened, only 11 infants need further studies to find the one infant with hypothyroidism.

## "ABNORMAL" TEST RESULTS—BAYES' THEOREM

Not all endocrine results that fall outside the reference range indicate disease. When such results occur, the physician must answer this question: What is the likelihood that this result indicates a particular disease in this patient? Several statistical models could be used to answer the question. The most widely publicized is Bayes' theorem.

Bayes' theorem answers the question directly, giving a numeric probability that the test result indicates a given disease. The principles of Bayes' theorem are given in Figure 237-4. The information needed to answer the question includes the frequency with which abnormal results are found in persons with the disease (sensitivity), the frequency with which normal results are found in persons without the disease (specificity), and the frequency of the disease in the population. The answer is called the *predictive value* of a positive result. Figure 237-5 illustrates the importance of disease prevalence on the predictive value. The percentage of abnormal results that indicate disease decreases as the frequency of the disease decreases.

Since the introduction of Bayes' theorem into medical use, it has found increasing application as a model for the diagnostic process, and several reviews highlighting it have appeared in the internal medicine literature.[1,57,58] The weaknesses of Bayes' theorem for medical decision making have not been emphasized. The first limitation is its use of a single decision level for predicting the presence of disease. For example, in the evaluation of hypercalcemia, a serum calcium level of 10.6 mg/dL would be treated the same as a calcium level of 12.1 mg/dL or a calcium level of 16.5 mg/dL. Few practicing endocrinologists would view such levels this way. A second obstacle is the difficulty of using Bayes' theorem for more than one variable. Although applications for multiple variables do exist, they are not commonly used, and they further compound the first limitation by looking at only a single decision level for each variable studied. Furthermore, equal emphasis is placed on each result. Physicians are well aware, however, that certain findings are virtually pathognomonic, whereas others are extremely nonspecific.

A further drawback lies not in the theorem itself, but in the way it has been used. In screening for rare diseases (e.g., neonatal hypothyroidism) or even in screening for relatively common endocrine disorders (e.g., primary hyperparathyroidism), most abnormal results from screening tests do not indicate the presence of disease. This has led many to criticize the screening of asymptomatic persons as worthless, because most abnormal results are false-positives.[17,18] The purpose of screening tests is not to make diagnoses, however, but to identify persons who are at high risk for having a disease. For example, as shown in Figure 237-5, only ~8% of infants with an elevated level of TSH have congenital hypothyroidism. What the screening program does, however, is virtually rule out hypothyroidism in 99.75% of the screened newborns. The task of finding affected infants is now much simpler because further tests can be performed only on the few infants with elevated TSH levels. Without screening, discovering infants with hypothyroidism would be like finding a needle in a haystack; screening puts the needle into a pincushion.

Bayes' theorem is an inadequate model for the diagnostic process. Although its popularization has focused attention on the inherent uncertainty in the interpretation of any data, other mathematical models and artificial intelligence systems (e.g.,

Internist) provide much closer approximations to the probability of diagnoses based on data obtained.[59]

# REFERENCE VALUES IN ENDOCRINOLOGY

Reference values should be used as a relative means of comparison, not as an absolute declaration of health or disease. Table 237-1 provides a context for the endocrinologist to interpret results for an individual patient.

Reference values are given first in the conventional units used in the United States. The conversion factor to transform these results to SI units and the reference range in SI units also are given. SI refers to the Système International, which is an attempt to create a universally accepted scientific nomenclature. This system is used widely in Europe and in other parts of the world. The SI recommends expressing concentration in moles (or fractions thereof) of a substance per liter, rather than in weight per volume. Young outlined the rationale for making this conversion. In summary, the major advantage of SI units is that they make interrelations between substances much easier to understand.[651] A good example is in the formula for calculated osmolality, in which glucose is divided by 18 and blood urea nitrogen by 2.8 to convert from weight units to moles (osmolality is related to moles of a substance in solution). In this example, expressing concentration in moles makes the calculation easy and eliminates the need for remembering the appropriate factors for conversion. Other advantages of using SI units include a better understanding of relationships between a compound and its target or receptor, and universality in the reporting system, which should improve the international usefulness of scientific studies.

The recommendation has been made that peptide hormone concentrations still be expressed in standard mass nomenclature. This decision is difficult to understand, because hormones with active forms of different molecular weights cannot be expressed accurately using such mass nomenclature. Hormone concentrations are reported in mass units; however, because all immunoassays detect molar concentrations of a substance, hormone immunoassays make use of some conversion factor. For the many hormones with multiple circulating forms, the conversion factor may be either an average molecular weight of all forms present, a weighted average, or the molecular weight of the most abundant or most physiologically important form (i.e., the immunoassay standard). Because the exact conversion factors may vary, Table 237-1 gives the conversion factor only for hormones with a single predominant circulating form.

The major disadvantage of conversion to SI units is that physicians in the United States would be required to learn a new set of reference ranges for all commonly ordered tests. Canada adopted SI units without major difficulty. In the late 1980s, several journals announced their intention to convert to SI units for all published scientific articles; however, most have returned to the use of conventional units.

The reference ranges given in Table 237-1 are those used in the author's laboratory or in the reference laboratories the author uses, employing the method listed first under "Methodologic Considerations." Reference ranges are for serum or plasma unless otherwise specified. For some tests, reference ranges published in the literature are included, with the reference number in superscript. Some of these reference ranges are based on results from fewer than 20 persons. These ranges may not be applicable to other methods or laboratories, and readers are urged to utilize reference ranges published by the laboratory they most commonly use. For tests in which reference ranges often differ by an order of magnitude (because of the lack of an acceptable standard or differences in reactivity of antibodies), the reference range carries the notation "method dependent."

For each test, the attempt has been made to define the common intraindividual, physiologic, drug-related, and methodologic factors influencing the results for a particular test. For each test, these comments apply to the specimen type (e.g., urine or serum) listed first, for the method given in the "Methodologic Considerations" column unless otherwise specified. Intraindividual variation includes day-to-day variation, within-day variation, and changes occurring during the menstrual cycle. Physiologic changes include commonly encountered alterations in expected physiology, such as exercise, obesity, pregnancy, and the effects of age, sex, and race. The effects of renal insufficiency and alcohol or tobacco use on test results also are given when indicated. This is not a comprehensive list of reference ranges for children; instead, the magnitude and direction of such changes is given. For more information on pediatric reference ranges, the reader should consult pertinent chapters of this book. In addition, two textbooks devoted to pediatric chemistry include endocrine values.[652,653] The column for drug effects includes only pharmacologic effects of drugs; cross-reactions are listed under "Methodologic Considerations," as are any special collection or handling requirements.

Several general references and a publication on drug effects are the sources of much of the data in this table.[47,48,652–659] In addition, specific references for each individual test are listed under the test name.

(see References on page 2216)

## Abbreviations

| | | | | | |
|---|---|---|---|---|---|
| ACE | = angiotensin-converting enzyme | hCG | = human chorionic gonadotropin | NCEP | = National Cholesterol Education Program |
| ACTH | = adrenocorticotropic hormone | HDL | = high-density lipoprotein | | |
| AMP | = adenosine monophosphate | 5-HIAA | = 5-hydroxyindoleacetic acid | NSAID | = nonsteroidal antiinflammatory drug |
| ANH | = atrial natriuretic hormone | HIV | = human immunodeficiency virus | PSA | = prostate-specific antigen |
| cAMP | = cyclic adenosine monophosphate | HMG-CoA | = 3-hydroxy-3-methylglutaryl coenzyme A | PTH | = parathyroid hormone |
| CEA | = carcinoembryonic antigen | HPLC | = high-performance liquid chromatography | PTHrP | = parathyroid hormone–related protein |
| DEC | = decreased | HVA | = homovanillic acid | RBC | = red blood cell |
| DES | = diethylstilbestrol | IGF-I | = insulin-like growth factor-I | RIA | = radioimmunoassay |
| DHEA | = dehydroepiandrosterone | IGFBP-3 | = insulin-like growth factor–binding protein-3 | SHBG | = sex hormone–binding globulin |
| EDTA | = ethylenediaminetetraacetic acid | INC | = increased | SI | = Système international d'Unités |
| ELISA | = enzyme-linked immunosorbent assay | IV | = intravenously | $T_3$ | = triiodothyronine |
| F | = females | LATS | = long-acting thyroid stimulator | $T_4$ | = thyroxine |
| FSH | = follicle-stimulating hormone | LDL | = low-density lipoprotein | TBG | = thyroxine-binding globulin |
| GAD | = glutamic acid decarboxylase | LH | = luteinizing hormone | THC | = tetrahydrocannabinol |
| GFR | = glomerular filtration rate | M | = males | TSH | = thyroid-stimulating hormone (thyrotropin) |
| GH | = growth hormone | MAO | = monoamine oxidase | | |
| GnRH | = gonadotropin-releasing hormone | N/A | = not applicable | VMA | = vanillylmandelic acid |

**TABLE 237-1.**
**Reference Values in Endocrinology**

| Test Name | Reference Range (Conventional Units) | Conversion Factor | Reference Range (SI Units) | Intraindividual Variation |
|---|---|---|---|---|
| α SUBUNIT[94–96] | 0–1.0 ng/mL | 1 | 0–1.0 µg/L | |
| ACE. See ANGIOTENSIN-CONVERTING ENZYME | | | | |
| ACETOACETATE[60,61,660] (see also KETONES) | 0.02–0.2 mmol/L | 1 | 0.02–0.2 mmol/L | Probably similar to ketones. |
| ACETONE. See KETONES | | | | |
| ACID PHOSPHATASE[62–64] | 0–0.5 U/L | 1 | 0–0.5 U/L | Highest in p.m. with nadir in a.m. Within-day variation 25–50%. Day-to-day variation 50–100%. |
| ACTH. See ADRENOCORTICO-TROPIC HORMONE | | | | |
| 3′,5′-ADENOSINE MONOPHOSPHATE. See CYCLIC ADENOSINE MONOPHOSPHATE | | | | |
| ADH. See VASOPRESSIN | | | | |
| ADRENOCORTICOTROPIC HORMONE[65–71] | 9–52 pg/mL | 0.22 | 2–11.5 pmol/L | INC: Highest shortly before waking, released in episodic spikes during the day, lowest in early sleep. |
| ALBUMINURIA, MINIMAL. See MICROALBUMIN, URINE | | | | |
| ALDOSTERONE[72–77,661] | Serum: Supine: 2–9 ng/dL Upright: 3–35 ng/dL | 27.7 | Supine: 50–250 pmol/L Upright: 80–970 pmol/L | While supine, decreases during day. Upright, increases progressively and remains elevated for 6 h. Day-to-day variation 40%. In women, higher in late luteal phase. |
| | Urine: High salt: 0–5 µg/d Normal salt: 2.3–31 µg/d Low salt: 17–44 µg/d | 2.77 | High salt: 0–13.9 nmol/d Normal salt: 6.4–86 nmol/d Low salt: 47–122 nmol/d | |
| ALKALINE PHOSPHATASE[78–82] | 30–130 U/L | 1 | 30–130 U/L | No diurnal variation. Day-to-day variation 5–10%. Higher in fall than in spring. |
| ALKALINE PHOSPHATASE BONE ISOENZYME[83–93,662] | M: 5.9–22.9 µg/L F: 3.9–15.1 µg/L Postmenopausal: 6.4–24.4 µg/L | 1 | M: 5.9–22.9 µg/L F: 3.9–15.1 µg/L Postmenopausal: 6.4–24.4 µg/L | Day-to-day variation 10%. Higher in fall than in spring. |
| ALKALINE PHOSPHATASE ISOENZYMES[83–93,662] | Bone: 12–84 U/L Liver: 13–92 U/L Intestine: 0–14 U/L Other: trace or less | 1 | Bone: 12–84 U/L Liver: 13–92 U/L Intestine: 0–14 U/L Other: trace or less | |
| ALUMINUM (Al)[97–100,174] | 0–6 µg/L | 0.0371 | <0.2 µmol/L | |
| AMP, CYCLIC. See CYCLIC ADENOSINE MONOPHOSPHATE | | | | |

| Physiologic Changes | Drug Effects | Methodologic Considerations |
|---|---|---|
| INC: renal failure<br>Gradually increases after age 50 years | INC: GnRH analogs | Immunometric assay: No interferences reported. |
| INC: fasting, obesity, ethanol | Same as for ketones | Enzymatic: No interferences reported.<br>Unstable on storage at room temperature. |
| INC: hemoconcentration. Other changes are seen that are method dependent; with prostatic acid phosphatase, increases after prostatic massage or prostatic biopsy for 24 h or more, slight elevations with benign prostatic hyperplasia. With total acid phosphatase assays, highest in children, marked increase at puberty, gradual decrease to adult levels by age 20. Higher in men than in women. Inversely related to sperm count. | INC: clofibrate, androgens (in women) | Spectrophotometry using thymolphthalein monophosphate as substrate; method relatively specific for prostatic acid phosphatase, agrees well with immunoassays. Heparin causes false decrease. Unstable at pH >7.0 at room temperature. Other chemical assays detect other isoenzymes of acid phosphatase from bone, platelet, and RBC; these assays may show falsely high values in hemolyzed specimens, and higher values in serum than in plasma. |
| INC: stress, pregnancy, exercise, hypoglycemia, hemoconcentration<br>DEC: weight loss, breast feeding<br>In neonates, values 2× normal during first 24 h of life. | INC: insulin, desipramine, erythropoietin, interferon-β, ketoconazole, L-dopa, mifepristone (RU-486), vasopressin<br>DEC: glucocorticoids, clonidine | Immunometric assay: Detects intact hormone, may not detect small fragments of ACTH in ectopic ACTH production, but usually reports increased levels. |
| INC: pregnancy, high temperature, prolonged fast, obesity<br>DEC: high altitude, ethanol, weight loss (in obesity), severe acute illness. Highest in neonates, adult levels by 3 mo, significantly lower over age 60.<br>Lower in blacks than in whites. | INC: volume-depleting agents, lithium, ethanol (acutely), spironolactone, verapamil<br>DEC: licorice, heparin, propranolol, ACE inhibitors, NSAIDs, ranitidine. Nifedipine decreases the response to the upright position. | RIA: A variety of steroids interfere in urine assays. β-adrenergic antagonists and calcium-channel blockers increase aldosterone/renin ratio but rarely cause significant elevation of aldosterone. Urine requires boric acid as a preservative. |
| INC: pregnancy, periods of bone growth, after meals, hemoconcentration, renal failure<br>Higher in blacks than in whites and higher in men than in women (until after menopause). Higher in persons of blood groups O and B, especially after meals.<br>Higher in children, rises during puberty and then falls to adult levels by age 20. Stable until age 50, then rises in both sexes. In adults, directly related to body mass, inversely related to height. In infants, transient marked elevations may occur after acute illness. | INC: drugs causing cholestasis, lithium, anticonvulsants (especially phenytoin)<br>DEC: oral contraceptives, clofibrate, tamoxifen, glucocorticoids | Spectrophotometric: Many anticoagulants (EDTA, fluoride, oxalate) inhibit the enzyme reaction and cause falsely decreased results. The method is zinc dependent; patients with zinc deficiency show falsely low values. Transiently low after blood transfusion, probably due to zinc chelation. Valproic acid causes slight overestimation in some methods, whereas methylxanthines inhibit alkaline phosphatase activity. |
| INC: renal failure, lactation<br>Higher in children, increases at puberty, declines to reach adult levels by age 20. Higher in men than in women until after menopause, when values become higher in women. Increases throughout pregnancy. Increases with age older than 50 yr. | INC: lithium, phenytoin<br>DEC: clofibrate | Immunoassay: Approximately 3% cross-reactivity with liver isoenzyme. Does not agree well with results of immunoinhibition assays in course of treatment of metabolic bone disease. |
| Bone: Higher in children, increase at puberty, decline to reach adult levels by age 20 yr. Higher in men than in women. Both bone and liver isoenzymes increase with age >50 yr. Bone isoenzyme increases throughout pregnancy and remains elevated during lactation. | Bone: INC: lithium, phenytoin<br>Bone: DEC: clofibrate<br>Liver: INC: anticonvulsants (especially phenytoin), drugs causing cholestasis<br>Liver: DEC: oral contraceptives | High-resolution electrophoresis: Resolves bone, liver, intestinal, placental isoenzymes. Standard electrophoresis resolves all isoenzymes except bone and liver. Heat fractionation is poorly reproducible and relatively inaccurate in most laboratories. |
| INC: hemoconcentration<br>Reflects recent exposure; returns to normal within months if only single exposure. Serum correlates poorly with total body aluminum. | INC: aluminum-containing antacids, sucralfate (in renal failure) | Atomic absorption: Contamination from glass, needles, and heparin a significant problem. |

(continued)

**TABLE 237-1.**
Reference Values in Endocrinology  (Continued)

| Test Name | Reference Range (Conventional Units) | Conversion Factor | Reference Range (SI Units) | Intraindividual Variation |
|---|---|---|---|---|
| ANDROSTANEDIOL GLUCURONIDE[101–105] | M: 270–1500 ng/dL<br>F: 60–300 ng/dL | 0.021 | M: 5.6–31.2 nmol/L<br>F: 1.2–6.2 nmol/L | Higher in a.m. than in p.m. In women, lower in follicular than in luteal phase. |
| ANDROSTENEDIONE[103–111] | 60–300 ng/dL | 0.0349 | 2.1–10.5 nmol/L | Highest in a.m., lowest in p.m. In women, highest at midcycle, 40% lower at onset of menses. Approximately 30–50% day-to-day variation. |
| ANGIOTENSIN I[76,112] | <25 pg/mL | 1 | <25 ng/L | INC: upright position, during sleep |
| ANGIOTENSIN II[76,113–115] | 10–60 pg/mL | 1 | 10–60 ng/L | INC: upright position |
| ANGIOTENSIN-CONVERTING ENZYME[75,76,116–120,663,664] | 18–55 U/L | 1 | 18–55 U/L | 10% day-to-day variation |
| ANION GAP | 7–14 mEq/L | 1 | 7–14 mmol/L | See sodium, bicarbonate, chloride. |
| ANP. See ATRIAL NATRIURETIC PEPTIDE<br>ANTIDIURETIC HORMONE. See VASOPRESSIN | | | | |
| ANTI–GLUTAMIC ACID DECARBOXYLASE[121–126] | 0–1.0 U/L | 1 | 0–1.0 U/L | |
| ANTI–21 HYDROXYLASE[127–130] | 0–1.0 U/L | 1 | 0–1.0 U/L | |
| ANTI–IA2[125,130,131] | 0–0.07 U/L | 1 | 0–0.07 U/L | |
| ANTI–ISLET CELL ANTIGENS[126,132–134] | Negative | | Negative | |
| ANTITHYROGLOBULIN[135] | 0–2.0 U/mL | N/A | 0–2.0 U/mL | |
| ANTI–THYROID MICROSOMES | 0–1.0 U/mL | N/A | 0–1.0 U/mL | |
| ANTI–THYROID PEROXIDASE[136–138,686–688] | 0–2.0 U/L | 1 | 0–2.0 U/L | |
| APOLIPOPROTEIN A-I[139–148] | 119–240 mg/dL | 0.01 | 1.2–2.4 g/L | Highest at 8 p.m., falls to lowest at 6 a.m. Day-to-day variation 7%. |

| Physiologic Changes | Drug Effects | Methodologic Considerations |
|---|---|---|
| Higher in younger than in older men. Higher in whites than in Asians. Decreases with increasing age >45 yr. | INC: DHEA | RIA: No interferences reported. |
| INC: obesity, smoking, after meals, exercise, pregnancy<br>DEC: chronic illness<br>Low in children; rises gradually with peak at puberty; gradual decrease throughout life, rapidly after menopause. Higher in whites than in blacks or Asians. | INC: clomiphene, metyrapone, cimetidine, DHEA (in women)<br>DEC: carbamazepine, ketoconazole, Norplant | RIA: Different antibodies give differing results. |
| Highest in neonates, decreases to adult levels by age 5. | INC: oral contraceptives | RIA: If plasma not separated and frozen immediately, levels rise due to renin action on angiotensinogen. |
| INC: first trimester of pregnancy<br>Highest in neonates, decreases to adult levels by age 5 yr. | INC: estrogens; volume-depleting agents<br>DEC: ACE inhibitors | RIA: Assay detects largely cross-reacting substances; venous levels 50–75% of arterial; hemolysis causes falsely low values; delay in separation causes increase due to renin action. |
| INC: hemoconcentration, HIV infection, ethanol<br>DEC: pregnancy, acute illness, smoking<br>Highest in newborns, falls to adult levels by 6 mo; rises after age 4 yr. Falls to adult levels during adolescence (later in boys than in girls). Levels directly related to $T_4$ concentration. | DEC: ACE inhibitors | Spectrophotometric: Heparin, EDTA cause artifactual decreases. Freezing of specimen causes 15% decrease in results. |
| See sodium, bicarbonate, chloride. | See sodium, bicarbonate, chloride. | Calculated using formula $Na - (Cl + HCO_3)$. Results vary from one instrument to another; individual laboratory reference values should be used. |
| Frequency of positive results higher in whites than in Asians. | | Immunoassay: No interferences reported. Positive in 60–80% of type 1 diabetes patients at time of diagnosis and persists for many years in 30–50%. Radiobinding assays have slightly higher sensitivity than ELISA methods. Also positive in a small percentage of patients with type 2 diabetes. |
| | | Immunoassay: No interferences reported. Rarely present in other autoimmune diseases in children, but may be seen with other endocrinopathies in adults. Titers decline with increasing duration of disease and are often negative after several years. |
| | | Immunoassay: no interferences reported. Positive in 50–70% of type 1 diabetes patients at time of diagnosis. Titers decline with increasing duration of disease but remain positive in a minority of patients, particularly those with onset at young age. |
| | | Immunofluorescence of tissue: Results from this method and ELISA methods do not always agree. Antibody titers and frequency of positive results fall with duration of disease and are more likely to become negative than anti-GAD. |
| Present in low titers in 10–15% of normal adults; prevalence increases with increasing age. | | Several methods; competitive protein-binding method gives false-positive results in persons after iodine-131 ($^{131}$I) administration. Elevated thyroglobulin causes false-positive in some assays. |
| Present in low titers in 10–25% of normal adults; prevalence increases with increasing age. | | Several methods; competitive protein-binding method gives false-positive results in persons after $^{131}$I administration. |
| INC: pregnancy<br>During pregnancy, falls during second and third trimesters. Increased prevalence with increasing age. More commonly found in women than in men. | | Immunoassay: No interferences reported. With thyroid disease, titers often decline with treatment. |
| INC: ethanol, hemoconcentration, pregnancy (30% increase), exercise<br>DEC: smoking, ethanol withdrawal, weight loss<br>Higher in women than in men, higher in blacks than in whites. In children, falls after puberty in boys but not girls. | INC: oral contraceptives, anticonvulsants, estrogen, clofibrate, HMG-CoA reductase inhibitors, gemfibrozil, niacin<br>DEC: estrogen/progesterone cycling, probucol, Norplant, phenytoin, valproic acid | Immunoassay: No interferences reported. |

(continued)

**TABLE 237-1.**
Reference Values in Endocrinology  (Continued)

| Test Name | Reference Range (Conventional Units) | Conversion Factor | Reference Range (SI Units) | Intraindividual Variation |
|---|---|---|---|---|
| APOLIPOPROTEIN B[139–148] | 52–163 mg/dL | 0.01 | 0.5–1.6 g/L | No diurnal variation. Day-to-day variation 10%. |
| ASCORBIC ACID. See VITAMIN C | | | | |
| ATRIAL NATRIURETIC HORMONE[149–158] | 30–77 pg/mL | 1 | 30–77 ng/L | Diurnal variation seen only in older individuals, with values highest around 4 a.m., lowest approximately noon. Within-day variation 10–20%. In women, similar in follicular and luteal phases with slight rise after menstruation begins. |
| β-ENDORPHIN[255–264] | 10–30 pg/mL | 1 | 10–30 ng/L | Highest in a.m., lowest in p.m.; changes parallel those of ACTH. In women, peaks at time of ovulation and again with onset of menses. |
| β-HYDROXYBUTYRATE[83,84,719] | <0.42 mmol/L | 1 | <0.42 mmol/L | Day-to-day variation 60%. Probably similar to that of ketone bodies. |
| β-HYDROXYBUTYRIC ACID. See β-HYDROXYBUTYRATE | | | | |
| BICARBONATE[159] | 22–30 mEq/L | 1 | 22–30 mmol/L | 30% day-to-day variation in normal individuals; highest in spring, lowest in summer; in women, lowest during menses. |
| BIOAVAILABLE TESTOSTE-RONE. See TESTOSTERONE, BIOAVAILABLE | | | | |
| BONE Gla PROTEIN. See OSTEOCALCIN | | | | |
| Ca. See CALCIUM | | | | |
| CADMIUM[160,161] | <0.5 µg/dL | 0.089 | <0.045 µmol/L | Values reflect recent exposure only. |
| CALCITONIN[162–168] | Serum: <10 pg/mL Urine: 40–370 pg/mg creatinine | 0.29 0.033 | Serum: <2.9 pmol/L Urine: 1.3–12.2 pmol/mmol creatinine | No diurnal variation |
| CALCIUM, IONIZED[171,175–181] | 4.7–5.2 mg/dL | 0.25 | 1.17–1.29 mmol/L | Highest at 8 a.m., 2% day-to-day variation |
| CALCIUM, TOTAL[171,182] | 8.9–10.5 mg/dL Urine: <250 mg/d | 0.25 0.025 | 2.23–2.63 mmol/L Urine: <63 mmol/d | 1–3% variation day-to-day; highest at 8 p.m., lowest at 4 a.m. Lowest in winter, highest in summer. |
| CARCINOEMBRYONIC ANTIGEN[183–185] | 0–5 ng/mL | 1 | 0–5 µg/L | 35% day-to-day variation (reported in individuals with elevated CEA). |

| Physiologic Changes | Drug Effects | Methodologic Considerations |
|---|---|---|
| INC: smoking, hemoconcentration, pregnancy (100% increase)<br>Higher in men than in women and in whites than in blacks; increases with age, especially after age 50. | INC: chlorthalidone, retinoids (>100%), progestational agents<br>DEC: HMG-CoA reductase inhibitors, phenytoin, phenobarbital, valproic acid | Immunoassay: No interferences reported. |
| INC: supine position, volume expansion, renal failure, pregnancy, starvation, ethanol<br>DEC: volume depletion<br>Higher in women than in men, increases with increasing age in adults. In children, highest in first week, falls to adult levels by 4–6 d. | INC: glucocorticoids, mineralocorticoids, catecholamines<br>DEC: ACE inhibitors | RIA: Probably labile, specimens should be collected in EDTA and plasma frozen immediately after separation. If plasma not extracted before analysis, overestimation of ANH occurs, possibly due to alteration of the iodine-labeled ligand. Hemolysis, heparin cause falsely low results. |
| INC: after meals, exercise, renal failure, ethanol, fasting, obesity, stress, caffeine<br>DEC: pregnancy, weight loss<br>High in neonates, falls to nadir by 5 d; gradually increases to adult levels by onset of puberty. | DEC: glucocorticoids, oral contraceptives | RIA: No interferences reported. |
| INC: starvation, obesity, ethanol | Same as for ketones | Enzymatic: No interferences reported. |
| INC: during sleep<br>DEC: exercise, prolonged fast | INC: volume-depleting agents, mineralocorticoids, carbenicillin, glucocorticoids<br>DEC: carbonic anhydrase inhibitors, spironolactone | Enzymatic: No interferences reported. $CO_2$ content usually measured in venous blood; this is 1–2 mmol/L higher than $HCO_3$. In arterial blood gases, $HCO_3$ is calculated; in acute illness, differences in ionic strength may make this calculation incorrect, whereas $CO_2$ content is accurate. With all methods, delay in analysis causes a decrease in concentration. With one ion-selective electrode, salicylate, ketones, and naproxen interfere, causing falsely high results. |
| INC: smoking | None known | Atomic absorption; Na salts may interfere. |
| INC: pregnancy, renal failure<br>DEC: exercise (acutely)<br>Higher in men than in women; decreases after menopause. Higher in children, values decrease with age. | INC: epinephrine, oral contraceptives, calcium (IV), pentagastrin | RIA: The most specific assays for mature calcitonin use a two-site immunoradiometric assay. For measurement of procalcitonin and calcitonin precursors, see Chapter 53. |
| INC: upright posture, meals, acidosis, tourniquet, exercise<br>DEC: alkalosis<br>Values highest in neonates, decrease through childhood to reach adult levels by mid to late teens.<br>Decreases with age. | INC: DES, thiazides, chlorthalidone, androgens, calcium carbonate, vitamin D, lithium<br>DEC: carbamazepine, phenytoin, estrogens, fluorides, foscarnet, furosemide, glucocorticoids, laxative abuse, octreotide, tetracycline | Ion-selective electrode: Differences in sodium and protein content may cause slight differences. Delay in measurement increases values, as glucose metabolism lowers pH and causes increase in ionized calcium in vitro. Use of nonbuffered or liquid heparin falsely decreases results. Nomograms for calculating ionized calcium from total calcium and protein are inaccurate, especially for acutely ill persons. |
| INC: hemoconcentration, upright posture, after meals, immobilization of patient, exercise<br>DEC: supine position, pregnancy, lactation, age >50 yr<br>Highest in neonates, reaches adult level by 1 yr; decreases in adults due to decrease in albumin. Urine calcium: higher in men than in women; directly related to dietary calcium. | Same as for ionized calcium | Spectrophotometric: No major interferences and correlates well with results from atomic absorption, the reference method, except in specimens contaminated with calcium-chelating anticoagulants, notably EDTA. In urine, calcium may precipitate and/or bind to plastic containers; addition of acid after collection prevents falsely decreased values. |
| INC: smoking, liver disease, hemoconcentration, renal failure | | Immunoassay: Heparin interferes in assays, causing falsely elevated results with one antibody and falsely decreased results with another. Because CEA is not a single substance but a family of compounds, immunoassays may differ in their ability to measure CEA in a patient and occasionally may be falsely negative. Results between two assays should be compared when a patient is going to be followed with a different CEA assay. |

(continued)

**TABLE 237-1.**
**Reference Values in Endocrinology  (Continued)**

| Test Name | Reference Range (Conventional Units) | Conversion Factor | Reference Range (SI Units) | Intraindividual Variation |
|---|---|---|---|---|
| CAROTENE[186–190] | 10–85 µg/dL | 0.0186 | 0.19–1.6 µmol/L | 5–10% day-to-day variation; no diurnal variation. Lowest in spring, 50% higher in fall. |
| CATECHOLAMINES[34,169,191–198, 666–678] | NOREPINEPHRINE<br>Plasma: 65–400 ng/L<br>Urine: 10–80 µg/d<br>EPINEPHRINE<br>Plasma: 0–70 ng/L<br>Urine: 0–20 µg/d<br>DOPAMINE<br>Plasma: 0–35 ng/L<br>TOTAL FREE<br>Urine: 0–100 µg/d | 5.91<br><br>5.46<br><br>6.53<br><br>5.91 | NOREPINEPHRINE<br>Plasma: 380–2365 pmol/L<br>Urine: 59–470 nmol/d<br>EPINEPHRINE<br>Plasma: 0–380 pmol/L<br>Urine: 0–109 nmol/L<br>DOPAMINE<br>Plasma: 0–230 pmol/L<br>TOTAL FREE<br>Urine: 0–591 nmol/d | Episodic release with marked diurnal variation; lowest at night; in women, highest at midluteal phase. Urine levels peak at 6 p.m., lower in a.m., lowest during sleep. Output directly related to emotional state at time of collection of urine. Day-to-day variation 10–20%, lowest variation is for dopamine. |
| **CCK. See CHOLECYSTOKININ**<br>**Cd. See CADMIUM**<br>**CEA. See CARCINOEMBRY-**<br>**ONIC ANTIGEN** | | | | |
| CERULOPLASMIN[199–200] | 25–65 mg/dL | 10 | 250–650 mg/L | Day-to-day variation 10–15%. |
| CHLORIDE | 100–109 mEq/L | 1 | 100–109 mmol/L | 1% day-to-day variation. Slight increase just before menses. |
| **CHOLECALCIFEROL. See**<br>**VITAMIN D** | | | | |
| CHOLECYSTOKININ[201–208] | <80 pg/mL | 1 | <80 ng/L | In women, higher in luteal than in follicular phase. |
| CHOLESTEROL[9–10,40,209,210] | NCEP recommended decision levels:<br>Borderline high: >200 mg/dL<br>High: >240 mg/dL | <br><br><br>0.0259 | NCEP recommended decision levels:<br>Borderline high: >5.18 mmol/L<br>High: >6.22 mmol/L | 7% day-to-day variation. 3–5% higher in winter, lowest in summer. In women, 10–20% lower in luteal phase of cycle, lowest during menstruation. |
| **CHOLESTEROL, HDL. See**<br>**HIGH-DENSITY LIPOPRO-**<br>**TEIN CHOLESTEROL**<br>**CHOLESTEROL, LDL. See LOW-**<br>**DENSITY LIPOPROTEIN**<br>**CHOLESTEROL** | | | | |
| CHORIONIC GONADOTRO-PIN, HUMAN[211–213,689,690] | Nonpregnant F: <5 mIU/mL<br>Pregnant F: <100,000 mIU/mL<br>See "Physiologic Changes" | 1 | Nonpregnant F: <5 IU/L<br>Pregnant F: <100,000 IU/L | Released in episodic spikes during first trimester of pregnancy. |
| CHROMIUM[214,215] | Serum: 0–1.4 µg/L<br>Urine: 0–2 µg/L | 19.2 | Serum: 0–27 nmol/L<br>Urine: 0–38 nmol/L | |
| CHROMOGRANIN A[691–694] | 1.6–5.6 ng/mL | 1 | 1.6–5.6 µg/L | |

| Physiologic Changes | Drug Effects | Methodologic Considerations |
|---|---|---|
| INC: pregnancy, after meals, hyperlipidemia, hemoconcentration<br>DEC: high fever, smoking, ethanol<br>Higher in women than in men. Low in neonates, transient rise from 6–12 mo, fall until 2 yr, slight rise to 6 yr and fall to adult levels by age 14. Gradual decrease in persons over age 40. | DEC: colestipol, estrogens | Spectrophotometric: Hemolysis causes falsely decreased values. Carotene is unstable in light, so specimens must be wrapped in foil after collection. |
| INC: stress (mental, physical; even stress of venipuncture), standing posture, exercise, smoking, ethanol, caffeine, parenteral nutrition<br>DEC: after meals<br>Norepinephrine is higher in persons over age 60, whereas epinephrine is lower in those over 60. In children, total values increase with age, but ratios of catecholamines to creatinine decrease progressively to age 12. | INC: calcium-channel blockers, methylxanthines, MAO inhibitors, phenothiazines, nitroglycerin, L-dopa (dopamine only), nifedipine, tricyclic antidepressants (norepinephrine only), nicotine patch<br>DEC: clonidine, reserpine, guanethidine, bretylium, bromocriptine, dexamethasone, radiographic contrast agents (urine) | Several different methods in use; all show poor reproducibility. Fluorometric assay worst, shows many cross-reacting substances (salicylate, erythromycin, ampicillin, chloral hydrate, quinine, quinidine, tetracycline). Chromatographic methods cross-react with α-methyl dopa, L-dopa, isoproterenol. Bananas cause increase in total but not free catecholamines. Other foods show somewhat less interference. Catecholamines are unstable on storage at room temperature unless the specimen is acidified to pH <3. |
| INC: pregnancy, smoking, exercise, acute illness, malignancies, hemoconcentration<br>Higher in women than in men; lower in newborns, rapidly rises to adult levels. | INC: androgens, oral contraceptives, estrogens, phenytoin, phenobarbital | Immunoassay: Ceruloplasmin unstable stored at room temperature; specimens must be frozen promptly. Hemolysis causes false decrease in assays measuring ceruloplasmin's enzymatic activity. |
| INC: response to renal bicarbonate loss, ethanol<br>DEC: after meals, renal bicarbonate retention<br>Lower in blind persons. | INC: drugs favoring renal bicarbonate loss<br>DEC: antacids, drugs favoring bicarbonate retention, drugs causing renal sodium loss | Electrochemical: Bromine cross-reacts with this and most other assay methods. |
| INC: After meals; response to meals is increased in diabetics, and abolished after vagotomy. | INC: caffeine<br>DEC: Response to meals abolished by atropine. | RIA: Specimen should be frozen promptly to prevent in vitro degradation. Assays not directed against cholecystokinin-specific epitopes show cross-reactivity with gastrin. Different molecular forms may show differing reactivity with antisera. |
| INC: pregnancy (75% increase in third trimester), smoking, hemoconcentration, mental stress, ethanol<br>DEC: major illness or surgery (falls by 40% after myocardial infarction), at puberty (in men only), exercise<br>Values higher in blind persons. Higher in whites than in blacks after puberty. Gradually rises after puberty in men and women of all races; in women, rises sharply after menopause. | INC: L-asparaginase, glucocorticoids, phenothiazines, phenytoin, chlorthalidone, thiazides, salicylates, retinoids, some oral contraceptives, β-adrenergic antagonists<br>DEC: chlorpropamide, haloperidol, estrogens, neomycin, thyroid hormones, ketoconazole, calcium-channel blockers | Enzymatic (95% of laboratories): α-Methyldopa, ascorbic acid, and bilirubin inhibit the reaction and cause underestimation of cholesterol; DHEA cross-reacts when markedly elevated. Specimens collected in EDTA are 3% lower due to dilution. Capillary blood, as used in satellite laboratory testing, may give different results than venous blood. Most laboratories now have standardized their methods with certified reference material from the Lipid Research Clinics to guarantee accuracy. |
| INC: pregnancy<br>DEC: smoking (20% lower in pregnant smokers)<br>During pregnancy, doubles in concentration every 1.5–2.5 d during the first 8–12 wk; peaks at 12 wk; falls to plateau at ~20 wk and remains constant to term. Higher in multiple gestations, higher with female than with male fetuses. | | RIA: The sera of some women contain substances that cross-react with antisera to hCG in some assays, but not in others; this appears to be due to varying detection of fragments of LH and hCG by different immunoassays. In urine, false-negative results occur with dilute specimens, and false-positive results with proteinuria. |
| DEC: pregnancy | | Atomic absorption: Steel needles cause marked contamination unless at least first 5 mL blood discarded; glass tubes cause mild contamination that increases on storage for as little as 1 h; hemolysis releases chromium from RBCs, causing increased values. |
| INC: renal insufficiency, hypertension, exercise, stress | | Immunoassay: Different tumors produce different-sized fragments that may react differently, depending on the epitope identified by the antibodies used in the assay. |

(continued)

TABLE 237-1.
Reference Values in Endocrinology  (Continued)

| Test Name | Reference Range (Conventional Units) | Conversion Factor | Reference Range (SI Units) | Intraindividual Variation |
|---|---|---|---|---|
| Cl. See CHLORIDE | | | | |
| CO$_2$ CONTENT. See BICAR-BONATE | | | | |
| COBALT[214–217] | Serum: 0–1.8 µg/L<br>Urine: 0–2 µg/L | 17 | Serum: 0–30.6 nmol/L<br>Urine: 0–34 nmol/L | |
| COLLAGEN TELOPEPTIDES, N AND C. See TELOPEPTIDE C and TELOPEPTIDE N | | | | |
| COPPER[218–223,669,670] | Serum: 70–155 µg/dL<br>Urine: <60 µg/d | 0.157<br>0.0157 | Serum: 11–24 µmol/L<br>Urine: <0.94 µmol/d | Highest after meals. Day-to-day variation 5%. Lowest in a.m., highest in midafternoon. |
| CORTICOSTERONE[224] | M: 1.0–4.6 ng/mL<br>F: 1.0–7.4 ng/mL | 2.89 | M: 2.9–13.3 nmol/L<br>F: 2.9–21.4 nmol/L | |
| 18-OH CORTICOSTERONE. See 18-HYDROXYCORTICO-STERONE | | | | |
| CORTICOTROPIN. See ADRENOCORTICOTROPIC HORMONE | | | | |
| CORTICOTROPIN-RELEASING HORMONE[695,696] | 24–40 pg/mL | 1 | 24–40 ng/L | |
| CORTISOL[70,225–234,697] | a.m.: 5–25 µg/dL<br>4 p.m.: <4–10 µg/dL<br>11 p.m.: <5 µg/dL<br>Urine free: 10–90 µg/d | 28<br><br><br>2.8 | a.m.: 140–700 nmol/L<br>4 p.m.: 96–280 nmol/L<br>11 p.m.: <250 nmol/L<br>Urine free: 28–250 nmol/d | Highest near time of rising, lowest around 4 a.m.; in individuals working nights, pattern changes. Day-to-day variation 15%.<br>Higher in upright position. Episodic release, difficult to evaluate a single result. |
| C PEPTIDE (INSULIN)[235–237] | Serum: 0.3–3.7 µg/L<br>Urine: 24–86 µg/d | 0.33<br>0.33 | Serum: 0.1–1.23 nmol/L<br>Urine: 8–29 nmol/d | Day-to-day variation 10–25%. |
| Cr. See CHROMIUM | | | | |
| CREATININE[46,671,672] | 0.6–1.4 mg/dL<br>Urine: 1–2 g/d | 88.4<br>8.8 | 53–124 µmol/L<br>Urine: 88–176 mmol/d | Highest in evening and at night; day-to-day variation 15–20%. |
| CRH. See CORTICOTROPIN-RELEASING HORMONE | | | | |
| Cu. See COPPER | | | | |
| CYCLIC ADENOSINE MONOPHOSPHATE[238–243] | Urine: 1.0–11.5 µmol/L<br>Plasma: 4–20 nmol/L | 1 | Urine: 1.0–11.5 µmol/L<br>Plasma: 4–20 nmol/L | Highest at noon, lowest at night.<br>Lower in upright position.<br>Highest in spring, lowest in winter.<br>Urine excretion higher in luteal than in follicular phase. |
| CYSTINE | Urine: 10–100 mg/d | 8.33 | Urine: 83–833 µmol/d | |
| DEHYDROEPIANDROSTER-ONE[71,103,108,226,244–248] | 160–700 ng/dL | 0.0347 | 5.6–24.3 nmol/L | Approximately 30% day-to-day variation; highest in a.m., lowest in p.m. |

| Physiologic Changes | Drug Effects | Methodologic Considerations |
|---|---|---|
| | INC: joint prostheses | Atomic absorption: Steel needles, glass tubes, hemolysis may cause artifactual increase. |
| INC: pregnancy, lactation, hemoconcentration, malignancies, ethanol, proteinuria (urine Cu)<br>DEC: heavy exercise, vegetarian diet<br>Lower in newborn infants, reaches adult levels by 4–5 mo.<br>Increases with age >60 yr; higher in women than in men. | INC: oral contraceptives, estrogens, carbamazepine, phenytoin, phenobarbital<br>DEC: penicillamine | Atomic absorption: Lower in heparinized plasma than in serum; rubber stoppers may be a source of contamination; freezing causes separation, may increase results if sample not well mixed. |
| INC: depression<br>Higher in premature than in term infants. | | RIA: No reported interferences. |
| INC: exercise, pregnancy<br>In pregnancy, rises after first trimester to levels 50 times higher at term. | | Immunoassay: No interferences reported. |
| INC: stress, pregnancy, short-term exercise, obesity, smoking, after meals, malnutrition, fasting, hemoconcentration, ethanol<br>INC (urine free cortisol): pregnancy, heavy exercise, malnutrition, stress, ethanol<br>Lower in blind persons.<br>Increases with age in women but not in men.<br>Urine free cortisol higher in men than in women.<br>Reference values are for ambulatory persons; mean levels approximately two-fold higher in acutely ill persons. | INC: amphetamines, carbamazepine, estrogens, interferon-β, oral contraceptives, mifepristone (RU-486), vasopressin, tricyclic antidepressants; licorice, oral contraceptives increase urine free cortisol.<br>DEC: glucocorticoids, lithium, L-dopa, megestrol acetate, oxazepam, ketoconazole, danazol, ephedrine; diuretics, ketoconazole decrease urine free cortisol. | Immunoassay: Results method dependent. Prednisone, prednisolone, cortisone cross-react in some assays. In competitive protein-binding methods, other corticosteroids also cross-react. |
| INC: obesity, meals<br>Increases with increasing age >60 yr. Higher in Hispanics than in whites. | Same as for insulin | RIA: Cross-reacts with proinsulin; different antibodies show considerable difference in cross-reactivity, which makes interlaboratory comparison difficult. |
| INC: exercise, after meat ingestion<br>DEC: pregnancy<br>Lower in vegetarians (also lower creatinine clearance).<br>Lowest in neonates; rises to adult levels by adolescence, remains stable throughout adult life (but with decreasing creatinine clearance and urine creatinine).<br>Higher in blind persons; higher in men than in women; higher in blacks than in whites. | INC: nephrotoxic agents; cimetidine, salicylate, trimethoprim-sulfamethoxazole (all inhibit tubular secretion of creatinine) | Spectrophotometric: Ketones, some cephalosporins cross-react; 5-fluocytosine cross-reacts with one enzymatic method, whereas lidocaine metabolites interfere in other enzymatic assays. |
| INC: exercise, manic disorders, caffeine, high-protein diet, obesity (ethanol increases urine)<br>DEC: depression, ethanol (plasma)<br>Highest in childhood; stable until age 16, gradual decrease until about age 50, then gradual increase.<br>Higher in blacks than in whites. | INC: epinephrine, theophylline<br>DEC: probenecid, THC | RIA: Different RIAs show different cross-reactions, making interlaboratory comparison difficult. Urine must be collected with acid in container. |
| INC: pregnancy, renal failure<br>Higher in vegetarians.<br>Higher in elderly. | INC: progesterone<br>DEC: penicillamine, ascorbic acid | Chromatographic separation: No interferences reported for urine assays. Plasma values falsely low in hemolyzed specimens. |
| DEC: pregnancy, dieting, malnutrition<br>Rise throughout childhood, peak in 20s, decrease with age.<br>In women, dramatic decrease after menopause. Higher in women who have never been pregnant. | INC: clomiphene, ACTH<br>DEC: danazol, androgens, ketoconazole; ampicillin decreases excretion in pregnancy. | RIA: No interferences reported. |

(continued)

**TABLE 237-1.**
Reference Values in Endocrinology  (Continued)

| Test Name | Reference Range (Conventional Units) | Conversion Factor | Reference Range (SI Units) | Intraindividual Variation |
|---|---|---|---|---|
| DEHYDROEPIANDROSTER-ONE SULFATE[71,103,105,226,244–248] | M: 800–5600 µg/L<br>F: 350–4300 µg/L | 0.0026 | M: 2.1–14.6 µmol/L<br>F: 0.9–11.2 µmol/L | Day-to-day variation 1% in men, 5% in women; highest in a.m., lowest in p.m. |
| 11-DEOXYCORTICOSTERONE (11-DESOXYCORTICOSTER-ONE)[249,250] | 3.5–11.5 ng/dL | 30.3 | 100–350 pmol/L | Highest in a.m., lowest in p.m.; in women, higher in luteal phase. |
| 18-OH DEOXYCORTICOSTER-ONE. See 18-HYDROXY-DEOXYCORTICOSTERONE | | | | |
| 11-DEOXYCORTISOL (11-DESOXYCORTISOL)[251,252] | 0.02–0.13 µg/dL | 29 | 0.6–3.8 nmol/L | Day-to-day variation 20–30%. |
| DEOXYPYRIDINOLINE[86,90,494, 495,503–511,698–702] | Urine: Units nmol/mmol creatinine<br>F: 3.0–7.4<br>M: 2.3–5.4 | 1 | Urine: Units µmol/mol creatinine<br>F: 3.0–7.4<br>M: 2.3–5.4 | Highest in early a.m.; lowest in evening; within-day variation 25–35%. Day-to-day variation 15%. Higher in autumn than in spring. |
| DHEA. See DEHYDROEPI-ANDROSTERONE | | | | |
| DHEAS. See DEHYDROEPI-ANDROSTERONE SULFATE | | | | |
| 1,25-DIHYDROXYCHOLECAL-CIFEROL. See VITAMIN D 1,25-DIHYDROXY | | | | |
| DIHYDROTESTOSTERONE[253,254] | M: 30–86 ng/dL<br>F: 4–22 ng/dL | 0.0344 | M: 1.0–2.9 nmol/L<br>F: 0.1–0.8 nmol/L | Probably similar to testosterone. |
| DOPAMINE. See CATECHOL-AMINES | | | | |
| ENDORPHIN, BETA. See β-ENDORPHIN | | | | |
| ENKEPHALIN (METHIO-NINE)[261–265,673,674] | 20–50 fmol/L | 1 | 20–50 fmol/L | Highest in late afternoon, lowest in a.m. In women, peaks at ovulation. |
| EPINEPHRINE. See CATE-CHOLAMINES | | | | |
| ERYTHROPOIETIN[264–269] | 0–27 mIU/mL | 1 | 0–27 U/L | Lowest in early afternoon, increases to peak around midnight; 60% within-day variation. |
| ESTRADIOL[71,225,226,248,253,270–273] | M and postmenopausal F: 10–60 ng/L<br>Menstruating F: <400 ng/L (see "Intraindividual Variation") | 3.67<br><br>0.0037 | M and postmenopausal F: 37–220 pmol/L<br>Menstruating F: <1.45 nmol/L (see "Intraindividual Variation") | In menstruating women, rises during follicular phase with sharp peak 2–3 d before ovulation, then later rise in midluteal phase. Marked diurnal variation (50%), highest in late afternoon, lowest around midnight; 25% day-to-day variation. |
| ESTRIOL[213,247,274,275,276] | Nonpregnant F: <2 ng/mL<br>Pregnant: see "Physiologic Changes" | 3.47 | Nonpregnant F: <7 nmol/L<br>Pregnant: see "Physiologic Changes" | High random diurnal variation (50%), even for samples 5–15 min apart. In nonpregnant women, parallels changes in estradiol. |
| ESTROGENS, TOTAL[277] | Urine: 4–25 µg/d | 3.67 | Urine: 15–92 nmol/d | In women, increases from nadir at menses to peak in late follicular and luteal phases, as with estradiol. |

| Physiologic Changes | Drug Effects | Methodologic Considerations |
|---|---|---|
| INC: exercise, fasting, smoking<br>DEC: pregnancy, dieting, ethanol, malnutrition, acute illness<br>Rise throughout childhood, peak in early teens, decrease with age after 45 yr.<br>Higher in women who have never been pregnant.<br>Higher in whites than in Asians. | INC: clomiphene, ACTH, danazol, DHEA<br>DEC: carbamazepine, phenytoin, ketoconazole, oral contraceptives; ampicillin decreases excretion in pregnancy. | RIA: Significantly higher if collected in tubes with barrier gels. |
| INC: pregnancy | INC: spironolactone, metyrapone | RIA: No interferences reported. |
| INC: pregnancy, rapid fall after delivery | DEC: phenytoin, megestrol | RIA: Some antibodies cross-react with cortisol, which may be major compound measured. |
| INC: acute illness, malignancy, heavy exercise, bed rest<br>Lowest in children, increases markedly (four- to five-fold) during puberty (higher in females than in males) and then falls to adult levels. Increases after age 40. In women, increases markedly after menopause.<br>Higher in whites than in blacks. | INC: estrogens<br>DEC: bisphosphonates | Immunoassay: No interferences reported. |
| INC: exercise, hemoconcentration, obesity<br>DEC: immobilization, after fatty meals, ethanol<br>Ratio of dihydrotestosterone to testosterone lower during puberty.<br>Decreases with age, especially over age 50; decreases after menopause. | DEC: finasteride<br>Otherwise same as for testosterone. | RIA: No interferences reported. |
| INC: exercise, renal failure<br>DEC: ethanol, pregnancy | | RIA: No interferences reported. |
| INC: pregnancy, high altitude, exercise<br>DEC: renal failure, malignancy, chronic inflammation<br>Highest in infants, decreases to adult levels by age 4 yr, increases in older persons. | INC: androgens<br>DEC: ACE inhibitors | Immunoassay: Increased levels of inactive cross-reactive substances in the serum of patients with renal failure; low levels are seen with bioassays in renal failure. |
| INC: pregnancy, smoking (in men), hemoconcentration<br>DEC: heavy exercise, malnutrition, acute illness<br>Increases with age >55 yr in men. In women, begins to decline after about age 35. | INC: clomiphene, tamoxifen<br>DEC: oral contraceptives, ketoconazole, megestrol; cimetidine decreases midcycle peak. | RIA: Background "blank" values may affect the results reported. Significantly lower if collected in tubes containing separator gels. |
| INC: hemoconcentration, pregnancy (see later)<br>DEC: high altitude<br>As with estradiol, peak levels occur before age 35. Lower in women who have never been pregnant.<br>In pregnancy, continuous slow rise in serum and urine levels in first two trimesters; higher with each week in third trimester. In pregnancy, lower in smokers and with chromosomally abnormal fetus. | INC: ACTH (in pregnancy), spironolactone (in men)<br>DEC: ampicillin, penicillin, aspirin, probenecid, $T_4$, albuterol (most effects seen only in pregnancy) | RIA: No interferences reported; however, several drugs cause falsely low urine estriol by spectrophotometric methods. |
| DEC: prolonged bed rest<br>Other changes similar to those for estradiol. | INC: digoxin, chlorpromazine<br>Other changes similar to those for estradiol. | Spectrophotometric: Cortisone, L-dopa, methenamine, and synthetic estrogens cross-react in the assay; acetazolamide, thiazides, and salicylate inhibit the reaction, causing falsely low results. Penicillin increases rate of hydrolysis, causing falsely high results, whereas acetazolamide and phenolphthalein cause the opposite effect. |

*(continued)*

TABLE 237-1.
Reference Values in Endocrinology (Continued)

| Test Name | Reference Range (Conventional Units) | Conversion Factor | Reference Range (SI Units) | Intraindividual Variation |
|---|---|---|---|---|
| ESTRONE[277] | Serum:<br>M and postmenopausal F:<br>15–65 pg/mL<br>Menstruating F: see "Intra-individual Variation"<br>Urine: 4–7 µg/d | 3.7<br><br><br><br>3.7 | Serum:<br>M and postmenopausal F:<br>55–240 pmol/L<br>Menstruating F: see "Intra-individual Variation"<br>Urine: 15–26 nmol/d | 10% day-to-day variation. In women, increases from nadir at menses to peak at time of ovulation. |
| F. See FLUORIDE | | | | |
| FATTY ACIDS, FREE[278] | 293–843 µEq/L | 1 | 293–843 µmol/L | In fasting individuals, lowest during sleep. Marked within-day differences (three-fold between highest and lowest). |
| Fe. See IRON | | | | |
| FLUORIDE[279,280] | Plasma: 0.01–0.20 mg/L<br>Urine: 0.2–1.0 mg/L | 52.6 | Plasma: 0.5–10.5 µmol/L<br>Urine:10.5–52.6 µmol/L | |
| FOLATE[186,281,282] | Serum: 2.8–21.8 ng/mL<br>RBC: 120–674 ng/mL | 2.27 | Serum: 6.4–49.5 nmol/L<br>RBC: 272–1530 nmol/L | Highest in winter, lower in summer. |
| FOLLICLE-STIMULATING HORMONE[213,225,226,283–294] | M: 0.6–8.6 mIU/mL<br>F: 4–13 mIU/mL<br>Postmenopausal F: 20–138 mIU/mL | 1 | M: 0.6–8.6 IU/L<br>F: 4–13 IU/L<br>Postmenopausal F: 20–138 IU/L | Pulsatile release during day (50% variation); spike at midcycle in menstruating women. Day-to-day variation 40%. |
| FREE THYROXINE. See THYROXINE, FREE | | | | |
| FRUCTOSAMINE[295–301] | 174–286 µmol/L | 1 | 174–286 µmol/L | Day-to-day variation 8%. |
| GAD ANTIBODIES. See ANTI–GLUTAMIC ACID DECARBOXYLASE | | | | |
| GASTRIN[302–309] | <100 ng/L | 1 | <100 ng/L | Lowest in early a.m., highest during day; 90% fall in values during night. |
| GH. See GROWTH HORMONE | | | | |
| GLUCAGON[170,310–319,676] | 20–200 pg/mL | 1 | 20–200 ng/L | Released in episodic spikes during day with amplitude up to 33%. |
| GLUCOSE[703,704] | 65–110 mg/dL | 0.055 | 3.6–6.1 mmol/L | Little variation other than meal related. |
| GLUTAMIC ACID DECARBOXYLASE ANTIBODIES. See ANTI–GLUTAMIC ACID DECARBOXYLASE | | | | |
| GLYCATED (GLYCOSYLATED) ALBUMIN[171,298–301,320,321,675] | 1.5–2.6% | 0.01 | 0.015–0.026 | Day-to-day variation 13%. |

| Physiologic Changes | Drug Effects | Methodologic Considerations |
|---|---|---|
| INC: pregnancy, puberty, obesity, smoking (in men)<br>DEC: acute illness<br>As with estradiol, peak levels occur before age 35. | INC: digoxin | RIA: No interferences reported. |
| INC: after meals (late), stress, exercise, prolonged fast, smoking, ethanol, obesity, caffeine<br>DEC: after meals (for 1–2 h), weight loss, refeeding<br>Higher in women than in men. | INC: amphetamines, desipramine, heparin, L-dopa, oral contraceptives, valproic acid, theophylline, catecholamines, prazosin<br>DEC: asparaginase, salicylate, β-adrenergic antagonists | Spectrophotometric: Values increase after collection due to hydrolysis of triglycerides; heparin not a suitable anticoagulant because it activates lipoprotein lipase. |
| INC: renal failure<br>Increases with increasing age. Levels related to recent intake. | INC: fluoride-containing toothpaste, mouthwash; anesthetic agents containing fluoride (halothane, methoxyflurane); flecainide | Electrochemical: Contamination from glassware is a major concern; specimens must be collected in plastic (but not Teflon). |
| DEC: smoking, ethanol, malnutrition, pregnancy<br>Decreases with increasing age >50 yr, but rises with age >90 yr. | INC: phenformin<br>DEC: anticonvulsants, folic acid antagonists, colchicine, oral contraceptives, isoniazid, triamterene, salicylate, estrogens, pentamidine, antacids, trimethoprim | Immunoassay: Unstable at room temperature, specimen must be frozen promptly. Microbiologic assays give falsely low results in patients receiving antibiotics (normally, folate causes growth of the indicator organism). |
| DEC: obesity, malnutrition<br>Follicular-phase levels increase with increasing age in menstruating women. | INC: L-dopa, clomiphene, ketoconazole<br>DEC: oral contraceptives, estrogens, phenothiazines | Immunoassay: With renal failure, values falsely increased due to increased α subunit. Values obtained cannot be compared with those obtained when different international standards are used. |
| In children, values lowest in infancy, rise to adult levels by age 6 yr.<br>INC: pregnancy (higher with increasing maternal age), renal failure<br>DEC: pregnancy (from nonpregnant values), obesity | | Spectrophotometric: Levels inversely related to half-life of protein; disorders increasing rate of turnover (nephrotic syndrome, hyperthyroidism) cause falsely low results. Values falsely low in patients with albumin <3 g/dL and falsely high in those with elevated immunoglobulin A. |
| INC: after meals, in presence of *Helicobacter pylori*<br>In children, values highest at birth and gradually decrease to adult levels. In adults, increases with age >50 yr. | INC: caffeine, calcium, catecholamines, insulin, omeprazole, ranitidine<br>DEC: atropine, lithium, octreotide | RIA: Different molecular forms show different reactions with each antiserum, which can cause difficulty in interpretation. High triglyceride may cause false increases. Gastrin is labile; specimens should be frozen promptly. Heparin alters binding to resins used in some assays. |
| INC: after meal (delay in rise), obesity, stress, fasting, exercise, renal failure<br>DEC: immediately after meal, especially if high in carbohydrate | INC: epinephrine, insulin, gastrin<br>DEC: propranolol | RIA: Much of immunoreactive material detected is not native glucagon, but glicentin, an intestinal peptide that contains glucagon within it. Different assays show differing reactions with glucagon, "big" glucagon, proglucagon, and intestinal glucagon. (Also see Chap. 134.) |
| INC: stress, after meals, mild exercise, emotional distress, ethanol, smoking<br>DEC: pregnancy, prolonged exercise, high altitude, fever, prolonged bed rest, prolonged fast<br>Lower in blind persons.<br>After meals glucose increases with increasing age. | INC: thiazides, phenothiazines, caffeine, estrogens, epinephrine, glucocorticoids, lithium<br>DEC: anabolic steroids, amphetamines, pentamidine, THC, MAO inhibitors, propranolol | Enzymatic (glucose oxidase): Falsely decreased with extremely high levels of ascorbic acid, α-methyl dopa. Values decrease 3–5%/h if serum not separated from cells; rate of fall is greater with leukocytosis. Arterial blood gives higher results than venous blood; capillary blood level (as in fingersticks) is considerably higher than venous level after eating, but not in fasting. With fingerstick glucose testing, results dependent on $P_{O_2}$ and hematocrit; results may be falsely high or low depending on method used (see Chap. 239). |
| INC: hemoconcentration, renal failure<br>DEC: pregnancy | | Same methods as for glycated hemoglobin, probably shows same difficulties. In addition, as for fructosamine, changes in albumin half-life affect results. |

(continued)

TABLE 237-1.
Reference Values in Endocrinology  (Continued)

| Test Name | Reference Range (Conventional Units) | Conversion Factor | Reference Range (SI Units) | Intraindividual Variation |
|---|---|---|---|---|
| GLYCATED (GLYCOSYLATED) HEMOGLOBIN. See HEMOGLOBIN A$_{1c}$ | | | | |
| GROWTH HORMONE[66,170,226,227,329–340] | Adult: 0–10 ng/mL<br>Child: 0–20 ng/mL | 1 | Adult: 0–10 µg/L<br>Child: 0–20 µg/L | Highest just after sleep; released in episodic spikes during the day. Highest in fall, lowest in spring. |
| hCG. See HUMAN CHORIONIC GONADOTROPIN | | | | |
| HDL CHOLESTEROL. See HIGH-DENSITY LIPOPROTEIN CHOLESTEROL | | | | |
| HEMOGLOBIN A$_{1c}$[321–328,677–680] | 4.9–6.2% | 0.01 | 0.049–0.062 | |
| Hg. See MERCURY | | | | |
| 5-HIAA. See 5-HYDROXYINDOLEACETIC ACID | | | | |
| HIGH-DENSITY LIPOPROTEIN CHOLESTEROL[142–145,341] | NCEP decision level: <35 mg/dL | 0.026 | NCEP decision level: <0.91 mmol/L | 5–8% day-to-day variation. |
| HISTAMINE[342–344] | 0–1 ng/mL<br>Urine: 0–118 µg/d | 9 | 0–9 nmol/L<br>Urine: 0–1062 nmol/d | Marked diurnal variation, highest in late a.m., lowest in afternoon at about one-third peak values. |
| HOMOCYSTEINE[173,705–718] | 2.8–18.5 µmol/L | 1 | 2.8–18.5 µmol/L | Day-to-day variation 10%. 30% higher in evening than in morning. |
| HOMOVANILLIC ACID[238,345–347] | Adults: <15 mg/d<br>Children: <16 µg/mg creatinine | 5.49<br>0.62 | Adults: <82 µmol/d<br>Children: <9.9 mmol/mol | No diurnal variation in HVA/creatinine ratio; excretion highest at night. |

| Physiologic Changes | Drug Effects | Methodologic Considerations |
|---|---|---|
| INC: after meals with protein, hypoglycemia, stress, starvation, exposure to heat or cold, exercise, renal failure, hemoconcentration, acute illness<br>DEC: obesity, glucose ingestion<br>Responsiveness to stimuli decreases with increasing age. | INC: amphetamines, estrogens, glucocorticoids (short term), indomethacin, interferon-β, L-dopa, propranolol, diazepam, ACTH, vasopressin, clonidine, desipramine, valproic acid, phenytoin<br>DEC: glucocorticoids (long term), octreotide, phenothiazines, probucol | RIA: Multiple circulating forms; specimen must be refrigerated after collection, unstable at room temperature. |
| INC: stress<br>DEC: hemolytic anemia (decreased life of RBC), pregnancy, acute caloric restriction<br>Lower in men with diabetes than in women with diabetes; increases with age. | INC: combination oral contraceptives | HPLC: Expressed as percentage of total hemoglobin A forms present. Cannot be used in absence of hemoglobin A (e.g., in sickle cell disease, SC disease, etc.); unaffected by presence of heterozygous abnormal hemoglobins. Column chromatographic and most electrophoretic methods measure total hemoglobin $A_1$, which includes forms other than $A_{1c}$ in presence of renal failure, salicylates, etc.; they also give falsely elevated values in persons with fast-migrating hemoglobins such as hemoglobin F. Because results are expressed as percentage of total hemoglobin, falsely low values occur with heterozygous presence of slow-migrating hemoglobins such as hemoglobin S or C. If preincubation step not used, column chromatography gives falsely high values when glucose is elevated at time of collection. Affinity chromatography measures total glycohemoglobin, and gives results that are ~15% higher than for hemoglobin $A_{1c}$; they are often expressed as $A_{1c}$ using a correction factor, but falsely underestimate $A_{1c}$ when elevated. Rare hemoglobin variants with substitutions at the same location as $A_{1c}$ may give falsely elevated results with HPLC methods, but not with immunoassays. All methods give falsely low results in patients with bleeding or hemolytic anemia due to decreased RBC life span, and falsely high results may occur with splenectomy or iron deficiency anemia. (Also see Chap. 239.) |
| INC: exercise, ethanol, obesity, hemoconcentration, pregnancy (peak 33% higher in second trimester)<br>DEC: acute infections, prolonged fasting, smoking<br>Higher in blacks than in whites and higher in women than in men.<br>In childhood, rises gradually during first decade, falls at puberty in boys but not girls, reaches adult levels by age 14. | INC: estrogens, phenytoin, cimetidine, fibric acids, HMG-CoA reductase inhibitors, niacin<br>DEC: thiazides, β-adrenergic blockers, progesterone, Norplant, probucol, phenothiazines, isotretinoin, danazol, spironolactone | Immunoprecipitation/enzymatic: Various methods are relatively imprecise and results often differ widely when different methods used. Precipitation methods often artifactually altered in specimens from nonfasting persons.<br>The recommendation is to measure at least twice. For some methods, results falsely low when triglycerides >400 mg/dL. |
| INC: ethanol, after meals, renal failure | INC: radiographic contrast agents<br>DEC: ascorbic acid, erythropoietin, glucocorticoids | Fluorometric: Serotonin shows 25% cross-reactivity in assay. |
| INC: after meals, caffeine, ethanol, exercise, renal failure<br>DEC: pregnancy<br>Higher in men than in women; in women, increases after menopause.<br>Increases with increasing age >40 yr. | INC: carbamazepine, cyclosporine, methotrexate, phenobarbital, phenytoin<br>DEC: estrogens, folic acid, pyridoxine, raloxifene, tamoxifen | HPLC: Homocysteine increases rapidly with storage of whole blood; serum should be rapidly separated from plasma, and frozen to −70°C quickly. Immunoassays agree relatively well with other methods. |
| Urine excretion decreases relative to creatinine during childhood, reaching adult levels by age 10–15. | INC: disulfiram (urine), L-dopa, reserpine, THC, amphetamines, verapamil | Spectrophotometric: Salicylate gives falsely elevated results. With fluorometric assay, salicylate falsely lowers results. |

(continued)

**TABLE 237-1.**
**Reference Values in Endocrinology (Continued)**

| Test Name | Reference Range (Conventional Units) | Conversion Factor | Reference Range (SI Units) | Intraindividual Variation |
|---|---|---|---|---|
| HUMAN CHORIONIC GONA-DOTROPIN. See CHORIONIC GONADOTROPIN, HUMAN | | | | |
| HUMAN PLACENTAL LACTO-GEN. See PLACENTAL LAC-TOGEN, HUMAN | | | | |
| HVA. See HOMOVANILLIC ACID | | | | |
| 25-HYDROXYCHOLECALCIF-EROL. See VITAMIN D, 25-HYDROXY | | | | |
| HYDROXYBUTYRATE, BETA. See β-HYDROXYBUTYRATE | | | | |
| 17-HYDROXYCORTICO-STEROIDS[348] | Urine:<br>M: 3–10 mg/d<br>F: 2–8 mg/d | 2.76 | Urine:<br>M: 8.3–27.6 μmol/d<br>F: 5.5–22.1 μmol/d | Urinary excretion parallels serum corti-sol; only 24-h or first morning urine collections should be used. |
| 18-HYDROXYCORTICO-STERONE[349] | Upright: 5–80 ng/dL<br>Supine: 4–37 ng/dL | 27.9 | Upright: 140–2230 pmol/L<br>Supine: 112–1030 pmol/L | |
| 18-HYDROXYDEOXY-CORTICOSTERONE[349] | 3–13 ng/dL | 29.2 | 88–390 pmol/L | |
| 5-HYDROXYINDOLEACETIC ACID[302,350–353] | <6 mg/d | 5.2 | <31.2 μmol/d | Highest in winter, 50% lower in summer. |
| 17-HYDROXYPREGNEN-OLONE[347] | M: 40–450 ng/dL<br>F: 20–400 ng/dL | 0.03 | M: 1.2–13.5 nmol/L<br>F: 0.6–12.0 nmol/L | In women, higher in luteal phase. |
| 17-HYDROXYPROGES-TERONE[70,120,294,353–357] | M: 0.5–2.5 μg/L<br>F: 0.2–5 μg/L<br>Postmenopausal F: 0.3–0.9 μg/L | 3.03 | M: 1.5–7.6 nmol/L<br>F: 0.6–15 nmol/L<br>Postmenopausal F: 0.9–2.7 nmol/L | Marked diurnal variation, highest in a.m., lowest in p.m.; in women, three-fold higher at midcycle, lowest in early follicular phase. Day-to-day variation 10% in men, 20% in women. |
| HYDROXYPROLINE[241,358–361] | Urine, total: 25–80 mg/d<br>Urine, free: 0–2.7 mg/d<br>Serum: 0–53 μmol/L | 0.0076<br>7.6<br>1 | Urine, total: 0.19–0.61 mmol/d<br>Urine, free: 0–20.5 μmol/d<br>Serum: 0–53 μmol/L | Day-to-day variation 20%; highest in spring, fall; lower in winter. |
| I. See IODIDE | | | | |
| IA-2 ANTIBODIES. See ANTI-IA2 | | | | |
| INHIBIN[720–727] | M: 0.5–3.7 U/mL<br>F: 0.8–3.2 U/mL | 1 | M: 0.5–3.7 U/mL<br>F: 0.8–3.2 U/mL | Inhibin A: higher in a.m. than p.m. In women, lowest in early follicular phase, rises to peak in midluteal phase.<br>Inhibin B: In women, high in follicular phase and falls during midluteal phase. |
| INSULIN[170,235,236,311–314] | 0–20 mIU/L | 7.18 | 0–144 pmol/L | Pulsatile secretion with values as much as 70% from mean values; decreases during sleep (in pregnancy). Day-to-day variation 15–25%. |

| Physiologic Changes | Drug Effects | Methodologic Considerations |
|---|---|---|
| INC: stress, pregnancy, obesity, acute illness, exercise, hyperthyroidism<br>DEC: hypothyroidism, prolonged fasting | INC: glucocorticoids, DES, estrogens<br>DEC: barbiturates, dexamethasone and other high-potency steroids, narcotic analgesics, phenothiazines, phenytoin, propoxyphene, medroxyprogesterone, megestrol acetate, oral contraceptives | Spectrophotometric: Nonspecific, cross-reacts with chloral hydrate, thiazides, digoxin, paraldehyde, cefoxitin, spironolactone, carbamazepine, ascorbic acid, phenothiazines, colchicine.<br>Salicylates and reserpine cause false-negative results. |
| DEC: severe acute illness<br>High in newborns, peaks on third day of life, gradually falls through childhood to reach adult levels by late teens. | INC: amiloride, metoclopramide, spironolactone | RIA: No interferences reported. |
|  | INC: amiloride | RIA: No interferences reported. |
| INC: smoking, pregnancy, ingestion of foods containing serotonin (bananas, avocado, plums, pineapple, walnuts, kiwi fruit, most nuts, tomatoes, eggplant)<br>DEC: malabsorption, especially after intestinal resection; depression, ethanol.<br>In children, decreases with increasing age.<br>Lower in persons older than age 60. | INC: reserpine<br>DEC: L-dopa, isoniazid, ranitidine, α-methyldopa, imipramine | Spectrophotometric: Acetaminophen, guaifenesin, naproxen, indomethacin, phenobarbital, sulindac, benzodiazepines, ephedrine cross-react in assay. Ketoacids, phenothiazines, and proteinuria produce falsely low results in most assays. Urine must be acidified, as 5-HIAA is unstable at neutral or alkaline pH. |
| DEC: obesity<br>Highest in neonates, falls through first year to ~60% of adult levels; slow rise after puberty to adult levels by late teens.<br>Decreases after menopause. | DEC: anabolic steroids | RIA: No interferences reported. |
| INC: pregnancy (three-fold higher near term), acute illness in neonates<br>Higher in premature infants, peaks at 3 mo, gradually decreases in late childhood, rises at puberty to adult levels.<br>Decreases after menopause. | INC: ACTH, ketoconazole, mifepristone (RU-486)<br>DEC: oral contraceptives, anabolic steroids | RIA: Cross-reacts with some antibodies. With some kits, falsely elevated values occur in neonates, due to cross-reacting steroid sulfates. |
| INC: protein in diet, especially gelatin; prolonged bed rest, severe burns, fractures, periods of growth, postpartum, postorchiectomy<br>DEC: malnutrition<br>Lower in children than in adults; lower in blacks than in whites. Total decreases with age from 20–60 yr, increase with age >60 yr. | INC: T$_4$, glucocorticoids<br>DEC: antineoplastic agents, salicylate, estrogens, mithramycin, omeprazole, propranolol (in hyperthyroidism) | Column chromatography: No interferences reported. |
| Inhibin A: INC: renal failure<br>In pregnancy, falls during second trimester and rises again after week 17. Higher in mothers of twins, infants with Down syndrome, and diabetic women.<br>Inhibin B: High in neonates, rises to peak at 4–12 mo before falling, and remains low until puberty. Peaks at age 20, then gradually decreases with increasing age.<br>In women, declines markedly after menopause. In pregnancy, rises third trimester to peak at term, returns to baseline within 24 h of delivery. |  | Immunoassay: No interferences reported. |
| INC: stress, obesity, pregnancy, after meals, renal failure<br>DEC: ethanol, fasting, exercise<br>In physically fit, lower response to meal as well as lower basal levels.<br>Higher in Hispanics than in whites. | INC: L-dopa, agents causing hyperglycemia, oral hypoglycemic agents, THC, oral contraceptives<br>DEC: asparaginase, diuretics, propranolol; fibric acids, nifedipine, phenytoin, calcitonin decrease postprandial release. | RIA: Heparin causes false elevations in double antibody methods. Hemolysis causes falsely low values. Insulin antibodies cause falsely low values in some assays, falsely high in others.<br>Proinsulin cross-reacts with most antibodies. |

(continued)

**TABLE 237-1.**
Reference Values in Endocrinology  (Continued)

| Test Name | Reference Range (Conventional Units) | Conversion Factor | Reference Range (SI Units) | Intraindividual Variation |
|---|---|---|---|---|
| INSULIN C PEPTIDE. See C PEP-TIDE | | | | |
| INSULIN-LIKE GROWTH FACTOR-I[225,327,362-367] | 123–463 ng/mL AGE RELATED | 1 | 123–463 µg/L | Approximately 15% variation during day, 30% fall at onset of sleep with rise to highest values at about 4:30 a.m. In women, higher in luteal than in follicular phase. |
| INSULIN-LIKE GROWTH FACTOR-II[368] | 405–1085 ng/mL | 1 | 405–1085 µg/L | |
| INSULIN-LIKE GROWTH FACTOR–BINDING PROTEIN-1[369-375] | 13–73 ng/mL | 1 | 13–73 µg/L | Highest at night, lowest during the day. |
| INSULIN-LIKE GROWTH FACTOR–BINDING PROTEIN-3[372-377] | 2–4 mg/L | 1 | 2–4 mg/L | Slightly lower at night. |
| IODIDE (INORGANIC)[378-381,728,729] | 0.5–2.0 mg/L Urine: 0.1–0.8 mg/L | 7.7 | 3.9–15.4 µmol/L Urine: 0.8–6.2 µmol/L | |
| IRON[38,382,383] | 44–160 µg/dL | 0.18 | 7.9–28.6 µmol/L | Marked diurnal variation, up to 40% variation within day, 25% day-to-day. Highest in p.m., lowest in a.m. In women, highest in luteal phase, lowest after menstruation. |
| IRON-BINDING CAPACITY[38,730] | 250–400 µg/dL | 0.18 | 44.8–71.6 µmol/L | Highest at 4–8 p.m., lowest at 8 a.m. Small diurnal variation. |
| ISLET CELL ANTIGEN ANTIBODIES. See ANTI–ISLET CELL ANTIGENS | | | | |
| K. See POTASSIUM | | | | |
| KETONES[384] (see also ACETOACETIC ACID, β-HYDROXYBUTYRATE) | <10 mg/dL (negative) | 0.1 | <1 mmol/L (negative) | |
| 17-KETOGENIC STEROIDS[385] | Urine: M: 4–14 mg/d F: 2–12 mg/d | 3.5 | Urine: M: 14–49 µmol/d F: 7–42 µmol/d | |
| 17-KETOSTEROIDS[385] | Urine: M: 7–20 mg/d F: 5–15 mg/d | 3.5 | Urine: M: 24.5–70 µmol/d F: 17.5–52.5 µmol/d | Highest in a.m., lowest at night. |
| LACTATE[386] | Venous: 3.6–18.9 mg/dL Arterial: 4.5–15.4 mg/dL | 0.11 | Venous: 0.4–2.1 mmol/L Arterial: 0.5–1.7 mmol/L | Day-to-day variation 25%. |

| Physiologic Changes | Drug Effects | Methodologic Considerations |
|---|---|---|
| INC: pregnancy, renal failure, hemoconcentration, exercise<br>DEC: malnutrition, liver disease, obesity, Down syndrome, acute illness, fasting<br>Values increase throughout childhood to peak in early teens, then decline gradually throughout adult life. Higher in women than in men. | INC: androgens, dexamethasone<br>DEC: estrogens, tamoxifen | RIA: Detects both native molecule and other compounds; some antibodies cross-react with insulin. |
| INC: exercise<br>DEC: severe illness<br>Values markedly reduced in neonates. | | RIA: Detects both native molecule and other compounds; some antibodies cross-react with insulin. In some assays, falsely increased in renal failure. |
| INC: pregnancy, renal failure, fasting<br>DEC: obesity, after meals<br>Gradual decrease during childhood.<br>Results inversely related to GH, insulin levels. | DEC: glucocorticosteroids, insulin | Immunometric assay: No interferences noted. |
| INC: renal failure<br>DEC: liver disease, fasting, pregnancy, acute illness<br>Rises gradually during childhood to sharp peak at puberty, falls gradually to adult levels by early 20s. Results directly related to GH and IGF-I levels. | INC: dexamethasone | RIA: No interferences noted. Although generally stable in vitro, increased activity of proteases that break down IGFBP-3 occurs in acute illness and in pregnancy, which can further reduce concentration after specimen collection. Generally advisable to place specimens in ice water and freeze serum quickly. |
| Serum and urine concentrations reflect recent intake. Urine excretion higher in men than in women. In women, urine iodide decreases during pregnancy. Urine concentration decreases with increasing age due to decreases in GFR; similar in all ages when expressed as I/creatinine ratio. | INC: amiodarone, after topical or vaginal applications of povidone-iodine, iodine-containing mineral supplements, radiopaque dyes, erythrosine<br>DEC: acetazolamide (urine) | Spectrophotometric: Ascorbic acid causes falsely increased results. Iodide present in urine dipsticks may contaminate specimens and give falsely high results. |
| INC: hemoconcentration, transfusions (for 24–36 h), hemolysis, ethanol, acute hepatitis<br>DEC: stress, malnutrition, pregnancy, acute illness<br>Decreases with increasing age >70 yr. | INC: salicylates, cisplatin, methotrexate, oral contraceptives, iron dextran<br>DEC: allopurinol, cholestyramine | Spectrophotometric: Cefotaxime causes falsely increased results; deferoxamine, EDTA falsely decrease results in most methods. Results falsely high by some assays in iron overdose. |
| INC: pregnancy, hemoconcentration, exercise<br>DEC: malnutrition, protein-losing states<br>Higher in trained athletes, higher in women than in men. Decreases with age >50 yr. | INC: estrogens, oral contraceptives<br>DEC: glucocorticoids, testosterone, chloramphenicol | Spectrophotometric: Falsely increased by iron dextran. Bears a constant relation to transferrin, as given by the equation: transferrin = (0.8 × total iron-binding capacity) – 43. |
| INC: fasting, exercise, ethanol | INC: salicylate, isopropanol toxicity, albuterol, nifedipine<br>DEC: valproic acid, salicylates | Semiquantitative colorimetric: L-dopa, paraldehyde, α-methyl dopa cross-react in urine; falls when stored at room temperature.<br>Test detects only acetoacetate (and in some assays acetone); in patients with ketoacidosis and extensive fatty acid metabolism, hydroxybutyrate predominates by as much as 16:1 early in ketoacidosis; with treatment, hydroxybutyrate is converted to acetoacetate and produces an increase in ketones. |
| INC: obesity, smoking<br>DEC: malnutrition<br>Low in children, rise to adult levels by puberty. Begin to fall after age 30, and values continue to decline with increasing age. | INC: glucocorticoids, ampicillin<br>DEC: oral contraceptives, estrogens, dexamethasone | Spectrophotometric: Many compounds cross-react or interfere with color development (see table in reference 385). |
| INC: stress, exercise, pregnancy<br>DEC: smoking<br>Gradually increase during childhood, peak at 20–30 yr, gradual decrease with increasing age.<br>Decreased in blind persons.<br>In women, decreased after menopause. | INC: androgens, ampicillin, danazol<br>DEC: morphine, phenothiazines, probenecid, propoxyphene, phenytoin, aminoglutethimide, dexamethasone, opiates, probenecid, propoxyphene, oral contraceptives | Spectrophotometric: Many compounds cross-react or interfere with color development (see table in reference 385). |
| INC: exercise, hyperventilation, ethanol, fasting<br>DEC: weight loss<br>Slightly higher in women than in men. | INC: catecholamines, oral contraceptives, carbamazepine, phenobarbital, valproic acid, albuterol, ritodrine<br>DEC: morphine | Enzymatic: Do not use tourniquet or allow patient to clench fist, as these increase lactate. Increases rapidly with storage at room temperature before analysis. Hemoglobin, bilirubin may falsely decrease results in some assays. |

(continued)

**TABLE 237-1.**
Reference Values in Endocrinology  (Continued)

| Test Name | Reference Range (Conventional Units) | Conversion Factor | Reference Range (SI Units) | Intraindividual Variation |
|---|---|---|---|---|
| LEAD[387] | <10 µg/dL | 0.048 | <0.48 µmol/L | Levels fluctuate from day to day; magnitude of fluctuation not reported. |
| LDL CHOLESTEROL. See LOW-DENSITY LIPOPROTEIN CHOLESTEROL | | | | |
| LEPTIN[731–737] | M: 1.2–9.5 ng/mL<br>F: 4.1–25 ng/mL | 1 | M: 1.2–9.5 ng/mL<br>F: 4.1–25 ng/mL | Highest at night, lowest at 8 a.m., gradually rises during the day. Little day-to-day variation in males or postmenopausal females. Increases during the follicular phase to peak in midluteal phase, 30% higher than baseline. |
| LIPOPROTEIN(a)[388–400] | 0–30 mg/dL | 10 | 0–300 mg/L | Day-to-day variation 8–10%; no diurnal variation. |
| LOW-DENSITY LIPOPROTEIN CHOLESTEROL[9–10,40,209,210] | NCEP decision levels:<br>Coronary artery disease,<br>  desirable: <100 mg/dL<br>Desirable: <130 mg/dL<br>Borderline: 130–160 mg/dL<br>High: >160 mg/dL | 0.0259 | NCEP decision levels:<br>Coronary artery disease,<br>  desirable: <2.6 mmol/L<br>Desirable: <3.4 mmol/L<br>Borderline: 3.4–4.1 mmol/L<br>High: >4.1 mmol/L | Day-to-day variation 10–15%. Higher in winter (2.5%) than in summer. In women, 10–20% lower in late luteal phase, lowest at menstruation. |
| LUTEINIZING HORMONE[170,226,283–296] | M: 0.5–11.2 mIU/mL<br>F: 1–18 mIU/mL<br>Postmenopausal F: 15–62 mIU/mL | 1 | M: 0.5–11.2 IU/L<br>F: 1–18 IU/L<br>Postmenopausal F: 15–62 IU/L | Released in episodic spikes during day; 30% variation day to day. Within day, values highest in early sleep, lowest in late afternoon. Highest in summer, lowest in winter. In women, sharp spike before ovulation. |
| MAGNESIUM[401–406,673] | 1.4–2.5 mg/dL<br>Urine: 14–290 mg/d | 0.41<br>0.041 | 0.6–1.0 mmol/L<br>Urine: 0.6–12 mmol/d | Seasonal variation (highest in winter, lowest in summer). In women, decreases with menses. Changes with an inverse relation to plasma glucose. Day-to-day variation 3–5%. |
| MANGANESE[294,295,407,408] | 0.1–1.0 µg/L | 18.2 | 1.8–18.2 nmol/L | |
| MELATONIN[270,409–416] | 0.17–0.43 nmol/L | 1 | 0.17–0.43 nmol/L | Highest at 4 a.m., falls gradually to nadir at 8 p.m.; circadian pattern abolished in renal failure.<br>In women, nocturnal melatonin higher in luteal phase.<br>Daytime melatonin higher in summer than in winter; nocturnal values similar throughout the year. |
| MERCURY[214,215] | Blood: <13.0 µg/L<br>Urine: <20 µg/L | 5 | Blood: <65 nmol/L<br>Urine: <100 nmol/L | |

| Physiologic Changes | Drug Effects | Methodologic Considerations |
|---|---|---|
| INC: smoking, ethanol<br>In children, decreases with age until 16 yr, then continuously increases throughout adult life.<br>Higher in men than in women; higher in blacks than in whites. | | Electrochemical: Some anticoagulants may complex with lead and cause falsely low values; heparin is anticoagulant of choice.<br>Because lead is intracellular, whole blood lead must be measured. |
| INC: after meals, ethanol, obesity, renal failure<br>DEC: exercise, fasting, smoking<br>High in newborns (lower in male than in female infants and lower in premature infants than in term infants). Increases during first decade, then falls to age 15 and gradually decreases with increasing age.<br>Higher in blacks than in whites.<br>In pregnancy, increases gradually and falls rapidly in the postpartum period. | INC: clozapine, glucocorticoids, insulin<br>DEC: GH | Immunoassay: No interferences reported. |
| INC: hemoconcentration, renal failure, acute illness, pregnancy (increases by 100%), ethanol withdrawal, hypothyroidism<br>DEC: hyperthyroidism<br>Lowest in neonates, gradually rises over first 6 mo of life. From ages 4–10, slightly higher in girls than in boys; at all other ages, similar in both sexes. Slight increase with increasing age.<br>Values highest in blacks, intermediate in whites and Asians, lowest in Hispanics. | INC: cyclosporine, some oral contraceptives<br>DEC: danazol, estrogens | Immunoassay: Specimens not stable on storage, even at –70°C in some assays. No standards are currently available, and the marked disparity in molecular size of different genetic variants makes standardization difficult. |
| INC: hemoconcentration, nephrotic syndrome, obesity, after meals, smoking<br>DEC: acute illness, ethanol, exercise<br>Low in neonates, rapidly rises to 80% of adult levels by age 4 d. Slight fall at puberty, then increases 5–10% per decade.<br>Increases by 100% during pregnancy.<br>Higher in whites than in blacks, higher in men than in women. | INC: androgens, β-adrenergic antagonists, cyclosporine, danazol, glucocorticoids, isotretinoin, progestational agents, thiazides<br>DEC: estrogens, lipid-lowering agents, interferon, $T_4$ | Calculated using Friedewald equation (values in mg/dL): LDL = total cholesterol – HDL – (triglycerides/5); results similar to those of direct LDL measurements when triglycerides are <400 mg/dL. Requires overnight fast for valid results. |
| INC: renal failure, psychological stress<br>DEC: obesity, starvation, high altitude, heavy exercise, acute illness | INC: clomiphene, propranolol (in men), ketoconazole<br>DEC: oral contraceptives, testosterone, estrogens, phenothiazines, digoxin, propranolol (in women), progesterones; THC | RIA: Cross-reacts with hCG in pregnancy, trophoblastic tumors; with renal failure, values falsely increased due to increased α subunit. Inactive fragments also detected by assay. As with FSH, results can only be compared with those from methods using the same international standard. |
| INC: dehydration, hemoconcentration, renal failure<br>DEC: pregnancy, malabsorption, ethanol | INC: lithium, estrogens, triamterene, progesterone, magnesium-containing antacids.<br>DEC: digitalis, cyclosporine, cis-platinum, diuretics, oral contraceptives, aminoglycosides, amphotericin B, citrate (in transfusions) | Spectrophotometric: Citrate cross-reacts. Serum does not reflect total body stores of magnesium. Falsely low in specimens contaminated with EDTA or oxalate. Hemolysis causes slight increase, because intracellular Mg is higher than serum. |
| INC: pregnancy<br>Highest in neonates, reach adult levels by 4 mo in females.<br>In males, values begin to decline gradually at puberty.<br>In older persons, values begin to rise again. | | Atomic absorption: Hemolysis causes slight increase. Specimens stored in glass tubes show artifactually high results that increase with time of storage. |
| INC: exercise, late pregnancy, renal failure<br>DEC: smoking, ethanol, fasting<br>Highest in young children, continues to fall throughout life.<br>Higher in women than in men. | INC: progesterone<br>DEC: β-adrenergic blockers | RIA: No interferences reported. |
| Higher in women than in men.<br>Higher in neonates (2×). | INC: penicillamine, penicillin(?)<br>DEC: iodine-containing products (urine) | Atomic absorption: Gold salts reported to cross-react. |

(continued)

TABLE 237-1.
Reference Values in Endocrinology  (Continued)

| Test Name | Reference Range (Conventional Units) | Conversion Factor | Reference Range (SI Units) | Intraindividual Variation |
|---|---|---|---|---|
| METANEPHRINES (METH-OXYCATECHOL-AMINES)[192,417,418,738] | Urine: 0.3–0.9 mg/d<br>Plasma:<br>Normetanephrine: 18–112 pg/mL<br>Metanephrine: 12–61 pg/mL | 5.07 | Urine: 1.5–4.6 μmol/d<br>Plasma:<br>Normetanephrine: 90–570 pmol/L<br>Metanephrine: 60–310 pmol/L | |
| MET-ENKEPHALIN. See ENKEPHALIN | | | | |
| Mg. See MAGNESIUM | | | | |
| MICROALBUMIN, URINE[170,739–750] | <40 mg/d<br><32 μg/mg creatinine | 1<br>0.11 | <40 mg/d<br><3.5 μg/μmol creatinine | Day-to-day variation 60% for total microalbumin and 50% for microalbumin/creatinine ratio; higher for first morning urine than for 24-h urine. |
| Mn. See MANGANESE | | | | |
| Na. See SODIUM | | | | |
| NATRIURETIC PEPTIDE. See ATRIAL NATRIURETIC HORMONE | | | | |
| NEUROTENSIN[414] | <140 pg/mL | 1 | <140 ng/L | |
| NICKEL[419] | Serum: <0.5 μg/L<br>Urine: 0–7 μg/L | 17 | Serum: <8.5 nmol/L<br>Urine: 0–119 nmol/L | |
| NOREPINEPHRINE. See CATE-CHOLAMINES | | | | |
| OSMOLALITY | 275–295 mOsm/kg | 1 | 275–295 mmol/kg | Highest in morning, lower by average of 7.5% in late afternoon or evening. Day-to-day variation 1–2%. |
| OSTEOCALCIN[90–92,361,366,420–431] | 8–52 ng/mL | 1 | 8–52 μg/L | Highest at night, falls to nadir in early afternoon; within-day variation 50–100%. Day-to-day variation >50%. In women, higher in luteal than in follicular phase. Higher in spring than in autumn. |
| OXALATE[432–437] | Urine: 0–40 mg/d<br>Serum: 1.0–2.4 mg/L | 11.4 | Urine: 0–456 μmol/d<br>Serum: 11.4–27.4 μmol/L | Higher in summer than in winter. Day-to-day variation 40% (urine). |
| 17-OXOGENIC STEROIDS. See 17-KETOGENIC STEROIDS | | | | |
| 17-OXOSTEROIDS. See 17-KETOSTEROIDS | | | | |
| OXYTOCIN[438–440] | 0–3.2 mU/mL | 1 | 0–3.2 U/L | In women, increases to peak near time of ovulation, nadir in late luteal phase. Episodic release occurs near term pregnancy, uncertain if release is episodic at other times due to lack of sensitivity of assays. |
| P. See PHOSPHATE | | | | |
| PANCREATIC POLYPEPTIDE[441–447] | 26–300 pg/mL | 0.24 | 6–72 pmol/L | Marked episodic fluctuation, average 200% within-day variation. |
| PANCREOZYMIN. See CHOLE-CYSTOKININ | | | | |

| Physiologic Changes | Drug Effects | Methodologic Considerations |
|---|---|---|
| Less subject to dietary cross-reactants than VMA. | INC: amphetamines, caffeine, hydrazines, MAO inhibitors, prochlorperazine<br>DEC: L-dopa | Spectrophotometric after chromatographic purification: α-Methyldopa and methylglucamine (radiopaque dye) cross-react to give false elevations in all assays; β-adrenergic blockers, imipramine, phenothiazines, phenacetin, and oxytetracycline cross-react in some assays; propranolol inhibits color formation. Acetaminophen interferes with plasma normetanephrine assay. |
| INC: acute illness, exercise, ethanol, smoking, stress, hypertension, high-fat meal, urinary tract bleeding or infection<br>DEC: high-fiber diet<br>Low in children, increases during puberty to peak in mid-teens, then declines to adult levels by age 30. Higher in blacks than in whites, lower in females than in males. | INC: lithium<br>DEC: heparin | Immunoassay: No interferences reported. Stable on storage at room temperature or in refrigerator up to 7 days. Dipsticks are less precise and accurate than quantitative immunoassays. |
| INC: renal failure; after meals, especially lipid containing | DEC: morphine | RIA: Must be frozen immediately. Different molecular weight forms may react differently. (Also see Chap. 182.) |
| INC: tissue necrosis (myocardial infarct, stroke, burns), renal failure, ethanol<br>Higher in women than in men. | | Atomic absorption: Elevated cadmium, gold may cause slight underestimation. |
| INC: dehydration, exercise, ethanol<br>DEC: at high altitudes, pregnancy | INC: steroids causing salt retention, mannitol<br>DEC: vincristine, cyclophosphamide, diuretics | Freezing point depression: When vapor pressure depression osmometers are used, volatile substances such as ketones, ethanol, isopropanol, and methanol do not increase osmolality, causing absence of "osmotic gap." |
| INC: renal failure, weight lifting<br>DEC: ethanol, acute illness, pregnancy<br>Highest in children, with peak values occurring during periods of bone growth; falls to adult levels by age 20 yr. In adults, increases throughout life.<br>Higher in men than in women, higher in whites than in blacks.<br>Decreases in early pregnancy, returns to normal by term; increased during lactation. | INC: calcitriol, omeprazole, phenytoin<br>DEC: glucocorticoids, warfarin, estrogen, oral contraceptives, tamoxifen, thiazides | RIA: Significantly lower if blood collected with anticoagulants, particularly oxalate and EDTA. RIA measures both active and inactive forms; active form is decreased by treatment with warfarin, so that RIA is falsely elevated. |
| INC: malabsorptive disorders, renal failure (serum), liver failure, ingestion of oxalate-containing foods (spinach, tomatoes, strawberries, rhubarb)<br>DEC: renal failure (urine)<br>Ratio of oxalate to creatinine highest in infancy, falls throughout childhood. | INC: vitamin C, especially in renal failure, methoxyflurane<br>DEC: pyridoxine | Spectrophotometric: Wide interlaboratory variation; methods are poorly reproducible, with most methods overestimating actual concentration. Oxalate concentration rises rapidly at room temperature, especially in serum; specimens must be frozen or, for urine, collected in acid. |
| INC: pregnancy, hemoconcentration<br>DEC: stress | INC: oral contraceptives | RIA: No interferences reported. |
| INC: after meals, acute stress, renal failure, especially with dialysis<br>Higher in men than in women, higher in children than in adults. Lowest values in persons <30 yr, slight increase from age 30–60 yr, rapid increase after age 60. | DEC: anticholinergic agents, morphine | RIA: No interferences reported. |

(continued)

**TABLE 237-1.**
Reference Values in Endocrinology  (Continued)

| Test Name | Reference Range (Conventional Units) | Conversion Factor | Reference Range (SI Units) | Intraindividual Variation |
|---|---|---|---|---|
| PARATHYROID HORMONE[163–165,170,181,238,361,426,448–461,751] | 10–65 pg/mL | 0.102 | 1.0–6.8 pmol/L | Highest at 4 p.m., gradually decreases to nadir at 8 a.m. Within-day variation 30%. In women, gradually increases to peak at midcycle. Values higher in summer than in winter. |
| PARATHYROID HORMONE–RELATED PROTEIN[462–464] | 0–1.5 pmol/L | 1 | 0–1.5 pmol/L | |
| Pb. See LEAD | | | | |
| PH | Arterial blood: 7.36–7.44 | 1 | Arterial blood: 7.36–7.44 | |
| PHOSPHATASE, ACID. See ACID PHOSPHATASE | | | | |
| PHOSPHATASE, ALKALINE. See ALKALINE PHOSPHATASE | | | | |
| PHOSPHATE[465,466] | Serum: 2.5–4.5 mg/dL<br>Urine: 0.4–1.3 g/d | 0.32<br>32.3 | Serum: 0.81–1.45 mmol/L<br>Urine: 12.9–42.0 mmol/d | Marked difference in pattern from person to person; some show peak at 8 a.m., some peak late morning, some show no diurnal rhythm. Overall day-to-day variation 5–10%. Highest in summer, lowest in winter. In women, lower during menstruation. |
| PHOSPHOETHANOL-AMINE[467,468] | Urine: <100 µmol/g creatinine | 113 | Urine: <11,300 µmol/mol creatinine | Highest at night, lowest in a.m. |
| PLACENTAL LACTOGEN, HUMAN[212,469] | Nonpregnant F: <0.5 µg/mL<br>26–30 wk of pregnancy: 2.8–7.1 µg/mL<br>>37 wk of pregnancy: 5–10 µg/mL | 46.3 | Nonpregnant F: <23 nmol/L<br>26–30 wk of pregnancy: 130–330 nmol/L<br>>37 wk of pregnancy: 230–460 nmol/L | Little diurnal variation (<5%). |
| POTASSIUM[53,54] | Serum: 3.5–5.0 mEq/L<br>Urine: 25–105 mEq/d | 1 | Serum: 3.5–5.0 mmol/L<br>Urine: 25–105 mmol/d | Highest 8 a.m., decreases during day. Within-day variation 20%, day-to-day variation 1–2%. |
| PREGNANEDIOL[470,471] | Urine:<br>M: 0.2–1.2 mg/d<br>F: 0.1–1.3 mg/d<br>First urine: 0.2–1.5 µg/mL | 3.12 | Urine:<br>M: 0.6–3.7 µmol/d<br>F: 0.3–4.0 µmol/d<br>First urine: 0.6–4.5 µmol/L | In women, increases markedly after ovulation to peak at midluteal phase. 50% day-to-day variation. |

| Physiologic Changes | Drug Effects | Methodologic Considerations |
|---|---|---|
| INC: after meals, malabsorption, obesity, early pregnancy, lactation, renal failure, liver disease (midmolecule fragment)<br>DEC: exercise, high protein diet, ethanol, late pregnancy<br>Higher in blacks than in whites. Increases with age >40 yr; similar in children and younger adults.<br>Low in neonates, rises markedly during first day of life. | INC: estrogens, glucocorticoids, octreotide, omeprazole, phosphate, lithium, phenytoin<br>DEC: pindolol, cimetidine (midmolecule only), thiazides | Immunometric assay for intact PTH: Some assays show falsely low results in persons with renal failure. Typically performed with antibodies to C-terminal epitopes as capture antibody and N-terminal epitopes as the indicator antibody. Immunoassays measure different portions of the molecule. Midregion and C-terminal assays are quite similar and measure inactive fragments that accumulate in renal insufficiency. N-terminal assays measure intact hormone and bioactive portion of molecule. Intact PTH is labile at room temperature; specimens should be frozen within 2–4 h of collection. |
| INC: lactation<br>Similar in neonates, children, and adults. | | Immunometric assay: A two-site assay that shows no cross-reactivity to PTH. PTHrP is extremely labile at room temperature; specimens must be collected with protease inhibitors and transported on ice water; plasma must be frozen after collection. Assays that measure inactive C-terminal fragments give falsely increased results in renal failure. |
| INC: after meals<br>DEC: fever (unless nomogram correction used) | INC: drugs causing alkalosis<br>DEC: drugs causing acidosis | Ion-selective electrode: No interferences reported. Delay in analysis causes false decreases, because metabolism of glucose produces acid. Exposure of specimens to air for prolonged time causes false increase due to loss of $CO_2$. |
| INC: after meals (immediately), starvation, acidosis, fracture healing, immobilization, cell lysis, pregnancy, renal failure<br>DEC: after meals (delayed), refeeding after starvation<br>In children, much higher than in adults, rises to peak in midteens and declines to adult levels. In men, decreases with increasing age.<br>Decreased in blind persons. | INC: anabolic steroids, clonidine, GH, vitamin D, phosphosoda (transient but may be marked)<br>DEC: acetazolamide, estrogens, insulin, calcitonin, oral contraceptives, lithium, phenytoin, mithramycin, aluminum-containing antacids | Spectrophotometric: Prolonged delay in separation of cells and serum causes false increases (phosphate higher in cells); citrate, oxalate may cause false decreases.<br>Methotrexate and cefotaxime may cause overestimation in some methods, and mannitol inhibits the reaction in other methods.<br>Markedly elevated immunoglobulins, either polyclonal or monoclonal, occasionally precipitate in dilute solutions used to measure phosphate; this may cause falsely high results in some assays and falsely low results in others. |
| INC: hypertension, high protein diets, metabolic bone diseases.<br>Markedly elevated in neonates, falls rapidly during first year of life and then more gradually to reach adult values by age 20.<br>In adults, higher in men than in women. | INC: ascorbic acid | Chromatographic separation: No interferences reported. |
| INC: with increasing mass of placenta, such as with infants of diabetic mothers, multiple pregnancies, hydrops fetalis<br>DEC: trophoblastic tumors (compared with normal pregnancy)<br>Higher with female than with male fetus. | | RIA: No interferences reported. |
| INC: acidosis (shift out of cells), insulin deficiency, renal failure<br>DEC: exercise, alkalosis (shift into cells), dehydration, malnutrition, ethanol, supine position<br>Higher in blind persons. | INC: drugs causing renal impairment, THC, heparin, histamine, isoniazid, lithium, propranolol, spironolactone, antineoplastic agents, salt substitutes, triamterene, amiloride, ACE inhibitors, cyclosporine, NSAIDs<br>DEC: diuretics, acetazolamide, aldosterone or other mineralocorticoids, glucocorticoids, antibiotics (aminoglycosides, carbenicillin), insulin, mithramycin, licorice, cisplatin, amphotericin | Ion-selective electrode: Artifactual hyperkalemia occurs (a) with refrigeration of whole blood; (b) with use of fluoride- or EDTA-containing tubes—even a small amount of contamination with EDTA during phlebotomy can cause marked elevation in potassium; (c) with hemolysis; (d) in serum of patients having extreme thrombocytosis (>1,000,000/$mm^3$), eliminated by using heparinized plasma; (e) in heparinized samples from patients with extreme lymphocytosis (>200,000/$mm^3$); (f) in serum or plasma from patients with extreme leukocytosis if delay of >1 h in analyzing specimen; (g) during collection if fist alternately clenched and relaxed while tourniquet in place. |
| INC: pregnancy (gradual rise to term), exercise<br>Highest in early 20s, gradual decrease; in women, marked decrease after menopause. | INC: ampicillin, gonadotropins, ACTH<br>DEC: medroxyprogesterone, phenothiazines, oral contraceptives | Gas chromatography: May adhere to glass and plastic, falsely decreasing results by ~15%. |

(continued)

TABLE 237-1.
Reference Values in Endocrinology  (Continued)

| Test Name | Reference Range (Conventional Units) | Conversion Factor | Reference Range (SI Units) | Intraindividual Variation |
|---|---|---|---|---|
| **PREGNANETRIOL** | Urine: 0.5–2.0 mg/d | 2.97 | Urine: 1.5–5.0 µmol/d | |
| **17-OH-PREGNENOLONE. See 17-HYDROXYPREG-NENOLONE** | | | | |
| **PROGESTERONE**[271,295,472–475] | M: 0–0.4 µg/L<br>F: cycle dependent:<br>Follicular phase: <1.5 µg/L<br>Luteal phase: 5.7–28.1 µg/L<br>Postmenopausal: <0.2 µg/L | 3.18 | M: 0–1.2 nmol/L<br>F: cycle dependent:<br>Follicular phase: <4.8 nmol/L<br>Luteal phase: 18.1–89.4 nmol/L<br>Postmenopausal: <0.6 nmol/L | Released in episodic spikes during day. In women, gradually increases after ovulation, peaks about 10 d later; 20% day-to-day variation. Highest at bedtime, lowest at 8 a.m. |
| **17-OH-PROGESTERONE. See 17-HYDROXYPROGESTER-ONE** | | | | |
| **PROINSULIN**[172,476–480] | <0.2 ng/mL | 1 | <0.2 µg/L | Probably similar to insulin. |
| **PROLACTIN**[170,226,227,230,270,275,336,378,481–493] | M: 1.6–18.8 µg/L<br>F: 1.4–24.2 µg/L | 44.4 | M: 71–835 pmol/L<br>F: 62–1075 pmol/L | Released in episodic spikes during day; 2–3× higher at night, lowest in early afternoon. Day-to-day variation 5–10% in men, 40% in women.<br>In women, increases during follicular phase to spike at time of LH surge.<br>Slightly higher in winter. 20% day-to-day variation. |
| **PROSTATE-SPECIFIC ANTI-GEN (PSA)**[496–502,752] | M: 0–4.0 ng/mL<br>F: 0–0.1 ng/mL | 1 | M: 0–4.0 µg/L<br>F: 0–0.1 µg/L | No diurnal variation. Day-to-day variation 15–20%. |
| **PROSTATE-SPECIFIC ANTI-GEN, FREE**[753–758] | High risk: <14%<br>Intermediate risk: 14–25%<br>Low risk: >25% | 0.01 | High risk: <0.14<br>Intermediate risk: 0.14–0.25<br>Low risk: >0.25 | Day-to-day variation 10–15%. |
| **PYRIDINIUM CROSS-LINKS. See DEOXYPYRIDINOLINE**<br>**PYRIDOXINE. See VITAMIN B₆** | | | | |
| **RENIN**[75–77,113,191,511–516,759] | Units: ng/mL/h<br>Normal sodium:<br>Supine: 0.5–1.6<br>Upright: 1.9–3.6<br>Low sodium:<br>Supine: 2.2–4.4<br>Upright: 4.0–8.1<br>After furosemide:<br>Upright: 6.8–15.0 | 0.278 | Units: ng/L/sec<br>Normal sodium:<br>Supine: 0.1–0.4<br>Upright: 0.5–1.0<br>Low sodium:<br>Supine: 0.6–1.2<br>Upright: 1.1–2.5<br>After furosemide:<br>Upright: 1.9–4.2 | Highest 4 a.m., lowest 4–6 p.m. In women, increases during menses. |
| **RETINOL. See VITAMIN A**<br>**RIBOFLAVIN. See VITAMIN B₂** | | | | |
| **SECRETIN**[517–520] | 12–75 pg/mL | 1 | 12–75 ng/L | |
| **SELENIUM**[521–527] | Whole blood: 110–430 µg/L<br>Serum: 100–170 µg/L | 0.0127 | Whole blood: 1.40–5.46 µmol/L<br>Serum: 1.30–2.16 µmol/L | |

| Physiologic Changes | Drug Effects | Methodologic Considerations |
|---|---|---|
| INC: exercise, smoking<br>Increases during childhood to peak at age 20, falls slightly with increasing age after 20 yr. | INC: gonadotropins | Gas chromatography: No interferences reported. |
| INC: pregnancy (gradual increase to peak at term)<br>DEC: bulimia, exercise, after meals<br>Luteal phase progesterone decreases with increasing age. | INC: clomiphene, ketoconazole<br>DEC: ampicillin, oral contraceptives, mifepristone (RU-486) | RIA: Shows some cross-reaction with 17-hydroxyprogesterone, pregnanediol. Use of serum separator tubes containing resins may cause false decreases, because progesterone adheres to these. |
| INC: (relative to insulin) after meals, hyperthyroidism, impaired glucose tolerance, type 2 diabetes; other probably similar to insulin | INC: (relative to insulin) glucocorticoids, GH; other probably similar to insulin | Immunometric two-site assay: Does not cross-react with insulin, C peptide. |
| INC: pregnancy, stress, exercise, after coitus(?), renal failure, smoking (in men), after meals, high altitude, hemoconcentration<br>DEC: smoking (in women), fasting, malnutrition, acute illness<br>Higher in children, falls during childhood to adult levels by age 12. Lower in women who have had children, decreases with increasing age in older adults. Increases near menopause in some women and may be above usual decision level for prolactinoma. After age 50, gradual decline in concentration. | INC: cimetidine, cocaine, estrogens, haloperidol, methadone, phenothiazines, tricyclic antidepressants, reserpine, MAO inhibitors, oral contraceptives, danazol, phenytoin, verapamil, opiates, propranolol (in men)<br>DEC: ergot alkaloids, L-dopa, bromocriptine, calcitonin, rifampin, valproic acid, tamoxifen, erythropoietin (in renal failure) | RIA: Measures both active and inactive forms; macromolecular form may cause false elevations. |
| INC: acute renal failure, exercise<br>DEC: hospitalization<br>In men, values usually <2.5 before age 40, gradually rise with increasing age. | DEC: GnRH analog, estrogen, finasteride | Immunometric assay: Falsely elevated results occur in some patients with renal cell carcinoma. Assays differ in their degree of measurement of free PSA and PSA complexed to antiproteases; results should always be compared to previous results using the same assay, and when laboratories switch assays, patients should be tested with both the old and new assay to determine comparability of results. |
| INC: renal failure<br>DEC: liver disease, chronic prostatitis<br>Increases with increasing age in men. | | Immunometric assay: Results must be correlated with a specific total PSA assay for accurate determination of risk. Delayed separation of serum cells or storage at 4°C causes false decrease in results. Stable with storage at −70°C for at least 2 yr. |
| INC: upright posture, stress, exercise, dehydration, pregnancy, hemoconcentration<br>DEC: volume overload, supine position, weight loss, fasting (in obese persons)<br>Highest in neonates, falls gradually during childhood. In adults both basal values and response to volume depletion decrease with increasing age. Lower at high altitude, lower in women than in men, lower in blacks than in whites. | INC: volume-depleting agents, estrogens, oral contraceptives, ACE inhibitors, nifedipine, albuterol, calcium-channel blockers<br>DEC: clonidine, licorice, guanethidine, digoxin, prazosin, β-blockers, α-methyldopa, NSAIDs | Renin activity measures generated angiotensin I from substrate in patient's serum. Prolonged storage at 0–6°C activates prorenin, which causes false increases in apparent renin activity.<br>States that cause increased production of renin substrate (such as pregnancy and oral contraceptive use) cause false increase in measured renin. Newly developed immunometric assay does not show the latter interference, and does not cross-react with prorenin. |
| INC: after meals, stress, exercise, renal failure, hemoconcentration | | RIA: Much of antigen measured appears to be nonsecretin cross-reacting substance(s). |
| INC: renal failure<br>DEC: smoking, ethanol, pregnancy, hemodialysis, malignancies, acute illness, malnutrition<br>Low in neonates, decreases during first month of life to approximately 10% of adult values, gradually increases during childhood. In boys, decreases at puberty. Levels decrease again after age 55. | INC: oral contraceptives, glucocorticoids<br>DEC: valproic acid | Atomic absorption: Significant decrease in serum concentration when stored as whole blood, even for as little as 1 h. |

(continued)

**TABLE 237-1.**
Reference Values in Endocrinology  (Continued)

| Test Name | Reference Range (Conventional Units) | Conversion Factor | Reference Range (SI Units) | Intraindividual Variation |
|---|---|---|---|---|
| SEROTONIN[302,528–537] | Whole blood: 90–340 µg/L | 0.057 | Whole blood: 0.51–1.93 µmol/L | Highest at noon, lowest at night; platelet serotonin shows no diurnal pattern. In women, lowest during menses. Highest in summer, 40% lower in fall and winter. |
| SEX HORMONE–BINDING GLOBULIN[429,538–547] | M: 0.2–1.4 µg/dL<br>F: 0.6–3.6 µg/dL | 10 | M: 2–14 µg/L<br>F: 6–36 µg/L | Day-to-day variation 10%; no changes during menstrual cycle. Highest in early afternoon, lowest around midnight. |
| SILICON[548,549] | 203–406 ng/mL | 0.036 | 7.23–14.45 nmol/L | |
| SODIUM | Serum: 135–143 mEq/L<br>Urine: 43–260 mEq/d | 1 | Serum: 135–143 mmol/L<br>Urine: 43–260 mmol/d | Little day-to-day variation (<1%); within day, peaks at noon, falls in evening, then rises during sleep; total diurnal variation is 1–2%. Highest in summer, lowest in winter. In women, lower by 1.5% during menses. |
| SOMATOMEDIN C. See INSULIN-LIKE GROWTH FACTOR-I | | | | |
| SOMATOSTATIN[305,442,518,550–554] | 5–25 pg/mL | 1 | 5–25 ng/L | 20% diurnal variation, increases during evening to peak at midnight, gradually decreases to low at 8 a.m. |
| SOMATOTROPIN. See GROWTH HORMONE<br><br>T₃. See TRIIODOTHYRONINE<br><br>T₃RU. See TRIIODOTHYRO-NINE RESIN UPTAKE<br><br>T₄. See THYROXINE | | | | |
| TELOPEPTIDE, C-TERMINAL[86,698–701] | M: 21–696 µg/mmol creatinine of urine<br>F: 34–992 µg/mmol creatinine of urine | 1 | M: 21–696 µg/mmol creatinine of urine<br>F: 34–992 µg/mmol creatinine of urine | Day-to-day variation 25%. 60% higher at night than in late afternoon. |
| TELOPEPTIDE, N-TERMINAL[86,698,700–702,760–763] | Serum:<br>M: 5.4–24.2 nmol/L<br>F: 6.2–19.0 nmol/L<br>Urine:<br>M: 7–68 nmol/mmol creat.<br>F: 11–48 nmol/mmol creat. | 1 | Serum:<br>M: 5.4–24.2 nmol/L<br>F: 6.2–19.0 nmol/L<br>Urine:<br>M: 7–68 nmol/mmol creat.<br>F: 11–48 nmol/mmol creat. | Urine: Day-to-day variation 20%. 40% higher at night than in late afternoon.<br>Serum: 40% higher in early a.m. than at nadir at noon. |
| TESTOSTERONE[111,170,225,226,253,283,555–558,580] | M: 300–1000 ng/dL<br>F: 15–60 ng/dL | 0.035 | M: 10.4–34.7 nmol/L<br>F: 0.52–2.08 nmol/L | Released in episodic spikes during day, 25% higher in a.m. than in p.m. In women, peaks at ovulation, 30% lower at menses. 10–20% day-to-day variation (highest in postmenopausal women). |
| TESTOSTERONE, BIOAVAILABLE[764,765] | M: 66–417 ng/dL<br>F: 0.6–5.0 ng/dL | 0.035<br>34.7 | M: 2.3–14.6 nmol/L<br>F: 21–174 pmol/L | Probably similar to testosterone. |
| TESTOSTERONE, FREE[170,225,226,253,555–558,580,766,767] | M: 50–210 pg/mL<br>F: 1.0–8.5 pg/mL | 3.47 | M: 175–730 pmol/L<br>F: 3.5–30 pmol/L | Same as for testosterone. |

| Physiologic Changes | Drug Effects | Methodologic Considerations |
|---|---|---|
| INC: schizophrenia, anxiety, some forms of mental retardation<br>DEC: migraine headaches, ethanol, renal failure<br>Higher in men than in women. In women, decreases after menopause. | INC: estrogens, MAO inhibitors<br>DEC: ranitidine, reserpine | Fluorometric: Ingestion of foods rich in serotonin (see list under 5-Hydroxyindoleacetic acid) does not alter platelet serotonin but increases whole blood and plasma levels. |
| INC: pregnancy, hemoconcentration, smoking, fasting<br>DEC: obesity, exercise<br>Highest in neonates, decreases to puberty, then gradually increases throughout adult years. In women, decreases after menopause. | INC: carbamazepine, phenytoin, estrogens, oral contraceptives, rifampicin, tamoxifen, thyroid hormones<br>DEC: androgens, danazol, glucocorticoids, insulin, Norplant | Immunoassay: No interferences reported. |
| INC: renal failure | | Atomic absorption: Siliconized test tubes or needles cannot be used. |
| INC: after meals (slight), exercise, dehydration<br>DEC: hyperglycemia or other osmotic stresses, pregnancy, ethanol<br>Lower in blind persons by 5 mmol/L. | INC: agents causing salt retention—mineralocorticoids, anabolic steroids, estrogens, oral contraceptives, phenylbutazone, licorice, guanethidine, clonidine, lithium<br>DEC: diuretics, heparin, chlorpropamide, aminoglutethimide, amphotericin, vincristine, cyclophosphamide, carbamazepine, miconazole | Ion-selective electrode: With instruments that require specimen dilution, falsely low values are obtained in specimens with extremely high lipids or protein; this also occurs with flame photometry instruments, but not with ion-selective electrodes without sample dilution (as is typically used on whole blood analyzers). |
| INC: after meals, renal failure, hemoconcentration, pregnancy<br>Low in newborns, rises rapidly over first 5 d of life, then falls throughout first year of life; results slightly higher in children than in adults. | DEC: oral contraceptives | RIA: Large-molecular-weight forms predominate, appear to be artifacts of assay. Theophylline may interfere with binding, causing falsely low results in some assays and falsely high results in others. (Also see Chap. 169.) |
| Highest in neonates, falls to low levels by age 2 yr and remains stable until onset of puberty, then increases in parallel to rate of increase in height, falls to adult levels by age 20 yr. In women, increases after menopause. | | Immunoassay: No interferences reported. Diurnal excretion pattern differs from that of creatinine; first or second voided specimens or 24-h urine should be used rather than random collections. |
| INC: bed rest, lactation<br>Highest in neonates, falls to low levels by age 2 yr and remains stable until onset of puberty, then increases in parallel to rate of increase in height (peak 4–5× adult levels), falls to adult levels by age 20 (age 30 in men). Higher in males than in females (before age 40), higher in whites than in blacks. In women, increases after menopause. | | Immunoassay: No interferences reported. Diurnal excretion pattern differs from that of creatinine; first or second voided specimens or 24-h urine should be used rather than random collections. |
| INC: pregnancy, fatty meals, exercise, after meals, hemoconcentration, obesity (in women)<br>DEC: stress, acute illness, immobilization, repeated heavy exercise, obesity (in men), ethanol<br>Higher in blacks than in whites.<br>In men, falls 1–2% per year at ages >30 yr, but in women increases after menopause. Diurnal variation is lost in older men.<br>Lower in blind persons. | INC: barbiturates, cimetidine, clomiphene, DHEA (in women), estrogens, oral contraceptives, rifampin, Norplant, phenytoin<br>DEC: androgens, DES, digoxin, danazol, glucocorticoids, nafarelin, spironolactone, thioridazine, phenothiazines, THC, ketoconazole | RIA: Cross-reacts with dihydrotestosterone; if extraction step not used, overestimates testosterone due to nonspecific cross-reactants in serum. Danazol cross-reacts to varying extent, usually causing falsely high results but producing falsely low results in some assays. |
| Probably similar to testosterone<br>Low in children, increases gradually during first decade. Decreases with increasing age >40 yr. | Probably similar to testosterone | Immunoassay after ammonium sulfate precipitation: No interferences reported. Measures testosterone not bound to SHBG, as ammonium sulfate precipitates SHBG-bound testosterone. |
| Same as for testosterone, although hemoconcentration does not affect results. | INC: barbiturates, clomiphene, danazol<br>DEC: androgens, antiepileptics, DES, digoxin, spironolactone, phenothiazines, THC, ketoconazole | Equilibrium dialysis: Results are generally similar to those calculated from total testosterone and SHBG levels. Variation in incubation temperature significantly affects results obtained. Analog immunoassays are widely used, but results are significantly lower and are affected by changes in the level of SHBG; factors affecting SHBG (see earlier) produce erroneous results. |

(continued)

**TABLE 237-1.**
Reference Values in Endocrinology  (Continued)

| Test Name | Reference Range (Conventional Units) | Conversion Factor | Reference Range (SI Units) | Intraindividual Variation |
|---|---|---|---|---|
| THIAMINE. See VITAMIN B[1] | | | | |
| THYROGLOBULIN[135,559–565,768] | <42 µg/L | 1 | <42 µg/L | Day-to-day variation 5%. In women, slight decline at time of ovulation. |
| THYROGLOBULIN ANTIBODIES. See ANTITHYROGLOBULIN | | | | |
| THYROID-BINDING GLOBULIN[556–572] | 17–36 mg/L | 1 | 17–36 mg/L | 5% day-to-day variation; no seasonal variation. |
| THYROID MICROSOMAL ANTIBODIES. See ANTI–THYROID MICROSOMES | | | | |
| THYROID PEROXIDASE ANTIBODIES. See ANTI–THYROID PEROXIDASE | | | | |
| THYROID-STIMULATING IMMUNOGLOBULINS[579] | <130% | 0.01 | <1.3 | |
| THYROTROPIN[560,573–578] | 0.3–5.0 µIU/mL | 1 | 0.3–5.0 mIU/L | Released in episodic spikes. Within day highest at midnight, falls to nadir (~40% of peak) at 4 p.m.; the magnitude of fluctuation decreases in older individuals. Day-to-day variation 20%. Highest in winter, lowest in summer. |
| THYROTROPIN-RECEPTOR ANTIBODIES[579] | <10% inhibition | 1 | <10% inhibition | |
| THYROXINE[170,222,581–590] | 4.5–12.5 µg/dL | 12.9 | 58–161 nmol/L | 15% day-to-day variation. Highest in winter, lowest in summer. Within day, may fluctuate as much as 50% in episodic spikes. |
| THYROXINE (T[4]), FREE[170,225,567–571,581–592,769–771] | 0.7–1.5 ng/dL | 12.9 | 9.0–19.4 pmol/L | 15% day-to-day variation; highest in winter, lowest in summer. |
| THYROXINE INDEX, FREE | 1.0–4.3 U | 1 | 1.0–4.3 U | Same as for free T[4]. |

| Physiologic Changes | Drug Effects | Methodologic Considerations |
|---|---|---|
| INC: hemoconcentration, pregnancy, after fine-needle aspiration biopsy, but not after thyroid palpation<br>Highest in neonates, higher in premature than in term infants; decreases in childhood to reach adult levels by adolescence. | DEC: neomycin | RIA: Antithyroglobulin antibodies cause interference with assay and result in either false elevation or false decrease depending on method used. Because these antibodies are present in ~50% of patients with thyroid cancer, their presence should be evaluated when measuring thyroglobulin. |
| INC: pregnancy, hemoconcentration<br>DEC: malnutrition/malabsorption, renal failure<br>Highest in children, progressively decreases with age throughout childhood and adult life. Higher in women than in men until after menopause. | INC: estrogens, oral contraceptives, phenothiazines, progestational agents, methadone, heroin, 5-fluorouracil, clofibrate, tamoxifen<br>DEC: androgens, high-dose glucocorticoids, phenytoin, danazol, propranolol, carbamazepine, colestipol | RIA: No interferences reported. With immunoradiometric assays, substances inhibiting $T_4$ binding to TBG cause falsely low values. |
| | | Bioassay, measuring cAMP by incubation of cultured thyroid cells with patient's serum: No interferences reported. Other assay systems include TSH displacement, LATS. |
| INC: smoking, pregnancy, renal failure, hemoconcentration, psychologic stress<br>DEC: fasting, prolonged malnutrition, acute illness<br>2× higher in neonates, gradually decreases during childhood to reach adult levels about age 20. Increases again in late adult life (? response to thyroid atrophy); however, a small percentage of elderly have low TSH. Higher in men than in women, higher in whites than in blacks. | INC: drugs decreasing $T_4$ production (see thyroxine for list), dopamine antagonists, prednisone<br>DEC: salicylates, thyroid hormones, dopamine, L-dopa, most glucocorticoids, somatostatin, danazol | Immunometric assay: Using monoclonal antibodies with sensitivity of <0.05 U/L can distinguish normal from hyperthyroid levels in virtually all cases, although low values also occur with acute illness. Assays with sensitivity of <0.005 have slightly better accuracy in separating hyperthyroid and acutely ill persons. With very sensitive assays, patients on replacement $T_4$ may have falsely suppressed TSH if specimens are drawn after daily $T_4$ dose. |
| | | Competitive binding assay: No interferences reported. Measures all classes of TSH-receptor antibodies, including stimulating immunoglobulins (see also thyroid-stimulating immunoglobulins), blocking antibodies, and growth-promoting antibodies. |
| INC: pregnancy, during recovery from hepatitis, hemoconcentration<br>DEC: protein malnutrition, protein-losing states, strenuous exercise, smoking, severe acute illness, renal failure<br>Higher in men than in women. | INC: propranolol, drugs increasing TBG (see earlier), $T_4$, amiodarone (most cases)<br>DEC: rifampin, lithium, isotretinoin, salsalate, drugs decreasing TBG (see earlier), drugs decreasing hormone binding to TBG (diazepam, heparin, trimethoprim-sulfamethoxazole, nitroprusside, carbamazepine, valproic acid, phenytoin, phenylbutazone) | Immunoassay: Hemolysis causes false decrease in some assays; radioiodine, technetium used in scans may cause false increases with radioimmunoassays. |
| INC: postoperatively, first trimester of pregnancy, acutely with fasting<br>DEC: hemodialysis<br>Higher in men than in women. Slight decrease with age >55 yr. | INC: heparin, propranolol, valproic acid<br>DEC: lithium, trimethoprim/sulfamethoxazole, nitroprusside, salsalate, phenytoin, carbamazepine, valproic acid, colestipol, rifampin | Labeled antibody immunoassay: Heparin causes falsely low values, whereas furosemide causes falsely high values. In normal patients, results agree with equilibrium dialysis. In patients with abnormal serum proteins or alteration in protein binding, results from the two methods diverge, and different immunoassays give differing results. Analog assays often disagree with results of equilibrium dialysis and extraction immunoassays in acute illness; in addition, phenytoin and carbamazepine produce falsely increased results with analog immunoassays. With virtually all assays, including equilibrium dialysis, results are falsely elevated (with room temperature incubation) in patients with decreased TBG or acute illness. |
| Same as for free $T_4$ | Same as for free $T_4$ | Calculated using formula ($T_4 \times T_3$ resin uptake) or ($T_4$/T-uptake). Agrees moderately well with results of measurement except in patients with acute illness or in patients with dysalbuminemic hyperthyroxinemia. |

(continued)

**TABLE 237-1.**
Reference Values in Endocrinology  (Continued)

| Test Name | Reference Range (Conventional Units) | Conversion Factor | Reference Range (SI Units) | Intraindividual Variation |
|---|---|---|---|---|
| TIBC. See IRON-BINDING CAPACITY | | | | |
| TOCOPHEROL. See VITAMIN E | | | | |
| TRIGLYCERIDES[209,593] | NCEP decision levels:<br>Normal: <200 mg/dL<br>Borderline: 200–400 mg/dL<br>High: 400–1000 mg/dL<br>Very High: >1000 mg/dL | 0.0113 | NCEP decision levels:<br>Normal: <2.26 mmol/L<br>Borderline: 2.26–4.52 mmol/L<br>High: 4.52–11.3 mmol/L<br>Very High: >11.3 mmol/L | 30% day-to-day variation. In women, highest at midcycle. Highest in winter, lowest in fall. |
| TRIIODOTHYRONINE[170,222,557–559,581–591] | 80–220 ng/dL | 0.0154 | 1.23–3.39 nmol/L | 20% day-to-day variation; highest in winter, lowest in summer. |
| TRIIODOTHYRONINE, FREE[170,225,567–571,581–592,594,682,770,771] | 230–420 pg/dL | 0.0154 | 3.5–6.5 pmol/L | Probably similar to $T_3$. |
| TRIIODOTHYRONINE, REVERSE[170,222,557–559,581–588] | 80–350 ng/L | 1.54 | 123–539 pmol/L | 25% diurnal variation; highest in winter, lowest in summer. |
| TRIIODOTHYRONINE RESIN UPTAKE[170,222,557–559,581–588] | 22–34% | 0.01 | 0.22–0.34 | In general, changes are proportional to changes in TBG but in a reciprocal fashion. |
| TSH. See THYROTROPIN | | | | |
| TSH-RECEPTOR ANTIBODIES. See THYROTROPIN-RECEPTOR ANTIBODIES | | | | |
| TSI. See THYROID-STIMULATING IMMUNO-GLOBULINS | | | | |
| T-UPTAKE | 0.78–1.24 | 1 | 0.78–1.24 | In general, changes are directly related to changes in TBG. |
| URIC ACID[595,596] | M: 4–8 mg/dL<br>F: 3–7 mg/dL | 0.059 | M: 0.24–0.47 mmol/L<br>F: 0.18–0.41 mmol/L | Slight diurnal variation (5%) with highest values in a.m., lowest in afternoon; day-to-day variation 10%. Higher in summer than in winter. |
| VANADIUM[410–411] | 14–230 ng/L | 0.0196 | 0.27–4.51 nmol/L | |
| VANILLYLMANDELIC ACID[345,352,416,599] | 1–8 mg/d | 5.05 | 5–44 µmol/d | Excretion highest at night. No reports on diurnal or intraindividual variation in normal individuals. |

| Physiologic Changes | Drug Effects | Methodologic Considerations |
|---|---|---|
| INC: marked increase (60%) after meals; stress, ethanol, hemoconcentration, smoking, pregnancy, renal failure, starvation<br>DEC: exercise, prolonged fast, physical training<br>Lower in children; higher in men than in women; higher in whites than in blacks. | INC: β-adrenergic antagonists, danazol, estrogens, furosemide, isotretinoin, ketoconazole, glucocorticoids, oral contraceptives, spironolactone, salicylates, tamoxifen, cholestyramine (in some patients)<br>DEC: androgens, amiodarone, ascorbic acid, bile salts, cholestyramine, fibric acids, glyburide, heparin, probucol, sulfonylureas | Enzymatic: In methods that do not use blanking, nitroglycerine, drugs containing propylene glycol, and endogenous glycerol (increased in ketoacidosis) may cause falsely high levels. Heparin causes decrease due to activation of lipoprotein lipase. Storage of specimen for >1 d is associated with spontaneous hydrolysis and artifactual decrease in values. |
| INC: parallel to $T_4$ (see earlier), obesity<br>DEC: acute stress, prolonged fasting, renal failure, smoking<br>Lower in neonates, decreases gradually over age 60. Higher in men than in women. | INC: rifampin, terbutaline, valproic acid; parallels $T_4$ (see earlier)<br>DEC: salsalate; as for $T_4$; in addition, drugs that inhibit conversion of $T_4$ to $T_3$ (propranolol, glucocorticoids, cimetidine, thiouracil) | RIA: No interferences reported. |
| INC: parallel to free $T_4$<br>DEC: parallel to $T_3$ | Should parallel free $T_4$ for increase, $T_3$ for decrease. | Immune absorption, RIA: Heparin causes falsely low values; carbamazepine, phenytoin, and fenoprofen may cause false increases.<br>Immunoassays often give discrepant results in pregnancy. |
| INC: decreased conversion of $T_4$ to $T_3$ (acute stress, prolonged fasting, renal failure), hemoconcentration<br>Higher in neonates, falls to adult levels by 1 mo of life. Higher over age 60. | INC: amiodarone, cimetidine, prednisone, propranolol, drugs inhibiting conversion of $T_4$ to $T_3$ (see earlier) | RIA: No interferences reported. |
| INC: similar to factors that decrease TBG<br>DEC: similar to factors that increase TBG | INC: similar to factors that decrease TBG<br>DEC: similar to factors that increase TBG | Indirect, measures residual labeled $T_3$ after mixing labeled $T_3$ with patient's serum. Changes in a reciprocal fashion to unoccupied binding sites on TBG. Heparin may cause decreased binding of $T_3$ to resin, causing falsely low values. |
| INC: similar to factors that increase TBG<br>DEC: similar to factors that decrease TBG | INC: androgens, high-dose glucocorticoids, phenytoin, danazol, propranolol, carbamazepine, colestipol<br>DEC: estrogens, oral contraceptives, phenothiazines, progestational agents, methadone, heroin, 5-fluorouracil, clofibrate, tamoxifen | Indirect, measures labeled $T_4$ bound to TBG; no interferences reported. Results normalized by dividing result obtained by the population mean value. Results change inversely to $T_3$ resin uptake. |
| INC: exercise, starvation, ethanol, renal failure<br>DEC: pregnancy, smoking, refeeding<br>Lower in children, rises to adult levels by adolescence. In women, increases after age 50.<br>Higher in blind persons. | INC: drugs impairing renal excretion (diuretics, aspirin), androgens, cisplatin, cyclosporine, ethambutol, disopyramide, piroxicam, propranolol, pyrazinamide, theophylline<br>DEC: warfarin, radiographic contrast agents, guaifenesin, glucocorticoids, allopurinol, azathioprine, lithium, THC, indomethacin | Enzymatic: No interferences reported. |
| INC: affective disorders, renal failure | | Neutron activation analysis: No interferences reported. |
| INC: caffeine, ketosis, exercise, starvation, factors that increase catecholamine output (see catecholamines), iron deficiency<br>DEC: renal insufficiency, ethanol<br>In children, excretion per mL decreases with increasing age; ratio of VMA to creatinine is unchanged during childhood. | INC: phenothiazines, lithium, drugs releasing catecholamines (see earlier)<br>DEC: drugs inhibiting catecholamine production (see earlier), radiographic contrast agents, disulfiram, phenothiazines, α-methyldopa | Spectrophotometric: A wide variety of substances that chemically resemble vanillin, the final product measured, can cause falsely elevated results. Ideally, patient should eliminate interfering foods (citrus fruits, bananas) and medications (salicylates, glyceryl guaiacolate, tetracycline, pyridine) for 3 days before urine collection; however, because of the wide range of normal, only large amounts of these substances or caffeine cause falsely low results. Clofibrate may cause falsely low results. VMA is unstable at alkaline pH; urine must be collected in container with acid. |

(continued)

**TABLE 237-1.**
Reference Values in Endocrinology (Continued)

| Test Name | Reference Range (Conventional Units) | Conversion Factor | Reference Range (SI Units) | Intraindividual Variation |
|---|---|---|---|---|
| VASOACTIVE INTESTINAL POLYPEPTIDE[600–604,683,684] | <50 pg/mL | 1 | <50 ng/L | |
| VASOPRESSIN[115,605–609] | 1–20 pg/mL | 0.93 | 1–18.6 pmol/L | Increases during night to maximum on rising, falls during day. In women, peaks at time of ovulation. |
| VITAMIN A[187,188,610–614] | 30–100 µg/dL | 0.03 | 0.9–3.0 µmol/L | 25% day-to-day variation; no diurnal pattern. |
| VITAMIN B$_1$[615,616] | Whole blood: 88–192 nmol/L | 1 | Whole blood: 88–192 nmol/L | |
| VITAMIN B$_2$ | 6.2–39 nmol/L | 1 | 6.2–39 nmol/L | |
| VITAMIN B$_6$[617–619] | 3.6–18 µg/L | 4.05 | 14.6–72.8 nmol/L | |
| VITAMIN B$_{12}$[620–624] | 180–1500 pg/mL | 0.74 | 133–1107 pmol/L | |
| VITAMIN C[625–627] | 0–2.0 mg/dL | 56.78 | 0–114 µmol/L | Day-to-day variation 25%. Highest in early a.m., falls during day; highest in summer, lowest in winter. In women, peaks at time of ovulation. |
| VITAMIN D, 1,25-DIHYDROXY[171,181,225,406,450–453,628–636] | 18–62 ng/L | 2.4 | 43–149 pmol/L | Higher in winter than in summer. In women, sharp increase (4–5×) at ovulation. Slightly higher in morning, 20% day-to-day variation. |
| VITAMIN D, 24,25-DIHYDROXY[171,225,406,450–453,628–633] | 0.2–2.2 µg/L | 2.4 | 0.5–5.3 nmol/L | Higher in summer than in winter; no data on diurnal variation. |
| VITAMIN D, 25-HYDROXY[171,225,406,450–453,628–641] | 10–55 µg/L | 2.4 | 24–132 nmol/L | Higher in summer than in winter; no data on diurnal variation. |
| VITAMIN E[188,642–644] | 5–20 mg/L | 2.32 | 12–46 µmol/L | 15% day-to-day variation; no diurnal pattern. |
| VMA. See VANILLYLMANDELIC ACID | | | | |
| ZINC[219–223,645–650,670] | Serum: 67–124 µg/dL Urine: 110–600 µg/d | 0.15 0.02 | Serum: 10.0–18.6 µmol/L Urine: 1.7–9.2 µmol/d | Highest at 9 a.m., lowest at 9 p.m.; day-to-day variation 15%. |

| Physiologic Changes | Drug Effects | Methodologic Considerations |
|---|---|---|
| INC: exercise, fat ingestion, chronic renal failure, obesity | | RIA: Extremely labile, must be collected in tubes containing protease inhibitor, and plasma frozen immediately after separation. Occasionally, large-molecular-weight forms cross-react. (Also see Chap. 182.) |
| INC: upright posture, dehydration, vasovagal reaction, premenstrual stress, smoking, exercise, fasting, renal failure<br>DEC: overhydration, ethanol, supine position, pregnancy (first and second trimesters), acute hypertension | INC: phenothiazines, cyclophosphamide, lithium, tricyclic antidepressants, vincristine<br>DEC: phenytoin, carbamazepine | RIA: Synthetic forms of vasopressin and arginine vasopressin from platelets cross-react. Vasopressin is unstable at room temperature; specimens should be placed in ice water, and plasma frozen as soon as possible. Platelet contamination of plasma causes falsely high values. |
| INC: pregnancy, renal failure, hemoconcentration, ethanol<br>DEC: malabsorption, malnutrition<br>Higher in men than in women. Decreases with increasing age >65 yr. Lower in infants and children below age 5 yr. | INC: oral contraceptives, estrogens, phenytoin<br>DEC: DES, cholestyramine, neomycin | Spectrophotometric: Carotene cross-reacts in some assays. Specimens must be protected from light to prevent falsely low results. |
| DEC: pregnancy, exercise<br>Serum levels reflect recent intake; return to normal rapidly with feeding.<br>Higher in infants, reach adult levels by age 1 yr. | | HPLC: No interferences reported. |
| DEC: pregnancy, ethanol<br>In children, falls during periods of bone growth. | | Enzymatic: No interferences reported. |
| DEC: pregnancy, ethanol, smoking, renal failure<br>Higher in men than in women; in men, decreases after age 50. | DEC: oral contraceptives, anticonvulsants, isoniazid, penicillamine, hydralazine, cycloserine, L-dopa, theophylline | RIA: No interferences reported. |
| INC: leukocytosis, liver disease, malignancies (all due to high binding protein levels), hemoconcentration<br>DEC: pregnancy<br>Highest in blacks, intermediate in Hispanics, lowest in whites.<br>Values decrease with age in men. | INC: valproic acid<br>DEC: most anticonvulsants, aspirin, neomycin, oral contraceptives, nitroprusside, colchicine | RIA: Current assays measure only active vitamin $B_{12}$ and do not cross-react with inactive analogs; in some sera, vitamin $B_{12}$ by RIA appears to be falsely low. Assay measures total $B_{12}$, which may falsely overestimate available $B_{12}$ in persons with high level of binding proteins. |
| DEC: pregnancy, ethanol, smoking, malabsorption, obesity<br>Higher in women than in men; levels fall with increasing age. | DEC: aspirin, oral contraceptives, estrogens | Spectrophotometric: No interferences reported. |
| INC: pregnancy, lactation, obesity, hemoconcentration<br>DEC: renal insufficiency, immobilization<br>Higher in blacks and Hispanics than in whites.<br>In children, highest in infancy; falls during childhood, but rises to second peak in teens. | INC: aluminum hydroxide, estrogens, octreotide, prednisone<br>DEC: isotretinoin, ketoconazole | Competitive protein binding after chromatographic separation: Assays tend to differ considerably from one another, and repeated measurements on the same specimen vary by ≥25%. |
| DEC: last trimester of pregnancy, renal insufficiency, hemoconcentration, after fractures<br>Higher in whites than in blacks. | | Competitive protein binding after chromatographic separation: Assays tend to differ considerably from one another, and repeated measurements on the same specimen vary by ≥25%. |
| INC: exercise<br>DEC: liver disease, malabsorption, hemoconcentration, ethanol<br>In children, values decrease slightly with increasing age. In adults, decreases with age after 65 yr.<br>Lower in Hispanics than in whites. | DEC: phenytoin, carbamazepine, glucocorticoids, rifampin | Competitive protein binding after chromatographic separation: Assays tend to differ considerably from one another, but assay reproducibility is better than for 1,25-dihydroxy form. |
| INC: renal failure, pregnancy<br>DEC: malabsorption<br>Extremely low in neonates, slowly rises to adult levels by puberty, decreases with increasing age >65 yr. Slightly higher in women than in men. | DEC: cholestyramine, clofibrate, anticonvulsants | Spectrophotometric: No interferences reported. Blood levels reflect recent intake. Specimens must be protected from light to prevent falsely low values. |
| INC: exercise<br>DEC: pregnancy, renal insufficiency, hepatic dysfunction, acute infections, ethanol, renal failure<br>Slightly higher in men than in women. Decreases with increasing age >60 yr. | INC: carbonic anhydrase inhibitors (whole blood), glucocorticoids<br>DEC: estrogens, oral contraceptives, captopril | Atomic absorption: Contamination, especially by rubber stoppers, is a major difficulty in assays, as is contamination from improperly cleaned glassware. |

# REFERENCES

1. Galen RS, et al. Beyond normality—the predictive value and efficiency of medical diagnoses. New York: John Wiley and Sons, 1975.
2. Murphy EA, et al. The normal range—a common misuse. J Chronic Dis 1967; 20:79.
3. Feinstein AR. Clinical biostatistics. XII. On exorcising the ghost of Gauss and the curse of Kelvin. Clin Pharmacol Ther 1971; 12:1003.
4. Grasbeck R, et al. Establishment and use of normal values. Scand J Clin Lab Invest 1969; 110(Suppl):62.
5. Statland BE, et al. Reference values: are they useful? Lab Med 1984; 4:61.
6. Enos WF, et al. Coronary disease among United States soldiers killed in action in Korea. Preliminary report. JAMA 1953; 152:1090 (reprinted in JAMA 1986; 256:2859).
7. Ross R, et al. The pathogenesis of atherosclerosis (first of two parts). N Engl J Med 1976; 295:369.
8. Rifai N. Lipoproteins and apolipoproteins. Composition, metabolism, and association with coronary heart disease. Arch Pathol Lab Med 1986; 110:694.
9. McManus BM. Reference ranges and ideal patient values for blood cholesterol. Can there be reconciliation? Arch Pathol Lab Med 1986; 110:469.
10. Summary of the second report of the National Cholesterol Education Program (NCEP) expert panel on detection, evaluation, and treatment of high blood cholesterol in adults (Adult Treatment Panel II). JAMA 1993; 269:3015.
11. Statland BE, et al. Response of clinical chemistry quantity values to selected physical, dietary, and smoking activities. Prog Clin Pathol 1981; 8:25.
12. Statland BE, et al. Factors contributing to intra-individual variation of serum constituents: 4. Effects of posture and tourniquet application on variation of serum constituents in healthy subjects. Clin Chem 1974; 20:1513.
13. Elveback LR, et al. Health, normality, and the ghost of Gauss. JAMA 1970; 211:69.
14. Reed AH, et al. Influence of statistical method used on the resulting estimate of normal range. Clin Chem 1971; 17:275.
15. Shultz EK, et al. Improved reference-interval estimation. Clin Chem 1985; 31:1974.
16. Feinstein AR. Clinical biostatistics. XXVII. The derangements of the "range of normal." Clin Pharmacol Ther 1974; 15:528.
17. Cebul RD, et al. Biochemical profiles. Applications in ambulatory screening and preadmission testing of adults. Ann Intern Med 1987; 106:403.
18. Berwick DM. Screening in health fairs. A critical review of benefits, risks, and costs. JAMA 1985; 254:1492.
19. Pickup JF, et al. Intra-individual variation of some serum constituents and its relevance to population-based reference ranges. Clin Chem 1977; 23:842.
20. Van Steirteghem AC, et al. Variance components of serum constituents in healthy individuals. Clin Chem 1978; 24:212.
21. Costongs GMPJ, et al. Short-term and long-term intra-individual variations and critical differences of clinical chemical laboratory parameters. J Clin Chem Clin Biochem 1985; 23:7.
22. Statland BE. Turning lab values into action. Diagn Med 1980; 3:56.
23. Statland BE. Clinical decision levels for lab tests, 2nd ed. Oradell, NJ: Medical Economics Company, 1987.
24. Sheps SB, et al. The assessment of diagnostic tests. A survey of current medical research. JAMA 1984; 252:2418.
25. Feinstein AR. Clinical biostatistics XXXI. On the sensitivity, specificity, and discrimination of diagnostic tests. Clin Pharmacol Ther 1975; 17:104.
26. Beck JR, et al. The use of relative operating characteristic (ROC) curves in test performance evaluation. Arch Pathol Lab Med 1986; 110:13.
27. Winkel P, et al. Using the subject as his own referent in assessing day-to-day changes of laboratory test results. Contemp Top Anal Clin Chem 1977; 1:287.
28. Dillon MC, et al. Diagnostic problem in acute myocardial infarction: CK-MB in the absence of abnormally elevated total creatine kinase levels. Arch Intern Med 1982; 142:33.
29. Hong RA, et al. Elevated CK-MB with normal total creatine kinase in suspected myocardial infarction: associated clinical findings and early prognosis. Am Heart J 1986; 111:1041.
30. Dufour DR, et al. Rapid serial enzyme measurements in evaluation of patients with suspected myocardial infarction. Am J Cardiol 1989; 63:652.
31. Fraser CG. Biological variation in clinical chemistry. An update: collated data, 1988–1991. Arch Pathol Lab Med 1992; 116:916.
32. Holzel WGE. Intra-individual variation of some analytes in serum of patients with insulin-dependent diabetes mellitus. Clin Chem 1987; 33:57.
33. Statland BE, et al. Factors contributing to intra-individual variation of serum constituents. 2. Effects of exercise and diet on variation of serum constituents in healthy subjects. Clin Chem 1973; 19:1380.
34. Levi L. The effect of coffee on the function of the sympatho-adrenomedullary system in man. Acta Med Scand 1967; 181:431.
35. Arendt J, et al., eds. Biological rhythms in clinical practice. Boston: Wright, 1989.
36. Touitou Y, Haus E, eds. Biologic rhythms in clinical and laboratory medicine. Berlin: Springer-Verlag, 1992.
37. Weitzman ED. Circadian rhythms and episodic hormone secretion in man. Annu Rev Med 1976; 27:225.
38. Statland BE, et al. Factors contributing to intra-individual variation of serum constituents. 1. Within-day variation of serum constituents in healthy subjects. Clin Chem 1973; 19:1374.
38a. Leppanen E, et al. When to collect blood specimens: midmorning vs fasting samples. Clin Chem 1998; 44:2537.
39. Nuttall FQ, Jones B. Creatine kinase and glutamic oxalacetic transaminase activity in serum: kinetics of change with exercise and effect of physical conditioning. J Lab Clin Med 1968; 71:847.
39a. De Souza MJ, et al. High frequency of luteal phase deficiency and anovulation in recreational women runners: blunted elevation in follicle-stimulating hormone observed during luteal-follicular transition. J Clin Endocrinol Metab 1998; 83:4220.
40. Tamir I, et al. Measurement of lipids and evaluation of lipid disorders. In: Henry JB, ed. Clinical diagnosis and management by laboratory methods, 16th ed. Philadelphia: WB Saunders, 1979:201.
41. Van der Poll T, et al. Tumor necrosis factor: a putative mediator of the sick euthyroid syndrome in man. J Clin Endocrinol Metab 1990; 71:1567.
42. Bhakri HL, et al. Longitudinal study of thyroid function in acutely ill elderly patients using a sensitive TSH assay-defer testing until recovery. Gerontology 1990; 36:140.
43. Weindling H, et al. Drug interactions and clinical laboratory data. Lab Med 1975; 6:24.
44. Fortman CS, et al. Serum 5'-nucleotidase in patients receiving anti-epileptic drugs. Am J Clin Pathol 1985; 84:197.
45. Blumberg AG, et al. The interference of chlorpromazine metabolites in the analysis of urinary methoxy-catecholamines. Clin Chem 1966; 12:803.
46. Kroll MH, et al. Reaction of picrate with creatinine and cepha antibiotics. Clin Chem 1984; 30:1664.
47. Young DS, et al. Effects of drugs on clinical laboratory tests, 4th ed. Washington: AACC Press, 1995.
48. Siest G, et al., eds. Drug effects on laboratory test results: analytical interferences and pharmacological effects. Littleton, MA: PSG Publishing, 1988.
49. Fisken RA, et al. Hypercalcaemia—a hospital survey. Q J Med 1980; 49:405.
50. Laessig RH, et al. The effects of 0.1 and 1.0 per cent erythrocytes and hemolysis on serum chemistry values. Am J Clin Pathol 1976; 66:639.
51. Laessig RH, et al. Changes in serum chemical values as a result of prolonged contact with the clot. Am J Clin Pathol 1976; 66:598.
52. Sazama K, et al. Is antiglycolysis required for routine glucose analysis? Clin Chem 1979; 25:2038.
53. Ingram RH, et al. Pseudohyperkalemia with thrombocytosis. N Engl J Med 1962; 267:895.
54. Dufour DR, et al. Artifactual hyperkalemia due to heparin in patients with extreme leukocytosis. Clin Chem 1987; 33:914.
55. Nicar MJ. Specimen processing and renin activity in plasma. Clin Chem 1992; 38:598.
56. Grannis GF, et al. Proficiency evaluation of clinical chemistry laboratories. Clin Chem 1972; 18:222.
57. Griner PF, et al. Selection and interpretation of diagnostic tests and procedures. Principles and applications. Ann Intern Med 1981; 94:557.
58. Sox HA. Probability theory in the use of diagnostic tests. An introduction to critical study of the literature. Ann Intern Med 1986; 104:60.
59. Myers JD. The computer as a diagnostic consultant, with emphasis on use of laboratory data. Clin Chem 1986; 32:1714.
60. Hansen JL, et al. Direct assays of lactate, pyruvate, beta-hydroxybutyrate, and acetoacetate with a centrifugal analyzer. Clin Chem 1978; 24:475.
61. Hall SEH, et al. Ketone body kinetics in humans: the effects of insulin-dependent diabetes, obesity, and starvation. J Lipid Res 1984; 25:1184.
62. Brenckman WD, et al. Unpredictable fluctuations in serum acid phosphatase activity in prostatic cancer. JAMA 1981; 245:2501.
63. Carson JL, et al. Diagnostic accuracy of four assays of prostatic acid phosphatase. Comparison using receiver operating characteristic curve analysis. JAMA 1985; 253:665.
64. Benvenuti M, et al. Circadian rhythm in prostatic acid phosphatase (PAP): a potential tumor marker rhythm in prostatic cancer (Pca). Chronobiologia 1983; 10:383.
65. Ohno Y, et al. Change of peripheral levels of pituitary hormones and cytokines after injection of interferon (IFN)-beta in patients with chronic hepatitis C. J Clin Endocrinol Metab 1998; 83:3681.
66. Yalow RS, et al. Change of peripheral levels of pituitary hormones and cytokines after injection of interferon (IFN)-beta in patients with chronic hepatitis C. J Clin Endocrinol Metab 1973; 36:415.
67. Schoneshofer M, et al. Corticotropin in human plasma. General considerations. Surv Immunol Res 1984; 3:55.
68. Farrell PA, et al. Plasma adrenocorticotropin and cortisol responses to submaximal and exhaustive exercise. J Appl Physiol 1983; 55:1441.
69. Laakman G, et al. Effects of psychotropic drugs (desimipramine, chlorimipramine, sulpiride and diazepam) on the human HPA axis. Psychopharmacology (Berl) 1984; 84:66.
70. Laue L, et al. Effect of chronic treatment with the glucocorticoid antagonist RU 486 in man: toxicity, immunological, and hormonal aspects. J Clin Endocrinol Metab 1990; 71:1474.
71. Venturoli S, et al. Ketoconazole therapy for women with acne and/or hirsutism. J Clin Endocrinol Metab 1990; 71:335.
72. Cugini P, et al. Toward a chronophysiology of circulating aldosterone. Biochem Med 1984; 32:270.
73. Saruta T, et al. Mechanism of age-related changes in renin and adrenocortical steroids. J Am Geriatr Soc 1980; 28:210.
74. Sancho JM, et al. Interference by ranitidine with aldosterone secretion in vivo. Eur J Clin Pharmacol 1984; 27:495.
75. Zipser RD, et al. Hyperreninemic hypoaldosteronism in the critically ill: a new entity. J Clin Endocrinol Metab 1981; 53:867.
76. Fiselier TJW, et al. Levels of renin, angiotensin I and II, angiotensin-converting enzyme and aldosterone in infancy childhood. Eur J Pediatr 1983; 141:3.
77. Saito I, et al. Effect of a calcium entry blocker on blood pressure, plasma renin activity, aldosterone and catecholamines in normotensive subjects. Clin Endocrinol (Oxf) 1986; 24:565.

78. Crofton PM. Biochemistry of alkaline phosphatase isoenzymes. Crit Rev Clin Lab Sci 1982; 16:161.

79. Broulik PD, et al. Alterations in human serum alkaline phosphatase and its bone isoenzyme by chronic administration of lithium. Clin Chim Acta 1984; 140:151.

80. Schoenau E, et al. "Fragmented" isoenzymes of alkaline phosphatase in the diagnosis of transient hyperphosphatasemia. Clin Chem 1986; 32:2211.

81. Stein P, et al. Transient hyperphosphatasemia of infancy and early childhood: clinical and biochemical features of 21 cases and literature review. Clin Chem 1987; 33:313.

82. Gordon T. Factors associated with serum alkaline phosphatase level. Arch Pathol Lab Med 1993; 117:187.

83. Schiele F, et al. Total bone and liver alkaline phosphatases in plasma: biological variations and reference limits. Clin Chem 1983; 29:634.

84. Rosalki SB, et al. Two new methods for separating and quantifying bone and liver alkaline phosphatase isoenzymes in plasma. Clin Chem 1984; 30:1182.

85. Valenzuela GJ, et al. Time-dependent changes in bone, placental, intestinal, and hepatic alkaline phosphatase activities in serum during human pregnancy. Clin Chem 1987; 33:1801.

86. Hannon R, et al. Response of biochemical markers of bone turnover to hormone replacement therapy: impact of biological variability. J Bone Miner Res 1998; 13:1124.

87. Withold W. Monitoring of bone turnover biological, preanalytical and technical criteria in the assessment of biochemical markers. Eur J Clin Chem Clin Biochem 1996; 34:785.

88. Kyd PA, et al. Clinical usefulness of bone alkaline phosphatase in osteoporosis. Ann Clin Biochem 1998; 35:717.

89. Romagnoli E, et al. Assessment of serum total and bone alkaline phosphatase measurement in clinical practice. Clin Chem Lab Med 1998; 36:163.

90. Douglas AS, et al. Seasonal differences in biochemical parameters of bone remodelling. J Clin Pathol 1996; 49:284.

91. Lau KH, et al. Phenytoin increases markers of osteogenesis for the human species in vitro and in vivo. J Clin Endocrinol Metab 1995; 80:2347.

92. Karlsson MK, et al. Indicators of bone formation in weight lifters. Calcif Tissue Int 1995; 56:177.

93. Panteghini M, et al. Biological variation in bone-derived biochemical markers in serum. Scand J Clin Lab Invest 1995; 55:609.

94. Medri G, et al. Pituitary glycoprotein hormones in chronic renal failure: evidence for an uncontrolled alpha-subunit release. J Endocrinol Invest 1993; 16:169.

95. Oppenheim DS, et al. Effects of chronic GnRH analogue administration on gonadotrophin and alpha-subunit secretion in post-menopausal women. Clin Endocrinol (Oxf) 1992; 36:559.

96. Madersbacher S, et al. Serum glycoprotein hormones and their free alpha-subunit in a healthy elderly population selected according to the SENIEUR protocol. Analyses with ultrasensitive time resolved fluoroimmunoassays. Mech Ageing Dev 1993; 71:223.

97. Taylor A, et al. Determination of aluminium in serum: findings of an external quality assessment scheme. Ann Clin Biochem 1985; 22:351.

98. Kostyniak PJ. An electrothermal atomic absorption method for aluminum analysis in plasma: identification of sources of contamination in blood sampling procedures. J Anal Toxicol 1983; 7:20.

99. De Broe ME, et al. Correlation of serum aluminum values with tissue aluminum concentration. Contrib Nephrol 1984; 38:37.

100. Cannata JB, et al. Effect of acute aluminium overload on calcium and parathyroid-hormone metabolism. Lancet 1983; 1:501.

101. Morimoto I, et al. Studies on the origin of androstanediol and androstanediol glucuronide in young and elderly men. J Clin Endocrinol Metab 1981; 52:772.

102. Greep N, et al. Androstanediol glucuronide plasma clearance and production rates in normal and hirsute women. J Clin Endocrinol Metab 1986; 62:22.

103. Lookingbill DP, et al. Clinical and biochemical parameters of androgen action in normal healthy Caucasian versus Chinese subjects. J Clin Endocrinol Metab 1991; 72:1242.

104. Gray A, et al. Age, disease, and changing sex hormone levels in middle-aged men: results of the Massachusetts Male Aging Study. J Clin Endocrinol Metab 1991; 73:1016.

105. Andre M, et al. Reference values for androstanediol glucuronide. Clin Chem 1994; 40:162.

106. Brody S, et al. Serum levels of 4-androstene-3,17-dione in menstruating and postmenopausal women. Evaluation of a radioimmunoassay and correlation with bone mineral content and endometrial pathology. Acta Obstet Gynecol Scand 1983; 62:531.

107. Hummer L, et al. An easy and reliable radioimmunoassay of serum androstenedione: age-related normal values in 252 females aged 2 to 70 years. Scand J Clin Lab Invest 1983; 43:301.

108. Siklosi G, et al. Episodic secretion of hormones and the diagnostic value of single blood estimates. III. Testosterone, androstenedione, dehydroepiandrosterone, dehydroepiandrosterone sulphate, cortisol. Acta Med Hung 1984; 41:213.

109. Long JP, et al. Prolactin and the hypothalamic-pituitary-testicular axis in cimetidine-treated men. Ir Med J 1985; 78:48.

110. Goldman J, et al. Contrast analysis for the evaluation of the circadian rhythms of plasma cortisol, androstenedione, and testosterone in normal men and the possible influence of meals. J Clin Endocrinol Metab 1985; 60:164.

111. Luppa P, et al. Serum androgens in intensive-care patients: correlations with clinical findings. Clin Endocrinol (Oxf) 1991; 34:305.

112. Workman RJ, et al. Circulating levels of angiotensin I measured by radioimmunoassay in hypertensive subjects. J Lab Clin Med 1979; 93:847.

113. Matthews PG, et al. Hormonal changes with long-term converting-enzyme inhibition by captopril in essential hypertension. Clin Sci 1979; 57(Suppl 5):135s.

114. Nussberger J, et al. True versus immunoreactive angiotensin II in human plasma. Hypertension 1985; 7(3 Pt 2):I1.

115. Crum R, et al. Neuroendocrinology of chronic renal failure and renal transplantation. Transplantation 1991; 52:818.

116. Studdy PR, et al. Angiotensin-converting enzyme and its clinical significance—a review. J Clin Pathol 1983; 36:938.

117. Smallridge RC, et al. Serum angiotensin-converting enzyme. Alterations in hyperthyroidism, hypothyroidism, and subacute thyroiditis. JAMA 1983; 250:2489.

118. Rasmussen AB, et al. The influence of normotensive pregnancy and pre-eclampsia on angiotensin-converting enzyme. Acta Obstet Gynecol Scand 1983; 62:341.

119. Pietila K, et al. Increase of serum angiotensin-converting enzyme activity after freezing. Scand J Clin Lab Invest 1984; 44:453.

120. Thompson PJ, et al. Angiotensin-converting enzyme. Investigation of diurnal variation, the effect of a large dose of prednisolone, and prednisolone pharmacokinetics in patients with sarcoidosis. Am Rev Respir Dis 1986; 134:1075.

121. Inukai T, et al. Clinical characteristics of patients with the initial diagnosis of NIDDM with positivity for antibodies to glutamic acid decarboxylase. Exp Clin Endocrinol Diabetes 1997; 105:327.

122. Zimmet PZ, et al. The ethnic distribution of antibodies to glutamic acid decarboxylase: presence and levels of insulin-dependent diabetes mellitus in Europid and Asian subjects. J Diabetes Complications 1993; 7:1.

123. Tuomi T, et al. Antibodies to glutamic acid decarboxylase reveal latent autoimmune diabetes mellitus in adults with a non-insulin-dependent onset of disease. Diabetes 1993; 42:359.

124. Schmidli RS, et al. Disease sensitivity and specificity of 52 assays for glutamic acid decarboxylase antibodies. The Second International GADAB Workshop. Diabetes 1995; 44:636.

125. Hermitte L, et al. Diverging evolution of anti-GAD and anti-IA-2 antibodies in long-standing diabetes mellitus as a function of age at onset: no association with complications. Diabet Med 1998; 15:586.

126. Imagawa A, et al. High prevalence of antibodies to glutamic acid decarboxylase in comparison to islet cell antibodies in patients with long-standing insulin-dependent diabetes mellitus. Res Commun Mol Pathol Pharmacol 1996; 92:43.

127. Betterle C, et al. II. Adrenal cortex and steroid 21-hydroxylase autoantibodies in children with organ-specific autoimmune diseases: markers of high progression to clinical Addison's disease. J Clin Endocrinol Metab 1997; 82:939.

128. Falorni A, et al. 21-hydroxylase autoantibodies in adult patients with endocrine autoimmune diseases are highly specific for Addison's disease. Belgian Diabetes Registry. Clin Exp Immunol 1997; 107:341.

129. Laureti S, et al. Levels of adrenocortical autoantibodies correlate with the degree of adrenal dysfunction in subjects with preclinical Addison's disease. J Clin Endocrinol Metab 1998; 83:3507.

130. Betterle C, et al. I. Adrenal cortex and steroid 21-hydroxylase autoantibodies in adult patients with organ-specific autoimmune diseases: markers of low progression to clinical Addison's disease. J Clin Endocrinol Metab 1997; 82:932.

131. Hawa M, et al. Value of antibodies to islet protein tyrosine phosphatase-like molecule in predicting type 1 diabetes. Diabetes 1997; 46:1270.

132. Savola K, et al. IA-2 antibodies—a sensitive marker of IDDM with clinical onset in childhood and adolescence. Childhood Diabetes in Finland Study Group. Diabetologia 1998; 41:424.

133. Bingley PJ. Interactions of age, islet cell antibodies, insulin autoantibodies, and first-phase insulin response in predicting risk of progression to IDDM in ICA+ relatives: the ICARUS data set. Islet Cell Antibody Register Users Study. Diabetes 1996; 45:1720.

134. Baron EJ, et al. Lack of agreement among two commercial enzyme-linked immunosorbent antibody assays and a conventional immunofluorescence-based method for detecting islet cell autoantibodies. Clin Diagn Lab Immunol 1996; 3:429.

135. Feldt-Rasmussen U. Serum thyroglobulin and thyroglobulin autoantibodies in thyroid diseases. Pathogenic and diagnostic aspects. Allergy 1983; 38:369.

136. Wilson R, et al. Thyroid antibody titer and avidity in patients with recurrent miscarriage. Fertil Steril 1999; 71:558.

137. Sundbeck G, et al. Prevalence of serum antithyroid peroxidase antibodies in 85-year-old women and men. Clin Chem 1995; 41:707.

138. Ogawa T, et al. Thyroid hormone autoantibodies in patients with Graves' disease: effect of anti-thyroid drug treatment. Clin Chim Acta 1994; 228:113.

139. Tyroler HA, et al. Apolipoprotein A-I, A-II and C-II in black and white residents of Evans County. Circulation 1980; 62:249.

140. Luoma PV, et al. Plasma high-density lipoproteins and hepatic microsomal enzyme induction. Relation to histological changes in the liver. Eur J Clin Pharmacol 1982; 23:275.

141. Matuchansky C, et al. Effects of cyclic (nocturnal) total parenteral nutrition and continuous enteral nutrition on circadian rhythms of blood lipids, lipoproteins and apolipoproteins in humans. Am J Clin Nutr 1985; 41:727.

142. Zeithofer J, et al. Changes of serum lipid patterns during long-term anticonvulsive treatment. Clin Investig 1993; 71:574.

143. Walsh BW, et al. Effects of postmenopausal estrogen replacement on the concentrations and metabolism of plasma lipoproteins. N Engl J Med 1991; 325:1196.

144. Piechota W, et al. Reference ranges of lipids and apolipoproteins in pregnancy. Eur J Obstet Gynecol Reprod Biol 1992; 45:27.

145. Rabe T, et al. Lipid metabolism in Norplant-2 users—a two-year follow-up study. Total cholesterol, triglycerides, lipoproteins and apolipoproteins. Contraception 1992; 45:21.

146. Lussier-Cacan S, et al. Cyclic fluctuations in human serum lipid and apolipoprotein levels during the normal menstrual cycle: comparison with changes occurring during oral contraceptive therapy. Metabolism 1991; 40:849.

147. Fulton-Kehoe DL, et al. Determinants of total high density lipoprotein cholesterol and high density lipoprotein subfraction levels among Hispanic and non-Hispanic white persons with normal glucose tolerance: the San Luis Valley Diabetes Study. J Clin Epidemiol 1992; 45:1191.

148. Naito HK. The clinical significance of apolipoprotein measurements. J Clin Immunoassay 1986; 9:120.

149. Cernacek P, et al. Atrial natriuretic peptide: blood levels in human disease and their measurement. Clin Biochem 1988; 21:5.

150. Richards AM, et al. Diurnal change in plasma atrial natriuretic peptide concentrations. Clin Sci 1987; 73:489.

151. Lijnen P, et al. Effects of haemolysis and prolonged cold storage of human plasma on the alpha-atrial natriuretic peptide concentration. Clin Chim Acta 1988; 171:333.

152. Hartter E, et al. Circadian variation and age dependence of human atrial natriuretic peptide levels in hospitalized patients. Horm Metab Res 1987; 19:490.

153. Rascher W, et al. Atrial natriuretic peptide in infants and children. Horm Res 1987; 28:58.

154. Saxenhofer H, et al. Corticosteroid-induced stimulation of atrial natriuretic peptide in man. Acta Endocrinol (Copenh) 1988; 118:179.

155. Sanfield JA, et al. Epinephrine increases plasma immunoreactive atrial natriuretic hormone levels in humans. Am J Physiol 1987; 252:E740.

156. Tan AC, et al. Atrial natriuretic peptide—the influence of various physiological and sampling conditions. Ann Clin Biochem 1987; 24:500.

157. Mann FE, et al. Effect of angiotensin I converting enzyme inhibition on circulating atrial natriuretic peptide in humans. Klin Wochenschr 1986; 64(Suppl 5):13.

158. Colantonio D, et al. A possible role of atrial natriuretic peptide in ethanol-induced acute diuresis. Life Sci 1991; 48:635.

159. Harrison SP. Naproxen interference with the ion-selective electrode in the RA-1000. Clin Chem 1987; 33:421.

160. Bernard A, et al. Cadmium in human population. Experientia 1984; 40:143.

161. Brockhaus A, et al. Levels of cadmium and lead in blood in relation to smoking, sex, occupation, and other factors in an adult population of the FRG. Int Arch Occup Environ Health 1983; 52:167.

162. Motté P, et al. Construction and clinical validation of a sensitive and specific assay for serum mature calcitonin using monoclonal antipeptide antibodies. Clin Chim Acta 1988; 174:35.

163. Ghillani PP, et al. Identification and measurement of calcitonin precursors in serum of patients with malignant diseases. Cancer Res 1989; 49:6845.

164. Born W, et al. Diagnostic relevance of the amino-terminal cleavage peptide of procalcitonin (PAS-57), calcitonin and calcitonin gene-related peptide in medullary thyroid carcinoma patients. Regulatory Peptides 1991; 32:311.

165. Snider RH Jr, et al. Procalcitonin and its component peptides in systemic inflammation: immunochemical characterization. J Investig Med 1997; 45:552.

166. Whang K, et al. Serum calcitonin precursors in sepsis and systemic infection. J Clin Endocrinol Metab 1998; 83:3296.

167. Snider RH Jr, et al. Radioimmunoassay of calcitonin in normal human urine. Anal Chem 1978; 50:449.

168. Silva OL, et al. Urine calcitonin as a test for medullary thyroid cancer: a new screening procedure. Ann Surg 1979; 189:269.

169. Wang Y, et al. A simple high performance liquid chromatography assay for simultaneous determination of plasma norepinephrine, epinephrine, dopamine, and 3,4-dihydroxyphenyl acetic acid. J Pharm Biomed Anal 1999; 21:519.

170. Roberts WL, et al. Comparison of four commercial urinary albumin (microalbumin) methods: implications for detecting diabetic nephropathy using random urine specimens. Clin Chim Acta 1998; 273:21.

171. Khuu HM, et al. Evaluation of a fully automated high-performance liquid chromatography assay for hemoglobin A1c. Arch Pathol Lab Med 1999; 123:763.

172. Nagi DK, et al. Hyperinsulinemia in nondiabetic Asian subjects using specific assays for insulin, intact proinsulin, and des-31, 32-proinsulin. Diabetes Care 1996; 19:39.

173. Nexo E, et al. Evaluation of novel assays in clinical chemistry: quantification of plasma total homocysteine. Clin Chem 2000; 46:1150.

174. Kausz AT, et al. Screening plasma aluminum levels in relation to aluminum bone disease among asymptomatic dialysis patients. Am J Kidney Dis 1999; 34:688.

175. Bowers GN, et al. Measurement of ionized calcium in serum with ion-selective electrodes: a mature technology that can meet the daily service needs. Clin Chem 1986; 32:1437.

176. Payne RB. Clinically significant effect of protein concentration on ion-selective electrode measurements of ionised calcium. Ann Clin Biochem 1982; 19:233.

177. Boink AB, et al. Recommendation on sampling, transport, and storage for the determination of the concentration of ionized calcium in whole blood, plasma, and serum. IFC Scientific Division, Working Group on Ion-Selective Electrodes (WGSE). J Int Fed Clin Chem 1992; 4:147.

178. Zaloga GP, et al. Assessment of calcium homeostasis in the critically ill surgical patient. The diagnostic pitfalls of the McLean-Hastings nomogram. Ann Surg 1985; 202:587.

179. Packer E, et al. Effects of estrogen on daylong circulating calcium, phosphorus, 1,25-dihydroxyvitamin D, and parathyroid hormone in postmenopausal women. J Bone Miner Res 1990; 5:877.

180. Jacobson MA, et al. Foscarnet-induced hypocalcemia and effects of foscarnet on calcium metabolism. J Clin Endocrinol Metab 1991; 72:1130.

181. Fredstorp L, et al. The short and long-term effects of octreotide on calcium homeostasis in patients with acromegaly. Clin Endocrinol (Oxf) 1993; 39:331.

182. Burritt MF, et al. Comparative studies of total and ionized serum calcium values in normal subjects and patients with renal disorders. Mayo Clin Proc 1980; 55:606.

183. Wu JT. Interference of heparin in carcinoembryonic antigen radioimmunoassays. Clin Chim Acta 1983; 130:47.

184. Lokich JJ, et al. Criteria for monitoring carcinoembryonic antigen: variability of sequential assays at elevated levels. J Clin Oncol 1984; 2:181.

185. Fletcher RH. Carcinoembryonic antigen. Ann Intern Med 1986; 104:66.

186. Witter FR, et al. Folate, carotene, and smoking. Am J Obstet Gynecol 1982; 144:857.

187. Vuilleumier JP, et al. Clinical chemical methods for the routine assessment of the vitamin status in human populations. Part I: The fat-coluble vitamins A and E, and beta-carotene. Int J Vitam Nutr Res 1983; 53:265.

188. Nierenberg DW, et al. Diurnal variation in plasma levels of retinol, tocopherol, and beta-carotene. Am J Med Sci 1987; 294:187.

189. Probstfield JL, et al. Carotenoids and vitamin A: the effect of hypocholesterolemic agents on serum levels. Metabolism 1985; 34:88.

190. Leung AK, et al. Serum carotene concentrations in normal infants and children. Clin Pediatr (Phila) 1990; 29:575.

191. Grossman E, et al. Diet and weight loss: their effect on norepinephrine renin and aldosterone levels. Int J Obes 1985; 9:107.

192. Moyer TP, et al. Analysis for urinary catecholamines by liquid chromatography with amperometric detection: methodology and clinical interpretation of results. Clin Chem 1979; 25:256.

193. Hjemdahl P. Inter-laboratory comparison of plasma catecholamine determinations using several different assays. Acta Physiol Scand Suppl 1984; 527:43.

194. Dunne JW, et al. The effect of ascorbic acid on plasma sulfate conjugated catecholamines after eating bananas. Life Sci 1983; 33:1511.

195. Zuspan FP, et al. The effect of smoking and oral contraceptives on the urinary excretion of epinephrine and norepinephrine. Am J Obstet Gynecol 1979; 135:1012.

196. Liebau H, et al. Diurnal and daily variations of PRA, plasma catecholamines and blood pressure in normotensive and hypertensive man. Contrib Nephrol 1982; 30:57.

197. Hoehe M, et al. Opiates increase plasma catecholamines in humans. Psychoneuroendocrinology 1993; 18:141.

198. Fitzgibbon M, et al. Reference values for urinary HMMA, HVA, noradrenaline, adrenaline, and dopamine excretion in children using random urine samples and HPLC with electrochemical detection. Ann Clin Biochem 1992; 29:400.

199. Wolf PL. Ceruloplasmin: methods and clinical use. Crit Rev Clin Lab Sci 1982; 17:229.

200. Galdston M, et al. Ceruloplasmin. Increased serum concentration and impaired antioxidant activity in cigarette smokers, and ability to prevent suppression of elastase inhibitory capacity of alpha 1-proteinase inhibitor. Am Rev Respir Dis 1984; 129:258.

201. Hopman WPM, et al. Plasma cholecystokinin response to a liquid fat meal in vagotomized patients. Ann Surg 1984; 200:693.

202. Rehfield JF. How to measure cholecystokinin in plasma? Gastroenterology 1984; 87:434.

203. Nakano I, et al. High plasma cholecystokinin response following ingestion of test meal by patients with non-insulin dependent diabetes mellitus. Regul Pept 1986; 14:229.

204. Radberg G, et al. Cholecystokinin secretion in pregnancy. Scand J Gastroenterol 1987; 22:687.

205. Maton PN, et al. Atropine inhibits meal-stimulated release of cholecystokinin. Scand J Gastroenterol 1984; 19:831.

206. Frick G, et al. Plasma levels of cholecystokinin and gastrin during the menstrual cycle and pregnancy. Acta Obstet Gynecol Scand 1990; 69:317.

207. Douglas BR, et al. Coffee stimulation of cholecystokinin release and gallbladder contraction in humans. Am J Clin Nutr 1990; 52:553.

208. Glasbrenner B, et al. Relationship between postprandial release of CCK and PP in health and in chronic pancreatitis. Regul Pept 1994; 50:45.

209. Blank DW, et al. The method of determination must be considered in interpreting blood cholesterol levels. JAMA 1986; 256:2867.

210. Friedlander Y, et al. Variability of plasma lipids and lipoproteins: the Jerusalem Lipid Research Clinic Study. Clin Chem 1985; 31:1121.

211. Hussa RO, et al. Discordant human chorionic gonadotropin results: causes and solutions. Obstet Gynecol 1985; 65:211.

212. Ayala AR, et al. Daily rhythm of serum human chorionic gonadotropin and human chorionic somatomammotropin in normal pregnancy. Int J Gynaecol Obstet 1984; 22:173.

213. Haning RV, et al. Effects of fetal sex and dexamethasone on preterm maternal serum concentrations of human chorionic gonadotropin, progesterone, estrone, estradiol, and estriol. Am J Obstet Gynecol 1989; 161:1549.

214. Versieck J, et al. Normal levels of trace elements in human blood, plasma, or serum. Anal Chim Acta 1980; 116:217.

215. Ong CN, et al. Concentrations of heavy metals in maternal and umbilical cord blood. Biometals 1993; 6:61.

216. Versieck J. Trace elements in human body fluids and tissues. Crit Rev Clin Lab Sci 22:96.

217. Hennig FF, et al. Nickel-, chrom- and cobalt-concentrations in human tissue and body fluids of hip prosthesis patients. J Trace Elem Electrolytes Health Dis 1992; 6:239.

218. Guillard O, et al. Diurnal variations of zinc, copper and magnesium in the serum of normal fasting adults. Biomedicine 1979; 31:193.

219. Kirsten GF, et al. Serum zinc and copper levels in the 1st year of life. S Afr Med J 1985; 67:414.

220. Helgeland K, et al. Copper and zinc in human serum in Norway. Relationship to geography, sex and age. Scand J Clin Lab Invest 1982; 42:35.

221. Wu C-T, et al. Serum zinc, copper, and ceruloplasmin levels in male alcoholics. Biol Psychiatry 1984; 19:1333.

222. Ghose K, et al. Hypercupraemia induced by antiepileptic drugs. Hum Toxicol 1983; 2:519.

223. Gallagher SK, et al. Short-term and long-term variability of indices related to nutritional status. I: Ca, Cu, Fe, Mg, and Zn. Clin Chem 1989; 35:369.

224. Seckl JR, et al. Diurnal variation of plasma corticosterone in depression. Psychoneuroendocrinology 1990; 15:485.

225. Feldman D. Ketoconazole and other imidazole derivatives as inhibitors of steroidogenesis. Endocr Rev 1986; 7:409.

226. Becker DJ. The endocrine responses to protein calorie malnutrition. Annu Rev Nutr 1983; 3:187.

227. Wilkins JN, et al. Nicotine from cigarette smoking increases circulating levels of cortisol, growth hormone, and prolactin in male chronic smokers. Psychopharmacology (Berl) 1982; 78:305.

228. Epstein MT, et al. Licorice raises urinary cortisol in man. J Clin Endocrinol Metab 1978; 47:397.

229. Halbreich U, et al. Effect of age and sex on cortisol secretion in depressives and normals. Psychiatry Res 1984; 13:221.

230. Ishizuka B, et al. Pituitary hormone release in response to food ingestion: evidence for neuroendocrine signals from gut to brain. J Clin Endocrinol Metab 1983; 57:1111.

231. Gram LF, et al. Suppression of plasma cortisol after oral administration of oxazepam in man. Br J Clin Pharmacol 1984; 17:176.

232. Wilke TJ, et al. The evaluation of five commercial serum cortisol kits regarding precision and accuracy. Clin Biochem 1984; 17:311.

233. Perini GI, et al. Effects of carbamazepine on pituitary-adrenal function in healthy volunteers. J Clin Endocrinol Metab 1992; 74:406.

234. Loprinzi CL, et al. Effect of megestrol acetate on the human pituitary-adrenal axis. Mayo Clin Proc 1992; 67:1160.

235. Osei K, et al. Decreased serum C-peptide/insulin molar ratios after oral glucose ingestion in hyperthyroid patients. Diabetes Care 1984; 7:471.

236. Boyko EJ, et al. Higher insulin and C-peptide concentrations in Hispanic population at high risk for NIDDM. San Luis Valley Diabetes Study. Diabetes 1991; 40:509.

237. Meistas M, et al. Correlation of urinary excretion of C-peptide with the integrated concentration and secretion rate of insulin. Diabetes 1981; 30:639.

238. Licata AA. Acute effects of increased meat protein on urinary electrolytes and cyclic adenosine monophosphate and serum parathyroid hormone. Am J Clin Nutr 1981; 34:1779.

239. Markianos M, et al. Effects of acute cannabis use on urinary neurotransmitter metabolites and cyclic nucleotides in man. Drug Alcohol Depend 1984; 14:175.

240. Gogel E, et al. Probenecid inhibits the secretion of nephrogenous adenosine 3',5'-monophosphate in normal man. J Clin Endocrinol Metab 1983; 57:689.

241. Kruse K, Kracht U. Urinary adenosine 3',5'-monophosphate excretion in childhood. J Clin Endocrinol Metab 1981; 53:1251.

242. Colin AA, et al. Effects of theophylline on urinary excretion of cyclic AMP, calcium, and phosphorus in normal subjects. Miner Electrolyte Metab 1984; 10:359.

243. Gennari C, et al. Seasonal variation in urinary excretion of cyclic AMP in healthy people. J Endocrinol Invest 1981; 4:323.

244. Sirinathsinghji DJS, et al. Concentration patterns of plasma dehydroepiandrosterone, delta 5-androstenediol and their sulphates, testosterone and cortisol in normal healthy women and in women with anorexia nervosa. Acta Endocrinol (Copenh) 1985; 108:255.

245. Parker LN, et al. Control of adrenal androgen secretion. Endocr Rev 1980; 1:392.

246. Levesque LA, et al. The effect of phenytoin and carbamazepine on serum dehydroepiandrosterone sulfate in men and women who have partial seizures with temporal lobe involvement. J Clin Endocrinol Metab 1986; 63:243.

247. Musey VC, et al. Long term effects of a first pregnancy on the hormonal environment: estrogens and androgens. J Clin Endocrinol Metab 1987; 64:111.

248. Mitchell E, et al. Evidence for an association between dehydroepiandrosterone sulfate and nonfatal, premature myocardial infarction in males. Circulation 1994; 89:89.

249. Brown RD, et al. Plasma deoxycorticosterone in normal and abnormal pregnancy. J Clin Endocrinol Metab 1972; 35:736.

250. Antonipillai I, et al. The origin of plasma deoxycorticosterone in men and in women during the menstrual cycle. J Clin Endocrinol Metab 1983; 56:93.

251. Kuwabara Y, et al. Plasma 11-deoxycortisol in normal and abnormal human pregnancy. Am J Obstet Gynecol 1983; 147:766.

252. Hosoda H, et al. The specificity of enzyme immunoassays for plasma 11-deoxycortisol. Chem Pharm Bull (Tokyo) 1983; 31:3595.

253. Drafta D, et al. Age-related changes of plasma steroids in normal adult males. J Steroid Biochem 1982; 17:683.

254. Rittmaster RS, et al. Effect of finasteride, a 5 alpha-reductase inhibitor, on serum gonadotropins in normal men. J Clin Endocrinol Metab 1992; 75:484.

255. Genazzani AR, et al. Proopiocortin-related peptide plasma levels throughout prepuberty and puberty. J Clin Endocrinol Metab 1983; 57:56.

256. Petraglia F, et al. Simultaneous circadian variations of plasma ACTH, beta-lipotropin, beta-endorphin and cortisol. Horm Res 1983; 17:147.

257. Matsumura M, et al. Effect of a test meal, duodenal acidification, and tetragastrin on the plasma concentration of beta-endorphin-like immunoreactivity in man. Regul Pept 1982; 4:173.

258. Laatikainen T, et al. Plasma beta-endorphin and the menstrual cycle. Fertil Steril 1985; 44:206.

259. Hoffman DI, et al. Plasma beta-endorphin concentrations prior to and during pregnancy, in labor, and after delivery. Am J Obstet Gynecol 1984; 150:492.

260. Aronin N, et al. Plasma immunoreactive beta-endorphin is elevated in uraemia. Clin Endocrinol (Oxf) 1983; 18:459.

261. Panerai AE, et al. Plasma beta-endorphin, beta-lipotropin, and met-enkephalin concentrations during pregnancy in normal and drug-addicted women and their newborn. J Clin Endocrinol Metab 1983; 57:537.

262. Howlett TA, et al. Release of beta endorphin and met-enkephalin during exercise in normal women: response to training. BMJ 1984; 288:1950.

263. Panerai AE, et al. Plasma beta-endorphin and met-enkephalin in physiological and pathological conditions. Adv Biochem Psychopharmacol 1982; 33:139.

264. Rahkila P, Laatikainen T. Effect of oral contraceptives on plasma beta-endorphin and corticotropin at rest and during exercise. Gynecol Endocrinol 1992; 6:163.

265. Govoni S, et al. Immunoreactive met-enkephalin plasma concentrations in chronic alcoholics and in children born from alcoholic mothers. Life Sci 1983; 33:1581.

266. Cotes PM, et al. Changes in serum immunoreactive erythropoietin during the menstrual cycle and normal pregnancy. Br J Obstet Gynaecol 1983; 90:304.

267. Pratt MC, et al. Effect of angiotensin converting enzyme inhibitors on erythropoietin concentrations in healthy volunteers. Br J Clin Pharmacol 1992; 34:363.

268. Schwandt HJ, et al. Influence of prolonged physical exercise on the erythropoietin concentration in blood. Eur J Appl Physiol 1991; 63:463.

269. Cahan C, et al. Diurnal variations in serum erythropoietin levels in healthy subjects and sleep apnea patients. J Appl Physiol 1992; 72:2112.

270. Martikainen H, et al. Circannual concentrations of melatonin, gonadotrophins, prolactin and gonadal steroids in males in a geographical area with a large annual variation in daylight. Acta Endocrinol (Copenh) 1985; 109:446.

271. Klaiber EL, et al. Serum estradiol levels in male cigarette smokers. Am J Med 1984; 77:858.

272. Boyden TW, et al. Sex steroids and endurance running in women. Fertil Steril 1983; 39:629.

273. Siklosi G, et al. Episodic secretion of hormones and the diagnostic value of single blood estimates. II. Progesterone, oestradiol and oestrone. Acta Med Hung 1984; 41:203.

274. Buster JE, et al. Subhourly variability of circulating third trimester maternal steroid concentrations as a source of sampling error. J Clin Endocrinol Metab 1978; 46:907.

275. Andersen AN, et al. Low maternal but normal fetal prolactin levels in cigarette smoking pregnant women. Acta Obstet Gynecol Scand 1984; 63:237.

276. Haning RV Jr, et al. Effects of fetal sex and dexamethasone on preterm maternal serum concentrations of human chorionic gonadotropin, progesterone, estrone, estradiol, and estriol. Am J Obstet Gynecol 1989; 161:1549.

277. MacMahon B, et al. Cigarette smoking and urinary estrogens. N Engl J Med 1982; 307:1062.

278. Golay A, et al. Effect of obesity on ambient plasma glucose, free fatty acid, insulin, growth hormone, and glucagon concentrations. J Clin Endocrinol Metab 1986; 63:481.

279. Singer L, Ophaug R. Ionic and nonionic fluoride in plasma (or serum). Crit Rev Clin Lab Sci 1982; 18:111.

280. Rimoli C, et al. Relationship between serum concentrations of flecainide and fluoride in humans. Boll Chim Farm 1991; 130:279.

281. Nakazawa Y, et al. Serum folic acid levels and antipyrine clearance rates in smokers and non-smokers. Drug Alcohol Depend 1983; 11:201.

282. Wickham C, et al. Seasonal variation in folate nutritional status. Ir J Med Sci 1983; 152:295.

283. Strain GW, et al. Mild hypogonadotropic hypogonadism in obese men. Metabolism 1982; 31:871.

284. Csako G. Causes, consequences, and recognition of false-positive reactions for ketones. Clin Chem 1990; 36:1388.

285. Haning RV Jr, et al. Effects of fetal sex and dexamethasone on preterm maternal serum concentrations of human chorionic gonadotropin, progesterone, estrone, estradiol, and estriol. Am J Obstet Gynecol 1989; 161:1549.

286. Dart AM, et al. The effect of propranolol on luteinising hormone and prolactin plasma concentrations in hypertensive women. Br J Clin Pharmacol 1982; 14:839.

287. Sawhney RC, et al. Hormone profiles at high altitude in man. Andrologia 1985; 17:178.

288. Siklosi G, et al. Episodic secretion of hormones and the diagnostic value of single blood estimates. I. LH, FSH, prolactin. Acta Med Hung 1984; 41:195.

289. Mendelson JH, et al. Effects of marijuana or neuroendocrine hormones in human males and females. Natl Inst Drug Abuse Res Monograph Ser 1984; 44:97.

290. MacNaughton J, et al. Age related changes in follicle stimulating hormone, luteinizing hormone, oestradiol and immunoreactive inhibin in women of reproductive age. Clin Endocrinol (Oxf) 1992; 36:339.

291. Gebhart SSP, et al. Reversible impairment of gonadotropin secretion in critical illness. Observations in postmenopausal women. Arch Intern Med 1989; 149:1637.

292. Valero-Politi J, et al. Within- and between-subject biological variations of follitropin, lutropin, testosterone, and sex-hormone-binding globulin in men. Clin Chem 1993; 39:1723.

293. Medri G, et al. Pituitary glycoprotein hormones in chronic renal failure: evidence for an uncontrolled alpha-subunit release. J Endocrinol Invest 1993; 16:169.

294. Glass AR. Ketoconazole-induced stimulation of gonadotropin output in men: basis for a potential test of gonadotropin reserve. J Clin Endocrinol Metab 1986; 63:1121.

295. Gebhart SSP, et al. Reversible impairment of gonadotropin secretion in critical illness. Observations in postmenopausal women. Arch Intern Med 1989; 149:1637.

296. Frandsen EK, et al. Serum fructosamine in diabetic pregnancy. Clin Chem 1988; 34:316.

297. De Schepper J, et al. Reference values for fructosamine concentrations in children's sera: influence of protein concentration, age, and sex. Clin Chem 1988; 34:2444.

298. Rodriguez-Segade S, et al. Effects of various serum proteins on quantification of fructosamine. Clin Chem 1989; 35:134.

299. Kurishita M, et al. Glycated hemoglobin of fractionated erythrocytes, glycated albumin, and plasma fructosamine during pregnancy. Am J Obstet Gynecol 1992; 167:1372.

300. Broussolle C, et al. Evaluation of the fructosamine test in obesity: consequences for the assessment of past glycemic control in diabetes. Clin Biochem 1991; 24:203.

301. Davie SJ, et al. Biological variation in glycated proteins. Ann Clin Biochem 1993; 30:260.

302. Cho CH, et al. Effects of eight-week treatment with oral ranitidine on plasma level changes of gastrin, histamine and serotonin in duodenal ulcer patients. Pharmacol Res Commun 1985; 17:525.

303. Sherbaniuk RW, et al. Gastrin, gastric emptying, and gastroesophageal reflux after ranitidine. J Clin Gastroenterol 1983; 5:239.

304. Feldman M, et al. Sex-related differences in gastrin release and parietal cell sensitivity to gastrin in healthy human beings. J Clin Invest 1983; 71:715.

305. Uvnas-Moberg K, et al. Nocturnal variation in plasma levels of gastrin and somatostatin-like immunoreactivity in man. Acta Physiol Scand 1984; 120:517.

306. Caldara R, et al. Effect of L-dopa with and without inhibition of extra cerebral dopa decarboxylase on gastric acid secretion and gastrin release in man. Gut 1985; 26:1014.

307. Lauritsen KB, et al. Lithium inhibits basal and food-stimulated gastrin secretion. Gastroenterology 1978; 75:59.

308. Jansen JB, et al. Effect of long-term treatment with omeprazole on serum gastrin and serum group A and C pepsinogens in patients with reflux esophagitis. Gastroenterology 1990; 99:621.

309. Romeo DP, et al. Misdiagnosis of the Zollinger-Ellison syndrome due to hyperlipidemia. Gastroenterology 1990; 99:1511.

310. Lacey RJ, et al. Evidence that the presence of arginine can lead to overestimation of glucagon levels measured by radioimmunoassay. Clin Chim Acta 1992; 210:211.

311. Lang DA, et al. Pulsatile, synchronous basal insulin and glucagon secretion in man. Diabetes 1982; 31:22.

312. LeBlanc J, et al. Daily variations of plasma glucose and insulin in physically trained and sedentary subjects. Metabolism 1983; 32:552.

313. Bergstrom J, et al. Influence of protein intake on renal hemodynamics and plasma hormone concentrations in normal subjects. Acta Med Scand 1985; 217:189.

314. Gossain VV, et al. Plasma glucagon in simple obesity: effect of exercise. Am J Med Sci 1983; 286:4.

315. Starke AAR, et al. Elevated pancreatic glucagon in obesity. Diabetes 1984; 33:277.

316. Naveri H, et al. Plasma glucagon and catecholamines during exhaustive short-term exercise. Eur J Appl Physiol 1985; 53:308.

317. Holst JJ, et al. Diurnal profile of pancreatic polypeptide, pancreatic glucagon, gut glucagon, and insulin in human morbid obesity. Int J Obes 1983; 7:529.

318. Lawrence AM, et al. Chronic propranolol administration impairs glucagon release during insulin-induced hypoglycemia in normal man. J Clin Endocrinol Metab 1984; 59:622.

319. Orskov C, et al. All products of proglucagon are elevated in plasma from uremic patients. J Clin Endocrinol Metab 1992; 74:379.

320. Dolhofer R, et al. Increased glycosylation of serum albumin in diabetes mellitus. Diabetes 1980; 29:417.

321. Willey DG, et al. Glycosylated haemoglobin and plasma glycoprotein assays by affinity chromatography. Diabetologia 1984; 27:56.

322. Goldstein DE, et al. Recent advances in glycosylated hemoglobin measurements. Crit Rev Clin Lab Sci 1984; 21:187.

323. Goldstein DE, et al. Glycated hemoglobin: methodologies and clinical applications. Clin Chem 1986; 32:B64.

324. Arnetz BB, et al. The influence of aging on hemoglobin A1c (HbA1c). J Gerontol 1982; 37:648.

325. Ktorza A, et al. Effect of slight plasma glucose decrease on glycosylated hemoglobin in healthy subjects during caloric restriction. N Engl J Med 1985; 313:958.

326. Cesana G, et al. Can glycosylated hemoglobin be a job stress parameter? J Occup Med 1985; 27:357.

327. Blum M, et al. Glycohemoglobin (Hb A1) levels in oral contraceptive users. Eur J Obstet Gynecol Reprod Biol 1983; 15:97.

328. Strickland MH, et al. Haemoglobin A1c concentrations in men and women with diabetes. BMJ 1984; 289:733.

329. D'Armiento M, et al. Diazepam-stimulated GH secretion in normal subjects: relation to oestradiol plasma levels. Horm Metab Res 1984; 16:155.

330. Duursma SA, et al. Changes in serum somatomedin and growth hormone concentrations after 3 weeks oestrogen substitution in post-menopausal women; a pilot study. Acta Endocrinol (Copenh) 1984; 106:527.

331. Baumann G, et al. Molecular forms of circulating growth hormone during spontaneous secretory episodes and in the basal state. J Clin Endocrinol Metab 1985; 60:1216.

332. Zadik Z, et al. The influence of age on the 24-hour integrated concentration of growth hormone in normal individuals. J Clin Endocrinol Metab 1985; 60:513.

333. Laakmann G, et al. Stimulation of growth hormone secretion by desimipramin and chlorimipramin in man. J Clin Endocrinol Metab 1977; 44:1010.

334. Lal S, et al. Effect of clonidine on growth hormone, prolactin, luteinizing hormone, follicle-stimulating hormone, and thyroid-stimulating hormone in the serum of normal men. J Clin Endocrinol Metab 1975; 41:827.

335. Meistas MT, et al. Integrated concentrations of growth hormone, insulin, C-peptide and prolactin in human obesity. Metabolism 1982; 31:1224.

336. Elwes RDC, et al. Prolactin and growth hormone dynamics in epileptic patients receiving phenytoin. Clin Endocrinol (Oxf) 1985; 23:263.

337. Monteleone P, et al. Growth hormone response to sodium valproate in chronic schizophrenia. Biol Psychiatry 1986; 21:588.

338. Jarrett DB, et al. Recurrent depression is associated with a persistent reduction in sleep-related growth hormone secretion. Arch Gen Psychiatry 1990; 47:113.

339. Schmitt JK. Indomethacin increases plasma growth hormone levels in man. Am J Med Sci 1990; 300:144.

340. Veldhuis JD, et al. Divergent effects of short term glucocorticoid excess on the gonadotropic and somatotropic axes in normal men. J Clin Endocrinol Metab 1992; 74:96.

341. Superko HR, et al. High-density lipoprotein cholesterol measurements. A help or hindrance in practical clinical medicine? JAMA 1986; 256:2714.

342. De Marchi S, et al. Relief of pruritus and decreases in plasma histamine concentrations during erythropoietin therapy in patients with uremia. N Engl J Med 1992; 326:969.

343. Johnston CS, et al. Antihistamine effect of supplemental ascorbic acid and neutrophil chemotaxis. J Am Coll Nutr 1992; 11:172.

344. Kong AN, et al. Pharmacokinetics and pharmacodynamic modeling of direct suppression effects of methylprednisolone on serum cortisol and blood histamine in human subjects. Clin Pharmacol Ther 1989; 46:616.

345. Tuchman M, et al. Assessment of the diurnal variations in urinary homovanillic and vanillylmandelic acid excretion for the diagnosis and follow-up of patients with neuroblastoma. Clin Biochem 1985; 18:176.

346. Brown GL, et al. Urinary 3-methoxy-4-hydroxyphenylglycol and homovanillic acid response to d-amphetamine in hyperactive children. Biol Psychiatry 1981; 16:779.

347. Martineau J, et al. Monoamines (serotonin and catecholamines) and their derivatives in infantile autism: age-related changes and drug effects. Dev Med Child Neurol 1992; 34:593.

348. Giacalone M, et al. Cefoxitin: another Porter-Silber chromogen. South Med J 1985; 78:493.

349. Williams FA, et al. Acquired primary hypoaldosteronism due to an isolated zona glomerulosa defect. N Engl J Med 1983; 309:1623.

350. Elghozi JL, et al. Pizotifen increases 5-HIAA urinary excretion in male healthy volunteers. Eur J Clin Pharmacol 1984; 27:191.

351. O'Leary PC, et al. Indomethacin therapy and the measurement of urinary 5-hydroxyindoleacetic acid. Clin Chim Acta 1982; 126:323.

352. Dzurik R, et al. Blood pressure, 5-OH indoleacetic acid, and vanilmandelic acid excretion and blood platelet aggregation in hypertensive patients treated with ketanserin. J Cardiovasc Pharmacol 1985; 7(Suppl 7):S29.

353. Ueshiba H, et al. Enzyme-linked immunosorbent assay (ELISA) method for screening of non-classical steroid 21-hydroxylase deficiency. Horm Metab Res 1994; 26:43.

354. Solyom J. Diurnal variation in blood 17-hydroxyprogesterone concentrations in untreated congenital adrenal hyperplasia. Arch Dis Child 1984; 59:743.

355. Akamatsu T, et al. Menopause related changes of adrenocortical steroid production. Asia Oceania J Obstet Gynaecol 1992; 18:271.

356. Murphy JF, et al. Plasma 17-hydroxyprogesterone concentrations in ill newborn infants. Arch Dis Child 1983; 58:532.

357. Whitworth JA, et al. Plasma 4-pregnene-17 alpha, 20 alpha-diol-3-one (17 alpha, 20 alpha-dihydroxyprogesterone) and 17 alpha-hydroxyprogesterone in man. Acta Endocrinol (Copenh) 1983; 102:271.

358. Yoneyama K, et al. The day to day variations of urinary hydroxyproline and creatinine excretions, and dietary protein intake. Nippon Eiseigaku Zasshi 1984; 39:587.

359. Minisola S, et al. Effects of age on the urinary excretion of total and non-dialyzable hydroxyproline. Ric Clin Lab 1984; 14:649.

360. Meier DE, et al. Racial differences in pre- and postmenopausal bone homeostasis: association with bone density. J Bone Miner Res 1992; 7:1181.

361. Mizunashi K, et al. Effect of omeprazole, an inhibitor of H+,K(+)-ATPase, on bone resorption in humans. Calcif Tissue Int 1993; 53:21.

362. Enberg G, et al. Immunoreactive IGF-II in serum of healthy subjects and patients with growth hormone disturbances and uraemia. Acta Endocrinol (Copenh) 1984; 107:164.

363. Hall K, et al. Somatomedin levels in childhood, adolescence and adult life. Clin Endocrinol Metab 1984; 13:91.

364. Clemmons DR, et al. Factors controlling blood concentration of somatomedin C. Clin Endocrinol Metab 1984; 13:113.

365. Kao PC, et al. Somatomedin C: an index of growth hormone activity. Mayo Clin Proc 1986; 61:908.

366. Nielsen HK, et al. Changes in biochemical markers of osteoblastic activity during the menstrual cycle. J Clin Endocrinol Metab 1990; 70:1431.

367. Miell JP, et al. Effects of dexamethasone on growth hormone (GH)-releasing hormone, arginine- and dopaminergic stimulated GH secretion, and total plasma insulin-like growth factor-I concentrations in normal male volunteers. J Clin Endocrinol Metab 1991; 72:675.

368. Daughaday WH, et al. Heterogeneity of serum peptides with immunoactivity detected by a radioimmunoassay for proinsulin-like growth factor-II E domain: description of a free E domain peptide in serum. J Clin Endocrinol Metab 1992; 75:641.

369. Weaver JU, et al. Decreased sex hormone binding globulin (SHBG) and insulin-like growth factor binding protein (IGFBP-1) in extreme obesity. Clin Endocrinol (Oxf) 1990; 33:415.

370. Lee PD, et al. Regulation and function of insulin-like growth factor-binding protein-1. Proc Soc Exp Biol Med 1993; 204:4.

371. Hall K, et al. IGFBP-1. Production and control mechanisms. Acta Endocrinol (Copenh) 1991; 124(Suppl 2):48.

372. Giudice LC, et al. Insulin-like growth factor binding proteins in maternal serum throughout gestation and in the puerperium: effects of a pregnancy-associated serum protease activity. J Clin Endocrinol Metab 1990; 71:806.

373. Argente J, et al. Normative data for insulin-like growth factors (IGFs), IGF-binding proteins, and growth hormone-binding protein in a healthy Spanish pediatric population: age- and sex-related changes. J Clin Endocrinol Metab 1993; 77:1522.

374. Miell JP, et al. The effects of dexamethasone treatment on immunoreactive and bioactive insulin-like growth factors (IGFs) and IGF-binding proteins in normal male volunteers. J Endocrinol 1993; 136:525.

375. Rutanen EM, et al. Assays for IGF binding proteins. Acta Endocrinol (Copenh) 1991; 124(Suppl 2):70.

376. Davenport ML, et al. Insulin-like growth factor-binding protein-3 proteolysis is induced after elective surgery. J Clin Endocrinol Metab 1992; 75:590.

377. Jorgensen JO, et al. Circadian patterns of serum insulin-like growth factor (IGF) II and IGF binding protein 3 in growth hormone-deficient patients and age- and sex-matched normal subjects. Acta Endocrinol (Copenh) 1990; 123:257.

378. Vorherr H, et al. Vaginal absorption of povidone-iodine. JAMA 1980; 244:2628.

379. Chanoine JC, et al. Iodine contamination of urine samples by test strips. Clin Chem 1987; 33:1935.

380. Ford HCE. Ascorbic acid interferes with an automated urinary iodide determination based on the ceric-arsenious acid reaction. Clin Chem 1991; 37:759.

381. Grasso L, et al. Iodine contamination in subjects admitted to a general hospital. J Endocrinol Invest 1992; 15:307.

382. Saxena S, et al. Effect of blood transfusion on serum iron and transferrin saturation. Arch Pathol Lab Med 1993; 117:622.

383. Fairbanks VF. Laboratory testing for iron status. Hosp Pract (Off Ed) 1991; 26(Suppl 3):17.

384. Touitou Y, et al. Seasonal rhythms of plasma gonadotrophins: their persistence in elderly men and women. J Endocrinol 1983; 96:15.

385. Rudd BT. Urinary 17-oxogenic and 17-oxosteroids. A case for deletion from the clinical chemistry repertoire. Ann Clin Biochem 1983; 20:65.

386. Panteghini M, Pagani F. Biological variation of lactate and pyruvate in blood. Clin Chem 1993; 39:908.

387. Vital health statistics, series 11, no 233. Rockville, MD: National Center for Health Statistics, 1984:1.

388. Panteghini M, Pagani F. Pre-analytical, analytical and biological sources of variation of lipoprotein(a). Eur J Clin Chem Clin Biochem 1993; 31:23.

389. Webb AT, et al. Does cyclosporin increase lipoprotein(a) concentrations in renal transplant recipients? Lancet 1993; 341:268.

390. de Bruin TW, et al. Lipoprotein(a) and apolipoprotein B plasma concentrations in hypothyroid, euthyroid, and hyperthyroid subjects. J Clin Endocrinol Metab 1993; 76:121.

391. Haffner SM, et al. Increased lipoprotein(a) concentrations in chronic renal failure. J Am Soc Nephrol 1992; 3:1156.

392. Huang CM, et al. The effect of alcohol withdrawal on serum concentrations of Lp(a), apolipoproteins A-1 and B, and lipids. Alcohol Clin Exp Res 1992; 16:895.

393. Cobbaert C, et al. Serum lipoprotein(a) levels in racially different populations. Am J Epidemiol 1992; 136:441.

394. Slunga L, et al. Lipoprotein (a) in a randomly selected 25-64 year old population: the Northern Sweden Monica Study. J Clin Epidemiol 1993; 46:617.

395. Marcovina SM, et al. Lipoprotein[a] concentrations and apolipoprotein[a] phenotypes in Caucasians and African Americans. The CARDIA study. Arterioscler Thromb 1993; 13:1037.

396. Soma MR, et al. The lowering of lipoprotein[a] induced by estrogen plus progesterone replacement therapy in postmenopausal women. Arch Intern Med 1993; 153:1462.

397. Crook D, et al. Lipoprotein Lp(a) levels are reduced by danazol, an anabolic steroid. Atherosclerosis 1992; 92:41.

398. Van Biervliet JP, et al. Lipoprotein(a) profiles and evolution in newborns. Atherosclerosis 1991; 86:173.

399. Kervinen K, et al. A rapid increase in lipoprotein (a) levels after ethanol withdrawal in alcoholic men. Life Sci 1991; 48:2183.

400. Maeda S, et al. Transient changes of serum lipoprotein(a) as an acute phase protein. Atherosclerosis 1989; 78:145.

401. Hollifield JW. Potassium and magnesium abnormalities: diuretics and arrhythmias in hypertension. Am J Med 1984; 77:28.

402. Schilsky RL, et al. Hypomagnesemia and renal magnesium wasting in patients receiving cisplatin. Ann Intern Med 1979; 90:929.

403. Whang R, et al. Frequency of hypomagnesemia in hospitalized patients receiving digitalis. Arch Intern Med 1985; 145:655.

404. Mather HM, et al. Diurnal profiles of plasma magnesium and blood glucose in diabetes. Diabetologia 1982; 22:180.

405. Thompson CB, et al. Association between cyclosporin neurotoxicity and hypomagnesaemia. Lancet 1984; 2:1116.

406. Fischer JA, Dambacher MA. Differential diagnosis of hypercalcitoninemia. Biomed Pharmacother 1984; 38:255.

407. Hatano S, et al. Erythrocyte manganese concentration in healthy Japanese children, adults, and the elderly, and in cord blood. Am J Clin Nutr 1983; 37:457.

408. Pleban PA, Pearson KH. Determination of manganese in whole blood and serum. Clin Chem 1979; 25:1915.

409. Theron JJ, et al. Effect of physical exercise on plasma melatonin levels in normal volunteers. S Afr Med J 1984; 66:838.

410. Attanasio A, et al. Circadian rhythms in serum melatonin from infancy to adolescence. J Clin Endocrinol Metab 1985; 61:388.

411. Cowen PJ, et al. Treatment with beta-adrenoceptor blockers reduces plasma melatonin concentration. Br J Clin Pharmacol 1985; 19:258.

412. Touitou Y, et al. Age- and sex-associated modification of plasma melatonin concentrations in man. Relationship to pathology, malignant or not, and autopsy findings. Acta Endocrinol (Copenh) 1985; 108:135.

413. Webley GE, et al. The circadian pattern of melatonin and its positive relationship with progesterone in women. J Clin Endocrinol Metab 1986; 63:323.

414. Rojdmark S, Wetterberg L. Short-term fasting inhibits the nocturnal melatonin secretion in healthy man. Clin Endocrinol (Oxf) 1989; 30:451.

415. Kivela A. Serum melatonin during human pregnancy. Acta Endocrinol (Copenh) 1991; 124:233.

416. Viljoen M, et al. Melatonin in chronic renal failure. Nephron 1992; 60:138.

417. Juan D. Pheochromocytoma: clinical manifestations and diagnostic tests. Urology 1981; 17:1.

418. Elia J, et al. Stimulant drug treatment of hyperactivity: biochemical correlates. Clin Pharmacol Ther 1990; 48:57.

419. Wills MR, et al. Serum and lymphocyte, aluminum and nickel in chronic renal failure. Clin Chim Acta 1985; 145:193.

420. Gundberg CM, et al. Measurements of gamma-carboxyglutamate and circulating osteocalcin in normal children and adults. Clin Chim Acta 1983; 128:1.

421. Epstein S, et al. Differences in serum bone GLA protein with age and sex. Lancet 1984; 1:307.

422. Gundberg CM, et al. Osteocalcin in human serum: a circadian rhythm. J Clin Endocrinol Metab 1985; 60:736.

423. Reid IR, et al. Low serum osteocalcin levels in glucocorticoid-treated asthmatics. J Clin Endocrinol Metab 1986; 62:379.

424. Menon RK, et al. Impaired carboxylation of osteocalcin in warfarin-treated patients. J Clin Endocrinol Metab 1987; 64:59.

425. Cole DEC, et al. Changing osteocalcin concentrations during pregnancy and lactation: implications for maternal mineral metabolism. J Clin Endocrinol Metab 1987; 65:290.

426. Napal J, et al. Stress decreases the serum level of osteocalcin. Bone Miner 1993; 21:113.

427. Perry HM 3d, et al. The effects of thiazide diuretics on calcium metabolism in the aged. J Am Geriatr Soc 1993; 41:818.

428. Karlsson R, et al. Osteocalcin 24-hour profiles during normal pregnancy. Gynecol Obstet Invest 1992; 34:197.

429. Kakonen SM, et al. Development and evaluation of three immunofluorometric assays that measure different forms of osteocalcin in serum. Clin Chem 2000; 46:332.

430. Power MJ, Fottrell PF. Osteocalcin: diagnostic methods and clinical applications. Crit Rev Clin Lab Sci 1991; 28:287.

431. Karlsson R, et al. Oral contraception affects osteocalcin serum profiles in young women. Osteoporos Int 1992; 2:118.

432. Elomaa I, et al. Seasonal variation of urinary calcium and oxalate excretion, serum 25(OH)D$_3$ and albumin level in relation to renal stone formation. Scand J Urol Nephrol 1982; 16:155.

433. Zerwekh JE, et al. Assay of urinary oxalate: six methodologies compared. Clin Chem 1983; 29:1977.

434. Balcke P, et al. Ascorbic acid aggravates secondary hyperoxalemia in patients on chronic hemodialysis. Ann Intern Med 1984; 101:344.

435. France NC, et al. In vitro oxalogenesis, and measurement of oxalate in serum. Clin Chem 1985; 31:335.

436. Leumann EP, et al. Urinary oxalate and glycolate excretion in healthy infants and children. Pediatr Nephrol 1990; 4:493.

437. Balchin ZE, et al. Biological variation of urinary oxalate in different specimen types. Ann Clin Biochem 1991; 28:622.

438. Otsuki Y, et al. Serial plasma oxytocin levels during pregnancy and labor. Acta Obstet Gynecol Scand 1983; 62:15.

439. Amico JA, et al. Oxytocin in human plasma: correlation with neurophysin and stimulation with estrogen. J Clin Endocrinol Metab 1981; 52:988.

440. Kumaresan P, et al. Human ovulation and plasma oxytocin. Int J Gynaecol Obstet 1983; 21:413.

441. Zaccaria M, et al. Effects of pirenzepine on plasma insulin, glucagon and pancreatic polypeptide levels in normal man. Eur J Clin Pharmacol 1985; 27:701.

442. Lugari R, et al. Human pancreatic polypeptide and somatostatin in chronic renal failure. Proc Eur Dial Transplant Assoc Eur Ren Assoc 1985; 21:614.

443. Hansen BC, et al. Fluctuations in basal plasma levels of pancreatic polypeptide in monkeys and humans. Am J Physiol 1985; 248:R739.

444. O'Hare MMT, et al. Radioimmunoassay for pancreatic polypeptide, and its age-related changes in concentration. Clin Chem 1983; 29:1923.

445. Cho CH, et al. Serum concentration of pancreatic polypeptide in normal subjects and in peptic ulcer patients. Horm Metab Res 1985; 17:215.

446. Jorde R, et al. Fasting and postprandial plasma pancreatic polypeptide (PP) levels in obesity. Int J Obes 1984; 8:393.

447. Hanukoglu A, et al. Human pancreatic polypeptide in children and young adults. Horm Metab Res 1990; 22:41.

448. Hackeng WHL, et al. Clinical implications of estimation of intact parathyroid hormone (PTH) versus total immunoreactive PTH in normal subjects and hyperparathyroid patients. J Clin Endocrinol Metab 1986; 63:447.

449. Bell NH, et al. Evidence for alteration of the vitamin D-endocrine system in obese subjects. J Clin Invest 1985; 76:370.

450. Bell NH, et al. Evidence for alteration of the vitamin D-endocrine system in blacks. J Clin Invest 1985; 76:470.

451. Petersen MM, et al. Parathyroid hormone and 25-hydroxyvitamin D concentrations in sick and normal elderly people. BMJ 1983; 287:521.

452. Specker BL, et al. Calcium-regulating hormones and minerals from birth to 18 months of age: a cross-sectional study. II. Effects of sex, race, age, season, and diet on serum minerals, parathyroid hormone, and calcitonin. Pediatrics 1986; 77:891.

453. Marcus R, et al. Age-related changes in parathyroid hormone and parathyroid hormone action in normal humans. J Clin Endocrinol Metab 1984; 58:223.

454. Kitamura N, et al. Episodic fluctuation in serum intact parathyroid hormone concentration in men. J Clin Endocrinol Metab 1990; 70:252.

455. Rudnicki M, et al. Effects of age, sex, season and diet on serum ionized calcium, parathyroid hormone and vitamin D in a random population. J Intern Med 1993; 234:195.

456. Frolich A, et al. Serum concentrations of intact parathyroid hormone during late human pregnancy: a longitudinal study. Eur J Obstet Gynecol Reprod Biol 1991; 42:85.

457. Saggese G, et al. Determination of intact parathyrin by immunoradiometric assay evaluated in normal children and in patients with various disorders of calcium metabolism. Clin Chem 1991; 37:1999.

458. Specker BL, et al. Changes in calcium homeostasis over the first year postpartum: effect of lactation and weaning. Obstet Gynecol 1991; 78:56.

459. Saggese G, et al. Intact parathyroid hormone levels during pregnancy, in healthy term neonates and in hypocalcemic preterm infants. Acta Paediatr Scand 1991; 80:36.

460. Prince RL, et al. Effects of transdermal estrogen replacement on parathyroid hormone secretion. J Clin Endocrinol Metab 1990; 71:1284.

461. Armitage EK. Parathyrin (parathyroid hormone): metabolism and methods for assay. Clin Chem 1986; 32:418.

462. Grill V, et al. Parathyroid hormone-related protein: a possible endocrine function in lactation. Clin Endocrinol (Oxf) 1992; 37:405.

463. Bucht E, et al. Parathyroid hormone-related peptide, measured by a mid-molecule radioimmunoassay, in various hypercalcaemic and normocalcaemic conditions. Acta Endocrinol (Copenh) 1992; 127:294.

464. Mallette LE. The parathyroid polyhormones: new concepts in the spectrum of peptide hormone action. Endocr Rev 1991; 12:110.

465. Sonnenblick M, et al. Paraprotein interference with colorimetry of phosphate in serum of some patients with multiple myeloma. Clin Chem 1986; 32:1537.

466. Uza G. Effect of clonidine on serum inorganic phosphorus in patients with essential arterial hypertension. J Hum Hypertens 1990; 4:687.

467. Licata AA, et al. The urinary excretion of phosphoethanolamine in diseases other than hypophosphatasia. Am J Med 1978; 64:133.

468. Eastman JR, Bixler D. Urinary phosphoethanolamine: normal values by age. Clin Chem 1980; 26:1757.

469. Houghton DJ, et al. Relationship of maternal and fetal levels of human placental lactogen to the weight and sex of the fetus. Placenta 1984; 5:455.

470. Shaw MA, et al. Adsorption of pregnanediol-3 alpha-glucuronide by plastics and glass. J Steroid Biochem 1983; 19:1681.

471. Metcalf MG, et al. Indices of ovulation: comparison of plasma and salivary levels of progesterone with urinary pregnanediol. J Endocrinol 1984; 100:75.

472. Junkermann H, et al. Circadian rhythm of serum progesterone levels in human pregnancy and its relation to the rhythm of cortisol. Acta Endocrinol (Copenh) 1982; 101:98.

473. Smith RL. Effect of serum-separating gels on progesterone assays. Clin Chem 1985; 31:1239.

474. Healy DL, et al. Pulsatile progesterone secretion: its relevance to clinical evaluation of corpus luteum function. Fertil Steril 1984; 41:114.

475. Spitz IM, et al. Response to intermittent RU486 in women. Fertil Steril 1993; 59:971.

476. Cohen RM, et al. A radioimmunoassay for circulating human proinsulin. Diabetes 1985; 34:84.

477. Deacon CF, et al. Measurement of circulating human proinsulin concentrations using a proinsulin-specific antiserum. Diabetes 1985; 34:491.

478. Beer SF, et al. The effect of thyroid disease on proinsulin and C-peptide levels. Clin Endocrinol (Oxf) 1989; 30:379.

479. Kahn SE, et al. Effect of glucocorticoid and growth hormone treatment on proinsulin levels in humans. Diabetes 1993; 42:1082.

480. Davies MJ, et al. Insulin deficiency and increased plasma concentration of intact and 32/33 split proinsulin in subjects with impaired glucose tolerance. Diabet Med 1993; 10:313.

481. Christensen SE, et al. Body temperature elevation, exercise and serum prolactin concentrations. Acta Endocrinol (Copenh) 1985; 109:458.

482. Jackson RD, et al. Macroprolactinemia presenting like a pituitary tumor. Am J Med 1985; 78:346.

483. Djahanbakhch O, et al. Changes in plasma levels of prolactin, in relation to those of FSH, oestradiol, androstenedione and progesterone around the preovulatory surge of LH in women. Clin Endocrinol (Oxf) 1984; 20:463.

484. Govoni S, et al. Plasma prolactin concentrations in a large population of healthy old people. BMJ 1983; 287:1107.

485. Mendelson J, et al. Acute effects of marihuana smoking on prolactin levels in human females. J Pharmacol Exp Ther 1985; 232:220.

486. Verbeelen D, et al. Effect of 1,25-dihydroxyvitamin $D_3$ and nifedipine on prolactin release in normal man. J Endocrinol Invest 1985; 8:103.

487. Lindstedt F, et al. "Hyperprolactinemia" in healthy women. Clin Chem 1984; 30:165.

488. Musey VC, et al. Long-term effect of a first pregnancy on the secretion of prolactin. N Engl J Med 1987; 316:229.

489. Maestri E, et al. Effects of five days verapamil administration on serum GH and PRL levels. Horm Metab Res 1985; 17:482.

490. Mendelson JH, et al. Cocaine effects on pulsatile secretion of anterior pituitary, gonadal, and adrenal hormones. J Clin Endocrinol Metab 1989; 69:1256.

491. Yeksan M, et al. Effect of recombinant human erythropoietin (r-HuEPO) therapy on plasma $FT_3$, $FT_4$, TSH, FSH, LH, free testosterone and prolactin levels in hemodialysis patients. Int J Artif Organs 1992; 15:585.

492. Willenbring ML, et al. Psychoneuroendocrine effects of methadone maintenance. Psychoneuroendocrinology 1989; 14:371.

493. Maestri E, et al. Effects of five days verapamil administration on serum GH and PRL levels. Horm Metab Res 1985; 17:482.

494. Bettica P, et al. Bone-resorption markers galactosyl hydroxylysine, pyridinium crosslinks, and hydroxyproline compared. Clin Chem 1992; 38:2313.

495. Schlemmer AE. Marked diurnal variation in urinary excretion of pyridinium cross-links in premenopausal women. J Clin Endocrinol Metab 1992; 74:476.

496. Oesterling JE. Prostate specific antigen: a critical assessment of the most useful tumor marker for adenocarcinoma of the prostate. J Urol 1991; 145:907.

497. Pummer K, et al. False positive prostate specific antigen values in the sera of women with renal cell carcinoma. J Urol 1992; 148:21.

498. Oesterling JE, et al. Serum prostate-specific antigen in a community-based population of healthy men. Establishment of age-specific reference ranges. JAMA 1993; 270:860.

499. Ruckle HC, et al. Prostate-specific antigen: critical issues for the practicing physician. Mayo Clin Proc 1994; 69:59.

500. Glenski WJ, et al. Prostate-specific antigen: establishment of the reference range for the clinically normal prostate gland and the effect of digital rectal examination, ejaculation, and time on serum concentrations. Prostate 1992; 21:99.

501. Zhou AME. Multiple forms of prostate-specific antigen in serum: differences in immunorecognition by monoclonal and polyclonal assays. Clin Chem 1993; 39:2483.

502. Price A. Abrupt changes in prostate-specific antigen concentration in acute renal failure. Clin Chem 1993; 39:161.

503. Lipton A, et al. Increased urinary excretion of pyridinium cross-links in cancer patients. Clin Chem 1993; 39:614.

504. Peel N, et al. Sulfasalazine may interfere with HPLC assay of urinary pyridinium crosslinks. Clin Chem 1994; 40:167.

505. Uebelhart D, et al. Effect of menopause and hormone replacement therapy on the urinary excretion of pyridinium cross-links. J Clin Endocrinol Metab 1991; 72:367.

506. Eastell R, et al. Nyctohemeral changes in bone turnover assessed by serum bone Gla-protein concentration and urinary deoxypyridinoline excretion: effects of growth and ageing. Clin Sci 1992; 83:375.

507. Hetland ML, et al. Low bone mass and high bone turnover in male long distance runners. J Clin Endocrinol Metab 1993; 77:770.

508. Harris ST, et al. The effect of short term treatment with alendronate on vertebral density and biochemical markers of bone remodeling in early postmenopausal women. J Clin Endocrinol Metab 1993; 76:1399.

509. Lipton A, et al. Increased urinary excretion of pyridinium cross-links in cancer patients. Clin Chem 1993; 39:614.

510. McLaren AM, et al. Physiological variations in the urinary excretion of pyridinium crosslinks of collagen. Br J Rheumatol 1993; 32:307.

511. Goldhaber SZ, et al. Plasma renin substrate, renin activity, and aldosterone levels in a sample of oral contraceptive users from a community survey. Am Heart J 1984; 107:119.

512. Sealey JE, et al. Changes in active and inactive renin throughout normal pregnancy. Clin Exp Hypertens [A] 1982; 4:2373.

513. Fiselier J, et al. The basal levels of active and inactive plasma renin concentration in infancy and childhood. Clin Sci 1984; 67:383.

514. Higaki J, et al. A new sensitive direct radioimmunoassay for human plasma renin and its clinical application. J Lab Clin Med 1984; 104:947.

515. Pessina AC, et al. Digitalis glycosides and plasma renin activity. Pharmacol Res Commun 1982; 14:629.

516. Sealey JE. Plasma renin activity and plasma prorenin assays. Clin Chem 1991; 37:1811.

517. Oektedalen O, et al. Basal hyperchlorhydria and its relation to the plasma concentrations of secretin, vasoactive intestinal peptide, and gastrin during prolonged strain. Regul Pept (Netherlands) 1983; 5:235.

518. Oektedalen O, et al. Secretin—a new stress hormone? Regul Pept 1982; 4:213.

519. Grekas DM, et al. Plasma secretin, pancreozymin, and somatostatin-like hormone in chronic renal failure patients. Uremia Invest 1984; 8:117.

520. Beglinger C, et al. Pancreatic enzyme response to a liquid meal and to hormonal stimulation. Correlation with plasma secretin and cholecystokinin levels. J Clin Invest 1985; 75:1471.

521. Subotzky EF, et al. Plasma zinc, copper, selenium, ferritin and whole blood manganese concentrations in children with kwashiorkor in the acute stage and during refeeding. Ann Trop Paediatr 1992; 12:13.

522. Lloyd B, et al. Effect of smoking, alcohol, and other factors on the selenium status of a healthy population. J Epidemiol Community Health 1983; 37:213.

523. Hurd RW, et al. Selenium, zinc, and copper changes with valproic acid: possible relation to drug side effects. Neurology 1985; 34:1393.

524. Dworkin B, et al. Diminished blood selenium levels in renal failure patients on dialysis: correlations with nutritional status. Am J Med Sci 1987; 293:6.

525. Marano G, et al. Increased serum selenium levels in patients under corticosteroid treatment. Pharmacol Toxicol 1990; 67:120.

526. Hawker FH, et al. Effects of acute illness on selenium homeostasis. Crit Care Med 1990; 18:442.

527. Marano G, et al. Changes of serum selenium and serum cholesterol in children during sexual maturation. J Trace Elem Electrolytes Health Dis 1991; 5:59.

528. Anderson GM, et al. Effect of a meal on human whole blood serotonin. Gastroenterology 1985; 88:86.

529. Davis DD, et al. Biological stress responses in high and low trait anxious students. Biol Psychiatry 1985; 20:843.

530. DeLisi LE, et al. Increased whole blood serotonin concentrations in chronic schizophrenic patients. Arch Gen Psychiatry 1981; 38:647.

531. Sanz Alaejos M, Diaz Romero C. Urinary selenium concentrations. Clin Chem 1993; 39:2040.

532. Flachaire E, et al. Determination of reference values for serotonin concentration in platelets of healthy newborns, children, adults, and elderly subjects by HPLC with electrochemical detection. Clin Chem 1990; 36:2117.

533. Hindberg I, et al. Serotonin concentrations in plasma and variations during the menstrual cycle. Clin Chem 1992; 38:2087.

534. Eynard N, et al. Platelet serotonin content and free and total plasma tryptophan in healthy volunteers during 24 hours. Clin Chem 1993; 39:2337.

535. Pietraszek MH, et al. Alcohol-induced depression: involvement of serotonin. Alcohol Alcohol 1991; 26:155.

536. Steyn ME, et al. Whole blood serotonin levels in chronic renal failure. Life Sci 1992; 51:359.

537. Gonzales GF, Carrillo C. Blood serotonin levels in postmenopausal women: effects of age and serum oestradiol levels. Maturitas 1993; 17:23.

538. Anderson DC. Sex-hormone-binding globulin. Clin Endocrinol (Oxf) 1974; 3:69.

539. Uriel J, et al. Maternal serum levels of sex steroid-binding protein during pregnancy. Br J Obstet Gynaecol 1981; 88:1229.

540. Maruyama Y, et al. Variation with age in the levels of sex-steroid-binding plasma protein as determined by radioimmunoassay. Acta Endocrinol (Copenh) 1984; 106:428.

541. Beastall GH, et al. Hormone binding globulins and anticonvulsant therapy. Scott Med J 1985; 30:101.

542. Belgorosky A, Rivarola MA. Progressive decrease in serum sex hormone-binding globulin from infancy to late prepuberty in boys. J Clin Endocrinol Metab 1986; 63:510.

543. Grenman S, et al. Sex steroid, gonadotropin, cortisol, and prolactin levels in healthy, massively obese women: correlation with abdominal fat cell size and effect of weight reduction. J Clin Endocrinol Metab 1986; 63:1257.

544. Lonning PE, et al. Plasma levels of estradiol, estrone, estrone sulfate and sex hormone binding globulin in patients receiving rifampicin. J Steroid Biochem 1989; 33:631.

545. Caballero MJ, et al. Effects of physical exercise on sex hormone binding globulin, high density lipoprotein cholesterol, total cholesterol and triglycerides in postmenopausal women. Endocr Res 1992; 18:261.

546. Dibbelt L, et al. Group comparison of serum ethinyl estradiol, SHBG and CBG levels in 83 women using two low-dose combination oral contraceptives for three months. Contraception 1991; 43:1.

547. Isojarvi JI. Serum steroid hormones and pituitary function in female epileptic patients during carbamazepine therapy. Epilepsia 1990; 31:438.

548. Berlyne GM, Caruso C. Measurement of silicon in biological fluids in man using flameless furnace atomic absorption spectrophotometry. Clin Chim Acta 1983; 129:239.

549. Mauras Y, et al. Increase in blood silicon concentration in patients with renal failure. Biomedicine 1980; 33:228.

550. Saito H, et al. Plasma somatostatin level during natural and interrupted nocturnal sleep in man. Acta Endocrinol (Copenh) 1983; 104:129.

551. Burhol PG, et al. Diurnal profile of plasma somatostatin in man. Acta Physiol Scand 1984; 120:67.

552. Conlon JM, et al. The nature of big plasma somatostatin: implications for the measurement of somatostatin-like immunoreactivity in human plasma. Anal Biochem 1982; 125:243.

553. Uvnas-Moberg K, et al. Plasma levels of gastrin, somatostatin, VIP, insulin and oxytocin during the menstrual cycle in women (with and without oral contraceptives). Acta Obstet Gynecol Scand 1989; 68:165.

554. Holst N, et al. Plasma concentrations of motilin and somatostatin are increased in late pregnancy and postpartum. Br J Obstet Gynaecol 1992; 99:338.

555. Bertello P, et al. Circadian patterns of plasma cortisol and testosterone in chronic male alcoholics. Alcohol Clin Exp Res 1982; 6:475.

556. Sharp AM, et al. Further studies on danazol interference in testosterone radioimmunoassays. Clin Chem 1983; 29:141.

557. Guglielmini C, et al. Variations of serum testosterone concentrations after physical exercises of different duration. Int J Sports Med 1984; 5:246.

558. Wheeler GD, et al. Reduced serum testosterone and prolactin levels in male distance runners. JAMA 1984; 252:514.

559. Buergi U, et al. Serum thyroglobulin before and after palpation of the thyroid. N Engl J Med 1983; 308:777.

560. Penny R, et al. Thyroid-stimulating hormone and thyroglobulin levels decrease with chronological age in children and adolescents. J Clin Endocrinol Metab 1983; 56:177.

561. Nakamura S, et al. Serum thyroglobulin (Tg) concentration in healthy subjects: absence of age- and sex-related differences. Endocrinol Jpn 1984; 31:93.

562. Nakamura S, et al. Serum thyroglobulin concentration in normal pregnancy. Endocrinol Jpn 1984; 31:675.

563. Catania A, et al. Circulating thyroglobulin and antithyroglobulin antibodies after fine needle aspiration of thyroid nodules. Horm Metab Res 1985; 17:49.

564. Aiello DP, Manni A. Thyroglobulin measurement vs iodine 131 total-body scan for follow-up of well-differentiated thyroid cancer. Arch Intern Med 1990; 150:437.

565. Ross HA, et al. Is free thyroxine accurately measurable at room temperature? Clin Chem 1992; 38:880.

566. Kojima N, et al. Age- and sex-related differences of serum thyroxine binding globulin (TBG) in healthy subjects. Acta Endocrinol (Copenh) 1983; 104:303.

567. Franklyn JA, et al. The effect of propranolol on circulating thyroid hormone measurements in thyrotoxic and euthyroid subjects. Acta Endocrinol (Copenh) 1985; 108:351.

568. Bentsen KD, et al. Serum thyroid hormones and blood folic acid during monotherapy with carbamazepine or valproate. A controlled study. Acta Neurol Scand 1983; 67:235.

569. Harrup JS, et al. Circannual and within-individual variation of thyroid function tests in normal subjects. Ann Clin Biochem 1985; 22:371.

570. Ramsay I. Drug and non-thyroid induced changes in thyroid function tests. Postgrad Med J 1985; 61:375.

571. Cashin-Hemphill L, et al. Alterations in serum thyroid hormonal indices with colestipol-niacin therapy. Ann Intern Med 1987; 107:324.

572. Benvenga S, et al. Effect of free fatty acids and nonlipid inhibitors of thyroid hormone binding in the immunoradiometric assay of thyroxin-binding globulin. Clin Chem 1987; 33:1752.

573. Spencer CA, et al. Dynamics of serum thyrotropin and thyroid hormone changes in fasting. J Clin Endocrinol Metab 1983; 56:883.

574. O'Malley BP, et al. Circadian rhythms of serum thyrotrophin and body temperature in euthyroid individuals and their responses to warming. Clin Sci 1984; 67:433.

575. Weeke J, et al. A longitudinal study of serum TSH, and total and free iodothyronines during normal pregnancy. Acta Endocrinol (Copenh) 1982; 101:531.

576. Greenspan SL, et al. Pulsatile secretion of thyrotropin in man. J Clin Endocrinol Metab 1986; 63:661.

577. Ain KB, et al. Thyroid hormone levels affected by time of blood sampling in thyroxine-treated patients. Thyroid 1993; 3:81.

578. Schedlowski M, et al. Acute psychological stress increases plasma levels of cortisol, prolactin and TSH. Life Sci 1992; 50:1201.

579. Jiang N-S, et al. Assay for thyroid stimulating immunoglobulin. Mayo Clin Proc 1986; 61:753.

580. Mielke AW, et al. Effects of a fat-containing meal on sex hormones in men. Metabolism 1990; 39:943.

581. Hugues JN, et al. Effects of cimetidine on thyroid hormones. Clin Endocrinol (Oxf) 1982; 17:297.

582. Guillaume J, et al. Components of the total serum thyroid hormone concentrations during pregnancy: high free thyroxine and blunted thyrotropin (TSH) response to TSH-releasing hormone in the first trimester. J Clin Endocrinol Metab 1985; 60:678.

583. Bellastella A, et al. Circannual rhythms of plasma growth hormone, thyrotropin and thyroid hormones in prepuberty. Clin Endocrinol (Oxf) 1984; 20:531.

584. Borowski GD, et al. Effect of long-term amiodarone therapy on thyroid hormone levels and thyroid function. Am J Med 1985; 78:443.

585. Sepkovic DW, et al. Thyroid activity in cigarette smokers. Arch Intern Med 1983; 144:501.

586. Franklyn JA, et al. Measurement of free thyroid hormones in patients on long-term phenytoin therapy. Eur J Clin Pharmacol 1984; 26:633.

587. Franklyn JA, et al. The influence of age and sex on tests of thyroid function. Ann Clin Biochem 1985; 22:502.

588. Ohnhaus EE, et al. The effect of antipyrine, phenobarbitol and rifampicin on thyroid hormone metabolism in man. Eur J Clin Invest 1981; 11:381.

589. McConnell RJ. Abnormal thyroid function test results in patients taking salsalate. JAMA 1992; 267:1242.

590. Ramaker J, Wood WG. Transthyretin—an explanation of "anomalous" serum thyroid hormone values in severe illness? J Clin Chem Clin Biochem 1990; 28:155.

591. Docter R, et al. Free thyroxine assessed with three assays in sera of patients with nonthyroidal illness and of subjects with abnormal concentrations of thyroxine-binding proteins. Clin Chem 1993; 39:1668.

592. Wang Y-S, et al. Comparison of a new ultrafiltration method for serum free T$_4$ and free T$_3$ with two RIA kits in eight groups of patients. J Endocrinol Invest 1985; 8:495.

593. Ng RH, et al. Falsely high results for triglycerides in patients receiving intravenous nitroglycerin. Clin Chem 1986; 32:2098.

594. Price A, et al. Comparison of methods for the determination of unbound triiodothyronine in pregnancy. Clin Endocrinol (Oxf) 1992; 37:41.

595. Nanji AA, et al. Increase in serum uric acid level associated with cisplatin therapy. Correlation with liver but not kidney platinum concentrations. Arch Intern Med 1985; 145:2013.

596. Burritt MF, et al. Pediatric reference intervals for 19 biologic variables in healthy children. Mayo Clin Proc 1990; 65:329.

597. Simonoff M, et al. Vanadium in human serum, as determined by neutron activation analysis. Clin Chem 1984; 30:1700.

598. Naylor GJ. Vanadium and affective disorders. Biol Psychiatry 1983; 18:103.

599. Robins AH, Barron JL. The effect of disulfiram on the urinary excretion of catecholamine metabolites in alcoholic males. S Afr Med J 1983; 63:41.

600. Hill P, et al. VIP and prolactin release in response to meals. Scand J Gastroenterol 1986; 21:958.

601. Bloom SR, et al. Vasoactive intestinal peptide secreting tumors. Pathophysiological and clinical correlations. Ann N Y Acad Sci 1988; 527:518.

602. Henriksen JH, et al. Circulating endogenous vasoactive intestinal polypeptide (VIP) in patients with uraemia and liver cirrhosis. Eur J Clin Invest 1986; 16:211.

603. Woie L, et al. Increase in plasma vasoactive intestinal polypeptide (VIP) in muscular exercise in humans. Gen Pharmacol 1986; 17:321.

604. Barreca T, et al. Plasma somatostatin and vasoactive intestinal polypeptide responses to an oral mixed test meal in obese patients. Horm Res 1989; 31:234.

605. Stromberg P, et al. Vasopressin and prostaglandins in premenstrual pain and primary dysmenorrhea. Acta Obstet Gynecol Scand 1984; 63:533.

606. Soelberg Sorensen P, Hammer M. Effects of long-term carbamazepine treatment on water metabolism and plasma vasopressin concentration. Eur J Clin Pharmacol 1984; 26:719.

607. Dietz R, et al. Vasopressor systems during smoking in humans. Klin Wochenschr 1984; 62(Suppl 2):11.

608. De Vane GW. Vasopressin levels during pregnancy and labor. J Reprod Med 1985; 30:324.

609. Punnonen R, et al. Plasma vasopressin during normal menstrual cycle. Horm Res 1983; 17:90.

610. Stewart WK, et al. Plasma retinol and retinol binding protein concentrations in patients on maintenance haemodialysis with and without vitamin A supplements. Nephron 1982; 30:15.

611. Mejia LA, Arroyave G. Determination of vitamin A in blood. Some practical considerations on the time of collection of the specimens and the stability of the vitamin. Am J Clin Nutr 1983; 37:147.

612. Kozlowski BW. Anticonvulsant medication use and circulating levels of total thyroxine, retinol binding protein, and vitamin A in children with delayed cognitive development. Am J Clin Nutr 1987; 46:360.

613. Ito Y, et al. Effects of the consumption of cigarettes, alcohol and foods on serum concentrations of carotenoids, retinol and tocopherols in healthy inhabitants living in a rural area of Hokkaido. Nippon Eiseigaku Zasshi 1991; 46:874.

614. Lewis CJ, et al. Relationship between age and serum vitamin A in children aged 4-11 y. Am J Clin Nutr 1990; 52:353.

615. Leigh D, et al. Erythrocyte transketolase activity in the Wernicke-Korsakoff syndrome. Br J Psychiatry 1981; 139:153.

616. Wyatt DT, et al. Age-dependent changes in thiamin concentrations in whole blood and cerebrospinal fluid in infants and children. Am J Clin Nutr 1991; 53:530.

617. Leinert J, et al. Methods and their evaluation for the estimation of vitamin B6 levels in man. 5. Serum pyridoxal-5-phosphate determination: method and comparison of methods. [In German]. Int J Vitam Nutr Res 1983; 53:156.

618. Shideler CE. Vitamin B6: an overview. Am J Med Technol 1983; 49:17.

619. Ubbink JB, et al. Relationship between vitamin B-6 status and elevated pyridoxal kinase levels induced by theophylline therapy in humans. J Nutr 1990; 120:1352.

620. Fahmy NR. Consumption of vitamin B12 during sodium nitroprusside administration in humans. Anesthesiology 1981; 54:305.

621. Fairbanks VF, Elveback LR. Tests for pernicious anemia: serum vitamin B12 assay. Mayo Clin Proc 1983; 58:135.

622. Hjelt K, et al. Oral contraceptives and the cobalamin (vitamin B12) metabolism. Acta Obstet Gynecol Scand 1985; 64:59.

623. Fernandes-Costa F, et al. A sex difference in serum cobalamin and transcobalamin levels. Am J Clin Nutr 1985; 41:784.

624. Saxena S, Carmel R. Racial differences in vitamin B12 levels in the United States. Am J Clin Pathol 1987; 88:95.

625. Sasaki R, et al. Influences of sex and age on serum ascorbic acid. Tohoku J Exp Med 1983; 140:97.

626. Sinha R, et al. Determinants of plasma ascorbic acid in a healthy male population. Cancer Epidemiol Biomarkers Prev 1992; 1:297.

627. MacRury SM, et al. Seasonal and climatic variation in cholesterol and vitamin C: effect of vitamin C supplementation. Scott Med J 1992; 37:49.

628. Rosen JF, Chesney RW. Circulating calcitriol concentrations in health and disease. J Pediatr 1983; 103:1.

629. Halloran BP, et al. Serum concentration of 1,25-dihydroxyvitamin D in the human: diurnal variation. J Clin Endocrinol Metab 1985; 60:1104.

630. Bikle DD, et al. Free 1,25-dihydroxyvitamin D levels in serum from normal subjects, pregnant subjects, and subjects with liver disease. J Clin Invest 1984; 74:1966.

631. Jongen MJM, et al. An international comparison of vitamin D metabolite measurements. Clin Chem 1984; 30:399.

632. Lichtenstein P, et al. Calcium-regulating hormones and minerals from birth to 18 months of age: a cross-sectional study. I. Effects of sex, race, age, season, and diet on vitamin D status. Pediatrics 1986; 77:883.

633. Glass AR, Eil C. Ketoconazole-induced reduction in serum 1,25-dihydroxyvitamin D. J Clin Endocrinol Metab 1986; 63:766.

634. Van der Wiel HE, et al. Biochemical parameters of bone turnover during ten days of bed rest and subsequent mobilization. Bone Miner 1991; 13:123.

635. Villa ML, et al. Effects of aluminum hydroxide on the parathyroid-vitamin D axis of postmenopausal women. J Clin Endocrinol Metab 1991; 73:1256.

636. Rodland O, et al. Serum levels of vitamin D metabolites in isotretinoin-treated acne patients. Acta Derm Venereol (Stockh) 1992; 72:217.

637. Reasner CA 2nd, et al. Alteration of vitamin D metabolism in Mexican-Americans. J Bone Miner Res 1990; 5:13.

638. Ala-Houhala M, et al. Serum 25-hydroxyvitamin D levels in Finnish children aged 2 to 17 years. Acta Paediatr Scand 1984; 73:232.

639. Tjellesen L, et al. Serum vitamin D metabolites in epileptic patients treated with 2 different anti-convulsants. Neurol Scand 1982; 66:335.

640. Goldray D, et al. Vitamin D deficiency in elderly patients in a general hospital. J Am Geriatr Soc 1989; 37:589.

641. Scragg R, et al. Plasma 25-hydroxyvitamin D$_3$ and its relation to physical activity and other heart disease risk factors in the general population. Ann Epidemiol 1992; 2:697.

642. Haga P, et al. Plasma tocopherol levels and vitamin E/beta-lipoprotein relationships during pregnancy and in cord blood. Am J Clin Nutr 1982; 36:1200.

643. Stein G, et al. Serum vitamin E levels in patients with chronic renal failure. Int J Artif Organs 1983; 6:285.

644. Ogunmekan AO. Plasma vitamin E (alpha tocopherol) levels in normal children and in epileptic children with and without anticonvulsant drug therapy. Trop Geogr Med 1985; 37:175.

645. Markowitz ME, et al. Circadian variations in serum zinc (Zn) concentrations: correlation with blood ionized calcium, serum total calcium and phosphate in humans. Am J Clin Nutr 1985; 41:689.

646. Walker AM, et al. Carbonic anhydrase inhibitors induce elevations in human whole-blood zinc levels. Arch Ophthalmol 1984; 102:1785.

647. Zumkley H, et al. Zinc metabolism during captopril treatment. Horm Metab Res 1985; 17:256.

648. Ohno H, et al. Exercise-induced changes in blood zinc and related proteins in humans. J Appl Physiol 1985; 58:1453.

649. Swanson CA, King JC. Reduced serum zinc concentration during pregnancy. Obstet Gynecol 1983; 62:313.

650. Aggett PJ. Zinc metabolism in chronic renal insufficiency with or without dialysis therapy. Contrib Nephrol 1984; 38:95.

651. Young DS. SI units for clinical laboratory data. JAMA 1978; 240:1618.

652. Soldin SJ, et al. Biochemical basis of pediatric disease, 3rd ed. Washington: AACC Press, 1998.

653. Soldin SJ, et al. Pediatric reference ranges, 2nd ed. Washington: AACC Press, 1997.

654. Ladenson JH. Nonanalytical sources of variation in clinical chemistry results. In: Sonnenwirth AC, Jarrett L, eds. Gradwohl's clinical laboratory methods and diagnosis, 8th ed. St. Louis: CV Mosby, 1980:149.

655. Teitz NW, ed. Clinical guide to laboratory tests, 3rd ed. Philadelphia: WB Saunders, 1995.

656. Dufour DR. Causes and control of preanalytic variation. In: Kaplan LA, Pesce AJ, eds. Clinical chemistry: theory, analysis, and correlation, 3rd ed. St. Louis: CV Mosby, 1996:65.

657. Young DS. Effects of preanalytical variables on clinical laboratory tests, 2nd ed. Washington: AACC Press, 1997.

658. Siest G, et al., eds. Interpretation of clinical laboratory tests. Foster City, CA: Biomedical Publications, 1985.

659. Tryding N, et al., eds. Drug effects in clinical chemistry 1992, 6th ed. Stockholm: Apoteksbolaget, Lakemedelsverket and Svensk Forening for Klinisk Kemi, 1992.

660. Yamanishi H, et al. Stability of acetoacetate after venesection. Clin Chem 1993; 39:920.

661. Pratt JH, et al. Racial differences in aldosterone excretion and plasma aldosterone concentrations in children. N Engl J Med 1989; 321:1152.

662. Prummel MF, et al. The course of biochemical parameters of bone turnover during treatment with corticosteroids. J Clin Endocrinol Metab 1991; 72:382.

663. Beneteau-Burnat B, et al. Serum angiotensin-converting enzyme in healthy and sarcoidotic children: comparison with the reference interval for adults. Clin Chem 1990; 36:344.

664. Colantonio D, et al. A possible role of atrial natriuretic peptide in ethanol-induced acute diuresis. Life Sci 1991; 48:635.

665. Fibiger W, et al. Cortisol and catecholamines changes as functions of time-of-day and self-reported mood. Neurosci Biobehav Rev 1984; 8:523.

666. Weeke J, et al. The effect of heating and central cooling on serum TSH, GH, and norepinephrine in resting normal man. Acta Physiol Scand 1983; 117:33.

667. Chen M, et al. Plasma catecholamines, dietary carbohydrate, and glucose intolerance: a comparison between young and old men. J Clin Endocrinol Metab 1986; 62:1193.

668. Cryer PE. Phaeochromocytoma. Clin Endocrinol Metab 1985; 14:203.

669. Tietz NW, et al. Laboratory values in fit aging individuals—sexagenarians through centenarians. Clin Chem 1992; 38:1167.

670. Gallagher SK, et al. Short-term and long-term variability of indices related to nutritional status. I: Ca, Cu, Fe, Mg, and Zn. Clin Chem 1989; 35:369.

671. Perrone RD, et al. Serum creatinine as an index of renal function: new insights into old concepts. Clin Chem 1992; 38:1933.

672. Lew SQ, Bosch JP. Effect of diet on creatinine clearance and excretion in young and elderly healthy subjects and in patients with renal disease. J Am Soc Nephrol 1991; 2:856.

673. Saad EA, et al. Peripheral plasma met-enkephalin levels in ovulatory and anovulatory human menstrual cycles. Fertil Steril 1992; 58:307.

674. Mozzanica N, et al. Association between circadian rhythms of endogenous hypothalamic opioid peptides and of natural killer cell activity. Int J Immunopharmacol 1991; 13:317.

675. Lamb E, et al. Serum glycated albumin and fructosamine in renal dialysis patients. Nephron 1993; 64:82.

676. Atkin SH, et al. Fingerstick glucose determination in shock. Ann Intern Med 1991; 114:1020.

677. Weykamp CW, et al. Interference of carbamylated and acetylated hemoglobins in assays of glycohemoglobin by HPLC electrophoresis, affinity chromatography, and enzyme immunoassay. Clin Chem 1993; 39:138.

678. Phillipou G, Phillips PJ. Intraindividual variation of glycohemoglobin: implications for interpretation and analytical goals. Clin Chem 1993; 39:2305.

679. Weykamp CW, et al. Influence of hemoglobin variants and derivatives on glycohemoglobin determinations, as investigated by 102 laboratories using 16 methods. Clin Chem 1993; 39:1717.

680. Kilpatrick ES, et al. Increased fetal hemoglobin in insulin-treated diabetes mellitus contributes to the imprecision of glycohemoglobin measurements. Clin Chem 1993; 39:833.

681. Panteghini M, Pagani F. Biological variation of lactate and pyruvate in blood. Clin Chem 1993; 39:908.

682. Isojarvi JI, et al. Thyroid function with antiepileptic drugs. Epilepsia 1992; 33:142.

683. Cugini P, et al. Vasoactive intestinal peptide fluctuates in human blood with a circadian rhythm. Regul Pept 1991; 34:141.

684. Cugini P, et al. The circadian rhythm of atrial natriuretic peptide, vasoactive intestinal peptide, beta-endorphin and cortisol in healthy young and elderly subjects. Clin Auton Res 1992; 2:113.

685. May RB, Sunder TR. Hematologic manifestations of long-term valproate therapy. Epilepsia 1993; 34:1098.

686. Massoudi MS, et al. Prevalence of thyroid antibodies among healthy middle-aged women. Findings from the thyroid study in healthy women. Ann Epidemiol 1995; 5:229.

687. Engler H, et al. Anti-thyroid peroxidase (anti-TPO) antibodies in thyroid diseases, non-thyroidal illness and controls. Clinical validity of a new commercial method for detection of anti-TPO (thyroid microsomal) autoantibodies. Clin Chim Acta 1994; 225:123.

688. Romaldini JH, et al. Effect of L-thyroxine administration on antithyroid antibody levels, lipid profile, and thyroid volume in patients with Hashimoto's thyroiditis. Thyroid 1996; 6:183.

689. Iles RK, et al. Cross-reaction with luteinizing hormone beta-core is responsible for the age-dependent increase of immunoreactive beta-core fragment of human chorionic gonadotropin in women with nonmalignant conditions. Clin Chem 1999; 45:532.

690. Cole LA. Immunoassay of human chorionic gonadotropin, its free subunits, and metabolites. Clin Chem 1997; 43:2233.

691. Jensen TB, et al. Library of sequence-specific radioimmunoassays for human chromogranin A. Clin Chem 1999; 45:549.

692. Boomsma F, et al. Sensitivity and specificity of a new ELISA method for determination of chromogranin A in the diagnosis of pheochromocytoma and neuroblastoma. Clin Chim Acta 1995; 239:57.

693. Takiyyuddin MA, et al. Chromogranin A in human hypertension. Influence of heredity. Hypertension 1995; 26:213.

694. Canale MP, Bravo EL. Diagnostic specificity of serum chromogranin-A for pheochromocytoma in patients with renal dysfunction. J Clin Endocrinol Metab 1994; 78:1139.

695. Inder WJ, et al. Prolonged exercise increases peripheral plasma ACTH, CRH, and AVP in male athletes. J Appl Physiol 1998; 85:835.

696. Sorem KA, et al. Circulating maternal corticotropin-releasing hormone and gonadotropin-releasing hormone in normal and abnormal pregnancies. Am J Obstet Gynecol 1996; 175:912.

697. Papanicolaou DA, et al. A single midnight serum cortisol measurement distinguishes Cushing's syndrome from pseudo-Cushing states. J Clin Endocrinol Metab 1998; 83:1163.

698. Zaninotto M, et al. A proposal for standardizing urine collections for bone resorption markers measurement. J Clin Lab Anal 1998; 12:145.

699. Aoshima H, et al. Circadian variation of urinary type I collagen crosslinked C-telopeptide and free and peptide-bound forms of pyridinium crosslinks. Bone 1998; 22:73.

700. Ju HS, et al. Comparison of analytical performance and biological variability of three bone resorption assays. Clin Chem 1997; 43:1570.

701. Bollen AM, et al. Circadian variation in urinary excretion of bone collagen cross-links. J Bone Miner Res 1995; 10:1885.

702. Mora S, et al. Urinary markers of bone turnover in healthy children and adolescents: age-related changes and effect of puberty. Calcif Tissue Int 1998; 63:369.

703. Rotblatt MD, Koda-Kimble MA. Review of drug interference with urine glucose tests. Diabetes Care 1987; 10:103.

704. Chance JJ, et al. Technical evaluation of five glucose meters with data management capabilities. Am J Clin Pathol 1999; 111:547.

705. Ubbink JB, et al. Comparison of three different plasma homocysteine assays with gas chromatography-mass spectrometry. Clin Chem 1999; 45:670.

706. Schwaninger M, et al. Elevated plasma concentrations of homocysteine in antiepileptic drug treatment. Epilepsia 1999; 40:345.

707. Mijatovic V, et al. Randomized, double-blind, placebo-controlled study of the effects of raloxifene and conjugated equine estrogen on plasma homocysteine levels in healthy postmenopausal women. Fertil Steril 1998; 70:1085.

708. Wright M, et al. Effect of acute exercise on plasma homocysteine. J Sports Med Phys Fitness 1998; 38:262.

709. Lakshmi AV, Ramalakshmi BA. Effect of pyridoxine or riboflavin supplementation on plasma homocysteine levels in women with oral lesions. Natl Med J India 1998; 11:171.

710. Bonnette RE, et al. Plasma homocyst(e)ine concentrations in pregnant and nonpregnant women with controlled folate intake. Obstet Gynecol 1998; 92:167.

711. Cattaneo M, et al. Tamoxifen reduces plasma homocysteine levels in healthy women. Br J Cancer 1998; 77:2264.

712. Clarke R, et al. Variability and determinants of total homocysteine concentrations in plasma in an elderly population. Clin Chem 1998; 44:102.

713. Nygard O, et al. Coffee consumption and plasma total homocysteine: The Hordaland Homocysteine Study. Am J Clin Nutr 1997; 65:136.

714. Arnadottir M, et al. Hyperhomocysteinemia in cyclosporine-treated renal transplant recipients. Transplantation 1996; 61:509.

715. Cravo ML, et al. Hyperhomocysteinemia in chronic alcoholism: correlation with folate, vitamin B-12, and vitamin B-6 status. Am J Clin Nutr 1996; 63:220.

716. Wouters MG, et al. Plasma homocysteine and menopausal status. Eur J Clin Invest 1995; 25:801.

717. Guttormsen AB, et al. Plasma concentrations of homocysteine and other aminothiol compounds are related to food intake in healthy human subjects. J Nutr 1994; 124:1934.

718. Ubbink JB, et al. The effect of blood sample aging and food consumption on plasma total homocysteine levels. Clin Chim Acta 1992; 207:119.

719. Widjaja A, et al. Within- and between-subject variation in commonly measured anthropometric and biochemical variables. Clin Chem 1999; 45:561.

720. Watt HC, et al. The pattern of maternal serum inhibin-A concentrations in the second trimester of pregnancy. Prenat Diagn 1998; 18:846.

721. Petraglia F, et al. Changes of dimeric inhibin B levels in maternal serum throughout healthy gestation and in women with gestational diseases. J Clin Endocrinol Metab 1997; 82:2991.

722. Yamoto M, et al. Serum levels of inhibin A and inhibin B in women with normal and abnormal luteal function. Obstet Gynecol 1997; 89:773.

723. Watt HC, et al. Maternal serum inhibin-A levels in twin pregnancies: implications for screening for Down's syndrome. Prenat Diagn 1996; 16:927.

724. Wald NJ, et al. Maternal serum inhibin-A in pregnancies with insulin-dependent diabetes mellitus: implications for screening for Down's syndrome. Prenat Diagn 1996; 16:923.

725. Tenover JS, Bremner WJ. Circadian rhythm of serum immunoreactive inhibin in young and elderly men. J Gerontol 1991; 46:M181.

726. Byrd W, et al. Regulation of biologically active dimeric inhibin A and B from infancy to adulthood in the male. J Clin Endocrinol Metab 1998; 83:2849.

727. Welt CK, et al. Female reproductive aging is marked by decreased secretion of dimeric inhibin. J Clin Endocrinol Metab 1999; 84:105.

728. Liberman CS, et al. Circulating iodide concentrations during and after pregnancy. J Clin Endocrinol Metab 1998; 83:3545.

729. Hollowell JG, et al. Iodine nutrition in the United States. Trends and public health implications: iodine excretion data from National Health and Nutrition Examination Surveys I and III (1971–1974 and 1988–1994). J Clin Endocrinol Metab 1998; 83:3401.

730. Siff JE, et al. Usefulness of the total iron binding capacity in the evaluation and treatment of acute iron overdose. Ann Emerg Med 1999; 33:73.

731. Ertl T, et al. Postnatal changes of leptin levels in full-term and preterm neonates: their relation to intrauterine growth, gender and testosterone. Biol Neonate 1999; 75:167.

732. Castracane VD, et al. Serum leptin concentration in women: effect of age, obesity, and estrogen administration. Fertil Steril 1998; 70:472.

733. Kristrom B, et al. Short-term changes in serum leptin levels provide a strong metabolic marker for the growth response to growth hormone treatment in children. Swedish Study Group for Growth Hormone Treatment. J Clin Endocrinol Metab 1998; 83:2735.

734. Johansen KL, et al. Leptin, body composition, and indices of malnutrition in patients on dialysis. J Am Soc Nephrol 1998; 9:1080.

735. Mantzoros CS, et al. Circulating insulin concentrations, smoking, and alcohol intake are important independent predictors of leptin in young healthy men. Obes Res 1998; 6:179.

736. Dubuc GR, et al. Changes of serum leptin and endocrine and metabolic parameters after 7 days of energy restriction in men and women. Metabolism 1998; 47:429.

737. Saad MF, et al. Diurnal and ultradian rhythmicity of plasma leptin: effects of gender and adiposity. J Clin Endocrinol Metab 1998; 83:453.

738. Lenders JW, et al. Plasma metanephrines in the diagnosis of pheochromocytoma. Ann Intern Med 1995; 123:101.

739. Reinartz JJ, et al. Plastic vs glass SST evacuated serum-separator blood-drawing tubes for endocrinologic analytes. Clin Chem 1993; 39:2535.

740. Metcalf PA, et al. Albuminuria in people at least 40 years old: effect of alcohol consumption, regular exercise, and cigarette smoking. Clin Chem 1993; 39:1793.

741. Metcalf PA, et al. Dietary nutrient intakes and slight albuminuria in people at least 40 years old. Clin Chem 1993; 39:2191.

742. Roberts WL, et al. Comparison of four commercial urinary albumin (microalbumin) methods: implications for detecting diabetic nephropathy using random urine specimens. Clin Chim Acta 1998; 273:21.

743. James MA, et al. Microalbuminuria in elderly hypertensives: reproducibility and relation to clinic and ambulatory blood pressure. J Hypertens 1994; 12:309.

744. Taskiran M, et al. Urinary albumin excretion in hospitalized patients with acute myocardial infarction. Prevalence of microalbuminuria and correlation to left ventricle wall thickness. Scand Cardiovasc J 1998; 32:163.

745. Jensen HV, et al. Urinary excretion of albumin and transferrin in lithium maintenance treatment: daily versus alternate-day lithium dosing schedule. Psychopharmacology 1995; 122:317.

746. Myrup B, et al. Effect of low-dose heparin on urinary albumin excretion in insulin-dependent diabetes mellitus. Lancet 1995; 345:421.

747. Collins AC, et al. Storage temperature and differing methods of sample preparation in the measurement of urinary albumin. Diabetologia 1993; 36:993.

748. Yokoyama H, et al. Changes of albumin concentrations in the first morning urine according to age and sex in 2990 healthy children and adults. Diabetes Res Clin Pract 1993; 21:167.

749. Gerber LM, et al. Differences in urinary albumin excretion rate between normotensive and hypertensive, white and nonwhite subjects. Arch Intern Med 1992; 152:373.

750. Shin SJ, et al. The variability of 24-hour, overnight 12-hour, and morning one-hour, urinary albumin excretion in normoalbuminuric and microalbuminuric hospitalized diabetics. Kao Hsiung I Hsueh Ko Hsueh Tsa Chih 1990; 6:511.

751. Slag MF, et al. Free thyroxine levels in critically ill patients. A comparison of currently available assays. JAMA 1981; 246:2702.

752. Oremek GM, Seiffert UB. Physical activity releases prostate-specific antigen (PSA) from the prostate gland into blood and increases serum PSA concentrations. Clin Chem 1996; 42:691.

753. Sasagawa I, et al. Serum levels of total and free prostate specific antigen in men on hemodialysis. J Urol 1998; 160:83.

754. Jung K, et al. Ratio of free-to-total prostate specific antigen in serum cannot distinguish patients with prostate cancer from those with chronic inflammation of the prostate. J Urol 1998; 159:1595.

755. Ornstein DK, et al. The effect of prostate volume, age, total prostate specific antigen level and acute inflammation on the percentage of free serum prostate specific antigen levels in men without clinically detectable prostate cancer. J Urol 1998; 159:1234.

756. Ornstein DK, et al. Biological variation of total, free and percent free serum prostate specific antigen levels in screening volunteers. J Urol 1997; 157:2179.

757. Nixon RG, et al. Variation of free and total prostate-specific antigen levels: the effect on the percent free/total prostate-specific antigen. Arch Pathol Lab Med 1997; 121:385.

758. Woodrum D, et al. Stability of free prostate-specific antigen in serum samples under a variety of sample collection and sample storage conditions. Urology 1996; 48(6A Suppl):33.

759. Deinum J, et al. Improved immunoradiometric assay for plasma renin. Clin Chem 1999; 45:847.

760. Orwoll ES, et al. Collagen N-telopeptide excretion in men: the effects of age and intrasubject variability. J Clin Endocrinol Metab 1998; 83:3930.

761. Gertz BJ, et al. Application of a new serum assay for type I collagen cross-linked N-telopeptides: assessment of diurnal changes in bone turnover with and without alendronate treatment. Calcif Tissue Int 1998; 63:102.

762. Sone T, et al. Urinary excretion of type I collagen crosslinked N-telopeptides in healthy Japanese adults: age- and sex-related changes and reference limits. Bone 1995; 17:335.

763. Aloia JF, et al. Biochemical and hormonal variables in black and white women matched for age and weight. J Lab Clin Med 1998; 132:383.

764. Nahoul K, Roger M. Age-related decline of plasma bioavailable testosterone in adult men. J Steroid Biochem 1990; 35:293.

765. Belgorosky A, et al. Progressive increase in non-sex-hormone-binding globulin-bound testosterone from infancy to late prepuberty in boys. J Clin Endocrinol Metab 1987; 64:482.

766. Winters SJ, et al. The analog free testosterone assay: are the results in men clinically useful? Clin Chem 1998; 44:2178.

767. Rosner W. Errors in the measurement of plasma free testosterone. J Clin Endocrinol Metab 1997; 82:2014.

768. Spencer CA, et al. Serum thyroglobulin autoantibodies: prevalence, influence on serum thyroglobulin measurement, and prognostic significance in patients with differentiated thyroid carcinoma. J Clin Endocrinol Metab 1998; 83:1121.

769. Hawkins RC. Furosemide interference in newer free thyroxine assays. Clin Chem 1998; 44:2550.

770. Wilke TJ. Estimation of free thyroid hormone concentrations in the clinical laboratory. Clin Chem 1986; 32:585.

771. Chopra IJ. Thyroid function in nonthyroidal illnesses. Ann Intern Med 1983; 98:946.

CHAPTER 238

# TECHNIQUES OF LABORATORY TESTING

D. ROBERT DUFOUR

The endocrinologist must be cognizant of the common methods used to measure the concentration of endocrine compounds in blood and/or body fluids. A single substance often can be measured by more than one method. In some laboratories, two or three different methods may be used to measure the same analyte. The choice of method may depend on the time of day at which the specimen is received, because some methods may be easier to perform and, thus, may be used for emergency or near-patient testing. Occasionally, this may lead to differing results, because interfering substances commonly do not react identically to the compound of interest and, thus, do not have the same effect on apparent concentrations. For example, one method for measuring bicarbonate shows a positive interference from salicylate, but salicylate does not affect results obtained with most other methods. If bicarbonate were determined using the former method, either no anion gap or, possibly, a negative anion gap, would be present, which would lead to markedly different interpretations of the patient's condition.

No method is completely free of all interferences or is absolutely specific for the compound of interest. This chapter reviews the most common techniques used in laboratories and their limitations. Methods using nucleic acid measurement are not discussed in this chapter but are covered in Chapter 240. In this chapter, in contrast to their use in Chapter 237, the terms *sensitivity* and *specificity* refer to *analytic sensitivity* (ability to detect a small amount of a substance) and *analytic specificity* (ability to detect a substance in the presence of interfering compounds).

## SPECTROPHOTOMETRY

Spectrophotometry and its variants are used for the majority of simple analyses in the clinical laboratory. A spectrophotometer is an instrument that allows light of a specific wavelength to pass through a solution to a detector. Spectrophotometric techniques rely on a direct linear relationship between the concentration of a substance and the amount of light absorbed when passing through the solution. This relationship, called *Beer's law*, holds true when substances are present in pure form in an aqueous solution. In biologic fluids, the multitude of substances present poses a difficult problem for the analyst. If a substance is strongly colored and is present in high concentration, the amount of light absorbed can be directly measured; this is the technique used for hemoglobin determinations and for bilirubin measurement on some instruments.

For most substances, however, this simple approach does not work, because many compounds in addition to the substance of interest absorb light at the same wavelength. The most common approach to eliminate these interferences is to combine the substance of interest with another compound to give a highly colored reaction product that absorbs light at an order of magnitude greater than that of any interfering substances. For many analytes, such as glucose, calcium, and phosphate, this step is enough to give the measurement adequate specificity. For example, glucose combines with *o*-toluidine to give a product with an intense blue color. The apparent concentration of glucose measured by this reaction is within 10% of the value obtained using

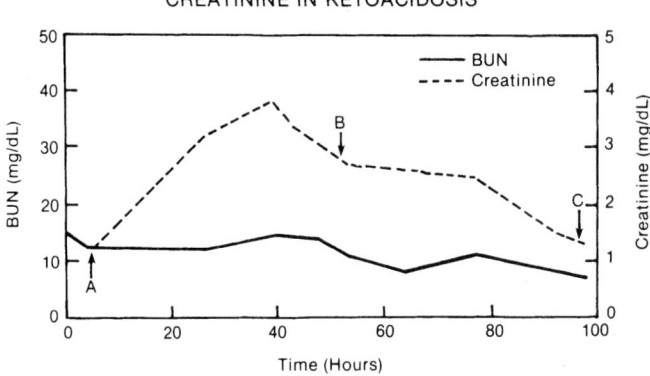

**FIGURE 238-1.** Changes in blood urea nitrogen (*BUN*) and creatinine in a patient with diabetic ketoacidosis. Point A represents the time at which serum ketones began to rise, and point B represents the last time that serum ketones were positive at a dilution of 1:32 or greater. At point C, ketones were no longer detectable. Changes in serum creatinine parallel changes in ketones, but BUN remains virtually unchanged during the entire episode. Because the chemical reaction used in most creatinine assays is nonspecific, ketone bodies produce the same colored product.

the accepted reference method.[1] For other substances, the method is specific enough to use for routine analyses, but some commonly encountered compounds also react. An example of such a reaction is that of creatinine with picrate, the Jaffe reaction, a method used by the great majority of laboratories to measure creatinine.[2] In urine and in most sera, the method provides an accurate approximation of the creatinine concentration. Ketone bodies cross-react in the most commonly used application of this method[3]; in patients with alcoholic or diabetic ketoacidosis, it is not uncommon for the apparent concentration of creatinine to be markedly elevated, leading to a false perception of renal insufficiency (Fig. 238-1). For other substances (e.g., urinary steroid and catecholamine metabolites), a large number of drugs and, for vanillylmandelic acid, food substances, cross-react, so that the interpretation of simple spectrophotometric methods is difficult at best. A number of modifications can increase the specificity of spectrophotometry, allowing its use for measurement of a larger number of compounds.

## ENZYMATIC METHODS

Enzymatic reactions can be used to confer added specificity to chemical reactions. Enzymes are similar to antibodies, in that they have a reactive site which recognizes a specific structural or chemical sequence. Occasionally, other compounds with a similar structure may be cleaved by the enzyme. An example is the cross-reaction of isopropanol, commonly used to prepare the skin for venipuncture, in the measurement of ethanol by alcohol dehydrogenase.[4] In an enzymatic assay, the rate of appearance of a product of the enzyme-catalyzed reaction is directly related to the concentration of the compound of interest, provided all other components of the reaction are present in standardized amounts. The assumption that only the compound of interest is in variable concentration is often not correct, causing erroneous results for some enzymatic measurements. As is discussed later, oxygen is an important variable in the measurement of glucose by glucose oxidase, and changes in the oxygen content of blood can affect measurement of glucose.[5] Most enzyme measurements involve a sequence of reactions, with only the final product being measured. If another substance reacts in one of the steps, or interferes with

one of the reactions, the result will be inaccurate. This is an occasional problem with urine containing large amounts of ascorbic acid, an antioxidant that prevents production of the colored final product used for detecting glucosuria.[6]

## ATOMIC ABSORPTION SPECTROPHOTOMETRY

The most specific spectrophotometric method is atomic absorption spectrophotometry, which uses a lamp containing a strip of the metal being measured. Atomic absorption is both extremely sensitive and specific for the elements that are measured, and is a reference technique for the assay of metals such as calcium and magnesium. It can be used only for metals, limiting its applicability, and the lengthy preparation time limits the number of specimens that can be analyzed. The extremely low concentrations of some trace metals make their measurements very dependent on careful technique to prevent contamination, which can occur from such diverse sources as collection tubes, wooden applicator sticks, and even the glass used in the collection of blood or the preparation of the specimens.[7]

## ELECTROCHEMISTRY

Another common technique is electrochemistry, in which molecules or ions either produce a chemical reaction that generates electrons, or interact with a selective membrane and create a difference in electrical potential. Electrochemical methods are commonly used to measure blood gases and electrolytes. They are highly specific for the substance being measured. To avoid interferences, most sodium electrochemical methods dilute specimens before measurement; thus, they measure the sodium concentration in plasma. The body regulates osmolality, which is related to the sodium concentration in water rather than to the total plasma concentration. In normal individuals, plasma is composed of 93% water and 7% solids (e.g., proteins and lipoproteins). In situations in which protein or lipid comprises a larger percentage of plasma (e.g., in multiple myeloma or severe hypertriglyceridemia), methods that measure the plasma sodium concentration produce falsely low results, termed *pseudohyponatremia*. (This phenomenon is also observed with older flame photometric techniques, which also required specimen dilution.) Some newer instruments, especially those using whole blood measurements (as are commonly found in critical care settings) measure sodium activity (related to the sodium concentration in water) directly without dilution; pseudohyponatremia is not observed with such methods.[8]

## IMMUNOLOGIC METHODS

The use of antibodies as reagents has allowed measurement of many compounds that cannot be assayed by other methods. Antibodies have high specificity in their reactions, minimizing (but not eliminating) cross-reactions. Antibody techniques can detect extremely small concentrations of substances, far below what can be measured with other methods. Detection of a reaction between antigen and antibody is based on labels that are placed on either the antibody or the antigen. Among the more common labels are radioactive isotopes, enzymes, fluorescent compounds, and chemiluminescent molecules.

Two basic forms of assay use antibodies to measure compounds. *Immunoassays* use a small amount of antibody that can bind either labeled antigen (from the reagents) or unlabeled antigen in the specimen. This technique is useful for measuring

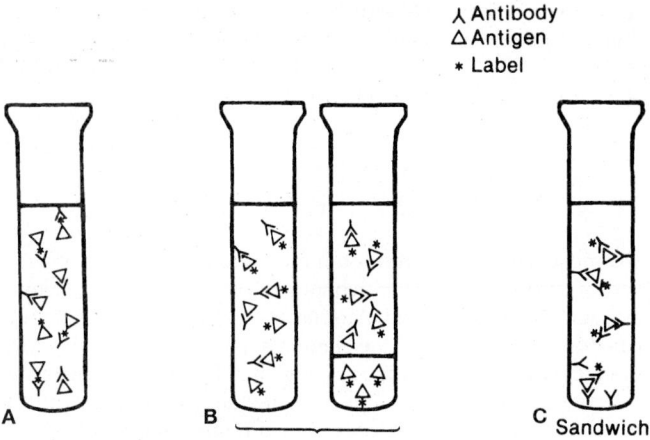

⅄ Antibody
△ Antigen
* Label

**FIGURE 238-2.** The common feature of all *immunoassays* is that a limited amount of labeled antigen competes for antibody binding sites with unlabeled antigen present in the standards or in a patient's serum. **A,** In *homogeneous immunoassays*, the label behaves differently if bound to antibody or if free within solution; therefore, no separation step is necessary, simplifying the measurement. This is the principle of enzyme-multiplied immunoassays and fluorescence polarization inhibition assays, which are the simplest immunoassay techniques to perform. **B,** In *heterogeneous immunoassays*, the remaining free labeled antigen must be separated from that bound to antibody before measurement. This is most often accomplished by precipitating unbound antigen by binding it to a nonspecific absorbent, such as charcoal or a resin. Alternative methods include precipitating antigen–antibody complexes and fixing antigen or antibody to a solid medium, such as the sides of a test tube or small beads. This methodology is typical of radioimmunoassay and fluorescence immunoassay. **C,** Antibody may be labeled instead of labeling the antigen. This is the principle of *immunometric methods*, such as enzyme-linked immunosorbent assay and immunoradiometry. The major advantages are that antibodies are generally easier to label, and sensitivity and specificity can be improved by using two antibodies.

small compounds (such as thyroid and steroid hormones). *Immunometric assays* use antibodies to form "sandwiches" with antigen in the middle. Typically, immunometric assays use two different antibodies that recognize different parts of the molecule, markedly improving specificity. Label is placed on the second antibody; thus, the amount of label bound is directly proportional to the amount of antigen in the sample. This type of assay is used with larger antigens that have more than one antibody-binding site (e.g., peptide hormones). An illustration of these two different principles of immunoassay is given in Figure 238-2.

## IMMUNOASSAYS

The basic principle underlying immunoassays is that a labeled compound competes with unlabeled compound present in the patient's serum for a limited number of binding sites on the antibody molecules. In *radioimmunoassay* (RIA), the label is a radioactive isotope, usually iodine or tritium; however, the label can also be a fluorescent compound (as in *fluorescence immunoassays [FIA]* or *fluorescence polarization inhibition assays [FPIA]*), or an enzyme (as in *enzyme-multiplied immune technique [EMIT]* or *enzyme-linked immunosorbent [ELISA]* assays), or a *chemiluminescent* compound. Generally, chemiluminescent and radioisotopic methods have the highest sensitivity. The higher the concentration of unlabeled compound in the patient's serum, the less labeled compound will bind to the antibody. After an incubation period to allow for equilibrium to be reached, the amount of label attached to the antibody is measured. In many methods, a

separation step is required to remove any residual free labeled compound; such methods are called *heterogeneous*, because they measure label in only one of (at least) two separate specimens. With some labels, the bound and free labeled compounds behave differently, so that no separation step is required; such methods are termed *homogeneous* assays.

## IMMUNOMETRIC ASSAYS

In immunometric assays, typically the first antibody is bound to a solid support. The sample is incubated with the bound antibody; after equilibrium is reached, the solid support is washed. A second, labeled antibody is then added and becomes bound to the solid support only if antigen is bound to the first antibody. After washing, the amount of labeled antibody bound to the solid is measured. Typically, this technique is used for large molecules that have more than one different antigenic site (*epitope*) that can be recognized by antibodies. By using antibodies against two different epitopes, immunometric assays are highly specific and typically show few interferences.

## METHODS OF DEVELOPING ANTIBODY

Antibodies are typically obtained by immunizing animals with the substance of interest. For small molecules, such as drugs, steroid hormones, and thyroid hormones, the molecule often must be attached to another substance (*hapten*) to make it more immunogenic. For larger molecules, immunization with the compound itself is usually adequate to provoke synthesis of antibodies. If serum from the animal injected with the compound is absorbed with human specimens lacking the compound, the antibody can be obtained in relatively pure form. With large molecules, the antibody typically consists of a mixture of antibodies (produced by different plasma cells) against different epitopes on the molecule; such a mixture is termed *polyclonal*. Different animals from the same species may make antibody of differing mixtures that react differently with the molecule of interest. This may cause significant variation in measurements from one lot of immunoassay reagent to the next. This is particularly problematic for molecules that have multiple antigenic sites, such as peptide hormones.[9]

An alternative method to develop antibodies is typically used with mice. After immunizing the mouse, the animal is sacrificed and the spleen is taken to isolate plasma cells. Single plasma cells are fused with myeloma cells to make a new cell line, termed a *hybridoma*, which produces antibody against a single epitope in a reproducible fashion. The hybridomas are grown in tissue culture, and the *monoclonal antibody* produced by each is tested for reactivity against the molecule of interest. Once a hybridoma producing a monoclonal antibody of suitable specificity is identified, a virtually limitless supply can be produced with identical reactivity against the molecule of interest.

Although antibody methods are usually quite accurate, they are prone to several types of interferences and inaccuracies that may cause difficulty in interpreting their results.

## ANTIBODY SPECIFICITY

Although some antibodies are highly specific and can differentiate compounds that vary only in the presence of a single constituent atom (e.g., triiodothyronine [$T_3$] and thyroxine [$T_4$]), many antibodies lack specificity in reactivity. Three common examples are the antibody for cortisol, which cross-reacts with endogenous and exogenous glucocorticoids[10]; the antibody used to detect amphetamine in urine, which cross-reacts with any number of prescription and over-the-counter drugs having a structure similar to amphetamine[11]; and the antibody to digoxin, which cross-reacts with inactive digoxin metabolites and endogenous digoxin-like substances.[12] Such *cross-reactivity* is not typically seen with immunometric assays.

Some patients' sera contain antibodies that react with immunoglobulins from other species. These are termed *heterophile antibodies*. This is most commonly seen in patients who have been treated with monoclonal antibodies (for example, in tumor localization or for treatment of malignancy), such that antibodies develop against mouse proteins.[13,14] These *human antibodies against mouse antibodies (HAMA)* may also be found in those working with laboratory mice and in a small percentage of the general population. HAMAs are a major cause of interference in immunometric assays if they are present in high titers and may cause falsely elevated results by binding the labeled indicator antibody to the solid support. This may affect any substance measured by immunometric assays, including most peptide hormones, tumor markers, and other substances.

Less commonly, *rheumatoid factor* (an autoantibody that reacts with the Fc portion of antibody molecules) may be able to react with immunoglobulins from other species, producing falsely elevated results in immunometric assays.

Finally, *autoantibodies* may be present in serum that compete with the antibody in the reagent for binding to the molecule of interest. Common examples of autoantibodies are *antibodies to thyroglobulin*, a major source of interference in the use of thyroglobulin as a tumor marker[15]; *antiinsulin antibodies* (present in many diabetics) that interfere in insulin assays; and *anti–thyroid hormone antibodies*, which are found in a small percentage of patients with autoimmune thyroid disease.[16] Such autoantibodies typically produce falsely elevated results in immunoassays and falsely low results in immunometric assays.

### ANTIGENICITY VERSUS BIOACTIVITY

Although antibodies detect the presence of an antigen, they indicate nothing about the bioactivity of the antigen being measured. Although this is not likely to pose a problem for small hormones such as $T_4$, it is of considerable importance in the measurement of peptide hormones, which may circulate as large-molecular-weight, and often inactive, prohormones, or which may be cleaved to metabolites that have little or no bioactivity. This problem became apparent early in the development of immunoassays, when it was noted that most patients with lung carcinomas had elevated serum adrenocorticotropic hormone levels but usually had no evidence of adrenal hyperfunction. This is due to the presence of a larger, inactive form of the hormone that cross-reacts in the assay.[17] Other hormones (e.g., calcitonin, insulin, and glucagon) also have inactive precursors in the circulation. The now seldom-used midmolecule assays for parathyroid hormone (PTH) predominantly measure an inactive fragment that accumulates whenever renal function is impaired.[18] Other hormones also may have *inactive metabolites* that lead to overestimation of the amount of active hormone present. Occasionally, with immunometric assays, such circulating inactive fragments may cause *falsely low* results for a hormone. For example, the immunometric assay for intact parathyroid hormone uses a bound antibody that recognizes epitopes in the C-terminal portion of the hormone, whereas the labeled second antibody recognizes epitopes in the N-terminal end of the molecule. In renal failure, high circulating levels of inactive fragments may compete for binding sites with parathyroid hormone, reducing its binding. Because the inactive fragments lack the N-terminal epitope, falsely low PTH values may be seen.[19,20]

## COMPETITIVE PROTEIN BINDING AND RADIORECEPTOR ASSAYS

Two other techniques are similar in principle to radioimmunoassay. Competitive protein binding uses a natural serum carrier protein such as corticosteroid-binding globulin or thyroid-binding globulin, and a labeled hormone that competes for the same binding sites as hormone in the patient's serum. An example is the formerly used Murphy-Patee test for $T_4$. This technique is virtually limited to steroid and thyroid hormones, because most peptide hormones do not have carrier proteins. Competitive protein-binding assays are subject to much the same interferences as are immunoassays; in addition, many are less specific, showing cross-reactions with a larger number of related compounds than is true for immunoassay. Competitive protein-binding techniques are still widely used for measurement of vitamin $B_{12}$ and folic acid, and in preparation for measurement of vitamin D metabolites. In the case of vitamin $B_{12}$, the use of intrinsic factor is necessary to assure that the assay measures only the active vitamin and not a number of inactive related cobalamins.

In radioreceptor assays, the binder is a cellular receptor, either in intact cells or purified in some subcellular fraction. Radioreceptor assays have the theoretical advantage of recognizing only the active part of the hormone, thereby eliminating one of the limitations of immunoassays. Radioreceptor assays can be used for steroid, peptide, and catecholamine classes of hormones. Thus, they virtually have the same applicability as immunoassays. Furthermore, both naturally occurring and synthetic hormones can be measured with radioreceptor techniques. The basic principle is the same as in immunoassay, namely, competition for binding sites between radioactively labeled hormone and unlabeled hormone in the patient's serum. Radioreceptor assays have not found widespread applicability because of their lack of specificity. For example, thyroid-stimulating hormone (TSH), luteinizing hormone, and human chorionic gonadotropin all combine with TSH receptors, and prolactin, growth hormone, and human placental lactogen all bind to cellular prolactin receptors. In addition, the small number of binding sites often reduces sensitivity below what can be achieved with immunoassays.

## ASSAYS FOR FREE HORMONE

Because the free hormone often is the bioactive form and, commonly, protein-bound hormones are an inactive reservoir, a great deal of attention has been paid to the development of assays for free hormone. This has led to a search for other body fluids that might accurately reflect free hormone levels. Salivary hormone levels have been noted to correlate extremely well with free plasma levels for most steroid hormones analyzed. *Salivary hormone concentrations* are independent of the rate of production of saliva and show the same circadian and other rhythmic variations as do plasma hormone concentrations. To date, these assays have not gained wide acceptance, but they likely will become more important in the future. (For more details, see the excellent review in ref. 21.)

## CHROMATOGRAPHY

Chromatographic methods use differences in the solubility of compounds to achieve their separation (Fig. 238-3; Table 238-1). In typical chromatography, a solid support medium is used, usually made of a polar material. Relatively nonpolar liquid is passed over or through the solid support, and compounds separate based on their relative solubility in the stationary or mobile

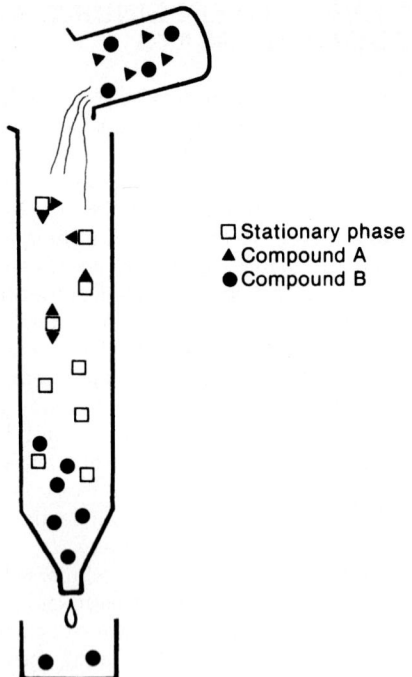

□ Stationary phase
▲ Compound A
● Compound B

**FIGURE 238-3.** In all chromatographic methods, substances are separated based on whether they have a greater affinity for the stationary or the mobile phase. Compound A is similar to the stationary phase in one physical property ("straight sides") and is separated from compound B as the mobile phase passes over the stationary phase.

phases. The time for a compound to be removed from the solid support (eluted) is characteristic for each compound. Variants of chromatography include *reversed-phase chromatography*, in which the stationary phase is nonpolar and the liquid phase is polar; *affinity chromatography*, in which the stationary phase contains chemical sequences that bind only to specific molecules (for example, boronate binds glucose-protein linkages and is used for total glycohemoglobin measurement); and *gas-liquid chromatography*, in which the stationary phase is a liquid and the mobile phase is an inert gas, so that compounds are separated on the basis of their volatility. Chromatographs can be connected to *mass spectrometers*, allowing separated compounds to be identified based on their masses and pattern of fragmentation by electrons.

Chromatography can both separate and quantify structurally related substances. Although such methods are reliable, accurate, specific, and highly sensitive (orders of magnitude more sensitive than immunoassays when coupled to mass spectrographic detectors), they are not commonly used in clinical laboratories because of their relatively high cost per test, the often extensive sample preparation required before analysis, and the small number of specimens that can be analyzed per day. They are commonly used in the measurement of catecholamine and serotonin and their metabolites, steroid hormone metabolites, vitamin D metabolites, and glycated hemoglobins.

## ELECTROPHORESIS

Electrophoretic techniques separate compounds on the basis of differences in their charge density and, particularly with poly-

**TABLE 238-1.**
**Types of Chromatographic Separation**

| Type of Chromatography | Stationary Phase | Mobile Phase | Advantages | Disadvantages | Endocrine Applications |
|---|---|---|---|---|---|
| THIN LAYER | Polar | Nonpolar | Easy to use; little expertise needed; can be used to purify compounds | Limited resolution and limited applications | Amino acids; lecithin/ sphingomyelin ratio |
| COLUMN | Polar | Nonpolar | Easy to use, little expertise needed; may be used as an initial preparation step to eliminate interfering substances | Slow separation, which limits the number of specimens that may be analyzed | Purification steps for vanillylmandelic acid, fractionation of urine androgens |
| AFFINITY | Specific adsorbent | Varies | Can be highly specific for compound of interest, because the binding site recognizes a unique structure | Limited applications; more expensive than simple column chromatography | Glycated hemoglobin |
| ION EXCHANGE | Cation exchange: polyanions Anion exchange: polycations | Varies | Separates compounds based on differences in charge; compounds of charge differing from the type of resin elute most rapidly | Limited applications in clinical laboratories | Glycated hemoglobin |
| MOLECULAR SIEVE | Sephadex resins | Varies | Separates compounds based on differences in size; larger compounds elute most rapidly | Limited applications | Separation of different-sized forms of peptide hormones (e.g., gastrin, glucagon) |
| HIGH-PERFORMANCE LIQUID (HPLC) | Normal: polar Reversed: nonpolar | Nonpolar Polar | Relatively rapid separation; may be automated; can be used to separate most compounds; can separate parent compound and metabolites; can be used to purify compounds; more sensitive than any procedures given earlier | More expensive than first two; requires some degree of experience in performing assays | Catecholamines, catecholamine metabolites, preparatory separation of vitamin D metabolites |
| GAS-LIQUID (GLC) | Liquid adsorbed to inert support | Inert gas | Can resolve substances indistinguishable by other methods; relatively rapid, compared with other chromatographic methods; may be coupled to mass spectrometry for positive identification and sensitivity much greater than other chromatographic methods | Requires high capital outlay and expert technical assistance; compounds must be volatile or able to be made volatile by derivitization | Estrogens, progestogens |

acrylamide gel, also on the basis of molecular weight. The basic technique of electrophoresis involves a usually inert supporting gel on which the sample is applied in the presence of a buffer to control pH. When the sample is placed in an electrical field, any charged compounds migrate, with their distance of migration primarily determined by charge density. After separation of the compounds is complete, a variety of reactive chemicals can be applied to the gel to detect the presence of the compounds of interest. For example, in *protein electrophoresis*, a protein stain is used; for *lipoprotein electrophoresis*, an enzymatic assay measuring cholesterol is used; and in *alkaline phosphatase isoenzyme electrophoresis*, the chemical reaction for measuring alkaline phosphatase in serum is used. Quantification of the amount of each of the separated forms uses a spectrophotometric technique termed *densitometry*, in which the intensity of each separate band of reactivity is measured. Quantification by electrophoresis is not highly accurate or reproducible; when available, more specific methods are typically used.

## BIOASSAY

Although bioassay was one of the first modes of testing used in endocrinology, more easily performed techniques such as immunoassay have almost totally replaced this method. Interest has been renewed, however, in new and highly sensitive in vitro bioassays for hormones. In a typical in vitro bioassay for a hormone-activating adenylate cyclase, the change in cyclic adenosine monophosphate (cAMP) in the cell culture medium is used as an indicator of active hormone concentration. The advantage of bioassays is that they *directly measure active hormone*. In vitro bioassays have been developed for most hormones. An example is a bioassay for PTH using cells from an osteosarcoma. The test for thyroid-stimulating immunoglobulins is, in effect, a bioassay, because the final product measured is cAMP induced by the antibody–TSH receptor interaction. Such assays are not yet commercially available for most hormones but, conceivably, could replace immunoassays after they have been validated by wider use. Their main theoretical advantage is that they should detect only a specific active hormone; however, at least in the case of PTH, PTH-related peptide also binds to the PTH receptor and activates adenylate cyclase.[22,23]

## COMMON INTERFERENCES IN ENDOCRINE TESTING

Although a few specific methodologic interferences have been discussed, for several common tests the endocrinologist must have a clear understanding of the differences between methods of analysis or the reliability of results obtained by specific methods. Although summaries of interferences with different methods are given in Table 237-1, a few of the more common assays that may produce misleading results are given below.

### GLUCOSE

As discussed earlier, most methods for measuring glucose use enzymatic assays. The most widely used of these is the glucose oxidase assay. The chemical reactions for glucose oxidase are shown below.

*SPECTROPHOTOMETRIC METHOD*

$$glucose + O_2 \xrightarrow{glucose\ oxidase} gluconic\ acid + H_2O_2$$

$$H_2O_2 + indicator \rightarrow colored\ reaction\ product$$

*ELECTROCHEMICAL METHOD*

$$glucose + electron\ acceptor\ (+O_2) \xrightarrow{glucose\ oxidase} electrical\ signal\ (+H_2O_2)$$

In serum, the amount of oxygen is trivial and primarily based on the oxygen content of air at the time of measurement; as such, it is constant from one specimen to another. In whole blood, as commonly used in fingerstick glucose measurement, however, the amount of oxygen in the specimen is dependent on the $P_{O_2}$ of the specimen and its hematocrit. With spectrophotometric methods, the amount of the colored reaction product is directly related to both the amount of glucose and the amount of oxygen, whereas with electrochemical methods the amount of the electrical signal is directly related to glucose and inversely related to the oxygen content of blood. In patients tested at home, usually little day-to-day variation exists in either hematocrit or oxygen content of blood, and results are fairly reliable. In hospitalized patients, particularly those critically ill, significant abnormalities of both oxygen content and hematocrit are often present; this frequently causes significant differences in measured glucose between serum specimens and whole blood specimens. Many manufacturers of glucose-testing strips have moved away from using glucose oxidase for this reason. A remaining limitation of whole blood assays for glucose is the difference between water content of whole blood and plasma. As mentioned earlier, plasma is 93% water, whereas whole blood is only ~80% water. The glucose content of whole blood is, thus, lower than that of serum. Manufacturers have calibrated their assays to give results similar to those for serum specimens by putting in a correction factor that is based on presence of a normal hematocrit. In patients with an abnormal hematocrit, the correction factor is erroneous, and glucose results diverge from those of serum. When the hematocrit is high, results are falsely low, whereas anemia causes falsely high results.[24]

## HEMOGLOBIN A$_{1c}$

A number of different methods are used in laboratories to measure glucose attachment to hemoglobin. When glucose attaches to the N-terminal valine on the β chain of hemoglobin A, it produces hemoglobin A$_{1c}$. Other substitutions at the same position produce other variants of hemoglobin A (collectively termed total hemoglobin A$_1$). Glucose can also attach to other amino groups on hemoglobin, particularly lysine residues; all such substitutions produce glycohemoglobin molecules. Normally, hemoglobin A$_{1c}$ represents ~80% of total glycohemoglobin.

Different assays for "hemoglobin A$_{1c}$" measure different modifications of hemoglobin; formerly, results from different assays were not easily compared to each other. The *Glycohemoglobin Standardization Program* has significantly improved agreement between laboratories, making differences in methods less obvious for most diabetic patients.[25] Because some situations exist in which differences between methods do occur, endocrinologists still must be aware of these differences and know the method used by their laboratory.

The most commonly used methods are high-performance, ion-exchange chromatography (HPLC) techniques. Although HPLC methods are generally the most reproducible and were used in the Diabetes Control and Complications Trial, rare situations exist in which results are not reliable. The most common is the lack of hemoglobin A, as occurs most commonly in persons with SS, SC, or CC hemoglobinopathies. Less commonly, congenital variants of hemoglobin (such as hemoglobin Raleigh[26]) have substitutions on the N-terminal valine that lead to a pattern of elution identical to that of hemoglobin A$_{1c}$. Assays for total glycohemoglobin are used by many laboratories, particularly those in smaller hospitals, because of their ease of automation. A mathematical conversion is used to approximate the *true hemoglobin A$_{1c}$* concentration from *total glycohemoglobin* results. The conversion formula appears to underestimate hemoglobin A$_{1c}$ values in patients with poorly controlled diabetes. In situations in which HPLC methods are not useful, total glycohemoglobin assays may still provide clinically useful information. Immunoassays for hemoglobin $A_{1c}$ do not produce inaccurate results in the rare hemoglobin variants with substitutions at the N-terminal valine.[26] Data are inadequate to assess their utility in patients with homozygous hemoglobin variants, but they appear to produce reliable results in patients with heterozygous hemoglobin variants. A few laboratories still use simple ion-exchange chromatography or electrophoretic techniques; these typically measure other hemoglobin $A_1$s, and often give falsely elevated results in patients with high levels of hemoglobin F.

## FREE THYROXINE

Several different methods are used to measure free $T_4$. The accepted reference method is equilibrium dialysis, in which a sample of serum is placed inside a dialysis bag, free $T_4$ is allowed to diffuse out of the bag and establish an equilibrium with the amount inside the bag, and the free $T_4$ concentration on the outside is measured. This technique assumes an equilibrium constant for the binding of thyroid hormone to its binding proteins. If the affinity of binding proteins were reduced, then this technique could overestimate free $T_4$. Free $T_4$ values measured by this technique are significantly higher in patients with acute, nonthyroidal illness than in normal individuals, perhaps reflecting this mechanism. The most widely used free $T_4$ assay involves use of an analog of $T_4$ in an immunoassay. The proprietary analog is said not to bind to thyroid-binding globulin, although evidence suggests that it does bind to albumin. In acute illness, a high percentage of patients have low free $T_4$ results by this assay. An increasing number of laboratories use a technique termed *immune extraction*, in which serum is briefly incubated with an antibody. After washing, labeled $T_4$ is added, and the amount of label bound to the antibody is inversely related to free $T_4$ in the sample. Such methods agree better with equilibrium dialysis results, although elevated levels are virtually never seen in acute illness.[27]

The foregoing are three of the more common examples of how *methodology may cause significant variations in results in patients with different clinical findings.* A more complete listing of such methodologic considerations can be found in Table 237-1.

## REFERENCES

1. Passey RB, Gillum RL, Fuller JB, et al. Evaluation and comparison of 10 glucose methods and the reference method recommended in the proposed product class standard (1974). Clin Chem 1977; 23:131.
2. College of American Pathologists' Comprehensive Chemistry Survey. College of American Pathologist: Northfield, IL 1986.
3. Watkins PJ. The effect of ketone bodies on the determination of creatinine. Clin Chim Acta 1967; 18:191.
4. Vasiliades J. Emergency toxicology: the evaluation of three analytical methods for the determination of misused alcohols. Clin Toxicol 1977; 10:399.
5. Maser RE, Butler MA, DeCherney GS. Use of arterial blood with bedside glucose reflectance meters in an intensive care unit: are they accurate? Crit Care Med 1994; 22:595.
6. Rotblatt MD, Koda-Kimble MA. Review of drug interference with urine glucose tests. Diabetes Care 1987; 10:103.
7. Ericson SP, McHalsky ML, Rabinow BE, et al. Sampling and analysis techniques for monitoring serum for trace elements. Clin Chem 1986; 32:1350.
8. Ladenson JH, Apple FS, Koch DD. Misleading hyponatremia due to hyperlipemia: a method-dependent error. Ann Intern Med 1981; 95:707.
9. Fuentes-Arderiu J, Navarro-Moreno MA. Errors in interpreting hormonal assays. Ann Intern Med 1986; 105:798.
10. Nolan GE, Smith JB, Chavre VJ, Jubiz W. Spurious overestimation of plasma cortisol in patients with chronic renal failure. J Clin Endocrinol Metab 1981; 52:1242.
11. Budd RD. Amphetamine EMIT—structure versus reactivity. Clin Toxicol 1981; 18:91.
12. Soldin SJ. Digoxin—issues and controversies. Clin Chem 1986; 32:5.
13. Boscato LM, Stuart MC. Incidence and specificity of interference in two-site immunoassays. Clin Chem 1986; 32:1491.
14. Kricka LJ. Human anti-animal antibody interferences in immunological assays. Clin Chem 1999; 45:942.
15. Spencer CA, Takeuchi M, Kazarosyan M, et al. Serum thyroglobulin autoantibodies: prevalence, influence on serum thyroglobulin measurement, and prognostic significance in patients with differentiated thyroid carcinoma. J Clin Endocrinol Metab 1998; 83:1121.
16. Despres N, Grant AM. Antibody interference in thyroid assays: a potential for clinical misinformation. Clin Chem 1998; 44:440.
17. Ayvazian LF, Schneider B, Gewirtz G, Yalow RS. Ectopic production of big ACTH in carcinoma of the lung. Its clinical usefulness as a biologic marker. Am Rev Respir Dis 1975; 111:279.
18. Freitag J, Martin KJ, Hruska KA, et al. Impaired parathyroid hormone metabolism in patients with chronic renal failure. N Engl J Med 1978; 298:29.
19. Dilena BA, White GH. Interference with measurement of intact parathyrin in serum from renal dialysis patients. Clin Chem 1989; 35:1543.
20. Blind E, Raue F, Reichel H, Schmidt-Gayk H. Validity of intact plasma parathyrin measurements in chronic renal failure as determined by two-site immunoradiometric assays with N- or C-terminal capture antibodies. Clin Chem 1992; 38:2345.
21. Riad-Fahmy D, Read GF, Walker RF, Griffiths K. Steroids in saliva for assessing endocrine function. Endocr Rev 1982; 3:367.
22. Mundy GR, Ibbotson KJ, D'Souza SM, et al. The hypercalcemia of cancer. Clinical implications and pathogenic mechanisms. N Engl J Med 1984; 310:1718.
23. Merendino JJ Jr, Insogna KL, Milstone LM, et al. A parathyroid hormone-like protein from cultured human keratinocytes. Science 1986; 231:388.
24. Chance JJ, Li DJ, Jones KA, et al. Technical evaluation of five glucose meters with data management capabilities. Am J Clin Pathol 1999; 111:547.
25. Weykamp CW. Effect of calibration on dispersion of glycohemoglobin values determined by 111 laboratories using 21 methods. Clin Chem 1994; 40:136.
26. Chen D, et al. Hemoglobin Raleigh as the cause of a falsely increased hemoglobin $A_{1c}$ in an automated ion exchange HPLC method. Clin Chem 1998; 44:1296.
27. Wong TK, Pekary AE, Hoo GS, et al. Comparison of methods for measuring free thyroxin in nonthyroidal illness. Clin Chem 1992; 38:720.

---

# CHAPTER 239

# EFFECTS OF DRUGS ON ENDOCRINE FUNCTION AND VALUES

MEETA SHARMA

A great number of drugs may *suggest, mimic, or cause disorders of endocrine or metabolic function.* Some of these are negligible and relatively well tolerated; others may be severe or even life-threatening. With some drugs, the disorder occurs rarely; with others, it occurs very frequently.

Moreover, a great number of drugs, although they do not affect endocrine function, *influence the analysis of one or several endocrine-metabolic tests.* This can cause an increase or decrease in the apparent value or may render the test difficult or impossible to perform. Such effects may lead to the erroneous diagnosis of an endocrine-metabolic disorder when none is present or may mask the bona fide presence of such a disorder.

This chapter consists of an extensive alphabetical list of many of the drugs that exert one or several of the previously described effects. Most of the drugs are not hormonal. However, if some hormonal agents exert effects on endocrine function or values other than the purpose for which they are prescribed, they may be listed as well. Note that some of the apparent drug effects are based on clinical or laboratory information that may have been reported in the literature only once or twice, and data may be insufficient to prove causality.

Table 239-1 includes findings that suggest or indicate endocrine-metabolic dysfunction (e.g., gynecomastia caused by spironolactone), effects on laboratory values (e.g., hyperkalemia caused by spironolactone), and/or interferences with a test on an analytical basis (e.g., an increase of urinary 17-hydroxycorticosteroids by a metabolite of spironolactone). Most of the drugs listed have been approved by the Food and Drug Administration. A few, however, are in use only in nations other than the United States. In addition, several agents are included that are only investigational. Although most of the signs and symptoms are endocrine-metabolic in nature, other clinically relevant findings are included to assist the clinician in making the correct diagnosis. Several of the drugs are grouped into chemical categories, but some of the constituent drugs within these categories are listed separately if they have been individually associated with certain reported effects.

Unless otherwise specified, tests are of the blood. Urine tests are specified as "**ur**," analytical effects are specified as "**an**." The analytical effect *often depends on the method used to perform the test*. The term "**exp**" indicates an effect in experimental animals. The term "**inc**" refers to an increase of a laboratory value, and "**dec**" indicates a decrease of a laboratory value.

For references or further information, contact Dr. Meeta Sharma, Washington Hospital Center, 110 Irving St. NW, Washington, DC 20010.

**TABLE 239-1.**
**Alphabetical List of Drugs with Effects on Endocrine Function and Values***

| ABBREVIATIONS | |
|---|---|
| ABG = arterial blood gases | IV = intravenous |
| ACE = angiotensin-converting enzyme | LDH = lactic dehydrogenase |
| ACTH = adrenocorticotropic hormone | LDL = low-density lipoproteins |
| ADH = antidiuretic hormone | LFT = liver function test |
| AIP = acute intermittent porphyria | LH = luteinizing hormone |
| ALB = albumin | NADH = reduced form of nicotinamide-adenine dinucleotide |
| alk = alkaline | NSAID = nonsteroidal antiinflammatory drug |
| an = analytical interference | PP = pancreatic polypeptide |
| ANH = atrial natriuretic hormone | PPG = postprandial glucose |
| BMD = bone mineral density | ppt = precipitation of an effect |
| BMR = basal metabolic rate | PRA = plasma renin activity |
| BPH = benign prostatic hyperplasia | preg = pregnancy |
| BUN = blood urea nitrogen | PSA = prostate-specific antigen |
| cAMP = cyclic adenosine monophosphate | pt = patient |
| CBG = corticosteroid-binding globulin | PTH = parathyroid hormone |
| chol = cholesterol | RBC = red blood cells |
| conc = concentrated | RBF = renal blood flow |
| CPK = creatine phosphokinase | RIA = radioimmunoassay |
| Cr = creatinine | RTA = renal tubular acidosis |
| CRF = chronic renal failure | SHBG = sex hormone–binding globulin |
| CS = corticosteroids | SIADH = syndrome of inappropriate ADH |
| dec = decreased | $T_3$ = triiodothyronine |
| DHEA = dehydroepiandrosterone | $T_4$ = tetraiodothyronine (thyroxine) |
| DHEAS = dehydroepiandrosterone sulfate | TBG = thyroxine-binding globulin |
| DHT = dihydrotestosterone | TBPA = thyroxine-binding prealbumin |
| DI = diabetes insipidus | TC = total cholesterol |
| EDTA = ethylenediaminetetraacetic acid | TFT = thyroid function tests |
| esp = especially | TG = triglycerides |
| ESRD = end-stage renal disease | tot = total |
| exp = experimental in animals | TRH = thyrotropin-releasing hormone |
| FFA = free fatty acids | TSH = thyroid-stimulating hormone |
| FPG = fasting plasma glucose | $TT_4$ = total thyroxine |
| FSH = follicle-stimulating hormone | ur = urine |
| G6PD = glucose-6-phosphate dehydrogenase | vit = vitamin |
| GFR = glomerular filtration rate | VLDL = very-low-density lipoproteins |
| GH = growth hormone | VMA = vanillylmandelic acid |
| GHRH = growth hormone–releasing hormone | vol = volume |
| GIP = gastric inhibitory peptide | w/ = with |
| GT = glucose tolerance | w/o = without |
| GTT = glucose-tolerance test | xs = excess; toxic dose |
| HDL = high-density lipoproteins | $1,25(OH)_2D_3$ = 1,25 dihydroxyvitamin $D_3$ |
| HMG-CoA = 3-hydroxy-3-methylglutaryl coenzyme A | 5-FU = 5-fluorouracil |
| HPA = hypothalamic–pituitary–adrenal axis | 5-HIAA = 5-hydroxyindoleacetic acid |
| HPG = hypothalamic–pituitary–gonadal axis | 11-(OH)CS = 11-hydroxycorticosteroids |
| HVA = homovanillic acid | 17-(OH)CS = 17-hydroxycorticosteroids |
| IGF-I = insulin-like growth factor-I | 17-KGS = 17-ketogenic steroids |
| IL = interleukin | 17-KS = 17-ketosteroids |
| inc = increased | $25-(OH)D_3$ = 25-hydroxyvitamin $D_3$ |
| inc/dec = either increased or decreased | ? = suspected but undocumented effect |
| I/T = intrathecal | |

*The author and editor appreciate the assistance of Roberta L. Brown, Pharm. D., in the verification of the data in this table and other pertinent pharmaceutical information in this textbook.

$\alpha_1$-**ADRENERGIC BLOCKERS:** dec fertility (exp), testicular atrophy (exp).

$\alpha$-**D-GALACTOSIDASE ENZYME:** inc galactose.

$\alpha$-**METHYLDOPA:** dec libido, gynecomastia, breast enlargement, galactorrhea, hyperprolactinemia, failure to ejaculate, dec 5-HIAA (ur), dec PRA, inc Na$^+$, inc BUN, dec GH, inc Cl$^-$, inc alk phosphatase, dec VMA (ur), inc porphyrins (ur), inc coproporphyrin (ur), inc tot metanephrines (ur) (an), inc VMA (ur) (an), inc catecholamines (an), inc catecholamines (ur) (an), inc triglycerides, dec LDL chol, dec HDL chol, dec chol (an), inc apolipoprotein C-III, inc ketones (ur) (an), inc or dec glucose (an), inc creatinine (an), uric acid (ur) (an).

**ACARBOSE:** inc transaminases, inc bilirubin, dec Ca$^{2+}$, dec vit B$_6$.

**ACEBUTOLOL (also see $\beta$-blockers):** dec chol, dec LDL chol, dec FFA, slight dec HDL chol (HDL/chol ratio unchanged), dec GT.

**ACE INHIBITORS:** hyperkalemia, dec angiotensin II, dec aldosterone, inc PRA, sodium and fluid loss, dec ANH, inc prostaglandins synthesis, transient inc in BUN/creatinine, inc bilirubin, inc uric acid, inc glucose, dec glucose.

**ACETAMINOPHEN:** inc alk phosphatase (xs), dec glucose (effect of metabolite), inc 5-HIAA (ur) (an), inc metanephrines (ur) (an), hypoglycemia, jaundice.

**ACETAZOLAMIDE (also see carbonic anhydrase inhibitors):** dec Ca$^{2+}$, inc Ca$^{2+}$ (ur), inc estrogens (ur), dec estrogens (ur) (an), inc glucose (in prediabetics), inc 17-(OH)CS (ur) (an), inc 17-KGS (ur) (an), inc 17-KS (ur) (an), inc Mg$^{2+}$, inc/dec Mg$^{2+}$ (ur), dec PO$_4$$^{3-}$, dec PO$_4$$^{3-}$ (ur), dec K$^+$, inc K$^+$ (ur), inc Na$^+$ (ur), dec pH, inc iodide (ur).

**ACETOHEXAMIDE (also see sulfonylureas):** mild diuresis, inc uric acid (ur), inc alk phosphatase, inc glucose, inc insulin, inc chol.

**ACETOPHENAZINE: (also see phenothiazines):** inc alk phosphatase, inc chol.

**ACETYLSALICYLIC ACID:** inc chol, inc glucose (an), inc triglycerides, dec TT$_4$, inc T$_3$ uptake, inhibits binding of T$_4$ and T$_3$ by TBG and TBPA.

**ACTH:** Cushingoid state (xs), osteoporosis (xs), hyperpigmentation (xs), thin fragile skin (xs), acne (xs), adrenal hemorrhage, sodium and fluid retention, suppression of skin test reactions, menstrual irregularities, suppression of growth in children (xs), hirsutism, dec carbohydrate tolerance, inc insulin requirements/oral hypoglycemics in diabetics, secondary adrenocortical and pituitary unresponsiveness (esp during stress), embryocidal effects, hyperadrenalism in fetus, dec $^{131}$I uptake, inc D IEA, inc DHEAS, inc cortisol, inc estriol (in preg), inc GH, inc 17-(OH)progesterone, inc pregnanediol, hypokalemic alkalosis, inc K$^+$ (ur), inc Ca$^{2+}$ (ur), dec estradiol (ur) (an), dec estriol (ur) (an), dec estrogen (ur) (an).

**ACYCLOVIR:** testicular atrophy (exp), inc BUN, inc creatinine, anuria, edema, anorexia, inc sediment (ur), dec K$^+$, renal failure (xs).

**ADENOSINE:** inc epinephrine, inc norepinephrine, dec spermatogenesis (exp), inc abnormal sperm (exp).

**ALANINE:** inc glucose, inc GH, inc insulin, inc PO$_4$$^{3-}$, dec K$^+$.

**ALBUTEROL (also see sympathomimetics):** mild dec aldosterone, dec Ca$^{2+}$, inc HDL chol, dec CS, dec Mg$^{2+}$, dec PO$_4$$^{3-}$, dec K$^+$, inc PRA, given IV aggravates diabetes and ketoacidosis.

**ALDESLEUKIN (IL-2):** hypothyroidism, inc bilirubin, inc BUN, inc creatinine, inc alk phosphatase, dec Mg$^{2+}$, acidosis, inc/dec Ca$^{2+}$, inc/dec PO$_4$$^{3-}$, inc/dec K$^+$, inc uric acid, dec ALB, dec protein, inc/dec Na$^+$, alkalosis, hypoglycemia, hyperglycemia, dec chol, anorexia, pancreatitis, oliguria, anuria, proteinuria, dysuria, alopecia, fatigue, weight gain, weight loss, malignant hyperthermia.

**ALDOSTERONE:** inc HCO$_3$$^-$, dec Cl$^-$, inc Mg$^{2+}$ (ur), dec K$^+$, inc K$^+$ (ur), dec Na$^+$ (ur), inc CS (an).

**ALENDRONATE:** dec bone turnover, dec osteoclast activity, inc BMD, bone pain, dec Ca$^{2+}$, dec PO$_4$$^{3-}$.

**ALFENTANIL (also see narcotic analgesics):** hypercarbia.

**ALGLUCERASE:** catalyzes hydrolysis of glucocerebroside to glucose and ceramide, improved mineralization in pts w/ type I Gaucher disease.

**ALLOPURINOL:** ppt of gout, cholestatic jaundice, inc alk phosphatase, hepatitis, uremia, alopecia, renal failure, infertility(?), gynecomastia(?), hyperlipidemia(?), salivary gland swelling(?), hypercalcemia(?), impotence, dec libido, albuminuria(?).

**ALPRAZOLAM. See benzodiazepines.**

**ALSEROXYLON. See *Rauwolfia* derivatives.**

**ALTRETAMINE:** inc alk phosphatase, anorexia, fatigue, inc creatinine, inc BUN, alopecia.

**ALUMINUM:** inc aluminum (in renal failure), inc alk phosphatase, dec 1,25(OH)$_2$D$_3$ (in renal failure), dec PTH (in renal failure), dec PO$_4$$^{3-}$ (in renal failure).

**ALUMINUM-MAGNESIUM HYDROXIDE (also see antacids):** aluminum intoxication (in renal failure), osteomalacia (xs), osteoporosis (in uremic pts), dec PO$_4$$^{3-}$, milk-alkali syndrome.

**AMANTADINE:** inc alk phosphatase, anorexia, edema, urinary retention.

**AMIKACIN. See aminoglycosides.**

**AMILORIDE:** dec libido, impotence, polyuria, alopecia, dec Ca$^{2+}$ (ur), inc Mg$^{2+}$, inc K$^+$, dec Na$^+$, dec Cl$^-$, inc BUN, inc aldosterone, inc angiotensin II, natriuresis (at start of therapy), inc PRA, inc uric acid.

**AMINOCAPROIC ACID:** impairment of fertility (exp), kidney concretions (in renal disease), inc CPK, rhabdomyolysis, inc K$^+$ (esp in renal disease), dry ejaculation (in one hemophiliac).

**AMINOGLUTETHIMIDE:** goiter, hypothyroidism, adrenal insufficiency (esp during stress), pseudohermaphroditism in fetus, masculinization and hirsutism in women, precocious sex development in men, inhibits conversion of chol to $\Delta^5$ pregnenolone, dec glucocorticoids, dec mineralocorticoids, dec estrogens, dec androgens, dec Na$^+$, inc alk phosphatase, dec T$_4$ by RIA, inc TSH.

**AMINOGLYCOSIDES:** dec Mg$^{2+}$, dec vit B$_{12}$, dec Ca$^{2+}$, dec Na$^+$, dec K$^+$, inc creatinine, inc BUN, inc casts (ur), dec pH, inc alk phosphatase, inc bilirubin, malabsorption syndrome, alopecia, oliguria, proteinuria, Fanconi-like syndrome.

**AMIODARONE:** hyperthyroidism, hypothyroidism, inhibits peripheral conversion of T$_4$ to T$_3$, thyroid follicular adenoma, thyroid carcinoma, congenital goiter/hypothyroidism/hyperthyroidism in babies of mothers taking amiodarone, dec fertility, dec libido, alopecia, blue discoloration of skin, inc T$_4$ by RIA (most cases), inc/dec TSH response to TRH, inc reverse T$_3$, inc TG, inc/dec chol, inc glucose, inc alk phosphatase.

**AMITRIPTYLINE. See tricyclic antidepressants.**

**AMLODIPINE:** hair loss, polyuria, anorexia, sexual difficulties, nocturia.

**AMOBARBITAL. See barbiturates.**

**AMOXAPINE. See tricyclic antidepressants.**

**AMPHETAMINES:** impotence, anorexia, changes in libido, inc cortisol, inc FFA, dec glucose inc GH, inc HVA (ur), inc epinephrine (ur), inc norepinephrine (ur), inc CS (greatest in evening), reversible inc T$_4$, inc T$_3$.

**AMPHOTERICIN:** dec Na$^+$, inc alk phosphatase (xs), inc chol (an), dec Mg$^{2+}$ (xs), inc/dec K$^+$, inc BUN, nephrocalcinosis, hyposthenuria, RTA.

**AMPICILLIN:** dec urinary excretion of DHEA and DHEAS (in preg), dec estriol (ur), dec 17-KGS (ur), dec 17-KS (ur), dec pregnanediol (ur), dec progesterone.

**AMPICILLIN-SULBACTAM:** inc LDH, inc alk phosphatase, dec ALB, dec tot proteins, inc BUN, inc creatinine, inc hyaline casts (ur).

**AMRINONE LACTATE:** anorexia, dec K$^+$.

**ANABOLIC STEROIDS:** acne, oligospermia, priapism, epididymitis, gynecomastia, testicular atrophy, change in libido, impotence, inc risk of prostatic hypertrophy and prostate cancer (in elderly), more rapid acceleration of epiphyseal maturation than of linear growth (in children), virilization (in women), male pattern baldness (in men), masculinization of female fetus, inc chol/HDL chol ratio, inc LDL chol, dec creatinine, dec glucose, inc PO$_4^{3-}$, inc Na$^+$, inc lean muscle mass (however, muscle tissue may be deficient in PO$_4^{3-}$ and structurally flawed), edema, inc Ca$^{2+}$, inc glucose in diabetics, altered metyrapone test, inc alk phosphatase, dec LH, dec FSH, dec T$_4$, dec TBG, inc T$_3$ resin uptake, dec radioactive iodine uptake, retention of Na$^+$, Cl$^-$, H$_2$O, K$^+$, PO$_4^{3-}$, and Ca$^{2+}$.

**ANDROGENS:** priapism, excessive sexual stimulation, virilization, clitoromegaly, hirsutism, male-pattern baldness, acne, amenorrhea, menstrual irregularities, polycythemia, precipitation of AIP, edema, gynecomastia, male contraception(?), oligospermia and dec ejaculatory vol (xs), virilization of external genitalia of female fetus, acceleration of linear growth rate, advance of bone maturation, prostatic hypertrophy, prostatic carcinoma, inc libido, inc tot Ca$^{2+}$ (in immobilized pts and pts w/ metastatic breast cancer), stimulation of osteolysis, inc acid phosphatase (in women), inc ceruloplasmin, dec LH, dec FSH, dec testosterone, dec free testosterone, dec DHT, dec SHBG, inc 17-KS (ur), dec TBG, dec T$_4$ by RIA, dec T$_3$ by RIA, inc T$_3$ resin uptake, inc TSH, inc uric acid, inc chol, dec TG, retention of N$_2$, Na$^+$, K$^+$, H$_2$O, PO$_4^{3-}$, and Cl$^-$, dec Ca$^{2+}$ (ur), inc protein anabolism, dec protein catabolism.

**ANISINDIONE:** albuminuria.

**ANTACIDS:** Aluminum containing—constipation, aluminum intoxication, osteomalacia, hypophosphatemia. Magnesium-containing—hypermagnesemia in pts w/ renal failure. Magnesium oxide—milk-alkali syndrome. Calcium carbonate—milk-alkali syndrome (xs). Sodium bicarbonate—milk-alkali syndrome (xs). Soluble bismuth salts—milk-alkali syndrome (xs).

**ANTICHOLINERGIC AGENTS:** suppression of lactation, impotence, prostatic hypertrophy, dec PP, difficulty in achieving or maintaining an erection.

**ANTICONVULSANTS:** inc alk phosphatase, inc SHBG, inc apolipoprotein A-I, dec folate, dec vit B$_6$, dec vit B$_{12}$, dec vit E.

**ANTIHISTAMINES:** anorexia, early menses, induced lactation, gynecomastia, inhibition of ejaculation, dec libido, impotence, high or prolonged glucose-tolerance curves, inc glucose (ur), inc chol, excessive perspiration.

**ANTINEOPLASTIC AGENTS:** inc K$^+$, dec hydroxyproline.

**ANTISPASMODICS. See anticholinergic agents.**

**APROBARBITAL. See barbiturates.**

**ARGININE:** When given IV induces pronounced inc in human GH (intact pituitary function).

**ASPARAGINASE:** dec insulin, dec C peptide, hyperglycemia, glycosuria, polyuria, dec FFA, azotemia, proteinuria, inc alk phosphatase, inc bilirubin, dec T$_4$, dec ALB, inc/dec chol (xs), inc/dec tot lipids, edema, malabsorption syndrome, anorexia, pancreatitis, weight loss.

**ASPIRIN (also see salicylates):** dec vit C.

**ATENOLOL. See β-adrenergic blockers.**

**ATORVASTATIN:** impotence, hyperglycemia/hypoglycemia, inc CPK, gout, weight gain.

**ATOVAQUONE:** inc alk phosphatase, inc amylase, dec Na$^+$, hyperglycemia, hypoglycemia, anorexia, inc creatinine.

**ATROPINE (also see anticholinergic agents):** dec gastrin, abolishes cholecystokinin response to meals.

**AZATADINE. See antihistamines.**

**AZATHIOPRINE:** inc uric acid (rapid tissue destruction), dec uric acid (in pts w/ gout), dec uric acid (ur), inc alk phosphatase, dec chol, inc K$^+$, dec sperm count.

**AZITHROMYCIN:** inc CPK, inc K$^+$.

**AZTREONAM:** diaphoresis, hepatitis, jaundice, breast tenderness, vaginitis, inc alk phosphatase, inc creatinine.

**β-ADRENERGIC BLOCKERS:** dec melatonin, dec PRA, sexual dysfunction, blunt premonitory signs and symptoms of acute hypoglycemia, mask signs of hyperthyroidism, inc TG, inc chol, inc LDL chol, inc VLDL chol, dec HDL chol, hypoglycemia, hyperglycemia, interfere w/ GTT, cause unstable diabetes, impotence, dec libido, alopecia, acne, gout.

**BACITRACIN:** albuminuria, cylindruria, azotemia.

**BACLOFEN:** ovarian cysts, weakness, dizziness, lethargy/fatigue, urinary frequency, palpitations, anorexia, taste disorder, enuresis, urinary retention, dysuria, impotence, inability to ejaculate, nocturia, hematuria, rash, pruritus, ankle edema, excessive perspiration, weight gain, inc alk phosphatase, inc glucose, dec appetite (I/T), dehydration (I/T), urinary incontinence (I/T), sluggish bladder (I/T), bladder spasms (I/T), sexual dysfunction (I/T), alopecia (I/T), facial edema (I/T), weight loss (I/T).

**BARBITURATES:** inc metabolism of vit D via enzyme induction, rickets, osteomalacia, skin rashes, oliguria (xs), inc steroid requirements in adrenal insufficiency, inc alk phosphatase (xs), dec BMR, inc CPK (xs), inc creatinine (xs), dec glucose, dec 17-(OH)CS (ur), inc $^{131}$I uptake, inc porphyrins (ur), acute attack of porphyria, inc T$_3$ uptake, dec T$_4$, competes w/ T$_4$ for TBPA, inc testosterone, inc free testosterone, inc DHT.

**BECLOMETHASONE DIPROPIONATE (inhalation):** suppression of HPA function.

**BELLADONNA ANTICHOLINERGICS. See anticholinergic agents.**

**BENAZEPRIL (also see ACE inhibitors):** impotence, dec libido, hyponatremia.

**BENDROFLUMETHIAZIDE (also see thiazide diuretics):** metabolic acidosis (in diabetics), false-negative phentolamine and tyramine tests (an).

**BENZODIAZEPINES:** anorexia, excessive salivation, palpitations, sweating, changes in libido, menstrual irregularities, hair loss, hirsutism, gynecomastia, galactorrhea, inc alk phosphatase.

**BENZQUINAMIDE:** sweating, shivering, flushing, salivation, fatigue, anorexia, inc temperature.

**BENZTHIAZIDE. See thiazide diuretics.**

**BEPRIDIL:** follicular adenomas of thyroid (exp), anorexia, sexual difficulties.

**BETAMETHASONE. See glucocorticoids.**

**BETAXOLOL. See β-adrenergic blockers.**

**BILE ACID SEQUESTRANTS:** inc fecal loss of bile acids, inc chol, inc LDL chol, inc/dec TG, malabsorption of fat-soluble vits (A, D, E, K), hyperchloremic acidosis, osteoporosis, diuresis, anorexia, inc libido, inc phosphorus, inc chloride, dec Na$^+$, dec K$^+$.

**BISMUTH SALTS. See antacids.**

**BISOPROLOL (also see β-adrenergic blockers):** inc uric acid, inc creatinine, inc BUN, inc K$^+$, inc glucose, inc phosphorus.

**BITOLTEROL (also see sympathomimetics):** proteinuria.

**BLEOMYCIN:** hyperpigmentation, hyperkeratosis, alopecia, nail changes, skin tenderness, anorexia, weight loss.

**BRETYLIUM:** dec catecholamines, dec VMA (ur).

**BROMOCRIPTINE:** dec catecholamines, dec VMA (ur), dec prolactin, inc testosterone, dec T$_4$ (in hypothyroid pts), inc alk phosphatase, inc CPK (transient), inc BUN (transient).

**BROMPHENIRAMINE. See antihistamines.**

**BUMETANIDE (also see loop diuretics):** inc alk phosphatase, chloruresis, natriuresis, no effect on GT, premature ejaculation, difficulty maintaining erection.

**BUPRENORPHINE:** fatigue, loss of appetite, sweating, urinary retention, flushing, malaise.

**BUPROPION:** weight loss, weight gain, anorexia, inc appetite, menstrual complaints, impotence, urinary frequency, urinary retention, excessive sweating, inc salivary flow, cutaneous temperature disturbance, palpitations, dec libido, fatigue, edema, alopecia, acne, hirsutism, gynecomastia, glycosuria, jaundice (xs), inc libido, dec sexual function, nocturia, vaginal irritation, testicular swelling, painful erection, retarded ejaculation, dysuria, dyspareunia, painful ejaculation, menopause, ovarian disorder.

**BUSPIRONE HCl:** fatigue, palpitations, sweating, cold intolerance, galactorrhea, thyroid abnormality, anorexia, inc appetite, salivation, urinary frequency, urinary hesitancy, menstrual irregularity, amenorrhea, spotting, dysuria, nocturia, inc/dec libido, delayed ejaculation, impotence, edema, hair loss, acne, thinning of nails, weight gain, weight loss, malaise.

**BUSULFAN:** ovarian suppression, amenorrhea, menopausal symptoms, sterility, azoospermia, testicular atrophy, hyperpigmentation, alopecia, porphyria cutanea tarda, dry and fragile skin, syndrome resembling adrenal insufficiency, gynecomastia, cholestatic jaundice.

**BUTABARBITAL. See barbiturates.**

**BUTORPHANOL:** sweating, lethargy, sensation of heat, impaired urination, palpitations, anorexia, edema.

**BUTYROPHENONE:** inc prolactin.

**CABERGOLINE:** dec prolactin, hot flushes, breast pain, dysmenorrhea, weight loss/weight gain.

**CAFFEINE:** inc chol, inc LDL chol, inc dopamine (ur), inc epinephrine (ur), inc glucose, inc/dec GT, inc 5-HIAA (ur), inc VMA (ur) (an), diuresis, inc uric acid (an), inc catecholamines (acute), inc PRA (acute), inc linoleic acid, severe acidosis in infants (xs).

**CALCIFEDIOL. See vitamin D.**

**CALCITONIN:** dec $PO_4^{3-}$, inc $PO_4^{3-}$ (ur), dec alk phosphatase, dec hydroxyproline (ur), dec bone resorption, dec elevated $Ca^{2+}$ in pts w/ carcinoma, multiple myeloma, and primary hyperparathyroidism, nocturia, inc urinary frequency, mild tetanic symptoms (rare), dec C peptide, inc glucagon, dec GT(?), dec insulin, inc $Mg^{2+}$ (ur), inc $K^+$ (ur), dec prolactin, inc $Na^+$ (ur), inc $Ca^{2+}$ (ur).

**CALCITRIOL. See vitamin D.**

**CALCIUM:** inc calcitonin (if given IV), inc gastrin, hypercalcemia (xs) (and in ESRD), hypercalciuria (xs), inc 11-(OH)CS, dec 17-(OH)CS (ur), inc insulin (newborns), dec $^{131}I$ uptake, dec $Mg^{2+}$ (an), dec $Mg^{2+}$ (ur) (an).

**CALCIUM CARBONATE. See antacids.**

**CALCIUM EDTA:** proteinuria, microscopic hematuria, renal tubular necrosis.

**CAPREOMYCIN:** hypokalemia, inc BUN, abnormal urine sediment, Bartter syndrome (one pt), renal injury, inc creatinine.

**CAPTOPRIL (also see ACE inhibitors):** proteinuria (clears in 6 months), nephrotic syndrome, in diabetic nephropathy may improve proteinuria, false-positive acetone (ur) (an), anorexia, alopecia, impotence, polyuria, hyponatremia, gynecomastia, dec catecholamines, glycosuria.

**CARBAMAZEPINE:** dec tot $Ca^{2+}$, inc Cu, dec DHEAS, dec free $T_4$ index, inc/dec TBG, inc/dec TSH, dec $T_4$, dec free $T_4$, dec $T_3$, dec free $T_3$, dec vasopressin, dec 25-(OH)vit D, dec androstenedione, osteomalacia, inc cortisol (an), inc glucose (ur), inc 11-(OH)CS (an), inc 17-(OH)CS (ur) (an), dec 17-KS (ur) (an), dec $PO_4^{3-}$, false-negative preg tests (ur), inc SHBG, dec $Na^+$, dec testosterone, dec free testosterone, inc BUN, inc ALB (ur), anorexia, jaundice, hepatitis, oliguria, impotence, SIADH.

**CARBIDOPA:** neuroleptic malignant syndrome, dec BUN, dec creatinine, dec uric acid.

**CARBINOXAMINE. See antihistamines.**

**CARBONIC ANHYDRASE INHIBITORS:** dec $HCO_3^-$, inc $Zn^{2+}$ (whole blood), hypokalemia, inc $Na^+$ (ur), inc $K^+$ (ur), inc $HCO_3^-$ (ur), inc $H_2O$ (ur), alkaline diuresis, anorexia, glycosuria, renal calculi, crystalluria, polyuria, phosphaturia, acidosis, dec libido, impotence.

**CARBOPLATIN:** inc alk phosphatase, inc BUN, inc creatinine, inc bilirubin, dec $Mg^{2+}$, dec $Ca^{2+}$, dec $K^+$, dec $Na^+$, alopecia.

**CARMUSTINE:** impaired fertility, progressive azotemia, inc alk phosphatase, inc bilirubin.

**CARTEOLOL. See β-adrenergic blockers.**

**CARVEDILOL:** hyperglycemia, weight gain, gout, inc BUN, hypercholesterolemia, dehydration, hypervolemia.

**CASCARA. See laxatives.**

**CASTOR OIL. See laxatives.**

**CATECHOLAMINES:** inc ANH, inc gastrin, inc lactate.

**CELECOXIB:** weight gain, water retention, inc BUN, hypophosphatemia, inc CPK, inc TC, inc glucose, dec $K^+$, inc alb (ur), renal calculus, breast pain.

**CELLULOSE SODIUM PHOSPHATE:** inc PTH, hyperparathyroid bone disease, dec intestinal $Ca^{2+}$ absorption, hypomagnesiuria, hyperoxaluria, dec $Mg^{2+}$, dec $Cu^{2+}$, dec $Zn^{2+}$, dec $Fe^{2+}$.

**CEPHALOSPORIN:** false-positive glucose (ur) (an), inc protein (ur) (an), inc 17-KS (ur) (an), inc creatinine (an), anorexia, inc alk phosphatase, inc bilirubin, inc LDH, hepatitis, inc BUN (transient), dec creatinine clearance, vaginitis, flushing.

**CHENODEOXYCHOLIC ACID:** dec hepatic synthesis of chol and cholic acid, inc chol, inc LDL chol, dec TG, inc alk phosphatase, inc/dec HDL chol.

**CHLORAL HYDRATE:** ppt of AIP, malaise, ketonuria, jaundice (xs), albuminuria (xs), interferes w/ $CuSO_4$ test for glycosuria, interferes w/ fluorometric tests for urine catecholamines, interferes w/ urine 17-(OH)CS determinations.

**CHLORAMBUCIL:** jaundice, sterility, azoospermia, amenorrhea.

**CHLORAMPHENICOL:** inc alk phosphatase (xs), inc bilirubin (xs), dec glucose(?), inc 17-KS (ur) (an), inc sugar (ur) (an), dec uric acid (an).

**CHLORDIAZEPOXIDE. See benzodiazepines.**

**CHLORMEZANONE:** flushing, edema, inability to void, reversible cholestatic jaundice.

**CHLORPROMAZINE (also see phenothiazines):** inc chol, photosensitization.

**CHLORPROPAMIDE (also see sulfonylureas):** inc/dec chol, dec $Na^+$, disulfiram-like syndrome w/ alcohol, SIADH, treatment of neurogenic DI, inc alk phosphatase, inc ADH (ur), inc $Ca^{2+}$ (an), HDL chol, dec $HDL_3$ chol, dec LDL chol, dec glucose, inc insulin, inc $T_3$ uptake, dec $T_4$, dec free $H_2O$ clearance (ur), dec urobilinogen (ur), inc uroporphyrin (ur), may ppt cutaneous porphyria, dec serum osmolality, inc urine osmolality, water retention, dilutional hyponatremia.

**CHLORPROTHIXENE. See thiothixene.**

**CHLORTHALIDONE. See thiazide diuretics.**

**CHLOROTHIAZIDE (also see thiazide diuretics):** alopecia.

**CHLORZOXAZONE:** urine discoloration, hepatitis.

**CHOLECALCIFEROL. See vitamin D.**

**CHOLESTYRAMINE (also see bile acid sequestrants):** dec folate, dec bile acids, inc $Ca^{2+}$ (ur), dec tot phospholipids, inc $Na^+$, dec tot lipids, dec $T_4$ (dec intestinal absorption of $T_4$), inc/dec TG, inc vit A, dec vit E.

**CHORIONIC GONADOTROPIN:** inc production of gonadal steroids (Leydig cells—androgens; corpus luteum—progesterone), ovarian hyperstimulation, fluid retention, multiple births, dec LH, dec FSH, precocious puberty, gynecomastia.

**CHROMIUM:** inc glucose-tolerance factor needed for activation of insulin-mediated reactions, improved GT.

**CIMETIDINE (also see H$_2$ antagonists):** inc alk phosphatase, inc HDL chol, dec estradiol, inc FSH, inc gastrin, dec glucose, inc HDL$_2$ chol, dec insulin, dec PTH, inc prolactin, dec sperm count, inc/dec testosterone, dec T$_3$, inc reverse T$_3$, inc BUN, inc uric acid, dec vit B$_{12}$ (ur), inc androstenedione, inc creatinine, inc estradiol (in males), antiandrogenic effect, gynecomastia, alopecia (rare), impotence, galactorrhea, inhibits cytochrome, P450 oxidase system.

**CIPROFLOXACIN:** gynecomastia, inc alk phophatase, inc creatinine, inc BUN, crystalluria (rare), inc LDH, inc bilirubin, hematuria, proteinuria, albuminuria, inc amylase, inc uric acid, inc/dec glucose, inc/dec K$^+$, inc TG, inc chol, acidosis, polyuria, renal calculi, anorexia, hyperpigmentation, exacerbation of myasthenia gravis.

**CISAPRIDE:** inc PP, inc cholecystokinin.

**CISPLATIN:** dec Mg$^{2+}$, inc uric acid, dec Ca$^{2+}$, inc Cu$^{2+}$ (ur), dec creatinine clearance, dec K$^+$, dec Na$^+$, inc Na$^+$ (ur), inc BUN, inc Zn$^{2+}$ (ur), dec PO$_4^{3-}$, tetany, SIADH, anorexia.

**CITALOPRAM:** somnolence, ejaculation disorder.

**CITRATE:** dec Mg$^{2+}$ (in transfusions), inc Al$^{3+}$, dec Ca$^{2+}$, dec chol (an), inc glucose (an), dec pH (an), dec PO$_4^{3-}$ (an), inc K$^+$ (ur), dec selenium (an), dec α-tocopherol (an), dec TG (an), inc uric acid, dec uric acid (ur), dec vit A (an), inc urine vol, dec Zn (an).

**CLADRIBINE:** fatigue, diaphoresis, malaise, dec appetite, edema, hyperuricemia.

**CLARITHROMYCIN:** tooth discoloration, inc alk phosphatase, inc LDH, inc BUN.

**CLEMASTINE. See antihistamines.**

**CLINDAMYCIN (also see lincosamides):** anorexia, inc alk phosphatase, inc bilirubin.

**CLOFAZIMINE:** skin pigmentation, acne, anorexia, hepatitis, jaundice, inc glucose, discolored urine/sweat/sputum, bone pain, edema, inc ALB, inc bilirubin, inc K$^+$.

**CLOFIBRATE:** inc or dec alk phosphatase, dec chol, dec LDL chol, dec VLDL chol, inc HDL chol, dec FFA, dec tot lipids, inc apolipoprotein A-I, dec TG, dec VMA (ur) (an), inc CPK, dec glucose, inc/dec GT, dec insulin, inc/dec T$_4$, dec TSH, dec T$_3$ uptake, inc TBG, dec free T$_4$, dec $^{131}$I uptake, alopecia, impotence, dec libido, proteinuria, polyphagia, weight gain, inc perspiration, gynecomastia(?), dec uric acid, inc uric acid (ur).

**CLOMIPHENE:** inc androstenedione, inc DHEA, inc DHEAS, inc DHT, inc estradiol, inc estrogens (ur), inc FSH, inc LH, inc progesterone, inc testosterone, inc free testosterone, inc sperm count, dec chol, inc TBG, inc/dec T$_4$, dec T$_3$, inc TSH, dec free T$_4$ index, induction of ovulation in selected anovulatory women, inc output of pituitary gonadotropins, dec number of available estrogenic receptors, ovarian stimulation, inc multiple pregnancies, vasomotor flushes, abnormal uterine bleeding, breast tenderness, reversible hair loss, abnormal ovarian enlargement, inc mid-cycle ovarian pain, ovarian cyst formation, prolonged luteal phase of menstrual cycle, birth defects.

**CLOMIPRAMINE (also see tricyclic antidepressants):** ejaculatory failure, impotence.

**CLONAZEPAM (also see benzodiazepines):** inc salivation.

**CLONIDINE:** dec catecholamines, dec catecholamines (ur), dec VMA (ur), dec epinephrine (ur), dec norepinephrine (ur), dec aldosterone (ur), dec PRA, inc Na$^+$, inc GH, inc IGF-I (in children w/ GH deficiency), dec cortisol, dec corticotropin, transient inc glucose, weight gain, transient inc CPK (rare), gynecomastia, hair thinning and alopecia, impotence, dec sexual activity, loss of libido, nocturia, anorexia.

**CLOPIDOGREL:** hypercholesterolemia, gout, inc uric acid, menorrhagia.

**CLORAZEPATE. See benzodiazepines.**

**CLOZAPINE:** fatigue, weakness, lethargy, sweating, salivation, anorexia, incontinence, abnormal ejaculation, urinary urgency, urinary frequency, urinary retention, weight gain.

**CODEINE (also see narcotic analgesics):** inc amylase, inc lipase, oliguria, antidiuretic effect, inc LDH, inc protein (ur), inc BUN.

**COLCHICINE:** dec folate, dec vit B$_{12}$, inc alk phosphatase, inc bilirubin, dec chol, inc CS (ur) (an), inc 17-(OH)CS (ur) (an), dec sperm count, loss of hair, reversible azoospermia.

**COLESTIPOL (also see bile acid sequestrants):** dec carotene level, dec chol, dec TBG, inc TSH, dec T$_4$, dec free T$_4$, dec T$_3$, inc T$_3$ uptake, dec CBG, inc/dec TG, inc alk phosphatase.

**COLISTIMETHATE SODIUM:** dec urine output, inc BUN, inc creatinine.

**CORTISONE. See glucocorticoids.**

**CROMOLYN SODIUM:** dec 17-(OH)CS.

**CURARE PREPARATIONS:** inc histamine release, excessive salivation, flushing, respiratory paralysis in myasthenia gravis.

**CYANIDE:** dec alk phosphatase (an), inc protein (an), dec uric acid (an).

**CYCLOBENZAPRINE:** malaise, anorexia, thirst, urinary frequency/retention, hepatitis, jaundice, inc alk phosphatase, sweating, edema, SIADH(?), inc/dec glucose(?), weight changes(?), change in libido(?), alopecia(?), impotence(?), testicular swelling(?), gynecomastia(?), galactorrhea(?), breast enlargement(?).

**CYCLOPHOSPHAMIDE:** dec osmolality, dec Na$^+$, inc ADH, SIADH, inc alk phosphatase, inc bilirubin, inc chol, dec $^{131}$I uptake, inc osmolality (ur), inc LH (in males), dec testosterone, testicular atrophy, inc plasma vol, dec urine vol, interferes w/ oogenesis and spermatogenesis, sterility, amenorrhea, dec estrogen, dec LH (in males), dec FSH (in females), ovarian fibrosis, oligospermia, azoospermia, anorexia, alopecia, pigmentation of skin and nails, renal function impairment, hemorrhagic cystitis.

**CYCLOPROPANE:** inc alk phosphatase, inc bilirubin, inc catecholamines, dec catecholamines (an), inc glucose, dec pH, malignant hyperthermia.

**CYCLOSERINE:** dec vit B$_6$, inc alk phosphatase, inc bilirubin, dec $^{131}$I uptake, renal function impairment, dec vit B$_{12}$, dec folate.

**CYCLOSPORINE:** inc chol, inc LDL chol, inc apolipoprotein B, dec HDL chol, inc TG, dec Mg$^{2+}$, inc Mg$^{2+}$ (ur), dec aldosterone, inc alk phosphatase, inc bilirubin, inc chloride, inc creatinine, dec GFR, dec RBF, inc K$^+$, inc protein (ur), dec PRA, inc BUN, inc uric acid, development of diabetes in kidney transplant pts, preserves B-cell function and may ameliorate newly diagnosed type 1 diabetes, hirsutism, acne, anorexia, gynecomastia, inc glucose, weight loss.

**CYPROHEPTADINE:** inc alk phosphatase, inc amylase, inc bilirubin, dec glucose, antiserotonin effect.

**CYPROTERONE (also see antihistamines):** inc androstenedione, inc/dec chol, dec DHEAS, dec estradiol, dec estrone, dec glucose, dec GT, inc insulin, insulin resistance (when given w/ ethinyl estradiol), inc/dec tot phospholipids, inc TG, dec progesterone, dec sperm count, dec testosterone, dec free testosterone.

**CYTARABINE:** hyperuricemia, acute pancreatitis, bone pain, anorexia, hepatic dysfunction, jaundice, alopecia, renal dysfunction.

**DACARBAZINE:** anorexia, malaise, alopecia, facial flushing, inc BUN, inc creatinine, abnormal LFTs (rare).

**DACTINOMYCIN:** anorexia, hepatitis, alopecia, acne, inc pigmentation of previously irradiated skin, malaise, hypocalcemia, renal toxicity.

**DANAZOL:** inc androstenedione, dec HDL chol, inc LDL chol, inc TG, dec cortisol, inc/dec cortisol (an), inc free cortisol, dec DHEA, inc DHEAS, dec estradiol, dec FSH, dec LH, inc glucagon, dec GT, dec HDL$_2$, dec HDL$_3$, inc 17-KS (ur), inc K$^+$, dec progesterone, inc prolactin, dec SHBG, inc/dec testosterone, inc/dec testosterone (an), inc free testosterone, dec TSH, dec T$_4$, dec T$_4$ (an), dec TBG, inc free T$_4$, dec T$_3$, direct enzymatic inhibition of sex steroid synthesis, competitive inhibition of binding of steroids to their cytoplasmic receptors, fluid retention, dec GT, inc insulin requirements (in diabetics), acne, hirsutism, testicular atrophy, hair loss, changes in libido, carpal tunnel syndrome, virilization, clitoral hypertrophy (in female fetus), labial fusion (in female fetus).

**DANTROLENE SODIUM:** malignant hyperthermia, malaise, anorexia, hepatitis, inc alk phosphatase, inc bilirubin, inc crystals (ur), difficult erection, nocturia, acne, abnormal hair growth.

**DAPSONE:** anorexia, proteinuria, nephrotic syndrome (xs), male infertility, hypoalbuminemia, inc methemoglobin.

**DAUNORUBICIN:** testicular atrophy (exp), hyperuricemia, red discoloration of urine, reversible alopecia.

**DEMECLOCYCLINE (also see tetracycline):** nephrogenic DI.

**DESERIPIDINE. See *Rauwolfia* derivatives.**

**DESICCATED THYROID. See thyroid hormone.**

**DESIPRAMINE (also see tricyclic antidepressants):** inc alk phosphatase, inc bilirubin, inc FFA, inc/dec glucose, inc GH, inc norepinephrine, inc prolactin, dec urine vol, inc ACTH.

**DESLANOSIDE. See digoxin.**

**DEXAMETHASONE (also see glucocorticoids):** dec catecholamines, dec VMA (ur), dec ACTH, dec 17-(OH)CS (ur), inc amylase, dec androsterone (ur), inc Ca$^{2+}$, dec CS, dec CS (ur) (an), dec cortisol, dec DHEA (ur), dec DHEAS, dec β-endorphin, dec estrogens (ur), inc glucose, inc glucose (ur), dec GT, dec 17-KGS (ur), inc 17-KS (ur) (an), negative nitrogen balance, dec K$^+$, inc K$^+$ (ur), dec prolactin, inc SHBG, inc Na$^+$ (ur), dec testosterone, dec T$_4$, dec T$_3$.

**DEXCHLORPHENIRAMINE. See antihistamines.**

**DEXTRAN 40:** dilutional acidosis, hypernatremia (w/ edema), inc glucose (an), dec protein (an).

**DEXTRAN 70. See dextran 40.**

**DEXTROTHYROXINE SODIUM:** dec chol, inc glucose (in diabetics), dec $^{131}$I uptake, dec LDL chol, dec tot lipids, dec β-lipoproteins, dec TG, inc T$_4$, inc T$_4$ (an), hair loss, exophthalmos, lid lag, diuresis, menstrual irregularities, changes in libido.

**DEZOCINE:** sweating, flushing, edema, inc alk phosphatase, urinary frequency, urinary hesitancy, urinary retention.

**DIAZEPAM (also see benzodiazepines):** inc GH, inc TSH, dec T$_3$ uptake, dec T$_4$, inc alk phosphatase, inc bilirubin, positive dopa screening test (ur) (an), inc estradiol, dec glucose (ur) (an), inc 5-HIAA (ur) (an), dec $^{131}$I uptake, inc porphyrins (ur).

**DIAZOXIDE:** inc glucose, dec pancreatic insulin release, inc alk phosphatase, azotemia, dec creatinine clearance, dec NaCl (ur), dec H$_2$O (ur), fluid retention, dec HCO$_3^-$ (ur), inc uric acid, dec uric acid (ur), dec urinary output, nocturia, inc ALB (ur), inc glucose (ur), inc FFA, ketoacidosis, nonketotic hyperosmolar coma, inc I$^-$, dec Cl$^-$ (ur), dec K$^+$ (ur), inc Na$^+$, dec Na$^+$(ur), inc plasma vol, inc PRA, dec cortisol, dec cortisol (ur) (an), dec glucagon-stimulated insulin release, dec libido, inc catecholamines, fetal or neonatal hyperbilirubinemia, altered carbohydrate metabolism in neonates, alopecia and hypertrichosis lanuginosa in infants of mothers taking drugs in last 19–60 days of preg, galactorrhea, gout, lanugo-like hirsutism (on forehead, back, and limbs), loss of scalp hair, advance in bone age.

**DICHLORPHENAMIDE. See carbonic anhydrase inhibitors.**

**DICLOFENAC SODIUM (also see NSAIDs):** inhibition of bone resorption, inc chol, inc glucose (an), inc BUN.

**DIDANOSINE (DDI):** pancreatitis, inc amylase, phenylketonuria, hyperuricemia, anorexia, inc alk phosphatase, inc bilirubin, edema, dec K$^+$, impotence, kidney calculus, nocturia, renal failure, diabetes mellitus (in children), DI (in children).

**DIETHYLSTILBESTROL:** inc tot Ca$^{2+}$, inc bilirubin, inc coproporphyrin (ur), inc CBG, dec estradiol (ur) (an), dec estriol (ur) (an), dec FSH, dec LH, dec GT, inc 17-(OH)CS (ur), inc 6-β(OH)cortisol (ur), inc prolactin, inc SHBG, dec DHT, dec testosterone, dec free testosterone, inc TBG, dec uric acid, inc uric acid (ur), dec vit A.

**DIFLUNISAL (also see salicylates):** anorexia, hepatitis, dysuria, renal dysfunction, light-headedness, pruritus, diaphoresis, fatigue, edema.

**DIGITOXIN. See digoxin.**

**DIGOXIN:** dec DHT, dec testosterone, dec free testosterone, inc estrone, inc estrogens, dec LH, dec PRA, dec Mg$^{2+}$, dec $^{131}$I uptake, inc 17-(OH)CS (ur) (an), 17-KS (ur) (an), dec glucose (ur) (an), anorexia, gynecomastia.

**DIGOXIN IMMUNE FAB:** hypokalemia.

**DIHYDROTACHYSTEROL. See vitamin D.**

**DILTIAZEM:** inc HDL chol, inc PRA, hyperglycemia, inc CPK, inc alk phosphatase, anorexia, polyuria, hair loss, gynecomastia, sexual difficulties, fetal skeletal abnormalities (xs).

**DIMENHYDRINATE:** lassitude, anorexia, palpitations, difficult/painful urination.

**DIMERCAPROL:** salivation, burning sensation in penis (xs).

**DIPHENHYDRAMINE (also see antihistamines):** dec $^{131}$I uptake.

**DISOPYRAMIDE:** hypokalemia, inc chol, inc TG, inc BUN, inc creatinine, hypoglycemia, inc uric acid, inc alk phosphatase, inc lactate, anorexia, impotence, gynecomastia (rare).

**DISULFIRAM:** inc acetone, inc acetoacetate, inc alk phosphatase, inc chol, inc β(OH)butyrate, dec $^{131}$I uptake, dec norepinephrine, dec VMA, impotence.

**DOBUTAMINE:** inc norepinephrine, inc PRA.

**DOCUSATE. See laxatives.**

**DOMPERIDONE:** gynecomastia, inc prolactin, inc TSH.

**DONEPEZIL:** diabetes (rare), goiter (rare), dehydration, gout, dec K$^+$.

**DOPAMINE:** inc catecholamines (ur) (an), inc dopamine (ur), inc epinephrine (ur), inc glucose, inc GH, dec LH, inc norepinephrine, inc K$^+$ (ur), dec prolactin, inc Na$^+$ (ur), dec TSH, dec TSH response to TRH, dec T$_4$, inc uric acid (an), inc urine vol.

**DOXAPRAM:** inc epinephrine, inc BUN, proteinuria.

**DOXAZOSIN (also see α$_1$-adrenergic blockers):** dec chol, dec LDL chol, inc HDL chol, dec VLDL chol, dec triglycerides, inc norepinephrine, inc PRA, gout, dec libido, sexual dysfunction, polyuria, alopecia.

**DOXEPIN. See tricyclic antidepressants.**

**DOXORUBICIN:** hyperuricemia, red discoloration of urine, reversible complete alopecia, hyperpigmentation of nail beds and dermal creases, onycholysis, anorexia, facial flushing.

**DOXYCYCLINE. See tetracycline.**

**DRONABINOL:** dec seminal fluid vol (exp), dec spermatogenesis (exp), palpitations, anorexia, hepatitis, flushing, sweating, urinary retention (xs).

**EDTA:** hypocalcemia, hyperuricemia, dec alk phosphatase, dec ACE (an), dec HCO$_3^-$, dec chol, inc glucose (an), dec glucose (ur), inc BUN, dec K$^+$ (an), inc K$^+$ (ur), inc Na$^+$ (an), inc sugar (ur) (an), dec tot lipids.

**ENALAPRIL (also see ACE inhibitors):** anorexia, alopecia, impotence, glycosuria, hypoglycemia (rare).

**ENCAINIDE:** inc glucose, inc insulin/oral hypoglycemic requirements in diabetics, anorexia.

**EPHEDRINE (also see sympathomimetics):** dec cortisol, inc epinephrine (ur), inc glucose, inc 5-HIAA (ur) (an), dec $^{131}$I uptake.

**EPINEPHRINE (also see sympathomimetics):** inc calcitonin, inc cAMP, inc glucagon, inc glucose, inc dose of insulin/oral hypoglycemics in diabetics, inc thyrotoxic symptoms in hyperthyroid pts, inc BMR, inc catecholamines, inc chol, inc FFA, inc gastrin, dec $Fe^{2+,3+}$, inc lactate, inc lipoproteins, dec $PO_4^{3-}$, inc tot phospholipids, inc/dec $K^+$, dec $Na^+$ (ur), inc TBG, dec tyrosine, inc uric acid, inc VMA (ur), dec urine vol, metabolic acidosis (xs).

**ERGOCALCIFEROL. See vitamin D.**

**ERGONOVINE:** proteinuria, inc BUN, renal damage (xs), inc porphyrins (ur), acute porphyria, inc aminolevulinic acid (ur).

**ERGOT ALKALOIDS:** dec prolactin, inc porphyrins (ur), ppt of acute porphyria, inc BUN, proteinuria (xs).

**ERYTHRITYL TETRANITRATE. See nitrates.**

**ERYTHROMYCIN:** inc alk phosphatase, inc amino acids (ur) (an), inc bilirubin, inc catecholamines (ur) (an), dec chol (xs), dec glucose (xs), dec $^{131}$I uptake, inc 17-(OH)CS (ur) (an), inc 17-KS (ur) (an), dec folate (an).

**ERYTHROPOIETIN:** exacerbation of porphyria (in CRF), hyperkalemia(?) (in CRF).

**ESMOLOL. See β-adrenergics blockers.**

**ESTAZOLAM (also see benzodiazepines):** dec libido, inc/dec appetite, acne, frequent urination, menstrual cramps, urinary hesitancy/urgency, vaginal discharge/itching, hematuria, nocturia, oliguria, penile discharge, urinary incontinence, thirst, swollen breast, thyroid nodule(?), weight gain/loss.

**ESTRAMUSTINE PHOSPHATE SODIUM:** dec GT, worsening of diabetic control, fluid retention, edema, anorexia, thirst, thinning hair, breast tenderness, breast enlargement, inc bilirubin, changes in $Ca^{2+}$ and phosphorus metabolism.

**ESTROGENS:** inc angiotensin II, inc PRA, inc $Ca^{2+}$, dec carotene, inc ceruloplasmin, inc HDL, inc TG, inc phospholipids, dec chol, inc Cu, inc cortisol, inc DHT, dec folate, dec FSH, dec LH, inc glucose, dec GT, worsening of diabetic control(?), inc GH, inc 17-(OH)CS (ur), dec (OH)proline (ur), dec IGF-I, dec 17-KGS (ur), inc $Mg^{2+}$, inc prolactin, inc SHBG, inc $Na^+$, inc testosterone, inc TBG, inc $T_4$, inc $T_3$, dec $T_3$ resin uptake, free $T_4$ unaltered, inc vit A, dec vit C, dec $Zn^{2+}$, dec pregnanediol (ur), dec response to metyrapone tests, hypercalcemia (in breast cancer w/ bone metastases), breakthrough bleeding, spotting, change in menstrual flow, dysmenorrhea, premenstrual syndrome, amenorrhea during and after treatment, chloasma, alopecia, hirsutism, ppt of AIP, changes in libido, mastodynia, fluid retention, edema, protein anabolism, thinning of cervical mucus, inhibition of ovulation, prevention of postpartum breast discomfort, maintenance of tone and elasticity of urogenital structures, shaping of skeleton, conservation of $Ca^{2+}$ and $PO_4^{3-}$, promotion of bone formation.

**ETHACRYNIC ACID (also see loop diuretics):** acute symptomatic hypoglycemia w/ convulsions in uremic pts (xs).

**ETHAMBUTOL:** inc uric acid, inc creatinine, dec creatinine clearance, inc BUN, dec uric acid (ur), ppt of acute gout, anorexia, abnormal liver function.

**ETHCHLORVYNOL (PLACIDYL):** cholestatic jaundice (hypersensitivity).

**ETHIONAMIDE:** hepatitis, worsening of diabetic control, jaundice, acne, alopecia, pellagra-like syndrome, impotence, gynecomastia, menorrhagia.

**ETHOSUXIMIDE. See succinimides.**

**ETHOTOIN. See hydantoins.**

**ETHYL NOREPINEPHRINE. See sympathomimetics.**

**ETIDRONATE:** dec $Ca^{2+}$, inc BUN, inc creatinine, dec bone turnover, dec $PO_4^{3-}$, dec $Mg^{2+}$, dec mineralization of osteoid during bone accretion, focal osteomalacia, inc pain at pagetic sites.

**ETODOLAC. See NSAIDs.**

**ETOPOSIDE. See podophyllotoxin derivatives.**

**FAMCICLOVIR:** dysmenorrhea, inc creatinine, inc lipase.

**FAMOTIDINE (also see $H_2$ antagonists):** alopecia, impotence, loss of libido, anorexia, acne, dec gastric HCl.

**FELODIPINE:** inc PRA, inc aldosterone (ur), inc norepinephrine, polyuria, sexual difficulties, dose-dependent inc in benign Leydig cell tumors and testicular hyperplasia (exp).

**FENCLOFENAC:** dec $T_4$, dec $T_3$, free $T_4$ normal, dec reverse $T_3$, (most potent drug that interferes w/ thyroid hormone binding).

**FENFLURAMINE:** dec blood glucose, inc GT, impotence, polyuria, menstrual upset, hair loss, gynecomastia, inc cortisol (an), inc GH, inc ketones, dec β-lipoproteins, dec TG.

**FENOFIBRATE:** pancreatitis, polyuria, dec libido, inc CPK, inc creatinine, inc BUN, dec uric acid.

**FENOLDOPAM:** dec $K^+$, flushing.

**FENOPROFEN (also see NSAIDs):** inc $T_3$ (an), inc free $T_3$ (an) (Amerlex-MKit), inc creatinine, dec creatinine clearance (ur), inc protein (ur).

**FENTANYL (also see narcotic analgesics):** diaphoresis.

**FILGRASTIM (G-CSF):** inc uric acid (reversible), inc alk phosphatase (reversible), anorexia, worsening of preexisting alopecia, proteinuria (xs), osteoporosis (xs).

**FINASTERIDE:** inhibits 5α-reductase, dec DHT in prostate, liver, skin, inc FSH, inc LH, inc testosterone, improvement in symptoms of BPH, dec PSA, regression in size of enlarged prostate, inc urinary flow, impotence, dec libido, dec vol of ejaculate.

**5-FLUOROURACIL:** inc 5-HIAA (ur), inc TBG, inc $T_4$ by RIA, inc $T_3$, dec $T_3$ resin uptake, inhibition of spermatogonial differentiation (exp), fetal teratogenicity, anorexia, alopecia, inc skin pigmentation, inc alk phosphatase, inc bilirubin.

**FLECAINIDE:** inc alk phosphatase, anorexia, impotence, dec libido, polyuria, alopecia.

**FLUCONAZOLE:** nausea, salivation (xs), urinary incontinence (xs), adrenal insufficiency(?), hepatitis.

**FLUCYTOSINE:** inc alk phosphatase (xs), inc bilirubin (xs), inc creatinine (an), anorexia, jaundice, azotemia, crystalluria, hypoglycemia, hypokalemia.

**FLUDARABINE:** anorexia, malaise, tumor lysis syndrome (hyperuricemia, hyperphosphatemia, hypocalcemia, metabolic acidosis, hyperkalemia, hematuria, urate crystalluria, renal failure), edema, hyperglycemia, proteinuria, osteoporosis.

**FLUDROCORTISONE:** dec aldosterone (ur), inc amylase, inc $HCO_3^-$, inc glucose, dec GT, dec $K^+$, inc $Na^+$, inc renal tubular reabsorption of $Na^+$, inc $K^+$ (ur), inc $H^+$ (ur), dec ACTH, dec adrenal cortical secretion, inc liver glycogen, negative nitrogen balance, edema, hypokalemic alkalosis (xs), weight gain (xs), hemorrhagic pancreatitis (xs).

**FLUMAZENIL:** inc sweating, fatigue, hot flushes, shivering, flushing.

**FLUORIDES:** hypocalcemia (xs), hypoglycemia (xs), delayed hyperkalemia (xs), tetany (xs), dec alk phosphatase, dec chol (an), inc $Na^+$(an), inc BUN, inc uric acid.

**FLUOXETINE HCl:** rash, urticaria, edema, carpal tunnel syndrome, proteinuria, serum sickness, dec appetite, significant weight loss, hyponatremia, SIADH, hypoglycemia, hyperglycemia (after drug discontinuation), fatigue, sweating, pelvic pain, hypothermia, hirsutism, acne, alopecia, skin discoloration, thirst, inc appetite, inc salivation, jaundice, hyperchlorhydria, dec libido, inc libido, hot flushes, palpitations, bone necrosis, painful menstruation, sexual dysfunction, frequent micturition, abnormal ejaculation, amenorrhea, breast pain, dysuria, impotence, fibrocystic breast, menorrhagia, vaginitis, urinary incontinence, dyspareunia, albuminuria, galactorrhea, kidney calculus, polyuria, urolithiasis, vaginal hemorrhage, pyuria, salpingitis, generalized edema, hypothyroidism, weight gain, goiter, gout, hypercholesterolemia, hyperlipemia, hyperthyroidism, dec $K^+$, dehydration.

**FLUOXYMESTERONE. See androgens.**

**FLUPHENAZINE. See phenothiazines.**

**FLURAZEPAM (also see benzodiazepines):** inc bilirubin, inc alk phosphatase.

**FLUTAMIDE:** hot flushes, loss of libido, impotence, gynecomastia, hepatitis, edema, anorexia, inc creatinine, inc bilirubin (xs), breast tenderness, inhibits androgen uptake, inhibits nuclear binding of androgen in target tissues.

**FOLIC ACID:** inc folate (an), dec $^{131}$I uptake.

**FOSCARNET SODIUM:** hypothermia, anorexia, inc amylase, dec $K^+$, dec $Ca^{2+}$, dec $Mg^{2+}$, inc/dec $PO_4^{3-}$, dec $Na^+$, dec weight, inc alk phosphatase, inc BUN, acidosis, cachexia, thirst, hypercalcemia, dehydration, glycosuria, inc CPK, diabetes mellitus, abnormal GT, hypervolemia, hypochloremia, dec protein, acne, alopecia, inc creatinine, dec creatinine clearance, inc ALB (ur), polyuria, ADH disorders, dec gonadotropins, gynecomastia, penile inflammation, perineal pain (in females).

**FOSINOPRIL (also see ACE inhibitors):** dec libido, sexual dysfunction, gout.

**FUROSEMIDE (also see loop diuretics):** renal calcifications in premature infants (if mother taking drug), inc aldosterone, inc angiotensin II, inc ADH, inc PRA, dec $Ca^{2+}$, dec $Cl^-$, inc chol, inc LDL, inc VLDL, inc TG, inc dopamine (ur), inc glucose, dec GT, dec insulin, dec $Mg^{2+}$, inc norepinephrine, inc norepinephrine (ur), inc PTH, inc $PO_4^{3-}$, dec $K^+$, inc prolactin, dec $Na^+$, inc $T_3$ uptake, dec $T_4$, dec $T_3$, inc BUN, dec plasma vol.

**GALLIUM NITRATE:** dec $Ca^{2+}$, dec $Ca^{2+}$ resorption from bone, dec bone turnover, inc BUN, inc creatinine, transient dec $PO_4^{3-}$, dec $HCO_3^-$, dec (OH)proline (ur), dec PTH.

**GANCICLOVIR:** anorexia, alopecia, hematuria, inc creatinine, inc BUN, edema, dec glucose.

**GASTRIN:** dec $Ca^{2+}$, dec ionized $Ca^{2+}$, inc glucagon.

**GEMFIBROZIL:** dec chol, inc HDL, dec LDL, dec VLDL, dec TG, inc apolipoprotein A-I, inc apolipoprotein A-II, inc alk phosphatase, inc CPK, inc glucose, alopecia, dec libido, myopathy, impotence, dec male fertility, weight loss, benign Leydig cell tumors (exp).

**GENTAMICIN (also see aminoglycosides):** pseudotumor cerebri.

**GH:** inc $PO_4^{3-}$, inc $Ca^{2+}$ (ur), inc intestinal $Ca^{2+}$ absorption, retention of $Na^+$ and/or $K^+$, inc tubular reabsorption of $PO_4^{3-}$, inc glucose, glucosuria, linear growth, skeletal growth, inc alk phosphatase, inc cellular protein synthesis, dec $N_2$ excretion (ur), nitrogen retention, dec BUN, impaired GT, inc insulin levels, insulin resistance, dec insulin sensitivity, dec body fat stores, lipid mobilization, inc FFA, inc synthesis of chondroitin $SO_4^{2-}$ and collagen, inc protein, inc (OH)proline (ur), gynecomastia, carpal tunnel syndrome, dec $T_4$, dec TSH response to TRH, hyperthyroidism(?), pseudotumor cerebri, inc GH antibodies, slipped capital epiphyses, acromegaly (xs).

**GLIMEPIRIDE:** hyponatremia, inc release of ADH, augments peripheral action of ADH, hypoglycemia.

**GLIPIZIDE (also see sulfonylureas):** mild diuresis.

**GLUCAGON:** dec $Ca^{2+}$, dec chol, dec dopamine (ur), dec gastrin, inc glucose, inc lipolysis, inc hepatic gluconeogenesis, inc glycogenolysis, inc FFA, dec GT, inc GH, inc insulin, dec TG, dec tot lipids, dec $Mg^{2+}$, inc norepinephrine (ur), inc $K^+$, inc VMA (ur), counteracts severe hypoglycemia in diabetics.

**GLUCOCORTICOIDS:** $Na^+$ and fluid rentention, hypokalemia alkalosis, metabolic alkalosis, thin fragile skin, hirsutism, acne, amenorrhea, postmenopausal bleeding, menstrual irregularities, suppression of growth in children, dec carbohydrate tolerance, inc insulin/sulfonylurea requirements in diabetics, protein catabolism, negative $N_2$ balance, exophthalmos(?), dec motility and number of spermatozoa, Cushing syndrome (xs), osteoporosis (xs), sexual dysfunction (xs), diabetes (xs), dec ACTH, inc ANH, dec $Ca^{2+}$, inc $Ca^{2+}$ (ur), dec $K^+$, inc chol, inc TG, inc glucose, inc glucose (ur), dec GH, inc 17-(OH)CS (ur), dec (OH)proline (ur), inc 17-KGS (ur), dec osteocalcin, inc PTH, dec TBG (high dose), dec TSH (high dose), dec $T_3$, dec $T_4$ (minimal), dec $^{131}$I uptake, dec TSH response to TRH, dec 25-(OH)vit D, inc $Zn^{2+}$.

**GLUTETHIMIDE:** edema, nocturnal diaphoresis, porphyria.

**GLYBURIDE (also see sulfonylureas):** mild diuresis.

**GLYCERIN. See osmotic diuretics.**

**GLYCERIN SUPPOSITORY. See laxatives.**

**GLYCYRRHIZA:** pseudoaldosteronism, dec aldosterone, inc estrogens (ur) (an), inc pH, alkalosis, dec $K^+$, inc $K^+$ (ur), dec PRA, inc BUN, nephropathy (xs).

**GOLD COMPOUNDS:** inc alk phosphatase (xs), inc aminolevulinic acid (ur), inc bilirubin (xs), inc chol, inc coproporphyrin (ur), dec creatinine clearance (ur), proteinuria (xs), inc BUN, alopecia, anorexia, chrysiasis.

**GONADORELIN ACETATE:** inc LH, inc FSH, inc gonadal steroids, induction of ovulation in female w/ hypothalamic amenorrhea, ovarian hyperstimulation, multiple preg.

**GONADOTROPINS:** inc androsterone (ur), inc estrogens (ur), inc etiocholanolone (ur), 17-(OH)CS (ur), inc 17-KS (ur), inc pregnanediol (ur), inc pregnanetriol (ur), inc testosterone, inc testosterone (ur).

**GOSERELIN ACETATE:** hot flushes, sexual dysfunction, dec erections, lethargy, edema, sweating, anorexia, gout, hyperglycemia, inc weight, breast swelling, breast tenderness, inc bone pain (transient), inc testosterone (transient), impairment of fertility (exp), gonadal suppression.

**GRISEOFULVIN:** inc alk phosphatase, inc aminolevulinic acid (ur), inc coproporphyrin (ur), inc porphyrins, ppt of acute porphyria attack, proteinuria (transient), inc creatinine, inc BUN, dec uric acid, dec creatinine clearance (ur), menstrual irregularities.

**GUAIFENESIN:** dec uric acid, inc VMA (ur) (an), inc 5-HIAA (ur) (an).

**GUANABENZ:** natriuresis, dec chol, dec TG, dec norepinephrine, dec PRA, dec apolipoprotein E, inc glucagon, gynecomastia, disturbances of sexual function.

**GUANADREL:** salt and $H_2O$ retention, anorexia, nocturia, impotence, ejaculation disturbances, weight gain or loss.

**GUANETHIDINE:** dec catecholamines (ur), inc epinephrine (ur), dec norepinephrine (ur), dec PRA, inc $Na^+$, $Na^+$ retention, inc VMA (early) (ur), dec VMA (late) (ur), inc BUN, dec glucose, inc GT, inc chloride, antidiabetic activity, hypoglycemia, priapism, inhibition of ejaculation, impotence, scalp hair loss, inc response to tyramine test.

**GUANFACINE:** dec chol, dec TG, dec PRA, dec catecholamines, inc GH, impotence, dec libido, testicular disorder.

**$H_2$ ANTAGONISTS:** dec gastric acid secretion.

**HALAZEPAM. See benzodiazepines.**

**HALOPERIDOL:** inc alk phosphatase, inc bilirubin, dec chol, inc glucose, dec glucose, inc prolactin.

**HALOTHANE:** inc alk phosphatase, positive antimicrosomal antibodies, inc fluoride, inc glucose, inc GH(?), dec testosterone, inc $T_4$, inc free $T_4$ index, inc BUN, inc uric acid.

**HEMIN:** dec aminolevulinic acid (ur), dec uroporphyrinogen (ur), dec porphobilinogen (ur).

**HEPARIN:** dec aldosterone, dec TG, inc FFA, inc $K^+$, dec $Na^+$, inc TSH, dec $T_4$, inc free $T_4$, dec hormone binding to TBG, induced hypoaldosteronism (esp in CRF and diabetes), adrenal hemorrhage leading to acute adrenal insufficiency, ovarian (corpus luteum) hemorrhage, osteoporosis (chronic xs), transient alopecia, priapism. If heparin is 10% of tot vol of a sample for ABG analysis, can cause errors in $HCO_3^-$, base excess, and $CO_2$ pressure; inc/dec $Ca^{2+}$ (an), inc chol (rebound after stopping drug), inc CS (an), inc glucose, dec 5-HIAA, inc/dec insulin (an), inc $PO_4^{3-}$.

**HEROIN:** inc alk phosphatase, inc chol, dec creatinine clearance (ur), inc $K^+$, rhabdomyolysis, proteinuria, inc TBG, inc $T_4$, inc free $T_4$, inc $T_4$ binding to TBG, mild inc $T_3$.

**HISTAMINE** (in vitro diagnostic aid for gastrointestinal function): inc epinephrine, inc GH, inc 17-(OH)CS (ur), inc norepinephrine, inc $K^+$, inc VMA (ur), dec plasma vol, dec urine vol.

**HISTRELIN:** inc LH (acute), inc FSH (acute), inc gonadal steroids (acute), dec LH (chronic), dec FSH (chronic), dec gonadal steroids (chronic), regression of secondary sexual characteristics in children w/ precocious puberty, dec linear growth velocity, dec skeletal maturation, dec testicular steroidogenesis, dec testicular vol, dec estradiol, cessation of menses, hypogonadism (if HPG axis does not reactivate after drug discontinuation), vaginal dryness, metrorrhagia, mastodynia, breast edema, breast discharge, dec breast size, dyspareunia, polyuria, nocturia, glycosuria, libido changes, hot flushes, vaginal bleeding, vaginitis, dysmenorrhea, goiter, hyperlipidemia, acne, alopecia.

**HMG-CoA REDUCTASE INHIBITORS:** inc HDL, dec LDL, dec chol, dec VLDL, dec TG, inc transaminases, inc CPK, myopathy, rhabdomyolysis, inc myoglobin (ur), gynecomastia, loss of libido, erectile dysfunction, alopecia.

**HYDANTOINS (also see phenytoin):** hyperglycemia, dec insulin release, worsening of glucose control in diabetics, ppt of AIP, hepatitis, interference w/ metyrapone and 1-mg dexamethasone tests, gynecomastia, weight gain, edema, goiter, hypothyroidism, dec $T_4$, dec free $T_4$, jaundice (xs), Peyronie disease.

**HYDRALAZINE:** inc aldosterone, inc/dec PRA, inc BUN, inc uric acid (an), inc alk phosphatase, inc $Ca^{2+}$ (an), inc catecholamines (ur) (an), dec chol, inc/dec glucose (an), dec 17-(OH)CS (ur) (an), inc 17-KGS (ur) (an), dec vit $B_6$, anorexia, impotence.

**HYDRAZINES:** inc alk phosphatase (xs), inc bilirubin (xs), dec glucose, potentiate action of insulin in diabetics, dec 5-HIAA (ur), inc tot metanephrines (ur), inc normetanephrine (ur), dec VMA (ur).

**HYDROCHLOROTHIAZIDE (also see thiazide diuretics):** alopecia.

**HYDROCODONE. See narcotic analgesics.**

**HYDROCORTISONE. See glucocorticoids.**

**HYDROFLUMETHIAZIDE. See thiazide diuretics.**

**HYDROMORPHONE. See narcotic analgesics.**

**HYDROXYCHLOROQUINE SULFATE:** retinopathy, alopecia, bleaching of hair, anorexia, weight loss, lassitude, ppt of porphyria.

**HYDROXYUREA:** dec TG (an), inc BUN, inc uric acid, inc creatinine, renal dysfunction, anorexia, alopecia, inc hepatic enzymes.

**HYDROXYZINE:** inc CS (ur) (an), inc 17-(OH)CS (ur) (an), inc 17-KGS (ur) (an).

**IBUPROFEN. See NSAIDs.**

**IDARUBICIN:** hyperuricemia, hair loss, alopecia, testicular atrophy (exp), inhibition of spermiogenesis and sperm maturation (exp).

**IFOSFAMIDE:** hemorrhagic cystitis, alopecia, anorexia, RTA, inc BUN, inc creatinine, metabolic acidosis, inc bilirubin.

**IMIPENEM-CILASTATIN:** hepatitis, inc salivation, palpitations, facial edema, oliguria, anuria, polyuria, acute renal failure, hyperhidrosis, inc alk phosphatase, inc bilirubin, dec $Na^+$, inc $K^+$, inc $Cl^-$, inc BUN, inc creatinine, inc protein (ur), inc casts (ur).

**IMIPRAMINE (also see tricyclic antidepressants):** dec 5-HIAA (ur), inc bilirubin, inc chol, dec $^{131}$I uptake, inc metanephrines (ur) (an), dec VMA (ur).

**IMMUNE SERUMS:** nephrotic syndrome (rare).

**INDAPAMIDE (also see thiazide diuretics):** frequent urination, polyuria.

**INDINAVIR:** nephrolithiasis, inc bilirubin.

**INDOMETHACIN (also see NSAIDs):** dec aldosterone, inc alk phosphatase (xs), inc glucose (rare), inc $K^+$, dec PRA, dec $Na^+$, dec $Na^+$ (ur), inc TSH response to TRH, inc BUN, renal insufficiency, dec uric acid, inc urine vol.

**INOSIPLEX:** inc uric acid, uricosuria.

**INSULIN:** inc ACTH, inc gastrin, inc glucagon, dec $PO_4^{3-}$, dec $K^+$, dec $Ca^{2+}$, dec chol, inc CS, inc cortisol, inc epinephrine, inc norepinephrine, dec FFA, dec glucose, inc GH, dec $Mg^{2+}$, inc prolactin, dec $Na^+$ (ur), inc $T_4$, inc $T_3$, dec reverse $T_3$, inc VMA (ur), hypoglycemia (xs), lipoatrophy, lipohypertrophy, insulin allergy, inc insulin antibodies causing insulin resistance.

**INTERFERON α-2a:** proteinuria, anovulation (exp), menstrual cycle irregularities (exp), fatigue, anorexia, loss of libido, hot flushes, partial alopecia, weight loss, transient impotence, excessive salivation, inc alk phosphatase, inc uric acid, inc BUN, inc creatinine, hypocalcemia, inc fasting glucose, inc phosphorus, fertility impairment (exp), dec estradiol, dec progesterone, edema, aggravation of diabetes mellitus, gynecomastia, virilism, thyroid disorder, bone pain, amenorrhea, leukorrhea, menorrhagia, nocturia, polyuria, acne, frequent micturition.

**INTERFERON α-n3:** dec estradiol, dec progesterone, menstrual irregularities (exp), sweating, malaise, anorexia, thirst, inc salivation, hot flushes, dysuria, inc alk phosphatase, inc bilirubin.

**INTERFERON β-1b:** malaise, generalized edema, pelvic pain, palpitations, inc salivation, pancreatitis, salivary gland enlargement, Cushing syndrome, diabetes, SIADH, inc alk phosphatase, inc BUN, hypercalcemia, glycosuria, hypoglycemia, ketosis, thirst, goiter, inc bilirubin, proteinuria, weight loss, weight gain, sweating, alopecia, dysmenorrhea, menstrual disorder, metrorrhagia, menorrhagia, urinary urgency, breast pain, urinary retention, dec libido, hirsutism, anuria, breast engorgement, gynecomastia, impotence, kidney calculus, nocturia, oliguria, polyuria, urinary incontinence.

**INTERFERON γ-1b:** irregular menstrual cycles (exp), fatigue, weight loss, anorexia, hyponatremia, hyperglycemia, pancreatitis, reversible renal insufficiency.

**IODIDE $^{131}$I (therapeutic):** inc in clinical symptoms of hyperthyroidism, acute thyroid crisis, sialoadenitis, temporary thinning of hair, thyroid destruction, hypothyroidism.

**IODIDES:** inc $Cl^-$ (an), inc chol (an), inc 17-(OH)CS (ur) (an), inc ionized $Ca^{2+}$ (an), dec $^{131}$I uptake, inc TSH, inc $T_4$, dec $T_3$.

**IODINE-CONTAINING PRODUCTS:** overactivity/underactivity of thyroid gland, goiter, thyroid adenoma, myxedema, dec $^{131}$I uptake, inc TSH, fetal goiter w/ or w/o hypothyroidism (in pregnant women), inc acne, hyperkalemia (KI), inc $Cl^-$ (an), inc chol (an), inc 17-(OH)CS (ur) (an), inc ionized $Ca^{2+}$ (an).

**IOPANOIC ACID:** dec $^{131}$I uptake, inc TSH, inc $T_4$, dec $T_3$, dec uric acid, inc uric acid (ur).

**IPODATE (also see iopanoic acid):** inc BUN, inc urobilin (ur).

**IPRATROPIUM:** alopecia.

**IRON DEXTRAN:** hemosiderosis (xs), inc glucose (an), inc protein (ur).

**ISOCARBOXAZID. See monoamine oxidase inhibitors.**

**ISOETHARINE. See sympathomimetics.**

**ISONIAZID:** inc bilirubin, dec pyridoxine, dec folate, pellagra, hyperglycemia, metabolic acidosis, gynecomastia, hypocalcemia/hypophosphatemia due to altered vit D metabolism, inc alk phosphatase, dec chol (xs), dec $^{131}$I uptake, inc ketones (ur), inc sugar (ur) (an), inc uric acid (an), dec 5-HIAA (ur), inc $K^+$.

**ISOPROTERENOL (also see sympathomimetics):** inc catecholamines (ur), inc catecholamines, inc cAMP, dec urine vol, inc epinephrine (ur), inc FFA, inc glucose, inc VMA (ur).

**ISOSORBIDE (also see nitrates):** inc $Cl^-$ (ur), inc $K^+$ (ur), inc $Na^+$, inc $Na^+$ (ur), inc BUN (xs), inc urine vol, inc creatinine clearance.

**ISOSORBIDE DINITRATE. See nitrates.**

**ISOSORBIDE MONONITRATE. See nitrates.**

**ISOTRETINOIN:** inc alk phosphatase, inc apolipoprotein B, inc chol, dec HDL chol, inc LDL chol, inc VLDL chol, inc TG, dec $T_4$, dec free $T_4$, dec $T_3$, worsening of diabetic control, thinning of hair, hirsutism, proteinuria, abnormal menses, inc fasting glucose, inc uric acid, inc CPK, PTH deficiency in fetus.

**ISRADIPINE:** polyuria, sexual difficulties, dose-dependent inc in benign Leydig cell tumors and testicular hyperplasia (exp).

**ITRACONAZOLE:** hepatitis, hypercholesterolemia (exp), nausea, anorexia, edema, fatigue, malaise, dec libido, impotence, gynecomastia, mastalgia (in males), hypokalemia, albuminuria, adrenal insufficiency.

**KANAMYCIN (also see aminoglycosides):** inc granular casts (ur), malabsorption syndrome.

**KETAMINE HCl:** anorexia, hypersalivation.

**KETOCONAZOLE:** dec chol, dec cortisol, dec DHT, dec estradiol, inc FSH, inc 17-(OH)progesterone, inc LH, dec testosterone, dec free testosterone, inc TG, dec $1,25(OH)_2D_3$, dec acid phosphatase (xs), dec free cortisol (ur), dec osmolality, dec $Na^+$, dec sperm count, dec ACTH-induced corticosteroid levels, impotence, gynecomastia, oligospermia.

**KETOPROFEN. See NSAIDs.**

**KETOROLAC. See NSAIDs.**

**LABETALOL (also see β-blockers):** inc/dec aldosterone (ur), inc catecholamines (ur) (an), inc epinephrine (an), inc epinephrine (ur) (an), inc glucose, inc HDL, inc tot metanephrines (ur) (an), inc norepinephrine, inc prolactin, inc/dec PRA, inc TG, transient inc BUN, transient inc creatinine, blocks signs and symptoms of acute hypoglycemia, ejaculation failure, impotence, priapism, reversible alopecia.

**LACTULOSE (also see laxatives):** worsening of diabetic control(?) (syrup contains galactose and lactose).

**LAMIVUDINE:** inc amylase.

**LANSOPRAZOLE:** diabetes mellitus, goiter, glycosuria, hyperglycemia/hypoglycemia, gout, weight loss, albuminuria, kidney calculus, weight gain, hyperlipemia, impotence, abnormal menses.

**LAXATIVES:** In excess most laxatives can cause inc PRA, inc aldosterone, inc $HCO_3^-$, inc pH, dec $Ca^{2+}$, dec $Cl^-$, dec $Na^+$, dec $K^+$, dec protein, steatorrhea, osteomalacia (xs), and vit and mineral deficiencies. Saline laxatives include magnesium sulfate, magnesium hydroxide, magnesium citrate, and sodium phosphate. (In renal failure the latter may cause dec $Ca^{2+}$, inc $PO_4^{3-}$, inc $Na^+$, acidosis.) Irritant/stimulant laxatives include cascara, senna, phenolphthalein, bisacodyl, casanthranol, castor oil. Bulk-producing laxatives include methylcellulose, psyllium, polycarbophil. Lubricant laxative: mineral oil. Surfactant: docusate. Miscellaneous: glycerin suppository, lactulose.

**LEFLUNOMIDE:** alopecia.

**LEUCOVORIN/5-FLUOROURACIL:** alopecia, anorexia.

**LEUPROLIDE ACETATE:** inc pituitary hyperplasia (exp), inc benign pituitary adenoma (exp), dec bone density, suppression of pituitary-gonadal system, dec testicular size, impotence, dec libido, gynecomastia, breast tenderness, hot flushes, sweating, anorexia, bone pain, vaginitis, acne, weight gain, weight loss, testicular pain, diabetes, inc $Ca^{2+}$, alopecia, hair growth, inc uric acid, body odor, accelerated sexual maturity, inc alk phosphatase, inc chol, inc LDL, inc TG, dec HDL, penile swelling, prostatic pain, hypoglycemia, inc BUN, inc creatinine, inc libido, dec protein, thyroid enlargement.

**LEVAMISOLE:** inc copulation period (exp), dec fertility (exp), alopecia, fatigue, renal failure, inc creatinine, inc alk phosphatase, inc bilirubin, anorexia, urinary infection.

**LEVODOPA:** inc ACTH, inc dopamine (ur), dec cortisol, inc insulin, inc C peptide, inc FFA, inc FSH, inc GH, inc HVA (ur), dec 5-HIAA (ur), dec prolactin, dec vit $B_6$, inc alk phosphatase, inc catecholamines (an), inc estrogens (ur) (an), inc/dec glucose, dec 17-(OH)CS (ur), dec $^{131}$I uptake, inc ketones (ur) (an), inc tot metanephrines (ur), inc norepinephrine (ur), dec normetanephrine (ur), dec $K^+$, inc $Na^+$(ur), inc sugar (ur) (an), dec TSH, dec TSH response to TRH in hypothyroidism, inc $T_4$, dec TG, inc/dec BUN, inc/dec uric acid (an), inc/dec VMA (ur), dec VMA (ur) (an), dark sweat/urine, change in weight, priapism, edema, hair loss.

**LEVONORGESTREL:** irregular menstrual bleeding, intermenstrual spotting, amenorrhea, fluid retention, dec insulin sensitivity in diabetics, dec chol, inc LDL chol(?), inc/dec HDL chol, dec TG, dec SHBG, slight dec $T_4$, inc $T_3$ uptake, acne, mastalgia, weight gain, hirsutism, hypertrichosis, scalp hair loss, inc/dec androstenedione, inc apolipoprotein B, dec estradiol, inc glucose, dec $PO_4^{3-}$, inc/dec testosterone.

**LEVORPHANOL. See narcotic analgesics.**

**LEVOTHYROXINE SODIUM. See thyroid hormone.**

**LICORICE:** inc $Na^+$, dec $K^+$, dec aldosterone, dec renin, inc free cortisol (urine).

**LIDOCAINE:** metabolic acidosis (xs), malignant hyperthermic crisis (xs), inc creatinine (an).

**LINCOMYCIN (also see lincosamides):** vaginitis, inc alk phosphatase (xs), inc bilirubin (xs), dec chol (xs), dec folate (an), dec glucose (xs), dec $^{131}$I uptake.

**LINCOSAMIDES:** jaundice, azotemia, oliguria, proteinuria.

**LIOTHYRONINE SODIUM. See thyroid hormone.**

**LIOTRIX. See thyroid hormone.**

**LISINOPRIL (also see ACE inhibitors):** anorexia, impotence, dec libido, gout.

**LITHIUM:** inc aldosterone (ur), inc alk phosphatase (bone isoenzyme), inc ADH, inc $HCO_3^-$ (ur) (on 1st day of therapy), inc $Ca^{2+}$, dec $Ca^{2+}$ (ur), inc chol, dec cortisol, inc creatinine, dec creatinine clearance (ur), inc glucose, dec GT, inc/dec $^{131}$I uptake, inc $Mg^{2+}$, inc $Mg^{2+}$ (ur), dec norepinephrine (ur), dec osmolality (ur), inc PTH, dec $PO_4^{3-}$, inc $K^+$, dec $Na^+$, inc $Na^+$ (ur), dec specific gravity (ur), dec free $T_4$, inc/dec $T_4$ by RIA, dec $T_3$ by RIA, dec $T_3$ resin uptake, dec free $T_4$ index, inc TSH, dec uric acid, inc uric acid (ur), mild inc VMA (ur), inc urine vol, acquired nephrogenic DI, glycosuria, transient hyperglycemia, hypothyroidism, euthyroid goiter, hyperthyroidism (rare), $Na^+$ depletion, thinning of hair, alopecia, impotence, sexual dysfunction.

**LOMUSTINE:** inc alk phosphatase, inc bilirubin, azotemia, alopecia.

**LOOP DIURETICS:** dec $Na^+$, dec $K^+$, dec $Mg^{2+}$, dec $Ca^{2+}$, tetany (xs), hypochloremic alkalosis, dehydration, azotemia, inc BUN, inc Cr, inc $Na^+$ (ur), inc $Mg^{2+}$ (ur), inc $Cl^-$ (ur), inc uric acid, gout (xs), inc glucose, dec GT, ppt of diabetes, inc chol, inc LDL chol, inc TG, slight dec HDL chol.

**LORATADINE (also see antihistamines):** menorrhagia, dysmenorrhea.

**LORAZEPAM. See benzodiazepines.**

**LOSARTAN:** hyperkalemia, inc BUN, inc Cr, gout, impotence.

**LOVASTATIN (also see HMG-CoA reductase inhibitors):** inc alk phosphatase, abnormalities in TFTs, testicular atrophy, dec spermatogenesis (exp).

**LOXAPINE:** inc prolactin, galactorrhea, amenorrhea, impotence, false-positive preg tests, neuroleptic malignant syndrome, gynecomastia, inc LFTs.

**LYMPHOCYTE IMMUNE GLOBULIN:** hyperglycemia (in renal transplantation), inc alk phosphatase (in aplastic anemia), edema, hepatitis, abnormal renal function tests.

**MAGNESIUM-CONTAINING DRUGS:** hypermagnesemia (xs) (and in renal disease), inc $Ca^{2+}$ (an), inc alk phosphatase (an), dec ACE.

**MANNITOL (also see osmotic diuretics):** inc osmolality, inc $Ca^{2+}$ (ur), dec $Cl^-$, dec $PO_4^{3-}$ (an), inc $K^+$, inc/dec $Na^+$, inc $Na^+$ (ur), dec uric acid, inc uric acid (ur), acidosis, marked diuresis, edema, urinary retention, dry mouth, thirst, dehydration.

**MAZINDOL:** dec glucose, testicular pain, polyuria, impotence, menstrual upset, gynecomastia.

**MECAMYLAMINE:** anorexia, dec libido, impotence, inc uric acid.

**MECHLORETHAMINE:** anorexia, delayed menses, oligomenorrhea, amenorrhea, impaired spermatogenesis, azoospermia, tot germinal aplasia.

**MECLIZINE:** anorexia, urinary frequency, difficult urination, urinary retention, palpitations, cholestatic jaundice (cyclizine).

**MECLOFENAMATE. See NSAIDs.**

**MEDROXYPROGESTERONE:** fluid retention, inc glucose, dec GT (esp in diabetics), inc insulin, dec progesterone, dec estradiol, dec pregnanediol (ur), dec testosterone, dec cortisol, dec gonadotropins, dec 17-(OH)CS (ur), dec SHBG, inc $Mg^{2+}$, inc $PO_4^{3-}$, may dec $T_3$ uptake, inc/dec chol, inc/dec TG, inc/dec LDL chol, inc/dec HDL chol, prolonged contraceptive effect, hirsutism, sensation of preg, lack of return of fertility, changes in breast size, breast lumps, nipple bleeding, prevention of lactation, irregular menstrual bleeding, spotting, heavy menstruation, amenorrhea, dec libido, anorgasmia, acne, pelvic pain, mastalgia, alopecia, bloating, hot flushes, galactorrhea, melasma, chloasma, dyspareunia, inc libido, inc bone loss initially, risk factor for osteoporosis(?).

**MEFENAMIC ACID (also see NSAIDs):** inc bile (ur) (an).

**MEFLOQUINE:** hair loss, telogen effluvium, loss of appetite, fatigue.

**MEGESTROL:** dec 11-deoxycortisol (in breast cancer), dec estradiol, dec FSH, dec LH, dec glucose, inc insulin, inc prolactin, dec SHBG, weight gain, inc appetite, fluid retention, nausea, vomiting, edema, breakthrough bleeding, galactorrhea, tumor flare (w/ or w/o hypercalcemia), hyperglycemia, alopecia, carpal tunnel syndrome, rash.

**MELPHALAN:** inc bilirubin (xs), inc 5-HIAA (ur), inc BUN (xs), nausea, vomiting, anorexia, skin ulceration, skin necrosis (at injury site), oral ulceration.

**MENOTROPINS:** ovarian follicular growth/maturation, abnormal ovarian enlargement (xs), hyperstimulation syndrome (xs), multiple births.

**MEPERIDINE (also see narcotic analgesics):** inc creatinine kinase, inc glucose, inc histamine, dec ACTH, dec 17-(OH)CS (ur), dec 17-KS (ur), inc LDH, inc lipase, inc amylase, inc $PCO_2$, dec $PO_2$, dec urine vol, inc ADH, sweating, nausea, anorexia, taste alterations, facial flushing, urinary retention or hesitancy, oliguria, antidiuretic effect, dec libido, dec potency, edema, interference w/ thermal regulation, pruritus.

**MEPHENYTOIN. See hydantoins.**

**MEPHOBARBITAL. See barbiturates.**

**MEPROBAMATE:** inc alk phosphatase (xs), inc aminolevulinic acid (ur), ppt of acute porphyria, inc bilirubin (xs), inc chol (xs), inc estrogens (ur) (an), inc 17-(OH)CS (ur) (an), inc/dec 17-KGS (ur) (an), inc/dec 17-KS (ur) (an), inc porphyrins (ur), urticaria, stomatitis, hyperpyrexia, oliguria.

**MERCAPTOPURINE:** inc alk phosphatase (xs), inc bilirubin (xs), inc glucose (an), inc uric acid (ur), hyperuricemia, pancreatitis.

**MERCURY COMPOUNDS:** dec $HCO_3^-$ (xs), dec $Ca^{2+}$ (xs), red urine, inc glucose (ur), Fanconi syndrome (xs), dec $Mg^{2+}$, dec pH (xs), inc $PO_4^{3-}$ (ur), dec $K^+$ (xs), dec protein, albuminuria, dec $Na^+$ (xs), dec BUN (an), dec uric acid (xs), inc uric acid (ur) (xs).

**MESALAMINE:** acne, dysmenorrhea, menorrhagia, hair loss, anorexia, inc appetite, inc alk phosphatase, inc BUN, inc Cr.

**MESCALINE:** inc free fatty acids.

**MESNA:** inc ketones (ur) (an), bad taste, fatigue, nausea, vomiting.

**MESORIDAZINE. See phenothiazines.**

**METAPROTERENOL. See sympathomimetics.**

**METARAMINOL:** metabolic acidosis (xs).

**METFORMIN:** dec $HCO_3^-$, lactic acidosis (xs), dec carotene, inc formiminoglutamic acid (ur), dec TG, dec vit $B_{12}$, megaloblastic anemia (xs), dec xylose (ur).

**METHACHOLINE:** inc amylase, inc bilirubin, inc lipase, inc norepinephrine (ur), itching, nausea, vomiting, worsening of thyrotoxicosis.

**METHACYCLINE. See tetracycline.**

**METHADONE (also see narcotic analgesics):** inc cortisol, false-positive preg tests (an), inc $T_4$, inc TBG, dec free $T_4$, inc $T_3$, inc $PCO_2$, nausea, anorexia, urinary retention, oliguria, antidiuretic effect, dec libido, dec potency, interference w/ thermal regulation.

**METHANOL:** inc acetone (ur) (xs), inc amylase (xs), dec $HCO_3^-$ (xs), acidosis (xs), dec ionized $Ca^{2+}$ (an), inc ketones (xs), proteinuria (xs), inc BUN (xs), inc uric acid (xs).

**METHAZOLAMIDE. See carbonic anhydrase inhibitors.**

**METHDILAZINE. See antihistamines.**

**METHENAMINE:** inc catecholamines (an), crystalluria, inc/dec estrogens (ur) (an), inc 17-(OH)CS (ur) (an), dec 5-HIAA (ur) (an), dec $^{131}I$ uptake, dec urine pH, proteinuria (xs), inc sugar (ur) (an), inc urobilinogen (ur)(an), inc VMA (ur) (an), nausea, stomatitis, anorexia, dysuria, hematuria, frequency, urgency, pruritus, urticaria.

**METHERGOLINE:** dec TSH.

**METHICILLIN:** dec $HCO_3^-$ (xs), dec $Ca^{2+}$(?), inc 17-KS (ur) (an), inc $PO_4^{3-}$ (xs), inc $K^+$ (xs), proteinuria (xs), inc TG (an), inc BUN (xs), inc uric acid (xs), glossitis, stomatitis, abnormal taste, oliguria (xs), hematuria (xs), pyuria (xs), hyaline casts (xs), nephropathy (xs), vaginitis, anorexia, hyperthermia, inc alk phosphatase, hypernatremia, dec tot proteins, dec ALB.

**METHIMAZOLE:** inc alk phosphatase, inc chol, inc glucose (an), dec $^{131}I$ uptake, inhibits synthesis of thyroid hormone, dec $T_4$, dec $T_3$, dec $T_3$ uptake, inc TSH (xs), insulin autoimmune syndrome (may cause hypoglycemic coma), aplasia cutis (in fetus), goiter (in fetus), cretinism, skin pigmentation, hair loss.

**METHIONINE:** inc insulin, dec urine pH.

**METHOCARBAMOL (ROBAXIN):** brown/green/blue urine, inc 5-HIAA (ur) (an), inc VMA (ur) (an), pruritus, rash, flushing, metallic taste, light-headedness.

**METHOTREXATE:** inc alk phosphatase (xs), nausea, vomiting, rash, pruritus, alopecia, anorexia, dysuria, fever, sweating, vaginal discharge, inc BUN (xs), inc creatinine (xs), renal failure, inc chol (an), dec folate, inc $PO_4^{3-}$ (an), dec sperm count, dec TG (an), inc/dec uric acid.

**METHOXAMINE:** inc cortisol, inc ACTH, uterine hypertonus.

**METHOXYFLURANE:** inc fluoride, inc oxalate, inc alk phosphatase (xs), dec $Ca^{2+}$, inc $Cl^-$ (xs), inc osmolality, inc $Na^+$, inc BUN, inc uric acid, inc urine vol.

**METHSUXIMIDE. See succinimides.**

**METHYCLOTHIAZIDE (also see thiazide diuretics):** SIADH.

**METHYLCELLULOSE. See laxatives.**

**METHYLDOPA:** inc alk phosphatase (xs), inc porphyrins (ur), ppt of acute attack of porphyria, inc coproporphyrin (ur), inc apolipoprotein C-III, inc catecholamines, dec catecholamines (ur), inc chloride, dec chol (an), dec HDL, dec LDL, dec VLDL, inc/dec glucose (an), dec GH, dec 5-HIAA (ur), inc ketones (ur) (an), inc metanephrines (ur) (an), inc prolactin, inc $Na^+$, salt retention, edema, inc glucose (ur) (an), inc triglycerides, dec TG (an), inc BUN, inc/dec uric acid (an), inc VMA (ur) (an), inc plasma vol, gynecomastia, galactorrhea, dec libido, dec potency, breast enlargement, lactation, amenorrhea, impotence, failure to ejaculate.

**METHYLPHENIDATE:** inc epinephrine (ur), urticaria, anorexia, weight loss, scalp hair loss, palpitations.

**METHYLPREDNISOLONE (also see glucocorticoids):** inc amylase (xs), dec ACE (an), inc $HCO_3^-$, dec ACTH, dec cortisol, inc creatinine clearance, dec GT, inc lipase (xs), inc lactate (xs), dec $K^+$, dec $PO_2$, dec testosterone, dec GnRH, inc trypsin (xs), inc plasma vol.

**METHYLTESTOSTERONE (also see androgens):** inc alk phosphatase (xs), inc bilirubin (xs), inc $Ca^{2+}$ (in females w/ breast cancer), inc chol (xs), dec sperm count, dec TBG, dec urobilinogen (ur).

**METHYLTHIOURACIL:** inc alk phosphatase (xs), inc bilirubin (xs), dec $T_4$ (dec iodination of tyrosine).

**METHYLXANTHINES:** inc catecholamines, inc VMA (ur).

**METHYPRYLON:** inc aminolevulinic acid (ur), inc 17-(OH)CS (ur) (an), inc 17-KGS (ur) (an), inc 17-KS (ur) (an), inc porphyrins (ur), inc ppt of acute porphyria, inc sugar (ur) (an), pyrexia, pruritus.

**METHYSERGIDE:** dec serotonin, inc BUN (xs), penile fibrotic plaques (simulating Peyronie disease), facial flush, localized brawny edema, hair loss, weight gain.

**METOCLOPRAMIDE:** inc aldosterone (transient), inc ACTH, inc cortisol, inc GH, inc 18-(OH)corticosterone, dec $K^+$, inc prolactin, inc TSH, hypoglycemia, galactorrhea, amenorrhea, gynecomastia, impotence, fluid retention, porphyria, nipple tenderness (in males), neuroleptic malignant syndrome, inc catecholamines (in hypertensives), hypertensive crisis in pts w/ pheochromocytoma.

**METOLAZONE. See thiazide diuretics.**

**METOPROLOL. See β-adrenergic blockers.**

**METRONIDAZOLE:** gynecomastia, inc/dec glucose (an), dec 17-KS (ur), dec LDH (an), dec TG (an), nausea, anorexia, polyuria, dyspareunia, dec libido, dryness of vagina, dysuria.

**METYRAPONE:** inc androstenedione, dec aldosterone, inc 11-deoxycortisol, dec cortisol, inc ACTH, inc 11-deoxycorticosterone, dec corticosterone, inhibits endogenous adrenal corticosteroid synthesis, mild natriuresis, may induce acute adrenal insufficiency in pts w/ low adrenal secretory capacity, dec $Na^+$, dec $Cl^-$, inc $K^+$, inc 17-(OH)CS (ur), 17-KGS (ur), dec 17-KS (ur) (an), inc porphyrins (ur), ppt of AIP, dec testosterone.

**METYROSINE:** dec catecholamines, therapy of pheochromocytoma, crystalluria, urolithiasis (exp), inc catecholamines (ur) (an), impotence, failure to ejaculate, galactorrhea, slight breast swelling.

**MEXILETINE:** hair loss, impotence, dec libido.

**MICONAZOLE:** inc CPK, dec $Na^+$, pruritus, nausea, anorexia, flushing, hyperlipemia (due to vehicle).

**MIDAZOLAM HCl:** excessive salivation, hives.

**MIFEPRISTONE (RU-486):** heavy bleeding, uterine pain.

**MILRINONE:** hypokalemia.

**MINERAL OIL (also see laxatives):** dec absorption of vits A, D, E, K.

**MINERALOCORTICOIDS:** inc ANH, inc $HCO_3^-$, dec $K^+$, inc $Na^+$.

**MINOCYCLINE. See tetracycline.**

**MINOXIDIL:** hypertrichosis (but may exacerbate hair loss), alopecia, light-headedness, fractures, edema, facial swelling, weight gain, urinary tract infections, renal calculi, urethritis, prostatitis, epididymitis, vaginitis, vulvitis, vaginal discharge, itching, sexual dysfunction, fatigue, menstrual changes, fluid retention, breast tenderness, inc alk phosphatase, inc BUN, inc creatinine, inc HDL chol, dec LDL chol.

**MISOPROSTOL:** menstrual spotting, hypermenorrhea, dysmenorrhea, postmenopausal vaginal bleeding.

**MITHRAMYCIN:** inc alk phosphatase, dec $Ca^{2+}$, inc $Ca^{2+}$ (ur), inc creatinine (xs), dec hydroxyproline (ur), inhibition of bone resorption, dec $PO_4^{3-}$, dec $K^+$, inc protein (ur) (xs), inc BUN (xs), inhibition of spermatogenesis (exp), anorexia, nausea, inc bilirubin.

**MITOMYCIN:** alopecia, inc creatinine, anorexia, fatigue, edema, hemolytic uremic syndrome.

**MITOTANE:** inc alk phosphatase (xs), dec 17-(OH)CS (ur), inc 6β-(OH)cortisol (ur), proteinuria (xs), hematuria (xs), renal damage (xs), inc $T_3$ uptake, competes for sites on TBG, dec $T_4$, lactic acidosis, adrenal insufficiency, anorexia, nausea, hyperpyrexia, generalized aching, dec glucocorticoids.

**MITOXANTRONE:** hyperuricemia, jaundice, alopecia.

**MOLINDONE:** inc FFA, inc prolactin, galactorrhea, amenorrhea, gynecomastia, impotence, neuroleptic malignant syndrome.

**MONOAMINE OXIDASE INHIBITORS:** inc catecholamines, inc epinephrine, inc norepinephrine, dec glucose, inc metanephrines (ur), inc prolactin, inc dopamine, galactorrhea, inc serotonin, inc VMA (ur), hypertensive crisis, nausea, edema, hyperhidrosis, inc transaminases, anorexia, weight changes, palpitations, dysuria, incontinence, urinary retention, sexual disturbances, hypernatremia, hypermetabolic syndrome, impaired $H_2O$ excretion compatible w/ SIADH, acidosis (xs), hyperpyrexia (xs), hepatitis (xs), jaundice (xs), inc alk phosphatase (xs), dec chol (xs), dec glucose (xs), inc GT, dec 5-HIAA (ur).

**MORICIZINE:** impotence, anorexia, dec libido.

**MORPHINE (also see narcotic analgesics):** inc alk phosphatase, dec BMR, dec cortisol, inc CPK, dec enteroglucagon, inc epinephrine, dec GIP, inc gastrin, inc glucose, inc histamine, dec 17-(OH)CS (ur), dec insulin, dec 17-KS, dec lactate, inc lipase, dec motilin, dec norepinephrine, dec PP, inc prolactin, galactorrhea(?), gynecomastia(?), inc sugar (ur) (an), inc TSH, dec VMA (ur), dec urine vol, stimulates ADH release, sweating, nausea, taste alterations, facial flushing, ureteral spasm, urinary retention or hesitancy, oliguria, dec libido, dec potency, pruritus, edema, interference w/ thermal regulation.

**MUMPS VIRUS VACCINE (LIVE):** parotitis, orchitis.

**MUROMONAB-CD3:** flushing, diaphoresis, hepatitis, inc BUN, inc creatinine, inc cellular casts (ur).

**NABUMETONE. See NSAIDs.**

**NADOLOL. See β-adrenergic blockers.**

**NAFARELIN ACETATE:** inc LH, inc FSH, inc ovarian steroidogenesis at onset of therapy; repeated dosing leads to dec LH, dec FSH, and dec secretion of gonadal steroids; arrests secondary sexual development, slows linear growth and skeletal maturation, estrogen withdrawal bleeding (within 6 weeks after initiation of therapy) then ceasing of menstruation, dec pelvic pain, dec dysmenorrhea, dec dyspareunia, arrests breast development in females, arrests genital development in males, dec pubic hair growth, slight dec in bone density/bone mass, inc ovarian cysts, acne, transient breast enlargement, body odor, seborrhea, hot flushes, asymmetry and enlargement of pituitary gland, pituitary microadenoma(?) (children), inc/dec libido, vaginal dryness, hirsutism, chloasma, lactation, breast engorgement, inc TG, inc chol, inc $PO_4^{3-}$, dec $Ca^{2+}$.

**NALIDIXIC ACID:** inc alk phosphatase (xs), inc bilirubin (xs), inc creatinine, inc glucose (an), inc BUN, inc 17-KGS (ur) (an), inc 17-KS (ur) (an), inc sugar (ur) (an), inc VMA (ur) (an), pruritus, cholestatic jaundice (xs), metabolic acidosis (xs).

**NALOXONE:** inc cortisol, inc FSH, inc LH, nausea, sweating, palpitations.

**NALTREXONE:** edema, loss of appetite, delayed ejaculation, dec potency, inc/dec sexual interest, acne, alopecia, oily skin, inc thirst, weight loss, weight gain.

**NANDROLONE. See anabolic steroids.**

**NAPROXEN (also see NSAIDs):** inc 17-KGS (ur) (an), inc 5-HIAA (ur) (an), inc alk phosphatase (an), inc $HCO_3^-$ (an), dec $Cl^-$ (ur), inc $PO_4^{3-}$ (an), dec TG (an), inc $Zn^{2+}$ (ur).

**NARCOTIC ANALGESICS:** inc amylase, dec BMR, inc CPK, dec 17-(OH)CS (ur), inc glucose, inc lipase, sweating, nausea, vomiting, taste alterations, anorexia, facial flushing, ureteral spasm, spasm of vesical sphincters, urinary retention or hesitancy, oliguria, antidiuretic effect, dec libido, dec potency, pruritus, diaphoresis, edema, interference w/ thermal regulation.

**NEFAZODONE:** priapism, impotence, dec libido, amenorrhea, polyuria, abnormal ejaculation, kidney calculus, anorgasmia (rare), weight loss, gout, dehydration, inc chol (rare), hypoglycemia (rare).

**NELFINAVIR:** inc glucose, new-onset diabetes mellitus.

**NEOMYCIN:** inc amino acids (ur) (an), dec ammonia ion, dec $Ca^{2+}$ (ur), inc $Ca^{2+}$ (feces), dec carotene, inc casts (ur) (xs), dec TG, dec FFA, dec chol, dec LDL, dec estrogens (ur), dec lactose tolerance, dec $Mg^{2+}$, dec $K^+$, dec thyroglobulin, dec $T_3$, inc BUN (xs), dec vit A, dec vit $B_{12}$, inc fecal fat, malabsorption syndrome.

**NETILMICIN (also see aminoglycosides):** hyperkalemia.

**NIACIN:** dec chol, dec LDL, dec TG, dec VLDL, inc action of lipoprotein lipase, dec lipolysis in adipose tissue, inc histamine, dec FFA, dec β lipoproteins, dec phospholipids, dec pre-β lipoproteins, inc ketones (ur), hyperglycemia, inc/dec GT, inc insulin, hyperuricemia, dec uric acid clearance, inc alk phosphatase, inc apolipoprotein A-I, inc catecholamines (an), inc GH, dec $K^+$ (ur), inc $Na^+$ (ur), inc sugar (ur) (an).

**NICARDIPINE:** dec $T_4$, inc TSH, polyuria, sexual difficulties, inc $Na^+$ (ur), dose-dependent inc in thyroid hyperplasia or neoplasia (follicular adenoma, carcinoma) (exp).

**NICOTINE:** inc ADH, inc catecholamines (ur), inc epinephrine, inc FFA, inc glucose, inc 11-(OH)CS, inc 5-HIAA (ur), inc neurophysin, inc norepinephrine, inc catecholamine release from adrenal medulla, inc cortisol, impaired fertility (exp), anorexia, excessive salivation, taste perversion, dysmenorrhea, sweating, edema.

**NITRATES:** dec chol (an), inc appetite, impotence, methemoglobinemia (xs), inc urine vol.

**NITRAZEPAM:** inc $HCO_3^-$ (an), dec glucose (an), inc 5-HIAA (ur), fatigue, pruritus.

**NITROFURANTOIN:** inc alk phosphatase (xs), inc antithyroglobulin antibodies, dec $HCO_3^-$ (xs), inc BUN (xs), dec GT, inc $Na^+$ (an), inc sugar (ur) (an), methemoglobinemia (xs), anorexia, pruritus, transient alopecia, dec glucose, inc bilirubin, inc creatinine.

**NITROGLYCERIN (also see nitrates):** inc catecholamines, inc VMA (ur), inc epinephrine (ur), inc norepinephrine (ur), inc TG (an).

**NITROPRUSSIDE:** inc TSH, inc $T_4$, dec hormone binding to TBG, dec free $T_4$, hypothyroidism, dec vit $B_{12}$, cyanide toxicity (xs), methemoglobinemia (xs), thiocyanate toxicity (xs).

**NIZATIDINE (also see $H_2$ antagonists):** gynecomastia (rare), impotence, loss of libido, inc uric acid, inc alk phosphatase.

**NORTRIPTYLINE (also see tricyclic antidepressants):** inc alk phosphatase (xs), inc/dec glucose.

**NOVOBIOCIN:** inc alk phosphatase (xs), dec $^{131}$I uptake, pseudojaundice, inc bilirubin, alopecia, jaundice (xs).

**NSAIDs:** dec aldosterone, inc creatinine, reversible acute renal failure, inc $K^+$, proteinuria, dec PRA, dec $Na^+$, $H_2O$ retention, interstitial nephritis, papillary necrosis, inhibition of prostaglandin synthesis, jaundice (xs), anorexia, hematuria, inc BUN, dec creatinine clearance, change in taste, skin discoloration, hyperpigmentation, inc/dec appetite, inc/dec weight, glycosuria, hyperglycemia, hypoglycemia, flushing, sweating, menstrual disorders, impotence, vaginal bleeding, diabetes mellitus, thirst, pyrexia, breast changes, gynecomastia, facial edema, libido changes, mastodynia, renal calculi(?), leukorrhea(?), displaces $T_4$ from TBG.

**NYSTATIN:** inc amino acids (ur) (an).

**OCTREOTIDE:** dec serotonin, dec gastrin, dec vasoactive intestinal polypeptide, dec insulin, dec glucagon, dec secretin, dec motilin, dec PP, dec GH, cholelithiasis, mild transient hypoglycemia/hyperglycemia, dec insulin requirements in diabetics, aggravation of fat malabsorption, dec libido, frigidity(?), hair loss, galactorrhea(?), secondary hypothyroidism, urine hyperosmolarity, hyperdipsia, inc CPK, dec $Ca^{2+}$ (?).

**OLSALAZINE:** alopecia(?), impotence(?), menorrhagia(?), proteinuria(?).

**OMEGA-3 POLYUNSATURATED FATTY ACIDS:** inc fasting glucose and/or inc mean glucose in type 2 diabetes, impaired insulin secretion/inc insulin sensitivity.

**OMEPRAZOLE:** dec gastrin, dec gastric acid secretion, dec cyanocobalamin (malabsorption), gynecomastia, hypoglycemia, weight gain, alopecia, electrolyte disturbances(?), hepatitis, jaundice, hypoglycemia(?), glycosuria, testicular pain.

**ONDANSETRON HCl:** hepatitis, hypokalemia.

**OPIATES:** inc aldosterone, inc cortisol, inc epinephrine, inc norepinephrine, inc PRA.

**ORAL CONTRACEPTIVES** (effects vary w/ contents): dec 17-(OH)progesterone, dec 17-KGS (ur), dec pregnanediol (ur), dec progesterone, inc lactate, inc oxytocin, inc PRA, inc renin substrate, inc $Na^+$, inc testosterone, inc SHBG, dec free testosterone, inc DHT, inc $TT_4$, inc TBG, dec $T_3$ uptake, inc vit A, dec vit $B_6$, dec vit $B_{12}$, dec vit C, dec $Zn^{2+}$, dec folate, dec $Mg^{2+}$, inc aminolevulinic acid (ur), inc amylase, inc coproporphyrin, inc CBG, dec DHEAS, inc GH, inc lipase, inc/dec $PO_4^{3-}$, inc uroporphyrin (ur), inc menstrual cycle regularity, dec blood loss, dec dysmenorrhea, dec ovarian cysts, dec ectopic preg, dec fibrocystic disease of breasts, breast enlargement, dec lactation (postpartum), fluid retention, premenstrual-like syndrome(?), changes in libido, hirsutism, loss of scalp hair, breakthrough bleeding, spotting, amenorrhea, fertility impairment, ppt of porphyria, melasma, breast tenderness, dec alk phosphatase, dec ALB, inc angiotensin I, inc aldosterone, inc amylase, inc calcitonin, inc glucose, dec GT, inc Cu, inc ceruloplasmin, dec $PO_4^{3-}$, inc selenium, inc cortisol, inc transcortin, inc CS, inc C peptide, inc insulin, dec response to metyrapone test, inc prolactin, galactorrhea(?), growth factor for prolactinomas(?), dec FSH, dec LH, inc FFA, inc TG, inc tot phospholipids, may inc LDL, inc chol, dec HDL (low-dose estrogen), inc apolipoprotein A-I (high-dose estrogen), dec apolipoprotein A-I (low-dose estrogen), inc glycosylated hemoglobin.

**ORLISTAT:** fatigue, menstrual irregularity, inc oxalate (ur), dec vit D, dec vit A, dec vit E, dec β-carotene, dec TC, dec LDL, inc HDL, inc TG, dec FPG, dec insulin.

**OSMOTIC DIURETICS:** inc $Na^+$ (ur), inc $Cl^-$ (ur), hypovolemia (xs), dilute urine, hypernatremia, hyponatremia, hyperkalemia, hypokalemia, acidosis, inc BUN (xs), electrolyte loss (xs).

**OUABAIN:** dec catecholamines (ur).

**OXACILLIN (also see penicillins):** inc alk phosphatase (xs), inc bilirubin (xs), inc creatinine, inc 17-KS (ur) (an), inc protein (an), proteinuria (xs), inc BUN (xs), hyperkalemia (xs).

**OXANDROLONE. See anabolic steroids.**

**OXAPROZIN. See NSAIDs.**

**OXAZEPAM (also see benzodiazepines):** inc cortisol, inc alk phosphatase (xs), inc bilirubin (xs), inc glucose (an), dec $^{131}$I uptake, inc sugar (ur) (an).

**OXYBUTYNIN:** dec sweating, impotence, suppression of lactation, dec lacrimation.

**OXYCODONE. See narcotic analgesics.**

**OXYMETAZOLINE:** dec CS.

**OXYMETHOLONE. See anabolic steroids.**

**OXYMORPHONE. See narcotic analgesics.**

**OXYPHENBUTAZONE (also see phenylbutazone):** inc alk phosphatase (xs), inc amylase, inc bilirubin (xs), inc Cl$^-$, inc Na$^+$, marked salt retention, inc creatinine, dec creatinine clearance, inc uric acid crystals (ur), inc glucose, dec glucose (an), dec $^{131}$I uptake, dec T$_4$, inc T$_3$ uptake, inc BUN, kidney damage, inc uric acid (an), dec uric acid, inc plasma vol, dec urine vol, edema, salivary gland enlargement, metabolic acidosis, respiratory alkalosis, proteinuria (xs), thyroid hyperplasia(?), goiters associated w/ hyperthyroidism/hypothyroidism(?), pancreatitis(?), excessive perspiration (xs).

**OXYPHENISATIN:** dec ALB (xs), inc alk phosphatase (xs), positive antimitochondrial antibodies, inc bilirubin (xs), dec $^{131}$I uptake.

**OXYTETRACYCLINE. See tetracycline.**

**OXYTOCIN:** contraction of lacteal glands, milk ejection (in lactating females), uterine stimulation, antidiuresis, inc plasma vol, water intoxication (xs), dec Na$^+$ (xs), hypertonic uterine contractions (xs), uterine rupture (xs), insulin-like action during labor(?).

**PACLITAXEL:** impaired fertility (exp), alopecia, inc bilirubin, inc alk phosphatase.

**PAMIDRONATE:** hypocalcemia, hypophosphatemia, hypomagnesemia, hypokalemia, hypothyroidism (90-mg dose), bone pain.

**PANCREATIN. See pancreozymin.**

**PANCRELIPASE. See pancreozymin.**

**PANCREOZYMIN:** inc amylase, inc glucose (IV), inc insulin (IV), inc lipase (an), hyperuricosuria (xs), hyperuricemia (xs).

**PANCURONIUM:** inc epinephrine/norepinephrine (if given w/ halothane anesthesia), salivation, rash.

**PAPAVERINE:** inc alk phosphatase (xs), metabolic acidosis (xs), hyperglycemia (xs), hypokalemia (xs), erections (intracavernous).

**PARA-AMINOSALICYLATE SODIUM:** crystalluria, dec vit B$_{12}$, jaundice, hepatitis, goiter w/ or w/o myxedema.

**PARALDEHYDE:** inc alk phosphatase (xs), dec HCO$_3^-$ (xs), metabolic acidosis (xs), inc bilirubin (xs), inc CS (ur) (an), inc glucose (transient), inc 17-(OH)CS (ur) (an), inc 17-KGS (ur) (an), inc ketones (transient), proteinuria (xs), inc BUN (xs), strong unpleasant breath.

**PARAMETHADIONE:** inc alk phosphatase (xs), inc bilirubin (xs), dec Ca$^{2+}$, inc chol (xs), inc creatinine (xs), dec 25-(OH)D$_3$, proteinuria (xs), inc BUN (xs), nephrosis (xs), myasthenia gravis–like syndrome (xs), nausea, anorexia, weight loss.

**PAROMOMYCIN. See aminoglycosides.**

**PAROXETINE:** hypercholesterolemia, hypocalcemia, hypoglycemia, hypokalemia, hyponatremia, diabetes mellitus, hyperthyroidism, hypothyroidism, thyroiditis, dec preg rate (exp), inc pre- and postimplantation preg losses (exp), atrophy of seminiferous tubules (exp), arrested spermatogenesis (exp), abnormal ejaculation, sweating, dry mouth, adrenergic syndrome, pelvic pain, salivary gland enlargement, urinary frequency, abortion, amenorrhea, breast pain, cystitis, dysmenorrhea, dysuria, menorrhagia, nocturia, polyuria, urethritis, urinary incontinence/retention/urgency, vaginitis, breast atrophy/carcinoma/neoplasm, female lactation, hematuria, renal calculus/pain, abnormal kidney function, mastitis, nephritis, oliguria, prostatic carcinoma, vaginal moniliasis, acne, alopecia, photosensitivity, skin discoloration, edema, weight gain/loss, hyperglycemia, thirst, inc alk phosphatase, inc bilirubin, gout, dehydration.

**PECTIN:** dec chol.

**PEMOLINE:** anorexia, weight loss, inc acid phosphatase, prostatic enlargement, hepatitis, jaundice, growth suppression (w/ long-term use in children), hyperpyrexia (xs), sweating (xs), flushing (xs).

**PENBUTOLOL. See β-adrenergic blockers.**

**PENICILLAMINE:** dec Cu , dec Hg, dec cystine, dec vit B$_6$, inc alk phosphatase (xs), inc amino acids (ur) (an), positive antinuclear antibodies, positive anti-DNA antibodies, inc bilirubin (xs), inc chol, dec chol (an), inc CPK, proteinuria (xs), inc BUN (xs), inc Zn$^{2+}$, myasthenic syndrome, skin rashes, oral ulcerations, hypoglycemia (rare), antiinsulin antibodies, skin friability, generalized pruritus, thyroiditis (rare), altered/blunted/loss of taste, pancreatitis, inc alk phosphatase, hematuria, hyperpyrexia, falling hair/alopecia, mammary hyperplasia, elastosis perforans serpiginosa, hot flushes, excessive wrinkling, inc excretion of Zn$^{2+}$, Hg, and Pb, nephrotic syndrome (xs).

**PENICILLINS:** dec ALB (an), inc α-levulinic acid (ur) (an), inc CPK when given as intramuscular injection (as occurs w/ other drugs administered by this route), dec estrogens (ur), inc 17-(OH)CS (ur) (an), dec $^{131}$I uptake, inc 17-KGS (ur) (an), inc 17-KS (ur) (an), inc Hg (ur), inc/dec K$^+$, proteinuria (xs), inc protein (ur) (an), inc sugar (ur) (an), inc T$_3$ uptake (competes for TBPA sites), dec T$_4$, inc BUN (xs), inc uric acid (an), dec uric acid, inc alk phosphatase, hypernatremia, dec ALB, dec tot proteins, vaginitis, anorexia, hyperthermia, oliguria (xs), hematuria (xs), hyaline casts (xs), pyuria (xs), nephropathy (xs), glossitis, stomatitis, abnormal taste.

**PENTAERYTHRITOL TETRANITRATE. See nitrates.**

**PENTAGASTRIN:** inc calcitonin, slight inc GH, inc histamine (ur), inc pepsin (gastric juice), inc prolactin, flushing, light-headedness, sweating, warmth.

**PENTAMIDINE:** dec folate, hypoglycemia, hyperglycemia, inc creatinine (xs), inc BUN (xs), renal toxicity (xs), pancreatic islet cell necrosis, inc insulin, diabetes mellitus, hypocalcemia, anorexia, rash, bad taste, hyperkalemia, dec appetite, hypersalivation, pancreatitis.

**PENTAZOCINE:** inc porphyrins (ur), attack of acute porphyria, inc epinephrine, dec 11-(OH)CS (ur), dec 17-(OH)CS (ur), inc lipase, inc norepinephrine, dec pH, anorexia, edema of face, urinary retention, change in rate/strength of uterine contractions in labor.

**PENTOBARBITAL. See barbiturates.**

**PENTOSTATIN:** seminiferous tubular degeneration (exp), anorexia, sweating, skin discoloration, weight loss, inc BUN, inc creatinine, jaundice, hepatitis, pelvic pain, acidosis, inc CPK, dehydration, diabetes mellitus, inc gamma globulins, gout, abnormal healing, dec chol, weight gain, hyponatremia, bone pain, acne, alopecia, inc ALB (ur), glycosuria, fibrocystic breast disease, inc gynecomastia, polyuria, oliguria, vaginitis, inc LFTs.

**PERCHLORATE:** inc ionized Ca$^{2+}$ (an), proteinuria (xs), inc BUN (xs), nephrotic syndrome (xs).

**PERGOLIDE:** dec prolactin, uterine neoplasms (exp), impaired fertility (xs) (exp), facial edema, palpitations, nausea, anorexia, malaise, pelvic pain, hypothyroidism, diabetes mellitus, SIADH, thyroid adenoma, weight loss, dehydration, dec K$^+$, inc/dec glucose, gout, inc chol, acidosis, inc uric acid, cachexia, skin discoloration, alopecia, hirsutism, urinary incontinence, dysmenorrhea, dysuria, mastalgia, menorrhagia, impotence, vaginitis, priapism, kidney calculus, lactation, fibrocystic breast disease, pyuria, amenorrhea, uricaciduria, withdrawal bleeding, urethral pain, breast engorgement, urolithiasis.

**PERPHENAZINE. See phenothiazines.**

**PHENACEMIDE:** inc alk phosphatase, inc bilirubin, dec creatinine (an), proteinuria (xs), anorexia, weight loss, skin rash, hepatitis, inc creatinine, nephritis, fatigue, palpitations.

**PHENAZOPYRIDINE HCl (PYRIDIUM):** yellowish tinge of skin/sclera, interferes w/ urine determinations by spectrometry, rash, pruritus, methemoglobinemia, renal toxicity (xs), hepatic toxicity (xs), red-orange urine.

**PHENELZINE (also see monoamine oxidase inhibitors):** pyridoxine deficiency, weight gain.

**PHENFORMIN:** inc folate, lactic acidosis, dec glucose.

**PHENINDAMINE. See antihistamines.**

**PHENMETRAZINE:** inc epinephrine (ur), inc 5-HIAA (ur), dec $^{131}$I uptake.

**PHENOBARBITAL (also see barbiturates):** dec creatinine, inc alk phosphatase, osteomalacia, inc aminolevulinic acid, inc bilirubin (xs), hypocalcemia, inc ceruloplasmin, inc Cu, dec folate, dec glucose (ur) (an), inc amino acids (ur) (an), dec 17-(OH)CS (ur), inc 6β-(OH)cortisol (ur), inc 5-HIAA (ur) (an), inc hydroxyproline (ur), dec 25-(OH)D$_3$, inc lactate, dec PO$_4^{3-}$, dec T$_4$, dec free T$_4$ index.

**PHENOTHIAZINES:** acne, lactation, breast enlargement (in females), SIADH, mastalgia, menstrual irregularities, changes in libido, hyperglycemia/hypoglycemia, hyponatremia, glycosuria, pituitary tumor correlated w/ hyperprolactinemia, heavy menses, dry mouth, anorexia, salivation, perspiration, urinary retention/frequency/incontinence, polyuria, enuresis, priapism, ejaculation inhibition, hyperpyrexia, enlarged parotid glands, inc appetite, polyphagia, inc weight, polydipsia, chromosomal aberrations in spermatocytes (exp), abnormal sperm (exp), severe neurotoxicity in thyrotoxic pts, gynecomastia; interferes w/ urinary ketone determinations, preg tests, and steroid determinations; inc catecholamines, dec HDL chol, inc chol, inc glucose, dec VMA (ur), inc vasopressin, dec FSH, dec LH, dec DHT, dec testosterone, dec free testosterone, dec GH, dec 17-(OH)CS (ur), dec 17-KS (ur), dec pregnanediol (ur), inc prolactin, inc TBG, inc TT$_4$, dec T$_3$ uptake, dec BUN (xs), inc/dec uric acid, inc alk phosphatase (xs), dec estrogens (ur), block ovulation, dec GT, dec gonadotropins (ur), dec 5-HIAA (ur) (an), inc $^{131}$I uptake, dec 17-KGS (ur) (an), inc tot metanephrines (ur) (an), dec PO$_4^{3-}$ (an), inc bilirubin (xs), renal dysfunction (xs), galactorrhea, amenorrhea, impotence, inc in mammary neoplasms (exp), neuroleptic malignant syndrome, tardive dyskinesia, alterations in LFTs, discoloration of urine to pink/red-brown, hair loss, papillary hypertrophy of tongue.

**PHENOXYBENZAMINE:** inhibition of ejaculation, dec Na$^+$, inc ADH.

**PHENSUXIMIDE. See succinimides.**

**PHENTOLAMINE:** inc catecholamines, inc 5-HIAA (ur) (an), dec glucose (xs).

**PHENYLBUTAZONE:** inc sodium, salt retention, inc alk phosphatase (xs), inc bilirubin (xs), inc Cl$^-$, inc chol (one pt), inc glucose, dec 17-(OH)CS (ur), inc 6β-(OH)cortisol (ur), dec $^{131}$I uptake, respiratory alkalosis, proteinuria (xs), dec T$_4$, dec free T$_4$, inc T$_3$ uptake, dec free T$_4$ index, inc TSH, inc BUN (xs), inc uric acid (low dose), dec uric acid (high dose), inc plasma vol, dec urine vol, edema, salivary gland enlargement, metabolic acidosis, hyperglycemia, thyroid hyperplasia, goiters associated w/ hyperthyroidism and hypothyroidism, pancreatitis.

**PHENYLEPHRINE:** inc glucose, inc tot metanephrines (ur) (an), inc amino acids (ur) (an).

**PHENYLPROPANOLAMINE:** inc amino acids (ur) (an), palpitations, renal failure (xs), rhabdomyolysis (xs), dysuria.

**PHENYTOIN (also see hydantoins):** inc alk phosphatase, dec Ca$^{2+}$, inc Cu, inc ceruloplasmin, inc chol, inc HDL chol, inc CS, inc apolipoprotein A-I, dec calcitonin, dec DHEAS, dec cortisol, dec 11-deoxycortisol, inc GH, dec 17-(OH)CS (ur), dec 17-KS (ur), dec PO$_4^{3-}$, inc prolactin, inc PTH (in epileptic children), inc FSH, inc LH, inc glucose, dec insulin, inc/dec GT, inc/dec free T$_4$, inc T$_3$ uptake, inc/dec T$_3$, dec free T$_3$, inc SHBG, inc testosterone, dec free testosterone, inc transcortin, dec 25-(OH)D$_3$, dec ADH, inc vit A, hyperglycemia, gynecomastia, goiter, clinical hyperthyroidism (rare), hirsutism, alopecia, dec binding of T$_4$ and T$_3$ by TBG (xs).

**PHOSPHATES:** inc PTH, dec alk phosphatase (an), dec Ca$^{2+}$ (an), crystalluria (xs), dec ionized Ca$^{2+}$ (slight), dec Mg$^{2+}$ (ur), dec K$^+$.

**PHOSPHORUS REPLACEMENT PRODUCTS:** weight gain, low urine output, unusual thirst, bone/joint pain (xs), osteomalacia (xs), extraskeletal calcifications (xs), inc alk phosphatase (xs), inc bilirubin (xs), inc creatinine (xs), dec glucose (xs), proteinuria (xs), inc BUN (xs).

**PHYTATE:** dec Ca$^{2+}$, dec Fe$^{2+,3+}$, dec PO$_4^{3-}$, dec Zn$^{2+}$.

**PIMOZIDE:** neuroleptic malignant syndrome, thirst, inc appetite, inc salivation, anorexia, impotence, nocturia, urinary frequency, sweating, weight gain, weight loss, loss of libido, menstrual disorder, breast secretions.

**PINDOLOL. See β-adrenergic blockers.**

**PIPECURONIUM BROMIDE:** hypoglycemia, hyperkalemia, inc creatinine, anuria.

**PIPERIDINES:** inc 17-(OH)CS (ur) (an), dec ionized Ca$^{2+}$ (an), inc 17-KS (ur) (an).

**PIRBUTEROL. See sympathomimetics.**

**PIROXICAM. See NSAIDs.**

**PIZOTIFEN:** inc 5-HIAA (ur).

**PODOPHYLLOTOXIN DERIVATIVES:** anorexia, alopecia, pigmentation, renal dysfunction, hepatic dysfunction.

**POLYMYXIN B:** albuminuria, cylindruria, azotemia, facial flushing, inc amino acids (ur) (an), inc creatinine (xs), dec K$^+$ (xs), proteinuria (xs), inc BUN (xs).

**POLYTHIAZIDE. See thiazide diuretics.**

**POTASSIUM CHLORIDE:** inc Cl$^-$, dec glucose, inc K$^+$, dec vit B$_{12}$.

**POTASSIUM IODIDE:** inc amylase, parotitis, inc CS (ur) (an), inc 17-(OH)CS (ur) (an), inc TSH, dec T$_4$, dec T$_3$.

**POVIDONE-IODINE:** inc glucose (an) (if swab used w/ fingerstick).

**PRAVASTATIN. See HMG-CoA reductase inhibitors.**

**PRAZEPAM. See benzodiazepines.**

**PRAZOSIN (also see α$_1$-adrenergic blockers):** dec chol, inc HDL, dec VLDL, inc FFA, inc glucose, dec GT, inc insulin, inc lipoprotein lipase, dec PRA, inc TSH (slight), inc T$_4$ (slight), dec TG, inc VMA (ur) (an), inc metabolites of norepinephrine (ur) (an), impotence, alopecia.

**PREDNISOLONE. See glucocorticoids.**

**PREDNISONE (also see glucocorticoids):** dec alk phosphatase, inc amylase, pancreatitis (xs), dec ACE, inc HCO$_3^-$, hypokalemic alkalosis, dec bilirubin, dec Ca$^{2+}$, inc chol, inc HDL, inc cortisol (an), dec creatinine clearance, dec 1,25-(OH)$_2$D$_3$, inc glucose, dec GT, inc PTH, dec K$^+$, inc Na$^+$, dec T$_3$-binding capacity, dec testosterone, inc TSH, dec TBG, dec TG, dec T$_3$, inc/dec reverse T$_3$, inc uric acid.

**PRILOCAINE:** dose-dependent methemoglobinemia.

**PRIMAQUINE:** inc bilirubin, rusty yellow/brown urine, dec RBC-reduced glutathione, hemolysis in G-6-PD deficiency, methemoglobinemia in NADH methemoglobin reductase deficiency.

**PRIMIDONE:** inc amino acids (ur) (an), crystalluria (xs), dec folic acid, dec free testosterone, dec T$_4$, dec free T$_4$ index, fatigue, anorexia, skin eruptions, impotence.

**PROBENECID:** inc alk phosphatase (xs), urinary calculi, dec estriol (ur), dec glucose, dec 17-KS (ur), proteinuria (xs), inc sugar (ur) (an), inc BUN (xs), dec uric acid, inc uric acid (ur), anorexia, urinary frequency, ppt of gout.

**PROBUCOL:** dec chol, dec LDL, dec HDL, dec TG, dec GH, inc HCO$_3^-$, dec Ca$^{2+}$, inc BUN, inc glucose, inc uric acid, inc CPK, inc alk phosphatase (xs), impotence, nocturia, hyperhidrosis, enlargement of multinodular goiter.

**PROCAINAMIDE:** anorexia, inc K$^+$ (an), worsening of myasthenia gravis, inc alk phosphatase (xs), positive antinuclear/antihistone antibodies, inc bilirubin (xs).

**PROCAINE:** inc porphobilinogen (ur) (an), inc urobilinogen (ur) (an).

**PROCARBAZINE:** anorexia, nocturia, hematuria, gynecomastia in prepubertal and early pubertal boys, flushing, hyperpigmentation, alopecia, jaundice, hepatic dysfunction, diaphoresis, inc bilirubin.

**PROCHLORPERAZINE. See phenothiazines.**

**PROGESTERONE:** (effects vary according to the progestational agent) inc aldosterone (ur) (an), inc alk phosphatase (xs), dec chol, inc CS (an), dec HDL, inc cortisol (an), dec glucose, dec 17-(OH)CS (ur), dec LH, inc $Mg^{2+}$, dec pregnanediol (ur), inc protein, sodium retention, inc TBG, inc cystine, inc melatonin, inhibits secretion of pituitary gonadotropins, prevents follicular maturation and ovulation, fluid retention, dec GT (esp in diabetics), amenorrhea, breast tenderness, acne, melasma, chloasma, alopecia, hirsutism, masculinization of female fetus (during preg).

**PROGESTINS. See progesterone.**

**PROGESTOGENS:** inc aminolevulinic acid (ur), inc porphyrins (ur), acute porphyria.

**PROMAZINE (also see phenothiazines):** inc alk phosphatase (xs), inc bilirubin (xs), inc chol (xs), dec 17-(OH)CS (ur), dec 5-HIAA (ur) (an), dec $^{131}$I uptake, 17-KS (ur) (an), inc prolactin, inc protein (ur).

**PROMETHAZINE (also see antihistamines):** false-negative or false-positive preg tests, inc blood glucose, inc alk phosphatase, inc bilirubin, inc catecholamines, dec CS (ur) (an), dec 17-(OH)CS (ur) (an), dec 5-HIAA (ur) (an), dec $^{131}$I uptake, dec $PO_4^{3-}$ (an).

**PROPAFENONE:** fertility impairment (exp), dec spermatogenesis (exp), anorexia, alopecia, inc alk phosphatase, hyponatremia, SIADH, impotence, inc glucose.

**PROPOFOL:** hypersalivation, enlarged parotid, metabolic acidosis, flushing, diaphoresis, green urine, oliguria, urine retention, hyperkalemia, hyperlipemia, inc BUN, inc creatinine, inc osmolality, dehydration, hyperglycemia, inc TG.

**PROPOXYPHENE (also see narcotic analgesics):** reversible jaundice, abnormal liver function tests, inc alk phosphatase (xs), dec glucose, dec 17-(OH)CS (ur), dec 17-KS (ur), dec $^{131}$I uptake, reversible jaundice.

**PROPRANOLOL (also see β-adrenergic blockers):** dec aldosterone, dec C peptide, dec FFA, dec glucagon, dec glucose, inc GH, dec insulin, inc LH (in males), dec LH (in females), inc $K^+$, inc prolactin (in males), dec TBG, dec $T_4$, inc free $T_4$, inc TSH, dec $T_3$, inc reverse $T_3$, inc BUN (xs), inc alk phosphatase (xs).

**PROPYLTHIOURACIL:** inhibits synthesis of thyroid hormone, dec $T_4$, dec $T_3$, dec peripheral conversion of $T_4$ to $T_3$, inc TSH (xs), pituitary adenomas(?), thyroid hyperplasia(?), goiter/cretinism in fetus, skin pigmentation, hair loss, insulin autoimmune syndrome (can cause hypoglycemic coma), inc alk phosphatase (xs), inc amylase, inc bilirubin (xs), dec FFA, inc glucose (an), dec $^{131}$I uptake, inc BUN (anaphylactic nephritis), inc uric acid (an), inc antinuclear antibodies.

**PROSTAGLANDIN E$_2$:** stimulation of uterus, uterine evacuation, hot flushes, breast tenderness, excessive thirst, uterine sacculation (xs), uterine rupture (xs), dehydration (xs), proliferation of bone, cervical ripening, inc $T_4$, inc $T_3$.

**PROTAMINE:** inc catecholamines (an), dec lipase, inc tot lipids, dec lipoprotein lipase.

**PROTEASE INHIBITORS:** new-onset diabetes mellitus, hyperglycemia, inc insulin resistance, Cushingoid habitus.

**PROTRIPTYLINE. See tricyclic antidepressants.**

**PSEUDOEPHEDRINE:** inc amino acids (ur) (an), palpitations, dysuria, weakness (xs).

**PSYLLIUM. See laxatives.**

**PTH (TERIPARATIDE ACETATE):** hypercalcemia (xs), hypertensive crisis, inc hydroxyproline (ur), inc prolactin, inc pH (ur), inc $HCO_3^-$ (ur), inc $Cl^-$ (ur), inc $Mg^{2+}$, dec $PO_4^{3-}$, inc urine vol.

**PYRAZINAMIDE:** dec ALB (xs), inc alk phosphatase (xs), inc bilirubin (xs), dec globulin (xs), inc ketones (ur) (an), inc 17-KS (ur), dec protein (xs), inc uric acid, gout, fever, porphyria, dysuria, anorexia, inc $Fe^{2+,3+}$ conc , rashes, pruritus, acne, photosensitivity, interstitial nephritis, worsening of glucose control in diabetics(?).

**PYRIDOSTIGMINE:** inc GH secretion, inc GH response to GHRH, urinary frequency, incontinence, urinary urgency, diaphoresis, rash, urticaria, flushing, alopecia.

**PYRIDOXINE:** dec oxalate, dec folic acid (xs), prolactin suppression(?), inhibition of lactation(?).

**PYRILAMINE. See antihistamines.**

**PYRIMETHAMINE:** dec folate, hemolysis in G-6-PD deficiency, anorexia, atrophic glossitis, malaise, light-headedness, dermatitis, abnormal skin pigmentation, hyperphenylalaninemia.

**QUATERNARY ANTICHOLINERGICS. See anticholinergic agents.**

**QUAZEPAM. See benzodiazepines.**

**QUINACRINE:** inc alk phosphatase (xs), inc bilirubin (xs), yellow skin, deep yellow urine, inc cortisol (an), inc cortisol (ur) (an), inc 11-(OH)CS (an), hemolysis in G-6-PD deficiency, acute porphyria attack, anorexia, dermatitis, yellow pigmentation of skin (xs).

**QUINAPRIL. See ACE inhibitors.**

**QUINETHAZONE. See thiazide diuretics.**

**QUINIDINE:** anorexia, abnormalities of pigmentation, inc CPK, acidosis (xs), inc alk phosphatase (xs), false inc catecholamines (an), inc catecholamines (ur) (an), inc CS (ur) (an), inc 17-(OH)CS (ur) (an), inc 17-KS (ur) (an), dec $^{131}$I uptake, inc antinuclear antibodies.

**QUININE:** inc bilirubin, inc catecholamines (an), inc CS (ur) (an), dec glucose, inc insulin, inc 17-(OH)CS (ur) (an), inc 17-KGS (ur) (an), hepatitis.

**RADIOGRAPHIC AGENTS:** inc histamine, dec VMA (ur), inc inorganic iodide, dec uric acid, inc amylase, dec catecholamines (ur), inc creatinine (xs), crystalluria, dec 17-KGS (ur) (an), dec $PO_4^{3-}$ clearance (ur), proteinuria, interferes w/ serum protein electrophoresis (an), inc specific gravity (ur), inc sugar (ur) (an), inc TSH, inc $T_4$ (an), dec $T_3$, inc reverse $T_3$, inc BUN, azotemia (xs), renal failure (xs).

**RALOXIFENE:** dec TC, dec LDL, dec lipoprotein(a), dec fibrinogen, hot flushes, weight gain, edema, breast pain.

**RAMIPRIL (also see ACE inhibitors):** anorexia, impotence, inc $Na^+$, dec $Na^+$(ur).

**RANITIDINE (also see H$_2$ antagonists):** impotence, loss of libido, inc creatinine, gynecomastia (rare), dec aldosterone, dec cortisol, inc/dec prolactin, dec $T_4$, dec free $T_4$, inc $T_3$, inc free $T_3$, dec TSH response to TRH, dec vit $B_{12}$, inc gastrin, dec serotonin, dec 5-HIAA (urine).

*RAUWOLFIA* **DERIVATIVES:** mammary fibroadenomas (exp), malignant tumors of the seminal vesicles (exp), malignant adrenomedullary tumors (exp), inc serum prolactin, inc/dec catecholamines (ur), dec 17-KS (ur), dec 17-(OH)CS (ur), dec VMA (ur), anorexia, pseudolactation, galactorrhea, amenorrhea, impotence, gynecomastia, dec libido, breast engorgement, weight gain, inc $Na^+$, edema.

**REPAGLINIDE:** hypoglycemia, dec FPG, dec PPG.

**RESCINNAMINE. See *Rauwolfia* derivatives.**

**RESERPINE (also see *Rauwolfia* derivatives):** dec catecholamines, inc/dec catecholamines (ur), inc HVA (ur), inc 5-HIAA (ur), inc prolactin, dec serotonin, inc/dec VMA (ur), inc CS (ur) (an), inc FFA, inc glucose, dec norepinephrine (ur), dec $T_4$, false-negative tyramine test, galactorrhea, amenorrhea, gynecomastia, impotence, dec libido.

**RESORCINOL:** green-blue urine, inc creatinine (an), dec $^{131}$I uptake, inc methemoglobin.

**RIBOFLAVIN:** inc catecholamines (an), inc catecholamines (ur) (an), yellow-orange urine, inc urobilin (ur) (an).

**RIFABUTIN:** fertility impairment (exp), rash, anorexia, discolored urine, taste perversion, inc alk phosphatase, hepatitis, skin discoloration.

**RIFAMPIN:** inc alk phosphatase (xs), inc bilirubin, inc casts (ur), dec chol (an), red-orange saliva/sweat/urine, dec CS, dec cortisone, inc C peptide, inc glucose, dec hydrocortisone, dec 25-(OH)$D_3$, inc insulin, inc $PO_4^{3-}$ (an), inc prolactin, dec protein, inc testosterone, inc TSH, dec $T_4$, dec free $T_4$, inc $T_3$, inc BUN, renal failure, inc uric acid, porphyria exacerbation, anorexia, pancreatitis, hepatitis, rash, pruritus, fatigue, osteomalacia, hematuria, hemoglobinuria, menstrual disturbances, edema of face and extremities, inhibits assays for folate and $B_{12}$ (an).

**RISEDRONATE:** dec $Ca^{2+}$, dec $PO_4^{3-}$, peripheral edema, bone pain.

**RISPERIDONE:** hyperprolactinemia, priapism, erectile dysfunction, ejaculatory dysfunction, weight gain, dec $Na^+$, gynecomastia (rare), male breast pain.

**RITODRINE:** dec contractility of uterine smooth muscle, inc insulin (IV), inc glucose (IV), dec $K^+$ (IV), inc FFA (IV), inc cAMP (IV), glycosuria, lactic acidosis, hypoglycemia (neonatal), hypocalcemia (neonatal).

**RITONAVIR:** inc uric acid, inc TG, inc CPK.

**ROFECOXIB:** fluid retention, edema, appetite change, inc chol, weight gain, menopausal symptoms, breast mass.

**ROSIGLITAZONE:** inc insulin sensitivity, dec insulin levels, dec FFA, inc TC, inc LDL, inc HDL, resumption of ovulation in anovulatory women, inc plasma vol, edema, hypoglycemia.

**SALICYLATES:** inc creatinine, dec estriol (ur), dec FFA, dec folate, dec hydroxyproline (ur), inc ketones (xs), dec TSH, dec $T_4$, inc uric acid, dec vit $B_{12}$, inc bilirubin, dec $T_3$, dec renal function, compete w/ thyroid hormone for binding sites on TBPA and TBG, dec glucose (ur) (an), interfere w/ 5-HIAA (ur) (an), inc VMA (ur) (an), dec VMA (ur) (an) (Pisano method), anorexia, hepatoxicity, rashes, thirst, respiratory alkalosis (xs), metabolic acidosis (xs), dehydration (xs), hyperthermia (xs), hypokalemia (xs), slight inc glucose, hypoglycemia (xs).

**SALSALATE (also see salicylates):** dec ALB, nephrotic syndrome, inc creatinine, proteinuria, dec $T_4$, dec $T_3$, displaces $T_4$ from TBG.

**SALT SUBSTITUTES (potassium-containing):** inc $K^+$ (xs).

**SAQUINAVIR:** new-onset diabetes mellitus, hyperglycemia, nephrolithiasis, dec glucose.

**SARGRAMOSTIM (GRANULOCYTE-MACROPHAGE COLONY-STIMULATING FACTOR):** fluid retention, anorexia, alopecia, inc creatinine (in preexisting renal dysfunction), inc bilirubin (in preexisting hepatic dysfunction).

**SCOPOLAMINE. See anticholinergic agents.**

**SECOBARBITAL. See barbiturates.**

**SECRETIN:** inc $HCO_3^-$ (ur), inc $Ca^{2+}$, dec gastrin, inc glucose, inc insulin, inc lipase, inc $Na^+$ (ur), dec titratable acidity (ur).

**SELEGILINE (also see monoamine oxidase inhibitors):** hair loss, weight loss, prostatic hyperplasia, facial hair, anorgasmia (xs), dec penile sensation (xs).

**SENNA (also see laxatives):** red/orange/rust urine, inc estradiol (ur) (an), inc estrogens (ur) (an), dec estrone (ur) (an).

**SERTRALINE:** significant weight loss, dec uric acid, uricosuria, inc sweating, male sexual dysfunction, ejaculatory delay, anorexia, fatigue, inc salivation, flushing, palpitations, edema, acne, alopecia, hypertrichosis, anorexia, inc appetite, dysmenorrhea, intermenstrual bleeding, amenorrhea, mastalgia, menorrhagia, micturition frequency, dysuria, nocturia, polyuria, fatigue, hot flushes, thirst, dehydration, inc chol, inc TG, hypoglycemia, exophthalmos, gynecomastia.

**SIBUTRAMINE:** weight loss, thirst, generalized edema, dysmenorrhea, metrorrhagia.

**SILDENAFIL:** flushing, edema, inc uric acid, inc $Na^+$, hyperglycemia.

**SILVER:** dec chloride, inc pH, proteinuria (xs), nephrotoxicity (xs), dec $Na^+$, inc BUN (xs).

**SIMVASTATIN (also see HMG-CoA reductase inhibitors):** dec vital sperm, inc abnormal sperm, dec fertility (exp).

**SODIUM BICARBONATE (also see antacids):** inc pH, alkalinization of urine, dec $K^+$, inc protein (ur) (an), inc urobilinogen (ur).

**SODIUM CHLORIDE:** dec bilirubin (an), inc cortisol (ur), inc ionized $Ca^{2+}$ (an).

**SODIUM NITROPRUSSIDE:** dec $^{131}$I uptake, dec $T_4$, thyroidal inhibition (in renal dysfunction).

**SODIUM POLYSTYRENE SULFONATE:** hypokalemia, hypocalcemia/hypercalcemia, sodium retention.

**SODIUM SALTS:** dec aldosterone, inc $HCO_3^-$, inc $Ca^{2+}$ (an), inc/dec $Ca^{2+}$ (ur), dec $Cl^-$, inc ionized $Ca^{2+}$, inc pH, dec $K^+$, dec PRA, inc $Na^+$.

**SOMATOSTATIN (also see octreotide):** dec $Na^+$, water intoxication, dec TSH, dec TSH response to TRH, inhibitor of TSH release, dec $T_4$, dec $T_3$, dec free $T_3$.

**SOMATROPIN:** hyperglycemia (mild), glycosuria, skeletal growth, cell growth, organ growth, inc $PO_4^{3-}$, inc hydroxyproline (ur), dec nitrogen excretion (ur), dec BUN, inc insulin, blocks insulin action, impaired GT, dec fat stores, inc FFA, inc TC, inc TG, inc $Ca^{2+}$(ur), retention of $K^+$, $PO_4^{3-}$, and $Na^+$.

**SORBITOL:** inc glucose, hyperglycemia in diabetics, dec intestinal absorption of $B_{12}$, acidosis, electrolyte loss, marked diuresis, edema, urinary retention, dry mouth, thirst, dehydration, inc bilirubin, inc lactate, dec pyruvate.

**SOTALOL (also see β-blockers):** inc chol, dec HDL, inc LDL, dec FFA, inc tot metanephrines (ur) (an), inc TG.

**SPECTINOMYCIN:** inc alk phosphatase, dec creatinine clearance (ur), inc BUN, inc urine vol, urticaria, dizziness.

**SPINAL ANESTHESIA:** dec $Cl^-$ (ur), dec effective renal plasma flow, dec GFR, dec $Na^+$ (ur), dec urobilinogen (ur), dec urine vol.

**SPIRONOLACTONE:** hyperkalemia, hyponatremia, gynecomastia, reversible hyperchloremic metabolic acidosis, inability to achieve or maintain erection, amenorrhea, irregular menses, postmenopausal bleeding, inc aldosterone, inc $Cl^-$ (ur), inc angiotensin II, inc $Ca^{2+}$, inc/dec chol, dec HDL, inc LDL, inc 18-(OH)corticosterone, inc insulin, inc 17-(OH)CS (ur) (an), inc 17-KGS (ur) (an), inc 17-KS (ur) (an), inc PRA, dec testosterone, inc/dec TG, inc/dec uric acid, inc CS (an), inc cortisol (an), inc 11-deoxycorticosterone, dec GT, inc estradiol (ur), inc 11-(OH)CS (an), sexual dysfunction, dec plasma vol, inc LH, displaces DHT from receptors, inc BUN.

**STANOZOLOL. See anabolic steroids.**

**STREPTOKINASE:** inc alk phosphatase, inc CPK, inc creatinine, nephrotoxicity (xs), proteinuria (xs), inc BUN.

**STREPTOMYCIN (also see aminoglycosides):** inc bilirubin, hemolytic anemia, nephrotoxicity, proteinuria (xs), inc sugar (ur) (an), inc BUN (xs).

**STREPTOZOCIN:** inc acetoacetate, dec $HCO_3^-$, polyuria, dec FFA, dec gastrin, inc glucose (ur), inc insulin, inc lactate, hypokalemia, inc pyruvate, polydipsia, nephrotoxicity, dec fertility (exp), hypoalbuminemia, abnormalities of GT, hypoglycemia, nephrogenic DI, lethargy.

**STRONTIUM:** inc $Mg^{2+}$ (ur) (an).

**SUCCIMER:** inc ketones (ur) (an), dec uric acid (an), dec CPK (an), appetite loss, inc alk phosphatase, inc chol, proteinuria.

**SUCCINIMIDES:** inc aminolevulinic acid (ur), inc porphyrins (ur), ppt of acute porphyria, anorexia, weight loss, inc libido, alopecia, hirsutism, urinary frequency, renal damage, hematuria, vaginal bleeding, microscopic hematuria, proteinuria (xs), nephrosis (xs).

**SUCCINYLCHOLINE:** inc CPK, inc histamine, inc ionized $Ca^{2+}$, inc myoglobin, inc $K^+$, malignant hyperthermia, metabolic acidosis (xs), inc salivation, hyperkalemia, myoglobinuria.

**SUCRALFATE:** aluminum toxicity (in renal failure), aluminum osteodystrophy, osteomalacia, encephalopathy; in conjunction w/ other aluminum-containing products may inc $Al^{3+}$ levels; dec $PO_4^{3-}$ (in renal failure).

**SUFENTANIL (also see narcotic analgesics):** chills.

**SULFACYTINE. See sulfonamides.**

**SULFADIAZINE (also see sulfonamides):** inc alk phosphatase, dec $Ca^{2+}$ (an), inc chol (xs), crystalluria, dec [131]I uptake, proteinuria (xs), hematuria, dec urine vol.

**SULFAMETHIZOLE. See sulfonamides.**

**SULFAMETHOXAZOLE (also see sulfonamides):** inc alk phosphatase, inc $T_4$ (an).

**SULFASALAZINE (also see sulfonamides):** oligospermia, infertility in men, inc alk phosphatase.

**SULFATE-CONTAINING DRUGS (if present in high concentration):** dec $Ca^{2+}$ (an), dec $Ca^{2+}$, inc $Ca^{2+}$ (ur), dec $K^+$, kaliuresis, dec $Na^+$, natriuresis.

**SULFHYDRYL COMPOUNDS:** dec alk phosphatase (an).

**SULFINPYRAZONE:** renal failure (xs), inc uric acid (ur), ppt of acute gouty arthritis, urolithiasis, renal colic, jaundice (xs).

**SULFISOXAZOLE (also see sulfonamides):** false-positive urinary protein.

**SULFONAMIDES:** ppt of acute porphyria, false-positive urinary glucose, methemoglobinemia, anorexia, pancreatitis, dec folic acid, crystalluria, hematuria, proteinuria, inc creatinine, nephrotic syndrome, toxic nephrosis, oliguria, anuria, alopecia, goiter production, diuresis, hypoglycemia, acidosis (xs), dec $Ca^{2+}$ (an), inc alk phosphatase (xs), inc chol (xs), dec [131]I uptake, dec $T_4$, inc $T_3$ uptake, inc BUN (an), dec uric acid, uricosuric effect, uremia.

**SULFONYLUREAS:** inc acetaldehyde, inc alk phosphatase, inc bilirubin, hypoglycemia, dec [131]I uptake, dec $Na^+$, inc $T_3$ uptake, dec $T_4$, dec TG, dec glucose, hypoglycemia (xs), SIADH, porphyria cutanea tarda, hepatic porphyria, inc BUN, inc creatinine, dec TG, inc insulin, inc C peptide, potentiation of effect of ADH, dec glucagon release from the liver.

**SULINDAC (also see NSAIDs):** inc alk phosphatase (xs), dec creatinine clearance, dec prostaglandin $F_{2\alpha}$, dec PRA, dec thromboxane $B_2$.

**SUMATRIPTAN SUCCINATE:** malaise, flushing, sweating, warm/hot sensation, thirst, polydipsia, dehydration, hunger, dec appetite, dysuria, dysmenorrhea, renal calculus, urinary frequency.

**SYMPATHOMIMETICS:** hypokalemia (xs), anorexia, alopecia.

**TAMOXIFEN:** dec alk phosphatase, inc $Ca^{2+}$, dec chol, dec LDL, inc VLDL, inc estradiol, dec FSH, inc/dec LH, dec prolactin, inc sperm count, inc $T_4$, inc TBG, inc free $T_4$, inc $T_3$, inc TG, endometrial hyperplasia, endometrial polyps, hyperlipidemia, hot flushes, vaginal bleeding, vaginal discharge, menstrual irregularities, ovarian cysts, loss of appetite.

**TAMSULOSIN:** dec libido, ejaculation failure, retrograde ejaculation.

**TEMAZEPAM. See benzodiazepines.**

**TENIPOSIDE. See podophyllotoxin derivatives.**

**TERAZOSIN (also see $\alpha_1$-adrenergic blockers):** dec chol, dec LDL chol, dec VLDL chol, impotence, dec libido, sexual dysfunction, gout, hemodilution, weight gain.

**TERBINAFINE:** malaise, hair loss, taste disturbance, loss of taste, abnormal liver function.

**TERBUTALINE (also see sympathomimetics):** inc HDL, inc glucose, inc insulin, inc/dec $K^+$, dec $T_4$, inc $T_3$.

**TERFENADINE (also see antihistamines):** alopecia, galactorrhea, dysmenorrhea.

**TESTOLACTONE:** anorexia, alopecia, edema, nail growth disturbances, dec estradiol, inc $Ca^{2+}$, inc 17-KS (ur), inc creatinine (ur).

**TESTOSTERONE (also see androgens):** inc aldosterone (ur) (an), inc alk phosphatase, inc androstenedione, inc $Ca^{2+}$, inc chol, dec CBG, inc CS (an), dec DHEA, inc estradiol, inc 17-(OH)CS (ur) (an), dec 17-(OH)progesterone, dec 17-(OH)pregnenolone, dec progesterone, dec SHBG, dec TBG, $Na^+$ retention, $H_2O$ retention, inc urine vol.

**TETRACYCLINE:** dec $Ca^{2+}$, inc alk phosphatase (xs), aminoaciduria (xs), inc amylase (xs), inc Bence-Jones protein (ur) (xs), dec $HCO_3^-$ (xs), acidosis (xs), inc catecholamines (an), dec chol (xs), inc estrogens (ur) (an), dec folate, inc/dec glucose (an), [131]I uptake, inc/dec $PO_4^{3-}$, Fanconi syndrome (outdated product), inc/dec $K^+$, proteinuria (xs), hypernatremia (xs), inc sugar (ur) (an), dec testosterone, dec free testosterone, inc BUN (xs), inc/dec uric acid (an), inc urine vol, anorexia, pseudotumor cerebri, brown-black microscopic discoloration of thyroid gland.

**TETRAHYDROCANNABINOL:** inc epinephrine (ur), inc norepinephrine (ur), dec testosterone, dec DHT, dec free testosterone, dec uric acid, inc C peptide, dec cAMP, dec glucose, inc insulin, dec LH (in women), inc $K^+$.

**THALLIUM:** inc BUN (xs), proteinuria (xs), inc casts (ur) (xs).

**THEOPHYLLINE:** inc cAMP, diuresis, inc catecholamines (ur), hyperglycemia (xs), proteinuria (xs), SIADH, alopecia, hypokalemia (xs), hypercalcemia (xs), dec $HCO_3^-$ (xs), acidosis (xs), dec alk phosphatase (an), inc FFA, dec $PO_4^{3-}$, dec $Na^+$, inc/dec somatostatin (an), inc uric acid, inc urine vol.

**THIABENDAZOLE:** inc alk phosphatase (xs), inc chol (xs), inc glucose, proteinuria (xs), inc crystals (ur) (an), anorexia, hematuria, enuresis, facial flush.

**THIAMINE:** inc uric acid (an), inc urobilinogen (an).

**THIAZIDE DIURETICS:** dec free cortisol (ur), dec C peptide, dec insulin, dec $Mg^{2+}$, dec osmolality, inc BUN, inc creatinine, dec $K^+$, dec $Na^+$, hypochloremic alkalosis, inc uric acid, inc $Ca^{2+}$, hyperglycemia, inc chol, inc LDL chol, inc TG, inc $Na^+$ (ur), inc $Cl^-$ (ur), inc $K^+$ (ur), inc $HCO_3^-$ (ur), dec $Ca^{2+}$ (ur), dec uric acid (ur), dec formation and recurrence of calcium nephrolithiasis, dec incidence of osteoporosis in postmenopausal women, dec urine vol (therapy of nephrogenic DI), impotence, dec libido, inc insulin or oral hypoglycemic requirement in diabetics, azotemia (xs), fetal/neonatal jaundice, fetal/neonatal hypoglycemia and electrolyte imbalances.

**THIOCYANATE:** proteinuria (xs), inc BUN (xs), nephrosis (xs).

**THIOGUANINE:** jaundice, inc alk phosphatase, anorexia, hyperuricemia.

**THIOPENTAL (also see barbiturates):** inc histamine, salivation, shivering, nausea.

**THIORIDAZINE (also see phenothiazines):** dec LH, dec testosterone.

**THIOTEPA:** inc uric acid, nephropathy (xs), anorexia, amenorrhea, interferes w/ spermatogenesis, chemical/hemorrhagic cystitis.

**THIOTHIXENE:** inc alk phosphatase (xs), inc bilirubin (xs), reversible cholestasis, inc/dec glucose, false-positive urine preg tests, inc prolactin, galactorrhea, amenorrhea, gynecomastia(?), impotence, neuroleptic malignant syndrome.

**THIOURACIL:** dec $T_3$, inc reverse $T_3$, inc alk phosphatase (xs), inc bilirubin (xs), inc chol (xs).

**THYROID HORMONE:** dec chol, dec HDL, dec LDL, inc SHBG, dec TSH, inc metabolic rate of body tissues; exacerbation of intensity of symptoms if given in diabetes mellitus, DI, or adrenal insufficiency; ppt of hyperthyroid state, dec bone density (xs), weight loss, menstrual irregularities, partial loss of hair in first few months of therapy, inc glucose, inc (OH)proline (ur), dec [131]I uptake, inc protein, dec catechol O-methyltransferase, dec estriol (ur), dec monoamine oxidase, dec norepinephrine, inc $T_4$, inc $T_3$, inc free $T_4$ index.

**THYROTROPIN:** inc [131]I uptake, inc $T_4$, inc $T_3$.

**THYROXINE. See thyroid hormone.**

**TICLOPIDINE:** inc chol, inc TG, anorexia, hyponatremia, inc alk phosphatase (xs), inc bilirubin (xs).

**TILUDRONATE:** vit D deficiency, hyperparathyroidism.

**TIMOLOL. See β-adrenergic blockers.**

**TIOPRONIN:** wrinkling and friability of skin, proteinuria, nephrotic syndrome (xs), dec vit $B_6$.

**TOBRAMYCIN (also see aminoglycosides):** cylindruria.

**TOCAINIDE:** anorexia, alopecia, myasthenia gravis, polyuria, positive antinuclear antibodies.

**TOLAZAMIDE (also see sulfonylureas):** mild diuresis.

**TOLBUTAMIDE (also see sulfonylureas):** false-positive reaction for ALB in urine (metabolite precipitates when acidified after boiling test).

**TOLMETIN (also see NSAIDs):** inc protein (ur) (an).

**TOSYLATE BRETYLIUM:** dec catecholamines (ur).

**TRAMADOL:** menopausal symptoms, proteinuria, inc Cr, menstrual disorder.

**TRANYLCYPROMINE. See monoamine oxidase inhibitors.**

**TRAZODONE:** priapism, inc/dec libido, impotence, retrograde ejaculation, early menses, missed periods, breast enlargement and engorgement, lactation, hypersalivation, SIADH, methemoglobinemia, inc bilirubin, hematuria, delayed urine flow, inc urinary frequency, urinary incontinence/retention, inc/dec appetite, sweating, weight gain/loss, malaise, alopecia.

**TRH:** inc epinephrine, inc norepinephrine, inc prolactin, inc TSH, inc $T_4$, inc $T_3$.

**TRIAMCINOLONE (also see glucocorticoids):** inc amylase, inc $Ca^{2+}$ (ur), dec cortisol, inc glucose, dec GT, negative nitrogen balance, hypokalemic alkalosis, inc $K^+$ (ur) (xs), inc $Na^+$ (ur).

**TRIAMTERENE:** hyperkalemia, mild $N_2$ retention, renal stones(?), metabolic acidosis, inc glucose, azotemia (xs), inc creatinine (xs), inc uric acid, gout(?), inc aldosterone, dec $HCO_3^-$, dec catecholamine (ur) (an), inc $Cl^-$, green-blue color of urine, dec creatinine clearance, crystalluria, dec folate, dec GFR, inc $Mg^{2+}$, dec $Na^+$, sexual dysfunction(?).

**TRIAZOLAM (also see benzodiazepines):** dec cortisol (ur).

**TRICHLORMETHIAZIDE (also see thiazide diuretics):** false-positive phentolamine and tyramine tests (an).

**TRICYCLIC ANTIDEPRESSANTS:** neuroleptic malignant syndrome, inc arrhythmias in hyperthyroid pts, inc/dec glucose, acne, inc alk phosphatase, gynecomastia, testicular swelling, breast enlargement, menstrual irregularity, galactorrhea (in females), inc/dec libido, painful ejaculation, impotence, nocturia, urinary frequency, dysuria, lactation (nonpuerperal), vaginitis, leukorrhea, mastodynia, amenorrhea, inc prolactin, inc ADH, SIADH, inc norepinephrine, inc cortisol.

**TRIFLUOPERAZINE. See phenothiazines.**

**TRIFLUPROMAZINE. See phenothiazines.**

**TRILOSTANE:** dec glucocorticoids, dec aldosterone, dec cortisol (ur), inc 17-KS (ur), inc ACTH, adrenal hypertrophy, inc adrenal adenoma(?), adrenal cortical hypofunction (in stress).

**TRIMEPRAZINE. See antihistamines.**

**TRIMETHADIONE (also see paramethadione):** attack of acute porphyria.

**TRIMETHAPHAN:** inc histamine.

**TRIMETHOPRIM-SULFAMETHOXAZOLE:** inc TSH, dec $T_4$, dec free $T_4$, inc alk phosphatase, inc BUN, inc creatinine, crystalluria, dec folate, dec $Na^+$, impairs free water clearance, anorexia, pancreatitis, oliguria (xs), anuria (xs).

**TRIMIPRAMINE. See tricyclic antidepressants.**

**TRIPELENNAMINE. See antihistamines.**

**TRIPROLIDINE. See antihistamines.**

**TROGLITAZONE:** inc insulin sensitivity, dec insulin levels, dec TG, dec lactate, dec ketone body formation, hypoglycemia, severe idiosyncratic hepatocellular injury, resumption of ovulation in anovulatory women.

**TROVAFLOXACIN:** thirst, hyperglycemia, inc alk phosphatase, dec $Na^+$, dec $HCO_3^-$.

**TRYPSIN:** dec ionized $Ca^{2+}$ (an).

**TRYPTOPHAN:** inc amino acids (an), inc chol (an), phosphaturia, inc uric acid (an), eosinophilia myalgia syndrome.

**TUBOCURARINE:** inc creatinine kinase, inc histamine, respiratory alkalosis, excessive salivation.

**TYRAMINE:** inc amino acid (an), inc glucose, inc tyrosine (an), inc uric acid (an), inc urobilinogen (an).

**TYROPANOIC ACID:** impairs conversion of $T_4$ to $T_3$, inc $T_4$, dec $T_3$.

**TYROSINE:** inc bilirubin (an), crystalluria, inc uric acid (an), inc urobilinogen (an).

**URACIL MUSTARD:** amenorrhea, impaired spermatogenesis, azoospermia, hair loss, inc alk phosphatase, inc bilirubin.

**UREA (also see osmotic diuretics):** dec bilirubin (an), inc chol (an), inc creatinine (an), inc creatinine (ur) (an), inc ionized $Ca^{2+}$ (an), inc osmolality (an), inc urine osmolality (an), dec porphobilinogen (ur) (an), hypokalemia, hyponatremia, inc BUN, dec urobilinogen (ur) (an), inc urine vol, dehydration (xs), inc aldosterone, inc angiotensin II, inc PRA.

**UROFOLLITROPIN:** stimulation of ovarian follicular growth, abnormal ovarian enlargement, multiple preg, breast tenderness, ectopic preg, hair loss.

**URSODEOXYCHOLIC ACID:** hair thinning.

**VALPROIC ACID:** inc GH, dec selenium, inc TSH, dec $T_4$, dec free $T_4$, inc alk phosphatase (xs), inc amylase, inc FFA (an), dec β-(OH)butyrate, dec ketones, inc ketones (ur) (an), inc lactate, inc organic acids (ur), dec prolactin, inc pyruvate, dec free testosterone, hyperammonemia, dec spermatogenesis (exp), testicular atrophy (exp), anorexia, weight loss, inc appetite, weight gain, transient hair loss, irregular menses, secondary amenorrhea, galactorrhea, parotid gland swelling, breast enlargement, hyperglycemia, hypocarnitinemia, edema, acute pancreatitis (xs).

**VANCOMYCIN:** inc casts (ur), inc creatinine, nephrotoxicity (xs), dec creatinine clearance (xs), proteinuria, red man syndrome.

**VASOPRESSIN:** inc ACTH, inc cortisol, inc GH, inc reabsorption of water, water intoxication (xs), SIADH (xs), inc CS, inc CPK, inc creatinine (xs), rhabdomyolysis (xs), dec $Na^+$ (xs), inc BUN (xs), dec urine vol.

**VIDARABINE (ADENINE ARABINOSIDE):** fluid overload, anorexia, inc bilirubin, weight loss.

**VINBLASTINE:** dec uric acid, aspermia, amenorrhea, anorexia, malaise, SIADH (xs).

**VINCRISTINE:** dec osmolality, dec $Na^+$, inc vasopressin, inc $Na^+$ (ur), SIADH (xs), water intoxication (xs), inc uric acid, inc osmolality (ur), azoospermia, amenorrhea, uric acid nephropathy (xs), pain in the parotid gland, bone pain, anorexia, polyuria, dysuria, urinary retention, weight loss, alopecia.

**VINDESINE SULFATE:** parotid pain, SIADH, alopecia, transient hepatic dysfunction.

**VINYL ETHER:** inc bilirubin (xs), inc glucose, inc BUN (xs).

**VITAMIN A:** inc alk phosphatase (xs), inc bilirubin (an), dec $^{131}I$ uptake, inc $Ca^{2+}$, alopecia (xs), hypomenorrhea (xs), polydipsia (xs), polyuria (xs), hypercalcemia.

**VITAMIN $B_{12}$:** hypokalemia (xs), inc RBC requirements of $K^+$ w/ conversion of megaloblastic to normal erythropoiesis.

**VITAMIN B COMPLEX:** inc catecholamines (an), dec estrogens (ur) (an).

**VITAMIN C:** false-positive urine glucose (xs), ppt of cystine/oxalate/urate renal stones (xs), dec triglycerides, inc oxalate (esp in renal failure).

**VITAMIN D:** inc $Ca^{2+}$, inc $PO_4^{3-}$, inc calculi (ur), inc chol (an), proteinuria (xs), inc BUN (xs), inc creatinine (xs), hypercalcemia (xs), metastatic soft-tissue calcification (xs), generalized vascular calcification (xs), nephrocalcinosis (xs), hypercalciuria (xs), hyperphosphatemia (xs), muscle pain, bone pain, polyuria, polydipsia, anorexia, nocturia, mild acidosis, dec libido, hypercholesterolemia (xs).

**VITAMIN E:** dec aminolevulinic acid (ur), dec uroporphyrin (ur), gynecomastia.

**VITAMIN K:** inc bilirubin (in neonates or G-6-PD deficiency), inc catecholamines (an), inc 17-(OH)CS (ur) (an), inc porphyrins (ur), inc protein (ur).

**XANTHINE:** inc chloride (ur), crystalluria, inc $K^+$ (ur), inc protein (an), inc $Na^+$ (ur), diuresis, inc urine vol.

**YOHIMBINE HCl:** antidiuresis, skin flushing, sweating, penile erectile stimulation.

**ZALCITABINE:** pancreatitis, anorexia, fatigue, dec weight, edema, inc amylase, jaundice, salivary gland enlargement, diabetes mellitus, hyperglycemia, dec $Ca^{2+}$, impotence, hot flushes, hepatitis, jaundice, acne, alopecia, gout, polyuria, renal calculus, inc alk phosphatase.

**ZIDOVUDINE (AZT):** diaphoresis, anorexia, acne(?), polyuria(?), urinary frequency(?), lactic acidosis.

**ZINC:** significant dec HDL (xs), Cu deficiency, dec alk phosphatase (an), inc $Ca^{2+}$ (an), inc $Mg^{2+}$ (ur) (an).

**ZOLPIDEM TARTRATE:** fatigue, lethargy, anorexia, palpitations, inc sweating, flushing, impotence, edema, hot flushes, dec weight, inc appetite, dec libido, hyperbilirubinemia, hyperglycemia, gout, hypercholesterolemia, hyperlipidemia, inc BUN, periorbital edema, thirst, menstrual disorder, vaginitis, breast pain, breast fibroadenosis, acne, dysuria, polyuria, renal pain, acute renal failure, micturition frequency.

# CHAPTER 240

# DNA DIAGNOSIS OF ENDOCRINE DISEASE

J. FIELDING HEJTMANCIK AND HARRY OSTRER

The dramatic progress in molecular genetics over the last two decades has made diagnosis possible for a variety of inherited diseases by direct analysis of DNA. Patients with many of these diseases are seen routinely by endocrinologists and primary care physicians, who are likely to have use for these diagnostic tests. Although these tests are extremely powerful diagnostic tools, their use and interpretation often are not straightforward. A confusing and rapidly changing array of laboratory techniques, each with particular strengths and weaknesses, confront the practitioner. In this chapter, the nature of these tests, the genetic principles on which they are based, and the types of information they provide are discussed. Finally, a list of diseases for which DNA diagnostic tests are available and suggestions for their practical use are provided.

## SITUATIONS APPROPRIATE FOR DNA DIAGNOSIS

In general, DNA analysis is used when more classic diagnostic tests cannot be applied. Although DNA diagnosis is extremely powerful and highly accurate, it tends to be more labor intensive and expensive than the diagnostic tests used routinely in most hospitals. This may change with the advent of powerful new technology to screen for DNA sequence changes using oligonucleotide probes arrayed on silicon chips (see later). Presently, however, cases are found in which the more routine diagnostic tests cannot be used or have marked limitations, often when the aberrant gene product is unknown or cannot be detected in readily accessible tissues. One particularly important example likely to come to the attention of an endocrinologist is multiple endocrine neoplasia, in which presymptomatic DNA diagnosis allows persons at risk to be observed closely for the development of tumors or undergo presymptomatic intervention.[1] Both multiple endocrine neoplasia type 1, the gene for which is located on chromosome band 11q13,[2] and multiple endocrine neoplasia type 2, which includes medullary thyroid carcinoma and is caused by mutations in the c-*ret* protooncogene on chromosome band 10q11, can be identified by direct screening for causative mutations or, if necessary, diagnosed by linkage (see later and Chap. 188).

Other examples include prenatal and postmortem testing. In these cases, DNA analysis is preferred because it relies on detection of changes in the DNA complement of the patient, which is (mostly) identical in all cells and at all stages of development and disease progression. Thus, a blood sample or even a saline mouth rinse might be collected rather than a biopsy sample from difficult-to-obtain tissues, such as the liver or those of the central nervous system.

Prenatal diagnosis, although it provides prospective parents with information about the disease status of a pregnancy at risk, can also confront them with the difficult decision of whether to continue with a pregnancy in the face of a potentially devastating illness or undergo pregnancy termination. This decision can be avoided now that preimplantation diagnosis of genetic disease is possible. In this procedure, which is available at a small number of specialized centers, women use fertility drugs to produce hyperovulation; the oocytes are collected by vaginal ultrasonography and then inseminated in vitro. One or two blastomeres are harvested, usually at the eight-cell stage, and analyzed for genetic defects. Whereas initial cases were limited to sexing for X-linked diseases, the polymerase chain reaction technique has allowed reliable detection of single gene defects, including those for cystic fibrosis, Lesch-Nyhan disease, Tay-Sachs disease, and Duchenne muscular dystrophy.[3]

DNA analysis falls into two categories: *direct detection of mutations* and diagnosis by *linkage to genetic markers*. In some situations, such as with familial male precocious puberty, specific mutations produce the disease phenotype.[4] These can be identified most efficiently by testing for the presence of the specific mutation in the affected gene. In other cases, the disease-causing gene and its product have not been identified, or disease-causing mutations cannot be identified readily. For example, maturity-onset diabetes of youth (MODY) is known to be a genetic condition with an autosomal dominant pattern of transmission. In some families, mutations of the glucokinase gene on chromosome 7 have been demonstrated.[5,6] In other families with MODY, mutations in the hepatic nuclear factor 1 gene on chromosome 12 or the hepatic nuclear factor 4 gene on chromosome 20 have been demonstrated.[7,8] When MODY is first identified in a family, which gene harbors the causative mutation is not obvious. By studying the transmission of anonymous DNA markers linked to the causative genes on chromosomes 7, 12, and 20 in MODY families, linkage to one of these three genes can be established and the likelihood that any individual has inherited a MODY-causing gene can be determined with a high degree of reliability.

DNA diagnostic techniques also have been used to determine a person's risk for developing tumors (as with familial medullary carcinoma of the thyroid) and to type tumors once they have occurred. Analysis of tumor tissue can provide information about both the stage and the probable natural history of the tumor. For example, marked increases in the copy number of the N-*myc* gene in pheochromocytoma is an indication of poor prognosis.[9]

Because of its broad applicability, DNA diagnosis is useful throughout the human life cycle. Persons who contemplate having children can be tested for carrier recessive gene status to determine their risk. Pregnant women can have prenatal (or preimplantation) diagnosis to determine whether the fetus is affected with a genetic condition. Persons with a family history of disease can undergo testing to determine their risk of developing the disease. DNA diagnostic methods can be applied to postmortem tissue samples and, thus, can be used to determine whether other family members are at risk for the development of a given disorder.[10]

# DIRECT DETECTION OF MUTATION

## TYPES OF MUTATIONS

Inherited disease results from mutations of many different types. Some mutational events involve whole chromosomes. These include *deletions, duplications, translocations,* and *insertions.* Deletions and duplications occur from unequal crossing over. Normally, two chromosomes pair during meiosis, and crossing over occurs between the two chromosomes at homologous sites. Sometimes, two or more members of a gene family occur as a tandem array, and pairing occurs between nonidentical members of the gene family. As a result of crossing over, there is a net gain of information on one chromosome, and a net loss of information on the other chromosome. Both can be disruptive.

Translocations are exchanges between nonidentical chromosomes. The chromosomes may pair at short regions that have similar sequences. After breaks at these sites, a region from one chromosome is joined to the other. Translocations can disrupt genes, cause novel chimeric genes to be formed, or put a gene under the control of a novel regulatory mechanism.

Other mutations involve individual genes. *Point mutations* result from the substitution of one base for another. *Insertion* is a process whereby pieces of extraneous DNA are integrated into a gene, disrupting the gene or adding novel coding sequences. In *gene conversion,* a certain stretch of one gene is lost and is replaced by a region from another gene. One means by which gene conversion may occur is from two unequal recombinational events. A novel form of mutation takes place when a trinucleotide sequence (e.g., CTG) is present as a tandem repeat in a gene.[11] DNA polymerase can slip during replication of the repeat region. As a result, the number of repeats either increases or decreases. Alternatively, the polymerase may cycle many times through the trinucleotide repeat, resulting in a marked increase in the number of repeats to hundreds or even thousands of copies. Diseases caused by unstable trinucleotide repeats are often associated with anticipation, in which increasing severity or decreasing age of onset occurs in affected individuals in subsequent generations of a family.[12]

The effect of these mutations is to alter the sequence, processing, or quantity of RNA transcripts and, thus, to alter the resulting *protein products.* In some cases, the stability or activity of the protein product is diminished, whereas in other cases, the quantity of the product may be increased or it may gain novel functions. The effect of a mutation on the protein product determines the number of copies of a gene that must carry the mutation to cause disease and, hence, the inheritance pattern for that disease. If inheritance of a single copy of the mutated gene is suffi-

cient to produce disease, it is dominant. If inheritance of two mutated copies of the gene is required to produce disease, it is recessive. Finally, deletions of DNA stretches including several genes may produce phenotypes that are composites of the genetic conditions caused by the individual genes. These are called *contiguous gene syndromes.*[13] When large, these deletions can be detected through cytogenetic analysis as chromosomal deletions. Otherwise, molecular analysis is required.

## METHODS OF DETECTING MUTATIONS

When the specific mutation causing an inherited disease is known, the disease may be diagnosed by detecting the mutation directly. The choice of test is determined by the relative frequency of the mutation. Some methods are efficient for detecting *single prevalent mutations,* whereas others are more efficient for identifying *multiple mutations* that may cause a genetic disease. In some cases, the disease is caused by a wide variety of mutations, no single one of which is prevalent. Some mutations may not be detectable using the commonly available techniques. These mutations must be detected by *direct sequencing* of the affected person's DNA or by techniques designed to screen for unknown mutations. If the disease-causing mutation cannot be identified but nevertheless is known to be present in a particular gene or genomic region, individuals of unknown genetic status within a family can be tested by using the technique of *genetic linkage analysis.*

Most contemporary DNA diagnostic techniques rely on the *polymerase chain reaction (PCR)*[14] (Fig. 240-1). Primers that are specific for a region of the genome are used to amplify short stretches of DNA. Two primers are used, priming the synthesis

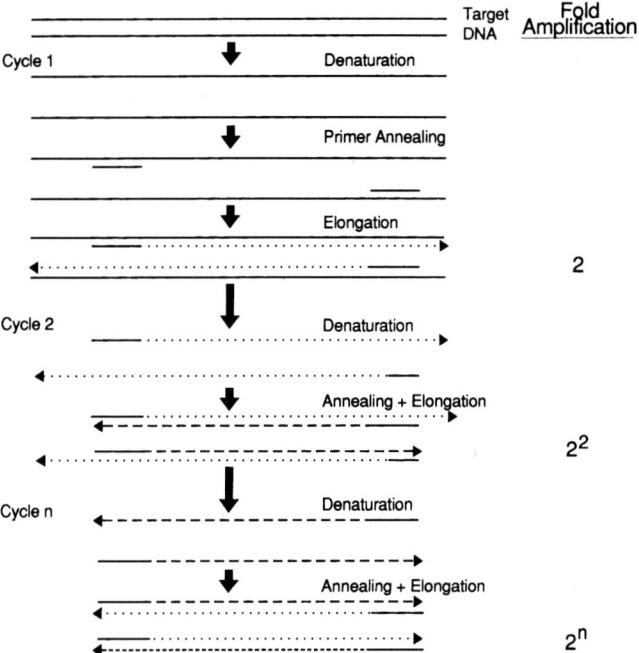

**FIGURE 240-1.** The polymerase chain reaction. The reaction is carried out in cycles, with several different temperatures used in each cycle. First, the double-stranded DNA template is denatured or melted into single strands. Next, the oligonucleotide primers are annealed to the melted DNA. Third, a new DNA strand is synthesized as the polymerase elongates from the primer and copies the template strand. Initially, each cycle doubles the amount of the target region, although the reaction loses efficiency at higher cycle numbers. Usually, 25 to 40 cycles are sufficient to synthesize enough DNA for easy visualization of the product, which has a discrete allele size, by staining with ethidium bromide.

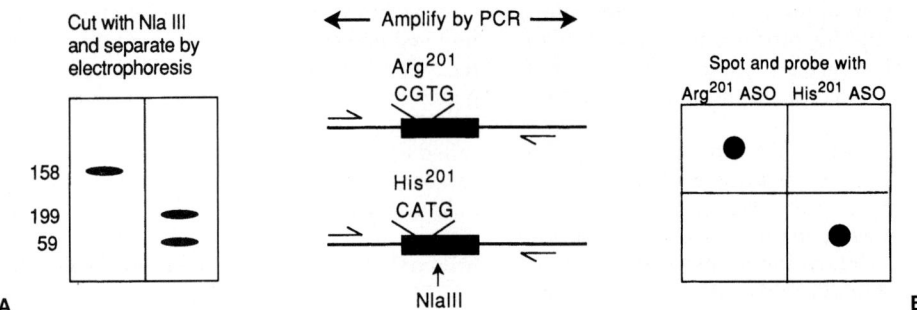

**FIGURE 240-2.** Analysis of known mutations or polymorphisms (diagnosis of Arg[201] His mutation in McCune-Albright syndrome). A single base change from G to A in codon 9 of the normal $G_s\alpha$ gene is one of the causes of the McCune-Albright syndrome. This base change also creates a recognition site for NlaIII (*CATG*), so that the enzyme now cuts at this site. The region encompassing the mutation is amplified using the polymerase chain reaction (*PCR*). **A,** The PCR product is digested with NlaIII and electrophoresed. The His[201] allele gives two fragments, whereas the Arg[201] allele is not cut and gives a single, larger band. **B,** The PCR product is spotted on a membrane and used as a target for hybridization with two labeled allele-specific oligonucleotide (*ASO*) probes. The Arg[201] and His[201] oligonucleotides are each 19 bases long and differ by a single base. Stringent washing that will melt a hybrid with a single mismatch is carried out. A hybridization signal results when at least one copy of the allele homologous to the labeled oligonucleotide probe is present.

of opposite strands of the DNA molecule and "pointing" toward each other. DNA synthesis is initiated from these primers in rounds, with each round of DNA synthesis doubling the number of copies of the template DNA included between the primers. After the first few rounds of synthesis, most of the amplified fragments are products of earlier DNA synthesis reactions rather than of the sample DNA. Hence they are a single discrete size, having the two primers as common ends. The length of the amplified fragment is determined by the distance between the two primers. Amplification of as little as a single DNA molecule, such as from a single blastomere, can be carried out.[15] PCR amplification may be applied simultaneously to many regions of a single gene or to multiple different genes. The presence of a PCR product itself is diagnostic for an intact target region on at least one chromosome. Alteration in the size of a PCR product may indicate the presence of insertions or deletions.

One way the PCR product can be analyzed is by restriction endonuclease analysis (Fig. 240-2). *Restriction enzymes* cleave DNA at sites with specific recognition sequences. For example, the restriction enzyme *Eco*RI cleaves DNA at the six-base sequence GAATTC, referred to as the *restriction site* for that enzyme. When this sequence is altered by a point mutation, the enzyme no longer cleaves at the site, resulting in a longer DNA fragment. Sometimes, point mutations create new restriction sites. Gain or loss of a restriction enzyme recognition site in a DNA sequence is indicative of the presence of a mutation.

The fragments that are generated by restriction enzyme digestion of PCR products or other DNA can be separated on the basis of size by electrophoresis in an agarose gel. Small fragments migrate more rapidly than larger ones. The fragments of DNA in the gel are identified by staining with a specific dye, such as ethidium bromide or silver. The sizes of the fragments depend on the location of the restriction sites. The occurrence of a restriction site is indicated by the presence of two fragments whose sizes sum to that of the uncut DNA molecule. *Homozygotes* for the presence of the restriction site have only the smaller DNA fragments, whereas *heterozygotes* have both smaller and larger fragments.

A potential pitfall in restriction endonuclease analysis is *incomplete cutting by a restriction enzyme*. As a result, a homozygote for the presence of a restriction site may be inappropriately labeled as a heterozygote. To correct for such possible inaccuracies, controls are built into the restriction endonuclease digestions. These may

include (a) choosing a restriction enzyme that cuts at more than one site in the PCR product, with one site being constant and the other being at a location where mutations are sometimes found; (b) cutting with more than one restriction enzyme, where one enzyme tests for the presence of the mutation and the other tests for the ability to obtain complete cleavage at a second site; and (c) doping the restriction endonuclease reaction with a second DNA molecule whose restriction site is known, to test for the completeness of digestion in the reaction.

Sometimes, restriction endonuclease analysis is performed on intact genomic DNA that has not been amplified by PCR. The fragments that are generated from the restriction enzyme digestion are separated in an agarose gel. These fragments are denatured to single-stranded molecules, then transferred to a nitrocellulose or a nylon membrane. This process is known as *Southern blotting*. To detect the sequences of interest, labeled molecular probes are used. These probes anneal to molecules with complementary sequences on the membrane. The location of the probes is then visualized, either by autoradiography for a radioactively labeled probe, or by an enzymatic reaction or fluorescence for molecules that have been labeled by other means. The sizes of the molecules on the Southern blot are indicative of whether cleavage by the restriction enzyme has taken place.

Because restriction enzymes have not been identified that recognize all possible mutations, other methods have been developed to identify single base changes. PCR products can be tested for their ability to anneal to short, single-stranded DNA probes that are complementary to either the normal or the mutant gene (see Fig. 240-2). These *allele-specific oligonucleotide (ASO) probes* can be used to determine the occurrence of specific mutations, because as little as a single base mismatch prevents the probe from annealing to the target DNA. Several different PCR products, corresponding to different regions of a gene, can be tested with many different ASO probes concurrently. The ability to screen for 32 different mutations in a single annealing reaction has been readily demonstrated.[16] The ASO probes are labeled radioactively or chemically. The annealing of a specific ASO to a PCR product is detected by methods similar to those used for Southern blot analysis, that is, by fixing the PCR product to a filter before the annealing. Control PCR products that contain each of the mutations for which the ASO reaction is screening are included in the sample tested to demonstrate that the expected reactions actually have occurred.

*Mismatch PCR*, or the *amplification refractory mutation system*, is another diagnostic method to test for the presence of a particular mutation.[17] Ordinarily, the PCR reaction tolerates a mismatch in the middle or the 5' end of a primer; however, the 3' end of the primer must be completely complementary to the genomic DNA sequence for the reaction to proceed efficiently. When primers are chosen for which the 3' ends correspond either to the normal or to the mutant sequence, the presence of a PCR product can be indicative of the sequence that was present in the genomic DNA. Thus, for a normal homozygote, amplification would occur only with the normal primer but not with the mutant primer. In contrast, in a mutant homozygote, amplification would occur only with the mutant primer. In a heterozygote, amplification would occur with both the normal and the mutant primers.

The *ligase chain reaction* is conceptually similar to mismatch PCR. Ligation, the process by which two DNA molecules are joined together, occurs efficiently only if the two DNA strands to be ligated are annealed to an intact strand of homologous DNA, closely approximating the ends to be joined.[18] For ligation to occur, the molecules must be completely complementary to the partner strands to which they are annealed. A mismatch between the template strand and the end of a DNA molecule that is to be ligated prevents the reaction from occurring. To detect the precursors and products of this reaction, one of the two DNA molecules can be labeled with a radioactive tracer or with a fluorochrome. When the labeled molecule is ligated to the other DNA molecule, the resulting molecule is larger and has altered mobility on polyacrylamide gel electrophoresis. To obtain sufficient numbers of molecules for analysis, many cycles of the ligase chain reaction may be performed. These cycles involve denaturation of the DNA molecules, annealing of the labeled and unlabeled target DNA molecules, and ligation (if possible) of these two molecules. This method lends itself readily to automation, both for ligation of DNA molecules and for analysis of the ligated products using a DNA sequencer. Simultaneous detection of many different mutations can be performed by using pairs of oligonucleotides that correspond to different regions of a gene or to different genes.

Solid-phase techniques that use high-density arrays of oligonucleotides immobilized on a silicon chip have been developed to increase the number of mutations that can be screened for simultaneously.[19] In the simplest version, a PCR product that has been labeled with a fluorochrome is hybridized to the chip, with specificity being determined by whether the match between PCR product and oligonucleotide is perfect or incomplete.[20] This technique has been used to screen for mutations in *BRCA1* and the reverse transcriptase and protease genes of human immunodeficiency virus 1. Variants of this technique have been developed to enhance both sensitivity and specificity. In the version known as *solid-phase minisequencing*, the PCR product is hybridized to the oligonucleotide array and the mutant site is queried by testing for incorporation of a fluorochrome-labeled oligonucleotide.[21,21a] As the use of this technology expands, it should enable cost-efficient screening for large numbers of genetic diseases.[22]

## SCREENING FOR MUTATIONS

When the specific mutations causing a disease are not known in a family being studied, they can be identified by a variety of techniques. The gold standard is direct sequence analysis of the gene or of a complementary DNA (cDNA) copy of its RNA transcript. Two general methods are used to screen for mutations, usually in PCR products. One depends on the dramatic effect

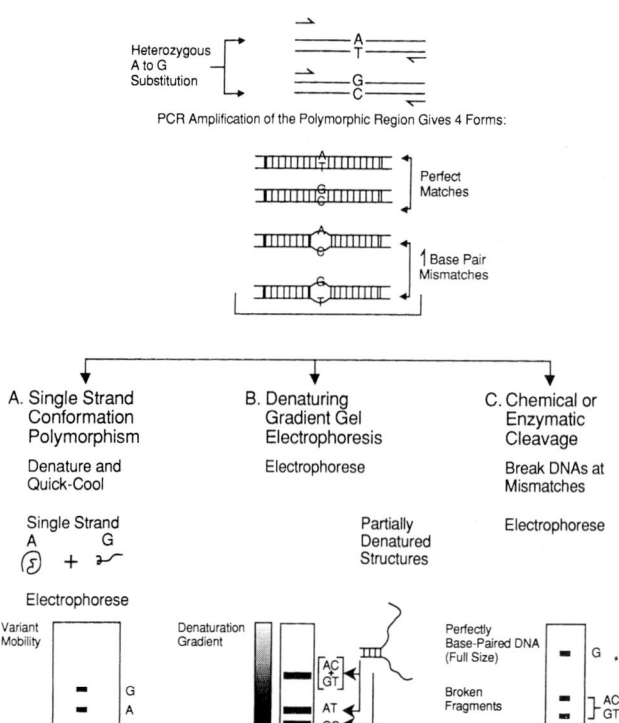

**FIGURE 240-3.** Screening for sequence changes. A segment of DNA suspected to contain a mutation (e.g., an exon of a candidate gene) is amplified by the polymerase chain reaction (*PCR*). Then, if two alleles are present, the amplification product will contain a mixture of the two perfectly matched homologous hybrids and the two heterologous hybrids derived from mixing and reannealing of melted PCR products during amplification. **A,** Single-strand conformation polymorphism analysis. The PCR products are denatured and quick-cooled to prevent legitimate annealing of complementary strands, favoring rapid "snap back" annealing of single strands. Single base changes cause major variation in secondary structure of the single strands, with the A allele having a more compact structure and electrophoresing farther in this example. **B,** Denaturing gradient gel electrophoresis. The products are electrophoresed on a denaturing gradient gel. The GC base pair gives the most stable structure and migrates the farthest before partially denaturing to form relatively immobile Y-like structures. The AT base pair is the next most stable. Fragments containing mismatches are least stable. **C,** Chemical or enzymatic mismatch cleavage. Hybrids containing mismatches are preferentially cleaved by deoxyribonuclease or chemical degradation, as used in Maxam-Gilbert sequencing reactions. Broken fragments are identified by resulting size differences on gel electrophoresis.

that small sequence changes can have on the secondary structure of single- and double-stranded polynucleotide chains, and the second depends on the greater sensitivity of single-stranded than of double-stranded DNA or RNA to both chemical and enzymatic cleavage.

The first technique, known as *denaturing gradient gel electrophoresis*, takes advantage of the alteration of the melting temperature of a double-stranded DNA molecule resulting from the mutation (Fig. 240-3). In this technique, a PCR product is subjected to electrophoresis in an acrylamide gel through increasing concentrations of denaturants, usually formamide and urea.[23] The concentration at which a given DNA molecule is denatured is determined by its sequence. When one end of a DNA fragment is less stable than the other, it tends to separate into single strands, forming a Y-shaped structure. When partial denaturation occurs, the mobility of the DNA molecule in the gel is greatly retarded. The identification of molecules whose migration in the denaturing gradient gel is altered compared with that of wild-type molecules suggests the presence of a mutation. If necessary, one end of the molecule can be stabilized or "clamped" by attaching a guanine-cytosine–rich sequence to one primer, allowing detection of almost all single base changes.[24]

Another conformational technique to identify mutations is *single-stranded conformation polymorphism analysis*.[25] In this technique, a mixture of DNA molecules that were generated by PCR is denatured and then rapidly cooled so that the single strands do not have sufficient time to reanneal to their complementary partners. Instead, they form secondary structures of their own. The secondary structures can be altered dramatically by the presence of even a single point mutation in the mixture of DNA molecules. The resulting conformational change of the molecule alters its electrophoretic mobility in a neutral acrylamide gel. Bands corresponding to each of the single-stranded DNA molecules as well as the double-stranded DNA molecule are observed.

The second group of techniques relies on cleavage of single-stranded regions of DNA or DNA-RNA hybrid molecules. In some of these techniques, a single-stranded RNA or DNA molecule of known sequence is annealed to a PCR product in which a mutation is suspected. The region at which the mismatch occurs creates a single-stranded bubble. This can be detected either by digestion with the enzyme ribonuclease A or by cleavage with a chemical that preferentially attacks single-stranded regions of DNA, such as hydroxylamine.[26] The cleaved products are recognized as fragments of smaller size on a denaturing acrylamide gel. Another technique combines the formation of single-stranded DNA molecules with defined stem and loop structures with enzymatic cleavage using an enzyme that cuts at the 3'-most base of these structures ("cleavase").[27] Mutation of even a single base can change the stem and loop structure, leading to a different cutting pattern with cleavase. These cutting patterns can be recognized as a characteristic set of bands (or "bar code") by acrylamide gel electrophoresis. The use of these indirect techniques for detecting mutations requires confirmation by direct sequencing of the DNA products.

## DIAGNOSIS USING LINKED MARKERS

### PRINCIPLES OF LINKAGE

Although diagnosis by linkage is required for fewer diseases as the knowledge of genetic diseases increases and the technical capabilities to identify mutations improve, it remains a useful tool in some situations.[28–30] The genes causing some diseases have been mapped but have not yet been identified and cloned. The genes causing some other diseases are known, but such a wide variety of mutations can cause the diseases that no efficacious means of testing for all of them has been developed. For these diseases, diagnosis still can be made using linked polymorphic genetic markers.[28] A genetic marker is said to be polymorphic if it occurs in more than one distinguishable form (called an "allele") in a reasonable fraction of the population; usually it does not affect an individual's ability to survive and reproduce. In the past, markers such as blood groups, soluble enzyme variants, or benign structural chromosome variants were used as polymorphic genetic markers. The DNA sequence variations described later have been found to be much more useful and have largely replaced these classic markers.

Linkage results when genes or DNA markers ("loci") are positioned in close physical proximity on the same chromosome. Genetic loci are said to be linked if their alleles tend to be coinherited within families. Genetic linkage should be distinguished from genetic association, which is the nonrandom occurrence together of alleles in populations, rather than in families. Inheritance of a pathologic allele at a disease locus thus can be predicted by the inheritance of an associated allele at a second closely linked polymorphic locus.

## TYPES OF POLYMORPHIC MARKERS

Three basic types of polymorphic markers are commonly used in diagnosis today (Table 240-1). *Restriction fragment length polymorphisms* (RFLPs) were the first DNA sequence variations to be used in diagnosis. These markers result from the natural sequence variation that occurs every 100 to 500 bases in the human genome.[31] These alterations change the recognition sequences for restriction endonucleases. When a DNA probe from the region of interest is annealed to a Southern blot of genomic DNA that has been cut with a given restriction enzyme, a larger fragment (indicative of no restriction site) or two smaller fragments (indicative of an internal restriction site) are observed. Single nucleotide polymorphisms (SNPs) might also be analyzed using ASO technology and oligonucleotide probe arrays, as described for mutation analysis, although this is not yet commonly done.

Other markers are based on short sequences of DNA that are duplicated in tandem a variable number of times. These duplicated sequences occur many times throughout the genome. When the reiterated sequence is 10 to 15 base pairs in length, the markers are called *variable number of tandem repeat (VNTR) markers*.[32] The number of tandem repeat units in the repetitive

**TABLE 240-1.**
**Summary of Commonly Used Polymorphic Markers***

| Type of Polymorphism | Molecular Basis | Repeat Length | Method of Detection | Maximum Number of Alleles* | Notes |
|---|---|---|---|---|---|
| VNTR | Reiterated short sequences | 10–15 bases | Southern blots, some PCR | Many | Same repeat elements as "DNA fingerprints" |
| RFLP and SNP | Single base change | — | Southern blots, some PCR or PCR with ASO or ARMS, oligonucleotide probe arrays | 2 | Classic polymorphism for linkage and diagnosis, possibly expanding role in future analyses as array technology becomes more widely available |
| Microsatellite or STR | Reiterated short sequences | 2–4 bases | PCR with sequencing gels | Many | Most commonly used markers for genetic mapping and diagnostic testing; STS (sequence tagged sites†) |

*VNTR*, variable number of tandem repeats; *PCR*, polymerase chain reaction; *RFLP*, restriction fragment length polymorphism; *SNP*, single nucleotide polymorphism; *ASO*, allele-specific oligonucleotide; *ARMS*, amplification refractory mutation system; *STR*, short tandem repeat.
*The likelihood that an individual will be heterozygous for a polymorphic marker increases as the number of equally frequent alleles for that marker increases.
†Sequence tagged sites are markers that can be analyzed with only knowledge of the sequence. Use of cloned DNA probes is not necessary.

sequence varies, providing an extremely informative marker. The size of a given VNTR sequence can be determined by Southern blot analysis. To identify only one of the many VNTR loci in the genome, the hybridization probe contains a unique sequence that flanks the marker.

The repeat unit for other markers, called *microsatellite* or *short tandem repeat (STR) markers*, is two to four bases in length.[33] The size varies with the number of repeat units in the repetitive sequence. These markers are more useful than others, not only because they tend to be highly polymorphic, but also because they can be analyzed as discrete alleles by PCR and acrylamide gel electrophoresis. Because of their ease of analysis and their highly informative nature, STR markers are used for most molecular diagnostic and mapping linkage studies.

## REQUIREMENTS FOR LINKAGE-BASED DIAGNOSIS

Although diagnosis by linkage analysis does not require detailed knowledge of the causative mutation or even the specific gene causing a disease, some conditions must be met for this type of diagnosis to be used. First, availability and cooperation of certain critical family members is required for diagnosis. For example, to predict whether a patient has inherited the gene for multiple endocrine neoplasia type 1 from his affected father using linked markers, at least one additional affected family member (e.g., the patient's sibling, father's sibling, or parent) must be tested to determine which paternal chromosome is associated with the disease (called "setting the phase"). In addition, the polymorphic markers must be sufficiently variable within a family to identify the parental chromosome that carries the disease-causing mutation. In this example, the father must be heterozygous for the markers tested. The allele that he has transmitted to the patient can then be determined. That allele marks the disease-bearing or normal chromosome.

The accuracy of the diagnosis is best when the markers are close to (or actually within) the disease-causing gene. In this case, crossing over (or recombination) between the marker and disease gene is unlikely and can be discounted. The greater the recombination frequency between the marker and disease locus, the less accurate is the diagnosis. For example, the accuracy of a linkage-based diagnosis using a marker having a recombination frequency of 10% with a disease locus is, at best, 90%. Because of this, the information obtained using linked markers often is probabilistic in nature and must be considered in light of all that is known of the patient's risk for disease, including both laboratory and clinical data. A patient's risk for carrying a disease-producing gene can be calculated by hand or with the LINKAGE program package[34] and can be combined with clinical and other laboratory data using Bayesian analysis.[28]

Accurate diagnosis, however, can be accomplished with linked markers that are some distance from the disease locus if two markers flanking the disease locus contain polymorphisms that can be distinguished in a family (i.e., they are informative). In this case, a recombination event between one marker and the disease would result in a crossover that could be detected between the two markers, unless a second recombination event also occurred between the disease locus and the second marker. Such double recombinations would be rare between two closely spaced markers. One must also remember that, when linked markers are used for diagnosis, the accuracy of the DNA diagnosis is completely dependent on the quality of the clinical diagnosis of the proband. If a proband is misdiagnosed, a "correct" DNA diagnosis may yield absolutely wrong information. Diagnosis using linked markers is potentially complex and has been reviewed in detail.[35]

## PRACTICAL CONSIDERATIONS

In addition to the technical and scientific issues discussed earlier, many practical and counseling issues exist that are equally challenging and important for obtaining a sound diagnosis. The first and most crucial principle is that genetic diagnosis is not an isolated service but should always be provided with appropriate counseling and support. This is perhaps best illustrated by the example of familial medullary carcinoma of the thyroid, in which provision of support to individuals determined to be at risk can be critical.[36] In general, patients should be counseled before testing regarding the types of information that probably will result, the benefits to their care, and any risks inherent in the testing (e.g., possible discovery of mistaken paternity in linkage studies). After the testing is completed, patients should undergo a second counseling session in which the results and their implications are explained in detail and patients are assisted in selecting among therapeutic choices. In practice, this is most often carried out by referral to a local genetics center at which the geneticists and counselors are experienced in providing these services. These specialists also can be of great help in selecting the laboratory to perform the tests and providing current information about which tests are available.

Optimally, a diagnostic test should be carried out in a service-oriented laboratory with a rapid response time and extensive experience in diagnosing the disease in question. Many diagnostic laboratories, both academic and commercial, now meet this description and provide high-quality, dependable service. A list of diseases for which such services are available is provided in Table 240-2. For some conditions, however, the genetic basis of the disease has only recently been recognized. As a result, the methods of testing for mutations in these conditions have not moved from the research laboratory. The genetic bases of other conditions have been recognized for some time, but because they are relatively rare, the market for the test is too small to attract service laboratories. A list of endocrine diseases for which molecular genetic testing is feasible is provided in Table 240-3. Sometimes, only one or two laboratories may be available for the diagnosis of a specific genetic disorder. Because they operate in a research rather than a service mode, the analyses may be performed only periodically, so that waiting times are long. When novel mutations are identified (i.e., rare mutations whose occurrence may be limited to individuals in only one family), their significance may not be known, especially if a functional test is not available. Moreover, the laboratories may be interested in studying affected persons but not in evaluating unaffected relatives or in performing prenatal diagnosis. Unless care is exercised, these circumstances may result in frustration both for the patients and for the physicians and genetic counselors caring for them.

Many resources are available for identifying laboratories that perform genetic tests for specific conditions. A computerized database called Gene Tests is maintained at the Children's Hospital and Medical Center in Seattle, Washington, and can be accessed on the internet at http://www.genetests.org. Gene Tests can also be accessed by telephone at (206) 527-5742 or by facsimile at (206) 527-5743. It offers health care providers current listings of clinical and research laboratories performing disease-specific molecular genetic testing useful in the diagnosis of heritable disorders, as well as a listing of regional clinical genetic service networks and organizations. The New York State Department of Health maintains its own registry of approved laboratories, because the state requires that tests be sent only to laboratories that have been licensed by the state or approved for compassionate use by the state. For conditions for which the genetic basis has only recently become understood, information about the investigating laboratories can be obtained from annual

**TABLE 240-2.**
**Diseases and Other Conditions Diagnosed in Service Laboratories**

α₁-Antitrypsin deficiency
Achondrogenesis type II
Achondroplasia
Acid phosphatase deficiency
Adenomatous polyposis (familial)
Adenosine monophosphate deaminase 1 (AMPD1), deficiency of
Adrenoleukodystrophy, recessive, X-linked
Adult polycystic kidney disease
Agammaglobulinemia, Bruton and Swiss (XSCID)
Alzheimer disease, apolipoprotein E and type 3
Amyloidosis (familial)
Angelman syndrome
Apert syndrome
Aspartylglycosaminuria (glycosylasparaginase deficiency)
Ataxia telangiectasia, Louis-Bar, and Nijmegen breakage syndrome
Azoospermia
Basal cell nevus syndrome (Gorlin syndrome, nevoid basal cell carcinoma)
Beckwith-Wiedemann syndrome
Bone marrow transplantation
*BRCA1, BRCA2* mutations (breast cancer)
Canavan disease
Carbamyl phosphate synthetase I deficiency
Carnitine deficiency
Carnitine-acylcarnitine translocase deficiency
Carnitine palmitoyltransferase (CPT) deficiency, CPT I, CPT II deficiency
Charcot-Marie-Tooth disease type 1, X-linked (CMTX)
Chorea and dementia, transfer RNA mitochondrial myopathy
Chronic granulomatous disease
Citrullinemia
Coffin-Lowry syndrome
Congenital adrenal hyperplasia (21 OH deficiency)
Congenital bilateral absence of the vas deferens (CBAVD)
Craniosynostosis, nonsyndromic, coronal
Cri du chat syndrome
Crouzon syndrome
Cystinosis, infantile, juvenile, and adult
Cytochrome C oxidase deficiency
Cystic fibrosis
Deafness, nonsyndromic
Dentatorubral-pallidoluysian atrophy (DRPLA)
Diabetes insipidus, nephrogenic, X-linked
Diabetes mellitus, type 2
DiGeorge syndrome
Duchenne/Becker muscular dystrophy
Dystonia type 1
Ehlers-Danlos syndrome types I, II, III, IV, VII
Epidermolysis bullosa
Fabry disease, α-galactosidase deficiency
Farber disease, lipogranulomatosis
Factor II mutation (prothrombin, hypercoagulability)
Factor V deficiency, Leiden mutation
Factor VIII deficiency (hemophilia A)
Factor IX deficiency (hemophilia Bl)
Familial adenomatous polyposis (APC, Gardner syndrome)
Familial colorectal cancer
Familial gastric cancer
Familial glucocorticoid deficiency, ACTH resistance
Familial Mediterranean fever
Fanconi anemia
Fascioscapulohumeral muscular dystrophy (FSH)
Fragile X syndrome

Fragile XE (FRAXE) syndrome
Friedrich ataxia
Fructose 1,6-biphosphatase deficiency
Fucosidosis
Galactosemia (galactose-1-phosphate uridyl-transferase deficiency)
Galactosialidosis
Gaucher disease (glucocerebrosidase deficiency)
Genotyping
Glutaric acidemia type II
Glycerol kinase deficiency
Glycogen storage disease types I/Ia, II, III, IV, V, VI, VII, VIII
GM₁ gangliosidosis
Hemochromatosis
Hemoglobin C, E, S disease (SC disease and sickle cell disease)
Hereditary fructose intolerance
Hereditary neuropathy with liability to pressure palsies (HNPP)
Hereditary nonpolyposis colon cancer (HNPCC), Lynch syndrome
Hereditary pancreatitis
Huntington disease
Hydrocephalus, X-linked
Hypochondroplasia
Hypokalemic periodic paralysis (periodic paralysis I)
I-Cell disease (ML II, ML2, mucolipidosis II)
Ichthyosis, X-linked
Jackson-Weiss syndrome
Kell antigen genotyping
Kennedy disease
Kniest dysplasia
Krabbe disease, globoid cell leukodystrophy
Leber hereditary optic neuropathy
Lesch-Nyhan disease
Li-Fraumeni syndrome
Long-chain acyl-CoA dehydrogenase deficiency (LCAD)
Long-chain 3-hydroxyacyl-CoA dehydrogenase deficiency (LCHAD)
α-Mannosidosis
β-Mannosidosis
Marfan syndrome
Medium-chain acyl-CoA dehydrogenase deficiency (MCAD)
Medullary thyroid carcinoma (MTC)
Metachromatic leukodystrophy (MLD)
Miller-Dieker syndrome (lissencephaly)
Mitochondrial myopathy (Kearns-Sayre syndrome, Leigh disease, MELAS, MERRF, NARP)
Metaphyseal chondrodysplasia, Schmid type
MTHFR deficiency (homocystinuria, methylene-tetrahydrofolate reductase deficiency) and thermolabile variant (cardiovascular and neural tube defect risk factors)
Mucopolysaccharidosis types I, II, III, IIIB, IIIC, IIID, IVA, IVB, VI, VII (Hurler, Hunter, Morquio, arylsulfatase B/Maroteaux-Lamy, Sly syndrome)
Multiple endocrine neoplasia types 1, 2A, 2B/3
Myotonic dystrophy
Myotubular myopathy, X-linked
Nail-patella syndrome
Narcolepsy
Neurofibromatosis types I, II
Niemann-Pick disease
Norrie disease

Oculocutaneous albinism type 1 (OCA1, tyrosinase negative)
Oculopharyngeal muscular dystrophy
Ornithine transcarbamylase deficiency (OTC)
Osteogenesis imperfecta types I, II, III, IV
Papillary renal carcinoma
Paraganglioma (carotid body tumor, glomus jugulare tumor)
Parentage (maternity, paternity)
Pearson syndrome
Pelizaeus-Merzbacher disease
Pfeiffer syndrome
Phenylketonuria (PKU)
Phosphoglycerate kinase deficiency (PGK)
Phosphoglycerate mutase deficiency
Platelet antigen genotyping
Polycystic kidney disease, dominant (ADPKD), recessive (ARPKD)
Prader-Willi syndrome
Precocious puberty, male
Preeclampsia (toxemia of pregnancy)
Pseudoachondroplasia
Pseudocholinesterase deficiency
Pseudo–Hurler polydystrophy (ML III, mucolipidosis III)
Retinoblastoma
Rh C, D, E genotyping
Rubinstein-Taybi syndrome
Russell-Silver syndrome
Saethre-Chotzen syndrome
Salla disease, sialic acid storage disease
Sandhoff disease
Sialidosis, ML1, mucolipidosis I, glycoprotein neuraminidase deficiency
Sialuria, French type
Schindler disease
Short-chain acyl-CoA dehydrogenase deficiency (SCAD)
Smith-Magenis syndrome
Spinal muscular atrophy types I, II, III
Spinocerebellar ataxia types I, II, III, VI, VII
Spondyloepimetaphyseal dysplasia, Strudwick type
Spondyloepiphyseal dysplasia (SED)
SRY detection
Stickler syndrome
Sulfatidosis, juvenile, Austin type (mucosulfatidosis, multiple sulfatase deficiency)
Tay-Sachs disease
α-Thalassemia
β-Thalassemia
Thanatophoric dysplasia types I and II
Thyroid hormone resistance (thyroid hormone β-receptor deficiency)
Uniparental disomy
Velocardiofacial syndrome
Very long chain acyl-CoA dehydrogenase deficiency (VLCAD)
Von Hippel-Lindau syndrome
Waardenburg syndrome type I
Williams syndrome
Wilson disease
Wiskott-Aldrich syndrome
Wolf-Hirschhorn syndrome (4p–)
Wolman disease, cholesterol ester storage disease
X-linked lymphoproliferative disease
X inactivation
Y chromosome detection
Zellweger syndrome
Zygosity (twinning)

*APC*, adenomatous polyposis of the colon; *ACTH*, adrenocorticotropic hormone; *CoA*, coenzyme A; *MELAS*, mitochondrial myelopathy, encephalopathy, lactic acidosis, and stroke-like episodes; *MERRF*, myoclonic epilepsy associated with ragged red fibers; *NARP*, neuropathy, ataxia, and retinitis pigmentosa; *SRY*, sex-determining region y.

**TABLE 240-3.**
**Endocrine Diseases and Conditions for Which DNA Studies Are Possible**

| | |
|---|---|
| Adrenal hyperplasia (CYP21B deficiency) | Hypoparathyroidism |
| Aldosteronism, sensitive to dexamethasone | Hypothyroidism |
| Adrenal hypoplasia congenita | Immunodeficiency syndrome, X-linked (diarrhea, autoimmunity, polyendo-crinopathy |
| Androgen resistance | Iodide transport defect |
| Angioneurotic edema types 1 and 2 | Kallmann syndrome, hypogonadotrophic hypogonadism/anosmia |
| Antimüllerian hormone deficiency | LCAT deficiency |
| Apolipoprotein deficiencies (A-I, B, E) | LDL deficiency |
| Breast cancer (early onset, *BRCA1, BRCA2*)* | Leydig cell hypoplasia/agenesis |
| Chylomicronemia | Liddle syndrome; pseudoaldosteronism |
| Congenital adrenal hyperplasia, X-linked (AHC) | Lipoprotein lipase deficiency |
| Congenital adrenal hyperplasia (21-OH, 11β OH deficiency)* | McCune-Albright syndrome |
| Congenital lipoid adrenal hyperplasia (lipoid CAH) | Multiple endocrine neoplasia types 1, 2A, 2B/3* |
| Corticosterone methyl oxidase II deficiency | Ovarian cancer (familial)* |
| Denys-Drash syndrome*; Wilms tumor and pseudohermaphroditism | Osteopetrosis |
| Diabetes insipidus (nephrogenic, neurohypophysial)* | Osteoporosis |
| Diabetes mellitus (autosomal dominant, maturity-onset diabetes of youth [MODY]) | Pearson syndrome*; sideroblastic anemia with marrow cell vacuolization and exocrine pancreatic dysfunction |
| Diabetes-deafness syndrome | Pendred syndrome*; goiter-deafness syndrome; thyroid hormonogenesis defect IIB |
| DiGeorge syndrome* | Porphyria |
| Dwarfism (Laron type) | Precocious puberty, male* |
| Euthyroid hyperthyroxinemia | Preeclampsia* |
| Follicle-stimulating hormone deficiency | Premature ovarian failure |
| Gastrinoma | Pseudohermaphroditism |
| Glucocorticoid receptor deficiency | Pseudohypoparathyroidism |
| Gonadal dysgenesis | Steroid hydroxylase 2β, 5α, 17α, 18, 21; see CAH* |
| Growth hormone deficiency | Swyer syndrome; 46,XY gonadal dysgenesis* |
| Hepatic lipase deficiency | Thyroid carcinoma (medullary)* |
| Hyperaldosteronism, familial | TBG deficiency |
| Hyperalphalipoproteinemia | TSH deficiency |
| Hypercalcemia (hypercalciuric) | Thyroid hormone–receptor defects* |
| Hypercholesterolemia | Vas deferens, congenital bilateral aplasia* |
| Hyperinsulinism (nesidioblastosis) | Vitamin D–resistant rickets |
| Hyperlipidemia (combined, type 1) | Y chromosome detection* |
| Hyperproinsulinemia | |
| Hypobetalipoproteinemia | |
| Hyperparathyroidism, primary familial (multiple endocrine neoplasia type 1 region) | |

*LCAT*, lecithin-cholesterol acyltransferase; *LDL*, low-density lipoprotein; *CAH*, congenital adrenal hyperplasia; *TBG*, thyroxine-binding globulin; *TSH*, thyroid-stimulating hormone.
*Listed clinically in Helix database.

reviews listing papers on molecular genetic diagnosis[37]; through Medline at the National Library of Medicine (URL http://igm.nlm.nih.gov); or through databases such as Online Mendelian Inheritance in Man, a database maintained at the National Center for Biotechnology Information (URL http://www.ncbi.nlm.nih.gov/Omim). This database is a catalog of single-gene conditions and includes a listing of mutations that have been identified in specific genes. It is updated on a regular basis.

In summary, although the availability of DNA analysis for the diagnosis of inherited diseases provides a powerful tool for the practitioner, pitfalls are also present in its use. Because the technology is advancing rapidly, with new diseases being diagnosed and new techniques used monthly, only general suggestions can be provided. The best approach is to understand the principles on which the tests are based and to apply them on a disease-by-disease basis. This is much more straightforward with the help of an experienced medical geneticist or genetic counselor. Careful application of DNA analysis in the proper setting can improve patient care dramatically, often in cases that are refractory to classic diagnostic techniques.

# REFERENCES

1. Calender A, Giraud S, Schuffenecker I, et al. Genetic testing in presymptomatic diagnosis of multiple endocrine neoplasia. Horm Res 1997; 47:199.
2. Lemmens I, Van de Ven WJ, Kas K, et al. Identification of the multiple endocrine neoplasia type 1 (MEN1) gene. The European Consortium on MEN1. Hum Mol Genet 1997; 6:1177.
3. Lissens W, Sermon K, Staessen C, et al. Review: preimplantation diagnosis of inherited disease. J Inherit Metab Dis 1996; 19:709.
4. Laue L, Chan WY, Hsueh AJ, et al. Genetic heterogeneity of constitutively activating mutations of the human luteinizing hormone receptor in familial male-limited precocious puberty. Proc Natl Acad Sci U S A 1995; 92:1906.
5. Stoffel M, Patel P, Lo YM, et al. Missense glucokinase mutation in maturity-onset diabetes of the young and mutation screening in late-onset diabetes. Nat Genet 1992; 2:153.
6. Hager J, Blanche H, Sun F, et al. Six mutations in the glucokinase gene identified in MODY by using a nonradioactive sensitive screening technique. Diabetes 1994; 43:730.
7. Yamagata K, Furuta H, Oda N, et al. Mutations in the hepatocyte nuclear factor-4 alpha gene in maturity-onset diabetes of the young (MODY1). Nature 1996; 384:458.
8. Yamagata K, Oda N, Kaisaki PJ, et al. Mutations in the hepatocyte nuclear factor-1 alpha gene in maturity-onset diabetes of the young (MODY3). Nature 1996; 384:455.
9. Joshi VV, Cantor AB, Brodeur GM, et al. Correlation between morphologic and other prognostic markers of neuroblastoma. A study of histologic grade, DNA index, N-myc gene copy number, and lactic dehydrogenase in patients in the Pediatric Oncology Group. Cancer 1993; 71:3173.
10. Mies C. Molecular pathology of paraffin-embedded tissue. Current clinical applications. Diagn Mol Pathol 1992; 1:206.
11. Caskey CT, Pizzuti A, Fu YH, et al. Triplet repeat mutations in human disease. Science 1992; 256:784.
12. Ashley CT Jr, Warren ST. Trinucleotide repeat expansion and human disease. Annu Rev Genet 1995; 29:703.
13. Schmickel RD. Contiguous gene syndromes: a component of recognizable syndromes. J Pediatr 1986; 109:231.
14. Saiki R, Scharf S, Faloona F, et al. Enzymatic amplification of B-globin genomic sequences and restriction site analysis for diagnosis of sickle cell anemia. Science 1985; 230:1350.
15. McGowan KD. Preimplantation prenatal diagnosis. X. Obstet Gynecol Clin North Am 1993; 20:599.
16. Shuber AP, Skoletsky J, Stern R, Handelin BL. Efficient 12-mutation testing

in the CFTR gene: a general model for complex mutation analysis. Hum Mol Genet 1993; 2:153.

17. Newton CR, Graham A, Heptinstall L, et al. Analysis of any point mutation in DNA. The amplification refractory mutation system (ARMS). Nucleic Acids Res 1989; 17:2503.

18. Barany F. Genetic disease detection and DNA amplification using cloned thermostable ligase. Proc Natl Acad Sci U S A 1991; 88:189.

19. Lipshutz RJ, Morris D, Chee M, et al. Using oligonucleotide probe arrays to access genetic diversity. Biotechniques 1995; 19:442.

20. Hacia JG, Brody LC, Chee MS, et al. Detection of heterozygous mutations in BRCA1 using high density oligonucleotide arrays and two-colour fluorescence analysis. Nat Genet 1996; 14:441.

21. Pastinen T, Kurg A, Metspalu A, et al. Minisequencing: a specific tool for DNA analysis and diagnostics on oligonucleotide arrays. Genome Res 1997; 7:606.

21a. Suomalainen A, Syvanen AC. Quantitative analysis of human DNA sequences by PCR and solid-phase minisequencing. Mol Biotechnol 2000; 15:123.

22. Shuber AP, Michalowsky LA, Nass GS, et al. High throughput parallel analysis of hundreds of patient samples for more than 100 mutations in multiple disease genes. Hum Mol Genet 1997; 6:337.

23. Myers RM, Maniatis T, Lerman LS. Detection and localization of single base changes by denaturing gradient gel electrophoresis. Methods Enzymol 1987; 155:501.

24. Myers RM, Fischer SG, Lerman LS, Maniatis T. Nearly all single base substitutions in DNA fragments joined to a GC-clamp can be detected by denaturing gradient gel electrophoresis. Nucleic Acids Res 1985; 13:3131.

25. Orita M, Iwahana H, Kanazawa H, et al. Detection of polymorphisms of human DNA by gel electrophoresis as single-strand conformation polymorphisms. Proc Natl Acad Sci U S A 1989; 86:2766.

26. Cotton RG, Rodrigues NR, Campbell RD. Reactivity of cytosine and thymine in single-base-pair mismatches with hydroxylamine and osmium tetroxide and its application to the study of mutations. Proc Natl Acad Sci U S A 1988; 85:4397.

27. Rossetti S, Englisch S, Bresin E, et al. Detection of mutations in human genes by a new rapid method: cleavage fragment length polymorphism analysis (CFLPA). Mol Cell Probes 1997; 11:155.

28. Hejtmancik JF, Ward P, Tantravahi U, et al. Genetic analysis: a practical approach to linkage, pedigrees, and Bayesian risk. In: Rowland LP, Wood DS, Schon EA, DiMauro S, eds. Molecular genetics in diseases of brain, nerve, and muscle. New York: Oxford University Press, 1989:191.

29. Ekelund J, Lichterman D, Hovatta I, et al. Genome-wide scan for schizophrenia in the Finnish population: evidence for a locus on chromosome 7q22. Hum Mol Genet 2000; 9:1049.

30. Paterson AD, Petronis A. Age of diagnosis-based linkage analysis in type 1 diabetes. Eur J Hum Genet 2000; 8:145.

31. Botstein D, White RL, Skolnick M, Davis RW. Construction of a genetic linkage map in man using restriction fragment length polymorphisms. Am J Hum Genet 1980; 32:314.

32. Nakamura Y, Leppert M, O'Connell P, et al. Variable number of tandem repeat (VNTR) markers for human gene mapping. Science 1987; 235:1616.

33. Weber JL, May PE. Abundant class of human DNA polymorphisms which can be typed using the polymerase chain reaction. Am J Hum Genet 1989; 44:388.

34. Lathrop GM, Lalouel JM. Easy calculations of lod scores and genetic risks on small computers. Am J Hum Genet 1984; 36:460.

35. Ostrer H, Hejtmancik JF. Prenatal diagnosis and carrier detection of genetic diseases by analysis of deoxyribonucleic acid. J Pediatr 1988; 112:679.

36. Giuffrida D, Gharib H. Current diagnosis and management of medullary thyroid carcinoma. Ann Oncol 1998; 9:695.

37. Cooper DN, Schmidtke J. Diagnosis of human genetic disease using recombinant DNA: fourth edition. (Review). Hum Genet 1993; 92:211.

# CHAPTER 241

# DYNAMIC PROCEDURES IN ENDOCRINOLOGY

D. ROBERT DUFOUR AND WILLIAM A. JUBIZ

## WHY PERFORM DYNAMIC ENDOCRINE STUDIES?

Because of the complex interrelationships in the endocrine system, evaluating the actual status of an endocrine organ by determining the concentration of a hormone produced by that organ at a certain time is often difficult. As emphasized in Chapter 237, many factors can affect the results of endocrine tests. Early changes in endocrine function may go undetected because a patient's results are compared with published reference ranges rather than with the patient's regular values. For example, a common reference range for calcium is 8.5 to 10.5 mg/dL; a patient who usually has a serum calcium concentration in the lower range of normal, and who now has a calcium concentration of 10.4, may have a disturbance of calcium homeostasis, even though both values are within the reference range.

The endocrine system is characterized by an ability to adjust quickly to changes in hormone concentrations or requirements. In some endocrine organs or tissues, rising concentrations of a substance regulated by a hormone result in decreased production of the hormone, a phenomenon known as *feedback inhibition* (see Chap. 5). Similarly, decreased concentrations of the regulated substance often stimulate hormone production. In endocrine disease, a regulatory system is disordered, either due to the failure of production of a hormone, as in *deficiency states,* or due to autonomous overproduction of a hormone, as in *hyperfunctional states*. In primary hypothyroidism, for example, low plasma thyroid hormone concentrations are accompanied by overproduction of thyroid-stimulating hormone (TSH). In established disease conditions, the diagnosis often is obvious because of abnormal circulating concentrations of these affected hormones. In the early stages of disease, however, the normal diurnal and individual differences in hormone concentrations may make it difficult to tell whether a person actually has normal or abnormal endocrine function. By studying the endocrine organ's response to one or more stimuli, a physician can gain additional information about its functional state. In the case of early hypothyroidism, measuring the response to thyrotropin-releasing hormone (TRH) can demonstrate the hyperfunctional state of the pituitary thyrotropes.

Dynamic evaluation of the function of the endocrine system has become widespread and often provides the key to recognizing the presence of an underlying endocrine disease. The limitations of dynamic endocrine procedures, however, are rarely emphasized. Many references imply that these procedures are highly sensitive and specific "tests" for a particular endocrine disease. As might be expected from the information provided in Chapter 237, such assumptions usually are not valid. Many physiologic and pharmacologic factors can affect the results of dynamic endocrine procedures, and these should be considered before deciding to perform the procedure as well as when interpreting its results.

## OVERVIEW OF DYNAMIC ENDOCRINE PROCEDURES

All endocrine organs are under the control of regulatory and counterregulatory mechanisms that allow the body to respond quickly to changing hormonal requirements. The amount of hormone produced by an organ or tissue depends on the balance between stimulatory and inhibitory factors. In the normal state, some cells may be actively producing hormone, whereas others are inactive. In many endocrine tissues, a hormone produced by the secretory cells is stored.

When the body requires the hormone, stimulatory or trophic factors may cause increased hormonal output by two mechanisms: increased release of hormone from cells that already are producing it, and recruitment of additional cells for active hormone synthesis. Because hormone synthesis may require several hours, the recruitment of inactive cells may not produce an immediate increase in blood hormone concentrations. In this simplistic view, if a stimulatory factor is administered as part of a dynamic test, the logical assumption would be that only those cells actively producing hormone would be able to respond initially. If the stimulatory factor has a short half-life, the increase in hormone concentration is related to the number of cells actively producing hormone at the time of the test. If a long-acting trophic factor is administered, or if the concentration of the stimulatory substance is maintained at an elevated level by repeated administration, the hormonal response is related directly to the total number of cells capable of producing the hormone. Similar considerations pertain for inhibitory factors.

Several assumptions are implicit in the use of dynamic endocrine procedures. The stimulatory or inhibitory factor must reach the target organ or tissue and, in the cells, the substance must be able to combine with the appropriate receptors to stimulate or inhibit hormone production. The method used to measure the response should be specific and sensitive enough to detect small changes in hormone concentrations, and no concurrent factors must be present that affect the rate of hormone production. Provided all these assumptions are correct, the status of an endocrine organ should be able to be evaluated by the nature of its response.

## POTENTIAL PITFALLS OF DYNAMIC ENDOCRINE PROCEDURES

Situations exist in which one or more of the required assumptions are not met. Evaluating the exact effects of failure to meet these assumptions is difficult, because many dynamic procedures are relatively new and the factors affecting the interpretation of their results are not well studied. Nevertheless, evidence is accumulating that dynamic procedures are subject to an impressive variety of confounding factors that may make interpretation difficult or impossible.

### ARRIVAL AT THE TARGET ORGAN OR TISSUE

Failure of the stimulatory or inhibitory factor to arrive at the target organ is an important cause of unexpected dynamic test results. For example, one of the first dynamic procedures was the dexamethasone suppression test, in which the potent glucocorticoid decreases adrenocorticotropic hormone (ACTH) output, which then decreases cortisol production by the adrenal gland. However, abnormal dexamethasone suppression test results have been reported in patients receiving diphenylhydantoin, because of an increased rate of metabolism of dexamethasone.[1]

### INTERACTION WITH THE TARGET ORGAN OR TISSUE

Once the influencing factor reaches the target organ, it must be able to interact with cellular receptors. Many endocrine cells can respond to more than one influencing factor, and inhibition of the receptors for one factor may block the response to other factors as well. For example, pituitary somatotropes can secrete growth hormone (GH) in response to numerous stimuli, including hypoglycemia and growth hormone–releasing hormone (GHRH). Hyperglycemia decreases GH output and inhibits the response to GHRH.[2]

Once the influencing factor has combined with its receptor, cell activation usually is mediated by a "second messenger" (e.g., calcium, cyclic adenosine monophosphate [cAMP]). Compounds that alter the concentration of intracellular calcium (e.g., calcium-channel blockers) or of cAMP (e.g., methylxanthines such as theophylline) may block or enhance the response of an organ or tissue to an influencing factor. Thus, calcium-channel blockers decrease cortisol production in response to ACTH stimulation, decrease the response of many pituitary hormones to their respective hypothalamic releasing factors, and decrease

insulin release in response to glucose and glucagon.[3–5] Theophylline, which augments cellular cAMP concentrations, increases the TSH response to TRH, but decreases the GH response to GHRH.[6,7]

## SENSITIVITY AND SPECIFICITY OF THE ASSAY TO MEASURE THE RESPONSE

To detect a change in hormone concentrations, the assay used must be sensitive and specific enough to indicate that an appropriate change has occurred. For example, interferences in the TSH assay using monoclonal immunoglobulins result in falsely elevated values for the TSH concentration, which do not change in response to TRH infusion.[8] Assays also should have the necessary sensitivity to detect an appropriate change in hormone concentrations. This is critical in suppression testing, in which the hormone concentration must fall below a certain value for a response to be recognized. Many of the cortisol assays used to measure the response to dexamethasone suppression may give a false indication of either suppression or nonsuppression because of problems with sensitivity, specificity, or both.[9] Similar problems with other assays may become apparent as dynamic procedures become more popular.

## OTHER FACTORS AFFECTING THE RESULTS OF DYNAMIC ENDOCRINE PROCEDURES

The major causes of uncertainty in interpreting the results of dynamic endocrine procedures are the same ones that can yield unexpected results in all other laboratory tests, as outlined in Chapter 237. These include normal variations within a given individual at different times of the day, month, or year; physiologic differences such as age, sex, and nutritional status; and use of medications that directly or indirectly affect test results. In addition, evidence is found that other disorders, endocrine and nonendocrine, may affect the results of dynamic endocrine procedures.

### INDIVIDUAL VARIATIONS

Just as basal concentrations of a hormone may differ in a given individual from day to day or at different times of the day, so may the responses to normal stimuli. For example, probably the most commonly used dynamic procedure for evaluating the pituitary-thyroid axis is TRH stimulation, which measures the change in serum TSH after the administration of TRH. The serum TSH response is slightly greater in the evening than in the morning, and the response is significantly higher in the winter months than in the summer.[10] In women, the TSH response is higher during the follicular phase of the menstrual cycle than at other times.[6] In addition, considerable day-to-day variation in the TSH response is found, with the peak TSH response varying by as much as 5 IU/L in a given individual.[11] Similar variations have been found for other dynamic procedures.

### PHYSIOLOGIC FACTORS

Physiologic factors are important contributors to the results of dynamic procedures. The TSH response to TRH is greater in women than in men, and the response decreases in older individuals, especially men.[12] In pregnancy, the TSH response is decreased in the first trimester, probably because of increased serum free thyroxine concentrations.[13] The serum TSH response to TRH decreases during prolonged fasting, an important consideration for persons who are not eating normally.[14] Obesity alters several endocrine responses, including those of insulin, GH, and cortisol to hypoglycemia.[15]

## DRUG EFFECTS

Drugs may alter the results of dynamic procedures by several different mechanisms. First, drugs may block the interaction of the influencing factor with its receptor or interfere with the effect of this interaction by altering cellular concentrations of the second messenger. Some drugs affect endocrine responsiveness by altering basal hormone concentrations. Many drugs decrease the production of thyroid hormone (see Chap. 237), thereby increasing the TSH response to TRH by producing a mild hypothyroidism. With other drugs, the cause of the abnormal results remains unexplained. For example, diphenylhydantoin has been shown to decrease serum free thyroid hormone concentrations, apparently due to an increased fractional metabolic rate. Although this may be expected to cause a subclinical hypothyroidism, making the pituitary more responsive to the effects of TRH, a blunted response to TRH actually is seen in patients receiving the drug.[16]

## EFFECTS OF OTHER DISEASES

Many disease processes can affect the results of dynamic endocrine procedures. Other endocrine disorders may cause hormonal abnormalities that directly interfere with test interpretation. For example, because TRH is known to be a stimulus for prolactin release, it has been used as a test of lactotrope function. In persons with coexisting thyroid disease, however, TRH concentrations may be affected by the normal feedback loop. Thus, in persons with hypothyroidism, low concentrations of thyroid hormone may result in increased hypothalamic production of TRH. If so, the endogenous TRH could stimulate the lactotrope cells to produce prolactin, raising the serum concentrations of this hormone. This would further augment the prolactin response to exogenous TRH. The opposite change would occur in persons with hyperthyroidism.[17] Cases of patients with hypothyroidism who initially were thought to have prolactin-producing adenomas, partly on the basis of abnormal results of dynamic procedures, have been reported.[18] Similar unexpectedly abnormal test results have been reported for aldosterone responsiveness in patients with hypopituitarism, for GH responses in patients with hypothyroidism, and for calcitonin responses in patients with hyperparathyroidism.[19–21]

Evidence is increasing that psychiatric disorders are caused by an imbalance in the levels of neurotransmitters in the brain. Because many neurotransmitters are important in determining the responsiveness of the pituitary and hypothalamus, the fact that an extremely high frequency of abnormal results of dynamic procedures is seen in patients with psychiatric disorders is not surprising. A series of studies[22–24] showed that almost any dynamic procedure may have abnormal results in patients with a variety of psychological problems.

Nonendocrine diseases also may affect the results of dynamic endocrine procedures. Probably the best-known example is dexamethasone suppression testing. Because stress is a known stimulus for ACTH secretion, the fact that a high percentage of hospitalized patients have "abnormal" dexamethasone suppression test results (i.e., decreased suppression) is not surprising.[25,26] Other disorders are associated with abnormal results of dynamic procedures that are not easy to explain. For example, suppressibility of insulin secretion by hypoglycemia is decreased in patients with cirrhosis.[27] Persons with chronic renal failure may show enhanced calcitonin release in response to calcium infusion.[28] In patients with autonomic nerve dysfunction, the response of vasopressin to acute volume depletion is diminished.[29] Because dynamic procedures are performed in individuals with suspected endocrine disease, these and other unreported effects of nonendocrine disease must be kept in mind when interpreting the results.

# UNRESOLVED ISSUES

## DYNAMIC RESPONSES AND BASAL HORMONE CONCENTRATIONS

The relationship between basal hormone concentrations and endocrine responsiveness has been evaluated for only a few endocrine systems. Because the assumption that basal hormone concentrations are important in feedback inhibition (or lack thereof) seems reasonable, a relationship between basal hormone concentrations and dynamic response should be expected. In the typical hypothalamic–pituitary–endocrine organ system, the amount of hormone produced by an endocrine organ represents the degree of stimulation by the pituitary. Thus, high circulating concentrations of a hormone represent near-maximal functioning of the organ. In this situation, administration of an influencing substance should have little additional effect. This predicted result is observed with the serum cortisol response to ACTH infusion, which is inversely related to basal serum cortisol concentrations.[30] On the other hand, high endogenous plasma ACTH concentrations may indicate the presence of cells that are hyperactive due to lack of feedback inhibition. Rapid infusion of a hypothalamic releasing hormone may lead to a larger increase in plasma concentrations of the pituitary hormone than in patients with low basal concentrations. This predicted response also is observed in the TRH infusion test.[12]

Published data do not indicate such a relationship for most dynamic endocrine procedures. This probably represents a lack of research on this subject rather than a lack of such relationships. Caution should be used in applying published reference ranges for endocrine response to patients whose basal hormone concentrations are at the low or high ends of reference ranges, because an "average" response should be expected only in patients with "average" basal hormone concentrations. In addition, published reference ranges often are based on results obtained from study of a handful of normal individuals.

## METHOD FOR QUANTIFYING THE RESPONSE

Considerable confusion exists about how best to express the response to a dynamic challenge to the endocrine system. The simplest method would be to measure the *peak hormone concentration* observed after stimulation, with the implication that any value above a certain cutoff represents adequate hormone production. This approach commonly leads to erroneous interpretations if responses are related to basal concentrations. The same criticism could be applied to the use of an *absolute difference* in hormone concentrations between the pretest and posttest samples (Δ value). A more appropriate approach would be to express the increase as a fraction of the basal concentration (*percentage change*). This has the advantage of correcting the response for the physiologic factors of the specific patient. For some dynamic tests, such as the prolactin and TSH responses to TRH and the insulin response to hyperglycemia, comparative studies[12,17] have shown that this method of reporting provides more reliable data than do the first two methods. Other investigators have recommended the use of an *integrated response*. This method involves measuring hormone concentrations at several times after stimulation, drawing a curve connecting these points, and integrating the area under the curve.

Although each of the four methods of reporting results has some advantage, no consensus exists about which is best. The different methods of evaluating a response often give divergent interpretations. For example, in one study[31] in which gastrin responses to secretin were evaluated before and after parathyroidectomy, the gastrin response was expressed in three different ways. Compared with the preoperative response, an increased responsiveness was seen if the gastrin response was expressed as a percentage of the basal concentration, an unchanged responsiveness if absolute change was used, and a decreased integrated responsiveness. This points out the need for uniform reporting of dynamic testing. Percentage change probably is the most useful reporting format for most procedures.

## RESPONSIVENESS OF ENDOCRINE TUMORS

In contrast to the situation in hyperplasia, in which the change in the number of functional cells is an appropriate response to a changing need for the hormone, neoplasia represents a somewhat autonomous proliferation of cells. Nevertheless, in most cases, the autonomy is not absolute. A tumor depends on the host for its blood supply, and in many cases, an endocrine tumor still may be somewhat responsive to changes in the concentration of normal stimulatory and inhibitory factors. Neoplasms are not identical; the same histologic type of tumor may have a totally different behavior in different individuals. All endocrine tumors do not show the same degree of autonomy or the same pattern of responsiveness to different influencing factors (see Chap. 219).

Although most endocrine tumors do not show the same degree of feedback inhibition or stimulation as do normal, nonneoplastic endocrine cells, they often retain limited responsiveness to normal control mechanisms. For example, cells from parathyroid adenomas decrease their production of parathyroid hormone in response to increasing calcium concentrations, although they do not show maximal feedback inhibition unless serum calcium concentrations are well above the reference range.[32] Similar results have been observed for other endocrine tumors, and this observation has proved beneficial in their treatment, as in the treatment of prolactinomas with bromocriptine, an agent similar in action to the normal prolactin inhibitory factor (see Chap. 21).

These observations suggest that caution may be necessary in interpreting the results of dynamic procedures in patients with endocrine tumors, because not all tumors behave in the same way. For example, in a study of patients with GH-producing tumors of the pituitary,[33] most had diminished responses to all commonly used GH stimuli (e.g., L-dopa, insulin-induced hypoglycemia, GHRH, and clonidine), but some had increased responses to all stimuli, and a few responded to some stimuli but not to others. In patients with elevated serum prolactin concentrations, stimulatory tests cannot reliably distinguish those with pituitary tumors from those with elevated prolactin levels due to other causes.[17] Thus, to make a diagnosis of neoplasia on the basis of an apparent autonomy demonstrated by a dynamic procedure, or to rule neoplasia out based on its absence, is unwise.

## USE AND ABUSE OF DYNAMIC PROCEDURES

Dynamic endocrine procedures are subject to many of the same limitations as are other forms of endocrine laboratory investigation. Although dynamic procedures may suggest that the response to a challenge appears to be adequate, the interpretation must take into consideration the physiologic, individual, and pharmacologic factors that affect the results. Although these usually are not considered in the initial evaluation of diagnostic procedures, one review[34] has documented the errors that may result from failure to consider them before a test is adopted for diagnostic use. As further research assesses these interactions, the role of dynamic procedures should become clearer.

For the present, the following approach is suggested. Ideally, dynamic evaluation should be performed in the morning in persons who have stopped taking all medications for at least 3 to 4 days (longer for medications with a long half-life). If a patient normally works nights, the procedure should be done shortly after awakening, because diurnal variation in endocrine responses often is determined by time of awakening.[35] Studies should be performed on acutely ill individuals only if absolutely necessary, because stress often alters normal endocrine responses. In general, in postoperative patients, many endocrine responses return to preoperative baseline levels within 24 hours of surgery.[36]

If studies are performed in this controlled fashion, and if no other concurrent illnesses are present, the results of dynamic procedures may be useful in evaluating the endocrine system. Unfortunately, it is in situations in which these conditions cannot be met that the greatest need usually exists to evaluate endocrine function. The results of dynamic procedures should be interpreted with great caution, because they may be affected by medications, concurrent illnesses, or the physiologic changes accompanying stress.

*Dynamic endocrine procedures are not diagnostic tests.* The fact that they are dynamic neither implies that they are accurate nor suggests that they are appropriate. Several of these procedures have been shown to be of little value in the evaluation of endocrine disease; they are included, with their appropriate references, for those who wish to perform them for nonclinical, investigative purposes. *All these pharmacologic challenges must be evaluated with due consideration for their intrinsic limitations, the possible presence of any interfering factors, and the overall clinical picture.*

## REFERENCE RANGES FOR DYNAMIC ENDOCRINE PROCEDURES: EXPLANATION OF TABLE 241-1

Although many dynamic endocrine procedures are listed in Table 241-1, no attempt has been made to be exhaustively complete. The reference ranges given are derived from published studies, and the dosages of stimulatory or inhibitory factors are those used by the authors of this chapter or by the authors of the references cited. For the categories of individual variation, physiologic changes, and drug effects, an attempt has been made to provide the most complete information available. For modifications of the procedures, for other opinions concerning their utility, and for additional alternative procedures, consult the indicated chapters.

The procedures in Table 241-1 are arranged to make them easier to locate and to allow comparison among several alternative procedures. All procedures are listed *under the end organ evaluated*, with the organs listed in alphabetical order. The subheadings list the regulatory axis evaluated, the particular organ in that axis whose function is being studied, and whether the procedure is used to stimulate or inhibit function. For example, the first organ listed is the adrenal gland. Separate subheadings are given for the hypothalamic–pituitary–adrenocortical axis, the renin–angiotensin–aldosterone axis, and the adrenal medulla; additional subheadings are found under these categories.

Table 241-1 begins on page 2268.

# REFERENCES (For this chapter, including Table 241-1.)

1. Jubiz W, et al. Effect of diphenylhydantoin on the metabolism of dexamethasone. N Engl J Med 1970; 283:11.
2. Masuda A, et al. The effect of glucose on growth hormone (GH)-releasing hormone-mediated GH secretion in man. J Clin Endocrinol Metab 1985; 60:523.
3. Guthrie GP, et al. Effects of intravenous and oral verapamil upon pressor and adrenal steroidogenic responses in normal man. J Clin Endocrinol Metab 1983; 57:339.
4. Barbarino A, et al. Calcium antagonists and hormone release. II. Effects of verapamil on basal, gonadotropin-releasing hormone- and thyrotropin-releasing hormone-induced pituitary hormone release in normal subjects. J Clin Endocrinol Metab 1980; 51:749.
5. De Marinis J, et al. Calcium antagonists and hormone release. I. Effects of verapamil on insulin release in normal subjects and patients with islet-cell tumor. Metabolism 1980; 29:599.
6. Scanlon MF, et al. In: Griffiths EC, Bennett GW, eds. Thyrotropin releasing hormone. New York: Raven Press, 1983:303.
7. Losa M, et al. Theophylline blunts the GH-response to growth hormone releasing hormone in normal subjects. Acta Endocrinol (Copenh) 1986; 112:473.
8. Brennan MD, et al. Heterophilic serum antibodies: a cause for falsely elevated serum thyrotropin levels. Mayo Clin Proc 1987; 62:894.
9. Ritchie JC, et al. Plasma cortisol determination for the dexamethasone suppression test. Comparison of competitive protein-binding and commercial radioimmunoassay methods. Arch Gen Psychiatry 1985; 42:493.
10. Harrop JS, et al. Circannual and within-individual variation of thyroid function tests in normal subjects. Ann Clin Biochem 1985; 22:371.
11. Sawin CT, et al. The TSH response to thyrotropin-releasing hormone (TRH) in young adult men: intra-individual variation and relation to basal serum TSH and thyroid hormones. J Clin Endocrinol Metab 1976; 42:809.
12. Enfurth E, et al. Normal reference interval for thyrotropin response to thyroliberin: dependence on age, sex, free thyroxin index, and basal concentrations of thyrotropin. Clin Chem 1984; 30:196.
13. Guillaume J, et al. Components of the total serum thyroid hormone concentrations during pregnancy: high free thyroxine and blunted thyrotropin (TSH) response to TSH-releasing hormone in the first trimester. J Clin Endocrinol Metab 1985; 60:678.
14. Vinik AI, et al. Fasting blunts the TSH response to synthetic thyrotropin-releasing hormone (TRH). J Clin Endocrinol Metab 1975; 40:509.
15. Vizner B, et al. Effect of l-dopa on growth hormone, glucose, insulin, and cortisol response in obese subjects. Exp Clin Endocrinol 1983; 81:41.
16. Surks MI, et al. Diphenylhydantoin inhibits the thyrotropin response to thyrotropin-releasing hormone in man and rat. J Clin Endocrinol Metab 1983; 56:940.
17. Barbieri RL, et al. Prolactin response to thyrotropin-releasing hormone (TRH) in patients with hypothalamic-pituitary disease. Fertil Steril 1985; 43:66.
18. Grubb MR, et al. Patients with primary hypothyroidism presenting as prolactinomas. Am J Med 1987; 83:765.
19. Bakiri F, et al. Aldosterone in panhypopituitarism: dynamic studies and therapeutic effects in Sheehan's syndrome. Acta Endocrinol (Copenh) 1986; 112:329.
20. Williams T, et al. Blunted growth hormone (GH) response to GH-releasing hormone in hypothyroidism resolves in the euthyroid state. J Clin Endocrinol Metab 1985; 61:454.
21. Becker KL, et al. Limited calcitonin reserve in hyperparathyroidism. Am J Med Sci 1980; 280:11.
22. Winokur A, et al. Variability of hormonal responses to a series of neuroendocrine challenges in depressed patients. Am J Psychiatry 1982; 139:39.
23. Amsterdam JD, et al. A neuroendocrine test battery in bipolar patients and healthy subjects. Arch Gen Psychiatry 1983; 40:515.
24. Roy-Byrne PP, et al. Reduced TSH and prolactin responses to TRH in patients with panic disorder. Am J Psychiatry 1986; 143:503.
25. Connolly CK, et al. Single-dose dexamethasone suppression in normal subjects and hospital patients. BMJ 1968; 2:665.
26. Crapo L. Cushing's syndrome: a review of diagnostic tests. Metabolism 1979; 28:955.
27. Cavallo-Perin P, et al. Feedback inhibition of insulin secretion is altered in cirrhosis. J Clin Endocrinol Metab 1986; 63:1023.
28. Mulder H. Enhanced calcitonin release in chronic renal failure depending on the absence of severe secondary hyperparathyroidism. Nephron 1982; 31:123.
29. Grimaldi A, et al. Antidiuretic hormone response to volume depletion in diabetic patients with cardiac autonomic dysfunction. Clin Sci 1985; 68:545.
30. May ME, et al. Rapid adrenocorticotropic hormone test in practice. Retrospective review. Am J Med 1985; 79:679.
31. Gogel HK, et al. Gastric secretion and hormonal interactions in multiple endocrine neoplasia type I. Arch Intern Med 1985; 145:855.
32. Brown EM, et al. Secretory control in normal and abnormal parathyroid tissue. Recent Prog Horm Res 1987; 43:337.
33. Karashima T, et al. Comparison of growth hormone responses to human pancreatic growth hormone releasing factor and other pharmacological stimuli in acromegalic patients. Endocrinol Jpn 1984; 31:343.
34. Nierenberg AA, et al. How to evaluate a diagnostic marker test. Lessons from the rise and fall of dexamethasone suppression test. JAMA 1988; 259:1699.
35. Zaloga GP, et al. A longitudinal evaluation of thyroid function in critically ill surgical patients. Ann Surg 1985; 201:456.
36. Tietz N, ed. Clinical guide to laboratory tests, 3rd ed. Philadelphia: WB Saunders, 1994.
37. Inder WJ, et al. A comparison of the naloxone test with ovine CRH and insulin hypoglycaemia in the evaluation of the hypothalamic-pituitary-adrenal axis in normal man. Clin Endocrinol (Oxf) 1995; 43:425.
38. Facchinetti F, et al. Changes of opioid modulation of the hypothalamo-pituitary-adrenal axis in patients with severe premenstrual syndrome. Psychosom Med 1994; 56:418.
39. Torpy DJ, et al. Diurnal effects of fluoxetine and naloxone on the human hypothalamic-pituitary-adrenal axis. Clin Exp Pharmacol Physiol 1997; 24:421.
40. Boushaki FZ, et al. Hypothalamic-pituitary-adrenal axis in abdominal obesity: effects of dexfenfluramine. Clin Endocrinol (Oxf) 1997; 46:461.
41. Jackson RV, et al. New diagnostic tests for Cushing's syndrome: uses of naloxone, vasopressin and alprazolam. Clin Exp Pharmacol Physiol 1996; 23:579.
42. Blevins LS, et al. Naloxone-induced activation of the hypothalamic-pituitary-adrenal axis in suspected central adrenal insufficiency. Am J Med Sci 1994; 308:167.
43. Inder WJ, et al. Elevated basal adrenocorticotropin and evidence for increased central opioid tone in highly trained male athletes. Clin Endocrinol Metab 1995; 80:244.
44. Dessi-Fulgheri P, et al. Blunted adrenocorticotrophic hormone release during captopril treatment. J Hypertens Suppl 1985; 3:S125.
45. Alevizaki-Harhalaki MC, et al. Intravenous insulin tolerance test: criteria for evaluation of the growth hormone and cortisol response. Acta Endocrinol (Copenh) 1984; 265(Suppl):31.
46. Berman JD, et al. Diminished adrenocorticotropin response to insulin-induced hypoglycemia in nondepressed, actively drinking male alcoholics. J Clin Endocrinol Metab 1990; 71:712.
47. Kathol RG, et al. Blunted ACTH response to hypoglycemic stress in depressed patients but not in patients with schizophrenia. J Psychiatr Res 1992; 26:103.
48. Schoneshofer M, et al. Suppressive effect of metyrapone on plasma corticotrophin immunoreactivity in normal man. Clin Endocrinol (Oxf) 1983; 18:363.
49. Meikle AW, et al. Effect of diphenylhydantoin on the metabolism of metyrapone and release of ACTH in man. J Clin Endocrinol Metab 1969; 29:1553.
50. Carpenter PC. Cushing's syndrome: update of diagnosis and management. Mayo Clin Proc 1986; 61:49.
51. Wand GS, Dobs AS. Alterations in the hypothalamic-pituitary-adrenal axis in actively drinking alcoholics. J Clin Endocrinol Metab 1991; 72:1290.
52. Torpy DJ, et al. Clin Exp Pharmacol Physiol 1995; 22:441.
53. Malchoff CD, et al. Ectopic ACTH syndrome caused by a bronchial carcinoid tumor responsive to dexamethasone, metyrapone, and corticotropin-releasing factor. Am J Med 1988; 84:760.
54. Ross JL, et al. Ovine corticotropin-releasing hormone stimulation test in normal children. J Clin Endocrinol Metab 1986; 62:390.
55. Pavlov EP, et al. Responses of plasma adrenocorticotropin, cortisol, and dehydroepiandrosterone to ovine corticotropin-releasing hormone in healthy aging men. J Clin Endocrinol Metab 1986; 62:767.
56. Tsukada T, et al. Plasma adrenocorticotropin and cortisol responses to intravenous injection of corticotropin-releasing factor in the morning and evening. J Clin Endocrinol Metab 1983; 57:869.
57. Tanaka K, et al. Effects of synthetic ovine corticotropin-releasing factor (CRF) on plasma ACTH and cortisol in 31 normal human males. Endocrinol Jpn 1983; 30:689.
58. Chrousos GP, et al. The corticotropin-releasing factor stimulation test. An aid in the evaluation of patients with Cushing's syndrome. N Engl J Med 1984; 310:622.
59. Gold PW, et al. Responses to corticotropin-releasing hormone in the hypercortisolism of depression and Cushing's disease. Pathophysiologic and diagnostic implications. N Engl J Med 1986; 314:1329.
60. Kamilaris TC, et al. Effect of altered thyroid hormone levels on hypothalamic-pituitary-adrenal function. J Clin Endocrinol Metab 1987; 65:994.
61. Linnoila M, et al. NIH conference. Alcohol withdrawal and noradrenergic function. Ann Intern Med 1987; 107:875.
62. Yanovski JA, et al. Differences in the hypothalamic-pituitary-adrenal axis of black and white women. J Clin Endocrinol Metab 1993; 77:536.
63. Reincke M, et al. The hypothalamic-pituitary-adrenal axis in critical illness: response to dexamethasone and corticotropin-releasing hormone. J Clin Endocrinol Metab 1993; 77:151.
64. Gisslinger H, et al. Interferon-alpha stimulates the hypothalamic-pituitary-adrenal axis in vivo and in vitro. Neuroendocrinology 1993; 57:489.
65. Grant AC, et al. Hypothalamo-pituitary-adrenal axis in uraemia: evidence for primary adrenal dysfunction? Nephrol Dial Transplant 1993; 8:307.
66. Greenspan SL, et al. The pituitary-adrenal glucocorticoid response is altered by gender and disease. J Gerontol 1993; 48:M72.
67. Schulte HM, et al. The corticotrophin releasing hormone test in late pregnancy: lack of adrenocorticotrophin and cortisol response. Clin Endocrinol (Oxf) 1990; 33:99.

68. Loriaux DL, Nieman L. Corticotropin-releasing hormone testing in pituitary disease. Endocrinol Metab Clin North Am 1991; 20:363.

69. Dahl RE, et al. Corticotropin releasing hormone stimulation test and nocturnal cortisol levels in normal children. Pediatr Res 1992; 32:64.

70. Oldfield EH, et al. Petrosal sinus sampling with and without corticotropin-releasing hormone for the differential diagnosis of Cushing's syndrome. N Engl J Med 1991; 325:897.

71. Yanovski JA, et al. The limited ability of inferior petrosal sinus sampling with corticotropin-releasing hormone to distinguish Cushing's disease from pseudo-Cushing states or normal physiology. J Clin Endocrinol Metab 1993; 77:503.

72. Yanovski JA, et al. Corticotropin-releasing hormone stimulation following low-dose dexamethasone administration. A new test to distinguish Cushing's syndrome from pseudo-Cushing's states. JAMA 1993; 269:2232.

73. Oliverio PJ, et al. Bilateral simultaneous cavernous sinus sampling using corticotropin-releasing hormone in the evaluation of Cushing disease. Am J Neuroradiol 1996; 17:1669.

74. Doppman JL, et al. The hypoplastic inferior petrosal sinus: a potential source of false-negative results in petrosal sampling for Cushing's disease. J Clin Endocrinol Metab 1999; 84:533.

75. Teramoto A, et al. Cavernous sinus sampling in patients with adrenocorticotrophic hormone-dependent Cushing's syndrome with emphasis on inter- and intracavernous adrenocorticotrophic hormone gradients. J Neurosurg 1998; 89:762.

76. Yanovski JA, et al. The dexamethasone-suppressed corticotropin-releasing hormone stimulation test differentiates mild Cushing's disease from normal physiology. J Clin Endocrinol Metab 1998; 83:348.

77. Modell S, et al. Hormonal response pattern in the combined DEX-CRH test is stable over time in subjects at high familial risk for affective disorders. Neuropsychopharmacology 1998; 18:253.

78. Schmider J, et al. Combined dexamethasone/corticotropin-releasing hormone test in acute and remitted manic patients, in acute depression, and in normal controls: I. Biol Psychiatry 1995; 38:797.

79. Heuser I, et al. The combined dexamethasone/CRH test: a refined laboratory test for psychiatric disorders. J Psychiatr Res 1994; 28:341.

80. Chrousos GP, et al. Late-onset 21-hydroxylase deficiency mimicking idiopathic hirsutism or polycystic ovarian disease. Ann Intern Med 1982; 96:143.

81. Ramirez G, et al. Evaluation of the hypothalamic hypophyseal adrenal axis in patients receiving long-term hemodialysis. Arch Intern Med 1982; 142:1448.

82. Wallace EZ, et al. Pituitary-adrenocortical function in chronic renal failure: studies of episodic secretion of cortisol and dexamethasone suppressibility. J Clin Endocrinol Metab 1980; 50:46.

83. Weller RA, et al. A comparison of the cortisol suppression index and the dexamethasone suppression test in prepubertal children. Am J Psychiatry 1985; 142:1370.

84. Rosenbaum AH, et al. The dexamethasone suppression test in normal control subjects: comparison of two assays and effect of age. Am J Psychiatry 1984; 141:1550.

85. Tyrrell JB, et al. An overnight high-dose dexamethasone suppression test for rapid differential diagnosis of Cushing's syndrome. Ann Intern Med 1986; 104:180.

86. Cameron OG, et al. Hypothalamic-pituitary-adrenocortical activity in patients with diabetes mellitus. Gen Psychiatry 1984; 41:1090.

87. Uhde TW, et al. Caffeine-induced escape from dexamethasone suppression. Arch Gen Psychiatry 1985; 42:737.

88. Burch EA, et al. Drug intake and the dexamethasone suppression test. J Clin Psychiatry 1986; 47:144.

89. Kyriazopoulou V, et al. Abnormal overnight dexamethasone suppression test in subjects receiving rifampicin therapy. J Clin Endocrinol Metab 1992; 75:315.

90. Kaye TB, et al. Effect of glycemic control on the overnight dexamethasone suppression test in patients with diabetes mellitus. J Clin Endocrinol Metab 1992; 74:640.

91. Reincke M, et al. The hypothalamic-pituitary-adrenal axis in critical illness: response to dexamethasone and corticotropin-releasing hormone. J Clin Endocrinol Metab 1993; 77:151.

92. Flack MR, et al. Urine free cortisol in the high-dose dexamethasone suppression test for the differential diagnosis of the Cushing syndrome. Ann Intern Med 1992; 116:211.

93. Al-Saadi N, et al. A very high dose dexamethasone suppression test for differential diagnosis of Cushing's syndrome. Clin Endocrinol (Oxf) 1998; 48:45.

94. Thomas S, et al. Response to ACTH in the newborn. Arch Dis Child 1986; 61:57.

95. Ohasi M, et al. Adrenocortical responsiveness to graded ACTH infusions in normal young and elderly human subjects. Gerontology 1986; 32:43.

96. McDermott MT, et al. The effects of theophylline and nifedipine on corticotropin-stimulated cortisol secretion. Clin Pharmacol Ther 1990; 47:435.

97. Azziz R, et al. Acute adrenocorticotropin-(1-24) (ACTH) adrenal stimulation in eumenorrheic women: reproducibility and effect of ACTH dose, subject weight, and sampling time. J Clin Endocrinol Metab 1990; 70:1273.

98. Harracksingh C, et al. Comparison of the adrenocorticotropic hormone stimulation test in the follicular and luteal phases of the menstrual cycle. Int J Fertil 1992; 37:123.

99. Dickstein G, et al. Adrenocorticotropin stimulation test: effects of basal cortisol level, time of day, and suggested new sensitive low dose test. Clin Endocrinol Metab 1991; 72:773.

100. Crowley S, et al. Reproducibility of the cortisol response to stimulation with a low dose of ACTH(1-24): the effect of basal cortisol levels and comparison of low-dose with high-dose secretory dynamics. J Endocrinol 1993; 136:167.

101. Dickstein G, Shechner C. Low dose ACTH test—a word of caution to the word of caution: when and how to use it. J Clin Endocrinol Metab 1997; 82:322.

102. Weintrob N, et al. Standard and low-dose short adrenocorticotropin test compared with insulin-induced hypoglycemia for assessment of the hypothalamic-pituitary-adrenal axis in children with idiopathic multiple pituitary hormone deficiencies. J Clin Endocrinol Metab 1998; 83:88.

103. Murphy H, et al. The low dose ACTH test—a further word of caution. J Clin Endocrinol Metab 1998; 83:712.

104. Thaler LM, et al. The low dose (1-microg) adrenocorticotropin stimulation test in the evaluation of patients with suspected central adrenal insufficiency. J Clin Endocrinol Metab 1998; 83:2726.

105. Oelkers W. The role of high- and low-dose corticotropin tests in the diagnosis of secondary adrenal insufficiency. Eur J Endocrinol 1998; 139:567.

106. Ambrosi B, et al. The one microgram adrenocorticotropin test in the assessment of hypothalamic-pituitary-adrenal function. Eur J Endocrinol 1998; 139:575.

107. Streeten DHP. Shortcomings in the low-dose (1 microg) ACTH test for the diagnosis of ACTH deficiency states. J Clin Endocrinol Metab 1999; 84:835.

108. Abdu TAM, et al. Comparison of the low dose short synacthen test (1 microg), the conventional dose short synacthen test (250 microg), and the insulin tolerance test for assessment of the hypothalamo-pituitary-adrenal axis in patients with pituitary disease. J Clin Endocrinol Metab 1999; 84:838.

109. Lyons DC, et al. Single dose captopril as a diagnostic test for primary aldosteronism. J Clin Endocrinol Metab 1983; 57:892.

110. Brown RD, et al. Evaluation of a test using saralasin to differentiate primary aldosteronism due to an aldosterone-producing adenoma from idiopathic hyperaldosteronism. Metabolism 1984; 33:734.

111. Anderson GH, et al. Acute effects of saralasin on plasma aldosterone in different pathophysiological conditions. J Clin Endocrinol Metab 1980; 50:529.

112. Sancho JM, et al. Interference by ranitidine with aldosterone secretion in vivo. Eur J Clin Pharmacol 1984; 27:495.

113. Weinberger MH. Primary aldosteronism: diagnosis and differentiation of subtypes. Ann Intern Med 1984; 100:300.

114. Tunny TJ, et al. Diagnosis of unilateral renovascular hypertension: comparative effect of intravenous enalaprilat and oral captopril. J Urol 1988; 140:713.

115. Naomi S, et al. Effects of sodium intake on the captopril test for primary aldosteronism. Jpn Heart J 1987; 28:357.

116. Muratani H, et al. Single oral administration of captopril may not bring an improvement in screening of primary aldosteronism. Clin Exp Hypertens [A] 1987; 9:611.

117. Hambling C, et al. Re-evaluation of the captopril test for the diagnosis of primary hyperaldosteronism. Clin Endocrinol (Oxf) 1992; 36:499.

118. Fallo F, et al. Effect of captopril on aldosterone response to potassium infusion in primary aldosteronism. Miner Electrolyte Metab 1991; 17:185.

119. Iwaoka T, et al. The usefulness of the captopril test as a simultaneous screening for primary aldosteronism and renovascular hypertension. Am J Hypertens 1993; 6:899.

120. Bravo EL, et al. Clonidine-suppression test: a useful aid in the diagnosis of pheochromocytoma. N Engl J Med 1981; 305:623.

121. Halter JB, et al. Clonidine-suppression test for diagnosis of pheochromocytoma. N Engl J Med 1982; 306:49.

122. Sjoberg RJ, et al. The clonidine suppression test for pheochromocytoma. A review of its utility and pitfalls. Arch Intern Med 1992; 152:1193.

123. Bellastella A, et al. Influence of blindness on plasma luteinizing hormone, follicle-stimulating hormone, prolactin, and testosterone levels in prepubertal boys. J Clin Endocrinol Metab 1987; 64:862.

124. Dana-Haeri J, et al. Pituitary responsiveness to gonadotrophin-releasing and thyrotrophin-releasing hormones in epileptic patients receiving carbamazepine or phenytoin. Clin Endocrinol (Oxf) 1984; 20:163.

125. Ronkainen H. Depressed follicle-stimulating hormone, luteinizing hormone, and prolactin responses to the luteinizing hormone-releasing hormone, thyrotropin-releasing hormone, and metoclopramide test in endurance runners in the hard-training season. Fertil Steril 1985; 44:755.

126. Perez-Lopez FR, et al. Gonadotrophin hormone releasing tests in women receiving hormonal contraception. Clin Endocrinol (Oxf) 1975; 4:477.

127. Ramirez G, et al. Hypothalamo-hypophyseal thyroid and gonadal function before and after erythropoietin therapy in dialysis patients. J Clin Endocrinol Metab 1992; 74:517.

128. Tenover JS, et al. The effects of aging in normal men on bioavailable testosterone and luteinizing hormone secretion: response to clomiphene citrate. J Clin Endocrinol Metab 1987; 65:1118.

129. Lamberts SWJ, et al. The effects of bromocriptine, thyrotropin-releasing hormone, and gonadotropin-releasing hormone on hormone secretion by gonadotropin-secreting pituitary adenomas in vivo and in vitro. J Clin Endocrinol Metab 1987; 64:524.

130. Daneshdoost L, et al. Recognition of gonadotroph adenomas in women. N Engl J Med 1991; 324:589.

131. Kwekkeboom DJ, et al. Gonadotropin release by clinically nonfunctioning and gonadotroph pituitary adenomas in vivo and in vitro: relation to sex and effects of thyrotropin-releasing hormone, gonadotropin-releasing hormone, and bromocriptine. J Clin Endocrinol Metab 1989; 68:1128.

132. Persani L, et al. Thyrotropin alpha- and beta-subunit responses to thyrotropin-releasing hormone and domperidone in normal subjects and in patients with microprolactinomas. Neuroendocrinology 1991; 53:411.

133. Bonora E, et al. Insulin and C-peptide responses to 75 g oral glucose load in the healthy man. Diabetes Metab 1986; 12:143.

134. Minaker KL, et al. Influence of age on clearance of insulin in man. Diabetes 1982; 31:851.

135. Roti E, et al. Basal and glucose- and arginine-stimulated serum concentrations of insulin, C-peptide, and glucagon in hyperthyroid patients. Metabolism 1986; 35:337.

136. Metz R, et al. Potentiation of the plasma insulin response to glucose by prior administration of alcohol. An apparent islet-priming effect. Diabetes 1969; 18:517.

137. Nelson RL, et al. Oral glucose tolerance test: indications and limitations. Mayo Clin Proc 1988; 63:263.

138. Pontiroli AE, et al. Different effects of histaminergic H1 and H2 antagonists on basal and stimulated insulin and glucagon release in humans. Horm Metab Res 1986; 14:496.

139. Golander A, et al. Inhibition of the insulin response to glucose after treatment with cyproheptadine. Acta Paediatr Scand 1982; 71:485.

140. Kaplan EL, et al. Endocrine tumors of the pancreas and their clinical syndromes. Surg Annu 1986; 18:181.

141. Gentile S, et al. The role of ranitidine infusion on glucose, insulin and C-peptide serum levels induced by oral glucose tolerance test in healthy subjects. Acta Diabetol Lat 1986; 23:165.

142. Zavaroni I, et al. Effect of age and environmental factors on glucose tolerance and insulin secretion in a worker population. J Am Geriatr Soc 1986; 34:271.

143. Reid RL, et al. Oral glucose tolerance during the menstrual cycle in normal women and women with alleged premenstrual "hypoglycemic" attacks: effects of naloxone. J Clin Endocrinol Metab 1986; 62:1167.

144. Irjala K, et al. Interpretation of oral glucose tolerance test: capillary-venous difference in blood glucose and the effect of analytical method. Scand J Clin Lab Invest 1986; 46:307.

145. Propranolol or hydrochlorothiazide alone for the initial treatment of hypertension. IV. Effect on plasma glucose and glucose tolerance. Veterans Administration Cooperative Study Group on Antihypertensive Agents. Hypertension 1985; 7:1008.

146. Berntorp K, et al. Relation between plasma insulin and blood glucose in a cross-sectional population study of the oral glucose tolerance test. Acta Endocrinol (Copenh) 1983; 102:549.

147. Verrillo A, et al. Circadian variation in glucose tolerance and associated changes in plasma insulin and somatostatin levels in normal volunteers. Boll Soc Ital Biol Sper 1984; 60:2261.

148. Report of the Expert Committee on the Diagnosis and Classification of Diabetes Mellitus. Diabetes Care 1997; 20:1183.

149. Gottsater A, et al. Pancreatic beta-cell function evaluated by intravenous glucose and glucagon stimulation. A comparison between insulin and C-peptide to measure insulin secretion. Scand J Clin Lab Invest 1992; 52:631.

150. Miki H, et al. Glucagon-glucose (GG) test for the estimation of the insulin reserve in diabetes. Diabetes Res Clin Pract 1992; 18:99.

151. Viikari J, et al. Glucagon-C-peptide test as a measure of insulin requirement in type 2 diabetes: evaluation of stopping insulin therapy in eleven patients. Ann Clin Res 1987; 19:178.

152. Madsbad S, et al. Outcome of the glucagon test depends upon the prevailing blood glucose concentration in type I (insulin-dependent) diabetic patients. Acta Med Scand 1987; 222:71.

153. Vahlkamp T, et al. The glucagon-stimulated C-peptide test: an aid in classification of patients with diabetes mellitus. Neth J Med 1990; 36:196.

154. Nyberg G, et al. Glucagon-stimulated serum C-peptide levels in the early period following pancreas transplantation. Transplant Proc 1990; 22:647.

155. Gjessing HJ, et al. Fasting plasma C-peptide, glucagon stimulated plasma C-peptide, and urinary C-peptide in relation to clinical type of diabetes. Diabetologia 1989; 32:305.

156. Pun KK, et al. The use of glucagon challenge tests in the diagnostic evaluation of hypoglycemia due to hepatoma and insulinoma. J Clin Endocrinol Metab 1988; 67:546.

157. Arnold-Larsen S, et al. Reproducibility of the glucagon test. Diabet Med 1987; 4:299.

158. Sherbaniuk RW, et al. Gastrin, gastric emptying, and gastroesophageal reflux after ranitidine. J Clin Gastroenterol 1983; 5:239.

159. Feldman M, et al. Sex-related differences in gastrin release and parietal cell sensitivity to gastrin in healthy human beings. J Clin Invest 1983; 71:715.

160. Skogseid B, et al. A standardized meal stimulation test of the endocrine pancreas for early detection of pancreatic endocrine tumors in multiple endocrine neoplasia type 1 syndrome: five years experience. J Clin Endocrinol Metab 1987; 64:1233.

161. Lamers CBH, et al. Comparative study of the value of the calcium, secretin, and meal stimulated increase in serum gastrin to the diagnosis of the Zollinger-Ellison syndrome. Gut 1977; 18:128.

162. Schrumpf E, et al. Effect of cholinergic, adrenergic, and dopaminergic blockade on gastrin secretion in healthy subjects. Scand J Gastroenterol 1982; 17:29.

163. Florent C, et al. Effect of two-week treatment with enprostil (35 micrograms twice a day) on 24-hour serum gastrin levels. Dig Dis Sci 1990; 35:1352.

164. Frucht H, et al. Prospective study of the standard meal provocative test in Zollinger-Ellison syndrome. Am J Med 1989; 87:528.

165. Lauritsen KB, et al. Lithium inhibits basal and food-stimulated gastrin secretion. Gastroenterology 1978; 75:59.

166. Primrose JN, et al. Differences between peptic ulcer and control patients on the basis of the response to secretin. Digestion 1985; 32:249.

167. Feldman M, et al. Positive intravenous secretin test in patients with achlorhydria-related hypergastrinemia. Gastroenterology 1987; 93:59.

168. Anderson J, et al. Lancet 1954; 267:720.

169. Watson L, et al. Hydrocortisone suppression test and discriminant analysis in differential diagnosis of hypercalcaemia. Lancet 1980; 1:1320.

170. Caroff SN, et al. Hormonal response to thyrotropin-releasing hormone following rest-activity reversal in normal men. Biol Psychiatry 1984; 19:1015.

171. Carlson HE. Carbidopa plus L-dopa pretreatment inhibits the prolactin (PRL) response to thyrotropin-releasing hormone and thus cannot distinguish central from pituitary sites of prolactin stimulation. J Clin Endocrinol Metab 1986; 63:249.

172. Donders SHJ, et al. Disparity of thyrotropin (TSH) and prolactin responses to TSH-releasing hormone in obesity. J Clin Endocrinol Metab 1985; 61:56.

173. Gahl WA, et al. Blunted prolactin response to thyrotropin-releasing hormone stimulation in cystinotic children receiving cysteamine. J Clin Endocrinol Metab 1985; 60:793.

174. Arnetz BB. Age-related differences in the pituitary prolactin response to thyrotropin-releasing hormone. Life Sci 1986; 39:135.

175. Rojdmark S, et al. Prolactin and thyrotropin responses to thyrotropin-releasing hormone and metoclopramide in men with chronic alcoholism. J Clin Endocrinol Metab 1984; 59:595.

176. Verbeelen D, et al. Effect of 1,25-dihydroxyvitamin $D_3$ and nifedipine on prolactin release in normal man. J Endocrinol Invest 1985; 8:103.

177. Kamal TJ, et al. Effects of calcium channel blockade with verapamil on the prolactin responses to TRH, L-dopa, and bromocriptine. Am J Med Sci 1992; 304:289.

178. Vance ML, et al. Role of dopamine in the regulation of growth hormone secretion: dopamine and bromocriptine augment growth hormone (GH)-releasing hormone-stimulated GH secretion in normal man. J Clin Endocrinol Metab 1987; 64:1136.

179. Kopelman PG, et al. Impaired growth hormone response to growth hormone releasing factor and insulin-hypoglycaemia in obesity. Clin Endocrinol (Oxf) 1985; 23:87.

180. Chihara K, et al. Augmentation by propranolol of growth hormone-releasing hormone-(1-44)-NH$_2$-induced growth hormone release in normal short and normal children. J Clin Endocrinol Metab 1985; 61:229.

181. Williams T, et al. Impaired growth hormone responses to growth hormone-releasing factor in obesity. A pituitary defect reversed with weight reduction. N Engl J Med 1984; 311:1403.

182. Krassowski J, et al. Exaggerated growth hormone response to growth hormone-releasing hormone in type I diabetes mellitus. Acta Endocrinol (Copenh) 1988; 117:225.

183. Smals AEM, et al. Human pancreatic growth hormone releasing hormone fails to stimulate human growth hormone both in Cushing's disease and in Cushing's syndrome due to adrenocortical adenoma. Clin Endocrinol (Oxf) 1986; 24:401.

184. Burguera B, et al. Dual and selective actions of glucocorticoids upon basal and stimulated growth hormone release in man. Neuroendocrinology 1990; 51:51.

185. Ramirez G, et al. Response to growth hormone-releasing hormone in adult renal failure patients on hemodialysis. Metabolism 1990; 39:764.

186. Tulandi T, et al. Effect of estrogen on the growth hormone response to the alpha-adrenergic agonist clonidine in women with menopausal flushing. J Clin Endocrinol Metab 1987; 65:6.

187. Coiro V, et al. Nicotine from cigarette smoking enhances clonidine-induced increase of serum growth hormone concentrations in men. J Clin Pharmacol 1984; 18:802.

188. Matussek N, et al. The dependence of the clonidine growth hormone test on alcohol drinking habits and the menstrual cycle. Psychoneuroendocrinology 1984; 9:173.

189. Gil-Ad I, et al. Effect of aging on human plasma growth hormone response to clonidine. Mech Ageing Dev 1984; 27:97.

190. Schittecatte M, et al. Tricyclic wash-out and growth hormone response to clonidine. Br J Psychiatry 1989; 154:858.

191. Tancer ME, et al. Blunted growth hormone responses to growth hormone-releasing factor and to clonidine in panic disorder. Am J Psychiatry 1993; 150:336.

192. Zanoboni A, et al. Inhibitory effect of cimetidine on L-dopa-stimulated growth hormone release in normal man. Clin Endocrinol (Oxf) 1984; 21:535.

193. Seki K, et al. Absence of growth hormone response to L-dopa and bromocriptine in hyperprolactinemic women with pituitary microadenoma. J Clin Endocrinol Metab 1986; 62:783.

194. Bellastella A, et al. Blindness impairs plasma growth hormone response to L-dopa but not to arginine. J Clin Endocrinol Metab 1990; 70:856.

195. Miell JP, et al. Effects of dexamethasone on growth hormone (GH)-releasing hormone, arginine- and dopaminergic stimulated GH secretion, and total plasma insulin-like growth factor-I concentrations in normal male volunteers. J Clin Endocrinol Metab 1991; 72:675.

196. Bartolotta E, et al. The GH-releasing effect of Hexarelin, a synthetic hexapeptide, in newborns is lower than in young adults. J Pediatr Endocrinol Metab 1997; 10:491.

197. Loche S, et al. Acute administration of hexarelin stimulates GH secretion during day and night in normal men. Clin Endocrinol (Oxf) 1997; 46:275.

198. Loche S, et al. The growth hormone response to hexarelin in children: reproducibility and effect of sex steroids. J Clin Endocrinol Metab 1997; 82:861.

199. Arvat E, et al. Influence of beta-adrenergic agonists and antagonists on the GH-releasing effect of Hexarelin in man. J Endocrinol Invest 1996; 19:25.

200. Maccario M, et al. Metabolic modulation of the growth hormone-releasing activity of hexarelin in man. Metabolism 1995; 44:134.

201. Arvat E, et al. Arginine and growth hormone-releasing hormone restore the blunted growth hormone-releasing activity of hexarelin in elderly subjects. J Clin Endocrinol Metab 1994; 79:1440.

202. Arvat E, et al. Effects of dexamethasone and alprazolam, a benzodiazepine, on the stimulatory effect of hexarelin, a synthetic GHRP, on ACTH, cortisol and GH secretion in humans. Neuroendocrinology 1998; 67:310.

203. Grottoli S, et al. Reduction of the somatotrope responsiveness to GHRH and Hexarelin but not to arginine plus GHRH in hyperprolactinemic patients. J Endocrinol Invest 1997; 20:597.

204. Arvat E, et al. Oestrogen replacement does not restore the reduced GH-releasing activity of Hexarelin, a synthetic hexapeptide, in post-menopausal women. Eur J Endocrinol 1997; 136:483.

205. Arvat E, et al. Effects of histaminergic antagonists on the GH-releasing activity of GHRH or hexarelin, a synthetic hexapeptide, in man. J Endocrinol Invest 1997; 20:122.

206. Arvat E, et al. Adrenocorticotropin and cortisol hyperresponsiveness to hexarelin in patients with Cushing's disease bearing a pituitary microadenoma, but not in those with macroadenoma. J Clin Endocrinol Metab 1998; 83:4207.

207. Bellone J, et al. Hexarelin, a synthetic GH-releasing peptide, is a powerful stimulus of GH secretion in pubertal children and in adults but not in prepubertal children and in elderly subjects. J Endocrinol Invest 1998; 21:494.

208. Merimee TJ, et al. Studies of the sex based variation of human growth hormone secretion. J Clin Endocrinol Metab 1971; 33:896.

209. Schopohl J, et al. Combined pituitary function-test with four hypothalamic releasing hormones. Klin Wochenschr 1986; 64:314.

210. Kaltenborn KC, et al. Quadruple injection of hypothalamic peptides to evaluate pituitary function in normal subjects. West J Med 1985; 142:37.

211. Sandler LM, et al. Combined use of vasopressin and synthetic hypothalamic releasing factors as a new test of anterior pituitary function. BMJ 1986; 292:511.

212. Abboud CF. Laboratory diagnosis of hypopituitarism. Mayo Clin Proc 1986; 61:35.

213. Barbarino A, et al. Corticotropin-releasing hormone inhibition of growth hormone-releasing hormone-induced growth hormone release in man. J Clin Endocrinol Metab 1990; 71:1368.

214. Sensi S, et al. Circadian time structure of pituitary and adrenal response to CRF, TRH and LHRH. Prog Clin Biol Res 1990; 341A:535.

215. Lee YJ, et al. Anterior pituitary functions in patients with uremia tested by stimulation with four combined hypothalamic releasing hormones. Taiwan I Hsueh Hui Tsa Chih 1989; 88:1091.

216. Gold PW, et al. Carbamazepine diminishes the sensitivity of the plasma arginine vasopressin response to osmotic stimulation. J Clin Endocrinol Metab 1983; 57:952.

217. Zerbe RL, et al. A comparison of plasma vasopressin measurements with a standard indirect test in the differential diagnosis of polyuria. N Engl J Med 1981; 305:1539.

218. Willenbring ML, et al. Psychoneuroendocrine effects of methadone maintenance. Psychoneuroendocrinology 1989; 14:371.

219. Loosen PT, et al. The TRH test in normal subjects: methodological considerations. Psychoneuroendocrinology 1982; 7:147.

220. Nathan RS, et al. Diurnal hormonal responses to thyrotropin-releasing hormone in normal men. Psychoneuroendocrinology 1982; 7:235.

221. Tarditi E, et al. Impaired TSH response to TRH after intravenous ranitidine in man. Experientia 1983; 39:109.

222. Kaptein EM, et al. Thyroxine metabolism in the low thyroxine state of critical nonthyroidal illnesses. J Clin Endocrinol Metab 1981; 53:764.

223. Hugues JN, et al. Effects of cimetidine on thyroid hormones. Clin Endocrinol (Oxf) 1982; 17:297.

224. Emmanouel DS, et al. Pathogenesis of endocrine abnormalities in uremia. Endocr Rev 1980; 1:28.

225. Isojarvi JI, et al. Thyroid function in epileptic patients treated with carbamazepine. Arch Neurol 1989; 46:1175.

226. Spencer CA, et al. Thyrotropin (TSH)-releasing hormone stimulation test responses employing third and fourth generation TSH assays. J Clin Endocrinol Metab 1993; 76:494.

227. Paunovic VR, et al. Neuroleptic actions on the thyroid axis: different effects of clozapine and haloperidol. Int Clin Psychopharmacol 1991; 6:133.

228. Panidis DK, et al. TRH test before, during, and after long-term danazol treatment in patients with endometriosis. Hum Reprod 1989; 4:903.

229. Deftos LJ, et al. Influence of age and sex on plasma calcitonin in human beings. N Engl J Med 1980; 302:1351.

230. Muse KN, et al. Calcium-regulating hormones across the menstrual cycle. J Clin Endocrinol Metab 1986; 62:1313.

231. Linehan WM, et al. Analysis of pentagastrin and calcium as thyrocalcitonin secretagogues in the early diagnosis of medullary carcinoma of the thyroid gland. Surg Forum 1977; 28:110.

232. Wells SA, et al. Provocative agents and the diagnosis of medullary carcinoma of the thyroid gland. Ann Surg 1978; 188:139.

**TABLE 241-1.**
Dynamic Endocrine Procedures*

| Name of Procedure | How Performed | Substance Measured | Expected Response | Intraindividual Variation |
|---|---|---|---|---|
| **ADRENAL GLAND** | | | | |
| HYPOTHALAMIC–PITUITARY–ADRENOCORTICAL AXIS | | | | |
| *STIMULATORY: HYPOTHALAMUS* | | | | |
| 1. Naloxone[37–43] | 125 µg/kg IV bolus | ACTH at 0, 30, 60 min<br>Cortisol at 0, 30, 60 min | Two to 4 times increase at 30 min<br>Peak >20 µg/dL | No significant diurnal variation |
| 2. Insulin-induced hypoglycemia[15,44–47] | 0.05–0.1 U/kg IV bolus | ACTH at 0, 30, 60, 90, 120 min<br>Cortisol at 0, 30, 60, 90, 120 min | Three to 5 times increase at peak<br>Peak >20 µg/dL, and increase of 10 µg/dL | |
| 3. Metyrapone[26,48–52] | Overnight: 3 g PO at midnight, with a glass of milk and a snack<br>Two-day: 750 mg PO q4h × 6 | Overnight: 11-deoxycortisol at 8 a.m.<br>Urine 17-OH steroids, basal and each day of test | >7 µg/dL<br>Increase of 3 to 5 times over basal level | Response greater in p.m. than in a.m. |
| *STIMULATORY: PITUITARY* | | | | |
| 1. CRH[43,52–69] | 100 µg IV bolus, or 1 µg/kg | ACTH at 0, 30, 60 min<br>Cortisol at 0, 30, 60 min | Two to 4 times increase at 30 min<br>Peak >20 µg/dL | Slightly greater response in a.m. than in p.m. Response inversely related to basal serum cortisol and plasma ACTH concentrations. |
| 2. CRH with inferior petrosal sinus sampling[70–75] | 100 µg IV bolus, or 1 µg/kg | ACTH from each petrosal sinus and peripheral vein at 0, 2, 3, 5, 10 min | Petrosal sinus/peripheral ACTH ratio <3<br>No ACTH gradient between right and left petrosal sinus | |

*The methodology, interpretation, and utility of some of these procedures are disputed; for further information and clinical recommendations, see the indicated chapters.

| Physiologic Factors | Drug Effects | Methodologic Considerations | Special Considerations/Interpretation |
|---|---|---|---|
| INC: exercise, obesity. DEC: premenstrual syndrome. | DEC: alprazolam, dexfenfluramine. | Because ACTH is extremely labile in vitro, proper specimen collection and handling is vital (see Table 237-1). Results from different assays are not directly comparable. | Responses usually less than those to CRH or insulin hypoglycemia, but side effects less common than with insulin. Occasional normal individuals fail to respond to naloxone. A blunted response is seen in most patients with Cushing syndrome, regardless of cause. (See Chap. 75.) |
| DEC: ethanol, depression. No difference in response between adults and children, men and women, or young and old individuals. Response inversely related to basal serum cortisol and plasma ACTH concentrations. A variation in response is seen in normal subjects. | DEC: captopril. | Because ACTH is extremely labile in vitro, proper specimen collection and handling is vital (see Table 237-1). Results from different assays are not directly comparable. | Blunted response is seen in all forms of Cushing syndrome but normal response is usually seen in depressed individuals. Clinical and laboratory evidence of hypoglycemia should be documented; a glucose <40 mg/dL ensures an adequate challenge. Insulin hypoglycemia may produce significant complications, including seizures and, rarely, cardiac arrest; contraindications to use of this test are a history of seizures or coronary artery disease. Should be performed only if a physician and 50% dextrose are immediately available. (See Chap. 75.) |
| DEC: ethanol. | DEC: phenytoin, barbiturates, glucocorticoids, valproic acid. | Urine 17-OH steroid levels may be falsely low in patients with renal failure; therefore, in such persons, serum 11-deoxycortisol should be measured. Estrogens and estrogen-containing oral contraceptives decrease urinary 17-hydroxysteroid response but increase 11-deoxycortisol response. | An exaggerated response occurs in Cushing disease, but often no response occurs in other forms of Cushing syndrome. No response occurs in adrenocortical insufficiency; however, a slight increase in 11-deoxycortisol above basal concentration occurs even in ACTH deficiency due to the blockage of cortisol synthesis. The test should not be performed if basal cortisol is <2 μg/dL, because ACTH already is maximally stimulated. Metyrapone may cause gastrointestinal symptoms, dizziness, and light headedness. May precipitate adrenal crisis in persons with borderline adrenal function. Metyrapone is no longer manufactured in the United States. (See Chaps. 74 and 78.) |
| INC: acute illness, ethanol withdrawal, chronic illness. DEC: pregnancy, obesity (ACTH response), renal failure (cortisol response), exercise. No apparent difference in ACTH response between children and adults, men and women, or young and old individuals; response greater in blacks than in whites. Cortisol response greater in older women than in older men, and in boys than in girls. Some normal subjects show minimal response. | INC: interferon-α. DEC: glucocorticoids, valproic acid. | Because ACTH is extremely labile in vitro, proper specimen collection and handling is vital (see Table 237-1). Results from different assays are not directly comparable. | An exaggerated response occurs in Cushing disease; a blunted response is seen in other forms of Cushing syndrome. Response is increased in persons with hypothyroidism, whereas many depressed patients have blunted responses. CRH of ovine and human sources may give dissimilar responses. Some batches of CRH are inactive. Human CRH is not yet approved for use in the United States. (See Chap. 75.) |
| Most normal subjects show response and have a gradient between the right and left petrosal sinuses; thus, both an increase in ACTH ratio of >3 times and a gradient must be seen. | | Because ACTH is extremely labile in vitro, proper specimen collection and handling is vital (see Table 237-1). Results from different assays are not directly comparable; in a small percentage of patients, a hypoplastic inferior petrosal sinus is present, producing falsely negative results. Some have suggested sampling from the cavernous sinus to avoid this problem and simplify the procedure; the gradient in ACTH seems to be higher than with IPS sampling, but no reference values are available. | Requires anticoagulation of patient and skilled interventional radiology to simultaneously catheterize both inferior petrosal sinuses. An exaggerated response occurs in Cushing disease; a blunted response is seen in other forms of Cushing syndrome. A similar response is seen in patients with pseudo-Cushing disease. Human CRH is not yet an approved drug for use in the United States. (See Chap. 75.) |

(continued)

**TABLE 241-1.**
**Dynamic Endocrine Procedures\*  (Continued)**

| Name of Procedure | How Performed | Substance Measured | Expected Response | Intraindividual Variation |
|---|---|---|---|---|
| 3. Dexamethasone/ CRH[72,76–79] | 1.5 mg dexamethasone PO at 11:00 p.m.<br>100 µg CRH IV bolus or 1 µg/ kg at 8:00 a.m. | ACTH at 0, 30, 60 min<br>Cortisol at 0, 30, 60 min | No increase in either ACTH or cortisol; cortisol <1.5 µg/dL | Little day-to-day variation |

*INHIBITORY: PITUITARY*

| | | | | |
|---|---|---|---|---|
| 1. Dexamethasone suppression[1,25,26, 50,51,53,80–93] | All doses given PO<br>Overnight:<br>Low dose: 1 mg at 11 p.m.<br>High dose: 8 mg at 11 p.m.<br>Two-day:<br>Low dose: 0.5 mg q6h × 2 d<br>High dose: 2 mg q6h × 2 d | Overnight:<br>Serum cortisol at 8 a.m.<br>Two-day:<br>Urine 17-OH steroids, basal and each day of test<br>*or* Urine free cortisol, basal and each day of test | Overnight:<br>Low dose: <2 µg/dL<br>High dose: <50% of basal<br>Two-day:<br>Low dose: <4 mg/24 h<br>High dose: <50% of basal<br>Two-day:<br>Low dose: <20 µg/24 h<br>High dose: <50% of basal secretion | Response greater in p.m. than in a.m. |

*STIMULATORY: ADRENAL*

| | | | | |
|---|---|---|---|---|
| 1. ACTH (1–24) infusion[3,30,94–108] | Rapid: 250 µg IV bolus<br>Low dose: 1 µg IV bolus<br>Prolonged: 250 µg IV over 6 h; some suggest repeat daily for 3 days<br>If adrenal insufficiency is being considered, give dexamethasone 1 mg PO before ACTH. | Cortisol at 0, 30, 60 min<br>Cortisol at 0, 30 min<br>Cortisol at 0 and 6 h<br>*or* Urine 17-OH steroids/24 h, basal and each day of test | >18 µg/dL<br>>18 µg/dL<br>Two to 5 times basal values | Response greater in p.m. than in a.m.; day-to-day variation 20–30% |

**RENIN-ANGIOTENSIN-ALDOSTERONE AXIS**

*STIMULATORY*

| | | | | |
|---|---|---|---|---|
| 1. Sodium restriction[109–113] | 10–20 mmol sodium diet until urine Na <6 mmol/12 h | Plasma renin activity<br>Plasma aldosterone<br>Urinary aldosterone | >5 ng/mL/h<br>>25 ng/dL<br>>100 µg/d | |

\*The methodology, interpretation, and utility of some of these procedures are disputed; for further information and clinical recommendations, see the indicated chapters.

| Physiologic Factors | Drug Effects | Methodologic Considerations | Special Considerations/Interpretation |
|---|---|---|---|
| INC: depression, bipolar disorder. | INC (cortisol, ACTH): phenytoin. | Because ACTH is extremely labile in vitro, proper specimen collection and handling is vital (see Table 237-1). Results from different assays are not directly comparable; many cortisol assays have poor reproducibility at such low values. | Absent response is seen in normal individuals and pseudo-Cushing syndrome. Most patients with psychiatric disorders, particularly affective disorders, will fail to show suppression of response to CRH despite administration of dexamethasone. Some have suggested use of dexamethasone 0.5 mg q6h for 2 days before administration of CRH. |
| DEC: acute illness, obesity, pregnancy, acute stress (for overnight and 2-d low-dose tests). In renal failure and alcohol abuse, lack of suppression is common with low-dose overnight and 2-d tests. Nonsuppression is more common in children and in those >age 65 yr, especially if cortisol is measured at 4 p.m. as is recommended in psychiatric uses of the test. | INC: amphetamines, carbamazepine, nonsteroidal antiinflammatory agents, benzodiazepines. DEC: phenytoin, barbiturates, estrogens (high doses), rifampicin. | Cortisol assay is important in interpreting results of overnight testing because some assays may be imprecise at low levels (near the 5 μg/dL decision level). Urine 17-OH steroids or free cortisol may be inaccurate in patients with renal failure. | The overnight low-dose test shows lack of suppression in 98% of cases of Cushing syndrome, regardless of cause. The low-dose test has better specificity for Cushing syndrome than the overnight test but is normal in a significant minority of patients with Cushing syndrome. The high-dose tests show suppression with Cushing disease, but usually not with other causes of Cushing syndrome; occasional patients with Cushing disease require higher doses of dexamethasone to show a fall in cortisol production. With the 1 mg overnight test, lack of suppression is common in affective psychiatric disorders, alcohol abuse, and acute illness. Lack of suppression in low-dose tests is common in patients with diabetes mellitus, but is not related to diabetic control. Some have suggested using larger doses of dexamethasone (32 mg/day) to improve ability to differentiate Cushing disease from other causes of Cushing syndrome. Poor dexamethasone absorption has been reported in patients with chronic renal failure. Ingestion of dexamethasone should be verified; in doubtful cases, plasma dexamethasone concentration is useful. (See Chaps. 74, 78, and 201.) |
| Response is similar in newborn infants, children, adults, and the elderly. | INC: estrogens, theophylline. DEC: calcium-channel blockers, glucocorticoids, ketoconazole, megestrol acetate. | If assays that show cross-reactivity with prednisone and cortisone are used (competitive protein binding and some immunoassays), a high basal value with no response to infusion may be seen in patients receiving the medications. | With 250 μg, diminished or no response is seen in patients with primary adrenal insufficiency or severe secondary adrenal insufficiency, and in patients treated with high-dose glucocorticoids in whom normal pituitary-adrenal responsiveness has not returned. Low-dose ACTH shows diminished response in patients receiving even low-dose long-term corticosteroids and, in one review, in 95% of patients with secondary adrenal insufficiency. It agrees better with results of insulin-induced hypoglycemia or metyrapone procedures in such cases than does the higher-dose test in some studies, although others suggest it is less sensitive than tests evaluating hypothalamic or pituitary response. Response to synthetic ACTH persists for at least 3–4 weeks following onset of secondary adrenal insufficiency; these tests should not be used in the first month after pituitary surgery. Patients with Cushing disease often hyperrespond, and those with adrenal carcinoma or ectopic ACTH production usually do not. As many as 50% of patients with adrenal adenomas show a response to ACTH. In normal individuals, the response decreases as basal serum cortisol increases. (See Chaps. 74 and 78.) |
| Response decreases with increasing age. | Drugs that alter aldosterone excretion also affect dynamic responses (see Table 237-1). | This degree of sodium restriction often is not achieved in practice, particularly in children. Appropriate sample collection is essential, because renin activity increases if specimens are not kept at room temperature until plasma is frozen; aldosterone is labile (see Table 237-1 for additional information on collection). | In persons with aldosteronoma, typically no change occurs in aldosterone, whereas an increase may be seen in persons with hyperplasia of the zona glomerulosa. In primary or secondary hypoaldosteronism, a blunted aldosterone response is seen; renin increases only in primary hypoaldosteronism. Hypokalemia and hypopituitarism blunt the response to volume depletion; in hypopituitarism, cortisol alone does not correct the response, but cortisol plus thyroxine does. (See Chaps. 79–81, and 183.) |

(continued)

TABLE 241-1.
Dynamic Endocrine Procedures* (Continued)

| Name of Procedure | How Performed | Substance Measured | Expected Response | Intraindividual Variation |
|---|---|---|---|---|
| 2. Diuretic/ posture[109–113] | 80 mg furosemide PO; have patient stand upright for 2 h, starting 2 h after diuretic administration | Plasma renin activity at 4 h<br>Plasma aldosterone at 4 h | >5 ng/mL/h<br>>25 ng/dL | |
| *INHIBITORY* | | | | |
| 1. Sodium loading[109–113] | Oral: 120 mmol Na diet until urine Na >60 mmol/12 h<br>Intravenous: 2 L normal saline IV over 4 h | Plasma renin activity<br>Urinary aldosterone<br>Plasma renin activity at 4 h<br>Plasma aldosterone, basal and at 4 h | <5 ng/mL/h<br><20 µg/d<br><5 ng/mL/h<br><5 ng/dL, or <50% of basal | |
| 2. Captopril infusion[114–119] | 25-50 mg PO | Plasma renin activity and aldosterone at 0, 60, 120 min | Aldosterone <15 ng/dL, renin <1 ng/L/h, and aldosterone/renin ratio <50 at 120 min | |
| **ADRENAL MEDULLA** | | | | |
| *INHIBITORY* | | | | |
| 1. Clonidine[120–122] | 0.3 mg PO | Plasma norepinephrine at 3 h | <320 ng/L | |
| **GONADS** | | | | |
| **HYPOTHALAMIC–PITUITARY–GONADAL AXIS** | | | | |
| *STIMULATORY: PITUITARY* | | | | |
| 1. GnRH [123–127] | 100 µg IV bolus | LH and/or FSH at 0, 30 min | Two to 3 times increase over basal LH; minimal increase in FSH | In women, response is greatest at ovulation, and greater in luteal than in follicular phase. |
| 2. Clomiphene citrate[128] | Men: 100 mg PO twice daily for 10 d<br>Women: 50-100 mg/d PO for 5 d | LH and/or FSH, basal and at end of administration | 50% increase over basal LH | |

*The methodology, interpretation, and utility of some of these procedures are disputed; for further information and clinical recommendations, see the indicated chapters.

| Physiologic Factors | Drug Effects | Methodologic Considerations | Special Considerations/Interpretation |
|---|---|---|---|
| Response decreases with increasing age. | Drugs that alter aldosterone excretion also affect dynamic responses; in addition, ranitidine decreases response to posture (see Table 237-1). | | The pattern of change is similar to that in sodium restriction.<br>Hypokalemia and hypopituitarism blunt the response to volume depletion; in hypopituitarism, cortisol alone does not correct response, but cortisol and thyroxine do. (See Chaps. 79–81, and 183.) |
| | Drugs that alter aldosterone excretion also affect dynamic responses. | | With both primary hyperplasia and aldosteronoma, sodium loading typically will not suppress aldosterone by >50%; suppression is seen in secondary hyperaldosteronism.<br>Converting-enzyme inhibitors decrease aldosterone in hyperplasia but not in aldosteronoma. This test may precipitate or worsen congestive heart failure, and may worsen hypokalemia; thus, sodium loading should be performed with caution in persons with either of these findings. In persons with renal failure, the inability to excrete a sodium load regularly leads to fluid overload.<br>Other procedures to inhibit aldosterone secretion include administration of fluorohydrocortisone or deoxycorticosterone. (See Chaps. 79–81, and 183.) |
| Salt intake has no effect on response. | Drugs that alter aldosterone excretion also affect dynamic responses. | | Patients with aldosteronoma typically have a high basal aldosterone that does not fall after captopril administration, as well as a high aldosterone/renin ratio. Patients with essential hyperaldosteronism may have a normal response. Patients with renal vascular hypertension show increased renin but decreased aldosterone in response to the test. Dynamic testing is only slightly superior to the supine renin/aldosterone ratio. (See Chaps. 79–81, and 183.) |
| Stressful situations may increase plasma norepinephrine concentration. | Drugs that alter catecholamine secretion also affect dynamic response, especially diuretics, β-adrenergic blockers, and antidepressants (see Table 237-1). | Specimen collection and processing is critical for assay of norepinephrine, because catecholamines are extremely labile in vitro (see Table 237-1). | Typically, suppression does not occur in pheochromocytoma; however, an insufficient number of patients have been evaluated. The absolute decrease is dependent on the basal norepinephrine concentration; the lower the level, the more likely that suppression will occur in patients with pheochromocytoma. (See Chaps. 85–87.) |
| INC: renal failure.<br>DEC: heavy exercise, blind persons.<br>Decreased or blunted response before puberty. | INC: carbamazepine (LH response only).<br>DEC: estrogens, oral contraceptives (LH response only). | Response criteria are dependent on standard used in validating FSH and LH method. | This procedure lacks dependability and reproducibility. A blunted response occurs in pituitary hypogonadism, whereas an exaggerated response occurs in primary hypogonadism. The initial response is blunted in hypothalamic hypogonadism, but a normal response may be seen with repeated testing. A blunted response also occurs in persons with elevated prolactin. (See Chaps. 16 and 115.) |
| In prepubertal and peripubertal individuals, clomiphene causes a paradoxic fall in LH and FSH. | Probably similar to GnRH. | Response criteria are dependent on standard used in validating FSH and LH method. | This procedure lacks dependability and reproducibility. If testosterone is used as indicator, response decreases with increasing age. Responses are otherwise similar to those in GnRH test, as given above. (See Chaps. 16 and 115.) |

*(continued)*

**TABLE 241-1.**
Dynamic Endocrine Procedures* (Continued)

| Name of Procedure | How Performed | Substance Measured | Expected Response | Intraindividual Variation |
|---|---|---|---|---|
| 3. TRH[129–132] | 500 µg IV bolus | α Subunit and LH β subunit at 0, 20, 30, 60 min (some also measure intact FSH and LH) | <30% increase in α subunit and <40% increase in LH β subunit | |
| *STIMULATORY: GONADAL* | | | | |
| 1. Human chorionic gonadotropin[128] | Men: 2000 U IM daily for 4 d<br>Women: 2000 U IM daily for 2 d | Testosterone, basal and at end of administration | Men: 2 times increase over basal, with peak at least 200 ng/dL<br>Women: up to 5 times increase over basal | |

## PANCREAS

### PANCREATIC B CELLS

*STIMULATORY*

| | | | | |
|---|---|---|---|---|
| 1. Glucose-tolerance test[133–148] | 75 g glucose PO<br>In pregnancy, 100 g glucose PO | Serum glucose at 2 h<br>In pregnancy, serum glucose at 0, 1, 2, 3 h | ADA criteria:<br>Diabetic: 2 h >200 mg/dL<br>Impaired: 2 h 140–200 mg/dL<br>Diabetes in pregnancy:<br>0 h >105 mg/dL<br>1 h >190 mg/dL<br>2 h >165 mg/dL<br>3 h >145 mg/dL<br>2 or more must be present to diagnose gestational diabetes | Serum glucose concentrations higher when glucose given in p.m., even after fasting. In women, response is similar in luteal and follicular phases. |
| 2. Glucagon-stimulated C peptide[149–157] | 1 mg IV bolus | Plasma C peptide at 0 and 6 min | Two to 4 times increase | Little day-to-day variation if glucose control maintained stable. |

*INHIBITORY*

| | | | | |
|---|---|---|---|---|
| 1. 72-h fast | No intake of food for 72 h; may ingest water or diet soft drinks without caffeine | Insulin and glucose at 0, 12, 24, 36, 48, 72 h; also, at any time that patient has symptoms of hypoglycemia<br>Perform analyses for insulin on specimens with glucose <50 mg/dL only | Glucose >50 mg/dL<br>Insulin <4 µU/mL<br>Insulin/glucose ratio <0.3 | |

### GASTRIN PRODUCTION

*STIMULATORY*

| | | | | |
|---|---|---|---|---|
| 1. Meal[158–163] | 180 g roast beef PO | Gastrin at 0, 30, 60 min | Increase of 50–100% over basal | |
| 2. Calcium[158–162] | 15 mg calcium/kg in 500 mL normal saline; infused IV over 3 h | Gastrin at 0, 1, 2, 3 h | <50% increase over basal | |

*The methodology, interpretation, and utility of some of these procedures are disputed; for further information and clinical recommendations, see the indicated chapters.

| Physiologic Factors | Drug Effects | Methodologic Considerations | Special Considerations/Interpretation |
|---|---|---|---|
| | | For maximum information, assays must show little cross-reactivity to other components and have good reproducibility, because of the low amplitude of response in most patients; this is particularly important for intact LH and LH-β. | No response in normal individuals; rare responses seen, particularly for α subunit, in patients with pituitary tumors producing prolactin or somatotropin. Up to 80% of patients with "nonsecretory" pituitary adenomas show response of one or both subunits. Limited information exists on effects of other diseases on this response, particularly the effect of secondary hypothyroidism, and little information is available on "normal" values. TRH causes flushing and, occasionally, hypertension; it should be used with caution in persons with a history of cardiac disease. (See Chaps. 16 and 115.) |
| Response in men decreases with increasing age. | INC: barbiturates, estrogens. DEC: in women—dexamethasone; in men—digoxin, metyrapone, spironolactone. | If basal serum gonadotropin concentrations are elevated, test not indicated. | Lack of response typically is seen in primary hypogonadism but may occur with other forms of hypogonadal states. (See Chaps. 16, 93, and 115.) |
| INC (in glucose): obesity, pregnancy, low-carbohydrate diet, stress, ethanol. DEC (in glucose): smoking. Glucose concentrations increase with increasing age, obesity. | INC (in glucose): oral contraceptives, estrogens, glucocorticoids, thiazides, phenytoin, lithium, ranitidine, propranolol, tetrahydrocannabinol. DEC (in glucose): guanethidine, clofibrate, salicylates. | Glucose concentration is considerably higher in capillary blood than in venous blood in postprandial specimens, but not in fasting specimens; criteria are based on venous serum glucose. | Test should not be continued if patient has vasovagal symptoms. Test is not needed to diagnose diabetes if fasting hyperglycemia is present, except in pregnancy. Glucose administration also can be used as a stimulus to insulin release. Other agents, such as tolbutamide and glucagon, induce an exaggerated insulin response in persons with insulinoma. Because of the unreliability and nonspecificity of response, and the potential danger of hypoglycemia, their use is not recommended. (See Chaps. 136–140, 158, and 161.) |
| Response directly related to basal glucose concentration between 55 and 125 mg/dL (3–7 mmol/L); even short-term changes in diabetic control alter response. | Medications that alter plasma glucose alter response. | | The test can be used to determine islet cell reserve in patients with diabetes; absent response is seen in most patients with type 1 diabetes, whereas a reduced response occurs in most patients with type 2 diabetes. Some overlap is seen in results for patients with type 1 and type 2 diabetes. The test cannot be used to predict need for insulin in those with type 2 diabetes. An exaggerated response occurs with insulinoma. (See Chaps. 136–140, 158, and 161.) |
| Previous starvation may magnify the response. | Insulin, oral hypoglycemic agents, and diazoxide may worsen hypoglycemia. | Many commercial RIA procedures for insulin do not have sensitivity adequate to differentiate low normal from decreased insulin concentrations. Insulin antibodies may produce falsely high or falsely low insulin concentration. | In patients with insulinoma, hypoglycemia develops and insulin production is not inhibited by the low serum glucose concentration. Severe liver disease may impair ability to maintain plasma glucose concentrations. The test should be terminated if a patient has severely symptomatic hypoglycemia; many normal persons, especially women, become hypoglycemic. (See Chaps. 158 and 161.) |
| Response is greater in women than in men. | INC: cimetidine, ranitidine, atropine, haloperidol. DEC: lithium. Drugs affecting basal gastrin also may affect response (see Table 237-1). | | Although, typically, gastrinomas show no or minimal response, some studies suggest that hyperresponsiveness is common in the early stages of gastrinoma. In one detailed study of gastrinoma, approximately half the patients showed a 50% increase and one-fifth showed a 100% increase. (See Chap. 220.) |
| | Drugs affecting basal gastrin also may affect response (see Table 237-1). | | An exaggerated response is seen in patients with gastrinoma, as well as in ~50% of patients with achlorhydria. (See Chap. 220.) |

(continued)

**TABLE 241-1.**
**Dynamic Endocrine Procedures\*  (Continued)**

| Name of Procedure | How Performed | Substance Measured | Expected Response | Intraindividual Variation |
|---|---|---|---|---|
| 3. Secretin[158–167] | 2 U/kg IV bolus | Gastrin at 0, 2, 5, 10, 15 min | <50% increase over basal | |

**PARATHYROID GLANDS AND BONE**

*STIMULATORY*

| | | | | |
|---|---|---|---|---|
| 1. Parathyroid hormone | 200 U parathyroid hormone IV over 5–10 min | 1 h timed urine collections for 3 h before and 1 h after PTH administration for $PO_4$ or cAMP | >100% increase in either $PO_4$ or cAMP | |

*OTHER*

| | | | | |
|---|---|---|---|---|
| 1. Cortisone[168,169] | 120 mg/d × 10 d | Serum calcium at 0, 5, 8, 10 d | <10.5 mg/dL | |

**PITUITARY GLAND**

**HYPOTHALAMIC-PITUITARY LACTOTROPE AXIS**

*STIMULATORY*

| | | | | |
|---|---|---|---|---|
| 1. Thyrotropin-releasing hormone[17,18,24,170–177] | 400–500 µg IV bolus | Prolactin at 0 and 30 (some say 15) min | Men: 3 to 5 times increase over basal level<br>Women: 5 to 8 times increase over basal level | Response greatest in evening; response greatest in winter, lowest in summer. |

**HYPOTHALAMIC-PITUITARY SOMATOTROPE AXIS**

*STIMULATORY*

| | | | | |
|---|---|---|---|---|
| 1. Growth hormone–releasing hormone[2,7,20,33,178–185] | 100 µg IV bolus | Growth hormone at 0, 30, 60 min | Five to 10 times increase over basal levels | In women, response is greatest at ovulation and lowest at menses. |
| 2. Clonidine[184–191] | 4 µg/kg PO | Growth hormone at 0, 60, 90, 120 min | Three to 6 times increase over basal levels | In women, response is greatest at ovulation and lowest at menses. |
| 3. L-dopa[189–194] | 0.5 g PO | Growth hormone at 0, 60, 90, 120 min | Peak >7 ng/mL or increase of 5 ng/mL over basal level | |

\*The methodology, interpretation, and utility of some of these procedures are disputed; for further information and clinical recommendations, see the indicated chapters.

| Physiologic Factors | Drug Effects | Methodologic Considerations | Special Considerations/Interpretation |
|---|---|---|---|
| | Drugs affecting basal gastrin also may affect response (see Table 237-1). | | In gastrinoma, an exaggerated response to secretin is the most consistently found change in gastrin secretion. Increases in gastrin of 30–50% are commonly seen in patients with active peptic ulcers; no significant change in gastrin is seen in those with achlorhydria. (See Chap. 220.) |
| | | | In hypoparathyroidism, a normal or increased response to PTH is seen, whereas the response is blunted in pseudohypoparathyroidism. A synthetic PTH is available in the United States; data given are for an older preparation, and new, normative data are needed. (See Chap. 60.) |
| | | | A decrease in serum calcium occurs in most cases of sarcoidosis, multiple myeloma, and lymphoma, and in hypervitaminosis D. In approximately two-thirds of patients with other malignancies, a fall in serum calcium is seen. In hyperparathyroidism, calcium seldom is decreased. (See Chap. 59.) |
| DEC: alcohol abuse, obesity, malnutrition, renal failure, severe acute illness. Response decreases with increasing age. | INC: dopamine antagonists, phenytoin, amiodarone, verapamil. DEC: dopamine agonists, cysteamine, salicylates. | | Stimulatory procedures, including TRH and chlorpromazine, and inhibitory procedures, such as L-dopa, are seldom used and have little, if any, clinical utility. This is because a blunted response is seen in virtually all patients with prolactinoma, as well as in most of those with other causes of hyperprolactinemia. The increase in prolactin is dependent on thyroid function; response is increased in hypothyroidism and blunted in hyperthyroidism. TRH causes flushing and, occasionally, hypertension; it should be used with caution in persons with a history of cardiac disease. (See Chap. 13.) |
| | | | **GENERAL COMMENTS:** Nonpharmacologic stimulants of GH release include sleep, exercise, and stress. Many normal persons show lack of response to one or more stimulants; to diagnose pituitary GH deficiency, lack of response to at least two different stimuli should be found. In acromegaly, response to stimulating agents may produce a paradoxic decrease in GH; in a given patient, response may differ, depending on the agent used. |
| INC: renal failure. DEC: obesity, alcohol abuse, hyperglycemia. Response does not change with increasing age and is similar in men and women. | INC: propranolol, dopamine agonists. DEC: theophylline, glucocorticoids, tamoxifen, estrogens (in men). | | In pituitary GH deficiency, no response is seen; in hypothalamic causes of deficiency, response is present but delayed. Response may be blunted in other endocrine disorders, including hypothyroidism and Cushing disease, and returns to baseline with treatment of the underlying disease. GHRH is not yet licensed for use in the United States. (See Chaps. 12, 18, and 198.) |
| INC: smoking. DEC: obesity, alcohol abuse, stress. Decreases with age over 60 yr in men; in women, decreases after menopause. | DEC: glucocorticoids, tricyclic antidepressants. Probably similar to GHRH. | | A blunted response occurs in hypothalamic-pituitary dwarfism. See general comments above. (See Chaps. 12, 18, and 198.) |
| DEC: hyperglycemia, obesity, blind persons. Decreases with increasing age; response is greater in women than in men. | DEC: phenothiazines, dopamine antagonists. | | A blunted response occurs in hypothalamic-pituitary dwarfism. A significant percentage of normal persons do not respond to L-dopa stimulation. In addition, response is blunted in persons with prolactinoma or hypothyroidism. Nausea and vomiting are common side effects. (See Chaps. 12, 18, and 198.) |

(continued)

**TABLE 241-1.**
**Dynamic Endocrine Procedures\*** (Continued)

| Name of Procedure | How Performed | Substance Measured | Expected Response | Intraindividual Variation |
|---|---|---|---|---|
| 4. Arginine[189,195] | 0.5 g/kg (maximum of 30 g) IV over 30 min | Growth hormone at 0, 60, 90, 120 min | Peak >7 ng/mL or increase of 5 ng/mL over basal level | |
| 5. Hexarelin[196–207] | 1–2 µg/kg IV bolus | Growth hormone at 0, 30, 60, 90, 120 min | Peak >7 ng/mL | Day-to-day variation in peak 20%; no diurnal variation in peak response, but values remain elevated longer at night. |
| 6. Insulin[179,189,208] | 0.05-0.1 U/kg IV bolus | Growth hormone at 0, 60, 90, 120 min | Peak >7 ng/mL or increase of 5 ng/mL over basal level | Day-to-day variation: 35–40%. In women response is greatest at ovulation, least during menses. |
| *INHIBITORY* | | | | |
| 1. Hyperglycemia | 75 g glucose PO | Growth hormone at 90, 120 min | <5 ng/mL (some say <2 ng/mL) | |
| **COMBINED HYPOTHALAMIC-PITUITARY PROCEDURE** [209–215] | | | | |
| | 200 µg TRH; 100 µg each of GHRH, CRH, and GnRH, IV bolus | TSH, ACTH, GH, LH, and prolactin at 0, 30, 60 min | See individual tests and Special Considerations. | See individual tests. |
| **HYPOTHALAMIC–POSTERIOR PITUITARY AXIS** | | | | |
| *STIMULATORY* | | | | |
| 1. Water deprivation[29,216–218] | Restrict all oral water intake starting in a.m. | Urine for osmolality and total volume, patient weight every hour; continue test until weight falls by 3% and/or osmolality does not change by >30 mOsm/kg between two specimens. | Urine osmolality >500 mOsm/kg | |

\*The methodology, interpretation, and utility of some of these procedures are disputed; for further information and clinical recommendations, see the indicated chapters.

| Physiologic Factors | Drug Effects | Methodologic Considerations | Special Considerations/Interpretation |
|---|---|---|---|
| DEC: hyperglycemia, obesity. Decreases with increasing age; response is greater in women than in men. | INC: diethylstilbestrol, propranolol, indomethacin, gluco-corticoids. DEC: cimetidine. | | A blunted response occurs in hypothalamic-pituitary dwarfism. Lack of response also is found in persons with hypothyroidism. Response is inversely proportional to basal GH; no response may be seen if basal level is >5 ng/mL. Arginine may exacerbate acidosis in patients with renal failure and may be hazardous in patients with liver disease; other stimulatory agents should be used in persons with these disorders. (See Chaps. 12, 18, and 198.) |
| DEC: glucose ingestion, increased prolactin. Low in newborns and children, increases at puberty; declines in older adults. In women, declines significantly after menopause. | DEC: alprazolam, diphenhydramine, salbutamol. | | A blunted response occurs in hypothalamic-pituitary dwarfism. Results are not always concordant with those of GHRH, especially in patients on medications and in children and the elderly. An exaggerated response of cortisol and ACTH to hexarelin is seen in Cushing disease due to microadenoma, but not in other forms of Cushing syndrome or Cushing disease due to macroadenoma. (See Chaps. 12, 18, and 198.) |
| DEC: obesity, renal failure. Decreases with increasing age. | INC: propranolol, estrogen (in men). DEC: cyproheptadine, phentolamine. | | A blunted response occurs in hypothalamic-pituitary dwarfism but also is seen in persons with Cushing syndrome, or in the presence of hypothyroidism or hyperthyroidism. Glucose should fall to <40 mg/dL to ensure an adequate challenge; however, the rise in growth hormone is not directly related to the magnitude of the fall in glucose. Insulin hypoglycemia may produce significant complications, including seizures and, rarely, cardiac arrest. Contraindications are a history of epilepsy or coronary artery disease. This procedure should be performed only if a physician and 50% dextrose are immediately available. (See Chaps. 12, 18, and 198.) |
| | | | A lack of suppression occurs in pituitary tumors secreting GH or in ectopic GHRH production. Lack of suppression also is common in patients with Cushing syndrome, affective disorders, and anorexia nervosa. In acute illness, acromegaly, or chronic renal failure, a paradoxic rise in GH may occur. (See Chaps. 12, 18, and 198.) |
| See individual tests. | See individual tests. | See individual tests. | Human CRH and GHRH are not approved for clinical use. The test is most useful in evaluating patients with possible panhypopituitarism; a lack of response to all hormones is expected in this disease. Although most responses are similar to those seen with administration of agents singly, increase in TSH and prolactin appears to be greater with combined testing. CRH decreases the GH response to GHRH. In some protocols, ADH also is included to enhance the ACTH response to CRH; this enhancement occurs only if ovine CRH is used. The risks are similar to those encountered with individual factor use; flushing and hypertension due to TRH are the most frequent. Because diurnal variation is seen in the response of different hormones, testing ideally should be performed in the morning. Most responses are blunted in renal failure, but GH response is augmented. |
| DEC: starvation, exercise, pregnancy, low-sodium intake. | Drugs affecting ADH likely affect results of dynamic testing (see Table 237-1); in addition, methadone produces a response similar to nephrogenic diabetes insipidus. | Proteinuria and glucosuria will increase osmolality, more so for glucosuria; this may cause high basal osmolality. Administration of iodine-containing contrast materials before initiation of water deprivation may increase osmolality. For all the above-mentioned sub- | A lack of response typifies persons with complete nephrogenic or central diabetes insipidus; urine osmolality between 300 and 500 mOsm/kg is seen in patients with partial forms. Patients with psychogenic water drinking may not respond. Patients with central diabetes insipidus will concentrate their urine when given an injection of arginine vasopressin. Patients must be monitored closely because those with ADH deficiency can become dehydrated. |

(continued)

**TABLE 241-1.**
**Dynamic Endocrine Procedures\* (Continued)**

| Name of Procedure | How Performed | Substance Measured | Expected Response | Intraindividual Variation |
|---|---|---|---|---|

## THYROID GLAND

### HYPOTHALAMIC–PITUITARY–THYROID AXIS

#### *STIMULATORY: PITUITARY*

| Name of Procedure | How Performed | Substance Measured | Expected Response | Intraindividual Variation |
|---|---|---|---|---|
| 1. TRH[4,6,10–14,16,219–228] | 500 µg IV bolus | TSH at 0, 30 (some also say 60) min | Two- to four-fold increase at peak | As much as 5 U/L day-to-day variation in peak response. Response greatest in the evening; in women, response higher in follicular than in luteal phase. Response greater in winter than in summer. |

### C CELLS (CALCITONIN)

#### *STIMULATION*

| Name of Procedure | How Performed | Substance Measured | Expected Response | Intraindividual Variation |
|---|---|---|---|---|
| 1. Calcium[229–231] | 15 mg calcium/kg in 500 mL normal saline; infused IV over 3 h<br>Rapid: 2 mg/kg IV push | Calcitonin at 3, 4 h<br><br>Calcitonin at 1, 2, 5, 10 min | Men: <265 pg/mL<br>Women: <120 pg/mL | In women, response similar in luteal and follicular phases. |
| 2. Pentagastrin[229,230] | 0.5 µg/kg IV push | Calcitonin at 1, 2, 5, 10 min | Men: <210 pg/mL<br>Women: <105 pg/mL | |
| 3. Combined calcium/ pentagastrin[232] | 2 mg calcium/kg IV push, immediately followed by pentagastrin, 0.5 µg/kg IV push | Calcitonin at 1, 2, 5, 10 min | <300 pg/mL | |

*ACTH*, adrenocorticotropic hormone; *ADA*, American Diabetes Association; *ADH*, antidiuretic hormone; *cAMP*, cyclic adenosine monophosphate; *CRH*, corticotropin-releasing hormone; *DEC*, decrease; *FSH*, follicle-stimulating hormone; *GH*, growth hormone; *GHRH*, growth hormone–releasing hormone; *GnRH*, gonadotropin-releasing hormone; *IM*, intramuscularly; *INC*, increase; *IPS*, inferior petrosal sinus; *IV*, intravenously; *LH*, luteinizing hormone; *17-OH*, 17-hydroxy; *PO*, orally; *PTH*, parathyroid hormone; *RIA*, radioimmunoassay; *TRH*, thyrotropin-releasing hormone; *TSH*, thyroid-stimulating hormone; *WHO*, World Health Organization.

\*The methodology, interpretation, and utility of some of these procedures are disputed; for further information and clinical recommendations, see the indicated chapters.

*(See References on page 2264.)*

| Physiologic Factors | Drug Effects | Methodologic Considerations | Special Considerations/Interpretation |
|---|---|---|---|
| | | stances, the effect is more marked if specific gravity is used as a measure of urine concentration. Measurement of plasma vasopressin at the end of the procedure enhances the diagnostic capabilities of the procedure, but reliable vasopressin assays are not widely available. | rapidly. Water restriction may worsen renal function in persons with dehydration and in the diuretic phase of acute tubular necrosis. If plasma vasopressin is measured, the concentration is elevated in nephrogenic forms, persistently low in the complete central form, and subnormal with partial central diabetes insipidus. (See Chaps. 25–27.) |
| INC: obesity.<br>DEC: acute illness, starvation, chronic renal failure, alcohol abuse.<br>Response greater in women than in men. In men, response decreases after age 50. | INC: carbamazepine, danazol, dopamine antagonists, estrogens, theophylline, lithium, drugs inhibiting thyroid hormone production.<br>DEC: clozapine, dopamine agonists, glucocorticoids, phenytoin, salicylates, somatostatin, propranolol, opiates, ranitidine, drugs increasing thyroid hormone production or release (see Table 237-1). | Interfering substances in TSH immunoassays that use monoclonal antibodies may cause a falsely elevated serum TSH before and after TRH administration. The procedure is invalidated under these conditions. | A blunted response is seen in hyperthyroidism and in some cases of hypopituitarism. An initial lack of rise with a delayed and prolonged response may be seen in hypothalamic hypothyroidism. In primary hypothyroidism, an exaggerated and prolonged response is seen. Many persons with secondary hypothyroidism show a normal or exaggerated response. The degree of response is directly proportional to basal TSH in normal individuals as well as in those with disease, although the proportional increase is blunted if TSH is >50 mU/L; thus, the most useful criterion for quantifying response is the percentage change. Occasionally, flushing and hypertension accompany TRH administration. (See Chaps. 15 and 33.) |
| Response decreases with increasing age in both sexes. | Drugs affecting basal calcitonin also may affect response (see Table 237-1). | Normative data vary with immunoassay used. | An exaggerated response is seen in the presence of medullary thyroid carcinoma and in C-cell hyperplasia. An exaggerated response also has been seen in persons with renal failure and extensive bone disease, and in those with pseudohypoparathyroidism. A blunted response occurs in primary hyperparathyroidism. (See Chaps. 40, 53, and 188.) |
| | Drugs affecting basal calcitonin also may affect response (see Table 237-1). | Normative data vary with immunoassay used. | See data under calcium above. Chest pain often is present after pentagastrin administration. (See Chaps. 40, 53, and 188.) |
| | Drugs affecting basal calcitonin also may affect response (see Table 237-1). | Normative data varies with immunoassay used. | See data under calcium, pentagastrin above. This appears to be the most reproducible stimulus of calcitonin release. (See Chaps. 40, 53, and 188.) |

Note: Page numbers followed by *f* indicate figures; those followed by *t* indicate tabular material. Page numbers in **boldface** indicate main text discussions.

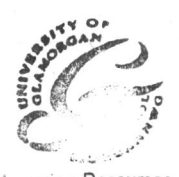